ELEVENTH Edition

APPLIED THERAPEUTICS

The Clinical Use of Drugs

ELEVENTH Edition

APPLIED THERAPEUTICS

The Clinical Use of Drugs

Caroline S. Zeind, PharmD

Associate Provost for Academic and International Affairs
Chief Academic Officer
Worcester, Massachusetts and Manchester,
New Hampshire Campuses
Professor of Pharmacy Practice
Academic Affairs
MCPHS University
Boston, Massachusetts

Michael G. Carvalho, PharmD, BCPP

Assistant Dean of Interprofessional Education
Professor and Chair
Department of Pharmacy Practice
School of Pharmacy–Boston
MCPHS University
Boston, Massachusetts

Wolters Kluwer

Philadelphia • Baltimore • New York • London
Buenos Aires • Hong Kong • Sydney • Tokyo

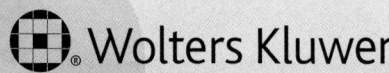

Acquisitions Editor: Matt Hauber
Development Editor: Andrea Vosburgh
Editorial Coordinator: Annette Ferran
Editorial Assistant: Brooks Phelps
Marketing Manager: Michael McMahon
Production Project Manager: Kim Cox
Design Coordinator: Steve Druding
Manufacturing Coordinator: Margie Orzech
Prepress Vendor: S4Carlisle Publishing Services

Eleventh edition

9 8 7 6 5 4 3 2

Printed in China

Library of Congress Cataloging-in-Publication Data

Names: Zeind, Caroline S., editor. | Carvalho, Michael G., editor.
Title: Applied therapeutics : the clinical use of drugs / [edited by]
Caroline S. Zeind, Michael G. Carvalho.
Other titles: Applied therapeutics for clinical pharmacists.
Description: Eleventh edition. | Philadelphia : Wolters Kluwer Health, [2018]
| Includes bibliographical references and index.
Identifiers: LCCN 2017045052 | ISBN 9781496318299
Subjects: | MESH: Drug Therapy
Classification: LCC RM262 | NLM WB 330 | DDC 615.5/8—dc23 LC record available at
https://lccn.loc.gov/2017045052

LWW.com

Dedication

The editors wish to express their sincere thanks to Dr. Mary Anne Koda-Kimble and Dr. Lloyd Young who created Applied Therapeutics, the gold standard textbook used in the teaching of patient-centered drug therapeutics. Their vision and legendary contributions have inspired generations of health profession students, faculty, and clinicians. We are grateful to the past editors and current editorial team and contributors, as well as faculty colleagues and clinicians across the globe for their tremendous dedication to their patients and their communities. They have shaped and inspired the next generation of health care professionals through innovative teaching, mentoring, and dissemination of their scholarship. Finally, we wish to thank our families for their patience and understanding as we embarked on this journey and completed this eleventh edition of the textbook.

Preface

It has been over forty years since the first edition of *Applied Therapeutics: The Clinical Use of Drugs* was published, and the landscape of health care has changed dramatically. While we have seen tremendous scientific and technologic advancements transform personalized medicine, we also realize the significant challenges that we face within our increasingly complex health care delivery system. More than ever, we are in need of health professionals who are able to think critically and to utilize problem-solving skills to improve patient outcomes. Approximately four decades later, the founding principle for this textbook—a patient-centric, case-based approach to learning—remains the cornerstone of health professions education. Our authors present approximately 900 patient cases that stimulate the reader to integrate and apply therapeutic principles in the context of specific clinical situations. Health profession students and practitioners gain a glimpse into the minds of clinicians as they work to assess and solve therapeutic problems and develop their own critical-thinking and problem-solving skills.

Readers familiar with past editions of the book will notice that the overall design of the book is consistent with the tenth edition, which incorporates a Core Principles section at the beginning of each chapter, providing the most important "take home" information from the chapter. Each Core Principle is mapped to specific cases within the chapter where the principle is discussed in detail. Key references and websites are listed at the end of each chapter, whereas the full reference lists for each chapter have been moved online.

Building upon the excellent foundation of case-based learning provided in previous editions, the eleventh edition has incorporated changes to meet the evolving educational needs of health profession educators and students across the globe. The editors and contributors have utilized the five Institute of Medicine (IOM) core competencies as a broad framework for proposing case studies and questions within the textbook: patient-centered care; interdisciplinary teams; evidence-based practice; quality improvement; and informatics. In addition, the Accreditation Council for Pharmacy Education (ACPE) Accreditation Standards 2016, the Center for the Advancement of Pharmacy Education (CAPE) Educational Outcomes, and the North American Pharmacist Licensure Examination (NAPLEX) revised competency statements have served as road maps for the editorial team and contributors in designing the eleventh edition.

Featuring contributions from more than 200 experienced clinicians, every chapter has been revised and updated to reflect our ever-changing knowledge of drugs and the application of this knowledge to the individualized therapy of patients. Content within several sections has been extensively reorganized, with new chapters introduced to expand important topics. Among these are seven new chapters within the General Principles, Immunologic Disorders, Rheumatic and Musculoskeletal Diseases, Neurologic Disorders, Psychiatric Disorders & Substance Abuse, and Hematology and Oncology sections. Of particular note are featured new chapters in the General Principles section on Drug Interactions, Pharmacogenomics and Personalized Medicine, and Interprofessional Education and Practice. In addition, a chapter has been redesigned to focus on Care of the Critically Ill Adult, which now complements the chapter on Care of the Critically Ill Child.

Given the importance of incorporating Interprofessional Education (IPE) within the didactic, practicum, and clinical settings, we have added an array of IPE case studies prepared by contributors that are representative of various sections of the textbook. These IPE cases, along with answer guides, will be available for instructors on the textbook's website (see the "Additional Resources" section).

We welcome your feedback as we undertake planning for the next edition. The authors have drawn on information from the literature, current standards, and their own clinical experiences to share the process involved in making sound and thoughtful therapeutic decisions. *However, it remains the responsibility of every practitioner to evaluate the appropriateness of a particular opinion in the context of the actual clinical situation, bearing in mind any recent developments in the field. We strongly urge students and practitioners to consult several appropriate information sources when working with new and unfamiliar drugs.*

Acknowledgments

We are deeply indebted to the many dedicated people who have given of themselves to complete the eleventh edition of *Applied Therapeutics: The Clinical Use of Drugs*. We are grateful to our contributing authors who have worked tirelessly to provide the highest quality of work, while balancing numerous responsibilities as educators, clinicians, and researchers. We are grateful for the exceptional work of our twenty-six section editors, who provided critical feedback necessary both in the organizational structure of the textbook and in the individual editing of chapters; without their dedication and support, this edition would not be possible. In particular, we wish to recognize those returning section editors as they have been a guiding force for the eleventh edition: Drs. Jean M. Nappi, Timothy J. Ives, Marcia L. Buck, Judith L. Beizer, and Myrna Y. Munar. We sincerely thank the past editorial team of *Applied Therapeutics*, with special thanks to Dr. Brian K. Alldredge and Dr. B. Joseph Guglielmo for their guidance and support and contributions to the eleventh edition. We would also like to thank Facts and Comparisons for allowing us to use their data for the construction of some of our tables.

The team from Wolters Kluwer, Matt Hauber, Andrea Vosburgh, and Annette Ferran, deserve special recognition for their efforts. Their exceptional patience, attention to detail, and guidance have been critical to the success of this project. We sincerely thank Tara Slagle (project management) and Samson Premkumar (production) for their assistance in completing this edition. Most importantly, we wish to acknowledge the love, understanding, and unwavering support of our spouses and families. They selflessly gave to us early mornings, late nights, weekends, and vacation time that we spent writing and editing.

Consistent with past editions, we continue to dedicate our work to our students who inspire us and to the many patients we have been privileged to care for and who have taught us invaluable lessons. We also dedicate the eleventh edition to those clinicians and educators who have served as pioneering leaders and role models in the delivery of patient-centered care using team-based approaches.

Additional Resources

The eleventh edition of *Applied Therapeutics: The Clinical Use of Drugs* includes additional resources for both instructors and students, available on the book's companion website at http://thepoint.lww.com/AT11e.

STUDENT RESOURCES

Students who have purchased *Applied Therapeutics: The Clinical Use of Drugs*, Eleventh Edition have access to the following additional resources for each chapter:

- A full online reference list for that chapter

INSTRUCTOR RESOURCES

Approved adopting instructors will be given access to the following additional resources:

- Interprofessional Education (IPE) Case Studies and Answer Guides
- Each chapter will map which NAPLEX competency statements are addressed within it, which will be a helpful resource for instructors.

Section Editors

Michael C. Angelini, PharmD, MA, BCPP
Associate Professor of Pharmacy Practice
School of Pharmacy–Boston
MCPHS University
Boston, Massachusetts

Judith L. Beizer, PharmD, CGP, FASCP
Clinical Professor
Department of Clinical Pharmacy Practice
College of Pharmacy & Allied Health Professions
St. John's University
Jamaica, New York

Marcia L. Buck, PharmD, FCCP, FPPAG
Professor
Department of Pediatrics
School of Medicine
Clinical Coordinator, Pediatrics
Department of Pharmacy
University of Virginia
Charlottesville, Virginia

Michael G. Carvalho, PharmD, BCPP
Assistant Dean of Interprofessional Education
Professor and Chair
Department of Pharmacy Practice
School of Pharmacy–Boston
MCPHS University
Boston, Massachusetts

Judy W. Cheng, PharmD, MPH, BCPS, FCCP
Professor of Pharmacy Practice
School of Pharmacy–Boston
MCPHS University
Boston, Massachusetts

R. Rebecca Couris, PhD, RPh
Professor of Nutrition Science and Pharmacy Practice
Department of Pharmacy Practice, School of Pharmacy–Boston
MCPHS University
Boston, Massachusetts

Steven Gabardi, PharmD, BCPS, FAST, FCCP
Abdominal Organ Transplant Clinical Specialist & Program Director
PGY-2 Organ Transplant Pharmacology Residency
Brigham and Women's Hospital
Departments of Transplant Surgery / Pharmacy / Renal Division
Assistant Professor of Medicine
Harvard Medical School
Boston, Massachusetts

Jennifer D. Goldman, BS, PharmD, CDE, BC-ADM, FCCP
Professor of Pharmacy Practice
School of Pharmacy–Boston
MCPHS University
Boston, Massachusetts

Christy S. Harris, PharmD, BCPS, BCOP
Associate Professor of Pharmacy Practice
School of Pharmacy–Boston
MCPHS University
Boston, Massachusetts

Timothy R. Hudd, PharmD, AE-C
Associate Professor of Pharmacy Practice
School of Pharmacy–Boston
MCPHS University
Boston, Massachusetts

Timothy J. Ives, PharmD, MPH, FCCP, BCPS
Professor
Eshelman School of Pharmacy
The University of North Carolina at Chapel Hill
Chapel Hill, North Carolina

Susan Jacobson, MS, EdD, RPh
Associate Professor of Pharmacy Practice
School of Pharmacy–Boston
MCPHS University
Boston, Massachusetts

Maria D. Kostka-Rokosz, PharmD
Assistant Dean of Academic Affairs
Professor of Pharmacy Practice
School of Pharmacy–Boston
MCPHS University
Boston, Massachusetts

Trisha LaPointe, PharmD, BCPS
Associate Professor of Pharmacy Practice
School of Pharmacy–Boston
MCPHS University
Boston, Massachusetts

Michele Matthews, PharmD, CPE, BCACP
Associate Professor of Pharmacy Practice
School of Pharmacy–Boston
MCPHS University
Boston, Massachusetts

Susan L. Mayhew, PharmD, BCNSP, FASHP
Professor and Dean
Appalachian College of Pharmacy
Oakwood, Virginia

William W. McCloskey, BA, BS, PharmD
Professor and Vice-Chair
Department of Pharmacy Practice
School of Pharmacy–Boston
MCPHS University
Boston, Massachusetts

Myrna Y. Munar, PharmD
Associate Professor
Department of Pharmacy Practice
College of Pharmacy
Oregon State University
Oregon Health and Science University
Portland, Oregon

Jean M. Nappi, PharmD, FCCP, BCPS AQ-Cardiology
Professor
College of Pharmacy
Medical University of South Carolina
Charleston, South Carolina

Kamala M. Nola, PharmD, MS
Professor and Vice-Chair
Department of Pharmacy Practice
Lipscomb University College of Pharmacy
Nashville, Tennessee

Dorothea C. Rudorf, PharmD, MS
Professor of Pharmacy Practice
School of Pharmacy–Boston
MCPHS University
Boston, Massachusetts

Carrie A. Sincak, PharmD, BCPS, FASHP
Assistant Dean for Clinical Affairs and Professor
Department of Pharmacy Practice
Midwestern University Chicago College of Pharmacy
Downers Grove, Illinois

Timothy E. Welty, PharmD, FCCP
Professor
Department of Pharmacy Practice
University of Kansas School of Pharmacy
Lawrence, Kansas

G. Christopher Wood, PharmD, FCCP, FCCM, BCPS
Associate Professor of Clinical Pharmacy
University of Tennessee Health Science Center
College of Pharmacy
Memphis, Tennessee

Kathy Zaiken, PharmD
Professor of Pharmacy Practice
School of Pharmacy–Boston
MCPHS University
Boston, Massachusetts

Caroline S. Zeind, PharmD
Associate Provost for Academic and International Affairs
Chief Academic Officer
Worcester, Massachusetts and Manchester, New Hampshire Campuses
Professor of Pharmacy Practice
Academic Affairs
MCPHS University
Boston, Massachusetts

Contributors

Steven R. Abel, PharmD, FASHP
Professor of Pharmacy Practice
Associate Provost for Engagement
Purdue University
West Lafayette, Indiana

Jessica L. Adams, PharmD, BCPS, AAHIVP
Assistant Professor of Clinical Pharmacy
HIV and Infectious Diseases Specialist
Department of Pharmacy Practice and Pharmacy Administration
Philadelphia College of Pharmacy
University of the Sciences
Philadelphia, Pennsylvania

Brian K. Alldredge, PharmD
Professor and Vice Provost
University of California–San Francisco
San Francisco, California

Mary G. Amato, PharmD, MPH, BCPS
Professor of Pharmacy Practice
School of Pharmacy–Boston
MCPHS University
Boston, Massachusetts

Jaime E. Anderson, PharmD, BCOP
Oncology Clinical Pharmacy Specialist
MD Anderson Medical Center
University of Texas
Houston, Texas

Michael C. Angelini, PharmD, MA, BCPP
Associate Professor of Pharmacy Practice
School of Pharmacy–Boston
MCPHS University
Boston, Massachusetts

Albert T. Bach, PharmD
Assistant Professor of Pharmacy Practice
School of Pharmacy
Chapman University
Irvine, California

Jennifer H. Baggs, PharmD, BCPS, BCNSP
Clinical Assistant Professor
University of Arizona
Tucson, Arizona

David T. Bearden, PharmD
Clinical Professor and Chair
Department of Pharmacy Practice
Clinical Assistant Director
Department of Pharmacy Services
College of Pharmacy
Oregon State University
Oregon Health and Science University
Portland, Oregon

Sandra Benavides, PharmD, FCCP, FPPAG
Professor
Assistant Dean for Programmatic Assessment and Accreditation
Interim Chair
Department of Clinical and Administrative Sciences
Larkin Health Sciences Institute College of Pharmacy

Paul M. Beringer, PharmD, FASHP, FCCP
Associate Professor
Department of Clinical Pharmacy
University of Southern California
Los Angeles, California

Snehal H. Bhatt, PharmD, BCPS
Associate Professor of Pharmacy Practice
School of Pharmacy–Boston
MCPHS University
Clinical Pharmacist
Beth Israel Deaconess Medical Center
Boston, Massachusetts

Jeff F. Binkley, PharmD, BCNSP, FASHP
Administrative Director of Pharmacy
Maury Regional Medical Center and Affiliates
Columbia, Tennessee

Marlo Blazer, PharmD, BCOP
Assistant Director
Xcenda, an AmerisourceBergen Company
Columbus, Ohio

KarenBeth H. Bohan, PharmD, BCPS
Professor and Founding Chair
Department of Pharmacy Practice
School of Pharmacy and Pharmaceutical Sciences
Binghamton University
Binghamton, New York

Suzanne G. Bollmeier, PharmD, BCPS, AE-C
Professor of Pharmacy Practice
School of Pharmacy–Boston
St. Louis College of Pharmacy
St. Louis, Missouri

Laura M. Borgelt, PharmD, BCPS
Associate Dean of Administration and Operations
Professor
Departments of Clinical Pharmacy and Family Medicine
University of Colorado Anschutz Medical Campus
Skaggs School of Pharmacy
Aurora, Colorado

Jolene R. Bostwick, PharmD, BCPS, BCPP
Clinical Associate Professor
Department of Clinical, Social, and Administrative Sciences
University of Michigan College of Pharmacy
Ann Arbor, Michigan

Nicole J. Brandt, PharmD, MBA, CGP, BCPP, FASCP
Executive Director
Peter Lamy Center on Drug Therapy and Aging
Professor
University of Maryland School of Pharmacy
Baltimore, Maryland

Marcia L. Buck, PharmD, FCCP, FPPAG
Professor
Department of Pediatrics
School of Medicine
Clinical Coordinator, Pediatrics
Department of Pharmacy
University of Virginia
Charlottesville, Virginia

Deanna Buehrle, PharmD
Infectious Diseases Clinical Specialist
University of Pittsburgh Medical Center Presbyterian
Pittsburgh, Pennsylvania

Sara K. Butler, PharmD, BCPS, BOCP
Clinical Pharmacy Specialist, Medical Oncology
Barnes-Jewish Hospital
Saint Louis, Missouri

Beth Buyea, MHS, PA-C
Assistant Professor
Tufts University, School of Medicine
Boston, Massachusetts

Charles F. Caley, PharmD, BCCP
Clinical Professor
School of Pharmacy
University of Connecticut
Storrs, Connecticut

Joseph Todd Carter, PharmD
Assistant Professor of Pharmacy Practice
Appalachian College of Pharmacy
Oakwood, Virginia
Primary Care Centers of Eastern Kentucky
Hazard, Kentucky

Michael G. Carvalho, PharmD, BCPP
Assistant Dean of Interprofessional Education
Professor and Chair
Department of Pharmacy Practice
School of Pharmacy–Boston
MCPHS University
Boston, Massachusetts

Jamie J. Cavanaugh, PharmD, CPP, BCPS
Assistant Professor of Clinical Education, Pharmacy
Assistant Professor of Medicine
University of North Carolina at Chapel Hill
Chapel Hill, North Carolina

Michelle L. Ceresia, PharmD, FACVP
Associate Professor of Pharmacy Practice
School of Pharmacy–Boston
MCPHS University
Boston, Massachusetts
Adjunct Associate Professor
Department of Clinical Sciences
Cummings Veterinary School of Medicine at Tufts University
North Grafton, Massachusetts

Laura Chadwick, PharmD
Clinical Specialist in Pharmacogenomics
Boston Children's Hospital
Boston, Massachusetts

Michelle L. Chan, PharmD, BCPS
Clinical Pharmacy Specialist
Infectious Diseases
Methodist Hospital of Southern California
Arcadia, California

Lin H. Chen, MD, FACP, FASTMH
Associate Professor of Medicine
Harvard Medical School
Boston, Massachusetts
Director of the Travel Medicine Center
Mount Auburn Hospital
Cambridge, Massachusetts

Steven W. Chen, PharmD, FASHP, FNAP
Associate Professor and Chair
Titus Family Department of Clinical Pharmacy
William A. Heeres and Josephine A. Heeres Endowed Chair in Community Pharmacy
University of Southern California School of Pharmacy
Los Angeles, California

Judy W. Cheng, PharmD, MPH, BCPS, FCCP
Professor of Pharmacy Practice
School of Pharmacy–Boston
MCPHS University
Boston, Massachusetts

Michael F. Chicella, PharmD, FPPAG
Pharmacy Clinical Manager
Children's Hospital of The King's Daughters
Norfolk, Virginia

Jennifer W. Chow, PharmD
Director of Professional Development and Education
Pediatric Pharmacy Advocacy Group
Memphis, Tennessee

Cary R. Chrisman, PharmD
Assistant Professor
Department of Clinical Pharmacy
University of Tennessee College of Pharmacy
Clinical Pharmacist, Department of Pharmacy
Methodist Medical Center
Memphis and Oak Ridge, Tennessee

Edith Claros, PhD, MSN, RN, APHN-BC
Assistant Dean and Associate Professor
School of Nursing
MCPHS University
Worcester, Massachusetts

John D. Cleary, PharmD, FCCP, BCPS
Director of Pharmacy
St. Dominic-Jackson Memorial Hospital
Schools of Medicine and Pharmacy
University of Mississippi Medical Center
Jackson, Mississippi

Michelle Condren, PharmD, BCPPS, AE-C, CDE, FPPAG
Professor and Department Chair
University of Oklahoma College of Pharmacy
University of Oklahoma School of Community Medicine
Tulsa, Oklahoma

Amanda H. Corbett, PharmD, BCPS, FCCP
Clinical Associate Professor
Eshelman School of Pharmacy and School of Medicine
Global Pharmacology Coordinator
Institute for Global Health and Infectious Diseases
University of North Carolina
Chapel Hill, North Carolina

Mackenzie L. Cottrell, PharmD, MS, BCPS, AAHIVP
Research Assistant Professor
UNC Eshelman School of Pharmacy
University of North Carolina at Chapel Hill
Chapel Hill, North Carolina

R. Rebecca Couris, PhD, RPh
Professor of Nutrition Science and Pharmacy Practice
Department of Pharmacy Practice, School of Pharmacy–Boston
MCPHS University
Boston, Massachusetts

Steven J. Crosby, MA, BSP, RPh, FASCP
Assistant Professor of Pharmacy Practice
School of Pharmacy–Boston
MCPHS University
Boston, Massachusetts

Jason Cross, PharmD
Associate Professor Pharmacy Practice
School of Pharmacy–Worcester/Manchester
MCPHS University
Worcester, Massachusetts

Sandeep Devabhakthuni, PharmD, BCPS–AQ Cardiology
Assistant Professor of Cardiology/Critical Care
University of Maryland School of Pharmacy
Baltimore, Maryland

Andrea S. Dickens, PharmD, BCOP
Clinical Pharmacy Specialist
MD Anderson Cancer Center
University of Texas
Houston, Texas

Lisa M. DiGrazia, PharmD, BCPS, BCOP
Director, Medical Affairs
Amneal Biosciences Bridgewater, New Jersey

Suzanne Dinsmore, BSP, PharmD, CGP
Assistant Professor of Pharmacy Practice
School of Pharmacy–Boston
MCPHS University
Boston, Massachusetts

Betty J. Dong, PharmD, FASHP, FAPHA, FCCP, AAHIVP
Professor of Clinical Pharmacy and Family and Community Medicine
Department of Clinical Pharmacy
Schools of Pharmacy and Medicine
University of California, San Francisco
San Francisco, California

Richard H. Drew, PharmD, MS, FCCP
Professor and Vice-Chair of Research and Scholarship
Campbell University College of Pharmacy and Health Sciences
Buies Creek, North Carolina
Associate Professor of Medicine (Infectious Diseases)
Duke University School of Medicine
Durham, North Carolina

Robert L. Dufresne, PhD, PhD, BCPS, BCPP
INBRE Behavioral Science Coordinator and Professor
College of Pharmacy
University of Rhode Island
Kingston, Rhode Island
Psychiatric Pharmacotherapy Specialist
PGY-2 Psychiatric Pharmacy Residency Program Director
Providence VA Medical Center
Providence, Rhode Island

Kaelen C. Dunican, PharmD
Professor of Pharmacy Practice
School of Pharmacy–Worcester/Manchester
MCPHS University
Worcester, Massachusetts

Brianne L. Dunn, PharmD
Associate Dean for Outcomes Assessment & Accreditation
Clinical Associate Professor
Department of Clinical Pharmacy and Outcomes Sciences
University of South Carolina College of Pharmacy
Columbia, South Carolina

Robert E. Dupuis, PharmD, FCCP
Clinical Professor of Pharmacy
Eshelman School of Pharmacy
University of North Carolina at Chapel Hill
Chapel Hill, North Carolina

Cheryl R. Durand, PharmD
Associate Professor of Pharmacy Practice
School of Pharmacy–Worcester/Manchester
MCPHS University
Manchester, New Hampshire

Megan J. Ehret, PharmD, MS, BCPP
Behavior Health Clinical Pharmacy Specialist
United States Department of Defense
Fort Belvoir Community Hospital
Fort Belvoir, Virginia

Carol Eliadi, EdD, JD, NP-BC
Professor and Dean of Nursing
MCPHS University
School of Nursing–Worcester, Massachusetts and Manchester, New Hampshire Campuses

Shareen Y. El-Ibiary, PharmD, FCCP, BCPS
Professor of Pharmacy Practice
Department of Pharmacy Practice
Midwestern University College of Pharmacy–Glendale
Glendale, Arizona

Katie Dillinger Ellis, PharmD
Clinical Specialist
Neonatal/Infant Intensive Care
Department of Pharmacy
The Children's Hospital of Philadelphia
Philadelphia, Pennsylvania

Justin C. Ellison, PharmD, BCPP
Clinical Pharmacy Specialist–Mental Health
Providence Veterans Affairs Medical Center
Providence, Rhode Island

Rachel Elsey, PharmD, BCOP
Clinical Pharmacist
Avera Cancer Institute
South Dakota State University
Sioux Falls, South Dakota

Gregory A. Eschenauer, PharmD, BCPS (AQ-ID)
Clinical Assistant Professor
University of Michigan
Ann Arbor, Michigan

John Fanikos, MBA, RPh
Executive Director of Pharmacy
Brigham and Women's Hospital
Adjunct Associate Professor of Pharmacy Practice
MCPHS University
Department of Pharmacy Practice, School of Pharmacy–Boston
Boston, Massachusetts

Elizabeth Farrington, PharmD, FCCP, FCCM, FPPAG, BCPS
Pharmacist III–Pediatrics
Department of Pharmacy
New Hanover Regional Medical Center
Wilmington, North Carolina

Erika Felix-Getzik, PharmD
Associate Professor of Pharmacy Practice
School of Pharmacy–Boston
MCPHS University
Boston, Massachusetts

Jonathan D. Ference, PharmD
Assistant Dean of Assessment and Alumni Affairs
Associate Professor of Pharmacy Practice
Director of Pharmacy Care Labs
Nesbitt School of Pharmacy
Wilkes University
Wilkes-Barre, Pennsylvania

Kimberly Ference, PharmD
Associate Professor
Department of Pharmacy Practice
Nesbitt College of Pharmacy and Nursing
Wilkes University
Wilkes-Barre, Pennsylvania

Victoria F. Ferraresi, PharmD, FASHP, FCSHP
Director of Pharmacy Services
Pathways Home Health and Hospice
Sunnyvale, California

Joseph W. Ferullo, PharmD
Associate Professor of Pharmacy Practice
School of Pharmacy–Boston
MCPHS University
Boston, Massachusetts

Christopher K. Finch, PharmD, BCPS, FCCM, FCCP
Director of Pharmacy
Methodist University Hospital
Associate Professor
College of Pharmacy
University of Tennessee
Memphis, Tennessee

Douglas N. Fish, PharmD, BCPS–AQ ID
Professor and Chair
Department of Clinical Pharmacy
Skaggs School of Pharmacy and Pharmaceutical Science
University of Colorado
Clinical Specialist in Critical Care/Infectious Diseases
University of Colorado Hospital
Aurora, Colorado

Jeffrey J. Fong, PharmD, BCPS
Associate Professor of Pharmacy Practice
School of Pharmacy–Worcester/Manchester
MCPHS University
Worcester, Massachusetts

Andrea S. Franks, PharmD, BCPS
Associate Professor, Clinical Pharmacy and Family Medicine
College of Pharmacy and Graduate School Medicine
University of Tennessee Health Science Center
Knoxville, Tennessee

Kristen N. Gardner, PharmD
Clinical Pharmacy Specialist–Behavioral Health
Highline Behavioral Clinic
Kaiser Permanente Colorado
Denver, Colorado

Virginia L. Ghafoor, PharmD
Pharmacy Specialist–Pain Management
University of Minnesota Medical Center
Minneapolis, Minnesota

Brooke Gildon, PharmD, BCPPS, BCPS, AE-C
Associate Professor of Pharmacy Practice
Southwestern Oklahoma State University College of Pharmacy
Weatherford, Oklahoma

Ashley Glode, PharmD, BCOP
Assistant Professor
Department of Clinical Pharmacy
Skaggs School of Pharmacy and Pharmaceutical Sciences
University of Colorado Anschutz Medical Campus
Aurora, Colorado

Jeffery A. Goad, PharmD, MPH, FAPhA, PCPhA, FCSHP
Professor and Chair
Department of Pharmacy Practice
School of Pharmacy
Chapman University
Irvine, California

Jennifer D. Goldman, BS, PharmD, CDE, BC-ADM, FCCP
Professor of Pharmacy Practice
School of Pharmacy–Boston
MCPHS University
Boston, Massachusetts

Joel Goldstein, MD
Assistant Clinical Professor
Harvard Medical School
Division of Child/Adolescent Psychology
Cambridge Health Alliance
Cambridge, Massachusetts

Luis S. Gonzalez, III, PharmD, BCPS
Manager
Clinical Pharmacy Services
PGY1 Pharmacy Residency Program Director
Conemaugh Memorial Medical Center
Johnstown, Pennsylvania

Larry Goodyer, PhD, MRPharmS, BCPS
Professor, School of Pharmacy
De Montfort University
Leicester, United Kingdom
Medical Director
Nomad Travel Stores and Clinic
Bishop's Stortford, United Kingdom

Mary-Kathleen Grams, PharmD, BCGP
Assistant Professor of Pharmacy Practice
School of Pharmacy–Boston
MCPHS University
Boston, Massachusetts

Philip Grgurich, PharmD, BCPS
Associate Professor of Pharmacy Practice
School of Pharmacy–Boston
MCPHS University
Boston, Massachusetts

B. Joseph Guglielmo, PharmD
Professor and Dean
School of Pharmacy
University of California, San Francisco
San Francisco, California

Karen M. Gunning, PharmD, BCPS, BCACP, FCCP
Professor (Clinical) and Interim Chair of Pharmacotherapy
Adjunct Professor of Family and Preventive Medicine
PGY2 Ambulatory Care Residency Director
Clinical Pharmacist–University of Utah Family Medicine Residency/Sugarhouse Clinic
University of Utah College of Pharmacy and School of Medicine
Salt Lake City, Utah

Mary A. Gutierrez, PharmD, BCPP
Professor of Pharmacy Practice
Chapman University School of Pharmacy
Irvine, California

Justinne Guyton, PharmD, BCACP
Associate Professor of Pharmacy Practice
Site Coordinator
PGY2 Ambulatory Care Residency Program
St. Louis College of Pharmacy
St. Louis, Missouri

Matthew Hafermann, PharmD, BCPS
Medical ICU/Cardiology Clinical Pharmacist
Harborview Medical Center
PGY1 Pharmacy Residency Coordinator
Medicine Clinical Instructor
University of Washington School of Pharmacy
Seattle, Washington

Jason S. Haney, PharmD, BCPS, BCCCP
Assistant Professor
Department of Clinical Pharmacy and Outcome Sciences
South Carolina College of Pharmacy
Medical University of South Carolina
Charleston, South Carolina

Christy S. Harris, PharmD, BCPS, BCOP
Associate Professor of Pharmacy Practice
School of Pharmacy–Boston
MCPHS University
Boston, Massachusetts

Mary F. Hebert, PharmD, FCCP
Professor
Department of Pharmacy
Adjunct Professor of Obstetrics and Gynecology
University of Washington
Seattle, Washington

Emily L. Heil, PharmD, BCPS-AQ ID
Assistant Professor
Infectious Diseases
University of Maryland School of Pharmacy
Baltimore, Maryland

Erika L. Hellenbart, PharmD, BCPS
Clinical Assistant Professor
University of Illinois at Chicago College of Pharmacy
Chicago, Illinois

David W. Henry, PharmD, MS, BCOP, FASHP
Associate Professor and Chair
Pharmacy Practice
University of Kansas School of Pharmacy
Lawrence, Kansas

Christopher M. Herndon, PharmD, BCPS, CPE
Associate Professor
Department of Pharmacy Practice
School of Pharmacy
Southern University Illinois Edwardsville
Edwardsville, Illinois

Richard N. Herrier, PharmD, FAPhA
Clinical Professor
Department of Pharmacy Practice and Science
College of Pharmacy
University of Arizona
Tucson, Arizona

Karl M. Hess, PharmD, CTH, FCPhA
Vice Chair of Clinical and Administrative Sciences
Associate Professor
Certificate Coordinator for Medication Therapy Outcomes
Keck Graduate Institute Claremont, California

Curtis D. Holt, PharmD
Clinical Professor
Department of Surgery
University of California, Los Angeles
Los Angeles, California

Evan R. Horton, PharmD
Associate Professor of Pharmacy Practice
School of Pharmacy–Worcester/Manchester
MCPHS University
Worcester, Massachusetts

Priscilla P. How, PharmD, BCPS
Assistant Professor
Director of PharmD Program
Department of Pharmacy
Faculty of Science
National University of Singapore
Principal Clinical Pharmacist
Department of Medicine
Division of Nephrology
National University Hospital
Singapore, Republic of Singapore

Molly E. Howard, PharmD, BCPS
Clinical Pharmacy Specialist
Central Alabama Veterans Health Care System
Montgomery, Alabama

Timothy R. Hudd, PharmD, AE-C
Associate Professor of Pharmacy Practice
School of Pharmacy–Boston
MCPHS University
Boston, Massachusetts

Bethany Ibach, PharmD, BCPPS
Assistant Professor of Pharmacy Practice
School of Pharmacy, Pediatrics Division
Texas Tech University Health Sciences Center
Abilene, Texas

Gail S. Itokazu, PharmD
Clinical Associate Professor
Department of Pharmacy Practice
University of Illinois, Chicago
Clinical Pharmacist
Division of Infectious Diseases
John H. Stroger Jr. Hospital of Cook County
Chicago, Illinois

Timothy J. Ives, PharmD, MPH, FCCP, CPP
Professor of Pharmacy
Adjunct Professor of Medicine
Eshelman School of Pharmacy
University of North Carolina at Chapel Hill
Chapel Hill, North Carolina

Nicole A. Kaiser, RPh, BCOP
Oncology Clinical Pharmacy Specialist
Children's Hospital Colorado
Aurora, Colorado

James S. Kalus, PharmD, FASHP
Director of Pharmacy
Henry Ford Health System
Henry Ford Hospital
Detroit, Michigan

Marina D. Kaymakcalan, PharmD
Clinical Pharmacy Specialist
Dana Farber Cancer Institute
Boston, Massachusetts

Michael B. Kays, PharmD, FCCP
Associate Professor
Department of Pharmacy Practice
Purdue University College of Pharmacy
West Lafayette and Indianapolis, Indiana

Jacob K. Kettle, PharmD, BCOP
Oncology Clinical Pharmacy Specialist
University of Missouri Health Care
Columbia, Missouri

Rory E. Kim, PharmD
Assistant Professor of Clinical Pharmacy
University of Southern California School of Pharmacy
Los Angeles, California

Lee A. Kral, PharmD, BCPS, CPE
Clinical Pharmacy Specialist, Pain Management
Department of Pharmaceutical Care
The University of Iowa Hospitals and Clinics
Iowa City, Iowa

Donna M. Kraus, PharmD, FAPhA, FPPAG, FCCP
Pediatric Clinical Pharmacist/Associate Professor of Pharmacy Practice
Departments of Pharmacy Practice and Pediatrics
Colleges of Pharmacy and Medicine
University of Illinois at Chicago
Chicago, Illinois

Susan A. Krikorian, MS, PharmD
Professor of Pharmacy Practice
School of Pharmacy–Boston
MCPHS University
Boston, Massachusetts

Andy Kurtzweil, PharmD, BCOP
Pharmacy Supervisor–Adult Hematology and Oncology/BMT
University of Minnesota Health
Minneapolis, Minnesota

Benjamin Laliberte, PharmD, BCPS
Clinical Pharmacy Specialist, Cardiology
Massachusetts General Hospital
Boston, Massachusetts

Jerika T. Lam, PharmD, AAHIVP
Assistant Professor of Pharmacy Practice
School of Pharmacy
Chapman University
Irvine, California

Trisha LaPointe, PharmD, BCPS
Associate Professor of Pharmacy Practice
School of Pharmacy–Boston

MCPHS University
Boston, Massachusetts

Alan H. Lau, PharmD
Professor
Director, International Clinical Pharmacy Education
College of Pharmacy
University of Illinois at Chicago
Chicago, Illinois

Elaine J. Law, PharmD, BCPS
Assistant Clinical Professor of Pharmacy Practice
Thomas J. Long School of Pharmacy and Health Sciences
University of the Pacific
Stockton, California

Kimberly Lenz, PharmD
Clinical Pharmacy Manager
Office of Clinical Affairs
University of Massachusetts Medical School
Quincy, Massachusetts

Russell E. Lewis, PharmD, FCCP
Associate Professor of Medicine, Infectious Diseases
Department of Medical and Surgical Services
Infectious Diseases Unit, Policlinico S. Orsola-Malpighi
University of Bologna
Bologna, Italy

Rachel C. Long, PharmD, BCPS
Clinical Staff Pharmacist
Carolinas HealthCare System
Charlotte, North Carolina

Ann M. Lynch, BSP, PharmD, AE-C
Professor of Pharmacy Practice
School of Pharmacy–Worcester/Manchester
MCPHS University
Worcester, Massachusetts

Matthew R. Machado, PharmD
Associate Professor of Pharmacy Practice
School of Pharmacy–Boston
MCPHS University
Boston, Massachusetts

Emily Mackler, PharmD, BCOP
Clinical Pharmacist and Project Manager
Michigan Oncology Quality Consortium
University of Michigan
Ann Arbor, Michigan

Daniel R. Malcolm, PharmD, BCPS, BCCCP
Associate Professor and Vice-Chair
Clinical and Administrative Services
Sullivan University College of Pharmacy
Louisville, Kentucky

Shannon F. Manzi, PharmD, NREMT, FPPAG
Director, Clinical Pharmacogenomics Service
Manager, Emergency and ICU Pharmacy Services
Boston Children's Hospital
Boston, Massachusetts

Joel C. Marrs, PharmD, FCCP, FASHP, FNLA, BCPS-AQ Cardiology, BCACP, CLS, ASH-CHC
Associate Professor
Department of Clinical Pharmacy
University of Colorado Anschutz Medical Campus
Skaggs School of Pharmacy and Pharmaceutical Sciences
Clinical Pharmacy Specialist
Department of Pharmacy
Denver Health and Hospital Authority
Aurora, Colorado

John Marshall, PharmD, BCPS, BCCCP, FCCM
Clinical Pharmacy Coordinator–Critical Care
Beth Israel Deaconess Medical Center
Boston, Massachusetts

Darius L. Mason, PharmD, BCPS, FACN
Clinical Pharmacist
Methodist South Hospital
Memphis, Tennessee

Susan L. Mayhew, PharmD, BCNSP, FASHP
Professor and Dean
Appalachian College of Pharmacy
Oakwood, Virginia

James W. McAuley, RPh, PhD, FAPhA
Associate Dean for Academic Affairs and Professor
Departments of Pharmacy Practice and Neurology
The Ohio State University College of Pharmacy
Columbus, Ohio

Sarah E. McBane, PharmD, CDE, BCPS, FCCP, FCPhA, APh
Professor and Chair
Department of Pharmacy Practice
West Coast University
Los Angeles, California

William W. McCloskey, BA, BS, PharmD
Professor of Pharmacy Practice
School of Pharmacy–Boston
MCPHS University
Boston, Massachusetts

Chephra McKee, PharmD
Assistant Professor of Pharmacy Practice
School of Pharmacy
Pediatrics Division
Texas Tech University Health Sciences Center
Abilene, Texas

Molly G. Minze, PharmD, BCACP
Associate Professor of Pharmacy Practice
Ambulatory Care Division
School of Pharmacy
Texas Tech University Health Sciences Center
Abilene, Texas

Amee D. Mistry, PharmD
Associate Professor Pharmacy Practice
School of Pharmacy–Boston
MCPHS University
Boston, Massachusetts

Katherine G. Moore, PharmD, BCPS, BCACP
Executive Director of Experiential Education
Associate Professor of Pharmacy Practice
Presbyterian College School of Pharmacy
Clinton, South Carolina

Jill A. Morgan, PharmD, BCPS, BCPPS
Associate Professor and Chair
Department of Pharmacy Practice and Science
University of Maryland School of Pharmacy
Baltimore, Maryland

Anna K. Morin, PharmD
Professor of Pharmacy Practice and Dean
School of Pharmacy–Worcester/Manchester
MCPHS University
Worcester, Massachusetts

Pamela B. Morris, MD, FACC, FAHA, FASPC, FNLA
Director, Seinsheimer Cardiovascular Health Program
Co-Director, Women's Heart Care
Medical University of South Carolina
Charleston, South Carolina

Oussayma Moukhachen, PharmD, BCPS
Assistant Professor Pharmacy Practice
School of Pharmacy–Boston
MCPHS University
Boston, Massachusetts
Clinical Care Specialist
Mount Auburn Hospital
Cambridge, Massachusetts

Kelly A. Mullican, PharmD
Primary Care Clinical Pharmacy Specialist
Kaiser Permanente–Mid-Atlantic States
Washington, District of Columbia

Myrna Y. Munar, PharmD
Associate Professor of Pharmacy
College of Pharmacy
Oregon State University
Oregon Health and Science University
Portland, Oregon

Yulia A. Murray, PharmD, BCPS
Assistant Professor of Pharmacy Practice
School of Pharmacy–Boston
MCPHS University
Boston, Massachusetts

Milap C. Nahata, MS, PharmD, FCCP, FAPhA, FASHP
Director, Institute of Therapeutic Innovations and Outcomes
Professor Emeritus of Pharmacy, Pediatrics, and Internal Medicine
Colleges of Pharmacy and Medicine
The Ohio State University
Columbus, Ohio

Richard S. Nicholas, PharmD, ND, CDE, BCPS, BCACP
Assistant Professor of Pharmacy Practice
Appalachian College of Pharmacy
Oakwood, Virginia

Stefanie C. Nigro, PharmD, BCACP, BC-ADM
Assistant Professor of Pharmacy Practice
School of Pharmacy–Boston
MCPHS University
Boston, Massachusetts

Cindy L. O'Bryant, PharmD, BCOP, FCCP, FHOPA
Professor
Department of Clinical Pharmacy
Skaggs School of Pharmacy and Pharmaceutical Sciences
Clinical Pharmacy Specialist in Oncology
University of Colorado Cancer Center
Aurora, Colorado

Kirsten H. Ohler, PharmD, BCPS, BCPPS
Clinical Assistant Professor of Pharmacy Practice
College of Pharmacy
University of Illinois at Chicago
Clinical Pharmacy Specialist–Neonatal ICU
University of Illinois at Chicago Hospital and Health Sciences System
Chicago, Illinois

Julie L. Olenak, PharmD
Assistant Dean of Student Affairs
Associate Professor
Department of Pharmacy Practice
Nesbitt College of Pharmacy and Nursing
Wilkes University
Wilkes-Barre, Pennsylvania

Jacqueline L. Olin, MS, PharmD, BCPS, CDE, FASHP, FCCP
Professor of Pharmacy
School of Pharmacy
Wingate University
Wingate, North Carolina

Neeta Bahal O'Mara, PharmD, BCPS
Clinical Pharmacist
Dialysis Clinic, Inc.
North Brunswick, New Jersey

Robert L. Page, II, PharmD, MSPH, FHFSA, FCCP, FASHP, FASCP, CGP, BCPS (AQ-Cards)
Professor
Departments of Clinical Pharmacy and Physical Medicine
School of Pharmacy and Pharmaceutical Sciences
University of Colorado
Aurora, Colorado

Louise Parent-Stevens, PharmD, BCPS
Assistant Director of Introductory Pharmacy Practice Experiences
Clinical Assistant Professor
Department of Pharmacy Practice
University of Illinois at Chicago College of Pharmacy
Chicago, Illinois

Dhiren K. Patel, PharmD, CDE, BC-ADM, BCACP
Associate Professor of Pharmacy Practice
School of Pharmacy–Boston
MCPHS University
Boston, Massachusetts

Katherine Tipton Patel, PharmD, BCOP
Clinical Pharmacy Specialist
The University of Texas
MD Anderson Cancer Center
Houston, Texas

Jennifer T. Pham, PharmD, BCPS, BCPPS
Clinical Assistant Professor, Department of Pharmacy Practice
University of Illinois at Chicago College of Pharmacy
Clinical Pharmacy Specialist, Neonatal Clinical Pharmacist
University of Illinois Hospital and Health Sciences System
Chicago, Illinois

Jonathan D. Picker, MBChB, PhD
Assistant Professor
Harvard Medical School
Clinical Geneticist
Boston Children's Hospital
Boston, Massachusetts

Brian A. Potoski, PharmD, BCPS
Associate Professor
Departments of Pharmacy and Therapeutics
University of Pittsburgh School of Pharmacy
Associate Director, Antibiotic Management Program
University of Pittsburgh Medical Center
Presbyterian University Hospital
Pittsburgh, Pennsylvania

David J. Quan, PharmD, BCPS
Health Sciences Clinical Professor of Pharmacy
Department of Clinical Pharmacy
School of Pharmacy
University of California, San Francisco
Pharmacist Specialist–Solid Organ Transplant
University of California, San Francisco Medical Center
San Francisco, California

Erin C. Raney, PharmD, BCPS, BC-ADM
Professor of Pharmacy Practice
Midwestern University College of Pharmacy–Glendale
Glendale, Arizona

Valerie Relias, PharmD, BCOP
Clinical Pharmacy Specialist
Division of Hematology/Oncology
Tufts Medical Center
Boston, Massachusetts

Lee A. Robinson, MD
Instructor
Department of Psychiatry
Harvard Medical School
Boston, Massachusetts
Associate Training Director
Child and Adolescent Psychiatry Fellowship
Primary Care Mental Health Integrated Psychiatrist
Cambridge Health Alliance
Cambridge, Massachusetts

Charmaine Rochester-Eyeguokan, PharmD, BCPS, BCACP, CDE
Associate Professor of Pharmacy Practice and Science
University of Maryland School of Pharmacy
Baltimore, Maryland

Carol J. Rollins, PharmD, MS, RD, CNSC, BCNSP
Clinical Associate Professor
Department of Pharmacy Practice and Science
College of Pharmacy
The University of Arizona
Tucson, Arizona

Melody Ryan, PharmD, MPH, GCP, BCPS
Professor
Department of Pharmacy Practice and Science
College of Pharmacy
University of Kentucky
Lexington, Kentucky

David Schnee, PharmD, BCACP
Associate Professor of Pharmacy Practice
School of Pharmacy–Boston
MCPHS University
Boston, Massachusetts

Eric F. Schneider, BS Pharm, PharmD
Assistant Dean for Academics
Professor
School of Pharmacy
Wingate University
Wingate, North Carolina

Sheila Seed, PharmD, MPH
Professor of Pharmacy Practice
School of Pharmacy–Worcester/Manchester
MCPHS University
Worcester, Massachusetts

Timothy H. Self, PharmD
Professor of Clinical Pharmacy
College of Pharmacy
University of Tennessee Health Science Center
Memphis, Tennessee

Amy Hatfield Seung, PharmD, BCOP
Senior Director of Clinical Development
Physician Resource Management/Caret
Cary, North Carolina

Nancy L. Shapiro, PharmD, FCCP, BCPS
Operations Coordinator
University of Illinois Hospital and Health Sciences System
Clinical Associate Professor of Pharmacy Practice
Director, PGY2 Ambulatory Care Residency
College of Pharmacy
University of Illinois at Chicago
Chicago, Illinois

Iris Sheinhait, PharmD, MA, RPh
Certified Poison Information Specialist
Adjunct Assistant Professor
Regional Center for Poison Control Serving Massachusetts and Rhode Island
Boston Children's Hospital and MCPHS University
Boston, Massachusetts

Greene Shepherd, PharmD, DABAT
Clinical Professor and Vice-Chair
Division of Practice Advancement and Clinical Education
Director of Professional Education, Asheville Campus
Eshelman School of Pharmacy
University of North Carolina at Chapel Hill
Asheville, North Carolina

Devon A. Sherwood, PharmD, BCPP
Assistant Professor
Psychopharmacology
College of Pharmacy
University of New England
Portland, Maine

Richard J. Silvia, PharmD, BCCP
Associate Professor of Pharmacy Practice
School of Pharmacy–Boston
MCPHS University
Boston, Massachusetts

Carrie A. Sincak, PharmD, BCPS, FASHP
Assistant Dean for Clinical Affairs and Professor
Department of Pharmacy Practice
Midwestern University Chicago College of Pharmacy
Downers Grove, Illinois

Harleen Singh, PharmD, BCPS-AQ Cardiology, BCACP
Clinical Associate Professor of Pharmacy Practice
Oregon State University
Oregon Health and Science University
Portland, Oregon

Jessica C. Song, MA, PharmD
Clinical Pharmacy Supervisor
PGY1 Pharmacy Residency Coordinator
Department of Pharmacy Services
Santa Clara Valley Medical Center
San Jose, California

Suellyn J. Sorensen, PharmD, BCPS, FASHP
Director
Clinical Pharmacy Services
St. Vincent Indianapolis
Indianapolis, Indiana

Linda M. Spooner, PharmD, BCPS (AQ-ID), FASHP
Professor of Pharmacy Practice
School of Pharmacy–Worcester/Manchester
MCPHS University
Clinical Pharmacy Specialist in Infectious Diseases
Saint Vincent Hospital
Worcester, Massachusetts

Karyn M. Sullivan, PharmD, MPH
Professor of Pharmacy Practice
School of Pharmacy–Worcester/Manchester
MCPHS University
Worcester, Massachusetts

David J. Taber, PharmD, MS, BCPS
Associate Professor
Division of Transplant Surgery
College of Medicine
Medical University of South Carolina
Charleston, South Carolina

Candace Tan, PharmD, BCACP
Clinical Pharmacist
Kaiser Permanente
Los Angeles, California

Yasar O. Tasnif, PharmD, BCPS, FAST
Associate Professor
Cooperative Pharmacy Program
University of Texas at Austin and University of Texas, Rio Grande Valley
Clinical Pharmacist Specialist
Doctor's Hospital at Renaissance–Renaissance Transplant Institute
Edinburg, Texas

Daniel J. G. Thirion, BPharm, MSc, PharmD, FCSHP
Professeur Titulaire de Clinique
Faculté de Pharmacie
Université de Montréal
Pharmacien
Centre Universitaire de Santé McGill
Montréal, Québec, Canada

Angela M. Thompson, PharmD, BCPS
Assistant Professor
Department of Clinical Pharmacy
Skaggs School of Pharmacy and Pharmaceutical Sciences
University of Colorado
Aurora, Colorado

Lisa A. Thompson, PharmD, BCOP
Clinical Pharmacy Specialist in Oncology
Kaiser Permanente Colorado
Lafayette, Colorado

Toyin Tofade, MS, PharmD, BCPS, CPCC
Dean and Professor
Howard University College of Pharmacy
Washington, District of Columbia

Tran H. Tran, PharmD, BCPS
Associate Professor
Midwestern University, Chicago College of Pharmacy
Downers Grove, Illinois

Dominick P. Trombetta, PharmD, BCPS, CGP, FASCP
Associate Professor
Department of Pharmacy Practice
Nesbitt School of Pharmacy
Wilkes University
Wilkes-Barre, Pennsylvania

Toby C. Trujillo, PharmD, FCCP, FAHAH, BCPS-AQ Cardiology
Associate Professor
Department of Clinical Pharmacy
Skaggs School of Pharmacy and Pharmaceutical Sciences
University of Colorado
Aurora, Colorado

Sheila K. Wang, PharmD, BCPS (AQ–ID)
Associate Professor of Pharmacy Practice
Chicago College of Pharmacy
Midwestern University
Downers Grove, Illinois
Clinical Pharmacist, Infectious Disease
Program Director, Rush University Medical Center
Chicago, Illinois

Brian Watson, PharmD, BCPS
Pharmacist
University of Maryland Medical System
St. Joseph's Medical Center
Baltimore, Maryland

Kristin Watson, PharmD, BCPS-AQ Cardiology
Associate Professor, Vice-Chair of Clinical Services
University of Maryland School of Pharmacy
Baltimore, Maryland

Lynn Weber, PharmD, BCOP
Clinical Pharmacy Specialist, Oncology/Hematology
Pharmacy Residency Coordinator and PGY-1 Residency Director
Hennepin County Medical Center
Minneapolis, Minnesota

Kellie Jones Weddle, PharmD, BCOP, FCCP, FHOPA
Clinical Professor of Pharmacy Practice
College of Pharmacy
Purdue University
Indianapolis, Indiana

C. Michael White, PharmD, FCP, FCCP
Professor and Head
Department of Pharmacy Practice
School of Pharmacy
University of Connecticut
Storrs, Connecticut

Natalie Whitmire, PharmD, BCPS, BCGP
Pharmacist Specialist
University of California, San Diego Health

Barbara S. Wiggins, PharmD, BCPS, CLS, AACC, FAHA, FCCP, FNLA
Clinical Pharmacy Specialist–Cardiology
Medical University of South Carolina
Charleston, South Carolina

Kristine C. Willett, PharmD, FASHP
Associate Professor of Pharmacy Practice
School of Pharmacy–Worcester/Manchester
MCPHS University
Manchester, New Hampshire

Bradley R. Williams, PharmD, CGP
Professor of Clinical Pharmacy and Clinical Gerontology
School of Pharmacy
University of Southern California
Los Angeles, California

Casey B. Williams, PharmD, BCOP, FHOPA
Director, Center for Precision Oncology
Director, Department of Molecular and Experimental Medicine
Avera Cancer Institute
Sioux Falls, South Dakota

Dennis M. Williams, PharmD, BCPS, AE-C
Associate Professor and Vice-Chair for Professional Education and Practice
Division of Pharmacotherapy and Experimental Therapeutics
Eshelman School of Pharmacy
University of North Carolina at Chapel Hill
Chapel Hill, North Carolina

Katie A. Won, PharmD, BCOP
Clinical Pharmacist
Hennepin County Medical Center
Minneapolis, Minnesota

Annie Wong-Beringer, PharmD, FIDSA
Professor of Pharmacy
School of Pharmacy
University of Southern California
Los Angeles, California

Dinesh Yogaratnam, PharmD, BCPS, BCCCP
Assistant Professor of Pharmacy Practice
School of Pharmacy–Worcester/Manchester
MCPHS University
Worcester, Massachusetts

Kathy Zaiken, PharmD
Professor of Pharmacy Practice
School of Pharmacy–Boston
MCPHS University
Boston, Massachusetts

Caroline S. Zeind, PharmD
Associate Provost for Academic and International Affairs
Chief Academic Officer
Worcester, Massachusetts and Manchester, New Hampshire, Campuses
Professor of Pharmacy Practice
MCPHS University
Boston, Massachusetts

Sara Zhou, PharmD
Certified Poison Information Specialist
Adjunct Assistant Professor
Regional Center for Poison Control Serving Massachusetts and Rhode Island
Boston Children's Hospital and MCPHS University
Boston, Massachusetts

Kristin M. Zimmerman, PharmD, CGP, BCACP
Associate Professor
Department of Pharmacotherapy & Outcomes Science
Virginia Commonwealth University
Richmond, Virginia

Brief Table of Contents

SECTION 5: RENAL DISORDERS 556

Section Editor: Myrna Y. Munar

SECTION 6: IMMUNOLOGIC DISORDERS 679

Section Editor: Steven Gabardi

SECTION 7: NUTRITION ISSUES 746

Section Editors: R. Rebecca Couris and Susan L. Mayhew

SECTION 8: DERMATOLOGIC DISORDERS 807

Section Editor: Timothy J. Ives

SECTION 9: RHEUMATIC AND MUSCULOSKELETAL DISEASES 865

Section Editor: Kamala M. Nola

SECTION 10: WOMEN'S HEALTH 929

Section Editor: Trisha LaPointe

SECTION 11: ENDOCRINE DISORDERS 1038

Section Editor: Jennifer D. Goldman

SECTION 12: EYE DISORDERS 1148

Section Editor: Susan Jacobson

SECTION 13: NEUROLOGIC DISORDERS 1170

Section Editors: Michele Matthews and Timothy E. Welty

SECTION 14: INFECTIOUS DISEASES 1319

Section Editors: Dorothea C. Rudorf, G. Christopher Wood, and Caroline S. Zeind

SECTION 15: PSYCHIATRIC DISORDERS AND SUBSTANCE ABUSE 1731

Section Editors: Michael C. Angelini and Michael G. Carvalho

SECTION 16: HEMATOLOGY AND ONCOLOGY 1926

Section Editor: Christy S. Harris

SECTION 17: PEDIATRICS 2127

Section Editor: Marcia L. Buck

SECTION 18: GERIATRIC THERAPY 2216

Section Editor: Judith L. Beizer

Detailed Table of Contents

SECTION 18: GERIATRIC THERAPY 2216

Section Editor: Judith L. Beizer

SECTION 1 | General Principles

Section Editors: William W. McCloskey and Maria D. Kostka-Rokosz

1 Medication Therapy Management and Assessment of Therapy

Matthew R. Machado, Amee D. Mistry, and Joseph W. Ferullo

CORE PRINCIPLES

	CORE PRINCIPLES	CHAPTER CASES
1	Medication Therapy Management Services (MTMS) are a service or group of services that optimize therapeutic outcomes for individual patients.	**Case 1-5 (Questions 1–4)**
2	A successful MTMS encounter includes medication reconciliation and a comprehensive medication history.	**Case 1-1 (Questions 1–3)**
3	Sources of patient information for MTMS include the patient, the electronic health record, the paper chart, and the pharmacy information system.	**Case 1-5 (Questions 1, 5), Table 1-1**
4	A careful and complete patient interview should include medical, medication, and social histories, and it must be provided in a culturally sensitive manner.	**Case 1-1 (Questions 1–3), Table 1-2, Online Content**
5	A successful MTMS encounter must be well documented following the Problem Oriented Medical Record (POMR). Documentation involves collecting subjective and objective data to identify the primary problem.	**Case 1-5 (Question 1), Table 1-4 Case 1-2 (Question 1), Case 1-3 (Question 1), Case 1-4 (Question 1)**
6	The clinician must assess the drug therapy or disease-specific problem and create a treatment plan.	**Case 1-5 (Questions 1, 2)**
7	The final step in documenting the MTMS encounter is developing the medication action plan and processing any billing requirements.	**Case 1-5 (Questions 1, 2, 4)**
8	Accurate and complete communication of the MTMS encounter to the patient's health care team is vital.	**Case 1-5 (Question 3)**

This chapter discusses medication therapy management services (MTMS) with a focus on the assessment of drug therapy. The illustrations in this chapter primarily focus on the pharmacist; however, the principles used to assess patient response to drug therapy are of value to all health care providers.

As defined by the American Pharmacists Association, medication therapy management (MTM) is a term used to describe a broad range of health care services provided by pharmacists, the medication experts on the health care team. A consensus definition created by 11 pharmacy associations, adopted by the pharmacy profession in 2004, defines MTM as a service or group of services that optimize therapeutic outcomes for individual patients.[1] Pharmacists provide MTM to help patients get the best benefits from their medications by actively managing drug therapy and by identifying, preventing, and resolving medication-related problems.

MTM has a direct relationship to pharmaceutical care. Pharmaceutical care has been described as *the responsible provision of drug therapy to achieve definite outcomes that are intended to improve a patient's quality of life.*[2,3] In fact, MTM has been described as a service provided in the practice of pharmaceutical care.[4] However, unlike pharmaceutical care, MTM is recognized by payers, has current procedural terminology (CPT) codes specifically for pharmacists, and has several clearly defined interventions. Therefore, MTMS will be the term used to describe the activity of MTM in various patient populations.

With the passage of the Patient Protection and Affordable Care Act and the Health Care and Education Reconciliation Act of 2010, pharmacists have tremendous opportunities in the implementation of health care reform.[5,6] One of the hallmarks of this law is delivery system reform. As health care delivery systems change, pharmacists have an opportunity to improve overall quality of care, to become involved in coordinated health care approaches such as medical home teams and accountable care organizations, and to collaborate to improve care for high-risk patients and those with chronic conditions in primary-care settings. In the United States, there are an estimated 133 million people that have at least one chronic medical condition.[7] In 2010, 86% of all health care spending was for people with one or more chronic health condition(s).[8] Pharmacists will have additional opportunities as hospitals will have financial incentives to improve quality, reduce costs, and decrease hospital-acquired conditions.[5,6]

Both patient self-care and medication reconciliation are critical aspects of any MTMS encounter regardless of the setting (i.e., inpatient, community, ambulatory, or institutional). Patient self-care requires the patient to take responsibility for the illness; however, the help of a professional to structure healthy self-care is important. For example, patients with diabetes who monitor their blood glucose levels regularly and adjust their diet according to the guidelines published from the American Diabetes Association (ADA) would be practicing self-care. Self-care is often the work that the patient performs between visits with the provider. The patient should be involved in his or her own care to ensure the best outcomes.

Medication reconciliation is the comprehensive evaluation of a patient's medication regimen any time there is a change in therapy in an effort to avoid medication errors such as omissions, duplications, dosing errors, or drug interactions, as well as to observe compliance and adherence patterns. This process should include a comparison of the existing and previous medication regimens and should occur at every transition of care in which new medications are ordered, existing orders are rewritten or adjusted, or when the patient has added nonprescription medications to his or her self-care.[9] Although not a new concept to the profession of pharmacy, there has been heightened awareness and intensified effort in this area of practice as a result of the Joint Commission. In 2005, the Joint Commission announced its National Patient Safety Goal (NPSG) 8A and 8B to *accurately and completely reconcile medications across the continuum of care*. This goal requires institutions to develop and test processes for medication reconciliation in ambulatory and acute care settings.[10] In 2015, the Joint Commission's NPSG 3 has continued its focus on improving the safe use of medications, in particular by *maintaining and communicating accurate patient medical information.*[11]

The Centers for Medicare & Medicaid Services (CMS), the largest purchaser of health insurance in the United States, is directly connecting reimbursement for Medicare services to patient outcomes. CMS developed star ratings as a means to move away from the Pay-for-Service Model of healthcare and move toward a new quality based or Pay-for-Performance Model. CMS annually rates Medicare health plans on a scale of 1 to 5 stars, with 5 stars representing the highest quality. The overall scores are based on more than 50 care and service quality measures across five categories, including staying healthy, managing chronic conditions, member satisfaction, customer service, and pharmacy services. Specific to pharmacy services, CMS assesses Medicare prescription drug plans (MA-PD's or PDPs) using its rating scale, focusing on five quality measures. Two of those quality measures assess medication safety, while the other three evaluate adherence. The quality measures that focus on safety look at decreasing the amount of high-risk medications (HRMs) in patients 65 and older and whether diabetic patients who also have hypertension are taking an ACE Inhibitor, Angiotensin Receptor Blocker (ARB), or Direct Renin Inhibitor. (To view complete list of HRM's visit website: https://www.cms.gov/Medicare/Medicare-Fee-for-Service-Payment/PhysicianFeedbackProgram/Downloads/Elderly-High-Risk-Medications-DAE.pdf) CMS will monitor adherence through three separate measures that focus on evaluating the level of adherence of patients who are on medications for diabetes, hypertension, or hypercholesterolemia, specifically statins.[12] In August 2013, CMS released a study demonstrating that in 2010 Medicare Part D MTM programs improved therapy outcomes, most notably adherence, on patients who had congestive heart failure (HF), chronic obstructive pulmonary disease, and diabetes compared to those who did not receive such services.[13]

It is important for pharmacists to realize that MTMS are integral to improving health outcomes and are continuing to gain acceptance from payers, in both the private and public sectors. The opportunity for pharmacists to continue to expand their role, while offering high level care, along with the potential for improvement in pharmacy compensation is in line with the CMS star ratings.

The general approach to an MTMS patient encounter in various clinical settings will be discussed in the next sections. Figure 1-1 provides a visual representation of a systematic process for a comprehensive and effective approach for delivering MTMS.

SOURCES OF PATIENT INFORMATION

Successful patient assessment and monitoring requires gathering and organizing relevant information.[3,14] The patient (or family member or representative) is always the primary source of

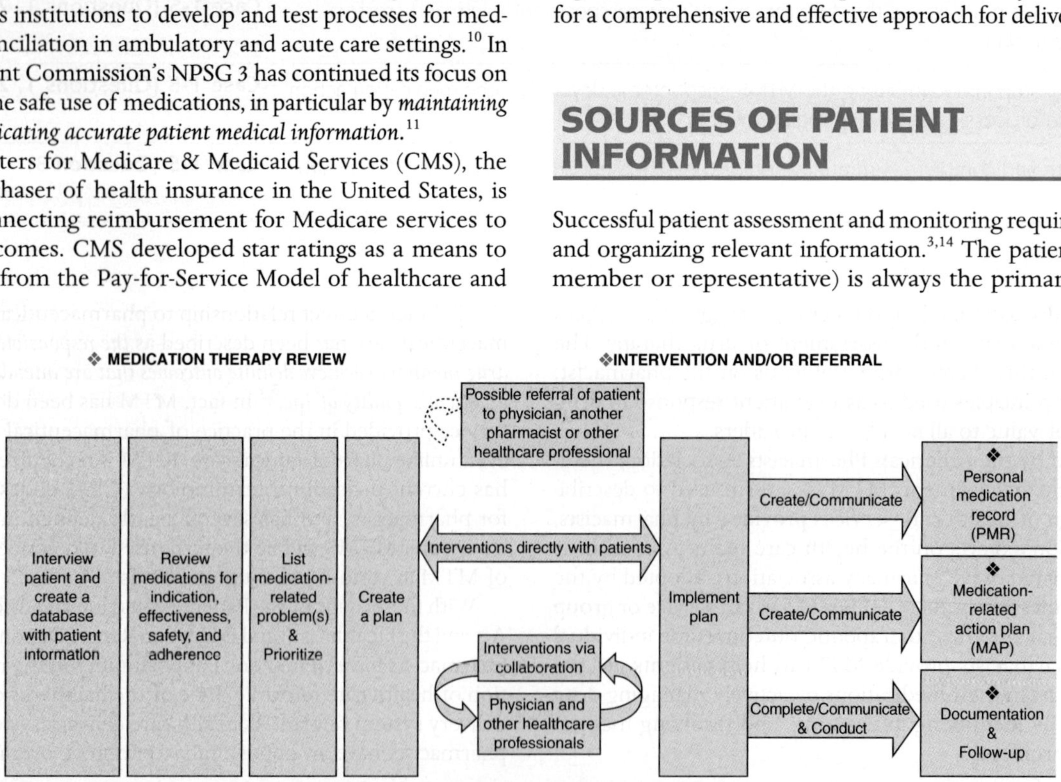

Figure 1-1 General approach to an MTMS patient encounter. (Reproduced from the American Pharmacists Association [APhA], with permission.)

information. The provider asks the patient a series of questions to obtain subjective information that is helpful in making a diagnosis or evaluating ongoing therapy. Likewise, providers without direct access to patient data must also obtain subjective data or measure objective physical data to guide recommendations for therapy and to monitor previously prescribed therapy.

Data-Rich and Data Poor Environments

In a "data-rich environment," such as a hospital, long-term facility, or outpatient medical clinic, a wealth of information is available to practitioners from the medical record, pharmacy profile, and medication administration record (MAR). In these settings, physicians, nurses, other health care providers, and patients are readily available. This facilitates timely, effective communication among providers involved in the drug therapy decision-making process. Objective data (e.g., diagnosis, physical examination, laboratory and other test results, vital signs, weight, medications, medication allergies, intravenous flow rates, and fluid balance) are readily available. The patient record provides information that is needed to identify and assess medical problems, which is necessary to design patient-specific care plans and document MTMS. In some settings, patient insurance information is important to help understand the formulary choices and access to medications.

In a "data-poor environment," such as a community pharmacy, clinicians are often required to make assessments with limited information. Although the information may be limited to (a) the medication profile, (b) patient demographic data, (c) medication allergy history, and (d) the patient's insurance coverage, it is still valuable.

The information in Table 1-1 is an illustrative summary of sources of patient information.

Table 1-1
Sources of Patient Information

Data-Rich Environment	Data-Poor Environment

Paper Charts
■ Decreasing use across the practice continuum
■ Limitations
  ■ Not consistent from site to site
  ■ Difficult to access, if more than one user
  ■ Delays in data entry
	Pharmacy Information Systems (PIS)—Outpatient and Inpatient
	■ Mainly focus on pharmacy billing, inventory management, production of medication labels
	■ Limited documentation of clinical pharmacy

Electronic Health Record (EHR) ■ Electronic version of a paper chart ■ Differs across practice settings ■ One of the most complete sources of reliable information ■ Can interface with other software systems in the pharmacy, laboratories, etc. ■ Data shared between systems in real time	

Pharmacy information systems (PIS) are generally considered data poor. Early PIS were established for pharmacy billing and inventory management. These initial systems provided fill lists, generated patient profiles, and produced medication labels, which were valuable to institutional pharmacies as the profession moved toward a unit dose medication distribution system. More modern functionalities allow for some limited documentation of clinical pharmacy activities, but still PIS is considered to be data poor.

An initiative by the US Department of Health and Human Services, called the EHR Incentive Program, exemplifies the importance of the integration of PIS with other computerized systems.[15] This initiative, the "Meaningful Use of an EHR," allows Medicare and Medicaid to provide incentive payments to providers and hospitals for the "meaningful use" of certified health information technology products. Eligibility for these incentive payments involves transitioning PIS to a more data-rich clinical information system (CIS), which includes direct computerized physician order entry, clinical decision support, an EHR, an electronic medication administration record (eMAR), and integration of various information systems, such as pharmacy and laboratory services. Additional functionality incorporates the use of bar code technology, which allows the ability to track and promote quality assurance during the medication administration process. Information generated by the CIS is electronically transmitted to the pharmacy in real time, eliminating lost, illegible, or incomplete medication orders.

In a data-poor environment, the clinician must be a proactive interviewer and may become an investigator. The investigative approach is direct and requires strong problem-solving abilities and active listening skills. Questions should be formulated to obtain information such as the medication history, actual medication use, patient perception of care, use of over-the-counter (OTC) and natural or herbal products, and health beliefs (cultural or otherwise). This approach can help to verify and ensure the accuracy of other data sources. Clinicians should be mindful that not all patients are reliable historians, and some are poor sources of information. Even when the patient is a poor historian, the interview provides critical information (e.g., indicator of poor adherence, need for a caregiver or interpreter) that cannot be obtained from other sources.

EFFECTIVE COMMUNICATION AND THE PATIENT INTERVIEW

The ability to use effective communication principles and history-taking skills is crucial to a successful patient interaction.[3,14] The importance of interviewing the patient, how to set the stage for the interview, general interview rules, and the essential information to be obtained from the interview are outlined in Table 1-2. Information obtained from the patient is critical for assessment and planning in MTM.

Motivational Interviewing (MI) is another useful method created by Miller and Rollnick that can be utilized during patient counseling to improve patient adherence to therapy. It is an empathetic and collaborative style of counseling based on five key principles: expressing empathy, developing discrepancy, adapting to resistance, avoiding arguments, and supporting self-efficacy, as seen in Table 1-3. The basis of MI is aimed to improve a patient's ambivalence to drug therapy through behavioral changes. It should be noted that motivational interviewing does not require a long-standing pharmacist–patient relationship to be effective, because individual sessions have been shown to be helpful.[16,17]

Table 1-2
Interviewing the Patient

Importance of Interviewing the Patient

Establishes professional relationship with the patient to:

- Obtain subjective data on medical problems
- Obtain patient-specific information on drug efficacy and toxicity
- Assess the patient's knowledge about, attitudes toward, and pattern of medication use
- Formulate a problem list
- Formulate plans for medication teaching and pharmaceutical care

How to Set the Stage for the Interview

- Have the patient complete a written health and medication questionnaire, if available
- Make the setting as private as possible
- Maintain eye contact
- Encourage the patient to be descriptive
- Clarify by restatement or patient demonstration (e.g., of a technique)

General Interview Rules

- Read the chart or patient profile first
- Ask for the patient's permission to conduct an interview or make an appointment to do so
- Begin with open-ended questions
- Move to close-ended questions
- Document interaction

Information to be Obtained

- History of allergies
- History of adverse drug reactions
- Weight and height
- Drugs: dose, route, frequency, and reason for use
- Perceived efficacy of each drug
- Perceived side effects
- Adherence to prescribed drug regimen
- Nonprescription medication use (including complementary and alternative medications)
- Possibility of pregnancy in women of childbearing age
- Family or other support systems

Source: Teresa O'Sullivan, PharmD, University of Washington.

Table 1-3
Principles of Motivational Interviewing

Expressing empathy	Convey to your patient that you understand their condition. This will allow the patient to be more open minded.
Develop discrepancy	Point out to the patient that there is a difference between current behavior and being able to reach their goals.
Adapt to resistance	Use different approaches to encourage the patient to channel their resistance into positive change.
Avoid arguments	Do not argue with your patient or force them to view things as you do.
Support self-efficacy	Assist the patient with believing that their own decisions will make a difference to behavioral change. Instead of telling the patient what to do, empower them to figure out what will be effective.

Adapted from Miller WR, Rollnick S. *Motivational Interviewing: Preparing People to Change Addictive Behavior*. New York, NY: Guilford Press; 1991. Center for Substance Abuse Treatment. Enhancing motivation for change in substance abuse treatment. Rockville, MD: substance abuse and mental health services administration (US); 1999. (Treatment Improvement Protocol (TIP) Series, No. 35.) Chapter 3—Motivational Interviewing as a Counseling Style. Available from: **http://www.ncbi.nlm.nih.gov/books/NBK64964/**

OBTAINING A PATIENT HISTORY

Those who provide MTMS should develop standardized forms to record patient information obtained from the patient interview. Standardization facilitates quick retrieval of information, minimizes the inadvertent omission of data, and enhances the ability of other practitioners to use shared records.[3,14]

The patient interview and record can be divided into sections with subjective and objective data as well as an assessment and plan (including expected outcomes). Components of subjective and objective data are the medical history, medication history, and social history. In some situations, histories can be supplemented by the generation of flowchart diagrams to monitor changes in specific variables with time. These charts and documentation systems may be incorporated into the EHR, PIS, or a similar electronic platform.

Medical History

A medical history is essential to the provision of MTMS. It can be as extensive as the medical records that are maintained in an institution or physician's office, or it can be a simple patient profile that is maintained in a community pharmacy. The purpose of the medical history is to identify significant past medical conditions or procedures; identify, characterize, and assess current acute and chronic medical conditions and symptoms; and gather all relevant health information that could influence drug selection or dosing (e.g., function of major organs such as the gastrointestinal tract, liver, and kidney; height and weight, including recent changes in either; age and sex; pregnancy and lactation status; and special nutritional needs). Not all interviews require the interviewer to ask for this much general information; however, in a data-poor environment, more information is required directly from the patient. A more focused interview may be appropriate in settings in which the information required is available electronically or is specific to a single disease state.

CASE 1-1

QUESTION 1: P.J., a 45-year-old woman of normal height and weight, states that she has diabetes. What questions might the practitioner ask P.J. to determine whether type 1 or type 2 diabetes should be documented in her medical history?

Patients usually can enumerate their medical problems in a general way, but the practitioner often will have to probe more specifically to refine the diagnosis and assess the severity of the condition. Diabetes mellitus is used to illustrate the types of questions that can be used to gather important health information and assess drug therapy. The following questions should generate information that will help to determine whether P.J. has type 1 or type 2 diabetes.

- How old were you when you were told you had diabetes?
- Do any of your relatives have diabetes? What do you know of their diabetes?
- Do you remember your symptoms? Please describe them to me.
- What medications have you used to treat your diabetes?

When questions such as these are combined with knowledge of the pathophysiology of diabetes, appreciation of the typical presenting signs and symptoms of the disease, and understanding of the drugs generally used to treat both forms of diabetes, meaningful MTM can be provided.

Medication History

In the community pharmacy setting, patients generally present themselves in one of four ways: (a) with a self-diagnosed condition for which nonprescription drug therapy is sought, (b) with a newly diagnosed condition for which a drug has been prescribed, (c) with a chronic condition that requires a refill of a previously prescribed drug or the initiation of a new drug, or (d) upon referral from their health plan or provider, or self-referral for focused medication therapy review (MTR).

In the first and second situations, the practitioner must confirm the diagnosis by using disease-specific questions as illustrated in Question 1. In the third situation, the practitioner uses the same type of questioning as in the first two situations; however, this time the practitioner needs to evaluate whether the desired therapeutic outcomes have been achieved. The practitioner must evaluate the information gleaned during follow-up visits in the context of the history and incorporate it into his or her assessment and medication action plan (MAP). In the fourth situation, in which patients require a focused MTR, the medication and medical history information are equally important. Without the medical history, it is not possible to evaluate whether the drug therapy is appropriate, and without an accurate medication history, it is not possible to determine whether the patient has reached the desired goals of therapy for her condition.

The goal of the medication history is to obtain and assess the following information: the specific prescription and nonprescription drugs that the patient is taking (such as OTC medications, botanicals, dietary supplements, recreational drugs, alcohol, tobacco, and home remedies); the intended purpose or indications for each of these medications; how it is taken (e.g., route, ingestion in relation to meals), how much, and how often these medications are used; how long these agents have been taken or used (start and stop dates); whether the patient believes that any of these agents are providing therapeutic benefit; whether the patient is experiencing or has experienced any adverse effects that could be caused by each of these agents (idiosyncratic reactions, toxic effects, adverse effects); whether the patient has stopped taking any of the medications for any reason; and allergic reactions or history of hypersensitivity or other severe reactions to drugs. This information should be as specific as possible, including a description of the reaction, the treatment, and the date of its occurrence.

A successful medication reconciliation process consists of a standardized systematic approach, with the initial step in this process involving the collection of the best medication history possible from every patient that enters any point in the health care system. Although pharmacists are uniquely qualified and have demonstrated increased accuracy in acquiring the medication history,[18] medication reconciliation requires a multidisciplinary effort in which all available resources are integrated into each step of the process when appropriate.[19] Shared accountability by using key members of the health care team such as nurses, pharmacy technicians, pharmacists, and prescribers is essential in this process. Once an accurate medication history is obtained, this information is used to ensure that as the patient moves through the health care system, any deviation from prescribed regimen is deliberate and based on acute changes in the patient's condition. If an observed discrepancy is the result of an intended therapeutic decision by the prescribing clinician, appropriate documentation with either the reason for or intention to change, hold, or discontinue the medication should be completed in a manner that is clear to all members of the health care team. Unintentional variances in the medication lists should be considered as potential medication errors pending clarification from the prescribing clinician.

Medication errors most commonly occur during transitions of care. It is essential to conduct medication reconciliation when a patient is admitted to or discharged from a health care facility.[20,21] A crucial final step in the reconciliation process, and a vital piece of MTMS, occurs at discharge to avoid therapeutic duplication, drug interactions, and omissions of medications that may have been discontinued or placed on hold during hospitalization. On departure from a health care facility, a complete list of the patient's medications must be communicated to the patient and the next provider of service regardless of the setting. This process allows for informed prescribing decisions and creates a safer environment for patients by improving the accuracy of medication administration throughout the continuum of care.

Perhaps the most important aspect of the medication history is to ensure that no assumptions related to medication use go unverified with the patient. The provider should ask questions related to how the current medication therapy is actually taken by the patient. The interviewer should then compare the use of medications as defined by the patient to the prescription information on the prescription bottle or in the PIS/EHR. This information may identify discrepancies or misunderstandings between the prescriber and the patient. The patient may not have adequate health literacy, and the interpretation of the medication instructions printed on the bottle or described by a health professional may not be understandable to a patient. The review of the medication history is an ideal time to identify and clarify such misunderstandings.

CASE 1-1, QUESTION 2: P.J. has indicated that she is injecting insulin to treat her diabetes. What questions might be asked to evaluate P.J.'s use of and response to insulin?

The following types of questions, when asked of P.J., should provide the practitioner with information on P.J.'s understanding about the use of and response to insulin.

DRUG IDENTIFICATION AND USE

- What type of insulin do you use?
- How many units of insulin do you use?
- When do you inject your insulin?
- Where do you inject your insulin?
- Please show me how you usually prepare your insulin for injection. (This allows the patient to demonstrate a skill.)
- What, if anything, keeps you from taking your insulin as prescribed?

ASSESSMENT OF THERAPEUTIC RESPONSE

- How do you know your insulin is working?
- What blood glucose levels are you aiming for?
- What foods or meals do you find affect your blood sugar most?
- How often and when do you test your blood glucose level?
- Do you have any blood glucose readings that you could share with me?
- Please show me how you test your blood glucose.
- What is your understanding of the hemoglobin A_{1c} blood test?
- When was the last time you had this test done?
- What were the results of the last hemoglobin A_{1c} test?

ASSESSMENT OF ADVERSE EFFECTS

- Do you ever experience reactions from low blood glucose?
- What symptoms warn you of such a reaction?
- When do these typically occur during the day?
- How often do they occur?

- What circumstances seem to make them occur more frequently?
- What do you do when you have low blood glucose?
- The patient's responses to these questions on drug use, therapeutic response, and adverse effects will allow a quick assessment of the patient's knowledge of insulin and whether she is using it in a way that is likely to result in blood glucose concentrations that are neither too high nor too low. The responses to these questions should also provide the practitioner with insight about the extent to which the patient has been involved in establishing and monitoring therapeutic outcomes. Based on this information, the practitioner can begin to formulate the patient's therapeutic plan.

Social History

The social history is used to determine the patient's occupation and lifestyle; important family relationships or other support systems; any particular circumstances (e.g., a disability) or stresses in her life that could influence the MAP; and attitudes, values, and feelings about health, illness, and treatments.

CASE 1-1, QUESTION 3: A patient's occupation, lifestyle, insurance status, ability to pay, and attitudes often can determine the success or failure of drug therapy. Therefore, P.J.'s prescription drug coverage, nutritional history, her level of activity or exercise in a typical day or week, the family dynamics, and any particular stresses that may affect glucose control need to be documented and assessed. What questions might be asked of P.J. to gain this information?

WORK

- Describe your typical workday and a typical weekend day.

INSURANCE/COST

- What type of prescription drug coverage do you have? How much do you pay for your insulin and diabetic supplies? How often do you go without your insulin or supplies because of cost?

EXERCISE

- Describe your exercise habits. How often, how long, and when during the day do you exercise? Describe how you change your meals or insulin when you exercise.

DIET

- How many times per day do you usually eat? Describe your usual meal times.
- What do you usually eat for each of your main meals and snacks?
- Are you able to eat at the same time each day?
- What do you do if a meal is delayed or missed?
- Who cooks the meals at home? Does this person understand foods to prepare for someone with diabetes?
- How often do you eat meals in a restaurant?
- How do you order meals in a restaurant to maintain a proper diet for your diabetes? (*Note:* This is asked to patients who frequently dine in restaurants.)

SUPPORT SYSTEMS

- Who else lives with you? What do they know about diabetes? How do they respond to the fact that you have diabetes? How do they help you with your diabetes management? Does it ever strain your relationship? What are the issues that seem to be most troublesome? (*Note:* These questions apply equally to the workplace or school setting. Often, the biggest barrier to multiple daily injections is refusal of the patient to inject insulin while at work or school.)

ATTITUDE

- How do you feel about having diabetes?
- What worries or bothers you most about having diabetes? (*Note:* Participate in the patient's care. This approach is likely to enhance the patient–provider relationship, which should translate into improved care.)

APPROACH TO AND ASSESSMENT OF PATIENT THERAPY

The provider–patient encounter will vary based on the location and type of services provided and access to necessary information. However, the general approach to the patient encounter should follow the problem-oriented medical record (POMR). Organizing information according to medical problems (e.g., diseases) helps to break down a complex situation (e.g., a patient with multiple medical problems requiring multiple drugs) into its individual parts.[1,2] The medical community has long used a *POMR* or *SOAP note* to record information in the medical record or chart by using a standardized format (Table 1-4). Each medical problem is identified, listed sequentially, and assigned a number. *Subjective* data and *objective* data in support of each problem are delineated, an *assessment* is made, and a *plan* of action identified. The first letter of the four key words (subjective, objective, assessment, and plan) serves as the basis for the SOAP acronym.

Table 1-4
Elements of the Problem-Oriented Medical Record

Problem name: Each "problem" is listed separately and given an identifying number. Problems may be a patient complaint (e.g., headache), a laboratory abnormality (e.g., hypokalemia), or a specific disease name if prior diagnosis is known. When monitoring previously described drug therapy, more than one drug-related problem may be considered (e.g., lack of adherence, an adverse drug reaction or drug interaction, or inappropriate dose). Under each problem name, the following information is identified:

Subjective	Information that explains the reason for the encounter. Information that the patient reports concerning symptoms, previous treatments, medications used, and adverse effects encountered. These are considered nonreproducible data because the information is based on the patient's interpretation and recall of past events.
Objective	Information from physical examination, laboratory test results, diagnostic tests, pill counts, and pharmacy patient profile information. Objective data are measurable and reproducible.
Assessment	A brief but complete description of the problem, including a conclusion or diagnosis that is supported logically by the above subjective and objective data. The assessment should not include a problem or diagnosis that is not defined above.
Plan	A detailed description of recommended or intended further workup (laboratory tests, radiology, consultation), treatment (e.g., continued observation, physiotherapy, diet, medications, surgery), patient education (self-care, goals of therapy, medication use, and monitoring), monitoring, and follow-up relative to the above assessment.

Sometimes referred to as the *SOAP* (subjective, objective, assessment, plan) note.

The POMR is a general approach and helps to focus on the encounter, which provides a structure for the documentation of the services provided. The following section will describe the POMR and SOAP note in more detail.

Problem List

Problems are listed in order of importance and are supported by the subjective and objective evidence gathered during the patient encounter. Each problem in the list can then be given an identifying number. All subsequent references to a specific problem can be identified or referenced by that number (e.g., "problem 1" or simply "1"). These are generally thought of in terms of a diagnosed disease, but they also may be a symptom complex that is being evaluated, a preventive measure (e.g., immunization, contraception), or a cognitive problem (e.g., lack of adherence). Any condition that requires a unique management plan should be identified as a problem to serve as a reminder to the practitioner that treatment is needed for that problem. Different settings and activities or clinical services will determine the priority of the problems identified.

Medical problems can be *drug related*, including prescribing errors, dosing errors, adverse drug effects, adherence issues, and the need for medication counseling. Drug-related problems may be definite (i.e., there is no question that the problem exists) or possible (i.e., further investigation is required to determine if the problem really exists). The most commonly encountered types of drug-related problems are listed in Table 1-5.[3,14]

The distinction between medical problems and drug-related problems sometimes is unclear, and overlap can exist. For example, a medical problem (i.e., a disease, syndrome, symptom, or health condition) can be prevented, cured, alleviated, or exacerbated by medications. When assessing drug therapy, several situations could exist: treatment is appropriate and therapeutic outcomes have been achieved; drugs that have been selected are ineffective or therapeutic outcomes are partially achieved; dosages are subtherapeutic or medication is taken improperly; an inappropriate drug for the medical condition being treated has been prescribed or is being used; or the condition is not being treated.

Likewise, a drug-related problem can cause or aggravate a medical problem. Such drug-related problems could include hypersensitivity reactions; idiosyncratic reactions; toxic reactions

Table 1-5
Drug-Related Problems

Drug Needed
Drug indicated but not prescribed; a medical problem has been diagnosed, but there is no indication that treatment has been initiated (maybe it is not needed)
Correct drug prescribed but not taken (lack of adherence)
Wrong or Inappropriate Drug
No apparent medical problem justifying the use of the drug
Drug not indicated for the medical problem for which it has been prescribed
Medical problem no longer exists
Duplication of other therapy
Less expensive alternative available
Drug not covered by formulary
Failure to account for pregnancy status, age of patient, or other contraindications
Incorrect nonprescription medication self-prescribed by the patient
Recreational drug use
Wrong Dose
Prescribed dose too high (includes adjustments for renal and hepatic function, age, body size)
Correct prescribed dose but overuse by patient (overadherence)
Prescribed dose too low (includes adjustments for age, body size)
Correct prescribed dose but underuse by patient (underadherence)
Incorrect, inconvenient, or less-than-optimal dosing interval (consider use of sustained-release dosage forms)
Adverse Drug Reaction
Hypersensitivity reaction
Idiosyncratic reaction
Drug-induced disease
Drug-induced laboratory change
Drug Interaction
Drug–drug interaction
Drug–food interaction
Drug–laboratory test interaction
Drug–disease interaction

secondary to excessive doses; adverse reactions (e.g., insulin-induced hypoglycemia or weight gain); drug–drug, drug–disease, drug–laboratory test, and drug–lifestyle interactions; or polypharmacy, which may increase the risk of adverse drug events.[22]

Subjective and Objective Data

Subjective and objective data in support of a problem are important because assessment of patients and therapies requires the gathering of specific information to verify that a problem continues to exist or that therapeutic objectives are being achieved. Subjective data refer to information provided by the patient or another person that cannot be confirmed independently. This is the data most commonly obtained during a patient interview. Objective data refer to information observed or measured by the practitioner (e.g., laboratory tests, blood pressure [BP] measurements). Objective data are most commonly obtained from the EMR or paper chart (data-rich environment). However, some objective data can be obtained in data-poor environments. In the absence of a medical record, weight, height, pulse, BP, blood glucose readings, and other objective information can be gathered during the provider–patient encounter.

CASE 1-2

QUESTION 1: P.N., a 28-year-old man, has a BP of 140/100 mm Hg. What is the primary problem? What subjective and objective data support the problem, and what additional subjective and objective data are not provided but usually are needed to define this particular problem?

The primary problem is hypertension. No subjective data are given. The objective data are the patient's age, sex, and BP of 140/100 mm Hg. Each of these is important in designing a patient-specific therapy plan. Because hypertension often is an asymptomatic disease (see Chapter 9, Essential Hypertension), subjective complaints such as headache, tiredness or anxiety, shortness of breath (SOB), chest pain, and visual changes usually are absent. If long-term complications such as rupturing of blood vessels in the eye, glomerular damage, or encephalopathy were present, subjective complaints might be blurring or loss of vision, fatigue, or confusion. Objective data would include a report by the physician on the findings of the chest examination (abnormal heart or lung sounds if secondary HF has developed), an ocular examination (e.g., presence of retinal hemorrhages), and laboratory data on renal function (blood urea nitrogen, creatinine, or creatinine clearance). To place these complications in better perspective, the rate of change should be stated. For example, the serum creatinine has increased from a level of 1 mg/dL 6 months ago to a value of 3 mg/dL today. Vague descriptions such as "eye changes" or "kidney damage" are of little value, because progressive damage to these end organs results from uncontrolled high BP, and disease progression needs to be monitored more precisely.

CASE 1-3

QUESTION 1: D.L., a 36-year-old construction worker, tripped on a board at the construction site 2 days ago, sustaining an abrasion of his left shin. He presents to the emergency department with pain, redness, and swelling in the area of the injury. He is diagnosed as having cellulitis. What is the primary problem? What subjective and objective data support the problem? What additional subjective and objective data are not provided but usually are needed to define this particular problem?

The primary problem is cellulitis of the left leg. Useful pieces of subjective information are D.L.'s description of how he injured his shin at a construction site and his current complaints of pain, redness, and swelling. The fact that he was at a construction site is indirect evidence of a possible dirty wound. Further information must be obtained about how he cleaned the wound after the injury and whether he has received a booster dose of tetanus toxoid within the past 10 years. Objectively, the wound is on the left shin. No other objective data are given. Additional data to obtain would be to document the intensity of the redness on a one-to-four-plus scale, the size of the inflamed area as described by an area of demarcation, the circumference of his left shin compared with his right shin, the presence or absence of pus and any lymphatic involvement, his temperature, and a white blood cell count with differential.

CASE 1-4

QUESTION 1: C.S., a 58-year-old woman, has had complaints of fatigue, ankle swelling, and SOB, especially when lying down, for the past week. Physical examination shows distended neck veins, bilateral rales, an S_3 gallop rhythm, and lower extremity edema. A chest radiograph shows an enlarged heart. She is diagnosed as having HF and is being treated with furosemide and digoxin. What is/are the primary problem(s)? What subjective and objective data support the problem(s)? What additional subjective and objective data are not provided but usually are needed to define this (these) particular problem(s)?

The primary problem is systolic HF. Subjectively, C.S. claims to be experiencing fatigue, ankle swelling, and SOB, especially when lying down. She claims to have been taking furosemide and digoxin. An expanded description of these symptoms and her medication use would be helpful. The findings on physical examination and the enlarged heart on chest radiograph are objective data in support of the primary problem of HF. In addition, other objective findings that would help in her assessment would be the pulse rate, BP, serum creatinine, serum potassium concentration, digoxin blood level, a more thorough description of the rales on lung examination, extent of neck vein distension, and degree of leg edema. Pharmacy records could be screened to determine current dosages and refill patterns of the medications.

In this case, a second primary problem may be present. Current recommendations for the management of HF include use of an angiotensin-converting enzyme (ACE) inhibitor before or concurrent with digoxin therapy. Thus, a possible drug-related problem is the inappropriate choice of drug therapy ("wrong drug"). The patient or prescriber should be consulted to ascertain whether an ACE inhibitor has been used previously, any contraindications exist, or possible adverse effects were encountered.

Assessment

After the subjective and objective data have been gathered in support of specific listed problems, the practitioner should assess the acuity, severity, and importance of these problems. He or she should then identify all factors that could be causing or contributing to the problem. The assessment of the severity and acuity is important because the patient expects relief from the symptoms that are of particular concern at this time. During the initial encounter with a patient, it might be discovered that the medical problem is only a symptom complex and that a diagnosis is needed to more accurately identify the problem and further define its severity.

The assessment is usually performed during or immediately after the data gathering, while the provider keeps in mind evidence-based practices. For example, if diabetes is assessed and pertinent subjective data (medication history, social history, diet, exercise, etc.) and objective data exist (laboratory test results like hemoglobin A_{1c}, low-density lipoprotein cholesterol [LDL-C], BP, etc.), then the assessment of diabetes may be to determine whether the patient is meeting the goals for the disease as defined by the ADA. If the patient is not at goal, then the explanation of the reasons why would be described in the assessment, and the plan would then be centered on helping that patient get to goal. Sometimes, the distinction between subjective information provided by the patient and assessments made by the practitioner are confused in the POMR. What the patient reveals belongs in the subjective data, and how the provider interprets it belongs in the assessment. For example, a patient stating that she is having difficulty affording her medications belongs in the subjective information. However, a patient appearing to have cost-related lack of adherence belongs in the assessment, because it is the provider's interpretation of what the patient has stated.

DRUG THERAPY ASSESSMENT

A responsibility of the practitioner is to monitor the response of patients to prescribed therapeutic regimens. The purpose of drug therapy monitoring is to identify and solve drug-related problems and to ensure that all therapeutic objectives are being achieved. Unless proven otherwise, the medical diagnosis should be assumed to be correct. On occasion, the diagnosis may not be readily apparent, or a drug-induced problem may have been diagnosed incorrectly as being a disease entity.

Health care practitioners share the responsibility to assess and monitor patient drug therapy. For the pharmacist, medication reconciliation and the drug therapy assessment may occur in many practice settings, including the community pharmacy while dispensing or refilling prescriptions or counseling patients, during MTMS encounters in the home or in the clinic, while assessing therapy for the hospitalized patient, or as part of routine monthly evaluations of patients residing in long-term care facilities. Many states have enacted legislation allowing pharmacists to develop collaborative drug therapy agreements with physicians for disease state management of common disorders such as asthma, diabetes, dyslipidemia, and hypertension. Additional services commonly provided by pharmacists through collaborative drug therapy agreements include anticoagulation monitoring, emergency contraception, and immunizations.[5] These services often involve more detailed drug therapy evaluation and assessment and may occur within or outside the traditional pharmacy setting. Regardless, the patient's need, time constraints, working environment, and practitioner's skill level govern the extent of monitoring. Similarly, the exact steps used to monitor therapy and the order in which they are executed need to be adapted to a practitioner's personal style. Thus, the examples given in this chapter should be used by the reader as a guide rather than as a recipe in a cookbook.

Plan

The next step in the problem-oriented (i.e., SOAP) approach is to create a plan, which at the minimum should consist of a diagnostic plan and a MAP that includes patient education. The plan is the action that was justified in the assessment. The plan is clear and direct and does not require explanation (this should be explained in the assessment). For example, if a patient is experiencing constipation while taking an opioid pain reliever, the plan would be to recommend a stool softener or stimulant laxative such as docusate sodium. The plan should also include any follow-up that would be necessary as a result of the action taken.

Patient Education

Educating patients to better understand their medical problem(s) and treatment is an implied goal of all treatment plans. This process is categorized as the development of a patient education plan. The level of teaching has to be tailored to the patient's needs, health literacy, willingness to learn, and general state of health and mind. The patient should be taught the knowledge and skills needed to achieve and evaluate his or her therapeutic outcome. An important component of the patient education plan emphasizes the need for patients to follow prescribed treatment regimens.

The POMR will allow the provider to focus on the interview and encounter independent of the site or service offered. The POMR facilitates documentation of the provision of MTMS across multiple sites and services (across the continuum of care).

The next few sections will discuss how to approach MTMS in various clinical settings.

MEDICATION THERAPY MANAGEMENT SERVICES IN THE COMMUNITY PHARMACY OR AMBULATORY SETTING

The core elements of MTMS have been described by the American Pharmacists Association (APhA) and the National Association of Chain Drug Stores (NACDS).[19] According to these organizations, the core elements of MTMS should include the following components:

1. Medication therapy review (MTR)
2. Personal medication record (PMR)
3. Medication action plan (MAP)
4. Intervention or referral
5. Documentation and follow-up

Medication Therapy Review

The MTR may be a comprehensive review, including medication reconciliation, in which the provider reviews all of the medications the patient is currently taking, or it may be a focused review of one medication-related issue such as an adverse event. Examples of services provided during the MTR are described in Table 1-6. MTR is dependent on the information that is available from the patient or other data sources.

Table 1-6
Examples of Services Provided During a Medication Therapy Review

- Assess the patient's health status
- Assess cultural issues, health literacy, language barriers, financial status, and insurance coverage or other patient characteristics that may affect the patient's ability to take medications appropriately
- Interview the patient or caregiver to assess, identify, and resolve actual or potential adverse medication events, therapeutic duplications, untreated conditions or diseases, medication adherence issues, and medication cost considerations
- Monitor medication therapy, including response to therapy, safety, and effectiveness
- Monitor, interpret, and assess patient laboratory values, especially as they relate to medication use/misuse
- Provide education and training on the appropriate use of medications
- Communicate appropriate information to other health professionals, including the use and selection of medication therapy

Source: American Pharmacists Association; National Association of Chain Drug Stores Foundation. Medication therapy management in pharmacy practice: core elements of an MTM service model (version 2.0). *J Am Pharm Assoc (2003)*. 2008;48(3):341–353.

My Medication Record

Name: MC ____________ Birth Date: May 28, 1939 ____________

Include all of your medications on this record: prescription medications, nonprescription medications, herbal products, and other dietary supplements. Always carry your medication record with you and show it to all your doctors, pharmacists, and other health care providers.

Drug	Take for...	When do I take it? Start Stop Doctor Special Instructions					
Lisinopril	40 mg	High blood pressure	Once daily	1/2/15		Sara Smith, MD	
Metoprolol	50 mg	High blood pressure	Twice daily	1/2/15		Sara Smith, MD	9 A.M. and 9 P.M.
Glipizide	5 mg	Diabetes	Once daily	1/2/15		Sara Smith, MD	9 A.M.
Indomethacin	50 mg	Back Pain	Up to 3 times daily if needed	1/2/15		Sara Smith, MD	Take with food. Do not take this medicine with other anti-inflammatory medicines (e.g., ibuprofen, naproxen). Do not take this medication unless you have pain.
Crestor (rosuvastatin)	40 mg	Cholesterol	Once daily	4/2/15		Ted Hart, MD	

This sample Personal Medication Record (PMR) is provided only for general informational purposes and does not constitute professional health care advice or treatment. The patient (or other user) should not, under any circumstances, solely rely on, or act on the basis of, the PMR or the information therein. If he or she does so, then he or she does so at his or her own risk. While intended to serve as a communication aid between patient (or other user) and health care provider, the PMR is not a substitute for obtaining professional health care advice or treatment. This PMR may not be appropriate for all patients (or other users). The National Association of Chain Drug Stores Foundation and the American Pharmacists Association assume no responsibility for the accuracy, currentness, or completeness of any information provided or recorded herein.

This form is based on forms developed by the American Pharmacists Association and the National Association of Chain Drug Stores Foundation. Reproduced with permission from APhA and the NACDS Foundation.

Figure 1-2 Example of a Personal Medication Record (PMR).

Personalized Medication Record

Regardless of the setting, a necessary tool to help with the gathering of the medication information is the PMR. This medication record should be updated after any change in medication therapy and should be shared with other health care providers. The goal of this record is to promote self-care and ownership of the medication regimen.[23] The PMR should be used at all levels of care, thereby facilitating the medication reconciliation process required across the continuum of care. An example of a PMR is shown in Figure 1-2.

Once the patient interview has occurred and the PMR has been updated, the provider may still require information to make an assessment. In such cases, the provider must do his or her best with the available information, or he or she may obtain missing information such as the medical history or objective data from other providers. In some encounters, obtaining the necessary information and medication reconciliation may take the entire visit, necessitating a follow-up encounter.

Medication Action Plan

If adequate information is available to assess the current problem, a MAP should be developed. Because the MAP is patient centered and is prioritized according to the urgency of need, the provider and the patient should develop the plan together. An example of a MAP can be seen in Figure 1-3.

Intervention and Referral

The MAP often describes the intervention performed in an MTM encounter and may serve as documentation that can be shared with the patient and other health care providers (like the PMR). The primary purpose of the MAP is to make the action plan patient centered and to provide the patient with documentation of what they need to do next in the action plan. It also provides space for the patient to document what he or she did related to this action and when it was done. In some instances, the MAP may involve referral to another provider (a physician or pharmacist with additional qualifications) if the issue is beyond the scope of the intervening pharmacist.

Coordination of care is a key element of MTMS and MTR.[1] This may include improving the communication between the patient and other health care providers, enhancing the patient's understanding of his or her health issues or concerns, maximizing health insurance coverage, advocating on behalf of the patient to get needed medications using available resources and programs, and various other functions that will improve the patient's understanding of his or her health care environment and promote self-care. Coordination of care may be the primary action taken on behalf of the patient and may be included in the MAP.

Documentation and Follow-up

The development of a documentation process is a necessary component of MTMS.[23] Documentation should be standardized and based on the POMR format. All appropriate records, including the PMR and MAP, should be shared with other providers to promote communication and continuity of care. If the encounter requires follow-up, the documentation should reflect the timing of the follow-up care, and any expectations of the patient and providers should be included. Thorough documentation of the encounter allows all providers to quickly assess the progress of the patient and determine that the desired outcome has been achieved.

An important aspect of documenting the encounter is to submit billing for the encounter when appropriate. Although billing for MTMS is not universally accepted by all payers, the introduction of the national provider identifier (NPI) and pharmacist-specific

CPT codes may soon make this a reality.[4,24] The implementation of Medicare Part D in 2006 allowed pharmacists in pharmacies contracted with prescription drug plans to provide MTMS to plan-identified Medicare recipients. Pharmacists bill these plans through the contracted pharmacy by using an NPI and one of three CPT codes. The NPI number designates the provider to be paid, and the CPT determines the amount of payment based on the services rendered. The CPT codes specific to pharmacists providing MTMS include the following:

CPT 99605: Initial face-to-face assessment or intervention by a pharmacist with the patient for 1 to 15 minutes

CPT 99606: Subsequent face-to-face assessment or intervention by a pharmacist with the patient for 1 to 15 minutes

CPT 99607: Each additional 15 minutes spent face-to-face by a pharmacist with the patient; used in addition to 99605 or 99606

Although the NPI number and CPT codes allow pharmacists to bill for MTMS, the reimbursement varies by plan and negotiated contract and is beyond the scope of this text. Pharmacists have also developed patient self-pay reimbursement strategies as well as contracts with self-insured employers and state-run Medicaid programs to provide services.[25,26]

The Patient Protection and Affordable Care Act of 2010 and the Health Care and Education Reconciliation Act of 2010 describe the need for payment reform that promotes improved quality of care. Other providers also see these laws providing new opportunities for pharmacists to participate in care teams such as the patient-centered medical home and pay-for-performance programs to improve medication-related care coordination, quality scores, and patient outcomes.[27,28] The enhanced payment for improving quality in medication-related areas could be used to fund the pharmacist in this activity.

CASE 1-5

QUESTION 1: M.C. is a 76-year-old woman who comes to an appointment at the community pharmacy with her daughter for a focused MTR. She has a Medicare Part D prescription drug plan and is asking for help with her medication costs. She indicates that she has type 2 diabetes, hypertension, back pain, and hyperlipidemia. Her medications include lisinopril 40 mg once daily, metoprolol 50 mg twice daily, glipizide 5 mg once daily, indomethacin 50 mg up to 3 times daily as needed for pain, and rosuvastatin 40 mg once daily. M.C. tells you that she has trouble paying for her rosuvastatin (tier 3, $60 copayment) and would rather have something generic that costs less (tier 1, $5 copayment). Further, she complains of muscle soreness and weakness during the last 3 weeks.

What is the primary problem? What objective information can be obtained in a community pharmacy setting? What additional information is necessary to determine the cause of her problem? How would a clinician assess and document her problem(s) in a SOAP format?

Although the patient presented for a MTR, the primary complaint is the patient's self-reported muscle weakness and soreness during the last 3 weeks. Assuming that M.C. is a patient of this pharmacy, the practitioner could gather the necessary medication history from the PIS. Because the patient is present, this is a good opportunity to develop a PMR with M.C. This process will help to quickly identify any medication discrepancies between the pharmacy computer system and the patient's understanding of medication administration. If discrepancies are noted, the practitioner can clarify them with M.C. right away as part of the intervention. The PMR should also include a section to list medication allergies. The type of reaction should also be included on the PMR so that other providers will know the severity of the medication allergy (i.e., intolerance vs. anaphylactic reaction). Based on the data gathered from the pharmacy computer and M.C., a PMR (depicted in Fig. 1-3) could be developed.

Reviewing the medications alone often does not provide enough information to determine whether M.C. is experiencing a medication-related event. Further questioning related to the onset of her symptoms of muscle soreness and weakness may help to determine whether this is a medication-related problem.

The practitioner can develop an assessment from this questioning and the PMR of the current problem that she is experiencing. As indicated on the PMR, M.C. started rosuvastatin most recently. The initiation of this medication corresponds to the onset of her recent soreness and weakness. β-Hydroxy-β-methylglutaryl-CoA (HMG-CoA) reductase inhibitors like rosuvastatin are known to cause myositis, or muscle breakdown, which may lead to weakness and muscle soreness. Furthermore, the prescribed dose is high for a woman of M.C.'s age. Based on this information, an assessment of the problem can be pursued. If rosuvastatin is the suspected agent, the plan would include actions necessary to solve the problem or to determine whether rosuvastatin is the cause of her muscle soreness and weakness. Unfortunately, not all of the necessary information is available (e.g., her baseline cholesterol, serum creatinine, liver function tests, or creatine kinase levels) to develop a formal plan of action to resolve the adverse medication event. However, part of the plan may be to obtain the laboratory test results necessary to identify or act on the adverse medication event. An example of the documentation of the SOAP note follows.

Primary Problem:

Muscle soreness and weakness (possible adverse medication event).

Subjective:

M.C. reports weakness and soreness, predominantly in her legs during the past 3 weeks. She has difficulty rising from her chair after sitting for long periods and describes the pain as aching. The patient reports taking her medications as prescribed and rarely misses a dose.

Objective:

Total cholesterol: 137 mg/dL; LDL-C: 56 mg/dL;
HDL: 54 mg/dL; Triglycerides: 136 mg/dL
Temperature: 98.5°F
Blood pressure: 144/68 mm Hg

Assessment:

M.C. has muscle weakness and soreness in her large muscle groups. According to the American College of Cardiology and the American Heart Association M.C. is considered to be at risk of heart disease because of her age and concurrent disease states.[29] Her current lipid therapy is rosuvastatin 40 mg once daily, which was started by her cardiologist 6 weeks ago. The initiation of rosuvastatin 40 mg correlates to the timing of her muscle soreness and weakness. HMG-CoA reductase inhibitors (i.e., rosuvastatin) are known to cause myositis or myalgias, and this patient is at particular risk given her age, sex, and starting dose. It is possible that the rosuvastatin could be causing her muscle soreness and weakness. Other lipid-lowering agents could be tried or the dose of rosuvastatin could be reduced, which might eliminate or reduce this adverse event. A creatine kinase level should be obtained to determine the severity of the myositis. A serum creatinine should also be measured, as myositis can lead to renal damage and rhabdomyolysis in severe cases; however, this is usually accompanied by fever and other symptoms that the patient is not currently experiencing.

Plan:

Drug-Related Adverse Event:

- Discussed the possibility of an adverse medication event with the patient, which included the signs and symptoms of myalgias and myositis.

My Medication-Related Action Plan

Patient:	MC
Doctor (Phone):	Sara Smith, MD
Pharmacy/Pharmacist (Phone):	Rite Mart/Mary John, PharmD
Date Prepared:	May 10, 2015

The list below has important Action Steps to help you get the most from your medications. Follow the checklist to help you work with your pharmacist and doctor to manage your medications AND make notes of your actions next to each item on your list.

Action steps → What I need to do...	Notes → What I did and when I did it....
☐ **For your muscle weakness and soreness** Stop Crestor (rosuvastatin) 40mg. We asked Dr. Hart to change to a lower dose or different agent such as simvastatin. Obtain blood test from Dr. Hart's office. Follow-up with Dr. Hart in 2 days.	
☐ **Medicine Cost** We have asked Dr. Hart to stop Crestor (rosuvastatin) as it is too expensive. A generic medicine such as simvastatin will cost you less and was recommended to Dr. Hart as an alternative. Continue to ask your pharmacist and doctor whether the medications you are taking are covered by your Medicare Part D plan and whether there are any alternatives that may be less expensive.	
☐ **For Pain** Take to Dr. Sara Smith about other pain medications, because the indomethacin may not be the best choice for you due to its side effects/ Some choices might include other medications such as Vicodin (hydrocodone and acetaminophen), over-the-counter acetaminophen, or naproxen or ibuprofen.	

My next appointment with my pharmacist is on: ________ (date) at ________ ☐ AM ☐ PM

This sample Medication-Related Action Plan (MAP) is provided only for general informational purposes and does not constitute professional health care advice or treatment. The patient (or other user) should not, under any circumstances, solely rely on, or act on the basis of, the MAP or the information therein. If he or she does so, then he or she does so at his or her own risk. While intended to serve as a communication aid between patient (or other user) and health care provider, the MAP is not a substitute for obtaining professional health care advice or treatment. This MAP may not be appropriate for all patients (or other users). The National Association of Chain Drug Stores Foundation and the American Pharmacists Association assume no responsibility for the accuracy, currentness, or completeness of any information provided or recorded herein.

This form is based on forms developed by the American Pharmacists Association and the National Association of Chain Drug Stores Foundation. Reproduced with permission from APhA and the NACDS Foundation.

Figure 1-3 Example of a Medication Action Plan (MAP).

- Contacted Dr. Hart (M.C.'s cardiologist) to discuss the current problem with rosuvastatin.
- Per discussion with Dr. Hart, will obtain a creatine kinase level and serum creatinine.
- Discontinue rosuvastatin per the pharmacist's recommendation. Dr. Hart agreed that M.C. should temporarily stop her rosuvastatin until her laboratory values are reviewed.
- Alternative dosing of rosuvastatin 5 mg or another equivalent agent (atorvastatin 10 mg or simvastatin 20 mg) was discussed with Dr. Hart.
- M.C. is to see Dr. Hart in the cardiology clinic in 2 days to discuss the laboratory values and alternative therapies.
- Discussed the entire plan with M.C., and she verbalized understanding of steps that she is to take with respect to her current medication-induced problem.

CASE 1-5, QUESTION 2: From M.C.'s medication profile, what other problems can be identified with her medication therapy? What can be done to address these issues?

There are two remaining issues that may need to be addressed. The first issue relates to the pain medicine (indomethacin) that M.C. is taking. It is suggested that indomethacin may have a higher rate of central nervous system side effects in the elderly compared with other agents in the same class.[30] Furthermore, the American Geriatric Society guidelines on the management of mild-to-moderate persistent pain caution the use of nonsteroidal anti-inflammatory agents in older adults, preferring acetaminophen as a first-line agent.[31] Other prescription medications or nonprescription medication such as acetaminophen alone could be used to help treat M.C.'s pain (see Chapter 55, Pain Management, and Chapter 107, Geriatric Drug Use).

Second, it is not clear from the current information whether the various providers are communicating. It is the responsibility of the pharmacist to help coordinate care among multiple prescribers as described by the APhA MTMS consensus document.[1] Therefore, it is important to be sure that both providers (Drs. Smith and Hart) receive a copy of the documentation of the issues addressed during the visit (SOAP note).

CASE 1-5, QUESTION 3: What additional information can be provided to M.C. at this time?

Finally, M.C. came into the pharmacy asking for help with her medication costs. To assess this problem, it is important to ask whether there are specific cost issues with a particular drug or whether it is her overall medication regimen that causes her concern. Another question to ask is whether she has stopped taking any medications or changed the way she takes them because of cost. Many patients will discuss cost and adherence issues with their pharmacist, because the point of sale for medications occurs at the pharmacy. However, they may not discuss this problem with the prescriber. Cost and lack of adherence because of cost are medication-related problems that the pharmacist must communicate to the prescriber on behalf of the patient. In assessing drug cost, there are several steps that can be taken. First, determine the patient's ability to pay for medications; implement low-cost, medically appropriate interventions targeted to patient needs; facilitate enrollment into relevant benefit programs; and confirm medication changes with the patient and prescribers.

For M.C., the rosuvastatin is her biggest concern, as it costs $60 per month and her Medicare Part D plan lists it as a non-preferred (tier 3) agent on the formulary. With the possible discontinuation of her rosuvastatin, it is important for the pharmacist to anticipate an alternative lipid-lowering agent and determine a cost-effective alternative that may be appropriate. This information can then be relayed to the prescriber. Furthermore, the alternative lipid-lowering formulary choice can be integrated into the plan developed for the primary issue of muscle soreness and weakness (see Case 1-5, Question 1). The integration of multiple problems is a complicated but an important aspect of the MAP.

As discussed previously, an important part of MTMS involves the MAP. The MAP is a document that may empower the patient and promote self-care. The information on the MAP is important for both the patient and the provider, and it facilitates communication among multiple providers. When a patient presents the PMR and MAP to all providers, complex medication information can be shared across the continuum of care. An example of M.C.'s MAP is included in Figure 1-3.

Because extensive information was communicated to the patient and other providers, follow-up (phone or face-to-face) would be appropriate and necessary to determine the resolution to the medication-related issues identified. Follow-up should occur in a timely manner, likely after M.C. has obtained the necessary laboratory test results and has been evaluated by her cardiologist as outlined in the plan. The follow-up should include questions related to the changes that were (or were not) made based on the practitioner recommendations and any new issues that have surfaced. Follow-up should be considered after any encounter in which an action plan is developed to determine whether the medication-related problem has been resolved. Additionally, problems may be identified and prioritized during the initial visit but, because of time constraints, may not be addressed. A follow-up visit allows for assessment of these problems.

CASE 1-5, QUESTION 4: Assuming that the pharmacy provider had an NPI number and a contract with M.C.'s Medicare Part D prescription drug plan, how could the 30 minutes spent with M.C. be billed to her insurance?

Provided that M.C. was identified by her Medicare prescription drug plan as eligible for MTMS, the practitioner could bill for the 30-minute encounter. Using the practitioner's NPI number and the appropriate CPT codes, the practitioner could bill for one CPT 99605 (for the first 15 minutes of initial face-to-face MTM encounter) and one CPT 99607 (for an additional 15 minutes spent with the patient in a face-to-face MTM encounter). M.C.'s Medicare Part D plan may require the practitioner to bill the prescription drug plan initially, and then the plan would pay the community pharmacy directly instead of reimbursing the individual pharmacist. Documentation of the visit would need to be stored at the site of the encounter in case any information was requested from M.C.'s prescription drug plan.

CASE 1-5, QUESTION 5: M.C. has just been hospitalized in a large medical center for renal failure and urosepsis. The pharmacist has access to the medical chart, nursing record, MAR, and a computer that directly links to the clinical laboratory. The pharmacists at this facility assess the patient's drug therapy and routinely provide clinical pharmacokinetic monitoring. How would the pharmacist approach M.C. differently in this inpatient setting compared with the pharmacist in Question 1 who worked in a community pharmacy?

MEDICATION THERAPY MANAGEMENT IN THE ACUTE CARE SETTING

Similar to the outpatient setting, the SOAP format is often used when documenting the encounter of the hospitalized patient; however, obtaining the information needed poses unique challenges. In this setting, subjective information may be more difficult to obtain at the time of assessment in those patients presenting with cognitive impairment resulting from their acute condition, such as the seriously ill or injured patient. Objective data, on the other hand, are more readily available and retrievable with access to pharmacy, laboratory, and other medical record information. On admission to the health care facility, the medication reconciliation process should be initiated to identify any variances in the admission orders when compared with the patient's home medication list. With acute medical problems superimposed on chronic conditions, it is not unusual to have new medications added and home medications held, changed, or discontinued.

Assessing the appropriateness of drug therapy requires a basic understanding of both pharmacokinetic (e.g., absorption, distribution, metabolism, and elimination) and pharmacodynamic (e.g., relief of pain with an analgesic or reduction of BP with an antihypertensive agent) principles. This detailed assessment and monitoring is dependent on the availability of robust patient and laboratory data. The inpatient setting is a relatively data-rich environment in which access to needed information is readily available. Knowledge of the patient's height, body weight, and hepatic and renal function are essential for proper dosage considerations. The type of hospitalized patient will vary from the short-stay elective surgery patient to the critically ill hemodynamically compromised patient. The pharmacist must be aware of how pharmacokinetics and pharmacodynamics can be altered throughout the hospitalization or disease-state process in each patient evaluated. This heightened awareness will allow for timely interventions and minimize medication errors resulting from improper or delayed dosage adjustments because the clinical status of the patient changes. Drug level monitoring may be suitable for certain medications and is of great clinical value; nevertheless, it is important to take into consideration clinical response to drug therapy along with the assessment of a specific laboratory value. Accurate interpretation of any drug level requires review of the nursing MAR (or eMAR), evaluating time of drug administration to serum sample acquisition. When serum drug levels are obtained, they must be reviewed for validity before alterations in medication regimens are made. If a serum drug concentration seems unusually high or low, the clinician must consider all of the various factors that might influence the serum concentration of the drug in that particular patient. When the reason for an unexpected abnormal serum drug concentration is not apparent, the test should be repeated before considering a dose change that may cause supratherapeutic or subtherapeutic concentrations resulting from erroneous data (see Chapter 2, Interpretation of Clinical Laboratory Tests).

When M.C. was seen in the community pharmacy, the pharmacist assessed her chronic conditions, her cost issues, and her drug therapy. Monitoring in the community pharmacy–based MTM program occurs at regular time intervals and is less sensitive to the day-to-day changes of the patient. However, in the inpatient setting, M.C. has acute conditions (renal failure and urosepsis) in addition to her chronic conditions. Monitoring of medication therapy will occur frequently, resulting in a dynamic treatment plan for her acute and chronic conditions.

Although the inpatient setting is relatively data rich, the information gathered and the assessment and plan formulated in the facility must be communicated to other providers once the patient is discharged. At discharge, it is critical to ensure that the patient has follow-up with his or her primary care physician or coordinated care team in a timely fashion. At this point, it is again critical for the pharmacist to perform medication reconciliation to determine exactly what did happen once the patient returned home. This closes the loop at a critical time when the patient is prone to medication errors and readmission.

MEDICATION THERAPY MANAGEMENT AND PHARMACOGENOMICS

The use of genetic information to predict an individual's response to a drug, known as pharmacogenomics, is currently factoring into drug design and development. Using genetic information to tailor drug therapy to an individual will reduce the risk of adverse events, potentially improve patient outcomes, and create a more efficient drug development process. By transforming drug therapy into a patient-specific approach, the health care community is one step closer to achieving the new medical paradigm of personalized health care.[32]

MTM can be the vehicle to allow pharmacists to serve an integral role in applying pharmacogenomics into clinical practice to improve the quality and safety of health care. Incorporating pharmacogenomics into MTMS allows pharmacists to lend their expertise to the treatment planning process to optimize treatment outcomes. Pharmacists, working collaboratively with prescribers and laboratory facilities, could review medications prescribed for a patient as well as the patient's genomic data to then offer an assessment on whether a prospective drug would provide the best fit for the condition and patient. Through MTMS and pharmacogenomics, pharmacists can optimize drug choice and maximize therapy outcomes (see Chapter 4, Pharmacogenomics and Personalized Medicine).

In order to successfully integrate a pharmacogenomic component within the clinical decision making process, key pharmacogenomic data must be identified. The challenge is complex, and research has begun to bring the application of pharmacogenomics to patients as part of the health care delivery system. The pharmacy profession must define a process for the application of pharmacogenomic data into pharmacy clinical practice that is aligned with MTMS delivery. A viable business model should be developed for these practices that encourages and promotes the use of the clinical expertise of pharmacists working in collaboration with other health care providers and laboratories. The development of technology solutions that support the pharmacist's role in this emerging field should also be encouraged and directed.[32]

CONCLUSION

MTMS are intended to be applicable to patients in all care settings where the patients or their caregivers can be actively involved with managing their medication therapy. The goals of all pharmacists providing MTMS are to confirm that the patient's medication therapy is ideal and that the best possible outcomes from treatment are achieved. The MTM process needs to be properly documented and accurately shared with all providers that are part of the patient's health care team. As drug therapy and technology options continue to evolve, pharmacists are encouraged to provide and optimize MTMS to improve patient outcomes and medication use.

ACKNOWLEDGMENT

The authors acknowledge Mary Anne Koda-Kimble, Wayne Kradjan, Robin Corelli, Lloyd Young, B. Joseph Guglielmo, Brian Alldredge, Marilyn Stebbins, Timothy Cutler, and Patricia Parker for their contributions to the version of this chapter found in previous editions.

KEY REFERENCES AND WEBSITES

A full list of references for this chapter can be found at http://thepoint.lww.com/AT11e. Below are the key references and websites for this chapter, with the corresponding reference number in this chapter found in parentheses after the reference.

Key References

American Pharmacists Association; National Association of Chain Drug Stores Foundation. Medication therapy management in pharmacy practice: core elements of an MTM service model (version 2.0). *J Am Pharm Assoc (2003)*. 2008;48(3):341. (23)

Bluml BM. Definition of medication therapy management: development of professionwide consensus. *J Am Pharm Assoc (2003)*. 2005;45(5):566. (1)

Cipolle RJ et al., eds. *Pharmaceutical Care Practice: The Clinician's Guide*. 2nd ed. New York, NY: McGraw-Hill; 2004. (14)

Health Information Technology: Initial Set of Standards, Implementation Specifications, and Certification Criteria for Electronic Health Record Technology. *Fed Regist*. 2010;75(144):44589. (15)

Health Care and Education Reconciliation Act of 2010. Pub L No. 111-152, 124 Stat 1029. (6)

Hepler CD, Strand LM. Opportunities and responsibilities in pharmaceutical care. *Am J Hosp Pharm*. 1990;47(3):533. (3)

Patient Protection and Affordable Care Act (PPACA). Pub L No. 111-148, 124 Stat 119. (5)

Rovers JP, Currie JD, eds. *A Practical Guide to Pharmaceutical Care: A Clinical Skills Primer*. 3rd ed. Washington, DC: American Pharmacists Association; 2007. (3)

Key Websites

National Patient Safety Goals. Joint Commission on Accreditation of Healthcare Organizations. http://www.jointcommission.org/standards_information/npsgs.aspx. Accessed June 17, 2015. (11)

Section 1 General Principles

2 Interpretation of Clinical Laboratory Tests

Erika Felix-Getzik, Yulia A. Murray, and Stefanie C. Nigro

CORE PRINCIPLES

		CHAPTER CASES
1	Laboratory findings should be used to complement other subjective and objective findings and must not be evaluated in isolation. The values must be assessed in context of the clinical situation and incorporate understanding of human physiology.	**Case 2-3 (Question 1), Case 2-4 (Question 1), Table 2-2 Case 2-5 (Questions 1, 2), Table 2-3, Case 2-6 (Questions 1, 2)**
2	Lack of availability, expense, or inconvenience may limit the usefulness of some clinical laboratory tests. Estimations by means of equations or nomograms may be used in clinical practice to overcome these barriers.	**Case 2-1 (Question 1), Table 2-2**
3	Test reliability is impacted by various factors including statistical and preanalytical variations, accuracy, and precision.	**Case 2-1 (Question 1), Case 2-2 (Question 1), Case 2-4 (Question 1), Table 2-1, Table 2-2**
4	Laboratory findings can be helpful in assessing clinical disorders, establishing a diagnosis, assessing drug therapy, or evaluating disease progression.	**Case 2-1 (Question 1), Table 2-2 Case 2-2 (Question 1), Table 2-3 Case 2-3 (Question 1), Case 2-4 (Question 1), Case 2-5 (Questions 1, 2), Case 2-6 (Questions 1, 2)**

This chapter provides the reader with an overview of laboratory tests commonly used in clinical practice. Specialized laboratory tests, which are used to monitor specific disease states or specific drug therapies, are integrated into the case histories, questions, and answers in the disease-specific chapters of this textbook. Over-the-counter or patient-directed laboratory tests are briefly discussed at the end of this chapter because of their increased availability and use. All stated laboratory ranges were obtained from the key references listed at the end of this chapter.[1–3]

GENERAL PRINCIPLES

Generally, laboratory tests should be ordered only if the results of the test will guide decisions about the care of the patient. Serum, urine, and other bodily fluids can be analyzed routinely, however, the economic cost and impact on the quality of life related to obtaining these data must always be balanced by benefit to patient-specific outcomes.

Reference Ranges

The term *reference range* is typically preferred in clinical practice rather than *normal range* because there are several factors that contribute to the "normal" value for each individual. Laboratory findings, within and outside the reference range, can be helpful in assessing clinical disorders, establishing a diagnosis, assessing drug therapy, or evaluating disease progression. In addition, baseline laboratory tests are often necessary to evaluate disease progression and response to therapy or to monitor the development of toxicities associated with therapy.

When assessing laboratory findings, it is important to be mindful that values outside the reference range may not require clinical intervention. Values must be assessed in context of the clinical situation and incorporate understanding of human physiology. Likewise, values that fall within the reference range may need further assessment secondary to limitations of the test or impact of biologic or physiologic considerations. Laboratory findings should also be used to complement other subjective and objective findings and must not be evaluated in isolation.

Laboratory test results are specific to the clinical laboratory conducting the test and can vary based on the type of equipment and testing methods used. Consequently, clinicians should rely on reference ranges listed by their own clinical laboratory when assessing laboratory tests.

Evaluating Laboratory Results

The reference ranges provided in this chapter are for general illustrative purposes. When applying this information to the clinical setting, appropriate clinical assessment and judgment should be applied. Patient-specific attributes such as the individual's age, sex, race, clinical presentation, and lifestyle are factors that may influence reported laboratory results and, therefore, must be taken into consideration. Statistical and preanalytical variations are common and must also be evaluated in context of the result obtained. Refer to Table 2-1 for examples of common preanalytical variables.

Test Reliability

As a result of probability, if the same test is completed multiple times on the same sample, typically 1 of 20 results or 5% will be reported outside of the provided reference range. Indicators of test reliability include accuracy, precision, sensitivity, and specificity. Precision refers to the repeatability of a laboratory test (i.e., test results fall within a similar value when repeated), whereas accuracy is the ability of a test to provide a result that is reflective of the "true" value (i.e., the test result matches the actual real value).

Table 2-1
Preanalytical Variation: Factors Affecting the Test Result from the Time the Test Is Ordered Until It Arrives at the Laboratory

Variable	Example(s)
Incorrect test ordered	Albumin ordered to assess impact of recent dietary change (prealbumin better marker for acute changes)
Sample incorrectly labeled	Sample obtained from one patient and labeled with another name
Improper preparation for test	Fasting indicated but not followed: fasting glucose, complete lipid panel Pretest medications not administered in the appropriate manner Pretest diet restrictions not met: rare meat ingested before guaiac test
Medication	Medication interfered with testing procedure or by pharmacologic effect: β-agonist can reduce serum potassium concentrations, thiazides can increase serum uric acid levels
Improper timing of test	Vancomycin trough taken after first dose (rather than before the fourth dose) aPTT measured 2 hours after initial dose (rather than 6 hours after start) Fasting glucose test completed shortly after a meal, TSH measured 2 weeks after dose change (rather than 4–6 weeks after change)
Collection incomplete or improper	Abnormal 24-hour urine collection secondary to patient forgetting to void in provided container, blood specimen obtained from extremity with IV infusion site resulting in dilutional effect of glucose, BUN, and electrolytes, specimen collected in incorrect container
Improper handling or storage	Hyperkalemia because of hydrolysis of blood specimen
Poor accuracy or precision	Faulty or outdated laboratory reagents in use
Technical	Result incorrectly read, computer keying error
Sex	Many laboratory findings are sex dependent
Age	Neonatal, pediatric, adult, and geriatric populations have unique reference ranges for numerous laboratory tests
Pregnancy	Gestational status impacts numerous laboratory findings: alkaline phosphatase, cholesterol, iron, etc.
Posture	Being in upright position during laboratory sampling can increase albumin, calcium, iron, etc.
Exercise	Strenuous exercise before testing can impact lactate, creatine kinase, ALT, AST, uric acid, etc.
Normal physiologic fluctuations	Circadian rhythm can impact cortisol, serum iron, serum creatinine, WBC count, etc.
Medical procedures	Blood transfusion with red blood cells before hemoglobin A_{1c} measured results in normal A_{1c} for poorly controlled individual with diabetes, creatine kinase elevated secondary to recent cardioversion

A_{1c}, hemoglobin A_{1c} (also glycosylated hemoglobin); ALT, alanine aminotransferase; aPTT, activated partial thromboplastin time; AST, aspartate aminotransferase; BUN, blood urea nitrogen; IV, intravenous; TSH, thyroid-stimulating hormone; WBC, white blood cell.

Quality control and assurance practices at each laboratory are monitored regularly to ensure reliability of results. Typically, if a result is obtained that is significantly outside the reference range, the laboratory will repeat the test to confirm or refute the finding.

Research studies generally establish the sensitivity and specificity of laboratory tests. Clinically, these are essential to distinguish the presence or absence of a disease or condition. Sensitivity is the ability of the test to correctly identify the disease or condition. If a test is 95% sensitive, then 95% of the individuals will be correctly identified as having the disease or condition, but 5% will have a negative test result even though they have the disease or condition (false negative). Specificity is the ability of the test to rule out individuals who do not have the disease or condition. If a test is 95% specific, then 95% of the individuals without disease will have a correct negative result, but 5% will be identified as having the disease or condition even though they are negative (false positive).

Units of Measure

The International System of Units (SI) reports clinical laboratory values using the metric system. The basic unit of mass for the SI system is the *mole*, which is not influenced by the added weight of salt or ester formulations. Therefore, the mole is technically and pharmacologically more meaningful than the gram because each physiologic reaction occurs on a molecular level. Efforts to implement the SI system internationally for laboratory test reports have been resisted in the United States. Despite adopting SI transition policies in the late 1980s, major American medical journals have since reverted back to the traditional units for laboratory test reporting.[4,5] In this chapter, reference ranges for common laboratory tests are presented in both conventional and SI units, along with "conversion factors" to interchange traditional and SI units (Tables 2-2 and 2-3).

Table 2-2
Blood Chemistry Reference Values

	Normal Reference Values			
Laboratory Test	**Conventional Units**	**SI Units**	**Conversion Factor**	**Comments**
Electrolytes				
Sodium	135–147 mEq/L or mmol/L	135–147 mmol/L	1	Low sodium is usually caused by excess water (e.g., ↑ serum antidiuretic hormone) and is treated with water restriction. ↑ in severe dehydration, diabetes insipidus, significant renal and GI losses
Potassium	3.5–5 mEq/L	3.5–5 mmol/L	1	↑ with renal dysfunction, acidosis, K-sparing diuretics, hemolysis, burns, crush injuries. ↓ by diuretics, alkalosis, severe vomiting and diarrhea, heavy NG suctioning
CO_2 content	21–32 mEq/L	21–32 mmol/L	1	Sum of HCO_3^- and dissolved CO_2. Reflects acid–base balance and compensatory pulmonary (CO_2) and renal (HCO_3^-) mechanisms. Primarily reflects HCO_3^-
Chloride	95–110 mEq/L	95–110 mmol/L	1	Important for acid–base balance. ↓ by GI loss of chloride-rich fluid (vomiting, diarrhea, GI suction, intestinal fistulas, overdiuresis)
BUN	8–20 mg/dL	2.8–7.1 mmol/L	0.357	End product of protein metabolism, produced by liver, transported in blood, excreted renally. ↑ in renal dysfunction, high protein intake, upper GI bleeding, volume contraction
Creatinine	≤1.5 mg/dL	≤133 μmol/L	88.4	Major constituent of muscle; rate of formation constant; affected by muscle mass (lower with aging and gender); excreted renally. ↑ in renal dysfunction. Used as a primary marker for renal function (GFR)
CrCl	90–130 mL/minute	1.5–2.16 mL/s	0.01667	Reflects GFR; ↓ in renal dysfunction. Used to adjust dosage of renally eliminated drugs
Estimated GFR	90–120 mL/minute/1.73 m^2	n/a	n/a	Possibly a more accurate reflection of renal function than CrCl. Still influenced by muscle mass

(continued)

Table 2-2
Blood Chemistry Reference Values (*Continued*)

Laboratory Test	Normal Reference Values: Conventional Units	Normal Reference Values: SI Units	Conversion Factor	Comments
Electrolytes				
Cystatin C	<1.0 mg/dL	<0.749 μmol/L	0.749	Indicator of renal function—not influenced by patient muscle mass, age, or sex. May also help predict patients at risk for cardiovascular disease
Glucose (fasting)	65–115 mg/dL	3.6–6.3 mmol/L	0.05551	↑ in diabetes or by adrenal corticosteroids
Glycosylated hemoglobin	3.8%–6.4%	3.8%–6.4%	1	Used to assess average blood glucose over 1–3 months. Used to diagnose diabetes, monitor disease progression, and/or assess the efficacy of drug therapy
Calcium—total	8.6–10.3 mg/dL	2.2–2.74 mmol/L	0.250	Regulated by body skeleton redistribution, parathyroid hormone, vitamin D, calcitonin. Affected by changes in albumin concentration. Total calcium ↓ when albumin ↓ (the serum total calcium concentration falls by 0.8 mg/dL for every 1-g/dL fall in serum albumin concentration). ↓ by hypothyroidism, loop diuretics, vitamin D deficiency; ↑ in malignancy and hyperthyroidism
Calcium—unbound (ionized)	4.4–5.1 mg/dL	1–1.3 mmol/L	0.250	Physiologically active form. Unbound "free" calcium remains unchanged as albumin fluctuates
Magnesium	1.3–2.2 mEq/L	0.65–1.1 mmol/L	0.51	↓ in malabsorption, severe diarrhea, alcoholism, pancreatitis, diuretics, hyperaldosteronism (symptoms of weakness, depression, agitation, seizures, hypokalemia, arrhythmias). ↑ in renal failure, hypothyroidism, magnesium-containing antacids
Phosphate (inorganic phosphorus)	2.5–5 mg/dL	0.8–1.6 mmol/L	0.323	↑ with renal dysfunction, hypervitaminosis D, hypocalcemia, hypoparathyroidism. ↓ with excess aluminum antacids, malabsorption, renal losses, hypercalcemia, refeeding syndrome
Uric acid	3–8 mg/dL	<0.42 mmol/L	0.06	↑ in gout, neoplastic, or myeloproliferative disorders, and drugs (diuretics, niacin, low-dose salicylate, cyclosporine)
Proteins				
Prealbumin	19.5–35.8 mg/dL	195–358 mg/L	10	Indicates acute changes in nutritional status, useful for monitoring TPN
Albumin	3.6–5 g/dL	36–50 g/L	10	Produced in liver; important for intravascular osmotic pressure. ↓ in liver disease, malnutrition, ascites, hemorrhage, protein-wasting nephropathy. May influence highly protein-bound drugs
Globulin	2.3–3.5 g/dL	23–35 g/L	10	Active role in immunologic mechanisms. Immunoglobulins ↑ in chronic infection, rheumatoid arthritis, multiple myeloma
CK	Female: 20–170 IU/L Male: 30–220 IU/L	Female: 0.33–2.83 μkat/L Male: 0.5–3.67 μkat/L	0.01667	In tissues that use high energy (skeletal muscle, myocardium, brain). ↑ by IM injections, MI, acute psychotic episodes. Isoenzyme CK-MM in skeletal muscle; CK-MB in myocardium; CK-BB in brain. MB fraction >5%–6% suggests acute MI
CK-MB	<6%	<6%	0.01667	
cTnI	0–0.04 ng/mL	0–0.04 mcg/L	1	More specific than CK-MB for myocardial necrosis; cTnI >0.04 suggests acute myocardial necrosis

Table 2-2
Blood Chemistry Reference Values (*Continued*)

	Normal Reference Values			
Laboratory Test	**Conventional Units**	**SI Units**	**Conversion Factor**	**Comments**
Electrolytes				
Myoglobin	Female: 12–76 mcg/L Male: 19–92 mcg/L	Female: 12–76 mcg/L Male: 19–92 mcg/L	1	Early elevation (within 3 hours) may suggest myocardial injury, but less specific than CK-MB or troponin
Homocysteine	4–12 μmol/L	4–12 μmol/L	1	Damages vessel endothelial, which may increase the risk for cardiac disease. Associated with deficiencies in folate, vitamin B_6, and vitamin B_{12}
LDH	100–250 IU/L	1.67–4.17 μkat/L	0.01667	High in heart, kidney, liver, and skeletal muscle. Five isoenzymes: LD1 and LD2 mostly in heart, LD5 mostly in liver and skeletal muscle, LD3 and LD4 are nonspecific. ↑ in malignancy, extensive burns, PE, renal disease
BNP	<100 pg/mL	<100 ng/L	1	BNP >500 ng/L indicates congestive heart failure. Released from ventricles with ↑ workload placed on heart
NT-proBNP	<60 pg/mL males <150 pg/mL females	<60 ng/L males <150 ng/L females	1	NT-proBNP has similar clinical utility to BNP as a marker for CHF
CRP	0–1.6 mg/dL	0–16 mg/L	1	Nonspecific indicator of acute inflammation. Similar to ESR, but more rapid onset and greater elevation. CRP >3 mg/dL increases risk of cardiovascular disease
hs-CRP	0–2.0 mg/L	0–2.0 mg/L	1	More sensitive measure of CRP; concentrations from 0.5 to 10 mg/L; hs-CRP <1.0 mg/L low risk for cardiovascular disease; 1.0–3.0 mg/L average risk; and >3.0 mg/L high risk for cardiovascular disease
Liver Function				
AST	0–35 units/L	0–0.58 μkat/L	0.01667	Large amounts in heart and liver; moderate amounts in muscle, kidney, and pancreas. ↑ with MI and liver injury. Less liver specific than ALT
ALT	0–35 units/L	0–0.58 μkat/L	0.01667	From heart, liver, muscle, kidney, pancreas. ↑ negligible unless parenchymal liver disease. More liver specific than AST
ALP	20–130 units/L	0.33–2.17 μkat/L	0.01667	Large amounts in bile ducts, placenta, bone. ↑ in bile duct obstruction, obstructive liver disease, rapid bone growth (e.g., Paget disease), pregnancy
GGT				Sensitive test reflecting hepatocellular injury; not helpful in differentiating liver disorders. Usually high in chronic alcoholics
Male	9–50 units/L			
Female	8–40 units/L			
Bilirubin—total	0.1–1 mg/dL	2–18 μmol/L	17.1	Breakdown product of hemoglobin, bound to albumin, conjugated in liver. Total bilirubin includes direct (conjugated) and indirect bilirubin. ↑ with hemolysis, cholestasis, liver injury
Bilirubin—direct	0–0.2 mg/dL	0–4 μmol/L	17.1	
Miscellaneous				
Amylase	35–118 units/L	0.58–1.97 μkat/L	0.01667	Pancreatic enzyme; ↑ in pancreatitis or duct obstruction

(*continued*)

Table 2-2
Blood Chemistry Reference Values (*Continued*)

Laboratory Test	Normal Reference Values		Conversion Factor	Comments
	Conventional Units	SI Units		
Electrolytes				
Lipase	10–160 units/L	0–2.67 μkat/L	0.01667	Pancreatic enzyme, ↑ acute pancreatitis, elevated for longer period than amylase
PSA	0–4 ng/mL	0–4 mcg/L	1	↑ in BPH and also in prostate cancer. PSA levels of 4–10 ng/mL should be worked up. Risk of prostate cancer increased if free PSA/total PSA <0.25
TSH	0.5–4.7 μunits/mL	0.5–4.7 munits/L	1	↑ TSH in primary hypothyroidism requires exogenous thyroid supplementation; ↓ TSH in hyperthyroidism
Procalcitonin	<0.5 ng/mL	<0.5 mcg/L	1	↑ Bacterial infections—low risk of sepsis if <0.5 ng/mL; high risk of severe sepsis if >2.0 ng/mL
Total cholesterol	<200 mg/dL	<5.2 mmol/L	0.02586	Current guidelines do not recommend a target level; consult current guidelines
LDL	<100 mg/dL	<2.58 mmol/L	0.02586	Current guidelines do not recommend a target level, but rather starting moderate- to high-intensity statin therapy based on current risk factors; consult current guidelines
HDL	Female: >50 mg/dL Male: >40 mg/dL	Female: >1.29 mmol/L Male: >1.03 mmol/L	0.02586	Current guidelines do not recommend a target level; consult current guidelines
Triglycerides (fasting)	<150 mg/dL	<1.70 mmol/L	0.0113	↑ by alcohol, saturated fats, drugs. Obtain fasting level. Current guidelines do not recommend a target level

ALP, alkaline phosphatase; ALT, alanine aminotransferase; AST, aspartate aminotransferase; BNP, brain natriuretic peptide; BPH, benign prostatic hypertrophy; BUN, blood urea nitrogen; CHF, congestive heart failure; CK, creatine kinase (formerly known as creatine phosphokinase); CrCl, creatinine clearance; CRP, C-reactive protein; cTnI, cardiac troponin I; ESR, erythrocyte sedimentation rate; GFR, glomerular filtration rate; GGT, γ-glutamyl transferase; GI, gastrointestinal; HDL, high-density lipoprotein; IM, intramuscularly; LDH, lactate dehydrogenase; LDL, low-density lipoprotein; MI, myocardial infarction; NG, nasogastric; PE, pulmonary embolism; PSA, prostate-specific antigen; SI, International System of Units; TPN, total parenteral nutrition; TSH, thyroid-stimulating hormone.

Table 2-3
Hematologic Laboratory Values

Laboratory Test	Normal Reference Values		Comments
	Conventional Units	SI Units	
RBC count			
▪ Male	$4.3–5.9 \times 10^6/\mu L$	$4.3–5.9 \times 10^{12}/L$	
▪ Female	$3.5–5.0 \times 10^6/\mu L$	$3.5–5.0 \times 10^{12}/L$	
Hct			↓ with anemias, bleeding, hemolysis. ↑ with polycythemia, chronic hypoxia
▪ Male	40.7%–50.3%	0.4–0.503	
▪ Female	36%–44.6%	0.36–0.446	
Hgb			Similar to Hct
▪ Male	13.8–17.5 g/dL	138–175 g/L	
▪ Female	12.1–15.3 g/dL	121–153 g/L	
MCV	80–97.6 μm^3	80–97.6 fL[a]	Describes average RBC size; ↑ MCV = macrocytic, ↓ MCV = microcytic
MCH	27–33 pg	1.66–2.09 fmol/cell	Measures average weight of Hgb in RBC

Table 2-3
Hematologic Laboratory Values (*Continued*)

Laboratory Test	Normal Reference Values		Comments
	Conventional Units	SI Units	
MCHC	33–36 g/dL	20.3–22 mmol/L	More reliable index of RBC hemoglobin than MCH. Measures average concentration of Hgb in RBC. Concentration will not change with weight or size of RBC
Reticulocyte count (adults)	0.5%–1.5%	0.005–0.015	Indicator of RBC production; ↑ suggests ↑ number of immature erythrocytes released in response to stimulus (e.g., iron in iron-deficiency anemia)
ESR	0–30 mm/hour	0–30 mm/hour	Nonspecific; ↑ with inflammation, infection, neoplasms, connective tissue disorders, pregnancy, nephritis. Useful monitor of temporal arteritis and polymyalgia rheumatica
WBC count	3.8–9.8 × $10^3/\mu L$	3.8–9.8 × $10^9/L$	Consists of neutrophils, lymphocytes, monocytes, eosinophils, and basophils; ↑ in infection and stress
ANC	2,000 cells/μL		ANC = WBC × (% neutrophils +% bands)/100; if <500 ↑ risk infection, if >1,000 ↓ risk infection
Neutrophils	40%–70%	0.4–0.7	↑ in neutrophils suggests bacterial or fungal infection. ↑ in bands suggests bacterial infection
Bands	0%–10%	0–0.1	
Lymphocytes	22%–44%	0.22–0.44	
Monocytes	4%–11%	0.04–0.11	
Eosinophils	0%–8%	0–0.08	Eosinophils ↑ with allergies, parasitic infections, and certain neoplasms
Basophils	0%–3%	0–0.03	
Platelets	150–450 × $10^3/\mu L$	150–450 × $10^9/L$	<100 × $10^3/\mu L$ = thrombocytopenia; <20 × $10^3/\mu L$ = ↑ risk for severe bleeding
Iron			
■ Male	45–160 mcg/dL	8.1–31.3 μmol/L	Body stores two-thirds in Hgb; one-third in bone marrow, spleen, liver; only small amount present in plasma. Blood loss major cause of deficiency
■ Female	30–160 mcg/dL	5.4–31.3 μmol/L	↑ needs in pregnancy and lactation
■ TIBC	220–420 mcg/dL	39.4–75.2 μmol/L	↑ capacity to bind iron with iron deficiency

ANC, absolute neutrophil count; ESR, erythrocyte sedimentation rate; Hct, hematocrit; Hgb, hemoglobin; MCH, mean corpuscular hemoglobin; MCHC, mean cell hemoglobin concentration; MCV, mean cell volume; RBC, red blood cell; SI, International System of Units; TIBC, total iron-binding capacity; WBC, white blood cell.
[a]fL, femtoliter; femto, 10^{-15}; pico, 10^{-12}; nano, 10^{-9}; micro, 10^{-6}; milli, 10^{-3}.

FLUIDS AND ELECTROLYTES

Please refer to Chapter 27, Fluid and Electrolyte Disorders, for more detailed information.

Sodium

Reference Range: 135–147 mEq/L or mmol/L

Sodium is the predominant cation of the extracellular fluid (ECF), and human cells reside in salt water. Along with chloride, potassium, and water, sodium is important in establishing serum osmolarity and osmotic pressure relationships between intracellular fluid (ICF) and ECF. Osmoregulatory system regulates the plasma sodium concentrations to remain in a normal range by controlling water intake and excretion.[6] An increase in the serum sodium concentration could suggest either impaired sodium excretion or volume contraction. On the contrary, a decrease in the serum sodium concentration to less-than-normal values could reflect hypervolemia, abnormal sodium losses, or sodium starvation. Although healthy individuals are able to maintain sodium homeostasis without difficulty, patients with kidney failure, heart failure, or lung disease often encounter sodium and water imbalances. In adults, changes in serum sodium concentrations most often represent water rather than sodium imbalance. Therefore, serum sodium concentrations are more reflective of a patient's fluid status rather than sodium balance. Clinical manifestations of hyponatremia or hypernatremia are mostly neurologic, and rapid changes in serum sodium concentrations can lead to severe and sometimes fatal brain injury.[6]

HYPONATREMIA

Hyponatremia can result from dilution of the sodium concentration in serum or from a total body depletion of sodium. The finding of hyponatremia implies that sodium has been diluted throughout all body fluids because water moves freely across cell membranes in response to oncotic pressures. Hyponatremia can denote low, high, or normal tonicity. Dilutional hyponatremia is the most common form and results from water retention.[7] Some clinical conditions such as cirrhosis, congestive heart failure (CHF), the syndrome of inappropriate antidiuretic hormone secretion (SIADH), and renal impairment, as well as the administration of osmotically active solutes (e.g., albumin and mannitol) are commonly associated with dilutional hyponatremia. Drugs that can induce SIADH, thereby causing a reversible hyponatremia (especially in the elderly), include cyclophosphamide, carbamazepine, desmopressin, oxcarbazepine, oxytocin, serotonin selective reuptake inhibitors, and vincristine.[7,8] Hyponatremia that results from sodium depletion presents as a low serum sodium concentration in the absence of edema. Sodium-depletion hyponatremia can be caused by mineralocorticoid deficiencies, sodium-wasting renal disease, or replacement of sodium-containing fluid losses with nonsaline solutions.[7] Therapy with thiazide diuretics may also lead to the development of severe hyponatremia. Hyponatremia can be frequently seen in hospitalized patients; however, morbidity varies significantly in severity, and serious complications can be due to the disorder itself or due to the inappropriate management and rapid correction of the sodium levels.

HYPERNATREMIA

Hypernatremia represents a state of relative water deficiency in relation to the body's sodium stores. Because sodium contributes to the cell's tonicity, hypernatremia denotes hypertonicity and at least transient cellular dehydration.[9] Some of the causes of hypernatremia are loss of free water, loss of hypotonic fluid, or excessive sodium intake. Free water loss is uncommon, except in the presence of diabetes insipidus. Diarrhea is the most common cause of hypotonic fluid loss in infants and the elderly. Increased retention of sodium in patients with hyperaldosteronism can also increase serum sodium concentrations. Excessive salt intoxication is usually accidental or iatrogenic and most commonly results from inappropriate intravenous administration of hypertonic salt solutions. Some β-lactam antibiotics (e.g., ticarcillin) contain a modest sodium load and can cause fluid overload when high dosages are administered.

The primary defense against hypertonicity is thirst and subsequent fluid intake. Hypernatremic syndromes, therefore, usually occur in patients who are unable to drink sufficient fluids. For example, demented elderly patients are at increased risk because they depend on others for their water requirements. Similarly, patients who are vomiting, comatose, or not allowed oral fluids are at risk for hypernatremia.

Potassium

Reference Range: 3.5–5.0 mEq/L or mmol/L

Potassium is the most abundant intracellular cation in the body responsible for regulating enzymatic function and neuromuscular tissue excitability. Approximately 90% of the total body potassium is found in the ICF, with the majority in muscle, and only about 10% available in the ECF. The potassium ion in the ECF is filtered freely at the glomerulus of the kidney, reabsorbed in the proximal tubule, and secreted into the distal segments of the nephron. Because the majority of potassium is sequestered within cells, a serum potassium concentration is not a good measure of total body potassium. Intracellular potassium, however, cannot be measured easily. Fortunately, the clinical manifestations of potassium deficiency (e.g., fatigue, drowsiness, dizziness, confusion, electrocardiographic changes, muscle weakness, and muscle pain) correlate well with serum concentrations. The serum potassium concentration is buffered and can be within normal limits despite abnormalities in total body potassium. During potassium depletion, potassium moves from the ICF into the ECF to maintain the serum concentration. When the serum concentration decreases by a mere 0.3 mEq/L, the total body potassium deficit is approximately 100 mEq. Serum potassium concentrations, therefore, can be misleading when interpreted in isolation from other considerations, and assumptions should not be made as to the status of total body potassium concentration based solely on a serum concentration measurement. Disorders of potassium are commonly the result of (1) alterations in intake, (2) alterations with excretion, and/or (3) unbalanced transcellular shifting of potassium (e.g., metabolic acidosis/alkalosis).

HYPOKALEMIA

The kidneys are responsible for about 90% of daily potassium loss (~40–90 mEq/day), and the remaining 10% of potassium is excreted in the stool and a negligible amount in sweat. The kidneys, however, have only a limited ability to conserve potassium. Even when potassium intake has ceased, the urine will contain at least 5 to 20 mEq of potassium per 24 hours. Therefore, prolonged intravenous therapy with potassium-free solutions in a patient unable to obtain potassium in foods (e.g., nothing by mouth) can result in hypokalemia. Hypokalemia can also be induced by osmotic diuresis (e.g., mannitol and glucosuria), use of thiazide or loop diuretics (e.g., hydrochlorothiazide, furosemide, respectively), excessive mineralocorticoid activity, or protracted vomiting. Although the fluid secreted along most of the upper gastrointestinal (GI) tract contains only a modest amount of potassium (i.e., 5–20 mEq/L), vomiting can induce hypokalemia because of the combined effect from decreased food intake, loss of acid, alkalosis, and loss of sodium. The loss of large amounts of colonic fluid through severe diarrhea and/or laxative abuse can cause potassium depletion because fluid in the colon is high in potassium content (i.e., 30–40 mEq/L). Insulin and stimulation of β_2-adrenergic receptors can also induce hypokalemia because both increase the movement of potassium into cells from the ECF. The magnitude of a potassium deficiency is difficult to establish because of the limited presence of potassium in the ECF. Equation 2-1 can be used to estimate the potassium deficit with hypokalemia:

$$\text{Kdeficit (mmol)} = (K_{normal} - K_{measured}) \times \text{kg of body weight} \times 0.4 \qquad \text{(Eq. 2-1)}$$

It is also important to note that hypomagnesemia often accompanies hypokalemia, because magnesium is necessary for the shifting of sodium, potassium, and calcium in and out of cells. As a result, hypokalemic individuals not responding to potassium therapy may be refractory to treatment until hypomagnesemia is corrected. Some laboratories omit magnesium from the general electrolyte panel, so this test may need to be specially ordered.

HYPERKALEMIA

Hyperkalemia most commonly results from decreased renal excretion of potassium (e.g., renal failure, renal hypoperfusion, and hypoaldosteronism), excessive exogenous potassium administration, or excessive cellular breakdown (e.g., hemolysis, burns, crush injuries, surgery, and infections). Drug-induced causes include angiotensin converting enzyme inhibitors, angiotensin receptor blockers, aldosterone antagonists, and nonsteroidal antiinflammatory drugs, to name a few. Metabolic acidosis can also induce hyperkalemia because hydrogen ions move into cells in exchange for potassium and sodium. Abnormal potassium concentrations in the serum primarily affect excitability of nerve and muscle tissue (e.g., myocardial tissue). As a result, arrhythmias can be induced by hyperkalemia or hypokalemia. Potassium also affects some enzyme systems and acid–base balance, as well as carbohydrate and protein metabolism.

Carbon Dioxide Content

Reference Range: 21–32 mEq/L or mmol/L

The carbon dioxide (CO_2) content in the serum represents the sum of bicarbonate (HCO_3) and dissolved CO_2 concentrations. The dissolved CO_2 represents a relatively small component of total CO_2 content, making CO_2 essentially a measure of the serum bicarbonate. Chloride and bicarbonate are the primary negatively charged anions that offset the positively charged cations (i.e., sodium and potassium).

Although several buffer systems (e.g., hemoglobin [Hgb], phosphate, and protein) participate in regulating pH within physiologic limits, the carbonic acid–bicarbonate system is the most important. From a clinical standpoint, most disturbances of acid–base balance result from imbalances of the carbonic acid–bicarbonate system. The importance of bicarbonate in maintaining physiologic pH is presented in Chapter 26, Acid–Base Disorders.

Chloride

Reference Range: 95–110 mEq/L or mmol/L

Chloride (Cl^-) is the principal inorganic anion of the ECF; changes in chloride concentration are usually related to sodium concentration in an effort to maintain a neutral charge. Serum chloride has no real diagnostic significance. The relationship between serum concentrations of sodium, bicarbonate, and chloride is described by Equation 2-2, where *R* represents the anion gap (AG):

$$Cl^- + HCO_3^- + R = Na^+ \qquad \text{(Eq. 2-2)}$$

As with bicarbonate, chloride contributes to maintaining acid–base balance. A decreased serum chloride often accompanies metabolic alkalosis, whereas an increased serum chloride may indicate a hyperchloremic metabolic acidosis. The serum chloride, however, can also be slightly decreased in acidosis if organic acids or other acids are the primary cause of the acidosis. *Hyperchloremia*, absence of metabolic acidosis, is seldom encountered, because chloride retention is usually accompanied by sodium and water retention. *Hypochloremia* can result from excessive GI loss of chloride-rich fluid (e.g., vomiting, diarrhea, gastric suctioning, and intestinal fistulas). Because chloride ions are excreted with cations by the kidneys, hypochloremia may also result from significant diuresis.

Anion Gap

Reference Range: 7–16 mEq/L or mmol/L

The *R* factor, or AG, represents the contribution of unmeasured acids, such as lactate, phosphates, sulfates, and proteins. As displayed in Equation 2-2, a patient's AG is determined by subtracting the primary anions (Cl^- and HCO_3^-) from the primary cation (Na^+). Some clinicians include potassium in this determination and subtract the anions from both major cations (Na^+ and K^+). If potassium is not incorporated in the calculation, a normal AG is typically 5 to 12 mEq/mL. If potassium is considered, a normal AG would be less than 16 mEq/mL.

An elevated AG may be indicative of a metabolic acidosis caused by an increase in lactic acids, ketoacids, salicylic acids, methanol, or ethylene glycol. A low AG may be the result of reduced concentrations of unmeasured anions (e.g., hypoalbuminemia) or from systematic underestimation of serum sodium (e.g., hyperviscosity of myeloma). See Chapter 26, Acid–Base Disorders, for a more detailed discussion of the clinical use of the AG.

Blood Urea Nitrogen

Reference Range: 8–20 mg/dL or 2.8–7.1 mmol/L

Urea nitrogen is a waste product that comes from protein breakdown. It is produced solely by the liver, transported in the blood, and excreted by the kidneys. The serum concentration of urea nitrogen (i.e., BUN) is reflective of renal function because the urea nitrogen in blood is filtered completely at the glomerulus of the kidney and then reabsorbed and tubularly secreted within nephrons. Acute or chronic renal failure is the most common cause of an elevated BUN. Although the BUN is an excellent screening test for renal dysfunction, it does not sufficiently quantify the extent of renal disease. In addition, several nonrenal factors such as unusually high protein intake, disease states that increase protein catabolism (or upper GI bleeding), and glucocorticoid therapy can increase the BUN concentration. Liver disease and low protein diet will lead to lower BUN concentration. A patient's hydration status will also influence BUN; a water deficit tends to concentrate the urea nitrogen, and a water excess dilutes the urea nitrogen. The ratio of BUN to SCr can also be of clinical use. A normal ratio is roughly 15:1. Ratios greater than 20:1 are observed in patients with decreased blood flow to the kidney (e.g., prerenal disease such as dehydration or conditions involving reduced cardiac output) or conditions involving increased protein in the blood (e.g., dietary intake or an upper GI bleed). Situations in which the BUN:SCr ratio is less than 15:1 are seen in patients with renal failure, significant malnourishment (decreased intake of protein), or severe liver disease in which the liver is no longer able to form urea. It is important to note that BUN can change independent of the renal function and therefore SCr is more useful in estimating renal function.

Creatinine

Reference Range: ≤1.5 mg/dL or ≤133 μmol/L

Creatinine is derived from the creatine and phosphocreatine metabolism in the skeletal muscle. Its rate of formation for a given individual is remarkably constant and is determined primarily by an individual's muscle mass or lean body weight. Therefore, the SCr concentration is slightly higher in muscular subjects, but unlike the BUN, it is less directly affected by exogenous factors or liver impairment. Once creatinine is released from muscle into plasma, it is excreted renally almost exclusively by glomerular filtration and is not reabsorbed or metabolized by the kidney. A decrease in the glomerular filtration rate (GFR) results in an increase in the SCr concentration. Thus, careful interpretation of the SCr concentration is used widely in the clinical evaluation of patients with suspected renal disease. However, SCr concentration on its own should not be utilized to assess the level of kidney function in an individual.

A doubling of the SCr level roughly corresponds to a 50% reduction in the GFR. This general rule of thumb only holds true for steady-state creatinine levels.[10]

Of importance, as patients become older, there is a reduction in muscle mass and creatinine production is progressively decreased. Furthermore, the SCr concentration in female patients is generally 0.2 to 0.4 mg/dL (85%–90%) less than for males because females have less muscle mass.

Creatinine Clearance

Reference Range: 90–130 mL/minute

Because creatinine is cleared almost exclusively through the glomerulus in the kidney, creatinine clearance (CrCl) can be used as a clinically useful measure of a patient's GFR. CrCl serves as a valuable clinical parameter because many renally eliminated drugs are dose-adjusted based on the patient's renal function. To determine actual CrCl, the patient's urine is collected for a 24-hour period, and the concentration of urine creatinine (mg/dL), total volume of urine collected during the 24-hour period (mL/minute), and SCr (mg/dL) are determined. The patient-specific measured CrCl is determined using Equation 2-3:

$$CrCl = U_{creatinine} \times U_{volume} / SCr \times Time\ (minutes) \quad (Eq.\ 2\text{-}3)$$

Unfortunately, urine collections are time consuming and expensive, and incomplete collections can substantially underestimate renal function. In lieu of measuring actual CrCl, simplistic equations are commonly used to estimate a patient's CrCl. The following Cockcroft–Gault formula incorporates age, body weight, and SCr.[11] This formula can be utilized to estimate renal function when SCr is stable. Typically, clinicians use ideal body weight (IBW) in the calculation of estimated CrCl; however, actual body weight (ABW) may be used when ABW is less than IBW. Equation 2-4 has the highest correlation and the greatest accuracy in patients with SCr concentrations less than 1.5 mg/dL[12]:

$$\text{Estimated CrCl for males (mL/minute)} = (140 - \text{Age})\,(\text{Body weight in kg}) / (72)(SCr_{(mg/dL)}) \quad (Eq.\ 2\text{-}4)$$

The Cockcroft–Gault formula must be multiplied by 85% to calculate CrCl for females to account for the fact that females have less muscle mass.

Another commonly used approach to estimating CrCl is the Jelliffe method[13], shown in Equation 2-5:

$$\text{Estimated CrCl for males (mL/minute/1.73 m}^2) = 98 - [(0.8)(\text{Age} - 20)] / SCr_{(mg/dL)} \quad (Eq.\ 2\text{-}5)$$

This Jelliffe formula must be multiplied by 90% to calculate CrCl for females. The use of this method substantially underestimates CrCl for patients with SCr values less than 1.5 mg/dL,[13] whereas Cockcroft–Gault appears to have the highest correlation and greatest accuracy in patients with SCr values less than 1.5 mg/dL.[12] For patients with liver dysfunction, all methods of calculating CrCl from an SCr value are associated with significant overpredictions of CrCl.[14] Thus, methods for predicting CrCl should be used cautiously when attempting to adjust drug dosages in patients with liver disease. These equations should not be utilized in patients with rapidly changing GFR (e.g., acute kidney injury) because they will not provide accurate estimates of the GFR.

CASE 2-1

QUESTION 1: A 24-hour CrCl determination was ordered for D.B., a 72-year-old, 62-kg white man. The following data were returned from the clinical laboratory (total collection time was 24 hours):

Total urine volume: 1,000 mL
Urine creatinine concentration: 42 mg/dL
SCr: 2.0 mg/dL

Determine both the measured and the estimated CrCl for D.B. based on the given data, and compare and contrast these results.

Using Equation 2-3, D.B. has a 24-hour measured CrCl of approximately 15 mL/minute. His estimated CrCl is 29.2 mL/minute using the Cockcroft–Gault method (Eq. 2-4). Based on both methods, D.B.'s ability to clear renally eliminated drugs is impaired and adjustments to the dose/frequency will need to be made. An incomplete collection of urine during the 24-hour period or possible mishandling of the specimen can be explanations for the lower value seen with the measured CrCl. Because D.B. had an elevated SCr of 2.0 mg/dL, the accuracy of the Cockcroft–Gault estimation might also be compromised. D.B's baseline SCr will need to be established and if it is determined that SCr of 2.0 mg/dL is corresponding with D.B's baseline, then Cockroft–Gault estimation will hold true; if SCr of 2.0 mg/dL represents an acute change, then Cockroft–Gault equation should not be used to estimate renal function in D.B.

Estimated Glomerular Filtration Rate

An alternative approach to the Cockcroft–Gault method of estimating an adult patient's clearance was developed as part of the Modification of Diet in Renal Disease (MDRD) study and has been referred to as the MDRD Equation.[15] The originally described equation has been modified into an abbreviated format (Eq. 2-6) as follows:

$$\text{Estimated GFR}_{\text{(mL/minute per 1.73 m}^2)} = 186 \times (SCr)^{-1.154} \times (\text{Age})^{-0.203} \times (0.742 \text{ if female}) \times (1.212 \text{ if African American}) \quad (Eq.\ 2\text{-}6)$$

where SCr is the serum creatinine in mg/dL, age is in years, and the appropriate additional components are included for female or African-American patients. The above equation is applicable to laboratories reporting SCr values that have not been standardized. Starting in 2005, laboratories began standardizing their SCr values using an isotope dilution mass spectrometry to minimize the variation observed in SCr results from different clinical laboratories. In settings in which the SCr results have been standardized, the initial parameter in the MDRD equation is adjusted downward. The following is used to estimate GFR:

$$\text{Estimated GFR}_{\text{(mL/minute per 1.73 m}^2)} = 175 \times (SCr)^{-1.154} \times (\text{Age})^{-0.203} \times (0.742 \text{ if female}) \times (1.212 \text{ if African American}) \quad (Eq.\ 2\text{-}7)$$

When compared with the Cockcroft–Gault approach, MDRD estimations of GFR were more consistent with actual measurements of GFR. However, because both approaches rely on SCr, the influence of muscle mass and dietary intake still must be taken into consideration. In certain patient populations (e.g., obese patients and elderly patients), use of the MDRD can be less accurate, because the MDRD study equation was primarily derived from white subjects with a mean age of 51 years who had nondiabetic renal disease. A more detailed description of the MDRD equation to estimate GFR is addressed in Chapter 28, Chronic Kidney Diseases.

Cystatin C

Although SCr has long been the primary marker for renal function, cystatin C is a relatively new biomarker being investigated as a more precise measure of GFR. Cystatin C is cleared predominantly through the kidneys and is not reabsorbed, and elevated levels are observed in patients with declining renal function. Reference ranges for cystatin C are similar to SCr (≤1.0 mg/L). In contrast to SCr, which is produced from muscle cells, cystatin C is produced by the blood cells and was not expected to be significantly influenced by factors such as muscle mass, diet, age, sex, and race; however, higher levels of cystatin C have been observed in males and patients with higher height and weight, and higher lean body mass. It was also observed that cystatin C levels are increased with age.[16] In addition, increases in serum cystatin C levels tend to occur earlier than increases in SCr, making it possible to detect renal insufficiency in patients at an earlier stage. This is particularly desirable in patients with diabetes, hypertension, or cardiovascular disease who may be at higher risk for the development of renal disease. Cystatin C is also being evaluated as a potential predictor of cardiovascular disease, and preliminary research has also been directed at the role of cystatin C in Alzheimer disease and demyelinating conditions like multiple sclerosis.

Glucose

Reference Range: 65–115 mg/dL or 3.6–6.3 mmol/L (fasting)

The glucose concentration in the ECF is tightly regulated by homeostatic mechanisms to provide body tissues and cells with a ready source of energy. Two endocrine hormones, insulin and glucagon, work synergistically to maintain normal glucose concentrations. Insulin lowers blood glucose concentrations whereas glucagon, along with the counterregulatory hormones epinephrine, cortisol, and growth hormone, raises glucose levels. Because plasma glucose concentrations fluctuate in response to ingestion of meals, most glucose concentrations are measured in either the fasting state or the postprandial state, depending on the type of information desired. Generally, normal glucose values refer to the plasma glucose concentration in the fasting state. The specific laboratory assay of blood sugar determinations must also be considered because different assay methods vary in their specificity and sensitivity to glucose. Glucose testing using whole blood from capillary finger sticks is used in conjunction with blood glucose metering devices for patients with diabetes. Whole blood measurements using these devices are typically 10% to 15% lower than corresponding plasma glucose levels.

GLYCOSYLATED HEMOGLOBIN

Reference Range: 3.8%–6.4%

Hgb is the oxygen-carrying component of the red blood cell (RBC). During the functional life span of RBCs (~4 months), glucose molecules irreversibly bind to Hgb, which results in glycosylated Hgb A1c (A1c). The concentration of A1c reflects a patient's average blood glucose concentration for the life span of circulating RBCs. As a result, measurement of A1c concentrations is useful to diagnose diabetes, monitor disease progression, and/or assess the efficacy of drug therapy. In a patient without diabetes, about 5% of Hgb is glycosylated. To diagnose diabetes, two confirmatory A1c ≥6.5% are needed.[17] Both fasting plasma glucose (FPG) and postprandial glucose contribute variably to the A1c measurement. One study suggests that the higher the A1c (>8.5%), the greater the contribution of FPG to the A1c.[18] As such, the contribution of FPG decreases as the A1c decreases. The American Diabetes Association suggests an A1c of 7% correlates to an estimated average glucose (eAG) of 154 mg/dL. Estimated average glucose can be calculated using the following equation: eAG (mg/dL) = (28.7 − A1c) − 46.7.[17] It has been estimated that for every 1% reduction in A1c, the risk of microvascular complications is reduced by 37% and the risk of acute myocardial infarction (MI) by 14%.[19]

HYPERGLYCEMIA AND HYPOGLYCEMIA

Hyperglycemia and hypoglycemia are nonspecific signs of abnormal glucose metabolism. Diabetes mellitus is the most common cause of hyperglycemia along with suboptimal use of insulin and/or other antidiabetic agents, high carbohydrate dietary intake, physical inactivity, recent illness or infection, and increased emotional stress. Hyperglycemia may be caused or worsened by certain medications such as corticosteroids, niacin (doses >2 g/day), thiazide and loop diuretics, protease inhibitors, atypical antipsychotics, and 3-hydroxy-3-methylglutaryl-coenzyme A (HMG-CoA) reductase inhibitors (statins). Insufficient carbohydrate intake because of a missed meal is the most common cause of hypoglycemia in a patient receiving insulin or another hypoglycemic medication. In addition to insulin, drug-induced hypoglycemia includes insulin secretagogues, fluoroquinolone antibiotics, and select herbal products.

CASE 2-2

QUESTION 1: T.C., a 68-year-old man, visits his primary care provider to assess control of his type 2 diabetes. His average blood sugar over the past 90 days recorded by his blood glucose monitor is 195 mg/dL. However, T.C.'s Hgb A1c is 9%, which correlates with an eAG of 240 mg/dL. T.C. is confused that these values are different because he routinely ensures his blood glucose machine is calibrated and coded properly. Why is the laboratory average different?

T.C. should not be alarmed with the difference in these values. His blood glucose monitor is likely working properly and adequately measuring his plasma glucose concentrations. However, the monitor may be reflecting a lower average glucose concentration because of the timing of his daily testing for glucose. For example, measuring blood glucose in a fasting state more frequently than after mealtime could contribute to lower average concentrations because fasting values are typically lower than postprandial concentrations. The A1c is more indicative of his average blood sugar control during the past 90 days than the 90-day average recorded by his blood glucose monitor.

Please refer to Chapter 53, Diabetes Mellitus, for more detailed information regarding glucose and Hgb A1c.

Osmolality

Reference Range: 280–300 mOsm/kg or mmol/kg

The osmolality of a solution is a measure of the number of osmotically active ions (i.e., particles present) per unit of solution. It is the total number of particles in the solution, not the weight of the particle or the nature of the particle that determines osmolality. Because 1 mole of a substance contains 6×10^{23} molecules, equimolar concentrations of all substances in the undissociated state exert the same osmotic pressure. A mole of an ionized compound such as $Na^{+}Cl^{-}$ contributes twice as many particles in solution as 1 mole of an undissociated compound such as glucose. In most situations, the primary determinants of serum osmolality in the ECF are sodium (and its accompanying anions), glucose, and BUN. If one corrects for the concentrations of glucose and BUN, the serum concentration of sodium closely mirrors the serum osmolality. A useful formula (Eq. 2-8) is as follows:

$$\text{Osmolality} = (2 \times \text{Na+}) + (\text{Glucose}/18) + (\text{BUN}/2.8) \quad \text{(Eq. 2-8)}$$

Serum osmolality is helpful when evaluating fluid and electrolyte disorders, particularly sodium imbalances. The difference between the measured serum osmolality and the calculated serum osmolality is commonly referred to as the "osmol gap." Please note that in practice, osmolality and osmolarity are often used interchangeably. The reader is referred to Chapter 27, Fluid and Electrolyte Disorders, for a more detailed discussion of osmolality.

MULTICHEMISTRY PANELS

Frequently, multiple laboratory tests are needed for a given patient. Common clinical laboratory panels include a basic metabolic panel (BMP), comprehensive metabolic panel, electrolyte, hepatic function, and renal function panels (Table 2-4). Clinicians will often use the following abbreviated method to report a BMP in written medical records:

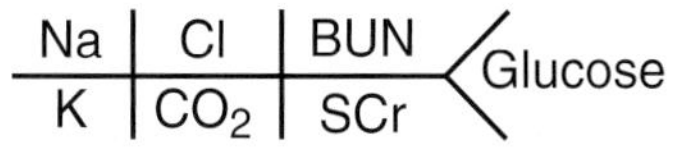

Table 2-4
Common Multichemistry Panels

Laboratory Panels	Electrolyte	BMP	CMP	Hepatic	Renal
Sodium	✓	✓	✓		✓
Potassium	✓	✓	✓		✓
Chloride	✓	✓	✓		✓
CO_2	✓	✓	✓		✓
Glucose		✓	✓		✓
Creatinine		✓	✓		✓
BUN		✓	✓		✓
Calcium		✓	✓		✓
Phosphorous					✓
Albumin, total			✓	✓	✓
Total protein			✓	✓	
Alkaline phosphatase (ALP)			✓	✓	
Alanine aminotransferase (ALT, SGPT)			✓	✓	
Aspartate aminotransferase (AST, SGOT)			✓	✓	
Bilirubin, total			✓	✓	
Bilirubin, direct				✓	

BMP, basic metabolic panel; BUN, blood urea nitrogen; CMP, comprehensive metabolic panel; SGOT, serum glutamic:oxaloacetic transaminase; SGPT, serum glutamic:pyruvic transaminase.

Multichemistry tests have become routinely used because they quickly provide basic information concerning organ function at relatively low cost. In addition, laboratory automation frequently makes it more cost effective to order a battery of tests within a panel versus a single test. A potential disadvantage of obtaining a battery of tests, however, is that clinicians may be inclined to pursue further laboratory testing when "abnormalities" are not clinically relevant. It is important to note that the individual laboratory tests included in a particular multichemistry panel may vary among clinical laboratories.

Calcium

Reference Range: 8.6–10.3 mg/dL or 2.2–2.74 mmol/L

Calcium has two key physiologic functions within our body; it is an essential intracellular messenger in cells and tissues and a key component of hydroxyapatite, which provides strength, rigidity, and elasticity to the skeleton. All calcium in the body resides primarily in the skeleton, with only about 1% freely exchangeable with that in the ECF. This reservoir of calcium in bones maintains the concentration of calcium in the plasma constant despite pronounced changes in the external balance of calcium. If the homeostatic factors (i.e., parathyroid hormone, vitamin D, and calcitonin) that regulate the calcium content of body fluid are intact, a patient can lose 25% to 30% of total body calcium without a change in the concentration of calcium ion in the plasma.

About 40% of the calcium in the ECF is bound to plasma proteins (especially albumin); 5% to 15% is complexed with phosphate and citrate; and about 45% to 55% is in the unbound, ionized form. Most laboratories measure the total calcium concentration; however, it is the free, ionized calcium concentration that is important and closely regulated physiologically. Most laboratories are also able to measure the ionized form of calcium, which has a reference range of 4.5 to 5.6 mg/dL (1.13–1.4 mmol/L). It is important to obtain an albumin level in patients in order to calculate a corrected calcium level that would account for hypoalbuminemia.

CASE 2-3

QUESTION 1: P.M. is a 61-year-old man admitted status post (s/p) fall because of alcohol intoxication. He has no known drug allergies. P.M's past medical history is significant for alcohol-induced seizures, alcohol abuse × 20 years, and hypertension. P.M's laboratory tests revealed the following:

Albumin: 2.0 g/dL
Ca: 6.8 mg/dL
Total bilirubin: 10.8 mg/dL
Serum AST: 280 units/L
Alkaline phosphatase: 240 units/L

Would P.M. be considered hypocalcemic, and how should he be managed?

This case presentation provides insufficient patient data to make a conclusion concerning treatment. However, it does illustrate the importance of treating the patient as a whole, not as a specific laboratory value. Because calcium in the serum is partially bound to plasma proteins (mostly albumin), the serum calcium concentration is affected by the concentration of these plasma proteins. If the albumin concentration is low, the reported serum calcium will generally be less than the lower limit of normal. A useful method to estimate a corrected value for serum calcium in the presence of a low serum albumin is to use the following guideline: the total serum calcium will decrease by 0.8 mg/dL for each decrease of 1.0 g/dL in serum albumin concentration. Thus, evaluating P.M.'s corrected calcium is indicated: $(4 - \text{albumin}_{\text{patient}} \times 0.8) + \text{calcium} = \text{corrected calcium}$. For P.M., his "corrected" serum calcium is 8.4 mg/dL, which is just below the reference range and probably does not warrant treatment with calcium supplementation unless his serum calcium continues to decline. Direct measurement of ionized calcium is independent of albumin concentration, making it unnecessary to correct calcium concentrations in the presence of hypoalbuminemia.

Unfortunately, some clinical laboratories do not have the capability of measuring ionized calcium.

Magnesium

Reference Range: 1.3–2.2 mEq/L or 0.65–1.1 mmol/L

Magnesium is primarily an intracellular electrolyte principally stored in bone and, together with potassium and calcium, helps maintain a neutral charge within the cell. Magnesium also serves an important metabolic role in the phosphorylation of adenosine triphosphate (ATP). Magnesium is necessary for the formation of bone and teeth and for normal nerve and muscle function.

A primary cause of hypomagnesemia is malnourishment. Some other factors associated with hypomagnesemia are use of proton pump inhibitors, chronic diarrhea, alcoholism, and diuretic use. Toxemia in pregnancy is associated with hypomagnesemia. Hypomagnesemia needs to be corrected before attempting to correct hypokalemia or hypocalcemia. Attempts to replace potassium or calcium in patients with hypomagnesemia will be ineffective until the low magnesium concentrations are adequately addressed. Excessive ingestion of magnesium-containing antacids can lead to hypermagnesemia. Increased concentrations of magnesium are also observed in patients with reduced renal function. Hypermagnesemia can slow conduction in the heart, prolong PT intervals, and widen the QRS complex.

Phosphate

Reference Range: 2.5–5 mg/dL or 0.80–1.6 mmol/L

The extracellular concentration of phosphate as inorganic phosphorus is the prime determinant of the intracellular concentration, which in turn is the source of phosphate for ATP and phospholipid synthesis. Intracellular phosphate is also important in the regulation of nucleotide degradation.

The ECF concentration of phosphate is influenced by parathyroid hormone, intestinal phosphate absorption, renal function, bone metabolism, and nutrition. Moderate hypophosphatemia is encountered by malnourished patients (especially when anabolism is induced), patients who excessively use antacids (aluminum-containing antacids bind phosphorus in the GI tract), chronic alcoholics, and septic patients. Clinical consequences of severe hypophosphatemia involve nervous system dysfunction, muscle weakness, rhabdomyolysis, cardiac irregularities, and dysfunction of leukocytes and erythrocytes. Hyperphosphatemia is most commonly caused by renal insufficiency, although increased vitamin D, hypoparathyroidism, and advanced malignancies are also significant causes.

Uric Acid

Reference Range: 3–8 mg/dL or 179–476 μmol/L

Uric acid is an end product of the metabolic breakdown of purines. It is commonly referred to as a metabolically inert compound offering little biologic role. The renal system is responsible for 60% to 70% of total body uric acid excretion. Most uric acid is freely filtered with approximately 90% reabsorbed via the nephron.

Increased serum uric acid concentrations can result from either a decrease in urate excretion (e.g., renal dysfunction) or excessive urate production (e.g., increased purine metabolism resulting from cytotoxic therapy of neoplastic or myeloproliferative disorders). Gout, a common arthritic condition characterized by hyperuricemia, is usually associated with increased serum concentrations of uric acid along with deposits of monosodium urate crystals in joints. Low serum uric acid concentrations are inconsequential and are usually reflective of drugs that have hypouricemic activity (e.g., high dosages of salicylates).

PROTEINS

Prealbumin

Reference Range: 19.5–35.8 mg/dL or 195–358 mg/L

Prealbumin is an important serum protein, but in comparison with other proteins, it accounts for a relatively small percentage of all circulating proteins. It is also referred to as thyroxine-binding prealbumin owing to its role as a transport mechanism for triiodothyronine (T_3) and thyroxine (T_4). However, it is most frequently used to monitor patients at risk for poor nutrition (e.g., patients with eating disorders, patients with human immunodeficiency virus, or patients receiving total parenteral nutrition). Compared with the long half-life of albumin (about 3 weeks), the half-life of prealbumin is only 1 to 2 days. This shorter half-life provides a more accurate reflection of acute changes in protein synthesis, catabolism, and ultimately immediate nutrition status. Hepatic disease and malnutrition are associated with decreases in prealbumin (and albumin). Hodgkin lymphoma, pregnancy, chronic kidney disease, and corticosteroid use can increase prealbumin serum concentrations.

Albumin

Reference Range: 3.6–5 g/dL or 36–50 g/L

Albumin, produced by the liver, contributes approximately 80% to serum colloid osmotic pressure. As a result, hypoalbuminemic states are commonly associated with edema and third spacing of ECF. A lack of essential amino acids from malnutrition or malabsorption, or impaired albumin synthesis by the liver, can result in decreased serum albumin concentrations. Most forms of hepatic insufficiency are associated with decreased synthesis of albumin. It can be lost directly from the blood because of hemorrhage, burns, or exudates or it may be lost directly into the urine because of nephrosis. Serum albumin concentrations seldom increase, but increases may be noted in volume depletion, in shock, or immediately after the administration of large amounts of intravenous albumin. In addition to its diagnostic value, albumin concentration is an important consideration in the therapeutic monitoring of drugs and electrolytes that are highly protein bound (e.g., phenytoin, digoxin, and calcium). In cases of severe hypoalbuminemia, determination of the "free" or unbound concentration of these entities might be necessary for an accurate assessment of drug therapy.

Globulin

Reference Range: 2.3–3.5 g/dL or 23–35 g/L

In addition to albumin, globulin is another primary plasma protein. Whereas albumin principally functions to maintain serum oncotic pressure, globulins play an active role in immunologic processes. The globulins can be separated into several subgroups such as α, β, and γ. The γ-globulins can be separated further into various immunoglobulins (e.g., IgA, IgM, and IgG). Chronic infection or rheumatoid arthritis can increase immunoglobulin levels, and fractionation of immunoglobulins can provide useful information in the evaluation of immune disorders. Because globulin is not manufactured solely by the liver, the ratio of albumin to globulin (the A/G ratio) is changed in patients with liver disease. Changes in this ratio result from decreased albumin concentration and a compensatory increase in globulin concentration.

CARDIAC MARKERS

Cardiac biomarkers are useful for the evaluation, diagnosis, and monitoring of patients with suspected heart damage. These markers, which include some enzymes, are often released into the blood when the myocardium becomes damaged or dies. Enzyme activity is typically expressed in terms of international units, where 1 international unit (IU) is the enzyme amount needed to catalyze the conversion of 1 μmol of substrate per minute. The analogous expression in SI terms involves the term katal (kat). One katal is the amount of enzyme to catalyze 1 mole of substrate per second, making 1.0 μkat the amount for 1.0 μmol/second. Based on this information, the conversion between μkat and IU is 1 μkat = 60 IU.

Creatine Kinase

Reference Range: Female 20–170 IU/L or 0.33–2.83 µkat/L; Male 30–220 IU/L or 0.5–3.67 µkat/L

Creatine kinase (CK), formerly known as creatine phosphokinase, catalyzes the transfer of high-energy phosphate groups in tissues that consume large amounts of energy (e.g., skeletal muscle, myocardium, and brain). The serum concentration of CK can be increased by strenuous exercise, intramuscular injections of tissue-irritating drugs (e.g., diazepam and phenytoin), crush injuries, myocardial damage, rhabdomyolysis, or high doses of certain HMG-CoA reductase inhibitors.

CK is composed of M and B subunits, which are further divided into three isoenzymes: MM, BB, and MB. The CK-MM isoenzyme is found predominantly in skeletal muscle, the CK-BB is predominantly in the brain, and the CK-MB is predominantly in the myocardium. Myocardial CK activity consists of 80% to 85% CK-MM and 15% to 20% CK-MB. Noncardiac tissues that contain large amounts of CK have either CK-MM or CK-BB. The MB fraction is rare in tissues other than the myocardium, making it a more specific cardiac marker.

CK-MB typically begins to increase 3 to 6 hours after an acute MI, peaks at 12 to 24 hours, and accounts for about 5% or more of the total CK.[20] Myocardial damage appears to correlate with the amount of CK-MB released into the serum (i.e., the higher the amount of CK-MB, the more extensive the myocardial injury). Although CK-MB levels greater than 25 units/L are usually associated with an MI, the absolute amount can vary, depending on the assay method.[21] Generally, if the amount of CK-MB exceeds 6% of the total CK, myocardial injury has presumably occurred. Analysis of CK-MB provides a rapid, sensitive, specific, cost-effective, and definitive means of detecting MI.[22]

Troponin

Reference Range: Cardiac Troponin T (cTnT) 0–0.01 ng/mL or mcg/L; Cardiac Troponin I (cTnI) 0.04 ng/mL or mcg/L

Troponins are proteins that regulate the calcium-mediated interaction of actin and myosin within muscles. There are two cardiac-specific troponins, cardiac troponin I (cTnI) and cardiac troponin T (cTnT). Whereas cTnT is present in cardiac and skeletal muscle cells, cTnI is present only in cardiac muscle.[23,24] Compared with the detection of CK-MB, the presence of troponin I is a more sensitive and specific indicator of myocardial necrosis.[25] The concentration of cTnI increases within 2 to 4 hours of an acute MI, enabling clinicians to quickly initiate appropriate therapy. Troponin also remains elevated for about 10 days compared with the 2- to 3-day elevation typically observed with CK-MB. cTnI levels >0.04 ng/mL are suggestive of acute myocardial tissue necrosis, but this value may vary slightly by assay (because of lack of standardization) and by institution. The reader is referred to Chapter 13, Acute Coronary Syndrome, for a more detailed discussion of the use of cardiac markers.

CASE 2-4

QUESTION 1: K.J., a 55-year-old man, with a history of stable angina presents to a hospital emergency department. He complains of sudden-onset chest pressure and tightness, diaphoresis, and nausea that has been waxing and waning for the last few hours. K.J. describes his discomfort as severe at times and not relieved by position change, antacids, or sublingual nitroglycerin. An electrocardiogram reveals ST segment depressions consistent with myocardial ischemia. His cardiac biomarkers reveal: CK 200 IU/L, CK-MB 5%, and cTnI 0.67. K.J. is diagnosed with an MI (non–ST segment-elevation MI) and is admitted for a cardiac catheterization. Why are the total CK and CK-MB serum concentrations within the reference range despite clear evidence, including elevated cTnI, supporting an acute MI?

Although CK and CK-MB are very helpful laboratory values for identifying and assessing myocardial damage/necrosis, the utility of these values alone can be quite limited. Troponin levels are very sensitive and specific to myocardial cell death and can become positive sooner than CK and CK-MB and will remain elevated for a much longer time frame (up to 10 days). So even if the CK and CK-MB are not elevated, the troponin can pick up even the smallest amount of myocardial cell death. Based on the clinical picture and the elevated troponin, the patient would be classified as having a non–ST segment-elevation MI.

Myoglobin

Reference Range: Female 12–76 mcg/L; Male 19–92 mcg/L

Myoglobin, a protein in heart and skeletal muscle cells, provides oxygen to working muscles. Damaged muscle releases myoglobin into the bloodstream. As a cardiac biomarker, myoglobin concentrations in serum rise within 3 hours of insult to the myocardial tissue, peak in about 8 to 12 hours, and return to normal in about a day. Because myoglobin serum concentrations rise more quickly than CK-MB after myocardial injury, they can be of value in helping rule out MI in the emergency department. Myoglobin serum concentrations, however, tend to be less specific for myocardial tissue compared with CK-MB and troponin; trauma or ischemic injury to noncardiac tissue can also increase serum myoglobin.

Homocysteine

Reference Range: 4–12 µmol/L

Patients with deficiencies in folate, vitamin B_6, or vitamin B_{12} tend to have elevated serum levels of homocysteine. Homocysteine is believed to have a destructive effect on vascular epithelium. With time, patients with elevated homocysteine levels (>12 μmol/L) are believed to be at increased risk for cardiac disease.[26] Screening individuals with a positive family history for elevated homocysteine or those with premature atherosclerosis without typical risk factors has been advocated. Understanding the association between increased homocysteine levels and specific vitamin deficiencies, supplementation of folate, vitamin B_6, and vitamin B_{12} has been used clinically. However, data are too limited to suggest that this approach reduces the incidence of acute MI or stroke.

Lactate Dehydrogenase

Reference Range: 100–250 IU/L (adult) or 1.67–4.17 µkat/L

The enzyme lactate dehydrogenase (LDH) is present in the heart, kidney, liver, and skeletal muscle. It is also abundantly present in erythrocytes and lung tissue. Because increased serum concentrations of LDH can be associated with diseases in many different organs and tissues, the diagnostic usefulness of an LDH determination is somewhat limited. There are, however, five isoenzymes of LDH. Although most tissues contain all five isoenzymes, some tissues have a predominance of one of the isoenzymes. LDH_1 and, to a lesser extent, LDH_2 predominate in the heart. Skeletal muscle and the liver have a predominance of LDH_5. LDH_3 and LDH_4 are found in a variety of tissues, including the lungs, RBCs, kidneys, brain, and pancreas. Consequently, identifying specific isoenzymes can increase the diagnostic usefulness of serum LDH determinations.

Brain Natriuretic Peptide

Reference Range: *<100 pg/mL or <100 ng/L: >500 pg/mL or >500 ng/L is considered elevated*

Brain natriuretic peptide (BNP) is released from the ventricles because of increased myocardial demand. Elevations in BNP are indicative of patients with CHF and volume overload. In an effort to reduce workload on the heart, BNP counteracts the renin–angiotensin–aldosterone system and causes vasodilatory effects, along with natriuresis (increased excretion of sodium), all geared at reducing blood volume. Patients with some degree of CHF typically have BNP levels greater than 100 ng/L. BNP levels greater than 500 ng/L represent definite CHF, but further evaluation is warranted to more fully characterize the extent of impaired cardiac function.[27] More recently, N-terminal proBNP (NT-proBNP), a by-product from the cleaving of pro-BNP to form BNP, is also being used in the clinical setting. BNP has also been used as a tool for patients presenting to the emergency department with severe dyspnea; however, studies have not demonstrated additional benefits associated with using BNP to guide therapy or to use BNP as a criterion for admission. The reader is referred to Chapter 14, Heart Failure, for a more detailed discussion of the use of BNP.

C-Reactive Protein

Reference Range: 0–1.6 mg/dL or 0–16 mg/L

C-reactive protein (CRP) is a nonspecific, acute-phase reactant helpful in the diagnosis and monitoring of inflammatory processes (e.g., rheumatoid arthritis and bacterial infections). CRP is produced by the liver in response to inflammation. Although an elevation in CRP indicates the presence of an acute inflammatory event, the nonspecific nature of the test does little to identify the cause or location of the inflammation. CRP is similar to an older test, the erythrocyte sedimentation rate (ESR), but it tends to be more sensitive than ESR and is also associated with a more rapid and greater response to acute inflammation. A potential use of CRP is as a novel risk factor for cardiovascular disease.[28] A more sensitive test for CRP is now available and is referred to as hs-CRP or high-sensitivity CRP. The hs-CRP test measures the same acute-phase reactant, but it is able to detect much lower levels of CRP, making it useful for early detection of patients at risk of cardiovascular diseases. Cardiovascular risk assessment is stratified based on the following criteria: patients with hs-CRP values less than 1.0 mg/L have a low risk; patients with an hs-CRP between 1.0 and 3.0 mg/L have an average risk; and patients with an hs-CRP greater than 3.0 mg/L are considered to be at high risk. It is important to realize that although hs-CRP is a new indicator for cardiovascular disease risk, evaluation of other well-established patient risk factors are still the gold standard and must be taken into consideration to determine the patient's overall risk of cardiovascular disease. CRP has also been used to assess chronic inflammatory diseases such as rheumatoid arthritis and Crohn disease. Additionally, because viral infections do not typically increase CRP serum concentrations, the use of CRP as a diagnostic tool to differentiate viral from bacterial infections might be clinically helpful.

LIVER FUNCTION TESTS

Aspartate Aminotransferase

Reference Range: 0–35 units/L or 0–0.58 μkat/L

The aspartate aminotransferase (AST) enzyme is abundant in heart and liver tissue and moderately present in skeletal muscle, kidney, and pancreas. In cases of acute cellular injury to the heart or liver, the enzyme is released into the blood from the damaged cells. In practice, AST determinations have been used to evaluate myocardial injury and to diagnose and assess the prognosis of liver disease resulting from hepatocellular injury. The serum AST level is increased in more than 95% of patients after an MI. However, the increase in AST does not occur until 4 to 6 hours after the onset of myocardial injury. Peak AST concentrations are seen in the serum after 24 to 36 hours, returning to the normal range in about 4 to 5 days.

Serum AST values are elevated significantly in patients with acute hepatic necrosis, whether caused by viral hepatitis or a hepatotoxin (e.g., carbon tetrachloride). In these situations, the serum concentrations of both AST and alanine aminotransferase (ALT) will be increased, even before the appearance of clinical symptoms (e.g., jaundice). The AST and ALT serum concentrations can be increased by as much as 100 times the usual upper limits of normal in the presence of parenchymal liver disease. Patients with intrahepatic cholestasis, posthepatic jaundice, or cirrhosis usually experience more moderate elevations of AST, depending on the extent of cell necrosis. The AST serum concentration is usually higher than that of ALT in patients with cirrhosis, and the AST increase is usually about four to five times greater than the upper limit of normal.

Alanine Aminotransferase

Reference Range: 0–35 units/L or 0–0.58 μkat/L

The ALT enzyme is found in essentially the same tissues that have high concentrations of AST. However, elevations in serum ALT are more specific for liver-related injuries or diseases. Although ALT is relatively more abundant in hepatic tissue versus cardiac tissue than AST, the liver still contains 3.5 times more AST than ALT. Serum concentrations of both AST and ALT increase when disease processes affect liver cell structure, but ALT concentrations are not significantly increased as a result of an acute MI. Evaluating the ratio of ALT to AST can be potentially useful, particularly in the diagnosis of viral hepatitis. The ALT/AST ratio frequently exceeds 1.0 with alcoholic cirrhosis, chronic liver disease, or hepatic cancer. However, ratios less than 1.0 tend to be observed with viral hepatitis or acute hepatitis, which can be useful when diagnosing liver disease.

Alkaline Phosphatase

Reference Range: 20–130 units/L or 0.33–2.17 μkat/L

The alkaline phosphatases (ALPs) constitute a large group of isoenzymes that play important roles in the transport of sugar and phosphate. These isoenzymes of ALP have different physiochemical properties and originate from different tissues (e.g., liver, bone, placenta, and intestine). In normal adults, ALP is derived primarily from liver and bone. Although only small amounts of ALP are present in the liver, this enzyme is secreted into the bile, and substantially elevated ALP serum concentrations can be seen with mild intrahepatic or extrahepatic biliary obstruction. Thus, the presence of early bile duct abnormalities can result in elevated ALP before increases in the serum bilirubin are observed. Drug-induced cholestatic jaundice (e.g., chlorpromazine or sulfonamides) can increase serum ALP concentrations. In mild cases of acute liver cell damage, ALP levels are seldom elevated. Even in cirrhosis, ALP concentrations are variable and depend on the degree of hepatic decompensation and obstruction.

The osteoblasts in bone produce large amounts of ALP, and marked serum elevations can be seen in Paget disease of the bone, hyperparathyroidism, osteogenic sarcoma, osteoblastic cancer metastatic to bone, and other conditions of pronounced osteoblastic activity. The serum ALP is increased during periods of rapid bone growth (e.g., infancy, early childhood, and healing bone fractures) and during pregnancy because of the contributions of the placenta and fetal bones.

Gamma-Glutamyl Transferase

Reference Range: male 9–50 units/L, female 8–40 units/L

Although the enzyme γ-glutamyl transferase (GGT) is found in the kidney, liver, and pancreas, its major clinical value is in the evaluation of hepatobiliary disease. An increase in the serum concentration of GGT parallels the increase of ALP in obstructive jaundice and infiltrative disease of the liver. However, increased ALP in the presence of a normal GGT is more suggestive of muscular or bone-related issues. GGT is one of the more sensitive liver enzymes for identifying biliary obstruction and cholecystitis. Because GGT is a hepatic microsomal enzyme, tissue concentrations increase in response to microsomal enzyme induction by alcohol and other drugs (e.g., carbamazepine, phenobarbital, and phenytoin). As a result, GGT is a sensitive indicator of recent or chronic alcohol exposure.

Bilirubin

Total Bilirubin—Reference Range: 0.1–1.0 mg/dL or 2–18 μmol/L
Direct (Conjugated) Bilirubin—Reference Range: 0–0.2 mg/dL or 0–4 μmol/L

Bilirubin is primarily a breakdown product of Hgb and is formed in the reticuloendothelial system (Fig. 2-1, step 1). It is then transferred into the blood (step 2), where it is almost completely bound to serum albumin (step 3). When bilirubin arrives at the sinusoidal surface of the liver cells, the free fraction is rapidly taken up into the cell (step 4) and converted primarily to bilirubin diglucuronide (step 5). A monoglucuronide is also formed that is metabolized predominantly to the diglucuronide. The conjugated bilirubin diglucuronide is then excreted into the bile (step 6) and appears in the intestine, where bacteria convert most of it to urobilinogen (step 7). The majority of urobilinogen is destroyed or excreted in the feces (step 13), but a small portion is reabsorbed into the blood (step 8) and either reabsorbed into the liver (step 9) and subsequently excreted into the bile (step 12) or excreted into the urine (step 10). Urobilinogen is responsible for the straw color of the urine and the yellowish-brown color of the feces. The mechanism by which conjugated bilirubin in the liver cell is transferred to the blood (step 14) is not well understood. However, in many types of liver disease, conjugated (direct) bilirubin is present in increased concentrations in the blood. When this concentration exceeds 0.2 to 0.4 mg/dL, bilirubin will begin to appear in the urine (step 11). Unconjugated (indirect) bilirubin is water insoluble and is highly bound to serum albumin; both factors account for its lack of excretion in the urine.[29]

MISCELLANEOUS TESTS

Amylase and Lipase

Amylase (reference range: 35–118 units/L or 0.58–1.97 μkat/L) and lipase (reference range: 10–160 units/L or 0–2.67 μkat/L) are enzymes produced by the pancreas and secreted into the duodenum to assist in the digestive process. Small amounts of both enzymes are also found in the saliva and stomach. Significantly elevated levels of either enzyme are suggestive of pancreatic damage.

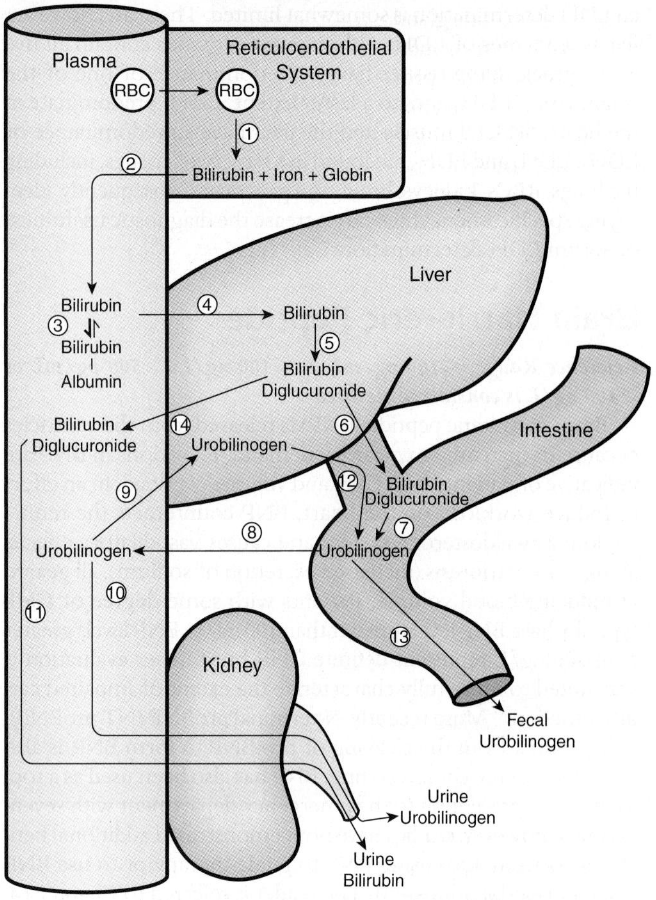

Figure 2-1 Bilirubin metabolism.

Amylase is responsible for breaking down complex carbohydrates into simple sugars. Significant elevations in serum amylase are observed in patients with acute pancreatitis or pancreatic duct obstruction. Amylase levels tend to rise 6 to 48 hours after onset of the disease and usually return to normal 3 days after the acute event. In chronic pancreatitis or obstruction, amylase levels may remain elevated for longer periods. Other nonpancreatic conditions (e.g., bowel perforation, biliary disease, perforated peptic ulcer, ectopic pregnancy, and mumps) can be associated with elevated serum amylase levels.

Lipase is responsible for breaking down triglycerides into fatty acids. Elevated serum lipase levels are also suggestive of pancreatic disease and tend to be more specific for pancreatic disease than amylase. Nonpancreatic conditions such as gallbladder disease or biliary cirrhosis can also lead to elevated lipase levels. The onset of lipase elevation is similar to amylase; however, lipase typically remains elevated for 5 to 7 days and can be useful in diagnosing patients in later stages of pancreatic disease. Narcotics (e.g., morphine) can constrict the sphincter of Oddi and increase serum concentrations of both amylase and lipase.

Prostate-Specific Antigen

Reference Range: 0–4 ng/mL or 0–4 mcg/L

Prostate-specific antigen (PSA) is a protease glycoprotein produced almost exclusively by prostate epithelial cells. Large quantities of PSA are carried in semen; only low levels are found in the blood. Serum concentrations of PSA are increased when the normal prostate glandular structure is disrupted by benign or malignant tumor or inflammation (prostatitis). More than half of men with benign prostatic hyperplasia (BPH) have elevated serum PSA concentrations. PSA is also a valuable parameter for staging and monitoring the progression and response to therapy of prostate cancer.[30]

The prostate gland increases in size with age; therefore, it is expected that older men will have higher PSA levels compared with younger men. PSA serum concentrations can also increase after prostatic manipulation such as digital rectal examination (DRE), catheter placement, transrectal ultrasound, cystoscopy, or biopsy of the prostate. In addition, serum PSA will increase 24 to 48 hours after ejaculation. Although elevated serum concentrations of PSA can occur in men with BPH, concentrations tend to be higher and encountered more often in men with cancer. Men with PSA levels between 4 and 10 ng/mL should be evaluated further for potential prostate cancer.

The serum half-life of PSA is 2 to 3 days, but serum PSA concentrations can remain high for several weeks after manipulation of the prostate. Circulating serum PSA is bound to plasma proteins, and the capability exists to measure both total and free (unbound) PSA concentrations. Increased risk of prostate cancer has been observed in men with a free PSA to total PSA ratio of less than 0.25.[31] An aggressive approach to localize prostate cancer for men with life expectancies more than 10 years is now favored.[30,32]

Thyroid-Stimulating Hormone

Reference Range: 0.5–4.7 μunits/mL or munits/L

Thyroid-stimulating hormone (TSH, also known as thyrotropin) is secreted by the pituitary gland to stimulate the thyroid gland to produce the thyroid hormones T_4 and T_3. TSH is measured, often in conjunction with the thyroid hormones, to diagnose thyroid disorders and to monitor exogenous thyroid supplementation therapy. The reader is referred to Chapter 52, Thyroid Disorders, as it provides a more detailed discussion of the clinical implications of altered thyroid laboratory findings.

Procalcitonin

Procalcitonin is a precursor for calcitonin and is typically undetectable in healthy individuals. Elevations in procalcitonin occur in patients with inflammation secondary to bacterial infections; however, a similar increase is not observed in patients with inflammation secondary to viral infections or noninfectious conditions. Interestingly, increases in calcitonin are not seen in patients with elevated procalcitonin. In patients with sepsis or sepsis syndrome, procalcitonin levels $<$0.5 ng/mL have been associated with a low risk of progression to severe sepsis and levels $>$2.0 ng/mL represent a high risk for severe sepsis. Trials involving lower respiratory tract infections have suggested that antibiotic therapy should be discouraged in patients with procalcitonin levels $<$0.25 ng/mL, but encouraged for those with levels $\geq$0.5 ng/mL. These criteria have also been used as a guide for discontinuing therapy as infections resolve; however, the exact role for the use of procalcitonin levels has not been clearly characterized. Additional trials will help to accurately define the role of procalcitonin testing.

Cholesterol and Triglycerides

A detailed discussion of hypercholesterolemia and lipid disorders is provided in Chapter 8, Dyslipidemias, Atherosclerosis, and Coronary Heart Disease. For convenience, the current range of desired values for total cholesterol (TC), low-density lipoproteins (LDLs), high-density lipoproteins (HDLs), and fasting triglycerides (TGs) has been incorporated in Table 2-2.

HEMATOLOGY

There are several different hematologic cell types that originate from the hematopoietic stem cell. Each cell line has a defined role and unique contribution to the overall homeostatic process and may be found in the bone marrow, lymph system, or blood. Typically, routine clinical laboratory testing involves measuring concentrations of mature myeloid cells found in the blood. Figure 2-2 illustrates the various lineages derived from the hematopoietic stem cell.[33] The cells derived from the myeloid linage are the focus of the following discussion. Readers are encouraged to refer to Section 16, Hematology and Oncology, to gain further understanding of the clinical relevance of lymphoid and myeloid cells (Fig. 2-2).

Complete Blood Count

The complete blood count (CBC) is one of the most commonly ordered clinical laboratory tests. A CBC measures the RBCs, Hgb, hematocrit (Hct), mean cell volume (MCV), mean cell Hgb concentration (MCHC), and total white blood cells (WBCs). Depending on the laboratory, an order for a CBC may also include platelets, reticulocytes, or leukocyte differential. An abbreviated method of noting hematologic parameters in clinical practice is noted in the following figure.

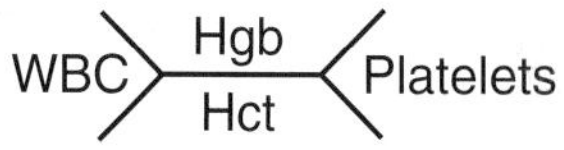

Red Blood Cells (Erythrocytes)

Males—Reference Range: 4.3–5.9 × 10^6/μL or 4.3–5.9× 10^{12}/L
Females—Reference Range: 3.5–5 × 10^6/μL or 3.5–5 × 10^{12}/L

Erythrocytes or RBCs are produced in the bone marrow, released into the peripheral blood, circulated for approximately 120 days, and cleared by the reticuloendothelial system. The primary function of RBCs is to transport oxygen linked to Hgb from the lungs to tissues. The concentration of RBCs in the blood can be measured to detect anemia, calculate RBC indices, or calculate the Hct. Hct and Hgb concentrations are generally used to monitor quantitative changes in RBCs.

Hematocrit

Males—Reference Range: 40.7%–50.3% or 0.4–0.503
Females—Reference Range: 36%–44.6% or 0.36–0.446

Hct (packed cell volume) is the percentage of RBCs to the total blood volume and is determined by centrifuging a capillary tube of whole blood and comparing the height of the settled RBCs to the height of the column of whole blood. A decrease in Hct may result from bleeding, the bone marrow suppressant effects of drugs, chronic diseases, genetic alterations in RBC morphology, or hemolysis. An increase in Hct may result from hemoconcentration, polycythemia vera, or polycythemia secondary to chronic hypoxia.

Hemoglobin

Males—Reference Range: 13.8–17.5 g/dL or 138–175 g/L
Females—Reference Range: 12.1–15.3 g/dL or 121–153 g/L

Hgb is the major oxygen-carrying compound contained in RBCs. Therefore, total Hgb concentration primarily depends on the number of RBCs in the blood sample. As mentioned with Hct, medical conditions that impact the number of RBCs will also affect Hgb concentration. As discussed previously, glycosylated Hgb (A_{1c}) is a related test used to monitor diabetes mellitus.

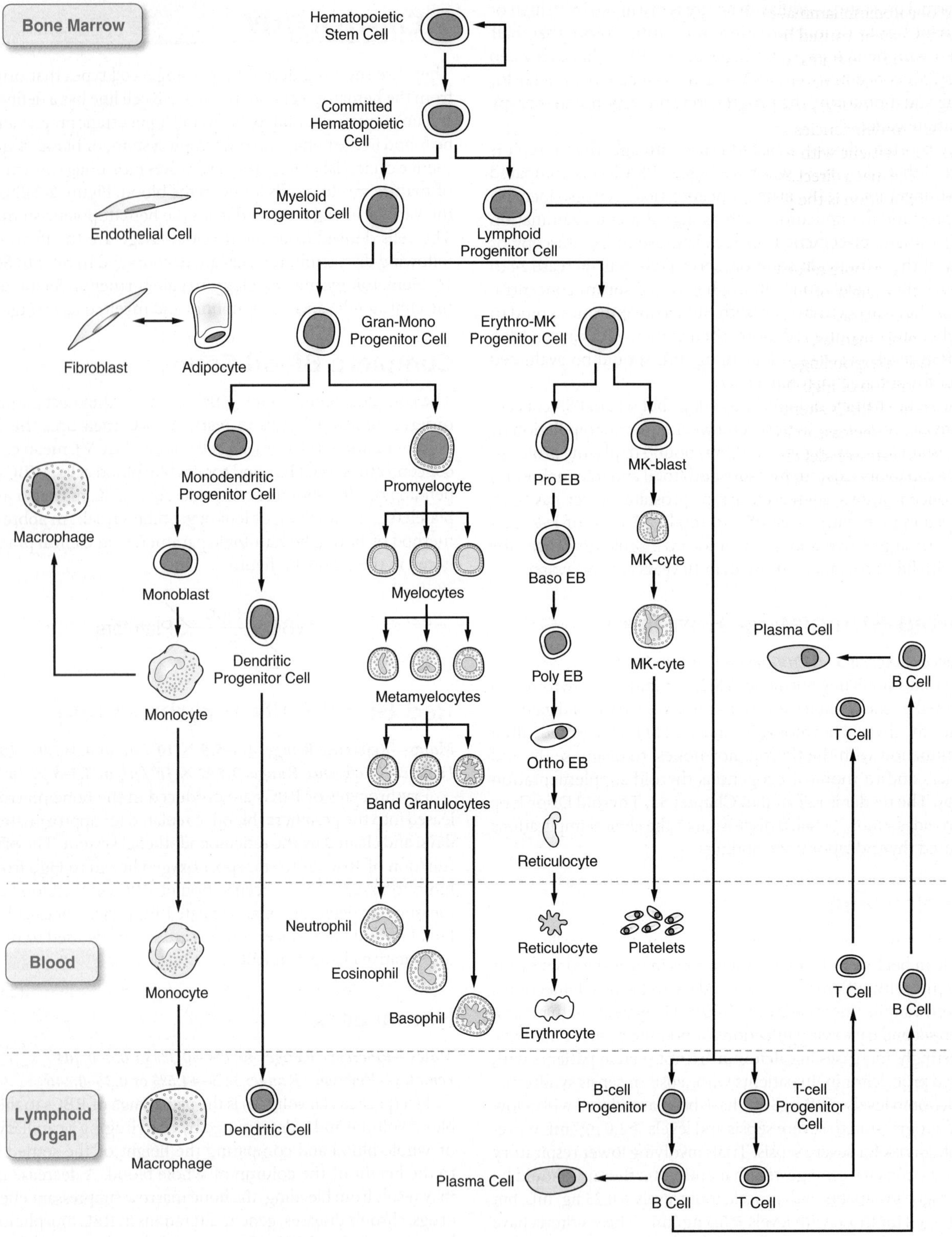

Figure 2-2 Hematopoietic stem cell lineage. (Adapted with permission from Greer JP et al, eds. *Wintrobe's Clinical Hematology*. 12th ed. Philadelphia, PA: Lippincott Williams & Wilkins; 2009:80.)

Red Blood Cell Indices

RBC indices (also known as Wintrobe indices) are useful in the classification of anemias. These indices include the MCV, the mean cell Hgb (MCH), and the MCHC. These indices are calculated in Equations 2-9 to 2-11:

$$\text{MCV} = \text{Hct (\%)} \times 10 \,/\, \text{RBC (in millions}/\mu\text{L)} = 80 - 97.6 \text{ (in } \mu\text{m}^3 \text{ or fL)} \quad \text{(Eq. 2-9)}$$

$$\text{MCH} = \text{Hgb (in g/dL)} \times 10/\text{RBC (in millions}/\mu\text{L)} = 27 - 33 \text{ (in pg)} \quad \text{(Eq. 2-10)}$$

$$\text{MCHC} = \text{Hgb (in g/dL)} \times 100/\text{Hct (\%)} = 33 - 36 \text{ (in g/dL)} \quad \text{(Eq. 2-11)}$$

MEAN CELL VOLUME

The MCV detects changes in cell size. A decreased MCV indicates a microcytic cell, which can result from iron-deficiency anemia or anemia of chronic inflammation. A large MCV indicates a macrocytic cell, which can be caused by a vitamin B_{12} or folic acid deficiency. Underlying disease states (e.g., habitual alcohol ingestion, chronic liver disease, anorexia nervosa, hypothyroidism, reticulocytosis, and hematologic disorders) may also present with an elevated MCV secondary to deficiencies in these vitamins.[34] The MCV can be normal in a patient with a "mixed" (microcytic and macrocytic) anemia. Note that a direct assessment of a blood smear by a microscopic examination is the gold standard for confirming RBC size.

MEAN CELL HEMOGLOBIN

The MCHC is a more reliable index of RBC Hgb than MCH. MCH measures the weight of Hgb in the RBCs in a sample and MCHC measures concentration of the RBCs contained within a sample. In normochromic anemias, changes in the size of RBCs (MCV) are associated with corresponding changes in the weight of Hgb (MCH), but the concentration of Hgb (MCHC) remains normal. Changes in the Hgb content of RBCs alter the color of these cells. Thus, hypochromic refers to a decrease in RBC Hgb, reflected by reduced MCHC, and may indicate iron-deficiency anemia. Conversely, hyperchromic RBCs have an elevated MCHC because of the presence of greater amounts of Hgb. Hyperchromic cells are not commonly encountered.

Reticulocytes

Adults—Reference Range: 0.5%–1.5% of RBCs or 0.005–0.015

Reticulocytes are young, immature erythrocytes and typically comprise about 1% of the RBCs. The reticulocyte count measures the percentage of these new cells in the circulating blood. An increase in the number of reticulocytes implies an increased number of erythrocytes are being released into the blood in response to a stimulus. Reticulocyte count is a good indicator of bone marrow activity because it represents a recent production. Because erythrocytes regenerate rapidly, reticulocytosis can be noted within 3 to 5 days after hemolysis or after a hemorrhagic episode. Appropriate treatment of anemias caused by iron, vitamin B_{12}, or folic acid deficiencies should result in an increased reticulocyte count. Caution must be exercised in the interpretation of reticulocyte counts. Changes in the number of RBCs will result in proportional changes in the reticulocyte count because the latter is reported as a percentage of the number of RBCs.

Erythrocyte Sedimentation Rate

Reference Range: 0–30 mm/hour

The ESR is the rate (expressed in mm/hour) at which erythrocytes settle to the bottom of a test tube through the forces of gravity and in response to fibrinogen levels in the blood. The ESR is a nonspecific value and may be increased abnormally in acute and chronic inflammatory processes, acute and chronic infections, neoplasms, infarction, tissue necrosis, rheumatoid-collagen disease, dysproteinemias, nephritis, and pregnancy. However, ESR can also be affected by changes not related to the inflammation (e.g., change in erythrocyte size, shape, or number). Laboratory technique can also affect the sedimentation rate substantially. Because many factors can enhance the settling rate of RBCs, moderate to marked elevation of the ESR merely indicates an inflammatory component to a disease state. An increased ESR in the setting of a normal physical examination is usually transient and is rarely the harbinger of serious occult disease.[35]

White Blood Cells

Reference Range: 3.8–9.8 $\times$ $10^3/\mu L$ or 3.8–9.8 $\times$ $10^9/L$

Leukocytes or WBCs comprise five different types of cells. Neutrophils are the most abundant of the circulating WBCs, followed in order of frequency by lymphocytes, monocytes, eosinophils, and basophils. The neutrophils, eosinophils, basophils, and monocytes are formed from stem cells in the bone marrow. Lymphocytes are formed primarily in the lymph nodes, thymus, spleen, and, to a lesser extent, bone marrow (Fig. 2-2). Each WBC type has unique function, and it is best to consider them independently rather than collectively as "leukocytes."[36] Ultimately, all WBCs contribute to host defense mechanisms.

NEUTROPHILS

Reference Range: 40%–70% of WBC

The terms *polys, segs, polymorphonuclear neutrophils,* and *granulocytes* are synonymous with the term *neutrophil* in clinical practice. The number of neutrophils is commonly increased during bacterial or fungal infections, because these cells are essential in killing invading microorganisms. Whereas the bone marrow increases production of new leukocytes, there is also an increase in the number of circulating immature neutrophils (e.g., bands); this phenomenon is commonly referred to as a "left shift," which suggests acute bacterial infection.

However, neutrophils are also important in the pathogenesis of tissue damage in some noninfectious diseases, such as rheumatoid arthritis, inflammatory bowel disease, asthma, MI, or gout.[37] Increased neutrophils or neutrophilia can also be encountered during metabolic toxic states (e.g., diabetic ketoacidosis, uremia, and eclampsia) and during physiologic response to stress (e.g., physical exercise and childbirth). Drugs (e.g., epinephrine and corticosteroids) can also cause significant neutrophilia, primarily caused by demargination from blood vessel walls.

Agranulocytosis and Absolute Neutrophil Count

The condition involving decreased neutrophils, or neutropenia, is defined as a neutrophil count of $<$2,000 cells/μL; agranulocytosis refers to severe neutropenia. The most common causes of neutropenia are metastatic carcinoma, lymphoma, and chemotherapeutic agents. The degree of neutropenia is often expressed by the absolute neutrophil count (ANC). The ANC is defined as the total number of granulocytes (polymorphonuclear leukocytes and band forms) present in the circulating pool of WBCs and can be calculated as WBC $\times$ (% neutrophils + % bands)/100. Generally, the risk of infection is low when the ANC exceeds 1,000/μL; however, the risk of infection increases significantly when the ANC is less than 500/μL. The risk of developing bacteremia is increased further as the ANC decreases to less than 100/μL, a condition commonly referred to as "profound neutropenia." The most common causes of neutropenia are metastatic carcinoma, lymphoma, and chemotherapeutic agents. The reader is referred to Chapter 75, Prevention and Treatment of Infections in Neutropenic Patients, for a more detailed explanation.

LYMPHOCYTES

Reference Range: 22%–44% of WBC

Lymphocytes constitute the second most common WBC in circulating blood. These leukocytes respond to foreign antigens by initiating the immune defense system. The vast majority of lymphocytes are located in the spleen, lymph nodes, and other organized lymphatic tissue. The lymphocytes circulating in blood represent less than 5% of the total amount in the body.

There are two major types of lymphocytes. T lymphocytes (thymic dependent) participate in cell-mediated immune responses, and B lymphocytes (bone marrow derived) are responsible for humoral antibody responses. Therefore, diseases affecting lymphocytes primarily manifest themselves as immune deficiency disorders that render the patient unable to defend against normal pathogens (see Chapter 76, Pharmacotherapy of Human Immunodeficiency Virus Infection) or as autoimmune diseases in which immune responses are directed against the body's own cells.[36]

Increased numbers of lymphocytes on a white count differential sometimes accompany lymphoma (see Chapter 96, Adult Hematologic Malignancies) and viral infections. A relative lymphocytosis is sometimes encountered when the total lymphocytes have remained constant despite a decline in the total neutrophils.

MONOCYTES

Reference Range: 4%–11% of WBC

Monocytes are formed in the bone marrow and are the precursors to macrophages and antigen-presenting cells (dendritic cells), which are found in the body's tissues.[38] Macrophages and dendritic cells are phagocytic cells that engulf foreign antigens or dead or dying cells. Dendritic cells also present fragments of antigens to T and B lymphocytes. Monocytosis may be observed in mononucleosis, subacute bacterial endocarditis, malaria, and tuberculosis, as well as during the recovery phase of some infections.

EOSINOPHILS

Reference Range: 0%–8% of WBC

Because eosinophils have surface receptors that bind IgG and IgE, they can modify reactions associated with IgG- and IgE-mediated degranulation of mast cells. Primary lysosomal granules, small dense granules, and specific or secondary granules are the three types of granules found within eosinophils. The latter granules account for most of the biologic activity of eosinophils and are toxic to parasites, tumor cells, and some epithelial cells.[39]

Eosinophils have phagocytic activity, catalyze the oxidation of many substances, facilitate killing of microorganisms, initiate mast cell secretion, protect against various parasites, and play some role in host defense. Eosinophilia is probably most commonly associated with allergic reactions to drugs, allergic disorders (e.g., hay fever, asthma, and eczema), invasive parasitic infections (e.g., hookworm, schistosomiasis, and trichinosis), collagen vascular diseases (e.g., rheumatoid arthritis, eosinophilic fasciitis, and eosinophilic-myalgia syndrome), and malignancies (e.g., Hodgkin lymphoma).[40–42]

BASOPHILS

Reference Range: 0%–3% of WBC

During infection or inflammation, basophils leave the blood and mobilize as mast cells to the affected site and release granules. These granules contain histamine, serotonin, prostaglandins, and leukotrienes. Degranulation results in an increased blood flow to the site and may compound inflammatory processes. An increase in basophils commonly accompanies allergic and anaphylactic responses, chronic myeloid leukemia, myelofibrosis, and polycythemia vera. A decrease in the number of basophils is generally not readily apparent because of the small number of these cells in the blood.[36]

CASE 2-5

QUESTION 1: L.H., a 50-year-old female, is hospitalized with a sustained high fever of 39.2°C and severe back pain. The results of the CBC and leukocyte differential are as follows:

Total WBC count: 21,000/μL
Neutrophils: 74%
Bands: 6%
Lymphocytes: 14.6%
Monocytes: 8%
Eosinophils: 1%
Basophils: 0%

Imaging and other blood work was ordered. L.H. is diagnosed with an abscess in her lower back and *Staphylococcus aureus* bacteremia. How is L.H.'s laboratory report consistent with a systemic bacterial infection?

WBCs are the host's chief defense system, and the neutrophil is the main component of that system. During bacterial infections, the leukocyte count and the neutrophils are generally increased, and a left shift (increase in bands) may be noticeable. The percentage of other types of WBCs is decreased proportionately because the number of neutrophils is increased.

As the infection progresses, the percentage of band cells may decrease as a result of an increase in the number of neutrophils that have a longer half-life. This decrease in bands does not necessarily indicate improvement. A decrease in the percentage of neutrophils with a decrease in the total WBC count is characteristic of effective antibiotic therapy.

CASE 2-5, QUESTION 2: The *S. aureus* causing L.H.'s bacteremia is found to be methicillin sensitive, and she is started on oxacillin 2 million units IV q 4 hour for treatment. After about a week of therapy, L.H. develops a fine red rash all over her body, mild lymphadenopathy, low-grade fever, and generalized swelling. The CBC shows a total WBC count of 8,600/μL with 11% eosinophils. What is the significance of this eosinophil count?

In the clinical setting, absolute leukocyte counts may be used in conjunction with normal reference values. Absolute counts are calculated by multiplying the percentage of each individual cell by the total leukocyte count. Eosinophils are usually increased in allergic reactions; therefore, a drug-induced hypersensitivity reaction is a strong probability in L.H., with an absolute count of 946 eosinophils/μL (i.e., 11% of 8,600 leukocytes). The clinician should be suspicious of an allergic drug reaction when absolute eosinophil counts exceed 300 cells/μL. Eosinophils may increase before, after, or concurrent with other evidence of allergy (e.g., rash). Eosinophilia without evidence of allergy is not sufficient cause to discontinue a suspected medication unless the eosinophilia is significant (i.e., >2,000 cells/μL). In addition, the absence of eosinophilia certainly does not rule out an allergic diagnosis in a patient exhibiting clear clinical manifestations of an apparent allergic reaction.

Thrombocytes

Reference Range: 150–450 $\times$ 10^3/μL or 150–450 $\times$ 10^9/L

Thrombocytes, commonly referred to as platelets, are tiny fragments of cells that assist with normal blood clotting. Platelet testing is included as part of a CBC and is often ordered along with other coagulation studies to evaluate bleeding and/or clotting disorders. Decreased platelet counts or thrombocytopenia may lead to petechiae, ecchymosis, and spontaneous hemorrhage.

Causes include decreased platelet production, accelerated destruction, loss from excessive bleeding or trauma, dilution of blood samples secondary to blood transfusion, sequestration secondary to hypersplenism, disseminated intravascular coagulation, infection, or systemic lupus erythematosus. Malignancy, rheumatoid arthritis, iron-deficiency anemia, polycythemia vera, and postsplenectomy syndromes are the most common causes of elevated platelet counts or thrombocytosis.

Coagulation Studies

The control of bleeding depends on the formation of a platelet plug and the formation of a stable fibrin clot. The formation of this clot depends on the complex interactions of plasma proteins and clotting factors. The prothrombin time (PT), international normalized ratio (INR), and activated partial thromboplastin time (aPTT) are used to diagnose coagulation abnormalities or to monitor the effectiveness of patients receiving anticoagulation therapy. When used to assess drug therapy, achieving a value outside the reference range is in fact a therapeutically desirable outcome.

ACTIVATED PARTIAL THROMBOPLASTIN TIME

Reference Range: 22–37 seconds

aPTT measures the time it takes the body to form a clot. aPTT depends on the activity of factors VIII, IX, XI, and XII (intrinsic pathway) and the factors involved in the final common pathway of the clotting cascade (II, X, and V). aPTT is commonly measured to detect bleeding disorders and coagulation deficiencies and monitor unfractionated heparin therapy. The reader is referred to Chapter 11, Thrombosis, for more detailed information regarding the use of coagulation parameters in treating and monitoring thrombotic disorders.

PROTHROMBIN TIME

Reference Range: 10–13 seconds

Prothrombin is synthesized in the liver and is converted to thrombin during the blood clotting process. Thrombin formation is the critical event in the hemostatic process because thrombin creates fibrin monomers that ultimately assemble into a clot and stimulates platelet activation. The PT test evaluates the integrity of the extrinsic and common pathways and directly measures the activity of clotting factors VII and X, prothrombin (factor II), and fibrinogen. Automated laboratory instruments measure PT by recording the time required for the blood to clot after a reagent (i.e., tissue thromboplastin) has been added to the patient's blood sample.

INTERNATIONAL NORMALIZED RATIO

Because different labs use different reagents, the PT results obtained from one reagent cannot be reliably compared with another reagent. Therefore, the INR is used as a standard unit to report the result of a PT test. The INR is the recommended method to monitor both the initiation and maintenance of anticoagulant therapy, most notably warfarin. Individuals who have normal blood clotting and are not on anticoagulation therapy should have an INR of 1. For patients on anticoagulation therapy, the target INR (i.e., therapeutic range) is usually between 2.0 and 4.0 depending on the indication and other patient-specific factors. Outside of the therapeutic range, the higher the INR, the higher the likelihood of bleeding because the blood is taking longer to clot. Conversely, if the INR is lower, there is an increased risk of developing a clot. Many factors including medications, diet, alcohol intake, and certain medical conditions can influence the INR.

The INR is calculated using Equation 2-12, where the prothrombin ratio (PTR) is the ratio between the patient's PT and the laboratory's control PT, and the ISI is the international sensitivity index. Commercial manufacturers quantify the ISI for the specific thromboplastin reagent used in each lot and report this information in the product package insert:

$$\text{INR} = \{\text{PT (patient)}/\text{PT (control)}\}^{\text{ISI}} = \text{PTR}^{\text{ISI}} \quad \text{(Eq. 2-12)}$$

URINALYSIS

A standard urinalysis includes physical, chemical, and microscopic evaluations to assist with diagnosis of various urologic conditions. It begins with simple observation of the color and the gross general appearance of the urine specimen. The urine pH and specific gravity are then recorded. Formed elements in the urine are examined microscopically, and the urine is searched routinely for pathologically significant substances that are normally not present (e.g., glucose, blood, ketones, and bile pigments). Urine specimens should be evaluated quickly after collection to minimize unreliable results. The reader is referred to Chapter 71, Urinary Tract Infections, for a more detailed description of the use of urinalysis in the detection and monitoring of urinary tract infections (UTIs).

Gross Appearance of the Specimen

The concentrated, first-morning urine specimen is usually analyzed to eliminate effects of undue dilution as a result of water intake. The color should be slightly yellow, depending on the degree of dilution, and the appearance should be clear. The appearance of the urine may reveal clouds of crystals, bilirubin, blood, porphyrins, proteins, food or drug colorings, or melanin. Discolored urine is abnormal. A red coloration of the urine may be imparted by blood, porphyria, or ingestion of phenolphthalein. A brown urine color may be caused by the acid hematin of blood or from melanin pigments. Excessive excretion of urobilinogen or the effects of drugs such as rifampin or phenazopyridine may cause a dark orange urine color. A blue to blue-green color of the urine may result from the systemic administration of methylene blue.

Specimen pH

When freshly produced, urinary pH can range from 4.5 to 8 but is mostly acidic because of metabolic activity. Alkaline urine may indicate an aged specimen, systemic alkalosis, failure of renal acidifying mechanisms, or infection in the urinary tract.

Specific Gravity

Urinary specific gravity provides information regarding a patient's hydration status. A normal morning urine specimen should have a specific gravity of 1.003 to 1.030. The upper end of this range is close to the maximal concentrating ability of the kidney. A value of 1.010 or less supports relative hydration, whereas a value greater than 1.020 indicates relative dehydration.

Protein

Proteinuria is a classic sign of renal injury. If proteinuria is found during the evaluation of a patient with a nonrenal illness, it suggests that the disease may also involve the kidneys (i.e., hypertension and diabetes).[43] A healthy adult generally excretes 30 to 130 mg/day of protein into the urine.

Protein in a urine sample is generally tested qualitatively on a random urine sample by a dipstick method and is usually reported on a scale of 0 (<30 mg/dL), 1+ (30–100 mg/dL), 2+ (100–300 mg/dL), 3+ (300–1,000 mg/dL), and 4+ (>1,000 mg/dL). A positive qualitative test for urine protein should be repeated after a few days because transient proteinuria can accompany various physiologic and pathologic states, even when kidney function is normal. Therefore, patients with CHF, seizures, or febrile illnesses and normal renal function need not undergo invasive renal function tests if the proteinuria is modest and likely to be transient. Another qualitative evaluation of proteinuria can be performed in about 2 weeks to confirm the diagnosis of transient proteinuria.[44] If subsequent qualitative test results are positive, a 24-hour urine sample should be collected to quantitatively test for protein and creatinine (see Creatinine Clearance section). In patients with a normal 24-hour urinary protein concentration, previous positive qualitative test results probably represent either false-positive results or a transient phenomenon.[42] A laboratory parameter being used with increased frequency to assess proteinuria is the urine albumin to urine creatinine ratio (UACR). This measurement tends to be less influenced by fluctuations in urine concentration and may offer a more reliable indication of proteinuria. UACR values are typically less than 30 mg/g; patients with values between 30 and 300 mg/g are considered to have microalbuminuria, and UACR values greater than 300 mg/g indicate macroalbuminemia.

MICROSCOPIC EXAMINATION

The urine sediment is examined for RBCs, WBCs, casts, yeast, crystals, and epithelial cells.

RBCs should be absent in normal urine, although fewer than 4 to 6 RBCs per high-power field (HPF) would still be considered in the normal range. Bleeding or clotting disorders, some collagen diseases, and various bladder, urethral, and prostatic conditions may cause microscopic hematuria. In women, vaginal blood occasionally contaminates the urine specimen, but the presence of numerous squamous epithelial cells should be sufficient to alert clinicians to this artifact.

WBCs should be virtually absent in normal urine, although up to 5 WBCs/HPF would still be in the reference range. The presence of WBCs in the urine (pyuria) usually suggests an acute infection in the urinary tract. Some noninfectious inflammatory diseases of the kidney, ureter, or bladder may also contribute WBCs to the urine sediment.

Casts may be used to identify the location of disease in the genitourinary tract. Casts are composed of proteinaceous or fatty material that outlines the shape of the renal tubules where they are deposited. The presence of casts must be interpreted in light of other factors related to the kidney and its function; however, fatty casts, RBC casts, and WBC casts are always significant. RBC casts usually suggest glomerular injury, and WBC casts suggest tubular or interstitial injury. Lipid casts with proteinuria are characteristic findings in patients with nephrotic syndrome or hypothyroidism.[43] The finding of hyaline casts alone in the presence of proteinuria suggests a renal origin for the protein. Hyaline or granular casts alone, however, only suggest some defect in factors that affect cast formation and are therefore difficult to interpret.

Crystals may originally appear as a cloud in the urine. Their formation is pH dependent, and they often appear only as the urine cools to room temperature or in concentrated urine. In acidic urine, crystals may be uric acid or calcium oxalate; in alkaline urine, they may be phosphates. Crystals per se are not highly significant, although they may reflect a tendency toward the formation of renal calculi.

CASE 2-6

QUESTION 1: S.T. is a 33-year-old female with type 1 diabetes who presents to the urgent care clinic with a 3-day history of fever, malaise, dysuria, and flank pain. Upon interview, you learn that over the past few days, S.T. has been unable to keep down any food because of feelings of nausea. Because of this, she has not taken her insulin for 48 hours. Today, her finger stick blood glucose is 415 mg/dL, and a STAT midstream urinalysis and Gram stain indicate the following:

pH: 5.2
Appearance: cloudy
Specific gravity: 1.033
Urine protein: 3+
Urine glucose: 4+
Urine ketones: positive
Urine bacteria: 4+
Urine WBC: too numerous to count (TNTC)
Squamous epithelial: few per HPF
Urine nitrite: positive
Gram stain: numerous Gram-negative rods

What objective data from the urinalysis indicate a UTI?

The cloudy appearance of S.T.'s urine indicates the presence of bacteria, protein, and WBCs, which is supported by the urinalysis results. The lack of a significant amount of squamous epithelial cells, the presence of a significant amount of nitrite-producing bacteria, and the Gram stain indicate a clean-catch urine specimen and a UTI involving Gram-negative organisms (most likely *Escherichia coli* that causes a majority of UTIs).

CASE 2-6, QUESTION 2: What objective data from the urinalysis indicate uncontrolled diabetes?

Glucose is normally filtered in the glomerulus and a majority is reabsorbed in the proximal tubule of the kidney. S.T.'s glycosuria (4+ glucose) and fingerstick of 415 mg/dL indicate the filtered amount of glucose exceeds the capacity for reabsorption (~180 mg/dL). Additionally, the presence of positive ketones indicates the body is utilizing fat, not glucose, for energy. High levels of ketones can predispose S.T. to dehydration, resulting in diabetic ketoacidosis.

THERAPEUTIC DRUG MONITORING

Many drugs have a wide dosing range that can achieve efficacy with low risk of toxicity. Drugs that have a narrow dosing range with high risk of toxicity (narrow therapeutic index) often have their blood levels monitored. Results from therapeutic drug monitoring assist clinicians with appropriate dosing adjustments to prevent toxicity and achieve appropriate clinical outcomes. Pharmacokinetic parameters as well as drug interactions may significantly impact the laboratory results and must be integrated into the clinical assessment of the data. Similarly, for certain drugs and drug classes, there are recommended laboratory tests that should be performed to monitor their potential adverse effects on organ systems. Ideally, blood level monitoring should occur after the drug has reached steady state and at a consistent time within the dosing interval.

PATIENT-DIRECTED MONITORING AND TESTING

Often patient-directed self-monitoring is an essential component to successful management of certain disease states such as blood pressure monitoring for hypertension and blood glucose monitoring for diabetes mellitus. When used appropriately, data obtained from these monitoring devices can be used by health care providers and consumers to initiate or modify therapies accordingly.

Additional laboratory, self-monitoring tests or devices are also available for consumers to purchase for independent testing or screening purposes at home. Some products provide an immediate result, whereas others require submitting a completed kit to a laboratory for analysis. Samples may be obtained from various sources, including urine, blood, saliva, stool, or hair samples. The incidence of consumers using these products has significantly increased and likely will continue to climb because of increased access via the Internet as well as additional tests becoming available.

In the United States, some, but not all, patient-directed tests have been approved by the US Food and Drug Administration (FDA). A current listing of approved products is available through the FDA's Office of In Vitro Diagnostic Device Evaluation and Safety (OIVD) and can be accessed online at http://www.fda.gov/MedicalDevices/ProductsandMedicalProcedures/InVitroDiagnostics/default.htm. Consumers should be cautioned about the accuracy of tests that have not been approved and the validity of all test results, especially for diagnostic purposes, because many factors can impact or interfere with the sensitivity (probability of obtaining a positive result when sample is truly positive) and specificity (probability of obtaining a negative result when the sample is truly negative). Follow-up assessment with a health care provider should be encouraged to confirm or refute patient-directed test results.

KEY REFERENCES AND WEBSITES

A full list of references for this chapter can be found at http://thepoint.lww.com/AT11e. Below are the key references and websites for this chapter, with the corresponding reference number in this chapter found in parentheses after the reference.

Key References

Facts & Comparison® eAnswers. Reference values for blood, plasma, or serum laboratory tests. 2015 Clinical Drug Information, LLC. Updated March 24, 2015. (2)

Kratz A et al, eds. Laboratory reference values. *N Engl J Med.* 2004;351: 1548–1563. (1)

Lee M. *Basic Skills in Interpreting Laboratory Data.* 5th ed. Bethesda, MD: American Society of Health-System Pharmacists; 2013. (3)

Key Websites

Mayo Medical Laboratories Mobile App. http://www.mayomedicallaboratories.com/mobile-apps/

Merck Manual. http://www.merckmanuals.com/professional/appendixes/normal-laboratory-values/normal-laboratory-values

3 Drug Interactions

Michelle L. Ceresia, Caroline S. Zeind, John Fanikos, and Michael G. Carvalho

CORE PRINCIPLES

	CORE PRINCIPLES	CHAPTER CASES
1	A drug interaction is either the result of pharmacokinetic changes of a drug or its metabolites due to alteration in absorption, distribution, metabolism or excretion, or is the result of pharmacodynamic changes, impacting the effect or mechanism of action. There are several types of drug interactions. Whereas the classic interaction involves two drugs (DDI), a drug interaction can involve the interaction of a drug with a nutrient, chemical, food, herbal, disease, or laboratory test.	**Case 3-1 (Questions 2-6), Case 3-2 (Questions 2-3), Case 3-3 (Question 1); Tables 3-1, 3-3, and 3-4**
2	Some patient populations are more vulnerable to drug interactions because of age, gender, race, and comorbidities such as renal and hepatic insufficiency. Drugs that have a higher potential for an interaction are those with a narrow therapeutic index (NTI).	**Case 3-1 (Question 1), Case 3-2 (Question 1), Case 3-3 (Question 1); Table 3-2**
	PHARMACOKINETIC CHANGES	
1	Administration/Absorption: Drug interactions resulting from alterations in absorption are caused by (1) changes in gastric pH, (2) formation of complexes in the gastrointestinal (GI) tract, (3) changes in GI motility, and (4) modulation of P-glycoprotein (P-gp) intestinal absorption of drugs.	**Case 3-1 (Question 1), Case 3-2 (Question 3); Table 3-3**
2	Distribution: Drug interactions resulting from displacement of drug bound to protein sites (e.g., albumin), particularly with drugs with a high degree of plasma protein binding that are more likely to be displaced by a drug with greater affinity for the same binding site.	**Case 3-1 (Question 2); Figure 3-1, Table 3-3**
3	Metabolism: A common cause of clinically significant drug interactions during multiple drug therapy involves drug metabolism in which cytochrome P450 isoenzymes (CYPs) play a significant role. Many drug interactions occur as a result of inhibition or induction of CYP enzymes.	**Case 3-1 (Questions 3, 5, 6) Case 3-2 (Question 2), Case 3-3 (Question 1); Figure 3-2, Table 3-3**
4	Excretion/Elimination: Drugs are eliminated mainly through renal tubular excretion and biliary excretion. Drug interactions may occur during the elimination of drugs and their metabolites by the kidney as a result of competition at the level of active tubular secretion, interference with tubular transport, or during tubular reabsorption.	**Case 3-2 (Question 2); Table 3-3**
	PHARMACODYNAMICS CHANGES	
1	Pharmacodynamic interactions occur when the presence of one drug changes the effect of another drug without pharmacokinetic alterations. It may be due to competition at the drug receptor level by indirect systems, involving interference with physiologic mechanisms, resulting in additive or synergistic interactions or antagonistic interactions.	**Case 3-1 (Question 4), Case 3-2 (Questions 2, 3); Table 3-4**
	RESOURCES AND EVIDENCE FOR CLINICAL DECISION SUPPORT	
1	Patient safety initiatives have expanded in efforts to improve the healthcare delivery system with medication error prevention as a high-priority area. Healthcare providers have become increasingly challenged on devising optimal approaches to managing drug interactions. A key challenge is that computerized drug interaction screening systems detect a large number of drug–drug interactions of questionable clinical significance. Expert groups have provided recommendations to improve the usability of clinical decision support alerts for managing drug interactions.	**Case 3-1 (Question 6)**

Because healthcare professionals are committed to ensuring patient safety and preventing drug-related harm, it is important to understand drug interaction principles and how to apply drug interaction decision support tools to provide evidence-based clinical decisions. This chapter will introduce the reader to general principles and concepts of drug interactions. Case studies are incorporated to illustrate the application of key concepts and to highlight the importance of understanding the mechanisms by which drugs interact and how it impacts the clinical assessment and management of drug therapy. Disease-specific chapters within this textbook will also apply drug interaction concepts and incorporate case studies relevant to disease management.

DEFINITION

Drug interactions can be broadly categorized as either pharmacokinetic or pharmacodynamic in nature.[1,2] Pharmacokinetic drug interactions involve absorption, distribution, metabolism, and excretion, whereas pharmacodynamic interactions can be characterized into three subgroups: (1) direct effect at receptor function; (2) interference with a biologic or physiologic control process; and (3) additive or attenuated pharmacologic effect.[3] Another key area of consideration is the biologic variance in a given individual: genetics, age, disease, as well as the internal environmental factors (i.e., the patient's medications, dietary intake, and social habits such as smoking and alcohol consumption).[4]

A drug–drug interaction (DDI) is defined "as a clinically meaningful alteration in the exposure and/or response to a drug (object drug) that has occurred as a result of the coadministration of another drug (precipitant drug)."[1-2,5,6] Drug interactions may have beneficial effects because some drug interactions are used to enhance therapeutic outcomes, whereas other interactions may have deleterious effects that result in serious toxicity or may inhibit the effects of a drug, leading to suboptimal therapeutic outcomes. Whereas the classic interaction involves two drugs (DDI), a drug interaction can involve the interaction of a drug with a nutrient, chemical, food, herbal, disease, or laboratory test.[7,8] A potential drug interaction is defined "as the occurrence in which two drugs that are known to interact are concurrently prescribed, regardless of whether adverse events occurred."[8]

In 2015, consensus recommendations for evaluating drug–drug interactions were published by an expert group that included definitions of relevant terminology for evaluation of DDI evidence.[5] Table 3-1 highlights their recommendations for key terms of relevant terminology for evaluation of DDI evidence (The reader is referred to the complete list of definitions agreed upon by this expert group that are provided in their supplementary publication).[5] They emphasize the importance of consistent use of relevant terminology for evaluation of DDI evidence. For example, a clinically relevant DDI is defined as one that is associated with either toxicity or loss of efficacy that warrants the attention of healthcare professionals.[2]

Table 3-1
Terminology Related to DDI[5]

Terminology	
Drug–drug interaction (DDI)	Clinically meaningful alteration in the exposure and/or response to a drug (object drug) that has occurred as a result of the coadministration of another drug (precipitant drug)
Potential DDI	Coprescription of two drugs known to interact, and therefore, a DDI could occur in the exposed patient
Clinically relevant DDI	Drug–drug interaction associated with either toxicity or loss of efficacy that warrants the attention of healthcare professionals.
Narrow therapeutic index (NTI) drugs	Drugs for which even a small change in drug exposure may lead to toxicity or loss of efficacy

Source: Scheife RT et al. Consensus recommendations for systematic evaluation of drug-drug interaction evidence for clinical decision support. *Drug Saf*. 2015;38:197–206.

RISK FACTORS FOR DRUG INTERACTIONS

Some patient populations are more vulnerable to drug interactions because of age, gender, race, and comorbidities such as renal and hepatic insufficiency. Polypharmacy, defined as the concomitant use of multiple drugs or the administration of more medications that are indicated clinically, is a leading cause of DDIs, resulting in higher rates of adverse events, higher drug costs, and medication nonadherence.[9–11] Elderly patients are at an increased risk of drug interactions given the rates of polypharmacy (estimated at 20% to 50%) in the older population, along with multiple comorbidities.[12-14] Adverse drug reactions have been observed 2 to 3 times more frequently in older persons and account for 5% to 17% of all hospital admissions.[15] Age alone is a key risk factor in the elderly population as altered pharmacokinetics and pharmacodynamics may result in a slower intestinal transit time, diminished absorption capacity, decreased liver metabolism and renal excretion, and alterations in volemia and body fat distribution.[16,17] Within the older population, the frail elderly represents a subgroup in which comorbidities primarily account for the observed changes in pharmacokinetic and pharmacodynamic properties.[12] When considering the impact of aging, it is important to differentiate the subgroup of fit elderly from that of the frail elderly, as those who are frail are at increased risk of death, institutionalization, and worsening disability.[12,18,19] A number of studies have shown that females are at greater risk for drug interactions.[20-23] Further research is needed in this area to better understand gender differences with drug interactions.[20-23] The distribution of many drugs may be significantly altered due to marked increases in total body weight (TBW).[24] Drugs that are lipophilic will have an increased volume of distribution. Patients who are obese and those who are malnourished will have altered levels of metabolizing enzymes, increasing their susceptibility to drug interactions.[15,25] Critically ill patients, those with poor nutritional status, and immunocompromised patients are at greater risk of drug interactions. Cigarette smoking can affect drug therapy by both pharmacokinetic and pharmacodynamic mechanisms. It can affect drug therapy by enzyme induction of cytochrome P450; enzymes induced by tobacco smoking may also increase the risk of cancer by enhancing metabolic activation of carcinogens.[26] Drugs that have a higher potential for an interaction are ones with a narrow therapeutic index (NTI) because there are small differences between therapeutic and toxic doses. For example, lithium, a monovalent cation, is a drug with a NTI that is influenced by changes of serum sodium. Patients taking lithium and who are also receiving chronic treatment with thiazides are at risk of lithium toxicity because thiazides can cause a high excretion of sodium that may increase lithium reabsorption.[3]

An individual's genetic makeup determines his/her complement of metabolizing enzymes, and based on their genotype, patients may be classified as having a phenotype for ultrarapid metabolizer, extensive metabolizers, intermediate metabolizers, or poor metabolizers (Refer to Chapter 4, Pharmacogenomics and Personalized Medicine).[27] Individuals who use multiple providers and/or multiple pharmacies are more likely to have incomplete information available for both the providers and themselves; this impacts clinical decision-making and increases the likelihood that a drug interaction may go undetected. Individuals who self-prescribe and take over-the-counter (OTC) products (including dietary supplements, vitamins, minerals, and herbal agents) may not understand the potential risk for drug interactions. In addition, if they do not maintain a complete listing of OTC products for themselves and their providers, there is a greater likelihood for adverse drug reactions and drug interactions. Whereas disease-specific chapters in this textbook will provide a wide array of risk factors for drug interactions, Table 3-2 outlines examples of risk factors for drug interactions.

Table 3-2
Risk Factors for Drug Interactions[1,12–33]

Category	Risk Factor	Potential Effect
Patient characteristics Demographics	Age (< 5 years and ≥ 65 years)	Alterations in drug distribution; ↓ clearance which may result in drug accumulation
	Female gender	↓ ability to metabolize compared to males
Social factors	Nutrition	Affects cytochrome p450 activity (e.g., grapefruit juice inhibits CYP 3A4 activity)
	Smoking	Affects cytochrome p450 activity (i.e., induces CYP 1A2)
	Alcohol	Affects cytochrome p450 activity specifically CYP 2E1
Organ dysfunction	↓ renal function	↓ clearance, which may result in ↑ serum concentrations of drug and accumulation
	↓ hepatic function	↓ metabolism, which may result in ↑ serum concentrations and accumulation of the parent drug and/or metabolite
	Heart Failure (HF)	↑ risk due to number of medications prescribed with comorbidities
	Chronic obstructive pulmonary disease (COPD)	↑ risk due to number of medications prescribed with comorbidities
Metabolic and endocrine	Obesity	↑ distribution of lipophilic drugs
	Fatty liver	Altered metabolism
	Hypoproteinemia	↑ serum drug concentration
Genetic[a]	Genetic polymorphisms (ultrarapid, extensive, intermediate, or poor metabolizers)	Altered metabolism
Acute medical conditions	Dehydration	↑ serum drug concentrations
	Hypotension	↓ clearance
	Hypothermia	↓ clearance
	Infection	↑ catabolism
Drug characteristics	Narrow therapeutic index (NTI)	↑ risk of dose-related adverse drug events
	Highly protein bound	↑ free fraction (active drug) from protein displacement
	Small volume of distribution	Drug confined to the plasma
	Cytochrome p450 substrate	↓↑ serum drug concentration with coadministration inducer or inhibitor precipitant drug
	P-glycoprotein substrate	↓↑ serum drug concentration with coadministration inducer or inhibitor precipitant drug
Other factors	Polypharmacy	Risk of adverse drug interactions ↑ with increase in number of medicines
	Number of prescribers	Number of prescribed drugs ↑ with multiple prescribers
	Number of pharmacies utilized	Number of prescribed drugs ↑ with multiple pharmacies; Pharmacist may not have knowledge of all drugs prescribed to patient
	Self-prescribing	OTC medicines interacting with prescribed medicines
	Duration of hospital stay	Susceptible to hospital-acquired conditions and subsequent drug therapy

[a]Refer to Chapter 4 Pharmacogenomics and Personalized Medicine for further information.

CASE 3-1

Question 1: N.M. is a 68-year-old obese, Hispanic female who underwent a total knee replacement at a local teaching hospital. The medical team plans to start N.M. on warfarin therapy for venous thromboembolism prophylaxis with an international normalized ratio (INR) target range of 1.8 to 2.3 for a total duration of 3 weeks. The first dose will be administered in the evening on the day of surgery.

Her medical history includes epilepsy for the past 10 years, controlled with phenytoin; hypercholesterolemia for the past 15 years, for which she takes pravastatin; and hypertension for the past 20 years, for which she takes lisinopril. Her social history includes a 1-pack-year history of smoking. She does not drink alcohol. She takes acetaminophen for headaches and has taken other over-the-counter medicines as needed, but doesn't recall the names of the products. Her renal and hepatic functions are within normal range.

Describe N.M.'s risk factors for drug interactions with the addition of warfarin postsurgery.

N.M. has multiple factors including patient-specific and drug-specific ones that increase her risk for drug interactions. Her patient risk factors include obesity, age, gender, and smoking history.

Patient Risk Factors

- Female gender
- Metabolic: obesity—increased distribution of lipophilic drugs (phenytoin); comorbidities: hypertension; and hypercholesterolemia
- Age: 66 years old—altered pharmacokinetics and pharmacodynamics
- Smoking history—induces the cytochrome (CYP) P450 system

With regard to drug-specific factors, N.M. has been taking phenytoin, a drug with a NTI, for the past 10 years. She will be receiving warfarin, another agent with NTI. Both medications are metabolized via cytochrome P450 system. In addition, N.M. is at increased risk of additional drug interactions due to polypharmacy because she has chronic disease comorbidities (i.e., seizure disorder, hypertension, and hypercholesterolemia).

Drug Risk Factors

- Warfarin—NTI, highly protein bound to albumin, small volume of distribution, metabolized by cytochrome P450 system
- Phenytoin—NTI, highly protein bound to albumin, metabolized by CYP2C9 and CYP2C19 isoforms, and susceptible to drugs that inhibit hepatic microsomal enzymes
- Pravastatin—whereas pravastatin does not appear to interact with warfarin, other agents in this class (i.e., atorvastatin, fluvastatin, rosuvastatin and simvastatin) have been suspected or are known to alter the INR in patients who receive warfarin[34,35,36]
- Lisinopril—a concern when administered concomitantly with diuretics or potassium supplementation

Other Risk Factors

- Polypharmacy—prior to admission, she is already on 3 prescription drugs and also takes OTC products. She is a poor historian.

MECHANISMS OF DRUG INTERACTIONS

Pharmacokinetics

ADMINISTRATION/ABSORPTION

Following oral administration, most drug absorption occurs in the proximal small intestine.[37] However, drug interactions that alter absorption may occur throughout the gastrointestinal (GI) tract by a variety of different mechanisms, including complexation (adsorption or chelation), changes in pH, changes in GI motility, altered drug transport, and enzymatic metabolism. The net effect of one or more of these mechanisms is a change in the rate of absorption, the extent of absorption, or a combination of both. While interactions that result in a reduced rate of absorption are generally not clinically significant for drugs given over the long term in multiple doses, for acutely administered drugs, such as analgesics or hypnotics, this can lead to an unaccepted delay or therapeutic failure.[1,38]

With regard to changes in gastric pH, the majority of drugs orally administered must be dissolved and absorbed in a gastric pH between 2.5 and 3. Drugs, such as antacids, proton pump inhibitors (PPIs), or H2-antagonists, can alter the kinetics of coadministered drugs.[3] Antifungal agents, such as ketoconazole or itraconazole, require an acidic environment to be properly dissolved. Coadministration with drugs that increase gastric pH may cause a reduction in the dissolution and absorption of antifungal drugs. It is recommended that these antifungal agents be administered at least 2 hours after the administration of antacids.

Coadministration of medications around the same time can result in drug interactions that may be clinically significant. Some antibiotics, such as tetracyclines, will combine with metal ions (e.g., calcium, magnesium, aluminum, iron) to form complexes that are poorly absorbed. Antacids also reduce the absorption of fluoroquinolones (e.g., ciprofloxacin) and tetracyclines because the metal ions form complexes with the drug. Therefore, the antacids and fluoroquinolones should be administered at least 2 hours apart. These types of interactions can decrease clinical effectiveness of the antibiotic and can lead to the emergence of resistant organisms.[33] Drugs that are able to increase the gastric transit, such as metoclopramide due to its prokinetic properties, may accelerate gastric emptying, resulting in decreased absorption of drugs such as digoxin or theophylline.

Altered Drug Transport

Transport proteins, which are present in the intestinal mucosa, are important considerations in clinically relevant DDIs.[37] Some proteins are involved in the transport of compounds from the lumen of the intestine into the portal bloodstream, whereas others are involved in the efflux of compounds from the intestinal mucosa back into the gut lumen. The efflux transporters, particularly a specific glycoprotein, which resides in the cell membrane, P-glycoprotein (P-gp), are the most well known. P-gp is an ATP-dependent transporter that is genetically encoded and located on the apical surface of mucosal cells in the intestine, generally in increasing concentration from the stomach to the colon. In addition, P-gp is also present on a number of lymphocyte subsets and within the brain capillary endothelial cells. The primary role of P-gp is to limit systematic drug exposure, pumping compounds from the inside of the cell back into the gut lumen, into renal tubules in the kidney, and into bile in the liver. Given its presence in various anatomic locations, drug-induced modulation of P-gp activity may affect the absorption and/or distribution of a coadministered substrate medication. There are several drugs that are known to block the action of P-gp and are known as P-gp inhibitors, and there are drugs that have been shown to cause induction of P-gp. Coadministration of a P-gp substrate with an inhibitor increases the amount of substrate available for absorption and may result in an elevated serum drug concentration. For drugs such as rifampin that increase expression of P-gp (i.e., P-gp inducer), the coadministration of a substrate results in an enhanced efflux of the substrate into the gut lumen and lowers serum concentration of the substrate.

DISTRIBUTION

Case 3-1, Question 2: Describe the interaction of warfarin and phenytoin based on protein binding.

Following administration and absorption, drugs are distributed throughout the body.[37,38] While some drugs have near-complete dissolution in the plasma, drugs such as warfarin and phenytoin are highly bound to protein (primarily to albumin) with the same affinity binding sites (Figure 3-1). Drugs that are highly protein bound (>90%), those with a NTI, and those with a small volume of distribution are more likely to result in significant drug interactions.

Warfarin can be displaced from protein-binding sites by drugs such as phenytoin. Although this displacement occurs quickly with rapid changes in serum warfarin levels, typically this interaction is not clinically significant. Warfarin that is displaced from protein-binding sites is readily available for elimination by hepatic metabolism, resulting in increased clearance without a significant change in the free drug concentration. Because warfarin's anticoagulant action takes several days due to the long half-lives of some of the vitamin K-dependent clotting factors, warfarin equilibrium is re-established before a new steady state can be reached for these clotting factors.[32]

METABOLISM

Pharmacokinetic interactions that involve changes in metabolism are a common cause of clinically significant drug interactions. Drug metabolism is divided into two general categories: phase I and phase II reactions.[37,38] Phase I reactions involve intramolecular changes including oxidation, reduction, and hydrolysis, which increases the polar nature of the drug, generally making it less toxic. Phase II reactions generally involve combining a phase I product with an endogenous substance resulting in glucuronidation, sulfation, acetylation, and methylation, and primarily results in termination of biologic activity of the drug.[39,40] The main enzymes that are responsible for drug-metabolizing systems in phase I reactions are the cytochrome (CYP) 450 enzymes, which play a key role in many therapeutically important drug interactions.[1,2] Drugs that are metabolized by the same CYP450 enzyme family, when administered concurrently, may interact with each other as a result of induction or inhibition.[39,40] Of the human CYP450 enzyme family, the 6 isozymes CYP1A2, CYP2C9, CYP2C19, CYP2D6, CYP3A4, and CYP3A5 contribute to the metabolism of a vast majority of drugs compared with other enzymes (Figure 3-2).[6,41-43] Examples of drug that induce enzymes are rifampin, phenytoin, carbamazepine, St. John's-wort, and nevirapine. Enzyme inducers cause an increase in the synthesis of the enzyme(s) responsible for metabolism of the substrate drug. The mechanisms of induction are complex involving presystemic metabolism via induction of hepatic and/or intestinal drug-metabolizing enzymes, subsequently reducing serum concentrations with a loss of pharmacologic activity of the drug. In some cases, induction will increase the formation of metabolites that are pharmacologically or toxicologically active.[1,43,44] There are many drugs that are inhibitors of CYP450 including some drugs within these classes: statins, macrolide antibiotics, antifungal azoles, fluoroquinolones, and HIV protease inhibitors. Inhibition of drug metabolism slows down the rate of drug metabolism, resulting in an increase in the amount of drug in the body and potential toxicity. Grapefruit juice is an inhibitor of CYP3A4 and has been known to increase the bioavailability and reduce the clearance of many drugs including HMG-CoA reductase inhibitors (statins), calcium antagonists, HIV protease inhibitors, and immunosuppressant agents.[45-48] Inhibition can be described as reversible or irreversible, with the reversible ones being a more common process. There are three mechanisms of reversible inhibition: competitive inhibition (competition between the inhibitor and the substrate for the enzyme's active site); noncompetitive inhibition (binding of the inhibitor to a separate site on the enzyme, rendering the enzyme complex nonfunctional); or uncompetitive inhibition (binding of the inhibitor only to the substrate–enzyme complex, rendering it ineffective).[1,48,49] Irreversible inhibition occurs when the perpetrator drug forms a reactive intermediate with the enzyme that leads to a permanent inhibition of the enzyme. Irreversible drug interactions tend to be more profound than those caused by reversible mechanisms. Examples of drugs that are known to cause irreversible inhibition include macrolide antibiotics, erythromycin, clarithromycin, paroxetine, and diltiazem.[15,50,51]

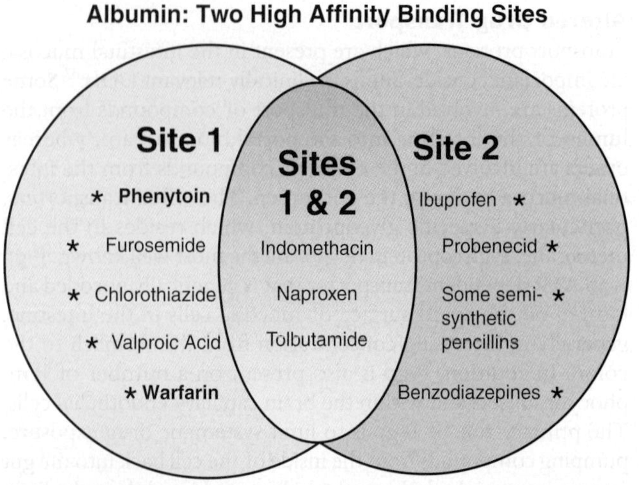

Figure 3-1 Examples of drugs that bind to and compete for one of two sites, designation I and II, on albumin. (Adapted from Drug Interactions. In: Rowland M et al, eds. *Clinical Pharmacokinetics and Pharmacodynamics: Concepts and Applications.* 4th ed. Baltimore, MD: Lippincott Williams & Wilkins; 2011:490.)

Case 3-1, Question 3: The medical team starts N.M. on warfarin therapy postsurgery for thromboembolism prophylaxis. The medical intern asks you to explain the mechanisms of drug interactions to consider with the use of warfarin and phenytoin because N.M has been on phenytoin for the past 10 years and her seizure disorder has been controlled on it.

There are two potential mechanisms for a warfarin (drug)–phenytoin (drug) interaction. In early therapy, there could be a displacement of warfarin from protein-binding sites by phenytoin (as described in the previous case question), and a possible enhancement of the anticoagulant effect and risk for bleeding. This is primarily a concern in patients with hepatic impairment. With prolonged therapy, there could be a phenytoin-induced, CYP enzyme induction thereby enhancing warfarin metabolism resulting in a decreased warfarin effect. INR monitoring on postoperative days 1 through 5 will provide information on the impact of the DDI and incorporation of a warfarin initiation guideline or algorithm will help adjust dosing until a stable regimen is established. After the initial period, weekly INR monitoring will provide information on enzyme induction and further adjustment of warfarin doses.

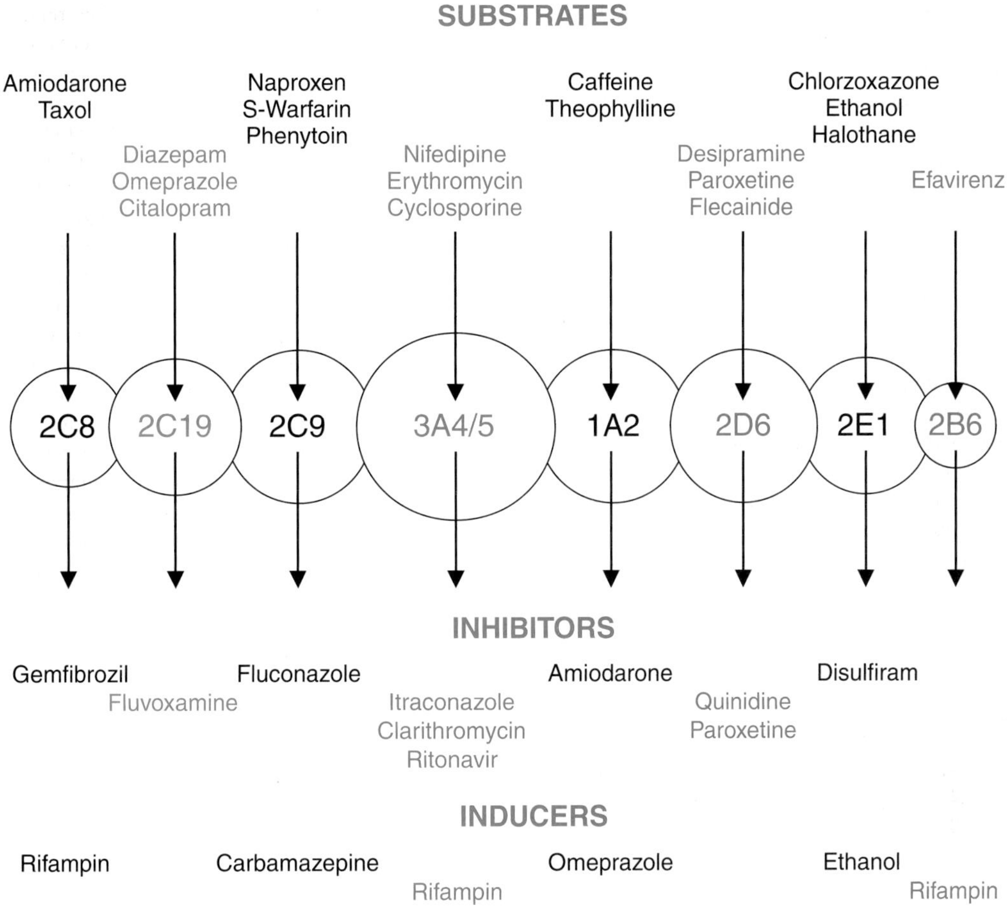

Figure 3-2 Graphic representation of the different forms of cytochrome-P450 (circles) in humans with different but some overlapping substrate specificities. The arrows indicate single metabolic pathways. Representative substrates are listed above for each enzyme. Also listed are relatively selective inhibitors and inducers of the enzymes. (Reprinted from Drug Interactions. In: Rowland M, Tozer TN, eds. *Clinical Pharmacokinetics and Pharmacodynamics: Concepts and Applications.* 4th ed. Baltimore, MD: Lippincott Williams & Wilkins; 2011, with permission.)

Warfarin is rapidly and completely absorbed after oral administration with the proximal duodenum appearing to be the most likely location of absorption. Case reports of warfarin malabsorption, whether acquired, related to surgery, or inflammatory conditions, are rare.[52]

The rate and extent of phenytoin absorption varies considerably among oral dosage forms.[53] Phenytoin suspension is poorly absorbed when administered via feeding tube with continuous enteral feedings.[54] The time to reach maximum plasma levels increases with increasing dose.[55] This is a reflection of low phenytoin solubility and capacity-limited metabolism. Therefore, a small change in the dosage form or bioavailability, coupled with limited metabolism, can produce a large change in plasma drug concentration.[56] GI surgery and GI inflammatory conditions (Crohn's disease, ulcerative colitis, scleroderma, etc.) can change the anatomy of the GI tract. Alterations to surface area, gastric emptying time, gastric pH, and inflammation of the intestinal lining may lead to abnormal plasma concentrations.[57]

N.M.'s GI function is still preserved after orthopedic surgery. Warfarin administration and absorption is unlikely to be impacted. She should continue on the same phenytoin dose and formulation that she has been taking at home with appropriate monitoring.

Pharmacokinetic interactions influencing the metabolism of warfarin and clinically significant interactions are likely with warfarin use when its metabolism is induced or inhibited.[48] Warfarin is a racemic mixture of R- and S-enantiomers. Interactions involving agents known to influence the hepatic microsomal enzyme systems responsible for the metabolism of the more potent S-enantiomer (CYP2C9) are more significant than those that influence the enzymes that metabolize R-enantiomer (CYP1A2, CYP3A4). Phenytoin is also predominately metabolized via the CYP2C9 enzyme and has been reported to interact with warfarin in a biphasic manner.[49-51]

Genetic polymorphism also is a significant factor affecting warfarin dosing and response. Nucleotide polymorphisms have been identified that influence warfarin metabolism and sensitivity, including variants of CYP2C9 and variants in vitamin K epoxide reductase complex (*VKORC1*).[58]

EXCRETION/ELIMINATION

Drugs are excreted and eliminated mainly via the kidneys (glomerular filtration, tubular reabsorption, and active tubular secretion); other important, though less common, routes are via biliary secretion, plasma esterases, and other minor pathways. Drug interactions may occur during the elimination of drugs and their metabolites by the kidney as a result of competition at the level of active tubular secretion, interference with tubular transport, or during tubular reabsorption.

Urinary alkalinization and acidification by some drugs can affect the excretion of other drugs changing their elimination rate. For example, the use of probenecid, a potent inhibitor of the anionic pathway of renal tubular secretion, increases the serum concentration of penicillins, which can be used for therapeutic purposes.

Pharmacodynamics

Pharmacodynamic interactions occur when the response of one drug is modified by the presence of another one without alterations in pharmacokinetics. These types of interactions may be predicted if the pharmacologic effects of a drug are known, and the patient response may be additive or antagonistic.[2,8] For example, there may be an interaction in which one drug, an ACE inhibitor, and another drug, a thiazide diuretic, each act by a different mechanism of action to lower blood pressure, producing an exaggerated hypotensive effect.

CASE 3-1, QUESTION 4: The intern asks you to explain the pharmacodynamic interactions that are clinically relevant to warfarin.

Pharmacodynamic interactions with warfarin are those that alter the physiology of hemostasis, particularly interactions that influence the synthesis or degradation of clotting factors or that increase the risk of bleeding through inhibition of platelet aggregation. In patients receiving warfarin, the addition of any drugs that increase or decrease clotting factor synthesis, enhance or reduce clotting factor catabolism, or that impair vitamin K production by normal flora will increase the risk of drug interactions.

Tables 3-3 and 3-4 provide examples of common mechanisms of pharmacokinetic and pharmacodynamic drug interactions, respectively.

MANAGEMENT OF DRUG INTERACTIONS

CASE 3-1, QUESTION 5: The medical intern on the team also plans to prescribe a combination analgesic (oxycodone/acetaminophen) in place of intravenous morphine for the pain management.

In a telephone conversation, N.M. expressed to a friend that she felt depressed. As a result, her friend brought her a bottle of St. John's-wort.

As the pharmacist on the multidisciplinary team your role is to assess therapy and make recommendations as needed. Provide appropriate recommendations regarding N.M.'s therapy, including the use of St. John's-wort.

Although acetaminophen is a commonly used nonprescription analgesic and antipyretic medication for mild-to-moderate pain and fever, its presence is often unrecognized in combination products containing opioids prescribed for moderate-to-severe pain. Several studies have identified acetaminophen as a culprit drug in potentiating the effects of warfarin.[66] Patients who take four 325-mg acetaminophen tablets per day for longer than a week were more likely to have an INR above 6.0 than those who did not take acetaminophen.

There is no evidence for a pharmacokinetic interaction between acetaminophen and warfarin.[67] However, acetaminophen is metabolized by CYP2E1 producing the metabolite N-acetyl-p-benzoquinone-imine (NAPQ1). NAPQ1 oxidizes vitamin K-hydroquinone (KH2), the "active" form of vitamin K, and directly inhibits vitamin K-dependent carboxylation. There may be other oxidative changes, producing enzymatic disruption, that impact vitamin k synthesis and activity. The end result is an exaggerated response to warfarin and an increased INR.

Therefore if N.M. is to be placed on oxycodone/acetaminophen therapy, her INR should be monitored more frequently and her dose adjusted accordingly. This is important particularly if she requires higher sustained doses of warfarin.

Dietary supplements, including herbal medicinals, amino acids, and other nonprescription products, are not tested before marketing for interactions with other medications, including warfarin. Little is known about their interactive properties, other than published case reports of varying quality. In addition, dietary supplements are not required to meet US Pharmacopeia standards for tablet content uniformity.

St. John's-wort, an herb whose yellow flowers and leaves are used to make herbal supplements, has been used for treatment of depression. It has also been shown to lower patient INR values and potentially decrease warfarin's effectiveness.[68,69] Although this interaction is probably due to the induction of CYP2C9, the degree of induction is unpredictable due to variable quality and quantity of the herbal constituent in the preparations. Similarly, St. John's-wort has been suspected of reducing phenytoin plasma concentrations through induction of CYP3A4.

The addition of St. John's-wort to N.M.'s current drug regimen would not be advisable because it would increase her risk for drug interactions. The implications for initiating St. John's-wort in N.M. would require measurement of phenytoin and more frequent INR testing to ensure a new steady state for each agent has been reached. At this point, it is important to assess N.M.'s depression and to evaluate therapeutic options that would provide the least risk of drug interactions, as well as psychosocial treatment.

CASE 3-1, QUESTION 6: Pravastatin, the medication that N.M. was taking prior to admission, is not available on the hospital's formulary list. Therefore, the medical intern prescribes the formulary-preferred agent rosuvastatin postsurgery. He receives an electronic health record drug interaction alert regarding the statin and warfarin and asks you how this should be managed.

Rosuvastatin is not metabolized extensively by the CYP 450 system (approximately 10% with CYP2C9 and CYP2C19 being the primary isoenzymes involved). However, the combination of rosuvastatin and warfarin has resulted in an increase in the INR and hence increasing risk of bleeding.[34-36] Each of the statin agents is metabolized by different CYP isoenzymes and to different degrees (Table 3-5). The goal of lipid management is to prescribe an agent with the least side effects and at the lowest effective dose. If a patient, such as N.M., requires a drug that interacts with statin metabolism (CYP), switching to a statin that has a more favorable elimination profile may be the best option. In this instance, pravastatin, which has limited CYP metabolism and is primarily excreted unchanged in the urine, may be the optimal choice. Otherwise, rosuvastatin may be used but more frequent monitoring of the INR is recommended until a stable INR has been reached. Table 3-5 provides a summary of the metabolism of HMG-CoA reductase inhibitors. Refer to Chapter 8 Dyslipidemias, Atherosclerosis, and Coronary Heart Disease for more information on the use of statins, including drug interactions.

CASE 3-2

QUESTION 1: J.A. is a 69-year-old previously healthy male who was admitted to the medical intensive care unit (ICU) with lower left lobe pneumonia, and he has developed septic shock. His hospital course for the first 18 days of admission consisted of a worsening bilateral pneumonia characterized by profound hypoxia and acute respiratory distress syndrome (ARDS). J.A. is currently deeply sedated and receiving neuromuscular blockade to manage his ARDS, high peak inspiratory pressures (PIPs), and low oxygen saturation (SaO_2).

Medications:

- Propofol IV infusion and fentanyl IV infusion for sedation and analgesia
- Cisatracurium IV infusion for neuromuscular blockade—goal is to improve oxygenation (PaO_2/ FiO_2 ratio)
- Pantoprazole IV for stress ulcer prophylaxis
- Heparin SC and pneumatic compression boots for Deep Venous thrombosis (DVT) prophylaxis

Table 3-3
Common Mechanisms of Pharmacokinetic Drug Interactions[1,3,6,16,31–33,37,59–64]

	Mechanism	Example
Pharmacokinetics: administration/absorption	Drugs that alter the pH of the stomach can affect absorption of other drugs	Itraconazole requires an acidic gastric pH to become soluble; absorption may be decreased if a patient is taking a drug that increases gastric pH such as a PPI or H_2-blocker
	Induction or inhibition of CYP enzymes in the gastrointestinal (GI) tract	Grapefruit juice inhibits intestinal CYP 3A4 potentially increasing the bioavailability of CYP 3A4 substrates such as nifedipine and verapamil
	Induction or inhibition of P-gp (an efflux pump that expels drugs) in GI tract	Dabigatran, a substrate for P-gp, peak concentrations may be increased by P-gp inhibitors (e.g., ketoconazole, clarithromycin, amiodarone) leading to a significantly increased risk of bleeding
	Increase or delay gastric emptying/motility	Erythromycin, a potent prokinetic agent, is a motilin receptor agonist that increases gastric motility; absorption of coadministered drugs may be affected
	Killing enteric bacteria	Antibiotics can kill bacteria that produce deconjugating enzymes; drugs that undergo enterohepatic circulation such as birth control pills may have decreased blood concentrations and half-life because of increased excretion in the feces
	Chelation	Cations such as aluminum or magnesium antacids decrease the GI absorption of tetracycline antibiotics by forming drug–metal complexes
	Physiochemical inactivation	Mixing a furosemide solution with an acidic solution (i.e., with midazolam) decreases the pH sufficiently to cause furosemide precipitation and reduced availability when administered intravenously
Pharmacokinetics: distribution	Interaction between two highly protein-bound drugs (e.g., a precipitant drug has stronger affinity for the same protein-binding site)	Sulfamethoxazole displaces warfarin from protein-binding sites increasing the free fraction. Sulfamethoxazole also inhibits the metabolism of warfarin. As a result, the body cannot compensate to increase the elimination of the high free (active) fraction of warfarin. The end result is likely an increase in the INR and potential risk for bleeding. See chapter 11 for detailed warfarin–sulfamethoxazole drug interaction
	Inhibition of carrier proteins such as P-gp located in blood–brain barrier and organic transporting peptides (OATPs) located in the liver	Cyclosporine may inhibit the transporter OATP1B1 decreasing the hepatic uptake of most statins; efficacy of the statin may be lost because the site of action is located in the liver
Pharmacokinetics: metabolism	Induction or inhibition of CYP enzymes in the liver	*Example 1:* Fluoroquinolones inhibit metabolism of theophylline via CYP 1A2 enzyme; the extent of the interaction varies between the different fluoroquinolones *Example 2:* Rifampin has a half-life of 4 hours; however, time to steady state induction with propranolol does not occur until 10–14 days
Pharmacokinetics: excretion/elimination	Administration of two drugs that use the same transport system and undergo active tubular secretion by the kidneys	Methotrexate clearance may be reduced in the presence of salicylates. Salicylates decrease renal perfusion via PGE_2, having the potential to cause renal impairment and competitively inhibit the tubular secretion of methotrexate
	Increased or decreased renal tubular absorption	*Example 1:* Quinidine reabsorption may be increased in alkalinized urine. *Example 2:* Thiazide diuretics initially cause sodium excretion followed by compensatory sodium reabsorption. Administered with lithium, a cation can cause increased lithium reabsorption and possible toxic concentrations

Table 3-4
Common Mechanisms of Pharmacodynamic Drug Interactions[65]

	Mechanism	Example
Pharmacodynamics	Additive—two or more medications with comparable pharmacodynamic effects result in an exaggerated and/or toxic response	Administration of thiopental and midazolam during induction. Midazolam reduces the amount of thiopental required for anesthesia
	Antagonistic—the effects of one drug oppose the actions of another drug	*Example 1:* Antagonism at the same receptor site: reversal of benzodiazepines with flumazenil. *Example 2:* Opposing pharmacodynamics actions: glucocorticoids cause hyperglycemia opposing the effects of hypoglycemic medications

- Hydrocortisone IV for corticosteroid insufficiency in critical illness
- Amikacin IV and imipenem/cilastatin IV for day 5 treatment of a multidrug resistant organism
- Norepinephrine and vasopressin IV infusions for septic shock secondary to pneumonia
- Ophthalmic ointment to lubricate eye while on prolonged neuromuscular blockade
- Lactated Ringer's IV infusion for hypotension secondary to septic shock

Vitals: T 101°F HR 105 RR 20 BP 95/60

Laboratory values: ABG: pH 7.30 /pCO_2 42/pO_2 80/CO_2 19/ SaO_2 90% on mechanical ventilation: Assist control RR 20 tidal volume 400 mL PEEP 10 FiO_2 50%

Na^+	138 mEq/L	WBC	14.600 × $10^3 \mu$/L
K^+	4.8 mEq/L	Poly	80 %
Cl^-	98 mEq/L	Bands	12 %
HCO_3^-	19 mEq/L	Hgb	9.0 g/dL
BUN	45 mg/dL	Hct	28 %
SCr	1.8 mg/dL (baseline SCr 1.0 mg/dL)	Platelets	202 × $10^3 \mu$/L
Glucose	142 mg/dL	AST	105 U/mL
Serum phosphate	0.9 mg/dL	ALT	85 U/mL

J.A.'s train-of-four (TOF) is 0/4. A peripheral nerve stimulator, the TOF, is a clinical tool used to monitor neuromuscular blockade. The TOF Scale includes the following: 0/4 indicates that no twitch elicited, neuromuscular blocker agent occupies 100% of postsynaptic nicotinic receptors, and a 100% blockade whereas 4/4 indicates that <75% of the postsynaptic nicotinic receptors are blocked. The goal of neuromuscular therapy is to achieve an adequate neuromuscular blockade, a TOF of 1/4 or 2/4 (80% to 90% of receptors blocked) or the desired clinical effect (e.g., accepting ventilation and not over breathing the ventilator), with the lowest dose of neuromuscular agent necessary.[71,72]

Describe J.A.'s risk factors for drug interactions.

There are several risk factors for drug interactions in critically ill patients. Critically ill patients are susceptible to drug interactions as a result of a debilitated condition and/or disease state (e.g., changes in physiologic pH and body temperature, electrolyte imbalances, organ failure, etc.), as well as the multitude of medications prescribed as treatment. ICU patients also have altered pharmacokinetics, placing them at an increased risk for an interaction. These changes include the following:

- Decreased GI absorption of enterally administered medications due to the following: hypoperfusion from shock; increased stomach pH from PPI and histamine blocker therapy; decreased GI motility; drug effect on carrier proteins, for example, P-gp;
- Decreased subcutaneous absorption due to the following: edema; vasopressor therapy; and disease-induced peripheral vasoconstriction;
- Increased volume of distribution (V_d) for hydrophilic medications due to increased total body water from fluid resuscitation and third spacing;
- Altered free drug fraction due to increased α-acid glycoprotein from systemic inflammation and decreased albumin plasma concentrations; and
- Half-life ($t_{1/2}$) and Clearance (CL) may be affected from decreased hepatic blood flow, renal or hepatic insufficiency, and induction or inhibition of hepatic enzymes by drugs. Patients without renal insufficiency may exhibit augmented clearance.[73,74]

Table 3-5
Metabolism of HMG-CoA Reductase Inhibitors (Statins)

Statins[a]	Isoenzyme	Comments
Lovastatin	CYP3A4 substrate	Caution drugs that significantly inhibit its metabolism (potent CYP 3A4 inhibitors)
Simvastatin	CYP3A4 substrate	Caution drugs that significantly inhibit its metabolism (potent CYP 3A4 inhibitors)
Atorvastatin	CYP3A4 substrate	Metabolized by CYP 3A4 but less than lovastatin and simvastatin
Fluvastatin	CYP2C9 substrate	Metabolized primarily by CYP2C9 and to a lesser extent by CYP3A4 and CYP2D6
Pravastatin	Excreted primarily unchanged in urine	Not significantly metabolized by cytochrome P450 system
Rosuvastatin	2C9/2C19	Not extensively metabolized by cytochrome P450 system

[a]Substrates for Pgp → drugs that inhibit Pgp may ↑ statin levels (e.g., cyclosporine, diltiazem).

Adapted from Pharmacist's Letter/Prescriber's Letter, "Clinically Significant Statin Drug Interactions," August 2009, Volume 25, Number 250812 and Pharmacist's Letter/Prescriber's Letter, "Characteristics of the Various Statins," June 2010, Volume 26, Number 260611.[70]

The mode of mechanical ventilation that is used most commonly today is positive pressure ventilation, whereby air is forced into the lungs to improve gas exchange. The use of mechanical ventilation may also affect drug pharmacokinetics by decreasing cardiac output secondary to reduced preload, which in turn may compromise perfusion to the liver and kidneys as well as GFR and urine output.[75] This effect is most pronounced in patients who are hypovolemic. These hemodynamic changes can result in a decrease of the clearance of several drugs.

J.A. has several risk factors for drug interactions. Many of his risk factors are patient-specific, including J.A.'s age, organ dysfunction, and acute medical conditions. Additional risk factors are the extended hospital stay in the ICU and multiple medications. J.A.'s specific risk factors are outlined below.

Patient Risk Factors

- Age: 69 years old—altered pharmacokinetic and pharmacodynamics
- Renal dysfunction: baseline SCr 1.0 mg/dL and current SCr 1.8 mg/dL—decreased renal clearance
- Mild hepatic dysfunction: AST 105 U/mL and ALT 85 U/mL—decreased metabolism
- Pneumonia: T 101°F, WBC 14.6 × $10^3 \mu$/L, poly 80%, bands 12%—increased catabolism
- Hypotension (result of shock): BP 95/60 on norepinephrine, vasopressin, and lactated Ringer's solution—decreased clearance
- Hyperthermia: T 101°F—increased clearance
- Hypophosphatemia: phosphate 0.9 mg/dL—increased neuromuscular blockade (see discussion Case 3-2 Question 2)

- Norepinephrine and vasopressin infusions: potential for decreased blood delivery to liver and kidneys
- Mechanical ventilation: decreased cardiac output

Other Risk Factors

- Polypharmacy: risk of adverse drug interaction increases with multiple medications
- Duration of hospital stay: 18 days—susceptible to hospital-acquired conditions and subsequent drug therapy

Case 3-2, Question 2: The medical team is concerned that J.A.'s condition may have worsened; he may have had a neurologic event (e.g., stroke) in the night. J.A. is clinically unstable to bring to computed tomography (CT). The team needs J.A. to be alert for purposes of conducting a neurologic examination. To undergo the examination, J.A. must have his neuromuscular blockade discontinued and sedation lightened. One and one-half hours after discontinuation of cisatracurium J.A. is still not moving (TOF 0/4). The medical team feels J.A.'s cisatracurium's paralytic effect should have worn off by now and is concerned about his prognosis. The medical team ask the clinical pharmacist to review J.A.'s case and affirm that the neuromuscular blockade has worn off.

After reviewing the case, the clinician identifies potential drug-condition/disease and drug–drug pharmacodynamic interactions that may contribute to the prolonged neuromuscular blockade. These interactions are discussed below.

Background: The incidence of ICU-acquired weakness (polyneuropathy and myopathy) in ARDS patients is 34% to 60%. This condition can last for months to years and can severely affect a patient's quality of life.[76] There are several risk factors for ICU-acquired weakness that includes prolonged mechanical ventilation, number of days with dysfunction in 2 or more organs before wakening, corticosteroids, female sex,[77] toxins (e.g., botulism), neuromuscular disease states (e.g., Guillain-Barre Syndrome), severe electrolyte imbalances, prolonged recovery from neuromuscular blockers, deconditioning, length of vasopressor support, and hyperglycemia just to name a few.[76,78,79] Neuromuscular blockade alone has been associated with ICU-acquired weakness. However, in a multicenter, double-blind trial, investigators found no statistical difference in ICU-acquired paresis between cisatracurium and placebo groups at day 28 or ICU discharge.[78,80] Prolonged recovery from neuromuscular blockade may occur in patients with organ failure and/or conditions that affect the overall clearance of the neuromuscular blocking agent (e.g., decreased metabolism of a parent drug, decreased elimination of the parent drug, and/or the active metabolite). In addition to that, certain disease states, conditions, or drugs that may potentiate a blockade may also lead to an increased recovery time.[78,79]

Drug-Condition/Disease Interactions

PHARMACOKINETICS—DRUG METABOLISM/ELIMINATION

The nondepolarizing agent, cisatracurium, is a benzylisoquinolinium compound. It is one of the ten isomers of the intermediate-acting neuromuscular blocker, atracurium. It is primarily eliminated by Hofmann degradation; optimal breakdown occurs at physiologic temperature (37°C or 98.6°F) and pH (7.40).[72] This process results in therapeutically inactive metabolites, monoquaternary alcohol, monoquaternary acrylate, and laudanosine.[81] Cisatracurium's organ-independent elimination is a benefit for J.A. because he has renal and hepatic insufficiency. However, because cisatracurium is degraded by the Hofmann process, alterations in pH and temperature will affect the elimination of the drug. For example, the neuromuscular blockade effect is prolonged with acidosis while elimination is enhanced with an increase in pH. Additionally, hypothermia decreases the elimination of cisatracurium whereas hyperthermia accelerates it. In ICU patients, the recovery rate from neuromuscular blockade is reported to range from 45 to 75 minutes after discontinuation of a prolonged cisatracurium infusion.[82-84] Because J.A. has both a fever (101°F) and metabolic acidosis (pH 7.30 and HCO_3^- 19), it is difficult to predict the clearance of the neuromuscular blocker.

PHARMACODYNAMIC INTERACTION

A second condition that may add to J.A.'s prolonged blockade is his low phosphate (phosphate 0.9 mg/dL). Phosphate is a building block of adenosine triphosphate (ATP). ATP produces energy via an enzymatic reaction by releasing a phosphate group. This reaction is necessary for physiologic and metabolic functions including muscle contraction. Therefore, a patient with hypophosphatemia is at risk for a myopathy.[85]

Drug–Drug Interaction

PHARMACODYNAMIC—ADDITIVE EFFECTS OF MEDICATIONS

J.A.'s medications may also have additive effects with cisatracurium. A rare adverse effect of amikacin is neuromuscular blockade. The mechanism of blockade involves inhibiting acetylcholine release by competing with Ca^{+2} at the preganglionic nerve terminal and to a smaller degree noncompetitive blocking of the receptor.[86] Corticosteroids (e.g., hydrocortisone) may also enhance blockade and increase recovery time. Proposed mechanisms for steroidal ICU-acquired weakness include increased muscle sensitivity to corticosteroids because of lack of movement and skeletal muscle atrophy from the steroid's catabolic actions. Additionally, corticosteroids may cause myopathy by denervation; corticosteroids have been shown to inhibit the nicotinic receptor; when combined with the neuromuscular blocking agent, vecuronium, this inhibition is potentiated.[76,87] It is thought that this interaction is more likely to occur with neuromuscular blockers that have a steroid structural ring, such as the aminosteroid (e.g., pancuronium, pipcuronium, vecuronium, and rocuronium). However, there have been case reports of prolonged paralysis with the benzylisoquinoliniums (e.g., atracurium, cisatracurium, doxacurium, mivacurium, and d-tubocurarine).[78,79,88]

J.A. may need a longer period than an hour and one-half to recover from his paralysis because of the following factors: decreased elimination of cisatracurium as a result of acidosis, hypophosphatemia, and medications (amikacin and hydrocortisone). J.A. should also have his phosphate slowly repleted.

Case 3-2, Question 3: The medical team asks you to explain the drug interactions affecting the antibiotic efficacy of J.A.'s regimen.

After reviewing the case, the clinician identifies potential drug–drug physiochemical interaction, as well as drug–condition and drug–drug pharmacodynamic interactions. The mechanism of action of these interactions is discussed below.

Drug–Drug Interaction

PHYSIOCHEMICAL INACTIVATION

It has been well documented that the coadministration of beta-lactam antibiotics with aminoglycoside antibiotics can lead to inactivation of the aminoglycoside. The mechanism involves the amino group of the aminoglycoside antibiotic forming an inactive amide with the beta-lactam ring of penicillin antibiotics.[89,90] Because penicillins have wide therapeutic index, this interaction primarily affects the efficacy of the aminoglycoside antibiotic.

This interaction has been shown to occur with the extended-spectrum penicillins (e.g., azlocillin, carbenicillin, mezlocillin, ticarcillin, and piperacillin). J.A. is currently on amikacin and imipenem–cilastatin antibiotics for treatment of a multiresistant organism. According to the literature, amikacin is the aminoglycoside that is least susceptible to this interaction.[90] Additionally, no inactivation of amikacin was observed when incubated in cilastatin 120 μg/mL human serum for 48 h at 37°C.[91]

This inactivation increases with contact time and is directly proportional to the concentration of penicillin.[92] The rate of elimination of aminoglycoside and imipenem–cilastatin may be increased because of J.A.'s renal dysfunction. This would increase the contact time of the medications.

Recommendations for J.A.'s antibiotic therapy include administration of medications separately; serum concentrations of aminoglycosides should be assayed immediately after drawn or if analysis is delayed freeze at −70°C; and because of his renal dysfunction, close monitoring of aminoglycoside serum concentrations is indicated.[92,93]

Drug-Condition/Disease Interaction

PHARMACODYNAMIC INTERACTION

The pharmacodynamic actions of amikacin may be decreased because J.A. is acidotic.

Amikacin enters the bacterial cell and reaches its site of action in three stages: ionic binding, energy-dependent phase I (EDP-I), and energy-dependent phase II (EDP-II) transport or uptake.

Ionic Binding to the Outer Membrane: At physiologic pH, amikacin (pKa 8.1) is a highly ionized basic cation. It binds to anionic lipopolysaccharides (LPSs), polar heads of phospholipids, and proteins on the outer cell membrane of Gram-negative bacteria and phospholipids and teichoic acids of Gram-positive bacteria.[94] This leads to displacement of cell wall Mg^{2+} and Ca^{2+} bridges that link LPS, and the result is the formation of pores in the cell wall where amikacin can enter into the periplasmic space.[95]

EDP-I: Amikacin is transported across the cytoplasmic membrane. EDP-I is dependent on pH and oxygen. Amikacin activity will decline in low pH and anaerobic conditions (e.g., abscesses).[95]

EDP-II: Amikacin is transported to the site of action, binding to the ribosomes.[95]

Drug–Drug Interaction

PHARMACODYNAMIC—ADDITIVE/SYNERGISTIC EFFECT OF MEDICATIONS

Penicillins form a covalent bond with the enzymes, the penicillin-binding proteins (PBPs) (specifically transpeptidase, endopeptidase, carboxypeptidase) inhibiting their action. These enzymes are needed for the final step of bacterial cell wall synthesis, the cross-linking between peptide side chains on the polysaccharide backbones of the peptidoglycan.[96] Cell wall inhibitors such as penicillins and vancomycin may expedite aminoglycoside entry into the bacterial cell resulting in synergistic effects when treating some organisms.[95]

J.A. is critically ill with renal failure, ARDS, pneumonia caused by a multiresistant organism, septic shock, and a metabolic acidosis. It is important to closely monitor his aminoglycoside therapy for efficacy (peaks) and toxicity (troughs).

This case illustrates the difficulties surrounding drug interaction identification, assessment, and follow-up intervention. Clinicians must recognize that literature to support the presence of a drug interaction is often scant and not always definitive and the optimal intervention may rely on clinical judgment. Refer to Chapter 56 for the Care of the Critically Ill Adult Patient.

CASE 3-3

QUESTION 1: D.T. is a 67-year-old Caucasian male who began taking imatinib about 10 years ago to treat a rare sarcoma: partially resected gastrointestinal stromal tumor (GIST). D.T. currently takes 600-mg imatinib daily, as well as rabeprazole and furosemide. He states that he is currently not taking any nonprescription medications. He continues to go to the cancer treatment center for continued monitoring. He contacts the cancer clinic to let them know that in 4 weeks he will be traveling to Africa to go on a safari. He mentioned that the friends that he will be traveling with told him that he will need malaria prophylaxis.

You are consulted regarding this request as the medical team wants to know whether there are any potential drug interactions and which antimalarial agent would be an appropriate selection.

Imatinib mesylate belongs to a class of drugs known as selective tyrosine kinase inhibitors (TKIs).[97] It inhibits the BCR-ABL tyrosine kinase, the constitutive abnormal tyrosine kinase created by the Philadelphia chromosome abnormality in chronic myeloid proteins.[97] It also inhibits the tyrosine kinase for platelet-derived growth factor (PDGF) and c-kit. TKIs, such as imatinib, are extensively metabolized via cytochrome P450 enzymes (with a large degree of interindividual variability).[98] Imatinib is metabolized primarily by CYP 3A4, whereas CYP1A2, CYP2C9, CYP2C19, CYP2D6, and CYP3A5 are reported to have a minor role in its metabolism.[99] In addition, imatinib is a substrate of human organic cation transporter type 1 (hOCT1), Pgp, and BCRP, though it is unclear whether imatinib is a substrate or inhibitor of BCRP.[100–103] Imatinib also competitively inhibits the metabolism of drugs that are CYP2C9, CYP2C19, CYP2D6, and CYP3A4 substrates.[104] It is also highly protein bound with approximately 95% bound to human plasma proteins.[99,105–107]

Drug–Drug Interaction

PHARMACOKINETICS—DRUG METABOLISM/ELIMINATION

There are several considerations of potential drug interactions with imatinib. Drug interactions should be considered when imatinib is administrated with other agents in the CYP3A family.[97] In particular, interactions are likely with inhibitors of CYP3A4, such as voriconazole or amiodarone, resulting in increases in the plasma concentration of imatinib. Concomitant use of rifampicin or other strong CYP3A4 inducers with imatinib should be avoided. In addition, concomitant administration of imatinib with agents that are both inhibitors of CYP3A4 and P-gp increases plasma and intracellular imatinib concentrations. Examples of dual CYP3A4 and Pgp inhibitors include verapamil, erythromycin, clarithromycin, ketoconazole, fluconazole, and itraconazole.[100,108,109] TKIs, such as imatinib, also can inhibit drug transporters and enzymes, resulting in changes in the exposure of coadministered drugs. St. John's-wort significantly altered the pharmacokinetic profile of imatinib with reductions of 30% in the medium area under the concentration–time curve (AUC). Patients should be cautioned regarding the concomitant use of products, such as St. John's-wort, as well as other inducers, that may necessitate an increase in imatinib dosing to maintain therapeutic efficacy.[110,111] Drug interactions involving protein binding of imatinib and other highly protein-bound drugs are not well understood.[97]

A study published in 2016 examined DDIs observed in patients treated with imatinib.[112] The investigators performed two observational studies to identify the medications that were most frequently dispensed simultaneously with imatinib through the French health insurance reimbursement database SNIIRAM (Systeme National d'Information Inter-Regimes Assurance Maladie), as well as the

ADRs related to DDIs involving imatinib using the French Pharmacovigilance Database. A sample of 544 patients from SNIIRAM with at least 1 reimbursement for imatinib were identified between January 2012 through August 2015. Of this cohort of 544 patients, 89.3% (486) of patients had at least 1 prescription medication that could potentially interact with imatinib based on mechanism of action (e.g., metabolism pathways). The results of the study also found that the most frequent DDI was with paracetamol (acetaminophen), (77.4%), which resulted in an increased risk of paracetamol toxicity. Other study findings with greater than 10% of patients with potential DDIs were with proton pumps inhibitors (33.3% for omeprazole) or dexamethasone (23.7%) that could reduce imatinib's effectiveness, and with levothyroxine (18.5%) that could decrease levothyroxine's effectiveness. The suspected mechanisms of this drug interaction with levothyroxine are an induction by imatinib of nondeiodination clearance or induction by imatinib of uridine diphosphate glucuronyl transferases.[113,114] Study results also found that the most frequently used drugs that could increase imatinib toxicity were ketoconazole and clarithromycin (respectively, 5.1% and 4.7%).[112] The overall findings of this study suggest that at least 40% of patients who are receiving imatinib are at risk of DDIs and may reach an even higher rate according to the results of the study performed in SNIIRAM. The highest rate of potential DDIs in this study with imatinib was with the following agents: paracetamol, PPIs, dexamethasone, or levothyroxine. Based on the study findings, the investigators provided recommendations regarding the use of imatinib with specific agents. It is recommended that the reader refers to the package insert of imatinib for drug interactions and dosing guidelines. Further study regarding DDIs with imatinib, as well as other TKIs, is warranted.

With regard to selection of an antimalarial agent for D.T., chloroquine, mefloquine, and atovaquone-proguanil (Malarone) may have potential interactions with imatinib. The proguanil component is metabolized via the 2C19 pathway. Given the options that can be used for malaria prophylaxis in D.T., doxycycline would be an appropriate antimalarial agent used for malaria prophylaxis that does not interact with imatinib or D.T.'s other medications (Refer to Chapter 81 Parasitic Infections for malaria prophylaxis options). The most commonly reported adverse effects with doxycycline are GI effects, including nausea, vomiting, abdominal pain, and diarrhea. Esophageal ulceration associated with doxycycline is a rare but well-described adverse event. D.T. should be counseled to take doxycycline with food and plentiful fluids, in an upright position in order to minimize GI adverse effects. Because doxycycline can cause photosensitivity and D.T. will be on a safari, the risk of photosensitivity can be reduced by the use of an appropriate sunscreen and wearing protective clothing, including a hat. D.T. should also be counseled regarding the use of paracetamol (acetaminophen) and also to check in advance with his pharmacist before taking any natural products that may be metabolized via cytochrome P450.

RESOURCES AND EVIDENCE FOR CLINICAL DECISION SUPPORT

Healthcare providers have become increasingly challenged on devising optimal approaches to managing drug interactions. Patient safety initiatives have expanded in efforts to improve the healthcare delivery system with medication error prevention as a high-priority area. The consensus recommendations published by the expert group in 2015 have provided a road map for addressing the key concerns to improve the approach to evaluating DDI evidence for clinical decision-making.[5] As part of this process, it was important to review existing methods for evaluating DDIs. The Drug Interaction Probability Scale (DIPS), a 10-item scale, was developed to evaluate individual case reports for DDIs by assessing an adverse event for causality by a DDI.[115] This tool was developed to address limitations of previous assessment instruments, such as the Naranjo scale. The reader is referred to Appendix C of the consensus recommendations for further information regarding DIPS and other available instruments.[5] The expert group also discussed the current systematic approaches using clinical decision support (CDS) systems, their limitations, and the need for a new assessment instrument to objectively evaluate a body of evidence to establish the existence of a DDI. One of the key challenges of CDS systems is to determine what evidence is required for a DDI to be applicable to an entire drug class. Pharmacokinetic interactions are rarely generalizable to all agents within a drug class, and if there is class effect, the magnitude of the effect can often vary, which typically necessitates that each drug is reviewed individually. In some cases, pharmacokinetic interaction data may be extrapolated from one agent to other agents in the small class if the purported mechanism of interaction involves common pharmacologic effects.

To advance this important initiative, recently another group of experts convened to address the following: (1) to outline the process to use for developing and maintain a standard set of DDIs; (2) to determine the information that should be included in a knowledge base of standard DDIs; (3) to determine whether a list of contraindicated drug pairs can or should be established; and (4) to determine how to more intelligently filter DDI alerts.[116] Their recommendations for selecting drug–drug interactions for CDS were released in 2016. The reader is referred to both the 2015 and the 2016 recommendations.[5,116]

Because various avenues are examined to reduce the risk of drug interactions within society, it is essential as healthcare providers that we improve patient education regarding medication information. This strategy includes our communications with patients both verbal instructions and patient instruction leaflets given with the prescription. It is important to consider translation of information into different languages and to also promote culturally competent communication within every healthcare setting. The use of auxiliary warning labels placed on the medication package, books, and referring patients to quality health information on the internet. Pharmacists are uniquely positioned to provide important information regarding OTC medications, including herbal products when patients receive prescription information, and when they are seeking recommendations for OTC products.[117]

CONCLUSION

Given the complexities of data on drug interactions and the complexities within the healthcare systems, healthcare providers have become increasingly challenged on devising optimal approaches to managing drug interactions.[3] Patient safety initiatives have expanded in efforts to improve the healthcare delivery system with medication error prevention as a high-priority area. Medication errors may be related to professional practice, healthcare products, procedures, and systems, including prescribing, order communication, product labeling, packaging, nomenclature, compounding, dispensing, distribution, administration, education, monitoring, and use.[2,4] Because exposure to drug–drug interactions is a significant source of preventable drug-related harm, appropriate medication use, including drug interaction management, will avoid medication errors.[5]

Although the majority of drug interactions are clinically insignificant, in certain circumstances drug interactions are considered to be highly significant and can cause harm. Patients should be informed of the importance of maintaining a complete medication profile including over-the-counter medications, herbs, and dietary supplements. The incorporation of pharmacogenetic information into risk assessment of patients will improve our ability to prevent DDIs and to better evaluate interactions with biologic drugs.

More well-controlled studies are needed after drug approvals. Population-based studies are useful to determine the severity of, incidence of, and clinical importance of drug interactions. Pharmacogenetic research can further improve the precision of DDE evidence and CDS by identifying patient-specific predisposing factors. Future directives will identify the most appropriate process to rate the quality of DDI evidence and provided graded recommendations to reduce the risk of adverse consequences.[5]

KEY REFERENCES AND WEBSITES

A full list of references for this chapter can be found at http://thepoint.lww.com/AT11e. Below are the key references and websites for this chapter, with the corresponding reference number in this chapter found in parentheses after the reference.

Key References

Baxter K, Preston CL. Stockley's Drug Interactions. 10th ed London, Pharmaceutical Press, 2013.[Preston CL. Stockley's Drug Interactions Pocket Companion. Pharmaceutical press, 2015.] (61).

Caterina P, Antonello DP, Chiara G, et al. Pharmacokinetic drug-drug interaction and their implication in clinical management. *J Res Med Sci.* 2013;18:600-609.(3)

Scheife RT, et al. Consensus Recommendations for Systematic Evaluation of Drug-Drug Interaction Evidence for Clinical Decision Support. *Drug Saf.* 2015;38:197–206. (5)

Tilson H, Hines LE, McEvoy G, Weinstein DM, et al. Recommendations for selecting drug-drug interactions for clinical decision support. *Am J Health-System Pharm.* 2016;73(8):576-585.(116)

Key Websites

Hartshorn EA TD. Principles of drug interactions. *Facts & Comparisons* eAnswers Web site. http://online.factsandcomparisons.com.ezproxymcp.flo.org/Viewer.aspx?book=DIF&monoID=fandc-dif5444. Updated 2015. Accessed March 10, 2017.(60)

4 Pharmacogenomics and Personalized Medicine

Shannon F. Manzi, Laura Chadwick, and Jonathan D. Picker

CORE PRINCIPLES

		CHAPTER CASES
1	Pharmacogenomics is a single and important element of the broader concept of personalized medicine, which incorporates a variety of factors, both genetic and nongenetic, to guide targeted and individualized therapeutic decisions.	**Case 4-1 (Question 1), Figure 4-1, Tables 4-1, 4-2, 4-3**
2	Pharmacogenomic effects can be both pharmacokinetic and pharmacodynamic in nature. Pharmacokinetic effects are observed when variants affect the absorption, distribution, metabolism, or excretion of a drug. Pharmacodynamic polymorphisms may result in variable amounts of drug target enzymes or receptors as well as possible changes in the drug target shape. These variations may render therapy ineffective or necessitate dose changes in certain affected populations.	**Case 4-2 (Questions 1, 2)**
3	DNA polymorphisms in drug-metabolizing enzymes can result in gain of function, loss of function, or no effect on function of the enzyme produced. In some cases, significant toxicity can result.	**Case 4-3 (Question 1), Figure 4-2, Table 4-4, Case 4-4 (Question 1), Table 4-5**
4	Drug transport proteins and binding targets can also be affected by pharmacogenomic variants.	**Case 4-5 (Questions 1,2), Table 4-6**
5	HLA genes are unique in that the presence of a variant does not impact the metabolism of a drug, but instead may indicate the likelihood of the development of a serious or life-threatening reaction.	**Case 4-6 (Questions 1, 2), Table 4-7**
6	Test interpretation is crucial to the practical application of pharmacogenomic data. In particular, CYP2D6 is a well-described cytochrome P450 enzyme responsible for approximately 25% of all drug metabolism. However, *CYP2D6* is a complicated gene locus subject to multiple variants, pseudogene interference, and copy number variation.	**Case 4-7 (Questions 1, 2), Case 4-8 (Question 1), Table 4-8**
7	Age-based development adds a level of complexity when assessing pharmacogenomic markers in pediatric patients. Many of the pharmacogenomic dosing guidelines have not been validated in infants and children.	**Case 4-9 (Question 1), Figure 4-3**
8	Implementation of pharmacogenomics into practice currently faces many challenges including: the appropriate determination of when and whom to test; storage, analysis, and security of genetic data; and considerations for implementing pharmacogenomic data and recommendations into practice.	**Case 4-10 (Question 1), Case 4-11 (Questions 1, 2)**

"Pharmacogenomics" is the study and application of gene expression on drug pharmacokinetics and pharmacodynamics. This term is often used interchangeably with "pharmacogenetics." In the strictest of definitions, "pharmacogenetics" is used in the context of a drug response to a single gene, whereas "pharmacogenomics" refers to the broader study of the full genomic impact on drug behavior.[1] Because genetic variants are very specific to the individual, the use of pharmacogenomics in clinical practice has become a core component of the personalized medicine and precision medicine movements.[2,3] Ironically, the study of pharmacogenomics is not new. There are cases in the literature from the 1950s and 1960s describing the influence of a person's genetics on drug toxicity.[4,5] With the advent of newer, cheaper, faster deoxyribonucleic acid (DNA) sequencing techniques, the study of pharmacogenomics has exploded. In recent years, we have been able to begin transitioning that knowledge from the research realm to the clinic, although not without challenges.

A brief review of the basics of human genetics in the context of application to pharmacogenomics will be discussed in this chapter. Students are encouraged to utilize the selected references provided for this chapter for further review if needed. Although somatic "tumor" genetics, or the study of the mutations found in cancer cells, is a very timely and important consideration in antineoplastic drug selection and the treatment of oncologic processes, this chapter will primarily focus on the germline mutations in human DNA affecting drug absorption, distribution, metabolism, and excretion.

Human DNA is composed of 3 billion nucleotide base pairs, arranged on 46 chromosomes. There is significant variation in the genetic code from one person to another, creating what makes each of us unique—such as brown eyes, red hair, height, and heritable diseases. Included in the unique variations are changes in our ability to process medications. These differences are largely a result of variants in the nucleotide sequence on the genes responsible. The four nucleotides that make up the genes are adenine (A), guanine (G), cytosine (C), and thymine (T).

In most cases, but not all, two copies of each gene are present, one inherited from the mother and one from the father. Each copy is referred to as an "allele." If both the maternal and paternal alleles are the same, then the individual is considered homozygous for that allele or gene. If the parental copies differ, then the patient is considered to be heterozygous. Genes code for the production of proteins, such as enzymes, the structural components of cells, hormones, antibodies, and transport molecules. In pharmacogenomics, the gene and the enzyme often share the same name. For example, the gene that codes for cytochrome P450 CYP3A4 is known as *CYP3A4* and the gene that codes for thiopurinemethyltransferase (TPMT) is known as *TPMT*.

When there is a change in the sequence or code, it is referred to as a variant. A change in a single base pair is commonly referred to as a single-nucleotide polymorphism or SNP (pronounced "snip") (**Fig.4-1**). Although the formal definition requires the variant to occur in at least 1% of the population, common usage does not differentiate on the basis of population frequency. A SNP that changes the function of the gene product is referred to as a mutation, and although not all SNPs are mutations, the terms are often used interchangeably. The location of the SNP is designated by a reference sequence number abbreviated "rsID." Many of the pharmacogenetic variants discussed in this chapter are SNPs and were originally found through genome-wide association studies (GWAS). Most GWAS are usually constructed to find common SNPs in a group of patients with the condition of interest and then subsequently define a level of association. These SNPs are responsible for 90% of pharmacogenetic variability and can result in gain of function (greater production of enzyme, or higher enzyme activity, than normal) or loss of function (decreased or no production of enzyme compared to normal).[3] Other changes can include deletions or insertions of larger segments of DNA and are commonly referred to as "indels." In many cases, indels terminate production of the protein.

In some cases, a change in a single allele is sufficient to affect drug metabolism. This occurs in dominant disorders. These occur because new mutations are passed from one individual to the next. Whether the ancestors exhibited symptoms or not likely depends on their own history and, of course, may not be known. In other cases, both copies of the gene must be defective in order for there to be a functional consequence. This occurs in recessive disorders, in which the parents are typically unaffected heterozygous carriers. One in four of their children will be at risk for inheriting the change and potentially exhibiting symptoms. As discussed earlier, this child may be homozygous if both parents have the same SNP, or it may be as a compound heterozygote, if each parent has a different dysfunctional SNP or mutation in the specific gene. Typically, in recessive disorders, there is otherwise no family history of any affected individual.

The resultant call or read of the variants gives us a genotype. The phenotype refers to the expression of that genotype. In some cases, this is visible, such as skin color or another physical characteristic. In other cases it is invisible, such as blood type or a less than normal amount of a Human Cytochrome P450 (CYP450) metabolizing enzyme. In the context of pharmacogenomics and the metabolizing enzymes, patients are often classified as having a phenotype of ultrarapid metabolizer, extensive metabolizers, intermediate metabolizers, or poor metabolizers based on their genotype.[6] There are several other phenotypes that will be discussed in the chapter, particularly those that deal with drug targets or pharmacodynamic responses.

The vast majority of drug metabolism pathways are not simply, a single enzyme resulting in one inactive metabolite that is immediately excreted by the body. Instead, most drugs utilize multiple metabolizing enzyme pathways, rely on several drug transporters, and have many metabolites of varying activity. Each of these steps may be subject to variable gene expression, coupled with indirect genetic and environmental effects on variables such as disease, weight, nutrition, age, and others. Add this complexity and it becomes evident how complicated pharmacogenomic interpretations can be.

Pharmacogenomics is unique in the field of genetics in that the representation of a person's genotype is noted by a "*," known as a star allele in the literature. For example, in many situations, the text representation of normal or "wild-type" variant status is *1/*1.[7] As other alleles are discovered, they are numbered sequentially *2, *3, etc. Inevitably, as discoveries are sometimes reported simultaneously around the world, there is occasionally an overlap of star alleles and the variants represented. There are several worldwide databases for reporting new pharmacogenomic variants, including the CYP Allele Nomenclature Database http://www.cypalleles.ki.se/ and the Database of Genomic Variants http://dgv.tcag.ca/dgv/app/home.

During drug development and postmarketing analysis, it becomes clear that some patients will have severe adverse drug reactions (including nonresponse) after receiving the population-derived standard dose. These adverse reactions occur in the absence of medication error or lack of proper adherence to the drug. The Institute of Medicine "To Err is Human" report published in 2000 cited over 2 million reported adverse drug reactions in the United States per year, resulting in approximately 100,000 deaths at a cost of 20.6 billion annually.[8] It is estimated that 52% of U.S. adults are taking at least one prescription drug and 12% are taking more than five prescription drugs. If herbal products and over-the-counter drugs are included, then the estimates increase to over 80% and 29%, respectively.[6] It is well known that adverse drug reactions often go unnoticed and even more frequently unreported, making the actual numbers likely far higher. The clinical application of pharmacogenomics not only has allowed us to explain some of these historical reactions, but also helps clinicians predict who may be at higher risk for developing an adverse reaction if exposed to a drug or drug class.[9] Avoidance of adverse drug reactions has a measureable impact on a patient's quality of life, decreases overall health care costs, and lessens the time burden on health care providers managing the adverse reaction. However, acceptance

Figure 4-1 Example of a single-nucleotide polymorphism (SNP).

ACGTTGGATGTACTTTTGAGGAAATGAG: Wild type sequence initially described

ACGTTGGATGTGCTTTTGAGGAAATGAG: A>G variant

The change from A to G at position 12 in this gene sequence results in a SNP.

of clinical pharmacogenomic testing is not universal and there remains the challenge of conclusively validating the genetic variant associated with the adverse reaction.[10]

PHARMACOKINETIC IMPLICATIONS

CASE 4-1

QUESTION 1: A.S. is a 2-year-old diagnosed with active multidrug-resistant tuberculosis (TB). The Centers for Disease Control and Prevention treatment protocol recommends isoniazid, rifampin, ethambutol, and pyrazinamide for initial therapy. Her mother is concerned because several family members in their home country of China had developed serious "liver problems" when they took isoniazid and she insists on the "gene test" for A.S. What genetic testing is A.S.'s mother referring to and what are the risks of toxicity in relation to isoniazid therapy?

Isoniazid is part of the four-drug regimen used to treat active TB and latent TB infection because it is bactericidal against *Mycobacterium tuberculosis* organisms.[11] One of the most commonly reported side effects leading to premature discontinuation of the drug is drug-induced liver injury (DILI). Significantly elevated hepatic enzymes are seen in up to 20% of patients, with progression to hepatitis in a smaller percentage of those treated.[12]

The metabolism of isoniazid is complex, with a key enzyme within the pathway being *N*-acetyltransferase-2 (NAT2).[11] NAT2 acetylates both the parent drug and a hydrazine metabolite, converting the hydrazine metabolite to acetyl hydrazine (AcHz).[12] An alternative metabolic pathway for hydrazine results in a toxic reactive metabolite. When NAT2 function is decreased, this pathway dominates, resulting in increased DILI and toxicity.

The production of the NAT2 enzyme is generated from a gene of the same name, with several known polymorphisms leading to alleles associated with either slow or rapid acetylation rates. Individuals homozygous for alleles associated with loss of function are considered "slow acetylators," those homozygous for alleles associated with gain of function "rapid acetylators," and heterozygotes "intermediate acetylators" (**Table 4-1**). DILI has been found to be highest in patients who are slow acetylators.[12] In addition to isoniazid, NAT2 is also a known acetylator of other drugs and/or metabolites, although the clinical effects of *NAT2* genotype on these drugs are less well-studied, including: sulfonamides (sulfamethoxazole, metabolites of sulfasalazine), aromatic and aliphatic amines (procainamide, dapsone, metabolite of clonazepam, mescaline).[12]

The "gene test" mentioned by A.S.'s mother is likely a test for the *NAT2* gene. A variety of pharmacogenomic tests are available to examine SNPs in the *NAT2* gene and assign a patient's genotype, either as part of a more extensive gene panel or as a targeted assay. Preemptive *NAT2* testing prior to isoniazid therapy is not currently the standard of care; however, evidence suggests that in some populations with a high prevalence of DILI in slow acetylators, this may be beneficial.[14–18] Asian cohorts have been found to have the highest rates of DILI in the setting of a slow acetylator status (see summary of studies in **Table 4-2**). Although there are no formal dosing guidelines set for isoniazid therapy in the context of genotype or acetylator status, a study completed by Azuma et al. with 155 Japanese TB patients proposed a modified, genotype-based dosing regimen with successful clinically and statistically significant outcomes (results summarized in **Table 4-3**).[19]

There remain several pending questions as to how to most safely and appropriately incorporate *NAT2* genotype results into a widespread clinical application. For example, pediatric patients such as A.S. offer a unique set of challenges, because recommended isoniazid starting doses are within a higher range (10–15 mg/kg), and dose modifications based on genotype have not been studied in this population.[13] Genotype concordance with predicted phenotype has also been found to be lower in pediatric patients.[20] Additionally, ethnic variation among study results also suggests that testing may be more beneficial in certain groups, namely those with Asian ancestry. As is the case when using ethnicity to determine whether or not to complete any genetic test, self-reported ancestry is not always a reliable means of predicting someone's actual genetic lineage. With the generation of promising preliminary studies, a continued focus on *NAT2* genotype effects on isoniazid safety has the potential to result in institutions and organizations adopting policies to proactively test *NAT2* in the context of isoniazid treatment to both prevent adverse drug events and increase treatment success in the future.

PHARMACODYNAMIC IMPLICATIONS

CASE 4-2

QUESTION 1: E.F. is a 51-year-old male status post ST elevation myocardial infarction (STEMI) and atrial fibrillation with a residual left ventricular thrombus. Despite aggressive dose escalations of warfarin, his international normalized ratio (INR) will not budge above 1.7. His current dose of warfarin is 10 mg daily and he reports no dietary changes or excessive vitamin K intake. There are no drug–drug interactions identified in his regimen. The cardiology team asks about pharmacogenomic testing. What are the known genes involved in warfarin metabolism that would impact E.F.'s INR?

Table 4-1
NAT2 Genotypes and Phenotypes

***NAT2* Allele Activity**	
Slow	*5-7, *10, *12D, *14, *17, *19
Rapid	*4 (wild type), *11, *12A-C, *13, *18

***NAT2* Phenotype Summary**

Genotype	Acetylator Rate	Clinical Manifestation with Isoniazid Therapy
Homozygous slow	Slow	Increased risk of adverse drug events
Heterozygous	Intermediate	
Homozygous rapid	Fast/rapid	Possible increased risk of treatment

[a]Shown in a small number of studies.[13]

Table 4-2
Summary of *NAT2* Genotypes and Hepatotoxicity Risk with Isoniazid Studies

Study	Study Type	Population	Metric	Result
Sun et al.[14]	Meta-analysis ■ *N* = 5 case–control studies ■ 133 cases (hepatotoxicity) ■ 492 controls	Chinese Japanese East Indian Caucasian	Prevalence of SA status in hepatotoxicity cases vs. control	*Overall*: no significant finding *Asian subgroup analysis*: ↑ risk hepatotoxicity for SAs ■ OR 2.52 (CI 1.5–4.3)
Wang et al.[15]	Meta-analysis ■ *N* = 14 case–control studies 11 Asian, 3 non-Asian ■ 474 cases (hepatotoxicity) ■ 1,446 controls	Japan China Taiwan India Korea Turkey Switzerland USA (8%)	SA hepatotoxicity risk vs. RA	↑ risk hepatotoxicity for SAs ■ OR_Asian: 4.9 (CI 3.3–7.1) ■ OR_non-Asian: 3.7 (CI 1.3–10.5) ↑ risk hepatotoxicity in combination regimen
Ben Mahmoud et al.[16]	Observational Case–control ■ *N* = 65	Tunisian	SA hepatotoxicity risk vs. RA and IAs	↑ risk hepatotoxicity for SAs ■ OR 4.3; (CI 1.5–18)
Du et al.[17]	Meta-analysis ■ *N* = 26 studies ■ 1,198 cases ■ 2,921 controls	Asian Caucasian M.Eastern Brazilian	Prevalence of SA status in hepatotoxicity cases vs. control	*Overall:* ↑ risk hepatotoxicity for SAs ■ OR 3.1 (CI 2.5–3.9) *Caucasian:* no significant finding
Huang et al.[18]	Observational Case–control ■ *N* = 224	Taiwan	SA hepatotoxicity risk vs. RA	↑ risk hepatotoxicity for SAs ■ OR 2.8 (CI 1.3–6.2)
Pasipanodya et al.[13]	Meta-analysis ■ *N* = 3,471	UK Asia East Africa USA Prague	RA treatment failure risk vs. SA	↑ risk of treatment failure for RAs ■ RR 2 (CI 1.5–2.7)

SA, slow acetylator; RA, rapid acetylator; IA, intermediate acetylator; OR, odds ratio; CI, confidence interval.

Table 4-3
***NAT2* Genotype-Based Dosing Recommendations for Isoniazid**

Summary of Results from Azuma et al.[19]

	Genotype-Based Dosing Recommendation	AE	Standard (5 mg/kg)	Genotype-Based Dosing	*p*
Slow	50% dose decrease (~2.5 mg/kg)	DILI	78%	0%	0.003
		TF	22.9%[a]	0%	NR
Intermediate	Standard (5 mg/kg)	DILI	4.7%		NR
		TF	26.8%		NR
Rapid	50% dose increase (~7.5 mg/kg)	DILI	4.2%	4.6%	NS
		TF	38%	15%	0.013

DILI,drug-induced liver disease;TF,treatment failure; NR: no result; NS: nonsignificant.

Warfarin's mechanism of action is to inhibit the Vitamin K Epoxide Reductase Complex subunit 1 (VKORC1), a key enzymatic component in the vitamin K clotting pathway.[21] By inhibiting VKORC1, synthesis of the vitamin K–dependent clotting factors II, VII, IX, and X is reduced and anticoagulation is achieved in conditions where thrombosis is a concern, such as atrial fibrillation. The amount of VKORC1 present in a person is linked to the *VKORC1* gene, a key pharmacodynamic consideration. Patients with the GG genotype at *VKORC1* rs9923231 are considered warfarin insensitive, meaning they are likely to require larger doses of medication to effectively inhibit the VKORC1 pathway. The AA genotype has been associated with lesser amounts of VKORC1, and therefore, these patients are considered to be warfarin sensitive and may require lower doses of medication for inhibition and anticoagulation.[22]

Another significant factor affecting warfarin dosing and response is the effect of genetic variants on warfarin metabolism. Warfarin is taken orally as a racemic mixture of *R*- and *S*-enantiomers, and its subsequent metabolism is complex, involving multiple genes and pathways. The primary pathway of the *S*-enantiomer, the active form of the drug, is via the CYP2C9 enzyme.[22] CYP2C9 is the predominant enzyme pathway responsible for more than 25% of the variation in warfarin metabolism. *CYP2C9* is highly polymorphic, with several known variants within the population linked to reduced metabolic rates, including *CYP2C9* *2 and *3 alleles. Reduced warfarin metabolism leads to increased concentrations of the active form of the drug. These patients may require lower warfarin doses, and thus may be at increased risk of bleeding using standard dosing algorithms.[22]

A more recent gene of focus with limited evidence relating to warfarin sensitivity is *CYP4F2*.[23] CYP4F2 affects the metabolism and therefore physiologic levels of vitamin K. Patients with the TT genotype for *CYP4F2* rs2108622 are thought to maintain higher concentrations of vitamin K, and therefore require approximately 1 mg/day more warfarin than patients with the CC genotype.[23] Although current dosing models focus strictly on genotype for *CYP2C9* and *VKORC1* for warfarin initiation, *CYP4F2* has shown early promise as a potential factor for strengthening the effectiveness of dose prediction algorithms in some ethnicities.[24]

It is important to remember that many nongenetic factors such as age, weight, diet, smoking status, and medication interactions contribute to a great variability of warfarin dosing among patient populations. Drug–drug interactions in which the CYP2C9 enzyme may be induced or inhibited will affect the rate of warfarin metabolism. Additionally, a diet high in vitamin K will make warfarin less effective, because this facilitates increased synthesis of vitamin K–dependent clotting factors. Algorithms for determining appropriate starting doses for patients over the age of 18 years based on both nongenetic and genetic factors are available at www.warfarindosing.org. Close monitoring of INR is also typically recommended to ensure proper anticoagulation and reduced risk of bleeding.

Case 4-2, Question 2: What other drugs are significantly affected by the CYP2C9 pathway?

CYP2C9 is estimated to play a role in the metabolism of up to 20% of commonly used medications.[25] From these medications, several associations have been found linking variants in the CYP2C9 pathway due to both increased rates of adverse drug events and variable medication response. Examples of such drugs include phenytoin, certain nonsteroidal anti-inflammatory drugs (such as celecoxib and diclofenac), sulfonylureas, losartan, and certain statins (such as fluvastatin and simvastatin). Patients with *2 or *3 alleles may be at increased risk of toxicities at standard doses of drugs that are processed through the CYP2C9 pathway decreased due to metabolism and increased parent drug concentrations and may require reduced dosing or increased monitoring.

TOXICITY IMPLICATIONS

Many known variants exist within the genes that code for enzyme proteins, affecting the rate at which the enzyme is able to metabolize drugs through its pathway. These variants may result in either reduced enzyme function and increased concentration of parent drug, or increased enzyme activity with decreased concentrations of a parent drug. The clinical effects of the variants depend on whether the parent drug is pharmacologically active or a prodrug.

CASE 4-3

Question 1: T.B. is a 28 kg, 5-year-old male admitted for status epilepticus treated with IV lorazepam and IV fosphenytoin on presentation, aborting the seizures. Past medical history is significant for congenital hydrocephalus, a ventriculoperitoneal shunt and refractory epilepsy secondary to an in utero right middle cerebral artery stroke. On day 5 of his hospitalization, he is still extremely lethargic and his free phenytoin level is high, peaking at 3 mcg/mL on day 2 and 1.4 mcg/mL on day 5 (see **Fig. 4-2**). Looking at his records, he received an appropriate initial loading dose of IV fosphenytoin18 mg phenytoin sodium equivalents (PE)/kg (500 mg PE) followed by a single maintenance dose of IV fosphenytoin140 mg PE (5 mg PE/kg) 5 hours later on day 1 of the hospitalization. He has no clinically relevant drug–drug interactions and his albumin is normal. What is a possible reason for the toxicity T.B. is experiencing?

Phenytoin/fosphenytoin serum concentrations can be difficult to control and are complicated by multiple factors including Michaelis–Menton kinetics, also known as capacity limited metabolism. Drugs that follow Michaelis–Menton kinetics go from first to zero order, meaning that metabolism increases with increasing concentration until enzyme saturation takes place.[26] Once saturation is reached, drug plasma concentrations can increase to toxic levels in a fast and unpredictable manner. Additionally, many factors affect an individual's safe and effective phenytoin dose, including albumin levels, other medications in the patient's regimen, and pharmacogenetics.

Phenytoin has many chronic effects associated with long-term use, including hepatotoxicity, osteoporosis, megaloblastic anemia, gingival hyperplasia, hirsutism, and peripheral neuropathy.[27] In the acute setting of toxic plasma concentrations or an overdose, phenytoin toxicity can manifest with a variety of signs and symptoms, including CNS effects (dizziness, confusion, drowsiness, and ataxia) as well as GI upset and nausea. Phenytoin is also associated with severe cutaneous reactions such as Stevens–Johnson syndrome (SJS) and toxic epidermal necrolysis (TEN) (see section with Case 4-6).

Fosphenytoin is a prodrug, converted by plasma esterases to the active drug phenytoin. Phenytoin is further metabolized by CYP2C9 to phenytoin arene-oxide, which is then broken down to multiple metabolites that are eventually excreted.[27] The contribution of these various metabolites to toxicity and efficacy of phenytoin is not well understood.

T.B. is found to have a loss of function variant status in *CYP2C9* *1/*2. With loss of CYP2C9 enzyme function comes decreased breakdown of the active drug phenytoin at standard doses. Given the narrow therapeutic index of phenytoin and the drug's propensity to cause side effects, T.B. ultimately experienced drug toxicity and accompanying symptoms. The evidence relating genotypes such

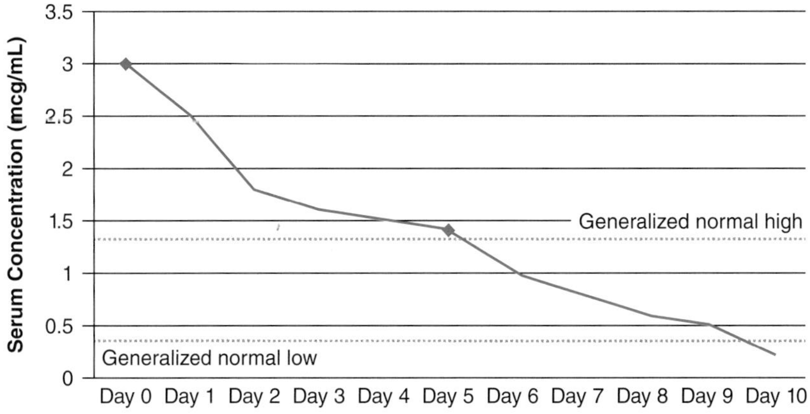

Figure 4-2 Free phenytoin levels (Case 4-3).

as T.B.'s to the development of adverse drug events is strong, and the Clinical Pharmacogenetics Implementation Consortium (CPIC, pronounced "See-Pick") has published dosing guidelines based on *CYP2C9* genotype summarized in **Table 4-4**.[28] Note that only the maintenance, not the loading dose, has adjustment recommendations ensuring that acute seizure activity can adequately be terminated.

CASE 4-4

QUESTION 1: J.P. is a 50-kg, 17-year-old female, status post kidney transplant. She is currently receiving azathioprine 100 mg PO daily to prevent rejection. She is brought to the emergency department 5 days after starting the medication complaining of lethargy, fever, and malaise. A white blood cell count comes back as a critically low value at 900 cells/μL (normal range,3.8–9.8 × $10^3/\mu$L), with an absolute neutrophil count (ANC) of 760 cells/μL (neutropenia defined as an ANC ≤ 2,000 cells/μL). What factors might explain the severe neutropenia and what test should be ordered for J.P.?

Azathioprine is an immunosuppressive agent in the thiopurine class, acting as a prodrug of 6-mercaptopurine. These drugs are purine analogs and antagonize purine synthesis, inhibiting synthesis of DNA, RNA, and proteins.[29] Thiopurines are used in a variety of conditions including renal transplant, rheumatoid arthritis, certain cancers, and inflammatory bowel disease.

Azathioprine is metabolized to an active drug 6-mercaptopurine via glutathione *S*-transferase (GST) reduction. 6-mercaptopurine is then converted into the active 6-methylmercaptopurine ribonucleotide (6-MMPR) and several inactive metabolites such as 6-methylmercaptopurine (6-MMP) through multiple pathways.[30] The two primary enzymes contributing to 6-mercaptopurine breakdown are TPMT and hypoxanthine-guanine phosphoribosyltransferase (HPRT). Although TPMT metabolism results in the generation of the inactive metabolite 6-MMP, HPRT contributes to a pathway that leads to the generation of active 6-MMPR and 6-thioguanine nucleotide (6-TGN) metabolites.[31] Furthermore, active 6-TGN metabolites are then inactivated by TPMT. The accumulation of active 6-TGN metabolites via HPRT is associated with myelosuppression with thiopurine therapy. In summary, TMPT acts as the detoxifying enzyme for drugs in the thiopurine class and its activity is directly linked to risk of drug toxicities.

The severe neutropenia J.P. experienced 5 days after beginning azathioprine is very likely the result of starting a full dose (2 mg/kg/day) in the setting of a homozygous variant *TPMT* genotype, such as *3B/*3C. Because of the near-absent enzyme level produced by homozygous variants, the TGN metabolites build up, resulting in severe and sometimes life-threatening neutropenia.

It is important to note that the genotype *3B/*3C is nearly impossible to distinguish from the less clinically impactful heterozygous genotype of *1/*3A on most commercially available *TPMT* assays. In cases of suspected homozygous variant status, parental studies may be necessary for absolute determination. Alternative therapy or a 90% reduction in the azathioprine dose is advised for J.P.'s *TPMT* genotype.[32] In the case of a heterozygous genotype such as *1/*3C, the dose would be decreased by 30%–70% (**Table 4-5**).[32]

Table 4-4
***CYP2C9* Genotype-Based Dosing Recommendations for Phenytoin/Fosphenytoin**

CYP2C9 Metabolizer Status	Sample Genotype(s)	Recommendation
Extensive metabolizer	*1/*1	Initiate therapy with recommended maintenance dose
Intermediate metabolizer	*1/*2, *1/*3	Consider 25% reduction of recommended starting maintenance dose and adjust according to therapeutic drug monitoring and response
Poor metabolizer	*2/*2, *3/*3, *2/*3	Consider 50% reduction of recommended starting maintenance dose and adjust according to therapeutic drug monitoring and response

DRUG TARGET IMPLICATIONS

CASE 4-5

QUESTION 1: L.K. is a 45-year-old woman referred for interpretation of pharmacogenomic results provided by a certified clinical lab as part of a research study. The report states that the called genotype for *SLCO1B1* is CC. L.K. asks if she is at risk for severe muscle pain, or myopathy, which she heard about on a recent television malpractice commercial. What information do you need to answer her question?

Table 4-5
Summary of CPIC Guidelines for TPMT Genotype-Based Thiopurine Dosing

Phenotype (Genotype)	Sample Genotype(s)	Implication for Thiopurine Pathway	Thiopurine Dosing Recommendations
Normal/High Activity (Homozygous wild-type)	*1/*1	Lower concentrations of TGN metabolites	Start with normal starting dose and adjust doses of thiopurine based on disease-specific guidelines. Allow 2 weeks to reach steady state after each dose adjustment.
Intermediate activity (Heterozygous)	*1/*2, *1/*3A, *1/*3B, *1/*3C, *1/*4	Moderate to high concentrations of TGN metabolites	Consider starting at 30-70% of target dose for azathioprine and 6-mercaptopurine and 30-50% of target dose for thioguanine. Titrate based on tolerance. Allow 2-4 weeks to reach steady state after each dose adjustment.
Low/deficient activity (Homozygous variant/mutant)	*3A/*3A, *2/*3A, *3C/*3A, *3C/*4, *3C/*2, *3A/*4	Extremely high concentrations of TGN metabolites	Consider alternative agents. If using thiopurine, start with drastically reduced doses (reduce daily dose by 10-fold and dose thrice weekly instead of daily) and adjust doses based on degree of myelosuppression and disease-specific guidelines. Allow 4-6 weeks to reach steady state after each dose adjustment.

Source: MV Relling, EE Gardner, WJ Sandborn, et al. Clinical Pharmacogenetics Implementation Consortium Guidelines for Thiopurine Methyltransferase Genotype and Thiopurine Dosing. *Clin Pharmacol Ther*. 2011 Mar;89(3):387–91.

Table 4-6
***SLCO1B1* Genotype-Based Dosing Recommendations for HMG-CoA Reductase Inhibitors**

***SLCO1B1* rs4149056 Genotype**	**Myopathy Risk with Simvastatin Use**	**Simvastatin Dosing Recommendation**
TT	Normal	Prescribe standard starting dose and modify based on tolerance and disease response
TC	Intermediate	Prescribe a lower dose or consider alternative statin (such as pravastatin or rosuvastatin). Routine monitoring of CK may be considered
CC	High	Prescribe a lower dose or consider alternative statin (such as pravastatin or rosuvastatin). Routine monitoring of CK may be considered

"Statins" or HMG-CoA reductase inhibitor drugs are associated with muscle toxicity, ranging from mild aches to the development of severe debilitating myopathy and rhabdomyolysis in a segment of the population.[33] Regardless of severity, this adverse drug event is a common cause for drug discontinuation.[34] Recent published literature links this risk of developing these muscle-related side effects to certain variants in the *SLCO1B1* gene.

Keeping in mind that a raw result from DNA analysis is essentially a string of A's, C's, T's, and G's within each individual gene, the CC genotype for SLCO1B1 information provided by L.K. is insufficient. In order to review available evidence, it is essential to know the actual variant location that the CC call was based upon. Although there are multiple polymorphisms that have been identified in the *SLCO1B1* gene, only few are linked to clinical effect.[35] The majority of laboratory interpretation will call out the relevant rs numbers needed to make a pharmacogenomic determination of drug selection and dose alteration. An rs number, or rsID, is used to point to a specific nucleotide location within a gene. Known SNPs within a gene are defined by rsID for the purpose of clinical guidelines and research reporting. This ensures standardization and proper assessment of variants. For *SLCO1B1*, the rsID most commonly associated with development of myopathy with HMG-CoA reductase inhibitors is rs4149056.[35] This rsID should be provided with any result in order to make the proper assessments and recommendations.

CASE 4-5, QUESTION 2: The clinical lab confirms the SLCO1B1 genotype CC call was based on rs4149056. What is your answer to L.K.'s question regarding her risk of developing severe myopathy?

The C allele at *SLCO1B1* rs4149056 has been associated with decreased statin intracellular transport and clearance.[34] SLCO1B1 is a transporter protein with a primary function of drug uptake into the liver. Variants affecting the hepatic uptake of drugs via SLCO1B1 ultimately increase overall area under the curve and drug exposure, resulting in higher risks of adverse drug events such as myopathy. Patients with homozygous variant status such as L.K. are at significantly increased risk of developing muscle toxicity with statin use. Although all statins may have adverse event profiles linked to this variant, the evidence is strongest for simvastatin. Published CPIC guidelines for simvastatin with *SLCO1B1* rs4149056 variant status are summarized in **Table 4-6**.

NONMETABOLISM IMPLICATIONS

CASE 4-6

QUESTION 1: J.C. is an 18-year-old female with a past medical history of epilepsy. Following a failed course of levetiracetam, her physician has decided to start her on carbamazepine therapy for seizure control. Approximately 2 months after starting the drug, J.C. is seizure free but feels as though she is coming down with what feels like a cold with accompanying headache and fever. She also begins to notice that her skin is becoming red and itchy in several locations. The rash quickly progresses to the point where she notes swelling and the formation of blisters on her nostrils, eyes and lips. J.C. realizes that she is experiencing something more than a common cold and rash, and calls the pharmacy in a panic to ask if it is possible that she is reacting to her medication, even though she has been on it for some time. Given the known side effects of carbamazepine, is it possible that J.C.is reacting to the medication?

Adverse drug reactions are often thought of as happening acutely following initial doses of medications; however, delayed hypersensitivities are also possible with certain drugs. In the case of carbamazepine, these reactions are linked to DNA changes within the human leukocyte antigen (HLA) genes. There is a strong association between positive *HLA-B*15:02* gene variant carrier status and increased risk of severe cutaneous adverse reactions.[36] A less established link has also been seen with carriers of the *HLA-A*31:01* variant, more common in Japanese and Caucasians.[37]

The HLA genes code for proteins that form an immunologic complex on all nucleated cells. This complex is responsible for presenting both self- and foreign peptides to immune cells, such as T-cells.[38] When a foreign peptide is presented and then recognized by a T-cell, an immunologic response results. Examples of peptides that may be recognized as foreign include viruses, bacteria, tumor antigens, and drugs. Although this may be the basis for the drug-induced reactions seen with the described HLA variants, there is still significant uncertainty that this is truly the only mechanism in play. Evidence has suggested that drug concentrations are also higher in patients who experience cutaneous reactions, meaning that CYP loss-of-function alleles as well as HLA variants may work synergistically to increase a patient's risk of SJS and TEN.[39] This is supported by the fact that not all patients who carry an HLA allele will experience a cutaneous reaction.[38]

HLA Class I genes are highly polymorphic.[40] Variants within these genes are thought to result in structural changes in the HLA complex that increase the recognition and subsequent response of the immune system to certain drugs, resulting in hypersensitivity. Reactions related to these variants tend to be dermatologic in nature with or without systemic involvement, ranging from a mild maculopapular rash or progressing to more severe cases of SJS and TEN.

CASE 4-6, QUESTION 2: What is the appropriate advice for the pharmacist to provide to J.C. given her presentation?

J.C. should be advised to seek care immediately at the closest and most accessible hospital emergency department. SJS and TEN have significant associated complications, and typically require inpatient treatment with fluids, corticosteroids, analgesics, nutritional supplementation, and antibiotics. Mortality rates with TEN are estimated to be higher than 30%.[38] In all cases, the suspected offending agent should be discontinued with no attempt to rechallenge.

CASE 4-6, QUESTION 3: In questioning J.C., the pharmacist learns that she has no prior history of adverse drug or food reactions.

Table 4-7
HLA Variants, Affected Drugs, and Population Incidence

HLAVariant	Drugs with Associated Adverse Cutaneous Reactions	Highest Variant Frequencies by Ethnicity
*HLA-B**57:01	Abacavir	Caucasian: 5%–8%
*HLA-B**58:01	Allopurinol	Han Chinese: 6%–8% Korean: 12%
*HLA-B**15:02	Phenytoin, Carbamazepine	Han Chinese: ~10%[44] Populations from Hong Kong, Thailand, Malaysia, Vietnam, Philippines, India, and Indonesia: >5%
*HLA-A**31:01	Carbamazepine	Northern European: 2%–5% Japanese: 9% Chinese: 3.7%[45]

She is of Chinese descent, and has never had genetic testing. What would have been the more appropriate course of action for a patient with J.C.'s history prior to starting carbamazepine therapy?

Carriers of certain HLA variants are at increased risk of cutaneous adverse drug reactions; however, recommendations and guidelines for preemptive testing are either nonspecific or lacking. Other HLA variants have been linked to liver injury, leading to the theory that the burden of HLA expression may be an important factor in the organ systems affected.[38] Much is left to the provider or institution-specific protocols to determine when and whom to test prior to therapy. An exception to this is the antiretroviral medication, abacavir, for which CPIC and FDA recommendations are in place stating that all patients should have *HLA-B**57:01 testing before initiating this regimen.[41]

Of note, HLA variants are reported as positive (at least one variant present) or negative (no variant present). Variants of the HLA genes are seen more commonly within certain ethnicities. In some cases, because of the high prevalence of allele carrier status in these populations, patients with particular ethnic backgrounds may be recommended for testing. Certain Asian populations in particular are known to have higher rates of certain variants, warranting caution when using particular therapies (see **Table 4-7**). In the case of carbamazepine and J.C., her physician may have justifiably ordered pharmacogenomic testing to determine her *HLA-B**15:02 carrier status on the fact that she identifies as Chinese. Relying on self-reported ethnicity can be problematic, however, as many people are not fully knowledgeable of their complete lineage.

Although recommendations for testing vary, for every drug with established clinical guidelines, if a patient is a known carrier of an HLA variant, it is recommended that they avoid the use of drugs for which there is an HLA variant–associated risk of adverse reaction.[38,42–44]

THE PECULIARITIES OF CYP2D6

CASE 4-7

Question 1: P.F. is a 37-year-old female with a history of depression and anxiety who presents to the local pharmacy with a printed report from a for-profit pharmacogenomic testing company. The report states that P.F. is an extensive metabolizer for CYP2D6 and she is concerned that her paroxetine is still not providing any relief of her depressive symptoms despite having taken the drug correctly for the past 3 months. What information do you want to know about the testing modality the company used prior to answering her question regarding the interpreted genotype?

There are several pharmacogenomic testing platforms available. The vast majority of panels that are available commercially are SNP based. The advantages to SNP-based platforms include a lower cost, faster turnaround time, vendor-provided interpretation software, and reliable calling for known variants. The main disadvantage to the SNP-based platforms is that the user is limited only to the genes and specific variants on the panel. If there are any unique or rare variants, the SNP-based panel will not detect them. Therefore, the patient's reported genotype will not match their phenotype (how they actually respond to the drug). Additionally, in the case of *CYP2D6*, it is a very polymorphic gene that frequently has more than two copies. This is referred to as copy number variation (CNV) and is extremely important in the interpretation of a patient's CYP2D6 genotype.[46,47] All of the copies should be typed, and this is not always possible on commercially available assays because it requires extra primers and interpretation algorithms. Another issue is that *CYP2D7* is a pseudogene (a gene with no function) that can be accidentally included in the *CYP2D6* assay if it has not been designed correctly.[48]

Pharmacogenetic data can be the by-product of other genetic assays as well. The exome is considered the workhorse or coding region of the DNA. Whole exome sequencing or sequencing of targeted regions of interest can provide significant pharmacogenomic data as long as the level of coverage of the genes of interest is adequate. This may include variants that may have only been reported once or twice before in the literature or variants of unknown significance (VUS). These findings become a challenge to manage and to provide meaningful interpretation to the patients. Additionally, in both exome and whole genome sequencing, incidental or secondary findings of disease state markers will become paramount to deal with making the case for pharmacogenomics (see section with Case 4-8). The hybrid test, a sequence-based targeted panel of pharmacogenes, has become a hot area of development, attempting to incorporate the best features of both sequencing and limited gene interrogation.

In the case of P.F., the report shows a genotype of *CYP2D6* *1/*2 but does not indicate the copy number of the *CYP2D6* gene. This is a red flag for interpretation and should prompt the

Table 4-8
CYP2D6 Genotypes, Phenotypes, and Activity Scores

Number of Copies	Genotype	Activity Score	Phenotype
≤2	*1/*2	1.0–2.0	Extensive metabolizer
>2	*1/*2	2.0	Ultrarapid metabolizer

pharmacist to call the company to obtain a detailed explanation of the assay used and how the interpretation of extensive metabolizer was determined.

Case 4-7, Question 2: Per the company, the copy number was equal to 3. Does this change the interpretation of P.F.'s phenotype?

With a copy number of 3, a genotype of *CYP2D6* *1/*2 is associated with an ultrarapid metabolizer phenotype.[49] Unique to *CYP2D6*, an activity score is calculated based on the number of copies of the gene present as all contribute toward drug metabolism. The activity score was described by Gaedigk[46] to better categorize the metabolism status of persons with multiple copies of the gene. An example of how this can change a phenotype is represented in **Table 4-8**.[46]

The lack of response demonstrated by P.F. to the standard dose of paroxetine fits the phenotype of an ultrarapid metabolizer. The recommendation per the CPIC guideline would be to choose another drug not primarily metabolized via the CYP2D6 pathway.[47] This case provides a prime example of how time can be wasted and patient morbidity increased due to lack of response when pharmacogenomic markers are not considered prior to initiating therapy.

CASE 4-8

Question 1: You have started work at a pediatric hospital and notice that codeine is not orderable in the electronic medical record. When you ask a coworker, they inform you that the black box warning placed on all codeine products by the FDA in 2012 has resulted in the majority of pediatric institutions removing the drug from the formulary. What genotype is correlated with the risk of life-threatening apnea?

Codeine is metabolized by CYP2D6 to the active metabolite morphine, which provides analgesic properties. For patients with the ultrarapid metabolizer status described earlier, the amount of morphine generated can exceed the body's ability to convert to less toxic metabolites, resulting in life-threatening apnea.[48] The ultrarapid metabolizer phenotype is found in up to 4% of the population.[49] In contrast, there are several loss-of-function variants with far-ranging incidence across ethnicities. For example, the *4 allele is found in 6% of African-Americans, 5% of Asians, and up to 18% of European-Americans/Europeans.[50] These variants confer little to no enzyme function, resulting in lack of morphine formation. Patients with these genotypes will not have the desired analgesic response to codeine.[50]

DEVELOPMENTAL IMPACT AND PHARMACOGENOMICS

CASE 4-9

Question 1: As part of a voluntary research study in the NICU, pharmacogenomic results are returned to the provider for a baby girl born at 30 weeks, who is now at corrected 36.5-week gestational age. The provider notes that the genotype is CYP2C19 *17/*17 gain of function, indicating she is an ultrarapid metabolizer. The provider states he would like to start her on voriconazole for a presumed fungal infection and asks what the dosing should be in context of her genotype. What other information would be necessary to recommend a voriconazole dose for this baby?

Voriconazole is metabolized by CYP3A4, CYP2C9, and CYP2C19, with the most significant contribution coming from CYP2C19.[9] The Royal Dutch Pharmacists Association has guidelines in place recommending monitoring of voriconazole serum concentrations for CYP2C19 poor and intermediate metabolizers, as these patients have been found to have higher concentrations of active drug and increased risk of toxicity. The consideration for a person with the *CYP2C19* *17/*17 is the potential for increased breakdown of active drug and treatment failure.[51]

Given this patient's age, there are multiple complex factors that need to be considered for dosing, both genetic and nongenetic. As voriconazole is dosed by body weight, the actual body weight of the child is necessary for an appropriate dose calculation.[52] Drug–drug interactions may also need to be considered in the event that the patient is receiving medications that induce or inhibit enzymes in the drug's pathway. Other variables also contributing to complicated infant dosing and clearance unpredictability include developing gastrointestinal and renal function and fluctuations in body fat and water composition affecting volume of drug distribution.[53] Additionally, although the patient's genotype suggests that she will have increased breakdown of the active drug, it is known that regardless of genotype, humans are not born with fully functional CYP enzymes.[53]

CYP enzyme development occurs at variable rates over time making it difficult to determine the contribution of pharmacogenomic variants on optimal dosing (see **Fig. 4-3**). An excellent summary review of enzyme maturation by Kearns and colleagues was published in the *NEJM* in 2003.[53] CYP1A2, for example, is virtually undetectable at birth, with initial development of low-level enzyme concentrations observed over the first month

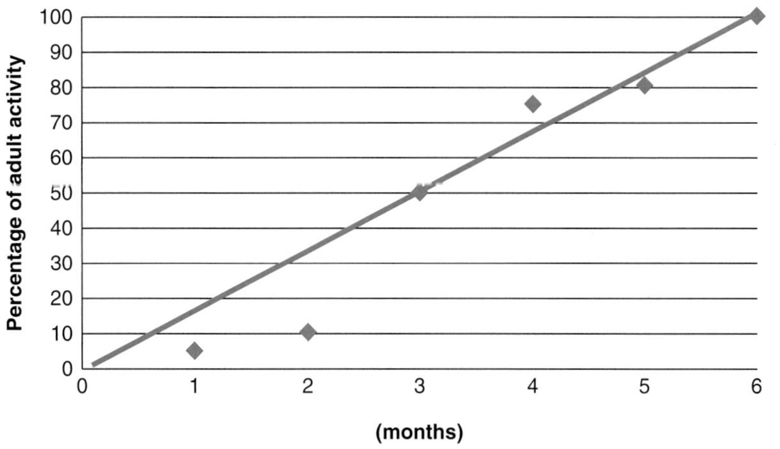

Figure 4-3 CYP2C19 enzyme activity by age.

of life.[54,55] Although general trends are observed, it is also understood that among individuals, development rates vary throughout childhood, particularly in the first year of life.[54] Given this consideration, pharmacogenomics in the infant population may be less of reliable factor than it is in adults, and its overall contribution remains unpredictable as few studies are dedicated to the effects of pharmacogenomic variants in younger individuals. Therefore, it is particularly important in children and infants to monitor for drug concentrations, response, and toxicities, and to adjust dose accordingly.[55] Voriconazole is of particular concern with this group, with evidence suggesting that current pediatric dosing recommendations may lead to subtherapeutic concentrations and a general increased risk of treatment failure.[55]

FAMILY IMPLICATIONS OF PHARMACOGENETICS

CASE 4-10

QUESTION 1: A 12-year-old-girl has an operation and develops malignant hyperthermia (MH) upon initiation of anesthesia. Subsequently, she is found to have a c. 7300G>A mutation in the *RYR1* gene, a common variant associated with predisposition for MH. Following her recovery and discussion of future medical and drug management, what else would be important to discuss?

Genes are inherited; therefore, any discussion of genetic variants must be undertaken with an awareness of the greater implications of any identified changes. In this case especially, because the consequences of the gene change are so profound and the mutation is a dominant one, it is likely that she inherited the change. An exploration of the family history may suggest that one parent is more likely to be the carrier than another, and counseling with a view toward testing may well be guided by such information. Furthermore, one must consider the potential for siblings, grandparents, and the extended family to be affected depending on the severity of the variant status and the clinical picture.

In the situation where the individual is being counseled for pharmacogenomic testing presymptomatically, it is important to raise the possibility that the results may have implications for the greater family before testing is undertaken.[58]

MAKING THE CASE FOR PHARMACOGENETICS

Pharmacogenomics has allowed pharmaceutical companies to design and develop drugs specifically targeted at certain mutations. In order to determine the right patient for the drug, companion tests (pharmacogenetic assays that target the variants of interest) are usually required. The pharmacist must understand which medications require companion testing and be able to interpret the results. Although up to 50% of drug companies are pursuing drug targets that would require companion genetic tests, there are several hindrances that must be addressed, including potential delays in companion test approval and potentially decreasing the patient base by eliminating those who would otherwise be prescribed the drug in the absence of knowledge of the genetic marker presence.[2] Additionally, several studies have shown that patients are more adherent with their medications after having personalized genotyping, even if the results show "normal" enzyme function.[59]

CASE 4-11

QUESTION 1: K.D. is a 22-year-old female with cystic fibrosis. Her pulmonologist is interested in the new drug ivacaftor, but is unsure what testing is required to start therapy. What testing is necessary and which variants qualify for ivacaftor therapy?

Ivacaftor (Kalydeco) is a drug for cystic fibrosis that targets ten specific variants in the Cystic Fibrosis Transmembrane Regulator (*CFTR*) gene. If a patient has a variant status other than G551D, G1244E, G1349D, G178R, G551S, R117H, S1251N, S1255P, S549N, or S549R, the drug will be ineffective.[60]

The *CFTR* gene codes for the CFTR protein on a variety of tissue surfaces, including the lungs. When functioning properly, the CFTR protein is a key component in maintaining intracellular salt balance.[61] In cystic fibrosis, because of a variety of possible genetic mutations the CFTR protein fails to function properly leading to fluid imbalances, the buildup of secretions, and several related complications. Ivacaftor acts as a CFTR potentiator increasing chloride ion transport, restoring electrolyte balance, reducing the buildup of secretions, and improving health outcomes such as pulmonary function and weight gain for affected patients.[62] The approval of this drug in 2012 for patients with the G551D mutation offered promise for continued future development of therapies targeting causes of disease that are genetically associated. This promise remains encouraging as the use of ivacaftor has since been approved in the treatment of several additional gene mutations, and new similar targeted therapies such as lumacaftor (Orkambi), a CFTR corrector, continue to enter the market.[63]

Another potential use of pharmacogenomics involves salvaging drugs with high toxicity profiles. Historically, drugs have been taken off the market after an unacceptable number of patients either suffered significant morbidity or mortality secondary to the use of the drug. In some cases, pharmacogenomic studies may be able to determine which patients could continue to benefit from the drug and which for patients' use must be avoided.

Despite all of the advances in testing and application, pharmacogenomic preemptive testing (testing prior to the development of an adverse effect or lack of response) is not currently in wide use. There are several reasons for this. The lack of knowledge by healthcare professionals, including pharmacists, is a large barrier. One recent study demonstrated that only 29% of the physicians surveyed had received any formal education and only 10.3% felt knowledgeable enough to prescribe or discuss the results of pharmacogenomic testing.[64] Another large impediment to implementation is the lack of consistent reimbursement by insurance providers. Consistent coverage by insurance companies will require regulatory effort and additional proof that pharmacogenomic testing improves outcome and decreases cost.[2]

Therefore, at this time, the majority of preemptive testing is being done in academic medical centers, in cancer centers, or by for-profit pharmacogenomic testing companies that can either institutionally support the development of the programs or can directly bill for the services not covered by insurance.

CASE 4-11, QUESTION 2: What references could be used to assist in interpretation of pharmacogenomic markers and subsequent drug dosing recommendations?

Currently, the FDA lists pharmacogenomic markers in 190 drug labels and the European Medicines Agency lists pharmacogenomic information in 78 drug labels.[65,66] In order to be included in the FDA labeling, the pharmacogenomic marker must have actionable data, such as an increase in adverse effects or reduction in efficacy in patients with certain variants. Guidelines for drug dosing and selection have been developed by the Clinical Pharmacogenomics Implementation Consortium (CPIC) and the Pharmacogenetics Working Groups of the Royal Dutch Pharmacists Association (DPWG). Each guideline is rated on the level of evidence available to support the recommendation. Currently, there are 36 CPIC Level I evidence published guidelines available on www.pharmgkb.org, a website supported by the NIH and hosted by Stanford University.[67] The site houses a wealth of information including pathway diagrams, annotated bibliographies, and lookup tables. It is important to note, the guidelines do not address who should be tested, but instead focus on what to do with the data if it is available.

Incorporating pharmacogenomic data into the electronic medical record systems used by many hospitals, clinics, pharmacies, and primary care offices is challenging at best. Result reports from the laboratories capable of running these tests are rarely in a machine-readable format and are generally scanned as pdf documents to the medical record.[68] This becomes a major challenge for the system to be able to provide relevant pharmacogenomic data at the time it is needed, usually during prescribing of a drug. Results of this type that persist throughout a person's lifetime and are relevant all along the continuum require significant bioinformatics expertise to house, retrieve, interpret, and present to the end user at the right time.[69] Additionally, understanding that the testing will evolve over time, either resulting in the need to sequence a new sample or ideally, reanalyzing the previously deep sequenced sample with new algorithms to apply the most recent variant knowledge. A payment model for reinterpretation without retesting is extremely uncommon in the field of laboratory medicine today.

Another extremely important consideration is data security and privacy. Data security refers to the ability to protect information from breaches and inadvertent dissemination. Data privacy refers to the ability to respect patient preference for data sharing, both with the patient themselves and with the larger health care community.

How is the decision made to offer and incorporate pharmacogenomic testing into practice? In some cases, it becomes forced upon the healthcare provider, such as a pharmacist or primary care physician, who is handed a printed report by a patient who has purchased direct to consumer pharmacogenetic testing services and insists that the information be considered when prescribing and dispensing decisions are made. Clearly, that is a less than ideal situation. Healthcare provider education has begun to incorporate pharmacogenomic science into the core curriculums, but it is often in the form of a single1-to 2-hour lecture. This will be inadequate preparation to deal with the era of personalized medicine and the eventual day when everyone will have access to their own genomic data.

When assessing a pharmacogenomic test for potential incorporation into practice, several factors impact the return on investment and clinical outcome. These include but are not limited to the number of patients needed to be tested in order to find one patient with an actionable variant (also known as the incidence of variant status) and the ethnic variation, being cognizant that we are becoming a very blended population without full knowledge of our entire ancestry. Additionally, institutions must investigate how much each test costs to run, if it will be reimbursed, and what are the cost savings offset by averting serious adverse reactions or the consequences of nonresponse.[2,70,71]

Genetic testing can introduce ethical questions that can be challenging, particularly when dealing with sequencing large portions of the DNA. Although most people want to know whether or not they should take a medication, many do not wish to know their risk of developing Alzheimer disease or breast cancer. This becomes a concern with some of the broader sequencing tests such as whole exome or whole genome. The American College of Medical Genetics and Genomics (ACMG) released a position statement in 2013, recommending mandatory reporting in 24 categories of diseases caused by genetic variants whenever a sequencing test is performed, regardless of patient preference around wanting to know that information and irrespective of age of the patient.[72] Arguments against this practice have included the patient's right to decide, informing the parents/caregivers of an adult-onset disease for a child, and insurance discrimination risks.[73,74] Although it is illegal for health insurance coverage to be denied due to genetic findings following the passage of the Genetic Information Nondiscrimination Act (GINA) in 2008, this is currently not true for life or long-term care insurance coverage.[75]

CONCLUSION

Pharmacogenomics is simultaneously an exciting and challenging component of personalized medicine and the practice of pharmacy. One of the most important points to remember is that pharmacogenomic information is an additional clinical marker, but is rarely the only answer. A patient's organ function, disease state, diet, smoking status, other environmental factors, and drug–drug interactions play a very large role in the disposition of drugs. Age-based maturation of enzyme function must also be accounted for when determining the impact of the genotype on drug metabolism.

Pharmacists are uniquely qualified to interpret and apply pharmacogenetic findings to medication recommendations. However, this will require adequate preparation, application of validated algorithms, access to continually updated literature, and a partnership with genetic experts, including geneticists and genetic counselors.[76]

KEY REFERENCES AND WEBSITES

A full list of references for this chapter can be found at http://thepoint.lww.com/AT11e. Below are the key references and websites for this chapter, with the corresponding reference number in this chapter found in parentheses after the reference.

Key References

Altman RB et al, eds. *Principles of Pharmacogenetics and Pharmacogenomics*. 1st ed. New York, NY: Cambridge University Press; 2012.

Gaedigk A. Complexities of CYP2D6 gene analysis and interpretation. *Int Rev Psychiatry*. 2013;25(5):534–553. (46)

Kearns GL et al. Developmental pharmacology—drug disposition, action, and therapy in infants and children. *N Engl J Med*. 2003;349:1157–1167. (53)

Samer CF et al. Applications of CYP450 testing in the clinical setting. *MolDiagn Ther*.2013;17:165–184. (6)

Key Websites

FDA Gene List. http://www.fda.gov/Drugs/ScienceResearch/ResearchAreas/Pharmacogenetics/default.htm.

NIH Precision Medicine Initiative. http://www.nih.gov/precisionmedicine/.

PharmGKB.org. http://www.pharmgkb.org.

Warfarin Dosing. http://www.warfarindosing.org/Source/Home.aspx.

5 Managing Drug Overdoses and Poisonings

Iris Sheinhait and Sara Zhou

CORE PRINCIPLES

	CHAPTER CASES
EPIDEMIOLOGY	
1 In 2013, 2.2 million poisonings were reported to the American Association of Poison Control Centers. Half of these exposures occur in children younger than 5 years of age and usually involve a single substance that is found in the home such as personal care items, analgesics, and cleaning agents. The most common exposures in descending order include cosmetic/personal care products, household cleaning agents, analgesics, toys and foreign bodies, and topical preparations.	**Case 5-1 (Questions 2, 3), Table 5-1**
GENERAL MANAGEMENT	
1 The most important aspect of patient management is to support airway, breathing, and circulation (the "ABCs"). There is no "cookbook" method to treat all poisoned patients, so it is important to treat the patient, not the poison or the laboratory values. The assessment and treatment of the potentially poisoned patient can be separated into seven functions: (a) gather history of exposure, (b) evaluate clinical presentation (i.e., "toxidromes"), (c) evaluate clinical laboratory patient data, (d) remove the toxic source (e.g., irrigate eyes, decontaminate exposed skin), (e) consider antidotes and specific treatment, (f) enhance systemic clearance, and (g) monitor patient outcome.	**Case 5-4 (Questions 1, 3, 5, 6)**
GASTROINTESTINAL DECONTAMINATION	
1 The most appropriate method for gastrointestinal (GI) tract decontamination is unclear because sound comparative data for different methods of GI decontamination are not available. Lavage, emesis, and cathartics are rarely performed as there is no evidence they improve patient outcome. Activated charcoal is generally safe to use, but it should not be administered if the benefit is not greater than the risk. Whole bowel irrigation using a polyethylene glycol–balanced electrolyte solution can successfully remove substances (iron, lithium, sustained-release dosage forms) from the entire GI tract in a period of several hours.	**Case 5-3 (Questions 6, 7), Case 5-4 (Questions 11, 12, 16), Case 5-5 (Question 3)**
ANTIDOTES	
1 An antidote is a drug that neutralizes or reverses the toxicity of another substance. Some antidotes displace drugs from receptor sites (e.g., naloxone for opioids, flumazenil for benzodiazepines), and some can inhibit the formation of toxic metabolites (e.g., *N*-acetylcysteine [NAC] for acetaminophen, fomepizole for ethylene glycol and methanol).	**Case 5-4 (Questions 2, 4)**
TOXICOLOGY LABORATORY SCREENING	
1 An antidote is a drug that neutralizes or reverses the toxicity of another substance. Some antidotes displace drugs from receptor sites (e.g., naloxone for opioids, flumazenil for benzodiazepines), and some can inhibit the formation of toxic metabolites (e.g., *N*-acetylcysteine [NAC] for acetaminophen, fomepizole for ethylene glycol and methanol).	**Case 5-4 (Questions 2, 4)**

Continued

Chapter 5

TOXICOLOGY LABORATORY SCREENING

1 Urine drug screens can be useful in a patient with coma of unknown etiology, when the presented history is inconsistent with clinical findings, or when more than one drug might have been ingested. Qualitative screening is intended to identify unknown substances involved in the toxic exposure. A benzodiazepine screen can detect oxazepam, a common benzodiazepine metabolite, but it will not detect alprazolam and lorazepam as they are not metabolized to oxazepam. Opioid screens may not detect synthetic opioids such as fentanyl and methadone. Quantitative testing determines how much of a known drug is present and can help determine the severity of toxicity and the need for aggressive interventions (e.g., hemodialysis in ethylene glycol, methanol, and salicylate).

Case 5-4 (Questions 1, 7, 8)

TOXIDROMES

1 A toxidrome is a consistent constellation of signs and symptoms associated with some specific classes of drugs. The most common toxidromes are those associated with anticholinergic activity, increased sympathetic activity, and central nervous system (CNS) stimulation or depression. Anticholinergic drugs increase heart rate and body temperature, decrease GI motility, dilate pupils, and produce drowsiness or delirium. Sympathomimetic drugs increase CNS activity, heart rate, body temperature, and blood pressure. Opioids, sedatives, hypnotics, and antidepressants depress the CNS, but the specific class of CNS depressant often cannot be easily identified.

Case 5-4 (Questions 1, 2, 5)

SALICYLATES

1 Acute ingestion of 150 to 300 mg/kg aspirin causes mild-to-moderate intoxication, greater than 300 mg/kg indicates severe poisoning, and greater than 500 mg/kg is potentially lethal. Symptoms of intoxication include vomiting, tinnitus, delirium, tachypnea, metabolic acidosis, respiratory alkalosis, hypokalemia, irritability, hallucinations, stupor, coma, hyperthermia, coagulopathy, and seizures. Salicylate intoxication mimics other medical conditions and can be easily missed. Patients with a chronic salicylate exposure, acidosis, or CNS symptoms and those who are elderly are at high risk and should be considered for early dialysis.

Case 5-1 (Questions 1, 3),
Case 5-2 (Questions 1–6)

IRON

1 Acute elemental iron ingestions of less than 20 mg/kg are usually nontoxic; doses of 20 to 60 mg/kg result in mild-to-moderate toxicity, and doses of greater than 60 mg/kg are potentially fatal. Symptoms of toxicity include nausea, vomiting, diarrhea, abdominal pain, hematemesis, bloody stools, CNS depression, hypotension, and shock. Patients with severe iron poisoning do not exhibit the second stage of so-called recovery but continue to deteriorate.

Case 5-3 (Questions 1, 2–14)

TRICYCLIC ANTIDEPRESSANTS

1 Severe toxicity has been associated with doses of 15 to 25 mg/kg. Symptoms include tachycardia with prolongation of the PR, QTc, and QRS intervals, ST and T-wave changes, acidosis, seizures, coma, hypotension, and adult respiratory distress syndrome. A QRS segment greater than 100 milliseconds is commonly seen in severe tricyclic antidepressant overdoses.

Case 5-4 (Questions 9–17)

ACETAMINOPHEN

1 Toxicity is associated with acute ingestions greater than 150 mg/kg or more than 7.5 g total in adults. Symptoms in patients with toxicity include vomiting, anorexia, abdominal pain, malaise, and progression to characteristic centrilobular hepatic necrosis. Acetaminophen induced hepatotoxicity is universal by 36 hours after ingestion, but patients who receive NAC within 8 to 10 hours after ingestion rarely exhibit hepatotoxicity. There is no consensus as to the best route of NAC administration, the optimal dosage regimen, or the optimal duration of therapy.

Case 5-5 (Questions 1–15)

This chapter reviews common strategies for the evaluation and management of drug overdoses and poisonings. Information for the management of specific drug overdoses is best obtained from a poison control center (reached by calling 1-800-222-1222 anywhere in the United States).

Epidemiologic Data

AMERICAN ASSOCIATION OF POISON CONTROL CENTERS AND DRUG ABUSE WARNING NETWORK

Toxicity secondary to drug and chemical exposure commonly occurs in children. The incidence of exposure to specific agents and the severity of outcomes varies based on the population studied (Table 5-1).[1–3] The number of reported toxic exposures in the United States in 2013 was approximately 2.2 million, according to the American Association of Poison Control Centers (AAPCC).[3] Approximately 70% of the reported cases were treated at home, saving millions of dollars in medical costs.

According to the Drug Abuse Warning Network, almost 5.1 million US emergency department (ED) visits involved drug misuse or abuse in the year 2011. Illicit drugs include cocaine, heroin, marijuana, ecstasy, gamma-hydroxyutyric acid, flunitrazepam (Rohypnol), ketamine, lysergic acid, phencyclidine, and hallucinogens. Of those cases, illicit drug use was mentioned more than 2.7 million times because many of the visits involved multiple drugs of abuse.[4]

AGE-SPECIFIC DATA

Stratifying patients by age can be useful in assessing the likelihood of severe toxicity from an exposure. Most unintentional ingestions by children 1 to 6 years of age occur because children are curious, becoming more mobile, and beginning to explore their surroundings, and they often put objects or substances into their mouths.[5] Severe toxicity in young children is relatively uncommon as exposures usually involve the ingestion of relatively small amounts of a single substance.[5,6] AAPCC epidemiologic data also report medication errors, which in the pediatric population commonly result from confusing units of measurement (e.g., teaspoons vs. milliliters or tablespoons vs. teaspoons), incorrect formulation or concentration administered, dispensing cup errors, and incorrect formulation or concentration dispensed from the pharmacy.[3]

In children older than 6 years of age, the reasons for toxic exposure to medications are less clear.[7] Adolescent children generally have poor knowledge of the toxicity of medications and can overdose themselves unintentionally.[5,8] The potential for suicide attempts or intentional substance abuse should not be ignored in older children. These intentional overdoses commonly involve mixed exposures to illicit drugs, prescribed medications, or ethanol and are associated with more severe toxicity and death than unintentional toxic exposures.

In geriatric patients, overdoses tend to have a greater potential for severe adverse effects compared with overdoses in other age groups.[9] Although the elderly constitute 13% of the population, they account for 33% of the drug use and 16% of the suicides.[10] Patients aged 65 or older take an average of 5.7 prescription medications along with 2 to 4 nonprescription drugs daily.[9,10] The elderly are more likely to have underlying illnesses and often have access to a variety of potentially dangerous medications. This results in higher rates of completed suicides than in other age groups.[10,11]

Information Resources

COMPUTERIZED DATABASES

A vast number of substances can be involved in a poisoning or overdose. Reliable data about the contents of products, toxicities of

Table 5-1
Substances Most Commonly Involved in Poisonings[a]

Children	Adults	Fatal Exposures (All Ages)
Personal care products	Analgesics	Sedatives/hypnotics/antipsychotics
Cleaning substances	Sedatives/hypnotics/antipsychotics	Cardiovascular agents
Analgesics	Antidepressants	Opioids
Topical products	Cardiovascular agents	Stimulants
Vitamins	Cleaning substances	Alcohols, acetaminophen-containing products
Antihistamines	Alcohols	Acetaminophen
Pesticides	Pesticides	Fumes/gases/vapors
Cough and cold products	Bites, envenomations	Antidepressants
Plants	Antiepileptic agents	Antihistamines
GI products	Personal care products	Tricyclic antidepressants, aspirin
Antimicrobials	Antihistamines	Muscle relaxants
Cardiovascular	Hormones and hormone antagonists	Antiepileptic agents
Arts and office supplies	Hydrocarbons	Nonsteroidal anti-inflammatory drugs
Hormones and hormone antagonists	Antimicrobials	
Alcohols	Chemicals	
	Fumes/gases/vapors	

[a]Poisoning exposures are listed in order of frequency encountered.
GI, gastrointestinal.
Source: Mowry et al. 2013 Annual report of the American Association of Poison Control Centers' National Poison Data System (NPDS): 31st Annual Report. *Clin Toxicol (Phila)*. 2014;52:1032.

substances, and treatment approaches need to be readily accessible. POISINDEX, a computerized database,[11] provides information on thousands of drugs by brand name, generic name, and street name, as well as foreign drugs, chemicals, pesticides, household products, personal care items, cleaning products, poisonous insects, poisonous snakes, and poisonous plants. Annual subscriptions to POISINDEX, updated quarterly, are expensive and are generally available only in large medical centers.[12]

PRINTED PUBLICATIONS

Textbooks and manuals also provide useful clinical information about the presentation, assessment, and treatment of toxicities. *Goldfrank's Toxicologic Emergencies*[13] and the pocket-size *Poisoning & Drug Overdose*[14] are valuable, less-expensive alternatives to computerized database programs. Books, however, are less useful than computerized databases because information must be condensed and cannot be updated as frequently. Some drug package inserts also refer to treatment of acute toxicities; however, the information can be inadequate or inappropriate.[15,16]

POISON CONTROL CENTERS

Poison control centers provide the most cost-effective and accurate information to health care providers and to the general public.[17,18] Poison centers are staffed by trained poison information specialists who have a pharmacy, nursing, or medical background. Physician backup is provided 24 hours a day by board-certified medical toxicologists. The nonphysician clinical toxicologists, pharmacists, and nurses who staff poison control centers are certified as specialists in poison information by the AAPCC or as clinical toxicologists by the American Board of Applied Toxicology.[19]

The poison information specialist must accurately and efficiently assess event-specific toxicity by telephone, without the benefit of direct observation of the patient. The specialist must communicate this assessment along with treatment information quickly, accurately, and professionally in a reassuring manner. Subsequent to telephone consultations, poison control center staff should initiate follow-up calls to determine the effectiveness of the recommended treatment and the need for additional evaluation or treatment.[20,21]

EFFECTIVE COMMUNICATION

Effective communication is essential to the assessment of potential poisonings. In most situations, the person seeking guidance on the management of a potentially toxic exposure is the parent of a small child who may have ingested a substance. The caller is usually anxious about the child and may feel guilty about the exposure. To calm the caller, the health care provider should quickly reassure the individual that telephoning for help was appropriate and that the best assistance possible will be provided.[21] If English is not the first language of the caller, or if there are other communication barriers (e.g., panic), solutions must be found to enhance outcomes. Most poison centers subscribe to translation services or have bilingual staff to communicate with non–English-speaking callers. Poison centers also have special equipment to serve the hearing- and speech-impaired populations.

Once calm, effective communication is established, the health care provider should first determine whether the patient is conscious and breathing and has a pulse. If life-threatening symptoms have occurred, the caller should call 9-1-1 for emergency services. If the health care provider does not have the knowledge or resources to provide poison information, he or she should refer the caller to the closest poison control center. Information on the location and phone number of the nearest poison control center can be found at http://www.aapcc.org or by calling 1-800-222-1222 in the United States.

GENERAL MANAGEMENT

Supportive Care and "ABCs"

Management of poisoned or overdosed patients is primarily based on symptomatic and supportive care. Specific antidotes exist only for a small percentage of the thousands of potential drugs and chemicals that can cause a poisoning.

The first aspect of patient management should always be basic support of airway, breathing, and circulation (the "ABCs"). The assessment and treatment of the potentially poisoned patient can be separated into seven primary functions: (a) gathering history of exposure, (b) evaluating clinical presentation (i.e., "toxidromes"), (c) evaluating clinical laboratory patient data, (d) removing the toxic source (e.g., irrigating eyes, decontaminating exposed skin), (e) considering antidotes and specific treatment, (f) enhancing systemic clearance, and (g) monitoring outcome.[22–24]

GATHERING HISTORY OF EXPOSURE

Comprehensive historical information about the toxic exposure should be gathered from as many different sources as possible (e.g., patient, family, friends, prehospital health care providers). This information should be compared for consistency and evaluated relative to clinical findings and laboratory results. The patient's history of the exposure is often inaccurate and should be confirmed with objective findings.[22,23,25] For example, a patient who presents to an ED with a supposed hydrocodone and carisoprodol overdose is expected to be lethargic or comatose. If the patient arrives wide awake with tachycardia and agitation, the clinician should suspect exposure to other substances.

Specific information should be sought concerning the patient's state of consciousness, symptoms, probable intoxicant(s), and maximal amount and dosage form(s) of substance ingested, as well as when the exposure occurred. Medications, allergies, and prior medical problems also should be ascertained to facilitate development of treatment plans (e.g., a history of renal failure may indicate the need for hemodialysis to compensate for decreased renal drug clearance).[22,23]

EVALUATING CLINICAL PRESENTATION AND TOXIDROMES

A thorough physical examination is needed to characterize the signs and symptoms of overdose, and it should be conducted serially to determine the evolution or resolution of the patient's intoxication. An evaluation of the presenting signs and symptoms can provide clues to the drug class causing the toxicity, confirm the historical data surrounding the toxic exposure, and suggest initial treatment.[22,26–28] The patient may be asymptomatic on presentation, even though a potentially severe exposure has occurred, if absorption of the drug or toxic substance is incomplete or if the substance has not yet been metabolized to a toxic substance.[29–31]

Characteristic toxidromes (i.e., a constellation of signs and symptoms consistent with a syndrome) can be associated with some specific classes of drugs.[23,27,28] The most common toxidromes are those associated with anticholinergic activity, increased sympathetic activity, and central nervous system (CNS) stimulation or depression. Anticholinergic drugs can increase heart rate and body temperature, decrease gastrointestinal (GI) motility, dilate pupils, and produce drowsiness or delirium. Sympathomimetic drugs can increase CNS activity, heart rate, body temperature, and blood pressure (BP). Opioids, sedatives, hypnotics, and antidepressants can depress the CNS, but the specific class of CNS depressant often cannot be easily identified.

Classic findings may not be present for all drugs within a therapeutic class. For example, opioids generally induce miosis, but meperidine can produce mydriasis. Furthermore, the association of symptoms with a particular class of toxic substances is difficult when more than one substance has been ingested. Practitioners should not focus only on the specific clinical findings associated with a toxidrome. Rather, they should consider all subjective and objective data gathered from the history of exposure, the patient's medical history, physical examination, and laboratory findings.[27]

INTERPRETATION OF LABORATORY DATA

Drug Screens

A urine drug screen can be useful in identifying the presence of drugs and their metabolites in selected patients but is not indicated in all cases of drug overdose. Urine drug screens can be useful in a patient with coma of unknown etiology, when the presented history is inconsistent with clinical findings, or when more than one drug might have been ingested.[32,33]

Pharmacokinetic Considerations

The absorption, distribution, metabolism, and elimination of drugs in the overdosed patient can be quite different than when the drug is taken in usual therapeutic doses.[29–31] The expected pharmacodynamic and pharmacokinetic features of drugs can be substantially altered by large drug overdoses, especially with drugs that exhibit dose-dependent pharmacokinetics. The rate of drug absorption is generally slowed by large overdoses, and the time to reach peak serum drug concentrations can be delayed.[32,34] For example, peak serum concentrations of phenytoin can be delayed for 2 to 7 days after an orally ingested overdose.[35,36] The volume of distribution of an overdosed drug can be increased, and when usual metabolic pathways become saturated, secondary clearance pathways can be important. For example, large overdoses of acetaminophen saturate glutathione mechanisms of metabolism, resulting in hepatotoxicity.[37]

When the pharmacokinetic parameters of an overdosed drug are altered, serial plasma concentration measurements can better define the absorption, distribution, and clearance phases of the ingested substance. Pharmacokinetic parameters that have been derived from therapeutic doses should not be used to predict whether absorption is complete or to predict the expected duration of intoxication caused by large overdoses.[31,38,39]

DECONTAMINATION

After the airway and the cardiopulmonary system are supported, efforts should be directed toward removing the toxic substance from the patient (i.e., decontamination).[22,40] Decontamination presumes that both the dose and the duration of toxin exposure are important in determining the extent of toxicity and that prevention of continued exposure will decrease toxicity.[29–31,40] This intuitive concept is clearly relevant to ocular, dermal, and respiratory exposures, when local tissue damage is the primary problem. Respiratory decontamination involves removing the patient from the toxic environment and providing fresh air or oxygen to the patient. Decontamination of skin and eyes involves flushing the affected area with large volumes of water or saline to physically remove the toxic substance from the surface.[22,23]

Gastrointestinal Decontamination

Because most poisonings and overdoses result from oral ingestions, measures to decrease or prevent continued GI absorption have commonly been used to limit the extent of exposure.[22,23,37] GI decontamination should be considered if the ingestion is large enough to produce potentially significant toxicity, or if the potential severity of the ingestion is unknown and the time since ingestion is less than 1 hour. The following methods have historically been used: (a) evacuation of gastric contents by emesis or gastric lavage, (b) administration of activated charcoal as an adsorbent to bind the toxic substance remaining in the GI tract, (c) use of cathartics or whole bowel irrigation (WBI) to increase the rectal elimination of unabsorbed drug, or (d) a combination of any of these methods.[41–46]

The efficacy of GI decontamination varies, depending on when the process is initiated relative to the time of ingestion, dose ingested, and other factors. Furthermore, ipecac-induced emesis, gastric lavage, cathartics, and activated charcoal are not directly associated with improved patient outcomes.[41–46]

The most appropriate method for GI tract decontamination remains unclear because sound comparative data for different methods of GI decontamination are not available. Clinical research in healthy subjects, by necessity, must use nontoxic doses of drugs. Studies using nontoxic doses are not applicable to the overdose situation because alterations in GI absorption can occur with large doses. In addition, low-dose studies generally rely on pharmacokinetic end points such as peak plasma concentrations, area under the plasma concentration–time curve, or quantity of drug recovered from the urine.[41,42,44–46] In contrast, clinical studies of GI decontamination methods in patients who have ingested toxic doses of a substance use clinical outcomes or a directional change in serum drug concentrations.[41,42,45,46] These latter trials are not standardized with respect to the dose ingested or to the time interval between drug ingestion and GI decontamination.[41–46]

Ipecac-Induced Emesis and Gastric Lavage

Ipecac-induced emesis and gastric lavage primarily remove substances from the stomach. Their efficacy is affected significantly by the time the ingested substance remains in the stomach. Gastric lavage and ipecac-induced emesis are most effective when implemented before the substance moves past the stomach into the intestine (usually within 1 hour).[41,42]

The commonly used adult gastric lavage tube (36F) has an internal diameter too small to allow recovery of large tablet or capsule fragments. An even smaller diameter lavage tube is used for children.[42] Gastric lavage may be useful only if large amounts of a liquid substance were ingested and the patient arrived within 1 hour of the ingestion.[45] However, patients usually arrive in the ED more than an hour after ingestion, when absorption of the toxin has most likely already occurred. As a result, the efficacy of these procedures in overdose situations is minimal, and no studies have confirmed that use of gastric lavage or ipecac-induced emesis improves the outcome of the patient.[41,42,47] For these reasons, ipecac is no longer used, and gastric lavage is used only in rare, specific situations.

Activated Charcoal

In 1963, a review article concluded that activated charcoal was the most valuable agent available for the treatment of poisoning.[48] This conclusion was based only on studies in fasting patients who had nontoxic exposures. Nevertheless, data from those studies were extrapolated to poisoned patients. Since then, activated charcoal has become the preferred method of GI decontamination for the treatment of toxic ingestions.[22,40,48]

The goal of the therapy is to decrease the absorption of the substance and reduce or prevent systemic toxicity.[43] Unfortunately, there are no satisfactorily designed clinical studies assessing benefit from the use of activated charcoal to guide the use of this therapy. There is also no evidence that the administration of activated charcoal improves clinical outcomes.[43]

The use of activated charcoal at a dose of 1 g/kg should be considered when the patient has ingested a toxic substance that is known to be absorbed by activated charcoal within 1 hour of the ingestion. The potential for benefit is unknown if the activated charcoal is given more than 1 hour after ingestion.[43] It should be noted that iron and lithium are not absorbed by activated charcoal. Other forms of GI decontamination must be used to remove those substances from the GI tract.[43]

Generally the use of activated charcoal is safe. Although there are relatively few reports of adverse effects from the use of activated charcoal, there are numerous reports of complications, usually involving aspiration. It is essential that the patient has an intact or protected airway (intubation) before activated charcoal is administered, especially in drowsy patients or patients who may rapidly become obtunded.[43]

Vomiting with aspiration of activated charcoal occurs in about 5% of patients who receive activated charcoal.[43,49–51] The resulting pulmonary problems can be caused by aspiration of acidic stomach contents or the charcoal. Decreased oxygenation can occur immediately, or pulmonary effects can occur later.[51–55] Adult respiratory distress syndrome has resulted after the unintentional instillation of charcoal into the lung.[51] Aspiration of charcoal can result in chronic lung disease or fatalities, whereas the toxic exposure, for which the charcoal was administered, is often not lethal or even serious.[52,56]

Cathartics

Historically, sorbitol (a cathartic) was often administered with activated charcoal to enhance passage of the charcoal–substance complex through the GI tract. However, decreased transit time through the bowel has not been proven to decrease absorption because drug absorption does not take place in the large bowel.[44] Sorbitol is also associated with vomiting and aspiration.[44] Hypernatremia can also develop subsequent to the administration of repeat doses of activated charcoal with sorbitol.[57,58] Currently, most EDs use aqueous activated charcoal mixtures rather than charcoal–sorbitol combinations. Because cathartics are not effective in reducing drug absorption or increasing patient outcome, their use is no longer advised.[44]

Whole Bowel Irrigation

WBI with a polyethylene glycol–balanced electrolyte solution (e.g., Colyte, GoLYTELY) can successfully remove substances from the entire GI tract in a period of several hours. WBI is effective with ingestions of sustained-release dosage forms, as well as substances that form bezoars (concretions of tablets or capsules), such as ferrous sulfate or phenytoin.[23,45,59] WBI is also indicated when the toxic agent is not adsorbed by activated charcoal (e.g., body-packer packets, lithium, iron, potassium).[22,23,45,59] This method of GI decontamination takes much longer to complete and is associated with poor patient compliance because large volumes of fluid (2 L/hour for adults until the effluent is clear) need to be ingested to be effective.[59] A nasogastric (NG) tube can be inserted, and the WBI fluid can be administered via NG tube so that lack of patient compliance is no longer a factor.[45]

ANTIDOTES AND SPECIFIC TREATMENTS

An antidote is a drug that neutralizes or reverses the toxicity of another substance. Some antidotes can displace a drug from receptor sites (e.g., naloxone for opioids, flumazenil for benzodiazepines), and some can inhibit the formation of toxic metabolites (e.g., *N*-acetylcysteine [NAC] for acetaminophen, fomepizole for methanol).[23,60,61] Some treatments are highly effective for the management of individual drug overdoses but do not meet the definition of an antidote. For example, sodium bicarbonate is used to treat the cardiotoxicity arising from tricyclic antidepressant (TCA) overdoses, and benzodiazepines are used to treat CNS toxicity associated with cocaine and amphetamine overdoses.[62–64] However, it is important to note that for antidotes to be effective, they must be readily available at the health care facility in adequate doses to treat the patient in a timely manner.[65]

ENHANCING SYSTEMIC CLEARANCE

Hemodialysis and manipulation of urine pH can enhance the clearance of substances. Hemodialysis can successfully treat some specific intoxications (e.g., methanol, ethylene glycol, aspirin, theophylline, lithium). Hemodialysis can also be used in patients with severe acid–base disturbances or renal dysfunction.[47] Alkalinization of the urine can enhance the elimination of drugs such as aspirin and phenobarbital.[66–68]

MONITORING OUTCOME

Selecting the appropriate parameters and length of time to monitor a patient who has been exposed to a toxic agent requires knowledge of toxic effects and the time course of the intoxication.[33,34] Most patients who are at risk for moderate or severe toxicity should be monitored in an intensive care unit (ICU) with careful assessments of cardiac, pulmonary, and CNS function.[69,70]

ASSESSMENT OF SALICYLATE INGESTION

Gathering a History

CASE 5-1

QUESTION 1: A.J., the mother of a 3-year-old child, states that her son, R.J., has ingested some aspirin tablets. What additional information should be obtained from or given to A.J. at this time?

Obtaining an initial assessment of the patient's status is essential. The caller's telephone number should be obtained in the event that the call is disconnected, initial recommendations need to be modified, or subsequent follow-up is needed. The health care provider should ask for patient-specific information with questions that are nonthreatening and nonjudgmental. The caller should be reassured that calling for help was the right thing to do.

Evaluating Clinical Presentation

CASE 5-1, QUESTION 2: On further questioning, A.J. states that R.J. is crying and complaining of a stomachache. Otherwise, the child appears to be acting normally. R.J. was found sitting on the bedroom floor with an aspirin bottle in his hand and some partially chewed tablets on the floor next to him. A.J. states that the child had the same look on his face that he has when he eats things that he does not like. A.J. reports that she can see white tablet material gummed on the child's teeth. The mother was gone no more than 5 minutes and had asked her 5- and 6-year-old sons to watch their brother. What additional information is needed to correctly assess the potential for toxicity in R.J.?

To determine the potential toxicity for an unintentional ingestion, it is important to assess the presence of symptoms and to identify the substance ingested. Inquiries should begin with open-ended questions to determine the facts that the caller is certain of versus what may have been assumed. The answers usually point to more specific information that is needed to accurately assess the exposure.[20]

R.J.'s symptoms presently are not life-threatening. His behavior is consistent with being scared in response to the mother's anxiety. Once it has been established that the child does not need immediate life-saving treatment, the caller is generally more willing and able to answer additional questions.

A.J. already has provided information about the child's symptoms. More information is needed to determine the identity of the ingested substance, the time of ingestion, the brand of aspirin (to ensure that the product is not an aspirin-combination or even an aspirin-free formulation), the dosage form, the number of dosage units in a full container, and the number of remaining dosage units in the container. The parent should be advised to look for tablets under beds, rugs, or other locations out of sight (e.g., wastepaper baskets, toilets, pet food dishes, pockets). The dosage forms in the container should be identical in appearance, and the contents should be what are stated on the label. Information concerning the child's weight and health status, as well as whether the child is taking other medications, is also important. The child's weight is useful in determining the maximum milligram per kilogram dose of aspirin that was ingested.

When more than one child is present during an ingestion, the caller should be questioned as to whether other children also could have participated in the ingestion. In this situation, the children could have shared equally in the missing medication, all of the drug could have been fed to one child, or all of the drug could have been ingested by the oldest or most aggressive child. When it is unclear how much is missing among a group of children, each child should be evaluated and managed as if he or she may have ingested the total missing quantity.

Triage of Call

Case 5-1, Question 3: A.J. has now determined that a total of seven tablets each containing 81 mg per tablet of aspirin are missing from the bottle. Because A.J. recalls having taken two aspirin tablets from this bottle, it is not likely that her son took more than seven tablets. A.J. states that R.J. weighs 42 pounds. What treatment is needed for this child?

The maximal dose of aspirin ingested by this child is likely to be much less than the minimal dose required to cause significant symptoms based on his weight for his age (i.e., 42 pounds or approximately 19 kg). A dose of 150 mg/kg of aspirin is the smallest dose at which treatment or assessment at a health care facility is necessary.[68,71] A.J. is likely to have ingested a maximum of 567 mg of aspirin (i.e., seven 81-mg tablets), which is about 29.8 mg/kg (567 mg divided by 19 kg). If this child is healthy, takes no medications, and is not allergic to aspirin, the child does not require any treatment. With this history of ingestion, the only adverse effect that might occur is some mild nausea. Providing information to the mother that her child had not ingested a toxic or dangerous amount will be reassuring.

For many years, aspirin was the most common cause of unintentional poisoning and poisoning deaths among children.[71–73] However, safety closure packaging and reduction of the total aspirin content in a full bottle of children's aspirin to approximately 3 g has steadily reduced the frequency of pediatric aspirin poisoning and deaths.[72–74] Although acute aspirin poisoning remains a problem, the largest percentage of life-threatening intoxications now results from therapeutic overdose.[68] Therapeutic overdoses occur when a dose is given too frequently, when both parents unknowingly dose the child with the drug, or when too large a dose is given. Therapeutic overdoses are especially problematic when excessive doses are given for a prolonged period and the drug is able to accumulate.[68]

Outcome for A.J.

Follow-up telephone consultation on toxic ingestions is important to identify children who unexpectedly develop symptoms that might need to be treated. A telephone call to A.J. 6 to 24 hours after her initial call would be appropriate to follow up on the child. On a call back to A.J., the parent stated that she gave R.J. lunch at the appropriate time. R.J. then watched cartoons, took his usual nap, and remained asymptomatic.

Acute and Chronic Salicylism

SIGNS AND SYMPTOMS

CASE 5-2

Question 1: A.S., a 71-year-old, 59-kg woman with a history of chronic headaches, has taken 10 to 12 aspirin tablets daily for several months. On the evening of admission, she became lethargic, disoriented, and combative. Additional history revealed that she ingested up to 95 aspirin tablets on the morning of admission (about 11 hours earlier) in a suicide attempt. She complained of ringing in her ears, nausea, and two episodes of vomiting. She is disoriented and lethargic. Vital signs were BP 148/95 mm Hg, pulse 114 beats/minute, respirations 38 breaths/minute, and temperature 101.2°F. A.S.'s laboratory data obtained on admission were as follows:

Serum sodium (Na), 144 mEq/L
Potassium (K), 2.5 mEq/L
Chloride (Cl), 103 mEq/L
Bicarbonate, 9 mEq/L
Glucose, 58 mg/dL
Blood urea nitrogen (BUN), 38 mg/dL
Creatinine, 2.5 mg/dL

Arterial blood gas (ABG) values (room air) were as follows: pH, 7.14; P_{CO_2}, 18 mm Hg; and P_{O_2}, 96 mm Hg. A serum salicylate concentration measured approximately 12 hours after the acute ingestion was 90 mg/dL. Her hemoglobin was 9.6 g/dL with a hematocrit of 28.9% and a prothrombin time (PT) of 16.4 seconds. Is A.S. at high risk because of her ingestion?

The symptoms and severity of salicylate intoxication depend on the dose consumed; the patient's age; and whether the ingestion was acute, chronic, or a combination of the two.[73,75,76] This case illustrates an acute ingestion in someone who has also chronically ingested aspirin. Acute ingestion of 150 to 300 mg/kg of aspirin is likely to produce mild-to-moderate intoxication, greater than 300 mg/kg indicates severe poisoning, and greater than 500 mg/kg is potentially lethal.[68,71] A.S., who ingested approximately 523 mg/kg, has taken a potentially lethal dose. Chronic salicylate intoxication is usually associated with ingestion of greater than 100 mg/kg/day for more than 2 days.[68,71] A.S. has been taking 66 mg/kg/day for her headaches in addition to her acute ingestion. A.S. demonstrates many of the findings typical of severe acute salicylism (see Pathophysiology of Salicylate Intoxication and Assessment of Toxicity sections). A.S.'s prognosis is potentially poor because she is elderly and has taken a potentially lethal overdose of aspirin.

Pathophysiology of Salicylate Intoxication

Case 5-2, Question 2: Describe the pathophysiology and clinical features of acute and chronic salicylism.

Toxicity from salicylate exposure results in direct irritation of the GI tract, direct stimulation of the CNS respiratory center, stimulation of the metabolic rate, lipid and carbohydrate metabolism disturbances, and interference with hemostasis.[68,71,73,75,76] Toxic doses of salicylate directly stimulate the medullary respiratory center leading to nausea, vomiting, tinnitus, delirium, tachypnea, seizures, and coma and influence several key metabolic pathways.[68,73–77] Direct stimulation of the respiratory drive increases the rate and depth of ventilation, which can result in primary respiratory alkalosis. The respiratory alkalosis causes increased renal excretion of bicarbonate, resulting in decreased buffering capacity. The patient usually presents with a partially compensated respiratory alkalosis.[68,74,75,77] Hypokalemia can result from increased GI and renal losses of potassium, as well as from systemic alkalosis.[68,75,76] Although marked metabolic and neurologic abnormalities are most commonly observed in young children with advanced salicylate intoxication, adolescents or adults acutely poisoned with a large dose of salicylates can exhibit these symptoms as well.[68,74,75] Acute salicylism in a young child often takes a more severe course than that typically seen in adults. After acute ingestion, children quickly pass through the phase of pure respiratory alkalosis. Renal bicarbonate loss secondary to respiratory alkalosis reduces the buffering capacity more profoundly in a child and facilitates the development of metabolic acidosis.[68,73,75,77]

Salicylates have toxic effects on several biochemical pathways that contribute to metabolic acidosis and other symptoms.[68,75,77] Mitochondrial oxidative phosphorylation is uncoupled and results in an impaired ability to generate high-energy phosphates, increased oxygen use and carbon dioxide production, increased heat production and hyperpyrexia, increased tissue glycolysis, and increased peripheral demand for glucose. Salicylates also inhibit key dehydrogenase enzymes within the Krebs cycle, resulting in increased levels of pyruvate and lactate. The increased demand for peripheral glucose causes increased glycogenolysis, gluconeogenesis, lipolysis, and free fatty acid metabolism. The latter results in enhanced formation of keto acids and ketoacidosis.[73,77]

The patient may become severely volume depleted through several mechanisms.[68,75,77] Hyperthermia and hyperventilation produce increased insensible water loss, vomiting may promote GI fluid losses, and the solute load caused by altered glucose metabolism results in an osmotic diuresis. Depending on the patient's acid–base balance and net fluid and electrolyte intake and output, serum sodium and potassium concentrations may be normal, elevated, or decreased. Hypernatremia and hypokalemia are most common.[73,75]

Blood glucose concentration is usually normal or slightly elevated, although hypoglycemia may accompany chronic salicylism (e.g., as illustrated by A.S.) or occur late in acute intoxication. CNS glucose levels can be markedly reduced in the presence of normal blood glucose concentrations because increased CNS glucose utilization to generate high-energy phosphate exceeds the rate at which glucose can be supplied.[68,73,75,77]

ASSESSMENT OF TOXICITY

CASE 5-2, QUESTION 3: What signs, symptoms, and laboratory values in A.S. are consistent with salicylate intoxication?

A.S. demonstrates many of the findings typical of severe acute salicylism. Hyperventilation has resulted from the direct respiratory stimulant effects of salicylate and as compensation for her metabolic acidosis (Pco_2, 18 mm Hg; pH, 7.14; serum bicarbonate, 9 mEq/L; respiratory rate, 38 breaths/minute). Hypokalemia (2.8 mEq/L) in the presence of metabolic acidosis represents severe potassium depletion because of increased renal and possibly GI losses. Hyperpyrexia caused by salicylate is present in A.S., although an infectious cause must also be considered. Her neurologic symptoms of lethargy, disorientation, and combativeness, as well as tinnitus, nausea, and vomiting, are commonly seen in severe salicylate intoxication. In addition, being elderly and taking a lethal amount of aspirin bodes ill for this patient's outcome.

LABORATORY EVALUATION

CASE 5-2, QUESTION 4: What objective evaluations should be assessed in a patient with presumed salicylate intoxication?

A.S.'s workup illustrates a thorough initial patient evaluation. Laboratory evaluation should include ABG values, serum electrolytes, BUN, serum creatinine, blood glucose, and a complete blood cell count.[73,74] Urine should be tested for specific gravity and pH.[73] In symptomatic patients, a PT or international normalized ratio (INR) and partial thromboplastin times are useful to assess the presence of salicylate-induced coagulopathy. Vitals signs should be monitored for an increased respiratory rate and hyperpyrexia.[74,75] Physical examination should include an evaluation of chest radiograph, cardiopulmonary and neurologic function, and measurement of urine output.[75]

A salicylate blood concentration should be obtained immediately and every 2 hours in patients.[24,64,73,75] Serum salicylate concentrations should be reassessed every 2 hours to verify that the original concentration represented a peak level and that the salicylate level is decreasing rather than increasing.[24,68,73,76,78] Obtaining the units of measurement on salicylate serum concentrations is essential because different laboratories report concentrations in different units (e.g., mg/dL, mcg/mL, mmol/L). An incorrect interpretation of the salicylate unit of measurement can result in overestimates or underestimates of the severity.[24]

Manifestations of severe acute salicylism include a variety of neurologic signs and symptoms: disorientation, irritability, hallucinations, lethargy, stupor, coma, and seizures.[69,73] Hyperthermia may be marked and can result in the inappropriate administration of aspirin as an antipyretic. Coagulopathy can occur because of impaired platelet function, hypoprothrombinemia, reduced factor VII production, and increased capillary fragility, especially when aspirin is taken chronically.[75–77] Pulmonary edema and acute renal failure also can occur, but the former occurs more commonly after chronic intoxication.[75,77,78]

Chronic salicylism symptoms are similar to acute intoxications. However, patients with chronic exposures may have fewer GI symptoms, but they generally appear more ill and have more CNS symptoms.[71,79] In both adults and children, the principal signs of chronic salicylism are a partially compensated metabolic acidosis, increased anion gap, ketosis, dehydration, electrolyte loss, hyperventilation, tremors, agitation, confusion, stupor, memory deficits, renal failure, and seizures.[73,75,76,80] The severity of CNS manifestations is related to the cerebrospinal fluid (CSF) salicylate concentration.[74,75] CSF concentrations may increase in the presence of systemic acidosis because a greater fraction of salicylate is not ionized and can cross the blood–brain barrier. Therefore, metabolic acidosis is especially dangerous in a salicylate-intoxicated patient.[73,75]

Unless the history of salicylate intake is specifically sought, the problem may not be immediately apparent, especially in the elderly in whom such findings are likely to be attributed to other causes (e.g., encephalitis, meningitis, diabetic ketoacidosis, myocardial infarction).[24,75,79] Delay in diagnosis has been associated with increased mortality.[24,68,75,79] Unfortunately, plasma salicylate concentrations do not correlate well with the degree of poisoning in chronically intoxicated patients. It is more important to treat the patient according to the clinical status rather than his or her salicylate concentration.[71] Death in patients with salicylism, whether acute or chronic, results from CNS or cardiac dysfunction, or pulmonary edema.[73,75,79]

MANAGEMENT

CASE 5-2, QUESTION 5: What would be a reasonable management plan for A.S.?

Management of salicylate intoxication depends on the degree of acid–base and electrolyte disturbances.[68,73,75] Activated charcoal is not indicated for A.S. because the ingestion occurred approximately 10 hours ago and she has a somewhat altered mental status.[46] The risk of aspiration is greater than the value of possibly adsorbing any remaining aspirin from the GI tract. In addition, A.S. already has symptoms of salicylate poisoning, indicating that the aspirin has already been absorbed. Others might argue that if she ingested 95 tablets, some of the drug may still be present in the GI tract and giving activated charcoal late may bind some of the drug still present. The benefit versus risk of giving activated charcoal must be assessed. A.S.'s hypokalemia, acidosis, and hypoglycemia must be corrected, and it is probably best accomplished through the administration of intravenous (IV) hypotonic saline–dextrose solutions combined with potassium supplementation. This solution is administered at a rate that replaces the patient's deficits and keeps pace with continued losses.[68,73,75–77] Care should be taken to avoid overzealous fluid therapy, which can predispose the patient to cerebral or pulmonary edema.[73,77] Administration of an IV dextrose bolus is also indicated because A.S. is hypoglycemic (60 mg/dL).[73,75–77]

Sodium Bicarbonate

It is important to correct A.S.'s acidosis because acidosis will increase CSF salicylate concentrations.[74,75] Correction of acidosis can be accomplished by adding sodium bicarbonate to her IV fluids.[68,73–76] A.S.'s serum sodium and potassium concentrations should be monitored closely as adding potassium to IV fluids will mostly likely be required.[82] Providing adequate ventilation to prevent respiratory alkalosis is essential. With a respiratory rate of 36 breaths/minute, placing the patient on a ventilator to assist with breathing might be considered. However, forced mechanical ventilation can interfere with the patient's need to compensate to maintain the serum pH. Patients on ventilators can become severely acidotic, which can result in death because of an inability to compensate adequately.[73,83]

Seizures

Seizures are not evident in A.S. but can be encountered in cases of severe salicylate poisoning. Seizures generally carry a poor prognosis and are indicative of severe salicylate intoxication that requires hemodialysis.[73] Other treatable causes of seizures (e.g., marked alkalosis, hypoglycemia, hyponatremia) can be present in individuals such as A.S. and should be ruled out. If seizures occur, benzodiazepines are the drugs of choice for treatment.[73]

Coagulopathy and Hyperthermia

Coagulopathy generally responds to vitamin K_1, which should be given if the PT or INR is prolonged.[73] GI bleeding or other hemorrhage can occur, but it is not common.[73,75,76] Mild hyperthermia usually does not require therapy, but cooling fans and mist may be required for extremely elevated temperatures.[73,77]

Pulmonary Edema

Noncardiogenic pulmonary edema commonly occurs in salicylate intoxications, especially when the overdose is attributable to chronic ingestions.[73,75,78] Pulmonary edema is associated with a high incidence of neurologic symptoms in patients and can occur even without fluid overload.[75,78] Increased alveolar capillary membrane permeability, prostaglandin effects, and a metabolic interaction with platelets releasing membrane permeability substances are the primary mechanisms for the cause of pulmonary edema associated with salicylate overdose. Treatment is aimed at reducing salicylate levels via alkalinization or hemodialysis.[78]

Alkalinization

Case 5-2, Question 6: What measures will enhance salicylate elimination? Which of these may be indicated in A.S.?

Alkalinization of the urine and hemodialysis can enhance the excretion of salicylate in overdose situations.[68,74] Hemodialysis is preferred because it can also correct fluid and electrolyte imbalances.[75,78,79] Sodium bicarbonate is recommended for alkalinization to increase the arterial pH with the goal of minimizing salicylate transport into the CNS.[74,75,77]

Although large doses of sodium bicarbonate can enhance the renal elimination of the weak acid and shorten its half-life, this treatment does not favorably influence the morbidity or mortality of patients with salicylism. Alkalinization with forced fluid diuresis can also place the patient at risk for sodium and fluid retention, as well as pulmonary edema if too much fluid is given too quickly.[76,78,79,81] Whether the urine can be adequately alkalinized (pH >7) in severely intoxicated pediatric patients has been questioned because of the large acid load that is excreted.[68,73,74] Nevertheless, urine alkalinization with sodium bicarbonate should be attempted in severely salicylate-intoxicated adult patients such as A.S.

Potassium replacement in patients receiving alkalinization is essential.[73,75,77] These patients may require large amounts of potassium supplementation as a result of renal wasting of potassium. The risk for pulmonary edema can be minimized if this is done without forcing fluids.[73,75–77]

Hemodialysis should be considered in patients who show progression of severe salicylate intoxication and seizure activity, renal failure, or plasma salicylate concentrations in the potentially fatal range.[68,75,76,78,80] Patients with a chronic exposure, acidosis, or CNS symptoms and those who are elderly or ill are high-risk patients and should be considered for early dialysis.[75,80] Because A.S. has many of the risk factors, she is a candidate for emergent hemodialysis.

CLINICAL OUTCOME OF PATIENT A.S.

A repeat salicylate level 6 hours later (18 hours after ingestion) had increased to 95 mg/dL. Her chemistry panel revealed serum sodium, 143 mEq/L; potassium, 2.2 mEq/L; chloride, 99 mEq/L; bicarbonate, 8mEq/L; glucose, 77 mg/dL; creatinine, 4.9 mg/dL; and BUN, 43mg/dL. Her hemoglobin was now 8.4 g/dL with a hematocrit of 23% and a PT of 16.6 seconds. A.S.'s pH on blood gases remained in the 7.2 to 7.3 range. Urinary alkalinization was attempted with a high-dose IV sodium bicarbonate infusion in an attempt to reach a urine pH of 7.5. However, her urine pH never increased above pH 5.7. A.S. became fluid overloaded and exhibited dyspnea. She was placed on a ventilator with worsening of her symptoms. A chest radiograph showed pulmonary edema. A.S. became confused and agitated, pulling at her IV lines and trying to get out of bed. Nephrology was consulted to provide emergent hemodialysis to correct the acidosis, electrolyte abnormalities, and fluid overload. As the catheter was being placed, the patient had a tonic–clonic seizure. Lorazepam 2 mg IV was administered and the seizure stopped. At this time, the patient was unresponsive. She had another tonic–clonic seizure, went into respiratory arrest, coded, and could not be resuscitated.

ASSESSMENT OF IRON INGESTION

Gathering History and Communications

CASE 5-3

Question 1: The babysitter of K.M., a 21-month-old girl, calls the ED because the child is vomiting and appears to have been playing with an open, unlabeled bottle of green tablets. The child was left alone in her room for about 20 minutes to take a nap. Why might the consultation with this babysitter be expected to be more difficult than the consultation in Case 5-1, Question 1?

In cases of unintentional pediatric ingestions, phone calls to a health care provider, a health care facility, or a poison control center made by individuals other than the parent are usually more difficult to manage as the caller is often unable to provide all patient-specific information needed (e.g., patient weight, chronic medications) to accurately assess the drug ingestion. Additional information is often needed from a parent. Nonparent callers also tend to be more upset about an unintentional ingestion and may have more difficulty than a parent in taking decisive action.

Triage of Call

Case 5-3, Question 2: Despite additional questioning, K.M.'s babysitter cannot identify the tablets. K.M. is still vomiting, and the vomitus is green like the color of the tablets. According to the babysitter, K.M. is the child of a single mother who is not known to have flu or any GI illness at this time. The child's mother is currently at work and is not answering her cell phone. What recommendations could be provided to K.M.'s babysitter at this time?

With this history, the practitioner should consider whether the information presented by K.M.'s babysitter is consistent with a drug ingestion and whether this incident is likely to be associated with a significant adverse outcome. Most 2-year-old children experience limited toxicity with unintentional drug ingestions because the amount of substance actually ingested is usually small.[5,6] Nevertheless, some substances (e.g., methanol, ethylene glycol, nicotine, caustic substances, camphor, chloroquine, clonidine, diphenoxylate-atropine, theophylline, oral hypoglycemic agents, calcium-channel blockers, TCAs, opioids) can produce significant toxicity even when small amounts are ingested.[6,84,85]

Although the history of drug ingestion in K.M. is somewhat vague, the description of green tablets and green-colored vomitus suggest possible ingestion of iron tablets. Because this is a possible exposure with a realistic potential for severe toxicity, K.M. should be brought to the ED for evaluation. Depending on the distance to the hospital and the anxiety level of the babysitter, the practitioner might want to instruct the babysitter to call for an ambulance. She should be instructed to bring the green tablets to the ED along with the child so the tablets can be identified. Other medications in the house should also be brought to the ED, and the mother should be contacted.

Substance Identification

Case 5-3, Question 3: K.M.'s mother has been reached and confirmed that the only green tablets in the house are her iron supplements. The babysitter was instructed to bring K.M. to the nearest Emergency Department, and the mother will meet them there. On arrival K.M. is still vomiting but is fully awake and alert with a heart rate of 122 beats/minute, a respiratory rate of 26 breaths/minute, a rectal temperature of 98.9°F, and pulse oximetry of 100%. How can the maximal potential severity of this ingestion be estimated at this time?

K.M.'s vital signs, when corrected for age, are normal. Attention should now focus on identifying the ingested substance and the maximal potential severity of the ingestion. Although this case involves an unknown ingestion, with a possibility of being a severe case of iron intoxication, the identity of the tablets still has not been verified. Therefore, K.M. must be carefully assessed, and the ingestion history reaffirmed.

All solid dosage prescription drugs are required by the US Food and Drug Administration (FDA) to have identification markings. Reference books (e.g., *Facts and Comparisons*,[86] *Physicians' Desk Reference*),[87] computerized databases (e.g., IDENTIDEX),[88] and the product manufacturers can assist in identifying solid dosage forms. Websites such as http://www.pharmer.org[89] and http://www.drugs.com[90] can also be useful in obtaining drug identification information.

The imprint code markings on the green tablet brought to the ED with K.M. and the mother's assistance should be sufficient to correctly identify the medication. Once the tablet has been identified, the maximal number of tablets ingested should be estimated.

In K.M.'s case, the bottle containing the green tablets was unlabeled. In most cases, the label on the medication container can provide information on the identity and number of tablets dispensed. The date the prescription was obtained, the number of estimated doses taken, and the number currently remaining in the medication container can be used to approximate the maximal number of tablets ingested.

K.M's vital signs and symptoms should be monitored closely to evaluate whether her clinical status is consistent with expectations based on the suspected ingestion. Nausea, vomiting, diarrhea, and abdominal pain are common early signs of iron intoxication.[91–96] The absence of symptoms, especially within a short time after the presumed ingestion, should not be interpreted as an indication that a poisoning has not occurred.[91,93–96]

Evaluating Severity of Toxicity

Case 5-3, Question 4: K.M. weighs 24.2 pounds, appears to be in no distress, and has stopped vomiting. About 25 mL of dark-colored vomitus was recovered, but no tablets are found. The vomitus tested negative for blood. A maximum of seven tablets was ingested based on the mother's recall. What degree of toxicity should be expected in K.M.?

The potential severity of toxicity can be estimated for commonly ingested drugs such as acetaminophen,[97] salicylates,[71] iron,[91] and TCAs[98] because of well-established dose–toxicity relationships. Acute elemental iron ingestions of less than 20 mg/kg are usually nontoxic, doses of 20 to 60 mg/kg result in mild-to-moderate toxicity, and doses greater than 60 mg/kg are potentially fatal.[92,94,96]

The independent verification of the tablet by K.M.'s mother and the tablet imprint indicate that each tablet contained 325 mg of ferrous fumarate in an enteric-coated formulation. Because the dose–toxicity relationship of iron is based on the amount of elemental iron ingested, knowledge of the specific iron salt is important in calculating the ingested dose. Ferrous fumarate contains 33% elemental iron, whereas ferrous gluconate contains 12%, and ferrous sulfate contains 20%.[91,92,94,95] Therefore, each 325-mg ferrous sulfate tablet contains 108 mg of elemental iron. K.M. ingested a maximum of seven enteric-coated ferrous fumarate 325-mg tablets and she weighs 24.2 pounds (11 kg). Her ingestion of approximately 69 mg/kg (108 mg per tablet $\times$ 7 tablets $=$ 756 mg total divided by 11-kg patient weight) of iron places her at risk of severe toxicity. Although K.M.'s only symptom is vomiting at this time, absorption could be delayed because she ingested an enteric-coated formulation.

Abdominal Radiographs

Case 5-3, Question 5: K.M. is expected to experience potentially severe toxicity from her iron ingestion. Why would an abdominal radiograph be useful to verify the number of iron tablets ingested?

In theory, radio-opaque substances (e.g., iron, enteric-coated tablets, chloral hydrate, phenothiazines, heavy metals) can be visualized in the GI tract by an abdominal radiograph.[99] The ability of a radiograph to detect the presence of a radiodense substance depends on the dosage form, concentration, and molecular weight of the substance. The intact dosage form can often be detected if the tablet has not already disintegrated or dissolved.[99]

Less than one-third of pediatric abdominal radiographs show positive evidence of tablets or granules after iron poisoning.[100] Children are more likely than adults to chew tablets rather than swallow them whole, and false-negative results can occur when whole tablets have not started to disintegrate. If the tablets were chewed, an abdominal radiograph is not likely to be useful for verifying the number of iron tablets ingested. However, an abdominal radiograph after the completion of GI decontamination can help assess whether additional decontamination is needed.[99]

Gastrointestinal Decontamination

CASE 5-3, QUESTION 6: Would gastric lavage or activated charcoal not be indicated for the management of K.M.'s iron ingestion? Why or why not?

When selecting a method of GI decontamination, consider the substance ingested, maximal potential toxicity expected from the drug dosage form, potential time course of toxicity, time elapsed between ingestion and the initiation of treatment, symptoms, and physical examination findings. Decontamination with activated charcoal is not indicated in K.M. because iron tablets are not adsorbed by activated charcoal.[49,91,99] Gastric lavage would also be ineffective because the removal of large undissolved iron tablets from the stomach is limited by the small internal diameter of the gastric lavage tube, especially in pediatric patients.[99,100]

Whole Bowel Irrigation

CASE 5-3, QUESTION 7: What other method of GI decontamination should be considered for K.M.?

Whole bowel irrigation with a polyethylene glycol electrolyte solution can be considered in this case. WBI fluid can be administered orally or by NG tube at a rate of 1.5 to 2 L/hour for adults and at a rate of 500 mL/hour for children.[59,101] Although the ingestion of a large volume of fluid over several hours and the likelihood of nausea and vomiting often result in poor patient compliance, K.M. is hospitalized and the fluid can be infused by NG tube. WBI should be continued until the rectal effluent is clear, which can take many hours.[59,101,102]

MONITORING EFFECTIVENESS OF TREATMENT

CASE 5-3, QUESTION 8: How should the effectiveness of GI decontamination be assessed in the ED?

In order to assess the effectiveness of GI decontamination, the return fluid from the WBI is visually inspected for tablets or tablet fragments. Increasing serum iron concentrations, deteriorating clinical status, or evidence of radiodense tablets in the GI tract on abdominal radiograph are all indications for more aggressive treatment.[92,94,102]

Serum Iron Concentrations

CASE 5-3, QUESTION 9: At this time, K.M. does not appear to be experiencing any CNS or cardiovascular symptoms associated with toxic iron ingestions. She did have one episode of diarrhea that tested negative for blood. A serum iron concentration, obtained about 4 hours after the ingestion, was 480 mcg/dL (normal, 60–160 mcg/dL). What conclusions as to severity or likely clinical outcome can be derived from this serum iron concentration?

The serum iron concentration provides an indication as to whether more aggressive therapy is needed.[96,100,103] The higher than normal serum iron concentration confirms the suspicion that K.M. has ingested iron tablets despite both her current lack of serious symptoms and the absence of tablet evidence in the rectal effluent or by abdominal radiograph.

The time course of absorption is probably the most difficult pharmacokinetic parameter to evaluate with toxic ingestions. Drug concentrations can continue to rise after an overdose despite GI decontamination.[93,95,96,103] This prolongation of absorption time is further complicated when sustained-release or enteric-coated dosage formulations have been ingested because the onset of symptoms is unpredictable.[94]

K.M.'s serum iron concentration of 480 mcg/dL suggests a serious ingestion because peak serum iron concentrations greater than 500 mcg/dL are usually predictive of significant toxicity.[93–96,100,103] This single serum iron concentration does not provide information as to whether the serum concentration is rising or declining or when the serum iron concentration will peak as a result of his iron ingestion.[104] Iron tablets may also clump together and form a bezoar, which can result in prolonged absorption and delay the onset of toxicity.[93,96] Samples for peak serum iron concentration should be obtained 4 to 6 hours after ingestion.[94–96,103] Although K.M.'s serum iron concentration was measured approximately 3 hours after ingestion, another serum iron level is needed in 2 to 4 hours because she ingested an enteric-coated formulation.

Blood Glucose, White Blood Cell Count, and Total Iron Binding Capacity

CASE 5-3, QUESTION 10: K.M. was administered WBI through the NG tube for several hours until the rectal effluent was clear. At this time, K.M. had three more episodes of vomiting and became drowsy and fussy. A repeat serum iron concentration was ordered at 6 hours after ingestion. What other laboratory tests could be helpful in assessing the potential toxicity of iron in K.M.?

Blood glucose concentrations and white blood cell counts usually are increased when serum iron concentrations are greater than 300 mcg/dL. A white blood cell count greater than 15,000/μL and a blood glucose concentration greater than 150 mg/dL within 6 hours of ingestion generally suggest a higher likelihood of severe toxicity.[93] These tests provide supplemental confirmation of iron intoxication and may be useful in medical facilities in which serum iron concentrations cannot be obtained. These laboratory tests are not routinely monitored in iron poisoning because of the poor sensitivity (about 50%).[94] Treatment should not be based on a white blood cell and glucose concentration alone.[93–95,100] If a patient with severe iron toxicity presents to a health care facility that cannot perform timely serum iron levels, either the blood iron sample must be sent to a laboratory that can do the testing quickly or the patient must be transferred to a health care facility that can do serum iron testing for patient monitoring.

It was once believed that if the serum iron concentration exceeded the total iron binding capacity concentration, it would indicate substantial iron toxicity. However, this theory has not held up, and the total iron binding capacity test is no longer used to monitor iron toxicity.[99]

Stages of Iron Toxicity

Case 5-3, Question 11: It is now 6 hours since K.M. ingested the iron tablets. Her second serum iron concentration is not yet available. She continues to be drowsy and fussy, and she has missed her usual nap. She is still vomiting. Why is K.M.'s relatively mild course at this time not particularly reassuring?

The time between the ingestion of an overdose of drugs and the development of severe toxicity can be delayed. It is unclear why there may be an asymptomatic period, but it may be secondary to delayed absorption of the ingested drug, the time required for the drug distribution, or the time needed to form a toxic metabolite. Consequently, K.M. may still exhibit further symptoms of severe toxicity. Four distinct stages of symptoms can be encountered with iron toxicity.[91–96]

STAGE I

Stage I symptoms usually take place within 6 hours of ingestion, during which nausea, vomiting, diarrhea, and abdominal pain occur, probably secondary to the erosive effects of iron on the GI mucosa. The caustic effects of free iron can cause bleeding as evidenced by blood in the vomitus and stool. In more severe intoxications, CNS and cardiovascular toxicity can be present during stage I.[93–96]

STAGE II

The second stage of iron toxicity has been suggested as a period of reduced symptoms and an apparent clinical improvement. This stage can last for up to 12 to 24 hours after the ingestion and could be misinterpreted as resolving toxicity. This stage may represent the time needed for the absorbed iron to distribute throughout the body before systemic symptoms develop.[91] In most severe cases, stage II does not occur and the patient's condition continues to deteriorate.[93–96]

STAGE III

Stage III generally occurs 12 to 48 hours after iron ingestion and is characterized by CNS toxicity (e.g., lethargy, coma, seizures) and cardiovascular toxicity (e.g., hypotension, shock, pulmonary edema). Metabolic acidosis, hypoglycemia, hepatic necrosis, renal damage, and coagulopathy can also happen during this stage.[93–96]

STAGE IV

The final stage is apparent 4 to 6 weeks after acute iron ingestion and consists of delayed-onset GI tract sequelae secondary to the initial local toxicity. In this stage, prior tissue damage can progress to gastric scarring and strictures at the pylorus, resulting in permanent abnormalities of GI function.[93–96]

Patients can present to the health care facility in any stage of iron toxicity and can have a fatal outcome in any stage. Determination of a stage of toxicity should be based on clinical symptoms rather than time of ingestion.[95]

Deferoxamine Chelation

Case 5-3, Question 12: The second serum iron concentration that was obtained 6 hours after ingestion has increased from 480 to 560 mcg/dL. The child has continued to vomit and appears pale. What criteria are most important in determining whether K.M. is a candidate for the antidote deferoxamine?

Deferoxamine (Desferal) chelates iron by binding ferric ions in plasma to form the iron complex ferrioxamine.[94] Deferoxamine prevents iron toxicity at a cellular level by removing iron from mitochondria.[92] Unfortunately, deferoxamine is not a very effective antidote because a relatively small amount of iron is bound (approximately 9 mg of iron to 100 mg of deferoxamine).[104,105] The iron–deferoxamine complex is primarily excreted renally as ferrioxamine.[92,94,95] Renal elimination of the ferrioxamine usually results in a pinkish-orange urine, often described as "vin rose."[92,94,95] Deferoxamine therapy should be initiated when serum iron concentrations exceed 500 mcg/dL and when symptoms of iron toxicity (e.g., GI symptoms, hemorrhage, coma, shock, seizures) are present.[92–95] K.M. is experiencing symptoms, she presumably ingested up to 69 mg/kg of elemental iron, and iron absorption appears to be ongoing based on the increase in her serum iron concentration. Therefore, K.M. should be treated with deferoxamine.

DEFEROXAMINE DOSE

Case 5-3, Question 13: What dose of deferoxamine should be prescribed for K.M., and how should it be administered?

Deferoxamine is most effective when administered intravenously as a continuous infusion because of its short half-life (76 ± 10 minutes).[95,104] Clinically, a slow IV infusion is preferred over intramuscular administration because the IV dose is better controlled, less painful, and better absorbed than an IM dose.[95,96] Deferoxamine is usually administered in a continuous IV infusion at a dose of 15 mg/kg/hour. However, doses up to 45 mg/kg/hour have been used in patients with severe iron poisoning.[93–96,104] Administering IV boluses of deferoxamine too rapidly can result in hypotension.[94,96,104,105] According to the manufacturer, the total deferoxamine dose should not exceed 6 g every 24 hours in children or adults, but adverse effects have not been seen in patients who received more than 6 g every 24 hours.[105]

Deferoxamine therapy should be initiated in K.M. at a lower rate of about 8 mg/kg/hour, and her clinical status should be monitored closely. If the dose is tolerated, the rate can be increased every 5 minutes until the desired rate of 15 mg/kg/hour is reached.[90]

MONITORING AND DISCONTINUATION

Case 5-3, Question 14: K.M. is admitted to the pediatric ICU shortly after the initiation of a deferoxamine infusion at 8 mg/kg/hour. How should deferoxamine therapy be monitored, and when should it be discontinued?

The rate of deferoxamine infusion should be increased with symptoms of severe iron toxicity, and decreased if patients experience adverse effects.[93,94,96,105] Treatment should continue until the serum iron concentration is less than 100 mcg/dL and symptoms of iron toxicity resolve.[105] Patients usually require chelation therapy for about 1 to 2 days, depending on the severity of symptoms.[93–95] Unnecessarily prolonged chelation therapy should be avoided because deferoxamine infusion for more than 24 hours has been associated with the development of acute respiratory distress syndrome.[93–98]

The urine color change to vin rose indicates ferrioxamine in the urine.[92,96] The lack of a color change is not a reliable indication of adequate deferoxamine therapy because not all patients experience vin rose urine.[92,96] There is also no correlation between amount of iron ingested, serum iron concentration, and the urine color change.[92]

Deferoxamine can interfere with some laboratory methods used to measure serum iron concentrations and cause falsely low values.[92,93,103,106] Atomic absorptive spectroscopy is a recommended method for monitoring serum iron concentrations once deferoxamine treatment has been started.[105] When initiating deferoxamine therapy, the clinical laboratory should be contacted to clarify whether deferoxamine will interfere with their serum iron analysis.

Outcome of Patient K.M.

K.M. was admitted to the pediatric ICU overnight and treated with a constant infusion of deferoxamine at 15 mg/kg/hour for 13 hours. Her GI symptoms resolved, she became more alert, and her vital signs were stable. Her serum iron level was 70 mcg/dL the next morning, and she was discharged home that afternoon.

ASSESSMENT OF CENTRAL NERVOUS SYSTEM DEPRESSANT VERSUS ANTIDEPRESSANT INGESTION

Validation of Ingestion

CASE 5-4

QUESTION 1: A.G., a 40-year-old man, was found unconscious in a pool of vomitus with a suicide note. The note stated that he had ingested 30 of his pills. A.G.'s 75-year-old mother called paramedics. When the paramedics arrived, A.G.'s heart rate was 150 beats/minute, BP was 115/70 mm Hg, and respirations were 14 breaths/minute and shallow. A.G. responded only to painful stimuli. The paramedics immediately started an IV line after completing their assessment of his ABCs. Why should the drug overdose information from this suicidal patient be validated?

Assessing the accuracy of historical information in adult drug exposures is difficult, and many health care professionals question the validity of information, especially from suicidal patients.[22–25,27] The ingestion history could be inaccurate because the patient's altered mental status might prevent accurate recollection of what occurred. He may also try to intentionally mislead health care providers to avoid appropriate care. Studies have demonstrated poor correlation between reported drug ingestions and urine drug test results.[23–25,27,32,33,107] There are also numerous false-positive results that can be misleading because of drug interference.[108,109]

Urine drug screens generally detect all recent drug and substance use, rather than just an overdosed drug. Urine drug screen results, therefore, are not reliable indicators of acute exposures. Every effort should be made to validate the history with information from other sources. In suicidal patients, one should consider all drugs that may have been available to the patient, as well as the patient's presenting symptoms, laboratory tests, and information obtained from family members, police, paramedics, and other individuals who know the patient.[22–25,27]

Interventions by Protocol

CASE 5-4, QUESTION 2: In addition to managing the ABCs, what pharmacologic interventions should be authorized for the paramedics to administer to A.G. in addition to the initiation of an IV solution?

GLUCOSE AND THIAMINE

Emergency medical service personnel often have protocols directing them to treat patients who are unconscious from an unknown cause. These protocols generally include administration of glucose, thiamine, and naloxone.[23,27,60,110] If paramedics cannot measure a blood glucose concentration immediately, A.G. should be given 50 mL of 50% dextrose to treat possible hypoglycemia. The risks of hyperglycemia from this dose of glucose are negligible relative to the significant benefits if the patient is hypoglycemic. Thiamine should be administered concurrently with glucose because glucose can precipitate Wernicke–Korsakoff complex in thiamine-deficient patients[111] (see Chapter 90, Substance Abuse Disorders). Wernicke encephalopathy is a reversible neurologic disturbance consisting of generalized confusion, ataxia, and ophthalmoplegia. Korsakoff psychosis is believed to be irreversible and is associated with a more prolonged deficiency of thiamine.[111,112] The unconscious patient should also be evaluated for blood loss, sepsis, hypoxia, and evidence of head trauma.[25]

NALOXONE

The pure opioid antagonist, naloxone, is indicated for the treatment of respiratory depression induced by opioids,[110,113] but many emergency medical service protocols authorize paramedics to routinely administer naloxone to all patients with any decreased mental status.[114] Naloxone reportedly has reversed coma and acute respiratory depression in intoxicated patients who have no evidence of opioid use.[60,112] The response of these patients to naloxone might have been secondary to opioids that were not detected by the urine toxicology screens (e.g., oxycodone, methadone, fentanyl). Reports of naloxone success in patients without opioid use could also have been the result of responses to other stimuli rather than a response to naloxone.

Administering naloxone to an opioid-addicted patient can precipitate withdrawal symptoms (e.g., agitation, combativeness, vomiting, diarrhea, lacrimation, rhinorrhea) that can further complicate the intoxication picture.[60] Small doses of naloxone should be administered initially to determine the patient's response to this medication. Violent and aggressive behavior can result when sudden increased consciousness is induced by naloxone.[27] This can complicate emergency care in an emergency transport vehicle and put caregivers and patients at risk for trauma.[60]

Initial Treatment

CASE 5-4, QUESTION 3: The paramedics arrive at the ED with A.G. 30 minutes after his mother called. A.G.'s heart rate in the ED is 155 beats/minute, BP is 89/50 mm Hg, and respirations have decreased from 14 to 9 breaths/minute, with assisted ventilation. A.G. remains unresponsive. The paramedics were unable to find any prescriptions or other medications in the house. The mother thinks her son was taking medication for depression. The medical team will try to obtain more details from A.G.'s pharmacy. What initial treatment should be provided for A.G. in the ED?

A.G. should be intubated and mechanically ventilated with 100% oxygen because of his shallow, slow respirations and the likelihood that vomitus could have been aspirated into his lungs. A bolus of IV fluid should be administered to A.G. to determine whether an increase in intravascular fluid volume will increase his BP and improve his mental status.[22,40]

Antidotes

CASE 5-4, QUESTION 4: A.G. fills his prescriptions at several pharmacies and it is taking a while to obtain his medication list. What antidotes can be administered in the ED for diagnostic purposes? Should flumazenil (Romazicon) be administered?

Theoretically, antidotes such as naloxone, flumazenil, deferoxamine, and digoxin-specific antibody-FAB fragments could be administered in a hospitalized setting to identify an unknown to xin.[22,26,27,113,115,116] However, the cost and time required for administration, and increased risks from these antidotes, preclude their use for diagnostic purposes without some plausible suspicion of a specific drug ingestion.[113,115]

Organ System Evaluations

CASE 5-4, QUESTION 5: How can the initial physical assessment, using an organ systems approach, help in identifying the drugs ingested by A.G.?

The patient's ABCs and CNS and cardiopulmonary functions should be assessed with special attention to clinical manifestations that suggest ingestion of a specific class of drugs.[27,40] A.G.'s history of depression suggests that antidepressants, antipsychotics, lithium, or benzodiazepines are candidates for ingestion. An organ system evaluation will help determine whether these (or other) drugs might have been ingested. Commonly used nonprescription medications such as aspirin, acetaminophen, decongestants, and antihistamines, should also be considered because adult drug ingestions usually involve more than one drug.

CENTRAL NERVOUS SYSTEM FUNCTION

Changes in CNS function are probably the single most common finding associated with drug intoxication.[27] CNS depression or stimulation, seizures, delirium, hallucinations, coma, or any combination of these can be seen in intoxicated patients. CNS changes can be the direct result of an ingested drug or may be attributed to other underlying CNS processes or medical conditions.[116] Clinical manifestations of drug overdoses may differ depending on where the patient is in the time course of the intoxication, and the amount of drug(s) ingested.[27,64]

Drugs with anticholinergic properties can produce disorientation, confusion, delirium, and visual hallucinations early in the course of the intoxication; coma can become apparent as toxicity progresses. Generally, overdoses with anticholinergic drugs do not produce true hallucinations, but rather pseudohallucinations. When a patient with an intact baseline mental status presents with psychosis, paranoia, or visual hallucinations, CNS stimulants such as cocaine or amphetamines should be considered.[30,65]

Drug intoxication–induced alterations in CNS function are initially difficult to distinguish from those caused by underlying psychiatric disorders, trauma, hypoxia, or metabolic disorders, such as hepatic encephalopathy or hypoglycemia. However, as time passes, decreased CNS function secondary to drug toxicity is more likely to wax and wane in severity in contrast to the persistent CNS depression that occurs with significant trauma or metabolic disorders. Drug toxicity also rarely produces focal neurologic findings. Changes in pupil size, reflexes, and vital signs can provide insights into the pharmacologic class of drug involved in the intoxication.[23,27,28]

CNS depression, seizures, disorientation, and other CNS changes that are commonly associated with psychiatric drugs should be evaluated carefully in A.G. For example, A.G.'s pupil size would most likely be dilated if he had ingested a TCA because of the anticholinergic effects of these drugs. TCA intoxications can also cause myoclonic spasms,[27] which are often difficult to differentiate from seizure activity caused by TCA overdoses, although the spasms are often asymmetric and more persistent.[117]

CARDIOVASCULAR FUNCTION

Assessment of heart rate, rhythm, conduction, and measurements of hemodynamic function can also be used to help identify the type of drug ingested. Overdoses of sympathomimetic drugs usually increase heart rate, while overdoses of cardiac glycosides or β-blockers can slow the heart rate. Although drugs can increase or decrease heart rate directly, indirect cardiac effects (e.g., reflex tachycardia in response to hypotension) also need to be considered. Abnormal heart rates produced by drug overdoses are usually not treated unless accompanied by hypotension or severe dysrhythmias.[27,40]

PULMONARY FUNCTION

Evaluating the rate and depth of respiration and the effectiveness of gas exchange in an intoxicated patient can also help identify drugs ingested. A decrease in respiratory rate is commonly associated with the ingestion of CNS depressants. An increased respiratory rate and depth is generally associated with CNS stimulant toxicity and can also be secondary to respiratory compensation for a drug-induced metabolic acidosis.[27] Aspiration of gastric contents after vomiting is common in drug ingestions. Aspiration pneumonitis is the most common pulmonary abnormality associated with significant intoxications.[43] Noncardiogenic acute pulmonary edema has been associated with salicylate overdoses[80] (especially with chronic intoxications) and drugs of abuse (e.g., cocaine and heroin).[114,118–124]

TEMPERATURE REGULATION

Body temperature is an important and sometimes overlooked parameter when assessing potential intoxications.[27,40] Decreased mental status is often associated with a loss of thermoregulation, resulting in a body temperature that falls or increases toward the ambient temperature. Increased body temperature (hyperthermia) caused by overdoses of CNS stimulants (e.g., cocaine, amphetamines, ecstasy), salicylates, hallucinogens (e.g., phencyclidine), or anticholinergic drugs or plants (e.g., jimsonweed) can have serious consequences.[27,29,40] Body temperature should be measured rectally to obtain an accurate representation of core body temperature.[125]

Hyperthermia caused by drug overdoses is commonly seen in hot, humid environments or when the intoxication is associated with physical exertion, increased muscle tone, or seizures. In these patients, it is important to obtain renal function tests (e.g., BUN, serum creatinine) and a serum creatine kinase measurement to determine whether rhabdomyolysis has occurred secondary to breakdown of muscle tissue.[27,40,125]

GASTROINTESTINAL FUNCTION

The GI tract should be assessed for decreased motility because drug absorption can be delayed or prolonged.[27,126,127] When this is the case, decontamination may be beneficial after an oral ingestion even if a long time has elapsed since the ingestion. The presence of blood in either emesis or stool may suggest ingestion of a GI irritant or caustic substance.[128]

SKIN AND EXTREMITIES

The physical examination should include a thorough examination of the body surface for causes of trauma that may also explain the patient's condition. Examination of the skin and extremities can provide evidence of drug intoxication, especially with IV or subcutaneous drug injection needle marks.[27] Drugs can be hidden in the rectum or vagina.[27] Drug patches (e.g., fentanyl) may be found in hidden areas of the body such as the back of the neck or scrotum. Fluid-filled bullae at gravity-dependent sites that have been in contact with hard surfaces for a long time suggest prolonged coma.[27] Muscle tone should also be assessed.[30] Increased tone or myoclonic spasms can be caused by some drug overdoses (e.g., TCAs) and can produce rhabdomyolysis or hyperthermia.[27,125] Dry, hot, red skin may also be an indication of anticholinergic toxicity.[27,40]

In summary, an organ system assessment of A.G. can provide useful insights into the identity of drugs that might have been ingested, the viability of organ function that might have been adversely affected, and the treatment needed.

Laboratory Tests

CASE 5-4, QUESTION 6: What laboratory tests should be ordered for A.G.?

The laboratory assessment of an intoxicated patient should be guided by the history of the events surrounding the ingestion, clinical presentation, and past medical history.[22,129] The status of oxygenation, acid–base balance, and blood glucose concentration must be determined, especially in patients with altered mental status such as A.G.[40] Oxygenation can be assessed initially by pulse oximetry and acid–base status by ABGs and serum electrolyte concentrations.[129,130] A.G. was given oxygen and a bolus of IV fluid on arrival at the ED, and paramedics administered glucose during transportation.

A medical history of organ dysfunction or medical disorders (e.g., diabetes, hypertension) that can damage organs of elimination (e.g., kidney, liver) will also guide the need for laboratory tests. A serum creatinine concentration and liver function tests (e.g., aspartate aminotransferase [AST], alanine aminotransferase [ALT]) should be ordered. Other more specific tests reflective of his past medical history can be ordered subsequent to dialogue with his psychiatrist. A complete blood cell count, complete chemistry panel, serum osmolality, and other baseline laboratory tests should be obtained.[27] Pregnancy tests should be considered in female patients of childbearing age because unwanted pregnancies are common causes of overdose.[131,132]

A baseline electrocardiogram (ECG) should be obtained when exposure to a cardiotoxic drug is suspected or whenever the cardiovascular or hemodynamic status is altered.[23,26,40,130] A 12-lead ECG should be ordered because A.G. is likely to have ingested a psychotropic agent. Continuous cardiac monitoring should be instituted because of the significant cardiotoxicity associated with overdoses of these agents. Patients with severe TCA overdoses frequently present with symptoms of coma, tachycardia with a widened QRS interval, seizures, hypotension, and respiratory depression.[133–136]

A chest radiograph is useful when the potential exists for either direct pulmonary toxicity or aspiration.[23,26] A chest radiograph is indicated because A.G. had vomitus in his mouth and TCAs are associated with the development of acute respiratory distress syndrome and pulmonary edema.[133,137,138]

Qualitative Screening

CASE 5-4, QUESTION 7: Should A.G.'s urine and blood be screened to assist in identifying the ingested substance? Explain your rationale.

Toxicology laboratory testing can be used to identify the substances involved in a toxic exposure, to exclude substances, or to measure the concentration of substances in serum or other biological fluids.[24,129,130] The identification and quantification of compounds should be considered as two distinct types of toxicologic testing.[24,139] *Qualitative* screening is used to identify which substance or class of substances is involved in the toxic exposure. *Quantitative* testing determines how much of a known substance is present.[24]

Screening of various biological fluids can identify unknown substances. Urine is screened much more commonly than blood, whereas gastric fluid is rarely evaluated. A urine drug screen is preferred to a blood drug screen because urine generally contains a higher concentration of a drug and its metabolites than other body fluids.[140]

When reviewing the results of urine screening panels for drugs and other substances, one must remember that the presence of a substance in urine is not necessarily related to a concurrent toxicity. A positive result on a urine screening panel merely indicates that the patient has ingested or has been exposed to the substance, but it does not differentiate between toxic and nontoxic doses. If a drug and its metabolites are eliminated slowly into the urine for a prolonged time, and if the testing methodology detects small concentrations of the substance, urine drug screening could identify the presence of a substance days, weeks, or even months after the exposure (e.g., marijuana).[24,130]

It is important to know which drugs or substances are tested at a given laboratory. Many laboratories restrict the number of drugs for which they test because 15 drugs account for more than 90% of all drug overdoses.[32] Some urine toxicology screens only detect common drugs of abuse (e.g., amphetamines, barbiturates, benzodiazepines, cocaine, marijuana, opioids).[130] Some drugs of abuse are not detected on routine drug screening (e.g., gamma hydroxybutyrate, ketamine, flunitrazepam).[24] Some analyses detect only antibodies to drug metabolites. For example, a benzodiazepine screen detects oxazepam, a common benzodiazepine metabolite. However, alprazolam and lorazepam are not metabolized to oxazepam and will not be detected in a urine screen. Likewise, an opioid screen may not detect the synthetic opioids such as fentanyl and methadone.[130]

Results of qualitative toxicology screening tests are difficult to interpret. False negatives, false positives, cross-reactivity with related drugs, chronicity of exposure, and length of time since last exposure all complicate results.[108,109,130] Urine toxicology screen results rarely change clinical management of the patient. Monitoring mental, cardiovascular, and respiratory status and other laboratory parameters provide better clues than the results of a urine toxicology screen.[23,24,129,130,139]

Toxicology screening can be appropriate when the history of a suspected toxic exposure is unavailable, inaccurate, or inconsistent with the clinical findings.[24] However, it is important to know which drugs are detected on a given toxicology screen.[130] A comprehensive qualitative urine drug screen can be considered for A.G. because information about the substance(s) he ingested is not yet known.

Quantitative Testing

CASE 5-4, QUESTION 8: Should a quantitative toxicology laboratory test be ordered for A.G. as well? Explain your rationale.

After a qualitative urine analysis for drugs, a quantitative analysis of drug concentration in blood can help determine the severity of toxicity and the need for aggressive interventions (e.g., hemodialysis).[24,33,130,139] Quantitative tests are especially useful when assessing the potential toxicity of drugs with delayed clinical toxicity or when the toxicity primarily is caused by metabolites (e.g., ethylene glycol, methanol). The concentration of a drug in serum is sometimes much more predictive of end-organ damage than clinical findings (e.g., acetaminophen effect on the liver).

Quantifying the amount of drug in serum is useful when (a) the concentration of the substance correlates with toxic effects, (b) the turnaround time for results is rapid, and (c) treatment can be guided by the serum concentration.[32,132,142] To aid in the care of poisoned patients, stat quantitative serum concentrations of acetaminophen, carbamazepine, carboxyhemoglobin, digoxin, ethanol, ethylene glycol, iron, lithium, methanol, methemoglobin, phenobarbital, salicylates, and theophylline should be available at laboratories of large health care facilities.[23,24,33,129,139]

When blood samples are collected to quantitate potentially intoxicating substances, as much information as possible should be obtained about the time course of events to determine whether absorption and distribution of the substance is complete. Serial samples may be needed to determine whether significant absorption is still occurring.[29,30] In contrast to the interpretation of therapeutic serum concentrations of chronically administered drugs, the serum concentration of a substance ingested in an overdose is not likely to be at steady state.

Quantitative toxicologic testing will likely not benefit A.G. at this point in time because the identity of the ingested substance is unknown. Nevertheless, a serum ethanol concentration could be obtained because alcohol is often ingested concurrently in overdose situations.[132] Most poison centers also recommend obtaining a quantitative acetaminophen level on all intentional ingestions because serious hepatotoxicity can occur if acetaminophen ingestion is missed.[24,129,130]

Assessment

CASE 5-4, QUESTION 9: A.G.'s clinical status has not changed in the past 10 minutes. A urine toxicology screen, blood acetaminophen, blood alcohol, and ABGs have been ordered. The 12-lead ECG shows a prolonged QRS interval of 0.13 seconds (normal, <0.1 seconds). No antidotes have been administered. A.G.'s physical examination did not detect any evidence of trauma to his head. His pupils were dilated and slowly responsive to light, and his bowel sounds were hypoactive. What conclusions can be made at this time with regard to the likely substance ingested by A.G?

Although the ingested substance still has not been specifically identified, the available data provide some clues as to the likely pharmacologic class of drug that was ingested. The presence of CNS depression (A.G. is unresponsive), slowed ventricular conduction (widened QRS on ECG), tachycardia (heart rate, 155 beats/minute), hypotension (BP, 89/50 mm Hg), and decreased GI motility (hypoactive bowel sounds), and the history of a possible depressive illness (history from mother) are all consistent with a TCA drug overdose. The antidepressant could have been ingested alone or with other agents.

Antidepressant Toxicities

CASE 5-4, QUESTION 10: How would the different toxicities of the many available antidepressants affect the treatment of A.G.?

The major pharmacologic effects and toxicities of the antidepressants are similar for all drugs within the same class. When a specific drug within a therapeutic class has not yet been identified, the overdose should be managed as if the ingested drug can produce the most severe toxicity of any drug in the class. Therefore, A.G.'s presumed antidepressant drug overdose should be evaluated and managed initially as TCA (e.g., amitriptyline) ingestion.[135,141] Antidepressants with different structures and actions (e.g., trazodone [Desyrel], fluoxetine [Prozac], sertraline [Zoloft]) generally do not produce toxicity as severe as that of the TCAs.[135,141,142]

Gastrointestinal Decontamination

CASE 5-4, QUESTION 11: If a TCA ingestion is presumed, why might GI decontamination be appropriate at this time?

The longer GI decontamination is delayed relative to the time of ingestion, the less effective it is likely to be because drug absorption will already have occurred. Because the time of ingestion is unknown and A.G. is unresponsive, he probably already has absorbed significant amounts of the drug, making him more vulnerable to aspiration. Additionally, A.G. might already have aspirated because he was found in a pool of vomitus. TCA overdoses can also cause seizures, which would be a relative contraindication to GI decontamination. In consideration of these concerns, many would not support GI decontamination for A.G.[41–44,51–54]

Others might support GI decontamination because TCAs have strong central and peripheral anticholinergic properties that slow GI emptying, which could result in erratic absorption and delayed toxicity, but A.G. would first need to be intubated to protect his airway. Furthermore, TCAs have a large volume of distribution (10–50 L/kg), and both the parent drug and its metabolite undergo enterohepatic recirculation. The half-life of TCAs in overdose situations is 37 to 60 hours. For those reasons, activated charcoal could be reasonably administered in an effort to adsorb any drug that may not yet be absorbed from the GI tract.[49]

Repeated doses of activated charcoal have been used to increase the elimination of TCAs because of the long half-life of TCAs and the enterohepatic recirculation. In clinical studies, multiple-dose activated charcoal has increased the elimination of amitriptyline, but the data are insufficient to support or exclude its use.[47]

MONITORING EFFICACY

CASE 5-4, QUESTION 12: How should the effectiveness of GI decontamination be monitored in A.G.?

If activated charcoal is administered, A.G. must first be intubated to protect his airway, and the charcoal must be administered via NG tube because he is unconscious. The insertion of the NG tube could stimulate the gag reflex, causing vomiting and possible aspiration. A.G.'s lung sounds should be monitored closely to determine whether aspiration pneumonitis is developing, particularly because AG. was found unconscious and had already vomited.

Activated charcoal, especially in multiple doses, can produce ileus, GI obstruction, or intestinal perforation, particularly when administered to patients who have ingested drugs that slow GI motility.[47,49,101] Bowel sounds must be monitored frequently to ensure that an ileus is not developing. Once the patient passes a charcoal-laden stool, the activated charcoal can be considered to have successfully passed through the GI tract.

Sodium Bicarbonate and Hyperventilation

CASE 5-4, QUESTION 13: According to A.G.'s psychiatrist, he prescribed amitriptyline 100 mg at bedtime for his severe depression. How does this new information alter A.G.'s treatment plan?

This information confirms the assumptions that a TCA was ingested. It also specifically identifies the drug ingested. In TCA ingestions, severe toxicity has been associated with doses of 15 to 25 mg/kg.[98] A.G. ingested a total of 3,000 mg based on his suicide note that said he took 30 tablets. If he weighs about 70 kg and was truthful about the amount taken, he ingested a significantly toxic dose (about 43 mg/kg).

On the ECG, TCA toxicity will manifest as tachycardia with prolongation of the PR, QTc, and QRS intervals, ST and T-wave changes, and abnormalities of the terminal 40-millisecond vector.[98,117,133,136,142–146] TCAs have anticholinergic, adrenergic, and quinidine-like membrane effects on the heart.[117,133,135,141,144] It is believed that the anticholinergic effect causes the tachycardia and the quinidine-like effect causes the ECG changes.

In addition, TCAs are sodium-channel blockers.[147] Sodium-channel blockade slows the maximum uptake stroke of phase 0 of the action potential and decreases automaticity. Blockade decreases conduction velocity in the Purkinje fibers, which increases the QRS interval.[144] Myocardial depression, ventricular tachycardia, and ventricular fibrillation are the most common causes of death from TCAs.[136] Therefore, admission to the ICU with continuous cardiac monitoring is essential for A.G.[143]

The primary therapy for reversing ventricular arrhythmias and conduction delays is alkalinization of the serum and sodium loading with IV hypertonic sodium bicarbonate.[117,133,135,136,144,145,148] Indications for sodium bicarbonate include hypotension, widened QRS interval (more than 100 milliseconds), right bundle branch block, and wide complex tachycardia.[135,145] Alkalinization increases serum protein binding of the TCAs and reduces the amount of free active drug (likely a minor consideration).[116,133,136,145] Correction of the serum pH is beneficial because underlying acidosis worsens TCA-induced cardiotoxicity.[145] Furthermore, sodium bicarbonate has been found useful even in patients with a normal pH because sodium bicarbonate purportedly overcomes the sodium-channel blockade and reduces cardiotoxicity.[145,147]

On the basis of A.G.'s tachycardia and a widened QRS segment on ECG, he should be treated with IV sodium bicarbonate with the goal of achieving an arterial pH of 7.5 to 7.55.[136,145] Sodium bicarbonate could have been administered earlier because the suspicion of an antidepressant overdose was strong initially, his ECG demonstrated QRS widening and worsening myocardial conduction, and his BP continued to decline from the time he was first seen by the paramedics. If not monitored closely, the use of IV sodium bicarbonate could introduce the risk of sodium overload and subsequent pulmonary edema.[98,146]

An alternative is to hyperventilate the patient to a pH of 7.5 by adjusting his ventilator setting, thereby reducing the cardiotoxicity of the TCA.[133,136,146] The combination of IV bicarbonate and mechanical ventilation is more likely to produce severe alkalemia. Careful and frequent monitoring of the serum pH of patients on dual therapy is essential.[133,147]

MONITORING EFFICACY

CASE 5-4, QUESTION 14: How should the sodium bicarbonate therapy in A.G. be monitored?

Patients intoxicated with TCAs often present with severe acidosis. Large doses of sodium bicarbonate may be required to normalize the arterial pH. The efficacy of sodium bicarbonate administration can be evaluated by monitoring acid–base status using ABGs, especially if the patient is also being ventilated mechanically.[133,147,148]

Sodium bicarbonate should be administered IV as a bolus of 1 to 2 mEq/kg for a 1- to 2-minute period. Continuous ECG monitoring is needed to monitor results of the bolus on cardiac abnormalities. Repeat bolus doses are administered as needed until the QRS interval narrows and tachycardia slows. Blood pH should be tested after several boluses to determine whether a target pH of 7.5 to 7.55 has been obtained.[145] At a minimum, ABGs should be determined within an hour of starting sodium bicarbonate therapy to determine pH response.[148] Bicarbonate boluses can be followed by a constant sodium bicarbonate infusion of 150 mEq/L to maintain an alkaline pH.[145] ABGs must be monitored frequently to ensure a response.[133,147,148] Serial ECGs to measure the QRS interval are useful for evaluating the efficacy of sodium bicarbonate therapy. A widened QRS interval will generally normalize after the systemic pH has been increased to about 7.5.[148]

Seizures

CASE 5-4, QUESTION 15: A.G. gradually developed more severely altered mental status and became comatose, not responding even to painful stimuli. He suddenly experienced a tonic–clonic seizure, which lasted about 1 minute and terminated spontaneously. Should anticonvulsant therapy be initiated for A.G. at this time?

CNS toxicity is common in TCA overdoses. Symptoms include agitation, hallucinations, coma, myoclonus, and seizures.[117,133–136] Seizures can cause significant increases in acidosis and increase cardiotoxicity. Seizures are often seen immediately before cardiopulmonary arrest. Because of the severe consequences of prolonged seizures, aggressive drug treatment with rapid onset of action is indicated, and benzodiazepines are the drugs of choice.[133,136]

Drug overdose–induced grand mal seizures are most commonly single seizures that terminate before drug therapy can be administered.[135] Seizure activity is not expected to persist, so instituting long-term anticonvulsant therapy is not indicated. However, if A.G.'s seizure did not stop within 1 to 2 minutes, a benzodiazepine would have been indicated.[117,133,136] The onset of action of phenobarbital is too slow for acute seizures, and phenytoin is usually ineffective in treating drug toxicity–related seizures.[117] After a seizure, the patient may become more acidotic and hypotensive.[136] Blood gases, creatine kinase, and ECG changes should be monitored immediately after a seizure.

Interpretation of Urine Screens

CASE 5-4, QUESTION 16: A.G.'s BP fell to 80/42 mm Hg, and dopamine was started. His pH on repeat ABGs was 7.20. A.G.'s ECG normalized after the administration of 150 mL of sodium bicarbonate by IV bolus. After dopamine, his BP increased to 100/56 mm Hg, and seizure activity ceased. The urine drug screen results were positive for amitriptyline and nortriptyline. Acetaminophen, salicylates, and ethanol were not detected in his blood. Does the presence of nortriptyline indicate that A.G. has ingested other drugs in addition to his amitriptyline?

Nortriptyline is a metabolite of amitriptyline and, therefore, was identified on the urine drug screen. Metabolites, as well as the parent compound, are often identified on comprehensive urine drug screens.[132]

Duration of Hospitalization

CASE 5-4, QUESTION 17: How long should A.G. be monitored?

A.G. should be admitted to the ICU and monitored until all evidence of CNS and cardiovascular toxicity has been reversed.[117] There is some controversy over how long symptomatic patients should be observed. Some believe symptomatic patients need cardiac monitoring for 24 hours after ingestion.[135] Others believe TCA overdose patients need to be monitored until they are symptom-free for 24 hours because of a few reports of late development of symptoms.[139] However, 98% of signs of cardiotoxicity and arrhythmias are seen within the first 24 hours after TCA ingestion.[117,134] Because the incidence of late-occurring symptoms is rare, most patients are discharged after they are fully awake.[133] After the toxicity has completely resolved, A.G. should be evaluated by a psychiatrist to determine whether he should be admitted for inpatient treatment of his suicidal ideation.[133–135]

Outcome of Patient A.G.

A.G. had no further seizure activity. He remained on a dopamine infusion for 8 hours and required several more boluses of IV sodium bicarbonate. The next afternoon, he started to awaken and expressed regret that his suicide attempt was not successful. Arrangements were made to transfer him to an inpatient psychiatric hospital once he was medically cleared.

ASSESSMENT OF ACETAMINOPHEN INGESTION

Mechanism of Hepatotoxicity

CASE 5-5

QUESTION 1: B.W., a 18-year-old woman who is about 30 weeks pregnant, presents to the ED 8 hours after ingesting 40 acetaminophen 500-mg tablets. She is depressed and hoped to end her pregnancy by ingesting acetaminophen. Her pregnancy was unplanned, and she has received no prenatal care. B.W. has vomited spontaneously 6 times since the ingestion and is complaining of abdominal pain; her heart rate is 95 beats/minute, BP is 110/74 mm Hg, and temperature is 98.5°F. B.W. does not have any chronic diseases, and the remainder of her medical history is unremarkable. How does an overdose of acetaminophen cause toxicity?

Acetaminophen is metabolized in the liver by glucuronidation and sulfation. The mixed-function oxidase system cytochrome P-450 (CYP) 2E1 metabolizes a portion of the acetaminophen to the highly reactive metabolite *N*-acetyl-*p*-benzoquinoneimine (NAPQI). In therapeutic doses, this metabolite is detoxified in the liver by glutathione. At toxic serum acetaminophen concentrations, the glucuronidation and sulfation metabolic pathways become saturated. Usually, NAPQI is detoxified by conjugation with glutathione, but increased amounts of the toxic metabolite deplete hepatic glutathione stores. When glutathione stores are decreased to about 30% of normal, the toxic metabolite binds to liver cells, resulting in the characteristic centrilobular hepatic necrosis seen in acetaminophen overdoses.[149–152]

Complication of Pregnancy

CASE 5-5, QUESTION 2: How does B.W.'s pregnancy change the management of her acetaminophen ingestion?

Pregnancy does not alter the initial approach to the assessment or treatment of potentially toxic ingestions, and assessment should focus initially on the mother.[153,154] Overdoses during pregnancy are often associated with attempted abortions, depression, prior loss of a child or children, potential loss of a lover, or economic reasons.[131,132,153,154] Intentional ingestions of analgesics, prenatal vitamins, iron, psychotropic agents, and antibiotics account for 74% of the overdoses during pregnancy.

The fetus is at risk when the mother overdoses on acetaminophen because acetaminophen crosses the placenta. The fetal liver can oxidize acetaminophen to its hepatotoxic metabolite by 14 weeks of gestation.[151] However, the fetal liver has only about 10% of the capability of the adult liver to metabolize acetaminophen. The fetal liver can conjugate acetaminophen with both glutathione and sulfate, but detoxification by glutathione conjugation appears to be decreased.[155,156]

In studies of maternal acetaminophen toxicity, most of the pregnant women survived without damage to themselves or their babies. However, there were also maternal and fetal deaths as a result of overdose.[155,157] Acetaminophen overdoses during pregnancy did not appear to increase the risk for birth defects or adverse pregnancy outcomes unless the mother suffered severe toxicity, emphasizing the need to treat the mother promptly.[149,155]

Gastrointestinal Decontamination

CASE 5-5, QUESTION 3: Should GI decontamination be initiated for B.W.? Justify your rationale.

B.W.'s acetaminophen ingestion occurred 8 hours ago; therefore, the drug is likely to be totally absorbed, and no GI decontamination should be initiated.

Estimating Potential Toxicity

CASE 5-5, QUESTION 4: How should the potential toxicity of the acetaminophen ingestion be assessed in B.W.?

Acetaminophen toxicity results from ingestions greater than 150 mg/kg or more than 7.5 g total in adults. However, serum acetaminophen concentrations better predict acetaminophen-induced hepatotoxicity than the dose of acetaminophen acutely ingested.[158,159] The Rumack–Matthew nomogram is used in the United States to assess the potential for hepatotoxicity from acute overdoses of acetaminophen.[160,161] The treatment line is defined by a serum acetaminophen concentration of 200 mcg/mL at 4 hours after acetaminophen ingestion and 30 mcg/mL at 15 hours after ingestion on a semilogarithmic graph.[152] Many prefer to be more conservative and use the bottom line of 150 mcg/mL at 4 hours to begin treatment as histories of ingestion are often inaccurate. The serum acetaminophen concentration is plotted on a graph against the time of ingestion.[159] The nomogram predicts the probability that the AST or ALT will be greater than 1,000 international units/L and can be used to guide therapy by indicating whether a specific acetaminophen concentration is in the toxic range.[162] The nomogram is useful only for acute ingestions because it underestimates the potential for toxicity in chronic acetaminophen ingestions. It should be noted that although the nomogram is used to plot acetaminophen concentrations for all patients, it has been validated only in healthy nonalcoholic adults.[152]

Acetaminophen Treatment Nomogram

CASE 5-5, QUESTION 5: When is the preferred time to measure a serum acetaminophen concentration?

Acetaminophen absorption generally is complete within 1.5 to 2.5 hours after ingestion of solid or liquid dosage forms.[159] The Rumack–Matthew nomogram is not applicable before 4 hours after ingestion because it is based on complete drug absorption.[159] Most clinical laboratories can complete their assays and report acetaminophen serum concentration results within 2 hours.

Stages of Acetaminophen Toxicity

CASE 5-5, QUESTION 6: What are the clinical signs and symptoms of acetaminophen toxicity?

Early detection of an acetaminophen overdose is difficult because there are no characteristic early diagnostic findings. Toxicity appears in stages that may overlap and are not clear-cut. About 30 minutes to 24 hours after ingestion, the patient may exhibit anorexia, nausea, vomiting, malaise, and diaphoresis that can easily be attributed to other causes. The second stage of acetaminophen toxicity occurs about 24 to 48 hours after ingestion and is the stage in which hepatotoxicity develops. Hepatotoxicity is universal by 36 hours after ingestion. An AST measurement is the most sensitive measure of hepatotoxicity as AST abnormalities always precede evidence of actual liver impairment.[152,160,163]

In the third stage, 72 to 96 hours after ingestion, maximal liver dysfunction is evident with the return of anorexia, nausea, vomiting, and malaise. Symptoms can range from mild to fulminant liver failure with hepatic encephalopathy, coma, and hemorrhage. AST and ALT serum concentrations can be greater than 10,000 international units/L. There are also increases in bilirubin and INR measurements, as well as abnormalities in glucose and pH readings. Death, if it occurs, is usually a result of multiorgan failure or hemorrhage caused by hepatic failure. Most deaths occur 3 to 5 days after exposure. Patients who survive this stage go into recovery.[152,160,163]

Antidotes

CASE 5-5, QUESTION 7: What antidote for acetaminophen ingestion should be considered in B.W.? How does the antidote work, and when is it most effective?

Toxicity is determined by the results of a serum acetaminophen concentration measured at least 4 hours after ingestion.[159] *N*-acetylcysteine, or NAC, is the antidote for acetaminophen toxicity. NAC is a sulfhydryl donor that converts to cysteine, which is subsequently converted to glutathione.[149,160,162,163] NAC acts as a glutathione substitute and directly combines with the toxic acetaminophen metabolite, NAPQI, reducing it to a nontoxic cysteine conjugate.[163] NAC can also substitute for sulfation, which increases the nontoxic metabolism through that route as well. NAC increases intrahepatic microcirculation and is believed to possess hepatoprotective properties, showing some value even after liver damage has already occurred.[149,160]

Instituting therapy early with NAC is essential. When NAC is started within 8 to 10 hours of the ingestion, hepatotoxicity resulted in only 1.6% of cases. In patients who were started on NAC more than 10 hours after ingestion, 53% developed liver damage.[152,160]

Safety of *N*-Acetylcysteine in Pregnancy

CASE 5-5, QUESTION 8: Is NAC safe to use during pregnancy?

Acetaminophen overdose in pregnant women should be managed in the same manner as in nonpregnant patients.[155–157] If the life of the mother is not saved, the fetus will not survive (unless the child is near term and is emergently delivered). NAC therapy is not contraindicated in pregnant patients and might be helpful because it crosses the placenta and can protect the fetus from hepatotoxicity.[155,157]

NAC therapy appears to be protective for both mother and fetus.[152,155,158-160,162,163] When used as an antidote for acetaminophen overdose in pregnancy, NAC did not appear to cause toxic effects to the fetus.[149,152,155,157] The probability of fetal death was increased with the delay in NAC treatment after acetaminophen overdose.[152,156,160]

Route of Administration of *N*-Acetylcysteine

CASE 5-5, QUESTION 9: The 9-hour acetaminophen concentration in B.W. was 170 mcg/mL. By what route should NAC be administered?

This concentration of acetaminophen at 6 hours is above the treatment line on the Rumack–Matthew nomogram.[161] Because there was some delay from the time of ingestion to presentation at the ED and B.W. was already vomiting, it will be more difficult for B.W. to tolerate oral NAC. For this reason, IV NAC is recommended.

An FDA-approved sterile, pyrogen-free formulation of NAC is available as Acetadote.[164–166] The use of IV NAC is not completely risk-free because of a possible anaphylactoid reaction during the first dose of the IV NAC. The incidence of adverse reactions ranges from 14.3% to 23%. Asthmatic patients and patients with ectopy should receive the drug slowly and carefully, while being watched for symptoms of a reaction.[166]

A majority of the adverse reactions include nausea, vomiting, urticaria, flushing, and pruritus. Bronchospasm, angioedema, hypotension, and death have rarely occurred and must be carefully monitored when the IV route is being used.[167,168] Most reactions occur during or just after the first 15 minutes of the initial antidote infusion and appear to be dose related.[168] Because of the timing issue, the first dose of IV NAC is usually administered for 60 minutes instead of 15 minutes, even though a study comparing adverse reactions in the two infusion rates did not show clinically significant differences.[166,169]

Intravenous *N*-Acetylcysteine

CASE 5-5, QUESTION 10: How should IV NAC be administered to B.W.?

The FDA-approved IV NAC protocol is the same 20-hour dosing regimen used in Europe, known as the Prescott protocol.[164,165,166] A 150 mg/kg loading dose of NAC in 5% dextrose is infused IV slowly for 60 minutes while watching for symptoms of a possible anaphylactoid reaction. This is followed by a maintenance dose of 50 mg/kg infused for 4 hours, and then followed with a 100 mg/kg dose infused for 16 hours. This regimen provides a total of 300 mg/kg NAC during the 20 hours after the loading dose.[166]

Oral *N*-Acetylcysteine

CASE 5-5, QUESTION 11: Once she is able to tolerate oral NAC treatment, what dosing regimen would be appropriate for B.W.?

The standard oral NAC protocol is based on the original clinical studies.[163] The loading dose of NAC is 140 mg/kg orally using either the 10% or 20% mucolytic solutions that were formulated for inhalation therapy. Seventeen additional maintenance doses of 70 mg/kg of NAC are administered at 4-hour intervals after the initial dose, for a total of 72 hours of therapy. This provides a total of 1,330 mg/kg NAC during 72 hours.[170] Because oral NAC contains a sulfhydryl group, the substance has a very disagreeable taste and smell (like rotten eggs) that commonly results in nausea and vomiting for the patient. To mask the unpleasant taste and odor, NAC is diluted to a concentration of 5% using a carbonated beverage or fruit juice.[163] Because the entire dose of oral NAC passes through the liver, high concentrations are produced, which is seen as an advantage of oral therapy.[164]

Shorter oral NAC regimens are currently being used based on the efficacy of IV therapy.[171,172] Short-course oral NAC follows the same 20-hour time course as IV NAC. Patients receive the usual 140 mg/kg oral loading dose of NAC, followed by 70 mg/kg every 4 hours for five additional doses (20 hours of therapy). Serum acetaminophen, liver function tests, and INR are repeated at 20 hours after the loading dose, which is after the fifth maintenance dose. If 20-hour liver function tests and coagulation studies are normal and the acetaminophen level is less than the lower limits of detection, NAC can be stopped. A repeat set of liver function tests is recommended at 36 hours after ingestion. In other versions of the 20-hour NAC therapy, the dosage regimen is the same, but the laboratory studies are measured initially, and then at 16, 36, and 48 hours after ingestion.[172]

Efficacy of *N*-Acetylcysteine

CASE 5-5, QUESTION 12: Which route of NAC administration is more effective?

There is no proven evidence that one route of NAC administration is superior to the other.[161,164,173–175] Patient outcome after an acetaminophen overdose depends more on the time after the ingestion that treatment begins rather than on the route of administration of NAC. Patients who are started on NAC within 8 to 10 hours after ingestion, regardless of the route, rarely develop hepatotoxicity. Patients who present late or have a delay in the time of NAC treatment have higher rates of hepatotoxicity.[150,161,164,170,174–176]

In one comparative study of IV NAC to oral NAC therapy, both were effective in reducing hepatotoxicity when therapy was initiated within 10 hours after ingestion. Vomiting delayed oral administration of the drug, but IV administration resulted in significantly longer delays in instituting therapy.[174] IV NAC avoids the problems of the vomiting patient, but oral NAC is safer. Oral NAC is associated with nausea and vomiting, whereas IV NAC is associated with bronchospasm, urticaria, and angioedema during administration.[149,160] In addition, oral therapy is much less expensive.[176]

Although the time of initiation of therapy is one of the key factors in reducing hepatotoxicity from acetaminophen ingestions, length of therapy has become another factor.[175,177] Because the duration of therapy with the IV formulation is 21 hours, patients with severe toxicity may be undertreated. It is essential that the patient be reevaluated at the end of the 21 hours to make sure that acetaminophen levels are not detectable and that liver enzymes are trending downward significantly. If there is still measurable acetaminophen and liver enzymes are still elevated, therapy with NAC must be continued.

Starting oral NAC may take less time to prepare than IV NAC therapy and is less expensive. If the patient presents early after an acetaminophen ingestion and does not have nausea and vomiting, oral therapy would be indicated. If the patient presents late (more than 10 hours after ingestion) with signs and symptoms of hepatotoxicity along with intractable nausea and vomiting, IV NAC should be instituted at once.[164,170]

Monitoring Efficacy of *N*-Acetylcysteine

CASE 5-5, QUESTION 13: How should the efficacy of NAC therapy be monitored in B.W.?

The effectiveness of NAC intervention in B.W. should be monitored by daily assessment of her acetaminophen concentration (as long as it is still measurable), AST, ALT, total bilirubin, glucose, and INR. The AST and ALT serum concentrations typically increase within 36 hours (range, 24–72 hours) after ingestion.[160,174] As the hepatic damage continues, the liver enzymes may peak at several tens of thousands units, even with NAC therapy. In most patients, AST and ALT begin to decline after 3 days and then return to baseline values.[160]

In a small number of patients, usually those who presented late after the ingestion, fulminant hepatic failure may develop. Symptoms of severe or persistent acidosis, coagulopathy, a significantly increased serum creatinine, and grade III to IV encephalopathy are consistent with fatal outcomes in patients with fulminant hepatic failure. Liver transplantation might be a consideration for these patients.[152,178–181]

Duration of *N*-Acetylcysteine Therapy

CASE 5-5, QUESTION 14: How long should NAC administration be continued?

The original NAC dosing protocol was based on an assumption that the half-life of acetaminophen was 4 hours. After five half-lives (20 hours), the acetaminophen should be metabolized and NAC could be discontinued. An NAC dose of 6 mg/kg/hour was determined to be necessary based on the rate of glutathione turnover relative to NAPQI production. To ensure that patients received an adequate NAC dose, the FDA recommended that this dose be changed to 18 mg/kg/hour for 72 hours.[182] This recommendation serves as the basis for the traditional 72-hour oral course of NAC therapy.

When using the traditional 72-hour oral course of NAC, therapy can be discontinued if the liver function tests are trending toward normal, other laboratory tests (i.e., coagulation studies, glucose, pH, bilirubin) are within normal ranges, and acetaminophen is no longer present in the serum. As long as acetaminophen is present, it can be metabolized to NAPQI and cause further toxicity.[162,171,182] Continued NAC will not be harmful to the patient and can be beneficial.

When using the shorter 20-hour course of oral NAC, if liver function tests and coagulation studies are normal and the 20-hour acetaminophen concentration can no longer be measured in the serum, NAC therapy can be stopped.[172] However, if 20-hour liver function tests or coagulation studies are abnormal, or if the 20-hour acetaminophen concentration measurement reveals acetaminophen still present in the serum, NAC therapy should be continued for at least another 24 hours.[173,174] Laboratory tests should be repeated every 24 hours, and the patient's progress must be monitored closely. If the patient is not improving, NAC should be continued until the patient recovers, receives a liver transplant, or dies.[152]

At this time, there is no consensus as to the best route of NAC administration, optimal dosage regimen, or optimal length of therapy.[160,164,182] There is consensus, however, that for optimal results, NAC therapy must be instituted within 10 hours after ingestion.[149,160,164,170,173,176] For patients who do not exhibit any signs of hepatotoxicity, shorter-course NAC therapy reduces the amount of NAC administered to the patient, decreases the quantity of laboratory tests, shortens hospital stay, and is less costly.[164,171,182]

N-Acetylcysteine Toxicity

CASE 5-5, QUESTION 15: How should the toxicity of NAC therapy be monitored in B.W.?

With the exception of vomiting, oral NAC is remarkably safe and has not been associated with toxicity.[149,161,164] Oral NAC must be retained for a minimum of 1 hour after ingestion to be successfully absorbed. If B.W. vomits within an hour after her oral NAC dose, the dose should be repeated. If she experiences protracted vomiting, administration of antiemetic drugs (e.g., ondansetron, metoclopramide) or placement of a duodenal feeding tube can improve GI tolerance.[164,183,184] If the patient cannot tolerate oral liquids, NAC therapy should continue via IV administration.

IV NAC therapy has been associated with anaphylactoid reactions in up to 14% of the patients. Although most reactions are not severe, bronchospasm, angioedema, and respiratory arrest have been reported.[149,160,164,182] Patients should be monitored for allergic and anaphylactoid reactions when NAC is administered IV. Most reactions can be avoided by infusing the NAC loading dose slowly for 60 minutes.[149,160,164]

Outcome of Patient B.W.

B.W. continued to have nausea and vomiting and had difficulty tolerating liquids. IV NAC was continued. An obstetrics consultation was requested to evaluate B.W.'s pregnancy. Fetal monitoring was instituted during her hospital admission. A sonogram was taken of the baby. Once B.W. saw her baby's image from the sonogram, her depressed mood seemed to lift. Approximately 36 hours after ingestion, her acetaminophen level was no longer detectable, and her liver function tests showed a mild elevation of her AST at 274 units/L and an ALT of 188 units/L. Her INR and total bilirubin values were normal at 0.7 seconds and 0.8 mg/dL, respectively.

B.W. was seen by a psychiatrist. She was scheduled for counseling and prenatal classes. B.W. seemed eager to attend the classes, and she talked enthusiastically about the baby when family members came to visit. Because of B.W.'s pregnancy, the decision was made to continue NAC for a full 72-hour course with the goal of protecting the fetal liver as much as possible. Six weeks later, she had a normal delivery of a healthy 6-pound, 1-ounce baby girl.

CONCLUSION

Unfortunately, there is no set formula to treat all poisoned patients. Each exposure is unique and patient-specific factors must be considered. Treatment of the poisoned patient often involves controversy because solid, evidence-based science to support a given decision is frequently lacking. When challenged with a poisoning exposure, consult with a poison control center by calling 1-800-222-1222, where consultation is available 24 hours a day in the United States.

KEY REFERENCES AND WEBSITES

A full list of references for this chapter can be found at http://thepoint.lww.com/AT11e. Below are the key references and websites for this chapter, with the corresponding reference number in this chapter found in parentheses after the reference.

Key References

Boyle JS et al. Management of the critically poisoned patient. *Scand J Trauma Resusc Emerg Med*. 2009;17:29. (26)

Mowry JB et al. 2013 Annual report of the American Association of Poison Control Centers' National Poison Data System (NPDS): 31st Annual Report. *Clin Toxicol (Phila)*. 2014;S2:1032. (3)

Chyka PA et al. Position paper: single-dose activated charcoal. *Clin Toxicol (Phila)*. 2005;43:61. (43)

Committee on Poison Prevention and Control, Board on Health Promotion and Disease Prevention, Institute of Medicine of the National Academies. Poison control center activities, personnel, and quality assurance. Forging a Poison Prevention and Control System. Chapter 5. Washington, DC: The National Academies Press; 2004. (19)

Forsberg S et al. Coma and impaired consciousness in the emergency room: characteristics of poisoning versus other causes. *Emerg Med J*. 2009;26:100. (113)

Kociancic T, Reed MD. Acetaminophen intoxication and length of treatment: how long is long enough. *Pharmacotherapy*. 2003;23:1052. (180)

Manoguerra AS et al. Iron ingestion: an evidence-based consensus guideline for out-of-hospital management. *Clin Toxicol (Phila)*. 2005;43:553. (89)

[No authors listed]. Position paper: cathartics [published correction appears in *J Toxicol Clin Toxicol*. 2004;42:1000]. *J Toxicol Clin Toxicol*. 2004;42:243. (44)

Höjer J et al. Position paper update: ipecac syrup for gastrointestinal decontamination. *J Clin Toxicol*. 2013;51:134. (3)

Thanacoody R. Position paper update: Whole bowel irrigation for gastrointestinal decontamination of overdose patients. *Clin Toxicol (Phila)*. 2015;53:5. (45)

Proudfoot AT et al. *Position paper on urine alkalinization*. *J Toxicol Clin Toxicol*. 2004;42:1. (64)

Rumack BH et al. Acetaminophen overdose: 662 cases with evaluation of oral acetylcysteine treatment. *Arch Intern Med*. 1981;141(3 Spec No):380. (158)

Shannon M, Liebelt EL. Targeted management strategies for cardiovascular toxicity from tricyclic antidepressant overdose: the pivotal role for alkalinization and sodium loading. *Pediatr Emerg Care*. 1998;14:293. (143)

Chyka PB et al. Salicylate poisoning: an evidence-based consensus guideline for out-of-hospital management. *Clin Toxicol (Phila)*. 2007;45:95 (69)

Benson BE et al. Position paper update: gastric lavage for gastrointestinal decontamination. *Clin Toxicol (Phila)*. 2013;51:140. (42)

Key Websites

American Association of Poison Control Centers. www.aapcc.org.

Centers for Diseases Control and Prevention Injury Prevention and Control: Data and Statistics (WISQARS). www.cdc.gov/injury/wisquars/index.html.

Drug Abuse Warning Network. www.dawninfo.samhsa.gov/data.

6 End-of-Life Care

Victoria F. Ferraresi

CORE PRINCIPLES

		CHAPTER CASES
1	End-of-life care consists of palliative and hospice care. It is ideally introduced early in the disease progression to provide support to patients of all ages with a serious chronic or life-threatening illness. Medicare patients who enter a hospice program agree to relinquish their regular Medicare benefits as they relate to the terminal illness and accept the palliative rather than curative approach that will be provided by hospice. The hospice provides all care related to the hospice diagnosis under a managed-care model at a fixed reimbursement.	**Case 6-1 (Question 1)**
2	In 2008, the Hospice Conditions of Participation were updated to include a review of the medication profile as part of the initial assessment of new patients. The medication regimens of hospice patients should be continually reviewed and updated, with unnecessary, ineffective, or duplicative medications discontinued.	**Case 6-1 (Question 2)**
3	Patients near end of life can experience a number of distressing symptoms. These should be anticipated and treated in a timely manner that is acceptable to the patients and their families.	**Case 6-1 (Question 3), Table 6-3**
4	Well-trained pharmacists can improve medication management for hospice patients, while helping the hospice manage their drug costs.	**Case 6-1 (Question 2)**
5	Many barriers exist regarding pain management and the use of opioids.	**Case 6-1 (Question 4)**
6	Effective pain management uses a variety of approaches.	**Case 6-2 (Question 1)**
7	Pain and symptom management may at times require an aggressive approach.	**Case 6-3 (Questions 1–3)**

HOSPICE AND PALLIATIVE CARE

Terminology

Hospice care and *palliative care* are similar, but distinct, terms sharing the common belief that the relief of suffering is a long-standing, central, and fully legitimate aim of medicine. *End-of-life care* refers to both hospice care and palliative care. The basic principle of end-of-life care is to optimize the quality of life for the patient and family in the last weeks and months of life, as well as to provide support for the family beyond the end of life into bereavement.

Palliative care, which includes hospice care, is ideally introduced early in the disease progression to provide support to patients of all ages with a serious chronic or life-threatening illness. It can be provided concurrently with other treatments to cure or reduce disease or it can be provided independently. The word *palliation*, derived from the Latin word *pallium* (a cloak), has been defined as "treatment to reduce the violence of a disease." The World Health Organization and the National Consensus Project define palliative care as an approach that improves the quality of life of patients and their families who are facing a life-threatening illness, by preventing and relieving suffering through early identification and impeccable assessment and treatment of pain and other physical, psychosocial, and spiritual problems.[1–4] Palliative care

- Affirms life and regards dying as a normal process;
- Provides relief from pain and other distressing symptoms;
- Intends neither to hasten nor postpone death;
- Integrates the psychological and spiritual aspects of patient care;
- Offers a support system to help patients live as actively as possible until death;
- Uses a multidisciplinary team approach to address the needs of the patient and his or her family during the patient's illness; and
- Provides bereavement counseling when indicated.[3]

Hospice and palliative medicine became a recognized subspecialty of internal medicine in 2006, awarded by the American Board of Medical Specialties.[5] The Joint Commission offers an Advanced Certification Program for Palliative Care to recognize hospitals that provide high-quality palliative care services.[6]

Hospice, originally a place or way station for people making a pilgrimage, is considered both a philosophy of care and a place to deliver care. *Hospice care* focuses on the palliation of pain and other symptoms when active treatment to cure a terminal illness ends. Hospice care can be delivered in a building designated as a hospice, in the patient's home, or in a facility where the patient resides. As a programmatic model for delivering palliative care, hospice care provides an interdisciplinary team approach to the individualized symptom management (e.g., pain), as well as psychosocial, emotional, spiritual, and bereavement support for the patient and his or her family and caregivers during the last months of life.[7]

Hospice Care in the United States

According to estimates of the National Hospice and Palliative Care Organization, there were approximately 5,800 hospice programs in the United States in 2013. In that year, 42.9% of all deaths in the United States occurred under hospice care.[7,8] Hospices provided care for patients with various terminal illnesses (e.g., cancer [36.5% of all admissions], heart disease [13.4%], dementia [15.2%], and lung disease [9.9%]).[7] During the Medicare demonstration project (1980–1982), 93% of home hospice patients had cancer of various types.[9]

Adults younger than 34 years of age and pediatric patients account for less than 1% of the hospice population. Although pediatric hospice programs are growing, and more pediatric patients receive hospice services, the percentage of patients in this population has not increased from 2006 to 2013.[10] Regulatory, financial, cultural, and educational barriers play a role in diminished access to hospice care for pediatric patients.[10,11] States are required to offer hospice care (under Medicaid and other state programs as part of the Affordable Care Act) to pediatric patients with expanded benefits to improve coordination of care.[12]

About 84% of hospice patients were 65 years of age or older, and 41.2% were 85 years or older and in 2013, 87.2% of hospice patients received this care as a benefit provided by Medicare. Almost all (92.7%) hospice programs are certified by the Centers for Medicare and Medicaid Services to provide care to beneficiaries under the Medicare Hospice Benefit.[7]

The Medicare Hospice Benefit

The Medicare Hospice Benefit is funded from Part A (the hospital portion) of Medicare.[13] Patients are eligible for this benefit if, in the opinion of two physicians (i.e., patient's primary-care physician and hospice medical director), the natural course of their disease will result in death within 6 months. The hospice medical director determines the terminal diagnosis and any other conditions related to the terminal prognosis. Eligibility for hospice can continue beyond the initial certification if the hospice medical director recertifies eligibility at defined intervals, called certification periods. Other insurance payers generally follow this criterion. In electing this benefit, patients agree to relinquish their regular Medicare benefits as they relate to the terminal illness and related conditions and accept the palliative rather than curative approach that will be provided by hospice. This benefit links all care related to these diagnoses to the selected Medicare-certified hospice program, which coordinates and provides all care. The regulatory framework for the provision of hospice care under Medicare is defined in 42 CFR Part 418, Medicare and Medicaid Programs: Hospice Conditions of Participation.[13]

Hospice care is provided (and reimbursed) under Medicare at four levels, all of which can be modified at any time based on a patient's condition or caregiving needs:

- Routine home care (day-to-day care in the home)
- Continuous home care (when more skilled care in the home is required owing to symptom management or a caregiving crisis)
- General inpatient care (reimbursement for an inpatient stay in a hospital or skilled nursing facility related to symptoms that cannot be managed in the home)
- Inpatient respite care (up to 5 days in a skilled nursing facility) to give the caregiver a break or respite

Most care, consisting of pain and symptom management and assistance with activities of daily living, as well as psychosocial support, is provided to hospice patients at the routine level of care.

Patients may freely visit their primary-care provider (i.e., physician or nurse practitioner) for any reason, including reasons unrelated to their terminal illness. The primary-care provider will be paid directly by Medicare. Patients may choose to use their regular Medicare benefits for other unrelated illnesses; visits to providers for care or treatments unrelated to the primary hospice diagnosis are not limited or restricted. Patients may revoke their election of the Medicare Hospice Benefit at any time (e.g., end hospice care to pursue curative treatment or seek treatment outside the hospice plan of care). Patients may, at a later date, choose to return to hospice care or change to a different hospice program, without restrictions or loss of benefits.[13]

It is common for patients to be referred to hospice when death is imminent. Median lengths of stay have declined, from 37.1 days during the Medicare demonstration project (1980–1982) to 26 days in 2005 and to 18.5 days in 2013.[7,9,14] Approximately 34.5% of patients admitted to a hospice program in 2013 died or were discharged within 7 days.[7]

Hospice programs have historically received a fixed daily payment to provide all care related to the terminal diagnosis (e.g., medications, supplies, durable medical equipment, procedures, home health aides, provider visits, spiritual care, bereavement services). The reimbursement rates for the four levels of hospice care under the Medicare Hospice Benefit are established each summer for the following fiscal year, effective October 1.[15] A baseline reimbursement rate is set, along with an adjustment for wage differentials (the wage index) based on the local cost of living.[15,16] As an example, Table 6-1 shows reimbursement

Table 6-1

Example of Hospice Daily Payment Rates for Routine Level of Care, 2016 Fiscal Year (October 1, 2015–September 30, 2016)[14,15]

	A Unadjusted Payment Rate (B + C)	B Nonlabor Portion	C Labor Portion	D Wage Index	E Adjusted Labor Portion (C × D)	F Total Daily Payment (B + E)
San Francisco, CA	$161.89	$50.66	$111.23	1.7260	$191.98	**$242.64**
Jefferson City, MO	$161.89	$50.66	$111.23	0.9366	$104.18	**$154.84**

rates for the provision of routine home care in San Francisco, CA, and Jefferson City, MO, for fiscal year 2016 up to December 31, 2015. Historically, hospice reimbursement rates have been low and have not kept pace with rising costs. The total unadjusted hospice daily payment rate increased from \$146.63 per day to \$161.89 per day from 2011 to 2016 (approximately 2.1% per year).[15,17]

Programs generally have high costs at the start of care because of personnel costs involved in the admission, assessment, and development of the initial plan of care, and obtaining medications, medical equipment, and medical supplies. High costs are also encountered nearer to the end of life, when new problems can appear and symptoms often intensify. The Centers for Medicare and Medicaid Services are implementing hospice payment reform beginning January 1, 2016, consisting of higher payments at the start of care (for days 1–60) and near the end of life via a service intensity add-on (SIA) to account for greater care needs during these periods.[15] It is anticipated that future reforms may include differing payments based on where the beneficiary resides (home versus a facility), including hospice care in Medicare Advantage plan coverage, or on the type of care provided, on quality outcomes, and on expanding the definition of what is related to the terminal prognosis.[18]

Drug costs continue to outpace increases in hospice reimbursement.[19] In 2014, overall drug spending in the United States increased 13.1% due primarily to increased prices for brand, niche ,and specialty drugs; increases in prices for compounded medications; and shortages resulting from industry consolidation. Prices for drugs for pain and inflammation increased by 15.7% in 2014. This is attributed by Express Scripts in part to new tamper-resistant formulations where there is no generic alternative.[19]

In reviewing hospice beneficiary use of Medicare Part D, CMS has reminded Medicare Part D Plans, pharmacies, and hospices that hospices are required to pay for virtually all care (including all related medications) for hospice patients (via Part A). An initiative to block Part D access to hospice patients was subsequently reversed by CMS with the clear expectation that hospices provide analgesics, antiemetics, laxatives, and anxiolytics and to coordinate drug coverage with the Part D plans.[20–22] Hospices are allowed to establish formularies, but if the hospice does not provide a related medication for any reason, the beneficiary may not use their Part D plan to obtain it. The result has been hospices paying for many more medications than in the past (i.e., covering medications used to treat rather than just palliate related conditions).

These variables (i.e., referrals to hospice later in the course of terminal illness, higher costs at the start of care, shortened lengths of stay, higher drug costs, providing more medications) have placed intense pressure on hospice programs to manage expenses. Because it is difficult to influence the time when patients are referred to hospice, the duration of time in hospice care, or the inherently higher costs when patients are first enrolled into hospice, the management of drug costs has taken a high priority in providing cost-effective hospice care.

Improving Patient Care and Managing Drug Costs

In 2008, the Hospice Conditions of Participation were updated to be more patient centered and outcome oriented.[13] Coverage of medications is mandated as described in 24 CFR §418.106 Drugs and biologicals, medical supplies, and durable medical equipment: ". . .drugs and biologicals related to the palliation and management of the terminal illness and related conditions, as identified in the hospice plan of care, must be provided by the hospice while the patient is under hospice care."

It also addresses medication management and the review of the medication profile specifying that "[t]he hospice must ensure that the interdisciplinary group (IDG) confers with an individual with education and training in drug management as defined in hospice policies and procedures and State law . . . to ensure that drugs and biologicals meet each patient's needs."

The regulations state that the comprehensive assessment must "take into consideration" the drug profile (24 CFR §418.54). This is defined as "[a] review of all of the patient's prescription and over-the-counter drugs, herbal remedies and other alternative treatments that could affect drug therapy" and is to include the following:

- Effectiveness of drug therapy
- Drug side effects
- Actual or potential drug interactions
- Duplicate drug therapy
- Drug therapy currently associated with laboratory monitoring

Although the regulations do not specify who is to perform the medication assessment, pharmacists are uniquely qualified to fill this role.

Well-trained pharmacists can improve patient care and positively affect the fiscal margins of hospice programs by discouraging inappropriate use of medications, establishing evidence-based formularies, promulgating prior authorization policies for specific targeted drugs, establishing policies for adhering to the use of generic drugs, and managing the quantities of medications to be dispensed. In addition to managing drug expenditures, pharmacists provide drug information both to patients and providers and work integrally with other members of the hospice health care team to improve the safe and effective use of medications.[23–37]

Referral to Hospice

ELIGIBILITY

CASE 6-1

QUESTION 1: M.P. is an 89-year-old woman referred to hospice for end-stage Alzheimer dementia. She lives in a residential care home for the elderly with a hired caregiver. Her husband has been unable to care for her at home for some time because she requires full assistance with all activities of daily living. She was recently hospitalized with aspiration pneumonia and a urinary tract infection (UTI) and completed a course of intravenous (IV) vancomycin and piperacillin/tazobactam. Her past medical history includes osteoporosis, coronary artery disease, chronic obstructive pulmonary disease (COPD), hypercholesterolemia, and hypothyroidism. She is not oriented to person, place, or date. Her speech is unintelligible or nonsensical. She cannot feed herself, but will eat the thick pureed food that is fed to her. She is bed-bound and incontinent of urine and stool. She is restless and irritable at times, especially at night. Her Palliative Performance Scale (PPS) is 30%. Weight is 112 pounds, decreased from 135 pounds a year ago, and a recent serum albumin is 2.2 g/dL. What criteria does M.P. meet for eligibility for hospice services under the Medicare Hospice Benefit?

Patients with chronic diseases (e.g., Alzheimer disease, Parkinson disease, stroke, heart failure, lung disease) can be sufficiently ill and debilitated to need custodial care, but might not be sufficiently ill to meet the definition of a terminal illness. This differentiation between terminally ill versus chronically ill requiring custodial care is important because to qualify for hospice services under the Medicare Hospice Benefit, patients must be at a stage where death is expected within the next 6 months. For cancer diagnoses, the presence of widespread metastatic disease may make this prognosis more easily evident. However, for other chronic diseases, this is not as clear.

The Medicare fiscal intermediaries have issued criteria to assist in the determination of eligibility for hospice care, as well as criteria to meet a 6-month terminal prognosis for a number of diseases. These criteria, or local coverage determinations (LCDs), provide guidelines for meeting an overall decline in clinical status, for meeting non–disease-specific data to establish a baseline, for establishing the effect of comorbidities (e.g., renal failure, liver disease), and for the submission of documentation for having met criteria. Criteria have been established for patients with cancer and non-cancer diagnoses, and these criteria are used in the determination of eligibility for service and reimbursement.[38] Criteria for the non-cancer diagnoses have been developed for amyotrophic lateral sclerosis, dementia as a result of Alzheimer disease and related disorders, heart disease, human immunodeficiency virus disease, liver disease, pulmonary disease, renal disease, stroke, and coma. Patients with cancer are eligible if they present with metastatic disease or progression from an earlier stage to metastatic disease with either a continued decline in spite of therapy or if they decline further disease directed therapy.

The determination of whether M.P. meets eligibility requirements for Medicare Hospice Benefits must be based on the established LCDs for dementia as a result of Alzheimer disease. These criteria include the following:

- Stage 7 or beyond, according to the Functional Assessment Staging Scale
  - Stage 7A: Can speak six or fewer intelligible words in a day or during an interview
  - Stage 7B: Speech ability limited to the use of a single intelligible word in a day or during an interview
  - Stage 7C: Cannot ambulate without assistance
  - Stage 7D: Cannot sit up without assistance
  - Stage 7E: Loss of ability to smile
  - Stage 7F: Loss of ability to hold head up independently
- Unable to ambulate without assistance
- Unable to dress without assistance
- Unable to bathe without assistance
- Urinary and fecal incontinence, intermittent or constant
- No consistently meaningful verbal communication; stereotypical phrases only or the ability to speak is limited to six or fewer intelligible words
- One of the following within the past 12 months: aspiration pneumonia, pyelonephritis, septicemia, decubitus ulcers (multiple, stages 3 and 4), fever (recurrent after antibiotic treatment)
- Inability to maintain sufficient fluid and caloric intake with 10% weight loss during the previous 6 months or serum albumin less than 2.5 g/dL

The Palliative Performance Score (PPS) (Table 6-2) gradates the extent of disability and can be used to assist in the determination of hospice eligibility.[39] M.P. meets the previous criteria and is eligible for hospice because of her Alzheimer disease. She clearly is debilitated. She is unable to speak intelligently, cannot feed herself, is not oriented to time or place, is incontinent of urine and stool, has lost about 20% of her weight during the past year, has a serum albumin of 2.2 g/dL, and has a PPS rating of 30% (i.e., totally bed-bound, unable to do any activity, confused). In addition, she has a number of comorbidities, experienced a recent episode of aspiration pneumonia, and finished a course of antibiotic therapy.

MEDICATION MANAGEMENT

CASE 6-1, QUESTION 2: M.P. has no known allergies. Her current medications are memantine 10 mg twice daily, aspirin 81 mg once daily, alendronate 70 mg weekly, esomeprazole 20 mg daily, lovastatin 20 mg with dinner, megestrol 40 mg/mL 5 mL (200 mg) twice daily, levothyroxine 0.1 mg daily, multivitamin daily, beclomethasone metered-dose inhaler one puff daily, albuterol 2.5 mg/ipratropium 0.5 mg via nebulizer every 4 hours as needed for wheezing or shortness of breath, acetaminophen 325 to 650 mg every 6 hours as needed for mild pain or fever, olanzapine 5 mg at bedtime as needed for restlessness and aggressive behavior, milk of magnesia 30 mL daily for constipation, and a bisacodyl suppository 10 mg every 3 days as needed if no bowel movement. The hospice medical director has determined that the aspiration pneumonia, UTI, and COPD are related to M.P.'s terminal prognosis. What is your assessment of M.P.'s medication regimen? Which medications are the hospice required to provide, and which might be discontinued?

Hospices are required to provide (pay for) all medications related to the terminal diagnosis and related conditions within the hospice plan of care (POC). The POC is the individualized plan of treatment developed for each patient formulated at the start of care and updated regularly by the IDG. The Conditions of Participation mandate that the IDG be composed of a physician, registered nurse, social worker, and a pastoral or other counselor.[13] A registered nurse coordinates the implementation of the POC. Some hospice program IDGs have incorporated a pharmacist into the group to review medication issues.

The large array of medications being taken by M.P. is similar to the medication lists of many hospice patients. These patients are often elderly and have a long history of several chronic medical conditions for which they have been taking multiple medications. In most cases, the medication lists of patients who are admitted into a hospice program have seldom been reviewed, updated, or modified in light of the present medical situation. Admission to a hospice program represents a change in the level of care and is a most appropriate time for a review and reconciliation of all medications to ascertain the necessity of each, with the goal of optimizing efficacy and minimizing the potential for adverse effects, medication errors, and inappropriate costs.

Because M.P. is to be enrolled into a hospice program, her care should not be focused on curative treatments, but rather on the management of discomforting symptoms and on improving her quality of life in the time remaining. M.P.'s medications should be analyzed with the goal of simplification. Unnecessary medications should be discontinued and alternatives added to manage two or more symptoms concurrently. The following changes should be considered:

Acetaminophen. This analgesic is often helpful in relieving mild pain, particularly in immobile elderly patients. A trial of around-the-clock acetaminophen could be helpful.

Albuterol/ipratropium combination. The hospice program is required to pay for medications related to M.P.'s aspiration pneumonia and COPD because the hospice medical director determined that these conditions are related to her terminal prognosis. This combination inhalation formulation should be continued if she is able to participate in her nebulizer treatments and it improves her breathing. (See Chapter 19, Chronic Obstructive Pulmonary Disease.)

Alendronate. This bisphosphonate drug can be discontinued because the treatment of osteoporosis is not an important consideration at this terminal stage of her life nor is it in the hospice POC. Thus, hospice would not cover it. Furthermore, M.P. is bed-bound; alendronate should be ingested in the upright position,

Table 6-2
Palliative Performance Score (PPS) Version 2

PPS Level (%)	Ambulation	Activity and Evidence of Disease	Self-Care	Intake	Conscious Level
100	Full	Normal activity and work No evidence of disease	Full	Normal	Full
90	Full	Normal activity and work Some evidence of disease	Full	Normal	Full
80	Full	Normal activity with effort Some evidence of disease	Full	Normal or reduced	Full
70	Reduced	Unable to do normal job/work Significant disease	Full	Normal or reduced	Full
60	Reduced	Unable to do hobby/housework Significant disease	Occasional assistance necessary	Normal or reduced	Full or confusion
50	Mainly sit/lie	Unable to do any work Extensive disease	Considerable assistance required	Normal or reduced	Full or confusion
40	Mainly in bed	Unable to do most activity Extensive disease	Mainly assistance	Normal or reduced	Full or drowsy ± confusion
30	Totally bed-bound	Unable to do any activity Extensive disease	Total care	Normal or reduced	Full or drowsy ± confusion
20	Totally bed-bound	Unable to do any activity Extensive disease	Total care	Minimal to sips	Full or drowsy ± confusion
10	Totally bed-bound	Unable to do any activity Extensive disease	Total care	Mouth care only	Drowsy or coma ± confusion
0	Death				

Instructions: PPS level is determined by reading left to right to find a "best horizontal fit." Begin at left column reading downwards until current ambulation is determined, then, read across to next and downwards until each column is determined. Thus, "leftward" columns take precedence over "rightward" columns.

Reprinted with permission from Victoria Hospice Society. *Palliative Performance Scale (PPSv2), version 2. Medical Care of the Dying*. 4th ed. Victoria, British Columbia, Canada: Victoria Hospice Society; 2006:120. http://www.victoriahospice.org/health-professionals/clinical-tools. Accessed April 13, 2016. Copyright © 2001 Victoria Hospice Society. The Palliative Performance Scale version 2 (PPSv2) tool is copyright to Victoria Hospice Society and replaces the first PPS published in 1996 [*J Pall Care* 9(4):26–32]. Victoria Hospice Society, 1952 Bay Street, Victoria, BC, V8R 1J8, Canada www.victoriahospice.org edu.hospice@viha.ca

and patients should remain upright after taking the medication to decrease the risk of alendronate-induced esophageal irritation (see Chapter 110, Osteoporosis). Pain that she may experience from osteoporosis can be treated with analgesics.

Aspirin. The low-dose aspirin is intended to decrease the risk of cardiovascular clotting. The aspirin will not increase M.P.'s comfort or quality of life. Although the aspirin would not be covered by her Medicare Hospice Benefit, it can be continued unless her primary-care provider prefers its discontinuation.

Beclomethasone. This patient is not functioning well cognitively (i.e., not oriented to time, person, or place) and would be unable to effectively time the inhalation of a breath to the actuation of her metered-dose inhaler. A systemic corticosteroid (e.g., prednisone) might improve her COPD symptoms and also improve her appetite and sense of well-being. The potential for adverse effects is modest with short-term corticosteroid use.

Bisacodyl, milk of magnesia. Constipation in patients with terminal illnesses is common, occurring in as many as 94% because of decreased gastrointestinal motility with advanced age, metabolic disturbances, decreased physical activity, lack of adequate fiber and fluid intake, and use of constipating medications (e.g., opioids, anticholinergics, psychotropic agents).[40–43] The milk of magnesia, with an occasional bisacodyl suppository, has been an adequate laxative regimen for this patient. If an opioid is later prescribed for M.P., a mild stimulant laxative (e.g., senna) can be added. Osmotic agents such as polyethylene glycol (PEG), oral sorbitol, or lactulose can be prescribed if needed. Mineral oil 30 mL daily is an option if the stool is hard; however, mineral oil should not be considered for M.P. because of her risk of aspiration. Bulk-forming laxatives should also be avoided in this population as they may not ingest adequate water to prevent a fecal impaction. In cases of refractory constipation, the use of methylnaltrexone bromide, an injectable opioid antagonist, can reverse opioid-induced constipation by antagonizing opioid effects within the gastrointestinal tract without affecting systemic analgesia.[44–46] This quaternary derivative of naltrexone does not cross the blood–brain barrier. Dosing is weight based; it is given subcutaneously as either 8 mg for patients weighing 38 to 62 kg (84–136 pounds) or 12 mg for patients weighing 62 to 114 kg (136–251 pounds) once a day. The most common adverse events are abdominal pain, flatulence, nausea, and dizziness.[43]

Esomeprazole. This proton-pump inhibitor would probably be unnecessary because alendronate-induced esophageal or gastrointestinal irritation would not be an issue subsequent to its discontinuation. However, if a proton-pump inhibitor is needed, nonprescription generic omeprazole or lansoprazole is preferred because they are more cost-effective.[47] If a patient such as M.P. cannot swallow intact tablets, a capsule formulation can be opened with the contents mixed with soft food and swallowed intact.

Levothyroxine. This thyroid medication should be continued until M.P. is no longer able to swallow. This medication, however, would not be covered under her Medicare Hospice Benefit, which is based on her Alzheimer disease, and was deemed not related to the terminal prognosis.

Lovastatin. Cholesterol-lowering agents are not necessary during the last 6 months of life and should be discontinued. Lovastatin would not improve the quality of life of M.P. at this stage of her terminal illness and would not be covered by her Medicare Hospice Benefit.

Megestrol. The progesterone derivative, megestrol, in doses of 400 to 800 mg daily, can substantially stimulate appetite.[48,49] If an undernourished hospice patient desires to eat more, the hospice may choose to provide an appetite stimulant. It is unclear whether stimulation of appetite in a cognitively impaired patient will result in weight gain or improved nutritional status. Because the benefits in this situation are unclear, the potential of adverse effects (e.g., venous thrombosis) of megestrol needs to be considered, especially in M.P., who is not ambulatory and had been taking low-dose aspirin for prevention of cardiovascular clotting.[50]

Memantine. Because the *N*-methyl-D-aspartate antagonist, memantine, has been modestly effective in improving performance in patients with moderate to severe Alzheimer disease,[51,52] but with decreasing effectiveness over time,[53] it is probably of limited utility for M.P. (See Chapter 108, Geriatric Neurocognitive Disorders.) It would be reasonable to discontinue M.P.'s memantine subsequent to discussion with appropriate hospice team members and M.P.'s family.

Multivitamins. Multivitamins and other nutritional supplements are unlikely to improve M.P.'s comfort or quality of life. The discontinuation of these drugs would simplify medication administration, decrease the potential for medication errors, and decrease costs.

Olanzapine. An antipsychotic (e.g., olanzapine, haloperidol, chlorpromazine) is often prescribed off-label to manage the agitation and confusion encountered by patients with dementia. Behavioral modifications can be tried (see Chapter 108, Geriatric Neurocognitive Disorders), but paranoid or delusional behavior may require drug therapy. At the time of admission to hospice, patients may be receiving atypical agents (e.g., olanzapine). Small doses of the first-generation antipsychotics, such as haloperidol and chlorpromazine, may offer a dual effect and be very useful in treating opioid-induced nausea and vomiting, although randomized clinical trials demonstrating efficacy are lacking.[54] They would be covered by M.P.'s Medicare Hospice Benefit. Chlorpromazine would be preferable when more sedation is desired.

SYMPTOM MANAGEMENT

The American College of Physicians has developed clinical guidelines, based on a systematic review of evidence and on a report by the Agency for Healthcare Research and Quality, to improve palliative care at the end of life. These guidelines provide strong recommendations for the regular assessment of patients at the end of life for symptoms of pain, dyspnea, and depression, and for therapies of proven effectiveness for these symptoms. For patients with cancer, these include the use of opioids, nonsteroidal anti-inflammatory drugs, and bisphosphonates for pain; tricyclic antidepressants, selective serotonin reuptake inhibitors, and psychosocial interventions for depression; and opioids for unrelieved dyspnea and oxygen for short-term relief of hypoxemia. The guidelines do not address other variables of palliative care at the end of life or the management of other matters (e.g., nutritional support) because the quality of evidence is limited rather than because other issues or symptoms are unimportant.[55] The National Consensus Project for Quality Palliative Care recommends the measurement and documentation of pain and other symptoms using available scales with timely assessment and symptom management acceptable to both the patients and their families as a preferred practice.[4]

CASE 6-1, QUESTION 3: As soon as the hospice admission and assessment is completed, the nurse in consultation with the IDG develops a plan for symptom management and orders a comfort kit for M.P. What are the components of this kit, and why is it useful?

Some hospices use a general comfort kit that contains specific medications to manage symptoms commonly encountered by most hospice patients, or they order medications to treat anticipated symptoms for a specific patient. These medications are placed in the home or facility where the patient resides. This facilitates the availability of medications to patients who encounter anticipated symptoms and is convenient when caregivers are instructed by the patient's primary-care provider to provide the medication to the patient. Patients living with cancer can encounter as many as 27 symptoms (median, 11), many of which occur together.[56] In one study, patients ($n = 176$) experienced an average of 6.6 to 6.8 distressing symptoms during the last week of life.[57] In general, the prevalence of each symptom is difficult to measure and demonstrates a high degree of variability. Pain (34%–96%), fatigue (32%–90%), and breathlessness (10%–95%) appear to be the most common in patients with a variety of terminal conditions, with the prevalence of pain in cancer patients reported as 35% to 96%.[58] Patients with terminal illnesses, including dementia as in M.P., also experience depression (3%–82%), anxiety (8%–79%), confusion (6%–93%), insomnia (9%–74%), nausea (6%–68%), constipation (23%–70%), diarrhea (3%–90%), and anorexia (21%–92%).[58] The disparity in symptom prevalence may be attributed to a host of variables (e.g., study design, patient population, underlying disease, inconsistent definitions, and where care was provided). The occurrence of symptoms, however, can vary significantly, even within the last week of life, and the need for frequent assessment of patients cannot be overemphasized. Morphine, lorazepam, haloperidol, prochlorperazine suppositories, and an anticholinergic agent are commonly ordered for hospice patients. Drugs that can palliate more than one symptom, such as morphine for pain or dyspnea, or haloperidol for agitation or nausea, are particularly suited to inclusion in a comfort kit.

Morphine. Every hospice patient should have a short-acting opioid available for the palliation of unrelieved dyspnea and pain. Although morphine can cause respiratory depression, small doses are very effective in controlling dyspnea by multiple mechanisms: vasodilation, reduced peripheral vascular resistance, inhibition of baroreceptor responses, reduction of brainstem responsiveness to carbon dioxide (the primary mechanism of opioid-induced respiratory depression), and lessened reflex vasoconstriction caused by increased blood Pco_2 levels. Opioids can also reduce the anxiety associated with dyspnea and might also act directly on opioid receptors present in the airways (Table 6-3).[59–64]

Hospice patients generally do not have IV access (i.e., an IV catheter) into which medications can be easily administered. As a result, medications are primarily administered orally and, occasionally, by sublingual, buccal, transdermal, rectal, or subcutaneous (if an infusion is warranted) routes of administration. When patients lose the ability to swallow near the end of life (or have a condition that precludes swallowing), the sublingual or buccal routes of administration are the most useful, especially

Table 6-3
Treatment of Dyspnea at End of Life[59,64]

Nonpharmacologic methods
Pursed-lip breathing
Upright position
Relaxation
Meditation
Use of a fan or open window to circulate air over the face
Pharmacologic therapy
Systemic opioids (short-acting) in small doses given orally, sublingually, or via injection can be given every 1–2 hours as needed
Long-acting agents can be added to supplement the routine use of short-acting opioids
Inhaled opioids deliver medication via nebulization directly into the airway, avoiding first-pass metabolism, allowing use of smaller doses, theoretically minimizing side effects such as drowsiness. May cause local histamine release, leading to bronchospasm. Use nonpreserved sterile injectable products. More cumbersome and expensive owing to use of nebulizer and nonpreserved parenteral products; evidence does not show that nebulized opioids provide greater benefit than nebulized saline
Agents: morphine 2.5–10 mg in 2 mL of 0.9% saline; hydromorphone 0.25–1 mg in 2 mL of 0.9% saline; fentanyl 25 mcg in 2 mL of 0.9% saline
Generally given every 2–4 hours as needed for breathlessness
Benzodiazepines are useful for the anxiety associated with breathlessness

if drugs are lipophilic. The use of orally disintegrating tablets (ODTs) may also be useful at this time. Morphine is hydrophilic, and although some of it might be absorbed across the mucous membranes, the primary clinical effect probably results from gastrointestinal absorption after the drug has trickled down the back of the throat.

Oral morphine sulfate, in a concentration of 20 mg/mL, is commonly packaged in a 30-mL bottle at the beginning of hospice care. This bottle of morphine can provide sixty 10-mg doses, and at this concentration, only 0.5 mL of morphine needs to be administered. Oxycodone or hydromorphone, in comparable adjusted doses, can be substituted for morphine when needed. There is no evidence demonstrating the superiority of any of these over the others in severe cancer pain.[65]

Lorazepam. A short-acting benzodiazepine (e.g., lorazepam 0.5 mg every 4 hours as needed) is useful for the treatment of anxiety. Patients, especially those with respiratory symptoms, can experience episodes of extreme anxiety near the end of life. Caution should be used to not overuse these drugs in the elderly because they can increase the risk of falling or cause paradoxical reactions and worsen delirium or restlessness.

Haloperidol. Small doses of haloperidol (e.g., 0.5–1 mg) are useful for the treatment of restlessness, delirium, or nausea and vomiting.

Prochlorperazine. When patients cannot take oral medications to manage nausea and vomiting, rectal suppositories of prochlorperazine are often effective. Although it is necessary to consider the etiology of the nausea and vomiting, prochlorperazine is generally a good initial agent.

Anticholinergic agent. As death approaches, patients can have difficulty in clearing pharyngeal secretions and, as a result, generate a sound commonly known as a death rattle.[66] Although patients are often unconscious at this point, this sound can be very distressing to those nearby. An anticholinergic agent (e.g., glycopyrrolate, hyoscyamine, scopolamine, atropine) can be administered in an attempt to prevent these pharyngeal secretions from forming. Patient positioning and gentle suctioning can remove secretions already present. This treatment modality is usually initiated after the patient has become obtunded; if begun too early, patients might develop problems with thickened bronchial or pulmonary secretions, tachycardia, delirium, dry mouth, urinary retention, or other adverse anticholinergic effects. However, efficacy is best if these agents are started earlier in the active dying process.[67] Glycopyrrolate, available in a tablet, injectable formulation and oral solution, is a good choice for an anticholinergic agent because it minimally crosses the blood–brain barrier. The 1-mg tablets could be crushed and placed under the tongue every 8 hours. Hyoscyamine is available as oral tablets, ODT, oral sustained-release tablets, sublingual tablets, oral liquid, oral solution, and injection. Either the ODT, sublingual tablets, or oral solution of hyoscyamine can be given in a 0.125- to 0.25-mg dose sublingually every 4 hours as needed. Scopolamine transdermal patches have a slow onset of action (blood levels are detected 4 hours after application)[68] and are of limited utility in this situation. The oral or sublingual administration of atropine ophthalmic solution 1% is convenient to administer. Recent shortages and price increases have made it less cost-effective. Assuming that 20 drops is approximately equivalent to 1 mL, patients can be given 0.5 to 1 mg (1–2 drops) of the atropine ophthalmic solution orally or sublingually every 4 hours as needed. Families and caregivers must be instructed not to use this in the eye.

CASE 6-1, QUESTION 4: The hospice nurse for M.P. has difficulty finding oral morphine sulfate available from a pharmacy and difficulty in finding a pharmacy willing to accept a faxed prescription. Why is morphine so difficult to obtain, and how should the nurse manage this problem?

Providing relief for pain or other symptoms with opioids is often difficult owing to numerous barriers. Patients and caregivers are often fearful of opioids, or mistakenly believe these medications will cause addiction or hasten death.[69] Pharmacists can create barriers by not having opioids in the pharmacy, sometimes because of the fear of robbery, fear of investigation by drug regulatory agencies, or insufficient appreciation of the usefulness of opioids in pain management and palliative care.[70] Pharmacists who are inexperienced in providing service to hospice patients might not be knowledgeable about federal regulations governing the provision of controlled substances to hospice patients. Federal statutes, as well as most state statutes, permit prescriptions for Schedule II controlled substances for hospice patients to be faxed. According to the Code of Federal Regulations (21 CFR 1306.11) paragraph (g): "A prescription prepared in accordance with 1306.05 written for a Schedule II narcotic substance for a patient enrolled in a hospice care program certified and/or paid for by Medicare under Title XVIII or a hospice program which is licensed by the state may be transmitted by the practitioner or the practitioner's agent to the dispensing pharmacy by facsimile. The practitioner or the practitioner's agent will note on the prescription that the patient is a hospice patient. The facsimile serves as the original written prescription for purposes of this paragraph (g) and it shall be maintained in accordance with 1304.04(h)."[71]

The process of ordering controlled substances for use by hospice patients at home can take many hours, and sometimes as much as an entire day. Hospice providers should anticipate possible difficulties when placing orders for Schedule II controlled substance medications. M.P.'s nurse should take the time to address any concerns M.P.'s caregivers and family may have about these medications (i.e., how they may affect her, any worries about addiction, side effects) and allow ample time to order them so that symptoms can be managed as they develop.

CASE 6-2

QUESTION 1: G.G., a 40-year-old woman, is admitted to hospice with stage IV ovarian cancer, metastatic to her pelvis, liver, and lungs. She was diagnosed after many months of nonspecific complaints of gastric distress and bloating. On laparotomy, she was evaluated as stage III and underwent a total abdominal hysterectomy and bilateral salpingo-oophorectomy and tumor debulking at that time. She has undergone subsequent chemotherapy and repeated tumor debulkings. In the past 6 months, her weight has decreased from 175 pounds to 153 pounds (she is 62 inches tall). Her primary complaints are constant nausea, constipation, and gripping abdominal pain, which she characterizes as burning and twisting. She quantifies the pain as 8 of 10 (on a 0-to-10-point scale) and describes the pain as one that moves into her groin and leg. Her family is unhappy about the drowsiness she experiences from her medications; they believe she is overmedicated. She is starting to have difficulty swallowing. She has no known allergies. Her current medications include fentanyl transdermal system 75 mcg/hour every 72 hours, extended-release morphine sulfate capsules 50 mg three times daily (usually intended for once-daily administration), docusate sodium 250 mg daily, lansoprazole 30 mg daily, and lorazepam 0.5 mg every 4 hours as needed for nausea and anxiety. What is the most accurate assessment of her pain management regimen?

G.G. is currently using two long-acting opioids (i.e., fentanyl transdermal, sustained-release morphine which is being dosed too frequently), but is still unable to achieve relief of her pain, which is probably neuropathic pain (described as burning and twisting). It is estimated that up to 39% of patients with cancer pain have neuropathic pain.[72–74] This may be caused by tumor growth around nerves, postoperative nerve damage, chemotherapy-induced neuropathy or following radiation therapy. Opioids alone may be of limited value or may require higher than usual dosing.[72] The addition of adjuvant analgesics such as antidepressants, anticonvulsants, and local anesthetics play an important role in treating neuropathic pain (see Chapter 55, Pain and Its Management).

The use of two long-acting agents is duplicative and should be replaced with one opioid. Methadone may be a better long-acting agent for G.G. because it has activity against neuropathic pain (see Chapter 55, Pain and Its Management) and can reduce the amount of medication she uses. Methadone affects the reuptake of serotonin and norepinephrine, and blocks the NMDA receptor.[75] Studies, however, do not show methadone to be superior to other opioids.[76] Advantages for G.G. include long half-life, high bioavailability, excellent absorption across mucous membranes, lack of active metabolites, and lower cost. Methadone liquid is long-acting which may be useful when patients lose the ability to swallow as death approaches. Disadvantages in using methadone are its long and variable elimination half-life, drug–drug interactions, prolongation of the QTc interval, and the variability of dosing equivalence with other opioids. Dosing methadone is complex and should be undertaken by experienced clinicians.[76,77]

When converting fentanyl and morphine to methadone, the following should be considered: (a) patient adherence and ability to follow prescription directions, (b) use of an appropriate conversion formula, (c) converting a transdermal formulation of fentanyl to an oral opioid formulation, and (d) a supplemental opioid for breakthrough pain.

Because of its long and variable elimination half-life, the dose of methadone should generally be adjusted only once every 4 to 6 days, and patients must be able and willing to precisely follow directions for its use. The methadone prescribing information should be used for the conversion, with a general rule of thumb being that the initial methadone dose should not exceed 30 mg (Table 6-4).[78,79]

New safety guidelines recommend electrocardiographic monitoring prior to and during methadone use[80]; the need for this is terminally ill patients should be balanced by life expectancy and goals of care. Caution should be used in patients with electrolyte abnormalities (hypokalemia or hypomagnesemia), impaired liver function, heart disease, prolonged QT syndrome, or the use of other QTc-prolonging drugs (e.g., amiodarone, azithromycin, citalopram, fluconazole, haloperidol, ondansetron).[81]

Once the conversion is made, the calculated dose is adjusted and the dosing interval is set at every 12, 8, or 6 hours, based on patient age, previous use of opioids, and current clinical status. Clinical judgment is vital in individualizing a regimen for each patient based on his or her needs.

Before calculating the conversion to methadone for G.G., an important consideration in patients using transdermal fentanyl is an assessment of its absorption.[82] Fentanyl from the transdermal system is absorbed through several layers of the skin and deposited in the subcutaneous fat, from which it is absorbed into the systemic circulation. It is generally observed that transdermal fentanyl is not effective in very thin, cachectic patients. In those cases, the conversion would be made without including the fentanyl. The patch would be removed at initiation of the first methadone dose and supplemented with medication for breakthrough pain if needed. In patients using multiple patches, one patch can be removed every 3 days. Despite weight loss, G.G. (62 inches and 153 pounds) is not cachectic, and the fentanyl should be included when calculating the conversion of her current opioid dose to a comparable methadone dose. In this patient, her sustained-release morphine formulation (50 mg three times daily) is equivalent to 150 mg/day of oral morphine. Her fentanyl transdermal system 75 mcg/hour is equivalent to about 150 mg/day of oral morphine. Her total morphine equivalents per day are 150 mg plus 150 mg, or 300 mg. Using a 1:5 to 1:10 ratio (10%–20%) for conversion of morphine equivalents to methadone, the calculated dose of oral methadone for this patient should be 30 to 60 mg/day.

Table 6-4

Conversion of Oral Morphine Dose to Oral Methadone Requirement[78,79]

Total Daily Baseline Oral Morphine Dose (i.e., Dose of Morphine Equivalents) (mg)	Estimated Daily Oral Methadone Requirement (as % of Total Daily Morphine Dose) (%)
<100	20–30
100–300	10–20
300–600	8–12
600–1,000	5–10
>1,000	<5

Although G.G. is relatively young, has been using opioids for some time, and has severe pain (quantified at 8 of 10), a methadone dose of 20 mg every 8 hours (i.e., 60 mg/day) might be excessive. She should be treated with 15 mg of methadone every 8 hours (45 mg/day), and the dose increased, if needed, based on her clinical response. This smaller initial dose would accommodate for some incomplete cross-tolerance from the morphine and fentanyl and for any fentanyl that remains in her system for the next several days. Patients who have been on much higher doses of opioids, alternatively, can be converted during a period of several days (e.g., converting one-third of the previous daily dose of opioid every 3 days). This is an especially useful method for converting opioid doses for thin, cachectic patients who have been on multiple transdermal patches. A clinician should be in touch with G.G. frequently during the first several days after her conversion to methadone. A telephone call should be made 2 to 4 hours after the first dose to assess for efficacy and toxicity (primarily somnolence, confusion, or nausea) and then every 3 to 5 days. If pain relief with the first dose does not last for the entire dosing interval, it can be adjusted, or G.G. can be instructed to take a one-time extra dose of methadone.

An added benefit in changing to methadone for G.G. is a financial one for the hospice. Outpatient prescription prices for long-acting opioids are very steep and significantly add to hospice costs. The prudent use of methadone can improve overall pain management and keep costs in check. When methadone is not appropriate, generic extended-release morphine is a good second choice. Transdermal fentanyl should be reserved for patients who cannot take oral medication or for when there are significant compliance issues. Extended-release oxycodone should be used only when patients cannot tolerate morphine, have significant renal impairment, or have other contraindications to its use. By converting to methadone, G.G.'s daily cost for the opioid alone will decrease substantially, while still providing appropriate and effective pain management.

G.G. will also need a supplemental analgesic for breakthrough pain. Some practitioners use small doses of methadone, 2.5 mg or 5 mg, as often as every 3 hours. This is a good choice in a well-supervised (i.e., inpatient) setting with nurses familiar with the use of methadone. However, if caregivers treat methadone as if it were morphine, which is much more commonly used for breakthrough pain, the risk of overmedicating the patient is very real. This can have disastrous consequences, especially in frail, elderly patients. Because G.G. is not in an inpatient setting and has tolerated morphine well in the past, 30 mg or 1.5 mL of morphine 20 mg/mL can be prescribed to be taken every 2 hours as needed for breakthrough pain.

G.G. should also start a bowel regimen; the use of a stool softener alone is inadequate.[42] The nurse should perform a rectal examination to determine if stool is present in the rectal vault. An enema or suppository can be given if needed and then senna or PEG can be taken on a routine basis.

Aggressive Symptom Management and Palliative Sedation

D.V.'s drug regimen is unnecessarily complicated for a patient at home. It may be possible to simplify it by looking at each problem anew. His pain is poorly managed as evidenced by his complaint of pain intensity at 7 of 10 (on a scale of 0–10), the use of multiple opioids, and the use of excessive PCA boluses. Once an infusion with PCA dosing is started, there is no need to continue other long-acting opioids (i.e., transdermal fentanyl) or oral agents for breakthrough pain. The PCA doses are serving as the rescue doses for breakthrough pain, and pain relief should be titrated using this method alone. Once pain is well controlled, an oral long-acting agent can be considered if the patient is able to swallow. To do otherwise creates a chaotic approach. Patients reporting allergic reactions to opioids should be carefully asked to describe the precise nature of the purported allergic reaction. True allergies to opioids are rare; patients often refer to an adverse reaction as an allergy or have experienced an effect from the histamine release that is associated with opioids. Hydromorphone, especially injectable hydromorphone, is much more expensive and no more effective than morphine and is best reserved for use in patients who have a genuine allergy or intolerance to morphine.

CASE 6-3

Question 1: D.V., a 35-year-old man with gastric cancer metastasized to the esophagus with periaortic involvement, is hospitalized. He was diagnosed 10 months ago, and his disease has progressed despite multiple courses of chemotherapy (most recently, irinotecan and cetuximab). A double-lumen, peripherally inserted central catheter line has been inserted. He has lost 65 pounds since diagnosis, weighs 150 pounds at 6 feet tall, and presents with abdominal pain, severe nausea, vomiting, obstipation (intractable constipation), and general malaise. D.V. describes his pain as a 7 of 10 in intensity and as "burning like a knife through my stomach." He uses 50 to 75 patient-controlled analgesia (PCA) bolus doses every 24 hours. He has no other medical problems. D.V. is referred to hospice care because he and his wife have agreed to stop chemotherapy and do not want to go back to the hospital. He states a history of allergic reactions to morphine, ondansetron, and diphenhydramine, although these reactions are not noted. He is presently receiving hydromorphone 2 mg/hour in an IV infusion with 1 mg PCA bolus dose every 5 minutes, hydromorphone 4 mg orally every 4 hours as needed for pain, fentanyl transdermal 275 mcg/hour every 3 days, ketamine 20 mg orally every 3 hours, senna two tablets twice daily, docusate sodium 250 mg twice, PEG 3350 17 g daily, lactulose 15 mL as needed for constipation, lorazepam 2 mg orally every 4 hours as needed for nausea or vomiting, metoclopramide 10 mg orally every 6 hours as needed for nausea or vomiting, promethazine 25 mg IV every 4 hours as needed for nausea or vomiting, baclofen 10 mg every 8 hours as needed for hiccups, and pantoprazole 40 mg once daily. What is your assessment of his medication regimen?

Although D.V. had been prescribed ketamine every 3 hours in the hospital, it is unrealistic to expect that this can be continued in the home setting. D.V. and his wife would probably be glad to discontinue it and replace it with an alternative because of his need to be dosed so often.

D.V.'s constipation is currently treated with multiple medications within the same therapeutic class. It would be more prudent to maximize the use of a single agent within a category, rather than using two products at less than the maximally recommended doses. D.V. can use a higher dose of senna (up to four tablets twice daily), and then, if necessary, continue to use the PEG 3350.

D.V. also takes multiple medications for his nausea and vomiting. Promethazine primarily blocks the histamine receptor and can be continued if there is a vertigo component to his nausea and vomiting. The injectable promethazine can be converted to suppositories for use at home. Ondansetron ODT can be a good option when patients or caregivers refuse to use suppositories. He had also been directed to take lorazepam for his nausea and vomiting; however, benzodiazepines are not effective antiemetics. They are given to manage the anxiety associated with nausea and vomiting and are particularly useful in managing the anticipatory nausea and vomiting that is commonly encountered during chemotherapy administration. Metoclopramide can be useful for D.V.'s nausea and vomiting if his physical examination reveals hypoactive bowel sounds. It is also useful for treating hiccups, and the need for baclofen can be reassessed.

In patients who are terminally ill, suffering may continue despite maximal palliative efforts. As a result, practitioners continually encounter patients' requests for the ending of their lives

CASE 6-3, QUESTION 2: A few days after arriving home, D.V. asks his hospice nurse, "Can't you just give me something to end it all?" He has not been sleeping well, is tired of taking so many medications, and wants to alleviate the burden he feels he is imposing on his wife.

because of overwhelming suffering. Clinicians may be averse to this practice both ethically and legally.[83–92] Although substantial numbers of clinicians can imagine situations in which assisted suicide would be acceptable, few are willing to actively participate in the ending of a patient's life.[93,94]

In a small number of patients, it may be desirable to reduce suffering by the thoughtful use of medications to induce sedation.[95–102] It is not appropriate to increase opioid doses to achieve the desired sedated state. Medications used successfully to induce sedation for these patients include benzodiazepines, barbiturates, and propofol, generally given in combination. Opioids are continued to manage pain and prevent withdrawal.

A trial of palliative sedation with intravenous midazolam could be initiated and managed by the hospice nurse at a rate of 1 mg/hour and gradually increased if needed to the desired effect.[88] For use in the home, compounded phenobarbital suppositories could be added if the desired effect is not attained with midazolam alone. Although palliative sedation has a small potential to shorten life, the need to relieve terminal agitation or other symptoms could justify this risk. Palliative sedation should only be initiated as a last resort in severe cases not responsive to other palliative measures, and only after thorough discussion of the important clinical and ethical issues with the patient, family, and other clinical team members.

Before considering palliative sedation, patients should be thoroughly assessed for insomnia, depression, pain, and other symptoms. Underlying reasons for insomnia should be explored

CASE 6-3, QUESTION 3: Repeated increases in the hydromorphone infusion basal rate (he is now at 25 mg/hour) had little effect on managing D.V.'s pain, and his consistent use of up to 120 PCA attempts in 24 hours reflects his continued pain. He describes the intensity of his pain as 8 of 10. Before considering palliative sedation, what other therapeutic interventions can be implemented for D.V.?

and treated. Poor pain management is often the cause for considering palliative sedation. As many as 10% to 20% of patients with cancer may have pain that does not respond to standard systemic analgesics.[103] Interventional techniques, including the administration of spinal opioids and/or local anesthetics may be useful, but may not be practical to initiate for the actively dying patient at home.[104,105] In D.V., lidocaine 0.5 to 1 mg/kg/hour administered IV or subcutaneously might be useful to assist in the management of his severe neuropathic pain.[106–110] Lidocaine purportedly interrupts pain transmission by blocking sodium channels (see Chapter 55, Pain and Its Management).

D.V. was started on lidocaine 1 mg/kg/hour IV. A bolus dose was not given because of the short half-life of lidocaine. Overnight, his use of hydromorphone boluses dropped to one. He now reports his pain as 1 of 10 and that he slept through the night for the first time in months. During the next 2 days, the hydromorphone basal rate was tapered to 5 mg/hour. He did not experience any lidocaine toxicity, such as perioral numbness, metallic taste, or somnolence. D.V. continued on lidocaine, using no hydromorphone boluses for the next 2 weeks, until he died at home surrounded by his family.

KEY REFERENCES AND WEBSITES

A full list of references for this chapter can be found at http://thepoint.lww.com/AT11e. Below are the key references and websites for this chapter, with the corresponding reference number in this chapter found in parentheses after the reference.

Key References

American Society of Health-System Pharmacists. ASHP statement on the pharmacist's role in hospice and palliative care. *Am J Health Syst Pharm*. 2002;59:1770. (24)

Atayee RS et al. Development of an ambulatory palliative care pharmacist practice. *J Palliat Med*. 2008;11:1077. (30)

Electronic Code of Federal Regulations. Title 42–Public Health, Part 418—Hospice Care. http://www.ecfr.gov/cgi-bin/text-idx?rgn=-div5;node=42%3A3.0.1.1.5. Updated July 23, 2015. Accessed July 26, 2015. (13)

Fass J, Fass A. Physician-assisted suicide: ongoing challenges for pharmacists. *Am J Health Syst Pharm*. 2011;68:846. (93)

Good G et al. Therapeutic challenges in cancer pain management: a systematic review of methadone. *J Pain Palliat Care Pharmacother*. 2014;28:197–206. (77)

Hill RR. Clinical pharmacy services in a home-based palliative care program. *Am J Health Syst Pharm*. 2007;64:806. (29)

Lee J, McPherson ML. Outcomes of recommendations by hospice pharmacists. *Am J Health Syst Pharm*. 2006;63:2235. (28)

Librach SL et al. Consensus recommendations for the management of constipation in patients with advanced, progressive illness. *J Pain Symptom Manage* 2010;40:761–773. (42)

Lycan J et al. Improving efficacy, efficiency and economics of hospice individualized drug therapy. *Am J Hosp Palliat Care*. 2002;19:135. (26)

National Consensus Project for Quality Palliative Care. *Clinical Practice Guidelines for Quality Palliative Care*. 3rd ed; 2009. http://www.nationalconsensusproject.org/NCP Clinical Practice Guidelines 3rd Edition.pdf. Accessed August 29, 2015. (4)

Oakman BN et al. Death with dignity: the developing debate among health care professionals. *Consult Pharm*. 2015;30:352–355. (92)

Portenoy RK et al. Opioid use and survival at the end of life: a survey of a hospice population. *J Pain Symptom Manage*. 2006;32:532. (69)

Smallwood N, et al. Management of refractory breathlessness with morphine in patients with chronic obstructive pulmonary disease. *Intern Med J*. 2015;45:898–904. (64)

Solano JP et al. A comparison of symptom prevalence in far advanced cancer, AIDS, heart disease, chronic obstructive pulmonary disease and renal disease. *J Pain Symptom Manage*. 2006;31:58. (58)

Victoria Hospice Society. *Palliative Performance Scale (PPSv2), version 2. Medical Care of the Dying*. 4th ed. Victoria, British Columbia, Canada: Victoria Hospice Society; 2006:120. http://www.victoriahospice.org/health-professionals/clinical-tools. Accessed April 13, 2016. (39)

Wilson S et al. Impact of pharmacist intervention on clinical outcomes in the palliative care setting. *Am J Hosp Palliat Care*. 2011;28(5):316–320. (36)

Key Websites

American Academy of Hospice and Palliative Medicine (AAHPM). http://www.aahpm.org/

American Academy of Pediatrics. Section on Hospice and Palliative Medicine. http://www.aap.org/sections/palliative

Center to Advance Palliative Care (CAPC). http://www.capc.org/

Centers for Medicare & Medicaid Services (CMS). https://www.cms.gov/Center/Provider-Type/Hospice-Center.html

Children's Hospice and Palliative Care Coalition. http://www.chpcc.org

End of Life Online Curriculum. http://endoflife.stanford.edu/M00overview/introlrnoverv.html

Hospice Foundation of America (HFA). http://www.hospicefoundation.org/

International Association for Hospice & Palliative Care (IAHPC). http://www.hospicecare.com/

MedlinePlus. Hospice Care. http://www.nlm.nih.gov/medlineplus/hospicecare.html

National Hospice and Palliative Care Organization (NHPCO). http://www.nhpco.org/

National Hospice and Palliative Care Organization (NHPCO). Pediatric Palliative Care and Hospice. http://www.nhpco.org/pediatric

Palliative Care Network of Wisconsin Fast Facts and Concepts. http://www.mypcnow.org/#!fast-facts/c6xb

Pallimed: A Palliative Medicine Blog. http://www.pallimed.org/

Society of Palliative Care Pharmacists. http://www.palliativepharmacist.org

The National Consensus Project for Quality Palliative Care. http://www.nationalconsensusproject.org

7 Interprofessional Education and Practice

William W. McCloskey, Edith Claros, Carol Eliadi, and Beth Buyea

CORE PRINCIPLES

	CHAPTER CASES
1 The Interprofessional Education Collaboration (IPEC) developed a report by an expert panel that highlighted what they believed are the 4 core competencies of interprofessional education (IPE): (1) values and ethics for interprofessional practice; (2) roles and responsibilities; (3) interprofessional communication; (4) teams and teamwork.	**Case 7-1 (Questions 1)**
2 The IPEC report considers communication a key competency but can be negatively impacted by demographic and professional differences that may exist between healthcare professionals. To address this issue, the IPEC report encourages all team members to be willing to speak up in a respectful way if they have a patient-related concern.	**Case 7-2 (Question 1)**
3 Although one should understand what IPE is, it is also important to clarify what does not constitute IPE. Experiences on Advanced Pharmacy Practice Experience (APPE) rotations that are directed by someone from another profession that do not include sharing of responsibility for patient care are not considered IPE.	**Case 7-3 (Question 1)**
4 Early exposure to IPE enhances students' confidence in their professional value, supports their respecting the contributions of other professions, and better prepares them for providing patient care. These early experiences also increase the appeal of collaborating with other professions, reduce any negative stereotypical attitudes toward these other professions, and strengthen communication skills.	**Case 7-4 (Question 1)**
5 One element of an IPE model is understanding that different professions may vary in how they approach patient care. Team-based care means a shared responsibility for patient care on the part of all team members and should not be dominated by any one profession.	**Case 7-5 (Question 1)**
6 It is important to understand that IPE models can place in a variety of settings, such a classroom, laboratory, and a patient care setting. Regardless of the environment, IPE-related activities should represent a "real-world" experience.	**Case 7-6 (Question 1)**
7 Despite the progress made in advancing IPE over the past few years, some barriers to implementing it exist on different levels, from the institution/organization level down to the individual level. Overcoming these barriers is important in order to continue to work toward preparing students to collaborate with other healthcare professionals.	**Case 7-7 (Question 1)**

Interprofessional education (IPE) is considered to be a major attempt to better prepare medical, pharmacy, nursing, and other health profession students to collaborate and deliver patient care as part of a team.[1] Despite the recent attention it has received, IPE is actually not new, and the idea behind it has been in existence for some time. The first phase was initially launched in the 1940s, and a second wave of IPE coinciding with a move to enhance primary care was described in the 1960s.[2] In the early 1970s, the Institute of Medicine (IOM) Report "Educating for the Health Team" addressed pharmacy as a component of the team as well as medicine, nursing, and dentistry.[3] However, there remains a concern that many practitioners, including pharmacists, are commonly trained in programs that are removed from other healthcare professionals. This educational separation could potentially have a detrimental effect on the beliefs and values that these practitioners may have on the contribution of other providers to patient care.[2] In 2003, the IOM addressed this matter in their report "Health Professions Education: A Bridge to Quality."[4]

The report stressed incorporating interprofessional experiences into healthcare education and establishing core competencies for IPE. The 2003 IOM report states "all health professionals should be educated to deliver patient-centered care as members of an interprofessional team, emphasizing evidence-based practice, quality improvement approaches, and informatics." These IOM recommendations generated the momentum for health professions to advance the need for IPE.[1] It is evident that with the increasing prevalence of chronic diseases and the complexities of delivering health care today, an interprofessional approach toward patient care is important.[2] In addition, new approaches to health care, including the Patient Protection and Affordable Care Act of 2010, have stimulated a movement toward team-centered health care, such as the patient-centered medical home (PCMH) concept which encourages interprofessional teamwork in providing primary care.[5,6] With the PCMH model, physicians share responsibility with nurses, pharmacists, social workers, and others to manage complex patient care cases.[7] The PCMH model puts the patient at the center of his/her health care and expands access and improves mechanisms for patient–provider communication, including the use of technology (e.g., email) for patients to interact with their healthcare provider.[7] Although studies have shown that collaboration of healthcare professionals can result in improved patient outcomes, more work needs to be done to examine the relationship between IPE and positive patient outcomes.[8]

The reader is encouraged to apply these concepts to subsequent chapters as many of the cases presented can be used as part of IPE activities. In addition, students are encouraged to apply these concepts to IPE activities at their own institution.

CORE IPE COMPETENCIES

CASE 7-1

QUESTION 1: You are enrolled in a IPE seminar with pharmacy, nursing, physician assistant, and medical students. Each week you will be assigned cases to work on in groups. Your initial impression is that these exercises are primarily designed to help foster teamwork, but are there any other areas that IPE helps develop as well?

The Interprofessional Education Collaboration (IPEC), a group representing schools of pharmacy, nursing, medicine, osteopathic medicine, dentistry, and public health convened an expert panel to develop core competencies for IPE. The expert panel report was originally published in 2011[5] and was recently updated in 2016.[6] The four major competencies that are highlighted in the report are as follows: (1) values and ethics for interprofessional practice; (2) roles and responsibilities; (3) interprofessional communication; and (4) teams and teamwork.[5,6] These competencies were identified in order to create a coordinated effort across the different healthcare professions to incorporate key content into their respective curricula and to guide curricular development. The competencies also provide a foundation for lifelong learning, as well as offer information to the different professions' educational program accrediting bodies that can be used to set common accreditation standards.[5,6]

Regarding the first competency, the IPEC report considers interprofessional values and ethics an important element of establishing a professional and interprofessional identity. These values and ethics are patient-centered and grounded in a shared purpose to providing patient care. Working in teams adds value by bring about patient/family and community outcomes that promote overall health, disease prevention, and treatment of disease. In addition to being patient-centered, competency in this area helps develop trusting relationships with patients, families, and other members of the healthcare team. There is also an expectation that one maintains competency in one's own profession relative to his/her area of practice.[5,6]

The second competency addresses the importance that the IPEC places on one understanding how professional roles and responsibilities complement each other in providing patient care and to advance the healthcare needs of patients and populations. It is this diversity of expertise that is the foundation of an effective healthcare team. Coordination of care occurs more effectively when each profession knows what the other can contribute to patient care.[5] Pharmacists should be able to effectively articulate to other team members what they can contribute to executing a treatment plan, especially when it comes to preventing and identifying any drug-related problems. Sharing roles has also been shown to enhance patient outcomes and reduce costs.[2] For example, a nurse, social worker, and pharmacist can collaborate to develop a discharge plan that reduces the potential for hospital readmission by addressing such issues as community resources that may be available for assistance, medication adherence, patient education, and healthcare provider follow-up.[2] The IPEC report notes that one should also understand the limitations of one's abilities, knowledge, and skills as well, and engage in continuous interprofessional development to improve team performance.[5,6]

The IPEC report also considers communication a key competency, and the expert panel states that one should communicate with patients, families, and both healthcare and non-healthcare professionals in a responsive and responsible manner. Characteristics such as being available, being well-informed, showing interest, and being receptive are key aspects of this communication area as well. Listening and encouraging the input of other members are also important attributes for this competency. Presenting information in a manner that patients, families, and other team members understand can help enhance the safety and effectiveness interprofessional care.[5,6]

CASE 7-2

QUESTION 1: You are on a medical team that includes a very intimidating attending physician. Your team is evaluating a patient presenting with an upper respiratory tract infection. You note from the medical record that the patient is on warfarin. The attending physician directs the medical resident to order an antibiotic that you know may interact with warfarin and possibly increase the risk of bleeding. How should you communicate your concerns to the attending?

Communication can be negatively impacted by demographic and professional differences that may exist between healthcare professionals (e.g., older attending physician and younger pharmacist). To address this issue, the IPEC report encourages all team members to be willing to speak up in a respectful way if they have a patient-related concern. You should politely and very clearly explain to the attending what your concern is and provide evidence-based literature to support the nature and severity of the interaction. Despite the attending's intimidating demeanor, failure to communicate the problem could possibly result in harm to the patient. Being able to provide and receive feedback with confidence helps promote team-based care.[5,6]

The fourth competency cited by the IPEC, teams and teamwork, means working together for a common shared goal for patient care. The IPEC report indicates that working in teams not only relates to shared problem-solving, but being able to constructively manage any disagreements that arise with other healthcare professionals as well and patients and family. Conflicts may occur when power is confused with expertise based on professional background. Staying patient outcome focused and addressing any potential conflict openly through shared problem-solving and utilizing effective communication skills can help establish a more effective team. The report also indicates that working in teams also means that giving up some professional autonomy. Healthcare teams function best when the knowledge and expertise of the different professions on the team are integrated to make patient care decisions.[5,6]

As a consequence of this shift toward teamwork, many healthcare profession-accrediting organizations, including pharmacy, nursing, and medicine, now incorporate interprofessional collaboration and teamwork as part of their standards.[9] Pharmacy school graduates, in addition to those from other healthcare professions, must be able to work effectively with other providers as part of a team. The basic principle of IPE is that if students from different healthcare professions learn together, they will be better positioned to work together in teams to provide optimal patient care.[10] As Brock and colleagues recently noted, "health care education must be more of a team sport."[11]

IPE TERMINOLOGY

The terminology related to IPE can be confusing as interpretation of multidisciplinary, interdisciplinary, and interprofessional may differ in the literature.[2] The Centre for the Advancement of Interprofessional Education (CAIPE) is an organization based in the United Kingdom that promotes and develops IPE initiatives. CAIPE defines IPE as occurring "when two or more professions learn with, from, and about each other to improve collaboration and the quality of care."[12] The term interdisciplinary is sometimes interchanged with interprofessional and may be the more appropriate term to use in those situations where individuals who are not health professionals (e.g., nursing aides) are part of the team.[2] However, the term multidisciplinary should not be confused with interprofessional. The former is simple and additive approach to patient care, with several healthcare providers providing independent services, and each responsible for their own specialty. As described earlier, IPE is a more coordinated approach in which there is an integration and collaboration to include the viewpoints of many different professions in order to optimize patient care.[2]

CASE 7-3

QUESTION 1: You are on an internal medicine APPE rotation and round with a patient care team that includes a medical student, nursing student, and dietetics student. The medical resident presents a case of an elderly patient recently admitted with worsening heart failure and determines what the treatment plan would be without actually involving anyone else on the team. Is your experience considered an example of IPE?

Although one should understand what IPE is, it is also important to clarify what does not constitute IPE. For example, students from different health professions learning the same topic in a classroom setting (e.g., pharmacology) without interacting and discussing the material as it pertains to their respective discipline are not considered IPE.[1] Nor is it IPE when a faculty member from another profession lectures pharmacy students unless that person incorporates some component on how the professions would interact in providing patient care.[1] Also, experiences on Advanced Pharmacy Practice Experience (APPE) rotations that are directed by someone from another profession that do not include sharing of responsibility for patient care are not considered IPE.[1] Consequently, the experience described in Case 7-3 is not considered IPE. Clearly the underlying theme of any IPE activity is that it should be a collaborative effort of students representing different professions.

INCORPORATING IPE IN THE CURRICULUM

CASE 7-4

QUESTION 1: In your first professional year in pharmacy school, you are in an introductory healthcare seminar course with other health profession students. A fellow classmate complains that she would prefer to be with only other pharmacy students until later in the curriculum. What are the possible benefits of having other healthcare students in an introductory-level course?

The goal of IPE is to develop knowledge, skills, and attitudes that result in interprofessional team competence.[9] This includes not only clinical skills but communication, conflict resolution, team building skills, in addition to respecting the roles and responsibilities of other health professions.[2] IPE is best when it is incorporated throughout the entire curriculum in a vertically and horizontally integrated fashion, in which collaboration, teamwork, and patient-centered care are introduced to students prior to their entering the professional phase of the curriculum.[9] It has been reported that early exposure to IPE approach enhances students' confidence in their professional value, supports their respecting the contributions of other professions, and better prepares them for providing patient care.[13] It has additionally been noted that early educational experiences within an IPE program increase the appeal of collaborating with other professions, reduce any potential negative stereotypical attitudes one may have toward these other professions, and enhance communication skills regardless of any specialized knowledge one may have.[14]

The pharmacy education accrediting body, the American Council for Pharmacy Education (ACPE), has included IPE in their 2016 Standards and Guidelines for Accreditation for the PharmD program.[15] The goal is to make sure that schools of pharmacy incorporate the IPE within the PharmD curriculum. Standard 11 of the 2016 ACPE Standards specifically covers IPE. In order to meet this standard, the PharmD curriculum of a particular pharmacy school should prepare "all students to provide entry-level, patient-centered care in a variety of settings as a contributing member of an interprofessional team."[15] The key elements of this standard include interprofessional team dynamics, interprofessional team education, and interprofessional team practice.

The interprofessional dynamics section of the standard addresses issues such as values and ethics, interprofessional communication, conflict resolution, and honoring interprofessional roles and responsibilities. The standard indicates that "these skills should be introduced, reinforced, and practiced in the didactic and Introductory Pharmacy Practice Experience (IPPE) components of the curriculum, and competency is demonstrated in the APPE practice settings."[15]

The interprofessional team education and team practice elements of the standard concern working together to improve patient care. Team education can include simulation exercises where pharmacy students can collaborate with medical, nursing, and other health professions students to better understand the contributions that each makes to the healthcare team. Team practice encompasses providing direct patient care as part of a shared decision-making process. It includes face-to-face interactions with individuals from other healthcare professions that are designed to improve interprofessional team effectiveness.[15]

Despite its merits, not every student may be initially understanding or accepting IPE. There are validated methods to evaluate an individual's ability to accept IPE. The Readiness for Interprofessional Learning Scale (RIPLS) has been used a research tool to assess attitudes and readiness for IPE.[16] It is a 19-item questionnaire that is designed to evaluate three primary areas: teamwork and collaboration, professional identity, and roles and responsibilities. The Interdisciplinary Education Perception Scale (IEPS) is another tool that assesses attitudes toward IPE.[17] This scale is an 18-item questionnaire that contains 4 subscale measures: competency and autonomy, perceived need for co-operation, actual cooperation, and understanding the value of others. Assessment instruments such as RIPLS and IEPS have been used to measure the impact that IPE experiences may have on students' pre-exposure acceptance and attitudes. Although these and some other tools may be useful for measuring change in behavior or attitudes concerning IPE, they do not assess the impact that IPE may have on patient outcomes.[2]

IPE MODELS

The creation of an effective model for IPE should start with the understanding that this is just the initial step in providing patient directed care.[2] An interprofessional environment helps students from one profession learning from individuals representing another discipline to better develop skills that will help improve their own professional specific skills and to more effectively work in team-based setting.[2] It is important that all representatives of a particular profession, including students and practitioners, be socialized to their own profession as well as to the interdisciplinary setting. There also needs to be a commitment that IPE be incorporated within the curricula of all programs within an institution to help sustain its viability for the future.[2]

In addition to other health profession students, pharmacy students should be considered essential to any IPE model. Pharmacists have not always been considered necessary on a healthcare team, and this needs to be addressed when developing IPE teams.[2] IPE teams should ideally include a pharmacy student, in addition to medicine, nursing, social work, and nutrition students.[2]

The stage of socialization within the specific profession must be considered when creating teams as well.[2] Socialization of healthcare students has been defined as "the acquisition of knowledge, skills, values, roles and attitudes of associated with the practice of that particular profession," and can be exhibited by the language, behavior, and demeanor that are representative of that specific discipline.[2] It is important that a student maintains his/her professional identity when participating in an IPE models. Also when creating student teams, one should try balance them with regard to what point they are in their professional socialization and education.[2] A medical student who is in the 4th year of his/her program who is paired with less experienced nursing or pharmacy student may negatively impact learning of the other students if the medical student assumes a more dominant role.[2]

CASE 7-5

QUESTION 1: M.M. is a 65-year-old retired man who presented to his provider three days ago with complaints of increasing shortness of breath (dyspnea) upon exertion. He reports noting swelling in his ankles for months that has started to get worse over the past 2 weeks, making it difficult to wear his shoes on toward the end of the day and going up the stairs to his apartment. In the past week, he has had a decreased appetite, some nausea and vomiting, and tenderness in the right upper quadrant of the abdomen. He reports that he has not taken his medications in the past month because he didn't think they were helping him. The patient lives alone with his dog in a small two-bedroom apartment on the second floor of a multifamily home. He has a daughter who lives in another state and who visits him during the holidays. The patient was hospitalized and treated for a diagnosis of exacerbation of CHF and is now being discharged home. A physician, nurse, social worker, and pharmacist are part of a discharge planning team working with M.M. How does the approach of the pharmacist to M.M.'s care differ from that of the other team members?

One element of an IPE model is understanding that different professions may vary in how they approach patient care. Medicine and pharmacy tend to focus on eliminating or "ruling-out" causes of a patient's complaint, whether it is medical- or drug-related.[2] While the physician will focus primarily on the medical evaluation of M.M., the pharmacist would determine whether any of his medications were causing any effects which may have contributed to his belief that they were not helping him. The pharmacist would also work with M.M. to develop a plan that would enhance adherence to his discharge medications. Some other members of the team, such as the nurse and social worker, may take a more holistic approach and address the patient from a broader perspective.[2] This would include considering any family or environment issues that may affect M.M.'s progress such as ability for self-care when living alone and not having a relative living close by. They could make arrangements to make sure M.M. has the proper support at home. The nurse can also educate the patient about the importance of adherence to proper diet and to recognize early signs and symptoms of exacerbation. Some professions such as social work or psychology tend to be more involved with the patient or family for a more prolonged period of time, particularly if change in behavior is warranted.[2] Another consideration with how different professions approach patient care is that medical students are typically trained to be decision-makers regarding clinical problem-solving, which has been a long-standing part of the culture of medicine.[18] As noted previously, team-based care means a shared responsibility for patient care on the part of all team members and should not be dominated by any one profession.

CASE 7-6

QUESTION 1: Your university has an IPE day where medical students, nursing students, pharmacy students, and physician assistant students work in teams on simulated patient cases using a manikin. Is this considered an appropriate strategy for delivering IPE?

It is important to understand that IPE models can take place in a variety of settings, such a classroom, laboratory, and a patient care setting. Regardless of the environment, IPE-related activities should represent a "real-world" experience.[2] Simulation activities (simulating a patient care setting) and case discussions in a seminar format, where participants can exchange information, are appropriate for the early professional education years. Students may also observe activities of health providers upon patient visits and reflect on the contributions of each to patient care. The patient care setting is more appropriate for students with more experience.[2] In addition to certainly being real world, it is more effective in developing the confidence and skills needed for students to function as part of the team. In this experiential setting, clinicians from multiple professions who are active and engaged as role models and mentors are critical to the success of the model.[2]

Bridges and colleagues describe three different practice models of IPE, representing a didactic program, a community-based experience, and an interprofessional simulation experience.[19] The didactic program focuses on developing interprofessional team building skills, understanding other professions, and how culture influences healthcare delivery. Students work in small groups and also engage in a community service project. There is also a clinical component where students from different professions form teams and attend a prescribed number of sessions at a practice site. The community model illustrates how collaboration by different professions can provide patient care services to many underserved individuals in their homes. Teams of students are assigned home visits in a manner so that they are exposed to a variety of family types (e.g., Medicaid family with multiple children, older adult living alone, hospice patient). Each team has a project that they present to their group at the end of the course. With the simulation model, students from different professions use simulation and not real patients to promote interprofessional teamwork. Even though there are a number of different strategies that may be used to deliver IPE, the common elements that lead to more successful experience include responsibility, assertiveness, accountability, coordination, communication, trust, respect autonomy, and cooperation.[19]

POTENTIAL BARRIERS TO IPE

CASE 7-7

Question 1: Although IPE is considered important, are there any barriers to implementing it?

Despite the progress made in advancing IPE over the past few years, some barriers to implementing it exist on different levels, from the institution/organization level down to the individual level. Overcoming these barriers is important in order to continue to work toward preparing students to collaborate with other healthcare professionals.

On the institutional/organizational level, academic calendars and requirements may differ between various healthcare disciplines. Also the requirements for assessing students may differ between professions due to accrediting body standards, and the timing of when topics are covered within the degree program may not be consistent. Finding a common time for students to meet is often a challenge, and there may not be available classroom space available to accommodate the increased number of students. In addition, the curricula of the different professions may also provide little flexibility in terms of incorporating IPE into the curriculum, although mandates by accrediting bodies such as ACPE dictate that this needs to happen for some professions. There may not be an adequate number of faculties trained in the area of IPE, and there may be insufficient faculty development efforts to address this issue. Collaboration with IPE efforts also may be negatively affected by geographic separation between disciplines that may exist within the institution.[2,20] It is important that the institution's administration commits the necessary financial and other resources necessary to address some of these potential obstacles to IPE.

There may also be barriers to IPE at the individual level. Differences in attitudes that exist between heath care professions can impact the implementation of IPE. It has been shown that healthcare providers may have negative opinions of each other's clinical knowledge and ability.[21] Michalec and colleagues surveyed over 600 first-year students from 6 different professions, including pharmacy, assessing their perceptions and stereotypes of their own as well as other healthcare professions.[21] The students rated the six professions based on nine distinct positive attributes (academic ability, professional competence, interpersonal skills, leadership ability, ability to work independently, ability to be a team player, ability to make decisions, practical skills, and confidence). Although medicine rated highest for most of these attributes, they rated lowest for ability to be a team player, which is contrary to the mission of team-based health care. Compared to the other professions (nursing, occupational therapy, physical therapy, couple and family therapy), pharmacy and medicine also scored low on interpersonal skills, which is a negative when it comes to working with others. Granted these are only perceptions of students about other health professions before any interaction, but they may represent potential barriers to providing team-based patient care.

Faculty also need to understand the value of IPE so they can be actively involved in implementing any program at their institution. Faculty may resist IPE if it results in an increase in workload and causes time constraints.[1]

FUTURE OF IPE

The first challenge is to sustain the IPE momentum that has been developed over the past several years and to provide the necessary resources to support it.[22] Expansion of IPE is also been identified as a future goal.[23] Further opportunities for collaboration between professions need to be identified, and the education of healthcare students needs to advance to the point where team-based learning is the norm, and that improved patient care is achieved.[23] It is believed that in the future, students and faculty will have multiple opportunities to interact with others, and that these experiences will further commit them to work together to improve patient outcomes.

There are still a number of issues concerning IPE that need to be addressed. There needs to be more objective evidence on the impact of IPE on improving patient outcomes.[24] In addition, there are still questions concerning how much IPE is needed to achieve learner competence, where in the curriculum does IPE have the greatest impact and what are the most effective formats for delivering IPE.[24]

CONCLUSION

The traditional model of practitioners working alone to provide patient care can result in communication failures and is detrimental to patient safety. A care plan that utilizes teams of healthcare providers, including pharmacists, to coordinate patient care can optimize patient outcomes. IPE can lead to better understanding of the roles and responsibilities of team members, improved communication and more effective teamwork.[8] Table 7-1 summarizes some suggested criteria for an organization to be engaged toward IPE.

Table 7-1
Suggested Criteria for Engagement for Interprofessional Education

1. A well-known, observable, measurable IPE philosophy that permeates the organization.
2. Faculty from different healthcare professions working together to develop the learning experiences.
3. Students having integrated didactic and experiential opportunities to learn how to build teams and to collaborate, and how working together can improve patient care.
4. IPE learning experiences being incorporated into to the curricula as a requirement.
5. Competence demonstrated by students with a defined set of competencies such as those outlined by the Interprofessional Education Collaboration.
6. Organization infrastructure that fosters and supports IPE including faculty time to develop IPE and having collaborative activities across the various professions.

Adapted from Barnsteiner JH. Promoting interprofessional education. *Nurs Outlook*. 2007;55:144–150.

KEY REFERENCES AND WEBSITES

A full list of references for this chapter can be found at http://thepoint.lww.com/AT11e. Below are the key references and websites for this chapter, with the corresponding reference number in this chapter found in parentheses after the reference.

Key References

Buring SM et al. Interprofessional education: definitions, student competencies, and guidelines for implementation. *Am J Pharm Educ.* 2009;73(4):59. (1)

American College of Clinical Pharmacy. Interprofessional education: principles and application. A framework for pharmacy. *Pharmacotherapy.* 2009;29(3):145e–164e. (2)

Key Websites

Interprofessional Education Collaboration. http://www.aacn.nche.edu/education-resources/ipecreport.pdf

Centre for the Advancement of Interprofessional Education. http://caipe.org.uk/resources/defining-ipe/

Section Editors: Jean M. Nappi and Judy W. Cheng

8 Dyslipidemias, Atherosclerosis, and Coronary Heart Disease

Barbara S. Wiggins and Pamela B. Morris

CORE PRINCIPLES

		CHAPTER CASES
1	The risk of atherosclerosis is directly related to increasing levels of serum cholesterol. Cholesterol, specifically lipoproteins, plays a central role in the pathogenesis of atherosclerosis. Thus, low-density lipoprotein cholesterol (LDL-C) is the primary target for intervention. The American College of Cardiology/American Heart Association (ACC/AHA) guideline and the National Lipid Association (NLA) recommend management for patients at high risk. This includes patients with atherosclerotic cardiovascular disease (ASCVD) as well as those with familial hypercholesterolemia (FH).	**Case 8-1 (Question 1)**
2	Every patient with dyslipidemia should be evaluated for secondary causes of elevated LDL-C, non–HDL-C, or triglycerides (TGs). These causes may be related to concomitant medications or due to a clinical condition.	**Case 8-1 (Questions 2, 3), Table 8-5**
3	LDL-C goals and the thresholds for instituting therapeutic lifestyle changes (TLC) and pharmacotherapy are guided by the presence of clinical atherosclerosis or based on cardiovascular risk.	**Case 8-2 (Questions 1, 2), Case 8-3 (Question 1), Case 8-4 (Questions 1, 2)**
4	An adequate trial of TLC should be used in all patients, but pharmacotherapy should be instituted concurrently in high-risk patients and patients should be monitored for adverse effects.	**Case 8-2 (Question 2), Case 8-5 (Question 1)**
5	In most cases, statins are the medications of choice to treat high LDL-C because of their ability to substantially reduce LDL-C, ability to reduce morbidity and mortality from atherosclerotic disease, convenient once-daily dosing, and low risk of side effects. Management of these adverse effects is necessary in order to optimize benefit.	**Case 8-2 (Question 3)**
6	Statins are the agents of choice to reduce LDL-C with low risk of adverse effects. However, drug interaction knowledge is needed in order to optimize efficacy without compromising safety.	**Case 8-4 (Question 3)**
7	Patients with high TGs are at increased risk of acute pancreatitis. The primary goal in these individuals is to lower their TG levels with diet, exercise, weight reduction, and TG-lowering drugs such as nicotinic acid, fibrates, and omega-3 fatty acids.	**Case 8-5 (Question 2), Case 8-6 (Question 1)**
8	Combination drug therapy is often needed in patients with severe lipid abnormalities, higher risk individuals with lower LDL-C goals, or patients with multiple lipid abnormalities such as those with the metabolic syndrome who have a secondary target of non–HDL-C.	**Case 8-6 (Question 2)**

Dyslipidemias (one or more abnormalities of blood lipids) play an important etiologic role in the pathogenesis of ASCVD, including coronary heart disease (CHD), cerebrovascular disease, and peripheral arterial disease.[1] Successful lifestyle changes and pharmacologic management of dyslipidemias have been shown to reduce the risk of ASCVD events such as heart attack and stroke.[2–4] For cardiovascular disease prevention, the clinician estimates the individual patient's ASCVD risk with available risk assessment tools, determines the intensity of lipid-modulating therapy to match the patient's level of risk, and implements appropriate treatments to meet and maintain treatment goals.[5–8]

LIPID METABOLISM

Knowledge of lipid and lipoprotein metabolism is essential to understanding therapeutic targets for pharmacologic agents. Lipids are small molecules that function in the body's storage of energy, in cellular signaling, and as components of cell membranes. Cholesterol, an essential lipid, is the precursor molecule for the formation of bile acids (which are required for absorption of nutrients), the synthesis of steroid hormones (which provide important modulating effects in the body), and the formation and integrity of cellular membranes. However, excess cholesterol plays a central role in atherogenesis and subsequent atherothrombotic complications.

Cells derive cholesterol in two ways: by intracellular synthesis or by uptake from the systemic circulation. Within each cell, cholesterol is synthesized through a series of biochemical steps, many of which are catalyzed by enzymes (Fig. 8-1). The irreversible and rate-limiting step in cholesterol production is the conversion of β-hydroxyl-β-methylglutaryl coenzyme A (HMG-CoA) to mevalonic acid, which is catalyzed by HMG-CoA reductase. One of the most effective lipid-lowering therapies developed to date for managing dyslipidemias, HMG-CoA reductase inhibitors or statins, competitively interferes with the binding of substrate to this critical enzyme, thereby reducing the cellular synthesis of cholesterol. The biosynthesis of cholesterol in humans follows a circadian rhythm with maximum cholesterol synthesis occurring near midnight and minimum synthesis at midday.[9]

Free cholesterol is esterified to cholesteryl esters for intracellular storage by the action of the enzyme acetyl CoA acetyl transferase (ACAT). Two forms of ACAT have been identified. ACAT1 is present in many tissues, including inflammatory cells, whereas ACAT2 is present in intestinal mucosa cells and hepatocytes. ACAT2 is required for the esterification and absorption of dietary cholesterol from the gut. In theory, inhibition of this enzyme could reduce the absorption of dietary cholesterol, the secretion of cholesterol by the liver, and even the uptake and storage of circulating cholesterol in inflammatory cells in the arterial wall. Several inhibitors of ACAT have been developed; however, in clinical trials they did not appear to reduce atherosclerosis and were possibly pro-atherogenic.[10] It is unlikely that there will be any further development of this class of drugs for cardiovascular prevention.

TGs are lipids that serve as an important source of stored energy in adipose tissue. TGs are synthesized from three molecules of fatty acids esterified to a glycerol backbone. Phospholipids

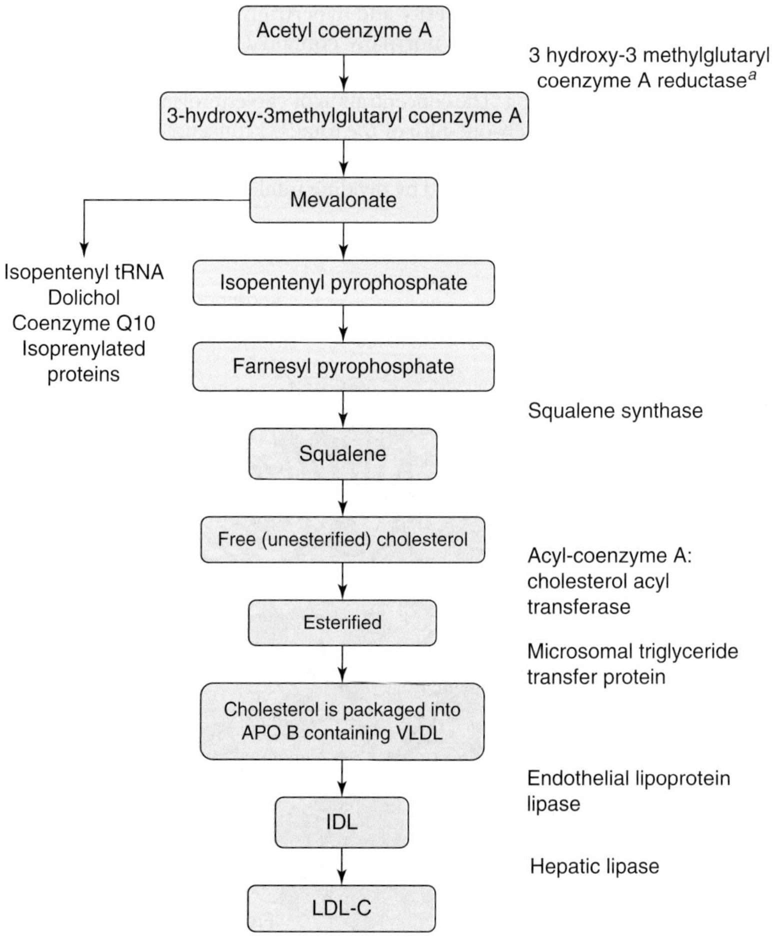

Figure 8-1 Biosynthetic pathway of cholesterol. *The rate limiting step in cholesterol biosynthesis. ApoB, apolipoprotein B; Coenzyme A, Ubiquinone 10; IDL, intermediate density lipoprotein; LDL-C, low density lipoprotein cholesterol.

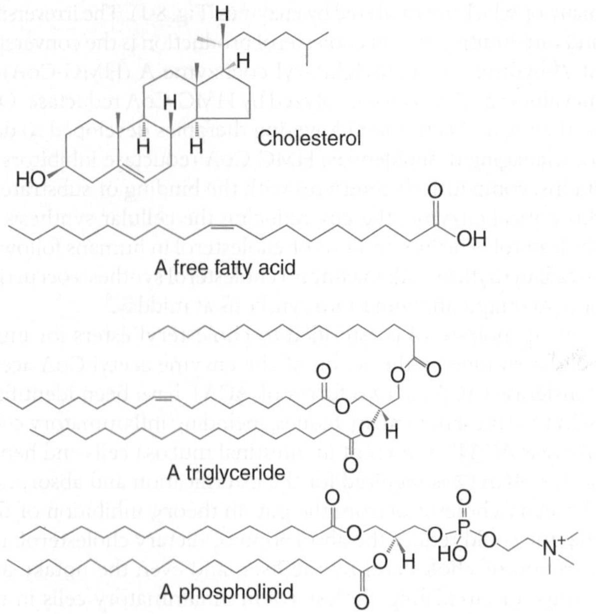

Figure 8-2 Chemical structure of lipids. At the top is cholesterol, followed by oleic acid. In the middle is a triglyceride comprised of an oleoyl, stearoyl, and palmitoyl chain attached to a glycerin backbone. At the bottom is a phospholipid.

(PLs) are a class of lipids formed from fatty acids, a negatively charged phosphate group, nitrogen-containing alcohol, and a glycerol backbone. PLs are essential for cellular function and the absorption, storage, and transport of lipids in the circulation. They form the monolayer on the surface of lipoproteins which function to transport neutral lipids throughout the body. PLs are amphipathic with a hydrophilic head and hydrophobic tail and form a membrane bilayer of lipoproteins to deliver hydrophobic cargo (cholesterol and energy in the form of fat) to other organs. PLs are also secreted into bile to aid in the digestion and absorption of dietary fat and lipid-soluble nutrients from the diet. They stabilize proteins within the membrane, function as cofactors in enzymatic reactions, and participate in the oxidation of lipoproteins in the arterial wall (Fig. 8-2).

Lipoproteins

Cells also obtain cholesterol by extracting it from the systemic circulation. The source of this cholesterol is the liver, where it is synthesized and secreted into the systemic circulation. As discussed above, cholesterol and other fatty substances are insoluble in water. Therefore, cholesterol, TGs, and PLs are packaged into water-soluble complexes called lipoproteins in the hepatocyte and enterocytes before being secreted into the aqueous medium of the blood. These lipoproteins contain an oily inner lipid core made up of cholesteryl esters and TGs and an outer hydrophilic coat made up of PLs and unesterified cholesterol (Fig. 8-3). The outer coat also contains at least one of a number of proteins known as "apoproteins," which provide the ligand for interaction with receptors on cell surfaces, act as cofactors for various enzymes, and add structural integrity.

The three major lipoproteins found in the blood of fasting (10–12 hours) patients are very low density lipoprotein (VLDL), low-density lipoprotein (LDL), and high-density lipoprotein (HDL).[11] These particles vary in size, cholesterol and TG composition, and accompanying proteins (Table 8-1 and Fig. 8-4).[12,13]

VERY LOW DENSITY LIPOPROTEINS

VLDL particles are formed in the liver (Fig. 8-1). Free fatty acids are taken up by the hepatocyte where the enzyme diglycerol acyltransferase (DGAT) catalyzes TG formation from diacylglycerol and the coenzyme AcylCoA. The enzyme microsomal triglyceride transfer protein (MTP) lipidates apoprotein B by transfer of cholesteryl esters (CE) and TG to form VLDL, which is then secreted by the liver into the circulation. Inhibitors of MTP reduce production of VLDL and downstream IDL and LDL. One of these agents, lomitapide, is currently approved for the treatment of the homozygous form of FH.[14] DGAT inhibitors which reduce TG synthesis are currently under investigation for management of obesity and hypertriglyceridemia.[15]

VLDL particles normally contain 15% to 20% of the total blood cholesterol concentration and most of the total blood TG concentration. The concentration of cholesterol in these particles is approximately one-fifth of the total TG concentration; thus, if the total TG concentration is known, the VLDL-cholesterol (VLDL-C) level can be estimated by dividing total TGs by 5. Newly secreted

Figure 8-3 Basic structure of lipoproteins. Lipoproteins vary in the amount of cholesterol esters and triglyceride content. Additionally, they have varying numbers and types of surface apolipoproteins.

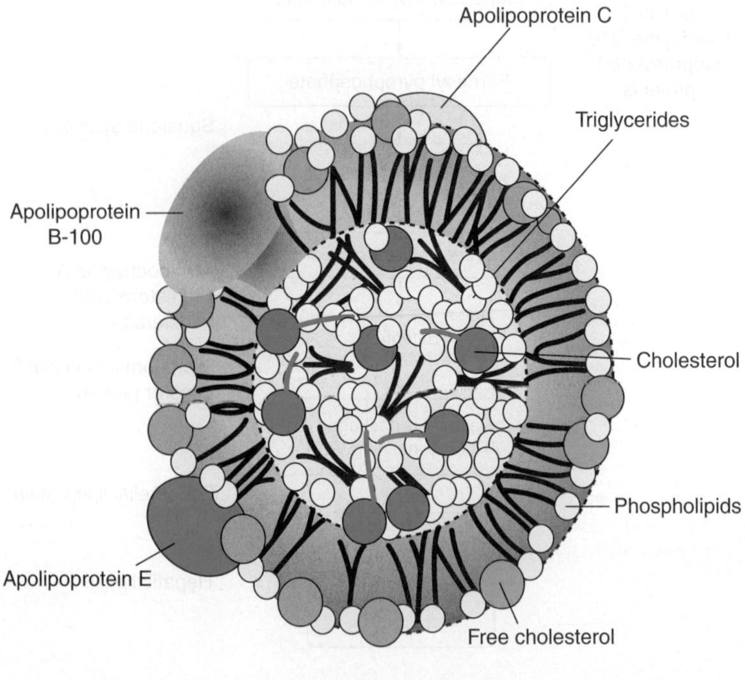

Table 8-1
Classification and Properties of Plasma Lipoproteins[12]

Lipoprotein	Origin	Density Range (g/mL)	Size (nm)	Cholesterol Concentration in plasma (mmol/L)[a]	Triglyceride Concentration in plasma (mmol/L)[b]	Major Apolipoprotein	Other Apolipoprotein
Chylomicrons	Intestine	<0.95	100–1,000	0.0	0	B-48	A-I, C
VLDL	Liver	<1.006	40–50	0.1–0.4	0.2–1.2	B-100	A-I, C
IDL	VLDL	1.006–1.019	25–30	0.1–0.3	0.1–0.3	B-100	
LDL	IDL	1.019–1.063	20–25	1.5–3.5	0.2–0.4	B-100	
HDL	Tissues	1.063–1.21	6–10	0.9–1.6	0.1–0.2	A-I	A-II, A-IV
Lp(a)	Liver	1.051–1.082	30–50			B-1, (a)	

[a]For mg/dL, multiply by 38.67.
[b]For mg/dL, multiply by 88.5.
HDL, high-density lipoprotein; IDL, immediate-density lipoprotein; LDL, low-density lipoprotein; Lp(a), lipoprotein A; VLDL, very low-density lipoprotein.
With kind permission from Springer Science+Business media: Genest J. Lipoprotein disorders and cardiovascular risk. *J Inherit Metab Dis*. 2002;26:267–287.

VLDL particles are too large to migrate into the arterial wall and appear to play only a small role in the pathogenesis of atherosclerosis.

VERY LOW DENSITY LIPOPROTEIN REMNANTS

In the circulation the enzyme lipoprotein lipase (LPL) hydrolyzes TGs in VLDL particles. The removed TGs are converted to fatty acids and stored as an energy source in adipose tissue. As TGs are removed, the VLDL particle becomes progressively smaller and relatively more cholesterol rich. The particles formed through this process include small VLDL particles (called remnant VLDL), intermediate-density lipoproteins (IDL), and LDL (Fig. 8-5). Approximately 50% of the remnant VLDL and IDL particles are removed from the systemic circulation by LDL or apolipoprotein (apo) B-100/apo E receptors on the surface of the liver; the other 50% are converted into LDL particles by further hydrolytic action of hepatic lipase. VLDL remnant particles are found in the arterial wall, though in smaller numbers than LDL. Drugs that enhance the activity of LPL, such as the fibrates, increase hydrolysis of TG in VLDL particles and lower blood TG levels.

LOW-DENSITY LIPOPROTEINS

LDL particles are cholesterol enriched and carry 60% to 70% of the total blood cholesterol. LDL plays a central role in the pathogenesis of atherosclerosis and is the primary target of lipid-lowering therapy. Approximately half of the LDL particles are removed from the systemic circulation by the liver; the other half may be taken up by peripheral cells or deposited in the intimal space of coronary, carotid, and other peripheral arteries, where atherosclerosis can develop. The probability that atherosclerosis will develop is directly related to the concentration of LDL-C in the systemic circulation and the duration of exposure to elevated LDL-C levels; thus, the cumulative risk of ASCVD in men and women with hypercholesterolemia increases with age.

HIGH-DENSITY LIPOPROTEINS

HDL particles transport cholesterol from peripheral, lipid-rich inflammatory cells in the arterial wall back to the liver, a process called *reverse cholesterol transport*.[16] In epidemiologic studies HDL cholesterol (HDL-C) concentrations are inversely associated with the risk of ASCVD, presumably because cholesterol is being removed from vascular tissue and is not available to contribute to atherogenesis. In peripheral cells, the adenosine triphosphate binding cassette transporter A-1 (ABCA-1) and adenosine triphosphate binding cassette transporter G-1 facilitate the efflux of both cholesterol and PLs to apo A1 to form nascent HDL particles. Cholesterol acquired from peripheral cells by HDL particles is

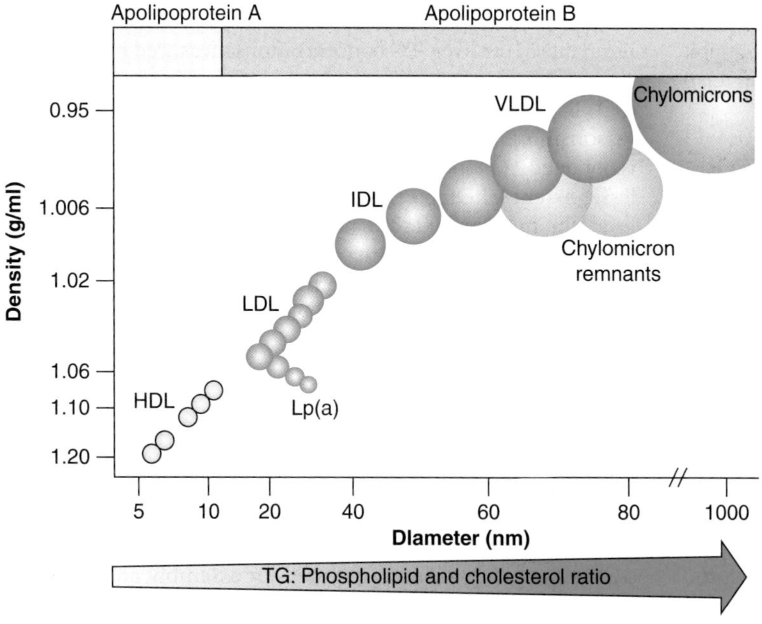

Figure 8-4 Relative lipoprotein sizes and densities.[13] Relative lipoprotein particle densities: In general, a subclass distribution of increased small LDL, decreased large HDL, and increased large VLDL particle size is most associated with increased CHD risk. Reprinted with permission from Bays H, Stein EA. Pharmacotherapy for dyslipdaemia—current therapies and future agents. *Expert Opin Pharmacother*. 2003;4:1901–1938.

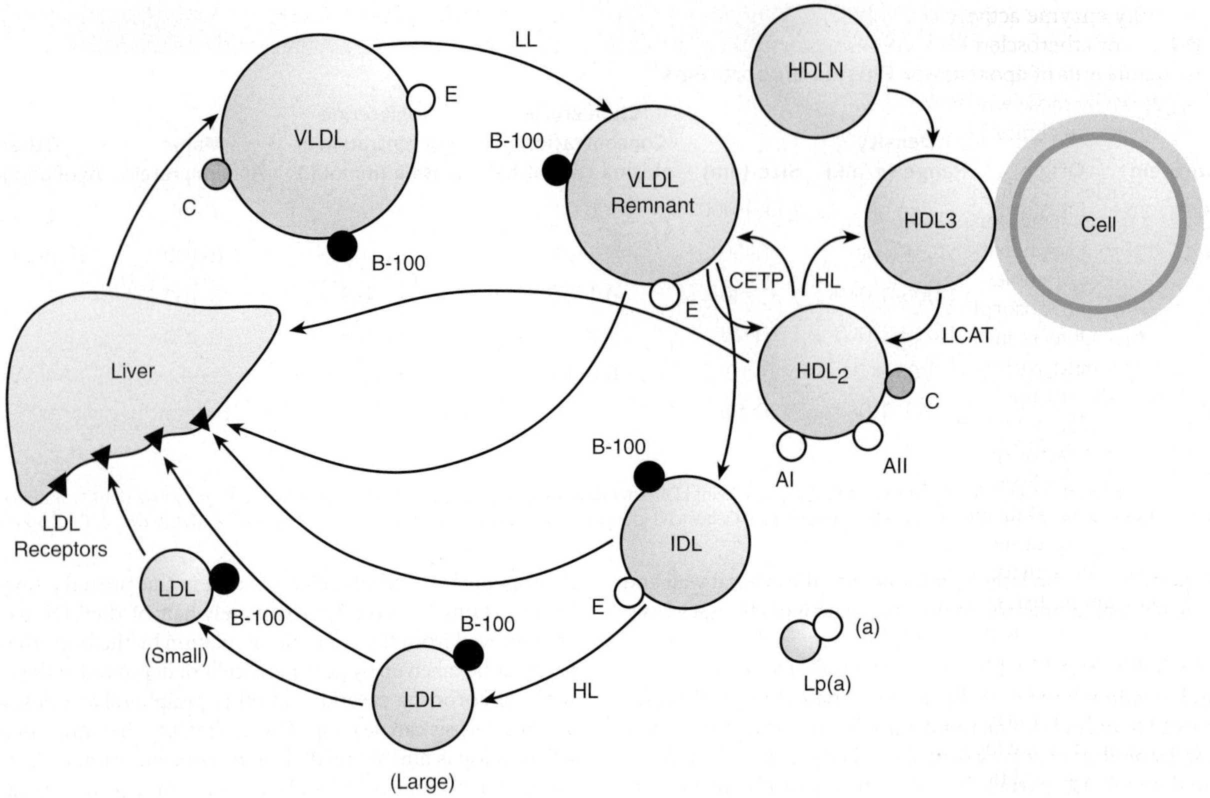

Figure 8-5 The lipoproteins, apolipoproteins, and enzymes involved in the transport of cholesterol and triglycerides. HDL, high-density lipoprotein; IDL, intermediate-density lipoprotein; LDL, low-density lipoprotein; VLDL, very-low-density lipoprotein; HDLN, nascent high-density lipoprotein; HL, hepatic lipase; LL, lipoprotein lipase; CETP, cholesterol ester transfer protein; LCAT, lecithin cholesterol acyltransferase; B-100, apolipoprotein B-100; C, apolipoprotein C; E, apolipoprotein E; AI, apolipoprotein AI; AII, apolipoprotein AII; Lp(a), lipoprotein (a).

converted into an esterified form through the action of the enzyme lecithin-cholesterol acyl transferase (LCAT). HDL particles may either transport cholesterol directly to the liver through interaction with the scavenger receptor, SR-B1, on the surface of hepatocytes or transfer it to circulating remnant VLDL and LDL particles by the action of cholesterol ester transfer protein (CETP). CETP transfers cholesterol from HDL particles to VLDL and LDL in exchange for TGs, making the HDL particle less cholesterol rich. If the latter occurs, cholesterol may be returned to the liver for clearance from the circulation or delivered back to peripheral cells. Patients have been identified who have a deficiency of CETP and high plasma concentration of HDL-C which appears to be associated with a low incidence of CHD. Drugs that inhibit CETP can raise HDL-C levels and are being studied in long-term cardiovascular outcomes trial.[17]

NON–HIGH-DENSITY LIPOPROTEIN CHOLESTEROL

Though elevated LDL-C is most commonly associated with ASCVD risk, in some patients the assessment of LDL-C alone may underestimate the risk of events. Non–HDL cholesterol (non–HDL-C), calculated by subtracting HDL-C from TC, provides a measure of cholesterol carried by all potentially atherogenic particles, including VLDL, VLDL remnants, IDL, and LDL particles. Also, in the presence of postprandial hypertriglyceridemia the calculation of LDL-C may be inaccurate, whereas non–HDL-C is reliable when measured in the non-fasting state.

CHYLOMICRONS

Unlike the lipoproteins that transport cholesterol from the liver to peripheral cells and back (endogenous lipid transport), chylomicrons transport TGs and cholesterol derived from the diet or synthesized in the enterocytes from the gut to the liver (exogenous lipid transport) (Fig. 8-5, Table 8-1). Chylomicrons are large, TG-rich lipoproteins. As they pass through capillary beds on the way to the liver, some of the TG content is removed through the action of LPL in a manner similar to that described for hydrolysis of TGs from VLDL particles. In the rare individual who has LPL deficiency, chylomicrons are inefficiently metabolized and TG levels in the blood may become severely elevated (e.g., 1,000–5,000 mg/dL).

After a fatty meal the number of TG-rich chylomicron particles is elevated and TG levels rise. Following a 10- to 12-hour period of fasting, chylomicrons will be removed from the blood by LPL-mediated hydrolysis of TGs and removal of chylomicron remnants in the liver. TG concentrations measured in the fasting state reflect primarily TGs that are produced by the liver as well as TGs carried in VLDL and other remnant particles. For this reason, most patients are asked to fast before a lipoprotein profile is obtained. A blood sample that is rich in chylomicrons (and to a lesser extent VLDL particles) appears turbid; the higher the TG level, the more turbid the sample. If the sample from a patient with hyperchylomicronemia is refrigerated, chylomicrons will float to the top and form a frothy white layer, whereas smaller VLDL particles stay suspended below.

Apolipoproteins

Each lipoprotein particle contains proteins on the outer surface called *apolipoproteins* (Fig. 8-5, Table 8-1). These proteins serve four main functions: (a) they serve as major structural components of lipoproteins, (b) they serve as cofactors for activation of enzyme systems, (c) they act as ligands for binding to receptors on cell surfaces, and (d) they are required for assembly and secretion of lipoproteins.[15] Abnormal metabolism of apolipoproteins can result in faulty enzyme activity or cholesterol transport and an increased risk of atherosclerosis. Clinicians may consider assessment of blood levels of apolipoproteins to evaluate dyslipidemic patients, especially those who have a family history of premature CHD. The five most clinically relevant apolipoproteins are B-100, C, E, A-I, and A-II.

VLDL particles contain apo B-100, E, and C (Fig. 8-5). The B and E proteins are ligands for LDL receptors (also called *B-E receptors*) on the surface of hepatocytes and peripheral cells. Linkage allows the transfer of cholesterol from the circulating lipoprotein into the cell through absorptive endocytosis and cellular uptake of the particle. Defects in these proteins reduce the ability of lipoproteins to bind with receptor proteins and may result in defective clearance of lipoproteins from the systemic circulation and increased levels of circulating cholesterol.

Apo C-II is a cofactor or activator of LPL. By activating LPL, apo C-II stimulates the hydrolysis of TGs from lipoprotein particles in the capillary beds. Deficiency of apo C-II may result in faulty TG metabolism and subsequent hypertriglyceridemia. Apo C-III downregulates LPL activity and interferes with the hepatic uptake of VLDL remnant particles. This leads to increased concentrations of small VLDL remnant particles, which are small enough to penetrate into the arterial wall and contribute to atherogenesis. Apo C-III is a marker of atherogenic dyslipidemia (elevated TGs, reduced HDL-C, near normal levels of LDL-C, and elevated LDL particle concentration), which is associated with an increased risk of ASCVD events. In addition, prolonged residence of VLDL and LDL particles in the systemic circulation results in the formation of small, highly atherogenic LDL particles and the atherogenic dyslipidemia (see below).[18]

Each VLDL, IDL, and LDL particle contains one molecule of apo B-100. Thus, the blood concentration of apo B-100 is an indication of the total number of VLDL, VLDL remnant, IDL, and LDL particles in the circulation. An increased number of lipoprotein particles and an increased apo B-100 concentration are strong predictors of ASCVD risk.[19] Remnant VLDL particles retain both apo B-100 and E during the delipidization process; LDL particles contain only apo B-100 (Fig. 8-5). Some patients have high levels of apo B-100 suggesting an increased number of atherogenic particles in the circulation, even though the LDL-C level is in the desirable range. These patients have an increased risk of atherosclerosis. Apo B-100 and the measurement of LDL particle concentrations by nuclear magnetic resonance spectroscopy are considered as recommended treatment targets by some guidelines for the management of dyslipidemia.[7,8]

HDL particles contain apo A-I, A-II, and C. Apo A-I is an activator of LCAT, which catalyzes the esterification of free cholesterol in HDL particles. Levels of apo A-I have a stronger inverse correlation with CHD risk than apo A-II levels. HDL particles that contain only A-I apolipoproteins are associated with a lower CHD risk than are HDL particles containing both A-I and A-II.[20]

Low-Density Lipoprotein Receptor

Cholesterol is taken up by peripheral and hepatic cells via binding of the ligands, apo B-100 and E, on circulating lipoproteins to cell-surface LDL receptors. The concentration of LDL receptors is mediated by intracellular cholesterol concentration. Synthesis of LDL receptors is stimulated by a low intracellular cholesterol concentration. Conversely, the concentration of cell-surface LDL receptors may be downregulated by the action of proprotein convertase subtilisin/kexin type 9 (PCSK9), which targets the LDL receptor for degradation within intracellular lysozymes.[21] Within the cell, the receptor protein is synthesized in the mitochondria and migrates to clathrin-coated pits on the cell surface. The LDL receptor may then bind to lipoproteins that contain apo E or B-100, including VLDL, remnant VLDL, IDL, and LDL. Because remnant VLDL and IDL particles contain both B-100 and E proteins, they may have a higher affinity for LDL receptors than do LDL particles, which contain only the B protein. Drugs that upregulate the synthesis of LDL receptors (e.g., statins), therefore, may increase the clearance of both VLDL remnant particles and LDL particles from the circulation. Thus, statins may reduce serum TG levels as well as cholesterol levels. Following binding of lipoproteins to the LDL receptor, the lipoproteins undergo endocytosis and are taken up by lysosomes, where they are metabolized into elemental substances for use by the cell. The cholesterol is transferred into the intracellular cholesterol pool. The LDL receptor may be returned to the cell surface, where it can bind with another circulating apo E- or apo B-containing lipoprotein.

ABNORMALITIES IN LIPID METABOLISM

Lipid synthesis and transport is complex with hundreds of possible steps that can malfunction resulting in a lipid disorder. However, there are only a few relatively common and important lipid disorders seen in clinical practice. The first two described subsequently, polygenic hypercholesterolemia and atherogenic dyslipidemia, are largely the result of an interaction between genes and lifestyle choices. Several prominent, but rarer, familial lipid disorders are subsequently described. Table 8-2 summarizes the characteristics of the most common lipid disorders.

POLYGENIC HYPERCHOLESTEROLEMIA

Polygenic hypercholesterolemia is the most prevalent primary disorder causing an increase in cholesterol. It is caused by a combination of environmental (e.g., poor nutrition, sedentary lifestyle) and multiple genetic factors. In patients with this disorder a diet high in saturated fatty acids can reduce LDL receptor activity, thus reducing the clearance of LDL particles from the systemic circulation. Patients with polygenic hypercholesterolemia have mild to moderate LDL-C elevations (usually in the range of 130–250 mg/dL), but no unique physical findings are usually present. A family history of premature CHD is present in approximately 20% of cases. These patients may often be effectively managed with dietary restriction of saturated fats and cholesterol and by drugs that lower LDL-C levels (statins, bile acid sequestrants (BASs), and ezetimibe).

Atherogenic Dyslipidemia

Atherogenic dyslipidemia is characterized by moderate elevations of TG (150–500 mg/dL, indicative of the elevated VLDL remnant particles), low HDL-C levels (<40 mg/dL), and mild to moderate elevations of LDL-C level.[22] These patients have increased concentrations of small, dense, cholesterol-poor LDL particles, non–HDL-C, and apo B-100. Most commonly, patients have increased visceral adiposity and are hypertensive and insulin resistant.

In the presence of increased visceral adiposity there is impaired glucose metabolism and/or diabetes with increased mobilization of fatty acids from adipose cells to the systemic circulation. The excess of free fatty acids leads to increased TG synthesis and secretion of TG-rich VLDL particles by the liver. These TG-rich particles contain apo C-III, which inhibits the action of LPL, thus retarding lipolysis of TGs from VLDL particles. This results in an excess of TG-rich VLDL remnant particles.[23] CETP mediates the exchange of TGs from these particles with cholesteryl esters from HDL, resulting in VLDL remnant particles that are enriched

Table 8-2
Characteristics of Common Lipid Disorders

Disorder	Metabolic Defect	Lipid Effect	Main Lipid Parameter	Diagnostic Features
Polygenic hypercholesterolemia	↓LDL clearance	↑LDL-C	LDL-C: 130–250 mg/dL	None distinctive
Atherogenic dyslipidemia	↑VLDL secretion ↑ApoC-III synthesis ↓LPL activity ↓VLDL removal	↑TG ↑Remnant VLDL ↓HDL ↑Small, dense LDL	TG: 150–500 mg/dL HDL-C: <40 mg/dL	Frequently accompanied by central obesity or diabetes
Familial hypercholesterolemia Heterozygous	Reduction in functional LDL receptor, defective apo B, gain-of-function mutations PCSK9	↑LDL-C	LDL-C: 250–450 mg/dL	Family history of premature CHD, tendon xanthomas, corneal arcus
Familial hypercholesterolemia Homozygous	Absent LDL receptors, defective apo B, gain-of-function mutations PCSK9	↑LDL-C	LDL-C: >450 mg/dL	Family history of premature CHD, tendon xanthomas, corneal arcus; affected individuals exhibit CHD by second decade of life
Familial defective apoB-100	Defective apoB on LDL and VLDL	↑LDL-C	LDL-C: 250–450 mg/dL	Family history of CHD, tendon xanthomas
Dysbetalipoproteinemia (type III hyperlipidemia)	ApoE2:E2 phenotype, ↓VLDL remnant clearance	↑Remnant VLDL, ↑IDL	LDL-C: 300–600 mg/dL TGs: 400–800 mg/dL	Palmar xanthomas, tuberoeruptive xanthomas
Familial combined hyperlipidemia	↑ApoB and VLDL production	↑CH, TG, or both	LDL-C: 250–350 mg/dL TGs: 200–800 mg/dL	Family history, CHD Family history, hyperlipidemia
Familial hyperapobetalipoproteinemia	↑ApoB production	↑ApoB	ApoB: >125 mg/dL	None distinctive
Hypoalphalipoproteinemia	↑HDL catabolism	↓HDL-C	HDL-C: <40 mg/dL	None distinctive

ApoB, apolipoprotein B; ApoC-III, apolipoprotein C-III; ApoE, apolipoprotein E; CH, cholesterol; CHD, coronary heart disease; HDL, high-density lipoprotein; HDL-C, high-density lipoprotein cholesterol; IDL, intermediate-density lipoprotein; LDL, low-density lipoprotein; LDL-C, low-density lipoprotein cholesterol; TGs, triglycerides; VLDL, very-low-density lipoprotein.

with cholesterol (Fig. 8-6). TGs are also exchanged from VLDL remnant particles with cholesteryl esters from LDL particles. Thus, VLDL remnants become even more cholesterol-enriched and LDL particles become TG-enriched. The cholesterol-enriched, small VLDL remnant particle is atherogenic. TG-rich LDL undergoes lipolysis catalyzed by hepatic lipase to remove TGs, resulting in small, cholesterol-poor LDL particles (called *small dense LDL*) that are highly atherogenic. Lipolysis of TG-rich HDL results in low HDL due to excretion of lipid-poor apo A-I by the kidneys.

Patients with atherogenic dyslipidemia may be effectively managed with weight reduction and increased physical activity. Pharmacologic agents that enhance the removal of remnant VLDL and small dense LDL particles (i.e., statins) and that lower TG levels (i.e., Omega 3 fatty acids or fibrates) may be effective in the management of these patients.

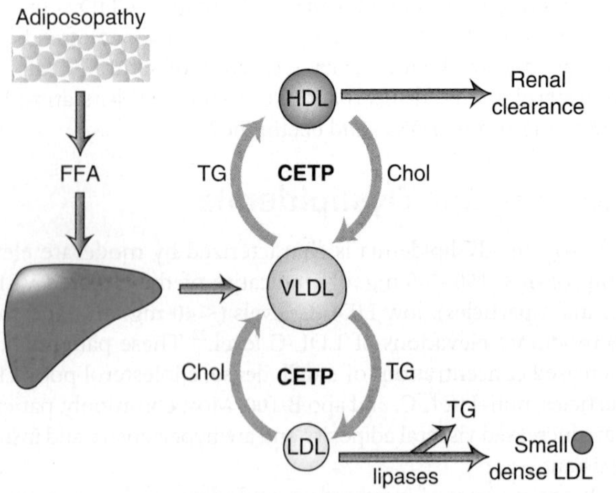

Figure 8-6 The role of CETP in creation of atherogenic dyslipidemia.[13] Role of cholesterol ester transfer protein (CETP) in the creation of an atherogenic lipid of someone with hypertriglyceridemia. Cholesterol-rich very low density lipoprotein (VLDL), low high-density lipoprotein cholesterol (HDL-C), as well as small dense low-density lipoprotein cholesterol (LDL-C) is a pattern often observed in patients with metabolic syndrome as well as those with type 2 diabetes. With permission from Bays H, Stein EA. Pharmacotherapy for dyslipdaemia—current therapies and future agents. *Expert Opin Pharmacother*. 2003;4:1901–1938.

Familial Hypercholesterolemia

FH is a disorder of defective LDL-C clearance. This autosomal dominant disorder is strongly associated with premature CHD.[24,25] Most recent estimates indicate that the prevalence of heterozygous FH (HeFH) ranges from 1 of 250 to 1 of 500 people in the United States.[26] Homozygous FH (HoFH) may occur in 1 of 1 million to 1 of 250,000 people in the United States. The most common cause of this disorder is a genetic mutation resulting in a defective or absent LDL receptor. Consequently, heterozygotes possess approximately half the number of functioning LDL receptors and double the LDL-C level of unaffected patients (LDL-C levels ranging between 250 and 450 mg/dL). Clinically, FH patients may exhibit excess cholesterol deposition in the iris, clinically manifested as arcus senilis. Cholesterol may also deposit in tendons, particularly the Achilles' tendon and extensor tendons of the hands, resulting in tendon xanthomas. The clinical diagnosis of FH is established by documenting a very high LDL-C level, a strong family history of hypercholesterolemia and premature CHD events, and the presence of tendon xanthomas. Untreated HeFH patients have approximately a 5% chance of a myocardial infarction (MI) by age 30, a 50% chance by age 50, and an 85% chance by age 60. The mean age of death in untreated male heterozygotes is in the mid-50s; for untreated female heterozygotes, it is in the mid-60s.[25]

Homozygotes generally have LDL-C levels greater than 500 mg/dL. This rare disorder results in CHD by age 10 to 20 years. Because these individuals have lost the ability to clear cholesterol-carrying lipoproteins from the circulation, combination pharmacotherapy and/or LDL-apheresis may be required to help remove atherogenic particles.

Familial Defective Apo B-100

Familial defective apo B-100 (FDB) is a genetic disorder clinically indistinguishable from HeFH. These patients have normally functioning LDL receptors, but defective apolipoprotein B-100, resulting in reduced binding of LDL particles to the LDL receptor and reduced clearance of LDL particles from the systemic circulation.[27–29] As with FH, LDL-C levels are usually 250 to 450 mg/dL. Presumably, the apo E and half of the apo B in heterozygous FDB patients function normally, providing mechanisms for removal of some lipoproteins from the systemic circulation. Clinical diagnosis of FDB is based on a very high LDL-C level, a family history of premature CHD, and tendon xanthomas. The definitive diagnosis requires molecular screening techniques.

Proprotein Convertase Subtilisin/Kexin Type 9 Gain-of-Function Gene Mutation

FH may also be caused by "gain-of-function" mutations in the gene encoding for proprotein convertase subtilisin/kexin type 9 (PCSK9), an enzyme that plays an important role in cholesterol homeostasis.[30] The frequency of these mutations in patients with FH is uncertain. When PCSK9 is secreted into the plasma, it binds to the epidermal growth factor-like repeat A (EGF-A) domain of the cell-surface LDL receptors. PCSK9 binding leads to endocytosis of the LDL–LDL receptor–PCSK9 complex into intracellular lysozymes for degradation, resulting in a reduced number of LDL receptors and increased LDL-C (to approximately 300 mg/dL). Drugs that inhibit PCSK9 have demonstrated significant reductions in LDL-C in patients with HeFH, HoFH, and polygenic hypercholesterolemia.[31]

Familial Combined Hyperlipidemia

Familial combined hyperlipidemia (FCHL) is caused by increased production of apo B-containing particles, VLDL, and LDL.[32] Patients with FCHL have an elevated apo B-100 level, hypercholesterolemia with LDL-C usually in the range of 250 to 350 mg/dL, elevated TGs (usually between 200 and 800 mg/dL), and reduced levels of HDL-C. First-degree relatives of these individuals frequently have a lipid disorder and often there is a family history of ASCVD. Patients with FCHL commonly are overweight, are hypertensive, and may have metabolic disturbances such as insulin resistance, diabetes, or hyperuricemia. The diagnosis of FCHL is presumed in patients who have increased cholesterol or TG levels, a strong family history of premature CHD, and a family history of dyslipidemia.

Familial Dysbetalipoproteinemia

Familial dysbetalipoproteinemia, also called type III hyperlipidemia or remnant disease, is caused by poor clearance of VLDL and chylomicron particles from the systemic circulation as a result of a defect in apo E.[33,34] Apo E is necessary for the normal clearance of chylomicrons and VLDL. It is inherited as an E2, E3, or E4 isoform from each parent. The E2 isoform has a low binding affinity for the LDL receptor. Thus, individuals with an apo E2/E2 phenotype have delayed clearance of VLDL remnant (and possibly chylomicron) particles from the circulation and a reduced conversion of IDL to LDL particles. However, a clinically significant lipid disorder usually does not result unless triggered by other metabolic problems such as diabetes, hypothyroidism, or obesity. Patients with this disorder have high cholesterol due to enrichment of cholesterol esters in VLDL remnant particles, high TGs in the range of 400 to 800 mg/dL, and a VLDL-C to TG ratio greater than 0.3. Patients may have palmar xanthomas (yellow-orange discoloration in the creases of the palms and fingers) and tuberoeruptive xanthomas (small, raised lesions in areas of pressure, particularly the elbows and knees). A personal and family history of premature atherosclerotic vascular disease often is present. As noted above, these patients often have diabetes mellitus, hypertension, obesity, and hyperuricemia.

Familial Disorders of Triglyceride Metabolism

Familial hypertriglyceridemia (FHTG) is associated with an increase in both TG-rich VLDL particles and chylomicrons. LDL-C is generally not significantly elevated (<130 mg/dL) and HDL-C is decreased (<40 mg/dL). FHTG is usually relatively mild and asymptomatic unless secondary causes of hypertriglyceridemia are present (poorly controlled diabetes, obesity, medications, etc.). TG levels are in the range of 200 to 500 mg/dL, but may be greater than 1,000 mg/dL. Patients with more marked TG elevations (>500 mg/dL) may present with eruptive xanthomas and/or acute pancreatitis.

Rare mutations in the LPL or cofactor apo CII genes may also be associated with severe hypertriglyceridemia.[35] Familial LPL deficiency usually presents in childhood with TG levels from 2,000 to 25,000 mg/dL and lipemic plasma, pancreatitis, eruptive xanthomas, and lipemia retinalis (creamy-white appearance of retinal blood vessels). The clinical presentation of familial deficiency in apo CII is similar to familial LPL deficiency in homozygotes, but heterozygous individuals may have normal plasma lipid concentrations. Patients with familial hepatic lipase deficiency may also present with severe hypertriglyceridemia (>500–1,000 mg/dL) associated with modest elevations in LDL-C and normal to increased HDL-C. This disorder is most common in individuals of Indian ancestry.

Hypoalphalipoproteinemia

Isolated low HDL-C (<40 mg/dL) without an increase in TG level is fairly uncommon, but is associated with increased ASCVD risk. The precise molecular defects causing this problem are uncertain, although genetic influences are likely involved.[36] Tangier disease, which is characterized by low HDL-C, orange tonsils, and hepatosplenomegaly, has been linked to a defect in the ABCA-1 transporter responsible for the efflux of cholesterol from peripheral cells (i.e., inflammatory cells in the arterial wall). The inherited tendency to have low HDL-C is accentuated by lifestyle factors such as obesity, smoking, and lack of exercise. Despite strong epidemiologic evidence showing an inverse relationship between HDL-C and CHD, clinical trials demonstrating a benefit of raising isolated low HDL-C with drugs are lacking. Therapy in patients with low HDL-C is, therefore, directed at lowering LDL-C to reduce ASCVD risk. Therapies to raise HDL-C by novel mechanisms are under investigation to determine if HDL-directed strategies can reduce CHD risk.[37]

LIPOPROTEINS AND ASCVD RISK

Epidemiologic studies have conclusively established a direct relationship between blood cholesterol concentrations in a population and the incidence of ASCVD events.[38–40] For every 1% increase in blood cholesterol levels, there is a 1% to 2% increase in the risk of CHD. In addition, using gene variants that exclusively affect a biomarker of interest (i.e., that do not have pleiotropic effects on other factors), investigators have confirmed LDL-C as a causal risk factor for CAD. HDL-C is inversely associated with CHD risk. For every 1% *decrease* in HDL-C levels, there is a 1% to 2% *increase* in the risk of CHD events.[41] However, gene variants that affect HDL-C have cast doubt on whether HDL-C directly influences risk for CAD.

The role of TGs in the pathogenesis of ASCVD continues to be a subject of important investigation.[23] Most epidemiologic studies have found that a high TG level is an independent risk factor for CHD when evaluated with univariate analysis. When other lipid abnormalities such as increased LDL-C or low HDL-C are included in a multivariate analysis, TGs may lose independent predictive power. This is, in part, because it is difficult to establish a causal relationship in observational epidemiology, especially given the correlations among TGs, LDL-C, and HDL-C. Patients with hypertriglyceridemia usually have low HDL-C (due to the action of CETP and increased renal clearance of apo AI) which is an important predictor of ASCVD risk. In addition, elevated TG levels are associated with increased levels of TG-rich lipoprotein remnants (remnant VLDL and chylomicron particles and IDL), increased LDL particle concentration, and small, dense LDL particles. These particles are all potentially atherogenic and mediate a higher CHD risk than that associated with an elevated LDL-C alone.[42–45] Recent meta-analyses of epidemiologic studies found that TGs independently predicted CHD risk, even after adjustment for other lipid-risk factors.[23] High TG levels are also found in certain familial disorders, including dysbetalipoproteinemia and FCHL, which carry increased CHD risk.[33,34] Additionally, hypertriglyceridemia is associated with a procoagulant state, which promotes coronary thrombosis.[45]

A recent analysis of 185 common genetic variants mapped for plasma lipids examined the role of TGs in risk for CAD. In a model accounting for effects on LDL-C and/or HDL-C levels, the strength of a polymorphism's effect on triglyceride levels was correlated with the magnitude of its effect on CAD risk.[46] These results suggest that triglyceride-rich lipoproteins causally influence risk for CAD.

Paradoxically, very high TG levels (>500 mg/dL) are not commonly associated with an increased CHD risk, but do cause an increased risk of pancreatitis, especially when levels exceed 1,000 mg/dL. Often, a genetic defect in LPL is present in these cases that impairs the removal of TGs from TG-rich particles (VLDL and chylomicrons). These particles do not become enriched with cholesterol and, therefore, are not often atherogenic.[47] If the blood sample is stored in the refrigerator overnight, a thick creamy layer often appears on the surface, indicating the presence of chylomicrons. Although most patients with very high TGs remain free of CHD throughout their lives, some do experience ASCVD events.

Pathogenesis of Atherosclerosis

Circulating cholesterol plays a central etiologic role in the pathogenesis of atherosclerosis.[1] Atherosclerotic vascular lesions begin in the first decade of life and may progress in the presence of elevated levels of cholesterol and other uncontrolled ASCVD risk factors.[48] Atherosclerosis is considered to be a chronic inflammatory process in response to injury of the vascular endothelium by factors such as glycoxidation products in diabetes, shear stress, excess free fatty acids released by adipocytes, bacterial products, and neurohormonal abnormalities, among other factors. The damaged endothelium becomes prothrombotic, has reduced release of nitric oxide and impaired vasodilatory capacity, and releases chemoattractants for inflammatory cells and platelets. Regulation of blood cholesterol levels and management of other risk factors can restore endothelial function, nitric oxide release, and the vasodilatory response.

In patients with excess apo-B-containing lipoproteins [VLDL remnants, IDL, LDL, and Lp(a)], atherogenic particles migrate through the endothelial junction into the subendothelial space or intima. The subsequent accumulation and retention of lipoproteins in the subendothelium (Fig. 8-7)[48] is the result of binding to subendothelial matrix molecules such as chondroitin sulfate proteoglycans.

Soon after taking up residence in the subendothelial space, lipoproteins are structurally modified primarily by oxidation. Modified lipoproteins stimulate dysfunctional endothelial cells to release cell adhesion molecules (intracellular adhesion molecule 1, vascular cell adhesion molecule 1, and E-selectin) and chemoattractants (monocyte chemotactic factor 1 and macrophage colony-stimulating factor) which promote adhesion and stimulate transmigration of monocytes and lymphocytes into the intimal space.[49–51] Thus, atherosclerosis is an inflammatory process in response to retained and modified lipoproteins. Once recruited, monocytes are converted to macrophages, which ingest oxidized lipoprotein particles via special scavenger or acetyl-LDL receptors on the surface of macrophage cells.[52] Further engorgement with oxidized lipoproteins inhibits mobility of resident macrophages and the cells become cytotoxic causing further damage to the vascular endothelium. As the uptake of modified lipoproteins into macrophage cells continues, the cells become laden with lipid and eventually become *foam cells* (Fig. 8-8). Monocytes and foam cells continue to secrete growth factors and cytokines establishing a chronic inflammatory process and progression to a more complex atherosclerotic plaque.

During plaque growth, smooth muscle cells from the media migrate upward and proliferate near the luminal surface.[53] Collagen synthesis is also increased. This leads to conversion of early atherosclerotic lesions that are lipid rich with a thin fibrous cap

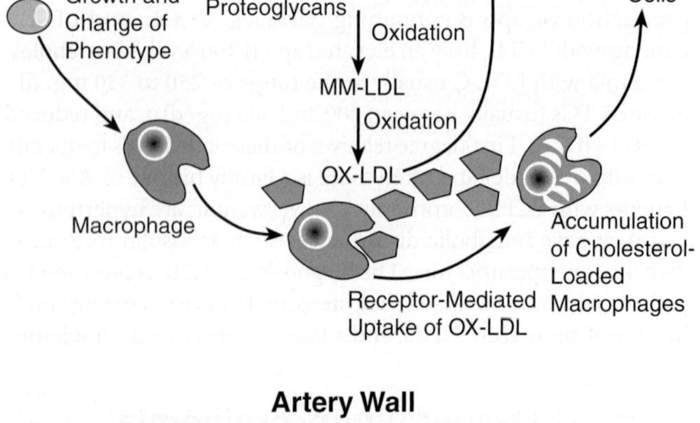

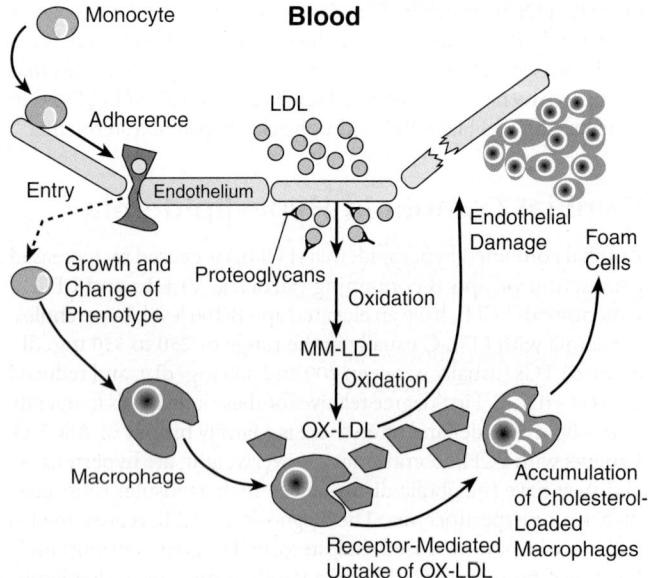

Figure 8-7 Pathogenesis of atherosclerosis and the role of oxidized LDL. LDL, low-density lipoprotein; MM-LDL, minimally oxidized low-density lipoprotein; OX-LDL, oxidized low-density lipoprotein.

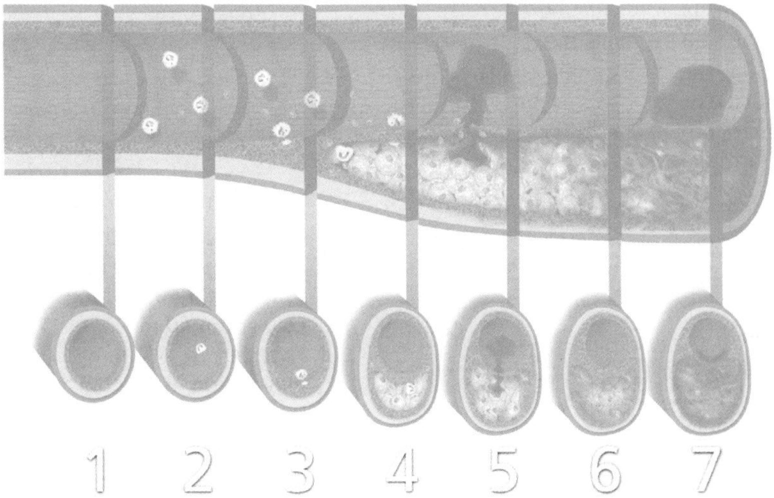

Figure 8-8 Initiation, progression, and complication of human coronary atherosclerotic plaque (numbers indicate order of progression).

to a potentially more stable lesion that has a small inner lipid core and more collagen and matrix proteins. At any given time, atherosclerotic lesions at various stages of development can be found all along the vascular arterial tree in high-risk patients (Fig. 8-7).

As atherosclerotic lesions grow, the coronary artery remodels to accommodate the lipid-rich core. Lesions initially enlarge away from the lumen toward the media/adventitia, thus preserving the vascular lumen and ensuring normal blood flow (positive remodeling). Late in the growth of the lesion, however, the luminal space is invaded and becomes progressively narrowed as the atherosclerotic lesion progresses (negative remodeling). Inflammatory cells secrete matrix metalloproteinases that degrade collagen and fibrin produced by arterial smooth muscle cells, causing a weakened fibrous cap and a lesion more vulnerable to plaque rupture.[54] Apoptosis (cell death) of smooth muscle cells in the shoulders of the atherosclerotic cap further weakens the lesion.[55] These processes increase the chance that the atherosclerotic lesion may rupture or erode, especially at the shoulders of the lesion, and expose the underlying tissue to circulating blood elements.[56] Collagen in the exposed plaque can trigger platelet activation, and tissue factor produced by macrophages and smooth muscle cells activates the coagulation cascade. Platelets may adhere and microthrombi may form. The resultant clot can occlude blood flow entirely, causing MI. More commonly, only partial occlusion of blood flow occurs, causing transient ischemic symptoms or unstable angina. The clot creates a barrier between the underlying tissue and circulating blood and allows healing of the plaque rupture. This process of fissuring and re-healing appears to lead to the more complicated lesions of atherosclerosis.

Atherosclerotic lesions exist along a continuum from vulnerable lipid-rich lesions that are prone to rupture and cause a thrombosis to more stable lipid-poor, fibrin- and collagen-rich lesions. Younger atherosclerotic lesions occupy only the intimal space, whereas the older lesions may protrude into the luminal space. In fact, the culprit lesion that results in acute MI is usually not at the site of the greatest stenosis, but distal to it.[55]

CLINICAL EVALUATION AND MANAGEMENT OF ASCVD RISK

Assessment of the Standard Lipid Panel and the Role of Advanced Lipid Testing

The routine lipid panel includes standardized measurements of total cholesterol (TC), HDL-C, and TGs. Although it is possible to measure LDL-C directly, it is common for most laboratories to calculate LDL-C. TC, HDL-C, and TGs are measured directly and then the Friedewald equation is applied to calculate LDL-C:

$$\text{LDL-C} = \text{total cholesterol} - (\text{HDL-C} + \text{VLDL-C}) \quad \text{(Eq. 8-1)}$$

Because the ratio of cholesterol to TGs in VLDL is 1:5, VLDL-C is estimated by dividing the total TG level by 5. Thus, the formula is rewritten as

$$\text{LDL-C} = \text{total cholesterol} - (\text{HDL-C} + \text{TG}/5) \quad \text{(Eq. 8-2)}$$

If the TG level is greater than 400 mg/dL the formula for estimating VLDL-C is not accurate and, therefore, LDL-C cannot be calculated. An accurate LDL-C calculation by the Friedewald equation also requires that the patient fast for 10 to 12 hours which provides sufficient time for exogenous TGs, carried by chylomicrons, to be cleared from the systemic circulation. Most laboratories can measure LDL-C directly but this is necessary only when the TG level is greater than 400 mg/dL or the patient has not fasted.

In the presence of cardiometabolic disturbances including the metabolic syndrome, insulin resistance, impaired glucose tolerance, diabetes, hypertriglyceridemia, as well as chronic kidney disease (CKD), the calculated or direct measurement of LDL-C may not provide a complete assessment of the lipid-related cardiovascular risk. Cardiometabolic disorders are often associated with the atherogenic dyslipidemia described above, in which there are near-normal to modest elevations of LDL-C, reduced HDL-C levels, elevations of TGs, and an excess of atherogenic small, dense LDL particles. When LDL-C levels are near-normal to modestly elevated and the LDL particle concentration (LDL-P) is elevated, the measures are considered to be "discordant."

There are a number of advanced lipid/lipoprotein tests to determine the concentration and/or the relative size distribution of both LDL and HDL particles. These include gradient gel electrophoresis, vertical automated profile, nuclear magnetic resonance spectroscopy, and ion mobility analysis. Data from both the Framingham Offspring Study and the Multi-Ethnic Study of Atherosclerosis demonstrated that patients with discordantly high LDL-P compared to LDL-C had higher CVD event rates, while patients with discordantly low LDL-P compared to LDL-C had lower CVD event rates.[57,58] CVD risk, therefore, tracked most closely with levels of LDL-P. Apo B is another measure of concentrations of atherogenic lipoproteins, including remnant VLDL particles and LDL particles and is strongly related to CVD risk.[59]

Non–HDL-C provides a simple and easily calculated estimate of the excess CVD risk associated with the atherogenic dyslipidemia.[7]

It is a single measurement of cholesterol carried by all potentially atherogenic particles, including VLDL, VLDL remnants, IDL, and LDL particles and can give the clinician information regarding the patient's CVD risk when LDL-C cannot reliably be calculated or in the presence of excess VLDL-C and excess LDL particle concentration. Non–HDL-C is calculated by the following formula:

$$\text{Non–HDL-C} = \text{total cholesterol} - \text{HDL-C} \quad \text{(Eq. 8-3)}$$

As mentioned previously, non–HDL-C can be calculated in both the fasting and non-fasting state because VLDL-C does not need to be estimated.

There are a number of guidelines for the management of lipid-related ASCVD risk and there is considerable variation in the recommended targets and goals of therapy, including LDL-C, non–HDL-C, LDL-P, and apo B. A recent review of guidelines from major US and international professional societies compares recommendations for lipid/lipoprotein targets and initiation of lipid-lowering therapies.[8]

Guidelines for the Management of Dyslipidemia to Reduce ASCVD Risk

In 2013 the ACC and the AHA published updated guidelines for management of blood cholesterol to reduce ASCVD risk.[5] Previous guidelines have focused on the fasting lipid panel as the initial evaluation of lipid-related risk. Within each category of ASCVD risk, lipid goals were then specified to achieve optimal risk reduction. In 2013 experts determined that current clinical trial data do not support the previous approach and that data are inadequate to indicate specific lipoprotein targets or goals of therapy. Therefore, the panel made no recommendation for or against specific targets (LDL-C or non–HDL-C) for primary or secondary ASCVD prevention. Instead, four groups of patients were identified in which there is the most extensive evidence of the benefit of statin therapy for prevention of ASCVD:

1. Individuals with clinical ASCVD,
2. Individuals with primary elevations of LDL-C ≥190 mg/dL,
3. Individuals 40 to 75 years of age with diabetes and LDL-C 70 to 189 mg/dL, and
4. Individuals without clinical ASCVD or diabetes who are 40 to 75 years of age with LDL-C 70 to 189 mg/dL and an estimated 10-year ASCVD risk of ≥7.5%.

For each risk group the guidelines recommend an intensity of statin therapy, either moderate or high intensity (Table 8-3). Low-intensity statins are recommended only in patients who have experienced or are at risk for adverse effects of treatment. The guidelines do not support dose titration to achieve specific levels of LDL-C, non–HDL-C, or apo B, as recommended in previous guidelines (Fig. 8-9). Measurement of the lipid panel is recommended at 4 to 12 weeks after initiation of statin therapy to assess compliance with lifestyle recommendations and medication, as well as response to therapy. Regular monitoring of the lipid panel is then recommended every 3 to 12 months as clinically indicated.

For primary prevention of ASCVD the recommended risk assessment tool is the new CV Risk Calculator based on the Pooled Cohort Equations as described in the 2013 ACC/AHA Guideline on the Assessment of Cardiovascular Risk.[6] The equations are derived from large, diverse, community-based cohorts that are generally representative of the US population of whites and African Americans. The calculator provides race- and sex-specific estimates of the 10-year risk of first hard ASCVD event (nonfatal MI, CHD death, fatal or nonfatal stroke) and should be used in non-Hispanic African American and non-Hispanic whites between 40 and 79 years of age. Lifetime- or 30-year risk is also provided for individuals aged 20 to 59 years who are not at high short-term risk. Variables considered in the risk calculation include age, sex, race, total cholesterol, HDL-C, systolic blood pressure, treatment for hypertension, tobacco use, and diabetes. To further refine risk assessment, optional factors that may be considered include family history of premature ASCVD, hs-CRP, LDL-C ≥160 mg/dL, coronary artery calcium scoring, and ankle brachial index. The National Lipid Association Patient-Centered Recommendations: Part 2 provide recommendations for risk assessment in non-Hispanic whites and other racial and ethnic groups which were not a part of populations used to derive the ACC/AHA Pooled Cohort Equations.[60]

Patients with a 10-year risk of ≥7.5% should be engaged in a patient–clinician discussion of the ASCVD risk reduction benefits of statin therapy, potential adverse drug effects, potential drug–drug interactions, and consideration of patient preferences to determine if statin therapy is appropriate (Fig. 8-10).

Table 8-3
Intensity of the Various Statins[5]

High intensity (when taken as prescribed will reduce LDL-C by ≥50%	Atorvastatin (40 mg)* – 80 mg Rosuvastatin 20 (40) mg
Moderate intensity (when taken as prescribed will reduce LDL-C by 30% < 50%)	**Atorvastatin 10** *(20)* **mg** **Rosuvastatin** *(5)* **10 mg** **Simvastatin 20–40 mg** **Pravastatin 40** *(80)* **mg** **Lovastatin 40 mg** *Fluvastatin XL 80 mg* **Fluvastatin 40 mg bid** **Pitavastatin 2–4 mg**
Low intensity (when taken as prescribed will reduce LDL-C by <30% on average	*Simvastatin 10 mg* **Pravastatin 10–20 mg** **Lovastatin 20 mg** *Fluvastatin 20–40 mg* *Pitavastatin 1 mg*

The doses listed in parenthesis were not evaluated in randomized controlled trials.

*Evidence is from one randomized controlled trial Bold—Doses of statins that were evaluated in randomized controlled trials

CASE 8-1

QUESTION 1: B.C. is a 46-year-old peri-menopausal white female who has recently relocated to the area and is establishing care with a gynecologist. As part of her annual evaluation a routine lipid panel is obtained. She takes no prescription medications but does take a number of dietary supplements and vitamins, including krill oil, multivitamin, B-complex, and vitamin D. She has no history of tobacco use, hypertension, or diabetes. She states she was told a number of years ago that her LDL "bad" cholesterol was elevated, but her HDL "good" cholesterol was high and no treatment was indicated. She has enjoyed jogging and spin classes but says that as she gets older she is more fatigued and sore with exercise. She follows a Mediterranean style diet and has a glass of red wine daily.

Her father is alive at age 72 and takes statin therapy for hyperlipidemia, though she is uncertain of the severity of his lipid disorder. He has no history of cardiovascular disease. Her mother is a 71-year-old diabetic and underwent coronary stent placement last year following the onset of angina and an abnormal stress test. She was started on statin therapy at the time of her procedure. Her brother is overweight, has hypertension and borderline diabetes, and is also on statin therapy and fenofibrate.

On physical exam the patient has the following: normotensive (128/76 mm Hg); carotid pulses with normal amplitude and no

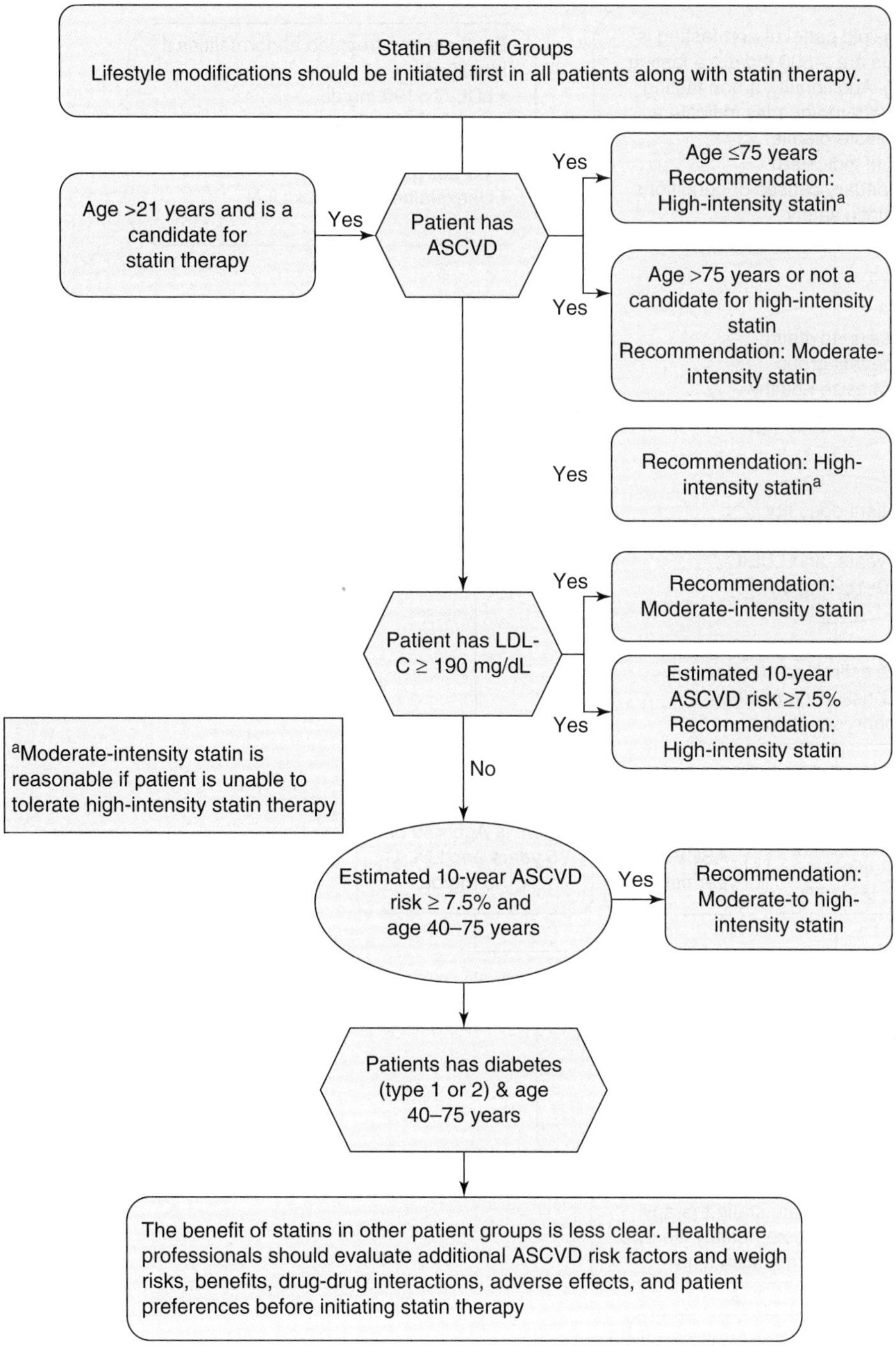

Figure 8-9 Recommendations for the intensity of statin therapy based on statin benefit group diagram. (Adapted from Stone NJ et al. 2013 ACC/AHA guideline on the treatment of blood cholesterol to reduce atherosclerotic cardiovascular risk in adults: A report of the American College of Cardiology/American Heart Association Task Force on Practice Guidelines. *J Am Coll Cardiol.* 2014;63:2889–2934. doi:10.1016/j.jacc.2013.11.002.)

bruits; 2/6 crescendo/decrescendo noted at the left sternal border; no abdominal bruit; peripheral pulses 2+; no tendon xanthomas, corneal arcus, or xanthelasmas.

Following a 12-hour fast the patient's lipid panel shows the following results:

Total cholesterol, 290 mg/dL
HDL-C, 56 mg/dL
LDL-C calculated, 218 mg/dL
TG, 132 mg/dL

What is your assessment of B.C.'s lipid panel results?

The NLA Recommendations for Patient-Centered Management of Dyslipidemia were published in 2014. Similar to NCEP ATP III Guidelines, these comprehensive recommendations for management of a variety of dyslipidemias continue to recommend lipoprotein targets (non–HDL-C and LDL-C) and titration to achieve goals of therapy (Table 8-4).[7]

The patient's LDL-C is very high and she would qualify for statin therapy as defined by both the ACC/AHA and NLA recommendations for management of hypercholesterolemia. Her HDL-C is near the average range for a woman and her TG level is considered normal (<150 mg/dL). There has been a misconception among some providers and patients that a normal or high HDL-C level is "protective" in the presence of hypercholesterolemia, based on a TC/HDL-C ratio of <3.5, and that statin therapy is not indicated. However, in the presence of very high elevations of LDL-C levels all current and previous guidelines recommend statin therapy regardless of baseline HDL-C.

In the presence of very high LDL-C levels it is important to consider a number of issues prior to initiation of therapy. The patient's lifestyle, including diet and exercise, may play an important role in B.C.'s new diagnosis of dyslipidemia. However, she

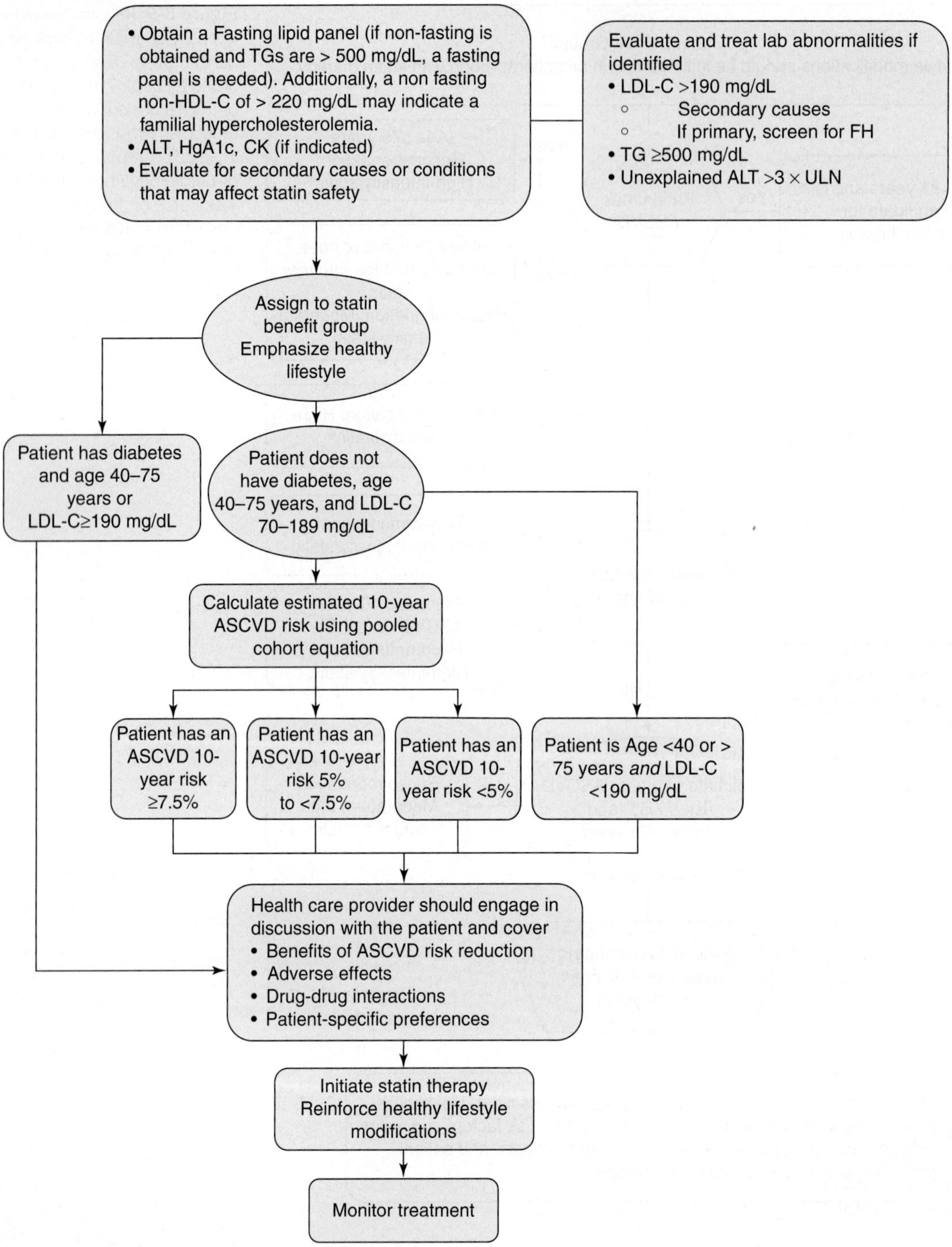

Figure 8-10 Recommendations for initiating statin therapy in patients *without* clinical ASCVD.(Adapted from Stone NJ et al. 2013 ACC/AHA guideline on the treatment of blood cholesterol to reduce atherosclerotic cardiovascular risk in adults: A report of the American College of Cardiology/American Heart Association Task Force on Practice Guidelines. J Am Coll Cardiol. 2014;63:2889–2934. doi:10.1016/j.jacc.2013.11.002.)

is actually quite compliant with lifestyle recommendations for optimal cardiovascular health and this is unlikely to be a factor in her lipid levels. Careful review of family history of hypercholesterolemia and ASCVD by construction of a detailed pedigree can identify patients with possible HeFH or HoFH. B.C.'s father has dyslipidemia of uncertain severity and is on statin therapy, but he has no history of premature ASCVD. Her mother developed ASCVD after age 65 and a long history of diabetes. Statin therapy was not prescribed until her stent placement and FH is unlikely. Her brother has a mixed dyslipidemia, most likely exacerbated by overweight and poorly controlled diabetes. Thus, based on this brief pedigree the diagnosis of FH is unlikely. Classic physical examination findings of tendon xanthomas, corneal arcus before age 45, and xanthelasmas are often, but not always present in FH. B.C. does not have these findings. The patient does have a systolic murmur on cardiac examination which may be indicative of aortic valvular disease, a very common problem in patients with HoFH.

Mean TC is typically lower in premenopausal women than in age-matched men. Premenopausal women have a less pro-atherogenic lipid profile with higher HDL-C levels (average 10 mg/dL) and lower LDL-C and non–HDL-C levels than age-matched men. Due to the hormonal alterations during the perimenopausal period, LDL-C levels rise and are often higher than in age-matched men. Postmenopausal women also have a higher incidence of high TG and low HDL-C levels, with an increase in small, dense LDL particles. It is not uncommon for women without a prior history of dyslipidemia to be newly diagnosed in the perimenopausal period and B.C. may be just such a patient.

Table 8-4

NLA Criteria for ASCVD Risk Assessment and Treatment Goals for Atherogenic Cholesterol, and Levels at Which Pharmacologic Therapy Should Be Considered[7]

Risk	Low	Moderate	High	Very High
Criteria	■ 0–1 Major ASCVD risk factor ■ Consider other known risk factors	■ Major ASCVD risk factors ■ Consider other risk factors ■ Consider quantitative risk scoring	■ ≥3 major ASCVD risk factors ■ Chronic kidney disease stage 3B or 4[a] ■ Quantitative risk score reaching the high-risk threshold ■ LDL-C ≥ 190 mg/dL (severe hypercholesterolemia ■ Diabetes mellitus[b] (type 1 or 2) with 0–1 major ASCVD risk factor and no evidence of end-organ damage	■ ASCVD diabetes[b] (type 1 or 2) and >2 major ASCVD risk factors or evidence of end-organ damage
Treatment Goal				
Non–HDL-C (mg/dL)	<130	<130	<130	<100
LDL-C (mg/dL)	<100	<100	<100	<70
Consider Pharmacologic Therapy				
Non–HDL-C mg/dL	≥190	≥160	≥130	≥100
LDL-C (mg/dL)	≥160	≥130	≥100	≥70

[a]Chronic kidney disease stage 3B or 4 = estimated glomerular filtration rate of 30 to 44 mL/minute and 15 to 29 mL/minute, respectively. Risk calculators should not be used in these patients as they underestimate risk.

[b]Diabetic patients plus 1 major ASCVD risk factor, treating to a non–HDL-C goal of <100 mg/dL (LDL-C).Adapted from Jacobson TA et al. National lipid association recommendations for patient-centered management of dyslipidemia: part 1—full report. *J Clin Lipidol*. 2015;9:129–169.

ASCVD, atherosclerotic cardiovascular disease; LDL-C, low-density lipoprotein cholesterol; non–HDL-C, non–high-density lipoprotein cholesterol.

Case 8-1, Question 2: Is there any evidence for other potential causes of B.C.'s dyslipidemia?

As a routine every patient with dyslipidemia should be evaluated for secondary causes of elevated LDL-C, non–HDL-C, or TG. Conditions that may be associated with lipid abnormalities include diabetes, CKD and nephrotic syndrome, obstructive liver disease, hypothyroidism, anorexia nervosa, polycystic ovarian syndrome, and pregnancy, among others (Table 8-5).[5] Average values of total-C, LDL-C, HDL-C, and TG steadily rise throughout pregnancy and levels peak near full-term. In uncomplicated or "normal" pregnancies, neither total-C nor TG exceeds 250 mg/dL at any time during pregnancy. A number of drugs are associated with dyslipidemia or worsening of baseline lipid abnormalities, including exogenous estrogen and progesterone therapy, and a careful review of the patient's medication regimen is necessary prior to initiation of lipid-lowering therapy. B.C. is currently perimenopausal and does not take any medications associated with exacerbation of dyslipidemia nor any form of exogenous hormone replacement therapy or oral contraception.

Table 8-5

Classification of Secondary Causes of Dyslipidemia[5]

Cause	Increased LDL-C	Increased TG
Drugs/medications	Glucocorticoids, amiodarone, diuretics, cyclosporine	Hormone therapy, glucocorticoids, bile acid sequestrants, protease inhibitors, retinoic acid, anabolic steroids, tamoxifen, sirolimus, atypical antipsychotics (predominately olanzapine and clozapine), raloxifene, β-blockers, thiazide diuretics
Dietary Influences	Anorexia, trans fats or saturated fats, weight gain	Very low fat diets, weight gain, high carbohydrate intake (refined), and excessive alcohol use
Disease states	Nephrotic syndrome, biliary obstruction	Nephrotic syndrome, chronic renal failure, lipodystrophies
Disorders of metabolism	Obesity, pregnancy, hypothyroidism	Hypothyroidism, poorly controlled diabetes, pregnancy, and obesity

Case 8-1, Question 3: Further review of B.C.'s laboratory studies showed the following:

Glucose, 92 mg/dL
Alanine aminotransferase (ALT), 24 mg/dL
Aspartate aminotransferase (AST), 18 mg/dL
Creatinine, 0.9 mg/dL

Thyroid-stimulating hormone (TSH), 57 international units (IU)/mL

Laboratory evaluation has revealed that B.C.'s fatigue and muscle soreness are likely due to hypothyroidism, which has also exacerbated her previous dyslipidemia. She is placed on thyroid replacement therapy and with normalization of her thyroid function her follow-up laboratory results show the following:

TSH, 1.254 IU/mL
TC, 215 mg/dL
HDL-C, 59 mg/dL
LDL-C calculated, 132 mg/dL
TG, 118 mg/dL

What is the next step in the evaluation of B.C.'s ASCVD risk?

B.C. has no other ASCVD risk factors or risk equivalents other than mild dyslipidemia. Using the ACC/AHA Pooled Cohort Equations or CV Risk Calculator her 10-year risk of ASCVD event is 0.9%. According to both the ACC/AHA and NLA recommendations for lipid management there is currently no indication for initiation of statin therapy.

The 2015 Standards of Diabetes Care of the American Diabetes Association (ADA) were revised to recommend initiation and intensification of statin therapy (high versus moderate) in patients with diabetes based on the individual patient's risk profile.[61] However, the ADA notes that the presence of diabetes confers significant risk of ASCVD and that the ACC/AHA CV Risk Estimator is of limited use in diabetics. Recommendations are made for patients <40, 40 to 75, and >75 years of age for moderate- or high-intensity statin therapy in the presence of ASCVD risk factors or overt ASCVD (Table 8-6).

The 2013 Clinical Practice Guideline for Lipid Management in Chronic Kidney Disease (CKD), published by the Kidney Disease: Improving Global Outcomes (KDIGO) Panel, notes that in nondialysis-dependent CKD patients the relationship between LDL-C and ASCVD events is weaker than in the general population.[62] This is likely related to lipoprotein metabolic abnormalities characterized by lower levels of LDL-C, elevated LDL-P, an increase in small dense LDL, reduced HDL-C, and elevated TG. Therefore, according to KDIGO guidelines the measured LDL-C may be less useful as a marker of coronary risk among people with advanced nondialysis-dependent CKD and does not serve as an indication for pharmacologic treatment. Instead, therapy is guided by the absolute risk of coronary events based on patient age and stage of CKD or estimated glomerular filtration rate (eGFR). Specific doses of individual statins are recommended for each stage of CKD or eGFR and dose titration is not indicated. Statin therapy or combination therapy with statin and ezetimibe is not recommended in adults with dialysis-dependent CKD due to lack of evidence of ASCVD risk reduction in patients with stage V CKD. However, therapy may be continued in patients already receiving therapy at the time of initiation of dialysis (Table 8-7).

CASE 8-2

Question 1: S.W. is a 51-year-old African American male with CKD due to polycystic kidney disease. He has no history of tobacco use or diabetes, but is treated for hypertension. He is very active and works in landscape maintenance, but does not have a program of consistent aerobic exercise. He follows a heart-healthy diet consistent with the DASH (Dietary Approaches to Stop Hypertension) recommendations and has maintained a normal BMI. He is referred for nephrology consultation and the following results are obtained:

eGFR, 42 mL/minute
TC, 187 mg/dL
HDL, 39 mg/dL
LDL-C calculated, 102 mg/dL
TG, 230 mg/dL
$HgbA_{1c}$, 6.8%
BP, 126/68 mm Hg

What is your assessment of S.W.'s ASCVD risk and his lipid panel results?

S.W. has stage 3b CKD defined as an eGFR between 30 and 44 mL/min/1.73 m^2. According to the NLA Recommendations for Patient-Centered Management of Dyslipidemia, patients with stage 3b to stage 4 CKD are at high risk for ASCVD and should be considered for drug therapy. Statin therapy with or without ezetimibe are recommended therapies in CKD patients who are

Table 8-6
ADA Recommendations for Statin Treatment in People with Diabetes[61]

Age	<40 years	40–75 years	>75 years
Risk factors	Zero risk factor(s) for CHD[a] Overt CHD[b]	Zero risk factor(s) for CHD Overt CHD	Zero risk factor(s) for CHD Overt CHD
Recommended dose of statin	■ No statin if zero risk factors ■ Moderate or high intensity in presence of CHD risk factor(s) ■ High if overt CHD	■ Moderate if no risk factors ■ High intensity in presence of CHD risk factor(s) ■ High if overt CHD	■ Moderate if no risk factors ■ Moderate or high intensity in presence of CHD risk factor(s) ■ High if overt CHD
Recommended monitoring of lipid panel	Annually or as needed	As needed to assess for adherence	As needed to assess for adherence

Statin therapy should be initiated as an adjunct to lifestyle modifications.
[a]CHD risk factors include hypertension, smoking, LDL-C ≥ 100 mg/dL, being overweight, and obesity.
[b]Overt CHD includes those who have had a previous cardiovascular event or an acute coronary syndrome.
CHD, coronary heart disease.
Adapted from Cromwell et al. LDL particle number and risk of future cardiovascular disease in the Framingham Offspring Study—implications for LDL management. *J Clin Lipidol*. 2007;1:583–592.

Table 8-7
KDIGO Clinical Practice Guideline for Lipid Management in Chronic Kidney Disease[62]

Chronic Kidney Disease Severity	Treatment Recommendations
Age ≥ 50 years of age with eGFR <60 mL/minute/1.73 m² not on HD or have a history of kidney transplant	Statin or statin/ezetimibe combination
Age ≥ 50 years with CKD and eGFR >60 mL/minute/1.73 m²	Statin
Age 18–49 years with CKD not on HD or history of kidney transplant with one or more of the following ■ Diabetes mellitus ■ Prior stroke ■ Known CAD ■ Estimated 10-year risk of CAD death or nonfatal MI > 10%	Statin
Dialysis-dependent CKD	No initiation of therapy

CHD, coronary heart disease; CKD, chronic kidney disease; eGFR, estimated glomerular filtration rate; HD, hemodialysis.

Adapted from Kidney Disease: Improving Global Outcomes (KDIGO) Lipid Work Group. KDIGO Clinical Practice Guideline for lipid management in chronic kidney disease. *Kidney Int Suppl*. 2013;3:259–305.

nondialysis dependent and the goals of therapy are non–HDL-C <130 mg/dL and/or LDL-C <100 mg/dL.

The 2013 ACC/AHA Blood Cholesterol guidelines do not consider CKD as a risk factor in ASCVD risk assessment and do not provide specific recommendations for statin or ezetimibe therapy in nondialysis-dependent patients. ASCVD risk assessment is performed by the CV Risk Calculator incorporating standard risk factors and pharmacotherapy is implemented according to the algorithm for primary prevention. For patients on maintenance peritoneal dialysis or hemodialysis the ACC/AHA experts felt that there was inadequate information to make a recommendation for or against the initiation or continuation of statin therapy.

CASE 8-2, QUESTION 2: Would this patient require treatment at this time?

The 2013 KDIGO Clinical Practice Guideline for Lipid Management in Chronic Kidney Disease provides guidance on lipid management and treatment for all patients with CKD (nondialysis dependent, dialysis dependent, kidney transplant recipients, and children). According to KDIGO experts, in patients with CKD who are nondialysis dependent, the relationship between LDL-C and ASCVD events is weaker than in the general population likely related to the atherogenic dyslipidemia characteristic in CKD. Thus, the measured LDL-C does not serve as an indication for treatment. KDIGO guidelines recommend that lipid therapy be guided by the absolute risk of coronary events based on patient age and stage of CKD or eGFR, regardless of baseline lipids. Statin or statin/ezetimibe therapy is recommended in nondialysis-dependent adults age ≥50 years with eGFR <60 mL/minute/1.73 m². In adults age ≥50 years with CKD and eGFR ≥60 mL/minute/1.73 m², only statin therapy is recommended. In adults age 18–49 years with CKD but not treated with chronic dialysis or kidney transplantation, statin treatment is suggested if one of the following is present: known CHD (MI or coronary revascularization), diabetes mellitus, prior ischemic stroke, or estimated 10-year incidence of coronary death or nonfatal MI >10% by the Framingham Risk Score. Statin therapy is also recommended in adult kidney transplant recipients. Therefore, according to KDIGO guidelines, S.W. may be treated with statin or statin/ezetimibe therapy.

PHARMACOLOGIC THERAPY

3-Hydroxy-3-Methyl-glutaryl Coenzyme A Inhibitors (Statins)

MECHANISM OF ACTION

Statins competitively inhibit HMG-CoA reductase, the enzyme responsible for converting HMG-CoA to mevalonate in an early, rate-limiting step in the biosynthetic pathway of cholesterol (Figs. 8-1 and 8-11). This causes decreased production of mevalonate and its subsequent conversion to cholesterol and a subsequent compensatory increase in the synthesis of LDL receptors. The increased LDL receptor density results in an increase in hepatic update of LDL-C, and to a lesser extent VLDL particles, and significantly lower levels of plasma LDL-C. In addition to the reduction in LDL-C, statins also reduce Apo B, triglyceride, and total cholesterol concentrations.[63–67]

EFFICACY

Lipid-lowering therapy for patients with ASCVD is now accepted as standard of care.[5] Beginning in the mid-1990s, the results of clinical trials with more potent statins were reported. Five of these (Scandinavian Simvastatin Survival Study (4S), Cardiovascular and Recurrent Events (CARE), the Long-Term Intervention with Pravastatin in Ischemic Disease Study (LIPID), Treating to New Targets (TNT), and Incremental Decrease in End Points through Aggressive Lipid Lowering (IDEAL)) were secondary prevention trials conducted in patients with known CHD.[68–72] In 4S, CARE, and LIPID, CHD death and nonfatal MI occurred in 13% to 22% of placebo-treated patients in the 5-year follow-up period, compared with event rates of 10% to 14% with patients on statin therapy.[68–70] Total mortality was reduced significantly in two of these trials, 4S and LIPID, that were powered to assess total mortality. Additionally, fewer revascularization procedures were required in patients receiving statin therapy and 31% fewer strokes occurred.[73] The TNT and IDEAL trials demonstrated additional cardiovascular benefit for high-intensity versus moderate-intensity statin therapy in patients with stable CHD. These trials randomly assigned patients to receive either high-dose atorvastatin 80 mg versus atorvastatin 10 mg or simvastatin 20 mg with an approximate follow-up period of 5 years. In both trials, more intensive lowering of LDL-C to significantly less than 100 mg/dL was associated with a reduction in CHD.[71,72] The further reductions in the incidence of heart attacks, revascularizations, and ischemic strokes with more intensive lowering of LDL-C with statins compared with less-intensive statin regimens was verified in a recent meta-analysis of randomized trials. An additional 38.6-mg/dL reduction of LDL-C in patients on high-intensity therapy was associated with a 38% relative reduction in major vascular events ($p < 0.0001$).[73]

The Heart Protection Study (HPS)[74] extended the results of earlier secondary prevention statin trials (4S,[68] CARE,[69] LIPID[70]). The HPS included 20,536 patients with a history of CHD or cerebrovascular disease (stroke or transient ischemic attacks), peripheral vascular disease, or diabetes not considered by their general practitioner to have a clear indication for statin therapy because of relatively low baseline cholesterol levels (mean LDL-C 131 mg/dL).[74] A reduction in CHD events was achieved in both men and women; in all age groups, including those aged 75 to

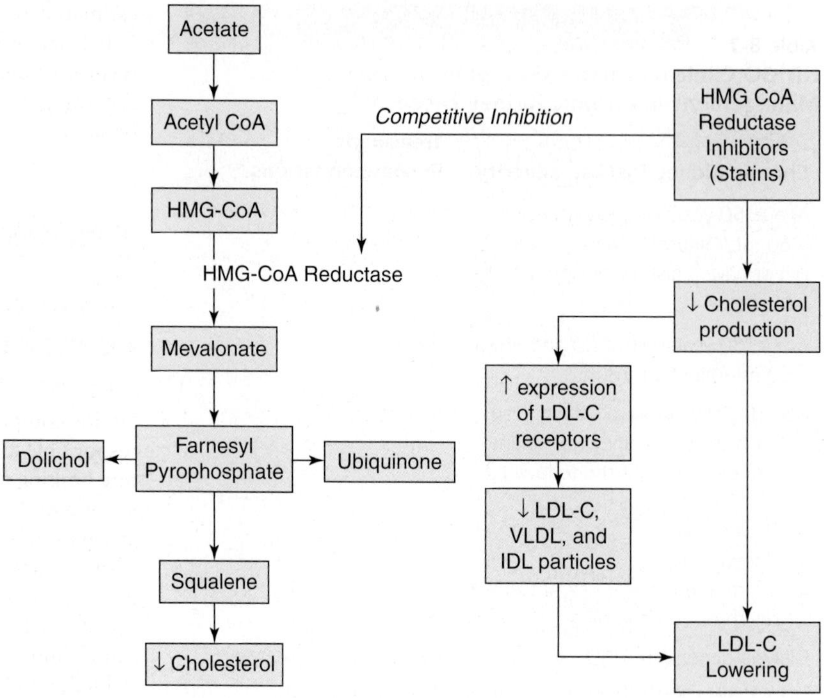

Figure 8-11 Reaction catalyzed by HMG-CoA reductase. HMG-CoA, 3-hydroxy-3-methylglutaryl coenzyme A; IDL, intermediate-density lipoprotein; LDL-C, low-density lipoprotein cholesterol; VLDL, very low-density lipoprotein.

85 years; and regardless of the baseline LDL-C, including those with initial levels less than 100 mg/dL.

Trials in patients with acute coronary syndromes (ACS) have also demonstrated CHD risk reduction. The Myocardial Ischemia Reduction with Aggressive Cholesterol Lowering (MIRACL) study randomly assigned patients presenting to the hospital with unstable angina or non–Q-wave MI to statin therapy or placebo for 4 months. This resulted in a 24% reduction in symptomatic ischemia requiring emergency hospitalization and a 60% reduction in nonfatal strokes in those receiving the statin.[75,76] More recently, the Pravastatin or Atorvastatin Evaluation and Infection Therapy—Thrombolysis in Myocardial Infarction (PROVE-IT) is considered a landmark trial that demonstrated superior cardiovascular event lowering when high-intensity statin therapy (atorvastatin 80 mg) was implemented within 10 days of ACS versus moderate-intensity (pravastatin 40 mg) statin therapy.[77] After 2 years of treatment, mean LDL-C levels in patients randomly assigned to receive atorvastatin 80 mg and pravastatin 40 mg were 62 and 95 mg/dL, respectively. The composite cardiovascular endpoint (death from any cause, MI, documented unstable angina requiring rehospitalization, revascularization, and stroke) was significantly reduced by 16% with high-intensity atorvastatin compared with moderate-intensity pravastatin.[77] Data from the National Registry of Myocardial Infarction 4 demonstrated that early initiation of statins in the acute setting (with the first 24 hours of an acute MI) was associated with a significantly lower rate of early complications and in-hospital mortality.[78] Additionally, discontinuation of statin in patients who present with an ACS is associated with increased event rates above those who are statin naive.[79,80]

PHARMACOKINETICS/PHARMACODYNAMICS

The currently available statins are atorvastatin, fluvastatin, lovastatin, pitavastatin, pravastatin, rosuvastatin, and simvastatin. These agents possess different pharmacokinetic properties that may play a role in their efficacy and safety.

Three statins are derived from fungi (simvastatin, pravastatin, and lovastatin),[81–83] while the others (atorvastatin, rosuvastatin, pitavastatin, and fluvastatin) are synthetic.[84–87] Lovastatin and simvastatin are prodrugs and must be converted to their active form to exert a pharmacologic effect. Rosuvastatin and atorvastatin have the longest half-lives of 19 and 14 hours, respectively, which enables longer inhibition of the HMG-CoA enzyme and greater LDL-C reductions compared to other agents.[84,86] Both of these agents lower LDL-C by a mean of approximately 60% at maximum doses (rosuvastatin 40 mg daily and atorvastatin 80 mg daily). The long half-life also allows for administration at any time of day rather than at bedtime for maximum effect, which is recommended for simvastatin, lovastatin, pravastatin, and fluvastatin.[81–83,85] Although pitavastatin has a shorter half-life (12 hours) than rosuvastatin and atorvastatin it may also be taken at any time of day.[84,86] The administration of the shorter acting agents at bedtime is important because cholesterol biosynthesis occurs at its highest rate in the evening hours, thus allowing these agents to have the greatest effect on HMG-CoA reductase inhibition and on lowering of LDL-C. However, with extended-release (ER) formulations of lovastatin and fluvastatin, bedtime administration is less important.[81–88]

The amount of statin that reaches the systemic circulation is relatively small. Bioavailability ranges from less than 5% with lovastatin and simvastatin to 51% with pitavastatin (oral solution). Pravastatin, fluvastatin, and rosuvastatin are hydrophilic agents and may have less tissue distribution and result in less muscle toxicity. However, this aspect is more theoretical than it is clinically valid. All statins are eliminated primarily by the liver, with substantial biliary excretion. However, several statins require dose adjustments in patients with significant renal insufficiency (Table 8-8).[81–88]

ADVERSE EFFECTS

Statins are generally well tolerated. The most common adverse effects reported include muscle pain and weakness (myalgias), headache, GI symptoms, including dyspepsia, flatus, constipation, and abdominal pain, and skin rashes.[81–91] These symptoms are usually mild and often dissipate with continued therapy. Less common adverse effects include myopathy, elevated hepatic transaminases, and diabetes. Cognitive dysfunction may be potentially associated with statin therapy but this has not yet been demonstrated to be causally related to statin treatment.

Muscle-related adverse effects associated with statins are divided into three different types based on symptoms and the presence or absence of creatine kinase (CK) elevations. These include myalgias,

Table 8-8
Dosing of Statins in Patients with Renal Insufficiency[81–88]

Statin	Creatinine Clearance 30–50 mL/minute	Creatinine Clearance 15–29 mL/minute	Creatinine Clearance <15 mL/minute or on Hemodialysis
Atorvastatin	Doses up to 80 mg may be used	Doses up to 80 mg may be used	Doses up to 80 mg may be used
Fluvastatin	Doses up to 80 mg may be used	Doses up to 40 mg may be used	Doses up to 40 mg may be used
Lovastatin	Doses up to 80 mg may be used	Doses up to 40 mg may be used	Doses up to 40 mg may be used
Pitavastatin	Doses up to 2 mg may be used	Doses up to 2 mg may be used	Doses up to 2 mg may be used
Pravastatin	Doses up to 40 mg may be used	Doses up to 40 mg may be used	Doses up to 40 mg may be used
Simvastatin	Doses up to 80 mg may be used	Doses up to 20 mg may be used	Doses up to 20 mg may be used
Rosuvastatin	Doses up to 40 mg may be used	Doses up to 10 mg may be used	No data

myopathy, and rhabdomyolysis. Myalgias are the most commonly reported muscle symptoms with an incidence of around 32%.[92] Myalgias are defined as muscle aches or weakness without CK elevations. This adverse effect is the most common reason for patients to discontinue statin therapy.[92]

Myopathy is defined as the presence of myalgias, including aches, soreness, or weakness, and an increase in serum CK more than 10 times the upper lipid of normal (ULN). Myopathy occurs in approximately 0.1% to 1% of patients and is a dose-dependent effect. If myopathy is present, a careful history is necessary to rule out usual causes (i.e., trauma, increased physical activity). Rhabdomyolysis is defined as a CK of at least 10 times the ULN with an elevated serum creatinine and symptoms requiring treatment.[93] Rhabdomyolysis is the least common of the muscle-related adverse effects, but can be life threatening with acute renal failure, cardiac arrest, or arrhythmias due to severe electrolyte abnormalities. Most cases of rhabdomyolysis have occurred with high doses of statins, in patients with impaired renal or hepatic function, in older individuals, or when statins are used in combination with interacting drugs. The most common areas affected are in the belly of larger muscles. It is important to distinguish between this and joint pain that may be associated with arthritis.

Simvastatin at a dose of 80 mg daily is associated with the highest incidence of rhabdomyolysis among the statins agents. However, this dose is no longer recommended by the US Food and Drug Administration (FDA) and the ACC/AHA cholesterol guideline.[5,81]

Management of statin-associated muscle adverse effects can be challenging. Routine monitoring of CK levels in asymptomatic patients is unnecessary. However, unexplained symptoms of muscle aches, weakness, or soreness should prompt evaluation of CK and other potential underlying etiologies. Myopathy is more likely to occur with high systemic concentrations of statin and when there are underlying risk factors (e.g., age > 80 years, severe CKD, hypothyroidism, trauma, interacting medications, or flu-like syndromes). If a patient develops signs and symptoms consistent with myopathy, statin therapy should be withdrawn until CK levels return to normal. If rhabdomyolysis is diagnosed, statin therapy should be discontinued immediately and etiology determined. Re-challenge of a statin may be considered if the cause was secondary to an interacting medication or other underlying cause that can be identified and corrected. Occasionally, symptoms of myalgia are bothersome or intolerable to the patient, even when the CK level is normal or elevated less than 10 times the ULN. In these cases, the statin should be discontinued. Once symptoms subside, statin therapy can be restarted at the same or reduced dose, or with a different statin. Alternate day and even once-weekly dosing of statins have been used in patients who have statin intolerance caused by myopathy.[94] However, these alternative regimens have not been evaluated in cardiovascular outcome trials.

Statins may also cause an elevation in transaminase enzyme levels of more than 3 times the ULN in 1% to 1.5% of patients in a dose-dependent manner. The transaminase level will often return to normal spontaneously in 70% of cases even with continued statin therapy.[93] Elevations in transaminases will also return to normal if the statin is discontinued. Rechallenge with the same or a different statin after enzymes have returned to normal limits is acceptable. If the medication is tolerated on rechallenge, it can be continued; recurrence of transaminase elevation warrants further evaluation of other potential causes. It is recommended that prior to initiating statin therapy patients should have baseline liver function tests performed. The report of the NLA Statin Safety Task Force recommends that if ALT or AST is 1 to 3 times the ULN during statin therapy, there is no need to discontinue the statin.[93] If ALT or AST exceeds 3 times the ULN during statin therapy, monitor the patient and repeat the transaminase measures. There is no need to discontinue the statin. If a patient's transaminase levels continue to rise or if there is further objective evidence (i.e., hepatomegaly, jaundice, elevated direct bilirubin, related symptoms) of liver injury, the statin should be discontinued. The estimated incidence of statin-associated liver failure is 1 per million person-years of use.[95] There is evidence that patients with chronic liver disease, nonalcoholic fatty liver disease, or nonalcoholic steatohepatitis may safely receive statin therapy.[96]

In 2012, the FDA required an update to the statin prescribing labeling to include information regarding a potential increased risk of reversible cognitive impairment, to include memory loss. Some case reports have suggested that the statins may cause cognitive impairment or memory loss.[97] However, data from randomized controlled trials have failed to show an association and some data even suggest a beneficial effect on the progression of Alzheimer disease.[74,98,99] Therefore, if a patient presents with cognitive deficits, he should first undergo an evaluation to identify other potential causes. If the statin is suspected, it is reasonable to consider discontinuing therapy for up to 3 months and monitor for improvment.[93] If improvement is noted, then a speculation may be made that the statin was the cause. However, one must carefully balance the decision to discontinue the statin due to the proven benefit of these agents. Consideration should be given to perhaps reintroduce a different statin or a different statin dose and monitor for recurrence of deficits. Additionally, because improvement in cognitive function is subjective, an objective test such as a Mini Mental State Exam (MMSE) should be considered prior to discontinuation and repeated after discontinuation to assess for any changes.

CASE 8-3

QUESTION 1: M.T. is a 56-year-old white female who presents for new patient evaluation with a 10-year history of type 2 diabetes and hypertension. Current medications include metformin, lisinopril, and chlorthalidone. She currently smokes about 1/2 pack of cigarettes/day, but is considering a quit date. She reports that she struggles with weight management (BMI 33.8 kg/m^2) and has difficulty with exercise due to previous knee injury and a torn rotator cuff. She has a strong family history of premature ASCVD, diabetes, hyperlipidemia, and obesity. Her father underwent coronary artery bypass grafting at age 51. Her mother suffered a mild stroke at age 62, but has no residual deficits. She has four siblings of which two have known CHD. On physical exam her BP is 148/88; bilateral carotid bruits; cardiac exam unremarkable; abdominal bruit; peripheral pulses 1+ bilaterally; no tendon xanthomas, corneal arcus, or xanthelasmas. Her initial laboratory results demonstrate the following:

Total cholesterol, 273 mg/dL
HDL-C, 43 mg/dL
LDL-C, 158 mg/dL
TGs, 360 mg/dL
HgbA$_{1c}$, 8.2%

What are your initial recommendations for lipid management for M.T.?

All available guidelines for the management of dyslipidemia and diabetes recommend lifestyle counseling as the foundation of therapy. M.T.'s BMI is consistent with obesity and she has inadequately controlled diabetes and hypertension. Nutrition counseling and weight management will be critical to improve control of these important ASCVD risk factors. Tobacco cessation counseling, referral to a cessation program, and possible pharmacotherapy and/or nicotine replacement therapy are important in this very high-risk patient with a strong family history of premature ASCVD. Given the patient's ongoing knee and shoulder pain, her ability to engage in significant aerobic activity may be limited until successful weight loss is achieved.

According to ACC/AHA, NLA, and ADA recommendations for management of dyslipidemia M.T. qualifies for statin therapy in a high-risk diabetic. Her 10-year ASCVD risk by the ACC/AHA CV Risk Calculator is 27.2% and high-intensity statin is indicated by the ACC/AHA treatment algorithm. Patients with diabetes and two or more other major ASCVD risk factors are considered to be at very high risk by the NLA and lipid-lowering therapy is recommended with treatment goals of non–HDL-C < 100 mg/dL and LDL-C < 70 mg/dL. The ADA recommends statin therapy in all patients between the ages of 40 to 75 with type 1 or type 2 diabetes. The intensity of statin therapy is based upon the patient's 10-year ASCVD risk by the ACC/AHA CV Risk Calculator. High-intensity statin is considered reasonable in patients with 10-year risk $\geq$7.5%. Thus, the recommendation for high-intensity statin therapy for M.T. is consistent across all three of these US guidelines.

CASE 8-3, QUESTION 2: M.T. is started on atorvastatin 40 mg but within the next 3 months returns to clinic complaining of joint and muscle symptoms, noting that her knees and shoulder are more painful. How would you approach the evaluation of possible statin-related muscle symptoms?

Statin-related muscle symptoms present a significant challenge to clinicians, though the prevalence of true statin intolerance is likely quite low. A systematic approach to possible statin intolerance is required to confirm the diagnosis, particularly in a very high-risk patient like M.T. The ACC/AHA guideline and NLA recommendations provide similar strategies for patient evaluation and management and these recommendations have been incorporated into the ACC Statin Intolerance app for all mobile devices as well as a web-based version.

It is important for clinicians to take a careful musculoskeletal history and review of systems and document patient complaints prior to initiation of statin therapy. As reported by M.T., patients may report baseline muscle and joint symptoms that have varied in severity and frequency prior to lipid management. Following initiation of statin therapy, patient's muscle symptoms should be compared to those at baseline evaluation to determine if complaints are new or merely coincidental exacerbations of prior existing symptoms. True statin-related myalgias are typically symmetric and are described as aching, soreness, stiffness, tenderness, weakness, or cramping of large proximal muscle groups. Tingling, numbness, sharp or stabbing pain, twitching, nocturnal cramps, arthralgias/arthritis, or unilateral symptoms are less likely to be statin related. Clinicians should consider factors that may increase the risk for statin-related muscle symptoms, such as heavy exercise or exertion, dehydration, substance abuse, frailty, low BMI, female gender, multiple or serious comorbidities, renal insufficiency, hepatic dysfunction, or drug interactions. Other potential primary causes of muscle symptoms should be evaluated such as hypothyroidism, vitamin D deficiency, trauma, previous or new primary muscle diseases, rheumatologic disorders, metabolic disorders (adrenal insufficiency, hypoparathyroidism, Cushing syndrome), or peripheral arterial disease.

CASE 8-3, QUESTION 3: What recommendations would you give the patient regarding continuation of statin therapy?

The ACC/AHA and NLA recommend temporary discontinuation of statin when a patient reports muscle symptoms that they believe are related to treatment. Statin-related complaints usually resolve within a few days to 2 weeks, though there have been rare case reports of persistent myopathy following discontinuation of statin therapy. When symptoms have resolved and the patient is asymptomatic, treatment with the same statin at original or lower dose is reinitiated to determine if the symptoms are definitively related to statin. If muscle complaints recur, it is assumed that symptoms may be related to drug therapy and statin should be discontinued. Most algorithms for evaluation and management of possible statin intolerance recommend a trial of at least two to three statins, with discontinuation and re-challenge if the patient again reports muscle-related symptoms.

The seven currently available statins differ in metabolism, half-life, and lipophilicity, and some providers recommend that the second (or third) statin prescribed in a patient with possible statin intolerance be chosen based on characteristics that differ from the initial agent. There is no trial evidence that this strategy is effective. There have been a number of smaller trials evaluating the potential benefits of ubiquinone or coenzyme Q10 in patients with possible statin-related muscle symptoms, but the results have been inconsistent.

If a patient has failed a systematic challenge/re-challenge approach with two to three statins, guidelines suggest consideration of non-statin therapies such as ezetimibe, BASs ,or PCKS9 inhibitors.[100]

DIABETES

Statins have been associated with an increased risk of type 2 diabetes. A review of 13 trials involving 19,140 patients showed a 9% relative increased risk for the incidence of diabetes in those taking statins compared to placebo. This equates to approximately one new case of diabetes for every 255 patients treated over a 4-year period.[101] A meta-analysis of five trials comparing high-dose versus low-dose statins showed a 12% increased relative risk for incident diabetes over a 2- to 5-year follow-up in those patients who received higher doses of statins.[102] Based on the data, there appears to be an increased risk of developing diabetes, albeit small. However, due to the demonstrated clinical benefit of statin therapy, the benefit clearly outweighs the risk of developing diabetes and statin therapy should not be avoided due to the concern for this adverse effect.

Overall, the incidence of adverse effects with statins varies with myalgia being the most common. When choosing a statin as well as a statin dose, one must consider the various pharmacokinetic characteristics of that statin, the patients' comorbid conditions, and concomitant medications to minimize risk.

PLACE IN THERAPY

Statins are considered first-line pharmacologic therapy for prevention of ASCVD events. They have demonstrated significant reductions in morbidity and mortality across many patient populations.[68–72,103,104] Statin therapy should be initiated before or simultaneously with therapeutic lifestyle modifications.[5]

The initial dose of statin is determined by certain criteria that then place them into any of the four statin benefit groups. The criteria are based on age, presence or absence of ASCVD, presence or absence of diabetes, LDL-C level, and their estimated risk based on the Pooled Cohort Equation.[5] High-intensity statin therapy is recommended in the following patient populations: patients <75 years of age who have clinical ASCVD; patients over 21 years of age and an LDL-C of >190 mg/dL; or patients with diabetes (type 1 or 2) between the ages of 40 and 75 with an estimated 10-year ASCVD risk of >7.5%. Moderate-intensity therapy is recommended in patients >75 years of age if not a candidate for high intensity; LDL-C > 190 mg/dL (if not a candidate for high intensity); type 1 or type 2 diabetes and age 40 to 75 years; or a 10-year ASCVD risk of >7.5% and age 40 to 75 years. The later population may be initiated on high-intensity therapy if clinically indicated. The intensity of doses of the various statins is outlined in Table 8-3.[5] Of note, in patients with LDL-C > 190 mg/dL, combination therapy with a non-statin agent may be needed to achieve additional LDL-C lowering if desired.

There are two patient populations for which there are limited data on the benefit of statin therapy. These include patients with ASCVD and heart failure (New York Heart Association Class II to IV) and patients on chronic hemodialysis. There are currently no recommendations to initiate statin therapy in these patient populations.[5]

In addition to their ability to lower LDL-C, statin also have many "pleiotropic" effects that play a role in patients with ASCVD, independent of their ability to lower LDL-C. These effects include improvement in endothelial function, plaque stabilization, antithrombotic effects, anti-inflammatory, antioxidant effects, increased nitric oxide bioavailability, and reduced plaque progression.[105]

Although well demonstrated as beneficial in patients with established CHD, this benefit in primary prevention is less well defined. In patients without CHD, statins have not been shown to reduce mortality. They have demonstrated a lowering of future vascular events over a time frame of 5 to 10 years, albeit small. As a result, prescribing statins in patients without ASCVD but who are between the ages 40 to 75 years with an estimated ASCVD risk of ≥7.5% remains controversial.

DRUG INTERACTIONS

Drug interactions with statins that result in higher blood levels of the statin or an active metabolite can increase the risk of myositis. Statins that depend on the cytochrome P-450 (CYP) 3A4 enzyme system to be metabolized are most vulnerable to this interaction (i.e., lovastatin, simvastatin, and to a lesser extent atorvastatin). Fluvastatin is primarily a substrate of the 2C9 isoenzyme and, to a lesser extent, 2C8 and 3A4 and, therefore, is more vulnerable to interactions with drugs that directly inhibit CYP2C9 or act as competitive inhibitors (substrates) for this alternative system. Pravastatin, pitavastatin, and rosuvastatin are not extensively metabolized by the CYP enzyme system.[85–87] Rosuvastatin is metabolized minimally (about 10%) with CYP2C9 and CYP2C19 being the primary isoenzymes involved. Pitavastatin is marginally metabolized by CYP2C9 and to a lesser extent by CYP2C8. The major metabolite in human plasma is lactone, which is formed via glucuronidation by uridine 5′-diphospho-glucuronosyltransferases UGTA3 and UGT2B7. Pravastatin undergoes isomerization in the gut to a relatively inactive metabolite. Variability of gastric metabolism has been shown to be associated with the LDL-C–lowering effects of pravastatin.[106] Therefore, rosuvastatin and pravastatin have the lowest potential for interaction with medications that inhibit the CYP metabolic pathways. Some of the most commonly encountered medications that interact with statins by inhibiting the CYP3A4 enzyme system are azole antifungals (itraconazole, ketoconazole, and miconazole), certain calcium-channel blockers (diltiazem and verapamil), macrolide antibiotics (clarithromycin and erythromycin), protease inhibitors (e.g., ritonavir), grapefruit juice (>1 quart), cyclosporine, and antidepressants (nefazodone). Drugs that are substrates for the CYP3A4 system include certain benzodiazepines (alprazolam, midazolam, triazolam), calcium-channel blockers (especially diltiazem), carbamazepine, cisapride, cyclosporine, estradiol, felodipine, loratadine, quinidine, and terfenadine. When these substrate drugs are used together with simvastatin or lovastatin (and to a lesser extent atorvastatin), systemic blood levels of the statin may be increased because of competitive inhibition of the CYP3A4 enzymes, and this may increase the risk for myositis.

Added caution should also be exercised when adding gemfibrozil with a statin to treat patients who also have elevated triglyceride levels. Gemfibrozil interferes with the glucuronidation of statins, thereby interfering with their renal clearance. This impact may be minimal or up to a three- to fourfold increase in statin levels depending upon the specific agent.[107–116] Due to the significance of this interaction, fenofibrate is the preferred fibric acid derivative to use in combination with statins. However, gemfibrozil may be used in combination with certain statins if clinically indicated.[86,109–114,117,118] A list of select statin drug interactions is presented in Table 8-9.

CASE 8-4

QUESTION 1: J.G. is a 63-year-old white woman who implemented lifestyle modifications for her dyslipidemia 7 months ago and is in clinic for follow-up. She has a history of gout, chronic nonischemic HF (LVEF 26%), and diabetes (diet controlled) as well as a 20 pack-year smoking history (quit 5 years ago). Her medications include lisinopril, furosemide, metoprolol succinate 25 mg once daily. Her vital signs include BP 124/80 mm Hg and HR 75 beats/minute. Her laboratory results are as follows: HDL-C 64 mg/dL, LDL-C 101 mg/dL, TG 98 mg/dL, and TC 185 mg/dL.

What is her 10-year ASCVD risk based on the calculator?

The components of the risk calculator that impact J.G. include her age, gender, total cholesterol, HDL cholesterol, and diabetes. She does not have hypertension and smoking does not count as a risk factor due to the fact that she is not a current smoker. Therefore, her 10-year ASCVD risk is 7.1%.

CASE 8-4, QUESTION 2: Based on her risk, what is the most appropriate next step for J.G.?

Table 8-9
Select Drug Interactions with Statins[81–88,118]

	Contraindicated Medications	Medications with Dose Limits	Maximum Dose of Statin When Used in Combination
Atorvastatin	Tipranavir plus ritonavir Telaprevir	Boceprevir Clarithromycin Itraconazole Nelfinavir Cyclosporine/tacrolimus/everolimus/sirolimus	Do not exceed 40 mg daily Do not exceed 20 mg daily Do not exceed 20 mg daily Do not exceed 40 mg daily Do not exceed 10 mg daily
Fluvastatin		Fluconazole Itraconazole Cyclosporine	Do not exceed 20 mg daily Do not exceed 20 mg daily Do not exceed 40 mg daily
Lovastatin	Boceprevir Clarithromycin Cyclosporine Erythromycin Gemfibrozil Ketoconazole Nifazodone HIV protease inhibitors Itraconazole Posaconazole Telaprevir Telithromycin Voriconazole	Amiodarone Danazol Diltiazem Verapamil Dronedarone Lomitapide	Do not exceed 40 mg daily Do not exceed 20 mg daily Do not exceed 20 mg daily Do not exceed 20 mg daily Do not exceed 10 mg daily Do not exceed 20 mg daily
Pitavastatin		Rifampin	Do not exceed 2 mg daily
Pravastatin		Clarithromycin Cyclosporine/tacrolimus/everolimus/sirolimus	Do not exceed 40 mg daily Do not exceed 20 mg daily
Rosuvastatin		Cyclosporine/tacrolimus/everolimus/sirolimus Gemfibrozil Lopinavir/ritonavir Atazanavir/ritonavir	Do not exceed 5 mg daily Do not exceed 10 mg daily Do not exceed 10 mg daily Do not exceed 10 mg daily
Simvastatin	Boceprevir Clarithromycin Cyclosporine Erythromycin Gemfibrozil Itraconazole Ketoconazole HIV protease inhibitors Itraconazole Posaconazole Telaprevir Telithromycin Voriconazole	Amiodarone Amlodipine Diltiazem Verapamil Dronedarone Lomitapide Ranolazine	Do not exceed 20 mg daily Do not exceed 20 mg daily Do not exceed 10 mg daily Do not exceed 10 mg daily Do not exceed 10 mg daily Do not exceed 20 mg daily Do not exceed 20 mg daily

J.G. falls into the statin benefit group of a diabetic with a 10-year risk of <7.5%. The guidelines recommend that she be initiated on moderate-intensity statin therapy. Therefore, any statin dose within this category that would lower LDL-C by 30% to <50% would be appropriate. At this time she is not a candidate for a high-intensity statin, despite having diabetes. The decision is made to initiate simvastatin 40 mg daily.

Case 8-4, Question 3: Four months later, J.G. is admitted to the hospital with atrial fibrillation and is started on amiodarone and apixaban 5 mg twice daily. What medication modifications should be done to J.G.'s medication regimen at this time?

The addition of amiodarone to her medication regimen necessitates a reduction in her dose of simvastatin to 20 mg daily. This dose is still within moderate-intensity range and is acceptable. The other option would be to switch her to different statin that is either not metabolized by CYP3A4 or metabolized to a lesser extent than simvastatin. Reasonable choices of statins would be pravastatin 40 to 80 mg daily, fluvastatin 40 mg BID or XL 80 mg daily, atorvastatin 10 to 80 mg daily, pitavastatin 2 to 4 mg daily, lovastatin 40 mg daily, and rosuvastatin 5 to 40 mg daily.

CLINICAL PEARLS

Approximately 50% of patients discontinue statin therapy within 6 months of initiation and only one-third are still adherent after a year. Therefore, it is important to minimize adverse effects and be able to identify if the statin may be the cause. The incidence of statin intolerance is estimated to be 5% to 10% among statin-treated patients. However, in light of the new AHA/ACC cholesterol guidelines, 13 million more individuals have become eligible for statin therapy and the overall prevalence of statin intolerance in the United States is likely to increase. Diagnosing statin intolerance is challenging as no universal definition exists. The NLA has several definitions of statin intolerance, but the one most clinically useful is the inability to tolerate at least two statins. The two statins should be one that was prescribed and taken at the lowest starting dose and another one that was taken at any dose. In addition to the two statins challenge, patients need to have either objectionable symptoms, or abnormal laboratory values, which are temporally related to statin therapy and reverse upon statin discontinuation and recur upon reinitiation. The ACC has also developed an application called "ACC Statin Intolerance App" designed to assist providers in making the diagnosis of true statin intolerance. The application provides the clinician with a systematic strategy for evaluation of symptoms, management recommendations, as well as information regarding statin characteristics and drug interactions. This application is available on the web at http://tools.acc.org/StatinIntolerance, via Itunes at https://itunes.apple.com/us/app/statin-intolerance/id985805274?mt=8 or via Google Play at https://play.google.com/store/apps/details?id=org.acc.StatinIntolerance&hl=en.

Routine monitoring of liver function tests is no longer recommended during statin treatment. However, patients should be made aware of symptoms that may indicate potential hepatic disease such as flu-like symptoms, fatigue, sluggishness, anorexia, weight loss, right upper quadrant pain, yellowing of eyes, or jaundice.

All patients should have a fasting lipid panel prior to statin initiation. The ACC/AHA guidelines for monitoring of statin therapy recommend a follow-up lipid panel in 4 to 12 weeks following statin initiation to assess patient adherence and response to therapy and then every 3 to 12 months as clinically indicated.[5]

Coenzyme Q10 is an isoprenoid that plays a unique role in cellular electron transport and energy synthesis. It is essential for the normal functioning of muscles. Statins have been shown to reduce blood levels of coenzyme Q10 but muscle tissue concentrations are unaffected. Evidence of the value of supplementing coenzyme Q10 in patients experiencing statin-induced myopathy has been mainly anecdotal. However, the risk of taking CQ10 is relatively small and may be considered in patients complaining of muscle aches in the absence of symptoms that are concerning for more serious muscle-related disease.

Cholesterol Absorption Inhibitor (Ezetimibe)

MECHANISM OF ACTION

Cholesterol that is ingested in the diet and circulated through the bile from the liver is actively reabsorbed in the intestines. Once transported across the intestinal lumen into the enterocyte, it is combined with TG and apo B-48 to form chylomicron particles that transport the lipids through the lymphatic system to the hepatocyte. The TG and cholesterol can then be packaged into VLDL particles and secreted into the systemic circulation (Fig. 8-12).

In the small intestine the Niemann–Pick C1L1 (NPC1L1) transporter is responsible for the uptake of dietary and biliary cholesterol into the small intestine. Ezetimibe interferes with the active absorption of cholesterol and plant sterols from the intestinal lumen into the enterocyte by binding to and inhibiting this transporter. By interfering with the absorption of cholesterol, about 50% less cholesterol is transported from the intestines to the liver by the chylomicrons. This causes an upregulation of hepatic LDL receptors and increased clearance of circulating VLDL and LDL particles. There is also an upregulation in hepatic cholesterol synthesis, which is diverted to the intestines via the bile to replenish the cholesterol available for intestinal absorption processes. The net effect of the inhibition of the NPC1L1 transporter is an approximate 70% increase in GI sterol excretion, a 50% reduction in hepatic cholesterol concentration, a 90% increase in hepatic cholesterol synthesis, and an approximate 20% increase in LDL-C clearance from the systemic circulation via upregulated LDL receptors.[119,120]

Ezetimibe also inhibits the absorption of sitosterol and other plant sterols from the gut, resulting in about a 40% reduction in blood sitosterol levels. The occurrence of sitosterolemia is rare, but is associated with a high CHD risk. Ezetimibe provides one of the first effective treatments for this rare disorder.

EFFICACY

The ENHANCE (Ezetimibe and Simvastatin in Hypercholesterolemia Enhances Atherosclerosis Regression) trial was a randomized, double-blind, placebo-controlled trial comparing simvastatin 80 mg combined with ezetimibe 10 mg versus simvastatin 80 mg alone administered once daily in 720 patients with HeFH.[121] The primary outcome was the change in mean carotid intima media thickness (CIMT) after 24 months of treatment. This trial was not statistically powered to determine differences in vascular disease event rates between treatments because of the short study duration and the small number of patients. Mean baseline LDL-C (319 vs. 318 mg/dL, respectively) and CIMT (0.69 vs. 0.70 mm, respectively) were similar between the treatment groups. The percent change in LDL-C was significantly ($p < 0.01$) greater in the simvastatin–ezetimibe group (−55.6%) compared with the simvastatin–placebo group (−39.1%). However, there was no regression in CIMT in either treatment group, and the mean changes in the CIMT were similar between the treatment groups ($p = 0.29$) after 24 months of treatment. Why was there not a greater change in CIMT in patients randomly assigned to the simvastatin–ezetimibe group compared with the simvastatin–placebo group given that these patients had a greater reduction in LDL-C? Before randomization, approximately 80% of the patients in both treatment groups were receiving statin therapy. Moreover, these patients had thinner or near-normal CIMT at baseline when compared with patients with HeFH studied in previously published statin trials[122,123] that did demonstrate

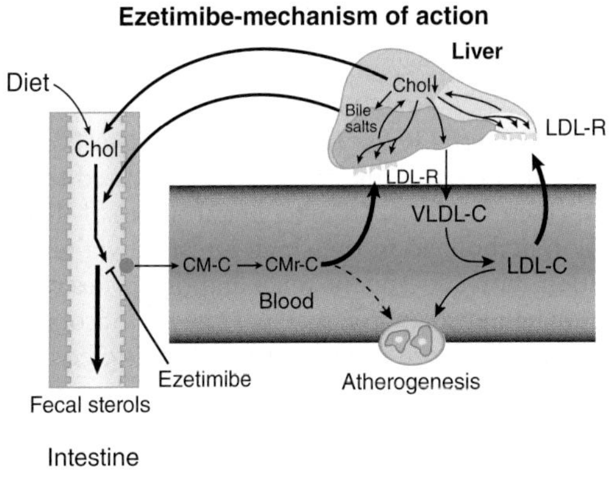

Figure 8-12 Mechanism of action of cholesterol absorption inhibitors. Chol, cholesterol; CM-C, chylomicron cholesterol; CMr-C, chylomicron remnant cholesterol; LDL-C, low-density lipoprotein cholesterol; LDL-R, low-density lipoprotein real; VLDL-C, very low-density lipoprotein cholesterol.

reduced CIMT with high-dose statin therapy. Collectively, this suggests that the patients studied in the ENHANCE trial were aggressively managed for their cholesterol for many years, resulting in the depletion of vascular wall lipids. Therefore, additional aggressive treatment would unlikely result in further regression of an already lipid-depleted carotid vascular wall. In contrast, Avellone et al.[124] recently demonstrated that ezetimibe combined with simvastatin caused a significant reduction in CIMT in FH patients with and without a history of MI. These patients had similar mean baseline LDL-C (301 mg/dL) to patients studied in the ENHANCE trial; however, baseline CIMTs in this trial were much larger (1.82 mm without a history of MI, and 1.98 mm with a history of MI) than those observed in the ENHANCE trial and were consistent with CIMTs in patients with FH who have not been aggressively treated.

When ezetimibe was combined with simvastatin versus placebo in 1,873 patients with mild to moderate, asymptomatic aortic stenosis and no previous history of vascular disease, diabetes mellitus, or any other indications for cholesterol-lowering therapy, significantly fewer patients treated with simvastatin–ezetimibe (15.7%) had ischemic cardiovascular events compared with the placebo group (20.1%), mainly related to a reduction in coronary artery bypass grafting ($p = 0.02$).[125]

The incremental benefits of adding ezetimibe to statin therapy were evaluated in the IMProved Reduction of Outcomes: Vytorin Efficacy International Trial (IMPROVE IT).[126] This was a multicenter, randomized, double-blinded trial involving 18,144 patients that sought to determine the clinical benefit and safety of combination therapy with ezetimibe and simvastatin compared to simvastatin monotherapy in high-risk patients presenting with ACS. This was the first large trial to evaluate the clinical efficacy of adding a non-statin (ezetimibe 10 mg/day + simvastatin 40 mg/day) to statin (simvastatin 40 mg/day) monotherapy. The primary endpoint was cardiovascular death, nonfatal MI, rehospitalization for unstable angina, coronary revascularization ≥30 days following randomization, or stroke. Over a median follow-up of 57 months, the addition of ezetimibe to simvastatin 40 mg reduced the primary endpoint by 6.4% when compared with patients who received simvastatin alone ($p = 0.016$). The absolute reduction in risk over 7 years was 2.0%. The reduction in the primary endpoint was largely driven by a statistically significant reduction in the risk of MI and ischemic stroke. Overall, there was a significant 10% reduction in the risk of cardiovascular death, nonfatal MI, or nonfatal stroke. However, there was no difference in all-cause mortality between the two treatment groups. The average LDL-C during the study was 53.7 mg/dL in the simvastatin–ezetimibe group, compared to 69.5 mg/dL in the simvastatin monotherapy group ($p < 0.001$). The results of this study support the "lower-is-better" premise for LDL-C.[126]

PHARMACOKINETICS/PHARMACODYNAMICS

Ezetimibe is a prodrug that is rapidly conjugated to an active phenolic glucuronide (ezetimibe-glucuronide).[120] The drug is primarily metabolized in the small intestine via glucuronide conjugation with subsequent renal and biliary excretion. The elimination half-life is approximately 22 hours. Absorption is not affected by food and ezetimibe may be administered at any time of day without regard to meals. There are no dose adjustments necessary for patients with renal impairment or with mild hepatic insufficiency.

ADVERSE EFFECTS

Ezetimibe is well generally well tolerated with minimal adverse effects. The adverse effects that are the most reported include diarrhea, arthralgias, cough, fatigue, abdominal pain, and back pain. However, the incidence is no more frequent with ezetimibe than with placebo. Elevations in serum transaminases have also been reported. When used as monotherapy, the incidence of consecutive elevations (≥3 times the ULN) in serum transaminases is similar between ezetimibe (0.5%) and placebo (0.3%); however, when combined with a statin, the incidence of consecutive elevations in serum transaminases is 1.3% and only 0.4% in patients taking a statin alone. These elevations are usually transient and return to baseline after discontinuation. Although very rare, cases of myopathy and rhabdomyolysis have been reported with ezetimibe monotherapy.

PLACE IN THERAPY

Ezetimibe may be used alone or in combination with a statin or fenofibrate along with diet for the management of dyslipidemia, specifically to lower LDL-C. Ezetimibe reduces LDL-C by 18% to 22%, but has little effect on TG or HDL-C.[127] In combination with a statin, it demonstrates an additive effect, enhancing LDL-C lowering by an additional 10% to 20%. In fact, when added to a low dose of a statin, the net LDL-C reduction can be similar to the lowering achieved with the maximal dose of the statin.[128] When added to the maximal dose of a statin, it causes further LDL-C reduction, an effect important in patients with very high LDL-C levels requiring substantial reduction to achieve treatment goals.

DRUG INTERACTIONS

Ezetimibe has been evaluated in combination with several other medications. When combined with statins or fenofibrate there is minimal impact on either drug in terms of an alteration in metabolism and increased bioavailability that requires any additional intervention.[120] Post-marketing data have shown that there are some elevations in the international normalized ratio (INR) when ezetimibe is added to warfarin. The exact mechanism of this interaction is not fully understood and no specific dose adjustments are necessary for either medication. However, when ezetimibe is initiated in a patient on warfarin, closer monitoring of the INR may be warranted. Cyclosporine in combination with ezetimibe results in increased exposure of both medications. When used in combination, serum concentrations of cyclosporine should be closely monitored and adjusted as clinically indicated. Additionally, the recommended initial dose of ezetimibe when used in combination with cyclosporine is 5 mg daily.

When cholestyramine or colestipol are in combination with ezetimibe there is an 80% reduction in the area under the curve of ezetimibe. Therefore, when these combinations are used ezetimibe should be administered at least 2 hours prior or 4 ounces following the administration of cholestyramine or colestipol.[120] The absorption of ezetimibe is not affected by colesevelam and this combination may be preferred.

CLINICAL PEARLS

Adding ezetimibe to a statin results in greater LDL-C reduction than increasing the dose of the statin. Doubling the dose of any statin provides only an additional 6% reduction in LDL-C. The addition of ezetimibe to statin therapy results in an approximate 18% additional reduction in LDL-C. However, maximally tolerated statin therapy is always recommended prior to consideration of the addition of non-statin therapy.

Due to a risk of increased hepatic serum transaminases, these laboratory values should be measured prior to the addition of ezetimibe to statin therapy and again following 6 weeks of combination therapy.

Ezetimibe monotherapy or combination therapy with statin should be avoided in patients with active liver disease or persistent elevations in serum transaminases that are otherwise unexplained.

Niacin

On the basis of currently available evidence of nonefficacy and potential harms, there are no clear indications for the routine use of niacin preparations and niacin is, therefore, not considered in this discussion.

CASE 8-5

QUESTION 1: RP is a 62-year-old male, with history of CHD (bypass 2 years ago), diabetes, end-stage renal disease (ESRD) on hemodialysis Monday, Wednesday, and Friday. He is on lisinopril 10 mg daily, atorvastatin 40 mg daily, aspirin 81, metoprolol succinate 50 mg daily, insulin, and calcium acetate 667 mg 3 times daily. His BP is 136/82 mm Hg; HgA_{1c} 11.6%; Wt 132 kg; Ht 5′10″; fasting lipid panel TC = 250 mg/dL, HDL-C = 30 mg/dL, TG = 450 mg/dL.

What would be the most appropriate treatment for RP and his dyslipidemia?

While RP does have elevated TGs, per the Endocrinology and AHA guidelines, pharmacologic therapy is not indicated at this time. The most important intervention for RP is lifestyle modifications. Controlling his diabetes and losing weight can successfully lower his TGs as much if not more than pharmacologic therapy.

CASE 8-5, QUESTION 2: If pharmacologic therapy were initiated on RP for his hypertriglyceridemia, which agent(s) would be the most appropriate?

All fibric acid derivatives undergo renal elimination and none of these agents are approved for patients on hemodialysis and are therefore not a good option in RP. Omega-3 fatty acids would be the best option to use in combination with atorvastatin that he is already taking.

Fibric Acid Derivatives

MECHANISM OF ACTION

Fibrates activate peroxisome proliferator-activated receptors α (PPARα) causing most of the beneficial effects on blood lipids.[129] PPARα are located in the nucleus of cells and are ligand-dependent transcription factors that regulate target gene expression. Stimulation of PPARα suppresses the gene responsible for the synthesis of apo C-III and stimulates the gene responsible for LDL receptor synthesis.[129,130] As a result, lipolysis of TGs from VLDL particles and the removal of these particles via hepatic LDL receptors are enhanced. Stimulation of PPARα also increases fatty acid oxidation, reducing the synthesis of TGs in the liver, reducing the TG content of secreted VLDL particles.[130] Stimulation of PPARα may increase the synthesis of apo A-I, the critical building block of nascent HDL, thereby enhancing reverse cholesterol transport. Research also suggests that fibrates stimulate the expression of ABCA-1 transporters in macrophage cells, which are responsible for bringing cholesterol from within the cell to the cell surface, where it can be taken up by nascent HDL particles and removed from the cell[129] (Fig. 8-13).

EFFICACY

The results of three major primary prevention trials have raised questions about the safety of fibrates. In the World Health Organization trial, clofibrate reduced nonfatal MI by 25%, but caused an increase in total mortality.[131,132] As a result, its use has declined markedly in the United States. Some of these deaths may have been related to gallstone disease.[131] In the Helsinki Heart Study (HHS), gemfibrozil reduced fatal and nonfatal MI by 37%, but was associated with a slight increase in non-CHD mortality such that there was no net reduction in total mortality.[133] Follow-up evaluations of therapies without gemfibrozil were associated with continued event reduction. In the Veterans Affairs High Density Lipoprotein Intervention (VA-HIT) trial, there was a significant 22% relative risk reduction in death from CHD with gemfibrozil ($p < 0.006$). There was also a 24% reduction in the combined endpoint of death from coronary revascularization, hospitalization due to angina, nonfatal MI, and stroke ($p < 0.001$). However, there was no significant effect on mortality.[134] In the Fenofibrate Intervention and Event Lowering in Diabetes (FIELD) study, fenofibrate did not significantly reduce CHD deaths and nonfatal MI compared with placebo. In addition, more patients receiving fenofibrate had pancreatitis or a pulmonary embolism compared with those given placebo.[135] Fenofibrate was also evaluated versus placebo in 418 patients with diabetes and at least one visible lesion on angiographic evaluation in the Diabetes Atherosclerosis Intervention Study (DAIS) trial.[136] The trial was not powered to examine clinical endpoints, but fewer events, including deaths, occurred in the fenofibrate group. In summary, the clinical trial evidence for cardiovascular benefit of the fibric acid derivatives is not as robust as for the statins. The data supporting the use of gemfibrozil in the primary and secondary prevention setting have been established. In contrast, clear improvements in CHD-related outcomes are still lacking for fenofibrate. Thus, these data support the use of fibric acid derivatives as second-line agents, with the exception of use in patients with severe hypertriglyceridemia. More recently, the incremental benefits of adding fenofibrate to background simvastatin therapy on CHD events in patients with

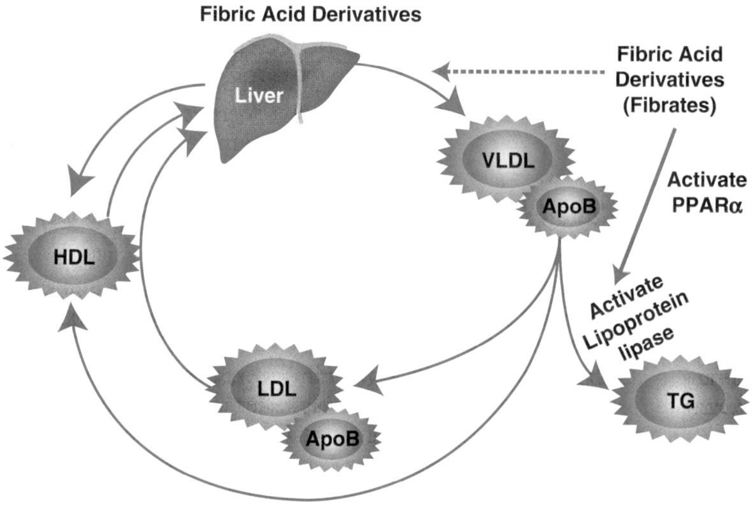

Figure 8-13 Mechanism of action of fibric acid derivatives. apo B, apolipoprotein B; HDL, high-density lipoprotein; LDL, low-density lipoprotein; PPAR-α, peroxisome proliferator-activated receptor alpha; TG, triglycerides.

diabetes were reported. Only patients with the highest tertile (≥204 mg/dL) of TGs and the lowest tertile (≤34 mg/dL) of HDL-C showed a benefit when fenofibrate was added to statin therapy. Overall, there was an insignificant 8% reduction in the composite cardiovascular endpoint, and fenofibrate appeared to be harmful in women compared with men.[137]

PHARMACOKINETICS/PHARMACODYNAMICS

Fenofibrate and fenofibric acids are well absorbed from the GI tract.[138–145] Fenofibrate is primarily metabolized by conjugation with peak plasma concentrations within 6 to 8 hours after administration. It is highly bound to plasma proteins, with an elimination half-life of 20 hours. The primary route of excretion is via the urine in the form of metabolites.

On the other hand, gemfibrozil is completely absorbed following administration and reaches peak plasma concentrations within 1 to 2 hours.[146] The rate and extent of absorption is optimal when taken 30 minutes prior to meals as food can result in a 14% to 44% reduction in the area under the curve. It is highly bound to plasma proteins, with an elimination half-life of 1.5 hours. It undergoes extensive hepatic metabolism via oxidation of the ring methyl group to form carboxyl and hydroxymethyl metabolites. Gemfibrozil relies significantly on renal excretion with approximately 70% being eliminated by the kidneys as a glucuronide conjugate.[146]

Dosing of fibric acid derivatives in patients with renal insufficiency is outlined in Table 8-10.

ADVERSE EFFECTS

Gemfibrozil, fenofibric acid, and fenofibrate are usually well tolerated. The most common adverse effects associated with fibric acid derivatives include, nausea, vomiting, dyspepsia, diarrhea, abdominal pain, flatulence, and constipation. Gemfibrozil causes mild GI symptoms (nausea, dyspepsia, abdominal pain) in about one-third of patients. Fenofibrate causes a rash in 2% to 4% of patients. Fibrate therapy can also cause muscle side effects, including myositis and rhabdomyolysis.[138–143] Most cases of muscle toxicity have been reported with gemfibrozil, especially when it is used in combination with a statin. Recent studies reveal that the area under the blood concentration curve of most statins is increased twofold to fourfold when given concurrently with gemfibrozil. These effects have not been observed with fenofibrate. The mechanism causing this interaction appears to be related to inhibition of glucuronidation by gemfibrozil, which is a metabolic pathway for statins, thereby reducing clearance of statins from the systemic circulation.[147]

Fibric acid derivatives have also been associated with abnormalities in liver function tests including bilirubin and alkaline phosphatase.[138–146] However, these elevations are often not worrisome and usually return to baseline levels upon discontinuation. Fenofibrate has been shown to cause a reversible increase in serum creatinine.[138–145] Although also observed with gemfibrozil, the incidence is lower. Despite this increase, there does not appear to be a resultant decrease in GFR and the mechanism for this effect has not been clearly defined. Gemfibrozil also increases biliary secretion of cholesterol, which increases the lithogenicity of bile and results in the development of cholesterol gallstones. Presumably, the same effect occurs with all fibrates.

PLACE IN THERAPY

Gemfibrozil, fenofibric acid, and fenofibrate are all indicated for the reduction of TG levels in patients with hypertriglyceridemia.[138–146] The NLA recommends a fibric acid derivative as one of several agents that may be initiated in patients who have TG levels > 1,000 mg/dL and are at risk for experiencing pancreatitis.[7] The AHA/ACC define hypertriglyceridemia at a TG level >500 mg/dL and make no formal recommendations on the use of fibric acid derivatives in this setting.[5] Similarly, in patients with familial

Table 8-10
Dosing of Fibric Acid and Fenofibric Acid Derivatives in Renal Insufficiency

Medication	Usual Dose	Creatinine Clearance 30–59 mL/minute	Creatinine Clearance 31–80 mL/minute	Creatinine Clearance ≤30 mL/minute or Hemodialysis
Gemfibrozil	600 mg twice daily		No specific recommendations	Not recommended
Fenofibrate (Fenoglide)	40–120 mg daily		Start at lowest dose of 40 mg daily	Contraindicated
Fenofibrate (Tricor)	48–145 mg daily	Start at lowest dose of 48 mg		Contraindicated
Fenofibrate (Fibricor)	35–105 mg daily		Start at lowest dose of 35 mg	Contraindicated
Fenofibrate (Liopfen)[a]	50–150 mg daily		Start at lowest dose of 50 mg daily	Contraindicated
Fenofibrate (Antara)	43–130 mg daily		Start at lowest dose of 43 mg daily	Contraindicated
Fenofibrate (Lofibra tablets)	54–160 mg daily		Start at lowest dose of 54 mg	Contraindicated
Fenofibrate (Lofibra micronized)	67–200 mg daily		Start at lowest dose of 67 mg	Contraindicated
Fenofibrate (Triglide)	160 mg daily		Avoid use	Contraindicated
Fenofibrate (Trilipix)	45–135 mg daily	Start at lowest dose of 45 mg		Contraindicated

[a]CrCl is 30–89 mL/minute.

dysbetalipoproteinemia, fibric acid derivatives are highly effective and are considered the drugs of choice. Fibrates also have a place in the management of combined or mixed hyperlipidemia. Support for this comes primarily from the results of the HHS and the VA-HIT trials, in which gemfibrozil combined with diet therapy was associated with a reduction in CHD deaths and nonfatal MI.[133,134] These positive outcomes are attributed to significant reductions in serum TGs (and, therefore, a reduction in TG-rich VLDL remnants and in small, dense LDL) and an increase in HDL-C. Persons most likely to benefit are those with diabetes or the lipid triad found in patients with the metabolic syndrome.

DRUG INTERACTIONS

Drug interactions associated with fibric acid derivatives are fairly well known and several of these drug interactions can be managed by careful monitoring. The most clinically significant interactions occur with statins, warfarin, repaglinide, cholestyramine, and colestipol. The combination of statins and gemfibrozil increases systemic concentrations of the statin and raises the risk for the development of myopathy and rhabdomyolysis. As previously mentioned, data suggest that there is less risk of a significant drug interaction with fenofibrate, and subsequently a lower risk of myopathy and rhabdomyolysis. The combination of gemfibrozil should be avoided with lovastatin, pravastatin, and simvastatin. The maximum dose of rosuvastatin should be 10 mg daily when combined with gemfibrozil. Although gemfibrozil does interact with atorvastatin and pitavastatin, the increase in statin concentrations is minor and the combination may be utilized if clinically indicated. However, there are no data demonstrating that adding a fibrate to a statin will reduce CHD risk. The co-administration of gemfibrozil with ezetimibe may cause increased cholesterol excretion into the bile, increasing the risk of cholelithiasis.[120,146] This does not appear to be a concern with fenofibrate and ezetimibe combination.

CASE 8-6

QUESTION 1: J.S. is a 46-year-old male with a history of hypertension and diabetes. He presented to his primary care physician with a chief complaint of abdominal pain that began 2 days ago and radiated to his mid-back. He also has some vomiting. All of his vital signs were within normal limits. On physical exam he has tenderness over his abdominal area that is more severe in the epigastric region. Pertinent laboratory values include an HgA_{1c} of 13.6% and the following cholesterol panel: total cholesterol 467 mg/dL, HDL-C 30 mg/dL, TG 1,872 mg/dL, LDL-C was unable to be calculated, amylase 325 U/L, and lipase 3,265 U/L.

Following acute management of his pancreatitis, what would be the most appropriate treatment for J.S.?

This is an individual that is high risk for pancreatitis as well as ASCVD. His risk score using the new risk calculator based on recent guidelines reveals a 10-year risk of about 18.6% and a statin is indicated. Additionally, the endocrinology guidelines define a triglyceride level of ≥1,000 mg/dL as severe and the AHA guidelines define a level ≥500 mg/dL as very high and that pharmacologic therapy should be initiated. J.S. should be initiated on a statin and a fibric acid derivative, or two different agents to lower TGs first such as omega-3 fatty acids plus fibric acid derivative to get TGs down and then consider the addition of a statin.

CASE 8-6, QUESTION 2: What are some considerations when using fibric acid derivatives in combination with statins?

The risk of adverse effects of statin–fibrate combination therapy is dependent on pharmacokinetic interactions that alter statin metabolism and clearance. One of the most significant drug interactions with statins and a fibric acid derivative is the combination of a statin with gemfibrozil. Gemfibrozil inhibits glucuronidation which is an elimination pathway of all statins with the exception of fluvastatin. This interaction can lead to increased concentrations of these statins, increasing the risk of toxicity. In contrast, fenofibrate appears to have a minimal effect and is considered a safer alternative. The use of gemfibrozil with simvastatin, pravastatin, or lovastatin should be avoided. The combination gemfibrozil with atorvastatin, pitavastatin, and rosuvastatin may be considered if fenofibrate is not an option.[118] However, lower doses of statins should be used to minimize adverse effects. Labeling for rosuvastatin suggests limiting the daily dose of rosuvastatin to 10 mg daily when used with gemfibrozil.

CLINICAL PEARLS

Many different formulations of fenofibrate are available with the dose ranging from 130 to 200 mg. All products are dosed once daily. For the treatment of hypertriglyceridemia, the initial dose may be at the lower end of the dosing range. If the initial dose chosen is lower than the maximum dose, it should be titrated upwards at 4- to 8-week intervals based on patient response up to the maximum dose.

Obtain a baseline serum creatinine prior to the initiation of therapy.
Gemfibrozil is preferred in renal insufficiency.
Consider discontinuation of fibric acid derivative or a dose reduction in the setting of otherwise unexplained increases in serum creatinine.
Fenofibrate is the preferred agent to use when combination with a statin is warranted.
Obtain a baseline CK prior to adding a fibrate to statin therapy and in those patients at high risk.

Patients who receive any fibric acid derivative therapy alone or in combination with a statin should be monitored for symptoms of muscle soreness and pain. If these symptoms emerge, a CK level should be obtained. CK level ≥10 times the ULN in combination with muscle symptoms supports a diagnosis of myositis. If other possible causes are not apparent, such as increased physical exercise or a recent trauma or fall, the presence of myositis is an indication to withdraw fibrate therapy.

Omega-3 Fatty Acids

MECHANISM OF ACTION

The exact mechanism by which the omega-3 fatty acids, dicosohexanoic acid (DHA) and eicosopentanoic acid (EPA), lower TGs is not fully understood. There are currently three prescription fish oil formulations available: combined EPA and DHA in ethyl ester form, EPA ethyl ester only, and EPA and DHA in carboxylic acid form.[148–150] The ethyl ester formulation may possibly work thru inhibition of acyl CoA:1,2-diacylglycerol acyltransferase and increased peroxisomal B oxidation. However, DHA and EPA inhibit the esterification of other fatty acids, and triglyceride lowering may be due to a reduction in hepatic TG synthesis.[148] The active metabolite of icosapent ethyl ester reduces hepatic VLDL-TG synthesis and/or secretion and increases TG clearance from circulating VLDL particles.[149] The potential mechanisms of action for the carboxylic acid formulation include inhibition of acyl-CoA:1,2-diacylglycerol acyltransferase, increased mitochondrial and peroxisomal oxidation in the liver, decreased lipogenesis in the liver, and increased plasma lipoprotein lipase activity. This agent may reduce the synthesis of TGs in the liver.[149]

EFFICACY

Consumption of foods rich in omega-3 fatty acids (e.g., fish) several times a week has been associated with a reduced risk of heart disease and is recommended as part of a low-fat diet. Supplements of fish oils demonstrated a reduction in CHD in patients with a recent MI[151] as well as patients taking statins.[152] Recently, however, other trials have failed to demonstrate the benefits of omega-3 fatty acids in addition to standard cardiovascular drugs, such as statins, angiotensin-converting enzyme (ACE) inhibitors, β-blockers, and antiplatelet agents.[153] Commercial sources of fish oils vary in their content. The omega-3 fatty acids used in the GISSI study, which demonstrated a CHD risk reduction, contained 850 mg of combined EPA and DHA. Currently two trials, the Reduction of Cardiovascular Events with EPA-Intervention trial (REDUCE-IT) and Outcome Study to Assess Statin Residual Risk Reduction with Epanova in Hypertriglyceridemia (STRENGTH), are underway to evaluate cardiovascular outcomes in patients with CHD or at high risk for CHD (REDUCE-IT) or high risk for CHD (STRENGTH) already taking statin therapy. The results of these trials will help to carve out the role of these agents in this patient population.[154,155]

PHARMACOKINETICS/PHARMACODYNAMICS

There is limited pharmacokinetic or pharmacodynamic data available for these agents. The combined EPA and DHA ethyl ester formulation (Lovaza®, Omtryg®) is well absorbed following oral administration. The EPA and DHA carboxylic acid preparation (Epanova®) is directly absorbed in the small intestines subsequently entering the systemic circulation mainly via the thoracic duct lymphatic system.[150] Steady-state concentrations of EPA and DHA in plasma are achieved within 2 weeks following repeat daily dosing. The omega-3 fatty acids in carboxylic acid form may be administered without regard to meals. They are mainly oxidized in the liver and do not undergo renal elimination.

Following oral administration, the EPA ethyl ester preparation (Vasepa®) is de-esterified during process and the active metabolite EPA is absorbed in the small intestine and enters the systemic circulation mainly via the thoracic duct lymphatic system.[149] Peak plasma concentrations of EPA are reached in approximately 5 hours. No studies on the effect of food on this product have been conducted. However, the recommendation is for it to be taken with or following a meal. The EPA ethyl ester is mainly metabolized by the liver via β-oxidation. This beta oxidation splits the long carbon chain of EPA into acetyl coenzyme A which is then converted into energy via the Krebs cycle. EPA ethyl ester does not undergo renal elimination.

ADVERSE EFFECTS

The most common adverse effects associated with Lovaza are eructation, dyspepsia, and taste perversion. In addition to eructation, Epanova has also been reported to cause diarrhea, nausea, and abdominal pain. The most common adverse effect reported with Vasepa is arthralgia.

PLACE IN THERAPY

Fish oils predominantly contain long-chain polyunsaturated (omega 3) fatty acids, EPA and DHA, which lower TG levels significantly (30%–60%) but have variable effects on cholesterol levels. They do not provide LDL-C reduction. All of the available prescription products may be used as an adjunct to diet to treat hypertriglyceridemia. The recommended dose of Lovaza is 4 g/day in either a single or divided dose. The dose for Vasepa is 2 g twice daily with food and Epanova is 2 to 4 g daily.

DRUG INTERACTIONS

No significant drug interactions have been reported with any of the prescription products. However, some studies suggest that the use of omega-3 fatty acids may prolong bleeding time. However, there have been no thorough clinical trials conducted to determine the magnitude of this interaction. Therefore, patients taking these along with other anticoagulants should be evaluated more closely for any signs of increased bleeding.

CLINICAL PEARLS

Omega-3 fatty acid capsules should be swallowed whole. Do not break open, crush, dissolve, or chew.

Administering fish oil before meals may decrease the fishy taste.

EPA has negligible effect on LDL-C Both EPA and DHA lower triglycerides but DHA as well as the combination of EPA/DHA is more effective than EPA-only preparations DHA-containing preparations may increase LDL-C, mechanism likely due to increase in apoC-III production.

Bile Acid Resins

MECHANISM OF ACTION

Bile acids are secreted into the intestines and are responsible for emulsifying fat and lipid particles in food. Most of the bile acids that are secreted are reabsorbed and returned to the liver by enterohepatic circulation. The BASs are anion-exchange resins that bind bile acids in the intestinal lumen and cause them to be eliminated in the stool.[156–159] By disrupting the normal enterohepatic recirculation of bile acids from the intestinal lumen to the liver, the liver is stimulated to convert hepatocellular cholesterol into bile acids. This results in a reduction in the concentration of cholesterol in the hepatocyte, prompting upregulation of LDL receptor synthesis. Finally, circulating LDL-C levels are lowered by binding to the newly formed LDL receptors on the liver surface (Fig. 8-14).

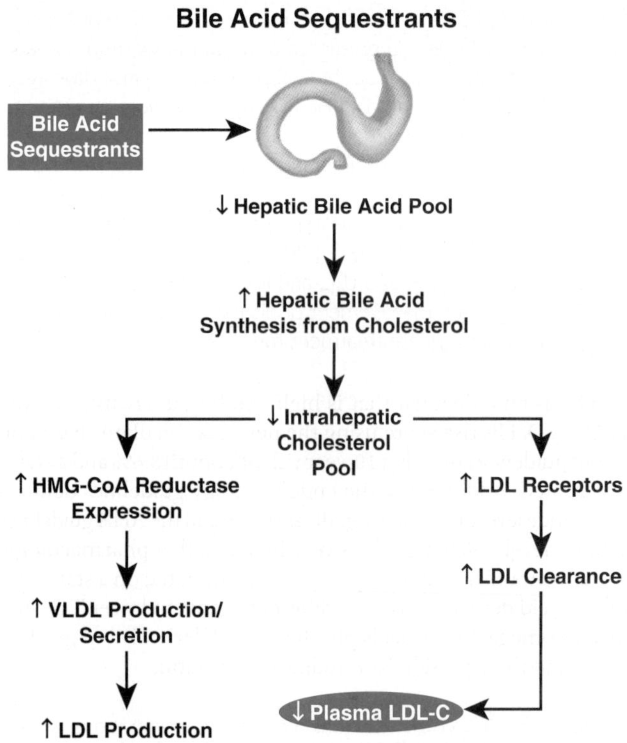

Figure 8-14 Mechanism of action of bile acid sequestrants. HMG-CoA, 3 hydroxy-3 methyl-glutaryl coenzyme A; LDL, low-density lipoprotein; LDL-C, low-density lipoprotein cholesterol; VLDL, very low-density lipoprotein.

EFFICACY

The BAS agents have demonstrated the ability to reduce CHD events in the Lipid Research Clinics Coronary Primary Prevention Trial (LRC-CCPT).[160] This was a randomized, multicenter trial evaluating the efficacy of cholesterol lowering in reducing coronary artery disease (CAD) risk in 3,806 men with primary hypercholesterolemia. In conjunction with diet, patients were randomized to cholestyramine 24 g/day or placebo. The mean follow-up was 7.4 years. The primary endpoint of combined CAD death and non-fatal MI was reduced by 19% in the patients treated with cholestyramine compared to placebo-treated patients ($p < 0.05$). This study also supports the "lower is better" hypothesis of LDL-C.[160,161] These agents reduce LDL-C between 12% and 27%, total cholesterol by 8% and 27%. HDL-C is increased minimally by around 3% to 10%. All of the BAS also may raise TG levels by 3% to 10% or more, especially in patients with high TG levels.

PHARMACOKINETICS/PHARMACODYNAMICS

Colesevelam is a nonabsorbable polymeric compound that binds to bile acids more strongly and more specifically than the other available BAS.[159] Colestipol and cholestyramine are nonabsorbable hydrophilic basic anion exchange resins. All of these agents are insoluble in water.[157,158]

ADVERSE EFFECTS

The most common adverse effect associated with these agents is constipation. Additional adverse effects include abdominal bloating, epigastric fullness, nausea, vomiting, steatorrhea, and flatulence.[157–160] The incidence of these GI symptoms is less with colesevelam.

PLACE IN THERAPY

BAS are indicated as an adjunct to diet and exercise to lower LDL-C. These agents may be used alone or in combination with statins. The BAS have appeal in the management of hypercholesterolemia because they have a strong safety record and they effectively lower LDL-C. They are not absorbed from the gastrointestinal (GI) tract and thus lack systemic toxicity. Older BAS (cholestyramine, colestipol) are not well tolerated due to numerous GI side effects and the unpleasant granular texture of the powder. Therefore, colesevelam is currently the preferred agent. Colesevelam is indicated as monotherapy or in combination with a statin to reduce LDL-C levels in boys and postmenarchal girls, 10 to 17 years of age, with HeFH. Therapy may be initiated following adequate trial of diet if LDL-C remains ≥190 mg/dL or LDL-C remains ≥160 mg/dL and there is a positive family history of premature ASVD or two or more other CVD risk factors. Colesevelam is also approved by the US FDA for use in type 2 diabetes to improve glycemic control.[159]

DRUG INTERACTIONS

Reduction in the absorption of fat-soluble vitamins and folic acid has been reported with high dosages of BAS, but this is rarely a problem in otherwise healthy patients consuming a nutritionally balanced diet. Cholestyramine and colestipol may reduce or delay the absorption of medications when co-administered.[157–159] This can be minimized by administering other medications 1 hour before or 4 hours after the resin dose. The resins may also reduce the absorption of warfarin, levothyroxine, thiazide diuretics, β-blockers, and presumably other anionic drugs. Colesevelam has been shown to reduce levels of glimepiride, glipizide, glyburide, levothyroxine, cyclosporine, olmesartan, and oral contraceptives containing esthynyl estradiol and norethindrone. To avoid these interactions, these agents should be administered 4 hours prior to colesevelam. Colesevelam has also been shown to increase metformin levels and patients should be monitored for clinical response. Post marketing reports have also shown an interaction with phenytoin. As with the other drug interactions, phenytoin should be administered 4 hours prior to colesevelam.

CLINICAL PEARLS

Use of BAS should be avoided in patients with complete biliary obstruction.

BAS are contraindicated if TGs are >500 mg/dL and in patients with a history of hypertriglyceridemia-induced pancreatitis.

Colesevelam for oral suspension should be mixed with 4 to 8 ounces of water, fruit juice, or diet soft drinks.

These agents should be initiated only when TG levels are <300 mg/dL.

Microsomal Triglyceride Protein Inhibitors (Lomitapide)

MECHANISM OF ACTION

Lomitapide is the first in a new class of antihyperlipidemic agents to improve lipoprotein profiles in patients with HoFH. Microsomal triglyceride protein (MTP) resides in the lumen of the endoplasmic reticulum. Inhibiting MTP production prevents the assembly of apoB-containing lipoproteins in enterocytes and hepatocytes. This subsequently inhibits the production and subsequent secretion of chylomicrons and VLDL, and subsequent production of LDL-C.[162]

EFFICACY

There is one pivotal phase III study that ultimately led to the approval of lomitapide. This was a multinational, single-arm, open-label, 78-week trial in 29 patients with HoFH.[163] Following a 6-week run in phase, patients were initiated on lomitapide 5 mg daily and titrated to doses of 10, 20, 40 mg, up to 60 mg, based on tolerability and liver enzymes levels.[163] Patients were also instructed to follow a low-fat diet (<20% of calories from fat) as well as to take dietary supplements to replace fat-soluble nutrients.

Initial efficacy was assessed after 26 weeks and then patients were continued on the study medication for an additional 52 weeks to assess for long-term safety. The primary endpoint was change in LDL-C from baseline at 26 weeks. The results showed that lomitapide, when added to the existing lipid-lowering therapy, significantly reduced LDL-C by an average of 40% from baseline at week 26.[163]

PHARMACOKINETICS/PHARMACODYNAMICS

Lomitapide undergoes extensive hepatic metabolism. Metabolic pathways include oxidative-*N*-dealkylation, glucuronide conjugation, oxidation, and piperidine ring opening. The CYP3A4 isoenzyme metabolizes lomitapide to its major metabolites. Lomitapide is highly bound to plasma proteins (99.8%) and has a mean terminal elimination half-life of 39.7 hours. Approximately 59.5% and 33.4% of the dose is excreted in the urine and feces, respectively.[162]

PLACE IN THERAPY

Lomitapide is approved as an adjunct to a low-fat diet and other lipid-lowering therapies, including LDL apheresis, to reduce LDL-C, TC, apo B, and non–HDL-C in patients with HoFH. Due to the concern for liver injury the drug is only available thru a Risk Evaluation and Mitigation Strategies (REMS) program. Given the risk of adverse effects, unknown effects on cardiovascular morbidity and mortality, as well as the absence of data in the non-HoFH population, lomitapide treatment should be restricted to patients with HoFH.

ADVERSE EFFECTS

The primary adverse effects associated with lomitapide include GI symptoms, elevated transaminases, and hepatic steatosis. The most common GI symptom report was diarrhea which occurred in 79% of patients, followed by nausea (65%), dyspepsia (38%), and vomiting (34%). Additional GI symptoms that have been reported include abdominal pain and discomfort, constipation, and flatulence. To minimize the risk of these adverse effects, patients should adhere to a diet that is low in fat (<20% of daily energy). Elevations in hepatic transaminases occurred in 34% of patients. The degree of elevation ranged from an ALT or AST of ≥3× the ULN to 5× the ULN. However, no patients in the clinical trial had to discontinue therapy due to elevated transaminases.

DRUG INTERACTIONS

The use of lomitapide in combination with strong inhibitors of CYP3A4 (boceprevir, clarithromycin, conivaptan, indivavir, itraconazole, ketoconazole, lopinavir/ritonavir, mibefradil, nefazodone, nelfinavir, posaconazole, ritonavir, saquinavir, telaprevir, voriconazole, telithromycin), moderate inhibitors of CYP3A4 (amprenavir, aprepitant, erythromycin, fluconazole, fosamprenavir, imatinib, verapamil, crizotinib, atazanavir, diltiazem, darunavir/ritonavir) as well as grapefruit juice is contraindicated. Strong CYP3A4 inhibitors in combination with lomitapide can result in an approximately 27-fold increase in exposure of lomitapide. Moderate CYP3A4 inhibitors in combination with lomitapide have not been fully evaluated but are expected to increase lomitapide levels. Even weak CYP3A4 inhibitors can increase lomitapide exposure by approximately twofold. When lomitapide is used in combination with warfarin, the INR may increase by as much as 22%. Lomitapide in combination with simvastatin leads to doubling of simvastatin exposure. When used in combination with statin therapy, the dose of statin should be reduced by 50% and the dose of simvastatin should be limited to 20 mg daily. A dose of simvastatin of 40 mg daily may be used if patients have previously tolerated simvastatin for at least a year at a dose of 80 mg daily. While specific drug interactions between lomitapide and lovastatin have not been studied, given that the metabolizing enzymes and transporters responsible for the disposition of these two agents are similar, a reduced dose of lovastatin should be considered. Lomitapide is also an inhibitor of P-glycoprotein (P-gp). The use of lomitapide in combination with P-gp substrates (aliskiren, fexofenadine, topotecan, sitagliptin, saxagliptin, imatinib, maraviroc, digoxin, dabigatran, ambrisentan, colchicine, everolimus, lapatinib, nilotinib, posaconazole, sirolimus, talinolol, tolvaptan, sirolimus, tolvaptan, talinolol) may lead to increased absorption of these agents and dose reduction should be considered. Although not tested, it is recommended that BAS be administered at least 4 hours apart from lomitapide. This is to avoid potential interference with absorption of lomitapide.[160]

CLINICAL PEARLS

The initial dose of lomitapide is 5 mg once daily with a full glass of water, and at least 2 hours following the evening meal.

Patients should adhere to a low-fat diet consisting of <20% of their dietary intake when prescribed lomitapide.

Patients should also consume supplements (provided by pharmacy with lomitapide prescription) that contain vitamin E (400 IU), linoleic acid (200 mg), alpha-linolenic acid (210 mg), EPA (110 mg), and DHA (80 mg).

The dose of lomitapide can be increased after 2 weeks to 10 mg once daily and then titrated upwards as follows: at 6 weeks increase the dose to 20 mg once daily, at 10 weeks increase to 40 mg once daily, and after 14 weeks the dose may be increased to the maximum dose of 60 mg.

The maximum dose in patients with ESRD on hemodialysis or mild hepatic impairment is 40 mg once daily.

The use of lomitapide is contraindicated in patients with active liver disease (unexplained persistent elevations of serum transaminases), moderate to severe hepatic impairment, pregnancy, as well in combination with moderate or strong CYP3A4 inhibitors as outlined above.

Patients on warfarin along with lomitapide should have their INR closely monitored and warfarin dosage adjusted as needed.

Obtain ALT, AST, and total bilirubin prior to initiation of therapy, prior to each dose increase, or monthly, whichever comes first.

After the first year of therapy, ALT, AST, and total bilirubin should be monitored at least every 3 months and prior to any dose increase. If the LFTs are >3× the ULN and <5× the ULN, repeat labs in 1 week to confirm the elevation. If the elevation is confirmed, reduce the dose and obtain additional liver-related tests. Repeat labs weekly and discontinue therapy if LFTs increase >5× the ULN and do not decrease to <3× the ULN within approximately 4 weeks.

Apo B Antisense Oligonucleotides

MECHANISM OF ACTION

Mipomersen is an antisense oligonucleotide targeted to human messenger ribonucleic acid (mRNA) for apo B-100. Mipomersen is complementary to the coding region of the mRNA for apo B-100 and binds by Watson and Crick (guanine–cytosine and adenine–thymine) base pairing. The hybridization of this agent to the cognate mRNA results in RNase H-mediated degradation of the cognate mRNA thereby inhibiting translation of the apo B-100 protein. This action leads to reduced apo B synthesis, the structural core for all atherogenic lipids, including LDL-C.[164–166]

EFFICACY

Mipomersen has been evaluated in two phase III studies. The first was a randomized, double-blind, placebo-controlled multicenter trial in 58 patients with FH. Patients were included if their LDL-C was ≥140 mg/dL or LDL-C ≥92 mg/dL plus CAD, on maximally tolerated lipid-lowering therapy. Patients were administered subcutaneous dose of 200 mg of mipomersen weekly for 26 weeks or placebo.[167] The results showed a 36% reduction in LDL-C versus a 13% increase with placebo ($p < 0.001$). Additionally, apo B and lipoprotein(a) were also significantly reduced ($p < 0.001$). ALT and AST were increased in 21% and 13% of patients, respectively. Hepatic steatosis was observed with an incidence of 13%. The second phase III study was also a randomized, double-blind, multicenter study evaluating 158 patients with baseline LDL-C ≥100 mg/dL with or at high risk for CAD and on maximum tolerated lipid-lowering therapy.[168] As with the previous study, mipomersen 200 mg was administered subcutaneously once a week for 26 weeks. The results revealed a 36.9% reduction in LDL-C compared to a 4.5% reduction with placebo ($p < 0.001$). Apo B was significantly reduced by 38% as was lipoprotein(a) by 24% ($p < 0.001$). Additionally, half of the patients achieved LDL-C levels of <70 mg/dL in the mipomersen group. Elevations in ALTs observed were similar to other studies and ALT > 3× the ULN occurred in 10% of patients.

PHARMACOKINETICS/PHARMACODYNAMICS

Mipomersen is administered via subcutaneous injection. The drug has a bioavailability ranging from 54% to 78%. Peak plasma concentrations are generally obtained within 3 to 4 hours. With weekly administration, steady state is reached within approximately 6 months. It is highly bound to human plasma (≥90%) and has an elimination half-life of 1 to 2 months following subcutaneous administration. Mipomersen is metabolized in tissues by endonucleases to form shorter oligonucleotides that are then substrates for additional metabolism by exonucleases. Mipomersen is not a substrate for the CYP450 enzyme system. Elimination occurs via metabolism in the tissues and urinary excretion.[164]

ADVERSE EFFECTS

The most common adverse effects associated with mipomersen with an incidence of ≥10% include injection site reactions, flu-like symptoms, nausea, headache, and elevated hepatic transaminases, specifically ALT. Injection site reactions occur in 84% of patients and consist of pain, tenderness, erythema, pruritus, and local swelling. Flu-like symptoms occur in 30% of patients and are usually noticed within 2 days after the injection. These symptoms include pyrexia, myalgia, chills, arthralgia, fatigue, and malaise. Elevations in hepatic transaminases occurred in approximately 12% of patients, with 9% having an ALT ≥ 3× the ULN. Hepatic steatosis has also been reported.

PLACE IN THERAPY

Mipomersen is indicated as an adjunct therapy to a low-fat diet and other lipid-lowering agents to reduce LDL-C, ApoB, TC, and non-HDL in patients with HoFH.[164] Due to concern for hepatotoxicity, mipomersen is also available only through a REMS program. Although mipomersen has only been studied in combination with simvastatin and ezetimibe therapies, its use with other non-statin lipid-lowering agents as well as in patients undergoing LDL-C apheresis is not recommended. The effect of mipomersen on cardiovascular morbidity and mortality is unknown. Additionally, the safety and efficacy of mipomersen has not been established in patients with hypercholesterolemia not secondary to HoFH. Maximum LDL-C reduction is usually seen after approximately 6 months of therapy.

DRUG INTERACTIONS

Secondary to the unique metabolism of mipomersen, there are no known clinically significant drug interactions. However, caution should be exercised when used with other medications known to have potential for hepatotoxicity, (e.g., isotretinoin, amiodarone, acetaminophen [>4 g/day for ≥3 days/week]), methotrexate, tetracyclines, and tamoxifen. If used in combination, more frequent monitoring of liver-related tests may be necessary.

CLINICAL PEARLS

Alcohol consumption should be limited to no more than 1 drink/day as it may increase hepatic fat and induce or exacerbate the risk of liver injury.

The recommended dose of mipomersen is 200 mg by subcutaneous injections once a week.

If a dose is missed, the injection should be given at least 3 days from when the next weekly dose is due.

Mipomersen should be stored in the refrigerator but removed from the refrigerator and allowed to reach room temperature for at least 30 minutes prior to administration.

Injection sites include the abdomen, thigh area, or outer area of upper arm.

Mipomersen should not be injected into any site that has injury to the skin such as sunburn, rash, skin infections, inflammation, or active areas of psoriasis, or in areas with tattoos or scars.

A full liver panel to include ALT, AST, total bilirubin, and alkaline phosphatase should be obtained prior to therapy initiation.

Mipomersen is contraindicated in patients with moderate or severe hepatic impairment or active liver disease.

For the first year, liver-related tests at least an ALT and AST should be checked monthly.

After the first year of therapy, liver tests should be checked at least every 3 months.

Discontinue therapy if persistent or clinically significant elevations occur.

If transaminase elevations are accompanied by clinical symptoms of liver injury, increases in bilirubin ≥2× the ULN, or active liver disease, therapy should be discontinued.

Lipid levels should be monitored at least every 3 months for the first year.

Proprotein Convertase Subtilisin/Kexin Type 9

MECHANISM OF ACTION

Proprotein Convertase Subtilisin/Kexin Type 9 (PCSK9) is a member of the proprotein convertase family, which consists of nine members. PCSK9 is thought to play a critical role in modulating the number of LDL receptors on the surface of the hepatocyte and consequently the amount of LDL-C in the plasma. PCKS9 binds irreversibly to LDL receptors on the hepatocyte and is internalized into the liver cells. This prevents the LDL receptor from being recycled back to the cell surface and the LDL-R/PCSK9 complex is degraded along with the LDL-C. Monoclonal antibodies to PCKS9, or PCSK9 inhibitors, neutralize PCSK9 and prevent PCSK9-mediated LDL receptor degradation, allowing more LDL receptors to return back to the cell surface. An increase in the number of LDL receptors leads to enhanced clearance of LDL-C and thus lower LDL-C levels (Fig. 8-15).[169,170]

EFFICACY

These agents have been evaluated in patients with HeFH and HoFH and in patients with ASCVD who have been on maximally tolerated statin doses and require further LDL-C reduction.

The LAPLACE-2 (LDL-C Assessment with PCSK9 Monoclonal Antibody Inhibition Combined with Statin Therapy) trial was a 12-week trial to evaluate the safety and efficacy of evolocumab in 2,067 patients with primary hypercholesterolemia and mixed dyslipidemia.[171] The study included 296 patients with clinical ASCVD. Patients were randomized to a specific, open-label regimen of three different statin doses (atorvastatin 80 mg daily, rosuvastatin 40 mg daily, or simvastatin 40 mg daily) and either fixed dose evolocumab 140 mg every 2 weeks, evolocumab 240 mg once a month, or placebo. The primary endpoint was change in baseline LDL-C at 12 weeks with a secondary endpoint of percent of patients achieving LDL-C of less than 70 mg/day. The results showed that in patients already on either moderate- or high-intensity statin therapy and clinical ASCVD, evolocumab demonstrated an additional mean reduction in LDL-C of 71% for the twice-weekly dose and 63% for the once-monthly dose compared to placebo ($p < 0.0001$). Additionally, 90% of evolocumab-treated patients achieved LDL-C < 70 mg/dL. The Durable Effect of PCSK9 Antibody Compared with Placebo Study (DESCARTES), was a randomized, double-blind, placebo-controlled 52-week trial comparing evolocumab versus placebo in 901 patients on background lipid-lowering therapy.[172] Background therapy included atorvastatin 80 mg with or without ezetimibe 10 mg daily. Of the entire study population, 139 patients had ASCVD. Evolocumab was administered 420 mg SQ once monthly. The results showed that in patients with ASCVD who received evolocumab, the mean percent LDL-C reduction was 54% ($p < 0.0001$). Alirocumab was evaluated in the COMBO study.[173] This was a multicenter, double-blind, placebo-controlled trial that randomly assigned patients to alirocumab or placebo in addition to maximally tolerated doses of statins with or without additional lipid-lowering therapy who required additional LDL-C lowering. The dose of alirocumab was 75 mg every 2 weeks. If additional LDL-C lowering was still needed at 12 weeks, the dose of alirocumab was increased to 150 mg every 2 weeks and continued for another 12 weeks. At 24 weeks, the mean reduction in LDL-C with alirocumab was 44% compared to 2% with placebo ($p < 0.0001$). A significant portion (84%) of the study population had ASCVD. After 12 weeks, the mean reduction in LDL-C from baseline was 45% versus 1% with placebo. Alirocumab has been evaluated in the Long-Term Safety and Tolerability of Alirocumab in High Cardiovascular Risk Patients with Hypercholesterolemia Not adequately Controlled with Their Lipid Modifying Therapy

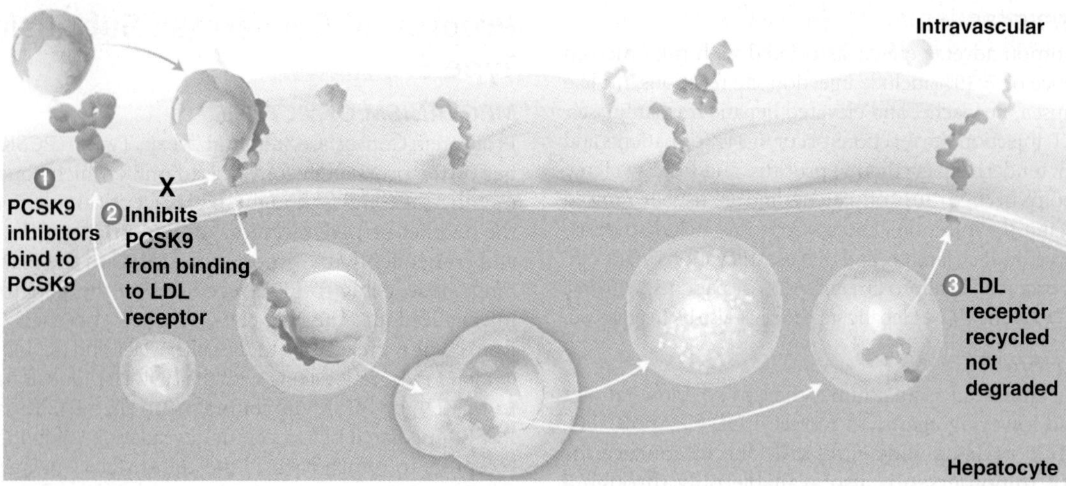

Figure 8-15 Mechanism of action of PCSK9 inhibitors. 1. PCSK9 inhibitors bind to PCSK9 made in the hepatocyte. 2. By binding to the PCSK9 receptor, PCKS9 inhibitors prevent PCSK9-mediated LDL receptor degradation. 3. Secondary to reduce degradation, more LDL receptors are recycled back to the cell surface that subsequently leads to lower LDL-C levels. Used with permission of Amgen.

(ODYSSEY LONG TERM) trial in 2,341 patients at high risk for CHD.[174] Patients were randomly assigned alirocumab 150 mg twice weekly to placebo in addition to maximum tolerated statin therapy with or without additional lipid-lowering therapy. Patients with ASCVD comprised 69% of the trial. At 24 weeks, the percent change in LDL-C reductions with alirocumab compared to placebo was 58% ($p < 0.0001$). This reduction in LDL-C was sustained over a 78-week treatment period.

The FOURIER (Further Cardiovascular Outcomes Research with PCSK9 Inhibition in Subjects with Elevated Risk) was the first trial published to demonstrate reduction in cardiovascular outcomes with the addition of a PCSK9 inhibitor.175 This was a randomized, double-blind, placebo-controlled trial that included 27,564 patients aged 40 to 85 years with clinical ASCVD. Patients were included if they had ASCVD defined as either MI, non-hemorrhagic stroke, or symptomatic peripheral arterial disease [PAD]). Study subjects were also required to have at least one major ASCVD risk factor or two minor risk factors. The minor risk factors were defined as a history of non-MI-related coronary revascularization, residual CAD with ≥40% stenosis in ≥2 large vessels, HDL-C <40 mg/dL for men and <50 mg/dL for women, high-sensitivity C-reactive protein [hs-CRP] >2 mg/L, LDL-C ≥130 mg/dL or non–high-density-lipoprotein cholesterol [non-HDL-C] ≥160 mg/dL, or metabolic syndrome). Patients also had to have a fasting LDL-C level >70 mg/dL or a non-HDL-C levels ≥100 mg/dL after ≥4 weeks of stable dose of atorvastatin 20, 40, or 80 mg daily, with or without ezetimibe, and fasting TG ≤400 mg/dL. The median LDL-C at baseline was 92 mg/dL. Patients were randomized to receive evolocumab administered subcutaneously at a dose of 140 mg every 2 weeks (or 420 mg monthly) or matching placebo. The median duration of therapy was 2.2 years. The results demonstrated that treatment with evolocumab significantly reduced the risk of the primary endpoint (composite of cardiovascular death, MI, stroke, hospitalization for unstable angina, or coronary revascularization) (hazard ratio, 0.85; 95% confidence interval [CI], 0.79 to 0.92, $P < 0.001$) and the key secondary endpoint (cardiovascular death, MI, or stroke) (hazard ratio, 0.80; 95% CI, 0.73 to 0.88; $P < 0.001$). The degree of risk reduction in cardiovascular death, MI, or stroke increased over time, from 16% in the first year of follow-up to 25% after 1 year. In terms of LDL-C reduction, at 48 weeks, the mean LDL-C was reduced by 59% (mean 56 mg/dL). Approximately 87% of patients achieved an LDL-C of <70 mg/dL. Additionally, 67% of patients had LDL-C levels <40 mg/dL, and 42% reached levels of <25 mg/dL. There was a slightly higher rate of injection-site reactions in the patients receiving evolocumab compared with placebo (2.1% vs. 1.6%).

Both alirocumab and evolocumab have been evaluated in patients with HeFH.[176–178] All patients in these studies were on maximally tolerated doses of statins. In the combined studies evaluating alirocumab, patients had an average baseline LDL-C of 141 mg/dL. Patients were treated for 12 weeks with alirocumab 75 mg every 2 weeks or placebo. At the end of the treatment period, the mean LDL-C reduction observed with alirocumab was 48%. As with other studies with alirocumab, if additional LDL-C lowering was needed patients were given an additional 12 weeks of therapy with an increased dose of 150 mg every 2 weeks. Following an additional 12 weeks of treatment, the mean LDL-C reduction from baseline was 54% ($p < 0.0001$). Almost half (42%) of the study population received the higher dose. Evolocumab was evaluated in the patient population in the RUTHERFORD-2 trial.[178] Patients were randomized to receive 140 mg every 2 weeks of evolocumab, or 420 mg once monthly or placebo. The mean baseline LDL-C was 156 mg/dL with 76% on high-intensity statin therapy. Following 12 weeks of therapy, evolocumab reduced baseline LDL-C by 61% with twice-weekly dosing and 62% with monthly dosing ($p < 0.0001$).

Evolocumab has been studied in patients with HoFH in the Trial Evaluating PCSK9 Antibody in Subjects with LDL Receptor Abnormalities (TESLA- Part B).[179] This was a multicenter, double-blind, randomized, placebo-controlled, 12-week trial in 49 patients. Patients received 420 mg monthly of evolocumab or placebo. The mean LDL-C at baseline was 349 mg/dL. All patients were on either atorvastatin or rosuvastatin with 92% also being on ezetimibe. Following 12 weeks of treatment with evolocumab, the mean decrease in LDL-C from baseline was 31% ($p < 0.0001$).

PHARMACOKINETICS/PHARMACODYNAMICS

Alirocumab and evolocumab are both human monoclonal IGg2 antibodies and therefore must be administered via subcutaneous injection to exert an effect. Maximum suppression of PCSK9 occurs in approximately 4 hours with evolocumab and 4 to 8 hours with alirocumab. Maximum serum concentrations reached in 3 to 4 days with evolocumab and 3 to 7 days with alirocumab. The volume of distribution for both agents is small; therefore, these agents are expected to stay in the extracellular space. Alirocumab is eliminated through degradation to small peptides and amino acids while evolocumab is cleared based on its concentration. At low concentrations it is cleared primarily thru saturable binding to PCSK9 and at higher concentrations it is eliminated via a non-saturable proteolytic pathway. The half-life of alirocumab is 17 to 20 days and 11 to 17 days for evolocumab.

ADVERSE EFFECTS

The most common adverse effects reported in the 52 weeks study with evolocumab were nasopharyngitis, upper respiratory tract infection, influenza, back pain, and injection site reactions. However, the difference in the incidence compared to placebo is relatively small. The most common injection site reactions were erythema, pain, and bruising. The most common adverse effect leading to discontinuation was myalgia that occurred in 0.3% of evolocumab patients and 0% in those receiving placebo. In pooled studies the types of adverse effects reported were relatively similar. Allergic reactions occurred in 5.1% of evolocumab-treated patients and 4.6% in those treated with placebo. Neurocognitive events were reported in less than 0.2% of patients. Hypersensitivity reactions such as rash and urticaria were also reported in 1% and 0.4%, respectively, with cases resulting in discontinuation of therapy. The adverse reactions reported with alirocumab were nasopharyngitis, injection site reactions, influenza, and urinary tract infection. The main adverse effects associated with discontinuation were allergic reactions (0.6% vs. 0.2% for placebo) and elevated liver enzymes (0.3% vs. <0.1% for placebo). Injection site reactions were similar to those reported with evolocumab. Neurocognitive events were reported in 0.8% of patients treated with alirocumab compared to 0.7% for placebo. Hypersensitivity reactions also occurred with alirocumab. However, hypersensitivity vasculitis as well as hypersensitivity reactions requiring hospitalizations were reported with alirocumab but not with evolocumab. Neutralizing antibodies were detected in 1.2% of patients treated with alirocumab, and no cases were reported in patients taking evolocumab. However, the long-term consequences from developing neutralizing antibodies are currently unknown.

PLACE IN THERAPY

Both alirocumab and evolocumab are indicated as an adjunct to diet and maximally tolerated statin therapy in patients with HeFH or clinical ASCVD, who require additional reductions in LDL-C. These agents should be considered as either add-on therapy to patients already on statin therapy who need additional LDL-C lowering, or in patients who are deemed statin intolerant.[100] Evolocumab is also indicated for use in combination with other lipid-lowering therapies including LDL apheresis in patients with HoFH who require additional lowering in LDL-C. Alirocumab is administered as a dose of 75 mg every 2 weeks and may be increased in 4 to 8 weeks to 150 mg every 2 weeks if additional LDL-C lowering is required. Evolocumab is dosed at 140 mg every 2 weeks or 420 mg once monthly for HeFH and those with primary hypercholesterolemia with clinical ASCVD. In patients with HoFH, the dose is 420 mg once monthly. Alirocumab has only been studied in patients over the age of 18, while evolocumab may be used in the adolescent population with HoFH aged 13 to 17. Neither agent requires a dose adjustment in patients with mild to moderate renal insufficiency. No data are available for patients with CrCl < 30 mL/minute. Since these proteins do not rely upon the kidneys as a method of excretion, they can likely be used in patients with low CrCl, including those undergoing hemodialysis. However, the PCSK9 inhibitors have not been studied in this patient population. Additionally, since they are large molecules, it is unlikely they would be removed by hemodialysis. No dose adjustment is necessary in patients with hepatic impairment.

CLINICAL PEARLS

Allow evolocumab injections to warm at room temperature for at least 30 minutes prior to use and alirocumab 30 to 40 minutes prior to use.

Do not warm evolocumab by any other means than setting at room temperature (e.g., rolling between hands).

If you miss a dose of evolocumab and the time to next dose is greater than 7 days, administer the dose. If less than 7 days, hold the dose and get back on usual schedule.

Evolocumab and alirocumab may be injected into the thigh, abdomen, or upper arm.

Evolocumab can remain at room temperature but expires in 30 days.

Alirocumab should not be left unrefrigerated for greater than 24 hours.

KEY REFERENCES

A full list of references for this chapter can be found at http://thepoint.lww.com/AT11e. Below are the key references and websites for this chapter, with the corresponding reference number in this chapter found in parentheses after the reference.

Key References

American Diabetes Association. 2015 standards of diabetes care. *Diabetes Care.* 2015;38(Suppl 1):S49–S57. doi:10.2337/dc15-S011. (61)

Brunzell JD et al. Lipoprotein management in patients with cardiometabolic risk: consensus conference report from the American Diabetes Association and the American College of Cardiology Foundation. *J Am Coll Cardiol.* 2008;51:1512–1524. doi:10.1016/j.jacc.2008.02.034. (22)

Goff DC Jr et al. 2013 ACC/AHA guideline on the assessment of cardiovascular risk: a report of the American College of Cardiology/American Heart Association Task Force on Practice Guidelines. *Circulation.* 2013. doi:10.1161/01.cir.0000437741.48606.98. (6)

Hopkins PN et al. Familial Hypercholesterolemias: prevalence, genetics, diagnosis and screening recommendations from the National Lipid Association Expert Panel on Familial Hypercholesterolemia. *J Clin Lipidol.* 2011;5:S9–S17. (26)

Jacobson TA et al. National lipid association recommendations for patient-centered management of dyslipidemia: Part 1—Full Report. *J Clin Lipidol.* 2015;9:129–169. (7)

Jacobson TA et al. National lipid association patient-centered recommendations for management of dyslipidemia: Part 2. *J Clin Lipidol.* 2015;9(Suppl 6):S1–S122. doi:10.1016/j.jacl.2015.09.002. (60)

Kidney Disease: Improving Global Outcomes (KDIGO) Lipid Work Group. KDIGO Clinical Practice Guideline for Lipid Management in Chronic Kidney Disease. *Kidney Int.* 2013;3:259–305. (62)

McKenney JM et al. Final conclusions and recommendations of the National Lipid Association statin safety assessment task force. *Am J Cardiol.* 2006;97:S89–S94. (93)

Morris PB et al. Review of clinical practice guidelines for the management of LDL-related risk. *J Am Coll Cardiol.* 2014;64:196–206. (8)

Stone NJ et al. 2013 ACC/AHA guideline on the treatment of blood cholesterol to reduce atherosclerotic cardiovascular risk in adults: A report of the American College of Cardiology/American Heart Association Task Force on Practice Guidelines. *J Am Coll Cardiol.* 2014;63:2889–2934. doi:10.1016/j.jacc.2013.11.002. (5)

9 Essential Hypertension

Judy W. Cheng

CORE PRINCIPLES

		CHAPTER CASES
1	A diagnosis of hypertension is based on the mean of two or more properly measured seated blood pressure (BP) measurements taken on two or more occasions.	**Case 9-1 (Questions 1, 2), Table 9-1, Table 9-4, Figure 9-1**
2	Most patients with hypertension have a recommended BP goal of less than 140/90 mm Hg (including those with diabetes or chronic kidney disease [CKD] under age 70 years). Elderly patients (age > 60 years) have a higher BP goal of less than 150/90 mm Hg (see core principle #7).	**Case 9-1 (Questions 6, 7, 8), Figure 9-2**
3	Lifestyle modifications are the foundation for preventing hypertension, and they are an important component of first-line therapy in all patients treated with antihypertensive drug therapy.	**Case 9-1 (Questions 11, 12, 13), Table 9-5**
4	Evidence supports the use of an angiotensin-converting enzyme inhibitor (ACEI), angiotensin receptor blocker (ARB), calcium-channel blocker (CCB), or thiazide diuretic as first-line therapy to prevent cardiovascular (CV) events for most patients.	**Case 9-1 (Questions 9, 14, 15), Case 9-3 (Question 2), Case 9-4 (Questions 1-9), Case 9-6 (Questions 1-3 and 6-10), Figure 9-2, Table 9-8, Table 9-9, Table 9-11, Table 9-12, Table 9-13**
5	In black population, including those with diabetes, evidence supports the use of thiazide diuretics and CCB.	**Case 9-1 (Questions 16, 17), Case 9-5 (Question 1) Case 9-6 (Question 4)**
6	Pharmacotherapy recommendations for patients with hypertension and other comorbidities are specifically based on evidence demonstrating reduced risk of CV events.	**Case 9-1 (Question 10), Case 9-3 (Questions 2, 4) Case 9-7 (Question 2), Table 9-7**
7	Elderly patients with hypertension should be managed using the same general treatment principles that apply to all patients with hypertension. However, their BP goal is higher (less than 150/90 mm Hg) unless they also have CKD and age younger than 70 years. In such case, their BP goal is less than 140/90 mm Hg.	**Case 9-2 (Questions 1, 2)**
8	In the population aged ≥18 years with CKD and age under 70 years, evidence supports initial (or add-on) antihypertensive treatment to include an ACEI or ARB to improve renal outcomes. This applies to all CKD patients with hypertension regardless of race or diabetes status.	**Case 9-3 (Questions 1, 3), Case 9-6 (Question 5)**
9	If goal BP is not attained within a month of treatment, increase the dose of the initial drug or add a second drug (ACEI, ARB, CCB, or thiazide diuretic). If goal BP cannot be reached with two drugs, add and titrate a third drug. If goal BP cannot be reached using only the drugs recommended as first line, because of a contraindication or the need to use more than three drugs to reach goal BP, antihypertensive drugs from other classes can be used. Referral to a hypertension specialist may be indicated.	**Case 9-4 (Question 10), Case 9-5 (Question 1) Case 9-8 (Questions 1–3) Case 9-9 (Questions 1–4) Case 9-10 (Questions 1–3) Case 9-11 (Questions 1–4) Case 9-12 (Questions 1–4) Table 9-2, Table 9-3, Table 9-10, Table 9-14, Table 9-15**

INTRODUCTION

Approximately 80 million Americans have hypertension, also called high blood pressure (BP).[1] It is estimated that approximately 33% of adult Americans have hypertension, making it the most frequently encountered chronic medical condition. About 77% of those are using antihypertensive medication, but only 54% of those are controlled (defined as both systolic BP [SBP] <140 mm Hg and diastolic BP [DBP] <90 mm Hg). It is also one of the most significant risk factors for cardiovascular (CV) morbidity and mortality resulting from target-organ damage to blood vessels in the heart, brain, kidney, and eyes. These complications can manifest as either atherosclerotic vascular disease or other forms of CV disease. The exact etiology of essential hypertension is unknown; however, lifelong management with lifestyle modifications and pharmacotherapy are usually needed.

Blood Pressure

During systole, the left ventricle contracts, ejecting blood systemically into the arteries causing a sharp rise in arterial BP. This is the systolic BP. The left ventricle then relaxes during diastole, and arterial BP decreases to a trough value as blood returns to the heart from the venous system. This is the diastolic BP. When recording BP (e.g., 120/76 mm Hg), the numerator is the SBP and the denominator is the DBP. BP has a predictable diurnal rhythm, with fluctuations throughout the day. Values are lowest during the nighttime, sharply rise starting in the early morning, and peak in the late morning to early afternoon.

Mean arterial pressure (MAP) is sometimes used to represent BP, especially in patients with hypertensive emergency. MAP collectively reflects both SBP and DBP, with one-third of the pressure from SBP and two-thirds from DBP. It is calculated using the following equation (Eq. 9-1):

$$\text{MAP} = (\text{SBP} \times 1/3) + (\text{DBP} \times 2/3) \qquad \text{(Eq. 9-1)}$$

Hypertension is defined as an elevated SBP, DBP, or both. A clinical diagnosis of hypertension is based on the mean of two or more properly measured seated BP measurements taken on two or more occasions. Since 1976, the National Heart Lung and Blood Institute has collaborated with researchers and practitioners to develop clinical practice guidelines focused on the management of hypertension (The Joint National Commission [JNC]). In late 2013, the eighth edition of the JNC guidelines were released.[2] Unlike previous editions of the JNC guidelines, definitions and staging of BP were not addressed, but thresholds for pharmacologic treatment were defined, which will be discussed here.

PATHOPHYSIOLOGY OF BLOOD PRESSURE REGULATION

Various neural and humoral factors are known to influence and regulate BP.[3] These include the adrenergic nervous system (controls α- and β-adrenergic receptors), the renin–angiotensin–aldosterone system (RAAS) (regulates systemic and renal blood flow), renal function and renal blood flow (influences fluid and electrolyte balance), several hormonal factors (adrenal cortical hormones, vasopressin, thyroid hormone, and insulin), and the vascular endothelium (regulates release of nitric oxide [NO], bradykinin, prostacyclin, and endothelin). Knowledge of these mechanisms is important in understanding antihypertensive drug therapy. BP is normally regulated by compensatory mechanisms that respond to changes in cardiac demand. An increase in cardiac output (CO) normally results in a compensatory decrease in total peripheral resistance (TPR); likewise, an increase in TPR results in a decrease in CO. These events regulate MAP, as is represented in the following equation (Eq. 9-2):

$$\text{MAP} = \text{CO} \times \text{TPR} \qquad \text{(Eq. 9-2)}$$

Adverse changes in BP can occur when these compensatory mechanisms are not functioning properly. It has been suggested that in hypertension an initial increase in fluid volume increases CO and arterial pressure. Eventually, with long-standing hypertension, it is believed that TPR increases so that CO returns to normal.

The kidney plays an important role in the regulation of arterial pressure, especially through the RAAS. Decreases in BP and renal blood flow, volume depletion or decreased sodium concentration, and an activation of the sympathetic nervous system can all trigger an increased secretion of the enzyme renin from the cells of the juxtaglomerular apparatus in the kidney. Renin acts on angiotensinogen to catalyze the formation of angiotensin I. Angiotensin-converting enzyme (ACE) converts angiotensin I to angiotensin II (see Figs. 14-2 and 14-6 in Chapter 14, Heart Failure). Angiotensin II is a potent vasoconstrictor that acts directly on arteriolar smooth muscle and also stimulates the production of aldosterone by the adrenal glands. Aldosterone causes sodium and water retention and the excretion of potassium. Several factors influence renin release, especially those that alter renal perfusion. The resultant increase in BP results in suppression of renin release through negative feedback.

Approximately 20% of patients with essential hypertension have lower-than-normal plasma renin activity (PRA), whereas approximately 15% have PRA concentrations that are higher than normal. Those with normal to high PRA (e.g., young and whites) should theoretically be more responsive to drug therapies that target the RAAS (e.g., ACE inhibitors and angiotensin receptor blockers [ARBs]). Patients with low PRA may be more responsive to diuretic therapy. However, routinely measuring PRA as a strategy to guide empiric drug selection has limited clinical utility and does not generally result in an outcome superior to careful selection of antihypertensive drug therapy.

Arterial BP is also regulated by the adrenergic nervous system, which causes contraction and relaxation of vascular smooth muscle. Stimulation of α-adrenergic receptors in the central nervous system (CNS) results in a reflex decrease in sympathetic outflow, causing a decrease in BP. Stimulation of postsynaptic α_1-receptors in the periphery causes vasoconstriction. The α-receptors are regulated by a negative feedback system; as norepinephrine is released into the synaptic cleft and stimulates presynaptic α_2-receptors, further norepinephrine release is inhibited. This negative feedback results in a balance between vasoconstriction and vasodilatation. Stimulation of postsynaptic β_1-receptors located in the myocardium causes an increase in heart rate and contractility, whereas stimulation of postsynaptic β_2-receptors in blood vessels results in vasodilation.

A direct association exists between sodium and BP. Although there is a considerably high degree of patient variability in BP sensitivity to sodium (likely affected by heredity and interactions with other environmental exposures), patients with a high dietary sodium intake generally have a greater prevalence of hypertension than those with a low sodium intake. The mechanism by which excess sodium intake contributes to hypertension is uncertain, but it is believed to involve an undetermined natriuretic hormone (not the A- and B-type natriuretic peptides associated with heart failure) that may be induced as a consequence of impaired renal sodium excretion. This natriuretic hormone might also cause an increase in intracellular sodium and calcium, resulting in increased vascular tone and hypertension. The consequences of impaired sodium excretion may have an underlying evolutionary basis. Human physiology evolved in a "hunter-gatherer" society with diets characterized by low sodium and high potassium. The relatively recent shifts in diet patterns brought about by the advent of modern food processing, coupled with increased survival beyond reproductive years, may not have made it possible for modern humans to adapt successfully to high sodium exposure.

Epidemiologic evidence and clinical trials have demonstrated an inverse relationship between calcium and BP. One proposed mechanism for this relationship involves an alteration in the balance between intracellular and extracellular calcium. Increased intracellular calcium concentrations can increase peripheral vascular resistance (PVR), resulting in increased BP.

A decrease in dietary potassium has been associated with an increase in PVR. In theory, diuretic-induced hypokalemia could counteract some of the antihypertensive effects of diuretic therapy, but this has not been seen in clinical trials. It is important, however, that potassium concentrations be maintained within the normal range because hypokalemia increases the risk of CV events, such as sudden death.

Insulin resistance and hyperinsulinemia also have been associated with hypertension. Kaplan[3] suggests that insulin resistance is responsible for the frequent coexistence of hyperglycemia, dyslipidemia, hypertension, and abdominal obesity (also called the *metabolic syndrome*).[4] The exact role of insulin resistance in the development of hypertension is still evolving.

The vascular epithelium is a dynamic system in which vascular tone is regulated by numerous substances. As noted previously, angiotensin II promotes vasoconstriction of the vascular epithelium. However, several other substances regulate vascular tone. NO is produced in the endothelium and is a potent vasodilatory chemical that relaxes the vascular smooth muscle. Hypothetically, some patients with hypertension have an intrinsic deficiency in NO release and inadequate vasodilation, which could contribute to hypertension and its vascular complications.

Factors that regulate BP are well understood and continue to evolve, but the cause of essential hypertension is still unknown. It is impossible to target therapy to specific abnormalities. Therefore, antihypertensive therapy should be selected based on evidence from clinical trials that have demonstrated reductions in hypertension-associated complications, as is discussed later in this chapter.

CARDIOVASCULAR RISK AND BLOOD PRESSURE

Direct correlations between BP values and risk of CV disease have been established based primarily on epidemiologic data. Beginning at a benchmark BP of 115/75 mm Hg, the risk of CV disease doubles with every increment of 20/10 mm Hg.[4] Clinically, it is important to note that incremental elevations in SBP are more predictive of CV disease than elevations in DBP, especially for patients older than 50 years of age. Therefore, SBP is the target of evaluation and intervention for most patients with hypertension. In younger patients with hypertension, elevated DBP may be the only BP abnormality present.

MEASURING BLOOD PRESSURE

Auscultatory Method

The measurement of BP should be standardized to minimize variability in readings. The American Heart Association (AHA) technique for auscultatory BP measurement (Table 9-1)[5] should be used in most patients.[6]

For a video demonstrating methods for measuring BP in adults (courtesy of the University of Colorado School of Pharmacy), go to **http://www.youtube.com/watch?v=-Blqei6_s6J0&list=UUPLXxewjAvEBrO9DuLERbbQ**.

Correct BP measurements require that the clinician listen through a stethoscope that is placed over the brachial artery for the appearance of the five phases of the Korotkoff sounds. Each sound has distinct features, which are depicted in Figure 9-1.[6] Examples of Korotkoff sounds can be found in the Thinklabs Medical Sound Library (http://www.thinklabsmedical.com/stethoscope_community/Sound_Library) under Blood Pressure—Korotkoff Sounds 1 and Blood Pressure—Korotkoff Sounds 2.

Table 9-1
Auscultatory Method for Blood Pressure Measurement in Adults as Recommended by the American Heart Association[5]

1. **PATIENT:** Patient should be seated for 5 minutes with arm bared, unrestricted by clothing, and supported at heart level. Smoking or food ingestion should not have occurred within 30 minutes before the measurement
2. **CUFF:** An appropriately sized cuff should be used. The internal inflatable bladder width should be at least 40% of the bladder length and cover at least 80% of the upper arm circumference. The cuff should be wrapped snugly around the arm with the center of the bladder over the brachial artery
3. **MONITOR:** Measurements should be taken with a correctly calibrated mercury sphygmomanometer, an aneroid manometer, or a validated electronic device
4. **PALPATORY METHOD:** SBP should be estimated using the palpatory method. The cuff is rapidly inflated in 10-mm Hg increments, while simultaneously palpating the radial pulse on the patient's wrist on the cuffed arm and observing the manometer. The pressure when the radial pulse is no longer palpable is the estimated SBP. The cuff is then deflated rapidly
5. **KOROTKOFF SOUNDS:** The head of the stethoscope, ideally using the bell, should be placed over the brachial artery, with each earpiece in the clinician's ear. The cuff should then be rapidly inflated to 20–30 mm Hg above the estimated SBP from the palpatory method. The cuff is slowly deflated at a rate of 2 mm Hg/second while the clinician simultaneously listens for phase 1 (the first appearance of sounds) and phase 5 (the disappearance of sounds) Korotkoff sounds while also observing the manometer. When the pressure is 10 to 20 mm Hg below phase 5, the cuff can be rapidly deflated
6. **DOCUMENTATION:** BP values should always be recorded. The BP values (SBP/DBP) should be recorded using even numbers (rounded up from an odd number)[a] along with the patient's position (seated, standing, or supine), arm used, cuff size, time, and date
7. **REPEAT:** A second measurement should be taken after at least 1 minute in the same arm. If the readings differ by more than 5 mm Hg, additional measurements should be obtained. The mean of these values should be used to make clinical decisions. BP should be taken in both arms at the initial visit with the BP measured in the arm with the higher reading at subsequent visits

[a]Terminal digit preference (i.e., tendency to report readings that end in 0 or 5) should be avoided.
BP, blood pressure; DBP, diastolic blood pressure; SBP, systolic blood pressure.

Out-of-Office Blood Pressure Monitoring

Home BP measurements can provide information on response to therapy and may help improve adherence to therapy and goal BP achievement in some patients.[7,8] Devices for home measurement should be validated for accuracy according to established protocols from either the British Hypertension Society or the Association

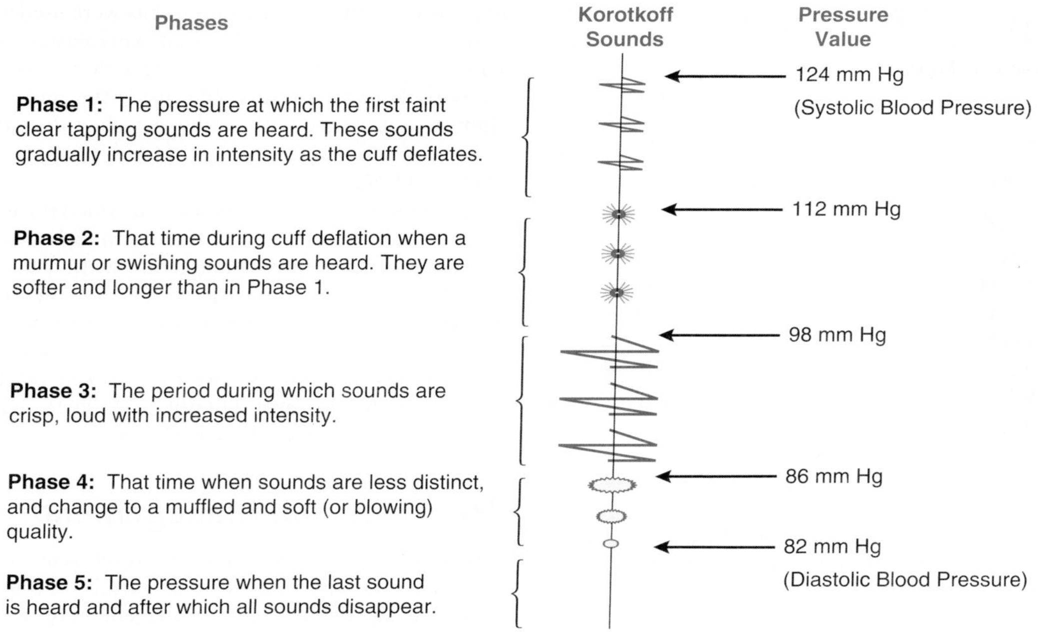

Phases
Korotkoff Sounds
Pressure Value
124 mm Hg
(Systolic Blood Pressure)
Phase 1: The pressure at which the first faint clear tapping sounds are heard. These sounds gradually increase in intensity as the cuff deflates.
112 mm Hg
Phase 2: That time during cuff deflation when a murmur or swishing sounds are heard. They are softer and longer than in Phase 1.
98 mm Hg
Phase 3: The period during which sounds are crisp, loud with increased intensity.
Phase 4: That time when sounds are less distinct, and change to a muffled and soft (or blowing) quality.
86 mm Hg
82 mm Hg
(Diastolic Blood Pressure)
Phase 5: The pressure when the last sound is heard and after which all sounds disappear.

Figure 9-1 Phases of the Korotkoff sounds heard when indirectly measuring blood pressure.

for Advancement of Medical Instrumentation. When placed in service, they should be routinely checked against office-based readings for accuracy, especially when readings between office and home are widely discrepant. Patients with average home BP values greater than 135/85 mm Hg are considered hypertensive.[7] Wrist or finger devices that measure BP are generally not accurate and should not be routinely used.

Ambulatory blood pressure monitoring (ABPM) typically measures BP every 15 to 30 minutes throughout the day and nighttime using a portable, noninvasive oscillometric device typically worn for 24 hours.[5] This form of specialized monitoring is indicated for patients with suspected white-coat hypertension and may also be helpful in patients with apparent drug resistance, hypotensive symptoms while receiving antihypertensive therapy, episodic hypertension, and autonomic dysfunction.[5] Similar to self-BP measurements, ABPM values are typically lower than office-based measurements. As a comparison, the normal upper limit for BP in most patients is 140/90 mm Hg for office-based measurement, 130/80 mm Hg for ABPM (135/85 mm Hg while awake and 120/75 mm Hg while asleep), and 135/85 mm Hg for self-BP measurements.[5] Therefore, the threshold for normal versus abnormal is lower than that obtained during office-based measurements.

Evidence indicates that ABPM recordings can predict clinical outcomes more strongly than office-based BP measurements, most likely because the device factors in BP throughout nighttime hours, which provides a more accurate reflection of the overall average pressure load.[9] However, in clinical practice ABPM is not recommended for routine evaluation of responses to treatment for a number of reasons, including lack of widespread availability, cost, and intrusiveness of performing multiple ABPM sessions in the same patient.[5]

BP values measured outside the office should be considered in the overall treatment of patients with hypertension. However, it is important to acknowledge that office-based BP measurements have been the source used in the major clinical trials establishing that treatment of hypertension reduces morbidity and mortality rates. Therefore, they are still considered the standard values that should guide evaluation of response to antihypertensive drug therapy in most patients.

The reliability and accuracy of automated BP monitors, whether they are used in the office or out of the office, can vary significantly. For a summary of commercially available automatic monitors and whether they have passed validation protocols, please refer to the dabl Educational Trust website (http://www.dableducational.org). The use of BP measurements from automated machines commonly found in grocery stores and pharmacies may have questionable reliability. Measurements using these publically available machines should not be relied on to make clinical decisions, but should be used to direct patients for follow-up with their medical provider as a screening tool.

Types of Hypertension

ESSENTIAL HYPERTENSION

Most patients with hypertension have essential hypertension (also known as primary hypertension), in which there is no identifiable cause for their chronically elevated BP.

SECONDARY HYPERTENSION

Patients with secondary hypertension have a specific identified cause for elevated BP (Table 9-2). Although only 5% to 10% of those among the hypertensive population have causes that are purely secondary, further diagnostic evaluation should occur if physical or laboratory findings suggest the possibility of a secondary cause (Table 9-3).[3,10,11] Some secondary causes are potentially reversible and may normalize BP (e.g., coarctation of the aorta), whereas others are more often superimposed on and worsen an already elevated BP (e.g., obstructive sleep apnea). The distinction is important because treatment of an underlying cause may not always be expected to completely normalize BP and allow discontinuation of antihypertensive therapies. In patients who have resistant hypertension (requiring three or more drugs for BP control) or who have a sudden and significant increase in BP, further diagnostic workup for secondary causes should be considered.

WHITE-COAT HYPERTENSION

White-coat hypertension describes patients who have consistently elevated BP values measured in a clinical environment in the

Table 9-2

Secondary Causes of Hypertension[10]

Alcoholism
Chronic kidney disease
Chronic steroid therapy and Cushing syndrome
Coarctation of the aorta
Drug induced or drug related: ■ Amphetamines (amphetamine, dexmethylphenidate, dextroamphetamine, lisdexamfetamine, methylphenidate, phendimetrazine, and phentermine) ■ Antidepressants (bupropion, desvenlafaxine, and venlafaxine) ■ Antihypertensive agents that are abruptly stopped (only β-blockers and central α_2-agonists) ■ Anabolic steroids (e.g., testosterone) ■ Calcineurin inhibitors (cyclosporine and tacrolimus) ■ Cocaine and other illicit drugs ■ Corticosteroids (cortisone, dexamethasone, fludrocortisone, hydrocortisone, methylprednisolone, prednisolone, prednisone, and triamcinolone) ■ Ephedra alkaloids ■ Erythropoiesis-stimulating agents (darbepoetin-alfa and erythropoietin) ■ Ergot alkaloids (ergonovine and methysergide) ■ Estrogen-containing oral contraceptives (ethinyl estradiol) ■ Licorice (including some chewing tobacco) ■ Monoamine oxidase inhibitors (isocarboxazid, phenelzine, tranylcypromine sulfate) when given with tyramine-containing foods or with an interacting drug ■ Nonsteroidal antiinflammatory drugs (all types) ■ Oral decongestants (e.g., pseudoephedrine) ■ Phenylephrine (ocular administration) ■ Vascular endothelial growth factor inhibitor (bevacizumab) ■ Vascular endothelial growth factor receptor tyrosine kinase inhibitor (sorafenib and sunitinib)
Pheochromocytoma
Primary aldosteronism
Renovascular disease
Sleep apnea
Thyroid or parathyroid disease

presence of a health care professional (e.g., physician's office), yet when measured elsewhere or with 24-hour ambulatory monitoring, BP is not elevated.[5,6] Home BP monitoring or 24-hour ABPM is warranted in patients suspected of having white-coat hypertension to differentiate this from true hypertension.[5] The commonly used definition is a persistently elevated average office BP of greater than 140/90 mm Hg and an average awake ambulatory reading of less than 135/85 mm Hg.[8] The label *white-coat hypertension* applies only to patients without target-organ disease who are not on antihypertensive therapy.

Significant controversies surround white-coat hypertension. Although this does not represent a clinical diagnosis, patients with white-coat hypertension are at risk for eventually developing essential hypertension. Moreover, patients with white-coat hypertension are at a higher risk for CV disease than normotensive patients.[12] The decision to treat or not treat white-coat hypertension is controversial. Many patients enrolled in the landmark clinical trials that demonstrated reductions in CV morbidity and mortality with antihypertensive therapy likely had white-coat hypertension because only office BP measurements were used for inclusion. At minimum, patients with white-coat hypertension should be treated with lifestyle modifications and need to be closely monitored with a device that can measure BP outside the clinic environment if they are not treated with antihypertensive drug therapy.

HYPERTENSIVE CRISES

Hypertensive crises are situations in which measured BP values are markedly elevated (>180/110 mm Hg). They are classified as either a hypertensive emergency (with acute or progressive target-organ damage) or urgency (without acute or progressive target-organ damage). Hypertensive emergencies require hospitalization for immediate BP lowering. Hypertensive urgencies do not require immediate BP lowering; instead, BP should be slowly reduced within 24 hours (but not generally to goal BP so quickly) (see Chapter 16, Hypertensive Crises).

Hypertension Management

Hypertension is treated with both lifestyle modifications and pharmacotherapy. The JNC-8 is considered the "gold standard" consensus guidelines for the management of hypertension in the United States.[2] The overall principle of the guideline is to implement lifestyle modifications in addition to pharmacotherapy to control BP in patients with hypertension. The presence of specific comorbidities in any given patient should be considered when selecting specific pharmacotherapy to treat hypertension. These issues are discussed later in this chapter.

GOALS

The overarching goal of treating patients with hypertension is to reduce associated morbidity and mortality (also called CV events). These manifest as hypertension-associated complications (Table 9-4), which include atherosclerotic vascular disease and other forms of CV disease.

Goal Blood Pressure Values

Achieving goal BP is an important step in the overall treatment of patients with hypertension. According to the JNC-8 guidelines, patients with hypertension of age greater than 18 and less than 60 should have a BP goal of less than 140/90 mm Hg (Figure 9-2).[2]

In contrary to previous editions of the JNC guidelines, where the BP goal for patients with diabetes or chronic kidney disease (CKD) is lower, JNC-8 recommends the same treatment goal for these patients (<140/90 mm Hg).

The change in recommendations is based on some more recent evidence failing to show that more aggressive BP lowering to goal of less than 140/90 mm Hg further improves clinical outcome. There is moderate-quality evidence from three trials (Systolic Hypertension in the Elderly Program [SHEP], Syst-Eur, and UKPDS) that treatment to an SBP goal of lower than 150 mm Hg improves CV and cerebrovascular health outcomes and lowers mortality in adults with diabetes and hypertension.[13–15] However, there are no randomized controlled trials addressing whether treatment to an SBP goal of lower than 140 mm Hg compared with a higher goal (e.g., <150 mm Hg) improves health outcomes in adults with diabetes and hypertension. In the absence of such evidence, the panel recommends a BP goal consistent with the BP goals in the general population younger than 60 years with hypertension. Use of a consistent BP goal in the general population in adults with diabetes of any age may facilitate guideline implementation. This recommendation for an SBP goal of lower than 140 mm Hg in patients with diabetes is also supported by the ACCORD-BP trial, demonstrating[16] no difference in the primary end point of major CV events when

Table 9-3
Clinical Findings Suggestive of Secondary Hypertension

Causes	Historical Findings	Physical Examination Findings	Laboratory Findings
Sleep apnea	Daytime fatigue and somnolence	Large neck circumference; overweight or obese	Abnormal sleep studies with frequent awakenings and anoxic episodes
Renovascular disease	Moderate or severe high BP before age 30 or after 55; rapidly progressive hypertension	Abdominal bruits; funduscopic hemorrhages	Suppressed or stimulated plasma renin activity; IVP (rapid sequence); digital subtraction angiography
Renoparenchymal disease	Dysuria, polyuria, nocturia; urinary tract infections; kidney stones; family history of polycystic or other types of kidney disease	Edema	Proteinuria; hematuria; bacteriuria
Coarctation of the aorta	Intermittent claudication	Diminished or absent femoral pulses compared with carotids; lower SBP in leg compared with arm	—
Pheochromocytoma	Paroxysmal headaches, palpitations, sweating, dizziness, and pallor	Nervousness, tremor, tachycardia, orthostatic hypotension	Clonidine suppression tests[a]; high urinary metanephrine or vanillylmandelic acid
Primary aldosteronism	Weakness, polyuria, polydipsia, intermittent paralysis	Orthostatic hypotension	Hypokalemia
Cushing syndrome	Menstrual irregularity	Moon face; truncal obesity; buffalo hump; hirsutism; violet striae	↑ serum glucose; ↑ plasma cortisol after suppression with dexamethasone

[a]Failure of plasma catecholamines to ↓ by 50% within 3 hours of administration of 0.3 mg clonidine highly suggests pheochromocytoma.
BP, blood pressure; IVP, intravenous pyelogram; SBP, systolic blood pressure

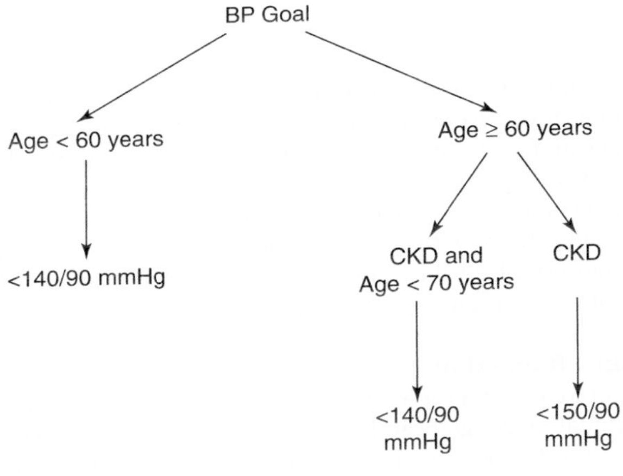

Figure 9-2 Goal blood pressure (BP) determination based on JNC-8, The Eighth Report of the Joint National Committee on Detection, Evaluation, and Treatment of High Blood Pressure.

patients with type 2 diabetes were treated to an SBP goal of less than 120 mm Hg compared with an SBP goal of less than 120 mm Hg after a mean of 4.7 years. There were also no differences in any of the secondary outcomes except for a reduction in stroke. However, the incidence of stroke in the group treated to lower than 140 mm Hg was much lower than expected, so the absolute difference in fatal and nonfatal stroke between the two groups was only 0.21% per year.

JNC-8 similarly recommends the same goal DBP in adults with diabetes and hypertension as in the general population (<90 mm Hg). There is no sufficient evidence to support such a lower goal.

Similarly, in patients with CKD, JNC-8 has recommended individuals younger than 70 years with an estimated glomerular filtration rate (GFR) or measured GFR less than 60 mL/minute/1.73 m^2 and people of any age with albuminuria defined as greater than 30 mg of albumin/g of creatinine at any level of GFR to have a BP goal for <140/90 mm Hg. This recommendation is less aggressive than previous JNC guidelines.

The new panel also felt that in adults younger than 70 years with CKD, the evidence is insufficient to determine if there is a benefit in mortality or CV or cerebrovascular health outcomes with antihypertensive drug therapy to a lower BP goal (e.g., <130/80 mm Hg) compared with a goal of lower than 140/90 mm Hg. There is evidence of moderate quality demonstrating no benefit in slowing the progression of kidney disease from treatment with antihypertensive drug therapy to a lower BP goal (e.g., <130/80 mm Hg) compared with a goal of lower than 140/90 mm Hg.[17–19]

It is important to note that the recommendation of BP goal for patients with CKD applies only to those younger than 70 years. Based on current available evidence, JNC-8 cannot make similar recommendation for a BP goal in people aged 70 years or older with GFR less than 60 mL/minute/1.73 m^2. The commonly used estimating equations for GFR were not developed in populations with significant numbers of people older than 70 years and have not been validated in older adults. No outcome trials included large numbers of adults older than 70 years with CKD.

Table 9-4
Hypertension-Associated Complications and Major Cardiovascular Risk Factors

Hypertension-Associated Complications
- Atherosclerotic vascular disease
  - Coronary artery disease (sometimes called coronary heart disease)
    - Myocardial infarction
    - Acute coronary syndromes
    - Chronic stable angina
  - Carotid artery disease
    - Ischemic stroke
    - Transient ischemic attack
  - Peripheral arterial disease
  - Abdominal aortic aneurysm
- Other forms of CV disease
  - Left ventricular dysfunction (systolic heart failure)
  - Chronic kidney disease
  - Retinopathy

Major CV Risk Factors
- Advanced age (>55 years for men, >65 years for women)
- Cigarette smoking
- Diabetes mellitus
- Dyslipidemia
- Family history of premature atherosclerotic vascular disease (men <55 years or women <65 years) in primary relatives
- Hypertension
- Kidney disease (microalbuminuria or estimated GFR <60 mL/minute/1.73 m^2)
- Obesity (BMI ≥ 30 kg/m^2)
- Physical inactivity

BMI, body mass index; CV, cardiovascular; GFR, glomerular infiltration rate.

The issue of whether more aggressive BP goals (i.e., <130/80 or <120/80 mm Hg) result in better reductions in risk of CV events than the standard goal of less than 140/90 mm Hg remains an ongoing clinical controversy. Until newer clinical data and newer consensus guidelines are published, it is reasonable for clinicians to follow the BP goals recommended in the JNC-8. The Systolic Blood Pressure Intervention Trial (SPRINT) is a randomized, multicenter clinical trial that is comparing intensive hypertension treatment (SBP goal <120 mm Hg) with standard treatment (SBP goal <140 mm Hg) in approximately 7,500 patients with hypertension and at least one other CV risk factor (patients with a history of diabetes or stroke are excluded). The SPRINT will not be completed until the year 2018 or later, but when completed it will provide further evidence regarding goal BP values.

Another area of controversy is the BP goal value in the very elderly, commonly defined as those 80 years of age or older. JNC-8 recommends that, in the general population aged 60 years or older, hypertension should be treated to a goal of <150/90 mm Hg.[2] However, within this population, the only clear prospective data supporting antihypertensive therapy is from the Hypertension in the Very Elderly Trial (HYVET), which used a BP goal of less than 150/80 mm Hg.[20] It is important to note that BP goals among the elderly are based primarily on expert consensus. BP treatment goal for individual elderly patients to a certain extent should be determined by their frailty and their ability in tolerating side effects of antihypertensive agents (such as orthostatic hypotension).

LIFESTYLE MODIFICATIONS

Lifestyle modifications are the cornerstone of management for preventing and treating hypertension. AHA guidelines for lifestyle modifications recommend both diet and exercise.[21,22] These recommendations are summarized in Table 9-5. Engaging in these modifications is encouraged for all persons to prevent the development of hypertension; however, they are recommended as a component of first-line therapy in all patients with prehypertension and in all patients with a diagnosis of hypertension regardless of whether their BP values are at goal or not.[2] Independent of BP lowering, CV risk may also be reduced.

Table 9-5
Lifestyle Modifications to Prevent and Treat Hypertension[20,21]

Modification	Recommendation
Weight management	Lose weight if overweight or obese, ideally attaining a BMI <25 kg/m^2 Maintain a desirable BMI (18.5–24.9 kg/m^2) if not overweight or obese
Adopt DASH-type dietary patterns	Consume a diet that is rich in fruits and vegetables (8–10 servings/day), rich in low-fat dairy products (2–3 servings/day), but has reduced amounts of saturated fat and cholesterol
Reduced sodium intake	Reduce daily dietary sodium intake as much as possible, ideally to <65 mmol/day (equal to 1.5 g/day sodium or 3.8 g/day sodium chloride)
Increased dietary potassium intake	Increase daily dietary potassium intake to 120 mmol/day (4.7 g/day), which is the amount provided in a DASH-type diet
Moderation of alcohol consumption	For patients who drink alcohol, limit consumption to no more than two drinks per day in men and no more than one drink per day in women and lighter-weight people.[a] Do not recommend alcohol consumption in patients who do not drink alcohol
Regular physical activity	Regular moderate-intensity aerobic physical activity; at least 30 minutes of continuous or intermittent 5 day/week, but preferably daily

[a]One drink is defined as 12 ounces of regular beer, 5 ounces of wine (12% alcohol), and 1.5 ounces of 80-proof distilled spirits.
BMI, body mass index; DASH, Dietary Approaches to Stop Hypertension.

Weight Reduction

Weight loss as small as 5% to 10% of body weight in overweight individuals may significantly lower CV risk. For most patients, an average weight loss of 10 kg can reduce SBP by 5 to 20 mm Hg, a reduction comparable to that achieved from the addition of an antihypertensive drug used as monotherapy.[2]

DASH Eating Plan

The DASH (Dietary Approaches to Stop Hypertension) diet is rich in fruits, vegetables, and low-fat dairy foods, coupled with reduced saturated and total fat.[23] The patient education publication entitled "Your Guide to Lowering Your Blood Pressure with DASH" can be found at **http://www.nhlbi.nih.gov/health/public/heart/hbp/dash/index.htm**. The DASH diet can substantially reduce BP (8–14 mm Hg in SBP for most patients) and yield similar results to single-drug therapy. The low-fat component of this diet is important because weight loss is more readily achieved by a reduced-calorie diet (fats contribute more calories per gram than do either carbohydrates or protein) and lowered fat intake also reduces the risk of CV disease by lowering cholesterol.

Dietary Sodium Restriction

The average American intake of sodium is more than 6 g/day. Restricting sodium should be encouraged for patients with prehypertension or hypertension, and the current recommendation to restrict daily sodium intake to no more than 1.5 g is lower than what has traditionally been suggested. Some clinicians may argue that the efficacy of implementing sodium restriction in patients with hypertension may vary. Evidence from clinical trials has shown, however, that sodium restriction provides mean reductions in BP of 5/2.7 mm Hg in patients with hypertension.[23] Restricting sodium to less than 1.5 g daily has been shown to decrease SBP by more than 20 mm Hg in patients with resistant hypertension.[24] Some populations (diabetic patients, blacks, and elderly persons) respond better to sodium restriction than the general population, but all patients with hypertension should be instructed to reduce their sodium intake. They should be counseled not to add salt to foods and to avoid or minimize ingestion of processed or packaged foods, foods with high sodium content, and nonprescription drugs containing sodium.

Increased Potassium Intake

Increasing dietary potassium intake is recommended, although it is not commonly identified by most patients as a dietary modification that will lower BP. Adhering to a DASH eating plan will usually assure an intake of the recommended 4.7 g daily. Dietary supplementation should be the primary strategy to increase potassium. Implementing potassium supplementation outside of dietary sources for the sole purpose of lowering BP should be avoided because of the potential harm from hyperkalemia. Moreover, potassium supplementation in patients with hypertension who are treated with a potassium-sparing diuretic, aldosterone antagonist, ACEI, or an ARB may cause hyperkalemia. This can also occur in patients with hypertension and CKD who are treated with potassium supplementation.

Moderate Alcohol Consumption

Explaining the need to limit alcohol consumption is complicated. Whereas data suggest that small daily doses of alcohol (e.g., one glass of red wine with dinner) are associated with lower CV risk, excessive alcohol intake can elevate BP, decrease the effectiveness of antihypertensive medications, and increase the risk of stroke. Patients who consume three to four drinks per day experience a 3- to 4-mm Hg increase in SBP and a 1- to 2-mm Hg increase in DBP compared with those who do not drink. These increases are even higher in patients who consume more alcohol. Moderate alcohol consumption of two or fewer drinks daily in men and one or fewer drinks daily in women or lighter-weight individuals can decrease SBP approximately 2 to 4 mm Hg. Patients should be instructed that one drink is equal to 1.5 ounces of 80-proof whiskey, 5 ounces of wine, or 12 ounces of beer.

Physical Activity

Regular physical activity can reduce SBP by 4 to 9 mm Hg in most patients.[2] Benefits include reducing the incidence of hypertension, assisting weight loss and weight loss maintenance, and improving overall CV fitness. Most patients with hypertension can safely increase their regular aerobic activity. Those with more severe forms of target-organ damage (e.g., angina and previous MI) may, however, need a medical evaluation before increasing their activity level. Physical activity should ideally occur for at least 30 minutes, at least 5 days of the week, but preferably daily. Walking, running, cycling, swimming, and cross-country skiing are examples of aerobic exercise that are recommended for physical activity.

PHARMACOTHERAPY

Numerous clinical trials have demonstrated that antihypertensive pharmacotherapy reduces the risk of hypertension-associated complications (e.g., CV morbidity and mortality). This evidence is the foundation for JNC-8 consensus guidelines, which provide specific evidence-based pharmacotherapy recommendations based on patient-specific medical history and CV risk.

JNC-8 guidelines recommend that in the general nonblack population, including those with diabetes, initial antihypertensive treatment should include a thiazide-type diuretic, calcium-channel blocker (CCB), ACEI, or ARB. In the general black population, including those with diabetes, initial antihypertensive treatment should include a thiazide-type diuretic or CCB. In the population aged ≥18 years with CKD, initial (or add-on) antihypertensive treatment should include an ACEI or ARB to improve kidney outcomes. This applies to all CKD patients with hypertension regardless of race or diabetes status. Evidence obtained since the 2003 JNC-7 guidelines demonstrates that, for first-line treatment in primary prevention patients, β-blocker therapy is not as effective in reducing CV events compared with ACEI, ARB, CCB, or thiazide diuretic therapy.[25] Therefore, unlike previous versions of the JNC guidelines, β-blocker is no longer recommended as one of the first-line treatment option. Moreover, newer evidence also suggests that the reductions in CV events with ACEI, ARB, CCB, or thiazide diuretic are comparable, so that one agent is not automatically preferred over another.[26] Unlike previous versions of JNC guidelines, JNC-8 guidelines also did not discuss selection of antihypertensive agents in patients with specific other comorbidities (aside from diabetes and CKD). Clinicians are to consult treatment guidelines of the specific comorbidities (e.g., heart failure and coronary artery disease) to help make treatment decisions.

First-Line Agents

Angiotensin-Converting Enzyme Inhibitors

The ACEIs directly inhibit ACE, blocking the conversion of angiotensin I to angiotensin II. This action reduces angiotensin II-mediated vasoconstriction and aldosterone secretion and ultimately lowers BP. Because additional pathways exist for the formation of angiotensin II, ACEIs do not completely block the production of angiotensin II. Aldosterone release is indirectly suppressed by ACEIs; thus, hyperkalemia is possible and potassium concentrations should be monitored. Patients with CKD or volume depletion may be more susceptible to hyperkalemia or to further kidney dysfunction owing to a higher dependence on the vasoconstriction provided by angiotensin II to support GFR among these patients.

Inhibiting ACE also prevents the breakdown and inactivation of bradykinin, which may lead to additive vasodilation by enhancing NO. However, bradykinin accumulation can also cause a nonproductive cough in some patients, which is the most frequent, yet harmless, side effect of ACEI therapy. ACEI therapy has been associated with angioedema, which is a rare, but serious, hypersensitivity reaction. Angioedema typically presents as swelling of the tongue, lips, and mouth, but can also involve the eyes and upper airway.

The development of angioedema requires discontinuation of the ACEI. These agents are metabolically neutral and may have a positive effect on insulin resistance and risk of progression to type 2 diabetes.[27]

Angiotensin Receptor Blockers

The ARBs modulate the RAAS by directly blocking the angiotensin II type 1 receptor site, preventing angiotensin II-mediated vasoconstriction and aldosterone release. Overall, ARBs are the best tolerated of the first-line agents.[28] They do not affect bradykinin and are therefore associated with less incidence of cough. Because aldosterone is indirectly suppressed, monitoring of potassium is important to avoid hyperkalemia. Similar to the ACEIs, patients with CKD or volume depletion may be more susceptible to hyperkalemia or to further kidney dysfunction. These agents are metabolically neutral and may have a positive effect on insulin resistance and risk of progression to type 2 diabetes.[27]

Calcium-Channel Blockers

The CCBs are pharmacologically complex. They reduce calcium entry into smooth muscles, which causes coronary and peripheral vasodilation and lowers BP. All decrease cardiac contractility (except amlodipine and felodipine). Dihydropyridine CCBs are primarily vasodilators that can cause a reflex tachycardia. This is in contrast to the nondihydropyridine CCBs (verapamil and diltiazem) that directly block the atrioventricular (AV) node, decrease heart rate, and decrease cardiac contraction, yet still have vasodilatory effects. Side effects depend on the type of CCB, but can include flushing, peripheral edema, tachycardia, bradycardia or heart block, and constipation.

Thiazide Diuretics

Diuretics, particularly thiazide and thiazide-like (e.g., chlorthalidone) diuretics, have been extensively studied in large landmark clinical trials for hypertension. When initially started, they induce a natriuresis that causes diuresis and decreases plasma volume and CO. With chronic use, diuresis usually dissipates, and CO gradually returns to near-normal levels. The long-term BP-lowering effect in the face of these changes suggests a sustained decrease in PVR as the primary mechanism responsible.

Dose-related electrolyte and metabolic alterations (e.g., hypokalemia, hyperuricemia, hyperglycemia, and hypercholesterolemia) can occur with thiazide diuretics. These effects were particularly problematic when high doses were used many years ago (e.g., hydrochlorothiazide [HCTZ] 100–200 mg/day), but are drastically minimized by using lower doses that are now considered the standard of care (e.g., HCTZ 12.5–25 mg/day).[26] Thiazide diuretics can be used in combination with a potassium-sparing diuretic (i.e., triamterene and amiloride) to minimize potential potassium depletion. Other biochemical changes in glucose and cholesterol are minimal and mostly transient with low-dose therapy.

Second-Line Agents

JNC-8 consensus statement recommends that first-line agents should be used when initiating antihypertensive therapy or when added on to existing antihypertensive therapy unless patients have contraindications to them.[2] In that case, second-line agents may be considered.

β-Blockers

β-Blockers have several direct effects on the CV system. They can decrease cardiac contractility and CO, lower heart rate, blunt sympathetic reflex with exercise, reduce central release of adrenergic substances, inhibit norepinephrine release peripherally, and decrease renin release from the kidney. All these contribute to their antihypertensive effects. Adverse metabolic effects include altered lipids and increased glucose concentrations. Similar to thiazide diuretics, these changes are generally temporary and have minimal to no clinical significance. These agents were considered first line for the treatment of most patients with hypertension in the JNC-7 guideline. However, evidence published after the 2003 JNC-7 has further defined their role.[25] Unless patients have other indication for β-blockers (e.g., CAD or left ventricular dysfunction), they should not be used as first-line agent for primary prevention of CV events in patients with hypertension.

Aldosterone Antagonists

Spironolactone and eplerenone are aldosterone antagonists. Potent blockade of the aldosterone receptor inhibits sodium and water retention and inhibits vasoconstriction. These agents are also considered potassium-sparing diuretics. Hyperkalemia is a known dose-dependent effect with aldosterone antagonists and is more prominent in patients with CKD or in patients taking a concurrent RAAS blocking agent (ACEI, ARB, or direct renin inhibitor). Gynecomastia is a side effect of spironolactone, usually more common with higher doses, that does not occur with eplerenone.

Other Agents

There are other antihypertensive drug classes, many of which are older agents, which should primarily be used to provide additional BP lowering only after first-line and second-line agents have been implemented.

Loop diuretics (e.g., furosemide and torsemide) can be used in some patients for hypertension.[26] When dosed appropriately, they can provide BP reductions similar to those seen with a thiazide diuretic. Because they are short-acting and subject to a significant postdose antinatriuretic effect, they should generally be reserved for patients with heart failure or severe CKD in whom their diuretic action remains prolonged. Significant edema usually accompanies these conditions, such that they generally require a loop diuretic instead of a thiazide diuretic for adequate diuresis and volume removal. Because they are more potent at inducing diuresis compared with thiazide diuretics, they can cause more electrolyte disturbances (e.g., hypokalemia).

Aliskiren, approved in 2007, is the only direct renin inhibitor. Similar to an ACEI or ARB, this agent is a RAAS blocker. It is approved for treatment of hypertension and has been studied in combination with an ACEI, ARB, or thiazide diuretic. It is the newest antihypertensive drug class; therefore, its exact role will continue to evolve as additional clinical data are generated.

α-Blockers (e.g., doxazosin, prazosin, and terazosin) attach to peripheral α_1-receptors, inhibiting the uptake of catecholamines in smooth muscle, and cause vasodilation. Although effective in lowering BP, they have more side effects than first-line or second-line agents. The most prominent side effect is hypotension, which is most evident after the first dose and with postural changes (arising from a lying position to a standing position).

Direct vasodilators (e.g., hydralazine and minoxidil) work on the arterial vasculature. They should be reserved for patients with specific conditions (e.g., severe CKD) or those with very difficult to control BP. Concomitant drug therapy with both a diuretic and an agent that lowers heart rate (a β-blocker, diltiazem, or verapamil) is usually needed to mitigate the associated fluid retention and reflex tachycardia that frequently occur.

Central α_2-agonists (e.g., clonidine and methyldopa) work in the vasomotor centers of the brain where they stimulate inhibitory neurons and decrease sympathetic outflow from the CNS. The resultant decrease in PVR and CO lowers BP. These agents commonly cause anticholinergic side effects (e.g., sedation, dizziness, dry mouth, and fatigue) and possibly sexual dysfunction. Although α_2-agonists lower BP, they often cause fluid retention and should be used in combination with a diuretic.

Adrenergic antagonists (e.g., reserpine, guanadrel, and guanethidine) are not frequently used to treat hypertension. Reserpine depletes catecholamines from storage granules to then decrease BP. High doses are associated with more side effects, but low-dose reserpine (0.05–0.1 mg/day), when used as an additive therapy, is well tolerated. Because of the potential for fluid retention, reserpine requires concurrent diuretic therapy. Guanadrel and guanethidine have numerous significant adverse effects and should be avoided.

CLINICAL EVALUATION

Patient Presentation

CASE 9-1

QUESTION 1: D.C. is a 44-year-old black man who presents to his primary care provider concerned about high BP. At an employee health screening last month, he was told he had hypertension. His medical history is significant for allergic rhinitis. His BP was 144/84 and 146/86 mm Hg last year during an employee health screening at work. D.C.'s father had hypertension and died of an MI at age 54. His mother had diabetes and hypertension and died of a stroke at age 68. D.C. smokes one pack per day of cigarettes and thinks his BP is high because of job-related stress. He does not believe that he really has hypertension. D.C. does not engage in any regular exercise and does not restrict his diet in any way, although he knows he should lose weight.

Physical examination shows he is 175 cm tall, weighs 108 kg (body mass index [BMI] 35.2 kg/m^2), BP is 148/88 mm Hg (left arm) and 146/86 mm Hg (right arm) while sitting, and heart rate is 80 beats/minute. Six months ago, his BP values were 152/88 mm Hg and 150/84 mm Hg when he was seen by his primary care provider for allergic rhinitis. Funduscopic examination reveals mild arterial narrowing and arteriovenous nicking, with no exudates or hemorrhages. The other physical examination findings are essentially normal.

D.C.'s fasting laboratory serum values are as follows:

Blood urea nitrogen (BUN), 24 mg/dL
Creatinine, 1.0 mg/dL
Glucose, 105 mg/dL
Potassium, 4.4 mEq/L
Uric acid, 6.5 mg/dL
Total cholesterol, 196 mg/dL
Low-density lipoprotein cholesterol (LDL-C), 141 mg/dL
High-density lipoprotein cholesterol (HDL-C), 32 mg/dL
Triglycerides, 170 mg/dL

An electrocardiogram (ECG) is normal except for left ventricular hypertrophy (LVH). Why does D.C. have hypertension?

D.C. has hypertension. He has had elevated BP values, measured in clinical environments, and meets the diagnostic criteria for hypertension because two or more of his BP measurements are elevated on separate days.

CASE 9-1, QUESTION 2: What is the proper assessment of D.C.'s BP?

D.C. has essential hypertension; therefore the exact cause is not known. He has several characteristics (e.g., family history of hypertension and obesity) that may have increased his chance of developing hypertension. Race and sex also influence the prevalence of hypertension. Across all age groups, blacks have a higher prevalence of hypertension than do whites and Hispanics.[1] Similar to other forms of CV disease, hypertension is more severe, more likely to include hypertension-associated complications, and occurs at an earlier age in black patients.

Patient Evaluation and Risk Assessment

The presence or absence of hypertension-associated complications as well as other major CV risk factors (Table 9-4) must be assessed in D.C. Also, secondary causes of hypertension (Table 9-2), if suggested by history and clinical examination findings, should be identified and managed accordingly. The presence of concomitant medical conditions (e.g., diabetes) should be assessed, and lifestyle habits should be evaluated so that they can be used to guide therapy.

HYPERTENSION-ASSOCIATED COMPLICATIONS

CASE 9-1, QUESTION 3: Which hypertension-associated complications are present in D.C.?

A complete physical examination to evaluate hypertension-associated complications includes examination of the optic fundi; auscultation for carotid, abdominal, and femoral bruits; palpation of the thyroid gland; heart and lung examination; abdominal examination for enlarged kidney, masses, and abnormal aortic pulsation; lower extremity palpation for edema and pulses; and neurologic assessment. Routine laboratory assessment after diagnosis should include the following: ECG; urinalysis; fasting glucose; hematocrit; serum potassium, creatinine, and calcium; and a fasting lipid panel. Optional testing may include measurement of urinary albumin excretion or albumin-to-creatinine ratio, or additional tests specific for secondary causes if suspected.

D.C. does not yet have hypertension-associated complications. He is exhibiting early signs, however, based on his physical examination that, if left untreated, will likely develop into such complications. These early signs have likely evolved from his longstanding, poorly controlled hypertension. D.C.'s ECG revealed LVH, indicating early cardiac damage. Although the gold standard for confirming LVH is echocardiography, this confirmatory procedure is not necessary unless symptoms are present indicating that LVH has progressed to left ventricular dysfunction (e.g., peripheral edema and shortness of breath). His funduscopic examination reveals mild arterial narrowing and arteriovenous nicking, which are early signs of retinopathy and atherosclerosis. D.C.'s serum creatinine is normal, ruling out overt CKD. Additional testing for microalbuminuria is needed, however, to confirm that he does not have early stage kidney disease.

CASE 9-1, QUESTION 4: What other forms of hypertension-associated complications is D.C. at risk for?

Hypertension adversely affects many organ systems, including the heart, brain, kidneys, peripheral circulation, and eyes. These are summarized in Table 9-4. Damage to these systems resulting from hypertension is termed *hypertension-associated complications*, *target-organ damage*, or *CV disease*. There are often misconceptions about the terms CV disease and CAD. CV disease encompasses the broad scope of all forms of hypertension-associated complications. CAD is simply a subset of CV disease and refers specifically to disease related to the coronary vasculature, including ischemic heart disease and MI. Hypertension-associated complications and major risk factors for developing such complications should be assessed by a thorough patient history, a complete physical examination, and laboratory evaluation.

Hypertension can affect the heart either indirectly, by promoting atherosclerotic changes, or directly, via pressure-related effects. Hypertension can promote CV disease and increase the risk for *ischemic events*, such as angina and MI. Antihypertensive therapy has been shown to reduce the risk of these coronary events. Hypertension also promotes the development of LVH, which is a myocardial (cellular) change, not an arterial change. These two conditions often coexist, however. It is commonly believed that LVH is a compensatory mechanism of the heart in response to the increased resistance caused by elevated BP. LVH is a strong and independent risk factor for CAD, left ventricular dysfunction, and arrhythmia. LVH does not indicate the presence of left ventricular dysfunction, but is a risk for progression to left ventricular dysfunction, which is considered a hypertension-associated complication. This may be caused by ischemia, excessive LVH, or pressure overload. Ultimately, left ventricular dysfunction results in a decreased ability to contract (systolic dysfunction).

Hypertension is one of the most frequent causes of cerebrovascular disease. Cerebrovascular signs can manifest as transient ischemic attacks, ischemic strokes, multiple cerebral infarcts, and hemorrhages. Residual functional deficits caused by stroke are among the most devastating forms of hypertension-associated complications. Clinical trials have demonstrated that antihypertensive therapy can significantly reduce the risk of both initial and recurrent stroke. A sudden, prolonged increase in BP can also cause hypertensive encephalopathy, which is classified as a hypertensive emergency.

The GFR is used to estimate kidney function, which declines with aging. This rate of decline is greatly accelerated by hypertension. Hypertension is associated with nephrosclerosis, which is caused by increased intraglomerular pressure. CKD, whether mild or severe, can progress to kidney failure (stage 5 CKD) and the need for dialysis. Studies have demonstrated that controlling hypertension is the most important strategy to slow the rate of kidney function decline,[29] but it may not be entirely effective in slowing the progression of renal impairment in all patients.

CKD is staged based on estimated GFR values.[30] Stage 3 CKD (moderate) is defined as a GFR 30 to 59 mL/minute/1.73 m^2, stage 4 CKD (severe) is 15 to 29 mL/minute/1.73 m^2, and stage 5 (kidney failure) is less than 15 mL/minute/1.73 m^2 or the requirement of dialysis. In hypertension, stage 3 CKD or worse is considered a hypertension-associated complication. An estimated GFR of less than 60 mL/minute/1.73 m^2 corresponds approximately to a serum creatinine concentration of greater than 1.5 mg/dL in an average man and greater than 1.3 mg/dL in an average woman. The presence of persistent albuminuria (>300 mg albumin in a 24-hour urine collection or 200 mg albumin/g creatinine on a spot urine measurement) also indicates significant CKD. (Note: These definitions of the stages of kidney disease and albuminuria will be used throughout the remaining cases in this chapter.) Assessment of kidney function is discussed in Chapter 2, Interpretation of Clinical Laboratory Tests, and Chapter 28, Chronic Kidney Disease.

Peripheral arterial disease, a noncoronary form of atherosclerotic vascular disease, is considered a hypertension-associated complication. It is equivalent in CV risk to CHD.[3] Risk factor reduction, BP control, and antiplatelet agent(s) are needed to decrease progression. Complications of peripheral arterial disease can include infection and necrosis, which in some cases require revascularization procedures or extremity amputation.

Hypertension causes retinopathies that can progress to blindness. Retinopathy is evaluated according to the Keith, Wagener, and Barker funduscopic classification system. Grade 1 is characterized by narrowing of the arterial diameter, indicating vasoconstriction. Arteriovenous nicking is the hallmark of grade 2, indicating atherosclerosis. Longstanding, untreated hypertension can cause cotton wool exudates and flame hemorrhages (grade 3). In severe cases (e.g., hypertensive emergency) papilledema occurs, and this is classified as grade 4.

MAJOR RISK FACTORS

CASE 9-1, QUESTION 5: Which major CV risk factors are present in D.C.?

Hypertension is one of nine major CV risk factors (Table 9-4). These are not risk factors for developing hypertension; rather, they increase the risk of hypertension-associated complications. D.C. has multiple CV risk factors: smoking, dyslipidemia, family history of premature CHD in a first-degree relative (father), hypertension, obesity, and physical inactivity.

D.C. is a primary prevention patient because he does not yet have any hypertension-associated complications. He has multiple major CV risk factors, so controlling his BP is of paramount importance to reduce the risk of developing hypertension-associated complications. The JNC-8 guidelines, considered the gold standard for treatment, recommend a BP goal of less than 140/90 mm Hg for D.C. because he is a primary prevention patient less than 60 years of age.

Many of D.C.'s risk factors are modifiable. He is a smoker and this significantly increases his CV risk and may reduce the efficacy of antihypertensive therapy. Smoking cessation may not independently lower D.C.'s BP, but it will decrease his overall risk of CV disease (see Chapter 91, Tobacco Use and Dependence). D.C. is obese based on his BMI. His lack of physical activity and dietary patterns have likely contributed to his obesity. A more focused patient interview on diet and exercise would be helpful to reinforce the assumption that he has a sedentary lifestyle. D.C.'s dyslipidemia increases his CV risk, and lipid-lowering therapy should be considered to further decrease the risk of CV disease (see Chapter 8, Dyslipidemias, Atherosclerosis, and Coronary Heart Disease).[31]

Advanced age is considered a major CV risk factor. Although CHD in the elderly is not considered premature, increasing age increases the risk of hypertension-associated complications. Premenopausal women are at low risk for CV disease. However, CV risk in women increases significantly after menopause, similar to the increased risk in men. Therefore, cutoff values for age as a risk factor in men and women are separated by 10 years (>55 years for men, >65 years for women). At age 50, D.C. does not yet have this risk factor.

CASE 9-1, QUESTION 6: What is D.C.'s BP goal?

The overarching goal of treating hypertension is to lower hypertension-associated complications. Control of BP is the most feasible clinical end point to guide therapy and should be viewed as a surrogate for attaining this goal. D.C.'s goal BP is less than 140/90 mm Hg according to JNC-8.

PRINCIPLES OF TREATMENT

Goals of Therapy

CASE 9-1, QUESTION 7: What are the goals of treating D.C.?

Pharmacotherapy principles to achieve these goals include selecting a treatment regimen with antihypertensive agent(s) that reduces risk of CV events, complemented by appropriate lifestyle modifications (Table 9-5).

Health Beliefs and Patient Education

CASE 9-1, QUESTION 8: What patient education should be provided to D.C. regarding his hypertension?

Patient education is needed to ensure that D.C. understands his disease and its complications (Table 9-6). This should comprehensively include information on disease, treatment, adherence, and complications. Several approaches can be effective, but all methods

Table 9-6
Patient–Provider Interactions for Hypertension

Patient Education

- Assess patient's understanding and acceptance of the diagnosis of hypertension
- Discuss patient's concerns and clarify misunderstandings
- When measuring BP, inform the patient of the reading both verbally and in writing
- Assure patient understands his or her goal BP value
- Ask patient to rate (1–10) his or her chance of staying on treatment
- Inform patient about recommended treatment, including lifestyle modification. Provide specific written information using standard brochures when available
- Elicit concerns and questions and provide opportunities for patient to state specific behaviors to carry out treatment recommendations
- Emphasize
  - the need to continue treatment
  - that control does not mean cure
  - that elevated BP is usually not accompanied by symptoms

Individualize Treatment Regimens

- Include the patient in decision making
- Simplify the regimen to once-daily dosing, whenever possible
- Incorporate treatment into patient's daily lifestyle
- Set realistic short-term objectives for specific components of the medication and lifestyle modification plan
- Encourage discussion of diet and physical activity, adverse drug effects, and concerns
- Encourage self-monitoring with validated BP devices
- Minimize the cost of therapy, when possible
- Discuss adherence at each clinical encounter
- Encourage gradual sustained weight loss

BP, blood pressure

should include direct communication between the clinician and the patient. Multidisciplinary approaches to disease-state management in hypertension can effectively use a team of different clinicians (e.g., physicians, nurse practitioners, physician assistants, and pharmacists). Providing face-to-face education is most common, but the key components in patient education can be delivered via indirect interactions (e.g., telephone).

Education should be tailored to the patient's specific needs. For example, some patients are able to comprehend the importance of achieving controlled BP by reading written materials, whereas others understand this only after implementing self-BP monitoring. The patient education process must be continuous throughout the duration of therapy. Not all aspects need to be discussed during each clinical interaction. Careful selection of both written and verbal information should be considered so that patients are not overwhelmed or intimidated. National Heart, Lung, and Blood Institute patient education materials are available at http://www.nhlbi.nih.gov/health/public/heart/index.htm#hbp. It is important that clinicians review all materials provided to patients to identify the source of information, assess ease of reading, and identify omitted information and sources of confusion or anxiety (e.g., drug side effects).

Patients such as D.C. often incorrectly explain BP elevation as stress related. Although certain patients (e.g., those with white-coat hypertension) may have BP that is more highly reactive, most patients with essential hypertension will have an elevated BP regardless of their stress level. D.C. should be informed about the cause of his disease and the lack of correlation between stress or symptoms and high BP. Importantly, D.C. needs to realize that elevated BP is almost always asymptomatic and that it can cause serious long-term complications. It is essential that he understand the chronic nature of hypertension and the need for long-term therapy. Otherwise, he may adhere to his treatment only when he "feels his BP is high" or during stressful events.

Some patients believe they can control their BP by stress management rather than with antihypertensive drug therapy and lifestyle modifications. Controlled trials have not consistently proven that stress management is beneficial in treating hypertension.[32] It is important to determine the patient's health beliefs and attitudes and to provide education about the etiology and management of hypertension to promote BP control.

Another common myth patients believe is that treating hypertension commonly leads to fatigue, lethargy, and sexual dysfunction. This misconception can compromise adherence and be a limiting factor in appropriate management. Clinical trials have repeatedly reported that quality of life is better with active medication than with placebo.[33–36] Data have indicated that as many as 27% of men with hypertension have erectile dysfunction.[5] Although many patients believe this to be a medication-related side effect and that incidence rates vary among antihypertensive agents and classes, erectile dysfunction is likely caused by penile arterial changes (probably atherosclerosis), which is related to uncontrolled or untreated hypertension.[37]

Benefits of Treatment

CASE 9-1, QUESTION 9: How can antihypertensive drug therapy reduce D.C.'s risk of hypertension-associated complications?

Without a doubt, antihypertensive therapy reduces the risk of CV disease and CV events in patients with hypertension. Numerous landmark placebo-controlled studies have clearly demonstrated these benefits. The first large-scale trial, published in 1967, was the Veterans Administration (VA) study in men with DBP between 115 and 129 mm Hg.[38] This study was prematurely stopped because benefits of treatment were so dramatic. Antihypertensive therapy significantly reduced cerebral hemorrhage, MI, left ventricular dysfunction, retinopathy, and kidney disease. Other landmark placebo-controlled studies have evaluated antihypertensive therapy in patients with less severe hypertension and have shown a reduced risk of CV events (stroke, ischemic heart disease, and left ventricular dysfunction) and even CV death.[29,31,39,40] Placebo-controlled studies evaluating morbidity and mortality in hypertension are now not only unnecessary, but considered unethical because of the well-established benefits of treatment. Even small reductions in BP have been associated with significant CV benefits. Based on prospective observational studies, a persistent 5 mm Hg reduction in DBP is associated with a 21% reduction in CHD and a 34% reduction in stroke.[41,42]

Most antihypertensive drugs reduce LVH through varying mechanisms. It is logical that regression of LVH is desirable, but this remains unproved.

CASE 9-1, QUESTION 10: Will D.C.'s early signs of hypertension-associated complications improve or reverse with appropriate BP control?

Reductions in BP can reverse many of the changes associated with D.C.'s retinopathy. Studies have demonstrated that the risk of retinopathy in diabetes increases significantly when BP is elevated and that BP lowering can slow this progression. Although D.C. has an elevated fasting glucose, he does not have diabetes. Regardless, lowering BP is desirable for anticipated beneficial effects on his retinopathy.

HYPERTENSION MANAGEMENT

Lifestyle Modifications

CASE 9-1, QUESTION 11: Should D.C. start antihypertensive drug therapy, or are lifestyle modifications alone sufficient?

It is reasonable to assume that lifestyle modifications can partially help D.C. achieve his BP goal. D.C. has multiple major CV risk factors and has early evidence of hypertension-associated complications. Lifestyle modifications are germane to the appropriate treatment of hypertension, but prospective clinical trials have not proven that this treatment approach prevents CV disease in patients with hypertension similar to what is proven antihypertensive drug therapy. Hence, initiation of drug therapy should not be delayed unnecessarily, especially for patients with CV risk factors.

MODALITIES THAT LOWER BP

CASE 9-1, QUESTION 12: Which lifestyle modifications can D.C. implement to lower his BP?

Weight reduction through dietary modifications and physical activity and sodium restriction are the most apparent lifestyle modifications for D.C. to lower his BP. A thorough patient interview (diet history to quantify total calories, sodium, fat, and cholesterol, and social history to determine alcohol consumption and confirm cigarette use) should be obtained. Based on this interview, customized recommendations can be made.

The DASH diet should be strongly encouraged in D.C. based on proven benefits.[23]

D.C.'s BMI of 30 kg/m^2 or more classifies him as obese. As little as a 5% to 10% loss in weight (5–11 kg) will provide global health benefits. Strategies that increase his aerobic activity, in addition to diet, can augment weight loss.

OTHER CARDIOVASCULAR RISK-REDUCTION STRATEGIES

CASE 9-1, QUESTION 13: Aside from treating hypertension, which other CV risk reduction strategies should be recommended in D.C.?

Smoking Cessation

Smoking is an important modifiable major CV risk factor. Cigarette smoking has been shown to independently increase CV and overall mortality, and cessation can decrease the incidence of CV disease.[43] Although smoking does not chronically lower BP, smoking cessation is strongly recommended to improve overall health. Hypertensive smokers should be continually educated about the risks associated with cigarette smoking and directed to behavior-modification programs that can assist smoking cessation efforts (see Chapter 91, Tobacco Use and Dependence).

Low-Dose Aspirin

Low-dose aspirin therapy (81 mg daily) is recommended by the US Preventive Services Task Force (USPSTF) for the primary prevention of MI in certain men 45 to79 years old and ischemic stroke in certain women 55 to 79 years old.[44] This recommendation is contingent on age and quantitative risk of CHD in men (e.g., Framingham risk scoring) and ischemic stroke in women. D.C. is not yet a candidate for low-dose aspirin based on his age.

Controlling Other Comorbid Diseases

In addition to treating hypertension and lowering BP to goal, controlling other comorbidities, which are themselves associated with increased CV risk, should be performed. When present, dyslipidemia, diabetes mellitus, obesity, and any other forms of CV disease should be diligently treated and controlled. D.C. has dyslipidemia and requires statin treatment (individuals without clinical atherosclerotic cardiovascular disease [ASCVD] or diabetes, who are 40–75 years of age with LDL-C 70–189 mg/dL, and have an estimated 10-year ASCVD risk of 7.5% or higher—D.C's calculated risk is 9.6%), and his CV risk would be reduced with better control of this condition (see Chapter 8, Dyslipidemias, Atherosclerosis, and Coronary Heart Disease).

Pharmacotherapy for Primary Prevention Patients

EVIDENCE-BASED RECOMMENDATIONS

CASE 9-1, QUESTION 14: Which treatment principles need to be considered when choosing an initial antihypertensive agent for D.C.?

Selecting an antihypertensive drug is complex. There are numerous choices, and all agents can effectively lower BP. Depending on the dose used, BP reductions are similar.[45] BP reduction, however, is only a surrogate end point of therapy and does not necessarily reflect overall effectiveness. Reducing hypertension-associated complications is the ultimate goal of treatment.

CASE 9-1, QUESTION 15: Which antihypertensive agents are appropriate first-line treatments for D.C.?

The JNC-8 report from 2013 outlines evidence-based pharmacotherapy recommendations accumulated from more than 50 years of clinical trials.[2] Because D.C. is black and does not have CKD, JNC-8 recommends thiazide-like diuretics or CCBs as first-choice antihypertensive therapy. This recommendation is based on the propensity of data showing reduced morbidity and mortality with these drug classes.[46]

Traditional landmark placebo-controlled hypertension studies (e.g., the SHEP,[39] Swedish Trial of Old Patients with Hypertension,[31] and Medical Research Council[29]) established that treating hypertension produces significant reductions in CV events (e.g., stroke and MI) and mortality. These traditional landmark trials used thiazide diuretic-based therapy, and thus thiazide diuretics have been the quintessential antihypertensive agent for most patients. Subsequently, several clinical trials evaluating newer agents (ACEI, ARB, and CCB) have provided additional evidence on CV event reduction.[12,40,47–67] Most of these trials do not include a placebo group (because it is unethical to use placebo in long-term studies); rather, they use an active antihypertensive agent as the comparator (often a thiazide diuretic or β-blocker or both). In those studies in which newer antihypertensive agents were compared with thiazide diuretics, very similar effects were seen. One of these studies was the Antihypertensive and Lipid-Lowering Treatment to Prevent Heart Attack Trial (ALLHAT).[48] In the ALLHAT, 33,357 patients with hypertension were randomly assigned in double-blind manner to thiazide diuretic (chlorthalidone), CCB (amlodipine), or ACEI (lisinopril)-based therapy. After a mean follow-up to 4.9 years, the incidence of the primary end point of fatal CHD or nonfatal MI was similar among all three treatment arms.

CASE 9-1, QUESTION 16: Should monotherapy or two-drug therapy be started in D.C. as his initial regimen?

A monotherapy approach is an option for D.C. Monotherapy with a CCB, or thiazide diuretic as recommended by JNC-8, will likely reduce his BP to less than 140/90 mm Hg. If D.C. is not black, ACEI and ARB would also be optimal alternatives.

SPECIAL POPULATIONS

Black Patients

CASE 9-1, QUESTION 17: How should D.C.'s race influence the selection of an antihypertensive regimen?

As monotherapy, it is well documented that a thiazide diuretic or a CCB is highly effective in lowering BP in black patients. This is likely because of the profile of low renin coupled with high plasma volume pattern of hypertension that is commonly seen in black patients with hypertension. Conversely, ACEI, ARB, or β-blocker monotherapy is less effective in lowering BP in blacks compared with white patients. However, when these agents are used in combination, especially with a thiazide diuretic, these race-based differences seen in BP lowering with monotherapy are abolished. This information may aid in selecting one drug option over another in a primary prevention patient, but does not apply to black patients with other comorbidities, in whom choice of therapy follows an evidence-based approach to selection based on the comorbidities.

D.C. does not have any other comorbidities for specific antihypertensive drug therapy. His first-line treatment option is CCB or thiazide diuretic. Monotherapy with either a thiazide diuretic or a CCB would be very effective in BP lowering; either of these two drugs is an acceptable treatment option for him.

Very Elderly Patients

CASE 9-2

QUESTION 1: B.D is an 83-year-old woman with a past medical history of hypertension, osteoporosis, and hypothyroidism. Her present medications are levothyroxine 100 mcg daily, alendronate 70 mg weekly, vitamin D 800 international units daily, and calcium carbonate 600 mg twice daily. She has been diagnosed with hypertension for 2 years, and it has been treated with lifestyle modifications (sodium restriction and exercise 3 times weekly). B.D. is 64 inches tall and weighs 55 kg. Her current BP is 160/78 mm Hg (160/80 mm Hg when repeated). All serum laboratory tests are normal. Her provider has been reluctant to start antihypertensive drug therapy because of B.D.'s age. How is treatment of B.D.'s hypertension different from that of a younger patient?

Older patients with hypertension (>65 years of age) have the lowest rates of BP control, and this rate decreases in even older populations.[1] Very elderly patients like B.D., similar to black patients, respond best to thiazides and CCBs and less to ACEIs, ARBs, and β-blockers when these are used as monotherapy. However, it is unclear whether these small differences in BP lowering among classes are clinically significant; thus they are all recommended as first choice per JNC-8 guidelines.

Isolated Systolic Hypertension

B.D. has isolated systolic hypertension (ISH), which is defined as an elevated SBP with a normal DBP.[2] This pattern of hypertension is most common in older patients and incurs a significant risk for CV disease. It was once thought that patients with ISH required high SBP to ensure normal perfusion of the heart and brain and that treating ISH would further lower DBP and worsen organ perfusion. Evidence clearly demonstrates, however, that treating ISH with antihypertensive drug therapy reduces the risk of CV events.[31,39,54] B.D.'s hypertension should be managed with drug therapy in addition to lifestyle modifications.

CASE 9-2, QUESTION 2: What data support antihypertensive drug therapy in patients who are very elderly, similar to B.D.?

The care of patients with ISH, including the very elderly, should follow the same general hypertension care principles that apply to all patients, with two exceptions. The first is that the BP goal is different. JNC-8 guideline recommends that BP goal of patients 60 years or older be <150/90 mm Hg.[2] Unless they also have CKD and are aged < 70 years, their BP goal would be similar to younger patient population, < 140/90 mm Hg. The second exception is that lower doses should be used when first starting therapy because of higher risk of developing orthostatic hypotension. Orthostatic hypotension occurs when standing upright results in an SBP decrease of more than 20 mm Hg (or a DBP decrease of more than 10 mm Hg) after 3 minutes of standing and is often accompanied by dizziness or fainting. This is a risk of rapid BP lowering. Orthostatic hypotension is more frequent in elderly patients (especially those with ISH), diabetes, autonomic dysfunction, volume depletion, and in patients taking certain drugs (i.e., diuretics, nitrates, α-blockers, psychotropic agents, and phosphodiesterase inhibitors). Antihypertensive dose increases should be gradual to minimize the risk of hypotension. Moreover, initial therapy with two drugs should probably be avoided in the elderly (age 80 years or older) owing to the increased risk of orthostatic hypotension.

The very elderly (i.e., patients 80 years or older) have traditionally been underrepresented in landmark placebo-controlled clinical trials. However, the HYVET was a placebo-controlled, randomized trial evaluating the effect of antihypertensive pharmacotherapy (ACEI with or without a thiazide-like diuretic) in patients with hypertension aged 80 years and older.[20] This trial was stopped prematurely, after 1.8 median years, owing to a significant reduction in overall mortality in the treatment arm. The HYVET provides compelling evidence that treatment of hypertension in the very elderly provides significant benefits. B.D. should be started on a low-dose thiazide diuretic or CCB for the treatment of her hypertension. For elderly patients with existing incontinence, diuretic therapy will be problematic. Under this circumstance, a CCB would be a more reasonable first-line option. Considering her advanced age, starting with monotherapy is appropriate to reduce her risk of orthostatic hypotension.

ADDITIONAL CONSIDERATIONS

CASE 9-3

QUESTION 1: You are developing a collaborative drug therapy management (CDTM) protocol for treatment of hypertension that will be used by clinical pharmacists. In your CDTM protocol, you include multiple pharmacotherapy options (ACEIs, ARBs, CCBs, and thiazide diuretics) as equally recommended in primary prevention patients. However, you wish to include additional guidance on how to select an individual drug class to treat hypertension. What additional factors should be considered in your protocol when selecting a first-line agent for a specific primary prevention patient?

It cannot be emphasized enough that selecting pharmacotherapy should follow an evidence-based philosophy. In patients with other comorbidities, certain antihypertensive drug classes are recommended in place of other options. In patients without other comorbidities, factors such as concomitant diseases, medication costs, serum electrolytes, and prior medication intolerances should be considered (Table 9-7). These are helpful when selecting initial therapy for a primary prevention patient who has more than one acceptable drug class as a first-line option or when selecting add-on therapy to further lower BP. These are discussed later in this chapter.

Table 9-7
Additional Considerations in Antihypertensive Drug Choice[a]

Antihypertensive Agent	Situations With Potentially Favorable Effects	Situations With Potentially Unfavorable Effects[b]	Avoid Use
ACEI	Low-normal potassium, elevated fasting glucose, microalbuminuria (with or without diabetes)	High-normal potassium or hyperkalemia	Pregnancy, bilateral renal artery stenosis, history of angioedema
ARB	Low-normal potassium, elevated fasting glucose, microalbuminuria (with or without diabetes)	High-normal potassium or hyperkalemia	Pregnancy, bilateral renal artery stenosis
CCB: dihydropyridine	Raynaud phenomenon, elderly patients with isolated systolic hypertension, cyclosporine-induced hypertension	Peripheral edema, left ventricular dysfunction (all except amlodipine and felodipine), high-normal heart rate or tachycardia	
CCB: nondihydropyridine	Raynaud phenomenon, migraine headache, supraventricular arrhythmias, high-normal heart rate or tachycardia	Peripheral edema, low-normal heart rate	Second- or third-degree heart block, left ventricular dysfunction
Thiazide diuretic	Osteoporosis or at increased risk for osteoporosis, high-normal potassium	Gout, hyponatremia, elevated fasting glucose (as monotherapy), low-normal potassium or sodium	

High-normal refers to patients in the high end of the normal range, but not above the range.
Low-normal refers to patients in the low end of the normal range, but not below the range.
[a]These considerations should never replace drug recommendations for a compelling indication.
[b]May use but requires diligent monitoring.
ACEI, angiotensin-converting enzyme inhibitor; ARB, angiotensin II receptor blocker; CCB, calcium-channel blocker.

The costs of treating hypertension and related complications are substantial to patients and health systems.[68] With expanding availability of generic agents, costs attributed to drug acquisition are small in comparison with expenses for laboratory evaluations, office visits, and medical care for hypertension-associated complications. Whenever possible, affordable regimens that do not compromise efficacy should be designed. Generic antihypertensive products are equally effective and less expensive than brand-name products, and all first- and second-line antihypertensive classes have generic alternatives. The frequency of administration can influence treatment. Once-daily administration assists adherence; all major drug classes contain agents that are either naturally long-acting or formulated in long-acting preparations.

Pharmacotherapy for Patients with Other Comorbidities

Case 9-3, Question 2: In your CDTM protocol, when should an ACEI or ARB be identified as first-line therapy ahead of other antihypertensive agents?

Unlike previous editions of JNC guidelines, JNC-8 guidelines did not specifically discuss how hypertension treatment should be managed in patients with other comorbidities (besides diabetes and CKD). However, there are other coexisting diseases or hypertension-associated complications in patients which may warrant the use of certain classes of antihypertensive because these agents show significant benefits in reducing CV morbidity or mortality in patients with those specific comorbidities.

DIABETES

Kidney disease and CV disease are both long-term hypertension-associated complications that are at high risk of occurring in patients with diabetes. JNC-8 recommends the same four classes of antihypertensive agents as first choice in nonblack patients with diabetes for primary prevention of CV events (ACEI, ARB, CCB, and thiazide diuretics) and thiazide diuretics and CCB in black patients.[2] When compared head to head, ACEIs are superior to dihydropyridine CCBs at reducing CV events.[57,58] Subgroup analyses of larger clinical trials further support CV event reduction with ACEIs and ARBs. Therefore, ACEI and ARB may be preferred initial antihypertensive therapy for a patient with diabetes if there is no other contraindication.

Case 9-3, Question 3: In your CDTM protocol, how should significant CKD be defined so that patients with CKD can be identified and treated appropriately?

CHRONIC KIDNEY DISEASE

It is common that CKD presents initially with microalbuminuria (30–299 mg albumin in a 24-hour urine collection) that can progress over the course of several years to overt kidney failure.[30] Progression is accelerated in the presence of both hypertension and diabetes. JNC-8 recommends ACEI or ARB therapy to be used as first-line therapy in CKD patients because both have been shown to reduce the progression of CKD in type 1 diabetes,[69] in type 2 diabetes,[61,62] and in those without diabetes.[65,70] Recently, ARB therapy has also been shown to decrease risk of developing microalbuminuria in patients with diabetes.[71]

Although many of the long-term benefits of ACEI or ARB therapy may be from BP lowering, their evidence base is robust enough to support their first-line use in CKD.[72,73] After ACEI or ARB therapy has been implemented, data support a CCB as the second drug because this has been shown to reduce progression of CKD better than a thiazide diuretic as the second drug added based on the Avoiding Cardiovascular Events through Combination Therapy in Patients Living with Systolic Hypertension (ACCOMPLISH) trial.[74]

Case 9-3, Question 4: In your CDTM protocol, although β-blocker is no longer considered as a first choice for primary prevention, are there any cases when β-blocker therapy would be identified as an appropriate first-line antihypertensive drug therapy?

CHRONIC AND ACUTE CORONARY ARTERY DISEASE

The American College of Cardiology (ACC)/AHA have guidelines for chronic CAD that recommend treatment with a β-blocker, followed shortly thereafter by the addition of an ACEI.[75] β-Blockers (those without intrinsic sympathomimetic activity [ISA]) decrease the risk of a subsequent MI or sudden cardiac death by decreasing the adrenergic burden on the heart, and progression of coronary atherosclerosis. ACEI therapy promotes cardiac remodeling, improves cardiac function, and reduces the risk of CV events. An ARB is an alternative in patients who do not tolerate an ACEI, because fewer data exist that assess the long-term impact of an ARB on CV events compared with an ACEI in chronic CAD.[76,77] A thiazide diuretic can be added to the core regimen of a β-blocker with an ACEI (or ARB) if additional BP reduction is needed. However, if an additional agent is needed to treat ischemic symptoms for patients with chronic stable angina, a dihydropyridine CCB can be added to this core regimen. If a β-blocker cannot be used because of intolerance or contraindication, a nondihydropyridine CCB can be used as an alternative to a β-blocker. Acute CAD, also called *acute coronary syndrome,* includes unstable angina, non–ST-segment elevation MI, and ST-segment elevation MI. The ACC/AHA guidelines for these conditions indicate a β-blocker as first-line pharmacotherapy.[78,79]

LEFT VENTRICULAR DYSFUNCTION

Pharmacotherapy for left ventricular dysfunction should include a three-drug combination of an ACEI, a β-blocker, and an aldosterone antagonist, plus loop diuretics depending on the need for diuresis.[79] ACEIs, β-blocker, and aldosterone antagonists, all have numerous landmark clinical trials showing reduced morbidity and mortality rates, whereas diuretics provide primarily symptomatic relief of edema.[79]

According to evidence-based medicine principles, only metoprolol, carvedilol, and bisoprolol are indicated for left ventricular dysfunction. Other β-blockers (e.g., atenolol) should not be used in patients with left ventricular dysfunction because they do not have supporting data demonstrating they reduce CV event rates in these patients. Patients should be clinically euvolemic and hemodynamically stable before adding a β-blocker. As discussed in Chapter 14 (Heart Failure), it is important to start with very low doses of a β-blocker, then slowly titrate upward over the course of several weeks to the recommended dosing range for left ventricular dysfunction. An ARB can be used as an alternative to an ACEI.[79]

Potassium serum concentrations must be carefully monitored in the situation when ACEI (or ARB) and aldosterone antagonist are used together. Alternatively, the combination of hydralazine with isosorbide dinitrate can be added in black patients.[80] This combination has been demonstrated to improve CV outcome in this patient population.

Monitoring Therapy

Four aspects of treatment must always be considered: (a) BP response to attain goal, (b) adherence with lifestyle modifications and pharmacotherapy, (c) progression to hypertension-associated complications, and (d) drug-related toxicity.

Reduction in BP should be evaluated 1 to 4 weeks after starting or modifying therapy for most patients. BP usually begins to decrease within 1 to 2 weeks of starting an agent, but steady-state antihypertensive effects can take up to 4 weeks. If patients are in hypertensive crisis, evaluation should occur sooner, within hours to days (see Chapter 16, Hypertensive Crises).

Two BP values separated by at least 1 minute should be measured during each clinical evaluation, with the average used to make a proper assessment. If dehydration or orthostatic hypotension is suspected, BP should be measured in both the seated and standing positions to detect orthostatic changes. For routine monitoring, measuring BP in the seated position is sufficient. Self-BP monitoring values should be considered if available. Normally, however, they are slightly lower (5 mm Hg) than clinical values even in patients without white-coat hypertension. For example, patients with a goal BP value of less than 140/90 mm Hg should have home measurements that are less than 135/85 mm Hg.[7]

All patients should be questioned in a nonthreatening manner regarding adherence with lifestyle modifications and drug therapy. This is especially important for complex regimens, when drug intolerance is likely, or when financial constraints hinder acquisition of medications. Evaluating hypertension-associated complications and drug side effects are essential. New hypertension-associated complications may necessitate changes to treat a compelling indication or attain a new BP goal. Drug-related side effects may similarly require therapy modifications.

CLINICAL SCENARIOS

Diuretics

CASE 9-4

Question 1: B.A. is a 58-year-old woman who is postmenopausal, does not smoke, and never drinks alcohol. Since being diagnosed with hypertension, she has modified her diet, begun routine aerobic exercise, and has lost 10 kg in the past 18 months. She now weighs 72 kg and is 165 cm tall. Her BP is now 150/94 mm Hg (150/92 mm Hg when repeated) and has consistently remained near this value for the past year. Her BP when first diagnosed was 156/96 mm Hg. Physical examination shows no LVH and no retinopathy. Urinalysis is negative for protein. Other laboratory tests are normal, except for dyslipidemia. B.A. has no health insurance and is concerned about the cost of therapy. She takes over-the-counter calcium with vitamin D, and her provider wants to start HCTZ 25 mg/day. Is HCTZ an appropriate agent for B.A.?

B.A. is a primary prevention patient with uncontrolled hypertension. According to the JNC-8, her BP goal is less than 140/90 mm Hg.[2] Initial monotherapy is reasonable. Appropriate first-line treatment options include an ACEI, ARB, CCB, or thiazide diuretic. All of these drug classes have generic options and should be easily affordable for B.A. A thiazide diuretic may also benefit her osteoporosis (Table 9-7) and is an appropriate choice. Several types of diuretics are used to manage hypertension (Table 9-8).[26] All lower BP, with differences being duration of action, potency of diuresis, and electrolyte abnormalities.

THIAZIDES

Thiazides are diuretics of choice for most patients with hypertension. Similar to loop diuretics, an initial diuresis is experienced. After approximately 4 to 6 weeks of thiazide diuretic therapy, diuresis dissipates, however, and is supplanted by a decrease in PVR, which is responsible for sustaining antihypertensive effects.

Case 9-4, Question 2: How should a thiazide diuretic be started in B.A.?

Table 9-8
Diuretics in Hypertension

Category	Selected Products	Usual Dosage Range (mg/day)	Dosing Frequency
Thiazide and thiazide-like	Chlorthalidone	12.5–25	Daily
	Hydrochlorothiazide	12.5–25	Daily
	Indapamide	1.25–5	Daily
	Metolazone	2.5–10	Daily
	Metolazone	0.5–1.0	Daily
Loop	Bumetanide	0.5–4	BID
	Furosemide	20–80	BID
	Torsemide	2.5–10	Daily
Potassium-sparing	Amiloride	5–10	Daily to BID
	Triamterene	50–100	Daily to BID
Potassium-sparing combination	Triamterene/HCTZ	37.5/25–75/50	Daily
	Spironolactone/HCTZ	25/25–50/50	Daily
	Amiloride/HCTZ	5–10/50–100	Daily
Aldosterone antagonist	Eplerenone	50–100	Daily to BID
	Spironolactone	12.5–50	Daily to BID

BID, 2 times daily; HCTZ, hydrochlorothiazide.

Hydrochlorothiazide Versus Chlorthalidone

HCTZ and chlorthalidone have been used in several major outcome trials, although only chlorthalidone-based regimens have proven to be of benefit in the low doses commonly used in practice today.[29,31,39,48,54,81,82] Both agents are inexpensive and dosed once daily, but HCTZ is most frequently used in the United States and is more widely available in fixed-dose combination products. The usual starting dose of HCTZ or chlorthalidone is 12.5 mg once daily. A maintenance dose of 25 mg once daily can effectively lower BP and has a low incidence of side effects (e.g., hypokalemia and hyperuricemia) that can be managed with routine monitoring.[33,45,46]

Significant controversy surrounds the comparative efficacy of HCTZ and chlorthalidone. Most clinicians, including the AHA, assume a class effect for these two drugs.[10] However, class effects can be legitimized only after assurance of equipotent dosing; for antihypertensives, when they are not directly compared in a CV event trial, it assumes that if two agents achieve similar BP lowering then both achieve similar reduction in CV events. With regard to HCTZ and chlorthalidone, this assumption is unproven. Chlorthalidone is more potent on a milligram per milligram basis and has a longer half-life than HCTZ (50–60 hours vs. 9–10 hours).[83] Based on a comparative study using 24-hour ABPM, it appears that the equipotent dose of chlorthalidone 25 mg daily is HCTZ 50 mg daily, but this dose of HCTZ is unpopular because of increased side effects. Consequently, it is believed by some that the antihypertensive efficacy of chlorthalidone is greater than HCTZ when contemporary doses are used; the 12.5- to 25-mg doses of chlorthalidone do not appear to significantly increase the risk of hypokalemia more so than HCTZ.[84] Complicating this issue is evidence demonstrating that office BP tends to overestimate the response to HCTZ, and the 24-hour BP lowering with HCTZ is only comparable to other common agents (ACEI, ARB, CCB, and even β-blocker) when 50 mg daily is used.[85] Recently, data from the Multiple Risk Factor Intervention Trial indicate that chlorthalidone reduces CV events more than HCTZ.[86] Although chlorthalidone is the most optimal and evidence-based thiazide diuretic for B.A., HCTZ remains currently accepted in the clinical environment as a reasonable thiazide diuretic for hypertension assuming her BP goal can be readily achieved with its use.

LOOP DIURETICS

Loop diuretics produce a more potent diuresis, but a smaller decrease in PVR, and less vasodilation than thiazide diuretics. They are subject to a significant postdose antinatriuretic period, which offsets their antihypertensive effect. Therefore, a thiazide is more effective at lowering BP than loop diuretics in most patients. Loop diuretics are usually considered only for patients with severe CKD (estimated GFR <30 mL/minute/1.73 m^2), left ventricular dysfunction, or severe edema. In these patients, potent diuresis is often needed. Furosemide has a short duration of effect and should be given twice daily when used in hypertension, whereas torsemide has a longer duration of action and can be given once daily.

POTASSIUM-SPARING DIURETICS

Potassium-sparing diuretics (triamterene and amiloride) should be reserved for patients who experience hypokalemia while on a thiazide diuretic. With low-dose thiazide diuretics, less than 25% of patients develop hypokalemia, and most cases are not severe. Triamterene and amiloride usually do not provide significant additional BP lowering when added to a thiazide diuretic. Several fixed-dose products are available that include HCTZ with triamterene or amiloride. Empirically starting all patients with hypertension treated with a thiazide diuretic on triamterene or amiloride to avoid hypokalemia is not rational or necessary unless baseline serum potassium is in the low-normal range.

A thiazide diuretic is an optimal first-line option in primary prevention in patients like B.A., and she has no contraindications (Table 9-9). Although B.A. has dyslipidemia, thiazide diuretics are unlikely to have a clinically significant effect on cholesterol when used in low doses.[87,88] An appropriate starting dose of HCTZ is 12.5 or 25 mg daily. B.A. has no additional risks for orthostatic hypotension, so starting at the higher 25-mg daily dose is safe and will have a better chance of lowering her BP to goal than the lower 12.5-mg dose because most antihypertensive agents

Table 9-9

Side Effects and Contraindications of Antihypertensive Agents

	Side Effects			
	Innocuous but Sometimes Annoying	**Potentially Harmful**	**Usually Requires Cessation of Therapy, at Least Temporarily**	**Contraindications**
Thiazide diuretics	Increased urination (at onset of therapy), muscle cramps, hyperuricemia (without gout)	Hypokalemia,[a] hyponatremia, hyperglycemia, hypovolemia, pancreatitis, photosensitivity, hypercholesterolemia, hypertriglyceridemia, hyperuricemia with gout, orthostatic hypotension (more frequent in elderly)	Hypercalcemia, azotemia, skin rash (cross-reacts with only certain sulfonamide allergies), purpura, bone marrow depression, lithium toxicity in patients on lithium therapy, hyponatremia	Anuria, kidney failure
Loop diuretics	Increased urination, muscle cramps, hyperuricemia (less than with thiazides)	Hypokalemia,[a] hyperglycemia, hypovolemia, pancreatitis, hypercholesterolemia, hypertriglyceridemia, hearing loss with large IV doses, orthostatic hypotension (more pronounced in elderly)	Hyponatremia, hypocalcemia, azotemia, skin rash (cross-reacts with only certain sulfonamide allergies), photosensitivity, lithium toxicity in patients on lithium therapy	Anuria
ACEI	Dizziness, dry cough	Orthostatic hypotension (more pronounced in elderly treated with a diuretic), increased serum creatinine, increased potassium	Angioedema, severe hyperkalemia, increase in serum creatinine >35%	Bilateral renal artery stenosis, volume depletion, hyponatremia, pregnancy, history of angioedema
ARB	Dizziness	Orthostatic hypotension (more pronounced in elderly treated with a diuretic), increased serum creatinine, increased potassium	Severe hyperkalemia, increase in serum creatinine >35%	Bilateral renal artery stenosis, volume depletion, hyponatremia, pregnancy
CCB: dihydropyridines	Dizziness, headache, flushing	Peripheral edema, tachycardia	Significant peripheral edema	Left ventricular dysfunction (not with amlodipine or felodipine)
CCB: nondihydropyridines	Dizziness, headache, constipation	Bradycardia	Heart block, left ventricular dysfunction, interactions with certain drugs	Left ventricular dysfunction, second- or third-degree heart block, sick sinus syndrome
β-Blocker	Bradycardia, weakness, exercise intolerance	Masking the symptoms of hypoglycemia in diabetes, hyperglycemia, aggravation of peripheral arterial disease, erectile dysfunction, increased triglycerides, decreased HDL-C	Left ventricular dysfunction (not with carvedilol, metoprolol, bisoprolol), bronchospasm in patients with asthma or COPD (more pronounced with nonselective agents)	Severe asthma, second- or third-degree heart block, acute left ventricular dysfunction exacerbation, coronary artery disease for agents with intrinsic sympathomimetic activity
Aldosterone antagonist	Menstrual irregularities (spironolactone only) or gynecomastia (spironolactone only)	Increased potassium	Hyperkalemia, hyponatremia	Kidney failure, kidney impairment (for eplerenone: CrCl <50 mL/min, or type 2 diabetes with proteinuria, and creatinine >1.8 in women, >2.0 in men), hyperkalemia, hyponatremia

[a]Routine addition of potassium supplementation or empiric concurrent potassium-sparing diuretics should be discouraged unless hypokalemia is demonstrated, the patient is taking digoxin, or potassium is in the low-normal range.

ACEI, angiotensin-converting enzyme inhibitor; ARB, angiotensin II receptor blocker; CCB, calcium-channel blocker; COPD, chronic obstructive pulmonary disease; CrCl, creatinine clearance; HDL-C, high-density lipoprotein cholesterol; IV, intravenous.

provide a 10-mm Hg reduction in SBP and 5-mm Hg reduction in DBP with a standard starting dose.[89]

PATIENT EDUCATION

CASE 9-4, QUESTION 3: B.A. is prescribed HCTZ 25 mg daily. How should she be counseled regarding this therapy?

Several counseling points are summarized in Table 9-6. Some patients disregard lifestyle modifications when they start antihypertensive therapy, so B.A. must be encouraged to continue lifestyle modification to maximize her response to drug therapy. B.A. should be informed that diuretics lower both BP and risk of CV events and that taking her dose at about the same time each morning to minimize nocturia and provide consistent effects is recommended. B.A. should expect to experience increased urination when starting HCTZ, but should be informed that this diminishes with time. Inform B.A. that missed doses should be taken as soon as possible within the same day, but doubling doses the next day is not recommended. The potential for hypokalemia, which is easily identified and managed, and the need for routine monitoring of serum potassium should be reviewed. She should be counseled on the signs and symptoms of electrolyte abnormalities (e.g., leg cramps and muscle weakness) and encouraged to report these to her health care provider if they occur. Increasing dietary intake of potassium-rich foods to minimize electrolyte depletion is an option to minimize potassium loss. This should be encouraged only with thiazide and loop diuretics, but not with potassium-sparing agents.

Despite improvements with lifestyle modifications and reported adherence with HCTZ, B.A.'s goal BP of less than 140/90 mm Hg has not been met (her BP average is 141/83 mm Hg). No new signs of hypertension-associated complications are seen. She should be encouraged to continue with her current efforts, but other interventions are warranted.

CASE 9-4, QUESTION 4: After 4 weeks of HCTZ 25 mg daily, B.A. has no complaints and has not missed a dose. She is exercising and is following the DASH diet. Her BP values are 142/86 mm Hg (140/84 mm Hg when repeated). Her fasting laboratory values are as follows:

Serum potassium, 3.8 mEq/L
Uric acid, 7.3 mg/dL
Glucose, 99 mg/dL

All other values are unchanged. Last month, potassium was 4.0 mEq/L, uric acid was 6.8 mg/dL, and fasting glucose was 95 mg/dL. What is your assessment regarding the efficacy and toxicity of B.A.'s antihypertensive therapy?

POTASSIUM LOSS

Adverse reactions with low-dose thiazide diuretics (e.g., HCTZ 12.5–25 mg daily) are minimal compared with higher-dose therapy (HCTZ > 25 mg daily). Moreover, side effects and tolerability with low-dose thiazide diuretic therapy are similar to other first-line drug therapy options and not much higher than what is seen with placebo.[33,35,36] Regardless, signs and symptoms of electrolyte and metabolic changes, such as hypokalemia, hyponatremia, hyperglycemia, or hyperuricemia, should be evaluated in all patients treated with thiazide diuretics. B.A. has experienced small changes in serum potassium and uric acid, which are typical thiazide-induced abnormalities. B.A. should be questioned about muscle cramps or weakness, which can be caused by decreased potassium.

CASE 9-4, QUESTION 5: Is B.A.'s potassium decrease concerning? If so, how should this be managed?

Most total body potassium is intracellular (~98%). Thiazide diuretics can cause potassium loss and can result in potassium serum concentrations in the low end of the normal range. However, with low-dose therapy, overt hypokalemia is not common. HCTZ in doses of 12.5, 25, and 50 mg daily can decrease serum potassium by an average of 0.21, 0.34, and 0.5 mEq/L, respectively.[33,87,88] This is usually considered mild, with serum potassium concentrations reaching a nadir within the first month of therapy and remaining stable thereafter. Restriction of dietary sodium in patients receiving diuretic therapy has been shown to reduce the loss of potassium and should be encouraged in B.A.[90]

Hypokalemia

CASE 9-4, QUESTION 6: When is potassium correction needed to manage diuretic-induced hypokalemia?

B.A.'s potassium is within the normal range. Potassium replacement is not indicated. Diuretic-associated hypokalemia should be treated when serum concentrations are below normal regardless of whether symptoms (e.g., muscle cramps) are present. Serum potassium should be measured at baseline and 2 to 4 weeks after initiating therapy or increasing the diuretic dose.

Potassium-rich foods (e.g., dried fruit, bananas, potatoes, and avocados) may help prevent small decreases in potassium, but they cannot be used as sole therapy to correct hypokalemia. For instance, one medium-size banana has only 11.5 mEq of potassium. The usual replacement dose of prescribed potassium chloride is 20 to 40 mEq/day but can range from 10 to more than 100 mEq/day. Potassium chloride, bicarbonate, gluconate, acetate, and citrate salts are available for potassium replacement therapy. Rather than supplement potassium, which does not effectively correct the underlying mechanisms responsible for hypokalemia, a more appropriate and effective strategy to manage diuretic-induced hypokalemia is to add a potassium-sparing diuretic. Hypomagnesemia often accompanies diuretic-induced hypokalemia and must be normalized before hypokalemia can be effectively reversed.

Other Metabolic Abnormalities

CASE 9-4, QUESTION 7: How should the increase in B.A.'s uric acid be managed?

Thiazide diuretics can increase serum uric acid concentrations in a dose-dependent fashion. Uric acid increases also occur with loop diuretics, but to a lesser extent. Increased proximal tubular renal reabsorption, decreased tubular secretion, or increased postsecretory reabsorption of uric acid contributes to diuretic-induced hyperuricemia. Thiazide-induced hyperuricemia is usually small (≤0.5 mg/dL) and is not clinically significant in patients without a history of gout.[89] For patients with a history of gout, diuretics are not contraindicated, but an increase in serum uric acid may require a decrease in dose or possibly discontinuation of the diuretic, especially for those not on preventive antihyperuricemic therapy (e.g., allopurinol and febuxostat). Acute gouty arthritis precipitated by diuretic therapy should be treated, and the diuretic should be discontinued, at least temporarily. Future use of the diuretic will depend on whether long-term antihyperuricemic therapy is to be added and the risk versus benefit for continuing the diuretic. B.A.'s serum uric acid concentration is elevated, but switching to a different agent or lowering the dose of HCTZ is unnecessary because she is not symptomatic of gout.

It should be noted that changes in parameters such as uric acid can be informative regarding dosing. When a given dose of a diuretic fails to lower BP, it is often unclear as to whether the failure is a result of mechanisms other than volume driving the hypertension or a result of the diuretic dose being insufficient to achieve the desired physiologic effect. For example, the absence of an increase in uric acid suggests that the administered dose was insufficient, and that a higher dose merits consideration. In B.A.'s case, the increase in uric acid confirms that the given dose was sufficient to have had a physiologic effect, so adding an antihypertensive agent from a different drug class would be preferable to increasing the diuretic dose if further BP lowering is necessary.

CASE 9-4, QUESTION 8: How much will HCTZ alter B.A.'s cholesterol values?

Small increases in LDL-C and triglycerides are potential side effects of diuretic therapy. Dietary fat restrictions help minimize, but do not necessarily prevent, these effects. Contrary to other biochemical disturbances, diuretic-induced changes in the lipid profile are not dose related, and overall changes are small. Many clinical trials lasting more than 1 year have shown that these alterations with diuretic therapy are not sustained with prolonged use.[87,88] Even if these changes are persistent, they are very small and are not clinically significant. The presence of dyslipidemia should never be a reason to avoid diuretic therapy.

CASE 9-4, QUESTION 9: What other potential electrolyte abnormalities should be evaluated in B.A. because of her thiazide diuretic therapy?

Hyponatremia is a serious, yet infrequent, adverse effect of diuretics. Changes in sodium concentrations are usually small, and the majority of patients are usually asymptomatic. Frail, elderly women appear more susceptible to experiencing severe hyponatremia (<120 mEq/L) from diuretics, which rarely occurs, but definitely requires discontinuation of therapy. Attention should be paid to the presence of other medications that can contribute to hyponatremia (e.g., selective serotonin reuptake inhibitors and psychotropic drugs), and patients should be counseled to avoid excessive free water intake.

Hypomagnesemia is an often overlooked metabolic complication of diuretic therapy. Both thiazide and loop diuretics increase urinary excretion of magnesium in a dose-dependent manner. Symptoms of significant hypomagnesemia include muscle weakness, muscle tremor or twitching, mental status changes, and cardiac arrhythmias. Presence of these symptoms would necessitate magnesium supplementation or use of a potassium-sparing agent as noted above if hypokalemia is also present.

Thiazide diuretics decrease urinary calcium excretion and can be used to prevent calcium-related kidney stones. The retention of calcium does not significantly increase serum calcium concentrations and does not place patients at risk for hypercalcemia. This effect, however, may be beneficial in women at risk for osteoporosis (e.g., postmenopausal) such as B.A. or in patients with osteoporosis. Conversely, loop diuretics increase renal clearance of calcium.

Reasons for Inadequate BP Control

CASE 9-4, QUESTION 10: What are common reasons for inadequate patient response to antihypertensive pharmacotherapy?

B.A. has been on her current dose of HCTZ for 4 weeks. The full antihypertensive effect of HCTZ has been achieved, but she still has uncontrolled hypertension. She has had a response, but it remains inadequate. Potential reasons for an inadequate response, or lack of attaining BP goal values, with an antihypertensive should be considered before modifying her drug therapy regimen (Table 9-10). A comprehensive medication history and medical evaluation is needed to rule out identifiable causes, in particular nonadherence to the prescribed regimen. Her BP reduction with HCTZ is typical. Her kidney function is good, and no evidence exists of edema, so volume overload is unlikely. There are no apparent secondary causes of elevated BP. It is reasonable to conclude that B.A. needs additional therapy to achieve her goal BP. It is very common that most patients require two or more agents to attain BP goal values.

Modifying Therapy

When patient cannot achieve optimal BP control with initial antihypertensive, JNC-8 recommends that the dose of the first drug may be increased (if patient has not yet achieved maximum dose of the agent), or low dose of a second agent may be added. Second agents of choice would be ACEI, ARB, CCB, or thiazide diuretics, whichever one the patient is not already taking.[2] B.A.'s present dose of HCTZ is appropriate and should not be increased to the maximal recommended dose of 50 mg daily (considered high-dose therapy) because it may increase risk of electrolyte and metabolic side effects. B.A.'s potassium dropped to 3.8 mEq/L with HCTZ, and further dosage increases may produce hypokalemia (<3.5 mEq/L) requiring correction. Her hyperuricemia may also be worsened. The slightly increased antihypertensive response expected from increasing to 50 mg/day is therefore not justified.[85] Discontinuing HCTZ and starting a different agent is an option, but it is not prudent to abandon the HCTZ; she tolerated the treatment and experienced a reasonable BP response, and the

Table 9-10
Reasons for Not Attaining Goal Blood Pressure Despite Antihypertensive Pharmacotherapy

Drug Related	Health Condition or Lifestyle Related	Other
Nonadherence	Volume overload	Improper blood pressure measurement
Inadequate antihypertensive dose	Excess sodium intake	Resistant hypertension
Inappropriate antihypertensive combination therapy	Volume retention from chronic kidney disease	White-coat hypertension
Inadequate diuretic therapy	Secondary disease causes (Table 9-2)	Pseudohypertension
Secondary drug-induced causes (Table 9-2)	Obesity	
Clinician's failure to intensify or augment therapy (i.e., clinical inertia)	Excessive alcohol intake	

HCTZ will augment the efficacy of nearly any other agent that may be added and may benefit her osteoporosis.

TWO-DRUG REGIMENS

The role of two-drug regimens in the treatment of hypertension is very clear. Most patients require multiple agents for BP control.

Adding a second agent to B.A.'s regimen is needed to reduce BP to her goal. She is a primary prevention patient, so three potential add-on antihypertensive agents that are considered first-line include an ACEI, ARB, or CCB. Ideally, a combination of two drugs with different mechanisms of action should be selected to produce a complementary effect to lower BP.

Adding an ACEI or ARB to B.A.'s HCTZ will result in additive antihypertensive effects that are independent of reversing fluid retention. Diuretics reduce BP initially by decreasing fluid volume, but maintain their antihypertensive effects by lowering PVR. BP lowering, however, can stimulate renin release from the kidney and activate the RAAS. This compensatory mechanism is an in vivo attempt to neutralize BP changes and regulate fluid loss. An ACEI or an ARB blocks the RAAS, explaining why combinations of these agents with diuretics are additive. Data from the ACCOMPLISH trial support combination therapy for hypertension. In this randomized, double-blind trial, 11,506 patients with hypertension were randomly assigned to the combination of an ACEI with thiazide diuretic or an ACEI with CCB.[74] After a mean follow-up of 3 years, the risk of CV events was significantly lower with the ACEI with CCB combination. Switching B.A.'s HCTZ to an ACEI with CCB may be more effective in lowering CV events than adding an ACEI to her current HCTZ. This would be an acceptable modification. However, considering her response to HCTZ, simply adding an ACEI is also reasonable.

Fixed-Dose Combination Products

Several fixed-dose combination products including two or three drugs are available.

Although individual dose titration is not simple with fixed-dose combination products, their use can reduce the number of tablets or capsules taken by patients. This has been demonstrated to improve adherence compared with using two separate single-drug products.[91] Improved adherence may increase the likelihood of achieving goal BP values.

Most fixed-dose combinations include a thiazide diuretic, and many are available generically. Other fixed-dose combination products combine a CCB with either an ACEI or ARB. These combinations, similar to a thiazide with an ACE or ARB, are highly effective in lowering BP. An economic advantage may even exist to using a fixed-dose combination if it allows the patient to receive two drugs for one medication copayment. The Simplified Treatment Intervention To Control Hypertension study demonstrated that initiating therapy with a fixed-dose combination product according to a treatment algorithm was superior in attaining goal BP values when compared with usual management according to national guidelines.[92] These data further support using a fixed-dose combination product for initial therapy.

B.A. is a candidate for fixed-dose combination product. If the combination of an ACEI with HCTZ is selected for her, many options exist. All of the products with an ACEI also include HCTZ at the dose she is currently on. If the combination of an ACEI with a CCB is selected, fewer options exist, but there are products that contain an ACEI with a dihydropyridine CCB or a nondihydropyridine CCB. Cost should be considered because this is a concern for B.A. Multiple ACEI with thiazide diuretic combinations are available generically, but there is only one generic ACEI with CCB combination. Many ARBs are gradually becoming generic, so those may be potential option as well; therefore a combination of ARB plus thiazide diuretic may be an option too eventually.

Step-Down Therapy

CASE 9-5

QUESTION 1: T.J. is a 58-year-old man with a 10-year history of hypertension. He has been treated with lisinopril/HCTZ 20/25 mg daily and amlodipine 10 mg daily for more than 2 years, and his BP has been well controlled during this time. His BP at an office visit today is 128/74 and 130/72 mm Hg. He has no significant past medical history and has no hypertension-associated complications, but he is a smoker. T.J. also has dyslipidemia, which is well controlled with simvastatin 40 mg daily. He denies dizziness or difficulties with his medications. Should T.J.'s antihypertensive therapy be changed to reduce his medication doses or possibly discontinue some of his medications?

Some patients with hypertension can have their BP medications slowly withdrawn, resulting in normal BP values for weeks or months after discontinuation of their medications. This is called *step-down therapy.* However, it is not a feasible option for most patients with hypertension. Primary prevention patients with no additional major CV risk factors who have very well controlled BP for at least 1 year might be eligible for a trial of step-down therapy. This option should not be considered for patients with other major CV risk factors or hypertension-associated complications. Step-down therapy consists of attempting to gradually decrease the dosage, the number of antihypertensive drugs, or both without compromising BP control. Abrupt or large dosage reductions should be avoided because of the risk of rapid return of uncontrolled BP and even rebound surges in BP (as is seen with rapid withdrawal of a β-blocker or an α_2-agonist).

Step-down therapy is most often plausible for patients who have lost significant amounts of weight or have drastically changed their lifestyle. Any attempt at step-down therapy must be accompanied by scheduled follow-up evaluations because BP values can rise over the course of months to years after drug discontinuation, especially if lifestyle modifications are not maintained. With adherence to lifestyle modifications (weight loss and reduction in sodium and alcohol), nearly 70% of patients remained free of antihypertensives for up to 1 year after being withdrawn from thiazide-based therapy in the Hypertension Control Program.[93]

Step-down therapy in T.J. is not an option. Although he does not have hypertension-associated complications, he has multiple major CV risk factors for development of CV disease.

Angiotensin-Converting Enzyme Inhibitor

CASE 9-6

QUESTION 1: A.R. is a 49-year-old black woman with type 2 diabetes. She started lisinopril 10 mg daily 2 weeks ago when her BP values were around155/90 mm Hg. Since then, she has had weekly BP measurements, and her values have averaged 145/85 mm Hg despite strict adherence to her lifestyle modifications. Her BP today is 144/84 mm Hg (142/88 mm Hg when repeated), and her heart rate is 78 beats/minute. She is not a smoker, and her BMI is 29 kg/m^2. All her laboratory test results, including kidney function, are within normal limits, except that her spot urine albumin-to-creatinine ratio is 80 mg/g (2 weeks ago it was 90 mg/g). Is 2 weeks of lisinopril therapy long enough to assess her antihypertensive response?

Table 9-11
Angiotensin-Converting Enzyme Inhibitors in Hypertension

Drug	Usual Starting Dose (mg/day)[a]	Usual Dosage Range (mg/day)	Dosing Frequency
Benazepril	10	20–40	Daily to BID
Captopril	25	50–100	BID to TID
Enalapril	5	10–40	Daily to BID
Fosinopril	10	20–40	Daily
Lisinopril	10	20–40	Daily
Moexipril	7.5	7.5–30	Daily to BID
Perindopril	4	4–16	Daily
Quinapril	10	20–80	Daily to BID
Ramipril	2.5	2.5–20	Daily to BID
Trandolapril	1	2–4	Daily

[a]Starting dose may be decreased 50% if patient is volume depleted, has acute heart failure exacerbation, or is very elderly (≥75 year).
BID, 2 times daily; TID, 3 times daily.

Several ACEIs are available (Table 9-11). Most ACEIs are dosed once daily in hypertension (Table 9-11). In general, most ACEIs, if used in equivalent doses, are considered interchangeable.

The time to reach steady-state BP conditions is similar to what is seen with other antihypertensive agents. It may take several weeks before the full antihypertensive effects of ACEIs are seen. Therefore, evaluating BP response 2 to 4 weeks after starting or changing the dose of an ACEI is appropriate. A.R. has been taking lisinopril for 2 weeks, and her present BP should be used to determine whether she has attained goal. Both her BP range during the past few weeks and today's average BP are above her goal of less than 140/90 mm Hg.

CASE 9-6, QUESTION 2: Why should A.R. have serum potassium and serum creatinine monitored while on lisinopril therapy?

Serum potassium can increase with ACEI therapy as a result of aldosterone reduction. Potassium increases with ACEI monotherapy are small (typically 0.1 to 0.2 mEq/L) and usually do not cause hyperkalemia. This risk is increased when ACEIs are used in patients with significant CKD (GFR <60 mL/minute/1.73 m^2) or when they are used in combination with other drugs that can also raise potassium.

ACEI therapy can also cause a small increase in serum creatinine owing to decreased vasoconstriction of the efferent arteriole in the kidney. This results in a minor decrease in GFR that may be evidenced by a small increase in serum creatinine. A common mistake is to discontinue an ACEI in response to this rise in serum creatinine. Increases in serum creatinine of up to 30% from the baseline creatinine value are safe and anticipated. In these patients, the ACEI should be continued because a strong association exists between acute increases in serum creatinine of up to 30% that stabilize within the first 2 months of ACEI therapy and long-term preservation of renal function.[94] Patients with an increase in serum creatinine of greater than 30% should have their ACEI therapy temporarily discontinued, as this may indicate other medical problems. Some of these problems can be underlying renal disease (such as bilateral renal artery stenosis) or other situations that may be compromising renal blood flow (e.g., volume depletion, concomitant nonsteroidal antiinflammatory drug therapy, and heart failure). Serum potassium and serum creatinine, in addition to BP, should be monitored in A.R. within 2 to 4 weeks after starting ACEI therapy or increasing the dose.

CASE 9-6, QUESTION 3: A.R.'s lisinopril dose is increased to 20 mg daily. Will this doubling of her dose place her at risk for significant hypotension?

The very elderly patients with volume depletion or patients with heart failure exacerbation may experience a significant first-dose response to an ACEI. This can manifest as orthostatic hypotension, dizziness, or syncope. The increased pretreatment activity of the RAAS, coupled with blockade of this system, explains this effect. In these patients, ACEI therapy should be initiated at half the normal dose (Table 9-11), followed by slow titration to standard doses.

Concurrent diuretic therapy may predispose some patients to first-dose hypotension. When ACEIs were first approved, dosing guidelines recommended starting at half the standard dose of the ACEI, decreasing the dose of the diuretic, or stopping the diuretic before initiating the ACEI. This was owing to fear that BP would sharply and acutely drop. These dosing recommendations are not necessary unless the patient is hemodynamically unstable (volume depleted, hyponatremic, or poorly compensated heart failure) or very elderly. A.R. does not have any of these characteristics and can safely increase her dose of lisinopril.

CASE 9-6, QUESTION 4: Is an ACEI an effective therapy in a black patient such as A.R.?

ACEI monotherapy is generally more effective at lowering BP in white patients than in black or elderly patients. In fact, JNC-8 guideline does not recommend the use of ACEI or ARB as first-choice antihypertensive in black patients for primary prevention, including those with diabetes (unless they have CKD).[2] Elderly and black patients are more likely to have low renin hypertension, which may partially explain some of the differences in response. Nevertheless, many of these patients still respond to ACEIs as monotherapy just to a less extent. Combination therapy, especially with a thiazide diuretic, usually mitigates this race- and age-related difference in BP response.

When an antihypertensive agent is being selected as initial monotherapy in a black patient, an ACEI should generally not be chosen unless the patient has CKD. A thiazide diuretic or CCB is otherwise preferred. In this case, considering switching to a different agent (thiazide and CCB) may be a good alternative to improve A.R.'s BP control. Of note, black patients have a twofold to fourfold increased risk of angioedema and cough with ACEIs compared with white patients.[95] This does not preclude ACEI use in black patients unless there is a prior history of angioedema.

CASE 9-6, QUESTION 5: A.R. has microalbuminuria, and lisinopril may help preserve kidney function. However, is there a risk that lisinopril can cause acute renal dysfunction?

The ACEIs are effective in patients with hypertension-associated renal disease. They are contraindicated, however, in several situations, including bilateral renal artery stenosis, pregnancy, and volume depletion (Table 9-9). In the case of bilateral renal artery stenosis or volume depletion, high angiotensin concentrations maintain renal blood flow, and acute renal dysfunction can occur when an ACEI is started. Because it is often not known whether a patient has bilateral renal artery stenosis, problems with ACEI can be minimized by starting with recommended doses and careful monitoring of serum creatinine within 2 to 4 weeks of starting therapy. Modest elevations in serum creatinine that are less than 30% (for baseline creatinine values <3.0 mg/dL) do not warrant adjustment in therapy.[94] If greater increases occur, ACEI therapy should be stopped, and further medical evaluation should occur. Patients with elevated serum creatinine at baseline (up to

3.0 mg/dL) may particularly benefit from the vasodilatory effects of ACEIs in the kidney, but require careful drug initiation and close monitoring. A.R.'s serum creatinine was normal after 4 weeks of lisinopril therapy. She is not experiencing any kidney-related adverse effects from lisinopril.

CASE 9-6, QUESTION 6: What are the risks of using ACEIs in women of childbearing age?

Because ACEIs are teratogenic in the second and third trimester,[96] their use in pregnancy is contraindicated. Moreover, their use in women of childbearing potential is discouraged. If used in this population, patient education should be explicitly clear regarding risks to the fetus, which include potentially fatal hypotension, anuria, renal failure, and developmental deformities. A highly effective form of contraception should be strongly recommended.

Angiotensin Receptor Blockers

CASE 9-6, QUESTION 7: A.R.'s lisinopril is increased to 20 mg daily, then to 40 mg daily during a period of 8 weeks. Her current BP is 136/78 mm Hg (134/76 mm Hg when repeated) at an office visit today. Her serum potassium and creatinine are unchanged from previous values. However, she reports a persistent dry cough for the past few months. She has no additional signs suggesting upper respiratory infection or left ventricular dysfunction. How should A.R.'s therapy be modified?

A well-known side effect of ACEIs is a nonproductive, dry cough, which can occur in up to 15% of patients, with some estimates of cough prevalence being higher.[97] Patients may describe this as a tickling sensation in the back of the throat that commonly occurs late in the evening. This is distinctly different from the cough associated with left ventricular dysfunction, which might be associated with crackles and rales (on auscultation) indicating possible pulmonary edema. ACEI-related cough resolves with discontinuation. Many agents have been used to treat an ACEI cough with poor results. The best treatment option for a patient with an intolerable ACEI cough is to switch agents.

CASE 9-6, QUESTION 8: How is an ARB different from an ACEI?

For A.R., switching to an ARB would likely eliminate the cough.[98] Although her first-choice antihypertensive should be CCB or thiazide diuretics, A.R. will also require the addition of a second agent, either a CCB or thiazide diuretic, because she has not achieved her goal BP of less than 130/80 mm Hg. ARBs are first line. There are eight ARBs (Table 9-12), and many are available as two-drug fixed-dose combination products (Online Table 9-1), as well as two different three-drug fixed-dose combination products (Online Table 9-2).

PHARMACOLOGIC DIFFERENCES BETWEEN AN ANGIOTENSIN-CONVERTING ENZYME INHIBITOR AND AN ANGIOTENSIN RECEPTOR BLOCKER

Unlike ACEIs, ARBs specifically bind to angiotensin II receptors in vascular smooth muscle, adrenal glands, and other tissues. Access of angiotensin II to its receptors is blocked, and angiotensin I-mediated vasoconstriction and aldosterone release is prevented, resulting in BP reduction. ARBs do not affect bradykinin; therefore dry cough does not occur.

Considerable investigation has focused on describing the pharmacologic differences between the angiotensin II type 1 and type 2 receptors. Stimulation of the type 1 receptor causes vasoconstriction, salt and water retention, and vascular remodeling.

Table 9-12
Angiotensin Receptor Blockers in Hypertension

Drug	Starting Dose (mg/day)[a]	Usual Dosage Range (mg/day)	Dosing Frequency
Azilsartan medoxomil	80	80	Daily
Candesartan cilexetil	16	8–32	Daily to BID
Eprosartan mesylate	600	600–800	Daily to BID
Irbesartan	150	75–300	Daily
Losartan potassium	50	25–100	Daily to BID
Olmesartan medoxomil	20	20–40	Daily
Telmisartan	40	20–80	Daily
Valsartan	80–160	80–320	Daily

[a]Starting dose may be decreased 50% if patient is volume depleted, very elderly, or taking a diuretic.
BID, 2 times daily.

Other deleterious effects from type 1 receptor stimulation include myocyte and smooth muscle hypertrophy, fibroblast hyperplasia, cytotoxic effects in the myocardium, altered gene expression, and possible increased concentrations of plasminogen activator inhibitor. Stimulation of the type 2 receptor results in antiproliferative actions, cell differentiation, and tissue repair.

CASE 9-6, QUESTION 9: Under what circumstances would an ARB be a more appropriate initial antihypertensive agent than an ACEI?

Theoretically, an ideal antihypertensive agent would block only type 1 and not type 2 receptors as is the case with ARBs. Therefore, it is possible that an ARB would be superior to an ACEI in reducing hypertension-associated complications because ACEIs ultimately decrease stimulation of both type 1 and type 2 receptors by decreasing production of angiotensin II. This argument is purely speculative and is not supported by clinical trial data. ONgoing Telmisartan Alone and in Combination With Ramipril Global Endpoint Trial (ONTARGET) was a prospective, double-blind, randomized controlled trial that directly compared ARB-based therapy, ACEI-based therapy, and the combination of an ACEI with ARB.[99] After a median of 56 months, the incidence of CV events was no different among all three treatment groups. Therefore, ARB therapy is as effective as, but no more superior than, ACEI therapy in the overall management of hypertension.

CASE 9-6, QUESTION 10: If A.R. experienced angioedema from lisinopril, would treatment with an ARB be appropriate?

A history of ACEI-induced angioedema does not preclude the use of ARB therapy. The cross-reactivity between angioedema with an ACEI and ARB is not exactly known. The Candesartan in Heart Failure: Assessment of Reduction in Mortality and Morbidity Alternative study prospectively included patients with a history of ACEI intolerance who were randomly assigned, in a double-blind manner, to placebo or candesartan. Of the 2,028 patients enrolled, 39 had a history of ACEI angioedema, and only 1 of these patients experienced repeat angioedema that required discontinuation of the ARB.[99] In the Telmisartan Randomised Assessment Study in ACE Intolerant Subjects with Cardiovascular Disease trial, 5,926 patients with a history of ACEI intolerance were randomly assigned in this double-blind trial to an ARB or placebo for a median duration of 56 months.[100] A total of 75 patients had a history of ACEI angioedema, and none of those patients who were randomly assigned to the ARB treatment arm experienced repeat angioedema. Therefore, cross-reactivity in angioedema between ACEIs and ARBs appears possible, but unlikely and very small. ARBs are an alternative for patients who experience ACEI angioedema but should be reserved for patients with a compelling indication for an ACEI. Of note, the ACC/AHA guidelines recommend an ARB in patients who have experienced angioedema from an ACEI.[79]

Calcium-Channel Blockers

CCBs effectively lower BP. Elderly and black patients generally have greater BP reduction with a CCB than with other agents (β-blockers, ACEIs, and ARBs). The addition of a diuretic to a CCB provides additive antihypertensive effects. CCBs do not alter serum lipids, glucose, uric acid, or electrolytes.

All CCBs inhibit the movement of extracellular calcium, but there are two primary subtypes: dihydropyridines and nondihydropyridines (i.e., diltiazem and verapamil). Each has distinctly different pharmacologic effects.

DIHYDROPYRIDINE CALCIUM-CHANNEL BLOCKERS

Dihydropyridines are potent vasodilators of peripheral and coronary arteries. They do not block AV nodal conduction and do not treat arrhythmias. Moreover, the potent vasodilation associated with most dihydropyridines can induce a reflex tachycardia. With the exception of amlodipine and felodipine, dihydropyridines decrease cardiac contractility and should be avoided in patients with left ventricular dysfunction. Side effects of dihydropyridines are related to their potent vasodilatory effects (e.g., tachycardia, headache, and peripheral edema).

Peripheral edema with CCB therapy, especially a dihydropyridine CCB, is a dose-dependent side effect. It is a direct result of the potent peripheral arterial vasodilation. When there is not equal vasodilation in the venous vasculature, a risk exists for leaking through the capillaries in the legs and, thus, an increased risk of peripheral edema. The best way to manage this side effect is to reduce the dose of the dihydropyridine or to add an agent that blocks the RAAS to decrease the effects of angiotensin II, which will result in a more balanced pressure gradient across her peripheral vasculature by providing vasodilation of both the arteries and veins. Adding either an ACEI or ARB can be used to accomplish this with the added benefit of further lowering BP. Clinicians should note that using diuretics for the primary purpose of treating peripheral edema that is secondary to CCB use is not recommended and is not effective.

NONDIHYDROPYRIDINE CALCIUM-CHANNEL BLOCKERS

The two nondihydropyridine CCBs, diltiazem and verapamil, are similar to each other. Relative to dihydropyridines, they are only moderately potent vasodilators, but they directly decrease AV nodal conduction and have greater decreases in cardiac contractility. The blockade of AV nodal conduction can slow heart rate and is the basis for their use in controlling supraventricular tachycardias associated with certain arrhythmias (e.g., atrial fibrillation). Most patients only have a modest decrease in heart rate. However, heart block (first, second, or third degree) is a potential adverse effect, especially with large doses. Both diltiazem and verapamil should be avoided in patients with an underlying second- or third-degree heart block. Under these circumstances, a dihydropyridine can be used if a CCB is needed. Verapamil and diltiazem should be avoided in patients with left ventricular dysfunction because they can significantly reduce cardiac contractility. When patients with left ventricular dysfunction require a CCB to treat another condition (i.e., angina or hypertension), amlodipine or felodipine may be used. They are the only CCBs that have been safely used in clinical trials of patients with left ventricular dysfunction. Unlike many other antihypertensive agents, they do not, however, protect against left ventricular dysfunction-related mortality. Diltiazem may have a lower incidence of constipation than verapamil. Verapamil is also an effective agent in migraine prophylaxis and can be used if patients also have migraine. Patients with Raynaud phenomenon can obtain symptomatic relief from the peripheral vasodilation associated with a dihydropyridine CCB. Lastly, CCBs are effective in treating cyclosporine-induced hypertension, but should be used cautiously because verapamil and diltiazem increase cyclosporine concentration.

OTHER CONSIDERATIONS

Formulations

Several CCBs are available for the treatment of hypertension. They are listed in Table 9-13. Immediate-release formulations should be avoided (see Chapter 16, Hypertensive Crises).

Sustained-Release Formulations

CASE 9-7

QUESTION 1: C.F. is a 60-year-old man with hypertension, asthma, and type 2 diabetes. His hypertension is treated with HCTZ 25 mg daily and ramipril 20 mg daily for many years. Today his BP is 148/74 mm Hg (144/72 mm Hg when repeated), and his heart rate is 90 beats/minute. C.F.'s physician would like to add a CCB to his regimen to improve BP control. What are the differences between controlled-onset, extended-release verapamil and sustained-release verapamil? Are they interchangeable?

All CCBs have short half-lives, except amlodipine. Immediate-release forms require multiple daily doses to provide 24-hour effects. Sustained-released formulations are preferred when a CCB is used to treat hypertension. Various sustained-release delivery devices are available. Serum drug concentrations differ among sustained-release CCBs, but overall BP lowering is usually similar. Nonetheless, most of these products that include the same drug are not rated by the US Food and Drug Administration as equivalent and identical. Insurance formularies often encourage therapeutic substitution between these agents. Therapeutic interchange between modified-release drug delivery formulations that allow for once- or twice-daily dosing (e.g., sustained-release, extended-release, and chronotherapeutic products), however, are not equivalent using a milligram-per-milligram conversion. Therapeutic substitution among these products may result in variable BP-lowering effects if not adjusted appropriately. BP and heart rate monitoring should occur within 2 weeks of interchanging sustained-release CCBs.

CASE 9-7, QUESTION 2: Is there any clinical evidence on the use of CCB in diabetic outcomes?

CALCIUM-CHANNEL BLOCKER AND DIABETES

CCBs have been shown to reduce risk of CV events in patients with diabetes,[98] although the evidence is not as convincing as that seen with an ACEI. The results of the Fosinopril versus Amlodipine

Table 9-13
Calcium-Channel Blockers in Hypertension[a]

Drug	Usual Dosage Range (mg/day)	Dosing Frequency
Nondihydropyridines[b]		
Diltiazem, sustained release	120–480	Daily
Diltiazem, extended release[c]	120–540	Daily
Verapamil, sustained release	180–480	Daily to BID
Verapamil, controlled-onset extended release[c]	180–480	QHS
Verapamil, chronotherapeutic oral drug absorption system[c]	100–400	QHS
Dihydropyridines		
Amlodipine	2.5–10	Daily
Felodipine, extended-release tablet	2.5–10	Daily
Isradipine, controlled-release tablet	5–20	Daily
Nicardipine, sustained-release capsule	60–120	BID
Nifedipine, sustained-release tablet[d]	30–90	Daily
Nisoldipine, extended-release tablet	17–34	Daily

[a]Immediate-release (IR) diltiazem, nifedipine, and verapamil should be avoided in hypertension.
[b]Many different long-acting products exist. Because their individual release characteristics vary, they are not exactly interchangeable using a milligram-per-milligram conversion.
[c]Chronotherapeutic agents are dosed primarily at bedtime and have a delayed drug release for a period of hours, followed by slow delivery of drug that starts just before morning, with no delivery during the early evening; because they use different delivery systems, they are not interchangeable products.
[d]Only sustained-release nifedipine is approved for hypertension. Immediate-release nifedipine should be avoided for the management of hypertension.
BID, 2 times daily; QHS, every night.

Cardiovascular Events Randomized Trial and Appropriate Blood Pressure Control in Diabetes trial suggest that ACEIs have more CV protection than CCBs.[56,57]

Nondihydropyridine CCBs (particularly diltiazem) may slow the progression of CKD, although evidence is not as extensive or definitive as it is with an ACEI or ARB. The proposed mechanism is dilation of both the afferent and efferent arterioles, which would decrease intraglomerular pressure. Dihydropyridines have unclear effects on progression of kidney disease. The prevailing opinion is that the renal protective effects of an ACEI and ARB are superior to that of a CCB.

Resistant Hypertension

CASE 9-8

Question 1: R.R. is a 52-year-old man with hypertension for 10 years. He has not yet experienced any hypertension-associated complications or target-organ damage. He does not have a history of diabetes and does not smoke. He has been treated with HCTZ 25 mg daily, amlodipine 10 mg daily, valsartan 320 mg daily, and carvedilol 12.5 mg twice daily for 1 year. He reports rarely missing a dose of his medications, measures his BP at home every day, and follows recommended lifestyle modifications as diligently as possible. He has tried other medications that resulted in intolerances (doxazosin, dizziness; clonidine, dry mouth). His BP has never been less than 140/90 mm Hg, which is his goal. His BP today is 150/90 mm Hg (152/92 mm Hg when repeated), his heart rate is 60 beats/minute, serum potassium is 4.2 mEq/L, and serum creatinine is 1.0 mg/dL. He is 183 cm tall and weighs 85 kg. Does R.R. have resistant hypertension? What are his treatment options?

R.R. has resistant hypertension. JNC-8 guidelines recommends that, if goal BP is not reached within a month of treatment of initial drug treatment, increase the dose of the initial drug or add a second drug from one of the first-choice classes of antihypertensives (thiazide diuretic, CCB, ACEI, or ARB). If goal BP cannot be reached with maximal tolerable doses of two drugs, add and titrate a third drug from the preferred provided. Do not use an ACEI and an ARB together in the same patient.[2] If goal BP cannot be reached using only the drugs in the preferred list, because of a contraindication or the need to use more than three drugs to reach goal BP, antihypertensive drugs from other classes can be used. Referral to a hypertension specialist may be indicated for patients in whom goal BP cannot be attained using the above strategy or for the management of complicated patients for whom additional clinical consultation is needed to rule out secondary causes of hypertension. R.R.'s treatment options are limited. Amlodipine and valsartan are both at the maximal doses. Carvedilol could be increased to 25 mg twice daily, but this should not be done because his heart rate is 60 beats/minute and increasing this dose would place him at risk for bradycardia. It is possible to increase HCTZ to 50 mg daily because this higher dose provides larger BP reductions than 12.5 or 25 mg daily based on 24-hour ABPM.[85] The limitation of this approach is an increased risk of electrolyte abnormalities and metabolic side effects.

Case 9-8, Question 2: How safe is it to add lisinopril 5 mg daily or spironolactone 25 mg daily in R.R.?

For resistant hypertension, three global treatment philosophies should be considered: (a) assuring appropriate diuretic therapy, (b) appropriate use of effective drug combination, and (c) use of alternative antihypertensive agents as appropriate.[13] Adding an ACEI to an already maximum dose of valsartan would not be recommended. The combination of an ACEI and ARB overall is not very beneficial. This combination should not be used specifically for the purpose of BP lowering, especially in primary prevention patients. When this combination was evaluated in the ONTARGET, the ACEI with ARB combination treatment arm provided only minimal additional reduction in BP compared with either agent alone and most importantly did not additionally lower risk of CV events. Moreover, there was a higher risk of adverse events (e.g., kidney dysfunction and hypotension) with the combination arm.

The combination of an ACEI with ARB has been used in patients with left ventricular dysfunction based on promising data of a reduced risk of heart failure hospitalizations.[101,102] However, the overall clinical benefits of an ACEI with an ARB versus an ACEI without an ARB are very small; addition of an aldosterone antagonist is the preferred next step in patients with left ventricular dysfunction who are already treated with the standard regimen of a diuretic, ACEI, and a β-blocker.[79] One potential niche for the use of an ACEI with an ARB is in the setting of CKD with significant proteinuria (300 mg albumin/day or 500 mg protein/day or per gram of urinary creatinine), in which the combination of an ACEI with an ARB seems to reduce progression of proteinuria better than either drug alone.[73]

Many patients with resistant hypertension have a significant component of volume expansion. Detecting this may not be easily observed using routine clinical examinations. However, identifying occult volume expansion using serial hemodynamic measurements from noninvasive bioimpedance testing, followed by enhancing diuretic therapy, has been shown to reduce BP better than treatment selected by an experienced hypertension specialist.[103] Options to assure appropriate diuretic therapy include switching diuretic agents, switching diuretic classes, increasing the dose, or adding a different class of diuretic. Instead of increasing HCTZ to 50 mg daily, switching HCTZ to the more long-acting chlorthalidone is another possible option to enhance BP lowering. This is an option in R.R. Another option is switching HCTZ to a loop diuretic (e.g., furosemide or torsemide). This should be considered for patients with stage 4 or 5 CKD (GFR <30 mL/minute/1.73 m^2) or for those who need diuresis because of edema. This is not a reasonable treatment option for R.R. because he does not have CKD. Another option is to add an aldosterone antagonist, which is considered an alternative antihypertensive agent. Patients with resistant hypertension often require the use of an agent(s) (Table 9-14) that is not widely used as either a first- or a second-line therapy. These therapies should not be used as monotherapy or a cornerstone of a multidrug regimen because there is less evidence to support their role in reducing CV events. It should be acknowledged, however, that some of these agents (e.g., reserpine and hydralazine) served as add-on agents to diuretics and β-blockers in early placebo-controlled, stepped-care approach trials in hypertension. R.R. has already failed to fully respond to, or tolerate, several drug classes that typically are associated with reductions in hypertension-associated complications. To attain his BP goal of less than 140/90 mm Hg, an alternative agent, other than clonidine, should be selected because he did not tolerate it in the past.

Table 9-14
Alternative Antihypertensive Agents

Drugs/Mechanism of Action	Usual Dosage Range (mg/day)	Dosing Frequency
Aldosterone Antagonists (see Table 14-9)		
α_1-Blockers		
Doxazosin	1–8	Daily
Prazosin	2–20	BID to TID
Terazosin	1–20	Daily to BID
Direct Renin Inhibitor		
Aliskiren	150–300	Daily
α2-Agonists (Central)		
Clonidine Clonidine	0.1–0.8 0.17–0.52	BID Daily
Clonidine transdermal	0.1–0.3	Once weekly
Methyldopa	250–1,000	BID
Arterial Vasodilators		
Hydralazine	25–100	BID to TID
Minoxidil	2.5–80	Daily to BID
Adrenergic Neuron Blockers		
Reserpine	0.05–0.25	Daily

BID, 2 times daily; TID, 3 times daily.

ALTERNATIVE ANTIHYPERTENSIVE AGENTS

Aldosterone Antagonists

Spironolactone and eplerenone are aldosterone antagonists that are especially useful as an add-on therapy in patients with resistant hypertension and would be a reasonable addition to R.R.'s regimen.[8,104] Many patients with resistant hypertension have increased activation of the RAAS, which can result in increased aldosterone. Moreover, up to 20% of patients with resistant hypertension have primary aldosteronism.[8] These characteristics of patients with resistant hypertension make the addition of an aldosterone antagonist very effective in lowering BP in resistant hypertension.

R.R.'s potassium is in the normal range, but could increase after adding spironolactone. Therefore, it should be monitored 2 to 4 weeks after therapy is started to assure R.R. does not experience hyperkalemia. Eplerenone is more specific than spironolactone in aldosterone blockade, although some data suggest that spironolactone is more effective in primary aldosteronism.[105] Compared with spironolactone, gynecomastia is less frequent with eplerenone. The incidence of hyperkalemia may be greater with eplerenone, however. When used for hypertension, eplerenone is contraindicated in populations at high risk for hyperkalemia including patients with an estimated creatinine clearance of less than 50 mL/minute or elevated serum creatinine (>1.8 mg/dL in women and >2.0 mg/dL in men).

CASE 9-8, QUESTION 3: How beneficial would more intensive lifestyle modifications be in R.R.?

In addition to nonadherence with drug therapy, lifestyle factors (obesity, sodium ingestion, and heavy alcohol intake) are a significant contributor to resistant hypertension.[8] Lifestyle modifications should continually be reinforced in patients, especially those with resistant hypertension. As previously discussed, these modifications should include dietary changes and physical activity. R.R should be instructed to restrict his daily sodium to less than 1.5 g because this has been shown to decrease SBP by more than 20 mm Hg in resistant hypertension.[23]

α-Blockers

CASE 9-9

QUESTION 1: J.L. is a 64-year-old man with hypertension. His BP is 158/84 mm Hg (156/86 mm Hg when repeated). His current antihypertensive regimen is HCTZ 25 mg daily, irbesartan 300 mg daily, and nifedipine extended-release 60 mg daily. J.L. is not completely adherent with lifestyle modifications, but insists he is doing the best he can. He has been experiencing frequent nocturia, difficulty in starting urination, and a decrease in his urinary flow for the past several months and is diagnosed with benign prostatic hyperplasia (BPH). J.L.'s physician is considering changing one of his antihypertensive agents to an α-blocker. How do α-blockers compare with other agents in reducing CV events?

α-Blockers are not first-line agents in the management of hypertension. The ALLHAT trial originally included an α-blocker (doxazosin) treatment arm.[48] Interim results after a mean follow-up of 3.3 years revealed that doxazosin had a statistically higher risk of combined CV disease and heart failure when compared with chlorthalidone.[106] Therefore, the ALLHAT data show that chlorthalidone was more effective in lowering some hypertension-associated complications than was doxazosin. This study did not include a placebo group; therefore, to conclude that doxazosin is harmful is inaccurate. For J.L., discontinuing HCTZ, irbesartan, or nifedipine to start an α-blocker is not prudent. It may be appropriate, however, to add an α-blocker to his regimen; an α-blocker will also have a benefit on his BPH (Table 9-7).

CASE 9-9, QUESTION 2: How can an α-blocker improve J.L.'s BPH?

The smooth muscle surrounding the prostate is innervated by α_1-receptors. By blocking these receptors, an α-blocker can improve the symptoms of BPH by reducing urethral tone and alleviating bladder outlet obstruction. Terazosin and doxazosin are both approved for the treatment of BPH. Prazosin should not be used because of the need for frequent dosing. Improvements in BPH symptoms with α-blockers are dose related. A high dose is often needed, and this increases the risk of side effects, such as orthostatic hypotension. In J.L., an α-blocker will lower his BP and improve his urinary symptoms.

CASE 9-9, QUESTION 3: J.L. prefers to try doxazosin rather than undergo surgery to relieve his symptoms of BPH. How should this agent be started?

For J.L., it would be best to add a low dose of doxazosin to his present regimen. Based on his BP response and tolerance, the dose can be titrated up. One of his other antihypertensive agents can be decreased if he becomes hypotensive. The initial dose of doxazosin should not exceed 1 mg daily and it should be given at bedtime. This can minimize orthostatic hypotension, which is the most frequent side effect of α-blockers. This complication is most pronounced with the first dose, but can persist in some patients. Moreover, if an α-blocker is selected as add-on therapy in patients like J.L. with resistant hypertension, nighttime administration of an α-blocker has been shown to be effective in further lowering BP.[107]

CASE 9-9, QUESTION 4: How should J.L. be counseled regarding side effects of doxazosin?

α-Blockers are well tolerated if dosed appropriately. J.L. could experience side effects, such as drowsiness, headache, weakness, palpitations from reflex tachycardia, and nausea, but these do not occur in all patients. Patients starting an α-blocker should be instructed to take the initial dose at bedtime and to anticipate the first-dose effect of orthostatic hypotension. Specifically, patients should be counseled to rise more slowly from a seated or supine position.

Miscellaneous Agents

ALISKIREN

CASE 9-10

QUESTION 1: R.P. is a 68-year-old man with hypertension and a history of ischemic stroke (1 year ago). Two months ago, his BP value was 164/94 mm Hg (162/98 mm Hg when repeated), with a heart rate of 62 beats/minute while on sustained-release diltiazem 240 mg daily. He was started on benazepril/HCTZ 10/12.5 mg daily 2 months ago. His BP today is 142/82 mm Hg (144/82 mm Hg when repeated). All his laboratory values are normal except his serum creatinine, which is 1.9 mg/dL. J.L. has implemented lifestyle modification to the best of his ability. His physician is wondering if aliskiren be added to his drug regiment considering he is also on ACEI.

DIRECT RENIN INHIBITORS

Aliskiren is a direct renin inhibitor. It inhibits the first step of the RAAS, which results in reduced PRA and BP lowering.

CASE 9-10, QUESTION 2: How is aliskiren different from an ACEI or ARB?

This is different from the decreased production of angiotensin II with ACEIs and the blocked angiotensin II receptor effects with ARBs; however, BP-lowering effects are similar to those with ACEIs and ARBs. Aliskiren has a 24-hour half-life and, similar to most ACEIs and ARBs, is dosed once daily.

Some similarities and some differences exist among the side effects associated with aliskiren when compared with ACEIs and ARBs. Aliskiren should not be used in pregnancy because of the known teratogenic effects from blocking the RAAS system. Increases in serum creatinine and serum potassium have been associated with aliskiren. These are similar to ACEI and ARB therapy and are mediated by the inhibition of angiotensin II vasoconstrictive effects on the efferent arterioles of the kidney and blocking of aldosterone. Monitoring of serum creatinine and serum potassium should be done in patients treated with aliskiren, particularly in those treated with the combination of aliskiren and an ACEI, ARB, potassium-sparing diuretic, or aldosterone antagonist. Angioedema has also been reported in patients treated with aliskiren.

CASE 9-10, QUESTION 3: What is the role of aliskiren in treating R.P.'s hypertension?

The exact role of aliskiren in treatment of hypertension is unclear. It is approved as monotherapy or in combination therapy. The BP reductions with aliskiren as monotherapy are similar to those seen with an ACEI, ARB, or CCB (specifically amlodipine). Aliskiren provides additive BP lowering when used in combination with HCTZ, ACEI, ARB, and CCB. Its efficacy in combination with maximal doses of ACEI is unknown, however. Aliskiren is an alternative antihypertensive agent at this time because of unknown long-term effects on CV events.

MIXED αβ-BLOCKERS AND NEBIVOLOL

Labetalol and carvedilol (Table 9-15) are nonselective β-blockers that also have α_1-receptor blocking activity. Their antihypertensive effects are only somewhat similar to a combination of a nonselective β-blocker with an α_1-antagonist.

These agents produce vasodilation because of the α-blocker effects. The only other β-blocker that provides vasodilation is nebivolol. However, nebivolol produces vasodilation without blockade of α-receptors. The same precautions and contraindications relevant to nonselective β-blockers apply to both carvedilol and labetalol because they block both β_1- and β_2-receptors (Table 9-9).

Carvedilol is approved for both hypertension and left ventricular dysfunction. Carvedilol has been shown to reduce morbidity and mortality in a wide range of patients with left ventricular dysfunction.[108,109] Labetalol and carvedilol have no clear advantage over other β-blockers in most patients with hypertension, with the exception that they offer a dual mechanism of action within a single drug formulation. In patients with type 2 diabetes, carvedilol

Table 9-15
Common β-Blockers in Hypertension

Drug	Usual Dosage Range (mg/day)	Dosing Frequency	Half-Life (hours)	β1-Selectivity	Lipid Solubility
Atenolol	25–100	Daily to BID	6–7	++	Low
Bisoprolol	5–20	Daily	9–12	+++	High
Carvedilol	12.5–50	BID	6–10	0	High
Carvedilol	10–80	Daily	6–10	0	High
Labetalol	200–800	BID	6–8	0	Moderate
Metoprolol tartrate	100–400	BID	3–7	+	Moderate to high
Metoprolol succinate	25–400	Daily	3–7	+	Moderate to high
Nebivolol	5–10	Daily	12–19	+++	High
Propranolol	40–180	Daily (LA and XL) or BID	3–5	0	High

BID, 2 times daily.

has been shown to have no significant effect on glucose in comparison with metoprolol, which may slightly increase glucose.[110]

CENTRAL α_2-AGONISTS

The antihypertensive effects of α_2-agonists (Table 9-14) are attributed to their central α_2-agonist activity. Stimulation of α_2-receptors in the CNS inhibits sympathetic outflow (via negative feedback) to the heart, kidneys, and peripheral vasculature, resulting in peripheral vasodilation. Although the α_2-agonists effectively lower BP, they have many potential side effects and have not been evaluated in trials focused on CV events.

Clonidine

CASE 9-11

QUESTION 1: T.M. is a 43-year-old man. He is a truck driver with a 5-year history of hypertension. He does not have hypertension-associated complications. Secondary causes have been ruled out. His regimen is losartan/HCTZ 100/25 mg daily and sustained-release diltiazem 240 mg daily. Other antihypertensive drugs have failed because of various side effects (captopril and lisinopril, dry cough; atenolol and carvedilol, fatigue; nifedipine and amlodipine, edema; terazosin, orthostasis). T.M. has been adherent with his present medications and lifestyle modification, but has been unable to quit smoking. His clinic values have been similar and averaged 150/95 mm Hg for the past 3 months. Clonidine 0.1 mg twice daily is added to his regimen. What problems might occur if T.M. is not adherent with clonidine therapy?

α_2-Agonists are most effective when used with a diuretic because they all can cause fluid retention. Ideally, they should be used with agents that have different mechanisms of action and with agents that do not affect other central adrenergic receptors. Clonidine can cause rebound hypertension when abruptly stopped. T.M.'s occupation may place him at risk for this complication if he misses doses because of unusual work hours or prolonged travel.

CASE 9-11, QUESTION 2: How should T.M.'s clonidine dose be titrated?

Clonidine should be started at a low dosage and gradually increased to achieve optimal BP lowering with minimal side effects. The immediate-release tablet is started as 0.1 mg twice daily, with 0.1- or 0.2-mg/day increases every 2 to 4 weeks until his BP goal is achieved or side effects appear. Clonidine is also available as an extended-release tablet and as a transdermal patch. The patch formulation releases drug at a controlled rate for 7 days and may have fewer side effects than the oral dosage form. The onset of initial BP effect may be delayed for 2 to 3 days after application; thus, rebound hypertension might occur when oral clonidine is switched to transdermal. To prevent this, an oral dose should be taken on the first day that the transdermal patch is used. Anticholinergic side effects, such as sedation and dry mouth, are the most frequent and bothersome side effects of clonidine. These are especially problematic in elderly patients.

CASE 9-11, QUESTION 3: After several months, T.M.'s BP is 148/84 mm Hg with clonidine 0.2 mg twice daily. However, he is now experiencing daytime somnolence and dry mouth. What other α_2-agonists are available?

Methyldopa

Methyldopa has been extensively evaluated and is considered safe in pregnancy. Therefore, it is recommended as a first-line agent when hypertension is first diagnosed during pregnancy.[111] Beyond that, little role exists for methyldopa in the management of hypertension. The usual initial dose is 250 mg administered twice daily up to 2,000 mg/day. Methyldopa causes side effects similar to those associated with clonidine, including sedation, lethargy, postural hypotension, dizziness, dry mouth, headache, and rebound hypertension. These may decrease with continued use. Other significant side effects include hemolytic anemia and hepatitis. Although these are both rare, they necessitate discontinuing the medication.

Others

Guanfacine and guanabenz have a high incidence of side effects. These agents can cause dry mouth, sedation, dizziness, orthostatic hypotension, insomnia, constipation, and impotence. Guanfacine has a long half-life and may have less rebound hypertension than other α_2-agonists. The adverse effects of other α_2-agonists (methyldopa, guanfacine, and guanabenz) are nearly identical to those of clonidine. In general, patients who do not tolerate one α_2-agonist will not tolerate the others. An antihypertensive agent from a different class (aldosterone antagonist, aliskiren, reserpine, or an arterial vasodilator) should be chosen for T.M.

RESERPINE

CASE 9-11, QUESTION 4: Would reserpine be a reasonable option for T.M.?

Reserpine is one of the oldest antihypertensive agents currently available. It is extremely effective in lowering BP when added to a thiazide diuretic. Reserpine is inexpensive and is dosed once daily. Several of the landmark trials that demonstrated reduced morbidity and mortality with BP lowering in hypertension used reserpine. The SHEP trial used reserpine as a second-step agent added to chlorthalidone in patients who could not take atenolol.[88]

Low-dose reserpine (0.05–0.1 mg once daily) is effective at lowering BP and has significantly fewer side effects compared with high doses. Reserpine can cause nasal stuffiness in many patients. Gastrointestinal ulcerations have been reported, but they are associated with either parenteral administration or very large doses. T.M. is a candidate for low-dose reserpine. He is already taking a thiazide diuretic, which should always be used with reserpine, and his therapeutic options are limited. Of all the agents remaining for T.M., other than aliskiren, reserpine has the most favorable side effect profile.

Many clinicians avoid reserpine because of the myth that it can cause depression. This fear was generated from case reports in the 1950s when high doses (0.5–1.0 mg/day) were used. Many of the patients described in these cases would not meet modern criteria for depression; rather, they would be considered oversedated. When reserpine is limited to a maximum of 0.25 mg daily, depression is no more frequent than with other antihypertensive agents.

ARTERIAL VASODILATORS

Hydralazine

CASE 9-12

QUESTION 1: C.M. is a 56-year-old woman with a history of hypertension and severe CKD (estimated GFR of 14 mL/minute/1.73 m^2). Her antihypertensive regimen consists of torsemide 40 mg daily, amlodipine/olmesartan 10/40 mg daily, and metoprolol succinate 200 mg daily. She started hydralazine 25 mg 3 times daily 4 weeks ago when her BPs were 148/92 and 146/90 mm Hg. She has been very compliant, and her BP is now 146/88 mm Hg with a heart rate of 82 beats/minute. Her lung fields are clear, with 1+ bilateral pitting edema. Serum electrolytes are within normal limits. Why was hydralazine used in C.M.?

Hydralazine causes direct relaxation of arteriolar smooth muscle. Arterial vasodilators are infrequently used, except for patients with severe CKD. In this population, hypertension is difficult to control and often requires four or five agents. Severe CKD results in increased renin release and increased fluid retention. Potent vasodilation, in combination with diuresis, is often effective in lowering BP under these conditions. This vasodilation, however, stimulates the sympathetic nervous system and results in a reflex tachycardia, increased PRA, and fluid retention. Thus, the hypotensive effects of direct arterial vasodilators can quickly diminish with time when used as monotherapy. To prevent this, arterial vasodilators need to be used in combination with agent that can slow down heart rate (e.g., β-blocker or nondihydropyridine CCB) to counteract reflex tachycardia, as well as a diuretic (often a loop diuretic if used in severe CKD) to minimize fluid retention.

CASE 9-12, QUESTION 2: After 18 months, C.M.'s hydralazine dose is 50 mg 3 times daily, and her BP is at goal. She now complains of joint pain in both her right and left hands, which extends to the wrists, and generalized weakness with frequent fevers. Laboratory findings for C.M. showed a positive antinuclear antibodies test (diffuse), a white blood cell count of 3,500/μL, and an erythrocyte sedimentation rate of 45 mm/hour, and she is diagnosed with drug-induced lupus (DIL). How should this be managed?

C.M.'s symptoms are consistent with DIL. Hydralazine is one of the most common agents reported to cause DIL. Musculoskeletal pains are the most frequent symptoms, but systemic symptoms and rash may also occur. Hydralazine doses as low as 100 mg/day can cause DIL, and the risk significantly increases when greater than 200 mg/day is used.

Hydralazine should be discontinued. Symptoms should subside within days or weeks, and complete resolution can be expected.

Minoxidil

CASE 9-12, QUESTION 3: What alternatives to hydralazine are available for C.M.?

C.M.'s BP responded to hydralazine, so she would likely benefit from another arterial vasodilator. Minoxidil, a potent arterial vasodilator, is similar to hydralazine with regard to reflex tachycardia, increased CO, increased PRA, and fluid retention. Therefore, concomitant β-blocker and diuretic therapy is still needed. Minoxidil should be reserved for patients such as C.M. who have severe CKD or possibly for resistant hypertension.

CASE 9-12, QUESTION 4: How should C.M. be counseled if minoxidil is started?

Hypertrichosis is a common adverse effect of oral minoxidil, occurring in 80% to 100% of patients. The hair growth is not associated with an endocrine abnormality and begins within the first few weeks. It commonly occurs on the temples, between the eyebrows, on the cheeks, and on the pinna of the ear. Hair growth can extend to the back of the legs, arms, and scalp with continued use. Some patients, especially women, find the hypertrichosis so intolerable that they stop treatment. Topical minoxidil is an approved therapy for male pattern baldness, but topical administration does not provide BP-lowering effects.

Fluid retention with minoxidil is common, presenting as edema and weight gain. If adequate diuresis is not maintained during minoxidil therapy, left ventricular dysfunction may be precipitated or worsened. This also occurs with hydralazine. The compensatory reflex tachycardia with minoxidil may also precipitate angina in patients who have, or are at risk for, CAD.

KEY REFERENCES AND WEBSITES

A full list of references for this chapter can be found at http://thepoint.lww.com/AT11e. Below are the key references and websites for this chapter, with the corresponding reference number in this chapter found in parentheses after the reference.

Key References

ACCORD Study Group et al. Effects of intensive blood-pressure control in type 2 diabetes mellitus. *N Engl J Med*. 2010;362:1575. (16)

ALLHAT Officers and Coordinators for the ALLHAT Collaborative Research Group. Major outcomes in high-risk hypertensive patients randomized to angiotensin-converting enzyme inhibitor or calcium channel blocker vs diuretic: The Antihypertensive and Lipid-Lowering Treatment to Prevent Heart Attack Trial (ALLHAT) [published corrections appear in JAMA. 2004;291:2196; *JAMA*. 2003;289:178]. *JAMA*. 2002;288:2981. (49)

Beckett NS et al. Treatment of hypertension in patients 80 years of age or older. *N Engl J Med*. 2008;358:1887. (20)

Calhoun DA et al. Resistant hypertension: diagnosis, evaluation, and treatment: a scientific statement from the American Heart Association Professional Education Committee of the Council for High Blood Pressure Research. *Circulation*. 2008;117:e510. (8)

Dahlof B et al. Cardiovascular morbidity and mortality in the Losartan Intervention For Endpoint reduction in hypertension study (LIFE): a randomised trial against atenolol. *Lancet*. 2002;359:995. (48)
Dahlof B et al. Prevention of cardiovascular events with an antihypertensive regimen of amlodipine adding perindopril as required versus atenolol adding bendroflumethiazide as required, in the Anglo-Scandinavian Cardiac Outcomes Trial-Blood Pressure Lowering Arm (ASCOT-BPLA): a multicentre randomised controlled trial. *Lancet*. 2005;366:895. (65)
Flack JM et al. Management of high blood pressure in Blacks: an update of the International Society on Hypertension in Blacks consensus statement. *Hypertension*. 2010;56:780. (95)
James PA et al. 2014 Evidence-based guidelines for the management of high blood pressure in adults: report from the panel members appointed to the Eighth Joint National Committee (JNC 8). *JAMA*. 2014;311(5):507–520. (2)
ONTARGET Investigators et al. Telmisartan, ramipril, or both in patients at high risk for vascular events. *N Engl J Med*. 2008;358:1547. (99)

Key Websites

Management of Blood Pressure in Adults: Systematic Evidence Review from the Blood Pressure Expert Panel. http://www.nhlbi.nih.gov/health-pro/guidelines/in-develop/blood-pressure-in-adults
National Kidney Foundation. Calculators for Health Care Professionals. http://www.kidney.org/professionals/KDOQI/gfr_calculator.cfm

10 Peripheral Vascular Disorders

Snehal H. Bhatt and Mary G. Amato

CORE PRINCIPLES

	CHAPTER CASES
1 Peripheral arterial disease (PAD) is stenosis or occlusion in the peripheral arteries of the legs, usually caused by atherosclerosis. A sometimes-painful complication called intermittent claudication (IC) can be associated with PAD and is described as aching, cramping, tightness, or weakness of the legs, which usually occurs during exertion.	**Case 10-1 (Question 1)**
2 Treatment for PAD should include therapeutic lifestyle changes and pharmacologic intervention based on risk factors present. Specific interventions may include smoking cessation; exercise; management of dyslipidemia, hypertension, and diabetes; antiplatelet therapy; and verapamil.	**Case 10-1 (Questions 2–11)**
RAYNAUD PHENOMENON (RP)	
1 RP is an exaggerated vasospastic response to cold or emotion, likely mediated through sympathetic response to the precipitating stimuli. RP is classified as primary or secondary, in which secondary causes include connective tissue diseases and occupational-related neural damage.	**Case 10-2 (Question 1)**
2 Treatment for RP should include therapeutic lifestyle changes and pharmacologic intervention based on clinical presentation and underlying etiology. First-line interventions may include avoidance of cold stimuli and medications associated with vasoconstriction and treatment with calcium-channel blockers (CCBs). Several other therapies may be emerging as possible therapeutic options, including renin–angiotensin–aldosterone inhibitors, topical nitroglycerin, statins, peripheral α-adrenergic blockers, intravenous prostanoids, endothelin antagonists, and oral phosphodiesterase inhibitors.	**Case 10-2 (Questions 2–4)**
NOCTURNAL LEG MUSCLE CRAMPS	
1 Nocturnal leg muscle cramps are idiopathic, involuntary contractions occurring at rest that cause a visible and palpable knot in the affected muscle, usually occurring in the early hours of sleeping.	**Case 10-3 (Question 1)**
2 The primary treatment goal of nocturnal leg muscle cramps is the prevention of episodes. Recommendations include stretching practices, alteration of sleeping position, and treatment of modifiable causes (i.e., electrolyte abnormalities).	**Case 10-3 (Questions 2–4)**

PERIPHERAL ARTERIAL DISEASE

Peripheral arterial disease (PAD) is a common and sometimes painful complication from stenosis or occlusion in the peripheral arteries of the legs, usually caused by atherosclerosis. Similar to coronary artery disease (CAD) resulting in chest pain, PAD pain can be classified as "angina" of the legs. When closely comparing the risk factors and pathology of both diseases, the association with CAD and IC becomes clear.

IC is described as aching, cramping, tightness, or weakness of the legs which usually occurs in the calves during walking and is relieved at rest. Tissue ischemia, resulting numbness or continuous pain in the toes or foot, may be present and can lead to ulceration. IC is a painful condition that can severely limit mobility and lead to tissue necrosis or amputation of the affected limb. Many patients with PAD, however, are asymptomatic or have atypical lower limb symptoms, such as leg fatigue, difficulty walking, or similar nonspecific complaints. Patients may not seek medical attention until the condition is advanced because of the gradual onset of symptoms associated with IC.

Table 10-1
Annual Incidence of Intermittent Claudication by Age[3]

Age Group (years)	Annual Incidence (%)
40–49	2.0
50–59	4.2
60–69	6.8
70	9.2

Epidemiology

PAD is a relatively common condition that affects men and women equally, with a prevalence of 12%,[1] although men have a twofold increased prevalence of symptomatic IC.[2] The annual incidence of IC increases dramatically with age (Table 10-1). Most patients with PAD are asymptomatic. In one study where the prevalence of IC symptoms was 2%, only 11.7% of patients had detectable large vessel atherosclerosis of the lower extremities.[3] This disparity between IC symptoms and the presence of PAD contributes to the observation that 50% to 90% of patients with IC do not mention PAD symptoms to their physician. Patients attribute the symptoms of IC to normal walking difficulties associated with aging, not a medical condition requiring treatment.[4] Public knowledge of the definition of PAD, risk factors for the development of the disease, associated symptoms and disease states, and amputation risk were evaluated in adults older than 50 years of age in a cross-sectional, population-based telephone survey. Unfortunately, only 25% of the population reported awareness of PAD.[5]

Risk factors for developing occlusive PAD are similar to those for CAD. Long-standing diabetes is the most significant risk factor, with 30% of patients with diabetes affected by PAD.[6] Each 1% increase in glycosylated hemoglobin is associated with a 28% risk of incident PAD.[7] Other atherosclerotic risk factors associated with PAD include cigarette smoking, hypertension, and dyslipidemia.[8] Hypertriglyceridemia is a more significant risk factor for PAD than for CAD, and this may partially explain the increased prevalence of PAD in patients with diabetes.[9]

Cigarette smoking is the strongest risk factor for PAD and the development of IC pain than any other risk factors, and the risk increases dramatically with the duration of smoking history and number of cigarettes smoked per day.[10] In patients with hypertension or diabetes, smoking further increases the rate of claudication development. Smoking confers a sevenfold increase in risk for PAD compared with not smoking.[11]

Epidemiologic studies following PAD patients over 4 to 9 years show that IC is nonprogressive in 75% of patients, whereas 25% of patients with IC will have worsening painful ischemic episodes. Ischemic tissue changes, ulceration, and gangrene can accompany advanced PAD. Amputation of the affected limb is rare, but can occur in up to 5% of patients with claudication.[12] The presence of two independent risk factors, such as diabetes and cigarette smoking, has an additive effect on the risk for the development of progressive IC and serious limb complications (Table 10-2). Finally, disease location in patients with severe disease may be associated with prognosis. Proximal disease may be associated with poor outcomes when compared with distal lesions, although further studies are needed to confirm these findings.[14]

Table 10-2
Long-Term Incidence of Outcomes in Patients with Intermittent Claudication[12,13]

Patient Population	Abrupt Limb Ischemia (%)	Amputation (%)
All patients	23	7
Diabetes	31	11
Smokers	35	21

During a relatively short 2-year follow-up of patients with IC, 3.6% of patients died, whereas 22% experienced a nonfatal cardiovascular event (defined as any cardiac, cerebral, or peripheral vascular event). Walking capacity declined in 26% during the same time frame, thus it is paramount to recognize that severe, short-term morbidity is highly likely in this patient population.[13,15]

Pathophysiology

IC is the predominant complication of occlusive PAD because of the resulting pain and subsequent decreased mobility. The major cause of occlusive PAD is arteriosclerosis obliterans, defined as the development of atherosclerotic plaques in the peripheral vasculature. These plaques develop as a result of

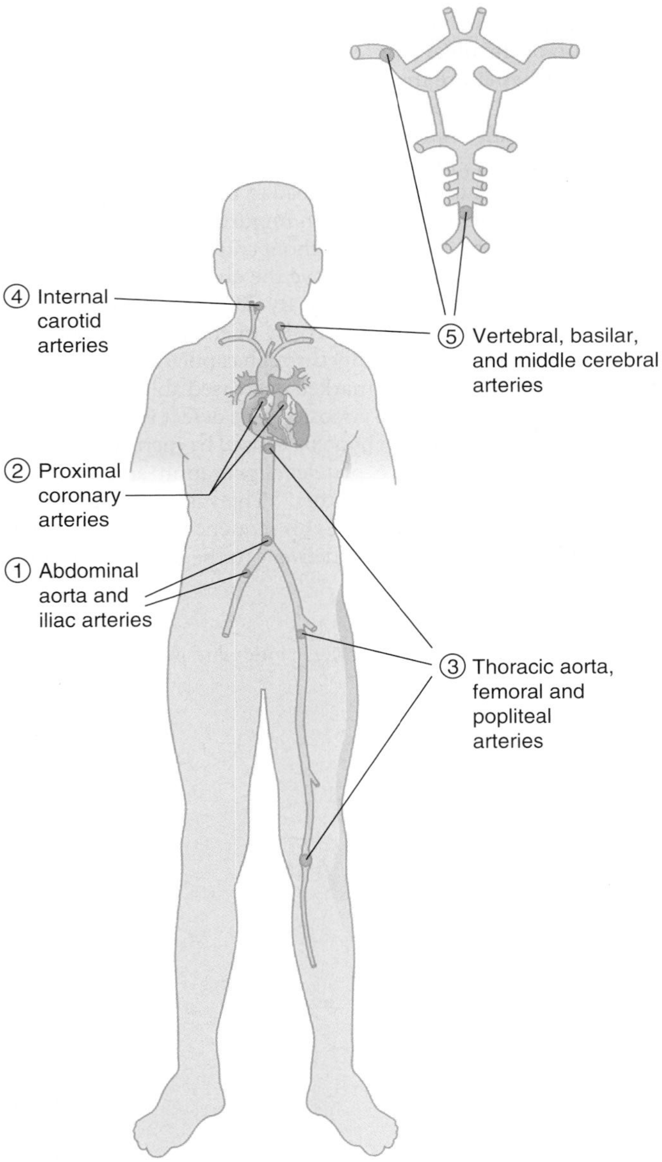

Figure 10-1 Sites of severe atherosclerosis in order of frequency. (Adapted with permission from Rubin R et al. *Rubin's Pathology: Clinicopathology Foundations in Medicine*. 6th ed. Philadelphia, PA: Wolters Kluwer, Lippincott Williams & Wilkins; 2012:452.)

endothelial activation in association with conditions such as dyslipidemia, diabetes mellitus, hypertension, and smoking. Plaques also result from the proliferation of vascular smooth muscle, with subsequent damage to the vascular structure. This damaged endothelium has impaired vasodilatory capabilities because secretion of nitric oxide is decreased and secretion of vasoconstrictive substances, such as endothelin, is increased, impeding blood flow to the extremities. Further growth of atherosclerotic lesions can physically limit blood flow. Exercise may induce IC symptoms in patients who have lesions with greater than 50% stenosis, whereas patients with lesions of greater than 80% stenosis can have pain at rest. The lesions themselves can become unstable and rupture, or adjacent smaller vessels experiencing high hemodynamic pressure caused by nearby plaques may rupture as well. Either situation can lead to acute vascular occlusion, analogous to unstable angina or acute myocardial infarction (MI) in coronary arteries.[16]

Figure 10-1 illustrates the common sites of atherosclerosis. Plaques that develop in central vessels (e.g., in the aorta and iliac artery) are primarily associated with buttock pain and erectile dysfunction. Those confined to the more distal femoral and popliteal arteries characteristically cause thigh and calf pain. Occlusion of the tibial arteries will produce claudication pain in the foot. When more than one arterial bed is affected by severe atherosclerosis, symptoms of IC will be diffuse. Symptoms of IC indicate an inadequate supply of arterial blood to peripheral muscles. Exercise, including walking, increases the metabolic demands of the muscles and can lead to claudication pain.

Erythrocyte deformability is an important factor for in vitro capillary perfusion.[17,18] In areas without compromised blood flow, normal red blood cells (RBCs) have the ability to deform when passing through a small capillary. By aligning themselves in a planar manner, RBCs reduce viscosity of the blood suspension, enabling them to pass smoothly through capillaries. In many patients with IC, RBCs have a marked decreased ability to deform, resulting in increased blood viscosity. This defect is promoted by chronic tissue ischemia and hypoxia caused by increased intracapillary leukocyte adherence, platelet aggregation, and activation of complement and clotting factors.[16] The vascular responses to hypoxia are detrimental because this sequence of events further inhibits blood flow and oxygen delivery to the tissues (Fig. 10-2).

Clinical Presentation

CASE 10-1

QUESTION 1: R.L. is a 60-year-old, 110-kg man with a history of type 2 diabetes mellitus, chronic stable angina, dyslipidemia, and smoking. His chief complaint today is right upper thigh pain while walking around the block. The pain has gradually increased during the past 12 months, but only recently has become intolerable. The pain is relieved within minutes after he stops walking. R.L. smokes 2 packs of cigarettes a day.

His most recent laboratory results are significant for the following results:

Total cholesterol, 290 mg/dL (SI units, 7.49 mmol/L)
Fasting triglycerides, 350 mg/dL (SI units, 3.95 mmol/L)
Low-density lipoproteins (LDL), 188 mg/dL (SI units, 4.86 mmol/L)
High-density lipoproteins (HDL), 32 mg/dL (SI units, 0.83 mmol/L)
Serum creatinine (SCr), 0.8 mg/dL (SI units, 61 mmol/L)
Blood urea nitrogen (BUN), 18 mg/dL (SI units, 6.4 mmol/L)
Hemoglobin (Hgb) A_{1c}, 10.5% (SI units, 91.3 mmol/mol)
Fasting glucose, 190 mg/dL (SI units, 10.5 mmol/L)
Blood pressure (BP), 170/95 mm Hg
Heart rate (HR), 89 beats/minute

His posterior tibial artery pulse is not palpable. A Doppler ultrasound study is performed, and his ankle-to-brachial index (ABI) is 0.7 (normal, >0.90).

R.L.'s medication list includes isosorbide mononitrate 60 mg daily, aspirin 81 mg daily, and ramipril 5 mg daily. His insulin doses have progressively increased to neutral protamine Hagedorn (NPH) insulin 40 units in the morning and 35 units in the evening. What risk factors and elements of R.L.'s presentation are consistent with a diagnosis of IC?

R.L.'s medical history illustrates classic risk factors for vascular occlusion and IC, including dyslipidemia, diabetes, hypertension, and smoking. His diabetes is not adequately controlled based on elevated Hgb A_{1c} and fasting glucose levels, and he is

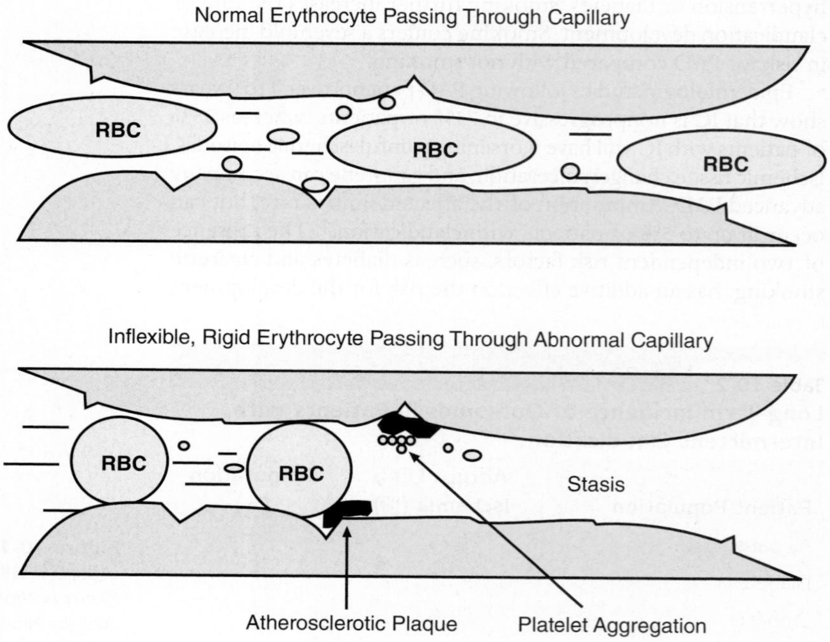

Figure 10-2 Erythrocyte inflexibility in intermittent claudication.

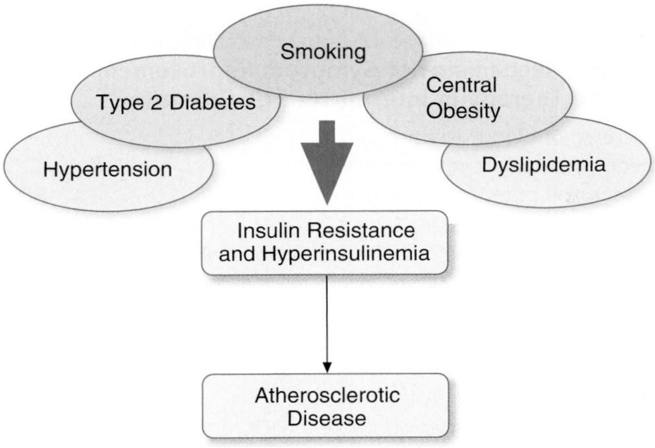

Figure 10-3 The metabolic syndrome in atherosclerosis.

obese. This constellation of disorders is known as the *metabolic syndrome*. These factors, along with smoking, are commonly seen together and have been linked with insulin resistance and accelerated atherosclerosis (Fig. 10-3).[19,20] The presence of angina indicates CAD, so it is not surprising that he has peripheral vascular occlusion as well.

The classic pain of IC described by R.L. is associated with exercise of the affected muscle group(s) and subsides with a few minutes of rest. Other common symptoms of extensive atherosclerosis include cold feet and persistent aching of the feet during rest or sleep. Restricted blood flow to the feet along with pooling of blood secondary to inadequate pressure needed to propel blood back up the leg can lead to rubor (red or purple color of the foot). Other indicators of peripheral atherosclerosis are the loss of hair from the top of the feet, thickening of the toenails, and absence of sweating of the lower legs and feet, all caused by poor circulation.[16]

The results of objective studies performed on R.L. are consistent with IC. Doppler ultrasound of the spine is helpful in excluding pseudoclaudication caused by spinal stenosis and other neurogenic or musculoskeletal causes of leg pain. Ultrasound is also useful to measure BP of the lower extremities. An ABI of 0.7 means that the ankle systolic BP reading is only 70% of the systolic pressure in the brachial artery supplying blood to the arm. In patients with IC, this is caused by atherosclerotic obstruction of blood flow in the lower limbs and subsequent decreased perfusion pressures in the ankle compared with the arm (Table 10-3). As the ABI decreases, blood flow to the extremities is reduced and the severity of symptoms is greater. An ABI less than 0.9 is diagnostic for PAD. Loss of the posterior tibial pulse, as seen in R.L., is common in those with peripheral vascular occlusion.

Table 10-3
Severity of Arterial Obstruction as Assessed by Ankle-to-Brachial Index[21]

Severity	Ankle-to-Brachial Index[a]
Normal	>0.90
Mild	0.70–0.89
Moderate	0.50–0.69
Severe	>0.50

[a]Ankle-to-brachial index is the systolic blood pressure in the ankle divided by the systolic blood pressure in the arm.

Treatment

THERAPEUTIC OBJECTIVES AND NONPHARMACOLOGIC INTERVENTIONS

CASE 10-1, QUESTION 2: What are the therapeutic goals in treating R.L.? What interventions should be initiated to prevent claudication pain and arrest progression of his disease?

Specific treatment goals include preventing further claudication pain, lessening his current pain, arresting the progression of underlying disease, and decreasing his risk of cardiovascular events. Achieving these goals will provide R.L. with the best chance of avoiding further mobility impairment, amputation, and cardiovascular events. An important concept that should be stressed when explaining these treatment goals to R.L. is that all his diseases are closely interrelated and that a beneficial intervention for one disease is beneficial for all. Interventions that can be initiated include diet modification; exercise and weight loss; and attainment of goal BP, lipids, Hgb A_{1c}, and fasting and postprandial blood glucose levels. The American College of Cardiology and American Heart Association (ACC/AHA) have published guidelines that thoroughly evaluate the interventions and medications that have been used to treat IC and PAD.[8] Table 10-4 summarizes these recommendations. The two most important things that R.L. can do for his IC are summed up in five words: "Stop smoking and keep walking."[23]

Smoking Cessation

The importance of smoking cessation cannot be overemphasized to patients with IC. It is the most important modifiable factor in preventing the development of rest pain, prolonged limb ischemia, need for amputation and reducing the risk for cardiovascular events. Several studies document improved survival and decreased amputation rates in patients with IC who stopped smoking compared with patients who continue to smoke.[24,25] Other benefits, such as improved treadmill walking distance, decreased disease progression, and decreased complications after vascular reconstructive surgery, have been shown in patients who quit smoking compared with patients who continue.[8,24,26–28] It is the one intervention that will decrease R.L.'s claudication pain most rapidly. He will also decrease his risk of MI and mortality by threefold and fivefold, respectively. Table 10-5 summarizes the risk of cigarette smoking and the value of smoking cessation on cardiovascular complications.

Many pharmacologic products and strategies are available to aid R.L. to stop smoking (see Chapter 91, Tobacco Use and Dependence).

Table 10-4
Medical Treatment of Peripheral Arterial Disease and Expected Outcomes[8,22]

Intervention	Improve Leg Symptoms?	Prevent Systemic Complications?
Smoking cessation	Yes	Yes
Exercise	Yes	No
Cilostazol	Yes	No
Statin drugs	Yes	Yes
Angiotensin-converting enzyme inhibitors	Yes	Yes
Blood pressure control	No	Yes
Antiplatelet therapy[a]	No	Yes

[a]Aspirin or clopidogrel.

Table 10-5
Patient Outcomes Based on Smoking Status After Intermittent Claudication Diagnosis[12,24]

Outcome	Length of Follow-Up (years)	Patient Population	
		Current Smokers (%)	Past Smokers(%)[a]
Rest pain	7	16	0
Myocardial infarction	10	53	11
Amputation	5	11	0
Mortality	10	54	18

[a]Quit after intermittent claudication diagnosis.

However, nicotine itself has harmful effects on the vasculature via catecholamine release and vasoconstriction; and it may play a role in endothelial damage and atherosclerosis progression.[29]

Exercise

An individualized and supervised exercise program is endorsed for patients with PAD and will benefit most of R.L.'s other risk factors as well.[8] IC pain results in decreased mobility, and because of deconditioning from lack of exercise, patients with IC may slowly become dependent on others for activities of daily living. An exercise program is the most effective way to both preserve and increase mobility. It is more effective than the best pharmacologic therapy currently available.[30] The ideal exercise program consists of walking for a minimum of 30 to 45 minutes at least 3 times a week, for a minimum of 12 weeks.[8] R.L. should walk as fast and far as he can until the pain becomes severe; he should then wait until the pain subsides, and then resume walking.[21] At first, R.L. may experience several painful episodes during each exercise session, but these should gradually decrease as the beneficial effects of exercise therapy begin to emerge. Studies have documented that this type of exercise program can more than double the pain-free distance a patient with IC is able to walk.[31] Lower extremity resistance training can provide improved functional performance measured by the following: quality of life, treadmill walking time, and ability to climb stairs.[32] An appropriate exercise program results in superior outcomes compared with angioplasty and stenting, and equal in terms of walking distance compared with surgery, but without any of the significant complications and mortality associated with surgery.[31]

Rheologic abnormalities of increased blood viscosity, impaired RBC filterability, hyperaggregation, and polycythemia (elevated hematocrit) have been shown to return to normal in many patients with IC who participate in a regular exercise program.[33] Exercise may offset the need for pharmacologic intervention. The potential mechanisms by which exercise benefits patients with IC are listed in Table 10-6.

Table 10-6
Primary Mechanisms of Symptom Improvement with Exercise Therapy in Intermittent Claudication[30]

- Decrease of blood viscosity
- Metabolic changes in the muscle
  - Improved muscle metabolism
  - Improved oxygen extraction
- Improved endothelial function and microcirculation
- Decreased occurrence of ischemia and inflammation
- Atherosclerosis risk factors improved via
  - Weight loss
  - Glycemic control
  - Blood pressure control
  - Increased high-density lipoprotein (HDL)
  - Decreased triglycerides
  - Decreased thrombotic tendency

Dyslipidemia Management

Case 10-1, Question 3: Is lipid-lowering therapy indicated for R.L.?

Because IC is a consequence of atherosclerosis, arresting the progression of R.L.'s atherosclerotic disease is important (see Chapter 8, Dyslipidemias, Atherosclerosis, and Coronary Heart Disease). Initiation of the nutritional and exercise recommendations should be recommended as outlined in 2013 ACC/AHA Lifestyle Management to reduce cardiovascular risk guidelines[34] and endorsed by the ACC/AHA Guideline on the treatment of blood cholesterol to reduce atherosclerotic cardiovascular risk in adults.[35] Therapeutic lifestyle changes and cholesterol-lowering agents are the cornerstones for attaining this goal. Considerable data suggest that aggressive dietary and pharmacologic management of dyslipidemia, particularly lowering low-density lipoprotein cholesterol (LDL-C), leads to regression of atherosclerotic lesions in the coronary and carotid vasculature.[36–38] In contrast, relatively few prospective data exist about the effect of successful lipid-lowering therapy on the regression or stabilization of peripheral lesions, or on clinical events in patients with PAD. A post hoc analysis of a large lipid-lowering study in subjects with known CAD treated with simvastatin demonstrated a significant decrease in new or worsening IC, suggesting that in high-risk patients, lipid lowering can prevent development of clinically symptomatic PAD.[39] The Heart Protection Study randomly assigned patients with known arterial disease of various types to simvastatin 40 mg daily or placebo. After 5 years, a 15% decrease was found in noncardiac revascularizations, including amputations, among the patients receiving simvastatin.[40] Short-term outcomes (e.g., 6 months to 1 year), such as improved walking distance and walking time, have also been documented with simvastatin 40 mg/day.[41,42]

A meta-analysis of 10,049 subjects from several randomized trials using a variety of lipid-lowering therapies in patients with PAD demonstrated reduced claudication severity and decreased disease progression as measured by angiography. A decrease in mortality did not reach statistical significance.[43] Limited data suggest high apolipoprotein [Lp(a)] concentrations may be particularly important in the development of PAD.[44]

Patients with PAD fall into one of the four major statin benefit groups, specifically falling into the group with known atherosclerotic cardiovascular disease (ASCVD). Since R.L. is less than 75 years old, he warrants high-intensity statin therapy, which is defined as statin therapy at doses that are expected to provide at least a 50% reduction in LDL cholesterol (see Chapter 8, Dyslipidemias, Atherosclerosis, and Coronary Heart Disease). There is a paucity of outcome data with other agents for dyslipidemia, as recent trials of omega-3 fatty acid, niacin, or fibric acid derivative have failed to demonstrate a reduction in cardiovascular events in patients with increased risk for cardiovascular events like R.L.[8,45–48]

Management of Hypertension

Case 10-1, Question 4: R.L.'s BP is elevated to 170/95 mm Hg despite ramipril therapy. Because he has angina, and his HR is 89, a β-adrenergic blocker is considered. Are there alternative antihypertensive therapies that might be preferable for R.L.?

R.L.'s hypertension has likely contributed to the development of his atherosclerosis and PAD. Hypertension (see Chapter 9, Essential Hypertension) has been associated with deficiencies in the synthesis of vasodilating substances, such as prostacyclin, bradykinin, and nitric oxide, by the endothelial cells lining the vasculature, along with increases in vasoconstricting substances like angiotensin II. Increased vascular tone can alter local hemodynamics, especially in the presence of a stenotic lesion. Although it has not been determined whether normalization of BP has a positive effect on IC, it is well established that uncontrolled BP results in vascular complications such as MI and stroke. In light of R.L.'s numerous risk factors for these complications, improvement in his BP is warranted.

β-Blockers are frequently cited as contraindicated in IC patients owing to the potential for unopposed α-adrenergic-mediated vasoconstriction during peripheral β-blockade. However, evidence to document worsening IC by β-blockade is lacking. Overall, controlled studies have been inconclusive and a meta-analysis of placebo-controlled trials and studies with control groups concludes that β-blockers do not worsen claudication.[49,50]

Angiotensin-converting enzyme (ACE) inhibitors are first-line agents in patients with PAD.[8] Compared with other antihypertensive agents, the data available support their beneficial effects in this population. Compared with placebo, walking distance is increased with both perindopril and ramipril in patients with PAD.[51,52] The Heart Outcomes Prevention Evaluation (HOPE) study compared ramipril versus placebo in over 9,000 patients who had evidence of vascular disease or diabetes. Impressively, they enrolled more than 4,000 patients with PAD, and similar to the overall trial population, patients with PAD derived a benefit in the composite endpoint of decreased mortality, MI, and stroke.[53] The ONTARGET trial compared telmisartan, ramipril, and the combination of the two in patients with vascular disease or high-risk diabetes without heart failure for a composite end point of cardiovascular death, MI, stroke, or hospitalization for heart failure. The results suggested equivalency of telmisartan to ramipril for the primary end point with similar BP reduction in both groups; however, the combination therapy group experienced more adverse events without any benefit.[54] Based on these data, ARBs may be a suitable substitute for ACE inhibitors, but combination therapy is not recommended.

R.L.'s. BP goal is less than 140/90 mm Hg.[55–57] His dose of ramipril could be increased, or a low-dose diuretic, such as hydrochlorothiazide or chlorthalidone,[55,56] could be added. Given his history of chronic stable angina, the addition of a CCB or a β-blocker would be an option as well. The ACCOMPLISH trial compared the combination of benazepril–amlodipine with benazepril–hydrochlorothiazide in patients with hypertension who were at high risk for cardiovascular events. Amlodipine therapy reduced cardiovascular events compared with hydrochlorothiazide, even though BP control was not significantly different.[58] While β-blockers are typically used in patients with CAD, the outcome data supporting their use are less clear.[59]

Management of Diabetes

Case 10-1, Question 5: Will improving R.L.'s diabetes control or slow the progression of his PAD? What changes in his diabetes management do you recommend?

Patients with type 2 diabetes mellitus (see Chapter 53, Diabetes Mellitus) are able to minimize macrovascular and microvascular complications of their disease with aggressive glucose control.[7,60,61] Insulin, sulfonylurea, or metformin therapies have a beneficial effect on slowing the development of the microvascular complications of diabetes, such as retinopathy and nephropathy. Metformin has specifically been shown to further reduce the occurrence of macrovascular complications such as stroke or MI compared with insulin or sulfonylureas in obese patients with type 2 diabetes.[60]

Table 10-7
Effect of Diabetes Mellitus on Intermittent Claudication Outcomes After 5 Years[11]

	Patients With Diabetes (%)	Patients Without Diabetes (%)
Mortality	49	23
Major amputation	21	3
Deterioration	35	19

R.L.'s diabetes is a significant risk factor for progression to further ischemic events (Table 10-7). He has a twofold greater risk of death and a sevenfold greater risk of amputation compared with a patient without diabetes. Although a specific benefit for IC has not been demonstrated, it seems prudent to initiate or continue aggressive diabetes management in patients with type 2 diabetes mellitus and IC. The addition of metformin to R.L.'s therapy could improve his blood glucose control and decrease his risk of vascular complications. It is hoped that R.L. can reach his Hgb A_{1c} goal of less than 7% and a fasting blood glucose of 80 to 130 mg/dL and 2-hour postprandial glucose of less than 180 mg/dL with diet and exercise, while adding metformin to his current therapy.[62,63]

R.L. also must take proper care of his feet to prevent ulcerative complications of IC. He should be encouraged to keep his feet warm, dry, and moisturized and to wear properly fitted shoes and perform daily foot inspections.[8] He should seek medical attention immediately for minor trauma to his feet or legs.[4] These measures can reduce the incidence of amputation in patients with diabetes.

PHARMACOLOGIC THERAPIES

Antiplatelet Therapies

Case 10-1, Question 6: Is R.L.'s aspirin therapy beneficial for preventing further complications of IC? Would alternative antiplatelet therapies offer advantages over aspirin?

Aspirin is one of several antiplatelet agents that may be considered for indefinite use in patients with PAD. There is limited data on the effects of aspirin on IC symptoms. Whether aspirin has any beneficial effects on walking distance or claudication pain has not been studied. Available data address the impact of aspirin on overall cardiovascular morbidity and mortality. Although aspirin has no direct effect on plaque regression, it does prevent and retard the role platelets play in the thrombogenic events that occur in the vicinity of atherosclerotic plaques.[64] Aspirin is an effective antithrombotic agent at dosages ranging from 50 to 1,500 mg daily. The lowest dosages proven to decrease cardiovascular events are 75 to 100 mg daily,[65] with the higher dosage showing benefit in active processes, such as acute ischemic stroke[66] and acute MI.[67] A dosage of 75 mg daily has demonstrated benefit in patients with hypertension[68] and stable angina.[69] No evidence indicates that these "low doses" are any more or any less effective than dosages of 900 to 1,500 mg daily.[70]

Aspirin is recommended in patients with vascular disease of any origin (this includes stroke, MI, PAD, and ischemic heart disease). At dosages of 75 to 162 mg/day, aspirin decreases vascular death by approximately 15% and all serious vascular events (MI, stroke, or vascular death) by approximately 20% in high-risk patients, including those with PAD.[62,65,69] In patients with PAD, aspirin can delay the progression of established lesions as assessed by angiography. When used for primary prevention of cardiovascular disease in men, aspirin decreased the need for arterial reconstructive surgery, which was needed because of PAD.[71] In a meta-analysis of 5,269 subjects with PAD, aspirin was associated with a significant reduction in nonfatal stroke with a statistically insignificant decrease of cardiovascular events.[72] However, in a recent large randomized, controlled trial in 3,350 patients 50 to 75 years of age without clinically evident cardiovascular disease but with a screening ABI of 0.95 or less, aspirin 100 mg/day was found to be no more effective than placebo in reducing the primary end point of fatal and nonfatal coronary events, stroke, or revascularization (13.7 events per 1,000 person-years in the aspirin group versus 13.3 in the placebo group; hazard ratio, 1.03; 95% confidence interval, 0.84–1.27).[73]

Because all dosages of aspirin are similarly efficacious in decreasing vascular events in this patient population, side effects influence the dose chosen. Although few studies have directly compared varying doses, side effects appear to be dose related. Aspirin 30 mg daily results in less minor bleeding compared with approximately 300 mg daily,[74] and 300 mg daily results in fewer gastrointestinal (GI) side effects compared with 1,200 mg daily.[75] Therefore, R.L. should take the lowest effective dose of aspirin: 75 mg to 100 mg daily. Of note, R.L.'s hypertension should be controlled before initiating aspirin therapy to decrease the small increased incidence of cerebral hemorrhage associated with its use.[76]

Ticlopidine is a thienopyridine derivative that blocks adenosine 5′-diphosphate (ADP) receptors on platelets and decreases platelet–fibrinogen binding.[77] Several studies document its efficacy in patients with PAD on end points such as walking distance, cardiovascular death, and the need for revascularization surgery.[78,79] However, hematologic toxicities (neutropenia and, rarely, thrombotic thrombocytopenic purpura) limit its use.[80,81]

Clopidogrel initially replaced ticlopidine largely because of its improved safety profile. The effects of clopidogrel on specific PAD outcomes are unknown, but it has been compared with aspirin in patients with known atherosclerotic disease. Dosages of 75 mg daily significantly reduced cardiovascular end points by approximately 25% compared with aspirin in this patient population.[82] The treatment effect was most pronounced in the PAD subgroup, leading to the suggestion that clopidogrel may be preferable in the patient population with PAD. No measure was taken of clopidogrel's effect on walking distance or claudication pain, however, and these results have not been confirmed by further studies.

The combination of aspirin and clopidogrel was compared with aspirin alone in more than 15,000 patients at high risk of vascular events, of whom greater than 20% had a history of PAD and approximately 10% had IC.[83,84] In this large study that assessed cardiovascular end points, no benefit was found for dual antiplatelet therapy with aspirin plus clopidogrel.[80] Thus, while clopidogrel has the same guideline recommendation as aspirin,8 clinically it is often used as an appropriate alternative to aspirin in patients unable to take aspirin therapy,[65] perhaps owing to a serious allergy.[8] It should not be used in addition to aspirin, however, because the risk of bleeding and increased cost outweigh any measurable vascular benefit.[84,85]

Ticagrelor was compared with clopidogrel in 13,885 patients with known symptomatic PAD but without documented CAD.[86] There was no difference between the two groups with regards to the primary composite endpoint of death, myocardial infarction and stroke. Based on these data, ticagrelor cannot be recommended to reduce the risk of cardiovascular events in PAD patients at this time. These data also question whether there are differences in cardiovascular risk in patients with both CAD and PAD versus those with PAD alone.

Cilostazol

CASE 10-1, QUESTION 7: Are there any medications that can be used to increase the walking abilities of patients with IC?

Cilostazol is one of the few agents approved by the US Food and Drug Administration (FDA) specifically for the treatment of IC. Several studies have confirmed that cilostazol 100 mg twice daily increases walking distance by approximately 50%[87–90] and that discontinuation of cilostazol results in a decline in function.[91] Cilostazol possesses antiplatelet and vasodilatory effects mediated by the inhibition of phosphodiesterase III.[92] In vitro observations suggest that these pharmacologic effects of cilostazol are particularly pronounced at the blood–vessel interface,[92] which may explain its particular efficacy in the patients with PAD. Studies that included quality-of-life measurements have found that cilostazol improved overall quality of life.[87,93] Small improvements in ABI with chronic cilostazol therapy have also been observed.[94] Two small studies indicate cilostazol is associated with a reduction in restenosis after endovascular therapy in femoropopliteal lesions.[95,96]

Despite these positive findings with cilostazol, several drawbacks exist. It is contraindicated in patients with heart failure based on data with other phosphodiesterase inhibitors demonstrating excess mortality, presumably due to increased arrhythmias.[97] Other common side effects include headache, occurring in up to one-third of patients, and loose stools or diarrhea.[88,98] Cilostazol is a cytochrome P-450 3A4 substrate; therefore, any inhibitor of this enzyme system may substantially increase cilostazol concentrations.

Cilostazol is an important advancement in the treatment of IC. It is the first pharmacologic agent to demonstrate a consistent effect on a significant source of IC disability: walking and mobility measures. While limited data address its impact on other important end points, such as amputation and revascularization procedures or cardiovascular events,[99] it should be added to R.L.'s existing medication regimen at a dosage of 100 mg twice daily to attenuate his symptoms of IC.

Rheologic Agents

CASE 10-1, QUESTION 8: Has pentoxifylline been shown to be efficacious in patients such as R.L.? How does this drug benefit patients with IC?

Pentoxifylline, a methylxanthine derivative, is another agent approved by the FDA for the treatment of IC. Pentoxifylline appears to decrease blood viscosity by decreasing fibrinogen, improving the deformability of both red and white blood cells, and eliciting antiplatelet effects, although the exact mechanism of action is unclear.[100] While the theoretic and in vitro data are unique and positive, data demonstrating its clinical usefulness are controversial. Improvements in walking distances from study to study are unpredictable, and the clinical importance of the sometimes minimal increases in walking distances is not clear (e.g., pain-free walking of approximately 30 m greater than with placebo).[101] Some experts assert that these potential benefits of questionable clinical significance are not worth the expense of drug therapy or the GI side effects.[102]

Pentoxifylline's role in IC therapy is limited. It may have a role in patients who are unable to engage in exercise therapy, or in patients with markedly reduced walking distances, or in whom any small increase in walking distance would greatly improve a patient's activity level.[103] It also may be tried in patients who have not gained the desired benefit from smoking cessation and exercise therapy, and in patients with contraindications, intolerance, or failure of cilostazol. A 2-month trial of pentoxifylline is adequate to determine whether the patient will benefit from therapy.[21] R.L. is not severely debilitated, and the benefits of smoking cessation, exercise therapy, and cilostazol have not been fully realized. Therefore, pentoxifylline should not be added until his response to these well-proven therapies has been determined and the need for further improvement in walking distance is established.

Vasodilators

CASE 10-1, QUESTION 9: R.L. is already taking isosorbide mononitrate for angina. Because IC is made worse by vasoconstriction, should another vasodilating agent be added to treat both his hypertension and IC?

The use of vasodilators for R.L. would at first appear to be a logical pharmacologic intervention to prevent claudication pain. Vasodilators, including isosorbide, directly or indirectly relax blood vessel walls and increase both skin and muscle blood flow as long as cardiac output is maintained. With obstructive arterial disease, however, vessels are sclerotic and unable to further dilate. As a result, healthy vessels dilate to a greater extent than diseased vessels, and blood flow is redistributed (shunted) away from areas that have the greatest need. BP and perfusion paradoxically drop even further in tissues affected by atherosclerosis, resulting in increased pain. If this process produces ischemia, it is known as the *steal phenomenon*. Thus, while nitrates are not contraindicated in patients like R.L, they may not be as helpful as their mechanism of action may suggest.

Numerous vasodilators (i.e., prostaglandin E_1, prostacyclin, isoxsuprine, papaverine, ethaverine, cyclandelate, niacin derivatives, reserpine, guanethidine, methyldopa, tolazoline, nifedipine) have been used to treat IC. None, however, has convincingly or consistently improved exercise performance, despite earlier beliefs that they were effective.[104,105] Limited data suggest L-carnitine 1 g twice daily may have benefit in walking distance and initial claudication distance.[106] ACE inhibitors are the exception to this rule, as their beneficial effects are likely independent of their vasodilator properties. One small, controlled study demonstrated improvement in walking distance with verapamil, a CCB, compared with placebo in patients with IC.[107] Further studies with verapamil are needed before its use can be recommended.

Smoking cessation, an exercise program, and cilostazol are the interventions that should reduce R.L.'s symptoms of IC to the greatest degree. Verapamil is a moderate cytochrome P-450 3A4 inhibitor and would be expected to increase concentrations of cilostazol. The magnitude of this interaction has not been characterized, nor has its impact on efficacy and bleeding events been assessed. Based on the necessity of cilostazol therapy in R.L., along with the poorly characterized benefits of verapamil in IC and the plethora of other antihypertensive and antianginal agents, avoidance of verapamil is prudent at this time. If additional BP or antianginal effects are needed, β-blockade or amlodipine can be initiated.

OTHER ANTITHROMBOTIC ALTERNATIVES

CASE 10-1, QUESTION 10: If R.L. was deemed as being high risk for a cardiovascular event while on aspirin, what other antithrombotic therapy options could be initiated?

While there is limited data regarding antithrombotic therapy in patients with PAD, recently one new agent has been approved with potential to provide a benefit in reducing cardiovascular events. Vorapaxar is a platelet protease-activated receptor (PAR)-1 antagonist, which inhibits thrombin-mediated plateletand recently received FDA approval for reducing thrombotic cardiovascular events in patients with PAD. The indication approval was based on a recent study, which enrolled 26, 449 patients with stable atherosclerotic vascular disease who were already receiving dual antiplatelet therapy, of which 14% had PAD.[108] The results showed that treatment with vorapaxar reduced the composite primary endpoint of cardiovascular death, MI stroke, although only the incidence of MI was reduced significantly. Importantly, major bleeding was increased significantly in the vorapaxar group, thus the true benefit of the addition of vorapaxar in these patients is unclear at this time.

Ongoing studies with the P2Y12 receptor antagonist ticagrelor and the direct factor Xa inhibitor oral anticoagulants rivaroxaban and edoxaban will further shed light on the risks and benefits of more potent, target-specific agents in patients with PAD.[109,110] The choice of antiplatelet therapy for R.L. in this scenario would be dependent upon what specific cardiovascular event he experienced, as the choice of therapy would be different if R.L. suffered a MI versus an ischemic stroke (see Chapter 12, Chronic Stable Angina and Chapter 13, Acute Coronary Syndrome).

CASE 10-1, QUESTION 11: Three years have passed, and R.L. stopped smoking 6 months ago. His current medications include isosorbide mononitrate 60 mg daily, aspirin 81 mg daily, and ramipril 10 mg daily; carvedilol 6.25 mg twice a day; NPH insulin 55 units in the morning and 40 units in the evening; and atorvastatin 80 mg daily. His symptoms of IC have remained fairly stable until the recent development of a nonhealing ulcer on his toe. What options are there for R.L. if nonpharmacologic and pharmacologic interventions are not sufficient?

Surgical intervention eventually may be necessary for persistent and complicated disease. Because success rates for preventing amputation and postsurgical complications vary from institution to institution, surgery should be considered only for severely ischemic limbs and should be performed in a hospital with a good record of success.[111] Arterial bypass grafting and percutaneous transluminal angioplasty of the femoral or iliac arteries, similar to cardiac revascularization, are two procedures that can be performed. Angioplasty is beneficial in patients with localized disease, especially in the iliac or superficial femoral arteries, and should be considered in patients who truly are incapacitated by their activity limitations.[112] Angioplasty with or without stent deployment, atherectomy, and the use of drug-eluting stents in the peripheral arteries are all options.[8] The more invasive reconstructive arterial (bypass) surgery can be used if diffuse lesions preclude the use of localized angioplasty. The true benefits and pitfalls of these skilled interventions remain unclear.[113]

Emergency surgical intervention may be required if acute, persistent ischemia develops. This is frequently due to thrombosis associated with advanced atherosclerosis, although other causes, such as cardiac emboli, cannot be excluded.[103] Both surgical thrombectomy and localized thrombolytic administration[114] with tissue-plasminogen activator or urokinase have equal success in alleviating acute limb-threatening ischemia.[115,116] After surgical intervention, patients are advised to resume and remain on antiplatelet therapy indefinitely to reduce the risk of future events.

RAYNAUD PHENOMENON

RP is a clinical syndrome caused by episodic vasospasm and ischemia of the extremities in response to cold, emotional, or physical stimuli.[117–122] Episodes include changes in color of the extremities from white, due to vasoconstriction, to blue, signaling tissue hypoxia and then red when reperfusion occurs.[118] It is usually limited to the skin of the fingers, and less often the toes, but can also occur on the nose, cheeks, and ears.[119] Between attacks, the digits may appear cool and moist or normal. In most cases, the ischemia produced by the phenomenon does not have important consequences; however, in severe cases, atrophy of the skin, irregular nail growth, and wasting or ulceration of the tissue pads can occur.[119] Although both IC and RP are disorders of the peripheral arterial circulation, they differ significantly in that IC results primarily from atherosclerotic obstruction, whereas Raynaud disease is caused by vasospasm.

Diagnosis

This disorder can be separated into primary RP, indicating an idiopathic origin, and secondary RP, which consists of signs and symptoms of RP in the presence of an associated disease or condition, most commonly a connective tissue disorder, such as scleroderma (also known as systemic sclerosis), mixed connective tissue disease, rheumatoid arthritis, or systemic lupus erythematosus. Primary RP is more common (89% of patients) and is more likely to occur in younger patients (<30 years), generally presents with less severe symptoms, normal erythrocyte sedimentation rate, negative antinuclear antibodies, and no associated signs of underlying disease. Patients with secondary RP are more likely to have severe disease with painful symptoms which can progress to ulceration or gangrene in extremities if untreated.[119] The diagnosis is generally a subjective one, consisting of clinical signs and symptoms, cold hands, feet, or both without normal recovery after a cold stimulus, emotional stress, or physical stress (such as vibrations) to the extremities.[121,122] In unaffected individuals, a cold provocation should result in some mottling and cyanotic changes in the hands, with recovery once the stimuli are removed. In patients with RP, however, the same cold provocation causes closure of the digital arteries, which produces a sharply demarcated pallor and cyanosis of the digits that persists despite removal of the stimulus.[121]

Epidemiology

In general, the prevalence of RP is about 3% to 5% across several ethnic groups[120]; however, it is higher in some geographically defined populations.[120] It is more common in women than men, is more frequent in non-Hispanic whites, and has a higher prevalence in patients with family members who also experience RP. An onset in the teenage years suggests primary RP, whereas an onset after 30 years of age suggests a secondary cause.[120] Secondary RP is usually associated with a connective tissue disorder, but several other conditions may predispose individuals to its development. These include occupational-related exposures to vibratory machinery (e.g., drills, grinders, chain saws) that cause neural damage,[120] vinyl chloride, or hand trauma.[122–124] Approximately 15% of patients diagnosed with primary RP will go on to develop a connective tissue disorder within10 years.[125]

RP can also be associated with medications, including β-adrenergic blocking agents, ergots, cytotoxic drugs, chemotherapy, amphetamines and other sympathomimetics, and interferon, all of which can induce vasoconstriction.[126–128] Although avoidance of β-adrenergic blocking agents in patients with RP appears prudent, no discernible effect, as measured by skin temperature and blood flow, was found with the administration of both selective and nonselective β-blockers to patients with RP.[129] RP not associated with a connective tissue disorder is often transient and does not interfere with daily activities.[129] The effect of smoking on RP has yielded conflicting results. Overall, there appears to be a negligible effect of smoking on the prevalence of RP and the incidence of attacks, although there is some evidence that the severity of attacks may be decreased with smoking cessation.[130,131]

Pathophysiology

The pathophysiology involved in the exaggerated, abnormally long-lasting vasoconstriction in response to stimuli seen in RP is complex and still not completely understood. Control of blood vessel reactivity involves a balance of mediators released from circulating cells, the vascular endothelium, hormones, and neurotransmitters.[118,122] Cold-induced vasospastic attacks in patients with primary RP involve a heightened vasoconstriction of digital arteries that is mediated by a subset of peripheral α_2-adrenergic receptors.[118,122,132]

Vascular abnormalities noted in RP can include a deficiency of the vasodilator nitric oxide (NO), an increase in endothelial production of the potent vasoconstrictor endothelin-1, and increased activity of the renin–angiotensin system resulting in vasoconstriction induced by angiotensin II.[122] In secondary RP, structural changes resulting from connective tissue disease may cause arterial damage that results in the α_2-adrenoreceptor aberrancy and endothelial injury that stimulates vasoconstriction, platelet activation, and impaired fibrinolysis.[118,122] It is also possible that serotonin receptors play a role in RP. Serotonin agonists have caused decreased finger blood flow, and, conversely, antagonists have increased digital blood flow.[133]

Clinical Presentation

CASE 10-2

Question 1: L.G., a 39-year-old man, presents today with a 4-day history of left hand pain. He notes that the third digit of his left hand is "cold and somewhat blue," especially in the distal area. The other areas of his hand have recovered, but the distal portion of the digit remains cyanotic and numb. He has used acetaminophen and warm-water soaks without success. He is a construction worker who uses his hands "quite a bit" in his work. He has a history of gastroesophageal reflux and has no allergies. His social history is significant for smoking 1.5 packs of cigarettes a day for 19 years. On physical examination, his extremities reveal appropriate sensation of the forearm and hand. Some blue areas are noted on the distal portion on the third phalanx, with no other signs and symptoms. When L.G.'s opposite hand was placed in cold water, several white splotches appeared, and he experienced tingling in this hand as a result of the cold-water exposure. He is diagnosed as having RP. Does L.G. present with primary or secondary RP?

L.G. presents with what is most likely secondary RP owing to one of several potential underlying causes. His clinical presentation is classic for RP, with vasospasm, pallor, and a cyanotic overtone. The diagnosis is confirmed by the cold-water test, which indicates that the vasospastic attack is precipitated by cold exposure. He has a work history that may easily include hand trauma and the use of vibrating machinery, and his age also suggests secondary RP. Because of its association with connective tissue disorders, other laboratory tests such as an antinuclear antibody and erythrocyte sedimentation rate should be checked.

Treatment

NONPHARMACOLOGIC MANAGEMENT

Case 10-2, Question 2: What conservative measures can be taken with L.G. to prevent or decrease the painful vasospasm of RP?

Most patients with either primary or secondary RP will respond to conservative management to reduce exposure to triggers such as cold and emotional stress.[119] L.G. should be instructed to protect his hands and fingers from exposure by using mittens and insulated wrappers when handling cold drinks, and to protect other parts of his body from cold exposure. He should also try to minimize emotional stress and occupational exposure to vibrating machinery, and avoid medications that can induce vasoconstriction, particularly sympathomimetics, clonidine, serotonin receptor agonists, and ergot preparations.[119,120] He should be encouraged to stop smoking, which may not affect occurrence of attacks but may decrease their severity and provide an overall positive health benefit.[130]

L.G. has new-onset and relatively mild RP. For others who have more severe symptoms and manifestations, especially patients with underlying connective tissue disorders, it is important to immediately and aggressively manage any ulcers that develop on the digits and to be extremely vigilant in detecting infected digits. Rarely, patients who have severe symptoms including ulceration or thrombosis may require surgical intervention such as peripheral sympathectomy, embolectomy, or ulcer debridement.[119,134,135]

CALCIUM-CHANNEL BLOCKERS

CASE 10-2, QUESTION 3: Nifedipine extended-release 30 mg every day is ordered for L.G. What is the rationale for using a CCB in this case?

Drugs can be used to treat primary and secondary RP if it interferes with the patient's ability to work or perform daily activities or if digital lesions develop. Most proposed treatments for RP are variably effective, and they introduce the risk for significant side effects.[136,137] Drug therapy should always be in addition to nonpharmacologic measures.

Dihydropyridine CCBs decrease calcium ion influx and prevent vascular smooth muscle contraction, especially vascular responses evoked by cold exposure. Nifedipine, a potent peripheral vasodilator, has been studied the most and has become the drug of choice in patients with RP not controlled by conservative measures. In primary RP, 10 or more episodes per week are common. A meta-analysis showed a decrease of 2.8 to 5 attacks per week and a decrease in severity by 33%.[137] Patients with secondary RP experience a similar decrease in attack severity and also achieve a decrease in number of attacks with nifedipine therapy. Because their baseline number of attacks per week often exceeds 20, the relative benefit is not as great as with primary RP, averaging approximately a 25% decrease in weekly episodes.[138] Doses of 10 to 30 mg 3 times daily of immediate-release nifedipine are beneficial,[137,138] although higher doses, if tolerated, may be required for maximal benefit.[137] Most clinicians administer nifedipine as an extended-release formulation to increase convenience and decrease side effects such as dizziness, headache, facial flushing, and peripheral edema, which can occur in up to 50% of patients,[119,122,137] and this practice is supported by clinical studies.[139,140]

Although less thoroughly studied than nifedipine, other vasoselective CCBs, such as amlodipine, felodipine, isradipine, and nisoldipine, decrease the frequency and severity of ischemic attacks.[141–144] Patients who do not benefit from nifedipine likely will not benefit by switching to another CCB. Patients who cannot tolerate the side effects of nifedipine (e.g., peripheral edema, headache) might benefit by switching to another CCB.

L.G. should be warned of the potential side effects with nifedipine therapy, especially dizziness associated with hypotension, and should return in 2 weeks for assessment. A 30-mg daily dose of extended-release nifedipine is a reasonable starting dose. He should be instructed to keep a diary documenting the number of attacks he experiences and details surrounding each attack, such as time course and precipitating factors. In addition to the usual side effects mentioned above, L.G. should be aware that his symptoms of gastroesophageal reflux could worsen with nifedipine therapy, which can cause a decreased lower esophageal sphincter pressure. This side effect should be specifically assessed at his follow-up appointment.

OTHER THERAPEUTIC AGENTS

CASE 10-2, QUESTION 4: What other drugs may be tried if L.G. cannot tolerate the CCB?

Other than CCBs, no proven therapy for RP exists. Many agents, however, have been used based on limited data. The α_1-adrenergic antagonist prazosin, 1 mg 3 times a day, yielded moderate benefit in two-thirds of patients in two small studies.[145,146] Side effects of prazosin are significant at maximal doses and include dizziness, edema, fatigue, and orthostasis. The longer acting α_1-adrenergic antagonist terazosin was evaluated in one small study, and it improved symptomatology as well as objective measures of blood flow.[147] Insufficient data with this class of drugs exist to routinely recommend their initial use in patients with RP. Topical nitrates have been used clinically for several years and newer formulations have recently been studied, but data showing efficacy is limited.[119]

Several therapeutic approaches are being vigorously investigated and show promise as future therapies for RP. These include the intravenous prostaglandin analogs iloprost and alprostadil, which enhance nitric oxide–mediated vasodilation[148]; endothelin antagonists, such as bosentan[149]; and oral phosphodiesterase inhibitors[150–152] which also promote vasodilation. A meta-analysis of phosphodiesterase inhibitors for the treatment of secondary RP showed a modest decrease in frequency and duration of attacks, although further larger trials are needed.[152] Botulinum toxin-A has also been studied.[153] Because of side effects, cost, and administration difficulties, these agents are primarily being studied in the most severe cases of secondary RP with digital ulcers or other systemic complications associated with connective tissue diseases. If benefit is proved, however, it will shed light on the pathogenesis of the disorder, and perhaps lead to therapies appropriate for the larger population with RP.

Statins may have promise in severe cases resulting in digital ulcers secondary to systemic sclerosis (SSc). Pleiotropic effects of atorvastatin 40 mg/day on endothelial function compared with placebo were investigated in 84 SSc patients who fulfilled the American College of Rheumatology criteria for classification of SSc with secondary RP despite ongoing vasodilator therapy. The study found a significant decrease in both new and the total number of digital ulcers in the atorvastatin group compared with placebo.[154]

The renin–angiotensin system mediators act as vasodilators and have been investigated in several small studies. ACE inhibitors and angiotensin receptor blockers, however, have yielded conflicting results with respect to beneficial effects in patients with RP.[155–158] Small beneficial effects have been realized, specifically with captopril 25 mg 3 times a day and losartan 12.5 to 25 mg/day; however, no benefit has been found with enalapril 20 mg once daily.[155] Fluoxetine, a selective serotonin reuptake inhibitor, was shown in one study to reduce the symptoms of RP.[159] It is hypothesized to exert its effect by depleting platelet serotonin, rendering the platelet unable to release a significant amount of the vasoconstrictive serotonin during activation and aggregation.

Alternative therapies, such as *Ginkgo biloba* and L-arginine, have also been studied in small trials with positive results; however, larger trials are needed to confirm the findings before these therapies can be recommended.[160–162]

All patients with RP should be counseled regarding cold avoidance and other protective measures. A CCB, extended-release nifedipine if tolerated, should be initiated if conservative measures are ineffective and titrated to the highest tolerated dose and symptom resolution. Combination therapies have not been investigated, but another agent, such as an α_1-adrenergic antagonist, may be considered in addition to the CCB if symptom resolution is not satisfactory and side effects permit.

NOCTURNAL LEG MUSCLE CRAMPS

Nocturnal leg muscle cramps are idiopathic, involuntary contractions occurring at rest that cause a visible and palpable knot in the affected muscle. This type of muscle cramp usually afflicts middle-aged to elderly persons and is a distressing and painful condition. Its cause is unknown. The two primary hypotheses that attempt to explain the pathophysiology propose neurologic impairments. One involves a central nervous system impairment of γ-aminobutyric acid,[163] and the other, an impaired peripheral response to muscle lengthening.[164] Although the incidence of nocturnal cramps is unknown, some data indicate it is very common. In a survey of veterans (95% men averaging 60 years of age), 56% complained of leg cramps, with 12% having cramping nearly every night[165]; 36% of these veterans were also attempting some type of drug treatment for their symptoms. A survey of the general population revealed that the prevalence of nocturnal leg cramps was 37% in people older than 50 years of age, and increased to 54% in people older than 80 years of age. The prevalence in men and women is equal.[166] Nocturnal leg cramps are associated with lower extremity atherosclerosis, CAD, and peripheral neurologic deficits.[166,167]

Clinical Presentation

CASE 10-3

QUESTION 1: H.C., a 62-year-old woman, complains of cramps in her left calf that began last night around 10 PM. The cramps occurred several times throughout the night and has resolved slowly this morning. These nighttime cramping episodes occur frequently, are very painful, and cause her calf muscle to become "knotted," but is not associated with walking. She denies any trauma, fever, or chills, has no other medical problems, and takes no medications. Her physical examination, extended chemistry panel, and thyroid function tests are unremarkable, and her vital signs are stable. H.C. works at an elementary school and walks up and down stairs throughout the day. Her physician associates the pain with nocturnal leg cramps. What characteristics differentiate H.C.'s nocturnal leg cramps from other pain syndromes?

Benign nocturnal leg cramps usually occur in the early hours of sleeping; they are asymmetric and primarily affect the calf muscle and small muscles of the foot. These cramps are not associated with exercise, electrolyte or laboratory abnormalities, or medications, although cramping requiring therapy was more likely in the first year of patients being prescribed long-acting β-agonists, thiazide, and potassium-sparing diuretics.[168]

For diagnosis and treatment of nocturnal cramps, other causes of muscle cramping, including drug-induced cramps, must be excluded (Table 10-8). The onset of cramps at rest is characteristic of ordinary leg cramps and is the primary symptom used for diagnosis. Clinical signs of sodium depletion, hyperthyroidism and hypothyroidism, tetany, and lower motor neuron disease should be evaluated. Laboratory measurements such as standard electrolytes and thyroid function tests can help rule out some of these other conditions.

Table 10-8
Other Causes of Muscle Cramps[169–171]

Drug-Induced Cramps	Biochemical Causes	Other
Alcohol	Dehydration	Contractures
Antipsychotics (dystonia)	Hemodialysis	Diabetes
β-Agonists (e.g., albuterol, terbutaline, salbutamol)	Hypocalcemia	Lower motor neuron disease
Cimetidine	Hypokalemia	Peripheral vascular disease
Clofibrate	Hypomagnesemia	Tetany
Diuretics	Hyponatremia	Thyroid disease
Lithium	Uremia	
Narcotic analgesics		
Nicotinic acid		
Nifedipine		
Penicillamine		
Statins		
Steroids		

Treatment

THERAPEUTIC OBJECTIVES AND NONPHARMACOLOGIC INTERVENTIONS

CASE 10-3, QUESTION 2: What are the therapeutic objectives in treating H.C.? What nonpharmacologic recommendations can be made?

The primary treatment goal is to prevent this uncomfortable condition. Given the limited evidence and potential side effects with drug therapy, nonpharmacologic therapy is the preferred initial therapy. Patients are commonly advised to stretch out the afflicted muscle or perform dorsiflexion of the feet throughout the day and before bedtime.[170] Patients are also warned to avoid plantar flexion while sleeping by hanging the feet over the edge of the bed when sleeping on the stomach. Once a cramp occurs, the goal is to relieve the cramp as quickly as possible. Acute therapy consists of dorsiflexion (grasping the toes and pulling them upward in the opposite direction of the cramp). This can be accomplished with the hands, by walking, or by leaning toward a wall while standing 2 feet away from it, maintaining the feet flat on the floor.[172]

PHARMACOTHERAPY

CASE 10-3, QUESTION 3: H.C. adopted the recommended stretching practices, and reduced plantar flexion during sleep. She returns 3 months later, and reports a minor decrease in the attack frequency, but not severity. Her sleep is affected 2 to 3 nights/week, and she feels it is affecting her performance as a teacher. She remembers her aunt taking a "pill" for her leg cramps. Are there any medications that may help relieve her symptoms?

A variety of medications have been reported to help treat nocturnal leg cramps, but all have limited, very limited, and inconclusive evidence. Vitamin B_{12}, vitamin E, diphenhydramine, gabapentin, diltiazem, and verapamil have limited effectiveness data, mostly via small single trials or case series. Quinine historically had been the most frequently prescribed medication for nocturnal leg cramps. The FDA, however, has clearly stated quinine should not be used for nocturnal leg cramps because of an unfavorable risk–benefit ratio.[173]

Quinine has been used to treat nocturnal leg cramps since the 1940s, when four patients having leg cramps experienced marked improvement in symptoms after being treated with quinine.[174] Despite its use, significant controversy exists about its benefit. Only a few small controlled trials have been conducted, with mixed conclusions. A meta-analysis was published in 1998 that included both published and unpublished data addressing the efficacy of quinine in the treatment of leg cramps.[175] Pooled data from 659 patients indicated that quinine, at 200 to 325 mg/day, reduced the severity and average number of cramps experienced in a 4-week period from 17.1 to 13.5. Of note, a recent study that randomly assigned patients to quinine cessation reported no effect on nocturnal leg cramp frequency (e.g., no worsening of symptoms).[176]

Cinchonism, a syndrome that includes nausea, vomiting, blurred vision, tinnitus, and deafness, is a dose-related side effect of quinine.[169] Tinnitus alone occurs in up to 3% of patients.[177] With overdose, central nervous system manifestations, such as headache, confusion, and delirium, can occur. Self-limiting rashes

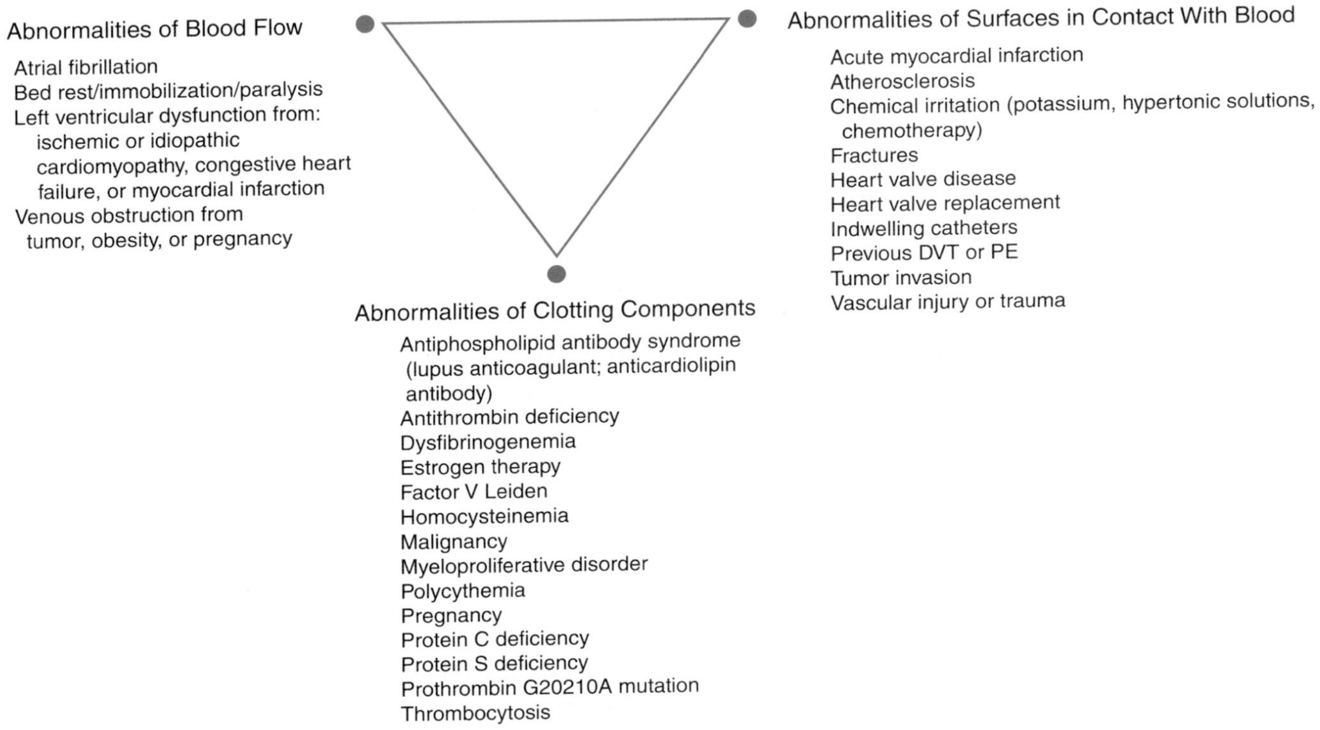

Abnormalities of Blood Flow
Atrial fibrillation
Bed rest/immobilization/paralysis
Left ventricular dysfunction from: ischemic or idiopathic cardiomyopathy, congestive heart failure, or myocardial infarction
Venous obstruction from tumor, obesity, or pregnancy
Abnormalities of Surfaces in Contact With Blood
Acute myocardial infarction
Atherosclerosis
Chemical irritation (potassium, hypertonic solutions, chemotherapy)
Fractures
Heart valve disease
Heart valve replacement
Indwelling catheters
Previous DVT or PE
Tumor invasion
Vascular injury or trauma
Abnormalities of Clotting Components
Antiphospholipid antibody syndrome (lupus anticoagulant; anticardiolipin antibody)
Antithrombin deficiency
Dysfibrinogenemia
Estrogen therapy
Factor V Leiden
Homocysteinemia
Malignancy
Myeloproliferative disorder
Polycythemia
Pregnancy
Protein C deficiency
Protein S deficiency
Prothrombin G20210A mutation
Thrombocytosis

Figure 11-1 Risk factors for thromboembolism.

Anticoagulant drug therapy is aimed at preventing pathologic clot formation in patients at risk and at preventing clot extension and/or embolization in patients who have experienced thrombosis. This chapter emphasizes arterial and venous thromboembolic disease and the use of the parenteral anticoagulants (unfractionated heparin, low-molecular-weight heparins, indirect factor Xa inhibitors, and injectable direct thrombin inhibitors) and oral agents (vitamin K antagonists, and direct oral anticoagulants [DOACs], which include the oral direct thrombin inhibitors, and the oral direct factor Xa inhibitors). Chapter 8, Dyslipidemias, Atherosclerosis, and Coronary Artery Disease; Chapter 13, Acute Coronary Syndrome, and Chapter 61, Ischemic and Hemorrhagic Stroke, provide more in-depth discussions of thrombolytic agents and antiplatelet therapy.

Etiology of Thromboembolism

Three primary factors influence the formation of pathologic clots and are described in a model referred to as Virchow's triad (Fig. 11-1).[1] Abnormalities of blood flow that cause venous stasis can result in DVT, which can progress to PE if embolization occurs. Intracardiac stasis of blood can also result in clot formation within the heart chambers, and embolization of intracardiac thrombi may lead to stroke or other systemic manifestations. Abnormalities of blood vessel walls, such as those that occur in injury or trauma to the vasculature, are a second source of thrombus formation. The presence of foreign material within the vasculature, including artificial heart valves and central venous catheters, is also thrombogenic and, like vascular injury, represents the presence of an abnormal surface in contact with blood. Finally, hypercoagulability resulting from alterations in the availability or the integrity of blood-clotting components or naturally occurring anticoagulants also represents a significant risk factor for thromboembolic disease.[2]

Clot Formation

The intact endothelial lining of blood vessels normally repels platelets and inhibits clot formation through secretion of numerous inhibitory substances. Damage to the endothelium leads to exposure of circulating blood to subendothelial substances, and this results in formation of a fibrin clot.[2]

PLATELET ADHESION, ACTIVATION, AND AGGREGATION

Endothelial damage leads to exposure of blood to subendothelial collagen and phospholipids, resulting in platelet adhesion to the surface. Von Willebrand factor serves as the binding ligand for platelet adhesion, via the glycoprotein I (GPI) receptor on the platelet surface. Adhered platelets become activated and release numerous compounds, including adenosine diphosphate and thromboxane A2, which stimulate platelet aggregation. Fibrinogen serves as the binding ligand for platelet aggregation, via the GPIIb/IIIa receptor on the platelet surface.[2]

CLOTTING CASCADE

Transformation of the relatively unstable platelet plug (i.e., the aggregated platelets) to a stable fibrin clot occurs as a result of an imbalance between other procoagulant and anticoagulant factors. In addition to stimulating the platelet response, endothelial damage results in activation of the extrinsic pathway of the clotting cascade by the release of thromboplastin (tissue factor) (Fig. 11-2). Tissue factor converts factor VII to factor VIIa, which mediates the activation of factor X. The intrinsic pathway of the clotting cascade is activated by exposure of factor XII to subendothelial components exposed during vessel injury. The intrinsic pathway mediates factor X activation via a chain of events initiated by factor XI. The distinction between these pathways is primarily an in vitro phenomenon; in vivo, the two pathways are activated simultaneously.

Once stimulated, both the extrinsic and intrinsic pathways activate the common pathway of the clotting cascade via factor X. Activated forms of factors V and VIII serve independently to accelerate this process. The final steps include conversion of factor II (prothrombin) to factor IIa (thrombin), with eventual formation of a stable fibrin clot.

Naturally occurring inhibitors of clotting factors play a role in localizing fibrin formation to the sites of injury and in maintaining the fluidity of circulating blood. Table 11-1 outlines these clotting inhibitors and their primary actions. In addition, the fibrinolytic system is involved in degradation of fibrin clots. The actions of both clotting inhibitors and the fibrinolytic system prevent excessive coagulation.

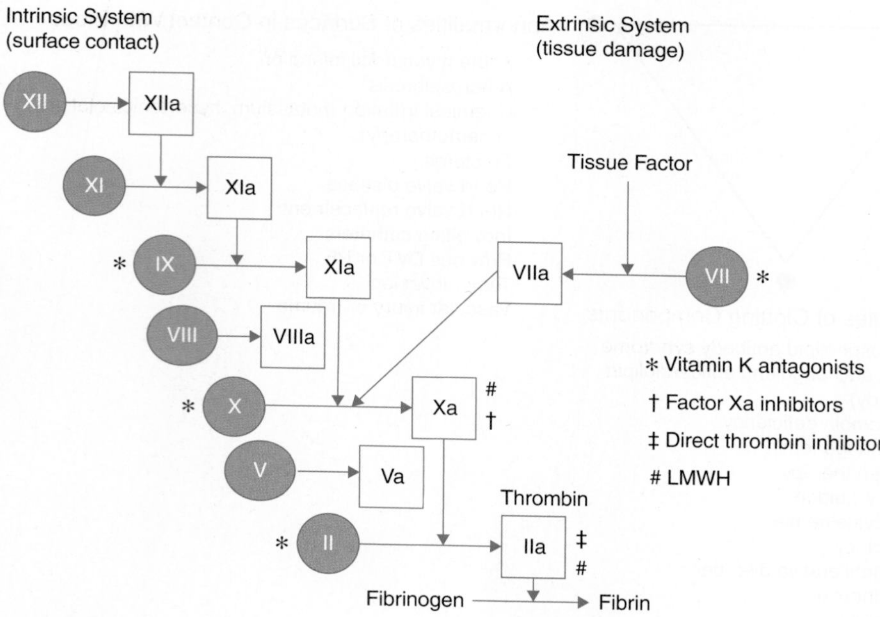

Figure 11-2 Simplified clotting cascade and respective anticoagulant targets.

Thus, the process of clot formation is dynamic and involves various factors that can stimulate, inhibit, and dissolve a fibrin clot.

PATHOLOGIC THROMBI

Pathologic thrombi are sometimes classified according to location and composition. Arterial thrombi are composed primarily of platelets, although they also contain fibrin and occasional leukocytes. Arterial thrombi generally occur in areas of rapid blood flow (i.e., arteries) and are typically initiated by spontaneous or mechanical rupture of atherosclerotic plaques followed by aggregation of platelets (see Chapter 8, Dyslipidemias, Atherosclerosis, and Coronary Heart Disease; and Chapter 13, Acute Coronary Syndrome). Venous thrombi are found primarily in the venous circulation and are composed almost entirely of fibrin and erythrocytes. Venous thrombi have a small platelet head and generally form in response to either venous stasis or vascular injury after surgery or trauma. The areas of stasis prevent dilution of activated coagulation factors by normal blood flow.

The selection of an antithrombotic agent is influenced by the type of thrombus to be treated. The anticoagulants heparin, low-molecular-weight heparins (LMWHs), indirect and direct factor Xa inhibitors, direct thrombin inhibitors, and warfarin are used in the treatment and prevention of both arterial and venous thrombi. Drugs that alter platelet function (e.g., aspirin, clopidogrel), alone and/or in combination with anticoagulants, are primarily used in the prevention of arterial thrombi. Fibrinolytic agents are used for rapid dissolution of thromboemboli, most notably during myocardial infarction (MI).

Table 11-1
Inhibitors of Clotting Mechanisms

Inhibitor	Target
Antithrombin	Inhibits factors IIa, IXa, and Xa
Protein S	Cofactor for activation of protein C
Protein C	Inactivates factors Va and VIIIa
Tissue factor pathway inhibitor	Inhibits activity of factor VIIa
Plasminogen	Converted to plasmin via tissue plasminogen activator
Plasmin	Lyses fibrin into fibrin degradation products

Pharmacology of Antithrombotic Agents

HEPARIN

Heparin is a rapid-acting anticoagulant that is administered parenterally. Standard heparin (unfractionated heparin [UFH]) is a heterogeneous mixture of glycosaminoglycans of varying molecular weights obtained from bovine lung or porcine intestinal mucosa (Table 11-2). The action of heparin is facilitated by its binding to the naturally circulating anticoagulant antithrombin (AT), a serine protease also referred to as heparin cofactor. Binding of heparin to AT accelerates the anticoagulant effect of AT. The heparin–AT complex attaches to and irreversibly inactivates factor IIa (thrombin) and factor Xa, as well as activated factors IX, XI, and XII.[3] Approximately one-third of the molecules present in UFH bind to AT and provide the anticoagulant properties of heparin. The remaining two-thirds of the heparin molecules bind to plasma proteins and to endothelial cells. In addition to its anticoagulant effects, heparin inhibits platelet function and increases vascular permeability; these properties contribute to the hemorrhagic effects of heparin.

In cases of acute DVT or PE, the clotting cascade has been activated, generating abnormal quantities of thrombin and fibrin. In these situations, thrombin must be inactivated directly, a process that may require relatively large doses of heparin. However, when the clotting cascade is in a normal balance, it is possible to indirectly inactivate thrombin with smaller heparin doses by complexing factor Xa. Because of the amplification effect of the clotting cascade, inactivation of relatively small amounts of factor Xa indirectly prevents the production of large quantities of thrombin. This phenomenon is the basis for low-dose heparin prophylaxis after surgery or in cases of prolonged bed rest or immobilization.

Heparin may be administered intravenously (IV) by continuous infusion, or subcutaneously (SC), although its bioavailability is significantly reduced by SC administration. Intramuscular administration of heparin (as well as intramuscular administration of other drugs in patients who are anticoagulated) should be avoided because of the potential for hematoma formation.

After IV administration, the anticoagulant effect of heparin is noted immediately. During active thromboembolism, the high concentration of clotting factors necessitates a higher concentration of heparin to neutralize them. This increased dosing requirement may also be related to continuing thrombin formation on the surface of the thrombus. Once endothelialization (localization and incorporation of the clot into the vascular endothelium) of the clot

Table 11-5
Approved Dosing of the DOACs for AF and VTE

	Atrial Fibrillation[a]	VTE Treatment
Dabigatran	CrCl > 30 mL/minute: 150 mg BID CrCl 30–50 mL/minute on dronedarone or ketoconazole: decrease to 75 mg BID CrCl 15–30 mL/minute: 75 mg BID or avoid if on P-gp inhibitor CrCl < 15 mL/minute or on dialysis: dosing recommendations cannot be provided	CrCl > 30 mL/minute: LMWH or UFH × 5–10 days then dabigatran 150 mg BID CrCl < 50 mL/minute and on P-gp inhibitor: avoid coadministration CrCl ≤ 30 mL/minute or on dialysis: dosing recommendations cannot be provided Extended treatment to prevent VTE recurrence (CrCl > 30 mL/minute): 150 mg BID
Rivaroxaban	Dosed with evening meal: CrCl > 50 mL/minute: 20 mg daily CrCl 15–50 mL/minute: 15 mg daily CrCl < 15 mL/minute: avoid	CrCl ≥ 30 mL/minute: 15 mg BID × 21 days then 20 mg daily CrCl < 30 mL/minute: avoid Extended treatment to prevent VTE recurrence: 20 mg daily
Apixaban	Most patients: 5 mg BID Any two of the following: 2.5mg BID: SCr ≥ 1.5mg/dL Age ≥ 80 years Weight ≤ 60 kg	10 mg BID × 7 days then 5 mg BID No dose adjustment recommended for renal function[b] Extended treatment to prevent VTE recurrence: 2.5 mg BID Strong dual inhibitors of CYP3A4 and p-glycoprotein (P-gp): reduce dose by 50% if taking 5 mg or 10 mg ■ If already taking 2.5 mg BID: avoid use Dual P-gp inducers and strong CYP3A4 inducers: avoid concomitant use
Edoxaban	CrCl > 95 mL/minute: do not use CrCl > 50–95 mL/minute: 60 mg daily CrCl 15–50 mL/minute: 30 mg daily CrCl < 15 mL/minute: use is not recommended	CrCl > 50 mL/minute: LMWH or UFH × 5–10 days then edoxaban 60 mg daily CrCl 15–50 mL/minute: 30 mg daily CrCl < 15 mL/minute: use is not recommended Pts ≤ 60 kg or on P-gp inhibitors: 30 mg daily

[a]DOACs are only indicated for nonvalvular AF.
[b]Patients with CrCl < 25 mL/minute excluded from clinical trials for apixaban.
BID, twice daily.
Source: *Pradaxa (dabigatran) [package insert]*. Ridgefield, CT: Boehringer Ingelheim Pharmaceuticals, Inc.; 2017; *Xarelto (rivaroxaban) [package insert]*. Titusville, NJ: Janssen Pharmaceuticals, Inc; 2017; *Eliquis (apixaban) [package insert]*. Princeton, NJ: Bristol-Myers Squibb Company; 2017; *Savaysa (edoxaban) [package insert]*. Parsippany, NJ: Daiichi Sankyo; 2017.

Table 11-6
Drug Interactions with the DOACs

Drug	Recommendation
Dabigatran	P-gp inhibitors: Reduced dose recommended with CrCl 30–50 mL/min and ketoconazole or dronedarone CrCl 15–30 mL/minute: AVOID concomitant use P-gp inducers: AVOID concomitant use with rifampin
Rivaroxaban	P-gp inhibitors and strong CYP3A4 inhibitors: Avoid concomitant use (e.g., ketoconazole, itraconazole, ritonavir, indinivir, conivaptan) P-gp inducers and strong CYP3A4 inducers: Avoid concomitant use (e.g., carbamazepine, phenytoin, rifampin, St. John's wort)
Apixaban	P-gp inhibitors and strong CYP3A4 inhibitors: Reduced dose recommended, or avoid concomitant use if currently on lowest dose (2.5mg) P-gp inducers and strong CYP3A4 inducers: Avoid concomitant use (e.g., carbamazepine, phenytoin, rifampin, St. John's wort)
Edoxaban	P-gp inhibitors (e.g., verapamil, quinidine, azithromycin, clarithromycin, erythromycin, itraconazole, or ketoconazole) AF: No dose reduction is recommended VTE: Reduced dose recommended P-gp inducers: AVOID concomitant use with rifampin
Betrixaban	P-gp inhibitors (e.g., amiodarone, azithromycin, verapamil, ketoconazole, clarithromycin) Medical prophylaxis: Reduced dose recommended P-gp inducers: no warnings at this time

Source: *Pradaxa (dabigatran) [package insert]*. Ridgefield, CT: Boehringer Ingelheim Pharmaceuticals, Inc., 2017; *Xarelto (rivaroxaban) [package insert]*. Titusville, NJ: Janssen Pharmaceuticals, Inc., 2017; *Eliquis (apixaban) [package insert]*. Princeton, NJ: Bristol-Myers Squibb Company, 2017; *Savaysa (edoxaban) [package insert]*. Parsippany, NJ: Daiichi Sankyo, 2017; *BEVYXXA (betrixaban) [package insert]*. South San Francisco, California: Portola Pharmaceuticals, Inc., 2017.

Table 11-7

Pharmacologic and Clinical Properties of Injectable Direct Thrombin Inhibitors

	Bivalirudin	Argatroban
Route of administration	IV	IV
FDA-approved indication	Patients with UA undergoing PTCA; PCI with provisional use of GPI; patients with or at risk of HIT/HITTS undergoing PCI	Treatment of thrombosis in patients with HIT; patients at risk for HIT undergoing PCI
Binding to thrombin	Partially reversible at catalytic site and exosite-1	Reversible at catalytic site
Half-life in healthy subjects	25 minutes	40–50 minutes
Monitoring	aPTT/ACT SCr/CrCl	aPTT/ACT Liver function
Clearance	Enzymatic (80%) Renal (20%)	Hepatic
Antibody development	May cross-react with antihirudin antibodies	No
Effect on INR	Slight increase	Increase
Initial dose for HIT	No bolus Infusion: 0.15 mg/kg/hour	No bolus Infusion: 2 mcg/kg/minute[a] In critically ill patients: consider lower infusion rate of 0.2–1 mcg/kg/minute
Initial dose for PCI	Bolus: 0.75 mg/kg Infusion: 1.75 mg/kg/hour	Bolus: 350 mcg/kg Infusion: 25 mcg/kg/minute

[a]In some cases, an initial infusion rates of < 1.5 mcg/kg/minute may be more appropriate.
ACT, activated clotting time; aPTT, activated partial thromboplastin time; BID, twice daily; CrCl, creatinine clearance; GPI, glycoprotein IIb-IIIa inhibitor; HD, hemodialysis; HIT, heparin-induced thrombocytopenia; HITTS, heparin-induced thrombocytopenia and thrombosis syndrome; IV, intravenous; PCI, percutaneous coronary intervention; PTCA, percutaneous transluminal coronary angioplasty; SC, subcutaneous; SCr, serum creatinine; UA, unstable angina.

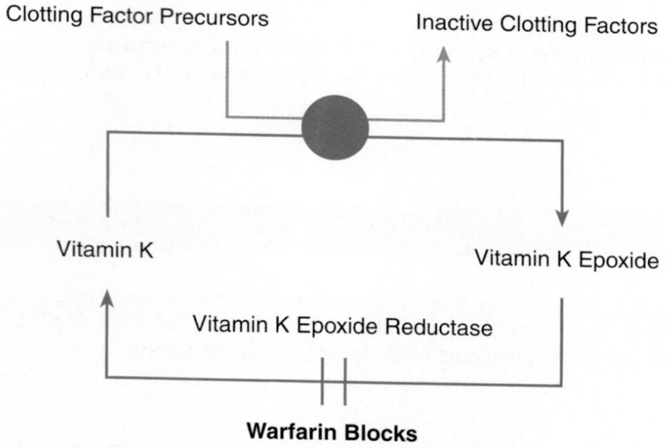

Figure 11-3 Mechanism of action of warfarin.

Table 11-8

Elimination Half-lives of Vitamin K-Dependent Clotting Factors

Clotting Factor	Half-Life (hours)
II	42–72
VII	4–6
IX	21–30
X	27–48
Protein C	9
Protein S	60

initiated or after dosing changes. Protein C and its cofactor protein S are also vitamin K dependent, and these proteins are depleted by warfarin at rates dependent on their elimination half-lives.

Warfarin is rapidly and completely absorbed in the upper gastrointestinal (GI) tract by passive diffusion, with nearly 100% bioavailability. Peak absorption of warfarin occurs in 60 to 120 minutes. It is approximately 99% bound to serum albumin. The volume of distribution for warfarin is 12.5% of body weight. This small volume of distribution is consistent with the extensive binding of warfarin to albumin. The primary laboratory test for monitoring warfarin therapy is the prothrombin time (PT). No correlation appears to exist between PT and the dose of warfarin, the total warfarin concentration, or the free warfarin concentration for any population of treated patients, although in individual patients an increasing dose of warfarin will increase the serum concentration (free and total) and the PT.

Warfarin is administered orally as a racemic mixture containing equal parts of the enantiomers R(+)-warfarin and S(−)- warfarin. The S(−)-isomer is 2.7 to 3.8 times more potent as an anticoagulant than the R(+)-isomer, has a longer elimination half-life, and is primarily metabolized by CYP2C9. Comparatively, R(+)-warfarin is metabolized primarily by CYP1A2 and CYP3A4. Many drugs interact with warfarin by stereoselectively inhibiting the metabolism of either the R(+)-isomer or the S(−)-isomer (see Drug Interactions section).

Genetic expression of CYP2C9 influences the rate of metabolism of warfarin and thus impacts dosing requirements to meet a particular therapeutic end point.[7] Variability in genetic expression of VKORC1 (the C1 subunit on the gene that codes for VKOR) also influences dosing requirements in patients taking warfarin. Genetic testing for CYP2C9 genotype and VKORC1 haplotype can be incorporated with clinical and demographic information to predict warfarin dose requirements in individual patients, using dosing algorithms that have been developed and investigated. A practical example is available online at www.warfarindosing.org. Routine pharmacogenomic testing of warfarin is not currently endorsed at this time.

Tests Used to Monitor Antithrombotic Therapy

Before the initiation of any antithrombotic therapy, an assessment of baseline hemostatic status is necessary. The clinician should obtain a baseline platelet count and hemoglobin (Hgb) and/or hematocrit (Hct), as well as evaluate the baseline integrity of the extrinsic and intrinsic coagulation pathways with PT and aPTT, the tests used to monitor warfarin and heparin, respectively. The DOACs do not require routine monitoring of laboratory tests to monitor their efficacy; however, because they have different doses based on renal function, baseline CrCl is needed with these agents.

PROTHROMBIN TIME/INTERNATIONAL NORMALIZED RATIO

The PT is prolonged by deficiencies of clotting factors II, V, VII, and X, as well as by low levels of fibrinogen and very high levels of heparin. It reflects alterations in the extrinsic and common pathways of the clotting cascade, but not in the intrinsic system.[8] The PT is measured by adding calcium and tissue thromboplastin to a sample of plasma from which platelets have been removed by centrifugation. The time to clot formation is detected by automated instruments using light scattering techniques that measure optical density. The mean normal PT, obtained by averaging a number of PT results from nonanticoagulated subjects, is approximately 12 seconds for most reagents.

The thromboplastins used in PT monitoring are extracted from various tissue sources by a number of techniques and prepared for commercial use as reagents. Unfortunately, thromboplastins are not standardized among manufacturers or among batches of reagent produced by the same manufacturer, leading to significant variability in PT results for anticoagulated patients. To standardize PT results, the World Health Organization developed a system by which all commercially available thromboplastins are compared with an international reference thromboplastin and then assigned an international sensitivity index (ISI). This value is used to mathematically convert PT to the international normalized ratio (INR) by exponentially multiplying the PT ratio to the power of the ISI of the thromboplastin being used in the laboratory to measure the test:

$$\text{INR} = (\text{PT patient}/\text{PT mean normal})^{\text{ISI}} \quad \text{(Eq. 11-1)}$$

The ISI of the international reference thromboplastin is 1.0.

The INR is the internationally recognized standard for monitoring warfarin therapy.[9] Current recommendations for intensity of oral anticoagulation therapy for accepted clinical indications are summarized in Table 11-9. Regular intensity therapy is defined as dosing warfarin to reach a goal INR of 2.5 (range, 2.0–3.0) and is appropriate for most settings that require the prevention and/or treatment of thromboembolic disease. High-intensity therapy is used in mechanical valve replacement and certain situations of thromboembolic recurrence, despite adequate anticoagulation, and is defined as dosing warfarin to reach a goal INR of 3.0 (range, 2.5–3.5).

ACTIVATED PARTIAL THROMBOPLASTIN TIME

The aPTT reflects alterations in the intrinsic pathway of the clotting cascade and is used to monitor heparin and injectable direct thrombin inhibitors.[8,9] The test is performed by adding a surface-activating agent (kaolin or micronized silica), a partial thromboplastin reagent (phospholipid; platelet substitute), and calcium to the plasma sample. Mean normal values vary among reagents, but typically fall between 24 and 36 seconds.

Like PT, the aPTT is a highly variable test based on differences among commercially available partial thromboplastin reagents. However, a system equivalent to the INR has not been developed for standardization of aPTT results. Heparinization to prolong the aPTT to 1.5 to 2.5 times the mean normal value historically was considered adequate to prevent propagation or extension of thrombus, but is no longer recommended because it is not appropriate for all reagents and testing systems. Instead, the aPTT should be calibrated for each reagent lot and coagulometer, and a reagent-specific therapeutic range in seconds should be determined that corresponds to therapeutic heparin levels of 0.3 to 0.7 international units/mL by factor Xa inhibition (anti-Xa activity).[3,9] For direct thrombin inhibitors, the same aPTT goal range is used.

Hospital-based and independent clinical laboratories that offer aPTT monitoring will report the reagent-specific therapeutic range in seconds and adjust it as new reagents are purchased and used clinically.

ANTI-FACTOR Xa ACTIVITY

Although LMWHs do not require coagulation monitoring to ensure an appropriate antithrombotic effect or to adjust dosing, certain clinical situations may require assessment of the anti-factor Xa activity of LMWHs.[3] Because these agents are eliminated renally, patients with renal failure may accumulate LMWHs, leading to an increased risk of hemorrhagic complications. Evaluation of trough anti-factor Xa activity at the end of the dosing interval can assess this accumulation of effect. LMWHs are dosed according to total body weight, but clinical trials have included only limited numbers of obese patients. Therefore, it may be appropriate to monitor anti-factor Xa activity in patients who weigh more than 150 kg. Anti-factor Xa activity may also be evaluated in patients who experience unexpected bleeding complications secondary to anticoagulation with LMWHs, and in pregnant patients in whom LMWHs are used for treatment or prevention of thrombosis.

Anti-factor Xa activity is measured using a chromogenic assay. If peak activity levels are used to assess dosing in obese and pregnant patients, they should be obtained once the patient has reached steady state, typically after three or four doses of LMWH. The anti-factor Xa level should be drawn approximately 4 hours after a SC dose of LMWH, with empiric dosing adjustments to maintain a level of roughly 0.5 to 1.0 international units/mL for therapeutic anticoagulation given every 12 hours, and slightly higher peaks up to 1.5 for therapeutic doses given every 24 hours.[3,9] However, there is little correlation between peak anti-factor Xa activity and therapeutic effect, and thus monitoring is not routinely recommended. Trough anti-factor Xa levels are expected to be less than 0.4 international units/mL at the end of the dosing interval. Like other measures of hemostasis, results vary considerably, requiring both instrument-specific and method-specific determination of therapeutic ranges.

DEEP VEIN THROMBOSIS

Clinical Presentation

SIGNS AND SYMPTOMS

CASE 11-1

QUESTION 1: J.T., a 60-year-old, overweight (92 kg, 6-foot tall) man, was admitted to the hospital 3 days ago for management of acute cellulitis of his left ankle that occurred after cutting himself with a lawn tool a week ago. He was started on intravenous antibiotics and had limited mobility in the hospital due to the pain at the wound site and is being evaluated by orthopedics for possible osteomyelitis and

Table 11-9

Optimal Therapeutic Range and Duration of Anticoagulation

Indication	INR Goal	Minimum Duration
Prophylaxis of VTE (DVT, PE)	2–3	~1–4 weeks depending on patient status and risk factors
Treatment of first VTE with transient risk factors	2–3	3 months
First episode of unprovoked VTE	2–3	3 months **Consider extended treatment** if first episode of VTE is PE or proximal DVT with no bleeding risk factors
Second episode of unprovoked VTE	2–3	Long term
VTE and cancer	2–3	Indefinitely or until cancer resolved[a]
VTE prophylaxis after hip or knee arthroplasty, hip fracture surgery	2–3	Up to 35 days after surgery
Atrial fibrillation (persistent or paroxysmal)/Atrial flutter $CHADS_2$ score ≥ 1	2–3	Long term
Acute MI: high risk (large anterior MI, significant heart failure, intracardiac thrombus visible on ECHO, AF, previous VTE)	2–3	3 months
Post-UA/NSTEMI (with or without stent placement): with AF requiring dual antiplatelet therapy and warfarin therapy	2–2.5	Variable
Bileaflet mechanical valve or tilting disc valve in aortic position in sinus rhythm	2–3	Long term
Bileaflet mechanical valve or tilting disc valve in mitral position	2.5–3.5	Long term
Caged-ball or caged-disc valve	2.5–3.5	Long term
Mechanical aortic heart valves with additional risk factors (AF, previous VTE, LV dysfunction, hypercoagulable conditions)[b]	2.5–3.5	Long term
Bioprosthetic valve in aortic position[c]	N/A	Aspirin 81 mg daily alone
Bioprosthetic valve in mitral position	2–3	3 to 6 months Followed by aspirin 81 mg daily
Bioprosthetic valves with additional risk factors (AF, previous VTE, LV dysfunction, hypercoagulable conditions)	2–3	Long term

Warfarin Use in Adults: Clinical Care Guideline, University of Illinois Hospital and Health Sciences System.
[a]Low-molecular-weight heparin preferred for patients with VTE and cancer.
[b]Higher goal INR recommended by the AHA/ACC. INR 2–3 recommended by ACCP.
[c]Warfarin (goal INR 2–3) for 3 to 6 months is also recommended by the AHA/ACC.
VTE, venous thromboembolism; DVT, deep vein thrombosis; PE, pulmonary embolism; $CHADS_2$, congestive heart failure, hypertension, age ≥ 75 years, diabetes mellitus, prior stroke or transient ischemic attack; MI, myocardial infarction; ECHO, echocardiogram; AF, atrial fibrillation; EF, ejection fraction.
Source: Nishimura RA et al. 2017 AHA/ACC focused update of the 2014 AHA/ACC guideline for the management of patients with valvular heart disease. *Circulation*. 2017; 70(2):252–289.

surgical intervention. On the third day of hospitalization, while the wound was improving, he noted progressive swelling and soreness of the left calf and around his left knee. He denied shortness of breath (SOB), cough, or chest pain. His medical history includes coronary artery disease, diabetes, and hypercholesterolemia. His medications are lisinopril 10 mg/day PO, isosorbide mononitrate 120 mg/day PO, atenolol 50 mg/day PO, aspirin 81 mg/day PO, metformin 1,000 mg PO twice daily, and atorvastatin 80 mg PO every evening. Initial laboratory values include:

Hct, 36.5%
PT, 10.8 seconds (INR, 1.0)
aPTT, 23.6 seconds
Platelet count, 255,000/μL

What signs and symptoms demonstrated by J.T. are consistent with DVT?

Patients with DVT typically present with unilateral leg swelling that often is accompanied by warmth and local tenderness or pain.[10] A tender, cordlike entity caused by venous obstruction can sometimes be palpated in the affected area. J.T. presented with the sudden onset of swelling along with soreness, but without evidence of a cord. Discoloration of the affected limb, including pallor from arterial spasm, cyanosis from venous obstruction, or a reddish color from perivascular inflammation, may also occur. The presence or absence of a positive Homans sign (pain behind the knee or calf on dorsiflexion of the foot) is rarely helpful in making the diagnosis because it is present in only about 30% of patients with DVT. Many patients (>50%) can present with asymptomatic disease, but even asymptomatic patients can have long-term complications such as recurrent DVT or post-thrombotic syndrome. Because symptoms of DVT are nonspecific, the diagnosis must be confirmed by objective testing.[10,11]

RISK FACTORS

CASE 11-1, QUESTION 2: What risk factors does J.T. exhibit that are associated with DVT?

The diagnosis of DVT depends not only on the presenting signs and symptoms but also on the presence of risk factors (Fig. 11-1). J.T. has presented with obesity and immobilization (i.e., prolonged bed rest), two important risk factors for thromboembolism, as well as an acute medical illness. It is common for more than one risk factor to be present in patients who exhibit DVT, and these factors are cumulative in their effect.[12]

DIAGNOSIS

CASE 11-1, QUESTION 3: How should the final diagnosis of DVT be made in J.T.?

After evaluation of the signs and symptoms of DVT and consideration of risk factors for the development of thrombus, a definitive diagnosis should be made. Diagnostic strategies should include an assessment of pretest clinical probability (clinical suspicion), D-dimer assay (an evaluation of the presence of fibrin degradation products, indicative of clot formation; see Chapter 2, Interpretation of Clinical Laboratory Tests), and noninvasive imaging tests.[10,11]

Despite its limitations as a single diagnostic tool, clinical assessment can improve the diagnostic accuracy of noninvasive testing. A clinical prediction rule, such as the Wells criteria, takes into account signs, symptoms, and risk factors to categorize patients as being at low, intermediate, or high probability of having DVT (Table 11-10).[13] The D-dimer test can be used in conjunction with clinical evaluation or a clinical prediction rule to help "rule out" DVT in patients with a low clinical suspicion and thus decrease the need for imaging tests in these patients.[14] If the clinical suspicion of DVT is high, diagnostic imaging is indicated, and if the imaging is negative, the D-dimer is helpful to rule out the diagnosis.[11]

The most common noninvasive test is duplex scanning, which combines B-mode imaging or color flow imaging with Doppler ultrasonography to visualize veins and thrombi while investigating flow patterns. Other noninvasive testing options include ^{125}I-fibrinogen leg scanning (injection of radiolabeled fibrinogen followed by scanning to detect areas of accumulation corresponding to thrombosis), impedance plethysmography (use of pneumatic cuffs to detect leg blood volume changes associated with thrombosis), and Doppler ultrasonography alone (use of a transducer to audibly detect venous flow changes indicative of thrombosis). Each option differs with respect to sensitivity, specificity, and cost. Venography (radiographic visualization of the involved vessels with injection of radiocontrast material), an invasive diagnostic test, is the most sensitive and specific method for diagnosis of DVT, but exposes patients to the risks associated with contrast material, and is not readily available in many hospitals.

Table 11-10
Clinical Model for Evaluating the Pretest Probability of Deep Vein Thrombosis

Clinical Characteristic	Score
Active cancer (cancer treatment within previous 6 months, or currently on palliative treatment)	1
Paralysis, paresis, or recent plaster immobilization of the lower extremities	1
Recently bedridden for ≥3 days, or major surgery within the previous 12 weeks requiring general or regional anesthesia	1
Localized tenderness along the distribution of the deep venous system	1
Entire leg swollen	1
Calf swelling at least 3 cm larger than that on the asymptomatic side (measured 10 cm below tibial tuberosity)	1
Pitting edema confined to the symptomatic leg	1
Collateral superficial veins (nonvaricose)	1
Previously documented deep vein thrombosis	1
Alternative diagnosis at least as likely as deep vein thrombosis	−2

Clinical probability of deep vein thrombosis: low, <0; moderate, 1–2; high, >3. In patients with symptoms in both legs, the more symptomatic leg is used. Source: Wells PS et al. Does this patient have deep vein thrombosis? *JAMA*. 2006;295(2):199–207.

Treatment

BASELINE INFORMATION

CASE 11-1, QUESTION 4: What additional baseline data should be obtained before administering anticoagulants to J.T.?

In addition to assessing the integrity of the clotting process with platelet count, Hgb/Hct, PT, and aPTT, the patient's baseline renal function should also be evaluated and documented because some anticoagulants are renally eliminated. Baseline values are used for comparison with the parameters that will be used in monitoring both therapeutic and adverse effects of anticoagulant therapy.

INITIATION OF THERAPY

CASE 11-1, QUESTION 5: Duplex scanning reveals clot formation in J.T.'s left calf extending to the left thigh. He does not exhibit signs of PE. What is the appropriate therapy for J.T., and how should it be initiated?

Prompt and optimal anticoagulant therapy is indicated to minimize thrombus extension and its vascular complications, as well as to prevent PE. Acute anticoagulation treatment options include injectable IV UFH initiated with a loading dose followed by a continuous infusion, adjusted-dose SC UFH, SC LMWH, or SC fondaparinux.[15] Alternatively, initial treatment with oral rivaroxaban or apixaban can be selected, without any initial parenteral anticoagulation. LMWH or UFH may be continued as monotherapy or transitioned to treatment with a VKA, dabigatran or edoxaban. Because J.T. is currently hospitalized and may need further surgical procedures, IV UFH is selected for initial treatment of his DVT.

HEPARIN

Loading Dose

CASE 11-1, QUESTION 6: J.T.'s medical resident ordered a heparin bolus dose of 5,000 international units IV, to be followed by a continuous infusion of 1,000 units/hour. Is this heparin dosing regimen appropriate?

A loading dose of heparin is required for several reasons. Based on pharmacokinetic principles, a therapeutic serum level will be achieved more quickly; thus, pharmacodynamic and therapeutic responses to help prevent progression of the clot will occur rapidly. Second, a relative resistance to anticoagulation exists during the active clotting process. Therefore, a larger initial dose generally is necessary to achieve a therapeutic effect.

Although standardized doses of heparin for initiation of therapy (i.e., 5,000 units loading dose; 1,000-units/hour maintenance dose) were used historically, this approach can result in significant delays in reaching a therapeutic intensity of anticoagulation. Body weight represents the most reliable predictor of heparin dosing requirement. For patients who do not have extremes of body weight (i.e., <165 kg), the use of the actual body weight (ABW) has been recommended to calculate the initial UFH dose.[16] For patients more than 165 kg, the use of the ABW is controversial, and the use of an adjusted-dosing weight is recommended by some experts.[16,17] Options include two different "dosing weight" calculations:

$$\text{Ideal Body Weight (IBW)} + 0.3 \times (\text{ABW} - \text{IBW}) \quad \text{(Eq. 11-2)}$$

Or

$$\text{IBW} + 0.4 \times (\text{ABW} - \text{IBW}) \quad \text{(Eq. 11-3)}$$

Compared with standardized dosing, weight-based dosing (80 units/kg loading dose; 18 units/kg/hour initial infusion rate) increases the frequency of therapeutic aPTT at 6 hours and at 24 hours, and decreases the risk of recurrent VTE.[18–20]

Initial heparin loading doses of 60 to 100 units/kg followed by an infusion rate of 13 to 25 units/kg/hour are commonly recommended.[21] Selection of the lower or upper dosage range is guided by the severity of the patient's symptoms and his or her potential sensitivity to adverse effects. For this 92-kg patient, a midrange loading dose of 7,400 units (92 kg × 80 units/kg), followed by a continuous infusion of 1,700 units/hour (92 kg × 18 units/kg/hour), is recommended. Loading doses are typically rounded to the nearest 500 units and maintenance infusion rates to the nearest 100 units for convenience of administration.

Dose Adjustments

CASE 11-1, QUESTION 7: The orders for J.T. were rewritten by his attending physician. Based on the data shown subsequently, explain the variability in laboratory results. (At this institution, aPTT values of 60–100 seconds correspond with heparin plasma concentrations of 0.3–0.7 units/mL determined by anti-factor Xa assay.)

Time	aPTT (seconds)	Heparin Dosage Order
0800	31 (baseline)	7,400 units bolus followed by 1,700 units/hour infusion
0900	130	Hold infusion for 30 minutes, then to 1,500 units/hour
1500	40	Rebolus with 2,400 units, then to 1,700 units/hour
2100	85	Continue at 1,700 units/hour; recheck aPTT every morning

Although the aPTT drawn 1 hour after the initiation of the maintenance infusion (9 AM) demonstrates excessive prolongation of the aPTT (130 seconds), this value is most likely explained by inappropriate timing of the test. When aPTT values are drawn too soon after a heparin bolus dose (i.e., before the maintenance infusion has achieved a steady state concentration in serum), they are predictably very high, but are not associated with a bleeding risk and do not accurately reflect the anticipated level of anticoagulation in the patient. To ensure accuracy, the clinician should obtain aPTT values no sooner than 6 hours after a bolus dose or any change in the infusion rate. Even results obtained at 6 hours may be excessively prolonged in some patients because of the dose-dependent pharmacokinetic characteristics of heparin.

J.T.'s heparin dose was decreased at 0900 based on this prolonged, yet inappropriately timed, value. A repeat aPTT at 3 PM was only 40 seconds. The decrease in the dosage to 1,500 units/hour and the repeat aPTT of 40 seconds reflect near steady state conditions because 6 hours has elapsed since the dosage change. Because the aPTT was subtherapeutic at 3 PM (40 seconds), administration of a smaller repeat bolus dose (2,000 units) and an increase in the maintenance infusion to 1,700 units/hour was the correct course of action. Subsequent aPTT values reflected therapeutic anticoagulation.

Dosing nomograms or protocols have been recommended for adjustment of heparin dosing based on aPTT results.[3,16] Nomogram-based dosing reduces the time to reach therapeutic range compared with empiric dosing.[22] Attaining a therapeutic aPTT in <24 hours has been shown to lower in-hospital and 30-day mortality rates.[23] After initiation based on patient weight, dosing adjustments may also be weight-based or may simply be made in international units per hour. A sample heparin dosing nomogram specific for a reagent with a therapeutic aPTT range of 60 to 100 seconds (and used in the adjustment of heparin doses for J.T.) is illustrated in Table 11-11.

Responses to changes in infusion rates of heparin are not always linear, and to some extent, heparin doses are adjusted by trial and error. As the patient's condition improves after several days and endothelialization of the clot occurs, heparin dosing requirements may decrease.

Therapeutic Monitoring

CASE 11-1, QUESTION 8: How should J.T.'s heparin therapy be monitored?

Once baseline clotting parameters have been established and a loading dose of heparin has been administered, the aPTT should be measured routinely to guide subsequent dosing adjustments. The aPTT should be evaluated no sooner than 6 hours after the loading dose or after any changes in infusion rate, as noted previously. If dosing is stable, the aPTT should be evaluated once daily (Table 11-11).

Additional monitoring parameters for heparin therapy include evaluation for potential adverse reactions and possible therapeutic failure. The Hgb and/or Hct and a platelet count should be checked every 1 to 2 days. J.T. should be examined for signs of bleeding, as well as for signs and symptoms associated with thrombus extension and PE. Finally, if unusual or unexpected aPTT results are reported, the clinician should consider the possible influence of solution preparation errors (see Chapter 2, Interpretation of Clinical Laboratory Tests), infusion pump failure, infusion interruption, and administration or charting errors in the assessment of J.T.'s heparin therapy.[24]

Duration of Therapy

CASE 11-1, QUESTION 9: How long should heparin therapy be continued in J.T. if the patient starts warfarin?

Adherence of a thrombus to the vessel wall and subsequent endothelialization usually takes 7 to 10 days. However, anticoagulation therapy must generally continue for 3 months to prevent recurrent thrombosis.[15] For many years, warfarin was preferred for this long-term anticoagulation because it can be administered orally, and it is generally initiated on the same day as heparin. The long elimination half-life of warfarin and the long elimination

Table 11-11
Sample Heparin Dosing Nomogram

1. Suggested loading dose
   - Treatment of DVT/PE: 80 units/kg (rounded to nearest 500 units)
   - Prevention, including cardiovascular indications: 70 units/kg (rounded to nearest 500 units)
2. Suggested initial infusion
   - Treatment of DVT/PE: 18 units/kg/hour (rounded to nearest 100 units)
   - Prevention, including cardiovascular indications: 15 units/kg/hour (rounded to nearest 100 units)
3. First aPTT check: 6 hours after initiating therapy
4. Dosing adjustments: per this chart (rounded to nearest 100 units)

aPTT[a] (seconds)	Heparin Bolus	Infusion Hold Time	Infusion Rate Adjustment	Next aPTT
<50	4,000 units	0	Increase by 200 units/hour	In 6 hours
50–59	2,000 units	0	Increase by 100 units/hour	In 6 hours
60–100	0	0	None	Every AM
101–110	0	0	Decrease by 100 units/hour	In 6 hours
111–120	0	0	Decrease by 200 units/hour	In 6 hours
121–150	0	30 minutes	Decrease by 200 units/hour	In 6 hours
151–199	0	60 minutes	Decrease by 200 units/hour	In 6 hours
>200	0	PRN	Hold until aPTT < 100	Every hour until <100

[a]Based on aPTT reagent-specific therapeutic range of 60–100 seconds corresponding to a plasma heparin concentration of 0.3–0.7 units/mL determined by anti-factor Xa activity.
aPTT, activated partial thromboplastin time; DVT, deep vein thrombosis; PE, pulmonary embolism; PRN, as necessary.

half-lives of clotting factors II and X necessitate a prolonged period of overlap between warfarin and heparin. Therefore, if warfarin is initiated, heparin is continued for a minimum of 5 days and until the INR is greater than 2.0 for 24 hours. If the INR exceeds the therapeutic range (i.e., INR > 3.0) prematurely, it is acceptable to stop parenteral therapy before the patient has received 5 days of treatment.[15]

Adverse Effects

Case 11-1, Question 10: On day 2 of heparin therapy, J.T.'s complete blood count reveals a platelet count of 180,000/μL, decreased from 255,000/μL at baseline. What is a reasonable explanation for this thrombocytopenia and how should it be managed?

Thrombocytopenia

Thrombocytopenia induced by heparin has two distinct presentations.[5] Heparin-associated thrombocytopenia (HAT) occurs as a direct effect of heparin on platelet function, causing transient platelet sequestration and clumping with reductions in platelet count, but usually remaining greater than 100,000/μL. This reversible form of thrombocytopenia occurs within the first several days of heparin therapy. Patients remain asymptomatic, and platelet counts return to normal even when heparin therapy is continued. J.T.'s reduction in platelet count is somewhat modest and likely represents HAT. His platelet count should be monitored daily, and heparin therapy should be continued.

Reductions in platelet count of greater than 50% from baseline suggest the development of heparin-induced thrombocytopenia (HIT), a more severe immune-mediated reaction with a typical delay in onset of 5 to 10 days after the initiation of heparin therapy. In contrast, "rapid-onset" HIT can occur rapidly (within 24 hours of UFH initiation) and is strongly associated with recent heparin exposure. And "delayed-onset" HIT is associated with an onset of thrombocytopenia that begins several days after heparin has been stopped.[5]

Heparin use leads to the formation of immunoglobulin G (IgG) antibodies that recognize multimolecular complexes of a platelet protein called platelet factor 4 (PF4) and heparin that form on the surface of platelets.[5] Antibodies against PF4/heparin complexes are responsible for the prothrombotic nature of HIT due to their capability to induce platelet activation by cross-linking platelet Fcc receptor IIa (CD32a),[25] and release procoagulant, platelet-derived microparticles, resulting in a large generation of thrombin and the formation of venous and arterial thromboses. The diagnosis of immune-mediated HIT is made based on clinical findings supplemented by laboratory tests confirming the presence of platelet-activating anti-PF4/heparin antibodies.[5,26] The 4-T score is the most common pretest probability test that can be used to estimate the likelihood of HIT based on extent and timing of platelet count reduction, the presence of thrombus, and the possibility of other causes of thrombocytopenia (Table 11-12).[5,27]

The overall incidence of HIT is less than 3% after 5 days of UFH use, but the cumulative incidence can be as high as 6% after 14 days of continuous heparin use. Despite its low incidence, HIT is a life-threatening condition with a reported mortality rate of 5% to 10%. Venous thrombosis is the most common complication secondary to HIT, with rates reported at 2.4 to 1 more common than arterial thrombosis (limb artery thrombosis, thrombotic stroke, and myocardial infarction).[28] Limb gangrene has been reported at 5% to 10%, with a resulting risk of amputation.[29]

In patients who develop HIT, heparin therapy should be stopped immediately, and treatment with an alternative anticoagulant should be initiated.[5,30] Although associated with a lower risk of HIT (<1%) than UFH, LMWH products are contraindicated in patients with HIT because of a high incidence of immunologic cross-reactivity with heparin.[5] The future use of heparin in patients with HIT, especially in the first 3 months after the diagnosis, should be avoided. Treatment options include the direct thrombin inhibitors argatroban and bivalirudin, although only argatroban is approved for this indication by the FDA. The dose of argatroban is administered as an IV infusion due to its short half-life and should be titrated based on aPTT testing. Bivalirudin also appears

Table 11-12

The 4T Score: Pretest Probability of Heparin-Induced Thrombocytopenia

Category	2 Points	1 Point	0 Points
1. Thrombocytopenia	Platelet count fall >50% and platelet nadir ≥20 × 10^9 L^{-1}	Platelet count fall 30%–50% or platelet nadir 10–19 × 10^9 L^{-1}	Platelet count fall <30% or platelet nadir <10 × 10^9 L^{-1}
2. Timing of platelet count fall	Clear onset between days 5 and 10 or platelet fall ≤1 day (prior heparin exposure within 30 days)	Consistent with days 5–10 fall, but not clear (e.g., missing platelet counts) or onset after day 10 or fall ≤1 day (prior heparin exposure 30–100 days ago)	Platelet count fall < 4 days without recent heparin exposure
3. Thrombosis or other sequelae	New thrombosis (confirmed) or skin necrosis at heparin injection sites or acute systemic reaction after intravenous heparin bolus	Progressive or recurrent thrombosis or nonnecrotizing (erythematous) skin lesions or suspected thrombosis (not proven)	None
4. Other causes for thrombocytopenia	None apparent	Possible	Definite

Total Score <3 = low probability of HIT 4–5 = intermediate probability of HIT >6 = high probability of HIT.
Source: Lo GK et al. Evaluation of pretest clinical score (4 T's) for the diagnosis of heparin-induced thrombocytopenia in two clinical settings. *J Thromb Haemost*. 2006;4:759.

to be a promising alternative for the treatment of HIT due to its short-half life, low immunogenicity, minimal effect on INR, and enzymatic metabolism. Various patient-related factors (such as the presence of renal or hepatic dysfunction; drug availability, cost, and institutional preference) should be used to select the most appropriate agent[5] (Table 11-7).

Case 11-1, Question 11: On day 3 of heparin therapy, J.T.'s Hct has dropped from a baseline of 37.5% to 28%, and the patient noted blood in his commode after urination. Describe an approach to evaluate and interpret this event.

Hemorrhage

Bleeding is the most common adverse effect associated with heparin. A summary of eight studies reporting heparin-associated bleeding found the absolute frequency of fatal, major, and all (major or minor) bleeding to be 0.4%, 6%, and 16%, respectively.[31] The corresponding average daily frequencies were 0.05% for fatal bleeding, 0.8% for major bleeding, and 2% for major or minor bleeding; cumulative risk increased with the duration of therapy. The most common sites for heparin-associated bleeding are soft tissues, the GI and urinary tracts, the nose, and the oral pharynx. The use of different criteria to define major versus minor bleeding accounts for much of the variability in reported frequency of bleeding among studies.

In addition to length of therapy, many factors influence the risk of bleeding during heparinization, including advanced age, serious comorbid illnesses (heart disease, renal insufficiency, hepatic dysfunction, cerebrovascular disease, malignancy, and severe anemia), and concomitant antithrombotic therapy.[31] The incidence of UFH-associated bleeding complications is minimal with SC prophylactic doses, but higher (2%–4%) with therapeutic doses given via IV infusion. Soft tissue bleeding commonly occurs at sites of recent surgery or trauma. Previously undiagnosed abnormalities, including malignancy and infection, may be identified in some patients with GI or urinary tract bleeding associated with heparin therapy.

The influence of the intensity of heparinization on bleeding risk is controversial. Although an elevated aPTT has historically been considered a risk factor for bleeding complications, several investigators have been unable to substantiate a relationship between supratherapeutic aPTT values and hemorrhagic effects.[3] In addition, bleeding episodes can occur when coagulation test results are within the therapeutic range. These conflicting results may be explained in part by the influence of additional risk factors for bleeding and by the effect of heparin on platelet function and vascular permeability.

J.T. has developed hematuria despite an acceptable intensity of anticoagulation. He should be questioned and examined for the presence of nose bleeding (epistaxis), increased tendency to bruise (ecchymosis), bright red blood in the stool (hematochezia), black or tarry stool (melena), or coughing up of blood (hemoptysis). Blood pressure and pulse, both sitting and standing, should be obtained to determine whether orthostasis representing blood loss is present. A thorough evaluation of the urinary tract may reveal a previously unknown abnormality that will explain the bleeding episode. Although his concurrent low-dose aspirin therapy may increase the risk of minor bleeding complications, aspirin therapy would not be discontinued due to his history of coronary artery disease.

Case 11-1, Question 12: What other side effects of heparin should be considered in J.T.?

Osteoporosis

The development of osteoporosis has been associated with administration of more than 20,000 international units/day of heparin for 6 months or longer.[32] Various mechanisms have been suggested, but the underlying pathophysiology of this rare adverse effect remains unclear. Affected patients may present with bone pain and/or radiographic findings suggestive of fractures. The possibility of osteoporosis should be considered in patients receiving long-term, high-dose heparin therapy such as pregnant patients, postmenopausal women, and elderly patients.

Hypersensitivity Reactions

Other rarely occurring adverse effects associated with heparin include generalized skin reactions that can progress to necrosis, alopecia, and hypersensitivity reactions, resulting in hypotension, nausea, and shortness of breath. In 2007, an increase in hypersensitivity reactions to heparin was attributed to oversulfated chondroitin sulfate in the heparin manufacturing process.[33]

Reversal of Effect

CASE 11-2

QUESTION 1: K.G. is a72-year-old woman with a DVT that occurred during her hospital stay. On day 4 of heparin therapy, she received a full bag of 25,000 units of heparin during a 1-hour period as a result of an infusion pump malfunction. The infusion was stopped and within 30 minutes, she became diaphoretic and hypotensive. Bright red blood was evident on rectal examination, and a large retroperitoneal mass was noted. How should the excessive heparin effect be reversed?

K.G. has definite signs of hemorrhage from the GI tract, a site of bleeding associated with considerable mortality. Heparin should be discontinued immediately, and treatment should include maintenance of fluid volume and replacement of clotting factors with whole blood, fresh frozen plasma, or clotting factor concentrates. If hemorrhage had not been present and the only manifestation of overdose had been a prolonged aPTT, administration of heparin simply could have been discontinued, permitting the effects to clear within a few hours.

Protamine can be used to neutralize heparin by forming an inactive protamine–heparin complex.[3] Protamine has a rapid onset of action, with effects lasting about 2 hours. Protamine sulfate is infused slowly over 3 to 5 minutes, as a 1% solution at a dose of 1 mg for each 100 international units of heparin administered in the last 2 to 3 hours. The maximum single recommended dose of protamine is 50 mg, but doses may be repeated if bleeding persists. Response to protamine therapy can be assessed by a return of the aPTT to baseline. Adverse effects associated with protamine include systemic hypotension secondary to rapid administration; anaphylaxis characterized by edema, bronchospasm, and cardiovascular collapse; and catastrophic pulmonary vasoconstriction[34] (see Chapter 32, Drug Hypersensitivity Reactions).

Outpatient Treatment of DVT

CASE 11-3

QUESTION 1: N.C. is a 32-year-old woman who presents to the emergency department (ED) complaining of right leg pain behind the right knee of 2-day duration. She denies recent injury, but her medication history reveals that she recently started combination oral contraceptive tablets. She has no significant medical history and has no family history of clotting disorders. A duplex ultrasound is positive for DVT and immediate anticoagulation is indicated. What therapeutic alternatives to hospitalization for IV UFH are available for this patient?

In the past, UFH was the initial treatment of choice for acute DVT; however, LMWHs and fondaparinux are now becoming more convenient and practical treatment alternatives to UFH.[15] These agents, administered SC and without the need for routine coagulation monitoring, allow patients to be treated at home while transitioning to therapeutic warfarin. In addition, meta-analysis data suggest that LMWH therapy for acute VTE results in fewer deaths, major hemorrhages, and recurrent VTE when compared to UFH.[35] Based on these advantages, outpatient use of LMWH has become the most common approach to treatment of uncomplicated DVT in patients that transition to warfarin. Home treatment is safe and effective and improves the overall physical and social functioning of patients being treated for DVT.[36] The drug costs associated with LMWH treatment are much higher than the costs of IV UFH, but overall costs to healthcare systems are significantly reduced when patients can be treated at home rather than in the hospital.[37,38] Fondaparinux can also be considered as an alternative treatment as it has been shown to be as effective and safe as LMWH in the treatment of DVT.[39] Additionally, weight-based SC UFH (initial dose of 333 international units/kg followed by 250 international units/kg every 12 hours) without routine aPTT monitoring while patients become therapeutic on warfarin is an alternative for the treatment of acute VTE.[40] Vials of UFH at a concentration of 20,000 international units/mL are used by the pharmacy or the patient to draw up the weight-based dose. Although routine aPTT monitoring is not necessary, platelet count monitoring during the first 2 weeks is required to evaluate the possible development of HIT.

For N.C. to be treated at home with LMWH, she or a family member must be willing and able to administer SC injections, and she must be able to return for frequent follow-up visits, particularly during the first few weeks while warfarin therapy is initiated. In addition, her healthcare insurance should cover the cost of the drug, or she must be able to pay out of pocket. Contraindications to outpatient treatment of VTE include a preexisting condition that requires hospitalization, clinical symptoms of PE with hemodynamic instability, and recent or active bleeding.

N.C. meets the eligibility requirements for home treatment of her DVT. She is also a suitable candidate for a DOAC and prefers to not have to perform self-injections of medication. Currently, there are two DOACs, rivaroxaban and apixaban, approved in the United States for monotherapy and do not require an initial period of parenteral anticoagulant. Advantages to the use of a DOAC compared to warfarin include the lack of routine monitoring for assessing drug efficacy, fewer drug and food interactions, and a lower rate of major bleeding compared to warfarin. Currently, only dabigatran has an FDA-approved agent for reversal, idarucizumab, and there are several other reversal agents in clinical trials. The lack of reversal agent leaves some providers and patients apprehensive to their use. When selecting a DOAC, it is important to know the patient's renal function because these agents have varying doses based on current renal function. A baseline CBC should also be checked, because all anticoagulants have the potential for bleeding, and it is important to know the baseline hemoglobin level in case bleeding occurs on treatment. In this case, N.C. received an injection of LMWH while in the emergency department, and rivaroxaban is selected for monotherapy, at 15 mg twice daily with food for 21 days, followed by 20 mg daily with food for the remainder of her 3-month duration of treatment. N.C. should be advised to follow up with her primary care provider regarding her new diagnosis, and it should be stressed to the patient the importance of proper transitioning of the dose from the twice a day to the once a day schedule. Anticoagulation clinics may also be involved in N.C.'s care to follow up and make sure she was able to obtain the medication without insurance barriers, that the DOAC dose was appropriate, that her DVT symptoms are improving, that she is tolerating the medication, and that she transitions to the correct dose appropriately.[41] Higher risk patients, such as those with lower health literacy and multiple medical problems, may benefit from face-to-face clinical visits if this information cannot be obtained by telephone. Centralized anticoagulation services are expanding beyond traditional monitoring to include patients on DOACs by prospectively following them to ensure optimal therapeutic outcomes. There are some cases where it may be necessary to test whether the DOAC is present, such as in a patient with acute stroke, need for urgent surgery, or in the case of major bleeding.[42] There is no current consensus on how best to do this, because the tests that correlate the best are not often readily available. Of those that are readily available, aPTT or thrombin time are often used to detect dabigatran presence,

Table 11-13

Dosing of Low-Molecular-Weight Heparin and Fondaparinux for the Treatment of Venous Thromboembolism

Dalteparin	Enoxaparin	Tinzaparin	Fondaparinux
100 international units/kg SC every 12 hours OR 200 international units/kg SC every 24 hours	1 mg/kg SC every 12 hours OR 1.5 mg/kg SC every 24 hours	175 international units/kg SC every 24 hours	5 mg SC every 24 hours if weight <50 kg 7.5 mg SC every 24 hours if weight 50–100 kg 10 mg SC every 24 hours if weight >100 kg

SC, subcutaneously.

and the prothrombin time or anti-factor Xa calibrated for the factor Xa inhibitors.[42]

Case 11-3, Question 2: During a follow-up call to N.C. from the anticoagulation clinic the next morning, it is discovered that N.C. was not able to get the rivaroxaban filled at her pharmacy last night because her insurance does not cover any DOAC therapy without first documenting a treatment failure to warfarin. What alternative treatment is available for N.C?

Before the DOACs, treatment with self-injected LMWH bridging to warfarin at home was the standard of care. Possible treatment options and doses for N.C. are listed in Table 11-13. In this case, enoxaparin is the LMWH preferred by her insurance because it is available generically. The usual dosing of enoxaparin for treatment of DVT is 1 mg/kg total body weight SC every 12 hours, rounded to the nearest 10-mg increment. Once-daily dosing at 1.5 mg/kg SC every 24 hours is also an option, but this strategy is inferior to twice-daily dosing in patients with malignancy or obesity.[43] N.C.'s medical history is suitable for the once-daily dose of enoxaparin, which is more convenient for administration. At 65 kg, a dose of 1.5 mg/kg would be 97.5 mg, which will be rounded to the nearest 10-mg increment. N.C. will therefore receive 100 mg SC every 24 hours. Warfarin therapy is initiated concurrently to expedite the conversion to oral treatment.

Because LMWHs are eliminated renally, patients with significant renal impairment require dose reductions to prevent drug accumulation and to minimize the risk of bleeding complications.[44] The degree of drug accumulation can vary between the various LMWH preparations, and thus specific guidelines for dose adjustments are agent specific (Table 11-14).[45] Some experts suggest monitoring of anti-factor Xa activity to rule out accumulation of LMWHs in patients with renal impairment who are on treatment for extended periods of time (i.e., greater than 1 week).[45,46] Fondaparinux is also renally excreted and is contraindicated in patients with creatinine clearance less than 30 mL/minute.

N.C. should be educated regarding the potential adverse effects of LMWH therapy (bleeding, thrombocytopenia, pain and bruising at the injection site), required laboratory monitoring, and the expected duration of anticoagulation. At baseline, Hgb and/or Hct, INR, serum creatinine (SCr), and platelet count should be determined. Platelets will continue to be monitored at least every 2 to 3 days while the patient is receiving LMWH therapy, to a maximum of 10 to 14 days. N.C. can expect to continue enoxaparin therapy for a minimum of 5 days. If by day 5 her INR is therapeutic and stable, enoxaparin can be discontinued. Oral anticoagulation with warfarin should be continued for 3 months.[15] N.C. should also be advised against further use of estrogen-containing contraceptives.[47]

To ensure the safety and efficacy of home treatment, N.C. should be provided with the names and telephone numbers of the healthcare providers who will assume responsibility for her care, including her primary physician and her anticoagulation management team. No patient should be sent home with LMWH without an adequate follow-up plan.

Table 11-14

Dosing of Low-Molecular-Weight Heparins in Patients with Renal Impairment (CrCl < 30 mL/minute)[a]

LMWH	Dalteparin	Enoxaparin	Tinzaparin
Product information recommendations	Use with caution	Prophylaxis—30 mg SC daily Treatment—1 mg/kg SC daily	Use with caution
Dosing suggestions based on agent-specific pharmacokinetic observations	CrCl < 30 mL/minute[a]: no dose adjustment needed up to 1 week with prophylactic doses For use longer than 1 week, consider monitoring of anti-Xa activity and adjust dose if accumulation is noted CrCl 30–50 mL/minute: no dose adjustment needed	CrCl <30 mL/minute[a]: Consider a 40%–50% dose decrease and subsequent monitoring of anti-Xa activity CrCl 30–50 mL/minute: Consider a 15%–20% dose decrease with prolonged use (longer than 10–14 days) and subsequent monitoring of anti-Xa activity	CrCl <30 mL/minute[a]: consider a dose decrease of 20% and subsequent monitoring of anti-Xa activity CrCl 30–50 mL/minute: no dose adjustment needed

[a]In patients with a CrCl <30 mL/minute, data are very limited and use of unfractionated heparin is suggested.

Prevention of Venous Thromboembolism

CASE 11-4

Question 1: M.G., a 63-year-old obese man, is to undergo elective abdominal surgery for treatment of an umbilical hernia. He has a medical history significant for hypertension, currently controlled by enalapril 10 mg daily (blood pressure, 130/80 mm Hg), and gout, controlled with allopurinol 300 mg daily. What therapeutic interventions might decrease the risk of DVT or PE in M.G.?

Surgical procedures represent a significant risk factor for DVT formation. However, all hospitalized patients, including both surgical and nonsurgical/medical patients, should be stratified for risk of VTE based on the presence of various factors.[12,48–50] Risk stratification is used to select the most appropriate therapeutic interventions to prevent DVT and thereby reduce the risk of fatal PE. These interventions include both mechanical and pharmacologic strategies.

NONPHARMACOLOGIC MEASURES

Mechanical interventions aimed at preventing venous stasis and increasing venous return include the use of elastic compression stockings, as well as leg elevation, leg exercises, and early postoperative ambulation. Intermittent pneumatic compression (IPC) of the leg muscles, using inflatable cuffs applied to the calf and thigh, represents another alternative for the prevention of DVT.[12] Because it is generally less effective than pharmacologic prophylaxis, mechanical prophylaxis is most commonly used in patients at high risk of bleeding, or as an adjunct to pharmacologic prophylaxis in patients at very high risk for VTE.

PHARMACOLOGIC MEASURES

Fixed, low-dose unfractionated heparin (LDUFH), administered as 5,000 units SC every 8 to 12 hours depending on the indication, is an inexpensive and effective pharmacologic approach to DVT prevention in the setting of venous stasis in patients with acute medical illness, or after certain surgical procedures. Because LDUFH inactivates factor Xa without a direct effect on factor IIa, the aPTT is not prolonged, and therefore aPTT monitoring is unnecessary. Bleeding complications are minimized using this dosing regimen.

Fixed-dose SC LMWH and fondaparinux are alternative approaches for preventing DVT. Enoxaparin 30 mg SC every 12 hours or 40 mg SC once daily, dalteparin 2,500 to 5,000 international units SC once daily, and fondaparinux 2.5 mg SC once daily are effective strategies, although enoxaparin has been studied for a larger number of indications. The DOACs rivaroxaban, apixaban, and dabigatran have been FDA-approved for DVT prophylaxis in orthopedic surgery patients. Betrixaban 160 mg as a single dose followed by 80 mg daily is approved for VTE prophylaxis in adult patients hospitalized for an acute medical illness. Current recommendations for prevention of VTE based on risk stratification are presented in Table 11-15.[12,48,49]

M.G. is at high risk for DVT and PE, not only because of general surgery but also because of his age (older than 40 years) and the presence of other risk factors for VTE (obesity, and probable postoperative immobilization). Options for DVT prevention include SC heparin at 5,000 international units every 8 hours or a LMWH (enoxaparin 40 mg SC daily, or dalteparin 2,500 international units initial dose followed by 5,000 international units SC daily). The first dose should be administered several hours preoperatively, and dosing should continue postoperatively until he is fully ambulatory. If bleeding risk is of concern, IPC could be used as an alternative. VTE prophylaxis is typically continued until hospital discharge, but may be continued for up to 30 days in certain high-risk populations, including patients with cancer, orthopedic surgery, bariatric surgery, or with a prior history of VTE.

PULMONARY EMBOLISM

Clinical Presentation

CASE 11-5

Question 1: A.W. is a 52-year-old, 70-kg woman. She recently returned from a 12-hour car ride where she only stopped to stretch twice. Yesterday she noticed a swollen right calf that is painful and warm. This swelling gradually increased, affecting the entire right leg to the groin, and prompted her to seek medical attention. In the ED, she also notes the recent onset of right-sided pleuritic chest pain without SOB or hemoptysis. Her medical history includes a gastric ulcer 4 years ago, treated with proton pump inhibitor therapy, that has not recurred. Physical examination reveals an enlarged right leg and moderate tenderness in the entire leg. Chest examination reveals labored respirations, equal breath sounds, and no wheezing or crackles. Vital signs include blood pressure, 160/90 mm Hg; heart rate, 100 beats/minute; and respiratory rate, 28 breaths/minute and regular. Laboratory data include the following:

Hct, 26.7%
SCr 1.1 mg/dL
Arterial blood gases (on room air)
Po_2, 72 mm Hg (normal, 75–100)
Pco_2, 30 mm Hg (normal, 35–45)
pH 7.48 (normal, 7.35–7.45)

Chest CT shows a pulmonary embolism in the distal right main pulmonary artery extending into the right lower lobe. The electrocardiogram (ECG) shows sinus tachycardia. The lower extremity duplex ultrasound is positive for acute occluding thrombus from the right femoral vein all the way down to the soleal vein. Coagulation test results include the following:

PT, 11.2 seconds (INR, 1.0)
aPTT, 28 seconds
Platelet count, 248,000/μL

What subjective and objective evidence in A.W. is consistent with PE?

SIGNS AND SYMPTOMS

The clinical diagnosis of PE is often difficult to make because of the nonspecificity of symptoms.[51,52] The most common symptoms of PE include tachypnea, cough, substernal and pleuritic chest pain, dyspnea, hemoptysis, fever, and unilateral leg pain. Signs and symptoms such as hypotension, tachycardia, presence of B-type natriuretic peptides (BNP) or NT-pro-BNP (N-terminal pro-brain natriuretic peptide), troponins (I or T), hypoxia, and electrocardiogram (ECG) changes suggestive of right ventricular strain are important to recognize as these may indicate more severe thromboembolism and increased risk for 30-day mortality.[53] DVT precedes PE in 80% or more of patients. A combination of these signs and symptoms provides further evidence for acute PE.

DEFINITIONS

There are varying ways to define the severity of a PE. Some define PE based on a patient's in-hospital or 30-day risk for mortality, whereas other literature will cite terms such as massive and submassive PE.[53,54] Low-risk PE is classified as the presence of thromboembolism without changes in hemodynamics, right ventricular function, or cardiac biomarkers. These types of patients can also be classified as small-to-moderate PE. High-risk PE is defined by the presence of shock (manifesting as tissue hypoperfusion, and hypoxia, cool clammy extremities, alterations in consciousness)

Table 11-15
Prevention of Venous Thromboembolism[12,48]

General and Abdominal–pelvic Surgery[a]	
Very low risk for VTE	Early and frequent ambulation
Low risk for VTE	IPC over no prophylaxis
Moderate risk for VTE not at high risk for MB	LMWH and LDUFH over no prophylaxis. IPC over no prophylaxis
Moderate risk for VTE & high risk for MB	IPC over no prophylaxis
High risk for VTE and not at high risk for MB	LMWH or LDUFH over no prophylaxis. IPC or elastic stockings can be added
High risk for VTE undergoing surgery for cancer and not otherwise at high risk for MB	Extended prophylaxis with LMWH (4 weeks) over limited duration
High risk for VTE and high risk for MB	IPC over no prophylaxis until bleeding risk diminishes then initiate pharmacologic prophylaxis
High risk for VTE unable to receive LMWH or LDUFH and not at high risk for MB	IPC over no prophylaxis
General and abdominal–pelvic surgery patients	IVC filter should not be used for primary VTE prevention Periodic surveillance with venous compression ultrasound should not be performed
Orthopedic Surgery	
Hip or knee replacement	Minimum of 10–14 days of one of the following: LMWH (preferred), fondaparinux, apixaban, dabigatran, rivaroxaban, LDUFH, warfarin (INR 2–3), or aspirin.
Hip fracture surgery	Minimum of 10–14 days of one of the following: LMWH, fondaparinux, LDUFH, warfarin (INR 2–3), or aspirin. LMWH preferred over warfarin or aspirin
Major orthopedic surgery	Dual prophylaxis with antithrombotic and IPC during hospital stay. Extended prophylaxis up to 35 days suggested.
Cardiac Surgery	Uncomplicated course: IPC over no prophylaxis Prolonged stay: add LDUFH or LMWH to IPC
Thoracic Surgery	
Moderate risk for VTE & not at high risk for MB	LMWH or LDUFH
High risk for VTE & not at high risk for MB	LMWH or LDUFH ±IPC
High risk for MB	IPC until bleeding risk diminishes, then pharmacologic prophylaxis
Trauma[b]	LMWH or LDUFH. Add IPC if high risk for VTE and use IPC if unable to take LMWH or LDUFH
Acutely Ill Hospitalized Medical Patients	
With increased risk of thrombosis	LMWH, LDUFH BID, LDUFH TID, fondaparinux, or betrixaban
With low risk of thrombosis	No pharmacologic or mechanical prophylaxis
With bleeding or at high risk of MB	No anticoagulant thromboprophylaxis
With increased risk of thrombosis and at high risk of MB	GCS, IPC. When bleeding risk decreases, start pharmacologic thromboprophylaxis instead of mechanical thromboprophylaxis

[a]includes gastrointestinal, urologic, gynecologic, bariatric, vascular, or plastic and reconstructive surgery.
[b]includes traumatic brain injury, acute spinal injury, and traumatic spine injury.
BID, twice daily; GCS, graduated compression stockings; INR, international normalized ratio; IPC, intermittent pneumatic compression; LDUFH, low-dose unfractionated heparin (5,000 international units subcutaneously every 8–12 hours); LMWH, low-molecular-weight heparin (enoxaparin 40 mg subcutaneously daily or 30 mg SC every 12 hours; dalteparin 2,500–5,000 international units subcutaneously daily); fondaparinux (2.5 mg subcutaneously daily); VTE, venous thromboembolism; MB, major bleeding; AC, anticoagulation.

or hypotension, specifically defined as: a systolic blood pressure < 90 mm Hg or a ≥ 40 mm Hg drop in systolic blood pressure for > 15 minutes which is not attributed to new onset arrhythmia, hypovolemia, or sepsis. These patients can also be classified as having massive PE.[54] Patients with right ventricular dysfunction characterized by echocardiographic evidence or by positive cardiac biomarkers (BNP > 90 pg/mL or NT-pro BNP > 500 pg/mL, Troponin I > 0.4 ng/mL, Troponin T > 0.1 ng/mL) are classified as having submassive PE if they are hemodynamically stable.[54]

DIAGNOSIS

Because the clinical signs and symptoms of PE are difficult to distinguish from many other medical conditions, further evaluation is necessary.[51,52] Chest radiograph, ECG, and arterial blood gas (alveolar-arterial oxygen gradient) abnormalities are often present in patients with PE, but like clinical signs and symptoms, they are somewhat nonspecific. Pulmonary imaging is necessary to diagnose or definitely rule out PE. Although many methods are clinically available for chest imaging, the computed tomographic (CT) pulmonary angiography and ventilation–perfusion lung scanning (V/Q scan) are the most common tests used for the diagnosis of PE, with the multi-detector CT (MDCT) being the imaging test of choice because of its ability to visualize the pulmonary arteries in the greatest detail. Lung scans that incorporate an assessment of perfusion, or regional distribution of pulmonary blood flow, and ventilation are referred to as V/Q scans; they involve both the injection and the inhalation of radiolabeled compounds. Test results are expressed as a high, intermediate, or low probability of PE. When ventilation (air movement) is normal over an area that shows abnormal perfusion (blood flow), a V/Q mismatch exists, and PE is highly probable. If a matched defect is noted (abnormal ventilation over an area of abnormal perfusion), another disease state, such as chronic obstructive airway disease, is more likely.

As in the case of DVT, clinical assessment of PE can improve the diagnostic accuracy of noninvasive tests such as CT, MRI, or V/Q scanning. Validated assessment tools can be used to stratify a patient's probability of a PE[55–58] (Table 11-16). In patients with a low clinical probability of PE, measuring a high-sensitivity D-dimer can be considered, and, if negative, PE can be ruled out, eliminating the need of further imaging studies.[59] In patients with a moderate-to-high clinical probability of PE, diagnostic imaging studies should be performed.

Table 11-16

Original and Simplified Pulmonary Embolism Severity Index (PESI) Scoring Systems

Parameter	Original Scoring Version (Points)	Simplified Scoring Version (Points)
Age	Points = age, (years)	1 (if age > 80 years)
Male sex	10	—
Cancer	30	1
Chronic heart failure	10	1[a]
Chronic pulmonary disease	10	1[a]
Heart rate > 110 BPM	20	1
Systolic blood pressure < 100 mm Hg	30	1
Respiratory rate > 30 breaths/minute	20	—
Temperature < 36°C	20	—
Altered mental status	60	—
Arterial oxygen saturation < 90%	20	1
30-Day Mortality Risk		
Very low: 0%–1.6%	Class I: < 65 points	0 points: 1%
Low: 1.7%–3.5%	Class II: 66–85 points	
Moderate: 3.2%–7.1%	Class III: 86–105 points	
High: 4%–11.4%	Class IV: 106–125 points	≥1 point: 10.9%
Very High: 10–24.5%	Class V: >125 points	

[a]only 1 point can be obtained for chronic heart failure and/or chronic pulmonary disease. Patients with both of these comorbidities can obtain only 1 point.
BPM, beats per minute; mm Hg, millimeters of mercury.
Source: Aujesky D et al. Derivation and validation of a prognostic model for pulmonary embolism. *Am J Respir Crit Care Med*. 2005;172:1041–1046; Jimenez D et al. Simplification of the pulmonary embolism severity index for prognostication in patients with acute symptomatic pulmonary embolism. *Arch Intern Med*. 2010;170:1383–1389.

Treatment

Case 11-5, Question 2: What anticoagulant strategy should be initiated for A.W.?

When the diagnosis of PE is suspected, anticoagulation should be initiated immediately while awaiting results of more definitive diagnostic procedures. There are several agents that can be used for the acute treatment of PE. IV UFH therapy initiated with a loading dose followed by a continuous infusion was the mainstay of therapy for many years. Alternatively, SC UFH can be used. However, if there is a concern about adequate SC absorption or in patients in whom fibrinolytic therapy is being considered, initial treatment with IV UFH is preferred to the SC route.[15] LMWHs are noninferior to UFH in the management of PE and are recommended over UFH in stable PE patients because of their ease of use, less major bleeding, and ability for outpatient management or early discharge.[60,61] Fondaparinux demonstrated noninferiority when compared with IV UFH for rate of recurrent PE, with similar rates of major bleeding.[62] More recently, the DOACs have been evaluated for both the initial and long-term management of VTE, with dabigatran, rivaroxaban, apixaban, and edoxaban all FDA-approved for the initial management of PE. All of the DOACs were compared to LMWH/VKA and found to be noninferior for the rate of recurrent VTE.[63–67] Rivaroxaban and apixaban were studied as monotherapy, whereas dabigatran and edoxaban patients were initially treated with at least 5 days of parenteral therapy prior to receiving a DOAC. If A.W. is being kept in the hospital for observation because of the severity of her symptoms, UFH therapy could be started at a loading dose of 5,600 units (80 international units/kg × 70 kg), followed by continuous infusion of 1,300 units/hour (18 units/kg/hour × 70 kg). Monitoring of the aPTT would be used to adjust dosing to maintain treatment within the therapeutic range (Table 11-11).

Alternatively, SC LMWH 70 mg every 12 hours (1 mg/kg every 12 hours × 70 kg) or SC fondaparinux 7.5 mg daily may be given while transitioning the patient to warfarin (Table 11-13). A.W. could receive fixed-dose enoxaparin 70 mg SC every 12 hours (1 mg/kg every 12 hours × 70 kg) or dalteparin 15,000 international units SC every 24 hours (200 international units/kg, rounded to nearest syringe size). Use of initial therapies such as LMWH, fondaparinux, and DOACs allows for outpatient therapy and early discharge in hospitalized patients with acute PE. For patients with low-risk PE and home circumstances that are adequate, early discharge is suggested over standard discharge.[15]

Fibrinolytic therapy reverses right ventricular dysfunction and restores pulmonary perfusion more rapidly than anticoagulant therapy alone. It is generally reserved for patients with a high risk for mortality and a low risk for bleeding.[53] Percutaneous catheter-directed treatment provides localized delivery of fibrinolytics to the pulmonary thrombi and is an alternative invasive method for removal of pulmonary emboli. It is a less invasive approach compared to surgical embolectomy in patients who are not candidates for systemic fibrinolytic therapy. For patients with moderate-to-high-risk PE, catheter-directed thrombolysis has emerged as a promising option for patients who would also be candidates for systemic fibrinolytic therapy.[53]

WARFARIN

Transition from Injectable Anticoagulant Therapy

CASE 11-5, QUESTION 3: If A.W. is to start on warfarin, rather than a DOAC, when should it be administered, and how should the transition from injectable anticoagulant therapy be accomplished?

As in the treatment of DVT, if warfarin is to be started, the use of heparin, LMWH, or fondaparinux therapy for PE treatment should be continued for at least 5 days and until warfarin therapy is therapeutic for at least 24 hours. Warfarin should be started on the first day of treatment and continued for 3 months, or longer if indicated. However, a delay in the initiation of warfarin may be acceptable in the setting of an anticipated extended hospitalization, recent or anticipated surgery or other invasive procedures, or a medical condition with the potential for uncontrolled bleeding.[15]

There are several reasons to overlap heparin/LMWH/fondaparinux and warfarin therapy.[6] The onset of warfarin activity depends not only on its inherent pharmacokinetic characteristics (half-life > 36 hours), but also on the rate of elimination of circulating clotting factors. Although warfarin inhibits production of the vitamin K dependent clotting factors, previously synthesized clotting factors must be eliminated at rates that correspond with their elimination half-lives (Table 11-8). Approximately four half-lives are required for these factors to reach a new steady state after their production is inhibited, so the effect of warfarin can be delayed for several days. Initial increases in the INR reflect only reductions in factor VII activity, but full anticoagulation with warfarin requires adequate suppression of factors II and X, which have significantly longer elimination half-lives. By overlapping a quick onset injectable anticoagulant such as heparin/LMWH/fondaparinux with warfarin therapy, adequate anticoagulation can be continued until warfarin therapy reaches a therapeutic intensity.

In addition to suppressing the synthesis of the vitamin K-dependent clotting factors, warfarin also inhibits the formation of the naturally occurring anticoagulant protein C and its cofactor, protein S. In patients with congenital protein C or protein S deficiency, initial warfarin therapy can suppress these proteins to concentrations that may result in hypercoagulability with possible thrombus extension, unless concurrent heparin therapy provides adequate anticoagulation. To prevent these complications, heparin/LMWH/fondaparinux and warfarin therapy should overlap.

Heparin therapy has been observed to prolong the INR,[68] and warfarin can prolong the aPTT by several seconds.[69] Thus, interference with laboratory tests should be considered in the evaluation of the intensity of anticoagulation during the overlap of heparin and warfarin therapy.

Initiation of Warfarin Therapy

CASE 11-5, QUESTION 4: In an effort to discharge A.W. from the hospital as soon as possible, an initial dose of warfarin 10 mg PO every evening for 3 days has been ordered. Is such a "loading dose" reasonable? What are more effective approaches to initiating therapy?

Initiation of warfarin dosing is complex because dosing requirements vary significantly among individuals. Daily doses as low as 0.5 mg and as high as 20 mg or more may be required in individual patients to reach a therapeutic INR.[70] Two primary methods for initiation of warfarin therapy are used.[71] The average daily dosing method relies on an understanding that although dosing requirements for warfarin vary significantly among patients, an average

Table 11-17
Factors that Increase Sensitivity to Warfarin

Age older than 75 years
Weight < 45 kg
Clinical congestive heart failure
Clinical hyperthyroidism
Decreased oral intake
Diarrhea
Drug–drug interactions
Elevated baseline INR (>1.4)
End-stage renal disease
Fever
Hepatic disease
Hypoalbuminemia
Known CYP2C9 or VKORC1 variant
Malignancy
Malnutrition
Postoperative status

INR, international normalized ratio.

dosing requirement of 4 to 5 mg/day of warfarin is necessary to maintain an INR of 2.0 to 3.0 in most patients. When average daily dosing is used for initiation of warfarin therapy, patients are typically started at 4 to 5 mg daily, with dosing adjustments as necessary until the therapeutic goal is reached. However, patients who may be more sensitive to the effects of warfarin (Table 11-17) are expected to require lower dosages of warfarin. In these patients, therapy should be initiated at 1 to 3 mg daily, with subsequent dosing adjustments as necessary. Several dosing algorithms, using a 4-mg to 5-mg initiation dose, have been developed to aid with dosing decisions after the first few doses of warfarin have been administered.[72–74] Another popular dosing algorithm recommended by the American College of Chest Physicians (ACCP) for outpatients uses a 10-mg initiation dose for the first 2 days, with the INR on day 3 measured to guide dosing on days 3 and 4, and the INR on day 5 used to guide the next three doses[21,75] (Fig. 11-4). Although using this dosing algorithm helps achieve a therapeutic INR more quickly than using a 5-mg initial dose, these findings may not be generalizable to all patient populations because the patients evaluated were relatively healthy, young outpatients.[76] The 10-mg initiation dose may lead to overanticoagulation and heightened bleeding risk in elderly and ill patients with multiple medical problems.[77] Average daily dosing is often used to initiate therapy in ambulatory patients; in this case, the first INR should be evaluated within 3 to 5 days of initiation of warfarin therapy (Table 11-18). In hospitalized patients, it is more common to evaluate the INR daily during initiation of therapy.

Flexible initiation of warfarin is an alternative approach for starting therapy that is based on evaluating the rate of increase in the INR and making daily dosing adjustments based on daily INR evaluation, with a goal of determining the eventual maintenance dosing requirement. A popular flexible initiation nomogram is presented in Table 11-19.[78,79] Using this nomogram, warfarin can be initiated with either a 10-mg or a 5-mg starting dose, with daily dosing adjustments based on the rate of increase in the INR. Flexible initiation does not necessarily shorten the time to reach the goal INR, and initiating therapy with a 10-mg dose as described in some protocols may be associated with an increased risk of early overanticoagulation in certain patients. Nonetheless,

Day-3 INR	Days/dose (mg) 3	4	Day-5 INR	Days/dose (mg) 5	6	7
<1.3	15	15	<2.0	15	15	15
1.3–1.4	10	10	2.0–3.0	7.5	5	7.5
			3.1–3.5	0	5	5
			>3.5	0	0	2.5
1.5–1.6	10	5	<2.0	7.5	7.5	7.5
1.7–1.9	5	5	2.0–3.0	5	5	5
			3.1–3.5	2.5	2.5	2.5
			>3.5	0	2.5	2.5
2.0–2.2	2.5	2.5	<2.0	15	5	5
2.3–3.0	0	2.5	2.0–3.0	2.5	5	2.5
			3.1–3.5	0	2.5	0
			>3.5	0	0	2.5
>3.0	0	0	<2.0	2.5	2.5	2.5
			2.0–3.0	2.5	0	2.5
			3.1–4.0	0	2.5	0
			>4.0	0	0	2.5

Figure 11-4 Warfarin initiation dosing algorithm based on starting with 10-mg doses on days 1 and 2. (Source: Kovacs MJ et al. Prospective assessment of a nomogram for the initiation of oral anticoagulant therapy for outpatient treatment of venous thromboembolism. *Pathophysiol Haemost Thromb*. 2002;32:131.)

these methods offer a more individualized approach to initiation of therapy.

The baseline INR for A.W. was 1.0. Using the flexible initiation protocol presented in Table 11-19, the first dose of warfarin should be 10 mg administered in the evening on the first day of hospitalization. Subsequent INR values obtained daily will guide dosing requirements until a therapeutic INR is reached. The order for warfarin 10 mg orally every evening for three doses should be discontinued and replaced with daily orders for warfarin and INR monitoring.

Table 11-18
Warfarin Initiation for Outpatients Using the Average Daily Dosing Method

	Nonsensitive Patients	Sensitive Patients[a]
Initial dose	5 mg daily	2.5 mg daily
First INR	3 days	3 days
<1.5	7.5–10 mg daily	5–7.5 mg daily
1.5–1.9	5 mg daily	2.5 mg daily
2.0–3.0	2.5 mg daily	1.25 mg daily
3.1–4.0	1.25 mg daily	0.5 mg daily
>4.0	Hold	Hold
Next INR	2–3 days	2–3 days
Subsequent dosing and monitoring	Continue dose escalation and frequent monitoring until lower limit of therapeutic range is reached.	

Warfarin Use in Adults: Clinical Care Guideline, University of Illinois Hospital and Health Sciences System.
[a]See Table 11-17 on factors that increase sensitivity to warfarin.

Table 11-19
Flexible Initiation Dosing Protocol for Warfarin Dosing, Including 10-mg and 5-mg Starting Dose Options

Day	INR	10-mg Initiation Dose (mg)	5-mg Initiation Dose (mg)
1		10	5
2	<1.5	7.5–10	5
	1.5–1.9	2.5	2.5
	2.0–2.5	1.0–2.5	1–2.5
	>2.5	0	0
3	<1.5	5–10	5–10
	1.5–1.9	2.5–5	2.5–5
	2.0–2.5	0–2.5	0–2.5
	2.5–3.0	0–2.5	0–2.5
	>3.0	0	0
4	<1.5	10	10
	1.5–1.9	5–7.5	5–7.5
	2.0–3.0	0–5	0–5
	>3.0	0	0
5	<1.5	10	10
	1.5–1.9	7.5–10	7.5–10
	2.0–3.0	0–5	0–5
	>3.0	0	0
6	<1.5	7.5–12.5	7.5–12.5
	1.5–1.9	5–10	5–10
	2.0–30	0–7.5	0–7.5
	>3.0	0	0

INR, international normalized ratio.
Source: Crowther MA et al. Warfarin: less may be better. *Ann Intern Med*. 1997;127:332.

Intensity and Duration of Therapy

CASE 11-5, QUESTION 5: What is the goal INR for A.W. and how long should anticoagulation be continued?

In patients with DVT or PE, warfarin doses that prolong the PT to an INR of 2.0 to 3.0 are defined as regular intensity therapy. This therapeutic range is recommended to maximize the antithrombotic effect of warfarin while minimizing potential bleeding complications associated with excessive anticoagulation.[6] Once formed, venous clots adhere to the blood vessel wall. Thus, the first step in resolution of a thrombus involves covering the clot with a layer of endothelial cells to prevent additional platelet aggregation at the site of vessel injury. This endothelialization process generally takes 7 to 10 days to be completed. Initial anticoagulant treatment is used to prevent clot extension while allowing adequate endothelialization to occur. Continued anticoagulation prevents further clotting.

The appropriate duration of warfarin therapy is based on the likelihood of a recurrent venous thromboembolic event and the risk of bleeding in each patient (Table 11-9). Patients with unprovoked (idiopathic) DVT or PE should be treated for at least 3 months, but considered for indefinite therapy as their likelihood of having a recurrent event can be as high as 30% over 5 years.[15] Patients with DVT or PE associated with transient or reversible risk factors (provoked VTE) are usually treated for 3 months, as in the case of A.W., whose VTE provoking risk factor was a prolonged car ride, as the risk of recurrence is lower (approximately 10% over 5 years). In cancer-associated thrombosis, first-line treatment consists of long-term LMWH based on improved clinical outcomes over warfarin; however, this needs to consider individual patient bleeding risk, patient preferences, tolerability, and drug costs.[80–86] The use of DOACs in patients with cancer is not currently endorsed; however, current data support its safety compared to other options.[87]

Adverse Effects

CASE 11-5, QUESTION 6: What possible adverse effects from oral anticoagulation therapy should be considered in A.W. and how should they be monitored?

Hemorrhage

Bleeding is the most common adverse effect associated with anticoagulation. A summary of experimental and observational inception cohort studies determined that the average annual frequency of fatal, major, and all (major or minor) bleeding in patients treated with warfarin was 0.6%, 3%, and 9.6%, respectively.[31] However, wide variation in bleeding frequencies has been reported, likely due to differences in patient characteristics, treatment protocols, and the definition and assessment of bleeding among trials.

The most common sites for anticoagulation-related bleeding are the nose, oral pharynx, and soft tissues, followed by the GI and urinary tracts. Hemarthrosis (bleeding into joint spaces) and retroperitoneal and intraocular bleeding represent less common hemorrhagic complications of anticoagulation therapy.[6] Gastrointestinal and urinary tract bleeding in anticoagulated patients is often caused by previously undiagnosed lesions. Menstrual blood flow may also be increased and prolonged in women taking anticoagulants. This problem may be clinically significant if there is an underlying pathologic condition (ovarian cysts, uterine fibroids, or polyps) resulting in abnormal vaginal bleeding.

For VTE treatment, the DOACs rivaroxaban and apixaban both showed significantly lower rates for major bleeding in clinical trials compared to warfarin, whereas edoxaban and dabigatran showed comparable rates. A recent meta-analysis demonstrated no statistically significant differences for efficacy and safety associated with most treatment strategies used to treat acute VTE compared with the LMWH/VKA combination.[88] However, it showed that the UFH/VKA combination is associated with a higher rate of recurrent VTE and that rivaroxaban and apixaban demonstrated a lower risk for major bleeding.

Although it is uncommon, intracranial bleeding resulting in hemorrhagic stroke represents the most common cause of fatal bleeding associated with warfarin therapy. Rates of intracranial hemorrhage associated with anticoagulants have been estimated to range from 0.3% to 2%, and up to 60% are fatal.[6] The DOACs have been shown to be as effective as warfarin for stroke prevention in patients with atrial fibrillation and are associated with lower rates of intracranial hemorrhage and reduced all-cause mortality. However, all of the DOACs, except for apixaban, are associated with a 25% increased risk of gastrointestinal bleeding.[89]

Many factors influence the risk of hemorrhagic complications associated with warfarin. The frequency of bleeding is higher in the first 3 months of therapy than during subsequent months.[90] Unlike heparin, the intensity of anticoagulation with warfarin directly influences the risk of bleeding, including intracranial hemorrhage.[91] Other patient-specific variables that influence the risk of warfarin-associated bleeding include a history of GI bleeding, serious comorbid disease (including malignancy), and concomitant therapy with aspirin, clopidogrel, or nonsteroidal anti-inflammatory drugs (NSAIDs).[6]

Several bleeding risk scores are available, including HAS-BLED (Hypertension, Abnormal renal or liver function, Stroke, Bleeding, Labile INR, Elderly, Drugs and alcohol) and ATRIA (Anticoagulation and Risk Factors in Atrial Fibrillation), which may identify patients at higher risk of bleeding; however, how best to use these tools remains in question.[92–94] None of these bleeding risk scores have been very effective at predicting risk for major or fatal bleeding in the first 3 months of anticoagulation for VTE, and none have performed well in the elderly in predicting major bleeding in the first 90 days of anticoagulation for VTE.[95–97]

Bleeding complications in A.W. can be minimized by careful attention to the signs and symptoms of bleeding by the patient and her caregivers, maintenance of the INR within the therapeutic range, avoidance of therapy with concomitant drugs known to increase the risk of bleeding or to increase the INR, and routine outpatient follow-up for INR monitoring and clinical assessment.

Skin Necrosis

Warfarin-induced skin necrosis is a rare but serious adverse effect of oral anticoagulation, occurring in approximately 0.01% to 0.1% of patients treated with warfarin.[98] Patients present within 3 to 6 days of the initiation of warfarin therapy with painful discoloration of the breast, buttocks, thigh, or penis. The lesions progress to frank necrosis with blackening and eschar. Skin necrosis appears to be the result of extensive microvascular thrombosis within subcutaneous fat and has been associated with hypercoagulable conditions, including protein C or protein S deficiency. In these patients, rapid depletion of protein C before depletion of vitamin K-dependent clotting factors during early warfarin therapy can result in an imbalance between procoagulant and anticoagulant activity, leading to initial hypercoagulability and thrombosis. Adequate use of injectable UFH, LMWH, or fondaparinux during initiation of warfarin can prevent the development of early hypercoagulability.

Warfarin therapy should be discontinued in patients who develop skin necrosis. However, subsequent warfarin therapy is not necessarily contraindicated if it is required for treatment or prevention of thromboembolic disease. In patients with protein C or protein S deficiency and a history of skin necrosis, warfarin therapy can be restarted at low dosages if given with UFH/LMWH/fondaparinux. Therapy is maintained until the INR has been within the therapeutic range for 72 hours. Supplementation of protein C through administration of fresh frozen plasma also may be indicated.

Purple Toe Syndrome

Purple toe syndrome is a rarely reported adverse effect that typically occurs 3 to 8 weeks after the initiation of warfarin therapy and is unrelated to intensity of anticoagulation.[99] Patients initially present with painful discoloration of the toes that blanches with pressure and fades with elevation. The pathophysiology of this syndrome has been related to cholesterol microembolization from atherosclerotic plaques, leading to arterial obstruction. Because cholesterol microembolization has been associated with renal failure and death, warfarin therapy should be discontinued in patients who develop purple toe syndrome.

Patient Education

CASE 11-6

QUESTION 1: E.N. is a 42-year-old man newly diagnosed with unprovoked DVT. He will be treated as an outpatient with enoxaparin 1.5 mg/kg SC daily and started on warfarin 5 mg PO daily using average daily dosing initiation. His primary care physician would like him to receive follow-up care in the medical center's pharmacist-managed anticoagulation clinic. What are the benefits of formal anticoagulation management services?

One of the keys to successful oral anticoagulant therapy is appropriate outpatient management. In comparison with routine medical care, management of warfarin therapy by anticoagulation clinics is associated with significant reductions in bleeding and thromboembolic complications, with reductions in the rates of warfarin-related hospital admissions and ED visits, and with outcome-based cost savings for healthcare organizations.[100] Pharmacist-managed anticoagulation clinics offer many benefits for the management of anticoagulation therapy, including improved dosing regulation, continuous patient education, early identification of risk factors for adverse events, and timely intervention to avoid or minimize complications.[101] E.N.'s referral to a pharmacist-managed anticoagulation clinic is likely to improve his overall satisfaction with care and to improve his clinical outcomes.

The availability of portable INR self-testing devices also allows the option of anticoagulation monitoring in the home setting. Patient self-testing of INRs has been shown to result in comparable outcomes to high-quality anticoagulation delivered via anticoagulation clinics.[6] For patients that may prefer this monitoring method, a structured education and follow-up program should be designed and integrated with the patient's provider or the anticoagulation management service.

CASE 11-6, QUESTION 2: At his initial visit to the anticoagulation clinic, E.N. will receive extensive education about his warfarin therapy. What information should be conveyed to him by his anticoagulation provider to ensure the safety and efficacy of warfarin therapy?

Successful warfarin therapy depends on the active participation of knowledgeable patients.[6] The anticoagulant effect of warfarin is influenced by various factors, and fluctuations in the intensity of the anticoagulant effect of warfarin can increase the risk of both hemorrhagic complications and recurrent thromboembolism. Pharmacists and other providers can improve adherence to the medication schedule, as well as ensure the safety and efficacy of warfarin therapy, by providing appropriate education to patients treated with this agent.

Key elements that form the basis of a thorough patient education program for anticoagulation therapy are listed in Table 11-20. This information may be conveyed through written teaching materials, recorded instruction, individual or group discussion, or a combination of these approaches. Many useful educational tools are available from the manufacturers of the oral anticoagulants and from other noncommercial sources.

E.N. should receive extensive education about warfarin therapy in an individual teaching session or an organized education program. A wallet card, medical bracelet, or alternative method of identifying him as a patient treated with warfarin should be provided. The healthcare provider who assumes responsibility for his outpatient warfarin therapy will need to provide continuing reinforcement of the essential elements of medication information at each follow-up visit.

Table 11-20
Key Elements of Patient Education Regarding Oral Anticoagulation

Identification of generic and brand names
Purpose of therapy
Expected duration of therapy
Dosing and administration
Visual recognition of drug and tablet strength
What to do if a dose is missed
Recognition of signs and symptoms of bleeding
Recognition of signs and symptoms of thromboembolism
What to do if bleeding or thromboembolism occurs
Potential for interactions with prescription and over-the-counter medications and natural/herbal products
Limiting use of alcohol
Avoidance of pregnancy
Significance of informing other healthcare providers that patient is taking anticoagulation, and when notify anticoagulation provider when invasive procedures are being scheduled
When, where, and with whom follow-up will be provided
Dabigatran only: swallow whole, keep in original container, caution about potential for GI upset
Rivaroxaban only: take with food (evening meal)
Warfarin only: importance of INR monitoring and expected frequency, consistency of vitamin K

INR, international normalized ratio.

Factors that Influence Warfarin Dosing

CASE 11-6, QUESTION 3: After receiving 6 days of enoxaparin therapy and six doses of warfarin 5 mg/day PO, E.N.'s INR is 2.4. Enoxaparin is discontinued and E.N. is instructed to continue his current dosage of warfarin. He is scheduled to return to the anticoagulation clinic in 1 week for re-evaluation. At that time, his INR is 1.7. What factors might account for this change in the intensity of anticoagulation?

Patients should always be questioned about their understanding of the prescribed dose and their adherence to the prescribed regimen. Questions might include, "What dose of the medication have you been taking?" "What time of the day do you take your medication?" and "How many times in the last week did you miss a dose of your medication?" If there is no evidence of misunderstanding of the correct dose or of noncompliance, numerous other factors should be considered that are known to influence warfarin dosing requirements in individual patients during both initiation and maintenance phases of therapy. Changes in dietary vitamin K intake, underlying disease states and clinical condition, alcohol ingestion, genetic factors, and concurrent medications can significantly change the intensity of therapy, resulting in the need for dosing adjustments to maintain the INR within the therapeutic range. In a dosing cohort of 1,015 patients on warfarin therapy, body surface area, age, target INR, amiodarone use, smoker status, race, current thrombosis, VKORC1 polymorphism 1639/3673 G.A, CYP2C9(*)3, and CYP2C9(*)2 were all independent predictors of warfarin therapeutic dose.[102]

Dietary Vitamin K Intake

The two primary sources of vitamin K in humans are the biosynthesis of vitamin K_2 (menaquinone) by intestinal bacteria and dietary intake of vitamin K_1 (phytonadione). The US-recommended daily allowance for vitamin K is 70 to 140 mcg/day, and the typical Western diet provides approximately 300 to 500 mcg/day.[103] Vitamin K is found in high concentrations in certain foods, including green leafy vegetables (asparagus, broccoli, Brussels sprouts, cabbage, cauliflower, collard greens, endive, kale, lettuce, parsley, spinach, and turnip greens), soy milk, certain oils, certain nutritional supplements, and multiple vitamin products.

Variations in vitamin K intake have been linked to INR fluctuations in patients taking warfarin.[104,105] In addition, diets high in vitamin K content have been associated with acquired warfarin resistance, defined as excessive warfarin dosing requirements to reach a therapeutic INR range.[106] Numerous cases have also been reported in which patients previously stabilized with warfarin experienced elevations in INR with or without hemorrhagic

Table 11-21
Warfarin Interactions with Disease States and Clinical Conditions

Clinical Condition	Effect on Warfarin Therapy
Advanced age	Increased sensitivity to warfarin due to reduced vitamin K stores and/or lower plasma concentrations of vitamin K-dependent clotting factors
Pregnancy	Teratogenic; avoid exposure during pregnancy
Lactation	Not excreted in breast milk; can be used postpartum by nursing mothers
Alcohol use	■ Acute ingestion: inhibits warfarin metabolism, with acute elevation in INR ■ Chronic ingestion: induces warfarin metabolism, with higher dose requirements
Liver disease	■ May induce coagulopathy by decreased production of clotting factors, with baseline elevation in INR ■ May reduce clearance of warfarin
Kidney disease	Reduced activity of CYP2C9, with lower warfarin dose requirements
Heart failure	Reduced warfarin metabolism due to hepatic congestion
Nutritional status	Changes in dietary vitamin K alter response to warfarin
Tube feedings	Decreased sensitivity to warfarin, possibly caused by changes in absorption or vitamin K content of nutritional supplements
Smoking and tobacco use	■ Smoking: may induce CYP1A2, increasing warfarin dosing requirements. ■ Chewing tobacco: may contain vitamin K, increasing warfarin dosing requirements
Fever	Increased catabolism of clotting factors, causing acute increase in INR
Diarrhea	Reduction in secretion of vitamin K by gut flora, causing acute increase in INR
Acute infection/inflammation	Increased sensitivity to warfarin

INR, international normalized ratio.

complications when dietary sources of vitamin K were eliminated. Conversely, reductions in INR with or without thromboembolic complications have been reported in patients in whom dietary sources of vitamin K have been added.

This data illustrate the potential clinical significance of dietary changes in patients taking warfarin. To minimize these potential effects, E.N. should be counseled to maintain a consistent intake of dietary vitamin K.[107] His final warfarin maintenance dose will be partially influenced by his typical diet. However, restriction of dietary vitamin K intake is unnecessary, except in cases of significant resistance to the anticoagulant effect of warfarin. E.N. should be aware of the types of foods and supplements that contain large quantities of vitamin K, and should be counseled to maintain a consistent diet, to avoid bingeing with foods high in vitamin K content, and to report significant dietary changes to his healthcare provider. Appropriate assessment and follow-up are essential to prevent hemorrhagic or thromboembolic complications that may arise from changes in INR resulting from dietary alterations.

Underlying Disease States and Clinical Conditions

The presence or exacerbation of various medical conditions can also influence anticoagulation status[71] (Table 11-21). Diarrhea-associated alterations in intestinal flora can reduce vitamin K absorption, resulting in elevations in INR. Fever enhances the catabolism of clotting factors and can increase INR. Heart failure, hepatic congestion, and liver disease can also cause significant elevations in INR because of a reduction in warfarin metabolism. End-stage renal disease is associated with decreased CYP2C9 activity, resulting in lower warfarin dose requirements.

The impact of changes in thyroid function on warfarin dose requirements is controversial.[108] It has been suggested that levothyroxine initiation accelerates clotting factor catabolism, enhancing warfarin's anticoagulation effect; however, there is conflicting evidence in whether a warfarin–levothyroxine interaction has an impact on the INR.[109,110] A recent retrospective review did not show a difference in the mean warfarin dose/INR ratios before and after levothyroxine initiation, suggesting that no clinical interaction exists, and additional monitoring may not be necessary.[111]

Acute physical or psychologic stress has been reported to increase INR. Increased physical activity has also been reported to increase the warfarin dosing requirement. Smoking can induce CYP1A2, which may increase warfarin metabolism in certain patients, resulting in increased dose requirements.[112] Due to its high vitamin K content, chewing smokeless tobacco can suppress the INR response.[113]

Thorough education of patients taking warfarin should include detailed attention to recognizing the signs and symptoms of changes in underlying disease states and clinical conditions that can influence warfarin dosing requirements. They should be instructed to contact their anticoagulation management program whenever changes occur that might influence INR and warfarin dose requirement.

Alcohol Ingestion

Chronic alcohol ingestion has been associated with induction of the hepatic enzyme systems that metabolize warfarin. Therefore, warfarin dosing requirements are sometimes higher in alcoholic patients. Conversely, acute ingestion of large amounts of alcohol can slow warfarin metabolism through competitive inhibition of metabolizing enzymes, leading to elevations in INR and an increased risk of bleeding complications.[6,107] Despite some reports linking low amounts of alcohol to an elevated INR,[114] in general it is believed that moderate intake of alcoholic beverages is not associated with alterations in the metabolism or the therapeutic effect of warfarin as measured by INR. Patients taking warfarin should be educated to limit their alcohol consumption to less than one to two alcoholic beverages per day. Chronic drinkers should be counseled to limit their drinking and maintain a regular pattern to avoid fluctuations in INR.[107] E.N. does not need to abstain from drinking alcoholic beverages in moderation, but he should be counseled to avoid the sporadic ingestion of large amounts of alcohol.

Conversely, alcoholic liver disease (i.e., cirrhosis) can alter multiple hemostatic mechanisms and reduces production of hepatic clotting factors. Decreased production and clearance of vitamin K-dependent clotting factors accounts for the prolonged PT and INR often seen in these patients. Therefore, an increased response to warfarin would be expected in patients with liver impairment. Worsening liver function is also a predictor for bleeding complications and patients with end-stage liver disease are at increased risk of bleeding. Before instituting warfarin therapy in these patients, the risks of bleeding associated with both the underlying liver disease and warfarin therapy must be weighed against the benefit of preventing thromboembolic events. If warfarin is indicated, the best approach would be to use a cautious initiation and dose titration approach by starting with lower doses and titrating up slowly to goal. Small increases in dosage should be made, if indicated, recognizing that the full effect of any dose adjustment may be delayed in patients with severe liver dysfunction. Monitoring for bleeding complications is essential, even at goal INR ranges, when warfarin is used in patients with liver dysfunction.

Genetic Factors

The cytochrome P450 (CYP) 2C9 and vitamin K epoxide reductase complex 1 (VKORC1) genotypes have been associated with warfarin dose requirements, and dosing algorithms incorporating genetic and clinical information have been shown to be predictive of stable warfarin dose.[115] However, dosing algorithms that incorporate CYP2C9 genotype and vitamin K epoxide reductase complex 1 (VKORC1) haplotype along with other patient characteristics to predict warfarin maintenance doses showed mixed results in randomized, prospective clinical trials, questioning the utility of this approach.[116,117] Based on current data failing to show a benefit, ACCP recommends against the routine use of pharmacogenetic testing for guiding doses of VKA (Grade 1B).[21] Further research is needed to determine the place of warfarin pharmacogenetic testing.

CASE 11-6, QUESTION 4: How should E.N. be assessed and evaluated at this clinic appointment?

At each clinic visit, E.N. should be assessed for signs and symptoms of bleeding, and for signs and symptoms of clot progression and/or recurrence. The accuracy and reliability of the INR test should be also considered. Additionally, E.N. should be asked about missed or extra doses of warfarin, dietary changes (increases or decreases in vitamin K, alcohol use), medication changes, recent illnesses (such as nausea/vomiting/fever/chills/diarrhea), any recent falls, and any known upcoming procedures. Regardless of the INR result, all factors that may influence E.N.'s anticoagulation status should be evaluated carefully.

Dosing Adjustments

CASE 11-6, QUESTION 5: After a thorough assessment, it is determined that E.N. has adhered to his prescribed warfarin dosage schedule and that there is no apparent explanation to account for his reduction in INR. How should his warfarin dosage be adjusted?

When overanticoagulation or underanticoagulation is verified, an adjustment in warfarin dosing may be necessary. Table 11-22 describes approaches to warfarin dosing adjustments for maintenance therapy. Typically, dosing adjustments of 5% to 20% of the total daily dose (or the total weekly dose) are appropriate to reach the therapeutic range.[118] Because warfarin does not follow linear kinetics, small adjustments in dose can lead to large INR changes, and thus large dose adjustments (i.e., greater than a 20% increase or decrease of the total weekly dose) are not recommended. These maintenance dosing guidelines should only be applied to patients who have reached a steady state dose and not in the initiation phase of therapy.

Because E.N. is currently taking 5 mg daily, an adjustment of 15% would increase his dosage to approximately 5.5 mg/day. This

Table 11-22
Warfarin Dose Adjustment Nomogram for Maintenance Therapy

INR (Goal 2–3)	Suggested change in total "weekly" dose
<1.5	Give extra one-time daily dose and increase weekly dose by 10%–20%
1.5–1.9	Increase weekly dose by 5%–15% (may give extra one-time daily dose)[a]
2.0–3.0	Maintain current dose
3.1–4.0[b]	Hold up to one daily dose and decrease weekly dose by 5%–20%[a]
4.1–5.0[b]	Hold up to two daily doses and decrease weekly dose by 10%–20%[a]

Warfarin Use in Adults: Clinical Care Guideline, University of Illinois Hospital and Health Sciences System.
[a]If transient cause identified, may need not to increase/decrease weekly dose.
[b]Assumes no active bleeding.

dosing adjustment can be made by having him take one 5-mg tablet and half of a 1-mg tablet each day (same daily dosing) or by having him take 7.5 mg 2 days per week and 5 mg all other days of the week (alternate-day dosing). Patient preference about breaking tablets in half, the likelihood of confusion about different tablet sizes, and potential confusion on taking different doses on different days of the week should be the primary considerations when selecting a dosing method.[119]

Frequency of Follow-Up

CASE 11-6, QUESTION 6: E.N. agrees to increase his warfarin dosage to 5.5 mg/day. A new prescription for 1-mg tablets is written for him, and he is instructed about the use of these tablets. When should his INR be reassessed and his anticoagulation status, including physical assessment, be re-evaluated?

It will take several days for his INR to reach a new steady state because of the long elimination half-lives of both warfarin and the vitamin K-dependent clotting factors. His INR should be rechecked approximately 1 week after a dosing adjustment has been made. Once a stable dose has been reached, patient assessment and INR monitoring typically occurs every 4 to 6 weeks. However, if E.N. displays any signs of medical instability or nonadherence, a follow-up schedule of every 1 to 2 weeks is indicated (Table 11-23). For carefully selected patients with well-controlled INRs, recall frequencies out to 12 weeks can be recommended.[21] For patients taking warfarin with previously stable therapeutic INRs who present with a single out-of-range INR of ≤ 0.5 below or above therapeutic, continuing the current dose and testing the INR within 1 to 2 weeks is suggested, rather than changing the overall daily dose.[21]

Management of Overanticoagulation

CASE 11-7

QUESTION 1: V.G., who has been taking warfarin for 3 years with good INR control, noted bright red blood after a bowel movement (hematochezia) that resolved and has not returned. In the ED, an INR of 5.6 was reported. Her Hct and Hgb were both within normal limits, as were her vital signs. A stool guaiac test was positive, and multiple external hemorrhoids were detected. How should this adverse effect of warfarin be treated in V.G.?

Management of overanticoagulation depends on the clinical presentation of the patient. In the case of an elevated INR without

Table 11-23
Frequency of International Normalized Ratio Monitoring and Patient Assessment during Warfarin Therapy

Initiation Therapy	
Inpatient initiation	Daily
Outpatient flexible initiation method	Daily through day 4, then within 3–5 days
Outpatient average daily dosing method	Within 3–5 days, then within 1 week
After hospital discharge	Within 3–5 days
First month of therapy	Every 1–4 days until therapeutic, then weekly
Maintenance Therapy	
Medically stable inpatients	Every 1–3 days
Medically unstable inpatients	Daily
After hospital discharge	If stable, within 3–5 days; If unstable, within 1–3 days
Routine follow-up in medically stable and reliable patients	Every 4–12 weeks
Routine follow-up in medically unstable or unreliable patients	Every 1–2 weeks
Dose held today for significant over-anticoagulation	In 1–2 days
Dosage change today	Within 1–2 weeks
Dosage change <2 weeks ago	Within 2–4 weeks

bleeding complications, interruption of warfarin therapy by holding one or two doses until the INR returns to the therapeutic range is usually sufficient.[21] Minor bleeding complications accompanied by an elevated INR can also be managed by withholding warfarin therapy for a short period until bleeding resolves. In either case, the patient should be questioned to determine a possible cause for overanticoagulation, including intake of extra doses of warfarin, changes in diet or alcohol intake, changes in underlying medical conditions, or the use of other medications. In some cases, no apparent explanation is identified. Depending on the cause, a reduction in the maintenance dosing of warfarin may be necessary.

The time required for INR to return to the therapeutic range after warfarin is withheld depends on several patient characteristics. Advanced age, lower warfarin maintenance dose requirements, and higher INR are associated with increased time for INR correction.[120] Other factors that can prolong the time for INR to return to the therapeutic range include decompensated heart failure, active malignancy, and recent use of medications known to potentiate warfarin.

Although previously recommended and commonly used, low-dose vitamin K in patients with elevated INR 4.5 to 10 and not bleeding is not associated with a reduction in major bleeding, and is no longer routinely recommended.[21] However, patients with INRs greater than 10 and not bleeding may benefit from small doses of oral vitamin K 1 to 2.5 mg. The decision on whether to give vitamin K in nonbleeding patients needs to consider the patient's individual risk for bleeding and thrombosis.[21] An oral dose of 1 to 2.5 mg can correct overanticoagulation in 24 to 48 hours without causing prolonged resistance to warfarin therapy, a problem commonly seen with larger (10 mg) doses of vitamin K. Intramuscular administration is contraindicated due to the risk of hematoma formation, and SC administration of vitamin K is not recommended because of variable absorption.[121]

IV doses of 0.5 to 1 mg of vitamin K can correct overanticoagulation within 24 hours.[6] This approach is also useful for reversal of therapeutic anticoagulation before invasive procedures and can be used to correct overanticoagulation in high-risk cases. Intravenous vitamin K should be diluted in a minimum of 50 mL intravenous fluid and administered with an infusion pump over a minimum of 20 minutes to prevent flushing, hypotension, and cardiovascular collapse.[6] Although these symptoms resemble anaphylaxis, the mechanism of this adverse response is unclear: It is not known whether it is caused by phytonadione or by the vehicle in which phytonadione is formulated. If this adverse reaction occurs, administration of epinephrine may be indicated, as well as other standard measures to support blood pressure and maintain the airway.

Rapid reversal of warfarin therapy is indicated in the setting of major, life-threatening bleeding (i.e., severe gastrointestinal bleeding, intracranial hemorrhage). Fresh frozen plasma or factor concentrates to replace clotting factors will decrease the INR for 4 to 6 hours and should be administered as needed with careful monitoring of volume status.[21] Supplementation with high-dose IV vitamin K (10 mg) may also be indicated. Administration of IV vitamin K will reverse the effects of warfarin within 6 to 12 hours. However, if continued warfarin therapy is indicated when bleeding resolves, anticoagulation with heparin may be necessary for as long as 7 to 14 days until the effect of high-dose vitamin K is diminished and warfarin responsiveness returns.

Hematochezia may be an early sign of more serious bleeding, but in many cases this condition is associated with minor bleeding episodes and identifiable causes such as hemorrhoids. In a reliable patient, holding the warfarin until the INR returns to a therapeutic level usually suffices, along with the addition of a bowel regimen to prevent straining with bowel movements, topical cream to minimize swelling and irritation, increased fluids, and/or increased fiber intake. Because V.G. appears to have only minor bleeding from the stool, is hemodynamically stable, and has a stable hemoglobin, withholding warfarin is appropriate. If the patient has never had a colonoscopy, then evaluation for the appropriateness of this test may be warranted.

Use in Pregnancy

CASE 11-8

Question 1: M.P., a 25-year-old woman, takes warfarin for chronic therapy for recurrent DVTs. She tells you today that she missed her menses and thinks she may be pregnant. A pregnancy test ordered today was positive. What effects might warfarin have on the fetus? Are UFH or LMWHs safer alternatives in this situation?

Warfarin and other coumarin anticoagulants cross the placental barrier and may place the fetus at risk for hemorrhage and teratogenic effects.[122] Up to 30% of pregnancies that involve exposure to coumarin result in abnormal liveborn infants, and up to 30% in spontaneous abortion or stillbirth. Congenital abnormalities such as stippled calcifications and nasal cartilage hypoplasia primarily occurred in infants born to mothers receiving warfarin during the first trimester of pregnancy, with the highest risk during weeks 6 to 12. Other abnormalities, involving the central nervous system and eyes, are more likely to occur when the mother is taking warfarin later in the pregnancy. In addition, because warfarin crosses the placenta, fatal bleeding complications may occur.

Women of childbearing age who require anticoagulation should be counseled about options for contraception. Patients who become pregnant while receiving warfarin should be informed of the risks of continued anticoagulation to the fetus, as well as the risk to themselves of discontinuing anticoagulation.

Other options for pregnant women who require anticoagulation include UFH and LMWHs.[122] Because these agents do not cross the placenta, they are preferred over warfarin for use in pregnancy. Many clinical trials have validated the safety and efficacy of UFH and LMWHs in the prevention and treatment of DVT and PE during pregnancy, with LMWH generally preferred to UFH for long-term management throughout pregnancy.[122,123] When used at full doses for the treatment of VTE during pregnancy, dosing must be adjusted throughout the pregnancy to account for the expected increase in the body weight of the mother and the reported increase in clearance of LMWH during pregnancy.[124,125] Selected current recommendations for use of anticoagulants in pregnancy are outlined in Table 11-24.

After being informed of the risks associated with warfarin, M.P. decided to continue her pregnancy and to begin anticoagulation with LMWH. Because pregnant women were excluded from clinical trials with the DOACs due to their increased risk for maternal and fetal bleeding, their use in pregnancy is not recommended at this time. Warfarin therapy should be discontinued immediately and LMWH initiated using SC treatment doses as previously described. Dosing adjustments may be required throughout pregnancy based on changes in body weight and clearance, possibly guided by anti-factor Xa monitoring. Potential adverse effects of LMWH use, including hemorrhage, thrombocytopenia, and osteoporosis, should be monitored appropriately.

For women desiring spinal anesthesia during delivery, treatment doses of LMWH should be discontinued a minimum of 24 hours before induction of labor, cesarean section, or placement of an epidural catheter, and restarted no sooner than 24 hours postoperatively, and with adequate hemostasis in place.[126] Neuraxial anesthesia should not be used in anticoagulated women (i.e., within 24 hours of the last treatment dose of LMWH, or for patients receiving IV UFH that have prolonged aPTTs). In patients not receiving epidural catheters, postpartum anticoagulation may be started 12 to 24 hours

Table 11-24

Selected Recommendations for Anticoagulation during Pregnancy

Clinical Situation	Antepartum Options	Postpartum
1. Prophylaxis: Prior VTE		
Low risk of recurrent VTE (single episode of VTE associated with transient RF not related to pregnancy or use of estrogen)	Clinical vigilance	Prophylactic or intermediate dose LMWH or VKA (INR 2–3) for 6 weeks over no prophylaxis
Moderate/high risk of recurrent VTE (single unprovoked VTE, pregnancy- or estrogen-related VTE, or multiple prior unprovoked VTE not receiving long-term AC)	Prophylactic or intermediate dose LMWH over clinical vigilance or routine care	Prophylactic or intermediate dose LMWH or VKA (INR 2–3) for 6 weeks over no prophylaxis
On long-term VKA	Adjusted-dose LMWH or 75% of a therapeutic dose of LMWH throughout pregnancy, over prophylactic dose LMWH	Resumption of long-term AC
2. Prophylaxis: No Prior VTE		
Homo-FVL or Prothrombin mutation and + FH for VTE	Prophylactic or intermediate dose LMWH	Prophylactic or intermediate dose LMWH or VKA (INR 2–3) for 6 weeks over no prophylaxis
All other thrombophilias who have + FH for VTE	Clinical vigilance	Prophylactic or intermediate dose LMWH or, in women who are not protein C or S deficient, VKA (INR 2–3) over routine care
Homo FVL or Prothrombin mutation and no positive FH for VTE	Clinical vigilance	Prophylactic or intermediate dose LMWH or VKA (INR 2–3) for 6 weeks over routine care
All other thrombophilias with no positive FH for VTE	Clinical vigilance	Clinical vigilance
Long-term oral anticoagulants for mechanical valve replacement	▪ Adjusted-dose SC UFH ▪ Adjusted-dose BID LMWH (adjusted to achieve manufacturer recommended 4-hour postdose peak anti-factor Xa concentration) ▪ UFH or LMWH (as above) until the 13th week, with substitution by VKA until close to delivery when UFH or LMWH is resumed	Long-term warfarin to prior INR goal with UFH/LMWH overlap until INR above lower limit of therapeutic range

Adjusted-dose UFH: UFH SC q12h in doses adjusted to target a mid-interval aPTT into the therapeutic range.
Prophylactic LMWH: dalteparin 5,000 units SC q24h, tinzaparin 4,500 units SC q24h, or enoxaparin 40 mg SC q24h (At extremes of body weight modification of dose may be required).
Intermediate-dose LMWH: dalteparin 5,000 units SC q12h, enoxaparin 40 mg SC q12h.
Adjusted-dose LMWH: weight-adjusted, full treatment doses of LMWH, given once or twice daily: dalteparin 200 units/kg daily, tinzaparin 175 units/kg daily, dalteparin 100 units/kg q12h, or enoxaparin 1 mg/kg q12h.
AC: anticoagulation; BID, 2 times daily; FH, family history; FVL, factor V Leiden mutation; INR, international normalized ratio; LMWH, low-molecular-weight heparin; RF: risk factor; SC, subcutaneous; UFH, unfractionated heparin; VKA: vitamin K antagonist; VTE, venous thromboembolism.
Source: Bates SM et al. 9th ed. ACCP guidelines. *Chest*. 2012;141(2)(Suppl):e691S–e736S.

after delivery as long as there are no bleeding concerns.[126] Consider IV UFH in women at high risk of bleeding, with LMWH reasonable for most women. Restart warfarin when hemostasis has occurred, bridging with UFH or LMWH until the INR is therapeutic. Warfarin, LMWH, and UFH do not accumulate in breast milk and do not induce anticoagulant effect in the infant and may be used in women who breastfeed[122]; therefore, M.P. can safely breastfeed. The DOACs are not currently recommended during breastfeeding.[122,123]

PREVENTION OF CARDIOGENIC THROMBOEMBOLISM

Atrial Fibrillation

ANTICOAGULATION BEFORE CARDIOVERSION

CASE 11-9

QUESTION 1: T.S., a 66-year-old woman with hypertension and no other significant past medical history, presents to the cardiology clinic complaining of several days of fatigue and a "racing heart." On physical examination, her pulse is irregularly irregular, and her heart rate is approximately 120 beats/minute. Using ECG, a diagnosis of atrial fibrillation is made and cardioversion planned. Should T.S. be anticoagulated before cardioversion?

In atrial fibrillation, atrial activity and atrial enlargement cause stasis of blood within the atria and the left atrial appendage, which can result in atrial thrombus formation. Atrial thrombus formation increases the risk of systemic embolization; clinical manifestations include arterial embolization of the extremities or embolization of the splenic, renal, or abdominal arteries. However, the most prevalent site of embolization is the cerebral arterial system, resulting in transient ischemic attack or stroke with potentially devastating neurologic and functional impairment. Atrial fibrillation carries a fivefold risk of ischemic stroke without thromboprophylaxis.[127]

Both direct current cardioversion and pharmacologic cardioversion using antiarrhythmic drugs expose patients to an initial short-term increase in stroke risk from embolization secondary to resumption of normal atrial mechanical activity (see Chapter 15, Cardiac Arrhythmias). Data from a prospective cohort study of 437 patients noted a stroke incidence of 5.3% in patients with atrial fibrillation who were cardioverted without prior anticoagulation, but a significant reduction in stroke incidence to 0.8% was noted if patients who had received cardioversion were anticoagulated.[128] In addition to preventing the development of new atrial thrombi, anticoagulation allows any thrombus that may be present to endothelialize and adhere to the atrial wall so that the thromboembolic risk is minimized. Based on the assumed time course of thrombus development, as well as the presumed time course of clot endothelialization, patients who have been in atrial fibrillation for 48 hours or longer should receive 3 weeks of therapeutic anticoagulation with warfarin to a target INR of 2.5 (range, 2.0–3.0) before cardioversion is attempted.[127,129] Direct oral anticoagulants such as dabigatran, rivaroxaban, and apixaban are alternative options to warfarin therapy.[129] Despite a lower risk of stroke than that associated with atrial fibrillation, patients with atrial flutter should be treated similarly.

Whether T.S. has been in atrial fibrillation for 48 hours is not known; therefore, she requires a 3-week course of oral anticoagulation before cardioversion is attempted. If T.S. cannot tolerate her heart symptoms despite control of the ventricular response rate, her medical team might consider immediate cardioversion without anticoagulation if transesophageal echocardiography (TEE) is used to rule out left atrial thrombi. TEE is much more sensitive than transthoracic echocardiography (TTE) to visualize the left atrium and the left atrial appendage.

In a clinical trial, 1,222 patients with atrial fibrillation for a duration of 2 days or more were randomly assigned to either cardioversion guided by TEE or to conventional anticoagulation prior to cardioversion.[130] Patients assigned to conventional treatment and patients in the TEE group in whom thrombus was detected received a 3-week course of warfarin before cardioversion. Patients without detectable thrombus by TEE were cardioverted without prior anticoagulation. All patients received 4 weeks of postcardioversion anticoagulation. Thromboembolic rates were identical between patients who received conventional treatment and those whose treatment was guided by TEE (0.5% vs. 0.8%, $p = 0.5$).[130]

ANTICOAGULATION AFTER CARDIOVERSION

CASE 11-9, QUESTION 2: After 3 weeks of regular intensity warfarin therapy, T.S. is successfully cardioverted to normal sinus rhythm. Should anticoagulation be discontinued?

Despite normalization of atrial electrical activity, restoration of effective atrial mechanical activity after cardioversion of atrial fibrillation can be delayed for up to 3 weeks. In addition, many patients who are cardioverted successfully will revert to atrial fibrillation during the first month. These factors contribute to the recognized delay in stroke presentation after cardioversion in patients with atrial fibrillation. Therefore, anticoagulation should be continued after cardioversion for a minimum 4 weeks. Longer duration of anticoagulation therapy should be based on the individual patient's thromboembolic risk profile.[127,129]

ANTICOAGULATION FOR PAROXYSMAL, PERMANENT, OR PERSISTENT ATRIAL FIBRILLATION

CASE 11-9, QUESTION 3: Two weeks after successful cardioversion, T.S. presents to the ED with chest palpitations and light-headedness. An ECG is performed and indicates atrial fibrillation again. What decisions regarding anticoagulation need to be made?

Anticoagulation in Valvular Atrial Fibrillation

Atrial fibrillation secondary to valvular heart disease has historically been recognized as a significant risk factor for stroke. Patients with atrial fibrillation who have a history of rheumatic mitral valve disease have a 17-fold higher incidence of stroke than in matched controls. Patients with valvular atrial fibrillation require long-term, regular intensity anticoagulation with warfarin to a target INR of 2.5 (range, 2.0–3.0) to prevent thromboembolism and stroke. DOACs have not been studied in this patient population and should be avoided at this time.[127,129]

Anticoagulation in Nonvalvular Atrial Fibrillation

Nonvalvular heart disease is the most common cause of atrial fibrillation and, like valvular heart disease, represents a significant risk for stroke in patients with atrial fibrillation. Five clinical trials have substantiated the role of warfarin in the primary prevention of systemic embolization and stroke in chronic, nonvalvular atrial fibrillation.[127,129,131] All five trials compared warfarin with a placebo and were terminated before completion because of the substantial benefit of warfarin. In comparison with a placebo, warfarin significantly reduced the risk of stroke from approximately 5% per year to approximately 2% per year, with an average relative risk reduction of 67%. Based on the results of these trials, long-term anticoagulation with warfarin to a goal INR of 2.5 (range, 2.0–3.0) is recommended in patients like T.S., who have atrial fibrillation secondary to nonvalvular heart disease.[127,129,131]

Several clinical trials have attempted to define the comparative efficacy of warfarin versus aspirin in the prevention of stroke associated with atrial fibrillation.[127,129,132] Compared with a placebo or control, aspirin decreases the risk of stroke in patients with atrial fibrillation. However, that reduction is not as substantial as the reduction seen with warfarin. In clinical trials comparing warfarin and aspirin, the risk reduction associated with warfarin is significantly larger than that of aspirin. However, aspirin may be appropriate in certain patients at low risk for stroke associated with atrial fibrillation based on individualized risk assessment using the $CHADS_2$ and CHA_2DS_2-VASc score (Table 11-9). The $CHADS_2$ score is currently endorsed by ACCP whereas the CHA_2DS_2VASc score is endorsed by the American Heart Association/American College of Cardiology/Heart Rhythm Society (AHA/ACC/HRS) and the European Society of Cardiology (ESC) (see Chapter 15, Cardiac Arrhythmias).

Subsequent trials have confirmed the superiority of warfarin over the combination of aspirin plus clopidogrel for stroke prevention in atrial fibrillation, and the increased risk of intracranial hemorrhage when aspirin and clopidogrel are combined.[133,134]

Direct Oral Anticoagulants

The direct thrombin inhibitor (dabigatran) and direct factor Xa inhibitors (rivaroxaban, apixaban, and edoxaban) have all been compared to warfarin for stroke prevention in patients with nonvalvular atrial fibrillation.[135–138]

Patient-specific characteristics such as age, renal function, weight, concomitant medications, and past medical history should be considered when selecting the most appropriate anticoagulant for initial therapy. Cost, insurance coverage and patient preference with regard to number of daily doses, frequency of monitoring, etc. must also be taken into account[139] (see Chapter 15, Cardiac Arrhythmias).

The decision to continue long-term anticoagulation with warfarin in T.S. should be based on an evaluation of the likelihood that her atrial fibrillation will become chronic with a paroxysmal, persistent, or permanent presentation, as well as an assessment of her risk of stroke compared with her risk of anticoagulant-associated bleeding complications. Because of her age and history of hypertension ($CHADS_2$ score of 2 and CHA_2DS_2-VASc score of 3), the appropriate strategy should be long-term anticoagulation, either with warfarin at a goal INR of 2.5 (range, 2.0–3.0) or full-dose DOAC therapy.

Cardiac Valve Replacement

MECHANICAL PROSTHETIC VALVES

CASE 11-10

QUESTION 1: P.B., a 59-year-old woman with a history of rheumatic mitral valve disease, has undergone mitral valve replacement. A St. Jude (bileaflet mechanical) valve has been implanted, and heparin therapy is initiated postoperatively. Does P.B. require continued anticoagulation with warfarin?

Mechanical prosthetic valves confer a significant thromboembolic risk by providing a foreign surface in contact with blood components on which platelet aggregation and thrombus formation can occur. Valvular thrombosis can impair the integrity of valve function and can lead to embolization with systemic manifestations, including stroke.[140] The incidence of thromboembolic complications depends on the type of artificial valve (caged ball [Starr-Edwards] > tilting disk [Medtronic-Hall; Bjork-Shiley] > bileaflet [St. Jude]), as well as the anatomic position of the replacement (dual valve replacement > mitral > aortic).[141]

Long-term anticoagulation is required in patients with mechanical valve replacement because it significantly reduces the risk of stroke and other manifestations of systemic embolization (Table 11-9). Trials comparing different intensities of oral anticoagulation with warfarin in mechanical valve replacement helped identify the intensity of anticoagulation that protects against thromboembolic risk, while reducing the incidence of hemorrhagic complications.[142] Patients with a mechanical aortic valve replacement (AVR) (St. Jude bileaflet or tilting disc) in the aortic position should receive long-term anticoagulant therapy with warfarin to a target INR of 2.5 (range, 2.0–3.0).[140,143] For all other mechanical valve types in the aortic position, and for any mechanical mitral valve replacement (MVR), chronic warfarin therapy with a target INR of 3.0 (range, 2.5–3.5) is recommended. The concurrent use of low-dose aspirin (81 mg daily) is recommended for patients with mechanical mitral or aortic valve at low-bleeding risk.

In 2012, the RE-ALIGN trial was halted early after demonstrating a significant increase in thromboembolic events such as valve thrombosis, myocardial infarction, transient ischemic attack and stroke as well as significant increase in bleeding when taking dabigatran versus warfarin in patients with mechanical prosthetic valves.[144] Based on these results as well as case reports reporting valve thrombosis following transition from warfarin to dabigatran, the FDA issued a MedWatch safety alert recommendation that dabigatran should not be used in any patient with a mechanical heart valve. Subsequently, dabigatran's product information was also updated to include this contraindication. Based on the results of this trial, it is unlikely any other DOAC will be tested in the population; thus, all DOACs should not be used in patients with mechanical prosthetic valves. Therefore, P.B. would be required to continue warfarin indefinitely to reduce the risk of stroke and other systemic embolism.

BIOPROSTHETIC VALVES

CASE 11-11

QUESTION 1: E.F., an 82-year-old woman with a history of symptomatic aortic stenosis, has received a bioprosthetic (mammalian) aortic valve replacement. Is anticoagulant therapy required in E.F.?

Prosthetic heart valves extracted from mammalian sources (porcine or bovine xenografts, homografts) are significantly less thrombogenic than mechanical prosthetic valves. The period of greatest thromboembolic risk appears to be during the first 3 months after implantation. Therefore, anticoagulation with warfarin to an INR goal of 2.5 (range, 2.0–3.0) is recommended for 3 to 6 months following implantation of a bioprosthetic aortic or mitral valve in patients at low risk of bleeding (Table 11-9). After this period, long-term aspirin therapy (75–100 mg) is indicated.[140,143] Alternatively, treatment with only aspirin 75 to 100 mg daily is also reasonable in patients with a bioprosthetic aortic or mitral valve. More about E.F.'s bleeding risk would need to be determined, however due to her age, long-term aspirin therapy only may be reasonable.[140] Transcatheter aortic valve replacement (TAVR) is a new technique that avoids the open chest approach. Initially, clopidogrel 75 mg daily for the first 3 to 6 months, followed by long-term aspirin was recommended following TAVR. However, the most recent AHA/ACC guidelines recommend either warfarin with a goal INR of 2.5 (range, 2.0–3.0) for at least 3 months or clopidogrel 75 mg daily for the first 6 months following TAVR in addition to life-long aspirin 75 to 100 mg daily.[143]

BRIDGE THERAPY

Management of Anticoagulation Around Invasive Procedures

CASE 11-12

QUESTION 1: L.P. is a 48-year-old woman with a history of valvular heart disease and a St. Jude mitral valve replacement. She is adequately anticoagulated with warfarin 7.5 mg once daily to a goal INR range of 2.5 to 3.5. Recently, she has complained of episodic rectal bleeding and is scheduled for a colonoscopy in several weeks. Her gastroenterologist calls the anticoagulation clinic to determine the most appropriate plan for reversal of her warfarin before the procedure. What are the options?

When an invasive procedure is planned, it is often necessary to reverse the effects of warfarin to minimize the risk of bleeding complications associated with the procedure, which can be worsened by the presence of an anticoagulant. It can take several days for the anticoagulant effect of warfarin to be reversed after discontinuation of the drug, but in that period of time, a patient may be at risk for thromboembolic complications associated with underanticoagulation. Bridge therapy is the term that refers to the use of a relatively short-acting injectable anticoagulant (UFH, LMWH) as a substitute for warfarin before and immediately after an invasive procedure to shorten the period of time a patient is without any anticoagulation.[145] Because UFH and LMWH have shorter elimination half-lives than warfarin, they can be stopped just before the invasive procedure without increasing the risk of bleeding associated with the procedure. The last dose of LMWH and SC UFH should be given at least 24 hours before the scheduled procedure, whereas IV UFH infusions are discontinued 6 hours before the procedure. The timing of the last dose of LMWH may need to be extended based on a patient's renal function because it is renally eliminated. Because of their faster onsets of effect, these agents are resumed after invasive procedures once hemostasis is achieved to establish an immediate degree of anticoagulation. Resumption of therapeutic injectable anticoagulants after a high-bleeding risk surgery should be delayed until at least 48 to 72 hours postoperatively, whereas patients undergoing lower-bleeding risk procedures can be restarted 24 hours later. Warfarin is resumed simultaneously, and the bridging anticoagulant is continued until the INR reaches the therapeutic range.[145]

Current guidelines for bridging are based on the results of case series, observational studies, and nonrandomized trials involving patients with various indications for anticoagulation, including valve replacement. The decision to use bridging depends on the risk of bleeding associated with continued anticoagulation for the surgery or procedure to be performed and on the risk of thromboembolism associated with underanticoagulation in the patient in question. Recently, a large registry called The Outcomes Registry for Better Informed Treatment of Atrial Fibrillation (ORBIT-AF) included patients with atrial fibrillation that underwent temporary interruption of oral anticoagulation therapy and showed that bridging was associated with higher risk of bleeding and adverse events.[146] Shortly after, the interim results of the BRIDGE trial (Bridging Anticoagulation in Patients who Require Temporary Interruption of Warfarin Therapy for an Elective Invasive Procedure or Surgery) that randomized patients with atrial fibrillation to receive bridging therapy with LMWH or placebo showed similar findings to the ORBIT-AF registry. The study showed no difference in the rate of arterial thromboembolism between the bridging and nonbridging group; however, the bridging group showed significantly higher rates of major bleeding. The mean $CHADS_2$ score was 2.3 and patients with mechanical heart valve or stroke, systemic embolism, and transient ischemic attack within the previous 12 weeks were excluded from the trial. Major surgical procedures associated with high rates of arterial thromboembolism and bleeding were also underrepresented. Therefore, the results from the BRIDGE trial should not be applied to patients that were underrepresented.[147]

Individualized risk assessment and bridge therapy planning are necessary for each patient who may require temporary discontinuation of warfarin. Current recommendations for risk stratification are outlined in Table 11-25. High-risk and moderate-risk patients typically receive bridge therapy if warfarin needs to be withheld, whereas in low-risk patients, warfarin is simply withheld before the invasive procedure, without the need for bridging. The bleeding risk of a performed procedure or surgery must also be weighed. Efforts should be made to continue oral anticoagulation in a patient with high thromboembolic risk undergoing a procedure with low-bleeding risk, such as a dental extraction or cataract surgery. Table 11-26 includes examples of high- versus low-bleeding risk surgeries.

Clinical outcomes in patients bridged with LMWH or UFH are similar and overall costs are lower for LMWH because of the avoidance of hospital admission for IV UFH administration;

Table 11-25
Risk Stratification for Determining the Need for Bridge Therapy

	Indication for VKA Therapy		
Risk Stratum	**Mechanical Heart Valve**	**Atrial Fibrillation**	**Venous Thromboembolism**
High	■ Any mitral valve prosthesis ■ Older (caged-ball or tilting disk) aortic valve prosthesis ■ Recent (within 6 months) stroke or transient ischemic attack	■ $CHADS_2$ score of 5 or 6 ■ Recent (within 3 months) stroke or transient ischemic attack ■ Rheumatic valvular heart disease	■ Recent (within 3 months) VTE ■ Severe thrombophilia (e.g., deficiency of protein C, protein S or antithrombin, antiphospholipid antibodies, or multiple abnormalities)
Moderate	■ Bileaflet aortic valve prosthesis and one of the following: atrial fibrillation, prior stroke or transient ischemic attack, hypertension, diabetes, congestive heart failure, age >75 years	■ $CHADS_2$ score of 3 or 4	■ VTE within the past 3 to 12 months (consider VTE prophylaxis rather than full intensity bridge therapy) ■ Nonsevere thrombophilic conditions (e.g., heterozygous factor V Leiden mutation, heterozygous factor II mutation) ■ Recurrent VTE ■ Active cancer (treated within 6 months or palliative)
Low	■ Bileaflet aortic valve prosthesis without atrial fibrillation and no other risk factors for stroke	■ $CHADS_2$ score of 0 to 2 (no prior stroke or transient ischemic attack)	■ Single VTE occurred greater than 12 months ago and no other risk factors

VTE, venous thromboembolism.
Source: Douketis JD et al. Perioperative management of antithrombotic therapy: 9th ed: American College of Chest Physicians Evidence-Based Clinical Practice Guidelines. *Chest*. 2012; 141(2)(Suppl):e326S–e350S.

Table 11-26
Bleed Risk of Selected Procedures

Low Risk (2-Day Major Bleed Risk of 0%–2%)	High Risk (2-Day Major Bleed Risk of 2%–4%)
Abdominal hernia repair	Abdominal aortic aneurysm repair
Cataract surgery	Any surgery lasting > 45 minutes
Cholecystectomy	Major cancer surgery
Colonoscopy	Major cardiac surgery (heart valve replacement & CABG)
Cutaneous biopsies	Major orthopedic surgery (joint replacement)
Cystoscopy	Major vascular surgery
Dilation and curettage	Transurethral prostate resection
Dental extractions	Neurosurgical procedures
GI endoscopy ± biopsy	Polypectomy, variceal treatment
Skin cancer excision	Renal biopsy

Adapted from Spyropoulos AC. Perioperative bridging therapy for the at-risk patient on chronic anticoagulation. *Dis Mon*. 2005;51:183–193.

therefore, the use of LMWH is recommended whenever possible.[145] UFH may be preferred in patients with significant renal impairment (CrCl < 30 mL/minute), and if LMWHs are used, reduced doses are suggested.[21] Monitoring anti-Xa levels for accumulation may be prudent if patients require a prolonged course of therapy (over 7 days). A guideline for bridge therapy based on the risk of thromboembolism and on renal function is presented in Table 11-27.

Because L.P. has a mechanical mitral valve replacement, her risk of thromboembolism associated with underanticoagulation is considered high. Therefore, she should receive bridge therapy with an injectable anticoagulant while warfarin is held. Her renal function is normal, and her healthcare insurance covers injectable drugs. Therefore, her plan will include early discontinuation of warfarin 5 days before the procedure and substitution with enoxaparin 1 mg/kg every 12 hours when the INR falls below the lower limit of the therapeutic range. The last dose of enoxaparin should be given 24 hours before the procedure to minimize the risk of bleeding at the time of the procedure. After the procedure, warfarin should be restarted at her usual dose, and enoxaparin should be continued until the INR is greater than 2.5, the lower limit of L.P.'s therapeutic range. For indications other than mechanical valves, enoxaparin 1.5 mg/kg every 24 hours may be used as an alternative to avoid twice-daily injections.

Table 11-27
Bridge Therapy Guidelines of Invasive Procedures

	Action		
Day	**Warfarin**	**LMWH**	**Laboratories**
−6	Last warfarin dose	N/A	INR; skip dose if supratherapeutic
−5	No warfarin	N/A	
−4	No warfarin	Start LMWH	
−3	No warfarin	LMWH	
−2 to −1	No warfarin	LMWH; last dose 24–36 hours prior to procedure	
0—day of procedure	Resume warfarin at usual dose if hemostasis is achieved[a]	No LMWH	Ensure INR is appropriate for surgery[b] CBC
1	Resume warfarin if not started day prior	LMWH; resume following minor surgery No LMWH following major surgery	
2–3	Warfarin	LMWH; resume following major surgery if bleeding controlled	
4	Warfarin	LMWH	
5–7	Warfarin	LMWH	INR; discontinue when therapeutic Consider CBC, CrCl, anti-Xa level with continued need for LMWH

[a]Consider giving 1.5 times usual warfarin dose for first 2 days when warfarin reinitiated.
[b]INR < 1.5 required for most surgical procedures.
INR, international normalized ratio; LMWH, low-molecular-weight heparin; CBC, complete blood count; CrCl, creatinine clearance.

DRUG INTERACTIONS

Interactions with Prescription Drugs

CASE 11-13

Question 1: P.T., a 48-year-old woman, received a mechanical mitral valve prosthesis 5 years ago and has been anticoagulated with warfarin 6 mg/day with good control. She asks to see you today in your anticoagulation clinic, after returning from an urgent appointment with her primary care physician for treatment of a skin infection that tested positive for community-acquired methicillin-resistant Staphylococcus aureus (MRSA), and was given a prescription for trimethoprim–sulfamethoxazole (TMP-SMX) twice a day for 10 days today. She is allergic to penicillin and has gastric intolerance to tetracycline. How will the combination of warfarin and TMP-SMX affect P.T.'s anticoagulation control? Should her warfarin dosage be adjusted or another drug substituted for TMP-SMX?

Drug interactions with warfarin occur by a number of different mechanisms and can have a significant impact on the anticoagulant effect of warfarin.[148,149] Elevations or reductions in INR have been observed when interacting drugs are added to or discontinued from the medication regimens of patients taking

Table 11-28
Warfarin Drug Interactions

Target	Effect	Response	Examples (Not Inclusive)			
Clotting factors	Increased synthesis	Decreased INR	Vitamin K			
	Decreased synthesis	Increased INR	Broad-spectrum antibiotics			
	Increased catabolism	Increased INR	Thyroid hormones			
	Decreased catabolism	Decreased INR	Methimazole		Propylthiouracil	
Warfarin metabolism	Inhibition	Increased INR	Acetaminophen	Allopurinol	Amiodarone	Azole antifungals
			Cimetidine	Fluoroquinolones	Macrolides	Metronidazole
			Propafenone	SSRIs	Statins	Sulfa antibiotics
	Induction	Decreased INR	Barbiturates	Carbamazepine	Doxycycline	Griseofulvin
			Nafcillin	Phenytoin	Primidone	Rifampin
Hemostasis	Additive antithrombotic effects	Increased bleeding risk	Aspirin	NSAIDs	Salicylates	GPIIb/IIIa inhibitors
	Additive anticoagulant response	Increased bleeding risk	Heparin	LMWH	Direct thrombin inhibitors	Thrombolytics
		Decreased INR	Cholestyramine	Colestipol	Sucralfate	
Absorption	Reduced	Decreased INR	Ascorbic acid	Azathioprine	Corticosteroids	Cyclosporine
Unknown		Increased INR	Androgens	Fenofibrate	Cyclophosphamide	Gemfibrozil

GP, glycoprotein; INR, international normalized ratio; LMWH, low-molecular-weight heparin; NSAIDs, nonsteroidal anti-inflammatory drugs.

warfarin or when used intermittently. Clinically significant hemorrhagic or thromboembolic complications can result. Careful selection of both prescription and nonprescription medications, appropriate INR monitoring, and detailed patient education regarding drug interactions are important interventions for pharmacists caring for patients taking warfarin. A selection of the hundreds of drugs that have been reported to interact with warfarin, including mechanisms of interaction and effect on INR, is provided in Table 11-28. Further information regarding the management of drug interactions can be found in Chapter 3, Drug Interactions.

Although warfarin is highly bound to protein (primarily to albumin), and can be displaced from protein-binding sites by a number of weakly acidic drugs, these interactions typically do not result in clinically significant elevations in PT/INR.[150] Warfarin displaced from protein-binding sites is readily available for elimination by hepatic metabolism, resulting in increased clearance without a significant change in the free drug concentration.

Other types of interactions with warfarin are much more significant. Pharmacodynamic interactions are those that alter the physiology of hemostasis, particularly interactions that influence the synthesis or degradation of clotting factors or that increase the risk of bleeding through inhibition of platelet aggregation. Pharmacokinetic interactions influence the absorption and metabolism of warfarin, and many clinically significant interactions with warfarin occur when warfarin metabolism is induced or inhibited. Interactions involving agents known to influence the hepatic microsomal enzyme systems responsible for the metabolism of the more potent S(−)-warfarin (CYP2C9) are more significant than those that influence the enzymes that metabolize R(+)-warfarin (CYP1A2, CYP3A4).

Sulfamethoxazole can increase the effect of warfarin significantly by stereoselectively inhibiting the metabolism of the more potent S(−)-enantiomer of warfarin. Potentiation of warfarin activity after inhibition of metabolism usually takes several days, and the effect may be slow to resolve once the offending agent is discontinued. In addition, fever associated with the infection for which TMP-SMX has been prescribed may enhance the catabolism of vitamin K-dependent clotting factors, resulting in an accentuated hypoprothrombinemic response. This effect will dissipate as the fever abates with antibiotic therapy.

For P.T., the ideal choice would be to discontinue TMP-SMX and use a noninteracting alternative. The decision of which agent to use must consider both the treatment(s) of choice for the clinical indication along with patient factors such as reported allergies or intolerances. In P.T.'s case, she has a penicillin allergy and intolerance to tetracyclines, both of which would prevent their use. If a noninteracting alternative is not clinically appropriate, the concomitant use of an interacting agent is not absolutely contraindicated in patients taking warfarin. Use of TMP-SMX in P.T. would be acceptable if she is monitored frequently and carefully, with adjustment of warfarin dosages as necessary to maintain her INR within the therapeutic INR range of 2.5 to 3.5 and with attention to potential hemorrhagic complications. No initial change in the dosage of warfarin should be made because it may take several days for the interaction to become apparent. The INR should be repeated within 3 days, with warfarin dosing adjustments and subsequent monitoring guided by initial INR results.

CASE 11-14

QUESTION 1: G.H. is a 54-year-old man on long-term anticoagulation for multiple, bilateral DVTs, most recently 1 year ago, for which he takes warfarin 7.5 mg daily. He had a knee replacement surgery 6 months ago and had a complication of infected hardware, for which he needs to start IV rifampin in a skilled nursing facility for several weeks. His orthopedic physician is asking about whether G.H. can be switched to an alternate anticoagulant, because he knows that there is a drug interaction with warfarin and rifampin. What options are available to him?

Although the DOACs are less prone to drug interactions than warfarin, all of them are P-glycoprotein substrates and can have their concentrations reduced by rifampin, which is a strong P-gp inducer.[151] At this time, dabigatran, rivaroxaban, apixaban, and edoxaban are all contraindicated with rifampin per package labeling and are not suitable options for G.H.

The interaction with warfarin and rifampin can be significant, with a potentially large dose increase (sometimes up to 3 times the original dose) of warfarin necessary to maintain G.H. in the therapeutic range. If G.H. is in a facility where his INRs can be measured frequently, such as every few days, it may be appropriate to maintain him on warfarin while continuing the rifampin, until the degree of the interaction can be detected, and a new stable dose can be determined. Alternatively, if G.H. is receiving the antibiotics at home, it may be appropriate for him to acquire a home INR meter and perform warfarin self-testing of his INRs. It has been shown that individuals performing patient self-testing (almost all testing weekly) had better time in therapeutic range (TTR) than those who underwent in-clinic testing every 4 weeks using high-quality anticoagulation management.[152] A substudy of this trial also showed that individuals on chronic anticoagulation who perform self-testing more often (i.e., weekly or twice weekly) had a modestly higher TTR compared to monthly testing.[153] The costs of the self-testing meter and supplies are often covered by the patient's insurance; however, sometimes the poor reimbursement for managing anticoagulation services this way can limit providers' willingness to offer patient-self testing. If reimbursement is not a concern (such as in a closed insurance system), then patient self-testing can be a way to empower patients to take more control of their warfarin management and reduce the burden of INR monitoring.

LMWH, UFH, and fondaparinux are also reasonable options for G.H. to use, especially if his INRs cannot be stabilized while receiving the rifampin. However, again, there could be barriers to self-injection and insurance limitations that may make it difficult to continue these agents for a prolonged length of time.

CASE 11-14, QUESTION 2: Can G.H. return to using his ibuprofen for pain control?

This question illustrates one of the most difficult therapeutic dilemmas for a patient taking warfarin. All NSAIDs have the potential to cause gastric irritation by inhibiting cytoprotective prostaglandins, thereby providing a focus for GI bleeding. In addition, most NSAIDs inhibit platelet aggregation, which compromises effective clotting and can lead to bleeding complications.[154]

These effects can increase the risk of hemorrhagic complications significantly in patients taking warfarin who are prescribed concurrent NSAID therapy. In a retrospective cohort study of patients age 65 years or older, the risk of hospitalization for bleeding peptic ulcer disease was approximately 3 times higher for patients taking concurrent warfarin and an NSAID versus patients taking either drug alone, and almost 13 times higher than in patients taking neither warfarin nor an NSAID.[155] Warfarin therapy is considered a relative contraindication to NSAID use.

In patients like G.H., routine use of NSAIDs with long-term anticoagulation should be avoided. Any patients requiring combined warfarin and NSAID therapy for limited periods of time should be followed closely and observed routinely for signs and symptoms of bleeding, with frequent stool testing for GI bleeding. Patients should be counseled to avoid additional NSAID use whenever possible, including use of aspirin, and to seek assistance from a pharmacist to prevent inadvertent NSAID use when selecting over-the-counter (OTC) medications, as some OTC cold preparations contain NSAIDs, aspirin, or aspirin-related compounds.

The analgesic and antipyretic of choice in patients taking warfarin is acetaminophen, which has not been consistently shown to increase the risk of bleeding. At doses greater than 2 g/day, acetaminophen can enhance the anticoagulant effect of warfarin.[156] It has been suspected of directly inhibiting CYP2C9 and CYP1A2, and toxic metabolites of acetaminophen have been suspected of inhibiting hepatic enzymes as well. Nevertheless, it can be used safely when used occasionally, and even when used routinely. INR monitoring is sufficient to detect any potential interaction. Other pain-relieving options to be considered that do not increase the bleeding risk include tramadol, gabapentin, pregabalin, topical lidocaine patches, and opiates.

KEY REFERENCES AND WEBSITES

A full list of references for this chapter can be found at http://thepoint.lww.com/AT11e. Below are the key references and websites for this chapter, with the corresponding reference number in this chapter found in parentheses after the reference.

Key References

Ageno W et al; American College of Chest Physicians. Oral anticoagulant therapy: Antithrombotic Therapy and Prevention of Thrombosis, 9th ed: American College of Chest Physicians Evidence-Based Clinical Practice Guidelines. *Chest*. 2012;141(2 Suppl):e44S–e88S. (6)

Cuker A et al. Laboratory measurement of the anticoagulant activity of the non–vitamin K oral anticoagulants. *J Am Coll Cardiol*. 2014;64:1128–1139. (42)

Douketis JD et al. Perioperative management of antithrombotic therapy: 9th ed: American College of Chest Physicians Evidence-Based Clinical Practice Guidelines. *Chest*. 2012;141(2)(Suppl):e326S–e350S. (145)

Falck-Ytter Y et al. Prevention of VTE in orthopedic surgery patients: Antithrombotic Therapy and Prevention of Thrombosis, 9th ed: American College of Chest Physicians Evidence-Based Clinical Practice Guidelines. *Chest*. 2012;141(2 Suppl):e278S–e325S. (48)

Garcia DA et al. Parenteral anticoagulants: antithrombotic therapy and prevention of thrombosis, 9th ed: American College of Chest Physicians evidence-based clinical practice guidelines. *Chest*. 2012;141: e24S–e43S. (3)

Gould MK et al. Prevention of VTE in nonorthopedic surgical patients: Antithrombotic Therapy and Prevention of Thrombosis, 9th ed: American College of Chest Physicians Evidence-Based Clinical Practice Guidelines. *Chest*. 2012;141(2 Suppl):e227S–e277S. (12)

Holbrook AM et al. Systematic overview of warfarin and its drug and food interactions. *Arch Intern Med*. 2005;165:1095. (148)

Holbrook A et al. Evidence-based management of anticoagulant therapy. *Chest*. 2012;141:e152S–e184S. (21)

January CT et al. 2014 AHA/ACC/HRS guidelines for the management of patients with atrial fibrillation: a report of the American College of Cardiology/American Heart Association Task Force on Practice Guidelines and the Heart Rhythm Society. *J Am Coll Cardiol*. 2014;64:e1–e76. (94)

Kahn SR et al. Prevention of VTE in nonsurgical patients: Antithrombotic Therapy and Prevention of Thrombosis, 9th ed: American College of Chest Physicians Evidence-Based Clinical Practice Guidelines. *Chest*. 2012;141(2 Suppl):e195S–e226S. (49)

Kearon C et al; American College of Chest Physicians. Antithrombotic therapy for VTE disease: Antithrombotic Therapy and Prevention of Thrombosis, 9th ed: American College of Chest Physicians Evidence-Based Clinical Practice Guidelines. *Chest*. 2012;141(2 Suppl): e419S–e494S. (15)

Kovacs RJ et al. Practical management of anticoagulation in patients with atrial fibrillation. *J Am Coll Cardiol*. 2015;65(13):1340–1360. (139)

Nutescu EA et al. Warfarin and its interactions with foods, herbs and other dietary supplements. *Expert Opin Drug Saf*. 2006;5:433. (107)

Whitlock RP et al. Antithrombotic and thrombolytic therapy for valvular disease. American College of Chest Physicians Evidence-Based Practice Guidelines (9th Edition). *Chest*. 2012;141(2)(Suppl):e576S–e600S. (140)

You JJ et al. Antithrombotic therapy for atrial fibrillation. American College of Chest Physicians Evidence-Based Practice Guidelines (9th Edition) *Chest*. 2012;141(2):e531S–e575S. (127)

12 Chronic Stable Angina

Angela M. Thompson and Toby C. Trujillo

CORE PRINCIPLES

	CHAPTER CASES
CHRONIC STABLE ANGINA—MEDICAL MANAGEMENT	
1 Chronic stable angina is a clinical syndrome resulting from an imbalance in myocardial oxygen supply and demand. The supply–demand imbalance is typically a result of coronary atherosclerosis.	**Case 12-1 (Questions 1–3)**
2 The modification of cardiovascular disease (CVD) risk factors and adoption of healthy lifestyles is a key strategy in both the primary prevention of coronary artery disease (CAD) and slowing the progression of established CAD.	**Case 12-1 (Questions 7–9)** **Case 12-2 (Question 2)**
3 Standard therapy for all patients with chronic stable angina includes sublingual nitroglycerin, antiplatelet therapy, and an anti-ischemic agent that either restores the appropriate balance of myocardial oxygen supply and demand (β-blockers, calcium-channel blockers, and long-acting nitrates), and/or interrupts the negative consequences of myocardial ischemia on myocardial energy consumption (ranolazine).	**Case 12-1 (Questions 10–14, 16)** **Case 12-3 Question 2)**
4 β-Blockers are the preferred initial agents for prevention of ischemic symptoms, especially in patients who have a history of myocardial infarction (MI) or heart failure.	**Case 12-1** **(Questions 11, 12, 13, 15)**
5 Although effective as monotherapy, long-acting calcium-channel blockers are typically added on to β-blocker therapy if additional control of ischemic symptoms is needed.	**Case 12-2 (Question 1)**
6 Long-acting nitrates should never be used as monotherapy but can be used as add-on therapy to other anti-ischemic options in chronic stable angina.	**Case 12-1 (Questions 16–19)**
7 Although ranolazine can be used as initial therapy for chronic stable angina, it is typically reserved as a second-line option. It is especially useful in patients who cannot tolerate further decreases in heart rate and blood pressure secondary to the use of traditional antianginal agents.	**Case 12-2 (Questions 3, 4)**
CHRONIC STABLE ANGINA—REVASCULARIZATION	
1 Myocardial revascularization can be accomplished either through percutaneous coronary intervention (PCI) or coronary artery bypass surgery (CABG). In most patients, both are equally effective in reducing myocardial ischemia.	**Case 12-3 (Question 5)**
2 Certain patients who are at high risk for morbidity and mortality from CAD derive a mortality benefit with CABG as compared to PCI or medical management.	**Case 12-3 (Question 5)**
3 In patients not at high risk, optimal medical management is as good as PCI in the long-term management of chronic stable angina, including the prevention of MI and death.	**Case 12-1 (Question 6)**
4 Patients who undergo myocardial revascularization either with PCI or CABG should still receive optimal pharmacotherapy for chronic stable angina.	**Case 12-3 (Question 6)**

Continued

	CHAPTER CASES
5 Appropriate pharmacotherapy for patients undergoing elective PCI plus myocardial stent implantation should include dual antiplatelet therapy with aspirin and a $P2Y_{12}$ antagonist, in most cases clopidogrel therapy, for a minimum of 1 month (bare-metal stent) and ideally up to 1 year (bare-metal and drug-eluting stents).	**Case 12-3 (Question 3)**
6 Antiplatelet nonresponsiveness has been demonstrated to be associated with an increased risk for cardiovascular events such as MI and death. An understanding of various testing modalities for antiplatelet response, as well as potential drug–drug interactions that may lead to reduced antiplatelet activity will facilitate optimal pharmacotherapy in each patient.	**Case 12-3 (Questions 6, 7)**
PRINZMETAL ANGINA/CARDIAC SYNDROME X	
1 Patients with Prinzmetal angina and cardiac syndrome X typically present with severe chest pain despite having coronary arteries that are free from atherosclerosis.	**Case 12-4 (Question 1)**
2 Vasodilators are the primary mode of therapy for patients with Prinzmetal angina, while standard anti-ischemic options should be used for cardiac syndrome X.	**Case 12-4 (Questions 2, 3)** **Case 12-5 (Question 1)**

CHRONIC STABLE ANGINA

Coronary heart disease (CHD) includes heart failure (HF), arrhythmias, sudden cardiac death, and ischemic heart disease (IHD) such as myocardial infarction (MI) as well as unstable and stable angina pectoris. Because angina is a marker for underlying heart disease, its management is of great importance. Typical angina pectoris is characterized by substernal chest, jaw, shoulder, back, or arm pain triggered by exertion or stress, and it is relieved by rest or nitroglycerin (NTG); however, its presentation is variable.[1,2]

Patients who have a reproducible pattern of angina that is associated with a certain level of physical activity have chronic stable angina or exertional angina. In contrast, patients with unstable angina experience new-onset angina or a change in their angina intensity, frequency, or duration.[3] Both chronic stable angina and unstable angina often reflect underlying atherosclerotic narrowing of coronary arteries on coronary angiography. In contrast, Prinzmetal variant angina is associated with normal findings on coronary angiography and is thought to be caused by a spasm of the coronary artery that decreases myocardial blood flow. The presence of atherosclerosis also may lead to impairment of the normal vasodilatory function of the coronary arteries. As such, coronary artery disease (CAD) patients who experience ischemia produced by an increase in myocardial oxygen demand (increased exertion) may also experience vasospasm at the site of atherosclerosis, further worsening the ischemic state. As such, patients with CAD likely experience angina due to both increased demand (exertion) and decreased supply (vasospasm), a phenomenon known as mixed angina.[3]

Silent (asymptomatic) myocardial ischemia can result in transient changes in myocardial perfusion, function, or electrical activity, and is detected on an electrocardiogram (ECG).[3] The patient, however, does not experience chest pain or other signs of angina during these episodes.

Epidemiology

It is estimated that 85.6 million adults in the United States have cardiovascular disease (CVD),[1] and 15.5 million of these adults have CHD.[4] Chronic stable angina is the first clinical sign of CHD in approximately 50% of patients.[1] Current estimates indicate 8.2 million American adults have angina pectoris, although the prevalence of angina is likely underestimated due to limited population-based data and because it is often unrecognized in patients.[4]

CVD is the leading cause of death in the United States responsible for one of every three deaths[4] Although CHD accounts for one of every seven deaths in the United States, individual mortality varies according to the patient's age, sex, cardiovascular risk profile, myocardial contractility, coronary anatomy, and specific anginal syndrome.[4]

In addition to the high morbidity and mortality associated with CHD, the economic cost to the US health care system is substantial. Total direct and indirect costs associated with CHD were estimated to be $204.4 billion in 2010, and direct medical costs for CHD are expected to increase by 100% between 2013 and 2030.[4]

Pathophysiology

A brief review of coronary anatomy will facilitate a thorough understanding of the pathophysiology of chronic stable angina. Figure 12-1 illustrates the normal distribution of the major coronary arteries, although variation is common between individuals.

Angina pectoris typically occurs from myocardial ischemia. Ischemia in the myocardium develops when there is a mismatch between myocardial oxygen supply and demand. The underlying pathologic condition of this mismatch invariably is the presence of atherosclerosis in one or more of the coronary arteries.[3]

MYOCARDIAL OXYGEN SUPPLY AND DEMAND

The oxygen demand of the heart is determined by its workload. The major determinants of myocardial oxygen consumption are heart rate, contractility, and intramyocardial wall tension during systole (Fig. 12-2).[3,5] Intramyocardial wall tension, the force the heart is required to develop and sustain during contraction, is affected primarily by changes in ventricular pressures and volume. Both enlargement of the ventricle and increased pressure within the ventricle increase the systolic wall force and consequently myocardial oxygen demand. Increases in contractility and heart rate also increase oxygen demand.[6] Pharmacologic control of angina is directed toward decreasing the myocardial oxygen demand by decreasing heart rate, myocardial contractility, or ventricular volume and pressures.[3,5]

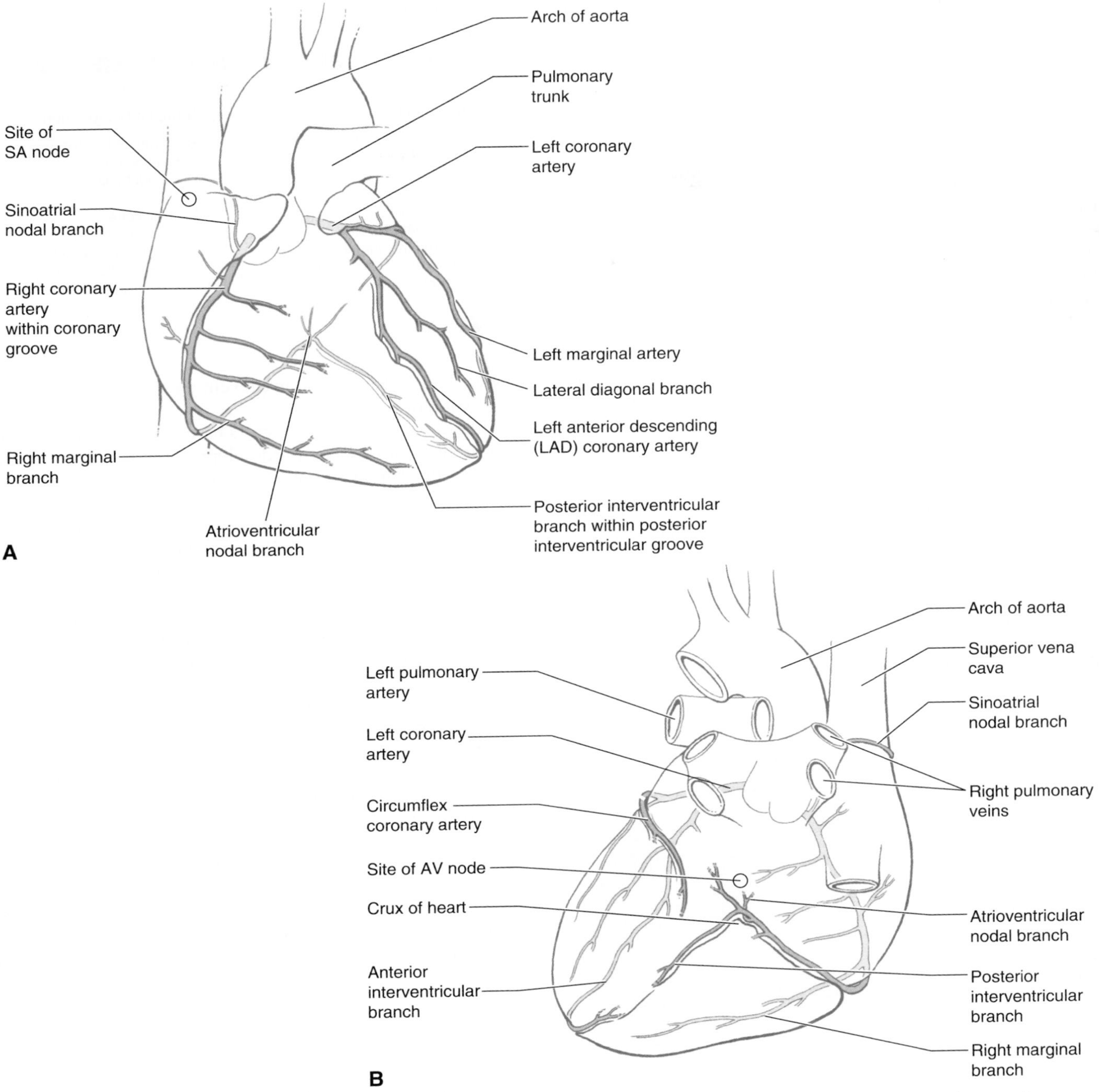

Figure 12-1 Coronary arteries. The right coronary artery (RCA) originates from the aorta and courses in the atrioventricular (coronary) groove to reach the posterior surface of the heart. The left coronary artery splits into the circumflex branch that supplies blood to the lateral and posterior walls of the left ventricle, and a left anterior descending (LAD) branch that supplies blood to the anterior wall of the left ventricle. **A:** Anterior view. **B:** Posteroinferior view.

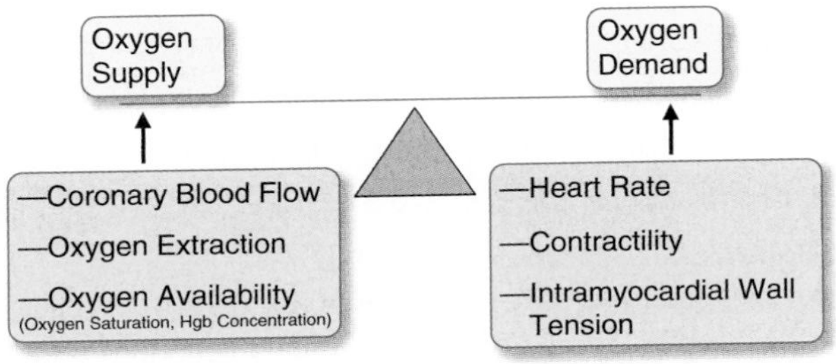

Figure 12-2 Determinants of myocardial oxygen supply and demand.

Oxygen supply to the heart is impacted by many factors including coronary blood flow and oxygen extraction (Fig. 12-2). Oxygen extraction by heart cells is high (~70%–75%) even at rest. When extra demand is placed on the heart, myocardial oxygen extraction increases slightly and plateaus at approximately 80%. Because oxygen extraction is increased only modestly when the heart is stressed, high oxygen demands must be met by increases in coronary blood flow.[7] The oxygen content of arterial blood also is important. Therefore, the hematocrit (Hct), hemoglobin (Hgb), and arterial blood gases should be monitored. In a similar fashion to targeting determinants of myocardial oxygen demand, pharmacologic control of angina is directed at improving oxygen supply through vasodilation of the epicardial coronary arteries.[5]

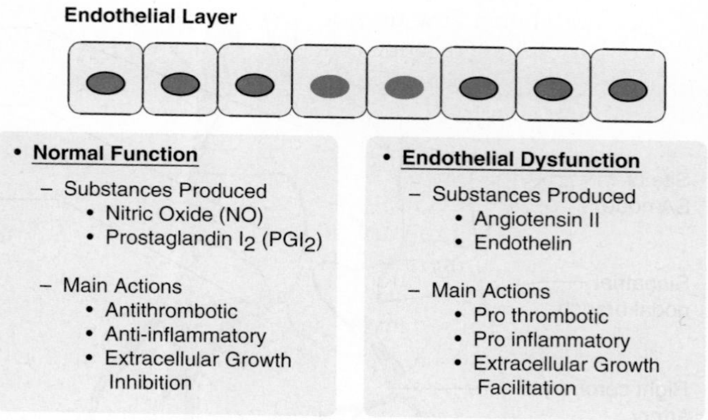

Figure 12-4 Endothelial function.

ATHEROSCLEROTIC VASCULAR DISEASE

Although understanding the determinants of myocardial oxygen supply and demand is important in treating CHD, of equal importance is understanding how atherosclerotic plaques develop because the underlying pathologic condition of this mismatch invariably is the presence of atherosclerosis in one or more of the coronary arteries. Understanding how the process of atherosclerosis unfolds, as well as the primary pharmacologic and non-pharmacologic interventions that help prevent progression of atherosclerosis, is an important piece in treating a patient with chronic stable angina (Fig. 12-3). (See Chapter 8, Dyslipidemias, Atherosclerosis, and Coronary Heart Disease.)

If an atherosclerotic plaque occludes less than 50% of the diameter of the vessel, coronary blood flow can be augmented sufficiently during exertion by the intramyocardial arterioles (resistance vessels), and the patient is pain free. In patients with chronic stable angina, most coronary artery stenoses are greater than 70%.[3,5]

Traditional risk factors, such as smoking, hypertension, hyperlipidemia, diabetes, and obesity, are linked to the process of atherosclerosis by producing oxidative stress within the vasculature. Increased oxidative stress leads to progressive decreases in nitric oxide (NO) levels and endothelial dysfunction, enhancing atherosclerosis (Fig. 12-4).[8] In addition, diets typically seen in western industrialized countries have been linked to increased oxidative stress within the vasculature. This may partially explain the link between diet and atherosclerosis.[9] The role of a healthy lifestyle and diet is crucial in preventing the development or progression of CAD.

Although traditional risk factors have long been appreciated as the underlying cause for the development of CAD, continuing research efforts have attempted to identify novel risk factors to refine risk assessment for the development of CAD. Potential candidates have included highly-sensitive C-reactive protein, homocysteine, fibrinogen, and lipoprotein (a), among others.[10,11] Findings from the INTERHEART study indicate little may be gained from identifying additional risk factors.[12] In this large case–control study, nine clinical risk factors were strongly associated with the development of first-ever MI and accounted for greater than 90% of the risk for developing CAD (Table 12-1). The results were consistent across sex, geographic regions, and ethnic groups, suggesting that strategies to reduce the incidence of CAD can be applied universally. Subsequent studies have verified the findings of INTERHEART, and many of these potential risk factors may indeed more accurately reflect the presence of CAD and be considered markers, as opposed to predicting who will subsequently exhibit CAD.[10,11,13]

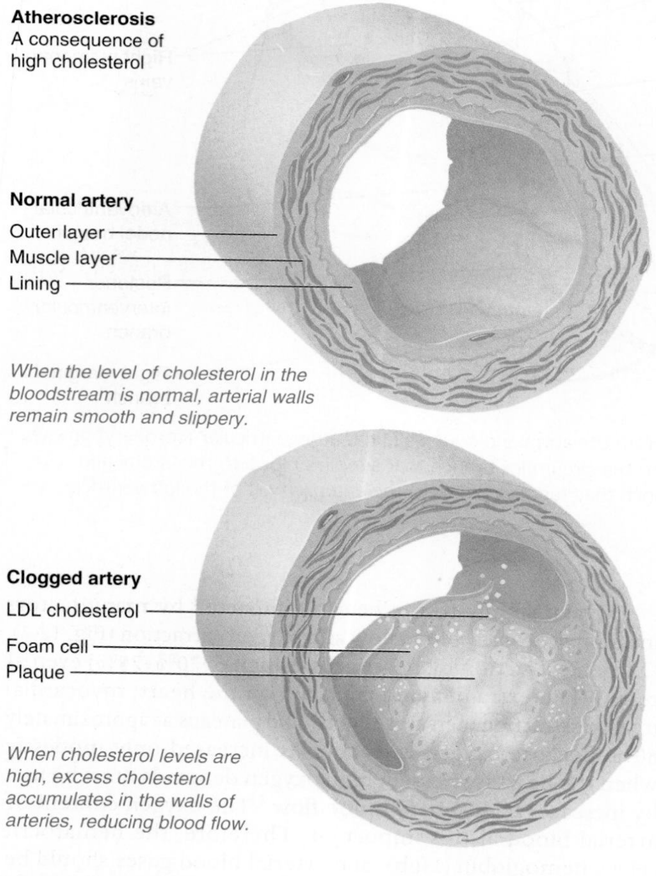

Figure 12-3 Process of atherosclerosis. (*Source:* Anatomical Chart Company. **http://www.anatomical.com/**.)

PLATELET AGGREGATION AND THE FORMATION OF THROMBI

Although coronary atherosclerosis is the underlying mechanism for most patients with anginal syndromes, thrombotic factors commonly play a key role in the pathogenesis of myocardial

Table 12-1
Risk Factors for First-Time Myocardial Infarction from the INTERHEART Study[12]

Risk Factor	Adjusted Odds Ratio (99% Confidence Interval)
ApoB to apoA-1 ratio[a]	3.25 (2.81–3.76)
Current smoking	2.87 (2.58–3.19)
Psychosocial	2.67 (2.21–3.22)
Diabetes	2.37 (2.07–2.71)
Hypertension	1.91 (1.74–2.10)
Abdominal obesity	1.62 (1.45–1.80)
Moderate alcohol intake	0.91 (0.82–1.02)
Exercise	0.86 (0.76–0.97)
Vegetables and fruits daily	0.70 (0.62–0.79)
All combined	129.2 (90.2–185.0)

Apo, apolipoprotein.
[a]Risk of MI increases with increased ratio.

ischemia. Both blood flow turbulence and stasis can cause intermittent platelet aggregation or intermittent coronary artery thrombosis. Thus, platelet-active agents are used in the treatment of chronic stable angina.[14]

INTRACELLULAR SODIUM AND CALCIUM HANDLING

Recently, an appreciation has emerged for the role of the late sodium current (I_{Na}) in the development and maintenance of myocardial ischemia. Most sodium enters the myocardium in phase 0 of the action potential. Under normal conditions, however, a small amount of sodium will enter the cell during phase 2 (plateau phase) of the action potential. When ischemia is present, sodium handling is altered such that a substantial increase occurs in the late I_{Na}. The increase in intracellular sodium triggers an increase in the influx of calcium through the reverse mode of the sodium–calcium exchanger. The net result of the alterations in intracellular ion handling is intracellular calcium overload.[5] Increases in intracellular calcium impair myocardial relaxation, increase intramyocardial wall tension, decrease perfusion to the myocardium owing to compression of the small arterioles feeding the myocardium, and increase myocardial oxygen demand.[15] Ultimately, these pathologic changes in sodium and calcium handling perpetuate and worsen ischemia once it develops. Targeting this pathologic process has led to the development of new antianginal medications (e.g., ranolazine) with a distinct, novel mechanism of action compared with traditional antianginal agents (i.e., nitrates, β-blockers, and calcium-channel blockers [CCBs]).[5]

Clinical Presentation

A detailed description of chest pain is vital in order for the clinician to determine whether chest pain represents chronic stable angina, Acute Coronary Syndrome (ACS), or is noncardiac in origin. Five key components commonly used to characterize chest pain include the location, duration, severity, and quality of pain, as well as any factors that provoke and relieve the pain (Table 12-2). Chest pain stemming from myocardial ischemia is often described as a sensation of pressure or heavy weight located over the sternum. Patients may also complain of shortness of breath (SOB), nausea, vomiting, or diaphoresis. Pain may also occur in the neck, jaw, shoulder, or arm. The precipitation of pain is typically associated with exertion and rapidly resolves with rest or the administration of NTG. Chest pain that occurs at rest, prolonged in duration, or increased in severity is likely reflective of unstable disease and warrants immediate medical attention to prevent complications such as MI, HF, and death. Importantly, some patients (women, people with diabetes) may present with atypical symptoms such as indigestion or gastric fullness, or may present with diaphoresis alone without concomitant chest pain. Last, many episodes of ischemia are asymptomatic and termed as "silent ischemia."[1–3]

Physical findings in patients with chronic stable angina are often absent or nonspecific.[1]

Diagnosis and Risk Assessment

The evaluation of a patient presenting with chest pain suspected to be due to CAD should begin with a detailed history of ischemic symptoms and physical examination. Once this information is available, an estimate can be made of the probability of CAD being present (low, intermediate, high).[1] The probability estimate will often help direct which diagnostic tests are appropriate. Given that many symptoms associated with chronic stable angina are nonspecific, several noninvasive and invasive testing modalities are available to assist in the diagnosis and risk assessment of CAD.[1,2] It is important to discern as soon as possible whether the patient's reported chest discomfort is consistent with chronic stable angina, or represents the presence of ACS. Patients presenting with ACS often are at high short-term risk of MI or death and warrant hospitalization with aggressive treatment strategies.[16,17] Lipid parameters, renal function, and fasting blood glucose levels should be obtained in all patients with suspected or established CAD to screen for metabolic abnormalities. Other biochemical markers such as high-sensitivity C-reactive protein, lipoprotein(a), lipoprotein-associated phospholipase A_2, and apolipoprotein B are not routinely recommended.[3]

A 12-lead ECG reading should be obtained in all patients with symptoms suggestive of angina pectoris. Although not useful

Table 12-2
Characteristics of Angina Pectoris[1–3]

Symptoms
Sensation of pressure or heavy weight on chest alone or with pain
Pain described variably as feelings of tightness, burning, crushing, squeezing, vicelike, aching, or "deep"
Gradual increase in intensity followed by gradual fading away (distinguished from esophageal spasm)[a]
Shortness of breath with feeling of constriction about the larynx of upper trachea
Duration of Symptoms
0.5–30 minutes
Location of Pain or Discomfort
Over the sternum or very near to it
Anywhere between epigastrium and pharynx
Occasionally limited to left shoulder and left arm
Rarely limited to right arm
Lower cervical or upper thoracic spine
Left interscapular or suprascapular area
Radiation of Pain
Medial aspect of left arm
Left shoulder
Jaw
Occasionally, right arm
Electrocardiogram
ST-segment depression >2 mm
T-wave inversion
Precipitating Factors
Mild, moderate, or heavy exercise, depending on patient
Effort that involves use of arms above the head
Cold environment
Walking against the wind
Walking after a large meal
Emotions: fright, anger, or anxiety
Coitus
Nitroglycerin Relief[a]
Relief of pain occurring within 45 seconds to 5 minutes of taking nitroglycerin

[a] Esophageal spasm and other gastrointestinal disorders occasionally mimic anginal pain and also can be relieved by nitroglycerin.

in establishing a definitive diagnosis of CAD, the ECG will be useful at detecting important information regarding conduction abnormalities, left ventricular hypertrophy, ongoing ischemia, or evidence of a previous MI. Chest radiography is not routinely recommended except in patients with an abnormal ECG, history of MI, symptoms of HF, or ventricular arrhythmias.[1] Cardiac computed tomography angiography (CCTA) is a reasonable option to determine risk in patients whose ECG cannot be interpreted, who are unable to exercise to an appropriate workload, unable to perform stress testing, or alternatively to invasive coronary angiography in moderate- to high-risk patients with unknown coronary anatomy.[1]

STRESS TESTING

The induction of stress via exercise or pharmacologic means is a common and highly useful procedure in the diagnosis of CAD. The test would be indicative of CAD if angina, ECG signs of ischemia, arrhythmias, abnormal heart rate, or abnormal blood pressure (BP) response develops. The product of the heart rate and systolic BP (i.e., the rate–pressure or double product) correlates well with myocardial oxygen demand. The rate–pressure product normally rises progressively during exercise, with the peak value best describing the cardiovascular response to stress. Often, patients with stable angina experience chest pain at a consistent rate–pressure product.[18]

Abnormal responses of either BP or heart rate may signal CAD. A normal BP response to exercise is a gradual rise in systolic BP with the diastolic BP remaining unchanged. A rise or fall of diastolic BP greater than 10 mm Hg is considered abnormal. A fall in systemic BP during exercise is especially ominous because this indicates that the cardiac output cannot increase sufficiently to overcome the vasodilation in the skeletal muscle vascular bed.[18]

Stress imaging studies, either echocardiographic or nuclear, are preferred over the exercise tolerance test in patients with left bundle-branch block, electronically paced ventricular rhythm, prior revascularization (percutaneous coronary intervention [PCI] or coronary artery bypass surgery [CABG]), preexcitation syndrome, greater than 1 mm ST-segment depression at rest, or other ECG conduction abnormalities. In addition, many patients are not able to exhibit an appropriate level of cardiac stress through exercise; pharmacologic stress testing is preferred in these patients.[1,18]

Pharmacologic stress may be achieved through the use of dipyridamole, adenosine, or dobutamine. Each of these agents is used to induce changes in the balance between myocardial oxygen supply and demand, similar to walking on a treadmill during the exercise stress test. Vasodilators (dipyridamole and adenosine) promote vasodilation in normal coronary segments, but have no effect in arteries affected by atherosclerosis. The net result is shunting of blood away from diseased coronary arteries and the development of ischemia that may be detected by changes in BP, heart rate, or ECG changes. These agents are typically used in conjunction with myocardial perfusion scintigraphy. Stress thallium-201 myocardial perfusion imaging provides a dynamic picture of the heart. The radionuclide is injected at peak stress and an image is obtained within several minutes. A defect in myocardial uptake of the thallium indicates an area of ischemia or possible infarction.[19]

Dobutamine is a positive inotrope and typically is used with echocardiography. Administration of dobutamine leads to an increase in myocardial oxygen demand secondary to increases in heart rate and contractility. If demand exceeds available oxygen supply, ischemia develops. Subsequent to the infusion of dobutamine, defects or decreases in the wall motion or thickening of the left ventricle are indicative of ischemia.[19]

CARDIAC CATHETERIZATION

CAD can be diagnosed definitively by coronary catheterization and angiography. In addition, angiography is the most accurate means of identifying less common causes of chronic stable angina, such as coronary artery spasm.[1] Cardiac catheterization is a procedure used to provide vascular access to the coronary arteries. Once access is gained with an intravascular catheter, a number of procedures (angiography, ventriculography, PCI) can be performed. Access to the vasculature is usually obtained percutaneously through the radial, brachial, or femoral arteries. From this point, the catheter is advanced through the vasculature until the coronary arteries are accessible. After the tip of the catheter is advanced into the coronary arteries, dye is injected into the coronary arteries and the location and extent of atherosclerosis can be determined. Approximately 75% of patients with chronic stable angina are noted to have one-vessel, two-vessel, or three-vessel disease by this procedure (equally divided).[3]

The results of angiography can be useful in determining the risk of death or MI in patients with CAD and, subsequently, the course of needed treatment. For example, patients who have a significant stenosis in the left main coronary artery are at high risk of death and should undergo CABG.[20,21]

OVERVIEW OF DRUG AND NONDRUG THERAPY

The goals of therapy for chronic stable angina are to reduce or eliminate the symptoms of angina, to maintain or improve the quality of life, halt the progression of atherosclerosis and prevent complications of the disease, such as MI and death while minimizing healthcare costs. Both pharmacologic and non-pharmacologic interventions, in addition to myocardial revascularization procedures, are utilized simultaneously to achieve each of these goals.[1]

Vasculoprotective Therapy

LIFESTYLE MODIFICATIONS

Lifestyle modifications should always constitute a significant portion of any treatment plan for patients with chronic stable angina. Lifestyle modification should include adoption of a heart-healthy diet, smoking cessation/avoidance of second-hand smoke, adequate physical activity, weight control, and maintenance of an acceptable waist circumference.[1,22,23] Dietary recommendations typically consist of limiting saturated fat, total fat, cholesterol, sodium, sugar-sweetened beverages, and red meat while consuming a diet high in fruits, vegetables, whole grains, omega-3 fatty acids, and fiber[22] (see Chapter 8, Dyslipidemias, Atherosclerosis, and Coronary Heart Disease). Adoption of a healthy dietary pattern reflective of these components has been demonstrated to have positive effects on cardiovascular risk factors.[1,22]

Smoking cessation is a crucial intervention as cigarette smoking (including second-hand smoke exposure) has been identified as the single most preventable cause of death due to CAD.[24] Clinicians should routinely assess the smoking status of patients with chronic stable angina and provide information regarding effective options to aid in smoking cessation. Nicotine replacement products, bupropion, and varenicline have been demonstrated as effective in assisting cessation efforts (see Chapter 91, Tobacco Use and Dependence). In addition to the avoidance of cigarette smoke, it is reasonable to recommend the avoidance of air pollution in patients with chronic stable angina. Unless contraindicated, it is appropriate to recommend one alcoholic beverage in women and one to two alcoholic beverages in men.[1]

A body mass index (BMI) of 18.5 to 24.9 kg/m^2 and a waist circumference less than 40 inches in men and 35 inches in women should be achieved or maintained. Adequate exercise facilitates both weight loss and better control of cardiovascular risk factors. Patients with chronic stable angina should be encouraged to engage in moderate-intensity exercise for 30 to 60 minutes/day for at least 5 days/week, but ideally each day. Weight loss can be facilitated through appropriate caloric restriction, as well as the adoption of healthy dietary eating patterns.[1]

RISK FACTOR MODIFICATION

In addition to appropriate lifestyle modifications, optimization of cardiovascular risk factors should be achieved. Although the lifestyle modifications may help improve risk factor control, pharmacotherapy may be required. Table 12-3 provides appropriate targets for risk factor optimization. Appropriate identification and treatment of risk factors helps prevent the development of CAD and disease progression in patients with existing CAD. Select drug therapies for each risk factor may be preferred due to their positive effects on the pathophysiology of atherosclerosis. Although several different classes of lipid-modifying drugs exist, 3-hydroxy-3-methylglutaryl co-enzyme A inhibitors (HMG-CoA reductase inhibitors, or statins) have been demonstrated in multiple trials to significantly reduce the progression of atherosclerosis, as well as reduce the incidence of death and MI.[25] In patients who require additional BP control after antianginal therapy has been optimized, angiotensin-converting enzyme (ACE) inhibitors may be preferred due to their theoretical potential to reduce the progression of CAD by improving endothelial function. Data suggest that angiotensin receptor blockers (ARBs) may provide similar benefits in patients who cannot tolerate ACE inhibitors.[1,26] The presence of diabetes has been shown to be a significant risk factor for the development and progression of atherosclerosis; however, the majority of clinical trials demonstrate that tight glycemic control did not have a positive effect on the progression of atherosclerosis or reduce the risk of hard end points such as MI.[27] Information from the Diabetes Control and Complications Trial indicates that tight glycemic control with intensive insulin therapy in patients with type 1 diabetes significantly reduces the risk for MI and cardiovascular death.[28] Similar effects have not been seen in large randomized trials in patients with type 2 diabetes. In one large trial involving patients with CVD and type 2 diabetes, the use of intensive insulin therapy reduced nonfatal MI at 5 years, but total mortality was increased.[29] Given the available information, intensive glucose lowering cannot be recommended for patients with CAD and type 2 diabetes. Patients with type 2 diabetes should target a glycosylated hemoglobin (Hgb A_{1c}) less than 7%.[27]

Table 12-3

AHA/ACC Guidelines for Secondary Prevention for Patients with Coronary and Other Atherosclerotic Vascular Disease[23,25,26]

Risk Factor	Intervention and Goal
Smoking	Complete cessation
	No exposure to environmental tobacco smoke
Blood pressure	<140/90 mm Hg
Lipid management	High intensity statin
Diabetes	Hemoglobin A_{1c} <7%
Physical activity	At least 30 minutes of moderate-intensity aerobic activity (e.g., brisk walking) for minimum of 5 days/week
Weight management	BMI between 18.5 and 24.9 kg/m^2
	Waist circumference, men <40 inches
	Waist circumference, women <35 inches
Influenza vaccination	Patients with CAD should have an annual influenza vaccination

BMI, body mass index; CAD, coronary artery disease; HDL-C, high-density lipoprotein cholesterol; LDL-C, low-density lipoprotein cholesterol.

ANTIPLATELET THERAPY

Antiplatelet therapy has a central place in the treatment of patients with CAD. Aspirin (acetylsalicylic acid [ASA]) therapy has demonstrated a reduction in the incidence of MI and sudden cardiac death in patients with chronic stable angina. Aspirin's clinical efficacy in chronic stable angina, coupled with its minimal cost and demonstrated efficacy after MI, have made it the gold standard for antiplatelet monotherapy in patients with CAD. Current national guidelines from the American College of Cardiology (ACC)/AHA recommend an ASA dose of 75 to 162 mg daily for the prevention of MI and death. Although higher doses have been investigated in clinical studies, they have not shown increased efficacy, but do increase the risk for adverse effects.[23]

Clopidogrel represents a suitable alternative antiplatelet agent to prevent MI and death in chronic stable angina patients unable to take ASA. The Clopidogrel versus Aspirin in Patients at Risk of Ischemic Events trial (CAPRIE) demonstrated that clopidogrel significantly reduced the incidence of stroke, MI, or vascular death in patients with atherosclerotic vascular disease (previous MI, stroke, or peripheral arterial disease [PAD]) compared with ASA. In addition, clopidogrel was well tolerated with the major adverse effects noted to be gastrointestinal (GI) intolerance and rash. Despite the significant results, the absolute difference in the primary outcome between the two strategies was quite small (0.4%, number need to treat = 200).[30] As such, clopidogrel remains a second-line choice behind ASA in patients with CAD. Clopidogrel should be administered at a dosage of 75 mg/day.

The approach of dual antiplatelet therapy (DAPT), combining ASA with a $P2Y_{12}$ antagonist (clopidogrel, prasugrel, or ticagrelor), has been demonstrated to improve morbidity and mortality in a number of high-risk patients with CVD.[16,17] Given the different mechanisms of antiplatelet effect, combining aspirin with a $P2Y_{12}$ antagonist might be expected to provide additional protection from MI and death in patients with stable CAD as compared to monotherapy. The Clopidogrel for High Atherothrombotic Risk and Ischemic Stabilization, Management, and Avoidance trial assessed the utility of long-term DAPT in patients with documented CAD or with multiple cardiovascular risk factors. The combination of ASA plus clopidogrel for 28 months did not reduce the risk of death, MI, stroke, or coronary revascularization as compared to ASA alone. However, dual therapy did increase the risk of bleeding.[31]

A post hoc analysis revealed a reduction in ischemic risk in patients with prior MI suggesting that some patients may benefit from long-term DAPT.[31] The Pegasus-TIMI 54 trial evaluated the role of DAPT (low-dose ASA plus either ticagrelor 90 mg BID or 60 mg BID vs. ASA alone) in patients with a prior MI in the previous 1 to 3 years.[32] The median time from MI to randomization was 1.7 years. In over 21,000 patients with a median follow-up of 33 months, ASA plus both doses of ticagrelor reduced the primary end point (cardiovascular death, MI, stroke) compared to ASA monotherapy. This reduction came at the expense of an increased risk of bleeding, with TIMI major bleeding occurring at a rate of 2.6% and 2.3% in the groups receiving ticagrelor 90 mg and 60 mg BID, as compared to 1.06% in patients receiving placebo.[32]

In a separate investigation, patients who received an additional 18 months of DAPT as compared to the standard duration of 12 months in patients who received drug-eluting stents (DES) had a lower rate of stent thrombosis (0.4% vs. 1.4%, $p < 0.001$) and major adverse cardiovascular and cerebrovascular events (4.3% vs. 5.9%, $p < 0.001$), which included a reduction in MI.[33] There was an increase in moderate to severe bleeding (2.5% vs. 1.6%, $p = 0.001$). Up to 40% of the 9,961 patients underwent PCI due to chronic stable angina, and DAPT either consisted of ASA plus clopidogrel, or ASA plus prasugrel.[33]

Given these results, some patients may receive extended durations of DAPT if they have a previous history of prior MI, or are post-PCI and have received a DES.

Anti-Ischemic Pharmacotherapy

Historically, agents used in the treatment of patients with chronic stable angina primarily affected either determinants of myocardial oxygen supply, myocardial oxygen demand, or both. Within this paradigm, β-blockers, CCBs, and chronic nitrate therapy have demonstrated effectiveness in the prevention of ischemic symptoms. In January 2006, the US Food and Drug Administration (FDA) granted approval to ranolazine, representing the first new class of agents to be approved for the treatment of chronic stable angina in the last 20 years. Unlike traditional anti-anginal medications, ranolazine does not affect heart rate or BP. The selection of specific anti-ischemic pharmacotherapy for patients with chronic stable angina should take into account relevant patient characteristics as well as guideline recommendations.

β-BLOCKERS

β-Blockers lower myocardial oxygen demand primarily by lowering heart rate and myocardial contractility. Neither β-selectivity nor the presence of α-1 blockade appear to vary efficacy at preventing ischemia and, therefore, the choice of a specific agent for a given patient will likely depend on cost, number of daily doses, and the presence of other comorbid conditions. β-Blockers with intrinsic sympathomimetic activity are not routinely used in patients with stable angina due to reduced efficacy. The dose of the β-blocker should be titrated to a goal resting heart rate of 55 to 60 beats/minute and therefore will be patient specific.[34] β-Blockers should be avoided in patients with primary vasospastic angina and may worsen symptoms in patients with reactive airway disease or PAD. The most common side effects observed with chronic therapy include bradycardia, hypotension, fatigue, and sexual dysfunction. Other conditions that may prevent the use of β-blocker therapy include severe bradycardia or atrioventricular (AV) nodal conduction defects.[35–37]

NITRATES

Nitrates are available in a number of different formulations and available options are listed in Table 12-4. Regardless of the formulation, all nitrate options are effective at preventing or relieving ischemic symptoms if used appropriately, including the use of a nitrate-free interval. Nitrates can increase myocardial oxygen supply through vasodilation of the coronary arteries, as well as reduce myocardial oxygen demand through the reduction of preload. Nitrates produce vasodilation through the biotransformation and the release of NO.[38] Long-acting nitrates are effective agents for the prevention of anginal symptoms. Sublingual NTG is a vital agent to treat acute anginal attacks. Common side effects of nitrate therapy include hypotension, dizziness, and headache. Headache often will resolve with continued therapy and may be treated with acetaminophen. Concomitant administration with phosphodiesterase type 5 inhibitors (within 24 hours for sildenafil and vardenafil, 48 hours for tadalafil) is contraindicated due to the risk of life-threatening hypotension.[38,39]

CALCIUM-CHANNEL BLOCKERS

CCBs are highly diverse compounds. They differ markedly in chemical structure as well as specificity for cardiac and peripheral tissue. Using these characteristics, it is possible to classify CCBs into several major types (Table 12-5).[40]

Both non-dihydropyridine CCBs (non-DHP CCBs), diltiazem and verapamil, exert similar effects on myocardial and peripheral tissue. They slow conduction and prolong the refractory period in the AV node (see Chapter 15, Cardiac Arrhythmias). Both agents can depress myocardial contractility and are moderate peripheral vasodilators and potent coronary artery vasodilators.[40]

In contrast to diltiazem or verapamil, the dihydropyridines (DHPs) such as nifedipine, amlodipine, felodipine, isradipine, and nicardipine do not slow cardiac conduction. They are more potent peripheral vasodilators and may be associated with a reflex increase in the heart rate. All DHPs have negative inotropic effects in vitro, but these effects, clinically, are overshadowed by the reflex sympathetic activation and decreased afterload. The net effect of these actions results in no or minimal depression of myocardial function (see Chapter 14, Heart Failure).[40]

Both DHP and non-DHP CCBs produce an increase in myocardial oxygen supply through vasodilation of the coronary arteries, as well as reduce myocardial oxygen demand through lowering of intramyocardial wall tension (by lowering systemic BP). However, non-DHP CCBs would be expected to lower myocardial oxygen demand to a greater degree because of additional reductions in heart rate and contractility. Although defined as being within the same pharmacologic class, it is important to consider DHPs and non-DHPs separately when considering their use in patients with chronic stable angina. The reductions in heart rate and contractility with non-DHPs may be beneficial for some patients, although detrimental in others such as patients with compromised left ventricular (LV) function or bradycardia at baseline. Conversely, amlodipine and felodipine have been shown to be safe to use in patients with LV dysfunction and to provide a reasonable option for the prevention of ischemic symptoms in those patients.[40] CCB should be used cautiously when used in combination with cyclosporine, carbamazepine, lithium, amiodarone, and digoxin. Non-DHP CCB should be avoided in most situations due to the duplicate effects on heart rate and cardiac contractility.[1] Side effects of CCB therapy depend on the specific agent used. Use of non-DHP CCBs may result in bradycardia, hypotension, and AV block. Patients receiving DHP CCBs may experience reflex tachycardia, peripheral edema, headache, and hypotension.[40]

RANOLAZINE

Ranolazine is an anti-ischemic agent that inhibits the late sodium current, thereby reducing intracellular sodium. During myocardial ischemia, sodium influx is increased, leading to intracellular calcium overload through the sodium/calcium exchanger. An excess of intracellular calcium leads to changes that promote and worsen ischemia, such as increased intramyocardial wall tension and reduced microvascular perfusion. By inhibiting sodium influx, ranolazine prevents ischemia-induced contractile dysfunction and delays the onset of angina. A key distinction between ranolazine and traditional antianginal agents is that it has no appreciable effect on heart rate and BP. The lack of significant hemodynamic effects makes the drug useful in patients in need of further antianginal therapy but who have low BP or heart rates preventing titration of conventional antianginal agents.[41]

Table 12-4
Commonly Prescribed Organic Nitrates

Drug	Dosage Form	Duration	Onset (minutes)	Usual Dosage
Short-Acting				
NTG	SL	10–30 minutes	1–3	0.4–0.6 mg[a,b]
NTG	Translingual spray	10–30 minutes	2–4	0.4 mg/metered spray[a,b]
NTG	IV	3–5 minutes[c]	1–2	Initially 5 mcg/minute. Increase every 3–5 minutes until pain is relieved or hypotension occurs
Long-Acting[d]				
NTG	SR capsule	4–8 hours	30	6.5–9 mg every 8 hours
NTG	Topical ointment[e]	4–8 hours	30	1–2 inches every 4–6 hours[f]
NTG	Transdermal patch	4–>8 hours	30–60	0.1–0.2 mg/h to start; titrate up to 0.8 mg/hour[f]
NTG	Transmucosal	3–6 hours	2–5	1–3 mg every 3–5 hours[f]
ISDN	SL	2–4 hours	2–5	2.5–10 mg every 2–4 hours[f]
	Chewable	2–4 hours	2–5	5–10 mg every 2–4 hours[f]
	Oral	2–6 hours	15–40	10–60 mg every 4–6 hours[f]
	SR capsule	4–8 hours	15–40	40–80 mg every 6–8 hours[f]
ISMN[g]	Tablet (ISMO, Monoket)	7–8 hours	30–60	10–20 mg BID (morning and midday) to start; titrate to 20–40 mg BID[f]
	Extended-release tablet (Imdur)	8–12 hours	30–60	60 mg every day to start; titrate to 30–120 mg every day

[a]When using sublingual or translingual spray forms of NTG, patients should administer the dose while sitting to minimize tachycardia, hypotension, dizziness, headache, and flushing. The optimal dose relieves symptoms with <10- to 15-mm Hg drop in systolic blood pressure or <10-beats/minute rise in pulse. Pain relief is rapid (onset 1–2 minutes; relief in 3–5 minutes), but up to three doses at 5-minute intervals may be given. After this, medical assistance should be summoned.
[b]Sublingual NTG tablets are degraded rapidly by heat, moisture, and light. They should be stored in a cool, dry place; do not leave the lid open or refrigerate. Tablets should be stored in the original manufacturer's container or a glass vial because the tablets volatilize and bind to many plastic vials and cotton. Previously, stinging of the tongue was an indicator of fresh tablets, but newer formulations only cause stinging in ~75% of patients.
[c]Duration after infusion discontinued.
[d]Longer-acting forms of nitrates are effective drugs, but it is important to understand their limitations to optimize effectiveness. Sublingual ISDN tablets display an onset and duration intermediate between that of sublingual NTG and oral ISDN. Because of high presystemic (first-pass) metabolism of the oral forms of both NTG and ISDN, very large doses may be required compared with SL or chewable dosage forms. Small oral doses (2.5 mg NTG, 5 mg ISDN) are probably not effective; doses as large as 9 mg NTG and 60 mg ISDN are not uncommon. Despite claims for longer activity, ointments and oral forms are often only effective for 4–8 hours, even when given as SR preparations. Also, continued daily use leads to rapid development of tolerance (see note *f*).
[e]Squeeze 1–2 inches of ointment onto the calibrated paper enclosed in the package with tube. Carefully spread the ointment on chest in a thin layer ~2 inches by 2 inches in size. Keep area covered with applicator paper. Wipe off previous dose before adding new dose or if hypotensive. If another person applies the ointment, avoid contact with fingers or eyes to prevent headache or hypotension.
[f]Dosage regimens should maintain a nitrate-free interval (e.g., bedtime) to decrease tolerance development. Give last oral dose or remove ointment or transdermal patch at 7 PM. Give last dose of SR ISDN in early afternoon.
[g]Major active metabolite of ISDN; 100% bioavailable; no first-pass metabolism, but tolerance may still occur. Rapid-release form (ISMO, Monoket) as 10- and 20-mg tablets. Extended-release form (Imdur) as 60-mg tablets. Okay to cut Indur in half, do not crush or chew.
BID, 2 times daily; ISDN, isosorbide dinitrate; ISMN, isosorbide monohydrate; IV, intravenous; NTG, nitroglycerin; SL, sublingual; SR, sustained-release.

Initial clinical trials demonstrated that ranolazine was an effective agent at reducing anginal episodes when added to existing therapy with CCBs or long-acting nitrates. Subsequent investigations demonstrated long-term safety and efficacy, and the agent may be considered at any stage in the treatment of chronic stable angina. Common adverse effects include headache, constipation, dizziness, and nausea. The drug is extensively metabolized in the liver through both cytochrome P-450 enzymes CYP3A4 and CYP2D6; therefore, attention should be paid to potential drug interactions. CYP3A4 appears to be the major pathway for metabolism and use of ranolazine is contraindicated in patients with significant hepatic dysfunction and in those receiving potent inhibitors and inducers of CYP3A4 such as ketoconazole or rifampin, respectively. Ranolazine is contraindicated in patients receiving many of the available antiretroviral agents.[41]

Myocardial Revascularization

Revascularization of the myocardium, with CABG or PCI, is a mainstay in the treatment of patients with CAD. The goals of revascularization do not differ from the overall goals in treating patients with chronic stable angina, namely, to relieve symptoms, improve quality of life, and prevent MI and death. Historically, a great deal of focus was devoted to comparing CABG, PCI, and medical management and their relative efficacy in relieving symptoms and improving prognosis. In a broad population of patients with CAD, revascularization with either CABG or PCI was found to be superior to medical management therapy alone at relieving symptoms at 1 year, although there was no difference in overall mortality between the treatment strategies.[42] However, CABG therapy tended to be superior at providing long-term relief of

Table 12-5

Calcium-Channel Blockers in Anginal Syndromes

Drug Name	FDA Approved[a]	Usual Dose for Chronic Stable Angina[b]	Product Availability
Dihydropyridines			
Amlodipine	Angina, hypertension	2.5–10 mg every day	2.5, 5, 10 mg tab
Felodipine	Hypertension	5–20 mg every day	5, 10 mg ER tab
Isradapine	Hypertension	2.5–10 mg BID	2.5, 5 mg IR cap
		5–10 mg every day	5, 10 mg CR tab
Nicardipine	Angina (IR only), hypertension	20–40 mg TID	20, 30 mg IR cap
		30–60 mg BID	30, 45, 60 mg SR cap
Nifedipine	Angina, hypertension	10–30 mg TID	10, 20 mg IR cap
		30–180 mg every day	30, 60, 90 mg ER tab
Nisoldipine	Hypertension	20–60 mg every day	10, 20, 30, 40 mg ER tab
Diphenylalkylamines			
Verapamil	Angina, hypertension, SVT	30–120 mg TID/QID	40, 80, 120 mg IR tab
		120–240 mg BID	120, 180, 240 mg SR tab
		120–480 mg every HS	180, 240 mg DR, ER tab
			120, 180, 240, 360 mg ER cap
			100, 200, 300 mg DR, ER tab
Benzothiazepines			
Diltiazem	Angina, hypertension, SVT	30–120 mg TID/QID	30, 60, 90, 120 mg IR tab
		60–180 mg BID	60, 90, 120, 180 mg SR cap
		120–480 mg every day	120, 180, 240, 300, 360 mg cap
			120, 180, 240 mg ER cap
			120, 180, 240, 300, 360, 420 mg ER cap

[a]FDA-approved indications vary among IR and ER products. However, most all have been used clinically for both angina and hypertension. Avoid IR products in hypertension.

[b]Because of short half-lives, most of these drugs are given TID if using IR tabs or caps. Amlodipine has a long half-life and is given once daily.

BID, 2 times a day; cap, capsules; CD, controlled diffusion; CR, controlled-release; DR, delayed-release; ER, extended-release; FDA, US Food and Drug Administration; HS, bedtime; IR, immediate-release; QID, four times a day; SR, sustained-release; SVT, supraventricular including atrial fibrillation, atrial flutter, and re-entry; tab, tablets; TID, three times a day.

symptoms, as well as providing a lower need for repeat revascularization therapy compared to PCI. When considering subgroups of patients with more severe disease or who have manifested left ventricular dysfunction, differences in long-term mortality can be observed among the different treatment strategies. In patients with double-vessel or triple-vessel disease, significant disease of the left main artery, or left ventricular dysfunction, CABG therapy has been demonstrated to provide a reduced 5-year mortality rate compared with PCI or medical therapy alone.[21]

Despite the availability of data regarding the relative effects of PCI, CABG, and medical management on morbidity and mortality, there has been a dramatic increase in the use of PCI in recent years. CABG remains the preferred strategy for patients with three-vessel disease or who have multi-vessel disease plus left ventricular dysfunction. In patients with less severe CAD, PCI can be expected to provide similar benefits in mortality as compared to CABG, but may not be as effective at reducing symptoms or the need for repeat revascularization procedures. Recent investigations have indicated that aggressive medical treatment, including intensive lipid-lowering therapy, may be as effective as PCI at improving prognosis over the long term, but may be inferior at reducing symptoms of angina.[1,43,44] These trials are significant in that they highlight the importance of implementing effective strategies, which reduce the progression of CAD, regardless of whether revascularization therapy is utilized. Relevant issues facing pharmacists today not only include optimizing the medical management of CAD but also providing effective pharmacotherapy to prevent complications of PCI.

CLINICAL PRESENTATION OF CHRONIC STABLE ANGINA

CASE 12-1

Question 1: J.P., a 62-year-old dairy farmer, is hospitalized for evaluation of chest pain. About 3 weeks before admission, he noted substernal chest pain brought on by lifting heavy objects or walking uphill. He describes a crushing or viselike pain that never occurs at rest and is not associated with meals, emotional stress, or a particular time of day. When J.P. stops working, the pain subsides in about 5 minutes.

J.P.'s mother and brother died of a heart attack at ages 62 and 57, respectively; his father, who is alive at age 86, has survived one heart attack and one stroke. Family history (except for J.P.)

is negative for diabetes mellitus. J.P. is 5 feet 10 inches tall and weighs 235 pounds; he drinks two or three beers a day and does not smoke or chew tobacco.

J.P.'s other medical problems include a 10-year history of hypertension and diabetes for 4 years. Until 3 weeks ago, J.P. could perform all his farm chores without difficulty, including heavy labor. He follows a no-added-salt diet, but consistently eats at fast-food establishments with his favorite meal consisting of two cheeseburgers and French fries.

J.P.'s medication history reveals the following: lisinopril 10 mg once daily, metformin 500 mg BID and hydrochlorothiazide 25 mg once daily. He rarely uses over-the-counter medications. He has an allergy to sulfamethoxazole.

On admission to the cardiac ward, J.P. appears his stated age and is in no apparent distress. Resting vital signs include supine BP, 145/95 mm Hg (last ambulatory visit, 130/85 mm Hg); regular pulse, 84 beats/minute (last ambulatory visit, 78 beats/minute), and respiratory rate, 12 breaths/minute. He has no peripheral edema or neck vein distension, and lung auscultation is within normal limits. Abdominal examination is unremarkable and he is alert and oriented × 3. Cardiac auscultation reveals a regular rate and rhythm with a normal S_1 and S_2; third or fourth heart sounds and murmurs are not noted. A 12-lead ECG reveals normal sinus rhythm at a rate of 84 beats/minute without evidence of previous MI. All intervals are within normal limits.

Admitting laboratory values include the following:

Hct, 43.5%
White blood cell (WBC) count, 5,000/μL
Sodium (Na), 140 mEq/L
Potassium (K), 4.7 mEq/L
Magnesium (Mg), 1.9 mEq/L
Random blood glucose, 132 mg/dL
Hgb A_{1c} 7.4%
Blood urea nitrogen, 27 mg/dL
Serum creatinine, 1.4 mg/dL
Urinary albumin–creatinine ratio, 27 mg/mmol
Chest radiograph is within normal limits.

What signs and symptoms does J.P. exhibit that are consistent with the diagnosis of chronic stable angina?

J.P.'s description of his chest pain includes several common characteristics of angina pectoris (Table 12-2).[1–3] The substernal location of J.P.'s chest pain is typical, although some patients describe pain radiating down the left arm or pain that is referred to the shoulder area or jaw. J.P.'s pain is described as crushing or viselike in quality, which also is common; a fullness in the throat or jaw may occur simultaneously or in lieu of chest pain. In some cases, the patient may not consider these sensations as pain, describing them instead as a sense of pressure or heaviness. Many patients complain of SOB. J.P.'s symptoms are related to exercise and exertion—both known precipitating factors of angina. Most episodes of exertional angina last several minutes in duration and are relieved with rest. Because J.P. has never sought medical attention for his chest pain, his response to NTG cannot be determined.

After getting a detailed description of J.P.'s symptoms, his physician can characterize his chest pain and make a global assessment. Initially, the chest pain should be classified as either typical angina, atypical angina, or noncardiac chest pain. Furthermore, angina should also be classified as either stable or unstable. This distinction is important because it indicates whether his short-term risk of an acute coronary event could be life-threatening. Attempts to categorize J.P.'s anginal symptoms on an objective measurement scale (e.g., Canadian Cardiovascular Society Grading Scale) can be misleading.[45] For example, a sedentary 65-year-old patient's class II symptoms may be tolerable, but the same symptoms could significantly disable an active 50-year-old patient.

J.P.'s chest pain is of a quality and duration characteristic of angina, provoked by exertion, and relieved by rest; therefore, J.P.'s constellation of symptoms can be classified as typical chest pain. J.P.'s symptoms do not occur at rest; however, they should be classified as stable angina.[1–3]

CASE 12-1, QUESTION 2: Assess J.P.'s physical examination. What signs and symptoms are relevant to the angina?

The physical examination typically provides little information about the presence of CAD. The most useful findings pertain to the cardiovascular system where heart rate and BP can be increased during an acute anginal episode. J.P.'s physical examination is characteristic of a man of his age with angina.[3] He is obese and hypertensive, but his cardiac examination is normal. The presence of murmurs would have required further workup; the absence of a third heart sound suggests that the left ventricle may be functioning normally. (See Chapter 14, Heart Failure, for a description of third heart sounds.) The absence of a fourth heart sound in J.P. is indicative of a low probability of cardiac end-organ damage resulting from systemic hypertension. His chest radiograph, which is normal, does not present evidence of other complications commonly associated with myocardial ischemia (e.g., enlarged heart, HF).

J.P.'s physical examination should also evaluate the possibility of the presence of atherosclerosis in other major vascular beds (peripheral vascular disease, cerebrovascular disease, abdominal aortic aneurysm). The presence of xanthomas would suggest severe hypercholesterolemia, but these were not noted in J.P.

Diagnostic Procedures

CASE 12-1, QUESTION 3: What other objective diagnostic procedures are helpful to confirm CAD and angina in J.P?

A 12-lead ECG indicates there is no ongoing ischemia at this time. As such, it does not help confirm the diagnosis of CAD. An echocardiogram could be used to better assess cardiac structure and function, including ruling out other potential causes for myocardial ischemia such as valvular dysfunction or pericardial disease, but would not definitively confirm the presence of CAD. Electron bean computed tomography or CCTA could be used to detect the presence of coronary atherosclerosis, but in J.P. would not offer vital prognostic information available with other testing modalities.[1]

Given J.P's current lifestyle and activity level, he would likely be able to tolerate exercise treadmill testing. Treadmill testing would be an appropriate initial diagnostic modality in J.P. due to its noninvasive nature, reliability with established protocols, as well as the ability to offer prognostic information regarding the risk of MI and death for J.P. Therefore stress testing, in this case with exercise treadmill versus pharmacologic means, is an excellent initial diagnostic modality to use in J.P.

CASE 12-1, QUESTION 4: Should J.P. undergo cardiac catheterization? How will the results of this invasive procedure influence future therapy?

Coronary catheterization and angiography is the best test for the definitive diagnosis of CAD. In addition, angiography is the most accurate means of identifying less common causes of chronic stable angina, such as coronary artery spasm.[1]

Although angiography is effective at identifying flow-limiting atherosclerotic plaques in the coronary vasculature, it cannot provide information on whether those lesions are causing clinical symptoms. Stress testing is often a more appropriate initial modality to first characterize the myocardial ischemia that takes place with exertion. Patients with significant ischemia via stress testing should then undergo cardiac catheterization to determine the nature and extent of disease. The results of angiography will be useful in determining the risk of death or MI in J.P. and, subsequently, the course of needed treatment. For example, patients who have a significant stenosis in the left main coronary artery are at high risk of death and should undergo CABG.[20]

Risk Stratification and Prognosis

CASE 12-1, QUESTION 5: After having a positive treadmill stress test and undergoing subsequent cardiac catheterization, J.P. is found to have two-vessel CAD with obstructive lesions of 55% and 70% in the right coronary artery (RCA) and circumflex arteries, respectively; the LAD coronary artery is not involved. What is his prognosis?

The prognosis of patients with stable angina is variable and dependent on the presence of other factors and comorbid conditions. The extent of CAD, quantification of ventricular function, the response to stress testing, as well as the initial clinical evaluation all help to provide an estimate of risk in a given patient. Developing a level of risk for a particular patient helps determine the appropriate treatment strategy.[1,2]

J.P.'s history and physical examination suggest he does not have HF; poor LV function would be an ominous concurrent finding. J.P. also does not have three-vessel disease or blockage of the LAD artery. J.P. does have type 2 diabetes, which elevates his risk for future cardiovascular events. The absence of other major comorbid conditions, myocardial dysfunction, along with the current extent of CAD indicates that J.P.'s prognosis at this time is favorable provided he initiate appropriate treatment strategies demonstrated to reduce morbidity and mortality in patients with CAD.[1,2]

Medical Management of Chronic Stable Angina

CASE 12-1, QUESTION 6: How should J.P. be managed at this time? Should he undergo revascularization with PCI or CABG, or be managed medically?

As discussed previously, goals for managing CAD and angina in J.P. include relief of symptoms and reduction of myocardial ischemia to improve quality of life, as well as prevention of major complications of CAD such as acute MI and death.[1] Depending on the patient, both goals may be accomplished through surgical revascularization, medical management, or both. Regardless of the treatment strategy chosen to relieve ischemic symptoms, therapies that prevent death (vasculoprotective agents) should receive priority.

Presently, CABG is not the best option for J.P. because the usual indications for surgical therapy include presence of left main CAD, presence of three-vessel disease (especially if LV function is impaired), or ineffectiveness of medical therapy.[1,20] However, revascularization with PCI is a potential option along with medical management alone. Although PCI would offer no mortality advantage over medical therapy at this time, it has been shown to decrease the incidence of recurrent symptoms in the short term (1 year).[1] If J.P. can implement aggressive lifestyle modifications and control of risk factors, progression of CAD and control of ischemic symptoms will be similar to PCI within a 5-year time frame.[42] Both strategies, including the pros and cons of PCI or medical management alone, should be offered to J.P. so that an informed decision can be made in accord with his wishes. Overall, J.P. will probably do well with medical therapy. His life expectancy depends on progression of the disease and development of other complications of CHD (HF, MI, sudden cardiac death).

RISK FACTORS AND LIFESTYLE MODIFICATIONS

CASE 12-1, QUESTION 7: What independent risk factors for CAD are present in J.P.? Which of these may be altered?

The first step in the treatment of any patient with chronic stable angina or CAD should be the modification of any existing risk factors and the adoption of a healthy lifestyle. By addressing the underlying circumstances, which likely led to the development of CAD, a significant impact can be made at halting the progression of the disease and preventing complications of CAD. Current recommendations for the goals for risk factor management are listed in Table 12-3.[23,25,26] In addition to specific risk factor goals, attention should be paid to evidence that favors specific drug therapies that have evidence supporting reductions in morbidity and mortality. Examples would include the use of HMG-CoA reductase inhibitors in the treatment of hyperlipidemia,[1,2] as well as the use of ACE inhibitors for the treatment of hypertension.[25,26]

J.P. has several risk factors for CAD, some of which cannot be altered, such as middle age, male sex, and a strong family history of CAD. Risk factors, such as hypertension, obesity, hypercholesterolemia, smoking, and possibly stress, can potentially be modified to decrease the likelihood of adverse sequelae for J.P. His hypertension should be controlled and statin therapy should be initiated (see Chapter 8, Dyslipidemias, Atherosclerosis, and Coronary Heart Disease). A fasting Hgb A_{1c} should be drawn with a goal of less than 7% (see Chapter 53, Diabetes Mellitus). Dietary modification and weight reduction for J.P. are mandatory, because they positively influence several risk factors. J.P., however, does not smoke cigarettes, which would significantly increase his cardiovascular risk.[1,22] J.P.'s active lifestyle may influence his prognosis favorably.[1]

DIETARY INTERVENTIONS

CASE 12-1, QUESTION 8: Are there any dietary patterns that J.P. can adopt that have demonstrated reductions in cardiovascular end points?

Although the positive effects of lifestyle modifications on cardiovascular risk factors are well recognized, the effect of specific lifestyle interventions on reducing hard cardiovascular end points can be underappreciated. The adoption of a healthy dietary pattern is one such example. Randomized controlled trials have demonstrated that the adoption of the Mediterranean Diet (diets emphasizing whole grains, fruit, vegetables, nuts and legumes, moderate dairy intake, moderate amounts of lean protein, and polyunsaturated fats) reduced the relative risk of MI or cardiac death by 50% to 73% as compared to a diet similar in composition to the AHA Step I diet.[46] It is important to note that in one of these studies, the Lyon Diet Heart Study, the improvements in cardiovascular morbidity and mortality occurred without significant changes in the lipid profiles of study subjects.[46] One trial found the Mediterranean Diet supplemented with either nuts or olive oil reduced cardiovascular events in patients at high risk of CVD when compared to a low fat diet.[47] Several additional trials demonstrated that patients with a history of MI who increased their intake of either fatty fish or ingested omega-3 fatty acid fish oil supplements also had reductions in cardiovascular death and

MI as compared to control patients without dietary intervention.[48] Lastly, epidemiologic studies have confirmed the results from randomized controlled trials showing that adherence to a Mediterranean diet significantly reduces cardiovascular morbidity and mortality.[46] A Mediterranean diet reduces systemic inflammation as measured by C-reactive protein, reduces the incidence of insulin resistance, and improves endothelial function. Although a great deal of attention has been directed at the increased intake of omega-3 polyunsaturated acids (eicosapentaenoic acid and docosahexaenoic acid derived from fish or α-linoleic acid derived from plants) being responsible for the observed benefits in each of these trials, multiple dietary alterations were likely in play. The results should be interpreted as the result of the adoption of a healthy dietary pattern.[22]

CASE 12-1, QUESTION 9: J.P. states he had heard that antioxidants such as vitamin E could benefit him along with a daily B vitamin. Would these supplements offer significant cardiovascular benefit for J.P.?

Because oxidation of LDL in the arterial wall is a key step in the atherosclerotic process, considerable interest exists in the theory that supplementation with high doses of antioxidants such as vitamin E, vitamin C, and β-carotene might mitigate this process and slow the progression of atherosclerosis. Early observational studies of antioxidants seemed to confirm this theory. Multiple large randomized studies, however, have shown no positive effect from supplemental intake of antioxidants such as vitamin E on the incidence of cardiovascular outcomes including MI or death.[1,49] These findings were observed in both primary and secondary prevention of cardiovascular events. J.P. should be informed that supplemental intake of vitamin E will not have any positive effect on his CVD.

Interest in the use of supplemental intake of folic acid and B vitamins stems from their ability to lower homocysteine levels. It is well established that elevated levels of homocysteine are associated with a higher incidence of CVD.[50] Despite this association, the great majority of appropriately designed, randomized, placebo-controlled studies have demonstrated that supplemental ingestion of folic acid and B vitamins has no impact in reducing cardiovascular outcomes such as MI or death[1,51] Therefore, similar to the advice for vitamin E, J.P. should be counseled that folic acid and B vitamin supplementation will not provide any tangible cardiovascular benefit.

Anti-Ischemic Drug Therapy

SUBLINGUAL NITROGLYCERIN

CASE 12-1, QUESTION 10: Should J.P. receive a prescription for SL NTG on discharge from the hospital?
If so, what education should J.P. receive with regard to the use and storage of SL NTG?

All patients with CAD, especially those with chronic stable angina, should receive a prescription for SL NTG for the treatment of acute anginal attacks.[38,39] NTG leads to vasodilation of both veins and arteries which reduces myocardial oxygen demand, thereby relieving angina. Because response to NTG varies among patients, the dosage should be individualized (Table 12-4). Most patients, however, use a dose of 0.4 mg. The administration of sublingual NTG is also useful in patients who have a good understanding of what level of exertion produces their chest pain. About 5 to 10 minutes before J.P. is about to undergo heavy exertion, he can take a sublingual NTG tablet to prevent angina.[1]

Patient education is a crucial component of ensuring SL NTG is used appropriately to treat acute anginal attacks. When angina occurs, J.P. should sit down immediately and utilize his SL NTG. If using tablets, he should place the NTG tablet under his tongue; he should not swallow it. If using the NTG spray, he should apply the spray on or under the tongue and not swallow or inhale it. Many patients experience dizziness and light-headedness, which is minimized by sitting. The onset of action is within 1 to 2 minutes, and pain usually is relieved within 3 to 5 minutes. If the pain persists or is unimproved 5 minutes after the first dose of NTG, the patient should call 9-1-1 as they may be experiencing an MI.[1] If he needs more than one dose, he can take a maximum of 1.2 mg in 15 minutes.

The tablets should be dispensed in the original, unopened manufacturer's container and stored in the original brown bottle. Because sublingual NTG tablets are degraded by heat, moisture, and light, they should be stored in a cool, dry place, but not refrigerated. The bottle should be closed tightly after each opening. Safety caps should not be used, although patients should be cautioned to keep all medications out of the reach of children. The cotton plug sometimes is difficult to remove. Therefore, it should be discarded on initial receipt of the prescription and should not be replaced. Use of cotton other than that supplied by the manufacturer should be discouraged because NTG tablets are volatile and are adsorbed by household cotton. This results in a significant loss in tablet effectiveness. Expiration dating should be monitored closely, and tablets should be replaced immediately if they are exposed to excessive light, heat, moisture, or air. Once a container is opened, the tablets should be used for only a limited time—usually from 6 months to 1 year.[1]

ADRENERGIC BLOCKERS

CASE 12-1, QUESTION 11: Given J.P.'s active lifestyle and recent history of frequent anginal attacks, the medical team wishes to optimize chronic preventative therapy for chronic stable angina. J.P. currently is receiving metformin 500 mg BID, lisinopril 10 mg once daily, and hydrochlorothiazide 25 mg once daily. His current resting heart rate and BP are 78 beats/minute and 135/90 mm Hg, respectively. Is a β-blocker the best initial option for chronic stable angina in J.P.?

Options for chronic prevention of anginal episodes include β-blockers, CCBs, long-acting nitrates, and ranolazine. Although each of these options is considered relatively equivalent in terms of ischemia prevention, current guidelines recommend that β-blockers should be administered before a nitrate or a CCB when long-term therapy is indicated.[1,2] β-Blockers are very effective at reducing anginal symptoms and ischemia, including silent myocardial ischemia.[1,2] β-Blockers also significantly increase exercise tolerance and time to ST-segment depression during exercise testing.[36] Several cohort and case–control studies have shown that β-blockers improve clinical outcomes, including reductions in mortality in patients with chronic stable angina or CAD.[52–56] In addition, recent evidence indicates that β-blockers may also slow the progression of atherosclerosis.[57] In a meta-analysis of clinical trials that compared the three classes of anti-ischemics, no differences in long-term mortality were noted. β-Blockers, however, were more effective in lowering the incidence of anginal episodes.[58] β-Blockers are generally considered the most effective class of agents at preventing silent myocardial ischemia.[3] In addition, β-blockers clearly lower morbidity and mortality in patients with CAD[17,19] and HF.[36] Overall, the body of literature available supports the recommendation that all patients with angina should receive a β-blocker as initial therapy unless contraindicated.[59] J.P. at this time does not appear to have any contraindications to β-blocker therapy, and β-blocker therapy should be initiated.

CASE 12-1, QUESTION 12: How should therapy with a β-blocker be optimized in J.P.?

All patients receiving antianginal drugs should be monitored for frequency of angina attacks and SL NTG consumption. Traditionally, clinicians have monitored the reduction in resting heart rate and have progressively increased the β-blocker dose until the resting heart rate was 55 or 60 beats/minute.[36] J.P. currently has a heart rate of 78 beats/minute and preserved BP. If J.P. continues to have preserved BP and his heart rate remains above 55 to 60 beats/minute after the initiation of β-blocker therapy, a doubling of his dose would be a reasonable increase, with close monitoring of heart rate and BP. Additional goals with β-blocker therapy include a maximum heart rate of 100 beats/minute or less with exercise. Resting heart rate less than 50 beats/minute may be acceptable, provided the patient is asymptomatic and heart block is not present. Variations in resting heart rate are normal and subject to the influence of the endogenous sympathetic nervous system and other exogenous factors, such as drugs, tobacco, and caffeine-containing beverages. β-Blockers with intrinsic sympathomimetic activity (e.g., pindolol) will not reduce the resting heart rate as much as β-blockers lacking this activity.[35]

Exercise stress testing is probably the most accurate, but least practical, method of documenting the adequacy of β-blocker therapy. During an exercise tolerance test, a β-blocker should substantially increase the time J.P. walks before developing angina. There also may be a reduction in ST-segment depression during exercise, indicating less myocardial ischemia. The rate–pressure product probably will be markedly lower, reflecting a decrease in both heart rate and systolic wall tension.[34] An alternative to conducting a formal stress test is to repeat the physical activity which produced angina during this hospitalization, namely, walking a few flights of stairs.

CASE 12-1, QUESTION 13: Would the decision to use β-blockers initially in J.P. be altered if he had a history of reactive airway disease such as asthma or PAD?

Although all β-blockers are equally effective in the treatment of angina, the addition of reactive airway disease or PAD to J.P.'s medical history would pose several relative contraindications to the use of some β-blockers. The concern directly relates to the potential for β-blockers to worsen either bronchoconstriction in the case of asthma by blunting β_2 receptors, or worsening vasoconstriction in the peripheral arteries, again, through blunting vasodilation through β_2 receptors. Although not absolute contraindications, the presence of these disease states warrants careful monitoring of β-blocker therapy during initiation and titration.[34]

Cardioselective β-blockers, such as metoprolol, are often considered in patients with reactive airway disease or PAD with the hope that β_2 receptors will be unaffected. In one meta-analysis, cardioselective β-blockers were better tolerated than nonselective β-blockers in patients with asthma.[60] Cardioselective β-blockers also are less likely to inhibit β_2-mediated vasodilation in the peripheral arterioles. Therefore, cardioselective β-blockers are preferred over nonselective β-blockers for patients with PAD and Raynaud disease.[61]

Unfortunately, cardioselectivity is not an all-or-none response; instead, it is a dose-dependent phenomenon. As the dose is increased, cardioselectivity is lost. The dose at which cardioselectivity will be lost in any given patient cannot be predicted, and even a very small dose (e.g., metoprolol 50–100 mg) could cause wheezing.[35,61] If β-blocker therapy is to be initiated in a patient with reactive airway disease or PAD, close monitoring for worsening of symptoms should occur and an alternative anti-ischemic medication should be used if symptoms worsen.

In the event that β-blocker therapy is not tolerated or considered too risky, initial therapy with a heart-rate–controlling CCB is the next best option, provided there is adequate heart rate and BP to tolerate therapy. In patients who already have low heart rate and/or marginal BP, ranolazine may be considered as an initial option. Long-acting nitrates are typically reserved for add-on therapy for reasons that will be subsequently discussed.[1]

CASE 12-1, QUESTION 14: J.P. is being discharged from the hospital today with prescriptions for SL NTG 0.4 mg tablets, metoprolol succinate 100 mg once daily, metformin 500 mg BID, and lisinopril 20 mg once daily, and education regarding diet and exercise. Is there anything else J.P. should receive for his chronic stable angina?

Antiplatelet therapy is a cornerstone in the management of a patient with atherosclerotic vascular disease. Antiplatelet therapy reduces the incidence of CVD events such as MI, stroke, and death. Although newer antiplatelet options are available, aspirin is still the first-line choice for patients with atherosclerotic vascular disease due to well-established efficacy and cost-effectiveness.[1]

The mechanism of action for aspirin's antiplatelet effect is inhibition of cyclooxygenase (see Chapter 11, Thrombosis). By acetylating the active site of cyclooxygenase, aspirin blocks the formation of prostaglandin endoperoxides from arachidonic acid. This inhibits the formation of both thromboxane and prostacyclin. Thromboxane A_2 is a potent vasoconstrictor and facilitates further activation of platelets. Prostacyclin (PGI_2) counterbalances the effect of thromboxane A_2, because it is a potent inhibitor of platelet aggregation and a vasodilator.[62]

Although it has been theorized that higher doses of aspirin would produce a higher level of efficacy than low doses, all available literature indicates that low dosages of aspirin (75–325 mg/day) are as effective as higher dosages (625–1,300 mg/day) in the treatment of patients with angina.[62] Conversely, as the aspirin dosage increases, the incidence of adverse effects, especially GI bleeding, increases. Therefore, current guidelines recommend a daily dosage of 75 to 162 mg orally for the prevention of MI and death in patients with CAD.[1] Given this information, J.P. should be advised to take aspirin at a dose of 81 mg/day to maintain efficacy but decrease the risk of adverse effects.

CASE 12-1, QUESTION 15: J.P. returns to the hospital with recurrent angina 8 weeks after he was discharged. He mentioned he stopped his metoprolol 36 hours ago when he forgot to get his prescriptions refilled. He is transported to the hospital emergency department for treatment of angina unresponsive to 3 NTG tablets. How could J.P.'s situation have been avoided?

The β-blocker withdrawal syndrome is a rebound phenomenon resulting from heightened β-receptor density and sensitivity (i.e., upregulation) subsequent to receptor blockade. It places patients with CAD at high risk for adverse cardiovascular events, which may include acute MI and sudden cardiac death. An "overshoot" in heart rate, as a consequence of sympathoadrenal activity from abrupt β-blocker withdrawal increases myocardial oxygen demand and platelet aggregation. Withdrawal syndromes may be less severe in patients taking β-blockers with partial agonist activity.[34–36]

If β-blockers are to be discontinued, a gradual tapering schedule (preferably for 1–2 weeks) should be used. Shorter periods for β-blocker withdrawal (e.g., 2–3 days) have been proposed, although the optimal strategy for discontinuation is not known. Ensuring that β-blockers are tapered and that the patient is reasonably monitored for adverse events for the duration of the taper is imperative. Patients should limit physical activity throughout the β-blocker withdrawal period and seek prompt medical attention when angina symptoms become apparent. Patients should be warned not to precipitously discontinue their β-blockers. Failure to renew prescriptions and financial hardship are common reasons for abrupt discontinuation, and clinicians need to have sufficient professional rapport with patients to understand when patients encounter difficulties in obtaining medications.

LONG-ACTING NITRATES

CASE 12-1, QUESTION 16: J.P. recovers quickly and is discharged from the hospital after 48 hours. He does well during the next several months, but he is still bothered by occasional angina episodes, two to four times a week. The attacks usually are precipitated by strenuous work and are relieved by rest and two or three NTG tablets. The quality and location of the pain are unchanged, although the duration has increased by 1 or 2 minutes. He follows a low-cholesterol, no-added-salt diet.

Physical examination is unchanged except for a 20-lb weight loss. Vital signs include the following: supine BP, 119/76 mm Hg; heart rate, 60 beats/minute; and respiratory rate, 12 breaths/minute. J.P.'s cardiologist elected to start a long-acting prophylactic nitrate (isosorbide mononitrate) as well as continuing his metoprolol succinate (100 mg daily), lisinopril (20 mg daily), aspirin (81 mg daily), and metformin (500 mg twice daily). Is a long-acting nitrate the best add-on option for J.P.'s chronic stable angina?

Long-acting nitrates occupy a key role in the prevention of angina of all types. The goals of therapy are to decrease the number, severity, and duration of J.P.'s anginal attacks. A CCB could be prescribed for J.P. instead of isosorbide mononitrate because he has no contraindications to this class of drugs. A CCB would have been a good alternative if his BP had remained elevated, but for now, J.P.'s BP and pulse are within a desired range. Nitrates can also affect BP, but will likely do so to a lesser extent than CCBs. Because sublingual nitrates were well tolerated by J.P., a long-acting nitrate would be acceptable. If a CCB is considered at this point, a DHP should be used because they have no effect on heart rate, unlike diltiazem or verapamil. Lastly, ranolazine would be an option for add-on therapy, especially if J.P. experiences any adverse hemodynamic effects from either a CCB or long-acting nitrate. Ultimately, the decision for additional therapy is based on the prescriber's personal choice and past experience, as well as the entire spectrum of the patient's disease complex.[63]

CASE 12-1, QUESTION 17: Will J.P. develop tolerance to the long-acting nitrate?

Although not completely understood, several mechanisms of nitrate tolerance have been proposed, including the increased production of catecholamines, plasma volume expansion, and activation of the renin-angiotensin-aldosterone system.[64]

All organic nitrates exhibit similar hemodynamic effects through a common pharmacologic mechanism; yet, the differing pharmacokinetic profiles of the nitrate delivery systems lead to a variation in the development of tolerance.[65] Short-acting formulations (e.g., SL NTG, oral NTG spray, and SL isosorbide dinitrate) are not likely to induce tolerance given their rapid onset of action and short duration of effect. Oral nitrates and transdermal products, both having an extended duration of action, are likely to induce tolerance.

Intermittent application of transdermal NTG can limit tolerance development in patients with both chronic stable angina and HF. The effects of continuous (24 hours/day) and intermittent (16 hours/day) transdermal NTG (10 mg/day) were compared in 12 men with chronic stable angina who also were being treated with β-blockers or CCB.[66] Nitrate efficacy was maintained with intermittent treatment and an 8-hour nitrate-free interval. Tolerance to the antianginal effects occurred, however, with continuous treatment. Twelve-hour intermittent patch therapy also prevents tolerance.[67] The minimal time necessary for a nitrate-free interval is unknown. Nitrate dosing schedules should be arranged to permit a nitrate-free interval during which time the patient may receive angina protection from β-blockers, CCBs, or ranolazine. Most often, this nitrate-free interval is arranged during the night because angina is more likely to occur during the workday. Patients with nocturnal or early morning angina should arrange their nitrate-free interval during the day.[68]

Despite the availability of nitrate preparations that can be dosed once or twice a day (isosorbide mononitrate), oral isosorbide dinitrate is still commonly used in a variety of settings for the treatment of angina. Isosorbide dinitrate needs to be dosed three times a day, and presents a challenge in ensuring patients have a nitrate-free interval. If J.P. were to receive isosorbide dinitrate, he should take his oral nitrate at 7 AM, noon, and 5 PM because his exercise-induced angina is likely to occur during daylight hours. If he were to take isosorbide dinitrate on a more traditional three-times-a-day or every-8-hours schedule, he would be in danger of not having an adequate nitrate-free interval. Because long-acting nitrates must be dosed intermittently to avoid tolerance, metoprolol therapy will provide J.P. with continuous protection, even during the nitrate-free interval. Although J.P. uses a long-acting nitrate, he still will respond favorably to sublingual NTG. No evidence indicates that use of long-acting nitrates leads to resistance or tolerance to the effects of sublingual NTG.

CASE 12-1, QUESTION 18: Does isosorbide mononitrate offer any distinct advantages over other nitrate preparations for angina prophylaxis?

Isosorbide mononitrate is the primary metabolite of isosorbide dinitrate. In fact, most of the clinical activity of isosorbide dinitrate is due to the mononitrate. Therefore, both drugs share a similar pharmacology. Isosorbide mononitrate does not undergo first-pass metabolism and has no active metabolites. Its oral bioavailability is almost 100%, and its overall elimination half-life is about 5 hours.[65] Maximal serum concentrations are observed 30 to 60 minutes after a dose. To minimize the potential development of nitrate tolerance, isosorbide mononitrate should be used in a twice-daily, asymmetric dosing regimen in which the first dose is taken on awakening and the second dose about 7 hours later. Because of this unconventional dosing pattern and the availability of the extended-release product, which can be taken once a day, most use of isosorbide mononitrate is in the form of the extended-release preparation. Pharmacists must be sure to recognize the difference between these two products.

General precautions and adverse reactions for isosorbide mononitrate are similar to those for the other nitrates. Potential advantages for the clinical use of isosorbide mononitrate are less dosage fluctuation because of the absence of presystemic clearance and an effective once-daily or twice-daily dosing schedule, which could perhaps lead to improved patient adherence. Nevertheless, isosorbide dinitrate is effective clinically when administered two or three times a day and is a viable alternative.

CASE 12-1, QUESTION 19: J.P. likes the idea of using topical nitrates instead of an oral agent. Are the transdermal patches a viable alternative?

Transdermal NTG patches were originally designed to provide anti-ischemic protection with once-daily application. The concept of a compact, easy-to-apply transdermal NTG patch prompted pharmaceutical manufacturers to design a number of products, which the FDA subsequently approved based on plasma level data, not clinical efficacy studies. Subsequently, the shortcomings of plasma level data have become apparent and prompted numerous clinical efficacy studies.

Transdermal NTG therapy has been shown to increase exercise duration and maintain an anti-ischemic effect for 12 hours after patch application. These beneficial responses remained consistent throughout 30 days of therapy. No significant nitrate tolerance or rebound was noted when the patch was applied for not more than 12 of 24 hours.[65]

Although the various patches use different pharmaceutical delivery systems, clear-cut advantages of one over another are not apparent. Despite variations in surface area and NTG content, the most important common denominator of the transdermal NTG systems is the amount of drug released per hour expressed as the release rate (e.g., 0.2 mg/hour). Each product label includes this information. Low dosages (0.2–0.4 mg/hour) may not produce sufficient plasma and tissue concentrations to produce a clinically significant effect[3]; however, it is still recommended to start with a low-dose patch and titrate upward as needed. Because the skin is the major factor influencing NTG absorption rate, product release characteristics do not favor one system over another. Contact dermatitis has been reported with the transdermal patches. Patient instructions are included with the patches and should be reviewed with the patient, emphasizing the appropriate time for application of the patch, removal of the patch, as well as the appropriate sites on the body where the patch should be placed.

CALCIUM-CHANNEL BLOCKERS

CASE 12-2

QUESTION 1: B.N., a 56-year-old man, has just undergone cardiac catheterization, which showed two-vessel CAD with obstructions of 55% and 65% in the right coronary and circumflex coronary arteries, respectively. Before catheterization he had a 2- to 3-month history of exertional angina for which his primary care physician prescribed sublingual NTG tablets (0.4 mg) and oral isosorbide mononitrate (60 mg once daily). B.N. discontinued the use of isosorbide mononitrate after a few weeks due to intolerable headaches. His medical history includes asthma, hypertension, and hyperlipidemia. Currently, his other medications include losartan 100 mg once daily, fluticasone inhaler two puffs twice daily, albuterol inhaler two puffs as needed, aspirin 81 mg daily, and atorvastatin 20 mg daily. Current vital signs include a resting heart rate of 75 beats/minute, BP of 125/80 mm Hg, and respiratory rate of 14 breaths/minute. His physician begins antianginal therapy with oral diltiazem 120 mg once daily. Is this a good option for B.N. and his chronic stable angina?

CCBs are effective in both vasospastic and classic exertional angina. These drugs relieve vasospasm of the large coronary arteries and, as a result, are effective in treating Prinzmetal variant angina. Their beneficial effect in chronic stable (effort-induced) angina is the result of multiple factors. Their vasodilatory effects in the coronary circulation increase myocardial oxygen supply, whereas dilation of the peripheral arterioles leads to a reduction in myocardial oxygen demand. Because coronary vasospasm can occur at the site of an atherosclerotic plaque, a CCB is particularly useful in patients who have a vasospastic component to their angina.[40,69]

Although β-blockers are considered the drugs of choice when instituting antianginal therapy[1], data indicate that the selection of a heart rate–lowering CCB may also be a reasonable first-line choice. CCBs and β-blockers appear to provide equivalent efficacy in head-to-head trials of chronic stable angina.[70,71] In addition, the available head-to-head trials with sufficient numbers also suggest that CCBs and β-blockers produce similar effects on cardiovascular outcomes and mortality in patients with chronic stable angina.[72,73] In addition, several trials in the setting of hypertension with CAD have demonstrated that CCBs can produce meaningful reductions in mortality.[74–77] It would appear that either a heart rate–lowering CCB, or a β-blocker, may be considered relatively equal options and initial therapy for chronic stable angina. The selection of a particular class will likely be dictated by patient characteristics.

In the case of B.N., his asthma may be worsened by the addition of a β-blocker. Although a cardioselective β-blocker could be tried to see if B.N. could tolerate it, a heart rate–lowering CCB is a good alternative to a β-blocker for the treatment of angina in this situation. The choice of a CCB as initial therapy in this patient is appropriate due to B.N.'s previous intolerance to nitrates and because nitrate therapy requires a nitrate-free period.[1]

Given B.N.'s current heart rate and BP, the selection of a heart rate–lowering CCB seems most appropriate. However, the distinct pharmacologic and adverse event profiles of the various classes may dictate agent selection from patient to patient. Some side effects of CCBs reflect an extension of their hemodynamic and electrophysiologic profiles and, therefore, are predictable (Table 12-6). DHP-induced hypotension and dizziness occur in approximately 15% of patients. Patients also may complain of light-headedness, facial flushing, headache, and nausea. Swelling of the lower legs and ankles (peripheral edema) is related to the potent peripheral vasodilating effects of these agents. The non-DHPs, verapamil and diltiazem, have similar side effect profiles, although diltiazem appears to be better tolerated. The lower incidence of side effects reported with diltiazem, compared with verapamil, may reflect a true difference or, perhaps, less aggressive dosing regimens. Both drugs can cause sinus bradycardia and worsen already existing conduction defects and heart block.[40,69] Neither should be used in patients with sick sinus syndrome or advanced degrees of heart block unless a functioning ventricular pacemaker is present. Patients should be monitored for signs of worsening HF, such as SOB, weight gain, and peripheral edema. Verapamil-induced constipation can be particularly troublesome to the elderly.[40,64]

Appreciation for the individual side effect profiles helps determine preference for one CCB over another. B.N. is not likely to experience major side effects with either verapamil or diltiazem.

CASE 12-2, QUESTION 2: On questioning, B.N. does not report any previous adverse events or tolerance issues with an ACE inhibitor. Is an ARB appropriate to use in B.N, or should he be switched to an ACE inhibitor for his CAD?

As discussed previously, the totality of available evidence supports the role of ACE inhibitors in reducing total mortality, cardiovascular mortality, nonfatal MI, and stroke in patients with stable IHD and preserved ventricular function. Although in theory ARBs should produce the same beneficial effects as ACE inhibitors in patients with atherosclerosis, there are far fewer clinical trials with ARBs. The best supporting evidence comes from the TRANSCEND and ONTARGET trials, both of which suggest ARBs produce similar benefits as ACE inhibitors in preventing CVD events.[78,79] Based on these trials, it would be reasonable to continue ARB therapy in B.N. at this time given he has demonstrated the ability to tolerate the medication. It would not be unreasonable though to discuss with B.N. the possibility of switching to an ACE inhibitor given the substantial body of evidence that exists for patients with CAD. The combination of an ACE inhibitor and ARB does not offer any increased benefit but does increase the risk of hyperkalemia and renal insufficiency.[79]

Table 12-6

Calcium-Channel Blocker Hemodynamic and Electrophysiologic Profile[40,69]

Effect	Dihydropyridine Derivatives[a]	Diltiazem	Verapamil
Peripheral vasodilation[b]	+++	++	++
Coronary vasodilation[b]	+++	+++	++
Negative inotropes[c]	±	++	+++
AV node suppression[c]	±	+	++
Heart rate	Increase (reflex)	Decrease or unchanged	Decrease or unchanged
Pharmacokinetics[d]			
Dosing[e]			
Side Effects			
Nausea, vomiting	+ (most)	+/1	±
Constipation	Not observed	±	+
Hypotension, dizziness[f]	++	+	+
Flushing, headache	++	+	+
Bradycardia, HF symptoms	±	+	++
Reflex tachycardia, angina	+[f]	Not observed	Not observed
Peripheral edema	+	±	±

[a]Dihydropyridine derivatives that are US Food and Drug Administration approved for angina: amlodipine (Norvasc), nicardipine (Cardene), and nifedipine (Adalat, Procardia).
[b]Peripheral and coronary vasodilation helpful for angina, hypertension, and possibly HF, but peripheral dilation is the basis for side effects of flushing, headache, and hypotension.
[c]AV node suppression is helpful for controlling supraventricular arrhythmias, but this property plus the negative inotropic effect may worsen HF. Nifedipine has less negative inotropic effect than verapamil and diltiazem, but still may worsen HF. Amlodipine may have the least negative inotropic effect.
[d]All have poor bioavailability owing to high first-pass metabolism and all are eliminated primarily by hepatic metabolism; intradivisional and interindividual variability in bioavailability and metabolism is extensive. Diltiazem, nifedipine, nicardipine, and verapamil have a short half-life (<5 hours) requiring frequent dosing or use of sustained-release products. Amlodipine, isradipine (8 hours), and felodipine (10–20 hours) have longer half-lives.
[e]See Table 12-5
[f]Hypotension and reflex tachycardia most with immediate-release nifedipine, occasional with immediate-release diltiazem and verapamil, minimal with sustained-release products or intrinsically long-acting agents.

CASE 12-2, QUESTION 3: Six months later, B.N. returns to see his physician. His current therapy consists of SL NTG 0.4 mg tablets, losartan 100 mg once daily, fluticasone inhaler two puffs twice daily, albuterol inhaler two puffs as needed, aspirin 81 mg daily, atorvastatin 20 mg daily, and diltiazem 180 mg once daily. Current vitals include a resting heart rate of 55 beats/minute, BP of 115/65 mm Hg, and respiratory rate of 10 breaths/minute. B.N. states he still is having roughly three to four anginal attacks per week when he exerts himself doing yard work. Would ranolazine be a therapeutic option for his chronic stable angina at this time?

Although higher doses of diltiazem might be attempted in B.N., his current heart rate and BP would likely prevent further titrating of therapy. β-Blocker therapy is not a good option due to the potential reduction in heart rate and asthma. Thus, ranolazine represents a good option for B.N. at this time due to the absence of heart rate and BP-lowering effects with ranolazine. Several large, randomized studies with ranolazine have been conducted, all demonstrating its effectiveness at reducing ischemia and angina when added to existing therapy. The Monotherapy Assessment of Ranolazine in Stable Angina (MARISA) trial randomly assigned patients in a crossover fashion who had met screening criteria to either escalating doses of ranolazine (500 mg BID, 1,000 mg BID, 1,500 mg BID) or placebo. All other antianginal agents, except for SL NTG, were discontinued. Ranolazine significantly increased exercise duration, time to onset of angina, and 1-mm ST-segment depression during exercise treadmill testing.[80] Similar results were seen in the Combination Assessment of Ranolazine in Stable Angina (CARISA) trial in which ranolazine (500 mg BID, 750 mg BID, 1,000 mg BID) was added to antianginal monotherapy that consisted of atenolol, diltiazem, or amlodopine.[81] The Efficacy of Ranolazine in Chronic Angina (ERICA) trial assessed the effects of ranolazine added to amlodipine 10 mg/day. Up to one-half of the patients enrolled in ERICA were also on a long-acting nitrate. Patients were randomly assigned to either placebo or ranolazine 500 mg/day for 1 week and then to 1,000 mg/day for an additional 6 weeks. Patients receiving 1,000 mg/day of ranolazine had a significant reduction in both the number of weekly anginal attacks, as well as the number of SL NTG tablets used.[82] A reduction in the frequency of angina was also seen in patients with CAD and diabetes mellitus when ranolazine was added in the Type 2 Diabetes Evaluation of Ranolazine in Subjects with Chronic Stable Angina (TERISA) study.[83] Ranolazine was well tolerated in all four of these trials with the most common side effects being dizziness, constipation, nausea, and headache. The incidence of adverse effects increased with increasing doses. No other significant adverse effects were noted, although it is important to note that the duration of these trials was limited.[41]

Information regarding the safety of ranolazine in patients with longer drug exposure came from the Ranolazine Open Label Experience (ROLE) program,[84] which followed patients from the MARISA and CARISA trials who continued in an open-label extension program. A total of 746 patients initially entered the 6-year run-on safety program. At the time of publication, the mean duration of therapy was 2.82 years, with 23.3% of patients discontinuing therapy. One-half of the withdrawals were because of adverse events, but the incidence of common adverse effects did not seem to change from that seen in the randomized portions of the clinical trials. Mortality rates at both 1 year (2.8%) and 2 years (5.6%) indicate no adverse risk of ranolazine on overall mortality.

The Metabolic Efficiency with Ranolazine for Less Ischemia in Non–ST-Elevation Acute Coronary Syndrome (MERLIN)-TIMI 36 trial[85] randomly assigned patients to ranolazine or placebo in the setting of ACS. Ranolazine was administered as an intravenous (IV) infusion for 12 to 96 hours, then converted to 1,000 mg twice daily. Patients were assessed for clinical end points during the acute hospitalization, then every 4 months thereafter. The incidence of recurrent ischemia was significantly reduced with ranolazine providing additional support for the efficacy of ranolazine in treating chronic stable angina. Although ranolazine appeared to offer no benefit in the setting of ACS, significant long-term safety data were seen in the trial. Importantly, the risk of mortality, sudden cardiac death, or symptomatic arrhythmias was not increased with ranolazine versus placebo. In fact, the incidence of arrhythmias in the first 7 days, as documented by Holter monitor, was significantly lower with ranolazine than with placebo.[86] This was an important finding given ranolazine produces a dose-dependent increase in the QT interval.[15,41] As QT prolongation activity has been associated with proarrhythmia in other medications, results from the MERLIN trial are reassuring that ranolazine appears to be safe to use for chronic treatment of patients with stable angina.

B.N. is at goal heart rate, and his BP is well controlled on his current regimen, but he continues to have anginal symptoms. Given the demonstrated efficacy in relieving anginal symptoms, as well as the safety profile in a patient like B.N., ranolazine would be an excellent option for him for additional angina control.

Case 12-2, Question 4: How should ranolazine be dosed in B.N.?

Ranolazine is marketed as an extended-release tablet formulation that should be dosed twice daily. Maximal plasma concentrations are observed 4 to 6 hours after administration of the extended-release formulation with a terminal half-life of 7 hours. With twice-daily dosing of the extended-release preparation, a more favorable peak-to-trough fluctuation of 1.6 is observed.[41] Steady-state is typically reached within 3 days and oral bioavailability is 30% to 55%. Ranolazine is primarily metabolized by the liver through CYP3A4 (70%–85%) and CYP2D6 (10%–15%). Ranolazine also is a substrate for P-glycoprotein.[15,41] Patients should initially be started at an oral dose of 500 mg twice daily, which can be titrated up to a maximal dose of 1,000 mg twice daily.[120]

Although ranolazine is an option in the treatment of chronic stable angina, careful patient selection is required for the drug to be used safely and effectively.[120] Table 12-7 summarizes significant issues, which should be evaluated when the drug is being considered for a patient. For B.N., the main issue is the drug–drug interaction with diltiazem, and the maximum dose of ranolazine that should be used in patients receiving diltiazem is 500 mg twice daily. B.N. should be monitored closely for possible increased adverse effects with ranolazine.

CASE 12-3

Question 1: E.R. is a 58-year-old woman with a history of chronic stable angina for the last several years that has been managed primarily with medical therapy. Her current medications include oral isosorbide mononitrate 120 mg daily, oral metoprolol succinate 200 mg daily, ranolazine 1,000 mg twice daily, fluticasone two puffs BID, albuterol two puffs as needed, NTG spray 0.4 mg as needed for chest pain, and enteric-coated aspirin 81 mg/day. Today she returns to your pharmacy to obtain refills of her medications with her 64-year-old brother who wants to know if he should be taking an aspirin a day to prevent heart disease. His only medical history consists of hypertension for which he is taking oral hydrochlorothiazide 25 mg every day. Is primary prevention of CAD with aspirin appropriate for E.R.'s brother?

Table 12-7

Considerations for the Use of Ranolazine in Patients with Chronic Stable Angina[15,41,120]

Clinical Issue	Recommended Management Strategy
Renal insufficiency	Ranolazine plasma levels may increase up to 50%. Caution with dose titration to maximal recommended dose
Hepatic insufficiency	Ranolazine is contraindicated in patients with clinically significant hepatic impairment
Drug Interactions: Effects on Ranolazine	
Strong CYP3A4 inhibitors	Plasma concentrations of ranolazine are significantly elevated when combined with potent inhibitors of CYP3A4. Ranolazine is contraindicated in patients receiving strong CYP3A4 inhibitors (ketoconazole, clarithromycin, nelfinavir, etc.)
Moderate CYP3A4 inhibitors	Limit the dose of ranolazine to 500 mg twice daily in patients receiving moderate inhibitors of CYP3A4 (diltiazem, verapamil, erythromycin, fluconazole, etc.)
CYP3A4 inducers	Coadministration of ranolazine with CYP3A4 inducers is contraindicated and should be avoided
P-glycoprotein inhibitors	Caution should be exercised when coadministering ranolazine with P-glycoprotein inhibitors, and the dose of ranolazine may need to be lowered based on clinical response
Drug Interactions: Effects on Other Medications	
Simvastatin	Plasma levels of simvastatin are increased twofold with coadministration with ranolazine through CYP3A4 inhibition by ranolazine; closely monitor for adverse effects (e.g., myositis) from simvastatin
Digoxin	Ranolazine coadministration increases plasma concentrations of digoxin by 1.5 times. Adjust dose of digoxin accordingly to maintain desired therapeutic level and response
CYP2D6 substrates	Ranolazine can inhibit the activity of CYP2D6, and plasma concentrations of 2D6 substrates (β-blockers, tricyclic antidepressants, antipsychotics) may be increased and lower doses of these agents may be required
QT prolongation	Caution is recommended if the patient is on other QT prolonging drugs, or has QT prolongation as baseline

The question of whether aspirin is valuable in the primary prevention of cardiovascular events has been debated for more than 20 years. The absolute risk–benefit ratio for aspirin in primary prevention will depend on the overall absolute risk of vascular ischemic events. Several meta-analyses suggest that any benefit for aspirin in reducing ischemic events is offset by an increase in bleeding, resulting in no net clinical benefit.[87–90]

In 2009, the US Preventative Services Task Force developed updated guidelines for aspirin use in primary prevention incorporating at the time of the most recent published evidence.[91] Recommendations are differentiated initially by age and sex, recognizing that the ischemic benefit varies between men (reduction in nonfatal MI) and women (reduction in ischemic stroke). Aspirin for primary prevention may be considered for men aged 45 to 79 years, and in women aged 55 to 78 years. Because E.R.'s brother is 64 years of age, it is appropriate for him to consider the use of aspirin for primary prevention. The first step is to calculate what his risk is for developing CVD.[25] This can be done by using a validated risk assessment scoring system, such as the Framingham risk score (see Chapter 8, Dyslipidemias, Atherosclerosis, and Coronary Heart Disease). Based on his age, if his 10-year risk of CVD is greater than 9%, the CVD benefit with aspirin will outweigh any potential bleeding harm according to the US Preventative Service Guidelines.[91] Recognizing the existing controversy surrounding the use of aspirin for primary prevention, a thorough review of the potential risk and benefits should take place with E.R.'s brother so that he may make the most informed decision possible.

Case 12-3, Question 2: E.R also buys a bottle of over-the-counter ibuprofen. On further questioning, you learn that E.R. suffers from occasional back and knee pain and uses ibuprofen three to five times a week for pain relief. How should E.R. be educated regarding the use of ibuprofen and aspirin concomitantly?

In 2006, the FDA released a warning statement on the concomitant use of both aspirin and ibuprofen. The impetus for the statement was the growing recognition that nonsteroidal antiinflammatory drugs (NSAIDs), in particular ibuprofen, may attenuate the antiplatelet effects of low-dose aspirin. This FDA warning was then followed by an updated scientific statement, from the AHA.[92] The mechanism of this interaction is that both aspirin and nonselective NSAIDs bind to the same acetylation sites of the cyclooxygenase enzyme. Although aspirin does this in a nonreversible fashion, binding by an NSAID occurs in a reversible fashion. If an NSAID, such as ibuprofen, is present, aspirin will be unable to bind to its site of action, and will be rapidly cleared from the plasma. The result is the patient will not receive the antiplatelet benefit of aspirin.

E.R. should be counseled on the consequences of the interaction between her aspirin and ibuprofen. Additionally, if she can avoid or at least minimize (both dose and duration) the use of ibuprofen, the effect on her cardiovascular health would be optimized. If occasional use of ibuprofen cannot be avoided, it should be administered to minimize the potential for interacting with her aspirin. This would include taking ibuprofen at least 2 hours after her daily dose of aspirin, as well as taking her daily aspirin dose at least 8 hours after the last dose of ibuprofen. Although similar concerns exist for other nonselective NSAIDs (naproxen, diclofenac), no formal recommendations exist on how to manage concomitant use of these agents with aspirin.[92] Beyond the potential drug–drug interaction with aspirin therapy, there has emerged a large body of observational evidence that the use of NSAIDs in patients with underlying CVD may increase the risk of major adverse cardiovascular events. Although the underlying mechanisms remain to be determined, clinicians should minimize the use of NSAIDs if possible in patients with underlying CVD.[93]

REVASCULARIZATION

Percutaneous Coronary Intervention

Case 12-3, Question 3: Nine months later, E.R. returns to her cardiologist stating that her chronic angina has been worsening. She is experiencing chest pain more frequently and much sooner when she does any type of physical activity. Her current medications are the same as discussed previously and it is felt that her medical management has been optimized as much as possible. After discussions with her cardiologist, she elects to undergo revascularization with PCI for symptom relief. What is the current standard for prevention of acute complications during PCI?

PCI, also known as angioplasty, involves the percutaneous insertion of a balloon catheter into the femoral or brachial artery. The catheter is advanced up the aorta and into the coronary arteries at the coronary sinus. PCI initially involved the inflation of a catheter-borne balloon that mechanically dilated a coronary artery obstruction through arterial intimal disruption, plaque fissuring, and stretching of the arterial wall. Balloon inflations were repeated until the plaque was compressed and coronary blood flow resumed. Since then, alternative devices have been developed, including rotational blades designed to remove atheromatous material, lasers to ablate plaques, and intracoronary stents that are designed to maintain the patency of the vessel after it is reopened.[94] Stents can be of the bare-metal (BMS) variety, or contain a drug impregnated on the surface of the stent to prevent restenosis (DES). It is estimated that more than 1,265,000 PCI procedures are performed in the United States each year. An overwhelming majority of these procedures involve placement of a BMS or DES (Fig. 12-5). PCI is indicated in patients with single-vessel or multi-vessel disease and who are either symptomatic or asymptomatic.[20,94,95]

Because of mechanical disruption of the atherosclerotic plaques and exposure of plaque contents to the bloodstream during PCI, potent antiplatelet and antithrombotic strategies are needed to prevent acute thrombotic events such as MI and death. Current strategies in patients undergoing elective PCI involve the administration of aspirin, a $P2Y_{12}$ antagonist (clopidogrel, prasugrel, or ticagrelor), an antithrombin agent, and occasionally

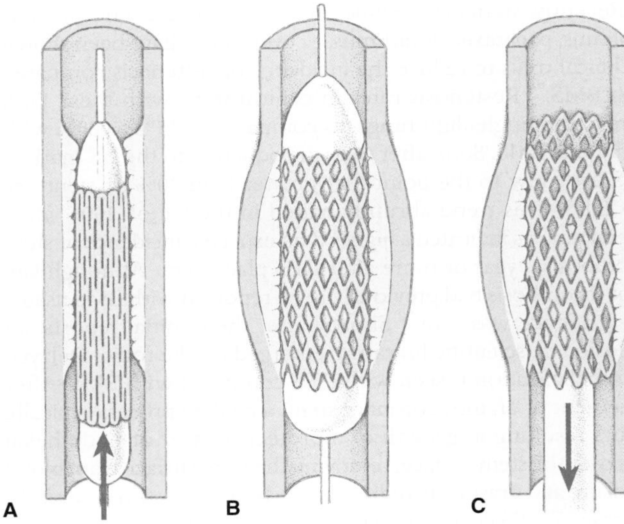

Figure 12-5 Vascular stent. **A:** A balloon catheter positions the stent at the site of arterial stenosis. **B:** Inflation of the balloon dilates the artery and expands the stent. **C:** The balloon is collapsed and withdrawn, leaving the expanded stent in position. (Illustration by Neil O. Hardy, Westpoint, CT.)

a glycoprotein (GP) IIb/IIIa receptor antagonist in selected patients. Although ticagrelor and prasugrel represent alternatives to clopidogrel in patients undergoing PCI, current ACC/AHA guidelines recommend their use only in patients undergoing PCI in the setting of ACS. In patients not taking aspirin on a daily basis, 300 to 325 mg of aspirin should be given at least 2 hours before the procedure. Patients currently on daily aspirin therapy should receive 75 to 325 mg of aspirin before PCI is performed. A 600-mg loading dose of clopidogrel on or before the time of the procedure is currently recommended, producing an antiplatelet action within 2 hours.[16,17,20,95] Adequate antithrombin therapy such as unfractionated heparin, the low-molecular-weight heparin enoxaparin, or the direct thrombin inhibitor bivalirudin should be used in patients having elective PCI.[20,95] (See Chapter 13, Acute Coronary Syndrome, for more information.)

CASE 12-3, QUESTION 4: E.R. undergoes PCI plus placement of a DES to address a 75% lesion in her proximal left circumflex artery. What advantages and disadvantages are there in the decision to place a DES versus a BMS?

The overall success of any procedure is directly related to the experience of the operator, patient factors (such as LV function or number of vessels treated), and the equipment used. In patients receiving balloon angioplasty alone (without stent placement), repeat revascularization procedures (either repeat angioplasty or surgery) may be required in as many as 32% to 40% of cases because of lesion recurrence at the angioplasty site. The process is known as restenosis.[94] Many pharmacologic strategies have been studied in an attempt to reduce the risk of restenosis. The outcome with most methods has been disappointing. The only strategy that has been associated with a decrease in restenosis is the use of intraluminal stents.[94] Stents are essentially metal scaffolding devices placed into the vessel after balloon inflation has taken place. They provide a physical barrier to the recurrence of a significant stenosis at the site. One of the early drawbacks of the use of stents was the need for complicated antithrombotic regimens, including aspirin, heparin, dipyridamole, and warfarin, to prevent in-stent thrombosis. DAPT—a combination of a $P2Y_{12}$ antagonist and aspirin—is effective at reducing in-stent thrombosis and is now recommended for use after stent placement.[20,95] The duration of DAPT will depend on the type of stent used, as well as other clinical characteristics of the patient.

Recently, stents that elude antiproliferative agents such as sirolimus, paclitaxel, zotarlimus, or everolimus have been shown in clinical trials to reduce the incidence of restenosis compared with BMS.[96] Restenosis rates in clinical trials with these DES were in the single-digit range, as compared to 15% to 20% with traditional BMS. Soon after their introduction to the US market, DES use grew to the point that greater than 90% of stent use was DES. This trend abruptly halted in the fall of 2006 when several reports indicated a higher than expected incidence of stent thrombosis a year or more after DES placement. Although late stent thrombosis had previously been reported with BMS usage, the incidence was rare.[20] Shortly after these initial reports, an explosion of scientific literature emerged on the topic. Delayed endothelialization is seen with DES compared with BMS. After placement of an intracoronary stent, a healing process typically occurs resulting in growth of a protective layer of endothelial cells over the stent surface, removing the stent surface from blood exposure and drastically reducing the stimulus for thrombosis. In the case of DES coated with paclitaxel, sirolimus, or everolimus, cellular growth may be inhibited, significantly impairing endothelialization of the stent surface. In a small number of patients, endothelialization does not seem to occur at all. In this scenario, the stent structure remains continually exposed to flowing blood and is a potent stimulus for thrombosis.[97] Because of the concerns of late stent thrombosis, the usage of DES has decreased. Some use of DES is likely to continue, however, owing to the tangible benefits in reduction of revascularization procedures in some patients. Therefore, practitioners will need to continue to stay abreast of evolving information regarding appropriate strategies to prevent late stent thrombosis.

One critical issue that has been identified as a cause of late stent thrombosis with DES is the premature discontinuation of DAPT. As such, consideration of whether the patient is likely to comply with aspirin and $P2Y_{12}$ antagonist therapy, or afford such therapy based on insurance status, has become a significant factor in the decision process between using a BMS or DES. Previous recommendations called for varying durations of combined therapy, depending on the type of stent used. Because of the recognition of a delayed healing response to DES, current guidelines recommend at least 1 year of DAPT in patients receiving a DES if patients are not at an elevated risk of bleeding. For BMS placement, DAPT should continue for a minimum of 1 month, and up to 1 year ideally, but this extended duration is not as critical as it is in the setting of DES placement. After PCI, it is reasonable to use aspirin 81 mg daily rather than higher doses.[20] The dose of clopidogrel should be 75 mg/day.[20,95]

CASE 12-3, QUESTION 5: Would revascularization therapy with coronary artery bypass grafting have been a better option for E.R. than PCI and stent placement?

Coronary artery bypass grafting is a complicated surgical procedure during which an atherosclerotic vessel is bypassed using either a patient's saphenous vein or internal mammary artery (IMA; Fig. 12-6). The graft (i.e., the saphenous vein or IMA) then allows blood to flow past the obstruction in the native vessel. The goals of antianginal therapy, whether medical (pharmacologic) or revascularization, remain unchanged: (a) to prolong life, (b) to prevent MI, and (c) to improve the quality of life.

The outcomes of medical therapy, PCI, and revascularization with CABG have been compared, and current guidelines are available.[1,21] When compared with medical treatment in patients who would not be considered high risk, PCI in general offers no improvement in the long-term incidence of MI or cardiovascular death, but significantly reduces symptoms.[1] Because of her escalating symptoms on triple drug therapy, the choice of PCI for E.R. is justified.

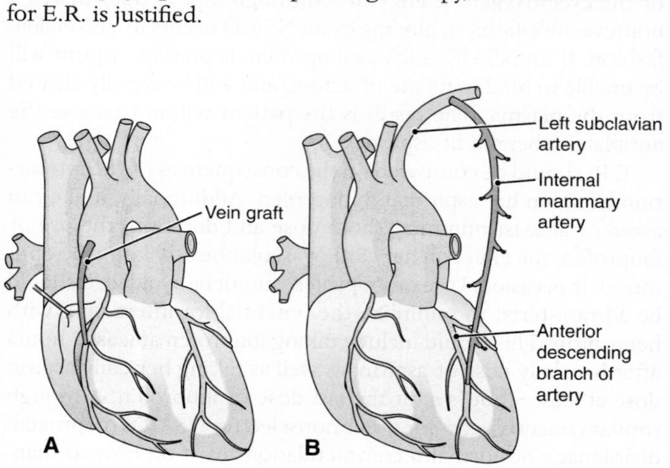

Figure 12-6 Coronary artery bypass graft (CABG). **A:** A segment of the saphenous vein carries blood from the aorta to a part of the right coronary artery that is distal to an occlusion. **B:** The mammary artery is used to bypass an obstruction in the left anterior descending (LAD) coronary artery. (Reprinted with permission from Cohen BJ. *Medical Terminology*. 4th ed. Philadelphia, PA: Lippincott Williams & Wilkins; 2003.)

Certain high-risk patient subgroups clearly have an improved outcome with CABG. These include (a) patients with significant left main coronary disease; (b) patients who have three-vessel disease, especially with LV dysfunction; (c) patients with two-vessel disease with a significant proximal LAD lesion; (d) patients who have survived sudden cardiac death; and (e) patients who are refractory to medical treatment. In patients who do not meet these criteria, either medical treatment or PCI is a viable option.[1,20] Because E.R. does not fall into one of these categories, PCI is preferable owing to the less invasive nature of the procedure and the equivalent outcomes that are seen. These results were recently confirmed in the Clinical Outcomes Utilizing Revascularization and Aggressive Drug Evaluation (COURAGE) trial.[43] Patients with CAD were randomly assigned to aggressive medical treatment with optimization of medical therapy and risk factors, or aggressive medical treatment plus PCI. During a 4.6-year period, no significant difference was noted between the groups in cardiovascular outcomes (death, MI, stroke, hospitalization for ACS). The only difference noted was better control of anginal symptoms early on with PCI, but that difference was no longer significant at the end of the study. These results highlight the crucial role of optimizing medical therapy (including diet, lifestyle changes, risk factor modification) for patients with CAD, regardless of whether revascularization is performed.[1]

CASE 12-3, QUESTION 6: E.R. undergoes PCI plus stent placement and returns to your pharmacy to have a new prescription filled. The prescription calls for clopidogrel at a dose of 150 mg once a day for 1 week, then 75 mg a day thereafter with 11 monthly refills. You have not seen clopidogrel dosed in such manner and are wondering what the rationale for the higher dose is, and whether there is evidence to support its use.

Clopidogrel, a thienopyridine, inhibits platelet function as a noncompetitive antagonist of the $P2Y_{12}$ platelet adenosine diphosphate receptor. Clopidogrel is dosed at 75 mg daily, and this dose has been demonstrated to be effective and safe as monotherapy, or as a component of DAPT with aspirin, in a wide variety of settings for patients with CAD.[98] Despite proven efficacy, patients continue to experience clinical events while receiving clopidogrel.[99] It is now understood that clopidogrel does not produce a consistent antiplatelet response in many patients.[100]

Although the term clopidogrel resistance was first used to describe patients who do not have the expected antiplatelet response to standard doses of clopidogrel, a better term to describe this phenomenon is clopidogrel nonresponsiveness. Alternatively, the phrase *high on-treatment platelet reactivity* is also used commonly in the literature, especially when characterizing the clinical consequences of decreased antiplatelet response.[100] The presence of high on-treatment platelet reactivity in patients who have undergone PCI has been linked to a higher rate of stent thrombosis, MI, repeat revascularization, and death. This link has been observed in both stable CAD patients undergoing elective PCI, and patients with ACS. Although nonresponsiveness identifies an elevated risk for ischemic events, not all patients with identified clopidogrel nonresponsiveness necessarily go on to have recurrent events.[99]

There is a lack of consistency of how clopidogrel nonresponsiveness is defined. It may be defined as the presence of a recurrent ischemic event while on therapy. But, thrombosis is a complex interplay of many different factors and recurrent clinical events do not necessarily imply a lack of antiplatelet effect. The identification of a lack of the expected biologic effect on platelet function is a more appropriate definition to work with. However, there are multiple tests available to assess the antiplatelet activity of clopidogrel (and other antiplatelet agents), and it is unclear which assay correlates best with clinical outcome and would be preferred to assess clopidogrel nonresponsiveness. Because of the variability in available platelet function tests, as well as definitions of nonresponsiveness, estimates for the incidence of clopidogrel nonresponsiveness range anywhere from 5% to 44%.[100] Table 12-8 lists some of the available laboratory testing modalities for antiplatelet agents, their pros and cons, as well as previously identified levels of high on-treatment platelet reactivity.[101]

Potential reasons for clopidogrel nonresponsiveness are multifactorial. One source of nonresponsiveness is in the decreased biotransformation of clopidogrel from its prodrug form to its active metabolite. Biotransformation is a multistep process through the cytochrome P-450 system, but the most important enzyme is CYP2C19, which exhibits variable metabolic capacity. Patients with the *1/*1 CYP2C19 alleles are considered extensive metabolizers and are capable of generating sufficient levels of clopidogrel's active metabolite. Patients with one or two copies of either the *2 or *3 alleles (considered loss of function alleles)

Table 12-8
Commonly Used Platelet Function Tests for Assessment of Antiplatelet Effects[121,122]

Test	Pros	Cons	Monitoring Key Points
Turbidimetric aggregometry, commonly referred to as light transmission aggregometry or LTA	Historical gold standard	Large blood volume Expensive Poor reproducibility Time-consuming Technical complexity	Whole blood assay Can be used for multiple antiplatelet agents with variable reagents
VASP phosphorylation	Whole blood assay Small blood volume needed	Technical complexity Expensive Requires a flow cytometer	Specific for thienopyridines Cutoff for antiplatelet nonresponsiveness ■ PRI > 50%
VerifyNow	True point-of-care assay Large number patients studied Whole blood assay Simple and rapid	Cartridge cost Limited ranges for hematocrit and platelet count	Can assess multiple antiplatelet agents Cutoff for antiplatelet nonresponsiveness ■ PRU >235–240
Thromboelastography	Whole blood assay Point of care	Limited clinical studies Substantial pipetting of reagents	Can assess multiple antiplatelet agents

PRI, platelet reactivity index; PRU, platelet reaction units; VASP, vasodilator-stimulated phosphoprotein.

are considered either intermediate or poor metabolizers, generate lower amounts of active metabolite, and generally produce a reduced antiplatelet effect as measured with available platelet function testing.[102] Conversely, patients with one or two copies of the *17 allele (considered a gain of function allele) are considered ultrarapid metabolizers and demonstrate a heightened antiplatelet response with clopidogrel. With the unraveling of pharmacogenomic factors related to clopidogrel response, a great deal of attention has been given to the idea of identifying patients with copies of either the *2 or *3 allele and adjusting antiplatelet therapy accordingly. The FDA added language to the clopidogrel package insert specifying that poor metabolizers have a higher cardiovascular event rate, and that tests are available to identify who those patients are who carry these genes.[103] Although the presence of either loss of function allele has been associated with an increased risk of clinical outcomes in some trials, this finding has not been uniformly observed. Additionally, there are no prospective trials evaluating a strategy of genetic testing with subsequent therapy changes. As such, genetic testing related to clopidogrel therapy is considered to be in the investigational stage.

An alternative approach to address the issue of clopidogrel nonresponsiveness is to assess platelet function in patients receiving clopidogrel. To date, trials conducted have indicated that increasing loading or maintenance doses of clopidogrel do have the potential to convert patients deemed nonresponders to responders.[104] However, not all patients can be converted and no trial has demonstrated that such an approach leads to improved clinical outcomes.[105] Additionally, data indicate no improvements in clinical outcomes from platelet function monitoring.[106]

Empirically using higher doses of clopidogrel in all patients undergoing PCI is an additional approach that has been considered in addressing clopidogrel nonresponsiveness. Although no trials have been conducted in the elective PCI setting, the CURRENT-OASIS 7 trial randomly assigned more than 25,000 ACS patients to either standard dosing of clopidogrel (300 mg load, then 75 mg daily) or a higher dosing regimen (600 mg load, then 150 mg daily for 7 days, then 75 mg daily).[107] Patients were also randomly assigned to either high-dose (300–325 mg daily) or low-dose (75–100 mg daily) aspirin. Approximately 17,000 of the 25,000 patients underwent PCI. Results showed that in PCI patients, the higher dosing regimen of clopidogrel reduced the risk of MI at the cost of a higher incidence of major bleeding.

Although the results of the CURRENT-OASIS 7 trial might be viewed in a positive light in relation to the prescription E.R. is presenting with today in your pharmacy, an important caveat is that the CURRENT-OASIS 7 trial was conducted in ACS patients, and it is unclear if the same benefits (and risks) can be expected in patients undergoing elective PCI for symptom management of chronic stable angina.

Case 12-3, Question 7: While you are filling her new clopidogrel prescription, E.R. mentions that she has been having some problems with heartburn lately and asks where she can find some over-the-counter omeprazole. Is omeprazole appropriate to use in a patient with clopidogrel therapy?

Another source of variable clopidogrel response is through potential drug–drug interactions involving the CYP2C19 enzyme. One class of agents that has generated substantial controversy in this area are the proton-pump inhibitors (PPIs), given the likelihood of coadministration to prevent GI bleeding as a result of antiplatelet therapy. Several studies indicate there is a pharmacokinetic interaction between PPIs, in particular omeprazole, with clopidogrel resulting in reduced levels of the active metabolite. Evidence that this interaction is clinically significant is variable. Several retrospective analyses suggest an increased risk for CVD events in patients taking PPIs with clopidogrel therapy.[108–112] However, the available evidence from randomized controlled trials does not support an increased clinical risk with this combination.[112–114] However, one study has identified that PPI use alone is associated with an elevated risk of CVD events.[115] Clinicians are faced with addressing this issue from a medical–legal aspect as the FDA has incorporated language into the clopidogrel package insert warning against the concomitant administration of omeprazole and esomeprazole with clopidogrel.[116] The recommendation applies to omeprazole and esomeprazole but not other PPIs. There is some evidence to suggest that alternative PPIs such as pantoprazole have a lower propensity to inhibit CYP2C19 and interact with clopidogrel. Until further information becomes available, clinicians should first validate the need for PPI therapy in clopidogrel patients. If acid suppressive therapy is needed, the use of a H_2 antagonist (excluding cimetidine which can inhibit CYP enzymes) or a PPI less likely to interact with clopidogrel would seem to be appropriate options to consider.[117]

VARIANT ANGINA (CORONARY ARTERY SPASM)

Clinical Presentation

CASE 12-4

Question 1: A.P., a 35-year-old woman, is hospitalized for evaluation of severe chest pain, which occurs almost daily at about 5 AM. A.P. ranks the severity of pain as 7 to 8 on a scale of 1 to 10. It is associated with diaphoresis and is not relieved by change in position. A.P. has no cardiovascular risk factors, and her hobbies include triathlon competition and rock climbing, neither of which has caused chest pain. She follows a strict vegetarian diet and takes no medications. Admission ECG reveals sinus bradycardia at 56 beats/minute. Serum electrolytes, chemistry panel, and cardiac enzymes are all within normal limits.

On day 1 of hospitalization, A.P. is awakened at 6 AM abruptly by severe chest pain. Her vital signs at this time include the following: heart rate, 55 beats/minute; supine BP, 110/64 mm Hg; and respiratory rate, 12 breaths/minute. An ECG shows sinus bradycardia with marked ST-segment elevation. The pain is relieved within 60 seconds by one NTG 0.4-mg sublingual tablet. During the day, she completes an exercise tolerance test without complication or evidence of CAD.

On the second day, A.P. undergoes cardiac catheterization, and no coronary atherosclerosis is visualized. A.P. is diagnosed as having Prinzmetal variant angina. Discharge medications include oral amlodipine 10 mg every day at 11 PM and NTG lingual spray 0.4 mg as needed for chest pain.

Is A.P.'s presentation typical for Prinzmetal variant angina?

A.P. presents with a classic picture of variant (Prinzmetal) angina, with transient total occlusion of a large epicardial coronary artery as a result of severe segmental spasm. Clinical manifestations include chest pain occurring at rest, often in the morning hours. As with A.P., patients with Prinzmetal variant angina generally are younger than patients with chronic stable angina and do not carry a high-risk profile. Other vasospastic disorders, such as migraine attacks or Raynaud's phenomenon, may be present; smoking and alcohol ingestion can be important contributing factors.[118]

The hallmark of variant angina is ST-segment elevation on the ECG, which denotes rapid and complete occlusion of the coronary artery. Many patients also have asymptomatic episodes of ST-segment elevation. Transient arrhythmias and conduction disturbances may be observed during pain, depending on the severity of the myocardial ischemia.[118]

As documented by angiography, A.P. has vasospasm of the large RCA. This transient, reversible narrowing is probably caused by increased coronary vascular resistance. It can occur in the absence of atherosclerosis, as illustrated by A.P., and also in the presence of CAD. One possible explanation for vasospasm occurring more commonly at night or during the early morning hours is increased vasomotor tone secondary to diurnal variations in catecholamines.

Therapy

Case 12-4, Question 2: Oral amlodipine 10 mg every day was ordered for A.P. Would long-acting nitrates or β-adrenergic blockers be reasonable alternatives to amlodipine for A.P.? Is one CCB preferable to another for treatment of Prinzmetal variant angina?

Because of their antispasmodic effects and low incidence of side effects, CCBs are generally selected over nitrates or β-blockers for nocturnal vasospastic angina. All CCBs appear equally effective in preventing Prinzmetal variant angina.[118] Intrinsically long-acting or sustained-release forms are preferred, however, and some patients may respond better to one agent than to another.

In patients who continue to experience pain using maximal CCB doses, combination therapy with a nitrate should be tried. Nitrates cause vasodilation by a different mechanism than CCBs and are effective in treating Prinzmetal variant angina.[118] To avoid tolerance, the nitrate-free interval for A.P. should be scheduled during the day so that the early morning hours when vasospasm occurs are covered by NTG. For example, A.P. could apply a transdermal NTG patch at bedtime and remove it on awakening. Statin therapy is indicated for A.P.[118]

Blockade of the β_2-receptors that mediate vasodilation may allow unopposed α_1-mediated vasoconstriction with worsening symptoms. Even a cardioselective β-blocker could worsen Prinzmetal variant angina.[118] Therefore, a CCB or nitrate is preferred.

Case 12-4, Question 3: Will A.P. require treatment for the remainder of her life?

During the first year of therapy, up to 50% of patients experience spontaneous remission by an unknown mechanism.[118] This occurs most often in patients who have had a short duration of symptoms or who have normal or mildly diseased coronary arteries (i.e., isolated vasospasm without atherosclerosis). If A.P. is pain free and not experiencing significant arrhythmias or silent ischemic episodes of Prinzmetal angina after 1 year, amlodipine could be tapered and discontinued. It is also possible, however, that she will require treatment indefinitely. Modification of smoking and ethanol ingestion may promote remission of Prinzmetal angina.[118]

CARDIAC SYNDROME X

CASE 12-5

Question 1: K.G., a 50-year-old female executive, has undergone an extensive cardiovascular workup for exertional angina associated with a 3-mm ST-segment depression. A recent cardiac catheterization did not reveal any atherosclerosis. The cardiologists believe K.G. has cardiac syndrome X. What drug therapy might be indicated for K.G.?

Cardiac syndrome X is a syndrome of angina or angina-like chest pain in the setting of a normal coronary arteriogram, and ST-segment depression during exercise. Several theories exist regarding the mechanism of pain production, including microvascular dysfunction producing ischemia or chest discomfort without ischemia in patients who may have an abnormal perception of pain. Half of patients with cardiac syndrome X present with chest pain induced by exercise followed by 15 to 20 minutes of chest discomfort.[119]

By symptoms alone, K.G.'s presentation does not significantly differ from that of a patient with exercise-induced angina secondary to atherosclerosis. Of concern is the finding of a 3-mm ST-segment depression on K.G.'s ECG, which raises concern of severe CAD. The negative findings from her cardiac catheterization, however, rule against both CAD and coronary artery spasm as a cause of her symptoms, and help to confirm the diagnosis of cardiac syndrome X.[119]

Treatment with a nitrate, CCB, or β-blocker all appear to offer some relief, but overall the response to therapy in these patients is poor. The choice of agent will likely depend on specific patient characteristics. Sublingual NTG is often ineffective at treating acute attacks, although it should still be prescribed. Often a combination of anti-ischemic therapy, analgesic therapy, and lifestyle modifications is necessary.[119]

KEY REFERENCES AND WEBSITES

A full list of references for this chapter can be found at http://thepoint.lww.com/AT11e. Below are the key references and websites for this chapter, with the corresponding reference number in this chapter found in parentheses after the reference.

Key References

Abraham NS et al. ACCF/ACG/AHA 2010 Expert Consensus Document on the concomitant use of proton pump inhibitors and thienopyridines: a focused update of the ACCF/ACG/AHA 2008 expert consensus document on reducing the gastrointestinal risks of antiplatelet therapy and NSAID use: a report of the American College of Cardiology Foundation Task Force on Expert Consensus Documents. *Circulation*. 2010;122(24):2619. (117)

Antithrombotic Trialists' (ATT) Collaboration. Aspirin in the primary and secondary prevention of vascular disease: collaborative meta-analysis of individual participant data from randomised trials. *Lancet*. 2009;373:1849. (87)

Chaitman BR. Ranolazine for the treatment of chronic angina and potential use in other cardiovascular conditions. *Circulation*. 2006;113:2462. (15)

Fihn SD et al. 2012 ACCF/AHA/ACP/AATS/PCNA/SCAI/STS guideline for the diagnosis and management of patients with stable ischemic heart disease: a report of the American College of Cardiology Foundation/American Heart Association Task Force on Practice Guidelines, and the American College of Physicians, American Association for Thoracic Surgery, Preventative Cardiovascular Nurses Association, Society for Cardiovascular Angiography and Interventions, and Society of Thoracic Surgeons. *Circulation*. 2012;126:e354–e471. (1)

Fox K et al. Guidelines on the management of stable angina pectoris: executive summary. The task force on the management of stable angina pectoris of the European Society of Cardiology. *Eur Heart J*. 2006;27:1341.

Hippisley-Cox J, Coupland C. Effect of combinations of drugs on all cause mortality in patients with ischaemic heart disease: nested case-control analysis. *BMJ*. 2005;330:1059. (52)

Kaul S et al. Thiazolidinedione drugs and cardiovascular risks: a science advisory from the American Heart Association and American College of Cardiology Foundation. *J Am Coll Cardiol*. 2010;55:1885.

Levine GN et al. 2011 ACCF/AHA/SCAI guideline for percutaneous coronary intervention: a report of the American College of Cardiology Foundation/American Heart Association Task Force on Practice Guidelines and the Society for Cardiovascular Angiography and Interventions. *J Am Coll Cardiol*. 2011;58:e44–e122. (95)

Mehta SR et al. Double-dose versus standard-dose clopidogrel and high-dose versus low-dose aspirin in individuals undergoing percutaneous coronary intervention for acute coronary syndromes (CURRENT-OASIS 7): a randomised factorial trial. *Lancet*. 2010;376(9748):1233. (107)

Parikh P et al. Diets and cardiovascular disease: an evidence-based assessment. *J Am Coll Cardiol*. 2005;45:1379. (48)

Pepine CJ, Wolff AA. A controlled trial with a novel anti-ischemic agent, ranolazine, in chronic stable angina pectoris that is responsive to conventional antianginal agents. Ranolazine Study Group. *Am J Cardiol*. 1999;84:46.

Windecker S et al. 2014 ESC/EACTS Guidelines on myocardial revascularization: the Task Force on Myocardial revascularization of the European Society of Cardiology (ESC) and the European Association for cardio-Thoracic Surgery (EACTS), developed with the special contribution of the European Association of Percutaneous Cardiovascular Interventions (EAPCI), *Eur Heart J*. 2014;35(37):2541–2619. (20)

Yusuf S et al. Effect of potentially modifiable risk factors associated with myocardial infarction in 52 countries (the INTERHEART study): case control study. *Lancet*. 2004;364:937. (12)

Key Websites

American College of Cardiology. CardioSource, http://www.cardiosource.org/acc.

American Heart Association, http://www.heart.org/HEARTORG/.

US Food and Drug Administration. Information for Healthcare Professionals: Update to the labeling of Clopidogrel Bisulfate (marketed as Plavix) to alert healthcare professionals about a drug interaction with omeprazole (marketed as Prilosec and Prilosec OTC), http://www.fda.gov/safety/medwatch/safetyinformation/ucm225843.htm.

13 Acute Coronary Syndrome

Brianne L. Dunn and Robert L. Page, II

CORE PRINCIPLES

	CHAPTER CASES
ACUTE CORONARY SYNDROME	
1 Acute coronary syndrome (ACS) is an umbrella term including unstable angina (UA) or acute myocardial infarction (MI) which consists of ST segment elevation MI (STEMI) and non–ST segment MI (NSTEMI). Diagnosis is based on patient presentation, electrocardiographic changes, and elevated cardiac biomarkers.	**Case 13-1 (Questions 1–5), Figures 13-1–13-4, Table 13-1**
2 Treatment objectives of ACS are to alleviate ischemic symptoms, restore blood flow to the infarct-related artery, arrest infarct expansion, and prevent mortality.	**Case 13-1 (Questions 6,7) Case 13-2 (Question 1)**
3 For both STEMI and NSTE-ACS, initial therapies may include oxygen, nitroglycerin (NTG), antiplatelet agents, β-blocker, angiotensin-converting enzyme (ACE) inhibitor or angiotensin receptor blocker (ARB), and morphine sulfate.	**Case 13-1 (Questions 8–11, 14–17), Table 13-2**
STEMI	
1 Treatment objectives of STEMI are to restore coronary blood flow by administering a fibrinolytic or performing percutaneous coronary intervention (PCI). Treatment strategy depends on availability of catheterization laboratory and skilled staff, time of initial medical contact, and contraindication for a fibrinolytic agent.	**Case 13-1 (Questions 12, 13), Figure 13-5, Table 13-4**
2 Regardless of reperfusion strategy, patients should receive aspirin in addition to a $P2Y_{12}$ inhibitor.	**Case 13-1 (Questions 8–10), Figure 13-5, Table 13-5**
3 For patients receiving fibrinolytic therapy, unfractionated heparin (UFH), enoxaparin, or fondaparinux should also be initiated.	**Case 13-1 (Question 8, 11), Figure 13-5**
4 For patients receiving PCI, an anticoagulant strategy consisting of either UFH with or without a glycoprotein IIb/IIIa inhibitor or bivalirudin alone should be administered.	**Case 13-1 (Question 11), Figure 13-5, Table 13-6**
NSTE-ACS	
1 For an invasive strategy, a $P2Y_{12}$ inhibitor (clopidogrel, prasugrel, or ticagrelor), anticoagulant (UFH, enoxaparin, bivalirudin, or fondaparinux with UFH) along with aspirin and/or a glycoprotein IIb/IIIa inhibitor is given before angiography.	**Case 13-2 (Question 2–5), Figure 13-6, Table 13-6**
2 For an ischemia-guided strategy, an anticoagulant (enoxaparin, fondaparinux, or UFH) along with dual antiplatelet therapy should be considered.	**Case 13-2 (Question 6), Figure 13-6**
LONG-TERM THERAPIES	
1 Potential long-term therapies include a β-blocker; statin; aspirin; clopidogrel, prasugrel, or ticagrelor; ACE inhibitor or ARB; aldosterone antagonist; and sublingual NTG. Unless contraindicated, ACE inhibitors or ARBs should be given to those with a left ventricular ejection fraction of less than 40%, hypertension, diabetes, or chronic kidney disease.	**Case 13-3 (Questions 1–9), Table 13-2**
2 Lifestyle modifications include smoking cessation, weight management through diet and exercise to reduce body weight by 10% if body mass index exceeds 25 kg/m^2, diabetic treatment to achieve a near-normal hemoglobin A_{1c}, and serum lipid control to achieve an optimal low-density lipoprotein concentration of 100 mg/dL or less.	**Case 13-3 (Question 10)**

ACUTE CORONARY DISEASE

Despite advances in medical intervention and pharmacotherapy, cardiovascular disease continues to be a leading killer in the United States. Acute coronary syndrome (ACS) is an umbrella term that includes patients who present with either unstable angina (UA) or acute myocardial infarction (AMI) which is further differentiated into ST segment elevation myocardial infarction (STEMI) or non–ST segment myocardial infarction (NSTEMI).[1–5] The terminology, non–ST segment elevation-ACS (NSTE-ACS) includes both UA and NSTEMI.[1] These two conditions are determined based upon the presence (NSTEMI) or absence (UA) of biomarkers associated with necrosis. The etiology of ACS originates from the erosion or rupture of an unstable plaque within the coronary artery leading to the formation of an occlusive or nonocclusive thrombus. Although NSTE-ACS and STEMI lead to hospitalization, patients presenting with STEMI are considered medical emergencies and warrant immediate intervention.[5] Today, the management of ACS is based on reperfusion and revascularization using both pharmacologic and nonpharmacologic interventions such as percutaneous coronary intervention (PCI) and coronary artery bypass grafting (CABG).[1–5] A committee composed of representatives from the American College of Cardiology (ACC) and the American Heart Association (AHA) periodically review the literature and publish practice guidelines to aid health care practitioners in selecting the most effective treatments for patients with ACS.[1–5] These guidelines consist of graded recommendations based on the weight and quality of the evidence. Although there are local variations in practice, these guidelines serve as the foundation for care of patients with ACS.

Epidemiology

According to AHA statistics, 652,000 hospital discharges in the United States were attributable to ACS as the primary diagnosis in 2010. Financially, the impact of ACS is also exceedingly high.[6] The cost of hospitalization for ACS is expensive and continues to rise. In terms of direct medical expenditures, ACS costs Americans more than $150 billion annually, with 60% to 75% of these costs related to hospital admission and readmission.[7–9] Approximately one-third of STEMI patients die within 24 hours of onset of ischemia compared with 15% of patients with NSTE-ACS who either die or experience reinfarction within 30 days of hospitalization.[10] Although these numbers are substantial, the risk-standardized 30-day in-hospital mortality for Medicare beneficiaries admitted for AMI have significantly dropped during the past decade.[11] In an analysis of Medicare data for all fee-for-service patients 65 years or older with a diagnosis of ACS, Krumholz et al. estimated that the length of hospitalization for STEMI/NSTE-ACS has decreased from 6.5 days in 1999 to 5.3 days in 2011. These trends may be reflective of application of evidence-based guidelines as well as aggressive treatment of hypertension and hypercholesterolemia.[11]

Pathophysiology

The majority of ACS results from occlusion of a coronary artery secondary to thrombus formation overlying a lipid-rich atheromatous plaque that has undergone fissuring or rupture (Fig. 13-1). Plaques that are susceptible to rupture have a thin fibrous cap, large fatty core, high content of inflammatory cells such as macrophages and lymphocytes, limited amounts of smooth muscle, and eccentric shape. Triggers such as surges in sympathetic activity with a sudden increase in blood pressure (BP), pulse rate, myocardial contractility, and coronary blood flow can lead to erosion, fissuring, or rupture of the fragile fibrous cap. Once ruptured, the thrombogenic components of the plaque consisting of collagen and tissue factor are exposed. This promotes activation of the platelet cascade, ultimately leading to the formation of a thrombus as well as ischemia in the corresponding myocardial area. The extent of intracoronary thrombosis and distal embolization determines the type of ACS (Fig. 13-1). In patients with UA, the coronary artery has enough blood flow such that the myocardial cells do not die. In patients with NSTEMI, there exists partial thrombotic occlusion with or without distal embolization or severe stenosis and some myocardial cells die. For STEMI, there exists total and persistent thrombotic occlusion leading to myocardial cell death.[12] Eighty percent of patients presenting with ACS have two or more active plaques.[12]

Most infarctions are located in a specific region of the heart and are described as such (e.g., anterior, lateral, inferior). Some patients exhibit permanent electrocardiographic (ECG) abnormalities (Q waves) after an AMI. In the past, patients with Q-wave infarctions were generally believed to have more extensive necrosis and a higher in-hospital mortality rate. Patients with a non–Q-wave infarct were believed to have a greater likelihood of experiencing postinfarction angina and early reinfarction. More recently these distinctions have come into question. Some cardiologists believe there is no difference in prognosis. The terminology has changed because most patients who have STEMI are treated emergently, preventing the development of Q waves. An anterior wall infarction carries a worse prognosis than an inferior or lateral wall infarction because it is more commonly associated with development of left ventricular (LV) failure and cardiogenic shock.

Clinical Presentation

An important part in establishing the diagnosis of ACS is obtaining the patient's "story," which can elicit crucial hallmark symptoms such as increasing the frequency of exertional angina or chest pain at rest, new-onset severe chest discomfort, or increasing angina with a duration exceeding 20 minutes. The pain is typically midline anterior chest discomfort that can radiate to the left arm, back, shoulder, or jaw, and may be associated with diaphoresis, dyspnea, nausea, and vomiting as well as unexplained syncope. Patients with STEMI will usually complain of unrelenting chest pain whereas patients with NSTE-ACS will present with either angina at rest, new-onset (2 months or less) angina, or chronic angina that increases in frequency, duration, or intensity. Presentation may differ by sex, age, and presence of various comorbidities. Men commonly complain of chest pain, whereas women often present with nausea and diaphoresis. Elderly patients may present with hypotension or cerebrovascular symptoms rather than chest pain. Additionally, onset of ACS does not occur at random, and many episodes appear to be triggered by external factors or conditions. MI occurs with increased frequency in the morning, particularly within the first hour after awakening; on Mondays; during winter months or colder days; and during emotional stress and vigorous exercise.[1–5]

The physical examination is important in guiding initial therapy. Signs of severe LV or right ventricular dysfunction may be present (see Chapter 14, Heart Failure). The patient may have severe hypertension as a result of pain or, conversely, may be hypotensive. Significant tachycardia (heart rate > 120 beats/minute) suggests a large area of damage. On cardiac auscultation, presence of a fourth heart sound (S_4) denotes an ischemia-induced decrease in LV compliance. New cardiac murmurs may be heard, resulting from papillary muscle dysfunction. The cerebral and peripheral vasculature should be

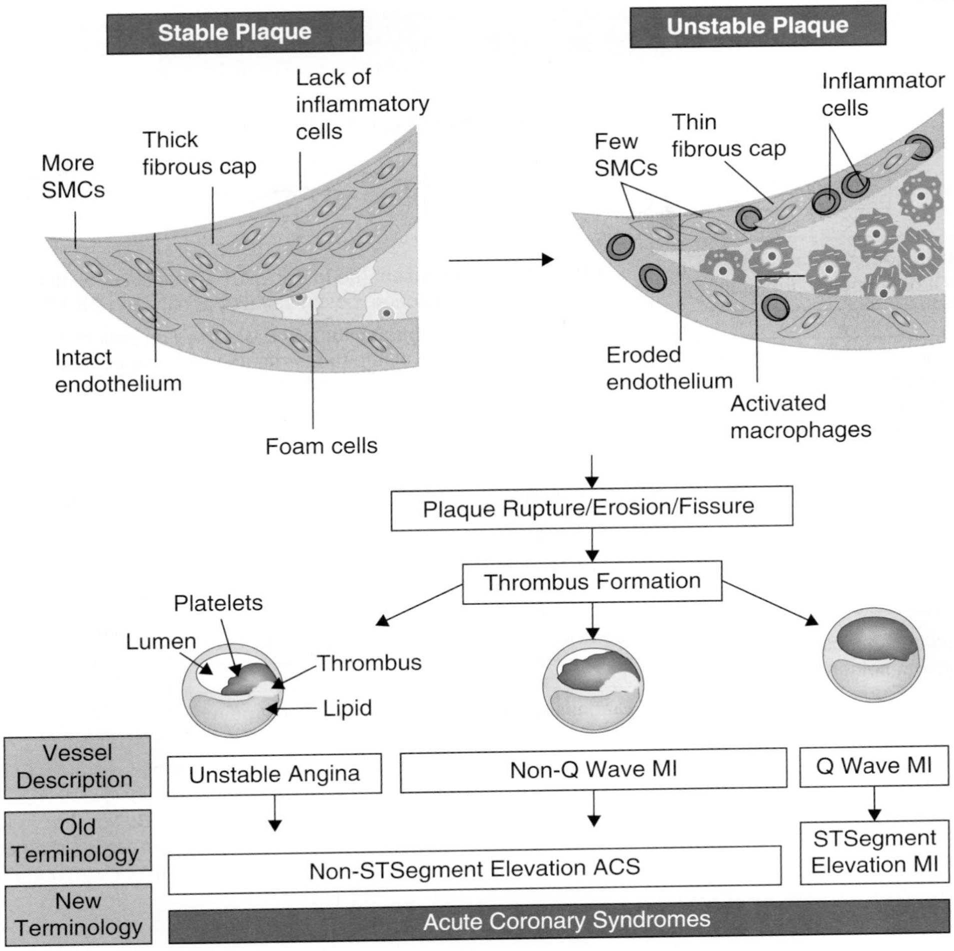

Figure 13-1 Thrombus formation and acute coronary syndrome definitions. MI, myocardial infarction; SMC, smooth muscle cells.

assessed. Patients with a history of cerebrovascular disease may not be eligible for fibrinolytic therapy. Peripheral pulses should be examined to assess perfusion and to obtain a baseline before invasive procedures are instituted.

Diagnosis

In addition to the patient's history and presentation, the diagnosis of ACS is based on the electrocardiogram (ECG) and laboratory results from a cardiac injury profile. A 12-lead ECG should be obtained within 10 minutes of presenting to the emergency department (ED). The ECG is an indispensable tool in the diagnosis of ACS and has become the key point in the decision pathway (Fig. 13-2). Key findings on ECG consist of ST segment elevation, ST segment depression, or T-wave inversion.[1–5] By definition, STEMI consists of ST segment elevation in two or more contiguous leads and either exceeding 0.2 mV (2 mm) in leads V_1, V_2, and V_3 or 0.1 mV (1 mm) or greater in other leads (Fig. 13-3). NSTE-ACS consists of ST segment depression exceeding 0.1 mV (1 mm) in two or more contiguous leads or T-wave inversions exceeding 0.1 mV (1 mm). Additionally, the 12-lead ECG is helpful in determining the location of an infarct. Q waves may be found in lead V_6 for a posterior infarct; in leads II, III, AVF for an inferior infarct; in lead I, AVL for a lateral infarct; and in the precordial leads V_1, V_2, V_3, or V_4 for an anterior infarction.[13]

Laboratory Changes

When a cardiac cell is injured, proteins are released into the circulation. The measurement of these sensitive and specific proteins (troponins T or I and creatine kinase [CK]) is routine in establishing the diagnosis of AMI (Fig. 13-4). There are three isoenzymes of CK, of which the MB band is the most specific for the myocardium. Troponin is the preferred biomarker for assessment of myocardial damage owing to its high cardiac specificity and sensitivity (90.7% and 90.2%, respectively) as well as the development of newer sensitive troponin assays. Troponins T and I are detectable in blood within 4 to 12 hours after the onset of MI, and peak values are observed at 12 to 48 hours. Troponin levels may also stay elevated for 7 to 10 days after myocardial necrosis. As seen in Figure 13-4, the horizontal line depicts the upper reference limit (URL) for the cardiac biomarker in the clinical chemistry laboratory.[1,2,5] The URL represents the 99th percentile of a reference control group without MI. Because cardiac troponin T and I are not normally detected in the blood of healthy people, the definition of an abnormally increased level is a value that exceeds that of 99% of a reference control group. For the diagnosis of NSTEMI or STEMI, the patient should have one troponin value or two CK-MB values greater than the URL. Cardiac biomarkers are not typically elevated in patients with UA. Presently, no current marker is detectable immediately upon onset of MI, and therefore repeated measurements of cardiac

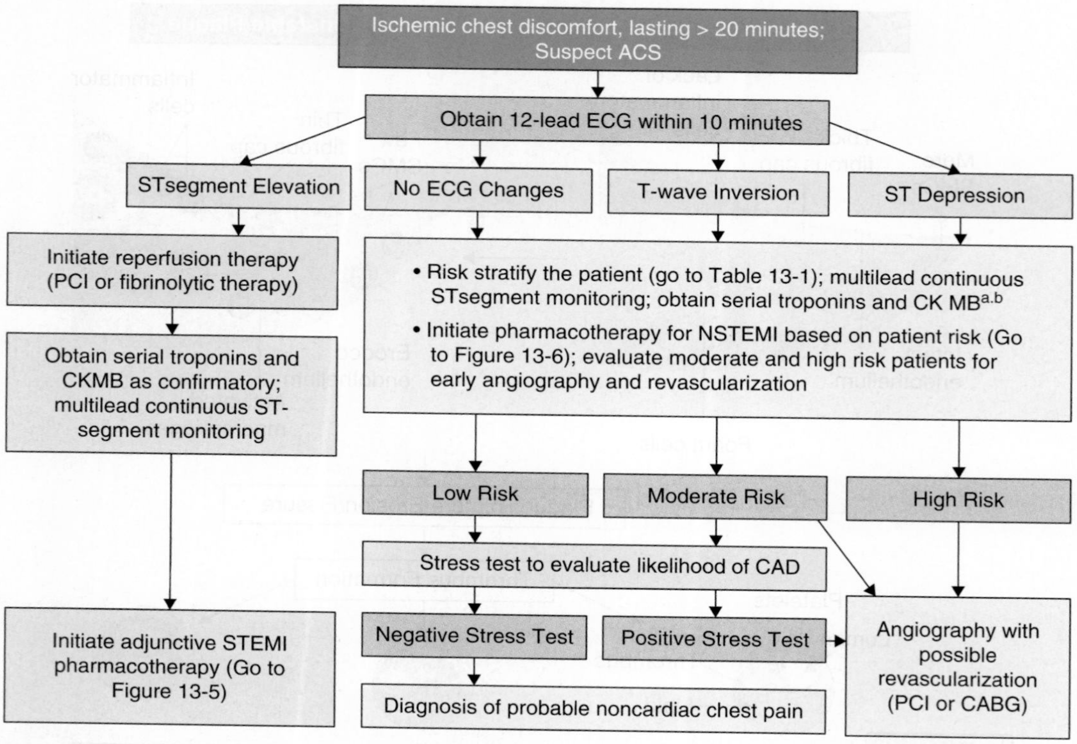

Figure 13-2 Evaluation algorithm for the patient presenting with acute coronary syndrome. ACS, acute coronary syndrome; CAD, coronary artery disease; CABG, coronary artery bypass graft; CK, creatinine; ECG, electrocardiogram; PCI, percutaneous intervention; NSTE-ACS, non-ST segment acute coronary syndrome; STEMI, ST segment myocardial infarction. **A:** Positive, above the myocardial infarction limit; **B:** Negative, below the myocardial infarction limit. (Adapted with permission from Spinler SA. Evolution of antithrombotic therapy used in acute coronary syndromes. In: Richardson M et al, eds. *Pharmacotherapy Self-Assessment Program. Cardiology*. 7th ed. Lenexa, KS: American College of Clinical Pharmacy; 2010:62.)

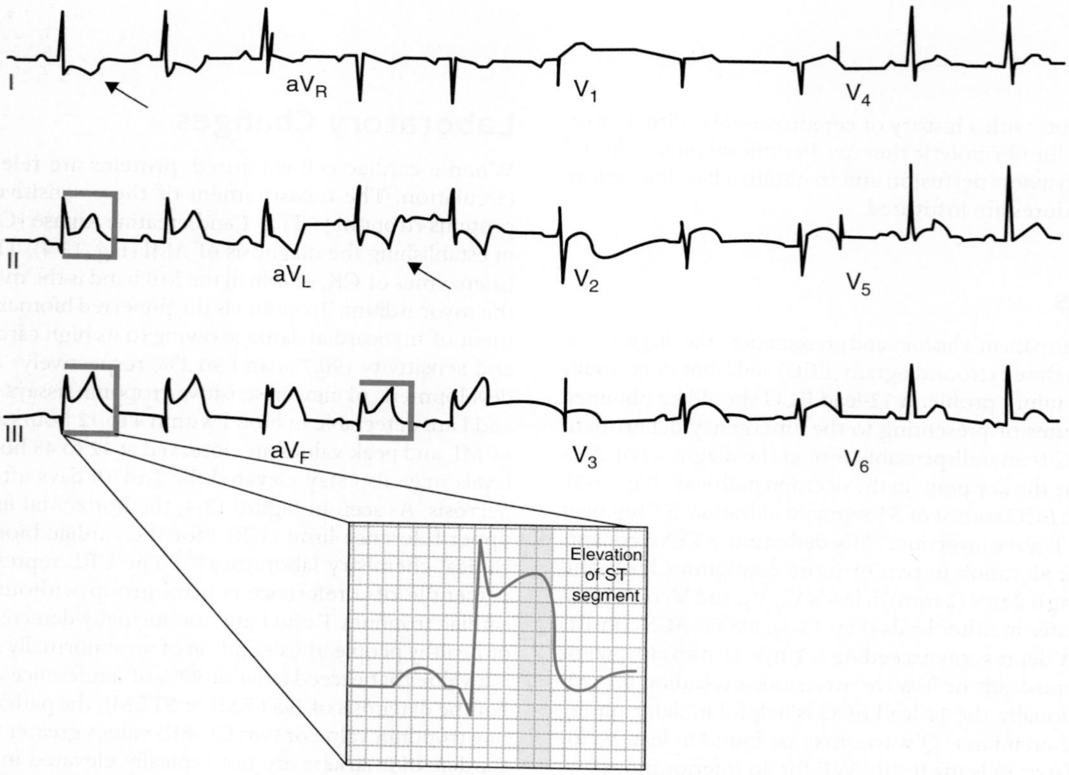

Figure 13-3 ECG changes related to STEMI. On this admission electrocardiogram (ECG), note the extensive ST segment elevation in leads II, III, and aV_F (*brackets*), indicating an inferior wall acute myocardial infarction (AMI). The patient also displays reciprocal ST segment depression in leads I and aV_L (*arrows*), which are the lateral ECG leads and are opposite the inferior leads.

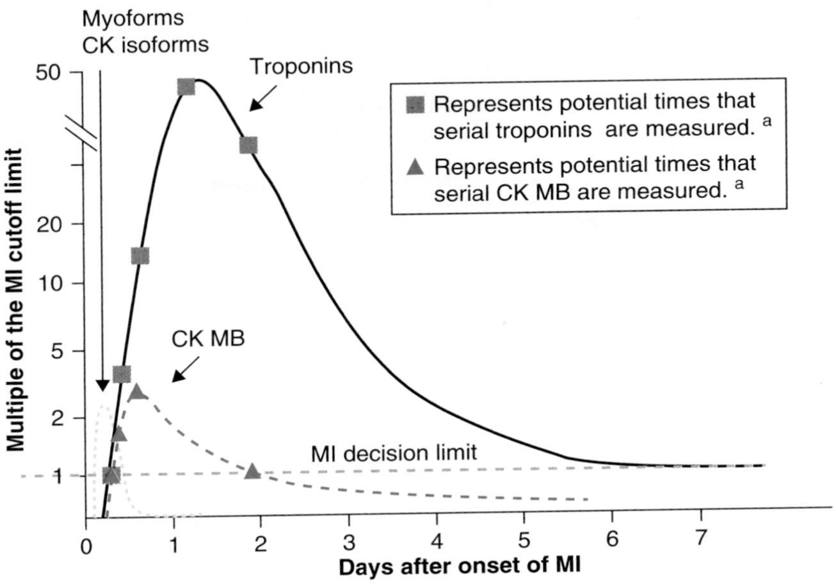

Figure 13-4 Cardiac biomarker elevation in acute coronary syndrome. CK, creatine kinase; MI, myocardial infarction. a. Serial troponins and CK-MB are initially measured during the first 12 to 24 hours of onset of chest pain and continued to be measured until the concentrations begin to decline. (Adapted with permission from Anderson JL et al. ACC/AHA 2007 guidelines for the management of patients with unstable angina/non-ST-Elevation myocardial infarction: a report of the American College of Cardiology/American Heart Association Task Force on Practice Guidelines (Writing Committee to Revise the 2002 Guidelines for the Management of Patients With Unstable Angina/Non-ST-Elevation Myocardial Infarction) developed in collaboration with the American College of Emergency Physicians, the Society for Cardiovascular Angiography and Interventions, and the Society of Thoracic Surgeons endorsed by the American Association of Cardiovascular and Pulmonary Rehabilitation and the Society for Academic Emergency Medicine. *J Am Coll Cardiol*. 2007;50(7):e1–e157.)

enzymes after admission are warranted. A cardiac injury profile will be measured at presentation and every 3 to 6 hours for the first 12 to 24 hours and periodically thereafter.[2–4] Unfortunately, several conditions other than AMI, such as tachyarrhythmias, heart failure (HF), myocarditis and pericarditis, hypotension or hypertension, acute pulmonary embolism, end-stage renal disease and cardiac trauma are associated with elevated troponin. As a result, it is important to assess other diagnostic criteria such as ECG changes, chest pain, presence of atherosclerotic risk factors, and echocardiographic findings.

Risk Stratification

The examination of a patient presenting with ACS begins with stratification for the risk of death and reinfarction, taking into account the presenting signs and symptoms, past medical history, ECG and cardiac biomarker changes. Patients can be stratified into low, medium, or high risk for mortality, and the need for urgent coronary angiography and PCI (Fig. 13-2). In 1967, Killip and Kimball introduced a useful, convenient tool for early risk stratification for patients with STEMI. Higher Killip class was found to be associated with increased in-hospital and 1-year mortality (Table 13-1).[14] The Thrombolysis in Myocardial Infarction (TIMI) risk score was introduced in 2000 and can be used with either STEMI or NSTE-ACS (Table 13-1).[15,16] For STEMI, a higher risk score indicates a greater 30-day mortality rate. Patients with STEMI are at the highest risk of death and reinfarction, and initial treatment should proceed with immediate revascularization regardless of their risk stratification score. "Time is tissue," means the sooner the thrombosed artery is opened, the lower the morality and greater amount of myocardium preserved. Reperfusion therapy should be initiated in all eligible patients with STEMI with symptom onset within the prior 12 hours. Primary PCI is the recommended method of reperfusion. The ACC/AHA guidelines define a target time to initiate reperfusion for STEMI within 30 minutes of hospital presentation for fibrinolytic therapy and within 90 minutes from presentation for PCI.[5]

In the case of NSTE-ACS, a TIMI risk score of 5 to 7, 3 to 4, and 0 to 2 reflect a high, moderate, and low risk for death, MI, or need for urgent coronary artery revascularization, respectively (Table 13-1). A low-risk patient with negative cardiac biomarkers may undergo a stress test or be discharged from the ED with a diagnostic test scheduled within 72 hours. Moderate and high-risk patients are often admitted to the hospital for pharmacologic treatment, further diagnostic tests, and angiography with possible intervention. Additional risk stratification tools such as the Platelet glycoprotein IIb/IIIa in Unstable angina: Receptor Suppression Using Integrilin Therapy (PURSUIT) risk score and Global Registry of Acute Cardiac Events (GRACE) risk score exist for in-hospital and 1-year morality.[1,5] Other risk scores are available to predict bleeding in patients with ACS.[17]

Complications

The primary complications of ACS can be divided into three major groups: pump failure, arrhythmias, and recurrent ischemia and reinfarction. Depression of cardiac function after AMI is related directly to the extent of LV damage. As a result of decreased cardiac output and decreased perfusion, a number of compensatory mechanisms become activated. The levels of circulating catecholamines increase in an attempt to increase contractility and restore normal perfusion. In addition, the renin-angiotensin-aldosterone system is enhanced, leading to an increase in systemic vascular resistance and sodium and water retention. These compensatory mechanisms can eventually worsen the imbalance between myocardial oxygen supply and consumption by increasing the myocardial oxygen demand.[18]

Table 13-1
Risk Stratification Tools for Acute Coronary Syndrome

TIMI Risk Score[a]			
STEMI		**NSTE-ACS**	
Risk Factor	**No. of Points**	**Risk Factor**	**No. of Points**
Age 65–74 years	2	Age ≥ 65 years	1
Age ≥ 75 years	3	≥3 risk factors for CAD[b]	1
SBP < 100 mm Hg	3	Prior history of CAD[c]	1
Heart rate > 100 beats/minute	2	Aspirin use in past 7 days	1
Killip class II–IV	2	≥2 anginal events in past 24 hours	1
Weight < 67 kg	1	ST segment deviation ≥ 0.5 mm	1
History of HTN, diabetes, or angina	1	Elevation of cardiac markers[d]	1
Time to reperfusion therapy >4 hours	1		
Anterior ST segment elevation or left bundle branch block	1		

Killip Class[e]		
Class	**Symptoms**	**In-Hospital and 1-Year Mortality (%)**
I	No heart failure	5
II	Mild heart failure, rales, S_3, congestion on chest radiograph	21
III	Pulmonary edema	35
IV	Cardiogenic shock	67

[a]TIMI risk score data from Antman EM et al. The TIMI risk score for unstable angina/non-ST elevation MI: a method for prognostication and therapeutic decision making. *JAMA*. 2000;284:835; Morrow DA et al. Application of the TIMI risk score for ST-elevation MI in the National Registry of Myocardial Infarction 3. *JAMA*. 2001;286:1356. A risk score is calculated by adding the total number of risk factors. Total points for STEMI are 0–14, in which risk scores of 0, 2, 4, 6, 7, and >8 correspond to a 30-day mortality rate of 0.8%, 2.2%, 7.3%, 16%, 23%, and 36%, respectively. Total points for NSTE-ACS are 0–7, in which scores of 0 or 1, 3, 5, and 7 correspond to a 3%, 5%, 12%, or 19% risk of death or repeat MI at 14 days, respectively. When risk stratifying, scores of 0 to 2, 3 to 4, and 5 to 7 represent low, moderate, and high risk for death or repeat MI at 14 days.
[b]Risk factors include smoking, diabetes, hypertension, family history of coronary artery disease, and hypercholesterolemia.
[c]Defined as a prior coronary stenosis ≥50%; history of previous myocardial infarction, percutaneous coronary intervention, or coronary artery bypass graft; or chronic stable angina pectoris associated with a positive exercise tolerance test or pharmacologically induced nuclear imaging or echocardiographic changes (positive nuclear imaging or echocardiographic changes required if female).
[d]Either troponin I or T or creatine kinase-MB.
[e]Killip class data from Killip T 3rd, Kimball JT. Treatment of myocardial infarction in a coronary care unit. A two year experience with 250 patients. *Am J Cardiol*. 1967;20:457.
CAD, coronary artery disease; HTN, hypertension; NSTE-ACS, non–ST segment elevation acute coronary syndrome; SBP, systolic blood pressure; STEMI, ST segment elevation myocardial infarction; TIMI, Thrombolysis in Myocardial Infarction.

Signs and symptoms of HF are common in patients who have abnormal wall motion affecting 20% to 25% of the LV. If 40% or more of the LV is damaged, cardiogenic shock and death may occur. Ischemia and scar formation after an AMI may lead to a decrease in ventricular compliance, resulting in abnormally high LV filling pressures during diastole. (See Chapter 14, Heart Failure, for further discussion on HF with reduced ejection fraction and preserved ejection fraction.)

Decreased contractility and a compensatory increase in LV end-diastolic volume and pressure lead to increased wall stress within the left ventricle. LV enlargement is an important determinant of mortality after AMI. During a period of days to months after an AMI, the infarcted area may expand as a result of dilatation and thinning of the LV wall. These changes are known as ventricular remodeling. In addition, hypertrophy of the noninfarcted myocardium occurs. Administration of oral angiotensin-converting enzyme (ACE) inhibitors, angiotensin receptor blockers (ARBs), or aldosterone antagonists may limit remodeling and will attenuate the progression of LV dilatation.[19,20]

During the peri-infarction period, the heart is irritable and subject to ventricular arrhythmias. The continuous monitoring of patients in a coronary care unit has reduced the in-hospital mortality rate related to ventricular arrhythmias. However, patients who have had an AMI have an increased risk of sudden cardiac death for 1 to 2 years after hospital discharge. The most important predictor for sudden cardiac death is an abnormal LV ejection fraction (LVEF). Other factors associated with an increased risk for sudden cardiac death are complex ventricular ectopy, frequent (>10/hour) premature ventricular complexes, and the identification of late potentials on a signal-averaged ECG.[18]

OVERVIEW OF DRUG AND NONDRUG THERAPY

Overlap exists regarding the pharmacotherapy for both STEMI and NSTE-ACS. According to the ACC/AHA guidelines, early therapies should consist of oxygen (if oxygen saturation is <90%), sublingual

(SL) and/or intravenous (IV) nitroglycerin (NTG), IV morphine, ACE inhibitor or ARB, aldosterone antagonist, antiplatelet agents, stool softener, β-blocker, statin, and anticoagulant. Adjunctive therapies such as analgesics and vasodilators can also be considered in selected patients. Table 13-2 summarizes the evidence-based pharmacotherapies for both STEMI and NSTE-ACS. Figure 13-5 provides an initial treatment algorithm for patients with STEMI, and Figure 13-6, for patients with NSTE-ACS. Administration of these pharmacotherapies serves as a performance measure for health systems to ensure effective, timely, safe, and efficient patient-centered care.[1,5]

Fibrinolytic Drugs

Because the majority of STEMI cases result from the sudden occlusion of a coronary artery, the priority is to open the occluded artery as quickly as possible. This is accomplished by administering a fibrinolytic agent that enhances the body's own fibrinolytic system or by mechanically reducing the obstruction with PCI.[5]

Large clinical trials have proven that administration of a fibrinolytic agent reduces mortality. Early mortality from STEMI was reduced by approximately one-third (from 10%–15% to 6%–10%) with fibrinolytic therapy.[5]

The fibrinolytic drugs currently used for STEMI patients in the United States are alteplase (t-PA), reteplase (r-PA), and tenecteplase (TNK). Alteplase is a naturally occurring enzyme produced by recombinant DNA technology. It cleaves the same plasminogen peptide bond that urokinase cleaves. However, t-PA has a binding site for fibrin, which allows it to bind to and preferentially lyse thrombin-bound instead of circulating plasminogen. Reteplase is a genetically modified plasminogen activator that is similar to t-PA. Reteplase has a longer half-life, allowing it to be administered as two bolus injections 30 minutes apart, rather than as a bolus plus infusion. TNK is a genetically modified form of t-PA. Compared with t-PA, TNK has a longer plasma half-life, better fibrin specificity, and higher resistance to inhibition by plasminogen-activator inhibitor.[21,22] The pharmacologic properties and dosing regimens are compared in Table 13-3.

Unfortunately, an ideal fibrinolytic agent does not exist. Three problems common to all fibrinolytic drugs are the inability to open 100% of coronary artery occlusions, inconsistent ability to maintain good blood flow in the infarcted artery after it is opened, and bleeding complications. When assessing coronary artery flow after reperfusion therapy, the TIMI flow grade is used. Flow in coronary arteries is classified as grade 0 (no flow), grade 1 (penetration without perfusion), grade 2 (partial perfusion), or grade 3 (complete perfusion).[23] When assessing an episode of bleeding, the TIMI bleeding criteria are used. TIMI major bleeding consists of overt clinical bleeding or documented intracranial or retroperitoneal hemorrhage that is associated with a drop in hemoglobin of at least 5 g/dL or hematocrit of at least 15% (absolute). TIMI minor bleeding is defined as overt clinical bleeding associated with a fall in hemoglobin of 3 to 5 g/dL or in hematocrit of 9% to 15% (absolute).[24]

To minimize the risk of bleeding complications, contraindications to the use of fibrinolytic drugs must be evaluated before administration (Table 13-4). There are relatively few absolute contraindications to fibrinolytic therapy, but each patient should be assessed carefully to ascertain whether the potential benefit outweighs the potential risk. Because of the serious nature of intracerebral hemorrhage, patients should be selected carefully before receiving these agents. Generally, the diagnosis of STEMI must be ensured, with a history consistent with ischemia, and presence of ST segment elevation in two contiguous leads, or a new left bundle branch block on the ECG. Once the diagnosis is made, the fibrinolytic agent should be administered immediately if there are no contraindications.[5]

Fibrinolytic therapy is indicated in patients with STEMI who present to the hospital within 12 hours of symptom onset and are unable to undergo primary PCI within 120 minutes from first medical contact.[5] The benefit derived from fibrinolytic therapy is directly related to the time from the onset of chest pain to the time of administration. Although the guidelines recommend initiation within 12 hours from the onset of chest pain, data from clinical trials suggest that mortality reduction is greater when fibrinolytic therapy is initiated within 0 to 2 hours of symptom onset compared with treatment initiated more than 2 hours after symptoms have begun. The guidelines recommend a "door-to-needle time" of 30 minutes, meaning the diagnosis of STEMI and initiation of fibrinolytic therapy should ideally take place within 30 minutes from the time the patient arrives at the hospital door. Once stabilized, the patient should be transferred to a facility capable of PCI in case reperfusion fails or reocclusion occurs.[5]

In patients with NSTE-ACS, fibrinolytic agents are not recommended. Thrombi in this population are primarily platelet-rich rather than fibrin-rich, and less responsive to fibrinolytic therapy.[25] Additionally, data from the TIMI IIIB trials suggest that compared with placebo, alteplase was not associated with any improvement in death, MI, or failure of initial therapy and was associated with an increased incidence in fatal and nonfatal MI.[26]

Antiplatelet and Anticoagulant Drugs

When thrombolysis occurs, whether because of the administration of a fibrinolytic agent or through activation of the body's own fibrinolytic system, the fibrin clot begins to disintegrate. As the clot dissolves, there is a paradoxical increase in local thrombin generation and enhanced platelet aggregability, which may lead to rethrombosis. Antiplatelet agents (aspirin, $P2Y_{12}$ receptor antagonists: clopidogrel, prasugrel, or ticagrelor, and the glycoprotein [GP] IIb/IIIa inhibitors), as well as parenteral anticoagulants (unfractionated heparin [UFH], low-molecular-weight heparins [LMWH] such as enoxaparin, and direct thrombin inhibitors [DTIs] such as bivalirudin), have been used to minimize rethrombosis. UFH has several limitations, including a highly variable anticoagulant effect necessitating frequent monitoring and development of heparin-induced thrombocytopenia (<0.2%). LMWH may offer advantages compared with heparin owing to its ease of administration, improved bioavailability, and need for less monitoring. Unlike UFH, the DTIs offer better protection against thrombin reactivation after therapy discontinuation.

The GP IIb/IIIa receptor inhibitors, which are tirofiban, eptifibatide, and abciximab are also used. Glycoprotein IIb/IIIa receptors are abundant on the platelet surface. Platelets become activated when patients are having an acute ischemic event or are undergoing PCI. With platelet activation, the GP IIb/IIIa receptor undergoes a conformational change that increases its affinity for binding fibrinogen. The binding of fibrinogen to receptors on platelets results in platelet aggregation, leading to thrombus formation. The GP IIb/IIIa receptor inhibitors prevent platelet aggregation by preventing fibrinogen from binding to GP IIb/IIIa receptor sites on activated platelets.[5]

Acute thrombocytopenia is a rare but recognized side effect of all three agents, but seen more often with abciximab.[27] The GP IIb/IIIa inhibitors are used in conjunction with other antiplatelet drugs and anticoagulants in patients with NSTE-ACS and in patients undergoing PCI. Although effective when used in conjunction with fibrinolytic agents for patients with STEMI, the benefit is offset by high rates of bleeding. Therefore, routine use of GP IIb/IIIa inhibitors is not recommended with fibrinolytics.[5]

Table 13-2
Evidenced-based Pharmacotherapies for Acute Coronary Syndromes[1,5]

Drug	Indication	Dose and Duration	Therapeutic End Points	Precautions	Comments
ACE inhibitors[a]	STEMI and NSTE-ACS within the first 24 hours of presentation for those with EF ≤40% or s/s of HF STEMI and NSTE-ACS for late hospital care for patients with hypertension, EF ≤ 40%, DM, or CKD STEMI and NSTE-ACS for indefinite use for all patients with EF ≤40%.	Usual captopril dose 12–50 mg TID, then start longer-acting ACE inhibitor. Duration indefinite.	Titrate to usual doses and maintain systolic BP > 90 mm Hg.	Avoid IV therapy within 48 hours of infarct. Avoid initiation with systolic BP <100 mm Hg, pregnancy, acute renal failure, angioedema, bilateral renal stenosis, serum potassium ≥ 5.5 mEq/L.	
Angiotensin receptor blockers[a]	STEMI and NSTE-ACS with ACE inhibitor intolerance.	Usual doses of ARBs (see Chapter 14, Heart Failure). Duration indefinite.	Same as for ACE inhibitors.	Same as for ACE inhibitors.	
Aldosterone antagonists[a]	STEMI and NSTE-ACS with EF ≤40% and either DM or HF symptoms already receiving therapeutic doses of an ACE inhibitor and β-blocker.	Spironolactone 12.5–50 mg daily or eplerenone 25–50 mg daily. Duration indefinite.	Titrate to heart failure symptom control without evidence of hyperkalemia	Hyperkalemia, hypotension Avoid if potassium ≥ 5 mEq/L or SCr ≥ 2.5 mg/dL for men and 2.0 mg/dL for women or CrCl ≤30 mL/minute	Dose can be increased every 4–8 weeks.
Aspirin[a]	STEMI and NSTE-ACS for all patients.	162–325 mg during AMI, then 81–325 mg daily indefinitely (81 mg daily is preferred).		Active bleeding, thrombocytopenia	Unless clear contraindication exists, aspirin should be given to all AMI patients.
Amiodarone	Treatment of VT, VF.	150 mg IV over 10 minutes, repeat for recurrence, follow with 1 mg/minute IV infusion for 6 hours, then 0.5 mg/minute (maximum: 2.2 g/24 hours).	Cessation of arrhythmia.	Bradycardia, hypotension.	
β-Blockers[a]	STEMI and NSTE-ACS in all patients without contraindications.	Variable. Titrate to HR and BP. It is reasonable to administer an IV β-blocker at the time of presentation to STEMI patients who are hypertensive and who do not have any of the following: (a) signs of heart failure, (b) evidence of a low output state, (c) increased risk for cardiogenic shock[b], or (d) other relative contraindications to β-blockade (PR interval > 0.24 second, second- or third-degree heart block, active asthma, or reactive airway disease). Duration indefinite.	Titrate to resting HR approx. 60 beats/minute, maintain systolic BP >100 mm Hg.	Observe HR and BP closely when given IV Contraindicated in patients with HR <50 beats/minute; PR ECG interval >0.24 second, second- or third-degree heart block, persistent hypotension, pulmonary edema, bronchospasm, risk of cardiogenic shock, severe reactive airway disease.	Unless clear contraindication exists, β_1-selective agents such as metoprolol and atenolol should be given to all AMI patients. In patients with systolic dysfunction, metoprolol, carvedilol, or bisoprolol can be considered.

Bivalirudin[a]	STEMI with primary PCI and NSTE-ACS with an early invasive strategy.	*STEMI with primary PCI*: 0.75 mg/kg IV bolus immediately prior to PCI, followed by 1.75 mg/kg/hour infusion with or without UFH. *NSTE-ACS with an early invasive strategy*: 0.1 mg/kg IV bolus followed by 0.25 mg/kg/hour infusion. Continue until diagnostic angiography or PCI is performed.		Avoid in patients with active bleeding.	Reduce infusion to 1 mg/kg/hour with estimated CrCl <30 mL/minute.
Cangrelor[a]	STEMI and NSTE-ACS before PCI in patients not treated with a $P2Y_{12}$ platelet inhibitor and are not being given a GP IIb/IIIa inhibitor.	30 μg/kg IV bolus prior to PCI followed immediately by a 4 μg/kg/minute IV infusion for at least 2 hours or duration of procedure, whichever is longer		Active bleeding	After discontinuation of infusion, an oral $P2Y_{12}$ platelet inhibitor should be administered: ticagrelor 180 mg load during or upon immediate discontinuation of infusion; prasugrel 60 mg or clopidogrel 600 mg upon immediate discontinuation of infusion.
Calcium-channel blockers	STEMI and NSTE-ACS for patients with ongoing ischemia who are receiving adequate doses of nitrates and β-blockers. Consider diltiazem or verapamil for patients with contraindication to β-blocker if EF normal.	Usual doses of calcium-channel blockers are used. Duration dictated by clinical scenario.	Titrate to usual doses and maintain systolic BP >90 mm Hg	Usual calcium-channel blocker contraindications. Avoid nondihydropyridines in patients with pulmonary congestion or EF <40% or AV block.	In patients with normal EF, most calcium-channel blockers will exert beneficial effects. Some data support use of verapamil or diltiazem for non–Q-wave AMI.
Clopidogrel[a]	STEMI and NSTE-ACS for patients allergic to aspirin.	75 mg daily.		Active bleeding, thrombotic thrombocytopenia purpura (rare).	
Clopidogrel + aspirin[a]	STEMI with fibrinolytic therapy, before PCI after fibrinolytic therapy, or before primary PCI. NSTE-ACS for early invasive or ischemia-guided strategies.	*STEMI with fibrinolytic therapy:* 300 mg load, then continue 75 mg daily, and continue for up to 1 year; aspirin 162–325 mg on first day, then 81–325 mg daily indefinitely (81 mg daily is preferred).		Active bleeding, thrombotic thrombocytopenia purpura (rare), avoid loading dose in patients ≥75 years of age, discontinue at least 5 days for CABG.	Whether administered before fibrinolytic or PCI, clopidogrel + aspirin reduced CV death, MI, or ischemia at 30 days. The 600 mg load should be considered if a GP IIb/IIIa is not used.

(continued)

Table 13-2
Evidenced-based Pharmacotherapies for Acute Coronary Syndromes (*continued*)

Drug	Indication	Dose and Duration	Therapeutic End Points	Precautions	Comments
		STEMI with fibrinolytic therapy with PCI: if PCI < 24 hours from fibrinolytic, then 300 mg load and for >24 hours from fibrinolytic, 600 mg load, then continue 75 mg daily if coronary stent deployed for at least 1 year; aspirin 162–325 mg on first day, then 81–325 mg daily indefinitely (81 mg is preferred). *STEMI before primary PCI:* 600 mg load, then continue 75 mg daily if coronary stent deployed for at least 1 year; aspirin 162–325 mg on first day, then 81–325 mg/day indefinitely. (81 mg daily is preferred.) *NSTE-ACS for early invasive or ischemia-guided strategy:* 300–600 mg load, then continue 75 mg daily for at least 1 year; aspirin 162–325 mg on first day, then 81–325 mg/day indefinitely. (81 mg daily is preferred).			
Enoxaparin[a]	STEMI (as an alternative for UFH) for patients receiving fibrinolytic therapy or for those not undergoing PCI. NSTE-ACS for early invasive or ischemia-guided strategies.	*STEMI with fibrinolytic therapy*: Age <75 years, administer 30 mg IV bolus followed by 1 mg/kg SQ every 12 hours (max dose of 100 mg for patients weighing ≥100 kg). Age ≥75, administer 0.75 mg/kg SQ every 12 hours (first two doses administer max dose of 75 mg for patients weighing ≥75 kg). Continue up to 8 days or until revascularization. *NSTE-ACS for early invasive or ischemia-guided strategies*: 1 mg/kg SQ every 12 hours. A supplemental 0.3 mg/kg IV dose should be administered at the time of PCI if the last dose of SC enoxaparin was given 8–12 hours before PCI. Continue for duration of hospitalization or until PCI.		Avoid in patients with active bleeding, history of HIT, planned CABG, SCr ≥ 2.5 mg/dL in men and ≥2.0 mg/dL in women, or CrCl <15 mL/minute.	For CrCl 15–29 mL/minute reduce to 1 mg/kg every 24 hours.

Fibrinolytic therapy[a]	STEMI presenting within 12 hours after onset of symptoms, can be considered in patients presenting within 12–24 hours after onset of symptoms with continuing s/s of ischemia.	See Table 13-3.	Improved TIMI grade flow.	See Table 13-4.	
Fondaparinux[a]	*STEMI:* alternative for UFH or LMWH in patients receiving fibrinolytic therapy or in those not undergoing PCI. *NSTE-ACS:* alternative for UFH or LMWH for early invasive or ischemia-guided strategies. Administer additional anticoagulant with factor IIa activity in patients undergoing PCI.	*STEMI:* 2.5 mg SQ daily starting on day 2 of hospitalization, continue for 8 days or until revascularization. *NSTE-ACS for early invasive or ischemia-guided strategies*: 2.5 mg SQ daily for the duration of the hospitalization or until PCI is performed.		Avoid with active bleeding or CrCl < 30 mL/minute.	In STEMI, fondaparinux reduced mortality and reinfarction without increased bleeding or strokes compared with UFH, but only in patients not undergoing PCI. In NSTE-ACS, fondaparinux was at least as effective as enoxaparin but exhibited less bleeding. Can possibly be used in HIT.
GP IIb/IIIa inhibitors[a]	*STEMI:* in patients undergoing PCI. *NSTE-ACS:* in patients treated with early invasive strategy and DAPT with intermediate/high-risk features.	See Table 13-6.		Avoid with active bleeding, thrombocytopenia, prior stroke.	In NSTE-ACS eptifibatide or tirofiban are FDA approved for PCI and ischemia-guided therapy. Abciximab is only for patients undergoing PCI.
Heparin[a]	*STEMI:* for patients undergoing PCI or treated with fibrinolytic therapy. *NSTE-ACS:* for early invasive or ischemia-guided strategies.	*STEMI with fibrinolytic therapy or NSTE-ACS with early invasive or ischemia-guided strategies*: 60 units/kg IV bolus (max 4,000 units) followed by 12 units/kg/hour (max 1,000 units/hour) for 48 hours or until revascularization. *STEMI with PCI:* 50–70 units/kg IV bolus if a GP IIb/IIIa inhibitor planned; or 70–100 units/kg IV bolus if no GP IIb/IIIa inhibitor. Continue for 48 hours or until end of PCI.	aPTT ratio 1.5–2.5× patient's control value, aPTT should be obtained 4–6 hours after initiation of infusion if not treated with fibrinolytic therapy or PCI and within 3 hours if treated with fibrinolytic therapy.	Avoid with active bleeding, thrombocytopenia, recent stroke.	Unless clear contraindication exists, UFH should be given to all AMI patients who do not receive fibrinolytic therapy.
Morphine and other analgesics	STEMI and NSTE-ACS for patients whose symptoms not relieved by NTG or adequate anti-ischemic therapy.	Morphine: 2–5 mg IV every 5–30 minutes PRN.	Decreased chest pain and HR.	Avoid morphine with bradycardia, right ventricular infarct, hypotension, confusion.	Has been associated with higher risk of death; discontinue nonselective NSAIDs and COX-2 selective agents.

(continued)

Table 13-2
Evidenced-based Pharmacotherapies for Acute Coronary Syndromes (*continued*)

Drug	Indication	Dose and Duration	Therapeutic End Points	Precautions	Comments
Nitroglycerin[a]	STEMI and NSTE-ACS with persistent ischemia, hypertension, or pulmonary congestion.	Variable; titrate to pain relief or systolic BP: 5–10 mcg/minute titrated to 200 mcg/minute. Usually maintain IV therapy for 24–48 hours after infarct.	Titrate to pain relief or systolic BP > 90 mm Hg	Avoid with systolic BP < 90 mm Hg, right ventricular infarction, sildenafil or vardenafil within 24 hours, or tadalafil within 48 hours.	Use acetaminophen or narcotics for headache. NTG should be tapered gradually in ischemic heart disease patients. Topical patches or oral nitrates are useful for patients with refractory symptoms.
Prasugrel + Aspirin[a]	*STEMI:* before PCI after fibrinolytic therapy or before primary PCI. *NSTE-ACS:* before PCI with coronary stenting.	60 mg loading dose, then 10 mg daily (if ≥60 kg) or 5 mg (if <60 kg) if coronary stent deployed for at least 1 year; aspirin 162–325 mg on day 1, then 81–325 mg daily indefinitely (81 mg daily is preferred).		Avoid with active bleeding, prior stroke or TIA, age ≥75 years Do not start if urgent CABG needed; discontinue 7 days before elective CABG or other surgery.	
Ticagrelor + Aspirin[a]	*ACS:* previous history of AMI *STEMI:* before primary PCI. *NSTE-ACS:* for early invasive or ischemia-guided strategies.	*ACS with previous history of MI:* Load with 180 mg oral loading dose following an ACS event, then continue treatment with 90 mg twice daily during the first year after an ACS event. After 1 year, administer 60 mg twice daily; aspirin 162–325 mg on day 1, then 81 mg daily indefinitely. *STEMI before primary PCI:* 180 mg load, then continue 90 mg BID if coronary stent deployed for at least 1 year; aspirin 162–325 mg on day 1, then 81 mg daily indefinitely. *NSTE-ACS with early invasive or ischemia-guided strategy*: 180 mg load, then continue 90 mg BID if coronary stent deployed or for both early invasive or ischemia-guided strategies for at least 1 year; aspirin 162–325 mg on day 1, then 81 mg daily indefinitely.	No firm end points	Avoid in patients with severe hepatic impairment or active bleeding. Maintenance doses of aspirin above 100 mg daily can decrease ticagrelor's effectiveness. Discontinue at least 5 days prior to CABG.	Monitor closely for dyspnea. For at least the first 12 months following ACS, ticagrelor was found to be superior to clopidogrel. Maximum dose of simvastatin is 40 mg with ticagrelor.

Vorapaxar	ACS for secondary prevention of thrombotic cardiovascular events.	1 tablet (2.08 mg) daily.		Contraindicated in history of stroke, TIA, ICH, or active bleeding.	Use with aspirin and/or clopidogrel according to their indications or standard of care. No data with ticagrelor or prasugrel or as use as a single antiplatelet agent.
Warfarin	STEMI and NSTE-ACS for left ventricular thrombus or for patients with AF with CHA_2DS_2VASc score ≥ 2.	Variable; titrate to INR. Duration usually dependent upon indication for warfarin.	INR goal 2–3. If receiving DAPT, then consider INR goal to 2.0–2.5 or discontinue aspirin.	Usual warfarin problems such as noncompliance and bleeding diathesis.	May be useful in the presence of a left ventricular thrombus or atrial fibrillation to prevent embolism.

ACE, angiotensin-converting enzyme; AF, atrial fibrillation; AMI, acute myocardial infarction; aPTT, activated partial thromboplastin time; ARBs, angiotensin receptor blockers; BID, twice daily; BP, blood pressure; CABG, coronary artery bypass graft; CHA_2DS_2VASc, risk score for atrial fibrillation comprising age, sex, HF, hypertension, stroke/TIA/thromboembolism, vascular disease, and DM; CKD, chronic kidney disease; CNS, central nervous system; COX-2, cyclooxygenase-2; CrCl, creatinine clearance; CV, cardiovascular; DAPT, dual antiplatelet therapy; DM, diabetes mellitus; ECG, electrocardiogram; EF, ejection fraction; FDA, Food and Drug Administration; GP IIb/IIIa, glycoprotein IIb/IIIa inhibitor; HF, heart failure; HIT, heparin-induced thrombocytopenia; HR, heart rate; INR, international normalized ratio; ICH, intracranial hemorrhage; IV, intravenous; LMWH, low-molecular-weight heparin; MI, myocardial infarction; NSAIDs, nonsteroidal antiinflammatory drugs; NSTE-ACS, non–ST segment elevation acute coronary syndrome; NTG, nitroglycerin; PCI, percutaneous coronary intervention; PRN, as needed; SCr, serum creatinine; SQ, subcutaneously; s/s, signs and symptoms; STEMI, ST segment elevation myocardial infarction; TIA, transient ischemic attack; TID, 3 times a day; TIMI, Thrombolysis in Myocardial Infarction; UHF, unfractionated heparin; VF, ventricular fibrillation; VT, ventricular tachycardia.

[a]Indicates specific drug therapies that are known to reduce morbidity or mortality.

[b]Risk factors for cardiogenic shock (the greater the number of risk factors present, the higher the risk of developing cardiogenic shock) are age >70 years, systolic BP < 120 mm Hg, sinus tachycardia >110 beats/minute, or HR < 60 beats/minute.

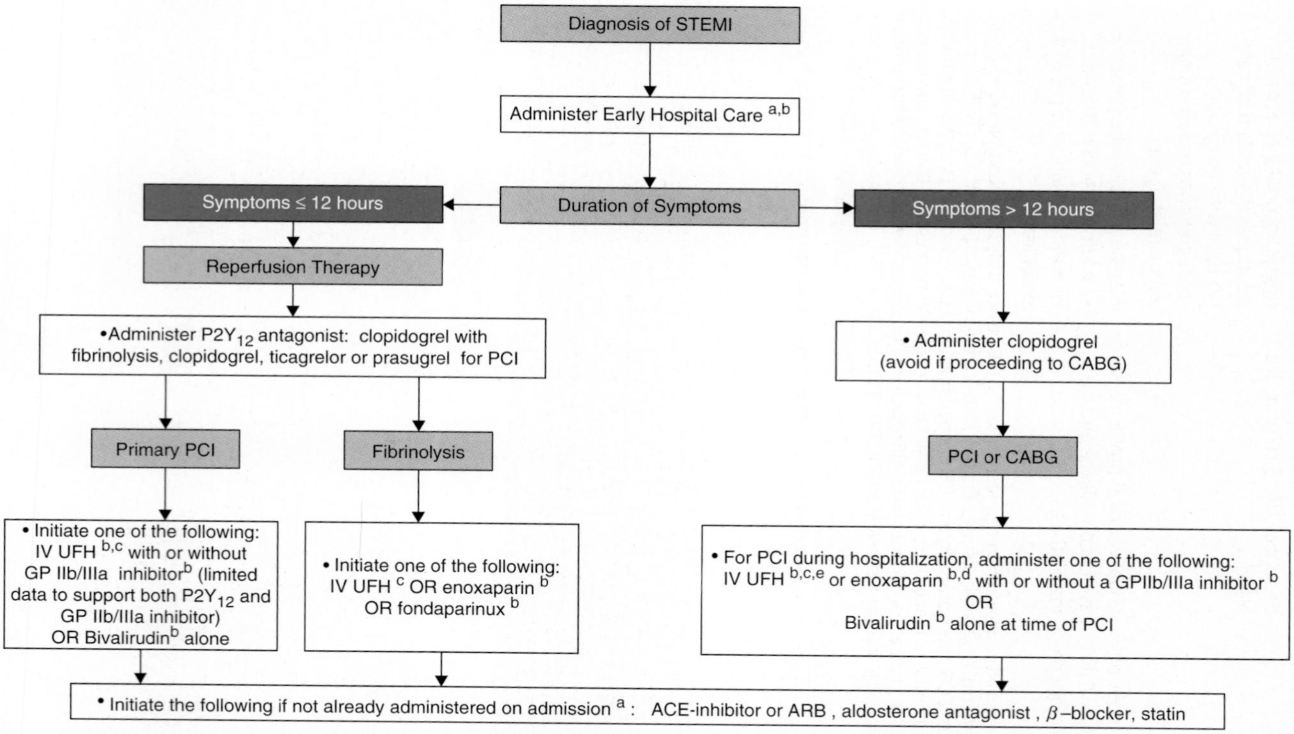

Figure 13-5 Initial treatment algorithm for STEMI. a: Early hospital care consists of oxygen for oxygen saturation <90%, SL nitroglycerin, IV nitroglycerin, IV morphine, β-blocker, ACE inhibitor or ARB, aldosterone antagonist, stool softener, and statin. b: Refer to Table 13-2 for indications, dosing, and contraindications. c: For at least 48 hours. d: For the duration of the hospitalization, up to 8 days. ACE, angiotensin-converting enzyme; ARB, angiotensin receptor blocker; CABG, coronary artery bypass graft; GP IIb/IIIa, glycoprotein IIB/IIIA; NTG, nitroglycerin; O_2, oxygen; PCI, percutaneous coronary intervention; SL, sublingual; STEMI, ST segment elevation myocardial infarction; UFH, unfractionated heparin. (Source: Kushner FG et al. 2009 focused updates: ACC/AHA guidelines for the management of patients with ST-elevation myocardial infarction (updating the 2004 guideline and 2007 focused update) and ACC/AHA/SCAI guidelines on percutaneous coronary intervention (updating the 2005 guideline and 2007 focused update) a report of the American College of Cardiology Foundation/American Heart Association Task Force on Practice Guidelines [published corrections appear in *J Am Coll Cardiol*. 2010;55:612 (dosage error in article text); *J Am Coll Cardiol*. 2009;54:2464]. *J Am Coll Cardiol*. 2009;54:2205; Anderson JL et al. ACC/AHA 2007 guidelines for the management of patients with unstable angina/non-ST-Elevation myocardial infarction: a report of the American College of Cardiology/American Heart Association Task Force on Practice Guidelines (Writing Committee to Revise the 2002 Guidelines for the Management of Patients With Unstable Angina/Non-ST-Elevation Myocardial Infarction) developed in collaboration with the American College of Emergency Physicians, the Society for Cardiovascular Angiography and Interventions, and the Society of Thoracic Surgeons endorsed by the American Association of Cardiovascular and Pulmonary Rehabilitation and the Society for Academic Emergency Medicine [published correction appears in *J Am Coll Cardiol*. 2008;51:974]. *J Am Coll Cardiol*. 2007;50:e1; O'Gara PT et al. 2013 ACCF/AHA guideline for the management of ST-elevation myocardial infarction: a report of the American College of Cardiology Foundation/American Heart Association Task Force on Practice Guidelines. *Circulation*. 2013;127(4):e362–e425.)

The $P2Y_{12}$ receptor antagonists, ticagrelor, prasugrel, and clopidogrel, have evolved to become an integral part in the management of ACS. By blocking the $P2Y_{12}$ adenosine diphosphate receptors, these agents decrease platelet activation and aggregation, increase bleeding time, and reduce blood viscosity.[1–5] Differences in antiplatelet potency, pharmacokinetics, pharmacodynamics, pharmacogenomics, and drug–drug interactions exist between the three agents (Table 13-5). Cangrelor is an intravenous agent recently approved to reduce the risk of thrombotic events in patients undergoing PCI. It is for patients who are not being treated with another $P2Y_{12}$ inhibitor or a GP IIb/IIIa inhibitor.[28] Compared with the oral agents, cangrelor has a very rapid onset (2 minutes) and offset of action (1 hour).[28] In the Cangrelor versus Standard Therapy to Achieve Optimal Management of Platelet Inhibition (CHAMPION) PHOENIX trial, the primary composite end point of death, MI, ischemia-driven revascularization, or stent thrombosis at 48 hours occurred in significantly fewer patients treated with IV cangrelor compared to oral clopidogrel (4.7% vs. 5.9%, $p = 0.005$). Although the benefit persisted at 30 days, it came at the expense of an increase in bleeding with rates of about one in 170 with cangrelor versus one in 275 with clopidogrel.[29] Controversy surrounds the use of pharmacogenomic and platelet function testing when determining whether a patient may be a "responder" or "nonresponder" to clopidogrel therapy.[30] At this time, the ACC / AHA guidelines do not recommend routine testing for genetic variants. See Chapter 12, Chronic Stable Angina, for greater detail about these controversies.

Vorapaxar is an oral antiplatelet that selectively inhibits the cellular actions of thrombin through antagonism of platelet protease-activated receptor-1. It is indicated for secondary prevention of cardiovascular events in patients who have a history of MI or peripheral vascular disease. In the Thrombin-Receptor Antagonist in Secondary Prevention of Atherothrombotic Ischemic Events (TRA2P–TIMI50) trial, patients with a history of MI, ischemic stroke, or peripheral arterial disease who received vorapaxar 2.5 daily had 13% reduction in the combined end point of death from cardiovascular causes, MI, or stroke ($p < 0.001$) and a 12% reduction in the combined end point of cardiovascular death, MI, stroke, or recurrent ischemia leading to revascularization ($p = 0.001$) compared to placebo.[31] However, patients receiving

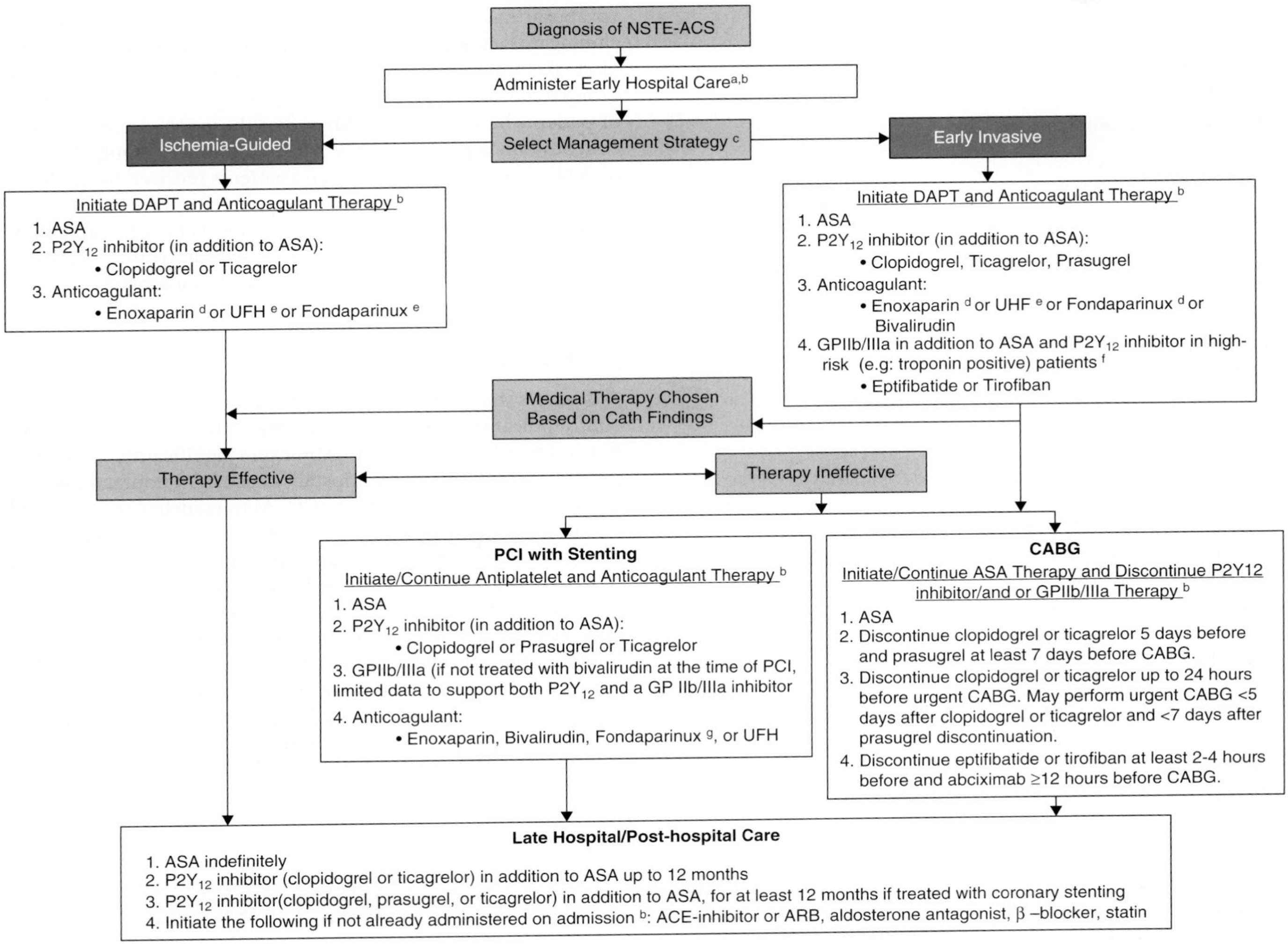

Figure 13-6 Initial treatment algorithm for NSTE-ACS. a: Early hospital care consists of oxygen for oxygen saturation <90%, SL nitroglycerin, IV nitroglycerin, IV morphine, *β*-blocker, ACE inhibitor or ARB, aldosterone antagonist, stool softener, and statin. b: Refer to Table 13-2 for indications, dosing, and contraindications. c: An early invasive strategy would be considered if one or more of the following occurs: recurrent angina or ischemia at rest, presence of elevated cardiac biomarkers, new or presumably new ST segment depression, signs or symptoms of HF or new worsening mitral regurgitation, hemodynamic instability, sustained ventricular tachycardia, PCI within 6 months, prior CABG, considered high risk per TIMI or GRACE risk score, LVEF < 40%. An ischemia-guided conservative strategy would be considered if the patient is classified as low-moderate risk per the TIMI or GRACE risk score or if the patient or clinician prefers this approach in the absence of high-risk features. d: For the duration of the hospitalization, up to 8 days. e: For at least 48 hours. f: Factors favoring administration of a GP IIb/IIIa in addition to a ASA and a $P2Y_{12}$ inhibitor are delay to angiography, high-risk features, and early recurrent ischemia. g: In patients who have been treated with fondaparinux (as upfront therapy) who are undergoing PCI, an additional anticoagulant with anti-IIa activity should be administered at the time of PCI due to the risk of catheter thrombosis. ACE, angiotensin-converting enzyme; ARB, angiotensin receptor blocker; ASA, aspirin; CABG, coronary artery bypass graft; Cath, catheterization; DAPT, dual antiplatelet therapy; GP IIb/IIIa, glycoprotein IIb/IIIa; HF, heart failure; GRACE, Global Registry of Acute Coronary Events; IV, intravenous; NSTE-ACS, non–ST segment elevation acute coronary syndrome; PCI, percutaneous coronary intervention; SL, sublingual; TIMI, Thrombolysis in Myocardial Infarction; UFH, unfractionated heparin. (Adapted with permission from Amsterdam et al. AHA/ACC 2014 guidelines for the management of patients with unstable angina/non-ST-elevation acute coronary syndromes: a report of the American College of Cardiology/American Heart Association Task Force on Practice Guidelines developed in collaboration with the Society for Cardiovascular Angiography and Interventions and the Society of Thoracic Surgeons endorsed by the American Association of Thoracic Surgeons. *J Am Coll Cardiol*. 2014;64:e1–e228.)

Table 13-3

Pharmacologic Properties of Approved Fibrinolytic Drugs[22]

Drug	Fibrin Specificity	Potential Antigenicity	TIMI Grade Flow at 90 Minutes (% of Patients)	Average Dose	Dosing Administration	Cost
Alteplase	Moderate	No	54	100 mg	15 mg IV bolus, 50 mg for 30 minutes, then 35 mg for 60 minutes[a]	High
Reteplase	Moderate	No	60	10 + 10 units	10 U IV bolus, second bolus 30 minutes later	High
Tenecteplase	High	No	63	30–50 mg (based on weight)[b]	Bolus for 5–10 seconds	High

IV, intravenous; TIMI, Thrombolysis in Myocardial Infarction.
[a]For patients = 65 kg; reduced doses for patients weighing <65 kg.
[b]For patients <60 kg, 30 mg; 60–69 kg, 35 mg; 70–79 kg, 40 mg; 80–89 kg, 45 mg; 90 kg, 50 mg.

Table 13-4
Risk Factors Associated with Bleeding Complications Secondary to Fibrinolytic Use[5]

Absolute Contraindications
Any prior intracranial hemorrhage
Known structural cerebral vascular lesion (e.g., arteriovenous malformation)
Known malignant intracranial neoplasm (primary or metastatic)
Active bleeding or bleeding diathesis (excluding menses)
Suspected aortic dissection
Significant closed-head or facial trauma within 3 months
Intracranial or intraspinal surgery within 2 months
Ischemic stroke within 3 months, EXCEPT acute ischemic stroke within 4.5 hours
Severe uncontrolled hypertension (unresponsive to emergency therapy)
Uncontrolled hypertension on presentation (SBP > 180 mm Hg, DBP > 110 mm Hg)
Chronic, severe, poorly controlled hypertension
Prior ischemic stroke > 3 months, dementia, or known intracranial pathology
Puncture of a noncompressible vessel
Major surgery (<3 weeks)
Recent internal bleeding within 2–4 weeks
Active peptic ulcer
Current use of anticoagulants (the higher the INR, the greater the risk for bleeding)
Pregnancy

DBP, diastolic blood pressure; INR, international normalized ratio; SBP, systolic blood pressure.

vorapaxar had an increase in moderate and severe bleeding including intracranial hemorrhage. Among patients with a history of stroke, the rate of intracranial hemorrhage in the vorapaxar group was 2.4% versus 0.9% with placebo ($p < 0.001$). About 67% of patients had a history of MI and of these 98% were receiving concomitant aspirin and 78% a $P2Y_{12}$ inhibitor.[31] Only 0.2% of patients received prasugrel and no patients received ticagrelor.[32] When considered for secondary prevention of thrombotic cardiovascular events in combination with aspirin and/or clopidogrel, vorapaxar is contraindicated in those with a history of stroke, transient ischemic attack, or intracranial hemorrhage.

β-Blockers

β-Blockers should be administered to patients with ACS unless a contraindication is present. In patients with ACS receiving either fibrinolytic therapy or PCI, β-blockers significantly decreased the rates of cardiovascular mortality, recurrent nonfatal MI, and all-cause mortality.[1–5] The 2014 ACC/AHA guidelines recommend that oral β-blocker therapy be initiated within 24 hours after the onset of symptoms for all patients without signs of HF, evidence of low output state, increased risk for cardiogenic shock or other contraindications. Both β-selective and nonselective agents have been evaluated; however, β-blockers with intrinsic sympathomimetic activity should be avoided as they lack efficacy data. For patients with tachycardia or hypertension without signs of HF, IV β-blockers followed by oral administration can be considered. Unless there are contraindications to their use, β-blocking agents should be prescribed for all patients after an AMI, and should be continued indefinitely.[5]

Table 13-5
Comparison of $P2Y_{12}$ Receptor Inhibitors[1,5,104]

Parameter	Clopidogrel	Prasugrel	Ticagrelor	Cangrelor
Class	Thienopyridine (second generation)	Thienopyridine (third generation)	Cyclopetyl triazolopyrimidine	Stabilized ATP analogue
Administration	Oral	Oral	Oral	Intravenous
Dose	300–600 mg LD 75 daily	60 mg LD 10 mg daily	180 mg LD 90 mg BID (60 mg BID for years 1–3)	30 μg/kg bolus 4 μg/kg/minute infusion
Age	–	If >75 years, not recommended unless history of DM or MI	–	–
Weight	–	If < 60 kg consider 5 mg daily	–	–
FDA Indications	ACS (NSTEMI, STEMI) Recent MI, stroke, PAD	*July 2009* NSTE-ACS + PCI STEMI + PCI	*July 2011* ACS (NSTE-ACS, STEMI)	*June 2015* PCI
Trials in ACS	CURE, PCI-CURE, CREDO, ACUITY, CLARITY, COMMIT	TRITON-TIMI 38 TRILOGY-ACS	PLATO PEGASUS TIMI-54	CHAMPION-PCI CHAMPION-PLATFORM CHAMPION-PHOENIX
Receptor Binding	Irreversible	Irreversible	Reversible	Reversible
Activation	Prodrug, limited by metabolism	Prodrug, *not* limited by metabolism	Active drug	Active drug
Interpatient variability	High	Low	Low	Low
Bioavailability	~50%	80%–100%	36%	NA
Onset of action	2–6 hours	30 minutes	0.5–2 hours	2 minutes

Table 13-5
Comparison of $P2Y_{12}$ Receptor Inhibitors (*continued*)

Parameter	Clopidogrel	Prasugrel	Ticagrelor	Cangrelor
Peak platelet inhibition	300 mg LD (6 hours) 600 mg LD (2 hours)	60 mg LD (1–1.5 hours)	180 mg LD (<1 hour)	30 μg/kg bolus (2 minutes)
Duration	3–10 days	5–10 days	1–3 days	1–2 hours
Half-life	6 hours	7 hours	7 hours	3–6 minutes
Metabolism	Hepatic via CYP450 (1A2, 3A4)	Minimal	Hepatic via CYP450 (main: 3A4, 2B6) (lesser: 2C9, 2C19)	Dephosphorylation by nucleotidases
Elimination	Urine 50% Feces 46%	Urine 68% Feces 27%	Urine 26% Feces 58%	Urine 58% Feces 35%
CYP2C19 Allele	Significant	Nonsignificant	Nonsignificant	Nonsignificant
Non-CABG major bleeding	Increased	>Clopidogrel	>Clopidogrel (overall) Similar in PCI	Similar (depending on definition)
CABG major bleeding	Increased	>Clopidogrel	=Clopidogrel Mortality benefit	Similar to placebo
Safe in stroke	Yes	Contraindicated	Similar stroke rate as clopidogrel Increased intracranial hemorrhage	Similar stroke rate as clopidogrel
Dyspnea/bradyarrhythmia	No	No	Yes	Yes
Platelet inhibition	~50%	~70%	>80%	100%
Drug–Drug Interactions	PPIs inhibit CYP 2C19 (concomitant use with omeprazole is discouraged per package labeling); enhanced bleeding with NSAIDs, oral anticoagulants, etc.	Minimal; enhanced bleeding with NSAIDs, oral anticoagulants, etc.	Strong CYP 3A4 inhibitors and inducers; max of simvastatin 40 mg; may increase digoxin concentrations; limit aspirin < 100 mg/day; enhanced bleeding with NSAIDs, oral anticoagulants, etc.	Enhanced bleeding with NSAIDs, oral anticoagulants, etc.
Drug–Disease Interactions	–	–	Careful with asthma, bradycardia, and possibly gout	Careful with asthma
Box warning	Genetic polymorphisms	Age-related bleeding Prior TIA/stroke	Prior intracranial hemorrhage Aspirin dosing > 100 mg	NA
CABG hold time	5 days	7 days	5 days	1 hour

ATP, adenosine diphosphate; CABG, coronary artery bypass graft; CYP, cytochrome P450; LD, loading dose; BID, twice daily; ACS, acute coronary syndrome; NSTEMI, non–ST elevation myocardial infarction; STEMI, ST-elevation myocardial infarction; MI, myocardial infarction; PAD, peripheral arterial disease; NSTE-ACS, non–ST elevation acute coronary syndrome; PCI, percutaneous coronary intervention; NA, not applicable; NSAIDs, nonsteroidal antiinflammatory drugs; PPIs, proton-pump inhibitors; TIA, transient ischemic attack.

Statins

β-Hydroxy-β-methylglutaryl-CoA (HMG-CoA) reductase inhibitors (statins) reduce long-term morbidity and mortality in patients with cardiovascular disease. Beyond their lipid-lowering properties, statins are believed to exhibit pleiotropic effects, which include plaque stabilization, anti-inflammation, antithrombogenicity, enhancement of arterial compliance, and modulation of endothelial function.[33] Data regarding early intensive statin therapy in patients with STEMI or NSTE-ACS exist with atorvastatin, simvastatin, pravastatin, rosuvastatin, and fluvastatin.[1,5,34] Recent ACC/AHA cholesterol guidelines shift away from specific low-density lipoprotein (LDL) targets, instead advocating for fixed doses of statins to reduce cardiovascular risk. Following an AMI, patients should receive a high-intensity statin such as atorvastatin 40 to 80 mg or rosuvastatin ≥ 20 mg daily. Lower doses could be considered in patients > 75 years of age or those unable to tolerate higher doses[34] (see Chapter 8, Dyslipidemias, Atherosclerosis, and Coronary Heart Disease).

Vasodilators

Other strategies for minimizing myocardial damage include the use of vasodilators in the peri-infarction period. Progressive LV dilatation ("remodeling") occurs in some patients after an AMI and has become an important marker for prognosis. Vasodilators reduce oxygen demand and myocardial wall stress by reducing afterload or preload and can attenuate the remodeling process. Some vasodilators may increase the blood supply to the myocardium by enhancing coronary vasodilatation.[1,5]

ACE inhibitors have been assessed in a large number of clinical trials, and all trials using oral agents have demonstrated a reduction in mortality.[1,5] Intravenous ACE inhibitors should be avoided because they cause excessive hypotension and do not improve survival. The benefit of ACE inhibitors is greatest in patients with anterior infarction, signs of HF, or a history of previous infarction. Ideally, oral ACE inhibitors should be started within 24 hours of diagnosis, after BP and renal function have stabilized. Initial doses should be low and then titrated as quickly as possible.[1,5] The ACC/AHA guidelines recommend an ARB in patients with ACS who cannot tolerate ACE inhibitors. The combination of an ACE inhibitor and ARB should be avoided because of an increase in adverse events such as hyperkalemia.

Aldosterone antagonists such as spironolactone and eplerenone have been associated with improved LV structural remodeling and performance by increasing LVEF and decreasing LV end-diastolic and end-systolic volumes. In the Eplerenone Post Acute Myocardial Infarction Heart Failure Efficacy and Survival Study (EPHESUS), patients with AMI and LV dysfunction (LVEF $< 40\%$) with or without HF were randomized 3 to 14 days after AMI to receive eplerenone (a selective aldosterone blocker). Eplerenone was found to decrease long-term mortality as an adjunct to ACE inhibitors and β-blockers.[35] Aldosterone blockade is recommended in post-MI patients with a LVEF $< 40\%$, diabetes or symptoms of HF, assuming they have no contraindications.[1]

Nitrates dilate venous capacitance vessels and peripheral arterioles. Their predominant effect is a decrease in preload, with a lesser effect on afterload. Consequently, nitrates lead to a decrease in both myocardial wall stress and oxygen demand. Intravenous NTG should be used in patients who have refractory ischemic discomfort (chest pain), acute HF, and/or hypertension. Hemodynamic targets are a systolic BP between 100 and 130 mm Hg with a heart rate less than 100 beats/minute.

Other vasodilators that have been investigated in the treatment of ACS are the calcium-channel blockers. There are several proposed mechanisms whereby a calcium-channel blocker might be beneficial. As a group, they dilate coronary and peripheral vessels. They also alleviate some of the coronary vasospasm present at the time of coronary thrombosis. In addition, they are effective anti-ischemic agents through their action in improving coronary blood supply and reducing myocardial oxygen demand.[1,5]

The ACC/AHA guidelines recommend calcium-channel blockers for patients with persistent or recurrent symptoms after treatment with full-dose nitrates and β-blockers, for patients with contraindications to β-blockade, and for patients with Prinzmetal or variant angina. For such patients, calcium-channel blockers that slow the heart rate (e.g., diltiazem or verapamil) are recommended. These nondihydropyridines should not be administered to patients with severe LV dysfunction or pulmonary edema. The Danish Verapamil Infarction Trial (DAVIT) evaluated the efficacy of verapamil for patients with ACS.[36] There was a trend toward lower MI and mortality rates when verapamil was given to patients with suspected ACS. Similar reductions in MI and refractory angina rates have been demonstrated with diltiazem.[37] The dihydropyridine calcium antagonists amlodipine and felodipine have not been evaluated specifically for administration to patients with ACS, but trials involving normotensive patients with coronary artery disease (CAD) or hypertensive patients with cardiovascular risk factors have demonstrated that these agents provide significant benefits in reducing cardiovascular events.[38,39]

Analgesics

It is important to abolish the patient's pain as quickly as possible because pain and anxiety associated with an AMI will contribute to increased myocardial oxygen demand. If the pain is not relieved by medications (e.g., nitrates, β-blockers), then additional analgesia may be necessary. Morphine sulfate (2 to 4 mg IV with increments of 2 to 8 mg IV repeated at 5 to 15 minute intervals) is the analgesic of choice for management of pain associated with STEMI. In addition to diminishing pain and anxiety, morphine also has beneficial hemodynamic effects. By reducing pain and anxiety, the release of circulating catecholamines is diminished, possibly reducing the associated arrhythmias. Morphine also causes peripheral venous and arterial vasodilatation, which reduces preload and afterload and, consequently, myocardial oxygen demand. However, retrospective studies have suggested the potential for increased mortality in patients with NSTE-ACS receiving morphine; thus, morphine carries a Class IIb recommendation in the 2014 ACC/AHA NSTE-ACS guidelines.[40] Clinicians should be aware of potential unwanted side effects of morphine such as hypotension, nausea, and respiratory depression.

The nonselective and cyclooxygenase (COX)-2–selective nonsteroidal antiinflammatory drugs (NSAIDs) have been associated with an increased risk of mortality, reinfarction, hypertension, HF, and myocardial rupture. These agents should be discontinued at the time a patient presents with ACS.[1,5]

Stool Softeners

It is common to administer agents such as docusate to prevent constipation in AMI patients because straining causes undesirable stress on the cardiovascular system.[1,5]

Oxygen

Many patients are modestly hypoxemic during the initial hours of an AMI. Supplemental oxygen should be administered to patients with ACS with an arterial saturation less than 90%, respiratory distress, or other high-risk features for hypoxemia. Patients with severe hypoxemia or pulmonary edema may require intubation and mechanical ventilation.[1,5]

Antiarrhythmic Agents

Ventricular arrhythmias, including ventricular fibrillation, are common complications associated with myocardial ischemia and AMI as well as a major cause of death. More than half of the episodes of ventricular fibrillation that occur with an AMI are within 1 hour of the onset of symptoms. If an antiarrhythmic agent is necessary, amiodarone is preferred over lidocaine (see Chapter 15, Cardiac Arrhythmias). The routine use of prophylactic lidocaine or other antiarrhythmic agents to prevent ventricular tachycardia and ventricular fibrillation is not recommended. Although lidocaine may reduce the number of episodes of ventricular fibrillation, it may contribute to an increased number of episodes of asystole.[5]

Suppression of ventricular ectopy after an AMI with the chronic use of oral antiarrhythmic agents is not recommended. Results of the Cardiac Arrhythmia Suppression Trial (CAST) showed an increase in mortality in asymptomatic patients with ventricular ectopy after an AMI who were treated with flecainide, encainide, or moricizine (see Chapter 15, Cardiac Arrhythmias).[41,42]

Nondrug Therapy

For STEMI, primary PCI is the preferred method for reperfusion as long as it can be performed in a timely fashion. Specific guidelines have been published by the ACC/AHA addressing PCI and stent use in AMI.[43]

For patients presenting to a PCI-capable hospital, PCI should be performed within 90 minutes after initial medical contact (also referred to as "door-to-balloon time"). If a patient is at a non-PCI facility, immediate transfer to primary PCI is preferred only if PCI can be performed within 120 minutes of first medical contact.[5] This threshold is based on a multivariant analysis of patients undergoing PCI in which an increased door-to-balloon time exceeding 120 minutes was associated with a higher mortality rate.[44] Fibrinolytic therapy should be given to patients when the 120-minute time goal cannot be met, unless a contraindication is present.[5]

The disadvantages of PCI include the longer amount of time needed to mobilize the personnel needed to prepare the catheterization laboratory and its initial higher cost. A potential advantage of PCI is the greater ability to achieve TIMI grade 3 flow in the affected vessel compared to fibrinolytic therapy (90% vs. 50%–60%, respectively).[5] PCI is associated with fewer major adverse cardiac events, irrespective of patient presentation time. Additionally, rates of major bleeding and intracranial hemorrhage are lower with PCI compared to fibrinolytic therapy. Unfortunately, many hospitals do not have the facilities or skilled personnel to complete this procedure in the necessary time frame.[5]

For NSTE-ACS, coronary angiography aids in defining the extent and location of coronary lesion and in directing the definitive care strategy (e.g., PCI with stent placement, CABG, or medical management). However, because angiography is an invasive procedure, there is a small risk of serious complications. Therefore, coronary angiography should be used only in patients for whom the procedure's benefits outweigh its risks. With this principle in mind, two pathways of treatment for NSTE-ACS patients have emerged: the early invasive strategy and the ischemia-guided strategy (Fig. 13-6). In the early invasive strategy, all patients without contraindications undergo coronary angiography with the intent to perform revascularization within 24 hours of hospital admission. The ischemia-guided strategy consists of aggressive medical therapy for all patients and coronary angiography only for those with certain risk factors or who fail medical therapy.

CLINICAL PRESENTATION OF ACS

CASE 13-1

QUESTION 1: P.H., a 68-year-old, 80-kg man, is being admitted to the ED after experiencing an episode of sustained chest pain while mowing his yard. After waiting 6 hours, he called 911 and was transported to the ED to a facility without the ability to conduct PCI. Physical examination reveals an anxious and diaphoretic man. Heart rate and rhythm are regular, and no S_3 or S_4 sounds are present. Vital signs include BP 180/110 mm Hg, heart rate 105 beats/minute, and respiratory rate 32 breaths/minute. P.H.'s chest pain radiates to his left arm and jaw, and he describes the pain as "crushing" and "like an elephant sitting on my chest." He rates it as a "10/10" in intensity. Thus far, his pain has not responded to five SL NTG tablets at home and three more in the ambulance. His ECG reveals a 3-mm ST segment elevation and Q waves in leads I and V_2 to V_4. Based on his history and physical examination, P.H. is diagnosed with an anterior infarction. Laboratory values include the following:

Sodium (Na), 141 mEq/L
Potassium (K), 3.9 mEq/L
Chloride (Cl), 100 mEq/L
CO_2, 20 mEq/L
Blood urea nitrogen (BUN), 19 mg/dL
Serum creatinine (SCr), 1.2 mg/dL
Glucose, 149 mg/dL
Magnesium (Mg), 2 mEq/L
CK, 1,200 U/L, with a 12% CK-MB fraction (normal, 0%–5%)
Troponin I-Ultra, 60 ng/mL (normal, <0.02 ng/mL)
Cholesterol, 259 mg/dL
Triglycerides, 300 mg/dL

P.H. has a prior history of CAD. A previous cardiac catheterization 2 years ago revealed lesions in his middle left anterior descending coronary artery (75% stenosis) and proximal left circumflex artery (30% stenosis). His echocardiogram at the time showed an EF of 58%. These lesions were deemed suitable for medical management. He also has a history of recurrent bouts of bronchitis associated with bronchospasm for 10 years, diabetes mellitus treated with insulin for 18 years with a hemoglobin A_{1c} of 6.8% obtained 6 months prior to admission, and hypertension with BPs usually 140/85 mm Hg. His father died of an MI at age 70. His mother and siblings are all alive and well. P.H. has smoked one pack of cigarettes a day for 30 years, and he drinks approximately one six-pack of beer a week. He has no history of IV drug use. On admission, P.H.'s medications include insulin glargine 40 units daily; albuterol inhaler as needed (PRN) for shortness of breath; hydrochlorothiazide 25 mg daily; NTG patch 0.2 mg/hour; and NTG SL 0.4 mg PRN for chest pain.

What signs and symptoms does P.H. have that are consistent with the diagnosis of AMI?

P.H. described his pain as a pressure sensation, which is common with ischemic heart disease. The chest discomfort associated with ACS often is described as pressure or as a tight band around the chest rather than pain. Although P.H. was involved in physical exertion when his chest discomfort began, this is not always the case. It can begin at rest and, frequently, in the early morning hours. At least 20% of patients with AMI have no pain or discomfort; these episodes are described as "silent" MIs.[5] Presentations range from no symptoms to shortness of breath, hypotension, HF, syncope, or ventricular arrhythmias. Silent or atypical infarctions occur more commonly in people with diabetes and in the elderly. P.H. is diaphoretic, a common finding, but other common symptoms such as nausea and anxiety are not present. He also describes his pain as "10/10" in intensity, or perhaps "the worst pain I've ever experienced," which is typical of a STEMI. The diagnosis primarily lies in the symptoms (e.g., the patient's "story"), the ECG, and the laboratory findings.

The history of diabetes, hypertension, smoking, and a positive family history in P.H. are all risk factors for coronary disease. His admission BP is high, which could indicate poor underlying control or anxiety and stress related to his ACS. The blood sugar of 149 mg/dL is high, again indicating either poor control or a stress response. Measurement of glycosylated hemoglobin is indicated during his hospitalization to better assess his diabetes control.

Laboratory Abnormalities

CASE 13-1, QUESTION 2: What laboratory abnormalities can you expect to see in P.H.?

P.H. demonstrates several laboratory abnormalities commonly seen with both STEMI and NSTEMI. Both his CK-MB and troponin are elevated, consistent with myocardial necrosis. With UA, cardiac biomarkers are not elevated. Several other nonspecific laboratory findings should be monitored in P.H. Hyperglycemia may develop because P.H. has diabetes, but this can also occur in patients without diabetes. ACS is also accompanied by an acute systemic inflammatory response manifested by fever, leukocytosis, and elevation of the erythrocyte sedimentation rate and C-reactive protein, as well as a drop in LDL, high-density lipoprotein, and total cholesterol. Specifically, these lipoprotein changes may begin to decrease within 24 to 48 hours after an ACS event, reaching a nadir within 5 to 7 days and then gradually recovering during the next 30 days.[45] Therefore, it is prudent to check serum lipid profiles within the first 24 hours of the AMI to get an accurate determination of the patient's lipid values.

ST Segment Elevation Myocardial Infarction Versus Non–ST Segment Elevation Myocardial Infarction

CASE 13-1, QUESTION 3: P.H. was noted to have ST segment elevation on the ECG. What are the implications of an ST segment elevation versus non–ST segment elevation MI?

Perhaps the most important diagnostic test in someone suspected of having an AMI is the ECG. The ECG is an important tool because it is noninvasive, can be performed rapidly, is readily available in most settings, and helps determine where the AMI is located (i.e., anterior, inferior, lateral). P.H. has classic ECG changes (ST segment elevation), and presence in the anterior ECG leads (V_2–V_4) points to the coronary artery likely to be blocked. P.H.'s previous left anterior descending lesion may have had a plaque rupture leading to thrombosis of the vessel.

The presence of ST segment elevation in two contiguous leads indicates severe ischemia and occlusion of the coronary artery. Every effort should be made to open the infarct-related artery as soon as possible, which could consist of PCI or fibrinolytic therapy. If the ECG showed ST segment depression (e.g., NSTE-ACS), instead of elevation, P.H. would not be eligible for fibrinolytic therapy because the risks of fibrinolytic therapy outweigh the benefits in NSTE-ACS.

Anterior Versus Inferior Infarction

CASE 13-1, QUESTION 4: What are the prognostic implications of an anterior versus an inferior MI?

Damage to the anterior section of the heart is more likely to be associated with increased morbidity (e.g., LV dysfunction) and mortality. The patients at highest risk of death are those with an anterior ACS, LV dysfunction, and complex ventricular ectopy. P.H. is at an increased risk because he has sustained an anterior infarction.

Risk Stratification

CASE 13-1, QUESTION 5: What is P.H.'s initial risk of mortality based on his presenting signs and symptoms?

Using the TIMI Risk Score for STEMI, P.H. has a score of 6 based on his age (2 points); history of angina, hypertension, and diabetes (1 point); heart rate (2 points); and location of his MI (1 point) (Table 13-1). P.H. has a 30-day mortality rate of 16%, thereby highlighting the serious nature of this event. If P.H. had experienced an NSTE-ACS with ST segment depression, he would have a TIMI risk score of 5 based on his age (1 point); at least three risk factors for CAD (1 point), prior CAD history (1 point), ST segment deviation (1 point), and elevated cardiac biomarkers (1 point). Based on this TIMI risk score, P.H. would be at high risk for death, MI, or need for urgent coronary artery revascularization within 30 days.

Therapeutic Objectives

CASE 13-1, QUESTION 6: What are the immediate and long-term therapeutic objectives in treating P.H.?

With both STEMI and NSTE-ACS, the immediate therapeutic objectives particularly as they apply to P.H. are to restore blood flow to the infarct-related artery, arrest infarct expansion, alleviate his symptoms, and prevent death. These objectives are achieved primarily by restoring coronary blood flow (administering a fibrinolytic or performing PCI for STEMI or performing PCI with NSTE-ACS) and lowering myocardial oxygen demand with nitrates and β-blockers. Any life-threatening ventricular arrhythmias that develop must be treated. The long-term therapeutic objectives are to prevent or minimize recurrent ischemic symptoms, reinfarction, HF, and sudden cardiac death. As P.H. is experiencing a STEMI, the specific therapeutic regimens are discussed in the questions that follow.

TREATMENT FOR ST SEGMENT ELEVATION MYOCARDIAL INFARCTION

Fibrinolytic Therapy

CASE 13-1, QUESTION 7: Is P.H. a candidate for fibrinolytic therapy? Is any one agent preferred?

STEMI is a medical emergency, and rapid administration of drug therapy is crucial to save myocardial tissue. The results of several major trials have shown unequivocally that if used appropriately, fibrinolytic agents can reduce the mortality associated with an AMI. Because mortality benefit is greatest when fibrinolytic therapy is administered within 2 hours of symptom onset, prehospital fibrinolytic therapy, in which trained paramedics administer the fibrinolytic in the field, is an attractive option to reduce total ischemic time.[46] If primary PCI cannot be performed within 120 minutes, fibrinolytic therapy should be given if no contraindications are present. For patients who present >12 hours after symptom onset, fibrinolytic therapy should be administered only if there is ongoing ischemia, hemodynamic instability or a large area of myocardium is involved. In the case of P.H., he is admitted to a hospital that is not PCI capable and cannot be transferred to a PCI-capable hospital within 120 minutes of first medical contact.

Controversy still exists about which fibrinolytic should be used, the best dosing regimen, the most appropriate adjunctive therapy, and whether the risk outweighs the benefit in some subpopulations of patients (e.g., those with an inferior AMI). P.H. has a history of hypertension, and at presentation his BP is 180/110 mm Hg. A BP this high is a relative contraindication to fibrinolytic therapy because of an increased risk of cerebral hemorrhage; however, P.H. has an anterior MI and is likely to benefit from fibrinolytic therapy. In this case, he should receive IV NTG immediately because the onset of BP control with this agent usually occurs within minutes. Once his systolic BP is less than 180 mm Hg and the diastolic is less than 110 mm Hg, a fibrinolytic can be administered. The NTG will also reduce the workload on his heart and may provide pain relief.

Because P.H. has severe pain and ECG changes consistent with an anterior AMI, he is at high risk for substantial morbidity or mortality. The argument for or against a specific fibrinolytic is probably less important than the decision to use an agent and to administer the medication as soon as possible after the onset of symptoms. P.H. is fortunate because he has presented within 1 hour of the onset of chest pain. Options in the United States include only fibrin-specific agents (Table 13-3).

Reteplase was compared with t-PA in the Global Utilization of Streptokinase and t-PA for Occluded Arteries (GUSTO)-III trial.[47] Reteplase has a slower clearance from the body, allowing the drug to be given as a bolus without the need for a constant infusion. In the GUSTO-III trial, reteplase was administered in two bolus doses of 10 million units, given 30 minutes apart. The mortality rate and incidence of stroke were the same in the two groups of patients. Tenecteplase (TNK) was compared with t-PA in the Second Assessment of Safety and Efficacy of a New Fibrinolytic (ASSENT-2) trial.[48] Tenecteplase was administered as a bolus of 30 to 50 mg for 5 to 10 seconds, based on body weight. No difference existed between TNK and t-PA in 30-day mortality and stroke and TNK had fewer bleeding complications. The 2013 guidelines do not explicitly endorse one fibrinolytic versus another, and all are acceptable first-line agents. Selection is usually based on clinician preference and hospital formulary.

ADJUNCT THERAPY

CASE 13-1, QUESTION 8: Orders are written for an infusion of t-PA along with UFH 4,000 units IV bolus, followed by 960 units/hour by continuous infusion. Aspirin 325 mg is ordered stat. Are both UFH and aspirin agents necessary?

The Second International Study of Infarct Survival (ISIS)-2 trial showed that the combination of aspirin and streptokinase reduced mortality in patients with an AMI by 42% compared to placebo.[49] In doses of 162 mg or more, aspirin generates a prompt clinical antithrombotic effect as a result of its inhibition of thromboxane A_2 production. Thus, immediate administration of 162 to 325 mg of aspirin in all patients diagnosed with ACS is indicated. In the acute setting, aspirin should be chewed because it is absorbed more quickly. All patients should receive low-dose aspirin indefinitely after a diagnosis of ACS. If patients have a contraindication to aspirin, clopidogrel can be substituted.[5]

The use of UFH as adjunct therapy to prevent reocclusion has been evaluated in many studies.[5] Because P.H. will receive t-PA, an IV UFH bolus followed by a continuous infusion should be started before the end of the t-PA infusion. The ACC/AHA guidelines recommend an initial UFH bolus of 60 units/kg (maximum of 4,000 units), followed by an initial infusion of 12 units/kg/hour (maximum of 1,000 units/hour) for 48 hours after fibrinolysis, with a targeted activated partial thromboplastin time (aPTT) of 1.5 to 2 times the upper limit of normal. UFH should always be considered in patients at high risk for systemic or venous embolism.

CASE 13-1, QUESTION 9: Would P.H. benefit from the addition of clopidogrel to his current drug regimen?

Two studies have evaluated the potential role of in-hospital clopidogrel as an integral part of fibrinolytic therapy in patients with STEMI.[50,51] The Clopidogrel as Adjunctive Reperfusion Therapy–Thrombolysis in Myocardial Infarction 28 (CLARITY-TIMI 28) evaluated patients with STEMI who received standard fibrinolytic therapy, aspirin, and UFH, and were scheduled for angiography within 2 days.[51] Patients received either clopidogrel (300 mg loading dose, followed by 75 mg daily) or placebo within 10 minutes of fibrinolytic administration. Clopidogrel was continued up to and including the day of angiography and then stopped. The primary end point was the composite of an occluded infarct-related artery on predischarge angiography or death or an MI up to the start of coronary angiography. Compared with placebo, patients receiving clopidogrel demonstrated a 36% reduction in the primary end point ($p < 0.001$). By 30 days, the clopidogrel treatment group had a 20% reduction in cardiovascular death, recurrent MI, or recurrent ischemia ($p = 0.03$). No difference in the rate of major bleeding was seen between groups. In a substudy of patients proceeding to nonemergent PCI after fibrinolytic therapy, patients receiving pretreatment with clopidogrel demonstrated a 66% reduction in 30-day mortality compared with those receiving placebo ($p = 0.034$).[52]

The Clopidogrel and Metoprolol in Myocardial Infarction Trial (COMMIT) evaluated the effect of clopidogrel 75 mg daily (with no loading dose) or placebo in 45,852 patients presenting with STEMI.[50] In the trial population, 93% had ST segment elevation or bundle branch block, 7% had ST segment depression, and 54% were treated with fibrinolytic therapy. The initial clopidogrel dose was given within 24 hours of symptom onset and continued until hospital discharge or up to 4 weeks in the hospital. Compared with placebo, clopidogrel was associated with a 9% reduction in death, reinfarction, or stroke ($p = 0.002$), and a 7% reduction in all-cause mortality ($p = 0.03$). No significant excess in bleeding was noted with clopidogrel, either overall or in patients who received concomitant fibrinolytic therapy or were older than 70 years. On the basis of these two studies, P.H. should receive clopidogrel as an inpatient.

CASE 13-1, QUESTION 10: What dose of clopidogrel should be considered?

According to the 2013 ACC/AHA guidelines, clopidogrel should be added to aspirin in patients who undergo reperfusion with fibrinolytic therapy.[5] A loading dose of clopidogrel 300 mg can be administered with fibrinolytic therapy followed by 75 mg/day for maintenance. The maintenance dose should be continued for 14 days and up to 1 year. The 1-year duration is extrapolated from experience with NSTE-ACS.[1] There are no studies evaluating a 600-mg loading dose in patients with STEMI treated with fibrinolytics. Additionally, uncertainty exists about the safety of giving a loading dose of clopidogrel in adults 75 years of age and older, particularly when they receive a fibrinolytic. Therefore, in this population, a loading dose should be avoided. A single loading dose of 300 mg of clopidogrel should be given to patients less than 75 years of age who receive a fibrinolytic agent and are subsequently proceeding to PCI within 24 hours.[5] If the patient received a fibrinolytic and then proceeds to PCI after 24 hours has lapsed, then a loading dose of 600 mg is preferred. For P.H., a loading dose of 300 mg of clopidogrel should be administered at the time of fibrinolytic administration followed by 75 mg/day for 14 days to 1 year. Because P.H. has already received 325 mg of aspirin in the ED, he should continue 81 mg of daily aspirin indefinitely.

CASE 13-1, QUESTION 11: What roles do the other anticoagulant and antiplatelet agents have in P.H.'s management?

Data available with the newer $P2Y_{12}$ inhibitors when used in the setting of fibrinolytic therapy are lacking. It would be prudent to avoid giving prasugrel and other potent $P2Y_{12}$ antagonists no sooner than 24 hours after administration of a fibrinolytic.[5] Coronary anatomy should be known to ensure the patient is not a candidate for CABG.

The replacement of UFH with a LMWH, factor Xa inhibitor, or the addition of a GP IIb/IIIa inhibitor to fibrinolytic therapy has been evaluated in patients with STEMI.

In the Enoxaparin and Thrombolysis Reperfusion for Acute Myocardial Infarction Study-25 (ExTRACT-TIMI 25), 20,506 patients with STEMI scheduled for fibrinolytic therapy were randomized to receive either enoxaparin or continuous infusion of UFH for 48 hours.[53] Enoxaparin was dosed according to age and renal function. UFH was dosed according to weight and adjusted to achieve an aPTT 1.5 to 2.0 times control. The composite end point of death or nonfatal MI through 30 days occurred in 12.0% in the UFH group and 9.9% in the enoxaparin group, representing a 17% risk reduction ($p < 0.001$). No difference was noted in mortality between the two groups. Major bleeding was higher in the enoxaparin group.

The Organization for the Assessment of Strategies for Ischemic Syndromes (OASIS) 6 was a randomized double-blind trial of 12,092 patients with STEMI assessing the effect of early initiation of fondaparinux with primary PCI and medical therapy.[54] The study compared the effects of fondaparinux with two different control arms. Patients with confirmed STEMI were assigned into one of the two following strata. Stratum 1: no indication for UFH (patients receiving streptokinase or those not receiving a thrombolytic agent) were assigned to this stratum. Stratum 2: indication for UFH (patients receiving alteplase, reteplase, or tenecteplase, and those undergoing primary PCI) were assigned to this stratum. Death or reinfarction at 30 days was significantly reduced in the fondaparinux group. However, fondaparinux did not benefit patients who were managed with primary PCI. Although the rates of death, MI, and severe bleeds did not differ in these patients, there was a higher rate of catheter thrombosis with fondaparinux.[54]

The TIMI-14 trial demonstrated enhanced reperfusion (TIMI 3 flow) using reduced-dose t-PA combined with abciximab compared with full-dose t-PA alone.[55] The GUSTO-V trial compared standard-dose reteplase to half-dose reteplase plus full-dose abciximab in STEMI patients.[56] The combination group had less reinfarction and recurrent ischemia, but more episodes of moderate and severe bleeding, especially in the elderly. Similar rates of enhanced reperfusion have also been observed with the combination of double-bolus dose eptifibatide (180/90 mcg/kg, 10 minutes apart) with a 48-hour infusion (2 mcg/kg/minute) plus half-dose t-PA (50 mg).[57] The ASSENT-3 trial assessed three regimens: (1) full-dose TNK plus enoxaparin or (2) full-dose TNK plus UFH or (3) half-dose TNK plus UFH with a 12-hour infusion of abciximab. The addition of either abciximab or enoxaparin to TNK reduced the composite end point of 30-day mortality, in-hospital reinfarction, or ischemia compared with UFH. More major bleeding complications were seen with abciximab compared with UFH.[58] In a meta-analysis of 11 trials involving 27,115 STEMI patients who received adjunctive abciximab in addition to either PCI or fibrinolytic therapy, use of abciximab was associated with a significant reduction in 30-day ($p = 0.047$) and 1- to 6-month mortality ($p = 0.01$) in patients undergoing PCI but not in those receiving fibrinolytic therapy.[59] Despite an improvement in patency rates, the combination of GP IIb/IIIa inhibitors with either full- or half-dose fibrinolytic should be avoided if at all possible, especially in the elderly.[5]

Based on data from ExTRACT-TIMI 25 and OASIS-6, the ACC/AHA guidelines allow for substitution of UFH with either enoxaparin or fondaparinux.[5] However, whereas fondaparinux appeared to be superior to control therapy in the OASIS-6 trial, relative benefit compared with placebo and UFH separately cannot be reliably determined.[60] If enoxaparin or fondaparinux are selected, anticoagulation should be continued for the duration of the hospitalization, up to 8 days or until revascularization. For P.H., enoxaparin would be the more appropriate choice; however, he will have a higher risk for bleeding and need to be monitored closely. Because P.H. is not undergoing PCI, the bleeding risks outweigh any benefit from the addition of a GP IIb/IIIa at this time.[5]

DETERMINATION OF REPERFUSION

CASE 13-1, QUESTION 12: How can you monitor for successful reperfusion in P.H. after he has received fibrinolytic therapy?

It is important to determine whether thrombolysis has been successful because the prognosis of the patient is related to the presence or absence of an open infarct-related artery. If fibrinolytic therapy fails to open the infarct-related artery, then the patient may benefit from PCI or a CABG. Although coronary angiography has been the standard for determining the success of reperfusion, this procedure is expensive and may be misleading, as some studies have suggested that microvascular perfusion may be impaired even when TIMI grade 3 flow has been achieved. A simple and readily available technique is evaluation of ECG ST segment resolution. A resolution of more than 50% of the ST segment elevation at 60 to 90 minutes after the initiation of fibrinolytic therapy is a good indicator of improved myocardial perfusion.[5] Relief of symptoms, maintenance or restoration of hemodynamic or electrical stability or both, and a reduction of >70% in the initial ST segment elevation are all suggestive of adequate reperfusion. P.H. should undergo a 12-lead ECG to evaluate reperfusion.[5]

CASE 13-1, QUESTION 13: P.H. continues to have chest pain, should the thrombolytic be readministered?

READMINISTRATION OF THROMBOLYTIC AGENTS

Reocclusion of the infarct-related artery after initial successful thrombolysis is a major setback. If reocclusion occurs, mechanical intervention (e.g., PCI) is often attempted. Several studies have evaluated whether to readminister the fibrinolytic or refer the patient for PCI. In a meta-analysis of eight trials of patients with STEMI who failed fibrinolytic therapy, those receiving rescue PCI showed no significant reduction in all-cause mortality, but had a 27% risk reduction in HF ($p = 0.05$) and 42% reduction in reinfarction ($p = 0.04$) when compared with standard medical therapy. Repeat fibrinolytic therapy was not associated with significant improvements in all-cause mortality or reinfarction. Both treatment strategies demonstrated a significant increase in minor bleeding, but PCI was associated with an increase in stroke.[61] The Rapid Early Action for Coronary Treatment (REACT) study found that patients who received rescue PCI compared to repeat fibrinolytic or conservative care had a significantly lower composite of death, reinfarction, stroke, or severe HF at 6 months (event-free survival rate: 84.6% vs. 70.1% vs. 68.7%, respectively, $p = 0.004$).[62] The ACC/AHA guidelines recommend that patients who have failed fibrinolytic therapy undergo catheterization with appropriate antithrombotic therapy if possible.[5] Patients best suited for catheterization consist of those with high-risk features such as cardiogenic shock, significant hypotension, severe HF, or ECG evidence of an extensive area of myocardial jeopardy.

In the case of P.H., a repeat infusion with t-PA would probably be safe, but it may not be effective. If a PCI-capable institution exists, P.H. should be transferred for an invasive strategy at this time.

USE IN THE ELDERLY

CASE 13-1, QUESTION 14: If P.H. had been 85 years of age, should he have still received fibrinolytic therapy?

Some of the early trials with fibrinolytic therapy excluded the elderly. Although the elderly may have a higher prevalence of relative contraindications such as severe hypertension or history of stroke at presentation, they also have a higher incidence of mortality after an AMI. The 30-day mortality rate after an AMI is 19.6% for patients between 75 and 84 years of age and 30.3% for those who are 85 years of age and older.[63] In the ISIS-2 trial, the greatest reduction in mortality occurred in the elderly subgroup. There are no controlled trials in which fibrinolytic therapy has increased mortality in the elderly. However, in a high-risk cohort of elderly female patients (older than 75 years, <67 kg), the ASSENT investigators demonstrated that TNK was associated with lower rates of major bleeding and intracerebral hemorrhage compared to t-PA. Another potential strategy to reduce intracranial hemorrhage risk is a reduced dose of fibrinolytic. The Strategic Reperfusion Early after Myocardial Infarction (STREAM) trial evaluated prehospital fibrinolytic therapy and reduced the dose of TNK by 50% in patients ≥75 years of age.[63] The intracranial hemorrhage rate was reduced to 0.5% and coronary patency rates were similar when compared to patients <75 years of age who received full-dose TNK. It is also important to ensure appropriate dosage adjustments are made for concomitant medications according to age (e.g., enoxaparin), weight (e.g., prasugrel), and renal function (e.g., enoxaparin and fondaparinux).

β-Blockers

CASE 13-1, QUESTION 15: The physician wishes to write a prescription for a β-blocker. What are the benefits of administering a β-blocker to P.H.? Should it be given as IV therapy or started as oral therapy a few days after the infarction?

β-Blockers offer significant benefits to the MI patient. Several large trials gave IV β-blockers (up to 24 hours after symptom onset) followed by oral therapy; other studies used oral therapy alone beginning days after the infarction. Early IV administration appears to be most beneficial, with a reduction in mortality of about 25% in the first 2 days when the results of these trials are pooled. However, late oral therapy alone, initiated up to 21 days after an MI in the β-Blocker in Heart Attack Trial, was also associated with a substantial reduction in mortality (around 10%).[5]

Early IV administration of propranolol, metoprolol, timolol, and atenolol has been studied. Typically, metoprolol is used in the acute setting because of its β_1 selectivity, ease of dosing and administration, and weight of evidence. Oral carvedilol, a nonselective β- and α-blocker, has been used in the peri-infarction period, specifically in patients with LV dysfunction. In the Carvedilol Post-Infarction Survival Control in Left Ventricular Dysfunction (CAPRICORN) trial, carvedilol 6.25 mg twice daily titrated to 25 mg twice daily reduced all-cause and cardiovascular mortality as well as recurrent nonfatal MI.[64]

It is important to tailor β-blockade therapy for each patient, as evidenced in the COMMIT trial.[65] In this study, patients were randomized to placebo or metoprolol (up to 15 mg IV of metoprolol, then oral 200 mg metoprolol succinate daily) within 24 hours of AMI. Although metoprolol reduced reinfarction and ventricular fibrillation rates compared with placebo, it was associated with a significant increase in cardiogenic shock. Patients with hemodynamic instability at randomization were at greatest risk of early cardiogenic shock associated with metoprolol. Given these concerns, oral β-blockers are generally preferred. If the patient is hypertensive or having ongoing ischemia, then IV metoprolol tartrate (5 mg IV every 5 minutes as tolerated up to three doses) can be considered (see Table 13-2). For all other patients without contraindications, oral metoprolol tartrate 25 to 50 mg every 6 to 12 hours should be initiated. Doses should be titrated on the basis of BP and heart rate. If a patient has transient cardiac decompensation or is at risk for cardiogenic shock during the acute infarction period, early IV β-blockers should be withheld. The patient's condition may be observed for a few days; if it stabilizes, oral therapy is initiated and titrated slowly. The ACC/AHA guidelines highlight the importance of an individualized approach, but do provide guidance on suggested dosing recommendations for both acute and long-term use.

In our case, P.H.'s situation is complicated by his history of intermittent pulmonary problems. In deciding whether to attempt use of β-blockers in patients with pulmonary disease, one must determine the nature of the pulmonary problem (i.e., reactive airway disease). It also would be helpful to determine P.H.'s need for routine use of β-agonists to help quantify the severity of his disease. By history, P.H. does not use β-agonist bronchodilators routinely. No history is given regarding his pulmonary function tests or the degree of reversibility of his airway disease with bronchodilators. β_1-selective antagonists are the drugs of choice in these patients, but at higher doses (e.g., metoprolol doses > 100 mg/day), the relative β_1-selectivity may be lost. A patient would need to experience significant worsening of the pulmonary disease to justify avoiding β-blockers. A better history of P.H.'s pulmonary problems should be obtained. If they are minor and as he has experienced an uncomplicated MI, P.H. may be a candidate for early therapy with metoprolol to reduce chest pain as well as decrease the risk of reinfarction and arrhythmias.

Nitroglycerin

CASE 13-1, QUESTION 16: Despite SL NTG, P.H. continues to have chest discomfort. Would he benefit from IV NTG?

Because P.H. is exhibiting refractory ischemic discomfort despite receiving SL and topical nitrates, symptomatic management with IV NTG is indicated. NTG lowers the LV filling pressure and systemic vascular resistance, thereby reducing myocardial oxygen consumption and myocardial ischemia. At lower doses (<50 mcg/minute), IV NTG preferentially dilates the venous capacitance vessels, which leads to a decrease in LV filling pressure. For patients who have signs of pulmonary congestion, IV NTG is of particular value.

CASE 13-1, QUESTION 17: How should IV NTG be administered to P.H.? How should it be monitored?

A continuous infusion of NTG is delivered in a controlled manner, starting with 5 to 10 mcg/minute, which is then increased by an additional 5 to 10 mcg/minute every 5 to 10 minutes if needed. Many cardiologists routinely give patients an infusion of NTG for the first 24 to 48 hours after an AMI. Increasing doses may be required during this period to maintain the desired hemodynamic effect owing to tolerance that occurs from prolonged nitrate exposure. However, if more than 200 mcg/minute is needed to achieve the desired response, another vasodilator may be needed. NTG is typically administered in combination with fibrinolytic agents in patients who require relief from myocardial ischemia.

Patients with an inferior or right ventricular infarct often develop hypotension (mean BP < 80 mm Hg) when given NTG. P.H.'s BP should be monitored closely during this infusion. After starting NTG, we would expect to see his BP decline; the pulse rate may or may not increase. The NTG dose should be titrated to relieve pain while avoiding symptomatic hypotension. In patients with evidence of HF, NTG can reduce LV filling pressure (preload), as well as improve orthopnea and pulmonary congestion. However, excessive doses of IV NTG can reduce LV filling pressure to excess, and potentially decrease cardiac output. The systolic BP should be maintained to at least 90 mm Hg. Once P.H.'s chest pain is controlled, he may be transitioned to either an oral agent or his transdermal delivery system increased. With either choice, a nitrate-free interval should be maintained (see Chapter 12, Chronic Stable Angina).

TREATMENT FOR UNSTABLE ANGINA OR NON–ST SEGMENT ELEVATION MYOCARDIAL INFARCTION

Invasive Versus Ischemia-Guided Strategy

CASE 13-2

QUESTION 1: J.W. is a 65-year-old man who presents to the ED with chest tightness and shortness of breath. He gives a history of similar symptoms the previous day that lasted 20 minutes. He was given aspirin 325 mg, intranasal oxygen, PO metoprolol tartrate, and started on an IV NTG infusion, which was increased to 80 mcg/minute; at that time, his BP was 130/60 mm Hg, and his heart rate was 88. His ECG revealed ST segment depression in the anterior leads. His shortness of breath was relieved, but he still complained of chest tightness. His past medical history includes hypertension for which he takes hydrochlorothiazide 25 mg daily. His mother died of a heart attack at age 62. He has smoked a pack of cigarettes per day for the past 30 years. Laboratory values include the following:

Na, 135 mEq/L
K, 4.0 mEq/L
Cl, 100 mEq/L
CO_2, 20 mEq/L
BUN, 15 mg/dL
SCr, 1.1 mg/dL
Glucose, 100 mg/dL
Mg, 2 mEq/L
CK-MB fraction, 1% (normal, 0%–5%)
Troponin I-Ultra, 0.05 ng/mL (normal, <0.02 ng/mL)
Hgb, 14 g/dL
Hct, 44%
Plt, 288 × 10^3/mm^3

Based on his symptoms and ECG, the diagnosis is presumed UA. Should J.W. receive an invasive or ischemia-guided strategy for management of his NSTE-ACS?

Although J.W. has negative biomarkers after 24 hours from his first episode of chest pain suggesting UA, the presence of new ST segment depression may prompt the clinician to choose an early invasive approach within 24 hours (see Fig. 13-6). If however, the patient is not at high or intermediate risk, then the invasive approach may be delayed and performed within 25 to 72 hours. A TIMI score would also be helpful to risk stratify the patient. J.W. has a score of 4 indicating a 19.9% risk at 14 days of all-cause mortality, new or recurrent MI, or severe recurrent ischemia requiring urgent revascularization. When risk stratifying, scores of 0 to 2, 3 to 4, and 5 to 7 represent low, moderate, and high risk for death or repeat MI at 14 days. So, based on his TIMI risk score, he is moderate risk. As an alternative, calculating a GRACE score would indicate 137 points representing an 11% risk of in-hospital death or MI and a 19% risk at 6 months. An ischemia-guided strategy might be selected based on patient or clinician preference in the absence of high-risk features such as elevated biomarkers. In this approach, pharmacotherapy would be initiated followed by a noninvasive stress evaluation. If J.W. were to have elevated cardiac biomarkers during his presentation, his diagnosis would be NSTEMI and an early invasive (within 24 hours) approach may be preferred. If during his hospitalization, J.W. were to experience any recurrent ischemia, arrhythmias, or signs and symptoms of HF, he would proceed directly to angiography and undergo possible PCI.

Anticoagulant Therapy

CASE 13-2, QUESTION 2: What anticoagulant regimen should J.W. receive?

The ACC/AHA guidelines recommend beginning anticoagulant therapy for all patients (without contraindications) with NSTE-ACS as soon as possible. The guidelines recommend one of four agents: UFH, enoxaparin, fondaparinux, or bivalirudin (approved only for patients managed according to an invasive strategy). Table 13-2 summarizes the dosing and contraindications for each of these agents.

In NSTE-ACS, UFH has been associated with lower rates of death or MI than aspirin alone.[1] Despite its limitations, UFH is preferred if the patient is to undergo CABG because of its rapid clearance. For an invasive strategy, the guidelines give a higher level of evidence for enoxaparin but do warn about an increase in bleeding.[1] When choosing an anticoagulant, renal function, bleeding risk, and concomitant therapy should be considered.

Data supporting LMWHs in this setting come from several studies. In the Efficacy and Safety of Subcutaneous Enoxaparin (ESSENCE) study, enoxaparin (1 mg/kg SQ twice daily) was compared with UFH (5,000 units IV bolus followed by continued infusion titrated to an aPTT of 55 to 86 seconds).[66] The composite outcome of death, MI, or recurrent angina at 14 days was reduced by 20% in the enoxaparin group. This benefit was maintained for 1 year.

In the Superior Yield of the New Strategy of Enoxaparin, Revascularization and Glycoprotein IIb/IIIa Inhibitors (SYNERGY) trial, 9,978 high-risk NSTE-ACS patients were randomized to enoxaparin (1 mg/kg SQ twice daily) or weight-based UFH (60 units/kg bolus followed by 12 units/kg/hour adjusted to an aPTT 1.5 to 2 times control) before undergoing an early invasive strategy.[67] Enoxaparin was found to be as efficacious as UFH in reducing 30-day all-cause mortality or nonfatal MI but was associated with a significant risk of major bleeding ($p = 0.008$). Bleeding was especially problematic in those patients who crossed over from one treatment to the other during the trial.

In the TIMI-11B trial, enoxaparin (30 mg IV bolus followed by 1 mg/kg SQ twice daily for 8 days) compared with UFH (70 units/kg bolus followed by 15 units/kg/hour for 3 to 8 days) reduced the composite end point of death, MI, or need for urgent revascularization.[68] The benefit of enoxaparin is greatest for high-risk subgroups such as those with ST segment changes, elevated troponins, and a high TIMI risk score.[1]

Finally, enoxaparin has been compared with fondaparinux. In the OASIS-5 trial, NSTE-ACS patients were randomized to fondaparinux (2.5 mg SQ daily) or enoxaparin (1 mg/kg SQ twice daily) for a mean of 6 days and evaluated at 9 days for the primary end point of death, MI, or refractory ischemia.[69] There was no difference between groups for the primary end point; however, compared with enoxaparin, fondaparinux had a significantly lower incidence of major bleeding at 9 days ($p < 0.001$) and a greater reduction in mortality at 30 days ($p = 0.05$). Based on these data, the guidelines give preference to fondaparinux compared with other anticoagulants for patients who are at an increased risk of bleeding and being treated with an ischemia-guided (conservative medical management) strategy. If fondaparinux is used for a patient undergoing PCI, an additional anticoagulant with factor IIa activity such as UFH is needed.[1]

Bivalirudin is given a Class I recommendation in the guidelines. In the Acute Catheterization and Urgent Intervention Triage

Strategy (ACUITY) trial, patients with NSTE-ACS managed with an early invasive strategy were randomly assigned to receive either UFH (or enoxaparin) plus a GP IIb/IIIa inhibitor, bivalirudin plus a GP IIb/IIIa inhibitor, or bivalirudin alone.[70] No differences in the primary end point (composite of death, MI, unplanned revascularization for ischemia, and major bleeding at 30 days) were observed between the group receiving UFH plus a GP IIb/IIIa inhibitor and the group receiving bivalirudin plus a GP IIb/IIIa inhibitor. However, compared with those receiving UFH plus a GP IIb/IIIa inhibitor, the 30-day composite of ischemia or major bleeding was significantly lower for those receiving bivalirudin alone. This difference was attributed to reduced major bleeding with bivalirudin.

The Unfractionated Heparin versus Bivalirudin In Primary Percutaneous Coronary Intervention (HEAT-PPCI) trial was a head to head comparison of bivalirudin versus UFH.[71] Patients who underwent emergent PCI were randomly assigned to receive either UFH or bivalirudin. At 28 days, the primary efficacy outcome of ≥1 major adverse cardiac events was significantly lower in the UFH group. When the individual components were evaluated, there was no difference in all-cause mortality or cerebrovascular accident. The driving factors favoring heparin were new MI or reinfarction and additional unplanned target lesion revascularization. The majority of these cases were related to stent thrombosis in the bivalirudin group (0.9% vs. 3.4%, $p = 0.001$). Major and minor bleeding events did not differ between the two groups.

Because J.W. is receiving an invasive strategy for his NSTE-ACS and he has adequate renal function, enoxaparin, UFH, or bivalirudin could be initiated and continued until the end of PCI.

Antithrombotic Therapy

CASE 13-2, QUESTION 3: What oral antithrombotic medications should be considered for J.W.?

For both an ischemia-guided and invasive strategy, aspirin along with a $P2Y_{12}$ antagonist (loading with maintenance dose) should be added as soon as possible to anticoagulant therapy unless the patient is to proceed to CABG. For an invasive strategy, prasugrel or ticagrelor can be considered in lieu of clopidogrel. The 2014 ACC/AHA guidelines recommend ticagrelor as the preferred agent (Class IIa). Prasugrel should only be used in patients undergoing PCI as long as they are not at high risk of bleeding complications.[1]

The use of clopidogrel in NSTE-ACS was evaluated in two studies.[72,73] In the Clopidogrel in Unstable Angina to Prevent Recurrent Ischemic Events (CURE) trial, patients with NSTE-ACS were randomized to placebo plus aspirin (75 to 325 mg) or clopidogrel (300 mg, immediately followed by 75 mg daily) plus aspirin.[72] The composite of cardiovascular death, MI, or stroke was significantly reduced with clopidogrel. However, compared with placebo, an increase in major and minor bleeding was seen. On the basis of these data, clopidogrel with aspirin should be administered immediately on admission and continued ideally for 1 year in patients with ACS.[1]

The PCI-Clopidogrel as Adjunctive Reperfusion Therapy (PCI-CLARITY) study was a planned subanalysis ($n = 1{,}863$) of the CLARITY-TIMI 28 study (see Case 13-1, Question 9) that evaluated the effects of pretreatment with aspirin plus clopidogrel, compared with aspirin plus placebo, in patients undergoing PCI with coronary artery stenting.[74] Compared with placebo, pretreatment with clopidogrel significantly reduced the incidence of cardiovascular death, MI, or stroke as well as recurrent MI or stroke before PCI with no significant excess in TIMI major or minor bleeding.

CASE 13-2, QUESTION 4: What loading dose should he receive and when should he receive it? What about his maintenance dose?

A loading dose of 600 mg of clopidogrel in patients undergoing PCI achieves greater platelet inhibition with fewer low responders and decreases the incidence of major cardiac events compared with a loading dose of 300 mg.[1] A 300-mg clopidogrel loading dose provides adequate antiplatelet activity in 6 hours whereas a 600-mg clopidogrel loading dose provides antiplatelet activity in 2 hours. Even after a loading dose, clopidogrel requires several hours to be metabolized to its active metabolite. The current guidelines prefer 600 mg because of a greater, more rapid, and more consistent degree of platelet inhibition. Patients undergoing PCI who have previously received a loading dose of 300 mg of clopidogrel and are on a 75-mg daily maintenance dose should receive another 300-mg loading dose. Data do not exist on additional loading doses for patients currently receiving maintenance doses of prasugrel or ticagrelor.

Prasugrel has been evaluated in patients with ACS undergoing PCI. In the Therapeutic Outcomes by Optimizing Platelet Inhibition with Prasugrel–Thrombolysis in Myocardial Infarction (TRITON-TIMI) 38 study, patients with moderate to high-risk ACS, 26% of whom had STEMI, were randomized to prasugrel (60 mg loading dose followed by 10 mg daily) or clopidogrel (300 mg loading dose followed by 75 mg daily).[75] All patients received aspirin (75 to 162 mg daily). The primary outcome of death from cardiovascular causes, nonfatal MI, or nonfatal stroke occurred in 9.9% of patients receiving prasugrel and in 12.1% of patients taking clopidogrel ($p < 0.001$). However, prasugrel was associated with a significant increase in TIMI—major, fatal, and life-threatening bleeding. A post hoc analysis found three subgroups that did not benefit from prasugrel: patients with a history of stroke or TIA, age of 75 years or older, or body weight less than 60 kg. Patients with at least one of these risk factors exhibited a higher rate of bleeding.[76] The Food and Drug Administration (FDA) recommends a 5-mg (rather than 10-mg) maintenance dose be considered for those patients weighing less than 60 kg, even though this dose has not been studied.[77]

In the Study of Platelet Inhibition and Patient Outcomes (PLATO) trial, patients with ACS, with or without ST segment elevation were randomized to receive ticagrelor (180 mg loading dose, 90 mg twice daily thereafter) or clopidogrel (300 to 600 mg loading dose, then 75 mg daily). Compared to clopidogrel, ticagrelor demonstrated a 16% reduced rate of mortality from MI, vascular causes, or stroke ($p < 0.001$) without an increase in the rate of major bleeding but an increased rate in CABG-related bleeding ($p = 0.03$).[78] However, the lowest 1-year rates of cardiovascular death, MI, or stroke were noted in patients with ACS treated with ticagrelor and maintenance low-dose aspirin (≤100 mg/day), whereas the highest rates occurred in those treated with ticagrelor and high-dose aspirin (>300 mg/day).[79] Based on these data, the maintenance dose of aspirin should not exceed 100 mg/day.[80]

When compared with clopidogrel, prasugrel and ticagrelor are more potent, exhibit a lower incidence of stent thrombosis, have fewer drug–drug interactions, and lack variable response based on pharmacogenomics (refer to Chapter 12, Chronic Stable Angina, about responders and nonresponders to clopidogrel). However, many providers have been concerned with the higher risk of bleeding. In the case of J.W., clopidogrel, prasugrel, or ticagrelor could be added, as he does not have a contraindication to any of these drugs. Ticagrelor may be preferred as long as cost is not a concern for the patient.

After PCI with coronary stent deployment with either a drug-eluting or bare metal stent, clopidogrel 75 mg, prasugrel 5 to 10 mg, or ticagrelor 90 mg twice daily should be administered for at least 12 months. It is important to highlight that clopidogrel and ticagrelor should be discontinued for 5 days and prasugrel for 7 days, prior to surgery.

As a rapid onset of action is needed, J.W. should receive a loading dose of 600 mg of clopidogrel as soon as possible, followed by 75 mg daily for at least 12 months. If prasugrel is chosen, a loading dose of 60 mg would be given followed by 10 mg daily as long as the patient is >60 kg. For ticagrelor, a loading dose of 180 mg is recommended following by 90 mg twice daily. Aspirin 81 mg daily should be continued indefinitely.

CASE 13-2, QUESTION 5: Should a GP IIb/IIIa inhibitor be added? If so, which one?

In patients with NSTE-ACS, the GP IIb/IIIa inhibitors are of benefit for patients considered high risk, those undergoing PCI, or both.[1] Analysis of GP IIb/IIIa studies suggest that those patients who obtain the greatest advantage from these agents are those who have elevated troponins, diabetes, ST segment changes, or a TIMI risk score of 4 or higher at presentation. The guidelines recommend that for patients with NSTE-ACS who will be treated initially according to an invasive strategy, either a GP IIb/IIIa inhibitor or a $P2Y_{12}$ inhibitor (clopidogrel or ticareglor), should be added to aspirin and anticoagulant therapy before diagnostic angiography is performed.[1] When used to treat patients medically, the GP IIb/IIIa inhibitors tirofiban or eptifibatide are generally given for 18 to 72 hours. Abciximab should be used only with PCI. (Table 13-6).[1]

The GUSTO-IV-ACS trial enrolled patients with NSTE-ACS in whom early (<48 hours) revascularization was not intended. All patients received aspirin and either UFH or LMWH.[81] They were randomized to placebo, abciximab bolus and 24-hour infusion, or abciximab bolus and 48-hour infusion. At 30 days, death or MI occurred in 8.0% of patients receiving placebo, 8.2% of patients receiving 24-hour abciximab, and 9.1% of patients receiving 48-hour abciximab (no significant difference). At 48 hours, death occurred in 0.3%, 0.7%, and 0.9% of patients in these groups, respectively (placebo vs. abciximab at 48 hours; $p = 0.008$). Based on these findings and those of other studies, abciximab is indicated only if angiography will not be appreciably delayed and PCI is likely to be performed; otherwise, IV eptifibatide or tirofiban is preferred (Fig. 13-6).

The guidelines recommend that in the setting of dual antiplatelet therapy used with UFH, the adjunctive use of a GP IIb/IIIa inhibitor administered at the time of PCI cannot be recommended as routine therapy. However, a GP IIb/IIIa inhibitor may be beneficial in those with a large thrombus burden or who have not received adequate $P2Y_{12}$ antagonist loading.[1]

J.W. has a TIMI risk score of 4; therefore, the addition of eptifibatide or tirofiban is a reasonable choice if a large thrombus burden is demonstrated on angiography. Administration prior to PCI ("upstream") is not indicated unless the administration of a $P2Y_{12}$ antagonist is delayed until time of PCI. Platelets and signs and symptoms of bleeding should be monitored closely.

Because J.W. is not at high risk for bleeding, dual antiplatelet therapy in addition to UFH should be adequate therapy. If a large thrombus burden is demonstrated on angiography, a GP IIa/IIIb could be initiated during PCI.

If J.W. had not received an oral $P2Y_{12}$ inhibitor or a GP IIb/IIIa inhibitor, consideration could be given to administering IV cangrelor, a direct-acting $P2Y_{12}$ platelet inhibitor, prior to PCI. Based on the results of the CHAMPION PHOENIX trial, cangrelor could be administered as a 30 mcg/kg bolus followed by a 4 mcg/kg/minute IV infusion for at least 2 hours or for the duration of the PCI.[29] After discontinuation of the infusion, an oral $P2Y_{12}$ inhibitor should be administered (ticagrelor 180 mg load during or upon immediate discontinuation of infusion; prasugrel 60 mg or clopidogrel 600 mg upon immediate discontinuation of infusion) followed by aspirin 81 mg daily along with a maintenance dose of the $P2Y_{12}$ inhibitor. If clopidogrel or prasugrel are administered during the infusion, they will have no antiplatelet effect until the next dose is administered.

CASE 13-2, QUESTION 6: What if an ischemia-driven strategy was decided for J.W. instead, would his antithrombotic therapy change?

Table 13-6
Dosing of Glycoprotein IIb/IIIa in Acute Coronary Syndromes[1,5]

Medication	Dosing for STEMI PCI	Dose for NSTE-ACS With or Without PCI	Comments
Abciximab	0.25 mg/kg IV bolus followed by 0.125 mcg/kg/minute infusion (max of 10 mcg/minute), continue for 12 hours at the discretion of the physician	Not recommended	
Eptifibatide	180 mcg/kg IV bolus, then begin 2 mcg/kg/minute infusion followed by second IV bolus of 180 mcg/kg 10 minutes after first bolus, continue infusion for 12–18 hours after PCI at the discretion of the physician	180 mcg/kg IV bolus, then begin 2 mcg/kg/minute infusion, continue infusion for 12–18 hours Repeat bolus dose after 10 minutes for PCI	Reduce infusion by 50% in patients with CrCl <50 mL/minute; not studied in patients with SCr >4.0 mg/dL; avoid in hemodialysis
Tirofiban	25 mcg/kg IV bolus followed by an infusion of 0.15 mcg/kg/minute, continue up to 18 hours at the discretion of the physician	25 mcg/kg IV bolus within 5 minutes followed by an infusion of 0.15 mcg/kg/minute (or 0.075 mcg/kg/minute for patients with CrCl ≤60 mL/minute), for up to 18 hours.	Reduce infusion by 50% in patients with CrCl < 30 mL/minute

CrCl, creatinine clearance; IV, intravenous; NSTE-ACS, non–ST segment elevation acute coronary syndrome; PCI, percutaneous coronary intervention; SCr, serum creatinine; STEMI, ST segment elevation myocardial infarction.

Management Strategy

ISCHEMIA-GUIDED STRATEGY

An ischemia-guided strategy avoids early invasive procedures, instead relying on the patient's symptoms to direct the need for intervention. Similarly, J.W. would be optimized on anti-ischemic and antithrombotic regimens. At this time, prasugrel and bivalirudin are only indicated in patients undergoing PCI. Additionally, the bleeding risk of GP IIb/IIIa inhibitors outweighs the benefit in this approach and therefore these medications should only be used if PCI is pursued. If during his hospitalization, the patient were to experience any recurrent ischemia, refractory angina despite medical therapy, or high-risk features (e.g., arrhythmias, signs or symptoms of HF, hemodynamic instability, elevated cardiac enzymes), an invasive approach would be pursued.[1]

LONG-TERM THERAPY

Angiotensin-Converting Enzyme Inhibitors, Angiotensin Receptor Blockers, and Direct Renin Inhibitors

CASE 13-3

QUESTION 1: J.S. is a 68-year-old man who presents with a STEMI along with signs and symptoms of HF. His past medical history includes hypertension treated with hydrochlorothiazide 25 mg daily and diabetes for which he takes metformin 500 mg twice daily. He has smoked a pack of cigarettes per day for the past 40 years. On admission, his BP was 145/86 mm Hg, and his heart rate was 90 beats/minute. His weight is 91 kg with a height of 5'9" and a body mass index (BMI) of 29.5 kg/m^2. Laboratory values include the following:

Na, 139 mEq/L
K, 4.2 mEq/L
Cl, 100 mEq/L
CO_2, 20 mEq/L
BUN, 15 mg/dL
SCr, 1.3 mg/dL
Glucose, 130 mg/dL
Hemoglobin A_{1c}, 6.9%
Mg, 2 mEq/L
CK-MB fraction, 35% (normal, 0%–5%)
Troponin I-Ultra, 10 ng/mL (normal, <0.02 ng/mL)

He is administered aspirin 325 mg, prasugrel 60 mg, IV NTG infusion, continuous infusion of UFH, and intranasal oxygen. J.S. is immediately sent to the catheterization laboratory in which he receives a drug-eluting stent in his left anterior descending artery. After stabilization of his HF symptoms, J.S. is started on oral metoprolol tartrate 25 mg every 6 hours. An echocardiogram is performed before discharge and shows an LVEF of 35% along with the appearance of a thrombus in the LV.

Is an ACE inhibitor appropriate for J.S.? When should an ARB be considered?

After an AMI, the heart undergoes processes that initially compensate for the loss of contractile function but may increase the long-term risk for development of HF. This is referred to as remodeling of the ventricle (see Chapter 14, Heart Failure). The increase in the number of survivors of AMI has led to an increase in the number of HF patients. A number of clinical trials with the use of ACE inhibitors have demonstrated reductions in HF symptoms and mortality after MI.[5]

For patients with ACS, oral ACE inhibitor therapy should be started within the first 24 hours of presentation for those with an LVEF of 40% or less (even if asymptomatic) or clinical evidence of HF. Additionally, ACE inhibitors should also be considered for patients with concomitant hypertension, diabetes, and/or chronic kidney disease.[5] The use of IV ACE inhibitor therapy is not recommended. Because of its short half-life, captopril could be given on postinfarction day 2 or 3, beginning with a test dose of 6.25 mg and then titrated as tolerated. Once it is established that the patient can tolerate an ACE inhibitor, he or she can be switched to a once daily agent such as lisinopril to simplify the regimen. The BP should be monitored closely, with systolic BP maintained greater than 90 mm Hg. Renal function and serum potassium levels should be monitored closely during the first few months of therapy. Because J.S. presents with clinical symptoms of HF, he is a candidate for an ACE inhibitor. Additionally, J.S. has an EF of less than 40%, hypertension, and diabetes, therefore the ACE inhibitor should be continued indefinitely (Table 13-2).

If the patient cannot tolerate an ACE inhibitor because of cough, an ARB may be an alternative. In the Optimal Therapy in Myocardial Infarction with the Angiotensin II Antagonist Losartan (OPTIMAAL) trial and Valsartan in Acute Myocardial Infarction Trial (VALIANT), losartan and valsartan demonstrated similar reductions in all-cause mortality compared with captopril.[82,83] Dual therapy of ACE inhibitors with ARBs offers no additional benefits but increases side effects.

Aldosterone Antagonists

CASE 13-3, QUESTION 2: Should J.S. receive an aldosterone antagonist?

Like angiotensin II, aldosterone plays an important role in LV remodeling. Inhibiting aldosterone directly in addition to ACE inhibitor therapy was first evaluated in HF patients in the Randomized Aldactone Evaluation Study (RALES) (see Chapter 14, Heart Failure). Another aldosterone antagonist, eplerenone, is a selective inhibitor of the mineralocorticoid receptor with fewer sexual side effects. In the Eplerenone Post Acute Myocardial Infarction Heart Failure Efficacy and Survival Study (EPHESUS), patients with AMI and EF less than 40% receiving optimal medical therapy were randomized to eplerenone or placebo.[35] Significant reductions in mortality (15%), sudden death (13%), and cardiovascular death or hospitalization (21%) were seen with eplerenone compared to placebo.

The ACC/AHA guidelines recommend an aldosterone antagonist in patients with NSTE-ACS or STEMI who are already receiving therapeutic doses of an ACE inhibitor, have an EF less than 40%, and have either symptomatic HF or diabetes.[1,5] Potential contraindications to the use of an aldosterone antagonist in this setting include significant renal dysfunction (creatinine > 2.5 mg/dL in men, >2.0 mg/dL in women, or creatinine clearance < 30 mL/minute) or hyperkalemia (potassium > 5 mEq/L).

Because J.S. has symptomatic HF with an EF less than 40% and diabetes, he is a candidate for an aldosterone antagonist. Serum potassium and renal function need to be checked in 2 to 3 days and 1 week after therapy initiation, then every month for the first 3 months. ACE inhibitor and potassium supplement doses may need to be adjusted.[84]

β-Blockers

CASE 13-3, QUESTION 3: Should J.S. receive a β-blocker on discharge?

The ACC/AHA guidelines recommend continued β-blocker therapy at discharge for all patients after ACS.[1,5] The benefits of β-blockers in reducing reinfarction and mortality outweigh the risk, even in patients with asthma, depression, insulin-dependent diabetes, severe peripheral vascular disease, first-degree heart block, and moderate LV dysfunction. Atenolol, propranolol, carvedilol, metoprolol tartrate, and metoprolol succinate are generic, making them cost-effective. Metoprolol succinate, carvedilol, and bisoprolol are considered first-line choices in patients with HF, whereas atenolol, metoprolol tartrate, or metoprolol succinate should be considered in patients with stable asthma or bronchospastic pulmonary disease. Being discharged on a β-blocker is a quality performance measure.[85] However, debate exists surrounding the duration of use, especially in low-risk patients without compelling indications.[86–89] Data suggest that the benefits from β-blockers emerge early following an AMI and are maintained out to 1 year. Although the exact duration of benefit is unknown, high-risk patients (e.g., GRACE score ≥ 121 and diuretic use) are likely to continue to derive benefit for up to 3 years. The 2011 AHA/ACCF secondary prevention guidelines recommend a 3-year treatment course for patients with normal LV function, with an option to continue indefinitely as long as the medication is well tolerated. Because J.S. has a low EF, he should be transitioned from oral metoprolol tartrate to metoprolol succinate, carvedilol, or bisoprolol, which should be continued indefinitely.

Lipid-Lowering Agents

CASE 13-3, QUESTION 4: Should J.S. be started on a lipid-lowering agent? If so, which one? When should it be initiated?

A complete fasting lipid profile would be helpful and should be completed within 24 hours of presenting with an AMI.[1,5] This is often overlooked or not done because the patient is not fasting. Most patients will require a low-cholesterol, low-saturated fat diet in addition to lipid-lowering therapy. The ACC/AHA STEMI and NSTE-ACS guidelines recommend that a high-intensity statin therapy be initiated or continued in all patients with ACS unless contraindications are present.[1,5] This would consist of atorvastatin 40 to 80 mg or rosuvastatin 20 to 40 mg daily.[34] When triglycerides are 500 mg/dL or more, drug therapy with niacin or a fibrate is beneficial.[89]

The Myocardial Ischemia Reduction with Aggressive Cholesterol Lowering (MIRACL) trial evaluated NSTE-ACS patients receiving atorvastatin 80 mg/day or placebo within 24 to 96 hours of hospitalization. A significantly lower rate of death and nonfatal major cardiac events at 4 months of follow-up was seen in patients receiving atorvastatin.[90] In the Pravastatin or Atorvastatin Evaluation and Infection Therapy (PROVE-IT)-TIMI 22 trial, patients with ACS who received atorvastatin 80 mg/day for 10 days exhibited a significantly lower risk of death, MI, UA hospitalization, stroke, and revascularization when compared with pravastatin 40 mg/day.[90] The A to Z trial showed a favorable trend toward major cardiovascular event reduction in AMI patients receiving an intensive simvastatin regimen (40 mg/day for 1 month followed by 80 mg/day thereafter) when initiated within 12 hours of stabilization compared to a less intensive regimen (placebo for 4 months followed by simvastatin 20 mg/day).[91] However, based on clinical trials, observational studies, adverse event reports, and prescription use data, simvastatin 80 mg may be associated with increased muscle injury (refer to Chapter 8, Dyslipidemias, Atherosclerosis, and Coronary Heart Disease).[34]

In the case of J.S., he should receive a high-intensity statin within 24 hours of his hospitalization and be discharged on a statin regardless of LDL cholesterol. This is a quality core performance measure.[85] Drug interactions, patient tolerability, and affordability should be considered. Currently, the LDL goal for patients with ACS remains controversial. The ACC/AHA STEMI and NSTE-ACS guidelines do not recommend a specific goal LDL. However, the National Lipid Association does recommend a goal LDL less than 100 mg/dL in patients with ACS.[92] For J.S. it would be reasonable to begin atorvastatin 80 mg daily and obtain an LDL of less than 100 mg/dL or a reduction of 50%.

Antiplatelet Therapy

CASE 13-3, QUESTION 5: How long should J.S. continue his aspirin and prasugrel?

Antiplatelet therapy with aspirin should be lifelong for J.S. because of aspirin's beneficial effects on reinfarction. There appears to be no difference in efficacy for a wide range of aspirin doses (75–1,500 mg/day), although higher doses may increase the incidence of side effects. The ACC/AHA guidelines recommend a dose of 81 to 325 mg daily indefinitely with a preferred maintenance dose of 81 mg daily.[1,5] Dual antiplatelet therapy with clopidogrel or ticagrelor and aspirin, compared with aspirin alone, reduces major cardiovascular events in patients with established ischemic heart disease.[93,94] The use of dual antiplatelet therapy with a $P2Y_{12}$ inhibitor for patients who have undergone coronary stenting reduces the risk of future stent thrombosis.[1,5] In ACS patients, ideally the $P2Y_{12}$ inhibitor should be continued for at least 1 year regardless of the type of coronary stent. Data from the Dual Antiplatelet Therapy (DAPT) trial found that dual antiplatelet therapy with clopidogrel or prasugrel continued for 30 months after placement of a drug-eluting stent significantly reduced the risk of stent thrombosis and major adverse cardiovascular and cerebrovascular events compared with 12 months of therapy, but was associated with an increased risk of bleeding.[95]

Because J.S. underwent PCI and received a coronary stent, his dose of aspirin will be 81 mg daily indefinitely. He should continue prasugrel 10 mg daily for at least 1 year. Aspirin should be prescribed at hospital discharge because it is a quality performance measure.[85]

CASE 13-3, QUESTION 6: If J.S. had received ticagrelor instead of prasugrel, how would his ticagrelor and aspirin been dosed?

In the Patients with Prior Heart Attack Using Ticagrelor Compared to Placebo on a Background of Aspirin–Thrombolysis in Myocardial Infarction 54 (PEGASUS TIMI-54) study, 21,162 patients who had an AMI 1 to 3 years earlier were randomized to ticagrelor 90 mg twice daily, ticagrelor 60 mg twice daily, or placebo plus low-dose aspirin.[94] Compared to placebo plus low-dose aspirin, both ticagrelor doses significantly reduced the rate of the composite of cardiovascular death, MI, or stroke with a 3-year rate of 7.85% in the group that received 90 mg of ticagrelor twice daily, 7.77% in the group that received 60 mg of ticagrelor twice daily, and 9.04% in the placebo group. Therefore, if J.S. were to receive ticagrelor, then he would have received 180 mg load following his ACS event, then 90 mg twice daily during the first year, then 60 mg twice daily after the first year for up to 3 years.[80] Aspirin 325 mg would be given on day 1 of his ACS event followed by 81 mg daily indefinitely.

Warfarin

CASE 13-3, QUESTION 7: Three days before J.S.'s anticipated discharge, the medical team is discussing the need to administer long-term warfarin in addition to his dual antiplatelet therapy with aspirin and prasugrel. Is warfarin indicated for J.S. at this time?

Long-term warfarin may be beneficial in some patients, but clinical judgment is needed to decide whether the benefit is likely to exceed the risk. Data suggest that the incidence of a LV thrombus and atrial fibrillation occurs between 7% to 46% and 2% to 22% respectively in patients following an AMI.[96,97] The ACC/AHA guidelines recommend warfarin for ACS patients with atrial fibrillation, mechanical heart valves, venous thromboembolism, hypercoagulable disorder, and LV mural thrombus.[5] In patients already receiving dual antiplatelet therapy, the guidelines recommend limiting the duration of triple antithrombotic therapy to minimize the risk of bleeding. Consideration can also be given to targeting a goal international normalized ratio (INR) of 2.0 to 2.5 for those patients whose usual goal INR is between 2.0 and 3.0; however, no prospective studies have demonstrated that a target INR of 2.0 to 2.5 reduces bleeding complications.[1,5] In the What is the Optimal Antiplatelet and Anticoagulant Therapy in Patients With Oral Anticoagulation and Coronary Stenting (WOEST) trial, use of clopidogrel without aspirin was associated with a significant reduction in bleeding complications and no increase in thrombotic events compared to clopidogrel with aspirin in patients undergoing PCI who were receiving oral anticoagulation.[98]

Triple antithrombotic therapy has limited information with the use of newer $P2Y_{12}$ inhibitors (prasugrel, ticagrelor); the DTI (dabigatran); or factor Xa inhibitors (rivaroxaban, apixaban, and edoxaban). Prasugrel and ticagrelor can produce a greater degree of platelet inhibition than clopidogrel and are associated with greater rates of bleeding. Therefore, caution is required when using these agents in patients who require an anticoagulant or who are at significantly increased risk of bleeding.[1]

In the case of J.S., due to the presence of a LV thrombus, he is probably a good candidate for 1 to 3 months of warfarin therapy titrated to an INR of 2 to 2.5. His dose of aspirin should be 81 mg/daily if warfarin is prescribed. It would also be reasonable to consider clopidogrel instead of prasugrel in J.S.

Proton-Pump Inhibitor

CASE 13-3, QUESTION 8: Should J.S. receive a proton-pump inhibitor (PPI)?

The ACC/AHA/American College of Gastroenterology recommend using a PPI in patients receiving dual antiplatelet therapy who have multiple risk factors for gastrointestinal bleeding such as advanced age; concomitant use of warfarin, steroids, or NSAIDs; or *Helicobacter pylori* infection.[99] The ACC/AHA NSTE-ACS guidelines recommend the use of a PPI in patients with a history of gastrointestinal bleeding who are receiving triple antithrombotic therapy (Class I) and for those without a history of gastrointestinal bleeding receiving triple antithrombotic therapy (Class IIa).[99] Because omeprazole and esomeprazole are known to inhibit the isoenzyme 2C19, the FDA recommends against the use of these with clopidogrel because of the possible reduced effectiveness of clopidogrel.[1,100] If J.S. receives triple antithrombotic therapy with prasugrel, any PPI can be used.

CASE 13-3, QUESTION 9: How would you summarize the long-term therapy needed by J.S. on discharge?

Appropriate discharge medications for J.S. include a β-blocker, ACE inhibitor, aldosterone antagonist, aspirin 81 mg/day, $P2Y_{12}$ inhibitor, PPI, and warfarin to achieve an INR of 2 to 2.5. He also should receive a prescription for sublingual NTG to carry with him for use as needed. These agents should be continued long term except for warfarin, which should be discontinued after a few months if his LV thrombus has resolved. Continuation of the $P2Y_{12}$ inhibitor beyond 1 year may be considered after careful assessment of the patient's ischemic and bleeding risk. J.S. should be started on a statin to achieve an LDL goal of less than 100 mg/dL or a 50% reduction from his baseline value. Routine liver function tests should be obtained before initiation of therapy and periodically thereafter. His previous hydrochlorothiazide may be discontinued because his hypertension will likely be controlled with the β-blocker, ACE inhibitor, and aldosterone antagonist. His metformin should be continued, and his blood glucose monitored closely. As J.S. will have several new medications, he will need education regarding his medications prior to discharge in order to optimize medication adherence.

LIFESTYLE MODIFICATIONS

CASE 13-3, QUESTION 10: What types of lifestyle modifications should J.S. be encouraged to pursue to reduce his risk factors?

J.S. must be encouraged to stop smoking; this may be the most important change he can make (see Chapter 91, Tobacco Use and Dependence).[101] For weight management, an initial goal weight loss should be to reduce body weight by approximately 10% from baseline if BMI exceeds 25 kg/m^2.[89] Other dietary modifications should be implemented so that J.S. can maintain a hemoglobin A_{1c} less than 7.0% and achieve a BP goal of less than 140/90 mm Hg (or possibly lower) because J.S. has diabetes, and a serum LDL less than 100 mg/dL.[89,102,103] (See Chapter 8, Dyslipidemias, Atherosclerosis, and Coronary Heart Disease; Chapter 9, Essential Hypertension; and Chapter 12, Chronic Stable Angina, for further information on antihypertensive and lipid-lowering drugs, as well as, diet therapy.)

SUMMARY

Although mortality and incidence rates for ACS appear to be on the decline, ACS still remains a major cause of morbidity and mortality in the United States. The use of PCI has significantly improved the survival of patients with STEMI. The major risk associated with thrombolysis is bleeding, especially intracerebral hemorrhage. Another problem associated with fibrinolytic therapy is reocclusion of the artery that was initially opened. PCI is more effective than fibrinolytic therapy; however, it is available only in hospitals with experienced invasive cardiologists, thereby limiting its availability to some patients.

Aspirin should be given to all patients with ACS; unless there is a contraindication, β-blockers and statins should be administered as well. $P2Y_{12}$ inhibitors are recommended with aspirin in all patients with ACS with or without stenting. ACE inhibitors, ARBs, and aldosterone antagonists have been shown to be beneficial in patients who have LV dysfunction (LVEF < 40%) and are also recommended for secondary prevention. Nitrates are useful, but care must be taken to maintain an adequate perfusion pressure. Secondary prevention emphasizing a healthy lifestyle and aggressive lipid lowering are important components to the overall treatment plan.

KEY REFERENCES AND WEBSITES

A full list of references for this chapter can be found at http://thepoint.lww.com/AT11e. Below are the key references and websites for this chapter, with the corresponding reference number in this chapter found in parentheses after the reference.

Key References

Abraham NS et al. ACCF/ACG/AHA 2010 Expert Consensus Document on the concomitant use of proton pump inhibitors and thienopyridines: a focused update of the ACCF/ACG/AHA 2008 expert consensus document on reducing the gastrointestinal risks of antiplatelet therapy and nsaid use. *Circulation*. 2010;24:2619. (99)

Amsterdam EA et al. 2014 AHA/ACC Guideline for the Management of Patients with Non-ST-Elevation Acute Coronary Syndromes: a report of the American College of Cardiology/American Heart Association Task Force on Practice Guidelines. *J Am Coll Cardiol*. 2014;64:e139. (1)

Levine et al. 2016 ACC/AHA Guideline Focused Update on Duration of Dual Antiplatelet Therapy in Patients With Coronary Artery Disease A Report of the American College of Cardiology/American Heart Association Task Force on Clinical Practice Guidelines. *J Am Coll Cardiol*. 2016;68:1082–1115.

O'Gara PT et al. 2013 ACCF/AHA guideline for the management of ST-elevation myocardial infarction: a report of the American College of Cardiology Foundation/American Heart Association Task Force on Practice Guidelines. *Circulation*. 2013;127:e362. (5)

Smith SC Jr et al. AHA/ACCF Secondary Prevention and Risk Reduction Therapy for Patients with Coronary and other Atherosclerotic Vascular Disease: 2011 update: a guideline from the American Heart Association and American College of Cardiology Foundation. *Circulation*. 2011;124:2458–2473. (89)

Stone NJ et al. 2013 ACC/AHA guideline on the treatment of blood cholesterol to reduce atherosclerotic cardiovascular risk in adults: a report of the American College of Cardiology/American Heart Association Task Force on Practice Guidelines. *J Am Coll Cardiol*. 2014;63:2889. (34)

Key Websites

American College of Cardiology. CardioSource. http://www.cardiosource.org/acc.

American Heart Association. http://www.heart.org/HEARTORG/HealthcareResearch/Healthcare-Research_UCM_001093_SubHomePage.jsp.

GRACE Model. https://www.mdcalc.com/grace-acs-risk-mortality-calculator.

TIMI Risk Score for NSTEMI. http://www.mdcalc.com/timi-risk-score-for-uanstemi/.

TIMI Risk Score for STEMI. http://www.mdcalc.com/timi-risk-score-for-stemi.

14 Heart Failure

Harleen Singh and Joel C. Marrs

CORE PRINCIPLES

	CORE PRINCIPLES	CHAPTER CASES
1	Heart failure (HF) "is a complex clinical syndrome that can result from any structural or functional cardiac disorder that impairs the ability of the ventricle to fill with or eject blood." This is further subdivided into HF with reduced left ventricular ejection fraction (HFrEF) or HF with preserved left ventricular ejection fraction (HFpEF), previously known as diastolic HF.	**Case 14-1 (Question 1)**
2	HF symptoms, including limitations in activity, can be quantified with the use of the New York Heart Association functional classification system and the American College of Cardiology–American Heart Association classification of chronic HF. The cardinal signs and symptoms (e.g., peripheral edema, dyspnea, fatigue) of HF must be evaluated in light of the patient's medical history, physical examination, and results of additional testing.	**Case 14-1 (Questions 2, 3)**
3	Coexisting medical conditions that lead to HF (e.g., ischemic heart disease, hypertension, atrial fibrillation [AF], diabetes mellitus, sleep apnea) or result from HF (e.g., AF, cachexia, depression) may influence the overall prognosis and treatment; therefore, these should be assessed on a routine basis.	**Case 14-1 (Question 4), Case 14-2 (Question 7), Case 14-5 (Question 3)**
4	Several categories of medications (such as nonsteroidal antiinflammatory drugs and "glitazones") may exert unfavorable hemodynamic effects and may precipitate HF symptoms in patients with previously compensated HF. In some patients, the occurrence of HF can be attributed to the cardiotoxic effect of a particular medication (cancer chemotherapeutic drugs).	**Case 14-1 (Question 5)**
5	Treatment goals are to improve symptoms, decrease hospitalizations, and prevent premature death in patients. The cornerstone of treatment for HFrEF is to optimize life-prolonging therapies (e.g., angiotensin-converting enzyme inhibitors, angiotensin receptor blocking agents, β-blockers, aldosterone antagonists) and promote healthy lifestyle choices (e.g., sodium restriction, exercise training).	**Case 14-1 (Questions 6–20), Case 14-2 (Questions 1–8), Case 14-3 (Questions 1,2)**
6	Prompt recognition of symptoms and appropriate treatment are critical in the management of acute decompensated HF. The mainstay of therapy in patients with volume overload is an intravenous loop diuretic. Other therapies (e.g., inotropic drugs) have failed to show long-term benefits in clinical trials.	**Case 14-4 (Questions 1–3), Case 14-5 (Questions 1, 2)**
7	An implantable cardioverter-defibrillator reduces the risk of sudden cardiac death in patients with reduced left ventricular function. Cardiac resynchronization therapy can be used in combination to improve symptoms and quality of life in patients with severe HF symptoms.	**Case 14-5 (Question 4), Case 14-6 (Questions 1, 2)**
8	There is little clinical trial evidence to guide which treatments are optimal to use in HFpEF.	**Case 14-7 (Question 1)**

Continued

	CHAPTER CASES
9 Although controversial, certain patients may respond differently to drug therapy (e.g., African American patients, women).	**Case 14-2 (Question 3), Case 14-3 (Question 2)**
10 HF is an extremely serious condition and requires careful diagnosis, ongoing monitoring, and the implementation of evidence-based therapy. Herbal remedies (e.g., hawthorn) have some evidence to support their role in improving symptoms of HF; however, they have no evidence demonstrating improvements in mortality. Herbals can also potentially interact with other heart medications.	**Case 14-8 (Question 1)**

Heart failure (HF) is "a complex clinical syndrome that results from any structural or functional cardiac impairment of ventricle filling or ejection of blood."[1] Congestive heart failure (CHF) is a subset of HF characterized by left ventricular (LV) systolic dysfunction and volume excess. However, some patients may lack symptoms of congestion and still have reduced cardiac output (CO) manifesting as fatigue and reduced exercise tolerance. Therefore, the term CHF has been replaced with HF.

The descriptive terminology, diagnostic techniques, and treatment of HF have undergone significant change in the past 20 years. Since 1994, a series of consensus and evidence-based practice guidelines have been published in an effort to standardize HF management. Guidelines from the Heart Failure Society of America,[2] American College of Cardiology (ACC), American Heart Association (AHA),[1] and the European Society of Cardiology[3] have been revised and updated to reflect ongoing changes in the management of HF. These guidelines use the four disease stages of HF first assigned by the ACC/AHA 2001 guidelines (Fig. 14-1).[4] This classification promotes the early identification of risk factors that are associated with the development of LV dysfunction and HF symptoms. It emphasizes that appropriate therapeutic interventions in the early stages (stages A and B) can prevent progression to overt HF symptoms. It does not replace the New York Heart Association (NYHA) functional classification, but reinforces that they should be used in combination to classify patients. The ACC/AHA guidelines[1,5,6] provide a comprehensive review on prevention, diagnosis, risk stratification, and treatment of HF in both outpatient and inpatient settings. The updates emphasize quality of care and adherence to performance measures. The terminology "guideline-directed therapy" (GDMT) is frequently used in lieu of optimal medical therapy.

Numerous programs and systems have been implemented in an attempt to decrease the cost and length of hospital stay for HF. It is recommended that practitioners look at least annually for the most recently published guidelines to be aware of the rapidly evolving treatment strategies for HF.

Incidence, Prevalence, and Epidemiology

It is estimated that there are 5.7 million people (1.5%–2% of the population) with HF in the United States, and approximately 23 million people with HF worldwide. The prevalence of HF continues to increase, with an estimated 46% increase in prevalence by 2030.[7] Every year, 870,000 people have a new diagnosis of HF, and at 40 years of age, one in five have a lifetime risk of developing this syndrome. After age 65, HF incidence approaches 10 per 1,000 person-years and is the most common cause of hospitalizations in the elderly population in the United States.

The incidence of HF is greater in men and in the elderly; however, the incidence in black women is as high as that in white men. In women, coronary artery disease (CAD) and diabetes are considered the strongest risk factors for HF. African Americans present with HF at a younger age compared with white individuals. Risk factors, such as ischemic heart disease, hypertension (HTN), smoking, obesity, and diabetes, among others, have been identified that predict the incidence of HF as well as its severity.[7]

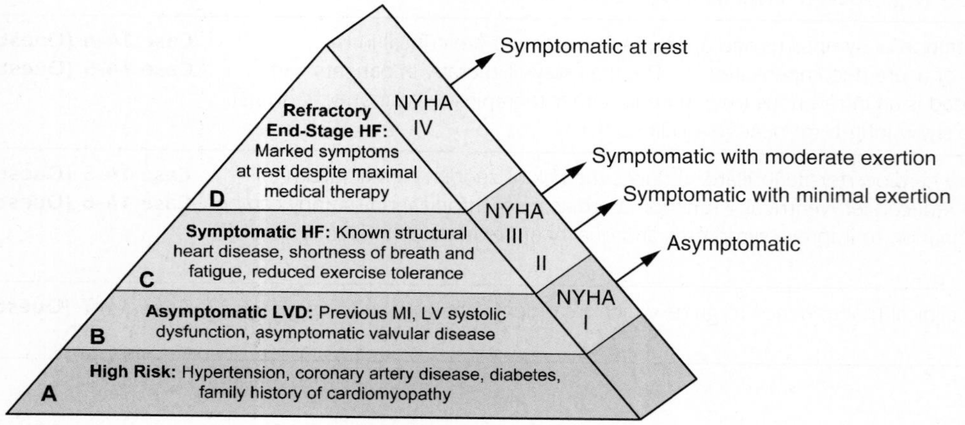

Figure 14-1 Staging and New York Heart Association (NYHA) classification of heart failure. (From Hunt SA et al. ACC/AHA Guidelines for the Evaluation and Management of Chronic Heart Failure in the Adult: Executive Summary. A Report of the American College of Cardiology/American Heart Association Task Force on Practice Guidelines (Committee to Revise the 1995 Guidelines for the Evaluation and Management of Heart Failure): Developed in Collaboration With the International Society for Heart and Lung Transplantation; Endorsed by the Heart Failure Society of America. *Circulation*. 2001;104:2996.)

In 2011, one in nine deaths has HF mentioned on the death certificate.[7] Evidence from national databases and community-based cohorts indicates that the incidence of HF seems to be stabilizing, if not decreasing, for women, and that the length of survival in patients with HF is increasing. However, the death rate remains high; almost 50% of people diagnosed with HF will die within 5 years.[5] The mortality risk steadily increases each year after the diagnosis of HF. The 6-month mortality rates are no different in patients with preserved versus reduced LV ejection fraction (EF).[8] Direct and indirect health care costs of HF in 2012 were estimated to be $30.7 billion.[7]

Various risk prediction models have been developed to predict HF outcomes. Given the heterogeneous nature of the HF population (ischemic vs. nonischemic, low vs. preserved EF), and multiple comorbid conditions, the validity of the risk prediction models is not consistent in all HF populations. Therefore, it is important to identify patients who are at high risk of HF and how various risks factors can predict outcomes.[9] Based on the strength of these associations, prevention measures need to be designed to decrease HF hospitalizations in targeted subpopulations. The 2013 guidelines[1] emphasize that validated multivariable risk scores can be useful to estimate subsequent risk of mortality in ambulatory or hospitalized patients with HF.

Etiology

LOW-OUTPUT VERSUS HIGH-OUTPUT FAILURE

HF has been described as being either *low-output* or *high-output failure,* with a predominance of cases being low-output failure (Table 14-1). In both types, the heart cannot provide adequate blood flow (tissue perfusion) to meet the body's metabolic demands, especially during exercise. The hallmark of classic low-output HF is a diminished volume of blood being pumped by a weakened heart in patients who have normal metabolic needs.

In high-output failure, the heart is healthy and pumps a normal or even higher than normal volume of blood. Because of high metabolic demands caused by other underlying medical disorders (e.g., hyperthyroidism, anemia), the heart becomes exhausted from the increased workload and eventually cannot keep up with demand. The primary treatment of high-output HF is amelioration of the underlying disease. Unless otherwise stated, this chapter focuses on the treatment of low-output HF.

LEFT VERSUS RIGHT VENTRICULAR DYSFUNCTION

Low-output HF is further divided into left and right ventricular dysfunction, or a combination of the two (biventricular failure). Because the left ventricle is the major pumping chamber of the heart, *left ventricular dysfunction* is the most common form of low-output HF and the major target for pharmacologic intervention. Right ventricular dysfunction may coexist with LV HF if damage is sustained by both sides of the heart or as a delayed complication of progressive left-sided HF.

Isolated right-sided ventricular dysfunction, which is relatively uncommon, is usually caused by either primary or secondary *pulmonary arterial hypertension.* In these conditions, elevated pulmonary artery pressure impedes emptying of the right ventricle, thus increasing the workload on the right side of the heart.[10,11] Primary pulmonary arterial HTN is idiopathic, caused by increased resistance of the pulmonary arterial vasculature of unknown etiology. Secondary causes of pulmonary HTN include collagen vascular disorders, sarcoidosis, fibrosis, exposure to high altitude, and drug and chemical exposure. Drug-induced causes include opioid overdoses (especially heroin), 5-hydoxytryptamine-2B (5HT-2B) agonists (e.g., dexfenfluramine, fenfluramine, and pergolide), and pulmonary fibrosis caused by intravenous (IV) injection of poorly soluble forms of methylphenidate. Right-sided heart disease that occurs as a result of a pulmonary process is known as cor pulmonale.

Table 14-1
Classification and Etiology of Left Ventricular Dysfunction

Type of Failure	Characteristics	Contributing Factors	Etiology
Low output, systolic dysfunction (dilated cardiomyopathy)[a]	Hypofunctioning left ventricle; enlarged heart (dilated left ventricle); ↑left ventricular end-diastolic volume; EF <40%; ↓stroke volume; ↓CO; S_3 heart sound present	1. ↓Contractility (cardiomyopathy) 2. ↑Afterload (elevated SVR)	1. Coronary ischemia,[b] MI, mitral valve stenosis or regurgitation, alcoholism, viral syndromes, nutritional deficiency, calcium and potassium depletion, drug induced, idiopathic 2. Hypertension, aortic stenosis, volume overload
Diastolic dysfunction	Normal left ventricular contractility; normal size heart; stiff left ventricle; impaired left ventricular relaxation; impaired left ventricular filling; normal EF; S_4 heart sound	1. Thickened left ventricle (hypertrophic cardiomyopathy) 2. Stiff left ventricle (restrictive cardiomyopathy) 3. ↑Preload	1. Coronary ischemia,[b] MI hypertension, aortic stenosis and regurgitation, pericarditis, enlarged left ventricular septum (hypertrophic cardiomyopathy) 2. Amyloidosis, sarcoidosis 3. Sodium and water retention
High-output failure (uncommon)	Normal or ↑contractility; normal size heart; normal left ventricular end-diastolic volume; normal or ↑EF; normal or increased stroke volume; ↑CO	1. ↑Metabolic and oxygen demands	1. Anemia and hyperthyroidism

[a]Same as congestive heart failure if symptoms also present.
[b]Heart failure caused by coronary artery ischemia or myocardial infarction classified as ischemic etiology. All other types combined classified as nonischemic.
CO, cardiac output; EF, ejection fraction; MI, myocardial infarction; SVR, systemic vascular resistance.

SYSTOLIC VERSUS DIASTOLIC DYSFUNCTION; ISCHEMIC VERSUS NONISCHEMIC HEART FAILURE

LV dysfunction is further subdivided into systolic and diastolic dysfunction, with mixed disorders also being encountered (Table 14-1). In systolic dysfunction, the *stroke volume* (SV) (the volume of blood ejected with each contraction; normal, 60–130 mL) and the subsequent CO (SV × heart rate; normal, 4–7 L/minute) are reduced. In diagnosing HF, a critical marker differentiating systolic from diastolic dysfunction is the *left ventricular ejection fraction* (LVEF), defined as the percentage of LV end-diastolic volume expelled during each systolic contraction (normal, 60%–70%).

In *systolic dysfunction,* the LVEF is less than 40%, dropping to less than 20% in advanced HF. Heart failure with reduced ejection fraction (HFrEF) is a result of factors causing the heart to fail as a pump (decreased myocardial contractility). The heart dilates as it becomes congested with retained blood, leading to an enlarged hypokinetic left ventricle.

HF caused by coronary ischemia or after MI is classified as *ischemic,* with all other types grouped as *nonischemic*. CAD is a common cause of HF in patients with LV systolic dysfunction. Other causes of LV pump failure include persistent arrhythmias, poststreptococcal rheumatic heart disease, chronic alcoholism (alcoholic cardiomyopathy), viral infections, or unidentified etiology (idiopathic dilated cardiomyopathy). Chronic HTN, as well as cardiac valvular disorders (aortic or mitral stenosis), also precipitate systolic HF by increasing resistance to CO (a high afterload state).

In contrast, LV diastolic dysfunction refers to impaired relaxation and increased stiffness of the left ventricle; the EF may or may not be abnormal, and the patient may or may not be symptomatic. Some patients have both systolic and diastolic dysfunction. The term *heart failure with normal or preserved left ventricular ejection fraction* (HFpEF) is used for patients who have symptoms of HF but a normal EF. These patients always have diastolic dysfunction.

Possible causes of diastolic dysfunction include: coronary ischemia, chronic uncontrolled HTN, LV wall scarring after an MI, ventricular wall hypertrophy, hypertrophic cardiomyopathy, restrictive cardiomyopathy (amyloidosis and sarcoidosis), and valvular heart disease (aortic stenosis). These factors lead to LV wall stiffness (reduced wall compliance), and inability of the ventricle to relax during diastole, which result in an elevated pressure within the ventricle despite a relatively low volume of blood. In turn, the elevated pressure impedes LV filling during diastole that would normally occur by passive inflow against a low-resistance pressure gradient. Heart size is usually (but not always) normal. It is estimated that 20% to 60% of patients with HF may have normal LVEF and reduced ventricular compliance.[12] Because coronary ischemia, MI, and HTN are contributors to both systolic and diastolic dysfunction, many patients have both systolic and diastolic dysfunction.

The pathology of systolic dysfunction most closely resembles what has historically been called "congestive heart failure." Tremendous variability exists in the clinical presentation of both systolic and diastolic dysfunction; however, both disorders can have similar symptoms.[4,11] Most patients exhibit exercise intolerance and shortness of breath (SOB) with either systolic or diastolic dysfunction. Some exhibit significant edema, whereas others may have no edema or symptoms of congestion. It is possible to be asymptomatic in the early stages of HF. For all these reasons, it is best to avoid the abbreviation *CHF*, because not all patients have congestion. CHF has also been used to denote "chronic heart failure." Clinicians are strongly encouraged to obtain an EF measurement in all patients. The diagnosis of HF should be based on a combination of symptoms and signs together with appropriate clinical tests.

CARDIAC WORKLOAD

A common finding of HF is increased cardiac workload. Four major determinants contribute to LV workload: preload, afterload, contractility, and heart rate (HR).

Preload

Preload describes forces acting on the *venous* side of the circulation affecting myocardial wall tension. The volume is maximal when filling finishes at the end of diastole (LV end-diastolic volume). An increased volume raises the pressure within the ventricle (LV end-diastolic pressure), which in turn increases the "stretch," or wall tension, of the ventricle. Peripheral venous dilation and decreased peripheral venous volume diminish preload, whereas peripheral venous constriction and increased peripheral venous volume increase preload.

Elevated preload can aggravate HF. Rapid administration of blood plasma expanders and osmotic diuretics or administration of large amounts of sodium or sodium-retaining agents increase preload. A malfunctioning aortic valve (aortic insufficiency), resulting in regurgitation of blood back into the left ventricle, can increase the volume of blood that must be pumped. A malfunctioning mitral valve (mitral regurgitation) can cause retrograde ejection of blood from the left ventricle back into the left atrium, with a resultant decrease in CO. In patients with systolic failure, ventricular blood is ejected less efficiently because of a hypofunctioning left ventricle; the volume of blood retained in the ventricle is thus increased, and preload becomes elevated. In HFpEF with a stiffened left ventricle, relatively small increases in end-diastolic volume from sodium and water overload can lead to exaggerated increases in end-diastolic pressure.

Afterload

Afterload is the tension developed in the ventricular wall as contraction (systole) occurs. This tension is affected by intraventricular pressure, ventricular diameter, and wall thickness. Afterload is affected by the systemic vascular resistance (SVR) or the impedance against which the ventricle must pump and is estimated by arterial blood pressure (BP). HTN, atherosclerotic disease, or a narrow aortic valve opening, increases arterial impedance (afterload), thereby increasing the workload of the heart. HTN is a major factor in the development of both HFrEF and HFpEF. The Framingham group found that 75% of patients who developed HF had a history of HTN.[13] The risk of developing HF was six times greater in hypertensive versus normotensive patients.

Cardiac Contractility

The terms *contractility* and *inotropic state* are used synonymously to describe the myocardium's ability to develop force and shorten its fibers independent of preload or afterload. Myocardial contractility is decreased when myocardial fibers are diminished or poorly functioning as may occur in patients with primary cardiomyopathy, valvular heart disease, CAD, or after a myocardial infarction (MI). Defects in contractility play a major role in systolic HF, but are not a factor for diastolic dysfunction. Drugs such as β-adrenergic blockers or anthracyclines precipitate HF by decreasing myocardial contractility.

Heart Rate

An increased HR is a reflex mechanism to improve CO as EF declines. The sympathetic nervous system is the major mediator of this response. The workload and energy demands of a rapid HR ultimately place strain on the heart and can eventually worsen HF.

Pathophysiology

When the heart begins to fail, the body activates several complex compensatory mechanisms in an attempt to maintain CO and oxygenation. These include increased sympathetic tone, activation of the renin–angiotensin–aldosterone system (RAAS), sodium and water retention, and other neurohormonal adaptations, which lead to cardiac "remodeling" (ventricular dilatation, cardiac hypertrophy, and changes in LV shape). The consequences of these adaptive mechanisms can create more harm than good (Fig. 14-2). The relative balance of each of these adaptive processes varies depending on the type of HF (systolic versus diastolic dysfunction) and from patient to patient with the same disorder. An understanding of the potential benefits and adverse consequences of these compensatory mechanisms is essential to understanding the signs, symptoms, and treatment of HF.[14]

SYMPATHETIC (ADRENERGIC) NERVOUS SYSTEM

The body's normal physiologic response to a decreased CO is generalized activation of the adrenergic (sympathetic) nervous system as evidenced by increased circulating levels of norepinephrine (NE) and other catecholamines. The inotropic (increased contractility) and chronotropic (increased HR) effects of NE initially maintain near-normal CO and perfusion of vital organs such as the central nervous system (CNS) and myocardium. Adverse consequences of NE activation include impaired sodium excretion by the kidneys, restricted ability of the coronary arteries to supply blood to the ventricle (myocardial ischemia), increased arrhythmias, hypokalemia, and oxidative stress triggering cell death (apoptosis).

Chronic high levels of catecholamines are harmful to the heart because they decrease β_1-receptor sensitivity and reduce β_1-receptor density on the surface of myocardial cells by 60% to 70% in severe HF.[14–20] The normal ratio of β_1- to β_2-receptors in the heart is ~80:20. As a response to overstimulation, this balance is shifted to a ratio of ~70:30 in the failing myocardium by downregulation of β_1-subtype receptors. This selective downregulation of β_1-receptors is accompanied by "uncoupling of the β_1- and β_2-receptor activity," whereby the number of β_2-receptors is unchanged but the responsiveness of these receptors can be reduced by 30%.[15] Over time, this leaves the myocyte less responsive to adrenergic stimuli and further decreases contractile function. β-Blockers cause the upregulation of the downregulated β_1 receptors and, the re-sensitization of the uncoupled β_2-receptors protecting the heart from the deleterious effects of catecholamines.[21]

Alterations in sympathetic adrenergic receptors are partially determined by genetic phenotype. Among African American patients with HF, a disproportionately high incidence of polymorphisms for variants of the β_1-receptor that are associated with increased function is seen. Additionally, the combined presence of a variant of the β_1-receptor (β_1Arg389) and α_{2C}-adrenergic receptor (α_{2c}Del322–325) results in adrenergic overstimulation and increases the risk of HF. These combined defects are found less often in whites, perhaps partially explaining a higher incidence of HF in African Americans. A better understanding of α- and β-receptor phenotypes may someday lead to improved prevention and treatment of HF.[22]

RENAL FUNCTION AND THE RENIN–ANGIOTENSIN–ALDOSTERONE SYSTEM

The reduced CO in HF leads to the stimulation angiotensin II, which is a potent vasoconstrictor. Angiotensin II is also a potent stimulator of the sympathetic nervous system, which increases SVR. Renal vascular resistance is increased, and the glomerular filtration rate (GFR) is decreased. As the GFR decreases, more sodium and water are reabsorbed. A diminished effective circulating plasma

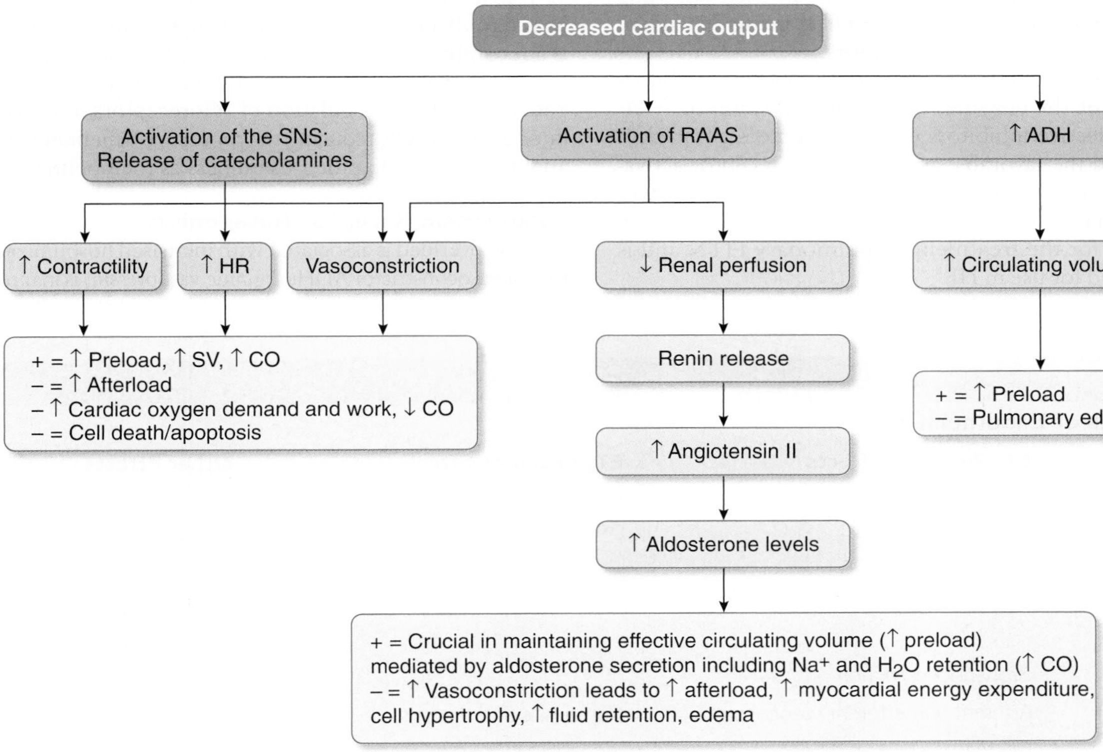

Figure 14-2 Adaptive mechanisms in systolic heart failure. +, beneficial results; –, negative (detrimental) effects; ADH, antidiuretic hormone; CO, cardiac output; HR, heart rate; H_2O, water; Na^+, sodium; RAAS, renin–angiotensin–aldosterone system; SNS, sympathetic nervous system; SV, stroke volume.

volume and angiotensin II also stimulate release of antidiuretic hormone (ADH) from the pituitary, resulting in the retention of free water in the collecting ducts.

The kidney releases renin when renal perfusion pressure is decreased. Renin converts *angiotensinogen* into *angiotensin I*. Angiotensin I is metabolized to *angiotensin II*, under the influence of angiotensin-converting enzyme (ACE) (Fig. 14-2). Angiotensin II has multiple effects favoring sodium and water retention. Its vasoconstricting effect decreases GFR, and it stimulates the adrenal glands to secrete aldosterone, which increases sodium reabsorption. Angiotensin II stimulates increased synthesis and release of vasopressin, thereby increasing free water retention and stimulation of thirst centers in the CNS. Finally, angiotensin II stimulates NE release. The net result of decreased renal perfusion is detrimental. Increased sodium and water retention increase preload, whereas angiotensin II–induced vasoconstriction increases SVR and afterload.

A chronic excess of aldosterone causes fibrosis in the myocardium, kidneys, and other organs.[23] Thus, aldosterone promotes remodeling of organs and fibrosis independent of angiotensin II.

OTHER HORMONAL MEDIATORS

Endothelins

Several other regulatory hormones and cytokines have been identified as playing a role in the pathogenesis and adaptation to HF. The first of these are the endothelins.[24,25] Endothelin-1 (ET-1) is the most active. ET-1 is synthesized by vascular and airway smooth muscle, cardiomyocytes, leukocytes, and macrophages. Serum concentrations of ET-1 are elevated in HF, pulmonary HTN, MI, ischemia, and shock, and cause vasoconstriction, potentiation of cardiac remodeling, and decreased renal blood flow (RBF). Although the effects of ET-1 are detrimental in HF, its pharmacology is complex and dependent on the relative balance of two distinct G protein–coupled receptor subtypes referred to as ET_A and ET_B. As illustrated in Table 14-2, ET-1 can elicit opposing effects from each receptor, with the net effect being dependent on the relative density of the two receptors.

Possible future therapeutic agents could be specific inhibitors of one or more of the enzymes to prevent activation of ET-1. Alternatively, selective inhibitors of ET_A receptors could shift responses toward the favorable aspects of ET_B receptor activation. Bosentan and tezosentan are nonselective dual ET_A/ET_B antagonists. Bosentan has U.S. Food and Drug Administration (FDA) approval for the treatment of pulmonary HTN and is being investigated for use in HF.[8,9]

Natriuretic Peptides

Natriuretic peptides (NPs) are a family of peptides containing a common 17–amino acid ring. A-type natriuretic peptide, previously referred to as atrial natriuretic peptide or atrial natriuretic factor, is secreted by the atria in response to dilatation. Similarly, B-type natriuretic peptide (BNP) is produced by the ventricular myocardium in response to elevations of end-diastolic pressure and volume. Type-C natriuretic peptide (CNP) is secreted by lung, kidney, and vascular endothelium in response to shear stress. Collectively, the NPs are considered to be a favorable form of neurohormonal activation. Among their positive attributes are antagonism of the renin–angiotensin system, inhibition of sympathetic outflow, and ET-1 antagonism. The net effect is peripheral and coronary vasodilation decreasing preload and afterload. As their name implies, they also have diuretic or natriuretic properties, with improved RBF and glomerular filtration resulting from afferent arteriolar dilation and possibly efferent arteriolar constriction. Sodium reabsorption is blocked in the collecting duct due to indirect aldosterone inhibition. NPs also inhibit vasopressin secretion and block salt appetite and thirst centers in the CNS which contributes to diuresis. CNP has minimal diuretic properties.[26]

The BNP precursor is cleaved to produce the biologically active C-terminal fragment (BNP) and an inactive N-terminal fragment (NT-proBNP). Plasma level measurement of either BNP or NT-proBNP can be used as a biologic marker to differentiate HF-induced dyspnea from other causes of respiratory distress.[27–29] BNP levels less than 100 pg/mL usually indicate absence of HF, whereas levels greater than 400 pg/mL are highly indicative of HF. However, the interpretation of BNP levels between 100 and 400 pg/mL can be challenging because elevated levels are also associated with renal failure, pulmonary embolism, pulmonary HTN, and chronic hypoxia.[30] Higher concentrations correlate with the severity of HF. Clinical resolution of symptoms is often accompanied by a decline in BNP concentration.

Natriuretic hormone analogs or inhibitors of their metabolism have been investigated for drug therapy of HF. Nesiritide is a recombinantly produced human BNP approved by the FDA for IV management of acute HF exacerbations in hospitalized patients.[31,32] Downregulation of NP receptors, however, occurs during chronic HF, reducing the protective benefit of their actions and possibly limiting their usefulness as therapeutic entities.

Vasopressin Receptor Antagonists

Volume overload is associated with increased hospitalization. The potent vasoconstrictor ADH (arginine vasopressin) is inappropriately

Table 14-2
Biologic Effects of Endothelin-1

Organ System	ET_A Receptor Effects	ET_B Receptor Effects	Other Effects
Blood vessels	Potent vasoconstrictor	Vasodilation mediated through nitric oxide and prostacyclin release	
	Collagen deposition		
Heart	Hypertrophy and remodeling		↑ HR
			+/– inotropic effects
Lungs	Bronchoconstriction		
Kidney	Afferent and efferent vasoconstriction	Natriuresis and diuresis	
	Decrease in RBF and GFR		
Neuroendocrine			Release of catecholamines, renin, aldosterone, and ANH

ANH, atrial natriuretic hormone; ET_A, endothelin A; ET_B, endothelin B; GFR, glomerular filtration rate; HR, heart rate; RBF, renal blood flow; +/–, positive/negative.
From Ergul A. Endothelin-1 and endothelin receptor antagonists as potential cardiovascular therapeutic agents. *Pharmacotherapy*. 2002;22:54.

elevated in HF. Early studies with tolvaptan (selective vasopressin subtype V2 receptor antagonist) demonstrated improvement in congestive symptoms of HF and overall hemodynamic profile but no improvement in long-term outcome.[33]

The EVEREST trial studied the efficacy of vasopressin antagonism in HF.[34,35] Tolvaptan was evaluated in 4,133 patients with acute decompensated heart failure (ADHF) with NYHA class III or IV and LVEF of less than 40%. All patients also received standard therapy (ACE inhibitors [ACEIs], angiotensin receptor blockers [ARBs], β-blockers, diuretics, nitrates, and hydralazine). The patients were randomly assigned within 48 hours of hospitalization to 30 mg/day tolvaptan or placebo. The trial was a composite of three distinct analyses. The primary end point for the two identical short-term trials was to assess the change in global clinical status and body weight at day 7 or the day of discharge. The primary outcome for the long-term trial was all-cause mortality and cardiovascular (CV) death or HF hospitalizations. The results of the short-term trial showed modest improvement in the global clinical score compared with placebo. The main clinical benefit was change in body weight. The long-term trial failed to show any significant difference between the study drug and placebo in the primary end points. Common side effects of tolvaptan were dry mouth and thirst. In a small number of patients, hyponatremia was corrected. Because long-term mortality benefits are lacking and the cost of the drug is high, the use of tolvaptan is restricted to patients with hypervolemic hyponatremia associated with HF despite fluid restriction and diuretic use.

Calcium Sensitizers

Calcium sensitizers represent another class of drugs investigated for the treatment of ADHF. They exert positive inotropic effects by stabilizing the calcium–troponin C complex and facilitating actin–myosin cross-bridging without increasing myocardial consumption of adenosine triphosphate.[36] Levosimendan, the prototype for this drug class, has a dual mechanism of action to increase myocardial contractibility and induce vasodilation. Unlike other inotropic agents, it does not affect the intracellular calcium concentrations and, therefore, has a lower potential for proarrhythmia. The safety and efficacy of levosimendan in ADHF has been evaluated in placebo-controlled trials and in comparative trials with dobutamine. In patients with decompensated HF, levosimendan significantly reduced the incidence of worsening HF and improved hemodynamic indices.[37–39] In addition, mortality was lower in the levosimendan group. These trials, however, were not powered to show a difference in mortality as an end point. A subsequent trial comparing levosimendan with dobutamine in ADHF, designed to confirm the beneficial effects on morbidity and mortality, did not reduce all-cause mortality, which contrasts with earlier studies.[40] The most common adverse effects associated with levosimendan are headache and hypotension. Currently, levosimendan is approved in Europe for ADHF.

Inflammatory Cytokines, Interleukins, Tissue Necrosis Factor, Prostacyclin, and Nitric Oxide

Vascular endothelial cells release pro-inflammatory cytokines, vasodilator and vasoconstrictor substances, including interleukin cytokines (IL-1β, IL-2, IL-6), tumor necrosis factor (TNF-α), prostacyclin, and nitric oxide (NO; also known as endothelium-derived relaxing factor).[41–43] The role of these mediators in the pathogenesis of HF is unclear. Recent studies have shown that patients with HF have elevated levels of the pro-inflammatory cytokines IL-1β, IL-6, and TNF-α that correlate with the severity of disease.[43–45] Initial enthusiasm for use of the TNF-α receptor antagonist etanercept as a treatment for HF has been abandoned after disappointing results in trials.[46] At least 47 adverse event reports were made to the FDA describing new-onset HF or exacerbation of existing HF with etanercept and infliximab in patients being treated for either Crohn's disease or rheumatoid arthritis.[47]

Other investigators have tried using either NO or prostacyclin (epoprostenol) as vasodilators with mixed success.[48–50] There was a trend toward increased death rates with prostacyclin despite improved hemodynamic status during the Flolan International Randomized Survival Trial (FIRST).[50]

CARDIAC REMODELING

Progression of HF results in *cardiac remodeling*, characterized by changes in the shape and mass of the ventricles.[51] The three primary manifestations of cardiac remodeling are chamber dilatation, LV myocardial hypertrophy, and a resulting spherical shape of the LV (Fig. 14-3). Cardiac remodeling, which starts before the appearance of clinical symptoms, contributes to the progression of the disease.

Cardiac Dilatation

Cardiac dilatation results from hypervolemia. End-diastolic volume increases, myocardial fibers are stretched, and the ventricle(s) become dilated. In the healthy heart, the end-diastolic volume is 110 to 120 mL. With an EF of 60%, the SV would be 70 mL, leaving an end-systolic residual volume in the ventricle of 40 to 50 mL. With HFrEF, the end-diastolic volume increases resulting in an enlarged heart. Cardiac dilatation is less evident in HFpEF because normal contractility is maintained and the stiffened LV is resistant to filling and less likely to dilate (Fig. 14-3).

Frank–Starling Curve

The Frank–Starling curve (Fig. 14-4) demonstrates a curvilinear relationship between LV myocardial muscle fiber "stretch" (wall tension) and myocardial work. As stretch increases, the volume of blood ejected (SV) with each contraction increases. In systolic HF, the work capacity for any degree of stretch is diminished. A simple analogy is drawn using a balloon. The greater amount of air blown into a balloon, the more it stretches and, if released, the farther it flies around a room. As the balloon gets old, it loses its elasticity and thus has less recoil. Similarly, dilatation of the ventricles initially may serve as an effective compensating mechanism in systolic failure, but becomes inadequate as the elastic limits of the muscle fibers are reached. HR also increases to maintain CO when SV is low. The disadvantage of cardiac dilatation is increased myocardial oxygen demand. Theoretically, as cardiac dilatation progresses beyond a certain point, CO could decrease (as visualized on the descending limb of the Starling curve), but this is rarely observed clinically.

Cardiac Hypertrophy

Cardiac hypertrophy represents an absolute increase in myocardial muscle mass and muscle wall thickness (Fig. 14-3). This is analogous to increased skeletal muscle mass in response to weightlifting. Cardiac hypertrophy should not be confused with cardiac dilatation.

FUNCTIONAL LIMITATION CLASSIFICATION AND STAGES OF HEART FAILURE

New York Heart Association Classification

The NYHA classification scheme identifies four categories of functional disability associated with HF. Patients in class I are well compensated with no physical limitations and lack symptoms with ordinary physical activity. In class II, ordinary physical activity results in mild symptoms and imparts slight limitations on exercise tolerance. Patients in class III are comfortable only at rest; even less than ordinary physical activity leads to symptoms. In class IV, symptoms of HF are present at rest and no physical activity can be undertaken without symptoms. Determination of class is subjective and will vary among observers.

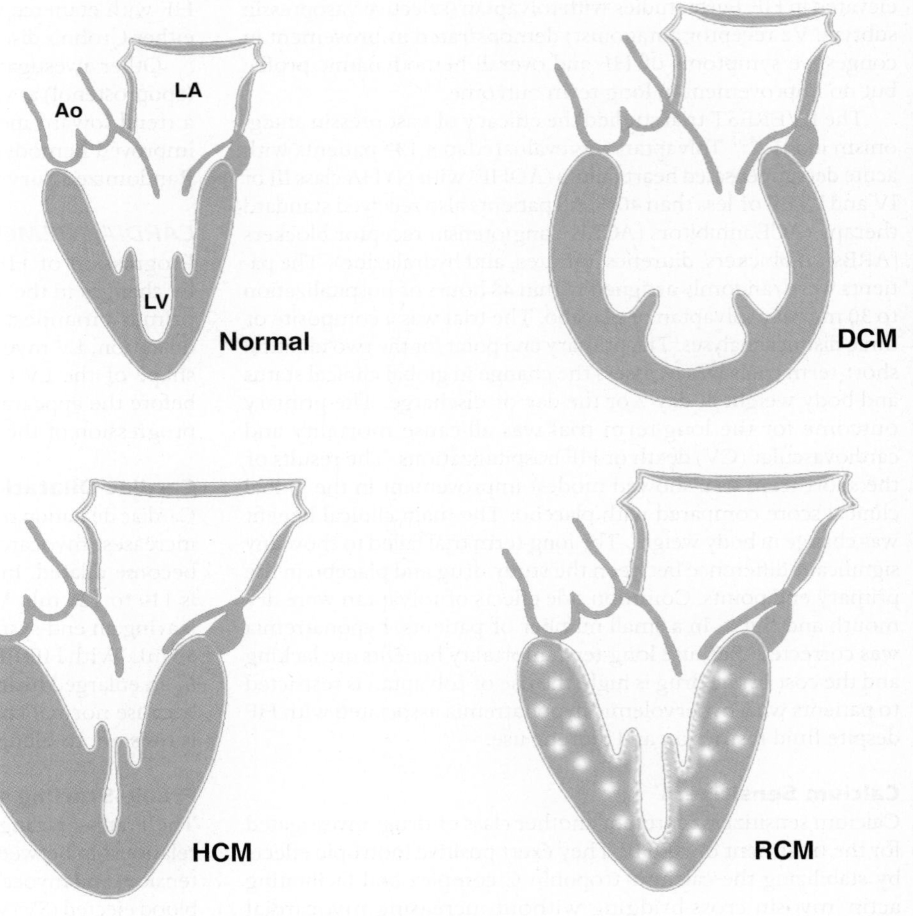

Figure 14-3 Cardiac remodeling. Dilated cardiomyopathy (DCM) results in thinning of the left ventricular walls and a decrease in systolic function; in hypertrophic cardiomyopathy (HCM), there is a marked thickening of the left ventricular walls leading to diastolic or systolic failure; and in restrictive cardiomyopathy (RCM), the left ventricular walls may be normal, hypertrophic, or slightly dilated, resulting in a decrease in diastolic compliance. Ao, aorta; LA, left articular; LV, left ventricular. (Adapted with permission from Topol EJ et al, eds. *Textbook of Cardiovascular Medicine*. 3rd ed. Philadelphia, PA: Lippincott Williams & Wilkins; 2006.)

A shortcoming of the NYHA classification scheme is that it does not include asymptomatic individuals who are at high risk for developing HF and may benefit from preemptive lifestyle changes and drug therapy. The 2001 ACC/AHA guidelines introduced a new staging system that can be used in conjunction with the NYHA classifications.[4] Patients in stage A have HTN, CAD, diabetes mellitus, or other conditions that, if left untreated, can result in the development of overt HF. HF symptoms or identifiable abnormalities of the myocardium or heart valves are absent in stage A. Patients in stage B remain asymptomatic but have structural defects within the heart (LV hypertrophy, dilatation, low EF, or valvular disease). Patients in stage C exhibit varying degrees of HF along with structural changes in the heart. Stage D in the ACA/AHA scheme roughly correlates with NYHA class IV. Patients in this latter category are frequently hospitalized, and are considered to have end-stage disease. Figure 14-1 summarizes these two classification schemes and how they overlap. The most recent guidelines[1] expand the definition of HF and add two subgroups to the HFpEF category: those with borderline EF (LVEF 41%–49%), and those with improved EF (patients with previously reduced EF, but now with an LVEF >40%).

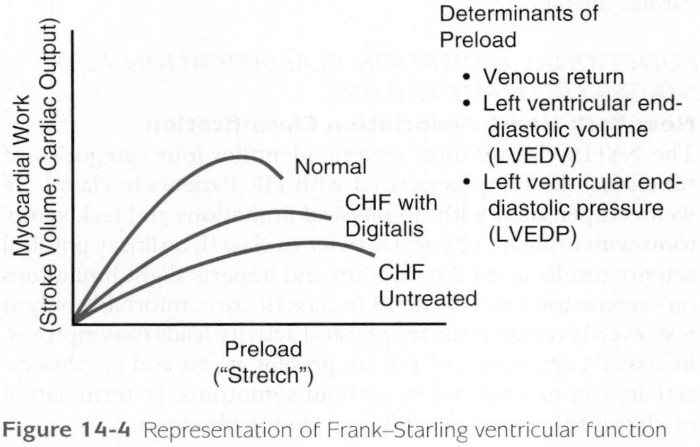

Figure 14-4 Representation of Frank–Starling ventricular function curve.

Overview of Treatment Principles

The ACC/AHA guidelines[1,5,6] updated their previous recommendations and expanded the role of both aldosterone antagonists and cardiac-resynchronization therapy (CRT) in patients with milder symptoms of HF. A clinical algorithm from the ACC/AHA guidelines is found in Figure 14-5.[1] The ACC/AHA Task Force recommends that most patients with HFrEF should routinely receive GDMT including an ACEI or an ARB, a β-adrenergic blocker, and an aldosterone receptor antagonist. Diuretics are recommended for patients with congestion. The combination of hydralazine and nitrate should be considered in in black patients with symptoms despite receiving other GDMT therapy or in patients unable to tolerate and ACEI or ARB. Digoxin is potentially beneficial in symptomatic patients with HFrEF already receiving optimal medical therapy to decrease HF hospitalizations.

The goals of therapy for HF are to abolish disabling symptoms, avoid complications such as arrhythmias, improve the quality of life, and prolong survival. Short of a heart transplant, none of the treatment measures are curative.

Nonspecific medical management of HF includes addressing CV risk factors, correcting underlying disease states (HTN, ischemic heart disease, arrhythmias, lipid disorders, anemia, or hyperthyroidism), performing moderate physical activity as tolerated, undergoing immunization with influenza and pneumococcal vaccines, and discontinuing possible drug-induced causes. The role of NPs, endothelin inhibitors, vasopressin receptor antagonists,

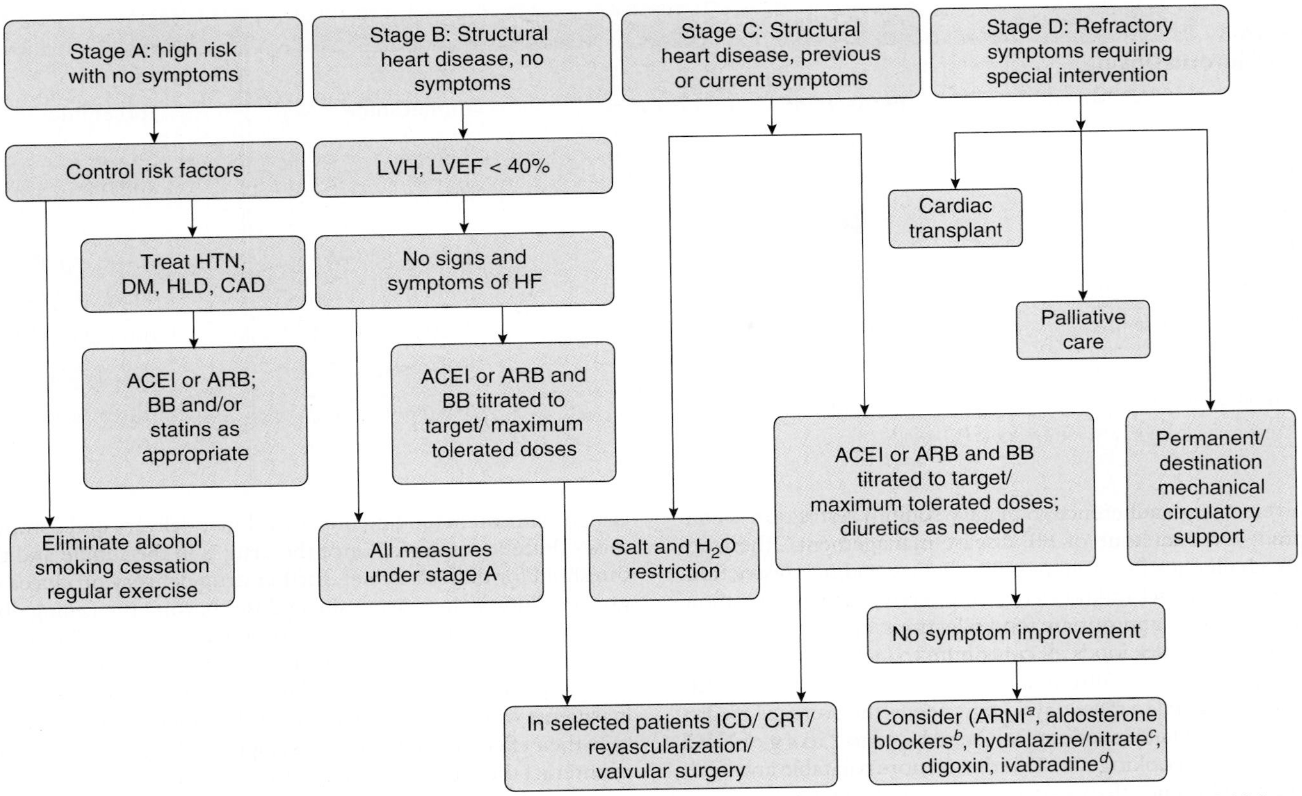

Figure 14-5 Stages in the development of heart failure and recommended therapy by stage. ACEI, angiotensin-converting enzyme inhibitors; ARB, angiotensin receptor blockers; BB, β-blockers; ARNI, angiotensin II receptor blocker neprilysin inhibitor; CAD, coronary artery disease; CrCl, creatinine clearance; DM, diabetes mellitus; EF, ejection fraction; HLD, hyperlipidemia; HTN, hypertension; ICD, implantable cardioverter-defibrillator; LVH, left ventricular hypertrophy.

[a]NYHA II or III who tolerate ACEI/ARB with adequate BP and no hx of angioedema – replace with ARNI to further reduce morbidity and mortality, must wait at least 36 hours of the last dose of ACEI
[b]NYHA II-IV unless est. CrCl < 30 mL/min and serum potassium > 5.0 mEq/L
[c]NYHA III or IV in black patients
[d]NYHA II or III, LVEF ≤ 35%, maximally tolerated dose of beta blocker, sinus rhythm, heart rate 70 bpm or greater

and calcium sensitizers continues to be investigated. Non-digitalis inotropic agents and TNF-α inhibitors, although theoretically valuable, have yielded disappointing results and significant complications, including arrhythmias and increased mortality rates.

Treatment of HFpEF is less well defined.[12,52–54] A sodium-restricted diet and diuretics are indicated for symptomatic relief of SOB or edema. Because these patients typically present with comorbid conditions (atrial fibrillation [AF], HTN, diabetes mellitus, and CAD), treatment of comorbidities with available therapies should aim to decrease CV events and improve survival.

PHYSICAL ACTIVITY

Patients should be encouraged to exercise to maintain physical conditioning. Treatment goals include prolonging life and improving quality of life. The results of The Effects of Exercise Training on Health Status in Patients with Chronic Heart Failure (HF-ACTION)[55] trial showed that a highly structured exercise program in HF patients did not reduce all-cause mortality or all-cause hospitalization when compared with patients who were getting the usual care in which exercise was simply encouraged. However, according to the HF-ACTION substudy, the structured exercise training program improved the overall Kansas City Cardiomyopathy Questionnaire (KCCQ) score (a test that includes questions on physical limitations, symptoms, quality of life, and social limitations). The improvement occurred early on and was sustained for 3 years. The ACC/AHA HF guidelines[1,5,6] recommend exercise training as safe and effective for patients with HF who are able to participate in symptom control.[1,5,6] However, during acute exacerbations, bed rest and restricted physical activity decrease the metabolic demands, and minimize gravitational forces contributing to edema. Renal perfusion is increased in the prone position, resulting in diuresis and mobilization of fluid.

SODIUM-RESTRICTED DIET

Dietary indiscretion (high salt intake) is often cited as the cause of HF exacerbations and hospital admissions. Several observational studies have demonstrated associations between lower dietary sodium intake and reduced hospitalizations and mortality.[56,57] In contrast, several randomized trials imply that dietary sodium restriction in patients with CV diseases may be deleterious. One of the largest meta-analysis in patients with HFrEF showed that compared with control groups (2,800 mg/day), the sodium-restricted groups (1,800 mg/day) had increased morbidity and mortality.[58] The trials included in this analysis had several limitations. High doses of diuretics were used in conjunction with strict fluid restriction, which could have resulted in intravascular volume depletion and adverse outcomes. Also, many patients were not on optimal doses of GDMT. There is limited evidence to support sodium restriction in the inpatient setting. In one trial, sodium restriction greater than the standard 2,000 mg/day in hospitalized HFrEF patients did not affect clinical stability or decrease length of stay.[59] For these reasons, further randomized trials are needed to elucidate the impact of sodium restriction on outcomes in HF patients. Because high sodium intake leads to HTN, LV hypertrophy, and CV disease, the ACC/AHA HF guidelines[1,5,6] recommend 1.5 g/daily sodium restriction for patients with stage A and B HF. In patients with advanced HF (stages C and D), <3 g/daily is recommended due to lack of sufficient data to support any specific degree of restriction.

Table 14-3
Loop Diuretic Dosing[1]

	Furosemide	Bumetanide	Torsemide
IV loading doses	40 mg	1 mg	20 mg
Maximum total daily dose	600 mg	10 mg	200 mg
Ceiling dose			
Normal renal function	80–160 mg (PO/IV)	1–2 mg (PO/IV)	20–40 mg (PO/IV)
Cl_{cr}: 20–50 mL/minute	160 mg (PO/IV)	2 mg (PO/IV)	40 mg (PO/IV)
Cl_{Cr}: <20 mL/minute	200 mg (IV), 400 mg (PO)	8–10 mg (PO/IV)	100 mg (PO/IV)
Bioavailability	10%–100%	80%–90%	80%–100%
Duration of action	6–8 hours	4–6 hours	12–16 hours

Cl_{Cr}, creatinine clearance; IV, intravenous; PO, oral.

Even though adherence to dietary sodium restriction is considered "a cornerstone of HF disease management," there are many challenges in implementing dietary sodium restriction. Barriers such as lack of knowledge, interference with socialization, limited access to appropriate food selections, and increased taste preference for salty foods all contribute to lack of adherence to low sodium diet.[60,61] Although less than 1 g of sodium chloride (NaCl) is required to meet physiologic needs, the average U.S. diet contains 10 g. Dietary sodium can be reduced to 2 to 4 g of NaCl by eliminating cooking salt. This diet is more palatable and leads to better adherence than a severely salt-restricted diet.

DIURETICS

Only those points salient to the treatment of HF are included in this chapter. Diuretic use is discussed in Chapter 9, Essential Hypertension and Chapter 27, Fluid and Electrolyte Disorders.

Diuretics are indicated in HF patients with congestion (pulmonary and/or peripheral edema). They produce rapid symptomatic relief. Because activation of the RAAS and sympathetic nervous system contributes to the progression of HF, diuretics should be combined with an ACEI and a *β*-blocker unless contraindications exist.[1]

Initially, the goal of diuretic therapy is symptomatic relief of HF by decreasing excess volume without causing intravascular volume depletion. Once excess volume is removed, therapy is aimed at maintaining sodium balance and preventing accumulation of new fluid, while avoiding dehydration. The rate at which volume can be removed is limited by its rate of mobilization from the interstitial to the intravascular fluid compartment. If diuresis is too vigorous, intravascular volume depletion, hypotension, and a paradoxical decrease in CO may result. Diuretic doses are titrated so that urine output increases and weight decreases, generally by 0.5 to 1.0 kg daily.[1]

The effectiveness of diuretics depends on the amount of sodium delivered to their site of action and the patient's renal function.[62,63] Proximal tubular reabsorption of sodium is increased in patients with severe HF when RBF is compromised, rendering thiazide and potassium-sparing diuretics (which act primarily on the distal tubule) minimally effective. Thiazides are believed to lose their effectiveness when creatinine clearance decreases to less than 30 mL/minute. Metolazone is an exception in that its activity may be preserved in these patients. The loop diuretics (furosemide, bumetanide, and torsemide) are more potent than thiazides, and retain their effectiveness in renal insufficiency. Thus, in most patients with HF, loop diuretics are preferred. In addition to having activity in the ascending limb of the loop of Henle, furosemide has vasodilating properties that decrease renal vascular resistance. The usual recommended doses for the loop diuretics are found in Table 14-3.[62]

The effectiveness of diuretics depends on active secretion of the drug in the proximal tubule. Slow absorption (even if bioavailability is high) or protein binding impairs tubular delivery and compromises diuretic response. Once the drug is in the tubule and the threshold for diuresis is met, further drug delivery produces no greater diuresis. Increasing single doses beyond the ceiling dose produces no additional diuretic response; however, improved diuresis may be obtained by giving the drug more frequently.

A combination of diuretics (a loop diuretic and thiazide) is used in patients who are refractory to high-dose loop diuretics.[62,63] Despite their effects on reducing HF symptoms, loop diuretics do not counteract the underlying cause of HF or modify mortality rates.

ALDOSTERONE ANTAGONISTS

The aldosterone antagonists eplerenone and spironolactone exert a mild diuretic effect by competitive binding to the aldosterone receptor site in the distal convoluted renal tubules. The Randomized Aldactone Evaluation Study (RALES) investigators found that spironolactone reduced both morbidity and mortality in patients in NYHA class III and IV.[64] The authors speculated that the beneficial effect of spironolactone was related to a reduction in aldosterone-induced vascular damage and myocardial or vascular fibrosis rather than its diuretic effect. Similarly, reduced mortality was observed in patients with LV dysfunction after a recent MI who were treated with eplerenone.[65] The ACC/AHA HF guidelines[1,5,6] recommend the addition of an aldosterone antagonist in all patients with HFrEF who are already on ACEIs (or ARB) and *β*-blockers irrespective of the severity of symptoms and in patients immediately after MI who have LV dysfunction or diabetes.[65] On initiating aldosterone receptor antagonists, GFR should be >30 mL/minute/1.73 m^2 and potassium levels <5 mEq/dL to avoid the risk of hyperkalemia or renal insufficiency.

ANGIOTENSIN-CONVERTING ENZYME INHIBITORS AND ANGIOTENSIN RECEPTOR BLOCKERS

Drugs with vasodilating properties are a primary treatment for HF. Arterial dilation provides symptomatic relief of HF by decreasing arterial impedance (afterload). Venous dilation decreases LV congestion (preload). The combination of these two properties provides additive benefits to alleviate the symptoms of HF and increase exercise tolerance. The first vasodilator drugs to be studied were hydralazine (an arterial dilator) and nitrates (predominately venous dilators). By combining these two drugs, significant reductions in HF symptoms can be achieved along with a reduction in mortality rates. With the advent of ACEIs, the use of hydralazine and nitrates has been relegated to a secondary role.

ACEIs possess both afterload- and preload-reducing properties and volume-reducing potential. They produce similar hemodynamic effects to the hydralazine–nitrate combination as a single agent, favorably modify cardiac remodeling, and have a more tolerable side effect profile. These advantages led to the recommendations that ACEIs are the drugs of choice for initial therapy, even in patients with relatively mild LV systolic dysfunction.[1]

The ACC/AHA guidelines[1,5,6] state that ACEIs should be prescribed to all patients with HFrEF unless they have a contradiction to their use or are unable to tolerate these drugs. In general, ACEIs are used with β-blockers. ACEIs should be initiated at low doses, and titrated to target doses if well tolerated. Fluid retention can blunt the therapeutic effects, and volume depletion can potentiate the adverse effects of ACEIs. Clinicians should attempt to use doses that have been shown to reduce CV events in clinical trials, but they should not delay the initiation of β-blockers in patients because of a failure to reach target ACEI doses.[1]

The pharmacologic actions of all the ACEIs are essentially identical, but some of them have not been studied or received FDA approval for use in HF (Table14-4). Their value in HFpEF still is unclear. A related class of drugs is the ARBs.[66,67] ARBs offer theoretic advantages compared with ACEIs by being more specific for angiotensin II blockade (preferentially bind to AT_1 receptors) and having a lower risk of drug-induced cough.

ARBs can be used as alternatives to ACEIs in patients who are intolerant (angioedema or cough). Triple combination of an ACEI, ARB, and an aldosterone receptor antagonist is potentially harmful for patients and therefore is listed as a class III (avoid) recommendation in the ACC/AHA guidelines.[1,5,6] Currently, only candesartan and valsartan are FDA-approved for the treatment of HF.

β-ADRENERGIC BLOCKING AGENTS

Until the mid-1990s, β-blockers were contraindicated in patients with HFrEF. This was based on the belief that sympathomimetic agonists and other positive inotropic drugs were the logical choices to counteract systolic failure and that negative inotropic drugs would exacerbate HF. A better understanding of the pathophysiology of HF led to a rethinking of this logic.[15–20,22] In combination with ACEIs, β-blockers are considered first-line agents in patients with HFrEF. The ACC/AHA guidelines state that β-blockers should be prescribed to all patients with HFrEF unless they have a contraindication to their use or are unable to tolerate the treatment. Intolerance or resistance to other HF therapies should not preclude or delay the initiation of β-blocker use in patients with HFrEF.[1] Although some patients can have a temporary worsening of symptoms, continued use results in improved quality of life, fewer hospitalizations, and most importantly, a reduction in mortality by approximately 34% when added to other HF therapies. Extended-release metoprolol succinate, carvedilol, and bisoprolol are FDA approved for use in HFrEF. Metoprolol and bisoprolol are both partially selective β_1-blockers, and carvedilol is a mixed α_1- and nonselective β-blocking agent.

DIGITALIS GLYCOSIDES (DIGOXIN)

Digoxin has several pharmacologic actions on the heart. It binds to and inhibits sodium-potassium (Na^+/K^+) adenosine triphosphatase (ATPase) in cardiac cells, decreasing outward transport of sodium and increasing intracellular concentrations of calcium within the cells. Calcium binding to the sarcoplasmic reticulum causes an increase in the contractile state of the heart.

At one time, the primary benefit of digoxin in HFrEF was assumed to be an increase in the force of contraction (positive inotropic effect). We now know that digoxin has beneficial neurohumoral and autonomic effects caused by reducing sympathetic tone and stimulating parasympathetic responses at serum concentrations below those associated with positive inotropism.[68,69] Inhibition of Na^+/K^+ ATPase in vagal afferent fibers sensitizes cardiac baroreceptors, resulting in reduced sympathetic outflow from the CNS. Similarly, inhibition of Na^+/K^+ ATPase in renal cells reduces renal tubular reabsorption of sodium and indirectly suppresses renin secretion. This has led to the suggestion that the positive benefits of digoxin can be obtained by using small doses.

Digoxin decreases the conduction velocity and prolongs the refractory period of the atrioventricular (AV) node. This AV node–blocking effect prolongs the PR interval and is the basis for use of digoxin in slowing the ventricular response rate in patients with AF and other supraventricular arrhythmias (see Chapter 15, Cardiac Arrhythmias).

Several studies have confirmed a clinical benefit for digoxin in reducing HF symptoms, independent of rhythm status, but there are no data that demonstrate a beneficial effect on survival. Digoxin is used for symptom management in patients optimally treated with ACEIs, β-blockers, and aldosterone antagonists. In symptomatic patients in stage C or stage D, digoxin can reduce HF-related hospitalizations.[1] Digoxin can also be considered in patients with HF who also have AF, although β-blockers are more effective than digoxin in controlling the ventricular response, especially during exercise.

OTHER VASODILATING DRUGS: HYDRALAZINE AND NITRATES

Although ACEIs are drugs of choice, the first vasodilators evaluated in HFrEF were hydralazine and nitrates. Hydralazine provides symptomatic relief of HF by decreasing afterload. Nitrates have venous dilating properties that decrease preload. Used in combination, these two agents have additive benefits in alleviating the symptoms of HF and increasing exercise tolerance. Importantly, the hydralazine–isosorbide dinitrate combination was the first treatment regimen to show improved survival in severe HF compared with placebo[70] (while patients continued their diuretic or digitalis therapy). The African American Heart Failure Trial (AHeFT)[71] showed that the addition of hydralazine combined with isosorbide dinitrate to standard HF therapy with an ACEI or a β-blocker improved survival and reduced HF hospitalizations. Based on the results of AHeFT, the FDA approved the combination product of hydralazine and isosorbide dinitrate (BiDil) for the treatment of HFrEF as an adjunct to standard HF therapy in African American patients. The combination of hydralazine and nitrate is reasonable in patients with current or prior HF symptoms and reduced LVEF who cannot tolerate ACEIs or ARBs, and is also recommended for patients self-described as African American with moderate to severe symptoms on optimal therapy with ACEIs, β-blockers, and diuretics.[1] IV NTG and nitroprusside (a mixed arterial and venous dilator) are also used in hospitalized patients with acute HF exacerbations. The role of these vasodilators in HFpEF is not well studied.

OTHER INOTROPIC AGENTS

IV dopamine and dobutamine, which are sympathomimetics, and milrinone (phosphodiesterase inhibitor) are used in acutely decompensated HF (see Chapter 17, Shock). They are associated with an increased incidence of mortality but frequently used short term for ADHF. Both dobutamine and milrinone are used chronically in some stage D patients.

Initial positive hemodynamic effects during the first few weeks to months of therapy are followed by increased mortality with continued therapy when compared with placebo. This is related to proarrhythmic effects. Inotropic drugs are contraindicated in HFpEF.

CALCIUM-CHANNEL BLOCKERS

Amlodipine, felodipine, isradipine, nifedipine, and nicardipine are examples of dihydropyridine calcium-channel blockers with arterial vasodilating effects. Compared with the nondihydropyridine calcium-channel blockers (verapamil and diltiazem), they have minimal negative inotropic properties. Only amlodipine[72] and felodipine[73] have been documented to be safe in HF, but only a small subset of patients with nonischemic dilated cardiomyopathy actually had a beneficial effect of improved survival with amlodipine.[72] Verapamil and diltiazem are safe to use in HFpEF and may improve symptoms by reducing HR and allowing more time to fill the ventricle, but should be avoided in patients with HFrEF due to their negative inotropic effects.

IMPLANTABLE CARDIOVERTER-DEFIBRILLATOR

Ventricular arrhythmias are common in patients with HF ranging from asymptomatic ventricular premature beats to sustained ventricular tachycardia, ventricular fibrillation, and sudden cardiac death (SCD). SCD is highest in patients with severe HF symptoms, or stage D HF.[1] Patients with previous cardiac arrest or documented sustained ventricular arrhythmias have a higher risk of future events. An implantable cardioverter-defibrillator (ICD) implantation is indicated for secondary prevention of SCD in HF patients who have good clinical function and prognosis and low EF and experience syncope of unknown origin, as well as in a small subset of HF patients who are awaiting a planned cardiac transplant. The ACC/AHA guidelines[1] also recommend ICD for primary prevention of SCD in patients with nonischemic dilated cardiomyopathy or ischemic heart disease at least 40 days after MI, EF of 35% or less despite optimal drug therapy, with mild to moderate symptoms of HF and in whom survival with good functional capacity is otherwise anticipated to extend beyond 1 year (see Case 14-5, Question 4, for detailed discussion).

CARDIAC RESYNCHRONIZATION

CRT is a therapeutic approach for treating patients with ventricular dyssynchrony (defined as a QRS duration of at least 120 ms). Selected HF patients benefit from simultaneous pacing of both ventricles (biventricular pacing), or of one ventricle in patients with bundle branch block. The rationale for using CRT is that dyssynchrony causes ventricular remodeling and worsens HF. CRT can be used alone or with an ICD device. Several clinical trials with CRT or CRT-D[74–77] (cardiac resynchronization defibrillator therapy) have demonstrated improvements in HF functional status, survival, and reduction in hospitalizations. The approved indication for cardiac CRT-D includes patients with NYHA class II or ischemic class I HF, with an EF of less than 30% and a QRS duration of longer than 130 ms, and left bundle branch block. These indications are based on results[75] which showed a significant reduction in HF events among patients with mild HF symptoms with CRT-D compared with ICD alone. Current guidelines[1] support the use of CRT in patients with NYHA class II, III or ambulatory IV symptoms on GDMT, LVEF of 35% or less, and LBBB with a QRS ≥150 ms (see Case 14-6, Questions 1 and 2).

LEFT VENTRICULAR ASSIST DEVICES

A left ventricular assist device (LVAD) is a battery-operated, mechanical pump that is surgically implanted to maintain the pumping ability of the heart. Clinical trials using LVADs have shown improvement in survival and quality of life. For patients with end-stage HF, LVADs are used as a bridge to transplant or as destination therapy, which is permanent device implantation for patients who are not candidates for a transplant.

The landmark trial REMATCH[78] (Randomized Evaluation of Mechanical Assistance for the Treatment of Congestive Heart Failure) found that end-stage HF patients who received an LVAD (HeartMate XVE) had a 52.1% chance of surviving 1 year, compared with a 24.7% survival rate for patients who received optimal medical therapy. At 2 years, the survival was 23% for the LVAD patients versus 8% for those receiving medical therapies. However, these survival rates were much lower than those seen with transplantation. Advances in technology led to the introduction of the second-generation devices, notably HeartMate II, which was approved as a bridge to transplant in 2008.[79] In January 2010, the HeartMate II (continuous flow), a smaller device, was approved for destination therapy. In a head-to-head comparison with the first-generation HeartMate XVE (pulsatile flow), 1- and 2-year survival rates were 68% and 58% with HeartMate II versus 55% and 24% with HeartMate XVE.[80] Adverse events were less frequent with the continuous-flow device and patients reported significant improvements in their quality of life. Recently, a new novel pump called HeartWare left ventricular assist device (HVAD) was tested in patients awaiting cardiac transplantation with refractory and advanced HF. This device is small and can be directly implanted into the pericardial sac. The nonrandomized ADVANCE trial[81] (Evaluation of the HVAD for the Treatment of Advanced Heart Failure) enrolled 140 patients who received HVAD compared with 499 patients who received an LVAD. The primary end points were survival and success rates at 180 and 360 days after implantation. At 180 days the survival was 92.0% for the HVAD group and 90.1% for the control group ($p < 0.001$). There was less bleeding and fewer infections reported with HVAD; however, the incidence of stroke was higher. New clinical trials are being designed and conducted to evaluate adverse events between HVAD and HeartMate II. Until further improvements are implemented and demonstrated, cardiac transplantation remains the gold standard for the treatment of end-stage HF.

NEW THERAPIES IN HFREF

Ivabradine

There is considerable evidence of an association between elevated HRs (HRs >80 beats/minute [bpm]) and increased risk of mortality in patients with HF. The HF trials with β-blockers demonstrated increased mortality with elevated baseline resting heart rates (RHR) >90 bpm.[82,83] Post hoc analysis of CHARM[84] showed that increased RHR was an independent predictor of mortality regardless of LV function or use of β-blockers. A subsequent meta-analysis of HF trials[85] showed an association between the magnitude of HR reduction and survival benefit.

Ivabradine is a selective I_f ("funny current") inhibitor which lowers HR by acting on the sinoatrial node. In 2010, the Systolic Heart Failure Treatment With the I_f Inhibitor Ivabradine Trial (SHIFT)[86] provided evidence for the benefit of HR lowering in patients with HF. SHIFT randomized 6,558 patients with symptomatic HF to ivabradine versus placebo. Patients had an EF ≤35%, normal sinus rhythm with a HR of ≥70 bpm, and at least one hospitalization for HF within the previous year. In addition to background treatment, which generally included a β-blocker, patients received either ivabradine to maintain a RHR between 50 and 60 bpm, or placebo. During a median 23 months of follow-up, patients in the ivabradine group had an 18% decrease in risk for CV death or hospitalization (hazard ratio, 0.82; $p < 0.0001$). Ivabradine significantly reduced the risk of hospitalization for worsening HF and death due to HF, but did not have a significant effect on all-cause mortality. Ivabradine was well tolerated with relatively few adverse events, although significantly more than placebo. The most common adverse events were bradycardia and visual disturbances.

In April 2015, the FDA approved ivabradine (*Corlanor*) for symptomatic chronic HF with LVEF ≤35%, to reduce the risk of hospitalization for worsening HF in adults. Because ivabradine did not reduce all-cause mortality, its broader application in clinical practice will emerge as more evidence becomes available. The 2016 ACC/AHA/HFSA update on 2013 HF guidelines notes that ivabradine can be beneficial to reduce HF hospitalization for patients with symptomatic (NYHA class II–III) stable chronic HFrEF (≤35%) who are receiving maximal GDMT, including a β-blocker at maximum tolerated dose, and in sinus rhythm with a heart rate of greater than or equal to 70 bpm at rest. It received a class IIa recommendation, level of evidence B-R.[5]

ANGIOTENSIN RECEPTOR-NEPRILYSIN INHIBITOR

The NP hormones are responsible for both natriuresis and diuresis and are broken down by the neutral endopeptidase neprilysin, which also degrades angiotensin II. Several neprilysin inhibitors (ecadotril, candoxatril, omapatrilat) have been developed to target this pathway in order to increase concentrations of NPs. Unfortunately, lack of efficacy and side effects led to discontinuation of their development. A new drug sacubitril/valsartan (Entresto) has shown improved outcomes with few adverse effects in patients with HFrEF. Sacubitril/valsartan is an angiotensin receptor-neprilysin inhibitor (ARNI), a unique combination with an ARB (valsartan) and a neprilysin inhibitor (sacubitril). Because neprilysin also breakdowns angiotensin II, a neprilysin inhibitor should be given in combination with a RAAS inhibitor. Sacubitril/valsartan provides a dual mechanism of action in HF by inhibiting the renin–angiotensin–aldosterone axis and augmenting several endogenous NPs. This mechanism has not been addressed by other HF therapies.

This was tested in a randomized, double-blind trial "**P**rospective comparison of **A**ngiotensin **R**eceptor neprilysin inhibitors with **A**ngiotensin converting enzyme inhibitors to **D**etermine **I**mpact on **G**lobal **M**ortality and Morbidity in **H**eart **F**ailure" (PARADIGM-HF)[83] that compared sacubitril/valsartan (400 mg daily) to enalapril (20 mg daily) in patients with a LVEF <35% and elevated BNP levels, almost all of whom were in NYHA class 2 to 3. At baseline, most patients in both groups were receiving the recommended pharmacologic treatment for HFrEF. At 3.5 years of follow-up, there was a significant reduction in the primary outcome of CV death or HF hospitalization in the sacubitril/valsartan group (21.8%) versus the enalapril group (26.5%). Patients receiving sacubitril/valsartan had lower rates of hyperkalemia, renal dysfunction, and cough, but higher rates of hypotension. Fewer patients in the sacubitril/valsartan group required treatment intensification and use of advanced therapies (inotropes, assist devices, cardiac transplantation) when compared with enalapril.

ACEIs have had a class I recommendation based on their magnitude of CV mortality prevention (18%) in HF. The finding that sacubitril/valsartan has a superior effect on CV mortality compared to enalapril lends support that an ARNI could replace ACEI and ARBs in patients with HFrEF who remain symptomatic despite being on optimal GDTM. However, it should be noted that fewer patients in both groups had CRT or ICD therapy compared to contemporary treatment in the United States. This is the first study which used substitution of an ACEI rather than an add-on strategy in chronic HF. Even though the ARNI clearly met the criteria for clinical superiority when compared with conventional therapy, the benefits have to be weighed against the side effect profile. In clinical practice, the frequency of the side effects (hypotension, angioedema) may be more pronounced due to a more complicated patient population. The drug was approved by FDA in 2015 for NYHA class I–IV. Post-marketing surveillance will determine the safety of sacubitril/valsartan. A cost–benefit analysis would also be of use.

The 2016 ACC/AHA/HFSA update on 2013 HF guidelines recommends an ARNI in patients with chronic symptomatic HFrEF (NYHA class II or III) who tolerate an ACE inhibitor or ARB, in order to further reduce morbidity and mortality. It has a class I, level of evidence B-R recommendation.[5] The guidelines also state that ARNI should not be combined with ACE inhibitors and a 36-hour washout period is required between these two therapies to minimize the risk of angioedema.

Given the positive results of the Paradigm trial, the benefit of sacubitril/valsartan in HFpEF patients is being evaluated in an ongoing study: "Efficacy and Safety of LCZ696 Compared to Valsartan, on Morbidity and Mortality in Heart Failure Patients With Preserved Ejection Fraction (PARAGON–HF)."[88] The primary end point is to determine whether sacubitril/valsartan can reduce CV death or total HF hospitalizations in patients with HFpEF.

PATIENT EVALUATION

Signs and Symptoms

CASE 14-1

QUESTION 1: A.J., a 58-year-old man, is admitted with a chief complaint of increasing SOB and an 8-kg weight gain. Two weeks before admission, he noted the onset of dyspnea on exertion (DOE) after one flight of stairs, orthopnea, and ankle edema. Since then, his symptoms have worsened. He has also noted episodic bouts of paroxysmal nocturnal dyspnea (PND), and he has been able to sleep only in a sitting position. A.J. reports a productive cough, nocturia (two to three times a night), and edema.

A.J.'s other medical problems include a long history of heartburn, a 10-year history of osteoarthritis, depression, and poorly controlled HTN. A family history of diabetes mellitus is also present.

Physical examination reveals dyspnea, cyanosis, and tachycardia. A.J. has the following vital signs: BP, 160/100 mm Hg; pulse, 90 bpm; and respiratory rate, 28 breaths/minute. He is 5 feet 11 inches tall and weighs 78 kg. His neck veins are distended. On cardiac examination, an S_3 gallop is heard; the point of maximal impulse is at the sixth intercostal space, 12 cm from the midsternal line. His liver is enlarged and tender to palpation, and a positive hepatojugular reflux is observed. He is noted to have 3+ pitting edema of the extremities and sacral edema. Chest examination reveals inspiratory rales and rhonchi bilaterally.

The medication history reveals the following current medications: hydrochlorothiazide (HCTZ) 25 mg every day, ibuprofen 600 mg 4 times a day (QID), ranitidine 150 mg every night at bedtime, and citalopram 20 mg every day. He has no allergies and no dietary restrictions.

Admitting laboratory values include the following:

Hematocrit, 41.1%
White blood cell count, 5,300/μL
Sodium (Na), 132 mEq/L
Potassium (K), 3.2 mEq/L
Chloride (Cl), 100 mEq/L
Bicarbonate, 30 mEq/L
Magnesium, 1.5 mEq/L
Fasting blood sugar, 100 mg/dL
Uric acid, 8 mg/dL
Blood urea nitrogen (BUN), 40 mg/dL
Serum creatinine (SCr), 0.8 mg/dL
Alkaline phosphatase, 44 units/L
Aspartate aminotransferase, 30 units/L
BNP, 1,364 pg/mL (normal <100 pg/mL)
Thyroid-stimulating hormone, 2.0 microunits/mL

The chest radiograph shows bilateral pleural effusions and cardiomegaly. What signs, symptoms, and laboratory abnormalities of HF does A.J. exhibit? Relate these clinical findings to the pathogenesis of the disease and to left-sided or right-sided HF.

Left-sided ventricular dysfunction primarily causes pulmonary symptoms, whereas right-sided ventricular dysfunction causes signs of systemic venous congestion. Although LV failure usually develops first, many patients present with signs of biventricular failure. The signs and symptoms of both left-sided and right-sided ventricular dysfunction are summarized in Table 14-4.

LEFT-SIDED HEART FAILURE (LEFT VENTRICULAR DYSFUNCTION)

Weakness, fatigue, and cyanosis result from decreased CO and compromised tissue perfusion. If the LV is not emptied completely, pulmonary congestion occurs. Dyspnea (labored or uncomfortable breathing) on exertion, a productive cough, rales (crackles in the

Table 14-4
Signs and Symptoms of Heart Failure

Left Ventricular Failure	Right Ventricular Failure[a]
Subjective	
DOE	
SOB	
Orthopnea (2–3 pillows)	
PND, cough	
Weakness, fatigue, confusion	Peripheral edema
Weakness, fatigue	
Objective	
LVH	Weight gain (fluid retention)
↓BP	
EF <40%[b]	Neck vein distension
RALES, S_3 gallop rhythm	Hepatomegaly
Reflex tachycardia	Hepatojugular reflux
↑BUN (poor renal perfusion)	

[a]Isolated right-sided failure occurs with long-standing pulmonary disease (cor pulmonale) or after pulmonary hypertension.
[b]Ejection fraction normal in patients with diastolic dysfunction.
BP, blood pressure; BUN, blood urea nitrogen; DOE, dyspnea on exertion; EF, ejection fraction; LVH, left ventricular hypertrophy; PND, paroxysmal nocturnal dyspnea; SOB, shortness of breath.

lung during auscultation), pleural effusions on chest radiograph, and hypoxemia all result from pulmonary congestion. Pulmonary symptoms are aggravated in the reclining position. Orthopnea or SOB in the supine position is quantified by the number of pillows the patient must lie on to sleep comfortably. A.J., for example, could sleep only sitting upright. PND is characterized by SOB that awakens the patient from sleep and is alleviated by an upright position.

Cardiac dilatation is observed on chest radiography as an enlarged cardiac silhouette. The point of maximal impulse corresponds to the apex of the LV and is visualized as an external pulsation on the left side of the chest. It is displaced laterally and downward from its normal location at the fifth intercostal space, less than 10 cm from the midsternal line. An S_3 gallop rhythm denotes a third heart sound often heard in close proximity to the second heart sound (closing of the aortic and pulmonary valves) in HF. Rapid filling of the ventricles causes the S_3 sound and, in an adult, usually indicates decreased ventricular compliance. In patients with mitral valve regurgitation, an S_3 heart sound is common and denotes systolic dysfunction and elevated filling pressure. Tachycardia is caused by compensatory increases in sympathetic tone.

Weight gain and edema reflect sodium and water retention resulting from decreased renal perfusion (see Pathogenesis section). As RBF and GFR decrease, a disproportionate amount of BUN may be retained. This phenomenon is termed *prerenal azotemia* and is detected by an elevated BUN to SCr ratio of greater than 20:1. A.J. has a ratio of greater than 40:1. Prerenal azotemia also can be caused by dehydration and overuse of diuretics. Frequency of urination at night (nocturia) is caused by improved perfusion of the kidney when the patient is lying down.

RIGHT-SIDED HEART FAILURE (RIGHT VENTRICULAR DYSFUNCTION)

The signs and symptoms of right ventricular dysfunction are related either to hypervolemia, valvular disease, or pulmonary HTN. The overall effect is elevation in central venous pressure.

Dependent edema results from increased venous and capillary hydrostatic pressure, causing a redistribution of fluid from the intravascular to interstitial spaces. Ankle and pretibial edema are common findings after prolonged standing or sitting because fluid tends to localize in the dependent portions of the body secondary to gravitational forces. Sacral edema can be present in patients at bed rest. Edema is subjectively quantified on a 1+ (minimal) to 4+ (severe) scale. A.J. has 3+ pitting edema.

Hepatomegaly, hepatic tenderness, and ascites (fluid in the abdomen) arise from hepatic venous congestion and increased portal vein pressure. Metabolism of drugs highly dependent on the liver for elimination can be impaired by both the retrograde venous congestion of the liver from right-sided HF and the decreased arterial perfusion of the liver from left-sided HF. Congestion of the gastrointestinal tract makes the patient anorectic.

Neck vein distension, primarily seen as internal jugular venous distension, denotes an elevated jugular venous pressure.

How high the neck veins are distended while the patient is lying down and how much the patient's head has to be raised before the jugular venous distension disappears gives the clinician a rough estimate of the patient's central venous pressure. Jugular distension in centimeters is measured as the vertical distance from the top of the venous pulsation down to the sternal angle. Neck vein distension of less than 4 cm when the patient is lying with the head elevated at a 45-degree angle is considered normal for an average, healthy adult. Applying pressure to the liver can cause further distension of the neck veins if hepatic venous congestion is present. This phenomenon is termed *hepatojugular reflux.*

EJECTION FRACTION MEASUREMENT

CASE 14-1, QUESTION 2: Does A.J. have LVSD?

SOB, crackles on auscultation, neck vein distension, edema, and nearly all of A.J.'s other signs and symptoms provide some important clues about the nature of the underlying cardiac abnormalities; however, they are limited in evaluating structural abnormalities. Some of these symptoms can be confused with other disorders, especially reduced exercise intolerance, which is often a gradual process that patients may fail to recognize and report. An enlarged heart on a chest radiograph increases the suspicion of LVSD, but this finding can be absent in some patients with LVSD and present in others with normal LV function. Some patients may be asymptomatic with structural abnormalities.

The most useful method to diagnose HF with LVSD is by measuring the LVEF. All patients with suspected HF should have an EF measured before beginning therapy because the treatment strategies between HFrEF and HFpEF differ. Two-dimensional echocardiography coupled with Doppler flow studies (Doppler echocardiogram) is the diagnostic test of choice for measuring EF. This procedure uses sound waves to visualize and measure ventricular wall thickness, chamber size, valvular function, and pericardial thickness. EF is estimated based on changes in ventricular chamber size between diastole and systole. This method of EF measurement is not as technically accurate as that provided by ventriculography, but the procedure is more comfortable for the patient and the correlation of the measured EF to that of the other methods is acceptable.

Radionuclide left ventriculography (also called a multiple gated acquisition scan) uses radiolabeled technetium as a tracer to measure LV hemodynamics. Although this method is the most accurate measurement of EF, it is moderately invasive because it requires venipuncture and radiation exposure. In addition, radionuclide scanning does not provide information on the architecture of the left ventricle. Magnetic resonance imaging and computed tomography are useful in evaluating ventricular mass but do not provide EF data.

Subsequently, A.J. underwent an echocardiogram. The results were reported as left ventricular hypertrophy (LVH) with mild to moderate depression of EF (30%–40%). Because he has systolic dysfunction and classic congestive signs, he fits the criteria for having congestive HF.

STAGES OF HEART FAILURE AND NEW YORK HEART ASSOCIATION CLASSIFICATION

CASE 14-1, QUESTION 3: What stage of HF does A.J. exhibit according the ACC/AHA criteria? How severe is A.J.'s disability according to the NYHA functional classification of HF?

The ACC/AHA staging scheme and the NYHA functional classification are summarized in Figure 14-1.[4,29]

Because A.J. has symptoms of HF and structural changes in cardiac architecture, he is in ACA/AHA stage C. On admission, A.J. is in NYHA functional class III as evidenced by a need to sleep upright and an inability to undertake even minimal physical activity. It is important to recognize that HF can progress very slowly in some patients and very rapidly in others. A patient with MI could move from stage A to stage C.

PREDISPOSING FACTORS

CASE 14-1, QUESTION 4: What factors contributed to the cause of A.J.'s HF?

Age, HTN, MI, diabetes, tachycardia-induced cardiomyopathy, valvular heart disease, and obesity are well-established major risk factors associated with the development of HF. Other risk factors associated with HF are smoking, excessive intake of alcohol, dyslipidemia, anemia, and chronic kidney disease.[89] There is interest in biochemical and genetic markers that are associated with HF. CAD, and in particular MI, is considered to be the most significant risk factor for HF in the elderly. During the past decades, there has been an increase in the incidence of HF after MI due to the increased survival after MI.[90]

A.J. is especially vulnerable to HF because of his poorly controlled HTN, which increases afterload. HTN can lead to LVH, which is a compensatory response to increased afterload. LVH is associated with a higher risk of HF, especially in younger individuals.[8] The lifetime risk for individuals developing HF with BP of at least 160/90 mm Hg is double that for those with BP less than 140/80 mm Hg.[91] Preventive strategies directed toward earlier and more aggressive BP control can reduce the incidence of HF by almost 50% and its associated mortality as well.[8]

NONSTEROIDAL ANTIINFLAMMATORY DRUGS AND SODIUM CONTENT

Nonsteroidal antiinflammatory drugs (NSAIDs) exert their antiinflammatory effects by inhibiting prostaglandins. Blocking prostaglandins leads to sodium reabsorption and counteracts the beneficial effects of diuretics and ACEIs. Ibuprofen used for A.J.'s arthritis contributes to sodium overload. Epidemiologic studies indicate that NSAIDs exacerbate HF symptoms, resulting in hospitalizations for HF.[92–94] ACC/AHA practice guidelines recommend avoiding NSAIDs whenever possible in patients with HF.[1]

Another potential source of excess sodium is in IV formulations. Sodium chloride is often used as a diluent for IV drug administration. Some parenteral antibiotics, particularly nafcillin and ticarcillin, have high sodium content. Most prescription and nonprescription drug labels carry a disclosure of sodium content.

A.J.'s HTN and HF are both poorly controlled and he has gained 8 kg. His clinical presentation (orthopnea, dyspnea, SOB, lower extremity edema, elevated jugular venous pressure) clearly indicates fluid overload. This could be a result of high-dose ibuprofen use. His HCTZ should be replaced by a loop diuretic to enhance diuresis. Also, an ACEI should be added to the current regimen for BP control. Once he is euvolemic, the addition of a β-blocker before discharge should be considered. Lowering the dose or preferably discontinuing all NSAIDs might reduce sodium retention and allow ACEI therapy to be more effective. Acetaminophen is an alternative for treating his osteoarthritis.

DIET

It is possible that A.J.'s diet contains a considerable excess of sodium from foods such as canned soups and vegetables, potato chips, or overuse of salt at mealtime. Dietary supplements and sports drinks can also be rich sources of sodium. He should follow a controlled-sodium (2–3 g/day) diet. If salt substitutes are used, he should be warned that they are high in potassium and could cause hyperkalemia if used concurrently with potassium supplements, an aldosterone antagonist, or other potassium-sparing diuretics.

Drug-Induced Heart Failure

CASE 14-1, QUESTION 5: What are the basic mechanisms by which drugs can induce HF, and how can an understanding of these mechanisms be predictive of drugs to avoid in A.J.?

Drug-induced HF is mediated by three mechanisms: inhibition of myocardial contractility (negative inotropic agents and direct toxins), proarrhythmic effects, or expansion of plasma volume (Table 14-5). The latter category includes drugs that act primarily on the kidney (to either alter RBF or increase sodium retention) or those that increase total body sodium and water because of their high sodium content.

The most recognized negative inotropic agents are the β-blockers, which decrease myocardial contractility and slow the HR. Both of these factors can compromise CO. Other well-documented negative inotropic drugs include the nondihydropyridine calcium-channel blockers (verapamil and diltiazem), and some antiarrhythmic agents (disopyramide, flecainide, and dronedarone). The anthracyclines (daunorubicin and doxorubicin) have a direct, dose-related cardiotoxicity that can be minimized by limiting total cumulative doses to 500 mg/m^2.[95,96] (See Chapter 94, Adverse Effects of Chemotherapy and Targeted Agents.) Cocaine and alcohol are cardiotoxins when used chronically in large quantities or after an overdose. Drugs that increase the incidence of arrhythmias will worsen HF if the abnormal rhythm compromises cardiac functioning or output.

Drugs that promote sodium and water retention include NSAIDs, certain antihypertensive drugs, glucocorticoids, androgens, estrogens, and licorice. Weight gain, peripheral and pulmonary edema has been observed in patients with pioglitazone and rosiglitazone.[97] Worsening of HF appears to be dose-dependent and presumed to be at least partly caused by fluid retention. As a consequence, the package inserts for pioglitazone and rosiglitazone recommend they not be administered to patients with NYHA class III or IV HF and that they be used cautiously in earlier stages of HF.[97] Saxagliptin has been also associated with an increased risk of HF hospitalizations. The FDA has initiated an investigation to further evaluate this risk.[98]

TREATMENT

Therapeutic Objectives

CASE 14-1, QUESTION 6: What are the therapeutic goals in treating A.J.?

Table 14-5
Drugs that May Induce Heart Failure

Negative Inotropic Agents	
β-Blockers[a]	Most evident with propranolol or other nonselective agents
	Less with agents with intrinsic sympathomimetic activity (acebutolol, carteolol, pindolol); can also be caused by use of timolol eye drops
Calcium-channel blockers[a]	Verapamil has most negative inotropic and AV-blocking effects; amlodipine has least
Antiarrhythmics	Disopyramide, flecainide, dronedarone
Direct Cardiotoxins	
Cocaine, amphetamines	Overdoses and long-term myopathy
Anthracycline cancer chemotherapeutic drugs	Daunorubicin and doxorubicin (Adriamycin); dose related; keep total cumulative dose <600 mg/m^2
Proarrhythmic Effects	
Class IA, Class III antiarrhythmic drugs	QT interval widening
	Probable torsades de pointes
	HF develops if disturbed rhythm compromises cardiac functioning
Nonantiarrhythmic drugs	Same mechanism as above
(See Crouch et al.[93] for a complete list)	Often associated with drug interactions that inhibit metabolism of the offending drug leading to higher than desired plasma levels
Expansion of Plasma Volume	
Antidiabetics	
	Na retention with pioglitazone and rosiglitazone
NSAID	Prostaglandin inhibition; Na retention
Glucocorticoids, androgens, estrogens	Mineralocorticoid effect; Na retention
Licorice	Aldosterone-like effect; Na retention
Antihypertensive vasodilators (hydralazine, methyldopa, prazosin, minoxidil)	↓Renal blood flow, activation of renin–angiotensin system
Drugs high in Na^+	Selected IV cephalosporins and penicillins
	Effervescent or bicarbonate-containing antacids or analgesics
	Also liquid nutrition supplements
Unknown Mechanism	
Tumor necrosis factor antagonists	Multiple case reports of new-onset HF or exacerbation of prior HF with etanercept and infliximab in patients with Crohn's disease or rheumatoid arthritis

[a]β-Blockers and verapamil may be beneficial in diastolic HF. Carvedilol and metoprolol counteract autonomic hyperactivity in systolic dysfunction.
AV, atrioventricular; HF, heart failure; IV, intravenous; Na, sodium; NSAID, nonsteroidal antiinflammatory drugs.

Cure is not a feasible therapeutic objective in patients with most forms of HF, exceptions being patients who are candidates for cardiac transplantation or who have certain forms of viral, alcohol-induced, or tachycardia-induced dilated cardiomyopathy. The immediate objective for A.J. is to provide symptomatic relief by reducing his complaints of SOB and PND, improve sleep quality, and increase exercise tolerance. Parameters to measure success include reduced peripheral and sacral edema, weight loss, slowing of the HR to less than 90 bpm, normalization of BP, reduction of BUN, reduction of heart size on chest radiograph, decreased neck vein distension, and loss of the S_3 heart sound. Long-range goals are to improve A.J.'s EF and quality of life including better tolerance of daily life activities, fewer future hospitalizations, avoidance of side effects of his therapy, and ultimately, an increased survival time. The achievement of these goals depends on the severity of A.J.'s disease, his understanding of his disease, and his adherence to prescribed interventions.

Diuretics

FUROSEMIDE AND OTHER LOOP DIURETICS

Case 14-1, Question 7: Bed rest and a 3-g sodium diet were ordered. The medical team decides to begin furosemide for A.J. What is the rationale for using diuretics and what route, dose, and dosing schedule should be used?

Excessive volume increases the workload of a compromised heart, and diuretics are an integral part of therapy. This is especially true if volume overload is symptomatic (dyspnea) as it is in A.J. Diuretics produce rapid symptomatic improvement. They relieve pulmonary and peripheral edema within hours, whereas the effects of ACEIs, β-blockers, and digoxin take days to months to be fully realized. Diuretics, however, should not be used alone. Even when they are initially successful in controlling symptoms and reducing edema, they are ineffective in maintaining clinical stability for long periods without the addition of other drugs.

More importantly, activation of the RAAS and sympathetic nervous system in response to diuresis could lead to HF progression.

All current guidelines recommend diuretic therapy, both acutely and chronically, if clinical volume overload is evident, but further state that patients without edema can be treated either intermittently or without diuretics.[1] Diuretics used on an intermittent (as-needed) basis are titrated based on changes in weight gain, neck vein distension, peripheral edema, or SOB. Patients with a good understanding of their disease can be instructed to weigh themselves daily and start taking their diuretic if they gain more than 1 to 2 lb in 1 day or 5 lb in 1 week or have leg or abdominal swelling. Diuretics can be withheld as long as patients are at their target dry weight. In other cases, diuretic-free intervals or weekends can be arranged. Even with these options, if the patient has experienced volume overload at some time during the course of his or her disease, either past or present, a diuretic should always be readily available.[99] Despite remarkable initial benefits, vigorous diuretic therapy carries the risk of volume depletion, electrolyte abnormalities, and diminished CO. Abrupt worsening of renal function (increased BUN or SCr) or hypotension indicates the need to temporarily withhold diuretics.

Route of Administration

Furosemide is a commonly used loop diuretic because of clinical experience and low cost. Bumetanide and torsemide are preferred in some settings because of more predictable absorption.[62,63,100,101] Ethacrynic acid, which is also a loop diuretic, is not preferred because of its ototoxic potential. However, unlike other loop diuretics, ethacrynic acid does not contain a sulfonamide moiety, and it is mainly reserved for patients with severe sulfonamide allergies to other loop diuretics.

According to one group of investigators, patients with HF treated with torsemide fare better than those receiving furosemide.[101] During a 1-year open-label trial, patients receiving torsemide were less likely to be admitted to the hospital for HF (17% torsemide vs. 32% furosemide). Admissions for all CV causes were also lower among patients taking torsemide (44%) than patients taking furosemide (59%). Fatigue scores improved to a greater extent in patients treated with torsemide, but no difference was found in the dyspnea score. Torsemide is more expensive than furosemide, and this may be an issue for some patients.

Erratic responses to furosemide are prevalent in persons with severe HF or diminished renal function. Some patients respond promptly and vigorously to small oral doses of furosemide, whereas others require large IV doses to achieve only minimal diuresis. Part of these differences can be explained by the drug's pharmacokinetics.[62,102] Loop diuretics are highly protein bound and have to be actively secreted into the proximal tubular lumen to elicit a response. Tubular secretion of loop diuretics can be compromised in the presence of increased levels of endogenous organic acids due to renal insufficiency and drugs (NSAIDs) that are competing for the same transporters. Also, oral absorption of furosemide is erratic and incomplete, averaging 50% to 60% in healthy subjects and 45% in those with renal failure. When taken with a meal, absorption is delayed, but the total amount absorbed does not differ. There are claims that the absorption and, therefore, effectiveness of furosemide are further diminished in patients with HF attributable to edema of the bowel and decreased splanchnic blood flow. This has been partially refuted by one investigator, who noted an average furosemide bioavailability of 61% in patients with HF, the same as in normal patients.[101] Total absorption in patients with HF varies widely (34%–80%); however, both the rate of absorption and the time to peak urinary excretion are delayed for furosemide and bumetanide.[62,63,103]

The rate and extent of absorption are not only different among individuals, but intraindividual variability also exists. Ingestion of the same brand of furosemide by the same individual on multiple occasions can show up to a threefold difference in bioavailability. These differences are evident with the innovator's brand (Lasix) or generic brands.[104,105]

Dosing

Typically, a patient's treatment is initiated with 20 to 40 mg of oral or IV furosemide given as a single dose and monitored for responsiveness (Table 14-3). If the desired diuresis is not obtained, the dose can be increased in 40- to 80-mg increments to a total daily dose of 160 to 240 mg, usually divided into two or three doses. For torsemide, a usual starting dose is 10 to 20 mg/day, but a ceiling effect is noted in patients with HF at a dosage of 100 to 200 mg/day.[106] Equivalent doses of bumetanide are 0.5 to 1.0 mg once or twice daily, titrated to a maximum of 10 mg daily. Because A.J. is not in acute distress, it could be argued that oral therapy would suffice. The decision, however, is to give a single 40-mg IV dose of furosemide for immediate symptom control. Further increases in the dose or frequency (i.e., twice-daily dosing) of diuretic administration may be required to maintain an active diuresis and sustain weight loss.

Another alternative in hospitalized patients is to administer loop diuretics via continuous infusion. Multiple studies have demonstrated the benefits of continuous infusions compared with intermittent infusions.[107–109] However, the results of these studies have been questioned because of a lack of methodological rigor, and the studies have been underpowered to address the primary end points. Recently, the DOSE trial[110] (Diuretic Optimization Strategies Evaluation) showed no difference in efficacy or safety between intermittent IV bolus or continuous infusion. There are potential benefits of continuous infusion when compared with intermittent bolus dosing. Bolus diuretic dosing can cause a higher rate of diuretic resistance owing to the postdiuretic phenomenon. Continuous IV infusion results in a constant delivery to the tubule, potentially reducing this phenomenon. Additionally, continuous infusions are also associated with a lower incidence of ototoxicity owing to lower peak concentrations. Patients who are candidates for continuous IV infusion should receive a loading dose before infusion to reach steady-state concentrations faster. However, if the patient has received one or more IV boluses within the previous few hours, then an infusion can be started without a loading dose. In case of inadequate response, the loading dose should be repeated and the infusion rate increased. The infusion rate depends on the patient's renal function and response.

ADVERSE EFFECTS

CASE 14-1, QUESTION 8: Examine A.J.'s laboratory values (see Question 1). Does A.J. have any abnormal values? What is the significance of these abnormalities?

Azotemia

A.J. has an elevated BUN (40 mg/dL) but a normal SCr (0.8 mg/dL). Worsening renal function is characterized by an elevation of BUN and creatinine. A disproportionately elevated BUN relative to creatinine is indicative of prerenal azotemia, secondary to poor renal perfusion from HF or overdiuresis. SCr will also rise in some patients with prerenal azotemia, but will quickly return to normal with rehydration.

A.J.'s laboratory values reflect prerenal azotemia. The most probable cause of his azotemia is decreased RBF secondary to decompensated HF. Diuretics should not be withheld and, in fact, judicious diuresis should improve his HF and help lower his BUN. Caution must be exercised because excessive diuresis and volume depletion can cause renal ischemia, leading to true renal damage. If this happens, the SCr also will rise.

Hyponatremia

A low serum sodium of 132 mEq/L is noted. Low serum sodium, however, is not necessarily a sign of overdiuresis. A person may be significantly overdiuresed with a body deficit of sodium, but if that sodium is lost isotonically, the serum sodium concentration will be normal. Conversely, a person such as A.J. can be hypervolemic, indicating excessive body sodium, but the serum sodium concentration may be normal or even low.

Hyponatremia (low serum sodium concentration) reflects the dilutional effect of extra free water in the plasma. The most common causes of dilutional hyponatremia are excess ADH production or excessive free water intake. Individuals on severely sodium-restricted diets can experience hyponatremia. Likewise, patients given too much diuretic and who are then given salt-free fluids or who have compensatory ADH release can become hyponatremic. Patients with HF or hepatic cirrhosis are more likely to develop diuretic-induced dilutional hyponatremia because of preexisting defects in free water excretion. The exact cause of hyponatremia in A.J. is unknown, but his marginally low serum sodium does not contraindicate continued diuretic therapy. In general, levels of serum sodium concentration less than 120 to 125 mEq/L are associated with adverse events in HF patients; chronic serum sodium concentrations of 130 mEq/L or less are associated with higher morbidity and mortality.[111] Asymptomatic hyponatremia can be treated with water restriction. In the setting of volume depletion, IV administration of normal saline may be effective. Vasopressin receptor antagonists can be used in patients with HF and hypervolemic hyponatremia.

Hypokalemia

A.J. has a serum potassium of 3.2 mEq/L. Hypokalemia is associated with an increased incidence of arrhythmias. Some studies showed increased ectopic activity with serum levels between 3.0 and 3.5 mEq/L.[112–114] It is estimated that the risk of arrhythmias increases by 27% with each 0.5 mEq/L reduction in the plasma potassium concentration less than 3.0 mEq/L.[115]

In chronic HF, potassium abnormalities are commonly seen. The risk of SCD in patients with HF may be lessened by using low doses of diuretics in combination with potassium-sparing agents, with the goal of maintaining serum potassium levels between 4.5 and 5.0 mEq/L.[116]

A.J. will be receiving increased doses of diuretics for the next several days and, therefore, may need additional potassium supplementation to prevent life-threatening hypokalemia. In addition, if he needs digoxin therapy in the future, low serum potassium levels can predispose him to digitalis toxicity. Potassium replacement is warranted for A.J. at this time. Long-term potassium supplementation may not be necessary with concomitant administration of ACEIs. If hypokalemia persists, A.J. can be started on an aldosterone antagonist.

Hypomagnesemia

A.J.'s serum magnesium level is 1.5 mEq/L. Severe hypomagnesemia can lead to somnolence, muscle spasms, a decreased seizure threshold, and cardiac arrhythmias, effects similar to those seen with hypokalemia. Some investigators have claimed that many of the arrhythmias previously ascribed to diuretic-induced hypokalemia were actually caused by diuretic-induced hypomagnesemia.[117] Concurrent hypokalemia and hypomagnesemia can be especially dangerous. A.J. should be given 1 g of magnesium sulfate IV and observed for changes in his magnesium level. If needed, he could be given chronic oral supplements of magnesium.

Hyperuricemia

Increases of 1 to 2 mg/dL in uric acid levels are common during thiazide administration. Rarely, 4- to 5-mg/dL elevations have been reported. A.J.'s uric acid level is 8 mg/dL, which is slightly elevated. It has been proposed that serum uric acid levels may be a valuable prognostic marker in HF patients. One study indicates a graded relationship between serum uric acid and HF survival.[118] In HF, xanthine oxidase is upregulated, which can lead to endothelial dysfunction. Therefore, treatment with allopurinol may improve endothelial function and promote reverse remodeling. The relationship between serum uric acid and CV disease is still controversial, and the guidelines do not recommend the use of xanthine oxidase inhibitors to prevent CV disease. In patients who experience symptomatic hyperuricemia, the addition of allopurinol or other urate lowering agent should be considered (Chapter 45, Gout and Hyperuricemia).

BNP

A.J.'s BNP is elevated (1,365 pg/mL). Various studies evaluating the diagnostic accuracy of BNP and NT-proBNP have used different lower limits to define normal values. The most commonly used plasma concentration to define the upper limit of normal for BNP is 100 pg/mL, with concentrations greater than 400 pg/mL being considered a strong indicator of HF. The age-related NT-proBNP diagnostic upper limit of normal is 125 pg/mL for patients younger than 75 years, and 450 pg/mL for patients older than 75 years of age. If the patient has a level below the upper limit of normal for the respective assay used, then the symptoms are most likely attributable to causes other than HF. In patients with renal impairment, the clearance of these peptides is reduced; therefore, the upper limit of normal is 200 pg/mL for BNP and the corresponding value for NT-proBNP is 1,200 pg/mL.[119] Moreover, concentrations of these biomarkers are influenced by age, sex, obesity, and other cardiac and noncardiac comorbidities. Asymptomatic patients with HF can also present with elevated BNP or NT-proBNP levels. This confounds the accurate interpretation of these markers and makes it challenging to integrate their usefulness into routine clinical practice. Elevated BNP and NT-proBNP have an established utility in ruling out HF in patients who present to the emergency department with SOB.[25] According to the ACC/AHA guidelines, measurement of BNP or NT-proBNP is useful for establishing prognosis or disease severity in chronic HF; however, the role of these biomarkers in reducing morbidity or mortality in HF is not well established. Several NP–guided therapy trials have been published.[120–122] The BNP- or NT-proBNP-guided HF therapy can be useful to achieve GDMT in selected clinically stable patients, but it is unclear if such an approach improves outcome. The Guiding Evidence Based Therapy Using Biomarker Intensified Treatment (GUIDE-IT) study,[123] designed to assess the effects of NP-guided therapy in high risk patients with left ventricular systolic dysfunction did not improve clinical outcomes between biomarker guided treatment strategy vs usual care. It is still not clear when to use biomarkers to adjust HF medications. BNP levels may be elevated in patients receiving ARNI, as BNP is a substrate for neprilysin. Therefore, the 2017 update states that the utility of natriuretic peptide biomarker levels should be cautiously interpreted in patients on ARNI.[6] A.J.'s elevated BNP level, along with his clinical presentation, is indicative of HF exacerbation.

POTASSIUM SUPPLEMENTATION

CASE 14-1, QUESTION 9: The physician gave A.J. one 1-g dose of magnesium sulfate and three 20-mEq doses of potassium chloride IV. This raised his serum magnesium to 2.0 mEq/L and his potassium to 3.9 mEq/L. Should he receive prophylactic magnesium or potassium supplementation? What is an appropriate dose?

At this time A.J. does not need further magnesium replacement, but his serum magnesium level should be measured again after he has received furosemide for a few days. If the level drops again, maintenance therapy with oral magnesium oxide tablets can be started.

A fall in serum potassium concentration can be seen within hours of the first dose of a diuretic, and the maximal fall usually is reached by the end of the first week of treatment. Potassium supplementation is not required in all patients receiving diuretics. They should be monitored frequently in the first few months of diuretic therapy to determine their potassium requirements. Similarly, when diuretics are stopped, it can take several weeks for serum potassium to return to baseline. Therefore, it is possible that A.J.'s admitting potassium level of 3.2 mEq/L reflects the nadir of his response to HCTZ. His initial response to potassium supplementation shows that his hypokalemia will be easily controlled. It might be argued that he should be observed for a few days and not given further supplements; however, because his diuresis is to be increased and if digoxin may later be considered, potassium supplementation is warranted. Long-term potassium supplementation may not be necessary with concomitant administration of ACEIs and aldosterone antagonists. Because A.J. is started on furosemide, HCTZ should be discontinued. If hypokalemia persists, the aldosterone antagonist dose can be uptitrated.

Dose Requirements

It is difficult to predict the dose of potassium chloride that will be required to maintain proper potassium balance. Many patients do well with 20 mEq/day, but it is questionable how many patients need any supplement at all. People with well-documented hypokalemia can require anywhere from 20 to 120 mEq of potassium chloride per day.[124–126] Those patients with disease states associated with high circulating aldosterone levels require doses of potassium in excess of 60 mEq/day. In patients who need long-term potassium supplementation, efforts should be made to increase doses of ACEIs to target doses or maximal tolerated doses, and appropriate addition of an aldosterone antagonist should be considered. However, a few selected patients may still need to take potassium supplementation, despite the addition of an aldosterone antagonist.

MONITORING

CASE 14-1, QUESTION 10: After a single 40-mg IV dose of furosemide, A.J. is begun on 40 mg of furosemide each morning and potassium chloride tablets 20 mEq BID. How should his therapy be monitored?

A.J. needs to be monitored for both an improvement in his HF and for side effects (Tables 14-4 and 14-6). Subjectively, the clinician should monitor for decreased pulmonary distress and an increased exercise tolerance, demonstrating control of HF. Objective monitoring parameters for disease control include weight loss (ideal, 0.5–1 kg/day until ideal dry weight is achieved), a decrease in edema, flattening of neck veins, and disappearance of the S_3 gallop and rales. Because A.J. has HTN, his BP also requires monitoring with a goal to reduce it to $<$130/80 mm Hg.

Patients are instructed to record their weight each day and are allowed to adjust their diuretic dose based on changes observed. If they are at their ideal "dry weight," they may reduce their dose of diuretic by 50% or even hold one or more doses. If weight increases more than 1 or 2 pounds in a day or 5 pounds per week, edema increases, or SOB returns, the dose of diuretic is temporarily increased.

Dizziness and weakness are subjective indices of volume depletion, hypotension, or potassium loss. Muscle cramps and abdominal pain could indicate rapid changes in electrolyte balance. Objectively, a lowering of BP, especially on standing, and a rising BUN (prerenal azotemia) signify overdiuresis. Serum sodium, potassium, and uric acid should be monitored routinely. Questioning the patient with regard to the onset of diuresis (relative to drug ingestion) and the duration of the diuretic effect helps develop the most convenient and effective schedule for the patient.

REFRACTORY PATIENTS: COMBINATION THERAPY

CASE 14-1, QUESTION 11: If A.J.'s furosemide dose was increased to 80 mg twice a day without much response, what should be the next step?

All loop and thiazide diuretics must reach the tubular lumen to be effective. Because these drugs are highly bound to serum proteins and endogenous organic acids, they cannot enter the tubular lumen by glomerular filtration. For diuresis to begin, they must be transported into the proximal tubule by active secretion from the blood into the tubule. If this active transport is blocked, diuretics will not reach their site of action. This can lead to a diminished diuretic response in patients with either renal insufficiency or decreased RBF associated with decompensated HF. Patients with renal insufficiency or poor RBF often require large doses of diuretics to achieve a desired response. Endogenous organic acids can accumulate during renal insufficiency, avidly binding the drug and preventing its access to the site of action.[62,63] Both the total amount of drug delivered to the tubule and the rate of delivery of the drug to the tubule determine the magnitude of diuretic response elicited.[62,63] This explains why 80 mg of furosemide yields more diuresis than a 40-mg dose and why an IV injection provides a more rapid and vigorous diuresis than an oral dose. Once a threshold concentration (ceiling dose) is achieved within the tubule, higher concentrations produce no greater intensity of effect, but the duration of action may be prolonged.

Many patients exhibit a blunted diuretic response with continued therapy for unknown reasons. Generally, alternative treatment plans are pursued when the dose given approaches the ceiling doses for each drug listed in Table 14-3. Continuous infusions of furosemide (5–15 mg/hour), bumetanide (0.5–1 mg/hour), or torsemide (3 mg/hour) can be more efficacious than intermittent bolus doses in patients with severe HF or renal insufficiency.[62,63,127–129] Even higher doses have been recommended: 0.25 to 1 mg/kg/hour for furosemide, 0.1 mg/kg/hour for bumetanide, and 5 to 20 mg/hour for torsemide.[130] An aggressive protocol of a 100-mg IV bolus of furosemide followed by a continuous IV infusion at a rate of 20 to 40 mg/hour, which is doubled every 12 to 24 hours in unresponsive patients, to a maximal infusion rate of 160 mg/hour to attain a diuresis rate of 100 mL/hour or greater has been described.[131]

In some instances, switching from one loop diuretic to another can overcome the problem.[131] For example, torsemide or bumetanide might work when furosemide fails because of more reliable absorption.[100,101] If this maneuver fails, a combination of diuretics can be tried. The most effective regimens combine drugs that work at two different parts of the tubule.[130] For example, a loop diuretic is used with metolazone, which blocks sodium reabsorption in the distal tubule. Various thiazide diuretics, including chlorthalidone, chlorothiazide, and HCTZ, have been reported to effectively enhance diuresis when combined with a loop diuretic. Triple-therapy regimens of metolazone, a loop diuretic, and an aldosterone antagonist are used to optimize diuresis and electrolyte control.

Most clinicians choose a combination of metolazone plus furosemide or bumetanide. A wide range of metolazone dosages has been investigated.[132] Typically, a low dose of metolazone (2.5–5 mg) is first added to the furosemide therapy. Metolazone can be given intermittently (2–3 times/week or as needed) to relieve congestion. The longer duration of action for metolazone can cause a greater than predicted diuresis and electrolyte loss when combined with a loop diuretic. Thus, careful monitoring of weight, urine output, BP, BUN, potassium, magnesium and SCr is required. Because no parenteral form of metolazone exists, chlorothiazide, at a dose of 500 to 1,000 mg once or twice daily, is an alternative to the thiazide diuretic that can be given intravenously. Although A.J.'s furosemide dose could be increased, metolazone 2.5 mg daily was added. A.J. may also require additional doses of potassium supplementation to avoid hypokalemia with the addition of metolazone.

Angiotensin-Converting Enzyme Inhibitors

AGENTS OF CHOICE

CASE 14-1, QUESTION 12: Along with furosemide, A.J. was started on 10 mg of lisinopril daily. Are there specific ACEIs approved for use in HFrEF patients?

As a general rule, formulary decisions are first based on comparative pharmacologic activity, efficacy, and drug safety. Other factors to consider are labeled (FDA approved) indications, convenience of dosing schedule, and—all else being equal—the cost to the institution and the patient. HTN is the primary indication for all of the ACEIs. Not all ACEIs have an indication for HF.

ACEIs inhibit ACE (also called kinase II), reducing the activation of angiotensin II, a major contributor to the undesired hemodynamic responses to HF. Decreased circulating levels of NE, vasopressin, neurokinins, luteinizing hormone, prostacyclin, and NO also have been noted after administration of ACEIs.

In addition, ACE is responsible for degradation of bradykinin, substance P, and possibly other vasodilatory substances unrelated to angiotensin II. Thus, part of the beneficial effects of ACEIs is caused by the accumulation of bradykinin (Fig. 14-6). After attaching to bradykinin-2 (B_2) receptors, vasodilation is produced by stimulating the production of arachidonic acid metabolites, peroxidases, NO, and endothelium-derived hyperpolarizing factor in the vascular endothelium. In the kidney, bradykinin causes natriuresis through direct tubular effects.

The net effect is that ACEIs regulate the balance between the vasoconstrictive and salt-retentive properties of angiotensin II and the vasodilatory and natriuretic properties of bradykinin. The effects of ACEIs are reduced pulmonary capillary wedge pressure (preload) and lowered SVR and systolic wall stress (afterload). CO increases without an increase in HR. ACEIs promote salt excretion by augmenting RBF and reducing the production of aldosterone and ADH. The beneficial effects on RBF, coupled with the drug's indirect inhibition of aldosterone, lead to a mild diuretic response, a distinct benefit compared to hydralazine.

Vasodilation and diuresis are not the only value of ACEIs in HF. Angiotensin II enhances vascular remodeling, whereas bradykinin impedes this process.[66,133] ACEIs impede ventricular remodeling by blocking the effects of angiotensin II on cardiac myocytes. Evidence as to whether preserving bradykinin levels affects remodeling is inconclusive, although it might attenuate the progressive deposition of collagen during the chronic phase of post-MI cardiac remodeling.

Table 14-6
Monitoring Parameters with Diuretics

↓CHF symptoms (see Table 14-4)
Weight loss or gain; goal is 1- to 2-lb weight loss/day until "ideal weight" achieved[a]
Signs of volume depletion
Weakness
Hypotension, dizziness
Orthostatic changes in BP[b]
↓Urine output
↑BUN[c]
Serum potassium and magnesium (avoid hypokalemia and hypomagnesemia)
↑Uric acid
↑Glucose

[a]Weight loss may be greater during the first few days when significant edema is present.
[b]A ↓ in systolic BP of 10 to 15 mm Hg or a ↓ in diastolic BP of 5 to 10 mm Hg.
[c]A rising BUN can be caused by either volume depletion from diuretics or poor renal blood flow from poorly controlled HF. Small boluses of 0.9% saline can be given cautiously to differentiate a rising BUN from volume depletion versus poor cardiac output. If volume depletion is present, saline will cause an ↑ in urine output and a ↓ in BUN. However, if the patient has severe HF, the saline could cause pulmonary edema.
BP, blood pressure; BUN, blood urea nitrogen; HF, heart failure.

Individual ACEIs with FDA-labeled approvals for the treatment of HF or LV dysfunction after MI are included in Table 14-7. There is no reason to favor one ACEI over another except in the case of optimizing dosing schedules for patients and trying to use once-daily dosing if possible to improve medication adherence rates.

Numerous placebo-controlled trials have documented the favorable effects of ACEI therapy on hemodynamic variables, clinical status, and symptoms of HF,[134,135] and demonstrated a consistent 20% to 30% relative reduction in HF mortality. ACEI therapy is generally better than other vasodilator regimens,

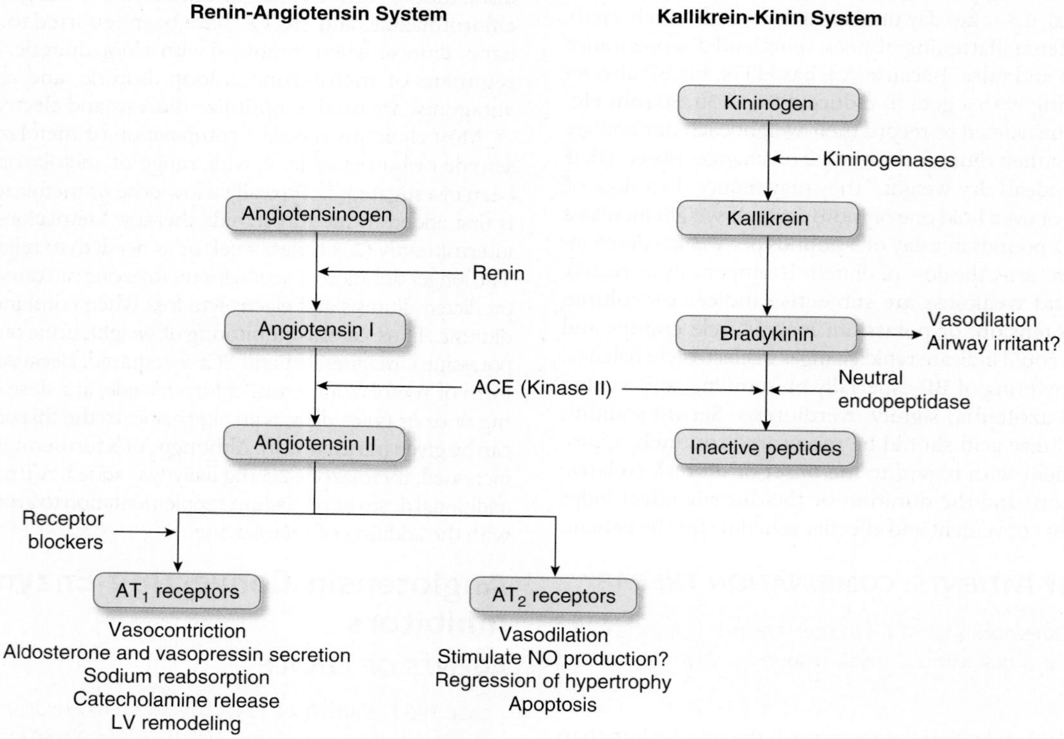

Figure 14-6 Angiotensin receptor blocker mechanism. ACE, angiotensin-converting enzyme; LV, left ventricular; NO, nitric oxide.

Table 14-7
ACE Inhibitor Dosing in HFrEF

Drug	Available Dosage Form	Initial Dose[a]	Maximal Dose
Captopril[b]	12.5, 25, 50, 100 mg tablets	6.25–12.5 mg TID	100 mg TID
Enalapril[c]	2.5, 5, 10, 20 mg tablets	2.5–5 mg every day	20 mg BID
Fosinopril	10, 20, 40 mg tablets	5–10 mg every day	40 mg every day
Lisinopril	2.5, 5, 10, 20, 40 mg tablets	2.5–5 mg every day	40 mg every day
Quinapril[c]	5, 10, 20, 40 mg tablets	5–10 mg every day	20 mg BID
Perindopril	2, 4, 8 mg tablets	2 mg every day	16 mg every day
Ramipril[c]	1.25, 2.5, 5, 10 mg capsules	1.25–2.5 mg every day	10 mg BID
Trandolapril	1, 2, 4 mg tablets	1 mg every day	8 mg every day

ACE, angiotensin-converting enzyme; BID, 2 times a day; TID, three times a day.
[a] Start with lowest dose to avoid bradycardia, hypotension, or renal dysfunction. All but captopril given every day in the morning at starting doses. Increase dose slowly at 2- to 4-week intervals to assess full effect and tolerance.
[b] Captopril is short acting. Start with a 6.25- or 12.5-mg test dose, then 6.25 to 12.5 mg TID.
[c] Enalapril, quinapril, and ramipril could possibly be given every day instead of BID based on half-life.
Benazepril, cilazapril, moexipril, perindopril, ramipril, and trandolapril not labeled for use in heart failure.

including the hydralazine–nitrate combination or ARBs after considering efficacy and tolerability.

Table 14-8 provides a brief summary of the results of the key ACEI HFrEF trials.[18,66,67,135–137] Of the five approved agents, the best evidence for improved survival is available for enalapril in both chronically symptomatic patients (NYHA classes II–IV) and asymptomatic patients with evidence of an impaired EF after an MI.[70,138–140]

The ACC/AHA guidelines recommend selecting an ACEI that has shown reductions in both morbidity and mortality in clinical trials in HFrEF. The following ACEIs are considered first-line options based on clinical trials: captopril, enalapril, fosinopril, lisinopril, perindopril, quinapril, ramipril, or trandolapril.[1,5,6]

Captopril and lisinopril are both active as the parent compound and do not have active metabolites. All other ACEIs are prodrugs

Table 14-8
Clinical Trials of ACE Inhibitors in HFrEF

Study	Patient Population	ACE Inhibitor	Time Started After MI	Treatment Duration	Outcome
Studies in LV Dysfunction					
CONSENSUS[138]	NYHA IV (n = 253)	Enalapril vs. placebo		1 day–20 months	Decreased mortality and HF
SOLVD-Treatment[136]	NYHA II/III (n = 2,569)	Enalapril vs. placebo		22–55 months	Decreased mortality and HF
V-HeFT II[247]	NYHA II/III (n = 804)	Enalapril vs. hydralazine, isosorbide		0.5–5.7 years	Decreased mortality and sudden death
SOLVD-Prevention	Asymptomatic LV dysfunction (n = 4,228)	Enalapril vs. placebo		14.6–62 months	Decreased mortality and HF hospitalizations
Studies in LV Dysfunction after MI					
SAVE[311]	MI, decreased LV function (n = 2,331)	Captopril vs. placebo	3–16 days	24–60 months	Decreased mortality
CONSENSUS II[312]	MI (n = 6,090)	Enalaprilat/enalapril vs. placebo	24 hours	41–180 days	No change in survival; hypotension with enalaprilat
AIRE[313]	MI and HF (n = 2,006)	Ramipril vs. placebo	3–10 days	>6 months	Decreased mortality
ISIS-4[314]	MI (n >50,000)	Captopril vs. placebo	24 hours	28 days	Decreased mortality
GISSI-3[315]	MI (n = 19,394)	Lisinopril vs. placebo	24 hours	6 weeks	Decreased mortality
TRACE[165]	MI, decreased LV function (n = 1,749)	Trandolapril vs. placebo	3–7 days	24–50 months	Decreased mortality
SMILE[166]	MI (n = 1,556)	Zofenopril vs. placebo	24 hours	6 weeks	Decreased mortality

ACE, angiotensin-converting enzyme; HF, heart failure; LV, left ventricular; MI, myocardial infarction; NYHA, New York Heart Association.
Source: Brown NJ, Vaughan DE. Angiotensin-converting enzyme inhibitors. Circulation. 1998;97:1411.

that require enzymatic conversion to active metabolites. Captopril has a short duration of action, necessitating three times daily administration in most patients. Although this characteristic may be advantageous when initiating therapy by allowing closer assessment of early side effects, for chronic maintenance, it is preferable to use a drug that can be given either once or twice daily. All other ACEIs meet this criterion. Package insert labeling and common standards of practice have led to twice-daily dosing, especially at higher doses, for enalapril, quinapril, and ramipril.

A.J.'s physician chooses to start lisinopril 10 mg daily based on evidence of clinical efficacy, improved survival, and availability as a generic medication. If there were concerns about hypotension, then captopril would be preferred during the initial 1 to 2 days of initiation therapy to avoid dropping the patient's BP too quickly.

Dose–Response Relationships

CASE 14-1, QUESTION 13: What is the target dose of lisinopril in A.J.? Do all patients need to be titrated to target doses?

Clinical evidence shows a relationship between the degree of improvement in HF symptoms and the dose of drug given. Larger doses are more likely to improve the patient's quality of life and reduce the incidence of hospital stays, but the impact of larger doses on mortality is less clear. At the same time, higher doses are associated with a greater risk of side effects. Based on these principles, proposed recommended starting and maximal doses for the ACEIs are listed in Table 14-7.[1]

The guidelines recommend that ACEIs be initiated at low doses, and titrated to the maximal tolerated target dose. Supporting this principle are the results of the Assessment of Treatment with Lisinopril and Survival trial.[141,142] Lisinopril 2.5 to 5 mg (low dosage) or 32.5 to 35 mg (high dosage) was given to over 3,000 patients. All-cause mortality did not differ significantly between the two groups. In the high-dose group, hospitalizations and the combined end point of death and hospitalization were reduced by 24% ($p = 0.003$) and 12% ($p = 0.002$), respectively. The higher dose was tolerated by 90% of patients assigned this dose.

Despite these recommendations for using the highest tolerated doses, evidence also suggests that lower doses are beneficial. The UK Heart Failure Network Study found that 10 mg of twice-daily enalapril was no more effective than 2.5 mg BID.[143] Mortality, evaluated separately, was 4.2%, 3.3%, and 2.9%, for low (2.5 mg BID), moderate (5 mg BID), and higher (10 mg BID) dosages respectively, and not significantly different. The guidelines recommend prescribing doses that have reduced the risk of CV events in clinical trials and if trial doses cannot be achieved, then lower doses should be used.

For lisinopril, the recommended starting dosage is 2.5 to 5 mg/day. For older patients or those with other risk factors (systolic BP <100 mm Hg, those taking large doses of diuretics, or those with preexisting hyponatremia, hyperkalemia, or renal insufficiency), the starting dose of 2.5 mg/day would be more appropriate. This dose, or an equivalent with one of the other drugs, should be considered if the patient is being started directly on a long-acting drug without prior titration on captopril. For a patient such as A.J. who has already been treated with captopril for 2 days with no evidence of intolerance, a 10-mg dose is appropriate.

The long-term target dosage of lisinopril for A.J. is 40 mg daily. No clear formula exists for deciding how quickly to titrate to this dose. It depends on the degree of reduction in his HF symptoms and side effects, and motivation to take the medication. Whenever dosage adjustments are made, it may take as few as 24 hours for the patient to perceive symptom reduction, but generally full hemodynamic affects are not reached for 1 to 2 months. Hypotension and other side effects are more immediate. A.J. should have his dose reassessed in 1 to 2 weeks to determine whether he can tolerate a dosage increase to 20 mg daily. A SCr and potassium should be ordered at this time to assess the safety of titrating the ACEI. Thereafter, a doubling of the dose could occur every 2 to 4 weeks. Thus, it could take 2 months to titrate upward to 40 mg daily. If A.J.'s symptoms do not improve, but he has no side effects, titration can occur more quickly either by shortening the assessment periods (e.g., every week) or by using larger dose increments.

ANGIOTENSIN RECEPTOR BLOCKERS

CASE 14-1, QUESTION 14: When should an ARB be used in A.J.?

Several clinical trials in HF have shown the therapeutic benefit of ARBs in modifying HF symptoms (Table 14-9).[144–151] A meta-analysis combined data on all-cause mortality and HF-related hospitalizations from a total of 17 clinical trials comparing an ARB with either placebo or an ACEI in patients with HF.[143] ARBs favorably improved exercise tolerance and EF compared with placebo. However, they were not superior to ACEIs in reducing all-cause mortality or hospitalizations for HF.

The first major clinical trial comparing an ARB with an ACEI in patients with HF was the Evaluation of Losartan in the Elderly (ELITE) study.[150] Losartan was compared to captopril. For the primary end point, a sustained increase in renal function decline, the two drugs performed identically with 10.5% of subjects in each group having a greater than 0.3 mg/dL rise in SCr. An unexpected finding was an insignificant trend toward more deaths from all causes in the captopril group (8.7%) compared with losartan (4.8%).

The follow-up ELITE II Trial was specifically designed to test the hypothesis that losartan was superior to captopril in terms of reduction in mortality and morbidity in patients 60 years of age or older.[148] No significant difference was seen in all-cause mortality, sudden death, or all-cause mortality plus hospitalization. Although ARB treatment was not superior to ACEI therapy, it was better tolerated. Specifically, significantly fewer patients experienced cough with the ARB.

The Valsartan Heart Failure Trial (Val-HeFT) was a double-blind, placebo-controlled study to measure the morbidity and mortality HFrEF patients given valsartan.[152] Patients were randomly assigned to receive valsartan or placebo twice daily. There was no significant difference in all-cause mortality between the valsartan group (19.7%) and the control group (19.4%). Nearly 93% of patients in both groups were receiving an ACEI. Dizziness, hypotension, and renal impairment all occurred more frequently in those treated with valsartan.

Further post hoc analysis found that within the 35% of subjects taking the combination of an ACEI and a β-blocker at baseline, the addition of valsartan as a third drug was associated with a trend toward increased morbidity and a statistically significant increase in the combined end point of mortality and morbidity. The overall study results suggested that a combination of valsartan and an ACEI reduces morbidity, but not mortality. More worrisome was the implication that the three-drug combination of valsartan, an ACEI, and a β-blocker adversely affects morbidity and mortality.[155]

The Valsartan in Acute Myocardial Infarction Trial (VALIANT) of stable patients after MI with LV dysfunction was designed to test the hypothesis that valsartan alone and in combination with captopril (ACEI) would improve survival. In VALIANT, 70% of the patients were also receiving β-blockers. All-cause mortality, the primary end point, was identical in all groups. In addition, an increased rate of side effects was seen in the combination ACEI/ARB group. Interestingly, among the subgroup of patients

Table 14-9
Clinical Trials of Angiotensin Receptor Blockers in Heart Failure

Trial	Patient Population	ARB	Treatment Duration	Outcome
ELITE[149]	NYHA II–IV (n = 722) EF ≤40%	Losartan (50 mg every day) or captopril (50 mg TID)	48 weeks	No significant difference observed for the primary end point (persistent renal dysfunction) or the secondary end point (composite of death/HF admissions). Losartan was associated with a lower mortality than captopril.
RESOLVD[151]	NYHA II–IV (n = 768) EF ≤40%	Candesartan (4, 8 or 16 mg), or candesartan (4 mg or 8 mg) + 20 mg enalapril, or 20 mg enalapril	43 weeks	Combination has greater benefits on LV remodeling. No difference in mortality. No difference in NYHA class, QoL, 6-minute walking distance.
ELITEII[150]	NYHA II–IV (n = 3,152) EF ≤40%	Losartan (50 mg every day) or captopril (50 mg TID)	48 weeks	Losartan was not superior to captopril in improving survival, but was significantly better tolerated. A subgroup analysis of ELITE II found a greater risk of death when losartan was used in addition to β-blockers.
Val-Heft[152]	NYHA II–IV (n = 5,010) EF <40%	Valsartan 160 mg BID or placebo BID	23 months	There was no difference in mortality between the two groups. In patients previously receiving both ACEI and a β-blocker (n = 1,610), the risk of death was increased with the addition of valsartan.
CHARM[154] Alternative	NYHA II–IV (n = 2,028) EF ≤40%	Candesartan (32 mg) vs. placebo	34 months	23% reduction in CV mortality or HF hospitalization favoring the candesartan group. More side effects in the candesartan group (hypotension, hyperkalemia, ↑ SCr) vs. placebo.
CHARM[155] Added	NYHA II–IV (n = 2,548) EF ≤40%	Candesartan (32 mg) + ACEI vs. placebo	41 months	15% risk reduction in CV mortality or HF admissions compared with placebo. However, there were more side effects in the candesartan group (hypotension, hyperkalemia, ↑ SCr) vs. placebo.
CHARM[157] Overall	NYHA II–IV (n = 7,599)	Candesartan (32 mg) vs. placebo	38 months	There was no overall difference in primary outcome of all-cause death.

ACEI, angiotensin-converting enzyme inhibitor; ARB, angiotensin receptor blocker; BID, 2 times a day; CV, cardiovascular; EF, ejection fraction; HF, heart failure; LV, left ventricular; NYHA, New York Heart Association; QoL, quality of life; SCr, serum creatinine; TID, three times a day.

taking β-blockers, no evidence was found of harmful interaction with triple therapy.[153] As a result of the VALIANT trial, the FDA approved the use of valsartan in patients at high risk after a heart attack, and in those with HF.

The best evidence addressing the efficacy and safety of ARB in HF comes from a series of three investigations known collectively as the Candesartan in Heart Failure Assessment of Reduction in Morbidity and Mortality (CHARM) trial. The individual components of the CHARM Program are (a) CHARM-Alternative, (b) CHARM-Added, and (c) CHARM-Preserved.[154–156] All three investigations were randomized, double-blind, placebo-controlled trials that enrolled adult patients (>18 years of age) with at least a 4-week history of symptomatic (NYHA class II–IV) HF. Subjects randomly assigned to candesartan were started on 4 mg and titrated to 32 mg once daily, as tolerated. Some standard therapy (diuretics, β-blockers, digoxin, spironolactone, and ACEI) was continued. For all three trials, the primary end point was the combined incidence of CV death, HF hospitalizations, or both. The differences in admission criteria and outcomes among the individual trials are discussed below.

CHARM-Alternative enrolled 2,028 subjects who met all of the inclusion criteria defined above plus two additional criteria: an EF of 40% or less and intolerance of ACEIs (cough, 72%; hypotension, 13%; renal dysfunction, 12%). Thus, subjects in this group received either an ARB alone or placebo without an ACEI. A 23% reduction was found in the primary outcome of CV death, hospital admission for HF, or both in the candesartan group compared with placebo. The overall incidence of drug discontinuations because of adverse events was not statistically different between candesartan and placebo, but there were significantly more reports of symptomatic hypotension, increased creatinine levels, and hyperkalemia in those treated with candesartan (Table 14-10).

The CHARM-Added trial attempted to determine whether the combination of an ACEI plus an ARB offered any clinical advantages compared with an ACEI alone in patients with symptomatic HF with an EF of 40% or less. At baseline, 55% of the patients were treated with β-blockers and 17% with spironolactone. The addition of candesartan to an ACEI and other usual HF treatments led to a 15% relative risk (p = 0.011) reduction in the primary outcome of CV death, hospital admission for HF in the combination group compared to the ACEI-alone group. It is interesting to compare the result of the CHARM-Added trial with those of the Val-HeFT study. In Val-HeFT, 93% of the subjects receiving the ARB valsartan were concurrently receiving an ACEI. The combined end point of morbidity and mortality was significantly reduced with combination therapy in Val-HeFT, but mortality alone was not reduced. A trend toward more deaths in the small

Table 14-10
Adverse Events that Lead to Permanent Drug Discontinuation

Trial	Outcomes	Candesartan (%)	Placebo (%)	*p* Value
CHARM-Alternative[152]	Any adverse event or laboratory abnormality	21.5	19.3	0.23
	Hypotension	3.7	0.9	<0.0001
	Increased creatinine	6.1	2.7	<0.0001
	Hyperkalemia	1.9	0.3	0.0005
CHARM-Added[153]	Any adverse event or laboratory abnormality			0.0003
	Hypotension	4.5	3.5	0.079
	Increased creatinine	7.8	4.1	0.0001
	Hyperkalemia	3.4	0.7	<0.0001
CHARM-Preserved[154]	Any adverse event or laboratory abnormality	17.8	13.5	0.001
	Hypotension	2.4	1.1	0.006
	Increased creatinine	4.8	2.4	<0.001
	Hyperkalemia	1.5	0.6	0.019
CHARM-Overall[155]	Any adverse event or laboratory abnormality	21	16.7	<0.001
	Hypotension	3.5	1.7	<0.0001
	Increased creatinine	6.2	3.0	<0.0001
	Hyperkalemia	2.2	0.6	<0.0001

subgroup receiving the triple combination of a β-blocker with an ACEI and ARB was observed, whereas β-blocker use had no adverse effect in CHARM-Added.

The combined results of all three CHARM components (CHARM-Added, CHARM-Alternative, and CHARM-Preserved; see discussion of CHARM-Preserved in Case 14-7, Question 1) were reported in the CHARM-Overall trial.[157] This composite analysis evaluates the benefits of candesartan in symptomatic patients with HF, regardless of LV systolic function. A different primary end point was chosen for the CHARM-Overall analysis: all-cause death. Although the combined results failed to detect a clinically significant reduction in all-cause death between candesartan and placebo (9% reduction; $p = 0.32$), significant reductions were seen in CV death (12%), hospital admission for HF (21%), and combined CV death or hospital admission for HF (16%), which was the primary end point for the individual trials.

The collective results of the CHARM program reinforce the conclusion that ARBs can reduce morbidity and mortality in symptomatic patients with HFrEF, and they can be safely used in patients who are intolerant of ACEI therapy. Combination therapy (ACEI plus ARB) with concomitant use of β-blockers appears to be beneficial and safe, as long as patients are closely monitored for adverse effects. Current guidelines recommend addition of an aldosterone antagonist over ARB in patients receiving an ACEI and β-blockers.

Because ELITE II failed to demonstrate any survival benefits of losartan 50 mg/day, over captopril 150 mg/day in HFrEF patients, the "Effects of high-dose versus low-dose losartan on clinical outcomes in patients with heart failure" (HEAAL) study was designed to compare the effect of two doses of losartan (50 mg daily versus 150 mg daily) on the combined end point of all-cause mortality and hospitalizations in HFrEF. A median follow-up of 4.7 years showed losartan 150 mg daily reduced the rate of death or HF admission when compared with losartan 50 mg daily. The high-dose group experienced more renal dysfunction, hypotension, and hyperkalemia, although these results did not lead to significantly more treatment discontinuations. Old age, concomitant aldosterone antagonist dose, and baseline levels of potassium and SCr were common predictors of adverse events and resulted in increased mortality among patients who experienced these adverse events. Therefore, dose titrations should be done with close monitoring especially in individuals at high risk of developing adverse events.[158]

In summary, ARB HF trials demonstrate survival benefits in HFrEF in ACEI–intolerant patients or as an add-on therapy to ACEIs and β-blockers. However, current guidelines do not recommend the routine use of triple therapy, and A.J. should not be started on an ARB in addition to his lisinopril. If A.J. develops a cough on lisinopril, he can be switched to an ARB such as candesartan.

Side Effects

ANGIOTENSIN-CONVERTING ENZYME INHIBITOR–INDUCED COUGH

CASE 14-1, QUESTION 15: A.J. presents to the outpatient HF clinic with an annoying productive cough after 6 weeks of lisinopril therapy. His chest examination reveals no evidence of wheezing, with only a few crackles, his neck veins are only minimally elevated over normal, his ankle edema is 1+, and his weight is stable. All laboratory values are normal. Could the cough be a symptom of his HF or is it ACEI–induced? What are the recommendations for managing an ACEI–induced cough?

Cough can be a sign of HF in patients with pulmonary congestion. In extreme cases, patients have "cardiac asthma" with severe air hunger, wheezing, and dyspnea. However, A.J.'s HF is much improved as evidenced by the objective data. The absence of wheezing and no prior history of asthma or smoking make an obstructive airways disease (asthma or chronic obstructive pulmonary disease) unlikely. It is possible that he does have bronchitis, but he does not report having a cold or other respiratory illness preceding the cough. Without other causes, an ACEI–induced cough is most likely.

This side effect occurs with all ACEIs.[159] Cough is a well-established complication of ACEIs and presents as dry and nonproductive; sometimes described as a "tickle in the back of the throat." This complication can arise within hours of the first dose, or it can present after weeks to months of treatment. Although resolution of the cough usually occurs within 1 to 4 weeks, in some patients it can persist up to 3 months after discontinuation of therapy.

Bradykinin accumulation within the upper airway and decreased metabolism of pro-inflammatory mediators such as substance P or prostaglandins are proposed mechanisms of ACEI–induced cough. These chemicals then act as irritant substances in the airways to increase bronchial reactivity and induce coughing.

Various case reports have found an incidence of cough in 5% to 35% of all patients. The incidence is dose-independent.[160] One investigator found a 5% to 10% incidence in white patients of European descent that rose to nearly 50% in Chinese patients.[161] There may also be a higher incidence in women and black populations.[158]

Because this is a pharmacologic effect rather than an allergic reaction, dose reduction or switching from one ACEI to another is generally not helpful. The only way to definitively diagnose the drug-induced cough is to discontinue therapy. Even then, false-positive results can occur if the patient had a mild case of bronchitis that spontaneously resolved at about the same time that the ACEI was discontinued. If the cough persists after drug discontinuation, other causes should be investigated such as coexisting gastroesophageal reflux disease or allergic rhinitis.

For patients with persistent cough, ARB or hydralazine–isosorbide are safe alternatives. Therefore, A.J. can continue taking lisinopril for another couple of weeks to determine whether the cough will resolve on its own. His symptoms of HF have abated since the initiation of ACEI therapy, and the cough may be no more than an annoyance. He is not at risk of experiencing asthma or other airway problems. If his cough persists, an ARB is probably the best alternative.

OTHER ANGIOTENSIN-CONVERTING ENZYME INHIBITOR AND ANGIOTENSIN RECEPTOR BLOCKER SIDE EFFECTS

Hyperkalemia

CASE 14-1, QUESTION 16: What other side effects of both ACEIs and ARBs need to be monitored? Does changing from an ACEI to an ARB reduce the risk of any of these side effects?

The ACEIs, and ARBs, have the potential to raise serum potassium concentrations via indirect aldosterone inhibition and other neurohormonal actions.[162,163] For most patients, the magnitude of increase in serum potassium concentration from ACEIs and ARBs alone is relatively small, but the risk of developing hyperkalemia is greater if the patient has compromised renal function or advanced HF. Combination therapy of an ACE or ARB with potassium supplements, or potassium-sparing diuretics, further accentuates the risk of hyperkalemia.

Several case reports and case series have reported hyperkalemia and hospitalizations secondary to spironolactone in patients with HF. This became more evident as prescribing patterns for spironolactone dramatically increased after publication of the RALES study.[164] Not only was there a significant increase in the number of prescriptions for spironolactone for patients with HF, but doses higher than those recommended by the clinical trials were often used, especially in patients with evidence of preexisting renal dysfunction. In addition, evidence indicated inadequate monitoring of serum potassium, renal function, and concomitant drug therapy. Although concurrent use of a potassium-wasting diuretic (thiazide or loop diuretic) may counteract potassium retention from spironolactone or other drugs (ACEIs, ARB), it is nearly impossible to predict who will exhibit hypokalemia, hyperkalemia, or remain normokalemic.[165,166] Each patient must be assessed individually for personal response to various drug combinations. Close monitoring of serum potassium is required; potassium levels and renal function should be checked in 3 days and at 1 week after initiation of therapy known to affect potassium and at least monthly for the first 3 months (Table 14-11).

Angioedema

Angioedema (angioneurotic edema) is a severe, potentially life-threatening complication of ACEI treatment.[167–169] Characterized by facial and neck swelling, with obstruction to air flow by laryngeal and bronchial edema, this reaction resembles anaphylaxis. The mechanism of ACEI induction of angioedema is unknown, but is thought to be hypersensitivity to accumulated vasodilating kinins.

Some, but not all, persons with drug-induced angioedema have a history of familial angioedema associated with a genetic defect in their complement system. ACEIs are contraindicated in this population. In one series of case reports, 22% of the reported angioedema reactions occurred within 1 month of starting therapy, with the remaining 77% arising from several months to years later.[168] Black patients and women may have a higher prevalence. Of concern is the observation that ACEI–induced angioedema is often misdiagnosed.[169] It is prudent to avoid all ACEIs in any patient with a history of angioedema from any cause.

Because the mechanism of ACEI–induced angioedema is thought to be caused by kinin accumulation, changing to an ARB might be an option.[170] Several case reports, however, have implicated candesartan, losartan, and valsartan as possible causative agents of angioedema.[167,171–174] In some cases, the subjects had previously experienced angioedema with an ACEI (indicating possible cross-reactivity), whereas others were ACEI–naïve. A small but potential risk for ARB-induced angioedema in patients who are ACEI–intolerant comes from the CHARM-Alternative trial.[154] Of 39 patients with a history of angioedema while taking an ACEI, three experienced angioedema on candesartan, although only one of the three actually discontinued taking candesartan. For now, it is prudent to assess risk–benefit, and ARBs should be used cautiously in the management of patients who have angioedema from ACEIs.

Effects of Angiotensin-Converting Enzyme Inhibitors and Angiotensin Receptor Blockers on Kidney Function

As seen in Figure 14-7, glomerular filtration is optimal when intraglomerular pressure is normal. The balance between afferent flow into the glomerulus and efferent flow exiting the glomerulus determines the intraglomerular pressure. A drop in afferent flow or pressure occurring as a result of hypotension, volume loss, hypoalbuminemia, decreased CO, or obstructive lesions such as renal artery stenosis can significantly lower intraglomerular pressure and lead to impaired renal function. Similarly, long-standing HTN can damage glomerular basement membrane capillaries and cause renal insufficiency.

In the case of low-pressure or low-flow states, the RAAS is activated to maintain intraglomerular pressure. A key factor in preserving glomerular pressure is *efferent vasoconstriction* mediated by angiotensin II. Increased efferent pressure helps to maintain intraglomerular pressure by impeding blood flow out of the glomerulus. When patients with low-pressure states are given ACEIs or ARBs, the protective mechanism of efferent vasoconstriction

Table 14-11
Various Causes of Hyperkalemia and Strategies to Minimize Risk

Cause	Mechanism	Strategies to Minimize Risk
Aldosterone blockers	Decreased levels of aldosterone and subsequent potassium retention.	GFR should be determined and aldosterone antagonist should be avoided if creatinine clearance is <30 mL/minute and baseline serum potassium is >5.0 mEq/L. An initial dose of spironolactone 12.5 mg or eplerenone 25 mg is recommended, after which the dose may be increased to spironolactone 25 mg or eplerenone 50 mg if appropriate. Close monitoring of serum potassium is required; potassium levels and renal function should be checked in 3 days and at 1 week after initiation of therapy and at least monthly for the first 3 months.
RAAS blockade by ACE inhibitors and ARBs Note: risk increases at higher doses (enalapril or lisinopril ≥10 mg/day)	Inhibition of angiotensin II production or receptor binding reduces the delivery of sodium and water to the distal nephron, which, in combination with hypoaldosteronism, promotes hyperkalemia.	Doses of drugs should be decreased as appropriate.
NSAIDs	Inhibit renal prostaglandin synthesis (PGE_2 and PGI_2), resulting in hyporeninemic hypoaldosteronism. Decreased availability of sodium for exchange with potassium at distal tubular sites.	NSAIDs and cyclooxygenase-2 inhibitors should be avoided.
Potassium-sparing diuretics, cyclosporine, tacrolimus, trimethoprim, and heparin	Decreased excretion of potassium.	Close monitoring of serum potassium is required. Doses of drugs known to cause hyperkalemia should be decreased as appropriate.
Patients who have increased dietary potassium intake, use salt substitutes (a rich source of potassium), or take potassium supplements in combination with aldosterone antagonists	In the presence of renal insufficiency, decreased potassium excretion occurs.	Potassium supplements should be discontinued or reduced. Patients should be educated on foods rich in potassium and to avoid salt substitutes.
HF patients with diabetes taking aldosterone antagonists	Hyporeninemic hypoaldosteronism leading to decreased levels of aldosterone and subsequent potassium retention. Insulin deficiency can stimulate the shift of potassium to the extracellular space.	Hyperglycemia should be monitored and appropriate drug therapy should be determined to treat diabetes.
Advanced age, low muscle mass, or renal insufficiency (serum creatinine >1.6 mg/dL)	Impaired release of renin resulting in hypoaldosteronism. SCr may not accurately reflect GFR. Risk of hyperkalemia increases progressively as SCr rises.	GFR should be determined and doses adjusted accordingly.

ACE, angiotensin-converting enzyme; ARBs, angiotensin receptor blockers; GFR, glomerular filtration rate; HF, heart failure; NSAIDs, nonsteroidal antiinflammatory drugs; PGE_2, prostaglandin E_2; PGI_2, prostaglandin I_2; RAAS, renin–angiotensin–aldosterone system.

is inhibited and GFR decreases to a modest degree, resulting in an increase in SCr.

By decreasing afterload, CO may improve after ACEI or ARB therapy, thus preserving or even enhancing RBF. If, however, starting ACEIs or ARB leads to a rapid decrease in systemic BP that is not followed by an increase in CO, worsening renal function may ensue. It is impossible to predict which event will occur. Therefore, ACEI or ARB therapy needs to be started with low doses, and careful monitoring of the BP and renal function should occur as dosages are increased. Renal function and BP should be checked before and 1 to 2 weeks after initiation or dose increase. Patients with risk factors such as preexisting renal insufficiency or concomitant treatment with NSAIDs or high-dose diuretics may require more frequent monitoring. Diuretics are not contraindicated, but the diuretic dosage may need to be reduced to avoid overly aggressive diuresis and the accompanying volume depletion and hypotension. The guidelines recommend caution when prescribing ACEIs/ARBs in patients who have low systolic BPs (80 mm Hg), increased SCr (>3 mg/dL), bilateral renal artery stenosis, or serum potassium >5.0 mEq/L.[1]

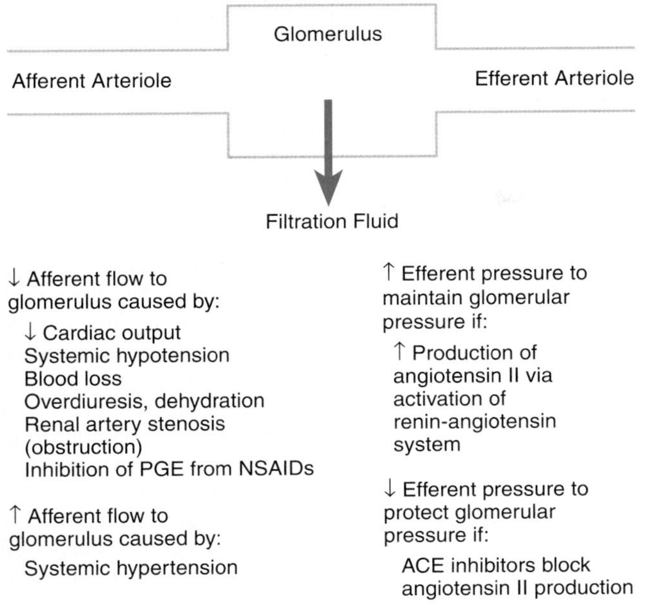

Figure 14-7 Factors affecting renal blood flow. Glomerular filtration is optimal when adequate hydrostatic pressure is maintained in the glomerulus. Governing factors include the blood flow rate to the glomerulus and the balance of afferent and efferent arteriole dilation and constriction. ACE, angiotensin-converting enzyme; NSAIDs, nonsteroidal antiinflammatory drugs; PGE, prostaglandin E.

Use of β-Blockers in HFrEF

CASE 14-1, QUESTION 17: After 3 days of furosemide and an ACEI, A.J.'s PND has resolved, but he still has difficulty walking without SOB and fatigue. His lower extremity edema has been significantly reduced. His current BP is 145/90 mm Hg, his pulse is 82 bpm, and his weight has dropped to 73 kg after diuresis. Repeat laboratory measurements include the following results:

Na, 139 mEq/L
K, 4.3 mEq/L
Cl, 98 mEq/L
CO_2, 27 mEq/L
BUN, 27 mg/dL
SCr, 0.6 mg/dL

The medical team has decided to discharge A.J. soon. You recommend that A.J. should be started on a β-blocker before discharge. What is your rationale?

β-Blockers have been evaluated during randomized clinical trials in more than 20,000 patients with varying degrees of HFrEF. Five meta-analyses have arrived at the same conclusions: the use of three β-blockers (bisoprolol, metoprolol succinate, or carvedilol) is associated with a consistent 30% reduction in mortality and a 40% reduction in hospitalizations in patients with HF.[175–179]

The ACC/AHA guidelines recommend bisoprolol, metoprolol succinate, or carvedilol for all patients with HFrEF unless there is a contraindication to their use or the patient is unable to tolerate treatment with a β-blocker.[1,5,6] They should be a part of the primary treatment plan with an ACEI or ARB. Patients should receive a β-blocker to slow the rate of disease progression and reduce the risk of sudden death. Patients do not need to be taking high doses of ACEIs before being considered for treatment with a β-blocker. To the contrary, in patients taking a low dose of an ACEI, the addition of a β-blocker produces a greater reduction in symptoms and in the risk of death than an increase in the dose of an ACEI. β-Blockers should be initiated before discharge in the vast majority of patients hospitalized for HF.[180] Only those clinically unstable patients who are hospitalized in an intensive care unit, require IV positive inotropic support, have severe fluid overload or depletion, have symptomatic bradycardia or advanced heart block that is not treated with a pacemaker, or have a history of poorly controlled reactive airways disease, are not candidates for a β-blocker.[181]

Based on all these factors, there is no question that A.J. should be started on a β-blocker. Treatment with a β-blocker should be initiated at low doses, followed by gradual increments in dose every 2 weeks as tolerated by the patient. Transient bradycardia, hypotension, and fatigue are common during the first 24 to 48 hours when β-blockers are first started or during subsequent increases in dosage. Thus, patients should be monitored daily for changes in vital signs (pulse and BP) and symptoms during this up-titration period. Bradycardia, heart block, and hypotension can be asymptomatic and require no intervention other than instructing the patient not to arise too quickly from a lying position to avoid postural changes. If either of these complications is accompanied by dizziness, lightheadedness, or blurred vision, it may be necessary to reduce the dose of β-blocker, the ACEI, or both or to slow the up-titration. In patients in whom benefits are especially apparent, but bradycardia or heart block is a concern, insertion of a pacemaker should be considered.

Because initiation of β-blocker therapy can also cause fluid retention, β-blockers should only be started or uptitrated when the patient is euvolemic. Patients should be instructed to weigh themselves daily and to adjust concomitantly administered diuretics as appropriate. Diuretic doses should be decreased temporarily if patients become hypotensive or their BUN begins to rise. Planned increments in the dose of a β-blocker should be delayed until any side effects observed with lower doses are tolerable or absent.

METOPROLOL AND BISOPROLOL

CASE 14-1, QUESTION 18: Metoprolol succinate (12.5 mg) is prescribed for A.J. Is this a good choice of agent and starting dose? What other similar drugs have been used to treat HF?

Several clinical trials substantiate the clinical benefits of metoprolol, a relatively selective β_1-receptor blocker, in HF.[182–185] By blocking β_1 receptors in the myocardium, HR, contractility, and CO are reduced at rest and during exercise, without a compensatory increase in peripheral vascular resistance. The relative sparing of β_2-receptors in the peripheral vasculature and lungs reduces vasoconstrictive and bronchospastic complications.

The Metoprolol CR/XL Randomized Intervention Trial in Heart Failure (MERIT-HF) showed a 35% reduction in all-cause mortality with sustained-release metoprolol succinate.[185] In this trial, 3,991 patients, most of whom had NYHA class II or III HF, were randomly assigned to receive metoprolol succinate controlled-release/extended-release (CR/XL) or placebo. The starting dose of metoprolol was 12.5 to 25 mg/day, which was gradually increased every 2 weeks to the target dose of 200 mg/day. Conventional therapy with diuretics, ACEIs, and digoxin was continued. At the end of the trial, 64% of subjects assigned to the active drug had reached the target dose. Although the number of subjects was too small to detect a statistical difference, patients with severe (class IV) HF seemed to benefit as well. Up to 15% of subjects had clinical worsening of HF, even at low metoprolol doses.

Positive results have also been seen with another relatively β_1-selective drug, bisoprolol fumarate.[186,187] In the first Cardiac Insufficiency Bisoprolol Study (CIBIS I), 641 subjects with moderate to severe HF were randomly assigned to placebo or bisoprolol (starting dose, 1.25 mg/day; maximal dose, 5 mg/day) added to conventional therapy for an average of 23 months.[186] A statistically significant reduction in HF-associated hospitalization with the active drug and an insignificant trend toward reduced mortality were noted. In the larger Second Cardiac Insufficiency Bisoprolol Study (CIBIS II), reduction in both hospitalization and mortality in the bisoprolol-treated group was significant.[187] A total of 2,647 patients were included in the second trial, and doses were increased to as high as 10 mg/day. The study was stopped prematurely because of a 34% reduction in total mortality with bisoprolol. As in the MERIT-HF study, the number of patients with severe (class IV) HF was inadequate to determine the value of β-blocker therapy in this population.

Two dosage forms of metoprolol are marketed: metoprolol succinate extended-release and metoprolol tartrate immediate-release. Only metoprolol succinate is approved for HF in the United States. It is indicated for patients with mild to moderate (NYHA class II or III) HFrEF. The starting dose of 12.5 mg of metoprolol succinate prescribed for A.J. is consistent with the clinical trials and manufacturer's labeling. If the initial dose is tolerated, the dose can be doubled to 25 mg daily for an additional 2 to 4 weeks. The final target dose is 200 mg daily either as 100 mg BID or 200 mg once daily.

When choosing among the various formulations of metoprolol, pharmacokinetic and bioavailability differences should be considered.[182,183] Metoprolol succinate is available as 25-, 50-, 100-, and 200-mg tablets. Each tablet is slowly released at a constant rate for 20 hours, and provides β-blockade for 24 hours. The extended-release formulation retains its release characteristics even if the scored tablet is divided in half, but it should not be crushed or chewed. Having the ability to split tablets is useful in the titration of metoprolol succinate when the goal is to reach target doses and sometimes patients require slower titrations.

Metoprolol has several metabolic routes of elimination that can affect dosing and drug interactions. The major routes of elimination are via α-hydroxylation, *O*-demethylation, and *N*-dealkylation.[182,183] A smaller portion is metabolized by cytochrome P-450 2D6 (CYP2D6), and drugs that inhibit metabolism of that isoenzyme may affect the drug's plasma levels. Approximately 10% of patients are poor metabolizers, resulting in higher drug plasma concentrations in these patients.

A.J. should be advised that the beneficial clinical response to metoprolol is usually delayed and may require 2 to 3 months to become apparent. Even if symptoms do not abate, long-term treatment should be maintained to reduce the risk of major clinical events. Abrupt withdrawal of treatment with a β-blocker can lead to clinical deterioration and should be avoided.[188]

Bisoprolol is FDA approved for treatment of HFrEF. Dosage size limitations, however, limit the clinical use of this drug. For example, the starting dose of bisoprolol is 1.25 mg/day, whereas the smallest commercially available dose in the United States is a 5-mg scored tablet. Attempting to break the tablet into quarters is not practical.

CARVEDILOL

Carvedilol is a β-blocker with some α-blocking acivity.[189] It is also theorized to possess antioxidant effects, which can protect against loss of cardiac myocytes and scavenge oxygen free radicals that are thought to potentiate myocardial necrosis. The correlation of these findings with clinical outcome is unknown.

Two pivotal studies support the use of carvedilol. The first was the U.S. Carvedilol Heart Failure Study.[190–194] Subjects were almost equally divided between NYHA class II and III HF and all had an EF of 35% or less despite diuretics, digoxin, and an ACEI. Subjects were stratified based on the severity of their HF and then randomly assigned to receive either placebo or carvedilol. The maximal dose given was 50 mg twice daily. During an average of 6.5 months, the mortality rate in the placebo group was 7.8% compared with 3.2% in the active treatment group, a statistically significant 65% risk reduction. The patients treated with carvedilol also had fewer HF-related hospitalizations. The most common side effect with carvedilol was dizziness.

In the Australia/New Zealand Carvedilol Study, 415 patients with chronic, stable HF were randomly assigned to receive placebo or carvedilol.[195] Those with severe symptoms were excluded. Maintenance doses in subjects randomly assigned to receive carvedilol ranged from 6.25 to 25 mg twice daily with an average follow-up of 19 months. After 12 months, EF had increased by 5.3%, and heart size was reduced in the carvedilol group. No differences between groups were found in treadmill exercise time, change in NYHA classification, or HF symptom scores, however. Most (58% in both groups) had neither improvement nor worsening of symptoms. The frequency of episodes of worsening HF was similar in the two groups. Total deaths in the carvedilol group were less than the placebo group, but most of the difference in mortality was attributed to non-CV deaths. There were 68% fewer hospital admissions for HF in the carvedilol group than for the placebo group. Overall, these findings could be interpreted as evidence for safety with either no overall benefit or a modest improvement with carvedilol.

The starting dose of carvedilol is 3.125 mg twice daily, with a doubling of the dose every 2 weeks or as tolerated up to a maximum of 25 mg twice daily in patients weighing less than 85 kg and 50 mg twice daily in larger patients. Hypotension, bradycardia, fluid retention, and worsening HF symptoms can occur in the first few weeks of therapy, necessitating additional diuretics, a reduction in dose, or discontinuation of carvedilol. Taking carvedilol with food slows the rate of absorption and reduces the incidence of orthostatic hypotension, which occurs in up to 10% of patients taking the drug. As with any β-blocker, carvedilol is not recommended for use in patients with asthma or poorly controlled diabetes.

Because carvedilol is metabolized by the CYP2D6 enzyme system, several potential drug interactions should be considered.[189,196] The best-documented ones are inhibition of metabolism by cimetidine and decreased carvedilol serum concentrations when taken with rifampin. Known inhibitors of CYP2D6 (quinidine, fluoxetine, paroxetine, and propafenone) might increase the risk of toxicity (especially hypotension). Carvedilol has been reported to increase serum digoxin levels by 15% by an unknown mechanism. Other sources of intrasubject variability in carvedilol response may be caused by differences in the extent or rate or absorption, stereospecific metabolism of the two isomers of the drug (carvedilol is a racemic mixture of *S*[–] and *R*[+] isomers), and impaired metabolism in the 10% of the population who lack CYP2D6 activity.[196]

CHOICE OF β-BLOCKER: METOPROLOL VERSUS CARVEDILOL

CASE 14-1, QUESTION 19: Would carvedilol be a better alternative than metoprolol for A.J.? What would be an appropriate dose and dosing schedule?

No consensus exists regarding the relative superiority of one β-blocker versus another. The additional α_1-blockade and antioxidant properties of carvedilol provide a theoretical basis for selecting carvedilol instead of metoprolol succinate or bisoprolol.

The Carvedilol or Metoprolol European Trial (COMET) was a multicenter, double-blind trial, where 3,029 patients with NYHA class II through IV HF and EF less than 35% were randomly assigned to receive either carvedilol (target dose, 25 mg BID) or metoprolol tartrate (target dose, 50 mg BID). Diuretics and ACEIs were continued in all subjects if tolerated. All-cause mortality was 34% for carvedilol compared with 40% with metoprolol ($p = 0.0017$).[197] The composite end point of mortality or all-cause hospital admissions was not significantly different. One major criticism of this study was the use of metoprolol tartrate instead of metoprolol succinate. Comparable doses between the two study groups have been questioned because the target dose of carvedilol was 25 mg twice daily compared with the target dose of metoprolol tartrate being 50 mg twice daily. Also, the trial used resting HR to determine comparable β-blockade among study groups rather than HR response to exercise. Exercise-induced HR changes are considered a better indicator of β-blockade.

Side effects and patient tolerability are similar among β-blockers in most trials. One investigator observed that carvedilol caused more hypotension and dizziness than metoprolol or bisoprolol, possibly owing to α_1-blockade or more rapid absorption.[198] Thus, metoprolol or bisoprolol may be preferred in patients with hypotension or with complaints of dizziness. Conversely, carvedilol may be preferred in patients with inadequately controlled HTN.

Whether carvedilol is a better choice for A.J. cannot be definitely answered. A starting dosage of 3.125 mg twice daily of carvedilol could be used in place of metoprolol succinate. Both drugs are generic, although the metoprolol sustained-release product is more expensive. A.J.'s provider decided to continue metoprolol and reserve use of carvedilol if he has difficulty tolerating metoprolol.

β-Blockers in Severe Heart Failure

Case 14-1, Question 20: The original clinical trials of β-blockers excluded patients with severe (NYHA class IV) HF at the time of randomization. For this reason, the FDA limited the original approval of carvedilol for use in NYHA class II and III HF. Likewise, the ACC/AHA guidelines strongly support the use of β-blockers in NYHA class II and III HF, but are less definitive about severe HF. If A.J. presented with NYHA class IV HF, what evidence supports or refutes the use of β-blockers in A.J.?

The COPERNICUS[199] study demonstrated clear benefit of carvedilol in patients with severe HF. COPERNICUS was a double-blind, placebo-controlled trial assessing the clinical benefits and risks of carvedilol in patients with advanced HF (NYHA class IIIB or IV).[199] Subjects were excluded who required intensive care, had significant fluid retention, were hypotensive, had evidence of renal insufficiency, or were receiving IV vasodilators or positive inotropic drugs. The starting dose of carvedilol was 3.125 mg twice daily, and increased every 2 weeks to a target dose of 25 mg twice daily. Of those in the carvedilol group, 65% achieved the target dose, with the mean dose being 37 mg at the end of the first 4 months of the trial. The trial was discontinued prematurely after an average patient follow-up of 10.4 months because of a significant survival benefit from carvedilol.

The BEST Investigators failed to demonstrate that bucindolol, a nonselective β-blocker with vasodilator properties, improved overall survival in patients with NYHA class III and IV HF.[200] They randomly assigned 2,708 patients to receive either bucindolol or placebo. Although the active drug yielded a significant decrease in NE levels and improvement in LV function, the study was stopped prematurely because of the low probability of showing any significant CV mortality benefit compared with placebo. A possible explanation is that bucindolol has intrinsic sympathomimetic activity that may counteract some of the benefits of β-blockade. Moreover, subgroup analysis suggested that black patients might have fared worse with bucindolol, raising concerns that β-blockers may not be effective therapy for black patients with advanced HF (see Case 14-3, Question 2, for further discussion of possible racial differences in drug response). Bucindolol has not been approved by the FDA.

Controversy still remains about the safe and effective use of β-blockers in class IV HF. There are data to support the safe and effective use of carvedilol. Clinically, the use of β-blockers is generally continued unless the patient requires inotropic therapy or if a dose increase of the β-blockers caused the ADHF episode. If the dose titration resulted in ADHF, then most patients should receive their previous β-blocker dose, but some may require acutely holding the β-blockers and reinitiating once stabilized.

Aldosterone Antagonists

CASE 14-2

Question 1: B.D. is a 65-year-old Caucasian man with an LVEF of less than 25% who presents to the HF clinic today for follow-up of his recent HF hospitalization. His BP is 120/85 mm Hg and his pulse is 70 bpm. His current medications include lisinopril 10 mg daily, metoprolol succinate 150 mg daily, and furosemide 20 mg daily. You have reviewed his chart and noted that these are the maximal tolerated doses of lisinopril and metoprolol owing to dizziness and near syncope with higher doses. Today his laboratory results show that his SCr is 0.9 mg/dL and his potassium level is 3.5 mEq/L. Is this patient a candidate for aldosterone antagonist therapy?

Aldosterone contributes to HF through the increased retention of sodium and water and contributes to the depletion of potassium. Likewise, the diuretic and potassium-sparing actions of spironolactone are attributed to inhibition of aldosterone.[201] At one time, it was believed that optimal doses of ACEIs fully suppressed the production of aldosterone. It is now recognized that aldosterone levels can remain elevated through a combination of nonadrenal production and reduced hepatic clearance. In addition, it has become clear that both angiotensin II and aldosterone have other negative effects on the CV system, including myocardial and vascular fibrosis, direct vascular damage, endothelial dysfunction, oxidative stress, and prevention of NE uptake by the myocardium.[23,202] This led the RALES investigators to test the hypothesis that low doses of spironolactone might impart a cardioprotective effect in patients with severe HF independent of diuresis or potassium retention. In this trial, 1,663 patients with a history of NYHA class IV HF were randomly assigned to receive either spironolactone 25 mg or placebo. The dose of spironolactone could be increased to 50 mg if HF worsened without evidence of hyperkalemia.

The study was discontinued prematurely after a mean follow-up of 24 months when a significant reduction in mortality was observed in the spironolactone group. Hospitalization rates were lower in the patients treated with spironolactone. Hyperkalemia developed in 2% of the patients on spironolactone and 1% of those on placebo. Gynecomastia was reported in 10% of men treated with spironolactone compared with only 1% of those receiving placebo.

Subsequently, the aldosterone receptor antagonist eplerenone was studied in 6,632 patients with LV dysfunction after MI. In the Eplerenone Post-Acute Myocardial Infarction Heart Failure Efficacy and Survival Study (EPHESUS), subjects were randomly assigned to receive either eplerenone or placebo.[65] Concurrent therapy included diuretics, ACEIs, β-blockers, and aspirin. During a mean follow-up of 16 months, there were 478 deaths (14.4%) in the eplerenone group compared with 554 deaths (16.7%) with placebo ($p = 0.008$). Most deaths were attributable to CV causes. More subjects experienced hyperkalemia with eplerenone than with placebo. Because eplerenone does not block progesterone and androgen receptors, gynecomastia and sexual dysfunction may be less.[65,202]

In 2011, the Eplerenone in Mild Patients Hospitalization and Survival Study in Heart Failure (EMPHASIS-HF) study was published. This study evaluated eplerenone in patients with NYHA class II HF and an EF of less than 35%.[203] In EMPHASIS-HF, subjects were randomly assigned to receive either eplerenone or placebo. The primary outcome of the trial was CV death or HF hospitalization. During a median follow-up of 21 months, 18.3% of eplerenone-treated patients versus 25.9% of placebo patients had a primary outcome event ($p < 0.001$). This study further supported the role of aldosterone antagonists in HFrEF and expanded the known effectiveness to NYHA class II HF patients.

B.D. has NYHA class II HF based on his current symptom control and fits the profile of the subjects in the EMPHASIS-HF study, although he is on a low dose of ACEI. Starting B.D. on an aldosterone antagonist is appropriate because of his relative intolerance to increasing the dose of ACEI and β-blocker. An initial spironolactone dose of 25 mg per day should be chosen for B.D. based on the dose studied in the RALES trial. Spironolactone is chosen based on the likely class effects of aldosterone antagonists in HF treatment and the lower cost compared with eplerenone. This dose is safe based on his current potassium of 3.5 mEq/L and SCr of 0.9 mg/dL. He will need to be followed to determine whether a larger dose of spironolactone will be tolerated and safe after a measurement of his potassium and SCr 2 weeks after initiation. Specific monitoring parameters for the management of hyperkalemia in patients treated with aldosterone antagonists can be found in Table 14-11.

Digitalis Glycosides

CASE 14-2, QUESTION 2: B.D. has tolerated spironolactone 25 mg daily for 2 months. His laboratory test results today show that his potassium is 4.4 mEq/L and his SCr is 1.0 mg/dL. His BP is 124/82 mm Hg and his pulse is 70 bpm. He has come to the clinic today for a follow-up appointment with his cardiologist who notes that B.D. has had four HF hospitalizations in the last year. B.D. also reports increased SOB, DOE, and PND, although his weight is stable and he takes all his medications as prescribed. The medical resident who is also staffing the clinic asks whether it would be appropriate to add digoxin to B.D.'s medical treatment of HF. He was told by a colleague that in clinical trials digoxin reduced both HF symptoms and hospitalizations for HF. What would you recommend?

Debates raged for years about whether digitalis glycosides or vasodilators should be the drug(s) of first choice for treating HFrEF. By the time the first ACC/AHA guidelines were published, a clear consensus was evident. Vasodilators are first-line therapy, with digoxin being added for patients with supraventricular arrhythmias, failure to achieve symptomatic relief with vasodilators alone, or intolerable side effects from vasodilators. ACEIs are preferred compared with other vasodilators because of proven efficacy, convenience of dosing, and fewer side effects. By 1999, experts also recommended starting β-blocker therapy earlier in the treatment plan. Digoxin, however, continues to be widely debated.

CONTROVERSY ABOUT EFFICACY OF DIGOXIN

Correction of the underlying defect is a rational approach to the treatment of any disease. When considering HF solely as "pump failure" with a weakened myocardial muscle, then digitalis is the logical choice to improve cardiac contractility, CO, and renal perfusion. If focusing on symptom relief and increased exercise tolerance as markers of benefit, digoxin is effective. Critics, however, raised concerns that symptom relief was less in patients with normal sinus rhythm than in those with supraventricular arrhythmias. The most vocal critics claimed that the risk of digitalis toxicity did not warrant using this class of drugs in patients with normal sinus rhythm.

Using multivariate analysis, one group of investigators concluded that a third heart sound (S_3 gallop rhythm), an enlarged heart, and a low EF best predict those patients with normal sinus rhythm who will derive a beneficial response from digoxin.[204] Several other meta-analyses and critical reviews of the literature concurred that digoxin therapy provides a beneficial effect, especially in patients with severe symptomatic ventricular systolic dysfunction.[205,206] However these opinions were based on historical data and when many current therapies were not available.

DIGOXIN WITHDRAWAL TRIALS

In 1993, two digoxin withdrawal trials, PROVED[207] and RADIANCE,[208] were published. Both attempted to determine whether patients with HF who were already treated with digoxin would show deterioration after discontinuation. In both studies, patients had documented HFrEF (LVEF <35%), mild to moderate symptoms, were in normal sinus rhythm and stable for at least 3 months with treatment of a diuretic and digoxin (baseline digoxin level, 0.9–2.0 ng/mL). Patients in the RADIANCE trial were also stabilized on an ACEI in addition to the diuretic and digoxin.[207] A 12-week, double-blind, placebo-controlled treatment period followed initial stabilization in both studies. Patients in the active treatment groups continued digoxin at their previous dose. Those in the placebo groups were withdrawn from digoxin and given placebo.

In PROVED,[207] 42 subjects continued digoxin and 46 were given placebo. There were 29% treatment failures in the withdrawal group compared with 19% in those taking digoxin. Exercise tolerance worsened in more patients taking placebo. Those taking digoxin tended to maintain lower body weight and HR as well as higher EF. In the RADIANCE study, 85 subjects continued digoxin therapy and 93 were switched to placebo.[208] During the 12-week follow-up period, 4.7% of the subjects taking digoxin experienced worsening symptoms compared with 24.7% of the placebo-treated patients. More of the placebo-treated patients had worsening of EF and lower quality-of-life scores. When comparing the two trials directly, fewer patients deteriorated in both arms in the RADIANCE study. Whether this is attributed to a greater benefit from combining an ACEI with a diuretic compared with using a diuretic alone (as in PROVED) cannot be established.

These studies establish a beneficial effect of digoxin, even in those patients receiving concurrent ACEIs. At least two factors, however, limit extrapolation to all patients with HF. First, the investigators only assessed the value of therapy indirectly by using a withdrawal design instead of initiating therapy in patients previously untreated with digoxin. Second, the patients had advanced disease as evidenced by NYHA class II or III symptoms despite triple-drug therapy. Thus, the benefit of digoxin as initial monotherapy in early disease remains an unanswered question.

EFFECT OF DIGOXIN ON MORTALITY

The seminal study to answer the question of whether treatment with digoxin improves survival in HF was the Digitalis Intervention Group (DIG) study.[209] In this study, 6,800 patients with HF were randomly assigned to receive either digoxin or placebo. Eligibility requirements included an EF of 45% or less (mean, 28% in both groups), normal sinus rhythm, and clinical evidence of HF. Most subjects were in NYHA class II or III HF, although a small number of class I and class IV subjects were included. Concurrent therapies included diuretics, ACEIs, and nitrates. In both groups, 44% were taking digoxin before randomization. The starting digoxin dose (or placebo) was based on age, weight, and renal function, with subsequent adjustments made according to plasma level measurements. Approximately 70% of subjects in both groups ended up taking 0.25 mg/day. By 1 month, 88.3% of patients receiving digoxin had serum levels between 0.5 and 2.0 ng/mL, with a mean of 0.88 ng/mL. Patients were followed for an average of 37 months.

For the primary outcome of total mortality from any cause, 34.8% of patients on digoxin and 35.1% of those on placebo died; corresponding CV deaths were 29.9% and 29.5%, respectively. Although neither of these differences is statistically significant, a trend was seen toward fewer HF-associated deaths and statistically fewer hospitalizations (risk ratio, 0.72) with digoxin. As would be expected, cases of suspected digoxin toxicity were greater in the active treatment group (11.9% vs. 7.9%), but the incidence of true toxicity was low.

The DIG trial improves on the PROVED and RADIANCE trials because it added digoxin to other therapy as opposed to being a withdrawal study and also because of the larger population. However, because nearly all patients were receiving concurrent vasodilator therapy, the value of digoxin as monotherapy on mortality rates remains unanswered.

The ACC/AHA guidelines indicate that patients with HF are unlikely to benefit from the addition of digoxin in stage A or stage B HF. In stage C patients, despite receiving optimal doses of ACEIs or β-blockers, digoxin may be beneficial to reduce HF hospitalizations.

Digoxin is prescribed frequently in patients with HF and concurrent AF, but β-blockers may be more effective in controlling the ventricular response, especially during exercise. Digoxin should be avoided if the patient has significant sinus or AV block, unless the block is treated with a permanent pacemaker. Digoxin should be used cautiously in patients taking other drugs that can depress sinus or AV nodal function (amiodarone or β-blockers), although patients usually will tolerate this combination.

Despite being on maximal tolerated doses of lisinopril and metoprolol, B.D. continues to have HF symptoms. In patients with persistent HF symptoms, especially like B.D. who also presents with an EF less than 25%, digoxin can be used as an additional agent. However, digoxin is not indicated as primary therapy for stabilization of patients with acutely decompensated HF. Such patients should first receive appropriate treatment, including IV medications.

SEX DIFFERENCES IN RESPONSE TO DIGOXIN

CASE 14-2, QUESTION 3: If B.D. had been a woman, would it have made any difference in the consideration to prescribe digoxin?

The retrospective post hoc analysis of the DIG study data reported that the death rate was lower among women in the placebo group as compared to men (28.9% vs. 36.9%; $p < 0.001$); however, this difference was not significant between women and men taking digoxin.[206] Women taking digoxin had a higher death rate than women taking placebo (33.1% vs. 28.9%), whereas death rates in men were similar in both groups. The authors speculate that a possible mechanism for the increased risk of death among women taking digoxin is an interaction between hormone-replacement therapy and digoxin. Progesterone might increase serum digoxin levels by inhibiting P-glycoprotein (PGP), thus reducing digoxin renal tubular excretion. Consistent with this hypothesis, digoxin serum concentrations after 1 month of therapy were higher in women than in men. The study investigators, however, did not gather data on estrogen and hormone-replacement therapy or consistently measure serum digoxin levels later in the trial. However, subsequent reanalysis[210] of the DIG data found lower serum concentrations (0.5–0.9 ng/mL) of digoxin associated with a decreased risk of hospitalizations and mortality in women. Serum concentrations greater than 1.2 ng/mL were associated with higher risk of death when compared with the placebo group. Higher digoxin concentrations resulted in worse clinical outcomes both in men and in women. Another analysis of patients treated with digoxin in the SOLVD trial failed to demonstrate a survival difference based on gender.[211] The available data suggest that serum digoxin concentrations in the range of 0.5 to 0.9 ng/mL are safe, improve LVEF, hemodynamics, and reduce hospitalizations irrespective of gender.

MAINTENANCE DOSE

CASE 14-2, QUESTION 4: What is the appropriate maintenance dose of digoxin for B.D.?

The usual maintenance doses of digoxin have traditionally ranged from 0.125 to 0.25 mg/day. With the increased emphasis on targeting lower serum concentrations (0.5–0.9 ng/mL), more patients are now empirically started at 0.125 mg/day. It is safer to start with a conservative dose and assess his needs after 1 to 2 weeks.

In all cases, smaller doses of digoxin are given to patients with impaired excretion rates (those with renal failure, older patients) or small-framed individuals. For example, a totally anuric patient may receive only 0.0625 mg 3 or 4 days/week.

Loading doses of digoxin are rarely necessary. Slow initiation of therapy with maintenance doses of digoxin is the method of choice for ambulatory or nonacutely ill patients with normal renal function. Even in the acute-care setting, no indication exists for loading doses of digoxin for HF alone. The exception might be if the patient has AF and it is desired to control ventricular response as quickly as possible. Even then, alternative drugs are likely to be used (see Chapter 15, Cardiac Arrhythmias).

MONITORING PARAMETERS

CASE 14-2, QUESTION 5: How should B.D.'s digitalis therapy be monitored? How useful are digoxin serum levels in monitoring therapy?

No clear therapeutic end point exists for digoxin therapy. Nonspecific electrocardiographic (ECG) changes (ST depression, T-wave abnormalities, and shortening of the QT interval) correlate poorly with both toxic and therapeutic effects of the drug.[212,213] Although digoxin serum levels are readily available from most clinical laboratories, no "therapeutic level" and corresponding "toxic level" are clearly defined.

A few patients, especially if they are hypokalemic or hypomagnesemic, will manifest apparent signs of toxicity when serum digoxin concentrations are less than 1 ng/mL. At the other extreme, some patients tolerate concentrations greater than 2 ng/mL with no signs of overt toxicity. Such overlap between therapeutic concentrations and toxic levels limits the value of serum level monitoring. Serum levels can be used as a guide in confirming suspected toxicity or in explaining a poor therapeutic response, but clinical evaluation ultimately remains the best therapeutic guide.

Clinical Evaluation

As with diuretic and vasodilator therapy, clinical monitoring is the key to evaluating adequacy of digitalis therapy. As B.D. begins to improve, he should have less dyspnea and complain less of PND, and a lower HR may be observed.

TREATMENT OF SUPRAVENTRICULAR ARRHYTHMIAS IN HEART FAILURE

CASE 14-2, QUESTION 6: B.D. did well for the next 6 months until he noted the onset of palpitations, which were diagnosed by ECG as AF. A month ago his primary care physician increased his digoxin dose to 0.25 mg every day. How should we treat his AF?

Supraventricular arrhythmias are frequently encountered in HF because volume or pressure overload can cause atrial distension and irritability. Specifically, AF is present in 10% to 30% of patients with advanced HF,[100] contributing to reduced exercise capacity, increased risk of pulmonary or systemic emboli, and worse long-term prognosis. Drug therapy should be aimed at controlling ventricular rate and preventing thromboembolic events. Cardioversion to normal sinus rhythm in patients with low EF and dilated cardiomyopathy is often unsuccessful.

Digoxin slows the ventricular response associated with AF and is a logical choice in patients with concurrent HFrEF. A potential limiting factor is that digoxin's AV-blocking properties are most evident at rest, and are less effective during exercise. Hence, digoxin may be ineffective at controlling exercise-induced tachycardia that limits the patient's functional capacity. β-Blockers are more effective than digoxin during exercise.[214–216] If digoxin, β-blockers, or both are ineffective, amiodarone is another useful alternative. Verapamil and diltiazem are not appropriate choices for rate control in patients with HFrEF due to their negative inotropic effects.

Some studies suggest that AF is an independent predictor of mortality in HF patients, and restoration of sinus rhythm may reduce mortality and prevent recurrences. Most patients who are electrically cardioverted revert to AF in a short time. In CHF-STAT (Congestive Heart Failure: Survival Trial of Antiarrhythmic Therapy),[217] a subset of patients who were converted to normal sinus rhythm with amiodarone treatment had significantly lower mortality than those who remained in AF. Similar results were observed in a substudy of the DIAMOND (Danish Investigations of Arrhythmia and Mortality on Dofetilide) trial,[218] in which HF patients with AF treated with dofetilide had significantly improved survival if the sinus rhythm was maintained. However, AF-CHF (Atrial Fibrillation in Congestive Heart Failure)[219] showed no mortality or morbidity benefits of rhythm control compared with rate control. The lack of mortality benefits seen in the AF-CHF might be explained by the high frequency of β-blocker use (88%). Antiarrhythmic agents are frequently unsuccessful in maintaining sinus rhythm.[220] Patients who benefit the most from conversion to sinus rhythm are the hemodynamically compromised. Maintaining sinus rhythm can potentially improve their quality of life.

The use of most antiarrhythmic agents, except amiodarone and dofetilide, is associated with worse prognosis due to proarrhythmic or negative inotropic effects and should be avoided in HF patients. Although amiodarone and dofetilide do not increase mortality in HF patients, they are associated with increased hospitalizations.[219] Current treatment guidelines do not support the routine use of anticoagulants in HF unless patients have concomitant AF or evidence of active thrombus. Finally, AV nodal ablation may be needed if tachycardia or bothersome symptoms persist despite aggressive pharmacologic intervention.

B.D. experienced AF while already taking a relatively high dose of digoxin (0.25 mg/day) and metoprolol. If his AF-associated palpitations persist, amiodarone should be started (see Chapter 15, Cardiac Arrhythmias). Amiodarone is a PGP inhibitor. The net effect of inhibition of gut PGP by amiodarone is increased bioavailability of digoxin. B.D.'s digoxin dose will need to be lowered by ~50% if amiodarone is started.[213,221] If digoxin is continued, serum levels should be closely monitored and patients observed for clinical evidence of toxicity.

DIGOXIN DRUG INTERACTIONS

CASE 14-2, QUESTION 7: What are other potential drug interactions with digoxin?

Two reviews of cardiac glycoside drug interactions have been compiled.[222,223] Since publication of these early reviews, a greater understanding of PGP-mediated drug interactions has evolved.[221,224] A brief summary of all digoxin interactions is found in Table 14-12. Drugs recently recognized as raising digoxin serum concentrations through PGP inhibition include atorvastatin.[225] CCBs (especially verapamil and diltiazem),[226] erythromycin and clarithromycin,[227,228] and cyclosporine. Conversely, rifampin[195] and St. John's wort[229] reduce oral digoxin bioavailability and serum concentrations via induction of intestinal PGP.

DIGITALIS TOXICITY

Signs and Symptoms

CASE 14-2, QUESTION 8: If B.D. presents with digoxin toxicity, what would be the common signs and symptoms of toxicity?

Digoxin has a narrow therapeutic index, and there is concern for morbidity and death associated with its use. The most important signs of digoxin toxicity are those relating to the heart. A common misperception is that gastrointestinal or other noncardiac signs will precede cardiac toxicity. To the contrary, cardiac symptoms precede noncardiac symptoms of digitalis toxicity in up to 47% of cases. Frequently nonspecific arrhythmias are the only manifestation of toxicity, with estimates that rhythm disturbances occur in 80% to 90% of all patients with digitalis toxicity.[230] Conversely, rhythm disturbances in patients taking digitalis are not always related to toxicity. In one study of 100 consecutive patients with suspected digitalis-induced arrhythmias, only 24 were confirmed as being toxic as defined by resolution of cardiac irritability after drug withdrawal. In the other 76 patients, the dysrhythmia persisted long after drug removal.[231]

Most arrhythmias can occur as a result of digoxin toxicity. Decreased conduction velocity through the AV node presents as a prolonged PR interval (first-degree AV block) and is seen in many patients with therapeutic concentrations of digoxin. However, higher concentrations of digoxin can impair conduction and result in bradycardia or a second-degree AV block. With severe toxicity, complete (third-degree) AV block can occur. AV block also may predispose patients to accelerated junctional rhythms. Increased automaticity of the atria can cause multifocal atrial tachycardia with block, paroxysmal atrial tachycardia with block, or AF.

Ventricular arrhythmias are among the most common rhythm disturbances caused by digoxin toxicity and include unifocal and multifocal premature ventricular contractions (PVCs), bigeminy, trigeminy, ventricular tachycardia, and ventricular fibrillation.[230,231] In the DIG trial, 11.9% of patients in the digoxin treatment group were found to have suspected digoxin toxicity compared with 7.9% in the placebo group. Comprehensive reviews are available on the topic of digitalis-induced arrhythmias.[213]

Hyperkalemia can develop as a consequence of massive digoxin ingestion by severely poisoning the Na^+/K^+ ATPase system, causing inhibition of the uptake of potassium by the myocardium, skeletal muscle, and liver cells.[232] The shift of potassium from inside to outside the cell can result in significant hyperkalemia, especially in patients with underlying renal insufficiency. These same patients also accumulate digoxin in the body because of decreased clearance of the drug.

Table 14-12
Digoxin Drug Interactions

Drug	Effect
Drugs Lowering Serum Digoxin Concentration	
Rifampin[195]	Probable induction of intestinal P-glycoprotein causing ↓bioavailability.
	↓Serum concentration after oral, but not IV digoxin. No change in digoxin renal clearance or half-life.
St. John's wort[229]	Possible induction of P-glycoprotein (33% reduction in digoxin trough concentrations).[316]
Sulfasalazine doses >2 g/day	Malabsorption of digoxin (decrease AUC of digoxin by 24%).[316]
Drugs Raising Serum Digoxin Concentration	
Amiodarone[213,221]	↑Serum digoxin levels inhibit intestinal P-glycoprotein (70% in 1 day).[316]
Atorvastatin[2,223]	20% increase in serum digoxin concentration with 80-mg dose, minimal effect with 20-mg dose. Speculated to inhibit intestinal P-glycoprotein, but not proven.
Calcium-channel blockers[213,221,226]	Inhibition of P-glycoprotein. Best documented with verapamil (70%–80%).[317] Diltiazem increases digoxin concentrations by 50% in some patients.[314]
Clarithromycin[227,316]	Inhibition of P-glycoprotein, decreased digoxin renal clearance. Digoxin clearance may be reduced by 60%, and plasma concentrations may increase by twofold.[316]
Cyclosporine[213,221]	Inhibition of P-glycoprotein, decreased digoxin renal clearance.
Erythromycin	↑Bioavailability in persons who normally metabolize digoxin in intestinal tract. May also inhibit P-glycoprotein in gut. Digoxin concentrations may increase by 100% in some cases.[316]
Itraconazole[318]	↑Serum digoxin levels by unknown mechanism. In one study, the AUC for digoxin was increased by 50% and renal elimination was decreased by 20%.[316]
Propafenone[213,319]	Inhibition of P-glycoprotein. Increases digoxin concentrations by 30%–60%.[316]
Quinidine[213,221,222,224,320–324] (usually doses above 500 mg/day may increase digoxin serum concentrations)	Inhibition of P-glycoprotein, decreased digoxin renal clearance, and increased bioavailability. Increases 25%–100% digoxin concentrations.[316]

References[213,221,223] include a discussion of many of these interactions that do not include a specific reference citation.
AUC, area under curve; IV, intravenous.

Vague gastrointestinal symptoms characteristic of digoxin toxicity are difficult to evaluate because anorexia and nausea are also part of clinical picture seen in patients with congestion.

CNS symptoms of digoxin are common, possibly associated with potassium depletion in neural tissue. Chronic digoxin intoxication can manifest as extreme fatigue, listlessness or psychic disturbances in the form of nightmares, agitation, and hallucinations.[233] Visual disturbances have been described as hazy vision and difficulties in both reading and red–green color perception. Other complaints included glitterings, dark or moving spots, photophobia, and yellow–green vision. Disturbances in color vision returned to normal 2 or 3 weeks after discontinuation of digitalis.

Digitalis-induced visual disturbances have been reported at serum concentrations below those considered to be toxic (all <1.5 ng/mL; range, 0.2–1.5 ng/mL).[234] Five of the reactions were described as photopsia (seeing lights not present in the environment), and one person had decreased visual acuity. The symptoms resolved in all but one subject when digoxin was discontinued.

Some prospective studies have shown a good correlation between serum digoxin serum concentration and toxicity,[233,235,236] whereas other investigators found a poor correlation.[237,238] Once levels exceed 6 ng/mL, the risk of mortality greatly increases.[239] Patients with hypokalemia can demonstrate digitalis toxicity at low serum digoxin concentrations.[240]

For many patients without life-threatening arrhythmias or major electrolyte imbalances, simple withdrawal of digoxin is the only treatment required. Potassium replacement should be considered in any patient with digoxin-induced ectopic beats who is hypokalemic. Digoxin-specific antibodies that bind digoxin molecules, rendering them unavailable for binding at receptors, are available.[241–246] The use of digoxin Fab products is restricted to potentially life-threatening intoxications (severe arrhythmias or hyperkalemia) that are either refractory to more conservative therapy or associated with extremely high serum digoxin concentrations.

Non–Angiotensin-Converting Enzyme Inhibitor Vasodilator Therapy

CASE 14-3

QUESTION 1: T.R. is a 57-year-old African American man (LVEF of 35%) who presents to the HF clinic for follow-up. His BP is 130/79 mm Hg and pulse is 65 bpm. Current medications include lisinopril 20 mg daily, metoprolol succinate 200 mg daily, spironolactone 25 mg daily, hydralazine 25 mg QID, and isosorbide dinitrate 20 mg TID. Why is the patient on hydralazine and isosorbide? What other forms of nitrates can be used in place of the isosorbide? Is combination therapy rational?

T.R. is treated with an ACEI, a β-blocker, and spironolactone. Despite this therapy, he is still having HF symptoms. He was started on hydralazine and isosorbide dinitrate, which is a possible next step in treating a patient with HFrEF.

Hydralazine's predominate action is as an arteriolar dilator. Decreasing afterload improves LV function. SVR is decreased, and this leads to an increase in CO.[140,247,248] Hydralazine is a direct-acting smooth muscle relaxant with significant arteriolar dilating effects in the kidneys and limbs. It has no effect on the venous system or on hepatic blood flow.

The reflex tachycardia and hypotension that accompany hydralazine in treating HTN are minimal or absent when treating HF. In patients with end-stage cardiomyopathy, significant hypotension can occur if the heart cannot respond appropriately by increasing CO. Because hydralazine is devoid of venous dilating properties, central venous pressure and pulmonary capillary wedge pressure (PCWP) are unchanged.[140,248]

The effect of a single dose of hydralazine occurs in about 30 minutes and lasts up to 6 hours. The average maintenance dose is 50 to 100 mg every 6 to 8 hours. T.R. is receiving an initial dose at this time and may warrant a higher dose in the future. Hydralazine used as monotherapy is not associated with long-term improvement in functional status.[248] Combination therapy of hydralazine with either nitrates or ACEIs is highly effective.

Although tachyphylaxis generally is not a significant problem with prolonged courses of hydralazine, some patients require increased diuretic doses to counteract hydralazine-induced fluid retention. This latter response reflects activation of the renin–angiotensin system after vasodilation of the renal vasculature. Other side effects with hydralazine include transient nausea, headache, flushing, tachycardia, and a lupus syndrome associated with prolonged, high doses (see Chapter 9, Essential Hypertension).

ORAL NITRATES

Nitrates have effects complementary to those of hydralazine.[140,247] They primarily dilate venous capacitance vessels. Venous dilation reduces preload, resulting in reductions in PCWP and right atrial pressure. They are especially effective in reducing the symptoms of pulmonary congestion. The lack of significant arterial dilation accounts for the observations that SVR is minimally reduced and CO remains unchanged.

Isosorbide

Because sublingual NTG has a short duration of action, more attention has been focused on isosorbide dinitrate. Sublingual isosorbide dinitrate is well absorbed and does not undergo first-pass metabolism. Its onset is rapid (5 minutes), but its effects are relatively short (1–3 hours). The usual starting dosage is 5 mg every 4 to 6 hours, but dosages may be titrated to 20 mg or more. Larger doses are associated with longer beneficial effects (approximately 3 hours), but also a high frequency of headaches and hypotension.

Oral isosorbide has a slower onset (15–30 minutes), but the duration of activity is longer (4–6 hours) than sublingual tablets. The smallest effective dose is 10 mg, with titration to dosages as high as 80 mg every 4 to 6 hours. The best dose for both sublingual and oral nitrates is that which provides the desired beneficial effect with the least side effects. Isosorbide mononitrate is frequently used as it is generally given once daily.

HYDRALAZINE–NITRATE COMBINATION

Combined afterload and preload reduction is clearly of benefit in improving symptoms and enhancing long-term survival. Compared with ACEIs, the hydralazine–isosorbide combination provides more improvement in exercise tolerance, but the side effect profile and survival statistics are better with ACEIs.[140] Generally, the use of the two drugs together is not accompanied by reflex tachycardia or hypotension.

Data supporting the use of combination hydralazine and nitrate vasodilator therapy come from two Veterans Administration Cooperative Studies (V-HeFT I and V-HeFT II).[70,140,247] These two studies confirmed symptomatic relief and improved exercise tolerance with combination therapy, and improved survival. (See Case 14-3, Question 2, for the discussion of the therapy in African American patients.)

In summary, nitrates alone are indicated for those patients with signs and symptoms of pulmonary and venous congestion. Use of an arterial dilator is beneficial in a patient with high SVR and low CO. Most patients, such as T.R., exhibit symptoms of decreased CO and elevated venous pressure, making combination therapy an attractive option. Although the hydralazine–isosorbide combination actually reduces symptoms slightly better than ACEIs, the data on survival are better with the ACEIs, probably owing to better adherence. A combination of an ACEI plus hydralazine, a nitrate, or both is common in patients with advanced disease.

Role of Race in the Pharmacotherapy of Heart Failure

CASE 14-3, QUESTION 2: Because T.R. is African American, would he be expected to respond differently to ACEIs or hydralazine–isosorbide dinitrate than a patient who is not African American?

In general, African American patients experience HF at an earlier age and are more likely to have HTN as a cause. The death rate of HF is higher for African American than for non–African American patients.

ANGIOTENSIN-CONVERTING ENZYME INHIBITORS AND HYDRALAZINE–ISOSORBIDE

Racial differences in response to drug therapy have been proposed, although this issue is far from resolved.[249–252] A post hoc analysis[250] of the V-HeFT trial data showed no difference in annual mortality between African American and non–African American patients receiving placebo. African American patients in the hydralazine–nitrate group had a significantly lower mortality rate than those in the placebo group. This implies that African American patients, but not non–African American patients, derive benefit from the treatment with hydralazine–isosorbide. These same investigators then reanalyzed the V-HeFT II trial results for possible racial differences between response to enalapril and the hydralazine–nitrate combination.[140,250] The outcome is difficult to interpret because of the absence of a placebo group. The all-cause annual mortality rate for African American patients was identical in the two drug groups (12.8% with enalapril and 12.9% with hydralazine–isosorbide). In non–African American patients, the corresponding mortality rates were 11% with enalapril and 14.9% with hydralazine–isosorbide. These data could be interpreted as either superior response to hydralazine–isosorbide in African Americans or inferior response to ACEIs in African Americans. The latter interpretation is consistent with the hypothesis that ACEIs might have a lesser BP-lowering effect in African American patients with HTN. A similar reanalysis of the SOLVD Prevention and Treatment trials,[136] which compared enalapril with placebo in patients with recent MI, concluded that enalapril is associated with a significant reduction in the risk for HF hospitalization among white patients (44% reduction) with LV dysfunction, but not among African American patients. Confounding variables contributing to all of these analyses include disproportionately low numbers of African American subjects in the trials, and possibly more underlying risk factors in African American subjects.

To address the effect of race on response to ACEIs, a meta-analysis of seven major ACEI studies with 14,752 patients, was conducted.[251]

The authors concluded that the relative risk for mortality when taking an ACEI compared with placebo was identical (0.89) for both African American and white patients. The authors urged that ACEIs not be withheld from African American patients. Although rare, there is a higher rate of angioedema with ACEIs in black patients compared to white patients.

The African American Heart Failure Trial (AHeFT) was a randomized comparison trial of hydralazine–isosorbide dinitrate versus placebo in African American patients with NYHA class III or IV HF who were receiving standard HF therapy (diuretics, β-blockers, ACEIs or ARB, digoxin, and aldosterone antagonists).[71] The primary end point was a composite of all-cause death, first hospitalization for HF, and quality of life scores at 6 months. Reduction in the primary end point events was statistically significant in favor of the active drug combination. All-cause mortality declined 43% with hydralazine–isosorbide dinitrate versus placebo ($p = 0.012$). The study also reported a 39% reduction in first hospitalization for HF with hydralazine–isosorbide dinitrate versus placebo ($p < 0.001$). The addition of hydralazine and isosorbide dinitrate is effective in African American patients with NYHA class III or IV HF already receiving ACEIs and β-blockers.[1] The results of AHeFT were also the primary factor leading the FDA to approve the combination product of hydralazine and isosorbide dinitrate (BiDil) for adjunctive treatment in self-identified African American patients. Using BiDil might improve compliance by using a combination tablet. Cost is lower using generic hydralazine and isosorbide as separate drugs.

β-BLOCKERS

A possible racial difference in response to β-blocker drugs has also been hypothesized based on effects observed in HTN.[249,251,252] A post hoc analysis of the U.S. Carvedilol Heart Failure trials[190–194] concluded that the benefit of carvedilol was similar in both black and nonblack patients.[252]

Contradictory evidence comes from BEST.[200] In this trial (discussed in Case 14-1 Question 20), 2,708 patients with NYHA class III or IV HF were randomly assigned to either bucindolol or placebo. Bucindolol is a nonselective β-blocker with partial agonist activity that imparts weak vasodilation. A unique characteristic of this study was a preplanned subgroup analysis for racial differences. Although there was a trend toward reductions in CV mortality and hospitalization with bucindolol, the trial was terminated after 2 years. A subgroup analysis showed a mortality benefit in nonblack subjects, but no benefit in black subjects. A meta-analysis of five major β-blocker in HF studies representing 12,727 patients has been conducted, suggesting that black patients will derive similar benefit from β-blockers as do white patients when given carvedilol, metoprolol, or bisoprolol.[251]

Critical Care Management of Heart Failure

CASE 14-4

QUESTION 1: L.M., a 62-year-old black man, was admitted several days ago with severe, progressive, and debilitating symptoms of HF. His family history is significant in that his father and two brothers died of heart attacks shortly after the age of 40. L.M. has a 5-year history of HF that is symptomatic despite treatment with furosemide 40 mg daily, lisinopril 10 mg daily, carvedilol 12.5 mg BID, digoxin 0.125 mg daily, and spironolactone 25 mg daily. His last echocardiogram showed an EF of 25%. He has a past medical history of HTN, CAD, and HF. During the last week, L.M.'s DOE became progressively worse, and he was confined to bed because of fatigue. He wakes once or twice nightly with PND. Physical examination revealed jugular venous distension, bilateral rales, hepatomegaly, and 3+ peripheral edema. Chest radiograph showed cardiomegaly and pulmonary congestion. His BP was 154/100 mm Hg and pulse was 105 bpm.

Laboratory test results include:

Serum Na, 134 mg/dL
K, 4.3 mg/dL
BUN, 15 mg/dL
SCr, 1.3 mg/dL
Glucose, 90 mg/dL
BNP, 944 pg/mL

Hemoglobin, hematocrit, troponin, and liver enzymes were within normal limits. L.M. was admitted to the hospital with ADHF. What factors are used to stratify risk for in-hospital mortality and morbidity?

ADHF is associated with high morbidity and mortality. It is the leading reason for hospitalizations among the elderly. Post discharge mortality among patients with HF is 11% at 30 days and 37% at 1 year.[253] The most common precipitants of HF hospitalization are noncompliance (dietary or medication), acute myocardial ischemia, uncontrolled comorbidities (HTN, diabetes mellitus, chronic kidney disease, arrhythmias), and prescribing of negative inotropic agents, NSAIDs, or other inappropriate agents. Regardless of the precipitating event, the common pathophysiologic state that perpetuates the progression of HF is complex. A cascade of hemodynamic and neurohormonal derangements provoke activation of adrenergic systems and RAAS, leading to volume overload and hypoperfusion—classic symptoms of ADHF. According to the ADHF National Registry, nearly half of the patients who present with ADHF have preserved EF (>50%).[254]

In-hospital mortality remains as high as 20% for patients who present with elevated BUN and creatinine, and low systolic BP (SCr >2.75 mg/dL, BUN >43 mg/dL, systolic BP <115 mm Hg[252]). Patients presenting with hyponatremia (serum sodium less than 135 mEq/L) have the worst outcomes and are more likely to receive inotropic agents. After discharge, patients who continue to be hyponatremic have an 8% risk of rehospitalization per 3 mEq/L decrease in serum sodium. Uric acid greater than 7 mg/dL in men and greater than 6 mg/dL in women is associated with a high admission rate for HF. Admission and discharge levels of BNP are also helpful in predicting rehospitalizations. According to studies, a 30% to 40% reduction in BNP levels during hospitalization may improve outcomes. Other biomarkers such as cardiac troponin levels, C-reactive protein, and apolipoprotein A-I levels are all linked to HF readmissions.[9] All these factors can be used to stratify risk for in-hospital mortality.

Another approach to risk stratification and therapeutic decision-making is based on hemodynamic profiles. Most patients with acute HF can be classified into one of four hemodynamic profiles using relatively simple assessment techniques (Fig. 14-8).[255–258] Patients are assessed for the presence or absence of elevated venous filling pressures ("wet" vs. "dry") and adequacy of vital organ perfusion ("warm" vs. "cold"). Elevated filling pressure can be assessed at the bedside by observing jugular venous distension, presence of a third heart sound (S_3), peripheral edema, and ascites. Presence or absence of rales on auscultation is not considered a reliable indicator.[258] Hypotension, weak peripheral pulse, a narrow pulse pressure, cool extremities, decreased mental alertness, and rising BUN and SCr are indicators of decreased organ perfusion. Continuous BP, ECG, urine output, and pulse oximetry measurements are standard noninvasive monitoring for all patients in an intensive care unit. Invasive hemodynamic monitoring is used in critically ill patients when more precise measurements of filling pressures, SVR, and CO or cardiac index are desired. The goals are to achieve a right atrial pressure of less than 8 mm Hg, pulmonary artery pressure of less than 25/10 mm Hg, pulmonary artery wedge pressure of 12 to 16 mm Hg, SVR 900 to 1,400 dyne second/m^5, and a cardiac index greater than 2.5 L/minute/m^2. (See Chapter 17, Shock, for more detailed discussion of hemodynamic monitoring.)

CASE 14-4, QUESTION 2: From his clinical presentation, what is L.M.'s hemodynamic profile? What are therapeutic goals for L.M.?

L.M.'s DOE, rales, peripheral edema, PND, and jugular venous pressure are consistent with ADHF and volume overload. L.M. does not have signs of hypoperfusion. His hemodynamic profile is "warm and wet" (subset II, Fig. 14-8). According to the guidelines, a rapid diagnosis of ADHF is necessary to initiate appropriate treatment. In patients who have established HF, precipitating factors should be identified and addressed. At the time of discharge, medications that decrease morbidity and mortality in HF should be optimized. BNP levels should be considered when the diagnosis is uncertain can be helpful in differentiating between cardiac and noncardiac causes of dyspnea.

Because volume overload is central to the pathophysiology of most episodes of ADHF, the primary goal is to relieve congestion. However, diuretics should be cautiously used in subset IV to avoid decreases in PCW less than 15 mm Hg as this can compromise preload and further reduce CO. Despite diuretics being the main therapy in reducing volume overload, their routine use in ADHF is associated with worsening renal function and mortality. Mortality rates are higher in patients receiving chronic diuretic therapy compared with those not receiving diuretics. These findings are based on retrospective data. Nevertheless, they suggest an association between mortality and diuretic use in patients with ADHF. (See Case 14-1, Question 7, for diuretic dosing.)

ULTRAFILTRATION

Ultrafiltration is an alternative approach for treating hypervolemia. It involves the use of a small device to rapidly remove fluid (up to 500 mL/hour). Typically, ultrafiltration for HF is reserved for patients with renal failure or those unresponsive to diuretics. Studies[259,260] in ADHF patients have shown that peripheral venovenous ultrafiltration results in greater weight loss and fluid removal, and reduced hospital length of stay and hospital readmissions compared with medical therapy. Significant reductions in neurohormonal activation and no significant changes in SCr or electrolytes were reported with ultrafiltration.[261] The Ultrafiltration versus Intravenous Diuretics for Patients Hospitalized for Acute Decompensated Heart Failure (UNLOAD trial)[262] randomly assigned 200 patients to either ultrafiltration or aggressive IV diuretic therapy. The study showed ultrafiltration significantly improved weight loss at 48 hours (5.0 vs. 3.1 kg; $p < 0.001$), decreased the need for vasoactive drugs (3% vs. 13%; $p = 0.02$), and reduced 90-day hospital readmission (18% vs. 32%; $p = 0.02$) compared with diuretics alone. Ultrafiltration has a class IIb recommendation for patients with refractory HF not responsive to medical therapy. Patients with fluid overload and some degree of renal insufficiency and those refractory to diuretic therapy are candidates for ultrafiltration.[1]

Intravenous Vasodilators

CASE 14-4, QUESTION 3: L.M. received a 40-mg IV furosemide dose with no improvement in symptoms. Then he received an 80-mg IV dose with only marginal improvement. The decision is made to start nitroprusside. What is the role of IV vasodilator therapy in someone with ADHF?

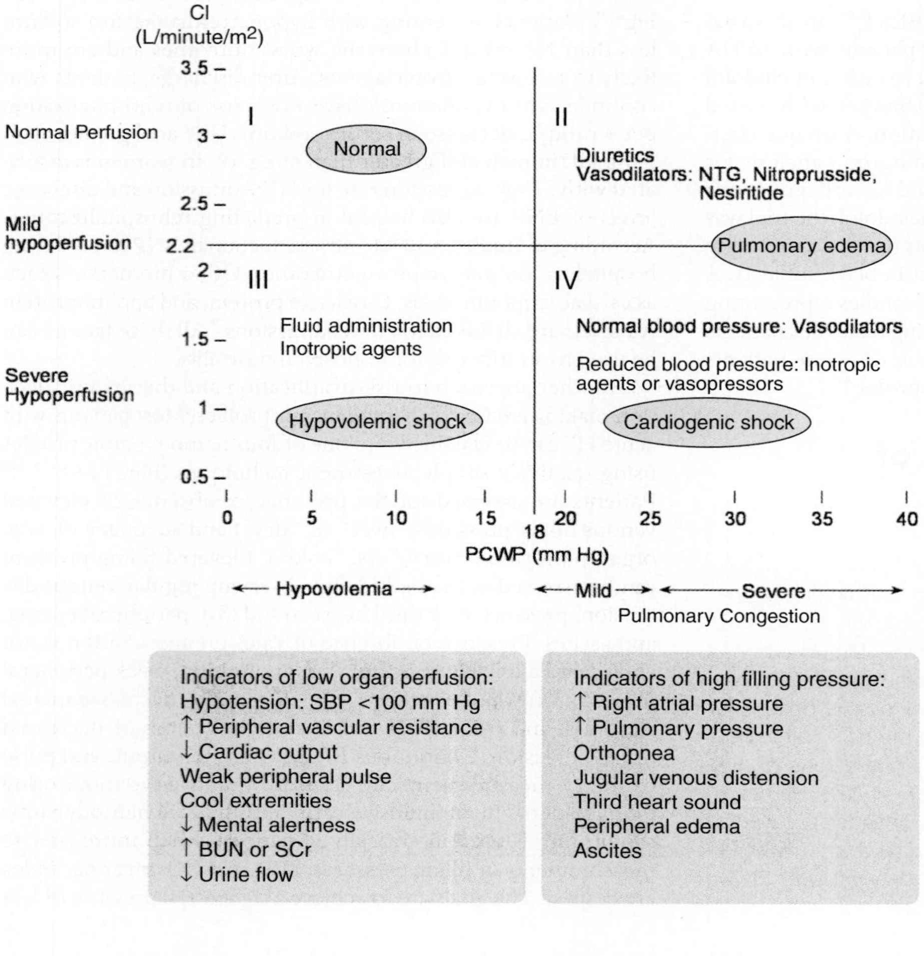

Figure 14-8 Hemodynamic profile of acute heart failure. BUN, blood area nitrogen; CI, cardiac index; NTG, nitroglycerin; PCWP, pulmonary capillary wedge pressure; SBP, systolic blood pressure; SCr, serum creatinine. (Adapted with permission from Forrester JS et al. Correlative classification of clinical and hemodynamic function after acute myocardial infarction. *Am J Cardiol*. 1977;39:137.)

The guidelines[1] recommend the addition of vasodilators in conjunction with diuretics to reduce congestion in patients with fluid overload. In the presence of asymptomatic hypotension, IV NTG, nitroprusside, or nesiritide may be considered cautiously in combination with diuretics. In the presence of low SVR, arterial vasodilators (e.g., nitroprusside, high-dose NTG, nesiritide) can further compromise perfusion and should be avoided, especially in patients who have preexisting hypotension.

NITROPRUSSIDE

Nitroprusside dilates both arterial and venous vessels, decreasing afterload and preload. Nitroprusside is valuable in severely congested patients with HTN or severe mitral valve regurgitation complicating LV dysfunction. Its major disadvantages include risk of hypotension, reflex tachycardia, "coronary steal" in CAD patients, and accumulation of toxic metabolites. Thiocyanate and cyanide toxicity are most likely seen in renal insufficiency and in patients who receive more than 4 mcg/kg/minute of nitroprusside for greater than 48 hours. When stopping nitroprusside therapy, a slow taper is recommended because a rebound increase in HF has been observed 10 to 30 minutes after drug withdrawal (see Chapter 16, Hypertensive Crises).

Nitroprusside must be given by continuous IV infusion, with arterial line placement and intensive care unit admission in most institutions. It is unstable if exposed to heat and light after reconstitution.

INTRAVENOUS NITROGLYCERIN

NTG primarily dilates the venous capacitance vessels with a slight effect on the arterial bed. Patients with acute MI and pulmonary edema are often considered ideal candidates for IV NTG. The resulting reduction in preload reduces PCWP. Because nitrates have minimal effect on afterload, CO will likely remain unchanged or increase slightly. In some patients, NTG could decrease CO if preload is reduced to less than 15 mm Hg. NTG is generally initiated at 10 mcg/minute and increased by increments of 10 to 20 mcg, until the patient's symptoms are improved or PCWP is less than 16 mm Hg. The most common side effect is headache, which can be treated with analgesics and often resolves after continuous therapy. Tachyphylaxis to NTG occurs within 24 hours after initiation of therapy. Approximately 20% of HF patients exhibit resistance to high doses of NTG.[1] Nitroprusside is a good choice for patients such as L.M. because he has elevated BP and no history of CAD.

NESIRITIDE

Nesiritide is recombinantly produced BNP.[31,32] BNP binds to guanylate cyclase receptors on vascular smooth muscle leading to expression of cyclic guanosine monophosphate and vasodilation. Other actions include inhibition of ACE, sympathetic outflow, and ET-1. Peripheral and coronary dilation coupled with improved RBF and increased glomerular filtration all contribute to the beneficial effects of nesiritide. Metabolic clearance of nesiritide is by a combination of binding to cell surfaces with cellular internalization and lysosomal proteolysis as well as proteolytic cleavage by endopeptidase. It undergoes minimal renal clearance. The elimination half-life is 8 to 22 minutes, necessitating a constant IV infusion.

In clinical trials of hospitalized patients with severe HF, nesiritide produced hemodynamic effects and reduction in dyspnea scores comparable to NTG when used in combination with IV diuretics and either dopamine or dobutamine.[31,32] Dose-dependent hypotension is the most common side effect with nesiritide, reported in 11% to 32% of patients. The incidence of PVC and nonsustained ventricular tachycardia is less with nesiritide than with dopamine, dobutamine, or milrinone. Nesiritide's side effects include headache, abdominal pain, nausea, anxiety, bradycardia, and leg cramps.

The use of nesiritide is generally restricted to those patients with acute HF exacerbations who are hypervolemic and have a PCWP greater than 18 mm Hg despite high doses of diuretics and IV NTG. In contrast to NTG, nesiritide has natriuretic properties that are additive to loop diuretics. It should be avoided in patients with a systolic BP less than 90 mg Hg or in cases of cardiogenic shock. Dobutamine or milrinone should be added or substituted in hypotensive patients or those with a cardiac index of less than 2.2 L/minute/m^2.

The IV infusion of nesiritide is prepared by diluting the contents of a 1.5-mg vial to 6 mcg/mL in 250 mL of 5% dextrose or 0.9% NaCl. An initial loading dose of 2 mcg/kg is sometimes given intravenously over 60 seconds, followed by a continuous IV infusion at a rate of 0.01 mcg/kg/minute. The desired response is a reduction of PCWP of 5 to 10 mm Hg at 15 minutes. The dose can be increased in 0.005 mcg/kg/minute increments at 3-hour intervals to a maximum of 0.03 mcg/kg/minute. Dosage should be titrated to a PCWP less than 18 mm Hg and a systolic BP greater than 90 mm Hg.

Although nesiritide is indicated in the treatment of ADHF, concerns were raised about its safety. A meta-analysis of randomized, controlled trials of nesiritide in ADHF suggests that nesiritide may be associated with worsening renal function and increased mortality.[263,264] The conclusions of the meta-analysis have been criticized, however. For example, the Vasodilation in the Management of Acute Congestive Heart Failure (VMAC) study was included in the meta-analysis but was not designed to evaluate renal end points, and therefore its inclusion may not be appropriate.[265] Differences in baseline characteristics of the treatment groups may have contributed to an increased risk of 30-day mortality seen in those patients treated with nesiritide.

The efficacy and safety of nesiritide have been evaluated in outpatients. The Follow-up Serial Infusions of Nesiritide (FUSION I) trial[266] included 202 patients with NYHA class III and IV who had been hospitalized for ADHF at least twice within the preceding year and once in the preceding month. Patients were randomly assigned to receive usual care with or without open-label nesiritide. A subgroup of patients was identified as high risk if they had at least four of the following: SCr greater than 2.0 mg/dL during the preceding month, NYHA class IV for the preceding 2 months, age greater than 65 years, history of sustained ventricular tachycardia, ischemic HF etiology, diabetes, or use of nesiritide or inotropic agents as outpatients within the preceding 6 months. These patients at high risk experienced fewer HF exacerbations and renal adverse effects with nesiritide infusions.

The benefit and safety in outpatients with severe HF was further explored in the Follow-Up Serial Infusions of Nesiritide for the Management of Patients With Heart Failure (FUSION II) trial.[267] This was a randomized, placebo-controlled, double-blind prospective trial of 911 subjects with advanced HF or chronic decompensated HF. Subjects were randomly assigned to receive a 2-mcg/kg nesiritide bolus followed by a 0.01-mcg/kg/minute infusion for 4 to 6 hours, or a matching placebo regimen, once or twice weekly for 12 weeks. Both groups also received optimal medical therapy and device therapy. Patients were required to have a creatinine clearance less than 60 mL/minute. No outpatient IV inotropic or vasodilator therapy was allowed. After 24 weeks, no difference was noted in the primary end point of either death or hospitalization for cardiac or renal causes. Significantly more drug-related adverse events (mainly hypotension) occurred in the nesiritide group (42.0%) compared with placebo (27.5%). The incidence of worsening renal function was significantly lower with nesiritide (32%) vs. placebo (39%).

The results of these studies alleviated some concerns regarding the safety of nesiritide; however, a group of independent cardiologists designed an "Acute Study of Clinical Effectiveness of Nesiritide in Decompensated Heart Failure" (ASCEND-HF)[268,269] trial to definitively answer the question of nesiritide safety and efficacy. This was a double-blind placebo trial, which enrolled 7,141 patients with ADHF. The participants were randomly assigned to receive an IV bolus (at the investigator's discretion) of nesiritide 2 mcg/kg or placebo followed by continuous IV infusion of nesiritide 0.01 mcg/kg/minute or placebo for 7 days in addition to standard therapy. The co-primary end points were the rate of HF hospitalizations or all-cause mortality through day 30 and a significant improvement in self-assessed dyspnea at 6 or 24 hours. Compared with placebo, nesiritide did not reduce 30-day mortality or rehospitalization. Nesiritide improved dyspnea at 6 and 24 hours compared with placebo. Nesiritide did not worsen renal function. Proponents of nesiritide argue that even though the ASCEND-HF trial failed to show a major benefit, it is the only vasodilator that has been well studied. The controversy regarding the safety of nesiritide can be put to rest.

L.M. responded well to nitroprusside and needed no other therapy. However, IV NTG and IV nesiritide are alternatives to nitroprusside in patients with "wet and warm" acute HF. NTG or nesiritide can either be a substitute for nitroprusside or be combined with nitroprusside. At the time of discharge, furosemide therapy should be continued, although the dose should be titrated to prevent DOE and peripheral edema. The dose of lisinopril and carvedilol should also be titrated to target or tolerated doses.

Inotropic Agents

CASE 14-5

QUESTION 1: B.J. is a 60-year-old man who presents to the emergency department with worsening DOE. He reports increased SOB during the last week. His medical history includes HTN, CAD, hyperlipidemia, and HF (EF 25%). His medications include metoprolol succinate 100 mg daily, enalapril 5 mg twice daily, furosemide 40 mg BID, aspirin 81 mg daily, and lovastatin 20 mg at bedtime. His vital signs on admission include BP 100/75 mm Hg, HR 92 bpm, respiratory rate 18 breaths/minute, and O_2 saturation 94% on room air. Laboratory values were BUN 20 mg/dL and SCr 1.4 mg/dL. Physical examination reveals pulmonary and peripheral edema and JVP 10 cm. He is given 80 mg IV furosemide with minimal response. His dose was increased to 120 mg IV furosemide and he still does not respond adequately. Within the last 24 hours his SCr has increased to 1.8 mg/dL and his BP is 92/70 mm Hg. The decision is made to admit him to the coronary care unit where a pulmonary artery catheter (Swan–Ganz catheter) is placed, and the following hemodynamic variables are: PCWP 21 mm Hg; CO 3.64 L/min (cardiac index 1.8 L/minute/m^2); SVR 1,489 dyne·second/cm^5. Is B.J. a candidate for inotropic therapy?

DOPAMINE AND DOBUTAMINE

The hemodynamic profile of B.J. is category IV (cold and wet) because of hypoperfusion and congestion. According to the ACC/AHA guidelines,[1] IV inotropic agents (dobutamine, dopamine, milrinone) are indicated in symptomatic patients with reduced LVEF, low CO, or end-organ dysfunction (i.e., worsening renal function) and in patients who are intolerant to vasodilators. They are recommended for patients with cardiogenic shock or refractory symptoms, and may be used in patients requiring perioperative support after surgery or for those awaiting transplantation. Dobutamine is usually preferred in patients with low-output HF. Dobutamine improves CO, decreases PCWP, and decreases total SVR with little effect on HR or systemic arterial pressure when compared with dopamine.[270] (See Chapter 17, Shock, for further information on dopamine and dobutamine.)

PHOSPHODIESTERASE INHIBITORS: MILRINONE

Although β-agonists, such as dobutamine, have been traditionally used in patients with ADHF, the phosphodiesterase inhibitor milrinone is an alternative to the catecholamines and vasodilators for the short-term parenteral treatment of severe congestive failure. This agent selectively inhibits phosphodiesterase III, the cyclic adenosine monophosphate (cAMP)-specific cardiac phosphodiesterase. Enzyme inhibition results in increased cAMP levels in myocardial cells and enhances contractility. The activity is not blocked by β-blockers. Phosphodiesterase inhibitors are also vasodilators. It has been suggested that at low doses they act more as unloading agents rather than as inotropic agents; others refute this viewpoint. Their overall hemodynamic effect probably results from a combination of positive inotropic action plus preload and afterload reduction.

Milrinone is structurally and pharmacologically similar to inamrinone, which is no longer used.[271–273] Besides inhibiting phosphodiesterase, it also may increase calcium availability to myocardial muscle. It has both inotropic and vasodilating properties. HR increase and myocardial consumption may be less with milrinone than with dobutamine[274,275] The half-life of milrinone is 1.5 to 2.5 hours, with renal clearance accounting for approximately 80% to 90% of total body elimination and is prolonged in patients with renal dysfunction. Although a loading dose of 50 mcg/kg is in the product labeling, it is rarely given due to resulting hypotension. Maintenance infusions are typically between 0.2 and 0.75 mcg/kg/minute. The infusion is adjusted according to hemodynamic and clinical responses and should be decreased in patients with renal insufficiency. The primary concern with milrinone is ventricular arrhythmias, reported in up to 12% of patients. Supraventricular arrhythmias, hypotension, headache, and chest pain also have been reported. Thrombocytopenia is rare.

The Outcomes of a Prospective Trial of Intravenous Milrinone for Chronic Heart Failure (OPTIME-CHF) trial assessed the in-hospital management of 951 patients with acute HF exacerbation (mean LVEF 23%) but not in cardiogenic shock.[274,275] In addition to standard diuretic and ACEI therapy, subjects were randomly assigned to receive either milrinone or placebo. The initial milrinone infusion rate was 0.5 mcg/kg/minute with no loading dose. The primary end point was total numbers of days hospitalized for CV causes from the time of the start of study drug infusion to day 60. No difference was found between milrinone and placebo with mortality at 60 days (10.3% with milrinone and 8.9% with placebo).[274] Follow-up analysis categorized subjects as ischemic vs. nonischemic.[275] Within the cohort of patients with ischemia, milrinone-treated patients tended to have worse outcomes than those treated with placebo. In contrast, nonischemic patients had a trend toward better outcomes with milrinone than with placebo. From these data, it can be concluded that the benefits of milrinone in patients with acute exacerbations of HF are minimal and more likely to be seen in patients with a nonischemic etiology of HF. Worse outcomes may be seen in patients with ischemic HF. However, short-term infusions of milrinone were not associated with excess mortality.

Few trials have compared dobutamine to milrinone in ADHF. One small retrospective analysis evaluated 329 patients admitted for ADHF (EF of less than 20%) who either received IV dobutamine or milrinone.[276] Hemodynamic response, need for additional therapies, adverse effects, length of stay, and drug cost were evaluated. Patients were similar in clinical presentation, but the milrinone group had higher mean pulmonary arterial pressure. A greater percentage of patients received dobutamine (81.7%)

versus milrinone (18.3%.). Only 19% of patients were taking β-blockers before admission. Clinical outcomes were similar and there was no significant difference in the in-hospital mortality rate, adverse effects, ventilator use, or length of stay. More patients in the dobutamine group required nitroprusside to achieve optimal hemodynamic response. The study concluded that both drugs have comparable efficacy.

Other factors to consider when deciding which inotropic agent should be used in ADHF are renal function, BP, and concomitant β-blocker use. Milrinone has a longer half-life than dobutamine, and accumulates in cases of renal dysfunction. Milrinone is also a vasodilator, which can limit its use in patients with hypotension. The concomitant use of β-blockers may antagonize the action of dobutamine.

B.J. has responded poorly to IV furosemide, his renal function has deteriorated, and his systolic BP is low. Patients with advanced HF and systemic hypoperfusion often will not tolerate vasodilator therapy. Inotropic agents may be necessary to maintain circulatory function in these patients. According to guidelines, IV inotropic drugs may be considered for patients who have symptomatic hypotension despite adequate filling pressure, who are unresponsive to diuretics and intolerant to vasodilators, or who have worsening renal function. Phosphodiesterase inhibitors are sometimes preferred over dobutamine for patients who are receiving concomitant β-blockers. For the abovementioned reasons, B.J. is a candidate for milrinone therapy. Patients should be on telemetry because milrinone has the potential to cause arrhythmias. Vital signs, SCr, symptom relief, and urine output should be monitored. Once the patient's hemodynamic profile improves, milrinone should be discontinued, and oral furosemide therapy can be resumed. At discharge, the outpatient HF medications should be optimized.

Outpatient Inotropic Infusions

CASE 14-5, QUESTION 2: Are there any indications for using repeated intermittent infusions of inotropic agents as part of a home-care regimen?

The long-term safety and efficacy of inotropic therapy is regarded with skepticism. There are few studies assessing intermittent (e.g., weekly) infusions of dobutamine or milrinone. Nearly all the data on this therapeutic approach are from open-label and uncontrolled trials that compare two inotropic agents without a placebo.[277–281] It is thought that long-term therapy may be cardiotoxic. The only placebo-controlled trial of intermittent infusion of dobutamine was terminated because of excess mortality with dobutamine.[278] Death occurred in 32% of patients treated with dobutamine versus 14% with placebo. Whether this was caused by progression of underlying heart disease, continued drug therapy, or was a cardiotoxic effect remains unknown. No corresponding data exist for milrinone, although a placebo-controlled trial with milrinone failed to support the routine use of IV milrinone as an adjunct to standard therapy in the treatment of patients hospitalized for an acute exacerbation of chronic HF.[274,275] For this reason, the ACA/AHA guidelines indicate that intermittent infusions of dobutamine and milrinone in the long-term treatment of HF, even in advanced stages, should be avoided.[4] Chronic continuous infusions of dobutamine and milrinone are sometimes administered in patients with refractory HF as palliative therapy or in those awaiting transplant. The lowest dose possible should be administered. The HFSA identifies the limited treatment options in advanced HF and proposes patient-centered outcomes (survival vs. quality of life, palliative and hospice care) to be incorporated into care plans.[282]

Ventricular Arrhythmias Complicating Heart Failure

AMIODARONE

CASE 14-5, QUESTION 3: B.J. was stabilized during the next several days and discharged home with furosemide 40 mg daily, enalapril 5 mg twice daily, metoprolol succinate 100 mg daily, aspirin 81 mg daily, and NTG 0.4 mg sublingual to be used as needed for chest pain. His EF is 23%. Laboratory values were normal. ECG monitoring during B.J.'s hospital stay showed normal sinus rhythm, with 15 to 20 asymptomatic PVCs/hour. At that time, it was decided not to treat his arrhythmia other than with metoprolol because he was asymptomatic. For the next several months, he continued to have frequent PVCs during follow-up examinations.

It has now been 5 months and he is still having up to 12 to 15 PVCs/hour. His exercise capacity is limited by SOB after walking about a block despite having enalapril increased to 20 mg/day, metoprolol succinate to 200 mg/day, and adding digoxin 0.25 mg/day. The furosemide is at 40 mg/day because he has edema. A repeat echocardiogram shows an EF of 20%. Is an antiarrhythmic agent indicated for B.J. at this time? What is the agent of choice, and what dose should be given?

PVCs and other arrhythmias are a common complication of LV dysfunction and may be present regardless of whether the patient has had an MI. Approximately 50% to 70% of patients with HF have episodes of nonsustained ventricular tachycardia on ambulatory monitoring.[4] This myocardial irritability may be a result of autonomic hyperactivity or ventricular remodeling. It is not clear whether these rhythm disturbances contribute to sudden death or simply reflect the underlying disease process. Recent studies suggest that bradyarrhythmia or electromechanical dissociation may be associated with sudden death in HF patients with nonischemic cardiomyopathy.[283,284] More importantly, suppression of ventricular ectopy in patients with HF has not been shown to lead to a reduction of sudden death in clinical trials. Neither prophylactic antiarrhythmic therapy nor treatment of asymptomatic PVC after an MI has been proven to improve outcome or survival. Because of concerns about the proarrhythmic effects of most class IA and class IC drugs, treatment with these agents is contraindicated.

Amiodarone has value in patients with HF with arrhythmias because it has antiarrhythmic and coronary vasodilating effects as well as α- and β-blocking properties. It may offer a dual benefit to reduce myocardial irritability and improve the hemodynamics of HF.

In the Grupo de Estudio de la Sobrevida en la Insuficiecia Cardiaca en Argentina (GESICA) study,[285] 516 patients with class II to IV HF symptoms (average EF 20%), and frequent PVCs were randomly assigned to receive either standard treatment (diuretics, vasodilators, digoxin) or a fixed dose of amiodarone plus standard treatment. The dose of amiodarone was 600 mg daily for 2 weeks, then 300 mg/day for at least 1 year. Fewer patients on amiodarone (33.5%) died compared with those receiving standard treatment (41.4%), a statistically significant difference. Similarly, the number of HF-related hospitalizations was reduced with amiodarone.

Somewhat different outcomes were noted in the Veterans Administration (VA) Cooperative Survival Trial of Antiarrhythmic Therapy in Congestive Heart Failure (CHF-STAT) study.[286,287] Entry criteria to this trial were similar to those in the GESICA study, with a primary indicator being more than 10 asymptomatic PVCs per hour on 24-hour monitoring, but without sustained ventricular tachycardia. A higher dose of amiodarone was used, 800 mg for 2 weeks, then 400 mg/day for 1 year. The dose was reduced to 300 mg/day after the first year, with the average follow-up being 45 months. No difference was found between groups for either all-cause mortality or SCD. EF improved more in the patients treated with amiodarone, rising from a baseline average of 24.9% to 33.7%. The corresponding change in the standard treatment group was from a baseline of 25.8% to 29.2% at follow-up. Despite the increase in EF, symptom scores did not differ between the two groups.

Amiodarone does not have a negative effect on mortality as seen with some of the other antiarrhythmic agents. Other factors to consider are the potential for significant side effects with amiodarone (see Chapter 15, Cardiac Arrhythmias) and the drug interaction with digoxin leading to the potential for digoxin toxicity.

The ACC/AHA guidelines do not recommend routine ambulatory ECG monitoring to detect asymptomatic ventricular arrhythmias, and recommend against treatment if such arrhythmias are inadvertently detected.[1,5,6] If symptomatic ventricular arrhythmias should arise or there is determined to be a high risk for sudden death, one of the following should be considered: a β-blocking drug, amiodarone, or an ICD. Nearly all patients with HF should have a β-blocker as part of their regimen because these drugs reduce all-cause mortality, not just sudden death. B.J. continued to have ectopy despite continued use of a β-blocker. Nonetheless, it is decided not to use amiodarone because he is asymptomatic.

IMPLANTABLE CARDIOVERTER-DEFIBRILLATOR

CASE 14-5, QUESTION 4: Is B.J. a candidate for an ICD implantation?

Although amiodarone is the preferred antiarrhythmic agent in patients with HF with reduced EF to prevent recurrent AF and symptomatic ventricular arrhythmias, it has not improved survival. Ventricular arrhythmias are associated with a high frequency of SCD in patients with HF. Numerous trials have established the role of ICDs in primary and secondary prevention of SCD. The earliest of the primary prevention trials was the Multicenter Automatic Defibrillator Implantation Trial (MADIT).[288] This study was terminated early because of the survival benefit seen in the ICD group compared with conventional therapy. There was no evidence that amiodarone, β-blockers, or any other antiarrhythmic therapy had a significant influence on the results. Unlike MADIT, the MADIT II[290] study enrolled patients with no documented arrhythmias but with previous MI and LVEF less than 30%. Patients received either an ICD or conventional medical therapy. The primary end point was death from any cause. There was a 31% relative reduction in the risk of death and an absolute reduction of 6% in the ICD group. This was the first trial to show mortality benefits of ICDs in patients with no documented history of abnormal heart rhythms.

The Sudden Cardiac Death in Heart Failure trial (SCD-HeFT) evaluated the efficacy of amiodarone in patients with LV dysfunction (EF $\leq$ 35%).[290] The patients (NYHA class II–III) were receiving conventional therapy and randomly assigned to placebo, amiodarone, or an ICD. Amiodarone was no better than placebo, whereas ICD decreased mortality by 23% ($p = 0.007$). A subgroup analysis showed that patients with class II HF had a greater drop in mortality with ICD use than class III patients, whereas amiodarone decreased survival in class III. The role of amiodarone in patients with NYHA class III needs to be further evaluated before it is routinely used in patients with LV dysfunction.

The ACC/AHA guidelines[1] recommend the use of ICDs in patients after MI with reduced LVEF and who have a history of ventricular arrhythmias. ICDs are also recommended for primary prevention in patients with nonischemic cardiomyopathy and ischemic heart disease who have an LVEF of 30% or less, those with NYHA functional class II or III symptoms while on optimal standard oral therapy, and patients who have reasonable expected survival with a good functional status of one or more years. Patients with ischemic heart disease should receive an ICD at least 40 days after MI. B.J. is currently on optimal HF drug regimen, and his EF is 20%. According to guidelines, B.J. would benefit from ICD implantation.

CARDIAC RESYNCHRONIZATION THERAPY

CASE 14-6

QUESTION 1: C.M., a 49-year-old woman with a history of cardiomyopathy (EF 25%), presents to the HF clinic with NYHA class III symptoms. She reports increased SOB, chest pain, and fatigue. She has been optimized on drug therapy for 3 months. Her medications include metoprolol succinate 200 mg daily, furosemide 40 mg BID, lisinopril 20 mg daily, and spironolactone 25 mg daily. An ECG showed sinus rhythm at a rate of 72 bpm and a QRS duration of 144 ms. Is she a candidate for CRT?

Approximately one-third of the patients with advanced systolic HF exhibit intraventricular or interventricular conduction delays that cause the ventricles to beat asynchronously.[291] Ventricular dyssynchrony is seen on ECG as a wide QRS complex with a left bundle branch block, and can lead to deleterious effects on cardiac function. Patients may present with reduced EF, decreased CO, and presence of NYHA class III or IV HF symptoms. These are all associated with increased mortality.

CRT is the use of cardiac pacing to coordinate the contraction of the left and right ventricles.[77] Initial randomized trials of CRT show reduced HF symptoms and improved exercise tolerance and quality of life. The Comparison of Medical Therapy, Pacing, and Defibrillator in Heart Failure (COMPANION) trial[77] enrolled 1,520 patients with NYHA class II or IV (QRS interval of at least 120 ms, and LVEF $\leq$35%) who were treated with optimal drug therapy (ACEIs, diuretics, β-blockers, and spironolactone). Patients were randomly assigned to receive optimal drug therapy alone, optimal drug therapy and CRT with a pacemaker, or optimal drug therapy and CRT with ICD (CRT-D). The primary end point was a composite of all-cause mortality and hospitalization. Both CRT and CRT-D groups were associated with a decreased risk of primary end point compared with optimal drug therapy alone. All-cause mortality at 1 year was decreased by 24% in the CRT group (which did not reach statistical significance) and 43% in the CRT-D group.

The results of the Cardiac Resynchronization in Heart Failure study (CARE-HF)[76] extended the findings of the COMPANION trial. CARE-HF demonstrated a significant all-cause mortality reduction for CRT pacing without defibrillator backup (CRT) in patients with HF who received similar medical treatment. The inclusion criteria were NYHA class III or IV, EF of 35% or less, and QRS duration of 120 ms or longer. The primary end point of all-cause deaths and hospitalizations for a CV reason occurred in fewer patients with CRT compared with the optimal drug therapy (39% vs. 55%; $p < 0.001$). Death or hospitalization for worsening HF was also significantly reduced with CRT.

The combined results of CARE-HF and COMPANION confirm the importance of CRT and CRT-D in improving ventricular function, HF symptoms, and exercise tolerance, while also reducing frequency of HF hospitalizations and death.[292] The role of CRT in patients with mild HF symptoms, narrow QRS, chronic AF, and right bundle branch block needs to be explored.

According to the ACC/AHA guidelines,[1] patients with NYHA class III and ambulatory patients with class IV HF should receive CRT (unless contraindicated) if they meet the following criteria: LVEF of 35% or less, presence of a wide QRS (>120 ms), and receiving optimal HF standard medical therapy. Despite optimal doses of HF medications, C.M. continues to have HF symptoms. CRT therapy could provide incremental benefits beyond what is provided with drug therapy.

CASE 14-6, QUESTION 2: If C.M. presented with NYHA class I or II symptoms, would she be a candidate for CRT therapy? What is the evidence to support CRT in NYHA class I and II patients?

As mentioned in Case 14-6, Question 1, the CARE-HF and COMPANION trials provide strong evidence that CRT induces reverse modeling in patients with symptomatic NYHA class III and ambulatory class IV HF. The next logical step was to evaluate the benefits of CRT therapy in HF patients with milder symptoms. The Multicenter InSynch ICD Randomized Clinical Evaluation (MIRACLE-ICDII)[293] trial randomized class II through IV HF patients but with separate specified end points for class II patients. In this trial, 186 patients with NYHA class II HF, an LVEF of less than 35%, and a QRS of more than 130 ms received a CRT-ICD device. Subjects were randomly assigned to active CRT group (ICD activated and CRT on) or control group (ICD activated and CRT off). The primary end point was progression of HF, defined as all-cause mortality, hospitalizations for HF, and ventricular tachycardia or ventricular fibrillation requiring device intervention. A 15% reduction in HF progression was observed with active CRT, but did not reach statistical significance. At 6 months, patients with active CRT had improved exercise tolerance, but this was not significantly different from the control group. However, there was a significant decrease in ventricular end-systolic volume and increased LVEF after 6 months of therapy. Even though the study results did not translate into improved exercise tolerance, it helped to set the stage for future trials in patients with less symptomatic HF.

The REVERSE trial[74] enrolled 610 participants with NYHA class I or II HF, LVEF less than 40%, and with a QRS duration of more than 120 ms who received a CRT device (with or without ICD) in combination with optimal drug therapy. The patients in the active CRT group had significant improvement in LV end-systolic volume index, LV end-diastolic volume index, and LVEF compared to control. The primary clinical end point (the percentage of patients with worsened clinical composite score) did not reach statistical significance at 12 months in patients enrolled in the United States, but in the European cohort[294] a significant difference was seen at 24 months, primarily driven by the time to first hospitalization The aggregate data from these two clinical trials provided overwhelming evidence that linked CRT with substantial reverse remodeling in mild HF patients.

The MADIT-CRT[75] was the largest randomized trial designed to determine whether CRT-D therapy would reduce the primary end point (all-cause mortality or HF events) when compared with patients receiving ICD-only therapy. The study population involved cardiac patients in NYHA functional class I or II with LVEF of 30% or less and QRS duration of more than 130 ms. There was a 34% ($p < 0.001$) reduction in the primary end point, and a 44% ($p < 0.001$) reduction in HF events when compared with ICD therapy. Patients with CRT-D therapy showed an 11% improvement in LVEF after 1 year, compared with 3% improvement for ICD-alone patients. Both MADIT-CRT and REVERSE excluded patients with AF. Both studies failed to show a benefit for CRT in patients with QRS duration less than 150 ms.

The Resynchronization/Defibrillation for Ambulatory Heart Failure Trial (RAFT)[295] confirmed that CRT benefited patients with a QRS duration of 150 ms or more and in those with left bundle branch block. The RAFT investigators randomly assigned 1,798 patients with NYHA class II or III HF, LVEF of 30% or less, and a QRS duration of at least 120 ms (or a paced QRS of at least 200 ms) to either ICD therapy alone or an ICD with CRT (CRT-D). The primary outcome was a combination of total mortality and HF hospitalization, which was significantly higher in the ICD group compared with the ICD-CRT group (40% vs. 33%, respectively). These findings demonstrate that earlier intervention with CRT-D, in addition to guideline recommended medical and ICD therapy, benefits this patient population.

HEART FAILURE WITH PRESERVED EJECTION FRACTION

CASE 14-7

QUESTION 1: D.F., a 72-year-old white woman, has a 5-year history of HF symptoms, including decreased exercise capacity, SOB, and distended neck veins. She has minimal peripheral edema. History is suggestive of rheumatic fever as a child, but she does not recall having any cardiac symptoms when she was younger, other than being told she had a murmur. Her symptoms are controlled with diuretics. She has HTN but no other medical problems, and all laboratory test findings are normal. Her BP is 155/85 mm Hg, and HR is 90 bpm. Cardiac examination reveals a prominent S_4 heart sound. Echocardiography reveals an EF of 50%. Prior treatment included furosemide, most recently at 40 mg BID. The physician is considering adding a β-blocker or CCB to control the BP and HR. Why might this consideration be appropriate?

This case exemplifies a patient with HF with preserved LVEF (HFpEF), previously referred to as diastolic HF. Risk factors for HFpEF include advanced age, female sex, HTN, and CAD. This diagnosis can be made on the basis of LVH, clinical evidence of HF, a normal EF, and echocardiography findings. The ideal treatment for HFpEF has not been extensively validated. A review of trials evaluating specific drug therapy in HFpEF is listed in Table 14-13. No drug selectively enhances myocardial relaxation without having associated effects on LV contractility or on the peripheral vasculature.[12,52–54,296]

Factors affecting HF control, such as adherence to medication and diet, including NSAID and herbal remedy use, should be appropriately managed along with drug therapy. Symptomatic HFpEF is initially treated similar to other forms of HF, by slow diuresis. Diuresis decreases preload and lessens passive congestion of the ventricles. Excessive lowering of ventricular filling pressures, however, can decrease CO and cause hypotension.

The most common cause of HFpEF is HTN that leads to LVH and decreased cardiac compliance.[297] The ACC/AHA/HFSA guidelines recommend a SPB goal of <130 mmHg in patients with HFpEF and persistent hypertension after management of fluid overload. Drugs that cause regression of LVH (e.g., ACEIs, ARBs, β-blockers) may also slow or reverse structural abnormalities associated with HFpEF.

In the Perindopril in Elderly patients with Chronic HF (PEP-CHF) trial,[298] the ACEI perindopril failed to reduce the incidence of the primary end point (all-cause mortality or HF hospitalizations), but did reduce symptoms and improved functional capacity. The CHARM-preserved trial[156] also failed to show any difference in CV mortality, but fewer hospitalizations were seen in the candesartan group (see Case 14-1, Question 13).

The Valsartan in Diastolic Dysfunction (VALIDD)[299] trial compared the effects of valsartan or placebo added to standard antihypertensive therapy (which included diuretics, β-blockers, CCBs, or α-blockers) in patients with mild HTN and diastolic dysfunction. The hypothesis of this trial was that RAAS inhibition with an ARB would be associated with greater improvement in diastolic function, due to more regression of LVH or myocardial fibrosis. Patients with a history of stage 1 or 2 essential HTN were randomly assigned to receive either valsartan 160 mg, titrated up to 320 mg, or matching placebo. Patients who did not achieve a target BP goal of less than 135/80 mm Hg received additional therapy starting with a diuretic followed by a CCB or a β-blocker, then an α-blocker. ARBs, ACEIs, and aldosterone blockers were excluded. The primary end point was the change in diastolic myocardial relaxation velocity from baseline to 9 months with a secondary end point of change in LV mass. During the study, the placebo group received more concomitant antihypertensive therapy compared with the valsartan group. A small, but significant, increase was seen in diastolic relaxation velocity in both groups from baseline to follow-up, but there was no significant difference between the treatment groups. BP reduction did not differ significantly between the two treatment groups, and was associated with significant improvement in diastolic function. The authors concluded that aggressive BP control—even in mild HTN—was associated with improvement in diastolic dysfunction, irrespective of whether BP reduction was achieved with a RAAS inhibitor or other antihypertensive agent.

CHARM-Preserved[156] investigated the role of candesartan in patients with HFpEF. The trial enrolled 3,023 subjects who met the overall CHARM trial inclusion criteria with an EF of more than 40% (mean, 54%). Subjects had symptomatic HF with normal (preserved) EF. They received either an ARB alone (n = 1,514) or placebo; only 20% of subjects in both groups were taking an ACEI at randomization, 56% a β-blocker, and 11% spironolactone.[156] After a median follow-up of 36.6 months, a trend was noted toward reduction in the primary outcome of CV death or hospital admission for HF in the candesartan group (22%) compared with placebo (24.3%; $p = 0.118$). CV deaths and all-cause mortality were nearly identical in both groups, but the total number of hospitalizations for HF was significantly reduced in the candesartan group. The most common side effects with candesartan were hypotension (2.4%), increase in creatinine (4.8%), and hyperkalemia (1.5%). Discontinuation because of an adverse event occurred in 17.8% of those treated with candesartan compared with 13.5% of placebo recipients ($p = 0.001$) (Table 14-13). Overall, in symptomatic patients with HFpEF, no significant improvement in mortality occurs with candesartan compared with placebo, but there was a significant reduction in HF-related hospitalizations.

I-PRESERVE evaluated irbesartan titrated to 300 mg daily or placebo for the management of HFpEF.[300] The patient population was 60 years of age or older with NYHA class II through IV symptoms, EF of at least 45%, and hospitalized for HF within 6 months prior, or have persistent class III or IV symptoms (n = 4,128). There was no difference in the primary end point (death from any cause or hospitalization for a CV cause) between irbesartan (36%) and placebo (37%). The irbesartan group had more patients experiencing hyperkalemia than placebo. One possible reason for the neutral results of I-PRESERVE included the high rate of dual RAAS blockade at baseline (39% ACEI use in the irbesartan group and 40% in the placebo group; 28% spironolactone use in

Table 14-13

Clinical Trials of Pharmacotherapy in Heart Failure with HFpEF

Study	Patient Population	Therapy Intervention	Outcome	Treatment Duration	Results
Aronow et al.[325]	NYHA III; Prior MI, EF >50%; (n = 21)	Enalapril vs. placebo	NYHA class, treadmill exercise time (seconds)	3 months	Enalapril: NYHA class from 3 ± 0 to 2.4 ± 0.5 (p = 0.005), exercise time from 224 ± 27 to 270 ± 44 (p <0.001) vs. no difference in placebo
Lang et al.[326]	HF symptoms >3 months; EF >50%; (n = 12)	Lisinopril vs. placebo crossover	Dyspnea and fatigue	5 weeks for each treatment arm	No significant differences
Cleland et al.[298] PEP-CHF	Diastolic dysfunction; CV admission within 6 months; EF >40%; n = 850)	Perindopril vs. placebo	Primary: composite of all-cause mortality or hospitalization for HF	Mean 26.2 months	Primary: 23.6% in perindopril group vs. 25.1% in placebo (HR 0.92 [0.70–1.21], p = 0.545)
Zi et al.[327]	NYHA class II or III; EF ≥40%; (n = 74)	Quinapril vs. placebo	6-minute walk test, QoL, NYHA class	6 months	No significant differences
Yusuf et al.[156] CHARM-Preserved	NYHA II–IV; hospitalization for CV causes; EF >40%; (n = 3,023)	Candesartan vs. placebo	Primary: CV death or hospital admission for HF	Median 36.6 months	Primary: 22% in the candesartan group vs. 24% in the placebo group (adjusted HR 0.86 [0.74–1.00], p = 0.051).
Massie et al.[300] I-PRESERVE	NYHA II–IV; hospitalized for HF in last 6 months; EF ≥45%; (n = 4,122)	Irbesartan vs. placebo	Primary: all-cause death or hospitalization for CV causes	Mean 49.5 months	Primary: 36% in the irbesartan group vs. 37% in the placebo group (HR 0.95 [95% CI 0.86–1.05], p = 0.35)
Yip et al.[328]	NYHA II–IV; history of HF in last 2 months; EF >45%; (n = 151)	Ramipril vs. irbesartan	QoL, 6-minute walk test, HF hospital admission	12 months	No significant differences

Table 14-13
Clinical Trials of Pharmacotherapy in Heart Failure with HFpEF (*continued*)

Study	Patient Population	Therapy Intervention	Outcome	Treatment Duration	Results
Warner et al.[329]	Diastolic dysfunction; DOE; EF >50%; SBP >150, <200 mm Hg (n = 20)	Losartan vs. placebo crossover	Exercise time, QoL	2 weeks for each treatment arm	Increase in exercise time (11.3 minutes at baseline, improved to 12.3 ± 2.6 minutes with losartan vs. 11.0 minutes with placebo, p <0.05) and improvement in QoL (25 at baseline, improved to 18 with losartan vs. 22 with placebo); p < 0.05 for both end points
Parthasarathy et al.[330]	Diastolic dysfunction; DOE; EF >40%; (n = 152)	Valsartan vs. placebo	Primary: exercise time	14 weeks	No significant differences
Takeda et al.[331]	NYHA II–III and stage C heart failure; EF ≥45%	Carvedilol vs. placebo	Plasma BNP, NYHA class, exercise capacity	12 months	NYHA class improved by 0.77 (carvedilol) vs. 0.25 (placebo) (p < 0.02), exercise capacity in METs improved 0.69 (carvedilol) vs. worsened by 0.07 (placebo) (p = 0.01).
Flather et al.[301] SENIORS	HF hospital admission in last year; EF ≤35%; subgroup EF ≥35%	Nebivolol vs. placebo	Primary: composite of all-cause mortality or hospitalization for a cardiovascular cause	Mean 21 months	EF >35%, primary event rate 17.6% in nebivolol and 21.9% in placebo (HR 0.86 [95% CI 0.74–0.99], p = 0.039).
Aronow et al.[332]	NYHA II–III; prior Q-wave MI; EF >40%; n = 158)	Propranolol vs. placebo	All-cause mortality, all-cause mortality plus nonfatal MI	32 months	All-cause mortality (56% propranolol group vs. 76% placebo group, p = 0.007) and all-cause mortality plus nonfatal MI (59% propranolol vs. 82% placebo, p = 0.002).
Setaro et al.[333]	Abnormal diastolic filling; EF >45%; (n = 20)	Verapamil vs. placebo	Exercise capacity	2 weeks for each crossover	Exercise capacity (10.7 minutes at baseline, improved to 13.9 minutes with verapamil vs. 12.3 minutes with placebo, p <0.05).
Ahmed et al.[334] DIG	NYHA I–IV; EF >45%; (n = 988)	Digoxin vs. placebo	Primary: composite of HF hospitalization or mortality	Mean 37 months	102 (21%) in the digoxin group vs. 119 (24%) in the placebo group (HR 0.82 [0.63–1.07], p = 0.136).
Pitt et al.[302] TOPCAT	Symptomatic HF; EF >45%; (n = 3445)	Spironolactone vs. placebo	Primary: composite of CV death, HF hospitalization, or aborted cardiac arrest	Mean 39 months	320 (18.6%) in the spironolactone group vs. 351 (20.4%) in the placebo group (HR 0.89 [0.77–1.04], p = 0.14).

BNP, B-type natriuretic peptide; CV, cardiovascular; DOE, dyspnea on exertion; EF, ejection fraction; HF, heart failure; HR, hazard ratio; METs, metabolic equivalents; MI, myocardial infarction; NA, not available; NYHA, New York Heart Association; QoL, quality of life; SBP, systolic blood pressure.

the irbesartan group and 29% in the placebo group). Based on this high use, the study is less likely to find benefit with ARBs in addition to other RAAS agents. Another potential limitation of the study included the high study discontinuation rate (34%). Overall, irbesartan showed no benefit in reducing morbidity or mortality in HFpEF patients.

β-Blockers or nondihydropyridine CCBs are other classes of drugs of interest in HFpEF. Part of their value is to control HTN, a risk factor for all forms of HF. More specific to HFpEF, *β*-blockers and CCBs (especially verapamil) possess negative inotropic properties that may favorably influence the pathophysiology of diastolic dysfunction by (a) slowing the HR to allow more time for complete ventricular filling particularly during exercise; (b) reducing myocardial oxygen demand; and (c) controlling BP. Both pharmacologic classes are beneficial in decreasing ischemia in patients with CAD.

Most HF trials with β-blockers demonstrating decreased morbidity and mortality have focused on HFrEF. The Study of the Effects of Nebivolol Intervention on Outcomes and Rehospitalization in Seniors with Heart Failure (SENIORS) study[301] evaluated β-blocker use in elderly HF patients irrespective of LV function. The trial randomly assigned patients to nebivolol or placebo. Nebivolol is a selective β_1-adernergic receptor blocker with vasodilator properties that are mediated through NO release. This effect may be beneficial in elderly patients who tend to have low reserves of endothelial vasodilation.

The primary end point of the study was the combination of all-cause mortality and CV hospital admissions. The end point was significantly reduced by 14% in the nebivolol group, regardless of the EF. Prospective subgroup analyses of the primary outcome by LVEF (≤35% or >35%), sex, or age (≤75 years or >75 years) showed benefits across all subgroups. Patients with EF greater than 35%, however, appeared to benefit a little more than those with low EF%, and all-cause mortality was lower in patients older than 75 years treated with nebivolol compared with placebo. The study reinforces the current recommendations that all HF patients with reduced EF should receive β-blockers. Only 35% of the patients had preserved LV function, and were mostly men. This is not typical of patients with HFpEF, who are frequently women. Further studies are required to define the role of β-blockers in HFpEF.

No randomized controlled trials have demonstrated mortality benefits with CCBs in HFpEF. Nondihydropyridine CCBs can be used in patients who have a contraindication to β-blockers to control BP and HR. Nondihydropyridine CCBs should not be used in patients with HFrEF.

The role of aldosterone antagonists in the management of patients with HFpEF has been evaluated in the Treatment of Preserved Cardiac Function Heart Failure with an Aldosterone Antagonist (TOPCAT) trial.[302] This trial evaluated the impact of spironolactone versus placebo on CV morbidity and mortality in patients older than 50 years of age with an EF greater than 45%. There was no difference in the primary end point (composite of CV death, aborted cardiac arrest, and hospitalization for HF) between the spironolactone and placebo treatment arms with a HR 0.89 (95% CI 0.77–1.04; $p = 0.14$). There was a significant reduction with spironolactone versus placebo in the secondary end point of hospitalization for HF (HR 0.83 [95% CI 0.69–0.99; $p = 0.04$]). There has also been a sub-analysis of the TOPCAT study evaluating differences in patients enrolled in the Americas compared to Russia/Georgia relative to the primary and secondary end points. When only looking at patients enrolled from North or South America, there was a significant reduction with the spironolactone-treated patients compared to placebo in the primary end point (HR 0.82 [95% CI 0.69–0.98]) and all secondary end points.[303] Based on these findings, the 2017 ACC/AHA/HFSA Focused Update recommend aldosterone receptor antagonists (class IIb) in HFrEF. An aldosterone receptor antagonist can be considered to decrease hospitalizations in patients with EF ≥ 45%, an elevated BNP or recent hospitalizations. If spironolactone is initiated, then potassium and renal function should be closely monitored (EGFR>30mL/min, creatinine, 2.5mg/dL, potassium <5.0mEq/L).[6]

D.F. fulfills the criteria for having HFpEF, based on her history of long-standing HTN, which has been poorly controlled. Her BP is not at goal, and her HR is elevated. Therefore, antihypertensive therapy is warranted. Tachycardia alone can compromise the ventricle filling time and cause myocardial ischemia. So far, no data support the use of one agent over another. β-Blockers and nondihydropyridine CCBs can each reduce BP and HR. β-Blockers are not considered first-line antihypertensive medications based on recent guidelines without a compelling indication. The use of a nondihydropyridine CCB would be supported in HFpEF patients to reduce both BP and HR. D.F. can be started on a nondihydropyridine CCB such as diltiazem sustained-release (120 mg daily).

Herbal Products and Nutritional Supplements

CASE 14-8

QUESTION 1: W.L., a 60-year-old man recently diagnosed by his naturopath with HF, is concerned about his decreasing exercise capacity and increasing SOB during his morning walks. The naturopath wants to initiate hawthorn and coenzyme Q10 to control his HF symptoms. The patient has uncontrolled HTN (170/85 mm Hg), and has 2+ ankle edema. He distrusts medical doctors because in the past he was given HCTZ for BP reduction, but stopped taking it after a few days because he did not tolerate the urinary urgency it caused. What is the role of herbal products and nutritional supplements in HF?

HAWTHORN

Hawthorn extracts from the leaves and flowers of *Crataegus monogyna* and *Crataegus oxyacantha* have been reported to have beneficial effects in mild HF.[304,305] Oligomeric procyanidins and flavonoids are considered the key active ingredients. Hawthorn extracts have shown positive inotropic effects, weak ACE inhibition, vasodilating properties, and increased coronary blood flow in vitro and in animal models. In short-term (8 weeks or less), placebo-controlled trials in patients with the equivalent of NYHA class II HF, modest improvements were noted in exercise tolerance and subjective symptoms as well as decreases in HR and BP. Patients with more advanced HF were excluded. A systematic review by Pittler et al. also concluded that hawthorn extract was efficacious in the treatment of HF when given with standard HF therapy.[306] Conversely, the results of the Hawthorne Extract Randomized Blinded Chronic Heart Failure (HERB-CHF) trial failed to provide any evidence that hawthorn was beneficial in patients with HF who were already receiving standard medical therapy.[307] In clinical trials, side effects of hawthorn include nausea, vomiting, diarrhea, palpitations, chest pain, and vertigo. These side effects are more common when doses exceed 900 mg/day, but in some trials they have not occurred more often than with placebo. The risks and benefits of using hawthorn and digoxin together, both of which have positive inotropic effects, are not known.

To further investigate the longer term benefits of hawthorn, additive effects to conventional therapy and effect on mortality were tested in the Survival and Prognosis: Investigation of Crataegus Extract WS 1442 in Congestive Heart Failure (SPICE) trial.[308] The trial enrolled 2,681 patients with NYHA class II or III, LVEF of 35% or less, who were randomly assigned to hawthorn or placebo for 2 years. Although the study failed to show any clear benefits in the treatment of chronic HF, hawthorn was well tolerated.

COENZYME Q

Coenzyme Q, also known as ubiquinone and ubidecarenone, is an endogenously synthesized provitamin that is structurally similar to vitamin E, serves as a lipid-soluble electron transport carrier in mitochondria, and aids in the synthesis of adenosine triphosphate.[309,310] It may also have membrane-stabilizing properties, enhance the antioxidant effects of vitamin E, and stabilize calcium-dependent slow channels. In animal models, it has positive inotropic effects, although weaker than those of digoxin. More than 18 open-label and double-blind, randomized clinical trials have been conducted of coenzyme Q in patients with HF ranging from NYHA classes II to IV.[309] Doses varied from 50 to 200 mg/day. Patients in many of these trials were also taking diuretics, ACEIs, and digoxin. Different trials used different end point measurements. Positive effects on subjective symptoms, NYHA class improvement, EF, quality of life, and hospitalization rates have all been observed. Two trials, however, failed to demonstrate significant changes in EF, vascular resistance, or exercise tolerance. None of the trials had sufficiently large samples sizes or adequate duration of assessment to detect reduction in mortality. Side effects were minimal, but included nausea, epigastric pain, diarrhea, heartburn, and appetite suppression. Mild increases in lactate dehydrogenase and hepatic enzymes have been rarely reported with coenzyme Q doses in excess of 300 mg/day.

Because no clinical trials have demonstrated improved survival with nutritional/herbal supplements, the current guidelines do not recommend these agents in patients with current or prior symptoms of HFrEF.

W.L. has poorly controlled systolic HTN and HF that is beginning to interfere with his activities of daily life. Although evidence indicates that patients with NYHA class II HF obtain symptomatic improvement with hawthorn and coenzyme Q, this does not address W.L.'s HTN. Conflicting data exist on the value of coenzyme Q in lowering BP.[309] The results of the SPICE trial did not demonstrate any mortality benefits, and no incremental benefits were seen when combined with standard therapy. Uncontrolled HTN in patients with HF leads to cardiac remodeling, and worsening HF. Currently W.L. is presenting with symptomatic HF; therefore, he should be started on a diuretic to alleviate his symptoms. Starting with a 20-mg dose of furosemide and titrating slowly may be one approach. For all of the reasons cited throughout this chapter, one must also argue strongly for starting an ACEI to control his HTN. He should be counseled that the urinary frequency he experienced previously should diminish after a few days. Once he is euvolemic, a β-blocker should be started.

The guidelines clearly state that natural products should not be used to treat symptomatic HF. Agents such as ephedra (which contain catecholamines), ephedrine metabolites, or imported Chinese herbs are contraindicated in HF because of increased risk of mortality and morbidity. No regulatory oversight, quality control, or regulations exist on the use of natural supplements. Because of the widespread use of nutritional supplements and herbal therapies and their potential to cause drug interactions, clinicians should routinely inquire about their use.

KEY REFERENCES AND WEBSITES

A full list of references for this chapter can be found at http://thepoint.lww.com/AT11e. Below are the key references and websites for this chapter, with the corresponding reference number in this chapter found in parentheses after the reference.

Key References

Bardy GH et al. Amiodarone or an implantable cardioverter-defi brillator for congestive heart failure [published correction appears in *N Engl J Med*. 2005;352:2146]. *N Engl J Med*. 2005;352:225. (290)

Barnes MM et al. Treatment of heart failure with preserved ejection fraction. *Pharmacotherapy*. 2011;31:312.

Felker GM et al. Diuretic strategies in patients with acute decompensated heart failure. *N Engl J Med*. 2011;364:797. (110)

Granger CB et al. Effects of candesartan in patients with chronic heart failure and reduced left-ventricular systolic function intolerant to angiotensin-converting-enzyme inhibitors: the CHARM-Alternative trial. *Lancet*. 2003;362:772. (154)

Heart Failure Society of America et al. HFSA 2010 Comprehensive Heart Failure Practice Guideline. *J Card Fail*. 2010;16:e1. (2)

Hunt SA et al. 2009 focused update incorporated into the ACC/AHA 2005 guidelines for the diagnosis and management of heart failure in adults: a report of the American College of Cardiology Foundation/American Heart Association Task Force on Practice Guidelines: Developed in collaboration with the international society for heart and lung transplantation. *Circulation*. 2009;119(14):e391–e479. (99)

McMurray JJ et al. Angiotensin-neprilysin inhibition versus enalapril in heart failure. *N Engl J*. 2014;371(11):993–1004. (87)

MERIT-HF Study Group. Effect of metoprolol CR/XL in chronic heart failure: Metoprolol CR/XL Randomised Intervention Trial in Congestive Heart Failure (MERIT-HF). *Lancet*. 1999;353:2001. (185)

Packer M et al. Comparative effects of low and high doses of the angiotensin-converting enzyme inhibitor, lisinopril, on morbidity and mortality in chronic heart failure. ATLAS Study Group. *Circulation*. 1999;100:2312. (142)

Packer M et al. The effect of carvedilol on morbidity and mortality in patients with chronic heart failure. U.S. Carvedilol Heart Failure Study Group. *N Engl J Med*. 1996;334:1349. (190)

Pitt B et al. Eplerenone, a selective aldosterone blocker, in patients with left ventricular dysfunction after myocardial infarction [published correction appears in *N Engl J Med*. 2003;348:2271]. *N Engl J Med*. 2003;348:1309. (65)

Pitt B et al. The effect of spironolactone on morbidity and mortality in patients with severe heart failure. Randomized Aldactone Evaluation Study Investigators. *N Engl J Med*. 1999;341:709. (64)

Pitt B et al. Spironolactone for heart failure with preserved ejection fraction. *N Engl J Med*. 2014;370:1383–1392. (302)

Rathore SS et al. Association of serum digoxin concentration and outcomes in patients with heart failure. *JAMA*. 2003;289:871.

Tang AS et al. Cardiac-resynchronization therapy for mild-to-moderate heart failure. *N Engl J Med*. 2010;363:2385. (295)

Writing Committee Members et al. 2013 ACCF/AHA guideline for the management of heart failure: a report of the American College of Cardiology Foundation/American Heart Association Task Force on practice guidelines. *Circulation*. 2013;128(16):e240–e327. (1)

Yancy et al. 2016 ACC/AHA/HFSA focused update on new pharmacological therapy for heart failur: an update of the 2013 ACCF/AHA guideline for the management of heart failure. *Circulation*. 2016;134:e282–293. (5).

Yancy et al. 2017 ACC/AHA/HFSA focused update of the 2013 ACCF/AHA guideline for the management of heart failure. *Circulation*. 2017;136:e137–e161. (6)

Zannad F et al. Eplerenone in patients with systolic heart failure and mild symptoms. *N Engl J Med*. 2011;364:11. (203)

15 Cardiac Arrhythmias

C. Michael White, Jessica C. Song, and James S. Kalus

CORE PRINCIPLES

		CHAPTER CASES
ATRIAL FIBRILLATION (AF)/FLUTTER		
1	Chest palpitations, light-headedness, and reduced exercise tolerance are the most common symptoms of AF, but stroke is among the severe complications. The goals of therapy are to control the ventricular rate and reduce the risk of stroke.	**Case 15-1 (Questions 1, 2)**
2	Digoxin, β-blockers, and nondihydropyridine calcium-channel blockers are appropriate rate-controlling medications. Digoxin is usually adjunctive therapy. Antiarrhythmic drugs are recommended in patients with symptoms but not needed in asymptomatic patients (no symptoms other than palpitations).	**Case 15-1 (Questions 3–7)**
3	Before converting AF to sinus rhythm, assurance of a lack of clot is important but not required if someone is unconscious or hemodynamically unstable. People with a CHA_2DS_2-VASc score of 2 or greater should receive chronic anticoagulant therapy with warfarin, dabigatran, rivaroxaban, edoxaban, or apixaban. Those with a score of 0 do not require antithrombotic therapy, and those with a score of 1 can receive no therapy, aspirin, or anticoagulant therapy based on patient and clinician preference.	**Case 15-1 (Questions 8, 13)**
4	Antiarrhythmic drugs convert patients out of AF 50% of the time, whereas electrical shock is successful 90% of the time. To maintain sinus rhythm after conversion, class Ib agents cannot be used, class Ic agents cannot be used in patients with structural heart disease (left ventricular hypertrophy, myocardial infarction, or heart failure), and class Ia and III agents can increase the risk of torsades de pointes. Propafenone, sotalol, dronedarone, dofetilide, and amiodarone are commonly used antiarrhythmic agents for AF.	**Case 15-1 (Questions 9–12)**
5	Atrial flutter is less common than AF, but similar rate control and antiarrhythmic strategies can be tried. Radiofrequency ablation can be used to terminate atrial flutter.	**Case 15-2 (Question 1)**
PAROXYSMAL SUPRAVENTRICULAR TACHYCARDIA (PSVT)		
1	PSVT is caused by reentry within the atrioventricular (AV) node. Palpitations and hypotension can occur. The Valsalva maneuver, adenosine, or nondihydropyridine calcium-channel blockers can be used to treat the arrhythmia.	**Case 15-3 (Questions 1–6)**
2	In Wolff–Parkinson–White syndrome patients with PSVT, the use of AV nodal blocking agents such as β-blockers, nondihydropyridine calcium-channel blockers, and digoxin can increase the risk of cardiac arrest. Ablation can destroy the bypass tract and cure the patient.	**Case 15-4 (Questions 1, 2)**
ATRIOVENTRICULAR (AV) BLOCK		
1	β-Blockers, digoxin, and nondihydropyridine calcium-channel blockers should be withheld in patients with type 1 second- or third-degree AV block. Atropine can be used to treat this disorder.	**Case 15-5 (Questions 1, 2)**
VENTRICULAR ARRHYTHMIAS		
1	In patients with premature ventricular complexes (PVCs) and myocardial infarction, β-blockers are the treatment of choice. Catheter ablation is recommended for those with ventricular compromise due to high PVC burden.	**Case 15-6 (Questions 1, 2)**

Continued

	CHAPTER CASES
2 Patients with myocardial infarction and nonsustained ventricular tachycardia (VT) should receive β-blockers and need to be evaluated to determine whether they should receive an implantable cardioverter-defibrillator (ICD).	Case 15-6 (Question 1)
3 Patients with sustained VT should be treated with intravenous antiarrhythmic agents unless they are hemodynamically unstable, in which case they should be electrically converted. To prevent death from arrhythmia recurrence, ICDs are superior to antiarrhythmic drugs, but to decrease the occurrence of painful shocks, both strategies may be used simultaneously.	Case 15-7 (Questions 1–3)
TORSADES DE POINTES (TDP)	
1 TdP occurs secondary to antiarrhythmic and nonantiarrhythmic medications that prolong the QTc interval. Class Ia and III antiarrhythmic agents, antipsychotic agents, citalopram, fluoroquinolones, macrolides, azole antifungals, and methadone can prolong the QTc interval. Magnesium is the treatment of choice for hemodynamically stable TdP with electrical cardioversion reserved for the hemodynamically unstable.	Case 15-8 (Questions 1–4)
CARDIAC ARREST	
1 Cardiac arrest should be treated with 2-minute cycles of aggressive cardiopulmonary resuscitation, electrical shock for VT or ventricular fibrillation (VF), epinephrine or vasopressin, and amiodarone for refractory VT or VF according to the Advanced Cardiac Life Support guidelines from the American Heart Association.	Case 15-9 (Questions 1–4), Case 15-10 (Question 1), Case 15-11 (Questions 1–3)

Adequate circulation depends on continuous, well-coordinated electrical activity within the heart. This chapter reviews and discusses cardiac electrophysiology, arrhythmogenesis, common arrhythmias, and antiarrhythmic treatment.

ELECTROPHYSIOLOGY

Understanding Electrophysiology

CELLULAR ELECTROPHYSIOLOGY

An electrical potential exists across the cell membrane, and the electrical potential changes in a cyclic manner that is related to the flux of K^+, Na^+, and Ca^{2+} ions across the cell membrane.[1] If the change in the membrane potential is plotted against time in a given cycle of a His-Purkinje fiber, a typical action potential results (Fig. 15-1).

The action potential can be described in five phases.[1] Phase 0 is related to ventricular depolarization resulting from sodium entry into the cell through fast sodium channels. On a surface electrocardiogram (ECG), phase 0 is represented by the QRS complex. Phase 1 is the overshoot phase in which calcium enters the cell and contraction occurs. During phase 2, the plateau phase, inward depolarizing currents through slow sodium and calcium channels are counterbalanced by outward repolarizing potassium currents. Phase 3 constitutes repolarization, which on the ECG is represented by the T wave. During phase 4, sodium moves out of the cell and potassium moves into the cell via an active pumping mechanism. During this phase, the action potential remains flat in some cells (e.g., ventricular muscle) and does not change until it receives an impulse from above. In other cells (e.g., sinoatrial [SA] node), the cell slowly depolarizes until it reaches the threshold potential and again spontaneously depolarizes (phase 0). The shape of the action potential depends on the location of the cell (see Fig. 15-1). In both the SA and atrioventricular (AV) nodes, the cells are more dependent on calcium influx than sodium influx, resulting in a less negative resting membrane potential, a slow rise of phase 0, and the capability of spontaneous (automatic) phase 4 depolarization (Fig. 15-1).

The upward slope of phase 0, referred to as V_{max}, is related to the conduction velocity. The steeper the slope, the more rapid the rate of depolarization. Another influence on V_{max} is the point at which depolarization occurs. The less negative the threshold potential, the slower V_{max} will be, and hence conduction velocity is slowed. Drugs can affect V_{max} and conduction velocity by blocking the fast sodium channels or by making the resting membrane potential less negative (e.g., class I agents).

The action potential duration (APD) is the length of time from phase 0 to the end of phase 3. The effective refractory period is the length of time that the cell is refractory and will not propagate another impulse. Both of these measurements can be obtained from intracardiac recordings of the action potential. Class Ia and III agents prolong the refractoriness of the heart.[1]

NORMAL CARDIAC ELECTROPHYSIOLOGY

Automaticity

Automaticity is the ability of cells (often called pacemaker cells) to depolarize spontaneously. These cells are located in the SA and AV nodes and the His-Purkinje system. The SA node is normally the dominant pacemaker because it reaches the threshold faster than other nodes in a normal heart, resulting in 60 to 100 depolarizations per minute.[2] The innate AV node and Purkinje rate of depolarization is 40 to 60 and 40 depolarizations per minute, respectively. In the healthy heart, the AV node and Purkinje fibers are prevented (overridden) from spontaneous depolarization by the more frequent impulses from the SA node.

Conduction

An impulse normally originates in the SA node and travels down specialized intranodal pathways to activate atrial muscle and the AV node. The AV node holds the impulse briefly before releasing it to the bundle of His. It then travels to the right and left bundle branches and out to the ventricular myocardium via the Purkinje

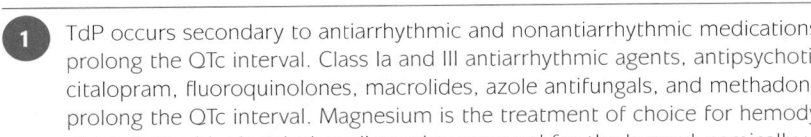

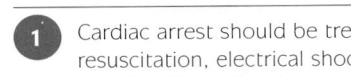

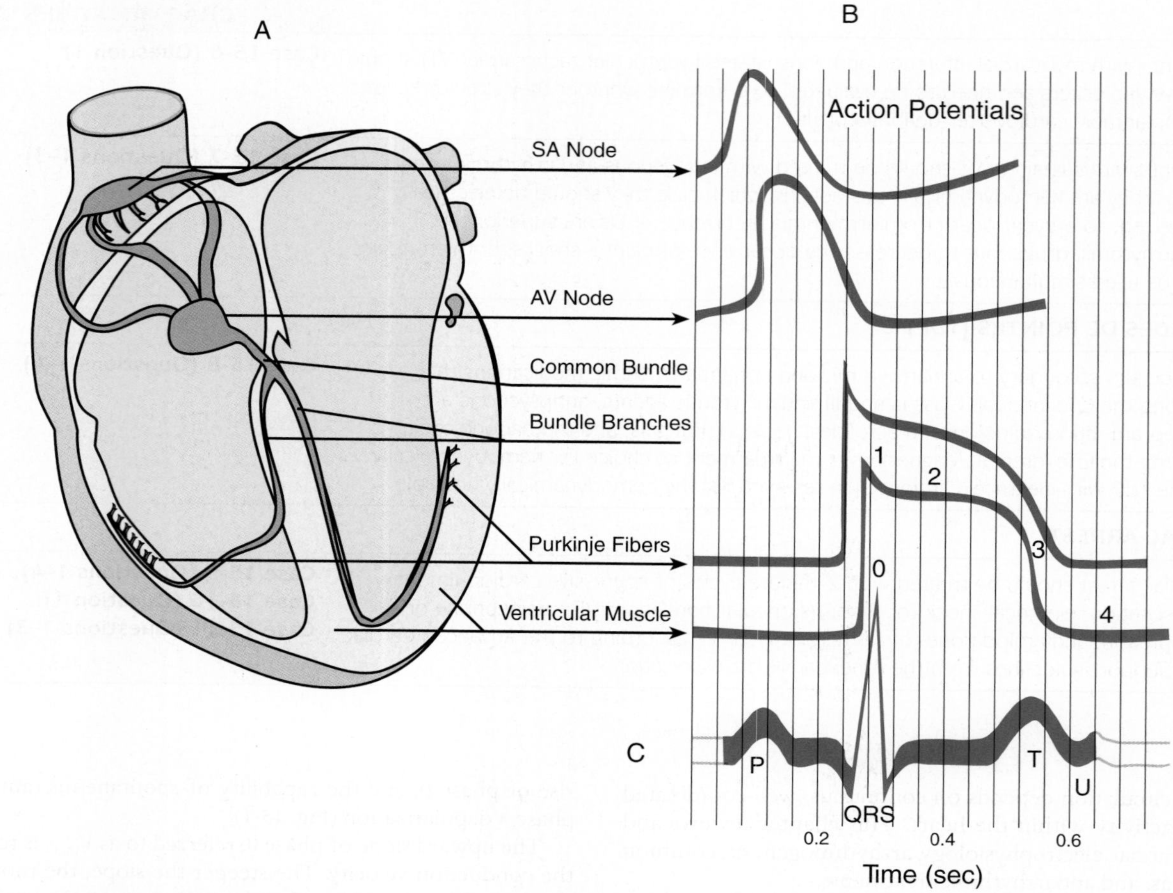

Figure 15-1 The cardiac conduction system. **A:** Cardiac conduction system anatomy. **B:** Action potentials of specific cardiac cells. **C:** Relationship of surface electrocardiogram to the action potential. SA, sinoatrial; AV, atrioventricular.

fibers. The ECG tracing consists of a series of complexes that correspond to electrical activity in a specific location or anatomic site. By convention, these electrical deflections have been labeled the P wave, QRS complex, and T wave. The P wave represents depolarization of the atria, whereas the QRS complex reflects ventricular depolarization. The T wave reflects repolarization of the ventricles. To evaluate the intact conduction system, conduction intervals at different sites can be obtained. The normal intervals as measured by ECG or intracardiac electrodes are shown in Table 15-1. Drugs and ischemia can alter the conduction and hence the ECG intervals. The effects of antiarrhythmic agents on the ECG are described in Table 15-2.

Table 15-1
Normal Electrocardiographic Intervals

Interval	Normal Indices (ms)	Electrical Activity
PR	120–200	Atrial depolarization
QRS	<140	Ventricular depolarization
QTc[a]	<400	Ventricular repolarization

[a]QTc interval is the QT interval corrected for heart rate. A common method for calculating QTc is the QT interval/(R-R interval)$^{1/2}$ (Bazett formula).

Pathophysiology

ABNORMAL IMPULSE FORMATION

Abnormal impulse formation can arise from abnormal automaticity or triggered activity originating from the SA node (e.g., sinus bradycardia) or other sites (e.g., junctional or idioventricular tachycardia). Causes of abnormal automaticity include hypoxia, ischemia, or excess catecholamine activity.

Triggered activity occurs when there is an attempted depolarization before or after the cell is fully repolarized, but not by a pacemaker cell. These after-depolarizations may occur in phase 2 or 3 (early) or phase 4 (delayed) of the action potential. Early after-depolarizations (EAD) arise from a reduced level of membrane potential and may require a bradycardic state. Torsades de pointes (TdP), a form of polymorphic ventricular tachycardia (VT), is thought to be initiated by EAD. Delayed after-depolarizations, often seen with digoxin toxicity, are thought to be secondary to an overload of intracellular free calcium.

ABNORMAL IMPULSE CONDUCTION

Reentry

The most common abnormal conduction leading to arrhythmogenesis is reentry. A reentrant circuit is formed as normal conduction occurs down a pathway that bifurcates into two pathways (e.g., AV node or left and right bundle branches). The impulse travels along one pathway (Fig. 15-2), but encounters unidirectional antegrade block in the other pathway (see Fig. 15-2). The impulse that passed through the

Table 15-2
Pharmacologic Properties of Antiarrhythmic Agents

	Surface ECG				
Type	**PR Interval**	**QRS Interval**	**QT Interval**	**Conduction Velocity**	**Refractory Period**
Ia	0/↑	↑	↑↑	↑↓[a]	↑[b]
Ib	0	0	0	0/↓	↓[b]
Ic	↑	↑↑	↑	↑[b]	0[b]
II	↑↑	0	0	↓[b]	↑[b]
III	0[c]	0	↑↑	0[b]	↑[b]
IV	↑↑	0	0	↓[b]	↑[b]

[a]Conduction increases at low dosages and decreases at higher dosages.
[b]On atrial and atrioventricular nodal tissue.
[c]May cause PR prolongation independent of class III antiarrhythmic activity.
ECG, electrocardiogram.

unblocked pathway propagates in a retrograde manner (i.e., moves backward) through the previously blocked pathway. This abnormal impulse can travel down the first pathway again when it is not refractory. Supraventricular and monomorphic VT are both examples of reentrant arrhythmias.

Block

Another form of abnormal impulse conduction occurs when the normal conducting pathway is blocked and the impulse is forced to travel through nonpathway tissues to cause depolarization. Common examples are left and right bundle branch blocks in the ventricles. A block in one path necessitates retrograde conduction through the opposite bundle to stimulate both ventricles. Nonpathway tissue conducts the electrical impulse more slowly than conduction tissues do.[1]

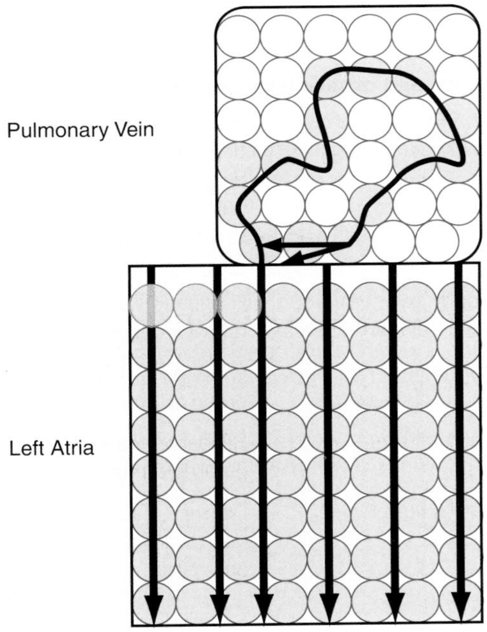

Figure 15-2 Reentrant circuit in the pulmonary vein. In the pulmonary vein there is a mixing of electrically active cells (*shaded circles*) and electrically inactive cells (*white circles*). Although the main wave of depolarization goes homogenously down the atria, a small depolarization stimulus enters the pulmonary vein and meanders through the electrically active tissue. In this case, there is a reentrant circuit formed where the impulse can continue to rotate through the pulmonary vein and a route for it to stimulate the atria as well.

Classification of Arrhythmias

All arrhythmias originating above the bundle of His are referred to as supraventricular arrhythmias. These may include sinus bradycardia, sinus tachycardia, paroxysmal supraventricular tachycardia, atrial flutter, atrial fibrillation (AF), Wolff–Parkinson–White (WPW) syndrome, and premature atrial contractions (PACs). All of these arrhythmias are characterized by normal QRS complexes (i.e., normal ventricular depolarization) unless there is a bundle branch block. Not all of these rhythm changes are necessarily a sign of pathology. For example, athletes with a well-conditioned heart and large stroke volume commonly have slow heart rates (sinus bradycardia). Vigorous exercise is accompanied by transient sinus tachycardia.

Arrhythmias originating below the bundle of His are referred to as ventricular arrhythmias. These include premature ventricular contractions (PVCs), VT, and ventricular fibrillation (VF). Conduction blocks often are categorized separately based on their level or location, which can be a supraventricular site (e.g., first-, second-, or third-degree AV block, see Case 15-6, Question 2) or in the ventricle (e.g., right or left bundle branch block). An alternative method of classifying arrhythmias is based on the rate: bradyarrhythmia (<60 beats/minute) or tachyarrhythmia (>100 beats/minute). There is a website with useful rhythm evaluation tutorials at http://www.blaufuss.org.

Antiarrhythmic Drugs

On the basis of their electrophysiologic (EP) and pharmacologic effects, there are four Vaughn-Williams antiarrhythmic drug classes. Class I drugs, sodium-channel blockers, are subdivided further depending on the duration of blockade (class Ia: intermediate; Ib: fast; and Ic: long). Class II drugs are β-adrenergic blockers, class III drugs are potassium-channel blockers, and class IV drugs are calcium-channel blockers. The classification, pharmacokinetics, and adverse effects of these agents are summarized in Table 15-3.

Class Ia and class III antiarrhythmic agents increase repolarization time, the QTc interval, and the risk of TdP. Class II and IV

Table 15-3
Vaughn-Williams Classification of Antiarrhythmic Agents

Drug and Classification	Pharmacokinetics	Indications	Side Effects
Class Ia (can cause torsades de pointes similar to class III agents)			
Quinidine sulfate (83% quinidine; SR) Quinidine gluconate (62% quinidine; SR)	$t_{1/2}$ = 6.2 ± 1.8 hours (affected by age, cirrhosis); V_d = 2.7 L/kg (↓ in HF); liver metabolism, 80%; renal clearance, 20%; C_p = 2–6 mcg/mL, CYP3A4 substrate, CYP2D6 inhibitor, P-glycoprotein inhibitor	AF (conversion or prophylaxis), WPW, PVCs, VT	Diarrhea, hypotension, N/V, cinchonism, fever, thrombocytopenia, proarrhythmia
Procainamide	$t_{1/2}$ = 3 ± 0.6 hours; V_d = 1.9 ± 0.3 L/kg; liver metabolism 40%; renal clearance (GFR + possible CTS) 60%; active metabolite (NAPA)[a] C_p = 4–10 mcg/mL, possible CTS substrate	AF (conversion or prophylaxis), WPW, PVCs, VT	Hypotension, fever, agranulocytosis, SLE (joint/muscle pain, rash, pericarditis), headache, proarrhythmia
Disopyramide (SR and CR forms)	$t_{1/2}$ = 6 ± 1 hours; V_d = 0.59 ± 0.15 L/kg; liver metabolism, 30%; renal clearance, 70%; C_p = 3–6 mcg/mL	AF, WPW, PSVT, PVCs, VT	Anticholinergic (dry mouth, blurred vision, urinary retention), HF, proarrhythmia
Class Ib[b] (cannot be used to treat atrial arrhythmias)			
Lidocaine	$t_{1/2}$ = 1.8 ± 0.4 hours; V_d = 1.1 ± 0.4 L/kg; liver metabolism, 100%; C_p = 1.5–6 mcg/mL	PVCs, VT, VF	Drowsiness, agitation, muscle twitching, seizures, paresthesias, proarrhythmia
Mexiletine	$t_{1/2}$ = 10.4 ± 2.8 hours; V_d = 9.5 ± 3.4 L/kg; liver metabolism, 35%–80%; C_p = 0.5–2 mcg/mL	PVCs, VT, VF	Drowsiness, agitation, muscle twitching, seizures, paresthesias, proarrhythmia, N/V, diarrhea
Class Ic (cannot be used in patients with structural heart disease)			
Flecainide	$t_{1/2}$ = 12–27 hours; CYP2D6 substrate, 75%; renal clearance, 25%; C_p = 0.4–1 mcg/mL	AF, PSVT, severe ventricular arrhythmias	Dizziness, tremor, light-headedness, flushing, blurred vision, metallic taste, proarrhythmia
Propafenone	$t_{1/2}$ = 2 hours (extensive metabolizer); 10 hours (poor metabolizer); V_d = 2.5–4 L/kg, CYP2D6 substrate/inhibitor, P-glycoprotein inhibitor	PAF, WPW, severe ventricular arrhythmias	Dizziness, blurred vision, taste disturbances, nausea, worsening of asthma, proarrhythmia
Class III (can cause torsade de pointes similar to class Ia agents, amiodarone, and dronedarone and have lower risk)			
Amiodarone	$t_{1/2}$ = 40–60 days; V_d = 60–100 L/kg; erratic absorption; liver metabolism, 100%; oral F = 50%, C_p = 0.5–2.5 mcg/mL, CYP1A2, 2D6, 2C9, 3A4 inhibitor, P-glycoprotein inhibitor	AF, PAF, PSVT, severe ventricular arrhythmias, VF	Blurred vision, corneal microdeposits, photophobia, skin discoloration, constipation, pulmonary fibrosis, ataxia, hypothyroid or hyperthyroid, hypotension, N/V
Sotalol[c]	$t_{1/2}$ = 10–20 hours; V_d = 1.2–2.4 L/kg; renal clearance, 100%	AF (prophylaxis), PSVT, severe ventricular arrhythmias	Fatigue, dizziness, dyspnea, bradycardia, proarrhythmia
Dofetilide	$t_{1/2}$ = 7.5–10 hours; V_d = 3 L/kg; renal elimination, 60% (GFR + CTS), CYP3A4 substrate	AF or atrial flutter conversion and prophylaxis	Chest pain, dizziness, headache, proarrhythmia
Ibutilide	$t_{1/2}$ = 6 (2–12) hours; V_d = 11 L/kg, C_p = undefined	AF or atrial flutter conversion	Headache, nausea, proarrhythmia
Dronedarone	$t_{1/2}$ = 13–19 hours; V_d = 20 L/kg, T_{max} = 3–6 hours, CYP3A4 substrate, CYP 2D6, 3A4 inhibitor, P-glycoprotein inhibitor, take with food for maximal absorption	AF or atrial flutter prophylaxis	Diarrhea, nausea, dermatitis or rash, bradycardia, hepatotoxicity, pregnancy category X

[a]NAPA is 100% renally eliminated and possesses class III antiarrhythmic activity.
[b]Phenytoin is classified as a class Ib antiarrhythmic.
[c]Possesses both class II and III antiarrhythmic activity.
AF, atrial fibrillation; C_p, steady-state plasma concentration; CR, controlled release; CTS, cation tubular secretion; CYP, cytochrome P-450; F, bioavailability; GFR, glomerular filtration rate; HF, heart failure; NAPA, *N*-acetylprocainamide; N/V, nausea and vomiting; PAF, paroxysmal atrial fibrillation; PSVT, paroxysmal supraventricular tachycardia; PVC, premature ventricular contraction; SLE, systemic lupus erythematosus; SR, sustained release; $t_{1/2}$, half-life; V_d, volume of distribution; VF, ventricular fibrillation; VT, ventricular tachycardia; WPW, Wolff–Parkinson–White syndrome.

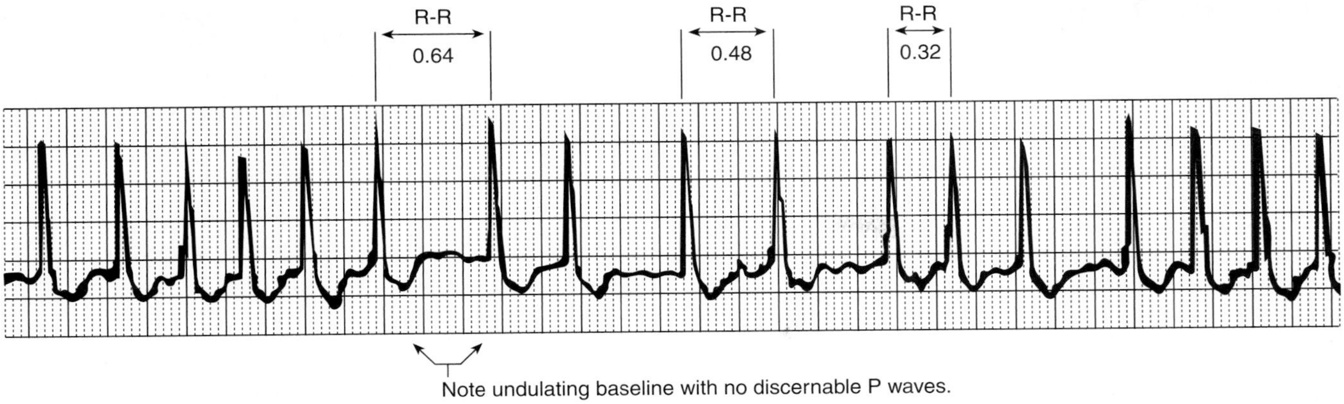

Figure 15-3 Atrial fibrillation. Note the irregularly irregular R-R intervals, undulating baseline without definitive P waves, normal width of the QRS complexes, and ventricular rate of 140 beats/minute.

antiarrhythmic agents may decrease heart rate (cause bradycardia), decrease ventricular contractility (decrease stroke volume), and prolong the PR interval (cause second- or third-degree AV block). Class Ib antiarrhythmic agents work only in ventricular tissue, so they cannot be used in AF or atrial flutter. Class Ic antiarrhythmic agents are useful, but should never be used after an MI or with systolic heart failure or severe left ventricular hypertrophy (classified as structural heart diseases) because increased mortality can result. These drugs are discussed in greater detail later.

SUPRAVENTRICULAR ARRHYTHMIAS

The specific arrhythmias include (a) those primarily atrial in origin, such as AF, atrial flutter, paroxysmal sinus tachycardia, ectopic atrial tachycardia, and multifocal atrial tachycardia; and (b) AV nodal reentrant tachycardia (AVNRT) and AV reentrant tachycardia (AVRT) involving accessory pathways within the atria or ventricle. AVNRT and AVRT often self-terminate and are paroxysmal (episodic) in nature; thus, they are commonly referred to as paroxysmal supraventricular tachycardias (PSVT). The most common supraventricular arrhythmias are AF, atrial flutter, and PSVT.

Atrial Fibrillation and Atrial Flutter

AF is usually initiated when a depolarization stimulus arising from an ectopic focus or reentrant circuit impacts the atria while the tissue is in the vulnerable period. The vulnerable period in the atria and ventricles occurs during the first half of the QRS complex; this period is vulnerable because the net charge is near normal but the ion concentrations of sodium, calcium, and potassium inside and outside the cells are radically different. Stimulation during the vulnerable period causes multiple ectopic foci to arise and attempt to pace the atria with no single pacemaker in control, eliminating discernable P waves on the ECG (Fig. 15-3) and eliciting a rapid, ineffective writhing of the atrial muscle with a classic "irregularly irregular" ventricular rate. In contrast, atrial flutter (Fig. 15-4) is characterized by typical sawtooth atrial waves, at a rate of 280 to 320 beats/minute, and a variable ventricular rate, depending on the nature of the AV block present (e.g., 2, 3, or 4 atrial beats for each ventricular beat or 2:1, 3:1, or 4:1 block). In most cases, the ventricular rate is approximately 150 beats/minute. Episodes of atrial flutter can progress to AF if the ectopic atrial depolarization stimulus impacts the surrounding atrial tissue in the vulnerable period. When patients initially experience AF, the episodes are usually short lived, and spontaneous conversion occurs. The pattern of erratic initiation and termination of AF is termed paroxysmal atrial fibrillation (PAF), and if enough AF events occur in close proximity to each other, the duration of subsequent AF events increases in length and the event degenerates into persistent AF. In persistent AF, the AF episode will continue until the heart is electrically or chemically converted out of the rhythm. With time, persistent AF degenerates into permanent AF, in which normal sinus rhythm cannot be achieved and sustained. An example of PAF is presented in the following section.

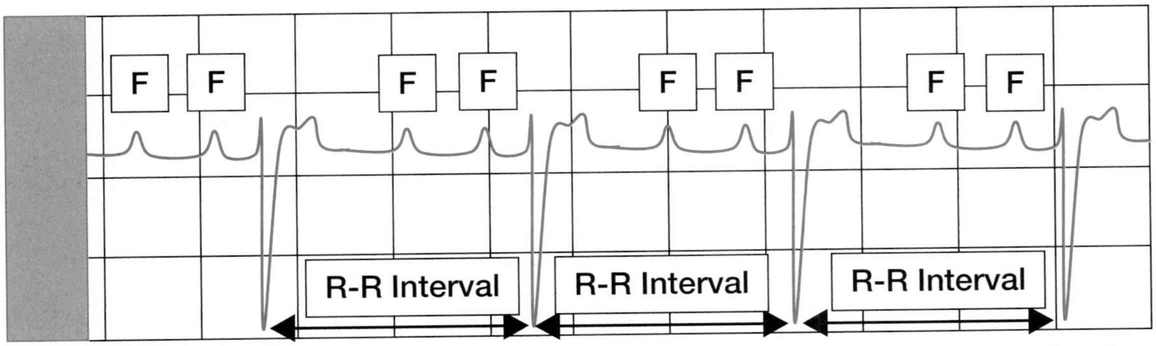

Figure 15-4 Atrial flutter. Note the sawtooth appearance of the rhythm strip. F denotes Flutter waves with consistent R-R spacing.

CASE 15-1

QUESTION 1: J.K., a 66-year-old man, presents for a routine checkup in the clinic. His medical history includes type 2 diabetes mellitus and systolic HF for the last 5 years, hypertension, and gout. There is no history of rheumatic heart disease, MI, pulmonary embolism, or thyroid disease. Medications include metformin 1 g twice daily, lisinopril 40 mg every day, furosemide 40 mg twice daily, metoprolol succinate 50 mg twice daily, and allopurinol 300 mg/day. J.K. does not smoke or drink alcohol. Physical examination reveals a blood pressure (BP) of 136/84 mm Hg, pulse of 70 beats/minute in normal sinus rhythm, respiratory rate of 12 breaths/minute, and temperature of 98.2°F. His body mass index is 32 kg/m^2. What factors in J.K.'s past medical history predispose him to development of AF? What is his 10-year risk of developing AF?

AF is commonly associated with, or a manifestation of, other diseases or disorders (Table 15-4).[3,3a] When treatable underlying causes are present, they should be corrected because this may resolve the AF. A risk prediction tool highlights common factors associated with the development of AF, particularly older age, male gender, hypertension, heart failure, obesity, and valvular disease.[4,5] In a small percentage of patients who do not have underlying heart disease, AF is called "lone" AF and usually has a more benign course.

J.K. has several risk factors for the development of AF within the next 10 years, including the presence of treated hypertension, heart failure, his age, and his sex. A detailed scoring system is described in the referenced manuscript but is beyond the scope of this chapter. Using his risk factors, his 10-year risk of developing AF would be greater than 30%.[4]

Table 15-4
Causes of Atrial Fibrillation and Flutter

Alcohol	Nonrheumatic Heart Disease
Atrial septal defect	Pericarditis
Cardiac surgery	Pneumonia
Cardiomyopathy	Pulmonary embolism
Cerebrovascular accident	Sick sinus syndrome
Chronic obstructive pulmonary disease	Stimulants Thyrotoxicosis
Fever	Trauma
Hypothermia	Tumors
Ischemic heart disease	Wolff–Parkinson–White syndrome
Mitral valve disease	

Consequences of Atrial Fibrillation

CASE 15-1, QUESTION 2: Two years later, J.K. presents with complaints of dyspnea on exertion (DOE) and palpitations for the last 2 weeks. He experienced palpitations of shorter duration three times in the last year, but these were not associated with DOE. On physical examination, he is found to have rales. Cardiac examination reveals an irregularly irregular rhythm without murmurs, gallops, or rubs. His jugular veins are distended 4 cm, but no organomegaly is found. His extremities have 1+ pitting edema. The ECG shows AF (see Fig. 15-3), and the chest radiograph is compatible with mild pulmonary congestion. A cardiac echocardiogram reveals the atrial size to be less than 5 cm (normal) and a left ventricular ejection fraction of 35%. What clinical findings demonstrated by J.K. are typically associated with AF? What are the likely consequences of his AF?

The most common complaint in patients with AF, as with J.K., is palpitations (the sensation of the heart beating rapidly or unusually in the chest). This is a result of the rapid ventricular rate, which typically ranges from 100 to 160 beats/minute. The R–R interval (time from the R wave in one QRS complex to the R wave in the next complex) is irregularly irregular (random irregularity). During AF, the atrial kick or the atria's contribution to stroke volume is lost. Because the atrial kick may account for 20% to 30% of the total stroke volume, this, coupled with rapid ventricular rates and irregular R–R interval spacing during AF, can cause symptoms of inadequate blood flow such as light-headedness, dizziness, or reduced exercise tolerance. However, some patients are asymptomatic except for the palpitations. Depending on the underlying ventricular function, signs of HF, such as DOE and peripheral edema, may develop, as experienced by J.K. Conversely, underlying HF may precipitate AF.

Patients with AF are at risk for thrombotic stroke (see Stroke Prevention section below).[6] With the chaotic movement of the atria, normal blood flow is disrupted, and atrial mural thrombi (usually in a pouch called the left atrial appendage) may form. The risk of stroke increases after restoration of normal sinus rhythm, which allows more efficient cardiac contractility and expulsion of the thrombus. Patients with nonvalvular AF have a fivefold increase in the risk of stroke; this risk increases as patients have an increased number of associated risk factors. Other concurrent diseases that may increase the risk of stroke are HF, cardiomyopathy, thyrotoxicosis, congenital heart disease, and valvular heart disease. Because of the high risk of stroke and significant impact of stroke on patient outcomes, pharmacologic stroke prophylaxis is often indicated. Selection of an appropriate antithrombotic regimen for the patient with AF must be based on assessment of the underlying stroke and bleeding risk. Risk stratification in AF is performed with the use of the CHA_2DS_2-VASc scoring system. A CHA_2DS_2-VASc score is calculated by assigning one point each for the presence of congestive heart failure, hypertension, diabetes, vascular disease, age of 65 to 74 years, or female gender and two points for age of 75 years or greater or a history of stroke. Points are totaled, and the subsequent score correlates with stroke risk.[7]

TREATMENT OF ATRIAL FIBRILLATION

Goals of Therapy

CASE 15-1, QUESTION 3: What are the therapeutic goals and general approaches used to treat AF in patients like J.K.?

The two primary goals of treatment are to control the ventricular response rate and to reduce the risk of stroke. In some cases, a third therapeutic goal may be conversion to normal sinus rhythm.

Ventricular Rate Control

Digoxin

CASE 15-1, QUESTION 4: J.K. is given a 1-mg loading dose of digoxin, followed by a 0.25-mg every day maintenance dose. What is the purpose of administering digoxin? What are the relative advantages and disadvantages of digoxin compared with other agents to control ventricular rate?

Table 15-5

Agents Used for Controlling Ventricular Rate in Supraventricular Tachycardias[a]

Drug	Loading Dose	Usual Maintenance Dose	Comments
Digoxin	10–15 mcg/kg LBW up to 1–1.5 mg IV or PO for 24 hours (e.g., 0.5 mg initially, then 0.25 mg every 6 hours)	PO: 0.125–0.5 mg/day; adjust for renal failure (see Chapter 14)	Maximal response may take several hours; use with caution in patients with renal impairment
Esmolol	0.5 mg/kg IV for 1 minute	50–300 mcg/kg/minute continuous infusion with bolus between increases	Hypotension common; effects additive with digoxin and calcium-channel blockers
Propranolol	0.5–1.0 mg IV repeated every 2 minutes (up to 0.1–0.15 mg/kg)	IV infusion: 0.04 mg/kg/minute PO: 10–120 mg TID	Use with caution in patients with HF or asthma; additive effects seen with digoxin and calcium-channel blockers
Metoprolol	5 mg IV at 1 mg/minute	PO: 25–100 mg BID	Use with caution in patients with HF or asthma; additive effects seen with digoxin and calcium-channel blockers
Verapamil	5–10 mg (0.075–0.15 mg/kg) IV for 2 minutes; if response inadequate after 15–30 minutes, repeat 10 mg (up to 0.15 mg/kg)	IV infusion: 5–10 mg/hour PO: 40–120 mg TID or 120–480 mg in sustained-release form daily	Hypotension with IV route; AV blocking effects are additive with digoxin and β-blockers; may increase digoxin levels
Diltiazem	0.25 mg/kg IV for 2 minutes; if response inadequate after 15 minutes, repeat 0.35 mg/kg for 2 minutes	IV infusion: 5–15 mg/hour PO: 60–90 mg TID or QID or 180–360 mg in extended-release form daily	Response to IV therapy occurs in 4–5 minutes; hypotension; effects additive with digoxin and β-blockers

[a]AV nodal ablation is a nonpharmacologic alternative to control the ventricular response, but the effect is permanent and may require chronic ventricular pacing afterward.
AV, atrioventricular; BID, 2 times a day; HF, heart failure; LBW, lean body weight; PO, orally; IV, intravenously; QID, four times a day; TID, three times a day.

The first treatment goal is to slow the ventricular response rate, which allows better ventricular filling with blood. Table 15-5 displays the agents commonly used to control the ventricular response and, provides typical loading and maintenance doses. Because of its direct AV node-blocking effects and vagomimetic properties, digoxin prolongs the effective refractory period of the AV node and reduces the number of impulses conducted through the AV node (negative dromotropy).[6]

There are several limitations associated with digoxin use in AF. Digoxin has a slow onset of action. After an intravenous (IV) dose, it will take more than 2 hours for the onset of effect and 6 to 8 hours for the maximal effect, which is markedly slower than other negative dromotropic agents.[8] Digoxin is also less effective than β-blockers and nondihydropyridine calcium-channel blockers during states of heightened sympathetic tone (e.g., exercise or emotional stress), a common precipitant of PAF.[7–11] The 2014 American Heart Association/American College of Cardiology/Heart Rhythm Society Guidelines for the management of patients with AF recommend that digoxin use be reserved for control of ventricular response rate in patients with impaired left ventricular function or HF or for use as an add-on therapy when treatment with a β-blocker or calcium-channel blocker provides inadequate rate control.[12] Patients who require rate control of AF and have a lower BP may also benefit from rate control with digoxin. It should also be noted that digoxin serum concentrations may be increased when combined with P-glycoprotein inhibitors such as verapamil, propafenone, quinidine, flecainide, and amiodarone.[13–15] Normally, P-glycoprotein in the brush border membrane of intestinal enterocytes pumps digoxin into the lumen of the gut reducing its bioavailability and pumps digoxin out of the body via the renal tubules (see Chapter 14, Heart Failure, for discussion of digoxin and digoxin drug interactions).

CASE 15-1, QUESTION 5: J.K. has diabetes, which increases the risk for diabetic nephropathy. Would the dosing be changed if J.K. had renal dysfunction?

J.K.'s renal function is normal. If he had significant renal dysfunction, both the loading and the maintenance doses of digoxin would need to be altered. A loading dose is used to achieve a therapeutic level and volume of distribution of digoxin is reduced in patients with renal dysfunction. The digoxin maintenance dose is highly dependent on renal clearance, because digoxin is eliminated 50% to 75% unchanged in the urine (see Chapter 14, Heart Failure, for further discussion of digoxin dosing in patients with normal and impaired renal function). Although the usual digoxin target range is generally 0.5 to 1.0 ng/mL in the management of patients with heart failure,[16] higher serum concentrations may be necessary when using digoxin as a rate control agent for J.K.

β-Adrenergic Blocking Agents

CASE 15-1, QUESTION 6: What other drugs can be used for ventricular rate control, and what are their relative advantages and disadvantages compared with digoxin?

β-Adrenergic blocking agents are another class of negative dromotropic agents used in AF. Propranolol, metoprolol, and esmolol are available for IV administration. Each agent rapidly controls the ventricular rate both at rest and during exercise. β-Blockers are the first choice in high catecholamine states such as thyrotoxicosis and postcardiac surgery. However, given their negative inotropic effects, β-blockers should be used cautiously to acutely control the ventricular response in patients with decompensated HF. Even though β-blockers are used to treat systolic HF (e.g., bisoprolol, carvedilol, and metoprolol), they need to be started at low doses and titrated slowly for several weeks to therapeutic doses[2] (see Chapter 14, Heart Failure). When trying to achieve rapid rate control, more aggressive dosing may be needed. β-Blockers should also be avoided in patients with asthma because of their β_2-blocking properties, and blood glucose levels should be monitored more closely in patients with diabetes mellitus because the signs and symptoms of hypoglycemia (except sweating) can be masked.

Calcium-Channel Blockers

Nondihydropyridine calcium-channel blockers are also effective in slowing ventricular rate at rest and during exercise. Both verapamil and diltiazem can be administered IV for a rapid (4–5 minutes) reduction in heart rate.[12] Nondihydropyridine calcium-channel blockers should not be used in patients presenting with decompensated HF.[7] They work through their effect on slow calcium channels within the AV node. Although the duration of action produced by bolus dosing is short, both agents can be administered either as a continuous drip or orally. Given the ability of calcium-channel blockers to cause arteriolar dilation, a transient decrease in BP may be seen. IV calcium pretreatment can be used to attenuate the BP decrease among patients with hypotension, near-hypotensive BP, or left ventricular dysfunction. Calcium pretreatment does not appear to diminish the negative dromotropic effects of nondihydropyridine calcium-channel blockers.[17–20] Verapamil is contraindicated in patients with an ejection fraction less than 35% and diltiazem should be used with caution in HF with a reduced EF. Verapamil increases the concentrations of other cardiovascular drugs such as digoxin, dofetilide, simvastatin, and lovastatin.[21] Verapamil and diltiazem are good alternatives to β-blockers in asthmatics.[7]

For chronic therapy, oral negative dromotropic agents (usually a β-blocker or nondihydropyridine calcium-channel blocker) are recommended. If higher dose monotherapy with one of these drugs is needed to control symptoms but is associated with intolerable side effects, adding lower dose digoxin to a β-blocker or calcium-channel blocker is recommended.[7,11,22–24]

J.K. has signs of mild HF, so digoxin is a reasonable choice, although short-term IV diltiazem is often used in this type of patient as well. IV verapamil and β-blockers may worsen the signs and symptoms of HF, and the β-blockers may mask signs of hypoglycemia in J.K. The goal of rate control should be a resting heart rate between 60 and 80 beats/minute and an exercising heart rate between 90 and 115 beats/minute.[7] A recent study has explored the use of a more lenient target resting heart rate (<110 beats/minute) and reported similar patient outcomes as compared with a more strict target heart rate (resting heart rate <80 beats/minute).[25] This study may suggest that it could be acceptable for a patient's heart rate to be greater than 80 beats/minute, if there is difficulty in achieving this level of heart rate control and in asymptomatic patients or those with HF and a preserved EF.[7,26]

Rate Control versus Rhythm Control

CASE 15-1, QUESTION 7: After loading of digoxin, J.K.'s heart rate is still 120 beats/minute and he continues to experience palpitations. His BP is 100/60 mm Hg, and his symptoms of heart failure are improving, but he still complains of mild shortness of breath. The decision is made to cardiovert J.K. to normal sinus rhythm. Is J.K. a good candidate for a rhythm control strategy and if so, why? What is the likelihood that J.K. will be successfully converted to normal sinus rhythm?

The use of a rhythm control strategy has become much less common during the last several years. This change is because of the completion of several studies comparing the effect of a rate or rhythm control strategy on patient outcomes.[27–32] The AFFIRM study (Atrial Fibrillation Follow-up Investigation of Rhythm Management), a randomized, multicenter study, was one of the largest to compare rate control with rhythm control for management of AF. AFFIRM enrolled 4,060 patients with AF and a risk of stroke.[27] The primary end point was all-cause mortality. Antiarrhythmic drugs were chosen at the discretion of the treating physician, but greater than 60% of the patients received amiodarone or sotalol as the initial antiarrhythmic agent. Rate control agents included digoxin, β-blockers, and nondihydropyridine calcium-channel blockers. After a mean follow-up of 3.5 years, there was a trend toward lower overall mortality ($p = 0.08$) with significant reductions in hospitalizations (10% lower; $p = 0.001$) and TdP (300% lower; $p = 0.007$) in the rate control group. Therefore, using rhythm control in patients with AF rather than rate control does not improve outcomes and increases the risk of hospitalizations and TdP.

The default long-term treatment strategy for most patients should be a rate control strategy, in which heart rate is controlled and anticoagulation is provided, if indicated. However, rhythm control is necessary when patients experience symptoms despite adequate rate control, when heart rate cannot be adequately controlled with currently available treatments, or if patients cannot tolerate the adverse effects of rate-controlling medications. J.K.'s heart rate is not adequately controlled with digoxin and an oral β-blocker. A nondihydropyridine calcium-channel blocker could be added or the β-blocker dose could be increased in order to better control his heart rate; however, his BP may not tolerate the increased dose of the β-blocker or the addition of a nondihydropyridine calcium-channel blocker. Therefore, pursuit of a rhythm control strategy is warranted.

Likelihood of successful conversion to, and maintenance of, normal sinus rhythm is determined by the duration of the arrhythmia, underlying disease processes, and left atrial size.[33] Duration of AF for more than 1 year significantly reduces the chances of maintaining a normal sinus rhythm.[34] When the atrial size exceeds 5 cm, there is less than a 10% chance of maintaining normal sinus rhythm at 6 months. J.K.'s chance of being maintained in normal sinus rhythm is good because the duration of his AF is short and the echocardiogram revealed only slight enlargement of his left atrium.

Conversion to Normal Sinus Rhythm

CASE 15-1, QUESTION 8: Warfarin treatment is begun and J.K.'s prothrombin time is to be maintained at an international normalized ratio (INR) of 2 to 3. J.K. is scheduled for a transesophageal echocardiogram (TEE) to determine whether cardioversion can be performed during this admission. How does a TEE help to determine whether cardioversion can be performed, and why is warfarin therapy being used?

When the onset of AF is less than 48 hours, the likelihood of atrial clot formation is low. However, if patients are at a high risk for stroke, they should receive an anticoagulant (unfractionated heparin, low-molecular-weight heparin, factor Xa, or direct thrombin inhibitor) as soon as possible surrounding the cardioversion, followed by long-term anticoagulation.[7] When the duration of AF is greater than 48 hours, or if duration is unknown, then an oral anticoagulant agent (warfarin, dabigatran, factor Xa inhibitor) should be given for 3 weeks before cardioversion at doses providing an INR between 2 and 3 if using warfarin.[7] Studies in patients with AF showed that those who were anticoagulated with warfarin before cardioversion had a lower incidence (0.8%) of emboli than those who were not anticoagulated (5.3%).[35] Alternatively, a TEE can be used to determine whether atrial clots have formed.[7,36] Atrial clots form most often in small side pouches on the atria called atrial appendages.[37] Because the frequency of right atrial appendage thrombosis is half that of left atrial appendage thrombosis in AF patients, the risk of stroke is enhanced much more than the risk of pulmonary embolism.[37]

If no clot is observed on TEE, then there is low risk for stroke with cardioversion of AF.[36] However, if an atrial clot is evident on TEE, J.K. would need to be adequately anticoagulated for

3 weeks before cardioversion to prevent embolization of the clot and stroke. If cardioversion is successful, patients should remain on an oral anticoagulant agent for at least 4 weeks after cardioversion because normal atrial contraction may not return for up to 3 weeks, and patients may be at risk of late embolization.[38] The decision to provide long-term oral anticoagulation is dependent on the patient's underlying stroke and bleeding risk. This will be discussed further below.

Chemical Conversion—Ibutilide, Propafenone, Flecainide

CASE 15-1, QUESTION 9: J.K. was found to be free of atrial clots. Chemical cardioversion with ibutilide is planned for tomorrow. If J.K. fails to convert with ibutilide, he will be electrically cardioverted later in the day. How does ibutilide therapy compare with the other therapeutic choices for chemical cardioversion?

The most effective method of cardioversion is by direct current (DC) cardioversion (see Electrical Cardioversion section below). However, the use of DC cardioversion may be undesirable if the patient is a poor candidate for conscious sedation or if the patient is not willing to undergo DC cardioversion. In these situations, pharmacologic cardioversion may be attempted. Many class I and III antiarrhythmic agents have been evaluated for efficacy in placebo-controlled trials for conversion of AF or atrial flutter to normal sinus rhythm. The available agents with the most positive data for chemical conversion include IV ibutilide, oral propafenone, oral flecainide, oral and IV amiodarone, and oral dofetilide. This section will focus on ibutilide, propafenone, and flecainide.

IV ibutilide, a class III antiarrhythmic agent with potassium-channel blocking and slow sodium-channel enhancing effects, was the first agent that the US Food and Drug Administration (FDA) approved for the termination of recent-onset AF and atrial flutter.[39] Ibutilide is administered as a 1-mg infusion for 10 minutes, followed by another 1-mg infusion for 10 minutes if conversion has not occurred by 10 minutes after the infusion. The conversion rate for recent-onset AF is 35% to 50%; the conversion rate is 65% to 80% in atrial flutter. In a retrospective study of hospital inpatients with either AF or atrial flutter, 50% of patients converted initially (41% conversion AF, 65% atrial flutter), but only 33% of patients left the hospital in sinus rhythm. If the duration of AF or atrial flutter before cardioversion was fewer than 15 days, significantly more patients remained in sinus rhythm at discharge compared with patients who had AF or atrial flutter for more than 15 days before cardioversion.[40] As is the case with most class III antiarrhythmic agents, the main adverse effect is TdP, which occurred in approximately 4% of patients. Ibutilide should be avoided in patients with hypokalemia, hypomagnesemia, QT prolongation, and a low ejection fraction (<30%). Aside from the risk of TdP, therapy is well tolerated.[41–43]

Propafenone is a class Ic agent with β-blocking properties. When given in doses of 450 to 750 mg orally (600 mg was the most common dose), the initial conversion rate in patients with AF ranged from 41% to 57%. In contrast to ibutilide, no patients experienced ventricular arrhythmias (including TdP), but a risk of hypotension, bradycardia, and QRS prolongation was noted.[44–46]

Oral flecainide is another class Ic antiarrhythmic agent. In one study, 300 mg oral flecainide converted 68% of patients to sinus rhythm within 3 hours and 91% of patients by 8 hours. The efficacy in atrial flutter has yet to be established. Sinus node dysfunction, prolongation of intraventricular conduction, dizziness, weakness, and gastrointestinal (GI) disturbances have been reported.[47,48]

A β-blocker or nondihydropyridine calcium-channel antagonist should be administered ≥30 minutes before administering the Vaughan Williams class Ic agent to prevent a rapid ventricular response due to 1:1 AV conduction during atrial flutter.[7] J.K. is not a candidate for these agents due to his structural heart disease.

Electrical Conversion

CASE 15-1, QUESTION 10: J.K. received two doses of IV ibutilide. After the second dose, he converted to normal sinus rhythm for only 5 minutes, then returned to AF. J.K. is scheduled for electrical cardioversion in 6 hours. What is electrical cardioversion? How efficacious and safe is it?

DC cardioversion quickly and effectively restores 85% to 90% of patients with AF to normal sinus rhythm.[38] If DC conversion alone is ineffective, it can be repeated in combination with antiarrhythmic drugs.[7,49] In one study, the success rate of electrical cardioversion was significantly higher in AF patients (duration of AF averaged 119 days) with ibutilide pretreatment (1 mg) compared with those without pretreatment (100% vs. 72%; $p = 0.001$).[49] This is because ibutilide pretreatment lowered the energy requirement for atrial defibrillation by 27% ($p = 0.001$). TdP occurred in 3% of patients receiving ibutilide, all of whom had an ejection fraction less than 20%. Flecainide, propafenone, amiodarone, and dofetilide could also be considered for enhancing DC cardioversion.[7]

DC cardioversion is clearly indicated for patients who are hemodynamically unstable. A reason one may wish to avoid DC conversion is because anesthesia (short-acting benzodiazepine, barbiturate, or propofol) is required for the procedure.

Maintenance of Sinus Rhythm

CASE 15-1, QUESTION 11: J.K. is discharged after successful DC conversion. However, when he returns for a follow-up visit 2 weeks later, he is found to be in AF again. He again reports frequent palpitations. His physician would like to initiate an antiarrhythmic drug to maintain normal sinus rhythm. Which agent(s) would be the best option for this patient?

To choose the best antiarrhythmic agent for J.K., the efficacy and adverse effect profiles for each agent should be reviewed. Class Ia, Ic, and III antiarrhythmic drugs (see Tables 15-2 and 15-3) prevent the recurrence of AF. Flecainide, sotalol, dofetilide, and dronedarone are approved by the FDA for maintenance of sinus rhythm. Propafenone and amiodarone are commonly used as well.

Flecainide and Propafenone

The class Ic agents flecainide and propafenone are effective in suppressing AF.[50–54] The efficacy rate may be as high as 61% to 92% for flecainide.[55,56] Flecainide and possibly other class Ic agents are proarrhythmic, especially in patients with structural heart disease, and they should be avoided in such patients. Propafenone, a class Ic agent with β-blocking properties, is as efficacious as flecainide and is relatively safe in patients without ischemic heart disease and an ejection fraction greater than 35%; it may be preferred in patients who require additional AV blockade to control ventricular response. In a direct comparison with flecainide (200–300 mg/day), propafenone (450–900 mg/day) was equally safe and effective. Over the course of 12 months, a similar percentage of patients (approximately 12% in each group) did not have adequate control of their arrhythmia. Adverse events were comparable and occurred in 10.3% of patients on flecainide and 7.7% of patients on propafenone. Of all the adverse events noted, only one patient who was receiving propafenone developed a ventricular arrhythmia. Another 1-year comparative study of propafenone versus flecainide demonstrated similar efficacy, but this study showed a trend toward better tolerability in the flecainide group.[57,58]

CASE 15-1, QUESTION 12: J.K. is to begin dofetilide today. He is admitted to the hospital for dofetilide initiation. Why would J.K. need to be admitted for dofetilide initiation? Is it necessary to initiate all antiarrhythmic medications in the hospital?

Class III agents (sotalol, dofetilide, amiodarone, dronedarone) prolong refractoriness in the atria, ventricles, AV node, and accessory pathway tissue and can prevent recurrence of AF. All of these agents act by blocking potassium channels; however, sotalol also has additional β-blocking properties.[59–61] Both amiodarone and dronedarone block sodium channels and calcium channels, and have antiadrenergic effects in addition to potassium-channel blocking properties.[59,61]

Sotalol, Amiodarone, Dofetilide, and Dronedarone

The efficacy of sotalol in delaying the recurrence of AF was evaluated in a double-blind, placebo-controlled, multicenter, randomized trial that enrolled 253 patients with AF or atrial flutter.[62] The median times to recurrence were 27, 106, 229, and 175 days with placebo, sotalol 160 mg/day (divided in two doses), sotalol 240 mg/day (divided in two doses), and sotalol 320 mg/day (divided in two doses), respectively. Sotalol is contraindicated in patients with a creatinine clearance (CrCl) of less than 40 mL/minute because of the fact that the drug is largely renally cleared and can cause TdP in high concentrations. In a comparative study versus propafenone, sotalol was similarly effective in producing at least a 75% reduction in AF recurrence (79% of patients on propafenone vs. 76% on sotalol). Bradycardia, dizziness, and GI disturbances were the most common intolerable side effects.[63] Sotalol should not be used in patients with systolic heart failure owing to the negative inotropic effects of the drug. It may be useful as a first-line agent in patients with AF and concomitant underlying coronary artery disease or in patients with no cardiovascular disease.[7]

Amiodarone is more effective at maintaining sinus rhythm than sotalol and propafenone.[64] The Canadian Trial of Atrial Fibrillation (CTAF) compared the ability of low-dose amiodarone (200 mg/day) versus propafenone (450–600 mg/day) and sotalol (160–320 mg/day) to prevent recurrence of AF.[64] After a mean follow-up of 16 months, 35% of the amiodarone-treated patients had a recurrence of AF versus 63% in the combined group with sotalol and propafenone ($p = 0.001$). In view of its unusual pharmacokinetics and potential serious adverse effects (see Table 15-3 and Case 15-7, Question 2), amiodarone is only recommended as a first-line choice for patients with HF, for which it has specific safety data, or for patients with significant left ventricular hypertrophy.[7] Amiodarone could also be used when other agents such as sotalol, propafenone, or dofetilide have failed.[7,65]

Dofetilide has been shown to be an effective pharmacologic agent for conversion to, and maintenance of, normal sinus rhythm. Two clinical trials, EMERALD (European and Australian Multicenter Evaluative Research on Atrial Fibrillation Dofetilide)[66] and SAFIRE-D (Symptomatic Atrial Fibrillation Investigation and Randomized Evaluation of Dofetilide),[67] have shown conversion rates of 30% in patients with AF or atrial flutter receiving higher doses of dofetilide. Patients failing chemical conversion received electrical conversion. If this conversion succeeded, they were continued on dofetilide for 1 year. At 1 year, 60% of those converted were still in sinus rhythm with the 500-mcg dose. Also, dofetilide appears to exert neutral effects on mortality rates in HF and post-MI patients.[68,69]

Dofetilide dose is based on the patient's CrCl; the doses are 500, 250, and 125 mcg twice daily with CrCl greater than 60, 40 to 60, and 20 to 39 mL/minute, respectively. Drug interactions pose a significant problem with dofetilide. Cimetidine, ketoconazole, prochlorperazine, megestrol, and trimethoprim (including in combination with sulfamethoxazole) inhibit active tubular secretion of dofetilide and can elevate dofetilide plasma concentrations.[60] Because the incidence of TdP is directly related to dofetilide plasma concentrations, concomitant use with these agents is contraindicated.[70] Concomitant administration of dofetilide with verapamil or hydrochlorothiazide increases the incidence of TdP by an unclear mechanism and is contraindicated as well.[60] Concurrent use of agents that can prolong the QTc interval is not recommended with dofetilide.[70] Dofetilide also undergoes metabolism by the cytochrome P-450 CYP3A4 isoenzyme to a minor extent. Therefore, inhibitors of this isoenzyme (e.g., azole antifungal agents, protease inhibitors, serotonin reuptake inhibitors, amiodarone, diltiazem, nefazodone, zafirlukast) should be coadministered with caution with dofetilide. Other agents that can potentially increase dofetilide levels (through inhibition of tubular secretion) include metformin, triamterene, and amiloride. Hence, these agents should be cautiously coadministered with dofetilide.[70]

Dofetilide is considered a first-line agent for patients with heart failure or coronary artery disease, as the impact on mortality in this patient population is neutral.[7] Dofetilide can also be considered as a first-line agent for patients without cardiovascular disease, but should be avoided in patients with severe left ventricular hypertrophy.[7]

Dronedarone is structurally and pharmacologically similar to amiodarone; however, it lacks iodine, and it has a much smaller volume of distribution than amiodarone. The lack of iodine may make dronedarone less likely to cause thyroid-related or other adverse effects.[61] Dronedarone has been shown to have modest efficacy in maintaining sinus rhythm when compared with placebo. The rate of recurrence of AF at 1 year is approximately 40%, and the number of days to recurrence is nearly doubled with dronedarone.[71] The major clinical trial evaluating dronedarone was the ATHENA study. The primary end point of ATHENA was a composite of death or cardiovascular hospitalization, and patients received either dronedarone 400 mg twice daily or placebo for at least 1 year.[72] The primary composite end point was significantly reduced from 39.4% with placebo to 31.9% with dronedarone. This reduction in the composite was completely attributable to the reduction in cardiovascular hospitalizations, most of which were related to AF recurrence. GI events were the most common type of adverse effect with dronedarone in this study. It should be noted that patients with recent decompensated HF or New York Heart Association (NYHA) class IV heart failure were excluded from this trial. The exclusion of patients with severe or unstable heart failure was related to negative findings that led to the early discontinuation of the ANDROMEDA study.[73] ANDROMEDA was designed as a safety study, to evaluate the impact of dronedarone on mortality in patients with HF. Patients admitted with NYHA class III or IV systolic HF were included in this study. The study was stopped early because of an approximate doubling in the risk of death with dronedarone as compared with placebo. Therefore, dronedarone is contraindicated in a patient with severe or recently decompensated HF. Based on the findings of the PALLAS study, dronedarone should be avoided in patients with permanent AF as well.[74] This study found that the rate of stroke, heart failure, and cardiovascular death was increased when dronedarone was used in this patient population. Dronedarone has also been compared directly with amiodarone.[75] In this study, dronedarone was less effective than amiodarone, but was less likely than amiodarone to cause thyroid, neurologic, skin, or ocular adverse effects. GI adverse effects were more common with dronedarone.[75] Dronedarone is appropriate as a first-line agent for patients with AF and concomitant coronary artery disease, and possibly left ventricular hypertrophy or in patients with no cardiovascular disease. Dronedarone should not be used in a patient with severe HF symptoms or a recent hospitalization for HF, but may be used with mild, well-controlled HF.[7,73]

In view of J.K.'s HF, sotalol, propafenone, and flecainide would not be indicated. Although dronedarone may be better tolerated than amiodarone, it would be contraindicated because J.K. was recently admitted with decompensated HF. Therefore, the only available options for J.K. would be either dofetilide or amiodarone, both of which have been proven safe in patients with HF. Selection between dofetilide and amiodarone could be based on renal function, the presence of any major drug interactions, or the desire to avoid adverse effects with amiodarone.

Dofetilide was approved with the requirement for in-hospital initiation because of the relatively high risk of TdP in clinical trials. ECG monitoring is required for patients being initiated on dofetilide for a minimum of 3 days in a properly equipped facility. The initial regimen is determined by the patient's estimated CrCl. The QTc interval must be measured (using a 12-lead ECG) 2 to 3 hours after the first dose and each subsequent dose while the patient is hospitalized. If the QTc interval increases by greater than 15% or if it surpasses 500 ms (>550 ms in patients with ventricular conduction abnormalities) after the first dose, the dofetilide regimen should be reduced by 50%. If the QTc interval exceeds the above parameters any time after the second subsequent dose, dofetilide should be discontinued.[76]

Sotalol may also be arrhythmogenic in high doses, and the risk of inducing TdP has prompted its manufacturer to mandate a minimum of 3 days of ECG monitoring in a properly equipped facility during therapy initiation as well.[76] Further, during initiation and titration, QTc intervals should be monitored 2 to 4 hours after each dose. In fact, most antiarrhythmic agents for AF should probably be initiated in the inpatient setting, with the exception of amiodarone owing to the low risk of proarrhythmia with this drug.[7]

STROKE PREVENTION

Antithrombotic Therapy

CASE 15-1, QUESTION 13: J.K. is discharged from the hospital on dofetilide 500 mcg twice daily, which is appropriate given his CrCl of 92 mL/minute. He has been doing fine for 2 weeks after discharge. Should J.K. remain on warfarin therapy? Could any other antithrombotic options be considered?

Patients with nonvalvular and valvular AF have a 5- and 17-fold increased risk for stroke compared with patients without AF, respectively.[4,5] Stroke can lead to death or significant neurologic disability in up to 71% of patients, with an annual recurrence rate as high as 10%.[77]

In three large, randomized trials, patients with nonvalvular AF benefited from antithrombotic therapy.[78–81] In the Stroke Prevention in Atrial Fibrillation (SPAF) study, both aspirin 325 mg/day and warfarin (titrated to an INR of 2.0–4.5) reduced the risk of stroke significantly with an acceptable level of hemorrhagic complications.[80] The results of SPAF II, a direct comparison of warfarin and aspirin, indicated that warfarin was more effective than aspirin in preventing stroke.[81] These results were verified by the Copenhagen AFASAK study, which found warfarin to be significantly better than aspirin and placebo at preventing cerebral emboli and overall vascular deaths (cerebral and cardiovascular).[78] An oral direct thrombin antagonist (dabigatran) and oral factor Xa antagonists (rivaroxaban, apixaban, edoxaban) are now available. These newer anticoagulant agents have been shown to have similar or better efficacy and safety compared to warfarin.[82–84]

Dabigatran is approved by the FDA to reduce the risk of stroke and systemic embolism in patients with nonvalvular AF.[85] In the Re-Ly trial, dabigatran 110 mg twice daily and 150 mg twice daily was compared with warfarin in patients with a $CHADS_2$ score of 1 or more (average $CHADS_2$ score of 2.1). The $CHADS_2$ score is a tool used to estimate stroke risk. In this study the lower dose of dabigatran was noninferior to warfarin for stroke prevention but was associated with less bleeding. High-dose dabigatran was superior to warfarin for stroke prevention but comparable in bleeding.[86] The most common nonbleeding adverse event in this study was GI upset. It should also be noted that dabigatran capsules should not be chewed or opened.

The three oral factor Xa inhibitors that are currently approved for prevention of stroke and systemic embolus in patients with AF include rivaroxaban, apixaban, and edoxaban. Each of these agents have been compared directly to warfarin using fairly similar study designs.[82–84] Rivaroxaban and edoxaban were found to be noninferior to warfarin in stroke/systemic embolus prevention, while apixaban was found to be superior to warfarin in efficacy. Major bleeding occurred less frequently with edoxaban and apixaban and at a similar rate with rivaroxaban, compared to warfarin. Although efficacy and safety of all of the new agents differed when compared with warfarin, there are no direct comparisons between any of the newer antithrombotic options. As such, no firm conclusions can be drawn regarding the optimal agent to choose. However, in a patient who is perceived to have a high bleeding risk, it is reasonable to select apixaban or edoxaban, given the bleeding risk advantage of these agents relative to warfarin.[83,84]

Some differences between the newer agents could be considered when selecting an anticoagulant regimen for a patient. For example, each agent has different recommendations for use with kidney dysfunction. None of the newer oral agents should be used in patients with a CrCl less than 15 mL/minute. The "renal doses" of rivaroxaban (15 mg/day with CrCl of 15–49 mL/minute) and edoxaban (30 mg/day with CrCl of 15–50 mL/minute) were evaluated in the ROCKET AF and ENGAGE AF TIMI 48 studies, whereas the renal dose adjustment recommended for dabigatran (75-mg twice daily dose for those with a CrCl of 15–30 mL/minute) was based on extrapolated pharmacokinetic data.[82,84,87] Apixaban does not require dosage adjustment based on a CrCl, but adjustment should occur if the patient has two or more high-risk characteristics (body weight <60 kg, serum creatinine >1.5 or age >80 years). Interestingly, edoxaban is less effective and should not be used when CrCl is greater than 95 mL/minute. Therefore, edoxaban, apixaban, or rivaroxaban may be a more evidence-based option than dabigatran for a patient with poor kidney function and edoxaban would be an inappropriate choice for the patient with very good kidney function.[82–85]

The drug interaction profiles of the oral direct thrombin inhibitor or oral factor Xa inhibitors are favorable compared to that of warfarin. All of the newer anticoagulant options interact with rifampin. Rivaroxaban and apixaban also interact with other strong inhibitors and inducers of both the P-glycoprotein and CYP 3A4 systems. Dabigatran interacts with inhibitors of P-glycoprotein (ketoconazole, dronedarone); however, no change in therapy is required unless the interacting drugs are used in a patient who also has a CrCl less than 50 mL/minute. At this time, no notable interactions have been identified with edoxaban, other than the interaction with rifampin. Although the number of interactions with the newer anticoagulants is fewer than with warfarin, it will still be important to evaluate for the presence of interactions at therapy initiation and when the drug therapy regimen is changed. An advantage of dabigatran and the oral factor Xa antagonists is that these agents do not require frequent monitoring and dosage adjustment in order to assure an appropriate level of anticoagulation. A potential disadvantage is that it is often not possible to monitor the extent of anticoagulation in the setting of bleeding or when an urgent procedure or surgery is needed. In addition, strategies for reversal of these agents are not well defined, in contrast to the reversal approach with warfarin. Best available evidence suggests that concentrated blood factor products (4-factor prothrombin complex concentrates and FEIBA) may be options for reversing the effects of these agents; however, specific reversal agents are likely to be commercially available in the near future.[88] Hemodialysis can also be used to remove dabigatran, in the setting of life-threatening bleeding.[88]

Generally, patients with a CHA_2DS_2-VASc score of 2 or greater should receive anticoagulant therapy for stroke prophylaxis.[7] Warfarin (INR target 2–3), dabigatran, rivaroxaban, apixaban are all recommended as antithrombotic agents for stroke prophylaxis.[7] Edoxaban was not approved at the time of publication of the 2014 guidelines for AF and is not currently included, but has FDA approval. No therapy, an antithrombotic agent, or aspirin alone could be used in patients with a CHA_2DS_2-VASc score of 1 and stroke prophylaxis is not required if a patient's CHA_2DS_2-VASc score is 0. If a patient's INR is difficult to control on warfarin, a direct thrombin inhibitor or oral Xa antagonist could be used.[7] It should be noted that patients with AF and valvular disease should only be treated with warfarin for stroke prophylaxis as data with valvular AF are either unfavorable or unavailable with the newer agents in this patient population.[89]

Even though J.K. is in normal sinus rhythm at this time, in the AFFIRM trial, only 73% and 63% of patients randomized to rhythm control remained in sinus rhythm at 3 and 5 years, respectively.[26] As such, the use of an antiarrhythmic drug does not eliminate the risk of stroke, and in fact, patients may return to AF and not be aware they are no longer in normal sinus rhythm. J.K. has a CHA_2DS_2-VASc score of 4 and does not appear to have any factors that would suggest a high bleeding risk (no recent history of GI bleeding, etc.). Therefore, he should continue to receive anticoagulation for stroke prophylaxis.[7] Although J.K. is currently taking warfarin, there would be no reason he could not receive any of the other available anticoagulants.

CASE 15-2

QUESTION 1: M.P. is a 38-year-old woman who has had frequent episodes of atrial flutter for the past 2 years. She has no other medical history and is taking metoprolol 50 mg twice daily. She does not want to take the drug any longer because it reduces her exercise tolerance. Does the treatment of atrial flutter differ from the treatment of AF and what is the role of radiofrequency catheter ablation for M.P.?

Atrial flutter is an unstable rhythm that often reverts to sinus rhythm or progresses to AF. If atrial flutter is episodic, its underlying cause should be identified and treated if possible. If a patient remains in atrial flutter, the treatment goals (control of ventricular rate, return to normal sinus rhythm) are the same as those for AF. Similar agents and doses can be used to control the ventricular response. Chemical conversion, low-energy (<50 J) DC cardioversion, or rapid atrial pacing may acutely convert atrial flutter back to sinus rhythm, but the recurrence of atrial flutter is high.

Radiofrequency catheter ablation therapy could be used as a nonpharmacologic treatment for atrial flutter and AF.[7] With both atrial flutter and AF, an EP study is performed to identify whether ablation can be performed. Various sections of the atria and pulmonary veins (where they intersect with the atria) are probed with a catheter that delivers cardiac pacing. If an area is stimulated with pacing and an atrial ectopic or reentrant focus is recognized, that area could be ablated. Ablation destroys tissue that is integral either to the initiation or to the maintenance of the arrhythmia by delivering electrical energy through electrodes on the catheter. If the focus of the arrhythmia is in the atrial tissue (typically for atrial flutter), then the focus itself is ablated. This procedure is successful in 75% to 90% of cases and can be recommended for patients with atrial flutter who are drug-resistant or drug-intolerant, or do not desire long-term therapy. In AF, an ectopic focus originating in the pulmonary veins can often initiate the arrhythmia. In this case, circumferential ablation, in which a circle of ablated tissue is made around the pulmonary veins, is performed. Circumferential ablation does not prevent the ectopic impulses from the pulmonary veins from occurring; however, it does prevent propagation of the impulse into the atria and may reduce the recurrence of AF. Recent data comparing ablation to antiarrhythmic drug therapy in patients with PAF suggest that ablation is more effective in preventing recurrence of AF than medications.[90]

Radiofrequency ablation therapy may be suitable for M.P. However, if exercise intolerance is her primary complaint, this might be relieved by switching M.P. to another drug, such as verapamil.[91,92]

Paroxysmal Supraventricular Tachycardia

CLINICAL PRESENTATION

CASE 15-3

QUESTION 1: B.J., a 32-year-old woman, presents to the emergency department (ED) complaining of fatigue and palpitations. She has had similar episodes approximately twice a year for the past 2 years, but has not sought medical attention for them. She is in no apparent distress and has a temperature of 98.0°F, heart rate of 185 beats/minute, BP of 95/60 mm Hg, and respiratory rate of 12 breaths/minute. Her ECG (Fig. 15-5) shows regular rhythm with a heart rate of 185 bpm. The P waves cannot be found, and the QRS complex is 110 ms (normal, <120 ms). She has no past medical history of note.

What is the clinical presentation of PSVT, and what are the consequences of this arrhythmia?

PSVT often has a sudden onset and termination. At the time of PSVT, the heart rate is usually 180 to 200 beats/minute. As illustrated by B.J., patients experience palpitations and often nervousness and anxiety. In patients with a rapid ventricular rate, dizziness, and syncope can occur, and the rhythm may degenerate to other serious arrhythmias. Angina, HF, or shock may be precipitated by underlying severe atherosclerosis or left ventricular dysfunction but this is not part of B.J.'s past medical history. There is no evidence that patients with episodes of PSVT are at an increased risk of stroke.

ARRHYTHMOGENESIS AND REENTRY

CASE 15-3, QUESTION 2: What is the arrhythmogenic mechanism of PSVT?

AV nodal reentry is the most common mechanism of paroxysmal supraventricular arrhythmias (see Fig. 15-2). Here AV nodal impulses

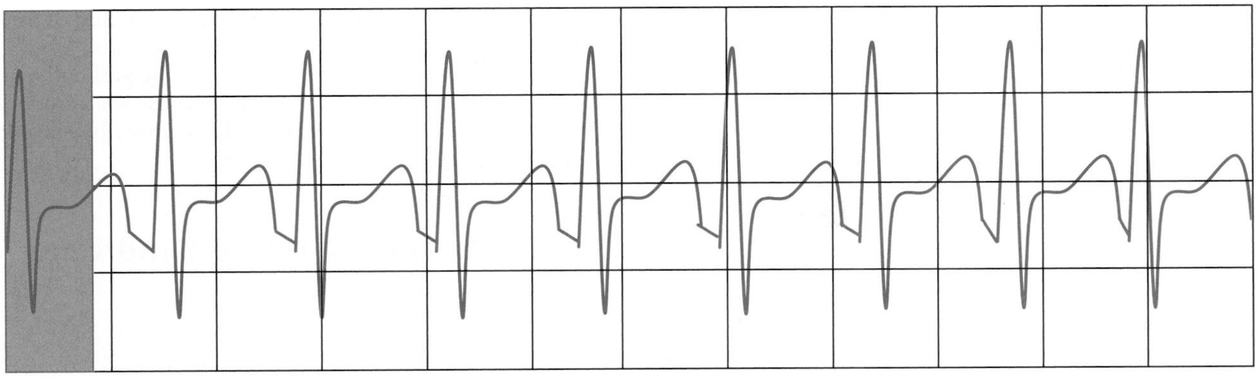

Figure 15-5 Supraventricular Tachycardia. Note the lack of P-waves, narrow QRS complexes, and rapid rate.

are blocked in one of two directions in an antegrade fashion but when reaching the end, conducts in a retrograde fashion setting up a circular reentrant circuit. Reciprocating tachycardias occur when there is an accessory pathway for conduction of impulses between the atria and ventricles, like with WPW syndrome, and PSVT results (Fig. 15-6).

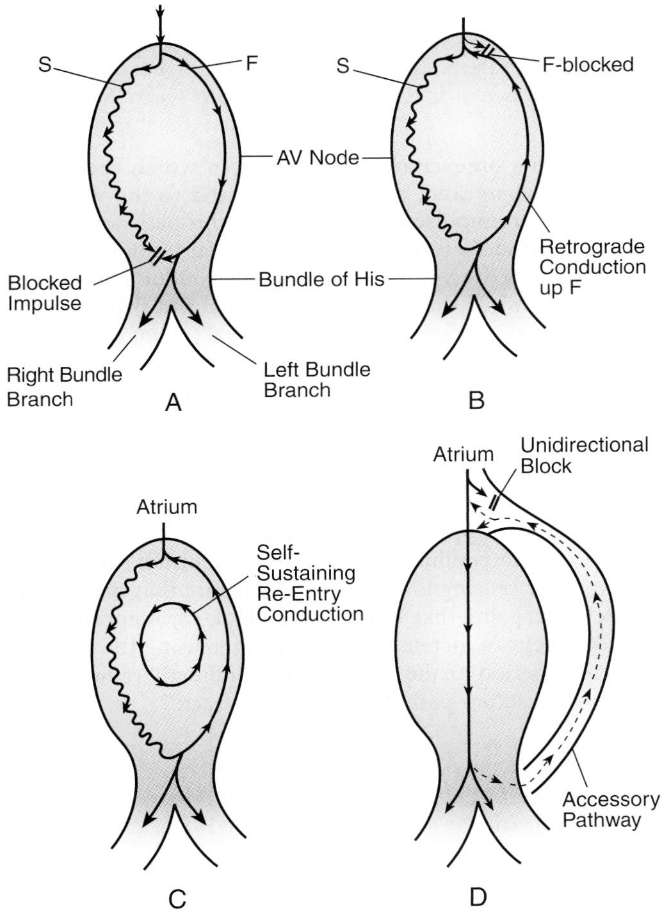

Figure 15-6 The atrioventricular (AV) node in paroxysmal supraventricular tachycardia and Wolff–Parkinson–White syndrome. **A:** A bifurcation of an impulse, one propagated fast and another slow. **B:** The slow impulse in **(A)** can send impulses in a retrograde fashion. **C:** The reentry from **(A)** to **(B)** can be self-sustaining. **D:** Normal impulse conduction through the AV node, but abnormal retrograde conduction up an accessory pathway, as would be seen in a patient with Wolff–Parkinson–White syndrome.

TREATMENT

CASE 15-3, QUESTION 3: B.J. tries the Valsalva maneuver, and her ventricular rate is reduced to 150 beats/minute; the other parameters are unchanged. She is given IV adenosine 6 mg, administered over 1 minute, with no effect on the PSVT rate. Another dose of adenosine 12 mg given over 1 minute has no effect. No side effects are noted from therapy. What treatment options can be used if B.J. is hemodynamically unstable? What is the Valsalva maneuver? What is the probable reason for B.J.'s unresponsiveness to adenosine? Are there any drug interactions that might diminish adenosine's effect?

Nondrug Treatment

Valsalva Maneuver

Although her BP is low at 95/60 mm Hg, B.J. is maintaining an adequate perfusion pressure, so vagal maneuvers should be attempted first. Two common vagal techniques are pressure over the bifurcation of the internal and external carotid arteries and the Valsalva maneuver (forcible exhalation against a closed glottis, similar to bearing down to have a bowel movement). The increase in pressure induced by these maneuvers is sensed by the baroreceptors, causing a reflex decrease in sympathetic tone and an increase in vagal tone. The increase in vagal tone will terminate in 10% to 30% of cases.[92] If B.J. was hemodynamically unstable or becomes hemodynamically unstable, she should receive synchronized DC cardioversion.

Drug Therapy

Adenosine

Because most PSVT episodes involve reentry in the AV node, drugs that block the AV node (negative dromotropic drugs) are generally effective. Adenosine, a purine nucleoside that exerts a transient negative chronotropic and dromotropic effect on cardiac pacemaker tissue,[93] is considered the drug of choice for the acute treatment of PSVT because of its rapid and brief effect. An initial 6-mg IV bolus is given; if this is unsuccessful within 2 minutes, it can be followed by one or two 12-mg IV boluses, up to a maximum of 30 mg. Because of its short half-life (9 seconds), adenosine should be administered as a rapid bolus (over 1–3 seconds), followed immediately by a saline flush. Adenosine begins to be metabolized immediately after entering the bloodstream; therefore, B.J.'s failure to respond is likely attributed to the prolonged (1-minute) infusion time.

Theoretically, adenosine may be ineffective or higher doses may be required in patients who are receiving theophylline because theophylline is an effective adenosine receptor blocker. Larger doses of other methylxanthines (caffeine, guarana) may also theoretically interact like theophylline. Conversely, concomitant use of dipyridamole may accentuate adenosine's effects because dipyridamole blocks the adenosine uptake (and subsequent clearance).

CASE 15-3, QUESTION 4: B.J. is given 12 mg adenosine IV during 2 seconds, followed by a 20-mL normal saline flush. Thirty seconds later, she complains of chest tightness and pressure. What is the explanation for these symptoms?

B.J. is experiencing a common side effect of adenosine. Patients receiving adenosine should be warned that they may feel transient chest heaviness, flushing, or a feeling of anxiety. Shortness of breath and wheezing may be observed in patients with asthma. The denervated heart of the patient who has undergone heart transplant is particularly sensitive to adenosine; therefore, lower doses of adenosine should be used.

Calcium-Channel Blockers

CASE 15-3, QUESTION 5: B.J. is still in PSVT. What other acute therapeutic options should be considered at this time?

Nondihydropyridine calcium-channel blockers, verapamil, and diltiazem, can be used in patients with PSVT. Verapamil (5–10 mg or 0.075–0.15 mg/kg IV given over 2 minutes) achieves peak therapeutic effects in 3 to 5 minutes after dosing and can be repeated at 10- to 15-minute intervals to a maximal dose of 20 mg if needed. The elderly should receive the verapamil infusion over 3 minutes to minimize the risk of adverse events. Diltiazem is given as a 0.25-mg/kg IV bolus over 2 minutes, and a second bolus of 0.35 mg/kg can be given 15 minutes later if the effect is inadequate. Both of these calcium-channel blockers have an 85% conversion rate.[94] However, verapamil should not be used in patients with wide complex tachycardia of unknown origin because it may lead to hemodynamic compromise and potentially VF. β-Blockers and digoxin can be used if calcium-channel blockers and adenosine fail.

CASE 15-3, QUESTION 6: B.J. is given 5 mg IV verapamil, followed by an additional 5 mg 10 minutes later. She converts to normal sinus rhythm 3 minutes after the second dose. Because she has experienced symptoms that could be attributed to PSVT in the past, she may be a candidate for chronic therapy to slow conduction and increase refractoriness at the AV node. Which agents have been evaluated for this indication? Is there a role for radiofrequency catheter ablation therapy for PSVT?

Radiofrequency catheter ablation is frequently used as a definitive treatment for PSVT. EP testing is used to determine the location of the reentrant tract, which then can be ablated, thereby interrupting accessory pathways and reentrant circuits. This treatment approach is potentially curative and is performed by an electrophysiologist. Patients who are not candidates for ablation, or who do not wish to undergo the procedure, can receive medications on a chronic basis. PSVT is managed with agents that slow conduction and increase refractoriness in the AV node, thereby preventing a rapid ventricular response. These include oral verapamil, diltiazem, β-blockers, or digoxin. Class Ic and III agents are used occasionally to slow conduction and increase refractoriness of the fast bypass tract to prevent triggering impulses such as premature atrial and ventricular contractions.

B.J. has had a few episodes of PSVT in the past and may be a candidate for ablation. Alternatively, because she responded to IV verapamil, oral SR verapamil could be prescribed at a dosage of 240 mg/day.

Wolff–Parkinson–White Syndrome

CASE 15-4

QUESTION 1: M.B., a 35-year-old man, presents to the ED with a chief complaint of chest palpitations for 4 hours with intermittent feeling of almost passing out (pre-syncope). M.B.'s vital signs are BP, 96/68 mm Hg; pulse, 226 beats/minute, irregular; respiratory rate, 15 breaths/minute; and temperature, 98.7°F. A rhythm strip confirms AF, with a QRS width varying from 0.08 to 0.14 seconds. To control the ventricular rate, 10 mg IV verapamil is administered over 2 minutes. Within 2 minutes of completing the infusion, VF is noted on the monitor. M.B. is defibrillated, and normal sinus rhythm is restored. A subsequent ECG demonstrates a P-R interval of 100 ms (normal, 120–200 ms) and delta waves, compatible with WPW. He relates a past medical history of many similar self-terminating episodes since he was a teenager but he has no atherosclerotic heart disease or HF. He took an unknown medication 5 years ago that decreased the occurrence of the palpitations, but he stopped taking it because of side effects. What is WPW syndrome?

WPW is a preexcitation syndrome in which there is an accessory bypass tract connecting the atria to the ventricles (Fig. 15-6). An impulse can travel down this pathway and excite the ventricle before the expected regular impulse through the AV node arrives. If there is antegrade conduction over the bypass tract while the patient is in normal sinus rhythm, the ECG will demonstrate a short P-R interval (<100 ms), a delta wave that represents a fused complex from preexcitation, and the regular QRS complex after AV conduction. PSVT and AF occur in these patients at a higher incidence than in the general population of the same age.[95] Similar to M.B., the rapid heart rate experienced during the tachycardia may cause palpitations, light-headedness, and fatigue. When patients with WPW develop AF, there is a danger that the rapid atrial impulses will be conducted directly to the ventricle through the bypass tract, causing a rapid ventricular rate that may evolve into VF. Verapamil (like diltiazem, β-blockers, adenosine, and amiodarone) can increase this risk by increasing the effective refractory period of the AV node and indirectly reducing the effective refractory period in the bypass tract.[96]

CASE 15-4, QUESTION 2: Why did verapamil cause VF in M.B.? What therapies would be appropriate for M.B., and what drugs should be avoided?

Because M.B. had AF, the rapid atrial impulses were conducted directly down the bypass tract to the ventricle, causing VF.[97,98]

The antiarrhythmic drugs used to chemically convert patients with AF who have WPW, such as M.B., include procainamide, propafenone, flecainide, and dofetilide.[99,100] DC cardioversion is an option for more emergent conversion of AF in patients with WPW and hemodynamic instability. Radiofrequency ablation of the bypass tract is curative for many patients with WPW and is indicated for people who maintain preexcitation during exercise stress testing, a shortest preexcited RR interval <250 ms, symptoms like syncope of palpitations, or preexisting structural heart disease. M.B. has symptoms associated with AF in WPW and should undergo evaluation from an cardiologist to determine if ablation is appropriate at this time.[101]

Further therapy for M.B. may not be useful at this time. However, if he has recurrent AF or other symptomatology associated with WPW, radiofrequency catheter ablation could be indicated.

CONDUCTION BLOCKS

Various arrhythmias can result from blockage of impulse conduction. These can occur above the ventricle, such as first-, second-, and third-degree (complete) AV block. Others, such as right or left bundle branch block (RBBB or LBBB) and trifascicular block, originate below the bifurcation of the His bundle. Although conduction blocks can be classified as either supraventricular or ventricular arrhythmias, they are discussed as a separate group because their mechanism of arrhythmogenesis is similar and their treatment is different from other arrhythmias.

CASE 15-5

QUESTION 1: H.T., a 63-year-old man, was admitted to the coronary care unit (CCU) 12 hours ago with an acute inferior wall MI. He has remained stable. On admission, he had developed left bundle branch block. Twelve hours later, it has changed to the rhythm strip shown in Figure 15-7 (Wenckebach or type I, second-degree AV block).

Are these rhythms potentially hazardous to H.T.? How is second-degree AV block different from first- or third-degree AV block?

H.T.'s rhythm strip initially revealed a diagnosis of LBBB. Bundle branch block occurs when the electrical impulse cannot be conducted along the left or right fascicle of the His-Purkinje system (see Fig. 15-1). In H.T., the impulse travels down the right bundle normally, and the right ventricle contracts at the normal time. The left bundle is blocked, and, therefore, the left side is depolarized from an impulse conducted from the right ventricle. This impulse must travel through atypical conduction tissues (with slower conduction), and hence the left side depolarizes later. This is revealed on the ECG by a widened QRS complex. Bundle branch blocks, particularly in the left fascicle, are associated with coronary artery disease, systemic hypertension, aortic valve stenosis, and cardiomyopathy.[102] Typically, they do not lead to clinical cardiac dysfunction on their own. Because H.T. has LBBB, he can develop complete heart block (third-degree block) if for any reason his right fascicle is damaged.

First-degree AV block usually is asymptomatic. The ECG will show P waves with a prolonged P-R interval (normal, <200 ms), but each P wave is followed by a normal QRS complex. First-degree AV block is a common finding in patients taking digoxin, verapamil, or other drugs that slow AV conduction.

Second-degree heart block consists of two types. Mobitz type I (Wenckebach) is characterized by progressive lengthening of the P-R interval with each beat until an impulse is not conducted; the cycle then starts over again. Mobitz type II (Fig. 15-8) impulse conduction is blocked in a fixed, regular pattern (e.g., 3:1 block, in which for every three P waves, only one is conducted). A major difference is that Mobitz type I can be drug induced or exacerbated by negative dromotropic drugs but not Mobitz type II.

Third-degree heart block (complete heart block) occurs when none of the impulses from the SA node are conducted to the ventricles. During third-degree block, the ventricle must develop its own pacemaker (escape rhythm), which may be too slow to provide adequate cardiac output, causing the patient to become symptomatic. A mechanical pacemaker is needed for treatment of third-degree AV block. AV blocks can be caused by drugs (β-blockers, calcium-channel blockers, digoxin), acute MI, amyloidosis, and congenital abnormalities.[102]

Atropine

CASE 15-5, QUESTION 2: How should H.T.'s heart block be treated?

H.T. is experiencing a Wenckebach rhythm, which often is transient after an inferior wall MI. As long as he is hemodynamically stable, he should be monitored closely. If his heart rate and BP drop, atropine 0.5 mg IV bolus (maximum 2 mg) or a temporary pacemaker can increase the heart rate. If the hemodynamic compromise persists, a permanent pacemaker must be inserted to initiate the impulse to control the heart rate.

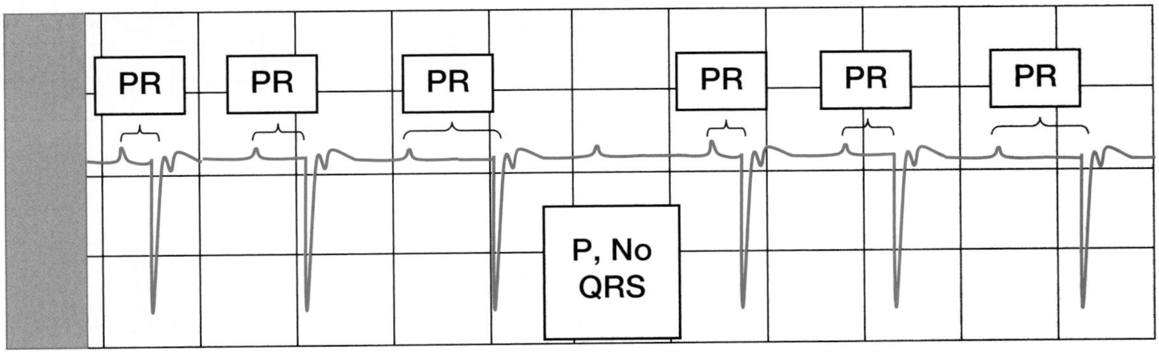

Figure 15-7 Second degree atrioventricular block type I. The P-R Interval progressively prolongs until a QRS complex is not conducted and then the cycle repeats.

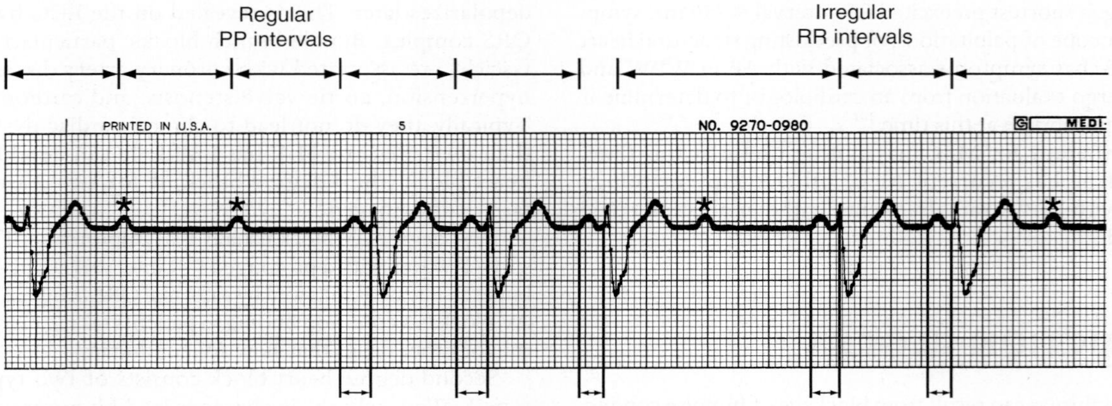

Figure 15-8 Sinus rhythm with second-degree AV block, Type II; note constant PR interval. (Reprinted with permission from Smeltzer SC, Bare BG. *Textbook of Medical-Surgical Nursing*. 9th Ed. Philadelphia: Lippincott Williams & Wilkins; 2000.)

VENTRICULAR ARRHYTHMIAS

Recognition and Definition

Impulses from ventricular ectopic foci or reentrant circuits generate wide, bizarre-looking QRS complexes leading to PVCs (Fig. 15-9). Three consecutive PVCs usually are defined as VT, which can be nonsustained or sustained. Ventricular flutter, VF, and TdP are other serious forms of ventricular arrhythmias. The presentation, etiology, treatment, and ion channels associated with TdP are discussed separately.

Nonsustained ventricular tachycardia (NSVT) (Fig. 15-10) commonly is defined as three or more consecutive PVCs lasting less than 30 seconds and terminating spontaneously. Sustained VT (SuVT) is defined as consecutive PVCs lasting more than 30 seconds, with a rate usually in the range of 150 to 200 beats/minute. P waves are lost in the QRS complex and are indiscernible. SuVT (Fig. 15-11) is a serious development because it can degenerate into VF. Ventricular flutter is characterized by sustained, rapid, regular ventricular beats (normal, >250 beats/minute) and usually degenerates into VF. VF (see Fig. 15-12) is characterized by irregular, disorganized, rapid beats with no identifiable P waves or QRS complexes. It is thought to be triggered by multiple reentrant wavelets in the ventricle. There is no effective cardiac output in patients with VF.[103,104]

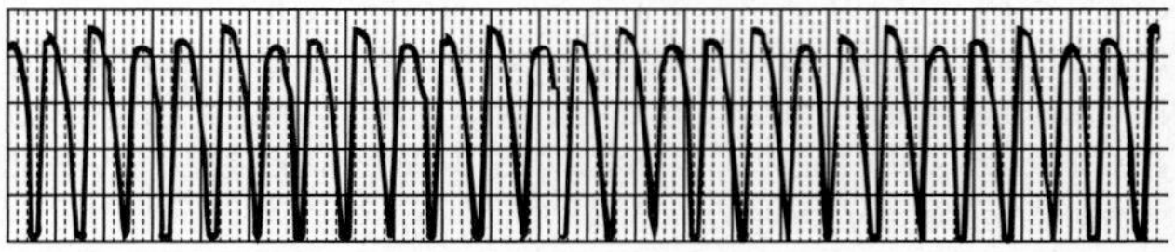

Figure 15-11 Sustained ventricular tachycardia.

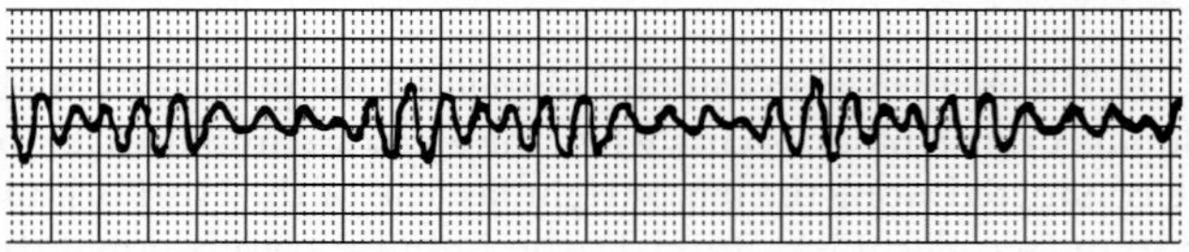

Figure 15-12 Ventricular fibrillation.

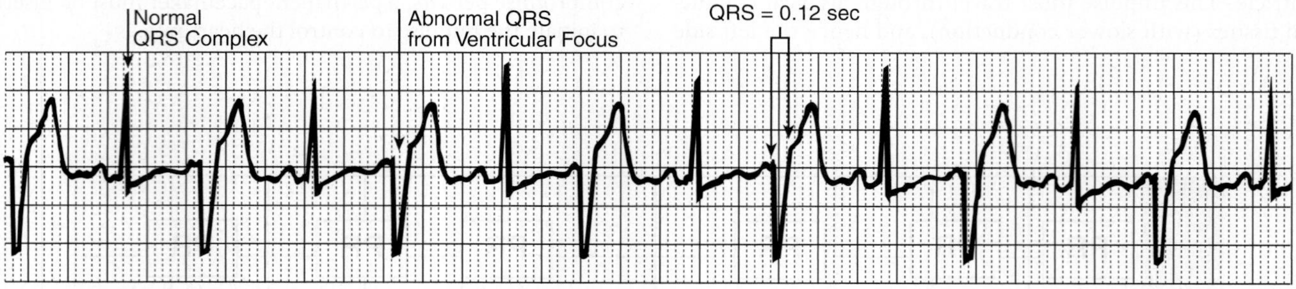

Figure 15-9 Premature ventricular contraction. Every other beat is a premature ventricular (ectopic) contraction.

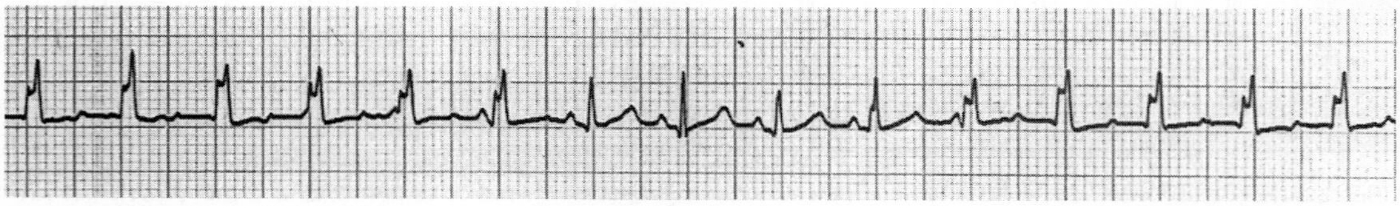

Figure 15-10 Nonsustained ventricular tachycardia. (Reprinted with permission from Mhairi G et al. *Avery's Neonatology Pathophysiology & Management of the Newborn*. 6th ed. Philadelphia: Lippincott Williams & Wilkins; 2005.)

Etiology

Common factors that cause ventricular arrhythmias are ischemia, the presence of organic heart disease, exercise, metabolic or electrolyte imbalance (e.g., acidosis, hypokalemia or hyperkalemia, hypomagnesemia), or drugs (digitalis, sympathomimetic amines, antiarrhythmic drugs). It is essential to identify and remove any treatable cause (e.g., metabolic or electrolyte imbalance and proarrhythmic drugs) before initiating antiarrhythmic drug therapy.

Evaluation of Life-Threatening Ventricular Arrhythmias

An episode of life-threatening ventricular arrhythmia (i.e., SuVT, TdP, VF) carries a significant risk of morbidity and mortality. Adequate documentation of the arrhythmia and its suppression by either drugs or a mechanical device are essential. Patients suspected of having, or documented to have, symptoms of a life-threatening arrhythmia (e.g., syncope, out-of-hospital cardiac arrest) should be admitted to the hospital and evaluated. At present, the European Heart Rhythm Association (EHRA)/Heart Rhythm Society (HRS)/Asia Pacific Heart Rhythm Society (APHRS) practice guidelines provided a class IIa recommendation for standard testing with a 12-lead ECG in all patients undergoing evaluation for ventricular arrhythmias, along with echocardiography (detects structural heart disease). Contrast-enhanced magnetic resonance imaging (MRI) may provide additional guidance in the management of certain forms of structural heart disease, such as dilated cardiomyopathy, hypertrophic cardiomyopathy, sarcoidosis, amyloidosis, and arrhythmogenic right ventricular cardiomyopathy.[103] Ambulatory monitoring and EP studies are two additional approaches used to evaluate the arrhythmia and the effectiveness of therapy.[103–105]

AMBULATORY MONITORING

The frequency of suspected ventricular arrhythmias determines the ambulatory monitoring device indicated for patients.[104,105] For more frequent occurrences (once daily) of arrhythmias, Holter monitoring during a 24- to 48-hour period represents the first-line ambulatory monitoring device. The patient wears a portable ECG monitoring device in a purse-like carrier, and electrodes connected to the monitor are taped to the patient's chest. The ECG is played back in the laboratory, correlating the presence of arrhythmias with a written patient activity and symptom log. In contrast, 30-day ambulatory event recorders are selected for patients presenting with arrhythmias that occur less frequently.[104,105] The event recorder (or loop recorder) is worn constantly for 30 days and stores and saves data upon activation by the patient. Whenever a patient experiences symptoms, a switch on the recorder is depressed, resulting in storage of a record of the patient's heart rhythm at the time of the event. A telephone can transfer event recorder data for analysis. On rare occasions, cardiologists will order mobile outpatient cardiac telemetry, which is the outpatient equivalent of continuous inpatient cardiac telemetry.[104] This wearable ambulatory device can be worn for up to 6 weeks, and offers the advantage of real-time automatic detection. However, because of its high cost, many third-party payers deny coverage for patients, thereby limiting more widespread use.

ELECTROPHYSIOLOGIC STUDIES

EP studies represent another approach to evaluating ventricular arrhythmias, especially in patients with sporadic ventricular arrhythmias that may be missed by short-term monitoring.[103] EP testing serves as a diagnostic tool for evaluating drug effects, assessing the inducibility of VT, determining the risks of recurrent VT or sudden cardiac death (SCD), guiding ablation, and assessing the need for an implantable cardioverter-defibrillator (ICD).

Premature Ventricular Contractions

CASE 15-6

QUESTION 1: A.S., a 56-year-old woman, is admitted to the CCU with a diagnosis of acute anterior wall MI. Her vital signs are BP, 115/75 mm Hg; pulse, 85 beats/minute; and respiratory rate, 15 breaths/minute. Auscultation of the heart reveals an S_3 gallop. Her electrolytes include potassium (K) 3.8 mEq/L, and magnesium (Mg) 1.2 mEq/L Otherwise, her examination is within normal limits. Two days later, an echocardiogram estimates her ejection fraction to be 35% (normal, >50%). During her stay in the CCU as well as the step-down unit, multiple PVCs (15/minute) were noted on the bedside monitor. No antiarrhythmic agent was ordered. Should A.S.'s multiple PVCs be treated with a class I antiarrhythmic drug?

Occasional PVCs are a benign, natural occurrence, even in a healthy heart, and are not an indication for drug therapy. Similarly, asymptomatic simple forms of PVCs, even in patients with other cardiac disease, usually do not need treatment. However, the presence of frequent PVCs may be associated with ischemia with impaired left ventricular function.[103] Of note, it is also possible that PVCs may emerge as a result of an underlying cardiomyopathy, thereby making it difficult to prospectively determine which of these sequences apply to a given patient.

TYPE IC ANTIARRHYTHMIC AGENTS

Because PVCs are a risk factor for SCD, the National Institutes of Health launched the Cardiac Arrhythmia Suppression Trial (CAST)[106,107] to assess the benefit of PVC suppression in survivors of MI. The CAST was a prospective, randomized, placebo-controlled trial that evaluated three antiarrhythmic agents: flecainide, encainide, and moricizine (all class Ic agents). The choice of these drugs was based on results of a pilot study of 1,498 patients that showed adequate suppression of arrhythmia (PVCs) in the target population. Ten months after initiation of the study, CAST was discontinued because of excess total mortality and cardiac arrests in patients receiving flecainide and encainide. Total mortality in the flecainide and encainide groups was 8.3% compared with 3.5% in the placebo group.[106] In the moricizine group, which was reported separately in CAST II, 16 of 660 patients in the drug group died compared with 3 of 668 patients in the placebo group in the initial 2 weeks. Subsequent long-term follow-up did not show a difference between moricizine and placebo.[107] It is believed that the excessive death rate in the drug-treated groups was attributable to the proarrhythmic effect of the drugs. Because the patients enrolled in CAST were asymptomatic and at low risk for the development of arrhythmias, they were at greater risk for drug toxicity (relative to benefit). Although many issues have been raised concerning CAST, one conclusion is that patients with a recent MI and the presence of asymptomatic PVCs should not be treated with encainide, flecainide, or moricizine. Whether other class I antiarrhythmic agents will produce similar results is unknown. Thus, the decision to avoid using a class I antiarrhythmic medication to treat A.S.'s PVCs was a sound one. The proarrhythmic effects of the drug may outweigh the potential danger of PVCs at this time.

CASE 15-6, QUESTION 2: What alternatives to class I antiarrhythmic drugs should be considered for A.S.?

β-BLOCKING AGENTS

Expert consensus from the EHRA/HRS/APHRS panel suggested the use of β-blockers in patients with structural heart disease who have higher burdens of PVCs (>10,000/24 hours) or in patients without structural disease who continue to experience symptomatic PVCs.[103] Despite the limited efficacy of this class of drugs with regard to PVC elimination (10%–15% achieve >90% PVC suppression), *β*-blockers represent the mainstay of medical suppression of PVCs. Blockade of β_1 receptors decreases automaticity in response to reduced intracellular cyclic adenosine monophosphate.[104] In addition, *β*-blockers exert negative chronotropic effects, lowering the resting sinus rate, along with slowing AV nodal conduction.

It is estimated that SCD accounts for 50% of all deaths among MI patients.[108] In a pooled analysis from 31 clinical trials evaluating *β*-blockers in MI, a 20% to 25% reduction in the risks of death and reinfarction during an average of 2 years of treatment was documented.[109] The beneficial effects of *β*-blockers on mortality were primarily attributed to a decrease in SCD, usually caused by arrhythmias such as VF.[110] Similarly, a meta-analysis of 28 randomized trials demonstrated that IV followed by oral *β*-blocker therapy resulted in a 15% to 20% decrease in the relative risks of reinfarction and cardiac arrest during the first 7 days of hospitalization for acute MI patients.[111]

The COMMIT/CCS2 (Clopidogrel and Metoprolol in Myocardial Infarction Trial/Second Chinese Cardiac Study) collaborative group assessed the effect of IV metoprolol (up to three 5-mg doses in the first 15 minutes) followed by oral metoprolol (200 mg/day in divided doses, then 200 mg once daily) or placebo on cardiovascular outcomes in 45,852 acute MI patients.[112] The two prespecified end points included the composite of death, reinfarction, or cardiac death, along with all-cause mortality. The mean duration of drug therapy was 15 days. *β*-Blocker therapy did not result in significant reductions in the rate of achieving the coprimary study outcomes, but five fewer episodes of VF for every 1,000 patients occurred during therapy with metoprolol (odds ratio [OR], 0.83; 95% confidence interval [CI], 0.75–0.93; $p = 0.001$). However, metoprolol-treated patients experienced 11 more episodes of cardiogenic shock for every 1,000 patients during the treatment period (OR, 1.30; 95% CI, 1.19–1.41; $p < 0.00001$).

The American College of Cardiology Foundation/American Heart Association Task Force group recommended the routine use of oral *β*-blocker therapy during the first 24 hours for patients who do not have contraindications (see Chapter 13, Acute Coronary Syndrome) to prevent the early occurrence of VF. Furthermore, the task force assigned a class I rating for the recommendation of long-term use of oral *β*-blockers for secondary prevention in patients with low ejection fraction, heart failure, or postshock.[113] Hence, in A.S. a *β*-blocker is an important first-line agent to initiate.

AMIODARONE

In high-risk patients with MI who are not candidates for *β*-blockade, alternative antiarrhythmic therapy with amiodarone can be considered.[104,105] Amiodarone is a class III antiarrhythmic agent, but also has antiadrenergic, class I, and class IV activity. However, given that cumulative exposure to this drug can result in damage to multiple organs, caution should be exercised before using it for PVC suppression.[103,105] An evaluation of amiodarone in post-MI patients with frequent PVCs (≥10/hour) or at least one run of VT was conducted in the Canadian Amiodarone Myocardial Infarction Arrhythmia Trial (CAMIAT).[114] In this trial, amiodarone significantly reduced the incidence of VF or arrhythmic death by 48.5% compared with placebo. Arrhythmic death alone was reduced by 32.6%, and all-cause mortality was reduced by 21.2%, but these differences were not statistically significant.

Similarly, the European Myocardial Infarct Amiodarone Trial (EMIAT), evaluated MI survivors with a reduced ejection fraction (<40%).[115] Amiodarone significantly reduced arrhythmic deaths by 35% compared with placebo, but this did not demonstrate any difference in mortality (13.86% with amiodarone vs. 13.72% with placebo). This suggests that amiodarone should not be used in all patients with a reduced ejection fraction after an MI, but that it could benefit patients in whom antiarrhythmic therapy is indicated. Hence, if A.S. reports problematic symptoms associated with the PVCs or develops additional risk factors for arrhythmia while on *β*-blockade, the first-line treatment option, antiarrhythmic therapy with amiodarone, can be given without an increased risk of overall mortality.[116,117]

If A.S. had nonsustained runs of VT instead of just PVCs, *β*-blockade would remain the first-line treatment option and amiodarone could similarly be considered if *β*-blockers are unsuccessful but in this scenario, A.S. would need to be assessed by a cardiologist to see if she would meet the criteria for receiving an ICD.[112–114]

Catheter Ablation

The EHRA/HRS/APHRS panel members recommend catheter ablation for patients with reversible left ventricular dysfunction associated with high PVC burden (>10,000/24 hours), who have failed, did not tolerate, or declined medical treatment.[103] The most commonly employed technique involves activation mapping, where electrophysiologists maneuver catheters to target the precise PVC origin in the heart, which is subsequently ablated.[104,105] Catheter ablation is not without risk, but has been shown to abolish PVCs in 74% to 100% of patients in numerous studies.[103–105]

Sustained Monomorphic Ventricular Tachycardia

TREATMENT

CASE 15-7

QUESTION 1: S.L., a 64-year-old woman, presents to the ED with a chief complaint of palpitations. Her medical history includes hypertension controlled with a diuretic, and an inferior wall MI 6 months ago. She is pale and diaphoretic but able to respond to commands. Her vital signs are BP, 95/70 mm Hg; pulse, 145 beats/minute; and respiratory rate, 10 breaths/minute. When telemetry monitoring is established, S.L. is found to be in SuVT (Fig. 15-11). S.L.'s echocardiography (6 months earlier) revealed a left ventricular ejection fraction (LVEF) of 35%.How should she be treated?

The majority of patients with SuVT have structural heart disease, and therefore require ICD placement with optimal programming. In addition to ICD placement, patients with SuVT and ischemic structural disease usually receive adjunctive therapy with antiarrhythmic drugs or undergo catheter ablation if they experience incessant SuVT. Patients with nonischemic structural disease may receive adjunctive therapy with an antiarrhythmic drug, but are less likely to undergo catheter ablation, unless they experience recurrent VT while receiving medications.[103]

The acute treatment of patients with SuVT depends on their hemodynamic stability and level of consciousness.[103] If unstable, patients should receive DC cardioversion synchronized to the QRS on the surface ECG. If the patient is conscious, but experiencing marked hypotension or excessive symptoms from SuVT, a short-acting benzodiazepine (e.g., midazolam) should be administered before undergoing cardioversion.

Antiarrhythmic Agents

To date, antiarrhythmic monotherapy has not been shown to improve mortality in patients with non-acute SuVT and structural heart disease.[117–119]

In the OPTIC study, amiodarone was superior to *β*-blocker monotherapy in lowering the frequency of recurrent appropriate ICD therapy (shocks) during 1-year follow-up of patients receiving secondary prophylaxis.[120] The OPTIC (Optimal Pharmacological Therapy in Cardioverter Defibrillator Patients) study enrolled 412 patients with St. Jude's Medical dual-chamber ICDs; LVEF <40% who had inducible VT or VF or prior; history of SuVT, VF, or cardiac arrest; or syncope of unknown cause with VF or VT. The effect of amiodarone plus β-blocker (metoprolol, carvedilol, or bisoprolol) compared with sotalol or β-blocker alone on the primary end point, first occurrence of any shock delivered by the ICD, was assessed for a median of 359 days. One-year shock rates were 10.3%, 24.3%, and 38.5%, respectively, in amiodarone/β-blocker–treated patients, in sotalol-treated patients, and in β-blocker–treated patients. Patients receiving amiodarone combined with β-blocker had significantly lower risk of shock compared with patients receiving β-blocker monotherapy and sotalol monotherapy. Of note, adverse effects such as pulmonary toxicity, thyroid effects, and symptomatic bradycardia contributed to an 18.2% discontinuation rate for amiodarone at 1 year. However, longer term studies assessing the safety and efficacy of amiodarone for secondary prophylaxis, showed higher rates of VT recurrence and major adverse effects, compared with placebo.[121,122] Dofetilide[123] (off-label use) and the combination of mexiletine and amiodarone, have shown reductions in recurrences of SuVT in other studies.[124]

The 2010 AHA guidelines for cardiopulmonary resuscitation (CPR) and emergency cardiovascular care addressed the potential efficacy of IV antiarrhythmic drugs in stable VT patients. A class IIa rating for the use of IV procainamide was recommended by the AHA guidelines, with amiodarone (class IIb) and sotalol (class IIb) representing alternative choices of antiarrhythmic therapy for wide complex regular tachycardias.[125] IV amiodarone should be administered as a 150-mg dose for 10 minutes, followed by a 6-hour infusion at a rate of 1 mg/minute, and finally a 0.5-mg/minute infusion for 18 hours. For recurrent or resistant arrhythmias, supplemental infusions of 150 mg can be repeated every 10 minutes, up to a maximal total daily IV dose of 2.25 g. Commonly seen adverse effects associated with IV amiodarone include hypotension and bradycardia, which can be prevented by slowing the drug infusion rate.[125] Per AHA 2010 recommendations, patients with monomorphic VT who receive IV sotalol should receive a 100-mg (1.5 mg/kg) dose infused for 5 minutes.[125] IV sotalol is approximately dose-equivalent to the oral formulation, because an IV dose of 75 mg equals an 80-mg oral dose.[126] The manufacturer suggests diluting sotalol in 100 to 250 mL of 5% dextrose, normal saline, or lactated Ringer's solution, and administering the drug using a volumetric infusion pump for a 5-hour period. Common adverse effects associated with sotalol include bradycardia and hypotension. The propensity of this agent to induce TdP is covered later in this chapter. The mean elimination half-life of sotalol is 12 hours. Because it is cleared by the kidneys, its clearance is reduced and its half-life prolonged in patients with renal dysfunction. Consequently, patients receiving sotalol should receive continuous BP, heart rate, and ECG monitoring. Patients who experience excessive QT prolongation while on sotalol should receive lower doses or the drug should be discontinued.

Implantable Cardiac Defibrillators (ICDs)

CASE 15-7, QUESTION 2: On hospital day 2, S.L. experiences a run of VT lasting about 2 minutes. The cardiology consult service has recommended placement of an ICD. What is an ICD, and how does it work?

Transvenous ICDs are devices implanted under the skin with wires or patches that are advanced or attached so they are in direct contact with the ventricular myocardium. The ICD is composed of a pulse generator, sensing and pacing electrodes, and defibrillation coils. The pulse generator consists of a microprocessor, a memory component capable of storing ECG data, a high-voltage capacitor, and a battery. The microprocessor controls the analysis of cardiac rhythm and delivery of therapy. An electrode is usually placed at the endocardium of the right ventricular apex, but in some rare cases, it is surgically placed on the epicardium. Patients with dual-chamber ICDs have a second electrode placed in the right atrial appendage. Biventricular ICDs have an additional electrode placed surgically on the epicardium of the left ventricle, or more commonly, placed transcutaneously in a branch off of the coronary sinus. Defibrillation coils are positioned on the right ventricular electrode at the level of the right ventricle and the superior vena cava. In most ICD systems, biphasic defibrillation current flows from the distal defibrillation coil to the pulse generator and to the proximal defibrillation coil.[127]

Since 2012, numerous advancements in ICD technology have occurred: (a) development of longer-lasting batteries (up to 12 years for Boston Scientific models); (b) emergence of quadripolar leads to optimize therapeutic efficacy through improved device programming; (c) development of subcutaneous ICDs (s-ICDs); and (d) development of MRI-safe ICDs (available in Europe).[128] The s-ICD system (model SQ-RX 1010, Cameron Health, Inc., San Clemente, California) consists of a subcutaneous pulse generator and a single subcutaneous electrode, comprised of sensing and defibrillating components.[129] The pulse generator is usually placed in the subcutaneous pocket created over the fifth intercostal space between the mid and anterior axillary lines. Placement of the subcutaneous lead is parallel to the left side of the sternum, with its upper pole situated at the level of the sternal notch and the lower electrode positioned beneath the level of the xiphoid process. Some of the advantages of using the s-ICD system include elimination of potential adverse events associated with venous access, minimal physical stress on leads associated with cardiac motion, and relative ease of device extraction. However, unlike transvenous ICDs, the currently marketed s-ICD has a larger pulse generator, along with having less data on long-term performance. Furthermore, the current s-ICD does not provide antitachycardia pacing for VT.[129] Multiple clinical trials have proved the superiority of ICD treatment over antiarrhythmic therapy for the secondary prevention of SCD. On the basis of evidence from numerous clinical trials of primary and secondary prevention of SCD, the American College of Cardiology/American Heart Association/Heart Rhythm Society 2012 guidelines for device-based therapy of cardiac rhythm abnormalities assigned a class Ia rating for ICD implantation in seven groups of patients. ICD therapy is indicated for (a) survivors of cardiac arrest caused by VF or hemodynamically unstable sustained VT (level of evidence [LOE] A); (b) patients with LVEF equal to or less than 35% caused by a prior MI who are at least 40 days after the event and are in NYHA functional class II or III (LOE A); (c) patients with LVEF equal to or less than 30% caused by prior MI who are at least 40 days after the event and are in NYHA functional class I (LOE A); (d) patients experiencing spontaneous SuVT in conjunction with structural heart disease, regardless of hemodynamic stability (LOE B); (e) hemodynamically compromised patients with electrophysiology study–induced SuVT or VF associated with syncope of undetermined origin; (f) patients with LVEF less than or equal to 35% associated with nonischemic dilated cardiomyopathy and are in NYHA functional class II or III (LOE B); and (g) patients with LVEF less than or equal to 40% in conjunction with NSVT secondary to prior myocardial infarction, who experience SuVT or inducible VF at EP study (LOE B).[130]

Although ICDs have been shown to improve survival in select patient populations, the benefit may be offset by diminished quality of life associated with painful shocks, increased mortality compared with ICD patients who do not require shocks, and incomplete protection from the occurrence of SCD (5% of patients fail to respond).[120,131,132] In recent years, investigators have examined various approaches to reducing the frequency of ICD shocks. Antiarrhythmic medications and prophylactic catheter ablation have been shown to reduce the incidence of ICD firing.[120,131,132] The EHRA/HRS/APHRS taskforce group assigned a class IIa rating for the strategies of programming ICDs to a delayed VT detection interval and a high VF detection rate in patients requiring primary prophylaxis.[103]

Defibrillation threshold is classified as the minimum amount of energy needed to result in successful defibrillation of the heart and restoration of normal sinus rhythm.[133] It is important for clinicians to be aware that antiarrhythmic agents have been associated with increases (amiodarone) or reductions (dofetilide) in ventricular fibrillation thresholds.[133–135]

Clearly, S.L. should have an ICD implanted. It is her best chance for prolonging long-term survival. Depending on the number of times the machine discharges per month and the patient's response, adjunctive antiarrhythmic drugs or prophylactic ablation may be needed, along with optimizing ICD programming.

Amiodarone

CASE 15-7, QUESTION 3: S.L.'s cardiologist would like to start amiodarone as adjunctive therapy because S.L. has expressed concern about the number of ICD discharges that may occur after ICD placement. If S.L. is to be treated with amiodarone, how should it be initiated and monitored?

Amiodarone exhibits properties of classes I, II, III, and IV antiarrhythmic agents. Although it has class II effects on the heart, amiodarone is virtually devoid of antiadrenergic effects outside the heart and is not contraindicated in patients with asthma. The antiadrenergic effects arise from inhibition of adenylate cyclase, the enzyme that catalyzes production of the second-messenger product cyclic adenosine monophosphate. Amiodarone can also cause a reduction in β_1-receptor density.[136,137]

Because of the extremely long half-life of amiodarone, loading doses are used to accelerate the onset of drug effect. The OPTIC trial used a loading dose of oral amiodarone 400 mg, given twice daily for 2 weeks, followed by a daily dose of 400 mg for the next 4 weeks, and a daily maintenance dose of 200 mg thereafter.[120] Although a concentration–effect relationship is hard to determine for amiodarone, levels greater than 2.5 mg/L are associated with an increased incidence of adverse effects.[138]

Amiodarone has many serious adverse effects involving a variety of organ systems, the most serious and life-threatening of which is pulmonary toxicity. Amiodarone-induced pulmonary toxicity (AIPT) has been shown to account for 11% of the sum total of all reported adverse events associated with this agent.[139] AIPT presents as an acute process or a chronic condition that develops several months after starting amiodarone therapy. The pathophysiologic mechanism for AIPT has not been fully elucidated, but may involve: (a) heightened extracellular expression of β-hexosaminidase; (b) imbalance between T-helper 1 and 2 cells, leading to a maladaptive immune response; (c) increased tumor necrosis factor-α activity; and (d) angiotensin-mediated apoptotic effects of amiodarone on alveolar epithelial cells. It has been suggested that higher doses of amiodarone, older age, and preexisting pulmonary disease may predispose patients to developing AIPT. However, AIPT has been shown to occur after patients received low doses of amiodarone (200 mg/day). Manifestations of chronic AIPT include cough, dyspnea, impaired diffusion capacity of carbon monoxide, infiltrates on chest radiograph, weight loss, and fever. In contrast, patients presenting with acute AIPT experience rapid decline in respiratory function, potentially culminating in the development of acute respiratory distress syndrome (ARDS) with alveolar opacities. Given the prolonged half-life of amiodarone, symptom resolution will be a slow process for patients with AIPT. Patients presenting with marked radiographic opacities and hypoxemia may need to receive prednisone 40 to 60 mg daily for several months. Mortality rates for patients with AIPT have been shown to approach 10%, with higher mortality rates seen in patients requiring hospitalization (20%–30%) or who develop ARDS (50%).[139]

A baseline chest radiograph and pulmonary function tests (diffusion capacity in particular) are recommended by the manufacturer.[140] The chest radiograph should be repeated at 3- to 6-month intervals, and patients should be specifically questioned about pulmonary symptoms because early detection can decrease the extent of lung damage.[140]

Liver toxicity can range from an asymptomatic elevation of transaminases (2–4 times normal) to fulminant hepatitis. The mean latent period between the start of amiodarone therapy and evidence of liver injury is 10 months (onset can be as short as 3–4 days), but with rapid IV loading of amiodarone, a Reye's-like fulminant hepatitis can occur as early as 1 day after starting therapy, most likely caused by the IV vehicle polysorbate-80. The precise mechanism of amiodarone-induced hepatotoxicity has not been fully elucidated. However, higher doses and prolonged drug use appear to place patients at higher risk of experiencing hepatotoxic effects of amiodarone. Thus liver enzymes should be monitored at baseline, 1, 3, 6 months, and semiannually afterward.[140,141] The most common GI complaints are nausea, anorexia, and constipation, which occur in 25% of patients receiving amiodarone.[140]

Both hypothyroidism and hyperthyroidism have been reported, although hypothyroidism is more common. The thyroid complications are a consequence of amiodarone's large iodine content and its ability to block the peripheral conversion of thyroxine (T_4) to triiodothyronine (T_3). In addition, amiodarone and its metabolite, desethylamiodarone, appear to be directly cytotoxic to the thyroid gland.[142]

Recent reports have indicated that photosensitive eruptions occur in 7% of amiodarone recipients.[143] Classical presentations of amiodarone photosensitivity involve a burning and tingling sensation in sun-exposed skin with accompanying erythema. Approximately 1% to 2% of patients receiving amiodarone for long-term use develop blue-gray pigmentation on sun-exposed skin. Resolution of amiodarone-associated photo-induced pigmentation may take up to 2 years, with gradual fading of skin discoloration.[143] In recent years, amiodarone-associated optic neuropathy has been highlighted in multiple case reports. A review of amiodarone-associated optic neuropathy (January 1993–May 2011) revealed a total of 214 cases from the FDA's Adverse Event Reporting System, 59 published cases, and 23 cases from clinical trials.[144] On average, patients received amiodarone for 9 months (range 1–84 months) before experiencing vision loss. In 20% of cases, patients progressed to legal blindness in at least one eye. Other bothersome side effects are corneal deposits (usually asymptomatic), exacerbation of heart failure, and central nervous system effects that include ataxia, tremor, dizziness, and peripheral neuropathy. Other than eye examination and pulmonary function tests, which should be repeated when the patient is symptomatic, other tests should be repeated every 6 months (thyroid and liver function) or annually (chest x-rays) for routine monitoring.[140,144] Amiodarone also blocks multiple cytochrome P-450 enzyme systems and P-glycoprotein pumps, resulting in clinically significant drug interactions.

Torsades de Pointes

PROARRHYTHMIC EFFECTS OF ANTIARRHYTHMIC DRUGS AND CLINICAL PRESENTATION

CASE 15-8

QUESTION 1: L.G. is a 69-year-old woman who is taking sotalol 80 mg twice daily for a previous episode of SuVT. L.G. was admitted to the hospital 3 days ago for altered mental status. She is also taking oral citalopram 40 mg every morning for major depressive disorder. At baseline, her QTc interval was 400 ms, and her CrCl was 50 mL/minute. Other laboratory values are as follows:

Sodium, 139 mmol/L
Chloride, 108 mmol/L
Potassium, 4.0 mmol/L
CO_2, 22 mmol/L
Blood urea nitrogen (BUN), 32 mg/dL
Serum creatinine, 1.5 mg/dL
Random glucose, 102 mg/dL
Calcium, 8.5 mg/dL
Albumin, 2.9 g/dL
Phosphorous, 3.3 mg/dL

Today, her ECG reveals a QT_c interval of 502 ms and TdP, with a ventricular rate of 110 beats/minute. What is QTc interval prolongation? Why does QTc interval prolongation indicate an increased risk of TdP? Could an antiarrhythmic agent such as sotalol cause this arrhythmia? How does CrCl affect this?

The QT interval denotes ventricular depolarization (the QRS complex in the cardiac cycle) and repolarization (from the end of the QRS complex to the end of the T wave). Certain ion channels in phases 2 and 3 of the action potential are vital in determining the QT interval (Fig. 15-1). An abnormal increase in ventricular repolarization increases the risk of TdP. TdP is defined as a rapid polymorphic VT preceded by QTc interval prolongation. TdP can degenerate into VF and as such can be life threatening (Fig. 15-13).[145]

Because there is tremendous variability in the QT interval resulting from changes in heart rate, the QT is frequently corrected for heart rate (QTc interval). Several correction formulas for the QT interval exist and give similar results at most heart rates. The most common correction formula uses QT and R-R intervals measured in seconds as follows: ($QTc = QT/[R\text{-}R^{0.5}]$). However, overcorrection of the QT interval may occur in persons with elevated heart rates (>85 beats/minute).[146,147] The Fridericia correction ($QT_c = QT/[R\text{-}R^{1/3}]$) represents an alternative correction method for patients with heart rates exceeding 85 beats/minute.

The ACC and AHA recently addressed the issue of the prevention of TdP in hospital settings. They stated that each 10-ms increase in QT_c confers an additional 5% to 7% TdP risk in patients with congenital long QT syndrome (LQTS).[147] The International Conference on Harmonization stated that prolongation of QT_c interval by more than 30 ms and in excess of 60 ms should be classified as a potential adverse effect and a definite adverse effect, respectively.[148]

Class Ia and class III antiarrhythmic agents have been shown to induce TdP in numerous literature reports.[149] Of note, class Ia antiarrhythmic agents do not exhibit dose-dependent association with TdP, whereas the incidence of TdP does appear to be dose-related with class III antiarrhythmic agents. QT prolongation associated with the use of class Ia antiarrhythmic agents is likely the result of blockade of outward potassium channels, but it is offset by concomitant blockade of inward sodium channels at increased drug concentrations.[150] TdP induced by class III antiarrhythmic agents arises from prolonged repolarization and cardiac refractoriness. All class III antiarrhythmic agents have been implicated in cases of TdP. A recent review of the US FDA Adverse Event Reporting System (AERS) database showed the following number of TdP cases that occurred during a 2-year time period: dronedarone (37), amiodarone (29), dofetilide (12), and sotalol (4).[150] Incidence rates could not be calculated because true denominators were not available and all events were self-reported. However, given the considerably larger prescriptive volume of amiodarone, this agent appears to have a relatively low propensity for inducing TdP.

Class Ic antiarrhythmic agents do not exert significant effects on repolarization, and therefore have rarely been shown to induce TdP. To date, eight cases of flecainide-induced TdP have been published, along with one report of propafenone-associated TdP.[151–153]

Sotalol is known to cause QTc interval prolongation in a dose-dependent manner. Total daily doses of 160, 320, 480, and >640 mg gave patients a steady-state QTc interval of 467, 473, 483, and 512 milliseconds, and the incidence of TdP was 0.5%, 1.6%, 4.4%, and 5.8%, respectively.[154]

It is likely that L.G.'s reduced renal function put her at high risk for sotalol accumulation and accentuated QTc interval prolongation. In patients with a CrCl greater than 60 mL/minute, the sotalol dose of 80 mg twice daily is appropriate, but in patients like L.G. with a CrCl less than 40 to 60 mL/minute, the manufacturer-recommended dose should be 80 mg daily or 40 mg twice daily owing to sotalol's predominant renal clearance.

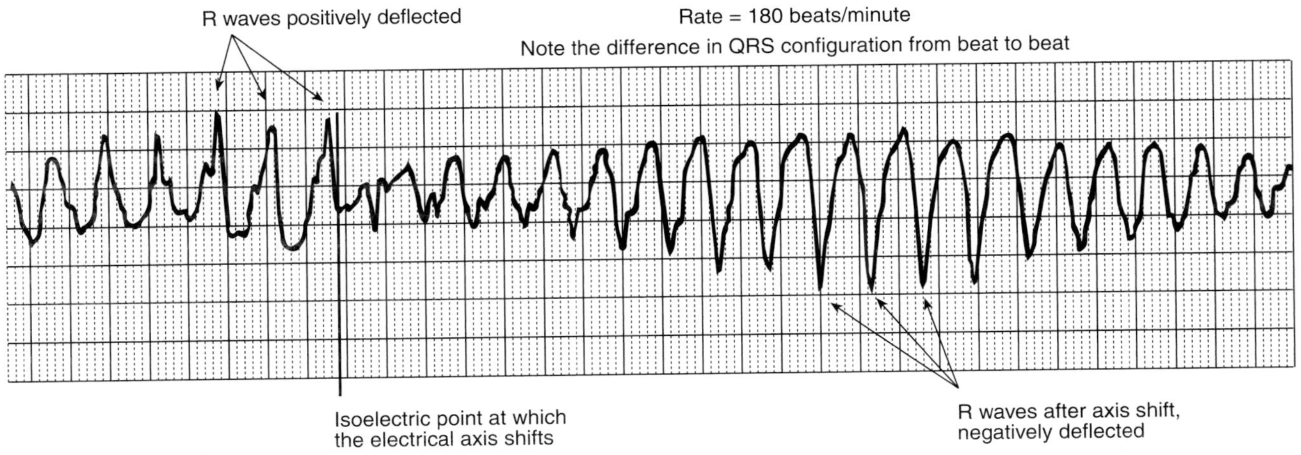

Figure 15-13 Torsades de pointes.

CASE 15-8, QUESTION 2: What transient conditions or other disorders can increase the risk of TdP in patients on class Ia or III antiarrhythmic agents?

Hypokalemia, hypomagnesemia, hypocalcemia (rare cases of TdP), concurrent use of more than one QT-prolonging drug, advanced age, female sex, heart disease (heart failure or myocardial infarction), treatment with diuretics, impaired hepatic drug metabolism, and bradycardia are important risk factors for TdP in hospitalized patients.[147] Hypokalemia may prolong QT interval by modifying the function of the inwardly rectifying potassium channel, resulting in heterogeneity and dispersion of repolarization. Prolonged ventricular cycle length can assume the form of complete AV block, sinus bradycardia, or a rhythm in which long cycles may progress to arrhythmogenic EAD.

Congenital LQTS occurs in 1 in 2,500 individuals, and is a channelopathy associated with mutations identified in genes encoding voltage-gated sodium and potassium channels.[147] Since 1995, approximately 1,000 individual LQTS-causing mutations have been detected in 12 distinct LQTS-susceptibility genes. The LQTS-susceptibility genes *KCNQ1* (encoded I_{Ks} α-subunit), *KCNH2* (encoded I_{Kr} α-subunit), and *SCN5A* (encoded Nav1.5 α-subunit) account for nearly 75% of all congenital LQTS cases.

Because L.G. did not have a family history of hereditary LQTS but was being treated with sotalol (an agent known to be associated with TdP) in renal dysfunction, it can be assumed that sotalol therapy was responsible for her arrhythmia.

CASE 15-8, QUESTION 3: Which nonantiarrhythmic agents cause TdP? What is the mechanism of TdP initiation in this situation?

PROARRHYTHMIC EFFECTS OF NONANTIARRHYTHMIC AGENTS

Nonantiarrhythmic agents can also exhibit potassium-channel inhibitory properties and can prolong the QTc interval. Most of these drugs, including arsenic trioxide, macrolide antibiotics, fluoroquinolones, azole antifungals, methadone, antidepressants, organophosphorus compounds, and antipsychotics, cause QTc interval prolongation by inhibiting the inwardly rectifying potassium ion channel, just like quinidine and sotalol.[155] Moreover, toxic concentrations of nonantiarrhythmic drugs can induce TdP as a result of large doses, impaired kidney or liver function, or other drug therapy that interferes with metabolism of nonantiarrhythmic drugs.

On August 24, 2011, the US FDA sent out an alert to health care providers and patients on new dosing recommendations for citalopram due to concerns of QT_c interval prolongation and TdP when using this agent at higher doses.[156] Key recommendations included: (1) prescribing citalopram at a dose of $\leq$20 mg/day for patients older than 60 years of age (also, in patients <60 years with hepatic impairment or taking cimetidine); and (2) prescribing citalopram at a dose of $\leq$40 mg/day for younger patients. Hasnain and associates recently conducted a comprehensive review of published literature on QT_c interval prolongation and/or TdP risk associated with antidepressants and second-generation antipsychotics (SGAPs).[157] The authors identified the highest number (16) of case reports implicating citalopram, relative to other antidepressants, including fluoxetine (9), escitalopram (6), venlafaxine (5), and sertraline (2). Case report material revealed quetiapine as the SGAP with the largest number of QT_c interval prolongation and/or TdP cases (16), followed by ziprasidone (13), risperidone (13), amisulpride, olanzapine (6), and clozapine (5). The authors of the review noted that patients had at least one additional risk factor for QT_c interval prolongation in 92% of the reports. In addition, they acknowledged that the information yielded by case reports did not allow for comparison between drugs and generalization to clinical practice.

During the past two decades, multiple case reports of methadone-induced TdP have been published. Guidelines recommend QT interval monitoring, but some experts have questioned the necessity of screening patients.[158] Kao et al.[158] reviewed the FDA Adverse Event Reporting System (FAERS) database for QT_c interval prolongation or TdP events linked with methadone compared to other agents, including antiarrhythmic drugs and other opioids. Between 2000 and 2011, the three most commonly implicated drugs included dofetilide (359 cases), methadone (211), and sotalol (119). The authors acknowledged limitations of their analysis (voluntary and selective reporting to FAERS, along with the inability to determine incidence rates), but suggested that a REMS specific to methadone may be warranted, in order to lower the risk of TdP. The recent emergence of methadone-associated TdP could be attributable to escalating doses used in recent years, given the preponderance of published cases of patients receiving very high doses of this agent.[159]

Currently, the utility of published cardiac risk data on anti-infective agents is limited, owing to underreporting, failure to completely eliminate contributory confounding variables (cardiac disease, electrolyte abnormalities, use of other QT-prolonging drugs), and the retrospective nature of some postmarketing studies.[148] However, the propensity of antimicrobial agents to induce QT prolongation appears to be especially marked with macrolide antibiotics.[160] All of the commercially available antifungal agents have been shown to induce TdP and QT_c prolongation, with a larger number of cases attributed to fluconazole, followed by voriconazole.[160] Among the marketed quinolones in the United States, ciprofloxacin appears to display the lowest potential for causing TdP.[161]

A list of nonantiarrhythmic agents implicated in causing QTc interval prolongation and known pharmacokinetic drug interaction increasing the blood concentrations of these drugs is given in Table 15-6.

Because L.G. was taking citalopram in combination with sotalol, it is likely that QTc-prolonging effects resulting from concomitant use contributed to the development of TdP.

TREATMENT

CASE 15-8, QUESTION 4: How should TdP be treated? What treatments should be considered for L.G.?

If the patient is significantly hemodynamically compromised (frequently associated with a ventricular rate >150 beats/minute and unconsciousness) while in TdP, electrical cardioversion is the therapy of choice and should be given immediately. Stepwise increasing shocks of 100 to 200, 300, and 360 J (monophasic energy) can be tried if earlier shocks are unsuccessful.

Magnesium

In a hemodynamically stable patient, magnesium is frequently considered the drug of choice to restore normal sinus rhythm. It benefits patients whether they have hypomagnesemia or normal serum magnesium levels. However, magnesium is not effective for patients with polymorphic VT without TdP and with normal QT intervals. Before administering magnesium, potassium levels should be supplemented to the high normal range of 4.5 to 5.0 mmol/L.[155] A common magnesium regimen is 2 g given for 60 seconds through the IV route, followed by an infusion of 2 to 4 mg/minute.[155] The exact mechanism of action for magnesium in TdP is not known, but it reduces the occurrence of triggered activity such as EAD. In addition, magnesium blocks L-type calcium channels in the membrane, and may stabilize the membrane gradient through activation of the sodium-potassium ATPase.[161]

Table 15-6

Nonantiarrhythmic Agents with Known Torsades de Pointes Risk[a]

Drug Class	Agent	Drugs That Increase Blood Concentrations of These QTc Interval–Prolonging Drugs
Anesthetic, general	Propofol, sevoflurane	
Antibiotics: macrolides	Azithromycin, clarithromycin, erythromycin (lactobionate and base)	
Antibiotics: fluoroquinolones	Ciprofloxacin, levofloxacin, moxifloxacin	
Antibiotics: other	Pentamidine isethionate	
Anti-cancer	Arsenic trioxide, vandetanib	
Antidepressants	Citalopram, Escitalopram	CYP3A4 or 2C19 inhibitors
Antiemetics	Chlorpromazine, droperidol, ondansetron	CYP3A4 (primary for ondansetron), 1A2 (primary for chlorpromazine), or 2D6 inhibitors
Antifungals	Fluconazole	
Antimalarials	Chloroquine, halofantrine	Cimetidine (chloroquine), CYP3A4 inhibitors (halofantrine)
Antipsychotics	Haloperidol, pimozide, thioridazine	CYP2D6 (thioridazine) or 3A4 (pimozide) inhibitors
Cholinesterase inhibitors	Donepezil	CYP3A4 or 2D6 inhibitors
Narcotics	Methadone	CYP3A4, 2B6, and 2C19 inhibitors
Phosphodiesterase 3 inhibitor	Anagrelide, cilostazol	CYP1A2 (anagrelide), 3A4 (primary for cilostazol), or 2C19 inhibitors

[a]An up-to-date list can be found at http://www.crediblemeds.org/everyone/

Other Treatment Options for TdP

Numerous other strategies have been utilized for patients who fail to respond adequately to standard therapeutic approaches, including calcium-channel blockers, αblockers, potassium-channel openers, lidocaine, and mexiletine.[162] However, the evidence supporting these alternative agents is not compelling enough to classify them as first-line options for abolishing TdP.

Cardio acceleration with isoproterenol (1–4 mcg/minute) or cardiac pacing has also been shown to be beneficial.[163–165] As described previously, the ability of sotalol, quinidine, and *N*-acetylprocainamide to prolong the APD is diminished at faster heart rates (reverse use dependence).[166] The more the inwardly rectifying potassium channels are activated, the less susceptible the channels are to inhibition by potassium-channel blocking drugs.

Transvenous pacing has been shown to be of some use in abolishing refractory TdP.[163] Before adjusting the ventricular rate to suppress ectopic ventricular beats, it is essential to ensure proper catheter placement and cardiac capture. In general, ventricular rates of 90 to 110 beats/minute can usually eliminate ventricular ectopy, but some patients may require rates as high as 140 beats/minute. Once control of TdP has been attained, the pacing rate can be gradually decreased to the lowest paced rate that suppresses further ectopy and dysrhythmia.

Because L.G. is hemodynamically stable, a bolus injection of 2 g of magnesium should be administered over 1 minute, followed by an infusion administered at a rate of 2 to 4 mg/minute. In addition, she should receive potassium supplementation (infusion) to achieve a potassium level of 4.5 to 5.0 mmol/L. If the arrhythmia recurs, cardiac pacing should be used.

CARDIOPULMONARY ARREST

Cardiopulmonary Resuscitation

Cardiac arrest from VF, pulseless VT, pulseless electrical activity (PEA), and asystole are life-threatening emergencies. Table 15-7[167–173] reviews commonly used drugs for these indications, and Figure 15-14 highlights key features of the management of pulseless arrest in the 2010 AHA Guidelines (2015 update to be released in October 2015). This section will review important aspects of therapy and will give clinical pearls, but the reader should also review the national consensus source document for these disorders, which includes more detail than can be given here.[167]

Treatment

CASE 15-9

QUESTION 1: M.N., a 52-year-old man, is visiting his wife, who is hospitalized for pneumonia. His past medical history is significant for hypertension and type 2 diabetes mellitus. He goes into the bathroom and 2 minutes later his wife hears a dull thud. She calls out for her husband, but he does not respond. After an additional 2 minutes, health care workers open the bathroom door and find M.N. unresponsive and pulseless. CPR is initiated and a code blue is called. The ECG shows VF (Fig. 15-12), and there is no BP. In addition to CPR, what initial therapy is available?

Determining the underlying rhythm disturbance is important because it directs health care workers to follow the Advanced Cardiac Life Support (ACLS) algorithm for pulseless VT or VF (Fig. 15-14). This algorithm calls for electrical defibrillation first, but other clinicians should work to establish IV access in case defibrillation fails.[167]

EXTERNAL DEFIBRILLATION

Although commercially available manual defibrillators provide monophasic or biphasic waveform shocks, the biphasic defibrillator has become the preferred device owing to its high first-shock efficacy.[167] Most commercially available biphasic defibrillators display the device-specific energy dose range that should be used. However, if a health care provider operating a manual biphasic defibrillator is uncertain of the effective energy dose to terminate

Table 15-7
Commonly Used Drugs in Cardiac Arrest

Drug	Formulation	Dosage/Administration	Rationale/Indications	Comments
Amiodarone	50 mg/mL Vials: 3, 9, 18 mL	300 mg diluted in 20–30 mL D5W or NS; additional 150 mg (diluted solution) can be given for recurrent or refractory VT or VF.	Exhibits antiadrenergic properties and blocks sodium, potassium, and calcium channels. First-line antiarrhythmic for pulseless VT and VF.	Excipients (polysorbate 80 and benzyl alcohol) can induce hypotension. Failing to dilute can induce phlebitis.
Epinephrine	0.1 mg/mL (1:10,000) or 1 mg/mL (1:1,000)	10 mL of a 1:10,000 solution of epinephrine (1 mg; dilute 1:1,000 solution in 0.9% sodium chloride) every 3–5 minutes.	Increases coronary sinus perfusion pressure through α_1 stimulation. Indicated in pulseless VT, VF, asystole, and PEA.	If administered through peripheral catheter, need to flush the line to get drug into the central compartment.
Vasopressin	20 units/mL Vials: 0.5, 1, 10 mL	40-unit dose can be used to replace first or second dose of epinephrine	Increases coronary sinus perfusion pressure through vasopressin receptor stimulation. Indicated in pulseless VT, VF, asystole, and PEA.	Vasopressin is an acceptable alternative to epinephrine, may work better if time from cardiac arrest to ACLS is delayed.

ACLS, Advanced Cardiac Life Support; D5W, 5% dextrose in water; NS, normal saline; PEA, pulseless electrical activity; VF, ventricular fibrillation; VT, ventricular tachycardia.

VF, using the maximal shock energy setting available is preferred. For second and subsequent shocks delivered by manual biphasic defibrillators, the same or higher energies should be used. For first and subsequent shocks, a shock of 360 J should be delivered if a monophasic defibrillator is used to terminate VF.

CASE 15-9, QUESTION 2: The initial shock fails to cause a return of spontaneous circulation in M.N. An IV catheter is established in a peripheral arm vein. The algorithm now calls for epinephrine or vasopressin, but which one should be used?

EPINEPHRINE AND VASOPRESSIN

Although epinephrine stimulates β_1-, β_2-, and α_1-adrenergic receptors, it is the α_1-adrenoceptor effects that are most closely associated with efficacy in VF or pulseless VT.[167] Applying α_1-adrenoceptor stimulation increases systemic vascular resistance (via vasoconstriction), which elevates coronary perfusion pressure. This increase in coronary perfusion pressure is most likely the key to enhancing the return of spontaneous circulation after subsequent electrical defibrillation. Epinephrine may convert fine VF to a coarse variety that may be more amenable to defibrillation.

The recommended dose of epinephrine is 1 mg (10 mL of a 1:10,000 dilution; refer to Table 15-7) given by IV push. The dosage can be repeated at 3- to 5-minute intervals during resuscitation. If the drug is given IV through a peripheral catheter, which in this case includes a peripherally inserted central catheter, then a 20-mL flush with normal saline is recommended to ensure delivery into the central compartment. Only chest compressions cause blood circulation in VF or pulseless VT, so movement of drugs from the periphery to the heart (where the benefit will occur) is severely impaired.

Vasopressin is an exogenously administered antidiuretic hormone. In supraphysiologic doses, vasopressin stimulates V1 receptors and causes peripheral vasoconstriction. Vasopressin use during CPR causes intense vasoconstriction to the skin, skeletal muscle, intestine, and fat, with much less constriction of coronary vascular beds. Cerebral and renal vasodilation occurs as well.

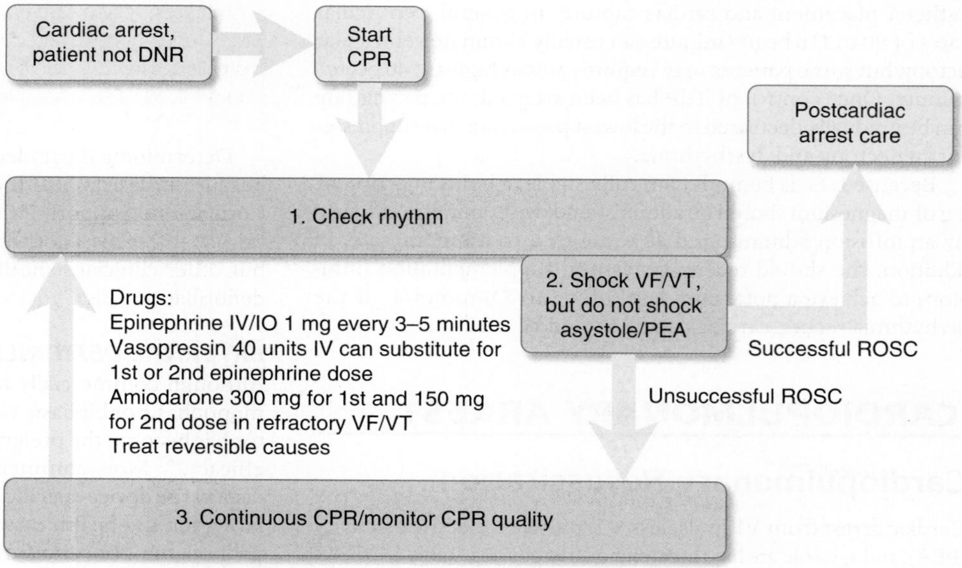

Figure 15-14 Cardiac arrest treatment algorithm. CPR, cardiopulmonary resuscitation; DNR, do not resuscitate; IO, intraosseous; IV, intravenous; PEA, pulseless electrical activity; ROSC, restoration of spontaneous circulation; VF, ventricular fibrillation; VT, ventricular tachycardia.

The results of a prospective, randomized, controlled, multicenter study ($n = 1{,}186$) that enrolled out-of-hospital cardiac arrest patients who presented with VF, PEA, or asystole showed that administration of vasopressin as adjunctive therapy resulted in similar survival to hospital admission rates (primary outcome measure) compared with adjunctive epinephrine therapy.[168] In this study, patients were randomly assigned to receive two ampules of 40 international units of vasopressin or two ampules of 1 mg of epinephrine. The second dose of vasopressor was injected if spontaneous restoration of circulation did not occur within 3 minutes after the first injection of the drug. If the absence of spontaneous circulation persisted, the physician administering CPR had the option of injecting epinephrine. The reported survival rates were similar between the two treatment groups for both patients with PEA and those with VF.

An in-hospital study of 200 cardiac arrest patients (initial rhythm: 16%–20% VF, 3% VT, 41%–54% PEA, 27%–34% asystole) showed no difference in 1-hour or hospital discharge survival for vasopressin 40 units versus epinephrine 1 mg.[169] Similarly, a meta-analysis of five randomized trials showed no survival advantage of vasopressin treatment versus epinephrine treatment at the time of hospital discharge or 24 hours after treatment.[170]

Since the publication of the 2010 ACLS guideline, some study investigators have focused on assessing long-term outcomes in out-of-hospital cardiac arrest patients.[174,175] Hagihara and associates[174] showed that out-of-hospital cardiac arrest patients who received epinephrine prior to hospital arrival had lower rates of 1-month survival and 1-month survival with favorable neurologic function, compared to patients who did not receive epinephrine ($p < 0.001$). Similarly, Goto et al.[175] showed significantly lower rates of 1-month survival and 1-month survival with favorable neurologic outcomes in out-of-hospital cardiac arrest patients with shockable rhythm, who received epinephrine before hospital arrival, relative to patients who did not receive epinephrine ($p < 0.001$).

On the basis of these trials, it would be reasonable to use a single dose of vasopressin 40 units as an alternative to either the first or second dose of epinephrine 1 mg in the treatment of VF (or pulseless VT).

CASE 15-9, QUESTION 3: One of the physicians delivering ACLS for M.N. wants to initiate corticosteroid therapy. What is the evidence supporting the use of corticosteroid therapy in patients experiencing cardiac arrest?

A randomized, double-blind, placebo-controlled, parallel-group trial performed by Mentzelopoulos et al.[176] assessed the impact of using two different strategies for managing in-hospital cardiac arrest patients on: (a) survival to hospital discharge with favorable neurologic status; and (b) probability for return of spontaneous circulation for 20 minutes or longer. One group of patients received epinephrine (1 mg/CPR cycle), vasopressin (20 IU/CPR cycle), and corticosteroid therapy (methylprednisolone 40 mg during first CPR cycle, then hydrocortisone 300 mg/day [for post-resuscitation shock] for up to 7 days, followed by taper). The control group received epinephrine in combination with saline placebo. Epinephrine–vasopressin–corticosteroid recipients exhibited superior rates of probability for return of spontaneous circulation for ≥20 minutes (83.9% vs. 65.9%; OR, 2.98; 95% CI, 1.39–6.40; $p = 0.005$), and survival to hospital discharge with favorable neurologic status (13.9% vs. 5.1%; OR, 3.28; 95% CI, 1.17–9.20; $p = 0.02$), compared to the control group.

CASE 15-9, QUESTION 4: Because M.N. has an IV site and the time from cardiac arrest to ACLS was brief, epinephrine was chosen and a 1-mg bolus was given, followed with a 20-mL normal saline flush. The arm was elevated for 20 seconds to ensure adequate delivery. Thirty seconds after administration a 200-J shock is given (via biphasic manual defibrillator), but it fails to convert VF. What can be done now?

The most recently updated ACLS guideline calls for the use of amiodarone in cases of VF or pulseless VT that do not respond to CPR, shocks, and a vasopressor.[167]

IV AMIODARONE AND LIDOCAINE

The effect of amiodarone on VF or pulseless VT was studied in the ARREST (Amiodarone for Resuscitation of Refractory Sustained Ventricular Tachyarrhythmias) trial.[171] This study was conducted in patients who experienced cardiac arrest in an out-of-hospital situation with therapy given by paramedics in the field. Patients who failed three stacked shocks and one dose of epinephrine with an electrical countershock were randomly assigned to amiodarone 300 mg IV bolus or placebo. This was followed by other antiarrhythmic agents historically used in ACLS (2,000 guidelines: lidocaine, procainamide, or bretylium) if the clinicians desired. Amiodarone significantly increased the chance of survival to hospital admission (44% vs. 34% of placebo group; $p = 0.03$), but survival to hospital discharge was not changed. Of note, 66% of patients received antiarrhythmic drug treatment for pulseless VT or VF after amiodarone administration.

The ALIVE (Amiodarone vs. Lidocaine in Ventricular Ectopy, $n = 347$) trial directly compared IV amiodarone 300 mg to lidocaine 1 to 1.5 mg/kg bolus.[173] In this trial, patients needed to fail three stacked shocks and epinephrine plus an additional shock to be eligible for randomization to either amiodarone or lidocaine. Amiodarone was given as an initial dose of 5 mg/kg followed by a shock. If unsuccessful, a dose of 2.5 mg/kg was given followed by a subsequent shock. Lidocaine was given as a 1.5 mg/kg bolus followed by a shock. If therapy failed, then a second bolus of 1.5 mg/kg was used with a subsequent shock. If the first antiarrhythmic drug failed, other routine antiarrhythmic drugs for cardiac arrest (per 2000 ACLS guidelines: e.g., procainamide, bretylium) could be tried. Patients given amiodarone were 90% more likely to experience the primary outcome, survival to hospital admission, than those given lidocaine ($p = 0.009$). Unfortunately, no significant advantage to hospital discharge occurred (5% vs. 3%).

On the basis of these findings, amiodarone is the only antiarrhythmic agent with proven ability to improve return of spontaneous circulation and short-term survival versus other antiarrhythmic therapy. However, it has not yet been shown to improve survival to hospital discharge.

M.N. is at serious risk of death as a result of VF. However, as long as M.N. remains in VF, it is appropriate to continue active therapy. If M.N. degenerates into asystole after this long period of VF, then the resuscitation efforts should be discontinued. However, if a patient only had a brief period of VF before having asystole, it is prudent to apply active therapy.

Pulseless Electrical Activity

CASE 15-10

QUESTION 1: J.D. is an 80-year-old woman who experiences cardiac arrest in the hospital. J.D. was in respiratory failure upon admission to the ED, where she underwent immediate intubation, had a peripheral IV placed, and upon transfer to the MICU, placed on assist/control mechanical ventilation with FiO_2 of 100%. A rhythm is noted on the monitor, but no femoral pulse is felt. M.N. is in PEA. How should J.D. be treated?

The clinical situation in which there is organized electrical activity on the monitor without a palpable pulse is called PEA. Although electrical activity is present, it fails to stimulate the contractile process. Virtually all patients in true PEA die. However, not all patients who present with a rhythm and no pulse are in true PEA. Therefore, it is important to rule out

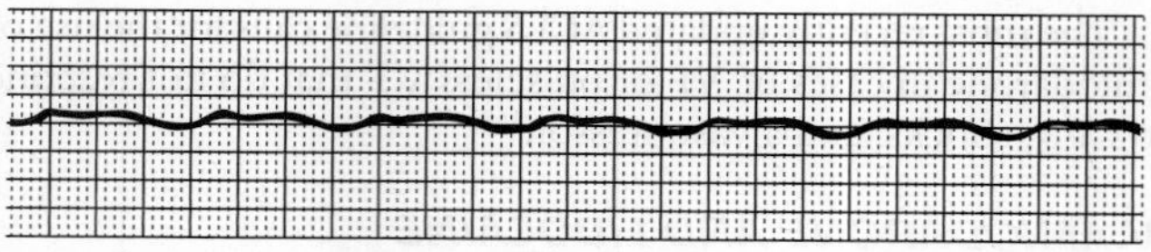

Figure 15-15 Asystole. There is no electrical activity detected in the heart resulting in a very low amplitude undulating waveform.

treatable causes in patients who appear to be in PEA. The major treatable causes are hypovolemia, hypoxia, acidosis, hyperkalemia, hypokalemia, hypothermia, cardiac tamponade, pulmonary embolism, acute coronary syndrome, trauma, and drug overdose. In the absence of an identifiable cause, the focus of resuscitation is to administer high-quality CPR, and after the initial rhythm check, resume CPR during the establishment of IV or IO (intraosseous) access.[167]

Once IV or IO access becomes available, administer epinephrine 1 mg every 3 to 5 minutes or give one dose of vasopressin 40 units in place of the first or second dose of epinephrine, as published studies have failed to demonstrate a survival advantage of either vasopressor for patients experiencing PEA.[167,169,170]

Asystole

CASE 15-11

QUESTION 1: K.K., a 73-year-old man, has a past medical history significant for hypertension and diverticulitis. Upon arrival at the OR for surgical correction of pericardial and pleural effusions, K.K. received etomidate, fentanyl, lidocaine, and succinylcholine. During placement of a double-lumen endotracheal tube, K.K. goes into cardiac arrest. The ECG shows a flat line, and the patient is determined to be in asystole (Fig. 15-15). Is this rhythm treatable?

Lack of electrical activity or asystole, like PEA, carries a grave prognosis. Its development usually indicates a prolonged arrest, which may explain its poor response to treatment. However, a few patients will go directly from a sinus rhythm into asystole and may be resuscitated. Enhanced parasympathetic tone, possibly attributable to a vagal reaction, manipulation of the airway from intubation, suctioning or insertion of an oral airway, or chest compression, may play a role in inhibiting supraventricular and ventricular pacemakers.[168]

A post hoc analysis performed by Wenzel et al.[168] demonstrated superior survival rates at the time of hospital admission in vasopressin-treated patients, compared with epinephrine-treated patients. However, no difference in intact neurologic survival was noted between the two treatment groups. Consequently, providers may choose to administer vasopressin 40 units IV (in place of the first or second dose of epinephrine) or epinephrine 1 mg IV every 3 to 5 minutes.

CASE 15-11, QUESTION 2: Does the timing of epinephrine dosing impact survival to hospital discharge in patients with non-shockable rhythms (asystole or PEA)?

A post hoc analysis of data from the Get With the Guidelines-Resuscitation study showed a stepwise reduction in survival to hospital discharge (primary study end point) with each 3-minute delay to epinephrine: (a) 1 to 3 minutes (OR 1.0, reference group); (b) 4 to 6 minutes (OR, 0.91; 95% CI, 0.82–1.00; $p = 0.055$); (c) 7 to 9 minutes (OR, 0.74; 95% CI, 0.63–0.88; $p < 0.001$); and (d) >9 minutes (OR, 0.63; 95% CI, 0.52–0.76; $p < 0.001$).[177]

CASE 15-11, QUESTION 3: What is the long-term prognosis for patients with non-shockable rhythms?

Goto et al.[175] assessed the impact of pre-hospital epinephrine administration on long-term outcomes seen in out-of-hospital cardiac arrest patients with non-shockable rhythms.[176] Epinephrine recipients showed superior 1-month survival rates compared to patients who did not receive pre-hospital epinephrine (3.9% vs. 2.2%; $p < 0.001$). However, pre-hospital administration of epinephrine did not result in improved 1-month favorable neurologic outcomes ($p = 0.62$).

KEY REFERENCES AND WEBSITES

A full list of references for this chapter can be found at http://thepoint.lww.com/AT11e. Below are the key references and websites for this chapter, with the corresponding reference number in this chapter found in parentheses after the reference.

Key References

Cohen MIet al. PACES/HRS expert consensus statement on the management of the asymptomatic young patient with a Wolff-Parkinson-White (WPW, Ventricular Preexcitation) Electrocardiographic pattern. *Heart Rhythm*. 2012;9:1006. (101)

Drew BJ et al. Prevention of torsade de pointes in hospital settings: a scientific statement from the American Heart Association and the American College of Cardiology Foundation [published correction appears in *Circulation*. 2010;122:e440]. *Circulation*. 2010;121:1047. (147)

Epstein AE et al. 2012 ACC/AHA/HRS focused update incorporated into the 2008 Guidelines for Device-Based Therapy of Cardiac Rhythm Abnormalities. *J Am Coll Cardiol*. 2013;61:e6. (130)

Giugliano RP et al. Edoxaban versus warfarin in patients with atrial fibrillation. *N Engl J Med*. 2013;369:2093. (84)

Granger CB et al. Apixaban versus warfarin in patients with atrial fibrillation. *N Engl J Med*. 2011;365:981. (83)

Hazinski MF, ed. *Highlights of the 2010 American Heart Association Guidelines for CPR and ECC*. Dallas, TX: American Heart Association; 2010. (167)

January CT et al. 2014 AHA/ACC/HRS guideline for the management of patients with atrial fibrillation. *Circulation*. 2014;130:e199–e267 (11).

Le Heuzey et al. A short-term, randomized, double-blind, parallel-group study to evaluate the efficacy and safety of dronedarone versus amiodarone in patients with persistent atrial fibrillation: the DIONYSOS study. *J Cardiovasc Electrophysiol*. 2010;21:597. (75)

Mentzelopoulos SD et al. Vasopressin, steroids, and epinephrine and neurologically favorable survival after in-hospital cardiac arrest: a randomized clinical trial. *JAMA*. 2013;310:270. (176)

Morillo CA et al. Radiofrequency ablation vs. antiarrhythmic drugs as first line treatment of paroxysmal atrial fibrillation (RAAFT-2). A randomized trial. *JAMA*. 2014;311:692. (90)

Pederson CT et al. HER/HRS/APHRS expert consensus on ventricular arrhythmias. *Heart Rhythm*. 2014;11:e166. (103)

Key Website

Blaufuss Medical Multimedia Laboratories ECG Tutorial. http://www.blaufuss.org.

16 Hypertensive Crises

Kristin Watson, Brian Watson, and Sandeep Devabhakthuni

CORE PRINCIPLES

	Core Principles	Chapter Cases
1	Hypertensive crisis is defined as a diastolic blood pressure greater than 120 mm Hg. This disorder can be further classified as hypertensive urgency or hypertensive emergency when there is evidence of acutely progressive end-organ damage.	**Case 16-1 (Question 1), Table 16-1**
2	Risk factors for the development of a hypertensive crisis include, but are not limited to, medication nonadherence, cocaine use, and drug–drug and drug–food interactions.	**Case 16-1 (Question 1)**
3	Hypertensive urgency can be treated with oral antihypertensive agents including clonidine, labetalol, or captopril. Caution must be taken to prevent rapid reductions in blood pressure.	**Case 16-1 (Questions 2–6) Table 16-3**
4	The organs primarily affected as a result of a hypertensive emergency are the central nervous system, eyes, heart, and kidneys.	**Case 16-2 (Question 1)**
5	Parenteral therapy should be used to manage hypertensive emergencies, and therapeutic options are dictated by the affected organ(s) and comorbidities. Mean arterial pressure should be reduced by no more than 25% initially, then subsequently reduced toward a goal of 160/100 mm Hg, for most patients, during the next 2 to 6 hours. Gradually reduce blood pressure to normal, for most patients, during the next 8 to 24 hours.	**Case 16-2 (Questions 2, 3, 4, 5, 9, 10), Case 16-3 (Questions 1–6), Case 16-4 (Questions 1, 2), Table 16-4, Figure 16-1, Table 16-2**
6	Nitroprusside, a therapeutic option for hypertensive emergencies, has been associated with cyanide and thiocyanate toxicity, and monitoring is required to minimize the risk of these toxicities, especially in patients with renal impairment.	**Case 16-2 (Questions 6–8)**
7	The most commonly used agents for the management of postoperative hypertension are nicardipine, nitroglycerin, nitroprusside, and labetalol.	**Case 16-5 (Questions 1, 2, 3)**
8	Management of aortic dissection requires prompt control of blood pressure without increasing the force of cardiac contraction or heart rate.	**Case 16-6 (Question 1)**

The term *hypertensive crisis* is defined as a diastolic blood pressure (DBP) greater than 120 mm Hg.[1] These disorders are divided into two general categories: *hypertensive emergency* and *hypertensive urgency* (Table 16-1). If these disorders are not treated promptly, a high rate of morbidity and mortality will ensue.[2–5]

The term *hypertensive emergency* describes a clinical situation in which the elevated blood pressure (BP) is immediately life-threatening and needs to be lowered to a safe level (not necessarily to normal) within a matter of minutes to hours.[1,3] Hypertensive emergencies are associated with acutely progressive secondary organ damage (e.g., stroke or myocardial infarction [MI]). *Hypertensive urgency* is not an immediately life-threatening situation; a reduction in BP to a safe level can occur more slowly in the next 24 to 48 hours.[1,6]

Acute, potentially life-threatening elevations of BP can occur in previously normotensive individuals with acute glomerulonephritis, head injury, or severe burns; during pregnancy (eclampsia); and with the use of recreational drugs such as cocaine. Other causes include abrupt medication withdrawal or medication nonadherence, drug–drug interactions (including herbal medications), erythropoietin administration, or drug–food interactions (i.e., patients receiving monoamine oxidase inhibitors who ingest foods rich in tyramine).[7–9] In addition, poor systolic BP control has been identified as an independent risk factor for the development of hypertensive crisis.[10] Despite improvements in the recognition and treatment of hypertension, there has been an increase in the number of hospitalizations for hypertensive emergencies in the United States from 2000 to 2007 (101–111 cases per 100,000 hospitalizations). Fortunately, in-hospital mortality associated with these admissions decreased from 2.8% to 2.6% in this time period.[11]

Table 16-1
Hypertensive Emergency versus Urgency

	Emergency	Urgency
Blood pressure criteria	Diastolic >120 mm Hg[a]	Diastolic >120 mm Hg[a]
Life-threatening	Potentially	Not acutely
End-organ damage	Acute or progressing	Chronic; not progressing
Clinical manifestations	CNS (dizziness, N/V, encephalopathy, confusion, weakness, intracranial or subarachnoid hemorrhage, stroke) Eyes (ocular hemorrhage or funduscopic changes, blurred vision, loss of sight) Cardiac (left ventricular failure, pulmonary edema, MI, angina, aortic dissection) Renal failure or insufficiency	Optic disc edema
Treatment strategy	Immediate reduction in blood pressure; administer parenteral therapy (Table 16-2)	Reduction in blood pressure over several hours to days; administer oral therapy (Table 16-3)

[a]Degree of blood pressure elevation less diagnostic than rate of pressure rise and presence of concurrent diseases or end-organ damage. See Chapter 9, Essential Hypertension, for staging of hypertension.
CNS, central nervous system; MI, myocardial infarction; N/V, nausea and vomiting.

CLINICAL PRESENTATION OF HYPERTENSIVE URGENCY

There are limited data describing the presentation and characteristics of those patients with a hypertensive urgency. Symptoms may include headache, dizziness, visual changes, chest discomfort, nausea, epistaxis, fatigue, and psychomotor agitation.[12] It should be noted that not all patients presenting with a hypertensive urgency will have symptoms.

CLINICAL PRESENTATION OF HYPERTENSIVE EMERGENCY

Similar to hypertensive urgencies, hypertensive emergencies typically occur in those with a history of hypertension. This suggests that hypertensive emergencies are almost entirely preventable.[13,14] Hypertensive emergencies tend to occur in patients with catecholamine-producing adrenal tumors (pheochromocytoma) or renal vascular disease. Additionally, hypertensive emergencies occur more often in African Americans than in Caucasians, among patients who have no primary care physician, and those who do not adhere to treatment regimens.[13,15]

Symptoms associated with hypertensive emergency are highly variable and reflect the degree of damage to specific organ systems. Rapid, severe BP elevation is not always the hallmark of a hypertensive emergency. The primary sites of damage are the central nervous system, heart, kidneys, and eyes. Although hypertensive emergencies are much less common than hypertensive urgencies, it is often difficult to know whether end-organ dysfunction is new or has progressed without a thorough patient history.

Central Nervous System

Central nervous system abnormalities are the most commonly reported complications in hypertensive emergencies. Symptoms may include a severe headache with or without dizziness, nausea, vomiting, and anorexia. Mental confusion with apprehension indicates more severe damage, as does nystagmus, localized weakness, or a positive Babinski sign (i.e., upward extension of the great toe and spreading of the smaller toes when moderate pressure is applied along a curve from the sole to the ball of the foot). Central nervous system damage may rapidly progress, resulting in coma or death. If a cerebrovascular accident has occurred, slurred speech or motor paralysis may be present.[13]

Other Complications

Cardiac consequences are the second most common complication of hypertensive emergency reported. Presentations may include heart failure (HF), acute pulmonary edema, and/or an acute coronary syndrome. Ocular symptoms of hypertensive emergency usually are related to changes in visual acuity. Complaints of blurred vision or loss of eyesight are often associated with funduscopic findings of hemorrhages, exudates (yellow deposits within the retina as a result of leaks from capillaries and microaneurysms), and occasionally papilledema (edema of the optic nerve). Acute kidney injury can also develop. Markers of renal dysfunction include hematuria, proteinuria, and elevated serum blood urea nitrogen and serum creatinine levels.

OVERVIEW OF TREATMENT

Oral versus Parenteral Therapy

Hypertensive urgency is not an indication for parenteral treatment; oral antihypertensive regimens are more appropriate. Practitioners should exercise caution in the treatment of patients with elevated BP in the absence of target organ damage. Aggressive dosing to rapidly lower BP is not without risk and can lead to hypotension and subsequent morbidity. Some have suggested that the term *hypertensive urgency* leads to overly aggressive treatment and should be discarded in favor of a less ominous term such as *uncontrolled BP*.[6] In contrast, hypertensive emergencies require immediate hospitalization, generally in an intensive care unit, and the administration of parenteral antihypertensive medications to reduce arterial pressure.[16] Effective therapy greatly improves the prognosis, reverses symptoms, and arrests the progression of end-organ damage.[17–19] Whether treatment can completely reverse end-organ damage is related to two factors: how soon treatment is initiated and the extent of damage at the initiation of therapy.

There are two fundamental concepts in the management of hypertensive emergencies. First, immediate and intensive therapy is required and takes precedence over time-consuming diagnostic procedures. Second, the choice of drugs will depend on how their time course of action and hemodynamic and metabolic effects meet the needs of the emergent situation. If encephalopathy, acute left ventricular failure, dissecting aortic aneurysm, eclampsia, or other end-organ damage is present, the BP should be lowered promptly with rapid-acting, parenteral antihypertensive medications such as clevidipine, esmolol, enalaprilat, fenoldopam, hydralazine, labetalol, nicardipine, nitroglycerin, or nitroprusside (Table 16-2).[1,3,4,20–24] If a slower BP reduction over the course of several hours or days is acceptable, as in the case of a hypertensive urgency, rapid-acting oral therapy using captopril, clonidine, labetalol, or minoxidil may be used (Table 16-3).[3,4,24–26] Figure 16-1 provides an overview of the management of a hypertensive crisis. A summary of treatment recommendations for acutely lowering BP for selected indications is listed in Table 16-4.

Table 16-2
Parenteral Medications Commonly Used in the Treatment of Hypertensive Emergencies

Medication (Brand Name)/ Class	Dose/Route	Onset of Action	Duration of Action
Clevidipine (Cleviprex)/calcium-channel blocker	Initial: 1–2 mg/hour; titrate dose to desired BP or to a max of 16 mg/hour	2–4 minutes	10–15 minutes after D/C infusion
Enalaprilat[a] (Vasotec IV)/ACE inhibitor	0.625–1.25 mg IV every 6 hours	15 minutes (max, 1–4 hours)	6–12 hours
Esmolol[b] (Brevibloc)/ β-adrenergic blocker	250–500 mcg/kg for 1 minute, then 50–300 mcg/kg/minute	1–2 minutes	10–20 minutes
Fenoldopam (Corlopam)/ dopamine-1 agonist	0.1–0.3 mcg/kg/minute	<5 minutes	30 minutes
Hydralazine[c] (generic) (20 mg/mL)/arterial vasodilator	10–20 mg IV	5–20 minutes	2–6 hours
Labetalol[d] (Normodyne)/α- and β-adrenergic blocker	2 mg/minute IV or 20–80 mg every 10 minutes up to 300 mg total dose	2–5 minutes	3–6 hours
Nicardipine[e] (Cardene IV)/ calcium-channel blocker	Initiate at 5 mg/hour IV increased by 2.5 mg/hour every 5 minutes to desired BP or a max of 15 mg/hour every 15 minutes, may decrease to 3 mg/hour after response achieved	2–10 minutes (max, 8–12 hours)	40–60 minutes after D/C infusion
Nitroglycerin[f] (Tridil, Nitro-Bid IV, Nitro-Stat IV)/arterial and venous vasodilator	IV infusion 5–100 mcg/minute	2–5 minutes	5–10 minutes after D/C infusion
Nitroprusside[g] (Nipride, Nitropress)/arterial and venous vasodilator	IV infusion.[a] Start: 0.5 mcg/kg/minute Usual: 2–5 mcg/kg/minute Max: 8 mcg/kg/minute	Seconds	3–5 minutes after D/C infusion
Medication	**Major Side Effects (All Can Cause Hypotension)**	**Avoid or Use Cautiously in Patients With These Conditions**	
Clevidipine	Atrial fibrillation, nausea, vomiting, headache, acute renal failure, reflex tachycardia, MI	Allergy to soybeans, soy products, eggs or egg products, severe aortic stenosis, defective lipid metabolism, HF	
Enalaprilat	Hyperkalemia, acute kidney injury in those who are volume depleted	Hyperkalemia, bilateral renal artery stenosis, pregnancy (teratogenic)	
Esmolol	Nausea, thrombophlebitis, painful extravasation	Asthma, bradycardia, decompensated HF, advanced heart block	
Fenoldopam	Tachycardia, headache, nausea, flushing	Glaucoma	
Hydralazine	Tachycardia, headache, angina	Angina pectoris, MI, aortic dissection	
Labetalol	Abdominal pain, nausea, vomiting, diarrhea	Asthma, bradycardia, decompensated HF	
Nicardipine	Headache, flushing, nausea, vomiting, dizziness, tachycardia; local thrombophlebitis change infusion site after 12 hours	Angina pectoris, decompensated HF, increased intracranial pressure	
Nitroglycerin	Methemoglobinemia, headache, tachycardia, nausea, vomiting, flushing, tolerance with prolonged use	Pericardial tamponade, constrictive pericarditis, or increased intracranial pressure	

(continued)

Table 16-2
Parenteral Medications Commonly Used in the Treatment of Hypertensive Emergencies (*continued*)

Medication	Major Side Effects (All Can Cause Hypotension)	Avoid or Use Cautiously in Patients With These Conditions
Nitroprusside	Nausea, vomiting, diaphoresis, weakness, thiocyanate toxicity,[h] cyanide toxicity (rare)[i] Chest pain, nausea, vomiting, dizziness, headache, nasal congestion, arrhythmia	Renal failure (thiocyanate accumulation), hepatic impairment (cyanide toxicity), pregnancy, increased intracranial pressure, acute coronary syndrome

[a]Not approved by the U.S. Food and Drug Administration for treatment of acute hypertension.
[b]Approved for intraoperative and postoperative treatment of hypertension.
[c]Parenteral hydralazine is an intermediate treatment between oral agents and more aggressive therapies such as nitroprusside. It can be given IV or intramuscularly, but there is no appreciable difference in onset of action (20–40 minutes) between the two routes. This slow onset minimizes hypotension.
[d]Labetalol is contraindicated in acute decompensated heart failure because of its β-blocking properties. Infusions start at 2 mg/minute and are titrated until a satisfactory response or a cumulative dose of 300 mg is achieved.
[e]Indicated for short-term treatment of hypertension when the oral route is not feasible or desirable.
[f]Requires special delivery system owing to drug binding to polyvinyl chloride tubing. Also see Chapters 12, Chronic Stable Angina, and Chapter 13, Acute Coronary Syndromes, for further information regarding nitroglycerin.
[g]The container should be wrapped with metal foil to prevent light-induced decompensation once reconstituted; the product will be a red-brown solution. Under these conditions, the solution is stable for 4 to 24 hours. A rising BP may indicate loss of potency. A change in color to yellow does not indicate effectiveness. The appearance of a dark brown, green, or blue color indicates loss in activity. When changing to a new bag, the administration rate may require adjustment.
[h]Thiocyanate levels rise gradually in proportion to the dose and duration of administration. The half-life of thiocyanate is 2.7 days with normal renal function and 9 days in patients with renal failure. Toxicity occurs after 7 to 14 days in patients with normal renal function and after 3 to 6 days in renal failure patients. Thiocyanate serum levels should be measured after 3 to 4 days of therapy, and the drug should be discontinued if levels exceed 10 to 12 mg/dL. Thiocyanate toxicity causes a neurotoxic syndrome of toxic psychosis, hyperreflexia, confusion, weakness, tinnitus, seizures, and coma.
[i]Signs of cyanide toxicity include lactic acidosis, hypoxemia, tachycardia, altered consciousness, seizures, and the smell of almonds on the breath. Concurrent administration of sodium thiosulfate or hydroxocobalamin may reduce the risk of cyanide toxicity in high-risk patients.
ACE, angiotensin-converting enzyme; BP, blood pressure; D/C, discontinued; HF, heart failure; IV, intravenous; MI, myocardial infarction.

Table 16-3
Oral Medications Commonly Used in the Treatment of Hypertensive Urgencies

Medication[a] (Brand Name)	Dose/Route	Onset of Action	Duration of Action	Major Side Effects[a]	Avoid or Use Cautiously in Patients With These Conditions
Captopril[b] (Capoten) 12.5-, 25-, 50-, 100-mg tablets ACE inhibitor	6.5–50 mg PO	15 minutes	4–6 hours	Hyperkalemia, angioedema, increased SCr if volume depletion, rash, pruritus, loss of taste	Renal artery stenosis, hyperkalemia, volume depletion, acute kidney injury, pregnancy
Clonidine (Catapres) 0.1-, 0.2-, 0.3-mg tablets Central α_2-agonist	0.1–0.2 mg PO initially, then 0.1 mg/hour up to 0.8 mg total	0.5–2 hours	6–8 hours	Sedation, dry mouth, bradycardia, constipation	Altered mental status, severe carotid artery stenosis
Labetalol (Normodyne, Trandate) 100-, 200-, 300-mg tablets α- and β-adrenergic blocker	200–400 mg PO repeated every 2–3 hours	30 minutes–2 hours	4 hours	Orthostatic hypotension, nausea, vomiting	HF, asthma, bradycardia
Minoxidil (Loniten) 2.5-, 10-mg tablets Arterial and venous vasodilator	5–20 mg PO	30–60 minutes; maximum response in 2–4 hours	12–16 hours	Tachycardia, fluid retention	Angina, HF

[a]All may cause hypotension, dizziness, and flushing.
[b]Other oral ACE inhibitors too slow in onset to be useful but should be used for maintenance therapy to improve adherence as captopril requires multiple daily doses.
ACE, angiotensin-converting enzyme; HF, heart failure, PO, orally; SCr, serum creatinine.

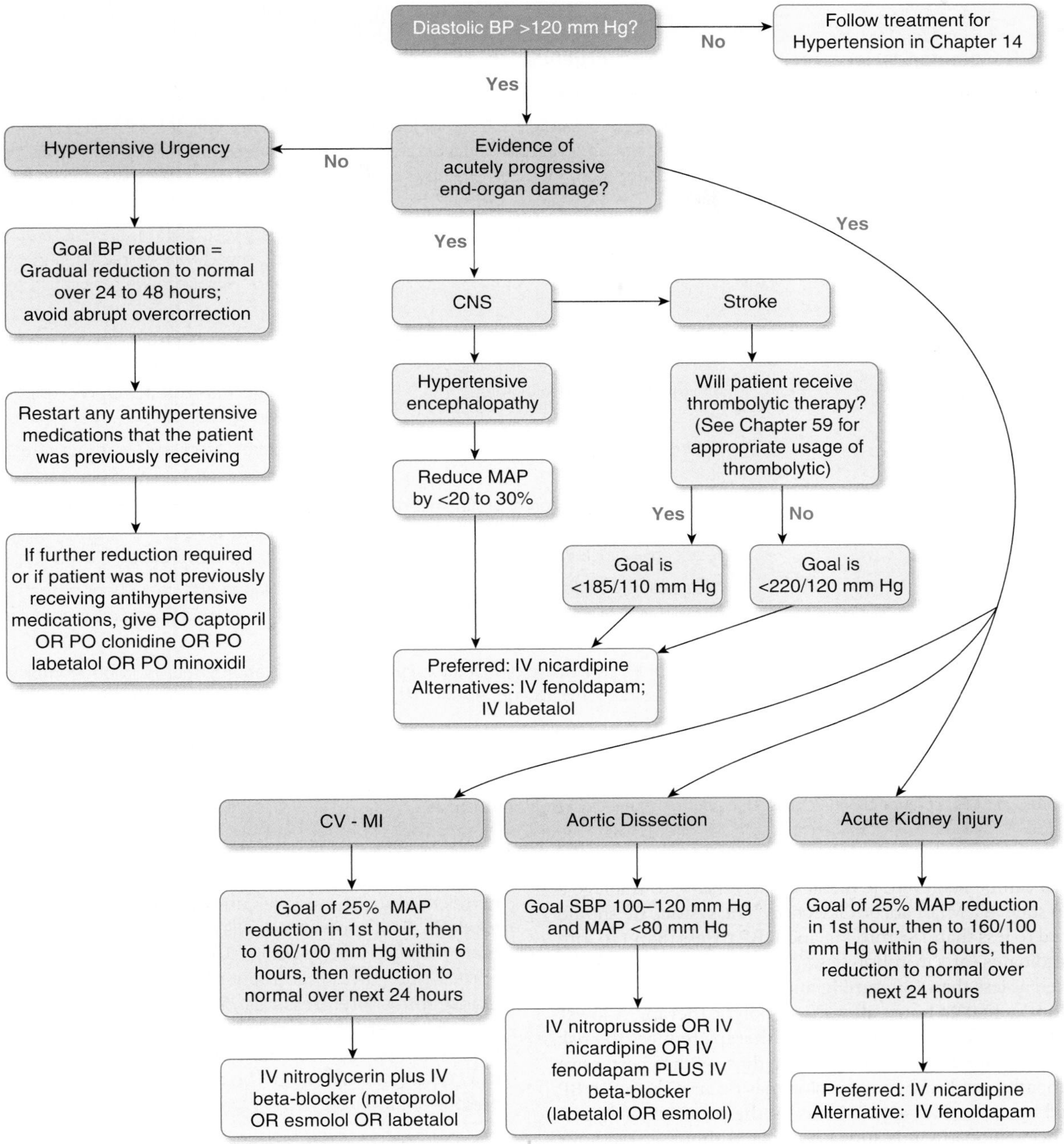

Figure 16-1 Overview of management for a hypertensive crisis. BP, blood pressure; CNS, central nervous system; IV, intravenous; MAP, mean arterial pressure; MI, myocardial infarction; SBP, systolic blood pressure.

Goals of Therapy

The rate of BP lowering must be individualized depending on whether the patient presents with a hypertensive urgency or emergency. Also, ischemic damage to the heart and brain can be provoked by a precipitous fall in BP.[26–30] As treatment is initiated, clinicians should recognize that the elderly and patients with severely defective autoregulatory mechanisms are at high risk for developing hypotensive complications. The latter group includes those with autonomic dysfunction or fixed sclerotic stenosis of cerebral or neck arteries.[31] In addition, patients who have chronically elevated BP are less likely to tolerate abrupt reductions in their BP, and the amount of reduction appropriate for those patients is somewhat less than for those whose BP is acutely elevated.

For hypertensive emergencies, it is recommended that the mean arterial pressure be reduced initially by no more than 25% (within minutes to 1 hour); then if stable, this should be followed by further reduction toward a goal of 160/100 mm Hg within 2 to 6 hours and gradual reduction to normal during the next 8 to 24 hours.[4] A DBP of 100 to 110 mm Hg is an appropriate initial therapeutic goal.[1] Lower pressures are typically indicated for patients with aortic dissection (Case 16-6).

Another exception to this rule applies in patients with acute cerebrovascular accidents. Cerebral autoregulation is disrupted in this setting, and the use of antihypertensives may cause a reduction in cerebral blood flow and increasing morbidity.[32] Current guidelines recommend lowering BP after acute ischemic stroke if the systolic BP is greater than 220 mm Hg or the DBP is greater than 120 mm Hg in patients ineligible for thrombolytic therapy; a lower

Table 16-4
Treatment Recommendations for Hypertensive Emergency

Clinical Presentation	Recommendation	Rationale
Aortic dissection	Nitroprusside, nicardipine, or fenoldopam plus esmolol or IV metoprolol; labetalol; trimethaphan. Avoid inotropic therapy.	Vasodilator will decrease pulsatile stress in aortic vessel to prevent further dissection expansion. β-blockers will prevent vasodilator-induced reflex tachycardia.
Angina, myocardial infarction	Nitroglycerin plus esmolol or metoprolol; labetalol. Avoid nitroprusside.	Coronary vasodilation, decreased cardiac output, myocardial workload, and oxygen demand. Nitroprusside may cause coronary steal.
Acute pulmonary edema, left ventricular failure	Nitroprusside, or nitroglycerin and a loop diuretic. Alternative: enalaprilat. Avoid nondihydropyridines, β-blockers.	Promotion of diuresis with venous dilatation to decrease preload. Nitroprusside, enalaprilat decrease afterload. Nicardipine may increase stroke volume.
Acute kidney injury	Nicardipine or fenoldopam. Avoid nitroprusside, enalaprilat.	Peripheral vasodilation without affecting renal clearance.
Cocaine overdose	Nicardipine, fenoldopam, verapamil, or nitroglycerin. Alternative: labetalol. Avoid β-selective blockers.	Vasodilation effects without potential unopposed α-adrenergic receptor stimulation. CCBs control overdose-induced vasospasm.
Pheochromocytoma	Nicardipine, fenoldopam, or verapamil. Alternatives: labetalol. Avoid β-selective blockers.	Vasodilation effects without potential unopposed α-adrenergic receptor stimulation.
Hypertensive encephalopathy, intracranial hemorrhage, subarachnoid hemorrhage, ischemic stroke, thrombotic stroke	Nicardipine, clevidipine or labetalol. Avoid nitroprusside, nitroglycerin, enalaprilat, hydralazine.	Vasodilation effects without compromised CBF induced by nitroprusside and nitroglycerin. Enalaprilat and hydralazine may lead to unpredictable BP changes when carefully controlled BP management is required.

BP, blood pressure; CBF, cerebral blood flow; CCB, calcium-channel blocker; IV, intravenous.

blood goal can be achieved, if medically necessary, to manage a condition such as a MI or aortic dissection. The systolic BP should be lowered to less than 185 mm Hg and DBP to less than 110 mm Hg in candidates for thrombolytics.[33] The systolic BP should be maintained at less than 180 mmHg and the DBP at less than 105 mmHg for the first 24 hours after thrombolytic therapy. A lower BP in patients undergoing thrombolytic therapy reduces the risk of intracerebral bleeding.[33] Additionally, in those with hypertensive encephalopathy, cerebral hypoperfusion may occur if the mean BP is reduced by more than 40%.[34] Thus, in the presence of hypertensive encephalopathy it is suggested that within the first hour of treatment the mean pressure be lowered by no more than 20% or to a DBP of 100 mm Hg, whichever is greater.[34,35]

HYPERTENSIVE URGENCIES

Patient Assessment

CASE 16-1

QUESTION 1: M.M. is a 60-year-old African American man with a long history of HF with a preserved ejection fraction (HFpEF), poorly controlled hypertension believed to be caused by nonadherence, and a history of MI. He was referred from a community health center this morning for a thorough evaluation of his elevated BP. He has not taken his enalapril, carvedilol, or amlodipine for the past 7 days. M.M. is completely asymptomatic. Physical examination reveals a BP of 180/120 mm Hg and a pulse of 92 beats/minute. Funduscopic examination is pertinent for mild arteriolar narrowing, without hemorrhages or exudates. The discs are flat. His lungs are clear, and the cardiac examination is unremarkable. The electrocardiogram indicates normal sinus rhythm at a rate of 90 beats/minute. The chest radiograph is interpreted as mild cardiomegaly. Serum electrolytes, blood urea nitrogen, and serum creatinine are within normal limits. A urinalysis is significant for 2+ proteinuria. How quickly should his BP be lowered, and what therapeutic options are available?

The absolute magnitude of BP elevation does not in itself constitute a medical emergency requiring an acute reduction in BP. There is no evidence of encephalopathy, cardiac decompensation, chest pain, or rapid change in renal function. Therefore, no evidence exists to indicate a rapid deterioration in the function of target organs. One would classify M.M.'s case as a hypertensive urgency.

As is often the case, M.M.'s lack of BP control is related to medication nonadherence. M.M.'s clinical presentation requires that his BP be lowered during the next 12 to 24 to 48 hours while being careful not to induce hypotension. Rapid-acting oral agents can be used for this purpose; parenteral therapy is not warranted. A number of different oral regimens using clonidine, captopril, labetalol, or minoxidil are available. Restarting his medications in a controlled manner so as not to drop his BP too rapidly may also be a reasonable option for treatment. Later, he can be converted to a regimen designed to enhance adherence by selecting medications with once-daily dosing. For example, lisinopril or another long-acting angiotensin-converting enzyme (ACE) inhibitor would be preferred for maintenance instead of the enalapril previously prescribed. One should also determine and address barriers to medication adherence with the patient including cost of therapy, lack of understanding of the benefits of therapy, misconceptions of the side effect profiles, and so forth. Timely follow-up within 1 week after treatment of hypertensive urgency is of paramount importance for the appropriate management of these patients.

Oral Drug Therapy

RAPIDLY ACTING CALCIUM-CHANNEL BLOCKERS

CASE 16-1, QUESTION 2: M.M.'s physician has ordered immediate-release nifedipine to be given 10 mg sublingually. Is this appropriate therapy to treat his hypertensive urgency?

Captopril, clonidine, labetalol, and minoxidil have all been used to lower BP acutely. These oral agents take several hours to adequately lower pressure and are therefore useful in treating hypertensive urgencies but not emergencies. Oral acting ACE inhibitors, other than captopril, are not useful for acutely lowering BP because of a slower onset of action.

The immediate-release calcium-channel blockers, including diltiazem, verapamil, and nicardipine, can rapidly lower BP; however, the most extensive experience is with nifedipine. Nifedipine, when given orally or by the "bite and swallow" method, was previously recommended as a rapid-acting alternative to parenteral therapy in the acute management of hypertension. However, its use has been associated with life-threatening adverse events related to ischemia, MI, and stroke.[26–30] The cavalier use of immediate-release nifedipine to acutely lower BP is potentially dangerous and should be discouraged.[36,37] M.M.'s BP can be managed safely using other oral medications. Captopril, clonidine, or labetalol can be used to lower his BP, and he can be restarted on his oral maintenance regimen with appropriate follow-up care.

CLONIDINE

CASE 16-1, QUESTION 3: A decision is made not to use nifedipine, but rather to give M.M. oral clonidine. What is an appropriate starting and maintenance dose?

Clonidine is considered a safe, effective first-line therapy for hypertensive urgency. It is a centrally acting, α_2-adrenergic agonist that inhibits sympathetic outflow from the central nervous system. BP can be lowered gradually over the course of several hours using oral clonidine. Traditional dosing regimens have included an initial oral loading dose (0.1–0.2 mg) followed by repeated doses of 0.1 mg/hour until the desired response is achieved or until a cumulative dose of 0.8 mg is reached.[38] Some authors, however, have cautioned against the use of sequential loading doses, citing lack of benefit over placebo and the potential for unpredictable adverse effects, particularly abrupt occurrences of hypotension.[39] If loading doses are to be used, it is especially important to reduce doses in patients with volume depletion, those who have recently used other antihypertensive drugs, and the elderly.[1,23,40]

The acute response to oral clonidine loading is not predictive of the daily dose required to maintain BP control. Maintenance oral therapy with clonidine is somewhat empiric; however, total daily doses should be spread between 2 and 3 times daily dosing owing to the drug's short half-life.

Adverse Effects and Precautions

CASE 16-1, QUESTION 4: What are the adverse effects and precautions that should be considered before recommending the use of clonidine?

Oral clonidine is generally well tolerated. Adverse effects include orthostatic hypotension, bradycardia, sedation, dry mouth, and dizziness. Clonidine can decrease cerebral blood flow by up to 28%; it should not be used in patients with severe cerebrovascular disease.[41] Clonidine also should be avoided in patients with HF, bradycardia, sick sinus syndrome, or cardiac conduction defects,[23] as well as in patients at risk of medication nonadherence because of the rebound hypertension.[42,43]

OTHER ORAL DRUGS

Captopril

CASE 16-1, QUESTION 5: M.M. has a history of HFpEF and normal renal function. Based on these findings, would captopril be a reasonable choice for initial treatment? How should it be given? What if his blood urea nitrogen or serum creatinine were elevated?

Captopril has been used both orally and sublingually to acutely lower BP.[44,45] Captopril decreases both afterload and preload, and lowers total peripheral vascular resistance.[23] For this reason, captopril and other ACE inhibitors are often considered the drugs of choice in patients with HF with reduced ejection fraction as they have been shown to reduce mortality in this patient population (see Chapter 14, Heart Failure, for further discussion). M.M has HFpEF; the evidence of using ACE inhibitors in improving cardiovascular outcomes in this patient population is not strong. However, given that M.M. appeared to be well controlled on his enalapril therapy before abruptly stopping his medications, it is reasonable to restart a rapid ACE inhibitor and reinforce medication adherence issues.

After oral administration, the onset of action of captopril occurs within minutes and peaks 30 to 90 minutes later.[46] Clinically, it reduces BP within 10 to 15 minutes, with effects persisting for 2 to 6 hours. Sublingual captopril is as effective as nifedipine but without reflex tachycardia in acutely reducing mean arterial pressure in both urgent and emergent conditions.[45–48]

Despite these beneficial effects, captopril, as well as long-acting ACE inhibitors, must be used with caution in patients with renal insufficiency or volume depletion. In most cases, an elevated blood urea nitrogen or serum creatinine will provide a clue to the existence of these conditions; however, captopril can also induce renal failure in patients with bilateral renal artery stenosis or renal artery stenosis in a solitary kidney. Such conditions may not be easy to detect in the context of an acute hypertensive emergency. Therefore, in patients in whom these conditions can be excluded, captopril can be considered for therapy. First-dose hypotension is a common limiting factor with captopril use. This complication is most likely to occur in the elderly and in patients with high renin levels such as those who are volume depleted or those receiving diuretics. Under these circumstances, initial doses should not exceed 12.5 mg, with repeat doses an hour or more later if necessary. Therefore, captopril would be a reasonable choice as initial therapy in M.M., which can later be replaced by a longer-acting ACE inhibitor.

Minoxidil and Labetalol

CASE 16-1, QUESTION 6: What other oral agents are used in the treatment of hypertensive urgency?

Minoxidil, a potent oral vasodilator, has been used successfully in the treatment of hypertensive urgencies.[49,50] An oral loading dose of 10 to 20 mg produces a maximal BP response in 2 to 4 hours and can be followed by a dose of 5 to 20 mg every 4 hours if necessary. Unfortunately, its onset of action is slower than that of clonidine or captopril. Another complicating factor is that β-blockers and loop diuretics generally must be used concomitantly to counteract minoxidil-induced reflex tachycardia and fluid retention.[50] Because of this, minoxidil should only be prescribed by those who have experience with prescribing this agent and managing these adverse effects. These adverse effects make this agent a less than ideal choice in M.M. because of his history of HF. Minoxidil should be used only in patients presenting with hypertensive urgency who are not responding to other antihypertensive therapies or who have previously been taking this agent.

Oral labetalol, a combined α- and β-receptor antagonist, is an alternative to oral clonidine or captopril for the treatment of severe hypertension, but the most appropriate dosing regimen remains to be determined.[51–54] Initial doses of 100 to 300 mg may provide a sustained response for up to 4 hours.[52] Labetalol (200 mg given at hourly intervals to a maximum dose of 1,200 mg) was comparable to oral clonidine in reducing mean arterial pressure.[54] An alternative regimen using 300 mg initially followed by 100 mg at 2-hour intervals to a maximum of 500 mg was also successful in acutely lowering BP.[53] Other literature has reported that a single loading dose of 200 to 400 mg does not appear to be effective in achieving an adequate BP response.[55] Because labetalol can cause profound orthostatic hypotension, patients should remain in the supine position and should be checked for orthostasis before ambulation. In addition, labetalol should be avoided in patients with asthma, bradycardia, or advanced heart block.

HYPERTENSIVE EMERGENCIES

Patient Assessment

CASE 16-2

QUESTION 1: M.R., a 55-year-old African American man, presents to the emergency department with a 3-day history of progressively increasing shortness of breath. During the past 2 days, he experienced a severe headache unrelieved by ibuprofen, as well as substernal chest pain, anorexia, and nausea. His medical history includes asthma and chronic stable angina. His medications include albuterol via metered-dose inhaler, furosemide, isosorbide dinitrate, felodipine, and lisinopril; however, he discontinued these medications on his own 3 weeks ago.

Physical examination reveals an anxious-appearing man who is alert, oriented, and in moderate respiratory distress. His vital signs include a heart rate of 125 beats/minute, respiratory rate of 36 breaths/minute, BP of 220/145 mm Hg without orthostasis, and a normal body temperature. Funduscopic examination shows arteriolar narrowing and arteriovenous nicking without hemorrhages, exudates, or papilledema. No jugular venous distention is observed, but bilateral carotid bruits are present. Chest examination reveals decreased breath sounds with bilateral rales extending to the tip of the scapula. M.R.'s heart is displaced 2 cm to the left of the midclavicular line with no thrills or heaves. The rhythm is regular with an S_3 and an S_4 gallop; no murmurs are noted. The remainder of M.R.'s examination is within normal limits.

Significant laboratory values include the following:

Sodium, 142 mEq/L
Potassium, 4.9 mEq/L
Chloride, 101 mEq/L
Bicarbonate, 23 mEq/L
Urea nitrogen, 30 mg/dL
Serum creatinine, 1.2 mg/dL
Hematocrit, 38%
Hemoglobin, 13 g/dL
White blood cell count and differential, within normal limits
Troponin—negative × 2

Urinalysis shows 1+ hemoglobin and 1+ protein. Microscopic examination of the urine reveals 5 to 10 red blood cells per high-power field and no casts. Pulse oximetry reveals an oxygen saturation of 88%. An electrocardiogram demonstrates sinus tachycardia and left ventricular hypertrophy. The chest radiograph shows moderate cardiomegaly and bilateral fluffy infiltrates.

What aspects of M.R.'s history and physical examination are characteristic of an emergent need to immediately lower his BP?

Hypertensive crisis occurs most often in African American men and in individuals between the ages of 40 and 60. Furthermore, many patients who present with hypertensive crisis have a recent history of discontinuing the use of their antihypertensives,[13,15] as is the case with M.R. in Case 16-2 and M.M. in Case 16-1.

Recent-onset severe headache, nausea, and vomiting are consistent with central nervous system signs of severe hypertension, as are the acute onset of angina (substernal pain) and acute HF (shortness of breath, increased pulse and respiratory rate, cardiomegaly, S_3, and chest radiographic findings of pulmonary edema). The absence of signs of right-sided HF such as jugular venous distention or hepatomegaly suggests an acute onset of HF caused by hypertension as opposed to a gradual worsening of chronic HF. M.R.'s urinary sediment is relatively unimpressive at this time, especially in light of his history, and his ocular complications are minimal. M.R.'s presentation is considered hypertensive emergency because of the presence of HF symptoms; M.R. should be admitted to the hospital as intravenous (IV) antihypertensive therapy is warranted.

Parenteral Drug Therapy

NITROPRUSSIDE

CASE 16-2, QUESTION 2: M.R. is to be started on nitroprusside. Is this an appropriate choice of drug? What alternatives to nitroprusside are available?

M.R.'s arterial pressure should be lowered with parenteral medications, which have a rapid onset of action. Nitroprusside, fenoldopam, and IV nitroglycerin all decrease total peripheral resistance rapidly with minimal effect on myocardial oxygen consumption and heart rate. Of these agents, either nitroprusside or fenoldopam would be preferred in patients with hypertension accompanied by decompensated HF in the absence of MI. Parenteral nitroglycerin is similar to nitroprusside except that it has a relatively greater effect on the venous circulation and less effect on arterioles. It is most useful in patients presenting with angina secondary to coronary insufficiency, ischemic heart disease, MI, or hypertension after coronary bypass surgery (also see Case 16-3, Question 6). In addition, nitroprusside and IV nitroglycerin may both decrease elevated left ventricular diastolic pressures in patients presenting with hypertensive emergency. Although nitroglycerin would be helpful for someone who is experiencing chest pain in the setting of an MI, this patient is not having an acute coronary syndrome, which is confirmed by negative troponins and electrocardiogram. Before considering nitroprusside, it is important to consider the etiology of the chest pain. As described above, the chest pain is likely due to acute-onset HF due to severe hypertension. Based on the signs and symptoms, it is not likely to have been caused by ischemic heart disease. In the setting of coronary ischemia, nitroglycerin has been shown to be more beneficial than nitroprusside; however, this patient does not have evidence of active coronary ischemia. Because the clinical presentation is more consistent with acute-onset HF, it is important to focus on reducing peripheral resistance and decreasing elevated left ventricular diastolic pressures. Nitroprusside provides an advantage here because it provides both arterial and venous vasodilation, allowing for further reduction in peripheral resistance and left ventricular diastolic pressures. Nitroglycerin has a relatively greater effect on venous circulation, especially at lower doses. Thus, nitroprusside would be preferred in this patient.

Fenoldopam and nitroprusside are equally efficacious in acutely lowering BP.[56–59] Both medications have an immediate onset, are easily titratable, have a short duration of action, and are relatively well tolerated.[60–63] Unlike nitroprusside, fenoldopam does not cause cyanide or thiocyanate toxicity. However, fenoldopam is associated with dose-related tachycardia and should be avoided in those with active coronary ischemia.

Therefore, in the absence of any significant renal or liver disease, nitroprusside is the preferred treatment for M.R.

Hemodynamic Effects

Nitroprusside has many pharmacologic effects that should improve M.R.'s condition. It dilates both venous and arterial vessels, thereby increasing venous capacitance and decreasing the venous return or preload on the heart (see Chapter 14, Heart Failure). A decrease in the pulmonary capillary wedge pressure and ventricular filling pressure will ultimately improve M.R.'s pulmonary edema. Afterload is also decreased as a result of arterial dilation. This action increases cardiac output, reduces arterial pressure, and increases tissue perfusion.

Concurrent Use of Diuretics

CASE 16-2, QUESTION 3: Should M.R. be given a diuretic before nitroprusside therapy is begun?

Administration of potent IV diuretics is relatively ineffective in the acute treatment of hypertensive crisis except in patients with concomitant volume overload or HF. Many patients with hypertensive emergencies are vasoconstricted and have normal or reduced plasma volumes; therefore, diuretics have little effect and may actually aggravate renal impairment or cause other adverse effects.[22,64] Furthermore, when diuretics are given acutely in combination with other antihypertensive agents, profound hypotension can occur.

The immediate value of diuretics in acute HF is related more to their hemodynamic effects (venodilation) than to diuresis. Venodilation after IV diuretic administration decreases right-sided cardiac filling pressures, decreases pulmonary artery and wedge pressures, and increases cardiac output before diuresis occurs.[65] The presence of HF and severely elevated BP in M.R. warrants IV administration of a loop diuretic (e.g., furosemide 40 mg, torsemide [Demadex] 10–20 mg, or bumetanide [Bumex] 1 mg).

Dosing and Administration

CASE 16-2, QUESTION 4: What dose of nitroprusside should be used initially?

Effective infusion rates range from 0.25 to 10 mcg/kg/minute.[66,67] For M.R., an infusion of nitroprusside should be initiated at a rate of 0.25 mcg/kg/minute. The dose should be increased slowly by 0.25 mcg/kg/minute every 5 minutes until the desired pressure is achieved. A maximum infusion rate of 10 mcg/kg/minute has been recommended. If adequate BP reduction is not achieved within 10 minutes after maximal dose infusion, nitroprusside should be discontinued.[4] The dosage must be individualized according to patient response using continuous intraarterial BP recording and observing for signs or symptoms of toxicity.

Nitroprusside decomposes on exposure to light, so the solution should be shielded with an opaque sleeve. It is not necessary to protect the tubing from light. Reconstituted solutions are stable for 24 hours at room temperature. A change in the solution's color from light brown to dark brown, green, orange, or blue indicates a loss in activity. The solution should be discarded if this change occurs.

Therapeutic End Point

CASE 16-2, QUESTION 5: A nitroprusside infusion is started. What is the goal of therapy?

For most patients BP should be reduced by no more than 25% within the first minutes to hour, then if stable, therapy can be titrated to achieve a goal BP of 160/100 mm Hg during the next 2 to 6 hours. BPs can be reduced to near-normal levels within 8 to 24 hours. However, because M.R. has cerebral occlusive disease (carotid bruits), excessive reduction of his BP should be avoided. Overly aggressive reduction of BP in the presence of major cerebral vessel stenosis may decrease cerebral blood flow and produce strokes or other neurologic complications.

Normal cerebral blood flow remains relatively constant over a wide range of systemic BP measurements through autoregulatory mechanisms.[40,68] The autoregulatory effects can prevent large alterations in cerebral blood flow from either slow or rapid changes in systemic arterial pressures. In addition, the arterial BP required to maintain cerebral perfusion is higher in hypertensive patients than in normotensive individuals. If M.R.'s BP is reduced excessively, cerebral blood flow may decrease sharply. Therefore, a DBP of 100 to 105 mm Hg would be a reasonable initial therapeutic goal for him in the first 6 hours. If hypotension occurs, nitroprusside should be discontinued and M.R. should be placed in the Trendelenburg position, in which the head is kept lower than the trunk.

Cyanide Toxicity

CASE 16-2, QUESTION 6: M.R. is being treated with nitroprusside. However, during the last 36 hours, dose titration to 7 mcg/kg/minute has been necessary to control his BP. His tachycardia angina have resolved. Is he at risk of developing cyanide toxicity? What indices of toxicity should be monitored? Are there agents available to prevent toxicity?

A major concern when using sodium nitroprusside is toxicity secondary to the accumulation of its metabolic by-products, cyanide, and thiocyanate. Sodium nitroprusside decomposes within a few minutes after IV infusion. Free cyanide, which represents 44% of nitroprusside by weight, is released into the bloodstream, producing prussic acid (hydrogen cyanide), which is responsible for the acute toxicity.[69] The amount of hydrogen cyanide released is dose related.[70] Endogenous detoxification of cyanide occurs through a mitochondrial rhodanese system, which, in the presence of a sulfur donor such as thiosulfate, converts cyanide to thiocyanate.[69] Theoretically, cyanide can be expected to accumulate in the body when the rate of the sodium nitroprusside infusion exceeds 2 mcg/kg/minute for a prolonged period. The presence of hepatic or renal impairment may also predispose the patient to cyanide toxicity.[71,72]

Symptomatic cyanide toxicity occurs infrequently; however, several deaths have been reported after the use of sodium nitroprusside.[73] Cyanide toxicity occurs most commonly when large doses (total dose 1.5 mg/kg) of nitroprusside are administered rapidly to patients undergoing a surgical procedure that requires induction of hypotension. However, cyanide toxicity and mortality associated with nitroprusside exceed 3,000 and 1,000 cases per year, respectively, according to two sources.[73,74]

Although concurrent sodium thiosulfate administration has been recommended in high-risk patients, no clinical data are available to indicate that it reduces overall mortality.[75] Furthermore, this intervention may result in the accumulation of thiocyanate, particularly if sodium thiosulfate is given at high infusion rates or to patients with renal insufficiency. Hydroxocobalamin has also been used to reduce the risk of cyanide toxicity secondary to nitroprusside infusions, but its use is limited because of poor availability and cost considerations.[72] With the availability of safer alternatives (e.g., fenoldopam, IV labetalol, IV nicardipine) for use in high-risk patients, the use of hydroxocobalamin or thiosulfate is rarely required.

Cyanide toxicity can be detected early by monitoring M.R.'s metabolic status. Lactic acidosis is an early indicator of toxicity because the progressive inactivation of cytochrome oxidase by cyanide results in increased anaerobic glycolysis.[76,77] A low plasma bicarbonate concentration and low pH, accompanied by an increase in the blood lactate or lactate-to-pyruvate ratio could indicate cyanide toxicity.[77] Additional signs of cyanide intoxication include tachycardia, altered consciousness, coma, convulsions, and the occasional smell of almonds on the breath.[70,77] Measuring serum thiocyanate levels is of no value in detecting the onset of cyanide toxicity. If toxicity develops, the infusion should be stopped and appropriate therapy for cyanide intoxication instituted. The need for such a high-dose infusion of nitroprusside to maintain M.R.'s pressure may increase his risk for cyanide toxicity, warranting close monitoring of his acid–base balance.

Thiocyanate Toxicity

CASE 16-2, QUESTION 7: Explain the difference between cyanide toxicity and thiocyanate toxicity. What is M.R.'s risk for thiocyanate toxicity if he is continued on a dose of 7 mcg/kg/minute? Is monitoring of serum thiocyanate concentrations necessary?

Sodium nitroprusside is more likely to produce thiocyanate toxicity. Although this complication is also rare, patients with renal impairment who receive infusions beyond 72 hours are particularly susceptible. Conversion of cyanide to thiocyanate, via sulfation by the liver, proceeds relatively slowly. The half-life of thiocyanate is 2.7 days with normal renal function and up to 9 days in patients with renal failure.[78] When sodium nitroprusside is infused for several days at moderate dosages (2–5 mcg/kg/minute), toxic levels of thiocyanate can occur within 7 to 14 days in patients with normal renal function and 3 to 6 days in patients with severe renal disease.[69]

Thiocyanate causes a neurotoxic syndrome manifested by psychosis, hyperreflexia, confusion, weakness, tinnitus, seizures, and coma.[71,78] Prolonged exposure to thiocyanate can suppress thyroid function through inhibition of iodine uptake and binding by the thyroid gland.[78] Measurement of blood levels of thiocyanate is only recommended in patients with renal disease or when the duration of the nitroprusside infusion exceeds 3 or 4 days. Nitroprusside should be discontinued if serum thiocyanate levels exceed 10 to 12 mg/dL.[79,80] Life-threatening toxicity is of concern when blood thiocyanate levels exceed 20 mg/dL. In emergency cases, thiocyanate can be readily removed by hemodialysis.[78]

For M.R., the potential for thiocyanate toxicity is low because his renal function is normal and the anticipated infusion duration is relatively short. Therefore, measurement of thiocyanate levels is not indicated.

Other side effects associated with nitroprusside therapy include nausea, vomiting, diaphoresis, nasal stuffiness, muscular twitching, dizziness, and weakness. These effects are usually acute and occur when nitroprusside is administered too rapidly. They can be reversed by decreasing the infusion rate.

CASE 16-2, QUESTION 8: M.R.'s serum chemistries and arterial blood gas values indicate a metabolic acidosis. Should the nitroprusside infusion be continued at 7 mcg/kg/minute? What alternatives are available?

Although the duration of M.R.'s nitroprusside therapy has been short, tolerance to the antihypertensive effect requires the use of a high-dose infusion to maintain BP control. Thus, acidosis may represent toxicity as a result of cyanide accumulation. The nitroprusside infusion should be discontinued at this time, and another rapidly acting, easily titratable parenteral antihypertensive such as fenoldopam or IV nicardipine should be initiated.

FENOLDOPAM

CASE 16-2, QUESTION 9: What are the advantages and disadvantages of fenoldopam compared with sodium nitroprusside?

Fenoldopam is a parenteral, rapidly acting, peripheral dopamine-1 agonist used to manage hypertensive crisis when a rapid reduction in BP is required.[81–84] Stimulation of the dopamine-1 receptors vasodilates coronary, renal, mesenteric, and peripheral arteries.[85,86] Fenoldopam has been used to control perioperative hypertension in patients undergoing cardiac bypass surgery.[87] The use of low-dose fenoldopam had been evaluated in those with acute kidney injury following cardiac surgery; therapy was not associated with a reduced risk of renal replacement therapy or 30-day mortality.[88] This refutes prior theories that dilation of the renal arteries with fenoldopam may reduce the risk of renal complications.[62,86]

Fenoldopam is as effective as sodium nitroprusside for treatment of hypertensive emergencies and does not cause either cyanide or thiocyanate toxicity.[57–59] Fenoldopam can be considered as an alternative to nitroprusside in patients who are at high risk for cyanide or thiocyanate toxicity. Over the past several years, the use of fenoldopam as an antihypertensive has decreased.[20]

Clearance of fenoldopam is not altered by renal or liver disease. Like nitroprusside, fenoldopam also has a short duration of action, with an elimination half-life of approximately 5 minutes, thus allowing for easy titration.[83,89] BP and heart rate should be frequently to avoid hypotension and dose-related reflex tachycardia. Flushing and headache may occur. Serum potassium should be monitored and repleted as necessary. Fenoldopam should be used cautiously in patients with glaucoma or intraocular hypertension due to a dose-dependent increase in intraocular pressure.[90,91]

CASE 16-2, QUESTION 10: Which antihypertensive agents should be avoided in M.R.? Why?

Labetalol, a potent, rapidly acting antihypertensive with both α- and β-blocking activity, is very effective in the treatment of hypertensive emergencies,[91–98] but it should not be used in M.R. Hemodynamically, labetalol reduces peripheral vascular resistance (afterload), BP, and heart rate, with almost no change in the resting cardiac output or stroke volume.[99]

M.R. was experiencing chest pain, and had tachycardia on admission; these signs and symptoms are most likely caused by his severely elevated BP and the presence of acute left ventricular failure. Even though labetalol may have alleviated M.R.'s angina, the negative inotropic action could acutely compromise his left ventricular dysfunction, an effect that outweighs the potential benefit of afterload reduction. In addition, even though labetalol is one of the safest β-blocking drugs when used in patients with asthma,[100] β-blocker therapy should be avoided as initial treatment in patients with asthma. Labetalol should be used only if alternative methods of reducing M.R.'s pressure fail.

LABETALOL

CASE 16-3

QUESTION 1: C.M., a 52-year-old Caucasian man, is admitted to the hospital with a 3-day history of increasing exertional substernal chest pain (without shortness of breath), diaphoresis, nausea, and vomiting. His history is significant for poorly controlled hypertension, glaucoma, and angina pectoris. Prior medications include dorzolamide ophthalmic drops, atenolol, hydrochlorothiazide, and oral nitrates. Physical examination reveals an anxious man who is alert and oriented. He has a BP of 210/146 mm Hg without orthostasis and a regular pulse of 115 beats/minute. Bilateral hemorrhages and exudates are present on funduscopic examination. The lungs are clear and the point of maximal impulse is displaced. There are no murmurs or gallops. Examination of the abdomen is unremarkable, and there is no peripheral edema. The neurologic examination is normal.

Significant laboratory values include the following:

Urea nitrogen, 49 mg/dL

Serum creatinine, 2.8 mg/dL

Serum creatinine was previously noted to be 1.2 mg/dL. Urinalysis shows proteinuria and hematuria. The electrocardiogram demonstrates sinus tachycardia with left-axis deviation, left ventricular hypertrophy, and nonspecific ST-T wave changes. The chest radiograph reveals mild cardiomegaly.

C.M. is given nitroglycerin sublingually and 1 inch of nitroglycerin ointment is applied topically. He is started on IV labetalol. Is this choice of treatment reasonable, considering C.M.'s angina and acute kidney injury?

The presence of chest pain, retinopathy, and new-onset renal disease, as well as the magnitude of the BP elevation in C.M., classifies his presentation as a hypertensive emergency that warrants a prompt reduction in BP. Sublingual and topical nitroglycerin may help in acutely and temporarily lower his BP and relieve his chest pain while waiting for more definitive treatment to be implemented.

IV labetalol has been used successfully in hypertensive emergencies.[92–98] Labetalol blocks both β- and α-adrenergic receptors and also may exert a direct vasodilator effect. The β-blockade is nonselective with β- to α-potency of 3:1 for oral and 7:1 for IV. Labetalol is advantageous in C.M. because the immediate onset of action will reduce peripheral vascular resistance without causing reflex tachycardia. Myocardial oxygen demand will be reduced and coronary hemodynamics will be improved, making this agent an excellent choice for patients such as C.M., with anginal symptoms or MI. In addition, IV labetalol does not significantly reduce cerebral blood flow; therefore, it may be useful in patients with cerebrovascular disease.[1,23]

Fenoldopam or nitroprusside could also be used to treat C.M. Fenoldopam could be considered, but C.M.'s history of glaucoma would preclude its use. Additionally, fenoldopam would not be preferred due to the potential for reflex tachycardia and risk of worsening ischemia. Treatment with nitroprusside would expose C.M. to the potential risk of cyanide and thiocyanate toxicity with his new-onset acute kidney injury. In contrast, labetalol has been used successfully in patients with renal disease without deleterious side effects.[101,102] Labetalol is eliminated by glucuronidation in the liver, with less than 5% of the dose being excreted unchanged in the urine.

Contraindications and Precautions

CASE 16-3, QUESTION 2: What cautions should be exercised when using labetalol in C.M.?

Labetalol's disadvantages are primarily related to its β-blocking effects. Therefore, it should not be used in patients with asthma, heart block greater than first degree, or sinus bradycardia, and it should be used with caution in patients with decompensated HF[93,97,103] (see Case 16-2, Question 10). None of these are present in C.M. Like other β-blockers, labetalol should also be used with caution in patients with β.[104] Labetalol has been effective in the treatment of hypertension associated with pheochromocytoma and excess catecholamine states as well as those with rebound hypertension from β-blocker withdrawal.[105] However, because labetalol is primarily a β-blocker, paradoxic hypertension may occur in patients with pheochromocytoma. These individuals have adrenal tumors that excrete high amounts of norepinephrine, which results in relatively unopposed α-receptor stimulation.[106] More clinical experience is required before labetalol can be recommended in patients with pheochromocytoma.[6,92]

CASE 16-3, QUESTION 3: How should parenteral labetalol be given to C.M.?

IV labetalol can be given by pulse administration or continuous infusion.[92–97] Bolus injections are administered, beginning with 20 mg given over 2 minutes, followed by 40 to 80 mg every 10 to 15 minutes until the desired response is achieved or a cumulative dose of 300 mg is reached. The desired response is usually achieved with a mean dose of 200 mg in 90% of patients.[93] The maximal effect occurs within 10 minutes,[95] and the antihypertensive response may persist for more than 6 hours.[107] Because the rate of BP reduction is accelerated with an increase in infusion rate,[95] a controlled continuous infusion may provide a more gradual reduction in arterial pressure with less frequent adverse effects.[97,108] The infusion can then be started at a rate of 2 mg/minute and titrated until a satisfactory response is achieved or until a cumulative dose of 300 mg is reached.

Parenteral to Oral Conversion

CASE 16-3, QUESTION 4: C.M. was treated with a labetalol infusion and required a cumulative dose of 180 mg to achieve a DBP of 100 mm Hg. His anginal symptoms resolved almost immediately, but 3 hours after the infusion, C.M. became faint and dizzy while ambulating. Should oral labetalol be withheld in C.M.?

Postural hypotension and dizziness are dose related and more commonly associated with the IV route of administration.[99,103] C.M. should remain in a supine position after the IV administration of labetalol, and his ability to tolerate an upright position should be established before permitting ambulation. Oral labetalol can be given to C.M. when his symptoms resolve. There is no correlation between the oral maintenance dose and the total initial IV dose. C.M. should be started on an empiric dose of 100 to 200 mg of oral labetalol 2 to 3 times per daily, and this should be titrated as necessary.

CASE 16-3, QUESTION 5: What other side effects can occur with labetalol therapy?

Other side effects commonly associated with labetalol include nausea, vomiting, abdominal pain, and diarrhea in up to 15% of the patients.[103] Scalp tingling is an unusual side effect that has been reported in a few patients after IV administration; it tends to disappear with continued treatment. Other side effects include tiredness, weakness, muscle cramps, headache, and skin rashes.

NITROGLYCERIN

CASE 16-3, QUESTION 6: Would parenteral nitroglycerin be an acceptable alternative to labetalol for C.M.?

Hypertensive emergencies in the setting of unstable angina or MI requires an immediate reduction in BP. Nitroprusside has been used successfully, but IV nitroglycerin can have more favorable effects on collateral coronary flow in patients with ischemic heart disease.[109] By diminishing preload, nitroglycerin decreases left ventricular diastolic volume, diastolic pressure, and myocardial wall tension, thus reducing myocardial oxygen consumption.[110] These changes favor redistribution of coronary blood flow to the subendocardium, which is more vulnerable to ischemia. At high dosages, nitroglycerin dilates arteriolar smooth muscles, and this reduction in afterload also decreases myocardial wall tension and oxygen consumption.[111]

IV nitroglycerin has a rapid onset of action and a short duration, and is easily titratable. It is generally appropriate to begin IV nitroglycerin in the dose range of 5 to 10 mcg/minute, increased as needed to control pressure and symptoms. The usual dose is in the range of 40 to 100 mcg/minute. The major limiting side effects are headache and the development of tolerance. In general, IV nitroglycerin is well suited for use in patients such as C.M. who have angina or in patients who have hypertensive emergency associated with MI or coronary artery bypass surgery.

HYDRALAZINE

CASE 16-4

QUESTION 1: T.M., a 30-year-old Caucasian man with a history of chronic glomerulonephritis and poorly controlled hypertension, came to the emergency department complaining of early morning occipital headaches during the past week. He has no other complaints. He has not taken any BP medication in a month. Physical examination revealed an afebrile man in no acute distress with a BP of 160/128 mm Hg without orthostasis and a regular pulse of 90 beats/minute. Funduscopic examination revealed bilateral exudates without hemorrhages or papilledema. The lungs were clear. Cardiac examination was pertinent for cardiomegaly and an S_4 gallop. The remainder of the physical workup was normal.

Laboratory results include the following values:

Hematocrit, 32%
Blood urea nitrogen, 40 mg/dL
Serum creatinine, 2.5 mg/dL (baseline serum creatinine 1.9 mg/dL)
Bicarbonate, 18 mEq/L

Urinalysis reveals 2+ protein, 2+ hemoglobin with 4 to 10 red blood cells per high-power field. The electrocardiogram demonstrates normal sinus rhythm with left ventricular hypertrophy. The chest radiograph is unremarkable.

T.M.'s presentation meets criteria for a hypertensive emergency (i.e., DBP >120 mm Hg and presence of worsening renal function). IV antihypertensive therapy is required for T.M. T.M. was given 20 mg hydralazine IV, and a repeat BP after 1 hour was 150/100 mm Hg. What are the advantages and disadvantages of parenteral hydralazine, and when should it be used to acutely lower BP?

Hydralazine is a direct vasodilator that reduces total peripheral resistance through relaxation of the arterial smooth muscle. It is rarely used to treat hypertensive emergencies because its antihypertensive response is less predictable than that of other parenteral agents. Additionally, hydralazine has a prolonged half-life, which can be problematic if too fast correction or hypotension occurs.[22] It is not consistently effective in controlling crises associated with essential hypertension.

Contraindications

Hydralazine should not be used in patients with coronary heart disease because the reflex tachycardia causes an increase in myocardial oxygen demand, which may result in the development or worsening of ischemic symptoms. In addition, hydralazine should be avoided in patients with aortic dissection because of its reflex cardiostimulating effect. In contrast, hydralazine can be useful in patients such as T.M., who have chronic renal failure because the reflex increase in cardiac output is accompanied by an increase in organ perfusion.[21]

Dosing and Administration

Parenteral hydralazine should be considered an intermediate treatment between oral agents and more aggressive therapy with such agents as fenoldopam or nitroprusside. It can be given IV or intramuscularly. The onset of action develops slowly over 20 to 40 minutes, thus minimizing the risk of acute hypotension. Parenteral doses are considerably lower than oral doses because of increased bioavailability.

OTHER PARENTERAL DRUGS

CASE 16-4, QUESTION 2: Are there alternatives to hydralazine for parenteral treatment of hypertensive crisis?

Intravenous Enalaprilat

Enalaprilat, the active metabolite of the oral prodrug enalapril, is approved by the U.S. Food and Drug Administration for the treatment of hypertension when oral therapy is not feasible. However, enalaprilat has been used to treat severe hypertension.[112–117] The initial dose is 0.625 to 1.25 mg IV and can be repeated every 6 hours, if necessary. To minimize the risk of hypotension, the initial doses should not exceed 0.625 mg in patients receiving diuretics or in patients with clinical evidence of hypovolemia. The onset of action is within 15 minutes, but the maximal effect may take several hours. Because only 60% of the patients respond to BP reduction within 30 minutes, it cannot be reliably used to acutely lower pressure in hypertensive emergencies.[115] Although higher initial doses have been successfully used to achieve BP control,[116] some evidence indicates that doses greater than 0.625 mg do not significantly alter the magnitude of enalaprilat's antihypertensive effect.[114] Enalaprilat is also beneficial in patients with HF. Precautions for the use of enalaprilat are similar to those of captopril (see Case 16-1, Question 5). Because of the prolonged time required to achieve an adequate response, limited clinical experience, and variable response rates (especially in African Americans), enalaprilat cannot be recommended for the routine treatment of patients with hypertensive emergencies.[115,117]

Intravenous Calcium-Channel Blockers

CASE 16-5

QUESTION 1: H.C. is a 71-year-old Caucasian man undergoing urgent coronary artery bypass graft surgery after a MI. H.C. has a history of a cerebrovascular accident and chronic kidney disease (serum creatinine is stable at 1.6 mg/dL). Two hours after surgery H.C.'s BP increased from 142/90 to 170/132 mm Hg. H.C. was administered IV nicardipine postoperatively for BP control. Is nicardipine an appropriate choice for H.C.?

Nicardipine

Postoperative hypertension is typically short lived and is most commonly seen after neurosurgical, head and neck, vascular, and cardiothoracic procedures (as is the case with H.C.). Treatment is typically only required for 6 hours postoperatively, and up to

24 to 48 hours for some who may have persistent hypertension. Adequate control of BP postoperatively is necessary to minimize the risk of cardiovascular, neurologic, or surgical-site complications such as bleeding.[118] When selecting an agent, one should consider therapies with a quick onset and short duration of action as well as established efficacy and safety in the postoperative setting.

Nicardipine is a potent cerebral and systemic vasodilator and a useful therapeutic option in the management of severe hypertension. Its onset of action is within 1 to 2 minutes, and its elimination half-life is 40 minutes.[119] Hemodynamic evaluations demonstrated that IV nicardipine significantly decreased mean arterial pressure and systemic vascular resistance and significantly increased cardiac index with little or no change in heart rate.[120] As a dihydropyridine, nicardipine has less negative inotropic activity compared with nondihydropyridines. Titratable IV nicardipine has been studied extensively for use in controlling postoperative hypertension[120–123] and hypertensive emergencies.[124–127]

In the treatment of postoperative hypertension,[120] IV nicardipine was administered as an infusion titrated in the following manner: 10 mg/hour for 5 minutes, 12.5 mg/hour for 5 minutes, and 15 mg/hour for 15 minutes, followed by a maintenance infusion of 3 mg/hour thereafter. The mean response time and infusion rate were 11.5 minutes and 12.8 mg/hour, respectively. The most commonly reported adverse effects included hypotension, tachycardia, and nausea and vomiting.

In studies of patients receiving nicardipine versus nitroprusside for postoperative hypertension after cardiac endarterectomy and coronary artery bypass grafting, breakthrough BP was controlled more rapidly with nicardipine and required fewer overall dose titrations. In addition, nicardipine was well tolerated and did not lead to an increased risk of complications.[128,129]

Nicardipine is an appropriate choice of therapy for H.C. in the postoperative setting because this agent has a rapid onset of action, and provides sustained BP control during the infusion period. It is easily titratable, with a predictable response, and is relatively free of severe adverse effects. Therapy should be titrated to achieve a BP approximately 10% higher than the patient's baseline. In addition to nicardipine, nitroprusside, nitroglycerin, and labetalol are most commonly used to manage postoperative hypertension.[118] Finally, nicardipine may be useful in patients with cerebral insufficiency or peripheral vascular disease. Because of the potential for reflex tachycardia, it should be used with caution in patients with ongoing coronary ischemia.

Nicardipine has been proven effective in multiple studies of populations with hypertensive emergencies, and, as a dihydropyridine, has less negative inotropic activity compared with nondihydropyridines.

In contrast, the nondihydropyridines parenteral verapamil and diltiazem, although clinically effective for prompt lowering of BP, have not been extensively studied in patients with hypertensive emergencies. Clevidipine, a third-generation dihydropyridine, has also been shown to be useful in controlling BP in hypertensive emergencies and in the perioperative setting.

CASE 16-5, QUESTION 2: What other IV forms of calcium-channel blockers are available? Would any of these agents be an appropriate choice of therapy for H.C.?

Nondihydropyridines

IV verapamil (5–10 mg) produces a significant reduction in BP, which occurs within 15 minutes and persists for 6 to 8 hours. As a cardiovascular drug, it is primarily used as a rate-controlling agent in the treatment of supraventricular tachycardias.

IV diltiazem is approved for temporary control of the ventricular rate in atrial fibrillation or atrial flutter and for rapid conversion of paroxysmal supraventricular tachycardia.[130–132] Parenteral diltiazem has also been used to control hypertension that occurs intraoperatively and postoperatively,[133,134] and in patients with an acute coronary syndrome.[135,136] However, published experience with the use of IV diltiazem for the treatment of severe hypertension is limited.[137,138]

Atrioventricular nodal conduction abnormalities can occur during administration of IV verapamil or diltiazem. Patients receiving either of these therapies require continuous monitoring by electrocardiogram and frequent BP checks. IV verapamil and diltiazem should be avoided in patients with sick sinus syndrome or advanced degrees of heart block. Until additional information is available, caution should be exercised in using either agent parenterally to lower BP acutely. In addition, use of nondihydropyridines should be avoided when acutely treating any hypertensive patient with concomitant systolic HF owing to their negative inotropic effects.

CASE 16-5, QUESTION 3: What factors should clinicians consider before recommending the use of clevidipine?

Clevidipine

Clevidipine is another IV dihydropyridine calcium-channel blocker with arterial-selective vasodilation properties.[139] Clevidipine is quickly metabolized in extravascular tissue and blood by esterases, leading to a short elimination half-life of 1 minute[140] and complete resolution of hemodynamic effects within 10 minutes after the end of a 24-hour continuous infusion.[141] Clevidipine demonstrates a quick onset of action of 1 to 2 minutes.[142] These pharmacokinetic and pharmacodynamic properties make it an attractive agent for managing hypertensive emergencies. Clevidipine demonstrated efficacy in the treatment of hypertension in both preoperative and postoperative cardiac surgery patients.[143,144] In this setting, therapy was initiated at a rate of 0.4 mcg/kg/minute. Target BP was a reduction of at least 15% from baseline. The dose was titrated every 90 seconds by doubling the dose up to an infusion rate of 3.2 mcg/kg/minute, then increasing the dose by 1.5 mcg/kg/minute to a maximum rate of 8 mcg/kg/minute. Clevidipine demonstrated a median time of effectiveness within 6 minutes in greater than 90% of the patients who received the study medication.

Clevidipine has been compared with nitroglycerin, nitroprusside, and nicardipine in the management of perioperative hypertension in cardiac surgery patients.[139] Clevidipine was more effective in maintaining patients within a predefined BP target range when compared individually with nitroglycerin and nitroprusside, but this did not translate to differences in clinical outcomes. Clevidipine was equivalent to nicardipine in keeping patients within a prespecified BP range. The incidence and severity of adverse events were similar among patients who received clevidipine and comparison agents.

Based on the limited data, nondihydropyridines would not be an appropriate choice of therapy for H.C. Additionally, IV verapamil has a long duration of action, which is not an ideal characteristic in the setting of postoperative hypertension. Clevidipine, however, has a rapid onset of action and short duration of action and is effective in controlling BP in the perioperative setting.

Clevidipine infusions can induce reflexive tachycardia with an increased heart rate by up to approximately 20 beats/minute.[141] Clevidipine is formulated in a 20% lipid emulsion, so it should be avoided in patients with serum triglycerides greater than 400 mg/dL, and any remaining drug should be discarded after 4 hours of use. Clevidipine is contraindicated in patients with allergies to soybeans, soy products, eggs, or egg products. This agent is also contraindicated in those with defective lipid metabolism or acute pancreatitis (if accompanied by hyperlipidemia), and in patients with severe aortic stenosis.[142]

TREATMENT

CASE 16-6

Question 1: B.S., a 68-year-old Caucasian man with a long history of hypertension and nonadherence, presents to the local emergency department complaining of the sudden onset of severe, sharp, diffuse chest pain that radiates to his back between his shoulder blades. Significant findings on physical examination include a pulse of 100 beats/minute, BP of 200/120 mm Hg, clear lungs, and an S_4 without murmurs. The laboratory data are unremarkable. The electrocardiogram results are interpreted as sinus tachycardia with left ventricular hypertrophy, but no acute changes are noted. The chest radiograph is significant for widening of the mediastinum. An emergency chest computed tomography scan reveals a dissection at the arch of the aorta. What antihypertensive medication(s) would be most appropriate for B.S., and why?

Dissection of the aorta occurs when the innermost layer of the aorta (the intima) is torn such that blood enters and separates its layers. The ultimate treatment for this type of hypertensive emergency depends on its location and severity; however, the first principle of therapy is to control any existing hypertension with agents that do not increase the force of cardiac contraction or heart rate. This lessens the force that the cardiac impulse transmits to the dissecting aneurysm.

The aim of antihypertensive therapy in aortic dissection is to lessen the pulsatile load or aortic stress by lowering the BP. Reducing the force of left ventricular contractions, and consequently the rate of rise of aortic pressure, retards the propagation of the dissection and aortic rupture.[145,146] The treatment of choice for aortic dissection has classically been a vasodilatory agent such as sodium nitroprusside, fenoldopam, or nicardipine in combination with a β-blocker titrated to a heart rate of 55 to 65 beats/minute.[145,147] Labetalol monotherapy has been used as an alternative.[148] These drugs decrease BP, venous return, and cardiac contractility, thus decreasing sheer stress to the aorta.

One common regimen is a combination of IV sodium nitroprusside (0.5–2 mcg/kg/minute) plus IV esmolol.[20,146] This combination can be used as initial therapy for B.S. The concurrent administration of a β-blocking agent with a vasodilator is desirable because the latter may induce reflex tachycardia in response to vasodilation.

Esmolol is a parenteral cardioselective β_1-blocker with a rapid onset and short duration of action. For the management of hypertension, esmolol should be given as a loading dose of 250 to 500 mcg/kg over 1 minute, followed by a maintenance infusion of 50 to 300 mcg/kg/minute. Irritation, inflammation, and induration at the infusion site occur in 5% to 10% of patients.

Hypotension is the most commonly reported adverse event and is directly related to the duration of esmolol administration.[149] However, because of the short half-life, resolution of hypotension occurs within 30 minutes of discontinuing the infusion. Direct vasodilators such as hydralazine should be avoided because they increase stroke volume and left ventricular ejection rate. These effects augment the pulsatile flow and accentuate the sharpness of the pulse wave. This increases mechanical stress on the aortic wall and may lead to further dissection.[20]

Depending on the location of the dissection, surgical intervention may be required.[147,150] However, until a definitive diagnosis is made, the primary goal is to reduce the BP and myocardial contractility to the lowest level compatible with the maintenance of adequate renal, cerebral, and cardiac perfusion.[20] Aggressive BP control is warranted to minimize target organ damage and to prevent further dissection or hemorrhage.[146] For aortic dissection, it is suggested that the systolic BP should be lowered to 100 to 120 mm Hg or a mean arterial pressure of less than 80 mm Hg within 5 to 10 minutes.[20]

KEY REFERENCES AND WEBSITES

A full list of references for this chapter can be found at http://thepoint.lww.com/AT11e. Below are the key references and websites for this chapter, with the corresponding reference number in this chapter found in parentheses after the reference.

Key References

Curran MP et al. Intravenous nicardipine: its use in the short-term treatment of hypertension and various other indications. *Drugs*. 2006;66:1755. (127)

Grossman E et al. Should a moratorium be placed on sublingual nifedipine capsules given for hypertensive emergencies and pseudoemergencies? *JAMA*. 1996;276:1328. (36)

Haas CE, LeBlanc JM. Acute postoperative hypertension: a review of therapeutic options. *Am J Health Syst Pharm*. 2004;61:1661. (118)

Jauch EC et al; on behalf of the American Heart Association Stroke Council, Council on Cardiovascular Nursing, Council on Peripheral Vascular Disease, and Council on Clinical Cardiology. Guidelines for the early management of patients with acute ischemic stroke: a guideline for healthcare professionals from the American Heart Association/American Stroke Association. *Stroke*. 2013;44:870–947. (33)

Khoynezhad A, Plestis KA. Managing emergency hypertension in aortic dissection and aortic aneurysm surgery. *J Card Surg*. 2006;21(Suppl 1):S3. (146)

Marik PE, Rivera R. Hypertensive emergencies: an update. *Curr Opin Crit Care*. 2011;17:569–580. (20)

Rodriguez M et al. Hypertensive crisis. *Cardiol Rev*. 2010;18:102. (3)

Key Websites

Barkis GL. Hypertensive Emergencies. Merck Manual Professional Version. http://www.merckmanuals.com/professional/cardiovascular-disorders/hypertension/hypertensive-emergencies. Accessed October 12, 2015.

Erbel R et al. 2014 ESC Guidelines on the diagnosis and treatment of aortic diseases. European Society of Cardiology. http://eurheartj.oxfordjournals.org/content/ehj/35/41/2873.full.pdf. Accessed October 12, 2015.

Jauch EC et al; on behalf of the American Heart Association Stroke Council, Council on Cardiovascular Nursing, Council on Peripheral Vascular Disease, and Council on Clinical Cardiology. Guidelines for the early management of patients with acute ischemic stroke: a guideline for healthcare professionals from the American Heart Association/American Stroke Association. American Heart Association/American Stroke Association. http://stroke.ahajournals.org/content/44/3/870. Accessed October 12, 2015.

17 Shock

Jason S. Haney

CORE PRINCIPLES

		CHAPTER CASES
1	Shock is a syndrome with multiple etiologies characterized by an impairment of tissue perfusion.	
2	The impairment of tissue perfusion, regardless of cause, can lead to cellular dysfunction, organ failure, and death.	
3	The diagnosis of shock is made by the findings of impaired tissue perfusion on physical examination, and hemodynamic and laboratory changes consistent with impaired perfusion. Hypotension may or may not be present. Hemodynamic monitoring is vital for the determination of the type of shock and assessment of response to interventions.	**Case 17-1 (Questions 1 and 6), Case 17-2 (Questions 1, 4 and 6), Case 17-3 (Questions 1-2), Tables 17-2 and 17-3, Figure 17-1**
4	Hypovolemic shock is caused by a reduction in intravascular volume, which results in changes in the hemodynamic profile such as decreases in blood pressure, central venous pressure, pulmonary capillary wedge pressure, and cardiac output, and a compensatory increase in heart rate, systemic vascular resistance, and myocardial contractility.	**Case 17-1 (Question 1), Case 17-2 (Questions 1-2)**
5	Resuscitation is required to treat hypovolemic shock to maintain adequate tissue perfusion and oxygenation. This can be achieved by administration of intravenous crystalloids, colloids, or blood.	**Case 17-1 (Questions 2-7), Case 17-2 (Questions 3-6)**
6	The physiologic response to fluid loss or gain is described by the Frank–Starling curve.	**Case 17-2 (Questions 3, 4), Figure 17-3**
7	Cardiogenic shock results from a decrease in the heart's ability to maintain cardiac output that is unrelated to hypovolemia.	**Case 17-3 (Questions 1-2)**
8	Treatment of patients in cardiogenic shock involves optimization of preload, increasing contractility, and reducing afterload if the blood pressure permits.	**Case 17-3 (Questions 3-8), Figure 17-4**
9	Septic shock is a type of distributive shock characterized by a profound vasodilatory response and decrease in blood pressure.	**Case 17-4 (Question 1)**
10	Treatment of septic shock involves stabilization with fluids, vasopressors, and inotropic agents and treatment of the underlying condition. Other therapies involve modification of the body's response to infection.	**Case 17-4 (Questions 2-7)**
11	Patients with sepsis can experience disseminated intravascular coagulation, which can lead to hemorrhagic and thrombotic complications.	**Case 17-4 (Questions 8-11), Figure 17-5**

INTRODUCTION

Shock is defined in simple terms as a syndrome of impaired tissue perfusion and oxygenation usually, but not always, accompanied by hypotension. This impairment of tissue perfusion eventually leads to cellular dysfunction, followed by organ damage and death if untreated. The most common causes of shock are situations that result in a reduction of intravascular volume (hypovolemic shock), myocardial pump failure (cardiogenic shock), or increased vascular capacitance (distributive shock). The type of treatment required depends on the etiology.

In recent years, medical support of patients with shock has improved because of better technologies for hemodynamic monitoring, recognition of the value of vigorous volume replacement, appropriate use of inotropic and vasoconstrictive agents, and the development of better ways to treat the underlying cause of the shock syndrome. Understanding the principles of shock should further enhance the prompt recognition of patients at risk, rapid initiation of corrective measures, and development of innovative treatment regimens.

CAUSES

Shock is common among intensive care unit (ICU) patients and is present in up to one-third of ICU admissions.[1] Table 17-1 outlines the classification of shock and precipitating events.[2] Recognition of the etiology and underlying pathology of the various forms of shock is essential for managing this condition. The distinctions among subtypes of shock only apply, however, in the relatively early stages. As the syndrome evolves and compensatory mechanisms are overwhelmed, it becomes increasingly difficult to determine the subtypes because the clinical and pathophysiologic features of advanced shock are the same for all. Also, different types of shock can occur at the same time (e.g., a patient with septic shock who is also hypovolemic). The mortality rate for shock remains quite high—as high as 60% to 80% in severe cases—despite recent improvements in its early recognition and management.[1]

PATHOPHYSIOLOGY

Tissue perfusion is a complex process of oxygen and nutrient delivery as well as waste removal. When perfusion is impaired, it sets up a cascade of events that can eventually end in death.

Table 17-1
Classification of Shock and Precipitating Events

Hypovolemic Shock
Hemorrhagic
Gastrointestinal bleeding (e.g., varices, peptic ulcer)
Trauma
Internal bleeding: ruptured aortic aneurysm, retroperitoneal bleeding, postoperative bleeding, hemorrhagic pancreatitis, postpartum hemorrhage
Nonhemorrhagic
Gastrointestinal losses: vomiting, diarrhea, external drainage
Renal losses: diabetes mellitus, diabetes insipidus, overuse of diuretics
Sequestration: ascites, third-space accumulation
Cutaneous: burns, nonreplaced perspiration, and insensible water losses
Cardiogenic Shock
Cardiomyopathic causes
Acute myocardial infarction (left or right ventricular infarction)
Low cardiac output syndrome
Myocarditis
End-stage cardiomyopathy or severe acute exacerbation of heart failure
Arrhythmogenic causes
Tachyarrhythmia (atrial fibrillation/flutter, reentrant tachycardia, ventricular tachycardia/fibrillation)
Bradyarrhythmia (Mobitz type II second-degree heart block, complete heart block)
Mechanical causes
Rupture of septum or free wall
Severe mitral or aortic valve insufficiency
Papillary muscle or chordae tendineae rupture or dysfunction
Critical aortic stenosis
Pericardial tamponade
Distributive Shock
Septic (bacterial, fungal, viral, parasitic, mycobacterial)
Non-septic
Anaphylactic
Neurogenic (spinal cord injury, traumatic brain injury, cerebral damage, severe dysautonomia)
Inflammatory (burns, trauma, pancreatitis, air/fat embolism, post-cardiopulmonary bypass)
Drug- or toxin-induced (anesthesia, ganglionic and adrenergic blockers, overdoses of barbiturates and narcotics, carbon monoxide, heavy metal, cyanide)
Endocrine (adrenal crisis, myxedema coma)

Adapted with permission from Gaieski D. Evaluation of and initial approach to the adult patient with undifferentiated hypotension and shock. In: Post TW, ed. *UpToDate*. Waltham, MA: Wolters Kluwer. Accessed July 1, 2015.

Although the etiology of shock is varied, the eventual progression (if untreated) to cell death and subsequent organ dysfunction results from a common pathway of ischemia, endogenous inflammatory cytokine release, and the generation of oxygen radicals. When cells are subjected to a prolonged period of ischemia, anaerobic metabolism begins. This inefficient process results in a decrease of adenosine triphosphate stores and causes the buildup of lactic acid and other toxic substances that can alter mitochondrial function and eventually result in cell death. In the advanced stages of shock, irreversible cellular damage leads to multiple organ system failure, also known as *multiple organ dysfunction syndrome*.

The body produces inflammatory cytokines in response to ischemia, injury, or infection. The phrase *systemic inflammatory response syndrome* (SIRS) is the recommended umbrella term to describe any acute, overwhelming inflammatory response, independent of the cause.[3] This syndrome has best been described in the sepsis literature; however, it can occur after a wide variety of insults, including hemorrhagic shock, infection (septic shock), pancreatitis, ischemia, multi-trauma and tissue injury, and immune-mediated organ injury. SIRS is usually a late manifestation of hypovolemic forms of shock. It is uncommon in cardiogenic shock but is the hallmark of septic shock. SIRS is clinically characterized by profound vasodilation, which impairs perfusion, increases capillary permeability, and can reduce intravascular volume.

CLINICAL PRESENTATION AND DIAGNOSIS

Independent of the pathophysiologic cause, the clinical syndrome of shock progresses through several stages. During each step, the body uses and exhausts various compensatory mechanisms to balance oxygen delivery ($\dot{D}O_2$) and oxygen consumption ($\dot{V}O_2$) in an effort to maintain perfusion of vital organs. Oxygen delivery is determined by the arterial concentration of oxygen multiplied by the blood flow (cardiac output [CO]) (Fig. 17-1 and Table 17-2). Normally, consumption is independent of supply, except at low rates of $\dot{D}O_2$. In some critically ill patients, perfusion is inadequate to meet metabolic demands and $\dot{V}O_2$ becomes dependent on the supply despite "normal" $\dot{D}O_2$ ranges.

Although hypotension is often described as the hallmark of shock, it is not necessarily present in all patients.

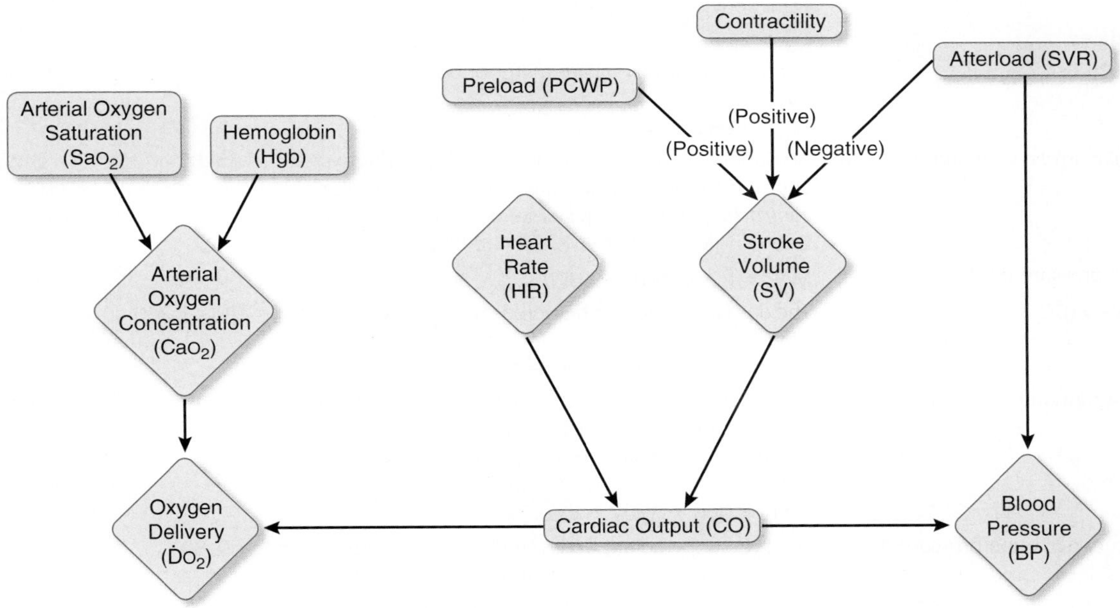

Figure 17-1 Determinants of blood pressure, cardiac output, and oxygen delivery.

Table 17-2
Normal Hemodynamic Values and Derived Indices

	Definition/Equation	Normal Value	Units
Directly Measured			
Blood pressure (BP) [systolic (SBP)/ diastolic (DBP)]	Pressure in the central arterial bed, determined by cardiac output and systemic vascular resistance.	120–140/80–90	mm Hg
Cardiac output (CO)	Amount of blood ejected from the left ventricle per minute; determined by stroke volume and heart rate. CO = SV × HR	4–7	L/minute
Central venous pressure (CVP)[a]	Measures mean pressure in right atrium and reflects right ventricular filling pressure and volume status. Primarily determined by venous return to the heart. The goal in most critically ill patients is 8–12 mm Hg.	2–6	mm Hg[b]
Heart rate (HR) (pulse)	Number of myocardial contractions per minute.	60–100	beats/minute

(continued)

Table 17-2
Normal Hemodynamic Values and Derived Indices (*continued*)

	Definition/Equation	Normal Value	Units
Directly Measured			
Pulmonary artery pressure (PAP)	*Systolic* (SPAP): Measures PAP during systole; reflects pressure generated by the contraction of the right ventricle. *Diastolic* (DPAP): Measures PAP during diastole; reflects diastolic filling pressure in the left ventricle. May approximate pulmonary capillary wedge pressure (PCWP); normal gradient <5 mm Hg between DPAP and PCWP. *Mean* (MPAP): Average measure of PAP during the entire cardiac cycle; mPAP ≥25 mm Hg at rest is defined as pulmonary hypertension.	20–30/8–12 (10–22)	mm Hg
Pulmonary capillary wedge pressure (PCWP)	Measures pressure distal to the pulmonary artery; reflects left ventricular filling pressures (*preload*). Usually lower than or within 5 mm Hg of pulmonary artery diastolic pressure (DPAP).	5–12[c]	mm Hg
Central venous oxygen saturation ($ScvO_2$)	The oxygen saturation of blood returning to the heart; a reflection of oxygen extraction from the upper body.	>70	%
Mixed venous oxygen saturation (SvO_2)	The oxygen saturation of blood in the pulmonary artery; a marker of the relationship between cardiac output and total body oxygen consumption.	>65	%
Derived Indices			
Cardiac index (CI)	Cardiac output per square meter of body surface area (BSA[d]). CI = CO/BSA	2.5–4.2	$L/minute/m^2$
Left ventricular stroke work index (LVSWI)	Amount of work the left ventricle exerts during systole; adjusted for body surface area (BSA[d]). A measure of *contractility*, the inotropic state of the myocardium. LVSWI = (MAP – PCWP) × SVI × 0.0136	35–85	$g/m^2/beat$
Mean arterial pressure (MAP)	MAP = [(2 × DBP) + SBP]/3	80–100	mm Hg
Oxygen delivery ($\dot{D}O_2$)	The amount of oxygen delivered by the body per unit time. $\dot{D}O_2 = CO \times CaO_2$ where $CaO_2 = Hgb \times SaO_2 \times 13.9$	700–1,200	mL/minute
Oxygen consumption ($\dot{V}O_2$)	The amount of oxygen consumed by the body per unit time. The product of cardiac output and the difference between the arterial and venous oxygen concentration. $\dot{V}O_2 = CO \times (CaO_2 - CvO_2)$ where $CvO_2 = Hgb \times SvO_2 \times 13.9$	200–400	mL/minute
Coronary artery perfusion pressure (CPP)	The pressure gradient between the coronary arteries and the pressure in either the right atrium or the left ventricle during diastole. A major determinant of coronary blood flow and oxygen supply to the heart. CPP = DBP – PCWP	60–80	mm Hg
Pulmonary vascular resistance (PVR)	Primary determinant of right ventricular *afterload*. PVR = [(MPAP – PCWP)/CO] × 74	20–120	$dynes \cdot s \cdot cm^{-5}$
Stroke volume (SV)	Amount of blood ejected from the ventricle with each systolic contraction. SV = CO/HR	60–130	mL/beat
Stroke volume index (SVI)	Stroke volume adjusted for body surface area (BSA[d]). SVI = SV/BSA	30–75	$mL/beat/m^2$
Systemic vascular resistance (SVR)	Measure of impedance applied by systemic vascular system to systolic effort of left ventricle; determined by autonomic nervous system and condition of vessels. Determinant of left ventricular *afterload*. SVR = [(MAP – CVP)/CO] × 74	800–1,440	$dyne \cdot s \cdot cm^{-5}$
Systemic vascular resistance index (SVRI)	SVR adjusted for body surface area (BSA[d]). SVRI = SVR × BSA	1,680–2,580	$dyne \cdot s \cdot cm^{-5} \cdot m^2$

[a]CVP is essentially synonymous with RAP.
[b]2–6 mm Hg = 3–6 cm H_2O (conversion: 1 mm Hg = 1.34 cm H_2O).
[c]May optimally ↑ PCWP to 16–18 mm Hg in critically ill patients.
[d]BSA, body surface area = 1.7 m^2 (average male).

The diagnosis of shock is based on the findings of impaired tissue perfusion on examination.[1] These findings may include the following:

- Systolic blood pressure (SBP) less than 90 mm Hg, mean arterial pressure (MAP) less than 65 mm Hg, or at least a 40 mm Hg decrease from baseline
- Tachycardia (heart rate [HR] greater than 90 beats/minute)
- Tachypnea (respiratory rate [RR] greater than 20 breaths/minute)
- Cutaneous vasoconstriction: cold, clammy, blue, mottled skin (although not typical of distributive shock)
- Abnormal mental status (agitation, confusion, stupor, or coma)
- Oliguria: urine output less than 0.5 mL/kg/hour
- Metabolic acidosis (usually because of an elevated blood lactate level)
- Decreased venous oxygen saturation (mixed [SvO_2], central [$ScvO_2$]) (reflects a mismatch between oxygen supply [$\dot{D}O_2$] and demand [$\dot{V}O_2$])

Not all these described findings are encountered in every patient with shock, and considerable variability exists in both the rapidity and the sequence of onset. This depends on the severity of the initiating event, the underlying mechanism, and the baseline condition of the patient, including medications that may alter the clinical presentation. It is important to consider the patient's medical and pharmacologic history, while monitoring for subtle clinical changes that may signal impending deterioration and necessitate immediate intervention.

TREATMENT OVERVIEW

The treatment of patients in shock requires both treatment of the underlying cause of shock, as well as early, aggressive measures to maintain adequate perfusion to vital organs. The general measures used are the restoration of volume in hypovolemic patients, the use of vasopressors or inotropic agents when volume resuscitation is inadequate to maintain perfusion, and careful monitoring of the hemodynamic status of the patient. In sepsis, specific hemodynamic goals have been determined.[4] In other types of shock, specific goals have not been established; however, the principles of ensuring adequate tissue perfusion are the same.

HEMODYNAMIC MONITORING

Hemodynamic monitoring in critically ill patients is mandatory to properly assess and manage various shock states. Both noninvasive and invasive monitoring techniques can be used to measure cardiovascular performance and differentiate the causes of various conditions that result in hypoperfusion and organ dysfunction. The values obtained with hemodynamic monitoring should always be used in conjunction with clinical judgment.

Noninvasive Monitoring

Noninvasive measures are an important part of hemodynamic monitoring. Clinical examination and vital signs (temperature, HR, blood pressure [BP], RR) provide valuable information regarding the cardiovascular system and organ perfusion. Other noninvasive techniques for monitoring the hemodynamic status of patients include pulse oximetry (for measuring arterial oxygen saturation [SaO_2]) and transthoracic echocardiography, which can estimate the functional status of the heart and heart valves. Cardiac telemetry and/or electrocardiogram may help identify a variety of causes for shock (e.g., arrhythmia, ischemia, pericarditis).

Although important, noninvasive measures have limitations, and certain hemodynamic values important for the diagnosis and assessment of illness, as well as the patient's response to therapy, must be measured invasively at the present time.

Invasive Monitoring

ARTERIAL PRESSURE LINE

The arterial line is a common tool in the ICU. It consists of a small catheter placed into an artery (usually the radial or femoral artery) under sterile conditions and attached to a pressure transducer. This allows for continuous measurement of BP and can be more accurate than a sphygmomanometer in patients with shock, cardiac arrhythmias, calcified arteries, or high systemic vascular resistance (SVR). It also provides for easy access for arterial blood gas (ABG) samples to be drawn and analyzed. Arterial lines should never be used for medication administration.

CENTRAL VENOUS CATHETER

Common in the ICU, the central venous catheter consists of a large-bore catheter usually inserted into either a subclavian or a jugular vein. It can be used for infusion of fluid and medications or frequent laboratory studies. When attached to a pressure transducer, it can be used to measure the central venous pressure (CVP), a reflection of right atrial pressure and volume status. In patients with sepsis, however, guidelines call for dynamic rather than static variables (e.g., CVP) to guide fluid resuscitation.[4] Central venous catheters are preferred to peripheral venous access for administration of large fluid volumes, blood products, or vasopressors in patients with shock, but resuscitative efforts should not be delayed if peripheral access is available. Central venous catheters that can continuously measure the central venous oxygen saturation ($ScvO_2$) have been developed and are becoming more common. These catheters allow for the assessment and monitoring of tissue perfusion and the response to interventions. Low $ScvO_2$ has been associated with worse outcomes.[5–7]

PULMONARY ARTERY CATHETER

The introduction of flow-directed, balloon flotation pulmonary artery (PA) catheters by Swan and colleagues[8] (Swan–Ganz catheter) in the 1970s represented a major advance in invasive bedside hemodynamic monitoring. The PA catheter is inserted via a central venous access and positioned into the PA; this enables clinicians to assess both right and left intracardiac pressures, determine CO, and obtain mixed venous blood samples. These capabilities allow one to evaluate volume status and ventricular performance, derive hemodynamic indices, and determine systemic $\dot{D}O_2$ and $\dot{V}O_2$. There are several versions of the PA catheter. Some provide additional lumens for intravenous (IV) infusions, temporary transvenous pacing, and continuous monitoring of SvO_2.[9] Catheters are available that can measure CO on a continuous basis. The essential components for hemodynamic monitoring are incorporated in the standard quadruple-lumen catheter pictured in Figure 17-2. This catheter is composed of multiple lumens, each terminating at different points along the catheter. When properly positioned, the proximal port (C) terminates in the right atrium and is used to measure right atrial pressure, to inject fluid for CO determination, and to administer IV fluids. The distal port (B), which terminates at the tip of the catheter (E), is positioned in the PA beyond the pulmonary valve and is used to measure PA and pulmonary capillary wedge pressure (PCWP; described in the following) and to obtain mixed venous blood samples. Intermittent inflation of the balloon is accomplished by inserting 1.5 mL of air into the balloon inflation valve (D). The thermistor (A) contains a temperature probe and electrical leads that connect to a computer, which calculates CO by the thermodilution technique.

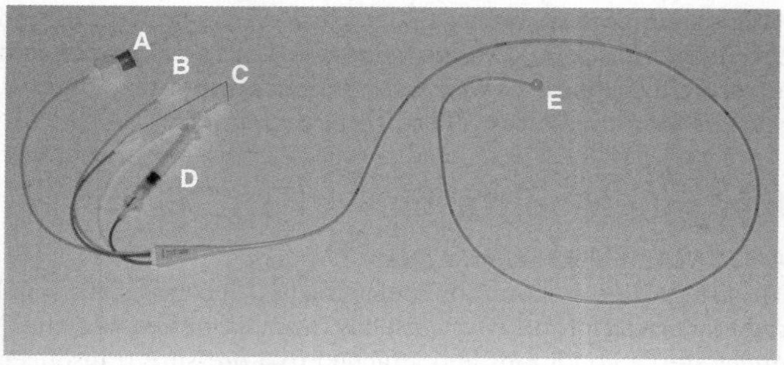

Figure 17-2 Pulmonary artery catheter. See text for definitions of A, B, C, D, and E.

Although the PA catheter is confined to the pulmonary vasculature, left ventricular (LV) pressure can be ascertained from the PCWP. When the balloon is inflated, the PA catheter becomes lodged or "wedged." Because forward flow from the right ventricle ceases beyond the wedged PA segment, a static fluid column exists between the LV and the PA catheter tip during diastole when the mitral valve is open. If no pressure gradients are present in the pulmonary vasculature beyond the balloon and if mitral valve function is normal, the PCWP then equilibrates with all distal pressures and thus indirectly reflects left ventricular end-diastolic pressure (LVEDP). Based on the relationship between pressure and volume, the LVEDP is equivalent to the left ventricular end-diastolic volume, or the left-sided *preload*. Because PCWP measurements are not always available, the diastolic pulmonary artery pressure (DPAP) may provide an estimate of left-sided preload in the absence of pulmonary hypertension or cardiac tamponade.

The use of PA catheters has potential complications. Arrhythmias, thrombotic events, infections, and, very rarely, PA rupture have been reported.[9] Several trials have questioned the routine use of PA catheters. A meta-analysis of 13 randomized, controlled trials found that use of a PA catheter did not have a significant effect on mortality, number of days in the ICU or hospital, or cost.[9] An international consensus conference recommends against the routine placement of the PA catheter in patients with shock.[1] Despite this, the PA catheter can provide essential diagnostic and hemodynamic information for specialists to utilize in certain patient populations. More studies are needed to determine the value of PA catheter data–driven treatment protocols. Because hypotension alone is not required to define shock, the presence of inadequate tissue perfusion on physical examination is more important than the numbers obtained by invasive monitoring.[1] The use of PA catheters has been decreasing in the ICU as newer and less invasive technologies become available. In most situations, the PA catheter is reserved for those patients who specifically require the monitoring of PA pressures and oxygenation parameters, such as patients with pulmonary hypertension, refractory shock, right ventricular (RV) dysfunction, or who are post-cardiac surgery.[1,4]

OTHER MONITORING TOOLS

New technologies to monitor a patient's perfusion status are being developed. End-tidal carbon dioxide monitors are used to determine $\dot{V}O_2$ and help guide therapies designed to improve $\dot{D}O_2$ and $\dot{V}O_2$. New devices that can measure CO and tissue perfusion noninvasively (or minimally invasively), such as gastric tonometry, esophageal Doppler monitoring, thoracic bioimpedance, and others, have been developed.[10–12] Devices (e.g., PulseCO, PiCCO, LiDCO) that can measure CO by pulse wave analysis are being increasingly used in ICUs as an alternative to the PA catheter.[10–12] An international consensus conference does not currently recommend the newer, less invasive technologies because of lack of validation in patients with shock.[1]

The effective interpretation and management of hemodynamic parameters requires a thorough understanding of the physiologic determinants of CO and arterial pressure. Assuming oxygen content of blood is adequate, CO and SVR are the ultimate determinants of $\dot{D}O_2$, adequate arterial pressure, and tissue perfusion. As outlined in Figure 17-1, CO may be quantified as the product of stroke volume (SV) and HR. SV is determined by preload, afterload, and contractility. Preload is defined as end-diastolic fiber length before contraction and is represented by left ventricular end-diastolic volume (LVEDV). It is approximated by left ventricular end-diastolic pressure (LVEDP) and pulmonary capillary wedge pressure (PCWP). Right ventricular preload is reflected by central venous pressure (CVP) or right atrial pressure (RAP). Afterload is defined as ventricular wall tension developed during contraction. It is determined by the resistance or impedance the ventricle must overcome to eject end-diastolic volume. Left and right ventricular afterload are determined primarily by systemic vascular resistance (SVR) and pulmonary vasular resistance (PVR), respectively. Contractility describes the inotropic state of the myocardium and affects the stroke volume (SV) and cardiac output (CO)independently of preload and afterload. The effects of these factors on hemodynamic parameters are interrelated and complex and must be assessed carefully when selecting therapeutic interventions that will produce the desired response. A review of the determinants of cardiac performance is found in Chapter 14, Heart Failure. Table 17-2 provides definitions of terms and normal hemodynamic indices.

ETIOLOGIC CLASSIFICATION OF SHOCK AND COMMON MECHANISMS

The most common clinical conditions associated with the major forms of shock are reviewed in the subsequent sections and detailed in Table 17-1. Table 17-3 describes the common hemodynamic findings for the various forms of shock.

HYPOVOLEMIC SHOCK

Shock secondary to reduced intravascular volume is referred to as *hypovolemic shock*. Whether the primary insult is the external loss of fluid (e.g., blood, plasma, or free water) or the internal sequestration of these fluids into body cavities (third spacing), the overall result is reduced venous return or preload (decreased CVP and PCWP) and decreased CO (Table 17-3). The severity of hypovolemic shock depends on the amount and rate of intravascular volume loss and each person's capacity for compensation. Although responses vary, a healthy person may tolerate an acute loss of as much as 30% of

Table 17-3
Hemodynamic Findings in Various Shock States

	Hypovolemic	Cardiogenic	Distributive (Septic)
Heart rate	↑	↑	↑
Blood pressure[a]	↓	↓	↓
Cardiac output	↓	↓	↑/↓[b]
Preload (PCWP)	↓	↑	↔/↓
Afterload (SVR)	↑	↑	↓

[a]Patients may be in a state of compensated shock in which blood pressure is normal, but clinical signs of hypoperfusion are evident.
[b]Cardiac output is increased early in sepsis but can be decreased in late or severe sepsis.
PCWP, pulmonary capillary wedge pressure; SVR, systemic vascular resistance.

his or her intravascular volume.[13] Compensatory mechanisms such as increased HR, myocardial contractility, and SVR are sufficiently effective for this loss in volume and measurable falls in SBP are not detected. Losses in excess of 40% generally overwhelm compensatory mechanisms, venous return decreases and the patient's condition can deteriorate to overt shock with hypotension and signs of hypoperfusion. If restorative measures are not taken immediately, irreversible shock and death may result. The most common and dramatic cause of hypovolemic shock is hemorrhagic shock in which intravascular volume depletion occurs as a result of bleeding. Trauma is responsible for most cases of acute hemorrhagic shock; other significant causes are listed in Table 17-1.

Acute Hemorrhagic Shock

CASE 17-1

QUESTION 1: N.G. is a 64-year-old woman with a history of peptic ulcer disease, who arrives to the emergency department (ED) complaining of diffuse abdominal pain and bright red blood in her stool over the past two days. She is confused and oriented only to person. Her skin is pale and cool, with HR 120 beats/minute, SBP 80 mm Hg, and RR 28 breaths/minute. Describe the physiologic changes in N.G. in response to her gastrointestinal (GI) bleeding. What are the goals of resuscitation in patients with hemorrhagic shock?

N.G. has lost a significant amount of intravascular fluid directly from her GI tract. She is hypotensive with a compensatory increase in both HR and RR. Her pale, cool skin indicates shunting of blood from the periphery to maintain perfusion of vital organs. Based on her clinical presentation, N.G. is in decompensated shock.

The major hemodynamic abnormality in hypovolemic shock is decreased venous return (preload) to the heart, resulting in a decrease in CO. $\dot{D}O_2$ to the tissues is reduced from this and the loss of oxygen-carrying hemoglobin (Hgb). The physiologic response of the body to a sudden decrease in volume (preload) is to activate the hypothalamic–pituitary–adrenal axis and autonomic nervous system to release catecholamines (epinephrine, norepinephrine). The subsequent increase in HR and contractility help maintain CO. The peripheral vasoconstriction caused by the sympathomimetic response helps maintain arterial pressure. In addition, fluid shifts from the interstitial spaces into the vasculature to increase preload. These responses are effective at maintaining BP in patients with a loss of up to approximately 30% of the total blood volume. N.G.'s increased HR and signs of peripheral vasoconstriction are consistent with these compensatory changes. Her SBP is still low, however, and she has signs of decreased perfusion to her brain, manifested by confusion and disorientation. Given the severity of her condition, if intravascular losses are not rapidly replaced, myocardial dysfunction may ensue and lead to irreversible shock.

The goals of resuscitation of patients in hypovolemic shock are the correction of inadequate tissue perfusion and oxygenation, and limiting secondary insults. HR, BP, and urine output have been traditional markers for the adequacy of resuscitation, but reliance on these end points alone is acceptable only in the initial management of hemorrhagic shock. One concern is that patients may persist in a state of compensated shock even after these parameters are normalized.[14] Ongoing deficiencies in $\dot{D}O_2$ to vital organs may progress, and if left untreated, organ dysfunction and death may result. Measurement of base (bicarbonate) deficit and lactate levels can be used to assess the global adequacy of perfusion by tracking trends, ensuring that the levels are decreasing. Metabolic acidosis can signal that resuscitation is incomplete despite normal vital signs.

TREATMENT

Choice of Fluid in Hypovolemic Shock

CASE 17-1, QUESTION 2: Is an IV saline solution adequate to compensate for N.G.'s blood loss? What other fluid options are available to resuscitate this patient?

Once an adequate airway is established and initial vital signs are obtained, the most important therapeutic intervention in hypovolemic shock is the infusion of IV fluids. Initially, crystalloids or colloids are used to restore blood volume as blood products are limited, costly, and transfusion of these products carries a risk.[15] Blood products may not be immediately available and are frequently unnecessary to manage mild shock (less than 20% blood loss).

Crystalloids Versus Colloids

Resuscitative *crystalloids* are isotonic solutions that contain either saline (0.9% sodium chloride; "normal saline" [NS]) or a saline equivalent (lactated Ringer's [LR] solution) (Table 17-4). *Colloidal solutions* contain high molecular weight molecules that are derived from natural products, such as proteins (albumin), carbohydrates (dextrans, starches), and animal collagen (gelatin), and largely remain in the intravascular space, thereby contributing to colloid oncotic pressure (COP) (Table 17-5). Healthy semipermeable capillary membranes are relatively impermeable to these large molecules.

The choice of a crystalloid versus a colloid solution to restore blood volume in hemorrhagic shock is controversial. The controversy primarily involves the ultimate distribution of these fluids in the extracellular compartment, which, in turn, depends on their composition. Isotonic solutions (NS or LR) freely distribute within the extracellular fluid compartment, which is divided between the interstitial and intravascular spaces at a ratio of 3:1. This distribution is determined by the net forces of COP and hydrostatic pressure, both inside and outside the capillary vascular space. Consequently, large volumes of crystalloid fluid are required to expand the intravascular space during resuscitation. In contrast, intact capillary membranes are relatively impermeable to colloids and, therefore, colloids effectively expand the intravascular space with little interstitial loss. Comparatively smaller volumes of colloids than of crystalloids are required for resuscitation, and

Table 17-4
Composition and Properties of Crystalloids

Solution	Sodium (mEq/L)	Chloride (mEq/L)	Potassium (mEq/L)	Calcium (mEq/L)	Magnesium (mEq/L)	Lactate (mEq/L)	Tonicity Relative to Plasma	Osmolarity (mOsm/L)
5% Dextrose	0	0	0	0	0	0	Hypotonic	253
0.9% Sodium chloride	154	154	0	0	0	0	Isotonic	308
Plasma-Lyte (Baxter)	140	103	10	5	3	8	Isotonic	312
Lactated Ringer's	130	109	4	3	0	28	Isotonic	273
7.5% Sodium chloride	1,283	1,283	0	0	0	0	Hypertonic	2,567

Table 17-5

Composition and Properties of Colloids

Solution	Colloid Type	MWw (KDaltons)	DS	Sodium (mEq/L)	Chloride (mEq/L)	Potassium (mEq/L)	Calcium (mEq/L)	Glucose (mg/L)	Osmolarity (mOsm/L)
Albumin	Blood-derived	67		130–160		≤2			300
Hespan 6%	Hetastarch	450	0.7	154	154				309
Hextend 6%[a]	Hetastarch	450	0.7	143	124	3	5	90	307
Voluven	Tetrastarch	130	0.4	154	154				308
Gentran 40	Dextran 40	40		154	154			50	308
Gentran 70	Dextran 70	70		154	154			50	308

[a]Hextend also contains magnesium 0.9 mEq/L and lactate 28 mEq/L

MWw, weight-averaged molecular weight (number of molecules at each weight multiplied by the particle weight divided by the total weight of all the molecules); MWn, arithmetic mean of all particle molecular weight; DS, proportion of substituted to non-substituted glucose moieties (higher DS is more resistant to hydrolysis)

their duration of action is longer. It is thought that 3 to 4 times as much volume of crystalloid compared to colloid is necessary to provide the same degree of volume expansion.

Proponents of crystalloids argue that both intravascular and interstitial fluids are depleted in hypovolemic shock because of the rapid shifts between the extracellular compartments. Volume replacement of both fluid spaces is best accomplished by using crystalloids. In addition, loss of capillary integrity in shock can cause the leak of larger molecules (including colloidal molecules) into the interstitium. This increase in the interstitial oncotic pressure would favor fluid movement out of the vascular space into the tissues, with resultant edema. Crystalloids do not produce allergic or hypersensitivity reactions like many of the colloidal agents. Colloids can also cause coagulopathies, have been associated with an increased incidence of acute kidney injury, and are much more expensive than crystalloids.

Proponents of colloids maintain that resuscitation with these solutions more rapidly and effectively restores intravascular volume after acute hemorrhage. For a given infusion volume, colloidal solutions (e.g., albumin) will expand the intravascular space 2 to 4 times more than crystalloids, and the intravascular effects persist longer. Traditionally, it has been contended that the larger volumes of crystalloids necessary to restore the vascular space will further dilute the plasma proteins, resulting in a decreased COP and promotion of pulmonary edema. However, clinical studies comparing colloids with crystalloids have failed to show any differences in the development of pulmonary edema. This is likely because of the relatively high alveolar capillary permeability to albumin causing a decreased transcapillary COP gradient. Research suggests that certain subgroups may be at greater risk for the development of pulmonary edema, but considerable variance remains because of differences in physiologic end points, criteria for assessing pulmonary edema, and the extent of shock.

Numerous meta-analyses have compared resuscitation with crystalloids or colloids in an effort to find a consensus among divergent clinical trial results. Two recent meta-analyses failed to show a mortality benefit for resuscitation with colloids compared to crystalloids in patients with sepsis, trauma, burns, or following surgery.[16,17] Patients receiving hydroxyethyl starch were at an increased risk of death and acute kidney injury. It is important to recognize that study inclusion criteria (heterogeneity), differences in fluid management, and dosages provide several limitations to these meta-analyses. Conversely, a more recent randomized, controlled trial found no difference in 28-day mortality or the need for renal replacement therapy in patients with hypovolemic shock who received crystalloid- or colloid-based resuscitation.[18] Any mortality difference between colloids and crystalloids at 90 days remains uncertain as trials have shown conflicting results.[18–21]

A Cochrane Database meta-analysis found that volume resuscitation with albumin in hypovolemic critically ill patients did not reduce mortality compared to crystalloids and was possibly associated with an increased risk of death in patients with burns or hypoproteinemia.[22] This meta-analysis was heavily influenced by the SAFE trial, the largest randomized, prospective trial to evaluate albumin versus NS solution resuscitation in the critically ill.[23] The primary end point of the SAFE trial was 28-day mortality, which showed no difference between albumin and NS solution. No statistical differences were identified in any of the predetermined subgroups (trauma, adult respiratory distress syndrome [ARDS], severe sepsis). A trend toward increased mortality in the trauma patients who received albumin led to a post hoc follow-up study in patients who had traumatic brain injury.[24] A higher mortality rate was seen in patients with severe traumatic brain injury (Glasgow Coma Scale 3–8), who received albumin versus those receiving saline for fluid resuscitation.

More certain differences between colloids and crystalloids are availability and cost. Crystalloid solutions are readily available and remain 20 to 100 times cheaper than colloidal solutions; therefore, treatment costs can be significantly different and must be considered when choosing between therapies with similar outcomes.[25] Given the lack of evidence for a significant clinical difference between crystalloids and colloids and the greater expense of using albumin, the guidelines for the use of resuscitation fluids developed by the University Hospital Consortium, a nonprofit alliance of US academic medical centers, remain unchanged.[26] Use of either NS or LR solution would be appropriate for N.G. Colloidal products are not needed at this time; instead, they should be reserved for persistent hypotension despite an appropriate crystalloid challenge.[26] Given the severity of N.G.'s hemorrhagic shock, blood transfusion is indicated and should be transfused as soon as available.[15]

Crystalloids

CASE 17-1, QUESTION 3: A large-bore IV catheter is inserted into N.G.'s arm and STAT blood samples are sent for type and cross-match, complete blood count (CBC), prothrombin time (PT), partial thromboplastin time (PTT), and serum chemistry (blood urea nitrogen [BUN], creatinine [SCr], Na, K, Cl, and bicarbonate). Warmed LR solution (2 L) is infused rapidly, and the GI endoscopy suite is notified. N.G.'s SBP has increased to 94 mm Hg, but the bleeding has not stopped. A Foley catheter is inserted to measure urine output. LR is continued, with 500- to 1,000-mL boluses ordered to maintain hemodynamic stability while waiting for fully cross-matched blood. Are the doses of LR given to N.G. appropriate? What clinical and objective parameters should be monitored to determine the success of fluid replacement?

Volume Requirements

Isotonic crystalloids equilibrate rapidly between the interstitial and the intravascular spaces at a ratio of 3:1. For every liter of fluid infused, approximately 750 mL will pass into the interstitium, whereas 250 mL will remain in the plasma. Based on estimated blood loss, the "three-to-one rule" may be applied as a general guideline: for each 1 mL of blood loss, 3 mL of crystalloid is infused. Because this determination of blood loss is based solely on clinical assessment and not on quantitative measurements, treatment is best directed by the response to initial therapy rather than the initial classification. Close observation of hemodynamic status with consideration of the patient's age, particular injury, and pre-hospital fluid therapy is essential to avoid inadequate or excessive fluid administration.

A safe and effective resuscitative approach for crystalloids in hemorrhagic shock is to give 2 L of fluid as an initial bolus as rapidly as possible for an adult or 20 mL/kg for a pediatric patient.[13] Additional fluid boluses may be necessary, depending on the patient's response. Between boluses, fluids are slowed to maintenance rates (150–200 mL/hour for adults, weight-based up to 100 mL/hour for children[27]), with ongoing evaluation of the patient's physiologic response for signs of continued blood loss or inadequate perfusion that would indicate the need for additional volume replacement. The fluid boluses given to N.G. are an appropriate initial measure, then assessment of her perfusion is vital to determine the need for additional boluses.

Normalization of BP, HR, and pulse pressure (difference between SBP and diastolic blood pressure [DBP]) indicate improved circulation. Signs that actual organ perfusion is normalizing and that fluid resuscitation is adequate include improvements in mental status, warmth and color of skin, improved acid–base balance, and increased urinary output. The minimal acceptable urine output is 0.5 mL/kg/hour for an adult, 1 mL/kg/hour for a child, and 2 mL/kg/hour in an infant under 1 year of age.[13] Persistent metabolic acidosis in normothermic shock usually indicates the need for additional fluid resuscitation; sodium bicarbonate administration is controversial but is not recommended unless the pH is less than 7.2.[14] Monitoring serum lactate and base deficit is important to determine adequate resuscitation. As perfusion improves, lactate and base deficit will decrease; thus, the actual values are not as important as the trend. It is important to note that resuscitation is not defined by just one value or number, such as BP, but by the constellation of indicators of overall perfusion.

Lactated Ringer's Versus Normal Saline

CASE 17-1, QUESTION 4: Is there an advantage to using LR solution versus NS solution?

The choice of replacement fluid varies widely in clinical practice. Normal saline solution has a supraphysiologic chloride content, while LR contains a more balanced chemical composition (Table 17-4). Large volumes of NS can cause hyperchloremic metabolic acidosis, thereby worsening the tissue acidosis from hypovolemic shock. This may also cause immune and renal dysfunction, but survival differences have not been seen and the clinical significance is unknown.[28,29] LR, in contrast, is a buffered solution designed to simulate the intravascular plasma electrolyte concentration. It contains 28 mEq/L of lactate, which is metabolized to bicarbonate in patients with normal circulation and liver function. In situations in which hepatic perfusion is reduced (20% of normal) or hepatocellular damage is present, lactate clearance may be significantly decreased, particularly in combination with hypoxia (SaO_2 50% of normal).[30] In patients with shock and those having cardiopulmonary bypass during surgery, the half-life of lactate, normally 20 minutes, increases to 4 to 6 hours and 8 hours, respectively. Because unmetabolized lactate can be converted to lactic acid, prolonged infusion of LR could cause tissue acidosis in predisposed patients. Concern about the high sodium and chloride content in NS has led to the first-line selection of more balanced resuscitative solutions (e.g., LR) in patients at high risk of acidosis, including those with trauma, burns, diabetic ketoacidosis, or undergoing surgery.[28] LR, however, should be avoided in patients with metabolic alkalosis, lactic acidosis, or hyperkalemia. In practice, NS and LR solutions typically are used interchangeably because neither solution appears to be superior to the other.

Hypertonic Saline

CASE 17-1, QUESTION 5: What is the role of hypertonic saline (HS) solution in the setting of hemorrhagic shock?

The advantage of HS (3% to 7.5% NaCl) solution as a resuscitative fluid is the smaller volume of fluid required to expand the intravascular compartment compared with isotonic solutions. This could be a particular advantage in the pre-hospital setting (e.g., field rescue by emergency medical technicians) given the large volumes of fluids necessary to restore ongoing blood loss.

With a high concentration of sodium, HS solution exerts an osmotic effect, translocating fluid from the interstitial and intracellular compartments to the intravascular space. Consequently, plasma volume is rapidly expanded to a greater extent than similar volumes of crystalloid solutions, and systemic BP, CO, and $\dot{D}O_2$ are readily increased. HS solution also improves myocardial contractility, causes peripheral vasodilation, and redistributes blood flow preferentially to the splanchnic and renal circulations. In addition, intracranial pressure is reduced, but to date HS has not been shown to improve outcomes in trauma patients with concomitant head injury.[31] Other recent studies have shown that HS may have beneficial effects on circulation, inflammation, and endothelial function, which may be beneficial in patients with septic shock and acute lung injury.[31,32] More robust clinical trials are needed to determine if these preliminary findings translate into improved clinical outcomes.

It is difficult to make conclusions about the utility of HS for fluid resuscitation because of the heterogeneity of studies and solutions. The majority of data regarding the use of HS in hypovolemic shock come from the trauma population. No high-quality trials are available in patients with GI bleeding. HS effectively raises BP in patients with hypovolemic shock, but as with isotonic saline the effects are transient and it has not been shown to improve mortality.[33]

These clinical trials suggest that HS solution may be safe and effective for the initial resuscitation of hemorrhagic shock. Despite these positive findings, HS solutions are not widely used. This is possibly because of its safety profile as a high-risk medication. HS is prone to dosing and administration errors, particularly when used by clinicians who are unfamiliar with the product. The osmolarity of HS can range from 1,026 to 2,567 mOsm/L (3%–7.5% NaCl), so infusion through a central line is preferred to minimize phlebitis. HS may cause hypernatremia and hyperchloremic metabolic acidosis, resulting in rapid fluid shifts between cellular compartments and potentially devastating effects such as osmotic demyelination syndrome. However, most studies have not reported such events, which may be because of a lack of power or the relatively small volumes of HS used for resuscitation.

Blood Replacement

CASE 17-1, QUESTION 6: N.G. has received 4 L of LR solution to maintain hemodynamic stability. Her current vital signs are BP 98/54 mm Hg, HR 108 beats/minute, and RR 30 breaths/minute. She is still confused and is becoming more agitated and combative. Urine output has been only 30 mL in the past 30 minutes. Laboratory results include the following:

Hematocrit (Hct), 21% (down from 26%)
Hemoglobin (Hgb), 7.1 g/dL (down from 8.9 g/dL)
pH, 7.14
PCO_2, 34 mm Hg
PO_2, 106 mm Hg
HCO_3^-, 16 mEq/L

Two units of packed red blood cells (PRBCs) are now available, and N.G. is being prepared for the GI endoscopy suite. Describe the current status of N.G.'s resuscitation and the need for blood products.

N.G. is still exhibiting signs of inadequate tissue perfusion. Although her BP has improved and her HR has decreased, her mental status has declined, she is oliguric, and her ABG indicates metabolic acidosis. N.G. has not been adequately resuscitated from her hemorrhage, is still actively bleeding, and should receive available blood at this point.

The prior conventional approach to the transfusion of critically ill patients was to maintain the hemoglobin greater than 10 g/dL or the hematocrit greater than 30%. It has been argued that these liberal transfusion goals are justified in acutely ill patients, particularly those with cardiovascular disease, because the compensatory mechanisms to maintain tissue $\dot{D}O_2$ are impaired. However, randomized, controlled trials have shown that a restrictive transfusion strategy (target hemoglobin 7 to 8 g/dL or transfused if symptomatic) is associated with equivalent or better outcomes in hemodynamically stable critical care, surgical, and medical patients.[34]

In acute hemorrhage, the actual degree of blood loss is not accurately reflected by the hemoglobin and hematocrit values, and it also does not take into account the body's ability to compensate for the loss of oxygen-carrying capacity. Because it takes at least 24 hours for all fluid compartments to come to equilibrium, a normal hematocrit (or hemoglobin concentration) in the setting of hemorrhagic shock does not rule out significant blood loss or indicate adequacy of transfusion. Only when equilibrium has been reached can these measures be used reliably to gauge blood loss. On the other hand, if cardiopulmonary function is normal and volume status is maintained, an increase in CO can compensate for a reduction in hemoglobin (O_2 content) to a certain degree (Fig. 17-1).

Because inadequacy of tissue perfusion, and hence $\dot{D}O_2$, is the primary abnormality in shock, the need for transfusion therapy is more accurately determined by the patient's symptoms and oxygen demand, rather than an arbitrary hematocrit or hemoglobin value.[15] Calculation of $\dot{D}O_2$ and $\dot{V}O_2$ can be used to determine the adequacy of perfusion. Although these values can be determined by use of a PA catheter and arterial and venous blood samples, for practical purposes the patient's response to initial fluid resuscitation and clinical signs of inadequate tissue perfusion are the primary determinants for blood transfusion. Patients who are not acutely bleeding and who do not respond to initial volume resuscitation or who transiently respond but remain tachycardic, tachypneic, and oliguric clearly are underperfused and will likely require blood transfusion. Patients who have acute bleeding or who demonstrate signs of underperfusion should be considered for transfusion much sooner; thus, N.G. should receive a transfusion.

Adverse Effects of Transfusion

Case 17-1, Question 7: After the transfusion, N.G. has a serum potassium concentration of 4.7 mEq/L compared with 4.2 mEq/L before the transfusion. Could this be a result of the blood product? What other potential acute transfusion-related complications are associated with PRBC administration?

Possible risks of blood transfusions include febrile and allergic reactions, hemolytic reactions, electrolyte abnormalities, infectious disease transmission, coagulopathies, and immunosuppression.[35] Febrile non-hemolytic and allergic transfusion reactions are the most common adverse reactions. Transfusions can also cause acute lung injury from activation of recipient neutrophils, which cause capillary endothelial damage. Transfusion-associated circulatory overload results in pulmonary edema in patients with limited cardiac reserve (elderly, infant, renal failure, heart failure) or after massive transfusions. Recognition of donor-recipient ABO incompatibility and the signs and symptoms of a transfusion reaction (e.g., anxiety, infusion site pain, chills, rigors, fever, hypotension, tachycardia, hemolysis, hemoglobinuria) can prevent unnecessary morbidity and mortality by stopping the infusion and providing supportive therapy.

Hemolytic transfusion reactions are the most common cause of fatalities from blood transfusions; however, it is unlikely that N.G. is having a true hemolytic reaction. Banked blood is stored with a citrate anticoagulant additive. With multiple transfusions, the large amount of citrate can cause hypocalcemia and acid–base abnormalities. Hyperkalemia also can occur because transfusion of stored blood causes the release of potassium from hemolyzed (ruptured) red blood cells. The increase in serum potassium observed in N.G. may be from the blood product; although, the average amount of extracellular potassium ranges from less than 0.5 to 7 mEq/unit of blood, so the transfusion is unlikely the culprit. The increased potassium may simply reflect hemolysis of blood cells in the test tube after the blood draw. In either case, the measured serum concentration of 4.7 mEq/L is not sufficiently high to warrant immediate treatment but should be monitored.

Blood products and donors are screened for disease; thus, transmission of bacterial or viral illness is rare. It is estimated that the transmission of hepatitis C is 1:1,149,000, and human immunodeficiency virus is 1:1,467,000.[36] Protozoan infection and prion disease are also transmissible through infusion but are an even lower risk. Hemostatic abnormalities, specifically coagulopathies and thrombocytopenia, may be transiently related to dilution from administration of large volumes of crystalloids, colloids, or banked blood, but they are more likely caused by the extent of injury and the development of disseminated intravascular coagulopathy (DIC). Banked whole blood is usually reserved for massive transfusions and contains sufficient coagulation factors (including labile factors V and VIII) to maintain hemostasis during the life span of the unit; however, it does not contain platelets because they do not survive the temperatures required for red blood cell storage.

Immunosuppression has also been associated with blood transfusions as evidenced by enhanced graft survival in renal transplant recipients, tumor recurrence in patients with colorectal carcinoma, and postoperative infections. Transfusion-related immunosuppression is multifactorial, but it is most likely caused by the infusion of donor white blood cells (WBCs), which creates a competition between the donor and the recipient leukocytes. Transfusion-related immunomodulation can be limited by leukoreducing PRBCs prior to transfusion. The majority of blood in the United States is leukoreduced, but it is not a universal practice primarily because of cost. Patients who are immunosuppressed, undergoing cardiac surgery, or receiving chronic transfusions should receive leukoreduced blood. This mechanism is not, however, the only cause because immunosuppression is associated with autologous blood transfusions as well as the infusion of plasma alone.

Because of the limited supply and potential adverse effects associated with blood, research is ongoing to develop blood substitutes. The ideal agent would have a longer shelf life, a reduced risk of disease transmission, and less risk of transfusion reactions. The agents in various stages of clinical research include the modified hemoglobins and the perfluorocarbons.[37] Problems have occurred with some of the products thus far, such as short half-life, vasoconstriction, GI disturbances, and flu-like symptoms. The exact role the blood substitutes would play in transfusions is unclear. No agents are approved, but research is continuing.

Postoperative Hypovolemia

HYPOVOLEMIA VERSUS PUMP FAILURE

CASE 17-2

QUESTION 1: P.T. is a 58-year-old man who arrives to the ED via ambulance after a motor vehicle accident. He has remained conscious during the event, but his mental status fluctuates between somnolent and agitated with a Glasgow Coma Scale of 10 (moderate injury). Chest CT reveals a type II proximal descending thoracic aortic injury. P.T. is taken for an emergent surgical repair of his aorta. He has been admitted to the ICU after surgery and is intubated and receiving 60% oxygen. His ABGs are adequate, and he is receiving 150 mL/hour of LR solution IV. His initial postoperative and 2-hour postoperative hemodynamic profiles are as follows (initial parameters in parentheses):

BP (S/D/MAP), 86/44/58 mm Hg (100/52/68 mm Hg)
HR, 96 beats/minute (88 beats/minute)
CO, 3.2 L/minute (4.8 L/minute)
CI, 1.9 L/minute/m^2 (3.3 L/minute/m^2)
CVP, 6 mm Hg (12 mm Hg)
PA pressure (S/D), 18/8 mm Hg (24/14 mm Hg)
PCWP, 13 mm Hg (18 mm Hg)
SVR, 1,080 dyne·s·cm^{-5} (1,560 dyne·s·cm^{-5})
Urine output, 0.4 mL/kg/hour (1.2 mL/kg/hour)
Temperature, 37.4°C (34.8°C)
Hct, 32% (31%)

From the hemodynamic profile, determine whether P.T. is hypovolemic or experiencing pump failure after his surgery.

Most of P.T.'s hemodynamic changes are consistent with hypovolemia. These include a drop in BP, CVP, PA pressure (PAP), PCWP, CO, and urine output. The decrease in CVP and PCWP suggest that preload is reduced, resulting in a lower CO. The pulse pressure is narrowed, suggesting either blood flow or ventricular contractility has decreased. (Decreases in pulse pressure correlate with decreases in SV or left ventricular stroke work index [LVSWI]). P.T.'s HR increased slightly, but it is unclear whether he was taking any medications, such as a β-blocker, before his injury. As body temperature rises postoperatively, vasodilation decreases SVR and increases the intravascular space. If intravascular volume is inadequate and increased sympathetic tone cannot generate a sufficient CO, mean BP falls. The decline in urine output reflects a compensatory drop in renal perfusion. The most likely explanation for the hemodynamic change in P.T. is hypovolemia. The PCWP would be higher if P.T. was in cardiogenic shock; although he also should be evaluated for the occurrence of a perioperative cardiac event (myocardial infarct). His ABG should be checked to assess oxygen requirements.

CAUSES

CASE 17-2, QUESTION 2: What are the most likely causes of hypovolemia in P.T.?

Common causes of hypovolemia in surgical patients are postoperative bleeding, third spacing, and temperature-related vasodilation. Postoperative bleeding can produce hypovolemia; however, P.T.'s initial and 2-hour postoperative Hct of 31% and 32%, respectively, do not support bleeding as a cause.

After major vascular or bowel surgery and in cases of burns or peritonitis, patients have an internal redistribution of fluids, called third spacing, which can result in intravascular volume depletion. It is not unusual for patients to third-space significant amounts of intravascular volume. The interstitial space and bowel walls can sequester large amounts of fluid, and this can produce a state of relative hypovolemia as is occurring with P.T. This is likely in the first 12 to 24 hours after the surgical procedure. P.T. is receiving 150 mL/hour of LR solution, but this is apparently not sufficient to maintain his intravascular volume.

Mild hypothermia is common during operative procedures. Vasodilation occurs as patients warm postoperatively, expanding the intravascular space. If the amounts of IV fluids administered are insufficient to compensate for the increased venous capacitance, BP and CO will decline during the rewarming phase, which can range from 1 to 6 hours. P.T. has rewarmed from 34.8°C to 37.4°C in 2 hours, which is not unusual after a major operative procedure. His temperature could conceivably rise to as high as 38°C to 38.5°C during the first 12 to 24 hours after surgery.

Other considerations include inadequate fluid administration during the operative procedure and the effects of drugs given in the operating room or in the immediate postoperative period (e.g., opioids, sedatives, inhaled anesthetics) that cause systemic vasodilation.

VOLUME REPLACEMENT AND VENTRICULAR FUNCTION

CASE 17-2, QUESTION 3: How will volume replacement improve P.T.'s CO and perfusion pressure?

The Frank–Starling mechanism indicates that the volume of blood returned to the heart is the main determinant of volume pumped by the heart. Therefore, as venous return is increased, the CO also will increase within physiologic limits until the optimal preload is achieved at which point further volume has minimal effect on SV (Fig. 17-1). The PCWP, the best indicator of LV preload, and the CVP, a marker of RV preload and overall estimate of volume status, are low because of declining venous return in P.T.

A ventricular function curve can be constructed by plotting a measure of cardiac pumping (CO, SV, or LVSWI) against a measure of preload (Fig. 17-3). Two hours after surgery, P.T.'s CVP has fallen from 12 to 6 mm Hg and his CO has fallen from 4.8 to 3.2 L/minute. Therefore, additional volume replacement is warranted.

CASE 17-2, QUESTION 4: P.T. is given a 500-mL bolus of NS solution in 10 minutes, and this results in the following hemodynamic profile:

BP (S/D/M), 96/54/68 mm Hg
HR, 88 beats/minute
CO, 3.9 L/minute
Cardiac Index (CI), 2.4 L/minute/m^2
CVP, 10 mm Hg
PCWP, 15 mm Hg

Assess P.T.'s response to the fluid challenge (see Table 17-2 for normal values).

According to the Frank–Starling curve, a small change in preload in response to a volume challenge with a minimal change in CO represents a ventricle on the flat portion of the ventricular function curve (Fig. 17-3). Additional fluid therapy given to these patients can increase their risk for pulmonary edema without improving

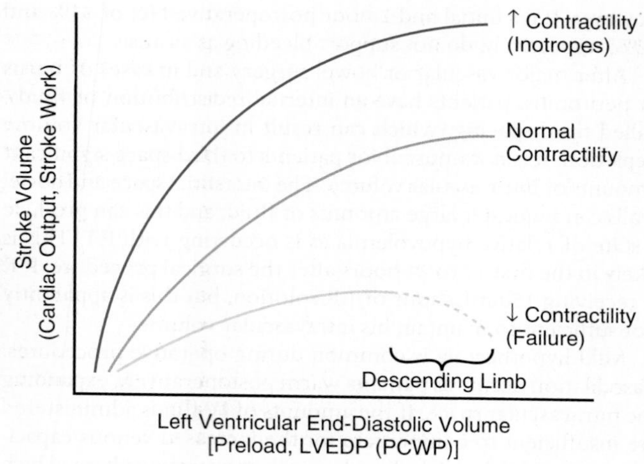

Figure 17-3 Ventricular function (Frank–Starling) curve. In the normal heart, as preload (left ventricular end-diastolic pressure [LVEDP]), measured clinically by pulmonary capillary wedge pressure (PCWP), increases, stroke volume (cardiac output, stroke work) increases until the contractile fibers reach their capacity, at which point the curve flattens. A change in contractility or afterload causes the heart to perform on a different curve. If the contractile fibers exceed their capacity, as with severe heart failure, the heart will operate on the descending limb of the curve.

CO. In contrast, a large change in preload in response to a fluid challenge with a significant increase in CO represents a ventricle on the steep portion of the curve. In P.T., the PCWP indicates he does not have pulmonary edema and the change in CVP from 6 to 10 mm Hg along with the increase in CO show that he is still responsive to fluid. Thus, it is reasonable to administer more fluid to enhance CO and renal perfusion.

FLUID CHALLENGE

CASE 17-2, QUESTION 5: One hour after the 500-mL NS bolus, P.T.'s hemodynamic profile returns to his postoperative state. ABGs are acceptable, and LR solution is infusing at 200 mL/hour. P.T. is continuing to "third-space" intravascular volume. Based on this information, develop a strategy for additional fluid challenges in P.T.

Acceptable strategies for administering additional fluid challenges to hypovolemic patients are based on the direction and degree of change in the various hemodynamic parameters in response to a fluid load rather than to their absolute values. CVP has a poor correlation with RV end-diastolic volume because it can be affected by changes in intrathoracic pressure, venous tone, and ventricular compliance (distensibility of the relaxed ventricle or stiffness of the myocardial wall).[38] PCWP and pulse pressure variation are more predictable markers of fluid status. Left ventricular SV (and thus pulse pressure) is inversely related to intrathoracic pressures during respiration; SV is maximally affected at lower filling pressures when the ventricles are operating on the steepest portion of the Frank–Starling curve. A SV that varies at least 12% during a respiratory cycle (between end inspiration and expiration) is highly predictive of a positive response to fluid challenge.[38]

Some practitioners argue that CVP is still an acceptable gauge of fluid responsiveness when used in conjunction with other parameters, including CO, BP, urine output, and tissue perfusion. Using CVP as a guide, an increase in the CVP of 5 mm Hg after a 250- to 500-mL fluid challenge in 10 minutes implies the LV is still functioning on the steep portion of the volume–pressure curve. If the CVP rises abruptly as fluid is given, with a small change in CO, the flat portion of the ventricular function curve has been reached and the IV infusion rate should be slowed. If signs and symptoms of inadequate tissue perfusion worsen or fail to improve and if the CVP remains greater than 10 to 14 mm Hg, fluid challenges should be stopped and inotropic therapy initiated.

Most critically ill patients require a CI above 2.5 L/minute/m^2 and a PCWP of 12 to 18 mm Hg, or a CVP of 8 to 14 mm Hg to maintain an acceptable MAP of 65 to 75 mm Hg. A downward trend in the lactate and base deficit and the change in hemodynamic parameters as well as vital signs and urine output should serve as indicators for whether additional fluid is required.

COLLOIDS

CASE 17-2, QUESTION 6: P.T. has received a total of 3.5 L of NS boluses during the past 6 hours and remains hemodynamically unchanged. His urine output has averaged 0.3 mL/kg/hour for the past 4 hours, indicating volume replacement is inadequate. Given his age and the lack of response to initial crystalloid administration, the decision is made to infuse a colloid solution. How do the colloids compare as a volume expander for P.T., and which agent should be used?

Albumin, the predominant protein in the plasma, accounts for approximately 80% of the COP, the force that maintains fluid in the intravascular space.[39] Human serum albumin is the colloidal agent against which all others are compared for volume-expanding properties. It is commercially prepared from pooled donor plasma that is heat-treated to eliminate the potential for disease transmission. Albumin 5% solution increases plasma volume by approximately 80% to 100% of the volume infused, with an initial duration of action of 16 hours.[39] At steady state (3–5 days), approximately 40% of albumin remains in the intravascular compartment while the rest is in the interstitial compartment. Side effects involve transient clotting abnormalities and anaphylactic reactions (0.5%), both of which are rare.[40] The anaphylactoid reaction is caused by the pasteurization process, causing albumin to polymerize, which produces an antigenic macromolecule. Albumin solutions also contain citrate, which can lower serum calcium concentrations and theoretically lead to decreased LV function. The effects on coagulation and serum calcium are possibly related to the volume of fluid infused rather than albumin administration.[39] Albumin is available as a 5% solution that is iso-oncotic with the plasma and as a 25% solution that is hyperoncotic. The 5% solution is generally preferred for routine volume expansion, whereas the 25% solution is most useful in correcting hypoproteinemia or intravascular hypovolemia in patients with excess interstitial water. Albumin is subject to availability, as approximately 1 L of pooled donor plasma is required to produce 20 to 25 g of albumin.

Hydroxyethyl starch (HES) is a synthetic colloid made from amylopectin, which closely resembles human serum albumin but is less expensive. Available as a 6% solution, HES expands the plasma volume by an amount greater than the volume infused because the high oncotic pressure draws water from the interstitial spaces. HES solutions have varying locations and degrees of substitutions on the glucose molecules, which slow enzymatic degradation and confer greater hydrolysis resistance (Table 17-5). HES solutions have complex pharmacokinetics because of their wide range of molecular weights; with an average molecular weight of 69,000 Da and a range of 1,000 to 3,000,000 Da. Numerous clinical studies have compared albumin and hetastarch for fluid resuscitation in patients with and without shock. However, most of these trials were underpowered and there were no significant differences in mortality.[41,42] Although HES has comparable efficacy to albumin, controversy exists regarding the use of HES owing to adverse effects seen with its use. These adverse effects include severe pruritus, coagulopathy, and renal dysfunction and appear to be class-related effects because the newer lower molecular weight and substitution products are similar.[20,21,43]

Dose-related reductions in platelet count and transient increases in PT, and PTT have been reported with moderate infusions of HES (up to 1,500 mL/day), and coagulopathies persist for up to 7 days with larger volumes.[21,42] HES causes factor VIII and von Willebrand factor levels to be lowered beyond that which can be attributed to hemodilution and also increases fibrinolysis.[42] This places patients with von Willebrand disease at greater risk of bleeding. In critically ill patients, particularly those with sepsis, HES is also associated with a dose-related increased risk of acute kidney injury and greater probability of needing renal replacement therapy.[20,21,44–46] HES now includes warnings of excessive bleeding when used in patients undergoing cardiopulmonary bypass as well as a boxed warning that states these products are contraindicated in critically ill patients. Experts argue that HES should not be used because of the potential adverse effects and that other alternatives are available.

Dextrans are colloidal solutions that are synthesized by bacteria from sucrose and are available in 40,000 and 70,000 Da average molecular weight solutions. These products lack adequately powered randomized trials to adequately examine their efficacy or safety.[42] Like HES, dextrans can cause renal dysfunction, bleeding, and anaphylactic reactions. Dextrans can cause acute kidney injury, possibly because of accumulation of dextran molecules within the renal tubules. They increase bleeding by causing dose-related decreased platelet adhesion, increased fibrinolysis, and decreased levels of factor VIII. Dextran solutions are associated with the highest incidence of anaphylactic reactions among all of the colloids.

Because of the lack of superior clinically important outcomes and less favorable safety profiles for HES and dextrans compared to albumin, it is decided to use albumin for further volume expansion in P.T.

CARDIOGENIC SHOCK

Shock arising primarily from an abnormality of cardiac function constitutes cardiogenic shock. The causes of cardiogenic shock can be separated largely into cardiomyopathic, arrhythmogenic, and mechanical (Table 17-1), although occasionally patients may have a combination of causes. Regardless of the source, the underlying problem in cardiogenic shock is a decrease in CO that is not caused by a reduction in circulating blood volume. This decrease in CO results in the syndrome of shock, organ dysfunction, and death if measures to restore perfusion are not successful.

The most common cause of cardiogenic shock is LV dysfunction and necrosis as a result of acute myocardial infarction (AMI) (see Chapter 13, Acute Coronary Syndrome). Necrosis of the left ventricle can be the result of a single massive myocardial infarction (MI), numerous smaller events, or severe global cardiac ischemia. Increases in sympathetic tone—seen clinically as increased HR and peripheral vasoconstriction—initially serve to increase CO and maintain arterial pressure. When necrosis exceeds approximately 40% of the LV, normal compensatory responses can no longer maintain CO, and hypotension and hypoperfusion results. In addition to decreased perfusion to vital tissues and organs, the decrease in CO leads to a reduction in the flow of blood through the coronary arteries, which can lead to infarct extension and a further worsening of cardiac performance.

Cardiogenic shock is the leading cause of death in patients hospitalized with AMI. It occurs in 5% to 10% of AMI cases and is more common with ST-elevation versus non-ST-elevation MI.[47] A registry of nearly 2 million patients admitted for ST-elevation MI in the United States from 2003 to 2010 found a 7.9% incidence.[48] The incidence was higher in patients at least 75 years of age, women, and Asian/Pacific Islanders versus less than 75 years of age, men, and other racial/ethnic groups, respectively. Patients with end-stage renal disease appear to be at a higher risk of cardiogenic shock and among those with ST-elevation MI that incidence increased three-fold from 2003 to 2011.[49] The in-hospital mortality for patients experiencing shock decreased 29% from 2003 to 2010, most likely because of coronary reperfusion strategies.[48] The overall mortality rate, however, has remained high (60%–80%).

Infarction involving the RV can cause cardiogenic shock, even with normal LV systolic function. In this situation, the volume of blood reaching the LV (preload) is reduced because of the inability of the RV to move blood to the left side of the heart. In most patients with cardiogenic shock and RV infarction, significant LV dysfunction is present as well. Arrhythmias are often associated with worsening perfusion, causing or worsening cardiogenic shock, and poor outcomes.

Patients with chronic heart failure (HF) (see Chapter 14, Heart Failure) usually compensate for their poor cardiac function, but acute exacerbations can cause cardiogenic shock with hypotension, hypoperfusion, and organ dysfunction. Cardiac dysfunction occasionally can be seen with severe sepsis because of increases in the production of inflammatory cytokines that have a depressant effect on the myocardium. However, the cytokine-mediated vasodilation and reduction in afterload usually negates the ability to detect the cardiac dysfunction. A similar picture occurs after cardiopulmonary bypass with heart surgery through activation of the inflammatory cascade.

Cardiogenic shock caused by mechanical problems occurs relatively infrequently. In this setting, the systolic function (contractility) of the heart may be normal, but other defects render the heart unable to eject a normal volume of blood. Pericardial tamponade (bleeding into the pericardial sac) and tension pneumothorax (air leakage from the lung into the chest) cause cardiogenic shock by compressing the heart and decreasing the diastolic filling. [Pericardial tamponade and tension pneumothorax are technically obstructive forms of shock as there is an extracardiac process that is impeding forward circulatory flow.] Acute valvular insufficiency or stenosis prevents the normal ejection of blood. Ventricular septal or free wall rupture can occur, often in the setting of AMI, with the reduction in CO related to the inability of the LV to eject a normal volume of blood during systole.

The symptoms of cardiogenic shock are largely the same as for other types of shock. Hypotension and signs of inadequate tissue perfusion, such as confusion, oliguria, tachycardia, and cutaneous vasoconstriction, are present in many patients. Differentiating cardiogenic shock from distributive or hypovolemic shock requires further examination. A history of coronary artery disease or symptoms of MI are important findings. Hypovolemia occurs in up to 20% of patients in cardiogenic shock, but patients frequently have signs of volume overload because the heart cannot move blood through the circulation. Peripheral edema can be seen in the extremities; lung sounds are diminished, and rales may be present as pulmonary edema develops with LV dysfunction. These findings are particularly evident in patients with severe HF.

Because the distinction between cardiogenic and other forms of shock can be difficult to make based on physical examination alone, further testing with invasive hemodynamic monitoring may be required to establish the diagnosis and guide therapy. Table 17-6 lists the common laboratory, electrocardiogram (ECG), and chest radiograph findings, and Table 17-3 lists the common hemodynamic findings in cardiogenic shock. CVP may be easily attained, particularly if the patient already has a central line; other hemodynamic findings will require further monitoring tools (e.g., PA catheter, echocardiography).

Table 17-6
Typical Findings of Early Cardiogenic Shock

- Arterial blood gas (ABG)
  - Hypoxemia secondary to pulmonary congestion with ventilation–perfusion abnormalities
  - Anion gap metabolic acidosis with a compensatory respiratory alkalosis
- Elevated blood lactate levels (which contributes to the acidosis)
- Complete bloodcount (CBC)
  - Leukocytosis
  - Thrombocytopenia (if disseminated intravascular coagulation is present)
- Elevated cardiac enzymes if myocardial infarction is present
- Electrocardiogram (ECG)–one or more of the following
  - T-wave changes indicating infarction
  - Left bundle branch block
  - Sinus tachycardia
  - Arrhythmia
- Chest radiograph
  - Pulmonary edema or evidence of adult respiratory distress syndrome (ARDS)
- Echocardiography
  - Valvular or mechanical problems if present
  - Normal or decreased ejection fraction
- Hemodynamic monitoring—one or more of the following:
  - Reduced cardiac output
  - Arterial hypotension
  - Elevated pulmonary capillary wedge pressure (PCWP) and central venous pressure (CVP)
  - Elevated pulmonary artery pressure (PAP)
  - Elevated systemic vascular resistance (SVR)

Acute Myocardial Infarction

IMMEDIATE GOALS OF THERAPY AND GENERAL CONSIDERATIONS

CASE 17-3

QUESTION 1: J.S. is a 43-year-old man who presents to the ED complaining of chest pain, tingling down his left arm, diaphoresis, nausea, vomiting, and shortness of breath. His pain has been ongoing for 3 hours and is not relieved by rest. He has no known history of cardiac disease and takes no home medications. His BP is 80/40 mm Hg (by cuff) with a weak pulse of 110 beats/minute. His RR is 24 breaths/minute, and his breathing is shallow. Heart sounds include S_3/S_4 gallops, but no murmurs are heard. The jugular venous pulse is normal. He has diffuse rales over the lower lung fields with moderate wheezing. J.S. is cold and clammy to touch; however, his temperature is normal. He is restless, anxious, and oriented only to person and place. A 3-mm ST-segment elevation is seen on 12-lead ECG in leads I and AVL. Cardiac biomarkers are pending. ABG measurements, on 4 L/minute oxygen via nasal cannula, are the following:

pH, 7.28
$PaCO_2$, 32 mm Hg
PaO_2, 94 mm Hg
HCO_3^-, 15 mEq/L
Hct, 31%

What immediate goals of therapy are necessary to stabilize and treat J.S.?

J.S. has signs of cardiogenic shock with decreased systemic perfusion. His BP is low, HR is elevated, and respiratory status is compromised. J.S. is restless, anxious, and confused, indicating poor cerebral perfusion. His ABG results indicate a component of metabolic acidosis secondary to poor systemic perfusion. The ST-elevation on the ECG is consistent with an acute anterior MI.

As discussed in Chapter 13, Acute Coronary Syndrome, most patients presenting with STEMI are routinely treated with aspirin, a β-blocker, and immediate percutaneous coronary intervention (PCI) if available or, if not, thrombolytic therapy (unless contraindicated).[50] The presence of cardiogenic shock can alter the interventional strategy, however. Patients presenting in cardiogenic shock after MI may progress rapidly to irreversible organ system dysfunction as the compensatory mechanisms fail to maintain tissue perfusion. Treatment of these critically ill patients involves two components: stabilization and definitive treatment. Initial stabilization of the patient must be attained before further evaluation and treatment of the cause of cardiogenic shock can proceed. The goals are to maintain adequate $\dot{D}O_2$ to the tissues and to prevent further hemodynamic compromise. Stabilization includes (a) establishing ventilation and oxygenation (arterial PO_2 should be greater than 70 mm Hg); (b) restoring arterial BP and CO with vasopressors and inotropic agents, if needed; (c) infusing fluids, if hypovolemic; and (d) treating pain, arrhythmias, and acid–base abnormalities, if present.

Administration of oxygen is appropriate for patients who have severe dyspnea, hypoxemia (oxygen saturation below 90%), or persistent or worsening acidemia (pH less than 7.3).[50,51] Improving oxygenation may contribute to improved ventricular performance; however, supplemental oxygen could potentially be harmful by causing increased coronary vascular resistance and infarct size, particularly in normoxic patients.[50,52] Invasive mechanical ventilation is indicated when arterial oxygen saturation cannot be maintained above 90% despite 100% oxygen per facemask. Once the patient is intubated, sedation should be provided to alleviate anxiety and discomfort while cautiously monitoring hemodynamic effects.

The arterial pressure must be increased to provide adequate coronary and systemic perfusion to meet oxygen requirements. Some areas of ischemia in the infarct zone may be depressed but viable, provided myocardial oxygen supply exceeds demand. If the myocardial oxygen demands are not met, however, myocardial tissue necrosis will expand into the area of ischemia. This results in further hemodynamic impairment and initiates a vicious cycle that can lead to intractable pump failure and irreversible shock. To be effective, treatment of cardiogenic shock should favorably influence the balance between oxygen supply and demand in the ischemic zone.

Optimizing preload to improve CO and systemic perfusion is crucial, especially in patients with RV infarction. In patients with severe LV impairment, increasing intravascular volume can worsen pulmonary congestion. J.S. currently has signs of pulmonary congestion and RV infarction is not evident; thus, a fluid challenge must be administered cautiously or withheld until hemodynamic monitoring can be established.

Inotropic agents or vasopressors should be used to increase systemic BP and reestablish coronary perfusion in patients with cardiogenic shock and hypotension. However, vasoactive agents have risk because they can exacerbate ventricular arrhythmias and increase $\dot{V}O_2$ in ischemic myocardium. Therefore, the minimal dose that will provide adequate perfusion pressure should be used. Achieving a MAP of 65 to 70 mm Hg is the immediate goal of therapy, but it should be adjusted based on adequate perfusion (e.g., warm extremities, adequate urine output, improved mental status).[51] Elevation of the MAP to more than 80 mm Hg is unnecessary because coronary blood flow is not significantly changed at this level, but energy expenditure is high.

Correction of metabolic acidosis is best accomplished by treating the underlying cause. Improving tissue perfusion by optimizing oxygen content and increasing CO can eventually restore aerobic metabolism and eliminate lactic acid production. The use of sodium bicarbonate to correct lactic acidosis in cardiogenic shock and other critically ill patients is controversial. Sodium bicarbonate can have numerous adverse effects, such as hypernatremia, paradoxical intracellular acidosis, and hypercapnia; conclusive data on its efficacy are lacking. Bicarbonate therapy is recommended only, if at all, when severe acidemia (pH below 7.2 or HCO_3^- less than 10–12 mEq/L) is present.

Inotropic agents and vasoconstrictors can increase myocardial $\dot{V}O_2$ and potentially extend the area of necrosis in patients with infarct-induced cardiogenic shock. Careful selection and titration of agents that will best preserve myocardium while sustaining systemic arterial pressure and tissue perfusion is essential. Although correction of volume deficits and early pharmacologic support may prevent the extension of myocardial damage, it must be emphasized that exclusive use of these measures does not improve survival. Therefore, drug therapy must be considered only an interim maneuver to preserve myocardial and systemic integrity while further therapeutic interventions and definitive therapy are being considered.

Cardiogenic shock after AMI occurs in only a small percentage of patients, but it carries a high mortality rate. Reperfusion of the occluded artery is of paramount importance in these patients. Two options are available for restoring patency of the artery: thrombolytic therapy and revascularization (PCI or coronary artery bypass grafting [CABG]) (see Chapter 13, Acute Coronary Syndrome).

Thrombolytic therapy in AMI may reduce the incidence of subsequent cardiogenic shock, but its value may be limited in patients who have already experienced shock.[53] The effectiveness of thrombolysis is reduced in this setting, possibly because of reduced delivery of the agent to the coronary artery thrombus as a result of hypotension.[54] The use of an intra-aortic balloon pump (IABP) to augment coronary artery blood flow may improve the efficacy of thrombolytic agents but has not been shown to improve mortality.[55,56]

Early revascularization with PCI or CABG is preferred in patients with cardiogenic shock complicating AMI, irrespective of time delay.[50] In the SHOCK trial, emergency revascularization, compared to immediate medical stabilization (fibrinolysis and IABP), resulted in significantly lower mortality at 1 and 6 years in patients with ST-elevation MI and cardiogenic shock.[53] Long-term mortality was positively correlated with time to revascularization from 0 to 8 hours, confirming that revascularization should be performed as soon as possible. However, a survival benefit for revascularization remains even as long as 54 hours after MI and 18 hours after shock onset.[53] Operator skill is also a consideration, and larger centers with greater experience may have better outcomes than smaller centers. In settings in which interventional cardiac procedures such as percutaneous transluminal coronary angioplasty or stenting are not readily available, insertion of an IABP and thrombolytic agents should not be delayed if indicated.

Postoperative Cardiac Failure

ASSESSMENT BY HEMODYNAMIC PROFILE

CASE 17-3, QUESTION 2: Cardiac catheterization reveals an acute occlusion of the proximal left circumflex artery, but a percutaneous coronary intervention was unable to be performed for J.S. He undergoes emergent CABG and arrives in the ICU sedated, intubated, and receiving mechanical ventilation with 50% inspired oxygen. Several hours after admission to the ICU his BP and urine output have fallen and his skin is mottled and cool. Urine output has fallen from 0.8 to 0.2 mL/kg/hour in the last hour. The chest tube output has been stable at 50 mL/hour. His current hemodynamic profile is as follows:

BP (S/D/M), 86/44/58 mm Hg
HR, 105 beats/minute
CO, 3.0 L/minute
CI, 1.7 L/minute/m^2
SvO_2, 48%
CVP, 14 mm Hg
PA pressure (S/D), 41/24 mm Hg
PCWP, 24 mm Hg
SVR, 1,570 dyne·s·cm^{-5}

What is your assessment of J.S.'s clinical status and hemodynamics?

Clinically, J.S. has signs of hypoperfusion manifested by low urine output; mottled, cool skin; and metabolic acidosis. His decreased SvO_2 shows that he has impaired perfusion owing to his low $\dot{D}O_2$. Evaluation of his hemodynamics will help determine a potential cause for his hypoperfusion and assist with the decision about appropriate therapeutic interventions to prevent his condition from worsening to serious organ dysfunction and death.

Possible causes of shock in cardiac surgery patients include blood loss, excessive vasodilation from medications or cardiopulmonary bypass-induced inflammation, cardiac ischemia-reperfusion injury, valvular dysfunction, tamponade, heart failure, or perioperative MI. Another concern is "stunning" of the myocardium caused by surgical trauma, which can take hours to days to resolve.

Hypovolemia should always be evaluated first when assessing hemodynamic profiles. Using vasopressor or inotropic agents in the setting of hypovolemia is rarely effective and could cause further hypotension or serious adverse effects (e.g., cardiac arrhythmias). Also, correction of hypovolemia is relatively straightforward and can be accomplished rapidly. Most patients require no more than 2 to 3 L of crystalloid after cardiac surgery, especially once rewarming is complete. J.S.'s tachycardia, low urine output, low BP, and low CO could indicate volume depletion. However, his Hct is adequate, and he has an elevated CVP, PAP, and PCWP, suggesting that he is not hypovolemic.

Excessive vasodilation is also unlikely in J.S., given that his calculated SVR (afterload) is above normal range. Cardiac tamponade should always be considered after cardiac surgery, and it is usually manifested by very high CVP, PCWP, and PA pressures, with significant decreases in CO and BP. Diminished or muffled heart sounds and an inappropriately fluctuating BP with respirations (pulsus paradoxus) will usually accompany an equalization of diastolic pressures during cardiac tamponade. J.S.'s CVP and PCWP are not as high as would be expected in pericardial tamponade, and his chest tube output has remained consistent, suggesting that blood is not accumulating.

Based on this hemodynamic profile, it appears that J.S. is in shock because of acute HF, most likely from postoperative myocardial dysfunction, although he should also be evaluated for myocardial ischemia or infarction and to rule out early cardiac tamponade. This evaluation should not delay the initiation of therapy.

Patients with cardiogenic shock from an acute event (such as an MI) are usually more critical than patients who have an acute exacerbation of chronic HF. Patients with HF have compensated with time for the increases in preload and reduced CO, but patients such as J.S. have not had time to develop compensatory mechanisms. His severely depressed CO should be treated immediately to prevent further decompensation.

CASE 17-3, QUESTION 3: The chest radiograph shows moderate pulmonary edema, and rales were heard on auscultation. His ABG measurements on mechanical ventilation with 50% inspired oxygen are pH 7.3, $PaCO_2$ 38 mm Hg, PaO_2 90 mm Hg, and HCO_3^- 18 mEq/L. Tamponade is not evident on the radiograph. The ECG shows ST-T-wave changes with some resolution of ST-elevation in leads I and AVL, but no indication is seen of a new AMI. Cardiac biomarkers are pending. BP and CO need to be improved to increase perfusion to vital organs. Three therapeutic interventions are available: fluid challenge, vasodilators, and inotropic agents. How would these choices affect J.S.'s ventricular function?

Fluid Challenge (Increase Preload)

Augmentation of preload with a fluid challenge to improve CO is the first option. However, J.S. has signs of pulmonary edema on chest radiograph, PCWP is 24 mm Hg, and PaO_2 is 90 mm Hg on 50% inspired oxygen. Increasing the PCWP above 18 mm Hg usually does not result in further benefit.[57,58] Therefore, giving volume might increase the pulmonary vascular hydrostatic pressure and worsen his pulmonary edema. If a fluid challenge is attempted to enhance preload, 250 to 500 mL of NS solution should be given over 20 to 30 minutes while continuously monitoring the hemodynamic profile and for volume overload. If the PCWP rises but the CO does not improve, fluid challenges should be discontinued. Elevating the preload without appreciably improving CO increases LV wall tension, which is a major determinant of myocardial $\dot{V}O_2$; consequently, myocardial ischemia could develop. Although J.S. has signs of pulmonary edema, diuretics to reduce his volume overload can be detrimental to his CO and BP and should not be used until J.S.'s hemodynamics and signs of hypoperfusion have improved.

Vasodilators (Preload and Afterload Reduction)

A peripheral venodilator will decrease pulmonary venous congestion by reducing preload (CVP and PCWP) and pulmonary vascular hydrostatic pressure. With myocardial ischemia, a reduction of the LV filling pressure may improve subendocardial blood flow, reduce the myocardial wall tension, and reduce the LV radius. The resultant decrease in myocardial $\dot{V}O_2$ will help prevent further depression of cardiac function.

In patients with LV failure, arterial resistance is also elevated because of a reflex increase in sympathetic tone in response to a fall in systemic arterial pressure. In LV failure, CO is inversely related to resistance to outflow from the LV. Lowering an elevated SVR (afterload) will decrease resistance to ventricular ejection and shift the ventricular function curve up and to the left, depending on whether an arterial, venous, or mixed vasodilator is used, thereby improving cardiac performance at a lower filling pressure (Fig. 17-4).

J.S. appears to have LV failure with elevations in PCWP and SVR. Vasodilator therapy in this setting will likely improve his CO and, therefore, increase the $\dot{D}O_2$ to the tissues and prevent organ dysfunction. The major risk of vasodilator therapy in J.S., however, is further reduction of an already low MAP. Although the reduction in BP may be offset by an increase in CO, a significant drop in arterial BP could occur, which could decrease perfusion to vital organ systems and exacerbate myocardial ischemia by reducing coronary perfusion pressure. Vasodilator therapy should be reserved for situations of LV failure with elevations in PCWP and SVR and a SBP greater than 90 mm Hg.

Inotropic Support

A rapid-acting inotropic agent also can be used to increase myocardial contractility if the CO remains low or inadequate with signs of tissue hypoperfusion after optimization of the volume

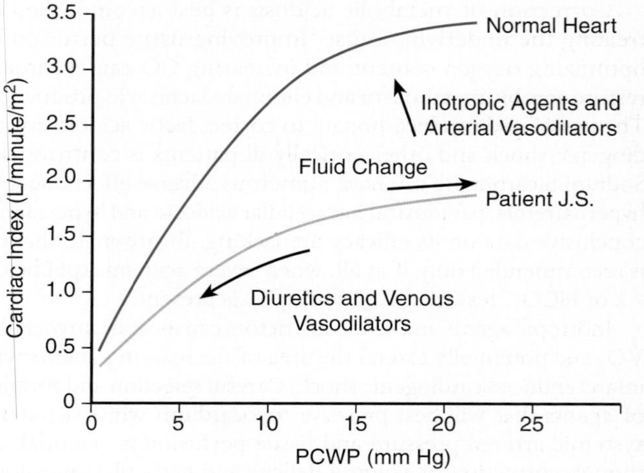

Figure 17-4 Ventricular function curve for J.S. PCWP, pulmonary capillary wedge pressure.

status.[1] This intervention shifts the ventricular function curve upward and slightly to the left (Fig. 17-4). The disadvantage of this intervention is that improved CO is accompanied by increased myocardial oxygen demand. Depending on the agent selected, three of the determinants of myocardial $\dot{V}O_2$ could be elevated: HR, contractility, and ventricular wall tension. Therefore, inotropic support is directed at establishing or maintaining a reasonable arterial pressure and ensuring adequate tissue perfusion by improving the CO.

In summary, the most appropriate therapeutic intervention for J.S. at this time would be inotropic support. The PCWP is elevated, suggesting that the preload has been maximized; therefore, fluid may worsen J.S.'s pulmonary edema. Although J.S.'s SVR is elevated (1,570 dyne·s·cm^{-5}), his BP is low; therefore, initial use of a peripheral vasodilator could jeopardize perfusion. Thus, an acceptable initial therapeutic intervention to improve CO and tissue perfusion is inotropic support. After a reasonable BP has been established, addition of a peripheral vasodilator could be considered to further enhance CO if needed, and diuretics added to reduce his pulmonary edema.

INOTROPIC AGENTS

CASE 17-3, QUESTION 4: Which inotropic agent is the best choice for J.S.?

Dopamine

Dopamine, a precursor of norepinephrine, has inotropic, chronotropic, and vasoactive properties, all of which are dose dependent (Table 17-7). The distinct ranges noted for dopamine activity are generalizations; responses noted in clinical practice will be patient specific. At less than 5 mcg/kg/minute, dopamine stimulates dopaminergic receptors primarily in the splanchnic, renal, and coronary vascular beds. The effect on dopaminergic receptors is not blocked by β-blockers, but is antagonized by dopaminergic-blocking agents such as the butyrophenones and phenothiazines. Depending on the clinical state of the patient, low dosages of dopamine may slightly increase myocardial contractility, but it usually will not alter HR or SVR significantly.

At 5 to 10 mcg/kg/minute, the improved cardiac performance produced by dopamine is through direct stimulation of β_1-adrenergic receptors and indirectly through release of norepinephrine from nerve terminals. Increased β_1-adrenergic receptor stimulation increases SV (inotropic effect), HR (chronotropic effect), and consequently CO. These cardiac effects can be blocked by β-blockers. As infusion rates increase above 5

Table 17-7
Inotropic Agents and Vasopressors

Drug	Usual Dose	Receptor Sensitivity			Pharmacologic Effect			
		$\alpha 1$	$\beta 1$	$\beta 2$	VD	VC	*INT*	*CHT*
Dobutamine	2–10 mcg/kg/minute	+	++++	++	+	+	+++[a]	+
	>10 mcg/kg/minute	++	++++	+++	++	+	++++[a]	++
Dopamine	<5 mcg/kg/minute[b]	0	+	0	+	0	++	+
	5–10 mcg/kg/minute[b]	0/+	++++	++	+	+	+++	++
	10–20 mcg/kg/minute[b]	+++	++++	+	0	+++	+++	+++
Epinephrine[c]	<0.1 mcg/kg/minute	+	++++	+++	+	+	++++[a]	++
	0.1–2 mcg/kg/minute	+++	++++	+++	0	+++	+++[a]	+++
	>2 mcg/kg/minute	++++	++	+	0	++++	++[a]	+++
Isoproterenol	0.01–0.1 mcg/kg/minute	0	++++	++++	+++	0	++++	++++
Milrinone	Possible 50 mcg/kg bolus, then 0.125–0.75 mcg/kg/minute	0	0	0	+++[d]	0	+++	0
Norepinephrine[c]	0.02–3 mcg/kg/minute[f]	++++	+++	+	0	++++	+[e]	++
Phenylephrine	0.5–5 mcg/kg/minute[f]	++++	0	0	0	++++	0	0
Vasopressin[g]	0.03–0.04 units/minute[h]	0	0	0	0	++++	0	0

[a]Dobutamine, milrinone, and epinephrine have more inotropic effect than dopamine.
[b]Dopamine stimulates dopaminergic receptors at all doses, causing vasodilation in the splanchnic and renal vasculature.
[c]Epinephrine has predominant inotropic effects; norepinephrine has predominant vasoconstrictive effect. Epinephrine may vasodilate at low dosages, vasoconstrict at high dosages.
[d]Milrinone inhibits phosphodiesterase-3, leading to increased contractility of the myocardium and vasodilation of vascular smooth muscle.
[e]Cardiac output unchanged or may decline because of vagal reflex responses that slow the heart.
[f]Highly variable, titrate to desired MAP
[g]Vasopressin stimulates V_{1a} receptors to cause vasoconstriction in the periphery.
[h]Dosing for sepsis; in other vasodilatory conditions, it may be titrated from 0.01 to 0.1 units/minute.
CHT, chronotropic; INT, inotropic; MAP, mean arterial pressure; VC, peripheral vascular vasoconstriction; VD, peripheral vascular vasodilation.

mcg/kg/minute, the α-adrenergic receptors are activated. At this dosage, the vasoactive effects on peripheral blood vessels are unpredictable and depend on the net effect of β_1-adrenergic stimulation, α-adrenergic stimulation, and reflex mechanisms. MAP and PCWP usually will rise. The increased HR, along with the elevated PCWP in J.S., could adversely affect the myocardial oxygen supply to demand ratio. However, it is hoped the increase in coronary blood flow (caused by the rise in arterial pressure) and the decrease in LV chamber size (associated with the increase in contractility) would tend to offset the increase in myocardial oxygen requirements.

At doses greater than 10 mcg/kg/minute, dopamine primarily stimulates peripheral α-adrenergic receptors. SVR increases, splanchnic and renal blood flow decreases, and LV filling pressure is raised. Cardiac irritability is a potential complication, and the overall myocardial $\dot{V}O_2$ is increased. The increase in SVR limits CO; thus, infusion rates should be limited to less than 15 mcg/kg/minute in patients with cardiac failure.[59]

In a recent trial of 1,679 patients with shock, who were randomized to dopamine or norepinephrine for blood pressure support, there was no significant difference in the primary outcome of 28-day mortality.[60] However, patients receiving dopamine had more arrhythmic events and a prespecified subgroup analysis showed an increased mortality rate in 280 patients with cardiogenic shock. Although these findings may have been because of chance and randomization was not stratified, these findings warrant consideration before selecting dopamine for J.S. and highlight the need for more studies comparing catecholamines in cardiogenic shock.

Dobutamine

Dobutamine, a synthetic catecholamine, is a potent positive inotropic agent with dose-dependent but predominant direct β_1-agonist effects and weak β_2- and α_1-adrenergic effects. With greater β_2-vasodilatory than α_1-vasoconstrictive actions, dobutamine reduces systemic and pulmonary vascular resistance. The reduction in SVR may be caused by a reflex decrease in vasoconstriction secondary to enhanced CO. Unlike dopamine, dobutamine does not release endogenous norepinephrine or stimulate renal dopaminergic receptors.[61]

Studies assessing dobutamine in cardiac failure demonstrate consistent increases in CO and SV, with reductions in PCWP and SVR. The reduction in filling pressures, as indicated by a lowered PCWP, results in a decrease in LV wall tension and myocardial $\dot{V}O_2$. Consequently, coronary perfusion pressure and myocardial oxygen supply is improved.

Compared with dopamine, dobutamine has equal or greater inotropic action. Dobutamine lowers PCWP and SVR with increasing doses, whereas dopamine may increase PCWP and SVR with increasing doses.[62] The effect on HR is variable; however, evidence suggests that dobutamine is less chronotropic than dopamine at lower infusion rates. In the clinical setting, dobutamine may be preferred in patients with depressed CO, elevated PCWP, and increased SVR with mild hypotension (SBP above 70 mm Hg) and no signs or symptoms of shock. The increase in CO may not be sufficient to raise the BP in a patient who initially is moderately to severely hypotensive (SBP below 70 mm Hg) or with signs or symptoms of shock. Dopamine may be recommended in patients with mild hypotension and symptoms of shock, whereas norepinephrine is reserved for patients with a SBP below 70 mm Hg.[63,64] Given the recent concerns of increased mortality with dopamine monotherapy in patients with cardiogenic shock, the combination of dopamine or norepinephrine with dobutamine may be preferred in patients with depressed CO, normal or moderately elevated PCWP, and moderate or severe hypotension.[59,60,64]

Epinephrine

Similar to dopamine and dobutamine, epinephrine has dose-dependent hemodynamic effects (Table 17-7). At lower infusion ranges (less than 0.1 mcg/kg/minute) epinephrine stimulates β_1-adrenergic receptors, causing increases in HR and contractility. As the dose increases, more α_1-receptor stimulation occurs, resulting in vasoconstriction and corresponding increases in SVR.

The favorable hemodynamic effects (increased CO and BP) make low-dose epinephrine an attractive option for J.S.; however, epinephrine can induce hyperglycemia through gluconeogenesis and has been shown to increase lactate levels compared with other vasopressors and inotropic agents.[65] J.S. already has signs of acidosis (pH 7.28, HCO_3^- 15 mEq/L), and increased lactic acid production by epinephrine could be detrimental to his organ function. Epinephrine should be reserved for patients with a markedly depressed CO in conjunction with severe hypotension.

In summary, very few comparable studies of inotropic agents in this setting have been conducted; thus, the selection of agent is often based on the expected clinical benefit as well as individual experience with the drugs.[66] None of the choices are without risk as they could adversely affect the myocardial oxygen supply to demand ratio and could further extend the area of ischemia or necrosis. J.S. would benefit from an increase in his CO, as well as in his MAP. The clinician elects to start J.S. on dobutamine and dopamine infusions.

SELECTION AND INITIATION OF THERAPY

CASE 17-3, QUESTION 5: At what doses should you initiate a dobutamine and dopamine infusion in J.S.? What therapeutic outcomes are anticipated at these doses and during what time? What adverse effects may be encountered with these infusions?

J.S. has a MAP of 58 mm Hg, CI of 1.7 L/minute/m², PCWP of 24 mm Hg, and HR of 105 beats/minute. Goals of therapy are to increase the CI to at least 2.5 L/minute/m², maintain a MAP of at least 70 mm Hg (preferably closer to 80 mm Hg, depending on clinical signs of hypoperfusion), reduce the PCWP to 12 to 18 mm Hg, and maintain an HR of less than 125 beats/minute. A urine output of at least 0.5 mL/kg/hour is desirable. Reasonable initial infusion rates would be dopamine 5 mcg/kg/minute and dobutamine 2 mcg/kg/minute. These doses should increase cardiac contraction and CO, resulting in an increase in renal blood flow. The onset of effect is rapid and the half-life short (approximately 2 minutes) for both agents, with steady-state conditions generally achieved within 10 minutes of initiation of therapy. This allows dose titration every 10 minutes based on patient tolerance.

Because the onsets of action are within minutes, J.S. can be reevaluated and the infusion rates can be alternately titrated upward by 1 to 2 mcg/kg/minute every 10 minutes, depending on the hemodynamic data. The response to both agents is highly variable among patients; thus, careful titration using the lowest effective infusion rates is advised.

Adverse effects encountered with both infusions include increased HR, angina, arrhythmias, headache, tremors, nausea, and vomiting. The increases in contractility and HR caused by dobutamine and dopamine pose additive risk of tachyarrhythmias and can increase myocardial $\dot{V}O_2$, leading to ischemia in patients with coronary artery disease.

Dobutamine could lower the MAP, adversely affecting coronary perfusion pressure. Another limiting factor to dobutamine is tolerance to its hemodynamic effects with long-term continuous use. A decline in CO and HR has been seen after prolonged infusion and is most likely caused by down-regulation of β_1-receptors. Of concern, evidence suggests that inotropic agents can be associated with an increased risk of mortality in patients with HF despite the improvement of symptoms and hemodynamic indices.[67]

Dopamine might elevate the PCWP, thereby decreasing coronary perfusion pressure. Extravasation of large amounts of dopamine during infusion can cause ischemic necrosis and sloughing. At higher dosages, α_1-adrenergic effects are more prominent, causing peripheral arterial vasoconstriction and increases in afterload, preload, and myocardial oxygen demand as well as ischemia.

CASE 17-3, QUESTION 6: Dobutamine and dopamine are titrated from 2 to 4 mcg/kg/minute and 5 to 6 mcg/kg/minute, respectively, in J.S. during the next 2 hours. A repeat chest radiograph shows slight worsening of pulmonary edema. The following hemodynamic profile is obtained (previous values are in parentheses):

BP (S/D/M), 105/60/75 mm Hg (86/44/58 mm Hg)
HR, 140 beats/minute (105 beats/minute)
CO, 5.3 L/minute (3 L/minute)
CI, 3 L/minute/m² (1.7 L/minute/m²)
CVP, 11 mm Hg (14 mm Hg)
PCWP, 22 mm Hg (24 mm Hg)
SVR, 1,493 dyne·s·cm^{-5} (1,570 dyne·s·cm^{-5})
Urine output, 0.4 mL/kg/hour (0.2 mL/kg/hour)
Hct, 33% (31%)

Do these data indicate a favorable or adverse hemodynamic effect from dobutamine and dopamine in J.S.?

Dobutamine at 4 mcg/kg/minute and dopamine at 6 mcg/kg/minute have established a trend in the desired direction for CI; however, the HR has increased significantly. The SVR and PCWP have not changed appreciably, and the urine flow has increased. The SV (CO/HR) has only increased from 28 to 38 mL/beat; thus, the increase in CO has resulted from both the chronotropic and the inotropic effects of these agents. As a net response, the dobutamine and dopamine have most likely adversely affected the myocardial oxygen supply to demand ratio; however, this cannot be established definitively. J.S. should be monitored closely for signs of myocardial ischemia.

CHANGING THERAPY

CASE 17-3, QUESTION 7: The clinician decides that an HR of 140 beats/minute is unacceptable in J.S., who presented with an AMI. Subsequent attempts to taper the dobutamine to lessen the induced tachycardia without dropping the CI and perfusion pressure are unsuccessful. Milrinone is suggested as an alternative to dobutamine. What hemodynamic changes would you expect with milrinone in J.S.? Does milrinone offer any advantages compared with dobutamine?

Milrinone increases intracellular AMP levels by inhibiting phosphodiesterase-3 within the sarcoplasmic reticulum of cardiac myocytes and vascular smooth muscle, leading to increased contractility of the myocardium and vasodilation of vascular smooth muscle. The increased CO and decreased SVR are accompanied by an increased lusitropic effect. Milrinone produces fewer chronotropic and arrhythmogenic effects than the catecholamines but, like dobutamine, can decrease SVR and cause hypotension. Moreover, milrinone has a longer half-life than dobutamine, making it difficult to use as monotherapy for cardiogenic shock. The combination of dopamine with milrinone would offset some of milrinone's hypotensive effects. Although milrinone has not been studied in patients who are post-AMI with cardiogenic shock, it could be beneficial in patients with adequate BP, who have down-regulated β receptors (chronic heart failure or beta agonist use), recently received β-blockade, or with catecholamine dose-limiting arrhythmias.

Dobutamine has equivalent or greater inotropic action than dopamine and, as mentioned above, dobutamine causes less tachycardia, so it may be better to remove dopamine in this patient. A decrease of 20% of the current dopamine infusion rate (1 to 2 mcg/kg/minute) every 10 to 15 minutes is reasonable. Just as with upward titration of therapy, steady state should be achieved within 10 minutes. When tapering vasoactive agents, it is prudent, however, to let the patient stabilize hemodynamically at new infusion rates for a period that exceeds the time to achieve a new steady-state plasma concentration. After each reduction in the infusion rate, hemodynamic data can be assessed. The major difference between the two agents is the effect of dopamine on α_1-receptors. With dobutamine's greater clinical effect on β_2-receptors compared to α_1-receptors, J.S. may experience a decrease in the SVR. A decreased SVR should allow for an increased CI, but J.S. should be monitored carefully as his MAP is relatively low and any major reduction in SVR could lead to further BP reduction.

CASE 17-3, QUESTION 8: Dopamine is tapered off and dobutamine is increased to 5 mcg/kg/minute for J.S. His HR decreased to 105 to 110 beats/minute within the next hour. Despite these changes and initiation of ventilatory support by tracheal intubation, J.S. continues to show signs of deterioration with progressive obtundation and loss of bowel sounds. His systemic arterial pressure has continued to decline. Preload reduction was attempted previously with nitroglycerin; however, the BP reduction was intolerable. A repeat hemodynamic profile shows the following values (previous values in parentheses):

BP (S/D/M), 86/40/55 mm Hg (105/60/75 mm Hg)
HR, 132 beats/minute (105 to 110 beats/minute)
CO, 3.2 L/minute (5.3 L/minute)
CI, 1.8 L/minute/m^2 (3 L/minute/m^2)
SvO_2, 42% (48%)
CVP, 16 mm Hg (11 mm Hg)
PCWP, 28 mm Hg (22 mm Hg)
SVR, 992 dyne·s·cm^{-5} (1,493 dyne·s·cm^{-5})
Urine output, 0.1 mL/kg/hour (0.4 mL/kg/hour)
PaO_2, 75 mm Hg (90 mm Hg)
$PaCO_2$, 42 mm Hg (38 mm Hg)
pH, 7.24 (7.3)
HCO_3^-, 17 mEq/L (18 mEq/L)

The ECG shows atrial tachycardia with occasional premature ventricular contractions. What therapeutic alternatives can be considered at this time?

J.S. is still in severe cardiogenic shock, and his tissue perfusion continues to deteriorate as evidenced by a further reduction in urine output, a loss of bowel sounds, continuing acidosis, and obtundation. Because his systemic arterial pressure and tissue perfusion have declined, additional support with a potent vasopressor and the insertion of an IABP or other percutaneous ventricular assist device are indicated. The combination of dopamine and dobutamine previously resulted in intolerable tachycardia, so other therapies should be considered.

Norepinephrine

Norepinephrine is a potent α-adrenergic agonist that vasoconstricts arterioles at all infusion rates, thereby increasing SVR. Thus, systemic arterial and coronary perfusion pressures both rise. Norepinephrine also stimulates β_1-adrenergic receptors to a lesser extent, resulting in increased contractility and SV. However, HR and CO usually remain constant or may decrease secondary to the increased afterload, and baroreceptor-mediated reflex increases in vagal tone. Although coronary perfusion pressure is enhanced as a result of the elevation in diastolic pressure, myocardial $\dot{V}O_2$ also is increased. Consequently, myocardial ischemia and arrhythmias may be exacerbated and LV function further compromised.

Infusions of norepinephrine are begun at 0.01 to 0.05 mcg/kg/minute and titrated upward to achieve a MAP of 65 to 70 mm Hg. Adverse effects of norepinephrine are related mostly to excessive vasoconstriction and compromise of organ perfusion. Administration should be through a central IV line because local subcutaneous necrosis and sloughing can result from peripheral IV extravasation. Prolonged infusion of larger doses will transiently exert a beneficial effect by diverting blood flow from the peripheral and splanchnic vasculature to the heart and brain; however, this ultimately can compromise capillary perfusion to the extent that end-organ failure, particularly renal failure, ensues.

Again, it must be emphasized that pharmacologic support for J.S., particularly the use of norepinephrine, is only an interim maneuver to temporarily maintain hemodynamic function. J.S. should continue to be monitored for signs of myocardial ischemia and the need for further revascularization procedures. Patients who cannot be stabilized with pharmacologic intervention, and in whom systemic or myocardial perfusion is becoming compromised, may require further support through insertion of a mechanical circulatory assist device.

Mechanical Circulatory Support

When drug therapy is ineffective at stabilizing patients in cardiogenic shock, mechanical intervention should be considered. Mechanical interventions can rapidly stabilize patients with cardiogenic shock, especially those with global myocardial ischemia or infarction complicated by mechanical defects, such as papillary muscle rupture or ventricular septal rupture. Sometimes combined inotropic support and intra-aortic balloon counterpulsation are required to maintain an acceptable BP (MAP above 65 mm Hg) and CI (greater than 2.2 L/minute/m^2).

The IABP has been in use for more than 40 years and remains the most commonly used mechanical assist device. It is designed to improve coronary arterial perfusion pressure and reduce afterload, providing short-term reperfusion of the ischemic myocardium.[68] A 20- to 50-mL balloon catheter is inserted into an artery (usually femoral) and advanced to the proximal descending aorta. Balloon inflation and deflation are synchronized with the ECG to inflate during diastole and deflate at the onset of systole. The inflated balloon in diastole increases coronary perfusion by elevating the mean aortic pressure. The rapid deflation of the balloon at the onset of systole decreases afterload and modestly improving CO.[68] The enhanced myocardial perfusion provided by IABP may reduce vasopressor requirements, thereby further decreasing myocardial $\dot{V}O_2$. Occasionally, IABP augmentation is sufficient to allow the institution of vasodilators (e.g., nitroprusside) or inodilators (e.g., milrinone). IABP support should be discontinued as soon as the patient stabilizes or complications develop. Complications associated with the IABP increase with longer duration of use and include vascular injury, thrombocytopenia from the mechanical destruction of platelets, and limb ischemia because of reduced blood flow in the artery into which the IABP catheter is inserted. Heparin anticoagulation is usually given with IABP because the device has a large, thrombogenic surface area. Infectious complications are uncommon when the use is limited to less than 7 days. Reviews of clinical studies investigating the use of the IABP in cardiogenic shock have found no differences in 30-day mortality and an increase in the risk of bleeding complications and stroke.[68,69] Despite the lack of evidence, this device is recommended as reasonable to consider for patients after ST-elevation MI and is commonly used to support patients with cardiogenic shock.[50]

Newer devices have been developed (TandemHeart, Impella) that augment CO directly and decrease the load on the LV.[68] These small pumps are placed percutaneously in the cardiac catheterization laboratory, avoiding major cardiac surgery. They are best used for temporary circulatory support until more definitive therapy is available. Systemic anticoagulation is required with these devices. Complications of the TandemHeart include vascular injury, limb ischemia, cardiac tamponade, thrombo- or air-embolism, and hemolysis. The most common adverse effects of the Impella include vascular injury, thrombosis, thrombocytopenia, bleeding, and hemolysis.

Advanced circulatory assist devices are evolving rapidly and are available in centers with access to cardiac surgical procedures. Most patients currently receive second- or third-generation, continuous flow devices (HeartMate II, Jarvik 2000, HeartWare) because of their superior survival rates and lower incidence of adverse events.[70] Mechanical assistance with these devices is used for patients with cardiogenic shock who need support while awaiting definitive, corrective therapy or as a bridging mechanism before cardiac transplantation. An improvement in survival rates with newer generation devices has allowed their long-term use as destination therapies in patients with severe cardiac failure despite optimal pharmacotherapy that are not transplant candidates. The high cost of these devices and need for experienced physicians will undoubtedly limit their use to only the most severely ill patients.

In summary, J.S.'s condition has continued to deteriorate since his admission to the ICU. Attempts at stabilizing his hemodynamic parameters with dopamine and dobutamine have failed. This is evidenced by inadequate tissue perfusion, which is reflected clinically by his continued lactic acidosis, decreased urine output, reduced bowel sounds, and central nervous system obtundation. Norepinephrine and epinephrine should be considered at this point to restore intra-arterial pressure and tissue perfusion. Intra-aortic counterpulsation can provide synergistic temporary support for J.S.

SEPTIC SHOCK

Distributive Shock

Distributive shock is characterized by an overt loss of vascular tone, causing acute tissue hypoperfusion. Although numerous events such as anaphylaxis or neurogenic causes can initiate distributive shock, most cases are readily reversed by supportive measures and treatment or elimination of the underlying cause.

SEPTIC SHOCK

Distributive shock secondary to sepsis, or septic shock, is associated with a high mortality rate, reflecting the limited therapeutic options available at this time. Over 1,500,000 cases of sepsis syndrome are seen annually in the United States. Mortality rates are as high as 50%.[71] The combination of degree of organ dysfunction and number of failing organs is the strongest predictor of death. Epidemiologic studies show that approximately 25% of cases of sepsis syndrome eventually result in septic shock. It has been projected that the incidence of sepsis will increase 1.5% per year mainly because of the disproportionate growth of the elderly in the US population, increasing burden of chronic health conditions, rising numbers of immunocompromised patients, and multidrug-resistant infections.[3,4,71–73]

The guidelines committee of the Surviving Sepsis Campaign—an international consortium of professional societies involved in critical care, infectious diseases, and emergency medicine—defines *sepsis* syndrome as life-threatening organ dysfunction caused by a dysregulated host response to infection (see Table 17-8 for definitions).[4] Organ dysfunction is identified as an acute change in total Sequential Organ Failure Assessment (SOFA) score by at least 2 points consequent to the infection (see Table 17-9 for SOFA calculation). In patients without preexisting organ dysfunction, the baseline SOFA score is assumed to be zero. Persons with an overall SOFA score of at least 2 may have a 25-times higher risk of mortality compared to those with a score less than 2. A new bedside clinical score termed quickSOFA (qSOFA) can easily identify persons that are more likely to have poor outcomes. Adults with suspected infection are expected to fare worse if they have at least two of three clinical criteria: RR of 22 breaths/minute or greater, altered mentation (Glasgow Coma Scale score <15), or SBP of 100 mm Hg or less. When hypotension persists despite adequate fluid resuscitation and requires vasopressor support to maintain a MAP of at least 65 mm Hg while also having a serum lactate level above 2 mmol/L, it is termed *septic shock*. Septic shock is associated with a higher risk of mortality. Persons most at risk for septic shock are those who are immunocompromised or have underlying conditions that render them susceptible to bloodstream invasion. Groups at risk include neonates, the elderly, patients with acquired immune deficiency syndrome, alcoholics, childbearing

Table 17-8
International Sepsis Definitions Task Force Definitions

Infection	Pathologic process caused by the invasion of normally sterile tissue or fluid or body cavity by pathogenic or potentially pathogenic microorganisms. (Noted exception: *Clostridium difficile* colitis does not occur in a sterile colon)
Bacteremia	The presence of viable bacteria in the blood.
Sepsis	Life-threatening organ dysfunction caused by a dysregulated host response to infection.
Organ dysfunction	Identified as an acute change in total SOFA score ≥2 points consequent to the infection.
Septic shock	A subset of sepsis in which underlying circulatory and cellular/metabolic abnormalities are profound enough to substantially increase mortality. Persistent sepsis-induced hypotension requiring vasopressors to maintain MAP ≥65 mm Hg and having a serum lactate level >2 mmol/L despite adequate fluid resuscitation. Patients who are on inotropic or vasopressor agents may not be hypotensive at the time that perfusion abnormalities are measured.
Multiple organ dysfunction syndrome	Presence of progressive organ dysfunction in an acutely ill patient, such that homeostasis cannot be maintained without intervention.

MAP, mean arterial pressure; SOFA, Sequential Organ Failure Assessment.
Source: Singer M et al. The third international consensus definitions for sepsis and septic shock (Sepsis-3). *JAMA*. 2016;315(8):801–810.

Table 17-9
Sequential Organ Failure Assessment Score

System	Score				
	0	1	2	3	4
PaO_2/FiO_2, mm Hg	≥400	<400	<300	<200 with respiratory support	<100 with respiratory support
Platelets, $\times 10^3/\mu L$	≥150	<150	<100	<50	<20
Bilirubin, mg/dL	<1.2	1.2–1.9	2–5.9	6–11.9	>12
Cardiovascular	MAP ≥ 70 mm Hg	MAP <70 mm Hg	DA < 5[a] or DOB (any dose)	DA 5.1–15 or Epi ≤0.1 or NE ≤0.1[a]	DA > 15 or Epi > 0.1 or NE > 0.1[a]
GCS score[b]	15	13–14	10–12	6–9	<6
Creatinine, mg/dL	<1.2	1.2–1.9	2–3.4	3.5–4.9	>5
Urine output, mL/day				<500	<200

DA, dopamine; DOB, dobutamine; Epi, epinephrine; FiO_2, fraction of inspired oxygen; GCS, Glasgow Coma Scale; MAP, mean arterial pressure; NE, norepinephrine; PaO_2, arterial partial pressure of oxygen.
[a]Catecholamine doses are expressed as mcg/kg/minute for at least 1 hour.
[b]GCS scores range from 3 to 15; higher score indicating better neurologic function.
Source: Singer M et al. The third international consensus definitions for sepsis and septic shock (Sepsis-3). *JAMA*. 2016;315(8):801–810.

women, and those undergoing surgery or who have experienced trauma. Other predisposing factors include coexisting diseases such as diabetes mellitus, malignancies, chronic hepatic or renal failure, and hyposplenism; exposure to immunosuppressant drugs and cancer chemotherapy; and procedures such as insertion of urinary catheters, endotracheal tubes, and IV lines.

Septic shock is characterized initially by a normal or high CO and a low SVR (Table 17-3). Hypotension is caused by the low SVR and alterations in macrovascular and microvascular tone, which result in maldistribution of blood flow and volume. Changes in the microvasculature can lead to loss of normal microvascular autoregulatory mechanisms, resulting in constriction of capillaries, changes in cellular rheology, fibrin deposition, and neutrophil adherence. This causes vascular "sludging" and, in some cases, arteriovenous shunts that bypass capillary beds. Loss of intravascular fluid caused by increased vascular permeability and third spacing of fluid further adds to hypovolemia.[74] In an effort to compensate for the changes in volume and SVR, the body goes into a hyperdynamic state and increases CO. Most patients exhibit myocardial dysfunction as manifested by decreased myocardial compliance, reduced contractility, and ventricular dilation, but they maintain a normal CO because of tachycardia and cardiac dilatation which increases or maintains preload.[75] Although the cause of, and mechanism for, this abnormality is not fully understood, it is not believed to be attributable to myocardial ischemia. Rather, it is thought to be caused by one or more circulating inflammatory mediators, such as cytokines (e.g., interleukin-1), tumor necrosis factor-α (TNF-α), platelet-activating factor, arachidonic acid, nitric oxide (NO), and reactive oxygen species. In late septic shock, the body is no longer able to compensate because of the cardiac effects of the inflammatory mediators and resultant myocardial edema, thus resulting in a decreased CO. The end product of this complicated pathway is cellular ischemia, dysfunction, and eventually cellular death unless the chain of events is interrupted.

The complex pathogenesis of sepsis is more fully understood now, but some of the exact mechanisms are still not completely clear. The changes that take place during sepsis are caused by the immunologic host response to infection, which involves inflammatory (SIRS) and immunodepressive (compensatory anti-inflammatory response) mediators that are present from the onset of the immune response.[76]

The inflammatory stage of sepsis is initiated by an infection with a microorganism, most commonly bacterial. Organisms can either enter the bloodstream directly (producing positive blood cultures) or may indirectly elicit a systemic inflammatory response by locally releasing their toxins or structural components at the site of infection. The lipopolysaccharide endotoxin of gram-negative bacteria is the most potent soluble product of bacteria that can initiate a response and is the most studied, but other bacterial products can initiate the response, including exotoxins, enterotoxins, peptidoglycans, and lipoteichoic acid from gram-positive organisms. The binding of these toxins to cell receptors promotes proinflammatory cytokine production, primarily TNF-α and interleukin-1 (IL-1). These toxins stimulate the production and release of numerous endogenous mediators that are responsible for the inflammatory consequences of sepsis. The cytokines act synergistically to directly affect organ function and stimulate the release of other proinflammatory cytokines, such as IL-6, IL-8, platelet-activating factor, complement, thromboxanes, leukotrienes, prostaglandins, NO, and others.[75]

The presence of these cytokines promotes inflammation and vascular endothelial injury, but it also causes an overwhelming activation in coagulation. Thrombin has potent proinflammatory and procoagulant activities, and its production is increased in sepsis. The human body normally counteracts these effects by increasing fibrinolysis, but the homeostatic mechanisms in the septic patient are dysfunctional. There are decreases in the levels of protein C, plasminogen, and antithrombin III as well as increased activity of plasminogen activator inhibitor-1 and thrombin-activatable fibrinolysis inhibitor, endogenous agents that inhibit fibrinolysis.[76] The patient is in a coagulopathic state, which promotes formation of microvascular thrombi, leading to hypoperfusion, ischemia, and, ultimately, organ failure. Multiple organ failure is responsible for about half the deaths caused by septic shock.[77]

The clinical features of sepsis are highly variable and depend on multiple factors: site of infection, causative organism, degree of organ dysfunction, baseline patient health status, and delay to initial treatment.[78] The working definition of sepsis accounts for the presence of systemic manifestations of infection and organ dysfunction, which may be subtle (Table 17-8). Serum biomarkers are the subject of intense research as they could aid the early diagnosis of sepsis, guide treatment, and predict outcomes. Most biomarkers have not been extensively studied and few are in clinical use (e.g., C-reactive protein, procalcitonin, sTREM-1, CD64, pancreatic stone protein).[79] Most of these biomarkers have high negative predictive values, but lack high specificity and positive predictive value.

Characteristic laboratory findings include leukocytosis or leukopenia, thrombocytopenia with or without coagulation abnormalities, and, often, hyperbilirubinemia. These features are usually readily detectable and occur within 24 hours after bacteremia develops, particularly if gram-negative organisms cause the bacteremia. In extremes of age (very young or very old) or in debilitated patients, hypothermia can be present and positive findings may be limited to unexplained hypotension, mental confusion, and hyperventilation.

Persons dying of septic shock often have a normal or elevated CO. Death within the first week after the onset of sepsis occurs as a result of intractable hypotension that is secondary to significantly depressed SVR. This causes extensive maldistribution of blood flow in the microvasculature, with subsequent tissue hypoxia and development of lactic acidosis. Death occurring beyond the first week usually is caused by multiple organ failure that began during acute circulatory failure. Severe, unresponsive hypotension as a result of a decreased CO occurs in a subpopulation of patients with septic shock; cardiogenic shock becomes superimposed on the distributive shock of sepsis, but this is a less common cause of death.[80]

Clinical and Hemodynamic Features

CASE 17-4

QUESTION 1: E.B., a 71-year-old woman, presents to the ED from a skilled nursing facility with a several day history of low-grade fever, rigors, and chills. She does not report a history of nausea or vomiting but had exceedingly poor oral intake for several days prior to admission.

E.B. has a history of diabetes mellitus type 2, hypertension, chronic kidney disease stage II, dyslipidemia, coronary artery disease, obesity, and peripheral arterial disease. She has a history of a transient ischemic attack and right lower extremity below-the-knee amputation.

Physical findings include a temperature of 38.7°C, BP 95/60 mm Hg, pulse 120 beats/minute, and RR 28 breaths/minute with oxygen saturation 95% on 2 L/minute nasal cannula. E.B. weighs 102 kg and is 65 inches tall. A Foley catheter is placed in her bladder and her urine output is 0.4 mL/kg/hour. The chest radiograph shows an enlarged heart, low lung volumes, and a distended, gas-filled stomach but no focal airspace disease, pneumothorax, or pleural effusion. Her left lower extremity has foul-smelling, purulent drainage from the posterior heel, surrounding erythema with macerated areas, and the heel is tender to the touch. E.B. has 3+ edema in the foot and lower extremity but no other significant findings aside from the heel ulcer. The patient also has a large stage III sacral decubitus ulcer with several open wound areas and serosanguinous drainage.

Pertinent laboratory values are as follows:

WBC count, 19,500 cells/μL
BUN, 58 mg/dL
SCr, 2.2 mg/dL
Na, 131 mEq/L
Glucose, 58 mg/dL
Albumin, 1.6 g/dL
ABG measurements on 2 L/minute nasal cannula (FiO_2 27%) are as follows:

PaO_2, 98 mm Hg
$PaCO_2$, 32 mm Hg
HCO_3^-, 16 mEq/L
pH, 7.31

Urine, sputum, blood, and deep tissue wound samples are sent for culture and sensitivity. A fluid bolus of 1,000 mL of normal saline solution is given. Arterial and pulmonary artery catheters are inserted, revealing the following hemodynamic profile:

BP (S/D/M), 90/48/62 mm Hg
HR, 122 beats/minute
CO, 7.1 L/minute
CI, 3.4 L/minute/m^2
PCWP, 10 mm Hg
SVR, 720 dyne·s·cm^{-5}

What hemodynamic and clinical features of E.B. are consistent with septic shock?

E.B. would not be classified in septic shock at this time because she has not been adequately fluid resuscitated. Though, she would be classified as having sepsis because of the manifestations of infection and organ dysfunction.

Hemodynamic signs consistent with sepsis include hypotension, tachycardia, elevated CO, low SVR, and low PCWP. Although the absolute value for CO is high or at the upper limits of the normal range, in septic shock it is inadequate to maintain a BP that will perfuse the essential organs in the face of a decreased SVR, evidenced by a low $\dot{D}O_2$ and $\dot{V}O_2$. E.B. has a metabolic acidosis (pH 7.31, $PaCO_2$ 32 mm Hg, HCO_3^- 16 mEq/L), indicating anaerobic metabolism and lactic acidosis most likely caused by decreased perfusion, and a CO that is inadequate to meet the oxygen requirements of the tissues.

Other features consistent with sepsis in E.B. include declining urine output indicating decreased renal perfusion, hypoglycemia, a rising WBC count, and a spiking fever.

Therapeutic Approach

The management of septic shock is directed toward three primary areas: (a) eradication of the source of infection, (b) hemodynamic support and control of tissue hypoxia, and (c) inhibition or attenuation of the initiators and mediators of sepsis.

ERADICATING THE SOURCE OF INFECTION

CASE 17-4, QUESTION 2: What factors should be considered in determining antimicrobial therapy in septic shock? What are the potential sources of infection in E.B.?

Systemic infection caused by either aerobic or anaerobic bacteria is the leading cause of septic shock. Fungal, mycobacterial, rickettsial, protozoal, or viral infections can also be encountered. Among sepsis syndromes caused by aerobic bacteria, gram-negative organisms (e.g., *Pseudomonas*, Enterobacteriaceae, and *Acinetobacter*, in decreasing order of frequency) are implicated slightly more often than gram-positive bacteria (e.g., *Staphylococcus aureus*, *Enterococcus*, *Staphylococcus* epidermidis, and *Streptococcus*, from highest to lowest frequency). Even these trends vary, however, depending on the infection site. For example, when an organism can actually be cultured in the blood, slightly more gram-positive infections (35% to 40%) than gram-negative infections (30% to 35%) are found. In non-bloodstream infections (e.g., respiratory tract, genitourinary system, and the abdomen, in descending order of frequency) 40% to 45% can be attributed to gram-negative organisms, and 20% to 25% are caused by gram-positive organisms.[71] Polymicrobial infections make up the next largest group, followed by fungi, anaerobes, and others. In up to 33% of sepsis syndrome cases, no organisms can be isolated. Careful consideration of the patient's history and clinical presentation often reveals the most likely cause.

Eradicating the source of infection involves the early administration of antimicrobial therapy, and, if indicated, surgical drainage. The use of an appropriate antibiotic regimen within 1 hour of the diagnosis of sepsis or septic shock is associated with a significant increase in survival. Appropriate cultures should be obtained before starting antibiotic therapy, unless this would result in a significant (greater than 45 minutes) delay in therapy.[4] The selection of antibiotics should take into account the presumed site of infection; whether the infection is community- or health care-associated; recent invasive procedures, manipulations, or surgery; any predisposing conditions; drug intolerances; and the likelihood of drug resistance. Ideally, the primary source of infection can be determined and therapy specifically tailored to the most likely organisms. If the source of infection is unclear, however, early institution of broad-spectrum antibiotics against all likely pathogens is generally recommended while awaiting culture results. Empiric broad-spectrum therapy usually requires combinations of antimicrobials because of the increasing frequency of polymicrobial infections and antimicrobial resistance. Even so, there are no data demonstrating better outcomes with combination therapy over adequate monotherapy, except in severely ill, septic patients with a high risk of death.[4,78] Empiric regimens must be determined by patient factors and broad enough to cover all likely pathogens. Mortality for septic shock may be as much as fivefold higher when an empiric regimen fails to cover the offending pathogen.[4] Because a wide range of variables must be considered in the selection of empiric regimens (e.g., anatomic site of infection, pathogen prevalence, resistance patterns), a specific regimen cannot be recommended for all episodes of sepsis or septic shock (see Chapter 62, Principles of Infectious Diseases). Generally, empiric regimens target gram-positive cocci, aerobic gram-negative bacilli, as well as anaerobes and include (1) an anti-pseudomonal penicillin, third- or fourth-generation cephalosporin, or carbapenem plus (2) vancomycin to cover methicillin-resistant *Staphylococcus aureus*. Combination gram-negative coverage (e.g., aminoglycoside, fluoroquinolone) is recommended for critically ill patients at risk of infection with difficult-to-treat, multidrug-resistant pathogens, such as *Pseudomonas* and *Acinetobacter* spp. Additional coverage should be considered based on the presence of other risk factors (e.g., *Candida* species, atypical pathogens).

Individuals with diabetes are presumed to be at an increased risk of infection because of multiple host factors, including hyperglycemia-induced immunosuppression, vascular insufficiency, peripheral neuropathies, and colonization with *S. aureus* and *Candida* species. The most likely potential sources of sepsis in E.B. are a combination of skin and soft tissue infections. E.B. has a severe diabetic foot infection involving her left heel with inflammation, purulence, and systemic manifestations of infection. She also has a large stage III sacral decubitus ulcer. A urinary tract infection and vulvovaginal candidiasis should be considered as well because of her history of diabetes. Other sources of infection are less likely based on her presentation. All IV catheters from the skilled nursing facility should be changed if possible.

Infected pressure ulcers and diabetic foot infections are usually polymicrobial wounds. These infections should be treated with parenteral broad-spectrum antibiotics to cover methicillin-sensitive and methicillin-resistant *S. aureus*, *Streptococcus* spp., Enterobacteriaceae, *Pseudomonas aeruginosa*, and obligate anaerobes (e.g., *Peptostreptococcus*, *Peptococcus*, *Bacteroides fragilis*, and *Clostridium perfringens*). As such, empiric therapy should include vancomycin in combination with one of the following: piperacillin–tazobactam, ceftazidime, ceftaroline, cefepime, aztreonam, or a carbapenem. If aztreonam or a cephalosporin is chosen then metronidazole or clindamycin should be considered to cover anaerobic organisms, particularly for ischemic or necrotic wounds.[81,82] Drainage, debridement, and wound dressing should accompany antibiotic therapy. Antimicrobial therapy should be adjusted once cultures are finalized.

INITIAL STABILIZATION

CASE 17-4, QUESTION 3: What are the immediate goals of therapy in E.B.? How can they be achieved and assessed?

The goals in treating septic shock, in addition to eradicating the precipitating infection, are to optimize $\dot{D}O_2$ to the tissues and to control abnormal use of oxygen and anaerobic metabolism by reducing the tissue oxygen demand. Tissue injury is widespread during sepsis, most likely because of vascular endothelial injury with fluid extravasation and microthromboses, which decrease oxygen and substrate utilization by the affected tissues. The mainstay of therapy is volume expansion to increase intravascular volume, enhance CO, and ultimately delay associated development of refractory tissue hypoxia.

Increasing CO with fluids will improve capillary circulation and tissue oxygenation by maintaining sufficient intravascular volume. At least 30 mL/kg of IV crystalloid fluid should be given within the first 3 hours of resuscitation.[4] If fluids do not correct the hypoxia or if filling pressures are increased, the sequential addition of vasopressors and inotropic agents is indicated. Blood transfusions should be used if the Hgb is less than 7 g/dL unless there is an active source of bleeding, severe hypoxemia, or a history of cardiac disease, in which case the Hgb value would be maintained at a higher value.[4] Crystalloids (with electrolytes to correct imbalances) should be initiated to maintain the CI goal as well as a MAP of 65 mm Hg. Although MAP is not an absolute measure of blood flow to all vital organs, it is considered the therapeutic end point that will sustain myocardial and cerebral perfusion. A higher MAP could be considered in septic patients with a history of hypertension or those who clinically improve with a higher BP.[1] After optimization with fluid therapy, vasopressor and inotropic agents are indicated if the patient remains hypotensive with a low CI or if signs of inadequate tissue perfusion persist.

The therapeutic goals used for hemodynamic resuscitation are controversial. The issue is whether therapy should be directed to physiologic end points of tissue perfusion or clinical end points, such as BP and urine output. The physiologic end points include clearance of blood lactate concentrations, base deficit, SvO_2, and increased CO. Serum lactate concentrations may be elevated through various mechanisms (e.g., tissue hypoxia, excessive beta-adrenergic stimulation, liver failure) but are associated with worse outcomes regardless of the source. Lactate-guided resuscitation of patients in septic shock is recommended because of its association with a significantly reduced mortality rate compared with usual care.[4]

Many institutions have developed "sepsis bundles" that incorporate these same variables and therapeutic end points as early as possible in the treatment of sepsis. Sepsis bundles often include many additional issues addressed in the Surviving Sepsis Campaign Guidelines,[4] such as ventilatory support, initial choice of antibiotics, glucose control, and stress ulcer prophylaxis.

One study by Rivers et al. combined physiologic and clinical end points of resuscitation during the early stages of sepsis.[83] CVP, MAP, Hct, and $ScvO_2$ were optimized during at least 6 hours of continuous care in the ED. This was compared to conventional therapy that targeted only CVP, MAP, and urine output. In-hospital mortality was significantly lower in the early goal-directed therapy

(EGDT) group (30.5% vs. 46.5%, $p = 0.009$). EGDT was adopted as the standard of care in the treatment of sepsis and septic shock. However, there are several limitations to the EGDT approach. As noted above, CVP is an unpredictable marker of fluid resuscitation,[38] and fluid overload is common after EGDT resuscitation. Furthermore, the Hct target of 30% is unnecessarily high because transfusions of PRBCs to achieve a Hgb above 7 g/dL do not increase $ScvO_2$. Finally, dobutamine could also be harmful if used to increase $ScvO_2$ in patients with unevaluated ventricular function.[84]

Several large, multicenter studies have shown no improvement in patient outcomes using EGDT for severe sepsis and septic shock. Protocol-based resuscitation did not improve in-hospital mortality among 1,341 patients in the ProCESS study.[85] In the ARISE and ProMISe studies, EGDT did not reduce all-cause mortality compared to usual care.[86,87] The mortality rates among the usual care groups from these trials (18.9%,[85] 18.8%,[86] 29.2%[87]) were similar to the EGDT group in the Rivers et al. study. These findings could be because of an improvement in our standard of care over that time period, chiefly the early identification and treatment. Nonetheless, the most recent Surviving Sepsis Campaign Guidelines[4] have departed from the EGDT-guided resuscitation strategy from the Rivers study.

E.B. should receive fluid boluses to maintain perfusion with a MAP of at least 65 mm Hg. Reassessment of E.B.'s hemodynamic status should include a thorough clinical examination as well as assessment of available physiologic variables (e.g., HR, BP, SaO_2, RR, temperature, urine output) and measurements from her PA catheter. A minimum of 30 mL/kg crystalloid fluid challenge is recommended within the first 3 hours of resuscitation. Albumin may be substituted if large volumes of crystalloids are required, but hydroxyethyl starches should be avoided because of an increased risk of acute renal dysfunction and potential increased mortality.[4] Continued, excessive fluid challenges to increase preload in E.B. must be approached cautiously because she has an enlarged heart on chest radiograph, coronary artery disease, and multiple risk factors for heart failure. In addition, patients in septic shock are susceptible to experiencing non-cardiogenic pulmonary edema or ARDS, which can cause severe deterioration in pulmonary function. Fluid boluses should be given with ongoing monitoring to determine the CVP and PCWP at which CO is maximal. This approach will avoid excessive CVP and PCWP beyond which CO is no longer increased, reducing potential pulmonary edema.

In summary, the immediate goal of therapy is to maximize $\dot{D}O_2$ to the tissues. Fluid resuscitation is the mainstay of therapy and improves $\dot{D}O_2$ by increasing CO; however, inotropic and vasopressor agents are often required for additional cardiovascular support. A favorable response to immediate resuscitative efforts will be reflected by a reversal or halt in the progression of the metabolic acidosis, improved sensorium, and increased urine output. In E.B., surgical evaluation and debridement and selection of appropriate antibiotics while maintaining hemodynamic support are the clinical goals of therapy.

HEMODYNAMIC MANAGEMENT

Fluid Therapy Versus Inotropic Support

CASE 17-4, QUESTION 4: E.B. is given three 1,000-mL fluid boluses, and norepinephrine is begun at a rate of 0.05 mcg/kg/minute. During the next 2 hours, she receives 4 L of fluid in boluses, and the norepinephrine is increased to 0.3 mcg/kg/minute to maintain her BP. She does not have signs of pulmonary edema. E.B. has the following hemodynamic profile (previous values in parentheses):

BP (S/D/M), 95/48/64 mm Hg (90/48/62 mm Hg)
HR, 124 beats/minute (122 beats/minute)
CO, 8 L/minute (7.1 L/minute)
CI, 3.8 L/minute/m^2 (3.4 L/minute/m^2)
CVP, 12 mm Hg (7 mm Hg)
PCWP, 16 mm Hg (10 mm Hg)
SVR, 550 dyne·s·cm^{-5} (720 dyne·s·cm^{-5})
Urine output, 0.25 mL/kg/hour (0.4 mL/kg/hour)
PaO_2, 85 mm Hg (98 mm Hg)
$PaCO_2$, 36 mm Hg (32 mm Hg)
HCO_3^-, 17 mEq/L (16 mEq/L)
pH, 7.3 (7.31)
$\dot{D}O_2$, 534 mL/minute (508 mL/minute)
$\dot{V}O_2$, 198 mL/minute (324 mL/minute)

Which of the following therapeutic considerations would be reasonable for E.B. at this time: additional fluid boluses, an increase in the norepinephrine infusion rate, or initiation of a different vasopressor?

E.B. continues to be hypotensive despite a PCWP of 16 mm Hg and a norepinephrine infusion rate of 0.3 mcg/kg/minute. The goals of therapy remain the same (i.e., maximize arterial oxygen content and $\dot{D}O_2$ to reverse cellular anaerobic metabolism).

E.B.'s PaO_2 of 85 mm Hg correlates with an oxygen–hemoglobin saturation of approximately 96%, which should provide an adequate arterial oxygen content. However, $\dot{D}O_2$ still may be inadequate despite the CI being above 3.5 L/minute/m^2 because $\dot{D}O_2$ and $\dot{V}O_2$ have not reached normal levels. E.B.'s Hgb and Hct should be checked to ensure adequate oxygen-carrying capacity in the blood. In addition, decreased tissue oxygen utilization can contribute to the continued acidosis. Further attempts to enhance the CI and, hence, $\dot{D}O_2$ are appropriate. E.B. has a dilated heart and a history of cardiovascular disease and chronic kidney disease that will influence the choice of therapeutic options.

Although fluid administration is the mainstay of therapy in septic shock, the elevation of E.B.'s PCWP to 16 mm Hg without a significant increase in CO suggests that an optimal PCWP has been reached. Therefore, additional fluid therapy to maintain BP may cause pulmonary edema and compromise pulmonary gas exchange. A plot of CO versus PCWP (ventricular function curve) would provide a more accurate assessment of the PCWP at which CO is maximal. Additional fluid boluses at this time should be used only to maintain the current level of intravascular volume status.

VASOPRESSORS AND INOTROPIC AGENTS

When fluid therapy fails to maintain a satisfactory MAP despite an elevated CO, the use of a vasopressor should be considered. Maintaining a goal MAP does not correlate with decreased mortality, but it helps sustain myocardial and cerebral perfusion. If it is necessary to increase CO, then inotropic agents should be used. Although the use of inotropic agents is well established, controlled comparative studies have not clearly determined which agent, or combination of agents, is most useful in the management of septic shock. Because differences among the inotropic agents are significant, however, selection of the most appropriate drug should be guided by careful consideration of the patient's hemodynamic status.

Norepinephrine and Dopamine

Norepinephrine is predominantly an α-adrenergic agonist (Table 17-7) and is the recommended first-line vasopressor for sepsis.[4] Norepinephrine has been titrated to 0.3 mcg/kg/min, but E.B.'s HR will likely limit the utility of further increases in the dose.

Dopamine has frequently been another initial pharmacologic agent chosen for the treatment of septic shock. A trial that randomized 1,679 patients with shock to dopamine or norepinephrine for BP support found no significant difference in the primary outcome of 28-day mortality but an increased risk of arrhythmic events with dopamine.[60] A meta-analysis of six randomized trials of septic patients found dopamine was associated with an increased risk of death and arrhythmias compared to norepinephrine.[88] Similarly, another meta-analysis that included six randomized trials found norepinephrine was associated with a lower in-hospital and 28-day mortality compared to dopamine as well as a lower incidence of arrhythmias.[89]

In light of these findings, the Surviving Sepsis Campaign relegated dopamine from a first-line to alternative vasopressor. Dopamine is now reserved for patients with absolute or relative bradycardia and a low risk of tachyarrhythmias, which is difficult to predict.[4] Accordingly, dopamine is not an appropriate therapeutic option for E.B.

Low-dose dopamine should not be used for renal protective purposes.[4] Despite the improvement in renal blood flow and a possible increase in urine output, dopamine does not decrease the time to recovery of renal function or the need for renal replacement therapy.

Epinephrine

Epinephrine stimulates α-, β_1-, and β_2-adrenergic receptors (Table 17-7). CO is augmented via increased contractility and HR, with the contribution of each being highly variable. Blood vessels in the kidney, skin, and mucosa constrict in response to α-adrenergic stimulation, whereas vessels in the skeletal muscle vasodilate because of β_2 effects. A biphasic response in SVR is observed as β_2-receptors are activated at the lower range and α_1-receptors are stimulated at higher infusion rates. The improvement in CO, therefore, may be negated by an increase in afterload at higher dosages.

Historically, epinephrine was reserved as a last-line therapy because of the studies that showed harmful splanchnic and renal vasculature effects and elevated lactate levels. Despite these effects, there are no clinical studies showing that epinephrine causes worse outcomes in sepsis. In fact, two prospective, double-blind, randomized controlled trials comparing epinephrine and norepinephrine in patients with septic shock found similar mortality rates, time to hemodynamic recovery, and time to vasopressor withdrawal.[90,91] Both studies showed lower arterial pH values associated with impaired serum lactate clearance in the epinephrine-treated groups. Therefore, lactate clearance would not be recommended to guide resuscitation when utilizing epinephrine.

Epinephrine is recommended as adjunctive therapy to norepinephrine to maintain adequate MAP.[4] However, if tachyarrhythmias are limiting the use or norepinephrine, epinephrine is likely to produce similar effects because it also stimulates β_1-receptors. Consequently, it is not appropriate to substitute epinephrine for norepinephrine at this time for E.B.

Vasopressin

Catecholamines have been the mainstay of treatment to support BP in septic patients once adequate fluid resuscitation has been achieved. Sepsis, however, can cause a decrease in responsiveness to catecholamines, resulting in refractory hypotension, possibly because of down-regulation of adrenergic receptors or altered receptor relative binding affinities in hypoxic and acidotic conditions.[59] Vasopressin is an endogenous hormone that has very little effect on BP under normal conditions, but it becomes important in maintaining BP when the baroreceptor reflex is impaired. In contrast to the catecholamines, vasopressin's effects are relatively preserved in hypoxic and acidotic states.[59]

Vasopressin's direct vasoconstricting actions are mediated by the vascular V_{1a} receptors coupled to phospholipase C.[59,92] When these receptors are activated, calcium is released from the sarcoplasmic reticulum in smooth muscle cells, leading to vasoconstriction. Vasopressin levels peak in early septic shock and decrease to low-normal levels in most patients within 48 hours. This phenomenon is coined a "relative vasopressin deficiency" because higher vasopressin levels would be expected in hypotensive states.

The VASST study compared norepinephrine to vasopressin in patients with septic shock, who were unresponsive to fluids and assessed mortality at 28 days.[93] Vasopressin 0.01 to 0.03 units/minute added to norepinephrine was compared to norepinephrine monotherapy. Vasopressin significantly decreased the amount of norepinephrine required; however, there was no difference in mortality between the treatment groups except when the patients were stratified according to severity of sepsis. The patients with less severe septic shock benefited from vasopressin therapy. This study evaluated vasopressin as a catecholamine-sparing drug rather than as rescue therapy for catecholamine-unresponsive shock, which was how it was studied in previous trials.

Small studies have shown vasopressin to be as effective as catecholamines in achieving blood pressure control with no difference in mortality, but vasopressin is not recommended as first-line therapy because of a delayed physiologic response.[4,92] Instead, low-dose vasopressin (up to 0.03 units/minute) is recommended to synergistically achieve the goal MAP with norepinephrine or allow norepinephrine dose reductions.[4] Doses higher than 0.03 to 0.04 units/minute are only recommended as salvage therapy.[4]

E.B. has a decreased MAP despite the increased titration of norepinephrine. The optimal time to consider additional or alternative therapies to norepinephrine is unknown. Because patients in septic shock have decreased endogenous levels of vasopressin, it would be reasonable to add vasopressin at 0.03 units/minute to increase the MAP and renal perfusion.

Phenylephrine

Phenylephrine is a pure α-adrenergic agonist (Table 17-7) and, thus, increases systolic, diastolic, and mean arterial pressures through vasoconstriction. Reflex bradycardia can occur secondarily because of the absence of β-adrenergic effects. The increase in afterload, while increasing myocardial $\dot{V}O_2$, correspondingly increases coronary blood flow because of increased perfusion pressure and autoregulation. In patients with myocardial hypoxia, or in those experiencing atrial or ventricular arrhythmias, phenylephrine can be beneficial because it has minimal direct cardiac effects. In situations in which the CO is decreased, phenylephrine can be detrimental. Preload is reduced as plasma fluid is lost owing to increased capillary hydrostatic pressure, forcing water and solutes from the vascular space into the interstitial spaces. This response, in addition to the increased afterload and reflex bradycardia, may significantly impair CO (Table 17-7). Therefore, phenylephrine should be reserved for treating septic shock in the following patients: (a) those with arrhythmias on norepinephrine, (b) those with high CO but persistent hypotension, or (c) those who fail to achieve the goal MAP on combination inotropes/vasopressors and low-dose vasopressin. Phenylephrine is a reasonable alternative therapy for E.B. if her hypotension and tachycardia persist despite the addition of vasopressin.

Dobutamine

Tissue $\dot{D}O_2$ may be impaired by a suboptimal CO or decreased oxygen-carrying capacity. If tissue hypoperfusion persists after optimizing fluid status, achieving the goal MAP, and assuring an adequate Hgb concentration, then CO should be assessed. Epinephrine and dopamine are inotropic therapies with vasoconstricting properties, but dobutamine is the recommended first-line inotropic agent in the management of septic shock.[4] Dobutamine produces a greater increase in CO than dopamine, but it also lowers SVR. In contrast to dopamine, dobutamine lowers PCWP and causes less pulmonary shunting. Because dobutamine can lower ventricular filling pressure, volume status must be monitored closely to avoid the development of hypotension and reduced MAP. Fluids should be administered as needed to maintain the PCWP at optimal and tolerated levels of 15 to 18 mm Hg. With the administration of greater amounts of fluid, CO, $\dot{D}O_2$, and systemic $\dot{V}O_2$ are significantly increased. Dobutamine increases $\dot{D}O_2$ and CI when given concurrently with or after volume resuscitation, and it may independently increase capillary perfusion regardless of systemic effects.[51] Decreases in PaO_2 and increases in venous PO_2, as well as adverse effects on myocardium, may be evident at higher dosages (above 6 mcg/kg/minute).[94]

Combinations of vasopressors and inotropic agents can also be used to achieve desired hemodynamic parameters. GI perfusion can be compromised owing to the vasoconstricting effects of catecholamines and may play a role in the pathogenesis of multiple organ dysfunction.[65] Currently, it is unknown whether a specific catecholamine regimen provides a significant benefit over others. There are conflicting data about which vasopressor can increase gastric perfusion and whether this increase can alter progression to organ dysfunction.

CASE 17-4, QUESTION 5: Given E.B.'s history of cardiovascular disease, what factors should you consider before initiating an inotropic or alternative vasopressor agent? Outline an overall approach to maintaining adequate hemodynamic status.

E.B. has a history of coronary artery disease and is susceptible to myocardial ischemia. Therefore, a careful balance must be achieved between myocardial $\dot{V}O_2$ and coronary perfusion pressure. Further attempts to optimize MAP and CI with norepinephrine alone could increase myocardial $\dot{V}O_2$ and precipitate ischemia. Evidence suggests that the goal of therapy in treating patients with septic shock, or any form of shock for that matter, is not to simply normalize BP but to optimize $\dot{D}O_2$ and $\dot{V}O_2$. Once anemia and hypoxia have been corrected, CO becomes the remaining parameter that can be adjusted to increase oxygen supply, but raising arterial BP and CO with inotropic agents or vasopressors before restoring adequate blood volume can actually worsen tissue perfusion. Therefore, the patient's current hemodynamic status and the individual properties of those agents that will most effectively maintain or increase the MAP and CO should be considered while selecting an inotropic agent. In many instances, because of individual variability and response, more than one inotropic agent or addition of a vasopressor is required to achieve these end points. These interventions must be made with strict monitoring of the patients' response to the interventions to prevent any adverse consequences, especially in those patients who are predisposed to an adverse event, such as E.B.

It is important to realize that the response to exogenous catecholamines in patients with septic shock is highly variable and a successful regimen in one patient may be unsuccessful in another. In addition, septic patients often require infusion rates in the moderate-to-high range. Therefore, the goal is to use one or more agents at the dosages necessary to achieve the desired end points without unduly compromising the patient's status. The use of catecholamines, however, is only a stabilizing measure. Strict attention to all other physiologic parameters—as well as nutritional support, antibiotic modification, respiratory support, and ongoing surgical intervention—cannot be overemphasized.

OTHER THERAPIES

Therapies directed against the initiators and mediators of sepsis are currently the focus of intense investigation. Numerous exogenous and endogenous substances are involved in the pathogenesis of sepsis within the cytokine and coagulation cascades. Strategies under development include antioxidants and free radical scavengers; anti-endotoxin therapy; and inhibition of leukocytes, secondary mediators (i.e., TNF-α, IL-1, cytokine pathway), coagulation and arachidonic acid metabolites, complement, and NO. The lack of development of successful new therapies over the past two decades is probably because of multiple factors, such as poor clinical trial design, oversimplification of the pathologic process in animal models, and suboptimal patient selection criteria.[79] Although several experimental therapies hold promise for the future, controlled human trials are still lacking.

Corticosteroids

CASE 17-4, QUESTION 6: What is the rationale for the use of glucocorticoids in the treatment of septic shock, and is there evidence to support their use for this indication in E.B.?

The use of corticosteroids in sepsis and septic shock has been a controversial topic for many years. Corticosteroids were originally proposed as a treatment option because of their anti-inflammatory properties with the hope of attenuating the body's response to infection. It has been shown that critically ill patients exhibit impaired cortisol secretion because of a relative adrenocortical insufficiency and a glucocorticoid peripheral resistance syndrome that can also be affected by multiple medications.[95] The Consensus Task Force from the American College of Critical Care Medicine has defined this dysfunction of the hypothalamic–pituitary–adrenal axis as *critical illness–related corticosteroid insufficiency*.[96]

Diagnosis of this condition is intensely debated. Some clinicians recommend a random cortisol level that is below a certain threshold during physiologic stress (i.e., shock) to diagnose adrenal insufficiency; however, this has only been shown to be useful in diagnosing absolute adrenal insufficiency.[4] The traditional assessment method has been the adrenal corticotropin hormone (ACTH) stimulation test with administration of either 1 mcg or 250 mcg of cosyntropin. Though, the ACTH tests only evaluates the adrenal function, not the entire hypothalamic–pituitary–adrenal axis, and lacks sensitivity and specificity in critical illness.[95] Random cortisol levels may be useful for evaluating absolute adrenal insufficiency but have not demonstrated a benefit in septic shock patients. The Surviving Sepsis Campaign does not recommend the ACTH stimulation test or random cortisol levels to identify patients who should receive glucocorticoids.[4]

Clinical trials investigating the use of steroids in septic shock have been performed with varying results. The trial by Annane et al.[97] showed a shortened time to shock reversal and mortality benefit with the use of low doses of hydrocortisone and fludrocortisone in patients with severe septic shock, who exhibited a relative adrenocortical insufficiency (serum cortisol increase less than or equal to 9 mcg/dL in response to ACTH stimulation). The CORTICUS trial[98] showed a faster resolution of shock for those patients on hydrocortisone as evidenced by faster time to weaning from vasopressors; however, those patients also had a higher incidence of superinfection and new episodes of sepsis or septic shock. There was no mortality benefit seen with the use of corticosteroids. The CORTICUS trial included patients with septic shock, whereas the study by Annane et al. only enrolled patients with severe septic shock unresponsive to vasopressor therapy. A recent retrospective study in patients with septic shock noted a neutral effect with corticosteroids, but a subgroup analysis revealed a 30-day mortality benefit in the patients with the highest severity of illness.[99] Additionally, refractory patients who have progressed to vasopressin therapy may have an even greater benefit. In a post hoc analysis of the VAAST trial, treatment with corticosteroids and vasopressin was associated with decreased organ dysfunction and mortality compared with corticosteroids and norepinephrine.[100] The results of these studies demonstrate that corticosteroid therapy may not have a role in the general population of patients with septic shock; however, it may be beneficial for those patients unresponsive to vasopressors who are treated early.

The optimal dose, duration, and method of administration are still unknown. The Surviving Sepsis Campaign recommends hydrocortisone 200 mg/day.[4] Continuous infusion of hydrocortisone may avoid significant fluctuations in glucose and sodium. Because E.B. is refractory to increasing doses of norepinephrine and is in severe sepsis, it was decided to start hydrocortisone 50 mg IV every 6 hours.

Statins

CASE 17-4, QUESTION 7: Should E.B. be started on a statin? Are there any differences in outcomes for patients taking statin therapy prior to developing sepsis?

Aside from their well-described lipid-lowering effects, statins appear to have immunomodulatory and anti-inflammatory effects. Statin therapy lowers C-reactive protein levels, inhibits endothelial cell dysfunction, causes up-regulation of endothelial NO synthase, and blocks immune cell receptors.[101] A recent meta-analysis of seven randomized, controlled trials comprising 1,720 septic patients did not show a decrease in mortality outcomes compared to placebo, regardless of the type of statin, dose, or observed mortality rates.[102] Statins are often discontinued in septic patients because of concern for adverse effects and further organ dysfunction. Presently, it is not clear whether statins should always be continued in septic patients. Recent studies in patients who were taking statin therapy prior to sepsis have not shown any difference in outcomes or rebound inflammation when discontinuing therapy.[103,104] More prospective, randomized trials are needed to further define the role of statins in sepsis.

DISSEMINATED INTRAVASCULAR COAGULATION

Pathophysiology

CASE 17-4, QUESTION 8: E.B. experiences sudden appearance of bright red blood per rectum and through her nasogastric tube; thus, a coagulation screen was ordered. Until this time, all coagulation parameters had been within normal limits. Now the results show the following:

Platelets, 43,000/μL
PT, 24 seconds
Activated PTT, 76 seconds
Thrombin time, 48 seconds (normal, 16–27 seconds)
Fibrinogen, 60 mg/dL
Fibrin degradation products, 580 ng/mL (normal, less than 250 ng/mL)

The diagnosis of disseminated intravascular coagulation (DIC) is made. How does the pathophysiology of DIC explain these hematologic abnormalities?

Thrombosis in response to endothelial damage or the presence of an altered surface in contact with blood components is a localized phenomenon. Thrombus formation occurs at the site of injury or abnormality, where procoagulant and anticoagulant mechanisms, as well as fibrinolytic and antifibrinolytic mechanisms, are regulated. The term *localized extravascular coagulation* describes the site-specific nature of venous and arterial thrombosis.

In contrast, DIC is a diffuse response secondary to an underlying disorder that causes systemic activation of the coagulation system (Fig. 17-5).[105] Circulating thrombin converts fibrinogen to fibrin, resulting in fibrin deposition within the microcirculation. Clinical manifestations of microvascular thrombosis are the result of tissue ischemia resulting from thrombotic occlusion of small and midsize vessels.

The presence of systemic circulating thrombin causes simultaneous systemic activation of the fibrinolytic system, resulting in circulating plasmin within the systemic circulation. Plasmin causes systemic lysis of fibrin to fibrin degradation products and results in hemorrhagic complications.

Bleeding manifestations of DIC occur not only as a result of systemic fibrinolysis but also secondary to thrombocytopenia, clotting factor deficiency, and platelet dysfunction. Circulating thrombin promotes platelet aggregation, resulting in thrombocytopenia as platelet aggregates deposit in the microcirculation. Circulating plasmin degrades clotting factors as well as fibrin, and the presence of fibrinogen degradation products from

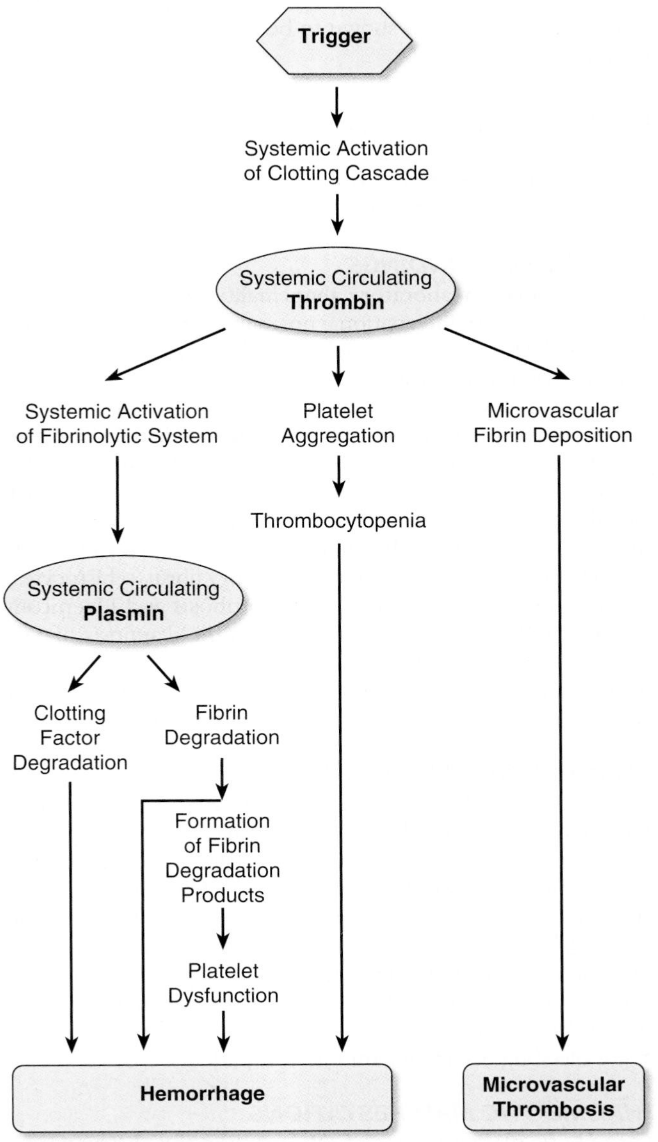

Figure 17-5 Pathophysiology of disseminated intravascular coagulation.

fibrinolysis inhibits platelet function. Normal mechanisms of platelet and clotting factor synthesis are unable to compensate for this consumption. In essence, the patient shows paradoxical bleeding secondary to overactivation and eventual consumption of available clotting factors and platelets.

Precipitating Events

CASE 17-4, QUESTION 9: What events may have precipitated the development of DIC in E.B.?

DIC is a pathologic syndrome triggered by disease states or conditions that activate coagulation systemically rather than locally.[105] The presence of thrombin within the systemic circulation can be triggered by systemic endothelial damage (e.g., bacterial endotoxin), systemic contact activation of the clotting cascade (e.g., cardiopulmonary bypass), or the release of procoagulants into the systemic circulation (e.g., malignancy). Table 17-10 presents an abbreviated list of disorders associated with the development of DIC. DIC complicates approximately 35% of severe sepsis cases.[105] Although sepsis is the most likely stimulus for DIC in E.B., both hypoxia and acidosis associated with respiratory compromise may also have contributed. Importantly, the development of DIC in septic patients has been shown to be an independent predictor of mortality.[76]

Clinical Presentation

CASE 17-4, QUESTION 10: What subjective and objective evidence in E.B. is consistent with the diagnosis of acute DIC?

LABORATORY FINDINGS

Many coagulation laboratory abnormalities occur in DIC.[105,106] The ratio of PT to international normalized ratio, the activated PTT, and the thrombin time are increased because clotting factors, as well as antithrombin and proteins C and S, are consumed more quickly than they can be replenished by hepatic synthesis. Platelet count is diminished secondary to thrombin-mediated platelet aggregation. Fibrinogen is reduced as a result of plasmin-mediated fibrinolysis, with an elevation in fibrinogen degradation products including D-dimer, indicative of a fibrinolytic state. A peripheral smear will often show thrombocytopenia and red blood cells fragmented by exposure to microcirculatory fibrin (schistocytes).

The International Society of Thrombosis and Haemostasis Overt DIC Scoring System is used in the diagnosis of DIC (Table 17-11).[107] The sensitivity and specificity of the DIC score is 93% and 98%, respectively.[108,109] There is a strong correlation between increasing DIC score and 28-day mortality.[108]

HEMORRHAGIC MANIFESTATIONS

As illustrated by E.B., hemorrhagic manifestations are the predominant clinical finding in DIC.[105] Bleeding can occur at sites of injury, including surgical incisions, venipuncture sites, nasogastric tubes, or gastric ulcers. However, spontaneous bleeding also occurs from intact sites or organ systems. Spontaneous ecchymosis, petechiae, epistaxis, hemoptysis, hematuria, and GI bleeding are commonly encountered. Intracranial, intraperitoneal, and pericardial bleeding may also occur. Critically ill patients with platelet counts less than 50,000/μL have a fourfold to fivefold higher risk of bleeding, but major bleeding occurs in a minority of patients.[105]

THROMBOTIC MANIFESTATIONS

Thrombotic manifestations of DIC result in the obstruction of blood flow to multiple organ systems. The resultant ischemic damage to end organs, including the skin, kidneys, brain, lungs, liver, eyes, and GI tract, can result in multisystem failure. Despite the severity of hemorrhagic complications, microvascular thrombosis represents a significant cause of morbidity and mortality in patients with acute DIC.

Table 17-10
Clinical Conditions Associated with Disseminated Intravascular Coagulation

Sepsis/Severe Infection (Any Microorganism)
Malignancy
Myeloproliferative/lymphoproliferative diseases
Solid tumors
Obstetric States
Abruptio placentae
Amniotic fluid embolism
Eclampsia
Retained dead fetus
Septic or saline abortion
Tissue Injury
Burns
Crush injuries
Extensive surgery
Fat embolism
Multiple trauma
Vascular Disorders
Giant hemangioma
Large vascular aneurysms
Kasabach–Merritt syndrome
Severe Toxic or Immunologic Reactions
Intravascular hemolysis (e.g., hemolytic transfusion reactions)
Recreational drugs
Severe allergic or anaphylactic reaction
Snake bites
Transplant rejection
Miscellaneous
Acidosis
Acute respiratory distress syndrome
Cardiopulmonary bypass
Heat stroke
Hypovolemia
Severe hepatic failure
Severe pancreatitis

Treatment

CASE 17-4, QUESTION 11: In the course of several hours, E.B. has exhibited more severe GI bleeding. Her Hct has fallen from 43% to 35%. What treatment course should be pursued? Should heparin therapy be given?

The most important element of treatment in patients with DIC is alleviation of the underlying cause to eliminate the stimulus for continued thrombosis and hemorrhage.[106] For E.B., this involves

Table 17-11

International Society on Thrombosis and Haemostasis Disseminated Intravascular Coagulation Scoring System

Does the patient have an underlying disorder known to be associated with DIC? (If YES, continue with scoring.)		
Laboratory Test	**Result**	**Point Score**
Platelet count	>100,000	0
	<100,000	1
	<50,000	2
Fibrin-related markers	No increase	0
	Moderate increase[a]	2
	Strong increase[a]	3
Prolonged PT (vs. baseline)	<3 seconds	0
	3–6 seconds	1
	>6 seconds	2
Fibrinogen	>1 g/L	0
	<1 g/L	1
TOTAL SCORE	≥5	Compatible with overt DIC (repeat daily)
	<5	Suggestive but not affirmative for non-overt DIC (repeat in 1–2 days)

[a]Most studies used D-dimer assays. Moderate increases were defined as a value above the upper limit of normal (0.4 mcg/L). Strong increases were defined as a value >10 times the upper limit of normal (4 mcg/L).
DIC, disseminated intravascular coagulation; PT, prothrombin time.
Source: Taylor FB Jr et al. Towards definition, clinical and laboratory criteria, and a scoring system for disseminated intravascular coagulation. *Thromb Haemost*. 2001;86:1327.

appropriate source control, antibiotic therapy, and supportive measures to correct or prevent the hemodynamic, respiratory, and metabolic manifestations of shock. Fluid replacement, maintenance of BP and CO, and adequate oxygenation are essential components of the treatment of patients with DIC.

The selection of other therapies aimed at correcting the hemorrhagic or thrombotic manifestations of DIC are controversial and to some extent depend on whether hemorrhagic manifestations or thrombotic complications predominate in the clinical presentation. Initial treatment in patients with hemorrhage involves replacement of clotting components that have been consumed in DIC, guided by coagulation laboratory data.[106] Transfusion of platelets, fresh-frozen plasma (containing all clotting factors), cryoprecipitate (containing factor VIII and fibrinogen), or prothrombin complex concentrate (containing factors II, IX, X, and factor VII for 4-factor products) may be necessary, with close monitoring of platelet count and fibrinogen level.

Several approaches to restoring the inherent anticoagulant pathways that are disrupted in DIC have been attempted. Transfusion of antithrombin concentrates may improve survival in DIC associated with sepsis.[106,110] Recombinant human thrombomodulin is a promising new adjuvant therapy that targets the protein C pathway in the pathogenesis of DIC. Recombinant thrombomodulin was associated with a higher degree of resolution of DIC compared with heparin in a randomized clinical trial, but it is not yet commercially available and additional clinical trials are being conducted to confirm its potential role.[111]

Anticoagulation with heparin in patients with DIC is controversial. In theory, because the initial pathologic event in DIC is activation of the clotting system with formation of intravascular thrombin, the antithrombin activity of heparin should prevent further fibrin deposition and subsequent activation of fibrinolysis. However, randomized trials have not been conducted to confirm this potential benefit, and the role of heparin remains controversial. The Scientific and Standardization Committee on DIC of the International Society on Thrombosis and Haemostasis recommends considering therapeutic doses of low molecular weight heparin in DIC cases with predominant thrombosis.[106] The committee also recommends venous thromboembolism prophylaxis with low molecular weight or unfractionated heparin in critically ill, non-bleeding patients with DIC.

Finally, the use of the antifibrinolytic agents such as tranexamic acid and aminocaproic acid to control bleeding is relatively contraindicated. These agents may worsen the thrombotic complications of DIC, particularly if heparin is not used concurrently. However, antifibrinolytic therapy or recombinant activated factor VII (NovoSeven) may be used in patients with life-threatening bleeding, who fail to respond to replacement of clotting components or to heparinization.

KEY REFERENCES AND WEBSITES

A full list of references for this chapter can be found at http://thepoint.lww.com/AT11e. Below are the key references and websites for this chapter, with the corresponding reference number in this chapter found in parentheses after the reference.

Key References

Angus DC, van der Poll T. Severe sepsis and septic shock. *N Engl J Med*. 2013;369:840. (78)

Cecconi M et al. Consensus on circulatory shock and hemodynamic monitoring. Task force of the European Society of Intensive Care Medicine. *Intensive Care Med*. 2014;40:1795. (1)

De Backer D et al. Comparison of dopamine and norepinephrine in the treatment of shock. *N Engl J Med*. 2010;362:779. (60)

Finfer S et al. A comparison of albumin and saline for fluid resuscitation in the intensive care unit. *N Engl J Med*. 2004;350:2247. (23)

Kenaan M et al. Hemodynamic assessment in the contemporary intensive care unit: A review of circulatory monitoring devices. *Crit Care Clin*. 2014;30:413. (12)

Mouncey PR et al. Trial of early, goal-directed resuscitation for septic shock. *N Engl J Med*. 2015;372:1301. (87)

Myburgh JA, Mythen MG. Resuscitation fluids. *N Engl J Med*. 2013;369:1243. (28)

Overgaard CB, Džavík V. Inotropes and vasopressors: Review of physiology and clinical use in cardiovascular disease. *Circulation*. 2008;118:1047. (59)

Patel GP, Balk RA. Systemic steroids in severe sepsis and septic shock. *Am J Respir Crit Care Med*. 2012;185:133. (95)

Russell JA et al. Vasopressin versus norepinephrine infusion in patients with septic shock. *N Engl J Med*. 2008;358:877. (93)

Vincent JL, De Backer D. Circulatory shock. *N Engl J Med*. 2013;369:1726. (51)

Wada H et al. Guidance for diagnosis and treatment of disseminated intravascular coagulation from harmonization of the recommendations from three guidelines. *J Thromb Haemost*. 2013;11:761. (106)

Key Websites

Dellinger RP et al. Surviving sepsis campaign: International guidelines for management of severe sepsis and septic shock: 2012. *Crit Care Med*. 2013;41:580. www.survivingsepsis.org (4)

SECTION 3 | Pulmonary Disorders

Section Editors: Timothy R. Hudd and Kathy Zaiken

18 Asthma

Timothy H. Self, Cary R. Chrisman, and Christopher K. Finch

CORE PRINCIPLES

		CHAPTER CASES
1	Asthma is a chronic inflammatory disorder of the airways in which many cells and cellular elements play a role. Airway inflammation also causes an increase in the existing bronchial hyperresponsiveness to a variety of stimuli. Bronchospasm is another key feature of asthma.	**Case 18-1 (Questions 1, 2), Case 18-5 (Question 6), Case 18-14 (Question 1)**
2	The clinical presentation of asthma includes recurrent episodes of wheezing, breathlessness, chest tightness, and cough, particularly at night and in the early morning. These episodes are usually associated with widespread but variable airflow obstruction that is often reversible either spontaneously or with treatment.	**Case 18-1 (Questions 1, 2), Case 18-2 (Questions 1, 7, 8), Case 18-3 (Question 1), Case 18-4 (Question 1), Case 18-7 (Question 1), Case 18-13 (Questions 1–3)**
3	Long-term management of persistent asthma according to national and international guidelines is aimed at reducing airway inflammation. Environmental control, inhaled corticosteroids, and management of comorbidities that worsen asthma are core management principles. Major treatments of acute exacerbations include frequent inhaled short-acting β_2-agonists and systemic corticosteroids.	**Case 18-1 (Questions 4–9), Case 18-2 (Questions 2–6, 9, 10, 12), Case 18-3 (Questions 2–4), Case 18-4 (Question 1), Case 18-5 (Questions 1–5), Case 18-6 (Question 1), Case 18-7 (Questions 1, 2), Case 18-8 (Question 1), Case 18-9 (Question 1), Case 18-10 (Questions 1, 2), Case 18-11 (Question 1), Case 18-13 (Question 3), Case 18-14 (Question 1)**
4	Monitoring parameters include spirometric measures such as forced expiratory volume in 1 second (FEV_1). Patient self-monitoring includes peak expiratory flow (PEF) as well as symptom assessment. Acute-care monitoring includes FEV_1, PEF, arterial O_2 saturation, and arterial blood gases.	**Case 18-1 (Questions 1–3), Case 18-2 (Questions 1, 4, 7, 8, 11)**
5	Based on current evidence, the number of therapeutic controversies is relatively small. Which patients should receive long-acting inhaled β_2-agonists is one topic of some debate.	**Case 18-5 (Questions 3, 4), Case 18-16 (Questions 1–4)**
6	Patient education is essential for optimal asthma management. Teaching patients with persistent asthma about daily use of preventive therapy is critical. Education regarding correct use of inhalation devices is frequently not done, but is absolutely necessary.	**Case 18-3 (Questions 2, 4), Case 18-5 (Question 2), Case 18-12 (Question 1)**
7	Improving outcomes, including reducing emergency department visits, hospitalizations, and unscheduled office visits, and enhancing quality of life are all achievable by use of the principles of national guidelines.	**Case 18-9 (Question 1), Case 18-15 (Question 1)**

ASTHMA

According to the National Institutes of Health (NIH); Expert Panel Report 3 (EPR-3): Guidelines for the Diagnosis and Management of Asthma,[1] *asthma* is defined as a chronic inflammatory disorder of the airways in which many cells and cellular elements play a role, in particular mast cells, eosinophils, T lymphocytes, neutrophils, and epithelial cells. In susceptible persons, this inflammation causes recurrent episodes of wheezing, breathlessness, chest tightness, and cough, particularly at night and in the early morning. These episodes are usually associated with widespread but variable airflow obstruction that is often reversible either spontaneously or with treatment. The inflammation also causes an increase in the existing bronchial hyperresponsiveness to a variety of stimuli.

In 2011, it was estimated that 25.9 million Americans have asthma.[2] It is an underdiagnosed and undertreated condition that is estimated to have overall costs of roughly $56 billion annually in the United States.[2] Asthma was the cause of 2.1 million emergency department visits in 2009, is the leading cause of lost school days in children, and is a common cause of lost workdays among adults.[2]

Mortality from asthma has decreased in the 21st century, from 4,657 deaths in 1999 to 3,447 deaths in 2007 in the United States according to the Centers for Disease Control and Prevention,[3,4] but morbidity and mortality are still unacceptably high, especially in inner-city minority populations. This chapter emphasizes the 2007 NIH EPR-3 guidelines.[1] Application of the principles of these recent guidelines by clinicians and patients is vital to further reducing asthma morbidity and mortality.

Etiology

Childhood-onset asthma is usually associated with atopy, which is the genetic predisposition for the development of immunoglobulin E (IgE)-mediated response to common aeroallergens. Atopy is the strongest predisposing factor in the development of asthma.[1] A very common presentation of asthma is a child with a positive family history of asthma and allergy to tree and grass pollen, house dust mites, household pets, and molds.

Adult-onset asthma may also be associated with atopy, but many adults with asthma have a negative family history and negative skin tests to common aeroallergens. Some of these patients may have nasal polyps, aspirin sensitivity, and sinusitis. In the British 1958 birth cohort study, participants were monitored for wheezing and asthma at periodic intervals from birth into their mid-forties.[5] In the subset of patients who were seemingly asymptomatic during late adolescence and early adulthood, the presence of asthma at 42 years of age was significantly higher in those patients who had a history of wheezing in childhood. Exposure to factors (e.g., wood dust, chemicals) at the workplace that may cause airway inflammation is also important in many adults. Inflammatory mechanisms are similar, but not the same, as in atopic asthma. Some clinicians may still refer to *intrinsic asthma* when referring to these patients and *extrinsic asthma* when discussing atopic asthma.

In addition to atopy and exposure to occupational chemical sensitizers being major risk factors for the development of asthma, several contributing factors may increase the susceptibility to the development of the disease in predisposed individuals.[1] These factors include viral infections, small size at birth, diet, exposure to tobacco smoke, and environmental pollutants.[1]

Recent literature has focused on the "hygiene hypothesis," an imbalance of T_H2 and T_H1 type T lymphocytes, to explain the marked increase in asthma in westernized countries.[1,6] Infants who have older siblings, early exposure to day care, and typical childhood infections are more likely to activate T_H1 responses (protective immunity), resulting in an appropriate balance of T_H1 to T_H2 cells and the cytokines that they produce. On the other hand, if the immune response is predominately from T_H2 cells (which produce cytokines that mediate allergic inflammation), development of diseases such as asthma is more likely. Examples of factors favoring this imbalance include the common use of antimicrobial agents, urban environment, and Western lifestyle. Further insights into the pathogenesis of asthma continue to be discovered.[1,6,7]

Pathophysiology

Asthma is caused by a complex interaction between inflammatory cells and mediators. As noted in the definition of asthma, mast cells, eosinophils, T lymphocytes, neutrophils, and epithelial cells are of central importance. The bronchial epithelium in asthmatic patients has been described as fragile, with various abnormalities including destruction of ciliated cells and overexpression of epidermal growth factors.[1,6] Figure 18-1 depicts the complex interaction of cells and mediators associated with airway inflammation.

After exposure to an asthma-precipitating factor (e.g., aeroallergen), inflammatory mediators are released from bronchial mast cells, macrophages, T lymphocytes, and epithelial cells. These mediators direct the migration and activation of other inflammatory cells, most notably eosinophils, to the airways.[1,6,7] Eosinophils release biochemicals (e.g., major basic protein and eosinophil cationic protein) that cause airway injury, including epithelial damage, mucus hypersecretion, and increased reactivity of smooth muscle.[1,6]

Research continues to determine the role of a subpopulation of T lymphocytes (T_H2) in asthmatic airway inflammation.[1,6] T_H2 lymphocytes release cytokines (e.g., interleukin [IL]-4 and IL-5) that at least partially control the activation and enhanced survival of eosinophils.[1,6] The complexity of airway inflammation is indicated by the fact that at least 27 cytokines may have a role in the pathophysiology of asthma.[6] In addition, at least 18 chemokines (e.g., eotaxins) have been identified that are important in delivery of eosinophils to the airways.[6] Studies have shown the efficacy of experimental humanized monoclonal antibodies against IL4, IL5, and IL13.[8–10] See Case 18-10 later in this chapter regarding anti-IgE therapy. Other potential targets for treatment of severe asthma continue to be discovered.[11,12] One biomarker of airway inflammation is exhaled nitric oxide (NO), which has been used as a treatment guide in chronic asthma.[1] Bronchial NO has been found to be elevated during periods of exacerbations and is measurably decreased with administration of inhaled steroids but not β_2-agonists.[1,13] Failure to adequately minimize severe and long-term airway inflammation in asthma may result in airway remodeling in some patients. Airway remodeling refers to structural changes, including an alteration in the amount and composition of the extracellular matrix in the airway wall, leading to airflow obstruction that eventually may become only partially reversible.[1]

Hyperreactivity (defined as an exaggerated response of bronchial smooth muscles to trigger stimuli) of the airways to physical, chemical, immunologic, and pharmacologic stimuli is pathognomonic of asthma.[1] Examples of these stimuli include inhaled allergens, respiratory viral infection, cold, dry air, smoke, other pollutants, and methacholine. Endogenous stimuli that can worsen asthma include poorly controlled rhinitis, sinusitis, and gastroesophageal reflux disease.[1] In addition, premenstrual asthma has been reported, but the exact hormonal mechanism is not known.[14]

Although patients with allergic rhinitis, chronic bronchitis, and cystic fibrosis also experience bronchial hyperreactivity, these patients do not experience bronchiolar constriction as severely as do patients with asthma. The degree of bronchial hyperreactivity

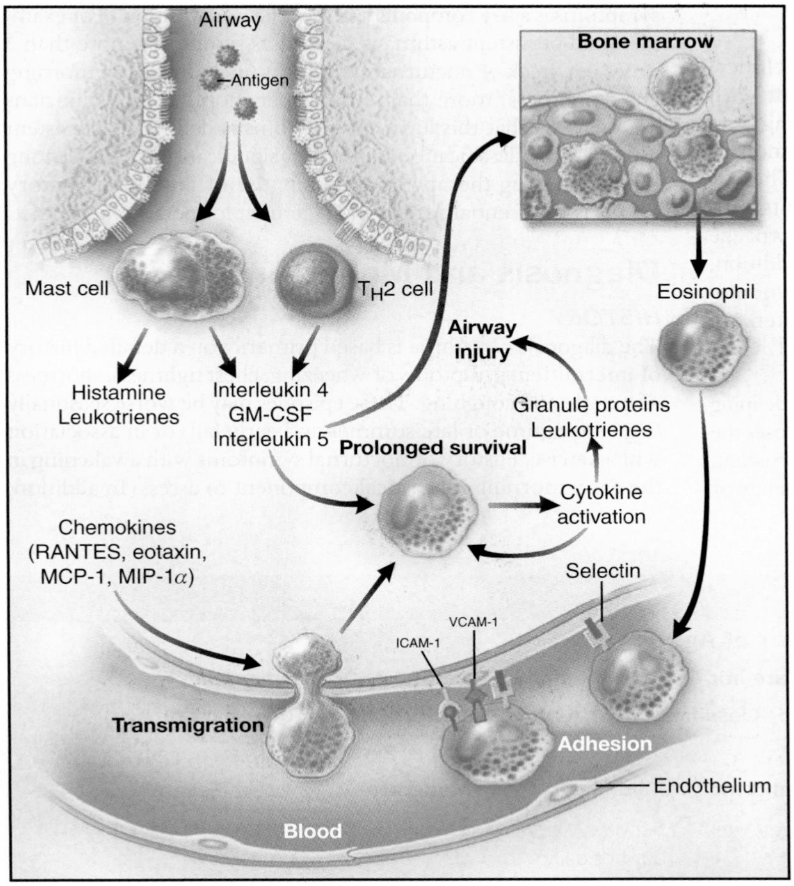

Figure 18-1 Airway inflammation. Inhaled antigen activates mast cells and T_H2 cells in the airway. They in turn induce the production of mediators of inflammation (such as histamine and leukotrienes) and cytokines including interleukin-4 and interleukin-5. Interleukin-5 travels to the bone marrow and causes terminal differentiation of eosinophils. Circulating eosinophils enter the area of allergic inflammation and begin migrating to the lung by rolling, through interactions with selectins, and eventually adhering to endothelium through the binding of integrins to members of the immunoglobulin superfamily of adhesion proteins: vascular cell adhesion molecule 1 (VCAM-1) and intercellular adhesion molecule 1 (ICAM-1). Because the eosinophils enter the matrix of the airway through the influence of various chemokines and cytokines, their survival is prolonged by interleukin-4 and granulocyte-macrophage colony-stimulating factor (GM-CSF). On activation, the eosinophil releases inflammatory mediators, such as leukotrienes and granule proteins, to injure airway tissues. In addition, eosinophils can generate GM-CSF to prolong and potentiate their survival and contribution to persistent airway inflammation. MCP-1, monocyte chemotactic protein; MIP-1α, macrophage inflammatory protein; RANTES, chemokine ligand 5. (Adapted from Busse WW, Lemanske RF, Jr. Asthma. *N Engl J Med*. 2001;344:350, with permission.)

of asthmatic patients correlates with the clinical course of their disease, which is characterized by periods of remissions and exacerbations. During times of remission, a more intense stimulus is required to produce bronchospasm than during times of increased symptoms. Numerous theories have been proposed to explain the bronchial hyperreactivity found in asthma, yet none fully explains the phenomenon. Inflammation appears to be the primary process in the pathogenesis of bronchial hyperreactivity; however, neurogenic imbalances in the airways also may play a significant role.[1] Hyperreactivity can be measured in the physician's office by having the patient inhale small concentrations of nebulized methacholine or histamine or by exercise (e.g., treadmill). The concentration of aerosolized methacholine or histamine that decreases the forced expiratory volume in 1 second (FEV_1) by 20% is referred to as the PD_{20} or the PC_{20} (provocative dose or concentration that decreases the FEV_1 by 20%).[2] An indicator of optimal anti-inflammatory therapy is an increase in the PD_{20} with time because the airways become less inflamed and therefore less hyperreactive.

Another concept related to inflammation is "late-phase" versus "early-phase" asthma (Fig. 18-2). The inhalation of specific allergens in atopic asthmatic patients produces immediate bronchoconstriction (measured by a drop in peak expiratory flow [PEF] or FEV_1) that spontaneously improves in an hour or is reversed easily by inhalation of a β_2-agonist. Although this early asthmatic response (EAR) is blocked by the preadministration of β_2-agonists or theophylline, a second response often occurs ~4 to 8 hours later. This late asthmatic response (LAR) often is more severe, more prolonged, and more difficult to reverse with bronchodilators than is the EAR. The LAR is associated with the influx of inflammatory cells and mediators as described previously. Bronchodilators do not block the LAR to allergen challenge; corticosteroids block the LAR but do not affect the EAR.[1]

Pathologic changes found at autopsy performed on asthmatic patients include (a) marked hypertrophy and hyperplasia of the bronchial smooth muscle, (b) mucous gland hypertrophy and excessive mucus secretion, and (c) denuded epithelium and mucosal edema owing to an exudative inflammatory reaction and inflammatory cell infiltration.[1] Hyperinflation of the lungs from air trapping with extensive mucous plugging is found at autopsy in patients who have died of acute asthma attacks, but these changes also are seen at autopsy in asthmatic patients dying of other causes. The bronchial smooth muscle hypertrophy and mucus hypersecretion are secondary to the chronic inflammatory response.[1,15]

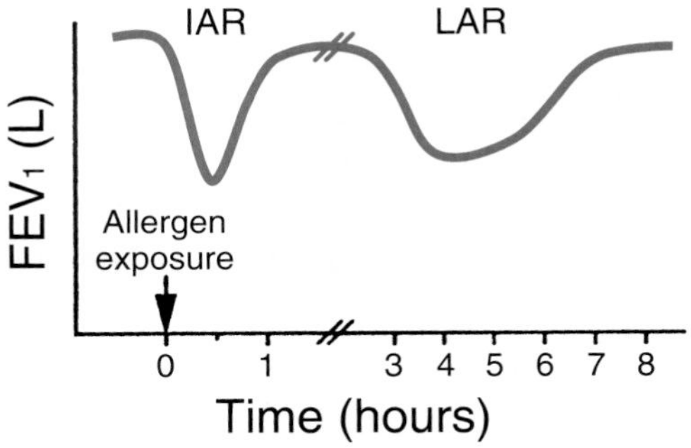

Figure 18-2 Typical immediate and late asthmatic responses seen after exposure to relevant allergen. Immediate asthmatic response (IAR) occurs within minutes, whereas late asthmatic response (LAR) occurs several hours after exposure. Patients may demonstrate isolated IAR, isolated LAR, or dual responses. FEV_1, forced expiratory volume in 1 second. (Adapted from Herfindal ET, Gourley DR, eds. *Textbook of Therapeutics Drug and Disease Management*. 7th ed. Baltimore, MD: Lippincott Williams & Wilkins; 2003, with permission.)

Symptoms

The heterogeneity of asthma is reflected best in its clinical presentation. Classically, patients with asthma present with intermittent episodes of expiratory wheezing, coughing, and dyspnea. Some patients, however, experience chest tightness or a chronic cough that is not associated with wheezing. There is a wide spectrum of disease severity, ranging from patients with occasional, mild bouts of breathlessness to patients who wheeze daily despite continuous high dosages of medication. In addition, the severity of asthma may be influenced by environmental factors (e.g., specific seasonal allergens). Symptoms often are associated with exercise and sleep (refer to Case 18-11, Case 18-12, and Case 18-14).

Classification of asthma severity is of major importance in defining initial long-term treatment. Within three age groups, EPR-3 uses the classifications of intermittent, mild-persistent, moderate-persistent, and severe-persistent asthma (Tables 18-1–18-3). The frequency of symptoms is a key component of asthma classification.[1] For example, mild-persistent asthma is defined as symptoms more than 2 times per week or nocturnal symptoms (including early morning chest tightness) more than 2 times per month. Many clinicians are unaware that this level of symptoms is defined as persistent asthma. This classification is of major significance when selecting long-term drug therapy in that daily use of anti-inflammatory agents is an essential part of management for persistent asthma.[1]

Diagnosis and Monitoring

HISTORY

The diagnosis of asthma is based primarily on a detailed history of intermittent symptoms of wheezing, chest tightness, shortness of breath, and coughing. These episodes may be worse seasonally (e.g., springtime or late summer and early fall) or in association with exercise. History of nocturnal symptoms with awakening in the early morning is a critical component to assess. In addition,

Table 18-1
Classifying Asthma Severity in Children 0 to 4 Years of Age

Classifying Severity in Children who are not Currently Taking Long-term Control Medication					
		Classification of Asthma Severity (Children 0–4 Years of Age)			
			Persistent		
Components of Severity		**Intermittent**	**Mild**	**Moderate**	**Severe**
Impairment	Symptoms	≤2 days/week	>2 days/week but not daily	Daily	Throughout the day
	Nighttime awakenings	0	1–2×/month	3–4×/month	>1×/week
	SABA use for symptom control (not prevention of EIB)	≤2 days/week	>2 days/week but not daily	Daily	Several times per day
	Interference with normal activity	None	Minor limitation	Some limitation	Extremely limited
Risk	Exacerbations requiring oral systemic corticosteroids	0–1/year	≥2 exacerbation in 6 months requiring oral corticosteroids or ≥4 wheezing episodes in 1 year lasting >1 day AND risk factors for persistent asthma		
		Consider severity and interval since last exacerbation. ← Frequency and severity may fluctuate with time. → Frequency and severity may fluctuate with time. Exacerbations of any severity may occur in patients in any severity category.			
Level of severity is determined by both impairment and risk. Assess impairment domain by caregiver's recall of previous 2–4 weeks. Assign severity to the most severe category in which any feature occurs.					
At present, there are inadequate data to correspond frequencies of exacerbations with different levels of asthma severity. For treatment purposes, patients who had ≥2 exacerbations requiring oral corticosteroids in the past 6 months, or ≥4 wheezing episodes in the past year, and who have risk factors for persistent asthma may be considered the same as patients who have persistent asthma, even in the absence of impairment levels consistent with persistent asthma.					
Classifying Severity in Patients After Asthma Becomes Well Controlled, by Lowest Level of Treatment Required to Maintain Control					
		Classification of Asthma Severity			
			Persistent		
		Intermittent	**Mild**	**Moderate**	**Severe**
Lowest level of treatment required to maintain control (See Fig. 18-6 for treatment steps.)		Step 1	Step 2	Step 3 or 4	Step 5 or 6

EIB, exercise-induced bronchospasm; SABA, short-acting inhaled β_2-agonist.
Reprinted from National Institutes of Health. *Expert Panel Report 3: Guidelines for the Diagnosis and Management of Asthma*. Bethesda, MD: National Heart, Lung, and Blood Institute; 2007. NIH publication 07-4051.

Table 18-2

Classifying Asthma Severity in Children 5 to 11 Years of Age

Classifying Severity in Children who are not Currently Taking Long-term Control Medication					
		Classification of Asthma Severity (Children 5–11 Years of Age)			
			Persistent		
Components of Severity		**Intermittent**	**Mild**	**Moderate**	**Severe**
Impairment	Symptoms	≤2 days/week	>2 days/week but not daily	Daily	Throughout the day
	Nighttime awakenings	≤2×/month	3–4×/month	>1×/week but not nightly	Often 7×/week
	SABA use for symptom control (not prevention of EIB)	≤2 days/week	>2 days/week but not daily	Daily	Several times per day
	Interference with normal activity	None	Minor limitation	Some limitation	Extremely limited
	Lung function	■ • Normal FEV_1 between exacerbations			
		■ • FEV_1 >80% predicted	■ • FEV_1 >80% predicted	■ • FEV_1 = 60%–80% predicted	■ • FEV_1 <60% predicted
		■ • FEV_1/FVC >85%	■ • FEV_1/FVC >80%	■ • FEV_1/FVC 75%–80%	■ • FEV_1/FVC <75%
Risk	Exacerbations requiring oral systemic corticosteroids	0–1 in 1 year (see note)	≥2 in 1 year (see note) →		
		Consider severity and interval since last exacerbation. Frequency and			
		← Severity may fluctuate with time for patients in any severity category. →			
		Severity may fluctuate with time for patients in any severity category.			
		Relative annual risk of exacerbations may be related to FEV_1.			
Level of severity is determined by both impairment and risk. Assess impairment domain by patient's or caregiver's recall of the previous 2–4 weeks and spirometry. Assign severity to the most severe category in which any feature occurs.					
At present, there are inadequate data to correspond frequencies of exacerbations with different levels of asthma severity. In general, more frequent and intense exacerbations (e.g., requiring urgent, unscheduled care, hospitalization, or ICU admission indicate greater underlying disease severity. For treatment purposes, patients who had ≥2 exacerbations requiring oral systemic corticosteroids in the past year may be considered the same as patients who have persistent asthma, even in the absence of impairment levels consistent with persistent asthma.					

Classifying Severity in Patients After Asthma Becomes Well Controlled, by Lowest Level of Treatment Required to Maintain Control				
	Classification of Asthma Severity			
		Persistent		
	Intermittent	**Mild**	**Moderate**	**Severe**
Lowest level of treatment required to maintain control (See Fig. 18-7 for treatment steps.)	Step 1	Step 2	Step 3 or 4	Step 5 or 6

EIB, exercise-induced bronchospasm; FEV_1, forced expiratory volume in 1 second; FVC, forced vital capacity; ICU, intensive care unit; SABA, short-acting β_2-agonist.

Reprinted from National Institutes of Health. *Expert Panel Report 3: Guidelines for the Diagnosis and Management of Asthma*. Bethesda, MD: National Heart, Lung, and Blood Institute; 2007. NIH publication 07-4051.

Table 18-3

Classifying Asthma Severity in Youths ≥12 Years of Age and Adults

Classifying Severity in Patients who are not Currently Taking Long-term Control Medication					
		Classification of Asthma Severity (Youths ≥12 Years of Age and Adults)			
			Persistent		
Components of Severity		Intermittent	Mild	Moderate	Severe
Impairment	Symptoms	≤2 days/week	>2 days/week but not daily	Daily	Throughout the day
	Nighttime awakenings	≤2×/month	3–4×/month	>1×/week but not nightly	Often 7×/week
	SABA use for symptom control (not prevention of EIB)	≤2 days/week	>2 days/week but not >1×/day	Daily	Several times per day
Normal FEV_1/FVC:					
8–19 years, 85% 20–39 years, 80% 40–59 years, 75% 60–80 years, 70%	Interference with normal activity	None	Minor limitation	Some limitation	Extremely limited
	Lung function	■ Normal FEV_1 between exacerbations			
		■ FEV_1 >80% predicted	■ FEV_1 ≥80% predicted	■ FEV_1 >60% but <80% predicted	■ FEV_1 <60% predicted
		■ FEV_1/FVC normal	■ FEV_1/FVC normal	■ FEV_1/FVC reduced 5%	■ FEV_1/FVC reduced >5%
Risk	Exacerbations requiring oral systemic corticosteroids	0–1 in 1 year (see note)	≥2 in 1 year (see note) →		
		← Consider severity and interval since last exacerbation. frequency and Severity may fluctuate with time for patients in any severity category. → Severity may fluctuate with time for patients in any severity category. Relative annual risk of exacerbations may be related to FEV_1.			

Level of severity is determined by assessment of both impairment and risk. Assess impairment domain by patient's or caregiver's recall of previous 2–4 weeks and spirometry. Assign severity to the most severe category in which any feature occurs.

At present, there are inadequate data to correspond frequencies of exacerbations with different levels of asthma severity. In general, more frequent and intense exacerbations (e.g., requiring urgent, unscheduled care, hospitalization, or ICU admission) indicate greater underlying disease severity. For treatment purposes, patients who had ≥2 exacerbations requiring oral systemic corticosteroids in the past year may be considered the same as patients who have persistent asthma, even in the absence of impairment levels consistent with persistent asthma.

Classifying Severity in Patients After Asthma Becomes Well Controlled, by Lowest Level of Treatment Required to Maintain Control				
	Classification of Asthma Severity			
		Persistent		
	Intermittent	Mild	Moderate	Severe
Lowest level of treatment required to maintain control (See Fig. 18-8 for treatment steps.)	Step 1	Step 2	Step 3 or 4	Step 5 or 6

EIB, exercise-induced bronchospasm; FEV_1, forced expiratory volume in 1 second: FVC, forced vital capacity; ICU, intensive care unit; SABA, short-acting β_2-agonist.

Reprinted from National Institutes of Health. *Expert Panel Report 3: Guidelines for the Diagnosis and Management of Asthma*. Bethesda, MD: National Heart, Lung, and Blood Institute; 2007. NIH publication 07-4051.

Table 18-4
Sample Questions for the Diagnosis and Initial Assessment of Asthma

A "yes" answer to any question suggests that an asthma diagnosis is likely.[a]

In the past 12 months

- Have you had a sudden severe episode or recurrent episodes of coughing, wheezing (high-pitched whistling sounds when breathing out), chest tightness, or shortness of breath?
- Have you had colds that "go to the chest" or take more than 10 days to get over?
- Have you had coughing, wheezing, or shortness of breath during a particular season or time of the year?
- Have you had coughing, wheezing, or shortness of breath in certain places or when exposed to certain things (e.g., animals, tobacco smoke, perfumes)?
- Have you used any medications that help you breathe better? How often?
- Are your symptoms relieved when the medications are used?

In the past 4 weeks, have you had coughing, wheezing, or shortness of breath

- At night that has awakened you?
- On awakening?
- After running, moderate exercise, or other physical activity?

[a]These questions are examples and do not represent a standardized assessment or diagnostic instrument. The validity and reliability of these questions have not been assessed.
Reprinted from National Institutes of Health. *Expert Panel Report 3: Guidelines for the Diagnosis and Management of Asthma*. Bethesda, MD: National Heart, Lung, and Blood Institute; 2007. NIH publication 07-4051.

history of symptoms after exposure to other common triggers (e.g., cats, perfume, secondhand tobacco smoke) is typical (Table 18-4). A positive family history and the presence of rhinitis or atopic dermatitis also are significant. After a careful history is obtained, skin testing may be useful in identifying triggering allergens, but it is only of supportive value in the diagnosis of asthma.

PULMONARY FUNCTION TESTS

The diagnosis of asthma is based in part on demonstration of reversible airway obstruction. A brief discussion of tests to detect reversibility of airway obstruction is important. Furthermore, a short summary of arterial blood gases (ABGs) is pertinent here in assessing the severity of asthma exacerbations.

Spirometry

Lung volumes often are measured to obtain information about the size of the patient's lungs because pulmonary diseases can affect the volume of air that can be inhaled and exhaled. The tidal volume is the volume of air inspired or expired during normal breathing. The volume of air blown off after maximal inspiration to full expiration is defined as the vital capacity (VC). The residual volume (RV) is the volume of air left in the lung after maximal expiration. The volume of air left after a normal expiration is the functional residual capacity (FRC). Total lung capacity (TLC) is the VC plus the RV. Patients with obstructive lung disease have difficulty with expiration; therefore, they tend to have a decreased VC, an increased RV, and a normal TLC. Classic restrictive lung diseases (e.g., sarcoidosis, idiopathic pulmonary fibrosis) present with decrements in all lung volumes.[16] Patients also may have mixed lesion diseases, in which case the classic findings are not apparent until the disease has advanced considerably.

The spirometer also can be used to evaluate the performance of the patient's lungs, thorax, and respiratory muscles in moving

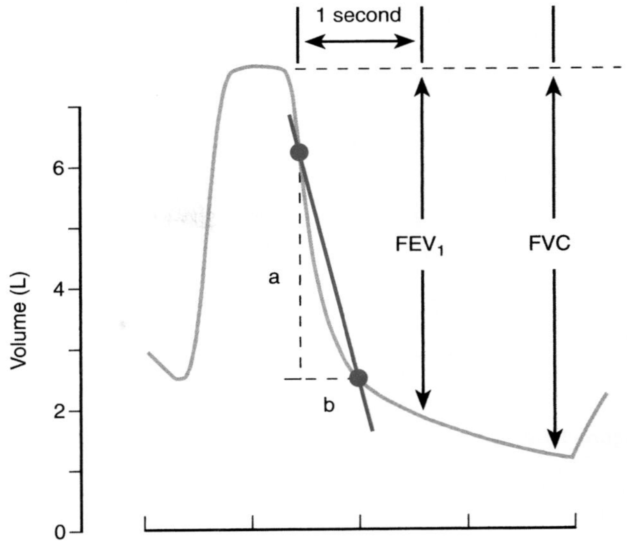

Figure 18-3 Volume–time curve from a forced expiratory maneuver. FEV$_1$, forced expiratory volume in 1 second; FVC, forced vital capacity.

air into and out of the lungs. Forced expiratory maneuvers amplify the ventilation abnormalities produced. The single most useful test for ventilatory dysfunction is the forced expiratory volume (FEV). The FEV is measured by having the patient exhale into the spirometer as forcefully and completely as possible after maximal inspiration. The resulting volume curve is plotted against time (Fig. 18-3) so that expiratory flow can be estimated.

For a video that shows how to take a lung function test, see http://www.european-lung-foundation.org/index.php?id=15411.

Standard spirometers contain pneumotachographs in the mouthpieces that can measure airflow directly. A number of important measures of lung function are made from the resulting flow–volume curves. The advantages of this technique include a display of simultaneous flows at any lung volume, visual estimation of patient effort and cooperation, high reproducibility within as well as across individuals, and an analysis of the distribution of flow limitation.[16,17] The FEV$_1$ of the forced vital capacity (FVC, the maximal volume of air exhaled with maximally forced effort from a position of maximal inspiration) commonly is measured to determine the dynamic performance of the lung in moving air. The FEV$_1$ usually is expressed as a percentage of the total volume of air exhaled and is reported as the FEV$_1$-to-FVC ratio. Healthy persons generally can exhale at least 75% to 80% of their VC in 1 second and almost all of it in 3 seconds. Thus, the FEV$_1$ normally is 80% of the FVC. The patient's breathing ability is compared against "predicted normal" values for patients with similar physiologic characteristics because lung volumes depend on age, race, sex, height, and weight. For example, an average-sized young adult man may have an FVC of 4 to 5 L and a corresponding FEV$_1$ of 3.2 to 4 L. The FEV$_1$ and the FVC are the most reproducible of the pulmonary function tests.

Peak Expiratory Flow

The PEF is the maximal flow that can be produced during the forced expiration. The PEF can be measured easily with various handheld peak flow meters and commonly is used in emergency departments (EDs) and clinics to quickly and objectively assess the effectiveness of bronchodilators in the treatment of acute asthma attacks. Peak flow meters also can be used at home by patients with asthma to assess chronic therapy. The changes in PEF generally parallel those of the FEV$_1$; however, the PEF is a less reproducible measure than the FEV$_1$.[1] A healthy, average-sized young adult

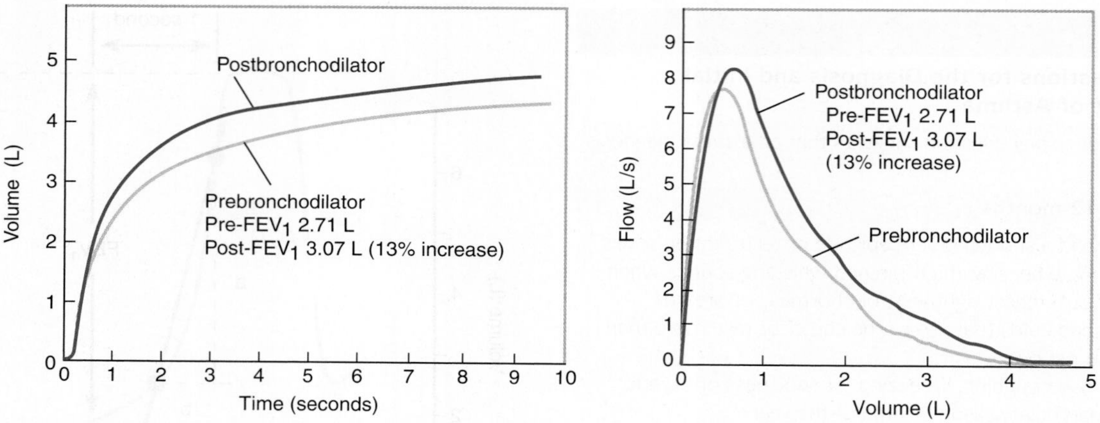

Figure 18-4 Interpretation of results of spirometry. The graphs depicted are for illustration only. The interpretation of flow rates may vary with the age of the patient. FEV_1, forced expiratory volume in 1 second. (Adapted from National Institutes of Health. *Expert Panel Report 2. Guidelines for the Diagnosis and Management of Asthma*. Bethesda, MD: National Heart, Lung, and Blood Institute; 1997. NIH publication 97-4051.)

man typically has a PEF of 550 to 700 L/minute. Commercial peak flow meters come with a chart for patients to determine their predicted normal PEFs based on their sex, age, and height.

OBSTRUCTIVE VERSUS RESTRICTIVE AIRWAY DISEASE

Generally, pulmonary disorders fall into two categories: those that restrict the lungs and thorax and those that obstruct them. In simplest terms, restrictive disease limits airflow during inspiration, and obstructive disease limits airflow during expiration. Restrictive disease results from a loss of elasticity (e.g., fibrosis, pneumonia) or physical deformities of the chest (e.g., kyphoscoliosis), with a consequent inability to expand the lung and a reduced TLC. Whereas restrictive airway diseases limit lung expansion, obstructive airway diseases (e.g., bronchitis, asthma) narrow air passages, create air turbulence, and increase resistance to airflow. In obstructive diseases, maximal expiration may begin at higher-than-normal lung volumes, and the expiratory flow is depressed.

REVERSIBLE AIRWAY OBSTRUCTION

Spirometry often is used to determine the reversibility of airway disease. Although many generally associate reversibility with bronchospasm, therapy can improve airflow by reversing any of the causative pathologic processes of asthma described previously. Significant clinical reversibility produced from bronchodilators is determined by the tests outlined in Figure 18-4. The FEV_1 is considered the gold standard test for determining reversibility of airway disease and bronchodilator efficacy. Significant clinical reversibility is defined as a 12% improvement in FEV_1 after administration of a short-acting bronchodilator.[1] An improvement of 20% in FEV_1 provides noticeable subjective relief of respiratory symptoms in most patients. For patients with a very low baseline FEV_1 (e.g., <1 L), an absolute improvement of 250 mL sometimes is considered a better indicator of therapeutic benefit than assessing percentage of change. In either case, the patient's subjective clinical impression also should be considered when using pulmonary function testing and drug challenges as predictors for future therapy.

BLOOD GAS MEASUREMENTS

The best indicators of overall lung function (ventilation and diffusion) are the ABGs (i.e., arterial partial pressure of oxygen [Pa_{O_2}], arterial partial pressure of carbon dioxide [Pa_{CO_2}], and pH). Although ABG measurements also are dependent on the patient's cardiovascular status, they are indispensable in assessing both acute and chronic changes in pulmonary patients. (See Chapter 26, Acid–Base Disorders, for a review of ABGs.) Another means of assessing the patient's ability to oxygenate tissues adequately is to measure oxygen saturation, which is described by the following equation:

$$O_2 \text{ saturation} = \text{Quantity of } O_2 \text{ actually bound to hemoglobin} / \text{Quantity of } O_2 \text{ that can be bound to hemoglobin} \times 100 \qquad \text{(Eq. 18-1)}$$

According to this equation, oxygen saturation is the ratio between the actual amount of oxygen bound to hemoglobin and the potential amount of oxygen that could be bound to hemoglobin at a given pressure. The denominator in the preceding equation is the oxygen capacity. The normal oxygen saturation of arterial blood at a Pa_{O_2} of 100 mm Hg is 97.5% and that of mixed venous blood at a P_{O_2} of 40 mm Hg is about 75%.[16]

Oxygen saturations can be measured continuously with transcutaneous monitors. This type of monitoring (pulse oximetry) is extremely helpful in determining whether supplemental oxygen therapy is indicated in patients with various chronic respiratory diseases. At a Pa_{O_2} of less than 60 mm Hg, oxygen saturation begins to drop precipitously (Fig. 18-5).

Goals of Therapy

The EPR-3[1] established the following goals of therapy to achieve control of asthma:

Reduce Impairment: (a) Prevent chronic and troublesome symptoms (e.g., coughing or breathlessness in the night, in the early morning, or after exertion); (b) maintain (near) "normal" pulmonary function; (c) maintain normal activity levels (including exercise, other physical activities, and attendance at work or school); (d) require infrequent use of short-acting inhaled β_2-agonists ([SABAs], ≤2 days a week for quick relief of symptoms); and (e) meet patients' and families' expectations of and satisfaction with asthma care.

Reduce Risk: (a) Prevent recurrent exacerbations of asthma and minimize the need for ED visits or hospitalizations; (b) prevent progressive loss of lung function—for children, prevent reduced lung growth; and (c) provide optimal pharmacotherapy with minimal or no adverse effects.

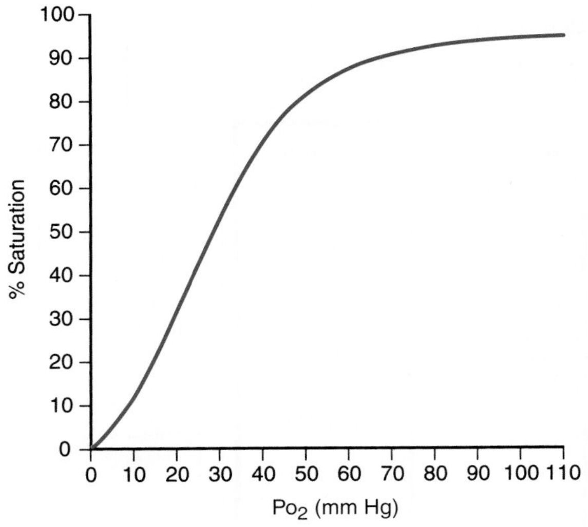

Figure 18-5 The oxygen dissociation curve reveals that the percent saturation of hemoglobin increases almost linearly with increases in the arterial O_2 tension until a partial pressure of arterial oxygen (Pao_2) of 55 to 65 mm Hg is reached. At Pao_2 values above this, the increase in hemoglobin saturation becomes proportionately less, and relatively little additional oxygen is added to the hemoglobin despite large increases in Pao_2. (Adapted from Guenther CA, Welch MH. *Pulmonary Medicine*. 2nd ed. Philadelphia, PA: JB Lippincott; 1982, with permission.)

MAJOR COMPONENTS OF LONG-TERM MANAGEMENT

To achieve these goals of therapy, EPR-3[1] also outlines some general treatment principles. Asthma management has four major components, including (a) measures of asthma assessment and monitoring, (b) education for a partnership in asthma care, (c) control of environmental factors and comorbid conditions that affect asthma, and (d) medications. Optimal long-term management requires a continuous-care approach, including each of these four major components, to prevent exacerbations and decrease airway inflammation. Early therapeutic interventions in managing acute exacerbations are very important in decreasing the chance of severe narrowing of the airways. Achieving the goals of asthma therapy also involves individualizing each patient's therapy. In addition, optimal care involves establishing a "partnership" between the patient, the patient's family, and the clinician.

For most patients with asthma, the condition can be well controlled by using the step-care approach recommended by EPR-3[1] (Figs. 18-6–18-8). A concerted effort in patient education as an integral part of state-of-the-art long-term management has been demonstrated to improve outcomes, including quality of life in patients with asthma. Because of the excellent outcomes associated with optimal long-term management, if a patient requires an ED visit or hospitalization, great care should be given to determining how the acute-care visit could have been prevented.

ACUTE ASTHMA

Assessment

SIGNS AND SYMPTOMS

CASE 18-1

QUESTION 1: Q.C., a 6-year-old, 20-kg girl, presents to the ED with complaints of dyspnea and coughing that have progressively worsened during the past 2 days. These symptoms were preceded by 3 days of symptoms of a viral upper respiratory tract infection (sore throat, rhinorrhea, and coughing). She has experienced several bouts of bronchitis in the last 2 years and was hospitalized for pneumonia 3 months ago. Q.C. is not being treated with any medications at present. Physical examination reveals an anxious-appearing young girl in moderate respiratory distress with audible expiratory wheezes; occasional coughing; a prolonged expiratory phase; a hyperinflated chest; and suprasternal, supraclavicular, and intercostal retractions. Bilateral inspiratory and expiratory wheezes with decreased breath sounds on the left side are heard on auscultation. Q.C.'s vital signs are as follows: respiratory rate (RR), 30 breaths/minute; blood pressure (BP), 110/83 mm Hg; heart rate, 130 beats/minute; temperature, 37.8°C; and pulsus paradoxus, 18 mm Hg. Her arterial oxygen saturation (Sao_2) by pulse oximetry is 90%. Q.C. is given O_2 to maintain Sao_2 greater than 90% and 2.5 mg of albuterol by nebulizer every 20 minutes for three doses. After the initial treatment, Q.C. claims some subjective improvement and appears to be more comfortable; however, wheezing on auscultation becomes louder. What signs and symptoms in Q.C. are consistent with acute bronchial obstruction? Does increased wheezing after albuterol indicate failure of the medication?

Asthma is an obstructive lung disease; therefore, the primary limitation to airflow occurs during expiration. This outflow obstruction leads to the classic findings of dyspnea, expiratory wheezes, and a prolonged expiratory phase during the ventilatory cycle.[1] Wheezing is a whistling sound produced by turbulent airflow through a constricted opening and usually is more prominent on expiration. Thus, the audible expiratory wheezing in Q.C. is compatible with bronchial obstruction. In fact, Q.C.'s obstruction is so severe that even inspiratory wheezes and decreased air movement were detected on auscultation. It is important to realize that the classic symptom of wheezing requires turbulent airflow; therefore, effective therapy of acute asthma actually may result in increased wheezing initially because airflow increases throughout the lung. As a result, Q.C.'s increased wheezing on auscultation is compatible with her clinical improvement after the albuterol nebulizer treatments.

The coughing experienced by Q.C. is another common finding associated with acute asthma attacks. The coughing may be caused by stimulation of "irritant receptors" in the bronchi by the chemical mediators of inflammation (e.g., leukotrienes) that are released from mast cells or from the mechanics of smooth muscle contraction.

In the progression of an asthma attack, the small airways become completely occluded during expiration, and air can be trapped behind the occlusion; therefore, the patient has to breathe at higher-than-normal lung volumes.[1] Consequently, the thoracic cavity becomes hyperexpanded, and the diaphragm is lowered. As a result, the patient must use the accessory muscles of respiration to expand the chest wall. Q.C.'s hyperinflated chest and her use of suprasternal, supraclavicular, and intercostal muscles to assist in breathing also are compatible with obstructive airway diseases.

Occlusion of the small airways, air trapping, and resorption of air distal to the obstruction can lead to atelectasis (incomplete expansion or collapse of pulmonary alveoli or of a segment of a lobe of the lung). Localized areas of atelectasis often are difficult to distinguish from infiltrates on a chest radiograph, and atelectasis can be mistaken for pneumonia.

Q.C.'s history of multiple bouts of "bronchitis" is significant and typical of many young asthmatic patients. In any patient with recurring episodes of bronchial symptoms (i.e., bronchitis, pneumonia), the possible diagnosis of asthma should be investigated.

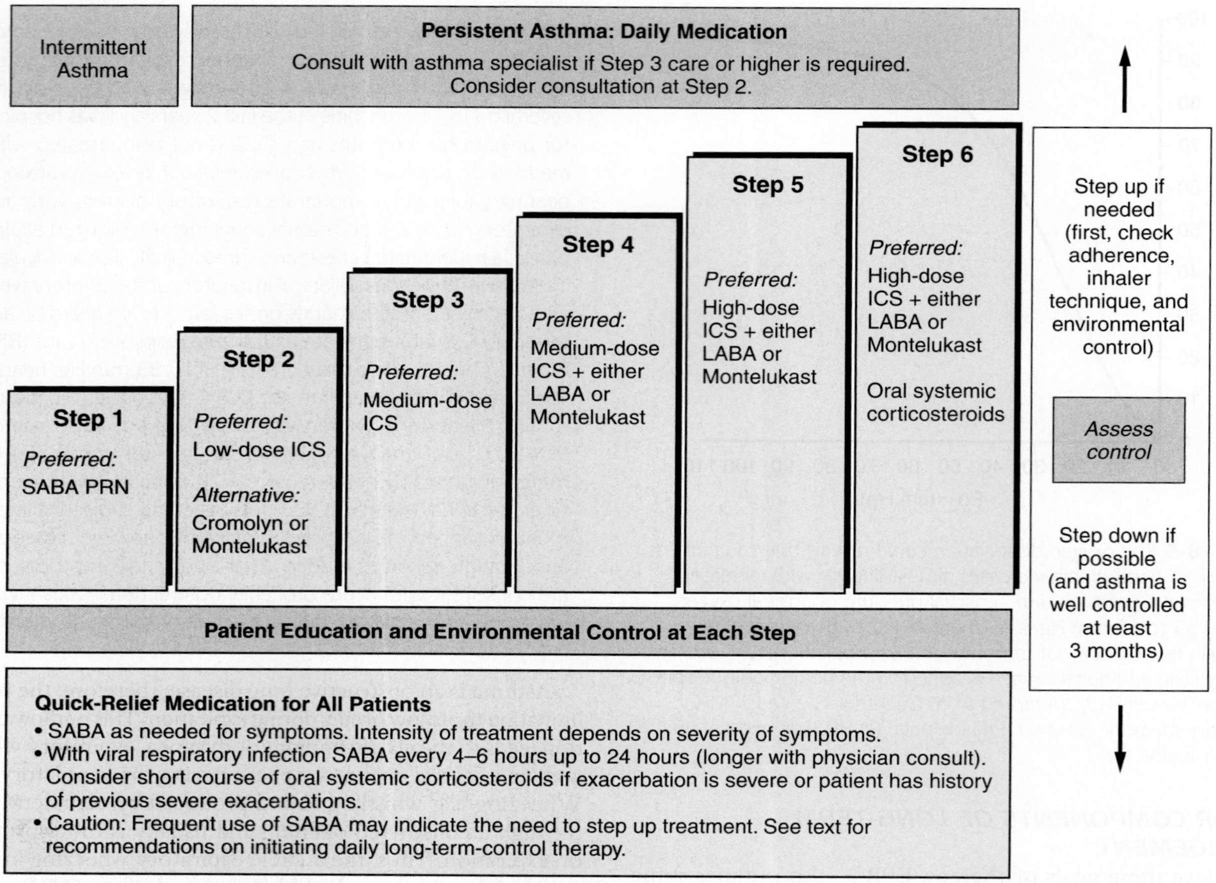

Key: **Alphabetical order is used when more than one treatment option is listed within either preferred or alternative therapy.** ICS, inhaled corticosteroid; LABA, inhaled long-acting β_2-agonist; SABA, inhaled short-acting β_2-agonist.

Notes:

- The stepwise approach is meant to assist, not replace, the clinical decision-making required to meet individual patient needs.
- If alternative treatment is used and response is inadequate, discontinue it and use the preferred treatment before stepping up.
- If clear benefit is not observed within 4–6 weeks and patient/family medication technique and adherence are satisfactory, consider adjusting therapy or alternative diagnosis.
- Studies on children 0–4 years of age are limited. Step 2 preferred therapy is based on Evidence A. All other recommendations are based on expert opinion and extrapolation from studies in older children.

Figure 18-6 Stepwise approach for managing asthma in children 0 to 4 years of age. (Reprinted from National Institutes of Health. *Expert Panel Report 3: Guidelines for the Diagnosis and Management of Asthma*. Bethesda, MD: National Heart, Lung, and Blood Institute; 2007. NIH publication 07-4051.)

The increased pulse, RR, and anxiety experienced by Q.C. can be attributed to both the hypoxemia and the feeling of suffocation. The hypoxemia in acute asthma is caused principally by an imbalance between alveolar ventilation and pulmonary capillary blood flow, also known as ventilation–perfusion mismatching.[16] Each alveolus of the lung is supplied with capillaries from the pulmonary artery for gas exchange. When ventilation is decreased to an area of the lung, the alveoli in that area become hypoxic, and the pulmonary artery to that region constricts as a normal physiologic response. As a result, blood flow is shunted to the well-ventilated portions of the lung because of the need to preserve adequate oxygenation of the blood. The pulmonary arteries, however, are not constricted completely, and when a small amount of blood flows to the poorly ventilated alveoli, mismatching is the result. Conditions of diffuse bronchial obstruction (i.e., acute asthma) increase the amount of mismatching. In addition, some mediators of acute bronchospasm (e.g., histamine) further worsen mismatching by constricting bronchial smooth muscle while concurrently relaxing vascular smooth muscle.

Q.C. also demonstrated a significant pulsus paradoxus. *Pulsus paradoxus* is defined as a drop in systolic BP of more than 10 mm Hg with inspiration. In general, pulsus paradoxus correlates with the severity of bronchial obstruction; however, it is not always present.[1]

EXTENT OF OBSTRUCTION

CASE 18-1, QUESTION 2: What additional tests would be helpful in assessing the extent of pulmonary obstruction in Q.C.?

Chest radiographs are not recommended routinely but should be obtained in patients who are suspected of having a complication (e.g., pneumonia).[1] Hyperinflated lungs and areas of atelectasis can be seen on a chest X-ray film; however, chest X-ray studies usually are negative and of little value in evaluating acute asthma attacks. The finding of a local decrease in breath sounds in Q.C.'s left lung may justify the need for a chest X-ray study, particularly if a significant differential in air movement persists after initial

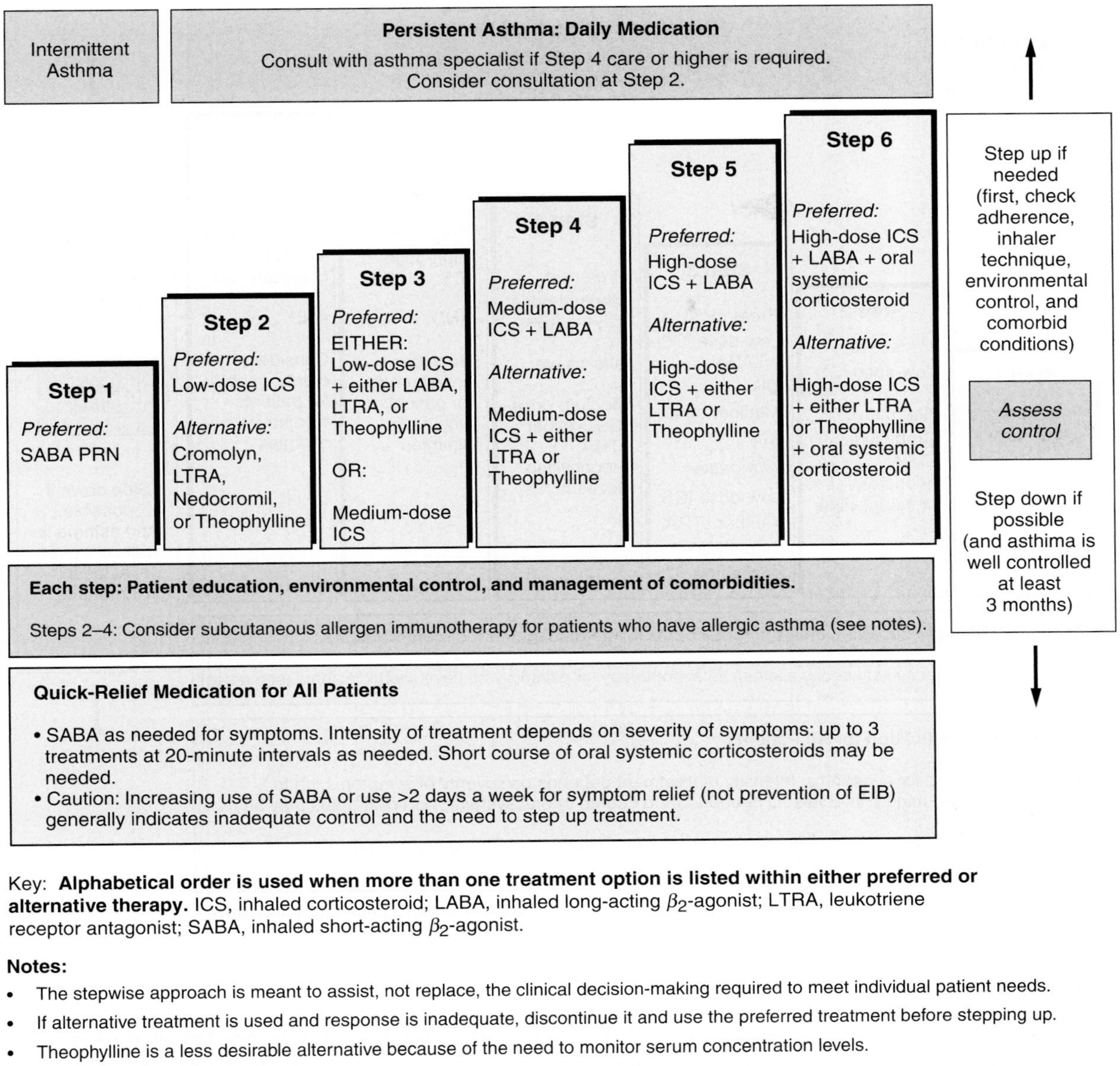

Figure 18-7 Stepwise approach for managing asthma in children 5 to 11 years of age. (Reprinted from National Institutes of Health. *Expert Panel Report 3: Guidelines for the Diagnosis and Management of Asthma*. Bethesda, MD: National Heart, Lung, and Blood Institute; 2007. NIH publication 07-4051.)

therapy. A local decrease in breath sounds may indicate pneumonia, aspiration of a foreign object, pneumothorax, or merely thickened mucous plugging of a large bronchus.

Pulmonary function testing (e.g., FEV_1, PEF) provides objective measurement of the degree of airway obstruction. Peak flow meters are helpful in the ED for assessing both the severity of airway obstruction and the response to bronchodilator therapy. Unfortunately, infants and many young children do not have the cognitive or motor skills necessary to perform pulmonary function tests. EPR-3 points out that in one study only 65% of children 5 to 16 years of age could complete either FEV_1 or PEF during an acute exacerbation. Because of Q.C.'s initial anxiety, the PEF should be measured after bronchodilator therapy has been initiated when she may be calmer. One disadvantage of pulmonary function tests in acute asthma is that the forced expiratory maneuver commonly triggers coughing. ABG measurements are the gold standard for assessing very severe airway obstruction.[1] EPR-3[1] suggests ABGs for evaluation of $Paco_2$ in patients who have suspected hypoventilation, severe distress, or FEV_1 or PEF less than 25% of predicted after initial treatment. ABG measurements are indicated in patients who fail to respond adequately to initial therapy or in patients requiring hospitalization; they are not indicated at this time for Q.C. A repeat pulse oximetry at 1 hour after treatment initiation is warranted in Q.C. to ensure adequate arterial oxygen saturation.

NEED FOR HOSPITALIZATION

CASE 18-1, QUESTION 3: Q.C. may require hospitalization. Which clinical test is predictive of the need for admission or whether Q.C. will relapse if sent home from the ED? Are Q.C.'s signs and symptoms predictive of whether she will relapse and return to the ED if not hospitalized?

The most useful predictive tool is the FEV_1 or PEF response to initial treatment. Patients who do not improve to at least 40% of predicted FEV_1 or PEF after initial intensive therapy are more likely to require hospitalization.[1] Although Q.C. is not able to perform spirometry, she is able to execute the PEF maneuver, and the plan is to check her PEF after 1 hour of therapy. Signs

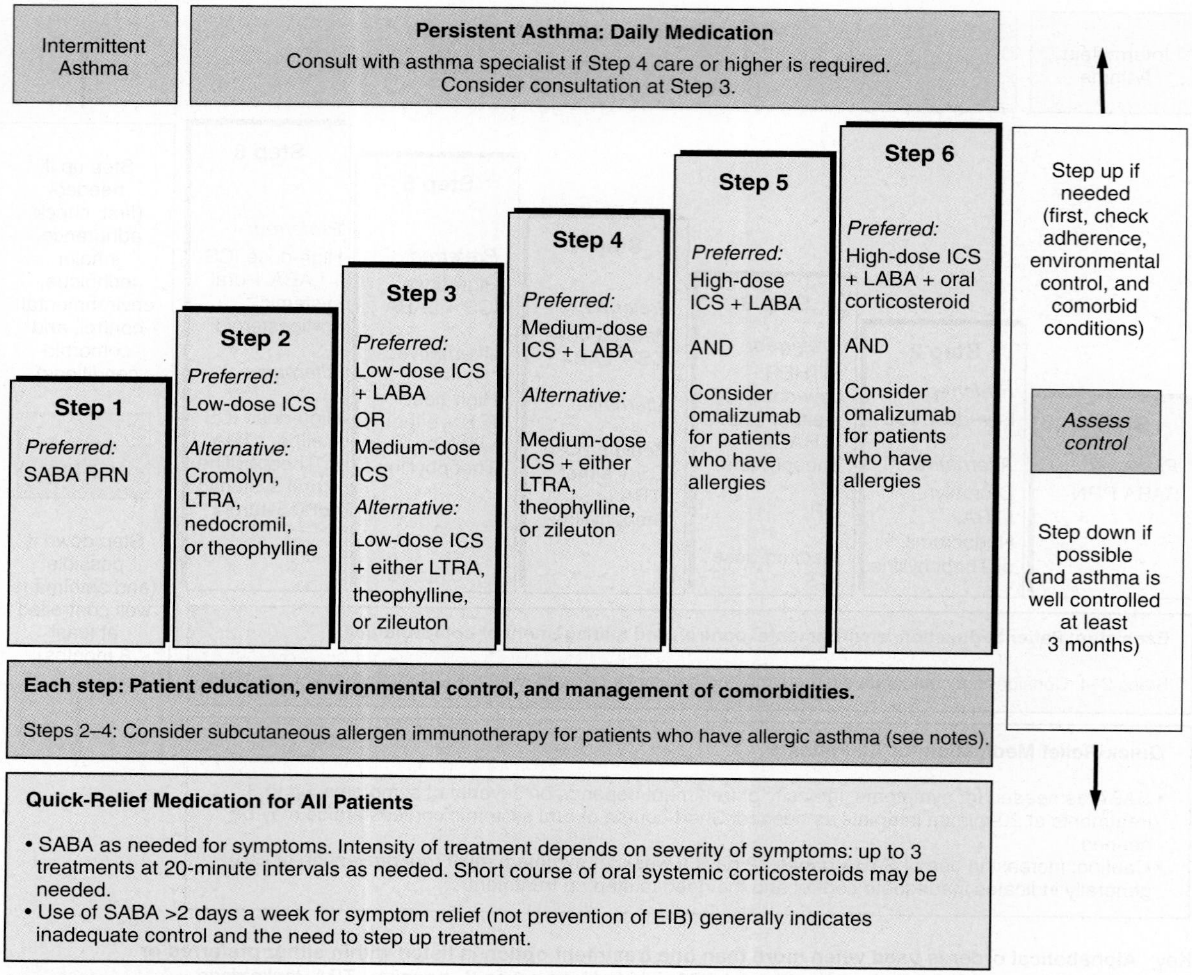

Key: **Alphabetical order is used when more than one treatment option is listed within either preferred or alternative therapy.** EIB, exercise-induced bronchospasm; ICS, inhaled corticosteroid; LABA, long-acting inhaled β_2-agonist; LTRA, leukotriene receptor antagonist; SABA, inhaled short-acting β_2-agonist.

Notes:

- The stepwise approach is meant to assist, not replace, the clinical decision-making required to meet individual patient needs.
- If alternative treatment is used and response is inadequate, discontinue it and use the preferred treatment before stepping up.
- Zileuton is a less desirable alternative because of limited studies as adjunctive therapy and the need to monitor liver function. Theophylline requires monitoring of serum concentration levels.
- In step 6, before oral systemic corticosteroids are introduced, a trial of high-dose ICS + LABA + either LTRA, theophylline, or zileuton may be considered, although this approach has not been studied in clinical trials.

Figure 18-8 Stepwise approach for managing asthma in youth 12 years of age or older and adults. (Reprinted from National Institutes of Health. *Expert Panel Report 3: Guidelines for the Diagnosis and Management of Asthma*. Bethesda, MD: National Heart, Lung, and Blood Institute; 2007. NIH publication 07-4051.)

and symptom scores alone are not adequate to predict outcome of ED treatment of asthma, but scores along with pulse oximetry and PEF or FEV_1 are helpful predictors.[1]

Short-Acting Inhaled β_2-Adrenergic Agonist Therapy

SHORT-ACTING INHALED β_2-AGONISTS COMPARED WITH OTHER BRONCHODILATORS

Case 18-1, Question 4: Why was a SABA selected as the bronchodilator of first choice in preference to other bronchodilators such as aminophylline or ipratropium for Q.C.?

Because of their potency and rapidity of action, short-acting inhaled β_2-agonists (SABAs) are considered the first choice for the treatment of acute asthma.[1] The bronchodilatory properties of SABAs are particularly effective in reversing early-phase asthma responses. Aminophylline (a theophylline salt) is not as efficacious and has more risks for serious adverse effects than inhaled albuterol.[1] Similarly, the bronchodilation from the anticholinergic drug ipratropium is of smaller magnitude than with inhaled SABAs.[1] However, two double-blind pediatric trials found that the sickest children had a reduced rate of hospitalization if given ipratropium with albuterol in the ED.[18,19] In one trial,[18] children with baseline FEV_1 less than 30% of predicted value had a reduced rate of admission with ipratropium, and in the other trial,[19] children with baseline PEF less than 50% had a reduced rate of hospital admission. Consequently, although early addition of inhaled ipratropium in adequate doses to SABAs will improve pulmonary function tests and reduce the rate of hospitalization in severely ill patients, Q.C.'s physician chose to use only inhaled SABAs initially because Q.C. was not severely ill.

PREFERRED ROUTES OF ADMINISTRATION

CASE 18-1, QUESTION 5: What is the preferred route of administration for short-acting bronchodilators?

It is well documented that SABAs administered by the inhaled route provide as great or greater bronchodilation with fewer systemic side effects than either the parenteral or oral routes.[1] In situations of acute bronchospasm, concerns about adequate penetration of aerosols into the bronchial tree led many clinicians to believe that the parenteral route of administration would be more effective than the inhaled route of administration. In clinical trials, however, inhaled SABAs were as effective as the standard treatment of subcutaneous epinephrine for ED treatment of acute asthma in adults and children.[1,20] Therefore, aerosolized SABAs now are considered the agents of choice for ED or hospital management of asthma.[1] β_2-Agonists should not be administered orally to treat acute episodes of severe asthma because of the slow onset of action, lower efficacy, and erratic absorption.[1]

CASE 18-1, QUESTION 6: Q.C. received albuterol by nebulization. Would metered-dose aerosol administration of the SABA have been preferred? Is the dose given by nebulization the same as that given by a metered-dose inhaler (MDI)?

Aerosols are mixtures of particles (e.g., a drug–lipid mixture) suspended in a gas. An MDI consists of an aerosol canister and an actuation device (valve). The drug in the canister is a suspension or solution mixed with propellant. The valve controls the delivery of drug and allows the precise release of a premeasured amount of the product. A second aerosol device, the air jet nebulizer, mechanically produces a mist of drug. The drug is placed in a small volume of solute (typically 3 mL of saline) and then placed in a small reservoir (nebulizer) connected to an air source such as a small compressor pump, oxygen tank, or wall air hose. Air travels from the relatively large-diameter tubing of the air source into a pinhole-sized opening in the nebulizer. This creates a negative pressure at the site of the air entry and causes the drug solution in the bottom of the nebulizer reservoir to be drawn up through a small capillary tube where it then encounters the rapid airflow. The drug solution is forced against a small baffle that causes mechanical formation of a mist. An ultrasonic nebulizer is a type of nebulizer that uses sound waves to generate the aerosol.

Studies that compared nebulization with pressurized metered-dose aerosols in stable chronic asthma patients have shown no advantage among these methods of administration when equivalent doses are administered.[1,21] Trials comparing metered-dose aerosols of inhaled SABAs with the nebulization of those same drugs in acute asthma also have shown no significant advantage for the nebulization method of administration when the metered-dose aerosolized administration was carefully supervised by experienced personnel and a spacer device was used.[22–24] However, in some younger acutely ill children, it is difficult (even with supervision) to administer an effective SABA with a metered-dose canister. Because many patients and clinicians *perceive* that nebulizers provide more intensive therapy, it often is important psychologically to give at least the first dose of a SABA via a nebulizer. Thereafter, it is more cost effective to use the therapeutically equivalent MDI plus spacer.[22]

The dose ratio for SABAs delivered by MDI plus spacer versus nebulizer has varied in the literature. For children with mild acute asthma, two puffs of albuterol MDI attached to a spacer were not different from 6 to 10 puffs of albuterol or via nebulizer 0.15 mg/kg.[23] In one double-blind trial in children with a severe exacerbation, investigators used a dose ratio of 1:5 (i.e., albuterol MDI spacer 1 mg [10 puffs]: nebulized albuterol 5 mg).[24] Nebulization of albuterol with compressed air or, preferably, oxygen was the preferred method of administration for Q.C. initially.

Dosing

CASE 18-1, QUESTION 7: Starting 20 minutes after the first albuterol dose, two more doses of 2.5 mg of albuterol were administered by nebulizer every 20 minutes during the next 40 minutes. After three treatments, Q.C.'s breath sounds became increasingly clear. She was no longer in distress and could speak in complete sentences. Her PEF was now 70% of predicted, her Sa_{O_2} was 97% on room air, and discharge to home was planned. Were the dose and dosing interval of albuterol appropriate for Q.C.?

Schuh et al.[25] demonstrated that a higher-dose albuterol regimen (0.15 mg/kg vs. 0.05 mg/kg every 20 minutes) produced significantly greater improvement with no greater incidence of adverse effects. Schuh et al.[26] subsequently reported greater efficacy of albuterol in a dose of 0.3 mg/kg (up to 10 mg) hourly compared with a dose of 0.15 mg/kg (up to 5 mg) hourly in children. The larger dose was tolerated as well as the 0.15 mg/kg dose. Therefore, Q.C.'s albuterol regimen of 2.5 mg (0.13 mg/kg) nebulized 20 minutes for 40 minutes subsequent to her first dose of aerosolized albuterol could have been even more aggressive but was appropriate. Figure 18-9 provides treatment guidelines for the ED and hospital management of asthma.[1] Drug dosing recommendations are listed in EPR-3.[1] In addition to EPR-3, a review of the emergency treatment of asthma has recently been published.[27]

Comparison of Short-Acting Inhaled β_2-Agonists

CASE 18-1, QUESTION 8: Would another SABA have been more effective in the initial therapy of Q.C.?

SABAs (e.g., albuterol) are preferred over nonspecific agonists (e.g., isoproterenol). Long-acting β_2-agonists (e.g., salmeterol) are not indicated for treatment of asthma in the ED. Levalbuterol (*R*-albuterol) is a single-isomer, higher-potency drug but does not offer any clinically significant advantages (i.e., improved outcomes) in most patients versus racemic albuterol to justify its higher cost.[1]

SYSTEMIC CORTICOSTEROIDS IN THE EMERGENCY DEPARTMENT FOR CHILDREN

CASE 18-1, QUESTION 9: Should Q.C. receive corticosteroid therapy as part of her ED management?

Yes. Because asthma is primarily an inflammatory airway disease, the degree of inflammation associated with Q.C.'s current exacerbation should be considered. Per EPR-3[1] (Fig. 18-9) if there is not an immediate response to inhaled β_2-agonist therapy, oral systemic corticosteroids should be administered (refer to further discussion of this subject in Case 18-2, Questions 4 and 5). Furthermore, if Q.C. had a peak flow meter at home, earlier objective detection of the development of this exacerbation might have prevented an ED visit. When the PEF is in the red zone ($<$50% of personal best) and poorly responsive to SABAs, early intervention with oral corticosteroids is associated with a reduction in ED visits[1] (Fig. 18-10); refer to the Outcomes section at the end of

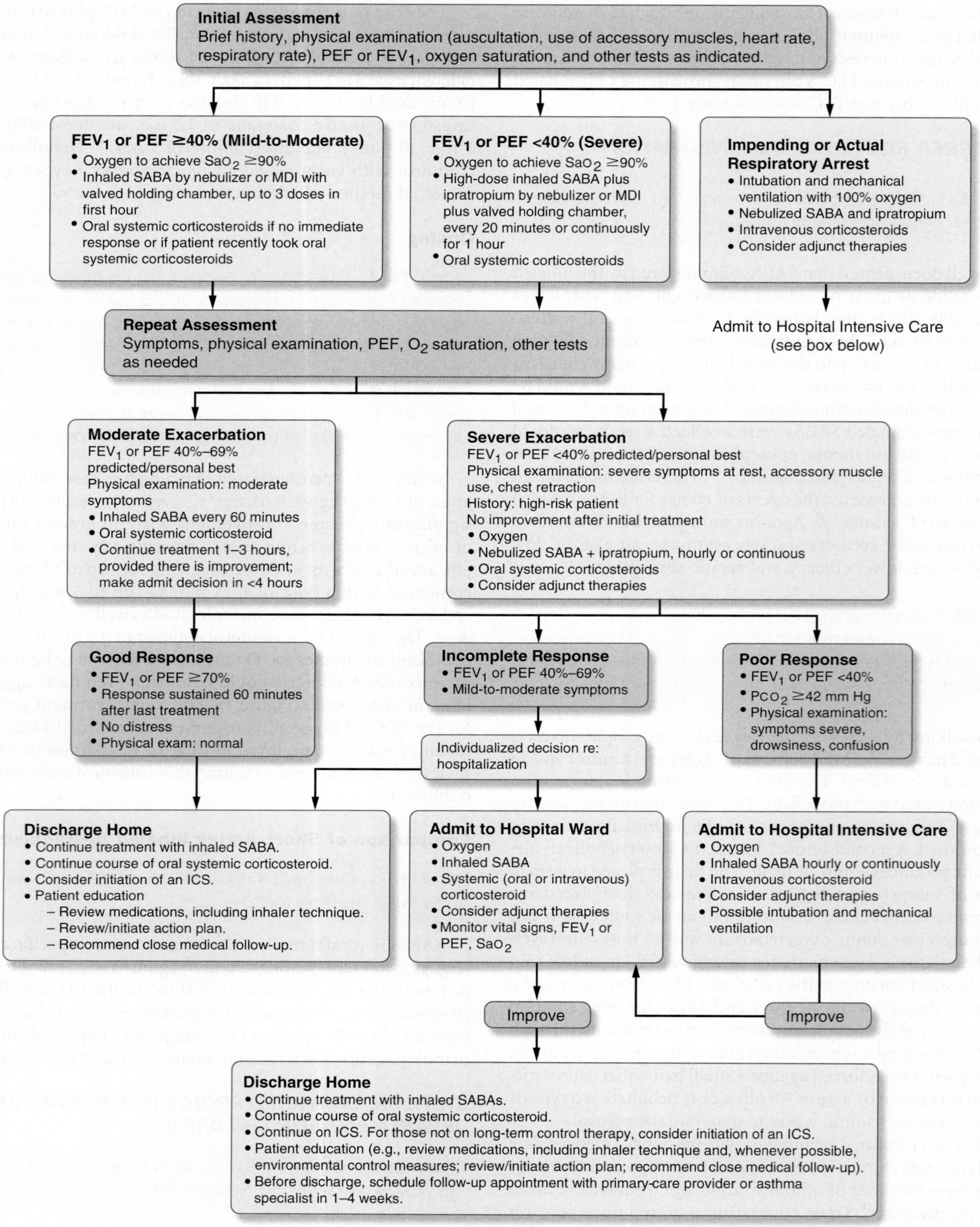

Initial Assessment
Brief history, physical examination (auscultation, use of accessory muscles, heart rate, respiratory rate), PEF or FEV1, oxygen saturation, and other tests as indicated.
FEV1 or PEF ≥40% (Mild-to-Moderate)
• Oxygen to achieve SaO2 ≥90%
• Inhaled SABA by nebulizer or MDI with valved holding chamber, up to 3 doses in first hour
• Oral systemic corticosteroids if no immediate response or if patient recently took oral systemic corticosteroids
FEV1 or PEF <40% (Severe)
• Oxygen to achieve SaO2 ≥90%
• High-dose inhaled SABA plus ipratropium by nebulizer or MDI plus valved holding chamber, every 20 minutes or continuously for 1 hour
• Oral systemic corticosteroids
Impending or Actual Respiratory Arrest
• Intubation and mechanical ventilation with 100% oxygen
• Nebulized SABA and ipratropium
• Intravenous corticosteroids
• Consider adjunct therapies
Admit to Hospital Intensive Care (see box below)
Repeat Assessment
Symptoms, physical examination, PEF, O2 saturation, other tests as needed
Moderate Exacerbation
FEV1 or PEF 40%–69% predicted/personal best
Physical examination: moderate symptoms
• Inhaled SABA every 60 minutes
• Oral systemic corticosteroid
• Continue treatment 1–3 hours, provided there is improvement; make admit decision in <4 hours
Severe Exacerbation
FEV1 or PEF <40% predicted/personal best
Physical examination: severe symptoms at rest, accessory muscle use, chest retraction
History: high-risk patient
No improvement after initial treatment
• Oxygen
• Nebulized SABA + ipratropium, hourly or continuous
• Oral systemic corticosteroids
• Consider adjunct therapies
Good Response
• FEV1 or PEF ≥70%
• Response sustained 60 minutes after last treatment
• No distress
• Physical exam: normal
Incomplete Response
• FEV1 or PEF 40%–69%
• Mild-to-moderate symptoms
Poor Response
• FEV1 or PEF <40%
• PCO2 ≥42 mm Hg
• Physical examination: symptoms severe, drowsiness, confusion
Individualized decision re: hospitalization
Discharge Home
• Continue treatment with inhaled SABA.
• Continue course of oral systemic corticosteroid.
• Consider initiation of an ICS.
• Patient education
– Review medications, including inhaler technique.
– Review/initiate action plan.
– Recommend close medical follow-up.
Admit to Hospital Ward
• Oxygen
• Inhaled SABA
• Systemic (oral or intravenous) corticosteroid
• Consider adjunct therapies
• Monitor vital signs, FEV1 or PEF, SaO2
Admit to Hospital Intensive Care
• Oxygen
• Inhaled SABA hourly or continuously
• Intravenous corticosteroid
• Consider adjunct therapies
• Possible intubation and mechanical ventilation
Improve
Improve
Discharge Home
• Continue treatment with inhaled SABAs.
• Continue course of oral systemic corticosteroid.
• Continue on ICS. For those not on long-term control therapy, consider initiation of an ICS.
• Patient education (e.g., review medications, including inhaler technique and, whenever possible, environmental control measures; review/initiate action plan; recommend close medical follow-up).
• Before discharge, schedule follow-up appointment with primary-care provider or asthma specialist in 1–4 weeks.

Figure 18-9 Management of asthma exacerbations: emergency department and hospital-based care. FEV_1, forced expiratory volume in 1 second; ICS, inhaled corticosteroid; MDI, metered-dose inhaler; Pco_2, partial pressure of carbon dioxide; PEF, peak expiratory flow; SABA, short-acting β_2-agonist; Sao_2, arterial oxygen saturation. (Adapted from National Institutes of Health. *Expert Panel Report 3: Guidelines for the Diagnosis and Management of Asthma*. Bethesda, MD: National Heart, Lung, and Blood Institute; 2007. NIH publication 07-4051.)

the chapter). Q.C. and her parents should also understand that if respiratory distress is severe and nonresponsive to treatment, they should proceed to an ED or call 9-1-1. Finally, before going home from the ED, Q.C. and her parents should receive some basic education regarding asthma and its acute and long-term management. It is important to follow up with more detailed education during future clinic visits. According to EPR-3,[1] Q.C. should receive a short course of systemic corticosteroids as part of her discharge plan, thereby reducing her risk of re-exacerbation. Typically, oral prednisolone solution at a dose of 1 to 2 mg/kg in

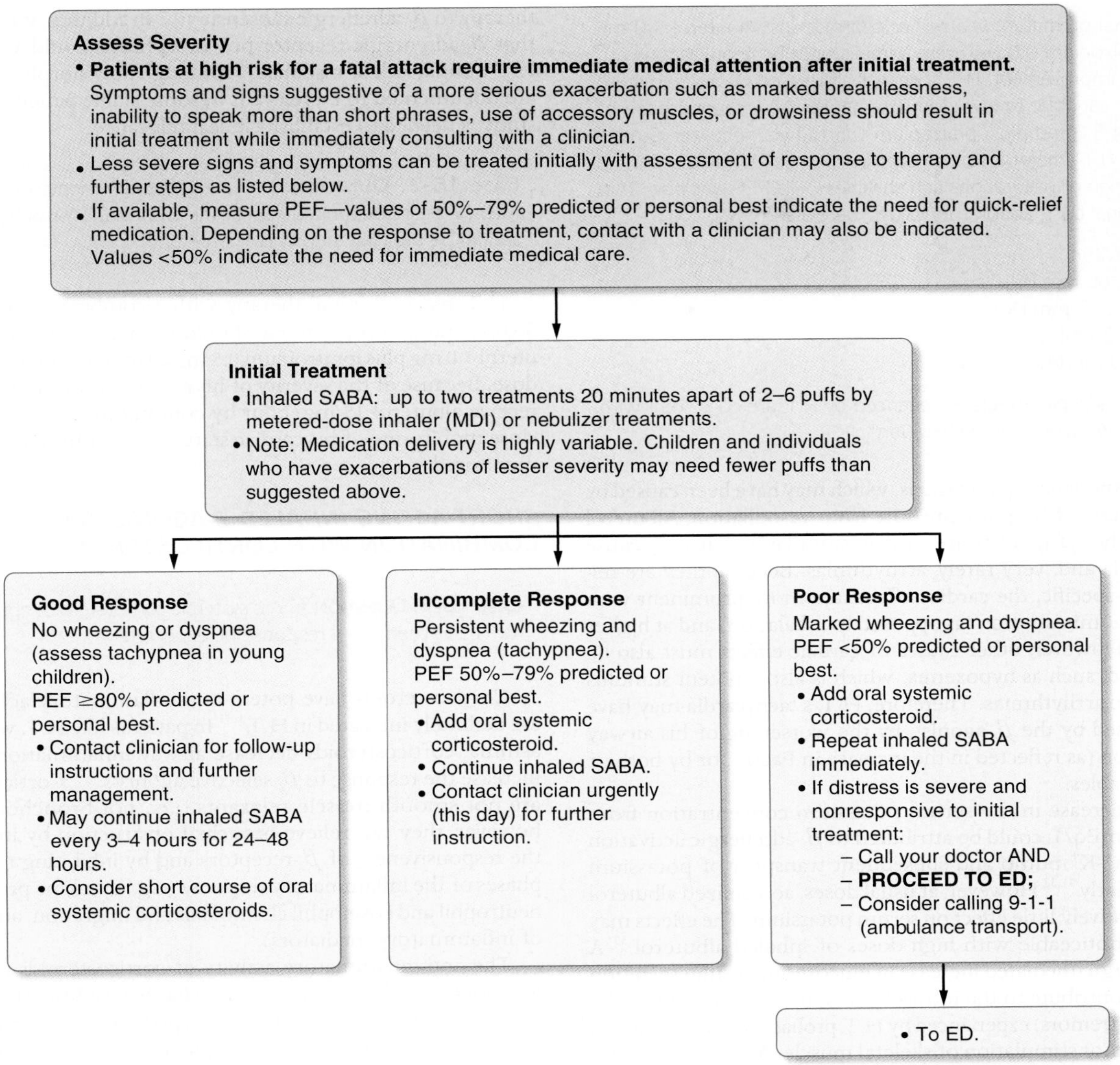

Assess Severity
• Patients at high risk for a fatal attack require immediate medical attention after initial treatment.
Symptoms and signs suggestive of a more serious exacerbation such as marked breathlessness, inability to speak more than short phrases, use of accessory muscles, or drowsiness should result in initial treatment while immediately consulting with a clinician.
• Less severe signs and symptoms can be treated initially with assessment of response to therapy and further steps as listed below.
• If available, measure PEF—values of 50%–79% predicted or personal best indicate the need for quick-relief medication. Depending on the response to treatment, contact with a clinician may also be indicated. Values <50% indicate the need for immediate medical care.
Initial Treatment
• Inhaled SABA: up to two treatments 20 minutes apart of 2–6 puffs by metered-dose inhaler (MDI) or nebulizer treatments.
• Note: Medication delivery is highly variable. Children and individuals who have exacerbations of lesser severity may need fewer puffs than suggested above.
Good Response
No wheezing or dyspnea (assess tachypnea in young children).
PEF ≥80% predicted or personal best.
• Contact clinician for follow-up instructions and further management.
• May continue inhaled SABA every 3–4 hours for 24–48 hours.
• Consider short course of oral systemic corticosteroids.
Incomplete Response
Persistent wheezing and dyspnea (tachypnea).
PEF 50%–79% predicted or personal best.
• Add oral systemic corticosteroid.
• Continue inhaled SABA.
• Contact clinician urgently (this day) for further instruction.
Poor Response
Marked wheezing and dyspnea.
PEF <50% predicted or personal best.
• Add oral systemic corticosteroid.
• Repeat inhaled SABA immediately.
• If distress is severe and nonresponsive to initial treatment:
– Call your doctor AND
– PROCEED TO ED;
– Consider calling 9-1-1 (ambulance transport).
• To ED.

Figure 18-10 Management of asthma exacerbations: home treatment. ED, emergency department; MDI, metered-dose inhaler; PEF, peak expiratory flow; SABA, short-acting β_2-agonist. (Adapted from National Institutes of Health. *Expert Panel Report 3: Guidelines for the Diagnosis and Management of Asthma*. Bethesda, MD: National Heart, Lung, and Blood Institute; 2007. NIH publication 07-4051.)

daily or divided doses twice daily is given for approximately 5 to 7 days. Although this regimen is very effective, to improve adherence several studies have examined shorter (1- to 2-day) courses of oral or intramuscular dexamethasone and have found similar results when compared with usual regimens of oral prednisone or prednisolone.[28–30]

Adverse Effects

CASE 18-2

Question 1: H.T., a 45-year-old, 91-kg man with a long history of severe-persistent asthma, presents to the ED with severe dyspnea and wheezing. He is able to say only two or three words without taking a breath. He has been taking four inhalations of beclomethasone hydrofluoroalkane (HFA; 80 mcg/puff) twice daily (BID) and two inhalations of albuterol MDI 4 times a day (QID) as needed (PRN) on a chronic basis. H.T. ran out of beclomethasone a week ago; since then, he has been using his albuterol MDI with increasing frequency up to every 3 hours on the day before admission. He is a lifelong nonsmoker. His FEV_1 was 25% of the predicted value for his age and height, and his Sao_2 was 82%. Vital signs are as follows:

Heart rate, 130 beats/minute
RR, 30/minute
Pulsus paradoxus, 18 mm Hg
BP, 130/90 mm Hg

ABGs on room air were as follows:

pH, 7.40
Pao_2, 55 mm Hg
$Paco_2$, 40 mm Hg
Serum electrolyte concentrations were as follows:
Sodium (Na), 140 mEq/L
Potassium (K), 3.9 mEq/L
Chloride (Cl), 105 mEq/L

Because of the severity of the obstruction, H.T. was monitored with an electrocardiogram that showed sinus tachycardia with occasional premature ventricular contractions. Albuterol 5.0 mg and ipratropium 0.5 mg were administered by nebulization with minimal improvement. H.T. then was started on O_2 at 4 L/minute by nasal cannula, followed in 20 minutes by a second dose of albuterol 5.0 mg plus ipratropium 0.5 mg via nebulizer. Subsequently, H.T.'s heart rate increased to 140 beats/minute, and he complained of palpitations and shakiness. His PEF was now 25% of personal best. Laboratory values were as follows:

pH, 7.39
Pao_2, 60 mm Hg
$Paco_2$, 42 mm Hg
Na, 138 mEq/L
K, 3.5 mEq/L

What adverse effects experienced by H.T. are consistent with systemic β_2-agonist administration?

H.T. experienced palpitations, which may have been caused by the widening of his pulse pressure from vasodilation. Albuterol and all other β-agonists are cardiac stimulants that may cause tachycardia and, very rarely, arrhythmias. Because they are relatively β_2-specific, the cardiac effects are more prominent with systemic administration (as opposed to inhalation) and at higher dosages. However, other causes of cardiac effects must also be considered, such as hypoxemia, which is also a potent stimulus for cardiac arrhythmias. Therefore, H.T.'s tachycardia may have been caused by the β_2-agonist, by the worsening of his airway obstruction (as reflected in the increase in $Paco_2$), or by both of these variables.

The decrease in the serum potassium concentration from 3.9 to 3.5 mEq/L could be attributed to β_2-adrenergic activation of the Na^+-K^+ pump and subsequent transport of potassium intracellularly.[31,32] However, at usual doses, aerosolized albuterol causes relatively little effect on serum potassium. The effects may be more noticeable with high doses of inhaled albuterol.[33] A β_2-adrenergic-mediated increase in glucose and insulin secretion also can contribute to the intracellular shift of potassium.[34] The shakiness (tremors) experienced by H.T. probably can be attributed to β_2-receptor stimulation of skeletal muscle. Again, this effect is most prominent with oral or parenteral administration, but some patients are very sensitive to even small doses of inhaled SABAs.

β-ADRENERGIC AGONIST SUBSENSITIVITY

CASE 18-2, QUESTION 2: Why did H.T. fail to respond to the initial therapy? Could tolerance to the β_2-agonists have contributed?

Although tolerance to systemic effects of β_2-agonists (e.g., tremor, sleep disturbances) is documented, tolerance to the airway response does not occur to a clinically significant extent.[33,34] Even with long-term use, the intensity of response to β_2-agonists is retained (i.e., the maximal percent increase in pulmonary function), but the duration of response with each dose may shorten. Such an effect is unlikely with intermittent use but may occur in patients who routinely use large, multiple doses daily. Possible explanations for this variability include downregulation of receptors, disease progression, or true drug tolerance. The exact contribution of each is not known. Therefore, H.T.'s failure to respond to the initial therapy most likely is attributable to the severity of his airway obstruction. H.T.'s history of severe chronic asthma, the slow progression of this attack, and the lack of response to his inhaled β_2-agonist also are largely owing to a significant inflammatory component to this attack. Thus, bronchodilators would not be expected to immediately reverse the airway obstruction in H.T. It would be difficult to attribute his lack of initial response to therapy to β_2-adrenergic subsensitivity. In addition, it is not likely that β_2-adrenergic receptor polymorphisms could account for H.T.'s initial lack of response.[34] Although polymorphic variations are documented to be relevant in some stable patients,[1] further study is needed to establish clinical relevance.

CASE 18-2, QUESTION 3: Repeat measurements of PEF and ABGs indicate continued significant bronchial obstruction. What should be the next step in H.T.'s therapy?

H.T. received initial therapy with a combination of inhaled SABAs and ipratropium. He should receive a third dose of albuterol 5.0 mg plus ipratropium 0.5 mg 20 minutes after the second dose. Because of the severity of his exacerbation, he should then receive albuterol 15 mg/hour by continuous nebulization with close monitoring of his cardiac status. H.T.'s PEF also should be monitored.

SHORT-ACTING INHALED β-AGONISTS IN COMBINATION WITH CORTICOSTEROIDS

CASE 18-2, QUESTION 4: Are systemic corticosteroids appropriate for H.T.? When can a response be expected?

Corticosteroids have potent anti-inflammatory activity and are definitely indicated in H.T.[1,35] In patients like H.T. with acute asthma, corticosteroids decrease airway inflammation[36–39] and increase the response to β_2-selective agonists.[1,36] Corticosteroids are not smooth muscle relaxants (i.e., not bronchodilators); however, they can relieve bronchial obstruction by improving the responsiveness of β_2-receptors and by inhibiting numerous phases of the inflammatory response (e.g., cytokine production, neutrophil and eosinophil chemotaxis and migration, and release of inflammatory mediators).[1]

The anti-inflammatory activity of corticosteroids is delayed for about 4 to 6 hours after the dose has been administered. Corticosteroid-induced restoration of responsiveness to endogenous catecholamines and exogenous β_2-agonists, however, occurs within 1 hour of administration of the corticosteroid in severe, chronic, stable asthmatic patients.[36] Significant improvement in objective measures (e.g., FEV_1) generally occurs 12 hours after administration.[38] Consequently, EPR-3[1] advocates early initiation of corticosteroids in cases of acute severe asthma. Corticosteroids also hasten the recovery of acute exacerbations of asthma[35,40–43] and decrease the need for hospitalization if given early in the initial management of acute asthma in the ED.[38]

On the basis of his initial presentation, H.T. should be started on systemic corticosteroid therapy immediately in the ED (Fig. 18-9). Preferably, oral corticosteroids would have been started at home before H.T.'s exacerbation escalated to this degree of severity (Fig. 18-10).

CASE 18-2, QUESTION 5: What would be an appropriate dosing regimen of corticosteroids for H.T. in the ED? Would the dose and route be the same if he were hospitalized?

Doses of corticosteroids used to treat acute asthma are largely empiric. Studies comparing very high dosages (e.g., intravenous [IV] methylprednisolone 125 mg every 6 hours in an adult) versus moderate dosages (40 mg every 6 hours) have shown no advantage with very high dosages.[1,44,45] In addition, oral therapy is as efficacious as the IV route.[1,44,45] Dosing recommendations for systemic corticosteroids in the management of asthma exacerbations in the ED or hospital are listed in EPR-3.[1] Higher corticosteroid dosages may be considered in patients with impending respiratory failure. When patients cannot take oral medication, IV methylprednisolone is preferred over hydrocortisone in patients with heart disease or fluid retention or when high dosages of corticosteroids are used; this is because it has less mineralocorticoid activity.

For patients who require IV corticosteroid therapy, the dosage can usually be reduced rapidly to 60 to 80 mg/day for adults (1–2 mg/kg/day for children) because the condition improves (usually after 48–72 hours). On discharge from the hospital, EPR-3[1] recommends, for example, prednisone 40 to 80 mg/day in one or two doses for 3 to 10 days. Although some clinicians may prescribe a tapering regimen, no taper is necessary in this situation. On the other hand, if the patient required long-term oral corticosteroid therapy before hospitalization, tapering the dose to the preadmission dosage is prudent. For patients who are discharged from the ED, up to 7 days of prednisone therapy usually is sufficient.

CASE 18-2, QUESTION 6: H.T. was given one dose of 60 mg of methylprednisolone (Solu-Medrol) IV and three doses of albuterol 5 mg/ipratropium 0.5 mg by nebulizer every 20 minutes in the ED). H.T. claimed slight subjective improvement after this therapy; yet, expiratory wheezes still were audible, and he still was using his accessory muscles for ventilatory efforts. His PEF improved only to 35% of predicted, and a repeat ABG measurement showed a $Paco_2$ of 40 mm Hg. What should be done at this time?

H.T. still is significantly obstructed despite intensive therapy in the ED. As a result, he should be admitted to the intensive care unit (ICU), where he can be monitored closely.

Respiratory Failure

SIGNS AND SYMPTOMS

CASE 18-2, QUESTION 7: What would be the best method of assessing the adequacy of therapy in H.T.? What are the signs of impending respiratory failure?

When patients continually must expand their chest wall with high lung volumes for a prolonged period, respiratory muscle fatigue may ensue, resulting in a decreased ventilatory effort. Clinical signs of impending respiratory failure include increased heart rate, decreased breath sounds, agitation from worsening hypoxia, or lethargy from increased CO_2 retention. These clinical signs and symptoms are relatively nonspecific and are affected by many variables. Thus, they should not be used to detect impending respiratory failure.

The best way to assess therapy is to monitor ABGs. The Pao_2 component of an ABG determination is not very helpful because of $\dot{V}/\dot{Q}$ mismatching and the administration of oxygen. The $Paco_2$ is the best indicator of hypoventilation in acute asthma[1]; however, there is no single value for $Paco_2$ that indicates impending respiratory failure, because different $Paco_2$ values are acceptable under different clinical circumstances. A $Paco_2$ of 55 mm Hg 1 to 2 hours after intensive bronchodilator therapy or an increase in $Paco_2$ of 5 to 10 mm Hg/hour during aggressive therapy is an ominous sign. The fact that H.T.'s $Paco_2$ is not rising with therapy is a good sign.

β_2-AGONISTS AND OTHER POTENTIAL THERAPIES

CASE 18-2, QUESTION 8: H.T. initially received three doses of albuterol 5 mg/ipratropium 0.5 mg by nebulizer every 20 minutes in the ED. He has also received IV methylprednisolone 60 mg. Would the IV administration of a β-agonist be indicated in H.T. at this time? What are other potential therapies in H.T.?

Although the use of IV β-agonists for asthmatic patients in the ICU formerly was advocated, current standards of care discourage the use of these agents.[1] H.T.'s response to inhaled albuterol also suggest that IV β-agonists are inappropriate at this time. Because standard therapies already administered were not sufficient, IV magnesium sulfate may benefit severely ill patients like H.T.[1,46] Recent research suggests that nebulized isotonic magnesium sulfate is a valuable adjunctive therapy to inhaled albuterol in the treatment of severe asthma exacerbations.[47] Further, heliox (a mixture of helium and oxygen) may also add benefit.[1,48]

THEOPHYLLINE

CASE 18-2, QUESTION 9: Intravenous theophylline is being considered for H.T. Is theophylline likely to be of benefit in impending respiratory failure?

Studies on the treatment of acute asthma in the ED have failed to demonstrate any benefit of adding theophylline to optimal, inhaled β-agonist therapy,[1,49] and the EPR-3 does not recommended this practice.[1] Furthermore, several double-blind, randomized, placebo-controlled studies have demonstrated that theophylline does not add benefit to intensive therapy with inhaled β_2-agonists and systemic corticosteroids in hospitalized adults[50] or children[51–54] who fail to respond to aggressive ED therapy with SABAs. Note in Figure 18-9 from EPR-3[1] that theophylline is not recommended for routine management of hospitalized patients with asthma. Although one study[55] has shown a slight benefit of theophylline in hospitalized adult asthmatic patients, one of the authors of that study has since noted that if adequate doses of SABAs and systemic corticosteroids are used, theophylline is probably not routinely indicated.[56] Although further research is needed to establish whether theophylline may add benefit to hospitalized adult patients who have impending respiratory failure, routine use of theophylline in hospitalized asthmatic patients no longer is justified.

Limited evidence suggests a potential benefit of theophylline for some pediatric patients in the ICU who have impending respiratory failure.[57] However, more recent study does not show any benefit and suggests longer ICU stays and time for symptom improvement.[58] EPR-3 does not recommend the use of theophylline in the hospital.[1] H.T.'s clinicians decide not to use theophylline. If a clinician decides to use theophylline in this setting, a current pharmacokinetics text should be consulted to help ensure safe and effective dosing and monitoring.[59]

Response to Therapy

CASE 18-2, QUESTION 10: H.T. has continued to improve slowly during the last 72 hours. The nebulizer treatments with albuterol are now administered every 4 hours, and he is taking oral prednisone 80 mg/day in two divided doses. PEF measurements taken before and after the last albuterol treatment were 65% of predicted and 80% of predicted, respectively. Is H.T.'s long duration of recovery unusual?

No. In a patient such as H.T., whose condition progressively deteriorated during a long period, a slow reversal should be expected. The prolonged deterioration reflects an increasing inflammatory response in the lung. These patients require prolonged, intensive bronchodilator and anti-inflammatory therapy before maximal improvement is noted in pulmonary function tests. Thus, H.T. should continue to receive systemic corticosteroids for approximately 10 days after such a severe acute exacerbation of asthma.[1]

Adverse Effects of Short-Term Corticosteroid Therapy

Case 18-2, Question 11: H.T. has been taking corticosteroids for a total of 6 days. Long-term corticosteroid use is associated with many adverse effects (e.g., adrenal suppression, osteoporosis, cataracts). What adverse effects are related to short-term corticosteroid use?

Short courses of daily corticosteroids are usually associated with minor side effects.[35,40–43] Facial flushing, appetite stimulation, gastrointestinal irritation, headache, and mood changes ranging from a mere sense of well-being to overt toxic psychosis are the most commonly encountered adverse effects of short-term corticosteroid therapy. Acne can be exacerbated in patients susceptible to this skin problem, and weight gain also can occur because of sodium and fluid retention. In addition, hyperglycemia, leukocytosis, and hypokalemia are possible. All of these problems are transient and will disappear with time after the corticosteroids are discontinued. These short-term adverse effects are less common when small corticosteroid doses are used; however, corticosteroid doses must be adequate to prevent disease exacerbation. The minor risks of short-term use are far outweighed by the marked benefits.

Overuse of Short-Acting Inhaled β-Agonists

Case 18-2, Question 12: H.T.'s history of increased use of his SABA inhaler during the early stages of this asthma attack suggests improper use of this medication. What are the risks from overuse of β_2-agonists?

The overuse of SABAs as a possible risk factor for asthma death has been debated for decades.[60] Because most deaths attributable to asthma occur outside the hospital setting before the patient can reach medical assistance, the primary cause of death in asthma most probably is an underestimation of the severity of the asthma attack by the patient and delay in seeking medical help. Overuse of quick reliever medication suggests inadequate asthma control and can lead to fatal asthma.[1,60]

The frequency of as-needed doses of albuterol is a good marker of the adequacy of inhaled anti-inflammatory therapy and environmental control measures. For example, if the patient needs the SABA more than 2 or 3 times a day, the clinician should reassess environmental control, increase the dose of inhaled anti-inflammatory therapy, or add other controller agents per EPR-3.[1]

Patients should be instructed verbally and in writing regarding the proper use of their inhalers during acute attacks and in recognizing when it is necessary to seek medical assistance (Fig. 18-10) Patients can continue using their short-acting β-agonist inhalers on an as-needed basis until they reach medical care. H.T. should be considered at high risk because of the severity of his latest attack and should be given oral corticosteroids to self-administer at the first sign of significant deterioration.[1] In addition, H.T. should have a home peak flow meter so that he can objectively determine the severity of his attacks. Finally, the β_2-agonist controversy does not extend to use of high dosages in the acute-care setting. High dosages are essential in the ED and hospital and, as discussed previously, usually are tolerated very well.

CHRONIC ASTHMA

Classification of Severity

CASE 18-3

Question 1: B.C. is a 3-year-old, 16-kg boy with a 1.5-year history of recurrent wheezing 3 days per week and nocturnal awakenings 4 times per month. His medications include albuterol syrup (2 mg/5 mL) one teaspoonful 3 times a day (TID) and albuterol metered-dose aerosol inhalation QID PRN for wheezing. B.C. demonstrates the use of the inhaler with his mother's assistance. The mother holds the inhaler in B.C.'s mouth and actuates it at the end of a deep inhalation. B.C.'s mother tells the clinician that he appears "jittery" after taking albuterol syrup. What is the first step in deciding how to improve B.C.'s long-term drug therapy?

While keeping in mind the goals of therapy defined by the NIH guidelines (EPR-3),[1] the first step here is to classify B.C.'s asthma severity (refer to Table 18-1) for infants to age 4 years). Because B.C. has symptoms 3 days per week and 4 nights per month, he should be classified as "moderate persistent." Note that the presence of even one of the features of severity places the patient in that category.

Selection of Appropriate Initial Long-Term Therapy

Case 18-3, Question 2: What would be a reasonable initial regimen for B.C.?

Because B.C.'s asthma is classified as moderate persistent, the clinician is now in a position to select appropriate long-term therapy. Using EPR-3[1] for very young children (Fig. 18-6), low- or medium-dose inhaled corticosteroids (ICS) with an as-needed SABA would be the choice for B.C.[1] In considering this decision, EPR-3 Figure 18-6 has "Notes" below the treatment steps. For example, it is noted that Step 2 (low-dose ICS) is preferred in this very young age group based on the strongest evidence (Evidence A). It is further noted that other recommendations are based on expert opinion and extrapolation from studies in older pediatric patients.[1] EPR-3 suggests an initial trial of low-dose ICS in very young children who have not previously been treated with ICS. B.C. could receive low-dose ICS treatments via nebulizer (budesonide) or MDI plus a spacer. Most children aged 3 years or younger cannot use dry powder inhalers because of inability to generate sufficient peak inspiratory flow (PIF). Because B.C. matures, he may be able to use some dry powder inhalers (e.g., Diskus). Because oral β_2-agonists are not recommended by EPR-3 and the albuterol syrup was not well tolerated, they should not be used. If concurrent inhaled albuterol is administered correctly, oral albuterol is not needed and would only be expected to add adverse effects. B.C.'s mother must be educated about asthma, its treatment, and the appropriate use of medications (e.g., proper use of inhaler devices; refer to Case 18-13, Questions 1 and 2).

Case 18-3, Question 3: It is anticipated that because of his young age, B.C. will find it difficult to use an MDI. What alternative inhalation devices are reasonable?

Children younger than 5 years of age generally have a difficult time coordinating the use of standard MDIs; therefore, the ICS and SABA should be administered by another mode of delivery. For example, the as-needed β_2-agonist and scheduled ICS could be administered with an inhalational aid ("spacer" or valved holding chamber), which is connected to an MDI. A nebulized corticosteroid preparation (budesonide) is available for very young children.[61] Inhalation aids significantly improve the efficacy of medications that are administered by MDI in very young children or other patients who are unable to coordinate the plain inhalers correctly.[1,62–64] The AeroChamber is a widely used valved holding chamber (the medication stays in the chamber for a few seconds until the patient inhales slowly and the inhalation valve opens). Studies have shown that many children as young as 2 and 3 years of age can use MDIs with spacer devices by modeling after a parent.[62,63] Spacer devices with face masks are required for some young children. Extender device-assisted delivery of aerosolized medications is as effective as nebulization in the home management of chronic severe asthma[65] and even in the ED treatment of asthma in children.[1,22–24,64] AeroChamber is an example of a device that contains a flow indicator whistle that sounds if the patient inhales rapidly. This whistle is particularly effective in teaching the patient the appropriate slow inhalation technique. As a 3-year-old, B.C. may not need a spacer with a face mask, but the clinician should verify correct use of the device by observation of the patient's or caregiver's administration technique.

Alternatively, the ICS could be administered to selected children by using a breath-activated dry powder inhaler (e.g., budesonide [Pulmicort Flexhaler] or fluticasone [combined with salmeterol in Advair Diskus]). In young children, the Diskus has the advantage of requiring a lower PIF than Flexhaler, and it has been used successfully in children as young as 4 years of age.[66] Another option is the Twisthaler used for delivery of mometasone (Asmanex), but it is approved for children 4 years of age and older.

Many pediatricians may choose a nebulizer to administer SABAs to a 3-year-old child. This method is certainly acceptable and very common, but it takes longer to administer the medication (about 15 minutes), and the device must be properly cleaned and maintained. Because B.C. recently turned 3 years old, therapy should be initiated with nebulized budesonide (Pulmicort Respules) in a low dose of 0.25 mg BID. As mentioned previously, EPR-3[1] suggests an initial trial of low-dose ICS in very young children who have not previously been treated with ICS. The plan is to switch B.C. to a dry powder inhaler or MDI spacer in 12 months, as soon as he and his caregiver can demonstrate correct use. B.C.'s clinician should assess the response to low-dose budesonide in 4 weeks. Therapy can be stepped up if necessary and subsequently stepped down in the coming months, if possible, so that optimal asthma control is achieved at the lowest ICS dose possible.

Case 18-3, Question 4: B.C.'s parents are wary of their son taking corticosteroids on a continual basis after having read about serious side effects attributed to corticosteroids on the Internet. How should the parents be counseled?

Corticosteroids reach the systemic circulation minimally via inhalation in part because they are largely inactivated through first-pass hepatic metabolism. However, a dose-dependent response is evident, and clinically significant adverse events resulting from systemic exposure can occur, albeit more commonly with doses at the high end of the range. Long-term studies in pediatric patients have examined the effects of ICS on growth reduction, bone density, and adrenal suppression.[1,67]

Although ICS can cause a mild and temporary reduction in growth velocity, final height attained in adulthood appears to be within normal limits.[1,67] Bone density and risk of fractures have not been found in the majority of investigations to be affected by ICS.[1] Although a measurable reduction in serum and urinary cortisol levels is not an uncommon finding in studies of ICS, clinically significant adrenal insufficiency solely caused by ICS is rare, although again it is more likely to occur with high doses.[1,67] In summary, these adverse effects are generally of minimal clinical significance, with the benefits of well-controlled asthma far outweighing the risks.

The most common local side effect with ICS therapy is oropharyngeal candidiasis (thrush), but this problem is rare with any delivery system. With MDIs, it can be further minimized by use of a spacer device. Rinsing the mouth with water after use of any ICS is also recommended. Another possible local side effect is hoarseness (dysphonia), and spacers may not effectively reduce this problem.[68] Dry powder devices (e.g., Flexhaler) may have less dysphonia associated with their use, but further study is required to verify this.[68]

Seasonal Asthma

CASE 18-4

Question 1: C.V., a 33-year-old woman, presents to the clinic with a history of asthma and seasonal allergic rhinitis (hay fever) each spring but not the rest of the year. She describes her asthma as "mild" and intermittent. Except during springtime, her daytime symptoms occur less than once per week, and she does not have nocturnal symptoms. Each spring, however, these symptoms worsen, and she requires her albuterol inhaler (her only asthma medication) TID or QID every day. During springtime, she takes a nonprescription antihistamine, which offers some relief. How can C.V.'s management be improved?

C.V. appears to have intermittent asthma during most of the year but converts to moderate-persistent asthma combined with worsening rhinitis symptoms in the springtime. This syndrome is consistent with a diagnosis of seasonal asthma and allergic rhinitis. Although as-needed albuterol is appropriate most of the year for C.V., she needs anti-inflammatory therapy during the spring.[1] Therapy to reduce airway inflammation should begin before the onset of tree and grass pollen season and continue throughout the spring (e.g., 3 months). Per the NIH guidelines, an excellent treatment option for C.V. is low-dose ICS combined with a long-acting inhaled β_2-agonist (LABA). Monotherapy with medium-dose ICS would also be an acceptable therapy. Not only are the causes and pathophysiology of allergic rhinitis and allergic asthma similar, poorly controlled rhinitis also serves as a major asthma trigger. In addition, C.V. should also ideally receive an intranasal corticosteroid if antihistamines (preferably nonsedating) do not provide optimal relief of her allergic rhinitis. Intranasal corticosteroid therapy not only offers excellent relief of nasal symptoms but also improves asthma control.[1] Good control of rhinitis is helpful in maintaining optimal asthma control[1] (see Chapter 20, Acute and Chronic Rhinitis). Despite precautions listed in manufacturer literature that older (sedating) antihistamines should be avoided in asthma, these agents are safe in patients with asthma.[1] Nevertheless, nonsedating antihistamines are preferred.

Corticosteroids

CASE 18-5

Question 1: S.T., a 12-year-old girl with severe-persistent asthma, has not been well controlled on mometasone 220 mcg (Asmanex) one inhalation daily (she admits to using it only when she feels as if she needs it) and uses as-needed inhaled albuterol MDI 5 or 6 times every day. When her symptoms worsen, she uses her "breathing machine" (nebulizer) at home. S.T. awakens most nights with wheezing. She has been hospitalized 4 times in the last 2 years and has required "bursts" of prednisone with increasing frequency. S.T. has missed many days of school in the past year and has withdrawn from physical education classes and her extracurricular sports activity after school. Her parents are concerned about her increased use of prednisone now that she is approaching puberty. S.T. is just finishing a 2-week course of prednisone 20 mg/day and has a round facies appearance typical of chronic oral corticosteroid use. On physical examination, S.T. has diffuse expiratory wheezes, and pulmonary function testing reveals significant reversibility. Her FEV_1 is only 60% predicted before use of albuterol in the physician's office and improves to 75% predicted 15 minutes after use of the SABA. What actions are needed to improve S.T.'s care?

Because S.T. is suffering needlessly and requiring frequent systemic corticosteroids, all efforts must be made to optimize other therapies and to minimize systemic corticosteroid toxicities. Although S.T. is receiving an ICS, she admits to poor adherence. Therefore, with her severe-persistent asthma, she initially needs higher-dose ICS therapy. Per EPR-3,[1] she should also receive a LABA. Although short bursts of prednisone (e.g., 40 mg/day for 3 days) are very helpful occasionally, frequent short courses often indicate the need to optimize other therapies. Some patients require courses of 1 to 2 weeks. S.T. is requiring longer frequent bursts and is showing signs of adverse effects. Obviously, S.T. and her parents also need a concerted and persistent effort in patient education as a partnership (refer to Patient Education and Outcomes sections).

ICS are chemically modified to maximize topical effectiveness while minimizing systemic toxicities. EPR-3[1] compares the dosages of ICS products. These differences in dosages (low, medium, and high) reflect differences among ICS in receptor-binding affinity and topical potency. There are also differences among these agents in oral bioavailability (i.e., absorption of drug that is swallowed after inhalation) and systemic availability via absorption from the lungs. Of these two variables, absorption from the lungs is the most likely contributor to possible hypothalamic–pituitary–adrenal (HPA) suppression or other systemic effects. Fortunately, the total absorption has not been shown to be clinically important except at the higher recommended dosages. Although the various ICS are not equipotent on a microgram-per-microgram basis, major differences in efficacy or adverse effects are not firmly established.[1] For patients with severe-persistent asthma, a logical choice would be a high-potency agent that would allow for a minimum number of inhalations per day, potentially improving treatment adherence. Furthermore, the delivery system used affects pulmonary deposition, but each available delivery system has established efficacy if used correctly.[1,69,70] The differences among the various dry powder inhalers are discussed later in this chapter. Addition of a spacer device to an MDI also enhances pulmonary deposition. In very high dosages (the equivalent of 1,600 mcg/day of beclomethasone dipropionate), all ICS produce some degree of HPA-axis suppression.[1] The clinical significance of this suppression has yet to be firmly established.

Although low-to-moderate dosages of ICS are accepted as being quite safe, very high dosages continue to be scrutinized regarding the potential adverse effects.[1] Clearly, for patients who require high dosages for optimal control of asthma, the benefits of therapy with these agents far outweigh the risks.[1] A possible association between prolonged, very high dosages of ICS and cataracts[71,72] and glaucoma[73] has been reported. EPR-3 has summarized research that has allayed concerns regarding use of ICS therapy and growth suppression in children (i.e., the decrease in growth velocity is small and not progressive, and appears to be quite minimal).[1,65,74]

CASE 18-5, QUESTION 2: How should S.T. be managed?

In the treatment of S.T., most clinicians would begin with a short course (e.g., 1 week) of systemic corticosteroids to maximally improve her pulmonary function. This approach is consistent with EPR-3,[1] which recommends gaining quick control. Using short-course systemic therapy is logical because it is inexpensive, efficacious, and associated with low risk. While gaining quick control with a short course of oral corticosteroids, it is logical to start ICS in many patients at a low[1,75]-to-moderate dosage. The evidence that ICS are highly effective in persistent asthma is unequivocal. Patients in this category who consistently take ICS are at a lower risk of hospitalization and death, and one study found an increased risk of death after discontinuation of ICS compared with patients who remained on these drugs.[76] ICS therapy should be initiated concomitantly with a short course of systemic corticosteroid therapy. Patient education at this time may have greater effectiveness because some patients are more attentive after having just experienced an exacerbation, and they know that change is needed to improve their health. Similar to adults, intensification of therapy with increasing the ICS dose, adding montelukast, or adding a LABA was found to be successful in pediatric patients, with the LABA being the most likely addition to be beneficial.[1,77–79] Because S.T.'s asthma is classified as *severe* persistent, it is reasonable to start her on a moderate-to-high dosage of an ICS in combination with a LABA (Fig. 18-8, Table 18-3). More aggressive therapy initially is especially important in S.T. because of her four hospitalizations in the last 2 years. In partnership with S.T. and her parents, her preference should be determined as to the delivery method (i.e., discuss options with her regarding breath-activated devices or MDI and spacer, including which spacer). Ideally, the clinician should recognize her emerging independence as a 12-year-old and talk with her alone and then with her parents. After S.T. is stabilized for 3 months, attempts should be made to slowly decrease the ICS dosage every 3 months until the lowest effective dosage is achieved. Administration of the total daily ICS dose is preferred twice daily or, in many patients with mild-persistent to moderate-persistent asthma, once daily.[1] Because adherence is a major determinant of success or failure with ICS and other therapies, simplified regimens and continued patient education and contact are essential.[1]

COMBINATION OF INHALED CORTICOSTEROIDS AND LONG-ACTING INHALED β_2-AGONISTS

CASE 18-5, QUESTION 3: Because S.T. is 12 years old, what options are appropriate to minimize the ICS dosage, realizing that aggressive therapy is needed? What are the risks associated with LABAs? Clinicians should monitor for which local side effects in S.T. with ICS therapy?

LABAs have been very successful in prevention of "stepping up" the dose of ICS while markedly enhancing overall asthma control,[77–79] and this fact is reflected in EPR-3.[1] A reasonable therapeutic option for S.T. would be the combination of fluticasone 250 mcg and salmeterol 50 mcg via Diskus (Advair 250/50) 1 inhalation BID, the budesonide/formoterol (Symbicort) combination inhaler (160/4.5 mcg; 2 inhalations BID), the mometasone/formoterol (Dulera) combination inhaler (100/5 mcg; 2 inhalations BID), or the fluticasone furoate/vilanterol (Breo Ellipta) combination inhaler (200/25 mcg; 1 inhalation once daily). S.T. should be re-evaluated in 2 weeks. The plan is to step down the dose of fluticasone after excellent asthma control is achieved.

Adverse Effects Associated with Long-Acting Inhaled β_2-Agonists

CASE 18-5, QUESTION 4: S.T.'s parents recently discovered an article in a national newspaper that addressed concerns of using LABAs because of an increased risk of death. Because S.T.'s parents have called and left a message for the clinician, what would be important information to share with her family regarding this issue? What other side effects should S.T. and her family be aware of?

Several randomized trials for more than a decade have demonstrated that LABAs have minimal adverse effects (e.g., tachycardia, tremor).[1,69,70,77–79] Although there are limited data, based primarily on one study (SMART),[80] there may be a very small increased risk of asthma-related death and asthma exacerbation in patients receiving LABAs. This small risk is likely attributable to patients receiving LABAs without concomitant ICS. In fact, EPR-3[1] recommends against the use of LABAs as monotherapy for long-term control of persistent asthma. SMART[80] data suggested that black patients may be at greater risk, but much more study is needed to confirm these data. LABA therapy should *only* be used in combination with ICS in patients with asthma. Both national[1] and international[81] asthma guidelines clearly state that combination ICS/LABA therapy for asthma is safe and effective. EPR-3[1] suggests giving equal consideration to a moderate dose of ICS alone or low-dose ICS combined with LABA for patients with moderate-persistent asthma. In 2010, the US Food and Drug Administration (FDA) offered recommendations regarding the use of LABA in patients with asthma, including always using combination products (ICS/LABA) versus two single-agent products to help ensure LABA are never used alone in asthma patients.[82] In response to the FDA, editorials by EPR-3 members and others question some aspects of the FDA recommendations.[83,84] For S.T., who has severe-persistent asthma, ICS/LABA combination therapy is preferred.[1]

Step-Down Treatment

CASE 18-5, QUESTION 5: After being adherent to her new therapy (fluticasone 250 mcg/salmeterol 50 mcg BID) for 1 month, S.T.'s asthma control has markedly improved. She required no ED visits or hospitalizations, was sleeping through the night, and began to exercise again. Her personal best PEF was 320 L/minute, and she was staying in her green zone (260–320 L/minute), requiring PRN albuterol no more than once per week. After 2 more months, S.T. continues to do well. Although S.T. clearly needs long-term ICS therapy, after 3 months of excellent response, her clinician is now ready to step down from high-dose fluticasone. What is a prudent approach to dosage reduction?

EPR-3[1] suggests stepping down the dose at a rate of 25% to 50% every 3 months to the lowest dose that maintains control. A step down to fluticasone 100 mcg/salmeterol 50 mcg (Advair 100/50) BID would be a reasonable reduction in therapy for S.T. If a single ICS product had been started in S.T. initially (e.g., budesonide, beclomethasone, fluticasone), the dosage reduction would normally proceed at a slower pace. However, fluticasone 100 mcg BID, especially in combination with salmeterol, will likely be an adequate dose for S.T. After S.T.'s dose of fluticasone was stepped down to 200 mcg/day, she started requiring only slightly more PRN albuterol (but still was symptom free most days). Another consideration for S.T. is that recent international evidence-based guidelines (Global Initiative for Asthma—GINA[81]) suggest an alternative approach for patients at risk of severe exacerbations. Patients receiving low-dose ICS combined with formoterol may be instructed to not only use their routine twice-daily scheduled doses, but also use the same combination for "as-needed" doses for quick relief instead of PRN albuterol.[81] Although this approach is not commonly used in the USA, it is an option per GINA.[81]

CASE 18-5, QUESTION 6: If symptoms recur during step-down, what management could possibly facilitate dosage reduction of the ICS in S.T.?

During follow-up evaluations, clinicians should carefully investigate factors that may contribute to poor asthma control, including exposure to inhalant allergens, indoor or outdoor irritants, medications, and tobacco smoke. Secondhand smoke exposure has been demonstrated to reduce the benefit of ICS in children and necessitate step-up therapy, and asthma patients who smoke have reduced response to ICS therapy.[85,86]

Leukotriene Modifiers

CASE 18-6

QUESTION 1: P.W. is a 52-year-old man with mild-persistent asthma. His asthma symptoms began when he was 2 years of age, and he has never smoked. P.W. has had numerous drug regimens for his asthma during the years, but he tells his physician that he wants the simplest regimen possible and that he prefers oral medication if at all possible. What is a good choice for controller therapy in P.W.?

In patients of any age with mild-persistent asthma, and certainly in children or adolescents, an oral agent such as montelukast with once-daily dosing at bedtime (or zafirlukast with twice-daily dosing) has obvious advantages. Zileuton is another leukotriene modifier, but it has more drug interactions and adverse effects than the other available agents. An ICS is the preferred treatment for mild-persistent asthma. Studies comparing ICS with leukotriene receptor agonists have consistently demonstrated the superiority of ICS for most asthma outcome measures,[1] but in patients (adults or children) who much prefer oral therapy to inhaling medication every day, leukotriene modifiers are a reasonable option. The simplest and safest possible oral controller regimen for P.W. is montelukast 10 mg at bedtime (with PRN inhaled albuterol). Bedtime dosing with montelukast is recommended because it will have peak activity late at night and in the early morning hours, when asthma symptoms tend to be more frequent. However, montelukast may be taken at any time of day as long as it is taken at a consistent time that is convenient for the patient. It is likely that this regimen will result in very good asthma control. If P.W. does not have good control of his asthma when he returns to the clinic in a few weeks, switching to a low-dose ICS in the evening only would keep the regimen simple while enhancing efficacy.

Theophylline

DOSING

CASE 18-7

QUESTION 1: K.J., a 14-year-old, 40-kg girl, has a history of recurring cough and wheezing. These symptoms worsen on vigorous running or when she has an upper respiratory infection. She has not required hospitalization for these symptoms but has missed a few school days. She has symptoms daily and uses her albuterol inhaler more than 2 times daily. K.J. has a family history of asthma. A diagnosis of moderate-persistent asthma is made. How should K.J. be managed?

Because K.J. has moderate-persistent asthma, treatment with an anti-inflammatory agent is indicated. A medium-dose ICS or a low-dose ICS plus a LABA is the preferred treatment in a 14-year-old child with moderate-persistent asthma.[1] However, not all healthcare professionals follow the latest evidence-based guidelines, and K.J.'s clinician opts to prescribe theophylline in combination with a low dose of budesonide via the Flexhaler.

CASE 18-7, QUESTION 2: What dosage of theophylline is appropriate for K.J.?

Low doses of budesonide combined with twice-daily theophylline that resulted in a median serum theophylline concentration of 8.7 mcg/mL were superior in efficacy to high-dose budesonide as single controller therapy.[87] Thus, it is wise to give a therapeutic trial with low-dose theophylline initially, aiming for serum concentrations between 5 and 10 mcg/mL. In the nonacute asthma patient in whom the theophylline dose requirement is unknown, dosages suggested for ages older than 1 year of age are listed in Table 18-5 and infant dosing is listed in Table 18-6. Accordingly, the initial dosage in K.J. would be 300 mg/day in divided doses (i.e., 150 mg every 12 hours). If tolerated, the dosage is increased at 3-day intervals by about 25% to the mean dose that usually is needed to produce a peak theophylline serum concentration between 5 and 10 mcg/mL. The final dosage can be adjusted by serum concentration monitoring. Serum theophylline concentrations should be obtained at steady state (i.e., when there have been no missed doses and no extra doses have been taken for at least 48 hours).

TOXICITY

CASE 18-7, QUESTION 3: K.J. now complains of headache and difficulty in getting to sleep. Why should a theophylline serum concentration be evaluated?

Theophylline side effects can be related to excessive serum concentrations, or adverse effects can be transient and unrelated to the amount in serum. Unfortunately, it is not always possible to determine which it might be. Side effects can include headache, nausea, vomiting, irritability or hyperactivity, insomnia, and diarrhea. With higher serum theophylline levels, cardiac arrhythmias, seizures, and death can occur.[88] Less severe symptoms may not be present before the onset of cardiac arrhythmias or seizures and cannot be relied on as a forewarning of these more serious adverse theophylline effects. It is important not to ignore any symptom consistent with theophylline toxicity. The insomnia and headaches experienced by K.J. may not be associated with excessive (i.e., out of the usual therapeutic range) serum theophylline concentrations, but a reduction in dosage should be contemplated because some patients experience toxicity when serum theophylline concentrations are within the therapeutic range. Guidelines for managing toxicity have been revised.[88]

Table 18-5
Theophylline Dosing Guide for Chronic Use

Starting dose for children 1–15 years <45 kg: 12–14 mg/kg/day to maximum of 300 mg/day[a,b]
Starting dose for adults and children 1–15 years >45 kg: 300 mg/day
Titrate dose upward after 3 days if necessary and if tolerated to:
■ 16 mg/kg/day to maximum of 400 mg/day in children 1–15 years <45 kg ■ 400 mg/day in adults and children >45 kg
Titrate dose upward after 3 more days if necessary and if tolerated to:
■ 20 mg/kg/day to a maximum of 600 mg/day in children 1–15 years <45 kg ■ 600 mg/day in adults and in children >45 kg

[a]Dose using ideal body weight or actual body weight, whichever is less. These dosages do not apply if liver disease, heart failure, or other factors documented to affect theophylline clearance are present. Doses must be guided by monitoring serum concentrations to ensure optimal safety and efficacy.
[b]Dosing schedule dependent on product selected; sustained-release products are much preferred, if at all possible.
Source: Hendeles L et al. Revised FDA labeling guideline for theophylline oral dosage forms. *Pharmacotherapy*. 1995;15:409.

Table 18-6
Food and Drug Administration Guidelines for Theophylline Dosing in Infants

Premature Neonates[a]
<24 days postnatal age: 1.0 mg/kg every 12 hours
≥24 days postnatal age: 1.5 mg/kg every 12 hours
Term Infants and Infants Up to 52 Weeks of Age
Total daily dose (mg) = ([0.2 × age in weeks] + 5.0) × (kg body weight)
■ Up to age 26 weeks; divide dose into 3 equal amounts administered at 8-hour intervals ■ >26 weeks of age; divide dose into 4 equal amounts administered at 6-hour intervals

[a]Final doses adjusted to a peak steady-state serum theophylline concentration of 5–10 mcg/mL in neonates and 10–15 mcg/mL in older infants.
Source: Hendeles L et al. Revised FDA labeling guideline for theophylline oral dosage forms. *Pharmacotherapy*. 1995;15:409.

DRUG INTERACTIONS

CASE 18-8

QUESTION 1: T.R., a 55-year-old woman with asthma, is well controlled on theophylline SR 300 mg BID, albuterol two puffs QID PRN, and mometasone 220 mcg (Asmanex) one inhalation at bedtime. A peak theophylline serum concentration obtained 3 months ago was 14 mcg/mL. Six months ago, on the same dose of theophylline, her serum concentration was 15 mcg/mL. T.R. presents with an upper respiratory tract infection, and clarithromycin 500 mg BID is prescribed. Is this antibiotic appropriate?

A large number of medications inhibit cytochrome P-450 (CYP) isoenzymes and are capable of inhibiting the metabolism of theophylline. Because theophylline is metabolized by CYP 1A2, 3A3, and 2E1, inhibitors of these isoenzymes can cause clinically significant interactions.[56,88] Cimetidine, clarithromycin, and some (but not all) of the quinolone antibiotics (e.g., ciprofloxacin) are well documented to inhibit theophylline metabolism.[1,56] Because numerous other drugs inhibit the metabolism of theophylline, all patients receiving this agent should be screened carefully for potential interactions. As with any drug interaction, the mechanism, time course, management, and clinical significance should be assessed before any interventions. For example, cimetidine decreases theophylline clearance within 24 hours, and this interaction should be circumvented by using another histamine H_2-blocker or a proton-pump inhibitor (Table 18-7). Classic inducers (e.g.,

Table 18-7
Factors Affecting Serum Theophylline Concentrations

Factor[a]	Decreases Theophylline Concentrations	Increases Theophylline Concentrations	Recommended Action
Food	↓ or delays absorption of some sustained-release theophylline (SR) products	↑ rate of absorption (fatty foods)	Select theophylline preparation that is not affected by food.
Diet	↑ metabolism (high protein)	↓ metabolism (high carbohydrate)	Inform patients that major changes in diet are not recommended while taking theophylline.
Systemic, febrile viral illness (e.g., influenza)		↓ metabolism	Decrease theophylline dose according to serum concentration level. Decrease dose by 50% if serum concentration measurement is not available.
Hypoxia, cor pulmonale, and decompensated congestive heart failure, cirrhosis		↓ metabolism	Decrease dose according to serum concentration level.
Age	↑ metabolism (1–9 years)	↓ metabolism (<6 months, elderly)	Adjust dose according to serum concentration level.
Phenobarbital, phenytoin, carbamazepine	↑ metabolism		Increase dose according to serum concentration level.
Cimetidine		↓ metabolism	Use alternative histamine H_2-antagonist (e.g., famotidine or ranitidine).
Macrolides: TAO, erythromycin, clarithromycin		↓ metabolism	Use alternative antibiotic or adjust theophylline dose.
Quinolones: ciprofloxacin, enoxacin, pefloxacin		↓ metabolism	Use alternative antibiotic or adjust theophylline dose.
Rifampin	↑ metabolism		Increase dose according to serum concentration level.
Ticlopidine		↓ metabolism	Decrease dose according to serum concentration level.
Smoking	↑ metabolism		Advise patient to stop smoking; increase dose according to serum concentration level.

[a]This list is not all inclusive; for discussion of other factors, see package inserts.
TAO, troleandomycin.
Modified from National Institutes of Health. *Expert Panel Report 3: Guidelines for the Diagnosis and Management of Asthma*. Bethesda, MD: National Heart, Lung, and Blood Institute; 2007. NIH publication 07-4051.

rifampin) of cytochrome P-450 also affect theophylline clearance, and patients should be monitored for decreased serum concentrations. In T.R., the interaction with clarithromycin can easily be circumvented by using azithromycin, which does not affect theophylline metabolism.

Anticholinergics

CASE 18-9

Question 1: R.K. is a 24-year-old African American graduate medical student with moderate-persistent asthma, which has been well controlled for 10 years with ICS therapy (beclomethasone HFA 80 mcg twice daily) and albuterol PRN. Recently, he has noticed that his asthma symptoms have worsened and he is requiring his albuterol inhaler 3 or 4 times per week, which causes him to have a resting tremor and feel anxious. One of his colleagues suggests that he should inquire about an anticholinergic medication in addition to his ICS. Is this appropriate?

Until now, anticholinergic agents have had limited use in asthma except in the ED[1,89] and a few other rare situations.[90] However, in a recent study of tiotropium, a long-acting once-daily anticholinergic agent, in persistent asthmatic patients poorly controlled on ICS alone, researchers demonstrated that the addition of tiotropium to ICS therapy was not inferior to the effects of adding salmeterol to ICS therapy and was superior to doubling the inhaled steroid dose.[91] The morning PEF and evening PEF were significantly higher in patients receiving tiotropium than those receiving a doubling of the ICS dose. A subsequent randomized, controlled trial found that tiotropium therapy added to combination ICS/LABA in suboptimally controlled adult asthma patients was superior to placebo.[92]

Although tiotropium is not identified in EPR-3 as an option for persistent asthma patients, a therapeutic trial in R.K. may be considered given these new data, especially given his anxiousness and tremor with the increased albuterol use. A similar response to LABAs may be seen. In 2015, Spiriva Respimat was approved for use as maintenance therapy in patients with asthma, ages >12-year-old, who remain symptomatic despite already receiving combination ICS/LABA treatment.

CASE 18-10

QUESTION 1: M.M. is a 30-year-old woman with severe-persistent asthma. Despite optimal assessment, drug therapy, environmental control, and patient education per the principles of management detailed in EPR-3, she has had two recent hospitalizations as a result of asthma. Her allergist is considering anti-IgE therapy. Is M.M. a good candidate for such therapy? How would it be given? M.M. has a pretreatment IgE level of 90 international units/mL, and she weighs 55 kg.

Omalizumab (Xolair) is a humanized monoclonal anti-IgE antibody that binds to free IgE in serum. Thus, binding of IgE to high-affinity receptors on mast cells is subsequently inhibited, and the initiation of the allergic inflammatory cascade is blocked.[1,93–96] Omalizumab is effective in reducing oral and ICS dose requirements in patients with severe asthma and in reducing exacerbations.[93–96] This novel therapy is administered as a 150- to 375-mg subcutaneous injection every 2 or 4 weeks. The dose and frequency of administration are based on the serum total IgE level (international units/mL) and the patient's body weight. Therefore, M.M.'s omalizumab dose is 150 mg subcutaneously every 4 weeks.

Common side effects associated with omalizumab include injection site reactions, upper respiratory tract infections, sinusitis, and headache. Less common but potentially serious adverse effects include anaphylaxis (0.2% in postmarketing spontaneous reports), which can occur after any dose even if previous doses have been well tolerated and 24 or more hours after administration, and the development of malignant neoplasms (0.5% of omalizumab-treated patients compared with 0.2% in control patients).

Because omalizumab is expensive and must be administered as a subcutaneous injection, it should be reserved for patients with severe asthma who are not adequately controlled with standard therapies. Despite the high cost, anti-IgE therapy might be cost effective in selected patients with severe disease (e.g., those with frequent ED visits and hospitalizations) because an estimated less than 5% of asthma patients (severe disease) account for greater than 50% of the dollars spent for asthma care.[97]

CASE 18-10, QUESTION 2: Because the nurse prepares the dose of omalizumab for M.M., what are some special considerations regarding administering and monitoring this drug?

After reconstitution of omalizumab, the drug must be administered within 4 hours if stored at room temperature and within 8 hours when refrigerated. As a result of its viscosity, the injection may take 5 to 10 seconds. No more than 150 mg is injected at each site. Although the risk of anaphylaxis is rare (0.2%),[98] patients should stay in the physician's office for at least 30 minutes after injection of omalizumab and be educated regarding the signs and symptoms of anaphylaxis. After leaving the physician's office, patients should seek emergency medical treatment at the first sign of anaphylaxis. Despite the low risk of severe allergic reactions, in 2010 the manufacturer added a black box warning about the risk of anaphylaxis.[98]

EXERCISE-INDUCED ASTHMA

CASE 18-11

QUESTION 1: T.W., a 33-year-old woman, presents to the clinic with a history of severe coughing and chest tightness after exercise. She recently joined an exercise club to lose weight but is unable to keep up with others of her own age and relative condition when jogging outside. She recalls having mild respiratory problems as a young child but has never taken any asthma medications. She has a positive treadmill test for exercise-induced asthma (EIA). How should T.W. be treated?

During sustained exercise, at least 90% of patients with asthma experience an initial improvement in pulmonary functions quickly followed by a significant decline (Fig. 18-11). This phenomenon may be the only symptom of subclinical asthma.[1,99] Patients can be diagnosed by measuring the FEV_1 or PEF before and after exercise (6- to 8-minute treadmill or bicycle exercise test). A reduction of FEV_1 by more than 15% of the baseline value is a positive test.

Hyperventilation of cold, dry air increases the sensitivity to EIA and induces bronchospasm.[99] The main stimulus for EIA is respiratory heat loss, water loss, or both,[99] while breathing heated, humidified air completely blocks EIA in many patients.[99] Masks are indicated for patients with EIA in the wintertime, and patients with severe asthma accompanied by EIA also should be encouraged to swim or engage in other indoor exercise that does not promote EIA. A warm-up period before strenuous exercise is helpful in some patients. With appropriate premedication, most EIA can be prevented, so virtually all patients with stable asthma should be encouraged to exercise. The mechanism of bronchoconstriction after airway heat and water loss is still incompletely understood.[99]

Although several drugs inhibit EIA, SABAs are generally the agents of choice for prophylaxis.[1,99] For typical periods of exercise (e.g., <3 hours), pretreatment with agents such as albuterol 5 to 15 minutes before exercise usually provides excellent protection from EIA.

For prolonged periods of exercise, LABAs (formoterol, salmeterol) provide several hours of protection.[1,100] Two differences in formoterol and salmeterol include the delivery systems for inhalation and the onset of action. If either of these agents is to be used to prevent EIA, it is important for the patient to inhale the medication at the proper time before exercise. Formoterol should be inhaled at least 15 minutes before exercise, and salmeterol administration should occur at least 30 minutes before vigorous activity. Patients who are receiving therapy every 12 hours with either drug concomitantly with ICS for long-term control of asthma should already be protected and therefore only use albuterol if symptoms occur after exercise. With maintenance therapy, as opposed to single doses before exercise, bronchoprotection from exercise may be reduced

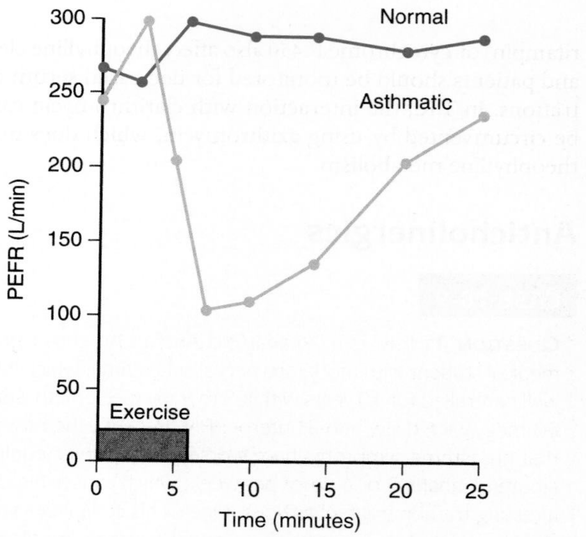

Figure 18-11 Changes in peak expiratory flow rate with exercise in an asthmatic and normal subject. PEFR, peak expiratory flow rate.

to 5 hours with LABAs.[1] Leukotriene receptor antagonists (e.g., montelukast once-daily chronic therapy) have also been demonstrated to prevent EIA.[101] Finally, it is important to point out that in persistent asthma, long-term anti-inflammatory therapy is helpful in reducing the response to most asthma triggers, including exercise.[1] For most patients who have EIA only, use of a SABA 15 minutes before exercise is the only therapy needed.

Because of the hyperventilation of relatively cool, dry air, jogging is a potent stimulus for EIA. A number of possible therapeutic interventions exist for T.W. She could be encouraged to swim because the inhalation of humidified warm air is less likely to produce EIA. However, if she wishes to continue jogging, two inhalations of a SABA (e.g., albuterol) from a metered-dose aerosol 15 minutes before exercise should provide adequate protection for 2 to 3 hours. If outdoor temperatures are quite cool or cold, T.W. should jog indoors. T.W. also should be counseled to take two additional inhalations if she "breaks through" the initial protection and experiences tightness.

CASE 18-12

QUESTION 1: W.L., a 17-year-old boy, presents to the clinic with a complaint of dyspnea and coughing that has limited his ability to keep up with his basketball teammates. He states that it is worse when playing outdoors unless the gym is cold and that it seems to be worse (occurring sooner during exercise) than a month ago. W.L. experienced several bouts of bronchitis as a young child but has not had any problems for the past 6 years. His symptoms are consistent with EIA. How should his EIA be treated?

W.L. presents a special problem in that he is a teenager. Both for adolescents and children, peer pressure usually is extremely significant. Optimal prophylaxis is important to allow W.L. to compete at his best level. Embarrassment about not keeping up with teammates can be very hurtful now, and it has implications for setting habits of exercise into adulthood. Many adults with asthma do not exercise because they think they cannot do so based on childhood experiences. Lack of exercise can have a negative impact on physiologic and psychologic well-being. W.L. should receive preventive treatment with an inhaled β_2-agonist. The question is whether he should receive a short-acting or a long-acting agent. The clinician should probe as to the duration of exercise. If W.L. exercises for longer than 3 hours, formoterol or salmeterol administered 15 to 30 minutes before exercise would be a logical choice. Finally, the clinician should verify that exercise is the only factor that precipitates asthma symptoms. It could be that further questioning of W.L. will reveal persistent asthma or mild intermittent asthma beyond EIA only. If that is the case, long-term ICS or montelukast therapy should be started to reduce overall airway hyperresponsiveness.

PATIENT EDUCATION

CASE 18-13

QUESTION 1: A.B., a 26-year-old woman, calls her clinician and states that she has run out of her albuterol MDI. She has a prescription for a budesonide dry powder inhaler but admits that she does not use this medication "because it doesn't seem to work as well as her albuterol MDI." A.B. has had asthma all of her life. She complains of symptoms most days but has not required visits to the ED or hospitalizations. The provider determines that A.B. is bothered most about daily shortness of breath and worries that her condition may get worse. What should the provider do in this situation?

Table 18-8
Key Educational Messages: Teach and Reinforce at Every Opportunity

Basic Facts About Asthma

- The contrast between airways of a person who has and a person who does not have asthma; the role of inflammation
- What happens to the airways in an asthma attack

Roles of Medications—Understanding the Difference Between the Following:

- Long-term control medications: prevent symptoms, often by reducing inflammation. Must be taken daily. Do not expect them to give quick relief.
- Quick-relief medications: Short-acting β_2-agonists relax muscles around the airway and provide prompt relief of symptoms. Do not expect them to provide long-term asthma control. Using quick-relief medication on a daily basis indicates the need for starting or increasing long-term control medications.

Patient Skills

- Taking medications correctly. Inhaler technique (demonstrate to patient and have the patient return the demonstration). Use of devices, such as prescribed valved holding chamber, spacer, nebulizer.
- Identifying and avoiding environmental exposures that worsen the patient's asthma (e.g., allergens, irritants, tobacco smoke).
- Self-monitoring to:
  Assess level of asthma control
  Monitor symptoms and, if prescribed, peak flow
  Recognize early signs and symptoms of worsening asthma.
- Using written asthma action plan to know when and how to:
  Take daily actions to control asthma
  Adjust medication in response to signs of worsening asthma
  Seek medical care as appropriate.

Reprinted from National Institutes of Health. *Expert Panel Report 3: Guidelines for the Diagnosis and Management of Asthma*. Bethesda, MD: National Heart, Lung, and Blood Institute; 2007. NIH publication 07-4051.

If optimal long-term drug therapy of asthma is prescribed, treatment may still fail or be suboptimal if the patient does not receive adequate education. Patients with asthma require special educational efforts because of the use of inhalation devices and peak flow meters. In addition, it often is a major challenge to have patients and parents understand the critical importance of long-term daily controller therapy and environmental control. Of course, an important first step in educating asthma patients is to be caring and a good listener. Rather than sharing your knowledge initially, it is important to help establish a "partnership" with the patient by first asking the following question: "What is bothering you the most about your asthma?" Really listening to the patient and then addressing patient concerns is extremely important to successful education and long-term management. EPR-3 lists several patient education activities in Table 18-8.[1]

Clinicians can be of invaluable assistance to the patient by repeatedly reinforcing education on the necessity of using anti-inflammatory (and combined ICS/LABA) therapies on a regular schedule. Many patients underuse long-term preventive therapy because no health professional took the time to adequately instruct them that most asthma symptoms are preventable. Although underusing the most important medicines for long-term control, many patients overuse "quick relievers" (i.e., SABAs). Healthcare providers must be able to detect these problems and intervene to enhance patient care.

Table 18-9

Steps to Correct Use of Metered-Dose Inhalers

1. Shake the inhaler well and remove the dust cap.
2. Exhale *slowly* through pursed lips.[a,b]
3. If using the "closed-mouth" technique, hold the inhaler upright and place the mouthpiece between your lips. Be careful not to block the opening with your tongue or teeth.
4. If using the "open-mouth" technique, open your mouth wide and hold the inhaler upright 1–2 inches from your mouth, making sure the inhaler is properly aimed.
5. Press down on the inhaler *once* as you *start* a *slow*, deep inhalation.
6. Continue to inhale slowly and deeply through your mouth. Try to inhale for at least 5 seconds.
7. Hold your breath for 10 seconds (use your fingers to count to 10 slowly). If 10 seconds makes you feel uncomfortable, try to hold your breath for at least 4 seconds.
8. Exhale *slowly*.[c]
9. Wait at least 30–60 seconds before inhaling the next puff of medicine.

[a] If using a spacer, see manufacturer's instructions. Same basic principles of slow, deep inhalation with adequate breath-hold apply. With spacers, put mouthpiece on top of your tongue to ensure that tongue does not block aerosol.
[b] As long as exhalation is slow, exhale can take place for several seconds. Some experts insist on exhaling only a tidal volume, but the key is to exhale *slowly*.
[c] If patient has concomitant rhinitis, exhaling through the *nose* may be of benefit when using corticosteroids or ipratropium (i.e., some medication may deposit in nose).

Because a large percentage of patients have difficulty using MDIs, teaching patients the correct use of MDIs (alone or in combination with spacers) and dry powder inhalers is absolutely essential.[1,102,103] In one study, 89% of patients could not perform all of the steps for MDI use correctly.[104] Competent teaching requires *observation* of the patient using the devices initially and again on repeat visits to the clinic, hospital, or community pharmacy. Telling the patient about correct use is inadequate. Health professionals must demonstrate use of the devices (live or with videotapes) for patients who cannot use the devices correctly. For videos that show proper use of many types of asthma inhalers, go to **http://www.nationaljewish.org/healthinfo/multimedia/asthma-inhalers.aspx** for a video of how to use a nebulizer, go to **http://www.nationaljewish.org/healthinfo/medications/lung-diseases/devices/nebulizers/instructions.aspx**.

Although there is more than one correct way to use an MDI, Table 18-9 summarizes two commonly accepted approaches.[1,102] Many asthma experts prefer to use spacers to help ensure optimal efficacy. Spacers should be used in virtually all patients receiving ICS via an MDI, even those with perfect MDI technique, because spacers enhance efficacy and reduce the risk of oropharyngeal candidiasis.[105,106] On the other hand, spacers do not add efficacy to *correct* use of a β_2-agonist MDI.[107] Although any spacer can be helpful, marketed devices that are valved holding chambers and have a flow indicator whistle when inhalation is fast are preferred (e.g., AeroChamber).

Studies have shown that health professionals, like some patients, generally are not competent in using MDIs.[108] Obviously, the clinician should practice with a placebo inhaler and gain competence before teaching a patient. Among clinicians who educate patients, pharmacists can be helpful in teaching correct use of MDIs.[109] Unfortunately, one study showed that community pharmacists commonly are not providing such teaching.[110]

In addition to teaching the correct use of MDIs and spacers, clinicians should help patients via education regarding the correct use of breath-activated dry powder inhalers (e.g., Twisthaler, Diskus, Aerolizer, HandiHaler, Flexhaler) and nebulizing machines.[1] When using the Flexhaler, for example, patients must clearly understand the need for a rapid (preferably 60 L/minute), deep inhalation (not slow as with an MDI).[111] Such rapid PIF is achievable by some young children, but many children younger than 8 years of age have difficulty reaching PIF greater than 60 L/minute.[111] With the Diskus, PIF does not have to be as rapid as with Flexhaler, but it should be greater than 30 L/minute.[112] In addition, patients need to breath-hold 10 seconds if possible, as with an MDI.

Asthma Self-Management Plans

Objective monitoring of lung function at home with the use of peak flow meters can be very helpful to patients and healthcare professionals. EPR-3 discusses the debates about PEF versus symptom-based action plans.[1] Use of peak flow meters may be valuable in patients who have had severe exacerbations and those who are "poor perceivers" of deteriorating asthma control. Instructing patients on the correct use of the devices, including use of the green, yellow, and red zones, is essential.[1] After establishing that optimal therapy has maintained the PEF in the "green zone" in the early morning, most patients can simply verify their values once daily in the early morning. Analogous to a traffic light, green, yellow, and red zones have been established to guide the patient and clinician. The *green zone* refers to a PEF that is 80% to 100% of "personal best" and generally indicates that therapy is providing good control. Before a course of optimal therapy to attain a personal best, the zones are set based on predicted values found in each peak flow meter package insert. The *yellow zone* indicates a PEF that is 50% to 79% of personal best. Patients should be instructed to call their physician or other healthcare provider for adjustment in preventive medication if the PEF stays in the yellow zone after using two puffs of a β_2-agonist. The *red zone* indicates a PEF that is less than 50% of personal best. The patient should know to call his or her healthcare provider immediately if the use of an inhaled β_2-agonist does not bring the PEF to the yellow or green zone. Figure 18-12 provides an example of PEF monitoring, and Figure 18-13 gives an example of a written action plan.

Correct use of the peak flow meter includes standing, inhaling completely, forming a tight seal with the lips around the mouthpiece, exhaling as hard and fast as possible (blast!), and repeating this maneuver twice.

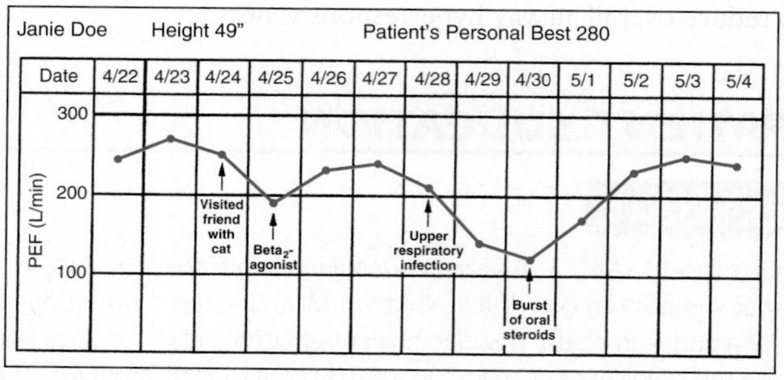

Figure 18-12 Asthma changes with time: patient monitoring and follow-up required. PEF, peak expiratory flow. (Adapted from National Institutes of Health. *Practical Guide for the Diagnosis and Management of Asthma*. Bethesda, MD: National Heart, Lung, and Blood Institute; 1997. NIH publication 97-4053.)

Asthma Action Plan

For: ______ Doctor: ______ Date: ______

Doctor's Phone Number ______ Hospital/Emergency Department Phone Number ______

GREEN ZONE

Doing Well

- No cough, wheeze, chest tightness, or shortness of breath during the day or night
- Can do usual activities

And, if a peak flowmeter is used,

Peak flow: more than ______
(80% or more of my best peak flow)

My best peak flow is: ______

Take these long-term control medicines each day (include an anti-inflammatory).

Medicine	How much to take	When to take it

Identify and avoid and control the things that make your asthma worse, like (list here):

______ ______ ______

______ ______ ______

Before exercise, if prescribed, take: ❒ 2 or ❒ 4 puffs ______ 5 to 60 minutes before exercise

YELLOW ZONE

Asthma Is Getting Worse

- Cough, wheeze, chest tightness, or shortness of breath, or
- Waking at night because of asthma, or
- Can do some, but not all, usual activities

-Or-

Peak flow: ______ to ______
(50% to 79% of my best peak flow)

First

Add: quick-relief medicine—and keep taking your GREEN ZONE medicine.

______ (short-acting β_2-agonist) ❒ 2 or ❒ 4 puffs, every 20 minutes for up to 1 hour
❒ Nebulizer, once

Second

If your symptoms (and peak flow, if used) return to GREEN ZONE after 1 hour of above treatment:
❒ Continue monitoring to be sure you stay in the Green Zone.

-Or-

If your symptoms (and peak flow, if used) do not return to GREEN ZONE after 1 hour of above treatment:

❒ Take: ______ (short-acting β_2-agonist) ❒ 2 or ❒ 4 puffs or ❒ Nebulizer

❒ Add: ______ (oral corticosteroid) mg per day For ______ (3–10) days

❒ Call the doctor ❒ before/ ❒ within ______ hours after taking the oral steroid.

RED ZONE

Medical Alert!

- Very short of breath, or
- Quick-relief medicines have not helped, or
- Cannot do usual activities, or
- Symptoms are same or get worse after 24 hours in Yellow Zone

-Or-

Peak flow: less than ______
(50% of my best peak flow)

Take this medicine:

❒ ______ (short-acting β_2-agonist) ❒ 4 or ❒ 6 puffs or ❒ Nebulizer

❒ ______ (oral corticosteroid) mg

Then call your doctor NOW. Go to the hospital or call an ambulance if:

- You are still in the Red Zone after 15 minutes AND
- You have not reached your doctor.

DANGER SIGNS
- **Trouble walking and talking because of shortness of breath**
- **Lips or fingernails are blue**

- **Take ❒ 4 or ❒ 6 puffs of your quick-relief medicine AND**
- **Go to the hospital or call for an ambulance** ______ (phone) **NOW!**

Figure 18-13 Sample asthma action plan. (Adapted from National Institutes of Health. *Expert Panel Report 3. Guidelines for the Diagnosis and Management of Asthma*. NIH Publication No. 08-4051.0; 2007.)

The best of three attempts should be recorded. Beyond giving maximal effort when using peak flow meters, patients should be instructed to place the instrument well into the mouth on top of the tongue to avoid acceleration of air in the mouth with the tongue and buccal musculature. In essence, "spitting" into the peak flow meter causes a dramatic false elevation in PEF.[113] Some data suggest that women need more initial coaching than men in giving maximal effort when using peak flow meters to ensure accurate assessments of PEF.[114]

A.B. needs education regarding the benefits of long-term inhaled anti-inflammatory therapy. The clinician should explain with enthusiasm that A.B.'s budesonide is an extremely effective medicine and that it is the cornerstone of her asthma management. The delayed onset and safety of ICS must be stressed as well as the requirement of regular use every day. Teaching A.B. the differences between preventers and quick relievers is essential. Showing her colored pictures, models, or a video of inflamed airways can be very helpful—these teaching aids are available from several pharmaceutical manufacturers. Likewise, a peak flow meter should be given to A.B. and correct use ensured by observing her use of it along with establishment of green, yellow, and red zones, coupled with a written action plan developed by her asthma-care provider.[1] A.B. needs to hear from the clinicians treating her that asthma is preventable, and in the words of a title to an NIH booklet for patients, "Your asthma can be controlled: Expect nothing less." As part of comprehensive education, such a positive message from all of her caregivers, as well as carefully listening to A.B.'s concerns, can have a major impact on A.B., who has not been managing her asthma optimally.

CASE 18-13, QUESTION 2: A.B. tells the provider that she was previously instructed to place the albuterol MDI in front of her open mouth and spray rather than put the MDI in her mouth. She says she is confused because the package insert shows placement of the inhaler in the mouth. What should the clinician tell A.B.?

A.B. is correct that this is a confusing issue to many patients and health professionals. A small number of studies show that the "open-mouth" technique is better, but several other studies with SABAs show that the "closed-mouth" technique is as good as or better than putting the MDI in front of the open mouth.[1,115] In addition, the correctly performed closed-mouth technique is as efficacious with a β_2-agonist as with a spacer[107] or nebulizer.[115] One caution with the open-mouth technique is that incorrect aiming of the MDI may result in the aerosol being sprayed onto the face or into the eyes. Because the open-mouth technique has not been studied with the currently available MDIs, it is recommended that the closed-mouth technique be used because the nonchlorofluorocarbon MDIs were FDA approved using this method. Finally, regarding the HFA MDIs, special care should be followed in cleaning the actuators.[116] Healthcare professionals should stress the importance of regular MDI actuator cleaning with their patients.

CASE 18-13, QUESTION 3: For patients who are using both a bronchodilator and an anti-inflammatory inhaler, is there a preferred sequencing of the inhalers?

For patients who have several inhalers, questions regarding sequencing of the inhalers are frequently asked. First, there is no well-documented evidence that outcomes are better using, for instance, a SABA or an anti-inflammatory agent first. A commonsense approach is that using a SABA first and then an anti-inflammatory second has some appeal (i.e., quick relief and theoretically enhanced penetration of the anti-inflammatory). However, as discussed previously, SABAs are preferred for as-needed use (and before exercise) and should not be used on a long-term scheduled basis. Thus, if a patient is not symptomatic at the time the anti-inflammatory is scheduled, current literature suggests that the patient inhales only the anti-inflammatory agent. Because time is limited in counseling patients and teaching them correct inhalation technique, the purpose of each medication (controllers vs. quick relievers) and the need for strict adherence to controller therapies are far more important than spending precious time on the sequencing of inhalers.

NOCTURNAL ASTHMA

CASE 18-14

QUESTION 1: R.R., a 41-year-old man, presents to the clinic with a history of coughing and shortness of breath that awakens him at least two nights a week. Most mornings on awakening, he complains of chest tightness. He has a history of asthma since childhood and currently is managed with beclomethasone HFA 160 mcg BID via a spacer and albuterol (90 mcg/puff) two puffs every 6 hours PRN and before exercise. R.R.'s morning PEF is consistently in the yellow zone, usually at about 400 L/minute (personal best, 600 L/minute), whereas the evening PEF is consistently 550 to 600 L/minute. What treatment should be recommended?

Many patients with asthma complain of symptoms that awaken them in the night or occur on awakening in the morning. Morning cough with or without bronchospasm may be a clue to nocturnal asthma. Although nocturnal asthma may be appropriately viewed as simply another manifestation of airway inflammation, it is so common and troublesome among asthmatic patients that it deserves special note. Circadian rhythm in PEF is exaggerated in patients with asthma. The difference in PEF in nonasthmatic patients averages about 8% between 4 PM (maximal airflow) and 4 AM (minimal airflow), but in patients with asthma, the average variation can be as high as about 50%.[117] Several mechanisms account for this diurnal variation in PEF. The following are examples of factors that contribute to nocturnal asthma: increased release of inflammatory mediators,[117] increased activity of the parasympathetic nervous system, lower circulating levels of epinephrine, and lower levels of serum cortisol (lowest at about midnight). In addition, for patients whose asthma is triggered by gastroesophageal reflux, this problem is worse at night, but treatment of this problem generally provides only minimal improvement in asthma management.[118]

The initial approach to managing nocturnal symptoms is the same as that for overall long-term therapy of persistent asthma, including adequate anti-inflammatory agents.[1,117] ICS are often effective in eliminating or reducing nocturnal asthma, including symptoms and the drop in PEF. If low-to-medium dosages (i.e., correctly inhaled every day) do not eliminate symptoms, combination therapy with LABA (salmeterol, formoterol) is indicated. Also, the basic asthma treatment principle of good control of concomitant rhinitis and environmental control, especially in the bedroom (e.g., house dust mites, household pets), should be considered in the patient with nocturnal asthma symptoms.

Because asthma is primarily an inflammatory disease and nocturnal symptoms are largely caused by airway inflammation, the first drug therapy concern in R.R. is to ensure that he is strictly adhering to his beclomethasone therapy and demonstrating excellent inhalation technique. If his use of the medication is optimal, a reasonable approach would be to add LABA therapy, because he is already at a medium ICS dosage.

As part of optimal management of nocturnal asthma, R.R. also should be asked about avoiding or minimizing exposure to

Key References

Bateman ED et al. Can guideline defined asthma control be achieved? The Gaining Optimal Asthma Control Study. *Am J Respir Crit Care Med*. 2004;170:836. (79)

Dolovich MB et al. Device selection and outcomes of aerosol therapy: evidence-based guidelines: American College of Chest Physicians/American College of Asthma, Allergy, and Immunology. *Chest*. 2005;121:335. (21)

Lemanske RF, Jr, Busse WW. The US Food and Drug Administration and long-acting beta$_2$-agonists: the importance of striking the right balance between risks and benefits of therapy. *J Allergy Clin Immunol*. 2010;126:449. (78)

Newman SP. Spacer devices for metered dose inhalers. *Clin Pharmacokinet*. 2004;43:349. (102)

Self TH et al. Reducing emergency department visits and hospitalizations in African Americans and Hispanic patients with asthma: a 15-year review. *J Asthma*. 2005;42:807. (142)

Suissa S et al. Low-dose inhaled corticosteroids and the prevention of death from asthma. *N Engl J Med*. 2000;343:332. (76)

Tan RA, Spector SL. Exercise-induced asthma: diagnosis and management. *Ann Allergy Asthma Immunol*. 2002;89:226. (99)

Key Websites

Global Initiative for Asthma (GINA) 2014 Update. http://ginasthma.org.

National Institutes of Health. *Expert Panel Report 3. Guidelines for the Diagnosis and Management of Asthma*. Bethesda, MD: National Heart, Lung, and Blood Institute; 2007. NIH publication 07-4051. http://www.nhlbi.nih.gov/guidelines/asthma/asthgdln.pdf. (1)

19 Chronic Obstructive Pulmonary Disease

Timothy R. Hudd and Kathy Zaiken

CORE PRINCIPLES

	Core Principle	CHAPTER CASES
1	Chronic obstructive pulmonary disease (COPD) is characterized by chronic airflow limitation and a range of pathologic changes in the lung, some significant extrapulmonary effects, and important comorbidities that may contribute to the severity of the disease in individual patients. Cigarette smoking is the major risk factor for COPD, and most cases of COPD are attributed to a current or past history of cigarette smoking.	**Case 19-1 (Question 1)**
2	Inhalation of noxious particles or gases, such as cigarette smoke, leads to the activation of resident immune and parenchymal cells, which in turn recruit additional inflammatory cells from the systemic compartment into the lung. The exact mechanisms responsible for the pathogenesis of COPD are not entirely clear, but likely involve activation of the innate and adaptive immune system, leading to chronic inflammation.	**Case 19-2 (Question 2)**
3	As COPD progresses, additional systemic consequences can arise, including cachexia, cardiac and skeletal muscle dysfunction, osteoporosis, depression, and anemia. Pulmonary rehabilitation is recommended to address these systemic manifestations.	**Case 19-2 (Question 5)**
4	The diagnosis of COPD is based on the presence of risk factors (usually including smoking), clinical symptoms, and airflow obstruction based on spirometric testing. Generally, COPD manifests in the sixth decade of life (or later) with symptoms of cough, wheeze, or dyspnea on exertion. The severity of disease is based on a grading system, which then guides therapy.	**Case 19-1 (Questions 1, 2)**
5	The only interventions that reduce mortality in COPD are smoking cessation, oxygen therapy for patients with severe hypoxemia at rest, and lung volume reduction surgery for very select patients with advanced emphysema. Medications are an important component of therapy and are aimed at alleviating symptoms and maximizing quality of life.	**Case 19-1 (Question 3)**
6	Bronchodilators are central to the symptomatic management of COPD and include short-acting and long-acting β_2-agonists, short-acting and long-acting anticholinergic agents, and theophylline.	**Case 19-2 (Questions 1, 3, 4), Case 19-3 (Questions 2, 3)**
7	Combination long-acting bronchodilator therapy or daily use of inhaled corticosteroid in combination with a long-acting β_2-agonist may be effective in patients with advanced COPD, whereas systemic corticosteroids are only advocated for short-term use owing to the risk of adverse effects.	**Case 19-2 (Question 3)**
8	Antibiotic use in the setting of an acute exacerbation should be made based on the presence of the following symptoms: increased dyspnea, sputum volume, and sputum purulence.	**Case 19-3 (Question 1)**
9	Supplemental oxygen is currently initiated for severe hypoxemia, defined as an oxygen saturation less than 88% or Pao_2 of 55 mm Hg or less (oxygen saturation < 90% or $Pao_2 \le 59$ mm Hg in the presence of polycythemia or clinical evidence of pulmonary hypertension, e.g., peripheral edema).	**Case 19-4 (Question 1)**
10	Lung volume reduction surgery, which involves the surgical removal of approximately 30% of the volume of each lung, can significantly improve quality of life, exercise tolerance, and mortality in selected patients with COPD.	**Case 19-4 (Question 2)**

Definitions

Chronic obstructive pulmonary disease (COPD) is a common preventable and treatable airway disorder characterized by symptoms such as dyspnea, chronic cough, and sputum production along with persistent airflow limitation that is not fully reversible.[1,2] Airflow limitation is often progressive and associated with an enhanced chronic inflammatory response in the airways and the lung to noxious particles or gases.[1] Emphysema and chronic bronchitis are two commonly used terms that reflect the spectrum of this disease and are often used as pathologic subtypes of COPD. More recent definitions have transitioned away from these terms, as both pathologic subtypes likely contribute to airflow limitation in patients with COPD.[1]

In 2001, the National Institutes of Health (NIH) and the World Health Organization (WHO) collaborated to develop the Global Initiative for Chronic Obstructive Lung Disease (GOLD) guidelines.[1] These guidelines address a wide variety of topics related to COPD, including current concepts of pathophysiology, and make recommendations regarding diagnosis and treatment. The guidelines are updated yearly, represent an international effort, and are based on the strength of the evidence supporting them.

Asthma is a separate obstructive airway disorder with features similar to COPD. However, airflow limitation and symptoms such as wheezing, cough, dyspnea, and chest tightness are usually episodic and reversible. Some patients may present with features from both conditions, with 15% to 20% of patients sharing a dual diagnosis of asthma and COPD.[3] The term "Asthma-COPD Overlap Syndrome" has been recently described to help clinicians better identify and manage these patients.[3]

Epidemiology

COPD affects an estimated 15 million Americans and is the fourth leading cause of death worldwide.[1,4,5] In 2010, associated US health care costs were approximately $49.9 billion dollars, including $29.5 billion in direct health care expenditures.[2] COPD exacerbations are the most significant contributor to the cost burden of the disease accounting for approximately 50% to 75% of all costs.[5]

COPD is also a leading cause of disability in the United States.[6] Surveillance data from the 2013 Behavioral Risk Factor Surveillance System found that patients with COPD were more likely to be unable to work (24.3% vs. 5.3%), have difficulty walking or climbing stairs (38.4% vs. 11.3%), and report limitations with daily activity because of health problems (49.6% vs. 16.9%) compared with adults without COPD.[4]

The prevalence of COPD and associated costs are expected to continue to rise over the next few decades, at least in part due to the increased life expectancy of the general population and advanced age of patients who began smoking earlier in life.[1,6–8] Historically, the prevalence of COPD and related mortality was reported to be greater in men than in women. However, COPD is now believed to affect both men and women equally.[1] In recent years, concerted efforts have been made to increase awareness around the rising prevalence of COPD among women.[9] Reason for this increase is likely multifactorial and may be due to changes in smoking patterns among women over the past century, and a growing body of evidence suggests women may be more vulnerable to the adverse effects of smoking.[10]

Risk Factors

Cigarette smoking is the major risk factor for COPD and most cases of COPD are attributed to a current or past history of cigarette smoking.[1] Importantly, with more severe disease, the relevance of cigarette smoking as a risk factor becomes even more pronounced. Evidence exists that among patients with severe emphysema approximately 99% have a history of regular cigarette smoking.[11] It should be noted that only a few smokers develop clinically significant COPD, suggesting that other risk factors may be important cofactors with smoking in COPD development. Such factors include occupational dusts and chemicals,[12–15] indoor and outdoor air pollution,[16–18] and certain infections, including respiratory viruses[19] as well as infection with human immunodeficiency virus.[20] It is possible that such factors may upregulate the inflammatory response of the lungs to cigarette smoke.[19,20] Genetic factors are also likely to be important, although precise genetic characteristics have not yet been elucidated.[21–23] One exception is α_1-antitrypsin deficiency, which affects less than 2% of patients with emphysema. Affected individuals have an inherited deficiency of this protective antiprotease and are at much greater risk of developing emphysema than the general population.[24]

The risk of COPD from cigarette smoking is related to an accelerated loss of lung function. After age 35, nonsmokers experience a decline in forced expiratory volume in the first second of expiration (FEV_1) of about 20 to 30 mL/year. In smokers, the decline may be 50 to 120 mL/year.[25] A model of the annual decline in lung function in nonsmokers, smokers, and susceptible smokers is illustrated in Figure 19-1.

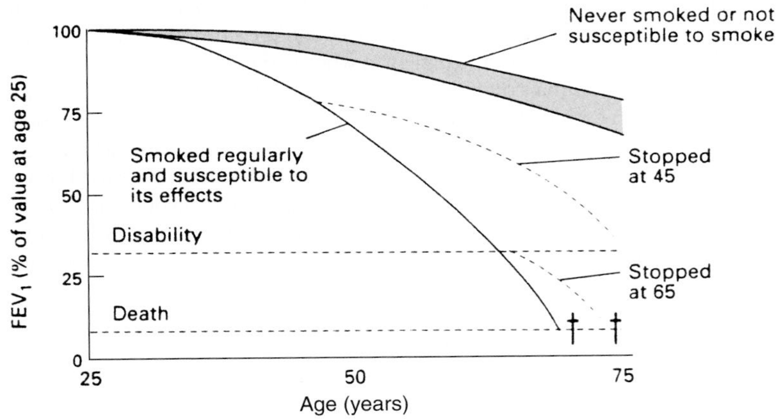

Figure 19-1 Model of annual decline in FEV_1 with accelerated decline in susceptible smokers. On stopping smoking, subsequent loss is similar to that in healthy nonsmokers. (Fletcher C, Peto R. The natural history of chronic airflow obstruction. *BMJ*. 1977;1:1645.)

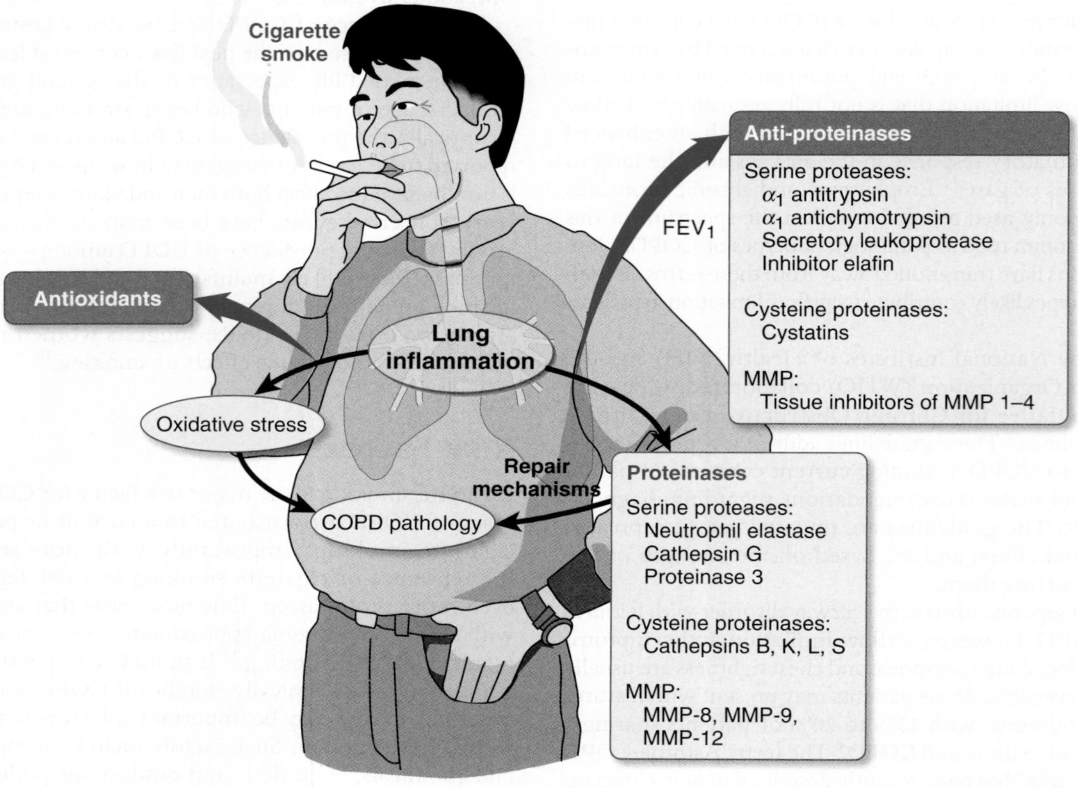

Figure 19-2 Pathogenesis of COPD. (Reference: Global Initiative for Chronic Obstructive Lung Disease (GOLD). Global Strategy for the Diagnosis, Management and Prevention of COPD. Updated 2010. **http://www.goldcopd.org**. Accessed July 27, 2015)

Pathogenesis

The exact mechanisms responsible for the pathogenesis of COPD are not entirely clear, but likely involve activation of the innate and adaptive immune system leading to chronic inflammation. In general, inhalation of noxious agents, such as cigarette smoke, leads to the activation of resident immune and parenchymal cells, which in turn recruit additional inflammatory cells from the systemic compartment into the resident tissue and airway (Fig. 19-2).

The activation and recruitment of immune cells is largely mediated through the production and release of cytokines and chemokines (Table 19-1). Recent evidence also supports a role for oxidant stress as a disease mediator.[26,27] The consequences of an oxidant-rich environment include the activation of inflammatory genes, inactivation of antiproteases, stimulation of mucus secretion, and increases in plasma exudate.

The most well studied cause of COPD, and particularly emphysema, relates to protease–antiprotease imbalance. In this setting, inflammation promotes the production and release of proteases from inflammatory and parenchymal cells. When the local concentration of antiproteases becomes overwhelmed, proteases go unchecked and destroy the major connective tissue components in the lung, such as elastin, leading to the irreversible loss of alveoli. The classic example of this occurs in patients with α_1-antitrypsin deficiency.

Although the traditional idea of disease pathogenesis focuses on smoking-related lung *injury*, more recent hypotheses suggest that another important component of disease pathogenesis may involve inadequate lung *repair*. Indeed, there is evidence that normal lung homeostatic mechanisms are altered in COPD. This may involve inadequate production of growth factors as well as altered regulation of apoptosis, or programmed cell death.[28]

Pathophysiology

The airflow obstruction caused by COPD is usually progressive and is attributed to pathologic changes in the lung that affect the proximal airways, peripheral airways, lung parenchyma, and pulmonary vasculature.[29] Alterations in tissue structure are caused by chronic inflammation that involves recruitment of inflammatory cells into the lung, as well as structural changes that result from repeated injury and tissue remodeling. The magnitude of structural changes and tissue dysfunction varies among patients and is often distinguished by two major phenotypes that include chronic bronchitis and emphysema. Chronic airflow limitation can result from both of these processes. The GOLD or most recent American Thoracic Society (ATS) and European Thoracic Society guidelines[30] do not distinguish between these two entities; however, the classic definitions and pathophysiologic features are described here to aid in a better understanding of the disease process.

In the simplest view, *bronchitis* is inflammation of the bronchioles. The clinical definition from the ATS for *chronic bronchitis* is "the presence of chronic productive cough for 3 months in each of two consecutive years in a patient in whom other causes of chronic cough (e.g., asthma, congestive heart failure, gastroesophageal reflux) have been excluded."[31] *Emphysema* is described as "abnormal permanent enlargement of the airspaces distal to the terminal bronchioles, accompanied by destruction of their walls and without obvious fibrosis." The degree of impairment of the small airways (bronchioles) or the lung parenchyma (alveoli and supporting structures) directly influences tissue dysfunction and the clinical symptoms of the patient.

LARGE (CENTRAL) AND SMALL (PERIPHERAL) AIRWAYS

The large airways, which include the trachea and first generations of the bronchi, are a major site of inflammation

Table 19-1
Inflammatory Cells and Mediators in Chronic Obstructive Pulmonary Disease (COPD)

Cell	
Neutrophils	↑ in sputum of normal smokers. Further ↑ in COPD and related to disease severity. Few neutrophils are seen in tissue. May be important in mucus hypersecretion and through release of proteases.
Macrophages	Greatly ↑ numbers in airway lumen, lung parenchyma, and bronchoalveolar lavage fluid. Derived from blood monocytes that differentiate within lung tissue. Produce increased inflammatory mediators and proteases in patients with COPD in response to cigarette smoke and may show defective phagocytosis.
T lymphocytes	Both $CD4^+$ and $CD8^+$ cells are increased in the airway wall and lung parenchyma, with ↑$CD8^+$:$CD4^+$ ratio. ↑$CD8^+$ T cells (Tc1) and Th1 cells that secrete interferon-γ and express the chemokine receptor CXCR3. $CD8^+$ cells may be cytotoxic to alveolar cells, contributing to their destruction.
B lymphocytes	↑ in peripheral airways and within lymphoid follicles, possibly as a response to chronic colonization and infection of the airways.
Eosinophils	↑ eosinophil proteins in sputum and ↑ eosinophils in airway wall during exacerbations.
Epithelial cells	May be activated by cigarette smoke to produce inflammatory mediators.
Mediators	
Chemotactic factors	Lipid mediators: e.g., leukotriene-B_4 (LTB_4) attracts neutrophils and T lymphocytes. Chemokines: e.g., interleukin-8 (IL-8) attracts neutrophils and monocytes.
Proinflammatory cytokines	Cytokines, including tumor necrosis factor-α (TNF-α), IL-1β, and IL-6 amplify the inflammatory process and may contribute to some of the systemic effects of COPD.
Growth factors	E.g., transforming growth factor-β (TGF-β) may induce fibrosis in small airways.

Source: Global Initiative for Chronic Obstructive Lung Disease (GOLD). Global Strategy for the Diagnosis, Management and Prevention of COPD (Updated 2010). **http://www.goldcopd.org**. Accessed July 27, 2015.

and mucus hypersecretion. This results from an increase in numbers (hyperplasia) and enlargement (hypertrophy) of the submucosal glands and mucus-producing goblet cells within the surface epithelium.[32,33] Overproduction of mucus in the large airways results in a chronic productive cough, as observed in chronic bronchitis, but this does not have a major impact on airflow limitation. Mucus hypersecretion coupled with impaired ciliary function reduces mucociliary clearance, increases the accumulation of secretions, and enhances the risk of bacterial colonization in an otherwise sterile environment.[34] As a result, recurrent infections often occur owing to the inability to clear pathogens.

The peripheral airway is composed of the smaller bronchi down to the terminal bronchioles, the smallest branches in the lung that are not involved in gas exchange. The extent of inflammation, fibrosis, and airway exudate in the peripheral airway correlates best with the reduction in airflow as measured by a decrease in FEV_1 or the FEV_1 to forced vital capacity (FVC) ratio.[35] Chronic obstruction of the peripheral airway also results in air-trapping on expiration, which contributes to hyperinflation. Hyperinflation places the respiratory muscles at a mechanical disadvantage and further reduces respiratory capacity. Hyperinflation can become more pronounced during exercise, leading to dyspnea and decreased exercise capacity. It is now known that hyperinflation can occur early in the course of COPD and is an important cause of exertional dyspnea.[36]

PARENCHYMAL DESTRUCTION

The terminal bronchioles lead directly to the alveolar ducts and sacs, the major site where gas exchange occurs. Emphysema is characterized by the destructive loss of alveolar walls and enlargement of the terminal airspaces, resulting in a loss of gas-exchanging surface area.[34,37] In advanced cases, large, balloon-shaped bullous lesions may develop. Rupture of these bullae (pneumothorax) can lead to collapse of lung segments (pneumothorax).

SIGNIFICANT COMORBID ILLNESS

In the later stages of disease, chronic hypoxemia causes persistent vasoconstriction in the lung vascular bed, particularly the small pulmonary arteries. This can result in permanent structural alteration of the blood vessels, causing intimal hyperplasia and smooth muscle hypertrophy.[38] The loss of pulmonary capillaries in emphysema can also contribute to increased pulmonary vascular pressures. The cumulative impact of vascular changes can result in progressive pulmonary hypertension and, eventually, right-sided cardiac failure (cor pulmonale).

As COPD progresses, additional systemic consequences can arise, including cachexia, skeletal muscle dysfunction, osteoporosis, depression, and anemia. The cause of these additional systemic disease processes is not entirely clear but likely involves the dynamic interplay of progressive respiratory dysfunction, lung and systemic inflammation, side effects from medication use, and physical debilitation. In summary, although COPD is primarily a disease of the large and small airways and adjacent alveolar structures, it also includes important systemic consequences. The clinical consequences of the morphologic and pathophysiologic alterations include progressive dyspnea on exertion, chronic cough and sputum production, increased risk for respiratory infections, deconditioning, and an overall reduction in quality of life.

COMPARISON WITH ASTHMA

COPD and asthma are common obstructive airway disorders, and both illnesses can coexist in the same patient. Nevertheless, these conditions should be considered as separate and distinct entities (Table 19-2). For example, although inflammation is a key component of both conditions, the pattern of inflammation differs significantly (Table 19-3). As a result, the pathophysiologic consequences, patient symptoms, and response to medications typically differ. Asthma is generally not progressive, and symptoms and airflow obstruction are often completely reversible. Patients with asthma respond well to antiinflammatory medication, including inhaled corticosteroids (ICS). Furthermore, in the absence of an acute exacerbation, significant gas exchange

Table 19-2
Clinical Features of Asthma, COPD, and ACOS

Clinical Feature	COPD	Asthma	Asthma-COPD Overlap Syndrome (ACOS)
Age of onset	>40 years of age	Childhood, but can occur at any age	Usually ≥40 years of age, but may have had symptoms in childhood or adolescence
Possible symptoms	Dyspnea, chronic cough, sputum production	Dyspnea, cough, wheeze, chest tightness	Mixed symptoms
Symptom pattern	Persistent and slowly progressive. Present daily, worse with exertion or exercise.	Vary day to day and may be episodic based on trigger exposure. Often worse at night or early morning.	Persistent and worse with exertion though variability may exist
Risk factors	History of chronic exposure to cigarette smoke, biomass fuels, or noxious particles and gases α_1-antitrypsin deficiency (<2% of cases)	Atopic conditions (i.e., allergies, eczema, etc.) Family history of asthma	History of asthma with chronic exposure to cigarette smoke, biomass fuels, or noxious particles and gases
Post-bronchodilator FEV_1 reversibility[a] FEV_1/FVC ratio	Usually little to no change FEV_1/FVC < 70%	Reversible and may be normal between symptoms	Airflow limitation is usually not fully reversible and often varies over time
Chest X-ray	Hyperinflation	Usually normal	Hyperinflation

[a]Reversibility defined as an increase in FEV_1 of >200 mL and 12% from baseline measure after inhalation of a short-acting β_2-agonist.
Source: GOLD (Global Initiative for Chronic Obstructive Lung Disease). Global strategy for the diagnosis, management, and prevention of chronic obstructive pulmonary disease. Updated 2015 [online]. Table 2a—Usual Features of Asthma, COPD and ACOS, p. 105. **http://www.goldcopd.org**. Accessed July 27, 2015.

abnormalities are uncommon. COPD, on the other hand, is a progressive and often fatal disorder. Although bronchodilators are helpful in COPD, the degree of bronchodilator reversibility is typically less than that seen in asthma. In addition, the beneficial effects of antiinflammatory medication, including ICS, are much more modest. Patients with COPD, particularly those with emphysema, have substantial derangements in pulmonary gas exchange even at baseline.

α_1-ANTITRYPSIN DEFICIENCY

The best-characterized antiprotease in the lung is α_1-antitrypsin. This serum glycoprotein is primarily produced in the liver and works by binding to and neutralizing proteases. As described previously, cigarette smoke can activate and attract inflammatory cells into the lung, thereby promoting the release of proteases such as elastase. Cigarette smoke can also inactivate endogenous protease inhibitors, including α_1-antitrypsin, further supporting protease activity and increasing the risk of tissue damage. This risk of tissue damage is greatly accentuated in patients with α_1-antitrypsin deficiency. α_1-Antitrypsin deficiency occurs in less than 2% of all COPD cases. Clinically significant disease is usually associated only with severe deficiency (i.e., serum α_1-antitrypsin levels < 45 mg/dL; normal > 150 mg/dL). The diagnosis of α_1-antitrypsin deficiency is made by measuring circulating serum α_1-antitrypsin levels, followed by phenotype analysis.[39] The PiM allele confers production of the fully functional protein. Accordingly, a homozygous PiMM individual will produce a functional protein with normal plasma concentrations. Other gene types include, but are not limited to, PiS (normal serum levels of a poorly functioning enzyme), PiZ (an active form but poorly secreted, leading to low circulating levels), and Pi null (gene polymorphism leads to production of a truncated protein and undetectable serum levels of functional protein). Different allele pairs can exist. PiMZ and PiSZ are heterozygous disorders, and PiSS is a homozygous phenotype, all with greater than 35% of normal enzyme activity and a relatively low risk of developing emphysema. PiZZ is a rare homozygous disorder characterized by accelerated lung destruction and serum α_1-antitrypsin levels approximately 15% of normal. In these rare patients, the disease develops as early as age 20, but more typically it occurs in the fourth to fifth decade of life.

Replacement therapy is available for patients with COPD with documented α_1-antitrypsin deficiency and emphysema. Patients who do qualify typically receive weekly intravenous infusions of α_1-antitrypsin to maintain acceptable antiprotease activity and minimize the progression of lung disease. This therapy is very expensive, and it is not well tolerated by some (fever, chills, allergic reactions, flulike symptoms). Currently, no placebo-controlled, randomized trials have documented the efficacy of replacement therapy. Case–control studies, however, suggest the replacement therapy may improve outcomes in patients with α_1-antitrypsin deficiency, documented emphysema, and an FEV_1 between 35% and 60% of predicted.[24] Three different formulations of α_1-antitrypsin are available: Aralast, Prolastin, and Zemaira. No clinically significant differences exist among these preparations. Because the α_1-antitrypsin products are derived from pooled human plasma, there are also associated risks for the transmission of infectious diseases (e.g., viral infections and Creutzfeldt–Jakob disease). Overall, use of the α_1-antitrypsin replacement therapy remains controversial, and some have argued that this therapy cannot be recommended based on a lack of proven clinical benefit and high cost of treatment.[40]

DIAGNOSIS AND PATIENT ASSESSMENT

The diagnosis of COPD is based on the presence of risk factors (generally smoking), clinical symptoms, and airflow obstruction on spirometric testing.[1] Generally, individuals with COPD present in the sixth decade of life (or later) with symptoms of cough, wheeze, or dyspnea on exertion.[30] Patients usually have at least a 10-pack-year history (e.g., averaging one pack of cigarettes a day for 10 years) of cigarette smoking. Because the severity of

Table 19-3
Differences in Pulmonary Inflammation Between Asthma and Chronic Obstructive Pulmonary Disease (COPD)

COPD	Asthma	Severe Asthma
Cells		
Neutrophils++	Eosinophils++	Neutrophils+
Macrophages+++	Macrophages+	Macrophages
$CD8^+$ T cells (Tc1)	$CD4^+$ T cells (Th2)	$CD4^+$ T cells (Th2)
		$CD8^+$ T cells (Tc1)
Key Mediators		
IL-8, TNF-α, IL-1β, IL-6, NO+	Eotaxin	IL-8
	IL-4, IL-5, IL-13	IL-5, IL-13
	NO+++	NO++
Oxidative Stress		
+++	+	+++
Site of Disease		
Peripheral airways	Proximal airways	Proximal airways
Lung parenchyma		Peripheral airways
Pulmonary vessels		
Consequences		
Squamous metaplasia	Fragile epithelium	
Mucous metaplasia	Mucous metaplasia	
Small airway fibrosis	↑Basement membrane	
Parenchymal destruction	Bronchoconstriction	
Pulmonary vascular remodeling		
Response to Therapy		
Small bronchodilator response	Large bronchodilator response	Smaller bronchodilator response
Poor response to steroids	Good response to steroids	Reduced response to steroids

IL, interleukin; NO, nitric oxide; TNF, tumor necrosis factor.

Source: Global Initiative for Chronic Obstructive Lung Disease (GOLD). *Global Strategy for the Diagnosis, Management and Prevention of COPD (Updated 2010)*. **http://www.goldcopd.org**.

COPD is related to the cumulative exposure to cigarette smoke, patients with more severe disease are likely to be older with a heavier smoking history. Cough and sputum production may be present for many years before airflow limitation develops, but not everyone with those symptoms will develop COPD. Dyspnea on exertion may not be present until the sixth or seventh decade.

On physical examination, patients with early COPD may not exhibit any changes.[30] Later, objective findings include the presence of a barrel chest (defined as an increase in the anteroposterior diameter of the chest), rales (defined as intermittent, nonmusical, brief crackle sounds), rhonchi (defined as continuous, musical high- or low-pitched sounds), prolonged expiratory phase, and cyanosis.[32] Symptomatic patients may present with decreased breath sounds, wheezes, or slight rales on auscultation. In advanced disease, cyanosis, edema, intercostal retractions, and pursed lip breathing may be present.[32]

Spirometry Testing

Spirometry is the gold standard measurement in assessing and monitoring obstructive lung disease and is required for a diagnosis of COPD.[1,30] In the evaluation of COPD, spirometry testing should be performed according to published guidelines, when the patient's condition is stable and after administration of two to four puffs (90 mcg/puff) of albuterol by metered-dose inhaler (MDI). During spirometry, a full breath is taken, followed by a forceful exhalation of all the air that can be exhaled (FVC). Flow rates and volumes of air that are expired at different time intervals can be recorded (Fig. 19-3). The FEV_1 is the volume of air that can be expired within the first second of an FVC maneuver. A decrease in the FEV_1/FVC ratio indicates airflow obstruction. Although the range of normal for FEV_1/FVC depends on the age, sex, and height of the patient, a value of less than 0.70 indicates airflow obstruction that is compatible with COPD.[1,30] Also, patients with COPD may have some improvement in spirometry testing with an acute bronchodilator challenge. The degree of reversibility is typically less than that seen with asthma, although up to 50% of patients with moderate to severe emphysema will have an increase in FEV_1 with acute bronchodilator challenge that meets ATS criteria as significant. In addition to being critical for making the diagnosis of COPD, spirometry also affords the best objective way to monitor disease progression and should be considered if there has been a persistent change in clinical symptoms (e.g., worsened dyspnea). Four "grades" are used to classify the degree of airflow limitation using post-bronchodilator spirometric results in patients with an FEV1/FVC $<$70%. The grades are as follows: GOLD 1 (Mild) FEV1 $\geq=$ 80% Predicted, GOLD 2 (Moderate) FEV1 between $\geq$ 50% to 80% Predicted,

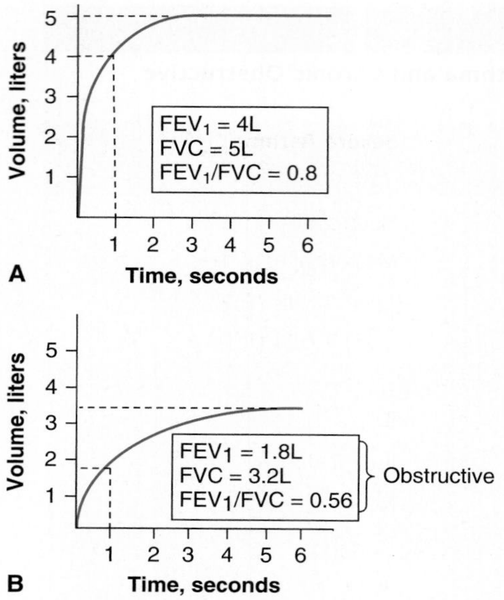

Figure 19-3 A normal spirometry tracing is shown in **A.** A spirometry tracing typical of a patient with obstructive disease is shown in **B.** Redrawn from Global Initiative for Chronic Obstructive Lung Disease (GOLD). Global Strategy for the Diagnosis, Management, and Prevention of COPD (Updated 2015). **http://www.goldcopd.org** Accessed July 27, 2015.

GOLD 3 (Severe) FEV1 between ≥ 30% to 50% Predicted, and GOLD 4 (Very Severe) FEV1 < 30% Predicted. Deteriorating lung function is associated with increased prevalence of hospitalizations, exacerbations, and associated mortality at the population level.[1] However, FEV1 is an unreliable clinical indicator when used alone to predict exacerbation or mortality risk at the individual patient level.[1] Although optimal frequency of spirometric testing for patients with COPD is not known, some groups recommend annual monitoring to identify patients whose lung function may be declining rapidly.[1]

Other pulmonary function testing is sometimes used to assess patients with COPD. The determination of lung volumes, including the total lung capacity (TLC) and residual volume (RV), as well as measurements of the diffusing capacity for carbon monoxide (DLCO) may provide more detail regarding lung physiology. For example, a reduction in DLCO indicates disruption or destruction of the alveolar capillary interface and correlates with the degree of emphysema. Determination of lung volumes may be used to assess the presence of concomitant restrictive lung disease (e.g., idiopathic pulmonary fibrosis) in the case of diagnostic uncertainty. Patients with COPD typically have normal or increased lung volumes; a reduction in TLC may indicate a superimposed restrictive process. Furthermore, lung volumes and diffusion capacity are used to assess patients for surgical procedures, such as lung volume reduction surgery.[11] In most cases, however, spirometric testing is adequate to make the diagnosis of COPD and follow the course of disease.[1,30]

A chest x-ray study (CXR) is often performed during the initial assessment of patients with COPD. Because the CXR lacks sensitivity and demonstrates minimal changes until COPD is moderately severe, its main utility is in ruling out other disease processes that may be contributing to the patient's symptoms. In severe disease, the chest radiograph may indicate hyperinflation manifested by a flattened diaphragm or evidence of pulmonary arterial hypertension characterized by enlarged pulmonary arteries.

Assessing the oxygen status of a patient with COPD can be done by pulse oximetry. This should be considered in patients with dyspnea and advanced disease, and patients with evidence of right ventricular pressure overload (e.g., peripheral edema or jugular venous distension). Although a decrease in pulse oximetry (normal, ≥ 97%) is common in COPD, values of 88% or less are consistent with chronic respiratory failure and qualify the patient for supplemental oxygen. Arterial blood gas (ABG) determination is generally reserved for patients with severe disease (i.e., an $FEV_1 < 50\%$ of predicted). ABGs can more precisely define the oxygen status of a patient and can be used to assess whether the patient has carbon dioxide retention (normal $P_{CO_2} = 35–45$ mm Hg). Determining the α_1-antitrypsin concentration is indicated for patients developing COPD before age 45, and for patients who have emphysema without a significant history of cigarette smoking or who have a family history of emphysema.

Classification of Severity and Clinical Presentation

A number of methods have been proposed to categorize the severity of COPD, many of which are based primarily on the degree of airflow obstruction as assessed by the FEV_1.[30,31] However, lung function has been found to be a poor indicator of disease severity when used alone. The most recent GOLD Report utilizes symptom severity and exacerbation risk to assess COPD (Table 19-4). Comorbidities are also considered when managing these patients.[1] Patients are assigned to one of the following four groups when classifying exacerbation risk and symptom burden: Group A Low Risk; Less Symptoms, Group B Low Risk; More Symptoms, Group C High Risk; Less Symptoms, and Group D High Risk; More Symptoms.

Two steps should be followed when using the ABCD Assessment tool. The first step is to assess patient symptoms. Several reliable questionnaires such as the Modified British Medical Research Council Questionnaire (mMRC), COPD Assessment Test (CAT), and COPD Control Questionnaire (CCQ) may be used to assess symptom burden and health status. The mMRC only assesses the impact of breathlessness on health-related quality of life. However, patients with COPD often exhibit additional symptoms such as cough, chest tightness, and mucus production. Therefore, scales that provide a more comprehensive assessment of symptoms, (e.g., CAT) may be preferred. Nevertheless, patients are considered to have a high level of symptoms when scoring ≥2 on the mMRC or ≥10 on the CAT. Of note, it is only necessary to use one of these scales when assessing symptom burden.

Table 19-4
Model of Symptom/Risk of Evaluation of COPD

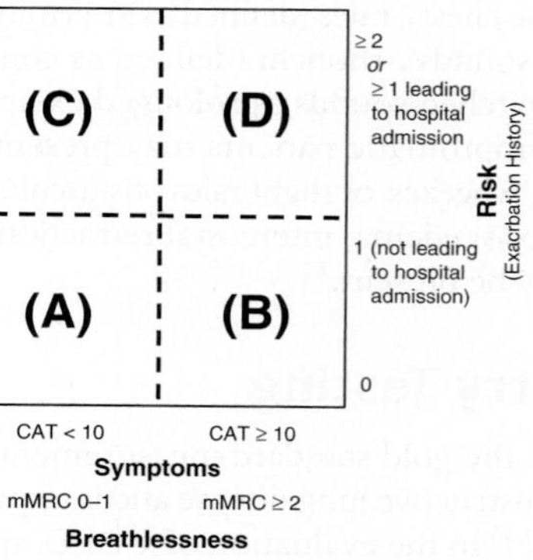

Source: Global Initiative for Chronic Obstructive Lung Disease (GOLD). Global Strategy for the Diagnosis, Management, and Prevention of COPD (Updated 2015). **http://www.goldcopd.org** Accessed July 25, 2017.

Table 19-5
The BODE Index Scoring System

Variable	Points 0	1	2	3
Body mass index (kg/m^2)	≥21	<21		
Obstruction of airflow (FEV_1% predicted)	≥65	50–64	36–49	≤35
Dyspnea?	None or only with strenuous exertion	Walking up a slight hill	Walking on the level	Getting dressed
Exercise capacity (6-minute walk distance, feet)	>1,148	820–1,149	492–819	<492

Approximate 4-year survival based on total BODE score:
- 0–2 points: 80%
- 3–4 points: 70%
- 5–6 points: 60%
- 7–10 points: 20%

BODE, body mass index, degree of airflow obstruction, dyspnea, and exercise capacity index.

Celli BR et al. The body-mass index, airflow obstruction, dyspnea, and exercise capacity index in chronic obstructive pulmonary disease. *N Engl J Med.* 2004;350:1005.

The second step involves an assessment of the patient's risk for future exacerbations. Patients are considered to be in the "high risk" category if the patient has experienced 2 or more exacerbations in the previous year or if the patient has had 1 exacerbation that led to a hospitalization within this time period.[1]

Although the GOLD management strategy can provide important prognostic information, other comprehensive assessment tools may too provide discriminating information with regard to survival in COPD. For example, a scoring system based on body mass index, obstruction on spirometry, dyspnea level, and exercise capacity (BODE) can predict survival in COPD better than the FEV_1 alone (Table 19-5).[41]

Natural Course

The natural course of COPD is highly variable, generally spanning 20 to 40 years and influenced by numerous factors, including genetic predisposition, exposure to inhaled irritants (tobacco smoke, workplace, or environmental pollutants), and repeated infections. The typical smoker who develops COPD remains asymptomatic for the first two decades of smoking, except for more frequent viral or bacterial upper respiratory tract infections. Clinical symptoms appear after significant irreversible lung damage occurs. After 25 to 30 years of smoking, mild dyspnea on exertion is commonly noted and can be accompanied by a morning cough; however, physical examination and chest radiograph are often unremarkable.[30] With continued exposure to risks (e.g., cigarette smoking), the disease progresses and patients develop increased airflow limitation and worsened dyspnea on exertion, and increased cough and sputum production. Ultimately, structural changes result in alveolar hypoxia and the secondary problems of pulmonary hypertension and cor pulmonale.

Exacerbations, or flares, of COPD are common and can be infectious or noninfectious. Moderate to severe exacerbations may require hospitalization. Acute or chronic respiratory failure can develop secondary to an acute infection, or other factors, including oversedation, heart failure, or pulmonary embolism.[42,43]

GENERAL MANAGEMENT CONSIDERATIONS

The overarching goals of COPD management involve two main principles. First, to reduce symptoms (i.e., relieve symptoms, improve exercise tolerance, and improve health status); and second, to reduce risk (i.e., prevent disease progression, prevent and treat exacerbations, and reduce mortality).[1] Unfortunately, the only interventions that have been proven to reduce mortality in COPD are smoking cessation, oxygen therapy for patients with severe hypoxemia at rest, and lung volume reduction surgery for very select patients with advanced emphysema.[11,44–46] As such, many of the interventions are aimed at alleviating symptoms and maximizing quality of life.

Because continued cigarette smoking is associated with accelerated progression of disease in susceptible smokers, smoking cessation is critical to disease treatment. Strategies for smoking cessation are detailed in Chapter 91, Tobacco Use and Dependence. The benefits of smoking cessation in COPD include decreases in respiratory symptoms, exacerbation rate, and lung function decline.[25,47] It should also be noted that cardiovascular complications, including coronary artery disease, are more common in patients with COPD and that smoking cessation may attenuate morbidity and mortality from this complication.

Immunizations provide protection against serious illness and death in patients with COPD.[48] The efficacy, benefit, and cost-effectiveness of vaccination against influenza among this population are significant.[49] In addition, the pneumococcal polysaccharide vaccine is recommended to all patients with COPD,[1] as well as, in adult patients 19 through 64 years of age who smoke cigarettes or have asthma.[50]

Pulmonary rehabilitation is an exercise-based program aimed at maximizing the patient's functional status and quality of life. Multiple studies have now documented the beneficial effects of pulmonary rehabilitation, particularly with respect to improved exercise tolerance and alleviation of dyspnea.[51] In addition, cost-effective analysis suggests that pulmonary rehabilitation programs are very cost-effective.[52] Pulmonary rehabilitation programs are multidisciplinary programs typically running for 6 to 12 weeks, two to three sessions per week. A number of interventions are used, including breathing retraining, psychosocial counseling, education, dietary counseling, and airway clearance techniques for patients with chronic sputum production. Arm strengthening and arm endurance exercises are important because patients with COPD commonly have excessive dyspnea when using their upper extremities.[51] The most important component of a pulmonary rehabilitation program is lower extremity endurance training, often using a treadmill or bicycle ergometer. Because the large muscle groups have diminished oxidative capacity,[53–55] likely related to deconditioning and chronic inflammation,[56,57] patients with COPD convert to anaerobic metabolism at low levels of exercise. This leads to increased lactate production for a given level of activity[58] and, subsequently, increased CO_2 production. Lower extremity endurance training can significantly improve mitochondrial oxidative capacity in patients with COPD.[53,59] This physiologic benefit is believed to be an important mechanism whereby pulmonary rehabilitation exerts its effect. Other important effects, such as alleviation of depression and anxiety, may be important as well.[51]

As mentioned, patients with severe resting hypoxemia have improved mortality with supplemental oxygen treatment. Based on studies published in the 1980s, it has been found that patients with a Pao_2 of 55 mm Hg or less (corresponding to an oxygen saturation of ~88%) have decreased mortality and evidence of better end-organ function when treated with supplemental oxygen.[45,46] Whether supplemental oxygen benefits subjects with moderate hypoxemia, corresponding to an oxygen saturation of 89% to 93%, is the objective of an ongoing, randomized, multicenter study, the Long-Term Oxygen Treatment Trial (LOTT).[60]

PHARMACOTHERAPY

The fundamental goals of medication use are to prevent or control symptoms, reduce the frequency and severity of exacerbations, and improve both health status and exercise tolerance. The currently available medications used to treat COPD, however, do not alter the natural course of this condition; therefore, pharmacotherapy should be individualized for each patient and focused on symptom management to improve quality of life.[25,61–63] Because of the potential for limited benefit with therapy, a specific set of desired goals must be defined for each patient before therapy is initiated. The initial outcomes should be realistic and developed jointly by the caregiver and the patient. In general, COPD is a progressive disease, and general guidelines will apply to most patients with COPD as they begin to require pharmacologic management.

- The number of medications will cumulatively increase as the disease worsens.
- Patients will eventually require daily maintenance therapy for sustained periods unless adverse effects of the medication(s) preclude further use.
- Interindividual variability in medication response is expected and requires careful monitoring over a continuum of time to ensure an acceptable benefit-to-risk ratio is achieved.

When medications are initiated or modified, a minimal trial period of several weeks to a few months is usually recommended before determining their full benefit. Single-dose challenges and frequent alterations in therapy do not allow adequate assessment and can compromise patient adherence. No consensus currently exists on the most appropriate outcome measure or degree of improvement needed to be determined clinically significant.

Although the standard for assessing benefit from treatment has been to measure spirometric improvement in FEV_1, many patients will not demonstrate noticeable changes after either an acute or extended therapeutic trial of any therapy. Increasingly, clinicians are considering other measures to determine the benefit of therapy. These include measuring improvements in quality of life, dyspnea, and exercise tolerance.[64] Other appropriate measures may include COPD exacerbation rates and utilization of health care resources. In most patients, it is important to consider the use of multiple outcome measures, both objective and subjective, to guide the therapeutic decision-making process.

Bronchodilators

Bronchodilators are central to the symptomatic management of COPD and include short-acting and long-acting β_2-agonists, short-acting and long-acting anticholinergic agents, and theophylline. These medications, although pharmacologically distinct, improve airflow primarily by reducing bronchial airway smooth muscle tone. In COPD, the spirometric response, as measured by FEV_1, can be variable and, in many cases, will demonstrate no change, although the patient may subjectively feel better. This can be attributed to treatment facilitating emptying of the lungs and a reduction in thoracic hyperinflation at rest and during exercise. No clear evidence exists for benefit of one bronchodilator over another in the chronic management of COPD, although inhaled therapy is generally preferred over oral therapy to achieve a more rapid onset of action and to minimize the risk of systemic exposure and adverse events. Generally, the choice of treatment should be individualized based on the frequency and severity of symptoms, as well as future exacerbation risk. The GOLD Report offers a systematic approach to initiating and adjusting pharmacotherapy in patients with COPD (Table 19-6). Additional factors such as product availability, cost, patient preference, and overall clinical response should be further tailored to the patient.[1]

Short-acting β_2-agonists (e.g., albuterol) with or without a short-acting anticholinergic (e.g., ipratropium) is usually preferred for exacerbations and acute symptoms because of their more rapid onset of action and relatively short duration of activity when compared with long-acting agents.[1] A short or long acting bronchodilator should be offered to patients who have few symptoms and are at a low risk for exacerbations (Group A). As disease progresses and the frequency of symptoms increases along with medication requirement, the patient should be transitioned onto daily maintenance bronchodilator therapy.[37] At this point, substitution of a short-acting agent with a long-acting agent is recommended because the bronchodilator effect will be sustained for a longer duration, thus reducing the number of daily inhalations. This strategy will also enhance patient adherence. The side effects of bronchodilators, particularly β_2-agonists, are predictable and dose dependent, even with excessive use of inhaled agents. The most common adverse effects are an extension of stimulation of β_2-adrenergic receptors that can produce resting sinus tachycardia or provoke cardiac dysrhythmias in predisposed individuals, especially the elderly. Precipitation of somatic tremors and hypokalemia can also occur with excessive use.

The relationship between β_2-agonist use and cardiovascular complications remains somewhat controversial. It is recognized that albuterol and long-acting inhaled β_2-sympathetic agents can induce systemic sympathetic states, hypokalemia, and other metabolic derangements that can contribute to cardiac rhythm disturbances. This has led to speculation that these abnormalities could contribute to an increase in cardiovascular death among patients with COPD using β_2-agonist inhalers.[65] Nevertheless, this speculation has been largely refuted by the TORCH (Towards a Revolution in COPD Health) study, in which more than 6,000 patients with COPD were randomly assigned to treatment with salmeterol, fluticasone, combination salmeterol–fluticasone, or placebo.[66] Overall mortality, cardiovascular mortality, and cardiovascular-related adverse events were no greater in the salmeterol group compared with any of the other groups.

Inhaled anticholinergic agents are generally well tolerated by virtue of their minimal systemic absorption. Excessive dry mouth is the most common complaint from patients who use inhaled anticholinergic agents, both short- and long-acting. It has been suggested that regular use of inhaled anticholinergic agents increases the risk of cardiovascular complications.[67,68] However, a recent large prospectively performed randomized trial found a decreased risk of cardiovascular complications among COPD patients using the long-acting anticholinergic tiotropium on a regular basis.[69]

It is not unusual to find reports in the literature that suggest superiority of one bronchodilator class versus another for COPD treatment.[70] It is difficult, however, to predict individual responses to treatment. For some patients, β_2-agonist bronchodilators will increase airflow, improve pulmonary function test results, and reduce symptoms of dyspnea.[71] Others may achieve greater improvement with an anticholinergic in comparison with a β_2-agonist.[72,73] Still others may not have a reversible component with either drug, but yet may perceive symptomatic benefit.[74,75] Thus, the therapeutic regimen should be reviewed with the patient at each follow-up visit to assess response. Careful review of adherence, technique, and response to therapy should be assessed before adjusting therapy.

Table 19-6

Therapeutic Selection by COPD Group

Group	Step	Therapy
GROUP A	• Initial Therapy:	Bronchodilator (short or long acting)
	• Evaluate Effect:	Continue, Stop, or Try Alternative Bronchodilator Class
GROUP B	• Initial Therapy:	LAMA or LABA
	• If Symptoms Persist:	LAMA + LABA
GROUP C	• Initial Therapy:	LAMA
	• If Further Exacerbation(s):	LAMA + LABA (*preferred*) ICS + LABA (*alternative*)
GROUP D	• Initial Therapy:	LAMA + LABA (*preferred*) LAMA (*alternative*) ICS + LABA (*alternative*)
	• If Further Exacerbation(s) /Persistent Symptoms:	LAMA + ICS +LABA (*preferred*) ICS + LABA (*alternative*)[a]
	• If Further Exacerbation(s):	Consider roflumilast[b] ***OR*** Consider macrolide (in former smokers)[b]

ICS = Inhaled Corticosteroid LABA = Long Acting b2-agonist LAMA= Long Acting Antimuscarinic (anticholinergic)

[a]If prior regimen consisted of LAMA monotherapy or combination long acting bronchodilator therapy

[b]Recommended "add-on" therapies

Theophylline or a Short-Acting β_2 Agonist ± Short-Acting Anticholinergic may be used alone or in combination with options listed above.

ICS, inhaled corticosteroid; → PDE 4 Inhibitor, phosphodiesterase 4 inhibitor.

Source: GOLD (Global Initiative for Chronic Obstructive Lung Disease). Global strategy for the diagnosis, management, and prevention of chronic obstructive pulmonary disease. Updated 2017 [online]. Figure 4.1, p. 85. http://www.goldcopd.org Accessed July 25, 2017.

Theophylline is a methylxanthine that induces bronchodilation by relaxing the smooth muscle of the bronchi. Although not fully understood, its pharmacologic activity has been attributed to nonselective inhibition of phosphodiesterase, inhibition of extracellular adenosine (a bronchoconstrictor), stimulation of endogenous catecholamines, and antagonism of prostaglandins PGE_2 and $PGF_{2\alpha}$.[76] Theophylline has been shown to provide greater symptomatic improvement when compared with placebo,[77] though it is considered to be less effective and usually less well tolerated than inhaled long-acting bronchodilators.[1] Theophylline may provide additional symptomatic improvement via stimulation of diaphragmatic contractility and antiinflammatory effects. However, the clinical significance of these findings remains to be determined.[1,77–79]

Currently, theophylline is reserved for patients who do not tolerate, or fail to adequately respond to, a combination of first-line bronchodilators. It is relatively inexpensive and studies showing clinical benefit have involved mostly slow-release preparations. The major limitation of theophylline is its relatively narrow therapeutic index, potential to cause significant adverse events, and requirement for blood monitoring of drug levels.[1]

Selective Phosphodiesterase 4 (PDE4) Inhibitors

In 2011, the US Food and Drug Administration (FDA) approved roflumilast (Daliresp) as an orally administered selective PDE4 enzyme inhibitor to reduce the risk of COPD exacerbations in patients with severe COPD associated with chronic bronchitis and a history of exacerbations.[80] Recent guidelines recommend the use of roflumilast in patients who are not adequately controlled by long-acting bronchodilators and continue to experience frequent exacerbations. It has been recommended to use this agent in combination with at least one long-acting bronchodilator.[1] Although roflumilast has been shown to improve FEV_1 by 40 to 60 mL compared to placebo, it is not a bronchodilator and is not indicated to relieve acute bronchospasm.[80,81] In comparison with theophylline, roflumilast has much less potential for drug–drug interactions and does not require drug level monitoring. Though it is metabolized to an active metabolite via CYP3A4 and CYP1A2 pathways, it be used with caution in patients receiving strong inducers or inhibitors of these enzymes and should be avoided in those with significant hepatic impairment. Significant adverse effects, including diarrhea, nausea, weight loss (~2 kg), and adverse psychiatric effects such as anxiety and depression have been reported.[1,80,81]

Corticosteroids

Historically, initiation of a short (2-week) course of oral corticosteroids was often advocated to identify patients with COPD who might benefit from long-term treatment. Recent evidence, however, indicates that a short-course challenge is a poor method to predict patients who will benefit from long-term ICS use.[63,82] Given the lack of evidence and risk for significant side effects that include steroid myopathy and loss of bone density, chronic systemic corticosteroid therapy is not generally recommended. For patients with COPD experiencing an acute exacerbation of their disease, the short-term use of systemic corticosteroids has proven efficacy.[83]

In contrast, inhalation of corticosteroids leads to substantially less systemic absorption, thereby minimizing many of the risks associated with systemic corticosteroid therapy. On the basis of this, several national and international studies have been conducted to evaluate the potential benefit of ICS maintenance therapy.[61–63,84] Well-conducted clinical trials have revealed that daily treatment with ICS does not delay the long-term decline in FEV_1 in patients with COPD. Daily use can result, however, in a reduction in the frequency of exacerbations and an improvement in overall health status, particularly in patients with more advanced disease.[85–88] The TORCH investigation demonstrated that ICS use in combination with a long-acting β_2-agonist is more effective than either agent alone or placebo in patients with advanced COPD.[66] Specifically, patients using combination therapy (one inhalation twice daily) experienced decreased exacerbations, improved spirometric values, and increased health status. Although no difference was seen in mortality or disease progression among treatment groups, some guidelines recommend ICS as a treatment option in symptomatic patients with COPD and an FEV_1 less than 60% predicted.[1,89] Most trials to date involving ICS have studied patients on moderate to high doses. Common adverse effects include oral candidiasis, dysphonia, and skin bruising. ICS either alone or in combination with a bronchodilator may increase the risk of pneumonia in some patients. However, risk estimates have varied due to inconsistencies related to how pneumonia is defined, reported, and diagnosed among trials.[90] Additionally, withdrawal from ICS therapy has led to exacerbations in some patients, but a more recent study found no increases in exacerbation risk among patients with moderate to severe COPD when the ICS dose was tapered over a 3-month period.[1,91] Given the paucity of data, patient symptoms and lung function should be monitored when stepping down therapy.

Triple therapy involving a long-acting β agonist and a long-acting anticholinergic with an ICS may further improve lung function, quality of life, and reduce exacerbations, but further study is needed.[92,93]

PHARMACOLOGIC THERAPY BY DISEASE SEVERITY

As described, it is expected that patients with COPD will require an increase in the dose and number of medications to effectively manage their disease with time. Patients with infrequent or intermittent symptoms who are at a low risk for a future COPD exacerbation (Group A) should be offered either a short or long acting bronchodilator. As the disease progresses and patients become more symptomatic, as-needed use of bronchodilators alone will not maintain adequate relief from these symptoms. Long-acting bronchodilators have been shown to be more effective and convenient for patients experiencing more persistent symptoms (Group B). These patients may also continue to use a short-acting bronchodilator as needed for additional symptomatic relief. The addition of an ICS may be recommended in patients who are classified as having a "high risk" for a future exacerbation (Group C or Group D).[1] Patients who have a history or underlying findings consistent with an asthma component (e.g., Asthma COPD Overlap Syndrome) or those with elevated eosinophil counts may be most likely to benefit, although further study is needed.

In general, nebulization of bronchodilators is primarily reserved for the acute-care setting for quick symptomatic relief and is not advocated routinely for home use. In select patients who are not achieving maximal benefit with standard inhalation delivery devices, a 2-week trial with nebulized therapy can be considered and then continued if a clear benefit is observed.[94]

COPD EXACERBATION

An exacerbation of COPD is defined as "an acute worsening of respiratory symptoms that results in additional therapy.[1] Acute exacerbations of COPD are important events in the natural history of this disease.[95,96] They are associated with considerable morbidity; severe exacerbations are associated with an increased mortality.[96] Furthermore, acute exacerbations are responsible for a high percentage of the health care costs associated with COPD.[1,5]

The cause of acute exacerbations is believed to be a result of respiratory tract infections, either viral or bacterial, air pollution, or other environmental exposures.[97,98] These triggers can initiate increased bronchospasm and airway resistance in an individual with already compromised lung function. Although mild exacerbations may be readily managed with outpatient therapy, severe exacerbations can result in respiratory failure and death, particularly if they occur in a patient with severe COPD.

Key therapeutic interventions for acute COPD exacerbations include regular bronchodilator therapy, a short course of systemic corticosteroid therapy, antibiotics, and supportive measures such as oxygen therapy. Bronchodilator therapy consisting of a short-acting β_2-agonist with or without a short-acting anticholinergic is given as needed by MDI or nebulizer every 3 to 4 hours.

For videos that show proper use of many types of inhalers, go to http://use-inhalers.com/ or http://www.nationaljewish.org/healthinfo/multimedia/asthma-inhalers.aspx. For a video of how to use a nebulizer, go to http://www.nationaljewish.org/healthinfo/medications/lung-diseases/devices/nebulizers/instructions.aspx.

Systemic corticosteroids shorten recovery time, improve lung function and hypoxemia when added to other treatments used to manage exacerbations. Although there are insufficient data to support the optimal duration of treatment, a 5-day course of prednisone has been shown as effective as a 14-day course for reducing the occurrence of a re-exacerbation within a 6-month follow-up period.[83] A prolonged 10-day course of prednisone 30 to 40 mg per day may be a reasonable option for some patients.[30,99] High-dose intravenous corticosteroids (methylprednisolone 125 mg every 6 hours) have been shown to be effective in hospitalized patients.[100] Such large doses, however, are associated with an increased risk of hyperglycemia, and it is not known whether this regimen is superior to lower dose oral regimens. A recent pharmacoepidemiologic study involving nearly 80,000 patients hospitalized for acute COPD exacerbations found no difference in treatment failure in patients receiving intravenous corticosteroids compared with those taking lower dosages of oral corticosteroids.[101]

Decisions about antibiotic use in the setting of an acute exacerbation should be made based on the presence of the following respiratory symptoms: increased dyspnea, sputum volume, and sputum purulence. Data suggest that if two of the three are increased, antibiotics are beneficial.[102] The optimal antibiotic regimen for acute COPD exacerbations has not been rigorously studied. For many outpatients, however, generic, low-cost antibiotics, including amoxicillin, trimethoprim–sulfamethoxazole, or doxycycline, may be very effective. Indeed, these agents can effectively cover the most common bacterial causes of acute exacerbations, including *Streptococcus pneumoniae, Haemophilus influenzae*, and *Moraxella catarrhalis*. Guidelines suggest that hospitalized patients in respiratory failure should receive broad-spectrum antimicrobials that include activity against *Pseudomonas aeruginosa*, because these patients have a higher risk for more resistant organisms.[30]

COPD GROUP A (LOW RISK; LESS SYMPTOMS)

Diagnosis

CASE 19-1

QUESTION 1: T.A., a 51-year-old white male smoker, presents with daily cough and mild dyspnea on exertion with strenuous activity. He has noticed that walking up two flights of steps bothers him, when previously it did not. He has had a slight amount of wheezing, but no chest pain. He has no known chronic medical problems. He has smoked 1.5 packs/day for 34 years and he continues to smoke that amount. His physical examination is unremarkable. COPD is suspected. What diagnostic test should be ordered?

A clinical diagnosis of COPD should be considered in any patient presenting with persistent dyspnea, chronic cough, or sputum production with a history of exposure to risk factors such as cigarette smoking. Spirometry is the gold standard diagnostic test and should be considered to confirm the diagnosis of COPD. The main values gleaned from spirometry will include the FVC, FEV_1, and the FEV_1/FVC ratio. An FEV_1/FVC ratio of less than 0.70 following a bronchodilator indicates obstruction to expiratory flow consistent with COPD. The FEV_1 can be used in conjunction with other clinical indicators to further determine disease severity.

CASE 19-1, QUESTION 2: Office spirometry demonstrates an FEV_1/FVC of 0.69 and an absolute FEV_1 of 81% of predicted. T.A. has a CAT score of 7 and has had one exacerbation in the past year, which was managed at home. Using GOLD criteria, which COPD risk group should T.A. be assigned and what other diagnostic tests would be necessary before initiating therapy?

Based on GOLD guidelines, this patient has clinical features most consistent with "Group A." A CXR study is often performed to exclude other respiratory diagnoses contributing to the patient's symptoms; however, the abnormal spirometry is sufficient to make the diagnosis of COPD and to initiate therapy.

In certain cases of diagnostic uncertainty or in patients with severe disease being considered for surgical intervention, such as lung volume reduction surgery, a complete set of pulmonary function tests, including the determination of lung volumes and DLCO, may be performed. Complete pulmonary function testing, however, is not necessary to make the diagnosis of COPD.

In patients with more severe symptoms or airflow obstruction, assessment of oxygen status by means of pulse oximetry or ABG may be necessary. Pulse oximetry should be used to assess stable patients if the FEV_1 is <35% of predicted or with clinical signs suggestive of respiratory failure or right heart failure. ABGs are recommended if peripheral saturation is <92%.[1] An α_1-antitrypsin level to rule out α_1-antitrypsin deficiency is generally reserved for patients with disease onset at a young age (<45 years of age), or in patients with a strong family history of COPD.[1]

Therapeutic Management

CASE 19-1, QUESTION 3: What therapeutic interventions should be recommended for T.A. at this point?

SMOKING CESSATION

A comprehensive smoking cessation plan with therapy should be initiated for T.A. because smoking cessation is the only intervention proven to decrease the decline in FEV_1 associated with COPD.[1,25] Although pharmacologic interventions for smoking cessation are covered elsewhere in the text (see Chapter 91, Tobacco Use and Dependence), it should be noted that a personalized message may be beneficial for this patient. Indeed, discussion of spirometry results with the patient can provide an important opportunity to deliver a personalized message.[103] It can be explained to T.A. that he is beginning to develop definite irreversible abnormalities in his pulmonary function and, therefore, is a "susceptible" smoker. It is critical for him to stop smoking and thereby prevent continued deterioration in lung function.

IMMUNIZATIONS

In addition to smoking cessation, this patient's immunization status should be evaluated.[104] According to the GOLD guidelines and in the absence of contraindications, T.A. is a candidate for vaccination against influenza and pneumococcal pneumonia, even though he is in the early stages of COPD.[1] Patients with COPD are at risk for increased morbidity and mortality if they develop either of these infectious complications.

Individuals at greatest risk for significant morbidity and mortality from influenza and pneumonia are those with chronic disease, including lung disease. Optimally, the influenza vaccine should be administered during the fall before the end of October.[105] This allows an adequate antibody response before the peak influenza season, which typically occurs within the first quarter of the year. Annual immunization is required to ensure adequate antibody protection against influenza virus and is effective in reducing morbidity and mortality from influenza.[106]

The pneumococcal polysaccharide vaccine (Pneumovax 23, PPSV23) is also recommended for patients with COPD.[1] The PPSV23 contains 23 *S. pneumoniae* serotypes and provides protection against *S. pneumoniae*.[107] The Advisory Committee on Immunization Practices (ACIP) now recommends a one-time dose of the PCV13 in addition to the PPSV23 in patients ≥65 years of age. These vaccines should be separated as indicated to ensure an optimal immune response.[108] To manage T.A.'s symptoms, treatment with an as-needed bronchodilator may be reasonable to start. Bronchodilators are the primary pharmacologic therapy used in the management of COPD.[1,30]

Available bronchodilator therapies include short or long acting β_2-agonists, short or long acting anticholinergics and methylxanthines (theophylline). For initial treatment, the most common choice for T.A. would be a short-acting, inhaled β_2-agonist, (e.g., albuterol), a short-acting inhaled anticholinergic (e.g., ipratropium), or a combination of these two agents. Either of these therapies has a relatively short onset of action and is effective in relieving symptoms. Table 19-7 summarizes inhaled therapeutic options for COPD.

SHORT-ACTING β_2-AGONISTS

β_2-Agonists produce bronchodilation by relaxing bronchial smooth muscle through activation of cyclic adenosine monophosphate (cAMP).[109] The inhalation route of delivery for bronchodilators is recommended over oral therapy based on safety and efficacy. The dose–response curve among all available bronchodilators is relatively flat and similar. No evidence suggests that one agent is superior to another.

Albuterol is the most frequently used agent in this class. It is available as an MDI or DPI 90 mcg/inhalation. It is also available as a premixed solution for nebulization (e.g., adult dose 2.5 mg/0.5 mL), as well as a concentrated solution 5 mg/mL (0.5%) that requires saline to be prescribed separately. The onset of action of short-acting β_2-agonists (e.g., albuterol, levalbuterol)

Table 19-7
Inhaled Therapeutic Options for COPD

Medication Brand Name and Strength (per inhalation)	Chemical Name	Device	No. of Doses[a]/ Device or Box
Short-Acting β_2 Agonists			
ProAir HFA 90 mcg, Proventil HFA 90 mcg, Ventolin HFA 90 mcg	Albuterol	MDI	200[b]
ProAir, RespiClick 90 mcg AccuNeb 0.63 mg/3 mL, 1.25 mg/3 mL	Albuterol	DPI	200
Proventil 2.5 mg/3 mL (0.083%), [d]5 mg/mL (0.5%) *concentrate*	Albuterol	Nebulizer	Varies
Xopenex HFA 45 mcg	Levalbuterol	MDI	200[b]
Xopenex 0.31 mg/3 mL, 0.63 mg/3 mL, 1.25mg/3 mL, [d]1.25 mg/0.5 mL *concentrate*	Levalbuterol	Nebulizer	Varies
Short-Acting Anticholinergic			
Atrovent HFA 17 mcg	Ipratropium	MDI	200[b]
Atrovent 0.02% (0.5 mg/2.5 mL) vial	Ipratropium	Nebulizer	25ct, 30ct, 60ct
Short-Acting Anticholinergic + β_2 Agonist Combination			
Combivent Respimat 20–100 mcg	Ipratropium + Albuterol	SMI	120[b]
DuoNeb 0.5–2.5 mg/3 mL vial	Ipratropium + Albuterol	Nebulizer	30ct, 60ct
Long-Acting β_2 Agonists			
Serevent Diskus 50 mcg	Salmeterol	DPI	60
Foradil Aerolizer 12 mcg	Formoterol	DPI	60 blister units
Brovana 15 mcg/2 mL vial	Arformoterol	Nebulizer	30ct, 60ct
Perforomist 20 mcg/2 mL vial	Formoterol	Nebulizer	30ct, 60ct
Long-Acting β_2 Agonists (Once Daily)			
Arcapta Neohaler 75 mcg	Indacaterol maleate	DPI	30 blister units
Striverdi Respimat 2.5 mcg	Olodaterol	SMI	60[b]
Long-Acting Anticholinergics			
Spiriva HandiHaler 18 mcg	Tiotropium	DPI	30 blister units
Spiriva Respimat 2.5 mcg	Tiotropium	SMI	60[b]
Tudorza Pressair 400 mcg	Aclidinium bromide	DPI	60
Incruse Ellipta 62.5 mcg	Umeclidinium	DPI	30 blister units
Seebri Neohaler 15.6 mcg	Glycopyrrolate	DPI	60 blister units
Inhaled Corticosteroid + Long-Acting β_2 Agonist Combination			
[c]Advair Diskus 250/50 mcg	Fluticasone + Salmeterol	DPI	60
[c]Symbicort HFA 160 mcg/4.5 mcg	Budesonide + Formoterol	MDI	120[b]
[c]Breo Ellipta 100–25 mcg	Fluticasone + Vilanterol	DPI	60 blister units
Long-Acting Anticholinergic + β_2 Agonist Combination			
Anoro Ellipta 62.5–25 mcg	Umeclidinium + Vilanterol	DPI	60 blister units
Stiolto Respimat 2.5–2.5 mcg	Tiotropium + Olodaterol	SMI	60[b]
Utibron Neohaler 15.6–27.5 mcg	Glycopyrrolate + Indacaterol	DPI	60 blister units
Bevespi Aerosphere 9–4.8 mcg	Glycopyrrolate + Formoterol	MDI	120[b]

[a]Institutional sizes not included.
[b]Number of doses after initial priming.
[c]Only FDA-approved strength for COPD other strengths may be commercially available.
[d]Nebulized solutions marked "0.5 mL concentrate" should be diluted with 0.9% sodium chloride solution.
DPI, dry-powder inhaler; MDI, metered-dose inhaler; SMI, soft mist inhaler.

is rapid (within 5 minutes) and generally reaches maximal effect in 15 to 30 minutes. The duration of action is approximately 4 hours. Although inhaled β_2-agonists are usually well tolerated, some patients experience adverse effects (tremors, tachycardia, or nervousness) with even low dosages. Although concern has been expressed about the safety of short-acting, inhaled β_2-agonists in patients with cardiac disease, a cohort study using the Saskatchewan Health Services database concluded that there was no increased risk for fatal or nonfatal myocardial infarction in patients using these agents.[110]

SHORT-ACTING ANTICHOLINERGICS

The parasympathetic (cholinergic) nervous system plays a primary role in the control of bronchomotor tone in COPD. By inhibiting cyclic guanosine monophosphate (cGMP) in the lung, aerosolized anticholinergic drugs are effective bronchodilators. The bronchodilation produced by anticholinergics in patients with stable COPD has been shown to be non-inferior to that achieved by inhaled β_2-agonists.

Ipratropium bromide is the primary short-acting anticholinergic agent used in COPD. It is marketed as both an MDI (17 mcg ipratropium per puff) and as a solution for nebulization (0.5 mg ipratropium/2.5 mL). Ipratropium has an average onset of effect within 15 minutes, with a maximal bronchodilator effect in 60 to 90 minutes, although some patients may experience more rapid symptom relief. The duration of action is approximately 6 hours. Although some reports suggest a quicker onset of action, patients should be advised that the relief of acute symptoms will be slower compared with an inhaled β_2-agonist. A typical dose of ipratropium is two inhalations four times daily.[111] Although well tolerated, some patients experience dry mouth, nausea, and blurred vision with use of ipratropium.

The anticholinergic actions of ipratropium are localized predominantly in the lungs, with an apparent specificity of action in the larger airways. Because it has minimal effects on sputum viscosity, there is little problem with drying of airway secretions. In addition, ipratropium's structure as a quaternary amine increases its polarity, thereby minimizing absorption from the lung and systemic side effects. These structural properties also reduce penetration across the blood–brain barrier, reducing the incidence of confusion and other central nervous system (CNS) side effects.

COMBINATION β_2-AGONISTS–ANTICHOLINERGICS

Combination therapy with two different classes of bronchodilators is appealing because it may decrease the cumulative dose of individual agents, thereby decreasing the risk of side effects while maintaining the benefits of each medication. In addition, anticholinergics and β-agonists have different mechanisms of action, and combining the two classes may provide additional benefit. Indeed, it has been demonstrated that combination therapy results in significantly greater increases in FEV_1 compared with use of either albuterol or ipratropium alone.[112] The Combivent Respimat contains both albuterol and ipratropium in a single inhaler.[113] The respimat is a novel propellant-free inhalation device that produces a slow moving mist from mechanical energy produced by the release of a compressed spring.

Umeclidinium plus vilanterol (Anoro Ellipta), and tiotropium plus olodaterol (Stiolto Respimat), are once-daily products that combine a long-acting anticholinergic plus a long-acting β_2-agonist in a single device.[114,115] Glycopyrrolate is available in combination with indacaterol (Utibron™ Neohaler) and in combination with formoterol (Bevespi® Aerosphere), but both dosed twice daily.[116,117] Each has been approved for the maintenance treatment of airflow obstruction in patients with COPD.[114–117]

COPD GROUP B (LOW RISK; MORE SYMPTOMS) WITH DISEASE PROGRESSION

Therapeutic Management

CASE 19-2

QUESTION 1: J.O., a 46-year-old woman with a 32-pack-year history of cigarette smoking, presents with increasing shortness of breath. She gets winded walking on level ground after about 100 yards. She quit smoking 2 years ago. The chronic cough that she previously had lessened after smoking cessation, but the dyspnea is now somewhat worse, despite use of an albuterol inhaler on an as-needed basis. On examination, mild wheezing is noted. A CXR is unremarkable. Office spirometry demonstrates an FEV_1/FVC ratio of 0.64 and an absolute FEV_1 of 2.0 L or 60% of predicted. J.O. has a CAT score of 20, and has had one exacerbation in the past year, which was managed at home. Post-bronchodilator treatment demonstrated an FEV_1 increase of 100 mL, a 5% increase. How should J.O. be treated?

J.O. would be considered to be in Group B. She has had progression of dyspnea despite smoking cessation and the addition of a short-acting β_2-agonist.She is still at a low risk for an exacerbation based on her exacerbation history. Because pharmacologic management of COPD involves a stepwise approach, regular use of a long-acting bronchodilator would be the next step in treatment.

The main classes of long-acting bronchodilators currently available include β_2-agonists and anticholinergics. Both classes can be further divided into two groups according to duration of activity—those producing bronchodilation for 12+ hours and those producing bronchodilation for 24+ hours. Both classes have been shown to improve quality of life and reduce dyspnea in patients with COPD.

LONG-ACTING β_2-AGONISTS

The role of inhaled, long-acting β_2-agonists in the chronic management of COPD has become well established in recent years. Available evidence with both salmeterol and formoterol shows improved pulmonary function, reduced dyspnea, and enhanced quality of life in patients with COPD.[30] Indacaterol, olodaterol, and vilanterol are dosed once daily and have a rapid onset of activity (e.g., >5 minutes) and produce bronchodilation for 24 hours or more. Their long duration of activity and comparable safety profile may offer an added convenience to some patients. A plateau in bronchodilation is achieved for most patients at the recommended dose for each agent, so no benefits exist in exceeding the recommended dose. In addition, higher doses will increase the risk of adverse events associated with β_2-agonist excess. Therefore, salmeterol should be prescribed as 42 mcg (50 mcg in a dry-powder device) twice daily and formoterol at 12 mcg twice daily.

LONG-ACTING ANTICHOLINERGICS

Vagal cholinergic tone is a reversible component of the airway limitation in COPD. Stimulation of the vagal parasympathetic nerves causes the release of acetylcholine, which then binds to muscarinic receptors to produce bronchoconstriction and secretion of mucus. Three muscarinic subtypes have been identified in human airways: the M_1, M_2, and M_3 receptors. Tiotropium is a long-acting anticholinergic that binds to the M_1, M_2, and M_3 muscarinic receptors of bronchial smooth muscle.[118] Although tiotropium dissociates rapidly from the M_2 receptor, it dissociates much more slowly from the M_1 and M_3 receptors. In fact, its dissociation from the M_1 and M_3 receptors is 100 times slower than that of ipratropium. M_1 receptors are located on parasympathetic ganglia, where they facilitate postganglionic transmission, thus enhancing cholinergic tone. M_3 receptors are found on airway smooth muscle and mucous glands, where activation leads to bronchoconstriction and mucus secretion. Conversely, M_2 receptors are located on postganglionic nerve endings, where they serve as autoreceptors regulating acetylcholine release and, thereby, cholinergic tone. Thus, anticholinergics, by virtue of antagonizing M_1 and M_3 receptors, relax airway smooth muscle, and can reduce mucus secretion. M_2 blockade, however, augments acetylcholine release and thus enhances cholinergic tone. Therefore, the slower dissociation rate from both the M_1 and M_3 receptors enhances bronchodilation and allows the convenience of once-daily dosing.

Tiotropium has a very long duration of action and can provide effective bronchodilation with once-daily dosing. Numerous studies have documented its beneficial effect on pulmonary function and quality of life. The UPLIFT (Understanding Potential Long-Term Impacts on Function with Tiotropium) compared 4 years of therapy with either tiotropium or placebo in nearly 6,000 patients with COPD. Tiotropium was associated with improvements in lung function, quality of life, and exacerbation risk, but did not impact the rate of decline of FEV_1 or mortality.[69] Tiotropium is also a quaternary amine with limited systemic absorption; therefore, the agent is well tolerated, with dry mouth being the major side effect. Concerns have been raised, however, about tiotropium's safety. In particular, disparate sources have identified stroke, cardiovascular events, and death as possible adverse outcomes. After completion of UPLIFT, which included 17,721 patient-years of drug exposure, the FDA recently concluded that the appropriate use of tiotropium in COPD patients does not place them at increased risk for stroke or adverse cardiovascular events.[119] In September 2014, tiotropium was also approved to be delivered via the Respimat device. The Tiotropium Safety and Performance in Respimat (TIOSPIR) Trial is the largest COPD trial to date involving more than 17,000 patients. This trial was designed to directly compare the safety of tiotropium respimat to tiotropium delivered via the HandiHaler device. The length of time to first COPD exacerbation was also followed to compare efficacy. Both the Respimat and HandiHaler were found to have comparable results for exacerbation frequency, as well as exacerbations associated with hospitalization. The incidence of adverse events was also similar between all treatment groups.[120]

Aclidinium bromide (Tudorza PressAir), umeclidinium bromide (Incruse Ellipta), and glycopyrrolate (Seebri Neohaler) are long-acting anticholinergics recently approved for the long-term maintenance treatment of COPD. These agents have been shown to improve lung function and appear to be well tolerated.[121–123]

J.O. should be started on a long-acting bronchodilator, such as salmeterol, formoterol, or tiotropium. Once-daily βagonists such as indacaterol or olodaterol are additional options to consider. Recently approved anticholinergics such as aclidinium bromide, glycopyrrolate, or umeclidinium bromide are other potential options. It should be noted that the tolerability and efficacy of the available long-acting bronchodilators are comparable. The choice of agent is largely based on considerations such as the frequency of drug administration, the patient's ability to use the inhalation device correctly, and any out-of-pocket costs incurred by the patient. J.O. should also be instructed to continue her albuterol two puffs every 4 hours as needed. A 3-month follow-up visit should be scheduled to assess her response.

CASE 19-2, QUESTION 2: J.O. is started on tiotropium Respimat, inhale 5 mcg daily and returns to the office for a check-up in 3 months as recommended. She has had significant benefit from the medication and has had decreased wheezing and a noticeable improvement in her exercise tolerance. She asks to have spirometry repeated to see whether her lung function has improved on the new medication. Spirometry is repeated, and no significant improvement is noted in her FEV_1. She asks how she can feel better, with improved exercise tolerance, without an improvement in her lung function.

Increasing evidence suggests that bronchodilators, including long-acting β_2-agonists and anticholinergics, may reduce exercise-related dyspnea in patients with COPD by decreasing dynamic hyperinflation.[124] This improvement may be independent of marked changes in spirometry performed at rest. Indeed, because of flow limitation, these patients who exercise can have significant worsening of air-trapping, which can worsen lung compliance and adversely affect respiratory muscle mechanics. A number of studies have shown that alleviation of such dynamic hyperinflation may be an important mechanism whereby bronchodilators improve exercise tolerance in patients with obstructive lung disease.[124]

CASE 19-2, QUESTION 3: J.O. seemed to do reasonably well for a number of years, but now, 3 years later, she has noticed progressive dyspnea on exertion. She is now having difficulty carrying laundry up from her basement, and she has noticed that her overall activity level has been curtailed. Repeat office spirometry now shows an FEV_1/FVC ratio of 0.49 and an absolute FEV_1 of 49% of predicted. She now has a CAT score of 22, and has had two exacerbations in the past year. J.O. has been adherent with her tiotropium regimen and has had no other significant changes to her medical history. She remains smoke free and is not exposed to second-hand smoke in her home and work environments. What therapeutic intervention(s) should be considered at this point?

INHALED CORTICOSTEROID THERAPY

J.O has had significant deterioration in status and repeated COPD exacerbations despite appropriate adherence to tiotropium. Patients with findings consistent with COPD risk Group D should be prescribed combination therapy consisting of either an ICS + LABA or LAMA + LABA. Fixed dose combination products are preferred and several options are commercially available. (Table 19-6.) LAMA + LABA therapy may be preferred given the lower incidence of pneumonia and adverse effects related to inhaled corticosteroids.[1] One LAMA + LABA combination was superior to ICS + LABA in preventing exacerbations, and other patient reported outcomes in those with a history of prior exacerbations.[125] However, a number of multicenter, randomized, controlled clinical trials have demonstrated the efficacy of ICS in COPD.[85–88] The data have supported the use of ICS in advanced COPD and in patients with frequent exacerbations. Regular use of ICS can decrease the frequency of acute exacerbations and improve health-related quality of life in patients with an FEV_1 <60% predicted.[1]

The TORCH study has defined the benefits and potential side effects of ICS in a broader patient population of COPD.[66] In this multicenter, randomized, placebo-controlled study, mean FEV_1 was 50% predicted, but entry criteria did not require a history of repeated exacerbations. More than 6,000 patients were randomly assigned to either an ICS (fluticasone 500 mcg BID), inhaled salmeterol (50 mcg BID), combination fluticasone 500 mcg and salmeterol 50 mcg BID, or placebo. Subjects were assessed for approximately 3 years. A significant benefit was seen as measured by decreased exacerbation rates in subjects taking either inhaled fluticasone or a combination of fluticasone–salmeterol therapy. Also, an improvement was found in mortality with combination therapy that approached, but did not reach statistical significance. Overall adverse side effects with ICS were similar to those with placebo. An increased risk, however, was seen for lower respiratory tract infections with inhaled fluticasone or fluticasone–salmeterol. Of note, patients did not experience an increased risk of ocular manifestations or decreased bone density with ICS treatment.

J.O. is already taking tiotropium, so a decision must be made regarding step-up therapy. A LAMA+LABA is the preferred regimen for this patient given findings consistent with COPD Group D. Tiotropium should be replaced with tiotropium + olodaterol fixed dose combination product. J.O. is already familiar with the Respimat device, which may help maintain adherence. However, other long acting bronchodilator combination products exist. A number of other potential interventions may be considered. One option would be to discontinue the tiotropium and initiate a combination ICS–long-acting β_2-agonist. Alternatively, an ICS–long-acting β_2-agonist product may be added to the tiotropium given the severity of her disease.[1,92,93] Lastly, an ICS could be added to the tiotropium, although less evidence is available to support this option.[1] Any of these choices is reasonable provided no other major contraindications in doing so exist. It should be noted that currently several corticosteroid–long-acting β_2-agonist inhalers are indicated for COPD, including Advair (fluticasone–salmeterol), Symbicort (budesonide–formoterol), and Breo Ellipta (fluticasone–vilanterol). No convincing data suggest that one preparation is superior to the other in the treatment of COPD.

The exact duration of treatment that ICS should be given before making an assessment of their benefit is not clear. Generally, an adequate trial is at least 4 to 6 weeks. One rationale for the use of ICS in COPD is, however, the prevention of acute exacerbations. As such, it can be very difficult to measure objectively the clinical benefit of the medication in individual patients.

SAFETY OF LONG-ACTING BRONCHODILATORS

Case 19-2, Question 4: J.O. calls the next day, having read something on the internet regarding possible increased risk of death in people with obstructive lung disease who take long-acting bronchodilators. She is reluctant to take it. What should you tell her?

Although some evidence in asthma indicates that use of long-acting bronchodilators may be associated with an increased risk of death, such evidence does not exist in patients with COPD. In fact, the TORCH study demonstrated no increased risk of death or adverse events among patients prescribed salmeterol compared with placebo.[66] The patient should be reassured that long-acting bronchodilators are safe in COPD.

PULMONARY REHABILITATION

Case 19-2, Question 5: J.O. also wonders whether anything else other than her medication can be done for her. What advice might be given?

At this point, pulmonary rehabilitation should be strongly considered. In fact, a comprehensive multidisciplinary pulmonary rehabilitation program should be considered in any patient with COPD experiencing persistent shortness of breath despite pharmacologic management.[51]

Increasing evidence points to COPD as a systemic process,[126] and pulmonary rehabilitation addresses the systemic nature of the disease. Although the proximate cause of disability involves the respiratory system, leading to dyspnea on exertion, this in turn has systemic consequences. Although the changes may be fairly subtle to start with, most patients will gradually manifest increasing limitations in their activity. This results in substantial deconditioning. It is likely that this deconditioning, in addition to other factors such as systemic inflammation, adversely affect skeletal muscle function. Indeed, evidence is clear that oxidative capacity is diminished in patients with COPD,[53–55] which results in overall decreased aerobic capacity and results in increased lactic acid production for a given level of activity.[56] The increased acid load will lead to a greater requirement for ventilation, which makes dyspnea more severe. The more dyspneic the patient is, the less activity he or she will do, leading to more deconditioning and recapitulation of the downward spiral.

Pulmonary rehabilitation is an exercise-based, multidisciplinary program that seeks to address this cycle.[51] Most programs generally last 8 to 12 weeks and involve two to three sessions per week. Education, particularly about medication use, as well as psychosocial counseling and breathing retraining are important components of the program. An important component of breathing retraining involves coaching patients how to use pursed lip breathing effectively. Pursed lip breathing involves pursing the lips together (as in whistling) during exhalation. This helps to slow down respirations and also provides a back-pressure in the small airways, preventing dynamic airway collapse and exercise-induced hyperinflation. The major intervention, however, is exercise training, especially endurance training of the lower extremities (e.g., using a treadmill or bicycle ergometer). Numerous studies have demonstrated that a rehabilitation program can significantly improve exercise capacity and quality of life, as well as decrease health care utilization.[51] This may partly be related to the beneficial effects of exercise on the oxidative capacity of the skeletal muscles.

J.O. should be referred to a local outpatient pulmonary rehabilitation program. A typical program involves 2-hour sessions, three times per week for 10 weeks. The sessions will involve education, breathing retraining, and strength and endurance exercise training.

COPD GROUP C (HIGH RISK; LESS SYMPTOMS)

Acute Exacerbation of COPD

ANTIMICROBIAL THERAPY

CASE 19-3

Question 1: R.L., a 66-year-old man with diabetes mellitus and severe (Group C) COPD, presents with increased cough with productive discolored sputum after a "cold." He had been hospitalized 6 weeks earlier with community-acquired pneumonia. He is a former smoker (quit 10 years ago); his current medications include tiotropium respimat 5mcg once daily, albuterol MDI two puffs every 4 hours as needed, and theophylline 200 mg BID. He also has increased dyspnea and chest tightness. On examination, he is in no acute distress and vital signs are stable. There is increased wheezing on chest examination, and the rest of the examination is unchanged. Room air pulse oximetry is 90%, and a CXR in the office shows no infiltrates. How should this patient be treated?

This patient has increased sputum purulence and increased dyspnea consistent with an exacerbation of COPD. It is not uncommon for such an exacerbation to be triggered by an upper respiratory viral infection. Given that the patient has increased dyspnea and purulent sputum production, a course of systemic corticosteroids (e.g., 40 mg of prednisone daily for 5 days) and a course of antibiotics is warranted. In outpatients with low risk factors, a low-cost antibiotic regimen is a reasonable option. Empirical treatment with an aminopenicillin with or without clavulanic acid, a macrolide, or tetracycline derivative such a doxycycline may be used.[1] Although other antibiotics are commonly given, no data support that they are superior in this setting when compared with these conventional, less-expensive agents. An acute exacerbation of COPD is one of the few instances in which antibiotic therapy is warranted to treat a respiratory infection in the absence of evidence of lower respiratory tract involvement (i.e., pneumonia).

Patients with COPD and risk factors for poor outcome (severe COPD, comorbid conditions, history of frequent exacerbations) may be more susceptible to resistant pathogens. As such, guidelines recommend that a broad-spectrum antibiotic regimen be considered, including β-lactam–β-lactamase inhibitor combinations, quinolone antibiotics, or second- or third-generation cephalosporins.[1,30]

Because of his recent hospitalization, R.L. is at increased risk for resistant pathogens, including *P. aeruginosa*. He also presents with increased sputum purulence and increased dyspnea, so a broad-spectrum antimicrobial regimen, such as oral ciprofloxacin 750 mg BID or oral levofloxacin 500 mg every day for 5 to 10 days would be appropriate. A course of oral prednisone 40 mg daily for 5 days is also indicated to improve R.L.'s lung function, reduce his hypoxemia, and hasten his recovery time.

CASE 19-3, QUESTION 2: R.L. was treated with oral ciprofloxacin 750 mg BID and demonstrated a decrease in sputum volume and purulence with less dyspnea after 3 days of therapy. However, 5 days later, he is feeling palpitations and has become nauseous. What laboratory value should be checked?

This patient has clinical evidence of theophylline toxicity. Both gastrointestinal complaints (e.g., nausea) and CNS symptoms, including sleep difficulty and nervousness, are consistent with theophylline toxicity. Other adverse reactions associated with methylxanthines are cardiac irritability (tachycardia or arrhythmias) and seizures. All these side effects are dose related. Gastrointestinal intolerance, nervousness, and insomnia can occur at any serum concentration, but increase in frequency when serum concentrations are greater than 15 mcg/mL.

In R.L., the addition of the antibiotic ciprofloxacin to his regimen most likely resulted in a drug interaction causing a rise in his theophylline concentration. The potential for an interaction with theophylline varies among the available fluoroquinolone antibiotics. Drug interactions are dependent on several factors, including the dose of each agent and the baseline serum theophylline concentration. Elevations in the theophylline concentration of 25% are typical with ciprofloxacin interactions, although elevations of 50% have been observed. In R.L., a theophylline concentration should be obtained and further doses withheld until results are known.

In general, theophylline metabolism is associated with significant interpatient and intrapatient variability. Patients should be monitored closely for early signs of toxicity, as well as for the initiation of drugs that potentially may interact. Understanding and recognizing the potential for drug interactions can allow safe and effective therapy with theophylline.

CASE 19-3, QUESTION 3: A theophylline serum concentration is measured for R.L. It is reported as 21 mcg/mL. What action should be taken?

The serum concentration is consistent with the interaction between theophylline and ciprofloxacin reported in the literature. His symptoms do not appear life-threatening at this point, so a conservative approach to treatment is appropriate. Theophylline should be withheld for one dose and then restarted at a lower dose (100 mg BID) until the ciprofloxacin therapy is completed. Alternatively, theophylline could be withheld until the antibiotic treatment is finished or discontinued. As mentioned, theophylline has a narrow therapeutic index and has the potential for serious toxicity as is evidenced by the current case. If the patient is unclear how beneficial the theophylline has been, a trial off of the medication is reasonable. After approximately 2 to 4 weeks, R.L. should be reassessed. If he feels that his chronic symptoms are no different without the drug, it should be discontinued. On the other hand, his symptoms may become more pronounced without the theophylline, and it could then be restarted. Alternatively, it would be reasonable to replace theophylline with an additional long-acting bronchodilator from a different class, in this case a long-acting β agonist. Evidence suggests that the combination of a long-acting anticholinergic and a long-acting β_2-agonist can increase lung function and reduce hyperinflation compared with either agent used alone.[127,128] Salmeterol and formoterol have a similar side effect profile and have similar effectiveness, the only significant difference being that formoterol has a more rapid onset of action. Either salmeterol, one inhalation (50 mcg) every 12 hours, or formoterol, one inhalation (12 mcg) twice daily, would be reasonable options for RL.

COPD has a progressive course, highlighted by a worsening of symptoms with time. Because stepwise therapy is recommended, it is not uncommon to find patients on multiple medications added on in an attempt to alleviate symptoms. Nevertheless, it is important periodically to assess the patient to determine whether all the medications are continuing to provide symptomatic benefit and are still needed. This may result in a step-down approach.

Oxygen Therapy

CASE 19-4

QUESTION 1: P.J., a 62-year-old man with long-standing COPD, presents with worsening dyspnea on exertion. He is currently prescribed combination fluticasone–salmeterol (Advair 250/50 one puff BID), tiotropium (Spiriva 18 mcg one puff every day), and as-needed albuterol (two to four puffs every 4 to 6 hours as needed). P.J. reports excellent adherence with his medications and an evaluation of his inhaler technique reveals he is able to use all three devices correctly. He has undergone pulmonary rehabilitation in the past with some benefit. He is no longer exercising, however. He has smoked 1.5 packs of cigarettes a day for 40 years (60 pack-years), but quit 1 year previously. His most recent FEV_1/FVC ratio is 0.41, and his FEV_1 is 1.25 L, or 38% of predicted. His room air oxygen saturation at rest is 85%. On examination, reduced breath sounds are noted in his chest and he has lower extremity edema. His physician recommended supplemental oxygen; however, he is resistant and wonders what kind of benefit he might receive.

The Nocturnal Oxygen Treatment Trial (NOTT), a randomized controlled study, studied patients with COPD and severe hypoxemia ($Pao_2 \leq 55$ mm Hg, or $Pao_2 \leq 59$ mm Hg associated with polycythemia or peripheral edema).[45] Patients were randomly assigned to receive continuous oxygen or nocturnal oxygen. The primary outcome variable was mortality. Subjects using continuous oxygen had a significantly greater survival and improved end-organ function, including improved cognitive function. The Medical Research Council Study published in 1981, using similar entry criteria, demonstrated a significant survival benefit with continuous supplemental oxygen compared with no oxygen.[46]

On the basis of these studies, supplemental oxygen is currently recommended for severe hypoxemia currently defined as an oxygen saturation less than 88% or Pao_2 equal to or less than 55 mm Hg (oxygen saturation $<$ 90% or $Pao_2 \leq 59$ mm Hg in the presence of polycythemia or clinical evidence of pulmonary hypertension; e.g., peripheral edema). These guidelines (Table 19-8) are used by Medicare and most insurance companies as criteria to determine coverage for supplemental oxygen. This patient should be encouraged to use supplemental oxygen because it is one of the few available interventions that has been associated with improved survival in COPD.

In addition to supplemental oxygen, the patient should be re-enrolled in pulmonary rehabilitation. As mentioned, existing data suggest that this intervention can improve quality of life and exercise tolerance and decrease health care utilization.

Table 19-8
Guidelines for Insurance Reimbursement of Oxygen Therapy in Chronic Obstructive Pulmonary Disease (COPD)

1. Severe hypoxemia at rest[a]:
   $Pao_2 \leq 55$ mm Hg
   Or
   $Pao_2 \leq 59$ mm Hg, with polycythemia or evidence of cor pulmonale
   Or
   Oxygen saturation ≤ 88%
2. Oxygen desaturation ≤ 88% with activity or during sleep[b]

[a]Proven to improve survival.
[b]Efficacy not proven.

Surgical Treatments for COPD

Case 19-4, Question 2: P.J. is prescribed supplemental oxygen and enrolls in a pulmonary rehabilitation program. These interventions are successful in improving exercise tolerance; however, he presents 12 months later complaining of worsening dyspnea. In addition, although he is compliant with the oxygen, he is wondering whether any other interventions available might improve his lung function and allow him to "get off" of oxygen.

He is reevaluated with pulmonary function studies, which demonstrate a reduced FEV_1/FVC ratio of 0.38 and an absolute FEV_1 of 29% of predicted. In addition, lung volume determinations show severe hyperinflation (TLC = 135% of predicted and air-trapping RV = 292% of predicted). His CXR shows a marked decrease in lung markings in the upper lung zones with vascular crowding in the lower lung fields. What therapeutic options are available for P.J.?

Lung volume reduction surgery, which involves the surgical removal of approximately 30% of the volume of each lung, can significantly improve quality of life, exercise tolerance, and mortality in selected patients with COPD. The National Emphysema Treatment Trial (NETT) demonstrated that patients with severe, upper lobe predominant emphysema who have lung volume reduction surgery have significant benefits in health-related quality of life as well as exercise tolerance.[11] Subjects who also had persistently poor exercise tolerance before surgery appeared to have the most benefit compared with control subjects with similar impairment. These patients also had a mortality benefit.[11] The rationale for the surgery is that removing the areas of the lung most involved with emphysema can improve the physiology of the remaining lung. This includes improvement in expiratory airflow and improved lung elastic recoil as well as improved ventilation–perfusion matching. The major patient selection criteria for lung volume reduction surgery are depicted in Table 19-9. After a successful surgery, patients can have improved gas exchange and may no longer require supplemental oxygen.

The CXR for this patient suggests upper lobe predominant emphysema. This would need to be confirmed with a high-resolution computed tomography scan of the chest. Furthermore, the patient would need to complete a comprehensive pulmonary rehabilitation program before surgery. Only a few centers within the United States are certified by Medicare to perform lung volume reduction surgery, and this could be an important issue for P.J., depending on where he lives. It should be stressed that lung volume reduction surgery is only appropriate for a select group of patients with advanced emphysema.

In patients with severe emphysema, another option is lung transplantation. This intervention has not been shown to decrease mortality, but can improve quality of life and exercise tolerance in carefully selected candidates.[129] Patients considered are those with severe disease, whose life expectancy is less than 5 years, and individuals with an FEV_1 less than 25% of predicted.

Table 19-9
Major Selection Criteria for Lung Volume Reduction Surgery

Moderate to severe airflow obstruction
Hyperinflation
Upper lobe predominant emphysema
Nonsmoker
Rehabilitation potential

KEY REFERENCES AND WEBSITES

A full list of references for this chapter can be found at http://thepoint.lww.com/AT11e. Below are the key references and websites for this chapter, with the corresponding reference number in this chapter found in parentheses after the reference.

Key References

Anthonisen NR et al. Effects of smoking intervention and the use of an inhaled anticholinergic bronchodilator on the rate of decline of FEV_1. The Lung Health Study. *JAMA*. 1994;272:1497. (25)

Calverley PMA et al. Salmeterol and fluticasone propionate and survival in chronic obstructive pulmonary disease. *N Engl J Med*. 2007;356:775. (66)

Celli BR et al. The body-mass index, airflow obstruction, dyspnea, and exercise capacity index in chronic obstructive pulmonary disease. *N Engl J Med*. 2004;350:1005. (41)

Fishman A et al. A randomized trial comparing lung-volume–reduction surgery with medical therapy for severe emphysema. *N Engl J Med*. 2003;348:2059. (11)

Leuppi JD et al. Short term versus conventional glucocorticoid therapy in acute exacerbations of chronic obstructive pulmonary disease: the REDUCE randomized clinical trial. *JAMA*. 2013;309(21):2223–2231. (83)

Lindenauer PK et al. Association of corticosteroid dose and route of administration with risk of treatment failure in acute exacerbation of chronic obstructive pulmonary disease. *JAMA*. 2010;303:2359. (101)

Nici L et al. American Thoracic Society/European Respiratory Society statement on pulmonary rehabilitation. *Am J Respir Crit Care Med*. 2006;173:1390. (51)

Nocturnal Oxygen Therapy Trial Group. Continuous or nocturnal oxygen therapy in hypoxemic chronic obstructive lung disease: a clinical trial. Nocturnal Oxygen Therapy Trial Group. *Ann Intern Med*. 1980;93:391. (45)

Tashkin DP et al. A 4-year trial of tiotropium in chronic obstructive pulmonary disease. *N Engl J Med*. 2008;359:1543. (69)

Wise RA et al. Tiotropium respimat inhaler and the risk of death in COPD. *N Engl J Med*. 2013;369:1491–1501. (119)

Key Websites

Diagnosis and Management of Stable Chronic Obstructive Pulmonary Disease: A Clinical Practice Guideline from the American College of Physicians, American College of Chest Physicians, American Thoracic Society, and European Respiratory Society. 2011 https://www.thoracic.org/statements/copd.php. Accessed July 25, 2017.

Global Initiative for Chronic Obstructive Lung Disease: Asthma, COPD, Asthma-COPD Overlap Syndrome (ACOS). 2015, http://goldcopd.org/asthma-copd-asthma-copd-overlap-syndrome/. Accessed July 25, 2017.

GOLD (Global Initiative for Chronic Obstructive Lung Disease). Global strategy for the diagnosis, management, and prevention of chronic obstructive pulmonary disease. Updated 2017 [online], http://www.goldcopd.org. Accessed July 25, 2017.

20 Acute and Chronic Rhinitis

Suzanne G. Bollmeier and Dennis M. Williams

CORE PRINCIPLES

		CHAPTER CASES
1	Rhinitis is a common disorder and refers generally to inflammation in the nasal cavity. Common manifestations can include nasal discharge, itching, sneezing, congestion, and postnasal drip. Rhinitis can be caused by allergic, nonallergic, or mixed allergic and nonallergic triggers. Distinguishing the subtype can be helpful in targeting symptomatic treatment and prevention.	**Cases 20-1 (Question 1)** **Cases 20-8 (Question 2)** **Cases 20-9 (Question 1)**
2	Oral antihistamines are the most common therapies used for treating allergic rhinitis. They are convenient and effective for most rhinitis symptoms, including rhinorrhea, sneezing, and itching.	**Cases 20-1 (Question 4)**
3	Second-generation antihistamines are preferred over first-generation agents based on a superior side-effect profile and convenience of dosing.	**Case 20-1 (Question 4)**
4	Intranasal antihistamines offer an alternative to oral agents, with the advantage of efficacy for congestion and for symptoms from some nonallergic causes. Side effects can challenge patient acceptance, however.	**Case 20-1 (Question 5)**
5	Intranasal corticosteroids are the most effective therapies available for treating a variety of rhinitis disorders. They are safe, well tolerated, and are highly effective in reducing itching, sneezing, rhinorrhea, and congestion.	**Cases 20-3 (Question 3)**
6	Proper administration technique is important for intranasal therapies in order to maximize effectiveness and minimize the risk of side effects and toxicities.	**Cases 20-1 (Question 5)** **Cases 20-2 (Question 3)** **Cases 20-3 (Question 7)**
7	Leukotriene modifiers have similar efficacy to oral antihistamines for seasonal allergic rhinitis and may be beneficial for selected patient populations (e.g., those with concomitant asthma or aspirin sensitivity).	**Cases 20-4 (Question 2)**
8	The duration of use of topical decongestants should be limited to 3 to 5 days.	**Case 20-7 (Question 1)**
9	Ophthalmic therapies may be indicated if ocular itching, tearing, and redness are the primary complaint or continue to be bothersome despite appropriate therapy for nasal symptoms associated with rhinitis.	**Case 20-1 (Question 5)**
10	Many patients seek complementary and alternative therapies to treat rhinitis conditions, despite limited evidence regarding their effectiveness.	**Cases 20-5 (Question 1)**

DEFINITION

Rhinitis is defined as an inflammatory condition affecting the mucous membranes of the nose and upper respiratory system. In clinical practice, however, the term is used broadly to encompass a heterogeneous group of nasal disorders characterized by periods of rhinorrhea (nasal discharge), pruritus (itching), sneezing, congestion, and postnasal drainage (postnasal drip). These nasal symptoms can be accompanied by ocular symptoms such as redness, itching, and discharge and can be exacerbated by the development or presence of sinusitis. The most common form of rhinitis occurs in response to an allergen, although a variety of other subtypes have been demonstrated.[1–3]

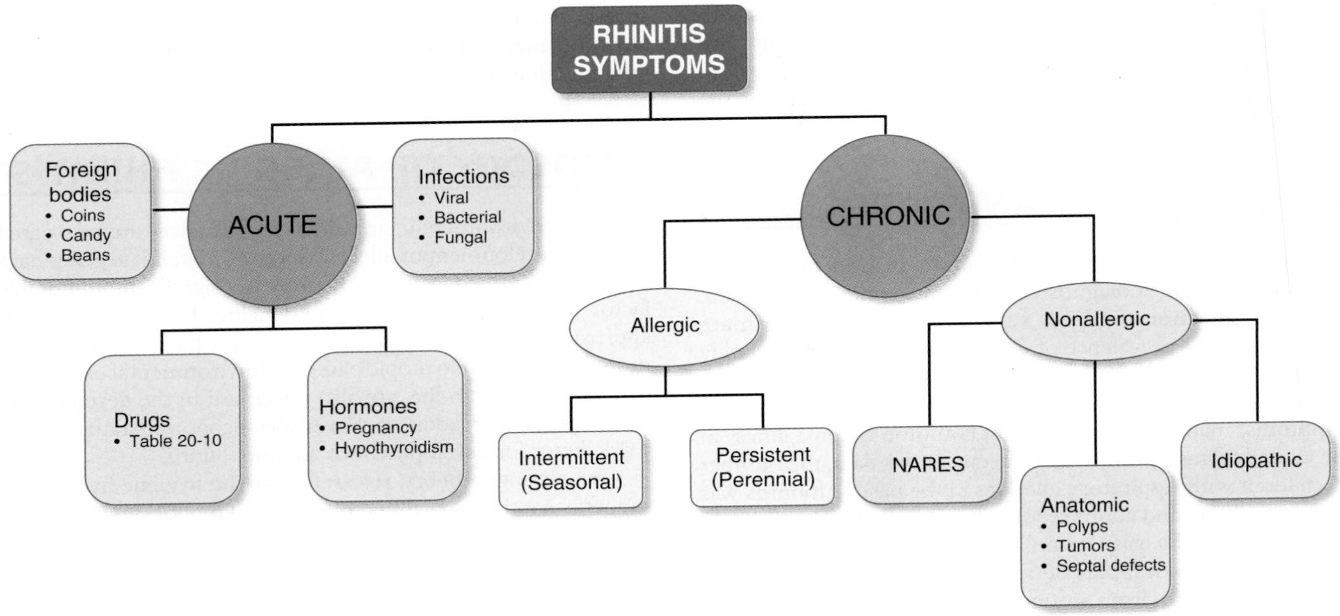

Figure 20-1 Possible causes of rhinitis symptoms. NARES, nonallergic rhinitis with eosinophilia syndrome.

CAUSES AND CLASSIFICATIONS

Rhinitis is not a single disease but rather has multiple causes and underlying pathophysiologic mechanisms.[2,4] Figure 20-1 depicts common causes of acute and chronic rhinitis symptoms, including some conditions that mimic rhinitis (e.g., nasal polyps). The most common cause of acute rhinitis is a viral upper respiratory infection, that is, the common cold.

In most patients, these viral infections are self-limited and require only symptomatic treatment.[2] Nasal foreign bodies are another frequent cause and should be suspected when a pediatric patient presents with acute, unilateral symptoms.[1,3] Hormonal, food, and medication-related rhinitis are also common acute syndromes.[3,5]

Chronic rhinitis can be classified as allergic, nonallergic, or mixed allergic and nonallergic.[2] Allergic rhinitis, the most common subtype, is typically associated with atopy, an inherited tendency to develop a clinical hypersensitivity condition, and its symptoms are a result of immunoglobulin E (IgE)–dependent events.[5] There is not a single, uniform standard for classifying allergic rhinitis. Traditionally, patients have been classified as having seasonal or perennial disease, based on frequency of symptoms and potential offending allergens.[1] An alternative classification system categorizes allergic rhinitis based on severity (e.g., mild, moderate, and severe) and frequency (e.g., intermittent or persistent) of symptoms.[1] This classification system is summarized in Figure 20-2. Clinicians are likely to encounter a combination of these classifications when evaluating the clinical literature and participating in patient care activities.

Several categories exist for nonallergic causes of rhinitis, including nonallergic rhinopathy (previously known as idiopathic rhinitis or vasomotor rhinitis), nonallergic rhinitis with eosinophilia syndrome (NARES), and anatomic abnormalities.[6] Nonallergic rhinopathy refers to symptoms associated with environmental stimuli, including temperature or barometric pressure changes, strong odors, tobacco smoke,[6] stress, or emotional factors.[7] NARES occurs frequently in middle-aged patients, who have no evidence of allergic disease excepting the presence of eosinophils in the nasal smear.[7] Mixed rhinitis is a subset of allergic rhinitis in which features of both allergic and nonallergic diseases are present, and

Intermittent[a] Disease	Persistent[b] Disease
Symptoms occur: Fewer than 4 days/week *or* for fewer than 4 weeks	**Symptoms occur**: At least 4 days/week *and* for at least 4 weeks

Mild	Moderate–Severe
All of the following:	At least *one* of the following:
• Normal sleep	• Impaired sleep
• No impairment of usual daily activities, sports, and leisure	• Impairment of daily activities, sports, and leisure
• No interference with work or school	• Interference at work or school
• No troublesome symptoms	• Troublesome symptoms

[a]Formerly "seasonal" symptoms.
[b]Formerly "perennial" symptoms.

Figure 20-2 ARIA classification of allergic rhinitis. ARIA, Allergic Rhinitis and its Impact on Asthma. (Source: Bousquet J et al. Allergic rhinitis and its impact on asthma [ARIA] 2008 update [in collaboration with the World Health Organization, GA(2)LEN and AllerGen]. *Allergy*. 2008;63[Suppl 86]:8.)

triggers include allergens as well as other irritants.[8] Patients with mixed rhinitis are difficult to differentiate but will typically have more nasal symptoms from nonallergic triggers.[8] The presence of mixed disease should not be overlooked when evaluating the presentation of a patient or assessing the response to therapy.

EPIDEMIOLOGY AND IMPACT

Prevalence rates for rhinitis are difficult to quantify because the condition is often undiagnosed, different definitions are used, and data collection methods vary.[9] A conservative estimate suggests that the prevalence of allergic rhinitis is approximately 15% (via physician diagnosis), but it may be as high as up to 30% in adults (and even more children), based on self-reported nasal symptoms[2] making it the fifth most common chronic illness in the United States.[1] According to recent survey data, the number of children with respiratory allergies in the past 12 months was nearly 8 million, and adults reporting a diagnosis of hay fever in the past 12 months was 17.8 million.[10]

In recent decades, prevalence in Western societies has increased, and studies from around the world are reporting similar trends.[5,11] Although studies have traditionally reported a 3:1 ratio of allergic to nonallergic rhinitis, recent data suggest that up to 87% of patients may experience symptoms from mixed causes.[7]

Rhinitis can lead to poor sleep,[12] decreased work productivity,[13] headache or fatigue,[14] irritability, and rhinitis patients are typically less attentive in school because of decreased concentration, and difficulty learning.[14] Although many patients will self-treat their rhinitis symptoms, visits to provider offices are common.[15] A patient with allergic rhinitis will visit the provider approximately three more times per year and fill nine more prescriptions yearly compared to a patient without rhinitis.[16]

Although rhinitis does not lead to the mortality associated with some illnesses, its prevalence and negative health impact make it an important health problem in the United States. Allergic diseases are a frequent contributor to health-related absenteeism.[17] It is estimated that 10.7 million workdays are missed because of allergic rhinitis in the United States per year.[17]

ANATOMY AND PHYSIOLOGY

The external nose is pyramidal and consists of paired nasal bones and associated cartilage. Its base has two elliptical-shaped openings called nares, or nostrils. Internally, a septum separates the nasal cavity into two halves and consists of bone and cartilage covered by a mucosal membrane.[18]

The membranes of the nasal cavity consist primarily of pseudostratified ciliated columnar epithelial cells with mucus-producing goblet cells interspersed among them.[18] The mucus lining serves as a protective shield against bacterial and viral infections.[18] The tiny cilia beat rhythmically to transport mucus across the upper airway membrane to the nasopharynx. In addition, respiratory secretions residing on these mucous membranes contain immunoglobulin A (IgA), which serves as an immunologic defense.[18]

The autonomic nervous system controls the vascular supply and the secretion of mucus to the nasal membrane. Sympathetic activation results in vasoconstriction, which decreases nasal airway resistance.[18] Parasympathetic stimulation results in glandular secretion and nasal congestion.[18] The mucosa is also innervated by the nonadrenergic–noncholinergic system. Neuropeptides from these nerves (e.g., substance P and neurokinins) play a role in vasodilation, mucus production, and inflammation,[18] although their significance is unclear. The trigeminal nerve also provides sensory innervation.[18] The primary functions of the nose and upper airway are smell, speech, and the exchange of air between the internal and external environments.[18] These processes are disrupted in the presence of inflammation, increased mucus, and congestion.

ETIOLOGY OF ALLERGIC RHINITIS

Genetic, environmental, and lifestyle influences are associated with the development of allergic rhinitis.[19] Candidate genes have not been identified;[19] however, atopy is a significant inheritable factor, and the risk of a child experiencing allergic symptoms is approximately 44% to 50% with one atopic parent[2,5] and is even more likely with two atopic parents.[5] Environmental exposures, particularly early in life, are also important in the development of symptoms.[20] In addition, lower socioeconomic status may be a risk factor for development of allergic rhinitis.[20]

One etiologic theory, referred to as the hygiene hypothesis, suggests that the initial differentiation of lymphocytes early in life has either positive or negative influences on the development of subsequent allergies. In the normal development of the immune system, the lymphocytes differentiate into helper T (either T_H1 or T_H2) cells based on environmental stimuli. Factors associated with a T_H1 (allergy protective) response include exposures to various bacteria and viruses, the presence of older siblings, and early attendance in day care. Factors associated with a T_H2 (predisposition to allergies) response include environmental exposures to house dust mites, cockroaches, or early, frequent antimicrobial use.[4,5]

In patients with seasonal or intermittent allergic rhinitis, grass and tree pollens and airborne mold spores are the most common allergens.[21] Although the pollen season varies with geographic location, types of grasses, trees, and weeds, it can be problematic for many people during active pollination. In the United States, ragweed is a primary cause of intermittent symptoms.[21]

In patients with persistent allergic rhinitis, the major allergens are house dust mites, indoor molds, animal dander, and cockroach antigen. Another common cause is occupational exposure, in which symptoms can be precipitated by agents such as flour, wood, paint, grain, latex, and detergents.[5]

PATHOPHYSIOLOGY

The pathogenesis of allergic rhinitis and asthma includes numerous areas of commonality. Inflammation is a central mechanism, and the role of cytokines is similar. This has led many scientists and clinicians to adopt the concept of "one airway, one disease."[4] Further evidence for this association includes the fact that rhinitis is a known risk factor for asthma,[5] some patients with rhinitis exhibit bronchial hyperresponsiveness,[4] and treating allergic rhinitis can improve asthma.[2,4] Consequently, some treatment strategies, including pharmacotherapy, have a role in both rhinitis and asthma.

Allergic rhinitis is characterized by an IgE-mediated response that involves three primary steps: sensitization, early-phase events, and late-phase events.[4] This process is depicted in Figure 20-3. The nonallergic pathogenic course is less well understood. It is not IgE-mediated, although in some subtypes inflammatory cells and mediators can cause similar effects to those seen in the allergic form.[6]

Sensitization

In atopic patients, sensitization to an allergen occurs after initial exposure causing production of IgE antibodies. These antibodies bind to receptors on mast cells. Upon subsequent exposure, activation of an inflammatory response is initiated because of the cross-linking of the allergen, IgE antibody, and the mast cell.[5]

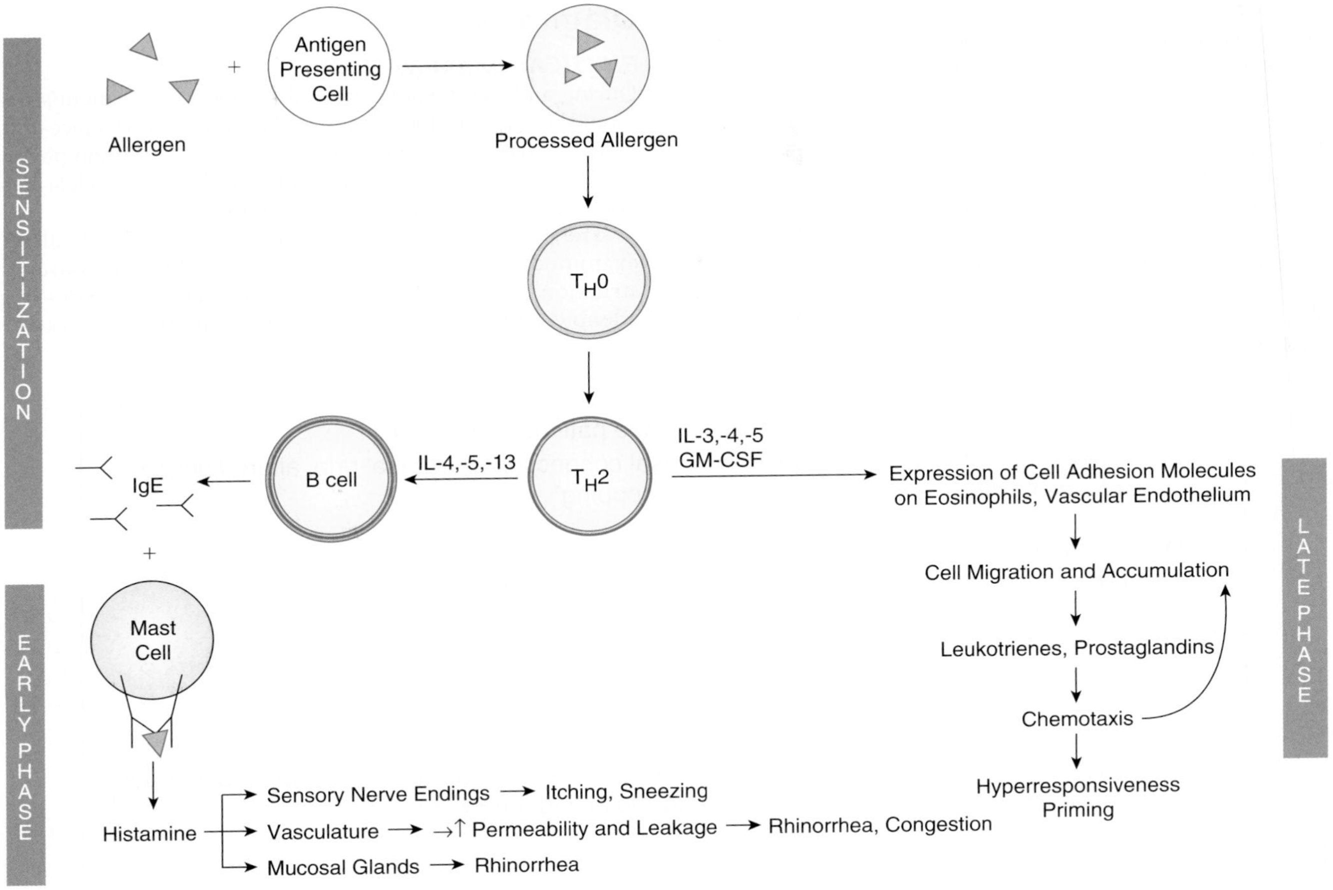

Figure 20-3 Pathophysiology of allergic rhinitis.

Early Response

After initial exposure, antigen-presenting cells of the immune system react to allergens deposited on the nasal mucosa.[5] Mast cells and other cells, such as basophils,[14] then release both new and preformed chemotactic[14] inflammatory mediators, such as histamine, which can cause localized inflammation.[4] Symptoms associated with this early response can occur within minutes, including sneezing, rhinorrhea, and nasal itching.[5] Histamine receptors (H_1) are present throughout the nasal mucosa and airway. Their activation results in vascular engorgement, leading to nasal congestion and rhinorrhea.[14] In addition, histamine stimulates sensory nerves of the parasympathetic nervous system in the upper airway causing other inflammatory mediators such as basophils,[5] eosinophils, lymphocytes, macrophages, and dendritic cells to migrate to the upper airway, contributing to a late-phase response.[14]

Late Response

Up to one-third of patients with allergic rhinitis also experience a late response that develops approximately 4 hours after initial exposure and may persist for up to 8 hours.[22] In this phase, the nature of inflammation is even more complex, and nasal congestion is a prominent feature.[4] Numerous cells and mediators, including T_H2 lymphocytes, cytokines, basophils, eosinophils, neutrophils, macrophages, and leukotrienes, play important roles.[4] These additional mediators, attracted to the area through chemotaxis, sustain the inflammatory response.[4] Also, some chemotactic proteins can cause damage to the airway epithelium and expose local nerve fibers.[4] Continued exposure to the offending allergen can also prolong the late-phase reaction.

CLINICAL PRESENTATION AND ASSESSMENT OF RHINITIS

The diagnosis of rhinitis is not defined by one specific laboratory test; rather, it is related to the coordinated results of a thorough patient interview, including medication history, pertinent physical examination, and a limited number of relevant laboratory assessments.

Risk Factors

Several elements increase the risk of developing allergic rhinitis. Parental history,[2] introduction of formula in infancy, exposure to maternal smoking at less than 1 year of age, serum IgE levels >100 IU/mL before 6 years of age, food allergies,[14] ethnic origin other than white European, environmental pollution, birth during pollen season, no older siblings, late entry into nursery or preschool, and exposure to indoor allergens such as animal dander and dust mites are risk factors.[5]

History, Signs, and Symptoms

A history should be obtained from the patient that includes details of the onset, character, frequency, duration, and severity of the patient's symptoms and any identifiable factors that provoke or relieve these symptoms.[5] Past medical history (including age of onset of symptoms) and family history (e.g., atopy) are also helpful.[5]

Both allergic and nonallergic forms of rhinitis are common and can potentially coexist.[2] Diagnostic criteria suggestive of allergic rhinitis include nasal itching, sneezing, nasal congestion, clear rhinorrhea, and occasionally a decreased sense of smell.[5] Symptoms of allergic conjunctivitis include itchy, watery eyes,[5] which occur in approximately 50% to 70% of allergic rhinitis patients. Their presence can be used to differentiate allergic rhinitis from other forms.[5] Persistent congestion and/or rhinorrhea[7] in response to nonallergic triggers like weather changes, perfumes/odors, and smoke/fumes[6] are consistent with nonallergic rhinitis. The negative impact of rhinitis on a patient's quality of life can be substantial, and it is important to assess this during the patient interview. Symptoms and symptom-induced interference with necessary (i.e., work, school) and enjoyable (e.g., hobbies, family events) activities can lead to patient anger, sadness, irritation, and withdrawal.[5] The questions listed in Figure 20-4 provide a guide to collecting the information needed to initiate and modify therapy based on the underlying causes of the rhinitis symptoms.

Diagnosis

PHYSICAL EXAMINATION

During a physical examination for rhinitis, the patient's nose should be inspected for position of the septum, appearance of the nasal mucosa, secretions, and any growths.[3] Common physical characteristics of patients with allergic rhinitis are clear nasal discharge and swollen nasal membranes.[4]

The patient's eyes, ears, throat, and chest should also be examined. Chronic mouth breathing because of nasal obstruction can cause recognizable facial characteristics (e.g., adenoid face, allergic shiners, and nasal crease) and dental abnormalities.[1,14]

1. Which of the common symptoms of rhinitis is the patient experiencing?
   - Sneezing, nasal itching, runny nose, nasal congestion, postnasal drip, altered sense of smell, watery eyes, itching eyes, ear "popping"
2. What color are the nasal secretions?
   - Clear, white, yellow, green, blood-streaked, rusty brown
3. When did the symptoms first appear?
   - Infancy, childhood, adulthood
4. Were the symptoms associated with a change in state/environment?
   - After a viral upper respiratory infection, after a traumatic blow to the head or face, upon moving into/visiting a new dwelling, after obtaining a new pet
5. How often do the symptoms occur?
   - Daily, episodically, seasonally, constantly
6. For how long has this symptom pattern persisted?
   - Days, weeks, months, years
7. Which factors or conditions precipitate symptoms?
   - Specific allergens, inhaled irritants, climatic conditions, food, drinks
8. Which specific activities precipitate symptoms?
   - Dusting, vacuuming, mowing grass, raking leaves
9. Are other members of the family experiencing similar symptoms?
10. Which of the following are prevalent in the household?
    - Carpeting, heavy drapes, foam or feather pillows, stuffed toys, areas of high moisture (basements, bathrooms), tobacco use (by patient or others), pets
11. Does the patient have other medical conditions that can cause similar symptoms?
12. Is the patient taking any medications that might cause or aggravate these symptoms?
13. What prescription and nonprescription medications have been used for these symptoms in the past? Were they effective? Did they cause any unwanted effects?
14. What is the patient's occupation?
15. What are the patient's typical leisure activities?
16. To what extent have the symptoms interfered with the patient's lifestyle (i.e., are they disabling or merely annoying)?
    - Greatly, somewhat, not much

Figure 20-4 Patient history interview.

Laboratory Tests

Several diagnostic tests are available for confirming a diagnosis of allergic rhinitis in patients who present with a suggestive history and symptoms. Microscopic examination of nasal secretions can be performed, but consensus on their usefulness is lacking.[1] In allergic conditions, the clinician would expect numerous eosinophils to be present in the sample; however, this could also be true of NARES or nasal polyps.[23]

Immediate hypersensitivity skin tests are used to demonstrate an IgE-mediated response of the skin to an allergen.[1] A variety of skin test methods are available; however, the skin-prick/puncture technique (in which the wheal-and-flare reaction is evaluated 15 to 20 minutes after allergen administration) is preferred.[1] A primary point of differentiation between pure allergic versus nonallergic disease is the presence of a serum IgE level greater than 100 international units/mL (especially before age 6), which is consistent with atopy.[5] However, a clinical diagnosis of either allergic or nonallergic disease is often made in the absence of a serum IgE and is based on the nature of symptoms and triggers.

OVERVIEW OF TREATMENT

There are two primary guideline resources available that summarize evidence and expert opinion regarding the diagnosis and management of allergic rhinitis. The first, from the America Academy of Otolaryngology, Head and Neck Surgery Foundation, was published in early 2015 by a panel consisting of 20 members representing experts in the field of allergy and immunology.[1] In addition, evidence linking asthma and allergic rhinitis epidemiologically, pathologically, and physiologically has been published, suggesting that upper respiratory allergic disorders and asthma represent components of a single inflammatory airway syndrome.[4] This prompted the development and subsequent update of the Allergic Rhinitis and Its Impact on Asthma (ARIA) guidelines in 2010, which provide direction for clinicians caring for patients with both conditions.[24] This document includes information about the use of complementary and alternative therapies, rhinitis in athletes, and grading the evidence used to establish the guidelines.[24]

The treatment goals for rhinitis are to prevent or relieve symptoms, and improve quality of life without adverse drug effects or excessive cost. These goals should be achievable through the establishment of a therapeutic partnership with a competent and caring clinician. With appropriate treatment, the patient should be able to maintain a normal lifestyle and perform desired activities. Common management strategies include patient education, allergen and irritant avoidance, and pharmacotherapy.[1,3,4,14] Figure 20-5 depicts an algorithm for the general management of allergic rhinitis.

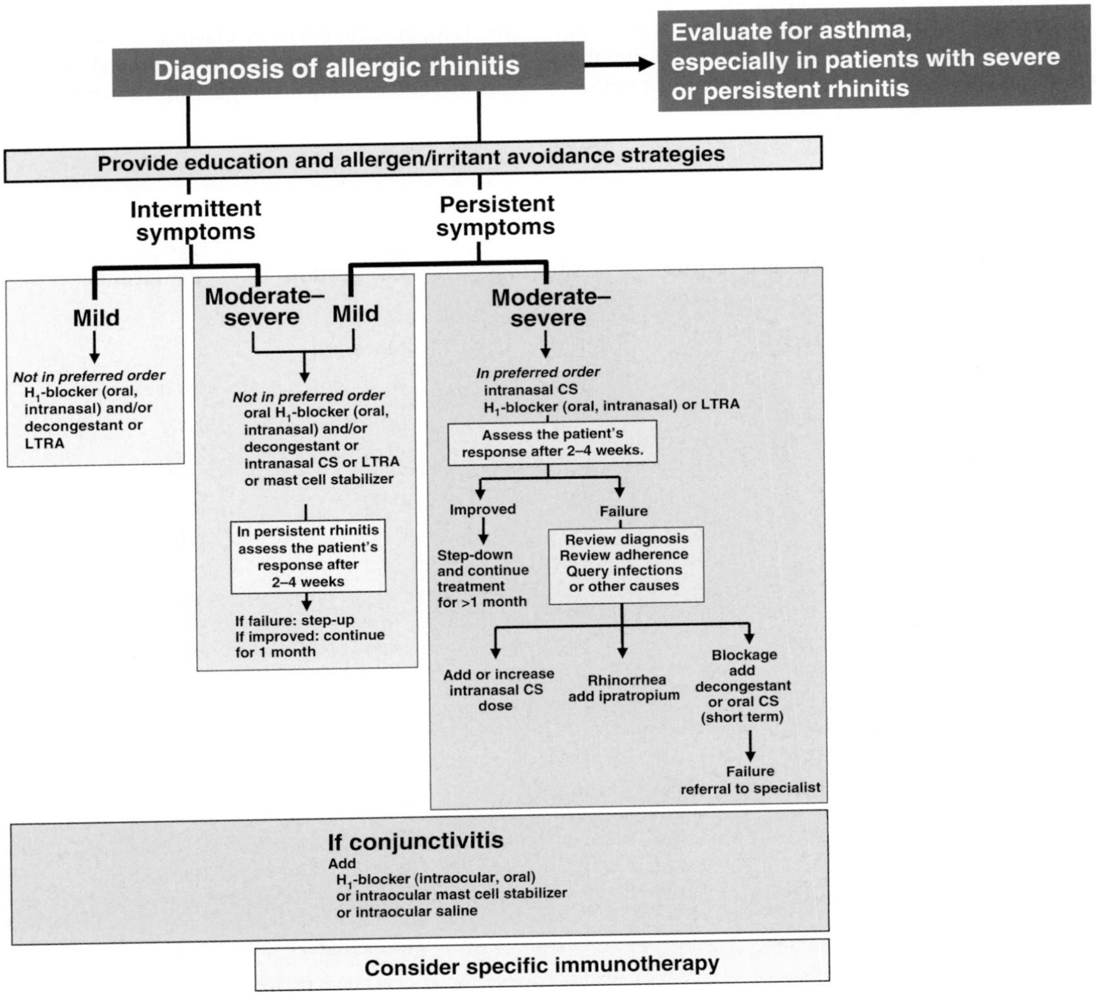

Figure 20-5 Treatment algorithm for allergic rhinitis. Treatment should be directed at predominant symptoms (i.e., for eye symptoms in the absence of other symptoms use ophthalmic preparation). Prevention strategies are more effective than treatment strategies. For intermittent symptoms, begin treatment several weeks before antigen exposure and discontinue when no longer needed. CS, corticosteroid; LTRA, leukotriene receptor antagonist (leukotriene modifier). (Source: Bousquet J et al. Allergic rhinitis and its impact on asthma [ARIA] 2008 update [in collaboration with the World Health Organization, GA(2)LEN and AllerGen]. *Allergy*. 2008;63[Suppl 86]:8.)

Patient Education

Patients should be educated about their rhinitis. Considerations for patient education include instruction about the disease and specific triggers, the range of symptoms, the role of various treatments, and suitable technique for nasal drug delivery.[5] A discussion of allergen and trigger avoidance is also important.

Allergen and Irritant Avoidance

Although the benefit of allergen avoidance has proved difficult to document, this strategy is considered central in a comprehensive management plan for allergic rhinitis.[1,5,6,14] Various strategies for minimizing exposure to known allergens (e.g., pollens, house dust mites, molds, animal dander, and cockroaches) are commonly used for prevention. Because little evidence supports a single physical or chemical intervention to reduce allergen exposure, a multifaceted approach should be used.[1] Efforts to reduce exposure to irritants (e.g., tobacco smoke, indoor, or outdoor pollutants) should also be recommended, because it is anticipated that this would have similar benefits as allergen avoidance.[3]

Pharmacotherapy

Several classes of medications are used in the management of rhinitis disorders. Choices should be based on goals of treatment, safety, efficacy, cost-effectiveness, adherence, severity, comorbidity, and patient preferences. Common therapies are administered either orally or topically and used on a regular schedule or on an as-needed basis.[1] Few cost-effectiveness data exist comparing the classes of therapy, except the second-generation antihistamines (SGAs),[25] nasal corticosteroids,[26] and subcutaneous immunotherapy,[27] which have been shown to be cost-effective. Table 20-1 summarizes the effectiveness of agents for specific symptoms used in the treatment of allergic rhinitis.

ANTIHISTAMINES

Antihistamines are the most common treatment for allergic rhinitis and are effective for relieving sneezing, itching, and rhinorrhea. They also diminish eye symptoms but, when taken orally, have minimal effects on nasal congestion.[2] Although first-generation antihistamines (FGAs) are efficacious, their use is limited by anticholinergic, sedative, and performance-impairing effects, which challenge their cost-effectiveness.[6] As a result, SGAs are preferred over FGAs in most cases where an antihistamine is desired.[1] Antihistamines are available in oral, ophthalmic, and intranasal formulations and can also be found in combinations with oral decongestants. They are most effective when administered before allergen exposure.

Although oral antihistamines (Table 20-2) represent the most commonly used therapy for allergic rhinitis, there is evidence that intranasal antihistamines are equal or superior in efficacy to oral agents. Further, they appear to relieve symptoms of mild congestion, which is not a feature of oral antihistamines.[1] Intranasal antihistamines work quickly; within 15 to 30 minutes but may be complicated by a bitter taste.[1] The improved efficacy of intranasal antihistamines over oral agents in certain rhinitis conditions may be because of direct administration to the affected site. Olopatadine 0.6%, Azelastine 0.1%, and 0.15% are Food and Drug Administration (FDA) approved for treatment of both seasonal and perennial allergic rhinitis in patients >6 years old.[1]

Table 20-1

Effectiveness of Agents[a] Used in the Management of Allergic Rhinitis

	Rhinorrhea	Nasal Pruritus	Sneezing	Nasal Congestion	Eye Symptoms	Onset
Antihistamines						
Nasal	Moderate	High	High	Moderate	0	Rapid
Ophthalmic	0	0	0	0	Moderate	Rapid
Oral	Moderate	High	High	0/Low	Low	Rapid
Decongestants						
Nasal	0	0	0	High	0	Rapid
Ophthalmic	0	0	0	0	Moderate	Rapid
Oral	0	0	0	High	0	Rapid
Corticosteroids						
Nasal	High	High	High	High	High	Slow (days)
Ophthalmic	0	0	0	0	High	Slow (days)
Mast-cell stabilizers						
Nasal	Low	Low	Low	0/Low	Low	Slow (weeks)
Ophthalmic	Low	Low	Low	Low	Moderate	Slow (weeks)
Anticholinergics						
Nasal	High	0	0	0	0	Rapid
Leukotriene Modifiers						
Oral	Low	0/Low	Low	Moderate	Low	Rapid

[a]Immunotherapy can lead to significant responses in all symptom categories; however, onset of action is delayed (months).

Source: van Cauwenberge P et al. Consensus statement on the treatment of allergic rhinitis. European Academy of Allergology and Clinical Immunology. *Allergy*. 2000;55:116; Bousquet J et al. Allergic rhinitis and its impact on asthma (ARIA) 2008 update (in collaboration with the World Health Organization, GA[2]LEN and AllerGen). *Allergy*. 2008;63(Suppl 86):8; and Facts & Comparisons eAnswers. **http://online.factsandcomparisons.com/index.aspx?** Accessed May 5, 2015.

High, significant effect; moderate, moderate effect; low, low effect; 0, no effect.

Table 20-2
Oral Antihistamines[a,b] Commonly Used in Allergic Rhinitis[29]

Generic Name (Example Brand Product)	Adult Dose	Pediatric Dose[c]	Other Effects		
First Generation			**Sedative**	**Antiemetic**	**Anticholinergic**
Chlorpheniramine (Chlor-Trimeton)	4 mg every 4–6 hours	Children 6–12 years: 2 mg every 4–6 hours Children 2–6 years: 1 mg every 4–6 hours	+	0	++
Clemastine (Tavist)	1 mg every 12 hours	Children 6–12 years: 0.67 mg every 12 hours	++	++ to +++	+++
Diphenhydramine (Benadryl)	25–50 mg every 6–8 hours	Children 6–12 years: 12.5–25 mg every 4–6 hours	+++	++ to +++	+++
Second Generation			**Sedative**	**Antiemetic**	**Anticholinergic**
Cetirizine (Zyrtec Allergy)	5–10 mg once daily	Children 6–12 years: 5–10 mg once daily Children 2–5 years: 2.5–5 mg once daily Children 12–23 months: 2.5–5 mg once daily	+	0	±
Fexofenadine (Allegra)	60 mg every 12 hours or 180 mg once daily	Children 2–11 years: 30 mg every 12 hours	±	0	±
Loratadine (Claritin)	10 mg once daily	Children 6–12 years: 10 mg once daily or 5 mg twice daily Children 2–5 years: 5 mg once daily	±	0	±
Levocetirizine[d] (Xyzal)	5 mg once daily in the evening	Children 6–11 years: 2.5 mg once daily in the evening Children 6 months–5 years: 1.25 mg once daily in the evening	±	0	±
Desloratadine[d] (Clarinex)	5 mg once daily	Children 6–11 years: 2.5 mg once daily Children 1–5 years: 1.25 mg once daily Children 6–11 months: 1 mg once daily	±	0	±

[a]Many oral antihistamines are sold as combination products with the oral decongestants pseudoephedrine and phenylephrine. The addition of the decongestant may alter the dosing scheme for the product. As of 2005, pseudoephedrine products have been placed behind the pharmacy counter in the United States. Federal law limits the quantity available for purchase and requires a signature and photo identification. Individual states may have additional restrictions regarding the sale of pseudoephedrine. Consult local boards of pharmacy for details.
[b]Some oral antihistamines are available in both short-acting and extended- or sustained-release formulations. Refer to package insert for specific dosing instructions for long-acting products.
[c]In 2008, the FDA issued an advisory alert recommending that OTC cough and cold agents (e.g., products containing antitussives, expectorants, decongestants, and antihistamines) not be used in infants and children younger than 2 years of age because of the potential for serious and possibly life-threatening adverse events (**http://www.fda.gov/ForConsumers/ConsumerUpdates/ucm048682.htm**). More recently, in October 2008, leading pharmaceutical manufacturers voluntarily modified product labels on OTC cough and cold preparations to state "do not use" in children younger than 4 years of age (**http://www.fda.gov/drugs/guidancecomplianceregulatoryinformation/enforcementactivitiesbyfda/selectedenforcementactionsonunapproveddrugs/ucm244478.htm#q1**). Furthermore, in 2011, the FDA removed unapproved prescription allergy products from the market because they had not been proven to meet standards for safety, effectiveness, and quality (**http://www.fda.gov/drugs/guidancecomplianceregulatoryinformation/enforcementactivitiesbyfda/selectedenforcementactionsonunapproveddrugs/ucm244478.htm#q1**).
[d]Currently available by prescription only.
Source: Facts & Comparisons eAnswers. **http://online.factsandcomparisons.com/index.aspx?** Accessed May 5, 2015.

INTRANASAL CORTICOSTEROID AGENTS

Intranasal corticosteroids are the most effective medication class for the treatment of allergic rhinitis, and are particularly useful for more severe or persistent symptoms.[1,6] Although achieving optimal outcomes depends on the patient's ability to use the device correctly, if administered as intended, these agents are appropriate for all symptoms, are generally well tolerated, and have few adverse effects.[24] They are most beneficial when dosed on a regular schedule; some evidence indicates, however, that they are effective when used on an as-needed basis.[1,6] Intranasal corticosteroids are also useful for treating nonallergic rhinitis[6] and some are available over-the-counter (OTC).

LEUKOTRIENE MODIFIERS

Leukotriene modifiers are effective in relieving many of the nasal symptoms of allergic rhinitis such as day-time congestion, rhinorrhea, pruritis, sneezing, and improves sleep as well as congestion on awakening.[4] Current guidelines recommend against utilizing this class of drugs as first-line.[1] They may have a role as an alternative option for preschool-aged children and adults with seasonal allergic rhinitis, but are not recommended for adult patients with perennial allergic rhinitis.[24] In addition, selected patients might benefit from the combination of an antihistamine and a leukotriene modifier,[14] such as those with concomitant asthma and allergic rhinitis.[1,28] There is no evidence that these agents are helpful for symptoms from nonallergic causes.

CROMOLYN

Intranasal cromolyn, a nonsteroidal agent, acts as a mast-cell stabilizer and, although safe, it is generally less efficacious than other therapies and only useful for symptoms related to allergic causes. It should be administered multiple times daily and requires several weeks to be effective.[5] It is best reserved for prophylaxis before exposure to a known allergen[14,28] and because of its excellent safety profile[28] for use by children or in pregnancy.[29]

DECONGESTANTS

Oral and nasal decongestants (Table 20-3) can effectively reduce nasal congestion by working on α-adrenergic receptors.[28] Oral agents are often combined with antihistamines and are generally well tolerated, but their use can lead to insomnia, nervousness, urinary retention, hypertension, and even palpitations which may be problematic for some patients.[30] Subsequently, these agents should be used with caution in elderly patients and in those with hyperthyroidism, cardiovascular disease, diabetes, glaucoma, or those who are pregnant.[30] Nasal agents are not typically associated with these effects, but should be limited to short-term use to avoid rebound nasal congestion.[28] Because pseudoephedrine is used in the illegal manufacture of methamphetamine, there are now restrictions on the sale of nonprescription formulations.[30] Also, questions regarding the efficacy of phenylephrine[30] have resulted in challenges to the optimal use of oral decongestants.

ANTICHOLINERGIC AGENTS

Intranasal ipratropium bromide is an anticholinergic agent effective in reducing watery, nasal secretions in allergic rhinitis, nonallergic rhinitis, and viral upper respiratory infections.[28] Anticholinergic agents have no significant effects on other symptoms.

OPHTHALMIC THERAPIES

Ophthalmic products used to treat symptoms of allergic conjunctivitis include antihistamines, decongestants, mast-cell stabilizers, and nonsteroidal anti-inflammatory agents. These agents are effective in reducing ocular symptoms and may be used in combination with oral and intranasal agents.

IMMUNOTHERAPY

Specific allergen immunotherapy (SIT) should be considered for patients with IgE-mediated disease,[3] who have severe symptoms despite optimal pharmacotherapy,[2,5] those who experience side effects from drugs restricting their treatment choices,[5] or those who cannot avoid allergen exposure.[3] The clinical efficacy of immunotherapy by subcutaneous injection (SCIT), sometimes

Table 20-3
Decongestants[a,b] Commonly Used in Allergic Rhinitis

Generic Name (Example Brand Product)	Adult Dose	Pediatric Dose[c]
Oral[a]		
Pseudoephedrine (Sudafed)	60 mg every 4–6 hours (max 240 mg/day)	Children 6–11 years: 30 mg every 4–6 hours (max 120 mg/day) Children 2–5 years: 15 mg every 4–6 hours (max 60 mg/day)
Phenylephrine (Sudafed PE)	10–20 mg every 4 hours (max 120 mg/day)	Children 6–11 years: 10 mg every 4 hours (max 60 mg/day)
Topical[d]		
Naphazoline (Privine)	0.05% solution: 1–2 drops or sprays/nostril every 6 hours	Children <12 years: avoid, unless under physician direction
Phenylephrine (Neo-Synephrine)	0.25%–1.0% solution: 2–3 sprays or drops/nostril every 3–4 hours	Children 6–11 years: 2–3 sprays or drops (0.25% solution)/nostril every 4 hours Children 2–5 years: 2–3 drops (0.125% solution) into each nostril not more than every 4 hours
Oxymetazoline (Afrin)	0.05% solution: 2–3 sprays/nostril every 10–12 hours	Children 6–12 years: 2–3 sprays/nostril every 12 hours
Xylometazoline	0.1% solution: 2–3 sprays into each nostril every 8–10 hours	Children 2–12 years: 1–2 sprays (0.05% solution) into each nostril every 8–10 hours

[a]Many oral decongestants are sold as combination products with the oral antihistamines. The addition of the antihistamine may alter the dosing scheme for the product. As of 2005, pseudoephedrine products have been placed behind the pharmacy counter in the United States. Federal law limits the quantity available for purchase to 9 g/month, 3.6 g/day with signature and photo identification. Individual states may have additional restrictions regarding the sale of pseudoephedrine. Consult local boards of pharmacy for details.
[b]Some oral decongestants are available in both short-acting and extended- or sustained-release formulations. Refer to package insert for specific dosing instructions for long-acting products. Note that some extended-release formulations are not recommended for children younger than 12 years of age.
[c]In 2008, the FDA issued an advisory alert recommending that OTC cough and cold agents (e.g., products containing antitussives, expectorants, decongestants, and antihistamines) not be used in infants and children younger than 2 years of age because of the potential for serious and possibly life-threatening adverse events(**http://www.fda.gov/ForConsumers/ConsumerUpdates/ucm048682.htm**). More recently, in October 2008, leading pharmaceutical manufacturers voluntarily modified product labels on OTC cough and cold preparations to state "do not use" in children younger than 4 years of age. Furthermore, in 2011, the FDA removed unapproved prescription allergy products from the market because they had not been proven to meet standards for safety, effectiveness, and quality(**http://www.fda.gov/drugs/guidancecomplianceregulatoryinformation/enforcementactivitiesbyfda/selectedenforcementactionsonunapproveddrugs/ucm244478.htm#q1**).
[d]Limit duration of treatment to less than 5 days to minimize risk of rebound congestion. Topical decongestants should never be used in preschoolers[24] or infants because of possible toxicity.[14]
Source: Facts & Comparisons eAnswers. **http://online.factsandcomparisons.com/index.aspx?**. Accessed May 7, 2015.

Table 20-4
Sublingual Tablet Immunotherapy

Drug Name	Allergen	Ages approved for (in years)	Dosing	Dosing considerations
Ragwitek	Ragweed pollen	18–65	1 tablet SL once daily	Initiate treatment at least 12 weeks before expected onset of each ragweed pollen season and continue throughout pollen season.
Oralair	Mixed grasses: Sweet Vernal, Orchard, Perennial Rye, Timothy, and Kentucky Bluegrass	10–65	Adults: 300 IR SL once daily 10 to 17 years of age: 100 IR sublingually on day 1, then 200 IR on day 2, and then 300 IR once daily thereafter Remove sublingual tablet from blister immediately prior to administration	Initiate treatment 4 months before expected onset of each grass pollen season and continue throughout pollen season
Grastek	Timothy grass	5–65	5 and older: 2,800 BAU SL once daily Remove sublingual tablet from blister immediately prior to administration	Initiate treatment at least 12 weeks before expected onset of each grass pollen season and continue throughout pollen season May be taken daily for 3 consecutive years (including intervals between grass pollen seasons) In clinical trials, treatment interruptions of up to 7 days were allowed

Administer first dose in a health care setting because of the potential for allergic reactions; monitor patient for 30 minutes after first dose. If well tolerated, subsequent doses may be taken at home. Auto-injectable epinephrine should be made available to patients.
Place tablet(s) under tongue until completely dissolved (at least 1 minute) and then swallow.
Wash hands after handling tablet. Avoid food or beverage for 5 minutes following dissolution of tablet (to prevent the swallowing of allergen extract).
SL, sublingual; IR, index of reactivity; BAU, bioequivalent allergy unit.
Source: Facts & Comparisons eAnswers. http://online.factsandcomparisons.com/index.aspx? Accessed May 7, 2015.

called "allergy shots," is well established[2] and is the only treatment that can offer the potential for disease remission.[1–3] Traditional SCIT presents some disadvantages, however, such as cost, adherence, and rare adverse systemic reactions.[1,31] Because regular injections can be unacceptable to some patients, alternative methods of delivering antigens, such as nasal, oral, bronchial, and sublingual immunotherapy (SLIT) have been investigated.[31] The oral, nasal, and bronchial routes have been abandoned because of lack of clinical efficacy or safety concerns.[31,32] Efficacy of immunotherapy given sublingually (SLIT) has been documented and the tablet form received FDA approval in April, 2014.[1,33] See Table 20-4 for details. There are potential adverse effects including local reactions such as oral itching[1] and swelling of the lips and mouth.[32] Systemic reactions can occur from both SCIT and SLIT and include urticaria, gastrointestinal upset, wheezing, and anaphylaxis.[1] Because of the potential for these reactions, SCIT is to be administered in the providers office; however, after the first dose of SLIT, it may be given at home (on a daily basis).[2] Providers are urged to prescribe and educate patients on how to use injectable epinephrine for emergency use and SLIT should not be given to patients with uncontrolled asthma or those on β-blocking agents.[29]

ANTI-IgE THERAPY

Omalizumab is a recombinant humanized monoclonal anti-IgE antibody that complexes free circulating IgE in the body. The complex cannot interact with mast cells and basophils, thus reduces IgE-mediated allergic reactions.[28] When administered as a subcutaneous injection once or twice monthly, omalizumab has been shown to decrease nasal symptoms[4] for both seasonal and perennial allergic rhinitis.[28] Currently, this therapy is approved only for people 12 years of age and older with moderate to severe allergy-related asthma inadequately controlled with inhaled corticosteroids. Omalizumab is also approved for patients with chronic idiopathic urticaria who remain symptomatic despite H_1 antihistamine treatment. This product has a high cost (estimated to be between $6,400 and $32,000 per patient per year).[28] The product has a boxed label warning to alert users that omalizumab can cause potentially life-threatening allergic reactions after any dose, up to 24 hours after the dose is given and even if there was no reaction to the first dose.[34] The FDA has also received reports regarding a slightly higher rate of heart and brain blood vessel problems as well as a potential increased risk of certain cancers, which needs to be monitored.[35]

Special Considerations of Medications in Pregnancy

The majority of data about the risks of various pharmacotherapies are derived from animal studies. There are limited human data; however, cohort and case control studies have been used to support therapeutic decision-making. Antihistamines, intranasal steroids, and cromolyn are considered safe to use during pregnancy.[3] Oral decongestants should generally be avoided,[3] although topical decongestants may be used on a short-term basis.[29] With limited human data available, oral montelukast is categorized as "probably compatible" with pregnancy;[29] however, generally, topical drugs are recommended over systemic therapy. Patients currently using immunotherapy may continue; however, initiation or an increased dose of immunotherapy is contraindicated.[3]

Nondrug Therapies

Supportive care is the foundation of treatment for patients with symptoms of rhinitis.[1] These strategies can be helpful during an acute worsening of symptoms as well as for the patient who suffers chronically. Supportive care can ameliorate discomfort, relieve mild symptoms, and assist with side effects from pharmacotherapies. Examples include the application of compresses to the sinuses or external nasal passages and humidification of mucous membranes with artificial tears or nasal saline solutions. Many patients with chronic symptoms of rhinosinusitis report subjective improvement with nasal saline douching,[3,5] or irrigation.

SPECIFIC THERAPEUTIC OPTIONS

Antihistamine Therapy

DIAGNOSIS OF ALLERGIC RHINITIS

CASE 20-1

QUESTION 1: L.B. is a 57-year-old man with a history of hypertension for 10 years and intermittent allergic rhinitis since childhood (confirmed sensitivity to birch tree pollen via skin testing). L.B. presents with complaints of nasal itching, sneezing, clear rhinorrhea, and stuffiness. He usually experiences similar symptoms, as well as ocular itching every spring, but has noticed that the problem has become persistent since he moved into an older home in the historic district of town. In the past, L.B. has successfully self-medicated his seasonal symptoms with an OTC antihistamine and decongestant (diphenhydramine 50 mg and pseudoephedrine 60 mg twice a day to 4 times a day as needed for symptoms), although "nothing seems to help much with the itchy eyes." L.B.'s hypertension has been well controlled with hydrochlorothiazide 25 mg every morning and amlodipine 10 mg every day. He denies any other medical problems, is afebrile, and his blood pressure is 128/82 mm Hg. He has no history of adverse drug reactions or drug allergies. He does not smoke, but drinks alcohol socially. What elements of L.B.'s presentation indicate a probable diagnosis of allergic rhinitis?

L.B. is exhibiting the classic symptoms of persistent (perennial) allergic rhinitis with intermittent (seasonal) exacerbations: nasal itching, sneezing, watery (often profuse) rhinorrhea, and congestion.[4] His history of positive skin tests and that his symptoms previously responded to antihistamine or decongestant[2] also support the diagnosis. In the past, L.B. has experienced symptoms predictably at the onset of the tree pollination season, with only minimal symptoms during the remainder of the year. Moving into an older home, however, has likely triggered latent sensitivities to dust mite allergens and mold spores. A treatment approach can be developed based on these presumptions. If this strategy is not effective, skin testing or additional laboratory assessments are warranted.

ALLERGEN AVOIDANCE MEASURES

CASE 20-1, QUESTION 2: What allergen avoidance strategies could L.B. use to minimize his exposure to triggers?

Allergen avoidance is important for reducing symptoms in patients with known sensitivities. Avoiding these triggers should lead to an improvement of symptoms; however, little evidence supports the effectiveness of a single physical or chemical method.[24] To achieve effective control, a multifaceted approach to the control of environmental triggers is usually needed.[24] Although total allergen avoidance is often impractical to implement, simple changes that can reduce exposure to many perennial triggers, such as house dust mites, animal dander, and mold, may assist with symptom control.[1,6]

Dust-mite avoidance (e.g., the use of impermeable covers on box springs, mattresses, and pillows) has traditionally been used as a method of reducing allergen exposure. Although this practice continues to be recommended frequently, it is controversial. Studies have shown less dust-mite levels in mattresses with impermeable covers, but this has not been correlated to improvement in symptoms.[1] Other methods of reducing antigen exposure include washing bedding at least weekly in hot water >130°F (>55°C) and dried under high heat in an electric dryer,[36] removing upholstered furniture, and washing floors daily.[1] Also, reducing humidity in the house to below 50% and replacing carpets with linoleum, tile, or wood floors are commonly recommended.[36]

Mold avoidance is difficult when outdoor humidity levels are high, but covering cold, moist surfaces such as water pipes with insulation and increasing ventilation can help reduce humidity. Also, visible mold should be removed from surfaces with detergent and water and any imbedded mold should also be removed.[36] Because L.B. has recently moved into an older home, he may not have used these avoidance strategies. These should be recommended and explained during the initial clinical consultation.

THERAPEUTIC OBJECTIVES FOR ALLERGIC RHINITIS

CASE 20-1, QUESTION 3: What are the therapeutic objectives in treating L.B.?

The therapeutic objectives for the treatment of allergic rhinitis are to control symptoms and permit all usual daily activities with no adverse effects of therapy. In patients with seasonal exacerbations, another objective is to prevent the onset of symptoms by anticipating the patient's season of sensitivity. In L.B.'s case, he should use environmental measures to reduce exposure and then begin chronic treatment with possible add-on therapy instituted 2 weeks before the start of pollen season.

CHOICE OF THERAPEUTIC AGENT

CASE 20-1, QUESTION 4: L.B. has used diphenhydramine for many years with good symptom relief and, as he recalls, only minimal daytime sedation. He asks your opinion regarding whether this is the best treatment for his allergic symptoms. He specifically requests the most cost-effective treatment available, because he must pay cash out-of-pocket for any medications. What therapy do you recommend and how should it be initiated?

Based on effectiveness and convenience, including nonprescription availability, oral antihistamines are the most frequent initial therapy recommended for patients with allergic rhinitis, particularly those with mild symptoms.[1] They reduce symptoms of nasal itching, sneezing, and rhinorrhea,[3] as well as ocular complaints but offer no benefit for nasal congestion. FGAs (e.g., diphenhydramine, brompheniramine, chlorpheniramine, and clemastine) lack specificity for the H_1 receptor and can cause significant sedation, various anticholinergic side effects, and can impair performance,[29] all of which limit their usefulness. Although at times these effects are considered desirable (e.g., to aid in sleep and dry nasal secretions), the SGAs (e.g., loratadine, fexofenadine, cetirizine, desloratadine, and levocetirizine)[28] are preferable in most instances.[1,2,3,37]

Antihistamines block the effects of histamine by one of two mechanisms: (i) as an H_1-receptor antagonist and (ii) as an inverse agonist of the H_1-receptor.[4] FGAs cross the blood–brain barrier (BBB) leading to unwanted adverse effects. The non-sedating antihistamines (second- and third-generation agents) do not cross the BBB[4] and therefore are less sedating and preferred for small children and the elderly. L.B. has experienced a good response to an FGA without complaints of excessive drowsiness. However, sedation includes both drowsiness (i.e., the subjective state of sleepiness or lethargy) and impairment (i.e., an objective decrease in specific physical or mental abilities),[4] and cognitive impairment can occur[4] even in the absence of overt drowsiness. Although patients can exhibit tolerance to sedative properties of FGAs, they may not perceive the performance impairment that is still present. This has led to a consensus opinion among experts that SGAs are preferred to FGAs when treating allergic rhinitis.[1,3,5,37]

Essentially, all the antihistamines listed in Table 20-2 are equally effective.[2] Therefore, the choice of agent is based on duration of action, side-effect profile (especially drowsiness and anticholinergic effects), risk of drug interactions, and cost.[1] Some patients claim that a kind of "tolerance" to the therapeutic effects occurs with antihistamines, in that with consistent use over time they perceive less symptomatic relief. Although no pharmacologic explanation exists to support these observations, patients may experience benefit from switching therapies if this perception presents.[1]

The major advantages of SGAs are their selectivity to the H_1-receptor and their reduced central nervous system sedative effects.[6,28] Desloratadine, fexofenadine, loratadine, and levocetirizine—at recommended doses—are reported to have no sedating effects.[6] Loratadine and desloratadine can cause sedation at higher than recommended doses.[6] Cetirizine[6] and levocetirizine[1] have more sedation potential than the other second- or third-generation agents.[6] Another advantage of SGAs is that most products can be dosed once daily[6] to improve patient adherence to therapy. Specific antihistamines are compared in Table 20-2. Maximum benefit is seen with continued use of oral antihistamines, but intermittent use may provide relief for many individuals.[1] In the case of L.B., it would be reasonable to begin therapy with loratadine 10 mg daily, because as an SGA it has demonstrated efficacy with minimal side effects and is also available without a prescription (as he requested) and as a generic formulation, which will further control costs.

INTRANASAL ANTIHISTAMINES

CASE 20-1, QUESTION 5: L.B. reports that a friend with similar symptoms had experienced relief from an antihistamine nasal spray. Is it possible to give antihistamines by this route, or is L.B. confusing this with other topical therapies, such as decongestants or corticosteroids? Are intranasal antihistamines appropriate for L.B.?

Topical formulations are available for intranasal use. These are considered to be equal in efficacy to oral SGAs[1,14] with a quicker onset of action.[37] Also, they may improve congestion.[1,6] The intranasal antihistamines (azelastine and olopatadine) have a faster onset of action than oral agents,[1] but unfortunately require twice daily dosing.[6] Early studies showed the side effects of intranasal antihistamines to be comparable to the FGAs in terms of somnolence; however, more recent data show much lower rates (0.4%–3%) similar to those of placebo and intranasal steroid groups.[1] Intranasal azelastine can also cause local side effects, including nasal irritation, dry mouth, sore throat, and mild epistaxis.[29] An objectionable bitter aftertaste is a significant problem, occurring in up to 20% of patients.[29] The original intranasal product (Astelin) was saline-based (and has since been removed from the market); but a newer formulation (Astepro) includes sorbitol and sucralose to mask this bitter taste.[38] Azelastine is also available generically. Patient complaints are fewer with the newer product, but still present.

A potential role for intranasal antihistamines is for patients who do not respond adequately to oral antihistamines.[1] In addition, some patients may prefer the intranasal route of administration or benefit from concomitant therapy with intranasal antihistamines and intranasal corticosteroids. As a prescription-only product, an intranasal antihistamine (even if available generically) would be more expensive than many oral alternatives. Because of the expense associated with prescription-only status, increased risk of side effects, and possibly objectionable taste, topical azelastine is not an optimal therapeutic option for L.B.

Decongestant Therapy

CASE 20-1, QUESTION 6: What role do decongestants have in L.B.'s treatment?

Nasal congestion is often much less severe in patients who experience only intermittent symptoms, but as L.B.'s symptoms have become persistent since his move, the exact frequency and severity of his nasal congestion should be assessed before recommending drug therapy. In patients with only mild, intermittent symptoms, saline irrigation (administered as frequently as needed) is helpful in soothing and moisturizing irritated nasal mucosa but may be impractical. Antihistamines do little to relieve nasal congestion; therefore, patients with moderate to severe congestion may require a combination of an antihistamine with a decongestant. The combination of an antihistamine and an oral decongestant is more effective than either component alone in the treatment of allergic rhinitis.[1]

Both the topical (intranasal) and the oral decongestants are sympathomimetics that directly stimulate α_1-adrenergic receptors, resulting in vasoconstriction.[28] Local effects on the nasal mucosa include reduced turbinate swelling and congestion,[4] and improved nasal airway patency.[1] Oral decongestants include phenylephrine and pseudoephedrine. Until 2005, pseudoephedrine was the more popular agent; however, because of the potential to use it in the manufacturer of illicit substances (e.g., methamphetamine), restrictions on the allowable quantity and methods for purchasing pseudoephedrine-containing products have been implemented at both the state and federal levels. These restrictions have resulted in the reformulation of many oral decongestant products to include phenylephrine as an alternative decongestant. These agents have no effect on sneezing, pruritis, or ocular symptoms.[4] A meta-analysis of phenylephrine used as a decongestant in doses approved for nonprescription use has raised concerns about its efficacy as an oral agent;[39] however, the FDA has determined that there are adequate data to support its continued use. The available oral and topical decongestants, some of which are available without prescription, are compared in Table 20-3.

Oral decongestants can cause systemic side effects, particularly those associated with central nervous system stimulation (e.g., nervousness, insomnia, tremor, anxiety, and panic attacks).[28] Cardiovascular stimulation (e.g., tachycardia, palpitations, increased blood pressure) can also occur, so patients with hypertension should be monitored carefully while taking oral decongestants.[28] Because oral decongestants are not associated with the development of rebound congestion, in most patients they are appropriate for intermittent short-term use; but not chronic use.[24] Topical administration of decongestants generally does not lead to systemic side effects; however, these agents are not appropriate for chronic use in rhinitis because of their potential for causing rebound congestion (see Case 20-7).

Because L.B. is complaining of nasal congestion, he will require a decongestant in addition to the loratadine. He may choose to use a once-daily fixed-dose combination product (e.g., loratadine 10 mg + pseudoephedrine extended-release 240 mg) or to supplement the daily loratadine with pseudoephedrine as needed. Although L.B. has used pseudoephedrine in the past without a problem, he may require education regarding the new procedures for purchasing this product, while assuring him that the new restrictions are not related to the drug's safety as a decongestant. In addition, although his hypertension is controlled, his blood pressure should be monitored regularly to detect any effect. If L.B. is ready to consider a prescription product, an intranasal steroid (discussed subsequently) would also be a reasonable option for him.

Ocular Therapies

RELATIONSHIP BETWEEN OCULAR AND NASAL SYMPTOMS

CASE 20-1, QUESTION 7: L.B.'s new therapies are effective for his persistent nasal symptoms; however, in the spring he complains that his eyes are itchy and watery and that the loratadine and pseudoephedrine do not seem to be helping. How are L.B.'s ocular symptoms related to his allergic rhinitis?

The most common forms of allergic ocular disorders are seasonal (intermittent) allergic conjunctivitis (SAC) and perennial allergic conjunctivitis (PAC).[40] The symptoms of both SAC and PAC are identical in that they are caused by allergic response in the conjunctiva to airborne allergens. SAC symptoms commonly occur in response to airborne pollens, whereas PAC is because of perennial allergens such as house dust mites.[40] The symptoms of allergic conjunctivitis are itchy eyes, redness, and swelling of the conjunctiva.[40]

Because of the potential for long-term damage to vision,[40] persistent ocular conditions should always be assessed by an eye care professional. Other ocular problems that can be confused with allergic conjunctivitis include atopic keratoconjunctivitis and vernal keratoconjunctivitis, and giant papillary conjunctivitis[40] (see Chapter 54, Eye Disorders).

CHOICE OF THERAPEUTIC AGENT

CASE 20-1, QUESTION 8: What are the treatment options for L.B.'s allergic conjunctivitis, and how does the clinician choose between the available options?

Seasonal and perennial allergic conjunctivitis are treated similarly with only the duration of the treatment course differing (i.e., episodic vs. chronic treatment). Nonpharmacologic treatment includes avoidance of aeroallergens to the extent possible, cold compresses,[41] and lubrication with frequent application of artificial tear substitutes to provide a barrier to and dilute various allergens and inflammatory mediators on the ocular surface.[40] The available therapeutic options for management of allergic conjunctivitis include topical ocular administration of antihistamines, decongestants (vasoconstrictors), mast-cell stabilizers, and nonsteroidal anti-inflammatory drugs (Table 20-5).[41] These ocular medications act by the same mechanisms as their nasal counterparts. In addition, topical ophthalmic corticosteroids have a limited role in the acute management of allergic conjunctivitis; however, they are not indicated for prolonged use because of the risk of serious infectious complications in the eye.[40]

In the case of L.B., a trial of antihistamine + vasoconstrictor combination eye drops (e.g., pheniramine maleate 0.3% + naphazoline hydrochloride 0.025%) one to two drops in the affected eye(s) up to 4 times a day for management of acute symptoms is an appropriate recommendation for short-term use. Note that the overuse of ocular vasoconstrictors can lead to rebound conjunctivitis, similar to that occurring with nasal decongestants (see Drug-Induced Nasal Congestion: Rhinitis Medicamentosa section). As a result, the use of a topical ophthalmic decongestant should be limited to 3 to 5 days. If the patient exhibits chronic symptoms, consider a switch to an intranasal corticosteroid (which may have better efficacy for combination symptoms)[1] or refer to specialist care.

Cromolyn Therapy

CASE 20-2

QUESTION 1: J.C. is a 10-year-old girl who has been experiencing rhinorrhea and sneezing during visits to her father's home in another state a couple of times each year. On questioning, J.C.'s mother reveals that although J.C. has not complained of symptoms previously, her father adopted a puppy from the local animal shelter about a year ago and the symptoms correspond to the times that the child spends with the dog. J.C. will be visiting her father again next month, and she is hoping to purchase something without a prescription to prevent her from "getting sick and missing out on her summer vacation." What options are available to treat J.C.'s intermittent symptoms of allergic rhinitis?

These symptoms may reflect mild allergic rhinitis triggered by exposure to animal dander. When it is possible to anticipate symptoms, as in J.C.'s case, initiating prophylactic therapy can help lessen the impact of allergen exposure.[36] Although intermittent use of antihistamines or intranasal corticosteroids are commonly selected options, intranasal cromolyn sodium, administered regularly beginning several weeks before each trip may also offer benefit in this situation. Because the mother indicates that she wants to select an OTC product, allergen avoidance strategies plus cromolyn nasal spray would be a reasonable choice for initial therapy. The drawbacks to this are its out-of-pocket cost, its technique-dependent administration, its multiple daily dosing requirements (up to 6 times daily),[24] and its reduced effectiveness compared with other treatments.[3]

CASE 20-2, QUESTION 2: What strategies should J.C.'s father use to minimize exposure to the allergic triggers?

To minimize J.C.'s exposure to allergens, the dog should be kept out of the child's bedroom at all times and, when possible, kept outside or confined to an uncarpeted area of the home. J.C.'s father should use a high-quality air purifier[42] and should vacuum the home with a double-filter system while J.C. is out of the house. Although evidence of benefit is unclear, it may be helpful to wash the dog at least twice a week while the child visits.[1] Similarly, after touching or playing with the dog, J.C. should wash her hands especially before touching her face.[42] The additional expense of regular, commercial cleaning of air ducts is not cost justified.

INSTRUCTIONS FOR USE

CASE 20-2, QUESTION 3: How should J.C. be advised to use cromolyn nasal spray to prevent her symptoms?

To be effective, cromolyn nasal spray must be dosed several times each day, which can hinder adherence.[37] The initial dose for the cromolyn sodium nasal spray (5.2 mg/actuation) is one spray in each nostril 3 to 4 times a day up to 6 times daily.[29] In some patients, symptom control can be maintained with dosing 2 to 3 times per day. J.C. should be instructed to begin therapy at least 2 weeks before her planned visit because of the delay in the onset of action for this agent.

Table 20-5
Topical Ophthalmic Medications Commonly Used for Allergic Conjunctivitis

Generic Name (Example Brand Product)	Available Dosage Forms/Strength	Dose
Antihistamines		
Azelastine (Optivar)	Ophthalmic solution: 0.05%	Adults and children ≥3 years: 1 drop in the affected eye(s) every 12 hours
Emedastine (Emadine)	Ophthalmic solution: 0.05%	Adults and children ≥3 years: 1 drop in the affected eye(s) up to 4 times daily
Epinastine (Elestat)	Ophthalmic solution: 0.05%	Adults and children ≥3 years: 1 drop in the affected eye(s) twice daily
Antihistamine/Decongestant Combinations		
Pheniramine + Naphazoline (Naphcon-A, Opcon-A, Visine-A)[a]	Ophthalmic solution: naphazoline HCl 0.025% + pheniramine maleate 0.3%	Adults and children ≥6 years: 1–2 drops in the affected eye(s) every 6 hours for up to 3 days
Antihistamine/Mast-Cell Stabilizers		
Ketotifen (various brand names)[a]	Ophthalmic solution: 0.025%	Adults and children ≥3 years: 1 drop in the affected eye(s) every 8–12 hours
Olopatadine (Pataday, Patanol, Pazeo)	Ophthalmic solution: 0.1%, 0.2%, 0.7%	0.1%: Adults and children ≥3 years 1 drop in affected eye(s) twice daily at an interval of 6–8 hours. 0.2% and 0.7%: Adults and children ≥2 years: 1 drop in the affected eye(s) once daily
Alcaftadine (Lastacaft)	Ophthalmic solution: 0.25%	Adults and children ≥2 years: 1 drop in the affected eyes(s) twice daily
Bepotastine (Bepreve)	Ophthalmic solution: 1.5%	Adults and children ≥2 years: 1 drop in the affected eyes(s) twice daily
Mast-Cell Stabilizers		
Cromolyn Sodium (Crolom)	Ophthalmic solution: 4%	Adults and children ≥4 years: 1–2 drops in the affected eye(s) 4–6 times daily
Lodoxamide (Alomide)	Ophthalmic solution: 0.1%	Adults and children ≥2 years: 1–2 drops in affected eye(s) 4 times daily for up to 3 months
Nedocromil (Alocril)	Ophthalmic solution: 2%	Adults and children ≥3 years: 1–2 drops in the affected eye(s) every 12 hours
Nonsteroidal Anti-Inflammatory Drugs[b]		
Ketorolac (Acular)	Ophthalmic solution: 0.5%	Adults and children ≥3 years: 1 drop in the affected eye(s) 4 times daily
Corticosteroids[c]		
Loteprednol (Alrex)	Ophthalmic suspension: 0.2%	Adults: 1 drop in the affected eye(s) 4 times daily

[a]Available without a prescription.
[b]Other ophthalmic nonsteroidal anti-inflammatory drugs (diclofenac, flurbiprofen, suprofen) indicated for intraoperative miosis and for postcataract surgery, but not approved for allergic conjunctivitis.
[c]Other ophthalmic corticosteroids (dexamethasone, difluprednate, triamcinolone, fluorometholone) indicated for ocular inflammation, but not approved for allergic conjunctivitis.
Source: Facts & Comparisons eAnswers. http://online.factsandcomparisons.com/index.aspx? Accessed May 8, 2015.

The clinician should ensure that both parent and child can demonstrate appropriate administration technique before therapy is initiated. On first use, the device should be primed until a consistent fine mist spray is achieved. J.C. should be instructed to gently blow her nose and then spray the cromolyn sodium solution into each nostril in a slightly upward direction, parallel to the nasal septum.

Topical nasal cromolyn has an excellent safety profile, including minimal incidence of adverse effects. Local irritation with burning, stinging, and sneezing being the most common manifestations. The safety of cromolyn[6,24] has made it widely used as initial therapy for children with allergic rhinitis and for treating rhinitis during pregnancy. Table 20-6 includes information about intranasal cromolyn dosing and availability.

Intranasal Corticosteroid Therapy

CASE 20-3

Question 1: A.R. is an 8-year-old girl with allergic rhinitis and asthma. She has been treated with orally inhaled budesonide for asthma and oral loratadine for rhinitis. Her mother reports that she frequently sneezes, complains of an itchy nose and eyes, and does not sleep well at night because of nasal congestion. She also reports that she cannot give her cetirizine on a daily basis because it "makes her drowsy at school." Her asthma has been well controlled in the past; however, she is concerned that she

Table 20-6
Additional Oral and Intranasal Agents for Rhinitis

Generic (Brand Product)	Available Dosage Forms/ Strength	Adult Dose	Pediatric Dose
Oral			
Leukotriene modifiers Montelukast (Singulair)	Tablets: 10 mg Tablets, chewable: 4 mg, 5 mg Oral granules: 4 mg	10 mg once daily	Children 6–14 years: 5 mg once daily Children 2–5 years: 4 mg once daily Children 6–23 months: 4 mg once daily
Intranasal			
Antihistamine Azelastine (Astepro)	Nasal spray: 0.1% 0.15%	Perennial: 0.15%: 2 sprays/nostril twice daily Seasonal: 0.1%: 1–2 sprays/nostril twice daily 0.15%: 1–2 sprays/nostril twice daily or 2 sprays/nostril once daily.	Perennial: Children 6 months–5 years (0.1%) 1 sp EN BID Children ≥2 years: 0.15%: 2 sprays/ nostril twice daily Children 6–11 years: 0.1% or 0.15%: 1 spray/nostril twice daily Seasonal: Children 6–11 years: 0.1% or 0.15%: 1 spray/nostril twice daily Children 2–5 years: 0.1%: 1 spray/ nostril twice daily
Olopatadine (Patanase)	Nasal Solution: 0.6%	Two sprays per nostril twice daily	6–11 years: 1 spray per nostril twice daily
Mast-cell stabilizer Cromolyn sodium (Nasalcrom)[a]	Nasal spray: 5.2 mg/spray	1 spray/nostril 3–4 times/ day (every 4–6 hours; max 6 times daily)	Children ≥2 years: 1 spray/nostril 3–4 times/day (every 4–6 hours; max 6 times daily)
Anticholinergic Ipratropium bromide (Atrovent)[b]	Nasal spray: 21 mcg/spray (for perennial symptoms), 42 mcg/ spray (for seasonal symptoms)	2 sprays/nostril up to 4 times daily (max = 672 mcg/day)	Children ≥6 years: 42 mcg/spray: 2 sprays/nostril 2–3 times/day Children 5–11 years: 84 mcg/spray: 2 sprays/nostril 3 times daily

[a]Available without a prescription.
[b]Optimum dosage varies with the response of the individual patient. It is always desirable to titrate an individual to the minimum effective dose to reduce the risk of side effects. In addition, the safety and efficacy of the use of ipratropium 42 mcg nasal spray beyond 3 weeks in patients with seasonal allergic rhinitis has not been established.
Source: Facts & Comparisons eAnswers. **http://online.factsandcomparisons.com/index.aspx?** Accessed May 8, 2015.

is experiencing some shortness of breath and that this might be related to her allergies. While you are talking to her, you note that A.R. breathes exclusively through her mouth, sniffs frequently, and rubs her nose. You also notice dark circles under her eyes. What signs and symptoms of allergic rhinitis is A.R. displaying?

A.R. is showing the classic signs of allergic airways disease in children. She is sniffing and snorting in response to nasal itching and discharge. The frequent upward rubbing of the nose (generally with the palm of the hand) is known as the "allergic salute"[1] and is caused by nasal itching. Long-standing symptoms can lead to facial abnormalities, including the formation of a transverse crease across the bridge of the nose.[3] Dark circles under the eyes are commonly known as "allergic shiners" and they can be further aggravated by the frequent rubbing of the eyes associated with severe ocular itching.[1,37]

CASE 20-3, QUESTION 2: Given her concomitant asthma, are there any special considerations for treating A.R.'s allergic rhinitis?

Based on the relationship between inflammation in the upper and lower airways, and the similar immunologic mechanisms involved in allergic rhinitis and asthma, it is a reasonable assumption that poor control of upper airway allergies can have a negative impact on asthma control.[24] In fact, rhinitis is a risk factor for asthma development,[37] and poorly controlled rhinitis can aggravate asthma control.[4] In a patient with asthma, like A.R., treatment of allergic rhinitis can also reduce airway hyperresponsiveness and symptoms of asthma.[1,37] Historically, the use of antihistamines (FGAs) was considered problematic for patients with asthma because of a theoretic concern about excessive drying of airway secretions caused by the anticholinergic properties of these agents. It is now clear that most patients with asthma can take any of the antihistamines without adverse pulmonary effects. Oral antihistamines (SGAs) would currently be a logical first addition to an asthma regimen because of their convenient dosing, but A.R.'s experience with these agents in the past has not been positive. For this reason, intranasal corticosteroids should be considered for A.R.

ROLE IN THERAPY

CASE 20-3, QUESTION 3: What would be the role of intranasal corticosteroids in A.R.?

Based on the frequency and severity of symptoms, and the lack of control / side effects with oral antihistamine therapy, intranasal corticosteroids are an appropriate consideration for A.R. Intranasal corticosteroids are the most effective therapy available for the treatment of allergic rhinitis. They are safe, well tolerated, and are highly effective in reducing itching, sneezing, rhinorrhea, and congestion in both adults and children.[1] In addition to improving all nasal symptoms, evidence also suggests that intranasal administration of corticosteroids effectively relieves ocular symptoms.[37]

Table 20-7
Intranasal Corticosteroids[a] Commonly Used for Rhinitis

Generic Name (Example Brand Product)	Available Dosage Forms/Strengths	Adult Dose[a]	Pediatric Dose[a]
Beclomethasone dipropionate (Beconase AQ) QNasal (HFA) QNasal (Children's)	42 mcg/spray 80 mcg/spray 40 mcg/spray	42 mcg: 1–2 sprays/nostril twice daily 80 mcg: 2 sprays/nostril once daily	Children 6–12 years: 42 mcg: 1 spray/nostril twice daily (max 2 sprays/nostril daily) Children 4–11 years: 40 mcg: 1 spray/nostril once daily (max 2 sprays/nostril daily)
Budesonide (Rhinocort Aqua) (Rhinocort Allergy) (Children's Rhinocort)	32 mcg/spray	1 spray/nostril once daily (max 4 sprays/nostril daily)	Children 6–12 years: 1 spray/nostril once daily (max 2 sprays/nostril daily)
Ciclesonide (Omnaris) Zetonna (HFA)	50 mcg/spray 37 mcg/spray	50 mcg: 2 sprays/nostril once daily 37 mcg: 1 spray/nostril once daily	50 mcg: Children 6–12 years: 2 sprays/nostril once daily (approved for seasonal symptoms in ages >6, and for perennial symptoms for ages >12) 37 mcg: do not use in children <12.
Fluticasone propionate (Flonase Allergy Relief) (Clarispray) (Children's Flonase) (GoodSense Nasoflow) (Ticaspray)	50 mcg/spray	2 sprays/nostril once daily or 1 spray/nostril twice daily	Children 4–11 years: 1 spray/nostril once daily (max 2 sprays/nostril daily)
Fluticasone furoate (Flonase Sensimist)	27.5 mcg/spray	2 sprays/nostril once daily	Children 2–11 years: 1 spray/nostril once daily (max 2 sprays/nostril daily)
Flunisolide (no brand product available)	0.025%	>15 years: 2 sprays/nostril 2 or 3 times daily (max 8 sprays/nostril daily)	Children 6–14 years: 1 spray/nostril 3 times daily or 2 sprays/nostril twice daily (max 4 sprays/nostril daily)
Mometasone furoate (Nasonex)	50 mcg/spray	2 sprays/nostril once daily	Children 2–11 years: 1 spray/nostril once daily
Triamcinolone acetonide (Nasacort AQ) (Nasacort Allergy)	55 mcg/spray	2 sprays/nostril once daily	Children 2–5 years: 1 spray/nostril once daily (max 1 spray/nostril daily) Children 6–11 years: 1–2 sprays/nostril once daily (max 2 sprays/nostril daily)
Azelastine HCl/fluticasone propionate (Dymista)	137/50 mcg/spray	1 spray/nostril twice daily	Children ≥6 years: 1 spray/nostril twice daily

[a]It is always desirable to titrate an individual patient to the minimum effective steroid dose to reduce the risk of side effects. When the maximum benefit has been achieved and symptoms have been controlled, reducing the steroid dose might be effective in maintaining control of rhinitis symptoms.
Source: Facts & Comparisons eAnswers. **http://online.factsandcomparisons.com/index.aspx?** Accessed May 11, 2015.

These agents also have demonstrated efficacy for nonallergic rhinitis,[6] rhinitis medicamentosa,[43] and nasal polyps.[44] The currently available intranasal corticosteroids are listed in Table 20-7.

Intranasal corticosteroids are the most effective agents available over other therapeutic options. They are frequently rated as more effective than antihistamines,[1] although the benefit from therapy requires correct use of the administration device.[3] Intranasal corticosteroids improve congestion, sneezing, rhinorrhea, and itching[36] with no difference in efficacy amongst the available options.[1]

MECHANISM OF ACTION

CASE 20-3, QUESTION 4: How do intranasal corticosteroids work to reduce the symptoms of allergic rhinitis?

Corticosteroids interact with a specific steroid receptor in the cytoplasm of a cell, and the steroid receptor complex then moves into the cell nucleus where it influences protein synthesis and inhibits the breakdown of phospholipids to arachidonic acid[45]; this, in turn, inhibits the formation of prostaglandins and leukotrienes. Topical corticosteroids reduce the number of eosinophils, basophils, and mast cells in the nasal mucosa and epithelium; directly inhibit the release of mediators from mast cells and basophils; reduce mucosal edema and vasodilation; and stabilize the endothelium and epithelium, resulting in decreased exudation.[1] Topical corticosteroids inhibit both the early-phase and late-phase reactions to antigen challenge,[28] and therefore pretreatment and continued use are recommended.[1]

CHOICE OF THERAPEUTIC AGENT

CASE 20-3, QUESTION 5: What intranasal corticosteroid products are appropriate to manage A.R.'s allergic rhinitis?

Currently marketed intranasal corticosteroid products vary in the pharmacologic characteristics that can influence patient acceptance and adherence; however, there do not appear to be significant advantages with regard to efficacy among them.[1] Primary differences among products include potency, dosing regimens, delivery systems, spray volume,[29] and patient preference. For sensitive patients, there may be some theoretical advantage to products that are preservative or alcohol-free.

The ideal intranasal corticosteroid agent should exhibit high topical potency and low systemic activity. After topical administration, the corticosteroid may reach the systemic circulation by absorption across the nasal mucosa or through gastrointestinal absorption of the swallowed portion of the dose.[44] Studies have shown that varying sensory attributes (e.g., aftertaste, nose runout, and smell) affect acceptability of, and preference for, particular nasal corticosteroid products.[1] Some degree of experimentation may be required to find the optimal product for A.R.

SAFETY

CASE 20-3, QUESTION 6: How safe are intranasal corticosteroids in this situation?

The corticosteroids currently available for intranasal administration are listed in Table 20-7. Among available products, intranasal corticosteroids have similar efficacy in clinical trials.[1] Budesonide, beclomethasone, ciclesonide, and flunisolide are indicated for ages 6 years or older. Beclomethasone HFA and fluticasone propionate are labeled for ages 4 and up, and mometasone and fluticasone furoate are indicated in children 2 years and older.[29] Triamcinolone (Nasacort Allergy 24 hour) and Fluticasone (Flonase Allergy Relief) are available OTC and approved in patients 2 and 4 years and older respectively. Because A.R. is 8 years old, theoretically she is a candidate for an OTC intranasal steroid; however, given her concomitant asthma, a prescription agent may be a better choice. Because poor control of upper airway allergies can have a negative impact on asthma control,[24] proper monitoring by her provider is important.

A common concern regarding the use of corticosteroids in children is the risk of growth suppression. Current US FDA labeling for inhaled and intranasal corticosteroid preparations include wording that use of these products in children may reduce their rate of growth. Although beclomethasone may be associated with reduced growth velocity,[44] numerous studies have shown no growth delay in children treated long term with newer intranasal steroids.[1] Specifically, studies with mometasone, fluticasone, budesonide, ciclesonide, and triamcinolone have shown no effect on growth at recommended doses for up to 1 year.[44] It is always judicious to recommended and utilize the lowest effective dose of intranasal corticosteroids especially in a pediatric population also on a concomitant inhaled corticosteroid agent. Because A.R. has concomitant asthma, this may be the case in this patient.

Other potential adverse effects of chronic intranasal corticosteroids have been investigated. Severe local effects such as nasal mucosal atrophy or septal ulceration are rarely seen and can be prevented with appropriate technique.[44] Changes in bone mineral density, intraocular pressure, or cataracts do not appear to be of a concern.[44]

INSTRUCTIONS FOR USE

CASE 20-3, QUESTION 7: A.R. is given a prescription for budesonide, two actuations in each nostril twice daily. How should she be counseled to use this drug?

Although intranasal corticosteroids have an excellent safety profile, some local adverse effects can occur. The currently available products are all aqueous solutions delivered via a manual spray pump; these are much less drying than the original propellant-based aerosol formulations of the same products. The most commonly reported side effect is epistaxis.[44] Local irritation, burning, stinging, and dryness are also possible.[1] Proper technique in using the nasal corticosteroid products can reduce the risks for these side effects.[1,6]

Patient education is important to ensure proper use of, and response to, the intranasal corticosteroids.[28] A.R. should be instructed to blow her nose gently before using the nasal spray as severe blockage of the nasal passage may prevent deposition of the drug at the intended site of action. The patient should be instructed to direct the spray away from the nasal septum.[36] This technique is facilitated by using the contralateral hand during administration to each nostril. This results in pointing the applicator nozzle straight and back to ensure application is parallel to the septum.[3]

Therapeutic benefit to intranasal steroids is generally evident in a few days,[37] although some newer agents may begin to relieve symptoms within hours because of a quick onset of effect.[1] Fluticasone has been effective when used on an as-needed basis.[1] Nonetheless, it is reasonable to advise patients that full benefit may not be realized for up to 2 to 3 weeks.[3]

Systemic Corticosteroids

CASE 20-3, QUESTION 8: What is the role of systemic corticosteroid therapy in the management of A.R.'s allergic rhinitis?

In contrast to the minimal side effects of the topical corticosteroids, systemic administration of these drugs can cause numerous, and at times serious, side effects. Systemic administration, therefore, must be reserved for only short-term, adjunctive therapy in cases of severe, debilitating rhinitis. In such cases, a short course of relatively high-dose corticosteroid, so-called burst therapy, can be administered. Prednisone 40 mg/day for adults or 1 to 2 mg/kg/day for children (or an equivalent dose of a comparable compound) every morning for up to 7 days effectively relieves acute, severe rhinitis symptoms. If A.R. were to have a particularly severe exacerbation of her allergic rhinitis such that it interfered with sleep or ability to attend school, an oral corticosteroid burst would be indicated. More likely, A.R. would require a short course of systemic corticosteroids for an acute asthma exacerbation, which should also result in improved nasal symptoms.

Combination Therapy

CASE 20-3, QUESTION 9: Would there be an advantage in combining various therapies for allergic rhinitis in A.R.?

The rationale for combining agents to treat allergic rhinitis is based on the theoretic benefit of additive or synergistic reactions. Various combinations have been studied. Concomitant use of antihistamines and decongestants has been shown to relieve individual nasal symptoms compared with either agent alone. Combining intranasal antihistamines and corticosteroids also is beneficial.[1] However, the combination of intranasal corticosteroids with oral antihistamines has not been shown to offer clinical benefit over use of intranasal steroids alone.[1] Similarly, the combination of oral antihistamines and leukotriene modifier therapy is generally not recommended.[1] When combination therapy of any kind is used, once symptoms are controlled, one agent should undergo a trial for discontinuation.

Leukotriene-Modifying Agent Therapy

CASE 20-4

QUESTION 1: K.H. is a 58-year-old man with allergic rhinitis. He has experienced symptoms during ragweed pollen season for several years. He has used various antihistamines for his symptoms during this time with moderate success. At times, K.H. has self-medicated with nonprescription medications, including clemastine and diphenhydramine. This year, he initiated therapy with diphenhydramine 1 week before the pollen season, but began experiencing symptoms of urinary retention after 10 days. His physician advised him that this might be related to the antihistamine aggravating his enlarged prostate and he was advised to use fexofenadine 60 mg twice daily.

After 1 week, K.H. complains that the medication is not working. After seeing an advertisement on television, he inquires about the use of a leukotriene modifier for his allergic rhinitis. What is the mechanism for the K.H.'s urinary discomfort attributed to the diphenhydramine?

K.H. is exhibiting symptoms of urinary outflow obstruction or prostatism. Common features of this are frequency, hesitancy, slow urine stream, dribbling, and bladder fullness after voiding. The most common cause of obstruction is benign prostatic hyperplasia (BPH). Because the prostate is located anatomically around the urethra, enlargement of the gland can obstruct urine flow.[46]

The bladder and urethra are made up of smooth muscle tissue that is innervated by the sympathetic and parasympathetic divisions of the autonomic nervous system. The detrusor musculature is predominantly innervated by β-adrenergic and cholinergic receptors, whereas the bladder neck (or outlet) is innervated predominately by α-adrenergic receptors.[47] Sympathetic stimulation causes relaxation of the detrusor muscle to allow bladder filling, closure of the urethra, and decreased bladder emptying. Cholinergic stimulation of the detrusor causes contraction of the detrusor to cause bladder emptying. Initially, the detrusor musculature can compensate for the urethral obstruction in BPH. Eventually, however, the detrusor muscle fibers hypertrophy and decompensate, resulting in urinary retention and detrusor hyperreflexia manifesting as urinary frequency, urgency, urge incontinence, and nocturia.[48]

When K.H. took diphenhydramine, the anticholinergic properties of the drug blocked detrusor contraction and precipitated acute urinary retention.[47] In this case, therapy with a SGA (i.e., fexofenadine) is more appropriate because these agents have little to no anticholinergic side effects.

EFFICACY

CASE 20-4, QUESTION 2: What is the rationale and evidence that a leukotriene modifier might be beneficial in the management of K.H.'s allergic rhinitis?

Leukotrienes are important inflammatory mediators in the upper and lower airways and are present in nasal secretions of patients with allergic rhinitis. They serve as inflammatory mediators that attract eosinophils, increase microvascular leakage, edema, and mucus gland secretion.[4] These actions lead to the symptoms of allergic rhinitis, as well as those of asthma.[24] In clinical trials, leukotriene modifiers relieve nasal symptoms in patients with allergic rhinitis however not as well as nasal corticosteroids.[1]

In actual use, the benefit of leukotriene modifiers has been modest; therefore, their role is typically adjunctive to the use of first-line agents for allergic rhinitis.[1] Clinical decisions about the value of combining treatments should be based on the specific clinical situation. Because K.H. has experienced intolerance to FGAs and a lack of efficacy with SGAs, a trial with an intranasal corticosteroid or a leukotriene-modifying agent is appropriate. Specifically, a patient with mild asthma and allergic rhinitis may benefit from therapy with a leukotriene modifier with or without an antihistamine.[28] If used, however, a risk exists of a rare complication known as Churg–Strauss syndrome, which is characterized by eosinophilia, vasculitic rash, worsening pulmonary symptoms, cardiac complications, and neuropathy.[49] Table 20-6 includes information about the use and availability of montelukast, which is currently the only leukotriene modifier approved for allergic rhinitis.

Complementary and Alternative Therapies

CASE 20-5

QUESTION 1: C.L., a 25-year-old woman, presents in mid-August complaining that her allergies are worsening daily. Symptoms are nasal discharge and obstruction, repetitive sneezing, and itching of the nose, eyes, and throat. She is fatigued and has difficulty concentrating. Her symptoms have been occurring in late spring and summer since high school, and she has used a variety of medications intermittently (clemastine, fexofenadine, beclomethasone nasal, ketotifen ophthalmic) over the years. C.L. is a competitive runner but has been unable to run as far or as often as usual because of bothersome symptoms. She is also reluctant to use medications as they may be prohibited by her race sponsors. A running partner mentioned that she could control her allergy symptoms with diet, exercise, and herbal remedies purchased at a local nutritional supplement shop. What, if any, alternative treatments have been shown to be efficacious in allergic rhinitis?

Alternative treatments such as yoga, massage, acupuncture, homeopathy, and herbal therapy are common among adults with rhinitis and should be taken into account by health care providers. Literature indicates that 25% to 50% of the general population and up to 70% of children have used an alternative method at least once.[50] A study in Americans showed that 29% had tried alternative treatments for rhinosinusitis.[50] Still, because allergic rhinitis is largely a self-managed disease, it is likely that reported use of these agents is underestimated. A survey found that only 43% of subject who had used alternative methods had informed their provider about it.[50] For these reasons, patients should always be questioned specifically about the use of alternative therapies during the patient interview. Although some alternative approaches such as acupuncture have been deemed to be safe,[1,51] the safety and efficacy of herbal remedies has not been clearly established and cannot be recommended at this time.[1] In addition, some complementary therapies have been associated with side effects and potential drug interactions.[50] Because of C.L.'s reluctance to use medications, other strategies are appropriate to consider to help manage her rhinitis symptoms.

PHYSICAL TECHNIQUES

Camphor and menthol-delivered rubs (Vicks VapoRub, Breathe Right Colds Nasal Strips) have been shown to have an ameliorating effect on nasal congestion;[52] however, the effects are short-lived.[29] Other forms of aromatherapy suggested to relieve nasal congestion are lacking data related to efficacy.[52] Saline nasal irrigation (e.g., neti pot) is simple, inexpensive, and has been shown to have some efficacy.[53]

HERBAL MEDICINES

It has been suggested that some herbs have antiallergy, anti-inflammatory, and improved immune system effects that may be helpful to ease symptoms of allergy.[51,54] With this in mind, echinacea has become one of the top-selling herbal products in the United States. Echinacea, also known as the purple cornflower, however, is a member of the daisy Compositae (Asteraceae) family.[55] Although Echinacea is often used for immune-related disorders, patients with known allergy to these plants should be cautioned regarding the use of Echinacea products.

A few herbal therapies, including butterbur, biminne, Chinese herbal mixture,[1] and spirulina[50] potentially hold some promise because of positive results in trials on clinical symptoms and quality of life in patients with AR, but more investigation is needed before they can be included in recommended treatment algorithms.[1] No good clinical data are available on the efficacy of supplements containing grapeseed extract, honey, lemon peel, stinging nettle, or red onions.[50]

OTHER

Reports regarding the use of intranasal zinc for upper respiratory symptoms, particularly those associated with the common cold, and congestion associated with allergies have been conflicting. Although zinc gels and sprays are popular OTC products, studies show inconsistent results[56] and may be associated in zinc-induced anosmia syndrome.[56] Some products have been removed from the market because of this problem. By giving patients minuscule amounts of allergen, homeopathic medicines are designed to mimic and augment a patient's own immune responses and natural defenses.[57] Some studies have shown that patients with allergic rhinitis who received homeopathic dilutions of allergens had significantly better nose running scores than those in the placebo group.[57] Further investigation is needed before homeopathy can be recommended for allergic rhinitis.

Although a variety of alternative remedies are widely available and used frequently in self-treatment, based on evaluation of these data, there is no firm recommendation for C.L. regarding the use of alternative therapies in allergic rhinitis.[1] C.L. should be advised to consult with the specific regulating agency that governs her sporting activities (e.g., the World Anti-Doping Agency for Olympic events) to gain a clear understanding of medicines that are banned in all cases as compared to those that may be used with medical exemptions or used outside of the competitive window. This may allow her to use many conventional treatments (e.g., intransal steroids) with confidence. Saline irrigation would also be a safe, noncontroversial option that may offer some efficacy.

Immunotherapy

EFFICACY

CASE 20-6

QUESTION 1: R.C. is a 25-year-old schoolteacher who has experienced allergic symptoms since childhood, but noticed a worsening after she graduated from college and moved to a new area of the country. Although she has mild symptoms year-round, she has severe exacerbations during April through June and August through October each year. During these periods, she feels that exposure to cut grass and weeds provoke profound nasal symptoms. She also notes that when she spends more time outdoors in spring and early fall, her regular therapy that she buys OTC, fluticasone (Flonase) nasal spray (two sprays per nostril once daily), is less effective. She has added loratadine (10 mg daily) during this time, but is frustrated by having to take so many medications while continuing to experience symptoms. R.C. asks your opinion about allergy shots, remarking that she started them as a child with some relief, but moved after a year and never resumed treatment. Is allergen immunotherapy effective for reducing symptoms of allergic rhinitis?

Allergen-specific immunotherapy has long-term efficacy, induces clinical and immunologic tolerance, and may prevent progression of allergic disease.[58,59] Immunotherapy is available via SCIT (sometimes called "allergy shots"),[58] sublingual aqueous drops[58] not FDA approved in the United States),[1] or sublingual tablets (SLIT).[60] Immunotherapy is unique and capable of changing the course of the disease.[1] By giving dilute solutions of allergen-containing extracts in repeated and increasing doses, immunologic tolerance is provided.[59] Therefore, subsequent exposure to those allergens elicits no or mild symptoms.

Immunotherapy administered via SCIT has been used empirically since the early 1900s, and its efficacy has been documented in many controlled trials.[61] SIT is effective in the treatment of allergic rhinitis and may even prevent the onset of asthma.[1] In addition, the benefit of immunotherapy is long-lived. Even after discontinuation, studies show continued beneficial effects up to 10 years later.[1] SCIT and SLIT should be considered a supplement to drug therapy in specific patients and possibly be used earlier in the course of allergic disease to achieve maximal benefit.[1,60]

ALLERGEN TESTING

CASE 20-6, QUESTION 2: How can the clinician determine R.C.'s specific sensitivities?

Skin testing using the modified prick test method or a prick-puncture method is used to confirm the diagnosis of allergic rhinitis and to determine specific allergen sensitivities. Skin testing is a highly sensitive and a relatively inexpensive objective measurement of allergen sensitivity. Small quantities of allergen are introduced into the skin by pricking or puncturing the skin in the immediate presence of the diluted allergen extract. Fifteen to 35 tests are placed on the upper portion of the back or the palmar surface of the forearms. A positive skin test produces a wheal-and-flare reaction at the site within 10 to 20 minutes of application and should be read after 15 minutes.[62] An experienced clinician, usually an allergist, should conduct skin testing using high-quality allergen extracts and should interpret the results.[62]

The allergens tested vary with geographic location, emphasizing the most common offending plant species that generate airborne particles. Pollen, the primary particle, is produced by trees, grasses, and weeds. Each of these plant groups generally pollinate at about the same time each year: trees in the spring, grasses from early to midsummer, and weeds from late summer into fall before the first killing frost. The onset and potency of the pollen season varies with geographic location and weather, particularly with respect to temperature and moisture. Seasonality can be misleading, however, because settled pollen particles from a previous season may be resuspended in the air following the spring snow melt or periods of heavy winds.

Mold spores are also common airborne allergens. The outdoor molds release their spores from early spring through late fall. Within this long season, spore counts increase and decrease, depending on the presence of local flora on which these molds grow (e.g., grain and other crops, forests, and orchards). Some perennial allergens (e.g., house dust mites, insect and animal dander, and some indoor molds) occur consistently across all geographic distributions.

In addition to skin-prick testing, clinicians can detect allergen-specific IgE antibodies in the blood.[63] Results are reported quantitatively and total serum IgE can be useful in determining if atopy is present.[63] In each case, skin test results[62] or IgE serum levels[63] must be correlated with the patient's clinical history. R.C.'s perennial symptoms with seasonal exacerbations indicate sensitivity to the common perennial allergens with a particular sensitivity to seasonal allergens such as tree, grass, and weed pollen, but these subjective relationships should be confirmed with skin testing.

CASE 20-6, QUESTION 3: R.C. is currently using medications (fluticasone nasal spray and loratadine) for her symptoms. Should these be discontinued before skin testing?

Antihistamines blunt the wheal-and-flare reaction by blocking the effects of histamine on capillaries. Different antihistamines vary in the extent to which they can inhibit wheal formation and in the duration of the inhibitory effect with older first-generation

Table 20-8

General Recommendations for Discontinuation of Antihistamines Before Allergen Skin Testing

1. Remind patient that allergic symptoms may return during the antihistamine-free period, but that reliable skin tests cannot be performed in a patient taking antihistamines.
2. Discontinue any short-acting antihistamine (i.e., those in Table 20-2 with a duration of suppression ≤4 days) 4 days before skin testing.
3. Discontinue longer-acting antihistamines (i.e., those in Table 20-2 with a duration of suppression >4 days) at an interval appropriate to their duration of effect (e.g., hydroxyzine should be discontinued 10 days before skin testing).
4. Before applying the full battery of skin tests, apply histamine (positive) control and glycerinated diluent (negative) control tests. Application of a 1 mg/mL histamine base equivalent should yield wheal-and-flare diameters of 2–7 mm and 4.5–32.5 mm, respectively, to be considered a normal histamine reaction. A normal cutaneous reaction to histamine control suggests that accurate skin testing can be performed.

From Bousquet J et al. Allergic rhinitis and its impact on asthma (ARIA) 2008 update (in collaboration with the World Health Organization, GA[2]LEN and AllerGen). *Allergy*. 2008;63(Suppl 86):8.

agents being the worst offenders.[62] Other agents that may interfere with skin-prick testing include long-term systemic corticosteroids, topical corticosteroids, tricyclic antidepressants, phenothiazine-type antipsychotics, and antiemetics.[62] Depending on the agent selected, antihistamines must be discontinued from 24 hours to 10 days before skin testing,[62] and even then considerable interpatient variability exists in blocking effects. For best results, R.C.'s loratadine should be discontinued 10 days before her skin testing. Recommendations for discontinuing antihistamines before allergen skin testing are listed in Table 20-8.

Other allergy medications, including cromolyn and nasal corticosteroids, have no effect on skin tests. Likewise, most asthma medications, including leukotriene modifiers, inhaled β_2-agonists, cromolyn, theophylline, and inhaled and short-course systemic (burst) corticosteroids have no effect on skin tests.[62] R.C. can continue the use of fluticasone nasal spray, although she waits to be skin tested.

CASE 20-6, QUESTION 4: Is R.C. a candidate for immunotherapy injections and/or sublingual tablets?

Immunotherapy via SCIT or SLIT should be offered to patients who have an inadequate response with pharmacologic treatment for AR with or without environmental controls.[1] Further considerations are the patient's preference, adherence, response to avoidance measures, adverse drug effects, and coexistence of allergic asthma.[1] It has also been shown that the clinical benefits of immunotherapy are similar if not better than standard therapy with intranasal steroids, montelukast, or antihistamines.[60] In the case of R.C., she has year-round symptoms with seasonal exacerbations, she has not experienced symptom relief when using appropriate therapies, and she is motivated to try immunotherapy. In addition, a previous trial in childhood was beneficial. For these reasons, skin-prick testing and a trial of immunotherapy with specific allergens are reasonable.

LENGTH OF THERAPY

CASE 20-6, QUESTION 5: If R.C. decides to proceed with immunotherapy, how long should her therapy continue and how long will the effects last?

After identifying the offending allergens via skin testing, subcutaneous immunotherapy is generally administered in two phases. During the build-up phase, increasing doses of allergen are given once or twice a week until a predetermined target or maintenance dose is achieved. Once this maintenance dose is reached, shots are usually administered every 2 to 3 weeks for the ensuing several years of treatment. Clinical improvement with immunotherapy usually occurs in the first year. In a small percentage of patients, there is no improvement and immunotherapy is discontinued. If symptoms are reduced, however, injections are usually continued for 3 to 5 years of maintenance therapy.[64]

Although immunotherapy can lead to long-term remission of symptoms, one drawback is the lengthy treatment period. SCIT alters the natural course of disease and evidence suggests that efficacy persists long after therapy ends.[1,64]

Immunotherapy via sublingual tablet involves placing the tablet under the tongue for 1 to 2 minutes before swallowing. There is no titration schedule. See Table 20-4 for dosing information and when best to initiate therapy in relation to the allergen season. A benefit of the sublingual tablet form of immunotherapy is only the first dose needs to be administered in the providers office, compared to every dose with SCIT.[64] Patients, however, need to be adherent because these sublingual tablets require daily dosing. RC would need to discuss with her provider her desire for daily dosing or travel to the clinic for routine injections.

RISKS

CASE 20-6, QUESTION 6: RC asks about the risks associated with either the shot or the sublingual tablet.

Local adverse reactions (i.e., redness, swelling) to SCIT can be common, but the risk of severe reaction (i.e., anaphylaxis) is low.[1] Sublingual tablets are FDA approved for administration after the first dose because of the perceived safety profile. Because of the risk of anaphylaxis, patients should have access to and be taught on the proper use of epinephrine autoinjector.[1] In view of the occasional occurrence of systemic side effects, it is important that if R.C. receives injections then it may be administered by personnel who are fully trained and experienced in the early recognition and treatment of such reactions.

CASE 20-6, QUESTION 7: Should R.C. also have a prescription for an epinephrine injector for use in case of anaphylaxis? If so, how should it be used?

Yes, if RC decides to use SLIT, she will need a prescription for and education on how to administer injectable epinephrine. She should be educated to use the injection of epinephrine if signs or symptoms (such as facial itching, tongue swelling, difficulty swallowing, or shortness of breath) occur after a dose of SLIT. The Auto injector is given intramuscularly into the thigh, through clothing if necessary. RC can repeat the injection with an additional epinephrine auto-injector as necessary.[29] See Table 20-9 for available injectable epinephrine products.

Table 20-9
Available Injectable Epinephrine Products

Product name	Dosage form and strength	Adult dose	Pediatric dose
EpiPen Jr 2-Pak	Solution Auto-injector 0.15 mg/0.3 mL	N/A	Dosage based on patient body weight: 15–29 kg: 0.15 mg IM or subcutaneously; ≥30 kg: 0.3 mg IM or subcutaneously
EpiPen 2-Pak Adrenaclick Auvi-Q	Solution Auto-injector 0.3 mg/0.3 mL	0.3 mg IM or subcutaneously into the anterolateral aspect of the thigh	

Source: Facts & Comparisons eAnswers. **http://online.factsandcomparisons.com/index.aspx?** Accessed June 9, 2015

DRUG-INDUCED NASAL CONGESTION: RHINITIS MEDICAMENTOSA

CASE 20-7

Question 1: L.K. is a 27-year-old man who has suffered intermittent symptoms of allergic rhinitis for several years. He reports that his symptoms are most bothersome in the spring and associated with blooming of various grasses. During these periods, he has typically used oral chlorpheniramine (4 mg every 6 hours), which relieves his symptoms but makes him drowsy at work. This season, he reports that his symptoms have been more severe, with sneezing, runny nose, and extreme itching in his nose. He tried oral loratadine (10 mg daily) with partial relief of symptoms. He also states that nasal congestion has been more of an issue with this episode and to address this he has used xylometazoline nasal spray (0.1% solution) for the past 3 weeks. Despite increasing the use of nasal spray from two sprays per nostril twice daily to three sprays per nostril 4 times a day, he reports that the congestion is getting worse. What might be an explanation for L.K.'s increasing need for nasal decongestant?

Selected medications and some drugs of abuse can cause nasal congestion through a variety of mechanisms.[65] Table 20-10 lists agents associated with drug-induced nasal symptoms. In this case, L.K. is likely experiencing rebound nasal congestion as a result of a specific form of drug-induced rhinitis called rhinitis medicamentosa (RM).

Topical decongestants are indicated for short-term use. When used acutely, sympathomimetic (adrenergic) agents stimulate α-adrenergic receptors on blood vessels, resulting in vasoconstriction (which serves to relieve nasal congestion associated with edematous, congested blood vessels).[65] But when these agents are used chronically, this can result in overstimulation of α-adrenergic receptors leading to tachyphylaxis, and decreased production of endogenous norepinephrine through a negative feedback mechanism.[65] RM has also been associated with the presence of benzalkonium chloride as a preservative in some nasal products.[66]

When RM occurs, many patients will attempt to treat the rebound congestion by using the offending topical decongestant more frequently and/or at increased doses, creating a vicious cycle. L.K.'s description of using the xylometazoline for an extended period of time (3 weeks), more frequently (from twice daily to 4 times daily) and at high doses (from two sprays per nostril to three sprays per nostril) support the diagnosis of RM.

Case 20-7, Question 2: How should L.K.'s rhinitis medicamentosa be managed?

Table 20-10
Drugs Capable of Causing Nasal Symptoms

Local Inflammatory Mechanisms
Aspirin
Nonsteroidal anti-inflammatory drugs
Neurogenic Mechanisms
Centrally Acting Sympatholytics
Clonidine
Methyldopa
Reserpine
Peripherally Acting Sympatholytics
Prazosin
Guanethidine
Doxazosin
Phentolamine
Vasodilators
Sildenafil
Tadalafil
Vardenafil
Idiopathic Mechanisms
Antihypertensives
Amiloride
Angiotensin-converting enzyme inhibitor class
β-Blocker class
Calcium-channel blockers
Chlorothiazide
Hydralazine
Hydrochlorothiazide
Hormonal Products
Exogenous estrogens

Table 20-10
Drugs Capable of Causing Nasal Symptoms (*continued*)

Oral contraceptives
Neuropsychotherapeutic Agents
Alprazolam
Amitriptyline
Chlordiazepoxide
Chlorpromazine
Gabapentin
Risperidone
Perphenazine
Thioridazine

Source: Dykewicz MS et al. Diagnosis and management of rhinitis: complete guidelines of the Joint Task Force on Practice Parameters in Allergy, Asthma and Immunology. American Academy of Allergy, Asthma, and Immunology. *Ann Allergy Asthma Immunol*. 1998;81(5, Pt 2):478; Ramey JT et al. Rhinitis medicamentosa. *J Investig Allergol Clin Immunol*. 2006;16:148; Varghese M et al. Drug-induced rhinitis. *Clin Exper Allergy*. 2010;40:381.

Strategies for Resolution

The best strategy for managing RM is prevention, by limiting the duration of topical decongestant use to no more than 3 to 5 days.[29] When these medications must be used for longer than 5 days, the patient should be advised to take a 1- to 2-day holiday during which the topical agent is not used before resuming treatment. Patients should be counseled about this whenever topical decongestants are recommended or purchased. When preventative strategies fail, several options for treatment exist.[66]

The first step is to discontinue the offending topical decongestant. L.K. should be counseled to stop the xylometazoline. Because abrupt discontinuation may cause discomfort or worsening of congestion,[66] L.K. should be educated to not restart the topical decongestant. Intranasal corticosteroids (any available product) should be recommended to patients with RM and may need 6 weeks to reach full effect.[65,66] Because L.K. is experiencing RM plus symptoms (sneezing, runny, and itchy nose) that occur seasonally, an IN corticosteroid such as mometasone nasal spray (two sprays in each nostril daily) should be recommended. Saline nose drops or spray can be added to moisturize and alleviate any nasal irritation. In refractory cases, a short course of systemic corticosteroids may be necessary.[66] Note that if the patient has used the topical decongestant continuously for many months or even years, the nasal mucosa may have undergone irreversible changes.

IDIOPATHIC RHINITIS

Diagnosis

CASE 20-8

Question 1: M.S., a 29-year-old man, complains of profuse watery rhinorrhea that has been a chronic and progressively worsening problem for the past 5 years. He also experiences some nasal congestion with the rhinorrhea, but denies nasal itching or sneezing. Although the symptoms tend to remit and exacerbate, they do not occur in any definable seasonal pattern. His symptoms are worsened by exposure to tobacco smoke, strong fumes such as paint or ammonia, and cold air. These often are associated with headaches. M.S. has no other medical problems and no family history of allergies. He does not smoke and rarely drinks alcohol. His only medication, mometasone (50 mcg/spray, two sprays in each nostril once daily as needed), only partially relieves the symptoms. M.S. sniffs and blows his nose several times during the medical history taking. Physical examination reveals a mildly erythematous nasal mucosa and a minimally edematous inferior turbinate. Copious nasal discharge is clear and watery and air movement through the nose is relatively good. There is no sinus tenderness. The remainder of his physical examination is normal. Microscopic examination of a nasal smear demonstrates only a few neutrophils and no eosinophils. What information about M.S. supports the diagnosis of idiopathic rhinitis?

Idiopathic rhinitis is a diagnosis of exclusion encompassing those patients with nasal mucous membrane inflammation with no proved immunologic, microbiologic, pharmacologic, hormonal, or occupational cause.[6] The syndrome is sometimes called nonallergic rhinitis or "vasomotor rhinitis", but using this terminology can be confusing because the cause of the symptoms has still not been clearly identified.[6] The prevailing theories involve local atopy, dysfunction of both or either the autonomic nervous system or nociceptive nerve sensor and ion channel proteins.[7] Theoretically, this is the reason that stimuli that normally increase parasympathetic activity in the nose, such as cold air and inhaled irritants, aggravate symptoms.[7] Still, substantial debate exists over whether idiopathic rhinitis represents a localized allergic response in the absence of systemic atopic markers as well as the evidence for inflammatory pathophysiology in the disease.[6]

Case 20-8, Question 2: M.S. asks what causes idiopathic rhinitis and what can be done to alleviate his symptoms.

The symptoms of idiopathic rhinitis are variable. Most patients experience perennial nasal obstruction accompanied by profuse, watery nasal, and postnasal discharge. Many patients complain of nasal obstruction as the primary symptom, whereas for others it is rhinorrhea. Sneezing, nasal itching, and conjunctival symptoms are rare.[7] Headache may occur and usually is frontal or localized over the bridge of the nose. Symptoms may also appear or worsen in response to climatic changes such as temperature, barometric pressure, and humidity.[7] Similarly, irritant triggers such as tobacco smoke, industrial pollutants, strong odors and perfumes, newsprint, and chemical fumes may worsen or aggravate symptoms.[7]

The appearance of the nasal mucosa also is variable. The turbinates are usually erythematous and, during an exacerbation, considerable quantities of nasal secretions, which can lead to crusting and dryness, may be present.[6] Nasal eosinophilia is not present and skin-prick testing results are usually negative.[7]

M.S.'s symptoms of bothersome watery rhinorrhea, nasal congestion, and headache without itching or sneezing are typical. His complaint of worsening symptoms with exposure to noxious inhalants and cold air supports the diagnosis of idiopathic rhinitis. The nasal smear, which notably lacks large numbers of eosinophils, initially differentiates this disease from nonallergic rhinitis with eosinophilia syndrome. This disorder has similar symptoms but also is marked by nasal eosinophilia (5%–20%) in the setting of negative skin-prick testing and negative IgE levels.[7]

Choice of Therapeutic Agent

Case 20-8, Question 3: What nonpharmacologic and pharmacologic treatments are appropriate to manage M.S.'s idiopathic rhinitis?

Patients should be instructed to avoid as many aggravating factors as possible, such as strong odors (perfumes, soaps, paints) and air pollutants (smoke and tobacco fumes).[6] Saline irrigation is valuable as a general soothing and moisturizing treatment.[6] Pharmacotherapy for idiopathic rhinitis should be directed toward the predominant symptoms of the individual patient. For patients with predominant nasal congestion and minimal rhinorrhea, the intranasal corticosteroids may be helpful.[6,67] The addition of oral decongestants may improve nasal obstruction in some patients with idiopathic rhinitis, but should be considered adjunctive therapy because side effects can be problematic and data regarding efficacy is lacking.[6]

M.S.'s case is typical of the often frustrating course in treating idiopathic rhinitis. Commonly, multiple therapeutic plans fail, and M.S. has responded incompletely and unsatisfactorily to intranasal corticosteroids. There is some older evidence suggesting topical nasal capsaicin may be effective, but this option has not garnered widespread support.[6] Surgical treatments have been attempted for patients in whom medical management fails, although it is typically reserved for patients with concomitant nasal septal deviation or turbinate hypertrophy.[6]

In patients such as M.S., who have rhinorrhea as their predominant symptom, FGAs may be helpful because of their anticholinergic drying effects.[6] The topical antihistamine, azelastine, has been shown to be efficacious for symptoms including congestion, postnasal drip, and sleeping difficulty in those with idiopathic rhinitis.[6] Another option for decreasing nasal secretions is nasal ipratropium bromide, a topical anticholinergic agent with minimal adverse effects[6] (see Table 20-6 for dosing information). In the case of M.S., because he has been comfortable using an intranasal product (mometasone) in the past, it would be reasonable to initiate a trial of ipratropium bromide 0.03% two sprays in each nostril 3 times daily. Once the rhinorrhea is controlled, he should be advised to reduce the dosage to twice daily. Nasal saline can also be used as needed if excessive dryness occurs during dosage optimization.

MIXED ALLERGIC–NONALLERGIC RHINITIS

CASE 20-9

QUESTION 1: D.W. is a 56-year-old woman with a longstanding history of allergic rhinitis related to triggers with seasonal ragweed. Her primary symptoms are rhinorrhea and sneezing, which she has relieved by using various oral antihistamines (clemastine 1 mg daily and, more recently, cetirizine 10 mg daily) that she takes several weeks each autumn. Recently (during winter), she has experienced new rhinitis symptoms associated with the weather and various odors that were not a problem in the past, specifically, perfumes and food spices. When she encounters these, she exhibits watery rhinorrhea and profound congestion. She has tried a combination of cetirizine with pseudoephedrine for these episodes, but reports that it "doesn't seem to help much and it makes me feel jumpy." Are D.W.'s new symptoms the result of breakthrough (uncontrolled) allergic rhinitis or do they represent something new?

Distinguishing between allergic rhinitis and nonallergic rhinitis may be difficult in clinical practice, and the presence of concomitant allergic and nonallergic rhinitis in some patients confounds the diagnosis further.[8] A careful history should be gathered from the patient and an assessment made of the temporal nature of the symptoms and various exposures. The Clinical Presentation and Assessment of Rhinitis section in this chapter can be helpful to review to help distinguish between allergic and nonallergic causes of rhinitis. When a patient presents with characteristics suggestive of both types, especially in the case of new symptoms or triggers despite optimized therapy, mixed rhinitis should be considered.

Although D.W. has a confirmed history of ragweed pollen sensitivity (supporting the allergic rhinitis diagnosis), the timing of the more recent symptoms and the new triggers (i.e., odors) suggest that she may have developed sensitivities of a nonallergic (non–IgE-based) nature. The patient's age also is consistent with the development of vasomotor rhinitis (nonallergic), which can present around the time of menopause. This, combined with the lack of efficacy from a previously successful therapy (i.e., oral antihistamine), suggest that D.W. may be exhibiting a mixed allergic–nonallergic rhinitis presentation.

CASE 20-9, QUESTION 2: How should D.W.'s mixed rhinitis be treated? How is this different from the management of allergic rhinitis?

The important point about nonallergic triggers, or new onset triggers such as those present in D.W., is that oral antihistamines and other therapies directed primarily at allergic responses may be ineffective in relieving all symptoms. Good clinical evidence suggests that intranasal steroids are an effective option, as well as intranasal antihistamine therapy or a combination of the two.[8] Avoidance or minimization of exposure to the triggers is also an important strategy. For D.W., a 4-week therapeutic trial of a benzalkonium chloride-free intranasal steroid (e.g., ciclesonide two sprays in each nostril once daily) with counseling about appropriate administration is warranted. Intransal steroid therapy may improve the response to both allergic and nonallergic triggers.[8]

SUMMARY

The initial management of rhinitis should be directed at preventing symptoms, which can be achieved through a variety of pharmacologic and nonpharmacologic methods. Treatment plans for allergic rhinitis, the most common subtype, should include patient education, allergen or irritant avoidance, and the appropriate medications, including immunotherapy, if indicated. Control of the disease process is the expected outcome, so that patients are able to live their lives comfortably without symptoms or impairment. Customizing therapy for each patient based on symptom history and response to treatments is important. Rhinitis can be controlled and effective management can greatly improve the quality of patients' lives.

KEY REFERENCES AND WEBSITES

A full list of references for this chapter can be found at http://thepoint.lww.com/AT11e. Below are the key references and websites for this chapter, with the corresponding reference number in this chapter found in parentheses after the reference.

Key References

Bousquet J et al. Allergic rhinitis and its impact on asthma (ARIA) 2008 update (in collaboration with the World Health Organization, GA(2) LEN and AllerGen). *Allergy*. 2008;63(Suppl 86):8. (19)

Brozek JL et al. Allergic rhinitis and its impact on asthma (ARIA) guidelines: 2010 revision. *J Allergy Clin Immunol*. 2010;126:466. (24)

Devillier P et al. A meta-analysis of sublingual allergen immunotherapy and pharmacotherapy in pollen-induced seasonal allergic rhinoconjunctivitis. *BMC Med*. 2014;12:71–90. (60)

Kern J, Bielory L. Complementary and alternative therapy (CAM) in the treatment of allergic rhinitis. *Curr Allergy Asthma Rep*. 2014;14: 479–485. (51)
Mandhane SN et al. Allergic rhinitis: an update on disease, present treatments and future prospects. *Int Immunopharmacol*. 2011;11:1646–1662. (4)
Seidman MD, et al. Clinical practice guideline: allergic rhinitis. *Otolaryngol Head Neck Surg*. 2015;152;15(1S):S1–S43. (1)
Scadding GK et al. BSACI guidelines for the management of allergic and non-allergic rhinitis. *Clin Exp Allergy*. 2008;38:19–42. (3)
Tran NP et al. Management of rhinitis: allergic and non-allergic. *Allergy Asthma Immunol Res*. 2011;3:148–158. (6)

21 Cystic Fibrosis

Paul M. Beringer and Michelle Condren

CORE PRINCIPLES

	Core Principle	CHAPTER CASES
1	Cystic fibrosis (CF) is a genetic disorder affecting approximately 30,000 individuals in the United States that is caused by a defect in the cystic fibrosis transmembrane conductance regulator protein, which is a chloride channel that regulates fluid and electrolyte transport within secretory epithelial cells throughout the body.	**Case 21-1 (Question 1), Figure 21-1, Figure 21-2**
2	The principal manifestations of CF include malnutrition secondary to pancreatic insufficiency and pulmonary dysfunction, resulting from chronic airway obstruction, infection, and inflammation.	**Case 21-1 (Question 1), Table 21-1, Figure 21-3**
3	Diagnosis of CF is based on newborn screening or presence of the typical signs and symptoms of the disease, and either documented abnormalities in ion transport or identification of two CF mutations.	**Case 21-1 (Questions 1, 2), Table 21-2**
4	Administration of pancreatic enzymes and fat-soluble vitamins are prescribed to correct malabsorption and vitamin deficiencies and improve nutritional status.	**Case 21-1 (Question 2), Table 21-3**
5	Key therapies for management of CF pulmonary disease include inhaled dornase alfa and hypertonic saline in combination with mechanical airway clearance techniques to combat airway obstruction, inhaled antibiotics to combat airway infection, and oral azithromycin for airway inflammation.	**Case 21-2 (Questions 1–3), Case 21-3 (Question 3)**
6	Periodically, patients will experience acute pulmonary exacerbations characterized by increased pulmonary symptoms, acute loss of lung function, and loss of weight, which require intensification of airway clearance, administration of systemic antibiotics, and nutritional supplements.	**Case 21-3 (Questions 1, 2, 4), Table 21-4**
7	Key monitoring parameters in patients with CF include trends in pulmonary function tests to determine response to therapies and identify possible acute pulmonary exacerbations, and body mass index to assess nutritional status.	**Case 21-1 (Question 3)**
8	Therapy for patients with CF should include attention to complications, including cystic fibrosis–related diabetes mellitus, osteoporosis, hepatobiliary disease, constipation, and depression. Future therapies directed against the basic defect offer a potential cure for CF.	**Case 21-3 (Question 5)**

Cystic fibrosis (CF) is a severe, complex, hereditary disease that affects 1 of every 3,200 Caucasian births, or approximately 30,000 children and adults in the United States. One in 31 Americans carries the autosomal recessive gene for CF, which arises from a mutation in coding for the cystic fibrosis transmembrane regulator protein (CFTR). This genetic mutational error results in the complex, multisystem disease of CF, which is characterized by malabsorption and a state of chronic lung obstruction, inflammation, and infection.

The course and severity of CF are variable and unpredictable. The median predicted survival age has increased from 28 to 41 years over the past two decades because of advances in the management of this disorder.[1] Although current therapy continues to rely on treatment of symptoms, several compounds in clinical development are directed at the basic defect and offer a potential cure. In the meantime, aggressive treatment with existing therapies can decrease the morbidity of this disease and increase the life expectancy of the patient.

GENETIC BASIS

CF is caused by mutations in the *CFTR* gene, which is a member of the ATP-binding cassette family. CFTR is dependent on cyclic adenosine monophosphate for chloride transport: defective coding for CFTR inhibits the normal regulation of ion transport in and out

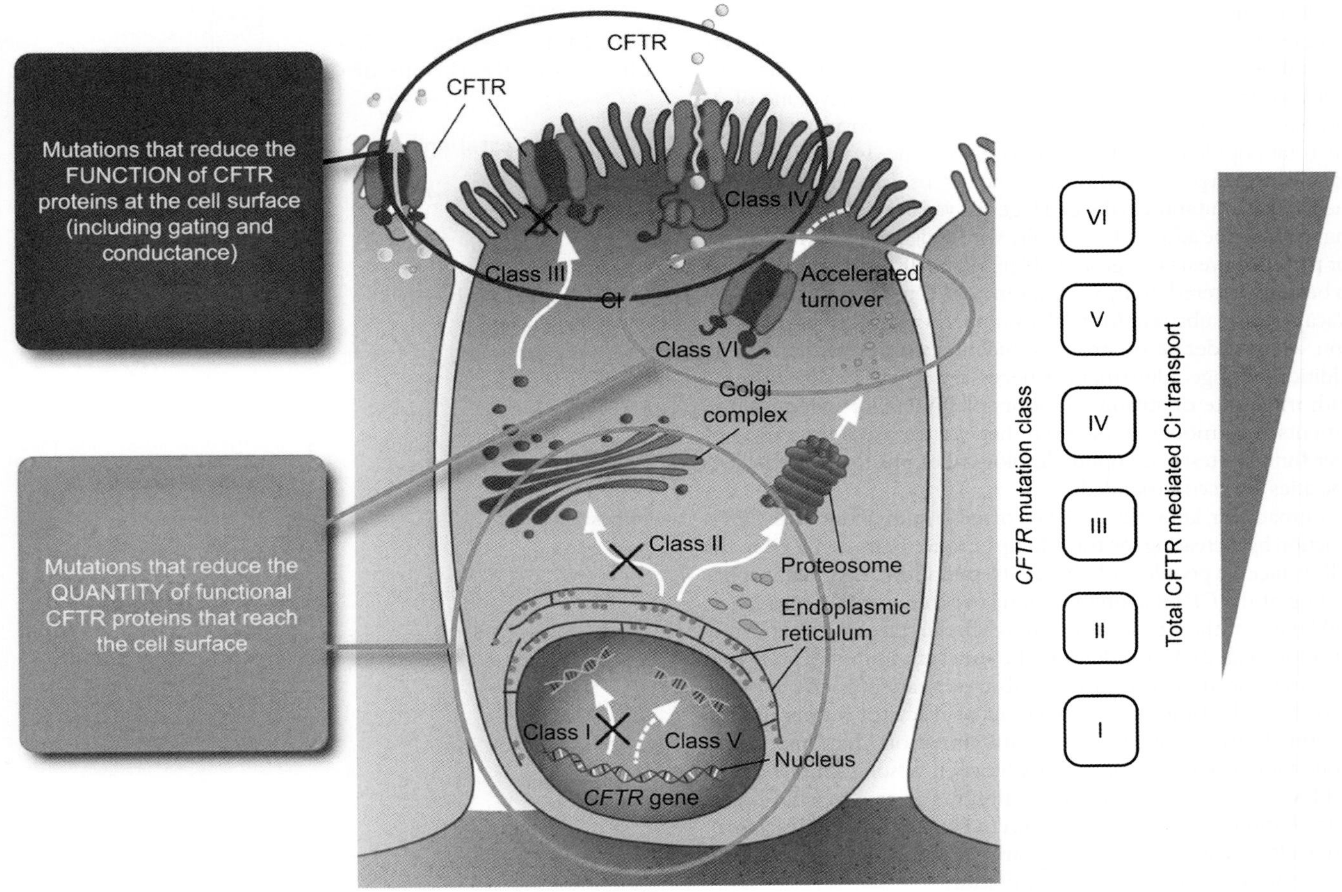

Figure 21-1 Classification of mutations. Cystic fibrosis transmembrane conductance regulator (*CFTR*) gene mutations are categorized into six classes. Mutation classes I, II, V, and VI result in an absence or reduced quantity of CFTR protein at the cell membrane, whereas mutation classes III and IV influence the function or activity of CFTR at the cell membrane. Class I mutations are associated with the greatest disruption to CFTR-mediated chloride transport; in general, chloride transport gradually increases through the remaining five classes, with the greatest activity being observed in class IV to VI mutations. (Reprinted with permission from Derichs, N. Targeting a genetic defect: cystic fibrosis transmembrane conductance regulator modulators in cystic fibrosis. *Eur Respir Rev*. 2013; 22: 58-65.)

of the cell on the apical surface of secretory epithelial cells.[2] CFTR also regulates the transport of bicarbonate and sodium ions, mucous rheology, pulmonary inflammation, and bacterial adherence.[3–7]

CF is an autosomal recessive disorder, which means there is a 25% chance of inheriting the malfunctioning genes from both parents and developing the disease, a 50% chance of inheriting one abnormal gene (i.e., carrier), and a 25% chance of inheriting two normal genes. Approximately 5% of whites are asymptomatic carriers of the CF mutation. More than two decades have passed since the identification and cloning of the gene responsible for CF, and nearly 2,000 *CFTR* mutations have been discovered (http://www.genet.sickkids.on.ca/cftr/app). These mutations have been grouped into six major classes according to the functional consequence of the defect (Fig. 21-1).[8–10] The most common variant is ΔF508, representing 66% of all mutations. Approximately 90% of all patients with CF have at least one copy of this mutation.

The importance of identifying the gene mutation relates to potential new therapies, currently, in various stages of clinical development. The greatest excitement and anticipation involves new therapies directed at the basic defect that offer a potential cure for CF. Replacement of the defective gene and repair of the dysfunctional CFTR protein are the two approaches actively being pursued.

Cystic Fibrosis Transmembrane Conductance Regulator Modulation

These therapies are designed to correct the function of the defective CFTR protein made by the *CFTR* gene, allowing normal chloride and sodium transport across epithelial cells lining the lungs and other organs. Several compounds are currently in clinical drug development for patients with different *CFTR* mutations, demonstrating a pharmacogenomic approach to CF treatment that is likely to be realized in the near future.

IVACAFTOR AND LUMACAFTOR

Ivacaftor, known as a CFTR potentiator, aims to increase the function of defective CFTR proteins by increasing the gating activity, or ability to transport ions across the cell membrane, of CFTR at the cell surface. In people with gating mutations (e.g., G551D mutation), CFTR proteins do not function normally at the cell surface (Fig. 21-1). A phase 3 trial of ivacaftor in CF patients with at least one copy of a G551D mutation demonstrated improvements in pulmonary function (absolute change of 10% in forced expiratory volume in 1 second [FEV_1]), and a 55% reduction is risk for acute pulmonary exacerbations over the 48-week study period.[11] Based on the positive results of this trial in patients with the G551D mutation as well as additional trials with patients with other gating/conductance abnormalities, ivacaftor received FDA approval. Ivacaftor is currently indicated in patients aged 2 years or above, who have one of 23 residual function mutations which represent approximately 5% of the total population of CF patients worldwide. Ivacaftor alone is not effective in patients who are homozygous (have two copies) for the F508del mutation in the *CFTR* gene. Ivacaftor is provided in 150 mg tablets to be administered orally with a high-fat meal twice daily for patients 6 years of age and older and as 50 and 75 mg granules to be administered orally in children between the ages of 2 and 5. Ivacaftor is a substrate for CYP3A, and, therefore, co-administration with moderate or strong inducers is not recommended. In addition, dosage adjustment is necessary when co-administered with moderate or strong inhibitors of CYP3A or when used in patients with moderate or severe hepatic disease. Monitoring of liver function tests and ophthalmological exams for potential lens opacities are recommended.

Lumacaftor, known as a CFTR corrector, aims to increase CFTR function by increasing the trafficking, or movement, of CFTR to the cell surface. In people with the ΔF508 mutation, there is improper folding of the CFTR protein, leading to proteosomal degradation and failure of the CFTR protein to reach the cell surface in normal amounts (Fig. 21-1). In addition, the small amount of protein that does make it to the cell surface fails to activate properly. A phase 3 study, evaluating the combination of ivacaftor/lumacaftor in patients homozygous for the ΔF508 mutation, demonstrated a modest improvement in pulmonary function (absolute improvement in FEV_1 of 2.6%–4%) and a reduction in the rate of pulmonary exacerbations (30%–39%).[12] The recent FDA approval of ivacaftor/lumacaftor is significant since nearly 50% of the CF population are homozygous for the ΔF508 mutation.

ATALUREN

Ataluren is a novel, small-molecule compound that promotes the read through of premature truncation codons in the CFTR mRNA. It aims to treat CF patients with nonsense mutations (nmCF). A nonsense mutation is an alteration in the genetic code that prematurely halts the synthesis of an essential protein (Fig. 21-1). About 10% of people with CF have nonsense mutations. Data from a phase 3 clinical trial of ataluren in pediatric and adult patients with nmCF did not demonstrate significant differences in pulmonary function or exacerbation frequency between ataluren and placebo over the 48-week study period.[13] Additional clinical studies in patients not receiving concurrent inhaled tobramycin are currently ongoing.

Gene Therapy

Since the discovery of the *CFTR* gene in 1989, there has been hope that a gene therapy treatment would soon be available as a potential cure to CF. Initial attempts at gene therapy using viral vectors were hampered by low transfer efficiency and short retention within the airways as a result of host immunogenicity. An alternative approach uses plasmid DNA encapsulated within cationic liposomes to deliver the gene to the airways. Potential advantages of nonviral approaches are that they are noninfectious and relatively nonimmunogenic, can accommodate a large DNA plasmid, and may be produced simply on a large scale. A multiple-dose phase 2b clinical trial of PGM169/GL67A conducted by the UK Gene Therapy Consortium demonstrated stabilization of FEV_1 in treated versus control patients (treatment effect 3.7%) over the 1-year study period.[14]

Interestingly, even among individuals with identical genotypes, a broad spectrum of disease severity is seen.[15,16] The contribution of genetic factors other than the misfunctioning CFTR can have a great influence on disease severity.[17] Screening for genetic modifiers is currently a research tool that will hopefully lead to the development of new potential therapies.[18]

Table 21-1
Clinical Manifestations of Cystic Fibrosis

Manifestation	Approximate Incidence (%) Children (Infants)	Adults
Pancreatic		
Insufficiency	85 (80–85)	90
Pancreatitis	1–2	2–4
Abnormal glucose tolerance	38	75
Diabetes mellitus	14	40–50
Hepatobiliary		
Biliary cirrhosis	10–20	>20
Cholelithiasis	5	5–10
Biliary obstruction	1–2	5
Intestinal		
Meconium ileus	20	
Meconium ileus equivalent	1–5	10–20
Rectal prolapse	10–15	1–2
Intussusception	1–5	1–2
Gastroesophageal reflux	1–5	>10
Appendiceal abscess	0–1	1–2
Respiratory		
Nasal polyps	4–10 (<1)	15–20
Pansinusitis		90–100
Bronchiectasis	30–50	>90
Pneumothorax	1–2	10–15
Hemoptysis	5–15	50–60
Reproductive		
Delayed puberty		85
Infertility		
Males		98
Females		70–80

CLINICAL MANIFESTATIONS

Genotype, environmental factors, and modifier gene status all contribute to the highly variable clinical course of CF. The linking of the loss of CFTR function to clinical manifestations of the disease, however, has been central to gaining an understanding of the disease and in the discovery of new therapies. Normally, CFTR is highly expressed on the membranes of epithelial cells of the lungs, sweat glands, salivary glands, male genital ducts, pancreas, kidney tubules, and digestive tract. The CFTR performs different functions in specific tissues; therefore, a dysfunctional or absent CFTR has different effects on different organs, resulting in the multiorgan clinical manifestations of CF (Table 21-1).

Sweat Glands

Fluid secreted by the sweat glands in patients with CF is normal, but a defect in the reabsorption of electrolytes leads to sweat

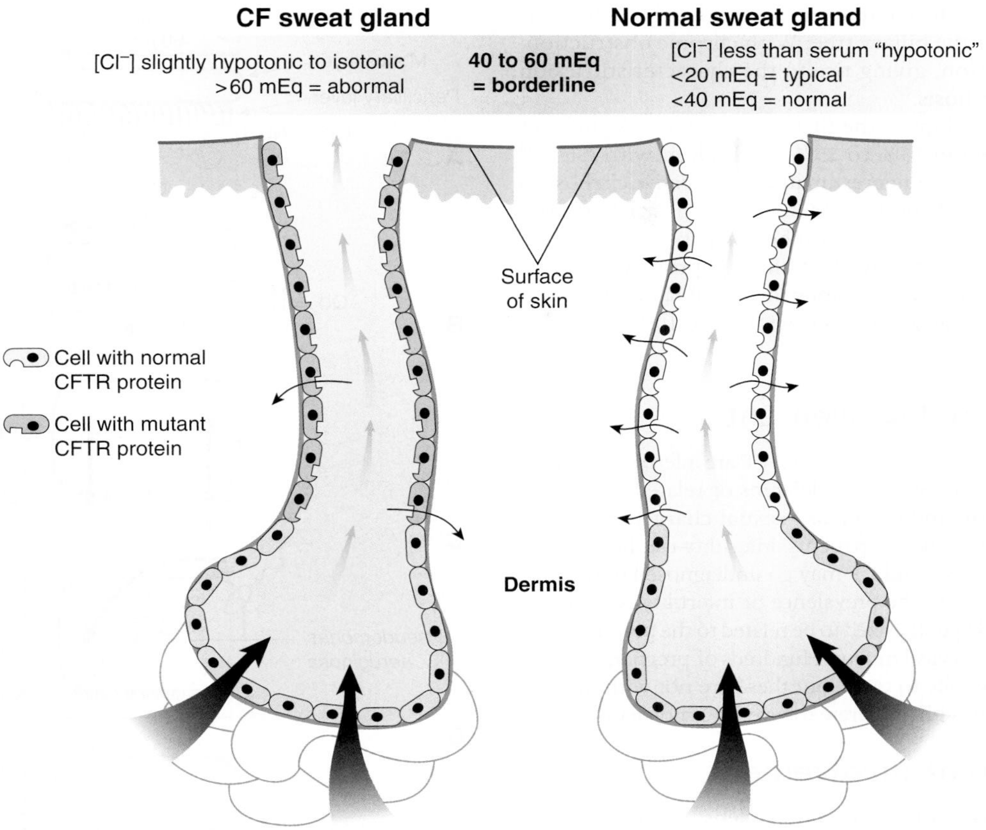

Figure 21-2 Chloride transport in sweat glands of normal and cystic fibrosis individuals. (Source: Lyczak JB, et al. Lung infections associated with cystic fibrosis. *Clin Microbiol Rev*. 2002;15(2):194–222.)

with a high salt content. CFTR, in the apical membrane of the resorptive area of the sweat gland, functions as an ion channel for chloride transport and also activates an associated epithelial sodium channel.[19] Normally, these channels efficiently reabsorb sodium chloride from sweat. In patients with CF, loss of these functioning channels blocks the ability of the sweat ducts to reabsorb salt, leading to elevated sweat sodium chloride concentrations (Fig. 21-2). The loss of these sodium and chloride ion channels serves as the basis for the diagnostic sweat chloride test.

Pancreatic Involvement

The exocrine and ultimately the endocrine functions of the pancreas are affected in CF. Pancreatic enzymes normally are secreted into bicarbonate-rich fluid from the pancreatic duct. The loss of CFTR function inhibits secretion of digestive enzymes and bicarbonate into the duodenum, resulting in ductal obstruction. With time, these enzymes (lipase, protease, and amylase) accumulate and eventually begin to digest the pancreatic tissue.[5,20] The term *cystic fibrosis* arises from the fibrotic scar tissue that replaces the destroyed pancreas. Without these enzymes, there is poor digestion of fats and, to a lesser extent, proteins and carbohydrates. As a result, 90% of patients with CF experience pancreatic insufficiency characterized by steatorrhea (fatty stools), decreased absorption of the fat-soluble vitamins (A, D, E, and K), malnutrition, and failure to thrive. Early in life, serum concentrations of amylase and lipase are increased secondary to pancreatic autodigestion. This destructive process can result in either painful or asymptomatic chronic pancreatitis.

Eventually, the progressive destruction of the pancreas affects its endocrine function, leading to cystic fibrosis–related diabetes mellitus in 15% to 20% of adolescents and nearly 40% of adults between the ages of 20 and 30.[21] The additional diagnosis of diabetes in CF is associated with more rapid decline in lung function and shortened survival. Early aggressive insulin therapy can result in improved clinical outcomes.

Gastrointestinal Involvement

Meconium ileus, an intestinal obstruction at birth, occurring in 20% of newborns with CF, is an inheritable trait of this disease.[22] Outside the neonatal period, distal intestinal obstruction syndrome (DIOS, also called *meconium ileus equivalent*) can occur at any age and results from the complete or partial obstruction of the intestine. Intestinal obstruction occurs in 10% to 20% of patients and results from the inspissation of intestinal secretions and incompletely digested intestinal contents. A right lower quadrant mass, abdominal distension, failure to pass stools, and vomiting can accompany DIOS.

Gastroesophageal reflux disease (GERD) is common in both children and adults with CF.[23–25] Children with CF should be screened for GERD and treated, if diagnosed. Other intestinal complications include rectal prolapse, intussusception, and appendiceal abscesses.

Hepatic Involvement

Located on the apical surfaces of the cells lining the intrahepatic and extrahepatic bile ducts and the gallbladder, CFTR functions to facilitate ion transport.[26] In patients with CF, the abnormal chloride efflux across the cells results in the reduction in water and sodium movement into the bile. The resulting decrease in the volume and flow of bile leads to stasis and obstruction of the biliary tree. With chronic obstruction, there is inflammation, giving rise to the characteristic lesion of focal biliary cirrhosis.[27]

Liver disease develops in the first decade of life. Significant liver disease is seen in 13% to 25% of children with CF.[28–30] Prevalence rates may be underestimated. Progressive cirrhosis is associated with portal hypertension, hypersplenism, esophageal varices, ascites, and, in a small number of patients, complete hepatic failure requiring transplantation. Approximately 30% of adult patients with CF have abnormal gallbladder function and size (absent or small gallbladder) with 5% to 10% of patients forming gallstones.[31]

Genitourinary Involvement

Approximately 98% of male patients with CF are infertile secondary to in utero obstruction of the vas deferens or related structures. Hormonal secretion and secondary sexual characteristics are normal. In a small number of patients, infertility can be the only manifestation of disease, and CF may go undiagnosed until fertility testing is performed. The prevalence of infertility is higher in women with CF and hypothesized to be related to the production of thick and tenacious cervical mucus. Hundreds of pregnancies have been carried successfully to term, but these are not without risk, especially for patients with moderate to severe pulmonary disease.[32]

Bone and Joint Involvement

Patients with CF have low bone mineral density, slower rate of bone formation, accelerated rate of bone loss, and arthritis.[33,34] Osteoclastic precursors are elevated during acute pulmonary exacerbation.[35] Although early, aggressive treatment of pulmonary exacerbations can improve bone health, sufficient intake and absorption of the fat-soluble vitamins, D and K, are important, and oral bisphosphonates may also be indicated.[36]

Patients with CF often suffer from intermittent arthritis symptoms, but only about 2% of patients have persistent symptoms. The three types of intermittent CF arthritis are (a) hypertrophic osteoarthropathy, (b) immunoreactive, and (c) CF arthropathy. The first two types are associated with pulmonary disease flare-up. The third type, CF arthropathy, affects large joints and may be accompanied by fever and erythema nodosum.[37–40]

Sinus Involvement

Nasal polyps, which are outgrowths of normal sinus epidermis, can be found in up to 20% of older patients with CF and may become sufficiently large to block nasal passages. The pathogenesis of these polyps is unknown, but the obstruction of nasal passages can lead to infection. The faulty ionic transport of chloride across the apical membrane of epithelial cells lining exocrine glands leads to dehydration of extracellular fluids and the development of inspissated mucus in nasal and sinus passages. Nearly all patients with CF (90%–100% of patients >8 months of age) develop sinus disease. On radiographic examination, greater than 90% of adult-age patients have pansinusitis, which can contribute to pulmonary exacerbations.[41,42] The impact of sinusitis on the CF population is significant.

Pulmonary Involvement

Respiratory disease is of major importance in patients with CF because it is the principal cause of repeated hospitalizations, decline in pulmonary function, and death. Although the exact pathophysiological mechanisms leading from the CFTR cellular defect to the development of bronchiectasis and loss of pulmonary function are not currently known, research in the past two decades since the discovery of the genetic defect has greatly expanded our understanding of this process.

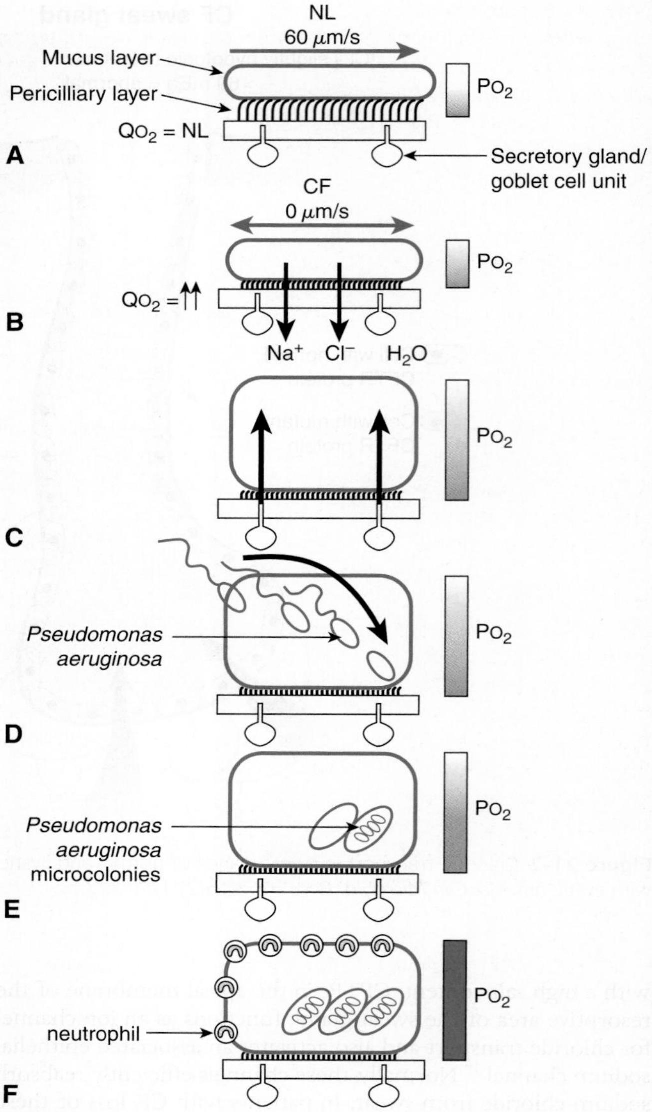

Figure 21-3 Pathophysiology of cystic fibrosis lung disease. Treatments in italics are investigational. **A:** Normal airway epithelia with functional CFTR demonstrates normal mucociliary clearance. **B:** CFTR defect leads to reduced periciliary liquid and loss of mucociliary clearance. Accelerated ion transport (sodium reabsorption) leads to increased oxygen consumption (QO_2) and hypoxic gradients (pO_2) in the airways. **C:** Impaired mucociliary clearance leads to accumulation of mucous within the airways causing airway obstruction. **D:** Retained secretions provide an optimal environment for initial infection. **E:** Chronic *P. aeruginosa* infections form microcolonies (i.e., biofilms) which resist host defenses as well as antibiotics. **F:** A chronic inflammatory response mediated by neutrophil recruitment to the airways leads to release of reactive oxygen species and proteases which damage the airways. (Reprinted with permission from Worlitzsch D et al. Effects of reduced mucus oxygen concentration in airway *Pseudomonas* infections of cystic fibrosis patients. *J Clin Invest*. 2002;109:317.)

AIRWAY OBSTRUCTION, INFECTION, AND INFLAMMATION

One of the leading theories regarding the pathogenesis of airway disease in CF is depicted in Figure 21-3.[43] The lower airways of a normal lung are maintained free of pathogens through various lung defense mechanisms. For example, a thin film of liquid on the airway surfaces called the *airway surface layer* (ASL) contains antimicrobials, antioxidants, proteases, and other substances that work to eliminate pathogens. In addition, the ASL can remove invading microbes from the lung by moving a mucous gel toward the mouth through ciliary motion. Mucociliary clearance of microbes and debris is aided by the cough reflex to keep the airways clear. Because coughing is an important defense mechanism, cough suppressants should not be used in patients with CF.

In patients with CF, the CFTR defect reduces the ASL, resulting in markedly thickened mucus and impaired mucociliary clearance. Continued mucus hypersecretion leads to mucus plugging and airway obstruction. Additionally, the CFTR defect causes acidification of the ASL secondary to reduced bicarbonate secretion, resulting in increased susceptibility to infection.[44] Accelerated ion transport increases oxygen consumption, leading to hypoxic gradients within the mucus. *Pseudomonas aeruginosa* adapts to the anaerobic environment by increasing alginate production and through the formation of biofilms. In response to infection, proinflammatory cytokines (e.g., tumor necrosis factor-α, interleukin [IL] 1), chemokines (e.g., IL-8), and other inflammatory mediators (e.g., leukotriene B_4) are released from airway epithelial cells and alveolar macrophages, resulting in neutrophil recruitment into the airways. Because the neutrophils undergo apoptosis, they release their DNA, which accumulates and contributes to airway obstruction. In the normal host, proteases (e.g., neutrophil elastase) are released in response to an infectious insult and digest the bacteria, while lung tissue is protected by the presence of antiproteases. In patients with CF the intense neutrophilic infiltration in response to IL-8 results in an imbalance between airway proteases and antiproteases.[45] The excess proteases cause degradation of elastin, a structural component of the airways. In addition, airway proteases degrade cell surface receptors (e.g., CXCR1 from neutrophils), leading to impaired bactericidal activity accounting for the persistence of *P. aeruginosa* within the airways despite a robust inflammatory response.[46] The chronic cycle of airway obstruction, infection, and inflammation leads to bronchiectasis, progressive loss of lung function with eventual respiratory failure, and death.

MICROBIOLOGY

The microbiology of airways in patients with CF changes as a function of age. In infants and toddlers, the principal organisms include nontypeable *Haemophilus influenzae* and *Staphylococcus aureus*. The prevalence of methicillin resistant *S. aureus* has increased dramatically in the last 5 years and has been associated with a more rapid decline in pulmonary function and increased mortality.[47,48] Clinical trials evaluating antibiotic therapy for eradication of MRSA as well as chronic suppressive therapy are currently ongoing. In older children and adults, *P. aeruginosa* becomes the predominant pathogen. Other unique pathogens in CF include *Burkholderia cepacia* and *Aspergillus fumigatus*.

Pseudomonas Aeruginosa

Infections with *P. aeruginosa* occur in three distinct phases. First, the patient acquires the organism and presents with an initial infection. Treatment often leads to eradication; however, reinfection eventually occurs and leads to chronic infection. Under pressure from hypoxic gradients within the mucus, *P. aeruginosa* within the airways converts to the mucoid phenotype. Observational studies have noted significant structural as well as functional changes within the lung in patients with sputum cultures that grow mucoid *P. aeruginosa* when compared with patients with nonmucoid strains or who are not infected with *P. aeruginosa*. Specifically, when compared with patients with nonmucoid *P. aeruginosa*, those with mucoid *P. aeruginosa* had significant abrupt declines in percentage of predicted FEV_1.[49] The median time to acquisition of nonmucoid and mucoid strains is 1 and 13 years, respectively; however, there is tremendous variability in the initial acquisition and development of chronic infection. Some patients avoid acquisition of *P. aeruginosa* until their adolescent years, whereas others acquire mucoid *P. aeruginosa* early in childhood (e.g., 5–6 years of age). Patients with delayed acquisition of *P. aeruginosa* typically have minimal lung disease and few hospital admissions when compared with children who acquire *P. aeruginosa* (in particular mucoid *P. aeruginosa*) earlier in life. The relatively long period between nonmucoid and mucoid *P. aeruginosa* offers an opportunity for intervention with pharmacologic therapy designed to eradicate the organism from the airways. The mucoid strains create a significant therapeutic challenge because they can develop into biofilms. A biofilm is a community of bacteria that adheres to tissues (e.g., airway epithelial cells) and secretes a slimy coating (mucoid exopolysaccharide), which protects it from the hostile environment within which it resides. *P. aeruginosa* biofilms create a therapeutic challenge when compared with their planktonic (freely motile) bacterial counterparts, because they evade local defense mechanisms, are slow growing, and can sequester β-lactamase.

Burkholderia Cepacia

Occasionally infections involve atypical organisms, including *B. cepacia* (2.8%). *B. cepacia* is actually a complex consisting of several distinct species. *Burkholderia cenocepacia* is the most frequently isolated and clinically relevant species in patients with CF. *B. cepacia* is easily transmitted via inhalation or contact with a reservoir of *B. cepacia*, including other patients with CF, health care professionals, or contaminated medical instruments. Colonization with *B. cepacia* can manifest as chronic asymptomatic carriage, progressive deterioration of lung function, or fatal decline during a short interval often associated with septicemia (known as *B. cepacia* syndrome), and is associated with a 50% reduction in life expectancy.[50] *B. cepacia* is intrinsically resistant to many antibiotics, including aminoglycosides and β-lactams, which limits treatment options. Because of the adverse health outcomes and limited treatment options, chronic infection with *B. cenocepacia* is a relative contraindication to lung transplantation at many centers, emphasizing the importance of preventing acquisition of this organism through active infection control measures.

Aspergillus Fumigatus

Aspergillus species present a unique challenge in patients with CF. The presence of this organism often ignites an immunologic response characterized by an increase in serum immunoglobulin E and eosinophilic infiltration of the alveoli. This syndrome is referred to as allergic bronchopulmonary aspergillosis. The typical symptoms of this syndrome include wheezing, shortness of breath, low-grade fever, and production of thick, brownish, or bloody sputum. This disease is not invasive; however, chronic eosinophilic infiltration can lead to bronchiectasis and lung scarring. Allergic bronchopulmonary aspergillosis is present in approximately 10% of patients with CF and accounts for 10% of acute pulmonary exacerbations. The diagnosis of allergic bronchopulmonary aspergillosis can be challenging owing to the overlap in clinical features with acute pulmonary exacerbations. A consensus conference sponsored by the Cystic Fibrosis Foundation provides guidelines for diagnosis and treatment of allergic bronchopulmonary aspergillosis in patients with CF.[51] The minimal diagnostic criteria include clinical deterioration, elevated total serum immunoglobulin E (greater than 500 international units/mL), positive immediate *A. fumigatus* skin test or serum immunoglobulin E antibodies, and *A. fumigatus* serum precipitins

Table 21-2
Phenotypic Features Consistent with Diagnosis of Cystic Fibrosis

Persistent colonization or infection with typical CF pathogens (e.g., *S. aureus*, nontypeable *H. influenzae*, *P. aeruginosa*, and *B. cepacia*
Chronic cough and sputum production
Persistent chest radiograph abnormalities
Airway obstruction manifested by wheezing and air trapping
Nasal polyps; radiographic or computed tomographic abnormalities of paranasal sinuses
Digital clubbing
Meconium ileus, distal intestinal obstruction syndrome, rectal prolapse
Pancreatic insufficiency, recurrent pancreatitis
Chronic hepatic disease
Failure to thrive, hypoproteinemia, and edema, complications secondary to fat-soluble vitamin deficiency
Salt loss syndromes: acute salt depletion, chronic metabolic alkalosis
Male urogenital abnormalities resulting in obstructive azoospermia (CBAVD)

CBAVD, congenital bilateral absence of the vas deferens.
Reprinted with permission from Farrell PM et al. Guidelines for diagnosis of cystic fibrosis in newborns through older adults: Cystic Fibrosis Foundation consensus report. *J Pediatr*. 2008;153:S4.

or immunoglobulin G antibodies or radiographic changes. Annual screening of serum immunoglobulin E concentrations is recommended for patients with CF older than 6 years of age.

DIAGNOSIS

The diagnosis of CF can be made soon after birth through newborn screening or later in life based on the presentation of symptoms. A newborn screening test based on measurement of trypsinogen concentrations in blood is performed for early diagnosis of CF. Trypsinogen is normally produced in the pancreas and is carried to the small intestine, where it changes from an inactive proenzyme to the active enzyme trypsin, which is used in digestion of proteins. In infants with CF, mucus can block the ducts from the pancreas into the small intestine. The mucus prevents trypsinogen from reaching the intestines, resulting in accumulation in the blood. This process can be detected and measured because immunoreactive trypsin (IRT) levels increase in the blood of the infant. The IRT testing is a screening test; confirmatory testing including a sweat chloride test and DNA analysis for CF mutations should be performed in infants with a positive IRT.[52]

When the pilocarpine iontophoresis test (i.e., sweat chloride test) is conducted at a certified CF center and is positive (≥60 mM), the diagnosis of CF can be applied. In infants younger than 6 months of age, a sweat chloride value of 30 to 59 mM indicates possible CF and should be repeated in conjunction with DNA analysis.[52] In infants older than 6 months of age, a value of 40 to 59 mM indicates possible CF and should be repeated in conjunction with DNA analysis.

DNA analysis is recommended and is expected to identify 90% of CFTR mutations. The DNA analysis used for population screening is not as sensitive at detecting CFTR mutations in non-white populations. Prenatal screening for the presence of a CF carrier state in the parents is recommended by the American College of Medical Genetics and the American College of Obstetrics and Gynecology.[53]

Symptoms Suggestive of Cystic Fibrosis

For those in whom CF may not have been detected by newborn screening, the suspicion for CF is raised by clinical symptoms. Infants born with meconium ileus, an intestinal obstruction attributable to thickened meconium, at birth are highly likely to have CF. Other clinical symptoms that require further diagnostic testing are listed in Table 21-2. Presence of these symptoms warrants obtaining a sweat chloride and DNA analysis.

CASE 21-1

Question 1: K.M. is a 1-week-old girl weighing 2.9 kg, who presents for routine follow-up. Her birth weight was 2.7 kg. She is growing well on breast milk every 3 hours. A review of systems reveals no abnormalities. K.M.'s newborn screening panel has returned with an elevated IRT concentration.

What further testing is recommended to determine whether this infant has CF?

At this time, it is recommended that K.M. have a sweat chloride test and DNA analysis performed. If K.M. has a positive sweat chloride, additional testing is recommended to determine whether she has pancreatic insufficiency. The preferred testing method is the fecal elastase, which is measured in a single stool sample. Fecal elastase is not degraded during intestinal transit and has been shown to correlate well with duodenal lipase, amylase, trypsin, and bicarbonate concentrations. A low value indicates the presence of pancreatic insufficiency necessitating enzyme supplementation. Although 25% of infants with CF are pancreatic sufficient at the time of diagnosis, most will become pancreatic insufficient in the first year of life.[52] For those at least 8 years of age, a serum trypsinogen may be used to assess pancreatic function.

EARLY INTERVENTIONS AND THERAPY

Case 21-1, Question 2: K.M. returns to the clinic 2 weeks later. Testing has revealed a sweat chloride of 84 mM and the presence of homozygous ΔF508 mutations. Fecal elastase is low, and the diagnosis of pancreatic insufficiency is made. What therapy should be initiated at this time?

K.M. now meets the diagnostic criteria for CF with pancreatic insufficiency. Early nutritional therapy to ensure appropriate growth is essential as good nutritional status has been associated with improved pulmonary outcomes.[54] CF patients are hypermetabolic and do not absorb fats and proteins normally. Therefore, the CF diet must be high in calories, fat, and protein. It is recommended that those with CF have an energy intake of 110% to 200% of that recommended for the general population.[55] If K.M. has difficulty gaining weight, the frequency of breast-feeding may need to increase or she will need to be changed to a high-calorie infant formula.

Vitamin and Mineral Supplementation

The malabsorption of fats in patients with CF with pancreatic insufficiency also results in decreased gastrointestinal absorption

Table 21-3
Daily Recommended Doses of Fat-Soluble Vitamins for Patients with Cystic Fibrosis and Vitamin Content in Specialty Vitamin Formulations

Age	Vitamin A (International Units)	Vitamin E (International Units)	Vitamin D (International Units)	Vitamin K (mg)
0–12 months	1,500	40–50	400	0.3–0.5
1–3 years	5,000	80–150	400–800	0.3–0.5
4–8 years	5,000–10,000	100–200	400–800	0.3–0.5
>8 years	10,000	200–400	400–800	0.3–0.5
Chewable Vitamins				
AquaDEK	9,083 (92% β carotene)	50	600	0.35
Choiceful	13,000 (88% β carotene)	180	800	0.6
Complete Formulation	16,000 (88% β carotene)	200	1,500	1
Complete Formulation D3000	16,000 (88% β carotene)	200	3,000	1
DEKAs Plus (per 1 mL)	18,167 (87% β carotene)	100	2,000	1
Libertas	16,000 (β carotene)	200	1,000	0.8
Liquid Vitamins				
AquADEK (per 1 mL)	5,751 (87% β carotene)	50	600	0.4
Complete Formulation (per 1 mL)	9,254 (75% β carotene)	100	1,500	1
Libertas	4,627 (as retinol)	50	500	0.4
DEKAs Plus (per 1 mL)	5,751 (87% β carotene)	50	750	0.5
Softgel Products				
Choiceful	14,000 (88% β carotene)	170	1,000	0.7
Complete Formulation	16,000 (88% β carotene)	200	1,500	0.8
Complete Formulation D3000	16,000 (88% β carotene)	200	3,000	0.8
Complete Formulation D5000	16,000 (88% β carotene)	200	3,000	0.8
DEKAs Plus	18,167 (92% β carotene)	150	3,000	1
Libertas	16,000 (88% β carotene)	200	1,000	0.8

of the fat-soluble vitamins (A, D, E, and K). Approximately 45% of the CF population is deficient in one of these vitamins, even when pancreatic enzymes are being used appropriately.[56] The current recommendations for replacement therapy are listed in Table 21-3.[57] Concerns about inadequate supplementation of vitamins D and K resulting in poor bone health have arisen.[58,59] Calcium supplementation will be needed for those receiving inadequate calcium in their diet. Iron supplements might also be needed if iron deficiency anemia occurs.

K.M. should be started on a CF-specific liquid multivitamin preparation at a dose of 1 mL once daily. Additional vitamins may be supplemented if laboratory monitoring reveals an abnormality. Additionally, K.M. should receive 1/8 teaspoon of table salt per day to account for sodium loss in sweat.[60] At 6 months of age, the dose increases to 1/4 teaspoon. For bottle-fed infants, a small amount of salt is added to each feeding. For K.M., who is breast-fed, the parents should attempt pumping and bottle-feeding with breast milk twice a day to add salt. If K.M. does not tolerate bottle-feeding, the salt is not supplemented, and they should ensure K.M. is not exposed to warm conditions for a prolonged time.

Enzyme Supplementation

The mainstay of treatment for pancreatic insufficiency is exogenous replacement of pancreatic digestive enzymes. The goals of pancreatic enzyme supplementation are to (a) improve weight gain, (b) minimize steatorrhea, and (c) eliminate abdominal cramping and bloating. Supplementation with currently available therapies does not fully restore fat absorption, and the absorption of sufficient fat-soluble vitamins continues to be problematic.[61] The digestive enzymes (lipase, protease, and amylase) are available in a mixture of approximately one part lipase to three parts protease and three parts amylase in capsules that contain enteric-coated microspheres of these enzymes. The enteric coating protects these enzymes from gastric acid. Because the breakdown of fat is the most important function of these enzymes, dosing is based on the lipase content, and the dose varies according to weight, age, dietary fat intake, and symptom severity. The initial dose for infants is 2,000 to 5,000 units of lipase per breast-feeding or per 120 mL of bottle-feeding. Infants eating solid food begin at a dose of 1,000 units/kg/meal.[60] For children older than 4 years of age, 500 units of lipase/kg/meal is the initial dose for enzyme supplementation.[55] A full dose is taken with meals, and half the prescribed dose is taken with snacks. Subsequent dosing adjustments are titrated to response. Lack of weight gain, smelly, greasy stools, and abdominal pain or bloating might be indicative of insufficient enzyme supplementation.[62,63]

High-strength pancreatic enzymes have been associated with colonic strictures, which are accompanied by symptoms similar to that of DIOS. Although cause and effect have not been firmly established, doses greater than 6,500 units of lipase/kg/meal have been associated with stricture formation. As a result, most recommend that the daily dose of lipase not exceed 10,000 units of lipase/kg or 2,500 units of lipase/kg/meal.[55]

When patients require unusually high doses of enzyme supplements, it sometimes can be attributable to high gastric acidity. The enteric coating on the pancreatic enzyme microspheres dissolves at a pH of 5.8, and the enzymes are destroyed at a pH of 4.0. Patients with CF have longer postprandial periods when the pH is less than 4.0 in the bowel and also have significantly less time when the pH is greater than 5.8. Because enzymes may be less effective when the bowel pH is very low,[64,65] adding a histamine type H_2 antagonist or a proton-pump inhibitor to increase gastric pH might help lower the enzyme dosing requirement.[66–68]

K.M. should receive a pancreatic enzyme supplement of 2,000 to 5,000 units per feeding. Even though K.M. is not yet eating solid food, the capsule may be opened and the contents sprinkled on a small amount (e.g., a baby's spoonful) of rice cereal, baby food, or applesauce and given before each feeding. K.M.'s caregivers should ensure that no beads are left in her mouth after the feeding is complete.

Pulmonary Interventions

Although data on the benefits of airway clearance and bronchodilator therapy in infants are sparse, these interventions are recommended by the Cystic Fibrosis Foundation.[60] Generally, albuterol may be administered before percussion and postural drainage (see Treatment of Cystic Fibrosis Airway Disease: Mechanical Methods section) once daily in infants with CF. The frequency of treatments may be increased if symptoms become evident. Respiratory syncytial virus affects most infants and may more adversely affect those with CF. Therefore, palivizumab is recommended in those with CF who are younger than 2 years of age.[60] K.M. should receive albuterol by nebulizer or metered-dose inhaler and spacer once daily before airway clearance. She should also receive palivizumab 15 mg/kg intramuscularly once a month during respiratory syncytial virus season.

CASE 21-1, QUESTION 3: What monitoring is recommended for K.M.?

K.M.'s head circumference, height, and weight should be plotted on standard growth charts every month for the first year. The goal is for her to have a weight-for-length status of the 50th percentile.[55] After the first year, quarterly growth evaluations are recommended. From 2 to 20 years of age, the goal for growth is to achieve at least the 50th percentile for body mass index. An experienced, knowledgeable registered dietitian should meet with the family to help them understand the importance of appropriate nutrition and help develop a plan for K.M. Fasting blood glucose, liver function tests, albumin, serum electrolytes, complete blood count, prothrombin time, and vitamins A, D, and E levels should be determined now, at 1 year of age, and at least annually. An abdominal examination should be done to determine liver and spleen size and consistency at each office visit.

Pulmonary status is monitored based on clinical symptoms, auscultation of the chest, and chest radiographs until about 5 years of age, when pulmonary function testing may be performed. Oropharyngeal cultures are recommended at least quarterly to detect the presence of pathogenic bacteria.

Those with CF are at risk for CF-related diabetes, warranting annual oral glucose tolerance testing starting at 10 years of age.[21] They are also at increased risk for osteoporosis and should be assessed annually for risk factors. Bone densitometry is recommended for all adults and starting at 8 years of age in those with risk factors including low vitamin D, FEV_1 less than 50%, oral corticosteroid use greater than 90 days in a year, diabetes, delayed puberty, and body mass index less than the 25th percentile.[69] K.M. currently does not have any known risk factors for osteoporosis and is too young for bone densitometry. Her risk should be re-evaluated annually starting at 8 years of age.

Treatment of Cystic Fibrosis Airway Disease

Treatment of CF airway disease involves the use of medications and techniques to mobilize pulmonary secretions, antibiotics to manage infection, and anti-inflammatory agents to reduce airway inflammation. A summary of the current evidence for specific therapies is described in the recently published pulmonary medication guidelines.[70]

MUCOCILIARY CLEARANCE

Sputum in patients with CF is difficult to mobilize because pulmonary secretions are thick as a result of the CFTR defect, the large amounts of viscous DNA from the breakdown of white blood cells, and the bacterial debris left over from chronic infections. Mechanical clearance methods, inhaled mucolytics, and airway hydration therapies can be helpful in mobilizing pulmonary secretions.

Mechanical Methods

Methods used to mechanically break up and mobilize mucus in the pulmonary tree include traditional hand percussion and postural drainage (P&PD), oscillating positive-end pressure (OPEP) with the flutter valve, high-frequency chest-wall oscillation (HFCWO), intrapulmonary percussive ventilation, and autogenic drainage (a technique of deep-breathing exercises).

For a video of how one of the HFCWO options, the Vest, works, see the last chapter at **http://www.thevest.com/resources/videos.asp**.

These mechanical approaches for mobilizing mucus are about equal in efficacy, and the selection of the most appropriate one for a patient depends on the ability, motivation, preference, and resources of the patient.[71] When the traditional P&PD was compared with HFCWO and OPEP, clinical efficacy and safety were comparable, but 50% of patients preferred the HFCWO, 37% preferred OPEP, and 13% preferred P&PD.[72]

Dornase Alfa

Dornase alfa is an inhaled recombinant form of human deoxyribonuclease I, which breaks up the extracellular DNA formed by apoptotic neutrophils that contributes to airway obstruction in patients with CF. The pivotal clinical trial demonstrated improvement in pulmonary function (FEV_1 5.8% vs. placebo, $p < 0.01$) and a reduction in exacerbation frequency (28% vs. placebo, $p = 0.04$) in patients receiving dornase alfa.[73] Based on these benefits, the use of dornase alfa is recommended in all patients 6 years of age and older.[70] Consideration can be given to treating infants and toddlers as well if their clinical symptoms support the presence of airway disease. Dornase alfa is expensive, with costs averaging about $3,000/month, and the cost–benefit ratio for its use continues to be debated.[74,75] A reasonable approach is to provide a brief trial of dornase alfa (1–2 months) to determine whether there is improvement in pulmonary function and the medication is well tolerated. A longer trial (up to 1 year) may be necessary to assess its effect on hospitalization rate.

Dornase alfa is available in 2.5 mg vials and is administered once daily via a vented jet nebulizer. The drug must be stored in the refrigerator and protected from light. Patients should be instructed in the proper use and maintenance of the nebulizer and compressor system. In addition, patients should be instructed not to dilute or mix dornase alfa with other drugs in the nebulizer.

Airway Hydration Therapies

Hypertonic Saline

Inhalation of hypertonic saline (IHS) improves mucociliary clearance.[76] Hypertonic saline rehydrates the airways through osmotic flow of water. When twice-daily inhaled normal saline was compared with 7% (hypertonic) sodium chloride, no difference was noted in the primary outcome, which was the linear rate of pulmonary function decline during the 48-week study period.[77] However, patients randomly assigned to receive IHS experienced a significant reduction in exacerbations (56% decrease vs. placebo, $p = 0.02$). In two small, randomized, crossover trials, dornase alfa provided a greater improvement in lung function, albeit at a much higher financial cost than IHS ($70/month). One approach is to consider the use of IHS in patients who are intolerant or do not respond to a trial of dornase alfa. In addition, IHS should be considered as add-on therapy in patients with airway congestion despite optimal standard therapy (i.e., dornase alfa and chest physiotherapy). A short-acting β_2-agonist should be given before IHS treatment because IHS has been associated with bronchospasm.[78] IHS is available commercially, and its use is recommended to improve lung function and reduce exacerbations in all patients 6 years of age or older.[70] If clinical symptoms warrant additional intervention, IHS may be considered for preschool children as well (Infant and pending preschool guidelines).

Bronchodilation

The chronic use of inhaled β_2-agonists improves lung function in patients with bronchial hyperresponsiveness or a positive bronchodilator response, and is recommended for use.[70] In addition, they may assist in airway clearance when administered before chest physiotherapy. No clear consensus exists for the use of other bronchodilators. Studies in support of inhaled anticholinergic medications for the treatment of CF also are limited, and the results have been mixed.[79]

CASE 21-2

QUESTION 1: J.P. is a 12-year-old girl who was seen for a routine quarterly visit at the CF center. J.P. was diagnosed with CF at age 7 months as a result of failure to thrive. Genotyping revealed she is homozygous for ΔF508. At this visit she has complaints of increased cough and chest congestion when compared with her visit 3 months ago. She has a history of hemoptysis, but has not had an episode recently. She has had no pulmonary exacerbations in the last 12 months. Her current medications include pancreatic enzymes (approximately 2,000 units of lipase/kg/meal) with all meals, a fat-soluble vitamin supplement, two puffs of albuterol inhaler before airway clearance treatment once daily, dornase alfa 2.5 mg via nebulization once daily, and fluticasone 44 mcg inhaler two puffs daily. She performs airway clearance using HFCWO for 30 minutes once daily and reports she is tolerating this therapy well. Microbiological cultures of her oropharyngeal tract grow *S. aureus*; she has not grown *P. aeruginosa* in the past. J.P.'s body mass index is in the 60th percentile (stable from last visit), and her lung function tests show an FEV_1 of 1.99 L (89% predicted), which is down from her baseline of 2.05 L (92% predicted). A recent chest computed tomography revealed mild bronchiectatic changes in all lobes as well as mucus plugging and air trapping. What steps should be taken to improve J.P.'s airway clearance?

Methods of mechanical assistance to remove pulmonary secretions are all equally effective, and the decision about which device to use should be individualized. J.P. is currently using HFCWO and appears to be tolerating this well. One advantage to this treatment is the independence it provides when compared with manual percussion and drainage, which requires the assistance of another individual. It is also efficient because the patient can perform some nebulization treatments while on the therapy vest (e.g., hypertonic saline).[70] This is especially an important consideration to improve adherence. The typical frequency and duration of treatment with HFCWO is 30 minutes twice daily. J.P. is currently using the therapy vest only once daily and could benefit from increasing the frequency of treatment to twice daily.

Dornase alfa improves sputum viscosity in patients with CF and provides benefit early in the course of the lung disease.[80] In the Pulmozyme Early Intervention Trial, the risk of pulmonary exacerbations was reduced by 34% in young patients with mild lung function abnormalities, and pulmonary function tests improved even in patients with close to normal pulmonary function. J.P. is currently receiving dornase alfa and should continue on this therapy to improve pulmonary function and reduce the risk of pulmonary exacerbations.

Hypertonic saline (7%) twice daily should also be considered for J.P. to enhance the mucociliary clearance and improve pulmonary function. The albuterol should be increased to twice daily to provide bronchodilation to prevent potential bronchospasm from the hypertonic saline. The recommended sequence of the treatments is albuterol for bronchodilation, hypertonic saline to hydrate the airways, and dornase alfa to liquefy the mucus, followed by airway clearance therapy to clear the mucus.[70] If adherence is an issue, the hypertonic saline can be administered during airway clearance treatment.

Control of Inflammation

The inflammatory response in CF airways contributes significantly to destruction of the airways and eventual pulmonary function decline. Pharmacological intervention to block the intense neutrophilic inflammatory response is a key strategy to reducing pulmonary disease progression. Corticosteroids, nonsteroidal anti-inflammatory drugs, and macrolides have all been used to control the inflammation seen in CF lung disease. Although leukotriene modifiers have improved lung function in small studies, the overall data are insufficient to support a recommendation for their use.[81] Cromolyn use is also not routinely recommended because of limited evidence of positive outcomes with this drug.[70]

CASE 21-2, QUESTION 2: Is J.P. a candidate for anti-inflammatory therapy?

CORTICOSTEROIDS

Oral corticosteroids are not recommended in the treatment of CF. Although prednisone 1 to 2 mg/kg every other day demonstrated a significant reduction in decline of lung function and decreased pulmonary exacerbations in patients with *Pseudomonas* infections, long-term use was associated with unacceptable adverse effects including cataracts, glucose intolerance, osteoporosis, and persistent growth retardation.[82–84] Although inhaled corticosteroids are widely prescribed to patients with CF, there are limited data supporting their use in this population. In particular, a randomized, controlled trial of withdrawal of inhaled corticosteroids demonstrated no change in pulmonary function after discontinuation; therefore, they are not recommended for routine use in patients with CF in the absence of concomitant asthma.[70,85] Fluticasone should be discontinued in J.P., and pulmonary function testing should be performed at the next clinic visit. In addition, J.P. should be questioned about wheezing or shortness of breath.

NONSTEROIDAL ANTI-INFLAMMATORY DRUGS

Nonsteroidal anti-inflammatory drugs have been used to slow lung function decline. High-dose ibuprofen (20–30 mg/kg twice daily with doses titrated to a peak concentration of 50–100 mg/L) can significantly slow the annual rate of FEV_1 decline in children between 5 and 13 years of age.[86] Ibuprofen serum concentrations must be measured and monitored closely to stay in the therapeutic range because lower concentrations can paradoxically increase neutrophil infiltration. Because these doses are much higher than the recommended doses to treat pain or fever, concerns about long-term side effects, including gastrointestinal bleeding and renal toxicity, together with the need for frequent blood draws have not made this method of treatment common. For patients at least 6 years of age with an FEV_1 greater than 60% of predicted, chronic oral ibuprofen is recommended to reduce the loss of lung function.[70] Considering J.P.'s history of hemoptysis, the use of high-dose ibuprofen is not recommended.

AZITHROMYCIN

Azithromycin is an antibiotic with anti-inflammatory properties. Although its use is established in patients with CF with chronic *P. aeruginosa* infection (see Case 26-3, Question 3), a recent study conducted in children and young adults who were not infected with *P. aeruginosa* demonstrated a significant reduction in exacerbation frequency (50%) and increased weight (0.58 kg) during the 24-week study period; however, no improvement in pulmonary function was noted.[87]

Because J.P. has not experienced any pulmonary exacerbations during the past year, there would be little advantage to adding azithromycin unless she becomes chronically infected with *P. aeruginosa*.[70]

ANTIBIOTIC THERAPY

Treatment of pulmonary infections in patients with CF has undoubtedly contributed to the improved survival observed in patients with CF in the past 30 years. Antibiotics are indicated in patients with CF for (a) early eradication of *P. aeruginosa* at the time of first detection with the intent to prevent or delay chronic infection, (b) treatment of acute pulmonary exacerbations, and (c) chronic maintenance therapy with inhaled antibiotics to control the bacterial burden within the airways with the goal of slowing the progression of pulmonary function decline.

Early Eradication of Pseudomonas Aeruginosa

CASE 21-2, QUESTION 3: J.P. returns to clinic 6 weeks later for a follow-up visit to evaluate response to changes made at the previous visit. Subjectively, she reports less chest congestion and cough. Spirometry demonstrates her FEV_1 has returned to baseline. A throat culture is obtained and reveals *P. aeruginosa*. What additional therapies should be considered for J.P. at this time?

Because of the increased rate of pulmonary function decline and shortened survival in patients chronically infected with *P. aeruginosa*, early treatment with the goal of eradication is recommended.[70] Results of two studies provide guidance on the optimal treatment approach. The Early Inhaled Tobramycin for Eradication trial demonstrated that treatment with inhaled tobramycin 300 mg twice daily for 28 or 56 days was similar in terms of eradication at 1 month (93% vs. 92%) and time to recurrence of *P. aeruginosa* (66% vs. 69% culture free at 27 months).[88] The Early Pseudomonas Infection Control trial demonstrated that therapy (inhaled tobramycin 300 mg twice daily for 28 days with or without ciprofloxacin twice daily for 14 days) initiated when quarterly respiratory cultures are positive for *P. aeruginosa* was not different in eradication or recurrence when compared with a similar antibiotic regimen cycled for 28 days followed by 56 days off for a period of six quarterly cycles.[89] Alternatively, results from a recent study conducted with aerosolized aztreonam 75 mg 3 times daily for 28 days in children older than 6 years with CF demonstrated eradication in 89.1% at the end of treatment and 58.2% remained culture negative at 28 weeks.[90] Based on the results of these two studies, it would be appropriate to start J.P. on inhaled tobramycin 300 mg twice daily or aztreonam 75 mg 3 times daily for 28 days. Cultures should be obtained on completion of the therapy to confirm eradication and quarterly thereafter to monitor for recurrence of *P. aeruginosa*.

Acute Pulmonary Exacerbation

Acute pulmonary exacerbations are an inevitable consequence of pulmonary disease in most patients with CF. A pulmonary exacerbation is defined as a change in respiratory signs and symptoms from the patient's baseline that necessitates treatment with antibiotics and augmented airway clearance. Key indicators include increased cough or sputum production, decreased exercise tolerance, loss of weight or appetite, decrease in FEV_1 or forced vital capacity (FVC) by more than 10%, or onset of new or increased crackles.[91] Approximately one-third of patients experience at least one pulmonary exacerbation annually; however, the onset and frequency varies widely in the population. The frequency of exacerbations is correlated with severity of pulmonary disease. Traditional management for an acute CF exacerbation includes nutritional repletion, antibiotics, and chest physiotherapy.[92] For mild exacerbations the patient can typically be managed in the outpatient setting using oral antibiotics and an intensification of airway clearance and nutritional therapies. For moderate to severe exacerbations, patients are typically hospitalized and receive a 14-day course of intravenous (IV) antibiotics, as well as airway clearance and nutrition therapies. If the patient demonstrates a significant improvement in signs and symptoms, he or she may be a candidate to complete treatment at home before completion of the 14-day course.[93]

ANTIBIOTIC DRUG SELECTION

Antibiotic drug selection is based on sputum or throat culture and susceptibility data. Combination therapy with two antibiotics with different mechanisms of action is often prescribed for treating acute pulmonary exacerbations involving *P. aeruginosa* to prevent the development of resistance and provide potential synergistic activity. Therefore, the combination of an antipseudomonal β-lactam and an aminoglycoside or fluoroquinolone is frequently used. Results of a controlled trial comparing β-lactam monotherapy versus β-lactam plus an aminoglycoside demonstrated similar improvement in pulmonary function, but greater reduction in bacterial density in sputum and a longer duration before readmission for a new pulmonary exacerbation in the patients receiving combination therapy.[94] Multidrug-resistant strains, defined as resistance to all agents within two of the three major classes of antipseudomonal therapies (e.g., β-lactams, aminoglycosides, and fluoroquinolones), are reported in 15% to 20% of patients. Treatment of infections involving these organisms may require the use of IV colistimethate. The use of IV colistin requires close monitoring as this drug exhibits both neurotoxic and nephrotoxic effects.

ANTIBIOTIC DOSING

The antibiotics used most commonly to treat acute pulmonary exacerbations and their dosage ranges are listed in Table 21-4. Typical dosage regimens used in other populations may not be adequate in patients with CF owing to reduced lung penetration, decreased activity in sputum, presence of bacteria within biofilms, heavy inocula, and reduced susceptibility. Altered pharmacokinetics of drugs in patients with CF is also frequently cited in the

Table 21-4
Antibiotic Doses for Cystic Fibrosis

	Systemic Antibiotics		
Drug	**Pediatric Dose**	**Adult Dose**	**Maximum Daily Dose**
Amikacin	30 mg/kg q24h	30 mg/kg q24h	TDM
Aztreonam	150 mg/kg/day divided q6-8h	2 gm q6h	8 g/day
Cefepime	150 mg/kg/day divided q6–8h	2 gm q6h	8 g/day
Ceftazidime	150 mg/kg/day divided q6–8h	2 gm q6h	8 g/day
Ciprofloxacin IV	30 mg/kg divided q8h	400 mg q8h	1.2 g/day
Ciprofloxacin PO	40 mg/kg divided q8-12h	750 mg q8–12h	2.25 g/day
Colistimethate	2.5–5 mg/kg/day divided q8h	2.5–5 mg/kg/day divided q8h	300 mg/day colistin base
Gentamicin	10 mg/kg q24h	10 mg/kg q24h	TDM
Imipenem	100 mg/kg/day divided q6h	1 g q6h	4 g/day
Meropenem	60–120 mg/kg/day divided q8h	2 g q8h	6 g/day
Piperacillin/tazobactam	400 mg/kg/day divided q6h	4.5 g q6h	16 g/day (piperacillin)
Ticarcillin/clavulanate	400 mg/kg/day divided q6h	3 g q6h	12 g/day (ticarcillin)
Tobramycin	10 mg/kg q24h	10 mg/kg q24h	TDM
TMP/SMZ	15–20 mg/kg/day divided q8h	15–20 mg/kg/day divided q8h	800 mg/day
	Inhaled Antibiotics		**Comments**
Drug	**Dosage (mg)**	**Interval**	
Aztreonam	75	TID	28 days on, 28 days off
Tobramycin nebulized	300	BID	28 days on, 28 days off
Tobramycin Podhaler	112 (4 × 28 mg capsules)	BID	28 days on, 28 days off
Colistin	37.5–75	BID	28 days on, 28 days off

BID, 2 times daily; TDM, therapeutic drug monitoring (gentamicin/tobramycin desired maximal concentration is 25–35 mg/L, AUC_{24h} = 70–100 mg/L × hour; once-daily dosing); TID, 3 times daily; TMP/SMZ, trimethoprim/sulfamethoxazole.
Adapted from Zobell et al. Optimization of anti-pseudomonal antibiotic for cystic fibrosis pulmonary exacerbations: VI. Executive summary. *Pediatr Pulmonol.* 2013;1.

published literature. In particular, both the volume of distribution and the clearance of a number of antibiotics (e.g., β-lactams and aminoglycosides) are reported to be higher in patients with CF when compared with healthy control subjects. Because many of the β-lactam antibiotics are cleared renally, it has been hypothesized that the enhanced renal clearance observed in patients with CF might be related to a higher tubular clearance as a result of upregulation of organic anion and cation transporters as a compensatory response to the CFTR defect.[95] However, subsequent controlled trials failed to confirm this hypothesis.[96,97] A more unifying explanation of the observed differences in pharmacokinetics in CF is related to differences in body composition. Patients with CF have reduced adipose tissue and lean mass owing to nutritional deficiencies. If the pharmacokinetic parameters are normalized to body weight (e.g., L/kg and L/kg/hour), then the parameters would appear to exceed that of normal healthy individuals. This observation was recently demonstrated in a clinical trial evaluating the pharmacokinetics of ceftazidime in CF. The intersubject variability in pharmacokinetic parameters was significantly reduced when the parameters were normalized to fat-free mass, indicating that fat-free mass is a better metric for normalization.[98] Importantly, the authors observed that the pharmacokinetic parameters appeared higher when normalized to body weight; however, when normalized to fat-free mass, there was no significant difference.

β-Lactam antibiotics can be administered as an intermittent, prolonged, or continuous infusion. Prolonged or continuous infusion are designed to maximize the time the concentrations exceed the minimum inhibitory concentration.[98] This is particularly important in patients with CF because of the rapid clearance (excellent renal function) and reduced susceptibility of the organisms within the airways.[99]

Extended-interval dosing of aminoglycosides (every 24 hours compared with every 8 hours) is easier and less costly to administer, and potentially limits toxicity. A randomized clinical trial in children and adults with CF ($n = 244$) demonstrated equivalent efficacy as evidenced by a change in FEV_1 in approximately 10% in patients receiving tobramycin 10 mg/kg/day either as a single dose or in three divided doses. However, the once-daily regimen provided improved renal safety in children as evidenced by serum creatinine and urinary *N*-acetyl-β-D-glucosaminidase, a biomarker of renal proximal tubular injury.[100] An evidence-based review conducted by the Cystic Fibrosis Foundation concluded that once-daily dosing of aminoglycosides is preferable to 3 times–daily dosing for treatment of an acute exacerbation of pulmonary disease.[93]

Routine monitoring of serum aminoglycoside concentrations is recommended to maximize efficacy and minimize the risk of toxicity. Because many patients with CF receive multiple courses of aminoglycosides, sometimes for extended durations, they are particularly predisposed to the toxicities. With once-daily dosing the trough concentrations are expected to be unmeasureable by design (e.g., dosing interval exceeds 5 half-lives). Therefore, serum concentrations are typically obtained between 1 to 2 and

6 to 8 hours after the end of the infusion. The two levels can then be used to determine the extrapolated peak concentration (target 20–30 mg/L) and the area under the serum concentration–time curve (target 72–100 mg/L × hour).[101]

CASE 21-3

QUESTION 1: B.W., a 19-year-old man, was diagnosed with CF at 3 years of age after a history of chronic pneumonias. He presents to the pulmonary clinic with increasing cough and sputum production during the past 2 weeks, with a change in sputum color from white to green. He was last admitted for treatment of an acute pulmonary exacerbation 6 months ago. He currently weighs 45.2 kg and states he has lost 4 pounds. B.W. is a slightly thin adult man whose breathing is labored. Pulmonary function tests reveal an FEV_1 of 75% of predicted and an FVC of 70% (his usual baselines are FEV_1, 85%, and FVC, 80%). *P. aeruginosa* grew out of his sputum sample taken at the clinic 4 weeks ago and demonstrated susceptibility to ceftazidime, piperacillin, imipenem, tobramycin, and colistin, and intermediate susceptibility to ciprofloxacin. Other pertinent laboratory findings are as follows:

White blood cell count, 17,000/μL, with 4% bands, 35% segmented neutrophils, 50% lymphocytes, and 11% eosinophils
Blood urea nitrogen (BUN), 7 mg/dL
Creatinine, 0.5 mg/dL

All other blood work, liver function tests, and electrolytes are within normal limits. Heart rate and blood pressure are normal. Temperature is 99.2°F, respiratory rate is 25 breaths/minute with an oxygen saturation of 95%. A number of new pulmonary infiltrates are seen on chest radiograph. His current medications include the following: one fat-soluble vitamin twice daily, two microencapsulated pancreatic enzyme capsules (16,000 units of lipase/capsule) with meals, and one or two capsules with snacks as needed, and dornase alfa 2.5 mg nebulized daily. What subjective and objective findings does B.W. exhibit that would lead to the diagnosis of a pulmonary exacerbation?

B.W. demonstrates an increase in sputum production (purulent), increased cough, dyspnea, weight loss, and a 10% decline in pulmonary function tests from baseline. B.W. also has a mild fever and elevated white blood cell count; however, an increase in white blood cell count, fever, or appearance of a new infiltrate on chest radiograph may or may not be present in all cases of pulmonary exacerbations.

CASE 21-3, QUESTION 2: B.W. is admitted to the hospital for treatment of an acute pulmonary exacerbation. What would be an appropriate antimicrobial treatment plan for B.W. based on his current laboratory data?

Based on these findings and the in vitro susceptibility results, it would be reasonable to initiate a regimen of ceftazidime or piperacillin in combination with tobramycin. Ciprofloxacin is not optimal in this instance because of reduced susceptibility. Imipenem and colistin are typically reserved for treatment of resistant *P. aeruginosa* infections.

Ceftazidime 2 g IV every 6 hours could be administered to B.W. by intermittent, 3 hour prolonged infusion, or a 2 g loading dose administered for 30 minutes followed by 6 g as a continuous infusion. Recent data from a large randomized trial demonstrated similar efficacy and safety between intermittent and continuous infusion ceftazidime in patients with CF; however, the continuous infusion treatment was associated with greater improvement in pulmonary function in those infected with resistant strains. In addition, continuous infusion resulted in a significantly prolonged interval between exacerbations.[99]

In B.W., the preferred initial dosing regimen of IV tobramycin would be 440 mg (10 mg/kg) every 24 hours. Target peak concentrations of 20 to 30 mg/L should be verified after the first or second dose. Target area under the concentration–time curve should be 72 to 100 mg/L × hour. Tobramycin concentrations should be measured at least every 7 days while B.W. is on therapy. In addition, serum concentrations of BUN and creatinine should be measured 3 times weekly for early detection of acute kidney injury.

The antibiotics should be administered for 2 weeks, and extended for an additional 7 days if B.W. fails to reach specified end points at day 14. After the initiation of antibiotics in this hospitalization, home IV antibiotic therapy should be a consideration for B.W.[102] The decision as to whether a patient is a good candidate for home IV antibiotic therapy is based on initial response as well as the expected level of support provided to the patient at home. In particular, the ability of the patient to maintain nutritional and intensive airway clearance programs established in the hospital needs to be assessed. The duration of B.W.'s antibiotic therapy should be based on his clinical response. Ideally, his pulmonary function (e.g., FEV_1) should improve by 10% to 20% and should be evaluated weekly. The purulent nature and volume of the sputum should decrease and a gradual overall improvement in subjective feeling should be noted. Improved appetite and increased weight gain should be assessed daily with the goal of reaching baseline weight (increase of 1–2 kg/week). For patients receiving repeated courses of IV aminoglycosides, periodic audiometric testing is recommended.

CHRONIC MAINTENANCE THERAPY WITH ORAL OR INHALED ANTIBIOTICS

Recognition of the progressive decline in pulmonary function despite aggressive treatment of acute exacerbations and the availability of oral and inhaled therapies with activity against typical CF pathogens have led to increased use of chronic maintenance antibiotic therapy. The goal of chronic maintenance therapy is to suppress bacterial infection to reduce the frequency and severity of pulmonary exacerbations and to slow the progressive deterioration in lung function. Inhaled antibiotics include tobramycin, aztreonam, and colistimethate. Inhaled antibiotics are desirable because of the relatively high sputum concentrations and low systemic bioavailability, which maximizes efficacy and minimizes toxicity.

Tobramycin for Inhalation

Results of phase 3 studies of inhaled tobramycin conducted during a 6-month interval demonstrated significant improvement in pulmonary function (relative difference in FEV_1 of 10%), a reduction in the risk of hospitalization (37%), and a reduced need for IV antipseudomonal antibiotics (32%).[103] A significantly greater proportion of patients in the treatment arm reported hoarseness; however, this did not require discontinuation and improved with time. In addition, some patients report a bitter taste to this preparation; however, this typically does not result in discontinuation of the medication. The recommended dosage of tobramycin nebulizer solution is 300 mg twice daily in a cycle of 28 days on and 28 days off. Tobramycin for inhalation is provided as a premixed solution contained in unit dose vials and requires refrigeration before use. Tobramycin for inhalation is administered via a vented jet nebulizer system (Pari LC Plus) to ensure consistent particle size and outflow characteristics. Based on the results of the phase 3 studies, inhaled tobramycin is indicated in patients older than 6 years of age with repeated sputum cultures demonstrating *P. aeruginosa* and FEV_1 between 25% and 75% of predicted.[70] Fortunately, there is a dry powder formulation of tobramycin for inhalation (TOBI podhaler) which offers the advantages of shortened administration time, no need for refrigeration, and easy portability. TOBI podhaler is provided in 28 mg capsules and is administered as four capsules twice daily in a cycle of 28 days on and 28 days off.

Aztreonam Lysine Solution for Inhalation

Two phase 3 trials evaluated the short-term safety and efficacy of aztreonam lysine solution for inhalation.[103,104] The results of these trials demonstrated a significant improvement in respiratory symptoms assessed using a patient-reported outcome instrument, and a significant delay in the need for inhaled or IV antipseudomonal antibiotics determined by the presence of pulmonary exacerbation symptoms. The most common adverse effects are cough and wheezing. Bronchodilator use is recommended before each dose to reduce these symptoms. The recommended dosage of aztreonam lysine is 75 mg 3 times daily for 28 days. Aztreonam is provided in a powder form that requires reconstitution with saline before administration. Aztreonam requires refrigeration before use. A special nebulizer device is required for administration (Altera), which delivers the drug in a relatively short time (e.g., 2–3 minutes). Based on the results of these studies, aztreonam lysine is indicated in CF patients older than 6 years of age with *P. aeruginosa* to improve respiratory symptoms. Aztreonam is particularly useful in patients who are intolerant of inhaled tobramycin, or as add-on therapy in those with frequent exacerbations or continued decline in pulmonary function.

Colistimethate

Colistimethate is a prodrug of colistin, an antibiotic in the polymyxin family. Colistimethate is available only in an IV powder formulation in the United States and requires reconstitution before nebulization. Clinical trials evaluating the safety and efficacy of colistimethate in CF are limited by the small number of patients enrolled in the trials. Based on the lack of data, colistimethate is not recommended for routine use.[70] Colistimethate may be useful in patients infected with multidrug-resistant *P. aeruginosa* or those intolerant to other inhaled antibiotics. Adverse effects associated with inhaled colistimethate include cough and bronchospasm. Bronchodilators should be used before each dose. In addition, colistimethate tends to foam on nebulization, resulting in incomplete drug administration. The typical dose of colistimethate is 75 mg twice daily.

The cost of inhaled antibiotics is relatively high (tobramycin solution for inhalation $7,000/month, aztreonam lysine solution for inhalation $7,000/month, colistimethate $1,800/month (http://www.walgreens.com/topic/pharmacy/cystic-fibrosis-services.jsp); however, use of inhaled antibiotics reduces hospital days, leading to substantial savings in direct medical costs that may offset its acquisition price. The cost-effectiveness of inhaled antibiotics would be expected to be greatest in patients experiencing relatively frequent exacerbations (two or more hospital admissions per year). A short-term trial (e.g., 1–2 months) is warranted in patients with CF chronically colonized with *P. aeruginosa* to assess improvement in pulmonary function. A longer trial period (e.g., up to 1 year) may be necessary to assess the impact on hospitalizations. Patients should be instructed in the proper use and maintenance of the nebulizer and compressor system used in its delivery. In particular, it is important to wash reusable nebulizers between uses to avoid buildup that can reduce their effectiveness. The nebulizers can be hand-washed with liquid dish soap or placed in the top rack of a dishwasher for cleaning. After each cleaning the nebulizer should be allowed to dry before reusing to reduce bacterial contamination. Regular sterilization is required to reduce the potential for bacterial contamination. In addition, the patient should be instructed not to dilute or mix antibiotic solutions with other drugs in the nebulizer, which can alter the delivery characteristics. Inhaled antibiotics are typically administered after the bronchodilator, dornase alfa, and airway clearance therapies to maximize retention time within the airways.

Azithromycin

Oral azithromycin is frequently prescribed to patients with CF owing to its anti-inflammatory and antivirulence properties. The macrolide antibiotics do not exhibit significant antibacterial activity against *P. aeruginosa* using conventional susceptibility testing methods; however, they do inhibit alginate production, the principal component of biofilms. Because of its favorable pharmacokinetics and reduced potential for drug interactions, most studies have evaluated azithromycin. Results of a multicenter randomized, controlled trial demonstrated treatment with azithromycin was associated with a significant improvement in FEV_1 (6%) and a reduction in hospitalizations for acute pulmonary exacerbations (44%).[105] The beneficial effect of azithromycin on pulmonary function was additive with other chronic therapies such as aerosolized tobramycin and dornase alfa. Azithromycin is generally well tolerated. Nausea, vomiting, and wheezing are the most common adverse effects reported. Based on current data, azithromycin is indicated in patients older than 6 years who are colonized with *P. aeruginosa*.[95] Based on the pivotal trial, the dose of azithromycin is 500 mg 3 times/week for patients weighing more than 40 kg and 250 mg 3 times weekly for patients weighing less than 40 kg. One contraindication to treatment with azithromycin is colonization with mycobacteria because of the potential for development of resistance.

CASE 21-3, QUESTION 3: B.W. comes to the outpatient clinic 2 weeks after hospital discharge for a follow-up visit and reports a significant reduction in cough and sputum production, and no shortness of breath. Spirometry reveals an FEV_1 of 85% of predicted. He has resumed his outpatient treatment regimen, which includes one multiple vitamin every day, two microencapsulated pancreatic enzyme capsules (16,000 units of lipase/capsule) with meals, and one or two capsules with snacks as needed, and dornase alfa 2.5 mg nebulized daily. What changes, if any, should be made to B.W.'s treatment regimen?

Because B.W. has had two exacerbations in the last 6 months, he would benefit from the addition of medications to reduce the frequency of exacerbations. In addition to the disruption to his life, frequent exacerbations are associated with more rapid decline in pulmonary function and reduced survival.[106] Key pharmacological therapies demonstrated to improve pulmonary function and reduce the frequency of pulmonary exacerbations include dornase alfa, inhaled tobramycin or aztreonam, IHS, and azithromycin. B.W. is already receiving dornase alfa, but is not on inhaled tobramycin or aztreonam, IHS, or azithromycin. One important consideration when adding new therapies is the treatment burden, particularly with inhaled therapies. Inhaled tobramycin 112 mg twice daily via the podhaler cycled for 28 days on and 28 days off and oral azithromycin 500 mg every Monday, Wednesday, and Friday would be appropriate additions to the treatment regimen because B.W. is chronically infected with *P. aeruginosa*, and these particular agents demonstrated the greatest improvement in pulmonary function when compared with IHS. In addition, azithromycin has a minimal effect on treatment burden as it can be administered orally 3 days a week. IHS would also be of benefit by reducing exacerbation frequency; however, it could be added in the future if B.W. demonstrates a decline in pulmonary function or increased frequency of exacerbations despite the new additions.

Oral Antibiotics

CASE 21-3, QUESTION 4: One year later, B.W. returns to the clinic exhibiting signs and symptoms of a mild exacerbation, but refuses IV antibiotics or hospitalization because he is in the middle of final examinations. What alternative to IV therapy is available to treat B.W.?

The quinolone family of antibiotics is currently the only option for oral treatment of *P. aeruginosa*. Emergence of resistant strains of *Staphylococcus* and *Pseudomonas* species have led the CF medical community to restrict the use of quinolones to the treatment of acute CF exacerbations.[107,108] Oral fluoroquinolones (e.g., ciprofloxacin) have become widely used in patients with CF because they are less expensive, easy to administer, and as effective as IV therapy in an acute exacerbation.[109,110]

Because of the past sensitivities of B.W.'s organisms and his refusal to be admitted to the hospital, ciprofloxacin 1,000 mg orally twice daily for 1 week can be initiated in addition to the aerosolized tobramycin and oral azithromycin.[111] After 1 week of the combined aerosol and oral therapies, B.W. should be re-evaluated for hospital admission if his condition worsens, or his therapy can be continued if his condition improves.

CASE 21-3, QUESTION 5: B.W. returns to the outpatient clinic 3 months later for his annual comprehensive visit. Results of laboratory studies, dual-emission x-ray absorptiometry (DXA) scan, spirometry, and an oral glucose tolerance test (OGTT) are as follows:

BUN, 10 mg/dL
Creatinine, 0.6 mg/dL
Urine microalbumin/creatinine, 12 mcg/mg
2-hour OGTT plasma glucose, 220 mg/dL
Glycosylated hemoglobin, 7.8%
DXA Z-score, −2.1 (pelvis)
FEV_1, 83% of predicted

How should these laboratory studies be interpreted and what new therapies would you recommend?

The elevated 2-hour OGTT plasma glucose indicates B.W. has CF-related diabetes mellitus. This is confirmed by the elevated glycosylated hemoglobin. The urine microalbumin testing indicates that B.W. is not spilling protein into the urine as a result of the CF-related diabetes mellitus. Treatment with insulin should be initiated in B.W. to improve nutritional status and prevent microvascular complications. The DXA scan results indicate B.W. has osteopenia and should be initiated on calcium 500 mg orally twice daily and his vitamin D status should be determined. Treatment of osteopenia is recommended to prevent progression to osteoporosis, which would put the patient at risk for fractures. In addition, osteoporosis is a relative contraindication for lung transplantation because of the risk for fractures after transplantation that may impair adequate recovery.

B.W.'s spirometry results indicate that his pulmonary function is stable and his current pharmacotherapeutic regimen should be continued.

LUNG TRANSPLANTATION

Pulmonary disease progression leading to eventual respiratory failure is an inevitable consequence of the chronic cycle of airway obstruction, infection, and inflammation. End-stage lung disease (defined by an FEV_1 of <30% of predicted) significantly affects the quality of life for patients with CF as a result of reduced exercise tolerance, heavy treatment burden, need for oxygen therapy, and frequent hospitalizations for pulmonary exacerbations. Lung transplantation is a potential therapeutic option for CF patients with end-stage lung disease.[112] The optimal time to refer a patient for lung transplantation is not precisely defined; however, patients are typically referred when their FEV_1 is approximately 40% to maximize the chances of obtaining new lungs before the patient experiences respiratory failure. Transplant evaluation includes assessments of pulmonary disease severity, patient adherence to therapies, and concomitant illnesses. Once accepted into the program, the patient is placed on the transplant list awaiting availability of potential organs. The waiting time to receive a lung transplant is highly variable and depends on the Lung Allocation Score, a score that distributes organs on the basis of model-predicted benefit from transplantation. The mean survival after lung transplantation is approximately 50% at 5 years. Importantly, the quality of life for many lung transplant recipients improves significantly.

KEY REFERENCES AND WEBSITES

A full list of references for this chapter can be found at http://thepoint.lww.com/AT11e. Below are the key references and websites for this chapter, with the corresponding reference number in this chapter found in parentheses after the reference.

Key References

Mogayzel PJ et al. Cystic fibrosis pulmonary guidelines: chronic medications for maintenance of lung health. *Am J Respir Crit Care Med.* 2013;7:280.

Stallings VA et al. Evidence-based practice recommendations for nutrition-related management of children and adults with cystic fibrosis and pancreatic insufficiency: results of a systematic review. *J Am Diet Assoc.* 2008;108:832. (80)

Key Websites

Cystic Fibrosis Foundation. Drug Development Pipeline. http://www.cff.org/research/DrugDevelopmentPipeline/.

Cystic Fibrosis Mutation Database. http://www.genet.sickkids.on.ca/cftr/app.

Johns Hopkins Cystic Fibrosis Center. http://www.hopkinscf.org/main/whatiscf/index.html.

Section Editor: Carrie A. Sincak

22 Nausea and Vomiting

Lisa M. DiGrazia and Joseph Todd Carter

CORE PRINCIPLES

		CHAPTER CASES
MOTION SICKNESS		
1	Motion sickness is caused by discordant information about body position or motion received from visual, vestibular, or body proprioceptors. Acetylcholine is thought to be the primary neurotransmitter involved.	**Case 22-1 (Question 1)**
2	Transdermal scopolamine is recommended for prophylaxis of motion sickness for moderate to severe stimuli. Dimenhydrinate or promethazine is recommended for treatment of breakthrough symptoms. The most common adverse effects of these agents include drowsiness, confusion, and dry mouth.	**Case 22-1 (Question 2), Table 22-1**
CHEMOTHERAPY-INDUCED NAUSEA AND VOMITING		
1	Nausea and vomiting are initiated by several stimuli and mediated by several neurotransmitters in the central nervous system, peripheral nervous system, and gastrointestinal tract. Because of the multiple neurotransmitter receptors involved, successful prophylaxis and treatment of chemotherapy-induced nausea and vomiting will almost always require medications with more than one mechanism of action.	**Case 22-2 (Question 1)**
2	The likelihood of nausea and vomiting depends on patient risk factors and, most importantly, on the emetogenicity of the chemotherapy agents prescribed. The antiemetic regimen should be appropriate for the chemotherapy agent with the highest emetogenicity level.	**Case 22-2 (Question 1), Table 22-2**
3	Patients receiving moderate to highly emetogenic chemotherapy should receive prophylaxis with an aprepitant-, netupitant-, or olanzapine-containing regimen. The backbone of these regimens includes a 5-hydroxytryptamine receptor type 3 (5-HT_3) antagonist and dexamethasone.	**Case 22-2 (Question 2), Tables 22-3, 22-4, Figures 22-2, 22-3**
4	For breakthrough symptoms, patients should receive rescue antiemetics with a different mechanism of action than the prophylactic medications and receive more aggressive antiemetics before the next cycle of chemotherapy.	**Case 22-2 (Question 3), Tables 22-3, 22-4, Figures 22-2, 22-3**
RADIATION-INDUCED NAUSEA AND VOMITING		
1	Radiation can cause nausea and vomiting by the same pathways as chemotherapy. The risk depends on the area and size of the radiation field as well as the fractional dose of radiation and whether the patient has had chemotherapy in the past.	**Case 22-3 (Question 1), Table 22-5**
2	The recommended prophylaxis for radiation-induced nausea and vomiting includes a 5-HT_3 antagonist with dexamethasone for high-risk patients and with or without dexamethasone for patients at moderate risk. Breakthrough symptoms may be treated with a 5-HT_3 antagonist or dopamine antagonist.	**Case 22-3 (Question 1), Table 22-5**

Continued

POSTOPERATIVE NAUSEA AND VOMITING	CHAPTER CASES
1 The risk of postoperative nausea and vomiting depends on several patient-related, surgical, and anesthetic factors. The antiemetic regimen should be proportional to the risk factors.	**Case 22-4 (Question 1), Table 22-6**
2 The most active agents in preventing postoperative nausea and vomiting are 5-HT_3 antagonists. For patients at moderate to high risk, a 5-HT_3 antagonist should be combined with dexamethasone or droperidol. Antiemetics used for rescue therapy should be of a different class than the prophylactic agents used.	**Case 22-4 (Question 1), Table 22-6**

DEFINITION

Nausea and vomiting are unpleasant symptoms caused by self-limiting disorders or serious conditions such as cancer. These symptoms can range from mild, short-lived nausea to continuing severe emesis and retching. The emetic response can be described in three phases: nausea, vomiting, and retching. *Nausea* is the subjective feeling of the need to vomit. It includes an unpleasant sensation in the mouth and stomach and can be associated with salivation, sweating, dizziness, and tachycardia. *Vomiting* is the forceful expulsion of the stomach contents through the mouth but is preceded by the relaxation of the esophageal sphincter, contraction of the abdominal muscles, and temporary suspension of breathing. *Retching* is the rhythmic contraction of the abdominal muscles without actual emesis. It can accompany nausea or occur before or after emesis.

EPIDEMIOLOGY AND CLINICAL PRESENTATION

Nausea and vomiting are caused by many disorders. Central nervous system (CNS) causes include increased intracranial pressure, migraine headaches, brain metastases, vestibular dysfunction, alcohol intoxication, and anxiety. Infectious disease causes include viral gastroenteritis, food poisoning, peritonitis, meningitis, and urinary tract infections. Metabolic causes include hypercalcemia, uremia, hyperglycemia, and hyponatremia. Gastrointestinal (GI) disorders, such as gastroparesis, bowel obstruction, distension, and mechanical irritation, can cause nausea and vomiting. Among the many medications that can cause nausea and vomiting are cancer chemotherapy, antibiotics, antifungals, and opiate analgesics.

In addition to the suffering involved, uncontrolled vomiting can lead to dehydration, electrolyte imbalances, malnutrition, aspiration pneumonia, and esophageal tears. Nausea and vomiting often reduces food intake and can impair a person's ability to care for himself or herself. Significant reductions in quality-of-life scores have been demonstrated in cancer patients with chemotherapy-induced nausea and vomiting (CINV) compared with patients who did not have those symptoms.[1]

PATHOPHYSIOLOGY

The CNS, the peripheral nervous system, and the GI tract are all involved in initiating and coordinating the emetic response. In the CNS, the vomiting center (VC) receives incoming signals from other parts of the brain and the GI tract, and then coordinates the emetic response by sending signals to the effector organs. The VC is located in the medulla oblongata of the brain, near the nucleus tractus solitarius (NTS). The VC is stimulated by neurotransmitters released from the chemoreceptor trigger zone (CTZ), the GI tract, the cerebral cortex, the limbic system, and the vestibular system (Fig. 22-1). The major neurotransmitter receptors associated with the emetic response include serotonin (the 5-hydroxytryptamine type 3 [5-HT_3]) receptors, neurokinin 1 (NK1) receptors, and dopamine receptors. Other receptors involved include corticosteroid, acetylcholine, histamine, cannabinoid, gabaminergic, and opiate receptors. Many of these receptors are targets for antiemetic therapy.

In the CNS, the CTZ is located in the area postrema on the floor of the fourth ventricle in the brainstem; it lies outside the blood–brain barrier. When the CTZ senses toxins and noxious substances in the blood or cerebrospinal fluid, it triggers the emetic response by releasing neurotransmitters that travel to the VC and NTS. The major neurotransmitter receptors include serotonin, dopamine, and NK1.

The GI system also plays a large part in the initiation of the emetic response. The GI tract contains enterochromaffin cells in the GI mucosa. When these cells are damaged by chemotherapy, radiation, anesthetics, or mechanical irritation, serotonin is released, which can stimulate the vagal afferents as well as directly stimulate the VC and NTS. The VC then initiates the emetic response.

The cerebral cortex and limbic system can stimulate the emetic center in response to emotional states, such as anxiety, pain, and conditioned responses (anticipatory nausea and vomiting). The neurotransmitters involved in this pathway are less well understood. Disorders of the vestibular system, such as vertigo and motion sickness, stimulate the VC through acetylcholine and histamine release.

DIAGNOSIS

The initial evaluation of the patient with nausea and vomiting should include the onset of symptoms, the severity and duration of symptoms, hydration status, precipitating factors, current medical conditions and medications, and food and infectious contacts. The etiology of the nausea and vomiting should be determined, if possible, so that underlying conditions can be treated specifically. Supportive treatment should be initiated, if needed, including fluid and electrolyte replacement. If the nausea and vomiting is mild and self-limited, antiemetic therapy may not be required. For others, however, the appropriate antiemetic therapy will depend on the patient and the etiology of the nausea and vomiting.

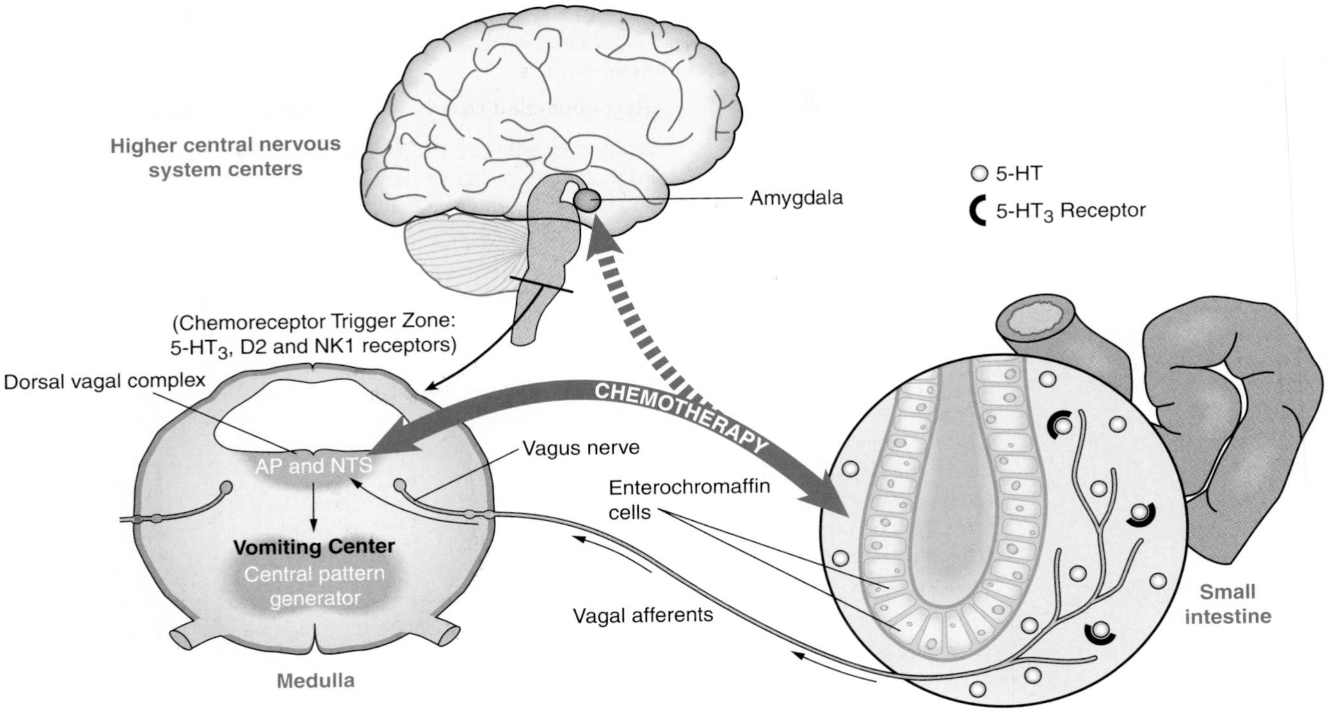

Figure 22-1 Pathways by which chemotherapeutic agents may produce an emetic response. AP, anterior pituitary; D, days; NTS, nucleus tractus solitarius; 5-HT, 5-hydroxytryptamine; 5-HT_3, 5-hydroxytryptamine type 3 receptor.

MOTION SICKNESS

Clinical Presentation and Risk Factors

CASE 22-1

QUESTION 1: P.C. is a 27-year-old woman who has no significant medical history, with the exception of moderate dysmenorrhea and motion sickness associated with travel by air. Previously, she has taken dimenhydrinate before airplane trips with moderate success. She is engaged to be married, and she and her fiancé have decided on a weeklong Caribbean cruise for their honeymoon. P.C. is concerned that she may also develop sea sickness and that dimenhydrinate may not control her symptoms, particularly in the event of rough weather at sea. Will P.C. be at higher risk for motion sickness?

The symptoms of motion sickness occur in response to an unusual perception of real or apparent motion. In these situations, there is sensory conflict about body position or motion through the visual, vestibular, or body proprioceptors. Acetylcholine is thought to be the primary neurotransmitter involved in signaling the VC, as is histamine, but to a lesser extent. Adrenergic stimulation can block this transmission. Symptoms begin with stomach discomfort and progress to salivation changes, sweating, dizziness, lethargy, retching, and emesis. The risk of motion sickness is low in children younger than 2 years. The risk is highest in children and adolescents compared with adults, and higher in women than men. In some individuals, sensitivity to motion sickness diminishes with time.[2] Travel by boat is most likely to cause symptoms; air, car, and train travel is less likely to cause them.[3,4] Severity of the motion sickness is highly dependent on the individual and also varies with the weather and position in the plane or boat. Because of P.C.'s history and her travel plans, she is at high risk for recurrence of her motion sickness symptoms.

Nonpharmacologic Measures

CASE 22-1, QUESTION 2: What nonpharmacologic methods could PC employ to reduce her chance of developing motion sickness?

Nonpharmacologic measures or natural remedies may be useful for reducing motion sickness.[2] These include riding in the middle of the boat or plane, where the motion is less dramatic, lying in a semirecumbent position, fixing the vision on the horizon, avoiding reading, and closing the eyes if below deck or in the cabin. Many people recommend keeping active on a ship to "get their sea-legs" faster through habituation. The effectiveness of acupressure at the P6 point of the wrist (about three finger-breadths above the wrist) is unclear. A controlled-stimulus trial compared two brands of wristbands with placebo; neither band was more effective than placebo in preventing symptoms of motion sickness.[5] Studies of ginger preparations also are equivocal. The action of ginger may be through enhanced gastric emptying and not on the vestibular system.[6,7]

Overview of Treatment

CASE 22-1, QUESTION 3: For P.C., what medications are available to prevent and treat motion sickness symptoms?

Anticholinergic agents and antihistamines that cross the blood–brain barrier effectively prevent and treat motion sickness.[3,4] In general, these medications are more effective in preventing than treating established symptoms. The 5-HT_3 receptor antagonists and NK1 receptor antagonists have not been shown to be effective in preventing motion sickness.[2,6] Nonsedating antihistamines are not as effective as other antihistamines because they do not sufficiently cross the blood–brain barrier.[2,3] Scopolamine has been well studied for the prevention of motion sickness and is highly effective.[2,8] In a controlled trial, scopolamine was more effective

Table 22-1

Medications for Prevention or Treatment of Motion Sickness in Adults

Medication (Trade Name)	Dosage	Recommended Use	Adverse Effects
Scopolamine (Transderm-Scop)	1.5 mg TOP behind the ear every 3 days. Apply at least 3 hours (preferably 6–8 hours) before exposure.	Long-term exposure (>6 hours) to moderate to intense stimulus. Alternative treatment for shorter or milder stimulus.	Dry mouth, drowsiness, blurred vision, confusion, fatigue, ataxia
Dimenhydrinate (Dramamine)	50–100 mg PO every 4–6 hours (max 400 mg/day). May be taken PRN or on scheduled basis if required.	Short- or long-term exposure to mild to moderate stimulus. Alternative for intense stimulus.	Drowsiness, dry mouth, thickening of secretions, dizziness
Promethazine (Phenergan)	25 mg PO every 4–6 hours. May be taken PRN or on scheduled basis if required. 25–50 mg IM every 4–6 hours for established severe symptoms. May be taken PRN or on scheduled basis if required.	In combination with dextroamphetamine for short exposure to intense stimulus. Alternative for longer or milder stimulus.	Drowsiness, orthostatic hypotension, dry mouth
Meclizine (Dramamine Less Drowsy, Bonine)	12.5–50 mg PO every 6–24 hours. May be taken PRN or on scheduled basis if required.	Alternative for mild stimulus or in combination for moderate to severe stimulus.	Drowsiness, dry mouth, thickening of secretions, dizziness
Dextroamphetamine (Dexedrine)	5–10 mg PO every 4–6 hours. May be taken PRN or on scheduled basis if required.	In combination with promethazine for short exposure of intense stimulus.	Restlessness, abuse potential, insomnia, overstimulation, tachycardia, palpitations, hypertension

IM, intramuscular; PO, oral; PRN, as needed; TOP, topically.

Source: Priesol AJ. Motion sickness. In: *UpToDate*. **http://www.uptodate.com/contents/motion-sickness**. Accessed September 9, 2015; Shupak A, Gordon CR. Motion sickness: advances in pathogenesis, prediction, prevention, and treatment. *Aviat Space Environ Med*. 2006;77:1213.

than promethazine, and both were more effective than placebo, meclizine, or lorazepam.[9] Scopolamine is available as a topical patch, which bypasses the problem of GI symptoms associated with motion sickness. Table 22-1 describes medications effective for motion sickness based on the intensity of the stimulus, adult doses, and potential adverse effects.

Because P.C. is susceptible in a moderate to severe stimulus situation, prevention with a scopolamine patch applied behind the ear every 3 days, starting 6 to 8 hours before departure, should be recommended. If she experiences breakthrough symptoms, dimenhydrinate or promethazine may be useful. She should be advised about the potential adverse effects of these agents, which include drowsiness, confusion, and dry mouth.

CHEMOTHERAPY-INDUCED NAUSEA AND VOMITING

CINV occurs in many patients receiving chemotherapy for cancer.[1] The mechanisms of the emetic response described at the beginning of this chapter apply to CINV as well. The major neurotransmitter receptors involved in these pathways include 5-HT_3, NK1, and dopamine receptors. CINV can occur in different phases. Acute-phase CINV symptoms occur within a few hours after the administration of the chemotherapy. These symptoms often peak several hours after administration and can last for the first 24 hours. Some antineoplastic agents can also cause nausea and vomiting symptoms for a longer time after chemotherapy administration. These delayed CINV symptoms peak in about 2 to 3 days and can last 6 to 7 days. Some patients may experience acute symptoms without delayed symptoms or delayed symptoms without acute symptoms, whereas others experience CINV in both the acute and delayed phases. Some patients who have received previous chemotherapy treatments may experience a conditioned response in which they have symptoms even before the chemotherapy starts. This is called anticipatory nausea and vomiting and is difficult to treat because it is primarily triggered by poor nausea and vomiting control in previous cycles. Breakthrough nausea and vomiting occur if the primary prophylactic antiemetics fail to work completely. Of course, regardless of the time course and cause, these are very distressing, unpleasant, and disruptive symptoms for the patient.

The likelihood of CINV depends on several factors.[1] Patient-related factors that increase the risk of acute-phase CINV include age under 50 years, female sex, poor control of symptoms in prior cycles, history of motion sickness or nausea with pregnancy, anxiety, or depression. A significant history of alcoholism actually protects against CINV. Delayed symptoms are more common in women, in those who have had poor emetic control in the acute phase, and in patients with anxiety or depression.

Chemotherapy-related factors also predict the likelihood of symptoms. Factors such as shorter infusion time, higher dose, and more chemotherapy cycles increase the risk of CINV. With multiday chemotherapy regimens, the symptoms usually peak around the third to fourth day of chemotherapy, when the acute symptoms caused by the later days' doses are overlapping with the delayed symptoms from the first days' doses. The most predictive factor, however, is the chemotherapy agent's inherent ability to cause CINV, or its emetogenicity.[1,10,11] Antineoplastics that are most likely (>90% of patients) to cause symptoms are classified as highly emetogenic chemotherapy. Agents that cause nausea and vomiting in 30% to 90% of patients are classified as moderate-risk agents. Low emetogenicity agents cause symptoms in 10% to 30% of patients. Other chemotherapy agents have a minimal risk, causing CINV in less than 10% of patients. Table 22-2 lists selected chemotherapy agents in the various emetogenicity classes, noting that references differ in the estimation of emetic risk for some antineoplastic agents. The emetogenicity risk also depends on the dosage used and the route of administration.

Table 22-2

Emetogenicity of Selected Intravenous and Oral Antineoplastic Agents with Prophylaxis Options

Potential	Chemotherapy		Prophylaxis Options
Intravenous high emetic risk >90% frequency of emesis	AC combination defined as anthracycline (either doxorubicin or epirubicin) with cyclophosphamide Carboplatin AUC ≥4 Carmustine >250 mg/m^2 Cisplatin Cyclophosphamide >1,500 mg/m^2 Dacarbazine Doxorubicin ≥60 mg/m^2 Epirubicin >90 mg/m^2 Ifosfamide ≥2 g/m^2 per dose Mechlorethamine Streptozocin		Aprepitant-containing regimen OR Olanzapine-containing regimen OR Netupitant-containing regimen OR Rolapitant-containing regimen
Intravenous moderate emetic risk 30%–90% frequency of emesis	Aldesleukin >12–15 million IU/m^2 Amifostine 7300 mg/m^2 Arsenic trioxide Azacitidine Bendamustine Busulfan Carboplatin AUC <4 Carmustine ≤250 mg/m^2 Clofarabine Cyclophosphamide ≤1,500 mg/m^2 Cytarabine >200 mg/m^2 Dactinomycin	Daunorubicin Dinutuximab Doxorubicin <60 mg/m^2 Epirubicin ≤90 mg/m^2 Idarubicin Ifosfamide <2 g/m^2 per dose Interferon alfa ≥10 million IU/m^2 Irinotecan Melphalan Methotrexate ≥250 mg/m^2 Oxaliplatin Temozolamide Trabectedin	Aprepitant-containing regimen OR Olanzapine-containing regimen OR Netupitant-containing regimen OR Rolapitant-containing regimen
Intravenous low emetic risk 10%–30% frequency of emesis	Ado-trastuzumab emtansine Aldesleukin ≤12 million IU/m^2 Amifostine ≤ 300 mg/m3 Atezolizumab Brentuximab vedotin Cabazitaxel Carfilzomib Cytarabine 100–200 mg/m^2 Docetaxel Doxorubicin (liposomal) Eribulin Etoposide 5-Fluorouracil Floxuridine Gemcitabine Interferon alpha >5 million <10 million IU/m^2 Irinotecan (liposomal)	Ixabepilone Methotrexate >50 mg/m^2–249 mg/m^2 Mitomycin Mitoxantrone Necitumumab Omacetaxine Paclitaxel Paclitaxel (albumin bound) Pemetrexed Pentostatin Pralatrexate Romidepsin Thiotepa Topotecan Ziv-aflibercept	Dexamethasone OR Metoclopramide OR Prochlorperazine OR 5HT$_3$ antagonist (choose one: dolasetron, granisetron, or ondansetron)
Intravenous minimal emetic risk <10% frequency of emesis	Alemtuzumab Asparaginase Bevacizumab Bleomycin Bortezomib Cetuximab Cladribine Cytarabine <100 mg/m^2 Decitabine Denileukin diftitox Dexrazoxane Elotuzumab Fludarabine Interferon alfa ≤5 million IU/ m^2 Ipilimumab Methotrexate ≤50 mg/m^2 Nelarabine Nivolumab	Obinutuzumab Ofatumumab Panitumumab Pegaspargase Peginterferon Pembrolizumab Pertuzumab Ramucirumab Rituximab Siltuximab Temsirolimus Trastuzumab Valrubicin Vinblastine Vincristine Vincristine (liposomal) Vinorelbine	No routine prophylaxis

(continued)

Table 22-2

Emetogenicity of Selected Intravenous and Oral Antineoplastic Agents with Prophylaxis Options (*continued*)

Potential	Chemotherapy		Prophylaxis Options
Oral moderate to high emetic risk ≥30% frequency of emesis	Altretamine Busulfan (≥4 mg/day) Ceritinib Crizotinib Cyclophosphamide ($\geq$100 mg/m^2/day) Estramustine Etoposide Lenvatinib Lomustine Mitotane Olaparib Panobinostat Procarbazine Rucaparib Temozolomide (>75 mg/m^2/day) Trifluridine/Tipiracil		5-HT_3 antagonist
Minimal to low emetic risk ≥30% frequency of emesis	Afatinib Alectinib Axitinib Bexarotene Bosutinib Busulfan (<4 mg/day) Cabozantinib Capecitabine Chlorambucil Cobimetinib Cyclophosphamide (<100 mg/m^2/day) Dasatinib Dabrafenib Erlotinib Everolimus Fludarabine Gefitinib Hydroxyurea Ibrutinib Idelalisib Imatinib Ixazomib Lapatinib Lenalidomide	Melphalan Mercaptopurine Methotrexate Nilotinib Palbociclib Pazopanib Pomalidomide Ponatinib Regorafenib Ruxolitinib Sonidegib Sorafenib Sunitinib Temozolomide (≤mg/m^2/day) Thalidomide Thioguanine Topotecan Trametinib Tretinoin Vandetanib Vemurafenib Venetoclax Vismodegib Vorinostat	As needed

5-HT_3, 5-hydroxytryptamine type 3; Intravenous high emetic risk, >90% frequency of emesis; intravenous moderate emetic risk, 30% to 90% frequency of emesis; intravenous low emetic risk, 10% to 30% frequency of emesis; intravenous minimal emetic risk, <10% frequency of emesis.

Source: Ettinger DS et al. Antiemesis: clinical practice guidelines in oncology. V2.2017. **http://www.nccn.org/professionals/physician_gls/pdf/antiemesis.pdf**. Accessed May 30, 2017; Grunberg SM et al. Evaluation of new antiemetic agents and definition of antineoplastic agent emetogenicity—an update. *Support Care Cancer*. 2005;13:80; American Society of Clinical Oncology et al. American Society of Clinical Oncology guideline for antiemetics in oncology: update 2011. *J Clin Oncol*. 2011;29:4189–4198; Roila F et al. Guideline update for MASCC and ESMO in the prevention of chemotherapy- and radiotherapy-induced nausea and vomiting: results of the Perugia consensus conference. *Ann Oncol*. 2010;21(Suppl 5):v232.

Certain antineoplastic agents are more likely to cause delayed CINV symptoms. These include cisplatin, carboplatin, cyclophosphamide, doxorubicin, epirubicin, ifosfamide, and, to a lesser degree, irinotecan and methotrexate. Patients receiving more than one of these agents are at high risk for delayed symptoms.

Most chemotherapy agents are given in combinations, rather than as single agents. Estimating the emetogenicity of chemotherapy combinations has always been difficult. The primary literature of the regimen should always be consulted to determine the emetic risk. Should that not be available, the antiemetic regimen should be geared toward the chemotherapy agent with the highest emetogenicity level given on that day.[1,12,13] For example, in a chemotherapy combination with one high-risk agent and one with a moderate risk, the antiemetic regimen should be appropriate for the high-risk chemotherapy agent.

Antiemetic efficacy, or complete emetic response, is usually defined as no emesis and no nausea or only mild nausea in the first 24 hours after chemotherapy administration. With currently recommended antiemetic regimens, most, but not all, patients will be protected from emesis in the acute phase (first 24 hours). Nausea, however, is more difficult to control. In addition, delayed CINV symptoms are more difficult to prevent.

Overview of Treatment

Appropriate antiemetic therapy is based on the emetogenicity of the chemotherapy regimen and patient risk factors. Because the pathophysiologic response of nausea and vomiting involves many neurotransmitters, combinations of antiemetics from different therapeutic classes will be more effective in most situations than a single agent. The predominant classes of antiemetics used for CINV include 5-HT_3 antagonists, the NK1 antagonist, and corticosteroids.

5-HT_3 ANTAGONISTS

The 5-HT_3 antagonists inhibit the action of serotonin in the GI tract and CNS, and thereby block the transmission of emetic signals to the VC. The 5-HT_3 antagonists are both highly effective and have minimal side effects. Several agents and dosage forms in this class are now available: ondansetron, granisetron, dolasetron, and palonosetron. Dosages of these agents are shown in Table 22-3. The route of administration should be matched to the clinical status of the patient. Oral tablets are appropriate for most patients, but intravenous (IV), topical, or oral dissolving tablet formulations may be needed in patients who cannot take oral medications.

These agents have been widely studied, and some commonalities have emerged. All of the 5-HT_3 antagonists are considered to have equivalent efficacy.[14–19] All of these agents have a threshold effect, and so a sufficiently large dose must be given to block the relevant receptors. In addition, the dose-response curve is relatively flat, such that escalating the dose beyond the threshold dose does not enhance efficacy. When given in appropriate doses, all of these agents have similar efficacy for acute CINV, with response rates of 60% to 80%, depending on study design.[1,12,14–19] The effectiveness of the 5-HT_3 receptor antagonists is enhanced by the addition of dexamethasone. The response rate increases by about 15% to 20% in regimens that include dexamethasone and a 5-HT_3 antagonist.[17,20] Oral and IV 5-HT_3 administration are equally effective assuming that the patient can take oral medications. The side effects of all the 5-HT_3 antagonists are similar and fairly mild and include headache, constipation, diarrhea, and transient elevations of liver function tests. The 5-HT_3 antagonists are one component of optimal antiemetic prophylaxis for acute CINV. However, they are not more effective than agents from other classes (notably dexamethasone, aprepitant, or prochlorperazine) for delayed CINV.[17,21–23] The 5-HT_3 antagonists, therefore, are not generally recommended for delayed CINV. The 5-HT_3 antagonists are metabolized by different cytochrome P-450 enzymes, including CYP1A2, CYP2D6, and CYP3A4. Differences in the metabolic rate of 5-HT_3 antagonists attributable to CYP2D6 polymorphisms might account for differences in efficacy among individual patients.[17] However, these differences are not used clinically to choose initial antiemetic therapy at this time.

Ondansetron, granisetron, and dolasetron have similar pharmacokinetic parameters. Palonosetron, the newest member of the 5-HT_3 antagonist family, is distinguished by a longer elimination half-life (approximately 40 hours) than others in its class.[24] One group of researchers described a three-drug combination of palonosetron, dexamethasone, and aprepitant in a noncomparative, phase II study with moderately emetogenic chemotherapy and found that the three-drug combination was safe and effective.[25]

Whether palonosetron is equivalent or superior to other 5-HT_3 antagonists should be determined by trials that compare palonosetron with another 5-HT_3 antagonist, with both treatment arms also containing dexamethasone and aprepitant in the acute and delayed phases. These trials have yet to be conducted. Currently, palonosetron is substantially more expensive than the generic forms of the other 5-HT_3 antagonists.

Palonosetron is normally administered as a single 0.25-mg IV before chemotherapy. Palonosetron has been studied in a three-dose regimen (administration on days 1, 3, 5) for multiday chemotherapy in an uncontrolled trial.[26] This regimen appeared to be safe and effective but was not compared with any other regimen. It is not clear that palonosetron would have superior activity compared with repeated doses of the other 5-HT_3 antagonists. In addition, palonosetron is given orally in combination with netupitant (see section on Neurokinin 1 Receptor Antagonist).

It is difficult to identify the 5-HT_3 antagonist with the highest overall cost-effectiveness because drug acquisition costs vary between the inpatient and outpatient clinics and from institution to institution. Costs of the different agents should be compared at each practice site to determine the preferred agent.

CORTICOSTEROIDS

The mechanism of action of corticosteroids as antiemetics has not been fully determined. Some suggest that corticosteroids may decrease serotonin release, antagonize 5-HT_3, or activate corticosteroid receptors in the NTS of the medulla in the CNS.[20] Many studies validate the effectiveness of corticosteroids in the prophylaxis of CINV symptoms. Efficacy with both dexamethasone and methylprednisolone has been described, but dexamethasone is much more widely studied and almost exclusively used. Dexamethasone improves the antiemetic control of 5-HT_3 antagonists by about 15% to 20%.[20] In addition to its use in the acute phase of CINV, dexamethasone is one of the cornerstone agents used to prevent delayed CINV. It is inexpensive and available in both IV and oral formulations.

The optimal dose of dexamethasone with different emetic stimuli has been studied in controlled trials.[20] For moderately emetogenic chemotherapy in the acute phase, a single 8-mg dose was as effective as larger 24-mg doses or prolonged administration. In the setting of highly emetogenic cisplatin-based chemotherapy, higher doses of 12 or 20 mg were superior to doses of 4 and 8 mg. If dexamethasone is used with aprepitant in the acute phase, the lower 12 mg prechemotherapy dose is recommended because of inhibition of steroid metabolism by aprepitant (see section on Neurokinin 1 Receptor Antagonist).[12] For prevention of delayed CINV symptoms, the most commonly used dose of dexamethasone is 8 mg twice daily on days 2 and 3 after chemotherapy without aprepitant. The dose for delayed CINV should be reduced to 8 mg daily when used with aprepitant.

Corticosteroids are sometimes underused because of the potential risk of side effects. The adverse effects of corticosteroids include insomnia, jitteriness, increased appetite, GI distress, and perineal irritation if the IV dexamethasone is infused too quickly.[18,20,27] For most patients, however, dexamethasone is well tolerated, especially because the therapy is typically short term at lower doses. Steroid-related hyperglycemia may occur, especially in patients with preexisting diabetes.[20] These patients should be advised to monitor their glucose levels more frequently and contact their practitioner if the levels remain elevated. In the nondiabetic patient, hyperglycemia is uncommon. Tapering the corticosteroid dose after the end of treatment for CINV is usually unnecessary because the duration of therapy is short. Rare patients who have steroid withdrawal-like symptoms may, however, benefit from a short taper on repeated corticosteroid courses.

Corticosteroids also have antitumor properties and are a part of the antineoplastic regimen for some malignancies, such as lymphoma, lymphoid leukemia, and myeloma, and additional dexamethasone for the antiemetic protection is not necessary. In these cases, the corticosteroid should be administered just before the rest of the chemotherapy to provide antiemetic activity. If aprepitant is part of an antiemetic regimen in a situation where the corticosteroid is given for antitumor reasons, the dose of the corticosteroid should not be reduced.[12]

NEUROKININ 1 RECEPTOR ANTAGONISTS

The potential use of NK1 receptor antagonists as antiemetics became apparent when the role of substance P in the peripheral nervous system and CNS was recognized in the emetic stimulus

Table 22-3
Antiemetic Agents for Chemotherapy-Induced Nausea and Vomiting

Medication (Trade Name)	Class	Indication	Dose in Adults (Doses Should be Given 30–60 Minutes Before Chemotherapy)
Aprepitant (Emend)	NK1 antagonist	Acute and delayed	PO: 125 mg on day 1, 80 mg on days 2 and 3
Dexamethasone (Decadron)	Corticosteroid	Acute (high emetogenicity)	PO/IV: 12 mg (with aprepitant) or 20 mg (without aprepitant)
		Acute (moderate emetogenicity)	PO/IV: 8–12 mg
		Acute (low emetogenicity)	PO/IV: 4–8 mg
		Delayed	PO/IV: 8 mg daily days 2–4 or days 2 and 3 or PO: 4 mg BID days 2–4
Dolasetron (Anzemet)	5-HT_3 antagonist	Acute	PO: 100–200 mg
Dronabinol (Marinol)	Cannabinoid	Breakthrough	PO: 2.5–10 mg PO TID to QID
Droperidol (Inapsine)	Butyrophenone	Breakthrough	IV: 0.625–1.25 mg every 4–6 hours PRN
Fosaprepitant (Emend)	NK1 antagonist	Acute	IV: 150 mg × 1 dose or 115 mg initial dose (followed by aprepitant 80 mg PO on days 2 and 3)
Granisetron (Kytril)	5-HT_3 antagonist	Acute	IV: 1 mg or 0.01 mg/kg PO: 2 mg TOP: 3.1 mg/24-hour patch applied 24–48 hours before chemotherapy and kept on until 24 hours after chemotherapy or up to 7 days
Haloperidol (Haldol)	Butyrophenone	Breakthrough	PO/IV/IM: 0.5–1 mg every 6 hours PRN
Metoclopramide (Reglan)	Dopamine antagonist	Breakthrough	PO/IV: 10–40 mg every 6 hours PRN
Lorazepam (Ativan)	Benzodiazepine	Breakthrough	PO/IV/IM/SL: 0.5–2 mg every 6 hours PRN
Nabilone (Cesamet)	Cannabinoid	Refractory symptoms	PO: 1–2 mg BID (max 2 mg TID)
Netupitant and palonosetron (Akynzeo)	NK1 antagonist + 5-HT_3 antagonist	Acute (moderate or high emetogenicity)	PO: netupitant 300 mg + palonosetron 0.5 mg
Olanzapine (Zyprexa)	Serotonin/dopamine antagonist	Acute (moderate or high emetogenicity)/delayed	PO: 10 mg on days 1–3 (moderate risk) or days 1–4 (high risk)
		Breakthrough	PO: 2.5–10 mg QHS or 2.5–5 mg BID–TID
Ondansetron (Zofran)	5-HT_3 antagonist	Acute (moderate or high emetogenicity) Delayed	IV: 8–12 mg or 0.15 mg/kg PO: 16–24 mg 8 mg PO BID or 8 mg IV daily
Palonosetron (Aloxi)	5-HT_3 antagonist	Acute/delayed	IV: 0.25 mg PO: 0.5 mg
Prochlorperazine (Compazine)	Dopamine antagonist	Breakthrough Acute	PO/IV/IM: 5–10 mg (up to 20 mg) every 4–6 hours PRN or PR: 25 mg every 12 hours PRN PO/IV: 10 mg
Promethazine (Phenergan)	Dopamine antagonist	Breakthrough	PO/IV/IM/PR: 12.5–25 mg every 4–6 hours PRN
Rolapitant (Varubi)	NK1 antagonist	Acute and delayed	PO: 180 mg on day 1

5-HT_3, 5-hydroxytryptamine type 3; BID, 2 times daily; IM, intramuscular; IV, intravenous; NK1, neurokinin 1; PO, oral; PR, rectal; PRN, as needed; QHS, at bedtime; QID, 4 times daily; SL, sublingual; TID, 3 times daily.
Source: Ettinger DS et al. Antiemesis: clinical practice guidelines in oncology. V2. 2017. **http://www.nccn.org/professionals/physician_gls/pdf/antiemesis.pdf**. Accessed May 30, 2017; American Society of Clinical Oncology et al. American Society of Clinical Oncology guideline for antiemetics in oncology: update 2011. *J Clin Oncol*. 2011;29:4189–4198; Roila F et al. Guideline update for MASCC and ESMO in the prevention of chemotherapy- and radiotherapy-induced nausea and vomiting: results of the Perugia consensus conference. *Ann Oncol*. 2010;21(Suppl 5):v232.

pathway. Aprepitant, the first NK1 receptor antagonist available, is active in both the acute and delayed phases of CINV caused by moderately and highly emetogenic chemotherapy. Aprepitant is usually given as a 3-day oral regimen, 125 mg on day 1 and 80 mg on days 2 and 3. Early trials determined that aprepitant could not replace a 5-HT_3 antagonist, but that it would be used best in conjunction with corticosteroids and a 5-HT_3 antagonist.[28]

Aprepitant has been studied in the prevention of CINV with highly and moderately emetogenic chemotherapy.[17,28] These studies showed improved response rates when aprepitant was added to antiemetic regimens containing a 5-HT_3 antagonist plus dexamethasone.

Although CINV symptoms tend to worsen from cycle to cycle, the effects of aprepitant seem to be maintained during four cycles of chemotherapy in patients receiving moderately emetogenic chemotherapy.[29] The addition of aprepitant to the antiemetic regimen during cycle 2 (even when omitted from cycle 1) also seems to improve control of CINV symptoms.[30,31] For patients who have had inadequate response to an antiemetic regimen that did not include aprepitant, it may be useful to add it in later cycles.

The efficacy of aprepitant for the control of delayed CINV symptoms was confirmed in a trial of 489 patients comparing a standard aprepitant regimen with a regimen without aprepitant in patients receiving highly emetogenic chemotherapy.[32] The aprepitant-containing regimen offered superior control of CINV in the acute, delayed, and overall periods. The study confirmed that the aprepitant-containing regimen is superior during the delayed phase of CINV.

There is growing evidence that the prechemotherapy dose of aprepitant (or fosaprepitant) provides the majority of benefit compared with postchemotherapy doses.[17,33] The first dose of aprepitant blocks about 80% of the NK1 receptors in the CNS.[17,33] One study compared a single 150-mg IV dose of fosaprepitant with the standard three-day oral regimen (along with ondansetron and dexamethasone) in patients receiving highly emetogenic chemotherapy. No difference was found in the antiemetic efficacy between the two groups.[34]

Aprepitant is generally well tolerated with mild side effects, including fatigue, hiccups, headache, and diarrhea.[28,32] The overall adverse effects in standard aprepitant-containing regimens are not appreciably different from regimens without aprepitant. NK1 antagonists are now available as an IV prodrug, fosaprepitant and an oral fixed combination capsule of a NK1-antagonist, netupitant plus palonosetron, which offer patients different dosage forms. Netupitant and palonosetron combination therapy is recommended as an option for patients receiving highly or moderately emetogenic regimens. Trials comparing its efficacy against aprepitant have not yet been studied. Rolapitant, the newest NKI antagonist, is an oral drug with an extended half life and should not be administered at less than 2-week intervals. "Studies investigating repeat dosing of fosaprepitant, netupitant and rolapitant are not available."

Aprepitant is metabolized by the CYP3A4 enzyme system. It is a moderate inhibitor and inducer of CYP3A4 and an inducer of CYP2C9.[1,28] Consequently, several drugs potentially interact with aprepitant. The most commonly encountered interaction is with corticosteroids. Aprepitant increases the area under the curve (AUC) of dexamethasone such that the dexamethasone dose (when used as an antiemetic) should be reduced by about one-half of the usual dose when these drugs are used together.[1,17,28] The interaction is greatest when the corticosteroid is administered orally. However, when the corticosteroid is also given as part of the antitumor regimen, the corticosteroid dose should not be reduced because of concern that the antineoplastic activity might be compromised.[12] Aprepitant, fosaprepitant and netupitant inhibit the metabolism of dexamethasone. Rolapitant does not share this interaction with dexamethasone. Aprepitant may also enhance warfarin metabolism by inducing CYP2C9. International normalized ratio (INR) values in patients treated with warfarin and the standard aprepitant regimen are significantly reduced, especially on day 8 of the chemotherapy cycle.[17,28,35,36] The patient's coagulation status after aprepitant administration should be monitored, especially during the 7- to 10-day period after aprepitant. The dosage of warfarin should be adjusted if the INR is out of range. Several chemotherapy agents (paclitaxel, etoposide, ifosfamide, irinotecan, imatinib, vinca alkaloids, and others) are metabolized by the CYP3A4 enzyme system, and the metabolism of these agents may be altered by aprepitant. Aprepitant was used in clinical trials with some of these agents. Caution is warranted because the clinical relevance of this potential interaction is not known.[28,37] In comparison of NKI antagonists, there are fewer drug interactions with rolapitant when compared with aprepitant, fosaprepitant and netupitant

OLANZAPINE

Olanzapine is an atypical antipsychotic agent that antagonizes several serotonin and dopamine receptors as well as other neurotransmitter receptors.[38] Its antiemetic action was first described in patients with refractory nausea or vomiting and advanced cancer. Olanzapine has activity both in the prevention of CINV in patients at high and moderate risk and in rescue treatment for patients with refractory nausea and vomiting. Studies have demonstrated its efficacy in preventing CINV in the setting of highly and moderately emetogenic chemotherapy. Newer, controlled trials show improved response rates when added to an antiemetic regimen of a 5-HT_3 antagonist plus dexamethasone, as well as comparable activity to aprepitant.[23,35,38,39] The typical dose of olanzapine used in these trials was 10 mg PO daily on days 1 through 5.

Olanzapine is also active as a rescue agent for patients with refractory CINV. In this setting, the usual dose of olanzapine is 2.5 to 10 mg daily in one to four divided doses. The common side effects of olanzapine include sleepiness, dry mouth, and dizziness, although these were not significant in preliminary reports.[23,35,38,39] Olanzapine is an option for the prevention of CINV in patients receiving highly to moderately emetogenic regimens and a good choice for control of highly refractory CINV symptoms.

OTHER ANTIEMETICS

Medications from other drug classes have also been used as antiemetics for CINV. These include dopamine antagonists (prochlorperazine, promethazine), benzodiazepines (lorazepam), butyrophenones (droperidol, haloperidol), benzamides (metoclopramide), and cannabinoids. Many of these agents were used widely until more effective antiemetic agents became available. These agents remain useful for breakthrough symptoms or for patients who are refractory to standard therapy. The dosages and indications for these agents are shown in Table 22-3. Many of these agents have more side effects than contemporary agents do, especially sedation and extrapyramidal side effects, such as dystonia and akathisia. Lorazepam is commonly used as a rescue antiemetic. Its mechanism of action as an antiemetic is not completely understood, but it may involve disruption of the cortical impulses to the VC, as well as anxiolytic activity.

Cannabinoids have long been used for refractory nausea and vomiting. This is based on the effect of the CNS cannabinoid receptors on the CTZ, the NTS, and the VC.[40] Small trials have shown conflicting effectiveness in the prevention of CINV.[41,42] An oral cannabinoid, nabilone, was approved for the treatment of CINV in patients who do not respond adequately to other antiemetics.[40] Cannabinoids are associated with side effects, such as drowsiness, dry mouth, dysphoria, vertigo, and euphoria.[40,41] Although some patients have a clear preference for, and good response to, cannabinoids, side effects and a lack of pronounced efficacy limit their use in the general population of chemotherapy patients. These agents are usually reserved for patients who do not have adequate relief from other rescue medications.

The optimal prophylactic antiemetic regimens depend on the emetic risk of the chemotherapy regimen. Treatment guidelines have been developed by several groups, including the American Society of Clinical Oncology (ASCO; http://jco.ascopubs.org/content/24/18/2932.full.pdf+html)[12]; the National Comprehensive Cancer Network (NCCN; http://www.nccn.org/professionals/physician_gls/PDF/antiemesis.pdf; guidelines can be accessed by creating a free login)[1]; and the Multinational Association of Supportive Care in Cancer (MASCC; http://annonc.oxfordjournals.org.floyd.lib.umn.edu/content/21/suppl_5/v232.full.pdf+html).[13] These evidence- and consensus-based guidelines, which are similar in regard to the roles of the various antiemetics, are summarized in Table 22-4 and Figure 22-2.

Many patients may benefit from nondrug therapy for CINV symptoms, especially for anticipatory nausea and vomiting and anxiety. Techniques include guided imagery, hypnosis, relaxation techniques, systematic desensitization, and music therapy.[43] Acupuncture and acupressure techniques have been investigated

Table 22-4

Recommended Antiemetic Regimens for Chemotherapy-Induced Nausea and Vomiting by Emetogenicity of Chemotherapy Regimen

Emetogenicity Potential	Acute-Phase CINV (Doses Should be Given 30–60 Minutes Before Chemotherapy)	Delayed-Phase CINV	Breakthrough CINV
High-risk IV chemotherapy regimens	**Aprepitant-containing regimen**		Two agents for PRN use
	Day 1: single dose 5-HT_3 antagonist + dexamethasone 12 mg PO/IV + aprepitant 125 mg PO once/fosaprepitant 150 mg IV once	Dexamethasone 8 mg PO/IV on days 2–4 + aprepitant 80 mg days 2–3 (not needed if fosaprepitant 150-mg dose used)	
	Netupitant-containing regimen		
	Day 1: netupitant 300 mg/palonosetron 0.5 mg PO once + dexamethasone 12 mg PO/IV once	Dexamethasone 8 mg PO/IV on days 2–4	
	Olanzapine-containing regimen		
	Day 1: Olanzapine 10 mg PO once + palonosetron 0.25 mg IV once + dexamethasone 20 mg IV once	Olanzapine 10 mg PO daily on days 2–4	
High risk	**Rolapitant-containing regimen** Day 1: Rolapitant 180 mg PO once + palonosetron 0.25 mg IV once + dexamethasone 12 mg PO/IV once	Dexamethasone 8 mg PO/IV twice daily on days 2–4	
Moderate risk	**Rolapitant-containing regimen** Day 1: Rolapitant 180 mg PO once + palonosetron 0.25 mg IV once + dexamethasone 12 mg PO/IV once	Dexamethasone 8 mg PO/IV daily on days 2–3	
Moderate-risk IV chemotherapy regimens	**Aprepitant-containing regimen**		Two agents for PRN use
	Day 1: single dose 5-HT_3 antagonist + dexamethasone ± aprepitant/fosaprepitant	Days 2–3: 5-HT_3 antagonist or dexamethasone or aprepitant	
	Netupitant-containing regimen		
	Day 1: netupitant 300 mg/palonosetron 0.5 mg PO once + dexamethasone 12 mg PO/IV once	Dexamethasone 8 mg PO/IV on days 2–3	
	Olanzapine-containing regimen		
	Day 1: Olanzapine 10 mg PO once + palonosetron 0.25 mg IV once + dexamethasone 20 mg IV once	Olanzapine 10 mg PO daily on days 2–3	
Low-risk IV chemotherapy regimens	Single dose dexamethasone or metoclopramide or prochlorperazine or 5HT_3 antagonist	None	Either none or one agent for PRN use
Minimal-risk IV chemotherapy regimens	None	None	Usually none
High- to moderate-risk PO chemotherapy regimens	5-HT_3 antagonist	None	One agent for PRN use
Low-risk PO chemotherapy regimens	None	None	One agent for PRN use

5-HT_3, 5-hydroxytryptamine type 3; CINV, chemotherapy-induced nausea and vomiting; IV, intravenous; PO, oral; PRN, as needed.

Source: Ettinger DS et al. Antiemesis: clinical practice guidelines in oncology. V2. 2017. **http://www.nccn.org/professionals/physician_gls/pdf/antiemesis.pdf**. Accessed May 30, 2017; American Society of Clinical Oncology et al. American Society of Clinical Oncology guideline for antiemetics in oncology: update 2011. *J Clin Oncol*. 2011;29:4189–4198; Roila F et al. Guideline update for MASCC and ESMO in the prevention of chemotherapy- and radiotherapy-induced nausea and vomiting: results of the Perugia consensus conference. *Ann Oncol*. 2010;21(Suppl 5):v232.

for use in CINV, and some patients benefit from their use. The use of acupressure devices that stimulate the P6 point on the wrist have been proposed; however, in a controlled trial in patients with breast cancer, it was not found to be helpful.[44] If patients are troubled by CINV symptoms, it is recommended that they refrain from heavy meals for 8 to 12 hours prior to chemotherapy. They should also avoid heavy, greasy foods and food with strong aromas. Chewing gum can mask the metallic

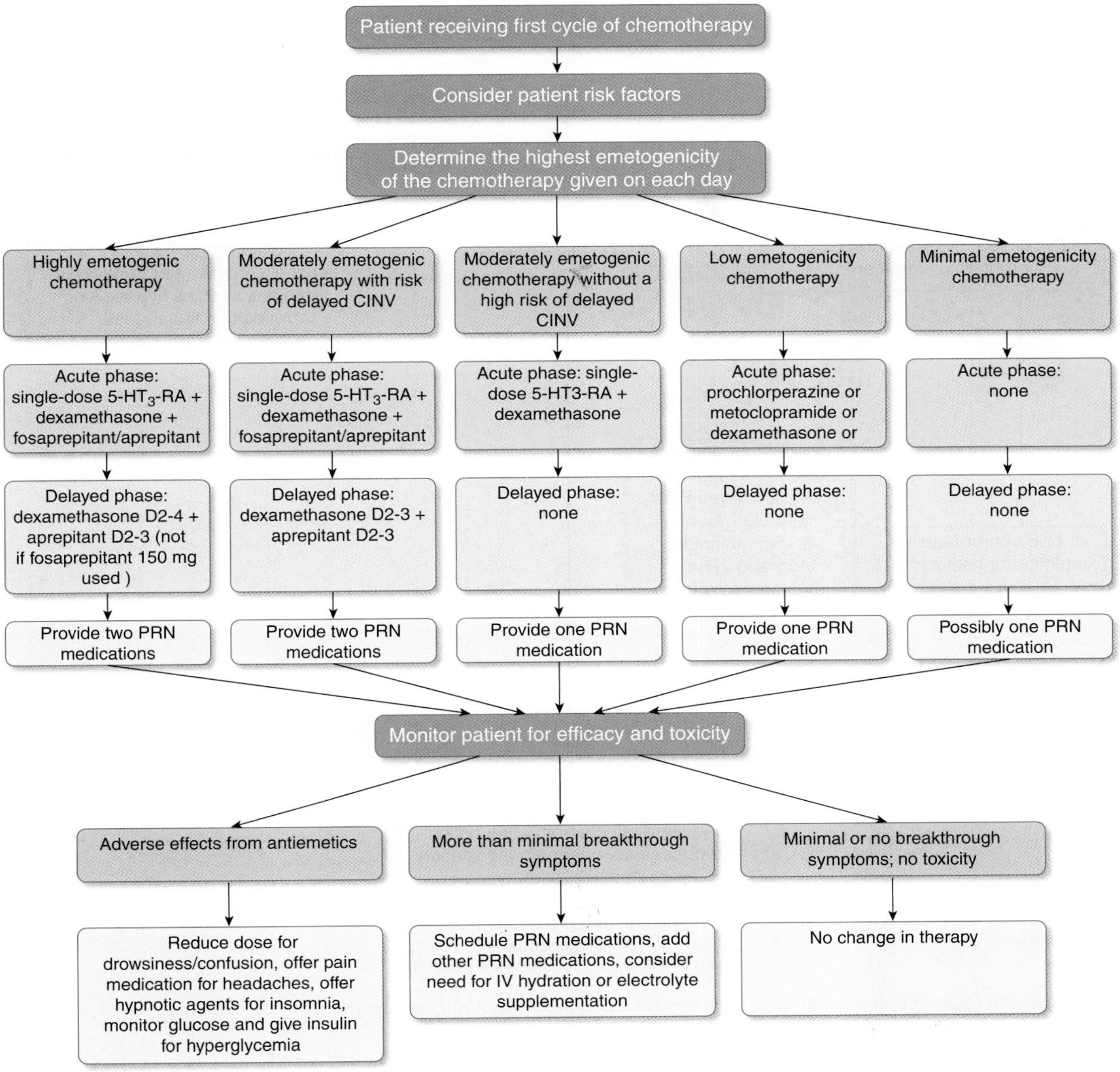

Figure 22-2 Algorithm for antiemetic selection of an *initial* chemotherapy cycle. CINV, chemotherapy-induced nausea and vomiting; PRN, as needed; 5-HT_3-RA, 5-hydroxytryptamine type 3 receptor antagonist.

taste that some patients perceive. Dry, salty foods can also help settle the stomach.

Clinical Presentation and Risk Factors

CASE 22-2

Question 1: M.C., a 54-year-old woman with breast cancer, is in the clinic today to receive her first cycle of chemotherapy. Her chemotherapy will consist of docetaxel 75 mg/m^2 IV, carboplatin dosed to achieve an AUC of 6 mg/mL × min. This will be repeated every 21 days. In addition, she will receive trastuzumab 4 mg/kg IV for one dose, then 2 mg/kg/week for 17 weeks. M.C. does not drink alcohol or smoke. Her only other medical condition is adult-onset diabetes, which is controlled with metformin and diet. She has had four children, now all grown, and had substantial morning sickness with each of her pregnancies. M.C.'s neighbor told her that all chemotherapy causes severe nausea and vomiting. How likely is M.C. to experience nausea and vomiting? What are her risk factors?

M.C. is at moderate risk for acute CINV. Her personal risk factors include female sex, history of morning sickness with pregnancy, and being a nondrinker. The docetaxel has a low risk of acute CINV, the carboplatin has a moderate risk of acute CINV with a high risk of delayed CINV, and the trastuzumab has a minimal risk of acute CINV. A moderate-risk prophylactic regimen should be recommended for M.C.

Case 22-2, Question 2: What antiemetics are available for M.C.?

For moderate-risk prophylaxis, an aprepitant-, netupitant-, rolapitant-, or olanzapine-containing regimen is recommended. For a single-day chemotherapy regimen, the aprepitant-containing regimen includes a single dose of 5-HT_3 antagonist plus dexamethasone 8 to 12 mg oral or IV plus oral aprepitant 125 mg on day 1, then oral dexamethasone 8 mg on days 2 through 4, and oral aprepitant 80 mg on days 2 and 3. The olanzapine-containing regimen includes olanzapine 10 mg oral on days 1 to 3, dexamethasone 20 mg IV once on day 1, and palonosetron

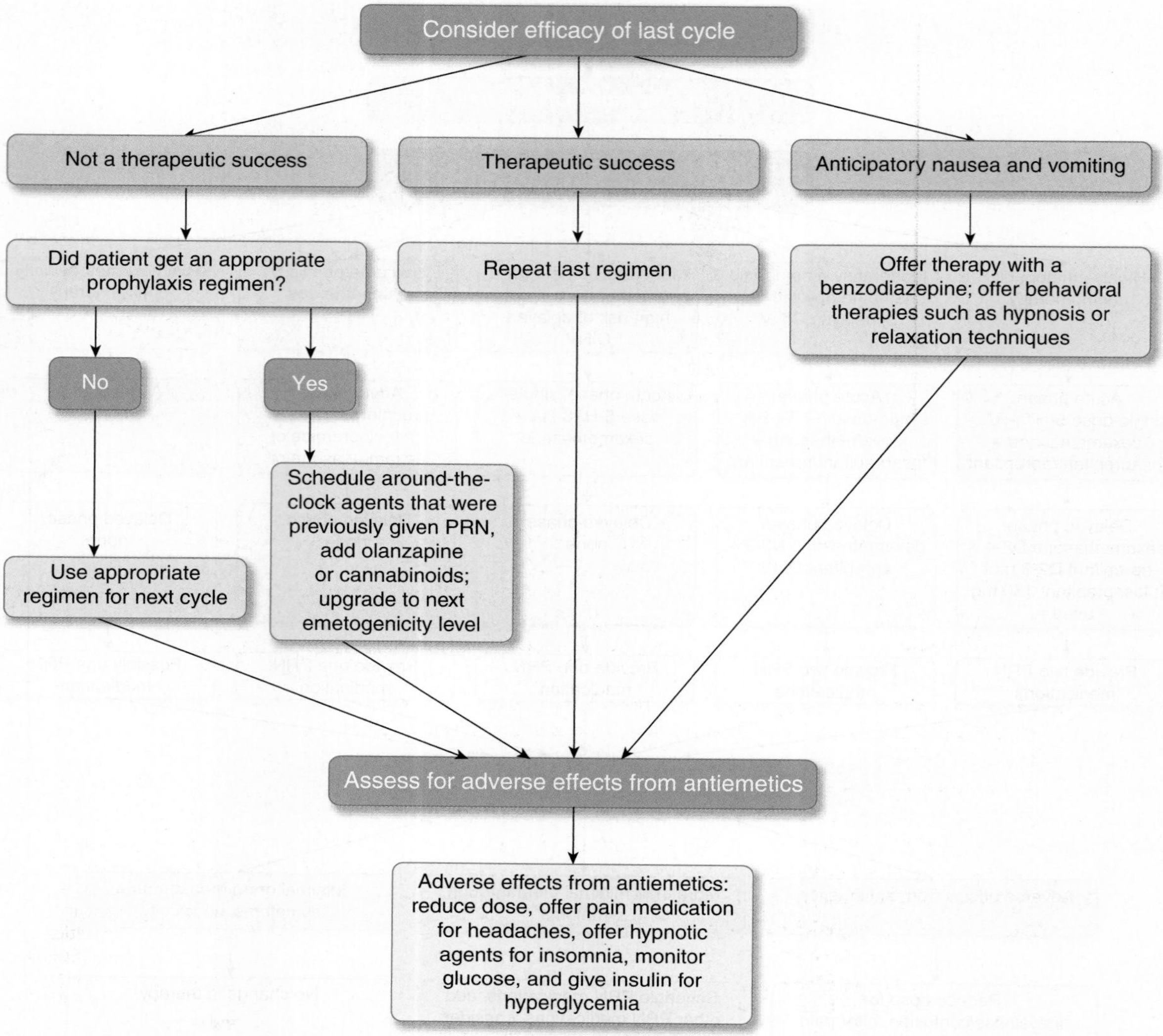

Figure 22-3 Algorithm for selection of antiemetic regimens for subsequent chemotherapy cycles. PRN, as needed.

0.25 mg IV once on day 1. The netupitant-containing regimen includes netupitant 300 mg plus palonosetron 0.5 mg oral on day 1, then oral dexamethasone 12 mg on day 1 and 8 mg oral or IV daily on days 2 to 3. The rolapitant-containing regimen includes rolapitant 180 mg PO, a 5HT3 antagonist & dexamethasone 12 mg oral on day 1, then oral dexamethasone 8 mg PO on day 2 and 3.

CASE 22-2, QUESTION 3: M.C. is at moderate risk for acute nausea and vomiting and at high risk for delayed CINV symptoms, as a result of her chemotherapy regimen of docetaxel, carboplatin, and trastuzumab. What would be the most appropriate antiemetic regimen for M.C.?

For M.C., the best regimen would be an aprepitant, netupitant, or rolapitant-containing regimen. The olanzapine-containing regimen is also an option but used cautiously in patients with diabetes mellitus. She should be offered medications for breakthrough CINV symptoms, such as prochlorperazine and lorazepam. She should be warned of the potential adverse effects of dexamethasone or olanzapine, especially hyperglycemia, and counseled to check her blood sugar levels more frequently and contact her physician if they remain elevated. M.C. should be advised to maintain a record of her symptoms and contact her physician if the breakthrough medications are not working or if she cannot keep fluids down.

If M.C. had been prescribed a multiday chemotherapy regimen, prophylaxis with a 5-HT_3 antagonist and dexamethasone should be offered for each day that moderately or highly emetogenic chemotherapy is administered.[1,12,13,45] If multiday chemotherapy regimens have a high risk of delayed symptoms, then therapy (e.g., dexamethasone plus prochlorperazine or metoclopramide, if aprepitant was already administered) for the delayed symptoms should be continued for at least 2 to 3 days after the last chemotherapy administration.

Modern antiemetic regimens achieve complete emetic control in about 70% to 90% of patients, but the response rate is lower for delayed CINV symptoms. If CINV symptoms are not adequately controlled, alterations in the prophylactic antiemetic regimen should be made for the next cycle (Fig. 22-3). Suggestions include upgrading to the next higher emetogenicity level recommendation, adding aprepitant if not already given, and scheduling antiemetic agents from other pharmacologic classes.

RADIATION-INDUCED NAUSEA AND VOMITING

Clinical Presentation and Risk Factors

CASE 22-3

Question 1: E.G. is a 54-year-old man with newly diagnosed head and neck cancer who will receive radiation therapy concurrently with chemotherapy containing cisplatin and fluorouracil. His daily (Monday through Friday) radiation treatments will last for 6 weeks. He has a heavy smoking history (35 pack-years) and "quit" last week, although it is not going well. After E.G.'s nausea and vomiting from the chemotherapy subsides, is he at risk for experiencing radiation-induced nausea and vomiting (RINV)? What antiemetic prophylaxis is appropriate?

Radiation therapy can cause nausea and vomiting through the same basic pathways that chemotherapy does. RINV affects 40% to 80% of patients receiving radiation therapy. The risk of RINV depends on several factors, namely, the size and area to be irradiated, larger fractional doses of radiation, and whether the patient has had previous chemotherapy.[1,46,47] Patients with radiation areas larger than 400 cm^2 are more likely to have significant RINV symptoms. The radiation therapy oncologist will determine the size of the radiation field and fractional doses of radiation to maximize the efficacy of the radiation therapy. The high dose used in total body irradiation (associated with hematopoietic stem cell transplantation) causes RINV in more than 90% of patients. Patients receiving radiation to the upper abdominal area experience nausea and vomiting about 50% to 80% of the time. Radiation to other areas of the body is less likely to cause nausea and vomiting.

Overview of Treatment

Just as with CINV, symptoms caused by radiation can be prevented with 5-HT_3 antagonists, corticosteroids, or both. Evidence- and consensus-based recommendations have been published by several multidisciplinary groups and are shown in Table 22-5. High-risk RINV is best treated with a combination of a 5-HT_3 antagonist and a corticosteroid.[1,46–50] Patients receiving concomitant chemotherapy and radiation should receive antiemetics appropriate for the chemotherapy regimen.[1] Patients receiving radiotherapy in the moderate RINV risk group can receive either prophylaxis or rescue therapy with a 5-HT_3 antagonist.

E.G. is at low risk for experiencing RINV because his radiation site will be in the head and neck region, his radiation site is not likely to be larger than 400 cm^2, and he will likely receive a smaller fractional dose, although he will be receiving concurrent chemotherapy. Because E.G. is at low risk for having RINV symptoms, he does not need prophylaxis with a 5-HT_3 antagonist. If he experiences symptoms, rescue therapy with a dopamine antagonist or a serotonin antagonist should be offered.

Table 22-5
Prophylaxis for Radiation-Induced Nausea and Vomiting for Adults

Emetic Risk	Radiation Area	Recommendation
High risk	Total body irradiation	Prophylaxis with a 5-HT_3 antagonist (e.g., ondansetron 8 mg PO BID–TID or granisetron 2 mg PO daily) ± dexamethasone 4 mg PO daily
Moderate risk	Upper abdomen	Prophylaxis with a 5-HT_3 antagonist (e.g., ondansetron 8 mg PO BID or granisetron 2 mg PO daily) ± dexamethasone 4 mg PO daily
Low risk	Lower thorax, pelvis, cranium, craniospinal region, head/neck	Prophylaxis or rescue with a 5-HT_3 antagonist
Minimal risk	Extremities, breast	Rescue with a dopamine antagonist or a 5-HT_3 antagonist

5-HT3, 5-hydroxytryptamine type 3; BID, twice daily; PO, oral; TID, 3 times daily.
Source: Ettinger DS et al. Antiemesis: clinical practice guidelines in oncology. V2. 2017. **http://www.nccn.org/professionals/physician_gls/pdf/antiemesis.pdf**. Accessed May 30, 2017; Grunberg SM et al. Evaluation of new antiemetic agents and definition of antineoplastic agent emetogenicity—an update. *Support Care Cancer*. 2005;13:80; Roila F et al. Guideline update for MASCC and ESMO in the prevention of chemotherapy- and radiotherapy-induced nausea and vomiting: results of the Perugia consensus conference. *Ann Oncol*. 2010;21(Suppl 5):v232; Feyer P et al. Radiotherapy-induced nausea and vomiting (RINV): MASCC/ESMO guideline for antiemetics in radiotherapy: update 2009. *Support Care Cancer*. August 10, 2010. [Epub ahead of print]; Abdelsayed GG. Management of radiation-induced nausea and vomiting. *Exp Hematol*. 2007;35(4 Suppl 1):34; Urba S. Radiation-induced nausea and vomiting. *J Natl Compr Canc Netw*. 2007;5:60.

POSTOPERATIVE NAUSEA AND VOMITING

Clinical Presentation and Risk Factors

CASE 22-4

Question 1: E.W. is a 48-year-old woman who is scheduled for a laparoscopic cholecystectomy. The scheduled duration of her surgery is less than an hour. Her medical history includes hypertension. She does not have a history of motion sickness, and she is a nonsmoker. E.W. has never had surgery before. Her sister-in-law had severe nausea and vomiting after an outpatient surgical procedure last year, and E.W. is worried that she too may have it. What is E.W.'s risk of having postoperative nausea and vomiting (PONV)? What can be done to reduce her risk, and how can symptoms be treated if they occur?

PONV is a common complication of surgery, affecting 25% to 30% of all patients but up to 80% of patients in high-risk groups.[51] In surgical patients, PONV can lead to hospitalizations, stress on the surgical closure, hematomas, and aspiration pneumonitis. Patient-related, surgical, and anesthetic factors can increase the risk of PONV.[51–55] Patient risk factors include female sex, history of motion sickness, nonsmoking status, obesity, and a history of PONV. Some surgical risk factors for PONV include long duration of surgery and type of surgical procedure (e.g., laparoscopy, ear–nose–throat procedures, gynecologic surgeries, and strabismus repair). Anesthetic risk factors include the use of volatile anesthetics or nitrous oxide (as opposed to IV propofol) and the use of intraoperative or postoperative opioids. Children are twice as likely to have PONV as adults.[52,56] The risk increases with the child's age but declines after puberty.

Certain anesthesia practices may reduce the risk of PONV. These include use of regional anesthesia (instead of general anesthesia); use

Table 22-6

Medications for Prevention and Treatment of Postoperative Nausea and Vomiting in Adults

Medication	Prophylactic Dose	Treatment or Rescue Dose
Aprepitant	40 mg PO within 3 hours before induction of anesthesia	None
Dexamethasone	4–10 mg at the start of induction of anesthesia	2–4 mg IV
Dolasetron	12.5 mg IV at end of surgery	12.5 mg IV
Droperidol	0.625–1.25 mg IV at end of surgery	0.625–1.25 mg IV or IM every 4–6 hours
Metoclopramide	10–20 mg IV at end of surgery	10–20 mg IV or IM every 6 hours
Granisetron	0.35–1 mg IV at end of surgery	0.1 mg
Ondansetron	4–8 mg IV at end of surgery	1 mg IV every 8 hours
Palonosetron	0.075 mg IV immediately prior to induction of anesthesia	None
Prochlorperazine	5–10 mg IV at end of surgery	5–10 mg IV or IM every 4–6 hours
Promethazine	12.5–25 mg IV at induction or end of surgery	12.5–25 mg IV or IM every 4–6 hours
Scopolamine	1.5 mg TOP evening before surgery or at least 4 hours before end of surgery	

IM, intramuscular; IV, intravenous; PO, oral; TOP, topical patch.
Source: Gan TJ et al. Consensus guidelines for managing postoperative nausea and vomiting. *Anesth Analg*. 2003;97:62; Golembiewski J et al. Prevention and treatment of postoperative nausea and vomiting. *Am J Health Syst Pharm*. 2005;62:1247; Kloth D. New pharmacologic findings for the treatment of PONV and PDNV. *Am J Health Syst Pharm*. 2009;66(1 Suppl 1):S11; Ignoffo RJ. Current research on PONV/PDNV: practical implications for today's pharmacist. *Am J Health Syst Pharm*. 2009;66(1 Suppl 1):S19; Kovac AL. Prevention and treatment of postoperative nausea and vomiting. *Drugs*. 2000;59:213; Gan TJ et al. Society for Ambulatory Anesthesia guidelines for the management of postoperative nausea and vomiting. *Anesth Analg*. 2007;105:1615; Wilhelm SM et al. Prevention of postoperative nausea and vomiting. *Ann Pharmacother*. 2007;41:68; Golembiewski J, Tokumaru S. Pharmacological prophylaxis and management of adult postoperative/postdischarge nausea and vomiting. *J Perianesth Nurs*. 2006;21:385.

of total IV anesthesia with propofol; use of intraoperative oxygen; adequate hydration; and avoidance of nitrous oxide, volatile anesthesia therapy, and intraoperative or postoperative opiates.[51–53,55–57]

Several risk factor models have been studied to correlate these factors into recommendations for prevention and therapy.[51,53] One model is both simple and practical and uses the following risk factors: female sex, history of PONV or motion sickness, nonsmoking status, surgery longer than 60 minutes in duration, and the use of intraoperative opioids. If the patient has zero or one risk factor, the risk of PONV is about 10% to 20%, and no prophylaxis is necessary unless there is a medical risk for emesis. If the patient has two or more risk factors, the incidence increases to 40% to 80%, and prophylaxis with one or two medications is warranted. E.W. has at least two risk factors (female, nonsmoker) and may have more if her surgery lasts longer than expected or if she receives intraoperative or postoperative opioids. She has a moderate to high risk of PONV.

Overview of Treatment

An optimal prophylactic regimen for PONV matches medication choice with the patient's risk level.[51–53,55,56,58] Patients with zero or one risk factor typically will not need prophylaxis. Patients with moderate risk (two to three risk factors) should receive one to two antiemetics. Appropriate choices for monotherapy include droperidol, a 5-HT_3 antagonist, or dexamethasone. Patients at the highest risk for PONV (at least four risk factors) should be given prophylaxis with a combination of two to three antiemetics. Dual-therapy choices include a 5-HT_3 antagonist plus either droperidol or dexamethasone. Triple therapy would combine a 5-HT_3 antagonist plus dexamethasone plus droperidol. Because E.W. has a moderate to high risk for PONV, a combination of a 5-HT_3 antagonist (such as ondansetron 4–8 mg at the end of surgery) and dexamethasone (4–8 mg at the start of anesthesia induction) would be a good choice for prophylactic therapy.

The most effective and commonly used medications for the prevention of PONV include 5-HT_3 antagonists, dexamethasone, droperidol, and combinations of these agents. No appreciable difference is found in efficacy or adverse effects between the 5-HT_3 antagonists; therefore, the costs of the different agents should be taken into consideration when selecting therapy.[51,59] Droperidol has long been used for PONV, but concerns have been raised about the rare occurrence of QT prolongation and torsades de pointes.[58,60] Most clinicians believe droperidol to be safe, especially when doses are not excessive (up to 1.25 to 2.5 mg/dose for adults).[52,60,61] The mechanism by which dexamethasone protects against PONV is unclear, but its efficacy has been shown in many trials.[52,56,58] Combinations of medications with different mechanisms of action are more effective than monotherapy. Aprepitant has been studied in the prevention of PONV.[28,51,52] Studies have shown similar activity of aprepitant compared with ondansetron.[28,51,52] Aprepitant, however, is significantly more expensive than generic ondansetron or dexamethasone, which is a consideration. The use of aprepitant is also limited by the potential for drug interactions.[55] Dexamethasone and 5-HT_3 antagonist combinations have been well studied and are highly effective.[51,52,56,58,61] Transdermal scopolamine is also effective but can have side effects.[51] Dosages for the prophylaxis and treatment of PONV are shown in Table 22-6. The 5-HT_3 antagonists and droperidol seem to be more effective when given at the end of surgery. Corticosteroids are best given before the induction of anesthesia.[52,60]

Several methods for nonpharmacologic techniques for the prevention of PONV have been studied and have been shown to be effective, at least in some patient populations. These include acupuncture, transcutaneous nerve stimulation, acupressure at the P6 wrist point, hypnosis, and aromatherapy with isopropyl alcohol. Ginger remedies were not found to be more effective than placebo for PONV.[52]

Even with appropriate prophylaxis for PONV, some patients will experience breakthrough symptoms and require rescue therapy.[51] Patients who have not received prophylaxis with a 5-HT_3 antagonist can be offered a low dose of a 5-HT_3 antagonist for rescue. For rescue, only about one-quarter of the prophylaxis dose is needed.[52] For all patients who have breakthrough symptoms, it is important to choose an antiemetic from a different pharmacologic class than the agents used for prophylaxis.[51,53,58] Droperidol, promethazine, metoclopramide, and prochlorperazine are commonly used as rescue medications. If E.W. had breakthrough nausea, droperidol (0.625–1.25 mg IV or intramuscular every 4–6 hours as needed) would be a good choice for rescue therapy.

KEY REFERENCES AND WEBSITES

A full list of references for this chapter can be found at http://thepoint.lww.com/AT11e. Below are the key references and websites for this chapter, with the corresponding reference number in this chapter found in parentheses after the reference.

Key References

American Society of Clinical Oncology et al. American Society of Clinical Oncology guideline for antiemetics in oncology: update 2011. *J Clin Oncol*. 2011;29:4189–4198 (12)

Feyer P et al. Radiotherapy-induced nausea and vomiting (RINV): MASCC/ESMO guideline for antiemetics in radiotherapy: update 2009. *Support Care Cancer*. 2011;19(Suppl 1):S5–S14. (47)

Gan TJ et al. Society for Ambulatory Anesthesia guidelines for the management of postoperative nausea and vomiting. *Anesth Analg*. 2007;105:1615. (57)

Golding JF, Gresty MA. Motion sickness. *Curr Opin Neurol*. 2005;18:29. (6)

Ignoffo RJ. Current research on PONV/PDNV: practical implications for today's pharmacist. *Am J Health Syst Pharm*. 2009;66(1 Suppl 1): S19. (55)

Roila F et al. Guideline update for MASCC and ESMO in the prevention of chemotherapy- and radiotherapy-induced nausea and vomiting: results of the Perugia consensus conference. *Ann Oncol*. 2010;21(Suppl 5):v232. (13)

Shupak A, Gordon CR. Motion sickness: advances in pathogenesis, prediction, prevention, and treatment. *Aviat Space Environ Med*. 2006;77:1213. (3)

Key Websites

Ettinger DS et al. Antiemesis: clinical practice guidelines in oncology. V2. 2017. http://www.nccn.org/professionals/physician_gls/pdf/antiemesis.pdf. Accessed May 30, 2017. (1)

Priesol AJ. Motion sickness. Up To Date. http://www.uptodate.com/contents/motion-sickness. Accessed September 9, 2015. (2)

23 Upper Gastrointestinal Disorders

Elaine J. Law and Jeffrey J. Fong

CORE PRINCIPLES

	CHAPTER CASES
PEPTIC ULCER DISEASE	
1 Chronic peptic ulcer disease (PUD) is causally linked to *Helicobacter pylori* (*H. pylori*) infection or the use of nonsteroidal anti-inflammatory drugs (NSAIDs) and is usually characterized by epigastric pain or discomfort, sometimes accompanied by heartburn, bloating, and belching.	**Case 23-1 (Questions 1, 2), Case 23-2 (Question 1), Case 23-4 (Question 3)**
2 Treatment for PUD is aimed at relieving ulcer symptoms, healing the ulcer, eradicating *H. pylori* (if positive), preventing ulcer recurrence, and reducing ulcer-related complications; eradication is recommended for all patients with an *H. pylori*–positive active ulcer or a history of a previous ulcer or ulcer-related complication; proton-pump inhibitors (PPIs) are the drugs of choice for healing and reducing the risk of an NSAID ulcer; patients with a peptic ulcer should stop or reduce cigarette smoking and NSAID use, reduce psychologic stress, and avoid foods and beverages that trigger symptoms.	**Case 23-1 (Questions 3–10), Case 23-2 (Questions 2–10)**
3 Treatment for an *H. pylori* ulcer should be initiated with a PPI-based three-drug eradication regimen; the regimen should be effective, well-tolerated, easy to comply with, cost-effective, and should take into consideration antibiotic resistance; if a second course of therapy is necessary, it should contain different antibiotics.	**Case 23-1 (Questions 3, 4, 6–10)**
4 PPIs are the preferred agents for healing an *H. pylori*–negative NSAID ulcer because they accelerate ulcer healing and provide more effective symptom relief; the duration of treatment should be extended if the NSAID is continued; if the patient is *H. pylori* positive, a PPI-based three-drug regimen should be used.	**Case 23-2 (Questions 2, 3, 10)**
5 Prophylactic risk-reduction therapy with a PPI or misoprostol or switching to an NSAID with greater cyclooxygenase-2 (COX-2) selectivity is recommended for patients at risk of exhibiting an ulcer or ulcer-related complication; when selecting a PPI, its gastrointestinal benefits must be weighed against the cardiovascular risks associated with COX-2 inhibitors and concomitant antiplatelet therapy.	**Case 23-2 (Questions 4–7), Case 23-5 (Question 2)**
6 Patients receiving an *H. pylori* eradication regimen, those undergoing treatment for an active NSAID ulcer, and individuals receiving prophylactic risk-reduction therapy require patient education regarding ulcer risk, potential ulcer complications, and drug therapy.	**Case 23-1 (Question 5), Case 23-2 (Questions 8, 9)**
GASTROESOPHAGEAL REFLUX DISEASE	
1 The classic symptoms associated with gastroesophageal reflux disease (GERD) are usually very specific and include heartburn and acid regurgitation; however, not all patients will present with these typical symptoms and may present with more serious "alarm symptoms" or extra esophageal manifestations, warranting referral for further evaluation.	**Case 23-3 (Question 1)**
2 Appropriate management of the patient with GERD is focused on the relief of symptoms, promotion of healing of the esophageal mucosa, and prevention of relapse or the development of complicated disease. This is accomplished with lifestyle modification and pharmacotherapy directed at reducing esophageal mucosal exposure to gastric acid.	**Case 23-3 (Questions 2–4)**

Continued

		CHAPTER CASES
3	Diagnostic testing strategies for patients with more severe GERD include empiric acid suppression test, upper endoscopy and biopsy, 24-hour continuous pH monitoring, radiologic testing, and esophageal manometry.	**Case 23-4 (Question 1)**
4	Mild to moderate GERD can be managed acceptably with antacids, sucralfate, and H_2RAs; however, for more severe, frequent, or complicated GERD, the drugs of choice are PPIs, which have demonstrated superiority over these other agents in terms of symptom relief and esophageal healing.	**Case 23-4 (Question 2)**
5	GERD can be associated with numerous manifestations that occur outside the esophagus, including noncardiac chest pain, asthma, hoarseness, laryngitis, and chronic cough.	**Case 23-5 (Question 1)**
	UPPER GASTROINTESTINAL BLEEDING	
1	Stress-related mucosal bleeding (SRMB) is a serious complication that can occur in critically ill patients under severe physiologic stress. Appropriate prophylactic management includes identification of risk factors for SRMB, such as mechanical ventilation and coagulopathy, and then implementation of an appropriate pharmacotherapy strategy (e.g., PPIs, H_2RAs) aimed at reducing the risk of exhibiting SRMB.	**Case 23-6 (Questions 1–4)**

UPPER GASTROINTESTINAL DISORDERS

Upper gastrointestinal (GI) disorders include a wide spectrum of maladies that range in importance from simple discomfort to life-threatening illness and include dyspepsia, peptic ulcer disease (PUD), gastroesophageal reflux disease (GERD), and upper GI bleeding. The majority of upper GI disorders are acid-related diseases in which gastric acid plays an important role in their development, progression, and treatment. In the United States, GI disorders add up to $142 billion in direct and indirect costs each year, with more than $10 billion of this amount spent on proton-pump inhibitors (PPIs), a primary pharmacotherapeutic option used to reduce gastric acid secretion.[1] These diseases place a substantial burden on both patients and the health-care system. Data from 2009 indicated that abdominal pain was the most common GI symptom reported by patients, leading to 15.9 million clinic visits, with GERD being the most frequent outpatient diagnosis, accounting for almost 9 million clinic visits.[1] Between 250,000 and 300,000 patients are hospitalized each year for upper GI bleeding, resulting in 15,000 to 30,000 deaths. Despite numerous advances in diagnostic techniques and management strategies, mortality rates of approximately 10% to 15% are reported with more than $2.5 billion spent each year to manage these patients.[2–4]

PHYSIOLOGY OF THE UPPER GASTROINTESTINAL TRACT

The upper GI tract consists of the mouth, esophagus, stomach, and duodenum (Fig. 23-1). Ingested food or liquids pass from the mouth through the esophagus and into the stomach. As these substances enter into the esophagus, the lower esophageal sphincter (LES), an area of smooth muscle near the distal end of the esophagus, relaxes to allow their entry into the stomach. The LES usually remains contracted to prevent the reflux of gastric contents into the esophagus. However, peristaltic contractions of the esophageal muscles allow the LES to remain open until all food has entered the stomach.[5] Although the LES is the primary barrier for the prevention of gastric refluxate entering the esophagus, healthy individuals reflux throughout the day and night without clinical consequences.[6]

The stomach consists of three distinct anatomic regions, each responsible for a variety of specialized functional processes (Fig. 23-1). The cardia (~5% of stomach surface area), which is the

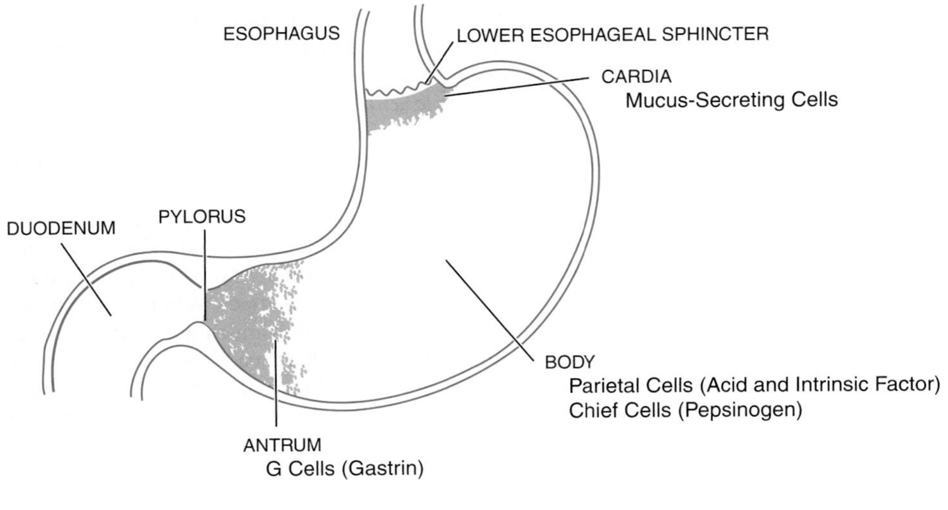

Figure 23-1 Gastrointestinal anatomic regions.

uppermost portion of the stomach, is at the junction between the esophagus and stomach and is responsible for the mucus secretion that protects against the stomach's acidic environment. The body, which makes up the majority of the surface area (80% to 90%) of the stomach, contains the parietal cells, which are responsible for gastric acid and intrinsic factor (required for vitamin B_{12} absorption) secretion. The body also contains the peptic (chief) cells, which secrete pepsinogen. Pepsinogen, under acidic conditions in the stomach, is converted to pepsin (a proteolytic enzyme), which is responsible for breaking down protein. The antrum makes up the final 10% to 20% of the stomach. It contains the G cells. The final portion of the upper GI tract is the duodenum, which begins just after the pylorus and extends to the ligament of Treitz. At this point, the jejunum begins the first portion of the lower GI tract.

The parietal cell is responsible for secreting gastric acid (Fig. 23-2). Three stimuli (neurologic, physical, and hormonal) trigger the parietal cell to secrete acid. Neurologic impulses, from the central nervous system (CNS) and initiated by the sight, smell, and taste of food, travel along cholinergic pathways to stimulate the release of acetylcholine, which arrives via nerve endings and activates the muscarinic receptor on the parietal cell.[7] Ingested food causes gastric distension, which triggers the release of acetylcholine and also stimulates G cells within the antrum to produce gastrin. Elevated intragastric pH also stimulates the production of gastrin. Gastrin works via a feedback mechanism that, although produced in response to elevated pH, can be inhibited by low gastric pH. The stomach is protected from overproduction of gastric acid by the release of somatostatin from antral D cells, which signal the G cell to stop the production of gastrin.[7,8] Gastrin enters the blood and arrives at the parietal cell, where it binds to the gastrin receptor. Acetylcholine and gastrin promote the release of histamine from

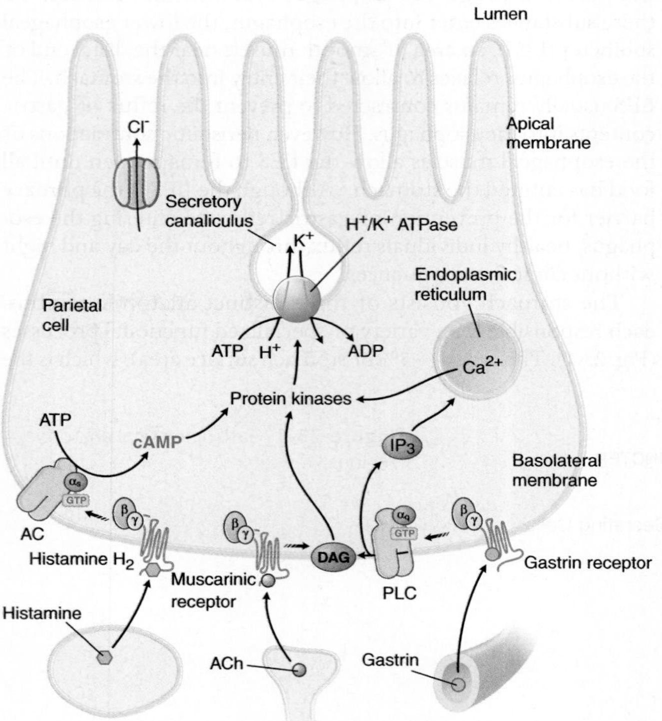

Figure 23-2 Parietal cell. ECL, enterochromaffin like. (Adapted with permission from Golan DE, et al. *Principles of Pharmacology: The Pathophysiologic Basis of Drug Therapy*. 3rd ed. Baltimore, MD: Wolters Kluwer Health; 2011.) DAG, diacylglycerol; PCL, phospholipase C.

the mast cell or enterochromaffin-like (ECL) cells, which then bind to the histamine H_2 receptor on the parietal cell. Histamine release is associated with both postprandial and nocturnal acid secretion. The gastrin, histamine H_2, and muscarinic receptors are located on the basolateral membrane of the parietal cell and binding of any of these receptors leads to a cascade of events stimulating gastric acid secretion (Fig. 23-2). Calcium influxes into the parietal cell, leading to increased intracellular levels of calcium. Levels of cyclic adenosine monophosphate also increase and activate intracellular protein phosphokinases. This, in turn, activates the hydrogen–potassium adenosine triphosphatase (H^+/K^+-ATPase) or proton pump to move into position in the secretory canaliculus located in the apical membrane of the parietal cell. The proton pump is an ion transport pathway that transports hydrogen ions out of the cytoplasm and into the secretory canaliculus, where they are exchanged for potassium ions that enter the parietal cell via the opposite ion channel. In the secretory canaliculus, hydrogen ions combine with chloride from the blood to form hydrochloric acid, which is then released into the gastric acid lumen.[7] The proton pump is the final common pathway for gastric acid secretion.[7]

PHARMACOTHERAPY OF DRUGS USED TO TREAT ACID-RELATED DISORDERS

The following section briefly reviews the pharmacotherapy of drugs used to treat acid-related disorders (Table 23-1). Their therapeutic use is discussed under each specific GI disorder.

Antacids and Alginic Acid

Antacids are widely used to relieve mild and infrequent symptoms associated with acid-related diseases. They act by neutralizing gastric acid and, thus, increasing intragastric pH.[9] The elevation of intragastric pH is dose-dependent and usually requires a substantial dose to raise the intragastric pH above 4 or 5.[9,10] Antacids are very quick acting and modestly elevate intragastric pH within minutes, but their duration of action is short (about 30 minutes on an empty stomach). The duration of action can be extended to 3 hours when given with or within 1 hour after a meal.[9] Antacids are available as individual salts or as combination of salts of magnesium, aluminum, calcium, or sodium. Aluminum salts may enhance mucosal protection by increasing mucosal prostaglandins, enhancing microvascular blood flow, stimulating mucus and bicarbonate secretion, and also by inhibiting the action of pepsin. These findings suggest that in addition to their acid-neutralizing capacity, antacids have other mechanisms by which they act. This helps to explain their many pharmacotherapeutic benefits.[9] A review of specific antacid products and their acid-neutralizing capacity is discussed elsewhere.[9] Antacids can also be combined with alginic acid. Alginic acid, however, is not an acid-neutralizing agent. It acts by forming a viscous solution that floats on top of the gastric contents and theoretically protects the esophageal mucosa from the potent acid refluxate.[11]

Antacids are generally well tolerated. The magnesium-containing antacids may cause a dose-related osmotic diarrhea but combining it with aluminum salts (which can cause constipation when used alone) can offset this side effect. When higher doses of combination of magnesium/aluminum antacids are used, the predominating side effect is diarrhea.[9,12] Small amounts of aluminum and magnesium are absorbed systemically and have the potential to accumulate in patients with renal insufficiency and lead to toxicity. Thus, magnesium-containing antacids should be avoided in patients with a creatinine clearance less

Table 23-1
Oral Medications Used to Treat Upper Gastrointestinal Disorders

	Gastric and Duodenal Ulcer Healing	Maintenance of Gastric and Duodenal Ulcer Healing	Reduction of Gastric Ulcer Risk Associated with NSAIDs	Relief of Heartburn and Indigestion (OTC Use)			Relief of GERD Symptoms (Rx Use)	Esophageal Healing[a]	Maintenance of Esophageal Healing[a]	Hypersecretory Diseases[a,b]
H_2 Receptor Antagonists										
Cimetidine	300 mg QID		400–800 mg at bedtime	Not indicated	200 mg BID PRN		300 mg QID	400 mg QID	400–800 mg at bedtime	[a]
	400 mg BID							800 mg BID		
	800 mg daily									
Famotidine	20 mg BID		20–40 mg at bedtime	Not indicated	10 mg BID PRN		20 mg BID	40 mg BID	20–40 mg BID	[a]
	40 mg at bedtime				20 mg BID PRN					
Nizatidine	150 mg BID		150–300 mg at bedtime	Not indicated	75 mg BID PRN		150 mg BID	300 mg BID	150–300 mg BID	[a]
	300 mg at bedtime									
Ranitidine	150 mg BID		150–300 mg at bedtime	Not indicated	75 mg BID PRN		150 mg BID	300 mg BID	150–300 mg BID	[a]
	300 mg at bedtime				150 mg BID PRN					
Proton-Pump Inhibitors										
Esomeprazole	20–40 mg daily		20 mg daily	20 mg daily	Not indicated		20 mg daily	20–40 mg daily	20 mg daily	60 mg daily
Dexlansoprazole	Not indicated		Not indicated	Not indicated	Not indicated		30 mg daily	60 mg daily	30 mg daily	Not indicated
Lansoprazole	15–30 mg daily		15–30 mg daily	15–30 mg daily	15 mg daily[c]		15–30 mg daily	30 mg daily	15–30 mg daily	60 mg daily
Omeprazole	20 mg daily		20 mg daily	20 mg daily	20 mg daily[c]		20 mg daily	20–40 mg daily	20 mg daily	60 mg daily
Pantoprazole	40 mg daily		40 mg daily	40 mg daily	Not indicated		20 mg daily	40 mg daily	40 mg daily	80 mg daily
Rabeprazole	20 mg daily		20 mg daily	20 mg daily	Not indicated		20 mg daily	20 mg daily	20 mg daily	60 mg daily
Other Agents										
Sucralfate	1 g QID		Not indicated	Not indicated		Not indicated	Not indicated	Not indicated	Not indicated	Not indicated
	2 g BID									
Misoprostol	Not indicated		Not indicated	200 mcg TID–QID		Not indicated	Not indicated	Not indicated	Not indicated	Not indicated

[a]Although FDA labeled for this indication, H_2RAs are not recommended even in higher dosages because they are not as effective as the PPIs.
[b]Initial starting dose; daily dosage must be titrated to gastric acid–secretory response.
[c]Duration of treatment should not exceed 14 consecutive days; if needed, repeat 14-day treatment every 4 months.

than 30 mL/minute, and chronic use of aluminum-containing antacids in patients with renal failure should be avoided.[9,12] Hypercalcemia has been described in patients taking prolonged, large doses of calcium carbonate (>20 g/day in patients with normal renal function and >4 g/day in patients with renal failure).[9] This issue is especially important when considering that many well-known over-the-counter (OTC) antacid products currently contains calcium.[12] High-dose regimens of calcium (4–8 g/day) in combination with alkalinizing agents (sodium bicarbonate) can produce the milk-alkali syndrome (i.e., hypercalcemic nephropathy with alkalosis).[9,12] Aluminum-containing antacids (with the exception of aluminum phosphate) binds to dietary phosphate within the GI tract to form insoluble salts that are excreted in feces. High dose or frequent administration may lead to hypophosphatemia.[12] Sodium bicarbonate should not be used for long periods of time (especially in the renally impaired patient) because systemic alkalosis can result from the accumulation of bicarbonate. Additionally, the high sodium content (274 mg sodium/g sodium bicarbonate) has been associated with sodium retention and may pose a problem in patients with hypertension, ascites, severe renal dysfunction, or heart failure.[9,12]

Antacids may lower the bioavailability of many orally administered drugs (e.g., digoxin, phenytoin, isoniazid, ketoconazole, itraconazole, iron preparations) that require an acidic environment for dissolution and absorption.[9,11,13] This may lead to potential therapeutic failures with these medications. Tetracyclines and fluoroquinolones are susceptible to interactions with antacids containing calcium, aluminum, or magnesium because they bind to divalent and trivalent cations.[12] The bioavailability of ciprofloxacin, for example, is reduced by more than 50% when concomitantly administered with an antacid, because aluminum and magnesium ions chelate with the antibiotic to form an insoluble and inactive complex. It is recommended to separate ciprofloxacin administration away from antacid use by 2 hours.[14] An increase in gastric pH may also result in the premature dissolution and altered absorption of enteric-coated dosage forms because the enteric coating is usually designed to dissolve at a pH greater than 6.0.[13] Urinary alkalinization may result in increased urinary excretion (salicylates) or decreased excretion (amphetamines and quinidine) leading to decreased or increased blood concentrations, respectively.[9,12] The majority of these drug interactions can be avoided by separating the antacid from the interacting drug by a minimum of 2 hours.[12]

Histamine-2 Receptor Antagonists

There are currently four H_2-receptor antagonists (H_2RAs) approved for use in the United States. These include cimetidine, ranitidine, famotidine, and nizatidine. All four agents are available in prescription and OTC dosage forms, as well as oral and parenteral formulations (nizatidine is not available parenterally in the United States). H_2RAs competitively and selectively inhibit the action of histamine on the H_2 receptors of the parietal cells, thus reducing both basal and stimulated gastric acid secretion (Fig. 23-2). Although the relative antisecretory potency on a milligram-per-milligram basis differs (famotidine has the greatest potency followed by nizatidine, ranitidine, and cimetidine), this is not an important factor because standard oral dosages of the four H_2RAs have been adjusted accordingly to have an equipotent antisecretory effect (Table 23-1).[15] Oral absorption from the small intestine is rapid, and peak drug concentrations usually are achieved within 1 to 3 hours after administration.[15] The bioavailability is lower for cimetidine, famotidine, and ranitidine because they are absorbed incompletely and undergo first-pass metabolism resulting in 40% to 65% bioavailability. The bioavailability of nizatidine is considered nearly 100% because this agent does not undergo first-pass metabolism.[15,16] All four drugs are eliminated by a combination of hepatic metabolism, glomerular filtration, and tubular secretion.[15] Hepatic metabolism is the principal pathway for the elimination of cimetidine, famotidine, and ranitidine, whereas renal excretion is the major route for elimination of nizatidine.[15–19] Dose reductions for all four agents are recommended for patients with moderate to severe renal insufficiency. The pharmacokinetics appear to be unaffected by hepatic dysfunction; however, in patients with combined hepatic failure and renal insufficiency, dosage reduction is likely necessary.[17]

H_2RAs are remarkably safe, and the frequency of severe adverse effects is low for all four drugs.[20] A meta-analysis of randomized placebo-controlled trials reported no difference in the incidence of adverse events of cimetidine versus placebo.[21] The most common adverse effects include GI discomfort (e.g., diarrhea, constipation), CNS effects (e.g., headache, dizziness, drowsiness, lethargy, confusion, psychosis, and hallucinations), and dermatologic effects (e.g., rashes).[20] The most frequent hematologic adverse effect is thrombocytopenia, which occurs in about 1% of patients but is reversible upon discontinuation of the H_2RA.[22] Although thrombocytopenia is more commonly reported with intravenous (IV) administration, it is likely that the overall incidence of H_2RA-associated thrombocytopenia is overestimated.[23] Hepatotoxicity, although uncommon, has been described primarily in patients receiving IV H_2RAs.[24] Cimetidine has demonstrated weak antiandrogenic effects, and its use in high doses (hypersecretory conditions) has been associated with gynecomastia and impotence in men. This effect is reversible with discontinuation of the medication or by switching to another H_2RA.[20,25] Patients at highest risk of experiencing any of these adverse effects include the elderly, those requiring higher doses (usually parenteral), and those with altered renal function.[25,26]

Similar to antacids, all four H_2RAs can potentially alter the absorption and reduce the bioavailability of drugs that require an acidic environment for absorption. The most important of these interactions is with ketoconazole, which requires an acidic pH for dissolution and absorption, potentially resulting in therapeutic failure of the antifungal.[13] Cimetidine has the greatest potential to cause drug interactions because of its ability to potently inhibit several hepatic cytochrome P-450 (CYP450) isoenzymes. The greatest concern is with those agents that have a relatively narrow therapeutic window (e.g., theophylline, lidocaine, phenytoin, quinidine, and warfarin).[13] Although ranitidine is more potent on a molar basis, it binds less intensely to the CYP450 isoenzyme system than cimetidine. Thus, when used in equipotent doses, there is less potential for interactions. Famotidine and nizatidine do not bind appreciably to the CYP450 system and do not interact with drugs that are metabolized through this hepatic system.[13] Because H_2RAs undergo renal tubular excretion, there is a potential for competition with other medications.[27] Cimetidine and ranitidine inhibit the tubular secretion of procainamide by as much as 44%, but famotidine does not have this effect.[28] Tachyphylaxis or tolerance has been described with all H_2RAs because of upregulation of the H_2 receptor site. It appears to occur more frequently with high-dose parenteral formulations but has also been described with oral therapy.[26,29] Tolerance to the antisecretory effect may develop after several days of regularly scheduled (continuous) use but can be avoided by taking the H_2RA only when needed.[30]

Proton-Pump Inhibitors

PPIs are highly specific inhibitors of gastric acid secretion and include omeprazole, lansoprazole, rabeprazole, pantoprazole, esomeprazole, and dexlansoprazole. These agents are substituted benzimidazoles and act by irreversibly binding to the H^+/K^+-ATPase (proton pump). PPIs are the most potent inhibitors of gastric acid secretion in that they inhibit the terminal step in the acid production cycle.[31–33] They inhibit both basal and stimulated gastric acid secretion in a dose-dependent and sustained fashion.[32] PPIs are prodrugs and require an acidic environment for conversion to the active sulfonamide. They are absorbed in the small intestine (protected from the acidic milieu of the stomach by enteric coating) and taken via the bloodstream to the acidic secretory canaliculus of the parietal cell for protonation to the active form (Fig. 23-2).[31,33] This conversion requires an actively secreting proton pump, and hence, these agents are most efficacious when taken 30 to 60 minutes before a meal on an empty stomach.[33] The most recent PPI, dexlansoprazole MR (modified release), differs from others in this class in that they use dual delayed-release technology, which extends the duration of their antisecretory effect. Dexlansoprazole MR contains two different pH-dependent granules. The first of these is initially released in the proximal duodenum similar to the other PPIs, followed by a second release of drug in the distal small intestine approximately 4 hours later. Given this broadened duration of drug exposure, dexlansoprazole MR may also be taken without regard to meal times.[34] Despite the short plasma elimination half-lives (~1–2 hours) of the other PPIs, the duration of their antisecretory effect is 48 to 72 hours because of covalent (irreversible) binding to the proton pump.[33,35] PPIs have similar acid-inhibitory effects and healing rates when used in equivalent doses (Table 23-1).[36–41] PPIs are superior to H_2RAs in reducing gastric acid secretion and mucosal healing.[35,41,42] Dosage reduction is not required in patients with renal insufficiency but is recommended for patients with severe hepatic impairment.[43]

The oral PPIs are formulated as delayed-release enteric-coated granules within capsules (omeprazole, lansoprazole, esomeprazole, dexlansoprazole MR), delayed-release enteric-coated tablets (pantoprazole, rabeprazole, OTC omeprazole), a rapidly disintegrating tablet (lansoprazole), delayed-release oral suspension (lansoprazole), and an immediate-release formulation (omeprazole and sodium bicarbonate capsules and powder for oral suspension).[36] IV formulations in the United States include pantoprazole and esomeprazole. Various methods of administration, specific dosage forms, and compounding options for patients with special needs (e.g., dysphagia, gastric tubes) will be discussed later in this chapter (see section on Upper Gastrointestinal Bleeding).

The short-term adverse effects of PPIs are relatively infrequent and comparable with H_2RAs or placebo. The most common side effects include GI discomfort (e.g., nausea, diarrhea, abdominal pain), CNS effects (e.g., headache, dizziness), and rare isolated reactions (e.g., skin rash, increased liver enzymes).[31,44] The immediate-release formulation of omeprazole contains sodium bicarbonate, and care should be taken in sodium-restricted patient populations, as discussed in the subsection Antacids and Alginic Acid of the Pharmacotherapy of Drugs Used to Treat Acid-Related Disorders. All PPIs are metabolized by the hepatic CYP450 microenzyme system. Omeprazole and esomeprazole have been described as inhibiting CYP2C19 and decreasing the clearance of diazepam, phenytoin, and R-warfarin, whereas lansoprazole increases the metabolism of theophylline by inducing CYP1A.[33,45] Although the clinical importance of these interactions is thought to be negligible, care should be taken when combining these agents to prevent possible toxicity or therapeutic failure.

The potential CYP2C19 interaction with the PPIs and the thienopyridine antiplatelet drug clopidogrel has generated a substantial amount of interest and debate. In 2008, consensus guidelines developed by the American College of Cardiology, the American Heart Association, and American College of Gastroenterology recommended the prophylactic use of PPIs in patients receiving concomitant dual antiplatelet therapy with aspirin and clopidogrel to reduce the risk of upper GI bleeding.[46] Since the publication of this document, there have been numerous reports suggesting an interaction between PPIs and clopidogrel, which attenuates the antiplatelet effects of clopidogrel and potentially increases the risk of adverse cardiovascular outcomes.[47–51] The hypothesis for this interaction is based on the requirement of clopidogrel to undergo biotransformation through CYP2C19 for conversion from prodrug to active metabolite. Because PPIs also require this metabolic pathway for metabolism, it has been suggested in pharmacokinetic and pharmacodynamic studies that concurrent use of PPIs may inhibit or compete for this enzyme, leading to a reduction in the conversion of clopidogrel to its active metabolite and, therefore, a reduction in its efficacy toward platelet inhibition.[48–51] Cardiovascular outcomes' studies involving a plethora of observational designs have suggested higher cardiovascular event rates (composite ischemic endpoints, all-cause mortality, nonfatal myocardial infarctions, stroke, and stent thrombosis).[51]

One important confounding variable involved in the evaluation of this interaction is the role played by genetic polymorphisms in CYP2C19—these can result in loss of functional alleles, which has been related to decreased clopidogrel effectiveness as a result of reduced ability to convert clopidogrel to the active metabolite responsible for platelet inhibition.[52] Upon review of this body of evidence, the US Food and Drug Administration (FDA) in 2009 issued a labeling change for clopidogrel and a safety warning recommending providers to avoid the coadministration of omeprazole, omeprazole/sodium bicarbonate, or esomeprazole with clopidogrel.[53] An update to the 2008 consensus document has attempted to critically evaluate the evidence regarding the interaction and give direction for health-care providers.[54] Although this document has taken a more cautious approach, suggesting that a likely interaction may exist especially between clopidogrel and omeprazole, data supporting definitive adverse clinical outcomes as a result of the interaction are limited to observational data. Also, the consensus document suggests there is no evidence to suggest switching from one PPI to another or that separating the timing of doses has any clear benefit on reducing the magnitude of the interaction.[54] A meta-analysis including more recently published, randomized controlled trials evaluating this drug interaction found conflicting results, whereas aggregate results from randomized controlled trials showed no difference in cardiovascular outcomes.[55] Until more comprehensive evidence becomes available, the most important aspects to consider are to ensure that patients have an appropriate indication for the use of a PPI, to determine that on a case by case basis the benefit outweighs the risk, and, if possible, to avoid concomitant use of omeprazole or esomeprazole with clopidogrel unless absolutely necessary.

An increase in intragastric pH may increase the bioavailability of orally administered medications (e.g., digoxin, nifedipine), leading to the possibility of toxicity, or it may decrease the absorption of ketoconazole and cefpodoxime, increasing the possibility of therapeutic failure.[33,45]

PPIs have been associated with a number of adverse effects when used long term and in high dosages.[56,57] However, in most cases, there is insufficient evidence to support a causal relationship between the PPI and the effect. There is evidence to suggest a relationship between elevated serum gastrin concentrations and ECL hyperplasia as a result of the PPIs' profound ability to inhibit gastric acid secretion. It has been hypothesized that this can progress to gastric carcinoid tumors (a precursor of gastric cancer). Although ECL hyperplasia has been described with the use of PPIs, there is no clinical evidence to suggest that long-term (>10 years) therapy progresses to a higher grade of hyperplasia or gastric ECL carcinoid.[58] Atrophic gastritis has been observed in gastric corpus biopsies from patients treated long term with omeprazole and positive for *Helicobacter pylori*. However, review of the data by the FDA has been inconclusive and not able to show causality among long-term use of PPIs, *H. pylori*, and atrophic gastritis.[56–58]

PPIs have been associated with an increased risk of infections (e.g., pneumonias, enteric infections) possibly because of the ability of the microorganisms to survive in a less acidic environment.[56–60] Acute nosocomial infections (pneumonia) associated with critically ill patients will be described later when discussing high-dose oral and parenteral PPI therapy (see section on Upper Gastrointestinal Bleeding). The risk of development of community-acquired pneumonia in patients treated with PPIs has also been evaluated in numerous retrospective studies; however, causality has been very difficult to establish and remains controversial.[57] Enteric infections and cancer have also been described as a result of potential bacterial overgrowth. The most common pathogens are *Clostridium difficile, Salmonella typhimurium, and Campylobacter jejuni*; however, data suggest that they rarely lead to illness.[59–60] A retrospective database study of PPI use describes a near threefold increase in the risk of *C. difficile*–associated diarrhea in patients receiving PPIs versus patients not on a PPI, but the overall risk remains low and should not be considered a contraindication to therapy.[61] Results from two published meta-analyses totaling ~300,000 patients enrolled into observational studies suggest that PPI users are at a greater than 65% risk increase of developing *C. difficile*–associated diarrhea.[61,62]

Long-term PPI use in older patients on high dosages has also been associated with an increased risk of hip fractures through the presumed inhibition of calcium absorption by PPI-induced hypochlorhydria or through inhibition of proton pumps within the osteoclastic vacuole resulting in decreased bone resorption.[56,63] Long-term PPI use has also been modestly associated with fractures of the spine, forearm, and wrist.[63] In a large retrospective cohort study of 8,400 patients, PPI therapy was not associated with any significant acceleration in bone-mineral density loss after 5 and 10 years of follow up. Additional studies are required to confirm a causal relationship between long-term PPIs and bone fractures, and at this time, additional bone density testing and calcium supplementation are not suggested beyond age-related recommendations.[60,64–67]

A decrease in vitamin B_{12} (cyanocobalamin) has been described in patients with long-term PPI use and may occur because gastric acid is required to liberate the vitamin from dietary sources.[56–58,67] In a large retrospective case-controlled study, long-duration PPI usage (greater than 2 years) was associated with an increased odds ratios of 1.65 (95% CI: 1.58–1.73). There was also a dose relationship, where high doses were associated an increased odds ratio of 1.95 (95% CI: 1.77–2.15).[67] Hypomagnesemia may occur in adults taking PPIs for longer than 1 year, but cases have been reported after 3 months of treatment.[68–70] This relationship has been confirmed in two retrospective studies in ambulatory care patients. The exact mechanism by which PPIs increase the risk of hypomagnesemia is uncertain but may be associated with altered intestinal absorption of magnesium. Malabsorption of iron secondary to long-term gastric acid suppression has been suggested but has not been confirmed in clinical trials.[56,57] PPIs have been associated with interstitial nephritis, but this is an extremely rare finding.[57,71] Although the long-term effects associated with PPIs are uncommon, the benefit of long-term use must always be weighed against potential risks in each individual patient.

Sucralfate

Sucralfate (an aluminum salt of a sulfated disaccharide) promotes gastric mucosal protection by shielding ulcerated tissue from aggressive factors, such as acid, pepsin, and bile salts.[72] At a pH of 2.0 to 2.5, sucralfate binds to damaged and ulcerated mucosa, forming a physical barrier against injury from these aggressive factors. The drug has minimal systemic absorption and does not possess antisecretory activity. Sucralfate may also have other protective actions related to the stimulation of mucosal prostaglandins.[72] The most common side effect associated with sucralfate is constipation, which occurs in approximately 1% to 3% of patients.[72] This is most likely attributable to the aluminum content of the compound, which can accumulate in patients with renal insufficiency. Therefore, long-term use should be avoided.[72] Additionally, aluminum salts can bind with dietary phosphate in the GI tract, the potential for hypophosphatemia exists (see subsection on Antacids and Alginic Acid of the section Pharmacotherapy of Drugs Used to Treat Acid-Related Disorders). Sucralfate tablets are large, and some patients, particularly the elderly, may have difficulty swallowing them. A liquid formulation is available for patients with swallowing difficulties. The bioavailability of oral fluoroquinolones, warfarin, phenytoin, levothyroxine, quinidine, ketoconazole, amitriptyline, and theophylline may be reduced when concomitantly administered with sucralfate.[13] The mechanism of these interactions is thought to be caused by binding of the medication with sucralfate in the GI tract, thus, limiting their absorption. Because of these interactions, sucralfate should be given at least 2 hours after these medications.

Misoprostol

Misoprostol, a synthetic prostaglandin E_1 analog, is the only prostaglandin analog approved for use in the United States. Misoprostol acts primarily by enhancing mucosal defense mechanisms.[73] It produces cytoprotective effects by stimulating the production of mucus and bicarbonate, improving mucosal blood flow, and reducing mucosal cell turnover similar to the effects of endogenous prostaglandin.[73] Misoprostol also produces a dose-dependent inhibition of gastric acid, but even at high doses, the inhibition is less than that of H_2RAs. The use of misoprostol is limited because of its potential to cause dose-dependent diarrhea (in up to 30% of patients) and abdominal cramping.[73] Taking the drug with meals may help to reduce the incidence of diarrhea. Decreasing the daily dose may also reduce diarrhea, but efficacy may be compromised[74] (see section on Peptic Ulcer Disease). Other troublesome side effects include nausea, flatulence, and headaches. Misoprostol is an abortifacient because of its uterotropic effects. Thus, it is contraindicated in pregnant women.[73,75] Use in women in their childbearing years requires a negative serum pregnancy test and adequate contraception.

Bismuth Salts

Bismuth subsalicylate has been used for years as an OTC option for many GI ailments. Although its mechanism of action is not completely understood, bismuth is thought to work by binding to and protecting mucosal lesions and enhancing cellular protective mechanisms. Bismuth also has an antimicrobial effect, primarily against *H. pylori*.[76] Bismuth salts have no acid-inhibitory effects. Bismuth-containing products have few side effects, but there is a decrease in drug elimination in patients with renal impairment. Bismuth subsalicylate should be used with caution in patients on concomitant salicylates because the potential exists for salicylate toxicity or increased bleeding risk. Patients with salicylate allergies or sensitivities should also be warned of the salicylate component. Long-term use is also not advised. Bismuth salts are associated with a harmless black coloring of the stools because of colonic conversion of bismuth to bismuth sulfide and a potential black discoloration of the tongue with liquid dosage forms.[8] Bismuth subcitrate potassium (biskalcitrate) is only available as a combination product with metronidazole and tetracycline for the treatment of *H. pylori* infection[77] (see section on Peptic Ulcer Disease). Although side effects are similar to bismuth subsalicylate, it has the advantage of not containing salicylate.

DYSPEPSIA

Dyspepsia refers to a subjective feeling of pain or discomfort located primarily in the upper abdomen and is a common problem that affects about 25% of the U.S. population.[78,79] The etiology of dyspepsia can be secondary to an organic disease, such as PUD, GERD with or without esophagitis, and gastric malignancy, or drug induced from medications such as nonsteroidal anti-inflammatory drugs (NSAIDs), antibiotics, such as erythromycin and tetracycline, iron and potassium supplements, digoxin, theophylline, and bisphosphonates. Smoking or a stressful lifestyle can also play a role in dyspepsia (Fig. 23-3). With chronic dyspepsia, patients usually have intermittent symptoms lasting a long time despite periods of remission. Heartburn may coexist with dyspepsia but is usually suggestive of GERD.

Patients who have not undergone diagnostic testing are referred to as having "uninvestigated" dyspepsia, whereas those who have undergone testing (usually upper endoscopy) are said to have "investigated" dyspepsia (Fig. 23-3). Functional dyspepsia, also known as idiopathic or non-ulcer dyspepsia (NUD), is a clinical syndrome in which there is no evidence of mucosal damage related to PUD, GERD, or malignancy found at endoscopy.

Functional dyspepsia is defined based on the ROME III diagnostic criteria. It includes the presence of one or more of the following symptoms for the last 3 months with symptom onset 6 months before diagnosis and no evidence of structural anatomic symptoms.[80,81]

- Postprandial fullness (classified as postprandial distress syndrome)
- Early satiation (inability to finish a normal-sized meal, also classified as postprandial distress syndrome)
- Epigastric pain or burning (classified as epigastric pain syndrome)

Pathophysiology

Acute, infrequent dyspepsia is most often related to food, alcohol, smoking, or stress. Chronic dyspepsia may be related to an underlying cause, such as PUD, GERD, or malignancy, or may not have any known cause (endoscopy-negative, functional, idiopathic dyspepsia). About 40% of patients with functional dyspepsia have pathophysiologic disturbances that involve delayed gastric emptying.[81] There is also evidence that the esophagus, stomach, duodenum, and other regions of the GI tract are hypersensitive and may be associated with irritable bowel syndrome, especially in women.[81] Others have failed to find a pathologic association between functional dyspepsia and gastroduodenal motility, hypersensitivity, or any other GI abnormality, and suggest that psychologic disturbances are an important contributing factor. Although *H. pylori* infection has been identified in 20% to 60% of patients with functional dyspepsia, its pathophysiologic relevance remains uncertain.[80]

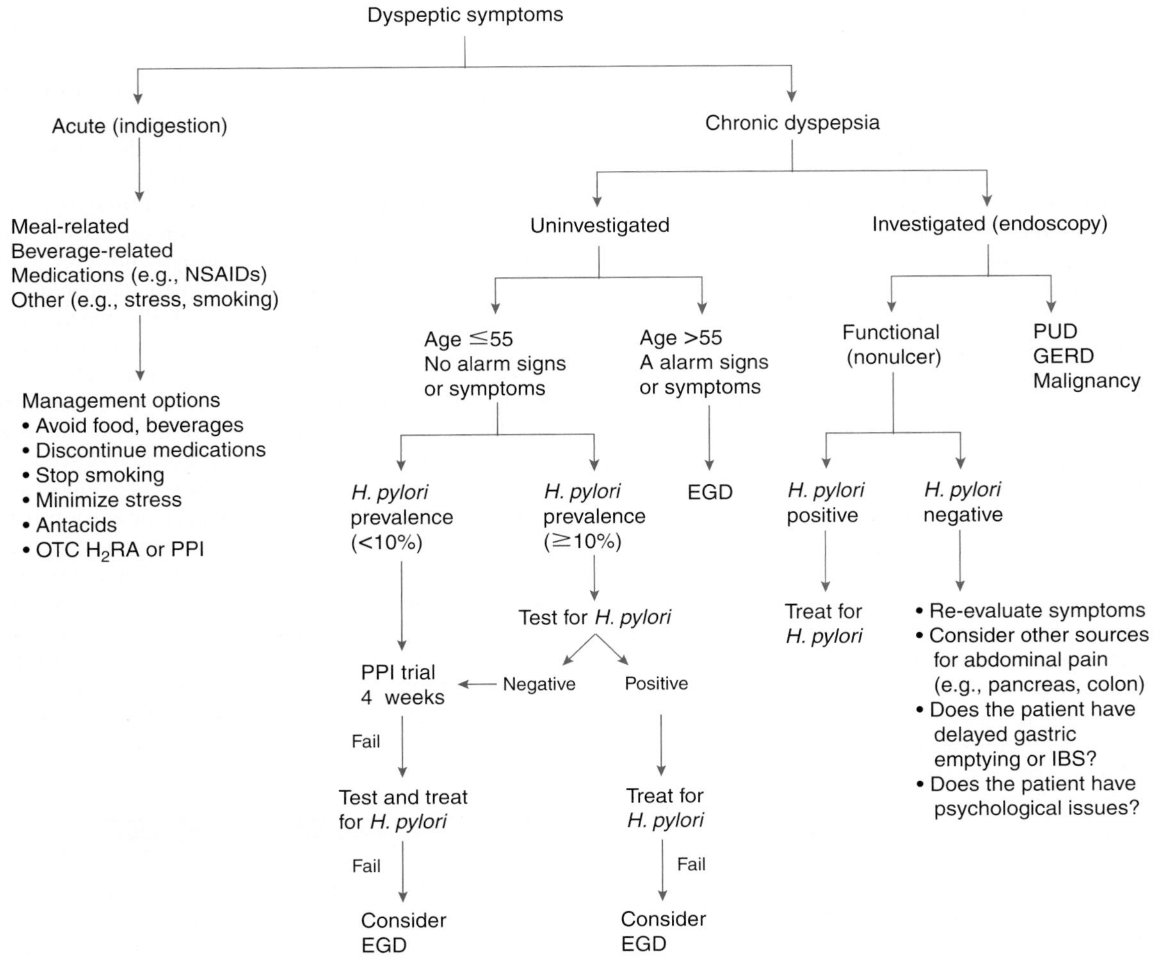

Figure 23-3 Management of dyspeptic symptoms. EGD, esophagogastroduodenoscopy; GERD, gastroesophageal reflux disease; *H. pylori*, *Helicobacter pylori*; H_2RA, H_2 receptor antagonist; IBS, irritable bowel syndrome; NSAID, nonsteroidal anti-inflammatory drug; OTC, over-the-counter; PPI, proton-pump inhibitor; PUD, peptic ulcer disease.

Clinical Assessment and Diagnosis

Acute, infrequent dyspepsia is usually self-limiting and generally requires no further investigation. Chronic dyspeptic symptoms cannot be used to predict endoscopic findings of PUD, GERD, or malignancy in patients with uninvestigated dyspepsia.[81–83] In addition, individual symptoms or symptom subgroups, such as PUD-like, GERD-like, or dysmotility-like dyspepsia are not useful in distinguishing organic disease from functional dyspepsia nor does it appear to aid in management. This is because there is considerable overlap of symptoms among patients with PUD, GERD, malignancy, and functional dyspepsia.

The clinical assessment of uninvestigated dyspepsia in patients younger than or 55 years of age with no alarm signs or symptoms includes a test-and-treat *H. pylori* option, which is preferable in geographic areas of moderate to high prevalence of *H. pylori* infection ($\geq$10%)[81] (Fig. 23-3). *H. pylori* testing should be conducted by using a nonendoscopic-validated test (see section on Tests for Detecting *Helicobacter pylori*). New-onset dyspepsia in an older individual is considered an independent risk factor for an underlying malignancy such as gastric cancer.[81] Dyspeptic patients older than 55 years of age or those with alarm signs or symptoms should undergo upper endoscopy (Fig. 23-3). Other alarm features that assist in identifying serious underlying diseases, especially malignancy, include early satiety, anorexia, worsening dysphagia or odynophagia, unexplained weight loss (>10% body weight), vomiting, anemia, GI bleeding, lymphadenopathy, jaundice, a history of PUD, a family history of upper GI tract cancer, previous gastric surgery, or malignancy.[81] Although a symptom duration threshold has not been established, a long history of symptoms or antisecretory drug use may suggest a serious underlying condition.

Table 23-2
Indications for Testing and Treating *Helicobacter pylori* Infection

Recommended (Evidence Established)
■ Uninvestigated dyspepsia (depending on *H. pylori* prevalence)
■ PUD (active gastric or duodenal ulcer)
■ History of PUD (confirmed ulcer not previously treated for *H. pylori*)
■ Gastric MALT lymphoma
■ After resection of early gastric cancer
■ Reduce the risk of recurrent bleeding from gastroduodenal ulcer
Controversial (Evidence Not Well Established)
■ NUD
■ Individuals using NSAIDs (no signs/symptoms of peptic ulcer)
■ GERD
■ Individuals at risk for gastric cancer
■ Individuals with unexplained iron deficiency anemia

GERD, gastroesophageal reflux disease; MALT, mucosa-associated lymphoid tissue; NUD, non-ulcer dyspepsia; NSAID, nonsteroidal anti-inflammatory drug; PUD, peptic ulcer disease.

From Talley NJ, Holtmann G. Approach to the patient with dyspepsia and related functional gastrointestinal complaints. In: Yamada T et al, eds. *Principles of Clinical Gastroenterology*. 5th ed. Hoboken, NJ: Wiley-Blackwell; 2008:38; Chey WD et al. American College of Gastroenterology guideline on the management of *Helicobacter pylori* infection. *Am J Gastroenterol*. 2007;102:1808; De Vries AC, Kuipers EF. *Helicobacter pylori* infection and nonmalignant diseases. *Helicobacter*. 2010;15(Suppl 1):29; Figura N et al. Extragastric manifestations of *Helicobacter pylori* infection. *Helicobacter*. 2010;15(Suppl 1):60.

Treatment

The recommended strategies for managing dyspepsia in adults are presented in Figure 23-3. Individuals with acute dyspepsia can be effectively treated with self-directed therapy using antacids or OTC antisecretory drugs if they are unable or unwilling to avoid offending foods and beverages, stop smoking, or discontinue troublesome medications. The initial management of patients younger than or 55 years of age with uninvestigated chronic dyspepsia and no alarm features depends on the prevalence of *H. pylori* and whether the patient is *H. pylori* positive or *H. pylori* negative (Table 23-2). Empiric therapy with a PPI for 4 weeks is considered first-line treatment and cost-effective in areas with a low prevalence of *H. pylori* and in patients who are *H. pylori* negative.[81–83] PPIs should be discontinued after 1 month if the patient's symptoms respond to treatment. If symptoms recur, then long-term PPI therapy may be considered, but the need for a PPI should be evaluated every 6 to 12 months.[80] Endoscopy is advocated for patients who fail to respond to an initial 4 to 8 weeks of empiric PPI therapy and those whose symptoms continue to recur after stopping the PPI (Fig. 23-3).[80,81] Patients who are *H. pylori* positive should receive a PPI-based eradication regimen[80–83] (see section on *Helicobacter pylori*–Related Ulcers).

Early endoscopy with biopsy for *H. pylori* is recommended for patients older than 55 years of age with uninvestigated chronic dyspepsia and those with alarm features. In the event that an abnormality (such as PUD, GERD, or malignancy) is found, it should be treated accordingly. The medical management of functional dyspepsia (e.g., NUD) is challenging and, when possible, should take into consideration the cost-effectiveness of treatment.[81–83] Although pharmacotherapy is considered for most patients, evidence of benefit is limited because of the lack of well-designed studies and an incomplete understanding of the disorder. Meta-analyses have demonstrated the efficacy of H_2RAs and PPIs, but there is no evidence to support the use of antacids, sucralfate, and misoprostol.[84] There appears to be no difference in efficacy between full-dose or double-dose PPIs.[84] An economic review suggests that PPIs are cost-effective for functional dyspepsia in the United States.[85] The impact of *H. pylori* eradication in functional dyspepsia remains limited, in part, because of the lack of short-term symptomatic benefit and because of the steadily declining prevalence of *H. pylori* in the United States.[82] An updated meta-analysis, however, reports a small therapeutic gain with eradication when compared with placebo at 12 months of follow up.[86] Although the benefit of prokinetics have been reported, most studies were conducted with cisapride, which was withdrawn from the U.S. market.[84] The use of available prokinetics (metoclopramide and erythromycin) should be reserved for difficult-to-treat patients because of their side effects and limited efficacy.[81,83] New guidelines also recommend against the combination of prokinetics and H_2RAs because the combination was not shown to be more effective than either agent alone and is usually not used unless there is the presence of gastroparesis. Antidepressants, especially the tricyclics, are often prescribed in functional dyspepsia and may have some benefit; however, the mechanism for this finding is unclear, and published clinical trials are small and of poor quality resulting in uncertain efficacy.[81,83,84] Alternative therapies, including herbal products, remain unproven.[81] Patients with persistent dyspepsia despite a negative endoscopy, in whom PPI therapy and *H. pylori* eradication fails, should have their diagnosis reevaluated.

PEPTIC ULCER DISEASE

PUD is one of the most common gastroenterologic diseases affecting the upper GI tract.[87] Chronic peptic ulcers are defects in the gastric (gastric ulcer) or duodenal (duodenal ulcer) mucosa that require gastric acid for their formation. Chronic peptic ulcers differ from erosions and gastritis in that the ulcer extends deeper into the muscularis mucosa.[87,88]

Stress ulcer is an acute form of peptic ulcer, but it occurs primarily in critically ill patients and differs in its underlying pathogenesis (see section on Stress-Related Mucosal Bleeding).

Epidemiology

It is difficult to estimate the epidemiology of PUD because of the different methods used to diagnose peptic ulcers (e.g., symptom-based, ulcer-related complications, radiology, or endoscopy) as well as differences in NSAID use, *H. pylori* prevalence, and cigarette smoking. Improved medical treatment, changes in the criteria and coding for hospitalizations and mortality, and the evolution from hospital-based to ambulatory care have also altered the epidemiology of PUD.[87] Current data suggest a shift in the prevalence of PUD in the United States from predominantly men to a comparable rate in men and women.[87] A declining ulcer rate in younger individuals and an increasing rate for older adults reflect a decline in *H. pylori* infection and an increased use of NSAIDs in the United States. Office visits, hospitalizations, and deaths have modestly declined during the last four decades, but deaths among older patients (>75 years) have increased and are most likely related to NSAID use.[87]

Etiology and Risk Factors

H. pylori and NSAIDs are the two most common causes of chronic PUD and influence the chronicity of the disease.[87] Less common causes include hypersecretory states, such as Zollinger–Ellison syndrome (ZES) (see section on Zollinger–Ellison Syndrome), viral infections (e.g., cytomegalovirus), radiation, and chemotherapy (e.g., hepatic artery infusion).[87] Factors that may increase the risk of a peptic ulcer include alcohol ingestion; cigarette smoking; psychologic stress; corticosteroids; and chronic diseases, such as renal failure, cirrhosis, pancreatitis, obstructive pulmonary disease, Crohn disease, or organ transplantation.[87]

HELICOBACTER PYLORI–RELATED ULCERS

H. pylori infection is causally linked to chronic gastritis, PUD, mucosa-associated lymphoid tissue (MALT) lymphoma, and gastric cancer (Table 23-2).[87–92] The lifetime risk of exhibiting an endoscopic ulcer in *H. pylori*–positive individuals is 10% to 20%, and the risk for developing gastric cancer is 1% to 2%.[87,88,92] Differences in strain variability and host-specific factors account for the variable pathogenesis of the organism.[88,91] There is an increasing evidence that iron deficiency anemia and idiopathic thrombocytopenia are associated with *H. pylori* infection, but cause and effect remain unproven.[89,93] The association between *H. pylori* and PUD bleeding remains unclear, but *H. pylori* eradication decreases recurrent bleeding[89] (see section on Upper Gastrointestinal Bleeding).

The prevalence of *H. pylori* varies by geographic location, socioeconomic status, ethnicity, and age and is more common in developing countries than in industrialized nations.[88] The overall prevalence in the United States is estimated to be 30% to 40% but is higher in older individuals (50%–60%) than in children (10%–15%).[88] The higher prevalence among older adults reflects acquisition during infancy and early childhood. However, infection rates in the United States have been declining in children because of improved socioeconomic conditions.[88,89]

Transmission occurs usually during childhood from the infected person by either the gastro-oral (vomitus) or fecal–oral (diarrhea) route or from fecal-contaminated water or food.[88,90] Individuals living in the same household with an *H. pylori*–positive person, especially when there is household crowding, are at increased risk for acquiring the infection.[88,90] *H. pylori* can also be transmitted through the use of inadequately sterilized endoscopes.

Nonsteroidal Anti-Inflammatory Drug–Induced Ulcers

There is a considerable evidence linking the chronic use of NSAIDs with GI injury.[87,94–97] Endoscopically confirmed gastric and duodenal ulcers develop in 15% to 30% of chronic NSAID users, and 2% to 4% experience ulcer-related bleeding or perforation.[94,95] Gastric ulcer is most common and develops primarily in the antrum. NSAIDs may also cause ulcers in the esophagus and the colon, but these ulcers occur less frequently and differ in their underlying pathogenesis.[94,97] It is estimated that NSAIDs account for about 100,000 hospitalizations and 7,000 to 10,000 deaths annually in the United States, but mortality may be overstated because of the recent decline in hospitalizations.[95] A national prescription audit in the United States revealed an annual NSAID cost of $4.9 billion, with additional nonprescription NSAID sales of $3 billion.[98] The risk factors for NSAID-induced ulcers and upper GI complications are listed in Table 23-3. Combinations of factors confer an additive risk.

Table 23-3
Risk Factors for Nonsteroidal Anti-Inflammatory Drug–Induced Ulcer and Ulcer-Related Upper Gastrointestinal Complications

Established

- Confirmed prior ulcer or ulcer-related complication
- Age >65 years
- Multiple or high-dose NSAID use
- Concomitant use of aspirin (including low cardioprotective dosages, e.g., 81 mg)
- Concomitant use of an anticoagulant, corticosteroid, bisphosphonate, clopidogrel, or SSRI
- Selection of NSAID (selectivity of COX-1 vs. COX-2)

Controversial

- *H. pylori*
- Alcohol consumption
- Cigarette smoking

COX-1, cyclooxygenase-1; COX-2, cyclooxygenase-2; NSAID, nonsteroidal anti-inflammatory drug; SSRI, selective serotonin reuptake inhibitor.
From Soll AH, Graham DY. Peptic ulcer disease. In: Yamada T et al, eds. *Textbook of Gastroenterology*. 5th ed. Hoboken, NJ: Wiley-Blackwell; 2009:936; Chey WD et al. American College of Gastroenterology guideline on the management of *Helicobacter pylori* infection. *Am J Gastroenterol*. 2007;102:1808; Scarpignato C, Hunt RH. Nonsteroidal anti-inflammatory drug-related injury to the gastrointestinal tract: clinical picture, pathogenesis and prevention. *Gastroenterol Clin North Am*. 2010;39:433; Lanza FL et al. Guidelines for prevention of NSAID-related ulcer complications. *Am J Gastroenterol*. 2009;104:728; Malfertheiner P et al. Peptic ulcer disease. *Lancet*. 2009:374:1449; Vonkeman H et al. Risk management of risk management: combining proton pump inhibitors with low-dose aspirin. *Drug Healthc Patient Saf*. 2010;2:191; Targownik LE et al. Selective serotonin reuptake inhibitors are associated with a modest increase in the risk of upper gastrointestinal bleeding. *Am J Gastroenterol*. 2009;104:1475; Dall M et al. There is an association between selective serotonin reuptake inhibitor use and uncomplicated peptic ulcers: a population-based case-control study. *Aliment Pharmacol Ther*. 2010;32:1383; Andrade C et al. Serotonin reuptake inhibitor antidepressants and abnormal bleeding: a review of clinicians and a reconsideration of mechanisms. *J Clin Psychiatry*. 2010;71:1565.

Pathophysiology

A physiologic balance exists in healthy individuals between gastric acid secretion and gastroduodenal mucosal defense. Peptic ulcers occur when the balance between aggressive factors (gastric acid, pepsin, bile salts, *H. pylori,* and NSAIDs) and mucosal defensive mechanisms (mucosal blood flow, mucus, mucosal bicarbonate secretion, mucosal cell restitution, and epithelial cell renewal) are disrupted.[87,96] Increased acid secretion may occur in patients with duodenal ulcer, but most patients with gastric ulcer have normal or reduced rates of acid secretion.[7] Pepsin is an important cofactor that plays a role in the proteolytic activity involved in ulcer formation. Mucosal defense and repair mechanisms protect the gastroduodenal mucosa from noxious endogenous and exogenous substances.[87] The viscous nature and near-neutral pH of the mucus–bicarbonate barrier protect the stomach from the acidic contents in the gastric lumen. The maintenance of mucosal integrity and repair are mediated by the production of endogenous prostaglandins. When aggressive factors alter mucosal defense mechanisms, back diffusion of hydrogen ions occurs with subsequent mucosal injury. *H. pylori* and NSAIDs cause alterations in mucosal defense by different mechanisms and are important factors in the formation of peptic ulcers.

HELICOBACTER PYLORI–RELATED ULCERS

H. pylori is a gram-negative, spiral-shaped bacillus that thrives in a microaerophilic environment. The bacterium resides between the mucus layer and surface epithelial cells in the stomach or any location where gastric-type epithelium is found.[88] Flagella enable it to move from the lumen of the stomach, where the pH is low, to the mucus layer, where the pH is neutral. Acute infection is accompanied by transient hypochlorhydria, which enables the organism to survive the acidic gastric juice. Although the exact method by which *H. pylori* induces hypochlorhydria is uncertain, it is hypothesized that its urease-producing ability hydrolyzes urea in the gastric juice and converts it to ammonia and carbon dioxide, which creates a neutral microenvironment that surrounds the bacterium.[88,96] Adherence pedestals attach to gastric-type epithelium and prevent the bacterium from being shed during cell turnover and mucus secretion.

Disease outcome depends on the patterns of *H. pylori* colonization and inflammation within the stomach.[88,96] Colonization of the antrum and acid-secreting body (corpus) of the stomach is associated with gastric ulcer and gastric adenocarcinoma and is typically accompanied by gastric atrophy and decreased acid secretion. When *H. pylori* colonizes, the antrum and the body of the stomach are spared, the risk for duodenal ulcer is increased, and gastric acid is normal or slightly increased. Ulcers in the duodenum arise from the colonization by antral organisms of gastric-type epithelium that develops in the duodenum in response to changes in duodenal pH.[88]

Direct mucosal damage is produced by virulence factors (e.g., cytotoxin-associated gene, vacuolating cytotoxin), elaborating bacterial enzymes (e.g., urease, lipases, proteases), and adherence.[88,96,99] Cytotoxin-associated gene A (CagA) protein occurs in about 60% of *H. pylori* strains in the United States and is associated with severe gastritis, peptic ulcers, and gastric cancer when compared with CagA-negative strains.[88,96,99] Although vacuolating cytotoxin A (VacA) is present in almost all *H. pylori* strains, differences in cytotoxic activity are related to variations in the *VacA* gene structure and are associated with an increased risk for PUD and possibly gastric cancer.[88,99] *H. pylori* infection may also cause alterations in the host immune response.[88,99] Host polymorphisms related to interleukin (IL)-1β and its receptor antagonist, tumor necrosis factor α (TNF-α), and IL-10, may be associated with increased gastric acid secretion and duodenal ulcer or acid suppression and gastric cancer.[88,99]

Nonsteroidal Anti-Inflammatory Drug–Induced Ulcers

Nonselective NSAIDs (Table 23-4), including aspirin, cause peptic ulcers and upper GI complications by systemically inhibiting protective prostaglandins in the gastric mucosa.[87,94,96] NSAIDs inhibit cyclooxygenase (COX), the rate-limiting enzyme in the conversion of arachidonic acid to prostaglandins. There are two COX isoforms: COX-1, which is found in the stomach, kidney, intestine, and platelets, and COX-2, which is induced with acute inflammation.[87,94] The inhibition of COX-1 is associated with upper GI and renal toxicity, and the inhibition of COX-2 is related to anti-inflammatory effects.[87,94] Nonselective NSAIDs, including aspirin, inhibit both COX-1 and COX-2 to varying degrees and decrease platelet aggregation, which may increase the risk for upper GI bleeding.[87,94] The coadministration of selected NSAIDs (e.g., ibuprofen) with aspirin also reduces the antiplatelet effects of aspirin.[46] Although prostaglandin inhibition is regarded as the major cause of gastric ulcers, diversion of arachidonate through the lipoxygenase pathway enhances leukotriene synthesis and results in vasoconstriction and release of oxygen free radicals, which may also contribute to impairment of mucosal defense.[94] There is an increasing evidence that NSAIDs may cause gastric damage by interfering with the mucosal synthesis of nitric oxide and hydrogen sulfide, important mediators in maintaining gastric mucosal intergrity.[94]

The relative COX selectivity among NSAIDs varies and is thought to be an important factor in determining the propensity for ulcer formation.[87,94] Thus, certain NSAIDs may be more COX-1–sparing than others (e.g., the partially selective NSAIDs; Table 23-4) and may be associated with less GI toxicity, but there are few controlled trials to support this claim.[87,94,100,101] COX-2 inhibitors, such as rofecoxib and valdecoxib (Table 23-4), do not inhibit gastric mucosal prostaglandin synthesis or serum thromboxane A_2, which accounts for their improved GI safety.[94,101] Unfortunately, both rofecoxib and valdecoxib were withdrawn from the U.S. market in 2004 because of concerns about cardiovascular safety.[87] Celecoxib, an NSAID initially marketed as a COX-2 inhibitor, currently remains available in the United States despite similar concerns about cardiovascular risk, especially at higher dosages.[87] However, the benefit of celecoxib in reducing the risk of gastric ulcer and upper GI complications may be lower than with rofecoxib and valdecoxib (Table 23-4).

Table 23-4

Selected Nonsteroidal Anti-Inflammatory Drugs

Salicylates
Acetylated: aspirin
Nonacetylated: trisalicylate, salsalate
Nonsalicylates[a]
Nonselective (traditional) NSAIDs: ibuprofen, naproxen, tolmetin, fenoprofen, sulindac, indomethacin, ketoprofen, ketorolac, flurbiprofen, piroxicam
Partially selective NSAIDs: etodolac, diclofenac, meloxicam, nabumetone
Selective COX-2 inhibitors: celecoxib[b], rofecoxib[c], valdecoxib[c]

[a]Based on COX-1/COX-2 selectivity ratio in vitro.
[b]Initially marketed as a COX-2 inhibitor, but current FDA labeling is consistent with nonselective and partially selective NSAIDs.
[c]Withdrawn from the U.S. market.
COX-2, cyclooxygenase-2; NSAID, nonsteroidal anti-inflammatory drug.

Aspirin and non-aspirin NSAIDs also have a topical (direct) irritating effect on the gastric mucosa, but the resulting inflammation and erosions usually heal within a few days. Gastric damage is associated with the acidic properties of aspirin and non-aspirin NSAIDs and their ability to decrease the hydrophobicity of the mucous gel layer in the gastric mucosa.[94,102] Thus, direct mucosal injury appears to correlate with the pK_a of a compound—suggesting the lower the acidity of the drug, the less the short-term topical damage.[94] Formulations, such as enteric-coated aspirin, buffered aspirin, NSAID prodrugs, and parenteral or rectal preparations, may spare topical effects on the gastric mucosa, but all have the potential to cause a gastric ulcer because of their systemic inhibition of endogenous prostaglandins.[87,103]

Clinical Presentation

SIGNS AND SYMPTOMS

The signs and symptoms associated with a peptic ulcer range from mild epigastric pain to life-threatening upper GI complications.[87,96] A change in the character of the pain may indicate an ulcer-related complication. The absence of epigastric pain, especially in older adults who are taking NSAIDs, does not exclude the presence of an ulcer or related complications. Although the reasons for this are unclear, they may be related to the analgesic effect of the NSAID. There is no one sign or symptom that differentiates an *H. pylori*–related ulcer from an NSAID-induced ulcer. Ulcer-like symptoms may occur in the absence of peptic ulceration in association with *H. pylori*–related gastritis or duodenitis.

COMPLICATIONS

The most serious life-threatening complications associated with chronic PUD are upper GI bleeding, perforation into the abdominal cavity or penetration into an adjacent structure (e.g., pancreas, liver, or biliary tract), and obstruction.[87,96,104,105] Ulcer-related bleeding is the most frequent complication and occurs with all types of ulcers (see section on Upper Gastrointestinal Bleeding). The incidence of ulcer-related upper GI bleeding and perforation is highest in individuals taking NSAIDs who are older than 60 years.[94,96] The bleeding may be occult (hidden), present as melena (black-colored stools), or hematemesis (vomiting of blood). Mortality is higher in patients who continue to bleed or who rebleed after the initial bleeding has stopped and in patients with a perforated ulcer.[4,5] The pain associated with perforation is typically sudden, sharp, and severe, beginning in the epigastric area but quickly spreading throughout the upper abdominal area. Gastric outlet obstruction, the least frequent complication, is caused by previous ulcer healing and scarring or edema of the pylorus or duodenal bulb and can lead to symptoms of gastric retention, including early satiety, bloating, anorexia, nausea, vomiting, and weight loss.

Clinical Assessment and Diagnosis

TESTS FOR DETECTING *HELICOBACTER PYLORI*

The detection of *H. pylori* infection can be made through gastric mucosal biopsies in patients undergoing upper endoscopy or by nonendoscopic tests (Table 23-5).[88,89,106] The selection of a specific method is influenced by the clinical circumstance and the availability and cost of the individual test. Endoscopic tests require a mucosal biopsy for the rapid urease test, histology, or culture. Medications that reduce urease activity or the density of *H. pylori* may decrease the sensitivity of the rapid urease test by up to 25%.[89] For this reason, when possible, antibiotics and bismuth salts should be withheld for 4 weeks, and H_2RAs and PPIs for 1 to 2 weeks before endoscopic testing. Patients who are taking these medications at endoscopy will require histology in addition to the rapid urease test. At least three biopsies are taken from different areas of the stomach because patchy distribution of *H. pylori* can result in false-negative results. Acute ulcer bleeding at the time of testing is likely to decrease the sensitivity of the rapid urease test and histology and increase the likelihood of false-negative results.[89,107]

Table 23-5
Diagnostic Tests for *Helicobacter pylori* Infection

Tests Using Gastric Mucosal Biopsy in Patients Undergoing Endoscopy
Rapid Urease Test
■ Tests for active *H. pylori* infection; >90% sensitivity and specificity. ■ In the presence of *H. pylori* urease, urea is metabolized to ammonia and bicarbonate resulting in an increase in pH, which changes the color of a pH-sensitive indicator. ■ Results are rapid (within 24 hours), and test is less expensive than histology or culture. ■ Withhold H_2RAs and PPIs 1–2 weeks before testing and antibiotics and bismuth salts 4 weeks before testing to reduce the risk of false negatives.
Histology
■ "Gold standard" for detection of active *H. pylori* infection; >95% sensitive and specific. ■ Permits further histologic analysis and evaluation of infected tissue (e.g., gastritis, ulceration, adenocarcinoma); tests for active *H. pylori* infection. ■ Results are not immediate; not recommended for initial diagnosis; more expensive than rapid urease test.
Culture
■ Permits sensitivity testing to determine antibiotic choice or resistance; 100% specific; tests for active *H. pylori* infection. ■ Use usually limited to patients who fail initial course of eradication therapy.
Polymerase Chain Reaction
■ Detects *H. pylori* DNA in gastric tissue; highly specific and sensitive. ■ High rate of false positives and false negatives; positive DNA does not correlate directly with presence of the organism; used primarily for research.

(continued)

Table 23-5
Diagnostic Tests for Helicobacter pylori Infection (*continued*)

Nonendoscopic Tests That Do Not Use Gastric Mucosal Biopsy

Urea Breath Test

- Tests for active *H. pylori* infection; >95% sensitive and specific.
- Radiolabeled urea with either C^{13} or C^{14} is given orally; urease secreted by *H. pylori* in the stomach (if present) hydrolyzes radiolabeled urea to produce radiolabeled CO_2, which is exhaled and then quantified from the expired breath; radiation exposure is minimal.
- Withhold H_2RAs and PPIs 1–2 weeks before testing and antibiotics and bismuth salts 4 weeks before testing to reduce the risk of false negatives.
- Used to detect *H. pylori* before treatment and to document posttreatment eradication.
- Results usually take about 2 days; less expensive than tests that utilize gastric mucosal biopsy but more expensive than serologic tests; availability and reimbursement is inconsistent.

Antibody Detection (In-Office or Near Patient)

- Qualitative test; detects IgG antibodies to *H. pylori* in whole blood or fingerstick.
- Effective for primary diagnosis, but not of benefit in confirming eradication because antibodies to *H. pylori* remain positive for years after successful eradication of the infection.
- Results obtained quickly (usually within 15 minutes) but reduced sensitivity and specificity compared with laboratory-based tests; widely available and inexpensive.
- Results not affected by H_2RAs, PPIs, or bismuth; antibiotics given for other indications may result in a positive antibody test.

Antibody Detection (Laboratory)

- Quantitative test; detects IgG antibodies to *H. pylori* in serum using laboratory-based ELISA tests and latex agglutination techniques.
- More accurate than in-office tests; similar sensitivity and specificity to rapid urease biopsy and urea breath tests.
- Unable to determine if antibody is related to active or cured infection; antibody titers vary between individuals and take up to 6 months to 1 year to return to the uninfected state.
- Results not affected by H_2RAs, PPIs, or bismuth; antibiotics given for other indications may result in a positive antibody test.

Fecal Antigen Test

- An enzymatic immunoassay test that identifies *H. pylori* antigen in stool; sensitivity and specificity comparable to the UBT for initial diagnosis.
- H_2RAs, PPIs, antibiotics, and bismuth may cause false-negative results but to a lesser extent than the UBT.
- Considered an alternative to detecting *H. pylori* before treatment and documenting posttreatment eradication; patients may have a reluctance to obtain stool samples.

ELISA, enzyme-linked immunosorbent assay; H_2RA, H_2 receptor antagonist; IgG, immunoglobulin G; PPI, proton-pump inhibitor; UBT, urea breath test.
Source: Washington MK, Peek RM. Gastritis and gastropathy. In: Yamada T et al, eds. *Textbook of Gastroenterology*. 5th ed. Hoboken, NJ: Wiley-Blackwell; 2009:1005; Chey WD et al. American College of Gastroenterology guideline on the management of *Helicobacter pylori* infection. *Am J Gastroenterol*. 2007;102:1808; Calvet X et al. Diagnosis of *Helicobacter pylori* infection. *Helicobacter*. 2010;15(Suppl 1):7.

Nonendoscopic tests either identify active infection or detect antibodies to *H. pylori*.[88,89,106] If endoscopy is not planned, these tests are a reasonable choice to determine *H. pylori* status as they are noninvasive, more convenient, and less expensive than the endoscopic tests. Testing should only be undertaken if eradication is planned in light of positive results. The urea breath test (UBT), the most accurate noninvasive test, detects active *H. pylori* infection and is also effective after eradication treatment.[88,89,106] The ^{13}carbon (nonradioactive isotope) and ^{14}carbon (radioactive isotope) tests require that the patient ingest radiolabeled urea, which is then hydrolyzed by *H. pylori* (if present in the stomach) to ammonia and radiolabeled bicarbonate. The radiolabeled bicarbonate is absorbed in the blood and detected in expired breath. The in-office and laboratory antibody tests are a cost-effective method to initially diagnose *H. pylori* infection, but because they do not differentiate between active infection and previously eradicated *H. pylori*, they should not be used to confirm eradication.[88,89,106] The fecal antigen test identifies *H. pylori* antigens in the stool and is less expensive and easier to perform than the UBT.[88,89,106] Although usually comparable with the UBT in the initial detection of *H. pylori*, the fecal antigen test may be less accurate when used to document eradication posttreatment. Salivary and urine antibody tests are under investigation.[106]

LABORATORY TESTS, RADIOGRAPHY, AND ENDOSCOPY

Generally, laboratory tests are not helpful in the diagnosis of PUD. Fasting serum gastrin concentrations are only recommended for patients who are unresponsive to therapy or those suspected of having a hypersecretory disease. Serum hematocrit (Hct) and hemoglobin (Hgb) and guaiac fecal occult blood tests assist in the evaluation of ulcer-related bleeding.

Gastric acid–secretory studies are not routinely performed for patients suspected of having an uncomplicated peptic ulcer. However, measurements of acid secretion are instrumental in the evaluation of patients with severe, recurrent PUD that is unresponsive to standard drug therapy. Acid secretion is expressed as basal acid output (BAO), in response to a meal (meal-stimulated acid secretion), or as maximal acid output (MAO).[7] These tests estimate the acid-secretory response under various circumstances and are measured by inserting a nasogastric tube into the stomach and aspirating the gastric contents.[7] The aspirate is estimated by titration with a basic solution of known concentration and expressed as milliequivalents of H^+ per hour. Results obtained for an individual patient is then compared with standard ranges for each test. The BAO, meal-stimulated acid secretion, and MAO vary according to age, sex, health, and time of day. The BAO follows a circadian rhythm, with the highest acid secretion occurring at night and the lowest in the morning. An increase in the BAO/MAO ratio suggests a basal hypersecretory state such as ZES.

Confirmation of a peptic ulcer requires visualizing the ulcer by either GI radiography or upper endoscopy.[87] Radiography is sometimes the initial diagnostic procedure because it is less expensive than endoscopy and more widely available, but small ulcers are often difficult to detect and false positives may result from trapped barium.[87] Fiber-optic upper endoscopy (esophagogastroduodenoscopy [EGD]) is the gold standard because it detects greater than 90% of peptic ulcers and permits direct inspection, biopsy, and visualization of superficial erosions and sites of active bleeding. Upper endoscopy is preferred if complications are suspected or if an accurate diagnosis is required. If a gastric ulcer is found on radiography, malignancy should be excluded by direct endoscopic visualization and histology.

Clinical Course and Prognosis

The natural history of PUD is characterized by periods of exacerbations and remissions unless the underlying cause is removed.[87] *H. pylori* and NSAIDs are the two most important risk factors for the development of peptic ulcer.[87] Successful eradication of *H. pylori* heals ulcers and dramatically decreases ulcer recurrence and GI complications.[87] The risk for NSAID-induced ulcer and life-threatening GI complications is greatest in the elderly and those with a history of PUD. Prophylactic co-therapy or the use of a selective COX-2 inhibitor markedly decreases ulcer risk and complications.[94,95] Gastric cancer in *H. pylori*–infected individuals develops slowly during 20 to 40 years and is associated with a slightly higher lifetime risk when compared with that in patients with duodenal ulcer or in the general population.[88,91,92]

Treatment

THERAPEUTIC GOALS

The therapeutic goals for treating PUD in adults depend on whether the ulcer is related to *H. pylori* or associated with an NSAID. Treatment goals may differ depending on whether the ulcer is initial or recurrent and whether complications have occurred. Treatment is aimed at relieving ulcer symptoms, healing the ulcer, preventing ulcer recurrence, and reducing ulcer-related complications. When possible, the most cost-effective drug regimen should be utilized.

NONPHARMACOLOGIC THERAPY

Patients with PUD should discontinue NSAIDs (including aspirin) if possible. Patients unable to tolerate certain foods and beverages (e.g., spicy foods, caffeine, and alcohol) may benefit from dietary modifications. Encourage lifestyle modifications like stress reduction and decreasing or stopping tobacco use.

Probiotics, especially strains of lactic acid–producing bacteria, such as *Lactobacillus* and *Bifidobacterium*; lactoferrin; and certain foods (e.g., cranberry juice, ginger, chili, oregano, some milk proteins) have been used to supplement *H. pylori* eradication.[87,108–110] Animal and in vitro data have shown that probiotics have both bactericidal and protective effects, but meta-analyses of clinical trials suggest only a slight improvement in eradication rates.[87,108,109] Lactoferrin, a member of the transferrin family, has been reported to inhibit *H. pylori* attachment to gastric epithelial cells.[110] Although certain strains of *Lactobacillus* and *Bifidobacterium* or lactoferrin may enhance eradication, they are not effective as single agents. Additional clinical trials are necessary before probiotics or lactoferrin are routinely recommended as supplements to *H. pylori* regimens.

Patients with ulcer-related complications may require surgery for bleeding, perforation, or obstruction.[105] Surgery for medical treatment failures (e.g., vagotomy with pyloroplasty or vagotomy with antrectomy) is rarely performed because of effective medical management and the risk of postoperative complications from surgery.

PHARMACOTHERAPY

Drug regimens used to eradicate *H. pylori* are identified in Table 23-6. Recommended first-line treatment in the United States includes PPI-based three-drug regimens or a bismuth-based four-drug regimen (Fig. 23-4). However, there is a controversy

Table 23-6
Oral Drug Regimens Used to Eradicate *Helicobacter pylori* Infection

Drug Regimen	Dose	Frequency	Duration
Proton-Pump Inhibitor–Based Three-Drug Regimens			
PPI	Standard dose[a]	BID[a]	14 days[b]
Clarithromycin	500 mg	BID	14 days[b]
Amoxicillin[c]	1 g	BID	14 days[b]
Or			
PPI	Standard dose[a]	BID[a]	14 days[b]
Clarithromycin	500 mg	BID	14 days[b]
Metronidazole[c]	500 mg	BID	14 days[b]
Bismuth-Based Four-Drug Regimens			
Bismuth subsalicylate[d]	525 mg	QID	10–14 days
Metronidazole	250–500 mg	QID	10–14 days
Tetracycline plus	500 mg	QID	10–14 days
PPI	Standard dose[a]	Daily or BID[a]	10–14 days
Or			
H_2RA[e]	Standard dose[e]	BID[e]	4–6 weeks
Sequential Therapy[f]			
PPI	Standard dose[a]	BID[a]	Days 1–10
Amoxicillin	1 g	BID	Days 1–5

(continued)

Table 23-6
Oral Drug Regimens Used to Eradicate *Helicobacter pylori* Infection (*continued*)

Drug Regimen	Dose	Frequency	Duration
Clarithromycin	250–500 mg	BID	Days 6–10
Metronidazole	250–500 mg	BID	Days 6–10
Secondary or Rescue Therapy			
Bismuth subsalicylate[d]	525 mg	QID	10–14 days
Metronidazole	500 mg	QID	10–14 days
Tetracycline	500 mg	QID	10–14 days
PPI	Standard dose[a]	Daily or BID[a]	10–14 days
Or			
PPI	Standard dose[a]	BID[a]	10–14 days
Amoxicillin	1 g	BID	10–14 days
Levofloxacin	500 mg	Daily	10–14 days

[a]Omeprazole 20 mg BID, lansoprazole 30 mg BID, pantoprazole 40 mg BID, rabeprazole 20 mg daily or BID, esomeprazole 20 mg BID or 40 mg daily.
[b]Although 7 to 10 day regimens may provide acceptable eradication rates, the preferred treatment duration in the United States is 14 days.
[c]Use amoxicillin in non–penicillin-allergic individuals; substitute metronidazole for amoxicillin in penicillin-allergic patients.
[d]Pylera, a prepackaged *H. pylori* regimen, contains bismuth subcitrate potassium (biskalcitrate) 140 mg as the bismuth salt in place of bismuth subsalicylate, metronidazole 125 mg, and tetracycline 125 mg per capsule. The patient is directed to take three capsules per dose with each meal and at bedtime. A standard dose of a PPI is added to the regimen and taken twice daily. All medications are taken for a 10-day period.
[e]See Table 23-1 for standard peptic ulcer healing dosage regimens.
[f]Requires validation in the United States.
BID, 2 times a day; H_2RA, H_2 receptor antagonist; PPI, proton-pump inhibitor; QID, 4 times a day.
From Soll AH, Graham DY. Peptic ulcer disease. In: Yamada T et al, eds. *Textbook of Gastroenterology*. 5th ed. Hoboken, NJ: Wiley-Blackwell; 2009:936; Washington MK, Peek RM. Gastritis and gastropathy. In: Yamada T et al, eds. *Textbook of Gastroenterology*. 5th ed. Hoboken, NJ: Wiley-Blackwell; 2009:1005; Malfertheiner P et al. Peptic ulcer disease. *Lancet*. 2009:374:1449; Gisbert JP et al. Sequential therapy for *Helicobacter pylori* eradication: a critical review. *J Clin Gastroenterol*. 2010;44:313; Gisbert JP et al. *Helicobacter pylori* first-line treatment and rescue options in patients allergic to penicillin. *Aliment Pharmacol Ther*. 2005;22:1041; Gisbert JP et al. *Helicobacter pylori* first-line treatment and rescue option containing levofloxacin in patients allergic to penicillin. *Dig Liver Dis*. 2010;42:287; Vergara M et al. Meta-analysis: comparative efficacy of different proton-pump inhibitors in triple therapy for *Helicobacter pylori* eradication. *Aliment Pharmacol Ther*. 2003;18:647; Gisbert JP et al. Meta-analysis: proton pump inhibitors vs. H_2-receptor antagonists—their efficacy with antibiotics in *Helicobacter pylori* eradication. *Aliment Pharmacol Ther*. 2003;18:757; Gisbert JP. Review: second-line rescue therapy of *Helicobacter pylori* infection. *Therap Adv Gastroenterol*. 2009;2:331.

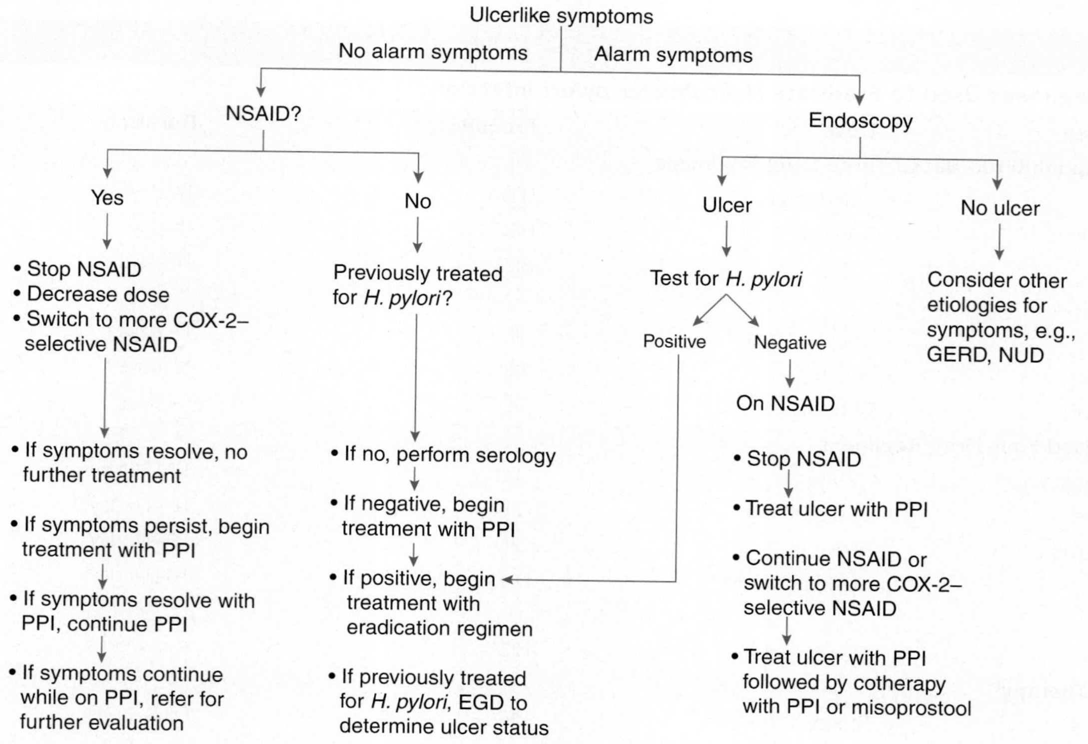

Figure 23-4 Management of peptic ulcer disease. COX-2, cyclooxygenase-2; EGD, esophagogastroduodenoscopy; GERD, gastroesophageal reflux disease; *H. pylori, Helicobacter pylori;* NSAID, nonsteroidal anti-inflammatory drug; NUD, non-ulcer dyspepsia; PPI, proton-pump inhibitor.

as to whether sequential therapy should replace the standard PPI-based triple drug regimen as first-line treatment. If initial eradication fails, a second course of therapy should be based on the selection of antibiotics that have not been previously used. Successful treatment eradicates the infection and heals the ulcer. Treatment for *H. pylori*–positive patients with a conventional antiulcer drug or combining an antisecretory drug with sucralfate is not recommended because of high rates of ulcer recurrence and complications. Maintenance therapy with a PPI or H_2RA (Table 23-1) should only be necessary in high-risk patients with a history of ulcer complications, those with *H. pylori*–negative ulcers, and patients with other concomitant acid-related diseases (e.g., GERD).

Drug regimens used to treat and prevent NSAID-induced ulcers are identified in Table 23-1. Patients with NSAID-induced ulcers should be tested to determine their *H. pylori* status. If the patient is *H. pylori* negative, the NSAID should be discontinued and treatment should be initiated with antiulcer medications. The duration of treatment should be extended if the NSAID is continued. Prophylactic co-therapy with a PPI or misoprostol or switching to an NSAID with greater COX-2 selectivity is recommended for patients at risk of exhibiting ulcer-related upper GI complications.

HELICOBACTER PYLORI–RELATED PEPTIC ULCER

CASE 23-1

QUESTION 1: R.L. is an otherwise healthy 45-year-old man who works in a high-stress job as an air traffic controller at a major airport. He complains of a 2-week history of "burning stomach pain" sometimes accompanied by "indigestion and bloating." The pain initially occurred several times a day, usually between meals, and sometimes awakened him at night, but it has increased in frequency during the last week. Initially, the pain was temporarily reduced by food or antacids. Last week, R.L. tried an OTC H_2 receptor antagonist that "lasted longer" but did not provide adequate symptom relief. R.L. states that he experienced a similar type of pain about 12 years ago when he was treated with omeprazole for a suspected peptic ulcer. He has smoked one pack of cigarettes daily for the past 20 years, has an occasional glass of red wine with dinner, and usually drinks 4 to 6 cups of caffeinated coffee throughout the day. R.L. takes acetaminophen when needed for occasional headaches and a daily multivitamin but denies the use of any other OTC or prescription medications, including NSAIDs and the previous use of clarithromycin or metronidazole. He denies nausea, vomiting, anorexia, weight loss, and changes in stool consistency or color. A review of other body systems is noncontributory. He has no known food or drug allergies.

Physical examination is normal except for epigastric tenderness on palpation of the upper abdomen. Vital signs include a temperature of 98.8°F, blood pressure of 132/80 mm Hg, and a heart rate of 78 beats/minute. Pertinent laboratory values include the following:

Hgb, 14.0 g/dL
Hct, 44%
Stool guaiac test, negative

All other laboratory values are within normal limits. What signs and symptoms are suggestive of a recurrent peptic ulcer?

The diagnosis of PUD cannot be made based on symptoms alone and requires visualization of the ulcer crater because the symptomology, severity of pain, and timing of the pain (e.g., seasonal, intermittent, or pain free periods lasting from weeks to years) can differ for each patient and encompass a wide variety of complaints. Most patients with PUD present with abdominal pain that is epigastric and often described as burning or gnawing, whereas others complain of abdominal discomfort, fullness, or cramping. Epigastric pain, however, does not necessarily correlate with an ulcer because patients with ulcer-like symptoms may have NUD and asymptomatic patients may have an NSAID-induced ulcer. Heartburn, bloating, and belching may accompany the pain. Ulcer pain typically occurs during the day but can also awaken the patient from sleep (nocturnal pain). In patients with a duodenal ulcer, epigastric pain frequently occurs between meals and is often relieved by food, but this varies from patient to patient. Alternatively, food may precipitate or accentuate pain in patients with a gastric ulcer.

Antacids and antisecretory medications usually provide relief of ulcer pain in most patients. Pain usually diminishes or disappears during treatment, but epigastric pain after healing often suggests an unhealed or recurrent ulcer. Changes in the character of the pain may suggest the presence of complications. Nausea, vomiting, anorexia, and weight loss are more common with gastric ulcer but may also be suggestive of ulcer-related complication.

CASE 23-1, QUESTION 2: R.L. underwent EGD, which revealed a single 0.5-cm ulcer in the duodenal bulb. The ulcer base was clear without evidence of active bleeding. Antral gastritis was biopsy positive for *H. pylori*. What risk factors may have contributed to ulcer recurrence in this patient?

R.L. indicates that he had a similar type of abdominal pain about 12 years ago, and he was treated with omeprazole for a suspected peptic ulcer. When conventional antiulcer therapy (e.g., PPI) is discontinued after ulcer healing, the ulcer tends to recur. The most important etiologic factors that influence ulcer recurrence are *H. pylori* infection and NSAID use. It is not known whether R.L. underwent testing for *H. pylori* 12 years ago. The patient denies the use of OTC and prescription NSAIDs. The long-term use of maintenance therapy (Table 23-1) to maintain remission after initial ulcer healing with a conventional antiulcer medication was standard practice for years and may have been an option for this patient at the time.[96] However, successful eradication of *H. pylori* (in an *H. pylori*–positive patient) cures the infection, heals the ulcer, and eliminates the need for long-term maintenance therapy in most patients.[89,96]

Other factors, such as cigarette smoking, psychologic stress, and diet, may have contributed to ulcer recurrence in this patient. There is strong epidemiologic evidence indicating that cigarette smoking is a major risk factor for PUD and that the risk is proportional to the number of cigarettes smoked per day.[87] Several mechanisms have been postulated, including delayed gastric emptying, inhibition of pancreatic bicarbonate secretion, promotion of duodenogastric reflux, reduction in mucosal prostaglandin production, and increased gastric acid secretion. Although cigarette smoking exacerbates PUD, there is insufficient evidence to conclude that it causes a peptic ulcer, but it is hypothesized that smoking or nicotine might provide an environment for *H. pylori* infection.

R.L. works as an air traffic controller, which is a high-stress job. The importance of psychologic stress and how it affects PUD is complex and multifactorial. Results from controlled trials are conflicting and have failed to demonstrate a cause-and-effect relationship.[87,96] However, the clinical observation of ulcer patients with high-stress jobs and a stressful lifestyle suggest that they are adversely affected.

Caffeine-containing coffee, tea, and cola beverages; constituents in decaffeinated coffee or tea; caffeine-free carbonated beverages; and alcoholic beverages, such as beer and wine, all increase gastric acid secretion, but there is no evidence that they increase the risk for PUD. Certain foods (e.g., spicy) may cause dyspepsia or worsen ulcer symptoms but do not cause peptic ulcers. In high concentrations, alcohol is associated with acute gastric mucosal damage and upper GI bleeding, but there is insufficient evidence to confirm that alcohol causes ulcers.[87] Dietary restrictions and bland diets do not alter the frequency of ulcer recurrence.

CASE 23-1, QUESTION 3: What are the goals of therapy when treating this patient?

The goals of therapy in an *H. pylori*–positive patient with an active ulcer, a previously documented ulcer, or a history of an ulcer-related complication are to render the patient asymptomatic, heal the ulcer, eradicate the infection, and cure the disease. Treatment should be effective, well-tolerated, easy to comply with, and cost-effective. Drug regimens should have an eradication rate of at least 80% (intention-to-treat, ITT) or 90% (per protocol analysis) and should minimize the potential for antimicrobial resistance.[111] The use of a single drug (antibiotic, bismuth salt, or antiulcer) does not achieve this goal. Two-drug regimens (PPI and amoxicillin or clarithromycin) are not recommended in the United States because of low and variable eradication rates and because of the inclusion of only one antibiotic.

Primary Treatment for *Helicobacter pylori* Infection

CASE 23-1, QUESTION 4: What factors should be taken into consideration when selecting a first-line eradication regimen? What are the therapeutic options for first-line *H. pylori* eradication in the United States? Which is the preferred *H. pylori* eradication regimen for R.L.?

The selection of a first-line *H. pylori* eradication regimen should be based on proven effectiveness and should take into consideration antibiotic combinations that permit second-line treatment (if necessary) with different antibiotics, treatment duration, the likelihood of antibiotic resistance, and the ability to adhere to the drug regimen. The antibiotics that have been most extensively studied in the United States and found to be effective in various combinations include clarithromycin, amoxicillin, metronidazole, and tetracycline.[87,89,96] A summary of treatments that will be discussed can be found in Table 23-6.

Current treatment guidelines in the United States and Europe recommend two first-line eradication therapies for patients with an *H. pylori*–positive peptic ulcer: standard PPI-based three-drug regimens or a PPI or H_2RA bismuth-based four-drug regimen (Table 23-6).[89,111] Despite these recommendations, there are recent concerns about the efficacy of these regimens because of declining eradication rates thought to be related to antibiotic resistance, particularly with clarithromycin, and the potential for nonadherence, especially with bismuth quadruple therapy (see Case 23-1, Question 8).[89,112–116] Controversy exists as to whether standard PPI triple therapy, in its present form, should remain as first-line treatment in the United States.[89,112–116] Some clinicians believe that sequential therapy should replace the standard PPI-based three-drug regimens because of superior eradication rates or that the bismuth-based four-drug regimen should be used exclusively as first-line treatment.[112,116] Others believe that more robust clinical trials involving a broader range of patients is needed before sequential therapy replaces the standard PPI three-drug regimens in the United States, and that medication adherence remains problematic with bismuth quadruple therapy.[89,113,114]

The most recommended treatment for *H. pylori* infection in the United States has been the standard PPI-based three-drug regimen. When combined with a PPI and clarithromycin, the inclusion of amoxicillin or metronidazole provides similar eradication rates.[89] Amoxicillin is usually preferred initially because it is associated with little or no bacterial resistance, has fewer adverse effects, and leaves metronidazole as an option for second-line therapies.[87] However, recent data suggest that eradication rates with traditional PPI triple therapy have been declining during the last decade from greater than 90% to 71% in the United States and down to 60% in Western Europe. Various strategies have been undertaken to enhance eradication rates, including lengthening treatment duration and increasing the antibiotic or antisecretory drug dosages. The recommended duration of treatment in the United States is 14 days, even though international guidelines recommend 7 to 10 days.[89] The superiority of the 14-day regimen over a 7-day or 10-day treatment course has been confirmed and is less likely to be associated with antimicrobial resistance.[89] A treatment duration of less than 7 days is not recommended and is associated with unacceptable eradication rates.[89] Increasing the antibiotic daily dose or extending antibiotic treatment beyond 14 days usually does not improve eradication rates. The PPI may be extended to 28 days if needed for ulcer healing. Twice-daily dosing of the PPI appears to be more effective than a single daily dose.[117] Pretreatment with a PPI before initiating *H. pylori* eradication does not decrease the rate of eradication.[118]

Bismuth-based quadruple therapy containing a bismuth salt, metronidazole, tetracycline, and either a PPI or H_2RA has been advocated as first-line treatment because it usually yields satisfactory eradication rates despite increased resistance to clarithromycin.[89,116] The complexity of this regimen and the potential for increased side effects often relegates it to preferred second-line status if not previously used. However, eradication rates, tolerability, and medication adherence were reported to be similar to PPI triple therapy when used as first-line treatment, although both regimens yielded eradication rates of less than 80% ITT.[119] Using a PPI instead of an H_2RA permits a shorter duration of treatment (10 days vs.14 days) and may provide increased efficacy in patients with metronidazole-resistant strains of *H. pylori*.[89] Increasing the duration of quadruple therapy to 1 month does not substantially increase eradication, although the antisecretory drug may be continued for an additional 2 (PPI) or 4 weeks (H_2RA) in patients with an active ulcer.

Small studies, primarily conducted in Italy, found that sequential therapy with a PPI and amoxicillin for 5 days followed by a PPI, clarithromycin, and an imidazole for an additional 5 days achieved eradication rates (>80% ITT). This made a compelling case to switch to sequential therapy as the preferred first-line treatment in the United States.[112–114] A recent meta-analysis of randomized controlled trials looking at previously untreated adults comparing sequential therapy with preexisting or emerging therapies demonstrated that sequential therapy is superior to a 7-day course of the standard PPI-based three-drug regimens containing clarithromycin.[89,112–116,120–122] However, sequential therapy was not superior when compared with standard three-drug regimens for therapy lasting 10 to 14 days.[115] An increased efficacy has also been reported with sequential therapy in patients with clarithromycin-resistant *H. pylori* strains.[112,120,123] The rationale for sequential therapy is to initially treat the patient with antibiotics that rarely promote resistance (e.g., amoxicillin) to reduce the bacterial load and preexisting resistant organisms, and then to follow with different antibiotics to eradicate the remaining organisms. Although the precise mechanism for the success of sequential therapy is uncertain, the increased efficacy may be related to the number of antibiotics to which the organism is exposed. In addition, sequential therapy is more complex than standard PPI triple therapy because it requires a mid-course change in medications. Lastly, sequential therapy has not been adequately compared with standard triple therapy containing a PPI–clarithromycin–metronidazole or bismuth-based quadruple therapy in the United States.

The therapeutic options available for the eradication of *H. pylori* should be carefully considered in each individual patient. The PPI–amoxicillin–clarithromycin regimen is an acceptable first-line management strategy for R.L., because he has not previously received clarithromycin and has no known allergies to penicillin. Posttreatment testing should be considered but may not be necessary if R.L. remains asymptomatic. Although sequential therapy may overcome clarithromycin resistance, it is unclear, at this time, whether it would provide any increased benefit in this patient.

Patient Education

CASE 23-1, QUESTION 5: R.L. is prescribed a 14-day PPI-based three-drug eradication regimen containing amoxicillin and clarithromycin. What instructions would you provide R.L. regarding his medications?

R.L. should be informed of the importance of taking his medications as prescribed to minimize treatment failure and the development of antibiotic resistance. He should be advised that the PPI is an integral part of the three-drug regimen and should be taken twice daily 30 to 60 minutes before breakfast and dinner (see section on Pharmacotherapy of Drugs Used to Treat Acid-Related disorders, Proton-Pump Inhibitors) along with amoxicillin and clarithromycin.

R.L. should also be informed of the most common side effects associated with his treatment regimen. All antibiotics included in the *H. pylori* eradication regimens are usually associated with mild side effects including nausea, abdominal pain, and diarrhea. *C. difficile*–associated diarrhea, a serious antibiotic-related complication, occurs occasionally. Oral thrush and vaginal candidiasis (in women) may also occur. Clarithromycin and metronidazole may cause taste disturbances.

R.L., as well as all other patients receiving *H. pylori* eradication therapy, should be advised of the risk for clinically important drug–drug interactions that may occur with the medications included in their eradication regimen. Special attention should be given to metronidazole and clarithromycin (inhibitors of CYP3A4), as well as to substrates of CYP2C9 (inhibited by metronidazole).[124] Drug–drug interactions may also occur with H_2RAs and PPIs (see section on Pharmacotherapy of Drugs Used to Treat Acid-Related Disorders).

Regimens for the Management of *Helicobacter pylori* Infection in Patients with Penicillin Allergies

CASE 23-1, QUESTION 6: What would have been the preferred initial *H. pylori* eradication regimen if R.L. had a documented allergy to penicillin?

There are two first-line treatment options if R.L. had a documented allergy to penicillin. Metronidazole can be substituted for amoxicillin in the PPI-based three-drug regimen, because similar eradication rates are achieved (Table 23-6).[89,125] Bismuth-based quadruple therapy may also be used, because it provides similar eradication rates to the PPI-based three-drug regimens.[89,119]

If R.L.'s medications included metronidazole, tetracycline, or a bismuth salt, he should be provided additional information on these medications. Metronidazole-containing regimens increase the frequency of side effects (especially when the dose is >1 g/day) and may be associated with a disulfiram-like reaction in patients who consume alcohol. Tetracycline may cause photosensitivity and should not be used in children because it may cause tooth discoloration. Bismuth salts may cause darkening of the tongue and stool.

Regimens that substitute levofloxacin for amoxicillin in PPI triple therapy have been used with success, but there are fewer studies to supporting their efficacy.[126] The most common sequential therapy contains amoxicillin and, therefore, is not suitable for a penicillin-allergic patient.

CASE 23-1, QUESTION 7: What drug substitutions are acceptable in the standard PPI-based three-drug and bismuth-based four-drug eradiation regimens?

There are insufficient data to support the substitution of ampicillin for amoxicillin, doxycycline for tetracycline, and azithromycin or erythromycin for clarithromycin. Substitution of clarithromycin 250 to 500 mg 4 times a day for tetracycline in the bismuth-based four-drug regimen (Table 23-6) yields similar results, but substitution of amoxicillin for tetracycline lowers the eradication rate and is not recommended.[87,96]

CASE 23-1, QUESTION 8: What are the most important predictors of *H. pylori* treatment outcomes, and how may they alter R.L.'s response to treatment?

The two most important factors in predicting *H. pylori* treatment outcomes are antibiotic resistance and medication adherence.[89,112,113,116] Antibiotic resistance rates are highly variable throughout the United States and the world and thus are difficult to compare.[89,113,116] However, there is evidence that clarithromycin resistance is increasing in North America and Europe and is thought to be the most important reason for the decreasing efficacy of clarithromycin-containing eradication regimens.[89,112,113,116] Because treatment with clarithromycin may increase the likelihood of *H. pylori* resistance, clinicians should ask about previous macrolide use when deciding upon an eradication regimen.[89]

The clinical importance of metronidazole resistance is unclear, because higher metronidazole doses and the synergistic effect of combining metronidazole with other antibiotics appear to render resistance to metronidazole more relative.[89,113,116,124] Resistance to amoxicillin and tetracycline is uncommon. Levofloxacin is emerging as a component of eradication therapy, but there are recent reports of increasing resistance to fluroquinolones.[112,113,116,124]

Medication adherence decreases with multiple medications, increased frequency of administration, increased duration of treatment, intolerable adverse effects, and costly drug regimens.[89,112] Although most eradication studies report greater than 95% adherence to medications, this high rate must be questioned because it is very difficult to accurately assess the level of compliance in clinical trials where patients take their own medications.[112] Additionally, medication adherence is usually more problematic in clinical practice. A longer treatment duration may contribute to nonadherence, but missed doses in a shorter regimen may also lead to failed eradication. Most bismuth-based four-drug regimens require the patient to take medications 4 times a day and as many as 18 tablets or capsules per day. The complexity of this regimen as well as a mid-treatment change in medications with sequential therapy should be considered when selecting an eradication regimen. Although mild side effects are common with all of the eradication regimens, some patients will experience clinically important effects that lead to discontinuation of a specific drug or of the entire regimen.

Other factors that may contribute to treatment failure include the high bacterial load, the specific *H. pylori* strain (e.g., CagA), low intragastric pH, and genetic polymorphism (e.g., CYP2C19 polymorphism) when PPIs are used as part of the eradication regimen.[89,113,116,124,127,128] There are limited data to suggest that smoking, alcohol consumption, and diet may negatively affect eradication.

CASE 23-1, QUESTION 9: What parameters should be monitored to determine R.L.'s response to treatment?

Posttreatment testing to confirm eradication is recommended for patients with an *H. pylori*–related ulcer, persistent dyspeptic symptoms, MALT lymphoma, or early gastric cancer.[89] However, posttreatment testing is neither practical nor cost-effective for all patients with an *H. pylori*–positive peptic ulcer.[89] When endoscopy follow up is not necessary, the UBT (Table 23-5) is the preferred test to confirm eradication of *H. pylori*. To avoid confusing bacterial suppression with eradication, the UBT must be delayed at least 4 weeks after the completion of treatment. The term eradication or cure is used when posttreatment tests conducted 4 weeks after the end of treatment do not detect the organism. Antibody tests should be avoided posttreatment, because antibody titers remain elevated for a long period of time (up to 1 year) before they return to the uninfected range after successful eradication.[88,89] If performed posttreatment, only a negative test is considered to be reliable.

Upper endoscopy should only be used to confirm eradication and ulcer healing if indicated (e.g., severe or frequent recurrent symptoms, current or previous ulcer complication), because the procedure is costly and invasive. When endoscopic follow up is necessary, testing to prove eradication includes a biopsy for the rapid urease test and histology (Table 23-5). Ulcer healing can also be confirmed at that time.

In clinical practice, the need for confirmation of ulcer healing and eradication in light of the declining success with the most commonly recommended eradication regimens must be weighed against the need, feasibility, availability, and cost of tests and procedures. Although posttreatment testing to confirm *H. pylori* eradication is recommended, patients like R.L., who present with an uncomplicated *H. pylori*–positive ulcer, are usually monitored for symptomatic recurrence 1 to 2 weeks after completion of drug therapy.[89] The absence of symptoms is considered a surrogate marker for successful ulcer healing and eradication. The persistence, or recurrence, of symptoms within 2 weeks after the end of treatment suggests failure of ulcer healing or eradication or an alternative diagnosis such as GERD.

Secondary or Rescue Therapy for *Helicobacter pylori* Infection

CASE 23-1, QUESTION 10: What other drug regimens can be used if R.L. fails initial eradication therapy with a PPI–amoxicillin–clarithromycin regimen? What regimens can be used when secondary treatment fails?

All initial eradication regimens require that there be an effective second-line treatment. Eradicating *H. pylori* is more difficult after initial treatment fails, and attempts to eradicate the organism are extremely variable.[89] Second-line regimens should (a) avoid using antibiotics that were used during initial therapy, (b) use antibiotics that have less problems with resistance, (c) use drugs that have a topical effect (e.g., bismuth), and (d) use a 10- to 14-day treatment duration.[89,112,116,129] If R.L. was not successfully eradicated initially with the PPI–amoxicillin–clarithromycin, he should receive second-line therapy with bismuth subsalicylate, metronidazole, tetracycline, and a PPI for 10 to 14 days.[89,112,116,129,130]

Bismuth-based regimens are the most frequently used second-line treatments in the United States when standard PPI-based three-drug regimens fail (Table 23-6).[89] A number of alternatives have been evaluated in small studies utilizing fluoroquinolone, rifabutin (an antibiotic used to treat tuberculosis), or furazolidone (no longer marketed in the United States).[89,112] The results from the levofloxacin-based clinical trials look promising and suggest that these regimens may be an alternative to second-line bismuth quadruple therapy, especially for patients who have no prior use of a fluoroquinolone.[89,112,126,129] However, increasing fluoroquinolone resistance, which appears to be easily acquired, is of concern and may limit the use of these agents for *H. pylori* eradication.[129] Various rifabutin-based regimens are effective in treating patients with *H. pylori* strains resistant to clarithromycin or metronidazole.[89,129] Regimens that include rifabutin should be the last option and only used for patients with multiple eradication failures because the drug is very expensive and there are concerns about major hematologic side effects and the possibility of resistance.[129]

NONSTEROIDAL ANTI-INFLAMMATORY DRUG–INDUCED PEPTIC ULCER

CASE 23-2

QUESTION 1: A.D. is a 70-year-old woman who retired from teaching 5 years ago. A few days ago, she noticed black "tarry" stools and was hospitalized for an upper GI bleed most likely secondary to NSAID use. She complains of "feeling tired" and occasionally dizzy for about 1 week. A.D. presents with a 5-year history of osteoarthritis for which she takes naproxen 250 mg in the morning and 500 mg in the evening. When questioned, she denies the use of corticosteroids, bisphosphonates, anticoagulants, clopidogrel, or a selective serotonin reuptake inhibitor (SSRI). She did not have a history of a previous ulcer or related complication. Other medications include hydrochlorothiazide 25 mg daily and lisinopril 20 mg daily for hypertension, self-directed treatment with enteric-coated aspirin 81 mg daily, calcium carbonate, and a multivitamin. A.D. does not use tobacco or drink caffeinated beverages but does have an occasional glass of wine. She denies epigastric pain, nausea, vomiting, anorexia, and weight loss but notes a recent change in stool color. A review of other body systems is noncontributory other than previously indicated. There are no known food or drug allergies.

Physical examination reveals a well-developed weak woman in no acute distress. The abdomen was normal with no pain on palpation. Bowel sounds were normal with no guarding, masses, hepatomegaly, or splenomegaly. The rectum was normal but with guaiac-positive stool. Vital signs include a temperature of 98.9°F, blood pressure of 100/65 mm Hg, and a heart rate of 90 beats/minute. Pertinent laboratory values include the following:

Hgb, 11.0 g/dL
Hct, 35%
Blood urea nitrogen (BUN), 40 mg/dL
Serum creatinine (SCr), 1.5 mg/dL
All other laboratory values are within normal limits.

What factors placed A.D. at increased risk for experiencing an NSAID-induced ulcer and related upper GI bleeding?

Risk factors for NSAID ulcers and related complications are presented in Table 23-3. The use of nonselective NSAIDs (e.g., naproxen) is linked to a threefold to fourfold increase in upper GI complications, and there is a twofold to threefold increase with

COX-2 inhibitors when partially and highly selective agents are evaluated as a group (Table 23-4).[101] The risk for upper GI events occur at any dosage, including low doses of OTC NSAIDs,[131] and can occur at any time during treatment.[94–96] A.D.'s self-treatment with cardioprotective dosages (81–325 mg/day) of aspirin in combination with an NSAID (naproxen) increases her risk of upper GI events to a greater extent than the use of either drug alone.[94–96] The use of buffered or enteric-coated aspirin does not confer added protection from ulcer or upper GI complications.[95,103,132] A.D.'s age (70 years) is an independent risk factor for NSAID-induced ulcers, because risk increases with the age of the patient (Table 23-3).[94,95] The increased incidence in older patients may be explained by age-related changes in gastric mucosal defense. Although A.D. did not have a history of an ulcer or ulcer-related complication before admission, a history of an NSAID-related upper GI event further increases the risk of NSAID-related GI injury.[94–96] Corticosteroids do not increase the ulcer risk when used alone, but the risk is increased twofold in corticosteroid users who are also taking concurrent NSAIDs.[94–96] The risk of upper GI bleeding is markedly increased when NSAIDs are taken with anticoagulants, bisphosphonates, or antiplatelet medications such as clopidogrel.[54,94–96,101] SSRIs independently increase the risk of upper GI bleeding, and although the magnitude of the risk is variable, it is increased in patients taking NSAIDs.[133–135] The pharmacologic mechanism underlying this adverse effect is thought to be related to SSRI inhibition of platelet aggregation, which may interfere with ulcer healing, but it remains unknown if SSRIs have a direct ulcerogenic effect.[133–135] It is uncertain whether *H. pylori* is a risk factor for NSAID-induced ulcers, but a higher incidence of PUD in *H. pylori*–positive patients taking NSAIDs suggests an additive effect, which may increase the risk of NSAID-related GI complications.[94–96] A.D.'s multiple risk factors convey an increased risk for an NSAID-related upper GI event (see Case 23-2, Question 4).

CASE 23-2, QUESTION 2: A.D. was admitted for further evaluation and treatment. An EGD revealed two bleeding antral ulcers (0.2 and 0.4 cm) and endoscopic hemostasis was performed. An antral biopsy was reported to be *H. pylori* negative. All medications were discontinued before endoscopy. Oral oxycodone was instituted after endoscopy at 5 mg every 6 hours when needed to control A.D.'s arthritic pain while she was hospitalized. Consideration was given to decreasing the naproxen dose and switching to acetaminophen, a nonacetylated salicylate, or a partially selective NSAID (Table 23-4) but none of these options were satisfactory for this patient. Treatment was initiated with a continuous infusion of IV pantoprazole for 3 days, and then switched to oral pantoprazole 40 mg twice a day (BID). A.D. was discharged on pantoprazole 40 mg daily and naproxen 250 mg in the morning and 500 mg in the evening. Hydrochlorothiazide, lisinopril, calcium carbonate, and the multivitamin were reinstituted upon discharge from the hospital. Will A.D.'s gastric ulcer heal if she continues to take the naproxen?

The naproxen should be discontinued, if possible, in the presence of an active ulcer.[87,96] If the NSAID was discontinued and A.D.'s treatment was continued with alternative therapy such as oxycodone, a PPI is the preferred treatment to heal the ulcer because it provides a more rapid rate of ulcer healing (4 weeks) and symptom relief than an H_2RA or sucralfate (6–8 weeks).[87,94,96] Because the naproxen was reinstituted at discharge in the presence of an active ulcer, a PPI is the drug of choice, because potent acid suppression is required to heal the ulcer and relieve the symptoms.[87,94,96] The duration of PPI therapy should be extended from 4 weeks to 8 to 12 weeks as continuing the offending NSAID will interfere with ulcer healing.[87,96] Cardiovascular risk and the need for low-dose aspirin must be determined by the patient's primary-care physician or cardiologist, and if not needed, the aspirin should be discontinued. However, low-dose aspirin should be continued after endoscopic hemostasis in patients at cardiovascular risk.[87,136] Clopidogrel should not be substituted for low-dose aspirin in order to reduce GI bleeding.[54,95]

CASE 23-2, QUESTION 3: Which ulcer-healing regimen would be recommended if A.D. was reported to be *H. pylori* positive?

All patients with NSAID-induced GI events should be tested for *H. pylori* (Figure 23-4). A PPI-based eradication regimen is recommended in an *H. pylori*–positive patient with an active ulcer who is also taking an NSAID. One reason for this is that it is not possible to determine whether the *H. pylori,* the NSAID, or both actually caused the ulcer. If an individual is tested and found to be *H. pylori* positive, he or she should be offered eradication therapy whether or not there is a documented ulcer. The selection of a specific regimen (Table 23-6) depends on a number of factors, including whether the individual is allergic to penicillin.

Strategies to Reduce the Risk of Nonsteroidal Anti-Inflammatory Drug–Induced Peptic Ulcers

CASE 23-2, QUESTION 4: Three months later, A.D. returned to her gastroenterologist for a follow up EGD, which confirmed that the gastric ulcers were healed. On return to her primary care physician, the pantoprazole was changed to famotidine 20 mg BID, and the patient was advised to discontinue low-dose aspirin. Current medications include naproxen 250 mg in the morning and 500 mg in the evening, hydrochlorothiazide 25 mg daily, lisinopril 20 mg daily, calcium carbonate, and multivitamins. What pharmacological options are available to reduce the risk of an NSAID ulcer now that A.D.'s initial ulcer is healed and she continues to take the naproxen?

Strategies to reduce the risk of NSAID (including aspirin) ulcers and upper GI complications include co-therapy with a PPI or misoprostol; the use of a COX-2 inhibitor; or various combinations of a PPI, misoprostol, and a COX-2 inhibitor.[46,87,94–96,98,104] All PPIs, when used in standard dosages (Table 23-1), are effective for this indication.[95] Standard H_2RA dosages (Table 23-1) should not be recommended as prophylactic co-therapy to reduce the risk of NSAID ulcers because they are not effective in reducing the risk of gastric ulcer, which is the most common ulcer associated with NSAIDs.[95,96] Higher H_2RA dosages (e.g., famotidine/ibuprofen 26.6/800 mg 3 times a day [DUEXIS]) reduce the risk of gastric and duodenal ulcer but are less effective than a PPI.[94,95] Famotidine 20 mg twice daily may be an alternative to a PPI in patients at risk who are taking low-dose aspirin,[137] but comparative trials with PPIs are needed to support the use of standard dose H_2RAs for this indication. There are no studies that have evaluated the use of H_2RAs in reducing the risk of ulcer-related upper GI complications. H_2RAs may be used when necessary to relieve NSAID-related dyspepsia.

Misoprostol reduces the risk of NSAID-induced gastric and duodenal ulcers,[94–96] as well as the risk of upper GI complications in high-risk patients.[136] Initially, the recommended dosage was 200 mcg 4 times a day, but diarrhea and abdominal cramping limited its use. A lower daily dosage of 600 mcg/day should be used because it reduces GI side effects and is comparable in efficacy.[95,96] Dosage reductions to 400 mcg/day or less minimize GI side effects but compromise gastroprotective effects. When used as co-therapy, misoprostol and PPIs have a similar efficacy in preventing gastric ulcer, but PPIs have few side effects.[95,96] A fixed dosage form containing misoprostol 200 mcg and diclofenac (50 mg or 75 mg) is available, but flexibility to individualize dosage is lost.

Two large randomized, placebo-controlled, multicenter, clinical trials compared the GI safety in patients taking COX-2 inhibitors with those taking nonselective and partially selective NSAIDs and reported a reduction of 50% to 60% in upper GI events with the COX-2 inhibitors.[138,139] A 6-month trial (CLASS) of celecoxib in patients who were not taking low-dose aspirin revealed a statistically lower rate of ulcer complications when compared with that of ibuprofen or diclofenac,[139] but evaluation at 1 year found no GI safety advantage among those taking celecoxib.[95] This explains why celecoxib contains the same GI warnings as the nonselective and partially selective NSAIDs (Table 23-4).[140] In addition, a post hoc analysis at 6 months indicated that patients taking celecoxib and concomitant cardioprotective doses of aspirin had a similar rate of upper GI events as those taking either diclofenac or ibuprofen, thus negating the beneficial effects of celecoxib.[139] Low-dose aspirin appears to have similar effects on other COX-2 inhibitors.

A.D. remains at high risk for another NSAID-related complication even though gastric ulcer healing was confirmed, because she continues to take naproxen. Co-therapy with a PPI or misoprostol is preferred for this patient because both are effective in reducing the risk of NSAID-related upper gastrointestinal events. A.D.'s osteoarthritis is well controlled with naproxen, so there is no need to switch her to celecoxib or another more costly NSAID. Combining PPI therapy with misoprostol is not necessary, but some physicians prefer to use combination therapy for older patients with multiple risk factors. Standard H_2RA dosages (e.g., famotidine 20 mg BID) should not be used as prophylactic co-therapy for A.D., because they are not effective in reducing the risk of NSAID-related gastric ulcer. Although higher H_2RA dosages (e.g., famotidine 40 mg BID) reduce the risk of gastric ulcer, they are less effective than a PPI. The famotidine should be discontinued, and prophylaxis should be instituted with a standard dose of a PPI (e.g., pantoprazole 40 mg daily). All PPIs, when used in standard dosages, are effective for this indication, but A.D.'s out-of-pocket cost should be taken into consideration when selecting a PPI.

Cyclooxygenase-2 Inhibitors and Cardiovascular Toxicity

CASE 23-2, QUESTION 5: What is the concern regarding the use of COX-2 inhibitors and the risk for cardiovascular toxicity?

The risk for cardiovascular events in patients taking COX-2 inhibitors increases with a number of factors, including increased COX-2 selectivity, higher dosages, a longer duration of treatment, and preexisting cardiovascular risk.[95,96,140–142] Although ulcers and related GI complications were less likely with rofecoxib than with naproxen in the VIGOR trial, the number of myocardial infarctions and thrombotic strokes were increased with rofecoxib.[138] Similar cardio thrombotic events were observed in other rofecoxib studies of longer duration.[143] In 2004, rofecoxib was withdrawn from the U.S. market and soon thereafter valdecoxib was withdrawn amid concerns about cardiovascular risk.[95]

The cardiovascular safety of celecoxib has been evaluated, but the risk of myocardial infarction and thrombotic stroke is less certain.[95] Although there was no difference in cardiovascular events when celecoxib was compared with diclofenac and ibuprofen in the CLASS trial,[139] cardiovascular events were significantly higher in a clinical trial where patients were taking higher dosages of celecoxib (400 mg twice daily).[144] Celecoxib remains available in the United States, but the underlying cardiovascular risk of the patient must be assessed when considering the use of this drug. The lowest effective celecoxib dose should always be used for the shortest duration of time.[140]

The risk for cardiovascular events is also increased in patients taking nonselective and partially selective NSAIDs, with the possible exception of naproxen.[95,96,145–147] Naproxen is usually the preferred NSAID, especially in patients with increased cardiovascular risk.[95,96 145–147] If possible, NSAIDs and COX-2 inhibitors should be avoided in patients at very high GI and cardiovascular risk.[95] Consideration should be given to using less risky therapeutic options including acetaminophen, tramadol, or narcotics.[148] Thus, the selection of a drug regimen to reduce the risk of NSAID ulcers and GI complications should not only be based on the GI safety of the NSAID or COX-2 inhibitor but must be weighed against the cardiovascular risk for each patient.[95,96,147]

Stratification of Future Risk for Nonsteroidal Anti-Inflammatory Drug–Induced Peptic Ulcers

CASE 23-2, QUESTION 6: How does a COX-2 inhibitor compare with a PPI and a nonselective or partially selective NSAID when used to decrease ulcer risk and related complications? Have any studies evaluated GI safety in patients taking a COX-2 inhibitor plus a PPI?

There have very few randomized controlled trials in *H. pylori*–negative patients at high risk for NSAID-related complications that compared the combined therapy of celecoxib with a PPI versus a partially selective NSAID with a PPI or celecoxib alone.[95,149,150] Results from these trials suggest that in high-risk, *H. pylori*–negative patients, combined therapy with a COX-2 inhibitor and PPI may be more efficacious than a partially selective NSAID plus a PPI or celecoxib monotherapy in reducing NSAID-related ulcer complications. Combining a COX-2 inhibitor with a PPI may be considered in very high-risk patients; however, long-term outcomes are unclear given the longest clinical trial follow up was 1 year.[95,149,150]

CASE 23-2, QUESTION 7: What factors should be considered when evaluating management strategies for patients at risk of experiencing an NSAID-induced ulcer? What risk-reduction strategies are considered acceptable for A.D.?

Strategies to reduce the risk of NSAID ulcers and related complications depend on the assessment of upper GI (Table 23-3) and cardiovascular risks. Although there are no universally accepted definitions, the levels of risk can be arbitrarily stratified into low, moderate, and high GI risk and low or high cardiovascular risk.[95,96] High cardiovascular risk implies a physician-recommended requirement for low-dose aspirin to prevent serious cardio thrombotic events.[95] In general, individuals younger than 65 years, and those taking NSAIDs in the short term who do not require low-dose aspirin, are considered to be at low GI and cardiovascular risk and usually do not require GI risk-reduction therapy.[95,96]

Patients at moderate GI risk typically have one to two risk factors that include age older than 65 years; a history of a prior uncomplicated ulcer; treatment with high-dose NSAIDs; or the concurrent use of aspirin (including low-dose), corticosteroids, or anticoagulants (Table 23-3). The recommended risk-reduction strategy in this group is co-therapy with either a PPI or misoprostol, but misoprostol is usually considered a secondary option because of GI adverse events and the need for more frequent daily dosing.[95,96] If the patient requires low-dose aspirin, naproxen is the NSAID of choice. Although a COX-2 inhibitor provides similar gastroprotective effects as a nonselective or partially selective NSAID plus a PPI or misoprostol, the use of COX-2 inhibitors (including celecoxib) has declined dramatically because they are typically more costly than the NSAID plus PPI and because of concerns related to myocardial infarction and thrombotic events.[95]

Patients at very high GI risk include those with a prior history of an ulcer-related complication or multiple (>2) risk factors.[95,96] If cardiovascular risk is low, alternative therapies such as oxycodone are preferred, but a COX-2 inhibitor plus a PPI or misoprostol may be used.[95] Although it is best to avoid an NSAID if the patient had a complicated ulcer, some physicians will continue the same NSAID that provided the most effective anti-inflammatory effect. This should be done with extreme caution and with maximally effective co-therapy. NSAIDs and COX inhibitors should be avoided in patients at high GI risk and high cardiovascular risk, and alternative therapy should be used.[95,96]

Patients like A.D., who have a history of a recent ulcer and related upper GI bleed, are at high risk for future NSAID-related ulcers and complications and require an effective risk-reduction strategy. Additionally, A.D. has other factors that contribute to her high-risk status, including her age (70 years) and the continued use of a nonselective NSAID (naproxen). Ranitidine should be discontinued immediately, and A.D. should be switched to an evidence-based risk-reduction regimen. If celecoxib is used, the risk of cardiovascular effects must be weighed against the gastroprotective benefits, especially because A.D. has a history of hypertension. If A.D. had renal dysfunction (creatinine clearance <30 mL/minute), NSAIDs and COX-2 inhibitors should be avoided, and the patient should be treated with other analgesics (e.g., tramadol, narcotics), keeping in mind that NSAIDs and COX-2 inhibitors are associated with fluid retention, hypertension, and renal failure. Although switching naproxen to celecoxib plus a PPI or continuing the oxycodone may be preferred by some, the selection of the optimal strategy for a high-risk patient like A.D. is debatable and should take into consideration the risks, benefits, patient preferences, continued analgesic relief, and cost of treatment. Co-therapy with a PPI or misoprostol is an acceptable risk-reduction strategy given A.D.'s GI and cardiovascular risk. Combination therapy of celecoxib and PPI may represent the greatest GI risk reduction and may be considered in this patient.

CASE 23-2, QUESTION 8: What information should be conveyed to A.D. regarding the combined use of OTC aspirin and NSAIDs?

Remind A.D. that her physician has recommended that she discontinue taking the enteric-coated aspirin and that she should not restart it without his/her consent. Explain to A.D. that enteric-coated aspirin may protect against the topical mucosal damage in the stomach and minimize dyspepsia, but the enteric coating does not prevent an ulcer. Even low-dose aspirin (e.g., 81 mg/day) is capable of causing an ulcer, especially when used in conjunction with an NSAID (naproxen). Buffered aspirin may cause less dyspepsia, but buffering does not prevent ulcers. Taking food, milk, or an antacid with aspirin or NSAIDs may minimize dyspepsia but does not prevent an ulcer. Inform A.D. that she should not take OTC NSAIDs in conjunction with her naproxen unless advised to do so by her physician, because combining NSAIDs will increase the risk for ulcers and GI bleeding. Advise A.D. that even though NSAIDs available for self-treatment may have different generic names (e.g., ibuprofen, naproxen) or brand names (e.g., Advil, Aleve), they all belong to the same drug class and have similar side effects.

CASE 23-2, QUESTION 9: A.D.'s physician decides to maintain her on naproxen but changes the famotidine to lansoprazole 30 mg daily. What instructions should you provide A.D. regarding her medications?

A.D. should be advised of the major signs and symptoms of upper GI bleeding and cardiovascular disease and what action should be taken if these signs or symptoms develop. She should be instructed to take the lansoprazole daily 30 to 60 minutes before breakfast and continue taking naproxen twice daily. The importance of adhering to PPI co-therapy must be stressed, especially because A.D. may not have accompanying dyspeptic or ulcer-like symptoms. There is a strong relationship between the level of adherence to gastroprotective medication and the risk for ulcers and serious GI complications in patients like A.D. who are high-risk NSAID users.[151] Older patients, like A.D., who are at risk for osteoporosis and hip fractures and who require long-term PPI therapy should be counseled to take age-related recommended dosages of a calcium salt and vitamin D and have periodic bone density examinations (see section on Pharmacotherapy of Drugs Used to Treat Acid-Related Disorders).

CASE 23-2, QUESTION 10: What parameters should be monitored to determine A.D.'s response to treatment?

High-risk patients like A.D. who continues to take an NSAID should be closely monitored for upper abdominal pain and signs or symptoms associated with bleeding, obstruction, or perforation. The presence of upper abdominal pain or a change in the severity of the pain may suggest an upper GI complication. Every effort should be made to monitor A.D.'s compliance to her PPI regimen because of the strong relationship between nonadherence and the risk of upper GI complications in high-risk NSAID users.

ZOLLINGER–ELLISON SYNDROME

ZES is an uncommon gastric acid hypersecretory disease characterized by severe recurrent peptic ulcers that result from a gastrin-producing tumor (gastrinoma).[130,152] The primary tumor is usually located in the duodenum or pancreas, but other locations (e.g., mesenteric lymph nodes, spleen, stomach, liver) have been described.[130,152] Although most gastrinomas occur sporadically, about 25% occur in association with multiple endocrine neoplasia type 1 (MEN 1), which is an autosomal dominant inherited syndrome.[152] Most gastrinomas are malignant and tend to be slow-growing, but a small number grow and metastasize rapidly to the regional lymph nodes, liver, and bone. Abdominal pain is the most predominant symptom and is usually related to persistent peptic ulcers, which are less responsive to antisecretory therapy. Duodenal ulcers occur most often, but ulcers may also occur in the stomach or jejunum. Diarrhea, which is present in more than half of patients, may precede ulcer symptoms and results from massive gastric acid hypersecretion, which activates pepsinogen and contributes to mucosal damage.[130,152] Steatorrhea may also occur and results from inactivation of pancreatic lipase by low duodenal pH resulting from excessive acid load.[152] This leads to the precipitation of bile acids, which, in turn, reduces micelle formation necessary for fatty acid absorption. Vitamin B_{12} deficiency may develop secondary to malabsorption related to reduced intrinsic factor activity. GERD often occurs and is complicated by esophageal ulcers and strictures. Other symptoms include nausea, vomiting, upper GI bleeding, and weight loss. Upper GI bleeding is related to duodenal ulceration and may be the presenting symptom.

Epidemiology

The incidence of ZES in the United States is 0.1% to 1.0% among patients with duodenal ulcers.[152] The majority of patients are diagnosed between the ages of 30 and 50 years, with men being slightly more affected than women.[152] The morbidity and mortality of ZES have decreased because of improved medical and surgical management.

Pathophysiology

The pathophysiology of ZES is related to a non-β islet cell gastrin-secreting tumor that stimulates the parietal cells of the stomach to hypersecrete gastric acid.[130,152] Large amounts of gastrin are produced by the gastrinoma cells, usually resulting in a profound hypergastrinemia. The gastric parietal cell mass is expanded in response to the trophic effects of hypergastrinemia and causes an increase in basal and stimulated acid output. Hypersecretion of gastric acid results in severe mucosal ulceration, diarrhea, and malabsorption, and is responsible for the signs and symptoms associated with ZES.

Clinical Assessment and Diagnosis

The diagnosis of ZES is established when the fasting serum gastrin is greater than 1,000 pg/mL and the BAO is greater than 15 mEq/hour in patients with an intact stomach (or >5 mEq/hour in the postgastric surgery patient) or when hypergastrinemia is associated with a gastric pH value less than 2.[152] When serum gastrin is between 100 and 1,000 pg/mL and gastric pH is less than 2, a provocative test (secretin or calcium) is recommended to assist in the diagnosis. Imaging techniques are performed to localize the tumor and are useful in evaluating metastatic disease. Upper endoscopy is performed to confirm mucosal ulcerations. The use of PPIs may mask the clinical presentation and complicate the diagnosis.[130]

Treatment

The goal of treatment for ZES is to pharmacologically control gastric acid secretion and to surgically resect the tumor, if possible. The oral PPIs are the drugs of choice for controlling acid secretion because of their potent and prolonged antisecretory effect. Treatment should be initiated with omeprazole 60 mg/day or an equivalent oral dose of lansoprazole, pantoprazole, esomeprazole, or rabeprazole (Table 23-1) and should be titrated to maintain a BAO less than 10 mEq/hour (1 hour before next dose) in uncomplicated patients or less than 5 mEq/hour in patients with complicated disease.[152] Once adequate control of acid secretion has been achieved, the daily PPI dose should be gradually reduced and administered every 8 to 12 hours. In most patients, an omeprazole dose of 60 to 80 mg/day reduces the BAO to target levels. IV PPIs should be reserved for those patients who are not able to take oral medications. H_2RAs are no longer used to treat ZES, even though they were initially proven to be effective (Table 23-1).

Somatostatin analogues are used with varying success to treat gastrinomas, but they are only available parenterally and rarely used as first-line treatment.[152] Octreotide, a synthetic somatostatin analogue, inhibits gastric acid secretion and decreases serum gastrin concentrations, but its subcutaneous route of administration, frequent dosing, and side effect profile (abdominal pain, diarrhea, gallstones, and pain at the injection site) make it less desirable for use in treating ZES. The long-acting depot formation of octreotide acetate for injection suspension can be administered less frequently and may be useful in controlling temporal growth. Patients with metastatic gastrinomas can be treated with chemotherapeutic agents to inhibit tumor growth or may require resection of the tumor. Localization and surgical removal of the gastrinoma should be considered in all patients unless widespread metastases exist.

GASTROESOPHAGEAL REFLUX DISEASE

GERD is a common acid-related GI disorder associated with a wide array of symptoms, the most frequent of which is heartburn and acid regurgitation. Gastroesophageal reflux (GER) is defined as the retrograde passage of gastric contents from the stomach into the esophagus. It is primarily the result of transient relaxation of the LES. When the LES is relaxed, the esophagus is exposed to small amounts of acidic stomach contents. This normal physiologic event occurs many times throughout the day in healthy individuals.[6,153,154] Protective mechanisms, such as esophageal peristalsis and bicarbonate-rich saliva, quickly return the acidic pH to normal. GERD develops when alterations in reflux result in symptoms, mucosal injury, or both.[65] Esophageal injury occurs with continued exposure of the mucosa to gastric acid and results in inflammation that can progress to ulceration (erosive esophagitis).[6,155] Complications associated with long-standing GERD include esophageal strictures, Barrett metaplasia (replacement of normal esophageal squamous epithelium by specialized intestinal-like columnar epithelium), and adenocarcinoma of the esophagus.[7]

Epidemiology

GERD is a chronic disease that affects patients across all age groups with equal distribution between men and women.[7] In the Western world, the prevalence of GERD is estimated to be about 10% to 20%, with lower prevalence in Asian countries. In Western populations, 25% of patients report heartburn monthly, 12% weekly, and 5% describe daily symptoms.[156,157] It has also been estimated that 7% of the U.S. population have complicated GERD associated with erosive esophagitis; however, this finding is difficult to validate, because most patients do not undergo diagnostic esophageal endoscopy.[7] Many patients with erosive esophagitis are asymptomatic on diagnosis, which suggests that symptoms do not correlate with the degree of esophageal injury. Up to 75% of patients who undergo endoscopic procedures as a result of symptoms associated with GERD have normal esophageal findings.[158] These patients are identified as having functional heartburn, nonerosive reflux disease (NERD), or endoscopy-negative reflux disease (ENRD). Other patients with GERD have symptoms that occur outside the esophagus, which are considered atypical or extraesophageal manifestations of GERD. Extraesophageal manifestations may be present with or without accompanying typical symptoms (e.g., heartburn). Extraesophageal manifestations have been estimated to occur in about 80% of patients with at least weekly symptoms of GERD (see section on Extraesophageal Manifestations).[159]

Childhood GERD appears to continue into adolescence and adulthood. Although most infants exhibit physiologic regurgitation, or spitting up, the majority (95%) will have abatement of symptoms by 1 year of age.[160] However, infants with persisting symptoms beyond 2 years of age are at risk of exhibiting complicated GERD.[161,162] One prospective study evaluated children with a prior diagnosis of complicated GERD (erosive esophagitis) made at approximately 5 years of age, and then reevaluated them 15 years later. This study revealed that 80% of the children reported monthly symptoms of heartburn and regurgitation, and 23% described weekly symptoms. In addition, 30% still required antisecretory therapy, and 24% underwent antireflux surgery[163] (see Chapter 104, Common Pediatric Illnesses). Pregnancy has also been associated with an increased incidence of GERD, with 30% to 50% of pregnant women complaining of heartburn, especially in the second and third trimesters; however, in individuals without a previous diagnosis of GERD, the symptoms resolve when the child is born.[6] The mechanisms for GERD in pregnancy are related to the hormonal effects of progesterone and estrogen, which lower LES pressure, and increase intra-abdominal pressure[6,164] (see Chapter 49, Obstetric Drug Therapy, for complete discussion related to the management as well as the risks and benefits associated with treating GERD in the pregnant patient).

Complications associated with GERD include esophageal erosions (5%), strictures (4%–20%), and Barrett metaplasia (8%–20%).[6] Male sex and advancing age (men and women) are associated with an increase in the prevalence of esophageal complications, presumably as a result of refluxed acidic contents damaging the mucosa over time.[6] When comparing quality of life in patients with GERD to those with other chronic medical diseases, the quality of life in GERD patients was between patients with psychiatric disorders and patients with mild heart failure.[165]

Etiology and Risk Factors

The causes of GERD are associated with factors that increase the frequency or duration of GER leading to increased contact of the acidic refluxate with the esophageal mucosa. Risk factors associated with GERD include dietary and lifestyle factors, drugs, and certain medical and surgical conditions[7,8,153–155,166,167] (Table 23-7). These factors may precipitate or worsen GERD symptoms by lowering the LES pressure (e.g., nitrates, progesterone, foods high in fat, mint, chocolate) or having a direct irritating effect on the esophageal mucosa (e.g., citrus, tomatoes, bisphosphonates). Stress reflux from increased intra-abdominal pressure has been associated with overeating, coughing, and bending or straining to lift heavy objects, as well as tight-fitting clothing.[6,8] Certain medical and surgical conditions, such as gastroparesis, scleroderma, ZES, and long-term placement of nasogastric tubes, may also be associated with GERD.[6]

Table 23-7

Risk Factors Associated With Gastroesophageal Reflux Disease[6,8,153–155,166,167]

Drugs	Dietary
α-Adrenergic agonists	Foods high in fat
Anticholinergics	Spicy foods
Aspirin	Carminatives (peppermint, spearmint)
Barbiturates	Chocolate
Benzodiazepines	Caffeine (coffee, tea, colas)
β_2-Adrenergic agonists	Garlic or onions
Bisphosphonates	Citrus fruits and juices
Calcium-channel blockers	Tomatoes and juice
Dopamine	Carbonated beverages
Estrogen	
Isoproterenol	**Lifestyle**
Iron	Cigarette/cigar smoke
Narcotics	Obesity
Nitrates	Supine body position
NSAIDs	Tight-fitting clothing
Progesterone	Heavy exercise
Potassium	
Prostaglandins	**Medical/Surgical Conditions**
Quinidine	Pregnancy
Tetracycline	Scleroderma
Theophylline	ZES
Tricyclic antidepressants	Gastroparesis
Zidovudine	Nasogastric tube intubation

NSAID, nonsteroidal anti-inflammatory drug; ZES, Zollinger–Ellison syndrome.

Pathophysiology

The pathophysiology of GERD is associated with defects in transient relaxations of the LES, esophageal acid clearance and buffering capabilities, anatomy, gastric emptying, mucosal resistance and with exposure of the esophageal mucosa to aggressive factors (gastric acid, pepsin, and bile salts) leading to esophageal damage.

TRANSIENT RELAXATIONS OF THE LOWER ESOPHAGEAL SPHINCTER

The LES, when in a resting state, remains at a high pressure (10–30 mm Hg) to prevent the gastric contents from entering into the esophagus.[6] Pressures are lowest during the day and with meals and highest at night.[6] Transient relaxations of the LES are short periods of sphincter relaxation that are different from those that occur with swallowing or peristalsis.[7,168,169] They occur as a result of vagal stimulation in response to gastric distension from meals (most common), gas, stress, vomiting, or coughing and can persist for more than 10 seconds.[7] These transient relaxations of the LES are associated with virtually all GER events in healthy individuals but account for 50% to 80% of occurrences in patients with pathogenic GERD.[7] Thus, not all transient relaxations of the LES are associated with GERD.

A small percentage of patients may also have a continuously weak and hypotensive LES (decreased LES resting tone). Stress reflux increases intra-abdominal pressure and may blow open the hypotensive LES.[7] When LES pressures remain constantly low, the risk for serious complications (e.g., erosive esophagitis) increases dramatically. Scleroderma, which is related to fibrosis of smooth muscle, may reduce LES tone and increase the potential for GERD.[170]

ESOPHAGEAL ACID CLEARANCE AND BUFFERING CAPABILITIES

Although the number of reflux events and quantity of refluxate are notable, it is the duration of time the mucosa is in contact with these noxious substances that determines esophageal damage and complications. More than 50% of patients diagnosed with severe esophagitis have decreased acid clearance from the esophagus.[6] Peristalsis is the primary mechanism by which acid refluxate is removed from the esophagus. Other mechanisms include swallowing, esophageal distension in response to refluxate, and gravity (which is only effective when the patient is in an upright position).

Saliva plays an important role in the neutralization of gastric acid within the esophagus. Its bicarbonate-rich content buffers the residual acid that remains in the esophagus after peristalsis.[6] However, saliva is only effective on small amounts of gastric acid, because patients with larger volumes of acid refluxate may not have the neutralizing capacity in saliva necessary to protect the esophagus.[6] Swallowing increases the rate of saliva production and esophageal acid clearance. The reduction of swallowing that occurs during sleep is associated with nocturnal GERD. Patients with decreased saliva production (e.g., elderly, patients taking medication with anticholinergic effects, and those with certain medical conditions such as xerostomia or Sjögren syndrome) may also be at increased risk of experiencing GERD.[6,171]

ANATOMIC ABNORMALITIES

Hiatal hernia (protrusion of the upper portion of the stomach into the thoracic cavity because of weakening in the diaphragmatic muscles) is frequently described as a cause of GERD, but its causal relationship remains uncertain.[6] Although hiatal hernia is associated with a greater degree of esophagitis, strictures, and Barrett metaplasia, not all patients with hiatal hernia exhibit symptoms or complications. This may be related to the size of the hiatal hernia and its effect on LES pressure.[6] An increase in the size of the hernia may decrease its ability to remain below the diaphragm during swallowing, and thus, reduces LES pressure. Hypotensive LES in combination with hiatal hernia increases the likelihood of reflux and complicated disease.[6]

GASTRIC EMPTYING

Delayed gastric emptying increases the volume of gastric fluid remaining within the stomach that is available for reflux and is associated with gastric distension.[6] Although delayed gastric emptying is present in up to 15% of patients with GERD, a causal relationship has not been established.[6,172] Because some patients, such as those with diabetic gastroparesis, also have GERD, the association between delayed gastric emptying and GERD cannot be overlooked.[6]

MUCOSAL RESISTANCE

The capability of the esophageal mucosa to endure contact with and withstand injury from gastric refluxate (acid and pepsin) is a substantial determinate for the development of GERD. When considering the mucosal resistance within the esophagus compared with that of the stomach and duodenum, the esophagus is less resistant to damage from gastric acid.[6] However, mucosal resistance in the esophagus is composed of many defensive factors working in tandem to prevent esophageal injury. An increase in mucosal cell thickness and intracellular junctional complexes prevents the diffusion of hydrogen ions from penetrating into the esophageal epithelium and leading to cell death.[6] The esophagus also secretes a protective mucous layer and bicarbonate.[6,173] Enhanced blood flow in response to an acidic environment within the esophagus improves tissue oxygenation, provides nutrients, and helps to maintain a normal acid–base balance.[6] Esophageal injury also occurs when the concentration of acid and pepsin exceed the protection afforded by mucosal resistance mechanisms.

AGGRESSIVE FACTORS ASSOCIATED WITH ESOPHAGEAL DAMAGE

The gastric refluxate, which is composed primarily of gastric acid and pepsin, is the primary aggressive factor associated with GERD. The development and degree of mucosal damage is dependent on the pH and contents of the refluxate as well as the total exposure time of refluxate with the esophageal mucosa. A pH less than 4 is usually required to produce injury to the esophageal mucosa, but as the refluxate becomes more acidic, the mucosal damage is accelerated.[6] The addition of pepsin (which is converted from secreted pepsinogen in an acidic pH) to the acidic refluxate will markedly increase the propensity of the refluxate to compromise mucosal resistance and increases the potential for esophageal bleeding.[6,172,174] Duodenogastric reflux or alkaline reflux containing bile acids and pancreatic juices may also contribute to esophagitis.[6] Because gastric and duodenogastric reflux are often concomitantly present, their actions may be additive in causing esophageal damage. The duration of total exposure time of the esophagus to the refluxate is the primary mechanism involved in the development of GERD and its complications. The longer the duration of exposure time, the greater the possibility of severe disease, including progression to Barrett metaplasia.

ERADICATION OF HELICOBACTER PYLORI

The relationship between *H. pylori* infection and GERD remains controversial.[175] Conflicting data from earlier studies suggested that *H. pylori* eradication is associated with increase gastric acidity and development of erosive esophagitis; however, this observation is not supported by the current treatment guidelines for *H. pylori* infection. Routine *H. pylori* testing in patients with GERD is not standard practice, if the patient is tested and found to be *H. pylori* positive, eradication is recommended[89] (see section on Primary Treatment for *Helicobacter pylori*).

Clinical Presentation

SIGNS AND SYMPTOMS

CASE 23-3

QUESTION 1: W.J. is a 39-year-old, 130-kg, 170-cm-tall man who presents with complaints of indigestion. He describes a burning sensation behind his breastbone and some belching that is often associated with an acid taste in the back of his mouth. He indicates that his symptoms began a few months ago, and they only occur a few times a month, especially after eating large or spicy meals. Also, if he eats too close to bedtime, the burning keeps him up at night. He has used liquid antacids in the past for these symptoms and states they work fairly well, but he has to take frequent doses, because the symptoms return quickly. He does not take any other medications. Which of W.J.'s symptoms are consistent with GERD?

Symptoms that are typically associated with GERD include heartburn, pyrosis (a retrosternal burning that occurs in the upper esophagus and travels up through the throat), regurgitation of gastric contents into the throat, or in many patients, the presence of both.[6,65,171] These symptoms may be episodic or meal related and are often alleviated by antacids.[6] Heartburn, the most frequent typical symptom, is caused by the contact of acidic refluxate with nerve endings within esophageal mucosa.[6] Other symptoms include water brash (salty or sour fluid occurring abruptly within the mouth), early satiety, belching, hiccups, nausea, and vomiting.[6] Worrisome symptoms (alarm signs or symptoms) include dysphagia (trouble swallowing), odynophagia (painful swallowing), vomiting of blood, bloody or tarry stools, unexplained weight loss, and anemia.[6,65] These symptoms suggest complicated disease, such as erosive esophagitis, esophageal stricture, malignancy, or GI bleeding, and require immediate evaluation by a health-care professional. Some patients, such as the elderly, may not have typical GERD symptoms but present initially with alarm symptoms.[6,176] This is attributable in part to older patients having a reduced pain perception and a possible reduction in the acidity of the refluxate.[6] Other patients may present with only extraesophageal or atypical symptoms (see section on Treatment for the Extraesophageal Manifestations of Gastroesophageal Reflux Disease). Despite the lack of esophageal symptoms, the potential for serious esophageal damage exists, because there is no correlation between symptoms and the degree of esophageal injury.[6] W.J.'s symptoms of a burning sensation (heartburn), regurgitation soon after eating spicy or large meals, and the association of symptoms with eating a meal near his bedtime are all consistent with GERD. The fact that his symptoms are relieved by his use of antacids is also suggestive of GERD.

Treatment

THERAPEUTIC GOALS

CASE 23-3, QUESTION 2: What are the therapeutic goals for the treatment of W.J.'s GERD?

The therapeutic goals for the management of GERD are to alleviate symptoms, promote esophageal healing, prevent recurrence, provide cost-effective pharmacotherapy, and avoid long-term complications.[6] One long-term consequence is Barrett esophagus, or Barrett metaplasia, which is identified in 10% to 15% of GERD patients on endoscopic evaluation.[6,177] This premalignant condition may predispose the patient to esophageal adenocarcinoma. Patients with Barrett esophagus have a risk of exhibiting esophageal cancer that is 30 to 40 times higher than patients without this disorder.[177] GERD is a chronic disease that carries the potential for serious complications.

NONPHARMACOLOGIC MEASURES AND SELF-DIRECTED TREATMENT

CASE 23-3, QUESTION 3: What lifestyle and dietary changes may potentially reduce W.J.'s GERD symptoms?

Lifestyle and dietary modifications comprise the initial step in managing patients with GERD[8,65,167,175,178] (Table 23-8). Strategies should be discussed with the patient and tailored to his or her specific needs. The paucity of evidence to date suggests that although many patients may benefit from these modifications, they are unlikely to completely alleviate symptoms in most patients.[65,171,178] Lifestyle modifications are aimed at reducing acid exposure within the esophagus by increasing LES pressure, decreasing intragastric pressure, improving esophageal acid clearance, and avoiding specific agents that irritate the esophageal mucosa. There is evidence to support several modifications that reduce esophageal gastric acid exposure and symptoms.[65,178] These include raising the head of the bed 6 to 8 inches by using blocks underneath the legs of the bed or using a foam wedge instead of traditional pillows; sleeping in a left lateral decubitus position; and weight loss, which also decreases intragastric pressure.[65,178]

Patients with GERD symptoms should avoid foods and beverages known to trigger symptoms (Table 23-7). However, the evidence suggesting benefit remains uncertain.[65,178] However, individualized lifestyle and dietary modifications should be recommended to all patients with GERD symptoms. When appropriate, OTC or prescription medications should be recommended.[8]

W.J. should be counseled to lose weight, wear loose-fitting clothing, and avoid eating spicy meals that he knows will exacerbate his symptoms. Recommend that he avoids eating at least 3 hours before bedtime as this may help decrease symptoms and consider raising the head of his bed 6 to 8 inches with wooden blocks.

CASE 23-3, QUESTION 4: Which OTC treatment options (if any) would you recommend for W.J.?

Many patients with mild, infrequent symptoms can be managed with OTC medications[6,8,179–181] (Fig. 23-5). First, a determination must be made as to the suitability of the patient for self-treatment. If the patient does not meet the criteria for self-treatment as described subsequently, he or she should be referred for further medical evaluation.[6,8,180,181] It is important to ensure that the following are not present: alarm signs or symptoms, severe or frequent (2 or more days a week) heartburn lasting greater than 3 months, presence of extraesophageal manifestations (see Case 23-5), or symptoms that persist despite appropriate drug therapy. OTC antacids and H_2RAs are the drugs of choice for patients with mild, infrequent heartburn. The nonprescription PPIs (omeprazole, immediate-release omeprazole with sodium bicarbonate, and lansoprazole) should be reserved for patients who experience frequent heartburn.[8]

Antacids remain an effective option for treating mild, infrequent heartburn, because they rapidly (within minutes) relieve symptoms, but the duration of symptom relief only lasts about 30 minutes when taken on an empty stomach.[7,8,180] The duration can be extended for several hours if taken within 1 hour after a meal.[8] Antacids are available in tablet and liquid form and are usually interchangeable when used in recommended dosages.[8] The dose can be repeated every 1 to 2 hours as needed, but the maximum recommended daily dose should not be exceeded. The addition of alginic acid to the antacid may improve symptom relief for some patients.[8,179] Patients requiring frequent or regular antacid use for more than 2 weeks should be reevaluated, because an OTC H_2RA or PPI may be needed.[8,180,181] About 20% of patients will achieve symptom relief with the use of antacids.[6] Antacids are not effective in healing erosive esophagitis.[7]

The OTC H_2RAs are indicated for mild to moderate infrequent GERD symptoms.[8,180] When compared with antacids, their onset of symptom relief occurs within 30 to 45 minutes, and they have a longer duration of action (up to 10 hours).[6,8] One benefit of the H_2RAs is that they can be taken before eating a heavy or spicy meal as prophylaxis for postprandial GERD symptoms.[6,8] They also have a beneficial effect on reducing nocturnal acid secretion.[8] Tachyphylaxis (tolerance) has been reported with continued use of H_2RAs, but this effect can be overcome with intermittent or as-needed use.[8] OTC H_2RAs

Table 23-8
Dietary and Lifestyle Modifications Used to Manage Gastroesophageal Reflux Symptoms[8,65,167,178]

Dietary	Medication	Lifestyle
Avoid foods listed in Table 23-7	Avoid medications with a potential to relax the lower esophageal sphincter or that have a direct irritant effect on the esophageal mucosa (Table 23-7)	Stop or decrease smoking/tobacco
Avoid eating large meals	Medications with the potential to irritate the esophagus should be taken with a full glass of water	Avoid alcohol
Avoid eating within 3 hours of bedtime		Lose weight[a]
		Elevate the head of bed 6–8 inches or use a foam wedge[a]
		Sleep in the left lateral decubitus position[a]

[a]Sufficient evidence exists to support lifestyle modification.

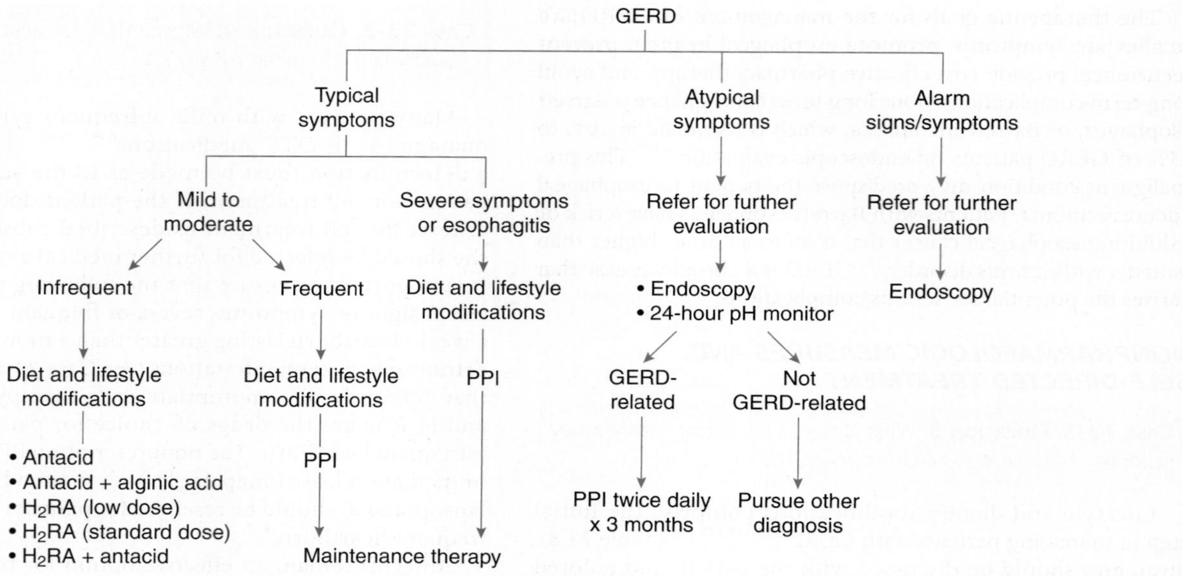

Figure 23-5 Management of GERD. GERD, gastroesophageal reflux disease; H_2RA, H_2 receptor antagonist; PPI, proton-pump inhibitor.

are available in one-half the original prescription low dose and as full prescription doses. Patients should use the lower OTC dose twice daily for mild, intermittent symptoms and the higher dose twice daily for moderate symptoms[8] (Table 23-1). The four OTC H_2RAs (cimetidine, famotidine, ranitidine, nizatidine) are interchangeable when used in recommended dosages.[8] Patients should avoid cimetidine if the potential for a clinically important drug interaction exists with drugs metabolized by the hepatic CYP450 enzyme system. When used for self-treatment, the H_2RA dose should not exceed two doses per day, and the treatment duration should not exceed 2 weeks. Use beyond 2 weeks should be under the care of a health-care provider.[6,8]

Esomeprazole, lansoprazole, and omeprazole are PPIs available OTC and are potent inhibitors of gastric acid and are indicated for use in patients with frequent heartburn (2 or more days a week).[8] The onset of symptom relief is slower (2–3 hours) than with H_2RAs, and complete relief may require up to 4 days after initiating therapy. PPIs are superior to H_2RAs with regard to symptom relief and duration of acid suppression.[8] Patients should take the OTC PPIs 30 to 60 minutes before a meal (breakfast is preferable) and not take more than one dose daily for up to 2 weeks. Another course of therapy should not be taken more than every 4 months unless directed by a health-care provider, because this may indicate more serious disease.[6,8,180,181]

W.J. is an appropriate candidate for self-treatment because his symptoms are mild and occur infrequently, and he has no alarm symptoms. Although antacids are an acceptable option for W.J., he has tried these and is unhappy with the frequency of dosing needed to relieve his heartburn. Because W.J. has requested a medication to specifically "prevent" meal-related symptoms, he should take an H_2RA 30 to 60 minutes before eating or drinking. If symptoms remain infrequent but are unrelated to meals, the use of an OTC H_2RA as needed for symptoms may be required. He can increase the dose to twice daily if symptom relief is not optimal and may consider an OTC PPI if symptoms occur more than 2 days a week. If he continues to have symptoms beyond 2 weeks, they become more severe, or they are accompanied by alarm symptoms, he should be referred for further evaluation.

SEVERE DISEASE WITH COMPLICATIONS

CASE 23-4

QUESTION 1: L.F. is a 48-year-old woman who presents to her primary-care provider complaining of recurrent heartburn occurring daily for the past 6 weeks. She states that the heartburn occurs frequently after meals and often wakens her at night. Lately, she has been experiencing difficulty swallowing solid foods. L.F. currently smokes two packs of cigarettes per day and likes to have two glasses of wine each night with her dinner. She states that she occasionally uses OTC ranitidine 150 mg orally up to twice daily, which temporarily relieves her symptoms. What diagnostic modalities are available for the evaluation of her GERD?

Clinical Assessment and Diagnosis

Numerous diagnostic options exist for the evaluation of the patient with presumed GERD. The medical history should include the identification of specific symptoms and an assessment of symptom frequency, severity, and duration as well as risk factors or triggers. An empiric diagnosis can be made in the majority of patients based on the symptoms of heartburn and regurgitation. However, patients who present with severe symptoms, alarm symptoms, or long-standing GERD or who do not respond to empiric therapy warrant further diagnostic evaluation.

ACID SUPPRESSION EMPIRIC TEST

A trial of a PPI is commonly used to empirically diagnose typical GERD-like symptoms in patients without alarm symptoms or symptoms of complicated disease. Doses used in clinical trials range from 20 to 80 mg of omeprazole (or equivalent) once daily for up to 4 weeks.[6,182] If symptoms are relieved after a short trial of a PPI (7 to 14 days), an empiric diagnosis of GERD may be made and other invasive and costly diagnostic methods may be avoided.[6,153,179,182,183] However, this methodology is not without its limitations. The test cannot differentiate between other acid-related disorders, such as PUD, and studies evaluating its ability to detect GERD versus other diagnostic options have been equivocal.[6,182,183] Despite these shortcomings, guidelines suggest that an empiric trial of a PPI is appropriate in selected patients given its ease of use and reduced cost.[65] The empiric use of a PPI may also be beneficial in identifying patients with extraesophageal manifestations of GERD[6] (see section on Treatment for Extraesophageal Manifestations of Gastroesophageal Reflux Disease). Further diagnostic evaluation is warranted in patients who do not respond to acid suppressive therapy, who present with alarm symptoms or symptoms suggestive of complicated disease, or who have long-standing GERD where the possibility of Barrett esophagus exists.

UPPER ENDOSCOPY AND BIOPSY

Upper endoscopy is the primary diagnostic method for evaluating the esophageal mucosa for injury or cellular changes. (To view a video of severe esophagitis, go to http://www.gastrointestinalatlas.com/english/esophagitis.html.) This test is highly specific, yet only moderately sensitive for the diagnosis of GERD, because many patients present with nonerosive disease. There are four primary reasons why endoscopy is performed in patients suspected of having GERD[6,184]: (a) to rule out significant disease (e.g., adenocarcinoma of the esophagus) or complications (e.g., stricture); (b) to screen for Barrett metaplasia; (c) to evaluate and grade the severity of esophagitis; and (d) to allow the provider to optimize treatment and predict the long-term course of the disease. The endoscope can be fitted with surgical instruments to allow the operator to perform procedures or obtain tissue specimens for biopsy. Endoscopic grading of the esophagus is based on the level of inflammation and mucosal damage. Two endoscopic classification systems are used for the grading of esophagitis[185,186] (Table 23-9). The Savary–Miller classification categorizes patients from grade 0 to grade 4 based on the severity of mucosal erosions of the esophagus.[185] The addition of a grade 5 was added to include the diagnosis of Barrett esophagus.[187] Although this classification system is no longer recommended in the United States, it is still used in many practices, as well as in Europe. The Los Angeles classification is preferred because it is more specific and categorizes patients from grades A to D based on the number of mucosal breaks, their size, and the amount of surface area with esophagitis involvement.[186] There is no classification for normal esophagus with this system and symptomatic patients are often classified with NERD.

Biopsy of the esophageal mucosa is performed during endoscopy, and tissue samples are evaluated by microscopy for evidence of Barrett metaplasia or neoplastic disease.[8] In patients with suspected Barrett metaplasia, the biopsy is obtained after the esophagus has healed to prevent misinterpretation of the inflammatory markers for dysplastic syndrome. Mucosal biopsy for inflammatory markers in nonerosive disease remains debatable.

TWENTY-FOUR–HOUR CONTINUOUS AMBULATORY pH MONITORING

Ambulatory pH monitoring is a valuable diagnostic test for evaluating GERD. It is especially helpful in patients who have not responded adequately to reasonable pharmacotherapy, in patients with nonerosive disease, and when there is a need to correlate reflux events with symptoms. A small (2–3 mm diameter) pH electrode is threaded through the patient's nostril (similar to placing a nasogastric tube), past the patient's larynx, to approximately 5 cm above the LES in the distal esophagus.[6] Once it is connected to a logging device, which documents pH measurements every few seconds, it allows for the determination of reflux events (defined as esophageal pH <4), duration of reflux events, and percentage of time within a 24-hour period that the patient's pH is less than 4. The patient is asked to keep a diary to record symptomatic events that can be correlated with a decrease in esophageal pH. This is especially important when correlating extraesophageal manifestations with reflux events.

RADIOLOGIC TESTING

The barium esophagram (barium swallow) is used primarily to identify suspected esophageal abnormalities, such as strictures, narrowing, and hiatal hernia, and to determine peristalsis disorders.[6] The procedure is relatively noninvasive and inexpensive when compared with endoscopy.

ESOPHAGEAL MANOMETRY

Esophageal manometry is used to evaluate the patient's LES pressure and esophageal peristalsis.[7] This procedure does not have a specific role in the diagnosis of GERD, because it does not detect the presence of acid within the esophagus. It is used primarily to evaluate patients before 24-hour continuous ambulatory pH monitoring and antireflux surgical procedures (e.g., Nissen fundoplication) to determine the location of the LES.[7,188]

CASE 23-4, QUESTION 2: L.F.'s frequent severe symptoms continue despite OTC ranitidine 150 mg orally twice daily, and the presence of warning signs warranted that she undergo endoscopy, which revealed moderate esophagitis (Los Angeles grade C), the presence of an esophageal stricture, and no evidence of Barrett metaplasia. Esophageal dilation was performed during the procedure to widen the lumen of the esophagus. What treatment options exist for L.F.?

Table 23-9
Classification Systems for Endoscopically Determined Esophagitis[185–187]

The Savary–Miller Classification System of Esophagitis	
Grade 0	Normal esophageal mucosa
Grade 1	Erythema or diffusely red mucosa, edema causing accentuated folds
Grade 2	Isolated round or linear erosions extending from the gastroesophageal junction upward, not involving entire circumference
Grade 3	Confluent erosions extending around entire circumference or superficial ulceration without erosions
Grade 4	Complicated cases; erosions as in grade 3 plus deep ulcerations, strictures, or columnar epithelium-lined esophagus
Grade 5	Presence of Barrett metaplasia
The Los Angeles Classification System of Esophagitis	
Grade A	One (or more) mucosal break no longer than 5 mm that does not extend between the tops of two mucosal folds
Grade B	One (or more) mucosal break more than 5 mm long that does not extend between the tops of two mucosal folds
Grade C	One (or more) mucosal break that is continuous between the tops of two or more mucosal folds but that involves <75% of the circumference
Grade D	One (or more) mucosal break that involves at least 75% of the esophageal circumference

ANTACIDS

Antacids are useful only in the relief of mild symptoms associated with GERD (see section on Nonpharmacologic Measures and Self-directed Treatment). Because of their short duration of action and inability to heal erosive esophagitis, they are not an option for treating moderate to severe GERD.[6,8]

HISTAMINE-2 RECEPTOR ANTAGONISTS

H_2RAs are effective in treating patients with mild to moderate GERD, but response rates vary with the severity of disease, the dose of the drug, and the duration of therapy. H_2RAs are considered equally effective when used in equipotent doses for symptomatic relief and esophageal healing (Table 23-1). They are effective in reducing nocturnal symptoms but only modestly effective in relieving meal-related symptoms, because they only block one mechanism of parietal cell activation (the H_2 receptor).[6] H_2RAs relieve symptoms in about 50% to 60% of patients treated after 12 weeks of continuous therapy and are superior to placebo.[189] Increasing the H_2RA dose may not improve symptoms in some patients.[190] Esophageal healing requires higher doses (e.g., famotidine 40 mg BID) compared with those used for symptom relief (Table 23-1). Esophageal healing rates with H_2RAs are reported to be about 50% after 8 to 12 weeks of treatment, but rates will vary depending on the degree of esophagitis.[189] For example, endoscopic healing rates in trials with high-dose H_2RAs were approximately 60% to 90% in patients with grades 1 and 2 esophagitis but were only 30% to 50% in patients with more severe disease (grades 3 and 4 esophagitis).[6,189] Some investigators have attributed inadequate esophageal healing to the development of tachyphylaxis.[179]

PROTON-PUMP INHIBITORS

PPIs are the drugs of choice for patients with frequent moderate to severe GERD symptoms and esophagitis because they provide more rapid relief of symptoms and esophageal healing than do H_2RAs. When used in recommended dosages, all of the PPIs provide similar rates of symptom relief and esophageal healing (Table 23-1). Their superior efficacy, when compared with H_2RAs, is related to their ability to maintain an intragastric pH less than 4 for a long duration time (up to 24 hours/day vs. up to 10 hours with a H_2RA).[8,191] Typically, PPIs are taken once daily 30 to 60 minutes before breakfast, but if a second dose is required, it should be taken before the evening meal.

A large meta-analysis of 16 trials confirms that PPIs are superior to H_2RAs for achieving rapid and complete relief of GERD symptoms. Complete symptom relief (within 4–12 weeks) was achieved in 77.4% of patients taking a PPI versus 47.6% of those taking an H_2RA ($p < 0.0001$).[189] PPIs have also been shown to heal esophagitis more quickly and effectively than H_2RAs. In the same meta-analysis, which evaluated 43 double-blinded or single-blinded, randomized studies (including patients with severe esophagitis), PPIs (83.6%) were more effective than H_2RAs (51.9%) at healing erosive esophagitis at 12 weeks.[189] Healing also occurred more quickly with PPI therapy in that by week 2, 63.4% of patients had healed with the PPI, whereas it took 12 weeks with the H_2RAs for 60.2% of patients to heal.[189] Another large meta-analysis, which evaluated more than 33 randomized trials, demonstrated similar results with 81.7% of patients healed at 8 weeks with a PPI versus 52.0% with an H_2RA.[42]

Esophageal healing among PPIs appears to be equivalent, because about 85% to 90% of patients achieve complete healing at 8 weeks in numerous head-to-head trials with equivalent doses.[37–40] One meta-analysis, which compared esophageal healing rates among omeprazole 20 mg, lansoprazole 30 mg, pantoprazole 40 mg, and rabeprazole 20 mg (each given once daily), reported no statistical difference.[36] However, all of the PPIs were superior to ranitidine 300 to 600 mg/day. Esomeprazole 40 mg once daily has been reported to be superior to omeprazole 20 mg once daily, at both 4 and 8 weeks, when used to heal erosive esophagitis.[192] However, the esomeprazole 40 mg and omeprazole 20 mg dosages are not equipotent, and this study has been heavily criticized based on this fact. Another study, which compared equipotent doses of esomeprazole (40 mg) and lansoprazole (30 mg), also suggests that esomeprazole has statistically significant greater healing rates (92.6% vs. 88.8%, respectively, $p = 0.0001$).[39] In contrast, a similar study comparing lansoprazole 30 mg with esomeprazole 40 mg showed no statistical difference in esophageal healing, albeit with a smaller population.[40] Dexlansoprazole MR 60 mg once daily has been compared with lansoprazole 30 mg once daily in randomized, double-blind clinical trials to assess healing of erosive esophagitis.[193] The results using life-table analysis reveal similar healing rates with dexlansoprazole MR 60 mg and lansoprazole 30 mg (92%–93% vs. 86%–92%, respectively), but the results were not statistically significant.[193] A higher dose of dexlansoprazole MR (90 mg daily) was superior to lansoprazole (30 mg daily) in patients with more severe disease (Los Angeles Classification grades C and D), but these are not equipotent doses. In spite of the lack of supportive evidence, some clinicians prefer to use esomeprazole 40 mg/day or dexlansoprazole MR 60 mg/day for patients with severe erosive esophagitis.

The ability of a high-dose PPI to reverse Barrett metaplasia remains controversial.[6,194] Although studies have demonstrated islands of normal squamous epithelium returning, no data have determined that this is associated with a risk reduction in adenocarcinoma.[6,194] In fact, others have suggested that this return of normal mucosa may actually mask carcinogenic changes occurring deeper in the gastric mucosa.[195]

Improvement in quality of life has also been evaluated in patients receiving PPI therapy in the management of GERD. A recent study comparing esomeprazole with ranitidine during a period of 6 months showed a significant improvement in both physical functioning and sleep with the PPI therapy.[196]

PROKINETIC AGENTS

Two prokinetic agents, metoclopramide and bethanechol, may be effective in the management of GERD. Both drugs increase LES pressure and stimulate the motility of the upper GI tract without altering gastric acid secretion.[6] Although these drugs may provide relief of symptoms, they are ineffective in healing erosive esophagitis unless they are combined with an H_2RA or PPI. Prokinetics are not widely used to treat GERD because they are not as effective as other treatments and are associated with numerous side effects (sedation, anxiety, extrapyramidal symptoms, etc.).[6,156] Prokinetics are reserved for patients who are refractory to other available treatment options or who have delayed gastric emptying.

SUCRALFATE

Sucralfate appears to be effective in treating mild cases of GERD and possibly mild esophagitis but is not effective in the management of severe disease.[197] Given more effective options at this time, sucralfate is rarely used in the management of GERD.

PPIs are considered the drugs of choice for patients with frequent or severe GERD symptoms, or who have complicated disease, because of their potent inhibition of gastric acid secretion[65,153,179–181] (Fig. 23-5). In this case, L.F., who presents with severe esophagitis (Los Angeles grade C), will require a PPI taken once daily in order to relieve her symptoms and heal the esophagus (Table 23-1). A reasonable option for L.F. would be lansoprazole 30 mg daily to be taken 30 to 60 minutes before breakfast each morning for the next 8 weeks; however, if the cost of therapy is an issue, generic omeprazole 40 mg daily would also be an acceptable alternative. L.F. should also be counseled regarding lifestyle and dietary modifications, including smoking cessation and abstinence from alcohol. She should avoid eating large meals before bedtime and may wish to elevate the head of her bed by 6 to 8 inches with wooden blocks.

Maintenance Therapy

CASE 23-4, QUESTION 3: L.F.'s symptoms resolved in about 2 weeks after starting PPI therapy, and she remained asymptomatic after 8 weeks. She then underwent endoscopy again, which revealed that the esophagus had healed completely. Her primary-care physician then stopped the PPI. Now, 2 weeks later, she is experiencing mild heartburn. Is L.F. a candidate for long-term maintenance therapy?

GERD is a chronic disease. Up to 80% of patients with severe esophagitis and 15% to 30% with less severe disease have a symptomatic relapse within 6 months after discontinuing treatment.[6] The goal of maintenance therapy is to keep the patient symptom-free and prevent potentially life-threatening complications. Continuous maintenance therapy with a daily PPI is more effective than an H_2RA, with reported relapse rates of 25% and 50%, respectively.[6] Thus, PPIs are the drugs of choice for maintaining remission in patients with healed esophagitis. An H_2RA may be considered for patients with mild nonerosive disease. Although one-half of the PPI dose used for esophageal healing has been suggested, guidelines indicate that the recommended maintenance dose should be the dose that is required to render the patient asymptomatic.[65,179] Maintenance therapy, to reduce the risk of morbidity associated with chronic, relapsing disease, should be initiated with lansoprazole 15 to 30 mg once daily or equivalent PPI dose given the severity of L.F.'s esophagitis and symptomatic recurrence after discontinuing the PPI.

On-Demand Pharmacotherapy

The use of intermittent (on-demand) courses of PPI therapy (2–4 weeks) has been suggested as being potentially beneficial in patients with GERD.[198–203] One trial, which compared continuous maintenance therapy with esomeprazole 20 mg daily versus on-demand therapy with the same drug and dose in patients with healed erosive esophagitis, reported that continuous therapy was superior to on-demand therapy (81% vs. 58%, respectively) in maintaining endoscopic remission at 6 months.[203] The ability to maintain remission with on-demand therapy was reduced as the severity in esophagitis increased. Although numerous studies with a variety of PPIs have demonstrated patient satisfaction with on-demand therapy,[199–202] a systemic review of 17 trials evaluating the use of on-demand therapy indicates that intermittent therapy should only be considered in patients with mild, nonerosive disease.[198]

Combination of a Proton-Pump Inhibitor and Histamine-2 Receptor Antagonists

The addition of an H_2RA at bedtime to a once or twice daily PPI regimen is sometimes used for patients who continue to have nocturnal symptoms, although the evidence to support this combination remains inconclusive and current guidelines do not endorse this type of antisecretory management strategy at this time.[65] The rationale for this practice is based on an evidence that suggests a period of nocturnal acid breakthrough (defined as intragastric pH <4 for longer than 1 hour during the night) in a significant number of patients despite twice-daily PPI therapy, suggesting that histamine release may have an important function in nocturnal acid secretion.[204] One study suggests that the addition of an H_2RA to a twice-daily PPI regimen resulted in a statistically significant reduction in nocturnal acid breakthrough during the sleeping hours.[204] This trial, however, evaluated only a single bedtime dose of an H_2RA and did not consider the tachyphylaxis that can occur with continuous use. A subsequent trial using a twice-daily PPI regimen with continuous use of an H_2RA for 4 weeks demonstrated no difference in nocturnal acid suppression, suggesting that tolerance does play an important role in the use of H_2RAs for this indication.[26] It has been theorized that one way to possibly avoid this occurrence is to use the H_2RA on only an as-needed basis when lifestyle and dietary modifications are not effective for preventing nocturnal symptoms.[6]

Nonerosive Reflux Disease

Up to 75% patients with typical GERD symptoms who undergo endoscopy will not have evidence of esophagitis or complicated disease.[158] These patients are described as having functional heartburn, NERD or ENRD, and often undergo 24-hour ambulatory pH monitoring to determine whether abnormal reflux is present despite a negative endoscopy. A trial of a PPI is usually indicated despite no esophageal findings, because many patients will respond to this therapy.[158] Further medical evaluation is required if a patient does not respond to PPI therapy despite a doubling of the daily dose.

Extraesophageal Manifestations

CASE 23-5

QUESTION 1: S.P. is a 71-year-old retired man who was eating dinner with his wife when he experienced a sudden onset of chest pain described as crushing, burning, and squeezing. His wife notified emergency personnel, who transported S.P. to the emergency department. His past medical history reveals some cardiovascular risk factors, including age, hypertension, hyperlipidemia, and a sedentary lifestyle. His medications before admission include aspirin 81 mg daily, hydrochlorothiazide 25 mg daily, and atorvastatin 40 mg at bedtime. He also takes OTC famotidine 20 mg daily as needed for dyspepsia. On examination, he complains of substernal crushing chest pain that has lasted more than 1 hour. He is diaphoretic and extremely anxious. He denies any shortness of breath, pain radiating to upper extremities or jaw, or cough. His vital signs include a temperature of 99.1°F, blood pressure of 155/95 mm Hg, and heart rate of 115 beats/minute. Pertinent laboratory results at this time are

White blood cell (WBC) count, 7,700/μL
Hgb, 14.2 g/dL
Hct, 45%
Platelets, 270,000/μL
SCr, 1.1 mg/dL
BUN, 11 mg/dL
Total cholesterol, 161 mg/dL
Low-density lipoprotein, 93 mg/dL
High-density lipoprotein, 30 mg/dL
Triglycerides, 190 mg/dL
Sodium, 141 mEq/L
Potassium, 4.1 mEq/L
Troponin I, 0.3 ng/mL

Electrocardiogram reveals sinus tachycardia with no evidence of ST-segment elevation, depression, or T-wave inversion or new left bundle branch block. Because of S.P.'s cardiovascular risk factors and indeterminate troponin, he underwent immediate diagnostic cardiac catheterization, which showed normal coronary angiography and an ejection fraction of 65%. S.P. was diagnosed with noncardiac chest pain (NCCP). Could S.P.'s chest pain be associated with an extraesophageal manifestation of GERD?

Extraesophageal (atypical) manifestations of GERD are those signs and symptoms that occur outside of the esophagus yet are presumed to be associated with GERD. The extraesophageal manifestations of GERD include NCCP; pulmonary symptoms; and complaints related to the ear, nose, and throat; as well as hypersalivation and dental erosions (Table 23-10). Interestingly, these symptoms are often the only complaint that a patient has when he or she presents to the health-care provider.[6,205]

NONCARDIAC CHEST PAIN

About 30% of patients with angina-like chest pain have normal coronary arteries or minimal microvascular disease as demonstrated by cardiac angiography.[206] Up to 60% of these patients will have concomitant GERD as demonstrated by an abnormal esophageal endoscopy or ambulatory pH monitoring.[6,206] The symptoms associated with NCCP are very similar to those associated with cardiac angina. The chest pain is usually described as crushing, squeezing, or burning; retrosternal in location; and with or without lateral radiation to the upper extremities, back, neck, or jaw. The pain is often temporarily related to a meal or occurs nocturnally, usually awakening the patient and continuing for hours. An appropriate workup for coronary artery disease must be performed in all patients presenting with chest pain before considering a GI cause or trial of antireflux therapy.[65,206] This is especially important in women, the elderly, and diabetic patients, because their initial presentation may be similar to GI complaints when in fact an acute coronary syndrome is present. Numerous trials have evaluated the use of acid suppression as a means to treat NCCP once cardiac etiology has been ruled out through appropriate evaluation.[206–208] Meta-analyses and guidelines have suggested the PPI test, in which a short course (4 weeks) of high-dose (twice-daily) PPI is used, is an effective diagnostic tool and is associated with a reduction in costs compared with other diagnostic methods of GERD.[65,207,208]

Table 23-10
Atypical Manifestations of Gastroesophageal Reflux Disease[6,205]

Noncardiac Chest Pain	Pulmonary
Ear, Nose, and Throat	Chronic cough
Laryngitis/pharyngitis	Nonallergic, nonseasonal asthma
Hoarseness	Aspiration
Globus sensation	Bronchiectasis/bronchitis
Laryngeal cancer	Sleep apnea
Sinusitis	Idiopathic pulmonary fibrosis
Otitis	Pneumonia
Other	
Hypersalivation	
Dental erosions	

ASTHMA AND GASTROESOPHAGEAL REFLUX DISEASE

Reports suggest that concomitant GERD occurs in up to 80% of the asthmatic population through two theoretical mechanisms that might work to exacerbate asthma symptoms.[209] One is the vagal reflex theory, which proposes that symptoms result from the direct irritation of the vagus nerve when refluxate comes into contact with the esophageal mucosa, resulting in reflex bronchospasm.[210,211] In contrast, the microaspiration or reflux theory proposes that aspiration of refluxed acid into the lungs causes caustic injury of tissue within the bronchial tree, resulting in asthmatic symptoms.[211,212] Significant controversy exists regarding the benefit of antireflux pharmacotherapy in patients with asthma, especially in those patients who do not endorse typical GERD symptoms. An important meta-analysis of trials that evaluated the effects of antireflux therapy on patients with asthma indicates that asthma symptoms improved in 69% of patients, that the use of asthma medications was reduced by 62%, and that only 26% of the subjects showed improvement in evening peak expiratory flow rate. All other pulmonary function tests showed little or no change with antireflux therapy.[213] However, this meta-analysis only evaluated studies of up to 8 weeks in duration. A large randomized, double-blind trial evaluated esomeprazole 40 mg twice daily versus placebo for 6 months in patients with poorly controlled asthma managed with inhaled corticosteroids, who lacked typical GERD symptoms. Results revealed no benefit in asthma control with the addition of a PPI, despite 40% of subjects demonstrating GERD by ambulatory pH monitoring.[214] Current American Thoracic Society/European Respiratory Society guidelines for the management of severe asthma suggest that GERD and antireflux therapy can be considered in patients with poorly controlled asthma, if they have GI symptoms consistent with GERD.[215] The American Gastroenterological Association position statement accepts the use of an empiric trial of twice-daily PPI for asthmatic patients with typical GERD symptoms, but that reflux monitoring should be considered before PPI trial in asthmatic patients with atypical GERD symptoms.[156]

OTOLARYNGOLOGY SYMPTOMS AND GASTROESOPHAGEAL REFLUX DISEASE

GERD is the most common etiologic factor in 60% of patients with chronic laryngitis and in 25% to 50% of patients with a globus sensation (the feeling that something is caught in the throat).[216] Symptoms relating to GERD are responsible for up to 10% of the patients seen by otolaryngologists.[216] The most likely mechanism for the pathophysiology of GERD-related laryngitis is that damage and inflammation occur at night while the patient is sleeping. It is during this time when upper esophageal sphincter pressures are especially low and the protective or neutralizing mechanisms of cough and salivation are suppressed.[217] This damage may be in addition to injury or laryngeal inflammation sustained from other causes, such as excessive voice usage, smoking, chronic throat clearing or cough, vomiting, or injury from endotracheal tubes.[205,218] The extent of injury in GERD-related hoarseness is directly related to the exposure time of the pharyngeal mucosa to the refluxate as well as the pH. Patients with GERD-related hoarseness usually do not have any other GERD-related symptoms.[205] The diagnostic procedure of choice is laryngoscopy and should be considered in all patients presenting with GERD-related hoarseness. Once the diagnosis of GERD-related hoarseness or laryngitis is established, the patient will likely require extended high-dose PPI therapy with the understanding that the majority of patients will relapse within 6 weeks once therapy is discontinued.[219]

TREATMENT FOR THE EXTRAESOPHAGEAL MANIFESTATIONS OF GASTROESOPHAGEAL REFLUX DISEASE

Experts suggest that treatment should be initiated with a high-dose (twice-daily) PPI for at least 3 months before considering drug therapy to be ineffective; however, data are lacking to support this recommendation with the exception of noncardiac chest pain.[65] Recent guidelines suggest this empiric strategy is acceptable if concurrent typical GERD symptoms are present.[65] Alternatively, it is possible that GERD may not be the cause of the patient's symptoms.

S.P.'s chest pain is not of cardiac origin based on angiographic findings. Therefore, it is reasonable to presume that he is having an extraesophageal manifestation of GERD. S.P.'s symptoms were meal related, and he has a history of dyspepsia for which he takes an OTC H_2RA. The H_2RA should be discontinued, and S.P. should be given a trial of empiric twice-daily PPI therapy for a period of 2 to 4 weeks. If symptoms are severe, the use of endoscopy (to determine if esophageal damage is present) or 24-hour esophageal pH monitoring (to correlate reflux events with symptomatic chest pain) is appropriate.

Antireflux Surgery

CASE 23-5, QUESTION 2: S.P. responded well to the trial of omeprazole 40 mg orally twice daily and has not had chest pain in 2 months. He has heard that surgical options exist that may eliminate his need for medications, as they are very expensive for him. Is S.P. a candidate for antireflux surgery?

Numerous surgical and endoscopic procedures exist for patients with GERD. These include, but are not limited to, Nissen fundoplication, Toupet partial fundoplication, Belsey Mark IV repair, and the Hill posterior gastropexy repair, as well as newer endoscopic techniques.[7] The primary goal of these procedures is to restore LES pressure by repairing a hiatal hernia or diaphragmatic hiatus. Appropriate candidates include patients who are in a good health and request another treatment option as a result of poor medication adherence, patients who are unable to afford their medication, patients who suffer from side effects or worry about risks with long-term therapy, patients with extraesophageal symptoms who have responded well to antireflux therapy, or patients experiencing volume regurgitation and aspiration of gastric contents who have not responded to PPI therapy.[6,65,148,188] Despite the availability of these surgical options, the consideration of antireflux surgery is one in which the benefits should be heavily weighed against the risks of such an invasive approach, because these procedures are not without potential complications. The effectiveness of these procedures has been questioned, because many patients will still require drug therapy.[6,65] S.P. has responded well to high-dose PPI therapy for his NCCP, but he describes some financial difficulties with affording his medications. Alternatively, he is 64 years of age, which may increase the risk associated with surgery. S.P. should be referred for further medical evaluation to determine whether he is a candidate for antireflux surgery.

UPPER GASTROINTESTINAL BLEEDING

Upper GI bleeding is a common medical emergency that occurs in up to 160 cases per 100,000 adults annually and is associated with increased morbidity and mortality as well as substantial costs to the health-care system.[220,221] Despite advances in endoscopic hemostatic therapy and pharmacotherapy, the mortality rate associated with upper GI bleeding remains at 5% to 15%, which is the same as it has been for the last 20 to 40 years.[2,3,220,221] Upper GI bleeding can be categorized as either variceal or nonvariceal bleeding (see Chapter 25, Complications of End-Stage Liver Disease). Nonvariceal bleeding describes bleeding associated with PUD or stress-related mucosal bleeding (SRMB). Other causes include erosive esophagitis, Mallory–Weiss tear (a tear near the gastroesophageal junction associated with retching or coughing), and malignancy.[4] Although PUD and SRMB are both acid-related disorders, their presentation and pathophysiology differ.

Peptic Ulcer Bleeding

EPIDEMIOLOGY

The majority of upper, nonvariceal GI bleeding is caused by PUD.[3,4,220,221] Bleeding ulcers account for more than 400,000 hospitalizations in the United States each year.[221] As mentioned, the mortality rate for peptic ulcer bleeding can be as high as 15%. It has been suggested that an older presenting patient population (>60 years of age) with a greater number of comorbidities may account for this continued high mortality rate.[2,220,221] Fortunately, the vast majority (80%) of upper GI bleeding events are self-limited and require only minimal intervention.[2] National data derived from an U.S. database demonstrate a decreasing mortality rate (3.54%) in complicated elderly patients during 2001 to 2009.[222] Length of stay has been dramatically reduced in the majority of patients who receive early endoscopy (within 24 hours of admission).[220,221] However, in the 20% to 25% of patients who continue to bleed or rebleed after appropriate intervention, mortality increases to nearly 40%.[4,223]

PATHOPHYSIOLOGY

The most common causes of upper GI bleeding in patients with PUD are NSAID use and *H. pylori* infection.[87] Bleeding occurs when an ulcer extends deeper into the mucosa and erodes the wall of a blood vessel.[224] The incidence of *H. pylori* infection in bleeding ulcers is 15% to 20% lower than in patients with nonbleeding ulcers.[224] Bleeding associated with PUD is generally not caused by the hypersecretion of gastric acid, with the exception of patients with ZES.[224] The pathophysiology and risk factors associated with PUD are described earlier in this chapter (see section on Peptic Ulcer Disease).

CLINICAL ASSESSMENT AND DIAGNOSIS

The clinical presentation of a patient with a bleeding peptic ulcer usually includes the presence of melena (dark, tarry stools), which occurs in 20% of patients, hematemesis (vomiting of blood) in 30%, and both in about 50% of patients. Up to 5% of patients present with hematochezia (bloody diarrhea) indicative of rapid and substantial blood loss.[224] The primary step in evaluating the patient is to assess the degree of urgency for rapid medical management.[224] Two validated prognostic scales exist for early risk stratification into high-risk or low-risk adverse outcomes for patients presenting with upper GI bleeding. The pre-endoscopy Rockall score and Glasgow–Blatchford score utilize laboratory and clinical characteristics of the patient to assist the clinician in determining the need for and emergent nature of endoscopy in the individual patient.[4,220,221] The complete Rockall score, which includes data from the endoscopy, is used to predict the likelihood of rebleeding after endoscopy and mortality.[4,220,221] Hypovolemia owing to substantial blood loss can rapidly lead to shock. The initial management of these patients should focus on volume resuscitation and improving the patient's hemodynamic status. Clinical features suggestive of high risk for rebleeding or mortality include patients older than 65 years, serious comorbidities (e.g., hepatic or renal dysfunction, cardiac or pulmonary disease), hemodynamic instability (e.g., hypotension, tachycardia), shock, poor health, continued bleeding, mental status changes, and prolonged prothrombin/activated partial thromboplastin time (aPTT) (or elevated international normalized ratio [INR]).[2,4,220,223–226] These patients should immediately be transferred to an intensive care setting.

Most patients should receive early diagnostic endoscopic evaluation within 24 hours of presentation to determine the source of the bleeding, to predict the risk for rebleeding, and when required, to perform endoscopic interventions directed at stopping the bleeding ulcer and restoring hemostasis.[220,221] Risk of rebleeding may be predicted based on the presenting lesion(s) identified on endoscopy.[4,224] The most common ulcer identified on endoscopy is a clean-base ulcer found in about 42% of patients. This ulcer has a very low risk of rebleeding (5%), and the patient can usually be discharged immediately after recovery from the endoscopy and managed with appropriate antisecretory therapy. Intermediate stigmata of bleeding include lesions identified as flat-spot ulcers and/or adherent clots, which have a risk of rebleeding of 10% and 22%, respectively. Although endoscopic procedures are not usually necessary with flat-spot ulcers, adherent clots remain an area of controversy and usually require the endoscopist to attempt to remove the clot and manage the underlying lesion.[220] Patients identified with high-risk ulceration (nonbleeding visible vessel or active bleeding) will require endoscopic intervention and have a high risk of rebleeding (43% and 55%, respectively) despite intervention. Nonbleeding visible vessel and active bleeding are associated with an 11% mortality on initial presentation.[224] Ulcer size is also predictive of mortality and rebleeding, because ulcers greater than 1 or 2 cm in diameter confer greater risk.[224] Despite appropriate endoscopic hemostasis, approximately 20% of patients with peptic ulcer bleeding will rebleed within 48 to 72 hours after treatment.[4,220,223,224] Mortality associated with rebleeding is about 30% to 37%.[223] Patients undergoing endoscopy should be tested for *H. pylori* infection with biopsy (rapid urease test), because infection with this organism is associated with an increased risk of rebleeding.[220,221] Because false negatives can occur in the presence of active bleeding, all *H. pylori*–negative patients should have a confirmatory follow up test with serologic antibody testing on discharge to ensure that the patient is not infected.[220]

TREATMENT

Patients with upper GI bleeding require rapid risk stratification based on the presenting signs and symptoms. Patients with hemodynamic instability require immediate institution of resuscitative measures.[4,220,221,227] IV access should be obtained with two large-bore (e.g., 16–18 gauge) catheters to facilitate the administration of fluids and blood products.[4,221] Intravascular volume should initially be replenished with normal saline to prevent the patient progressing into hypovolemic shock. During this time, blood can be typed and crossed in the event a transfusion is required. Guidelines recommend the transfusion of packed red blood cells for patients with a Hgb level of less than 7 g/dL; however, consideration is warranted in the patient with tachycardia or hypotension and a Hgb level of 10 g/dL.[220,221] A nasogastric tube should be placed to allow for lavage and determination of the upper GI tract as the source of the bleed and evaluation of continued bleeding.[4,220,221,227]

Endoscopic evaluation with hemostatic techniques (when required) should be performed as soon as safely possible.[220,221] Endoscopic hemostasis is the cornerstone of management of patients with serious bleeding ulcers, because it reduces the incidence of rebleeding, the need for surgery, and mortality when compared with placebo or drug therapy.[220,221] Endoscopic procedures include thermocoagulation, laser therapy, injection therapy (epinephrine, ethanol, or saline), injection with sclerosing agent, or placement of endoscopic clips. Combining thermocoagulation with injection therapy is superior to either therapy alone or hemoclipping alone in patients with serious ulcer bleeding.[4,220,221] Despite initial hemostasis, however, the potential for rebleeding remains high, especially in patients with high-risk lesions.[4,220–224]

Improvements in hemostatic parameters (e.g., platelet aggregation, inactivation of pepsin, and correction of coagulation) leading to clot stabilization correlate directly with an intragastric pH greater than 6.[221,222,225] Therefore, treatment with an antisecretory drug is beneficial in patients after endoscopy to promote healing of the lesion. After the acute phase, the patient should be placed on appropriate drug therapy to continue healing and prevent ulcer recurrence (see section on Peptic Ulcer Disease). Patients who are *H. pylori* positive should receive appropriate eradication pharmacotherapy and confirmation of eradication at a later time.[220]

Histamine-2 Receptor Antagonists

Once widely used to manage upper GI bleeding, H_2RAs are now considered inferior to PPIs for reducing the incidence of rebleeding and the need for surgery.[220,221] This is likely related to the inability of H_2RAs to achieve an intragastric pH greater than or equal to 6 (even with continuous IV administration) and the rapid development of tachyphylaxis (especially with high IV doses).[220,225,29] Thus, H_2RAs are no longer recommended for the prevention of rebleeding associated with a peptic ulcer.[220,221]

Proton-Pump Inhibitors

PPIs are the drugs of choice to reduce the incidence of PUD-related rebleeding and the need for surgical intervention.[4,220,221,228–230] However, no clinical trials were able to show a mortality benefit with PPIs when entire treatment cohorts were evaluated.[228–230] Two meta-analyses performed by the Cochrane Collaborative group evaluating PPIs administered IV or orally against H2RAs or placebo showed a reduction in rebleeding, surgery, and repeat endoscopic treatment. [228,229] Based on these available data, PPI therapy for peptic ulcer bleeding is superior to H_2RAs and placebo.[220] Although no reduction in the number of deaths were identified when all patients were considered, PPI treatment of patients at the highest risk of mortality, as evidenced by endoscopically determined active bleeding or nonbleeding visible vessel, did impart a mortality benefit.[229] All-cause mortality was also reduced in Asian trials, with a concomitant greater reduction in the incidence of rebleeding and need for surgery than in trials performed elsewhere in the world. This may be explained by the inclusion of a younger patient population, more potent acid suppression because of genetic polymorphism in CYP450 metabolism leading to a slower clearance of PPIs, a lower parietal cell mass, and a greater incidence of *H. pylori* infection.[228]

Despite the data, important questions remain as to the most appropriate dose and route of administration for PPIs in patients with peptic ulcer bleeding. Evidence suggests that most patients with low-to-intermediate risk lesions (clean-base or flat-spot ulcers) and who are hemodynamically stable may be treated with oral PPIs and immediately discharged after endoscopy, because rebleeding is infrequent in this population.[220,228,231] Patients with adherent clots and high-risk bleeding ulcers (active bleeding and nonbleeding visible vessels) are typically managed with high-dose bolus and continuous infusion of a PPI (omeprazole 80 mg or equivalent PPI followed by 8 mg/hour for 72 hours of omeprazole or an equivalent PPI) as recommended by the current treatment guidelines.[220] However, a recent meta-analysis has called into question the need for high-dose PPI therapy.[232] This meta-analysis evaluated over 1,300 patients enrolled into 10 randomized controlled trials treated with intermittent or continuous infusion PPIs. The risk ratio of rebleeding within 7 days of therapy was 0.72 with an upper boundary 1-sided 95% confidence interval of 0.97

suggesting non-inferiority of intermittent PPI dosing. These results will need to be confirmed with a carefully designed randomized controlled trial. Finally, another meta-analysis has also suggested that PPI therapy is associated with reduced blood transfusion requirements.[233] Some patients may be switched to an oral PPI if rapid stabilization occurs, but careful clinical assessment should be performed to ensure the patient is stable.[231] Early initiation of a PPI bolus infusion before endoscopy has been shown to reduce the proportion of patients with active bleeding once endoscopy is performed, reduce the requirements for endoscopy, and reduce hospital stay.[234] However, this strategy should not replace early endoscopic management in high-risk patients, because combination PPI therapy with endoscopic maneuvers has been proven to be more effective than monotherapy with an IV PPI.[220,221,235]

Once the high-risk patient has stabilized and is considered safe for discharge after endoscopy and 72 hours of IV PPI, the patient should be discharged with a prescription for at least once-daily PPI pharmacotherapy for continued healing of the lesion and further prevention of rebleeding.[220] The actual dose and duration, however, should be decided based on the patient's severity of disease and identified complications, with more severe disease warranting consideration of twice daily therapy.[220] Patients who are required to remain on cardioprotective aspirin or NSAID therapy may require long-term secondary prophylaxis in an attempt to prevent future upper GI bleeding events.[220]

Other Agents

The use of somatostatin or octreotide is not recommended for the treatment of patients with nonvariceal upper GI bleeding, because there is no evidence of benefit to support their use.[220,221] However, these agents are commonly used in the management of variceal bleeding (see Chapter 25, Complications of End-Stage Liver Disease).

Stress-Related Mucosal Bleeding

Acute SRMB is a type of erosive gastritis that occurs in critically ill patients with severe physiologic stress (e.g., surgery, trauma, organ failure, sepsis, severe burns, and neurologic injuries).[229,236–239] The term stress ulcer is a misnomer in that SRMB may range from numerous diffuse superficial erosive mucosal lesions (those that do not penetrate the muscularis mucosa) to major deep ulceration (penetration of the muscularis mucosa and potentially submucosa).[240,241] Initial lesions occur early (<24 hours) and appear as subepithelial petechiae that can develop into superficial erosions and ulcerations.[239,240] Early stress-related mucosal lesions are multiple, usually asymptomatic, without perforation, and commonly bleed from superficial mucosal capillaries.[238,240] The gastric fundus is the most likely anatomic region of the stomach to be involved. Distal lesions involving the gastric antrum and duodenum have also been described but tend to appear later in the hospital course and are often deeper and associated with a greater probability for bleeding.[240] SRMB from these lesions may be categorized into three distinct types based on clinical presentation.[238–241] Occult (hidden) bleeding is defined as aspirated gastric fluid or stool that is guaiac-positive for the presence of occult blood and without other signs or symptoms. Overt bleeding is defined as frank hemorrhage identified by hematemesis (bloody vomitus or the appearance of coffee grounds in gastric aspirates or vomitus), hematochezia (bloody diarrhea), or melenic stools. Clinically important bleeding or life-threatening bleeding is the presence of overt bleeding that is associated with hemodynamic changes (tachycardia, hypotension, orthostatic changes, or Hgb concentration decline of >2 g/dL) and the requirement of transfusion of blood products. Endoscopic therapy is generally not a viable option because of the extensive distribution of lesions associated with SRMB.[236]

EPIDEMIOLOGY

The majority (>75%) of the critically ill patients admitted to intensive care units (ICUs) will exhibit mucosal lesions consistent with SRMB within 24 hours of admission.[236,238–241] Only a small percentage (up to 6%) of these patients will progress to clinically important GI bleeding.[238–241] Clinically important SRMB has been associated with an increased length of stay in the ICU by up to 11 days and results in substantial increases in the cost of healthcare.[236,238–240,242] The mortality of clinically important SRMB approaches 50%, but mortality may also be associated with underlying comorbidities related to the critical illness.[229,239]

PATHOPHYSIOLOGY

Numerous factors have been identified in the pathogenesis of SRMB and resultant bleeding. These include gastric acid and pepsin secretion, disruptions to the normal homeostatic mechanisms that protect the gastric mucosa against the highly acidic environment (decreases in prostaglandin, bicarbonate, and GI mucus formation as well as impaired turnover of gastric epithelium), GI motility disturbances, and mucosal ischemia resulting from decreased blood flow.[236,238,239,241] Gastric acid is likely the central factor associated with development of SRMB.[236,240] Because of the absence of protective defenses, substantial amounts of acid are not required for the formation of lesions, but some acid is required for damage to occur.[241] Although some patients may have increased acid secretion (e.g., sepsis, CNS injuries, small bowel resections), the majority of critically ill patients have normal or decreased acid secretion.[237,240,241] Pepsin secretion is associated with the lysis of clots owing to its proteolytic action on fibrin.[236,243] Gastric prostaglandins play a key role in the cellular defense against gastric acid.[236] These prostaglandins are responsible for maintaining the integrity of the mucosal barrier by stimulating mucus and bicarbonate production; regulating blood flow; and, to some degree, inhibition of acid production. Mucosal ischemia secondary to splanchnic hypoperfusion also plays a large role in the pathogenesis of SRMB.[236,238,241] Mucosal ischemia is associated with reduced ability to neutralize hydrogen ions leading to intracellular acidosis within the mucosa and subsequent cell death. These factors all contribute to an imbalance by increasing injurious factors and reducing the protective mechanisms within the gastric fundus.

RISK FACTORS

CASE 23-6

QUESTION 1: J.S., a 58-year-old, 110-kg man was admitted to the medical ICU for severe necrotizing pancreatitis identified on abdominal computed tomography. The patient was immediately made "nothing by mouth" and started on imipenem/cilastatin 1,000 mg IV piggyback (IVPB) every 6 hours. He was given hydromorphone 1 mg IV every 3 hours as needed for pain. He subsequently exhibited shortness of breath on his third day after admission. He required intubation and was placed on a ventilator. A chest x-ray showed a left lower lobe infiltrate suggestive of hospital-acquired pneumonia. Antibiotic coverage was increased with the addition of ciprofloxacin 400 mg IVPB every 8 hours and linezolid 600 mg IV every 12 hours. He has a temperature of 103.5°F, heart rate of 115 beats/minute, and blood pressure of 70/40 mm Hg. Pertinent laboratory results at this time include the following:

WBC count, 38,000/μL
Hgb, 13.6 g/dL
Hct, 40%
Platelets, 150,000/μL
SCr, 1.3 mg/dL

BUN, 24 mg/dL
INR, 1.0
aPTT, 39 seconds
Aspartate aminotransferase, 292 units/L
Alanine aminotransferase, 305 units/L
Amylase, 508 units/L
Lipase, 624 units/L

In addition to the antimicrobials and initiation of fluid resuscitation, the critical care team is considering stress ulcer prophylaxis. What risk factors does J.S. have (if any) for SRMB, and is he a candidate for stress ulcer prophylaxis?

Numerous risk factors have been associated with SRMB[236–240] (Table 23-11). However, a large landmark, multicenter, prospective study involving more than 2,200 critically ill patients admitted to a medical ICU identified only the requirement of mechanical ventilation (respiratory failure) or coagulopathy as independent risk factors for development of clinically important bleeding.[244] Considering the cost associated with the reduction of risk related to SRMB, the authors concluded that only these two risk factors warrant the use of prophylactic therapy. Because not all risk factors impose the same level of risk, clinical guidelines and most practitioners recommend prophylaxis only when the patient is mechanically ventilated, has a coagulopathy, or when two or more of the remaining risk factors are present[236,237,239] (Table 23-11). J.S.'s risk factors include septic shock as evidenced by hemodynamic instability and mechanical ventilation. Therefore, a prophylactic regimen to reduce the risk of SRMB is appropriate.

TREATMENT

CASE 23-6, QUESTION 2: What options exist to prevent SRMB in J.S.?

Not all patients admitted to the critical care unit will require prophylaxis for SRMB. However, because mortality can be high in patients when bleeding occurs, evaluation of risk is of absolute importance to ensure that protective pharmacotherapy is initiated in appropriate patients.[236–241] Because acid is required for mucosal injury, the inhibition of gastric acid is the primary target when pharmacotherapy is used to reduce the risk of SRMB. An intragastric pH greater than 4 is the recommended goal of therapy.[229,236–241] Therapeutic options include the use of antacids, sucralfate, H_2RAs, and PPIs (Table 23-12).

Table 23-11
Risk Factors for Stress-Related Mucosal Bleeding[236–240]

- Respiratory failure
- Coagulopathy
- Hypotension
- Sepsis
- Hepatic failure
- Acute renal failure
- Enteral feeding
- High-dose corticosteroids[a]
- Organ transplant
- Anticoagulants
- Severe burns (>35% of body surface area)
- Head injury
- Intensive care unit stay >7 days
- History of previous GI hemorrhage

[a]Greater than 250 mg/day hydrocortisone or equivalent.

Antacids

The use of aggressive antacid therapy is superior to placebo in reducing clinically important SRMB when an intragastric pH greater than 3.5 is maintained.[236,238,239] Although antacids are effective in preventing SRMB, their use has fallen out of favor because of difficult administration regimens (every 1–2 hours) with the continuous requirement of intragastric pH monitoring for dose titration, electrolyte abnormalities (especially in patients with renal dysfunction), diarrhea, constipation, and the potential risk of aspiration pneumonia.[236,238–240] These issues, coupled with the fact that potent acid suppression is available in far more convenient dosage forms, have all but eliminated the use of antacids as SRMB prophylaxis.[236]

Sucralfate

Sucralfate is effective in preventing SRMB but does not have an important effect on intragastric pH.[245,246] Despite the fact that antisecretory therapy is preferred, sucralfate remains an available therapeutic option. Early studies suggested a reduction in nosocomial pneumonia with sucralfate when compared with ranitidine or antacids. However, a subsequent randomized trial involving 1,200 mechanically ventilated patients revealed no increase in pneumonia with H_2RAs when compared with sucralfate or antacids.[247] The usual dose of 1 g 4 times daily can present problems within the critical care setting because of multiple daily dosing, binding of other enterally administered drugs, and occlusion of nasogastric tubes (may be reduced with suspension formulation). Other potential issues include the risk for aluminum toxicity in patients with renal failure, constipation, and electrolyte imbalances. The concomitant use of sucralfate with antisecretory therapy may reduce the effectiveness of sucralfate as an intragastric pH less than 4 is needed for conversion to its active form, which binds to the gastric mucosa.[239]

Histamine-2 Receptor Antagonists

H_2RAs are effective in preventing SRMB and are the most widely used for this indication.[248,249] Although only cimetidine continuous infusion has been FDA labeled for the prevention of SRMB, continuous or intermittent infusions of ranitidine and famotidine are most often used for this indication.[225,236,238] Continuous infusions have been suggested as being more effective in maintaining a pH greater than 4, but there are no data comparing these two treatment options with respect to clinical outcomes.[236,240] Despite this, intermittent dosing is used more commonly than continuous infusions for the prophylaxis of SRMB.[225,238,248,249]

Numerous meta-analyses have evaluated the effectiveness of H_2RAs for prophylaxis of SRMB.[250,251] Cook et al. reviewed 63 randomized trials and determined that prophylaxis with H_2RAs was associated with a statistically significant reduction in overt and clinically important upper GI bleeding when compared with no therapy and a significant reduction in overt bleeding when compared with antacids.[250] A trend toward reduced clinically important bleeding was identified when H_2RAs were compared with sucralfate, but this was not statistically significant. In another meta-analysis, ranitidine was shown to be of no benefit in preventing SRMB and increased the risk of pneumonia.[251] However, neither of these meta-analyses included the large study involving 1,200 mechanically ventilated patients that compared sucralfate, ranitidine, and placebo.[247] Despite these conflicting results, H_2RAs remain a recommended option for the prophylaxis of SMRB.[248,249] One shortcoming of H_2RAs is that tolerance may develop (within 72 hours) and thus theoretically lead to potential prophylaxis failure.[29] H_2RAs are eliminated renally, and dosage reductions may be required in patients with renal failure.

Table 23-12
Stress-Related Mucosal Bleeding Prevention: Regimens and Doses

Agent	Dose and Frequency of Administration	FDA Approval[a]
Antacid	30 mL PO/NG every 1–2 hours	No
Cimetidine	300 mg IV loading dose, then 50 mg/hour continuous IV infusion[b]	Yes
Famotidine	20 mg IV every 12 hours or	No
	1.7 mg/hour continuous infusion	No
Ranitidine	50 mg IV every 6–8 hours or	No
	6.25 mg/hour continuous infusion	No
Sucralfate	1 g PO/NG every 6 hours	No
Omeprazole	20–40 mg PO/NG[c] every 12–24 hours	No
Omeprazole/sodium bicarbonate powder for oral suspension	40 mg PO/NG initially, followed by 40 mg 6–8 hours later, then 40 mg PO/NG every 24 hours	Yes
Lansoprazole	30 mg PO/NG[c,d] every 12–24 hours	No
Pantoprazole	40 mg IV/PO/NG[c] every12–24 hours	No
Esomeprazole	40 mg IV/PO/NG every 12–24 hours	No

[a]For prevention of stress-related mucosal bleeding.
[b]Not available in the United States
[c]Extemporaneously compounded in sodium bicarbonate.
[d]Oral disintegrating tablet.
IV, intravenous; NG, by nasogastric tube; PO, by mouth.

Proton-Pump Inhibitors

PPIs, because of their profound ability to inhibit gastric acid secretion and lack of tolerance to their antisecretory effect, would appear to be the preferred option for preventing SRMB. However, there is very little evidence to confirm their clinical superiority to H_2RAs for this indication. Numerous studies have compared PPIs with H_2RAs or placebo in critically ill patients in small populations using varied predetermined end points.[239,252] These studies suggest that PPIs provide greater acid suppression compared with H_2RAs and are likely to be as effective in preventing SRMB.[239,252] One study in 359 critically ill patients evaluated the use of immediate-release omeprazole suspension in bicarbonate given via nasogastric tube at a dose of 40 mg for two doses, then 40 mg/day versus IV cimetidine given as a 300-mg bolus and then infused at 50 mg/hour (dosing was adjusted for patients with renal dysfunction).[253] The results indicated that the PPI-bicarbonate suspension was associated with a greater mean time of intragastric pH greater than 4 than the cimetidine infusion but that the rate of clinically important bleeding did not differ between cimetidine (6.8%) and omeprazole (4.5%). The FDA considered the immediate-release omeprazole-bicarbonate suspension to be noninferior to cimetidine for the prevention of SRMB.[254] An extremely important analysis aimed at identifying the most appropriate dose for IV PPIs in SMRB prophylaxis was performed in more than 200 critically ill patients.[255] This analysis included five different dosing approaches of IV pantoprazole intermittent infusions (40 mg given every 8, 12, or 24 hours or 80 mg given every 12 or 24 hours) compared with cimetidine given as a 300-mg IV bolus immediately followed by a 50 mg/hour continuous infusion. The patients received a minimum of 48 hours of therapy with a maximum of 7 days. In all the study arms, pH control was achieved (defined as intragastric pH $\geq$ 4); however, in all the pantoprazole arms, pH control continued to improve from day 1 to 2, whereas a decline was noted in the cimetidine group, suggesting the occurrence of tachyphylaxis. No upper GI bleeding was noted in any patient during the trial regardless of treatment group assigned. The conclusions of this study demonstrated that patients may have adequate pH control with an initial IV dose of pantoprazole 80 mg followed by 40 mg IV every 12 hours. Finally, a recent meta-analysis that included 14 studies totaling ~1,700 patients evaluating the efficacy and safety of PPIs compared with H_2RAs demonstrated a statistically significant difference between the two options with respect to the important endpoints of overt or clinically important bleeding. There were no differences with regard to mortality or incidence of pneumonia.[252]

The incidence of nosocomial pneumonia in patients receiving PPI therapy undergoing cardiothoracic surgery has been evaluated in two retrospective cohort studies.[256,257] Patients receiving PPIs were at an increased risk for developing pneumonia even after data adjustments for various risk factors. Numerous alternative administration options exist for patients in the critical care setting who cannot take medications by mouth, have nasogastric tubes in place, or have difficulty swallowing[239,254,257] (Table 23-13). PPIs are becoming first-line therapy for the prevention of SRMB, but additional studies are needed to confirm the most effective dose and route of administration in order to obtain optimal clinical outcomes in patients at risk of SRMB.[238,248] The use of early enteral nutrition that is initiated within 48 hours of admission to the ICU has also been evaluated as a means of prophylaxis against SMRB.[258] This was demonstrated in a meta-analysis of 17 studies, which suggested that patients who require enteral tube feedings may not require additional forms of SRMB prophylaxis and may also have a reduced risk of pneumonia or death when compared with patients receiving an H_2RA-based SMRB prophylaxis regimen.[258] This meta-analysis, however, was only hypothesis generating and should be interpreted with care until a large controlled study is available to confirm these findings.

Table 23-13
Alternative Proton-Pump Inhibitor Administration Options[239,254,257]

	Omeprazole	Lansoprazole	Pantoprazole	Esomeprazole	Rabeprazole	Dexlansoprazole
Capsule granules sprinkled on selected soft foods (i.e., applesauce)		✓[a]		✓[a]	✓[a]	✓[a]
Capsule granules mixed in water and flushed down NG tube				✓		✓[a]
Capsule granules mixed in juice (can be administered via NG tube if required)	✓[a]	✓[a]		✓[a]	✓[a]	✓[a]
Extemporaneous compound of PPI in bicarbonate for NG tube	✓	✓	✓			
Package for oral suspension	✓[a,b]	✓[a,c]		✓[a]		
Oral disintegrating tablet		✓[a]				
IV formulation	Not available in the United States	Removed from US market	✓[a]	✓[a]		

[a]Labeled by the FDA for this administration option.
[b]Omeprazole suspensions available in 20- and 40-mg packets with bicarbonate (1,680 mg); both contain same amount of bicarbonate, and two 20-mg packets cannot be substituted for one 40-mg packet.
[c]Not to be administered via NG tube, because occlusion of tube is possible.
IV, intravenous; NG, nasogastric; PPI, proton-pump inhibitor.

MONITORING

CASE 23-6, QUESTION 3: J.S. has been started on famotidine 20 mg IV every 12 hours. How should this pharmacotherapy be monitored for safety and efficacy?

The famotidine dose should be adjusted to maintain an intragastric pH greater than 4 and should be based on severity of the patient's illness, renal function, and intragastric pH measurements. The intragastric pH can be determined with an indwelling probe or by measuring the pH of nasogastric aspirates. The patient should be monitored for signs of bleeding (e.g., presence of blood or coffee-ground material in nasogastric aspirates, hematemesis, hematochezia, or melena), hypotension, reductions in Hgb or Hct, and thrombocytopenia.

CASE 23-6, QUESTION 4: During the next 6 days, J.S. improves and is subsequently removed from mechanical ventilation and transferred to the medical ward. He is now able to eat normally. Should J.S. be continued on SRMB prophylaxis?

Patients receiving prophylaxis for SRMB should be evaluated for the continued presence of risk factors. As the patient improves, the risk factors should in turn be reversed, and the need for SMRB prophylaxis should diminish. Factors such as extubation, correction of coagulopathies, discharge from the intensive care setting, and the ability to take oral feeding advocate the discontinuation of prophylaxis. Numerous studies have suggested that up to 54% of patients were ordered SRMB prophylaxis outside the ICU setting and without a compelling indication.[259] Erstad and colleagues surveyed 153 institutions within the United States and found that in 65% of the hospitals, more than 25% of patients remained on SRMB prophylaxis after discharge from the ICU.[260] This can lead to increased costs, the potential of the patient being discharged on medication for which there is no indication, and future potential adverse effects from the medication.[259] Because J.S. does not possess any risk factors for SRMB, famotidine should be discontinued at this time.

KEY REFERENCES AND WEBSITES

A full list of references for this chapter can be found at http://thepoint.lww.com/AT11e. Below are the key references and websites for this chapter, with the corresponding reference number in this chapter found in parentheses after the reference.

Key References

ASHP Commission. ASHP therapeutic guidelines on stress ulcer prophylaxis. ASHP Commission on Therapeutics and approved by the ASHP Board of Directors on November 14, 1998. *Am J Health Syst Pharm.* 1999;56:347. (237)

Abraham NS et al. ACCF/ACG/AHA 2010 expert consensus document on the concomitant use of proton pump inhibitors and thienopyridines: a focused update of the ACCF/ACG/AHA 2008 expert consensus document on reducing the gastrointestinal risks of antiplatelet therapy and NSAID use: a report of the American College of Cardiology Foundation Task Force on Expert Consensus Documents. *Am J Gastroenterol.* 2010;105:2533. (54)

Ali T, Harty RF. Stress-induced ulcer bleeding in critically ill patients. *Gastroenterol Clin North Am.* 2009;38:245. (236)

Armstrong D, Sifrim D. New pharmacologic approaches in gastroesophageal reflux disease. *Gastroenterol Clin North Am.* 2010;39:393. (154)

Barkun AN et al. International consensus recommendations on the management of patients with nonvariceal upper gastrointestinal bleeding. *Ann Intern Med.* 2010;152:101. (220)

Chey WD et al. American College of Gastroenterology guideline on the management of *Helicobacter pylori* infection. *Am J Gastroenterol.* 2007;102:1808. (89)

Gisbert JP et al. Sequential therapy for *Helicobacter pylori* eradication: a critical review. *J Clin Gastroenterol*. 2010;44:313. (113)

Kahrilas PJ et al. American Gastroenterological Association Medical Position Statement on Management of gastroesophageal reflux disease. *Gastroenterology*. 2008;135:1383. (65)

Katz P et al. Guidelines for the diagnosis and management of gastroesophageal reflux disease. *Am J Gastroenterol*. 2013;108:308–328. (156)

Lanza FL et al. Guidelines for prevention of NSAID-related ulcer complications. *Am J Gastroenterol*. 2009;104:728. (95)

Napolitano L. Refractory peptic ulcer disease. *Gastroenterol Clin North Am*. 2009;38:267. (130)

O'Connor A et al. Treatment of *Helicobacter pylori* infection 2010. *Helicobacter*. 2010;15(Suppl 1):46. (112)

Scarpignato C, Hunt RH. Nonsteroidal anti-inflammatory drug-related injury to the gastrointestinal tract: clinical picture, pathogenesis and prevention. *Gastroenterol Clin North Am*. 2010;39:433. (94)

Tytgat GN et al. New algorithm for the treatment of gastro-oesophageal reflux disease. *Aliment Pharmacol Ther*. 2008;27:249. (180)

Yang YX, Metz DC. Safety of proton pump inhibitor exposure. *Gastroenterology*. 2010;139:1115. (57)

24 Lower Gastrointestinal Disorders

Toyin Tofade, Benjamin Laliberte, and Charmaine Rochester-Eyeguokan

CORE PRINCIPLES

		CHAPTER CASES
INFLAMMATORY BOWEL DISEASE		
1	Inflammatory bowel disease (IBD) is a generic classification for a group of chronic, idiopathic, relapsing inflammatory disorders of the gastrointestinal tract. Symptoms of IBD are thought to result from dysregulation of the mucosal immune system. By convention, IBD is divided into two major disorders, ulcerative colitis (UC) and Crohn's disease (CD).	**Cases 24-1, 24-2**
2	Ulcerative colitis (UC) is an inflammatory condition of the large intestine, but it can cause disturbances in other organ systems. It is typified by abdominal pain, chronic loose bloody stools, and fatigue.	**Case 24-1 (Questions 1, 2)**
3	Crohn's disease usually causes significant diarrhea without frank blood, abdominal pain, and weight loss. Extraintestinal symptoms such as skin lesions, arthralgias, and ocular inflammation occur more commonly with CD than UC. CD can affect any part of the gastrointestinal tract, but small and large bowel involvement is most common.	**Case 24-2 (Question 1)**
4	Treatment for both UC and CD are divided into two areas: induction treatment, which controls symptoms, and maintenance treatment, which prevents recurrences. Specific agents used for induction in IBD depend on the extent and location of disease.	**Case 24-1 (Questions 3–5, 8)**
5	Topically applied agents (suppositories, foams, enemas), specifically mesalamine products (5-aminosalicylic acid), are effective for induction in UC confined to the rectum (proctitis) or the distal colon.	**Case 24-1 (Question 6)**
6	Long-term use of corticosteroids for treatment of both UC and CD is not effective and can result in serious adverse effects; thus, other agents should be used for maintenance of remission.	**Case 24-1 (Questions 7, 9–11)**
7	Corticosteroids are used most often for induction in CD patients. Agents such as azathioprine, infliximab, or other agents are used to maintain remission.	**Case 24-2 (Questions 2, 3)**
8	Tumor necrosis factor blocking agents such as infliximab are used in patients who do not respond to less aggressive therapy. These agents have a high acquisition cost and carry significant risks for developing infections. However, clinical trials have shown that they are generally more effective than other therapies.	**Case 24-2 (Question 6)**
IRRITABLE BOWEL SYNDROME		
1	Irritable bowel syndrome (IBS) is a common and often debilitating condition that involves abdominal pain, bloating, and defecation associated with a change in bowel habits (usually constipation or diarrhea). It is benign and has no long-term complications.	**Case 24-3 (Question 1)**
2	The treatment goal is to improve global IBS symptoms, including abdominal discomfort, bloating, altered bowel habits, and overall well-being. Treatment for IBS is based on the predominant symptoms of the patient. For irritable bowel syndrome with constipation (IBS-C), an increase in dietary "soluble" fiber is recommended, such as psyllium followed by lubiprostone or linaclotide.	**Case 24-3 (Questions 2, 3)**

Continued

		CHAPTER CASES
3	Pain and bloating or visceral hypersensitivity associated with IBS may respond to antispasmodic agents such as peppermint oil, hyoscyamine, low-dose tricyclic antidepressants, or selective serotonin reuptake inhibitors.	Case 24-4 (Question 1)
4	Treatment for irritable bowel syndrome with diarrhea (IBS-D) includes antimotility agents such as loperamide. The Food and Drug Administration (FDA) also approved the antibiotic rifaximin and eluxadoline, a controlled substance with mixed opioid receptor activity.	Case 24-4 (Question 2)

OVERVIEW OF INFLAMMATORY BOWEL DISEASE

Definition and Epidemiology

Inflammatory bowel disease (IBD) is a generic classification for a group of chronic, idiopathic, relapsing inflammatory disorders of the gastrointestinal (GI) tract. IBD is common in developed countries.[1] It is estimated that more than 1.5 million people in the United States have IBD, and the prevalence of these disorders ranges from 100 to 200 per 100,000 people for CD and 205 to 240 per 100,000 for UC.[2,3] By convention, IBD is divided into two major disorders: ulcerative colitis (UC) and Crohn's disease (CD).[1,3,4]

However, approximately 10% to 15% of patients with IBD have symptoms that defy this schema.[5] Both UC and CD frequently affect a similar group of patients (Table 24-1).[2,6] Caucasians appear to have a higher incidence of IBD compared with Asians or African Americans. In particular, Jews of European descent may have up to a fourfold increase in the incidence of IBD. Studies have found trends toward an increased incidence of IBD with increased socioeconomic status and in urban compared with rural communities. Hypotheses for this trend include overcrowding, exposure to infectious agents, and lifestyle differences. Although both UC and CD are generally considered diseases of the young, with peak incidences from ages 15 to 30 years, there seems to be no significant sex preference for IBD.[3,7]

Etiology

The true cause of IBD is unclear; however, hypotheses for these disorders include a combination of genetic abnormalities, chronic infection, environmental factors (bacterial, viral, temperate climate, prior appendectomy, and dietary antigens), host or intestinal microbiome interactions, and other abnormalities of immunoregulatory mechanisms.[1] Whatever the mechanism, it is now generally agreed that the symptoms of IBD result from dysregulation of the mucosal immune system and from an interplay between genes and the environment.[3,8] A number of environmental exposures have been associated with IBD. Smoking has been the most consistent and most studied environmental factor associated with IBD. Interestingly, the effects of smoking are different between UC and CD, with smokers having a decreased risk of developing UC but an increased risk for CD.[9]

The theory of an infectious etiology for IBD remains controversial. Patients may be genetically predisposed to mucosal immune dysregulation, and either normal flora or bacterial pathogens may trigger the inflammatory response that leads to IBD. While no causal relationship has yet been found, further investigation on the role of gut flora is ongoing.[3,10]

Pathogenesis

Under normal conditions, the mucosal immune system interacts with luminal antigens and mucosal bacteria on a continuous basis to maintain a state of controlled inflammation. In IBD, genetic predisposition leads to immune response dysfunction, and an autoimmune cascade occurs. Thus, proinflammatory cytokines in the gut trigger an "attack" on the colonic mucosa by leukocytes and other factors, leading to edema, ulceration, and destruction of the tissue. Normal immune regulators fail to halt this process, and the disease progresses. This can be attributable to a lack of regulatory or suppressor cells, an enhanced numbers

Table 24-1
Pathophysiological Differences Between Ulcerative Colitis and Crohn's Disease[1,2,4,14,15,19]

Characteristic	Ulcerative Colitis	Crohn's Disease
Incidence (per year)	6–12/100,000	5–7/100,000
Anatomic location	Colon and rectum	Mouth to anus
Distribution	Continuous, diffuse, mucosal	Segmental, focal, transmural
Bowel wall	Shortened, loss of haustral markings, generally not thickened	Rigid, thick, edematous, and fibrotic
Gross rectal bleeding	Common	Infrequent
Crypt abscesses	Common	Infrequent
Fissuring with sinus formation	Absent	Common
Noncaseating granulomas	Absent	Common
Strictures	Absent	Common
Abdominal mass	Absent	Common
Abdominal pain	Infrequent	Common
Toxic megacolon	Occasional	Rare
Bowel carcinoma	Greatly increased	Slightly increased

of T cells, or both.[11] Studies have demonstrated that an increase of proinflammatory cytokines, chemokines, prostaglandin, and reactive oxygen species leads to increased inflammation and tissue destruction.[1]

Clinical Presentation

A careful patient history, physical examination, and endoscopic and radiologic studies are necessary to determine the severity of IBD. Laboratory studies such as an increased ESR or C-reactive protein can also aid in the diagnosis, but no single marker is pathognomonic.

Extraintestinal manifestations of IBD that can cause significant morbidity include reactive arthritis, uveitis, ankylosing spondylitis, pyoderma gangrenosum, and primary sclerosing cholangitis.[12] Although their incidence varies, many of the extraintestinal manifestations of UC and CD are similar.[12]

Patients with IBD often require surgery to control symptoms. For patients with UC, surgery is often curative. In contrast, in patients with CD, the frequency of recurrent disease after surgery is high and anatomically correlates with the original pattern of the disease.[13] Other similarities and differences in the pathophysiology of these disease states are outlined in Table 24-1.[1,4,14,15]

ULCERATIVE COLITIS

UC usually presents as a shallow, continuous inflammation of the colon ranging from limited forms of proctitis (rectal involvement only) to disease involving the entire colon. Crypt abscesses consisting of accumulations of polymorphonuclear neutrophil (PMN) cells, necrosis of the epithelium, edema, hemorrhage, and surrounding accumulations of chronic inflammatory cells are typical in UC.[15] Fistulas, fissures, abscesses, and small bowel involvement are not present. The inflammation is limited to the mucosa, which presents as friable, granular, and erythematous, with or without ulceration. Most patients with UC experience a chronic, intermittent course of disease. Chronic, loose, bloody stools are the most common symptom of UC.[4,15] Other common complaints include tenesmus (urge to defecate) and abdominal pain. Patients with pancolitis usually have more severe symptoms than those with disease limited to the rectum. Generally, in studies determining goals for UC management, clinical assessment, endoscopic or radiographic evidence, and a recognized scoring system (Trulove or Whitt) were used to determine severity, relapse, or remission induction.[3] Mild UC is defined as fewer than four stools a day, no systemic signs of toxicity, and a normal erythrocyte sedimentation rate (ESR). Moderate disease is characterized by more than four stools a day but minimal evidence of systemic toxicity. Severe disease is defined as more than six bloody stools a day, fever, tachycardia, anemia, or an ESR greater than 30.[14,15] Proctitis is usually considered a separate type of UC for treatment purposes. Constipation can occasionally be the presenting symptom with proctitis. Relapses and remissions are common in UC, with up to 70% of patients with active disease relapsing within 1 year after induction treatment.

CROHN'S DISEASE

CD is a chronic, transmural, patchy, granulomatous, inflammatory disease that can involve the entire GI tract, from mouth to anus, with discontinuous ulceration (so-called skip lesions), fistula formation, and perianal involvement. The degree of colonic involvement is variable; however, the terminal ileum is most commonly affected. Intestinal involvement is characteristically segmented and can be interrupted by areas of normal tissue.

Patients usually present with abdominal pain and chronic, often nocturnal, diarrhea.[16] Weight loss, low-grade fever, and fatigue are also common. Three patterns of disease exist predominantly: inflammatory, stricturing, or fistulizing. These patterns are the primary determinants of the disease course and the nature of complications.[14] Typically, inflammatory disease is observed early in the disease course. Stricturing or fibrostenotic disease is characterized by narrowing of the ileum because of growth of scar tissue from persistent inflammation. Fistulizing disease is particularly difficult to treat and is the source of significant morbidity in CD patients. Enterocutaneous and enterorectal fistulae are common, but other types, such as enterovaginal, can occur. Fistulae can be excruciatingly painful, can be a source of infection, and can also exert significant psychosocial distress.[1,4,14] Generally, in studies determining goals for CD management, clinical assessment, endoscopic or radiographic evidence, and a Crohn's Disease Activity Index (CDAI) score were used to determine severity, relapse, or remission induction. Defining the severity of CD is a difficult, yet important, step in successful treatment. Current guidelines from the American College of Gastroenterology define mild-to-moderate CD as ambulatory patients who are able to tolerate oral feeding without signs of systemic toxicity. Moderate-to-severe disease is defined as patients with symptoms of fever, weight loss, abdominal pain, nausea and vomiting, or significant anemia. Severe fulminant disease refers to patients with persistent symptoms despite standard induction regimens or those with signs of severe systemic toxicity.[16] The disease course of CD is variable. Years of frequent relapses may be followed by complete remission.

Treatment

Treatment of IBD depends on both the anatomic location of the disease and the patient-specific factors such as coexisting medical conditions, medication adherence, lifestyle and dietary factors, and patient health literacy. Furthermore, the goals of therapy include (a) relieving symptoms (induction and maintenance of remission or preventing relapse); (b) improving quality of life; (c) maintaining adequate nutritional status; (d) minimizing the risk of cancer; (e) attaining mucosal healing; and (f) reducing the need for surgery or chronic corticosteroid use.[16–18] Most drug therapies for IBD have been tested for both UC and CD (Table 24-2).

AMINOSALICYLATES

Aminosalicylates were the first class of drugs to show benefits in IBD. The prototypical agent is sulfasalazine, which is composed of sulfapyridine (a sulfonamide antibiotic) linked by an azo bond to 5-aminosalicylic acid, or mesalamine (5-ASA). Lower intestinal bacteria cleave the azo bond and release 5-ASA (the active moiety) for localized action in the colon. Systemic absorption of the sulfapyridine is responsible for most of the drug's adverse effects, but contributes nothing to the therapeutic benefit. A significant number of patients discontinue this medication because of dose-dependent adverse effects, including nausea, vomiting, headache, alopecia, and anorexia. Patients taking sulfasalazine may also experience an orange discoloration of their urine, tears, and sweat that may stain clothing or contact lenses. Other idiosyncratic adverse effects include rash, hemolytic anemia, hepatitis, agranulocytosis, pancreatitis, and male infertility. Additionally, patients with a sulfa or salicylate allergy should avoid sulfasalazine.

Safer sulfa-free compounds that contain only 5-ASA have been developed with techniques to decrease systemic absorption and maximize local drug delivery. Significant efficacy advantages of any 5-ASA drug versus another have not been demonstrated.[19–21] Mesalamine products have been developed for both oral and rectal administration. Administration of mesalamine by retention enemas

Table 24-2
Pharmacotherapy for Inflammatory Bowel Disease[3,12,13,17,19,21,78,79]

Drug	Indication	Quality of Evidence per ACG	Recommendation per ACG	Dose	Adverse Reactions	Comment
Sulfasalazine	UC: mild-to-moderate induction	Moderate	Strong	See Table 24-3	N/V, diarrhea, HA, rash, body fluid discoloration, anemia, hepatotoxicity, pancreatitis, nephrotoxicity, thrombocytopenia	High ADR rate has caused use to decline
	UC: mild-to-moderate maintenance	High	Strong			
	CD: Not recommended	Low	Weak			
Mesalamine	UC: mild-to-moderate induction	Moderate	Strong	See Table 24-3	N/V, diarrhea, HA, abdominal pain	Topical formulations more effective for proctitis and distal UC than oral formulations.
	UC: mild-to-moderate maintenance	High	Strong			
	CD: Not recommended	Low	Weak			
Olsalazine	UC: mild-to-moderate induction	Moderate	Strong	See Table 24-3	N/V, diarrhea, HA, abdominal pain	
	UC: mild-to-moderate maintenance	High	Strong			
	CD: Not recommended	Low	Weak			
Balsalazide	As above	As above	As above	See Table 24-3	As above	
Corticosteroids	UC: induction (all severities) CD: induction (all severities)	Low	Strong	Various	Hyperglycemia, dyslipidemia, hypertension, infection, osteoporosis, psychosis	Goal should be avoiding chronic use in UC and CD
Budesonide	CD: mild-to-moderate induction/maintenance	Low	Strong	9 mg daily, may taper to 6 mg daily for maintenance	As above for corticosteroids, with less short-term effects	Limited efficacy after 1 year; May be considered for patients who are steroid dependent
6-MP/azathioprine	UC: maintenance (all severities) CD: maintenance (all severities)	Low	Weak	6-MP: 1–1.5 mg/kg/day Azathioprine: 1.5–2.5 mg/kg/day	N/V, diarrhea, HA, rash, myelosuppression (esp. neutropenia), liver dysfunction, pancreatitis, teratogenicity	Pharmacogenomic testing for TPMT polymorphism now commonly performed prior to initiating drug Avoid use with xanthine oxidase inhibitors
Methotrexate	UC: not recommended CD: induction/maintenance (all severities)	Low	Weak	25 mg IM/SQ weekly induction dose, then 15 mg weekly for maintenance	N/V, alopecia, stomatitis, hepatotoxicity, pancreatitis, pulmonary fibrosis, pneumonitis, teratogenicity	Usually reserved for patients who have failed 6-MP/azathioprine
Cyclosporine	UC: induction (severe hospitalized) CD: not recommended	Low	Weak	4 mg/kg for 7 days followed by oral cyclosporine	Nausea, headache, hypertension, nephrotoxicity	IV route preferable in hospitalized patients

(continued)

Table 24-2
Pharmacotherapy for Inflammatory Bowel Disease[3,12,13,17,19,21,78,79] *(continued)*

Drug	Indication	Quality of Evidence per ACG	Recommendation per ACG	Dose	Adverse Reactions	Comment
Infliximab	UC: moderate-to-severe induction	Moderate	Strong	5 mg/kg IV at weeks 0, 2, and 6; then every 8 weeks thereafter	Infusion reactions (acute and delayed), respiratory infections, arthralgia, malignancy, reactivation of latent infection (TB, hepatitis B, histoplasmosis), may worsen neuromuscular disease and congestive heart failure	Scheduled treatment preferred to episodic treatment to maintain response and decrease delayed infusion reactions
	CD: moderate-to-severe induction	Moderate	Strong			
	CD: maintenance	High	Strong			
	CD: fistulizing disease	Low	Strong			
Adalimumab	UC: moderate-to-severe induction/ maintenance	None	None	160 mg SQ day 1, 80 mg SQ day 14, then 40 mg SQ every other week	Similar to infliximab	Available as a prefilled pen for self-administration Often used if infliximab is not effective or well tolerated
	CD: moderate-to-severe induction	Moderate	Strong			
	CD: maintenance	High	Strong			
	CD: fistulizing disease	Low	Strong			
Certolizumab pegol	CD: moderate-to-severe induction	Moderate	Strong	400 mg SQ at weeks 0, 2, and 4; then every 4 weeks thereafter.	Similar to infliximab	Available as a prefilled syringe for self-administration
	CD: maintenance	High	Strong			
	CD: cessation of fistula drainage	Low	Strong			
Natalizumab	CD: moderate-to-severe induction	Moderate	Weak	300 mg IV every 4 weeks	Injection site reactions, respiratory infections, arthralgia, reactivation of latent infection, hepatotoxicity, herpes encephalitis and meningitis, PML	Requires TOUCH Prescribing Program, which is a restricted distribution program because of cases of PML
	CD: maintenance	Low	Weak			
Vedolizumab	UC: moderate-to-severe induction/ maintenance CD: moderate-to-severe induction/ maintenance	None	None	300 mg IV at weeks 0, 2, and 6; then every 8 weeks thereafter.	Injection site reactions, respiratory infections, arthralgia, reactivation of latent infection, risk of PML	No cases of PML were observed in clinical trials, and does not currently require a restricted distribution program

ADR, adverse drug reaction; CD, Crohn's disease; CNS, central nervous system; HA, headache; IM, intramuscularly; IV, intravenously; N/V, nausea/vomiting; 6-MP, 6-mercaptopurine; PML, progressive multifocal leukoencephalopathy; SQ, subcutaneously; TB, tuberculosis; TPMT, thiopurine methyltransferase; UC, ulcerative colitis ACG, American College of Gastroenterology.

Table 24-3
Comparison of Aminosalicylate Compounds

Generic (Trade)	Delivery System	Intestinal Site of Release	Usual Dose and Frequency
Balsalazide (Colazal)	Bacterial cleavage of azo bond	Colon	2.25 g PO TID
Mesalamine (Apriso)	Polymer matrix/enteric coating that dissolves at pH 6	Ileum (distal), colon	1.5 g PO every morning
Mesalamine (Asacol HD)	pH-dependent coating (Eudragit S) dissolves at pH ≥7	Ileum (distal), colon	1.6 g PO TID
Mesalamine (Delzicol)	pH-dependent coating (Eudragit S) dissolves at pH ≥7	Ileum (distal), colon	800 mg PO TID 1 hour before or 2 hours after meals
Mesalamine (Lialda)	Multi-matrix (pH-sensitive coating and delayed-release)	Ileum (distal), colon	2.4–4.8 g PO every day with food
Mesalamine (Pentasa)	Controlled-release microspheres	Duodenum, jejunum, ileum, colon	1 g PO QID
Mesalamine suppository (Canasa)	Direct topical therapy	Rectum	1 g PR at bedtime after bowel movement, retain for at least 1–3 hours while sleeping
Mesalamine enema (Rowasa)	Direct topical therapy	Descending colon/rectum	4 g/60 mL enema PR at bedtime after bowel movement, retain for at least 8 hours while sleeping
Olsalazine (Dipentum)	Bacterial cleavage of azo bond	Colon	500 mg PO BID with food
Sulfasalazine (Azulfidine)	Bacterial cleavage of azo bond	Colon	Initially 500 mg PO BID; titrate dose over 1–2 weeks up to 4–6 g PO divided TID–QID with food

BID, 2 times daily; PO, orally; PR, per rectum; QID, 4 times daily; TID, 3 times daily.
Adapted with permission from Fernandez-Becker NQ, Moss AC. Improving delivery of aminosalicylates in ulcerative colitis: effect on patient outcomes. *Drugs*. 2008;68:1089; Drug Facts and Comparisons 4.0 [on-line] 2015. http://www.wolterskluwercdi.com/facts-comparisons-online/. Accessed August 26, 2015.

or suppositories is significantly more effective in the treatment of active distal colitis or ulcerative proctitis, respectively, than oral mesalamine or topical steroids.[17,19,22] Combination oral and rectal therapy for distal colitis or ulcerative proctitis are superior to either modality alone.[22] With the exception of abdominal pain, cramps, and discomfort, rectally administered mesalamine is well tolerated. Enemas or suppositories should be administered at bedtime, preferably after a bowel movement. Recent studies have confirmed that higher doses rather than a proprietary delivery system of mesalamine are associated with improved response.[23] New higher-dose formulations of 5-ASA (e.g., Lialda, Apriso) decrease the daily pill burden but may be expensive. Common adverse effects of the oral 5-ASA compounds are listed in Table 24-2. Interstitial nephritis has rarely been reported with chronic use of mesalamine, but the association remains controversial. A comparison of aminosalicylate compounds is provided in Table 24-3.

CORTICOSTEROIDS

Corticosteroids are the most commonly used agents in the treatment of acute flares in patients with moderate-to-severe IBD.[24] The anti-inflammatory actions of corticosteroids are well known, but how these translate into their full mechanism of controlling IBD is not completely understood. First-line treatment for moderate-to-severe active IBD includes doses of corticosteroid equivalent to 40 to 60 mg of prednisone.[25] Data are insufficient to demonstrate any difference between single versus divided oral doses or continuous versus intermittent bolus intravenous (IV) administration. IV doses should be equivalent to hydrocortisone 300 to 400 mg/day or methylprednisolone 48 to 60 mg/day.[25]

Topical steroids can serve as an adjunct in patients with proximal rectal disease who have failed topical 5-ASA therapy.[22] Oral enteric-coated budesonide is approved for the treatment of CD. Budesonide possesses a high degree of topical anti-inflammatory activity with low systemic bioavailability.[26] The Entocort EC formulation of budesonide delivers drug primarily to the ileum and ascending colon. Short-term corticosteroid-associated adverse effects may be less than with traditional agents, and its use up to 1 year seems to be well tolerated.[27] Compared with traditional corticosteroids, budesonide has a number of potential drug interactions owing to its metabolism via the cytochrome P450 3A4 system.[28] Studies suggest that budesonide is as effective as traditional corticosteroids for the treatment of mild-to-moderate CD localized to the right colon or ileum, and recent guidelines identify budesonide as the preferred agent in this situation.[17,29–31]

IMMUNOMODULATORS

Azathioprine (AZA) and 6-mercaptopurine (6-MP) may be used for the management of corticosteroid-dependent and quiescent IBD. AZA is converted to 6-MP, which is then metabolized to thioinosinic acid by thiopurine methyltransferase (TPMT), the active agent that inhibits purine ribonucleotide synthesis and cell proliferation. It also alters the immune response by inhibiting natural killer cell activity and suppressing cytotoxic T-cell function. AZA (1.5–2.5 mg/kg/day) and 6-MP (1–1.5 mg/kg/day) are used in the treatment of UC and CD in patients whose conditions have not responded to systemic steroids, or as "steroid-sparing" agents.[16,17,32] Because of the long onset of action of 6-MP and AZA, these agents should be reserved for maintaining remission. Adverse effects of 6-MP and AZA include rash, nausea, pancreatitis, alopecia, and diarrhea. Myelosuppression, especially neutropenia, may have a delayed onset, and clinicians should monitor the complete blood count monthly for the first 3 months of treatment, then every 3 months thereafter. Pharmacogenomic testing for TPMT before initiation is recommended.[16,19] Low levels of TPMT result in reduced AZA and 6-MP clearance, thereby increasing the risk of severe myelosuppression and hepatotoxicity.

Methotrexate (MTX), a folate antagonist, impairs DNA synthesis. Data suggest that MTX (15–25 mg intramuscular [IM] weekly) may have a role for both initial and chronic treatment of CD. The onset and degree of effect is comparable to that with 6-MP and AZA.[33] Most experts and recent guidelines suggest reserving MTX use for patients with CD intolerant of, or refractory to, 6-MP or AZA treatment.[17,34] Adverse effects with MTX include stomatitis, neutropenia, nausea, hypersensitivity pneumonitis, alopecia, and hepatotoxicity.

Cyclosporine (CSA), which selectively inhibits T-cell–mediated responses, has been used to treat severe, acute UC.[35] Because of serious adverse effects, CSA is usually reserved for patients with severe UC refractory to corticosteroids. A randomized controlled trial found equal efficacy (about 85% response) with a 2-mg/kg daily IV dose compared with the standard 4-mg/kg dose.[36] The emergence of the tumor necrosis factor drugs for IBD has caused CSA use to significantly decline.

ANTITUMOR NECROSIS FACTOR AGENTS

Infliximab

Infliximab is a recombinant chimeric monoclonal antibody that binds to human tumor necrosis factor (TNF) α, neutralizing its biological activity. Infliximab is indicated for inducing and maintaining remission in patients with moderate-to-severe active UC and CD refractory to other treatments.[37,38] Infliximab is effective for healing CD fistulae, with data showing that chronic treatment can maintain fistula closure and decrease the need for surgery.[39] The response to infliximab is usually rapid, often occurring within several days. Since infliximab is a monoclonal antibody, a number of immunologic-mediated adverse effects are associated with therapy. Antibodies to infliximab have been detected in up to 60% of CD patients using the drug, and emerging data suggest that patients who develop these antibodies may be at more risk, not only for infusion-related reactions but also for reduced efficacy over time.[40,41] Immediate infusion-related reactions such as fever, chills, pruritus, urticaria, and (rarely) severe cardiopulmonary symptoms can occur. Infectious complications, including pneumonia, cellulitis, sepsis, and cholecystitis have also been reported. All TNF α blockers carry black-box warnings for their risk of serious infections and malignancy, particularly lymphoma.[42]

Other Biological Therapies

Success with infliximab in IBD has led scientists to develop and test other biological therapies designed to either block pro-inflammatory mediators or enhance anti-inflammatory mediators in the gut. To date, four other biologic agents are approved in the United States: the fully humanized anti-TNF-α antibody adalimumab, pegylated humanized Fab′ fragments against TNF-α (certolizumab pegol), and the humanized α_4-integrin antibodies natalizumab and vedolizumab. Adalimumab is approved for the treatment of moderate-to-severe UC and CD and may be particularly useful in patients with an attenuated response to infliximab.[43] Certolizumab and natalizumab are approved for patients with moderate-to-severe CD, whereas vedolizumab was most recently approved for both moderate-to-severe UC and CD. These agents will be further discussed in Case 24-2.

The precise place in therapy of the newer biologic agents is controversial. Most experts consider infliximab the biologic agent of first choice with the other agents reserved for a loss or lack of efficacy or adverse effects.[44]

ANTIBIOTICS

Because an infectious etiology has been proposed for IBD, it stands to reason that antibiotics may have some utility.[4] However, most studies evaluating antibiotics have shown little benefit with the exception of ciprofloxacin or metronidazole in fistulizing disease and metronidazole in perianal or perhaps postoperative CD disease.[3,45,46] Common adverse effects with chronic, high-dose metronidazole include metallic taste and peripheral neuropathy.

NUTRITIONAL THERAPIES

Nutritional therapies for IBD have been used because dietary intraluminal antigens may stimulate a mucosal immune response.[4] Patients with active CD respond to bowel rest, total parenteral nutrition (TPN), or total enteral nutrition. Enteral nutrition, with elemental or peptide-based preparation, appears to be as efficacious as TPN, without its associated complications. Unfortunately, poor compliance often limits this modality. Such therapy is used more commonly in the pediatric population with mild-to-moderate CD.[47,48]

SUPPORTIVE THERAPY

Symptomatic management of IBD is important to the patient's quality of life. This includes pain relief and diarrhea control. Loperamide or diphenoxylate with atropine may be used to treat mild symptoms provided obstruction or toxicity is not evident.[49] Severe worsening of symptoms and abdominal distension may indicate toxic megacolon caused by the inability to empty rapidly produced secretory products of the bowel. Patients should be monitored for iron and vitamin B_{12} deficiencies, especially if ileal involvement is extensive or resection has been performed.

SURGERY

Surgery is indicated in the treatment of IBD when the patient fails to respond to medical management; demonstrates intestinal complications such as perforation, obstruction, hemorrhage, toxic megacolon, or fistula formation; fails to grow and develop at a normal rate; or exhibits carcinoma of the rectum or colon.[16,17,50] Furthermore, patients with UC for longer than 10 years or who demonstrate premalignant changes on rectal biopsy may be managed surgically as a prophylactic measure. In patients with CD, surgical intervention is common.

ULCERATIVE COLITIS

Pathophysiology and Clinical Presentation

CASE 24-1

QUESTION 1: A.C., a 24-year-old female college student, has had episodic, watery diarrhea, and colicky abdominal pain relieved by defecation for the past 9 months. Eight weeks before admission, the diarrhea increased to 3 to 5 semi-formed stools daily. The frequency of the stools gradually increased to 7 to 10 times a day 1 week ago. At that time, A.C. noted bright red blood in the stools. Stool frequency has now increased to 12 to 15 per day, although the volume of each stool is estimated to be only "one-half cupful." She feels a great urgency to defecate, even though the volume is small. She has not traveled outside the United States, has not been camping, and has not taken any antibiotics within the past 6 months. She is allergic to sulfa, and takes only occasional over-the-counter acetaminophen for body aches or headaches.

A.C. complains of anorexia and a 10-lb weight loss during the previous 2 months. For the past 4 months, she has had intermittent swelling, warmth, and tenderness of the left knee, which is unassociated with trauma. She denies any skin rashes or any difficulties with her vision. A review of other body systems and social and family history are largely noncontributory.

A.C. appears to be a slightly anxious and tired young woman of normal body habitus. She is 165 cm tall and weighs 51 kg. Her temperature is 100°F; her pulse rate is 105 beats/minute and regular. Physical examination is normal, except for evidence of acute arthritis of the left knee and tenderness of the left lower abdomen to palpation.

Stool examination shows a watery effluent that contains numerous red and white cells with no trophozoites. Stool cultures and an amebiasis indirect hemagglutination test are negative. Other laboratory values include the following results:

Hematocrit (Hct), 30%
Hemoglobin (Hgb), 8.1 g/dL
White blood cell (WBC) count, 17,500/μL with 82% PMNs
ESR, 72 mm/hour
Serum albumin, 2.8 g/dL
Alanine aminotransferase (ALT), 33 units/mL

Sigmoidoscopy showed evidence of granular, edematous, and friable mucosa with continuous ulcerations extending from the anus throughout the colon. What is the most likely cause of A.C.'s diarrheal illness, and what is the evidence for this?

A.C.'s presentation is typical of a patient with new-onset UC. Drug-induced (pseudomembranous colitis) and infectious (parasitic) causes of diarrhea have been ruled out by history (no travel outside the United States, no recent camping, no antibiotic use) and stool examination. As discussed previously, UC is an inflammation of the mucosal layer of the colon and rectum.[1] Characteristically, the inflammation does not extend beyond the submucosa, and transmural ulcers are rare. On examination, the mucosa appears erythematous and is friable. Differentiation from CD is made by endoscopic and radiologic evidence of continuous distribution of pathologic disease (as opposed to segmental), as well as the anatomic location (confined to colon and rectum).

A.C. presents with the classic triad of UC clinical symptoms: chronic diarrhea, rectal bleeding, and abdominal pain. Diarrhea is secondary to decreased colonic absorption of water and electrolytes and diminished colonic segmental contractions that normally serve to decrease the flow of bowel content. A good indication of the severity of a patient's disease is the volume of stool passed per day.[16] Because the severity of the disease increases, incontinence and nocturnal diarrhea commonly occur. Stools are usually soft, mushy, formed, and often contain small amounts of mucus mixed with blood. In addition to diarrhea, the malabsorption of water and electrolytes causes dehydration, weight loss (as observed in A.C.), and electrolyte disturbances.

A.C.'s rectal bleeding is secondary to colonic mucosal erosions and occurs in most patients with UC. Generally, bright red blood mixed in the stools indicates a colonic origin, whereas blood-streaked stools indicate an anal or rectal origin. The anemia associated with UC is generally secondary to this rectal bleeding. It presents as a hemorrhagic or iron-deficiency anemia, depending on the acuteness of the bleeding. Hemoglobin and hematocrit laboratory values often are decreased as in A.C.'s case. Chronic inflammatory disease–induced hypoalbuminemia is often exacerbated by malnutrition.

A.C.'s abdominal pain and cramping are caused by spasm of the irritated and inflamed colon. This abdominal pain is commonly associated with urgency to defecate. As illustrated by A.C., the pain is usually relieved with defecation, even though the stool volume may be small.

A.C.'s arthritis and elevated ALT are indicative of the extraintestinal manifestations that occur in IBD.[51] Her nonspecific symptoms (i.e., anorexia, fatigue, weight loss, anxiety, tachycardia) could become profound during an exacerbation of UC. Fever, leukocytosis, and increased ESR are also systemic manifestations of an inflammatory disease. Rehydration is important to assure fluid balance and maintain good renal function. Given her anemia, tachycardia, elevated ESR, and frequency of bloody stools, A.C.'s disease would be classified as severe.

CASE 24-1, QUESTION 2: How should A.C.'s diarrhea be managed?

Treatment of the diarrhea associated with UC is often difficult. In patients with mild-to-moderate disease, antidiarrheals, such as loperamide or diphenoxylate with atropine, may help minimize chronic diarrhea. Extreme caution must be used, however, especially in patients with severe disease because of the chance of inducing toxic megacolon, a life-threatening condition and medical emergency. For this reason, antidiarrheals are best avoided in patients with severe active disease, such as with A.C. Bulk-forming agents (i.e., psyllium) may be helpful for patients suffering from constipation caused by ulcerative proctitis.[52]

Remission Induction

CORTICOSTEROIDS

CASE 24-1, QUESTION 3: What agents can be used to induce disease remission in A.C.?

Corticosteroids are the most effective agents to induce remission of acute, severe exacerbations of UC. Clinical improvement or remission occurs in 45% to 90% of patients taking up to 60 mg/day of prednisone, with a recommended dose of 40 to 60 mg/day.[53] However, corticosteroids are not beneficial for maintaining remission. One strategy to minimize adverse effects of corticosteroid therapy is to taper them by 5 to 10 mg/week over 1 to 2 months after demonstrated improvement. Unfortunately, a subset of patients will experience a disease flare if the corticosteroid dosage is decreased or tapered too quickly. IV corticosteroids are an important option, especially in patients who have poor oral intake. Patients with active distal disease can be treated with hydrocortisone enemas; however, topical 5-ASA therapy is more efficacious. Biologic agents and cyclosporine may be considered for induction of remission in patients with fulminant disease or have failed other agents.[53] Given that A.C. is of childbearing age, a pregnancy test should be obtained and results taken into consideration when choosing current and future drug therapy, particularly if pregnant or breastfeeding[54] (see Chapter 49, Obstetric Drug therapy).

CASE 24-1, QUESTION 4: Methylprednisolone at a dosage of 40 mg IV every 6 hours is ordered. What are the treatment goals for A.C.?

The goal of parenteral corticosteroid therapy for A.C. is to achieve a rapid therapeutic response as measured by decreased frequency of stools, decreased pain, and decreased fever and heart rate. This goal may be attained with a high initial dose, followed by a gradual dosage reduction to minimize the development of corticosteroid adverse reactions.

Poorly nourished patients in whom oral intake is expected to be absent for more than 7 days should receive parenteral nutrition, and treatment should be continued until oral feeding is tolerated.[55] An adequate response is defined as resolution of fever and tachycardia, improved patient well-being, and less abdominal tenderness on palpation. Diarrhea is usually considered to be resolved with four or less bowel movements daily. Stools are rarely formed at this stage, but macroscopic bleeding has stopped. Patients can then receive oral prednisone, a 5-ASA drug, and a light diet. If the patient does not respond within 72 hours of starting high-dose corticosteroids, infliximab or surgery may be indicated. Once A.C.'s symptoms are controlled, the goal should be to switch to oral corticosteroids and discharge her from the hospital.

Oral Administration

CASE 24-1, QUESTION 5: A.C. is responding well to methylprednisolone. She is afebrile, her abdominal pain is reduced (to a score of 4 on a 1–10 scale), and her diarrhea is decreasing. When is the oral route of corticosteroid administration indicated in UC? What are the most appropriate dosages?

Oral corticosteroids are effective for the initial treatment of mild-to-moderate acute UC.[25] In addition, they should be substituted for parenteral corticosteroids once a satisfactory initial response of more severe exacerbations has been achieved. Prednisone of 40 mg/day was significantly more efficacious than 20 mg/day in controlling ambulatory patients with moderately severe acute UC, but prednisone doses of 60 mg/day had no additional therapeutic value, while causing more adverse effects.[17] In addition, a single 40-mg morning dose of prednisone was as effective as and more convenient than an equivalent divided dose (10 mg 4 times a day [QID]). Therefore, the initial dose of corticosteroid for a patient with moderately severe acute UC is 40 mg of prednisone or its equivalent administered once daily in the morning.

Although corticosteroids are effective for inducing remission in many cases of IBD, up to 50% of patients may not respond (steroid resistant) or will be steroid-dependent at 1 year.[24] Additionally, rates of mucosal healing with these drugs are less than those with other modalities.[56] This combined with the significant adverse effects of corticosteroids (e.g., hyperglycemia, osteoporosis) argue against their long-term use in IBD, as reflected in current practice guidelines.[16,17]

Topical Administration

CASE 24-1, QUESTION 6: What if A.C.'s UC was limited to the distal colon or rectum? Would topical corticosteroids be indicated? When should other topical agents be considered for A.C.?

Topically administered 5-ASA and corticosteroids, in the form of suppositories, foams, and retention enemas, are effective in the management of acute, mild-to-moderate UC that is limited to the distal colon and rectum.[22]

The desired outcome for medications administered via this topical route is to provide a higher concentration of drug to the diseased mucosal area, exerting a local anti-inflammatory effect, while minimizing systemic side effects. Unfortunately, variable but significant systemic absorption (up to 90%) and adrenal suppression occur from the topical administration of corticosteroid to the rectum and distal colon.[57] Therefore, the beneficial effects produced by topical use of these agents may accrue from both systemic and local effects. The relatively low incidence of corticosteroid side effects associated with topical administration may be related to both the low doses and the infrequent administration (daily to twice daily) needed to control mild acute UC.

5-ASA suppositories and enemas are preferred over topical corticosteroids for the treatment of distal UC and proctitis because they produce higher remission rates in proctitis and effectively maintain remission of distal UC.[57] For distal UC, therapy is initiated with a nightly enema (4 g of mesalamine), and the response should be evaluated in 3 to 4 weeks. For mild acute proctitis, administering one suppository of 5-ASA twice daily for 3 to 6 weeks is generally sufficient to induce disease remission. Improvement should be seen in 2 to 3 weeks, and therapy should be maintained until complete remission is achieved. If remission is attained, therapy can then be tapered to one suppository or enema, 2 to 3 times weekly. Therapy with oral plus topical mesalamine showed greater efficacy than either alone in achieving remission of distal UC or proctitis.[22]

Adverse Effects

CASE 24-1, QUESTION 7: What particular corticosteroid adverse effects should the clinician monitor in A.C.?

Corticosteroid side effects and precautions for use often limit the therapeutic effectiveness of these agents and should never be overlooked.[24] Certain glucocorticoid adverse effects are of particular importance in patients with IBD in that they may mimic, mask, or intensify symptoms and complications of this disease. For example, the symptoms of peritonitis, one of the major complications of intestinal perforation, may be masked by corticosteroids. Other deleterious effects of corticosteroids include hyperglycemia, avascular necrosis, cataract formation, and central nervous system effects, including mood disorders, insomnia, psychoses, and euphoria.

Patients with IBD are at risk for decreased bone mineral density, which is exacerbated by prolonged use of corticosteroids.[58,59] This is an often-overlooked side effect of these drugs. One study suggested that even budesonide, with its low overall bioavailability, causes this adverse effect.[60] Thus, calcium, vitamin D supplements, and possibly bisphosphonates are recommended to minimize metabolic demineralization in all IBD patients taking corticosteroids for longer than 3 months. Given the patient's family history (mother with osteoporosis) and her high risk of bone loss, alendronate 35 mg weekly with 1,500 mg daily of calcium and 800 international units of vitamin D intake should be initiated.

SULFASALAZINE AND 5-AMINOSALICYLIC ACID

CASE 24-1, QUESTION 8: A.C. is still responding well to oral prednisone; however, her blood glucose concentrations have ranged from 226 to 445 mg/dL (normal, 70–110 mg/dL). Her physician would like to try another modality for active treatment. What other drugs could be used for remission induction?

Previously, sulfasalazine was considered the drug of choice in UC exacerbation because of its demonstrated efficacy and reduced toxicity when compared with corticosteroids. However, controlled trials have shown that corticosteroids may act more promptly than sulfasalazine alone for severe acute UC.[4] Sulfasalazine use has declined significantly since the availability of better-tolerated 5-ASA formulations.[21] Additionally, as in the case of A.C., patients with a sulfa allergy should avoid sulfasalazine. Clinical improvement or remission of mild-to-moderate UC can be attained in 40% to 74% of patients treated with oral 5-ASA in doses ranging from 1.5 to 4.8 g/day with further improved response at dosages greater than 2 g/day.[61,62] In summary, oral 5-ASA compounds are considered first-line therapy for mild-to-moderate exacerbations of UC, with systemic corticosteroids reserved for more severe active UC or refractory disease. Because A.C. has improved symptomatically and is suffering significant adverse effects from corticosteroid treatment, switching to oral mesalamine is a reasonable option at this time.

Remission Maintenance

MESALAMINE

Case 24-1, Question 9: A.C. feels much better and claims to be "back to normal." Her abdominal pain is gone, and she currently has two formed, non-bloody stools daily. Most of her laboratory parameters have returned to normal (ESR, 19 mm/hour; blood glucose, 95 mg/dL; WBC, 8,300/μL). She is currently taking mesalamine 800 mg PO TID. What drug regimen should be used to maintain disease remission in A.C.?

5-ASA agents significantly reduce the incidence of relapse in UC patients who are in remission.[17,19] At 12 months, 65% to 70% of patients remain relatively symptom-free compared with placebo.[63] As discussed previously, the anatomic site of disease is an important consideration in the selection of a 5-ASA preparation.[20,21] Data also suggest that, if tolerated, higher doses have higher rates of treatment success. In contrast, oral and topical corticosteroids do not prevent relapse of UC once remission has occurred.

On the basis of this information, A.C.'s mesalamine should be titrated to a total dose of 4.8 g in divided doses. If she experiences a relapse, a course of oral corticosteroids may be needed to re-achieve remission. Prophylactic therapy should be continued indefinitely unless intolerable adverse effects develop. This is especially true in light of data that suggest that long-term mesalamine may be chemoprotective against colon cancer.[63]

Adverse Effects

Case 24-1, Question 10: A.C.'s mesalamine has been increased to 1,200 mg TID for UC maintenance therapy. Several days after starting this higher dose of mesalamine, A.C. experienced anorexia, nausea, and epigastric pain. What is the possible cause of A.C.'s symptoms? How can they be minimized?

A.C. appears to be experiencing adverse effects of mesalamine. Although usually better tolerated than sulfasalazine, unwanted adverse effects occur in 10% to 45% of patients. Most 5-ASA adverse reactions are dose related and tend to occur early in the course of therapy.

Dose-related 5-ASA adverse effects can be minimized by initiating the patient on a low dosage (1–2 g/day) and gradually increasing the amount to tolerated therapeutic doses.[62] If dose-related reactions do occur, the drug should be discontinued until the symptoms subside, then it may be reinstituted at a lower dosage. A.C.'s symptoms are probably dose-related adverse reactions to mesalamine. The dosage should be decreased, or the drug temporarily withheld. If tolerated, the dosage can be increased slowly as necessary, or she can be switched to another agent to maintain disease remission, such as an immunomodulator. An algorithm depicting treatment for UC is shown in Figure 24-1.

IMMUNOSUPPRESSIVE AND BIOLOGICAL AGENTS

Case 24-1, Question 11: A.C.'s dose of mesalamine was decreased to 800 mg TID. After 2 weeks, A.C. continued to have nausea, diarrhea, and headache severe enough to cause her to miss classes and call in sick from her part-time job. Objectively, she has lost 5 kg (now 46 kg) in the last week as a result of anorexia and nausea. What alternative therapies should be considered at this point?

The results of several trials suggest AZA and 6-MP are appropriate alternatives for patients with active UC that have not responded to systemic steroids, although their actual level of effectiveness is debated.[64,65] These drugs are also used to maintain remission, although they are probably used more in CD than UC for this purpose (see Case 24-2, Question 3).

Infliximab, adalimumab, and vedolizumab are approved in the United States for moderate-to-severe UC (both for induction

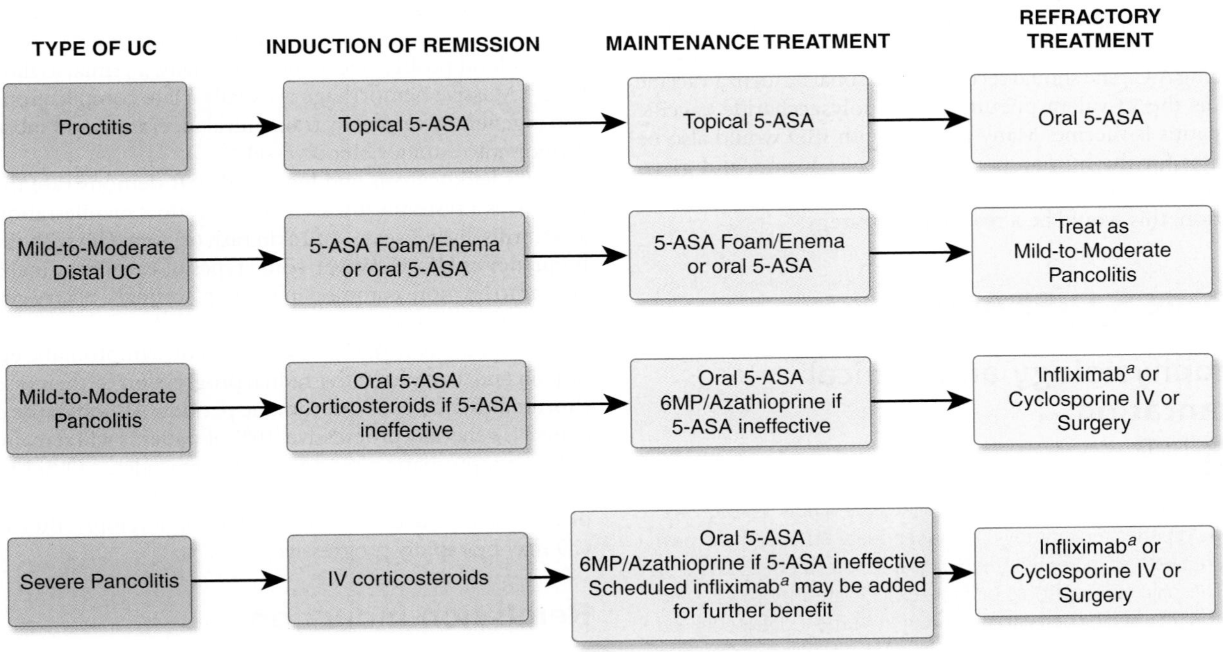

Figure 24-1 Treatment algorithm for ulcerative colitis. Pancolitis refers to extensive ulcerative colitis. 5-ASA, mesalamine products, including mesalamine (e.g., Asacol, Pentasa, Rowasa), olsalazine, and balsalazide (see text for selection guidelines); IV, intravenous; 6-MP, 6-mercaptopurine; UC, ulcerative colitis. [a]For UC adalimumab is an alternative option to infliximab. (Source: Bernstein CN et al. World Gastroenterology Organization Practice Guidelines for the diagnosis and management of IBD in 2010. *Inflamm Bowel Dis*. 2010;16:112; Carter MJ et al. Guidelines for the management of inflammatory bowel disease in adults. *Gut*. 2004;53(Suppl 5):V1; Kornbluth A et al. Ulcerative colitis practice guidelines in adults: American College of Gastroenterology, Practice Parameters Committee. *Am J Gastroenterol*. 2010;105:501.)

therapy and for maintenance of remission). Because of significant costs and adverse effects, they should be reserved for patients with refractory disease.

Cyclosporine (CSA) has also been used to treat active UC. In one retrospective review, IV CSA had a roughly 50% response rate even 2 years after acute therapy.[65] Many drug interactions and adverse effects are associated with CSA. Hypertension, gingival hyperplasia, hypertrichosis, paresthesias, tremors, headaches, electrolyte disturbances, and nephrotoxicity are common. In A.C., a reasonable choice would be AZA 115 mg (approximately 2.5 mg/kg/day). Monthly monitoring of WBC counts and liver function testing as well as periodic assessment for any signs and symptoms of pancreatitis would be appropriate.[66]

Vaccinations in the IBD Patient

Case 24-1, Question 12: One year has passed since A.C. last had an acute attack of UC. She has been taking AZA 2.5 mg/kg/day. Today she presented to her primary health care provider for her annual physical examination. She asked about receiving the yearly influenza vaccination as well as the pneumococcal vaccination she has been reading about online. Her primary care provider is unsure whether A.C. is a candidate for either vaccination. Should A.C. receive both vaccinations? What vaccinations, if any, is A.C. a candidate for?

Immunomodulators and biologic drugs are the mainstay of IBD treatment. However, one of the most important adverse effects are infectious complications. As mentioned above, serious and sometimes fatal infections have been reported with drugs such as AZA and infliximab.[42] Some of these infections are preventable with immunizations.[67] Unfortunately, data exist that immunization strategies are significantly underutilized in the IBD population.[68] Guidelines recommend that standard immunization schedules (see Chapter 64, Vaccinations) be adhered to; that serologic testing for varicella be performed on IBD patients without a clear history of chickenpox, and if negative, such patients should be vaccinated against this virus; and that live virus vaccinations should be avoided in patients, such as A.C., who are receiving AZA.[68] Specifically, concerning A.C., she should receive the seasonal influenza vaccine as well as the 23-valent pneumococcal polysaccharide vaccine and hepatitis B vaccine. Many patients with IBD would also be candidates for the human papilloma virus vaccine, and given the increased incidence of abnormal Papanicolaou tests in this population, this would be a reasonable strategy.[69]

CROHN'S DISEASE

Pathophysiology and Clinical Presentation

CASE 24-2

Question 1: C.J., a 30-year-old man, was well until 18 days ago when he experienced crampy right lower quadrant abdominal pain associated with an increased frequency of semiformed stools (4–5/day). The pain was episodic at first, exacerbated by meals, and somewhat relieved by defecation. During this time, C.J. experienced anorexia and a 10-pound weight loss. He denied any change in vision, joint pain, or the appearance of skin rashes. He has not traveled outside the United States or taken antibiotics recently.

Physical examination is essentially normal, except for soft, loose, watery stools that are streaked with fat and positive for occult blood. The abdomen is tender on palpation of the right lower quadrant. Vital signs include a temperature of 37.8°C, pulse of 100 beats/minute, and blood pressure of 135/75 mm Hg. He is 180 cm and weighs 80 kg. Pertinent laboratory values include the following:

Hct, 28%
Hgb, 9 g/dL
WBC count, 14.0 × 10^9/L
ESR, 60 mm/hour

Results of sigmoidoscopy and rectal biopsy are negative. Stool cultures and toxin studies for *C. difficile* are negative, as is the examination for signs of trophozoites. A barium enema shows an edematous ileocecal valve and a terminal ileum that has a nodular irregularity of the mucosa. Follow-up colonoscopy reveals a cobblestone-appearing terminal ileum with areas of normal tissue separated by diseased mucosa. Which of C.J.'s signs, symptoms, and laboratory data are consistent with CD? Describe the pathophysiological basis for C.J.'s clinical presentation.

C.J., like most patients with CD, presents with the classic symptom triad of abdominal pain, diarrhea, and weight loss.[11] His most frequent symptom is right lower quadrant abdominal pain, which is secondary to an indolent inflammatory process in the ileocecal area. Diarrhea is also a characteristic symptom; however, in contrast to UC, the stools are usually partly formed, and gross blood is generally not visible. If the disease is limited to the colon, the diarrhea may be of the same quality and quantity as that associated with UC. If the disease is limited to the ileum, as it appears to be with C.J., the diarrhea is generally moderate, with four to six stools daily. If ileal involvement is significant, bile salt malabsorption may occur, resulting in steatorrhea. Weight loss may be pronounced in patients with long-standing CD because of anorexia and malabsorption. Additionally, vitamin deficiencies, including vitamin B_{12} and vitamin D, are more common in CD patients than control subjects.[70]

Rectal bleeding often occurs in patients with CD, particularly those with colonic involvement, although it is not as common as that associated with UC. Slow blood loss may occur in patients with disease limited to the small intestine, which may cause occult blood-positive feces and, eventually, anemia, as illustrated by C.J. Massive hemorrhage is usually a late complication of CD and is generally caused by transmural ulceration and subsequent erosion into a major blood vessel.

C.J.'s leukocytosis and increased ESR demonstrate that, like UC, CD is a systemic disease. Extraintestinal manifestations such as arthritis, liver disease, and skin rash occur in CD with the same frequency as UC. However, some types of extraintestinal disease appear to be more common in UC (e.g., primary biliary cirrhosis) than CD (e.g., pyoderma gangrenosum).[71]

Most patients with CD have recurrent, symptomatic episodes of pain and diarrhea with gradual progression of their disease to shorter and shorter asymptomatic periods. Although the clinical course is generally progressive, 10% of patients will remain essentially asymptomatic after a few acute episodes.[72] Other patients may only manifest a slight fever for years until a late complication of the disease, such as fistula formation, develops. Alternatively, CD may be rapidly progressive.

Remission Induction

Case 24-2, Question 2: What agents can be used to induce a remission of C.J.'s CD?

Because the clinical course of CD varies among patients, the management of this disease must be individualized. The anatomic location of the disease is also an important determinant of therapy. Most investigations evaluating the treatment of acute symptomatic CD have ignored this factor and are therefore difficult to assess or compare.

CORTICOSTEROIDS

Corticosteroids are the most widely used therapeutic agents for the treatment of active, symptomatic CD.[16,24] A systematic review of the literature confirms that steroids have a valuable role in remission induction.[56] Landmark studies have demonstrated that approximately 60% to 80% of patients with active CD will respond to a course of corticosteroids.[24] These agents seem to be particularly effective in ileal and ileocolonic disease and can induce remission in even moderate-to-severe CD. Budesonide is also recommended in current CD guidelines for active mild-to-moderate ileocolonic CD.[16]

5-AMINOSALICYLIC ACID

Although previously used extensively for mild-to-moderate CD, current trial data and expert opinion have limited the role of 5-ASA drugs to mild active colonic CD. A large meta-analysis comparing 5-ASA (Pentasa) versus placebo found a small and probably clinically insignificant treatment benefit.[73]

OTHER INDUCTION AGENTS

The immunomodulators AZA, 6-MP, and MTX have an onset of action of weeks to months and are not usually appropriate monotherapy for treatment of a CD flare. Infliximab is effective for both active and quiescent disease.[74] It can be used alone owing to its rapid onset. A recent landmark study found that early aggressive use of infliximab, with or without AZA, was associated with both corticosteroid-free clinical remission and mucosal healing in patients with moderate-to-severe CD.[31,74] Newer agents have been approved. Clinical studies have suggested a roughly equivalent symptom response between adalimumab and infliximab, and because the former drug is also a potent TNF-α blocker, similar safety concerns and adverse effects have been shown between the two agents.[40] Efficacy has also been demonstrated in the treatment of fistulating Crohn's disease.[75] One potential advantage of adalimumab is its ability to be self-administered subcutaneously by patients. Certolizumab contains only the antibody receptor for TNF-α bound to polyethylene glycol to increase its duration in the body. Currently, it is only approved for both inducing and maintaining remission in CD.[76] A prefilled syringe is now available for self-administration. Infection and other adverse effects have been reported in clinical trials that are similar to other TNF-α blockers. Two randomized controlled trials have found that natalizumab may be beneficial for induction and maintenance of remission of moderate-to-severe CD in a small subset of patients, but at the increased risk of developing progressive multifocal leukoencephalopathy (PML), a potentially fatal adverse effect.[77] Thus, natalizumab should be reserved as a last-line agent. Furthermore, patients are required to be enrolled in a mandatory patient registry program (TOUCH) to receive the drug and should avoid concomitant immunosuppressive therapies.[78] In 2014, vedolizumab was approved for inducing and maintaining remission of moderate-to-severe UC and CD in patients who have failed TNF-α therapy. There were no cases of PML observed in clinical trials and the medication does not currently require a restricted distribution program.[79]

Certainly, the added expense and risk of using biologics earlier in this population needs to be weighed against the possibility of longer periods of remission and avoidance of surgery. An additional concern is reports of hepatosplenic T-cell lymphoma in young men receiving either AZA or 6-MP with or without concomitant infliximab, which is usually fatal.[80] An algorithm for the treatment of CD is depicted in Figure 24-2.

Remission Maintenance

CASE 24-2, QUESTION 3: After 4 weeks of prednisone 40 mg daily, C.J. experienced fewer symptoms of CD; he has one to two well-formed stools a day, increased appetite and weight, decreased abdominal pain and tenderness, and normal body temperatures. Should prednisone be discontinued? What agents are effective in maintaining remission of symptoms in patients with CD?

CORTICOSTEROIDS

Once prednisone has induced remission of active symptomatic CD, attempts should be made to taper the drug.[16] The tapering schedule is usually fairly slow (typically, a dose reduction of 5%–10%/week), taking several weeks to months to complete. Several studies have demonstrated that corticosteroids are ineffective in maintaining remission in CD, and many patients continue to have active disease while receiving therapy. However, a significant subset of patients (25%) with CD requires chronic administration of corticosteroids to prevent recurrence of symptoms (termed steroid-dependent CD).[81] Given the poor long-term adverse effect profile of steroids, many clinicians attempt treatment with other modalities to maintain remission.

6-MERCAPTOPURINE OR AZATHIOPRINE

Both 6-MP and AZA have a major role in maintenance treatment of CD, particularly as a steroid-sparing strategy. Recent guidelines recommend the use of 6-MP and AZA in most relapsing cases of CD, regardless of anatomic site, and for both severe and steroid-dependent disease. Provided patients are appropriately monitored, these agents are safe with a favorable risk–benefit ratio. Both 6-MP and AZA are the first-line immunomodulators used in CD. Should these agents be ineffective or not tolerated, either MTX or infliximab can be used to maintain remission.[15] The top-down strategy of starting TNF blockers earlier in the course of disease is currently under debate.[81–83] Recent findings have prompted experts to increasingly advocate initial therapy with biologic drugs in high-risk patients with moderate-to-severe CD ("top-down" therapy) rather than initiating after other agents have failed.[3,31,74] Some experts believe that infliximab should be used earlier in the course of relapsing disease, especially in patients with fistulae.[82]

In summary, C.J.'s prednisone should be tapered as suggested previously and then discontinued if possible. As the tapering regimen is begun, C.J. should start 6-MP 120 mg (approximately 1.5 mg/kg/day) or AZA 200 mg (approximately 2.5 mg/kg/day). This is because of the long onset of effect for the latter drugs (usually 3–6 months). C.J.'s WBC counts should be monitored regularly, and he should be counseled regarding the signs and symptoms of severe infection (e.g., fever, sore throat, or chills) and pancreatitis (e.g., severe epigastric pain and nausea).

Adverse Effects

CASE 24-2, QUESTION 4: Six weeks after starting to taper C.J.'s prednisone dosage (currently, 10 mg/day) and the initiation of AZA, he returns to the clinic for routine laboratory monitoring. His WBC count is 1,800/μL with an absolute neutrophil count of 1,100/μL. He is afebrile and without complaint. His physical examination is negative for any sign of infection. Why is C.J. experiencing leukopenia? What is the treatment for this side effect?

6-MERCAPTOPURINE AND AZATHIOPRINE MONITORING

AZA is a prodrug that is converted to the active moiety, 6-MP, in the liver. 6-MP is then metabolized by xanthine oxidase, hypoxanthine-guanine phosphoribosyltransferase, or

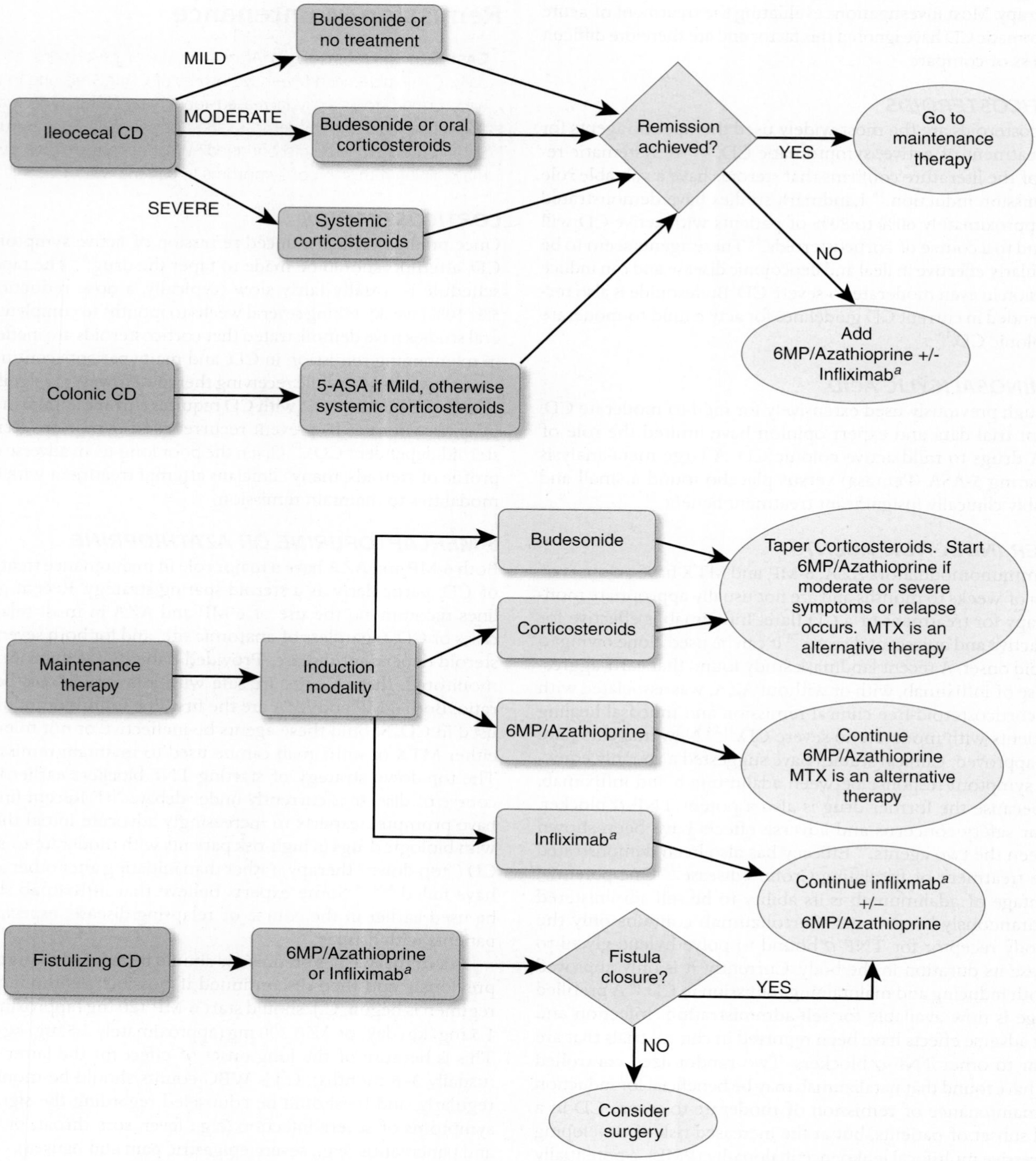

Figure 24-2 Treatment algorithm for Crohn's disease. KEY: CD, Crohn's disease; 5-ASA, aminosalicylate; 6MP, 6-mercaptopurine; MTX, methotrexate; [a]For nonfistulizing Crohn's disease adalimumab or certolizumab are alternative options to infliximab

thiopurine-*S*-methyltransferase (TPMT). Genetic polymorphism determines the extent of TPMT activity. In approximately 90% of whites, TPMT activity is considered high, but the remainder of the population has either intermediate or low TPMT activity.[83,84] These patients are predisposed to 6-MP or AZA myelosuppression because diminished TPMT activity leads to the metabolism of these compounds being shunted to the other enzymatic pathways. Accumulation of the 6-thioguanine byproducts is correlated with leukopenia. Pharmacogenomic testing to assess TPMT activity has been developed and found to be effective in guiding therapy with AZA or 6-MP, while minimizing the incidence of bone marrow suppression.[85] The CD guidelines note that no randomized controlled trials have compared pharmacogenomic guided dosing to usual care dosing in patients receiving AZA or 6-MP. However, the US Food and Drug Administration recommends such testing before initiating these medications.[85] Additionally, several retrospective studies have assessed the clinical utility of measuring AZA and 6-MP metabolites such as 6-thioguanine and 6-methylmercaptopurine.[86] Although some experts have used these data to suggest a therapeutic level for these metabolites (e.g., 6-thioguanine levels of 250–400 pmol/8 $\times$ 10^8 red blood cells have been considered optimal), the CD guidelines do not recommend their routine use.[16]

The optimal role for these tests remains to be fully determined, and data in this area are rapidly evolving.

In patients who have experienced neutropenia from AZA therapy, as C.J. has, the primary treatment is to discontinue AZA. In most cases, the WBC count will normalize over the course of several days to weeks. In extreme cases, the use of granulocyte colony-stimulating factor may be considered. C.J. should be monitored for signs and symptoms of infection, and the AZA should be withheld. Frequent, conceivably daily, WBC determinations should be made until the count is greater than 3,000/μL.

OTHER AGENTS

CASE 24-2, QUESTION 5: C.J.'s leukocyte count returned to normal after 2 weeks. Unfortunately, he experienced a flare of his CD symptoms, specifically, an increase in diarrhea and abdominal pain that C.J. has noted during the past 5 days. What other agents should be considered to maintain remission in C.J.?

A number of other immunosuppressive drugs have been examined in CD. MTX produces and maintains remission in patients with refractory disease. Clinical improvement or reduction in corticosteroid dosages have been observed with 15 mg/week oral MTX or 25 mg/week of intramuscular or subcutaneous MTX in roughly 40% of patients who had active bowel disease.[87,88] In clinical studies, GI toxicity was the most common reason for discontinuing treatment, but neutropenia and liver enzyme elevations were also reported.[89] Current guidelines recommend reserving MTX for patients who have failed or are intolerant of 6-MP or AZA. Some experts consider MTX to be inferior to 6-MP or AZA in CD, but no comparison studies have been published to date. Given an apparent therapeutic failure with AZA, a reasonable approach would be a short course of corticosteroids (prednisone 40 mg daily with a taper for 6–8 weeks) and MTX 25 mg weekly. Folic acid 1 mg daily should be initiated in patients started with the MTX. MTX use may result in a depletion of folate stores because of dihydrofolate reductase inhibition. Alternatively, biologic therapy could also be considered.

Metronidazole

CASE 24-2, QUESTION 6: C.J. has developed an enterocutaneous fistula with his latest disease exacerbation, and nothing is helping him achieve remission. What alternatives are appropriate for C.J.?

Recent guidelines recommend that antibiotics have little role in the maintenance of remission in CD, but they may be helpful in fistulizing disease or in patients with abscesses. Taste disturbances and peripheral neuropathy are the most commonly reported adverse effects associated with metronidazole treatment.

Infliximab

Infliximab is now firmly established as an important therapy in the treatment of CD, especially fistulizing disease. However, a number of concerns regarding this agent must be discussed with the patient before initiation of therapy. It is an expensive therapy (approximately $15,000/year), although it may be cost effective in CD.[90] Fistulizing disease seems to respond particularly well to infliximab, and its use may avert the need for surgery.[89] Acute and delayed hypersensitivity reactions can occur and are occasionally life threatening.[21] Some clinicians premedicate patients with a combination of diphenhydramine, acetaminophen, or corticosteroids before an infusion; however, the most effective strategy to avoid a serious reaction is to regularly monitor vital signs during infliximab infusion and slow the rate or stop the infusion if any symptoms develop. The majority of reactions consist of headache, flushing, itching, and dizziness, with anaphylactic reactions rarely occurring. Also of concern is the development of human antichimeric antibodies in some patients receiving infliximab, which may lead to either loss of response or immunologic adverse reactions.

Infliximab should be avoided in patients who have a serious active infection. Because of reports that infliximab treatment may reactivate tuberculosis, all patients considered for treatment must receive a tuberculin skin test to rule out the disease (see Chapter 68, Tuberculosis). If this test is negative and because C.J. does not appear to have any other contraindications, he would seem to be an appropriate candidate for infliximab. If latent tuberculosis is found, antitubercular treatment must be initiated before infliximab can be considered since patients with treated latent tuberculosis still have an increased risk of active disease.[91,92] In addition, screening for hepatitis B (and probably hepatitis C) is reasonable owing to the number of cases describing reactivation of these viral infections.[66] Current data concerning a link between TNF-α blockers use and malignancy are conflicting.[93] To date, the balance of data suggests a small but real risk of developing lymphoma in CD patients using TNF-α blockers, but despite this, its use is associated with an increase in quality-adjusted years of life.[94] Another problem commonly faced by clinicians and patients is loss of effectiveness in patients receiving TNF-α blockers. This may occur months or years after initiation of therapy. Common strategies to regain response may include increasing the dose of infliximab to 10 mg/kg per dose or switching to another TNF-α blocker. The success of these strategies is variable, and often comes with significantly increased treatment costs.[40] A recent paper has shed light on the possible causes of this loss of efficacy.[41] In 155 patients receiving infliximab, who had declining response to the drug, both trough serum infliximab levels and human anticlonal antibodies (HACA) were measured. The authors found that in patients with subtherapeutic trough infliximab levels, increasing the dose of the drug was a successful strategy to regain response, whereas those patients who were HACA-positive benefited more from changing to another TNF-α blocker. Such laboratory markers may have the potential to be routinely used to assess the effectiveness of infliximab, but more data on this issue are needed to make such a recommendation.

Surgery in Crohn's Disease

CASE 24-2, QUESTION 7: C.J. was initiated on infliximab 400 mg IV every 8 weeks, and it was successful at keeping him symptom free. However, after 2 years of remission, C.J. is hospitalized for an acute exacerbation of right lower quadrant pain associated with abdominal distension, lack of bowel movements, and vomiting during the past 24 hours. Radiographic studies indicate partial small bowel obstruction at the terminal ileum. Is surgery indicated at this time?

Because medical therapy of CD is often inadequate, 78% of patients with this disease will require surgery within 20 years of symptom onset.[4] In contrast to UC, surgical removal of the involved bowel in CD is not a definitive form of therapy. CD can recur even after extensive resections.[72] Various investigations have determined that cumulative recurrence rates after surgery for this disease are as high as 80%, depending on the surgical procedure and disease location. Therefore, multiple operations and their attendant risks are often necessary during the life of the CD patient. Depending on the amount and site of the bowel removed during surgery, specific malabsorption syndromes can occur (e.g., vitamin B_{12} malabsorption with removal of the terminal ileum). If an ileostomy is part of the surgical procedure, the patient will have to undergo significant psychological adjustments. Therefore, surgery is indicated only for specific complications that are unresponsive to medical therapy, and it should be avoided if possible.

IRRITABLE BOWEL SYNDROME

Irritable bowel syndrome (IBS) is one of the most common chronic, relapsing, but benign disorders causing patients to seek medical treatment. It exerts a significant economic burden and is responsible for considerable morbidity in Western countries. Until recently, little was understood about the pathophysiology or etiology of this disorder. Indeed, some controversy exists today as to whether IBS is a distinct syndrome or a grouping of several chronic GI disorders. Still, investigators have made strides in understanding IBS, particularly the role of the enteric nervous system in the etiology of this disorder. As a result, new pharmacotherapeutic options are emerging for patients experiencing this often bewildering condition.

IBS can be defined as "a functional bowel disorder characterized by abdominal pain associated with a change of bowel habit."[95] The incidence of IBS has been reported to be 3% to 20% in Western countries.[96] It is the most common disorder seen by gastroenterologists and is commonly seen by primary-care clinicians as well.[97] Prevalence rates are dependent on IBS diagnostic criteria, which have varied over the years. A female sex predominance of about 3:1 is evident in most epidemiologic studies of IBS.[96] Some studies have demonstrated a white predominance in IBS, whereas other studies have found no such association. Many patients with IBS never seek medical attention, and those who do tend to see their physician frequently.[98]

Many of these patients also have other functional disorders, such as fibromyalgia and interstitial cystitis; and psychiatric disorders, such as major depression and generalized anxiety disorder. It is estimated that IBS accounts for $33 billion in direct and indirect costs in the United States annually.[99]

Pathophysiology

Although knowledge of the cause of IBS remains incomplete, several theories have emerged to explain the underlying pathophysiology of this disorder. Previously, the primary cause of IBS was believed to be psychiatric or psychosomatic. This picture was at least partially validated by the finding that many IBS patients had psychiatric comorbidities. Today, it is believed that factors such as psychological stress may exacerbate the disease, but they are not the cause of IBS.[100] It has long been known that IBS patients tend to exhibit visceral hypersensitivity to colonic stimulation or manipulation. Although concomitant anxiety and hypervigilance undoubtedly played a role in such observations, it is now believed that the reaction to visceral stimuli in these patients results in the perception of abdominal pain, whereas patients without IBS would have no symptoms. The etiology of this hypersensitivity is the focus of intense research efforts. Theories have emerged suggesting that the activation of silent gut nociceptors owing to ischemia or infection may lead to increased abdominal pain in IBS.[100] Other experts propose that an increase in the excitability of neurons in the dorsal horn of the spinal cord lead to gut hyperalgesia. An abnormality in the processing of ascending signals from the dorsal horn may be responsible for a lower pain threshold in IBS patients. Similarly, findings suggest that neurotransmitter abnormalities may cause the symptoms of IBS. Of particular interest is the role of serotonin (5-HT) in the etiology of this disorder. Greater than 95% of the body's 5-HT is located in the GI tract and is stored in many cells, such as enterochromaffin cells, neurons, and smooth muscle cells. When released, this 5-HT can trigger both GI smooth muscle contraction and relaxation, as well as mediate GI sensory function.[101] Different 5-HT receptor subtypes may be responsible for these differing actions. A study examining rectal biopsy specimens in patients with IBS found defects in 5-HT signaling, supporting the theory of neurotransmitter abnormalities.[102] The primary 5-HT subtypes in the GI tract are 5-HT_3 and 5-HT_4. Some data suggest that IBS patients may have higher levels of 5-HT in the colon compared with control subjects.[103] Thus, these receptors have become the target of pharmacotherapeutic manipulation for IBS.

Another proposed pathological mechanism of IBS is altered colonic motility. Diarrhea, constipation, and abdominal bloating are common features of IBS. Patients with IBS are often categorized as having either IBS with diarrhea (IBS-D) or IBS with constipation (IBS-C).[95] About one-half of patients with IBS report increased symptoms postprandially, and patients with IBS-D have been shown to have an exaggerated response to cholecystokinin after eating, leading to increased colonic propulsions.[104] However, patients with IBS-C tend to have fewer colonic propulsions postprandially. Patients in whom bloating is the primary symptom of IBS may have gas production from poor fermentation of carbohydrates.[105] This has led investigators to search for a link between bacterial overgrowth of the small bowel (leading to an increase of gas production and pain and bloating symptoms) and IBS.

Etiology

The pathogenesis of IBS is poorly understood, although consensus theories are emerging. Some investigators believe that inflammation of the GI mucosa associated with infection may be the triggering factor that results in IBS.[98] The fact that symptoms associated with IBS can appear in up to 30% of patients who had an episode of bacterial gastroenteritis in the recent past lend credence to an infectious etiology.[106] Recent studies have also determined that a percentage of patients diagnosed with IBS may in fact have small intestinal bacterial overgrowth.[107] Diagnosis of the latter disorder is particularly important as treatment may involve a simple course of antibacterials. Also controversial is the possible association of a history of physical or sexual abuse and the development of IBS.[108] Most IBS patients under emotional or psychological stress will report an exacerbation of their symptoms, but this is not surprising considering that such stressors affect non-IBS patients' GI function as well.[109] Familial clustering of IBS patients suggests that both genetics and formative environments may play a role in the pathogenesis of this disorder.[110] Finally, food intolerances (e.g., lactose intolerance) may be misdiagnosed as IBS.

Diagnosis

One of the more challenging and frustrating aspects of IBS is its lack of biochemical or physical markers that are pathognomonic for the disorder. This lack of "objective" criteria for diagnosis can propagate the notion that IBS is a psychological or psychosomatic disorder. Many patients express frustration with the traditional medical establishment and individual providers.[111] Patients and providers often want expensive laboratory or imaging tests to rule out other diseases; however, guidelines suggest that extensive testing in IBS patients is usually unnecessary provided that patients are younger than 50 years and do not present with any alarm symptoms. Alarm symptoms include:

- Abdominal pain and cramping not relieved by a bowel movement
- Fatigue
- Rectal bleeding
- Iron-deficient anemia
- Weight loss (significant and unexplained)
- Fever
- Onset >40 years
- Family history of IBD or colon cancer
- Nocturnal symptoms (abdominal pain and cramping which awakes the sufferer from sleep)[112]

The presence of alarm symptoms or an unusual finding on routine examination (e.g., thyroid abnormality) may prompt further referrals and testing. Although several symptom-driven criteria have been published, including the different Rome Foundation systems and the Manning criteria, it is important to realize that such systems have rarely been validated in IBS patients and their use to confirm or exclude the disorder is controversial.[113] This may be why previous guidelines have focused on a simple and practical definition for IBS: abdominal pain or discomfort that is accompanied by a change in bowel habits for at least 3 months (without alarm symptoms).[114] Once IBS is diagnosed, it should be further differentiated by predominant symptom pattern into IBS with diarrhea (IBS-D), IBS with constipation (IBS-C), mixed IBS or alternating bowel patterns (IBS-M), or unclassified (IBS-U).[115] Symptoms are not always stable and patients may change from one IBS subtype to the next during different stages of life. Small intestinal bacterial overgrowth or celiac sprue may be tested for in selected patients, but routine screening is not currently recommended. Because there is no known cure for IBS, it is logical to use these subgroups to help direct symptomatic therapy. In most cases, the primary-care clinician can successfully manage the IBS patient using the treatment algorithm depicted in Figure 24-3.

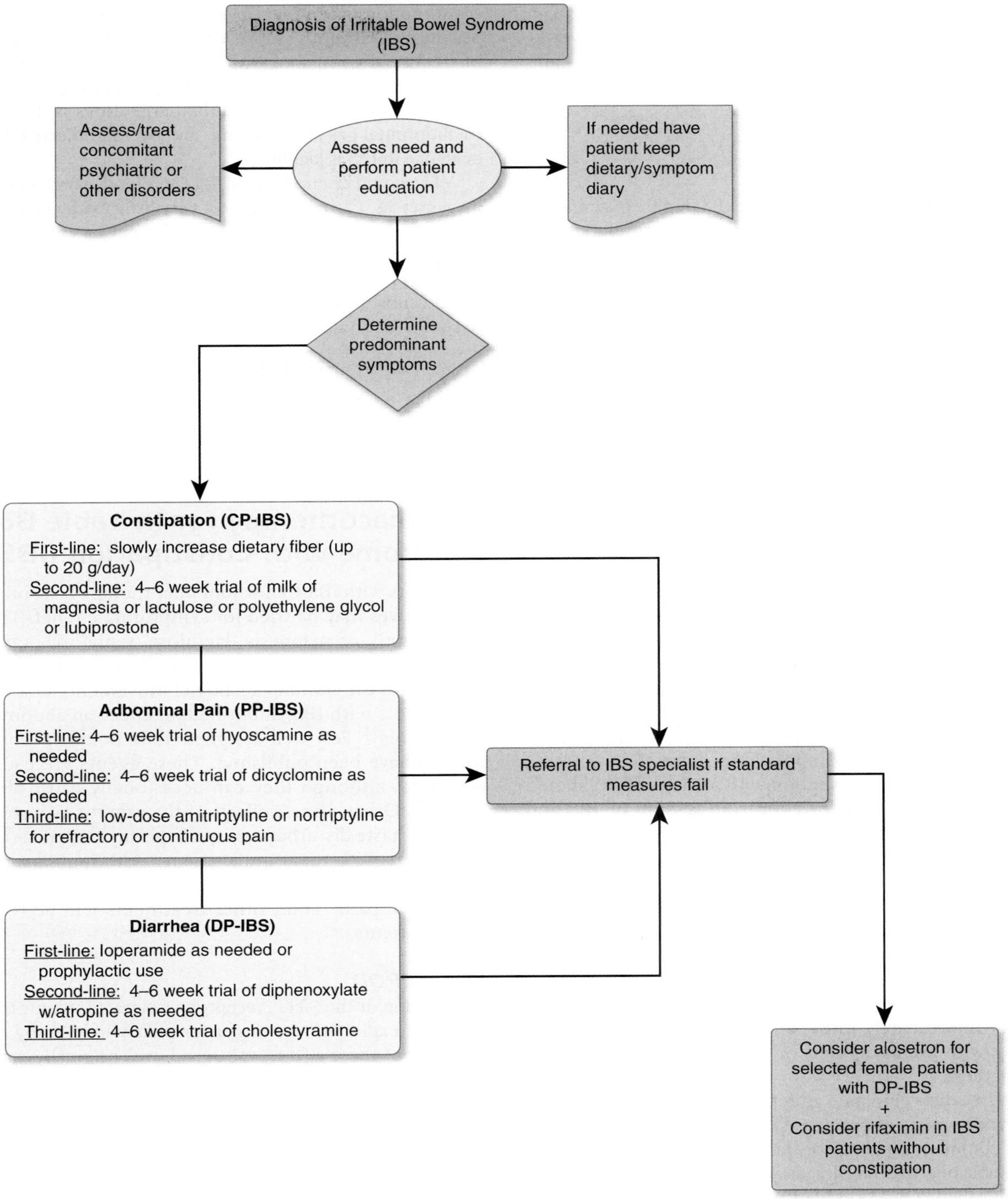

Figure 24-3 Treatment algorithm for irritable bowel syndrome. (Source: American College of Gastroenterology Task Force on Irritable Bowel Syndrome et al. An evidence-based position statement on the management of irritable bowel syndrome. *Am J Gastroenterol*. 2009;104(Suppl 1):S1; Pimentel M et al. Rifaximin therapy for patients with irritable bowel syndrome without constipation. *N Engl J Med*. 2011;364:22.)

There are limited data concerning the natural history of IBS. IBS is generally considered a benign disease with a good prognosis.[116] Patients' symptoms often wax and wane, and, in some cases, the syndrome resolves spontaneously.

Management

PATIENT EDUCATION

CASE 24-3

QUESTION 1: V.H. is a 33-year-old woman who presents with complaints of severe abdominal pain (rated 6 on a scale of 1–10), bloating, and the passage of hard pellet-like stools about every 3 days. This has gone on for about 6 months, and V.H. notices that an "attack" occurs usually after a large meal. Her past medical history is significant for a generalized anxiety disorder. Her current medications include buspirone and Yaz (drospirenone and ethinyl estradiol). She drinks socially and does not smoke or use illicit drugs. V.H. is concerned that her symptoms are indicative of cancer. How should the clinician respond to V.H.'s concerns?

Clinicians must reassure patients with IBS that their symptoms are real but benign. An effective physician–patient relationship is important for improved patient satisfaction, adherence to therapy, and symptom reduction.[117] Furthermore, patients should be thoroughly counseled concerning the prognosis of IBS. Many patients are fearful that their symptoms are indicative of severe pathology such as cancer. Reassurance and education are vital to assuage fears and to reinforce the generally benign nature of this disorder. Involving patients at the earliest stages in their treatment plan is vital for patient acceptance and to avoid "doctor shopping." Further, some patients exhibit a phenomenon known as *somatization*. This is defined as a tendency to experience and communicate somatic distress in response to psychosocial stress and is a factor in how often IBS patients seek health care for their condition.[118] Educational sessions and psychological techniques are thought to decrease the risk of developing somatization, but data to date are limited concerning these interventions.[119] Unfortunately, psychological disorders are present in a large segment of IBS patients. The clinician should again reinforce the notion that IBS is not "all in the patient's head." However, treatment of comorbid disorders, including the discovery of a history of physical or sexual abuse (and possible posttraumatic stress disorder), is an important component in successfully treating IBS.[116] Thus, the initial intervention with patients of IBS should include an interactive patient education session of IBS and earning the patient's trust.

DIET AND PROBIOTICS

Food intolerance may cause symptoms similar to those associated with IBS. Patients with lactose intolerance can experience pain, bloating, and diarrhea after ingesting milk-based products. A dietary and symptom diary may reveal such an intolerance, and avoidance of the implicated foods would constitute effective treatment. Unfortunately, most patients with IBS have difficulty complying with exclusion diets or will not achieve significant relief with them.

Gluten-free diets eliminate gluten found in wheat, barley, and rye and a wide variety of processed foods, while FODMAPs diets consist of eliminating a group of short-chain carbohydrates such as fermentable oligosaccharides, disaccharides, monosaccharides, and polyols called FODMAPs because they are unable to be properly absorbed by patients with IBS and cause fermentation by bacteria in the gut producing gas.[120,121] Recent guidelines suggest that gluten-free and low FODMAPs diets show promise, but their role is still questionable.[114] Guidelines also suggest there is not enough data to recommend prebiotics or synbiotics. However, probiotics have shown promise with a decrease in flatulence or bloating, although there are no comparative studies to suggest one product over another.[114]

CASE 24-3, QUESTION 2: V.H. has gradually increased her dietary fiber, mainly bran, during the past 6 weeks. She still feels constipated and did not experience any improvement. In addition, new symptoms of abdominal bloating have occurred in the past week. What is a reasonable strategy to treat V.H.'s IBS-C?

Patients with IBS-C may benefit from increased dietary consumption of soluble fiber; with a recent study finding that psyllium significantly improved IBS symptoms during 3 months of treatment compared with placebo.[122] Insoluble fiber such as bran can worsen symptoms of bloating, cramping, or flatulence.[114] Patients should be counseled that large doses of fiber can lead to abdominal gas and bloating, and overall objective long-term evidence in IBS is lacking.

V.H. should be encouraged to keep a food diary to identify food intolerances. Currently, there is very little evidence to suggest a gluten-free or a FODMAPs diet for this patient. She can consider probiotics, but there is insufficient evidence to suggest one probiotic over the other. When choosing fiber for constipation, she should substitute bran fiber for soluble fiber, such as psyllium, to reduce abdominal gas and bloating.

CASE 24-3, QUESTION 3: Several months have passed since V.H. was first diagnosed with IBS-C. She has had therapeutic trials of several over-the-counter agents that were either poorly tolerated or lacked effectiveness. What other options are available for treating V.H.'s IBS-C?

Pharmacotherapy for Irritable Bowel Syndrome with Constipation (IBS-C)

In patients with IBS-C in whom fiber therapy fails, other standard laxatives may be tried for symptomatic relief. These may include milk of magnesia, lactulose, senna, or polyethylene glycol without electrolytes (Miralax). This last agent was shown to improve the number of bowel movements in a cohort of adolescents with IBS-C, but had no effect on abdominal pain or bloating.[123] Few well-designed trials looking at any laxative for IBS have been published. These agents are usually well tolerated, although they can occasionally cause abdominal bloating. Other adverse effects of the osmotic laxatives include diarrhea, taste disturbances, and hypermagnesemia (especially in patients with renal impairment). Although laxatives may provide relief of constipation, they will not effectively treat abdominal pain. Thus, other treatments will be required in many patients.

TEGASEROD

Stimulation of the 5-HT_4 receptor accelerates colonic transit and has been exploited as a target for pharmacotherapy of IBS-C. The first of these agents, tegaserod, was originally approved in the United States for women with IBS-C. Tegaserod is a specific 5-HT_4 partial agonist that was evaluated in women with at least a 3-month history of IBS-C symptoms.[124] Clinical studies demonstrated a modest but significant benefit with tegaserod. Unfortunately, postmarketing analysis by the US Food and Drug Administration found an increased incidence of heart attack, stroke, and unstable angina in patients receiving the drug, and in April 2008, the manufacturer of tegaserod halted all sales and marketing of this agent.

LUBIPROSTONE

Lubiprostone, a GI chloride-channel activator (ClC-2 channels) that enhances intestinal fluid secretion and acts as a laxative, was approved in the United States for IBS-C in women older than 18 years of age. The drug has several actions on GI function including increased small and large bowel transit time and decreased gastric emptying.[125] The dose of lubiprostone for IBS-C is 8 mcg orally twice daily with food and water, which is a lower dose than used for chronic idiopathic constipation. Mechanical GI obstruction is a contraindication to lubiprostone's use.[126] A recent analysis of two randomized controlled studies of lubiprostone versus placebo in women with IBS-C found that the drug was moderately effective in improving patient perception of constipation symptoms (17.9% vs. 10.1% of placebo groups responded; $p = 0.001$).[127] Primary adverse effects of lubiprostone include nausea and vomiting, but the effects are less likely at the dose of the drug approved for IBS-C and can be somewhat ameliorated by taking the medication with food.[125] Too few men with IBS-C were enrolled in the clinical trials with lubiprostone to draw any conclusions about its effectiveness in this population. Because the drug is associated with teratogenic effects in animals, the manufacturer recommends that women who could become pregnant have a negative pregnancy test before beginning therapy and be able to comply with effective contraceptive measures during therapy.[126] The drug is significantly more expensive than traditional laxatives, and should generally be reserved for patients who have failed other therapy for IBS-C.

Linaclotide

Linaclotide (Linzess) is a guanylate cyclase-C (GC-C) agonist and together with its active metabolite bind to GC-C receptors acting locally on the luminal surface of the intestinal epithelium to increase intracellular and extracellular cyclic guanosine monophosphate (cGMP) concentrations.[128] Elevated cGMP stimulates chloride and bicarbonate secretions into the intestinal lumen, resulting in increased intestinal fluid and gastrointestinal movement with decreased response to pain.

Linaclotide's approval was based on two randomized, double-blind, placebo-controlled phase III trials.[129,130] Results from clinical trials show that patients receiving linaclotide reported small but statistically significant improvements in abdominal pain, discomfort, and bloating with some improvements in bowel straining, constipation, and stool consistency compared to placebo-treated patients.[129,130] On withdrawal of linaclotide therapy, abdominal pain returned and bowel movements decreased to levels similar to the placebo group, but there was no rebound effect noted.[130] Linaclotide is approved for use in male and female adult patients >18 years at a dosage of 290 mcg daily taken 30 minutes before breakfast. There is a boxed warning for contraindicated use in children less than 6 years old and patients with known or suspected mechanical GI obstruction. Use should be avoided in children 6 to 17 years because of deaths from dehydration in younger juvenile mice.[128] Because of low systemic exposure, drug interactions are unlikely. The main side effect is diarrhea, abdominal pain, and flatulence.[128]

Because there are no head-to-head comparative trials with lubiprostone and linaclotide, both of these agents are viable options for V.H. Therefore, a trial of lubiprostone 8 mcg orally twice daily with meals or linaclotide 290 mcg daily taken 30 minutes before breakfast would be reasonable.

Irritable Bowel Syndrome–Associated Pain and Bloating

CASE 24-4

QUESTION 1: L.K. is a 38-year-old woman who has a long history of abdominal pain and episodic diarrhea. L.K. works as a sales representative for a major software vendor and is called on periodically to make formal presentations. She finds that just before these presentations she experiences "attacks" of abdominal pain and diarrhea. Her past medical history is significant for fibromyalgia, which manifests as chronic tiredness and fatigue. She has no other medical problems and takes no medications. She has no known drug allergies. She does not drink, smoke, or use illicit drugs. She has undergone an extensive workup, including colonoscopy, upper GI endoscopy with small bowel follow-through, computed tomography abdominal scans, serum electrolytes, thyroid function tests, and stool studies. These procedures and tests were negative, and L.K.'s gastroenterologist has diagnosed her with IBS. L.K. currently has one to two loose stools daily. They are not greasy appearing or foul smelling. She has bouts of abdominal pain (severity of 7 on a 1–10 pain scale) with or without diarrhea several times daily. She describes the pain as "stabbing" and "cramping." She has not noted any temporal relationship to meals or that certain foods exacerbate her condition. What pharmacologic options are available for L.K.'s abdominal pain? What adverse effects are associated with these medications?

ANTISPASMODICS

Drugs that possess smooth muscle relaxation properties, usually by anticholinergic pathways, have long been used to treat IBS. In the United States, the two most commonly prescribed antispasmodics are hyoscyamine and dicyclomine, both of which possess significant anticholinergic properties.[98] Clinical trials that have examined the use of these agents in IBS have been plagued by small numbers and methodological problems, and recently several meta-analyses have been conducted to provide insight in this area. In general, these systematic reviews have found that, as a class, smooth muscle relaxants were superior to placebo in improving abdominal pain, although they are less effective at treating other IBS symptoms.[131] Unfortunately, there seems to be significant heterogeneity when looking at the efficacy of single agents in this class. Additionally, many agents studied in clinical trials are not available in the United States. Current treatment guidelines list antispasmodics as options for pain or bloating associated with IBS. If prescribed, an as-needed strategy of use has been advocated by some experts as opposed to continuous dosing owing to anticholinergic adverse effects.[109] Peppermint oil capsules also have smooth muscle relaxation properties and have been shown to be beneficial in IBS-related pain and cramping.[132]

ANTIDEPRESSANTS

Current treatment guidelines recommend the use of either tricyclic antidepressants or selective serotonin reuptake inhibitors (SSRIs) for patients with severe or continuous abdominal pain.[114] The analgesic effects of these agents are well known, and it is believed that these agents may work by a similar mechanism in IBS-associated pain and bloating as well as global well-being. One recent meta-analysis examined the class as a whole in IBS patients and found low-dose tricyclic antidepressants significantly improved pain, bloating, and IBS symptoms compared with placebo.[133] A dose–response relationship was not noted, and low doses of tricyclic antidepressants (e.g., amitriptyline 10–25 mg at bedtime) are often effective in relieving abdominal pain and diarrhea. A 3-month trial at a target dose of a drug (e.g., amitriptyline 50 mg) should be attempted before therapeutic failure is confirmed. Secondary amine tricyclic antidepressants (nortriptyline, desipramine) are better tolerated by many patients than tertiary amines (amitriptyline, imipramine) owing to decreased anticholinergic adverse effects such as sedation, dry mouth and eyes, urinary retention, and weight gain. SSRI use is more controversial in IBS patients as conclusive evidence of efficacy is lacking.[134] Still, practice guidelines note that these agents are also reasonable agents to consider in patients with pain or bloating associated with IBS.

Information on other antidepressants for IBS symptoms is limited. A recent pilot study suggested that duloxetine may improve pain and diarrhea in IBS patients, but more data are needed before this drug can be recommended.[135] Nortriptyline 10 mg orally at bedtime should be initiated with titration to symptom relief and lack of adverse effects.

Irritable Bowel Syndrome with Diarrhea

CASE 24-4, QUESTION 2: Two weeks after L.K. starts nortriptyline 25 mg at bedtime, she reports significant relief from both her abdominal pain and fatigue. She reports that she is sleeping better, and she now rates her pain as a 2 on a 1–10 scale. Her diarrhea has improved somewhat; however, she still suffers from a "diarrhea attack" before each presentation. What other treatments are available for IBS-D? What are the risks and benefits of these treatments?

STANDARD ANTIDIARRHEALS

Small bowel and colonic transit is accelerated in patients with IBS-D; thus, drugs that slow this process should be effective in relieving diarrhea.[136] Loperamide, an opioid agonist that penetrates poorly into the central nervous system, is the preferred agent for IBS-D. Meta-analyses have found loperamide to be an effective agent for improving diarrhea and, in some cases, improving patients' global well-being.[137] As with the antispasmodics, as-needed treatment is preferred to scheduled dosing (e.g., 2–4 mg PO up to QID as needed). Prophylactic dosing before a stressful situation or an event during which bathroom access is limited is particularly effective. Diphenoxylate with atropine is generally considered a second-line agent because of its increased risk of anticholinergic adverse effects. Finally, cholestyramine is occasionally used in refractory cases of IBS-D, especially when bile acid malabsorption is suspected or confirmed.[138] This agent is often poorly tolerated as a result of palatability problems. Cholestyramine also has a significant number of drug interactions of which the clinician must be aware.

ALOSETRON

Alosetron is a highly potent 5-HT_3 receptor antagonist that slows colonic transit time, increases intraluminal sodium absorption, and decreases small intestinal secretions.[139] Constipation is the most frequently reported adverse effect in clinical studies (approximately 30% of alosetron patients), with approximately 10% of patients withdrawing from studies for this reason. Postmarketing reports of severe constipation with cases of bowel obstructions and ischemic colitis were reported.[140] Bowel perforation and, rarely, death were also reported with alosetron use, and the drug was voluntarily withdrawn from the market in November 2000. After extensive lobbying by several patient groups, alosetron was reintroduced to the US market in June 2002, with restricted conditions for use. Prescribers must be registered with the drug manufacturer, and patients must sign a patient–physician agreement and be provided with a written medication guide. The starting dose and regimen for alosetron is 0.5 mg BID for 1 month. If, after 4 weeks, this is well tolerated but does not adequately control IBS symptoms, then the dosage can be increased to 1 mg BID.[141] It is imperative that patients not start alosetron if they have a history of problems with constipation, bowel obstruction or ischemic colitis, IBD, or a thromboembolic disorder. Patients must immediately discontinue alosetron if they become constipated or have symptoms of ischemic colitis, such as new or worsening abdominal pain, bloody diarrhea, or blood in the stool. A recent review of the mandatory postmarketing surveillance system designed to monitor the safety of the drug found an overall low rate of ischemic colitis.[142]

Newer Agents for IBS

In May 2015, the FDA approved two new drugs, rifaximin (Xifaxan) and eluxadoline (Viberzi), to treat IBS with diarrhea. Rifaximin was previously approved for traveler's diarrhea. Because some evidence exists concerning a possible association of bacterial GI infection and IBS symptoms, this has prompted some investigators to postulate that small bowel flora overgrowth may contribute to IBS symptoms. The nonabsorbable antibiotic rifaximin had been shown in two small studies to improve global symptoms in IBS for up to 10 weeks.[143,144] More recently a report of two randomized, double-blind, placebo-controlled trials of rifaximin in IBS (without constipation) was published.[145] In this trial a 14-day course of rifaximin 550 mg TID was found to significantly improve relief of global IBS symptoms during the first 4 weeks after treatment compared with placebo. The magnitude of improvement was small, but was considered clinically relevant. Rifaximin is approved for a dosage of 550 mg TID for 14 days for IBS-D. The patient can be treated 2 times with the same regimen if there is recurrence.[146] The most common side effects in patients treated with rifaximin for IBS-D include nausea and an increase in alanine aminotransferase (ALT). Caution should be used when using rifaximin in patients with severe liver impairment.[146]

Eluxadoline is a minimally absorbed μ-opioid receptor agonist and δ-opioid receptor antagonist. Studies have shown that when there is simultaneous μ-opioid receptor agonism and δ-opioid receptor antagonism, patients will experience decreased abdominal pain and diarrhea.[147]

The dosage approved for the treatment of IBS-D is 100 mg twice daily taken with food, but the dose is reduced to 75 mg BID in patients who are unable to tolerate 100 mg BID, have no gallbladder, have mild to moderate liver impairment, or are on organic anion transporting polypeptides (OATP1B1) inhibitors.[148] Patients treated with eluxadoline had better clinical response in phase 2 trials with decreased abdominal pain and increase stool consistency without significant risk of constipation.[147] The most common side effects in patients treated with eluxadoline include constipation, nausea, and abdominal pain.[148] The most serious known risk associated with eluxadoline is the risk of sphincter of Oddi spasm, which can result in pancreatitis. Eluxadoline should not be used in patients with a history of bile duct obstruction, pancreatitis, severe liver impairment, or severe constipation, and in patients who drink more than three alcoholic beverages daily.[148] Patients should be counseled to avoid alosetron or loperamide in combination with eluxadoline on a chronic basis, although it can be used on an acute as needed basis. If signs of constipation occur, the patient must be advised to discontinue loperamide immediately. They must discontinue eluxadoline if they experience constipation for more than 4 days. Patients should also be advised to avoid concomitant use of anticholinergics and other opioids with eluxadoline to avoid constipation. They should be reminded that eluxadoline has a potential for drug abuse.[148]

In L.K.'s case, initiation of loperamide 2 mg as needed before a stressful situation would be a cost-effective approach to her symptoms. Should her symptoms worsen or her current regimen lose effectiveness, eluxadoline 100 mg BID with food is an alternative, while a course of rifaximin 550 mg TID for 14 days would be considered an alternative strategy if she fails eluxadoline. The patient should be advised not to combine these therapies for chronic treatment and discontinue eluxadoline if she experiences constipation for 4 days.

KEY REFERENCES AND WEBSITES

A full list of references for this chapter can be found at http://thepoint.lww.com/AT11e. Below are the key references and websites for this chapter, with the corresponding reference number in this chapter found in parentheses after the reference.

Key References

Buchner AM et al. Update on the Management of Crohn's Disease. *Curr Gastroeterol Rep*. 2011;13:465. (31)

Colombel JF et al. Infliximab, azathioprine, or combination therapy for Crohn's disease. *N Engl J Med*. 2010;362:1383. (74)

Hoentjen F et al. Update on the Management of Ulcerative Colitis. *Curr Gastroenterol Rep*. 2011;13:475. (19)

Ford A et al. "American College Gastroenterology Monograph on the Management of Irritable Bowel Syndrome and Chronic Idiopathic Constipation" *Am J Gastroenterol*. 2014;109:S2–S26. (114)

Kornbluth A et al. Ulcerative colitis practice guidelines in adults: American College of Gastroenterology, Practice Parameters Committee. *Am J Gastroenterol*. 2010;105:501. (14)

Lichtenstein GR et al. American Gastroenterological Association Institute technical review on corticosteroids, immunomodulators, and infliximab in inflammatory bowel disease. *Gastroenterology*. 2006;130:940. (25)

Lichtenstein GR et al. Management of Crohn's disease in adults. *Am J Gastroenterol*. 2009;104:465. (16)

Pimentel M et al. Rifaximin therapy for patients with irritable bowel syndrome without constipation. *N Engl J Med*. 2011;364:22. (143)

Regueiro M et al. Clinical guidelines for the medical management of left-sided ulcerative colitis and ulcerative proctitis: summary statement. *Inflamm Bowel Dis*. 2006;12:972. (22)

Talley NJ et al. An evidence-based systematic review on medical therapies for inflammatory bowel disease. *Am J Gastroenterol*. 2011;106(Suppl 1):S2–25; quiz S26. doi: 10.1038/ajg.2011.58. (3)

25 Complications of End-Stage Liver Disease

Yasar O. Tasnif and Mary F. Hebert

CORE PRINCIPLES

		CHAPTER CASES
ASCITES		
1	Cirrhosis is defined as the fibrosis of the hepatic parenchyma, resulting in altered hepatic function, restricted venous outflow, and portal hypertension. Cirrhosis results in an overall vasodilated state, activation of the renin–angiotensin–aldosterone system, altered hepatic synthetic function, and development of complications such as ascites and other complications of cirrhosis.	**Case 25-1 (Question 2)**
2	Physical findings of ascites can include the presence of an enlarged fluid-filled abdomen, increased abdominal girth, a positive fluid wave, increased body weight and is often accompanied by peripheral edema. The goals of treatment for ascites are to mobilize ascitic fluid, diminish abdominal discomfort, as well as to prevent complications such as bacterial peritonitis and respiratory distress.	**Case 25-1 (Questions 1, 3)**
3	The treatment for ascites involves sodium restriction (2 g/day), water restriction for severe dilutional hyponatremia, and the use of spironolactone and furosemide (100:40 mg ratio). Management and monitoring of ascites includes ensuring adequate weight loss, maintaining electrolyte balance, and preventing complications of diuretic therapy.	**Case 25-1 (Questions 4–8)**
4	In cases of refractory ascites (diuretic-resistant), large-volume paracentesis, along with albumin replacement, is often indicated. Transjugular intrahepatic portosystemic shunt (TIPS), surgical shunts, and liver transplantation are the options for the treatment of refractory ascites when paracentesis is deemed ineffective, or in patients who are intolerant or who have a contraindication to paracentesis.	**Case 25-1 (Questions 9–11)**
5	Spontaneous bacterial peritonitis (SBP) is a common complication of ascites. Prophylactic regimens include the long-term administration of oral antibiotics such as fluoroquinolones (norfloxacin) or trimethoprim-sulfamethoxazole to prevent the recurrence of SBP. Recommendations also include the administration of antibiotic prophylaxis for prevention of SBP in patients with variceal hemorrhage.	**Case 25-2 (Question 4)**
ESOPHAGEAL VARICES		
1	Because esophageal varices are directly related to the severity of portal hypertension, the treatment is aimed at primary prevention of bleeding by reduction of portal pressure with the use of nonselective β-blockers, and/or elimination of the varices with endoscopic variceal ligation (EVL). Treatment approaches depend on the risk of hemorrhage.	**Case 25-2 (Question 5)**
2	Secondary prophylaxis to prevent recurrent bleeding episodes includes the combination of nonselective β-blockers and EVL. TIPS may be an option in patients who experience recurrent variceal hemorrhage despite combination of pharmacologic and endoscopic therapy.	**Case 25-2 (Question 6)**

Continued

	CHAPTER CASES
3 Acute variceal bleeding is considered a medical emergency and should be treated immediately. Treatment goals include volume resuscitation, acute treatment of bleeding, and prevention of recurrence of variceal bleeding. For the control and management of acute hemorrhage, the combination of pharmacologic therapy and variceal ligation is the preferred approach. In cases of acute variceal bleeding uncontrolled by pharmacologic and endoscopic therapy, TIPS can be an effective option.	**Case 25-2 (Questions 1–3)**
HEPATIC ENCEPHALOPATHY	
1 Hepatic encephalopathy is a metabolic disorder of the central nervous system that occurs in patients with either advanced cirrhosis or fulminate hepatic failure. The clinical features include altered mental state and asterixis. Several theories exist about the pathogenesis of hepatic encephalopathy; however, it is likely multifactorial. Precipitating causes can include GI bleeding, diuretic-induced hypovolemia and/or electrolyte abnormalities, metabolic alkalosis, as well as sedating drugs.	**Case 25-3 (Questions 1–3)**
2 After identifying and removing precipitating causes of hepatic encephalopathy, therapeutic management is aimed primarily at reducing the amount of ammonia or nitrogenous products in the circulatory system by limiting protein intake and by the use of lactulose. Other therapeutic options include rifaximin and neomycin.	**Case 25-3 (Questions 4, 5)**
3 Monotherapy with lactulose should be tried first. If satisfactory results do not occur, switching to another option (rifamixin or neomycin) or combination therapy should be considered.	**Case 25-3 (Question 6)**
HEPATORENAL SYNDROME	
1 Hepatorenal syndrome (HRS) is a complication of advanced cirrhosis and is diagnosed by exclusion of other known causes of kidney disease. The definitive treatment for type 1 and type 2 HRS is liver transplantation, which is the only treatment that assures long-term survival. The main goal of pharmacologic therapy is to reverse HRS sufficiently so that appropriate candidates for liver transplantation can survive until suitable donor organs can be procured.	**Case 25-3 (Questions 7, 8)**

OVERVIEW

According to the National Vital Statistics Report published by the Centers for Disease Control and Prevention, chronic liver disease and cirrhosis is the 12th leading cause of death in the United States, accounting for approximately **38,170** deaths each year.[1] Cirrhosis, or end-stage liver disease, can be defined as fibrosis of the hepatic parenchyma resulting in nodule formation and altered hepatic function, which results from a variety of causes. Although there are other common causes of cirrhosis, most cases of cirrhosis worldwide result from chronic viral hepatitis or chronic alcohol consumption.[2] This chapter describes the pathogenesis of cirrhosis and the associated complications of portal hypertension (esophageal varices, gastric varices, ascites, spontaneous bacterial peritonitis, hepatic encephalopathy, and hepatorenal syndrome) and their treatment.

PATHOGENESIS OF CIRRHOSIS

The liver consists of the hepatic parenchyma (hepatocytes) and a large proportion of nonparenchymal cells, including sinusoidal endothelial cells, Ito cells, and macrophages. Most of the liver's role in detoxification takes place within the hepatocytes. Also within the liver is the biliary tree in which bile drains from the liver and some substances are actively transported into the bile.[3] The liver has a strong capacity to regenerate; however, ethanol and hepatitis viruses can impair this.[4]

Liver injury leading to cirrhosis impairs hepatic function. Steatosis from ethanol is characterized by lipid deposition in the hepatocytes, which is followed by liver inflammation (steatohepatitis), hepatocyte death, and collagen deposition leading to fibrosis.[5] Oxidative stress appears to play a role in ethanol-induced liver injury. It is important to note that not all heavy drinkers experience liver cirrhosis.[6] Factors such as sex, genetic predisposition, and chronic viral infection also play a role in the development and progression of ethanol-induced liver disease.[7]

Hepatitis C virus (HCV) affects millions of people worldwide. Approximately a third of those chronically infected are predicted to progress to cirrhosis or hepatocellular carcinoma.[8] The progression of liver disease in patients with HCV is dependent on both patient and viral factors. Multiple mechanisms are proposed to play a role in liver injury associated with HCV infection, such as diminished immune clearance of HCV, oxidative stress, hepatic steatosis, increased iron stores, and increased rate of hepatocyte apoptosis.[9] Because not all patients infected with HCV experience cirrhosis, factors other than viral clearance, such as individual immune response, age, sex, hepatic iron content, and HCV genotype, are all implicated as cofactors in the development of cirrhosis.[10]

Among other causes, autoimmune hepatitis, primary biliary cirrhosis, primary sclerosing cholangitis, biliary atresia, metabolic disorders (e.g., Wilson disease and hemochromatosis), chronic inflammatory conditions (e.g., sarcoidosis), and vascular derangements can lead to hepatic fibrosis and cirrhosis.[2] Approximately 20% of Americans have nonalcoholic fatty liver disease (NAFLD), which in most cases have no symptoms. Risk factors commonly associated with the development of NAFLD include obesity, hyperlipidemia, and diabetes. Although corticosteroids can cause fatty liver, NAFLD diagnosis excludes corticosteroids and other causes of fatty liver. Nonalcoholic steatohepatitis (NASH) is a more serious form of NAFLD, which can lead to cirrhosis. Evidence suggests that insulin resistance and lipid peroxidation play a role in the pathogenesis of this condition.[11,12] Regardless of the cause of end-stage liver disease, the most frequent complications of portal hypertension are esophageal or gastric varices, ascites, hepatic encephalopathy, and hepatorenal syndrome.[13]

COMPLICATIONS OF CIRRHOSIS

Portal Hypertension

The portal vein begins as a confluence of the splenic, superior mesenteric, inferior mesenteric, and gastric veins and ends in the sinusoids of the liver (Fig. 25-1). Blood in the portal vein contains substances absorbed from the intestine and delivers these substances to the liver to be metabolized before entering the systemic circulation. Once the portal blood reaches the liver, it crosses through a high-resistance capillary system within the hepatic sinusoids.

In cirrhosis, increased intrahepatic resistance results from intrahepatic vasoconstriction that is hypothesized to be caused by a deficiency in intrahepatic nitric oxide (NO).[14] Increased intrahepatic resistance also results from an enhanced activity of vasoconstrictors and structural changes from liver regeneration, sinusoidal compression, and fibrosis.

Portal hypertension results from both an increase in resistance to portal flow and an increase in portal venous inflow because of splanchnic vasodilatation from increased NO production in the extrahepatic circulation.[15]

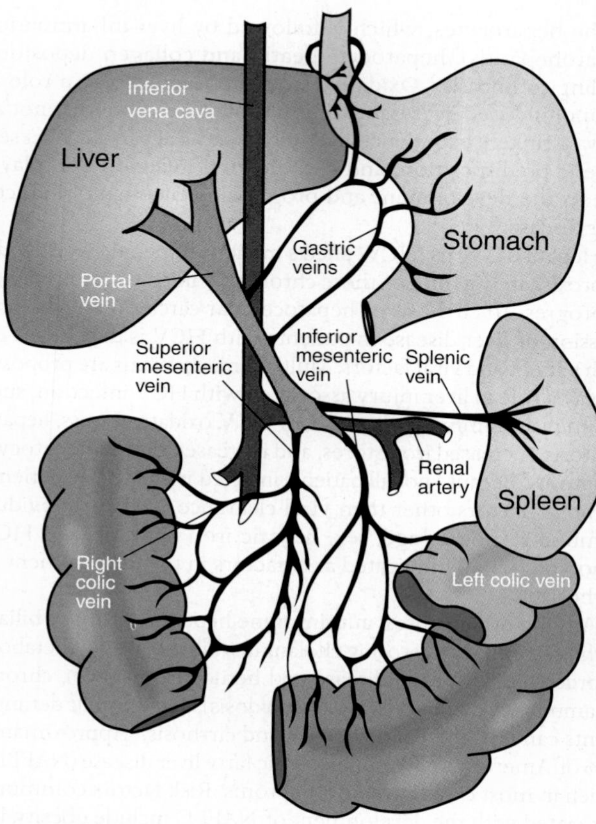

Figure 25-1 Schematic diagram of the portal venous system.

Direct portal pressure measurement is invasive and not routinely performed. The hepatic venous pressure gradient (HVPG), which reflects the gradient between the portal vein and vena cava pressure, is another accurate, safe, and less-invasive procedure, widely accepted as the portal venous pressure gradient.[16–18] Normal portal pressure is generally below 6 mm Hg, and in cirrhotic patients, it may increase to 7 to 9 mm Hg. Clinically significant portal hypertension develops when portal pressure exceeds 10 to 12 mm Hg, resulting in complications such as esophageal varices and ascites.[17,19] Portal hypertension can be further classified as prehepatic (e.g., splenic, portal vein thrombosis), intrahepatic (e.g., hepatic cirrhosis and fibrosis), or posthepatic portal hypertension (e.g., inferior vena cava obstruction, right-sided heart failure).[20–22] Persistent portal hypertension may (a) change both blood flow and the lymphatic circulation and lead to ascites formation; (b) increase pressure in the vessels that branch off the portal vein, such as the coronary veins, leading to the formation of esophageal varices; and (c) lead to the development of increased abdominal collateral circulation. Hepatic encephalopathy and hepatorenal syndrome are other complications associated with advanced cirrhosis and portal hypertension.[20–22] The American Association for the Study of Liver Diseases and European Association for the Study of the Liver Single-Topic Conference classified cirrhosis into two main categories, compensated and decompensated. Patients can be cirrhotic with a portal pressure less than 10 mm Hg and an absence of the complications of cirrhosis (e.g., ascites, variceal hemorrhage, or encephalopathy) and thus would be considered to be compensated. This is in contrast to a patient presenting with ascites, esophageal hemorrhage, hepatic encephalopathy, and/or hepatorenal syndrome, which are present in decompensated cirrhosis.[23] Patients with compensated cirrhosis are managed by treatment of the underlying cause as well as prevention (primary prophylaxis) and early diagnosis of the complications. For patients with decompensated cirrhosis, the aim is to treat the complications and prevent sequela (secondary prevention).[24]

LABORATORY FINDINGS

Laboratory evaluations in cirrhosis may not reflect the extent of the parenchymal necrosis, regeneration, and fibrotic nodular scarring. Conventional liver "function" tests, such as the serum aminotransferases (aspartate aminotransferase [AST, formerly known as SGOT], alanine aminotransferase [ALT, formerly known as SGPT]), and alkaline phosphatase, are actually better characterized as liver "injury" tests and are modestly helpful to the clinician screening for hepatobiliary disease and monitoring injury progression. These tests, however, do not quantitatively measure the functional capacity of the liver. The aminotransferases are released during the normal turnover of liver cells (see Chapter 2, Interpretation of Clinical Laboratory Tests). High serum concentrations of aminotransferases suggest enzyme release from injured hepatocytes. Serum concentrations of AST and ALT may initially rise very high with acute liver injury and then fall when the etiology is removed or necrosis is so severe that few hepatocytes remain.

Because alkaline phosphatase is present in high concentrations in biliary canaliculi (as well as bone, intestines, kidneys, placenta, and white blood cells [WBCs]), its concentration increases more with biliary than hepatocellular injury. High serum concentrations of gamma glutamyl transpeptidase and bilirubin are also suggestive of biliary injury. Elevated serum concentrations of alkaline phosphatase, AST, and/or ALT may suggest hepatic injury, but because they are also found in other tissues, their elevation is not diagnostic for liver disease.[25,26]

Serum concentrations of proteins (e.g., albumin), clotting factors, prothrombin time (PT), and international normalized

Table 25-1
Child-Turcotte-Pugh Classification of Severity of Liver Disease

	Score[a]		
	1 Point	**2 Points**	**3 Points**
Bilirubin (mg/dL)	<2	2–3	>3
Albumin (g/dL)	>3.5	2.8–3.5	<2.8
INR	<1.7	1.7–2.3	>2.3
Ascites	None	Mild to moderate	Severe
Encephalopathy (grade)	None	Mild to moderate (1 and 2)	Severe (3 and 4)

[a]Class A, 5–6 points; class B, 7–9 points; class C, 10–15 points. INR, international normalized ratio.
Sources: Garcia-Tsao G, Bosch J. Management of varices and variceal hemorrhage in cirrhosis [published correction appears in N Engl J Med. 2011;364:490]. *N Engl J Med*. 2010;362:823; Gitto S et al. Allocation priority in non-urgent liver transplantation: an overview of proposed scoring systems. *Dig Liver Dis*. 2009;41:700.

ratio (INR) provide insight into liver function. Albumin is synthesized entirely by the liver; therefore, concentrations reflect hepatocellular function to some degree. However, changes in albumin concentration are nonspecific, because they are influenced by other factors, including poor nutrition, renal wasting (proteinuria), and gastrointestinal (GI) losses. Prothrombin time is also nonspecific, since it is prolonged in vitamin K deficiency from poor nutrition or fat malabsorption as well as biliary obstruction (cholestasis).[27]

A number of the factors described above are included in the Child–Turcotte–Pugh classification of liver disease severity (Table 25-1).[28,29] This scoring system helps clinicians grade disease severity, and predicts the long-term risk of mortality and quality of life. A person with Child–Turcotte–Pugh class A cirrhosis may survive 15 to 20 years, whereas those with class C may survive only 1 to 3 years.[30] The main limitation of the Child–Turcotte–Pugh classification is the subjective nature of some factors, such as ascites and hepatic encephalopathy, which are subject to clinical interpretation and may be altered by therapy.[31,32] As a general guide, and not a rule, class A patients are considered to be compensated, and classes B and C decompensated.[24]

An alternate method for assessing survival in patients with liver disease is the Model for End-Stage Liver Disease (MELD) score, which is calculated by the formula[32]:

$$\text{MELD Score} = (0.957 \times \text{In}[\text{Creatinine mg/dL}] + 0.378 \times \text{In}[\text{total bilirunbin mg/dL}] + 1.120 \times \text{In}[\text{INR}] + 0.643 \times 10 \quad \textbf{(Eq. 25-1)}$$

Because of the good correlation between the MELD score and short-term (3-month) mortality as well as the objective nature of the system, it replaced the Child–Turcotte–Pugh score in the United Network for Organ Sharing (UNOS) prioritization of organ allocation of cadaveric livers for transplantation.[33–35] MELD scores range from 6 (less ill) to 40 (gravely ill) with highest scores given priority for organ allocation with the exception of Status 1A adult patients (acute and severe onset of liver failure, who have a life expectancy of hours to a few days without liver transplantation) who are given highest priority.[36]

CLINICAL PRESENTATION

CASE 25-1

QUESTION 1: R.W. is a 54-year-old man with a 2-week history of nausea, vomiting, and lower abdominal cramps without diarrhea. Despite chronic anorexia, he has managed to drink a fifth of vodka (750 mL) and eat about two meals a day for the past 2 years. During this time, he experienced a 30-lb weight loss. He began drinking 9 years ago when his wife became disabled after diagnosis of a brain tumor. Two years ago, his alcohol consumption increased from one pint to a fifth daily. Recently, he has noted bilateral edema of his legs, an increased tenseness and girth of his abdomen, jaundice, and scleral icterus. His medical history is noncontributory, other than a history of spontaneous bacterial peritonitis (SBP) 6 months ago. He is not taking any medications and has no known drug allergies.

Physical examination reveals an afebrile, jaundiced, and cachectic male in moderate distress. Spider angiomas were found on his face and upper chest. In addition, palmar erythema was noted.

Abdominal examination reveals prominent veins on a very tense abdomen. The liver edge is percussed below the right costal margin and ascites is noted by shifting dullness and a fluid wave. The spleen is not palpable. On neurologic examination, R.W. is awake and oriented to person, place, and time. Cranial nerves II to XII are grossly intact, but a decrease in vibratory sensation of the lower extremities is noted bilaterally. Admission laboratory data are as follows:

Sodium, 135 mEq/L
Chloride, 95 mEq/L
Potassium, 3.8 mEq/L
Bicarbonate, 25 mEq/L
Blood urea nitrogen (BUN), 15 mg/dL
Serum creatinine (SCr), 1.4 mg/dL
Glucose, 136 mg/dL
Hemoglobin (Hgb), 11.2 g/dL
Hematocrit (Hct), 33.4%
AST, 212 IU
ALT, 110 IU
Alkaline phosphatase, 954 IU
PT, 13.5 (INR, 1.1)
Total/direct bilirubin, 18.8/10.7 mg/dL
Albumin, 2.3 g/dL
Guaiac positive stools

On admission to the hospital, the impression is alcoholic cirrhosis, ascites, and heme-positive stools.

What subjective and objective evidence are compatible with alcoholic cirrhosis in R.W.?

R.W.'s liver function tests (elevated ALT, AST, alkaline phosphatase, and bilirubin) and physical findings (enlarged, palpable liver edge; jaundice; spider angiomas; palmar erythema; and cachexia) are consistent with advanced alcoholic cirrhosis in a patient with a history of chronic alcohol abuse. The prolonged PT and hypoalbuminemia suggest impaired hepatic synthesis of both albumin and vitamin K–dependent clotting factors. The low albumin contributes to both ascites and edema. The bilirubin of 18.8 mg/dL suggests that vitamin K absorption may be a factor in the prolonged PT. The presence of ascites (an enlarged fluid-filled abdomen) and prominent abdominal veins are suggestive of portal hypertension. A biopsy of the liver may establish the presence and severity of cirrhosis. R.W.'s prolonged PT, however, will increase the risk of bleeding from a liver biopsy. His positive guaiac finding could be indicative of bleeding esophageal varices or from another GI source. This needs to be confirmed by endoscopy. He is oriented to person, place, and time, but full hepatic encephalopathy evaluation is needed. R.W.'s calculated MELD score is 22, which predicts a 90-day mortality of approximately 20%.[33] A patient's MELD score may increase or decrease for a period of time depending on the patient's clinical status and treatment. A number of MELD scores will be calculated if R.W. is listed as a transplantation candidate to determine his status for organ allocation.[36] Muscle wasting and poor nutrition are the most common causes of weight loss in patients with alcoholic cirrhosis (see Chapter 90, Substance Abuse Disorders).

ASCITES

Pathogenesis of Ascites

CASE 25-1, QUESTION 2: What physiologic mechanism predisposes R.W. to fluid accumulation in the peritoneal cavity?

Ascites, or accumulation of fluid in the peritoneal cavity, is the most commonly encountered clinical symptom of cirrhosis.[24,37] This complication can be detected during physical examination when more than 3 L of fluid have accumulated. In addition to an obviously enlarged abdomen, R.W. was found to have a positive fluid wave and shifting dullness, indicating that the abdominal enlargement is not simply obesity. If the diagnosis is in doubt, which sometimes occurs in obese patients, ascites can be confirmed with ultrasound. Generally speaking, in obesity the abdomen enlarges over time (months to years), in contrast to ascites where abdominal enlargement can occur over a few weeks.[38] Once ascites develops, the 1-year patient survival rate falls to ~50%.[24]

In cirrhosis, high hepatic venous pressure leads to high intrasinusoidal pressure and development of ascites across the hepatic capsule.[39] The systemic compensation to the generalized vasodilation in cirrhosis is increased cardiac output as well as sodium and water retention through activation of the renin–angiotensin–aldosterone system (RAAS).[40] R.W.'s hypoalbuminemia (2.3 g/dL), RAAS activation, exudation of fluid from the splanchnic capillary bed and the liver surface when the drainage capacity of the lymphatic system is exceeded, and decreased ability of fluid to be contained within the vascular space owing to impaired hepatic albumin synthesis contributes to the development of ascites.

Goals of Therapy

CASE 25-1, QUESTION 3: What are the therapeutic goals in the treatment of R.W.'s ascites?

The goals of treatment for R.W.'s ascites are to treat the cause of cirrhosis by ceasing alcohol consumption; mobilize ascitic fluid; diminish abdominal discomfort, back pain, and difficulty in ambulation; as well as to prevent complications (e.g., bacterial peritonitis, hernias, pleural effusions, hepatorenal syndrome, and respiratory distress).[38] After the initial resolution of significant edema, the goal is a weight loss of 0.5 kg/day, which corresponds to a net fluid volume loss of about 0.5 L/day. Treatment of ascites in R.W. should be undertaken cautiously and gradually because acid–base imbalances, hypokalemia, or intravascular volume depletion caused by overly aggressive therapy can lead to compromised renal function, hepatic encephalopathy, and death.[41,42] The initial medical management of ascites involves restriction of sodium intake and the use of diuretics to promote salt and water excretion.[38]

Fluid and Electrolyte Balance

URINARY NA:K RATIO

CASE 25-1, QUESTION 4: The 24-hour urinary electrolytes for R.W. were as follows:

Na, 10 mEq/L
K, 28 mEq/L

Why would sodium or water restriction be appropriate (or inappropriate) for R.W.?

Normally, urine electrolytes mirror serum electrolytes (i.e., sodium concentration is greater than that of potassium). A reversal of this pattern (i.e., potassium exceeding sodium) may indicate a relative hyperaldosteronism secondary to diminished renal blood flow and low oncotic pressure. A small study by Trevisani et al.[43] evaluated renal sodium and potassium handling and plasma aldosterone in a 24-hour period in cirrhotic patients without ascites, with ascites, and healthy controls. Plasma aldosterone was significantly higher in patients with ascites, resulting in reduced renal sodium excretion, and more than doubling renal potassium excretion in comparison to healthy controls.[43] For urine electrolyte monitoring to be meaningful, the first sample must be obtained before initiating diuretics.[44,45]

SODIUM RESTRICTION

Although serum sodium in patients with ascites is often low, they are total body sodium overloaded. Sodium restriction has been shown to enhance mobilization of ascites, because fluid loss and weight change are directly related to sodium balance in patients with portal-hypertension–related ascites.[46] This finding has been incorporated into the American Association for the Study of Liver Diseases (AASLD) guidelines for the treatment of ascites. The AASLD recommends that dietary sodium should be restricted to 2,000 mg/day (88 mmol/day) and R.W. should be advised to limit his sodium intake accordingly.[38] Historically, bed rest has been advocated; however, no controlled trials support this practice.[38,42]

WATER RESTRICTION

A large prospective, observational study[47] reported that hyponatremia (sodium <135 mEq/L) is common in patients with cirrhosis, associated with poor ascites control and a greater frequency of hepatic encephalopathy, hepatorenal syndrome, and spontaneous bacterial peritonitis compared to patients with normal serum sodium concentrations.[47] In addition, very low serum sodium concentrations (<120 mEq/L) are independent from the MELD score in predicting 3- to 6-month mortality. The AASLD recommends that water restriction should be implemented in cirrhotic patients who have severe dilutional hyponatremia (serum Na <125 mEq/L).[38] Water restriction is not indicated for R.W. at this time because his serum sodium concentration is within normal limits (135 mEq/L).

VASOPRESSIN RECEPTOR ANTAGONISTS

A complete discussion of vasopressin receptor antagonists can be found in Chapter 27, Fluid and Electrolyte Disorders. The AASLD guidelines do not recommend the use of vasopressin (V2) receptor antagonists because of the lack of evidence of efficacy in patients with cirrhosis, side effects, as well as the low cost-effectiveness of these medications.[38] However, it is possible that with more evidence from clinical trials, this class of medications may find a niche in the treatment of hyponatremia in cirrhotic patients.

Diuretic Therapy

CHOICE OF AGENT

CASE 25-1, QUESTION 5: R.W. was prescribed sodium restriction after initial evaluation. Spironolactone 100 mg/day and furosemide 40 mg/day were ordered to induce diuresis. Why is spironolactone preferred over other diuretics in the treatment of ascites?

Most patients with cirrhosis have elevated plasma concentrations of aldosterone.[48] High serum concentrations of aldosterone may be attributed to both increased production and decreased excretion of the hormone. Increased portal pressure, ascites, depletion of intravascular volume, and decreased renal perfusion can lead to activation of the RAAS.[49] In addition, hepatic shunting also increases aldosterone production by decreasing renal blood flow.[50] The liver metabolizes aldosterone, and hepatic impairment prolongs the physiologic half-life of aldosterone.[51] The AASLD consensus guidelines recommend the use of spironolactone as the initial diuretic of choice in the treatment of ascites.[38] Although no large comparative studies have evaluated different diuretics as first-line treatment of ascites, spironolactone is a rational diuretic choice for R.W. based on its aldosterone antagonist activity. Perez-Ayuso et al.[52] conducted a small randomized trial to study the efficacy of furosemide versus spironolactone in non-azotemic cirrhotic patients with ascites. They reported a higher response to spironolactone than furosemide (18/19 vs. 11/21; $p < 0.01$). Of the 10 nonresponders to furosemide, 9 responded to spironolactone. The authors also found that patients with higher renin and aldosterone levels did not respond to furosemide and required higher doses of spironolactone to achieve a diuretic response.[52]

Some clinicians may initiate spironolactone at a dose of 25 mg once or twice daily; however, much larger doses (100–400 mg/day) are generally necessary to antagonize the high circulating levels of aldosterone in patients with ascites.[38] The diuretic effect is enhanced when spironolactone is combined with sodium restriction.[42] In addition, furosemide can be started to minimize the risk of hyperkalemia and enhance diuresis. The AASLD guidelines recommend starting spironolactone 100 mg and furosemide 40 mg/day simultaneously and maintaining a 100:40 mg ratio. The doses of both oral diuretics can be increased simultaneously every 3 to 5 days (maintaining the ratio) to achieve adequate response. Usual maximal doses are 400 mg/day of spironolactone and 160 mg/day of furosemide.[38] In patients without renal failure, sodium restriction and diuretic therapy are effective in 90% of patients with ascites.[38,53]

Triamterene and amiloride can be used as alternatives to spironolactone if intolerable side effects (e.g., gynecomastia) occur with spironolactone.[54,55] In a small trial,[56] non-azotemic, cirrhotic patients with ascites were randomly assigned to receive amiloride (20–60 mg/day) or potassium canrenoate (150–500 mg/day, an active metabolite of spironolactone not available in the United States). A higher response rate was seen in the canrenoate group versus the amiloride group (14/20 vs. 7/20; $p < 0.025$). The authors also assessed plasma aldosterone activity and found that all responders to amiloride had normal plasma aldosterone concentrations, and all nonresponders to amiloride who later responded to potassium canrenoate had increased levels of plasma aldosterone.[56]

Eplerenone (a selective aldosterone blocker, more specific for the aldosterone receptor with a lower affinity for progesterone and androgen receptors than spironolactone) has been studied in patients with heart failure, hypertension, and renal disease.[57,58] The usual dose for eplerenone is 25 to 50 mg/day,[59] with no dosage adjustment needed in mild-to-moderate liver disease. However, severe liver disease has not been studied.[60] Approximately 10% of patients treated with spironolactone develop gynecomastia or breast pain, with 2% requiring drug discontinuation.[61] In contrast, gynecomastia occurs at a similar rate with eplerenone as with placebo (0.5%).[62,63] Unfortunately, eplerenone is much more expensive than spironolactone.[63] The lower risk of gynecomastia with eplerenone may make it a useful alternative to spironolactone; however, given its higher cost and the lack of data in the treatment of ascites in patients with severe liver disease, its role in ascites treatment remains unclear.

R.W. should receive spironolactone 100 mg and furosemide 40 mg simultaneously (maintaining a 100:40 mg ratio) as recommended by the AASLD.[38] R.W. should be carefully monitored for diuretic complications and clinical response (see Case 25-1, Questions 6–8).

MONITORING

Clinical Responses

CASE 25-1, QUESTION 6: What clinical responses should be monitored to ensure the therapeutic effectiveness of spironolactone therapy for R.W.?

Because ascitic fluid is slow to re-equilibrate with vascular fluid, diuresis greater than 0.5 to 1 kg/day (>0.5–1 L) may be associated with volume depletion, hypotension, and compromised renal function.[38] Patients may tolerate a faster diuresis if peripheral edema is present. Once edema has resolved, a scaled-back weight loss, not to exceed 0.5 kg/day, can be used as a rule of thumb to minimize the risk of renal insufficiency induced by plasma volume contraction and other diuretic-induced complications.[38,64] Monitoring body weight and abdominal girth are routinely performed in both the inpatient and outpatient settings. Monitoring fluid intake and urine output are performed primarily for inpatients, owing to practical constraints in the outpatient setting. Ideally, urine output should exceed fluid intake by about 300 to 1,000 mL/day. These measurements do not account for nonrenal fluid losses; therefore, total fluid loss will be somewhat higher. Abdominal girth measurement (circumference around the abdomen) is subject to error, because of its dependence on patient position and measurement location on the abdomen.[65] Attempts should be made to standardize patient position (e.g., sitting at a 45-degree angle) and location of measurement (level of umbilicus) to minimize variability in abdominal girth measurements.

Laboratory Parameters

CASE 25-1, QUESTION 7: What laboratory parameters could be monitored to assess the therapeutic efficacy of R.W.'s spironolactone treatment?

Serum concentrations of creatinine and urine chemistries (sodium and potassium) can be monitored to define and guide the need for increasing dosage of spironolactone. A low baseline urine Na:K ratio (<1.0) suggests high intrinsic aldosterone activity and that larger dosages of spironolactone may be needed, as is the case for R.W. If necessary, the dosage of diuretic therapy may be doubled after a few days.[49] AASLD recommends increasing both spironolactone and furosemide simultaneously every 3 to 5 days (maintaining a 100:40 mg ratio) to achieve adequate diuresis and maintain a normal serum potassium.[38]

Case 25-1, Question 8: The spironolactone and furosemide dosages were increased to 200 and 80 mg/day (maintaining a 100:40 mg ratio). What potential complications from the diuretic therapy might arise in R.W. and how can they be minimized?

Electrolyte and Acid–Base Disturbances

Hyponatremia, hyperkalemia, metabolic alkalosis, and, uncommonly, hypokalemia occur as side effects of diuretic therapy in patients with ascites. Hyponatremia results from a reduction in free water clearance (dilutional hyponatremia). Diuresis exacerbates hyponatremia by causing volume depletion and antidiuretic hormone (ADH) release. Hyponatremia usually can be corrected by temporary withdrawal of diuretics and free water restriction.[53,66–68] Although serum sodium may be low, these patients are total body sodium overloaded. Hyperkalemia is common in patients with refractory ascites and impaired renal function requiring high doses of diuretics such as spironolactone. Hyperkalemia can be approached in multiple ways, depending on the clinical situation (see Chapter 27, Fluid and Electrolyte Disorders). Furosemide is added to spironolactone to maintain normal serum potassium.[38] Decreasing or holding spironolactone may be appropriate depending on the patient's renal function and serum potassium.[24] Metabolic alkalosis, a result of loop diuretics, occurs because of increased urinary hydrogen loss from enhanced distal hydrogen secretion. Hypokalemia often accompanies metabolic alkalosis owing to loop diuretics.[67] Furosemide can be temporarily withheld in patients presenting with hypokalemia.[38] R.W. has some degree of renal impairment (SCr, 1.4 mg/dL) and is receiving spironolactone and furosemide. Therefore, his electrolytes and renal function tests should be monitored daily while hospitalized. After hospital discharge, monitoring will be dictated by the stability of the patient and need for diuretic dosage adjustments. For example, outpatients may need electrolytes and renal function monitoring once or twice weekly early after hospital discharge to as infrequently as every 3 months for very stable patients.[38]

Pre-renal Azotemia

Pre-renal azotemia usually results from over diuresis with subsequent compromise of intravascular volume and decreased renal perfusion. In addition to looking for clinical signs of hypovolemia, such as dizziness, orthostatic hypotension, and increased heart rate, frequent measurements of BUN and serum creatinine concentrations provide a relatively simple means of assessing the intravascular volume. A gradual rise in serum creatinine, BUN, as well as the BUN:serum creatinine ratio can serve as a warning to slow the rate of diuresis.[69] In a small study,[64] serial measurements of plasma volume and ascites volume were made during treatment with diuretics in patients with cirrhosis. Patients with ascites and no edema were able to mobilize more than 1 L/day during rapid diuresis, but at the expense of plasma volume contraction and renal insufficiency. Patients with peripheral edema appear to be somewhat protected from these effects and may safely undergo diuresis at a more rapid rate (>2 kg/day) until edema resolves.[64] Others suggest, however, that the maximal daily fluid loss should not exceed more than 0.5 L/day (>0.5 kg/day) for patients with ascites alone or 1 L/day (>1 kg/day) for those with both ascites and edema to prevent plasma volume depletion and decreased renal perfusion. If faster removal of ascites is required because of respiratory distress, large-volume paracentesis may be more effective than rapid diuresis (see Case 25-1, Question 9).[38,45,70,71] In cirrhotic patients, azotemia may also occur because of nonsteroidal anti-inflammatory drugs (NSAIDs). All NSAIDs should be discontinued, except low dose aspirin in patients at high risk for a cardiac or neurological event.[38]

Because R.W. presented with both edema and ascites, an initial weight loss of up to 1 kg/day would be reasonable with slowing to 0.5 kg/day when the edema resolves. Gradual diuresis avoids diuretic-induced depletion of intravascular fluid volume by permitting ascitic fluid to equilibrate with intravascular fluid. Long-term management of ascites is done in the outpatient setting. Severe cases with respiratory distress or impaired ambulation as well as patients with spontaneous bacterial peritonitis (see Chapter 70, Intra-Abdominal Infections) require hospitalization. If outpatient therapy is an option, a weekly evaluation initially would be prudent to prevent over diuresis and electrolyte disturbances.[38]

Refractory Ascites

Case 25-1, Question 9: Over the next several days, R.W.'s spironolactone dosage was increased to 400 mg/day. Furosemide was simultaneously increased to 80 mg BID without major improvement in diuresis. Laboratory data revealed that R.W.'s SCr had increased to 3.2 mg/dL (estimated creatinine clearance: 26 mL/minute) and his BUN had increased to 45 mg/dL. Serum electrolytes were as follows:

K, 3.1 mEq/L
Na, 130 mEq/L
Cl, 88 mEq/L
Bicarbonate, 32 mEq/L

R.W. became progressively short of breath because of restricted diaphragmatic movement secondary to his significantly enlarged abdomen. What therapeutic measures are appropriate for R.W.'s refractory (diuretic-resistant) ascites?

The AASLD guidelines mention a few treatment options for refractory ascites. Midodrine 7.5 mg given 3 times daily to increase blood pressure in hypotensive patients could possibly convert diuretic-resistant patients to diuretic-sensitive. In addition, discontinuation of β-blockers is recommended since these drugs are associated with increased mortality in patients with refractory ascites. The guidelines also mention avoiding angiotensin converting enzyme inhibitors (ACEIs) and angiotensin receptor blockers (ARBs) because of the risk of hypotension.[38]

Because of the increase in SCr and respiratory distress, R.W.'s ascites treatment needs modification. Patients with cirrhosis experiencing respiratory distress despite diuretic therapy, sodium restriction, and appropriate management of hypotension (discontinuation of β-blockers and adding midodrine) may warrant more aggressive second-line treatment, including large-volume paracentesis, shunting procedures, or both.[38] Paracentesis involves the removal of ascitic fluid from the abdominal cavity with a needle or a catheter. Although paracentesis can remove large amounts of ascitic fluid (e.g., 10 L), removal of as little as 1 L of fluid may provide considerable relief from the painful stretching of skin and the respiratory distress that occurs with massive ascites. The ascitic fluid often re-accumulates rapidly after paracentesis. The major complications of overly aggressive, large-volume paracentesis include hypotension, shock, oliguria, encephalopathy, and renal insufficiency. Other potential complications of paracentesis are hemorrhage, perforation of the abdominal viscera, infection, and protein depletion.[38]

ALBUMIN

Case 25-1, Question 10: R.W. continues to re-accumulate ascitic fluid and is exhibiting signs of declining renal function. A 6-L paracentesis coupled with a 50-g albumin infusion is ordered. Why are albumin infusions used in conjunction with paracentesis?

Large-volume (>4 L) paracentesis should be performed for patients with tense ascites, resulting in respiratory distress or impaired ambulation. However, large-volume paracentesis is associated with paracentesis-induced circulatory dysfunction (PICD), which manifests clinically as worsening renal function 24 to 48 hours post-procedure.[72,73] Intravenous (IV) albumin infusions are commonly administered to prevent PICD after large-volume paracentesis.[38] Use of albumin in combination with large-volume paracentesis produces an expansion of circulating blood volume, increases cardiac output, and suppresses release of renin and norepinephrine.[73] Although albumin is costly and sometimes in short supply, for some patients it is appropriate with paracentesis.[74] In one study, patients requiring large-volume paracentesis (≥6 L/day) received either concomitant IV albumin (40 g) or saline. The incidence of PICD was significantly higher in the saline than the albumin group (33.3% vs. 11.4%, respectively). The prevalence of PICD after paracentesis depends on the volume of ascites removed such that albumin infusion may not be necessary for a single paracentesis <4 to 5 L.[38,74] For large-volume paracentesis greater than or equal to 6 L, 6 to 8 g of albumin is typically administered for each liter of ascites removed.[38]

Wilkes et al.[75] conducted a meta-analysis of 55 randomized, controlled trials evaluating the effects of albumin administration for a variety of indications on patient mortality. They found no improvement in mortality with albumin administration.[75] However, albumin administered to patients with spontaneous bacterial peritonitis lowered the incidence of renal impairment (10% vs. 33%; $p = 0.002$), overall mortality at 3 months (22% vs. 41%; $p = 0.03$), and hospital mortality (10% vs. 29%; $p = 0.01$) than the group that did not receive albumin.[76]

DEXTRAN 70 AND OTHER PLASMA EXPANDERS

The use of synthetic plasma expanders with large-volume paracentesis has also been explored in patients with refractory ascites.[77] Gines et al.[78] studied patients with ascites refractory to diuretic therapy, who required paracentesis. More patients treated with dextran 70 (34.4%) or polygeline (37.8%) experienced PICD than those receiving albumin (18.5%).[78] Hydroxyethyl starch, an effective colloid agent for intravascular volume expansion, should not be used in patients with cirrhosis, because repeated administration in this population has been reported to accumulate in the hepatocytes, causing severe portal hypertension and acute liver failure.[79]

R.W. should be given 50 g of 25% albumin administered at a rate of 3 mL/minute, for the 6 L of ascitic fluid removed. Albumin 25% infusion is preferred because 5% solution has fivefold the sodium load.[38] More rapid administration than 3 mL/minute in hypoproteinemic patients can cause circulatory overload and pulmonary edema. R.W. should be monitored for anaphylactic reactions (rare), hypotension, hypertension, and signs of pulmonary edema.[80–82]

Alternative Therapy

CASE 25-1, QUESTION 11: What alternative treatments are available for management of refractory ascites? How would these alternatives be applied in R.W.'s case?

TRANSJUGULAR INTRAHEPATIC PORTOSYSTEMIC SHUNT

Transjugular intrahepatic portosystemic shunt (TIPS) is another option for patients who are refractory to the pharmacologic interventions described previously. It is a nonsurgical technique for establishing a shunt in patients with portal hypertension (Fig. 25-2).[83] The TIPS procedure involves opening a conduit between the hepatic vein and the intrahepatic segment of the portal vein with an expandable metal stent placed during an angiographic procedure. This low-resistance channel allows blood to return to the systemic circulation and reduces portal pressure. In addition, TIPS may improve urinary sodium excretion. The major complications of TIPS include severe encephalopathy and shunt occlusion. Hepatic encephalopathy (see Case 25-3) occurs in approximately 20% of patients after TIPS.[83] Because of poor prognosis, liver transplantation should be considered for appropriate candidates refractory to pharmacologic treatment and/or shunt placement.[38] Selection of surgical shunt procedures may include evaluation of liver transplantation candidacy because some procedures may complicate the feasibility of a future liver transplantation procedure.

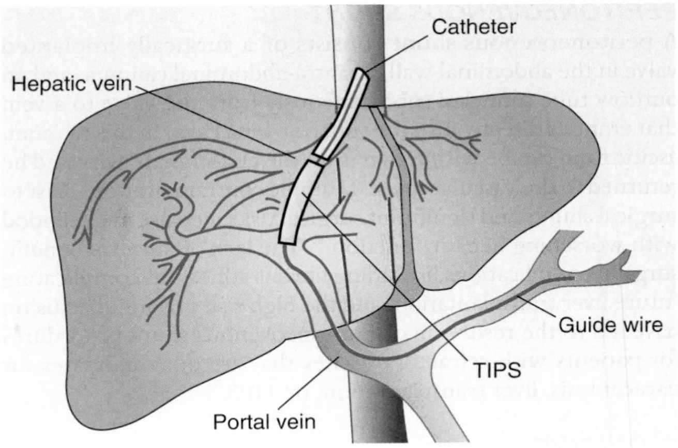

Figure 25-2 Transjugular intrahepatic portosystemic shunt (TIPS). A stent is inserted via catheter to the portal vein to divert blood flow and reduce portal hypertension. (Adapted with permission from Smeltzer SC, Bare BG. *Textbook of Medical-Surgical Nursing*. 9th ed. Philadelphia, PA: Lippincott Williams & Wilkins; 2000.)

In a small randomized study evaluating patients with cirrhosis and refractory ascites,[84] the probability of survival without liver transplantation was 41% at 1 year and 26% at 2 years in the TIPS group, as compared with 35% and 30%, respectively, in the paracentesis group (not significant [NS]). Recurrence of ascites and development of hepatorenal syndrome (49% and 9%, respectively) were lower in the TIPS group compared with the paracentesis group (83% and 31%, respectively; $p = 0.003$ and $p = 0.03$), whereas the frequency of severe hepatic encephalopathy was greater in the TIPS group ($p = 0.03$). The calculated costs of procedures performed per patient in the TIPS group were 103% greater than those in the paracentesis and albumin group.[84] Salerno et al.[85] conducted a meta-analysis of cirrhotic patients with refractory ascites and found that transplant-free survival was higher in the TIPS group (38.1% vs. 28.7% at 3 years; $p = 0.035$), and the recurrence of ascites was lower (42% vs. 89%; $p < 0.0001$) than in the large-volume paracentesis group. The average number of hepatic encephalopathy episodes was significantly higher in the TIPS group ($p = 0.006$). However, the probability of developing the first episode of hepatic encephalopathy was similar between the groups ($p = 0.19$).[85]

The AASLD guidelines mention that as the level of experience as well as technology with TIPS improves, the outcomes associated with TIPS in future trials may also improve.[38] Currently, the AASLD treatment guidelines continue to recommend TIPS for the treatment of refractory ascites in patients for whom paracentesis is contraindicated, ineffective as determined by the frequency of repeated paracentesis (more than 3 times per month), or intolerant of repeated large-volume paracentesis.[86]

PERITONEOVENOUS SHUNT

A peritoneovenous shunt consists of a surgically implanted valve in the abdominal wall, an intra-abdominal cannula, and an outflow tube tunneled subcutaneously from the valve to a vein that empties directly into the superior vena cava. In this manner, ascitic fluid can be withdrawn from the abdominal cavity and be returned to the vascular space. Multiple contraindications exist to surgical shunts and significant surgical risks increase in likelihood with worsening hepatic function.[87] The lack of survival benefit, surgical complications, including fibrous adhesions complicating future liver transplantation, and the high risk of shunt occlusion have led to the reserving of peritoneovenous shunt procedures for patients with refractory ascites that are not candidates for paracentesis, liver transplantation, or TIPS.[38]

CLONIDINE

It has been shown that the activation of the sympathetic nervous system leads to renal hypoperfusion and sodium retention. The activated sympathetic nervous system stimulates renal α_1-adrenoreceptors and causes decreases in renal blood flow and glomerular filtration rate. Additionally, norepinephrine increases proximal tubular reabsorption of sodium and enhances renin, aldosterone, and vasopressin secretions.[88–90] Preliminary evidence suggests that clonidine may be of benefit in refractory ascites and an activated sympathetic nervous system. Lenaerts et al.[91] conducted a very small study in patients randomly assigned to receive repeated large-volume paracentesis (4–5 L every 48 hours) plus IV albumin (7 g/L ascites) until ascites disappeared, or a combination of clonidine 0.075 mg BID for 8 days and then clonidine 0.075 mg BID with spironolactone 200 to 400 mg daily for 10 days. Both groups were discharged with spironolactone adjusted according to individual response. During the first hospitalization, the mean weight loss in the paracentesis group was higher than in the clonidine group, but the mean hospital stay was shorter in the clonidine group ($p \leq 0.01$). Clonidine decreased sympathetic activity and increased glomerular filtration rate. During the follow-up, the number of re-hospitalizations for ascites was higher and the mean time to the first readmission was shorter in the paracentesis group than in the clonidine group ($p \leq 0.01$).[91] In another trial, Lenaerts et al.[90] found that the time to first readmission for tense ascites was shorter in the placebo group than in the clonidine group. Both groups received spironolactone and furosemide.[90] The addition of clonidine to diuretic therapy may be an effective therapeutic modality; however, a large randomized trial is needed to establish the role of clonidine in the treatment of ascites. Currently, the use of clonidine is considered experimental by the AASLD guidelines.[38]

In consideration of R.W.'s increasing serum creatinine concentration, rising BUN, and the grave prognosis of hepatorenal syndrome, TIPS is a reasonable therapeutic alternative if R.W. cannot tolerate or requires frequent large-volume paracentesis. Patients with a history of spontaneous bacterial peritonitis (SBP) and ascites with advanced liver failure or renal impairment appear to benefit from SBP prophylaxis. R.W. would benefit from the addition of SBP prophylaxis because of his history of SBP (see Chapter 70, Intra-Abdominal Infections).

ESOPHAGEAL VARICES

Treatment

CASE 25-2

Question 1: C.V., a 55-year-old, pale-looking woman with alcohol-induced cirrhosis, was admitted for a chief complaint of hematemesis. C.V. has a history of recurrent upper GI bleeding and documented esophageal varices. She has no other significant medical history. She is not taking any medications and has no known drug allergies. On examination, her blood pressure (BP) was 78/40 mm Hg, pulse rate was 110 beats/minute, and respiratory rate was 22 breaths/minute. Her skin was cold; chest and cardiac examinations were within normal limits and abdominal examination revealed ascites and a palpable spleen. Bowel sounds were normal. Laboratory values included the following:

Hgb, 7 g/dL
Hct, 22%
Albumin, 3.0 g/dL
AST, 160 IU
ALT, 250 IU
Alkaline phosphatase, 40 IU
Creatinine, 2.0 mg/dL
PT, 18 seconds (INR, 1.5)
Serum electrolytes, all within normal limits

An electrocardiogram revealed sinus tachycardia. What are the immediate goals of therapy and treatment measures of the highest priority in managing C.V.'s hematemesis?

GOALS OF THERAPY

Most patients with cirrhosis develop portal hypertension, which in turn can progress to bleeding varices (dilated veins in the upper GI tract that protrude into the esophageal or gastric lumens). Of patients with Child–Turcotte–Pugh class A cirrhosis, 40% develop esophageal varices, as compared with 85% of those with Child–Turcotte–Pugh class C.[24,92] Unless varices bleed, they do not cause significant complications or symptoms.

The progression and severity of varices is directly related to the severity of portal hypertension. The major site of concern in portal hypertension is the coronary vein, draining the bottom of the esophagus and upper stomach. The scarring and fibrosis associated with cirrhosis initially leads to an increase in portal vein pressure (PVP), which may eventually rise, causing backflow of blood supply and subsequent increased pressure in the veins coming off the portal vein. Hyperkinetic circulation in the branches of the portal vein raises the esophageal trans-mural pressure and increases the risk of upper GI bleeding. Because the veins are designed for low-pressure circulation (5–8 mm Hg) and generally cannot tolerate a sustained hyperdynamic circulation, the shunting of high portal pressure blood results in gastric and esophageal varices. When PVP exceeds 12 mm Hg, patients are at increased risk of variceal hemorrhage.[93]

Varices can only be visualized during a diagnostic endoscopy. Esophageal varices are graded as small or large (>5 mm). The presence or absence of red signs (red wale marks or red spots) on varices is also noted.[92]

Despite improvement in the management of portal hypertension, massive bleeding from esophageal or gastric varices is the leading cause of death in patients with cirrhosis.[94] Prevention of variceal bleeding is critical because the mortality rate remains at 32% in Child–Turcotte–Pugh class C patients.[94] New varices develop at a rate of 5% to 10% per year in cirrhotic patients. Once varices develop, they enlarge by 4% to 10% each year.[95] Acute variceal bleeding is considered a medical emergency and should be treated immediately. Treatment goals include volume resuscitation, acute treatment of bleeding, and prevention of recurrence of variceal bleeding. Approximately 10% to 20% of patients are refractory to endoscopic and medical intervention and may require life-saving portal decompressive shunt surgery or TIPS.[24]

GENERAL MANAGEMENT

Resuscitation is the first priority in patients with acute bleeding episodes. An indwelling nasogastric tube (NG) should be placed, then saline or tap-water lavage of the stomach, with suctioning of the gastric contents, should be initiated promptly to prevent airway complications such as aspiration pneumonia.[83,96] Obtunded or unconscious patients should be intubated to maintain and protect the airway. Pharmacologic treatment should be initiated immediately to reduce bleeding and the risk of hypotension-induced renal failure. The patient should also be monitored for any abnormal electrolyte and metabolic chemistries (e.g., potassium, sodium, bicarbonate), hypoxia (e.g., Po_2, pH), serum creatinine, and decreased urinary output.[96]

Re-bleeding is most likely to occur within the first 2 to 5 days in patients with large varices and in patients with advanced liver disease (i.e., Child–Turcotte–Pugh class C, Table 25-1).[24,97] Factors associated with early re-bleeding include age greater than 60 years, acute renal failure, and severe initial bleeding defined by hemoglobin less than 8 g/dL at presentation. Risk factors for late re-bleeding are severe liver failure, continued alcohol abuse, large variceal size, renal failure, and hepatocellular carcinoma.[97]

HYPOVOLEMIA/BLOOD LOSS

Care should be taken when correcting hypovolemia so as not to increase the degree of portal hypertension by over-transfusion, which can increase the risk of further bleeding. Hypovolemia should be immediately managed to maintain a systolic blood pressure of 90 to 100 mm Hg and the hemoglobin at approximately 8 g/dL.[24,98] C.V.'s pallor, cold and clammy skin, rapid pulse, and a systolic BP less than 80 mm Hg suggest significant hypotension and hypovolemia needing correction with whole blood or packed red cell transfusion along with fresh frozen plasma.[92,97]

Patients with liver disease and elevated bilirubin frequently develop some level of vitamin K deficiency. Prolongation of the PT because of vitamin K deficiency usually improves within 24 hours after a 10 mg subcutaneous or oral dose of vitamin K (although evidence suggests parenteral repletion may be more reliable).[27] In contrast, a prolonged PT caused by poor liver function is not responsive to the administration of vitamin K. If the INR requires rapid correction because of bleeding or a planned invasive procedure, fresh frozen plasma should be transfused. Although vitamin K is often administered in the treatment of acute variceal bleeding, there is no data to support this practice.[99]

CASE 25-2, QUESTION 2: Three units of whole blood and two units of fresh frozen plasma were transfused initially. C.V.'s stomach was lavaged with saline, and the gastric aspirate from the NG tube continued to be strongly positive for blood. Four hours later, her bleeding still persisted. What other pharmacologic interventions can be used to control C.V.'s bleeding esophageal varices?

OCTREOTIDE

Octreotide is a synthetic analog of somatostatin, with similar pharmacologic properties and a slightly longer half-life. Somatostatin is available in Europe, but is substituted with octreotide or vapreotide (orphan drug status) in the United States (Table 25-2).[100–103] Octreotide is shown to be effective for controlling acute variceal bleeding and appears comparable in efficacy to vasopressin and balloon tamponade, with fewer side effects. Octreotide is administered as a 50 mcg bolus followed by an infusion of 50 mcg/hour for 3 to 5 days.[24] In one study, complete bleeding control was achieved in all patients receiving octreotide after 48 hours of therapy compared with 64% of vasopressin-treated patients, and 59% in the omeprazole groups ($p < 0.005$). Patients receiving vasopressin also experienced more side effects (abdominal cramps, nausea, tremor, decreased cardiac output, myocardial ischemia, and bronchial constriction) than those receiving octreotide or omeprazole ($p < 0.01$). In the patients with bleeding not controlled within 48 hours in the vasopressin and omeprazole groups, complete bleeding control was subsequently achieved by octreotide.[104] In a meta-analysis of octreotide and somatostatin versus vasopressin in the management of acute esophageal variceal bleeds, octreotide and somatostatin appeared to be more effective in controlling acute bleeding (82% vs. 55%; p = NS) and had fewer adverse effects requiring discontinuation than vasopressin (0% vs. 10%; $p = 0.00007$).[105] In general, octreotide is fairly well tolerated.[104] Although some centers may still initiate therapy with vasopressin, most will use octreotide as first-line therapy and reserve vasopressin for treatment failures.

VASOPRESSIN

Vasopressin, a naturally occurring hormone (also known as 8-arginine vasopressin, ADH), is produced by the posterior pituitary and was originally derived for the treatment of diabetes insipidus in persons with pituitary insufficiency.[100,101] Its use to control variceal bleeding is a non-FDA-labeled use that takes advantage of its intense smooth muscle vasoconstrictive properties. Vasopressin (Table 25-2) is effective in reducing or terminating bleeding in approximately 60% of patients with variceal hemorrhage.[100,101] Of concern are reports of patients developing hypertension, angina, arrhythmias, and, rarely, myocardial infarction while receiving vasopressin. Vasopressin is given as a continuous IV infusion because of its short half-life. To minimize dose-related adverse effects, the lowest effective dosage should be used. Vasopressin may be administered by peripheral IV infusion, but use of a central vein is preferred because of the risk of tissue necrosis if extravasation occurs. Most commonly, vasopressin is initiated as a continuous IV infusion of 0.2 to 0.4 units/minute, and increased every hour by 0.2 units/minute until control of bleeding is obtained (maximal dose 0.8 units/minute).[92] Approximately 12 hours after the control of bleeding, the infusion rate can be decreased by half. Higher doses should be avoided because dosages exceeding 1 unit/minute fail to control hemorrhage in patients who are unresponsive to lower dosages.[106] Because of the potential for serious cardiovascular and dermatologic complications caused by nonspecific vasoconstriction, vasopressin should be used only when necessary and for a duration necessary to control bleeding. The duration of infusion should not exceed 24 hours.[92] Interestingly, a meta-analysis of four randomized controlled trials comparing vasopressin for the acute treatment of variceal bleeding with non-active treatment or placebo found no difference in mortality.[100] Since efficacy of vasopressin for treatment of esophageal bleeding is limited and adverse effects (e.g., abdominal cramping, arrhythmias, and gangrene) are of great concern (Table 25-2), it has largely been replaced by octreotide. Nonetheless, some clinicians still prescribe vasopressin.

Nitroglycerin can help to minimize the adverse vascular and cardiac effects of vasopressin and enhance the reduction in portal pressure. When given by IV infusion, the nitroglycerin dosage is 40 to 200 mcg/minute.[100,102,107] A randomized trial by Gimson et al.[108] found a lower rate of complications in the vasopressin and nitroglycerin group compared with vasopressin alone. At the end of the 12-hour study period, variceal hemorrhage was controlled in 68% receiving combined therapy versus 44% in those given vasopressin alone ($p < 0.05$). Major complications requiring cessation of therapy were less common in those given nitroglycerin compared with those given vasopressin alone ($p < 0.02$).[108]

TERLIPRESSIN

Terlipressin, a synthetic analog of vasopressin and a pro-drug of lypressin (currently not available in the United States), effectively

Table 25-2
Treatment of Acute Bleeding

Therapy	Mechanism	Side Effects and Risks
Octreotide	Selective and potent vasoconstrictor that reduces portal and collateral blood flow by constricting splanchnic vessels	Diarrhea, hyperglycemia, hypoglycemia, constipation, rectal spasms, abnormal stools, headache, dizziness, fat malabsorption
Vasopressin	Nonspecific vasoconstrictor of all parts of the vascular bed	Abdominal cramping, nausea, tremor, skin blanching, phlebitis, hematoma at the site of the infusion, worsening of hypertension, angina, arrhythmias, myocardial infarction, bowel necrosis, gangrene, dilutional hyponatremia
Endoscopic variceal ligation (EVL)	An elastic band is placed around the mucosa and submucosa of the esophageal area containing the varix, leading to strangulation, fibrosis, and ideally obliteration of the varix	Moderate bleeding, hypotension, gastrointestinal discomfort, esophageal ulceration, perforation
Sclerotherapy	Injection of 0.5–5 mL of a sclerosing agent (e.g., concentrated saline: 11.5% NaCl or ethanolamine oleate) into each varix at points about 2 cm apart to induce immediate hemostasis (cessation of bleeding within 2 to 5 minutes)	Esophageal ulceration, stricture formation, esophageal perforation, retrosternal chest pain, temporary dysphagia
Balloon tamponade	Bleeding is controlled by direct compression of the varices at the gastroesophageal junction or at the bleeding site by a Sengstaken–Blakemore tube or Linton tube (gastric varices only). The tube is passed through the mouth and into the stomach. A balloon is then inflated, which applies direct compression to the varices	Aspiration (>10% incidence), pressure necrosis, pneumonitis, esophageal ulceration and rupture, bleeding on balloon deflation, chest pain, asphyxia (aspiration may be minimized by endotracheal intubation and continued aspiration of oropharyngeal secretions)
Transjugular intrahepatic portal systemic shunt (TIPS)	A conduit between the hepatic vein and the intrahepatic segment of the portal vein with an expandable metal stent is placed during an angiographic procedure. This channel allows blood to return to the systemic circulation and reduces portal pressure	Bleeding, thrombosis, stenosis, severe encephalopathy, hepatic failure, shunt occlusion, shunt migration

Sources: Goulis J, Burroughs AK. Role of vasoactive drugs in the treatment of bleeding oesophageal varices. *Digestion*. 1999;60(Suppl 3):25; Wao T et al. Effect of vasopressin on esophageal varices blood flow in patients with cirrhosis: comparisons with the effects on portal vein and superior mesenteric artery blood flow. *J Hepatol*. 1996;25:491; Law AW, Gales MA. Octreotide or vasopressin for bleeding esophageal varices. *Ann Pharmacother*. 1997;31:237; de Franchis R. Longer treatment with vasoactive drugs to prevent early variceal re-bleeding in cirrhosis. *Eur J Gastroenterol Hepatol*. 1998;10:1041.

controls acute bleeding from esophageal varices in 80% of patients. Fewer cardiovascular side effects have been associated with terlipressin than with vasopressin.[109] Octreotide, vapreotide, vasopressin, and terlipressin have been shown to be effective in the control of acute variceal hemorrhage.[110,111] Terlipressin, however, is the only medication for the acute treatment of variceal hemorrhage that has been shown to improve patient survival. In a meta-analysis of seven randomized, placebo-controlled trials, terlipressin led to significant reductions in mortality as compared with placebo (relative risk [RR], 0.66; 95% CI, 0.49–0.88).[112]

Pharmacologic therapy for C.V. (somatostatin or its analogs [octreotide or vapreotide] or terlipressin) should be initiated as soon as variceal hemorrhage is suspected and continued for 3 to 5 days after diagnosis is confirmed.[92]

ENDOSCOPIC VARICEAL LIGATION AND SCLEROTHERAPY

CASE 25-2, QUESTION 3: Octreotide and vasopressin are nonspecific vasoconstrictors that require continuous IV infusion and carry a risk of systemic side effects. What is the place of endoscopic variceal ligation and sclerotherapy in the management of C.V.'s hemorrhage? What is a balloon tamponade? Are alternative therapies such as TIPS appropriate?

After successful resuscitation, endoscopy should be performed within 12 hours to establish the cause of bleeding.[92] Fiberoptic endoscopy allows direct visualization of the esophagus and location of the bleeding. Those with actively bleeding varices can be treated with endoscopic variceal ligation (EVL), sclerotherapy, or balloon tamponade. EVL is a well-tolerated procedure (Table 25-2).[110,113–117] Villanueva et al.,[118] in a randomized, controlled trial, found that the use of variceal ligation instead of sclerotherapy had a lower failure rate (4% vs. 15%; $p = 0.02$) and a lower transfusion requirement ($p = 0.05$). No statistically significant differences were found in mortality. Adverse effects (e.g., aspiration pneumonia, esophageal bleeding, ulceration, and chest pain) occurred in 28% of patients receiving sclerotherapy and 14% with ligation (RR, 1.9; 95% CI, 1.1–3.5; $p = 0.03$).[118] In another similar but smaller study, Sarin et al.[119] found that the rate of re-bleeding was lower in the EVL group than in the sclerotherapy group (6.4% vs. 20.8%; $p < 0.05$). EVL is the recommended form of therapy for acute esophageal variceal bleeding, although sclerotherapy may be used in the acute setting if ligation is technically difficult. Endoscopic treatments are best used in combination with pharmacologic therapy, which preferably should be started before endoscopy.[111] The AASLD Practice Guidelines Committee and the Practice Parameters Committee of the American College of Gastroenterology (ACG) on the Prevention and Management of Gastroesophageal Varices and Variceal Hemorrhage in Cirrhosis recommend that for the control and management of acute hemorrhage, the combination of vasoconstrictive pharmacologic therapy and variceal ligation is the preferred approach.[92] Therefore, C.V. should immediately be treated with octreotide for 3 to 5 days, and EVL to control the esophageal variceal bleeding.[24,92]

BALLOON TAMPONADE

Balloon tamponade is used to control bleeding by direct compression to the site of origin in massive hemorrhage cases (Table 25-2). It is important to remember that balloon tamponade is only a temporary measure and can cause pressure necrosis after 48 to 72 hours. Thus, the balloon should be deflated after 12 to 24 hours. Deflation and removal of the tube can result in removal of the fibrin scab at the bleeding site, resulting in re-bleeding. Balloon tamponade will achieve temporary control of the bleeding and allow time for other measures (e.g., EVL or sclerotherapy) to be undertaken.[92,110,120,121]

ALTERNATIVE TREATMENT MODALITIES

Transjugular Intrahepatic Portal Systemic Shunt

Although the combination of pharmacotherapy (octreotide, terlipressin, or somatostatin) and endoscopic procedures (EVL or sclerotherapy) has been shown to be beneficial in controlling acute bleeding, re-bleeding episodes can occur.[92,110] Poor responders to initial therapy may require further intervention to lower portal pressure and control the bleeding.

Henderson et al.[122] conducted a prospective, multicenter trial comparing distal splenorenal shunt (DSRS) to TIPS for variceal bleeding refractory to medical treatment with β-blockers and endoscopic therapy. Patients with Child–Turcotte–Pugh class A and class B cirrhosis and refractory variceal bleeding were randomly assigned to DSRS or TIPS. No significant differences were found in survival at 2 and 5 years (DSRS, 81% and 62%; TIPS, 88% and 61%, respectively). Thrombosis, stenosis, and re-intervention rates were significantly higher in the TIPS group (DSRS, 11%; TIPS, 82%; $p < 0.001$). Re-bleeding, encephalopathy, ascites, need for transplantation, quality of life, and costs did not significantly differ between groups.[122] TIPS has the advantage of being less invasive and faster than surgical portal systemic shunts. Long-term patency of the TIPS remains problematic (Table 25-2). TIPS can be used as a bridge to liver transplantation, and might be an effective option for nonsurgical patients or those with advanced cirrhosis (Child–Turcotte–Pugh class C) with recurrent bleeding, uncontrolled by pharmacologic and endoscopic therapy.[86,92,110,123,124] TIPS would be an option for C.V. if EVL and pharmacologic therapy fail.

Surgery

Surgical creation of a portacaval shunt has been effective in reducing portal pressure and in preventing recurrent bleeding. These shunts, however, are associated with a high incidence of hepatic encephalopathy and may exacerbate hepatic parenchymal dysfunction by shunting blood away from the liver. Mesocaval shunts and distal splenorenal shunts are also effective in preventing variceal re-bleeding and may be associated with a lower incidence of hepatic encephalopathy.[125]

INFECTION PROPHYLAXIS: SHORT-TERM ANTIBIOTICS

CASE 25-2, QUESTION 4: Should C.V. receive prophylaxis for bacterial infections?

Variceal hemorrhage is a risk factor for the development of severe bacterial infections, which increase mortality.[92] Short-term administration of antibiotics for the prevention of bacterial infections in patients with variceal hemorrhage has demonstrated favorable results.[126,127] In a prospective, randomized trial comparing norfloxacin 400 mg BID for 7 days ($n = 60$) with no treatment controls ($n = 59$), the norfloxacin group had a significantly lower incidence of spontaneous bacterial peritonitis (SBP, 3.3% vs. 16.9%; $p < 0.05$); although the decrease in mortality (6.6% vs. 11.8%) did not reach statistical significance.[126] Because of the emergence of infections caused by quinolone-resistant bacteria, Fernandez et al.[127] compared oral norfloxacin versus IV ceftriaxone in the prophylaxis against bacterial infection in cirrhotic patients with GI hemorrhage. Patients were randomly assigned to oral norfloxacin 400 mg BID or IV ceftriaxone 1 g/day for 7 days. Antibiotics were initiated after emergency endoscopy and within 12 hours of hospital admission. The probability of developing proven infections (26% vs. 11%; $p < 0.03$), and bacteremia or spontaneous bacterial peritonitis (12% vs. 2%, $p < 0.03$) was significantly higher in patients receiving norfloxacin as compared with ceftriaxone. No significant difference was seen between groups in mortality at 10 days.[127] A Cochrane review of 12 trials evaluating the role of antibiotic prophylaxis with placebo or no antibiotic prophylaxis to prevent bacterial infections in cirrhotic patients with upper gastrointestinal bleeding reported that antibiotic prophylaxis was associated with a significant decrease in mortality from bacterial infections (RR, 0.43; 95% CI, 0.19–0.97).[128]

The AASLD guidelines recommend 7 days of antibiotic prophylaxis for prevention of SBP in patients with variceal hemorrhage with oral norfloxacin (400 mg BID) or ceftriaxone IV (1 g/day; when oral administration is not possible).[38] C.V. should be treated with norfloxacin 400 mg orally once daily (dose adjusted for creatinine clearance of 30 mL/minute), or ceftriaxone 1 g/day for 7 days to prevent SBP.

PRIMARY PROPHYLAXIS

CASE 25-2, QUESTION 5: All variceal hemorrhage interventions up to this point were aimed at terminating the acute bleeding episode. Could drug therapy have helped prevent the first episode of bleeding from C.V.'s esophageal varices?

Preventing the initial occurrence of variceal bleeding is referred to as primary prevention or primary prophylaxis. Pharmacologic prophylaxis is aimed at reducing the HVPG to $\leq$12 mm Hg, or a decrease from baseline of $\geq$20%.[129,130] In a small study by Vorobioff et al.,[129] none of the patients with HVPG $\leq$12 mm Hg bled from portal hypertensive-related causes as compared to 42% in the HVPG >12 mm Hg group. In addition, only one of the six patients with a HVPG less <12 mm Hg as compared with 16 (of 24) in the HVPG >12 mm Hg group died during the study period ($p < 0.06$).[129] In addition, Escorsell et al.[130] confirmed that a fall of HVPG by 20% or more from baseline was associated with a decreased risk of variceal bleeding (6% vs. 45%; $p = 0.004$).

β-Blockers

Nonselective β-adrenergic blockers decrease portal pressure through a reduction in portal venous inflow as a result of a decrease in cardiac output (β_1-adrenergic blockade) and splanchnic blood flow (β_2-adrenergic blockade). Only nonselective β-blockers have an adrenergic vasoconstrictive effect on mesenteric arterioles, resulting in a decrease in portal pressure. Usual starting dosages of propranolol are 10 mg 3 times a day, or nadolol 20 mg daily. Selective β-blockers (e.g., atenolol and metoprolol) have little effect on mesenteric arterioles and have not been shown to be effective in primary prophylaxis.[131]

Propranolol or nadolol, given in dosages to reduce the resting heart rate to 55 to 60 beats/minute or by 25%, have been shown to prevent or delay the first episode of variceal bleeding.[15] Nonselective β-blockers are considered first-line drug therapy in the prevention of variceal hemorrhage based on numerous randomized, placebo-controlled trials and meta-analyses.[110,132] For example, Pascal et al.[133] conducted a prospective, randomized, multicenter, single-blinded trial of propranolol compared with placebo in the prevention of bleeding in patients with large esophageal varices without previous bleeding. Patients received either propranolol or placebo, with the endpoints of the study being bleeding and death. The dosage of propranolol was progressively increased to decrease the heart rate by 20% to 25%. The cumulative percentages of patients free of bleeding 2 years after inclusion in the study (74% vs. 39%; $p < 0.05$) and cumulative 2-year survival (72% vs. 51%; $p < 0.05$) were higher in the propranolol compared to the placebo group.[133]

Sarin et al.[134] conducted a prospective, randomized, controlled trial comparing EVL plus propranolol with EVL alone as primary prophylaxis for prevention of first variceal bleeding among patients with high-risk varices. The mean duration of follow-up for both groups was about 12.2 months (±10.7 months). EVL was performed at 2-week intervals until obliteration of varices. Propranolol was administered at a dosage sufficient to reduce heart rate to 55 beats/minute or 25% reduction from baseline, and continued after obliteration of varices. No significant differences were seen in the rates of bleeding and survival between groups, although more patients in the EVL alone group had recurrence of varices ($p = 0.03$).[134]

In a prospective, randomized, double-blind, placebo-controlled trial of propranolol for the primary prevention of variceal hemorrhage, Abraczinskas et al.[135] found that when propranolol was tapered off, the risk of variceal hemorrhage increased from 4% (while on propranolol therapy) to 24% (after propranolol withdrawal), and was comparable to the risk of bleeding in an untreated population (22% in the placebo group from the previous study). Importantly, patients who abruptly discontinued β-blockers experienced increased mortality compared with the untreated population (48% vs. 21%; $p < 0.05$).[135] Therefore, avoiding sudden discontinuation of β-blockers in this population is essential.

The AASLD/ACG guidelines recommend nonselective β-blockers for primary prophylaxis in patients with small varices that have not bled, but are at increased risk of hemorrhage (Child–Turcotte–Pugh class B or C or presence of red wale marks on varices). Patients with medium or large varices that have not bled but are at a high risk of hemorrhage (Child–Turcotte–Pugh class B or C or variceal red wale markings on endoscopy), nonselective β-blockers or EVL may be recommended. In contrast, patients with medium or large varices that have not bled and are not at the highest risk of hemorrhage (Child–Turcotte–Pugh class A patients and no red signs), nonselective β-blockers are preferred and EVL should be considered in patients with contraindications, intolerance, or noncompliance to β-blockers. The β-blocker should be titrated to the maximal tolerated dose.[92]

Isosorbide-5-Mononitrate

Isosorbide-5-mononitrate monotherapy for primary prophylaxis for variceal hemorrhage has not proven to be effective.[136,137] Garcia-Pagan et al.[137] conducted a prospective, multicenter, double-blind, randomized, controlled trial evaluating whether isosorbide-5-mononitrate prevented variceal bleeding in cirrhotic patients with gastroesophageal varices, who had contraindications or could not tolerate β-blockers. Patients received isosorbide-5-mononitrate or placebo. No significant differences were noted in the 1- and 2-year actuarial probability of bleeding or survival between the two treatment groups.[137]

When combined with a β-blocker, isosorbide-5-mononitrate caused a greater reduction in the hepatic venous pressure gradient than propranolol alone.[138] Merkel et al.[139] examined the value of combining nadolol and isosorbide-5-mononitrate for primary prevention of variceal bleeding. Patients in the nadolol monotherapy group received between 40 and 160 mg/day titrated to achieve a 20% to 25% decrease in resting heart rate. Patients in the combination group received nadolol and isosorbide-5-mononitrate 10 to 20 mg orally BID. The overall risk of variceal bleeding was 18% in the nadolol group compared with 7.5% in the combined treatment group ($p = 0.03$). However, a higher number of patients had to be withdrawn from the combination therapy group compared with the nadolol monotherapy group (eight vs. four patients) because of side effects.[139] The AASLD and ACG guidelines suggest that nitrates (either alone or in combination with β-blockers), shunt therapy, or sclerotherapy should not be used in the primary prophylaxis of variceal hemorrhage.[92]

Depending on the size of C.V.'s varices on endoscopy and the risk of hemorrhage, C.V. should have been given propranolol 10 mg 3 times a day or nadolol 20 mg daily titrated to reduce the resting heart rate to 55 to 60 beats/minute (or by 25%), or EVL to prevent or delay the first episode of variceal bleeding.

SECONDARY PROPHYLAXIS

CASE 25-2, QUESTION 6: C.V.'s hepatologist would like to start treatment to prevent further variceal hemorrhage. What are the long-term objectives for the treatment of C.V.? What treatment approaches can be used to prevent a recurrence of bleeding (secondary prevention)?

Secondary prevention or secondary prophylaxis is when therapy is used to prevent re-bleeding once it has occurred. All patients who survive a variceal bleeding episode should receive therapy to prevent recurrent episodes. It is important that the initiation of β-blockers be delayed until after recovery of the initial variceal hemorrhage. Initiation of a β-blocker during the treatment of an acute bleed would block the patient's acute tachycardia in response to his or her hypotension, which may adversely impact survival. The benefit of nonselective β-blockers in the prevention of re-bleeding episodes has been demonstrated by a number of trials.[113,140,141] For example, Colombo et al.[140] randomized cirrhotic patients with a history of variceal hemorrhage to propranolol, atenolol, or placebo. Oral propranolol was titrated until the resting pulse rate was reduced by ~25%, and atenolol was given at a fixed dose of 100 mg daily. The incidence of re-bleeding was significantly lower in patients receiving propranolol than those receiving placebo ($p = 0.01$). Bleeding-free survival was higher for patients on active drugs than for those on placebo (propranolol vs. placebo, $p = 0.01$; atenolol vs. placebo, $p = 0.05$).[140]

Eradication of varices by endoscopic procedures is also effective in preventing recurrent variceal bleeding.[15,141] A study by de la Pena et al.[141] showed that nadolol plus EVL ($n = 43$) reduced the incidence of variceal re-bleeding compared with EVL alone ($n = 37$). Variceal bleeding recurrence rate was 14% in the EVL plus nadolol group and 38% in the EVL alone group ($p = 0.006$). Mortality was similar in both groups and the actuarial probability of variceal recurrence at 1 year was lower in the EVL plus nadolol group than in the EVL alone group (54% vs. 77%; $p = 0.06$). The adverse effects in the β-blocker group were higher, and led to the withdrawal of 20% to 30% of the patients.[141]

A meta-analysis of randomized trials[142] reported that compared with EVL alone, EVL combined with β-blockers ± isosorbide mononitrate reduced overall re-bleeding (32% vs. 17%, respectively; $p < 0.01$) with no significant difference in mortality or complications. When comparing drug therapy alone to combination therapy with EVL and β-blockers ± isosorbide mononitrate, combination therapy showed a trend toward lower re-bleeding (29% vs. 37%, respectively; NS), but no effect on mortality. Combination therapy with EVL plus β-blockers ± isosorbide mononitrate is effective in preventing re-bleeding. Drug therapy alone is an alternative.[142]

TIPS is an option for those patients who fail both EVL and prophylaxis with β-blocker therapy. In a randomized study of Child–Turcotte–Pugh class B and C cirrhotic patients surviving their first episode of variceal hemorrhage, Escorsell et al.[143] reported a lower rate of re-bleeding (13% vs. 39%; $p = 0.007$) and higher rate of encephalopathy (38% vs. 14%, $p = 0.007$) in patients treated with TIPS versus those treated with the combination of propranolol and isosorbide-5-mononitrate. The 2-year re-bleeding probability was also lower in the TIPS group (13% vs. 49%; $p = 0.01$). Of note, drug therapy improved the Child–Turcotte–Pugh class more frequently than with TIPS (72% vs. 45%; $p = 0.04$) and at lower costs.[143]

The AASLD/ACG guidelines suggest the use of a combination of nonselective β-blockers plus EVL for secondary prophylaxis. TIPS should be considered in patients who are Child–Turcotte–Pugh class A or B who experience recurrent variceal hemorrhage despite combination pharmacological and endoscopic therapy.[86,92]

Since C.V. has a history of recurrent upper GI bleeding, the best option to prevent further bleeding is to initiate a nonselective β-blocker and begin EVL. The β-blocker should be titrated to reduce the resting heart rate to 55 to 60 beats/minute or by 25%. EVL should be repeated every 1 to 2 weeks until obliteration with a repeat endoscopy performed 1 to 3 months after obliteration and then every 6 to 12 months to check for variceal recurrence.[92] If this combination fails to prevent variceal hemorrhage, then TIPS would be considered as a therapeutic option.[86]

HEPATIC ENCEPHALOPATHY

CASE 25-3

QUESTION 1: R.C., a 57-year-old man, was admitted to the hospital because of nausea, vomiting, and abdominal pain. He had a long history of alcohol abuse, with multiple hospital admissions for alcoholic gastritis and alcohol withdrawal. Physical examination revealed a cachectic male patient (weighing 55 kg) with clouded mentation, who was not responsive to questions about name and place. Tense ascites and edema were noted, and the liver was percussed at 9 cm below the right costal margin. The spleen was not palpated, and no active bowel sounds were heard. Laboratory results on admission included the following:

Na, 132 mEq/L
K, 3.7 mEq/L
Cl, 98 mEq/L
Bicarbonate, 27 mEq/L
BUN, 24 mg/dL
SCr, 1.4 mg/dL
Hgb, 9.2 g/dL
Hct, 24.1%
AST, 520 IU
Alkaline phosphatase, 218 IU
Lactate dehydrogenase (LDH), 305 IU
Total bilirubin, 3.5 mg/dL
PT, 22 seconds (INR, 1.8)

A 70-g protein, 2,000-kcal diet was ordered. Furosemide 40 mg IV every 12 hours was ordered in an attempt to reduce the edema and ascites. Morphine sulfate and prochlorperazine were ordered for his abdominal pain and nausea, respectively. Two days after admission, R.C. had an episode of hematemesis. He became mentally confused and at times nonresponsive to verbal command. An NG tube was inserted and coffee-ground material was produced on continuous suctioning. Saline lavage was continued until the aspirate became clear. The next morning, R.C. was still in a confused mental state. He demonstrated prominent asterixis, and fetor hepaticus was noted on his breath. On the second day of his hospitalization, laboratory data were as follows:

Hgb, 7.4 g/dL
Hct, 21.2%
K, 3.1 mEq/L
SCr, 1.4 mg/dL
BUN, 36 mg/dL
PT, 22 seconds (INR, 1.8)
Guaiac positive stool

Hepatic encephalopathy and upper GI bleeding were added to his problem list.

What aspects of R.C.'s history are compatible with a diagnosis of hepatic encephalopathy? What classification of hepatic encephalopathy does he fall into?

Hepatic encephalopathy (HE) is a spectrum of central nervous system (CNS) abnormalities ranging from subclinical alterations to coma and caused by advanced liver disease and/or portosystemic shunting of blood. According to the guidelines by the American Association for the Study of Liver Diseases (AALSD) and the European Association for the Study of the Liver (EASL) for HE in Chronic Liver Disease, HE is classified according to four criteria: (1) underlying disease (Acute Liver Failure [Type A]; resulting from portosystemic bypass or shunting [Type B]; from cirrhosis [Type C]), (2) severity of manifestations, (3) according to time course (episodic, recurrent, or persistent HE), and (4) according to precipitating factors (nonprecipitated or precipitated).[144]

The gold standard to measure the severity of HE is by the West Haven Criteria (WHC), and patients with significant altered consciousness by the Glasgow Coma Scale (GCS). For more detail on WHC criteria and GCS, please refer to the AASLD/EASL 2014 guidelines at aasld.org (https://www.aasld.org/sites/default/files/guideline_documents/141022_AASLD_Guideline_Encephalopathy_4UFd_2015.pdf). The ISHEN (International Society for Hepatic Encephalopathy and Nitrogen Metabolism) consensus classifies patients as having Minimal Hepatic Encephalopathy (MHE) and Grade I hepatic encephalopathy (WHC) as Covert Hepatic Encephalopathy (CHE), whereas those with apparent clinical abnormalities as Overt Hepatic Encephalopathy (OHE). The ISHEN consensus defines the onset of disorientation or asterixis as the onset of OHE.[145] This chapter will focus on the treatment of OHE in cirrhosis.

During the early phase of HE, the altered mental state may present as a slight derangement of judgment, and change in personality, sleep pattern, or mood. Drowsiness and confusion become more prominent as the HE progresses. Finally, unresponsiveness to arousal and deep coma ensue. Asterixis, or flapping tremor, is often present in the early to middle stages of HE that precede stupor or coma.[144]

The clinical features (as seen in R.C.) include altered mental state and asterixis. He is classified as having OHE, Type C, Grade III, Episodic, Precipitated (by upper GI bleed; see Question 3).

Asterixis can be demonstrated by having the patient hyperextend his or her wrist with the forearms outstretched and fingers separated. It is characterized by bilateral, synchronous, repetitive arrhythmic motions occurring in bursts of one flap (twitch) every

1 to 2 seconds. Asterixis is not specific for HE and may also be present in uremia, hypokalemia, heart failure, ketoacidosis, respiratory failure, and sedative overdose.[144]

As discussed in the questions that follow, the pharmacologic management of HE is guided by both an understanding of the pathogenesis of this disorder and the stage of severity demonstrated by the individual patient. In most cases, HE is fully reversible; therefore, it is likely a metabolic or neurophysiologic rather than an organic disorder.[144] Severe, progressive HE can lead to irreversible brain damage (caused by increased intracranial pressure), brain herniation, and death.[144,146,147]

Pathogenesis

CASE 25-3, QUESTION 2: What is the pathogenesis of hepatic encephalopathy?

Several theories exist about the pathogenesis of HE. The most widely referenced theories involve abnormal ammonia metabolism; altered ratio of branched chain to aromatic amino acids; imbalance in brain neurotransmitters, such as γ-aminobutyric acid (GABA) and serotonin; derangement in the blood brain–barrier; and exposure of the brain to accumulated "toxins."[148] The pathogenesis of HE is likely multifactorial.

AMMONIA

Ammonia is a byproduct of dietary protein metabolism or digestion of protein-rich blood in the GI tract (e.g., from bleeding esophageal varices). Bacteria present in the GI tract digest protein into polypeptides, amino acids, and ammonia. These substances are then absorbed across the intestinal mucosa. Ammonia is readily metabolized in the liver to urea, which is then renally eliminated. However, when blood flow and hepatic metabolism are impaired by cirrhosis, serum and CNS concentrations of ammonia are increased. The ammonia that enters the CNS combines with α-ketoglutarate to form glutamine, an aromatic amino acid. Ammonia has been considered central to the pathogenesis of HE. An increased ammonia level raises the amount of glutamine within astrocytes, causing an osmotic imbalance, cell swelling, and ultimately brain edema. Although high serum ammonia and cerebrospinal glutamine concentrations are characteristic of encephalopathy, they may not be the actual cause of this syndrome.[147,149] According to the AALSD/EASL guidelines, high ammonia levels alone may not add any diagnostic, staging, or prognostic value. However, if a level is normal, the diagnosis of HE should be questioned. In the case where ammonia-lowering drugs are used (e.g., lactulose), repeated measurements of ammonia would be beneficial to assess their efficacy.[144]

AMINO ACID BALANCE

In both acute and chronic liver failure, the ratio of the branched chain to aromatic amino acids is altered. Because of the higher permeability of aromatic amino acid across the blood–brain barrier and into the cerebrospinal fluid, some aromatic compounds can lead to production of "false neurotransmitters" that can lead to hepatic encephalopathy with altered mental status (see Chapter 38, Adult Parenteral Nutrition).[148,149]

γ-AMINOBUTYRIC ACID

Schafer et al.[150] proposed that in liver disease, gut-derived GABA escapes hepatic metabolism, crosses the blood–brain barrier, binds to its postsynaptic receptor sites, and causes the neurologic abnormalities associated with HE. Others hypothesize that endogenous benzodiazepine-like substances, via their agonist properties, contribute to the pathogenesis of hepatic encephalopathy by enhancing GABA-ergic neurotransmission. The role of GABA and endogenous benzodiazepines in HE is still not clearly defined.[151,152]

Of all the toxins suspected to cause hepatic coma, ammonia and certain aromatic amino acids are most commonly studied. Other precipitating factors include infections, electrolyte disorders, GI bleeding, constipation, and over diuresis. These factors may increase the serum ammonia and precipitate an exacerbation of HE.[144,153,154]

CASE 25-3, QUESTION 3: What are the probable precipitating causes of hepatic encephalopathy in R.C.?

The main precipitating cause of HE in R.C. was the sudden onset of upper GI bleeding. The bacterial degradation of blood in the gut results in absorption of large amounts of ammonia and possibly other toxins into the portal system. Other important contributory factors in this case are diuretic-induced hypovolemia (BUN:SCr ratio >20), hypokalemia (potassium, 3.1 mEq/L), and potentially metabolic alkalosis (continuous NG suctioning and furosemide). Overzealous diuretic therapy increases HE by inducing pre-renal azotemia, hypokalemia, and metabolic alkalosis. Alkalosis promotes diffusion of nonionic ammonia and other amines into the CNS. The associated intracellular acidosis "traps" the ammonia by converting it back to ammonium ion (NH_4^+).[155,156]

Sedating drugs such as opioids (e.g., morphine, methadone, meperidine, codeine), sedatives (e.g., benzodiazepines, barbiturates, chloral hydrate), and tranquilizers (e.g., phenothiazines) can also precipitate HE. Encephalopathy precipitated by most drugs can be explained by increased CNS sensitivity and decreased hepatic clearance with subsequent drug and, in some cases, active metabolite accumulation. For R.C., the morphine and prochlorperazine might have contributed to the worsening of his HE. Although not applicable to this case, excessive dietary protein, infections, and constipation can also contribute to excess nitrogen load and hepatic coma.

Treatment and General Management

CASE 25-3, QUESTION 4: What nondrug steps should be taken to manage R.C.'s hepatic encephalopathy?

Correcting the precipitating factor underlying the episode of OHE can improve mental status in 90% of patients.[144] After identifying and removing precipitating causes of HE, therapeutic management is aimed primarily at reducing the amount of ammonia or nitrogenous products in the circulatory system. The 2013 ISHEN guidelines recommend an energy intake of 35 to 40 kcal/kg of body weight/day and a protein intake of 1.2 to 1.5 g/kg of ideal body weight/day for cirrhotic patients and those awaiting liver transplantation surgeries.[157–160] A study conducted by Cordoba et al.[161] randomized patients with cirrhosis and HE to two dietary groups for 14 days. The first group followed a progressive increase in the dose of protein receiving 0 g of protein for the first 3 days, then the protein was increased progressively every 3 days (12, 24, and 48 g) up to 1.2 g/kg/day for the last 2 days. The second group received 1.2 g/kg/day from the first day. Results showed that the course of HE was not significantly different between groups. The patients in the first group, however, experienced a higher degree of protein breakdown.[161]

R.C. is a cachectic male, and care should be taken in providing nutrition to malnourished patients. The 70-g protein, 2,000-kcal diet ordered for R.C. is appropriate because it falls within the recommended weight-based ranges established by the ISHEN guidelines. R.C. should be offered small meals or liquid nutritional supplements evenly distributed throughout the day along with a late-night snack.[157,158]

Case 25-3, Question 5: Which pharmacologic interventions are appropriate to manage R.C.'s hepatic encephalopathy?

LACTULOSE

Lactulose is broken down by GI bacteria to form lactic, acetic, and formic acids, which acidify colonic contents converting ammonia into the less readily absorbed ammonium ion. Back diffusion of ammonia from the plasma into the GI tract can also occur. The net result is a lower plasma-ammonia concentration. The absorption of other protein breakdown products (e.g., aromatic amino acids) may also be reduced. Lactulose-induced osmotic diarrhea decreases intestinal transit time available for ammonia production and absorption, and it may help clear the GI tract of blood. Lactulose syrup (10 g/15 mL) has been used successfully for the treatment of HE. For OHE, lactulose 25 mL is administered every 1 to 2 hours until catharsis occurs. Doses are then titrated downward to maintain 2 to 3 bowel movements daily and clear mentation in order to avoid complications of overuse of lactulose (aspiration, dehydration, severe perianal skin irritation, and precipitation of HE).[144] When the oral route of administration is not possible, as in the treatment of a comatose patient, it may be necessary to administer the drug through an NG tube. Alternatively, a rectal retention enema compounded with 300 mL of lactulose in 700 mL water can be prepared. The lactulose water mixture (125 mL) is retained for 30 to 60 minutes, although this is difficult in patients with altered mental status. The beneficial clinical effect of lactulose occurs within 12 to 48 hours. Patients may need long-term administration of lactulose as maintenance therapy, especially in patients with recurring HE. For prevention of recurrence of OHE, oral daily prophylactic dosing of lactulose should be maintained. If precipitating factors have been removed or liver function improved, prophylactic therapy may be tapered and potentially discontinued.[144] The administration of lactulose permits better dietary protein tolerance and is well tolerated if dosages are kept sufficiently low to avoid diarrhea.[162]

Although lactulose is the mainstay of HE treatment,[144,163] very limited data exist evaluating its efficacy. Care should be taken not to induce excessive diarrhea that could lead to dehydration and hypokalemia, both of which have been associated with exacerbation of HE. Although lactulose is generally well tolerated, 20% of patients may complain of gaseous distention, flatulence, or belching. Dilution with fruit juice, carbonated beverages, or water can reduce the excessive sweetness of the syrup.[146]

RIFAXIMIN

Rifaximin is a synthetic antibiotic structurally related to rifamycin. It has a wide spectrum of antibacterial activity against gram-negative and gram-positive bacteria, both aerobic and anaerobic.[164] Of note, 96.6% of the drug is recovered in the feces as unchanged drug, and what is absorbed undergoes metabolism with minimal renal excretion of unchanged drug.[82,165] It was introduced in the United States for the treatment of travelers' diarrhea,[166] but also is indicated for HE.[165] Although dosages used in HE trials ranged from 550 mg twice daily to 400 mg every 8 hours,[167,168] the FDA-approved dose for HE is 550 mg twice daily.[165] Rifaximin is well tolerated, but can cause flatulence, nausea, and vomiting. Some urticarial skin reactions have been reported with prolonged use.[169] Bacterial superinfections (*Clostridium difficile*—associated diarrhea) with >2 months of rifaximin have also been reported.[82,165]

NEOMYCIN

Neomycin is also an antibiotic effective in reducing plasma-ammonia concentrations (presumably by decreasing protein-metabolizing bacteria in the GI tract). Approximately 1% to 3% of the neomycin dose is absorbed. Chronic use in patients with severe renal insufficiency can cause ototoxicity or nephrotoxicity. Routine monitoring of serum creatinine, presence of protein in the urine, and estimation of creatinine clearance are advisable for patients receiving high dosages for more than 2 weeks.[162] Neomycin therapy can also produce a reversible malabsorption syndrome that not only suppresses the absorption of fat, nitrogen, carotene, iron, vitamin B_{12}, xylose, and glucose but also decreases the absorption of some drugs, such as digoxin, penicillin, and vitamin K.[146] Typical HE dosage for neomycin ranges from 500 to 1,000 mg 4 times daily, or as a 1% solution (125 mL) given as a retention enema (retained for 30–60 minutes) 4 times daily.[162]

FLUMAZENIL

Based on the theory of accumulation of endogenous benzodiazepine-like substances in HE, flumazenil, a benzodiazepine antagonist, has been evaluated for its role in the treatment of HE. Several trials have demonstrated both clinical and electrophysiologic improvement in patients with HE.[170] However, an IV product with modest benefits in the treatment of HE is not an ideal treatment option.

Lactulose versus Rifaximin

An extensive review of rifaximin for the treatment of HE conducted by Lawrence et al.[171] found that rifaximin was equally effective, and in some studies superior to lactulose in mild-to-moderate disease. Patients treated with rifaximin required fewer, shorter and less costly hospitalization than lactulose-treated patients.[171]

Bucci et al.[172] conducted a double-blind study comparing rifaximin (1,200 mg/day) and lactulose (30 g/day) for 15 days in patients with moderate to severe HE. After 7 days, ammonia concentrations normalized and at the end of the treatment period, cognitive function test scores improved in both groups. Rifaximin therapy was better tolerated.[172] Although the data reported from these and other trials suggest a benefit with rifaximin for the treatment of HE, larger trials must be conducted to determine its superiority over lactulose. In addition, the current cost of rifaximin is considerably higher than both lactulose and neomycin (estimated cash price: lactulose [60–100 g daily] ~$170–280/month; neomycin [500 mg 4 times daily] ~$220/month; and rifaximin [550 mg twice daily] ~$2,000/month; data per goodrx.com).

Rifaximin versus Neomycin

Miglio et al.[173] conducted a randomized, controlled, double-blind study to evaluate the efficacy and tolerability of rifaximin (400 mg 3 times daily) in comparison to neomycin (1 g 3 times daily) treatment for 14 days each month over 6 months. During the study, blood ammonia concentrations in both the rifaximin and neomycin groups decreased a similar amount.[173] Pedretti et al.[174] compared rifaximin 400 mg every 8 hours to neomycin 1 g every 8 hours in patients with cirrhosis and reported a higher rate of adverse events (increases in BUN, creatinine, nausea, abdominal pain, and vomiting) in the neomycin group after 21 days of therapy. Both drugs significantly decreased blood-ammonia concentrations. However, rifaximin produced an earlier reduction of blood ammonia.[174] Because of the lower adverse-effect profile and considerable efficacy, rifaximin has taken over as second-line therapy for HE over neomycin at many institutions.

Lactulose versus Neomycin

Orlandi et al.[175] found that lactulose and neomycin appear to have similar efficacy for the acute treatment of HE. However, in the treatment of an acute exacerbation, particularly in an acute GI bleed, lactulose may produce a faster response than neomycin.

Interestingly, although lactose therapy is considered the standard of practice in OHE treatment and prevention, a meta-analysis evaluating the efficacy of lactulose in patients with HE questions its benefit.[176] Large randomized, controlled trials are needed to determine the optimal treatment for HE management.[147] The AASLD/EASL guidelines consider neomycin as an alternative choice for treatment of OHE.[144]

Lactulose would be the preferred option to treat R.C.'s HE because it would shorten the time to clear the blood from his GI tract and hopefully lead to a rapid resolution of his confusion. Although neomycin is not contraindicated for R.C., the potential for worsening of his coagulopathy (by interfering with vitamin K absorption) and risk of nephrotoxicity (SCr, 1.4 mg/dL) make this a less optimal choice. If R.C.'s renal function continues to decline, neomycin may become contraindicated. Lactulose can be initiated at 25 mL every 1 to 2 hours until at least two soft or loose stools per day are produced. The dose can then be reduced to maintain 2 to 3 soft stools per day and improved mental status. R.C. may receive lactulose by NG tube if necessary in the early treatment period.

COMBINATION THERAPY WITH LACTULOSE

CASE 25-3, QUESTION 6: Would combination therapy provide any additive beneficial effect for R.C.?

A randomized, double-blind, placebo-controlled trial by Bass et al.[167] compared rifaximin versus placebo in the prevention of HE and hospitalization in patients recovering from recurrent HE (≥2 episodes within the previous 6 months). Patients were assigned to either rifaximin at a dose of 550 mg twice daily or placebo for 6 months. The study allowed the use of lactulose (approximately 90% of patients received concomitant therapy). The results of the study showed that a breakthrough episode of HE occurred in 22.1% with rifaximin and 45.9% with placebo. Hospitalization involving HE was lower with rifaximin (13.6%) than with placebo (22.6%). Adverse events were similar amongst the two groups.[167] The AASLD/EASL considers rifaximin as an effective add-on therapy to lactulose for prevention of OHE recurrence.[144] Previous HE guidelines (American College of Gastroenterology) stated that combination therapy of lactulose and neomycin may be reasonable in patients who do not respond to monotherapy.[162] The current AASLD/EASL guidelines do not address this combination.[144] R.C. would not benefit from combination therapy at this time.

HEPATORENAL SYNDROME

CASE 25-3, QUESTION 7: Lactulose treatment was initiated at 25 mL every hour and titrated to effect with some improvement in R.C.'s mental status. A few days after resolution of his GI bleeding, his serum creatinine increased from 1.4 to 2.7 mg/dL and he became progressively oliguric. His BP was 85/65 mm Hg, pulse rate was 70 beats/minute, and respiratory rate was 16 breaths/minute. Furosemide was discontinued, and R.C. was treated with albumin infusions to allow volume expansion and improve urine output. A renal ultrasound did not reveal any specific abnormalities. Minimal improvement occurred in his blood pressure and urine output. Laboratory results included the following:

Na, 123 mEq/L
K, 3.6 mEq/L
Cl, 98 mEq/L
Bicarbonate, 25 mEq/L
BUN, 96 mg/dL
SCr, 2.7 mg/dL
Hgb, 8.4 g/dL
Hct, 27.1%
AST, 640 IU
Alkaline phosphatase, 304 IU
LDH, 315 IU
Total bilirubin, 4.1 mg/dL
PT, 22 seconds (INR, 1.8)

A 24-hour urinalysis showed the following:
Protein, 50 mg/day
Red blood cells, 1 to 2 per high power field
Negative for WBC, glucose, and ketones

After exclusion of other possible causes of kidney disease, R.C. is diagnosed with hepatorenal syndrome. What are potential treatment options for R.C.'s hepatorenal syndrome?

Pathogenesis

Hepatorenal syndrome (HRS) is a complication of advanced cirrhosis characterized by an intense renal vasoconstriction, which leads to a very low renal perfusion and glomerular filtration rate, as well as a severe reduction in the ability to excrete sodium and free water.[177] Cárdenas et al.[178] summarized the pathogenesis and the precipitating factors of HRS, which can be found on nature.com (http://www.nature.com/nrgastro/journal/v3/n6/fig_tab/ncpgasthep0517_F1.html). HRS is diagnosed by exclusion of other known causes of kidney disease in the absence of parenchymal disease. The revised criteria for the diagnosis of HRS as defined by the International Ascites Club (IAC) can be found at icascites.org (http://www.icascites.org/about/guidelines/).[179,180]

Hepatorenal syndrome can be classified into two categories. Type 1 HRS is characterized by an acute and progressive kidney failure defined by doubling of the initial serum creatinine concentrations to a level greater than 2.5 mg/dL in less than 2 weeks. Type 1 HRS is precipitated by factors such as SBP or large-volume paracentesis, but can occur without a precipitating event. This usually occurs within the setting of an acute deterioration of circulatory function characterized by hypotension and activation of endogenous vasoconstrictor systems. It may be associated with impaired cardiac and liver functions as well as HE. The prognosis of patients exhibiting type 1 HRS is very poor.[180,181] In contrast, type 2 HRS is a progressive deterioration of kidney function with a serum creatinine from 1.5 to 2.5 mg/dL. It is often associated with refractory ascites, and has a better survival rate than that of patients with type 1 HRS.[178,179,180]

Treatment

Treatments for HRS are still investigational. HRS is associated with a high mortality rate (within 2 weeks for type 1 HRS and 6 months for type 2 HRS). The definitive treatment for type 1 and type 2 HRS is liver transplantation, which is the only treatment that assures long-term survival.[68] The main goal of pharmacologic therapy is to manage HRS sufficiently so that the patient can survive long enough to obtain a suitable donor liver.[179,180] Diuretic therapy worsens HRS and should be discontinued.[178]

Solanki et al.[182] randomized patients with type 1 HRS to terlipressin 1 mg IV every 12 hours or placebo. Both groups also received albumin. Urine output, creatinine clearance, mean arterial pressures, and survival (42% vs. 0%) were significantly better with terlipressin than with placebo ($p < 0.05$). All survivors in the terlipressin group had a reversal of HRS.[182]

Sanyal et al.[183] conducted a prospective, double-blind, placebo-controlled clinical study in which patients with type 1 HRS were randomly assigned to terlipressin (1 mg IV every 6 hours) or placebo. If, after 3 days of therapy, the SCr level had not decreased by ≥30% from baseline, the dose was increased to 2 mg every 6 hours. All patients in this study also received albumin. The primary end point at day 14 was SCr ≤ 1.5 mg/dL on two occasions at least 48 hours apart, without dialysis, death, or recurrence of type 1 HRS. The primary end point was achieved twice as often with terlipressin than with placebo (25% vs. 12.5%, respectively), although this did not reach statistical significance. In addition, terlipressin did not improve survival. However, terlipressin was superior to placebo for type 1 HRS reversal as defined by SCr $\leq$ 1.5 mg/dL (34% vs. 13%; $p = 0.008$). Adverse events were similar between groups.[183] In 2009, the FDA accepted the final section of the New Drug Application seeking marketing approval for terlipressin for the treatment of type 1 HRS, and granted priority review and fast-track designation. In 2013, terlipressin was granted Orphan Drug Status.

Other nonrandomized studies suggest that vasoconstrictor therapy with norepinephrine (combined with albumin and furosemide) or midodrine (combined with octreotide and albumin) improve renal function in patients with type 1 HRS.[184–186] Esrailian et al.[187] conducted a retrospective chart review of type 1 HRS patients who received a combination of octreotide, midodrine, and albumin compared to untreated controls who received albumin only. Octreotide administration started at 100 mcg subcutaneously TID, with the goal to increase the dose to 200 mcg subcutaneous TID. Midodrine administration started at 5, 7.5, or 10 mg TID orally, with the goal to increase the dose to 12.5 or 15 mg if necessary. Adjustment in medication doses was based on a goal of increasing the mean arterial pressure by at least 15 mm Hg from baseline. All patients received intravenous expansion of plasma volume with 1.5 L of saline combined with an average of 120 g of human albumin after diuretic withdrawal. The authors found that at 30 days, 40% of treated patients had a sustained reduction in SCr, compared with 10% of the concurrent untreated controls ($p = 0.01$). In that same time period, 43% of patients in the treatment group had died, compared with 71% of controls ($p = 0.03$).[187]

Duvoux et al.[186] conducted a pilot study describing the efficacy and safety of norepinephrine in combination with IV albumin and furosemide in patients with type 1 HRS. Norepinephrine was given for 10 $\pm$ 3 days, at a mean dosage of 0.8 $\pm$ 0.3 mg/hour. Reversal of HRS was observed in 83% of patients after a median of 7 days, with a reduction in SCr (358 $\pm$ 161 to 145 $\pm$ 78 μmol/L; $p < 0.001$), a rise in creatinine clearance (13 $\pm$ 9 to 40 $\pm$ 15 mL/minute; $p = 0.003$), an increase in mean arterial pressure (65 $\pm$ 7 to 73 $\pm$ 9 mm Hg, $p = 0.01$), and a marked reduction in active renin and aldosterone plasma concentrations ($p < 0.05$).[186]

Two small, open-labeled, randomized, pilot studies evaluated the efficacy and safety of norepinephrine compared to terlipressin in the treatment of HRS.[188,189] All subjects also received albumin. Both drugs significantly improved renal function and had similar effects with respect to efficacy and safety. This preliminary data suggests that norepinephrine may be a safe, effective, and less costly alternative to terlipressin in the treatment of type 1 HRS. Further research is warranted.

The IAC guidelines recommend vasoconstrictors and albumin for first-line treatment of type 1 HRS. They advocate for the use of terlipressin (2–12 mg/day) in combination with albumin (20–40 g/day after 1 g/kg on the first day), and mention that about 60% of renal failure cases recover with this therapy. The IAC recommends midodrine (in addition to octreotide) and norepinephrine as two possible alternatives to terlipressin.[180] The latest AASLD recommendation is to consider the use of albumin plus octreotide and midodrine (largely because of the lack of availability of terlipressin in the United States).[38] Studies mention that the combination of both octreotide and midodrine are required to be effective.[190,191] The AASLD guidelines also recommend that albumin plus norepinephrine as a treatment option of type 1 HRS; however, this approach requires an intensive care unit.[38] Vasoconstrictor efficacy and safety requires further evaluation in large, randomized clinical trials.[184–186]

Type 2 HRS manifests itself as a progressive disease and, therefore, patients do not present acutely with deterioration in kidney function. No particular treatment exists for type 2 HRS. The main clinical problem in type 2 HRS is refractory ascites, which can be controlled by large-volume paracentesis along with IV albumin or TIPS.[178,184,192] Studies are needed to determine the place in therapy for vasoconstrictors and other potential treatments in patients with type 2 HRS.[180]

R.C. should continue to receive albumin 10 to 20 g IV per day, octreotide 100 mcg SC 3 times daily with a target dose of 200 mcg SC 3 times daily and midodrine 5 to 10 mg orally 3 times daily, with the goal to titrate up to 12.5 mg orally 3 times per day. The target increase in mean arterial pressure is 15 mm Hg.[38] Because of the poor prognosis associated with hepatorenal syndrome, R.C. should be evaluated for liver transplantation.

CASE 25-3, QUESTION 8: Why should liver transplantation be considered in patients with end-stage liver disease such as R.C.?

Liver transplantation for appropriate candidates may be the best option for end-stage liver disease and its complications leading to improved quality and duration of life. Transplantation is generally considered in patients with refractory ascites, severe hepatic encephalopathy, esophageal or gastric varices, and hepatorenal syndrome.[193] Because of the shortage of organs available and significant complications associated with transplantation, therapeutic alternatives should be considered to avoid the necessity for transplantation. For patients such as R.C., who are candidates for transplantation, therapeutic strategies to improve outcomes after transplantation should be considered in therapeutic decision-making before transplantation (see Chapter 34, Kidney and Liver Transplantation, for further information on the indications for liver transplantation).[192]

KEY REFERENCES AND WEBSITES

A full list of references for this chapter can be found at http://thepoint.lww.com/AT11e. Below are the key references and websites for this chapter, with the corresponding reference number in this chapter found in parentheses after the reference.

Key References

Amodio P et al. The nutritional management of hepatic encephalopathy in patients with cirrhosis: International Society for Hepatic Encephalopathy and Nitrogen Metabolism Consensus. *Hepatology*. 2013;58:325–336. (157)

Bajaj JS et al. Review article: the design of clinical trials in hepatic encephalopathy—an International Society for Hepatic Encephalopathy and Nitrogen Metabolism (ISHEN) consensus statement. *Aliment Pharmacol Ther*. 2011;33:739–747. (145)

Boyer et al. The Role of Transjugular Intrahepatic Portosystemic Shunt (TIPS) in the Management of Portal Hypertension: update 2009. *Hepatology*. 2010;51(1):306. (86)

Garcia-Tsao G et al. Prevention and management of gastroesophageal varices and variceal hemorrhage in cirrhosis [published correction appears in *Am J Gastroenterol*. 2007;102: 2868]. *Am J Gastroenterol*. 2007;102:2086. (92)

Runyon BA. Introduction to the revised American Association for the Study of Liver Diseases Practice Guideline management of adult patients with ascites due to cirrhosis 2012. *Hepatology*. 2013;57:1651–1653. doi:10.1002/hep.26359. (38)

Salerno F et al. Diagnosis, prevention and treatment of the hepatorenal syndrome in cirrhosis. A consensus workshop of the international ascites club. *Gut*. 2007;56:1310. (180)

Vilstrup H et al. Hepatic encephalopathy in chronic liver disease: 2014 Practice Guideline by the American Association for the Study of Liver Diseases and the European Association for the Study of the Liver. *Hepatology*. 2014;60(2):715–735. (144)

Section Editor: Myrna Y. Munar

26 Acid–Base Disorders

Luis S. Gonzalez, III

CORE PRINCIPLES

	CHAPTER CASES
1 Acid–base analysis should proceed in a stepwise approach to avoid missing complicated disorders that may not be readily apparent.	**Case 26-1 (Question 1), Case 26-2 (Question 1), Case 26-3 (Question 1), Case 26-4 (Question 2), Case 26-5 (Question 3), Case 26-6 (Question 1)**
2 A normal anion gap metabolic acidosis is most commonly found in patients who have either diarrhea or are receiving large amounts of isotonic crystalloid infusions. A less common cause of a normal anion gap metabolic acidosis occurs with patients who present with one of several types of renal tubular acidosis.	**Case 26-1 (Questions 2–6)**
3 A metabolic acidosis with an elevated anion gap is created by a disease process that produces an acid, which is buffered by the major extracellular buffer, bicarbonate. It is important to include a calculation of the anion gap in the workup of all patients considered for acid–base analysis.	**Case 26-2 (Questions 1–4)**
4 Metabolic alkaloses can be classified according to a patient's volume status and responsiveness to the administration of chloride-containing solutions. A contraction alkalosis, also called chloride-responsive alkalosis, is generally caused by diuretic administration whereas a chloride-nonresponsive alkalosis may be caused by glucocorticoid administration.	**Case 26-3 (Questions 1–4)**
5 A respiratory acidosis can be acute, chronic, or acute-on-chronic. The best way to differentiate these disorders is with a careful patient history and review of previous blood gas values looking for elevated carbon dioxide levels when a patient is at his or her baseline.	**Case 26-4 (Questions 1–4)**
6 Unlike respiratory acidosis, most patients presenting with a respiratory alkalosis do so acutely. There are a relatively small number of conditions that cause an acute respiratory alkalosis, which can aid in the diagnosis when it is not apparent.	**Case 26-5 (Questions 1–4)**
7 Mixed metabolic and respiratory acid–base disorders occur commonly in acutely ill patients. Acid–base analysis can assist in the diagnosis of clinically difficult cases. Following a stepwise approach in the analysis of acid–base disorders should identify all clinically important abnormalities.	**Case 26-6 (Questions 1–3)**

Understanding the etiology of a clinically important acid–base disturbance is important because therapy generally should be directed at the underlying cause of the disturbance rather than merely the change in pH. Severe acid–base disorders can affect multiple organ systems, including cardiovascular (impaired contractility, arrhythmias), pulmonary (impaired oxygen delivery, respiratory muscle fatigue, dyspnea), renal (hypokalemia, nephrolithiasis), or neurologic (decreased cerebral blood flow, seizures, coma).

ACID–BASE PHYSIOLOGY

To protect body proteins, acid–base balance must be tightly controlled in an attempt to maintain a normal extracellular pH of 7.35 to 7.45 and an intracellular pH of approximately 7.0 to 7.3.[1] This narrow range is maintained by complex buffer systems, ventilation to expel carbon dioxide (CO_2), and renal elimination of acids and reabsorption of bicarbonate (HCO_3^-).[2] At rest, about 200 mL of CO_2, and even more during exercise, is transported from the tissues and excreted in the lungs.[3] Although HCO_3^- is responsible only for about 36% of intracellular buffering, it provides about 86% of the buffering activity in extracellular fluid (ECF).[1] Extracellular fluid contains approximately 350 mEq of HCO_3^-, which buffers generated H^+.

$$HCO_3^- + H^+ \Leftrightarrow H_2CO_3 \quad \text{(Eq. 26-1)}$$

Hydrogen ion (H^+) combines with HCO_3^- and shifts the equilibrium of Eq. 26-1 to the right. In the proximal renal tubule lumen, carbonic anhydrase catalyzes the dehydration of H_2CO_3 to CO_2 and H_2O, which are absorbed into the tubule cell, as illustrated in Eq. 26-2 and in Figure 26-1. Within the tubule cell, H_2O dissociates into H^+ and OH^-. The H^+ is then secreted into the lumen by a Na^+–H^+ exchanger. Carbonic anhydrase then catalyzes the combination of OH^- and CO_2 to HCO_3^-, which is carried into the circulation by a $Na^+HCO_3^-$ cotransporter.[4]

$$HCO_3^- + H^+ \Leftrightarrow H_2CO_3 \overset{CA}{\Leftrightarrow} CO_2\,(\text{dissolved}) + H_2O \quad \text{(Eq. 26-2)}$$

To maintain acid–base balance, the kidney must reclaim and regenerate all the filtered HCO_3^-. The daily amount that must be reabsorbed can be calculated by the product of the glomerular filtration rate (GFR) and the HCO_3^- concentration in ECF (180 L/day GFR × 24 mEq/L HCO_3^- = 4,320 mEq/day).[1] The proximal tubule reabsorbs about 85% of the filtered HCO_3^-. The loop of Henle and the distal tubule reabsorb about 10%.[5] Acid salts, such as HPO_4^- (pK_a of 6.8), that have a pK_a greater than the pH of the urine (titratable acids) can accept a proton and be excreted as the acid, thus regenerating an HCO_3^- anion.[5] Sulfuric acid and other acids with a pK_a less than 4.5 are not titratable. Protons from these acids must be combined with another buffer to be secreted. Glutamine deamination in proximal tubular cells forms NH_3, which accepts these protons. In the collecting tubule, the NH_4^+ produced is lipid insoluble, trapping it in the lumen and causing its excretion, eliminating the proton, and allowing for regeneration of HCO_3^-.[4–6] Figure 26-2 is a simplified illustration of the buffering of these acids.

The daily metabolism of carbohydrates and fats generates about 15,000 mmol of CO_2. Although CO_2 is not an acid, it reversibly combines with H_2O to form carbonic acid (i.e., H_2CO_3). Respiration prevents the accumulation of volatile acid through the exhalation of CO_2. Metabolism of proteins and fats results in several fixed acids and bases. Amino acids such as lysine and arginine have a net positive charge and serve as acids. Compounds such as glutamate, aspartate, and citrate have a negative charge. In general, animal proteins contain more sulfur and phosphates, producing an acidic diet. Vegetarian diets consist of more organic anions, resulting in a more alkaline diet.[7] Normally, fatty acids are metabolized to HCO_3^-; however, during starvation or diabetic ketoacidosis, they may be incompletely oxidized to acetoacetate and β-hydroxybutyric acid.[6] The typical diet generates a net nonvolatile acid load of about 70 to 100 mEq of H^+ (1.0–1.5 mEq/kg)/day.[1,8] Renal excretion of 70 mEq in 2 L of urine each day would require a pH of 1.5. Because the kidney cannot produce a pH less than 4.5, most of this fixed acid load must be buffered. The primary buffers for renal net acid excretion are NH_3^-/NH_4^+ and titratable buffers, such as HPO_4^-/$H_2PO_4^{2-}$, as mentioned earlier.[7] The correct assessment of acid–base disorders begins with an evaluation of appropriate laboratory data and an understanding of the physiologic mechanisms responsible for maintaining a normal pH.

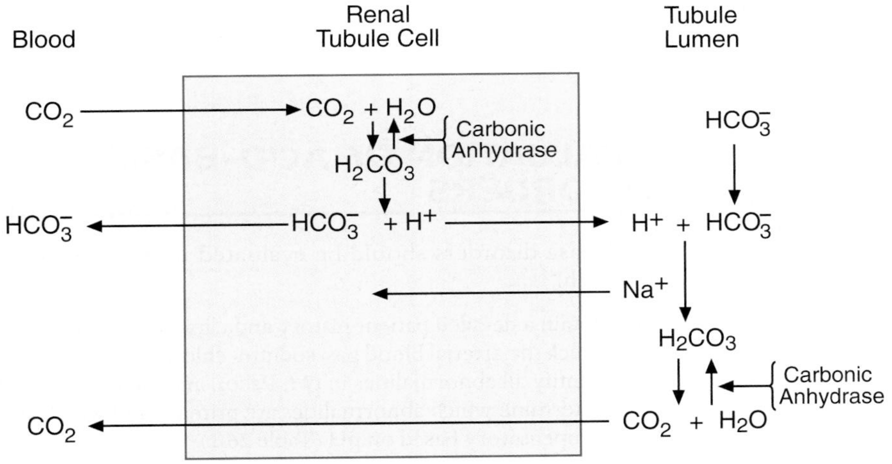

Figure 26-1 Renal tubular bicarbonate reabsorption.

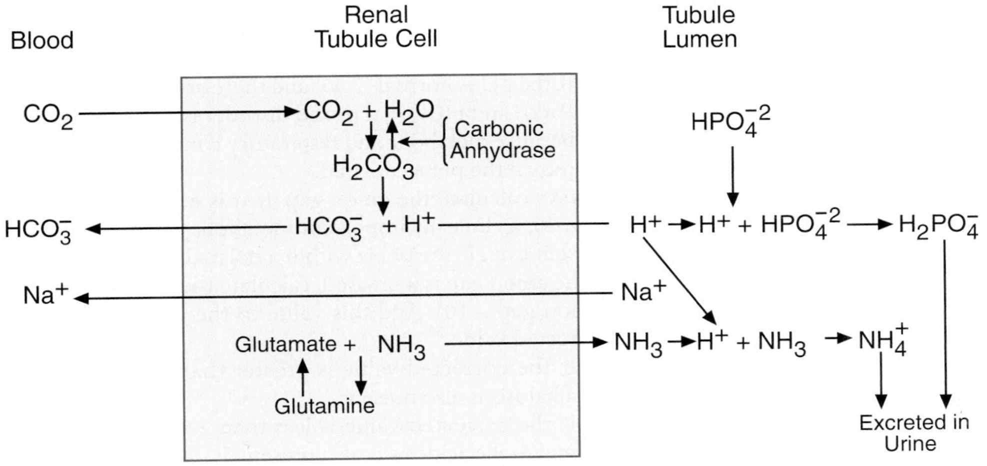

Figure 26-2 Renal tubular hydrogen ion excretion.

Laboratory Assessment

Laboratory data used to evaluate acid–base status are arterial pH, arterial carbon dioxide tension ($Paco_2$), and serum bicarbonate (HCO_3^-).[9–11] These values are obtained routinely with an arterial blood gas (ABG) determination. Acid–base abnormalities occur when the concentration of $Paco_2$ (an acid) or HCO_3^- (a base) is altered. ABG measurements also include the arterial oxygen tension (Pao_2); however, this value does not directly influence decisions regarding acid–base abnormalities. Normal ABG values are listed in Table 26-1. When arterial pH is less than 7.35, the patient is considered acidemic, and the process that caused acid–base imbalance is called acidosis. Conversely, when the arterial pH is greater than 7.45, the patient is considered alkalemic, and the causative process is alkalosis. The process is further defined as respiratory in cases of an inappropriate elevation or depression of $Paco_2$ or metabolic with an inappropriate rise or fall in serum HCO_3^-.

Acid–base balance is normally maintained by the primary extracellular buffer system of HCO_3^-/CO_2. Components of this buffer system are measured routinely to assess acid–base status. Other extracellular buffers (e.g., serum proteins, inorganic phosphates) and intracellular buffers (e.g., hemoglobin, proteins, phosphates), however, also contribute significant buffering activity.[1,7–10] Serum electrolytes are obtained to calculate the anion gap, an estimate of the unmeasured cations and anions in serum. The anion gap helps determine the probable cause of a metabolic acidosis.[6,10,12–21] Urine pH, electrolytes, and osmolality help to further differentiate among the possible causes of metabolic acidosis.[10,22–26]

Acid–Base Balance, Carbon Dioxide Tension, and Respiratory Regulation

In aqueous solution, carbonic acid (i.e., H_2CO_3 formed through the reaction described in Eq. 26-1) reversibly dehydrates to form carbon dioxide (CO_2) and water (H_2O) as shown in Eq. 26-2.

The enzyme carbonic anhydrase (CA), present in red blood cells, renal tubular cells, and other tissues, catalyzes the interconversion of carbonic acid and carbon dioxide. Some of the carbon dioxide produced by dehydration of carbonic acid remains dissolved in plasma, but most exists as a volatile gas:

$$HCO_3^- + H^+ \Leftrightarrow H_2CO_3 \overset{CA}{\Leftrightarrow} CO_2\,(\text{dissolved}) + H_2O$$
$$\uparrow\downarrow$$
$$k \times CO_2\,(\text{gas}) \qquad \text{(Eq. 26-3)}$$

In Eq. 26-3, k is a solubility constant that has a value of approximately 0.03 in plasma at body temperature.[2,26] Virtually, all the carbonic acid in body fluids is in the form of carbon dioxide. The $Paco_2$, a measure of carbon dioxide gas, is therefore directly proportional to the amount of carbonic acid in the HCO_3^-/H_2CO_3 buffer system. The normal range for $Paco_2$ is 35 to 45 mm Hg.

Table 26-1
Normal Arterial Blood Gas Values

ABGs	Normal Range
pH	7.35–7.45
Pao_2	80–105 mm Hg
$Paco_2$	35–45 mm Hg
HCO_3^-	22–26 mEq/L

ABG, arterial blood gas.

The lungs can rapidly exhale large quantities of carbon dioxide and thereby contribute significantly to the maintenance of a normal pH. Carbon dioxide formed through the reaction described in Eq. 26-3 diffuses easily from tissues to capillary blood and from pulmonary capillary blood into the alveoli where it is exhaled from the body.[3] Pulmonary ventilation is regulated by peripheral chemoreceptors (located in the carotid arteries and the aorta) and central chemoreceptors (located in the medulla). The peripheral chemoreceptors are activated by arterial acidosis, hypercarbia (elevated $Paco_2$), and hypoxemia (decreased Pao_2). Central chemoreceptors are activated by cerebrospinal fluid (CSF) acidosis and by elevated carbon dioxide tension in the CSF.[3] Activation of these chemoreceptors stimulates the respiratory control center in the medulla to increase the rate and depth of ventilation, which results in increased exhalation of carbon dioxide.

In clinical practice, the serum bicarbonate concentration usually is estimated from the total carbon dioxide content when the serum concentration of electrolytes are ordered on an electrolyte panel or calculated from the pH and $Paco_2$ on an ABG determination. These estimations of the serum bicarbonate concentration are more convenient than directly measuring serum bicarbonate. The total carbon dioxide content that is reported on serum electrolyte panels is determined by acidifying serum to convert all the bicarbonate to carbon dioxide and measuring the partial pressure of CO_2 gas. Approximately 95% of the total carbon dioxide content is bicarbonate. The serum bicarbonate concentration reported on ABG results is calculated from the patient's pH and $Paco_2$ using the Henderson–Hasselbalch equation (Eq. 26-4). This calculated bicarbonate concentration should be within 2 mEq/L of the measured total carbon dioxide. The normal range of serum bicarbonate using these methods is 22 to 26 mEq/L.[10]

$$\text{pH} = \text{pK} + (\text{base})/(\text{acid}) \qquad \text{(Eq. 26-4)}$$

EVALUATION OF ACID–BASE DISORDERS

Acid–base disorders should be evaluated using a stepwise approach.[24,25]

1. Obtain a detailed patient history and clinical assessment.
2. Check the arterial blood gas, sodium, chloride, and HCO_3^-. Identify all abnormalities in pH, $Paco_2$, and HCO_3^-.
3. Determine which abnormalities are primary and which are compensatory based on pH (Table 26-2).
   a. If the pH is less than 7.40, then a respiratory or metabolic acidosis is primary.
   b. If the pH is greater than 7.40, then a respiratory or metabolic alkalosis is primary.
   c. If the pH is normal (7.40) and there are abnormalities in $Paco_2$ and HCO_3^-, a mixed disorder is probably present because metabolic and respiratory compensations rarely return the pH to normal.
4. Always calculate the anion gap. If it is equal to or greater than 20, a clinically important metabolic acidosis is usually present even if the pH is within a normal range.[27]
5. If the anion gap is increased, calculate the excess anion gap (anion gap − 10). Add this value to the HCO_3^- to obtain corrected value.[28]
   a. If the corrected value is greater than 26, a metabolic alkalosis is also present.
   b. If the corrected value is less than 22, a nonanion gap metabolic acidosis is also present.

Table 26-2
Laboratory Values in Simple Acid–Base Disorders

Disorder	Arterial pH	Primary Change	Compensatory Change
Metabolic acidosis	↓	↓HCO_3^-	↓$Paco_2$
Respiratory acidosis	↓	↑$Paco_2^-$	↑HCO_3^-
Metabolic alkalosis	↑	↑HCO_3^-	↑$Paco_2$
Respiratory alkalosis	↑	↓$Paco_2^-$	↓HCO_3^-

6. Consider other laboratory tests to further differentiate the cause of the disorder.
   a. If the anion gap is normal, consider calculating the urine anion gap.
   b. If the anion gap is high and a toxic ingestion is expected, calculate an osmolal gap.
   c. If the anion gap is high, measure serum ketones and lactate.
7. Compare the identified disorders to the patient history and begin patient-specific therapy.

METABOLIC ACIDOSIS

Metabolic acidosis is characterized by loss of bicarbonate from the body, decreased acid excretion by the kidney, or increased endogenous acid production. Two categories of simple metabolic acidosis (i.e., normal anion gap and increased anion gap) are listed in Table 26-3. The anion gap (AG) represents the concentration of unmeasured negatively charged substances (anions) in excess of the concentration of unmeasured positively charged substances (cations) in the extracellular fluid. The concentrations of total anions and cations in the body are equal because the body must remain electrically neutral. Most clinical laboratories, however, measure only a portion of these ions (i.e., sodium, chloride [Cl^-], and bicarbonate). The concentrations of other negatively and positively charged substances, such as potassium (K^+), magnesium (Mg^+), calcium (Ca^{2+}), phosphates, and albumin, are measured less often. The concentration of unmeasured anions normally exceeds the concentration of unmeasured cations by 6 to 12 mEq/L, and the anion gap can be calculated as follows:

$$\text{Anion gap} = Na^+ - (Cl^- + HCO_3^-) \quad \text{(Eq. 26-5)}$$

Of the unmeasured anions, albumin is perhaps the most important. In critically ill patients with hypoalbuminemia, the calculated AG should be adjusted using the following formula: adjusted AG = AG + 2.5 × (normal albumin − measured albumin in g/dL), where a normal albumin concentration is assumed to be 4.4 g/dL.[16–19] For example, a hypoalbuminemic patient (serum albumin, 2.4 g/dL) with early sepsis and lactic acidosis might have a calculated AG of 11 mEq/L; however, after the calculation is corrected for the effect of the abnormal serum albumin concentration, the presence of elevated AG acidosis is more prominent (the calculated AG is adjusted: $AG_{(adjusted)}$ = 11 mEq/L + 2.5 × [normal albumin – measured albumin] = 16 mEq/L).

Metabolic acidosis with a normal AG (e.g., hyperchloremic metabolic acidosis) usually is caused by loss of bicarbonate and can be further characterized as hypokalemic or hyperkalemic.[5,23,26,29–36] Diarrhea can result in severe bicarbonate loss and a hyperchloremic metabolic acidosis. Elevated AG metabolic acidosis usually is associated with overproduction of organic acids or with decreased renal elimination of nonvolatile acids.[26,37–39] Increased production of organic acids (e.g., formic, lactic acids) is buffered by extracellular bicarbonate with resultant consumption of bicarbonate and appearance of an unmeasured anion (e.g., formate, lactate).[24,37,38] The decrement in serum bicarbonate approximates the increment in the AG, the latter being a good estimate of the circulating anion level. Prolonged hypoxia results in lactic acidosis. Uncontrolled diabetes mellitus or excessive alcohol intake with starvation can cause ketoacidosis. In the case of renal failure, the capacity for H^+ secretion diminishes, resulting in metabolic acidosis.[29] The accompanying increased AG results from decreased excretion of unmeasured anions such as sulfate and phosphate.[20]

Table 26-3
Common Causes of Metabolic Acidosis

Normal AG	Elevated AG
Hypokalemic	**Renal Failure**
Diarrhea	**Lactic Acidosis**
Fistulous disease	(see Table 26-4)
Ureteral diversions	**Ketoacidosis**
Type 1 RTA	Starvation
Type 2 RTA	Ethanol
Carbonic anhydrase inhibitors	Diabetes mellitus
Hyperkalemic	**Drug Intoxications**
Hypoaldosteronism	Ethylene glycol
Hydrochloric acid or precursor	Methanol
Type 4 RTA	Salicylates
Potassium-sparing diuretics	
Amiloride	
Spironolactone	
Triamterene	

AG, anion gap; RTA, renal tubular acidosis.

Normal Anion Gap (Hyperchloremic) Metabolic Acidosis

EVALUATION

CASE 26-1

Question 1: J.D., a 21-year-old, 75-kg woman, is hospitalized for evaluation of weakness. She has a history of bipolar affective disorder, pica, and reports recent ingestion of paint from the walls of her house. J.D.'s only current medication is lithium carbonate 300 mg 3 times a day (TID). On admission, she appears weak and apathetic and complains of anorexia. Laboratory tests reveal the following:

Serum Na, 143 mEq/L
K, 3.0 mEq/L
Cl, 121 mEq/L

Albumin, 4.4 g/dL
pH, 7.28
$Paco_2$, 26 mm Hg
HCO_3^-, 12 mEq/L
Urine pH, 5.5

J.D.'s urine pH after an ammonium chloride (NH_4Cl) 0.1 g/kg IV load is less than 5.1. A bicarbonate load of 1 mEq/kg infused intravenously (IV) for 1 hour induces bicarbonaturia (urinary pH, 7.0) and lowers the serum potassium to 2.0 mEq/L. Her blood pH only increased to 7.31. What type of acid–base disorder is present?

Using a stepwise approach, we see that J.D.'s history gives a clue to the cause for her acidosis. The low pH is consistent with a metabolic acidosis because her CO_2 and HCO_3^- are both reduced (Table 26-3). Alterations in pH resulting from a primary change in serum bicarbonate are metabolic acid–base disorders. Specifically, metabolic acidosis is associated with a decrease in serum HCO_3^- and decreased pH, whereas metabolic alkalosis is associated with an increase in serum HCO_3^- and increased pH. In respiratory disorders, the primary change occurs in the $Paco_2$. If J.D. had a decrease in pH and increase in $Paco_2$, a respiratory acidosis would be present. Because J.D. has a low $Paco_2$ and decreased serum HCO_3^-, she has a metabolic acidosis. In most cases of metabolic acidosis or alkalosis, the lungs compensate for the primary change in serum HCO_3^- concentration by increasing or decreasing ventilation. Most stepwise approaches would next suggest the evaluation of whether the decrease in $Paco_2$ of 14 mm Hg for J.D. is consistent with respiratory compensation (Table 26-4). A primary decrease in the serum bicarbonate to a level of 12 mEq/L should result in a compensatory decrease in the $Paco_2$ concentration by 12 to 14 mm Hg (Table 26-4). J.D.'s $Paco_2$ has fallen by 14 mm Hg (normal, 40 mm Hg; current, 26 mm Hg), confirming that normal respiratory compensation has occurred. When values for $Paco_2$ or serum HCO_3^- fall outside of normal compensatory ranges, either a mixed acid–base disorder, inadequate extent of compensation, or inadequate time for compensation should be suspected.

Nomograms, especially ones that are different for acute and chronic disorders, are inherently difficult to memorize, however, and are often not available to the clinician at the point of care. Following the stepwise approach advocated herein will enable clinicians to identify most clinically important disorders without needing to depend on tables or formulas.

Table 26-4
Normal Compensation in Simple Acid–Base Disorders

Disorder	Compensation[a]
Metabolic acidosis	$\downarrow Paco_2$ (mm Hg) = 1.0–1.2 × HCO_3^- (mEq/L)
Metabolic alkalosis	$\uparrow Paco_2$ (mm Hg) = 0.5–0.7 × $\uparrow HCO_3^-$ (mEq/L)
Respiratory acidosis	
Acute	$\uparrow HCO_3^-$ (mEq/L) = 0.1 × $\uparrow Paco_2$ (mm Hg)
Chronic	$\uparrow HCO_3^-$ (mEq/L) = 0.4 × $\uparrow Paco_2$ (mm Hg)
Respiratory alkalosis	
Acute	$\downarrow HCO_3^-$ (mEq/L) = 0.2 × $\downarrow Paco_2$ (mm Hg)
Chronic	$\downarrow HCO_3^-$ (mEq/L) = 0.4–0.5 × $\downarrow Paco_2$ (mm Hg)

[a]Based on change from normal HCO_3^- = 24 mEq/L and $Paco_2$ = 40 mm Hg.

CAUSES

Case 26-1, Question 2: What are potential causes of metabolic acidosis in J.D.?

Steps 4 to 7 of the stepwise approach in the evaluation of acid–base disorders are used to further determine the cause of the disorder. In patients with metabolic acidosis, calculation of the AG serves as a first step in classifying the metabolic acidosis and provides additional information about conditions that might be responsible. J.D.'s calculated AG is 10 mEq/L (Eq. 26-5). Thus, J.D. has hyperchloremic metabolic acidosis with a normal AG.

The common causes of metabolic acidosis are presented in Table 26-3.[5,10,37] Normal AG metabolic acidosis usually is caused by gastrointestinal loss of bicarbonate (diarrhea, fistulous disease, ureteral diversions); exogenous sources of chloride (normal saline infusions); or altered excretion of hydrogen ions (renal tubular acidosis). J.D. reports a history of both, pica resulting in paint ingestion (perhaps lead-based paint) and chronic use of lithium. Both lead and lithium have been associated with the development of renal tubular acidosis.[23,40]

Renal Tubular Acidosis

Case 26-1, Question 3: How do the results of NH_4Cl and sodium bicarbonate ($NaHCO_3$) loading help identify the type of renal tubular acidosis in J.D.?

Renal tubular acidosis (RTA) is characterized by defective secretion of hydrogen ion in the renal tubule with essentially normal GFR. Many medical conditions and chemical substances have been associated with RTA.[23,26] The recognized forms are type 1 (distal), type 2 (proximal), and type 4 (distal, hypoaldosterone). Type 1 RTA is caused by a defect in the distal tubule's ability to acidify the urine. The most common causes in adults are autoimmune disorders, toluene sniffing in recreational drug users, and marked volume depletion.[41] Type 2 RTA is caused by altered urinary bicarbonate reabsorption in the proximal tubule as can occur with the use of acetazolamide. Type 4 is characterized by hypoaldosteronism and impaired ammoniagenesis.[23,34]

Evaluation of bicarbonate reabsorption during bicarbonate loading and of response to acid loading by infusion of ammonium chloride is useful in distinguishing among the various types of RTA. In healthy subjects, approximately 10% to 15% of the filtered bicarbonate escapes reabsorption in the proximal tubule, but it is reabsorbed in more distal segments of the nephron. Urine bicarbonate excretion is therefore negligibly small, and urine pH is maintained between 5.5 and 6.5.

Type 2 RTA is associated with a decrease in proximal tubular bicarbonate reabsorption. The distal tubular cells partially compensate for this defect by increasing bicarbonate reabsorption, but urinary bicarbonate excretion still is increased. As occurred with A.B., serum HCO_3^- concentration in patients with type 2 RTA may acutely fall below a threshold of 15 but then stabilize around 15 mEq/L.[10,23] At this point, distal bicarbonate delivery no longer is excessive, allowing the distal nephron to acidify the urine appropriately and excrete acid in the form of titratable ammonia and phosphate.

In type 1 RTA, a defect in net hydrogen ion secretion results from a back-diffusion of H^+ from the tubule lumen to the tubule cell. Patients with type 1 RTA cannot reduce their urine pH below 5.5 even when systemic acidosis is severe.[34]

J.D.'s response to the acid (NH_4Cl) load demonstrates an ability to acidify the urine (i.e., pH < 5.1), which helps rule out type 1 RTA. During bicarbonate loading in patients with type 2 RTA, serum bicarbonate concentration is increased, and abnormally large amounts of bicarbonate are again delivered to the distal tubule. Its hydrogen secretory processes are overwhelmed, resulting in bicarbonaturia. Administration of bicarbonate to J.D. produced bicarbonaturia and an elevation in urine pH (7.0), with low blood pH (7.31). These findings indicate that the reabsorption of bicarbonate in the proximal tubule is impaired, which is characteristic of type 2 RTA. Type 4 RTA is unlikely given her initial serum potassium of 3.0 mEq/L.

Lead-Induced

CASE 26-1, QUESTION 4: What is the cause of J.D.'s proximal RTA?

The most likely cause of A.B.'s proximal RTA is her exposure to presumably lead-based paint. The pathogenesis of lead-induced type 2 RTA is unclear. Some studies suggest that carbonic anhydrase deficiency in the proximal tubule is the major factor, but these data are inconclusive.

CASE 26-1, QUESTION 5: Why is J.D. hypokalemic?

Bicarbonate wasting in proximal RTA is associated with sodium loss, extracellular fluid reduction, and activation of the renin–angiotensin–aldosterone axis. Aldosterone increases distal tubular sodium reabsorption and greatly augments potassium and hydrogen ion secretion. This results in potassium wasting, which explains J.D.'s hypokalemia.[42] When plasma bicarbonate achieves steady state, less bicarbonate reaches the distal tubule, and the stimulus for aldosterone release is removed. Therefore, J.D. experiences only a mild depletion of potassium body stores. When J.D. is exposed to bicarbonate loading, the renin–angiotensin–aldosterone axis is reactivated, and hypokalemia worsens. In addition, raising the concentration of bicarbonate in the blood drives potassium intercellularly and contributes to her hypokalemia.

TREATMENT

CASE 26-1, QUESTION 6: What treatment is indicated for J.D.?

Although it is rare for patients with type 2 RTA to develop severe acidosis and potassium depletion chronically, it is not uncommon in an acute situation such as this. J.D. has a bicarbonate deficit; thus, she should be treated with alkali replacement, and the offending agent, if confirmed to be lead, should be removed concurrently. Her serum potassium is also dangerously low, and bicarbonate correction could further decrease it. J.D. needs potassium supplementation. The clinician should obtain hourly blood samples for electrolytes until her potassium is greater than 3.5 mEq/L. In adults such as J.D., chronic treatment often is not needed because acidosis is self-limited. J.D., however, should be treated with sodium bicarbonate until proximal RTA resolves. Very large doses of bicarbonate (6–10 mEq/kg/day) would be required to increase serum bicarbonate to the normal range.[10] In adults with proximal RTA, however, the goal is to increase serum bicarbonate to no more than 18 mEq/L.[23] Bicarbonate can be provided as sodium bicarbonate tablets (8 mEq/600-mg tablet) or Shohl's solution. Shohl's solution, USP, contains 334 mg citric acid and 500 mg sodium citrate per 5 mL. Sodium citrate is metabolized to sodium bicarbonate in the liver. Shohl's solution provides 1 mEq of sodium and 1 mEq of bicarbonate per milliliter of solution. Therapy for J.D. should be initiated with 1 mEq/kg/day. The clinician should monitor A.B.'s lithium levels while she is receiving alkali therapy. Sodium ingestion might increase renal lithium excretion and exacerbate her bipolar disorder. Because of severe hypokalemia resulting from alkali administration, supplemental potassium as chloride, bicarbonate, acetate, or citrate salts also should be administered.

Metabolic Acidosis with Elevated Anion Gap

EVALUATION AND OSMOLAL GAP

CASE 26-2

QUESTION 1: G.D., a 64-year-old, 60-kg man, is brought to the emergency department (ED) by his family in a semicomatose state. He was found lying on the floor of his garage near a partially empty bottle of windshield wiper fluid 30 minutes ago. G.D. has a long history of alcohol abuse and recently diagnosed dementia. In the ED, supine blood pressure (BP) is 120/60 mm Hg, pulse is 100 beats/minute, and respiratory rate is 40 breaths/minute. G.D.'s pupils are reactive, and mild papilledema is noted. Laboratory tests reveal the following:

Serum Na, 139 mEq/L
K, 5.8 mEq/L
Cl, 103 mEq/L
Blood urea nitrogen (BUN), 25 mg/dL
Creatinine, 1.4 mg/dL
Fasting glucose, 150 mg/dL

ABG include pH, 7.16; $Paco_2$, 23 mm Hg; and HCO_3^-, 8 mEq/L. His toxicology screen is negative for alcohol, and his serum osmolality is 332 mOsm/kg. What acid–base disturbance is present in G.D., and what are possible causes of the disorder?

G.D. has an acidosis (pH, 7.16; HCO_3^-, 8 mEq/L) with a large AG (28 mEq/L). Subtracting 10 from the anion gap of 28 and adding this value to his serum bicarbonate concentration (see Step 5 in the section Evaluation of Acid–Base Disorders) yields a value of 26, suggesting no other metabolic abnormality is present.

An elevated AG metabolic acidosis often indicates lactic acidosis resulting from intoxications (e.g., salicylates, acetaminophen, methanol, ethylene glycol, paraldehyde, metformin) or ketoacidosis induced by diabetes mellitus, starvation, or alcohol.[14,21,25,38,43–48] Step 6 in the stepwise approach leads to the consideration of additional laboratory tests that may be helpful in the differential diagnosis of an elevated AG. These include serum ketones, glucose, lactate, BUN, creatinine, and plasma osmolal gap.[25] Osmolal gap is defined as the difference between measured serum osmolality (SO) and calculated SO using Eq. 26-6.

$$\text{Calculated SO (mOsm / kg)} = 2 \times \text{Na}^+ \text{ (mEq / L)} + \text{Glucose (mg / dL)}/18 + \text{BUN (mg / dL)}/2.8 \quad \text{(Eq. 26-6)}$$

When the difference between measured and calculated SO is greater than 10 mOsm/kg, the presence of an unmeasured osmotically active substance, such as ethanol, methanol, or ethylene glycol, should be considered.[25,49] G.D.'s calculated SO is 295 mOsm/kg, compared with the measured value of 332; therefore, his osmolal gap is 37 mOsm/kg. An increase in the anion gap and osmolal gap, without diabetic ketoacidosis or chronic renal failure, suggests the possibility of metabolic acidosis resulting from a toxic ingestion.[25] On the basis of G.D.'s presentation (papilledema, history of alcohol abuse, increased osmolal gap, increased AG metabolic acidosis), history of dementia, and partially empty bottle of windshield wiper fluid found at the scene, methanol intoxication should be considered.

CAUSES

Methanol-Induced

CASE 26-2, QUESTION 2: How would G.D.'s methanol intake induce metabolic acidosis with an elevated anion AG?

Methanol intoxication results in the formation of two organic acids, formic and lactic acids, which consume bicarbonate with production of an AG metabolic acidosis. Alcohol dehydrogenase in the liver metabolizes methanol to formaldehyde and then to formic acid. The formic acid contributes to the metabolic acidosis and also is responsible for the retinal edema and blindness associated with methanol intoxication.[25,26,48]

Serum lactic acid concentrations also are increased in patients with methanol intoxication.[25] Lactic acidosis classically has been divided into type A, which is associated with inadequate delivery of oxygen to the tissue, and type B, which is associated with defective oxygen utilization at the mitochondrial level (Table 26-5). Although these distinctions often are not clear, the lactic acidosis caused by methanol intoxication is most consistent with the type B variety.[50]

TREATMENT

CASE 26-2, QUESTION 3: How should G.D.'s methanol intoxication be managed acutely?

Antidotes

Because G.D.'s mental status is impaired and his respiratory rate is 40 breaths/minute, his airway was secured via endotracheal intubation and he was placed on mechanical ventilatory support. Even though both ethanol and fomepizole compete with methanol for alcohol dehydrogenase binding sites and could be used to treat G.D., fomepizole is chosen because it is easier to dose and does not need serum-level monitoring to ensure efficacy like ethanol.[26,48–52] Because ethanol and fomepizole have much greater affinity for alcohol dehydrogenase than methanol, these agents may reduce the conversion of methanol to its toxic metabolite, formic acid. The unmetabolized methanol is then excreted by the lungs and kidneys. Fomepizole can be given IV as a 15 mg/kg loading dose for 30 minutes, followed by bolus doses of 10 mg/kg every 12 hours. Because of induction of metabolism of fomepizole, doses should be increased to 15 mg/kg every 12 hours if therapy is required beyond 2 days.[48] Fomepizole is usually continued until the serum methanol concentration is less than 20 mg/dL (6.2 mmol/L). Adverse effects of fomepizole are relatively mild; G.D. should be monitored for headache, nausea, dizziness, agitation, metallic taste, abnormal smell, and rash. Cofactor therapy with folinic acid or folic acid at a dosage of 50 mg IV every 6 hours should be given to enhance the elimination of formate along with IV thiamine because of G.D.'s history of chronic alcoholism.

Because of its high cost and infrequent use, some hospitals might not have fomepizole readily available. In such cases, ethanol is an alternative. Administration of IV ethanol as an antidote can be technically difficult and may produce central nervous system (CNS) depression.[48,51] For G.D., an IV-loading dose of 0.6 g/kg ethanol solution should be administered over the course of 30 minutes, followed by a continuous infusion of about 150 mg/kg/hour if the patient has been drinking, or 70 mg/kg/hour for nondrinkers if the patient was not drinking. Serum ethanol concentration should be maintained at more than 100 mg/dL.[26,50] Charcoal may be considered to bind other agents that may be coingested.[26,53]

When other low-molecular-weight toxins, such as ethanol or ethylene glycol, are not present, the serum methanol level can be estimated by multiplying the patient's osmolal gap by a standardized conversion factor of 2.6. G.D.'s osmolal gap of 37 mOsm/L, therefore, may reflect a methanol level of approximately 96 mg/dL (37 mOsm/L × 2.6). When methanol blood levels are higher than 50 mg/dL, hemodialysis is indicated to rapidly reduce concentrations of methanol and its toxic metabolite. The dosage of fomepizole or ethanol should be increased in patients receiving hemodialysis to account for the increased elimination of these antidotes.[26,50] Ethylene glycol poisoning can also be treated by using fomepizole or ethanol.

Bicarbonate

In general, a severe acidosis causes reduced myocardial contractility, impaired response to catecholamines, and impaired oxygen delivery to tissues as a result of 2,3-diphosphoglycerate depletion. For this reason, some clinicians have judiciously administered IV sodium bicarbonate to patients with metabolic acidosis in an attempt to raise the arterial pH to about 7.20.[15,54,55] In G.D.'s case, bicarbonate therapy is indicated in an attempt to raise the pH to 7.3 which converts formic acid (unionized metabolite of methanol) to formate (ionized form) to decrease tissue penetration. If IV sodium bicarbonate is given, the amount required to correct serum HCO_3^- and arterial pH can be estimated using Eq. 26-7 as follows:

$$\text{Bicarbonate dose (mEq)} = 0.5\ (\text{L/kg}) \times \text{Body weight (kg)} \times \text{Desired increase in serum } HCO_3^-\ (\text{mEq/L}) \qquad \text{(Eq. 26-7)}$$

Bicarbonate distributes to approximately 50% of total body weight (thus, the factor of 0.5 L/kg in Eq. 26-7). To prevent overtreating, bicarbonate doses should only attempt to increase the bicarbonate concentration by 4 to 8 mEq/L (see Case 26-2, Question 4).[54] For G.D., the dose required to raise serum bicarbonate from 8 to 12 mEq/L amounts to 120 mEq of bicarbonate (0.5 L/kg × 60 kg × 4 mEq/L; Eq. 26-7). Clinical assessment of the effect of bicarbonate can be determined about 30 minutes after administration.[54] Arterial pH and serum bicarbonate concentrations should be obtained before any additional therapy.

RISKS OF BICARBONATE THERAPY

CASE 26-2, QUESTION 4: What are the risks of G.D. bicarbonate therapy?

Table 26-5
Common Causes of Lactic Acidosis

Type A	Type B
Anemia	Diabetes mellitus
Carbon monoxide poisoning	Liver failure
Congestive heart failure	Renal failure
Shock	Seizure disorder
Sepsis	Leukemia
	Drugs
	Didanosine
	Ethanol
	Isoniazid
	Metformin
	Methanol
	Salicylates
	Zidovudine

Concerns about the risks of bicarbonate administration and the failure of studies to demonstrate significant short-term benefits have raised questions about the appropriateness of bicarbonate therapy in metabolic acidosis, particularly in ketoacidosis and lactic acidosis caused by cardiac arrest or other hypoxic events.[55–61] Bicarbonate administration can result in overalkalinization and a paradoxical transient intracellular acidosis. Whereas arterial pH can increase rapidly after bicarbonate administration, intracellular pH increases more slowly because of slow penetration of the negatively charged bicarbonate ion across cell membranes. The bicarbonate in plasma, however, is converted rapidly to carbonic acid, and the carbon dioxide tension increases as a result (Eq. 26-2). Because CO_2 diffuses into cells more rapidly than HCO_3^-, the intracellular HCO_3^-/CO_2 ratio decreases, resulting in a decrease in intracellular pH. This intracellular acidosis will persist as long as bicarbonate administration exceeds the CO_2 excretion; therefore, adequate tissue perfusion and ventilation must be provided in patients with diminished CO_2 excretion (e.g., cardiac or respiratory failure).[56]

Overalkalinization also will cause a shift to the left in the oxygen–hemoglobin dissociation curve. This shift increases hemoglobin affinity for oxygen, decreases oxygen delivery to tissues, and potentially increases lactic acid production and accumulation.[26] Sodium bicarbonate administration also can cause hypernatremia, hyperosmolality, and volume overload; however, the excessive sodium and water retention usually can be avoided by the administration of loop diuretics.[26,49] Hypokalemia is another potential adverse effect of bicarbonate therapy. Acidosis stimulates movement of potassium from intracellular to extracellular fluid in exchange for hydrogen ions. When acidosis is corrected, potassium ions move intracellularly, and hypokalemia can occur. This translocation of potassium tends to reduce serum potassium levels by about 0.4 to 0.6 mEq/L for each 0.1 unit increase in pH, although wide interpatient variability in this relationship exists.[5,8] In G.D. and other patients with organic acid intoxications, raising extracellular pH helps to provide a gradient to shift the toxin from the CNS and "trap" it into the blood and urine, thus enhancing elimination. To prevent the risks of bicarbonate therapy, G.D.'s mental status, serum sodium and potassium levels, and ABG should be monitored.

METABOLIC ALKALOSIS

Metabolic alkalosis is associated with an increase in serum bicarbonate concentration and a compensatory increase in $Paco_2$ (caused by hypoventilation). The two general classifications of metabolic alkalosis, saline-responsive and saline-resistant (Table 26-6), are usually distinguishable based on an assessment of the patient's volume status, BP, and urinary chloride concentration.

Table 26-6
Classification of Metabolic Alkalosis

Saline-Responsive	Saline-Resistant
Diuretic therapy	Normotensive
Extracellular volume contraction	Potassium depletion
Gastric acid loss	Hypercalcemia
Vomiting	Hypertensive
Nasogastric suction	Mineralocorticoids
Exogenous alkali administration	Hyperaldosteronism
Blood transfusions	Hyperreninism
	Licorice

Saline-responsive metabolic alkalosis is associated with disorders that result in the loss of chloride-rich, bicarbonate-poor fluid from the body (e.g., vomiting, nasogastric suction, diuretic therapy, cystic fibrosis). Physical examination may reveal volume depletion (e.g., orthostatic hypotension, tachycardia, poor skin turgor), and the urinary chloride concentration often will be less than 10 to 20 mEq/L (although urine chloride levels may be >20 mEq/L in patients with recent diuretic use).[10,27,62]

Severe hypokalemia or excessive mineralocorticoid activity can result in a saline-resistant metabolic alkalosis, but this disorder is rare in comparison with saline-responsive metabolic alkalosis. Saline-resistant metabolic alkalosis should be suspected in alkalemic patients with evidence of increased ECF volume, hypertension, or high urinary chloride values (>20 mEq/L) without recent diuretic use.[10,62]

Evaluation

CASE 26-3

QUESTION 1: S.J., a 75-year-old, 60-kg woman, was admitted to the hospital 4 days ago with peripheral edema and pulmonary congestion consistent with a congestive heart failure exacerbation. Since admission, she has been treated aggressively with furosemide 80 to 120 mg IV daily, which has generated approximately 3 L of urine output each day. Today her lung sounds are clear and peripheral edema shows considerable improvement with diuresis; however, she now complains of dizziness when she gets out of bed to go to the bathroom. Physical examination reveals a tachycardic (heart rate [HR], 100 beats/minute), thin elderly woman with poor skin turgor and slight muscle weakness. S.J.'s electrocardiogram shows flattened T waves and U waves. Laboratory tests reveal the following:

Serum Na, 138 mEq/L
K, 2.5 mEq/L
Cl, 92 mEq/L
Creatinine, 0.9 mg/dL
BUN, 28 mg/dL
pH, 7.49
$Paco_2$, 46 mm Hg
HCO_3^-, 34 mEq/L

Urine Cl concentration is 60 mEq/L. What acid–base disorder is present in S.J.?

Using the stepwise approach to the evaluation of acid–base disorders as previously described, S.J.'s elevated pH is consistent with alkalosis.

Furosemide-induced diuresis may be a clue to her acid–base disorder. The increased serum HCO_3^- and increased $Paco_2$ suggest primary metabolic alkalosis with respiratory compensation. S.J.'s anion gap is 12, suggesting no additional metabolic acid–base abnormalities are present. A $Paco_2$ of 46 mm Hg suggests normal respiratory compensation for metabolic alkalosis. Appropriate treatment of the metabolic alkalosis should return her $Paco_2$ to normal if there is no underlying pulmonary disease.

Causes

DIURETIC-INDUCED

CASE 26-3, QUESTION 2: What is the most likely cause of S.J.'s acid–base imbalance?

Common causes of metabolic alkalosis are listed in Table 26-6. The hypokalemic, hypochloremic, metabolic alkalosis in S.J. most likely is the result of diuretic-induced volume contraction. The incidence of this adverse effect is influenced by the type, dose, and dosing frequency of the diuretic.

Diuretics cause metabolic alkalosis (sometimes referred to as a "contraction alkalosis") by the following mechanisms. First, they enhance excretion of sodium chloride and water, resulting in extracellular volume contraction. Volume contraction alone will cause only a modest increase in plasma bicarbonate; however, volume contraction also stimulates aldosterone release. Aldosterone increases distal tubular sodium reabsorption and induces hydrogen ion and potassium secretion, resulting in alkalosis and hypokalemia. In addition, hypokalemia induced by diuretics will stimulate intracellular movement of hydrogen ions to replace cellular potassium, producing extracellular alkalosis. Hypochloremia also is important in sustaining metabolic alkalosis. In a hypochloremic state, sodium will be reabsorbed, accompanied by bicarbonate generated by secreted hydrogen (Fig. 26-1).[62–64]

Treatment

CASE 26-3, QUESTION 3: How should S.J.'s acid–base imbalance be corrected and monitored?

Treatment of metabolic alkalosis depends on removal of the cause. S.J.'s diuretic therapy should be temporarily discontinued until her volume status and electrolytes can be restored. The initial goal is to correct fluid deficits and replace chloride and potassium by infusing sodium and potassium chloride. As long as hypochloremia exists, renal bicarbonate excretion will not occur and the alkalosis will not be corrected.[63] The severity of alkalosis dictates how rapidly fluid and electrolytes should be administered. In patients with hepatic or renal failure or congestive heart failure, infusion of large volumes of sodium and potassium salts can produce fluid overload or hyperkalemia. Thus, fluid and electrolyte replacement should proceed cautiously, and these patients should be monitored closely for these complications.

Potassium chloride should be administered to correct S.J.'s hypokalemia. The amount of potassium required to replace total body stores is difficult to determine accurately because 98% of the potassium in the body is intracellular. Although wide variation exists, for each 1 mEq/L decrease in K^+ from an ECF concentration of 4 mEq/L, the total body K^+ deficit is about 4 to 5 mEq/kg.[10] S.J.'s serum potassium is 2.5 mEq/L, which correlates with a decrease of about 350 mEq in total body potassium stores. S.J. should be treated with the chloride salt to ensure potassium retention and correction of alkalosis. Potassium replacement can be achieved over the course of several days with supplements of 100 to 150 mEq/day given either orally in divided doses or as a constant IV infusion. S.J.'s laboratory tests for BUN, creatinine, chloride, sodium, and potassium should be monitored during sodium and potassium chloride therapy. As noted earlier, hypercapnia should disappear after correction of the alkalemia, and can be confirmed with an ABG, if clinically indicated.

CASE 26-3, QUESTION 4: What other agents are available to treat S.J.'s alkalosis if fluid and electrolyte replacement does not correct the arterial pH?

Patients unresponsive to sodium and potassium chloride therapy or those at risk for complications with these agents can be treated with acetazolamide, hydrochloric acid (HCl), or a hydrochloric acid precursor. The most commonly used agent is acetazolamide, a carbonic anhydrase inhibitor that blocks hydrogen ion secretion in the renal tubule, resulting in increased excretion of sodium and bicarbonate. Although the serum bicarbonate concentration often improves with acetazolamide, metabolic alkalosis may not completely resolve. Other concerns with the use of acetazolamide include its ability to promote kaliuresis and its relative lack of effect in patients with renal dysfunction.[62,65,66]

A solution of 0.1 N HCl may be administered to patients who require rapid correction of alkalemia. The dose of HCl is based on the bicarbonate excess using Eq. 26-8, where the factor 0.5 × body weight (kg) represents the estimated bicarbonate space.[10,62,63,65]

$$\text{Dose of HCl (mEq)} = 0.5 \times \text{Body weight (kg)} \times (\text{plasma bicarbonate} - 24) \quad \text{(Eq. 26-8)}$$

Parenteral hydrochloric acid is prepared extemporaneously by adding the appropriate amount of 1 N HCl through a 0.22-μm filter into a glass bottle containing 5% dextrose or normal saline. The dilute solution should be administered through a central venous catheter in the superior vena cava to reduce the risk of extravasation and tissue damage. The infusion rate should not exceed 0.2 mEq/kg/hour.[65] ABG should be monitored at least every 4 hours during the infusion. HCl should not be added to parenteral nutrition solutions.[66]

RESPIRATORY ACIDOSIS

Respiratory acidosis occurs as a result of inadequate ventilation by the lungs. When the lungs do not excrete CO_2 effectively, the $Paco_2$ rises. This elevation in $Paco_2$ (a functional acid) causes a fall in pH (Eq. 26-3). Common causes of respiratory acidosis are listed in Table 26-7. They generally can be categorized into conditions of airway obstruction, reduced stimulus for respiration from the CNS, failure of the heart or lungs, and disorders of the peripheral nerves or skeletal muscles required for ventilation.[67]

Table 26-7
Common Causes of Respiratory Acidosis

Airway Obstruction	Cardiopulmonary
Foreign body aspiration	Cardiac arrest
Asthma	Pulmonary edema or infiltration
COPD	Pulmonary embolism
Adrenergic blockers	Pulmonary fibrosis
CNS Disturbances	**Neuromuscular**
Cerebral vascular accident	Amyotrophic lateral sclerosis
Sleep apnea	Guillain–Barré syndrome
Tumor	Myasthenia gravis
CNS depressant drugs	Hypokalemia
Barbiturates	Hypophosphatemia
Benzodiazepines	Drugs
Opioids	Aminoglycosides
	Antiarrhythmics
	Lithium
	Phenytoin

CNS, central nervous system; COPD, chronic obstructive pulmonary disease.

Evaluation

CASE 26-4

QUESTION 1: B.B., a 70-year-old man, is admitted to the hospital for treatment of an exacerbation of chronic obstructive pulmonary disease (COPD). He complains of worsening shortness of breath and increased production of sputum for the past 3 days. He has also noted a mild headache, a flushed feeling, and drowsiness within the past 24 hours. He has a history of COPD, hypertension, coronary artery disease, and low back pain. Current medications are tiotropium one inhalation daily, salmeterol dry powder inhaler one inhalation BID, chlorthalidone 12.5 mg daily, long-acting diltiazem 240 mg daily, and diazepam 5 mg TID as needed for back pain.

Vital signs include respiratory rate of 16 breaths/minute and HR of 90 beats/minute. Diffuse wheezes and rhonchi are heard on chest auscultation. Laboratory tests reveal the following:

Na, 140 mEq/L
K, 4.0 mEq/L
Cl, 100 mEq/L
pH, 7.32
$Paco_2$, 58 mm Hg
Pao_2, 58 mm Hg
HCO_3^-, 29 mEq/L

B.B.'s baseline ABG at the physician's office last month was pH, 7.35; $Paco_2$, 51 mm Hg; Pao_2, 62 mm Hg; and HCO_3^-, 28 mEq/L. Which of B.B.'s signs and symptoms are consistent with the diagnosis of respiratory acidosis?

A stepwise evaluation reveals a respiratory acidosis. A history of COPD and physical findings of dyspnea, headache, drowsiness, and flushing support the ABG evaluation. Respiratory acidosis also can cause more severe symptoms, including CNS effects, such as disorientation, confusion, delirium, hallucinations, and coma. These CNS abnormalities probably are partly caused by the direct effects of carbon dioxide. Hypoxemia (decreased Pao_2), which commonly accompanies respiratory acidosis, also contributes to these symptoms. Elevated $Paco_2$ causes cerebral vascular dilation, resulting in headache caused by increased blood flow and increased intracranial pressure. Cardiovascular effects typically include tachycardia, arrhythmias, and peripheral vasodilation.[68]

CASE 26-4, QUESTION 2: Is the respiratory acidosis present in B.B. consistent with an acute or a chronic disorder?

Following the stepwise approach, it is determined that B.B. has a respiratory acidosis. He has a normal AG. Comparing his current to previous values (e.g., pH, $Paco_2$, HCO_3^-), it appears B.B. has an acute-on-chronic respiratory acidosis because his baseline $Paco_2$ was 51 mm Hg with an acute worsening to 58 mm Hg. In respiratory acidosis, increased renal reabsorption of bicarbonate compensates for the increase in $Paco_2$; however, at least 48 to 72 hours are needed for this compensatory mechanism to become fully established.[10] Patients with COPD commonly present with an acute-on-chronic respiratory acidosis similar to B.B.

Causes

CASE 26-4, QUESTION 3: What potential causes of respiratory acidosis are present in B.B.?

Respiratory acidosis often is caused by airway obstruction, as shown in Table 26-6.[67,68] Chronic obstructive airway disease is a common cause of both acute and chronic respiratory acidosis. Upper respiratory tract infections, such as acute bronchitis, can worsen airway obstruction and produce acute respiratory acidosis.

DRUG-INDUCED

B.B.'s drug therapy also may be contributing to respiratory insufficiency. Many drugs (Table 26-7) decrease ventilation, but usually these drugs only significantly affect patients who are predisposed to respiratory problems because of underlying diseases. Because B.B. has COPD, he may be more sensitive to drugs affecting respiration. The benzodiazepines, barbiturates, and opioids minimally decrease respiration in normal subjects and in most patients with COPD when given in usual therapeutic doses. These drugs, however, can cause significant respiratory insufficiency when administered either in large doses or in combination with other respiratory depressant drugs.[68] B.B.'s diazepam may be contributing to hypoventilation and respiratory acidosis and should be withdrawn from his regimen. Nonselective adrenergic blocking drugs should be used cautiously in patients with COPD.

Treatment

CASE 26-4, QUESTION 4: How should B.B.'s respiratory acidosis be treated?

As with most cases of respiratory acidosis, treatment primarily involves correction of the underlying cause of respiratory insufficiency. In this case, treatment of acute bronchospasm with a β-adrenergic agent, such as inhaled albuterol, is warranted. Corticosteroids, such as methylprednisolone (60–125 mg every 6–12 hours initially), are commonly used in hospitalized patients with acute exacerbations of COPD.[69] Antibiotic therapy with a β-lactam with or without a β-lactamase inhibitor should be considered in hospitalized patients producing purulent, large-volume secretions.[70] B.B's respiratory status should be monitored closely during his hospitalization. If the acidosis, hypercarbia, or associated hypoxemia worsen, noninvasive positive-pressure ventilation or intubation with mechanical ventilation may be required.[54]

Treatment with IV sodium bicarbonate is not recommended in most cases of acute respiratory acidosis because of the risks associated with bicarbonate therapy (see Case 26-2, Question 4) and because an absolute deficiency of bicarbonate is not present. When the excess CO_2 is excreted, arterial pH should return to normal. Hypercapnia should not be overcorrected, because hypocapnia results in decreased lung compliance, increases dysfunctional surfactant production, and shifts the oxyhemoglobin dissociation curve to the left, restricting the release of oxygen to tissues.[60,61,71]

RESPIRATORY ALKALOSIS

Respiratory alkalosis usually is not a severe disorder. Excessive rate or depth of respiration results in increased excretion of carbon dioxide, a fall in $Paco_2$, and a rise in arterial pH. Common causes of respiratory alkalosis are presented in Table 26-8. Many conditions can cause respiratory alkalosis by stimulating respiratory drive in the CNS. In addition, pulmonary diseases can stimulate receptors in the lung to increase ventilation, and conditions that decrease oxygen delivery to tissues also can stimulate ventilation, causing respiratory alkalosis.[72,73]

Evaluation

CASE 26-5

QUESTION 1: S.P., a 50-year-old, 80-kg woman, is admitted for treatment of presumed bacterial pneumonia. She was in good health until 24 hours before presentation when she noted an abrupt onset of fever, a productive cough with thick, yellowish sputum;

and chest pain on deep inspiration. She has taken aspirin 650 mg every 3 hours since the onset of fever, with mild relief. Since arriving in the ED, she has become anxious and lightheaded and has developed tingling in her hands, feet, and lips. Vital signs include the following: temperature, 38°C; respiratory rate, 24 breaths/minute; HR, 110 beats/minute; and BP, 135/70 mm Hg. Physical examination reveals dullness to percussion, rales, and decreased breath sounds over the left lower lung field.

Laboratory findings include the following:
Serum Na, 135 mEq/L
Cl, 105 mEq/L
pH, 7.49
$Paco_2$, 30 mm Hg
Pao_2, 90 mm Hg
HCO_3^-, 22 mEq/L

Gram stain of sputum reveals 25 white blood cells per high-power field and many gram-positive diplococci. White blood cell count is 15,400 cells/μL with a left shift. A left lower lobe infiltrate is seen on chest radiograph. What acid–base disorder is present in S.P.?

Steps 1 to 3 in the evaluation of the ABG values, as described previously, indicate a respiratory alkalosis (increased pH, decreased $Paco_2$). The history and physical findings of deep, rapid breathing and tingling sensations are clues to the etiology. This disorder is most likely acute because her HCO_3^- concentration is normal. She does not have an AG. If a large AG were present, it would suggest she has a coexisting metabolic acidosis, possibly caused by salicylate intoxication (see Case 26-5, Question 3).

Case 26-5, Question 2: Which of S.P.'s signs and symptoms are consistent with the diagnosis of acute respiratory alkalosis?

S.P.'s paresthesias of the extremities and perioral region, lightheadedness, tachycardia, and increased rate and depth of respiration are common signs and symptoms of respiratory alkalosis. Confusion and decreased mental acuity also may be evident.[5,6,10] Simple respiratory alkalosis rarely produces life-threatening abnormalities.

Causes

Case 26-5, Question 3: What is the cause of the acid–base disorder in S.P.?

Table 26-8
Common Causes of Respiratory Alkalosis

CNS Disturbances	**Pulmonary**
Bacteremia	Pneumonia
Cerebrovascular accident	Pulmonary edema
Fever	Pulmonary embolus
Hepatic cirrhosis	
Hyperventilation	**Tissue Hypoxia**
Anxiety-induced	High altitude
Voluntary	Hypotension
Meningitis	CHF
Pregnancy	
Trauma	**Other**
Drugs	Excessive mechanical ventilation
Progesterone derivatives	Rapid correction of metabolic acidosis
Respiratory stimulants	
Salicylate overdose	

CHF, congestive heart failure; CNS, central nervous system.

Common causes of respiratory alkalosis are listed in Table 26-8.[5,6,10,72–74] Based on physical examination, laboratory findings, and chest radiograph, S.P. appears to have an acute bacterial pneumonia. Pneumonia and other pulmonary diseases can result in stimulation of ventilation and respiratory alkalosis, even with a normal Pao_2, as in this case. The anxiety S.P. is experiencing also may be contributing to respiratory alkalosis by producing the familiar anxiety–hyperventilation syndrome. Although salicylate intoxication is a potential cause of respiratory alkalosis because of the direct respiratory stimulant effect of salicylate,[74] S.P. displays few other symptoms of salicylate intoxication (e.g., nausea, vomiting, tinnitus, altered mental status, elevated AG metabolic acidosis). The total aspirin dose reportedly ingested (65 mg/kg in 24 hours) is not large enough to be associated with significant risk for toxicity.

Treatment

Case 26-5, Question 4: What is the appropriate treatment for S.P.'s respiratory alkalosis?

Similar to respiratory acidosis, treatment of respiratory alkalosis usually involves correcting the underlying disorder. Initiation of appropriate antibiotic therapy for a community-acquired pneumonia is indicated in this case (see Chapter 67, Respiratory Tract Infections). Simple respiratory alkalosis is unlikely to cause life-threatening symptoms, although mortality rates for critically ill patients with this disorder can be high.[68] The well-known remedy of rebreathing expired air from a paper bag for treatment of hyperventilation associated with anxiety appears to be effective for this cause of respiratory alkalosis and may be helpful for S.P.

MIXED ACID–BASE DISORDERS

Evaluation

CASE 26-6

Question 1: B.L., a 65-year-old man who was transferred from a long-term acute care facility 2 days previously, is disorientated and lethargic. He was doing well until 1 week before admission, when the staff noted that he was somnolent. He progressively became more lethargic and could no longer remember the names of other persons. B.L. has a history of alcoholic cirrhosis, type 2 diabetes mellitus, and hypertension. Medications before admission were nadolol 80 mg daily, isosorbide mononitrate 20 mg BID, glyburide 10 mg daily, and spironolactone 50 mg BID. On admission, B.L. was disoriented to person, place, and time and was difficult to arouse. Vital signs include the following: temperature, 37°C; respirations, 16 breaths/minute; HR, 70 beats/minute; and BP, 154/92 mm Hg. Physical examination revealed asterixis and mild ascites. Laboratory studies included the following:

Na, 133 mEq/L	Albumin, 3.2 g/dL
K, 4.3 mEq/L	Ammonia, 120 μmol/L
Cl, 106 mEq/L	pH, 7.43
BUN, 5 mg/dL	$Paco_2$, 30 mm Hg
Creatinine, 0.7 mg/dL	Pao_2, 90 mm Hg
Fasting glucose, 150 mg/dL	HCO_3^-, 19 mEq/L

On admission, spironolactone was increased to 200 mg daily and lactulose 60 mL orally QID was started for treatment of hepatic encephalopathy. Within the first 24 hours of lactulose therapy, B.L.

produced four loose, watery stools; however, his mental status worsened to the point of being unresponsive, his BP dropped to 100/60 mm Hg, and his breathing became labored and eventually required mechanical ventilation. At the time of intubation, his laboratory values were as follows:

Na, 137 mEq/L	Arterial pH, 7.06
K, 4.5 mEq/L	$Paco_2$, 48 mm Hg
Cl, 105 mEq/L	Pao_2, 58 mm Hg
BUN, 10 mg/dL	HCO_3^-, 13 mEq/L
Creatinine, 1.2 mg/dL	

Gram stain of peritoneal fluid revealed many WBC and gram-negative rods; the diagnosis of spontaneous bacterial peritonitis with septic shock is made. Describe B.L.'s acid–base status on admission and at the current time.

An evaluation of B.L.'s first ABG results using Steps 1 and 2 (in the section Evaluation of Acid–Base Disorders) reveals abnormal $Paco_2$ and serum bicarbonate values, suggesting the existence of an underlying acid–base abnormality. The direction of change in his $Paco_2$ and serum HCO_3^-, along with a pH of 7.43, suggests a respiratory alkalosis is the primary disorder. His calculated AG of 8 is not increased. Examination of the ranges of expected compensation in Table 26-3 reveals that these values are indeed consistent with chronic respiratory alkalosis (serum HCO_3^- decreased by 0.5 mEq/L for each 1 mm Hg drop in $Paco_2$). B.L.'s history of alcohol-induced liver disease is consistent with the diagnosis of chronic respiratory alkalosis (Table 26-8).[8,10]

The second set of ABG reveals severe acidosis. B.L.'s serum bicarbonate has fallen from 19 to 13 mEq/L, and his $Paco_2$ has increased acutely from 30 to 48 mm Hg. Because these values have changed in opposite directions, a mixed acid–base abnormality should be suspected.

The diagnosis of a mixed metabolic and respiratory acidosis can be confirmed by applying the stepwise approach outlined previously. If the acidosis were purely metabolic in nature, a serum HCO_3^- of 13 mEq/L should result in hyperventilation and a low $Paco_2$. B.L.'s $Paco_2$ of 48 mm Hg is high, which would be consistent with coexistent respiratory acidosis. The anion gap is 19, indicating an AG metabolic acidosis is present. The excess AG (AG − 10 = 9) added to B.L's HCO_3^- of 13 yields a corrected HCO_3^- of 22, which is normal. This suggests no additional metabolic disturbances are present.

Causes

Case 26-6, Question 2: What are possible causes for the mixed acidosis in B.L.?

The AG should be calculated in all patients with a metabolic acidosis. B.L.'s calculated AG has increased from 8 to 19 mEq/L (11 and 22 mEq/L, respectively, after adjusting for hypoalbuminemia), suggesting that an elevated AG acidosis is now present. Septic shock from bacterial peritonitis can produce profound hypotension, which leads to tissue hypoperfusion, generation of lactic acid, and a subsequent elevation in the AG. Other causes of elevated AG metabolic acidosis can be excluded with additional laboratory data (e.g., serum ketones, glucose, osmolal gap).

Although diarrhea and spironolactone should be considered in the differential diagnosis, these are usually associated with hyperchloremic, normal AG metabolic acidosis (Table 26-2).[75] The coexisting respiratory acidosis is most likely the result of B.L.'s altered mental status and his diminished respiratory drive.

Case 26-6, Question 3: During the next 6 hours, B.L.'s hepatic encephalopathy, peritonitis, and acid–base disorders are aggressively treated with lactulose, antibiotics, fluids, and mechanical ventilation. His most recent ABG reveals the following:

pH, 7.45
$Paco_2$, 24 mm Hg
Pao_2, 90 mm Hg
HCO_3^-, 16 mEq/L

Ventilator settings are assist-control mode at 16 breaths/minute, tidal volume 700 mL, and inspired oxygen concentration 40%. B.L. is noted to be more awake, anxious, and initiating 25 to 30 breaths/minute. What is the current acid–base status and probable cause?

Evaluation of the ABG reveals a pH at the upper limit of normal with significant decreases in both $Paco_2$ and serum HCO_3^- concentration. This clinical scenario is most consistent with a mixed acute respiratory alkalosis and ongoing metabolic acidosis. The time frame in which B.L.'s $Paco_2$ decreased from 48 to 24 mm Hg is consistent with acute respiratory alkalosis. B.L.'s low serum HCO_3^- suggests ongoing metabolic acidosis as a result of his septicemia. The metabolic acidosis should improve with time, given adequate antibiotic therapy and supportive measures that maintain BP and increase oxygen delivery to the tissues.

The acute respiratory alkalosis in this case is most likely caused by the mechanical ventilator, B.L.'s anxiety, or sepsis. In the assist-control mode, any inspiratory effort by B.L. results in the delivery of a fully assisted breath by the ventilator.[76] B.L.'s anxiety and resultant tachypnea are resulting in over ventilation, producing excessive CO_2 elimination and respiratory alkalosis. Appropriate changes in the therapy may include use of an anxiolytic, an analgesic if needed to treat pain, changing the ventilator settings, or probably a combination of these strategies.

KEY REFERENCES AND WEBSITES

A full list of references for this chapter can be found at http://thepoint.lww.com/AT11e. Below are the key references and websites for this chapter, with the corresponding reference number in this chapter found in parentheses after the reference.

Key References

Adrogue HJ, Madias NE. Management of life-threatening acid–base disorders: first of two parts. *N Engl J Med*. 1998;338:26. (54)

Adrogue HJ, Madias NE. Management of life threatening acid–base disorders: second of two parts. *N Engl J Med*. 1998;338:107. (55)

Rose BD, Post TW. Metabolic alkalosis. In: Rose BD, Post TW, eds. *Clinical Physiology of Acid–Base and Electrolyte Disorders*. 5th ed. New York: McGraw-Hill Medical; 2001:551. (62)

Rose BD, Post TW. Regulation of acid–base balance. In: Rose BD, Post TW, eds. *Clinical Physiology of Acid–Base and Electrolyte Disorders*. 5th ed. New York: McGraw-Hill Medical; 2001:325. (4)

Rose BD, Post TW. Introduction to simple and mixed acid–base disorders. In: Rose BD, Post TW, eds. *Clinical Physiology of Acid–Base and Electrolyte Disorders*. 5th ed. New York: McGraw-Hill Medical; 2001:535. (8)

Rose BD, Post TW. Metabolic acidosis. In: Rose BD, Post TW, eds. *Clinical Physiology of Acid–Base and Electrolyte Disorders*. 5th ed. New York: McGraw-Hill Medical; 2001:578. (26)

Rose BD, Post TW. Respiratory acidosis. In: Rose BD, Post TW, eds. *Clinical Physiology of Acid–Base and Electrolyte Disorders*. 5th ed. New York: McGraw-Hill Medical; 2001:647. (67)

Rose BD, Post TW. Respiratory alkalosis. In: Rose BD, Post TW, eds. *Clinical Physiology of Acid–Base and Electrolyte Disorders*. 5th ed. New York: McGraw-Hill Medical; 2001:673. (74)

27 Fluid and Electrolyte Disorders

Alan H. Lau and Priscilla P. How

CORE PRINCIPLES

CORE PRINCIPLES	CHAPTER CASES
FLUID AND SODIUM DISORDERS	
1 Plasma osmolality is maintained within normal limits through a delicate balance between water intake and excretion. Antidiuretic hormone (ADH) plays an important role in maintaining fluid balance in the body.	**Case 27-1 (Question 1), Figure 27-1**
2 Signs of volume depletion include orthostatic hypotension, dry mucous membranes, and poor skin turgor. Because water and sodium are inherently linked, the assessment of volume status and selection of replacement fluid require examination of sodium concentration.	**Case 27-2 (Questions 1, 2)**
3 Aldosterone is the main regulatory hormone for sodium homeostasis. A patient may have hypotonic, isotonic, or hypertonic hyponatremia depending on the plasma osmolality. Normal serum sodium concentration is 135–145 mEq/L.	**Cases 27-4 through 27-7, Figure 27-1**
4 Hypovolemic hypotonic hyponatremia can occur with volume depletion and decreased extracellular fluid. Calculation of sodium deficit will determine how much sodium replacement is required.	**Case 27-5 (Questions 1, 2)**
5 Hypervolemic, hypotonic hyponatremia is caused by a disproportionate accumulation of ingested water relative to sodium. It is also observed in patients with heart failure, liver and renal failure, and nephrotic syndrome. Management includes sodium and water restriction, as well as the use of diuretics.	**Case 27-6 (Question 1)**
6 Syndrome of inappropriate antidiuretic hormone is a common cause of normovolemic hypotonic hyponatremia. Persistent ADH secretion together with water ingestion results in hyponatremia.	**Case 27-7 (Question 1)**
7 Neurologic symptoms may be manifested in acute or severe hyponatremia. Low plasma osmolality causes water to move into the brain resulting in cerebral edema, increased intracranial pressure, and central nervous system symptoms. Rapid or overly aggressive correction of hyponatremia can result in osmotic demyelination.	**Case 27-7 (Questions 3, 4)**
POTASSIUM DISORDERS	
1 The sodium–potassium adenosine triphosphatase pump plays a pivotal role in maintaining potassium homeostasis. Normal serum potassium concentration is 3.5–5.0 mEq/L. Clinical manifestations of hypokalemia include muscle weakness and electrocardiography (ECG) changes.	**Case 27-8 (Questions 1, 2)**
2 Potassium repletion should be guided by close monitoring of serum potassium. Oral supplementation is usually preferred. Patients who cannot tolerate oral potassium or who have severe/symptomatic hypokalemia can receive intravenous potassium. In general, the rate of potassium infusion should not exceed 10 mEq/hour to prevent phlebitis.	**Case 27-8 (Question 3)**

Continued

	CHAPTER CASES
3 Hyperkalemia can be caused by chronic kidney disease and medications that inhibit the renin–angiotensin–aldosterone system. Intravenous calcium is administered to antagonize the cardiac effects (ECG changes and ventricular arrhythmias) of hyperkalemia. Other treatment strategies include the use of insulin and glucose, β_2-agonists, sodium polystyrene sulfonate, sodium bicarbonate, and dialysis.	**Case 27-9 (Question 1), Case 27-10 (Questions 1, 2), Table 27-3**
CALCIUM DISORDERS	
1 Normal serum calcium is 8.5–10.5 mg/dL (corrected for serum albumin as calcium is protein-bound). Hypercalcemia can be caused by dehydration, malignancy, hyperparathyroidism, vitamin D intoxication, sarcoidosis, and other granulomatous disease. Clinical presentation of hypercalcemia includes signs and symptoms involving the neurologic, cardiovascular, pulmonary, renal, gastrointestinal, and musculoskeletal systems. First-line treatment for hypercalcemia is hydration and diuresis. Calcitonin and bisphosphonates are alternative agents used in the management of hypercalcemia.	**Case 27-11 (Questions 1–3), Table 27-4**
PHOSPHATE DISORDERS	
1 Hypophosphatemia can develop as a result of impaired intestinal phosphorus absorption, increased renal elimination, or shift of phosphorus from extracellular to intracellular compartments. Normal serum phosphorus concentration is 2.7–4.7 mg/dL.	**Case 27-12 (Questions 1, 2)**
2 Clinical effects of hypophosphatemia can involve multiple organ systems and are attributed to impaired cellular energy stores and tissue hypoxia secondary to ATP depletion. Phosphorus supplementation can be administered orally or intravenously, depending on the signs and symptoms, and severity of hypophosphatemia. Renal function, serum phosphorus, calcium, and magnesium need to be monitored closely. Diarrhea is a common dose-related side effect of oral phosphorus replacement.	**Case 27-12 (Questions 3, 4)**
MAGNESIUM DISORDERS	
1 Magnesium depletion (normal serum magnesium, 1.8–2.4 mEq/L) can result in abnormal function of the neurologic, neuromuscular, and cardiovascular systems. Typical findings include Chvostek and Trousseau signs, muscle fasciculation, tremors, muscle spasticity, convulsions, and possibly tetany. As serum magnesium does not reflect total body stores, symptoms are more important determinants of the urgency and aggressiveness of magnesium replacement.	**Case 27-13 (Questions 1, 2)**
2 Oral magnesium replacement is indicated in asymptomatic patients with mild depletion. Urinary excretion of magnesium increases during intravenous replacement. Thus, replenishment of magnesium stores usually takes several days. After intravenous magnesium administration, the patient should be monitored for hypotension, marked suppression of deep tendon reflexes, ECG and respiration changes, as well as hypermagnesemia.	**Case 27-13 (Questions 3, 4)**
3 A common cause of hypermagnesemia is the use of magnesium-containing laxatives and antacids by patients with renal impairment. Potentially life-threatening complications of severe hypermagnesemia include respiratory paralysis, hypotension, and complete heart block. Intravenous calcium should be administered to antagonize the respiratory and cardiac manifestations of magnesium. Diuretics may be given to patients with good renal function to enhance urinary magnesium excretion.	**Case 27-14 (Questions 1–3)**

BASIC PRINCIPLES

Body Water Compartments and Electrolyte Composition

In newborns, approximately 75% to 85% of body weight is water. After puberty, the percentage of water per kilogram of weight decreases as the amount of adipose tissue increases with age.[1,2] Body water constitutes 50% to 60% of the lean body weight (LBW) in adult men but only 45% to 55% in women because of their greater proportion of adipose tissue. The water content per kilogram of body weight further decreases with advanced age. Total body water (TBW) is usually calculated as 0.6 × LBW in men and 0.5 × LBW in women.

Two-thirds of the total body water resides in the cells (intracellular water). The extracellular water can be divided into different compartments—the interstitial fluid (12% LBW) and the plasma (5% LBW) are the two major compartments. Other compartments of the extracellular fluid (ECF) include the connective tissues and bone water, the transcellular fluids (e.g., glandular secretions), and other fluids in sequestered spaces, such as the cerebrospinal fluid.[1]

The electrolyte composition differs between the intracellular and extracellular compartments. Potassium, magnesium, and phosphate are the major ions in the intracellular compartment, whereas sodium, chloride, and bicarbonate are predominant in the extracellular space.[2] Water travels freely across the cell membranes of most parts of the body. The cell membrane, however, is only selectively permeable to solutes. The impermeable solutes are osmotically active and can exert an osmotic pressure that dictates the distribution of water between fluid compartments. Water moves across the cell membrane from a region of low osmolality to one of high osmolality. Net water movement ceases when osmotic equilibrium occurs. Each fluid compartment contains a major osmotically active solute: potassium in the intracellular space and sodium in the ECF. The volumes of the two compartments reflect the asymmetrically larger number of solute particles or osmoles inside the cells.[2,3]

The capillary wall separates the interstitial fluid from plasma. Because sodium moves freely across the capillary wall, its concentration is identical across both sides of the wall. Therefore, no osmotic gradient is generated, and water distribution between these two spaces is not affected. Plasma proteins, which are confined in the vascular space, are the primary osmoles that affect water distribution between the interstitium and the plasma.[2] In contrast, urea, which traverses both the capillary walls and most cell membranes, is osmotically inactive.[2,3]

Plasma Osmolality

Osmolality is defined as the number of particles per kilogram of water (mOsm/kg). It is determined by the number of particles in solution and not by particle size or valence. Nondissociable solutes, such as glucose and albumin, generate 1 mOsm/mmol of particles; and dissociable salts, such as sodium chloride, liberate two ions in solution to produce 2 mOsm/mmol of salt. The osmolality of body fluid is maintained between 280 and 295 mOsm/kg. Because all body fluid compartments are iso-osmotic, plasma osmolality reflects the osmolality of total body water. Plasma osmolality can be measured by the freezing point depression method, or estimated by the following equation, which takes into account the osmotic effect of sodium, glucose, and urea[2,3]:

$$P_{osm} = 2(\text{Na})(\text{mmol/L}) + \text{Glucose (mg/dL)}/18 + \text{BUN (mg/dL)}/2.8 \quad \text{(Eq. 27-1)}$$

This equation predicts the measured plasma osmolality within 5 to 10 mOsm/kg. Although urea contributes to the measured osmolality, it is an ineffective osmole because it readily traverses cell membranes and, therefore, does not cause significant fluid shift within the body. Hence, the effective plasma osmolality (synonymous with tonicity, the portion of total osmolality that has the potential to induce transmembrane water movement) can be estimated by the following equation:

$$P_{osm} = 2(\text{Na})(\text{mmol/L}) + \text{Glucose (mg/dL)}/18 \quad \text{(Eq. 27-2)}$$

An osmolal gap exists when the measured and calculated values differ by greater than 10 mOsm/kg[4]; it signifies the presence of unidentified particles. When the individual solute has been identified, its contribution to the measured osmolality can be estimated by dividing its concentration (mg/dL) by one-tenth of its molecular weight. Calculating the osmolal gap is used to detect the presence of substances, such as ethanol, methanol, and ethylene glycol, that have high osmolality. Occasionally, the osmolal gap can also result from an artificial decrease in the serum sodium secondary to severe hyperlipidemia or hyperproteinemia.

CASE 27-1

QUESTION 1: J.F., a 31-year-old man, is admitted to the inpatient medicine service for methanol intoxication. Routine laboratory analysis reveals the following:

Sodium (Na), 145 mEq/L
Potassium (K), 3.4 mEq/L
Blood urea nitrogen (BUN), 10 mg/dL
Creatinine, 1.1 mg/dL
Glucose, 90 mg/dL

The blood methanol concentration was 108 mg/dL, and the measured plasma osmolality was 333 mOsm/kg. What is J.F.'s calculated osmolality? Are other unidentified osmoles present?

Using Equation 27-1, J.F.'s total calculated osmolality is

$$\begin{aligned} P_{osm} &= 2(145\ \text{mEq/L}) + 90\ \text{mg/dL}/18 + 10\ \text{mg/dL}/2.8 \\ &= 290 + 5 + 3.6 \\ &= 299\ \text{mOsm/kg} \end{aligned} \quad \text{(Eq. 27-3)}$$

$$\text{Osmolal gap} = 333\ \text{mOsm/kg} - 299\ \text{mOsm/kg} = 34\ \text{mOsm/kg} \quad \text{(Eq. 27-4)}$$

In J.F., the entire osmolal gap can be accounted for by the presence of the methanol (because 108 mg/dL of methanol will provide 108/3.2 = 33.7 mOsm/kg). It is unlikely, therefore, that other unmeasured osmoles are present (e.g., ethylene glycol, isopropanol, and ethanol). The laboratory determination of osmolality measures the total number of osmotically active particles but not their permeability across the cell membrane. Methanol increases plasma osmolality but not tonicity because the cell membrane is permeable to methanol. Therefore, no net water shift occurs between the intracellular and extracellular compartments. Conversely, mannitol, which is confined to the extracellular space, contributes to both plasma osmolality and tonicity.

Tubular Function of Nephron

The kidney plays an important role in maintaining a constant extracellular environment by regulating the excretion of water and various electrolytes. The volume and composition of fluid filtered across the glomerulus are modified as the fluid passes through the tubules of the nephron.

The renal tubule is composed of a series of segments with heterogeneous structures and functions: the proximal tubule, the medullary and cortical thick ascending limb of Henle's loop, the distal convoluted tubule, and the cortical and medullary collecting duct[2] (Fig. 27-1). The mechanism for sodium reabsorption is different for each nephron segment, but it is generally mediated by carrier proteins or channels located on the luminal membrane of the tubule cell.[2] Na^+/K^+ ATPase (sodium–potassium adenosine triphosphatase) actively pumps sodium out of the renal tubule cell in exchange for potassium in a 3:2 ratio. Hence, the intracellular sodium concentration is kept at a low level. The potassium that is pumped into the cell leaks back out through potassium channels in the membrane, rendering the cell interior electronegative. The low intracellular sodium concentration and a negative intracellular potential produce a favorable gradient for passive sodium entry into the cell.[3] Na^+/K^+ ATPase also indirectly provides the energy for active sodium transport and the reabsorption and secretion of other solutes across the luminal membrane of the renal tubule. The distal segments are mainly involved in the reabsorption of sodium and chloride ions and the secretion of hydrogen and potassium ions.[2]

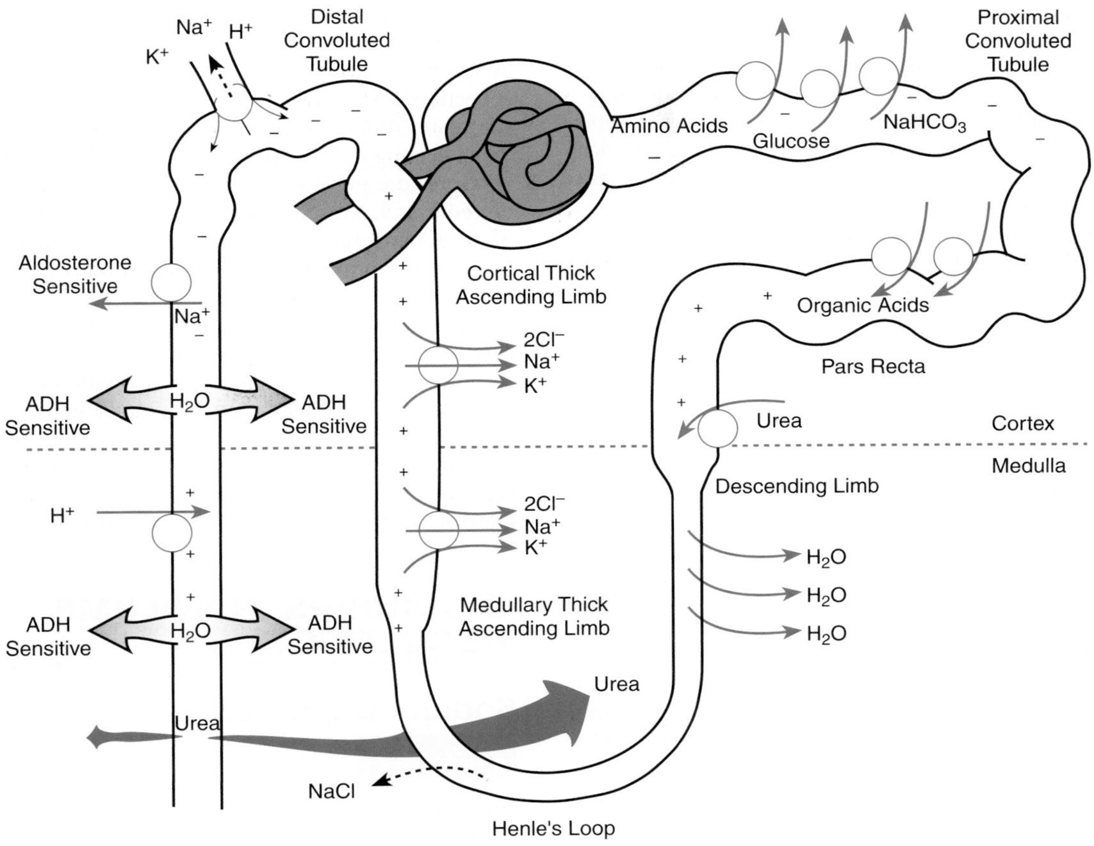

Figure 27-1 Sites of tubule salt and water absorption. Sodium is reabsorbed with inorganic anions, amino acids, and glucose in the proximal tubule against an electrical gradient that is lumen-negative. In the distal part of the proximal tubule (pars recta), sodium and water are reabsorbed to a lesser extent and organic acids (hippurate, urate) and urea are secreted into the urine. The electrical potential is lumen-positive in the pars recta. Water, but not salt, is removed from tubule fluid in the thin descending limb of Henle's loop, but in the ascending portion salt is reabsorbed without water, rendering the tubule fluid hyposmotic with respect to the interstitium. Sodium, chloride, and potassium are reabsorbed by the medullary and cortical portions of the ascending limb; the lumen potential is positive. Sodium is reabsorbed and potassium and hydrogen ions are secreted in the distal tubule and collecting ducts. Water absorption in these segments is regulated by antidiuretic hormone (ADH). The electrical potential is lumen-negative in the cortical sections and positive in the medullary segments. Urea is concentrated in the interstitium of the medulla and assists in the generation of maximally concentrated urine. (Reprinted with permission from Chonko AM et al. Treatment of edema states. In: Narins RG, ed. *Maxwell & Kleeman's Clinical Disorders of Fluid and Electrolyte Metabolism*. 5th ed. New York, NY: McGraw-Hill; 1994:545.)

Iso-osmotic reabsorption of the glomerular filtrate occurs in the proximal tubule such that two-thirds of the filtered sodium and water and 90% of the filtered bicarbonate are reabsorbed. The Na^+/H^+ antiporter (exchanger) in the luminal membrane is instrumental in the reabsorption of sodium chloride, sodium bicarbonate, and water. The reabsorption of most nonelectrolyte solutes, such as glucose, amino acids, and phosphates, are coupled to sodium transport.[2,5]

Both the thick ascending limb of Henle's loop and the distal convoluted tubule serve as the diluting segments of the nephron because they are impermeable to water. Sodium chloride is extracted from the filtrate without water. Sodium transport in both of these segments is flow-dependent and varies with the amount of sodium ions delivered from the proximal segments of the nephron. Decreased sodium ions in the tubular fluid will limit sodium transport in the thick ascending limb of Henle's loop and the distal convoluted tubule.[2,6]

Reabsorption of sodium in the thick ascending limb of Henle's loop accounts for approximately 25% of the total sodium reabsorption. Sodium, chloride, and potassium are reabsorbed by the medullary and cortical portions of the ascending limb, but the leakage of reabsorbed potassium ions back into the tubular lumen, via potassium channels, makes the tubular lumen electropositive. This electrical gradient promotes the passive reabsorption of cations, such as sodium, calcium, and magnesium, in the distal convoluted tubules. Because the thick ascending limb of Henle's loop is impermeable to water, it contributes to the interstitial osmolality in the medulla. This high osmolality is key to the reabsorption of water by the medullary portion of the collecting duct under the influence of antidiuretic hormone (ADH, vasopressin). Therefore, the thick ascending limb of Henle's loop is important for both urinary concentration and dilution.[6]

Because, as noted previously, the distal convoluted tubule is also impermeable to water, the osmolality of the filtrate continues to decline as sodium is being reabsorbed. In the distal convoluted tubule and collecting duct, sodium is reabsorbed in exchange for hydrogen ions and potassium. When sodium ions are reabsorbed, the tubule lumen becomes electronegative, which promotes potassium secretion in the lumen via potassium channels. Aldosterone enhances sodium reabsorption in the collecting duct by increasing the number of opened sodium channels.[2,7]

The collecting duct is usually impermeable to water. Under the influence of ADH, however, water permeability is increased through an increase in the number of water channels along the luminal membrane. The amount of water reabsorbed depends on the tonicity of the medullary interstitium, which is determined by the sodium reabsorbed in the thick ascending limb of Henle's loop and urea.[2,7,8]

Osmoregulation

A reduction of intracellular volume often increases effective plasma osmolality; conversely, decreased effective plasma osmolality is associated with cellular hydration. Water homeostasis is important in the regulation of plasma osmolality, and plasma tonicity is maintained within normal limits through a delicate balance between the rates of water intake and excretion.

The amount of daily water intake includes the volume of water ingested (sensible intake), the water content of ingested food, and the metabolic production of water (insensible intake).[2] To maintain homeostasis, these should be equal to the amount of water excreted by the kidney and the gastrointestinal (GI) tract (sensible loss) plus water lost from the skin and respiratory tract (insensible loss).[2,3]

Changes in plasma tonicity are detected by osmoreceptors in the hypothalamus, which also houses the thirst center and is the site for ADH synthesis.[9,10] When the plasma tonicity falls below 280 mOsm/kg as a result of water ingestion, ADH release is inhibited,[2] water is no longer reabsorbed in the collecting duct, and a large volume of dilute urine is excreted. Conversely, when the osmoreceptors in the hypothalamus sense an increased plasma osmolality, ADH is released to increase water reabsorption. A small volume of concentrated urine is then excreted. The threshold for ADH release is 280 mOsm/kg, and maximal ADH secretion occurs when the plasma osmolality is 295 mOsm/kg.[9] Thus, urine osmolality varies from 50 mOsm/kg in the absence of ADH to 1,200 mOsm/kg during maximal ADH release. The volume of urine produced depends on the solute load to be excreted, as well as the urine osmolality[2,3,9,10]:

$$\text{Urine volume (L)} = (\text{Solute load (mOsm)}/\text{Urine osmolality (mOsm/kg)}) \times (1/\text{Density of water (kg/L)}) \quad \text{(Eq. 27-5)}$$

Therefore, for a typical daily solute load of 600 mOsm:

$$= (600\ \text{mOsm}/50\ \text{mOsm/kg})(1/1\ \text{kg/L}) = 12\ \text{L (No ADH)} \quad \text{(Eq. 27-6)}$$

$$= (600\ \text{mOsm}/1{,}200\ \text{mOsm/kg})(1/1\ \text{kg/L}) = 0.5\ \text{L (Max ADH)} \quad \text{(Eq. 27-7)}$$

Although the kidney has a remarkable ability to excrete free water, it is not as efficient in conserving water. ADH minimizes further water loss, but it cannot correct water deficits. Therefore, optimal osmoregulation requires increased water intake stimulated by thirst. Both ADH and thirst can be stimulated by nonosmotic stimuli. For example, volume depletion is such a strong nonosmotic stimulus for ADH release that it can override the response to changes in plasma osmolality. Nausea, pain, and hypoxia are also potent stimuli for ADH secretion.[11]

Volume Regulation

Sodium resides almost exclusively in the ECF; the amount of total body sodium, therefore, determines the extracellular volume.[2,11] Because daily sodium intake varies from 100 to 250 mEq, the body must rely on adjustments in urinary sodium excretion to maintain the extracellular volume and tissue perfusion.[2,11] The ability of the kidney to retain sodium is so remarkable that a person can survive with a daily sodium intake of as low as 20 to 30 mEq.

The afferent sensors for the changes in the effective circulating volume are the intrathoracic volume receptors, the baroreceptors in the carotid sinus and aortic arch, and the afferent arteriole in the glomerulus.[11]

When the effective circulating volume is decreased, both the renin–angiotensin–aldosterone and the sympathetic nervous systems are activated.[2,11] Angiotensin type 2 (AT_2) and norepinephrine enhance sodium reabsorption at the proximal convoluted tubule. In addition, aldosterone stimulates sodium reabsorption at the collecting tubule. The decrease in effective arterial volume also stimulates ADH release, which enhances water reabsorption at the collecting duct. Conversely, after a salt load, the increases in atrial pressure and renal perfusion pressure suppress the production of renin and, subsequently, AT_2 and aldosterone. The release of atrial natriuretic peptide secondary to increased atrial filling pressure and intrarenal production of urodilators increase urinary excretion of the excess sodium.[12,13]

Although the kidney can excrete a 20-mL/kg water load in 4 hours, only 50% of the excess sodium is excreted in the first day.[3] Sodium excretion continues to increase until a new steady state is reached after 3 to 4 days, when intake equals output.[3,12] It is important to recognize that osmoregulation and volume regulation occur independently of each other.[2,3] The two homeostatic systems regulate different parameters and possess different sensors and effectors. Both systems can be activated simultaneously, however.

DISORDERS IN VOLUME REGULATION

Sodium Depletion

CASE 27-2

QUESTION 1: A.B., a 17-year-old girl, presented to the emergency department (ED) with complaints of anorexia, nausea, vomiting, and generalized weakness for the past 3 days. She denied other medical problems and had not used any medications. On examination, her supine blood pressure (BP) was 105/70 mm Hg, with a pulse of 80 beats/minute. Her standing BP was 85/60 mm Hg with a pulse of 100 beats/minute, and she complained of feeling dizzy when she stood up. Her mucous membranes were dry, but her skin turgor was normal. The jugular vein was flat, and peripheral or sacral edema was not present. Laboratory blood tests showed the following:

Serum Na, 134 mEq/L
K, 3.5 mEq/L
Chloride (Cl), 95 mEq/L
Total CO_2 content, 35 mEq/L
BUN, 18 mg/dL
Creatinine, 0.8 mg/dL
Glucose, 70 mg/dL

Random urinary sodium was 40 mEq/L, potassium was 40 mEq/L, and chloride was less than 15 mEq/L. The hemoglobin was 14 g/dL, and white cell and platelet counts were normal. Based on the clinical and laboratory data in A.B., what is the most probable explanation for her presentation?

The signs and symptoms in A.B. are consistent with volume depletion. The loss of gastric fluid owing to vomiting and decreased oral intake secondary to anorexia led to moderate-to-severe volume depletion. She exhibits orthostatic changes in both her BP (a drop in systolic BP of 20 mm Hg) and pulse (an increase of 20 beats/minute). The dry mucous membranes, the flat jugular vein, and the absence of edema support volume depletion as well, and dizziness on standing indicates extracellular volume depletion.[14] Her hypochloremic metabolic alkalosis was probably initiated by loss of acidic gastric contents through vomiting. Her volume depletion increased renal bicarbonate reabsorption, perpetuating the metabolic alkalosis. The decreased renal perfusion brought about by volume depletion enhanced proximal tubular reabsorption of urea, resulting in an increased BUN to creatinine ratio (prerenal azotemia). When renal perfusion is decreased and the renin–angiotensin–aldosterone system is activated, the proximal reabsorption of sodium and chloride is increased. A.B.'s urinary sodium is, therefore, less than 10 mEq/L.[15] Excretion of the poorly permeable bicarbonate ions, however, results in obligatory urinary sodium loss to maintain luminal electroneutrality. A.B.'s urinary sodium was therefore elevated (40 mEq/L). In this situation, the urinary chloride remained low, and this is a better index of volume status.[15] Both urinary sodium and chloride are elevated, however, in patients using diuretics, in those undergoing osmotic diuresis, and in those with underlying renal disease or hypoaldosteronism, even in the face of volume depletion. Physical examination should therefore be conducted as part of the volume status assessment. A.B.'s volume depletion increased the concentration of red blood cells, which could explain her slightly elevated hemoglobin concentration of 14 g/dL.

CASE 27-2, QUESTION 2: How should A.B.'s volume depletion be managed?

The etiology of A.B.'s vomiting should be sought and the cause removed. Because the patient is neither hypernatremic nor hyponatremic, normal saline should be administered intravenously to replenish the extracellular volume and improve tissue perfusion.[2,14] If the patient is hypernatremic (having a greater deficit of water than solute), half-isotonic saline or dextrose solution, which contains more free water, should be administered. In contrast, hyponatremic hypovolemic patients have a greater deficit of solute than water; isotonic or hypertonic saline should then be given. The amount of volume deficit is often difficult to ascertain. Because A.B. was severely orthostatic, 1 or 2 L of fluid can be given over the course of 2 to 4 hours. The subsequent rate of infusion will depend on A.B.'s response and the prevailing symptoms. The clinician should monitor her body weight, skin turgor, supine and upright BP, jugular venous pressure, urine output, and urine chloride concentration to assess the adequacy of volume repletion. Because the treatment goal is to achieve a positive fluid balance, the infusion rate should be 50 or 100 mL/hour in excess of the sum of urine output, insensible losses, and other losses, such as emesis and diarrhea.[2]

Sodium Excess

CASE 27-3

QUESTION 1: L.J., a 45-year-old man, presented to the clinic with complaints of swollen legs and puffy eyelids. He also noticed that his urine had been foamy recently. On examination, his BP was 180/100 mm Hg and his pulse was 80 beats/minute. Bilateral periorbital edema and 2+ bilateral pitting edema up to the thigh were noted. On auscultation, his heart was normal and his lungs had bilateral crackles. His jugular venous pressure was elevated at 10 cm H_2O. Laboratory tests revealed the following:

Serum Na, 132 mEq/L
K, 3.8 mEq/L
Cl, 100 mEq/L
Bicarbonate, 26 mEq/L
BUN, 40 mg/dL
Creatinine, 2.5 mg/dL
Glucose, 120 mg/dL
Albumin, 2 g/dL
Serum cholesterol, 280 mg/dL,
Triglycerides, 300 mg/dL

The serum transaminases, alkaline phosphatase, and bilirubin were within normal limits. Urinalysis showed the following:

Specific gravity, 1.015
pH, 7.0
Protein, >300 mg/dL
24-hour urinary protein excretion, 6 g
Creatinine clearance (CrCl), 40 mL/minute

Urinalysis also showed oval fat bodies and fatty casts. L.J. was taking no medications and he denied illicit drug use. Hepatitis B serology and human immunodeficiency virus (HIV) antibody were negative. The impression was anasarca (total body edema) secondary to nephrotic syndrome. What is nephrotic syndrome? What could be the cause of L.J.'s sodium excess state?

Nephrotic syndrome is characterized by hypoalbuminemia, urine protein excretion greater than 3.5 g/day, hyperlipidemia, lipiduria, and edema.[16,17] The heavy proteinuria is a result of damage to the selective barrier of the glomerulus. The causes of nephrotic syndrome are multiple and diverse.[16] The causes can be idiopathic (primary glomerular disease) or secondary to chronic systemic diseases (e.g., diabetes mellitus, amyloidosis, sickle cell anemia,[18] lupus), cancer (e.g., multiple myeloma, Hodgkin disease), infections (e.g., HIV,[19] hepatitis B, syphilis, malaria), intravenous (IV) drug abuse, and medications (e.g., gold, penicillamine, captopril, nonsteroidal anti-inflammatory drugs [NSAIDs][20]).

A heavy urinary protein loss results in various extrarenal complications.[16,17] Hypoalbuminemia reduces plasma oncotic pressure and contributes to the increased hepatic synthesis of both albumin and lipoproteins. This, coupled with the decreased catabolism of lipoproteins, resulted in L.J.'s hyperlipidemia.[16,21] Urinary loss of inhibitors of coagulation predispose these patients to thromboembolism.[16]

Specific therapy of nephrotic syndrome ranges from simple removal of the offending medication and treatment of the underlying comorbidities to the use of immunosuppressive agents in specific glomerular diseases.

L.J.'s anasarca results from changes in both capillary hemodynamics and renal sodium and water retention.[22] The hypoalbuminemia (2 g/dL) and proteinuria (>300 mg/dL) produce an imbalance in the Starling forces across the capillary wall, namely the hydrostatic and oncotic pressures in the capillary and interstitial compartments. The reduced capillary oncotic pressure favors movement of fluid from the vascular space into the interstitium.[23] This leads to contraction of the effective arterial blood volume, which in turn activates humoral, neural, and hemodynamic mechanisms that signal the kidney to retain sodium and water.[24,25] This underfill hypothesis has been challenged by data, suggesting that hypoalbuminemia plays a minor role in nephrotic edema[26,27] and the observation that patients with nephrotic syndrome can have increased, normal, or decreased plasma volumes.[23]

A defect in the intrarenal sodium handling mechanism that causes inappropriate sodium retention also contributes to nephrotic edema.[23,26] According to this overflow hypothesis, proteinuric renal disease leads to increased sodium reabsorption in the distal nephron. The mechanism is not well defined but may be related to cellular resistance to atrial natriuretic peptide.[23] Thus, a sodium excess state occurs and edema results. It is likely that the interaction between the underfill and overflow mechanisms results in the production of nephrotic edema.[28] Patients with severe hypoalbuminemia (i.e., serum albumin level < 1.5 g/dL), who have a severe reduction in plasma oncotic pressure, are most likely to exhibit evidence of the underfill phenomenon.[22]

CASE 27-3, QUESTION 2: How should L.J.'s sodium excess state be managed?

The etiology of L.J.'s nephrotic syndrome should be identified for specific treatment. Although L.J.'s serum sodium concentration of 132 mEq/L is low, it reflects dilution secondary to fluid excess. Salt restriction is therefore important to control L.J.'s generalized edema.[23] For most nephrotic patients, modest dietary sodium restriction to approximately 50 mEq/day may be sufficient to maintain neutral sodium balance.[22,23] For nephrotic patients who are very sodium avid (urine sodium concentration < 10 mEq/L), sufficient restriction is difficult to achieve. Thus, slowing the rate of edema formation rather than hastening its resolution should be the goal of therapy for these patients.[23] Bed rest reduces orthostatic stimulation of the renin–angiotensin–aldosterone and sympathetic systems, thereby favoring the movement of interstitial fluid into the vascular space.[23] The central blood volume is thus increased and natriuresis and diuresis are facilitated. Prolonged bed rest might, however, predispose these hypercoagulable patients to thromboembolism.[16] Similarly, use of support stockings may reduce the stimulation for sodium retention by redistributing blood volume to the central circulation.[23,29]

DIURETICS

Usually, loop diuretics are the mainstay of therapy in the management of nephrotic edema.[2,23] In most of these patients, the edema can be removed safely with rapid diuresis without compromising the systemic circulation, probably because of the rapid refilling of the plasma volume by interstitial fluid.[23] Nevertheless, as the edema resolves, the rate of fluid removal and weight loss should be decreased to avoid compromising the effective circulating volume. The patient should be monitored for the development of orthostatic hypotension.

Infusions of albumin can expand the plasma volume; however, it is expensive, the relief is temporary, and it should therefore be used only for resistant edema.[30] In patients who are resistant to the aforementioned measures, extracorporeal fluid removal, namely ultrafiltration, may be necessary.[23,31]

L.J. was initially treated with IV furosemide 60 mg twice daily and placed on a low-sodium (50 mEq), low-fat, high-complex carbohydrate diet that consisted of 0.8 g/kg protein of high biologic value with additional protein to match gram-per-gram of urinary protein loss. Fluid was restricted to 1,000 mL/day.[32] He had 5 L of diuresis in 2 days, with resolution of respiratory symptoms and a reduction in the anasarca. Parenteral furosemide was discontinued on the fifth day of hospitalization and oral furosemide 120 mg twice daily was started. After a total weight loss of 12 kg, he was then discharged with instructions to maintain the diet and oral furosemide.

DISORDERS IN OSMOREGULATION

Hyponatremia

Serum sodium concentration reflects the ratio of total body sodium to total body water and is not an accurate indicator of total body sodium. Both hyponatremia and hypernatremia can occur in the presence of a low, normal, or high total body sodium.[33,34]

Because the kidney can excrete greater than 12 to 16 L of free water daily, hyponatremia does not occur unless the water intake overwhelms the kidney's ability to excrete free water (e.g., psychogenic polydipsia),[35,36] or free-water excretion is impaired.[2,37]

Free-water formation requires a normal glomerular filtration rate (GFR), the reabsorption of sodium chloride without water in the thick ascending limb of Henle's loop and the distal convoluting tubule, and the excretion of a dilute urine in the absence of ADH[37] (Fig. 27-1). Therefore, hyponatremia can occur when the kidney's diluting ability is exceeded or impaired owing to volume depletion and nonosmotic stimulation of ADH release or inappropriate stimulation of ADH production.[2,37]

Although plasma sodium is the primary determinant of plasma tonicity, hyponatremia does not always represent hypotonicity.[2,37] In patients with severe hyperlipidemia or hyperproteinemia (e.g., multiple myeloma), pseudohyponatremia can occur because the increased amounts of lipids and proteins displace plasma water, in which sodium ions dissolve, resulting in a lower concentration of sodium per unit volume of plasma.[34,37,38] Normally, water accounts for 93% of the plasma volume, and lipids and proteins make up the rest.[37] The increase in plasma lipid and protein contents expands plasma volume, displaces water, and increases the percentage of solids in plasma.[34,37] Because sodium is distributed only in the aqueous phase, the sodium content per liter of the newly recomposed plasma is thus decreased and the plasma sodium concentration is reduced.[34,37,38] The sodium concentration in plasma water remains the same, however. Because osmolality depends on the solute concentration in plasma water, serum osmolality remains unchanged.[34] Indeed, the measured osmolality is normal. Another example of isotonic hyponatremia can be found when a large volume of isotonic mannitol irrigant is used during prostate surgery.[34,37] Absorption of the irrigation solution can result in severe hyponatremia but normal osmolality. In contrast, use of large amounts of isotonic sorbitol and isotonic, or slightly hypotonic, glycine solutions during urologic surgery can cause the hypotonicity as a late complication.[34,37] Similar to mannitol, sorbitol and isotonic glycine initially distribute only in the extracellular space, resulting in hyponatremia without a change in osmolality.[37] Unlike mannitol, both sorbitol and glycine are later metabolized, leaving water behind to result in hypotonicity. The severe hypotonic hyponatremia, in conjunction with the neurotoxic effects of glycine and its metabolites, puts the patient at significant risk for severe neurologic symptoms (Table 27-1).[37,39]

CASE 27-4

QUESTION 1: T.T., a 63-year-old man with end-stage renal disease caused by diabetic nephropathy, is receiving chronic ambulatory peritoneal dialysis. Because of dietary and fluid noncompliance, T.T. complained of shortness of breath (SOB) and his dialysis prescription was adjusted to include six cycles of 2.5% peritoneal dialysis solutions. Today, his laboratory values are as follows:

Na, 128 mEq/L
K, 4 mEq/L
Cl, 98 mEq/L
Total CO_2, 24 mM
BUN, 50 mg/dL
Creatinine, 6 mg/dL
Glucose, 600 mg/dL

Evaluate T.T.'s plasma osmolality. What is the etiology of T.T.'s hyponatremia?

Table 27-1
Clinical Presentation and Treatment of Hyponatremia

Na+ and H_2O Status	Clinical Presentation/Cause	Treatment
Edematous, Fluid Overload (Hypervolemic, Hypotonic)		
↑ Total body Na^+–↑↑ Total body H_2O	Cirrhosis/HF/nephrotic syndrome: A ↓ in renal blood flow activates renin–angiotensin system. ↑ Aldosterone leads to ↑ Na^+, and ↑ ADH leads to free H_2O retention. Urine Na^+ is low (0–20 mEq/L) and urine osmolality ↓. Diuretics can induce paradoxical effects on urine Na^+ and osmolality. This form can also occur in patients with renal failure who drink excessive amounts of water. Patients have symptoms of fluid overload (ascites, distended neck veins, edema).	Fluid and Na^+ restriction. Correct underlying disorder (e.g., paracentesis for ascites). Diurese cautiously[a]; avoid ↓ ECF and accompanying ↓ tissue perfusion. ↑ BUN may indicate overly rapid diuresis. Conivaptan: Loading dose of 20 mg IV for 30 minutes, followed by 20 mg IV as continuous infusion for 24 hours for an additional 1 to 3 days; may titrate up to maximal dose of 40 mg/day; maximal duration is 4 days after the loading dose. Dedicated IV line recommended and site of peripheral IV lines should be changed every 24 hours. Caution if used together with fluid restriction. Tolvaptan: Start 15 mg PO once daily. Dose may be increased at intervals of at least 24 hours to 30 mg PO once daily and then to a maximum of 60 mg PO once daily as needed. Caution if used together with fluid restriction. Initiate therapy in a hospital setting.
Nonedematous Hypovolemic (Hypotonic with ECF Depletion)		
↓↓ Total body Na^+ ↓ Total body H_2O	Occurs in GI fluid loss (e.g., diarrhea) with hypotonic electrolyte-poor fluid replacement, overdiuresis, "third spacing," Addison disease, renal tubular acidosis, osmotic diuresis. Replacement of fluid losses with solute-free fluid predisposes these patients to hyponatremia. Kidneys concentrate urine to conserve fluid (urine Na^+ <10 mEq/L). Symptoms: nonedematous; ECF depletion (collapsed neck veins, dehydration, orthostasis). Neurologic symptoms: (see Hyponatremia: Neurologic Manifestations in text).	Discontinue diuretics. Replace fluid and electrolyte (especially K^+) losses. 0.9% saline preferred unless Na^+ deficit[a] severe, then use 3%–5% saline.
Nonedematous, Normovolemic (Normovolemic, Hypotonic)		
↓ Total body Na^+ ↑ Total body H_2O	SIADH[b]: Hyponatremia, hypo-osmolality, renal Na^+ wasting (>40 mEq/L), absence of fluid depletion, $U_{osm} > P_{osm}$, normal renal and adrenal function. Free H_2O retained while Na^+ lost. *Causes:* (a) ADH production (infectious disease, vascular disease, cerebral neoplasm, cancer of lung, pancreas, duodenum); (b) exogenous ADH administration; (c) drugs; (d) psychogenic polydipsia.	See earlier for dosing of VRA (conivaptan and tolvaptan) Chronic treatment: Restrict fluids to less than urine loss. Demeclocycline (300–600 mg BID) induces reversible diabetes insipidus. Emergency treatment for unresponsive patients includes furosemide diuresis to achieve negative H_2O balance with careful replacement of Na^+ and K^+ using hypertonic saline solutions.[c]

[a]Remove estimated excess free water with IV furosemide (1 mg/kg). Repeat as necessary. Because furosemide generates a urine that resembles 0.5% NaCl, urine losses of sodium and potassium must be carefully measured and replaced hourly with hypertonic salt solutions. Correction rate: 1 to 2 mEq Na/hour in symptomatic patients; 0.5 mEq/hour in asymptomatic patients.
[b]Estimate sodium deficit: (mEq) = TBW (sodium desired − sodium observed). Rate of sodium and fluid repletion used depends on severity. Mild: replace with NS. First one-third for 6 to 12 hours at a rate of <0.5 mEq/L/hour, remaining two-thirds for 24 to 48 hours. Severe (e.g., seizures): Use 3% to 5% saline, rate gauged by patient's ability to tolerate sodium and volume load. Monitor central nervous system function, skin turgor, blood pressure, urine sodium, signs of sodium or water overload, especially in patients with cardiovascular, renal, and pulmonary disease.
[c]Total body water (TBW) = 0.6 L/kg × weight in kg (for men) and 0.5 L/kg × weight in kg (for women).
TBW excess = TBW − [TBW (observed serum NA)/(desired serum NA)].
ADH, antidiuretic hormone; BID, twice daily; BUN, blood urea nitrogen; HF, heart failure; ECF, extracellular fluid; GI, gastrointestinal; IV, intravenous; NS, normal saline (0.9% Na); PO, orally; SIADH, syndrome of inappropriate ADH; TBW, total body weight.

T.T.'s effective plasma osmolality is calculated to be 289 mOsm/L, of which 33 mOsm/L is contributed by the hyperglycemia. The slow utilization of glucose, because of the lack of insulin, causes water to move from the intracellular compartment into the plasma space because of the increased tonicity, thereby lowering the plasma sodium concentration.[34,37] Despite the lowered plasma sodium concentration, the plasma osmolality is normal because of hyperglycemia. Hence, no symptoms attributable to hypo-osmolality are observed. Indeed, when serum glucose is normalized with insulin and hydration, the serum sodium level will increase to approximately 136 mEq/L. For each 100-mg/dL increment in serum glucose, serum sodium decreases by 1.3 to 1.6 mEq/L.[34,37] Use of hypertonic mannitol or glycine solutions in patients with cerebral edema also results in a hyperosmolar hyponatremia.[34]

Hypotonic Hyponatremia with Decreased Extracellular Fluid

CASE 27-5

QUESTION 1: Q.B., a 30-year-old male athlete who has had multiple bouts of diarrhea for the last several days, has been drinking a sports drink to keep himself from getting dehydrated. His vital signs include supine BP, 145/80 mm Hg, and pulse, 70 beats/minute; standing BP, 128/68 mm Hg, and pulse, 90 beats/minute. Respiratory rate (RR) is 12 breaths/minute, and he is afebrile. His skin turgor is mildly decreased and laboratory data are the following:

Na, 128 mEq/L
K, 3.0 mEq/L
Cl, 100 mEq/L
Bicarbonate, 17 mEq/L
BUN, 27 mg/dL
Creatinine, 1.2 mg/dL

Urinary sodium and chloride were both less than 10 mEq/L. Assess Q.B.'s electrolyte and fluid status. What is the etiology of Q.B.'s hyponatremia?

Q.B. has true hypotonic hyponatremia with ECF depletion, suggesting that his total body sodium deficit is greater than that of total body water.[34] His poor skin turgor, orthostasis, prerenal azotemia, and low urinary sodium are consistent with volume depletion. The urinary sodium concentration helps distinguish between renal and nonrenal losses that result in the sodium and water deficits.[15,34,40] When the plasma volume is depleted, the urinary sodium concentration is less than 10 mEq/L, suggesting appropriate renal sodium conservation.[15] This is usually seen in patients such as Q.B. with GI fluid loss as in vomiting, diarrhea, or profuse sweating.[34,37,40]

Other causes of hypotonic hyponatremia are less likely in Q.B. They include surreptitious cathartic abuse and "third spacing," or accumulation of ECF in the abdominal cavity during acute pancreatitis, ileus, or pseudomembranous colitis.[37,40] If the urinary sodium is less than 20 mEq/L in the face of volume depletion, renal salt wastage should be considered.[15,37,40] The potential causes of this latter problem include diuretic use,[41–44] adrenal insufficiency,[44] and salt-wasting nephropathy[35] (e.g., chronic interstitial nephritis, medullary cystic disease, polycystic kidney disease, obstructive uropathy, and cisplatin toxicity[44,45]). In patients with renal insufficiency, neither the urinary sodium nor chloride concentration is a reliable index of volume status.[15]

Volume depletion leads to increased reabsorption of sodium and water in the proximal tubule and, thus, decreased sodium delivery to the diluting segments for free-water formation.[34,37,40] Decreased effective arterial volume is also a potent nonosmotic stimulus for ADH release.[9,10] These factors combine to dampen the ability of the kidney to form dilute urine and result in high urine osmolality despite a low serum sodium concentration.[34,37,40] Although the fluid lost in diarrhea is hypotonic, it is the replacement of fluid lost with an even more hypotonic fluid such as the sports drink or tap water that causes hyponatremia in patients such as Q.B.[37,40]

Q.B.'s diarrhea probably caused loss of potassium and bicarbonate through the GI tract, resulting in hypokalemia and hyperchloremic metabolic acidosis. The potassium depletion can sensitize ADH secretion in response to hypovolemic stimuli, and the hypokalemia can also lead to hyponatremia.[37] The cellular efflux of potassium causes cellular uptake of sodium, further reducing the serum sodium concentration.

CASE 27-5, QUESTION 2: How should Q.B.'s hyponatremia be treated?

The treatment of hypovolemic hyponatremia involves sodium replacement to correct the deficit. The sodium deficit can be estimated by the following formula:

$$\begin{aligned}\text{Na Deficit} &= \text{TBW} \times (\text{Desired} - \text{Current Na concentration})\\ &= 0.6\ \text{L/kg} \times 70\ \text{kg} \times (140 - 125\ \text{mEq/L})\\ &= 630\ \text{mEq} \qquad \text{(Eq. 27-8)}\end{aligned}$$

Recall that TBW = 0.6 L/kg × weight in kg for men and 0.5 L/kg × weight in kg for women.

Approximately one-third of the deficit can be replaced over the course of the first 12 hours at a rate of less than 0.5 mEq/L/hour. The remaining amounts can be administered over the course of the next several days.

The use of isotonic sodium chloride solution is ideal for the treatment of hyponatremia associated with volume depletion. As renal perfusion is restored, free water will be excreted with appropriate retention of sodium.[40] Because Q.B. has only mild volume depletion, oral replacement fluids can be given. Oral solutions containing both electrolyte and glucose[46] or rice-based solutions[47] are ideal for the management of persistent fluid loss. Glucose not only provides calories but also promotes the intestinal absorption of ingested sodium.[48] Because the rice-based solution provides more glucose and amino acids, both of which can promote intestinal sodium absorption, it is more effective than glucose alone.[2,48]

In patients with renal salt wasting, the ongoing daily sodium loss should also be taken into consideration when estimating the amount of replacement. Potassium should be given to correct hypokalemia, thereby reducing the hyponatremia as well. The serum sodium concentration may rise faster than expected because as tissue perfusion is restored, sodium delivery to the distal tubules will increase and ADH secretion will be suppressed appropriately.[34,37,40] In the absence of ADH, increased free-water excretion will improve the serum sodium concentration faster than initially estimated.

Hypervolemic Hypotonic Hyponatremia

CASE 27-6

QUESTION 1: T.W., a 55-year-old man with a longstanding history of alcoholic liver cirrhosis, is admitted to the hospital for worsening shortness of breath. His medical history includes portal hypertension, esophageal varices, and noncompliance with dietary restriction and medications. His BP is 120/60 mm Hg; pulse, 100 beats/minute; RR, 20 breaths/minute. He is afebrile. Physical examination reveals a jaundiced man in respiratory distress. His jugular vein is flat and lung examination reveals bilateral basal rales. Abdominal examination shows tense ascites with hepatomegaly and spider angiomas (telangiectasias resembling a spider). He has 1+ pedal edema bilaterally. Laboratory data on admission are as follows:

Na, 127 mEq/L
K, 3.4 mEq/L
Cl, 95 mEq/L
Total CO_2 content, 24 mEq/L
BUN, 10 mg/dL
Serum creatinine (SCr), 1.2 mg/dL
Albumin, 2.5 g/dL
Urine Na, <10 mEq/L
Osmolality, 380 mOsm/L

Identify the possible causes of hyponatremia in T.W. and discuss its pathophysiology. How should he be treated?

T.W. had no history of vomiting or diarrhea and had stopped using diuretics before admission. The physical findings of ascites and bilateral edema are not consistent with volume depletion but indicate a sodium-excess state. Both sodium and water retention occur, but the disproportionate accumulation of ingested water relative to sodium leads to hyponatremia.[34,37,40]

Cirrhotic patients who are susceptible to developing hyponatremia have a decreased effective arterial blood volume.[24,37,46,47] The low urinary sodium concentration suggests that the effective arterial blood volume was decreased.[15] The high urinary osmolality in the face of hypotonic hyponatremia suggests, however, that the release of ADH has been stimulated, impairing free-water excretion. Peripheral vasodilation causes decreases in systemic arterial BP despite a normal-to-high cardiac output. This, along with splanchnic venous pooling and decreased oncotic pressure secondary to hypoalbuminemia, decreases renal perfusion in patients with cirrhosis, such as T.W.[22,28,46] Decreased renal perfusion activates the renin–angiotensin–aldosterone system, the sympathetic nervous system, and the release of ADH. Reabsorption of sodium and water in the proximal tubules is enhanced, diminishing sodium and water delivery to the distal segments of the nephron. The diluting capacity of the kidney is thus impaired. Increased secretion of antidiuretic hormone also promotes free-water reabsorption at the collecting tubule and contributes to the hyperosmolality of urine and hyponatremia. The hypervolemic hyponatremia is also seen in patients with heart failure (HF) and nephrotic syndrome[24–28] and in patients with chronic renal disease who drink excessive amounts of water[37,40] (see Chapter 14, Heart Failure). As the GFR decreases, distal delivery of sodium is reduced and the ability to generate free water is impaired. In addition, the capacity to conserve sodium is impaired in these patients.[15]

Most patients who are edematous and hyponatremic are asymptomatic, but the degree of hyponatremia probably reflects the severity of the underlying disease.[46,47,49] Unless an acute decrease in serum sodium occurs, rapid therapeutic correction is not warranted.[37,40,46,47,50] Water restriction, the mainstay of therapy, is determined by the degree of hyponatremia and the severity of symptoms. Sodium restriction and judicious use of diuretics may help reduce the edematous state, but the patient must be monitored closely to avoid prerenal azotemia, which suggests overaggressive diuresis. Furthermore, diuretics can induce or worsen hyponatremia and volume depletion by impairing the diluting capacity of the kidney.[43–47]

T.W. had abdominal paracentesis to relieve respiratory discomfort with no sequelae. He was then prescribed a 1,000-mg sodium diet, and water was restricted to 500 mL/day. Diuretic therapy was resumed.

Normovolemic Hypotonic Hyponatremia

CASE 27-7

QUESTION 1: C.C., a 50-year-old man who was diagnosed recently with small-cell lung carcinoma, was brought to the ED by his family because he had become progressively lethargic and stuporous during the past week. Laboratory data revealed the following:

Serum Na, 110 mEq/L
K, 3.6 mEq/L
Cl, 78 mEq/L
Bicarbonate, 22 mEq/L
BUN, 10 mg/dL
SCr, 0.9 mg/dL
Glucose, 90 mg/dL
Serum osmolality, 230 mOsm/kg
Urine osmolality, 616 mOsm/kg
Urine Na, 60 mEq/L

Arterial blood gas (ABG) examination at room air showed pH, 7.38; P_{CO_2}, 38 mm Hg; and P_{O_2}, 80 mm Hg. On physical examination, C.C. was normotensive, appeared to be euvolemic, and had no edema detected. Review of his medical records showed normal adrenal and thyroid function. C.C. was currently not using any medications. On admission to the ward, C.C. weighed 60 kg and was given 1 L of normal saline, after which his serum sodium concentration was 108 mEq/L. Identify the cause of hyponatremia in C.C. and describe its pathophysiology.

In a patient with hypo-osmolar hyponatremia with a volume status that is apparently normal, the differential diagnosis[40] includes hypothyroidism,[51] cortisol deficiency,[52] a reset osmostat,[53] psychogenic polydipsia,[36,38] and the syndrome of inappropriate antidiuretic hormone secretion (SIADH),[54–56] which is a diagnosis of exclusion. C.C.'s normal thyroid and adrenal function tests exclude hypothyroidism and cortisol insufficiency as causes of his hyponatremia. The inappropriately elevated urine osmolality (>100 mOsm/kg) is inconsistent with psychogenic polydipsia or a reset osmostat, because free-water excretion is usually not impaired in these disorders. These findings, in addition to a urine sodium concentration greater than 40 mEq/L and a normal acid–base and potassium balance, are consistent with SIADH.[37,55,56]

In SIADH, the ADH secretion is considered inappropriate because of its persistence in the absence of appropriate osmotic and hemodynamic stimuli. Water ingestion is essential to the development of hyponatremia in SIADH because persistent ADH activity impairs water excretion, resulting in expansion of body fluids and hypo-osmolar hyponatremia. Edema rarely is apparent because only one-third of the retained water resides in the extracellular space and the sodium homeostatic mechanisms are intact.[34,40] The ECF expansion activates volume receptors and results in natriuresis. At steady state, urinary sodium excretion reflects sodium intake and is usually greater than 40 mEq/L, as in C.C.'s case. Nonetheless, if sodium intake is reduced severely, the urinary sodium concentration may become less than 40 mEq/L.[37]

The causes of SIADH are diverse and are shown in Table 27-1. Four different patterns of inappropriate ADH release have been identified.[37] No correlation has been found between these patterns and the underlying causes of SIADH, however. Mechanisms for drug-induced SIADH include ADH-like action on the collecting tubule, central stimulation of ADH release, and potentiation of the ADH effect.[37,57] Small-cell lung carcinoma is the most likely cause of C.C.'s SIADH.

CASE 27-7, QUESTION 2: Why was C.C.'s serum sodium concentration lower after the saline infusion?

Isotonic sodium chloride solution (154 mEq/L each of sodium and chloride ions, or 308 mOsm/L) initially will increase the plasma sodium concentration because its osmolality is higher than C.C.'s.[58] C.C., however, has a relatively fixed urine osmolality of 616 mOsm/kg owing to persistent ADH activity; thus, he must excrete an osmolar load of 616 mOsm in a volume of 1,000 mL of urine at steady state. Because a total of 1 L of fluid containing 308 mOsm was administered, all the solutes were excreted in 500 mL of urine output, and 500 mL of free water was retained to cause a further dilution of sodium and a reduction in serum sodium concentration.[37,58]

Neurologic Manifestations

CASE 27-7, QUESTION 3: Why are C.C.'s neurologic manifestations characteristic of hyponatremia?

As the plasma osmolality declines, the osmotic gradient created across the blood–brain barrier favors the movement of water into the brain and other cells.[37,40] Water movement from the cerebrospinal fluid into the cerebral interstitium results in cerebral edema. Brain swelling is limited by the meninges and cranium, however, giving rise to increased intracranial pressure and neurologic symptoms. The degree of cerebral overhydration and the rapidity of its development appear to correlate with the severity of symptoms.[37,40]

When hyponatremia develops in less than 2 to 3 days or the rate of decline in serum sodium is greater than 0.5 mEq/L/hour, the situation is regarded as acute.[37,59,60] The patient often becomes symptomatic when serum sodium concentration falls to 125 mEq/L; early complaints include nausea, vomiting, and malaise.[37,61] Severe symptoms occur more commonly when the serum sodium falls to less than 120 mEq/L and the rate of decline is greater than 0.5 mEq/L/hour. The patient may present with headache, tremors, incoordination, delirium, lethargy, and obtundation. As the serum sodium drops less than 110 to 115 mEq/L, seizure and coma may result.[37,61] On occasion, severe brain edema leads to transtentorial herniation and eventually death. Women, especially those who are premenopausal, apparently are more susceptible to the development of severe neurologic symptoms and irreversible neurologic damage than are men.[62,63]

In contrast to acute hyponatremia, patients who are chronically hyponatremic are usually asymptomatic.[37,59] If present, symptoms are usually vague and nonspecific and tend to occur at lower serum sodium concentrations than those associated with symptomatic acute hyponatremia.[37,59,61] The patient may experience anorexia, nausea, vomiting, muscle weakness, and cramps. Irritability, hostility, confusion, and personality changes may also be seen. At extremely low sodium levels, stupor and, rarely, seizures have been reported.

Brain Adaptation to Hyponatremia

The difference in symptoms between acute and chronic hyponatremia is related to cerebral adaptation to hypotonicity. Two adaptive mechanisms are important in minimizing cerebral edema.[37,40,64,65] First, cerebral overhydration increases the hydrostatic pressure in the cerebral interstitium, which results in the movement of fluid from the cerebral interstitial space to the cerebrospinal fluid. Second, the extrusion of intracellular solutes reduces cellular osmolality, which in turn enhances water movement out of the cells. Sodium and potassium ions are the initial solutes extruded, followed over a period of hours to days by osmolytes such as inositol, glutamine, glutamate, and taurine.[64] Therefore, when the serum sodium concentration falls faster than the onset of brain osmotic adaptation processes, serious and permanent neurologic damage can occur.[37,40,64,65] On the other hand, when hyponatremia develops over the course of 2 to 3 days, symptoms are not usually seen unless the serum sodium concentration is reduced markedly.

It is often difficult to determine the acuity and chronicity of hyponatremia. Unless an obvious cause for acute hyponatremia is found, assume that the condition is chronic.[37,59,60,65] A rapid decline in serum sodium concentration usually suggests that hypotonic fluid was administered to a patient with a condition that overwhelms or impairs renal water excretion. These conditions include psychogenic polydipsia[35,36]; postoperative hyponatremia[62,63,66,67]; postprostatectomy syndrome[39]; and administration of thiazide diuretics,[41,42] parenteral cyclophosphamide,[68] oxytocin,[69] and arginine vasopressin or its analogs.[57] C.C.'s symptoms appear to have developed over the course of 7 days and are consistent with chronic hyponatremia.

Rate of Correction of Hyponatremia

CASE 27-7, QUESTION 4: How should C.C.'s hyponatremia be managed?

C.C.'s water excess should be calculated to estimate the amount of water that should be removed to achieve the desired sodium concentration.

$$\text{Water excess} = \text{TBW} - \text{TBW (Observed serum Na/Desired serum Na)} = 36\ \text{L} - 36\ \text{L}\ (110\ \text{mEq/L}/120\ \text{mEq/L}) = 3.0\ \text{L} \quad \text{(Eq. 27-9)}$$

where

$$\text{TBW} = 0.6\ \text{L/kg} \times 60\ \text{kg} = 36\ \text{L} \quad \text{(Eq. 27-10)}$$

The treatment of hyponatremia has been controversial. Severe hyponatremia is associated with high rates of morbidity and mortality, but its treatment can also result in morbidity. The rate of correction has been implicated as the main cause of complications.[59–61,65,70–72]

It takes time for the brain to lose osmolytes to reduce cerebral swelling during hyponatremia; conversely, the rate of reaccumulation of these osmolytes must keep pace with the rise in serum sodium concentration to avoid brain dehydration and damage. Indeed, rapid correction of hyponatremia can cause a constellation of neurologic findings known as osmotic demyelination syndrome (ODS).[71,72] Clinical manifestations usually are delayed and occur one to several days after the treatment has been started. Neurologic findings include transient behavioral changes, seizures, akinetic mutism in mild cases, and features of a pontine disorder in severe cases (pseudobulbar palsy, quadriparesis, and coma). In some patients, the damage is irreversible, and central pontine myelinolysis can be documented in fatal cases. Patients at greatest risk for osmotic demyelination are those with severe hyponatremia lasting greater than 2 days and those in whom the rate of correction of hyponatremia is greater than 12 mEq/L in any 24-hour period.[65,71,72] Hypokalemia, which was found in about 90% of patients with ODS associated with rapid hyponatremia correction, has been suspected as a predisposing factor in the development of ODS.[72] Because the etiology of this complication is unclear, it may be beneficial to correct the hypokalemia before correcting the severe hyponatremia.[72]

Retrospective reviews suggest that acute hyponatremia can be treated safely at a rate of 1 mEq/L/hour initially, until the serum sodium concentration reaches 120 mEq/L. Thereafter, the rate of correction should be reduced to less than or equal to 0.5 mEq/L/hour, such that an increment in sodium concentration does not exceed 12 mEq/L in the first 24 hours.[59,73] Slow correction is indicated for severe chronic hyponatremia. No neurologic complications were seen in patients with severe hyponatremia when the average rate of correction to serum sodium was less than 0.55 mEq/L/hour or when the increase in serum sodium was less than 12 mEq/L in 24 hours or less than 18 mEq/L in 48 hours.[73]

In C.C., the serum sodium concentration should be raised to approximately 120 mEq/L at a correction rate of approximately 0.5 mEq/L/hour, using hypertonic saline and furosemide. Serum sodium concentrations should be monitored closely because the equation for calculating water excess does not take into account insensible loss, which can increase the rate of sodium correction.

The use of normal saline is not useful in C.C. because he excretes salt normally (urine sodium, 60 mEq/L). C.C.'s sodium deficit is as follows:

$$(0.6\ L/kg)(60\ kg)(120 - 110\ mEq/L) = 360\ mEq \quad \text{(Eq. 27-11)}$$

Because 1 L of 3% sodium chloride solution contains 513 mEq of sodium, approximately 700 mL of 3% saline solution, which contains 360 mEq of sodium, will be required to correct the sodium deficit. The recommended serum sodium concentration correction rate is 0.5 mEq/L/hour; therefore, a minimum of 20 hours will be needed to raise the serum sodium concentration by 10 mEq/L (from 110 to 120 mEq/L). The amount of sodium replacement to safely increase the serum sodium concentration can be determined by the product of the rate of replacement (0.5 mEq/L/hour) and TBW (36 L, Eq. 27-10)—that is, 18 mEq/hour. The maximal rate of infusion of 3% saline, which contains 0.513 mEq/mL of sodium, is therefore 35 mL/hour (18 mEq/hour)/(0.513 mEq/mL). A rate of 30 mL/hour, therefore, is appropriate to safely replace C.C.'s sodium deficit.

Because calculations for water excess and sodium deficits are only approximations, the patient's serum osmolality, serum sodium, and clinical response must be monitored closely. Urinary losses can be replaced with 3% sodium chloride solution and appropriate amounts of potassium.

Chronic Management of the Syndrome of Inappropriate Antidiuretic Hormone Secretion

Case 27-7, Question 5: How should C.C.'s SIADH be managed chronically?

SIADH is usually transient if the underlying cause can be removed. Chronic SIADH can occur, however, as illustrated by C.C. Water restriction sufficient to create a negative water balance is the primary therapy and should be attempted first.[37,40] In general, all fluids, not just water, should be included in the restriction. Salt intake, however, should not be reduced or solute depletion can occur. The extent of fluid restriction depends on urine output, the amount of insensible water loss, and urine osmolality. For a given amount of solute excretion, patients with a high urine osmolality require a smaller volume of urine (i.e., more water retained) than those with a lower urine osmolality (i.e., less water retained). Hence, more stringent water restriction is required in patients with a high urine osmolality. Commonly, several days of restriction are needed before a significant increase in plasma osmolality is observed.

When fluid restriction fails to reverse the hypo-osmolar state or when the patient is unwilling or unable to comply with the severe fluid restriction, drugs that antagonize the effect of ADH can be used.[37,40] These include loop diuretics,[74,75] demeclocycline,[76] and lithium.[77] Furosemide (20–40 mg/day) reduces urine osmolality by blocking the concentrating ability of the kidney.[74] Demeclocycline and lithium directly impair the response to ADH at the collecting tubule, inducing nephrogenic diabetes insipidus.[76,77] Demeclocycline (300–600 mg twice daily) is usually better tolerated than lithium. Its effect on water excretion is delayed for a few days, and it dissipates over a similar period of time after the drug is stopped. Nephrotoxicity has been reported with its use in patients with cirrhosis.[78] Limited data suggest that phenytoin may inhibit ADH secretion, but its effectiveness is questionable.[79] Urea can correct hypo-osmolality by increasing solute-free water excretion and reducing urinary sodium excretion.[80] It has been used effectively, at 30 to 60 g/day, both short term and long term, to reduce the need for fluid restriction.[81] An IV formulation of urea is available commercially; however, for oral administration, 30 g of urea crystals can be dissolved in 10 mL of aluminum–magnesium antacid and 100 mL of water. Orange juice or other strongly flavored liquids can be used to improve palatability.

VASOPRESSIN RECEPTOR ANTAGONISTS

Nonpeptide vasopressin receptor antagonists (VRAs), also known as the "vaptans" or "aquaretic agents," constitute a class of agents used for the treatment of hyponatremia. Arginine vasopressin (AVP), a neuropeptide hormone, plays an important role in maintaining serum osmolality, as well as circulatory and sodium homeostasis.[82,83] AVP exerts its physiologic effects by acting on V1A, V1B, and V2 receptors, causing effects such as vasoconstriction,[84,85] corticotropin release,[86] and water excretion,[87] respectively. V2 receptors are located in the renal collecting tubules and mediate the antidiuretic effects of AVP. Antagonism of the V2 receptors results in aquaresis, which is a unique solute-free and electrolyte-sparing (sodium and potassium) water excretion process in the kidneys. Because circulating levels of AVP are elevated in SIADH, cirrhosis, and HF, VRA can be beneficial in the management of hyponatremia associated with these conditions.

Conivaptan, a mixed V1A and V2 receptor antagonist, was the first VRA approved by the US Food and Drug Administration (FDA) for the treatment of euvolemic and hypervolemic hyponatremia in hospitalized patients.[88] Randomized, double-blind, placebo-controlled trials demonstrated its efficacy in increasing serum sodium concentrations in patients with euvolemic and hypervolemic hyponatremia associated with SIADH and HF, respectively.[88,89] It is administered as an IV infusion and its use is restricted to a short-term (4 days) inpatient use only. Close monitoring of serum sodium concentration is necessary to prevent overly rapid correction of hyponatremia and central pontine myelinolysis that may ensue. Because conivaptan is a potent inhibitor of the cytochrome P-450 3A4 (CYP3A4) enzyme, drug interactions with medications that undergo CYP3A4-mediated metabolism are possible.[82] In addition, patients may experience infusion-site reactions with conivaptan caused by the organic solvent, polypropylene glycol.

Tolvaptan, a selective oral VRA, was approved by the FDA in 2009 for the treatment of hypervolemic and euvolemic hyponatremia in patients with HF, cirrhosis, and SIADH. Because of its selectivity for the V2 receptor, tolvaptan increases urinary excretion of free water (aquaresis) and has less of a blood pressure–lowering effect. As such, it may be more suitable for use in patients with low to normal blood pressure, such as those with HF or cirrhosis. Tolvaptan has been shown to increase serum sodium concentration significantly and correct hyponatremia in patients with SIADH, chronic HF, or cirrhosis.[90] It has also been studied extensively in chronic HF where improvement in signs and symptoms such as reduction of edema and weight, as well as normalization of serum sodium concentrations, were shown.[91,92] However, the use of tolvaptan in HF had no effect on long-term cardiovascular mortality or hospitalization for HF.[93] More recent studies have shown the potential benefits of tolvaptan in patients with autosomal dominant polycystic kidney disease.[94,95] However, hepatic injury was noted in some patients, thus resulting in the release of a safety announcement by FDA to limit tolvaptan's use to no more than 30 days and the removal of the indication for use in patients with cirrhosis.[96] It should not be used also in patients with underlying hepatic disease.

Lixivaptan is another VRAs that is selective for the V2 receptor. Like tolvaptan, they are orally active and thus useful in patients who require chronic therapy or when oral therapy is preferred. Lixivaptan has been studied in patients with hyponatremia from HF, cirrhosis, and SIADH; the results showed significant increases in aquaresis and serum sodium concentrations in both in- and outpatients.[97–101] However, it has yet to receive FDA approval.

Common adverse effects of VRAs include thirst, dry mouth, polyuria, and blood pressure reduction. Aquaretics increase thirst by increasing blood tonicity and urine volume; orthostatic hypotension has been reported.[83,102] These agents are thus contraindicated in hypovolemic hyponatremia. The risk of excessive correction of hyponatremia and the resultant neurologic complications from osmotic demyelination exists with VRA, especially when used in combination with fluid restriction. These agents should therefore be initiated in the inpatient setting at the lowest possible dose and titrated slowly, with close monitoring of serum sodium concentrations and volume status. Additionally, the VRAs are substrates and inhibitors of the CYP3A4 enzyme. As a result, there is a potential for clinically significant drug interactions, particularly with concomitant administration of moderate or strong CYP3A4 inducers or inhibitors.

The VRAs should be used in hyponatremic patients with mild-to-moderate severe neurologic symptoms. Not only have they been shown to maintain normal serum sodium concentrations both short- and long-term but their aquaretic effect could also reduce or eliminate the need for fluid restriction normally required of patients.[90,103] The effectiveness of VRA to correct serum sodium concentration in euvolemic and hypervolemic hyponatremia has been shown. However, their long-term safety with chronic use and their potential benefits on morbidity and mortality still need to be assessed. The high cost of using these agents is also a major barrier to routine clinical use.

Hypernatremia

Hypernatremia can occur under the following conditions: (a) normal total body sodium with pure water loss, (b) low total body sodium with hypotonic fluid loss, and (c) high total body sodium as a result of pure salt gain.[104] Therefore, as in hyponatremia, it is important to assess the volume status of the ECF when evaluating hypernatremia.

Pure water loss can result from the inability of the kidney to conserve water (diabetes insipidus) or from extrarenal water loss through the respiratory tract or the skin.[105] Usually, pure water loss does not cause hypernatremia unless the thirst center is damaged or access to free water is limited.[104]

Hypotonic fluid loss can occur renally as a result of osmotic diuresis, use of loop diuretics, postobstruction diuresis, or intrinsic renal disease. Extrarenally, hypotonic fluid loss can result from diarrhea, vomiting, burns, and excessive sweating.

Pure salt gain can result from the use of hypertonic saline during abortion, sodium bicarbonate administration during cardiopulmonary resuscitation, hypertonic feedings in infants, and, rarely, mineralocorticoid excess.

The management of hypernatremia includes correcting the underlying cause of the hypertonic state, replacing the water deficits, and administering adequate water to match ongoing losses.[104] The pure water deficit can be estimated as follows:

$$\begin{aligned}\text{Water deficit} &= \text{TBW (Observed serum Na/Desired serum Na)} - \text{TBW}\\ &= \text{TBW (Observed serum Na/Desired serum Na} - 1) \quad \text{(Eq. 27-12)}\end{aligned}$$

where desired serum sodium is usually 140 mEq/L.

The rate at which hypernatremia should be corrected depends on the severity of symptoms and degree of hypertonicity. Too-rapid correction can precipitate cerebral edema, seizures, and irreversible neurologic damage, and can be fatal. For asymptomatic patients, the rate of correction probably should not exceed changes of 0.5 mEq/L/hour in plasma sodium. A rule of thumb is to replace half the calculated deficit with hypotonic solutions over the course of 12 to 24 hours. Any ongoing water loss, including insensible loss, should also be replenished while carefully monitoring the patient's neurologic status. The remaining deficit can then be replaced during the ensuing 24 to 48 hours. Concomitant solute deficits and ongoing solute losses should also be replaced as appropriate. If hypernatremia is caused only by pure water loss, free water can be administered as 5% dextrose in water. Half-normal saline or quarter-normal saline is used if a sodium deficit is also present. In patients with hypotension or shock, the effective arterial blood volume should be restored with normal saline or colloids before the plasma tonicity is corrected.

CLINICAL USE OF DIURETICS

Diuretics reduce sodium and chloride reabsorption in the renal tubules, thereby increasing urine volume. Enhanced solute and fluid excretion can be initiated through osmotic diuresis or inhibition of transport in the kidney tubules. Diuretics are categorized according to the sites within the kidney tubules where they inhibit sodium reabsorption (see Chapter 9, Essential Hypertension, and Chapter 28, Chronic Kidney Diseases).

Loop Diuretics

The loop diuretics—furosemide, bumetanide, torsemide, and ethacrynic acid—are the most potent diuretics available. They are also known as high-ceiling diuretics because they can inhibit the reabsorption of up to 20% to 25% of the filtered sodium load. The loop diuretics act in the medullary and cortical portion of the thick ascending limb of Henle's loop. Sodium and chloride transport through the $Na^+/K^+/2Cl^-$ carrier in the luminal membrane is inhibited. Reabsorption of calcium and magnesium is reduced secondary to the reduction in sodium chloride transport. The loop diuretics also possess a vasodilatory effect that can contribute to their diuretic activity.

Thiazide Diuretics

The thiazide diuretics are a group of structurally similar compounds that share a common mechanism of action. Several other sulfonamide diuretics that differ chemically, such as chlorthalidone, indapamide, and metolazone, also have diuretic effects similar to the thiazides. The primary site of action of these diuretics is at the proximal portion of the distal tubule. Sodium reabsorption via the Na^+/Cl^- cotransporter is blocked through competition with the chloride site of the transporter. Some of these agents, such as chlorothiazide, may also reduce sodium transport in the proximal tubule. The contribution of this effect toward net diuresis is negligible, however, because the sodium ions that are not reabsorbed in the proximal tubule will subsequently be reabsorbed in Henle's loop. Thiazide diuretics can enhance the reabsorption of calcium ion through a direct action on the early distal tubule. Therefore, these agents are useful to reduce calciuria in patients with kidney stones. In contrast, magnesium excretion is increased by the thiazides, which may result in hypomagnesemia.

Potassium-Sparing Diuretics

SPIRONOLACTONE, TRIAMTERENE, AND AMILORIDE

Spironolactone, triamterene, and amiloride are potassium-sparing diuretics that inhibit sodium reabsorption in the cortical collecting tubules through different mechanisms. Spironolactone is a competitive receptor-site antagonist of aldosterone in the distal segment of the renal tubule and is indicated especially for patients with hyperaldosteronism secondary to decreased renal perfusion. Patients with hyperaldosteronism can be identified by urinary electrolyte screening, which shows high urine potassium excretion with concomitant diminished or absent urine sodium excretion. By serving as an aldosterone antagonist, spironolactone inhibits sodium reabsorption and decreases the excretion of potassium and hydrogen ions. Dosages as high as 200 to 400 mg/day may be needed to induce natriuresis in patients with hyperaldosteronism.

In contrast to spironolactone, triamterene and amiloride reduce the passage of sodium ions through the luminal membrane, independent of aldosterone activity, by directly acting on sodium and potassium transport processes in the distal renal tubular cells. Triamterene and amiloride offer the advantage of a more rapid onset of action than spironolactone.

The initial effects of spironolactone are usually delayed for 2 or 3 days, and several additional days are needed to attain maximal diuretic effect. This delay is caused partly by the formation of an active metabolite, canrenone, which accounts for approximately 70% of the antimineralocorticoid activity of spironolactone. The elimination half-life of canrenone is 13.5 to 24 hours in normal subjects and is prolonged in patients with chronic liver disease (59 hours [range, 32–105 hours]) or HF (37 hours [range, 19–48 hours]).[106] Although the elimination half-life of canrenone is prolonged in these patients, plasma canrenone concentrations do not differ significantly from those in normal subjects because assay methods for canrenone are nonspecific and include measurement of both active and inactive metabolites.[107,108]

Triamterene is absorbed incompletely from the GI tract. The drug has a short half-life of 1.5 to 2.5 hours. The total body clearance is high because of rapid and extensive hepatic metabolism. Both the parent compound and the metabolite undergo biliary and renal excretion. As with spironolactone, the hepatic metabolism of triamterene can be altered in patients with cirrhosis.[109] The diuretic effect of triamterene begins within 2 to 3 hours of administration, with a maximal duration of 12 to 16 hours.

Amiloride does not undergo hepatic metabolism; approximately 50% of amiloride is excreted in the urine unchanged and the remainder is recovered in the stool as unabsorbed drug or through biliary excretion. Serum amiloride concentrations peak 3 hours after oral ingestion, and the half-life is 6 hours. Although commonly administered doses are in the range of 2.5 to 10 mg, diuresis increases over a much greater range. The onset of action is 2 hours, with maximal effects at 4 to 6 hours. Duration of action is dose dependent and ranges from 10 to 24 hours. Amiloride does not undergo hepatic metabolism, and the drug can accumulate in patients with renal insufficiency.

The maximal amount of filtered sodium that can be excreted through the action of potassium-sparing diuretics is approximately 1% to 2%. Their natriuretic activity, therefore, is relatively limited compared with the thiazide and loop diuretics. These agents are often used concurrently with thiazide and loop diuretics to reduce potassium loss. Spironolactone is especially useful in patients with liver cirrhosis and ascites, who are likely to have high levels of aldosterone.

Acetazolamide

Acetazolamide inhibits carbonic anhydrase, an enzyme that mediates the excretion of sodium, bicarbonate, and chloride ions in the proximal tubule. Use of the drug will increase urine pH owing to the increased excretion of bicarbonate ion. The net diuretic and natriuretic effects are limited, similar to those of the potassium-sparing diuretics. Because of the drug's proximal site of action, the sodium ions that are not reabsorbed will subsequently be reclaimed in Henle's loop and the distal tubule. In addition, metabolic acidosis associated with the use of acetazolamide diminishes its diuretic effect.

Osmotic Diuretics

Osmotic diuretics are nonresorbable solutes in the kidney tubule. They act primarily in the proximal tubule, where the osmotic pressure they generate impedes the reabsorption of water and solutes. Unlike other diuretics, the amount of water loss exceeds the concurrent loss of sodium and potassium. Mannitol has been used in the early treatment of oliguric postischemic acute renal failure to increase urine output. Urea, another osmotic diuretic, and mannitol are used to reduce intracranial pressure through cellular dehydration.

Complications of Diuretic Therapy

Disturbances in fluid, electrolyte, and acid–base balance are common side effects associated with diuretic therapy. These side effects, including hypokalemia, are discussed in detail in Chapter 9, Essential Hypertension; Chapter 14, Heart Failure; and Chapter 45, Gout and Hyperuricemia. Two complications, hyponatremia and metabolic alkalosis and acidosis, are, however, discussed in the subsequent section because of their specific relevance to fluid balance.

HYPONATREMIA

Thiazides induce diuresis by inhibiting sodium and water reabsorption in the kidney tubule. Because both sodium and water are lost, overdiuresis per se is not expected to cause hyponatremia. Instead, hyponatremia represents a dilution of plasma sodium by excess free water caused by volume-depletion–induced ADH activity. The enhanced ADH secretion increases free-water reabsorption, resulting in hyponatremia. Large doses of diuretic, excessive water drinking, and severe sodium-intake restriction all will accentuate the hyponatremia. Elderly patients are particularly susceptible to this diuretic-induced complication because of the age-associated loss of nephrons and consequent impairment of sodium–potassium exchange.

METABOLIC ALKALOSIS AND ACIDOSIS

Metabolic alkalosis often occurs in conjunction with potassium depletion secondary to diuretic use. The diuretic-induced contraction of ECF volume stimulates the secretion of aldosterone, which promotes the absorption of sodium and the retention of hydrogen ions in the kidney tubule. The net urinary loss of hydrogen ions into the urine results in metabolic alkalosis. Generally, reducing the dose of the diuretic will restore the acid–base balance.

Acetazolamide causes metabolic acidosis by inhibiting carbonic anhydrase, which results in urinary excretion of sodium bicarbonate. Spironolactone, amiloride, and triamterene can cause hyperchloremic metabolic acidosis because of their ability to decrease potassium and hydrogen ion tubular secretion. Patients with renal dysfunction or those taking potassium supplements or angiotensin-converting enzyme inhibitors, which reduce aldosterone secretion, are at increased risk for developing hyperkalemia and metabolic acidosis.

POTASSIUM

Homeostasis

The total amount of potassium stored in the body is approximately 45 to 55 mEq/kg and varies with age, sex, and muscle mass. Lower total body potassium is found in older adults, females, and individuals with a low lean-body-mass to fat ratio. Potassium is distributed unevenly between the intracellular and extracellular compartments; 98% of the total body potassium resides in the intracellular compartment, predominantly the muscle, and only 2% is found in the extracellular space.[34,110] The disproportionate intracellular distribution of potassium is maintained by the Na^+/K^+ ATPase pump, which transports sodium out of the cell in exchange for potassium.[110–113] The cell membrane resting potential is determined by the ratio of intracellular/extracellular potassium concentrations. As this ratio increases, hyperpolarization of the cell membrane occurs. Conversely, cellular depolarization results when the ratio decreases. In both situations, generation of the action potential is impaired.

The plasma potassium concentration is maintained within a narrow range of 3.5 to 5.0 mEq/L. Although the plasma potassium concentration can be affected by the total body potassium store, total body potassium excess or deficit cannot be estimated accurately based solely on the plasma concentration. In fact, a normal plasma potassium concentration does not imply normal total body potassium because multiple factors affect the plasma potassium concentration independent of total body potassium.[111]

Potassium homeostasis is maintained by both renal and extrarenal processes. The renal process regulates total body potassium by matching potassium excretion to dietary intake (external balance),[114] whereas the extrarenal process regulates potassium distribution across cell membrane (internal potassium balance).[111–112]

The normal daily intake of potassium ranges between 50 and 100 mEq. Approximately 90% of the ingested potassium is eliminated by the kidneys and approximately 10% is eliminated via the GI tract.[114] Potassium is filtered freely through the glomerulus and then reabsorbed. By the time the filtrate reaches the distal convoluted tubule, greater than 90% of filtered potassium has already been reabsorbed. The amount of potassium excreted is determined by distal tubular potassium secretion in the principal cells of the cortical collecting duct, which is under the influence of aldosterone. Hyperkalemia, increased potassium load, and AT_2 can all stimulate aldosterone secretion.[111]

Factors that affect renal potassium excretion include tubular flow, sodium delivery to the distal segments of the nephron, the presence of poorly absorbable anions that increase luminal electronegativity, acid–base status, and aldosterone activity.[114] Potassium excretion increases during hyperkalemia and decreases during potassium depletion. Excretion of an acute potassium load is a slow process, with only half the potassium load excreted in the first 4 to 6 hours. Lethal hyperkalemia would ensue were it not for the extrarenal process that regulates intracellular/extracellular potassium distribution.[111]

The Na^+/K^+ ATPase pump, which extrudes sodium from the cell in exchange for potassium, is pivotal in maintaining internal potassium balance.[114] Different hormonal factors regulate the activity of the Na^+/K^+ ATPase pump, namely insulin, catecholamines, and aldosterone. Insulin, the most important regulator, enhances potassium uptake by muscle, liver, and adipose tissue by stimulating Na^+/K^+ ATPase.[115] Indeed, basal insulin secretion is essential for potassium homeostasis.[111] Whereas β_2-adrenergic agonists activate the Na^+/K^+ ATPase pump via cyclic adenosine monophosphate and cause hypokalemia, α-adrenergic stimulation promotes hepatic potassium release and causes hyperkalemia.[116] Epinephrine, an α-agonist and β-agonist, causes a transient increase in plasma potassium (α-agonism) followed by a more sustained decrease in plasma potassium (β-agonism).[116,117] Besides its kaliuretic effect and enhanced potassium secretion in the colon, aldosterone also stimulates Na^+/K^+ ATPase.

Other factors that affect the transcellular distribution of potassium include systemic pH, plasma tonicity, and exercise.[111,113] The effect of acid–base balance on potassium distribution is not readily predictable and depends on both the nature and the direction of the underlying disorder. The concomitant effect of the acid–base disorder on renal potassium excretion further complicates the relationship between plasma potassium concentration and pH.[111,118] In acute inorganic acidosis, plasma potassium concentration increases by 0.2 to 1.7 mEq/L per 0.1-unit decrease in pH. Chronic inorganic metabolic acidosis usually is associated, however, with hypokalemia because of urinary potassium loss associated with both proximal (type 2) and distal (type 1) renal tubular acidosis.[111,118] In contrast, organic acidosis commonly has no effect on potassium distribution.[119]

Other associated factors in organic acidosis may, however, affect cellular potassium distribution.[118] For example, hyperglycemia in diabetic ketoacidosis may increase the serum potassium concentration because of the hypertonic effect of glucose.[120] Hypertonicity causes cell shrinkage and increases the intracellular to ECF potassium gradient, favoring potassium egress. Acute metabolic alkalosis only modestly decreases the plasma potassium concentration: 0.3 mEq/L for each 0.1-unit pH increment.[111,118] As with chronic metabolic acidosis, chronic metabolic alkalosis causes profound renal potassium wasting and is associated with hypokalemia. Respiratory acid–base disorders usually are associated with less significant changes in plasma potassium concentration than are metabolic acid–base disorders.[118] Exercise often causes an increase in the serum potassium concentration to a degree that varies with the intensity of the exercise.[121]

Hypokalemia

ETIOLOGY

CASE 27-8

QUESTION 1: J.P., a 60-year-old woman, presents to the ED with complaints of malaise, generalized weakness, nausea, and vomiting for 3 days. Her medical history includes hypertension for 20 years. J.P.'s current medications include hydrochlorothiazide 25 mg/day and nifedipine XL 30 mg/day. She has not been able to take her medications in the past few days, however, because of vomiting. J.P. denies recent diarrhea or use of laxatives. Her BP is 130/70 mm Hg with a pulse of 80 beats/minute while sitting, and 120/70 mm Hg with a pulse of 95 beats/minute on standing. Physical examination reveals a thin, older woman with poor skin turgor, dry mucous membranes, and a flat jugular vein. T-wave flattening is noted on the electrocardiogram (ECG). Laboratory tests show the following:

Serum Na, 138 mEq/L
K, 2.1 mEq/L
Cl, 100 mEq/L
Bicarbonate, 32 mEq/L
BUN, 30 mg/dL
Creatinine, 1.2 mg/dL
Glucose, 100 mg/dL

ABG shows pH, 7.50; Pco_2, 45 mm Hg; and Po_2, 70 mm Hg at room air. Urine electrolytes are sodium, 30 mEq/L; potassium, 60 mEq/L; and chloride, less than 15 mEq/L. The patient's presentation is consistent with gastroenteritis. What are the causes of J.P.'s hypokalemia?

When evaluating hypokalemia, the clinician should determine whether the hypokalemia is a result of low intake, increased cellular uptake of potassium, or excessive loss of potassium via the kidneys, GI tract, or skin.[34,122] History and physical evidence of potassium depletion, medication history (including use of over-the-counter medicines), and assessment of the patient's BP, extracellular volume, and concurrent acid–base status can provide clues to the causes of hypokalemia.[34,122]

Because J.P. has been unable to eat for the past few days, decreased oral intake may have contributed to her hypokalemia. Because most foods are rich in potassium, however, inadequate intake rarely is the sole cause of potassium depletion unless inappropriate and continued renal or extrarenal losses occur, or potassium intake is severely restricted to less than 10 to 15 mEq/day.[122] Alkalosis,[119] insulin administration,[111] hypertonic solution administration, periodic paralysis,[123] β_2-agonists,[124] barium poisoning,[125] and treatment of megaloblastic anemia with vitamin B_{12}[126] all have been associated with increased cellular potassium uptake (Table 27-2). Although the relationship between the degree of hypokalemia and increase in blood pH varies widely,[118] J.P.'s metabolic alkalosis probably enhances the cellular uptake of potassium. The transcellular shift of potassium should not result in total body potassium depletion, however.

The GI tract is an important site of potassium loss, particularly through vomiting and diarrhea. Because the potassium content of gastric secretion (5–10 mEq/L) is much less than that of the intestinal secretion (up to 90 mEq/L),[122] loss of a large volume of gastric secretion is needed to produce substantial potassium depletion. Potassium deficit induced by vomiting, however, is commonly secondary to renal potassium loss, especially within the initial 24 to 48 hours.[127] The loss of hydrogen ion in gastric juice results in an elevated plasma bicarbonate concentration. The increased amount of bicarbonate ion, as a nonresorbable anion, increases water delivery to the distal nephron and enhances sodium reabsorption and potassium secretion, resulting in hypokalemia. The potassium wasting is often transient, because increased proximal reabsorption of sodium and bicarbonate will result in diminished bicarbonate delivery to the distal site. Reduced potassium excretion will ensue, commonly within 48 to 72 hours. Subsequent potassium loss will then be primarily consequent to gastric secretion removal.

The absence of diarrhea in J.P. excludes the GI tract as the source of potassium loss. Potassium loss through the skin is also unlikely in J.P. because the potassium concentration of sweat is less than 10 mEq/L. Therefore, profuse sweating, such as that induced by vigorous exercise in a hot, humid environment, or severe burns are needed to cause substantial loss.

J.P.'s inappropriately high urinary potassium concentration indicates that the kidney is the source of the potassium loss.[34,122] The urinary potassium concentration is a good marker for differentiating various hypokalemic syndromes. A urinary potassium excretion of less than 20 mEq/day suggests extrarenal potassium loss. Renal potassium wastage cannot be excluded, however, unless the low urinary potassium excretion is accompanied by a sodium intake of at least 100 mEq/day, because a low-sodium diet can reduce renal potassium excretion.[34] In J.P., the metabolic alkalosis and hypovolemia promote renal potassium wastage.[34,122] The distal delivery of a large sodium bicarbonate load and increased aldosterone activity (from hypovolemia) enhance potassium secretion and severely impair the kidney's ability to conserve potassium. The hydrochlorothiazide, which J.P. had been taking until 3 days before admission, could also have induced hypokalemia through volume depletion, hypochloremic metabolic alkalosis, and renal potassium wastage. The diuretic is unlikely, however, to be the cause for J.P.'s hypokalemia because she has stopped taking the medication, and this is reflected by the low urinary chloride concentration.[15] Bartter syndrome, which presents as normotension, hypokalemia, hypochloremic metabolic alkalosis, and renal potassium wastage, is characterized by impaired renal sodium and chloride reabsorption. The low urinary chloride concentration in J.P. can rule out Bartter syndrome. Other causes of hypokalemia are listed in Table 27-2.

In an asymptomatic hypokalemic patient with no apparent causes for potassium depletion or transcellular redistribution, pseudohypokalemia should be excluded before pursuing an intensive evaluation.[106] Spurious hypokalemia can occur in leukemic patients whose leukocyte count ranges from 100,000 to 250,000 cells/μL.[128] The potassium in serum is taken up by the large number of leukemic cells when the blood specimen is allowed to stand at room temperature.

CLINICAL MANIFESTATIONS

CASE 27-8, QUESTION 2: What clinical manifestations of hypokalemia are evident in J.P.?

Table 27-2
Drugs that Most Commonly Induce Hypokalemia

Drug	Mechanism	Predisposing Factors
Acetazolamide	Marked ↑ in renal K^+ loss	Most profound with short-term therapy
Amphotericin	Renal K^+ loss (renal tubular acidosis)	Concurrent piperacillin, ticarcillin
β_2-Agonists	Intracellular shift of K^+	
Cisplatin	Renal K^+ loss secondary to renal tubular damage	May be dose related but can occur after a single 50-mg/m^2 dose
Corticosteroids	Renal K^+ loss. Enhanced Na^+ reabsorption at distal tubule and collecting ducts in exchange for K^+ and H^+	Supraphysiologic doses of agents with moderate to strong mineralocorticoid activity (e.g., prednisone, hydrocortisone)
Insulin with glucose	Intracellular shift of K^+	Predictable effect when insulin administered to patients with diabetic ketoacidosis' combination used to treat hyperkalemia
Penicillins (piperacillin, ticarcillin)	High Na^+ load and nonresorbable anions can ↑ K^+ loss	Was more common with carbenicillin when it was available; newer penicillins are used in lower doses; less likely to produce hypokalemia
Thiazide and loop diuretics	Renal K^+ loss. ↑ Na^+ delivery to the late distal tubule, resulting in Na^+ resorption in exchange for K^+	Patients with hyperaldosteronism (e.g., cirrhosis, HF) predisposed; may be dose related

HF, heart failure.

The clinical presentation of hypokalemia, which depends on the severity of potassium depletion, is a result of changes in cell membrane polarization.[122] Patients are usually asymptomatic when the plasma potassium level is 3.0 to 3.5 mEq/L, but they may complain of malaise, weakness, fatigue, and myalgia. J.P.'s muscle weakness and ECG changes reflect the muscular and cardiac manifestations of hypokalemia, respectively.[129,130]

Potassium depletion can lead to hyperpolarization of myocardial cells and a prolonged refractory period. When serum potassium concentrations fall below 3 mEq/L, T-wave flattening, straight tubule segment depression, and prominent U waves are seen on the ECG.[130]

Mild hypokalemia (potassium concentration of 3.0–3.5 mEq/L) is potentially arrhythmogenic in patients with underlying coronary artery disease. The incidence of ventricular arrhythmia increases with the degree of hypokalemia. Patients without underlying heart disease may be susceptible to these myocardial effects during exercise, especially if the patient's pre-exercise potassium concentration is less than 3.5 mEq/L, because the potassium concentration may drop to less than 3.0 mEq/L as a result of β_2-adrenergic receptor-mediated cellular potassium uptake.[122] Potassium depletion may also increase the BP,[123] which can be lowered with potassium supplementation.[131]

When the serum potassium concentration is less than 2.5 to 3.0 mEq/L, muscle weakness, cramps, general malaise, fatigue, restless leg syndrome, and paresthesia can occur, probably because potassium is necessary for vasodilation in skeletal muscle. In addition, severe potassium depletion (<2.5 mEq/L) can result in elevation of serum creatine phosphokinase, aldolase, and aspartate aminotransferase levels. Rhabdomyolysis can ensue when the serum potassium concentration falls below 2.0 mEq/L.[122,129]

Chronic potassium depletion can alter renal function and structure, which can manifest as decreased GFR and renal blood flow, disturbance in tubular sodium handling, impaired urinary concentrating ability with polydipsia, and ADH-resistant nephrogenic diabetes insipidus.[106,115] Reversible pathologic changes include renal hypertrophy and epithelial vacuolization of the proximal convoluted tubule. Interstitial scarring and tubular atrophy have been reported with prolonged potassium depletion.[122]

Other effects of hypokalemia and potassium depletion include decreased insulin secretion resulting in carbohydrate intolerance,[132] metabolic alkalosis, and increased renal ammoniagenesis, which may play a role in the development of hepatic encephalopathy.[133]

TREATMENT

CASE 27-8, QUESTION 3: How should J.P.'s hypokalemia be treated?

J.P.'s protracted vomiting should be corrected, and fluids and electrolytes (sodium, potassium, and chloride) should be replaced to correct the volume deficit, hypokalemia, and hypochloremic metabolic alkalosis. Hydrochlorothiazide should continue to be withheld.

The amount of potassium deficit and the rate of continued potassium loss should be determined to guide replacement therapy. It has been estimated that a 1-mEq/L fall in serum potassium from 4 to 3 mEq/L represents a total body deficit of approximately 200 mEq. When the serum potassium falls to less than 3 mEq/L, the total body deficit increases by 200 to 400 mEq for each 1 mEq/L reduction in serum concentration. Other data suggest that even greater degrees of potassium loss can occur—a deficit of 100 mEq per 0.27-mEq/L fall in the serum potassium concentration.[110] Transcellular redistribution of potassium may, however, significantly alter the relationship between serum concentration and total body deficit.[122] Therefore, potassium repletion should be guided by close monitoring of serum concentrations and analysis of J.P.'s urine for potassium content to help assess the need for additional replacement.

The route of potassium administration depends on the acuity and severity of hypokalemia,[134] but oral supplementation is usually preferred. The parenteral route is indicated for patients who cannot tolerate high dosages of oral potassium supplements and for those with severe or symptomatic hypokalemia. J.P.'s potassium deficit is estimated to be 300 to 500 mEq, but because she is only moderately symptomatic, aggressive therapy is not indicated. Potassium chloride can be added to her IV fluid in a concentration of 40 mEq/L and infused at a rate that does not exceed 10 mEq/hour. For patients with life-threatening, hypokalemia-induced arrhythmias or those with a serum potassium level less than 2.0 mEq/L, a more concentrated potassium solution (60 mEq/L) can be infused at a rate not exceeding 40 mEq/hour. A solution that is too concentrated or a rate of infusion that is too rapid would likely cause phlebitis in the peripheral veins and could cause arrhythmias, especially when administered through a central line. The potassium concentration should be monitored every 4 hours, more frequently in patients with severe potassium depletion or when a rapid infusion is given.[135] ECG monitoring is mandatory to identify life-threatening hyperkalemia that can result from over-correction.

Parenteral potassium can be given as chloride, acetate, or phosphate. The chloride salt is preferred in J.P., who has concurrent hypochloremic metabolic alkalosis. The acetate preparation is useful in cases of concomitant metabolic acidosis. Potassium phosphate is indicated if hypophosphatemia coexists. In the latter condition, the serum calcium concentration should also be monitored because hypocalcemia may ensue. Glucose solution should be avoided as the vehicle because glucose-induced insulin secretion will promote intracellular potassium uptake.[136]

Once J.P.'s potassium levels are replenished and she can take medicine by mouth, oral potassium chloride can be started (see Chapter 9, Essential Hypertension, and Chapter 14, Heart Failure).

Hyperkalemia

ETIOLOGY

CASE 27-9

QUESTION 1: A.B., a 25-year-old woman with type 1 diabetes and hypertension, returns to the clinic for follow-up. Her BP is 170/90 mm Hg with a pulse of 80 beats/minute, and her physical examination is remarkable for 2+ pedal edema. Laboratory tests show the following:

Plasma Na, 135 mEq/L
K, 5.8 mEq/L
Cl, 108 mEq/L
Total CO_2, 20 mEq/L
BUN, 28 mg/dL
Creatinine, 2 mg/dL
Glucose, 200 mg/dL

Current medications include oral captopril 25 mg 3 times daily, hydrochlorothiazide 25 mg/triamterene 37.5 mg one capsule daily, human isophane insulin 30 units subcutaneously (SC) every morning, and ibuprofen 200 mg as needed for menstrual cramps. She uses a salt substitute occasionally. What is the etiology of her hyperkalemia?

Before conducting any extensive evaluation to identify the etiology of hyperkalemia, the serum potassium concentration ought to be repeated to confirm the presence of hyperkalemia. Also to be ruled out are the different causes of spurious hyperkalemia, which can result from severe leukocytosis (>500,000/μL),[136] thrombocytosis (>750,000/μL),[137] or hemolysis within the blood collection tube.[138] Pseudohyperkalemia is a test-tube phenomenon that occurs when potassium is released from leukocytes, platelets, or erythrocytes during blood coagulation. These disorders can be confirmed easily by comparing serum (clotted) and plasma (unclotted) potassium concentrations from the same blood sample. The two values should agree within 0.2 to 0.3 mEq/L. Improper tourniquet technique, causing strangulation of the patient's arm before blood sampling, may also result in spurious hyperkalemia.[139]

Identifying the etiology of hyperkalemia can be approached systematically by considering possible disturbances in internal and external potassium balance. The former involves transcellular flux of potassium from the intracellular to the extracellular space, whereas the latter involves either increased intake, including increased endogenous potassium load (e.g., rhabdomyolysis,[140] tumor lysis syndrome[141]), or decreased elimination. A thorough medication history is important to identify drugs associated with hyperkalemia.[142–144] (Also see Chapter 28, Chronic Kidney Diseases, for additional information on hyperkalemia.)

A dietary history should ascertain whether A.B.'s consumption of potassium-rich foods, salt substitutes, or potassium supplements has increased. Dietary intake alone will not induce hyperkalemia unless renal excretion is impaired. Usually, the GFR must be less than 10 to 15 mL/minute, unless there is concurrent hypoaldosteronism or distal tubular potassium secretory defects.[1] A.B.'s renal insufficiency is mild, with an estimated CrCl of 40 mL/minute.

Conditions associated with low renin and aldosterone, which usually present as hyperkalemia and hyperchloremic metabolic acidosis, decrease potassium excretion by the kidneys. These include diabetes,[145] obstructive uropathy, sickle cell disease, lupus nephritis, and various tubulointerstitial diseases (e.g., gouty nephropathy, analgesic nephropathy). Adrenal insufficiency presents commonly with hyperkalemia because of mineralocorticoid deficiency.[146] A.B.'s hyperglycemia because of poorly controlled diabetes may cause movement of potassium-rich fluid from the intracellular space to the extracellular space because of the increased tonicity. Elevating the plasma tonicity by 15 to 20 mOsm/kg will increase the plasma potassium concentration by 0.8 mEq/L.[147] Patients with diabetes, mineralocorticoid deficiency, or end-stage renal failure, which commonly results in hyporeninemic hypoaldosteronism, are particularly susceptible.

A.B. is also taking several medications that may impair her ability to excrete potassium. Captopril indirectly decreases aldosterone secretion by decreasing the formation of AT_2.[148] Ibuprofen inhibits prostaglandin production as well as renin and aldosterone secretion.[149] Other drugs that cause hyperkalemia by impairing renin and aldosterone production include AT_2 receptor antagonists,[150] β-adrenergic blockers,[151] lithium,[152] heparin,[153,154] and pentamidine.[155] Triamterene, a component of her diuretic, inhibits tubular potassium secretion, as do amiloride, spironolactone, high-dose trimethoprim,[156,157] cyclosporine,[158] tacrolimus,[159] and digitalis preparations.[160] By inhibiting Na^+/K^+ ATPase, digitalis decreases tubular potassium secretion and reduces cellular potassium uptake. Arginine,[161] succinylcholine,[162] β-adrenergic blockers, α-adrenergic agonists, and hypertonic solutions also cause hyperkalemia by impairing transcellular potassium distribution into the intracellular space.

CLINICAL MANIFESTATIONS

CASE 27-10

QUESTION 1: V.C., a 44-year-old woman with chronic renal failure, returns to the outpatient unit for routine hemodialysis with complaints of severe muscle weakness. Her vital signs are BP, 120/80 mm Hg; pulse, 90 beats/minute; RR, 20 breaths/minute; and temperature, 98°F. Laboratory data are as follows:

Serum K, 8.9 mEq/L
Total CO_2, 15 mEq/L
BUN, 60 mg/dL
Creatinine, 9 mg/dL
Glucose, 100 mg/dL

The ECG reveals an increased PR interval and a widened QRS complex. What clinical manifestations of hyperkalemia are evident in V.C.?

Hyperkalemia decreases the intracellular/extracellular potassium ratio. Hence, the resting membrane potential becomes less negative and moves closer to the threshold excitation potential. Muscle weakness and flaccid paralysis result when the resting membrane potential approaches the threshold potential, rendering the excitable cells unable to sustain an action potential.

The cardiac toxicity of hyperkalemia is a major cause of morbidity and mortality, with ECG findings paralleling the degree of hyperkalemia. When plasma potassium is greater than 5.5 to 6.0 mEq/L, narrow, peaked T waves and a shortened QT interval are seen. As the plasma potassium concentration increases further, the QRS complex widens and the P-wave amplitude decreases. As the level reaches 8 mEq/L, the P wave disappears and the QRS complex continues to widen and merge with the T wave to form a sine wave pattern. If these ECG changes are not recognized and no treatment is initiated, ventricular fibrillation and asystole will ensue. Hyponatremia, hypocalcemia, and hypomagnesemia all reduce the threshold potential, thereby increasing the patient's susceptibility to the cardiac effects of hyperkalemia.[140] V.C.'s muscle weakness, ECG, chronic renal failure, and serum potassium concentration all are consistent with severe hyperkalemia.

TREATMENT

CASE 27-10, QUESTION 2: How should V.C.'s hyperkalemia be treated?

Hyperkalemia with ECG changes requires urgent treatment. Three therapeutic modalities are available: (a) agents that antagonize the cardiac effects of hyperkalemia, (b) agents that shift potassium from the extracellular into the intracellular space, and (c) agents that enhance potassium elimination. Considering V.C.'s severe ECG changes, 10% calcium gluconate IV should be administered at a dose of 10 to 20 mL over the course of 1 to 3 minutes. Calcium counteracts the depolarizing effect of hyperkalemia by increasing the threshold potential, thus making it less negative and moving it away from the resting potential. The onset of action occurs in a few minutes, but the effect is short-lived, lasting approximately 15 to 60 minutes. The dose can be repeated in 5 minutes if ECG changes do not resolve and as needed afterward for recurrence. With no response after the second dose, additional attempts, however, are not beneficial. When the hyperkalemia presents with a digitalis overdose, calcium should be used cautiously because it can worsen the cardiotoxic effects of digoxin.[140,163]

Because the serum potassium concentration is not affected by calcium administration, maneuvers should be used to shift potassium from plasma into the cells. Three modalities are available: insulin and glucose, β_2-agonists, and sodium bicarbonate.

Insulin rapidly shifts potassium into the cell in a dose-dependent fashion. The maximal effect occurs at insulin concentrations greater than 20 to 40 times the basal levels. Therefore, endogenous insulin secreted in response to dextrose administration is insufficient, and exogenous insulin must be administered.[111] Although high concentrations of dextrose may worsen hyperkalemia, particularly in diabetic patients because intracellular potassium may be shifted to the extracellular space owing to the elevated plasma tonicity,[164] it is always administered with insulin to prevent hypoglycemia. Regular insulin (5–10 units) can be given with 50 mL of 50% dextrose as IV boluses, followed by a continuous infusion of 10% dextrose at 50 mL/hour to prevent late hypoglycemia.[111] In dialysis patients susceptible to experiencing fasting hyperkalemia, 20 units of insulin can be added to 1 L of 10% dextrose and administered at a rate of 50 mL/hour to prevent the hyperkalemia.[165] The insulin–dextrose combination lowers serum potassium by direct stimulation of cellular potassium uptake and potentiates the potassium-lowering effect of β-adrenergic stimulation.[165] The reduction in potassium is apparent 15 to 30 minutes after the start of the therapy and persists for 4 to 6 hours.[140] In a diabetic patient who is both hyperkalemic and hyperglycemic, insulin alone may be insufficient. If the patient has end-stage renal disease, the insulin–glucose combination is more predictable in lowering plasma potassium concentrations than sodium bicarbonate.[110,163,165]

β_2-Agonists, by binding with the β_2-adrenoreceptor to activate adenylate cyclase, have an additive effect with the insulin–dextrose combination in decreasing serum potassium. When albuterol nebulization is used alone, the hypokalemic effect may be inconsistent.[166] Although side effects of albuterol nebulization are minimal, these agents can cause tachycardia and should be used cautiously in patients with underlying coronary artery disease.[167] Although not commercially available, IV albuterol has a faster onset of action (30 vs. 90 minutes).[168] In contrast, nebulization is easier to set up and is less likely to be associated with tachycardia, but multiple doses are often necessary to attain an adequate response. In conjunction with the insulin–dextrose combination, albuterol (20 mg dissolved in 4 mL of saline) can be administered by nebulization and inhaled over the course of 10 minutes to further decrease serum potassium, if necessary.[169]

Although sodium bicarbonate has long been recommended for the acute treatment of hyperkalemia, its efficacy in this setting has been questioned.[110,163] The usual dose, 44 to 50 mEq, is infused slowly over the course of 5 minutes and repeated in 30 minutes when necessary. Alternatively, it can be added to dextrose and saline solution to form an isotonic sodium bicarbonate infusion.[170] The hypokalemic effect is variable and may be delayed up to 4 hours, and it is reportedly ineffective in patients on maintenance hemodialysis. Although bicarbonate therapy is not a reliable option in the acute management of hyperkalemia, it may be beneficial in patients with severe metabolic acidosis (pH < 7.20).[110] Potential complications of sodium bicarbonate therapy are volume overload and metabolic alkalosis.

The definitive treatment of hyperkalemia is removal of potassium from the body. Sodium polystyrene sulfonate (SPS) with sorbitol is an ion-exchange resin that binds potassium in the bowel and enhances its excretion in the stools.[171] Each gram of SPS exchanges 0.5 to 1.0 mmol of potassium for an equal amount of sodium. SPS can be administered orally or rectally; the latter route is preferred in the symptomatic hyperkalemic patient because intestinal potassium exchange occurs mainly in the ileum and colon. A dose of 50 g of SPS in sorbitol can be given as an enema, retained for at least 30 to 60 minutes, at 4-hour to 6-hour intervals. For nonemergent removal of body potassium, 15 to 60 g of SPS with sorbitol suspension can be given orally, which can be repeated as needed. The onset of action is approximately 1 to 2 hours after administration. The major side effects are GI intolerance, including constipation, diarrhea, and sodium overload. Potentially fatal intestinal necrosis, though rare, have been reported with the use of SPS with sorbitol.[172] It is unclear if intestinal injury is caused by SPS or sorbitol, but FDA has released a safety warning against the use of SPS in individuals with impaired bowel function.[173]

Hemodialysis is the most efficient way to remove potassium; potassium clearance by peritoneal dialysis is lower than for hemodialysis.[174] The hypokalemic effect is immediate and lasts for the duration of dialysis[163]; however, the amount of potassium removed is variable.[175] Dialysis with a glucose-free dialysate will remove 30% more potassium than one containing 200 mg/dL of glucose.[176] Table 27-3 summarizes the treatment alternatives for hyperkalemia. Although V.C. is receiving chronic maintenance hemodialysis, the severe cardiac effects of hyperkalemia she experienced warrant immediate institution of the aforementioned measures while awaiting preparation for dialysis. Loop diuretics, which enhance kaliuresis, are rarely useful in managing severe hyperkalemia, especially in patients with renal dysfunction.

Two new oral agents, patiromer and sodium zirconium cyclosilicate, currently still under investigation, have been shown to be effective in reducing serum potassium concentrations in patients with mild-to-moderate hyperkalemia.[177,178] As the studies conducted thus far are short-term studies and excluded patients with severe hyperkalemia, the long-term beneficial and adverse effects of these agents need to be further evaluated.

After V.C.'s condition stabilized, she admitted to eating a lot of fruits in the past few days. Because noncompliance with dietary potassium restriction is the most common cause for acute and chronic hyperkalemia in a dialysis patient, V.C. should be counseled to consume potassium-rich foods in moderation. Medications that impair V.C.'s extrarenal potassium handling should be avoided. If V.C. remains chronically hyperkalemic, SPS will then be needed, probably 3 or 4 times weekly. If hyperkalemia is associated with metabolic acidosis, however, an alkalinizing agent should be added to maintain a serum bicarbonate concentration of about 24 mEq/L.

CALCIUM

Homeostasis

Healthy adults have approximately 1,400 g of calcium in the body, of which greater than 99% is stored in bone. Nonetheless, the 0.1% of the total body calcium that is in the plasma and extravascular fluid plays a critical role in many physiologic and metabolic processes. Calcium is important in maintaining nerve tissue excitability and muscle contractility. It regulates the secretory activities of exocrine and endocrine glands and serves as a cofactor for enzyme systems and the coagulation cascade. It is also an essential component of bone metabolism.

Plasma calcium concentration is normally maintained within a relatively narrow range: 8.5 to 10.5 mg/dL. This is accomplished through a complex interaction between parathyroid hormone (PTH), vitamin D, and calcitonin, as well as the effect of these hormones on calcium metabolism in bone, the GI tract, and the kidneys.

Normally, about 40% of the plasma calcium is protein-bound, primarily to albumin, and is nondiffusible.[126] Of the 60% that is diffusible, about 13% is complexed to various small ligands: phosphate, citrate, and sulfate. The remaining 47% is ionized, free, and physiologically active. Changes in serum protein concentration will alter the concentrations of both protein-bound and total calcium. Therefore, the serum albumin concentration needs to

Table 27-3
Treatment of Hyperkalemia

Drug	Mechanism	Dose	Comment
Calcium gluconate	Reverse cardiotoxicity caused by K^+	10 to 20 mL 10% calcium gluconate IV over 1 to 3 minutes; may repeat once	*Onset:* 1 to 3 minutes *Duration:* 30 to 60 minutes. (K^+) remains unchanged
Insulin and glucose	Redistribution of K^+ intracellularly	5 to 10 units regular insulin with 50 mL 50% dextrose, then $D_{10}W$ infused at 50 mL/hour[a]	*Onset:* 15 to 30 minutes *Duration:* several hours Watch for hypoglycemia and hypokalemia. Does not ↓ total body K^+
β_2-agonists (e.g., albuterol)	Redistribution of K^+ intracellularly	Oral: 2 or 4 mg TID–QID Inhalation: 20 mg in 4 mL saline via nebulizer	*Onset:* 30 to 60 minutes *Duration:* 2 hours
SPS	Cationic binding resin. 1 g of resin binds 0.5 to 1 mEq K^+ in exchange for Na^+	Oral: 15 to 20 g with 20 to 100 mL 70% sorbitol every 4 to 6 hours; PRN preferred Retention enema: 50 g in 50 mL (70% sorbitol and 150 mL H_2O). Retain 30 minutes and follow with nonsaline irrigation	*Onset:* Slow; 50 g will lower (K^+) by 0.5 to 1 mEq/L over 4 to 6 hours; watch for Na^+ overload (100 mg Na^+/1 g SPS)
$NaHCO_3$	Redistribution of K^+ intracellularly	50 mEq IV for 5 minutes. Repeat PRN	*Onset:* variable, ≈30 minutes May work best in acidosis Watch for Na^+ overload and hyperosmolar state No change in total body K^+
Dialysis	Removal of K^+		Use as last resort

[a]Glucose unnecessary in patients with high glucose concentrations.
BID, twice daily; IV, intravenous; PRN, as needed; QID, 4 times daily; SPS, sodium polystyrene sulfonate; TID, 3 times daily.

be monitored to adequately interpret the total serum calcium concentration. Each 1-g/dL increase in serum albumin concentration is expected to increase the protein-bound calcium by 0.8 mg/dL, thus increasing the total serum calcium concentration by the same amount. The total serum calcium therefore can be corrected by the following equation:

$$\text{Correct Ca} = \text{Observed Ca} + 0.8\,(\text{Normal albumin} - \text{Observed albumin}) \qquad \text{(Eq. 27-13)}$$

where normal albumin = 4 g/dL.

Calcium is also bound to plasma globulins at the rate of 0.16 mg of calcium for each gram of globulin. When the total globulin concentration exceeds 6 g/dL, moderate hypercalcemia may be seen. Changes in pH have an effect on calcium protein-binding; acidosis decreases calcium binding, resulting in an increase in free-calcium fraction, whereas an increase in pH reduces the amount of ionized calcium. Changes in serum phosphate and sulfate concentrations are expected to alter the fraction of ionized calcium because of the formation of calcium complexes with these anions. The presence of abnormal plasma proteins with a high affinity for calcium-binding, as in patients with multiple myeloma, also affects the preceding equation for serum calcium concentration correction.[179]

Serum calcium concentration is regulated by the combined effect of GI absorption and secretion, renal reabsorption, and turnover of the skeletal calcium pool. Several hormones, such as PTH, 1,25-dihydroxyvitamin D_3, and calcitonin, have significant effects on these processes. Balanced diets generally contain 600 to 1,000 mg of calcium, although the minimum daily requirement is 400 to 500 mg. Calcium is primarily absorbed in the duodenum and jejunum via saturable and nonsaturable processes.[180] The nonsaturable process is diffusive in nature and varies with luminal calcium concentration. The saturable carrier-mediated component is stimulated by 1,25-dihydroxyvitamin D_3. Absorption of calcium is enhanced when the calcium intake is low and also when the demand is increased, such as in pregnancy and when total body calcium is depleted. Conversely, protein deficiency can reduce intestinal calcium absorption, presumably because of the reduced amount of specific calcium-binding protein.[181] Calcium is also secreted into the bowel lumen, which may account for the presence of a negative calcium balance when there is no oral calcium intake.[182]

The portion of plasma calcium that is not bound to protein is filtered by the glomerulus. Approximately 97% to 99.5% of the filtered calcium is reabsorbed: 60% in the proximal tubule, 20% in the ascending limb, 10% in the distal tubule, and 3% to 10% in the collecting duct. Approximately 20% of the calcium in the kidney tubule is ionized, whereas the remainder is bound to anions such as citrate, sulfate, phosphate, and gluconate. The extent of calcium reabsorption depends on the presence of specific anions and also on the urine pH, which affects the fraction of calcium bound to anions. Passive reabsorption at the proximal convoluted tubule is linked closely to sodium transport and is increased by ECF contraction and decreased by volume expansion. At the proximal straight tubule, the transport process is active and dissociable from sodium and water transport. PTH increases the calcium reabsorption at the distal tubule and also at the collecting duct independent of sodium reabsorption. Acidosis can also increase renal calcium excretion by inhibiting tubular reabsorption and by increasing the ultrafiltrable calcium through reduced binding of calcium to plasma proteins. Conversely, alkalosis promotes calcium protein binding, thus reducing the amount of ultrafiltrable calcium. It also induces hypocalciuria independent of PTH. Phosphorus administration reduces renal calcium excretion, whereas phosphorus depletion increases urinary calcium elimination. Normally, approximately 50 to 300 mg of calcium is excreted by the kidneys daily, but this can be increased to 600 mg/day.[183]

The other important factor regulating plasma calcium concentration is bone metabolism. The rate of bone turnover and calcium resorption is influenced by PTH, 1,25-dihydroxyvitamin D_3, and calcitonin.

Hypercalcemia

ETIOLOGY

CASE 27-11

QUESTION 1: A.C., a 62-year-old woman, is brought to the hospital by family members because she has become increasingly lethargic and unresponsive during the past several days. Approximately 4 years ago she underwent a radical mastectomy and node dissection followed by radiation and chemotherapy for breast carcinoma. Despite several courses of chemotherapy, she developed metastasis to the bone. About 1 week before this admission, A.C. complained of fatigue, muscle weakness, and anorexia. Since then, she has spent most of her time in bed and has had very limited oral intake. Medications taken before admission included hydrochlorothiazide, oral morphine sulfate, and tamoxifen. Physical examination reveals a dehydrated, cachectic woman responsive only to painful stimuli. Vital signs include BP, 100/60 mm Hg, and RR, 16 breaths/minute. Pertinent laboratory values are as follows:

Na, 138 mEq/L
K, 4.5 mEq/L
Cl, 99 mEq/L
CO_2, 33 mEq/L
BUN, 40 mg/dL
Creatinine, 1.2 mg/dL
Calcium, 19 mg/dL
Phosphate, 4.5 mg/dL
Albumin, 3.0 g/dL

The ECG revealed a shortened QT interval. What are the common causes of hypercalcemia? Which of these might be responsible for the hypercalcemia seen in A.C.?

Malignancy

Malignancy and primary hyperparathyroidism are the most common causes of hypercalcemia. Hematologic malignancies, such as multiple myeloma, tend to be responsible for more hypercalcemia than are solid tumors. Cancer of the breast, lung, head and neck, and renal cell carcinoma are solid tumors commonly associated with hypercalcemia. Malignancy can cause paraneoplastic hypercalcemia secondary to bone metastasis, which results in increased bone resorption. Alternatively, patients may exhibit hypercalcemia in the absence of bone metastasis owing to the production of osteolytic humoral factors by the tumor. The mediators secreted may be PTH, PTH-like substances, prostaglandins, cytokines, transforming growth factor-α, and tumor necrosis factor.[184]

Hyperparathyroidism

Hyperparathyroidism is the other common cause of hypercalcemia. Although the etiology of primary hyperparathyroidism is unclear, women tend to experience the condition more frequently, especially in the fourth to sixth decades of life. Approximately 75% of patients have a single adenoma, whereas much smaller percentages of patients have multiglandular disease, hyperplasia, or carcinoma.[184] Other conditions that can result in hypercalcemia include postkidney transplantation, immobilization, vitamin A intoxication, hyperthyroidism, Addison disease, and pheochromocytoma. Hypercalcemia can also occur secondary to increased intestinal calcium absorption because of vitamin D intoxication, sarcoidosis, and other granulomatous diseases. Use of thiazide diuretics, lithium, estrogens, and tamoxifen, as well as excessive calcium ingestion together with alkali (milk-alkali syndrome), may result in hypercalcemia.

A.C.'s breast cancer bone metastasis, volume contraction, and use of hydrochlorothiazide and tamoxifen may all contribute to her hypercalcemia.

CLINICAL MANIFESTATIONS

CASE 27-11, QUESTION 2: How is hypercalcemia manifested in A.C.?

The clinical presentations of hypercalcemia vary substantially among patients, but the severity of the symptoms correlates well with free calcium concentrations.[185] The specific presentation depends on the rate of serum calcium concentration elevation, the presence of malignancy, the PTH concentration, and the patient's age. Concurrent electrolyte and metabolic abnormalities and underlying diseases will also have an effect. Because calcium is an important regulator of many cellular functions, hypercalcemia can produce abnormalities in the neurologic, cardiovascular, pulmonary, renal, GI, and musculoskeletal systems. As seen in A.C., the signs and symptoms can be nonspecific: fatigue, muscle weakness, anorexia, thirst, polyuria, dehydration, and a shortened QT interval on the ECG.

The effect of hypercalcemia on the central nervous system includes lethargy, somnolence, confusion, headache, seizures, cerebellar ataxia, altered personality, acute psychosis, depression, and memory impairment. The neuromuscular manifestations include weakness, myalgia, hyporeflexia or areflexia, and arthralgia.

Symptoms of impaired renal function include polyuria, nocturia, and polydipsia. These may reflect a defective concentrating ability, possibly because of resistance to the effects of ADH.[186] The GFR may be decreased because of afferent arteriolar vasoconstriction, and if hypercalcemia is prolonged, nephrolithiasis, nephrocalcinosis, chronic interstitial nephritis, and renal tubular acidosis may be present. Hypermagnesuria and metabolic alkalosis may also be observed.[183]

Calcium has a positive inotropic effect and reduces heart rate, similar to cardiac glycosides. ECG changes indicative of slow conduction, with prolonged PR and QRS intervals and shortened QT intervals, are commonly seen. In severe hypercalcemia, increased QT intervals, widened T waves, and arrhythmia may be present.[183,187]

The GI symptoms of hypercalcemia are related primarily to the depressive action of calcium on smooth muscle and nerve conduction. Constipation, anorexia, nausea, and vomiting result from reduced GI motility and delayed gastric emptying. Duodenal ulcer can occur because of increased acid and gastrin secretion. Pancreatitis can occur during acute hypercalcemia owing to the blockade of the pancreatic ducts caused by intraductal calcium deposits.[183] Proteolytic enzymes may also be activated by calcium to cause tissue damage. Both ulcer disease and pancreatitis are more common in hypercalcemia associated with primary hyperparathyroidism; they are less likely to be seen in patients with malignancy-induced hypercalcemia.[179]

Treatment

CASE 27-11, QUESTION 3: After vigorous fluid resuscitation with IV saline, combined saline and furosemide diuresis was instituted in A.C. Her serum calcium concentration declined very slowly, prompting the use of calcitonin. Despite initial success, the serum calcium concentration rose to pretreatment values within 24 hours. Higher dosages of calcitonin could have been attempted at this point; however, pamidronate was used instead. Her serum calcium concentration finally stabilized at 8 mg/dL after several days of therapy. What was the rationale for each of these regimens? What other agents are available for hypercalcemia treatment?

Several therapeutic approaches are used to lower serum calcium concentration: increasing urinary calcium excretion, inhibiting release of calcium from bone, reducing intestinal calcium absorption, and enhancing calcium complex formation with chelating agents. The underlying disease that causes the hypercalcemia should also be treated, if possible. The specific treatment used depends on the serum ionized calcium concentration, the presenting signs and symptoms, and the severity and duration of hypercalcemia. Immediate therapy was needed for A.C., who had symptoms consistent with severe hypercalcemia.

Specific interventions are described in the subsequent paragraphs, but as an overview, hydration and diuresis with furosemide generally are the first steps in the acute treatment of hypercalcemia. If these measures fail to reduce the serum calcium concentration adequately, several other agents can be added. Calcitonin provides a rapid onset of hypocalcemic effect, but its duration of action is relatively short. Thus, a bisphosphonate could be used to elicit a longer hypocalcemic response. Gallium nitrate is an alternative, but it is not commonly used. Other agents, such as inorganic phosphates, glucocorticoids, and prostaglandin inhibitors, also have been used to treat hypercalcemia with varying success (Table 27-4).

Hydration and Diuresis

As noted, the first-line emergency treatment for hypercalcemia is hydration and volume expansion. Most patients with hypercalcemia are volume-depleted because of the accompanying polyuria, nausea, and vomiting. Normal saline 1 to 2 L is commonly given to correct the fluid deficit and to expand extracellular volume, which will increase urinary calcium excretion by increasing the GFR and inhibiting calcium reabsorption in the proximal tubule. Because both sodium and calcium are reabsorbed at the same site in the proximal tubule, saline hydration will reduce the reabsorption of both cations simultaneously. A.C. was hypotensive and appeared dehydrated; therefore, saline hydration was used initially to treat the hypercalcemia. In patients who have renal failure or HF, saline hydration and forced diuresis should be avoided.

After adequate volume repletion has been established, IV furosemide can be administered to augment calciuresis. Furosemide blocks the reabsorption of sodium, chloride, and calcium at the thick ascending limb of Henle's loop. Doses of 80 to 100 mg every 2 to 4 hours can be used until a sufficient decline of the serum calcium concentration is attained.[188]

Table 27-4
Treatment of Hypercalcemia

Intervention	Dose	Comment
Saline and furosemide	1–2 L NS; then furosemide 80 to 100 mg every 2 to 4 hours. Establish and maintain normovolemia. Other electrolytes as needed.	Saline diuresis and volume expansion depresses Ca^{2+} reabsorption in tubules. Lowers (Ca^{2+}) within 24 hours. Treatment of choice in patients without HF or renal failure.
Calcitonin	Four international units/kg SC or IM every 12 hours. ↑ Dose or use another therapy if unresponsive after 24 hours (Max: 8 international units/kg every 6 hours).	Inhibits osteoclast resorption and renal reabsorption of calcium. Preferred second-line agent because it has a rapid onset (6 hours) and is nontoxic. It can be used safely in HF and renal failure. Nausea is the major adverse effect. Tolerance occurs in 24 to 72 hours. Concomitant plicamycin can lead to hypocalcemia. Only the salmon-derived product is available.
Biphosphonates (etidronate, pamidronate)	Etidronate: 7.5 mg/kg IV daily × 3 days over at least 2 hours. Maintenance: 20 mg/kg/day PO. Pamidronate: 60 to 90 mg IV for 4 hours × 1. Repeat in 7 days PRN.	Inhibits osteoclast reabsorption in malignancy state. Efficacy 75% to 100%. Onset 48 hours. Duration, days. Concomitant hydration is imperative. Do not use in renal failure. Adverse effects: ↑ phosphorus, ↑ SCr, N/V (oral).
Zoledronic acid	*Doses*: 4 mg IV administration for 15 minutes.	Potent effect on bone resorption. Preferred bisphosphonate for hypercalcemia of malignancy. May have promising effects on skeletal complications secondary to bone metastasis.
Gallium nitrate phosphate	100–200 mg/m²/day infused IV over 24 hours for 5 days (depending on severity of hypercalcemia). If calcium levels return to normal before 5 days, therapy may be discontinued. IV PO^-_4 not recommended PO PO^-_4 gradually titrate to 30 to 60 mmol/day (1–3 g/day in divided doses).	Inhibits bone resorption. Patients should be well hydrated during therapy. A urine output of ~2 L/day should be maintained owing to risk for nephrotoxicity (10%). Inhibits bone resorption; soft tissue calcification. IV onset 24 hours but not drug of choice. Oral agents used for chronic therapy. Contraindicated in renal failure.
Corticosteroids	Prednisone: 60–80 mg/day Hydrocortisone: 5 mg/kg/day IV × 2–3 days.	Impair GI absorption and bone resorption. Onset several days. Best in patients with multiple myeloma, vitamin D intoxication, granulomatous conditions. Can be used in HF, renal failure.
Indomethacin	75–150 mg/day.	Reports of efficacy are mixed.

GI, gastrointestinal; HF, heart failure; IM, intramuscularly; IV, intravenously; NS, normal saline; N/V, nausea and vomiting; PO, orally; PRN, as needed; SC, subcutaneously; SCr, serum creatinine.

Smaller doses (20–40 mg) commonly are given to avoid the significant loss of fluid and electrolytes caused by the more aggressive regimen. Adequate amounts of sodium, potassium, magnesium, and fluid should be used to replace any therapy-induced electrolyte abnormalities. Fluid balance as well as serum and urine concentrations of these electrolytes must be monitored closely. Urine flow must be maintained and the renal loss of sodium chloride must be replaced to preserve the calciuric effect of furosemide.[189] In A.C., the decline of serum calcium concentration was slow, possibly because of inadequate restoration of plasma volume, replacement of renal sodium loss, or both. More aggressive hydration with adequate sodium replacement ensures that the efficacy of furosemide is not compromised.

Calcitonin

Calcitonin can be used when saline hydration and furosemide diuresis fail to lower serum calcium concentration adequately or when their use is contraindicated. Calcitonin reduces serum calcium concentration by inhibiting osteoclastic bone resorption. It may also increase the renal excretion of calcium and phosphorus. Only the salmon-derived calcitonin product is available in the United States.

The serum calcium concentration is often reduced several hours after calcitonin is administered, and the response may last approximately 6 to 8 hours. The drug is relatively nontoxic compared with organic phosphates and may be used in patients with dehydration, HF, or renal failure.[189] Nausea, vomiting, diarrhea, and facial flushing are the more common side effects; soreness and inflammation at the injection site may also be seen.[184] Because of the potential for developing a hypersensitivity reaction to salmon calcitonin, the manufacturer recommends skin testing with 1 international unit of the salmon calcitonin before the first dose. As seen in A.C., tolerance to the hypocalcemic effect of calcitonin can develop after 24 to 72 hours of therapy. This "escape phenomenon" may be secondary to the altered responsiveness of the hormone receptors and might be prevented by concurrent use of corticosteroids.[190] After long-term therapy, antibodies may develop as well.

The dosage of salmon calcitonin is 4 international units/kg given SC or intramuscularly every 12 hours; the maximal dosage is 8 international units/kg every 6 hours. The hypocalcemic response is often limited, and serum calcium concentration seldom drops to the normal range.[191]

Bisphosphonates

Bisphosphonates are synthetic analogs of pyrophosphate that form stable bonds that are resistant to phosphatase degradation during osteoclast-mediated bone mineralization and resorption. The compounds adsorb to the hydroxyapatite crystals of the bone, inhibiting their growth and dissolution. In addition, the compounds may have a direct effect on osteoclasts. The two distinct pharmacologic classes of bisphosphonates that exist have different mechanisms of action. Etidronate, which does not contain any nitrogen atom, is metabolized to cytotoxic, nonhydrolyzable ATP analogs. In contrast, nitrogen-containing bisphosphonates, such as pamidronate and zoledronic acid, inhibit the prenylation of proteins and have potent inhibitory effects on osteoclast-mediated bone resorption.[192] In addition, they induce apoptosis of osteoclasts as well as certain tumor cells. Further antitumor activities may be mediated through their inhibitory effect on angiogenesis, stimulation of the γ-T-cell fraction in blood, and reduction of cancer cells' adherence to bone matrix. At present, etidronate, pamidronate, and zoledronic acid are approved in the United States for the treatment of hypercalcemia secondary to malignancy.

Etidronate

Etidronate is administered in doses of 7.5 mg/kg for 3 consecutive days by IV infusion over the course of 2 to 4 hours. Response may be seen after 1 to 2 days, and normocalcemia is expected to be attained in most patients, with response sustained for greater than 10 days.[193] Because of the inconvenient dosing schedule as well as variability in its duration of action, other bisphosphonates are now preferred for the treatment of hypercalcemia of malignancy. In addition, etidronate may inhibit bone mineralization, a property not shared by other bisphosphonates.

Pamidronate

Pamidronate is more potent than etidronate as an inhibitor of bone resorption, but it has negligible effect on bone mineralization. For moderate hypercalcemia (albumin-corrected serum calcium concentration of 12.0–13.5 mg/dL), a single dose of 60 to 90 mg of pamidronate is commonly infused over the course of 3 to 4 hours. For severe hypercalcemia (albumin-corrected serum calcium concentration >13.5 mg/dL), the dose is 90 mg. The advantages of pamidronate are that it requires only a single dose and produces a superior response compared with three doses of etidronate.[194]

If the hypercalcemia recurs, the etidronate or the pamidronate regimen may be repeated after an interval of greater than or equal to 7 days. Etidronate (20 mg/kg/day by mouth) may be given to prolong the normocalcemic duration, but nausea and vomiting are common with the oral therapy. Long-term treatment may result in osteomalacia; however, the limited life expectancy of most patients may diminish the significance of this adverse effect.

Etidronate use has resulted in renal failure,[195] which probably is caused by the formation of bisphosphonate–calcium complexes in the serum.[196] Because pamidronate requires a lower molar concentration to produce a comparable hypocalcemic effect, it is less likely to impair renal function. In fact, pamidronate has been given to a limited number of patients with end-stage renal disease without adverse consequence.[196]

Zoledronic Acid

Among the bisphosphonates approved for the treatment of hypercalcemia of malignancy, zoledronic acid has the most potent effect on bone resorption. It is superior to pamidronate with respect to the number of complete responses, time needed to attain calcium normalization, and duration of effect.[197] Because 8-mg doses are not superior to 4-mg dose, 4-mg doses are administered IV over the course of 15 minutes.[198] The drug is well tolerated at 4-mg doses. Zoledronic acid's superior efficacy and convenience of administration make it the preferred bisphosphonate for hypercalcemia of malignancy. Emerging studies show that zoledronic acid may also have promising effects in reducing skeletal complications secondary to bone metastasis associated with breast cancer, prostate cancer, non–small cell lung cancer, and multiple myeloma.[198]

Gallium Nitrate

Gallium is a naturally occurring group IIIa heavy metal. In addition to its antitumor activity and potential for use as a chemotherapeutic agent, it has been shown to be effective in the treatment of moderate-to-severe hypercalcemia of malignancy. Hypocalcemia is induced primarily via the inhibition of bone resorption and reduction in urinary calcium excretion.[199] Several clinical studies have shown the effectiveness of gallium nitrate in the treatment of cancer-related hypercalcemia when compared with agents such as calcitonin and bisphosphonates.[199–203] The recommended dose is 100 to 200 mg/m^2/day as a 24-hour continuous infusion for 5 days. Vigorous hydration is necessary to prevent nephrotoxicity. In general, its clinical use is limited by the inconvenient method of administration, significant risk of nephrotoxicity, and cost.

Phosphate

Inorganic phosphates lower the serum calcium concentration by inhibiting bone resorption. They also promote the deposition of calcium salts in the bone and soft tissue. If given orally, phosphate reduces intestinal calcium absorption by forming a poorly soluble complex in the bowel lumen and also by decreasing the formation of active vitamin D through enzyme inhibition.[204]

When given IV, phosphate is very effective, but renal failure and extensive extraskeletal calcifications are a concern. For these reasons, IV phosphate is not the agent of choice for acute treatment of hypercalcemia.

Oral phosphate (1–3 g/day in divided doses) may be used for long-term maintenance therapy, with the optimal dose determined by serum calcium concentrations. Nausea, vomiting, and diarrhea are common problems, especially when the daily dose exceeds 2 g. Soft tissue calcification is also a concern, and hyperphosphatemia and hypocalcemia can occur if the dose is not titrated appropriately. Phosphate therapy should not be given to patients with hyperphosphatemia or renal failure because it can cause further deterioration of renal function. Accumulation of the potassium and sodium salts in phosphate preparations may also present a therapeutic problem in certain patients.

Corticosteroids

Several possible mechanisms exist that may explain the hypocalcemic effect of corticosteroids. Vitamin D_3–mediated intestinal calcium absorption may be impaired[205] and the action of osteoclast-activating factor, which mediates bone resorption in malignancy, may be inhibited. Corticosteroids may also have a direct cytolytic effect on tumor cells and inhibit the synthesis of prostaglandins (see the subsequent section, Prostaglandin Inhibitors). Prednisone in daily doses of 60–80 mg is given initially, with subsequent dosage reduction based on the calcemic response. Alternatively, hydrocortisone (5 mg/kg/day for 2–3 days) may be given. The hypocalcemic effect will not be apparent for at least 1 to 2 days. Patients with hematologic malignancies and lymphomas tend to have a better response than those with solid tumors. Corticosteroids are also effective in treating hypercalcemia associated with vitamin D intoxication,[205] sarcoidosis,[206] and other granulomatous conditions. They are not generally used for long-term therapy because of their potential for serious adverse reactions.

Prostaglandin Inhibitors

Because prostaglandins of the E series, especially PGE_2, may be responsible for hypercalcemia associated with some malignancies, NSAIDs may be useful for a select group of patients with hypercalcemia.[207] For example, indomethacin is effective in lowering the serum calcium concentration in patients with renal cell carcinoma but not in patients with other types of malignancy.[194] Indomethacin, 75 to 150 mg/day, can be tried in patients unresponsive to other therapy, especially when it is used as part of palliative treatment for cancer pain.

PHOSPHORUS

Homeostasis

Phosphorus is found primarily in bone (85%) and soft tissue (14%); less than 1% of the total body store resides in the ECF. Virtually, all of the "free" or active phosphorus exists as phosphates in the plasma. Most clinical laboratories, however, measure and express the concentrations of elemental phosphorus contained in the phosphate molecules. Phosphate of 1 mmol contains 1 mmol of phosphorus, but 1 mmol of phosphate is 3 times the weight of 1 mmol of phosphorus. Therefore, it is incorrect to equate a certain milligram weight of phosphorus as the same milligram weight of phosphate. Of the total plasma phosphorus, 70% exists as the organic form and 30% as the inorganic form. Organic phosphorus, primarily phospholipids and small amounts of esters, is bound to proteins. About 85% of inorganic phosphorus, or orthophosphate, is unbound or "free." The relative amounts of the two orthophosphate components, $H_2PO_4^-$ and HPO_4^{2-}, vary with pH. At pH 7.40, the ratio of the two species is 1:4, giving rise to a composite valence of 1.8 for the orthophosphate. Serum phosphate concentrations reported by clinical laboratories reflect only the inorganic portion of the total plasma phosphate. To avoid confusion related to the pH effect on valence, phosphate concentrations are reported as mg/dL or mmol/dL rather than mEq/volume.

The normal range of serum phosphate concentration in healthy adults is 2.5 to 4.5 mg/dL. The value is higher in children, possibly because of the increased amount of growth hormone and the reduced amount of gonadal hormones.[208] In postmenopausal women, the range is slightly higher; it is lower in older men. The serum phosphate concentration is also affected by dietary intake. Phosphate-rich foods can transiently increase the serum phosphate concentration. In contrast, glucose decreases the serum phosphate concentration because of the flux of sugar and phosphate into cells and because of the phosphorylation of glucose. Similarly, administration of insulin and epinephrine decreases the serum phosphate concentration because of their effects on glucose. The serum concentration of phosphate is reduced in alkalosis and increased in acidosis.[209]

A balanced diet contains 800 to 1,500 mg/day phosphorus. Both the organic and inorganic forms of phosphorus are present in food substances. Most of the phosphorus in milk is the organic form; the phosphorus in meat, vegetable, and other nondairy sources represents organic forms bound to proteins, lipids, and sugars, which usually are hydrolyzed before absorption.[210] In general, 60% to 65% of the phosphorus ingested is absorbed, mostly in the duodenum and jejunum through an energy-dependent, saturable, active process.[211] Phosphorus absorption is linearly related to the dietary intake when the intake is 4 to 30 mg/kg/day. The amount of phosphorus ingested probably is the most important factor in determining net absorption. Phosphorus absorption is also stimulated during periods of increased demand, such as active growth and pregnancy.[212] Increased intake of calcium and magnesium and concurrent use of aluminum hydroxide antacids may reduce phosphorus absorption owing to formation of a nonabsorbable complex.[213] In addition, absorption is also affected by vitamin D, PTH, and calcitonin.[208]

Renal phosphorus excretion depends on the dietary phosphorus intake. Normally, greater than 85% of the filtered phosphate load is reabsorbed; however, the fractional urinary excretion can vary from 0.2% to 20%. Renal phosphate excretion is also affected by acid–base balance, ECF volume, and calcium and glucose concentrations.[208] In addition, PTH, thyroid hormone, thyrocalcitonin, vitamin D, insulin, glucocorticoid, and glucagon can also alter renal phosphate excretion.[7]

Hypophosphatemia

ETIOLOGY

CASE 27-12

QUESTION 1: M.R., a 72-year-old woman, was admitted to the hospital with a 1-week history of increasing malaise, confusion, and decreased activity. M.R. has a history of HF, hypertension, type 2 diabetes, and peptic ulcer disease. She was receiving hydrochlorothiazide, aluminum–magnesium antacid, sucralfate, and insulin. She is febrile and in significant respiratory distress. ABG results at admission were pH, 7.5; P_{O_2}, 42 mm Hg; and P_{CO_2},

20 mm Hg. Respiratory function continued to deteriorate, requiring intubation and mechanical ventilation. Serum electrolyte concentrations were as follows:

Na, 128 mEq/L
K, 3.6 mEq/L
Cl, 96 mEq/L
CO_2, 23 mEq/L
Glucose, 320 mg/dL
Phosphorus, 0.9 mg/dL

What may have contributed to the low serum phosphorus concentration in M.R.?

Hypophosphatemia can develop as the result of a phosphorus deficiency or secondary to a net flux of phosphorus out of the plasma compartment without a total body deficit. Moderate hypophosphatemia is defined as a serum phosphorus concentration of 1.0 to 2.5 mg/dL. A concentration of less than 1.0 mg/dL, as in M.R., is considered severe.[214] The extent of hypophosphatemia may not be assessed accurately by a single plasma phosphorus concentration determination because of diurnal variation.[215] Patients receiving large doses of mannitol may have pseudohypophosphatemia owing to the binding of mannitol with molybdate, which is used in the calorimetric assay for phosphorus.[216]

Hypophosphatemia is commonly caused by conditions that impair intestinal absorption, increase renal elimination, or shift phosphorus from the extracellular to the intracellular compartments. Hypophosphatemia secondary to low dietary phosphorus is exceedingly rare because phosphorus is ubiquitous.[208] In addition, renal phosphorus excretion is reduced and intestinal phosphorus absorption is increased to prevent a deficiency state.[217] Starvation in itself does not result in severe hypophosphatemia because the phosphorus content in plasma and muscles is often normal. Hypophosphatemia, however, can develop during refeeding with a high-calorie diet low in phosphorus. Therefore, hyperalimentation without phosphorus supplementation is likely to cause severe hypophosphatemia.[218]

Impaired phosphorus absorption secondary to malabsorptive conditions, prolonged nasogastric suction, and protracted vomiting can also result in hypophosphatemia. In M.R., the use of aluminum-containing and magnesium-containing antacids may further reduce phosphorus absorption. The antacids bind with endogenous and exogenous phosphorus in the GI tract and cause severe hypophosphatemia in patients with or without renal failure.[219] In addition, M.R. was taking sucralfate, which contains aluminum and can bind phosphorus in the GI tract.[220] Similarly, iron preparations can bind phosphorus.[221]

Hyperglycemia-induced osmotic diuresis and diuretic use may have increased the renal loss of phosphorus in M.R. Other conditions associated with renal phosphorus wasting include renal tubular acidosis, hyperparathyroidism, hypokalemia, hypomagnesemia, and extracellular volume expansion.[208] None of these situations, however, was evident in M.R. Shifting of phosphorus into the intracellular compartment by glucose or insulin and profound respiratory alkalosis may also have contributed to M.R.'s hypophosphatemic state.[222,223]

CASE 27-12, QUESTION 2: What other conditions are commonly associated with hypophosphatemia?

Diabetic ketoacidosis, chronic alcoholism, chronic obstructive airway disease, and extensive thermal burns are other conditions commonly associated with hypophosphatemia.[224,225] They are characterized by a combination of factors that result in phosphate loss and intracellular phosphate use. In patients with diabetic ketoacidosis, metabolic acidosis enhances the movement of phosphate from the intracellular compartment to plasma, whereas the concurrent osmotic diuresis secondary to hyperglycemia increases the renal elimination of extracellular phosphate.[226] The net result is a depletion of total body stores. Correction of the acidosis and administration of insulin then promotes the rapid uptake of phosphorus by tissues, and volume repletion dilutes the extracellular concentration. This sequence of events can ultimately lead to severe hypophosphatemia. The hypophosphatemia associated with chronic alcoholism and acute alcohol intoxication is also thought to be related to several factors, including reduced intestinal phosphorus absorption caused by vomiting, diarrhea, and antacid use; repeated acidosis that results in increased urinary phosphate excretion; and a shift of phosphorus into cells because of respiratory alkalosis. Renal phosphorus wasting can also result from hypomagnesemia or as a direct effect of alcohol.[226]

CLINICAL MANIFESTATIONS

CASE 27-12, QUESTION 3: What are the signs and symptoms associated with hypophosphatemia?

The clinical effects associated with chronic phosphorus depletion are often insidious and gradual in onset. In contrast, a rapid decline in plasma phosphorus concentrations results in sudden and serious organ dysfunction. Most of the effects can be attributed to impaired cellular energy stores and tissue hypoxia secondary to depletion of ATP or erythrocyte 2,3-diphosphoglycerate.[227] Severe hypophosphatemia can result in generalized muscle weakness, confusion, paresthesias, seizures, and coma. In addition, reduced cardiac contractility, hypotension, respiratory failure, and rhabdomyolysis have been observed with acute severe hypophosphatemia.[208] Chronic phosphorus depletion has been associated with decreased mentation; muscle weakness; osteomalacia; rickets; anorexia; dysphagia; cardiomyopathy; tachypnea; reduced sensitivity to insulin; and dysfunction of red blood cells, white blood cells, and platelets. Renal function is altered, as manifested by hypophosphaturia, hypercalciuria, hypermagnesuria, bicarbonaturia, and glycosuria. M.R.'s decreased mentation, weakness, and respiratory failure are consistent with severe hypophosphatemia.

TREATMENT

CASE 27-12, QUESTION 4: How can phosphate depletion be assessed? Outline a treatment regimen that would effectively and safely correct the phosphorus deficit in M.R. How should her therapy be monitored?

Phosphorus resides primarily in the intracellular space; the amount in the ECF is only a small percentage of the total body store. Because the patient's pH, blood glucose concentration, and insulin availability may affect phosphorus distribution, it is difficult to determine the magnitude of the phosphorus deficit based on the serum concentration alone. As discussed, a patient may have hypophosphatemia secondary to a rapid shift of phosphorus into the intracellular space without a total body deficit. The duration of the hypophosphatemia is often limited because it may be corrected by renal phosphorus conservation and oral intake of phosphorus-containing foods. Aside from serum phosphorus concentrations, urinary phosphorus excretion may be used to further assess the phosphorus deficit. Typically, renal phosphorus excretion is severely limited in patients with significant deficits. A phosphorus excretion of less than 100 mg/day (fractional phosphorus excretion $<10\%$) confirms appropriate renal phosphorus conservation when the serum phosphorus is less than 2 mg/dL. It also suggests a nonrenal etiology (e.g., impaired GI absorption) or some type of internal redistribution (e.g., respiratory alkalosis).[228]

Prophylactic supplementation should be used in situations that predictably increase the risk for developing hypophosphatemia. These include patients who are receiving total parenteral nutrition or large doses of antacids for an extended period, alcoholic patients, and those with diabetic ketoacidosis.

The specific treatment of hypophosphatemia depends on the presence of signs and symptoms, as well as the anticipated duration and severity of hypophosphatemia. In an asymptomatic patient with mild hypophosphatemia (1.5–2.5 mg/dL), who has no evidence of phosphorus depletion, phosphorus supplementation is generally not necessary because the condition is usually self-limited.[200] In other patients with mild and moderate hypophosphatemia, who have evidence of phosphorus deficit, oral supplementation is the safest and preferred mode of replacement. Skim or low-fat milk is a convenient source of phosphorus and calcium. Whole milk, because of its high fat content, can cause diarrhea if a large amount is consumed. Several oral phosphorus preparations can be used in patients who cannot tolerate milk products.

When hypophosphatemia is severe, as in M.R., or when the patient is vomiting or unable to take oral medication, parenteral phosphorus replacement is needed. Several empiric regimens have been evaluated. IV administration of 0.08 to 0.5 mmol/kg body weight of phosphorus over the course of 4 to 12 hours is safe and effective in restoring the serum phosphorus concentration.[228,229] More aggressive regimens, such as infusion over the course of 30 minutes to 2 hours, have also been suggested for critically ill and surgical patients.[230,231] Parenteral phosphorus replacement should be stopped once the serum phosphorus concentration reaches 2.0 mg/dL and also when oral supplementation is started. In general, no more than 32 mmol (1 g) of phosphorus should be administered IV in a 24-hour period. Regardless of the regimen used, serum phosphorus, calcium, and magnesium concentrations should be monitored closely because IV phosphorus administration can induce hyperphosphatemia quite rapidly, as well as hypocalcemia and hypomagnesemia. Monitoring of urine phosphorus concentration also helps determine the adequacy of therapy. Metastatic soft tissue calcification, hypotension, and, depending on the preparation used, potassium, sodium, or volume overload may occur. This could be significant in patients such as M.R. who have a history of HF and hypertension. Therefore, renal function and volume status should be monitored during therapy. Diarrhea, a common dose-related side effect of oral phosphorus replacement, can be minimized by diluting the supplement and slowly titrating the dose. Large doses can also result in metabolic acidosis.[228]

Phosphorus can be administered orally in doses of 30 to 60 mmol/day, usually given in two to four divided doses to minimize GI adverse events, using any commercially available oral supplement (e.g., Fleet or Neutra-Phos). Fleet Phospho-Soda (5 mL twice daily) delivers 40 mmol/day of phosphorus. Skim milk, the preferred agent for diluting the supplement, contains approximately 7 mmol of phosphorus/cup and provides calcium and potassium as well.

In M.R., oral supplementation was not feasible because she had intermittent diarrhea and vomiting. Potassium phosphate 15 mmol (providing 22 mEq of potassium) was therefore infused IV in 250 mL of 0.45% saline over the course of 12 hours. The regimen was repeated once until the serum phosphorus concentration reached 2 mg/dL. Oral supplementation with Fleet Phospho-Soda then was begun by adding one teaspoonful twice daily to her enteral tube feeding.

Hyperphosphatemia

Refer to the Mineral and Bone Disorders section in Chapter 28, Chronic Kidney Disease.

MAGNESIUM

Homeostasis

Magnesium is an intracellular cation found primarily in bone (65%) and muscle (20%). Only 2% of the total body store of 21 to 28 g (1,750–2,400 mEq) is located in the extracellular compartment. Serum magnesium concentrations, therefore, do not reflect the total magnesium body store accurately. In healthy adults, the serum magnesium concentration is 1.5 to 2.4 mEq/L, with approximately 20% of the serum magnesium bound to proteins.

Magnesium plays an important role in different metabolic processes, particularly in energy transfer, storage, and utilization. Cation deficiency can impair many ATP-mediated energy-dependent cellular processes as well as the action of phosphatases.[232] Magnesium is necessary for many enzymes involved in the metabolism of carbohydrate, fat, and protein, as well as RNA aggregation, DNA transcription, and degradation. The normal operation of many sodium, proton, and calcium pumps and the regulation of potassium and calcium channels are all dependent on the availability of intracellular magnesium.[233,234] In addition, adequate magnesium stores are needed to maintain normal neuronal control, neuromuscular transmission, and cardiovascular tone.

The average diet in North America contains about 20 to 30 mEq of magnesium.[235] The daily requirement is approximately 18 to 33 mEq for young persons and 15 to 28 mEq for women.[236] Normally, 30% to 40% of the elemental magnesium is absorbed, primarily in the jejunum and ileum. However, absorption may be increased to 80% in deficiency states and reduced to 25% during high magnesium intake. In patients with uremia, GI absorption of magnesium is decreased; however, absorption in the jejunum can be normalized by physiologic doses of 1α,25-dihydroxyvitamin D_3.[237] In addition, PTH also modulates magnesium absorption.[238]

Magnesium is eliminated primarily by the kidneys; only 1% to 2% of the endogenous magnesium is eliminated by the fecal route.[182] The magnitude of renal removal is determined by GFR and tubular reabsorption. Approximately 20% to 30% of the tubular reabsorption takes place in the proximal tubule, whereas Henle's loop, primarily the thick ascending limb, is responsible for up to 65% of the total reabsorption.[238] Only about 5% to 6% of the filtered magnesium is generally eliminated in the urine. The extent of magnesium reabsorption changes in parallel with sodium reabsorption, which is affected by the ECF volume. The renal threshold for urinary magnesium excretion is 1.3 to 1.7 mEq/L, which is similar to the normal plasma magnesium concentration. Slight changes in plasma magnesium concentration, therefore, may substantially alter the amount of magnesium excreted in the urine.[239]

Urinary magnesium reabsorption is affected by many factors, including sodium balance; ECF volume; serum concentrations of magnesium, calcium, and phosphate; and metabolic acidosis and alkalosis.[240] Concurrent use of loop and osmotic diuretics will also modulate the reabsorption.[241] Hormones, such as PTH, and possibly calcitonin, glucagon, and mineralocorticoids may affect the routine maintenance of magnesium balance as well.[242,243]

Hypomagnesemia

ETIOLOGY

CASE 27-13

QUESTION 1: R.J., a 61-year-old man, is admitted to the hospital because of trauma to his forehead after falling at home. He has a long history of conditions related to his alcohol abuse: liver disease, ascites, seizures, pancreatitis, and malabsorption. R.J. complained of abdominal pain, nausea, vomiting, and diarrhea for the past several days. At admission, R.J. was confused, apprehensive, and combative, and he had marked tremors. He also had delirium, as evidenced by hallucinations, screaming, and delusions, and he was having multiple tonic–clonic seizures. The medical record revealed that R.J. had been taking furosemide for the last 2 months. Pertinent laboratory test results obtained at admission were as follows:

K, 2.5 mEq/L
Magnesium, 0.8 mEq/L
Creatinine, 0.8 mg/dL

Phenytoin was administered for seizure control and R.J. was placed on nasogastric suction. Fluid restriction was instituted and furosemide therapy was continued to control his ascites. What are the circumstances that have contributed to R.J.'s hypomagnesemia?

Magnesium body stores are difficult to assess because magnesium is primarily an intracellular ion, and serum magnesium concentrations do not provide an accurate indication of the total body load. In fact, cellular magnesium depletion may be present with low, normal, or even high serum magnesium concentrations.[243,244] Conversely, hypomagnesemia may be seen without a net loss of body magnesium. Refeeding after starvation will result in increased trapping of magnesium by newly formed tissue, resulting in hypomagnesemia. Similarly, acute pancreatitis and parathyroidectomy can cause hypomagnesemia without a net loss of the cation.[245,246]

The prevalence of hypomagnesemia in ambulatory and hospitalized patients is approximately 6% to 12%.[247] The incidence increases to 42% in patients who are hypokalemic[248] and to 60% to 65% in those under intensive care.[249] Multiple risk factors and clinical conditions can contribute to the high rate of hypomagnesemia in critically ill patients.

Magnesium depletion and hypomagnesemia can develop owing to GI, renal, and endocrinologic causes. Depletion can occur in patients whose dietary magnesium intake is severely restricted[250] and in those who have protein calorie malnutrition.[251] Also at risk are patients who receive prolonged parenteral nutrition[252] and those who undergo prolonged nasogastric suction.[253] Hypomagnesemia may be present in patients who have increased magnesium requirements, such as pregnant women and infants.[254] Conditions associated with steatorrhea, such as nontropical sprue and short-bowel syndrome, can result in reduced GI magnesium absorption. Insoluble magnesium soaps may be formed in the GI tract because of the presence of unabsorbed fat.[255] Hypomagnesemia can also occur in patients with a bowel resection[256] and severe diarrhea.[257] A rare genetic disorder has also been reported in patients with defective GI magnesium absorption.[258] An impaired carrier-mediated magnesium transport system is believed to be responsible for the symptomatic deficiency, which requires high oral magnesium intake to overcome the defect.

Renal magnesium wasting can be caused by a primary defect or be secondary to systemic factors. A rare form of renal magnesium wasting is congenital.[259] Various drugs can induce hypomagnesemia through increased renal loss: cisplatin,[260] aminoglycosides,[261] cyclosporine,[262] and amphotericin B.[263] Use of loop and thiazide diuretics can also result in hypomagnesemia, which can be reversed with the concurrent use of amiloride or triamterene. Magnesium depletion can be associated with phosphate depletion,[264] calcium infusion,[265] and ketoacidosis.[266] Acute and chronic ingestion of alcohol will result in increased renal magnesium loss.[253,267] Various endocrinologic disorders, such as SIADH,[268] hyperthyroidism,[269] hyperaldosteronism,[244] and postparathyroidectomy,[271] are also associated with hypomagnesemia.

R.J. could be hypomagnesemic for many reasons. His long history of alcohol use, malnutrition, and malabsorption may all have contributed to his magnesium deficit. The vomiting and diarrhea that he experienced could have reduced GI magnesium absorption. Use of furosemide and nasogastric suction while in the hospital could also have exacerbated his magnesium depletion through renal and GI losses, respectively.

CLINICAL MANIFESTATIONS

CASE 27-13, QUESTION 2: What are the clinical manifestations of hypomagnesemia in R.J.?

Magnesium depletion can result in abnormal function of the neurologic, neuromuscular, and cardiovascular systems. Hypomagnesemia lowers the threshold for nerve stimulation, resulting in increased irritability. Typical findings include Chvostek and Trousseau signs, muscle fasciculation, tremors, muscle spasticity, generalized convulsions, and possibly tetany. The patient may experience weakness, anorexia, nausea, and vomiting, as seen in R.J. Hypokalemia, hypocalcemia, and alkalosis may be present as well. In patients who are moderately depleted, changes in the ECG include widening of the QRS complex and a peaking T wave.[272] In severe depletion, a prolonged PR interval and a diminished T wave may be seen. Ventricular arrhythmias have also been reported in some patients.[273]

TREATMENT

CASE 27-13, QUESTION 3: Outline a regimen to replenish the body stores of magnesium for R.J., and develop a monitoring plan to assess efficacy and potential adverse effects.

The specific regimen for magnesium replenishment depends on the clinical presentation of the patient. Symptomatic patients require more aggressive parenteral therapy, whereas oral replacement may suffice for asymptomatic hypomagnesemia. Patients with life-threatening symptoms, such as seizures and arrhythmias, need immediate magnesium infusion. Because serum magnesium concentrations do not reflect total body stores, symptoms are more important determinants of the urgency and aggressiveness of therapy.

The body stores of magnesium must be replenished slowly. Serum magnesium concentrations may return to the normal range within the first 24 hours, but total replenishment of body stores may take several days. Furthermore, approximately 50% of the administered IV dose of magnesium will be excreted in the urine.[273] Because the threshold for urinary magnesium excretion is low, the abrupt increase in serum magnesium after an IV dose will result in increased urinary magnesium excretion despite a total body magnesium deficit. Conversely, in patients with renal insufficiency, decreased excretion of magnesium will place the patient at risk for hypermagnesemia. A reduced rate of magnesium administration and frequent monitoring of serum magnesium concentrations are therefore necessary in patients with renal dysfunction.

Oral replacement of magnesium is indicated for asymptomatic patients with mild depletion. Magnesium-containing antacids, milk of magnesia, and magnesium oxide are effective choices for replacement. Sustained-release preparations, such as Slow Mag (magnesium chloride) or Mag-Tab SR (magnesium lactate), are preferred, however. With 5 to 7 mEq (2.5–3.5 mmol or 60–84 mg) of magnesium per tablet, six to eight tablets should be given daily in divided doses for severe magnesium depletion. For mild and asymptomatic disease, two to four tablets per day may be sufficient.[274] A diet high in magnesium (cereals, nuts, meat, fruits, fish, legumes, and vegetables) will also help replenish body stores and prevent depletion.[275]

For patients with symptomatic hypomagnesemia, such as R.J., parenteral magnesium replacement is indicated. The magnesium deficit in patients with chronic alcoholism is estimated to be 1 to 2 mEq/kg.[276] Because up to half of the IV magnesium dose will be excreted in the urine during replacement, approximately 2 to 4 mEq/kg will be needed to replenish R.J.'s body store.[277] Magnesium of 1 mEq/kg, as magnesium sulfate 10% solution, should be administered IV in the first 24 hours. Half of this amount is given in the first 3 hours, and the remaining half is infused over the course of the rest of the day. This dose may be repeated to keep the serum magnesium concentration greater than 1.0 mg/dL.[274] Later on, 0.5 mEq/kg of magnesium may be replenished daily for up to 4 additional days.[277,278] Magnesium can be given IM as 50% solution, but the injections are painful and potentially sclerosing, and multiple administrations are needed. Therefore, the IV route is the preferred mode of parenteral administration. For patients with symptomatic hypomagnesemia who are unstable, such as those experiencing seizures or life-threatening arrhythmias, 16 mEq of magnesium sulfate may be administered as a short IV infusion over the course of 2 minutes, followed by 16 mEq over the course of 20 minutes, then 16 to 24 mEq over the course of 2 to 4 hours.[278,279]

After IV magnesium administration, the patient should remain in a supine position to avoid hypotension. He should be monitored carefully for marked suppression of deep tendon reflexes (magnesium, 4–7 mEq/L); ECG, BP, and respiration changes; and high serum magnesium levels. Facial flushing, a sensation of warmth, and sweatiness may result from vasodilation secondary to a rapid magnesium infusion.[277] Particular caution is warranted in patients with renal impairment, in whom the rate of magnesium should be reduced. These patients should be monitored frequently to avoid toxicities related to hypermagnesemia. IV magnesium should also be administered cautiously in patients with severe atrioventricular heart block or bifascicular blocks because magnesium possesses pharmacologic properties similar to calcium channel blockers.[277,279]

In patients who exhibit hypomagnesemia secondary to a thiazide or loop diuretic, amiloride may be added to reduce renal magnesium loss by increasing reabsorption in the cortical collecting tubule.[274]

CASE 27-13, QUESTION 4: For the initial 2 days of hospitalization, R.J. received 3 mEq/kg of IV magnesium sulfate. However, his serum magnesium concentration remained less than 1.5 mEq/L. What might have contributed to the lack of favorable response to the magnesium therapy?

The total amount of magnesium administered to R.J. during the past 2 days was higher than the usual recommended rate (4–5 days) of magnesium replenishment, leading to renal excretion of a large portion of the dose.[280] Furthermore, the use of nasogastric suction and furosemide have increased the magnesium loss during the replacement period, and hypokalemia may have reduced the effectiveness of magnesium replacement. In a patient whose serum magnesium concentration does not increase after appropriate magnesium therapy, a 24-hour urine collection to assess magnesium renal excretion can be helpful. A low urinary magnesium concentration is consistent with magnesium depletion, whereas high urinary magnesium excretion in the presence of hypomagnesemia suggests renal magnesium wasting.

Hypermagnesemia

ETIOLOGY

CASE 27-14

QUESTION 1: J.O., a 63-year-old man with renal insufficiency, was admitted to the hospital because of increasing weakness during the past several days. J.O. began taking a magnesium–aluminum hydroxide antacid several times daily 2 weeks ago when he exhibited stomach upset. Physical examination reveals hypotension and depressed deep tendon reflexes. The ECG reveals prolonged PR and QRS intervals. The serum magnesium concentration is 6.5 mEq/dL. What is the most likely cause of hypermagnesemia in J.O.?

Because the kidney is the primary route of magnesium elimination, renal impairment is a virtual requisite for hypermagnesemia (see Chapter 28, Chronic Kidney Diseases). A common cause of hypermagnesemia is the use of magnesium-containing medications, such as antacids and laxatives, by patients with impaired renal function, including older adults. When a patient with renal failure, such as J.O., takes magnesium-containing medications, the serum magnesium concentration can increase substantially, resulting in toxicities. Hypermagnesemia may be seen when the creatinine clearance drops to less than 30 mL/minute; an inverse relationship is observed between the serum magnesium concentrations and the creatinine clearances.[281] Hypermagnesemia is also seen in patients with acute renal failure during the oliguric phase, but not the diuretic phase.[282] Other potential causes of hypermagnesemia include adrenal insufficiency,[232] hypothyroidism,[283] lithium,[283] magnesium citrate used as a cathartic for drug overdose,[284] and parenteral magnesium given for preeclampsia.[285]

CLINICAL MANIFESTATIONS

CASE 27-14, QUESTION 2: Describe the usual clinical presentation of a patient with hypermagnesemia.

An elevated magnesium serum concentration alters the normal function of the neurologic, neuromuscular, and cardiovascular systems. When the serum magnesium concentration is greater than 4 mEq/L, deep tendon reflexes are depressed; they are usually lost at greater than 6 mEq/L. Flaccid quadriplegia can develop when the concentration is greater than 8 to 10 mEq/L. Respiratory paralysis, hypotension, and difficulty in talking and swallowing may also be present. Changes in the ECG may include a prolonged PR interval and widening of the QRS complex. Complete heart block may be seen at concentrations of approximately 15 mEq/L. In mild hypermagnesemia, the patient may experience nausea and vomiting.

Drowsiness, lethargy, diaphoresis, and altered consciousness may be present at higher serum magnesium concentrations. J.O.'s increasing weakness, hypotension, depressed deep tendon reflexes, and ECG findings are consistent with hypermagnesemia.

TREATMENT

CASE 27-14, QUESTION 3: How should J.O.'s hypermagnesemia be treated?

If magnesium-containing medications are discontinued in patients with hypermagnesemia, the serum magnesium concentration will usually return to the normal range through renal elimination. When potentially life-threatening complications are present, as in J.O., 5 to 10 mEq of IV calcium should be administered to antagonize the respiratory and cardiac manifestations of magnesium.[285,286] The dose of the calcium can be repeated as necessary because its effect is short lived. In patients with good renal function without life-threatening complications, IV furosemide, plus 0.45% sodium chloride to replace lost urine volume, will enhance urinary magnesium excretion while preventing volume depletion. Hemodialysis or peritoneal dialysis is indicated for patients with significant renal function impairment and possibly for those with severe hypermagnesemia.

KEY REFERENCES AND WEBSITES

A full list of references for this chapter can be found at http://thepoint.lww.com/AT11e. Below are the key references for this chapter, with the corresponding reference number in this chapter found in parentheses after the reference.

Key References

Agus Z. Hypomagnesemia. *J Am Soc Nephrol*. 1999;10:1616. (274)

Alfrey AC. Normal and abnormal magnesium metabolism. In: Schrier RW, ed. *Renal and Electrolyte Disorders*. 6th ed. Philadelphia, PA: Lippincott Williams & Wilkins; 2003:278. (275)

Allon M. Hyperkalemia in end stage renal disease: mechanism and management. *J Am Soc Nephrol*. 1995;6:1134. (167)

Davidson TG. Conventional treatment of hypercalcemia of malignancy. *Am J Health Syst Pharm*. 2001;58(Suppl 3):S8. (189)

Gross P. Treatment of severe hyponatremia. *Kidney Int*. 2001;60:2417. (61)

Lehrich RW et al. Role of vaptans in the management of hyponatremia. *Am J Kidney Dis*. 2013;62:364–383. (83)

Morrison G et al. Hyperosmolal states. In: Narins RG, ed. *Maxwell & Kleeman's Clinical Disorders of Fluid and Electrolyte Metabolism*. 5th ed. New York, NY: McGraw-Hill; 1994:617. (104)

Rose BD. Introduction to disorders of osmolality. In: Rose BD et al, eds. *Clinical Physiology of Acid-Base and Electrolyte Disorders*. 5th ed. New York, NY: McGraw-Hill; 2000:682. (3)

Rose BD. Renal function and disorders of water and sodium balance. In: Rubenstein E, Federman DD, eds. *Scientific American Medicine*. New York, NY: Scientific American Inc., 1994; Section 10:1. (2)

Rubin MF, Narins RG. Hypophosphatemia: pathophysiological and practical aspects of its therapy. *Semin Nephrol*. 1990;10:536. (229)

Stanaszek WF, Romankiewicz JA. Current approaches to management of potassium deficiency. *Drug Intell Clin Pharm*. 1985;19:176. (134)

28 Chronic Kidney Disease

Darius L. Mason

CORE PRINCIPLES

		CHAPTER CASES
1	Chronic kidney disease (CKD) is progressive, irreversible kidney damage characterized by decreased estimated glomerular filtration rate (eGFR) or evidence of kidney damage for at least 3 months.	**Case 28-1 (Question 1)**
2	Classification of CKD staging should be determined on the basis of kidney function, defined by the Kidney Disease: Improving Global Outcomes (KDIGO). Each stage is associated with certain action plans.	**Case 28-1 (Question 1)**
3	Many equations exist for calculating creatinine clearance (CrCl) or eGFR. The Modification of Diet in Renal Disease (MDRD) equation is used to quantify GFR, to detect or stage the degree of CKD, and to follow progression. The Cockcroft–Gault (CG) equation is used to adjust the doses of medications that are eliminated by the kidneys.	**Equations 28-3–28-5**
4	Diabetes is the number one cause of CKD in the United States. Optimal control of blood glucose levels is essential to slow the progression of CKD and reduce morbidity and mortality.	**Case 28-1 (Questions 2–4)**
5	Fluid accumulation and electrolyte abnormalities secondary to CKD often complicate the treatment of hypertension and can have cardiotoxic effects.	**Case 28-1 (Questions 5–9)**
6	Metabolic acidosis presents in late stages of CKD from reduced hydrogen ion excretion and bicarbonate production. Metabolic acidosis can worsen bone disease and other metabolic processes.	**Case 28-1 (Question 8)**
7	Treating anemia of CKD is essential to reducing cardiovascular disease (CVD) complications. Management of anemia includes administration of iron supplementation and erythropoiesis-stimulating agents.	**Case 28-1 (Questions 10–12)**
8	CVD is the number one cause of morbidity and mortality in CKD. Cardioprotective measures should be addressed at all stages.	**Case 28-2 (Question 1)**
9	Hypertension is the second leading cause of CKD in the United States. Treating hypertension to target goals is necessary to slow the progression of CKD and reduce mortality.	**Case 28-2 (Question 2)**
10	Mineral and bone disorders (MBD) characterized by biochemical abnormalities, renal osteodystrophy, and vascular calcification become more common as CKD progresses. Biochemical abnormalities lead to the development of vascular calcifications and increase the risk for cardiovascular mortality.	**Case 28-3 (Questions 1, 2)**
11	Hyperphosphatemia is managed with dietary phosphorus restriction and phosphate-binding agents.	**Case 28-3 (Question 2)**
12	Activated forms of vitamin D (calcitriol, paricalcitol, and doxercalciferol) or a calcimimetic agent (cinacalcet) may be necessary to achieve proper biochemical balance and bone metabolism.	**Case 28-3 (Question 2)**
13	Glomerulonephropathies (GN) are a collection of glomerular diseases caused by a variety of immunologic mechanisms and the third leading cause of CKD. Patients with GN may present with nephrotic syndrome and require treatment with immunosuppressant therapy.	**Case 28-4 (Questions 1, 2), Case 28-5 (Questions 1, 2)**

INTRODUCTION

Chronic kidney disease (CKD) describes the continuum of kidney dysfunction from early to late-stage disease. Estimated glomerular filtration rates (eGFR) range from 90 mL/minute/1.73 m^2 in the early stages to less than 15 mL/minute/1.73 m^2 in the late stages of disease. The most advanced stage of CKD, known as end-stage renal disease (ESRD), occurs when chronic renal replacement therapy in the form of dialysis or kidney transplantation is necessary to sustain life.[1] Complications associated with CKD that increase the complexity of this condition include fluid and electrolyte abnormalities, anemia, cardiovascular disease (CVD), mineral and bone disorders (MND), and malnutrition. Optimal treatment of patients with CKD is best achieved using a multidisciplinary approach to address the concurrent medical problems and complex pharmacotherapeutic regimens. Alterations in drug disposition that occur with kidney impairment and the subsequent need for dosage adjustments are additional considerations when determining rational pharmacotherapy in this population.

Implementation of clinical practice guidelines leads to improved patient outcomes and reduced variability in patient care.[2] As a result many countries have developed evidence-based clinical practice guidelines for the treatment of kidney disease. In the United States, the National Kidney Foundation (NKF) established the Kidney Disease Outcomes Quality Initiative (K/DOQI) to provide evidence-based treatment guidelines for all stages of kidney disease and related conditions. However, because kidney disease is a worldwide public health issue and the problems faced by kidney disease around the world are universal, the Kidney Disease: Improving Global Outcomes (KDIGO) was established in 2003. The mission of KDIGO is to improve the care and outcomes of kidney disease patients worldwide by promoting coordination, collaboration, and integration of initiatives. KDIGO is managed by the NKF. Contact information for K/DOQI and KDIGO and corresponding web addresses for clinical practice guidelines can be found in Table 28-1.

Definition and Classification of CKD

CKD is characterized by a progressive deterioration in kidney function with time characterized by irreversible structural damage to existing nephrons. The KDIGO 2012 Clinical Practice Guideline for the Evaluation and Management of Chronic Kidney Disease defines CKD as abnormalities in kidney structure or damage (e.g., albuminuria) or function (e.g., decreased glomerular filtration rate or GFR) present for at least 3 months with implications for the patient's health (Table 28-2). CKD is classified by CGA categories (**c**ause of kidney disease, **G**FR, **a**lbuminuria) in the KDIGO guidelines. (Table 28-3 and Table 28-4).[1] The presence of the protein albumin in urine (defined as *albuminuria*) is an early and sensitive marker of kidney damage (Table 28-4). Unlike previous K/DOQI guidelines, KDIGO divides category three into two subcategories, 3a (GFR 45–59 mL/min/1.73 m^2) and 3b (GFR 30–44 mL/min/1.73 m^2), to better stratify patients based on the different outcomes and risks associated with these levels of GFR. Kidney damage is indicated by pathologic abnormalities of the kidneys or markers of kidney injury, including abnormalities in blood or urine tests and imaging studies.[1] Table 28-5 provides etiologic examples of CKD staging.

Table 28-1
Resources for Kidney Disease Clinical Practice Guidelines

National Kidney Foundation Kidney Disease Outcomes Quality Initiative 30 East 33rd Street New York, New York 10016 Phone: 1-800-622-9010 Website: **https://www.kidney.org/professionals/guidelines**
Kidney Disease: Improving Global Outcomes 30 East 33rd Street, Suite 900 New York, New York 10016 Phone: 212-889-2210 x288 Website: **http://kdigo.org/home/**

Table 28-2
Criteria for CKD[1]

Markers of Kidney Damage	Decreased GFR
■ Albuminuria (AER ≥30 mg/24 hours; ACR ≥30 mg/g [≥3 mg/mmol]) ■ Urine sediment abnormalities ■ Electrolyte and other abnormalities due to tubular disorders ■ Abnormalities detected by histology ■ Structural abnormalities detected by imaging ■ History of kidney transplantation	GFR<60 mL/minute/1.73 m^2

Must be at the defined GFR range or damage persisting for 3 months or greater.
AER, albumin excretion rate; ACR, albumin-to-creatinine ratio; CKD, chronic kidney disease; GFR, glomerular filtration rate.

Table 28-3
Staging of Chronic Kidney Disease Based on eGFR Category[1]

GFR Categories (mL/minute/1.73 m2)	Description	Range
G1	Normal or high	≥90
G2	Mildly decreased	60–89
G3a	Mildly to moderately decreased	45–59
G3b	Moderately to severely decreased	30–44
G4	Severely decreased	15–29
G5	Kidney failure	<15

CKD, chronic kidney disease; GFR, glomerular filtration rate.

Table 28-4
Albuminuria Categories: Description and Range[1]

	A1	A2	A3
Description	Normal to mildly increased	Moderately Increased	Severely Increased
Albumin-to-creatinine ratio (mg/g)	<30	30–300	>300
Albumin excretion rate (mg/24 h)	<30	30–300	>300

Table 28-5
Examples of CKD Staging[1]

Cause	GFR Category	Albuminuria Category	Criterion for CKD
Diabetic kidney disease	G5	A3	Decreased GFR, albuminuria
Idiopathic focal sclerosis	G2	A3	Albuminuria
Kidney transplant recipient	G2	A1	History of kidney transplantation
Polycystic kidney disease	G2	A1	Imaging abnormality
Vesicoureteral reflex	G1	A1	Imaging abnormality
Distal renal tubular acidosis	G1	A1	Electrolyte abnormalities
Hypertensive kidney disease	G4	A2	Decreased GFR and albuminuria
CKD presumed due to diabetes and hypertension	G4	A1	Decreased GFR
CKD presumed due to diabetes and hypertension	G2	A3	Albuminuria
CKD presumed due to diabetes and hypertension	G3a	A1	Decreased GFR
CKD cause unknown	G3a	A1	Decreased GFR

Patients above the thick horizontal line are likely to be encountered in nephrology practice. Patients below the thick horizontal line are likely to be encountered in primary care practice and in nephrology practice.
CGA, cause, GFR category and albuminuria category; CKD, chronic kidney disease; GFR, glomerular filtration rate.

A substantial decline in kidney function also leads to *azotemia*, the accumulation of nitrogenous wastes such as urea in the plasma, and an increased risk for developing complications of CKD. Uremic signs and symptoms from accumulation of nitrogenous wastes and other toxins manifest clinically as an elevated blood urea nitrogen (BUN) and lead to a myriad of complications affecting most major organ systems. Laboratory biochemical abnormalities include azotemia, hyperphosphatemia, hypocalcemia, hyperkalemia, metabolic acidosis, and worsening anemia. Clinical signs of CKD and its associated complications, including hypertension, uremic symptoms (e.g., nausea, anorexia), and bleeding, are observed as the disease advances to categories 3 through 5. Interventions to slow the progression of kidney disease are critical. Patients who reach an eGFR of less than 30 mL/minute/1.73 m^2 (category 4), in general, will ultimately progress to ESRD.

Epidemiology of Chronic Kidney Disease

INCIDENCE AND PREVALENCE

The United States Renal Data System (USRDS) is a national data system which collects, analyzes, and distributes information about all categories of CKD in the United States. Data describing CKD incidence and prevalence are made available annually by the USRDS and the USRDS provides data from approximately 2 years prior.[3] The 2014 USRDS report estimated CKD to affect 14% of the US population in 2012. Category 3 CKD reported the greatest increase in prevalence from 4.5% to 6.0%. The NKF's Kidney Early Evaluation Program (KEEP) screens high-risk individuals across the United States with high blood pressure (BP), diabetes, or a family history of kidney failure. Based on the high-risk participants from the KEEP screenings from 2000 to 2011, 24% of the participants had CKD.[4]

Based on the 2014 USRDS data from 2012, there were 114,813 new cases of ESRD; 102,277 of those cases started hemodialysis. This ESRD number includes peritoneal, hemodialysis, and transplant recipients. The rate of ESRD has declined each year since 2009. The 2012 adjusted incidence rate of 353/million/year was the lowest incidence rate since 1997. There were 449,342 patients receiving dialysis therapy (408,711 on hemodialysis and 40,631 on peritoneal dialysis) as of December 31, 2012. This was an increase in prevalence of 3.8% and 57.4% larger than in 2000. Prevalence was lowest in the New England and Northwest regions whereas it was highest in the Midwest regions. African Americans and Native Americans had a 3.3 and 1.85 times greater incidence rate of kidney failure, respectively, compared with white individuals. Hispanic patients had the highest ESRD incidence rate compared to the non-Hispanic population.[3]

In 2012, the majority of the increase in prevalence of ESRD occurred in patients aged 45 and over.[1] The age groups with the highest incidence of ESRD were those aged 65 to 74 years with 6,302 ESRD cases per million of the population. Those greater than age 75 had the greatest increase in cases at 50% since 2000. The African American population had the highest prevalence per million of the population that was 2-fold higher than Native Americans, 2.5-fold higher than Asians, and 4-fold higher than whites.[3]

CKD is a health priority identified as a disease prevention target for the Healthy People 2020 (HP2020) national health initiative; one of the specific CKD-related objectives is to reduce the number of cases of ESRD.[5] The HP2020 target rate of ESRD cases is 13.7% of the population. Currently, the adjusted prevalence from 1999 to 2004 is 15.2% of the population.[5] Additional objectives such as increasing awareness, improving cardiovascular care, and reduction of mortality in CKD patients can be found at the HealthyPeople.gov website.

ETIOLOGY

In CKD, the progressive loss or damage to functioning nephrons as a function of time is the result of a primary disorder or disease of the kidney, a secondary complication of certain systemic diseases (e.g., diabetes mellitus or hypertension), or an acute injury to the kidney that results in irreversible kidney damage. In 2012, the leading causes of ESRD in newly diagnosed American patients were diabetes mellitus (44%), hypertension (28%), and chronic glomerulonephritis (GN; 7%).[3] The remaining cases of ESRD can be attributed to a variety of other pathologies; examples include polycystic kidney disease, congenital malformations of the kidneys, nephrolithiasis, interstitial nephritis, renal artery stenosis, renal carcinoma, and human immunodeficiency virus–associated nephropathy.

RISK FACTORS

A variety of risk factors associated with development, initiation, and progression of CKD have been identified. Initiation factors

Table 28-6
Risk Factors for Chronic Kidney Disease

Susceptibility	Initiation	Progression
Advanced age	Diabetes mellitus	Glycemia
Reduced kidney mass	Hypertension	Hypertension
Low birth weight	Glomerulonephritis	Proteinuria
Racial/ethnic minority	Drug induced or toxicity	Smoking
Family history	Smoking	Obesity
Low income or education	Obesity	
Systemic inflammation		
Dyslipidemia		

KDOQI. KDOQI clinical practice guidelines for chronic kidney disease: evaluation, classification, and stratification. *Am J Kidney Dis*. 2002;39(2, Suppl 1):S73.

are medical conditions that directly cause kidney damage. Risk factors for the progression of CKD exacerbate kidney damage and are related to an accelerated decline in kidney function with time. The majority of susceptibility factors are not modifiable, but may identify people who are at high risk for developing CKD. In contrast, pharmacotherapy and lifestyle interventions have been shown to modify CKD-related initiation and progression factors (see Prevention and Diabetic Nephropathy section). A summary of risk factors associated with CKD can be found in Table 28-6.

MORBIDITY AND MORTALITY

Rates of hospitalizations and mortality are much greater in those with kidney disease compared with the non-CKD population. Not surprisingly, mortality rates increase with progressing stages of CKD, patient health complexity, and age. The mortality rate of non-dialysis patients with CKD was 36% higher compared with those without CKD, and the adjusted rates of all-cause mortality were 6 to 8 times higher for dialysis patients compared with the general population.[3]

Advances in dialysis and transplantation have improved patient care, and as a result, mortality rates continue to decline. From 2003 to 2012, the mortality rate fell by 25%, whereas from 1993 to 2002, there was only a 9% reduction in mortality.[3] Cardiovascular-related events, particularly cardiac arrest and myocardial infarction, remain the leading causes of hospitalizations and death in both the non–dialysis CKD and ESRD populations. This is not surprising given the high prevalence of coexisting cardiac disorders in patients with kidney disease and the elevated risk for mortality associated with these conditions. However, since 1999, the overall rate of cardiovascular mortality in the ESRD population has continued to decline. After CVD, infection (predominantly septicemia) is a substantial contributor to overall morbidity and mortality in patients with ESRD.[3]

The mortality rates during the first year of hemodialysis are the highest. However, reductions in the first year of hemodialysis have decreased by 19%, 30%, and 56% for all-cause, cardiovascular, and infection death as compared to 2001, respectively. Although improvements in mortality are acknowledged, only 54% and 65% of hemodialysis and peritoneal dialysis patients survive beyond 3 years after ESRD onset.[3]

Medication Use

Data regarding medication use in the kidney disease population reveal non–dialysis CKD patients are prescribed an average of 6 to 8 medications and HD patients are prescribed approximately 12 medications (10 home medications and 2 in-center medications).[5,6] These patterns of medication use are reflective of the higher prevalence of complications and comorbidities in the latter stages of CKD, which require additional drug therapies. The extent of medication use and the complexity of prescribed drug regimens contribute to nonadherence and medication-related problems (MRPs) in the ESRD population.[7]

To manage MRPs, some dialysis units use a clinical pharmacist as part of the multidisciplinary health care team to provide pharmaceutical care to ESRD patients. Services provided by a clinical pharmacist have been shown to be cost-effective and associated with maintenance of health-related quality of life.[8,9] Additionally, a randomized study of 104 ESRD patients investigated the impact of pharmaceutical care (individualized drug therapy reviews conducted by a clinical pharmacist) to standard care (brief drug therapy reviews conducted by a nurse) on drug use, drug costs, hospitalization rates, and MRPs. After a 2-year follow-up, patients who received pharmaceutical care were taking fewer medications and had fewer all-cause hospitalizations compared with those receiving standard care.[10]

Economics

The cost of treating both non–dialysis CKD patients and ESRD patients is substantial. In 2012, the overall per person per year cost of medical treatment for Medicare non–dialysis CKD patients was more than $20,162 and the cost of medical care for those with stages 4 to 5 CKD was 1.4 times higher than those with CKD stages 1 to 2.[3] Furthermore, the majority of the costs of medical care provided to those with ESRD are paid by the federal government. In 2012, the cost for ESRD was $28.6 billion dollars, corresponding to 5.6% of the Medicare budget.[3] This amount reflects a consistent increase from prior years. The increase is most likely associated with the higher prevalence of ESRD, changes in the standard of care, reimbursement structure, and types of patients being treated (e.g., diabetic patients versus nondiabetic patients).

The continually growing costs of ESRD care require careful attention, given the implementation of the Centers for Medicare and Medicaid Services' *bundled* payment system that changed how Medicare pays for dialysis services. Under the bundled system, Medicare provides a single payment to ESRD facilities to cover all dialysis-related services for each dialysis treatment.[10] In the prior reimbursement system, Medicare paid a composite rate to dialysis units to cover the costs of an individual's dialysis treatment, certain routine medications (e.g., heparin), laboratory tests, and supplies. In addition to the composite rate, Medicare was billed separately for other related dialysis services and billable items (e.g., erythropoietin [EPO]-stimulating agents).[8] The bundled payment system is likely to reduce the government reimbursement for dialysis services, but may increase barriers to care for some ESRD patients.[10]

Pathophysiology

Progression of kidney disease to ESRD generally occurs over the course of months to years and is assessed by the rate of GFR decline. Each kidney contains approximately 1 million nephrons (the functional units of the kidney), and every nephron maintains its own single-nephron GFR. In the face of nephron loss, the remaining functional nephrons maintain renal function by increasing their single-nephron GFR via compensatory glomerular hemodynamic changes.[9] With time, this compensatory increase in single-nephron GFRs eventually leads to hypertrophy and an irreversible loss of nephron function from sustained increases in glomerular pressure. Furthermore, glomerulosclerosis (glomerular arteriolar damage) develops from prolonged elevation of glomerular capillary pressure and increased glomerular plasma flow, resulting in a continuous cycle of nephron destruction. Regardless of the cause, a predictable and continuous decrease in kidney function occurs in patients when the eGFR drops below a critical value, approximately one-half of normal.[11] Usually, the rate of decline in kidney function remains fairly constant for an individual, but can vary substantially among patients and disease states. A rapid rate of decline in kidney function has been associated with black race, proteinuria, male sex, older age, and smoking.[12–14] Rapid progression of kidney disease is defined as persistent decline in GFR >5 mL/minute/1.73 m^2/year.[1] Although early changes in kidney function can be detected through routine laboratory monitoring (e.g., serum creatinine [SCr]), most patients do not develop signs and symptoms of uremia until they have reached the more severe stages of the disease (i.e., CKD categories 4, 5, and/or ESRD).

As the leading causes of ESRD in the United States, diabetes mellitus, hypertension, and glomerular diseases have been the focus of research to identify their associated mechanisms of kidney damage. In the case of diabetes mellitus, excess filtration of glucose, excessive glucose contact with the glomerular and tubular cells leads to increased cellular osmotic pressure and thickening of the capillary basement membrane and other anatomic changes. Systemic hypertension is a potent stimulus for the development and progression of kidney disease caused by the association with increased single-nephron GFRs.[9,14] Hypertension, whether the primary cause of kidney disease or a coexisting disease in the presence of other etiologies, can promote kidney damage through transmission of elevated systemic pressure to glomeruli. The result is glomerular capillary hyperperfusion and hypertension leading to progressive kidney damage as nephron destruction continues. Glomerular ischemia induced by damage to the preglomerular arteries and arterioles also occurs. People with coexistent diabetes mellitus and hypertension increase the risk of developing ESRD by fivefold to sixfold compared with those with hypertension alone.[11] Most glomerular diseases are mediated by immune mechanisms. The deposition and formation of immune complexes in the glomerulus cause injury, resulting in increased glomerular permeability to macromolecules (e.g., proteins).[15]

Proteinuria, one of the initial diagnostic signs of kidney disease, also contributes to the progressive decline in kidney function. A faster rate of progression is associated with higher protein excretion.[16] Immunologic and hemodynamic mechanisms have been identified to explain the glomerular injury. Increases in kidney plasma flow are associated with proteinuria and high protein intake. Inflammatory cytokines may be responsible for fibrosis and kidney scarring, ultimately resulting in loss of nephron function.

Dyslipidemias are common in patients with CKD and often observed concurrently with proteinuria. Increased low-density lipoprotein (LDL) cholesterol, total cholesterol, and apolipoprotein B, as well as decreased high-density lipoprotein (HDL) cholesterol, have been observed in patients with progressive kidney disease.[15] Hypercholesterolemia has been associated with loss of kidney function in patients with and without diabetes.[17,18] Accumulation of apolipoproteins in glomerular mesangial cells contributes to cytokine production and infiltration of macrophages and has been implicated in the progression of CKD, primarily in the presence of previous kidney disease or other risk factors such as hypertension.[17] LDL is thought to promote glomerular damage by initiating a series of cellular events in mesangial cells and through oxidation to a more cytotoxic derivative once within these cells. Although serum total cholesterol, triglycerides, and apolipoprotein B all correlate with the rate of decline in eGFR, it is not clear that they directly increase the rate of progression of kidney disease, particularly when present with concomitant conditions that also cause kidney damage. Some evidence, however, suggests that treatment of hypercholesterolemia with statin therapy in patients with CKD may reduce proteinuria and progression of CKD.[19]

Drug-Induced Causes of Chronic Kidney Disease

ANALGESIC NEPHROPATHY

Analgesic nephropathy results from habitual ingestion of analgesics for many years. Particularly, agents containing at least two antipyretic analgesics and usually caffeine or codeine are commonly associated with the development of analgesic nephropathy. It is a tubulointerstitial kidney disease characterized by renal papillary necrosis as a primary lesion and chronic interstitial nephritis as a secondary lesion.[20] Analgesic nephropathy is a slowly progressive disease, and the clinical signs and symptoms are similar to the nonspecific presentation of CKD attributable to any other etiology. Phenacetin, an acetaminophen prodrug, was the first agent to be identified as causing this syndrome.

Currently in the United States, most cases are caused by long-term use or misuse of compound analgesics containing acetaminophen and aspirin along with caffeine or codeine. Similar findings in terms of the effect on kidney function have also been observed with chronic nonsteroidal antiinflammatory drug (NSAID) therapy.[21] The uses of acetaminophen, aspirin, and NSAIDs have been associated with the progression of kidney disease in CKD patients in a dose-dependent manner.[22] The cumulative amount (at least 1–2 kg of acetaminophen), rather than the duration of analgesic intake, is a primary risk factor for developing chronic analgesic nephropathy.[23,24] Thus, analgesics should be used with caution in the CKD population, and chronic analgesic therapy should be discouraged. KDIGO guidelines recommend discontinuation of NSAIDs in people with a GFR <60 mL/minute/1.73 m^2.[1]

Analgesic nephropathy is more prevalent in female patients, with a female to male ratio of 5:1 to 7:1. The peak incidence occurs between the fourth and fifth decades of life.[20,24] Patients usually have a history or complaint of chronic pain syndromes. Often, patients who develop analgesic nephropathy are dependent on analgesic therapy and may exhibit psychiatric manifestations indicative of an addictive behavior. At presentation, patients may have a reduced GFR and findings consistent with CKD, such as elevated SCr, BUN, and proteinuria. However, during acute necrosis, patients may experience flank pain, pyuria, and hematuria. As necrosis progresses, cellular debris may cause ureteral obstruction. Kidney dysfunction is characterized as a salt-wasting nephropathy, with a substantial reduction in urine-concentrating and urine-acidifying capabilities. The exact mechanism for kidney damage is uncertain, but it is thought that because acetaminophen accumulates in the renal medulla, its oxidative metabolite produced by the medullary cytochrome P-450 enzyme system may bind to macromolecules, causing cellular necrosis. Although the reduced form of glutathione in the medulla can prevent this process, agents that reduce medullary glutathione content (e.g., aspirin) may promote kidney damage. This mechanism may explain a lack of analgesic nephropathy associated with acetaminophen alone. NSAIDs, which attenuate prostaglandin-mediated vasodilatation, may induce an ischemic state within the renal medulla, leading to papillary necrosis.[21]

Data on the chronic kidney effects of selective cyclooxygenase-2 (COX-2) inhibitors are limited compared to traditional NSAIDs. A meta-analysis of 114 randomized, double blind clinical trials evaluated the adverse kidney events of COX-2 inhibitors. The authors reported that, of the six agents evaluated, only rofecoxib was associated with adverse kidney effects, defined as significant changes in urea or creatinine levels, clinically diagnosed kidney disease, or kidney failure. In contrast, celecoxib was associated with a lower risk of kidney dysfunction.[21] A cohort study of 19,163 newly diagnosed CKD patients examined the association between analgesic use and the risk of progression to ESRD. Among the COX-2 inhibitors, only rofecoxib use was significantly associated with an increased risk of progression to ESRD.[22]

The long-term management of analgesic nephropathy is generally supportive and primarily involves discontinuation of the offending agent and subsequent abstinence from the use of NSAIDs and combination analgesics. If patients develop CKD or ESRD, treatment of kidney disease-related comorbidities should be treated in the same manner as those with kidney disease owing to any other cause. For patients requiring analgesics, aspirin taken alone may be a reasonable alternative. Acetaminophen as a single agent may be safe, although habitual use can contribute to progression of kidney disease as well as to liver toxicity.[23,24] CKD patients requiring chronic analgesic therapy should use the lowest dose to control pain, avoid combination products when possible, and maintain adequate hydration.

LITHIUM NEPHROPATHY

Lithium use has been associated with alterations in kidney function secondary to acute functional and histologic changes and has been associated with the development of chronic pathologic changes to the kidneys (e.g., chronic interstitial nephritis). The role of lithium as a causative agent in the development of CKD has been suggested in a variety of epidemiologic, clinical, and histopathologic studies.[25] The concentrating ability within the kidney and GFR have been shown to decline with long-term lithium use.[26] Lithium-induced chronic renal disease has a slow progression (average latency between onset of lithium use and ESRD is 20 years) in which the rate of progression is related to the duration of lithium therapy.

Patients with lithium nephropathy are generally asymptomatic. They typically present with an insidious decline in renal function over the course of many years, and proteinuria is usually absent or minimal.[25] Women are generally at greater risk than men.[26] In patients taking chronic lithium therapy, close monitoring of serum lithium concentrations is advised, and regular measurements of SCr should be obtained to detect changes in kidney function. Higher lithium concentrations are associated with increased renal risk.[26] Current clinical practice guidelines recommend monitoring SCr every 2 to 3 months during the first 6 months of chronic lithium therapy, followed by yearly measurements thereafter.[25] If patients develop CKD or ESRD, management of kidney disease–related comorbidities should be treated in the same manner as those with kidney disease owing to any other cause. The decision to discontinue lithium and to initiate another mood stabilizer should be a mutual decision made by the psychiatrist, the nephrologist, and the patient. The diuretic amiloride has been suggested to reduce lithium-induced renal adverse effects.[25]

Clinical Assessment

QUANTIFYING GLOMERULAR FILTRATION RATE

One of the most widely used clinical measures to determine baseline kidney function and monitor progression of kidney disease with time is eGFR. The ideal marker of eGFR should be a nontoxic substance that is freely filtered at the glomerulus and not secreted, reabsorbed, or metabolized by the kidney. Inulin and exogenous radioactive markers, such as ^{125}I-iothalamate or ^{51}CrEDTA, have been used to assess GFR because they meet these criteria; however, they are not readily available to clinicians, require intravenous (IV) administration, and are costly.

Creatinine is an endogenous substance that is produced at a relatively constant rate by nonenzymatic hydrolysis of muscle stores of the amino acid derivatives creatine and phosphocreatine. Under steady-state conditions, the urinary excretion of creatinine equals the creatinine production rate, and the SCr concentration remains relatively stable. Creatinine is excreted primarily by glomerular filtration—thus, creatinine clearance (CrCl) has been used as a reasonable surrogate for eGFR. There are limitations to consider when using methods to assess eGFR that incorporate creatinine. Creatinine is eliminated not only through glomerular filtration but also by tubular secretion. Consequently, the CrCl overestimates the true GFR by 10% to 20%. As nephron function declines, tubular secretion of creatinine contributes more substantially to overall elimination such that CrCl overestimates true GFR. Extrarenal elimination of creatinine in the gastrointestinal (GI) tract may also lead to overestimation of actual GFR.[27] As a result of these processes, disease progression may be underestimated. Commonly used drugs also need to be taken into consideration when interpreting SCr values. For example, trimethoprim can inhibit the secretion of creatinine, and increase SCr and decrease CrCl without affecting GFR. On the other hand, cimetidine has been administered to block tubular secretion of creatinine before measurement of CrCl for a more accurate assessment of GFR.[16]

SCr alone is used clinically as an index of kidney function; however, multiple limitations to this practice exist. In the initial stages of kidney disease, SCr may remain within the normal range. Consequently, SCr may be relatively insensitive in detecting early kidney disease and is not accurate for estimating the progression of the disease. Because generation of creatinine is proportional to total muscle mass, it is affected by diet (notably by the ingestion of meats), age, and sex. Generally, muscle mass declines with age and is lower in women. Thus, a SCr that is in the upper limit of normal (e.g., 1.2 mg/dL) for a young male athlete is likely to be associated with a high CrCl, whereas the same SCr in a 70-year-old woman could indicate compromised kidney function.

Use of SCr to assess kidney function in patients with liver disease may also lead to overestimation of GFR.[28] This may be attributed to decreased production of creatine (the precursor of creatinine) by the liver or increased tubular secretion of creatinine by the kidney. Also, substantial variation is seen in the calibration of SCr among laboratories that can result in differences in measured SCr. The National Kidney Disease Education Program Laboratory Working Group initiated the creatinine standardization program to improve and normalize SCr results, reduce interlaboratory variability, and enable more accurate eGFR determinations.[29] Although SCr can provide a rough estimate of kidney function, other markers of early kidney damage, such as proteinuria, should also be evaluated in patients at risk for kidney disease.

Several equations have been developed to calculate CrCl or eGFR.

The Cockcroft–Gault (CG) equation (Eq. 28-1). has been the most commonly used method to estimate kidney function for drug dosing, which provides an estimate CrCl in patients with stable renal function[27,30]:

$$\mathrm{CrCl} = \frac{(140 - \mathrm{Age})(\mathrm{IBW})}{(72)} \qquad \text{(Eq. 28-1)}$$

where age is in years, IBW is ideal body weight in kg (male IBW = 50 + [2.3 × height >60 inches]; female IBW = 45 + [2.3 × height >60 inches]), and SCr is the serum creatinine concentration (mg/dL). For women, the CG equation is multiplied by 0.85 to account for decreased muscle mass.

The CG equation should not be used to estimate GFR in patients with rapidly changing SCr concentrations because it was derived from normal, healthy subjects with stable kidney function. The CG equation is also inaccurate in populations that have low muscle mass—such as elderly, obese, or cachectic patients.

The Schwartz equation[31] is used in children (Eq. 28-2):

$$\mathrm{Cr\,Cl\,(mL/minute)} = \frac{(k \times \text{length [in cm]})}{\mathrm{SCr}} \qquad \text{(Eq. 28-2)}$$

where k is dependent on age (infant [1–52 weeks] $k = 0.45$; child [1–13 years] $k = 55$; adolescent male $k = 0.7$; and adolescent female $k = 0.55$), and SCr is the serum creatinine concentration (mg/dL).

The most commonly used method for kidney function assessment is the prediction equation developed using data from the Modification of Diet in Renal Disease (MDRD) study, a multicenter trial that evaluated the effects of dietary protein restriction and BP control on progression of kidney disease. This equation, referred to as the MDRD equation, was derived using GFR measured directly by urinary clearance of a radiolabeled marker (^{125}I-iothalamate) as opposed to creatinine, and included a relatively large and diverse population (>500 white and black individuals with varying degrees of kidney disease) for derivation and validation of the equation. The MDRD equation[32] is as follows (Eq. 28-3):

$$\begin{aligned}&\text{Estimated GFR}\\&(\mathrm{mL/minute/1.73\ m^2}) = 170 \times (\mathrm{SCr})^{-0.999}\\&\quad \times (\mathrm{Age})^{-0.176} \times (\mathrm{BUN})^{-0.170} \qquad \text{(Eq. 28-3)}\\&\quad \times (\mathrm{Alb})^{+0.318} \times (0.762 \text{ if female})\\&\quad \times (1.18 \text{ if black})\end{aligned}$$

where SCr is the serum creatinine concentration (mg/dL), age is in years, BUN is the blood urea nitrogen concentration (mg/dL), and Alb is the serum albumin concentration (g/dL).

An abbreviated version was developed and is referred to as the four-variable MDRD equation (Eq. 28-4)[1]:

$$\begin{aligned}&\text{Estimated GFR}\\&(\mathrm{mL/minute/1.73\ m^2}) = 186 \times (\mathrm{SCr})^{-1.154} \qquad \text{(Eq. 28-4)}\\&\quad \times (\mathrm{Age})^{-0.203} \times (0.742 \text{ if female})\\&\quad \times (1.21 \text{ if black})\end{aligned}$$

where SCr is the serum creatinine concentration (mg/dL) and age is in years. Subsequently, this equation was reexpressed in 2005 for use with a standardized SCr assay enabling consistent results across clinical laboratories to improve accuracy in eGFR determinations (Eq. 28-5).[27]:

$$\begin{aligned}&\text{Estimated GFR}\\&(\mathrm{mL/minute/1.73\ m^2}) = 175 \times (\text{standardized SCr})^{-1.154} \qquad \text{(Eq. 28-5)}\\&\quad \times (\mathrm{Age})^{-0.203} \times (0.742 \text{ if female})\\&\quad \times (1.21 \text{ if black})\end{aligned}$$

where SCr is the serum creatinine concentration (mg/dL) and age is in years. The National Kidney Disease Education Program recommends this equation for laboratories using a creatinine method that has its calibration standardized by isotope dilution mass spectrometry.

The MDRD equation was found to be biased and imprecise at higher GFRs with the potential of misidentifying patients with high GFR as having poor kidney function.[1,33] The Chronic Kidney Disease Epidemiology Collaboration (CKD-EPI) research group established by the National Institute of Diabetes and Digestive and Kidney Diseases pooled studies of different populations to develop and validate a new estimating equation for GFR that is more complex, but uses the same variables as the MDRD equation.[1,34] The CKD-EPI equation was found to be more accurate than the MDRD equation, especially at high GFRs and across a wider range of body mass index.

An important point is that the results from the MDRD and CG equations are not interchangeable. That is, the MDRD equations are used to quantify GFR, to detect or stage the degree of CKD, and to follow progression. The CG equation is most commonly used to evaluate the appropriate doses of drugs that are eliminated by the kidney[27] (see Chapter 31, Dosing of Drugs in Renal Failure).

Cystatin C is another endogenous marker of kidney function that is freely filtered at the glomerulus. Subsequently, it is reabsorbed and catabolized by proximal tubular epithelial cells. Unlike SCr, cystatin C is not influenced by gender, age, body mass, and nutritional status. Several equations based on serum cystatin C levels either alone or in combination with SCr and other demographic variables have been developed.[1,35] The KDIGO guidelines suggest the use of a Cystatin C–based equation test for confirmatory testing of GFR when eGFR based on SCr is less accurate.[1]

PROTEINURIA

Normally, proteins are not filtered at the glomerulus because of their relatively large molecular size. Thus, only trace amounts of protein are present in the urine in patients without kidney disease. However, with glomerular damage, proteinuria is commonly observed and may precede elevations in SCr. The amount of protein present in the urine has been shown to be a predictor of kidney disease progression. As a result, protein excretion should be monitored in patients at risk for kidney disease as well as those with existing kidney disease at routine checkups.

Proteinuria is defined as a total protein excretion rate >200 mcg/minute or >300 mg/24 hour (referred to as *albuminuria;* if albumin is the only protein measured). Measurement of total protein includes quantification of albumin plus other proteins, such as low molecular weight globulins and apoproteins. Assessment of albuminuria is a better indicator of early kidney disease because it is primarily indicative of glomerular damage as opposed to total protein, which is not specific for glomerular damage. Other tests, including urinalysis (UA), radiographic procedures, and biopsy, may also be valuable in further assessing kidney function.

Determination of albuminuria can be done using timed urine samples (Table 28-4). Typically, a 24-hour collection period termed albumin excretion rate (AER) is used, although a timed sample collected overnight may be more reliable because albumin excretion can vary throughout the day and with postural changes (i.e., orthostatic proteinuria). Untimed or "spot" urine samples for measurement of albumin-to-creatinine ratios (ACR) are more convenient. As opposed to measuring protein or albumin in a timed collection, this method corrects for variations in hydration status and may be more accurate because protein excretion is normalized to glomerular filtration. The albumin and creatinine concentrations in the urine are measured from a spot urine sample, preferably from first morning urine sample, because it correlates best with 24-hour albumin excretion. If a first morning urine sample is not available, a random sample is acceptable. Factors associated with albuminuria, such as ingestion of a high-protein meal and vigorous exercise, must be considered when evaluating urinary albumin. Measuring urinary protein after exercise will result in a falsely elevated urine protein level as a consequence of an increase in the membrane permeability of the glomeruli to protein and a saturation of the tubular reabsorption process of filtered protein. To minimize this risk, it is recommended to wait approximately 4 hours after exercise to test for proteinuria.[36] Screening for albuminuria can also be done using urine dipstick testing of a spot urine sample. Reagent strips are available from several commercial vendors and differ with regard to the specified testing procedure and the sensitivity and specificity for detecting albuminuria. Patients with a positive dipstick screening test should have a subsequent quantitative assessment of the ACR to confirm proteinuria. The KDIGO Guidelines for Evaluation and Management of CKD provide criteria for albuminuria categories (Table 28-4).[1]

COMPLICATIONS OF CHRONIC KIDNEY DISEASE

Complications specific to CKD begin to develop as kidney disease progresses, most often when patients reach CKD 3 (eGFR <60 mL/minute/1.73 m^2). These complications include fluid and electrolyte abnormalities, metabolic acidosis, anemia, MND, cardiovascular complications, and poor nutritional status. Often, these complications go unrecognized or are inadequately managed during the earlier stages of CKD, leading to poor outcomes by the time a patient is in need of dialysis therapy. Hypoalbuminemia and anemia were identified in more than 50% of a population of patients new to dialysis therapy, and these findings were associated with a decreased quality of life.[37] Late referral to a nephrologist to manage CKD and its associated complications has also been associated with increased mortality in the ESRD population.[37] The KDIGO guidelines recommend referral of patients to a nephrologist in any of the following circumstances: AKI or an abrupt fall in GFR, a GFR <30 mL/minute/1.73 m^2, persistent albuminuria (ACR ≥ 300 mg/g), progression of CKD, unexplained persistence of red blood cell (RBC) casts and >20 RBCs per high-power field in UA, persistent abnormalities in potassium, extensive nephrolithiasis, hereditary kidney disease, CKD with resistant hypertension on four or more antihypertensive agents, and in all patients in whom the risk of progression to CKD 5D (CKD category 5 receiving dialysis) in the next year is estimated at 10% to 20% or greater.[1] These and similar reports underscore the need for early and aggressive therapy to manage complications of CKD. Complications of CKD will be presented in more detail throughout this chapter, and complications associated with dialysis therapy are discussed in Chapter 30, Renal Dialysis.

Prevention

Appropriate management of CKD includes measures to slow progression of the disease and regular evaluation of kidney function to assess changes in disease severity and to monitor therapy. This includes aggressive strategies to manage the disorders that cause kidney disease or are known to accelerate the disease process, such as diabetes mellitus, hypertension, high protein intake, and dyslipidemias (see Chapter 8, Dyslipidemias, Atherosclerosis, and Coronary Heart Disease; Chapter 9, Essential Hypertension; and Chapter 53, Diabetes Mellitus).

DIETARY PROTEIN RESTRICTION

Proteinuria is a significant predictor of ESRD in patients with CKD.[38,39] Increases in protein ingestion are associated with a rise in eGFR, possibly as a result of structural changes of the glomerulus and changes in renal plasma flow with an increased protein load.[40] Evidence such as this has led to the investigation of methods to reduce the degree of proteinuria. In addition to controlling the primary causes of kidney disease (e.g., diabetes, hypertension, and glomerulopathies) and using angiotensin-converting enzyme (ACE) inhibitor and angiotensin receptor blocker (ARB) therapy, dietary protein restriction has been evaluated as a strategy for reducing proteinuria and delaying progression of kidney disease.

A number of studies have investigated the effect of protein restriction on disease progression with varying results.[40–42] These conflicting conclusions may be attributable to differences in study design, patient populations, methods to assess kidney function, degrees of protein restriction, and dietary compliance. The MDRD study evaluated the effects of protein restriction and strict BP control on the progression of kidney disease. There was no difference in renal function deterioration comparing patients who received a normal protein diet (1.3 g/kg/day) with those receiving a low-protein (0.58 g/kg/day) diet.[43] In contrast, patients receiving a low-protein diet (0.58 g/kg/day) compared with those receiving a very low-protein diet (0.28 g/kg/day plus keto and amino acid supplementation) had a faster decline in renal function. A secondary analysis of the MDRD study, which accounted for dietary compliance, suggested that patients with severe kidney disease (eGFR <25 mL/minute/1.73 m^2) could benefit from protein restriction of 0.6 g/kg/day.[44] However, a follow-up analysis of the MDRD study found no significant benefit.

KDIGO Guidelines for Evaluation and Management of CKD currently recommend lowering protein intake to 0.8 g/kg/day while avoiding high protein intake (i.e., >1.3g/kg/day) in adults at risk for progression.[1] Avoiding excessive accumulation of uremic toxins, loss of lean body mass, and malnutrition are benefits of appropriate dietary protein restrictions. The potential benefits of protein restriction in patients with CKD must be weighed against the potential adverse effect on overall nutritional status. Malnutrition is prevalent in patients with CKD starting dialysis and is a predictor of mortality in this population.[45]

ANTIHYPERTENSIVE THERAPY

Antihypertensive therapy prevents kidney damage and slows the rate of progression of CKD in both diabetic and nondiabetic patients.[46] In addition, the added benefit of reduced cardiovascular mortality further supports the use of antihypertensive therapy in patients at risk for progressive CKD. Despite what is known about the beneficial effects of BP control in patients with CKD, rates of hypertension control in the predialysis population remain suboptimal.[46]

The 2014 Evidence-Based Guideline for the Management of High Blood Pressure in Adults (commonly referred to as JNC-8) and the KDIGO/Management of Blood Pressure in Chronic Kidney Disease Guideline recommends is a BP less than 140/90 mm Hg in CKD.[46,47] Controversy exists as to the optimal BP target in CKD patients with albuminuria (>30 mg in 24 hours or equivalent). The KDIGO guidelines recommend a BP target of ≤130/80 mm Hg in CKD patients with albuminuria (>30 mg in 24 hours or equivalent) while JNC-8 suggest a target of 140/90 mm Hg for patients with albuminuria. Evidence for further reduction of BP in patients with albuminuria stems mostly from ancillary analysis of larger trials. Results from the MDRD study showed that further lowering of BP to less than 125/75 mm Hg (or a mean arterial pressure <92 mm Hg) was more beneficial than usual BP control in patients with higher rates of urinary protein excretion (>1 g protein/day).[48] The effects of more aggressive BP control on progression of kidney disease were also studied in the African American Study of Kidney Disease and Hypertension (AASK) trial.[49] African Americans aged 18 to 70 years with hypertensive kidney disease (eGFR 20–65 mL/minute/1.73 m^2) were included in this study. A post hoc analysis of the AASK trial found that patients with proteinuria greater than 1 g/day assigned to the low BP target had slower progression to ESRD.[50] Clearly, BP control is important to delay progression of kidney disease, and with the expanding data supporting more aggressive BP lowering in patients with more severe proteinuria, the importance of BP control in this patient population is pivotal in slowing progression of CKD. In light of the concerns with the presence of albuminuria, a target of <140/90 mm Hg is reasonable in the CKD patient with albuminuria.

Among the available classes of antihypertensive agents, ACE inhibitors (ACEIs; e.g., enalapril, captopril, lisinopril) and ARBs (e.g., losartan, irbesartan, candesartan) may afford additional benefits in preserving kidney function. As a result, ACEIs and ARBs are most commonly recommended as first-line treatment options for hypertension in those with CKD, those at risk for CKD (e.g., diabetics), and those with albuminuria by the KDIGO hypertension guidelines.[46] In conditions of decreased eGFR, angiotensin II primarily causes compensatory vasoconstriction of the efferent arteriole, thereby increasing glomerular capillary pressure (P_{GC}) and eGFR (Fig. 28-1). This effect is beneficial in conditions of acute renal failure; however, sustained increases in P_{GC} cause hypertrophy of individual nephrons and progressive kidney disease. ACEI and ARB therapy prevent the chronic increase in glomerular pressure mediated by angiotensin II. Benefits of ACEIs have been demonstrated in patients with diabetes with some degree of proteinuria, suggesting that ACEI use be considered in this population regardless of BP.[46] In patients without diabetes, ACEIs have been shown to reduce BP, decrease proteinuria, and slow the progression of kidney disease when compared with other agents. An initial and mild decrease in eGFR is expected with ACEI therapy; therefore, an increase in SCr of 30% within the first 2 months of therapy is acceptable.[51] Hypotension, acute kidney failure, and severe hyperkalemia are reasons to consider discontinuing therapy (also see Chapter 14, Heart Failure).

Angiotensin II receptor blockers offer similar benefits to ACEIs on the basis of their ability to decrease efferent arteriolar resistance by blockade of the angiotensin type 1 (AT_1) receptor. In patients with type 2 diabetes mellitus, losartan decreased the incidence of a doubling of SCr by 25% and of ESRD by 28% when compared with placebo after a mean of 3.4 years of therapy.[52] Similar effects were observed in the Irbesartan Diabetic Nephropathy Trial (IDNT), with a 23% decreased risk of ESRD observed in patients treated with irbesartan.[53] In both studies, these beneficial effects were independent of reduction in BP. Reduction in the degree of proteinuria has also been demonstrated with candesartan and valsartan.[54] Combination therapy with an ARB and ACEI increases the progression to ESRD, hyperkalemia events, and acute kidney injury risk and should be avoided.[55,56]

Aliskiren is the only available direct renin inhibitor. Its use as monotherapy is unclear and combination with ACEI or ARBs should be avoided.[57] Aliskiren has been associated with reduction in GFR and filtration fraction in patients receiving optimal heart failure therapy.[58]

Calcium-channel blockers have been considered for preventing progression of kidney disease owing to their effects on renal hemodynamics and cytoprotective and antiproliferative properties (prevention of mesangial expansion and renal scarring). Nondihydropyridine agents (e.g., diltiazem and verapamil) have been beneficial in reducing proteinuria when compared with dihydropyridines (e.g., amlodipine), which have been found to worsen proteinuria.[59,60] Dihydropyridine calcium-channel blockers have the effect of increasing albuminuria and should not be used alone in patients with proteinuria, but can be used safely in combination with an ACEI or ARB. Combination therapy with an ACEI and nondihydropyridine agents has resulted in greater reductions in proteinuria in patients with diabetes than with either agent alone, suggesting that it may be rational to use multiple agents in this population.[59]

β-Blockers may offer benefits in the treatment of diabetic nephropathy as demonstrated by the United Kingdom Prospective Diabetes Study, which showed similar effects of atenolol and captopril on decreasing the incidence of albuminuria in patients with diabetes.[61] β-Blockers offer several benefits to CKD patients such as attenuation of excessive sympathetic output and reduction in sudden cardiac death seen in dialysis patients.[62,63] β-Blocker selection should take into account the dialyzability of the drug and/or the risk for drug accumulation.[64]

TREATMENT OF DYSLIPIDEMIA

Low HDL levels, impaired HDL function, higher percentages of oxidized LDL (highly atherogenic LDL molecules), and elevated lipoprotein(a) (highly atherogenic lipoproteins) levels are characteristic alterations of dyslipidemia in CKD that vary from the general population.[65] Similar to the general population, very high cholesterol and elevated non-HDL lipoprotein cholesterol have been associated with increased hospitalizations and CVD mortality in CKD. A meta-analysis of trials have demonstrated an association of statin use with decreased proteinuria and uncertainty with preservation of eGFR.[66] Despite uncertainty of therapy with regard to delaying CKD progression, dyslipidemia should be treated in the kidney disease population. Abnormal lipid metabolism is present in these patients, which predisposes them to the development of atherosclerotic disease. Although the potential for elevated cholesterol profiles in CKD suggests a beneficial role for lipid-lowering therapies in CKD, a varying cardiovascular pathology (e.g., vascular calcification, sympathetic

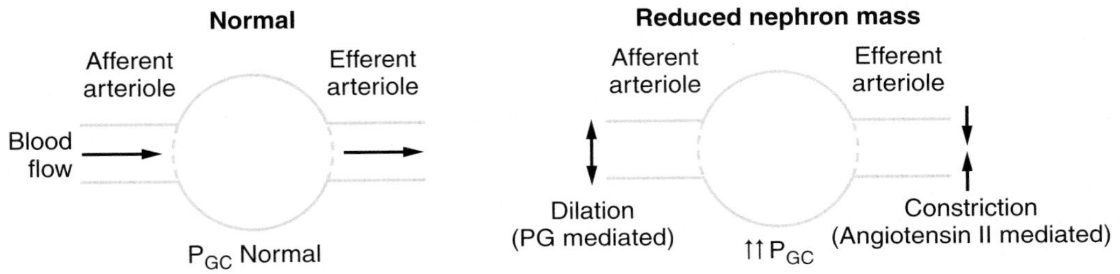

Figure 28-1 Renal hemodynamics are dependent on afferent and efferent arteriolar tone and glomerular capillary pressure (P_{GC}). With reduced nephron mass, afferent arteriolar vasodilation (mediated primarily by prostaglandins [PG] I_2 and E_2) and efferent arteriolar constriction (mediated primarily by angiotensin II) occur within remaining functioning nephrons to compensate. This leads to an increase in blood flow, intraglomerular capillary filtration pressure (P_{GC}), and hyperfiltration (increased single-nephron effective GFR). Sustained increases in plasma flow and hydrostatic pressure lead to hyperfiltration injury and glomerular sclerosis. With time, these changes contribute to continued loss of nephron function (i.e., progression of kidney disease). Angiotensin-converting enzyme inhibitors and angiotensin receptor blockers prevent vasoconstriction of the efferent arteriole and reduce the P_{GC}.

overactivity) in CKD limits the role of lipid-lowering therapies (i.e., statins) across stages of CKD.

The KDIGO Clinical Practice Guidelines for Lipid Management in CKD released guidance for the management of dyslipidemia. Similar to the general population, statin therapy is recommended irrespective of baseline LDL cholesterol levels in non-dialysis–dependent CKD patients.[67] For CKD patients ≥50 years and not on dialysis, KDIGO recommends treatment with a statin or statin/ezetimibe combination. CKD patients aged 18 to 49 years with additional CVD risk factors such as known coronary disease (MI or coronary revascularization), diabetes, prior ischemic stroke, or estimated 10-year coronary heart disease risk >10% are recommended to initiate statin therapy. A strategy of "fire-and-forget" is suggested for statin therapy where measurement of LDL cholesterol is avoided unless results would alter management. However, recent commentary of the KDIGO guidelines suggest measuring lipids 6 weeks to 3 months after initiation of a statin in order to identify patients with an inadequate response to moderate-intensity statins and who require dose titration as a reasonable approach to lipid monitoring.[68]

The Study of Heart and Renal Protection (SHARP) assessed the effect of lowering LDL cholesterol in 9,270 CKD patients with ezetimibe 10 mg daily and simvastatin 20 mg daily or matching dummy placebo tablets for an average of 5 years. Mean eGFR was 27 mL/minute/1.73 m^2; 3,023 (33%) were on dialysis and 2,094 (23%) had diabetes. Key outcomes were reductions in major atherosclerotic events and kidney disease progression. SHARP results showed a 25% risk reduction in major atherosclerotic events. However, there was no effect on the progression of kidney disease.[69] The significance found with the combined primary outcome was most likely driven by significant reductions in non-hemorrhagic stroke and coronary revascularization. Although the study was not powered to detect differences within subgroups, subgroup analysis did not find a statistically significant benefit in patients receiving dialysis.

The cardiovascular benefits of statin use observed in the general population have not consistently been demonstrated in the dialysis populations, possibly owing to the multifactorial pathogenic process of CVD in those with kidney disease (e.g., the presence of vascular calcification).[65] KDIGO lipid guidelines recommend against treatment with a statin in CKD 5D patients unless initiated prior to the start of dialysis.

The Die Deutsche Diabetes Dialyse Studie (4D) and AURORA are two large multicenter, double blind, placebo-controlled, randomized controlled trials that examined the effects of lowering the level of LDL-C on cardiovascular events and mortality with atorvastatin or rosuvastatin, respectively. Both studies with a combined patient population of greater than 4,000 demonstrated significant reductions in LDL cholesterol levels; however, neither produced statistically significant reductions in the primary outcome measure. The results of these studies along with the negative effects in dialysis patients from the SHARP study have largely driven KDIGO recommendations to avoid initiating statin therapy in dialysis patients.[67]

KDIGO recommend that statins be prescribed in preference to fibrates. Fibrates should be used cautiously in patients with CKD; all agents in this class are metabolized by the kidney and are eliminated primarily via the kidney, which may lead to an increased risk of rhabdomyolysis. However, fibric acid derivatives may be considered in patients presenting with very high triglycerides (>1,000 mg/dL). Gemfibrozil is cautioned in mild to moderate kidney dysfunction and not recommended in severe kidney impairment.[70]

END-STAGE RENAL DISEASE (CHRONIC KIDNEY DISEASE 5D)

Clinical Signs and Symptoms

During CKD 4 and 5, patients may develop the more severe signs and symptoms associated with advanced kidney disease, often referred to as *uremic syndrome.* The manifestations and metabolic consequences of advanced kidney disease are listed in Table 28-7. These manifestations certainly may develop in the earlier stages of CKD, underscoring the importance of early intervention, but they become more prominent as the disease worsens. The pathogenesis of these disorders has been attributed, in part, to the accumulation of uremic toxins. The search for uremic toxins has led to the identification of nitrogenous compounds that are consistently observed in the serum of patients with kidney disease. A cause and effect relationship between these compounds and the clinical manifestations of uremia has not been clearly established.[71]

Table 28-7
Metabolic Effects of Progressive Kidney Disease

Cardiovascular
Hypertension
Congestive heart failure
Pericarditis
Atherosclerosis
Arrhythmias
Metastatic calcifications
Dermatologic
Altered pigmentation
Pruritus
Endocrine
Calcium–phosphorous imbalances
Hyperparathyroidism
Metabolic bone disease
Altered thyroid function
Altered carbohydrate metabolism
Hypophyseal-gonadal dysfunction
Decreased insulin metabolism
Erythropoietin deficiency
Fluid, Electrolyte, and Acid–Base Effects
Fluid retention
Hyperkalemia
Hypermagnesemia
Hyperphosphatemia
Hypocalcemia
Metabolic acidosis
Gastrointestinal
Anorexia
Nausea, vomiting
Delayed gastric emptying
GI bleeding
Ulcers
Hematologic
Anemia
Bleeding complications
Immune suppression

Table 28-7

Metabolic Effects of Progressive Kidney Disease (*continued*)

Musculoskeletal
Renal bone disease
Amyloidosis
Neurologic
Lethargy
Depressed sensorium
Tremor
Asterixis
Muscular irritability and cramps (i.e., restless legs syndrome)
Seizures
Motor weakness
Peripheral neuropathy
Coma
Psychological
Depression
Anxiety
Psychosis
Miscellaneous
Reduced exercise tolerance

GI, gastrointestinal.

Treatment

DIALYSIS AND TRANSPLANTATION

As ESRD becomes inevitable, the appropriate dialysis modality must be selected on the basis of patient preference and options for vascular access for HD or peritoneal access for PD. Early planning for dialysis therapy and timely initiation may lower patient morbidity and mortality. (Indications for dialysis and considerations in selection of modality are discussed in Chapter 30, Renal Dialysis.) Kidney transplantation is an option for all patients with ESRD without specified contraindications if a suitable organ match is available (see Chapter 34, Kidney and Liver Transplantation).

PHARMACOTHERAPY

Pharmacotherapy in patients with ESRD requires interventions to manage comorbid conditions and secondary complications of CKD. The extent of medication use, including medications administered during dialysis therapy, contributes to the potential for drug interactions, adverse reactions, and nonadherence to therapy.[72] The effect of decreased kidney function on absorption, distribution, metabolism, and elimination of pharmacologic agents, in addition to the contribution of dialysis to drug removal, further complicates pharmacotherapy in this population (see Chapter 31, Dosing of Drugs in Renal Failure). Appropriate pharmacotherapeutic management includes choice of rational agents based on the indication, a regular comprehensive review of all medications, and frequent reevaluation to adjust regimens relative to kidney function.

DIABETIC NEPHROPATHY

CASE 28-1

QUESTION 1: G.B. is a 44-year-old, African American woman (weight, 175 lb; height, 5 ft. 5 inches) with a 20-year history of type 2 diabetes mellitus. She presents to the diabetes clinic for her quarterly checkup. She has been noncompliant with regular appointments, and her blood glucose has generally remained greater than 200 mg/dL on prior evaluations, with a hemoglobin A_{1c} of 10.1% (goal, <7%) 2 months ago. Lately G.B. complains of general nausea, malaise, and poor appetite. She has been treated for peptic ulcer disease for the past 6 months. The workup reveals the following pertinent laboratory values:

Serum sodium (Na), 143 mEq/L
Potassium (K), 5.3 mEq/L
Chloride (Cl), 106 mEq/L
CO_2 content, 18 mEq/L
SCr, 2.9 mg/dL
BUN, 63 mg/dL
Random blood glucose, 289 mg/dL

Physical examination reveals a BP of 160/102 mm Hg, 2+ pedal edema, and mild pulmonary congestion, and a 10-lb weight gain. Additional laboratory studies show the following results:

Serum phosphate, 6.6 mg/dL
Calcium (Ca), 8.8 mg/dL
Albumin (Alb), 3.6 g/dL
Magnesium (Mg), 2.8 mEq/L
Uric acid, 8.8 mg/dL

Hematologic studies show the following results:

Hematocrit (Hct), 28%
Hemoglobin (Hgb), 9.3 g/dL
White blood cell (WBC) count, 9,600/μL
Platelet count, 155,000/μL

RBC indices are normal. G.B.'s reticulocyte count is 0.5%. Her UA showed 4+ proteinuria, later quantified as a urinary albumin of 700 mg/24 hours. What subjective and objective data in G.B. are consistent with a diagnosis of advanced kidney disease?

G.B.'s abnormal values for SCr, BUN, serum potassium, magnesium, phosphate, uric acid, CO_2 content, hemoglobin, are all consistent with kidney disease and its associated complications. Assuming relatively stable kidney function (i.e., no acute changes in kidney function), her eGFR is approximately 21 mL/minute/1.73 m^2 based on the MDRD equation, placing her in CKD category 4 (eGFR 15–29 mL/minute/1.73 m^2). As the eGFR declines to the degree observed in G.B., normal regulation of fluids and electrolytes is impaired. Elevations in SCr, BUN, sodium, potassium, magnesium, phosphate, and uric acid as well as signs of fluid accumulation are observed. G.B.'s serum potassium is slightly elevated and the risk of hyperkalemia increases with CKD.[73] The substantial degree of proteinuria observed in G.B. is consistent with advanced glomerular damage. Volume overload from continued intake and decreased sodium and water excretion leads to weight gain, hypertension, and edema. Metabolic acidosis results from impaired synthesis of ammonia by the kidney, which normally buffers hydrogen ions and facilitates acid excretion. Anemia associated with CKD is caused primarily by decreased EPO production by the kidneys, but it also can be caused by shortened half-life of RBCs from uremia, and iron deficiency. G.B.'s recent onset of nausea and malaise may be a consequence of the accumulation of uremic toxins (azotemia) from the decline in kidney function.

CASE 28-1, QUESTION 2: What is the cause of G.B.'s advanced kidney disease?

Given G.B.'s presentation, her kidney disease is most likely caused by diabetic nephropathy from her 20-year history of type 2 diabetes mellitus. Poor compliance with regular appointments, elevated glucose concentration and hemoglobin A_{1c} values, and albuminuria serve as the primary cause. Diabetic nephropathy rarely develops within the first 10 years after the onset of type 1 diabetes; however, 5% to 20% of patients with type 2 diabetes have some degree of albuminuria at diagnosis. The annual incidence is greatest after approximately 20 years' duration of diabetes and declines thereafter. G.B. fits this pattern in that she has diabetic nephropathy after a 20-year history of diabetes, although her nephropathy was likely evident several years previously. African Americans, Native Americans, and Hispanics have an increased risk of developing ESRD from diabetes relative to whites.[5]

Diabetic nephropathy is a microvascular complication of diabetes resulting in albuminuria, hemodynamic changes in kidney microcirculation, glomerular structural changes, and a progressive decline in kidney function. Diabetic nephropathy develops in approximately one-third of all patients with type 1 and type 2 diabetes.[72] Because type 2 diabetes is more prevalent, these patients account for most diabetic patients starting dialysis. With the increased prevalence of diabetes and the increase in life expectancy of this population, it is likely that diabetic nephropathy will remain the leading cause of ESRD in the United States. Whereas most research has focused on the pathophysiology, prevention, and treatment of diabetic nephropathy in type 1 diabetes, it is reasonable to extrapolate available evidence on prevention of diabetic nephropathy to the population with type 2 diabetes.[74]

The exact mechanisms leading to the development of diabetic nephropathy are not clearly defined; however, several predictive factors for the development and progression of kidney damage have been identified. These include elevated BP, plasma glucose, glycosylated hemoglobin, and cholesterol; smoking; advanced age; male sex; and, potentially, high protein intake.[75] Insulin deficiency and increased ketone bodies have also been proposed as contributors to the pathogenesis. Advanced glycosylation end products (AGE) that form in conditions of hyperglycemia have also been implicated as a cause of end-organ damage. The accumulation of multiple AGE is associated with the severity of kidney disease in patients with diabetic nephropathy.[76] A genetic predisposition exists in that higher rates of diabetes and nephropathy, hypertension, cardiovascular events, albuminuria, and elevated BP have been observed in relatives of patients with type 2 diabetes.[77] Certain genes and polymorphisms have also been associated with the development of diabetic nephropathy, and further exploration into this area may prove beneficial in identifying high-risk patients.[78,79]

CASE 28-1, QUESTION 3: What is the significance of G.B.'s albuminuria?

Albuminuria, the earliest sign of kidney involvement in patients with diabetes mellitus, correlates with the rate of progression of kidney disease. Albuminuria not only indicates renal damage but is also a powerful predictor of cardiovascular morbidity and mortality.[1] For most patients, eGFR begins to decline once proteinuria is established. Because of this association, annual testing for the presence of microalbuminuria is indicated in patients who have had type 1 diabetes for more than 5 years and in all patients with type 2 diabetes starting at diagnosis.[75] The presence of albuminuria indicates irreversible kidney damage. G.B. has likely reached the point at which such damage is inevitable because her urinary protein exceeds ranges normally observed at the earlier stages of kidney disease. G.B.'s current laboratory data suggest that she has substantial kidney disease and has developed associated complications of the disease. Although progression to ESRD is generally beyond prevention at this stage, appropriate intervention can slow the progression to ESRD for G.B. Progressive diabetic nephropathy consists of proteinuria of varying severity occasionally leading to nephrotic syndrome with hypoalbuminemia, edema, and an increase in circulating LDL cholesterol as well as progressive azotemia.

CASE 28-1, QUESTION 4: How should G.B.'s kidney disease be managed?

Management

Because reversal of G.B.'s kidney disease is not possible, the primary goals are to delay the need for dialysis therapy as long as possible and to manage complications. The three main risk factors for the progression of incipient nephropathy to clinical diabetic nephropathy are poor glycemic control, systemic hypertension, and high dietary protein intake (>1.3 g/kg/day). G.B.'s current random blood glucose concentration of 289 mg/dL, history of elevated glucose on prior visits, and elevated hemoglobin A_{1c} indicate poorly controlled diabetes, which will accelerate the progression of diabetic nephropathy and time to ESRD. Thus, her blood glucose concentrations should be maintained within target goals while avoiding hypoglycemia. G.B.'s elevated BP is likely the result of kidney disease and changes in intravascular volume; reduction in BP may prevent further damage to functioning nephrons and slow the progression to ESRD. Similarly, reductions in dietary protein intake (dietary protein intake of approximately 0.8 g/kg body weight/day) should be initiated in an attempt to reduce the rate of further progression, although this needs to be evaluated in the context of her overall nutritional status.

INTENSIVE GLUCOSE CONTROL

Strict glycemic control can improve diabetic management, reduce proteinuria, and slow the rate of decline in eGFR. The Diabetes Control and Complications Trial (DCCT), a randomized clinical trial of type 1 diabetic patients ($n = 1{,}441$), demonstrated that maintaining fasting blood glucose concentrations between 70 and 120 mg/dL, with postprandial blood glucose concentrations less than 180 mg/dL, delayed the onset and progression of microvascular diseases such as diabetic nephropathy and reduced the risk of CKD. Patients were randomly assigned to receive either conventional insulin treatment (one to two insulin doses a day) or intensive treatment (three or more insulin doses a day). After a mean follow-up of 6.5 years, the intensive insulin regimen reduced the overall risk of moderately increased albuminuria by 39% and severely increased albuminuria by 54%. Unfortunately, stricter glycemic control was associated with an increased incidence of hypoglycemic episodes.[80]

The UK Prospective Diabetes Study (UKPDS) demonstrated the beneficial effects of intensive glycemic control in patients with type 2 diabetes ($n = 3{,}867$). During a 10-year treatment period, intensive glucose control (fasting glucose <108 mg/dL) with either insulin or an oral sulfonylurea reduced microvascular complications (e.g., retinopathy and nephropathy), including albuminuria by 33%, when compared with conventional dietary therapy (fasting glucose <270 mg/dL). Similar to the DCCT, intensive treatment groups in the UKPDS experienced more hypoglycemic reactions.[81]

Additionally diabetes trials such as Action to Control Cardiovascular Risk in Diabetes (ACCORD) and Action in Diabetes and Vascular Disease: Preterax and Diamicron MR Controlled Evaluation (ADVANCE) evaluated the macrovascular and microvascular outcomes associated with intensive glucose control in type 2 diabetics. The ACCORD trial showed a 21% reduction in the development of moderately increased albuminuria cases and a 32% reduction in severely increased albuminuria cases.[82] In the ADVANCE trial, there was a 9% reduction in moderately increased albuminuria and 30% reduction in progression to severely increased albuminuria.[83] Similar to other studies, severe hypoglycemia, although uncommon, was more common in the intensive-control group.[83]

KDIGO Guidelines for Evaluation and Management of CKD recommend a hemoglobin A_{1c} of approximately 7% to prevent or delay progression of the microvascular complications of diabetes including diabetic kidney disease. Targeting an A_{1c} less than 7% increases patients' risk of experiencing hypoglycemia and without improvements in cardiovascular outcomes and should be avoided. In CKD patients with diabetes and comorbidities or a limited life expectancy and risk of hypoglycemia, a target A1c above 7.0% is suggested.[1]

G.B. will benefit from a multifactorial approach addressing glycemic control and hypertension to slow her progression of CKD from DM. Appropriately dosed oral and/or insulin therapy can achieve these goals despite her advanced kidney disease. G.B. should be counseled on appropriate techniques for home glucose monitoring, particularly given her history of noncompliance. Compliance with this regimen will require motivation as well as encouragement from G.B.'s family and health care providers. (See Chapter 53, Diabetes Mellitus, for a more complete discussion of intensive insulin therapy and counseling.)

ANTIHYPERTENSIVE THERAPY

Systemic hypertension usually occurs with the development of normal to moderately increased albuminuria in patients with type 1 diabetes. It is also present in about one-third of patients at the time of diagnosis of type 2 diabetes, and hastens the progression of kidney disease in both groups. The coexistence of these disorders further increases the risk of cardiovascular events. Hypertension may be a result of underlying diabetic nephropathy and increased plasma volume or increased peripheral vascular resistance. Regardless of the etiology, virtually any level of untreated hypertension (either systemic or intraglomerular) is associated with a reduction in eGFR. As such, the control of systemic and intraglomerular BP is perhaps the single most important factor for retarding the progression of kidney disease and has been shown to increase life expectancy in patients with type 1 diabetes.[84]

Patients with diabetes and hypertension exhibit elevated systemic vascular resistance and increased vasoconstriction from angiotensin II, which are in large part responsible for the glomerular damage characteristic of diabetic nephropathy. Although the management of hypertension with virtually any agent can attenuate the progression of kidney disease, ACEIs, which inhibit the synthesis of angiotensin II, and ARB, which block angiotensin II AT_1 receptors, are preferred owing, in part, to the effects of these agents on renal hemodynamics (Fig. 28-1). KDIGO guidelines recommend ACEI or ARB for the treatment of hypertension in all CKD patients with AER >300 mg/24 hour and diabetic CKD adults with AER ≥30 mg/24 hour.[46] JNC-8 recommends ACEI or ARB for all CKD patients regardless of race and with an ACR >30 mg/g to improve kidney outcomes.[47] Reductions in proteinuria and a decreased rate of decline in eGFR have been observed with ACEIs and ARB in patients with type 1 and type 2 diabetes.[46] As a result of these and other studies, ACEIs or ARB should be considered for all patients with diabetes and AER >30 mg/24 hour, even if their BP is normal.[1,47] ACEI and ARBs have similar efficacy in BP reduction when dosed accordingly. Combination therapy is associated with an increased risk of dialysis and doubling of SCr and should be avoided.[56]

Additionally, spironolactone in combination with an ACEI or ARB lowers albuminuria independent of BP control in patients with type 2 diabetes.[85] However, the risk of hyperkalemia increases significantly limiting the benefit of this therapy. Aliskiren, an oral direct renin inhibitor, has demonstrated a reduction in albuminuria when added to losartan. However, additional studies have resulted in early termination because of increased risk of adverse events and lack of demonstrable benefits.[57] The role of aliskiren is uncertain and benefits do not appear to compare with ACEI and ARBs. The primary goal in G.B. is to delay development of ESRD and to reduce the risk of cardiovascular complications and death. Treatment with an ACEI (e.g., ramipril) should be initiated, because she has substantial albuminuria (700 mg/day) and an elevated BP. An ARB (e.g., losartan) is a reasonable alternative to an ACEI in patients with ACEI–induced cough or other adverse effects that do not cross-react with an ARB. The initial product selected is generally based on tolerance to therapy and cost. A goal BP for G.B., given the fact that she has diabetes and kidney disease, is a BP less than 130/80 mm Hg,[1] 140/90 mg may be reasonable goal as well.[46] Because the beneficial effects of ACEI therapy occur over the course of months to years, G.B. must be monitored on a long-term basis for changes in kidney function and albuminuria and for side effects of therapy, such as hyperkalemia. A moderate increase in SCr is acceptable with initiation of therapy with ACEIs or ARBs. Contraindications for the use of ACEIs and ARBs include bilateral kidney artery stenosis and pregnancy. The risk of hyperkalemia must also be weighed against the potential beneficial effects of these agents.

Some evidence suggests that a nondihydropyridine calcium-channel blocker (e.g., diltiazem, verapamil) may be beneficial alone or in combination with an ACEI.[51] Diuretics may be considered for patients with diabetic nephropathy and edema, depending on their degree of kidney function. For patients with kidney disease as extensive as that observed in G.B. (eGFR <30 mL/minute/1.73 m^2), loop diuretics are generally preferred because, unlike thiazide diuretics, they may retain their effect at this reduced eGFR level (see Chapter 27, Fluid and Electrolyte Disorders, and Chapter 9, Essential Hypertension). Other antihypertensive agents may be considered based on response to initial therapy and changes in kidney function. Currently, clinical studies are examining the use of an aldosterone blocker (spironolactone) and a selective aldosterone blocker (eplerenone) for use in patients with diabetic nephropathy and overt proteinuria on maximal doses of both an ACEI and an ARB. The antiproteinuric effect of these agents has been confirmed by several studies, but the potential increased risk for hyperkalemia when adding these agents to patients already taking an ACEI and ARB warrants further evaluation of their use. The effect on slowing progression of kidney disease has not been evaluated with these agents.[85] Additionally, G.B. should be counseled regarding an exercise program compatible with her cardiovascular health and tolerance.

DIETARY PROTEIN RESTRICTION

High protein consumption accelerates the progression of diabetic nephropathy, presumably because of increased glomerular hyperfiltration and intraglomerular pressure. In patients with overt albuminuria, some evidence indicates that the rate of decline in eGFR, as well as urinary albumin excretion, can be blunted by restricting protein intake to 0.8 g/kg/day and maintaining an isocaloric diet.[44] Limited evidence indicates, however, a beneficial role of dietary protein restriction in diabetic patients with microalbuminuria. Nonetheless, given the potential benefits to delay progression of kidney disease, G.B. should be advised to maintain an isocaloric diet with a protein intake of 0.8 g/kg/day (approximately 10% of daily calories).[1] Because the typical Western diet is high in protein, some patients may have difficulty complying with such a low-protein diet because of its perceived unpalatability. Intervention by a dietitian is recommended to design a feasible dietary regimen limited in protein, yet consistent with nutritional requirements in a diabetic patient.

FLUID AND ELECTROLYTE COMPLICATIONS

Sodium and Water Retention

CASE 28-1, QUESTION 5: Assess G.B.'s sodium and water balance. What interventions may be used to address this problem?

As illustrated in G.B., patients in the latter stages of CKD commonly retain sodium and water. This is supported by G.B.'s elevated BP, 2+ pedal edema, and mild pulmonary congestion. Sodium and water retention also lead to weight gain. Early in the course of CKD, glomerular and tubular adaptive processes develop as an increase in the fractional excretion of sodium (FE_{Na}). These mechanisms enable patients to maintain relatively normal sodium and water homeostasis. As G.B.'s normal serum sodium concentration indicates, this value is of little use in establishing the diagnosis of total body sodium and fluid excess because retention of sodium and water usually occurs in an isotonic fashion, leaving the serum sodium concentration relatively normal. Eventually, patients with advanced kidney dysfunction exhibit signs of sodium and fluid retention because sodium balance is maintained at the expense of increased extracellular volume, which results in hypertension. Expansion of blood volume, if not controlled, can cause peripheral edema, heart failure, and pulmonary edema. Thus, management of sodium and water retention is essential. To achieve control, most patients with advanced kidney disease are placed on sodium restriction (2 g/day) and fluid restriction (approximately 1–2 L/day). These restrictions will depend on the current dietary intake, extent of volume overload, and urine output, and should be altered according to the special needs of the patient.

Because some patients with advanced kidney disease produce normal amounts of urine, whereas others may produce less (or no urine for HD patients), fluid restrictions must be based on urine output. Diuretic therapy, usually with loop diuretics (e.g., furosemide, bumetanide, torsemide), is often required. Combination therapy with two different types of diuretics (i.e., loop and thiazide) may be successful in patients resistant to a single agent; however, limitations in efficacy of diuretics exist under certain conditions (e.g., a reduced eGFR and hypoalbuminemia), and these situations must be considered when designing a diuretic regimen. Thiazide diuretics as single agents are generally not effective when the eGFR is less than 30 mL/minute/1.73 m^2, as in G.B. The possible exception is use of the thiazide-like diuretic, metolazone, which may retain its effect at reduced eGFRs.[46] As kidney failure progresses, manifestations of excess fluid accumulation (i.e., edema, uncontrollable hypertension) develop that are resistant to more conventional interventions and dialysis will be required to control volume status.

Hyperkalemia

CASE 28-1, QUESTION 6: G.B. has a serum potassium concentration of 5.3 mEq/L. Describe the mechanisms by which potassium imbalance occurs in patients such as G.B. who have progressive CKD.

Hyperkalemia can result from a combination of factors, including diminished kidney potassium excretion, redistribution of potassium into the extracellular fluid owing to metabolic acidosis, and excessive potassium intake. In G.B., all these mechanisms are likely to be contributing to hyperkalemia.

Potassium normally is filtered at the glomerulus and undergoes nearly complete reabsorption throughout the kidney tubule. Distal tubular secretion is the primary mechanism by which potassium is excreted in the urine. A variety of factors affect this distal secretion of potassium, including aldosterone, sodium load presented to the distal reabsorptive site, hydrogen ion secretion, the amount of nonresorbable anions, urinary flow rate, diuretics, mineralocorticoids, and potassium intake.[86] Serum potassium concentrations are relatively well maintained within normal limits in patients with CKD. At eGFR greater than 10 mL/minute/1.73 m^2, hyperkalemia is rare without an endogenous or exogenous load of potassium. This balance is maintained despite a decreasing nephron population and an overall drop in eGFR because the remaining nephrons undergo adaptive changes to enhance the distal tubular secretion of potassium per nephron (i.e., increased fractional excretion of potassium, FE_K).[87] GI excretion of potassium is also important because increased GI excretion and fecal losses may account for up to 35% of the daily potassium loss in patients with severe kidney disease. G.B.'s eGFR of 21 mL/minute/1.73 m^2 is above the threshold value for adequate potassium homeostasis. G.B. should be carefully observed for manifestations of hyperkalemia as her kidney disease progresses.

Additional factors that alter potassium homeostasis include metabolic or respiratory acidosis. Acidemia can cause a redistribution of intracellular potassium to the extracellular fluid. G.B. has metabolic acidosis as indicated by serum bicarbonate of 18 mEq/L. This condition may account for her mildly elevated potassium concentration. Correction of metabolic acidosis could lower her potassium concentration. For each 0.1-unit change in blood pH, an inverse approximately 0.6-mEq/L change in the serum potassium concentration occurs (see Chapter 26, Acid–Base Disorders).

G.B. is not taking any drugs that could contribute to hyperkalemia, although the influence of ACEIs and ARB must be considered because they are now advocated for G.B. to delay progression of kidney disease. Potassium-sparing diuretics triamterene and amiloride should be avoided and spironolactone used with caution in patients with severe CKD because they decrease tubular secretion of potassium.

CASE 28-1, QUESTION 7: Is treatment of G.B.'s potassium indicated? How should severe hyperkalemia be managed?

Treatment of hyperkalemia depends on the serum concentration of potassium as well as the presence or absence of symptoms and electrocardiographic (ECG) changes. Manifestations of hyperkalemia include weakness, confusion, and muscular or respiratory paralysis. These symptoms may be absent, especially if hyperkalemia develops rapidly. Early ECG changes include peaked T waves, followed by decreased R-wave amplitude, widened QRS complex, and a prolonged P-R interval. These changes may progress to complete heart block with absent P waves and, finally, a sine wave. Ventricular arrhythmias or cardiac arrest may ensue if no effort to lower serum potassium is initiated. However, with a potassium level less than 6 mEq/L, G.B. is unlikely to be experiencing ECG changes.

G.B. has a mild elevation in potassium to 5.3 mEq/L; therefore, no specific treatment is required. Generally, treatment is unnecessary if the potassium concentration is less than 6.5 mEq/L and there are no ECG changes. Although this serum potassium concentration does not require immediate intervention, close monitoring for hyperkalemia and its manifestations is necessary. This would be particularly important after starting ACEI therapy, which can contribute to development of hyperkalemia by decreasing aldosterone production. If potassium concentrations rise above 6.5 mEq/L, and especially if they are accompanied by neuromuscular symptoms or changes in the ECG, treatment should be instituted.

Goals of therapy include prevention of adverse events related to excessive potassium and reduction of serum potassium concentrations to a relatively normal range. Chronic management involves prevention of hyperkalemia by limiting potassium intake and avoiding the use of agents that could elevate potassium levels. This requires regular monitoring of potassium concentrations. Acute management involves reversal of cardiac effects with calcium administration and reduction of serum potassium. The latter can be achieved by shifting potassium intracellularly with administration of glucose and insulin, β-adrenergic agonists, or alkali therapy (if metabolic acidosis is a contributing factor) and by removing potassium using exchange resins or dialysis (see Chapter 27, Fluid and Electrolyte Disorders).

Metabolic Acidosis

CASE 28-1, QUESTION 8: Assess G.B.'s acid–base status. How should her acid–base disorder be managed?

G.B.'s low blood CO_2 content and high chloride concentration are consistent with metabolic acidosis. Normal buffering of hydrogen ions by the bicarbonate–carbonic acid system as well as other extracellular and intracellular buffers, including proteins, phosphates, and hemoglobin, is essential for maintaining normal acid–base balance (i.e., normal pH). Normal metabolism of ingested food produces approximately 1 mEq/kg of metabolic acid daily, which must be excreted by the kidneys (primarily as ammonium ion) to maintain acid–base balance. The kidney is responsible for reabsorption of bicarbonate and excretion of hydrogen ions through buffering by ammonia (produced by the kidney) and filtered phosphates. Reduced bicarbonate reabsorption and impaired production of ammonia by the kidneys are the major factors responsible for development of metabolic acidosis in advanced kidney disease. As nephron function declines, production of ammonia is increased to compensate for a decrease in secretion of hydrogen ions; however, once the maximal capacity for ammonia production is reached, acidosis develops. Mild hyperchloremia is generally observed in the earlier stages. As kidney disease progresses, metabolic acidosis with an elevated anion gap is observed owing to accumulation of organic acids (see Chapter 26, Acid–Base Disorders). Bone carbonate stores serve as a source of alkali, but with time cannot compensate for changes in acid–base balance. Metabolic acidosis can contribute to bone disease by promoting bone resorption, and it may also influence nutritional status by decreasing albumin synthesis and promoting a negative nitrogen balance.[88]

G.B.'s mild acidosis should be treated with a goal of normalizing the plasma bicarbonate concentration or at least achieving bicarbonate levels of at least 22 mEq/L. Treatment includes use of preparations containing sodium bicarbonate or sodium citrate. Each 650-mg tablet of sodium bicarbonate provides 8 mEq of sodium and 8 mEq of bicarbonate. Shohl's solution and Bicitra contain 1 mEq of sodium and the amount of citrate or citric acid to provide 1 mEq of bicarbonate/mL. These latter agents may be used in patients who experience excessive GI distress with sodium bicarbonate because of production and elimination of carbon dioxide. If a patient such as G.B. is sodium and fluid overloaded, it is important to consider that sodium bicarbonate can exacerbate this problem. Polycitra, or potassium citrate, is a possible alternative; however, the potassium content limits its use in patients with more severe kidney disease. Citrate also promotes aluminum absorption and should not be used in patients taking aluminum-containing agents. The amount of bicarbonate supplementation to achieve a bicarbonate of 22 mEq/L can range from 0.3 to 1 mEq/kg/day.[89–91] Typical starting regimens can be two to four 650mg sodium bicarbonate tablets/days (divided into two to three doses). Afterwards, doses should be titrated to desired bicarbonate levels. Equations based on the serum bicarbonate level are available if an immediate correction of the metabolic acidosis is warranted.[88]

Once dialysis therapy is initiated in patients with kidney disease, IV and oral supplementation with bicarbonate or citrate or citric acid preparations is generally not required. At this point, dialysis therapy is used to chronically manage metabolic acidosis through use of dialysate baths containing bicarbonate. Bicarbonate is added to the dialysate solution and is delivered through the process of diffusion from the dialysate bath into the plasma (see Chapter 30, Renal Dialysis). If dialysis therapy is initiated in G.B., the continued need for oral bicarbonate supplementation should be reassessed.

Other Electrolyte and Metabolic Disturbances of Chronic Kidney Disease

CASE 28-1, QUESTION 9: What other electrolyte and metabolic disturbances are exhibited by G.B.?

G.B.'s hyperphosphatemia is a result of decreased phosphorus elimination by the kidneys (see Case 28-3, Question 2, for a more detailed discussion of hyperphosphatemia). The KDIGO guidelines for Diagnosis, Evaluation, Prevention, and Treatment of CKD Mineral and Bone Disorder recommend reducing dietary phosphorus to 800 to 1,000 mg/day while maintaining adequate nutritional needs.[92] Phosphorus-containing laxatives and enemas should also be avoided. Hyperphosphatemia is associated with low serum calcium concentrations.

The mild degree of hypermagnesemia seen in G.B. is a common finding in patients with CKD owing to decreased elimination of magnesium by the kidney. Magnesium is eliminated by the kidney to the extent required to achieve normal serum magnesium concentrations until eGFR is less than 30 mL/minute/1.73 m^2. Serum magnesium concentrations less than 4 mEq/L rarely cause symptoms. Higher concentrations can lead to nausea, vomiting, lethargy, confusion, and diminished tendon reflexes, whereas severe hypermagnesemia may depress cardiac conduction. The risk of hypermagnesemia can be reduced by avoiding magnesium-containing antacids and laxatives and by use of a magnesium-free dialysate in patients with CKD 5D.

G.B. also has mild hyperuricemia. Asymptomatic hyperuricemia frequently develops in patients with kidney disease owing to diminished urinary excretion of uric acid. In the absence of a history of gout or urate nephropathy, asymptomatic hyperuricemia does not require treatment.

ANEMIA OF CHRONIC KIDNEY DISEASE

CASE 28-1, QUESTION 10: What findings in G.B. are consistent with the diagnosis of anemia of CKD, and what is the etiology of this disorder?

G.B.'s hemoglobin of 9.3 g/dL is substantially lower than the normal range for premenopausal females, indicating that she has anemia. Her normal RBC indices suggest her red cells are of normal size, but the absence of an elevated reticulocyte count suggests an impaired bone marrow response for her degree of anemia. Her recent history of peptic ulcer disease may also have contributed to the observed drop in hemoglobin as a result of blood loss. Her complaint of general malaise is consistent with the symptoms of anemia.

Characteristics and Etiology

Anemia, which affects most patients with CKD, is caused by a decreased production of EPO, a glycoprotein that stimulates RBC production in the bone marrow and is released in response to hypoxia. Approximately 90% of the total EPO is produced in the peritubular cells of the kidney; the remainder is produced by the liver. EPO concentrations in patients with kidney failure are lower than in individuals with normal kidney function who have the same degree of anemia and the same stimulus for EPO production and release.[93]

Anemia appears as early as CKD 3 and is characterized by normochromic (normal color) and normocytic (normal size) RBCs unless a concomitant iron, folate, or vitamin B_{12} deficiency exists. A direct correlation between eGFR and hematocrit has been demonstrated, with a 3.1% decrease in hematocrit for every 10 mL/minute/1.73 m^2 decline in eGFR.[94] A higher prevalence of anemia occurs in the population with an eGFR less than 60 mL/minute/1.73 m^2.[1] Pallor and fatigue are the earliest clinical signs, with other manifestations developing as anemia progresses with declining kidney function. A significant consequence of anemia is development of left ventricular hypertrophy (LVH), further contributing to cardiovascular complications and mortality in patients with CKD. LVH has been observed in approximately 30% of patients with eGFR 50 to 75 mL/minute/1.73 m^2 (CKD 2 and 3) and in up to 74% of patients at the start of dialysis.[95] These findings support the need for early and aggressive treatment of anemia of CKD before the development of CKD 5.

A complete workup for anemia of CKD is recommended for patients with an eGFR of less than 60 mL/minute/1.73 m^2.[93] This workup includes a complete blood count including hemoglobin, assessment of iron indices with correction if iron deficiency is present, and evaluation for sources of blood loss, such as bleeding from the GI tract. This workup should be done at least twice per year for the stage of CKD because of the association between anemia and the progressive decline in eGFR.[93]

IRON STATUS

Iron deficiency substantially contributes to anemia development and is the primary cause of erythropoiesis-stimulating agent (ESA) hyporesponsiveness; thus, iron status assessment is essential before considering or initiating erythropoietic therapy. The two tests that best evaluate iron status are the transferrin saturation percent (TSAT) and serum ferritin.[93] Transferrin is a carrier protein, and its concentration depends on nutritional status. The TSAT indicates the saturation of the protein transferrin with iron and is determined as follows (Eq. 28-6):

$$\%\,\text{TSAT} = \frac{\text{serum iron (mcg/dL)}}{\text{TIBC (mcg/dL)}} \times 100 \qquad \text{(Eq. 28-6)}$$

where TIBC is the total iron-binding capacity of the transferrin protein. The TSAT is considered iron readily available for RBC production. Serum ferritin is a marker for iron reserves, which are stored primarily in the reticuloendothelial system (e.g., liver, spleen). The goal of iron replacement therapy is to maintain the TSAT greater than 30% and a serum ferritin greater than 500 ng/mL for CKD to provide sufficient iron for erythrocyte production. Values below these targets are indicative of absolute iron deficiency. A functional iron deficiency may exist when ferritin is greater than 500 ng/mL, TSAT is less than 20%, and anemia persists despite appropriate ESA therapy. In these cases, iron supplementation may lead to improved erythropoiesis. Other tests, including the percentage of hypochromic RBCs, reticulocyte hemoglobin content, serum transferrin receptor, RBC ferritin, and zinc protoporphyrin, have been proposed as indicators of iron status.[93] Although some of these markers have demonstrated predictive value in assessing iron status, either alone or in conjunction with other laboratory data, further investigation is warranted to determine their utility and to make such testing procedures readily available.

The availability of recombinant human EPO to directly stimulate erythrocyte production revolutionized the treatment of CKD-associated anemia. However, iron deficiency is the leading cause of ESA hyporesponsiveness and must be corrected before ESA therapy is initiated. Iron deficiency can develop as a result of increased requirements for RBC production with ESA administration and from chronic blood loss owing to bleeding or HD. Identification and management of iron deficiency through regular follow-up testing and iron supplementation is essential for adequate RBC production (see Case 28-1, Question 12, for Iron Therapy, and also Chapter 92, Anemias).[93]

Other factors that contribute to anemia include a shortened RBC life span secondary to uremia, blood loss from frequent phlebotomy and HD, GI bleeding, severe hyperparathyroidism, protein malnutrition, aluminum accumulation, severe infections, and inflammatory conditions.[93] Substances present in the plasma of patients with CKD, collectively termed *uremic toxins*, may inhibit the production of EPO, the bone marrow response to EPO, and the synthesis of heme. The negative effects of these substances on RBC production are supported by improvement in erythropoiesis with dialysis, which removes these uremic toxins. This uremic environment also causes a decrease in the RBC life span, from a normal life span of 120 days to approximately 60 days in patients with severe CKD. A shortened RBC life span has been observed in uremic patients transfused with RBCs from individuals with normal kidney function, whereas RBCs from uremic individuals maintain a normal survival time when transfused into patients without kidney failure.

Blood loss also contributes to anemia of CKD, particularly in patients requiring HD. With each HD session, generally performed 3 times a week, blood loss occurs. In addition, these patients are usually administered heparin during dialysis or antiplatelet drugs to prevent vascular access clotting, which further increases the risk of bleeding. Although a stool guaiac test was not performed in G.B., many patients with uremia and CKD will have a positive guaiac reaction because of the risk of bleeding from uremia itself. G.B. also has a peptic ulcer, which increases her potential for blood loss.

Other deficiencies can contribute to anemia of CKD. Deficiency of folic acid, as evidenced by low serum folate concentrations and macrocytosis, is relatively uncommon in patients with early kidney disease, but occurs most often in patients on dialysis because folic acid is removed by dialysis. Therefore, the daily prophylactic administration of the water-soluble vitamins, including 1 mg of folic acid, is recommended. Routine use of fat-soluble vitamin A is discouraged, because hypervitaminosis A may develop, contributing to anemia.[93] Several multivitamin preparations devoid of vitamin A (e.g., Nephrocaps) are available for patients with kidney failure. Pyridoxine (vitamin B_6) deficiency can also occur in both dialyzed and nondialyzed patients with CKD. Significant similarities are seen between this deficiency and the symptoms of uremia, which include skin hyperpigmentation and peripheral neuropathy. Current multivitamin products for patients with CKD 5D contain adequate amounts of pyridoxine to prevent deficiency.

Goals of Therapy

CASE 28-1, QUESTION 11: What are the goals of therapy for anemia of CKD in G.B.?

TARGET HEMOGLOBIN

Normalization of hemoglobin (i.e., ≥13 g/dL) in CKD should be avoided. In early 2007, an FDA-mandated black box warning was added to the safety labeling for all ESA products, which states that use of ESA therapy may increase the risk for death and for serious cardiovascular events when administered to achieve a hemoglobin greater than 12 g/dL. This came as a result of four completed cancer trials that evaluated new dosing regimens, use of ESA in a new patient population, and use of new unapproved ESA. Three trials have evaluated the efficacy and safety of hemoglobin targets in patients with CKD not on HD. In each study, the higher target hemoglobin groups (hemoglobin ≥13 g/dL) experienced increased cardiovascular events, stroke, or mortality rates; thus, observing these black box warnings in CKD is warranted.[96–98] Partial correction of anemia to approximately 11 g/dL is considered to offer improvements in quality of life, reduction in hospitalizations, and improvement in LVH.[99–101] It is at these targets that benefits such as increased survival, exercise capacity, quality of life, cardiac output, cognitive function, and decreased risk of LVH were observed in the CKD population. The KDIGO Clinical Practice Guideline for Anemia in Chronic Kidney Disease recommends a target hemoglobin of up to 11.5 g/dL.[93] Furthermore, for non-dialysis CKD patients with a hemoglobin <10.0 g/dL, the decision to start ESA therapy is based on the rate of fall of the hemoglobin.

Hemoglobin, rather than hematocrit, should be used to evaluate anemia in this population for several reasons. Hematocrit is dependent on volume status, which can be problematic for patients with fluctuations in plasma water (e.g., dialysis, volume overload). In addition, a number of variables can affect the hematocrit value including temperature, hyperglycemia, the size of the RBC, and the counters used for the test. These variables do not significantly affect hemoglobin, making it the preferred test for anemia.[93]

G.B.'s iron status should be evaluated first, and corrected if necessary. If achieving an adequate iron status does not improve anemia management, ESA therapy may be started (see Treatment section, and also Chapter 92, Anemias).

Treatment

CASE 28-1, QUESTION 12: Describe the options available to treat anemia of CKD and achieve the goals of therapy in G.B.

IRON THERAPY

Before initiating ESA therapy, G.B.'s iron indices should be determined. If G.B. is iron deficient, as indicated by the TSAT and serum ferritin and other supporting laboratory data (see Chapter 92, Anemias), supplemental iron therapy should be administered. If iron deficiency is the cause of anemia, G.B. may benefit from iron supplementation alone (i.e., without erythropoietic therapy) to increase hemoglobin. Peptic ulcer disease will need to be evaluated as a source of blood loss. Given the poor bioavailability of oral iron and patient noncompliance, oral iron is usually inadequate for repletion of iron in patients receiving HD who experience chronic blood loss.[102] For the population with early CKD and for patients receiving PD, an initial trial of oral iron may correct the deficiency because these patients do not have the same degree of blood loss. However, IV therapy will be required to replenish iron and meet the increased demands once erythropoiesis is stimulated with ESA therapy. Administration of IV iron requires IV access and frequent outpatient visits, which are drawbacks to therapy with IV iron in CKD 3 and 4. A trial examined an accelerated dosing regimen (500 mg given on two consecutive days) of IV iron sucrose to address these issues. This regimen was adequate to restore iron stores with only two patients experiencing hypotension related to iron therapy.[103] However, IV iron sucrose given 200 mg every 2 weeks for a total 1 g repletion in CKD 3 and 4 was associated with increased risk of cardiovascular causes and infectious diseases compared to oral ferrous sulfate.[104]

Common infusion-related effects associated with IV iron include hypotension, myalgias, and arthralgias. Despite the controversy about the best strategy for iron supplementation in patients with early CKD, current recommendations support reserving IV iron for patients in whom oral iron has failed.[93] Therefore, a trial of oral iron is reasonable for G.B. Oral iron supplementation with 200 mg/day of elemental iron should be started to address iron deficiency, if present, and this regimen should be continued to maintain sufficient iron status while receiving ESA therapy. Many oral iron preparations are available, and their iron content varies as will the number of tablets or capsules that must be taken per day to provide the required elemental iron (Table 28-8). Some oral formulations include ascorbic acid to enhance iron absorption. A heme iron product, Proferrin-ES, has recently been approved. Heme iron is more readily absorbed; however, a large number of tablets are required to supply the required 200 mg of elemental iron (Table 28-8). G.B. should be advised to take oral iron on an empty stomach to maximize absorption, unless side effects prevent this strategy. She also should be counseled on potential drug interactions with oral iron (e.g., antacids, quinolones) and GI side effects (e.g., nausea, abdominal pain, diarrhea, constipation, dark stools). Noncompliance with therapy as a result of side effects is a common cause of therapeutic failure with oral iron. An acidic environment is needed for adequate iron absorption, and acid-suppression therapies (e.g., proton-pump inhibitors) may limit the absorption of oral iron. Oral iron is a mucosal toxin, and her previous history of peptic ulcer disease requires caution with the use of oral iron.

Table 28-8
Oral Iron Preparations

Preparation	Common Brand Names	Commonly Prescribed Unit Size (Amount Elemental Iron in mg)[a]	Number of Units/Day to Yield 200 mg Elemental Iron
Ferrous sulfate	Slow FE, Fer-In-Sol	325 (65)	3 tablets
Ferrous gluconate	Feratab	325 (36)	5 tablets
Ferrous fumarate	Femiron, Feostat	200 (66)	3 capsules
Iron polysaccharide	Niferex, Nu-Iron	150 (150)	2 capsules
Heme iron polypeptide	Proferrin-ES	12 (12)	17 tablets
Carbonyl Iron	Fesol	45 (45)	4 tablets

[a]Unit size reflects common tablet or capsule sizes prescribed and not necessarily that of the brand names listed.

If G.B.'s condition does not respond to oral therapy, as indicated by either persistent iron deficiency based on iron indices or inadequate response to what is considered an adequate dose and duration of erythropoietic therapy, IV iron is necessary. The IV iron preparations currently available are iron dextran (INFeD, DexFerrum), sodium ferric gluconate complex in sucrose (Ferrlecit), iron sucrose (Venofer), ferumoxytol (Feraheme), and ferric carboxymaltose (Injectafer). Additionally, soluble ferric pyrophosphate citrate was approved by the FDA in 2015; this iron product is added to the dialysate used for hemodialysis. The dextran products have caused anaphylactic reactions and, as a result, have an FDA-mandated black box warning that requires administration of a 25-mg test dose followed by a 1-hour observation period before the total dose of iron is infused.[105] The dextran component is believed to be the cause of such reactions. The dose of IV iron recommended to correct absolute iron deficiency is a total dose of 1 g administered in divided doses or for a prolonged period to minimize the risk of adverse effects.[93] For iron dextran, the approved dose is 100-mg increments, administered during 10 dialysis sessions for patients on HD to provide a total of 1 g. Larger doses of 500 mg up to the total 1-g dose have been safely administered during a longer infusion period of 4 to 6 hours.

Sodium ferric gluconate and iron sucrose are the most widely used iron products in the CKD population. Both the ferric gluconate and iron sucrose products have been used successfully in patients who have experienced allergic reactions to the dextran products, and evidence indicates that they are safer: 8.7 adverse events per million doses for dextran versus 3.3 adverse events for gluconate.[102] To provide the recommended total dose of 1 g, ferric gluconate is administered as 125 mg (10 mL) during eight consecutive dialysis sessions for patients on HD. The dose can be administered as a slow IV injection at a rate of up to 12.5 mg/minute or diluted in 100 mL of normal saline and infused for 1 hour. Administration of 125 mg for 10 minutes (without a test dose) was determined to be a safer alternative to dextran preparations in patients on HD and is an approved dosing strategy. Doses up to 250 mg for 1 hour have been administered safely.[106] The flexibility of administering larger doses of iron is an important factor in achieving efficiencies in the outpatient setting for patients with early CKD and those receiving PD.

Iron sucrose (Venofer) is a polynuclear iron hydroxide sucrose complex. The recommended dose of iron sucrose is 100 mg (5 mL) during 10 consecutive HD sessions to provide the total dose of 1 g.[106] The dose can be administered by a slow IV injection for 5 minutes or diluted in 100 mL of normal saline and infused for at least 15 minutes. As with sodium ferric gluconate, a test dose is not required. Iron sucrose doses of 250 to 300 mg have been safely administered for 1 hour and found to be as effective as sodium ferric gluconate administration in maintaining hemoglobin in patients receiving epoetin.[106] Furthermore, iron sucrose has demonstrated the lowest anaphylaxis at first exposure and during total iron repletion.[107]

Smaller doses of IV iron, in increments of 25 to 200 mg, can be administered on a weekly, every 2-week, or monthly basis to patients without absolute iron deficiency. These doses will sustain adequate iron stores, maintain target hemoglobin values, and potentially reduce the required dose of the erythropoietic agent.[106] This regimen is most convenient for patients on HD who have regular IV access and increased iron needs because of chronic blood loss. Maintenance iron therapy replaces these losses and minimizes the need for the more aggressive 1-g total doses of IV iron required for absolute iron deficiency. If G.B. starts on HD in the future, regular dosing of IV iron during dialysis is the most reasonable way to maintain adequate iron required for sustained erythropoiesis. Iron indices should be monitored at least every 3 months to guide IV iron therapy. This strategy, however, could lead to increased exposure to free iron, which may place the patient at an increased risk of adverse effects (e.g., inflammation, oxidative stress).[108]

Ferumoxytol (Feraheme) is a semisynthetic carbohydrate-coated, superparamagnetic iron oxide nanoparticle approved for the treatment of iron deficiency anemia of CKD. The small content of free iron in the formulation allows for doses of 510 mg to be administered safely for 17 seconds, followed by a second 510-mg IV injection 3 to 8 days later. Contrary to previous IV iron formulations, a 1-g repletion regimen of ferumoxytol can be completed in two settings. Prospective, randomized studies in patients with CKD (categories 1–5) demonstrated the effectiveness of ferumoxytol in increasing hemoglobin levels in CKD patients compared with oral iron.[109] Ferumoxytol presents the same side effect profile as other IV iron preparations (i.e., hypotension or hypersensitivity reactions, including anaphylaxis or anaphylactoid reactions). The carbohydrate coating of ferumoxytol is suggested to reduce immunologic sensitivity, potentially resulting in less risk for anaphylactic type reactions compared with the other available high molecular weight IV iron products (e.g., iron dextran).[110] However, ferumoxytol has an adverse drug event rate of approximately 0.2% and the FDA has added a black box warning stating concern for fatal and serious hypersensitivity reactions particularly with the first dose.[111,112] Additionally, ferumoxytol can affect the diagnostic ability of magnetic resonance imaging for up to 3 months after the last dose.[111]

ERYTHROPOIESIS-STIMULATING AGENT THERAPY

Recombinant human EPO should be initiated for anemia of CKD in G.B. if there is no response in her hemoglobin to IV iron. Regular dialysis may improve an anemic condition, but it will not restore the hemoglobin concentrations to normal because the primary cause of anemia is reduced EPO production by the kidneys. Although blood transfusions were once the mainstay of treatment, they are now avoided, if possible, because they are associated with a risk for viral diseases (hepatitis, human immunodeficiency virus), iron overload, and further suppression of erythropoiesis. Transfusions may be required in certain patients with substantially low oxygen-carrying capacity or substantial blood loss, and in those patients exhibiting persistent symptoms of anemia (e.g., fatigue, dyspnea on exertion, tachycardia). Currently, G.B. is not a candidate for transfusions based on her hemoglobin of 9.3 g/dL and the absence of significant symptoms on presentation. Androgens raise EPO concentrations and were previously used to treat the anemia of CKD. However, inconsistent erythropoietic response, many adverse effects, and the availability of recombinant EPO have terminated the use of androgens as a treatment of anemia.

Human Erythropoetin-Epoetin Alfa

Human EPO or epoetin, the exogenous form of EPO, is produced using recombinant technology. Epoetin alfa is available in the United States, whereas epoetin beta is available primarily outside the United States. Since it became available in 1989, epoetin alfa (Epogen, Procrit) has provided an effective treatment option for anemia and has substantially decreased the need for RBC transfusions. Epoetin alfa stimulates the proliferation and differentiation of erythroid progenitor cells, increases hemoglobin synthesis, and accelerates the release of reticulocytes from the bone marrow.

For patients such as G.B. who do not yet require dialysis and for patients receiving PD, epoetin alfa is generally administered by subcutaneous (SC) injection. However, HD patients often receive epoetin alfa by IV administration because easy IV access is established. SC administration is preferred because lower doses can be administered less frequently and cost is lower than with IV administration. Starting doses for epoetin alfa administration are 50 to 100 units/kg 2 times weekly.[113] For patients being converted from IV to SC administration (half-life of epoetin alfa is 8.5 hours IV vs. 24.4 hours SC) whose hemoglobin is within the target range, the SC dose is usually two-thirds the IV dose. For patients not yet at the target hemoglobin, an SC dose equivalent to the IV dose is recommended. Patients receiving epoetin alfa SC should be instructed on the appropriate administration technique, which includes rotating the sites for injection (e.g., upper arm, thigh, and abdomen).

Darbepoetin Alfa

Darbepoetin alfa (Aranesp) was approved in 2001 for the treatment of anemia of CKD, regardless of dialysis requirements. Darbepoetin is a hyperglycosylated analog of epoetin alfa that stimulates erythropoiesis by the same mechanism. Instead of the three *N*-linked carbohydrate chains on epoetin alfa, darbepoetin has five, which increase the capacity for sialic acid residue binding on the protein. The increased protein binding slows total body clearance and increases the terminal half-life to 25.3 hours and 48.8 hours after IV and SC administration, respectively. Darbepoetin alfa's longer half-life relative to epoetin alfa offers the potential advantage of less frequent dosing to maintain target hemoglobin values.

Studies in patients with CKD 3 and 4 determined that starting SC doses of 0.45 mcg/kg administered once per week and 0.75 mcg/kg once every other week were effective in achieving target hemoglobin and hematocrit values in patients who had not previously received erythropoietic therapy.[114] In patients on dialysis converted from epoetin alfa to darbepoetin alfa (IV and SC), darbepoetin maintained target hemoglobin values when administered less frequently (i.e., one dose every week in patients previously receiving epoetin alfa 3 times/week, and one dose every other week in patients previously receiving epoetin once weekly).

The approved starting dose of darbepoetin alfa in patients who have not previously received epoetin therapy is 0.45 mcg/kg given either IV or SC once weekly.[115] Patients who are already receiving epoetin therapy may be converted to darbepoetin alfa based on the current total weekly epoetin dose (Table 28-9).[115] For patients currently receiving epoetin alfa 2 to 3 times a week, darbepoetin alfa may be administered once weekly. Patients who are receiving epoetin alfa once weekly should receive darbepoetin alfa once every 2 weeks. To calculate the once every 2-week darbepoetin dose, the weekly epoetin alfa dose should be multiplied by 2 and that value used in column 1 of Table 28-9 to find the corresponding darbepoetin dose from column 2 in Table 28-9. For example, a patient receiving epoetin 6,000 units/week should receive 40 mcg of darbepoetin alfa once every 2 weeks (6,000 units epoetin $\times$ 2 = 12,000 units, which corresponds to a weekly darbepoetin dose of 40 mcg).[115]

Epoetin alfa and darbepoetin alfa are generally well tolerated, with hypertension being the most common adverse event reported. Although elevated BP is not uniformly considered a contraindication to therapy, BP should be monitored closely so that changes in antihypertensive therapy and the dialysis prescription are made, if justified. Failure to elicit a response to erythropoietic therapy requires evaluation of factors that cause resistance, such as iron deficiency, infection, inflammation, chronic blood loss, aluminum toxicity, malnutrition, and hyperparathyroidism. Resistance to erythropoietic therapy has been observed in patients receiving ACEI, although data are conflicting.[116] Rare cases of antibody formation to epoetin therapy have been reported primarily with one epoetin alfa product manufactured outside the United States. Neutralizing anti-EPO antibodies were identified in 13 patients with pure RBC aplasia who required blood transfusions after a course of therapy with epoetin alfa or beta.[117]

Treatment of G.B.'s anemia must be initiated, given the chronic nature of her kidney disease and her current hemoglobin. In patients with hemoglobin values less than 10 g/dL, it is important to identify and correct any iron or folate deficiency and perform a stool guaiac test to rule out active GI bleeding. Iron supplementation is indicated, not only if G.B. is iron deficient but also to maintain iron status while receiving erythropoietic therapy (see Iron Therapy section). Although administration of iron alone may improve her anemia, epoetin alfa or darbepoetin alfa may likely be required, based on the severity of her anemia and the progressive nature of her kidney disease. G.B. may start darbepoetin alfa administered at a dose of 25 mcg (0.45 mcg/kg) SC once per week, assuming her iron status is appropriate (see Iron Status section). Another option would be epoetin alfa at a dose of 6,000 units (approximately100 units/kg) administered SC once per week or divided into two weekly doses of 3,000 units. She also should be instructed on how to administer SC epoetin alfa or darbepoetin alfa. Dose adjustments should not be made more frequently than once every 4 weeks for either agent because of the time course for response (i.e., the pharmacodynamic effects on RBC homeostasis). The time it takes to reach a new steady state, when RBC production is equal to RBC destruction, depends on the life span of the RBC, which is approximately 60 days in patients with kidney failure. Therefore, it will take approximately 2 to 3 months to reach a plateau in measured hemoglobin. Dose adjustments should be made on the basis of G.B.'s hemoglobin,

Table 28-9
Estimated Darbepoetin Alfa Starting Doses Based on Previous Epoetin Alfa Dose

Previous Weekly Epoetin Alfa Dosage (units/week)	Weekly Starting Darbepoetin Alfa Dosage (mcg/week)	
	Adults	Children
<1,500	6.25	[a]
1,500–2,499	6.25	6.25
2,500–4,999	12.5	10
5,000–10,999	25	20
11,000–17,999	40	40
18,000–33,999	60	60
34,000–89,999	100	100
≥90,000	20	200

[a]For children receiving a weekly epoetin alfa dosage of <1,500 units/week, the available data are insufficient to determine a darbepoetin alfa conversion dosage.
Reprinted with permission from Facts & Comparisons eAnswers.

which should be monitored every 1 to 2 weeks after initiation of therapy or after a dose change. If a rapid increase in hemoglobin is observed (hemoglobin >1.0 g/dL during any 2-week period) or approaching 11.5 g/dL, then doses of either agent should be decreased by approximately 25%. If response is inadequate (hemoglobin increase <1 g/dL in 2–4 weeks), then the doses should be increased by 25%. Once stable, the hemoglobin should be monitored every 2 to 4 weeks. If a response is not observed despite appropriate dose titration, G.B. should be evaluated for possible reasons for nonresponse (i.e., iron deficiency, bleeding, aluminum intoxication, hyperparathyroidism, infection).

Other ESA Agents

The ESA peginesatide, a pegylated peptide, was FDA approved for anemia treatment in dialysis patients in March 2012. However, peginesatide was withdrawn from the market by the manufacturer after serious hypersensitivity reactions, including anaphylaxis, were reported.

Continuous EPO receptor activator (Mircera) is a long-acting ESA. CERA is twice the molecular weight of EPO from the addition of a single 30-kDa polymer chain into the EPO molecule that results in a considerably longer elimination half-life compared with EPO (130 hours vs. 4–28 hours). This allows for extended-interval dosing of biweekly and once monthly. It has an efficacy and safety profile comparable to other available ESAs. Extended-interval dosing agents, such as CERA, have several advantages in patients with CKD 3 and 4, including improved patient compliance, less administration costs, reduced burden on patient from fewer injections given, and fewer outpatient visits to receive IV administration.[118]

CARDIOVASCULAR COMPLICATIONS

CASE 28-2

Question 1: H.B. is a 65-year-old white man with category 5 CKD who has just started chronic HD. He comes in today for his third HD session (dialysis scheduled 3 times/week, 4-hour duration). He has a history of hypertension, which has been poorly controlled during the past 4 months (BP ranges 150–190/85–105 mm Hg), and has experienced shortness of breath and a significant weight gain during the past month. His pertinent medical history includes hypertension for the past 14 years. H.B.'s current medications include metoprolol tartrate 50 mg BID, furosemide 80 mg BID, calcium carbonate 500 mg TID with meals, and Nephrocaps one by mouth (PO) every day. H.B.'s most recent predialysis BP was 195/100 mm Hg, and his postdialysis BP was 168/90 mm Hg. A recent ECG showed evidence of LVH.

Predialysis laboratory values were as follows:
Serum sodium (Na), 140 mEq/L
Potassium (K), 5.1 mEq/L
Chloride (Cl), 101 mEq/L
CO_2 content, 23 mEq/L
SCr, 8.8 mg/dL
BUN, 84 mg/dL
Phosphate, 6.5 mg/dL
Calcium, 8.6 mg/dL
Serum albumin, 3.0 g/dL
Cholesterol (nonfasting), 345 mg/dL
Triglycerides, 285 mg/dL
TSAT, 18%
Ferritin, 250 ng/mL
Hct, 27%
Hgb, 9.0 g/dL

H.B. has a urine output of 50 mL/day. What conditions evident in H.B. place him at increased risk of cardiovascular complications and mortality?

H.B. has uncontrolled hypertension that is not adequately managed with his current drug therapy or HD. Hypertension is associated with LVH, ischemic heart disease, and heart failure, all of which are contributing factors to overall mortality in patients with CKD 5D who are undergoing dialysis.[4] H.B.'s ECG evidence of LVH should trigger additional evaluation to determine the extent of cardiac involvement and diagnosis of heart failure, which is associated with increased mortality in both diabetic and nondiabetic patients (see Chapter 14, Heart Failure).[95] LVH develops early in the course of CKD and progresses as kidney disease progresses. H.B. is in the most severe stage of CKD and has the greatest likelihood of developing LVH. Anemia contributes substantially to the development of LVH and heart failure as well. H.B.'s hemoglobin of 9.0 g/dL is below the target value and requires treatment based on evaluation of his iron indices (see Anemia section).

Additional factors that increase the risk of cardiovascular complications and mortality in H.B. include elevated cholesterol and triglycerides levels as well as hypoalbuminemia (serum albumin, 3.0 g/dL). Increased levels of homocysteine are common in patients with kidney failure and have been associated with increased risk of coronary artery disease.[119] Because elevated concentrations of homocysteine have been observed in conjunction with decreased folate and vitamin B_{12} levels, more aggressive supplementation of these vitamins in this population has been suggested. Because H.B.'s total corrected calcium (corrected for hypoalbuminemia; see Case 28-3, Question 2, for an explanation of this correction) is 9.4 mg/dL, his calcium and use of a calcium-containing phosphate binder will need to be monitored frequently. Cardiac calcification is common in patients with kidney disease and also is associated with cardiovascular complications. It has been reported that approximately 80% of patients with ESRD have detectable coronary artery calcification.[120] CVD and complications continue to be the leading cause of mortality in patients with kidney failure.[1]

Hypertension

Case 28-2, Question 2: What options are available to treat H.B.'s hypertension considering his other cardiac complications and BP goal?

DIALYSIS

Hypertension is common in patients with CKD. Multiple factors are involved in the development of hypertension in the CKD population, including extracellular volume expansion from salt and water retention and activation of the renin–angiotensin–aldosterone system.[116] Additionally, the increase in uremic toxins leads to sympathetic nervous system stimulation and elevation of BP.[121]

Because H.B. is just beginning dialysis therapy, it is difficult to assess the degree to which volume removal will ultimately affect his BP. To control BP related to volume changes, dialysis therapy should be adjusted as needed to achieve H.B.'s *dry weight*, the postdialysis weight at which symptoms of hypervolemia and hypovolemia are absent (i.e., normovolemia and free from edema). H.B. has had recent findings consistent with worsening volume status (shortness of breath, weight gain) that should be considered when modifying his dialysis prescription; further workup is needed to determine whether H.B. has systolic or diastolic heart failure. It is also important to counsel H.B. on the importance of salt and fluid intake restriction between HD sessions to minimize weight gain, volume expansion, and hypertension. Restriction of salt intake to less than 2.4 g/day and fluid to 1 L/day is appropriate and will require regular follow-up by a dietitian.

ANTIHYPERTENSIVE THERAPY

Currently, there are no published guidelines for the management of hypertension in patients receiving hemodialysis. Although there are no published guidelines, control and management of hypertension is important. Antihypertensive therapy should be used in conjunction with dialysis therapy in H.B. to a target BP. In the absence of published guidelines targeting a BP of <150/90 mm Hg before HD is reasonable.

For some patients, initiation of dialysis alone may achieve this goal, and antihypertensive therapy may be withdrawn. The aim of the BP goal in patients with CKD 5D is to minimize cardiovascular complications, but it should not increase the risk for hypotension and its associated complications during dialysis. The choice of an agent is based on the patient's comorbid conditions because no single agent has a consistently proven mortality benefit in patients on HD. The complexity of managing hypertension in patients on HD is enhanced by the apparent U-shaped relationship between BP and mortality.[122] A study of patients on HD found an increased risk of cardiac-related death at a systolic BP less than 110 mm Hg and at a systolic BP greater than 180 mm Hg.[123] Another cohort study found a systolic BP between 100 and 125 mm Hg was associated with the lowest risk of death, and systolic BP >150 mm Hg associated with increased death.[122] The mortality risk with a low pre-HD BP may be indicative of severe cardiac disease at the initiation of HD. If patients experience hypotensive symptoms during HD, the goal BP can be increased, but they also should be evaluated for other cardiovascular disorders. Because the BP between dialysis sessions varies owing to volume changes, the ideal time to measure BP relative to dialysis (i.e., predialysis versus postdialysis) is unclear, but predialysis BP has been favored.

Diuretics are commonly used in patients in the early stages of CKD. As discussed previously, the effectiveness of diuretics depends on the amount of sodium delivered to their site of action in the kidney tubule and on the patient's kidney function. For example, a decrease in the eGFR from 125 to 25 mL/minute/1.73 m^2, theoretically, could result in an approximate 80% decrease in the amount of sodium filtered. Early in the course of kidney failure, thiazides or thiazide-like diuretics are effective antihypertensive agents. As eGFR is further reduced (eGFR <30 mL/minute/1.73 m^2), the thiazide diuretics become less effective. Potassium-sparing diuretics are also ineffective and may increase the risk of hyperkalemia. Loop diuretics (e.g., furosemide), which function more proximally, are indicated in patients with CKD 4 (eGFR 15–29 mL/minute/1.73 m^2).[124] These drugs can be effective for BP and volume control in patients with advanced kidney disease if residual kidney function is substantial (urine output >100 mL/day). Their effect must be frequently reevaluated on the basis of urine output and any effect on volume control. H.B.'s urine output should be assessed to determine the rationale for continued use of furosemide, and the current dose should be assessed because doses higher than his current dose of 80 mg BID are often required in patients with this degree of kidney dysfunction. It is likely that furosemide will need to be discontinued as H.B.'s residual kidney function declines.

Given the role of the renin–angiotensin system in the development of hypertension in patients with CKD, ACEIs are a logical choice for antihypertensive therapy. ACEIs are effective antihypertensive agents in patients with CKD and have been shown to reverse LVH.[125] ACEIs are underused in this population. Response must be assessed individually to determine whether renin–angiotensin–aldosterone activity is a predominant etiology of hypertension. Initiating therapy with low doses is prudent to evaluate patient response and tolerance. Use of these agents in combination with other antihypertensives is often required for adequate BP control. Most of these agents can be administered once daily; however, because of the kidney elimination of the parent drug or active metabolite, dosage adjustments are necessary in patients with CKD. ACEI use should be avoided in patients undergoing dialysis with the polyacrylonitrile (AN69) membranes. The AN69 dialyzer increases bradykinin production, whereas ACEIs decrease the breakdown of bradykinin, predisposing patients to systemic or immune-mediated reactions that can lead to anaphylactic reactions.

ARBs effectively lower BP and reverse LVH in patients without kidney disease.[126] These agents offer an alternative to ACEIs in patients experiencing kinin-mediated adverse effects; however, similar side effects have been reported with ARBs.

β-Adrenergic blockers (β-blockers) inhibit release of renin and may be useful in hypertension associated with CKD. β-Blockers can counteract the elevated sympathetic activity observed in dialysis patients, lower the risk of sudden cardiac death, and improve survival in heart failure.[127] Unfortunately, they are underutilized, and the mentioned benefits are understudied in the dialysis population.[128] Risk versus benefit should be evaluated when β-blockade is considered in conjunction with other comorbid conditions such as asthma, heart failure, and lipid abnormalities. Dosage adjustment is required for the less lipophilic agents (i.e., atenolol, nadolol).

Calcium-channel blockers are effective antihypertensive agents in patients with CKD. Because the nondihydropyridine agents (i.e., diltiazem, verapamil) have negative chronotropic and inotropic effects, they should be used with care in patients with heart disease. Generally, dosage adjustment is not required in patients with kidney disease.

Other agents used to treat hypertension in the CKD population include centrally acting agents (e.g., clonidine, methyldopa), vasodilators (e.g., minoxidil, hydralazine), and α_1-adrenergic blockers (prazosin, terazosin, doxazosin). However, these agents are generally reserved as last-line therapies.

H.B. is currently taking the β-blocker metoprolol and the loop diuretic furosemide. Metoprolol is a β-blocker considered to be removed by dialysis and should be monitored closely for H.B. clinical response to the therapy while starting dialysis. It is likely that his diuretic will need to be discontinued as his residual kidney function decreases and response to therapy is inadequate. If changes imposed in H.B.'s HD prescription are able to improve volume control and achieve his dry weight but do not reduce his BP, another antihypertensive regimen should be selected. A reasonable antihypertensive regimen would include an ACEI (e.g., ramipril). The selection will depend substantially on follow-up results of his cardiac disease, BP control with HD, and the development of adverse effects (see Chapter 9, Essential Hypertension, and Chapter 14, Heart Failure).

Dyslipidemia

CASE 28-2, QUESTION 3: How should H.B.'s lipid abnormalities be treated?

H.B. has elevated serum cholesterol and triglyceride concentrations, a common finding in patients with CKD. Dyslipidemia and increased oxidative stress contribute to premature atherogenesis in these patients. Several atherogenic factors in patients with CKD have been postulated, including arterial wall injury, platelet activation and adherence, smooth muscle cell proliferation, and intraarterial accumulation of cholesterol. Lowering of serum lipids has not been shown to improve morbidity and mortality in hemodialysis patients. Furthermore, current KDIGO Guidelines for Lipid Management in CKD do not recommend using cholesterol values to determine who to treat or as treatment targets. Currently, H.B. is not receiving a statin which has not demonstrated the ability to reduce mortality or morbidity in dialysis. If concern with treating H.B.'s dyslipidemia persists, a moderate-intensity statin may be considered. Dietary intervention successfully reduces triglyceride and cholesterol concentrations in patients with CKD 5D.

MINERAL AND BONE DISORDERS

CASE 28-3

QUESTION 1: W.K. is a 24-year-old Hispanic woman who has an 18-year history of type 1 diabetes mellitus with complications of diabetic nephropathy, retinopathy, and neuropathy. She was diagnosed with CKD 5 two years ago. She started PD at that time. Her current medications include metoclopramide (Reglan) 10 mg TID before meals, insulin aspart 10 units with meals, insulin glargine 25 units nightly, docusate 100 mg every day, calcium acetate 2001 mg PO TID with meals, EPO 5,000 units IV twice weekly, iron sucrose 100 mg IV 3 times a week, paricalcitol 4 mcg IV 3 times weekly, and Nephrocaps one capsule every day. At a recent clinic visit, findings on physical examination included a BP of 128/84 mm Hg, diabetic retinopathic changes with laser scars bilaterally, and diminished sensation bilaterally below the knees. Her laboratory values were as follows:

Normal serum electrolytes
Random blood glucose, 250 mg/dL
BUN, 45 mg/dL
SCr, 8.9 mg/dL
Hgb, 10 g/dL
WBC count, 6,200/μL
Calcium, 10.2 mg/dL
Phosphate, 6.8 mg/dL
Intact parathyroid hormone (iPTH), 950 pg/mL
Thyroid-stimulating hormone, 5 mIU/L
Total serum protein, 5.0 g/dL
Serum albumin, 3.1 g/dL
Uric acid, 8.9 mg/dL

Describe the etiology of W.K.'s abnormal bone, calcium, phosphorus, and parathyroid hormone (PTH) findings.

Etiology

MND of CKD (CKD-MBD) is the term used to collectively describe the mineral (e.g., phosphorus, calcium, PTH), bone (osteodystrophy), and soft-tissue calcification abnormalities that develop as a complication of CKD. The older collective term of renal osteodystrophy failed to adequately illustrate the broader clinical complications associated with the biomarker abnormalities and calcification, and is now only used to describe, specifically, the bone pathology.[92]

Hyperphosphatemia, hypocalcemia, hyperparathyroidism, decreased production of active vitamin D, and resistance to vitamin D therapy are all frequent problems in CKD that can lead to the secondary complications of CKD-MBD. Although the interrelationships among phosphorus, calcium, vitamin D, and PTH have been reviewed extensively, fibroblast growth factor 23 (FGF23), a phosphaturic hormone, has added some new insight.[129] Increased dietary phosphorus intake stimulates FGF23 secretion. FGF23 increases phosphorus excretion via the proximal tubules, inhibits vitamin D activation, increases activated vitamin D catabolism, and is associated with kidney disease progression.[130]

At a GFR above 30 mL/minute/1.73 m^2, elevations in FGF23 and PTH maintain normal serum phosphorus. This concept is referred to as the trade-off hypothesis, where the ability to maintain normal phosphorus concentrations occurs at the expense of developing secondary hyperparathyroidism (SHPT), the excessive secretion of PTH and elevated FGF23. However, FGF23 is not currently measured in the clinical setting. Clinically significant increases in serum phosphorus (or frank hyperphosphatemia) typically are not seen until late stages of CKD, GFR <30 mL/minute/1.73 m^2, when compensatory mechanisms within the kidney are compromised.

The kidney is the principal organ responsible for systemic vitamin D production, and, as such, vitamin D metabolism is altered in the presence of uremia. Persistent hyperphosphatemia stimulates the release of excessive FGF23, which inhibits the normal conversion of 25-hydroxyvitamin D_3 to its biologically active metabolite, 1,25-dihydroxyvitamin D_3, by the enzyme 1-α-hydroxylase (Fig. 28-2). This enzyme is present in proximal tubular cells of the kidney and is necessary for conversion of vitamin D to the active form. This active form of vitamin D, also known as *calcitriol*, increases gut absorption of calcium and interacts with vitamin D receptors on the parathyroid gland to suppress PTH release. As a result of decreased calcitriol production, the absorption of dietary calcium in the gut is diminished. Decreased suppression of PTH release by vitamin D in conjunction with hypocalcemia promotes continued stimulus for mobilization of calcium from bone. Furthermore, uremic patients require a higher extracellular calcium concentration to suppress secretion of PTH. This is also described as an increase in the calcium "set point" or the concentration of calcium required to inhibit 50% of maximal PTH secretion.[131]

The chronic effects of hyperparathyroidism on the skeleton lead to bone pain, fractures, and myopathy. In children, these effects may be particularly severe and usually retard growth. The metabolic acidosis of kidney disease also contributes to a negative calcium balance in the bone.

W.K.'s presentation is consistent with CKD-MBD based on the observed changes in bone architecture and abnormalities in serum phosphorus, calcium, and PTH; all can be attributed to her kidney disease.

Vitamin D levels (i.e., 25-hydroxyvitamin D) should be checked in CKD 3. Insufficient (<30 ng/mL) and deficient (<15 ng/mL)

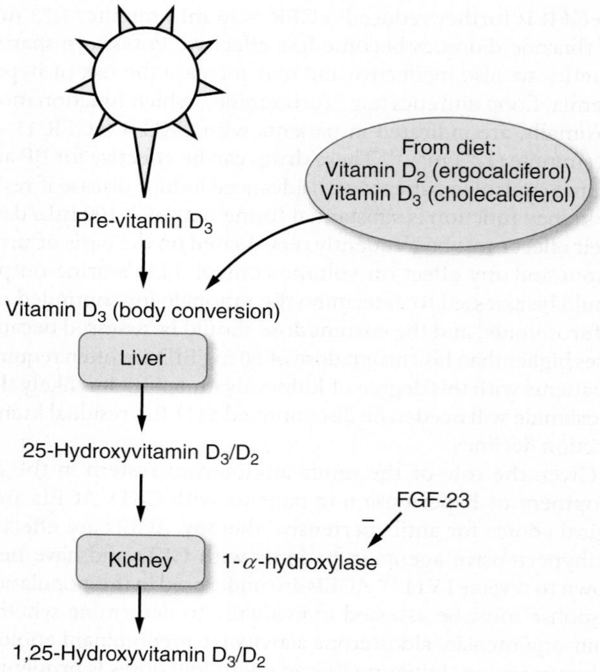

Figure 28-2 Vitamin D biotransformation.

vitamin D levels are prevalent in the majority of CKD and ESRD patients. Several studies have linked depressed vitamin D levels to increased vascular calcification, CVD, and mortality.[132]

Treatment

CASE 28-3, QUESTION 2: What are the goals of therapy for W.K.'s calcium, phosphorus, and PTH abnormalities? What options are available to treat these disorders?

The management objectives for W.K. are to (a) manage serum calcium and phosphorus concentrations, (b) prevent or manage SHPT, and (c) restore normal skeletal development without inducing adynamic bone disease (or low bone turnover). These goals are best achieved with dietary phosphorus restriction, appropriate use of phosphate-binding agents, vitamin D therapy, calcimimetics, and dialysis.

DIETARY RESTRICTION OF PHOSPHORUS

In general, serum phosphorus should be lowered toward near-normal levels. The KDIGO recommends normal levels for all stages of CKD. Dietary phosphorus restriction can prevent hyperphosphatemia and maintain target phosphorus concentrations. Dietary phosphorus should not exceed 800 to 1,000 mg/day.[92] Predominate sources of phosphorus are protein-rich foods, which presents a challenge in tailoring a diet that lowers dietary phosphorus intake while providing adequate nutrition. However, efforts should be made to distinguish between organic (e.g., plant seeds, nuts, legumes, and meats) and inorganic phosphorus (e.g., preservatives and additive salts found in processed foods) sources. Inorganic phosphorus sources are absorbed to a greater extent than organic phosphorus (90% vs. 50%, respectively) and should be minimized in the diet.[133] Dark carbonated beverages are a common culprit for elevated phosphorus levels; their consumption should be discouraged, and the beverages should be removed from vending machines in dialysis clinics. Additionally, the type of organic phosphorus sources, plant versus meat, has varying effects with plant sources associated with lower serum phosphorus levels and decreased FGF23 levels. Although phosphorus is removed to some extent by dialysis, neither conventional HD nor PD removes adequate amounts to warrant complete liberalization of phosphorus in the diet. Nocturnal HD is an exception where patients may require phosphate supplements because of the prolonged dialysis duration. Regular dietary counseling by a kidney dietitian specialist is necessary to reinforce the importance of phosphorus restriction and other dietary recommendations.

PHOSPHATE-BINDING AGENTS

A significant reduction in serum phosphorus is difficult to achieve with dietary intervention alone, particularly in patients with more advanced kidney disease (eGFR <30 mL/minute/1.73 m^2). For these patients, phosphate-binding agents used in conjunction with dietary restriction are necessary. Phosphate-binding agents limit phosphorus absorption from the GI tract by binding with the phosphorus present from dietary sources. Therefore, these agents must be administered with meals. Available binders include products that contain calcium, iron, lanthanum, aluminum, or magnesium cations or the polymer-based agent, sevelamer.

Calcium-Containing Preparations

Calcium-containing preparations, especially calcium carbonate and calcium acetate, are frequently used to prevent hyperphosphatemia in patients with kidney disease. The many preparations available vary in their calcium content (Table 28-10). Correction of hypocalcemia is an added beneficial effect of the calcium-containing preparations; however, a risk exists of hypercalcemia and cardiac calcification associated with the prolonged use of these agents.[134] Additionally, the higher bioavailable calcium in calcium carbonate may lead to positive calcium balance.[135] Calcium citrate is a calcium salt with a phosphate-binding capacity similar to that of calcium carbonate; however, because it also increases aluminum absorption from the GI tract, its use is not recommended in patients with kidney disease.

Simultaneous administration of vitamin D preparations and calcium also increases the risk of hypercalcemia. A corrected serum calcium should be determined before therapy is started and at regular intervals thereafter.

Many clinicians often correct calcium levels for low albumin. Although this practice is still very common, new Medicare Quality Improvements will be based on uncorrected total serum calcium levels. Calculating corrected calcium adjusts for the change in the ratio of free (unbound) versus protein-bound calcium owing to reduced serum albumin concentrations (Eq. 28-7).

$$\text{Corrected calcium (mg/dL)} = \text{measured Ca (mg/dL)} + 0.8 \times (4\ \text{g/dL} - \text{measured albumin [g/dL]}) \quad \text{(Eq. 28-7)}$$

Calcific uremic arteriolopathy (CUA) or calciphylaxis, is characterized by calcification of the arterioles and small arteries with intimal proliferation and endovascular fibrosis. CUA and manifests visually as necrosis of the skin and is most frequently seen in dialysis patients, affecting up to 5% of patients. Calcium-based phosphate binders are one of the triggering factors associated with the development of CUA.

If the patient experiences hypercalcemia or evidence of advance calcification, the patient should be switched to a non–calcium-based phosphate binder. Alternatives include sevelamer and cations, such as lanthanum carbonate or magnesium preparations. For patients requiring dialysis, reducing the calcium concentration of the dialysate bath may decrease the risk of hypercalcemia. Although avoiding hypercalcemia should reduce the risk of cardiac calcification, calcifications still can occur because of other contributing factors in the CKD population (e.g., hyperphosphatemia).

Nausea, diarrhea, and constipation are other side effects of calcium-containing products. Because calcium-containing phosphate binders may interact with other drugs, the timing of their administration relative to other agents must be considered. Fluoroquinolones and oral iron, for example, should be taken at least 1 or 2 hours before calcium-containing phosphate binders. Importantly, if the calcium products are being used as supplementation to treat hypocalcemia or osteoporosis, they should be taken between meals to enhance intestinal absorption. This is in contrast to their administration with meals if they are being used as phosphate binders. Starting doses of common calcium-containing phosphate binders are listed in Table 28-10.

Sevelamer

Sevelamer hydrochloride (Renagel) or carbonate (Renvela) is a nonabsorbed, polymer-based product that binds phosphorus in the GI tract.[136,137] The benefit of lowering phosphorus without significantly affecting serum calcium has led to the increased use of sevelamer in patients with CKD. Sevelamer also lowers LDL and total serum cholesterol, a benefit considering the increased risk of cardiovascular events in this population.[92]

Sevelamer has a potential benefit of attenuating the progression of coronary calcification, which may be related to its LDL and total serum cholesterol-lowering effects and a benefit from reduced calcium loading. The actual benefit of sevelamer on mortality is controversial. The post hoc analysis of the Renagel in New Dialysis (RIND) trial showed a survival advantage with sevelamer compared

Table 28-10
Available Phosphate Binders

Agent	Availability (Pill Burden)	Comments	Adverse Effects and Warnings
Aluminum-Based Binder			
Aluminum hydroxide	320 mg/5 mL suspension	OTC	Constipation and sodium overload Aluminum toxicity: CNS, anemia, and bone disease Warnings: perforation, fecal impaction, ileus
Calcium-Based Binders			
Calcium acetate	667 mg caplets (3–12 caplets) 667 mg/5 mL (15–20 mL with meal)	Oral solution associated with higher diarrhea risk	N/V/D; hypercalcemia; vascular calcification; oral solution associated with greater diarrhea
Calcium carbonate	500–1,250 mg tablets (3–6 tablets)	OTC	N/V/D; hypercalcemia; vascular calcification
Iron-Based Agents			
Ferric citrate	210 mg ferric iron tablet (6–12 tablets)	210 mg of ferric iron = 1 g ferric citrate	N/V/D; discolored feces; iron overload Precautions: gastric/hepatic disorders; CI: hemochromatosis
Sucroferric oxyhydroxide	500 mg chewable tablet (3–6 tablets)	500 mg ferric iron = 2,500 mg sucroferric oxyhydroxide	N/D; discolored feces; iron overload Precautions: gastric/hepatic disorders; hemochromatosis
Lanthanum-Based Binder			
Lanthanum	500, 750, and 1,000 mg chewable tablets (3–6 tablets)	Chewed and crushed have similar efficacy	Accumulation in bone, brain, and liver; visible on abdominal X-ray; hypercalcemia CI: bowel obstruction, ileus, and fecal impaction
Magnesium-Based Binder			
Magnesium hydroxide	311 mg tablets (1–6 tablets)	OTC; impair iron absorption	Hypermagnesemia; diarrhea very common
Resin Binders			
Sevelamer carbonate	800 mg caplet (3–12 caplets) 0.8 g/2.4 g powder packets	Reduces low-density lipoprotein cholesterol	N/V/D; hypercalcemia CI: bowel obstruction Warnings: perforation, fecal impaction
Sevelamer hydrochloride	400, 800 mg caplets 1–2 tablets TID (6–12 caplets)	Reduces low-density lipoprotein cholesterol	N/V/D; hypercalcemia CI: bowel obstruction Warnings: perforation, fecal impaction; risk of metabolic acidosis

CI, contraindications; N/V/D, nausea, vomiting, diarrhea.

with calcium acetate; however, the Dialysis Clinical Outcomes Revisited (DCOR) trial failed to show a difference in mortality between the two agents.[138] One explanation for the disparity in results may be the difference in the population of patients on HD between the two trials. The RIND trial included incident patients on HD, whereas the DCOR trial included prevalent HD patients who likely would have advanced CVD.

Sevelamer hydrochloride is available as 400- and 800-mg tablets. Sevelamer carbonate is available as 800-mg tablets and 0.8-g powder packets. The phosphorus-binding capacity remains equipotent between the two formulations. The starting dose is variable and depends on the baseline serum phosphorus concentration (800 mg TID with meals if serum phosphorus is <7.5 mg/dL; 1,600 mg TID with meals if serum phosphorus is >7.5 mg/dL).[136,137] Gradual adjustments can be made at 2-week intervals, based on serum phosphorus levels. Dosing guidelines for sevelamer are also available for patients being converted from calcium acetate. On the basis of studies showing similar reductions in serum phosphorus, 800 mg of sevelamer is considered equivalent to 667 mg of calcium acetate (169 mg of elemental calcium).[137]

The administration of sevelamer hydrochloride to patients on HD is associated with a lowering of serum bicarbonate; this effect should be taken into account when using this agent. Sevelamer carbonate avoids the metabolic acidosis seen with the hydrochloride formulation and raises the serum bicarbonate level.[139] Adverse reports of fecal impaction, ileus, intestinal obstruction, and perforation should caution the use in patients with GI disease. The current prescribing information recommends administering sevelamer 1 hour before or 3 hours after administration of other agents with narrow therapeutic indices.[136,137]

Lanthanum Carbonate

Lanthanum carbonate (Fosrenol) is a noncalcium, nonaluminum phosphate binder preparation. When ingested, it dissociates into a trivalent cation with similar binding capacity as aluminum salts. Lanthanum also has been found to be as effective and tolerable as standard treatment. Both calcium and iPTH were lower in the lanthanum group.[140] Lanthanum is mainly excreted via the biliary route, with minimal kidney elimination.

Studies have evaluated the deposition and toxicity of lanthanum in the bone, liver, and brain due to concerns of lanthanum accumulation. Although lanthanum accumulates in lysosomes in the liver, this has not been correlated with increased liver enzymes or hepatobiliary adverse events in patients receiving lanthanum for up to 6 years.[141] This is likely an excretory process through the biliary tract similar to that for iron and copper. A prospective trial of patients on HD receiving lanthanum for 1 year found minimal deposition of lanthanum within the bone and less likelihood of adynamic bone histology compared with patients receiving calcium carbonate.[142] During a 2-year period, patients receiving lanthanum were not found to accelerate the natural deterioration in cognitive function seen in patients on HD.[143]

Lanthanum is supplied as chewable tablets for oral administration in four strengths: 250, 500, 750, and 1,000 mg. The recommended initial total daily dose is 750 to 1,500 mg given with meals, and dosage titration up to a maximal dosage of 3,000 mg daily based on serum phosphate levels. Lanthanum retains the same phosphorus-binding capabilities irrespective of whether it is chewed or crushed into powder.[144] Drug interactions with lanthanum include a reduction in the bioavailability of ciprofloxacin (approximate 50% reduction) and levothyroxine. The most frequent adverse events reported in clinical trials are nausea and vomiting.[145]

Iron-Based Phosphate Binders

Sucroferric oxyhydroxide and ferric citrate are iron-based phosphate binders with proven efficacy at reducing serum phosphate levels in hemodialysis patients. The newer iron-based binder ferric citrate has the advantage of providing supplemental iron. Early studies of ferric citrate demonstrate a reduction in IV iron and EPO-stimulating agent use.[146] However, sucroferric oxyhydroxide as a chewable tablet is not systemically absorbed, thus not affecting anemia management.[147]

Other Phosphate Binders

Aluminum preparations are very potent dietary phosphorus binders. Although these products were once used as first-line agents to decrease phosphorus, aluminum accumulation and toxicities in patients with CKD have restricted their use. Aluminum toxicity occurs in dialysis patients because absorbed aluminum is not removed by the diseased kidney and enters various tissues where it binds to tissue and plasma proteins. Aluminum accumulation in the bone, brain, and other organs leads to toxicities such as osteomalacia (aluminum-related bone disease), microcytic anemia, and a fatal neurologic syndrome referred to as *dialysis encephalopathy*.[91] Treatment of aluminum toxicity requires chelation with deferoxamine. Aluminum-containing agents should only be considered on a short-term basis (up to 4 weeks) for patients with a severely elevated phosphorus[91]; however, high-dose lanthanum may generally be preferred in these situations. Sucralfate, used primarily for the treatment of ulcers, also contains aluminum and should be used cautiously in patients with kidney disease.

Magnesium agents (magnesium hydroxide, magnesium carbonate) may be beneficial, but as with aluminum, their use should be limited because at the high doses required to control serum phosphorus concentrations, severe diarrhea and hypermagnesemia invariably result. Magnesium may be considered in patients whose serum phosphorus concentrations cannot be controlled adequately by other phosphate-binding agents. In this instance, a magnesium-containing phosphate binder may be added in conjunction with a reduction in the dialysate magnesium concentration (in the dialysis population). These agents should not be considered first-line therapy for control of phosphorus, and careful monitoring of magnesium is warranted if therapy is started.

More aggressive control of W.K.'s serum phosphorus is needed to lower serum phosphorus toward normal levels. Currently, W.K. is taking a calcium-based phosphate binder. Although presumably much of this calcium will be bound to phosphorus in the GI tract, a potential exists for calcium absorption. Furthermore, her serum calcium levels are in the upper range of normal not corrected. Sevelamer should be started to limit her calcium exposure and decrease her phosphorus levels. The recommended starting dose is 800 mg TID with meals, titrated based on follow-up phosphorus values. Adjustments should also be considered in conjunction with vitamin D therapy (see Vitamin D section). W.K. should be instructed to take her phosphate binder with meals. This regimen should be implemented in conjunction with a restricted-phosphorus diet. Regular reinforcement of the importance of compliance is necessary because nonadherence with prescribed dietary phosphorus restriction and drug therapy is one of the most significant factors associated with treatment failure. Use of a low-calcium dialysate may also help decrease her risk of hypercalcemia.

VITAMIN D

Nutritional Vitamin D

Nutritional vitamin D (NVD) occurs naturally as ergocalciferol (vitamin D_2) obtained from dietary sources and as cholecalciferol (vitamin D_3) obtained from dietary sources and activated in the skin by sunlight in mammals, both of which are inactive precursors of active forms of vitamin D. An intermediate activation step (25-hydroxylation) occurs in the liver to produce 25-hydroxy vitamin D (25-hydroxycalciferol), which is also relatively inactive (Fig. 28-2). Final activation (1-hydroxylation) occurs in the kidney, yielding calcitriol (1,25-dihydroxycholecalciferol), the active form of vitamin D. Thus, the response to vitamins D_2 and D_3 in patients with compromised kidney function can vary, depending on the degree of kidney dysfunction and the ability of the kidney to metabolize 25-hydroxyvitamin D to calcitriol. Decreased levels of 25-hydroxyvitamin D occur in the early stages of CKD, reducing substrate for producing calcitriol.[91] Altered vitamin D metabolism that occurs in this population warrants measurement of 25-hydroxyvitamin D and supplementation with NVD. Oral therapy with active vitamin D (oral calcitriol) or an analog (oral doxercalciferol) is likely warranted only when PTH remains elevated despite normal 25-hydroxyvitamin D levels.[91] As the final, active metabolite of vitamin D, calcitriol (or another activated form of vitamin D) is usually required in patients with more severe kidney disease (CKD 4–5).

Several small studies have shown that the benefits of NVD administration extend beyond bone and mineral metabolism. Reduction in ESA doses, improved glycemic control, reduced activated vitamin D administration, and inflammation modulation are benefits observed from NVD supplementation in dialysis patients.[148,149] Although some effects have been repeated in different studies, randomized control trials are needed to confirm these benefits.

Vitamin D Receptor Agonist

Calcitriol

Administration of vitamin D receptor agonist (VDRA), active vitamin D, in conjunction with control of serum phosphorus and calcium, is necessary in many patients with CKD to manage CKD-MBD. Calcitriol interacts with the vitamin D receptor (VDR) located in the parathyroid gland, intestines, bone, and kidney. It is thought to decrease PTH messenger RNA, resulting in decreased PTH secretion. In addition, calcitriol stimulates calcium absorption from the GI tract to correct hypocalcemia and prevent SHPT. In order to avoid hypercalcemia, the lowest effective dose should be used, and the patient's serum calcium should be monitored at least every 2 weeks for 1 month and then monthly thereafter. Furthermore, control of serum phosphorus is critical before calcitriol is initiated, as vitamin D increases GI phosphorus absorption.

Calcitriol is available as an oral formulation (Rocaltrol) or IV formulation (Calcijex). Administration of calcitriol by either the oral or IV route may be based on conventional dosing (usually 0.25–0.5 mcg/day) or pulse dosing (intermittent dosing of 0.5–2.0 mcg 2–3 times/week). Higher doses (e.g., 4 mcg 3 times/week) are generally required to reduce PTH secretion in more severe SHPT (PTH >1,000 pg/mL). Daily dosing of 0.25 to 0.5 mcg may be preferred in patients with hypocalcemia because this regimen primarily works to stimulate calcium absorption from the GI tract. Intermittent dosing of IV calcitriol is routine in the HD population because administration is coordinated with dialysis. In contrast, oral dosing is more convenient in patients with CKD who are not having dialysis and the PD population. Intact PTH and serum calcium concentrations are used to determine starting doses and dosing adjustments for calcitriol. Changes in Medicare have resulted in more outpatient hemodialysis units utilizing oral activated vitamin D therapy.

Intact PTH (1–84 PTH) is the 84-amino acid biologically active form of this hormone. It is metabolized into smaller, less-active fragments (e.g., 7–84 PTH) with activity that is not well characterized. These fragments are cleared from the circulation by the kidney and may accumulate in patients with CKD. Assays used for iPTH measure the intact structure as well as the biologically active and inactive PTH fragments. Thus, proposed ranges for iPTH in current guidelines are based on these assays. Assays that measure only the biologically active form (1–84 biPTH) have become available (third-generation assays). When iPTH is measured using both methods, there is roughly a 2:1 ratio between the second- and third-generation assay results. An iPTH of 150 pg/mL would correspond to a biPTH 75 pg/mL.[150] These assays correlate very well and the third-generation assay offers no advantage over the widely used second-generation assay. Clearly, the clinician must know which assay has been used to appropriately interpret the results, establish the desired PTH range, and correctly adjust therapy.

The KDIGO guidelines vary as they recommend iPTH levels to be maintained within the normal limits in CKD 3 and 4. However, the CKD 5D iPTH target range is 2 to 9 times the upper normal limits, approximately 150 to 600 pg/mL.

Dose adjustments of calcitriol are generally made in 0.5- to 1.0-mcg increments every 2 to 4 weeks in the early stages of therapy until iPTH and serum calcium are maintained at target levels. If hypercalcemia develops, the decision to withhold therapy or to switch to a less hypercalcemic VDRA must be made. Serum iPTH should be monitored every 3 to 6 months, and adjustments of calcitriol doses made to maintain the goal iPTH and to prevent hypercalcemia and hyperphosphatemia.

Paricalcitol

The unique interactions of vitamin D with the VDR led to the development of designer vitamin D analogs, which vary in their affinity for the VDR. In the case of treatment for SHPT, some were developed to retain the suppressive effect on PTH release while decreasing the potential for hypercalcemia relative to calcitriol. Currently approved agents for managing SHPT in the United States are paricalcitol (Zemplar), also referred to as 19-nor-1,25-dihydroxyvitamin D_2, and doxercalciferol (Hectorol), or 1-α-hydroxyvitamin D_2. Doxercalciferol requires conversion to the active form (1-α-,25-dihydroxyvitamin D_2) by the liver.

In patients with SHPT, paricalcitol significantly decreases iPTH without significantly increasing calcium or phosphorus. Paricalcitol is approximately 10-fold less hypercalcemic and hyperphosphatemic than calcitriol.[151,152] The initial dose of IV paricalcitol is 0.04 mcg/kg to 0.1 mcg/kg (2.8–7 mcg) administered with each dialysis session or every other day.[153] Oral paricalcitol capsules are available in three strengths (1, 2, and 4 mcg) administered daily or 3 times weekly. The starting dose should be 1 mcg daily or 2 mcg 3 times weekly if the baseline iPTH level is 500 pg/mL or less, and 2 mcg daily or 4 mcg 3 times weekly if the iPTH is greater than 500 pg/mL. Some data have also suggested paricalcitol dosing based on initial PTH levels (paricalcitol dose = PTH/80) rather than weight as a reasonable dosing strategy.[153] Doses can be titrated every 2 to 4 weeks based on iPTH values.

The recommended conversion ratio for calcitriol to paricalcitol is 1:4 (i.e., for every 1 mcg of calcitriol, 4 mcg of paricalcitol should be administered). This information is based on similar efficacy observed when patients treated for SHPT with calcitriol were switched to paricalcitol using this dosing strategy.[151,152] A lower ratio of 1:3 also has been proposed in patients resistant to therapy with calcitriol.

Doxercalciferol

Doxercalciferol, another vitamin D analog, is an alternative to calcitriol and has been studied in patients with CKD 5D. Doxercalciferol has similar effects on PTH as the other vitamin D analogs; however, it increases phosphorus and calcium to a greater degree than paricalcitol.[154] Doxercalciferol is available as a capsule and IV injection. The doses were 4 mcg IV or 10 mcg orally 3 times a week with HD. Oral and IV therapy are both effective in reducing iPTH levels in patients with SHPT; however, some evidence indicated that intermittent IV therapy may result in less hypercalcemia and hyperphosphatemia than oral intermittent therapy.[155] The recommended starting dose of doxercalciferol for patients on dialysis is 4 mcg IV or 10 mcg orally administered 3 times a week with dosing titration based on changes in iPTH.[156,157]

Vitamin D analogs offer an alternative for patients in whom persistent hypercalcemia develops with calcitriol therapy. Use of these agents is increasing in clinical practice because of the concerns of hypercalcemia and its adverse consequences. Repeated observational reports indicate lower overall and cardiovascular-related mortality rates with activated vitamin D therapy, regardless of the agent received, than in those not receiving vitamin D therapy.[158] Two trials also examined survival advantages among the different forms of vitamin D in patients on HD. One report indicated that receiving paricalcitol for 36 months conferred a survival advantage starting at 12 months from initiation of therapy and increased with time compared with those receiving calcitriol. Another study reported that patients taking either paricalcitol or doxercalciferol had a significantly lower mortality rate than patients receiving calcitriol, although when adjusted for laboratory values and clinic standardized mortality, no difference was found between the products.[158]

Possible biologic reasons for vitamin D improving outcomes include its role in downregulating the RAAS and immunomodulatory properties. A prospective trial would be required to confirm a survival advantage associated with vitamin D therapy.

CALCIMIMETICS

Calcimimetic agents increase the sensitivity of the calcium-sensing receptors (CaSR) to extracellular calcium ions and inhibit the release of PTH, lowering PTH levels within hours after administration. The discovery of extracellular CaSR prompted research with calcimimetic agents that allosterically modulate CaSR. CaSR are located in the parathyroid gland, thyroid, nephron, brain, intestine, bone, lung, and other tissues.[159] The calcimimetic cinacalcet is the first agent in this class to be approved by the FDA to treat SHPT in ESRD.[160] Cinacalcet is an effective agent at reducing and sustaining iPTH within target concentrations in HD patients.[161] Cinacalcet offers an additional choice of agent to lower PTH when vitamin D cannot be increased because of elevated calcium or phosphorus. The EVOLVE trial was a randomized clinical trial comparing cinacalcet to placebo in 3,883 dialysis patients with a primary outcome of death, cardiovascular events, or hospitalizations. Patients were eligible to receive phosphate binders or vitamin D analogs in either arm. There was 7% nonsignificant reduction in primary end points in the cinacalcet group.[162] However, issues plagued the large trial as several patients in the placebo arm actually received cinacalcet therapy. The survival benefits of cinacalcet remained undetermined. Cinacalcet is not FDA approved for use in CKD patients not receiving dialysis because it is associated with frequent hypocalcemic episodes.[163]

Appropriate treatment for W.K. should be based on assessment of her serum calcium, phosphorus, and PTH values. She currently has an elevated PTH, phosphorus, and calcium; therefore, cinacalcet should be started in conjunction with her dietary phosphorus restriction, phosphate binder regimen, and vitamin D therapy. Cinacalcet should be initiated at a dose of 30 mg daily, with dosage titrations occurring every 2 to 4 weeks to 60, 90, 120, or a maximum of 180 mg daily to achieve target iPTH levels. Serum calcium and phosphorous levels should be drawn within 1 week after initiation or dosage increase, and plasma PTH levels drawn within 4 weeks after initiation of therapy or dosage adjustment. Nausea and vomiting are the most common adverse events associated with cinacalcet. Nausea is twice as likely to occur at any dose, while vomiting is more frequent at higher doses.[162] In phase III trials, 66% of patients receiving cinacalcet experienced at least one episode of hypocalcemia (serum calcium <8.4 mg/dL), although less than 1% of patients discontinued treatment.[164] The high incidence of hypocalcemia is not solely caused by lowered PTH activity but is also attributed to the mechanism of action of cinacalcet. It is thought that activation of CaSR in bone, intestine, and other tissues may contribute to hypocalcemia. Most episodes of hypocalcemia occur during the initiation of cinacalcet therapy, and slowly titrating the dose reduces the risk. Seizures caused by hypocalcemia have been reported. Vitamin D or calcium-based phosphate binders can be used to increase serum calcium levels between 7.5 and 8.4 mg/dL. If serum calcium falls below 7.5 mg/dL and is associated with symptoms of hypocalcemia and vitamin D cannot be increased further, cinacalcet should be withheld until serum calcium normalizes or the patient is asymptomatic. Cinacalcet is a strong in vitro inhibitor of cytochrome P-450 isoenzyme CYP2D6; therefore, dose adjustments of concomitant medications that are predominantly metabolized by CYP2D6 may be required. Cinacalcet is also a substrate of CYP3A4, and ketoconazole, a potent inhibitor of CYP3A4, has been shown to increase the area under the curve of cinacalcet 2.3 times. Thus, other inhibitors of the CYP3A4 isoenzyme should be used with caution in patients receiving cinacalcet.[160]

PARATHYROIDECTOMY

The parathyroid glands enlarge as a compensatory response to disturbances of phosphorus, calcium, and calcitriol metabolism in patients with CKD. Timely administration of vitamin D therapy to prevent parathyroid hyperplasia is crucial as treatment with vitamin D cannot adequately reverse established hyperplasia. A parathyroidectomy is often reserved for patients with severe hyperparathyroidism with PTH values greater than 1,000 pg/mL, concomitant hypercalcemia, and failure to respond to pharmacologic therapy.[91] Parathyroidectomy can be subtotal, total, or total with autotransplantation. One of the major complications of parathyroidectomy is the early development of postsurgical hypocalcemia.[165] Clinical symptoms of hypocalcemia include muscle irritability, fatigue, depression, and memory loss. Patients should be monitored closely after parathyroidectomy, and all patients with signs or symptoms of hypocalcemia should be treated with calcium supplementation (see Chapter 27, Fluid and Electrolyte Disorders). In patients who have had subtotal parathyroidectomy, the remaining parathyroid tissues will start functioning adequately, so the acute hypocalcemia is transient, lasting only a few days. Hypocalcemia is permanent in total parathyroidectomy and requires long-term treatment with calcitriol and oral calcium supplements (1–1.5 g/day of elemental calcium). Studies investigating SHPT management with cinacalcet report reduced rates of parathyroidectomy surgeries.[162,166]

OTHER COMPLICATIONS OF CKD

Endocrine Abnormalities Caused by Uremia

CASE 28-3, QUESTION 3: Does W.K.'s hypothyroidism have any relationship to her CKD? What other endocrine abnormalities are associated with uremia?

Disturbances in thyroid function are frequently encountered in patients with CKD because the kidney is involved in all aspects of peripheral thyroid hormone metabolism. Common laboratory abnormalities include reduced serum concentrations of total thyroxine (T_4) and 3,5,3′-triiodothyronine (T_3) and a low free thyroxine index (FTI). The thyroid-stimulating hormone (TSH) concentration is usually normal, but peripheral conversion of T_4 to T_3 is reduced in uremic patients.[167] Despite these abnormalities, clinical hypothyroidism does not occur solely as a result of kidney disease, probably because the amount of free (unbound to protein) thyroid hormone in serum remains normal. Hypothyroidism in patients with kidney failure should be confirmed by the presence of an elevated serum TSH concentration and a low serum concentration of free T_4.

Other endocrine abnormalities that have been observed in patients with CKD include gonadal dysfunction leading to impotence, diminished testicular size, menstrual abnormalities, and cessation of ovulation.[168] Decreased libido and infertility occur in both sexes. Uremic women of childbearing age should be counseled on the risk of becoming pregnant because of the multiple complications of pregnancy in ESRD, including high termination rates.[169]

Altered Glucose and Insulin Metabolism

CASE 28-3, QUESTION 4: Other than the obvious effect of W.K.'s diabetes mellitus on blood glucose, are there any effects of kidney disease itself on glucose metabolism?

Uremia often is associated with glucose intolerance early in the course of kidney disease in nondiabetic patients. Specifically, patients with CKD often exhibit an abnormal response to an oral glucose challenge and have sustained hyperinsulinemia.[170,171] The fasting blood glucose is typically within normal limits. Diminished tissue sensitivity to the action of insulin is also observed. Inflammation and oxidative stress are likely contributors predisposing CKD patients to insulin resistance.[172] Most nondiabetic patients with kidney disease do not require therapy for hyperglycemia, and dialysis can correct these abnormalities in glucose metabolism.

Patients with diabetes mellitus and advanced kidney disease may experience improved glucose control and decreased insulin requirements. This is because the kidney is responsible for a substantial amount of daily insulin degradation and, as the disease progresses, less insulin is cleared and its metabolic half-life is increased. A decreased clearance of insulin by muscle tissue also can occur in patients with uremia.[173] Thus, in diabetic patients with progressive kidney disease, blood glucose concentrations should be monitored and insulin doses adjusted to avoid hypoglycemia. W.K. has CKD 5D and is receiving her insulin in the peritoneal dialysate solution. Hyperglycemia is also a concern in W.K. because the glucose present in her continuous ambulatory peritoneal dialysis (CAPD) fluid to promote fluid removal will be absorbed systemically. Insulin dosage adjustments should be made on the basis of repeated home blood glucose measurements, changes in the CAPD prescription, and glycosylated hemoglobin determinations.

Gastrointestinal Complications

CASE 28-3, QUESTION 5: One month before her current clinic visit, W.K. complained of nausea and vomiting of partially digested food. Metoclopramide (Reglan) was begun at that time. Could W.K.'s nausea and vomiting have been caused by her kidney failure? Was the appropriate therapy selected?

GI abnormalities are extremely common in patients with CKD and include anorexia, nausea, vomiting, hiccups, abdominal pain, GI bleeding, diarrhea, and constipation. Diminished gastric motility can occur from uremia; however, this problem may improve with adequate HD. Dyspeptic complaints and gastroparesis may be more prevalent in the PD population than in the HD population and in the earlier stages of CKD.[174] W.K. has diabetes and diabetic neuropathy, which also contributes to the delayed gastric emptying (diabetic gastroparesis) and retention of food in the upper intestinal tract. This frequently causes distension, nausea, and vomiting. Metoclopramide is recommended to relieve these symptoms, although the risk for extrapyramidal side effects should be considered. A lower dose of 5 mg before meals may be warranted for W.K.

Severe uremia also causes nausea and vomiting, and these can be initial presenting symptoms of kidney failure. At this stage of clinical presentation, dialysis is the preferred therapy. Drug-induced nausea and vomiting always should be considered because patients with CKD often take multiple drugs and are at risk for drug toxicity because of diminished kidney function (e.g., digitalis intoxication).

BLEEDING

CASE 28-3, QUESTION 6: During her clinic visit, W.K. reports that her bowel movements have become black and tarry in appearance. A rectal examination reveals guaiac-positive stools. Is GI bleeding related to kidney failure?

W.K. should be evaluated for peptic ulcer disease and lower GI bleeding. Uremic patients are at risk for bleeding from mucosal surfaces such as the stomach. Angiodysplasia of the stomach and duodenum, as well as erosive esophagitis, are the most common causes of bleeding in patients with CKD.[175] Treatment of upper GI bleeding in uremic patients usually consists of cautious use of H_2-receptor antagonists, which should be given in reduced doses according to the degree of kidney function. Proton-pump inhibitors are primarily eliminated by nonkidney routes and can be administered at standard doses (see Chapter 23, Upper Gastrointestinal Disorders).

Dermatologic Complications

Several dermal abnormalities have been observed in patients with CKD, including hyperpigmentation, abnormal perspiration, skin dryness, and persistent pruritus. Of these, *uremic pruritus* can be the most bothersome for the patient and may lead to repeated scratching and skin excoriation. Hyperparathyroidism, hypervitaminosis A, and dermal mast cell proliferation with subsequent histamine release have been suggested as causes of pruritus.[176]

Treatment of pruritus often is a frustrating experience for the patient and clinician. Although many therapies have been advocated, few have provided sustained benefit. A trial-and-error approach is recommended. Efficient dialysis therapy relieves pruritus in some patients and pharmacologic therapy may be avoided. When necessary, initial pharmacologic treatment usually consists of oral antihistamines (e.g., hydroxyzine). Topical emollients or topical steroids may provide benefit if antihistamine therapy is not completely successful. If pruritus is still present, other treatment options can be tried. These include cholestyramine, ultraviolet B phototherapy, and oral administration of activated charcoal. Control of calcium, phosphorus, and PTH concentrations is also advocated to reduce pruritus in patients with CKD.[176]

GLOMERULAR DISEASE

Glomerular diseases lead to many complications that result from disruption of normal glomerular structure and function. Several clinical syndromes of glomerular disease exist; however, GN, characterized as proliferation and inflammation of the glomerulus, is observed most frequently. According to the most recent USRDS report, GN as a broad category remains the third leading cause of ESRD in the United States.[3] In developing countries, ESRD caused by GN is more common as a result of various infectious processes causing kidney failure.

Nephrotic Syndrome

Nephrotic syndrome is characterized by proteinuria greater than 3.5 g/day, hypoalbuminemia, edema, and hyperlipidemia. In more severe conditions, hypercoagulable conditions are increased from a loss of hemostasis control proteins, including antithrombin III, protein S, and protein C. This syndrome can occur with or without a change in GFR. Nephrotic syndrome may be caused by a primary disease, such as membranous glomerulopathy, which is characterized by deposition of immune complexes, or other systemic diseases including diabetic glomerulosclerosis and amyloidosis. Elevated serum cholesterol and triglycerides are observed in patients with this degree of proteinuria ($>$3.5 g/day). This hyperlipidemic condition also predisposes patients with nephrotic syndrome to accelerated atherosclerosis. Hyperlipidemia itself can also contribute to progression of kidney disease. Because nephrotic syndrome is associated with numerous causes, further evaluation of the patient for systemic causes is required to determine the course of therapy and prognosis.

Chronic Glomerulopathies

GN can occur as a primary disease that is idiopathic in origin (e.g., focal segmental glomerulosclerosis [FSGS]) or as a secondary manifestation of other systemic disease (e.g., lupus nephritis [LN], Wegener granulomatosis). Kidney biopsy is often required for definitive diagnosis. Glomerular lesions associated with glomerulopathies are characterized as diffuse, focal, or segmental, depending on the extent of involvement of individual glomeruli. Pathologic changes are characterized as proliferative, membranous, and sclerotic based on the pattern observed. Proliferative changes usually involve an overgrowth of the epithelium or mesangium, whereas membranous changes are typically described as a thickening of the glomerular basement membrane. Signs and symptoms of GN include hematuria, proteinuria, and decreased kidney function. An autoimmune reaction is the predominant pathogenic process leading to most forms of primary and secondary GN. Although a number of autoantibodies are associated with GN, their exact role in the pathogenesis of GN is still unclear.[177]

Glomerular damage generally occurs in two phases: acute and chronic. During the acute phase, immune reactions occur within glomeruli that stimulate the complement cascade, ultimately resulting in glomerular damage. Nonimmune mechanisms that occur in response to loss of nephron function and hyperfiltration of remaining nephrons are characteristic of the chronic phase.

GN often causes acute kidney failure. Patients with damage to more than 50% of glomeruli in the presence of rapid loss in kidney function (over the course of days to weeks) are classified as having rapidly progressive glomerulonephritis (RPGN).[178] If kidney involvement is severe, signs and symptoms of uremia may develop. RPGN may be classified based on the immunopathogenic etiology of the glomerular damage: (a) immune complex deposition (e.g., LN); (b) nonimmune deposit-mediated mechanism (e.g., Wegener granulomatosis); and (c) sclerotic lesions of the glomerulus (e.g., FSGS).[177] This chapter focuses on the treatment of the more common forms of chronic GN (i.e., LN, Wegener granulomatosis, FSGS).

LUPUS NEPHRITIS

Systemic lupus erythematosus (SLE) is a multisystem autoimmune disease characterized by abnormalities in cell-mediated immunity, such as B-cell hyperresponsiveness and defective T-cell–mediated suppressor activity. In certain predisposed individuals, SLE can lead to the development of LN, a secondary form of GN. LN is the prototypical immune complex–mediated kidney disease, characterized by deposition or in situ formation of autoantibody–antigen complexes along the glomerular capillary network. LN remains an important cause of mortality. Up to 60% of adults with SLE have some degree of kidney involvement later in the course of their disease, discernible from clinical evidence of kidney damage: heavy proteinuria, hematuria, decreased eGFR, and hypertension. Early in the disease, laboratory abnormalities indicative of kidney involvement are seen in approximately 25% to 50% of patients[177] (see also Chapter 33, Systemic Lupus Erythematosus).

CASE 28-4

QUESTION 1: S.L., a 34-year-old black woman with a 7-year history of SLE, presents to the nephrology clinic for follow-up of LN. BP of 160/95. Pertinent laboratory values are as follows:

Serum Na, 146 mEq/L
K, 4.2 mEq/L
Cl, 100 mEq/L
CO_2 content, 25 mEq/L
SCr, 2.0 mg/dL
BUN, 20 mg/dL
WBC count, 9,600/μL

RBC indices are normal. Platelet count is 175,000/μL. Her 24-hour urine contains 2.3 g of albumin (normal, <30 mg/day), and her urine analysis shows 12 RBCs/high-power field (HPF) (normal, 0–3). Compared with her visit of a week ago, S.L.'s kidney function and urinary indices (proteinuria, hematuria) show substantial worsening of her nephritis. S.L. was hospitalized, and a kidney biopsy showed inflammation of 40% of the glomeruli. What subjective and objective data in S.L. are consistent with a diagnosis of LN, and what is the stage of her nephritis?

S.L. has clinical evidence of kidney damage as demonstrated by her proteinuria, hematuria, and a slightly increased SCr concentration. Glomerular damage is most evident by the presence of RBC or red cell casts in the urine, a finding observed in S.L.

Classifications

The International Society of Nephrology and the Renal Pathology Society (ISN/RPS) classification system was developed in 2003 to replace the previous classification system published by the World Health Organization (Table 28-11).[179] This classification scheme provides a reasonable correlation among histopathology, outcome, and response to treatment. S.L. has proteinuria, hematuria, and inflammation of less than 50% of her glomeruli, and she is diagnosed as having class III/A (focal proliferative) GN.

Table 28-11
2003 International Society of Nephrology/Renal Pathology Society Classification of Lupus Nephritis[177]

Class	Histologic Characterization	Usual Clinical Presentation
I	Minimal mesangial lupus nephritis	Mild proteinuria
II	Mesangial proliferative glomerulonephritis	Mild proteinuria and urine sediment abnormalities
III	Focal and segmental proliferative glomerulonephritis A: active lesions; A/C: active and chronic lesions; C: chronic lesions	Proteinuria and hematuria
IV	Diffuse proliferative segmental (S) or global (G) glomerulonephritis A: active lesions; A/C: active and chronic lesions; C: chronic lesions	Heavy proteinuria; active sediment; hypertension; renal failure
V	Membranous glomerulonephritis	Proteinuria; often nephrotic syndrome
VI	Advanced sclerosing glomerulonephritis	Proteinuria; renal failure; nephrotic syndrome

Data from the 2003 International Society of Nephrology/Renal Pathology Society Classification of Lupus Nephritis.

Treatment

CASE 28-4, QUESTION 2: Should S.L.'s LN be treated?

Unlike nonkidney manifestations of SLE, serologic markers of disease correlate poorly with LN. Therefore, elevations in SCr, hypertension, proteinuria and hematuria, as seen in S.L., are used as primary markers of disease activity.

Treatment of LN must address both management of the acute disease process and maintenance therapy for the more stable chronic disease process. A general consensus is that patients, such as S.L., who present with focal or diffuse proliferative GN (class III or IV) should be treated aggressively, with the primary goal of preventing irreversible kidney damage. The prognosis of kidney function in patients with SLE has improved. However, the prognosis is worse in blacks when compared with the white population treated for SLE.[180] Elevated SCr, heavy proteinuria, anemia, and disease onset during childhood or in those older than 60 years of age are other predictors of a worse prognosis. Advances in pharmacologic therapy (i.e., safer immunosuppressive regimens and antihypertensives) have improved the prognosis for the population as a whole.

The treatment of LN is primarily empiric but is based, to some extent, on histologic findings. The KDIGO Clinical Practice Guideline for Glomerulonephritis provides recommendations for treatment based on disease activity.[177] Although appropriate treatment can improve patient outcomes, vigorous attempts to suppress SLE activity may lead to serious drug-related complications.

The primary strategy in the treatment of LN involves suppression of the immune system with corticosteroids and cytotoxic agents, such as cyclophosphamide (CYC), azathioprine (AZA), calcineurin inhibitor (CNI) therapy (cyclosporine or tacrolimus) and mycophenolate mofetil (MMF). Clinicians need to be aware of the potential complications associated with these therapies and carefully monitor patients to determine the indication for treatment and improved prognosis. Toxicities associated with immunosuppressive agents depend on both the dose and the duration of therapy. Abnormalities in hematopoiesis, such as neutropenia and thrombocytopenia, are the most common adverse effects associated with cytotoxic agents. Immunosuppression, in general, increases a patient's susceptibility to a vast array of infections and to lymphocytic malignancies. In addition, the alkylating agent CYC can cause nausea and vomiting, gonadal toxicity, hemorrhagic cystitis, and alopecia. The risk versus benefit of CYC use has to be seriously weighed in young women who are considering pregnancy in the future. The antimetabolite AZA can cause pancreatitis and abnormalities in liver function. The selective inhibitor of inosine monophosphate dehydrogenase, MMF, although relatively benign compared with the other agents, can cause GI disturbances.

Induction Therapy

Therapy for LN is usually not indicated in patients with normal kidney function and proteinuria less than 1 g, because these patients have a good prognosis. Corticosteroids represent the cornerstone of therapy in patients with a mild form of LN. Prednisone (1 mg/kg or methylprednisolone) should be initiated for patients with class II LN with proteinuria >3 g/day or CNI. In patients with a more severe form (class III and IV), prednisone 1 mg/kg/day combined with either CYC or MMF should be initiated. For the treatment of acute exacerbations of LN, high-dose pulse therapy with methylprednisolone may be warranted. Given that S.L.'s LN has worsened, she should receive pulse methylprednisolone (0.5–1 g IV, not to exceed 1 g) for 3 days in an attempt to reduce the degree of proteinuria and improve kidney function.[177] Although generally well tolerated, rapid methylprednisolone injections can cause transient tremor, flushing, and altered taste sensation. To reduce the risk of adverse effects associated with the rate of injection, S.L. should receive methylprednisolone for 30 minutes. After a course of pulse methylprednisolone therapy, oral prednisone at a dose 10 to 20 mg daily may be initiated.[177] Suppression of S.L.'s active LN should be demonstrated by a reduction in proteinuria and hematuria and an increase in her eGFR.

The addition of cytotoxic agents is reserved for patients who do not respond to corticosteroids alone, or those who have unacceptable toxicity to corticosteroids, worsening kidney function, severe proliferative lesions, or evidence of sclerosis on kidney biopsy. Induction therapy with six monthly pulse doses of IV CYC (0.5–1 g/m^2) or six doses of CYC given every 2 weeks at a dose of 0.5 g/m^2 along with steroid therapy was shown to have improved kidney outcomes with fewer flares and relapses.[177] Before and for 24 hours after initiating IV CYC, the patient must be well hydrated to prevent bladder toxicity. Alternatively, MMF (2,000–3,000 mg/day times 6 months) or TAC (0.06–0.1 mg/kg/day) has been proven to be as effective as CYC in the induction treatment for LN.[181,182] Given the significant toxicities associated with CYC (e.g., gonadal toxicity and hemorrhagic cystitis), MMF or tacrolimus are attractive options given their antiinflammatory properties and the lower side effect profile. Recently, rituximab, an anti-CD20 monoclonal antibody, has demonstrated similar efficacy as MMF and CYC.[183]

Maintenance Therapy

Once the acute flare resolves (generally in up to 12 weeks), low-dose, maintenance steroid therapy with 5 to 15 mg/day of prednisone can be initiated in combination with cytotoxic therapy, if indicated, based on the severity of LN. In a meta-analysis assessing the efficacy of therapeutic agents used to treat LN, improved outcomes (total mortality and ESRD) were associated with use of oral prednisone in combination with IV CYC. As a result, the National Institutes of Health recommends the use of IV CYC pulse therapy (0.5–1 g/m^2) every 3 months for up to 2 years for maintenance therapy of LN.[177] An additional benefit of combination therapy with immunosuppressive agents is their steroid-sparing effect and, potentially, lower risk of steroid toxicity.

Steroid and CYC free regimens are often desired to avoid steroid and CYC adverse events. Studies have evaluated other immunosuppressive agents (AZA, MMF) for maintenance therapy in light of the toxicities associated with CYC or steroids. The KDIGO Clinical Practice Guideline for Glomerulonephritis recommends AZA (1.5–2.5 mg/kg/day) or MMF (1–2 g/day) and low-dose corticosteroids (≤10 mg/day prednisone equivalent) for maintenance therapy.[177]

A multi-regimen trial compared maintenance therapy with AZA (1–3 mg/day) and MMF (500–3,000 mg/day) with CYC along with steroids after induction with CYC in patients with severe LN. Patients receiving AZA had a lower mortality rate than those treated with CYC, and the MMF treatment group had fewer relapses than the CYC treatment group.[184] MMF and AZA may be indicated in patients resistant to CYC therapy or with a more severe type of LN (class III and IV). The addition of AZA or MMF, along with corticosteroid therapy, should be considered in S.L. once the acute lupus flare resolves. Once suppression of S.L.'s LN is documented, initiation of either AZA or MMF and steroids is indicated because of the severity of her LN (class III). The duration of therapy is dictated by the individual's response, but typically patients will require up to 2 years of maintenance therapy.

Alternative Agents

The KDIGO practice guidelines recommend reserving CNI for those intolerant to MMF or AZA as maintenance therapy.[177] Rituximab, a monoclonal antibody that inhibits B-cell production, is being studied because B-cell hyperactivity is one of the major pathophysiologic mechanisms of LN. Small studies in patients with LN resistant to therapy have shown rituximab to be of benefit. Cyclosporine, in doses of 5 mg/kg/day, may also provide an alternative therapy to treat lupus in the maintenance phase in patients unresponsive to treatment.[177]

WEGENER GRANULOMATOSIS

CASE 28-5

QUESTION 1: J.M. is a 42-year-old white man who presents to the clinic with a 1-month history of cough, nasal congestion, facial pain with headache, fever, and lethargy. During the past week, he has noted bright red blood in his phlegm, which has worsened in the past 3 days. Pertinent laboratory values are as follows:

Serum Na, 143 mEq/L
K, 5.1 mEq/L
Cl, 102 mEq/L
CO_2 content, 24 mEq/L
SCr, 2.8 mg/dL
BUN, 41 mg/dL

This compares with last year's physical checkup visit when his SCr and BUN were within the normal range. Hematologic studies reveal an Hct of 35%, an Hgb of 11.7 g/dL, a mean corpuscular volume of 69 μL, a mean corpuscular Hgb concentration of 24%, and a reticulocyte count of 1.8%. RBC indices are normal, and the platelet count is 175,000/μL. His 24-hour urine contains 3.8 g of albumin (normal, <30 mg), and his eGFR is calculated to be 27 mL/minute/1.73 m^2. His urine also contains many RBC casts and 16 RBCs/HPF (normal, 0–3 RBCs/HPF). Chest radiograph shows alveolar shadowing spreading from the hilar region. The result of J.M.'s cytoplasmic-staining, antineutrophil cytoplasmic antibody (c-ANCA) is positive. On the basis of his subjective and objective data, which of the chronic glomerulopathies is J.M. likely to have?

Wegener granulomatosis is a primary systemic vasculitis characterized by granulomatous inflammation of the upper and lower respiratory tract and secondary GN. Primary systemic vasculitic syndromes, such as Wegener granulomatosis, often cause GN. Although vasculitis involves inflammation of blood vessels of any size, the small- and medium-size vessels are most commonly affected.[185] The etiology of Wegener granulomatosis is unclear; however, an autoimmune response is suspected for two reasons. First, Wegener granulomatosis is a systemic inflammatory disease without a known infectious etiology. Second, good treatment response can be obtained with immunosuppressive therapy.

The clinical features of Wegener granulomatosis include upper airway disease, such as sinusitis, epistaxis, and nasopharyngitis, as well as otitis media caused by blockage of the eustachian tube. Constitutional symptoms include fever, night sweats, arthralgia, anorexia, and malaise. After a few months, weakness may progress, severely limiting physical activity. Although the lungs are invariably affected, most patients remain asymptomatic; however, cough and hemoptysis may be present. J.M.'s presenting symptoms are consistent with the above clinical features. The laboratory signs also are nonspecific and indicate the presence of a systemic inflammatory process. They include an elevated erythrocyte sedimentation rate in virtually all patients, anemia of chronic disease, and thrombocytosis.[185] Hematuria and proteinuria can be prominent features of Wegener granulomatosis and are present on initial presentation in 80% of patients. The presence of severely diminished kidney function, seen in approximately 10% of patients, is an ominous sign, with nearly one-third of these patients progressing to ESRD. All patients with Wegener granulomatosis are at risk of developing irreversible, rapidly progressive kidney failure. Kidney histologic findings are nonspecific, with most patients exhibiting necrotizing crescentic GN.[185]

Wegener granulomatosis is diagnosed primarily by the presenting signs and symptoms. According to the American College of Rheumatology 1990 classification, a person is diagnosed with Wegener granulomatosis if any two of the following four criteria are present: (a) nasal or oral inflammation, (b) abnormal chest radiograph, (c) microhematuria (>5 RBCs/HPF) or RBC casts in the urine sediment, or (d) granulomatous inflammation on biopsy.[185] J.M. has satisfied three of the four criteria for diagnosing Wegener granulomatosis.

Treatment

CASE 28-5, QUESTION 2: How should J.M.'s Wegener granulomatosis be treated?

The discovery of c-ANCA and its strong association with Wegener granulomatosis has permitted a more certain diagnosis. Because of the substantial rise in titer that commonly precedes relapse of Wegener granulomatosis, the c-ANCA test is best used to follow the course of disease activity and guide induction of therapy. Treatment with CYC and corticosteroids results in improvement in kidney function in approximately 80% to 85% of patients, versus 75% with pulse steroids alone.[177] The main predictive factors for treatment success are the extent of kidney damage before therapy starts and how long therapy is delayed after symptoms develop.

Cyclophosphamide

Because Wegener granulomatosis is considered an autoimmune inflammatory disease, immunosuppressive therapy is the mainstay of treatment. Table 28-12 list KDIGO guidelines-recommended treatment regimens. Therapy is generally indicated for 6 months if remission occurs and up to 12 months in resistant cases.[185] J.M.

Table 28-12
Recommended Treatment Regimens for ANCA Vasculitis with GN[177]

Agent	Route	Initial dose
Cyclophosphamide[a]	IV	0.75 g/m^2 q 3–4 weeks. Decrease initial dose to 0.5 g/m^2 if age >60 years or GFR <20 mL/minute/1.73 m^2. Adjust subsequent doses to achieve a 2-week nadir leukocyte count >3,000/mm^3.
Cyclophosphamide[b]	PO	1.5–2 mg/kg/day, reduce if age >60 years or GFR <20 mL/minute/1.73 m^2. Adjust the daily dose to keep leucocyte count >3,000/mm^3
Corticosteroids	IV	Pulse methylprednisolone: 500 mg i.v. daily × 3 days.
Corticosteroids	PO	Prednisone 1 mg/kg/day for 4 weeks, not exceeding 60 mg daily. Taper down over 3–4 months.
Rituximab[c]	IV	375 mg/m^2 weekly × 4.
Plasmapheresis[d]		60 mL/kg volume replacement. Vasculitis: 7 treatments over 14 days. If diffuse pulmonary hemorrhage, daily until the bleeding stops, then every other day, total 7–10 treatments. Vasculitis in association with anti-GBM antibodies: Daily for 14 days or until anti-GBM antibodies are undetectable

[a]Given with pulse and oral steroids. An alternative IV cyclophosphamide dosing schema is 15 mg/kg given every 2 weeks for three pulses, followed by 15 mg/kg given every 3 weeks for 3 months beyond remission, with reductions for age and estimated GFR.
[b]Given with pulse and oral steroids.
[c]Given with pulse and oral steroids.
[d]Not given with pulse methylprednisolone. Replacement fluid is 5% albumin. Add 150 to 300 mL fresh frozen plasma at the end of each pheresis session if patients have pulmonary hemorrhage, or have had recent surgery, including kidney biopsy.
ANCA, antineutrophil cytoplasmic antibody; GBM, glomerular basement membrane; GFR, glomerular filtration rate; GN, glomerulonephritis; IV, intravenous; PO, orally.

should be started on oral CYC 2 mg/kg/day, as a single morning dose, and corticosteroids to prevent irreversible glomerular scarring. High fluid intake (>3 L/day) and mesna reduce the risk of hemorrhagic cystitis. Regular UA should be performed (every 3–6 months) to detect hematuria caused by hemorrhagic cystitis.

Corticosteroids

The main role of corticosteroids is to induce remission of the disease. J.M. should receive prednisone 1 mg/kg/day in addition to CYC. The combined regimen should be continued for 2 to 4 weeks until the immunosuppressive effect of CYC becomes evident. Then, during the next 2 months, the prednisone dose can be tapered to 60 mg every other day to reduce the risk of infection. Then, the dose can be tapered by 5 mg/week to discontinue prednisone over the course of 3 to 6 months. For patients with a more fulminant form of the disease, pulse methylprednisolone 500 mg/day for three doses is administered. The dose can be repeated in 1 to 2 weeks if disease progression is uncontrolled.

Alternative Therapies

Rituximab as an induction agent has been evaluated in two randomized controlled trials. The RITUXVAS randomized 44 subjects to rituximab (375 mg/m^2 weekly × 4) plus IV CYC or to IV CYC alone. Each group received IV methylprednisolone followed by oral corticosteroids. Remission rates were 76% for the rituximab group and 82% for CYC. The RAVE trial rituximab was compared to oral CYC (2 mg/kg/day) for up to 3 months plus AZA (2 mg/kg/day) for 4 to 6 months. IV methylprednisolone plus oral corticosteroid were given to both groups. Rituximab proved noninferior to the CYC regimen with similar rates, 64% versus 53%, respectively. There were no significant differences in adverse events rates in either trial. Although rituximab has performed well in comparison studies, the high cost limits it acceptance and applicability in clinical practice.

Azathioprine and Mycophenolate Mofetil

AZA (1–2 mg/kg/day) and MMF (up to 1 gram daily) are effective as maintenance therapy once remission has been achieved with CYC. However, a comparative study demonstrated mycophenolate to be less effective at maintaining remissions compared with AZA, thus AZA is the preferred maintenance therapy.[186] Maintenance therapy should be continued for a minimum of 18 months for patients in complete remission.

Alternative Agents

Methotrexate (MTX) may be beneficial for patients with milder disease, although one study demonstrated high relapse rates in patients treated initially with weekly MTX and daily prednisone; disease was controlled in only select patients.[187] However, MTX should be reserved for patients intolerant of AZA and MMF and GFR >60 mL/min/1.73 m^2. Use of trimethoprim-sulfamethoxazole for 1 year was evaluated for patients in remission or after treatment with CYC and prednisolone and is recommended for those with upper respiratory tract disease. A reduction in relapse rate was demonstrated compared with placebo; however, trimethoprim-sulfamethoxazole use is not supported.[187]

FOCAL SEGMENTAL GLOMERULOSCLEROSIS

CASE 28-6

QUESTION 1: A.G. is a 37-year-old morbidly obese (body mass index, 40 kg/m^2), black woman who presents to the clinic with complaints of increased swelling in her extremities for the last 2 weeks, decreased urine output, and pink-colored urine. Her medical history is significant only for hypertension, which is well controlled with amlodipine 5 mg PO every day. She takes no other prescription or over-the-counter medications. Pertinent laboratory values are as follows

SCr, 2.1 mg/dL (normal, 0.6–1.2 mg/dL)
Spot ACR, 1,200 mg/g (normal, <30 mg/g)
UA, 18 RBCs/HPF (normal, 0–3)
eGFR, 34 mL/minute/1.73 m^2

The nephrologist schedules a biopsy to obtain a definitive diagnosis for her new-onset kidney disease. Biopsy results are as follows: light micrograph shows a moderately large segmental area of sclerosis with capillary collapse on the upper left side of the glomerular tuft; the lower right segment is relatively normal. Electron micrograph shows diffuse epithelial cell foot process fusion with occasional loss of the epithelial cells. The other major finding is massive subendothelial hyaline deposits under the glomerular basement membrane. The pathologist's impression is FSGS. What is the relevance of FSGS, and what are the management strategies for FSGS?

FSGS is characterized by sclerotic lesions of the glomerulus, which can be either focal or segmental in nature. The development of FSGS may be idiopathic (primary) or secondary to other diseases (i.e., morbid obesity, sickle cell disease, congenital heart disease, AIDS). Currently, FSGS is the leading cause of idiopathic nephrotic syndrome and accounts for 15% to 20% of the cases. Black patients are 2 to 4 times more likely to experience idiopathic FSGS than white patients, and they have a higher incidence of ESRD caused by FSGS.[188] Genetic variants of the apolipoprotein L1 (APOL1) gene predominate in patients of African ancestry and have been identified as a major risk factor.[189]

Most patients with FSGS will present with proteinuria, but only about half of them will initially present with the nephrotic syndrome. Patients with the nephrotic syndrome will also likely present with hypertension, increased SCr levels, and hematuria. During the early stages of FSGS, the symptoms may be indistinguishable from minimal-change nephropathy, a glomerulopathy characterized by similar lesions within the glomeruli. A kidney biopsy is necessary for diagnosis. Predictors of increased risk of progression to ESRD include massive proteinuria (>10 g/day), higher SCr level (>1.3 mg/dL), and black race.[188,190]

Treatment

Corticosteroids

A.G. should be placed on steroids, in addition to an ACEI or ARB and a loop diuretic, because she has FSGS and nephrotic syndrome.[177] A course of corticosteroids 1 mg/kg/day (maximum 80 mg) or 2 mg/kg every other day (maximum 120 mg) for at least 4 weeks and for up to 4 months with tapering of the dose over the course of 6 months after complete remission is achieved. Complete remission is defined as reduction of albuminuria <0.3 g/day, normal urine and SCr, and serum albumin >3.5 g/dL.[177] The median time to remission is 3 to 4 months. Patients whose proteinuria does not respond after a 4-month trial of therapy should be considered resistant to steroids and be rapidly tapered off over the course of 6 weeks.[177]

Steroid-Resistant Treatment

Calcineurin Inhibitors

The addition of cytotoxic agents (CYC, TAC) may be considered for A.G. if she is steroid resistant, intolerant of long-term steroid therapy, severely nephrotic, frequently relapsing, or steroid dependent. The data supporting the use of these agents in FSGS are limited. Retrospective studies have shown that use of cytotoxic drugs can produce complete remission in 50% of cases. Length of therapy of these agents may predict the remission rates of FSGS. Recent prospective studies support a longer duration of therapy. Evidence supporting the efficacy and safety of cyclosporine in FSGS stems from randomized controlled trials. In addition to being options for steroid-resistant patients, CNIs provide a steroid-sparing effect in FSGS steroid-sensitive patients. Cyclosporine studies are the most prevalent of the CNIs. Cyclosporine response is highly dependent on the previous steroid response. Complete remission rates of 73% can be seen with cyclosporine in steroid-sensitive patients.[190] Conversely, therapy with cyclosporine doses of 5 mg/kg/day for 6 to 12 months has been found to be effective and can result in remission rates of up to 69% in patients resistant to steroids.[191] The current recommendation is CYC of 3 to 5 mg/kg/day in two divided doses. If remission is achieved, continue treatment for 1 year. However, if no remission is achieved by 6 months, discontinue cyclosporine. Limitations of cyclosporine therapy include high relapse rate (23%–100%) after withdrawal, side effect profile (nephrotoxicity, hypertension), and resistance to therapy. Studies evaluating tacrolimus as a treatment option for FSGS are few and lack randomized controlled trials. Current TAC therapy should be initiated at 0.1 to 0.2 mg/kg/day in two divided doses. Tacrolimus has a similar side effect profile to that of cyclosporine.[190] Sirolimus is associated with nephrotoxicity in FSGS and is not recommended for treatment.

Mycophenolate Mofetil

MMF has the potential for a steroid-sparing effect; however, relapses are common. MMF and high-dose dexamethasone are recommended for steroid-resistant patients intolerant to cyclosporine therapy. A small study of patients with FSGS resistant to steroids, cytotoxic agents, or both and cyclosporine received MMF for 6 months.[177] At the end of 6 months, 44% of patients had improved proteinuria, but no patient achieved complete remission. Other studies examining MMF therapy at doses of up to 2,000 mg/day have found no clinically significant effect on remission rates.[192]

KEY REFERENCES AND WEBSITES

A full list of references for this chapter can be found at http://thepoint.lww.com/AT11e. Below are the key references and websites for this chapter, with the corresponding reference number in this chapter found in parentheses after the reference.

Key References

Cardone KE et al. Medication-related problems in CKD. *Adv Chronic Kidney Dis*. 2010;17(5):404–412 (7)

Kalantar-Zadeh K et al. Understanding sources of dietary phosphorus in the treatment of patients with chronic kidney disease. *Clin J Am Soc Nephrol*. 2010;5(3):519–530. (133)

Kidney Disease: Improving Global Outcomes (KDIGO) CKD Work Group. KDIGO 2012 Clinical practice guideline for the evaluation and management of chronic kidney disease. *Kidney Int Suppl*. 2013;3(1):1–163 (1)

Kidney Disease: Improving Global Outcomes (KDIGO) CKD-MBD Work Group. KDIGO clinical practice guideline for the diagnosis, evaluation, prevention, and treatment of chronic kidney disease-mineral and bone disorder (CKD-MBD). *Kidney Int Suppl*. 2009;(Suppl 113):S1–S130. (92)

Kidney Disease: Improving Global Outcomes (KDIGO) Glomerulonephritis Work Group. KDIGO clinical practice guideline for glomerulonephritis. *Kidney Int Suppl*. 2012;2:139–274. (177)

Kidney Disease: Improving Global Outcomes (KDIGO) Lipid Work Group. KDIGO practice guideline for lipid management in chronic kidney disease. *Kidney Inter Suppl*. 2013;3:259–305. (67)

Larson DS, Coyne DW. Update on intravenous iron choices. *Curr Opin Nephrol Hypertens*. 2014;23(2):186–191. (106)

Key Websites

HealtyPeople2020, http://www.healthypeople.gov/.

Kidney Disease, Improving Global Outcomes: http://kdigo.org/home/.

National Kidney Disease Education Program, http://nkdep.nih.gov/.

US Renal Data System, http://www.usrds.org/.

29 Acute Kidney Injury

Susan A. Krikorian and Oussayma Moukhachen

CORE PRINCIPLES

		CHAPTER CASES
1	Acute kidney injury (AKI) is characterized clinically by an abrupt decrease in renal function over a period of hours to days, resulting in the accumulation of nitrogenous waste products (azotemia) and the inability to maintain and regulate fluid, electrolyte, and acid–base balance.	**Case 29-1 (Question 1), Table 29-1**
2	Risk factors for the development of AKI include older age, higher baseline serum creatinine (SCr), chronic kidney disease (CKD), diabetes, chronic respiratory illness, underlying cardiovascular disease, prior heart surgery, dehydration resulting in oliguria, acute infection, and exposure to nephrotoxins.	**Case 29-1 (Question 1), Case 29-2 (Questions 1, 2), Case 29-3 (Questions 2, 4) Tables 29-5, 29-6, 29-7, 29-8 Case 29-5 (Question 2), Case 29-6 (Question 1)**
3	The clinical course of AKI has three distinct phases: the oliguric phase—a progressive decrease in urine production after kidney injury; the diuretic phase—initial repair of the kidney insult with resultant diuresis of accumulated uremic toxins, waste products, and fluid; and the recovery phase—return of kidney function depending on the severity of injury.	**Case 29-1 (Questions 1–3)**
4	AKI is classified according to the physiologic event leading to AKI: prerenal azotemia—decreased renal blood flow; functional—impairment of glomerular ultrafiltrate production or intraglomerular hydrostatic pressure; intrinsic—damage to the kidneys; and postrenal—outflow obstruction in the urinary tract.	**Case 29-1 (Questions 1, 2), Case 29-2 (Question 1, 4), Case 29-3 (Question 1), Case 29-5 (Question 1), Case 29-6 (Question 1), Case 29-7 (Question 1), Case 29-8 (Question 1), Table 29-2**
5	The urinalysis is an important diagnostic tool for differentiating AKI into prerenal azotemia, intrinsic, or obstructive AKI. Urinary chemistries are used to differentiate between prerenal azotemia and intrinsic AKI.	**Case 29-1 (Question 2), Case 29-3 (Question 1), Case 29-6 (Question 1), Case 29-7 (Question 1), Case 29-8 (Question 1), Tables 29-3, 29-4, Equation 29-1**
6	Medications that affect renal function (e.g., angiotensin-converting enzyme [ACE] inhibitors, angiotensin II receptor blockers [ARBs], and aminoglycoside antibiotics) should be dosed according to renal function and monitored closely in patients with AKI. Nephrotoxic medications should be avoided.	**Case 29-1 (Question 3), Case 29-2 (Question 1, 4), Case 29-3 (Question 5), Case 29-6 (Question 2, 3), Case 29-9 (Question 1)**
7	Patients with nonoliguric renal failure have significantly better outcomes than those with oliguria; however, converting a patient from oliguria to nonoliguria through pharmacologic intervention does not improve patient outcomes.	**Case 29-9 (Question 1)**
8	Hydration therapy is useful in the following ways: to increase renal perfusion and avert the conversion of prerenal azotemia to acute tubular necrosis (ATN), to reduce the risk of contrast-induced nephropathy (CIN) in high-risk patients, and to prevent and treat kidney stones.	**Case 29-2 (Question 3), Case 29-5 (Question 3), Case 29-8 (Question 1), Case 29-9 (Question 1), Table 29-5**

Continued

	CHAPTER CASES
9 Few treatment options are available in established AKI, therefore prevention is key. Supportive therapy is aimed at preventing the morbidity and mortality of AKI: close patient monitoring; strict fluid, electrolyte, and nutritional management; treatment of life-threatening conditions, such as pulmonary edema, hyperkalemia, and metabolic acidosis; avoidance of nephrotoxic drugs; and initiation of renal replacement therapy (RRT).	**Case 29-1 (Question 3), Case 29-5 (Question 4), Case 29-7 (Question 2), Case 29-9 (Question 1)**
10 Although diuretics have not been shown to improve patient outcomes, they can be used to prevent complications from fluid overload. Sodium restriction, daily monitoring of volume status, laboratory chemistries, urine output, and gastrointestinal (GI) and insensible losses should be measured during diuretic therapy.	**Case 29-1 (Question 3), Case 29-3 (Question 3), Case 29-4 (Question 1), Case 29-9 (Question 1)**
11 RRT is reserved for patients with severe acid–base disorders, fluid overload, hyperkalemia, or symptomatic uremia as a result of AKI. Dosage adjustments are necessary for drugs that are removed during RRT.	**Case 29-9 (Question 2), Table 29-9**

DEFINITION

Acute kidney injury (AKI) is characterized clinically by an abrupt decrease in renal function over a period of hours to days, resulting in the accumulation of nitrogenous waste products, urea and creatinine (azotemia), and the inability to maintain and regulate fluid, electrolyte, and acid–base balance.[1] AKI is a devastating syndrome with multiple risk factors or causes. It is associated with multi-organ dysfunction, increased resource utilization, high cost, and increased mortality. Like chronic kidney disease (CKD), AKI is common, treatable, and is also largely preventable. Not only is underlying CKD a risk factor for AKI, but AKI also contributes to CKD development and may result in dialysis dependency. Minimizing causes of AKI and increasing awareness of the importance of early detection and treatment are associated with improved outcome in AKI. Clinicians recognize a rapid approach to treatment is essential because the causes and complications of AKI do not allow much time to initiate management and reversal.[2–6]

Many attempts have been made to objectively quantify AKI based on laboratory data, daily urine output, or the need for renal replacement therapy (RRT) (i.e., dialysis). Over the past decade the working definition of AKI has evolved. Currently, expert opinion and consensus recommend assessing quantitative serum creatinine (SCr) changes from baseline or urinary volume. They are considered important clinical pointers in the detection, diagnosis, and severity of AKI. Vigilant daily assessment of these markers continues while the patient is hospitalized. In 2004, the Acute Dialysis Quality Initiative created an international expert panel, which proposed a new classification system called RIFLE.[7] This system defines various stages of AKI, including risk, injury, failure, loss (defined as the need for dialysis at least 1 month after failure), and finally end-stage renal disease (ESRD). In 2007, the recognition that even smaller changes in SCr than defined in RIFLE might be associated with adverse outcomes and mortality led to newer definitions by the Acute Kidney Injury Network (AKIN).[8] The three AKIN stages map to, but are not identical to, the RIFLE classification. The RIFLE and AKIN are very useful for quantitating renal function for research purposes rather than clinical activities. In 2012, the Kidney Disease Improving Global Outcomes (KDIGO)[9] guidelines proposed a uniform practical clinical definition of AKI, essentially merging the RIFLE and AKIN criteria. AKI is defined as an increase in SCr $>$ 0.3 mg/dL within 48 hours, OR an increase in SCr $>$ 1.5 times baseline in 7 days or less OR a decrease in urine volume $<$0.5 mL/kg/hour for $>$6 hours. The most recent guideline provides a useful tool to assist clinicians for managing AKI (Table 29-1).

These new classification systems provide advantages over traditional definitions, and represent a significant step forward in detecting and preventing AKI. Future studies need to prospectively evaluate their application in diverse clinical settings on the basis of evidence rather than opinion or consensus and also their performance as prognostic predictors of patient outcome. Regardless of the definitions used, the clinician should suspect AKI when the kidney is unable to regulate fluid, electrolyte, acid–base, or nitrogen balance, even in the presence of a normal SCr concentration. Healthcare technology information systems are working on alerts to notify clinicians to warn of possible AKI during patient care.[3,10]

EPIDEMIOLOGY

Multivariable models have identified risk factors for the development of AKI, including older age, higher baseline SCr, underlying CKD, diabetes, chronic respiratory illness, underlying cardiovascular disease, prior heart surgery, dehydration resulting in oliguria, acute infection, and exposure to nephrotoxins.[11] The incidence of community-acquired AKI (development of AKI before hospitalization) is just 1%; approximately 75% of these admissions result from decreased kidney blood flow, termed prerenal azotemia. Other less-common causes include obstructive uropathy (17%) and intrinsic renal disease (11%).[12] Community-acquired AKI can usually be reversed by correcting the underlying problems of volume status or obstruction. Hospital-acquired AKI is much more common, and the incidence and severity vary based on intensive care unit (ICU) or non-ICU setting.[13] The incidence of AKI in general-medicine patients is approximately 5% to 7%, with the most common causes being prerenal azotemia, postoperative complications, or nephrotoxin exposure.[14,15] These patients can experience one or more of these renal insults throughout their hospitalization. Conversely, ICU-acquired AKI is more prevalent and severe. Data suggest the incidence of AKI in patients in the ICU approaches 25%, stemming from multiple risk factors including older age, sepsis, nephrotoxin exposure, male sex (gender), multi-organ dysfunction, and the need for mechanical ventilation.[16–18] Severe burns, rhabdomyolysis, chemotherapy, and open heart surgery are also considered risk factors. The natural history of patients who develop AKI includes (1) complete recovery of renal function, (2) development of progressive CKD, (3) increased rate of progression of preexisting CKD, or (4) irreversible loss of kidney function with dialysis-dependent ESRD.[19] Although many patients with stage 3 AKI will initially require dialysis, a small percentage will develop ESRD requiring long-term dialysis.

Table 29.1
Classification/Staging System for Acute Kidney Injury

Category	SCr and GFR Criteria	Urine Output Criteria
RIFLE Criteria		
Risk	Increased SCr × 1.5-fold or GFR decrease >25%	<0.5 mL/kg/hour × 6 hour
Injury	Increased SCr × 2-fold or GFR decrease >50%	<0.5 mL/kg/hour × 12 hour
Failure	Increased SCr × 3-fold or GFR decrease >75% or SCr ≥4.0 mg/dL with an acute increase of at least 0.5 mg/dL	<0.3 mL/kg/hour × 24 hour or anuria × 12 hour
Loss	Complete loss of kidney function (RRT) >4 weeks	
ESRD	RRT >3 months	
AKIN Criteria		
Stage 1	Increased SCr ≥0.3 mg/dL or × ≥1.5 to 2-fold	<0.5 mL/kg/hour × >6 hour
Stage 2	Increased SCr × >2 to 3-fold	<0.5 mL/kg/hour × >12 hour
Stage 3	Increased SCr × >3-fold or SCr ≥4 mg/dL with an acute increase of at least 0.5 mg/dL or need for RRT	<0.3 mL/kg/hour × 24 hour or anuria × 12 hour
KDIGO Criteria		
Stage 1	Increased SCr ≥0.3 mg/dL within 48 hours or increased SCr × 1.5 to 1.9-fold in 7 days or less	<0.5 mL/kg/hour × 6–12 hour
Stage 2	Increased SCr × 2 to 2.9-fold	<0.5 mL/kg/hour × ≥12 hour
Stage 3	Increased SCr × ≥3-fold or SCr ≥4 mg/dL or need for RRT or eGFR <35 mL/minute/1.73 m^2	<0.3 mL/kg/hour × ≥24 hour or anuria × ≥12 hour

SCr, serum creatinine; GFR, glomerular filtration rate.

PROGNOSIS

Despite recent advances in dialysis delivery and the development of sophisticated continuous renal replacement therapy (CRRT), patients with AKI continue to have a grim prognosis. A mild elevation of SCr in ICU patients is associated with a twofold increase in the risk of death.[20] Indeed, the occurrence of AKI in critically ill patients carries at least a 50% mortality rate. Worse yet, the mortality rate increases correspondingly by 10% with each additional failed organ system. The mortality rate of AKI has declined minimally during the last 50 years. This slow decline may be explained in part by three important factors. First, patients are older when they develop AKI. Second, patients are often afflicted with serious underlying medical illnesses beyond AKI. Third, the clinical severity status of the patient with AKI is much higher now than ever before. Before the widespread availability of RRT, the most common causes of death in patients with AKI were fluid and electrolyte disorders and advanced uremia. Today, the most common causes of death are sepsis, cardiovascular disease as a result of heart failure and ischemic heart disease, malignancy, and withdrawal of life support.[21]

CLINICAL COURSE

There are three distinct phases of AKI. The oliguric phase generally occurs over the course of 1 to 2 days and is characterized by a progressive decrease in urine production. Urine production of less than 400 mL/day is termed oliguria, and urine production of less than 50 mL/day is termed anuria. The oliguric stage may last from days to several weeks. Nonoliguric renal failure (>400 mL/day of urine output) carries a better prognosis compared with oliguric renal failure, although the exact reason remains unknown. Similarly, the shorter the duration of oliguria, the higher the likelihood of successful recovery. This is probably because the renal insults (e.g., dehydration, nephrotoxin exposure, postrenal obstruction) in these cases are less severe. Strict fluid and electrolyte monitoring and management are required during this phase until renal function normalizes.

After the oliguric phase, a period of increased urine production occurs for several days; this is called the diuretic phase. This phase signals the initial repair of the kidney insult. The diuretic phase can result, in part, from a return to normal glomerular filtration rate (GFR) before tubular reabsorptive capacity has fully recovered. The elevated osmotic load from uremic toxins and the increased fluid volume retained during the oliguric phase may also contribute to the diuretic phase. Despite the increased urine production, patients may remain markedly azotemic for several days. The increase in urine output may lead to volume depletion and electrolyte loss if patients are not given adequate replacement therapy. Daily modifications in the fluid and electrolyte requirements are necessary based on urine output.

The recovery phase occurs over the course of several weeks to months, depending on the severity of the patient's AKI. This phase signals the return to the patient's baseline kidney function, normalization of urine production, and the return of the diluting and concentrating abilities of the kidneys.

PATHOGENESIS

The production and elimination of urine requires three basic physiologic events:

- Blood flow to the glomeruli
- The formation and processing of ultrafiltrate by the glomeruli and tubular cells
- Urine excretion through the ureters, bladder, and urethra

Many conditions and drugs can alter these physiologic events leading to AKI. These are classified as prerenal azotemia, and functional, intrinsic, and postrenal AKI (Table 29-2). It is possible for more than one of these categories to coexist.[22,23]

Normal renal function depends on adequate renal perfusion. The kidneys receive up to 25% of cardiac output, which is greater than 1 L/minute of blood flow. Prerenal azotemia, the most common form of AKI, occurs when blood flow to the kidneys is reduced. Major causes include decreased intravascular volume (e.g., hemorrhage or dehydration [including overdiuresis]), decreased effective circulating volume states (e.g., cirrhosis or heart failure [HF]), hypotensive events (e.g., shock or medication-related hypotension), and renovascular occlusion or vasoconstriction. Because no structural damage occurs to the kidney parenchyma per se,

Table 29-2
Causes of Acute Kidney Injury

Classification	Common Clinical Disorders
Prerenal azotemia	**Intravascular Volume Depletion**
	Hemorrhage (surgery, trauma) Dehydration (gastrointestinal losses, aggressive diuretic administration) Severe burns Hypovolemic shock Sequestration (peritonitis, pancreatitis)
	Decreased Effective Circulating Volume
	Cirrhosis with ascites Heart failure
	Hypotension, Shock Syndromes
	Antihypertensive vasodilating medications Septic shock Cardiomyopathy
	Increased Renal Vascular Occlusion or Constriction
	Bilateral renal artery stenosis Unilateral renal stenosis in solitary kidney Renal artery or vein thrombosis (embolism, atherosclerosis) Vasopressor medications (phenylephrine, norepinephrine)
Functional acute kidney injury	**Afferent Arteriole Vasoconstrictors**
	Cyclosporine Nonsteroidal anti-inflammatory drugs
	Efferent Arteriole Vasodilators
	Angiotensin-converting enzyme inhibitors Angiotensin II receptor antagonists
Intrinsic acute kidney injury	**Glomerular Disorders**
	Glomerulonephritis Systemic lupus erythematosus Malignant hypertension Vasculitic disorders (Wegener's granulomatosis)
	Acute Tubular Necrosis
	Prolonged prerenal states Drug induced (iodinated contrast media, cisplatin, aminoglycosides, amphotericin B, adefovir, cidofovir, tenofovir, HMG CoA reductase inhibitors, pamidronate, gold salts)
	Acute Interstitial Nephritis
	Drug induced (penicillins, β-lactam antibiotics, fluoroquinolones, proton pump inhibitors, NSAIDs, sulfonamides)
Postrenal acute kidney injury	**Ureter Obstruction (Bilateral or Unilateral in Solitary Kidney)**
	Malignancy (prostate or cervical cancer) Benign prostate hypertrophy Anticholinergic drugs (affect bladder outlet muscles) Renal calculi Crystals (i.e., drugs such as methotrexate, acyclovir, indinavir, atazanavir, sulfonamide antibiotics, and ethylene glycol)

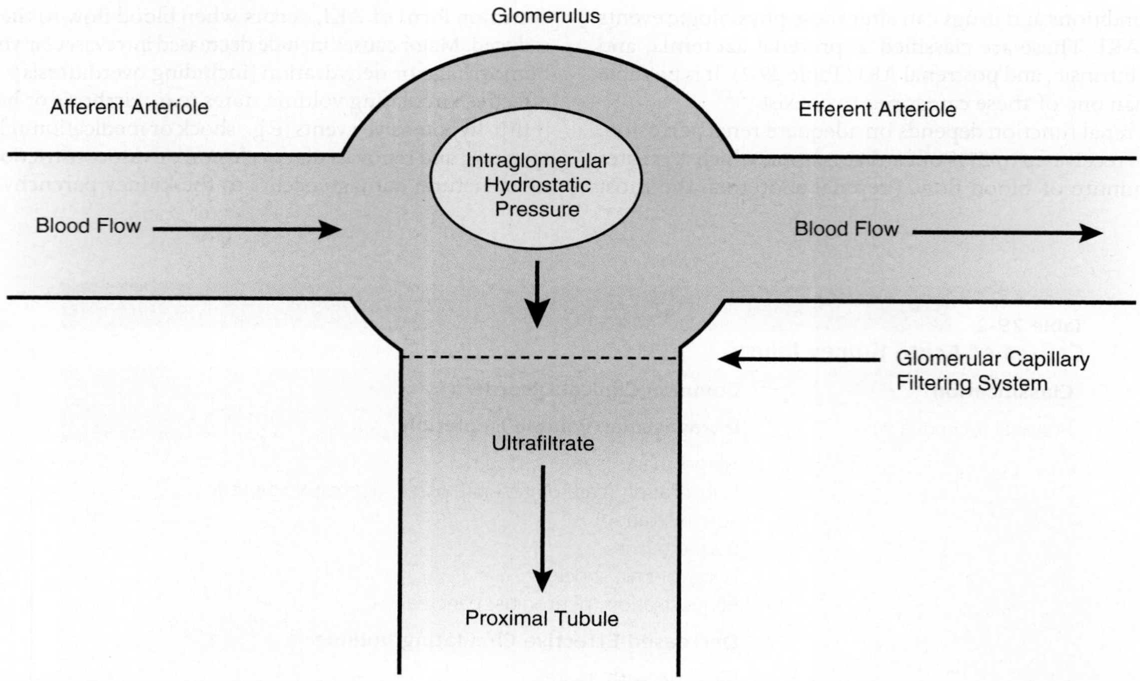

Figure 29-1 Schematic of renal blood flow. Blood enters the glomerulus via the afferent arteriole. The intraglomerular hydrostatic pressure leads to ultrafiltration across the glomerulus into the proximal tubule. The unfiltered blood leaves the glomerulus via the efferent arteriole. In conditions of decreased renal perfusion, efferent arteriolar vasoconstriction occurs to increase intraglomerular hydrostatic pressure and maintain ultrafiltrate production. Afferent arteriolar vasodilation also occurs to improve blood flow into the glomerulus.

correcting the underlying cause rapidly restores GFR. Sustained prerenal conditions can result, however, in glomerular ischemia causing acute tubular necrosis (ATN).

Functional AKI results when medical conditions or drugs impair glomerular ultrafiltrate production or intraglomerular hydrostatic pressure as a result of impaired autoregulation. Blood travels through the afferent arteriole and enters the glomerulus, where it is filtered, and exits through the efferent arteriole (Fig. 29-1). The afferent and efferent arterioles work in concert to maintain adequate glomerular capillary hydrostatic pressure to form ultrafiltrate. Many medications can drastically reduce intraglomerular hydrostatic pressure and GFR by producing afferent arteriolar vasoconstriction or efferent arteriolar vasodilation (Fig. 29-2).

Intrinsic AKI can occur at the microvascular level of the nephron, glomeruli, renal tubules, or interstitium. Vasculitic diseases (e.g., Wegener's granulomatosis, cryoglobulinemic vasculitis) involve the small vessels of the kidney. Glomerulonephritis and systemic lupus erythematosus, although relatively uncommon, result in glomerular damage. ATN is by far the most common cause of intrinsic AKI. In fact, the term acute tubular necrosis is often used

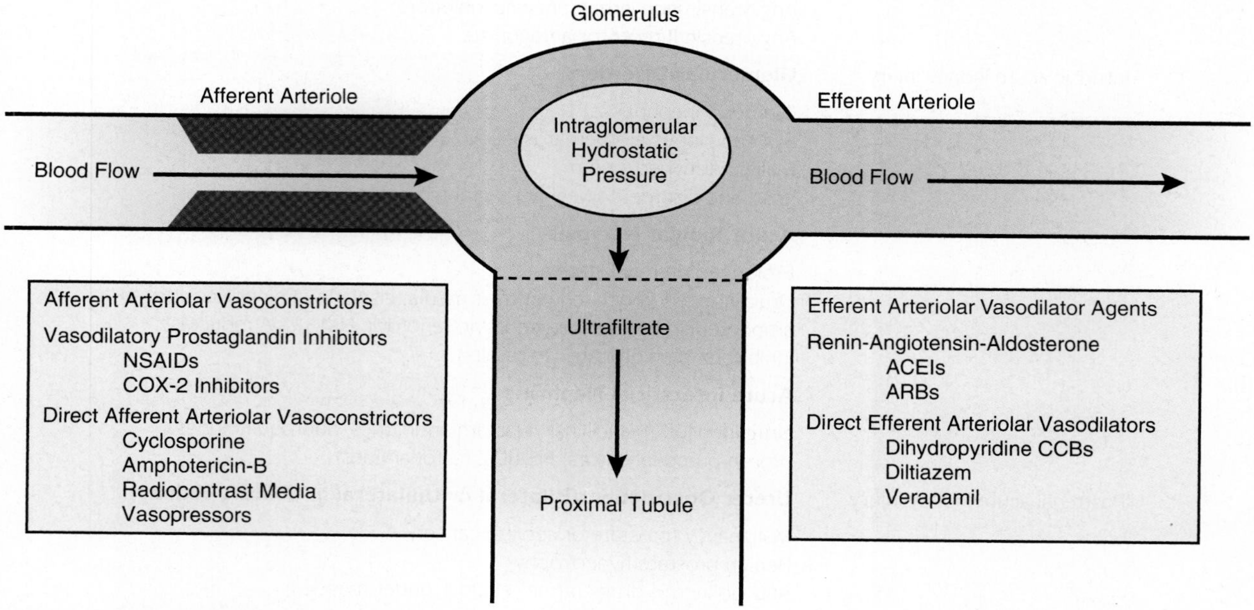

Figure 29-2 Drugs that alter renal hemodynamics by causing afferent arteriole vasoconstriction or efferent arteriole vasodilation. ACEIs, angiotensin-converting enzyme inhibitors; ARBs, angiotensin II receptor blockers; CCBs, calcium-channel blockers; COX-2, cyclo-oxygenase-2; NSAIDs, nonsteroidal anti-inflammatory drugs.

interchangeably with AKI. ATN occurs in part because the renal tubules require high oxygen delivery to maintain their metabolic activity. Consequently, any condition that causes ischemia to the tubules (e.g., hypotension, decreased blood flow) can induce ATN. Moreover, the tubules may be exposed to exceedingly high concentrations of nephrotoxic drugs (e.g., aminoglycosides). Interstitial nephritis or inflammation within the renal parenchyma is most often associated with drug administration (e.g., penicillins).

Postrenal AKI occurs when there is an outflow obstruction in the upper or lower urinary tract. Lower tract obstruction is most common and can be caused by prostatic hypertrophy, prostate or cervical cancer, anticholinergic drugs that cause bladder sphincter spasm, or renal calculi. Upper tract obstruction is less common and occurs when both ureters are obstructed or when one is obstructed in a patient with a single functioning kidney. Postrenal AKI usually resolves rapidly after the obstruction has been removed. Postobstructive diuresis can be dramatic (e.g., 3–5 L/day).[23]

CLINICAL EVALUATION

History and Physical Examination

A detailed history and physical examination often reveal the cause(s) of AKI. The clinician's responsibility is to ask specific, open-ended questions regarding the patient's chief complaint; history of present illness; medical history; family, social, and allergy history; and current prescription and nonprescription medication use. Probing for pertinent information regarding recent surgery, nephrotoxin exposure, or concurrent medical conditions can aid in rapidly determining the etiology of AKI. For example, does the patient have preexisting conditions that point toward prerenal azotemia, such as heart failure (HF) or liver disease? Did the patient receive prophylactic antibiotics before surgery? Did the patient hemorrhage or have protracted hypotension during surgery? Furthermore, assessment of the vital sign flowchart for documented weight loss, hypotensive events, fluid intake, and urine output may also prove useful.

A thorough physical examination, when used in conjunction with the history, can be invaluable in confirming the cause of AKI. The patient's volume status should be evaluated first. Evidence of dehydration (e.g., syncope, weight loss, orthostatic hypotension) or decreased effective circulating volume (e.g., ascites, pulmonary edema, peripheral edema, jugular venous distension) usually indicates prerenal azotemia. The presence of edema in a patient with normal cardiac function can, however, signal the early signs of nephrotic syndrome. A more detailed discussion of nephrotic syndrome is presented in Chapter 28, Chronic Kidney Disease. Concurrent rash and AKI associated with recent antibiotic exposure suggest drug-induced allergic interstitial nephritis. The clinician should suspect rhabdomyolysis in a patient with trauma or crush injuries and AKI. In a patient with suspected AKI the purpose of ultrasonography early in the diagnostic work-up is to rule out obstructive causes of oliguria. An enlarged prostate, painful urination, or wide deviations in urine volume can suggest obstructive AKI causes. Flank and lower abdominal pain suggest upper obstruction, whereas urinary frequency, hesitancy, dribbling, and abdominal fullness indicate lower obstruction.

Laboratory Evaluation

QUANTIFYING GLOMERULAR FILTRATION RATE

No estimating equations can provide an accurate estimate of GFR in AKI because the SCr is fluctuating and not at steady-state. In Chapter 28, Chronic Kidney Disease, the Modification of Diet in Renal Disease (MDRD) equation and the Cockcroft–Gault (CG) equation are reviewed, and both require a SCr value at steady-state. The MDRD equation is used to quantify baseline GFR, to detect or stage the degree of CKD, and to follow progression. The CG equation is most commonly used to evaluate the appropriate doses of drugs that are eliminated by the kidney.[9] CG may significantly overestimate the renal function in the early stages of AKI and may underestimate the renal function when AKI is resolving.[24] An example of this is a patient who develops ATN and anuria. Within the first few days, the SCr level may increase slightly because it takes time for the SCr concentration to achieve a new steady-state. In fact, the calculated creatinine clearance (ClCr) may even remain in the normal range, although the true GFR is substantially lower. The converse is true with patients recovering from ATN. As the diuretic phase of ATN begins, urine output can be dramatic, but patients may remain markedly azotemic for several days. Using the CG equation in this setting will produce a falsely low ClCr estimate. The CG equation is also inaccurate in populations that have low muscle mass—such as elderly, obese, or cachectic patients. Use of SCr to assess kidney function in patients with liver disease may also lead to overestimation of GFR.[25] This may be attributed to decreased production of creatine (the precursor of creatinine) by the liver or increased tubular secretion of creatinine by the kidney. Therefore, clinicians should be aware that estimating equations have potential limitations and pitfalls. In the past, many clinicians advocated the collection of timed urine specimens to calculate ClCr in AKI. Although this may seem relatively simple, it is susceptible to serious errors, particularly the timing of the collection and ensuring that the patient has not voided urine in the commode, resulting in an incomplete urine collection. For these reasons, the practice of collecting timed urine specimens is no longer routinely performed. Populations in whom estimation of GFR using a 24-hour urine collection is more reasonable include patients with variation in dietary intake of creatine sources (such as vegetarians) or persons with poor muscle mass (e.g., malnourished individuals or amputees).[26] Alternatively, shorter collection times or spot untimed urine samples are sometimes used to determine creatinine excretion.

Because an acute decline in kidney function may not be reflected by a rise in SCr for several hours, the recent emergence of novel serum and/or urinary AKI biomarkers is expected to aid in the early diagnosis of AKI. Neutrophil gelatinase-associated lipocalin (NGAL), Kidney Injury Molecule-1 (KIM-1), interleukin-18 (IL-18), and cystatin C have been shown to detect AKI in different patient cohorts. Future clinical trials are needed to identify and validate their prognostic role in AKI and estimating GFR.[27–31]

Many drugs are eliminated at least in part by the kidneys and must be dosed according to renal function. A more detailed discussion of drug dosing in the presence of compromised renal function is provided in Chapter 31, Dosing of Drugs in Renal Failure. Thus, standard doses and dosing intervals of many agents in the presence of AKI may lead to increased drug exposure of the active drug or metabolites. It is important to recommend appropriate drug doses in the presence of AKI. Some clinicians make renal dosing recommendations based on eGFR $<$15 mL/minute as an initial guide for drug therapy in an AKI patient not receiving CRRT when no other information is available. Drugs not essential for care should be discontinued to avoid potential drug-induced toxicity in the presence of AKI.

Careful monitoring of clinical and biochemical surrogate parameters associated with efficacy and toxicity and therapeutic drug monitoring (TDM), especially for drugs with a narrow therapeutic index eliminated by the kidneys, are required. High-risk medications such as aminoglycosides, vancomycin and calcineurin inhibitors (e.g., cyclosporine, tacrolimus), those with known nephrotoxicity, or other potential toxicities associated with supratherapeutic serum concentrations should be closely monitored. It is also important to note the volume of distribution (Vd) of drugs such as aminoglycosides, vancomycin, β-lactams (e.g., most cephalosporins, carbapenems) is dramatically increased in the presence of AKI. Therefore, larger loading doses may need to be administered to avoid subtherapeutic responses from lower than desired serum concentrations.[32–34] For most drugs, clinically useful serum drug assays are unavailable. Therefore, trends in renal function indices (e.g., SCr and urine output) along with volume status and response to therapy should be utilized to guide drug dosing. Further dose adjustments may be necessary when RRT is provided.

BLOOD TESTS

Assessment of blood urea nitrogen (BUN) and SCr concentrations is crucial for guiding the diagnosis, treatment, and monitoring of AKI. Measurement of BUN is discussed in Chapter 2, Interpretation of Clinical Laboratory Tests. The BUN:SCr ratio can delineate prerenal causes from intrinsic and postrenal causes. Urea reabsorption is inversely proportional to the urine flow rate. The normal steady-state BUN:SCr ratio is approximately 10:1. In prerenal conditions, the BUN:SCr ratio is greater than 20:1 because sodium and water are actively reabsorbed in the renal tubules to expand the effective circulating volume. Urea, an ineffective osmole, is reabsorbed as a result of increased water reabsorption, whereas creatinine is not reabsorbed. Although SCr may increase owing to decreased glomerular filtration, BUN increases to a greater degree as a result of increased proximal reabsorption.

The presence of hypercalcemia or hyperuricemia can indicate a hematologic malignancy. Tumor lysis syndrome is a condition that occurs in patients with leukemia after chemotherapy induction. The destruction of cancerous cells results in the release of large quantities of cellular contents (e.g., potassium, uric acid) into the bloodstream, which can overwhelm the kidney's functional ability, especially in dehydrated states.

Other elevated enzymes may also aid in the diagnosis of AKI. An increased level of creatine kinase or myoglobin in the face of AKI usually indicates rhabdomyolysis. Eosinophilia may suggest acute allergic interstitial nephritis from drug exposure. High levels of circulating immune complexes in the presence of AKI suggest glomerulopathies.[22]

URINALYSIS

The urinalysis is an important diagnostic tool for differentiating AKI into prerenal azotemia, intrinsic AKI, or obstructive AKI (Table 29-3). The presence of highly concentrated urine, as determined by elevated urine osmolality and specific gravity, suggests prerenal azotemia. During dehydrated states, vasopressin (antidiuretic hormone) is secreted, and the renin–angiotensin–aldosterone system (RAAS) is activated. These mechanisms promote the reabsorption of water and sodium at the collecting duct of the nephron, which serves to expand the effective circulating volume in an attempt to restore renal perfusion. As a result of diminished urine volume, the urine osmolality and specific gravity increase dramatically. Patients with prerenal azotemia and oliguria often have a urine osmolality greater than 500 mOsm/kg. The maximal urine osmolality can exceed 1,200 mOsm/kg.

The presence of proteinuria or hematuria can indicate glomerular damage. Nephrotic syndrome is characterized by urinary protein losses greater than 3.5 g/1.73 m^2/day. Proteinuria can also result from tubular damage; that protein loss is rarely over 2 g/day, however. The protein content can be used to differentiate glomerular versus tubular damage. The low-molecular-weight protein, β_2-microglobulin, is freely filtered at the glomerulus and reabsorbed at the proximal tubule. Therefore, the presence of excessive β_2-microglobulin in the urine suggests a tubular source of AKI, such as ATN. Conversely, albumin is not readily filtered at the glomerulus; hence, the presence of heavy albuminuria suggests a glomerular source of AKI.

Microscopic examination of the urine provides helpful clues for determining the source of AKI (Table 29-4). Pigmented granular casts are generally seen with ischemic or nephrotoxin-induced AKI. White blood cells (WBCs) and WBC casts can indicate an inflammatory process in the glomerulus, such as acute interstitial

Table 29-3
Urinary Indices in Acute Kidney Injury

Component	Prerenal Azotemia	Acute Tubular Necrosis	Postrenal Obstruction
Urine Na^+ (mEq/L)	<20	>40	>40
FE_{Na} (%)	<1	>2	>1
Urine/plasma creatinine	>40	<20	<20
Specific gravity	>1.010	<1.010	Variable
Urine osmolality (mOsm/kg)	Up to 1,200	<300	<300

Table 29-4
Clinical Significance of Urinary Sediment in Acute Kidney Injury

Cellular Debris	Clinical Significance
Red blood cells	Glomerulonephritis IgA nephropathy Lupus nephritis
White blood cells	Infection (pyelonephritis) Interstitial nephritis Glomerulonephritis Acute tubular necrosis
Eosinophils	Drug-induced acute interstitial nephritis Pyelonephritis Renal transplant rejection
Hyaline casts	Glomerulonephritis Pyelonephritis Heart failure
Red blood cell casts	Acute tubular necrosis Glomerulonephritis Interstitial nephritis
White blood cell casts	Pyelonephritis Interstitial nephritis
Granular casts	Dehydration Interstitial nephritis Glomerulonephritis Acute tubular necrosis
Tubular cell casts	Acute tubular necrosis
Fatty casts	Nephrotic syndrome
Myoglobin	Rhabdomyolysis
Crystals	Nonspecific

Note: Hyaline casts may also be detected in normal renal function.

nephritis (AIN) or pyelonephritis. Red blood cells (RBCs) and RBC casts can result from strenuous exercise or can indicate glomerulonephritis. Allergic interstitial nephritis can be detected by the presence of urinary eosinophils. Obstructive AKI causes, such as nephrolithiasis, can be identified by the presence of crystals in the urine. Cystine, leucine, and tyrosine crystals are considered pathologic. The presence of calcium oxalate crystals may suggest toxic ingestion of ethylene glycol.

URINARY CHEMISTRIES

Analyzing urine electrolyte concentrations and simultaneously comparing them with serum sodium and creatinine concentrations is useful for differentiating between prerenal azotemia and ATN (Table 29-3). The fractional excretion of sodium (FE_{Na}) is a measurement of how actively the kidney is reabsorbing sodium, and it is calculated as the fraction of filtered sodium excreted in the urine using creatinine as a measure of GFR. In normal conditions, the proximal tubule reabsorbs 99% of filtered sodium. The FE_{Na} formula is listed as follows:

$$FE_{Na^+}\ (\%) = \frac{(U_{Na})(SCr)}{(U_{cr})(S_{Na})} \times 100\% \qquad \text{(Eq. 29-1)}$$

where U_{Na} is the urine sodium concentration (mEq/L), SCr is the serum creatinine concentration (mg/dL), U_{Cr} is the urine creatinine concentration (mg/dL), and S_{Na} is the serum sodium concentration (mEq/L).[35] In prerenal azotemia, the functional ability of the proximal renal tubule remains intact. In fact, its sodium-reabsorbing abilities are markedly enhanced because of the effects of circulating vasopressin and activation of the RAAS. Both the FE_{Na} and urine sodium concentration become markedly low (<1% and <20 mEq/L, respectively) in prerenal conditions. In contrast, these indices are elevated in ATN because the renal tubules lose their ability to reabsorb sodium; the FE_{Na} is greater than 2%, and the urine sodium is greater than 40 mEq/L. FE_{Na} values between 1% and 2% are generally inconclusive. The clinician should ensure that the patient is not receiving scheduled thiazide or loop diuretic therapy when the FE_{Na} is calculated. These diuretics increase natriuresis, thereby making the results difficult to interpret. Urea excretion is not affected by diuretics. The FE_{Urea} appears more accurate in detecting prerenal azotemia, particularly in patients taking diuretics. Serum and urine creatinine concentrations are replaced by blood and urine urea concentrations in the FE_{Na} formula. A FE_{urea} of <35% and >50% are used to distinguish prerenal azotemia and ATN, respectively.[36]

PRERENAL AND FUNCTIONAL ACUTE KIDNEY INJURY

Chronic Heart Failure and Nonsteroidal Anti-Inflammatory Drug Use

CASE 29-1

QUESTION 1: A.W. is a 71-year-old white male (height = 6 feet; weight = 194 pounds), who had an ST-segment elevation myocardial infarction (STEMI) 2 months ago. His ejection fraction is currently 15% (normal, 50%–60%). He presents today for his 2-month follow-up clinic appointment complaining of shortness of breath, dyspnea on exertion, and inability to produce much urine. His medical history is significant for long-standing hypertension, coronary artery disease, osteoarthritis, and recent-onset HF after his MI. His home medications include furosemide 40 mg daily, lisinopril 20 mg daily, metoprolol succinate 100 mg daily, digoxin 0.125 mg daily, atorvastatin 40 mg daily, and naproxen sodium 550 mg twice daily (BID), all of which are taken orally (PO). With the exception of naproxen, A.W. often forgets to take his medications. Physical examination reveals lower leg 3+ pitting edema, pulmonary crackles and wheezes, positive jugular venous distension, and an S_3 heart sound. His vital signs are significant for a blood pressure (BP) of 198/97 mm Hg and a weight gain of 4 kg since his last visit 2 months ago. Last week, his BUN and SCr were 23 and 1.2 mg/dL, respectively. What are A.W.'s risk factors for AKI?

A.W.'s risk factors for AKI are heart failure (HF) with poor cardiac output (ejection fraction, 15%) that resulted from his STEMI and his medication, naproxen sodium. HF is a major cause of functional AKI.[37] A.W.'s diminished cardiac output has resulted in decreased effective circulating volume and activation of the RAAS, which are impairing his renal perfusion. In states of decreased renal perfusion, prostaglandins E2 and I2 compensate for the afferent arteriole vasoconstriction by stimulating afferent arteriole vasodilation, thereby enhancing renal blood flow. Prostaglandin synthesis is mediated predominantly by cyclo-oxygenase-1 (COX-1) and perhaps cyclo-oxygenase-2 (COX-2). Nonsteroidal anti-inflammatory drugs (NSAIDs), such as naproxen, are often overlooked as causes of AKI. NSAIDs exert their pharmacologic effect by inhibiting prostaglandin synthesis, thereby negating compensatory vasodilation. NSAIDs induce abrupt decreases in GFR in at-risk patient populations, specifically those with HF, liver disease, the elderly, or dehydrated patients. Figure 29-2 illustrates common medications that alter renal hemodynamics by causing either afferent arteriole vasoconstriction or efferent arteriole vasodilation. The term "triple whammy" refers to the risk of AKI when an ACE inhibitor or ARB is combined with a diuretic and NSAID. This combination might be seen in a patient with hypertension, congestive heart failure, or renal disease who has arthritis or other mild-to-moderate pain.[38,39]

COX-2 inhibitors also inhibit prostaglandin synthesis. A study comparing the effects of rofecoxib (voluntarily withdrawn from the market in 2004) and celecoxib to nonselective NSAIDs demonstrated similar renovascular effects.[40] In a large cohort of more than 1.4 million new NSAID users receiving care in the US Department of Veterans Affairs health care system, a greater risk of AKI (based on AKIN criteria) was found in nonselective versus COX-2 selective agents.[41] High-dose aspirin (defined as doses of at least 400 mg) was associated with the highest AKI risk. Naproxen, piroxicam, ketorolac, etodolac, indomethacin, sulindac, ibuprofen, and salsalate were also associated with a higher risk of AKI, whereas celecoxib, meloxicam, diclofenac, and other NSAIDs were not associated significantly with AKI. The highest risk was found in those using more than one NSAID, and in those switching from one agent to another. The lowest risk was found in those using the same agent continuously.[41,42] AKI risk was highest in the first 45 days of treatment initiation.[40] Sulindac may offer a "renal-sparing" effect. Sulindac is a prodrug that is converted to its active sulfide metabolite by the liver and then becomes reversibly oxidized back to its parent compound in the kidney; renal prostaglandin synthesis is essentially unaltered by sulindac. Cases of sulindac-induced renal dysfunction have been reported when the drug was administered to patients with cirrhosis and ascites.

CASE 29-1, QUESTION 2: A.W.'s cardiologist obtains a stat digoxin level, serum and urine electrolyte panels, and urinalysis. The digoxin level is reported as "not detectable" (target, 0.5–0.8 ng/mL). Other significant serum laboratory values include:

Na^+, 140 mEq/L
BUN, 56 mg/dL
SCr, 1.8 mg/dL

The urinalysis is significant for a urinary osmolality of 622 mOsm/kg, and specific gravity of 1.092. The urine electrolytes are significant for Na^+ of 12 mEq/L and creatinine of 102 mg/dL. What laboratory findings suggest functional AKI? Define the criteria used for the detection of AKI and staging of AKI in this patient.

A.W. has classic laboratory findings associated with poor renal perfusion (Table 29-3). It is important to compare the current and previous laboratory data to assess acute changes in renal function. Compared with last week, A.W.'s renal function has deteriorated based on substantial increases in BUN and SCr concentrations; BUN has increased nearly twofold and creatinine by 50% (SCr increased × 1.5-fold within 7 days). According to the AKIN/KDIGO criteria, the patient has stage 1 AKI. Renal demise is most likely due to functional AKI because the BUN:SCr ratio is greater than 20:1, suggesting poor renal blood flow, which is corroborated by other urinary indices such as the urinary Na^+ 12 mEq/L; specific gravity, 1.090 (elevated); urine osmolality, 622 mOsm/kg; and the calculated FENa, 0.1%. These values reflect the ability of the renal tubules to respond to vasopressin and aldosterone in an attempt to expand effective circulating volume and restore renal perfusion.

Another consideration is furosemide-induced volume depletion; however, the nondetectable serum digoxin level indicates likely noncompliance with his medications. A more likely explanation is poor renal perfusion because of his heart failure (i.e., low cardiac output).

CASE 29-1, QUESTION 3: How should A.W.'s prerenal azotemia be treated?

The presence of volume overload in the face of prerenal azotemia suggests a decreased effective circulating volume, most likely from poorly controlled HF. Restoring and improving A.W.'s cardiac output and renal perfusion will rapidly correct the prerenal azotemia. This can be achieved by (a) optimizing doses and assuring adherence to his heart failure medications (furosemide, lisinopril, metoprolol succinate, and digoxin); (b) controlling BP to a goal of lower than 140/90 mm Hg by decreasing both preload and afterload; and (c) modifying any drug therapy that has deleterious effects on the renal hemodynamics (e.g., NSAID). The specific therapies for controlling hypertension and improving cardiac output are presented in Chapter 9, Essential Hypertension, and Chapter 14, Heart Failure. Naproxen should be discontinued and substituted with acetaminophen to treat his osteoarthritis. Normal renal function should return in a few days after correction of the underlying causes.

Angiotensin-Converting Enzyme Inhibitor and Angiotensin Receptor Blocker–Induced Acute Kidney Injury

CASE 29-2

QUESTION 1: G.B. is a 53-year-old white woman (height = 5 feet, 3 inches; weight = 170 pounds) with hypertension, coronary artery disease, peripheral vascular disease, and diabetes, for which she had been taking hydrochlorothiazide 25 mg PO daily, atorvastatin 10 mg PO daily, aspirin 81 mg PO daily, and insulin glargine 30 units subcutaneously once daily every morning. At last week's clinic visit, she had two consecutive BP readings of 187/96 and 193/95 mm Hg, respectively, measured 20 minutes apart. At that time, G.B.'s primary-care physician started her on lisinopril 5 mg PO daily. Other notable laboratory values at the time included HgA_{1c} 7.5% and urine albumin to creatinine ratio (ACR) 50 mg/g. The region was in the midst of a protracted heat wave with temperatures above 95°F and she claims not drinking much liquids. She returns to the clinic today for her 1-week follow-up appointment complaining of dizziness, dry mouth, and very little urine production during the past week. Laboratory values and vital signs obtained at this visit include the following:

BP, 98/43 mm Hg
Hg, 15 g/dL
Hct, 45%
Na, 145 mEq/L
K, 5.2 mEq/L
BUN, 62 mg/dL
SCr, 2.7 mg/dL (baseline SCr, 1.0 mg/dL)
Why is G.B. experiencing AKI?

According to AKIN/KDIGO criteria, G.B. is diagnosed with stage 2 AKI most likely because of prerenal azotemia. Inhibition of the RAAS in patients with compromised renal blood flow is a common cause of functional AKI. A basic understanding of the effects of the RAAS on renal hemodynamics is necessary in this situation (Fig. 29-3). When renal perfusion is impaired, the juxtaglomerular cells of the kidney secrete renin into the plasma and lymph. Renin cleaves circulating angiotensinogen to form angiotensin I (AT I), which is further cleaved by angiotensin-converting enzyme (ACE) to form angiotensin II (AT II). AT II induces two physiologic events to improve renal perfusion. First, it directly causes systemic vasoconstriction, which shunts blood to the major organs, and indirectly increases intravascular volume through aldosterone- and vasopressin-mediated activity. Second, it preferentially vasoconstricts the efferent renal arteriole to maintain adequate intraglomerular hydrostatic pressure. Under conditions of decreased arterial pressure or effective circulating volume, the RAAS is activated and plasma renin and AT II activity are increased.[43,44]

CASE 29-2, QUESTION 2: Are there other factors that predispose patients to ACE inhibitor–induced AKI?

G.B. has extensive atherosclerotic disease indicated by the presence of coronary artery and peripheral vascular disease. Atherosclerosis not only affects major blood vessels but also the macrovasculature and microvasculature of the kidney; indeed, atherosclerosis is a major cause of renal artery occlusion and decreased renal perfusion. This activates the RAAS, which causes sodium and water reabsorption and AT II-mediated efferent arteriole vasoconstriction, in an attempt to restore normal renal perfusion and intraglomerular hydrostatic pressure.

The administration of ACE inhibitors directly inhibits the formation of AT II, which is necessary for efferent arteriole vasoconstriction. Consequently, the compensatory physiologic event that maintains G.B.'s renal blood flow is inhibited, thereby reducing her intraglomerular hydrostatic pressure and GFR. ACE inhibitors are contraindicated in patients with bilateral renal artery stenosis or unilateral stenosis in patients with a single functioning kidney.[45] In addition to the previous situation, three other general scenarios will result in the development of AKI with ACE inhibitors. First, conditions of sodium and water depletion (e.g., dehydration, overdiuresis, poor fluid intake, low-sodium diet) can increase the dependency of the efferent arteriole on AT II. Dehydration from diuretic use and decreased fluid intake during the heat spell may have compromised effective circulating volume and led to decreased renal blood flow in G.B. When ACE inhibitors are given in these situations, GFR can fall dramatically, and SCr rises. AKI can be averted by withholding the ACE inhibitor (or diuretic, or both) for a day and repleting the intravascular fluid volume with

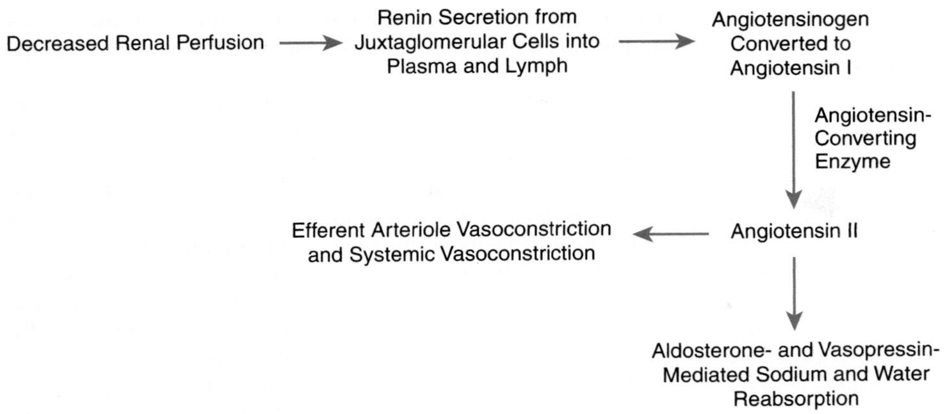

Figure 29-3 Compensatory hormonal mechanisms of decreased renal perfusion.

a saline-containing fluid (e.g., normal saline or 0.45% saline). The ACE inhibitor can be restarted at the same dose after adequate hydration when SCr returns to baseline. Second, ACE inhibitors can decrease the mean arterial pressure to such a degree that renal perfusion cannot be sustained. This is more likely to occur with long-acting agents or in situations in which the pharmacologic half-life of the ACE inhibitor is prolonged (e.g., preexisting renal disease). Finally, ACE inhibitors may precipitate AKI in patients who are taking concomitant drugs with renal afferent arteriole vasoconstricting effects, most notably cyclosporine and NSAIDs. In AKI, another important consideration is thiazides (except metolazone), which are less effective in the presence of ClCr <30 mL/minute and can be restarted when renal function improves.

CASE 29-2, QUESTION 3: How should G.B.'s ACE inhibitor–induced AKI be managed?

Patients who are receiving ACE inhibitors should be monitored judiciously with regard to their SCr and electrolyte concentrations. Once an ACE inhibitor is initiated, an increase in SCr of 20% to 30% can be expected.[44] This slight increase should not worry clinicians, because SCr typically normalizes within 2 to 3 months. SCr increases greater than this along with reduced urine output signal AKI, however. AKI related to ACE inhibitors is usually reversible, principally because the AKI is caused by inadequate glomerular capillary pressure, which is restored as soon as sufficient AT II is produced. This normally takes 2 to 3 days to re-equilibrate. Anecdotally, AKI appears to develop more commonly in hypotensive patients or in those with intravascular volume depletion (e.g., patients with HF receiving high-dose diuretics, inadequate fluid intake with diuretic use). In these conditions, it is prudent to replete the intravascular fluid volume or temporarily discontinue diuretic therapy until renal function improves. G.B.'s ACE inhibitor therapy should be temporarily discontinued and reinstituted when she has a normalized intravascular volume and is hemodynamically stable and kidney function has returned to baseline or stabile kidney function is established. See Chapter 14, Heart Failure, for a discussion on the use of ACE inhibitors and concurrent diuretic therapy in patients with heart failure.

CASE 29-2, QUESTION 4: Do angiotensin II–receptor blockers (ARBs) cause less AKI compared with ACE inhibitors?

The ARBs competitively inhibit the angiotensin II receptor. At least two subtypes of the angiotensin II receptors exist: AT1 and AT2. The ARBs exert their pharmacologic effect at the AT1 receptor subtype, which is responsible for most, if not all, of the cardiovascular effects of angiotensin II, such as vasoconstriction, aldosterone release, and β-adrenergic stimulation. Few differences are seen in the incidence of AKI between ACE inhibitors and ARBs[45] and one should not be interchanged with the other in an attempt to decrease AKI risk. See Chapter 14, Heart Failure, for further discussion.

HgA_{1c} and urine ACR are elevated. The patient may be at risk for diabetic nephropathy from uncontrolled diabetes. Initially, albuminuria (at least 2 out of 3 elevated ACR values >30 and <300 mg/g within 3 months) is considered a renal marker indicative of early stage CKD with or without an increase in baseline SCr. ACE inhibitors or ARBs are prescribed as anti-proteinuric agents to manage albuminuria and delay the progression of CKD with or without underlying hypertension. ACE inhibitors are the preferred anti-proteinuric agents in type 1 diabetes, whereas ARBs are preferred in type 2 diabetes and in patients intolerant to cough associated with ACE inhibitors. After AKI resolves in G.B., an ACE inhibitor is appropriate to consider treating hypertension and delay the progression of CKD.

INTRINSIC ACUTE KIDNEY INJURY

Intrinsic AKI is a general term that connotes damage at the parenchymal level of the kidney. The term acute tubular necrosis is often used to describe this type of AKI, but this is a histologic diagnosis that describes only one of several intrinsic disorders. Pragmatically, intrinsic AKI can be subdivided into vascular, glomerular, or tubular disorders.

Disorders involving the large renal vessels are relatively uncommon. Acute renal artery or vein occlusion can be caused by vasculitis, atheroembolism, thromboembolism, dissection, or clamping of the ascending aorta during surgery. To affect BUN and Scr, occlusion must be bilateral, or it can be unilateral in patients with concomitant renal insufficiency or one functioning kidney. Reduced blood flow to the renal microvasculature and glomeruli also can result in AKI. Common examples are rapidly progressing glomerulonephritis (RPGN) and vasculitis. If these conditions become sufficiently severe, they can cause ischemia, resulting in superimposed ATN. Any disorder that produces tubular ischemia, such as prolonged hypotension or shock syndromes, can result in ATN.

Nephrotoxic drugs are a common cause of ATN, especially when given in septic or volume-contracted patients. The various mechanisms by which drugs can cause ATN are explained in detail later in this chapter. Although relatively uncommon, drug-induced AIN is another type of intrinsic AKI. This is a hypersensitivity reaction that results from the formation of drug–antibody complexes that subsequently deposit in the glomerular membrane.

Acute Glomerulopathies

POSTSTREPTOCOCCAL GLOMERULONEPHRITIS

CASE 29-3

QUESTION 1: B.M. is an 18-year-old white male college freshman (height = 5 feet, 8 inches; weight = 150 pounds) in otherwise good health who recently developed strep throat. He received a 10-day course of amoxicillin, which cleared the infection. He returns to the student health center after completing his 10-day course complaining of "puffy eyes," swelling in his legs, a cough productive of clear sputum, and decreased urine output that appears "tea-colored." Other than the amoxicillin, he is not on any medication. Baseline records from a routine physical examination 2 months ago reveal a BUN and SCr of 10 and 0.8 mg/dL, respectively, and a BP of 120/80 mm Hg. Today, the physical examination is significant for a BP of 176/95 mm Hg, 2+ peripheral edema, and bilateral pulmonary rales. The urinalysis is significant for gross hematuria, nephritic-range proteinuria, RBC and WBC casts, and epithelial cells. B.M.'s SCr has increased to 7.1 mg/dL. Based on the history, physical examination, and laboratory findings, what is the most likely cause of AKI in this patient?

B.M.'s recent history of a streptococcal infection with the development of AKI suggests poststreptococcal glomerulonephritis (PSGN), which results from the formation of antibodies against streptococcal antigens. The streptococcal–antigen immune complexes are deposited in the glomerulus, resulting in complement, cytokine, and clotting cascade activation; neutrophils and monocytes attack the glomerulus causing glomerulonephritis. The onset of PSGN is usually 7 to 21 days after the start of the pharyngeal infection. PSGN is the most common acute-onset, immune-mediated, diffuse glomerulopathy. It primarily affects children, although it can affect any age group and is more prevalent in males than in females. Certain serologic subtypes of group A β-hemolytic streptococci, known as nephritogenic strains, cause PSGN. The M and T proteins located in the bacterial cell wall are used to classify streptococci. Nephritogenicity has been shown with certain M serotypes (e.g., 1, 2, 4, 12, 18, 25, 49, 55, 57, and 60).[46] Strains that follow pharyngeal infections (e.g., strep throat) include types 1, 3, 4, 6, 12, 25, and 49. Type 49 is the most prevalent strain worldwide. The overall risk of developing PSGN by the M type 49 subtype when present in the throat is about 5% and increases to 25% if it is found in the skin. Acute PSGN has also been described after infection with group C streptococci in epidemics outside of the United States.[47] Positive diagnosis of PSGN requires identification of a nephritogenic strain; objective urinalysis findings suggestive of glomerular damage, such as proteinuria, hematuria, and casts; and elevated streptococcal antibody titers.

B.M. exhibits the classic physical and laboratory findings associated with PSGN. The pertinent positive physical findings include periorbital, pulmonary, and peripheral edema; tea-colored urine; hypertension; and decreased urine output. Edema is a common manifestation, with periorbital edema typically being the first to appear. Reduced GFR, proteinuria, and sodium retention by the kidney all contribute to edema formation. When protein, principally albumin, is lost in the urine, the intravascular oncotic pressure declines, causing a shift of fluid into the extravascular space. The loss of intravascular volume stimulates sodium and water reabsorption by the kidney via aldosterone and vasopressin, which often produces stage 1 to 2 hypertension.

Pertinent laboratory data in B.M. include elevated SCr, and urinalysis positive for hematuria, proteinuria, WBC casts, and epithelial cells. Hematuria, which is found in almost all patients with PSGN, accounts for the reddish-brown, tea-colored urine. Other commonly found urine sediments include cellular casts and hyaline and granular casts. Oliguria is common in PSGN, but anuria is rare.

Given that B.M. has received a 10-day course of amoxicillin, it is unlikely that throat cultures for the nephritogenic group A hemolytic streptococcal strain will be positive. Cultures of close contacts may, however, be positive for the streptococcal strain, even if they are asymptomatic. The presence of circulating antibodies to the nephritogenic streptococcal strains indicates recent exposure. The antistreptolysin O (ASO), antihyaluronidase (AHase), antideoxyribonuclease B (ADNase B), and antinicotyladenine dinucleotidase (NADase) antibody titers can be measured clinically. ASO titers begin to rise 2 weeks after pharyngeal infection, peak at 4 weeks, and slowly decline over the course of 1 to 6 months. No correlation exists between degree of ASO rise and nephrogenicity. In fact, ASO titers may not be elevated at all if early antibiotic treatment is initiated or in cases of streptococcal skin infections. The use of ADNase and AHase titers is more specific to detect recent infection in these situations.

CASE 29-3, QUESTION 2: Are there other tests that can be used to confirm this diagnosis?

The streptozyme test, which can be used clinically for rapid screening purposes, uses several antistreptococcal antibody assays. False-positive and false-negative results are common, however, because of cross-reactivity between the antibody and normal collagen.

Serial complement determinations may be of value in diagnosing PSGN. Decreased levels of C3 protein and hemolytic complement activity (CH50) are observed in nearly all patients with active PSGN. Serum C3 levels can fall by nearly 50% of normal in the first weeks of infection and return to normal within 8 weeks after infection. No correlation, however, exists between the degree of C3 depression and severity of nephritis. Circulating antibody complexes of C3 can be found in patients with acute infection.

Renal biopsy is rarely needed, but it may be prudent in patients who present with atypical symptoms, such as anuria, prolonged oliguria, marked azotemia, hematuria for more than 3 weeks, or in those who have no streptococcal antibody titers.

CASE 29-3, QUESTION 3: What are the therapeutic goals and treatment options for PSGN?

The therapeutic goals are to minimize further kidney damage and to provide symptomatic relief for B.M. The underlying streptococcal infection should be treated with appropriate antibiotics, but as illustrated by B.M., this has no effect in preventing PSGN. Family members and close contacts of the infected patient should receive antibiotic prophylaxis as well. Restriction of protein to 0.8 g/kg/day may be beneficial in patients with marked proteinuria, and antihypertensive drugs can be used on a short-term basis to control BP. Sodium and water restriction is beneficial in reducing edema, and loop diuretics may be used as needed for symptomatic pulmonary or peripheral edema. Close monitoring of electrolytes is warranted if diuretics are used. Dialysis is rarely required. Given his age and previous health, B.M.'s prognosis is very good. In general, prognosis is excellent in youth, but significantly worse in the elderly and in patients with other risk factors for CKD, such as diabetes and hypertension.[47]

RAPIDLY PROGRESSIVE GLOMERULONEPHRITIS

CASE 29-3, QUESTION 4: Are there other glomerulopathies that cause AKI?

Yes. Rapidly progressive glomerulonephritis (RPGN), also called *crescentic glomerulonephritis*, is a clinical syndrome of rapid decline in renal function (from days to weeks) combined with the hallmark findings of gross hematuria, nephritic syndrome with proteinuria, and the presence of extensive glomerular crescents (>50% of glomeruli) on renal biopsy. It is not uncommon for patients with RPGN to have a 50% decline in GFR in only a few weeks. RPGN is a medical emergency, and treatment success depends on how early therapy is initiated. If left untreated, progression to end-stage renal disease or death is almost certain.

Idiopathic RPGN is divided into three categories based on immunofluorescence microscopy. Type I idiopathic RPGN is characterized by linear deposition of immunoglobulins, primarily IgG, along the glomerular basement membrane (GBM) indicating anti-GBM antibodies. Type II idiopathic RPGN is identified by granular immunoglobulin and complement depositions in the glomerular microvasculature and mesangium, suggesting immune complex deposition. Type III idiopathic RPGN is also called *pauci-immune* because there are no hallmark immunoglobulin or complement findings on immunofluorescence microscopy. Type III idiopathic RPGN is identified by the presence of circulating antineutrophil cytoplasmic antibodies (ANCA). Type IV, known as double-antibody disease, is characterized by anti-GBM antibodies and ANCA seen in Types I and III RPGN.[48]

Multisystem vasculitic disorders that result in glomerular capillary inflammation are the most common cause of RPGN.[49] Many of these patients present with nonspecific flulike symptoms such as fever, weight loss, myalgia, and malaise with proteinuria and hematuria.[50] Uremic symptoms can occur with severe disease. The presence of AKI with pulmonary congestion, cough, hemoptysis, or dyspnea suggests Wegener's granulomatosis. The treatment for autoimmune RPGN generally involves various regimens of immunosuppressive agents. Corticosteroid monotherapy (oral or "pulse" intravenous) or combined with either cyclophosphamide or rituximab have been investigated. Rituximab may improve renal outcomes in Type III idiopathic RPGN; in addition to anti–B-cell therapy, therapy directed at T cells may improve renal outcome.[51] Plasmapheresis is also a non-pharmacological treatment option in selected patients. A more detailed discussion of glomerulonephritis is presented in Chapter 28, Chronic Kidney Disease.

NONSTEROIDAL ANTI-INFLAMMATORY DRUG–INDUCED GLOMERULOPATHY

CASE 29-3, QUESTION 5: Which drugs cause glomerulonephropathy?

Minimal-change disease and membranous nephropathy have been associated with NSAID use.[52] The mechanism is probably related to NSAID-induced inhibition of the cyclo-oxygenase pathway, which leads to increased arachidonate catabolism and increased proinflammatory leukotriene production. The hallmark feature of NSAID-induced nephropathy is nephrotic-range proteinuria. The nephropathy resolves slowly over the course of several months once the NSAID is discontinued.

TUBULOINTERSTITIAL DISEASES

Acute Tubular Necrosis

ATN arises most often from ischemia or drug-induced causes.[53] Prolonged prerenal conditions, such as hypotension, surgery, overwhelming sepsis, or major burns, can lead to ischemic ATN. Unlike prerenal azotemia, tubular cell death occurs in ATN, and immediate volume resuscitation will not reverse the damage. The pathophysiology of ATN is complex and remains unclear. It is currently thought that when tubular cells die, they slough off into the tubule lumen and contribute to cast formation. The casts completely obstruct the tubule lumen and increase intratubular pressure, which causes a back leak of ultrafiltrate across the tubular basement membrane (Fig. 29-4). The aforementioned processes are mediated by a variety of substances, including calcium, phospholipases, and perhaps growth factors as well as free radical and protease activation.

TREATMENT WITH DIURETICS AND DOPAMINE

CASE 29-4

QUESTION 1: V.B. is a 86-year-old white man (height = 5 feet, 2 inches; weight = 138 pounds), who was admitted for elective aortic valve replacement secondary to severe aortic stenosis. He became hypotensive during surgery, requiring aggressive fluid resuscitation. He is now in the ICU and requires vasopressors for hemodynamic support. His BUN is 88 mg/dL and his SCr is 3.5 mg/dL today. His renal function tests have remained at these levels for the past 3 days. His baseline SCr before surgery was 1.2 mg/dL. Despite IV fluids, V.B. is oliguric with a urine output of 15 mL/hour (350 mL/day). Do diuretics and dopamine have a role in treating ATN?

It is well documented that patients with nonoliguric renal failure have significantly better outcomes compared with those with oliguria. This is probably because patients who are nonoliguric have less extensive renal damage and are better able to maintain fluid and electrolyte balance. Loop diuretics have been used in established ATN in an attempt to convert patients with oliguria to a nonoliguric state despite the lack of conclusive evidence for their benefits. Numerous clinical trials, however, have failed to demonstrate improved mortality or duration of azotemia in oliguric patients who receive loop diuretics, despite improved urine output.[9] Two large systematic reviews of the primary literature convincingly showed that diuretic therapy plays little role in altering the course of AKI, decreasing length of hospitalization, or helping recover renal function.[54,55] These data suggest that although patients who are nonoliguric generally have better outcomes, converting a patient from oliguria to nonoliguria through pharmacologic intervention does not improve patient outcomes. Currently, the only role that diuretic administration has in patients with established ATN is to increase urine output, which facilitates fluid, electrolyte, and nutritional support.[9]

Another controversy that has been debated extensively in the literature is the use of dopamine in patients with established ATN. Dopamine is a catecholamine that stimulates dopaminergic receptors at low dosages (1–3 mcg/kg/minute), and α- and β-receptors at higher dosages (5–20 mcg/kg/minute). Animal and human studies have demonstrated that low-dose dopamine improves renal blood flow by inducing afferent arteriolar vasodilation. No data, however, support the use of dopamine in the treatment of established AKI. A meta-analysis of 61 clinical trials including nearly 3,500 patients failed to detect any significant improvement in variables such as occurrence of AKI, need for renal replacement therapy, or mortality.[56] Unequivocally, dopamine has no role in preventing or treating AKI.

Other modalities such as fenoldopam or atrial natriuretic peptide (ANP) have not been shown to be conclusively beneficial to treat AKI and hence are not recommended to be used.[9] RRT would be the most appropriate to use if life-threatening changes in fluid, electrolytes, or acid–base balance are noted.

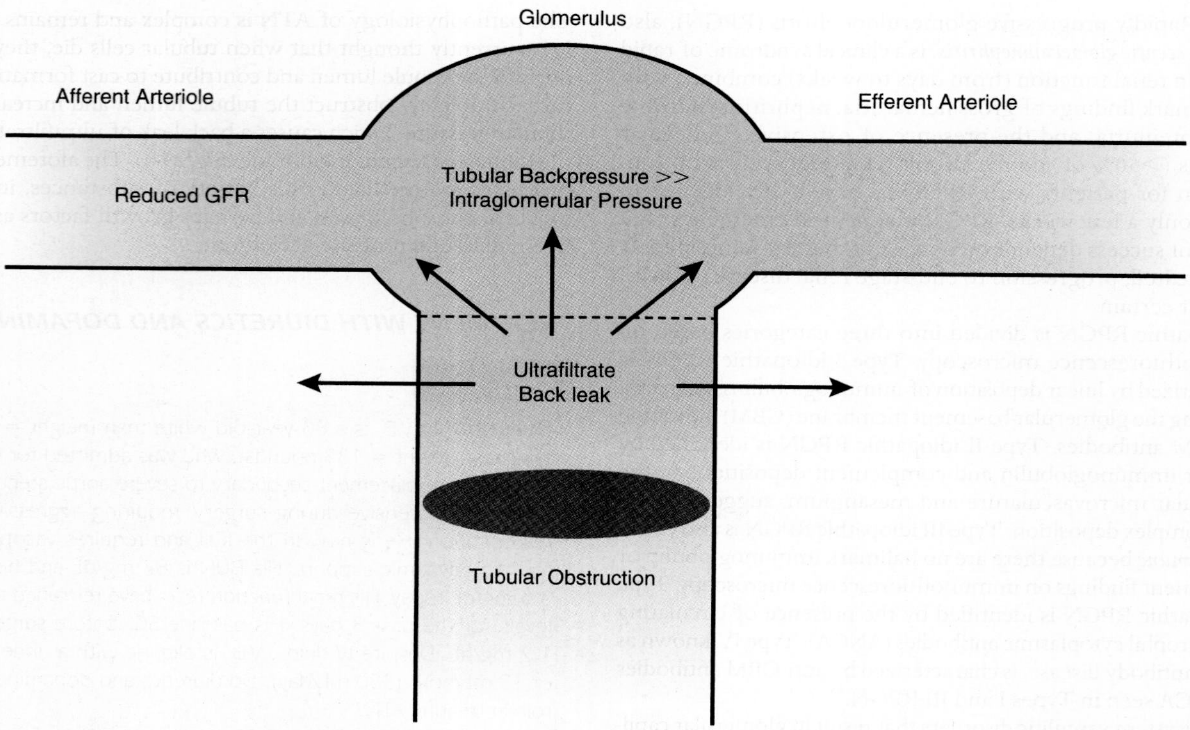

Figure 29-4 Schematic of acute tubular necrosis (ATN). The process is initiated by ischemia or nephrotoxin exposure that leads to tubular cell death. The cellular debris sloughs off and obstructs the proximal tubule lumen. Once the nephron is obstructed, a back leak of the glomerular ultrafiltrate occurs across the tubular basement membrane and impairment of glomerular filtration is seen. During the recovery phase of ATN, the obstructive cellular casts are released into the urine and filtration begins to normalize. GFR, glomerular filtration rate.

Radiocontrast Media–Induced Acute Tubular Necrosis

CASE 29-5

QUESTION 1: K.S., a 74-year-old black man (height = 5 feet, 9 inches; weight = 210 pounds), presents to the emergency department complaining of chest pain. His medical history is significant for advanced type 2 diabetes mellitus, with retinopathy, peripheral vascular disease, and advanced coronary artery disease. Based on cardiac enzymes, K.S. is ruled in for STEMI. He is taken to the cardiac catheterization laboratory for a percutaneous coronary intervention. Immediately before the procedure, K.S. is given iopamidol (Isovue, Bracco Diagnostics Inc., Princeton, NJ, USA) a nonionic, low-osmolar radiocontrast to enhance visualization of his cardiac arteries. His admission BUN is 37 mg/dL and SCr is 1.5 mg/dL. Two days later, pertinent laboratory findings include a BUN and SCr of 60 and 2.0 mg/dL, respectively, and his urine output is 700 mL/day. Why did AKI develop in K.S.? How is his diagnosis substantiated by his clinical findings?

Radiocontrast media administration is one of the most common causes of drug-induced ATN. Although no set criteria exist for its diagnosis, it is generally considered after radiocontrast exposure when an increase in SCr of 0.5 mg/dL or 25% greater than baseline occurs in 24 to 48 hours, peaks at 3 to 5 days, and returns to baseline in 1 to 3 weeks.[57,58] The American College of Radiology has recommended using the AKIN criteria requiring smaller changes in serum creatinine occurring within 48 hours after the administration of iodinated contrast media to define contrast-induced nephropathy (CIN) in order to standardize the varying definitions found in the literature.[59] CIN usually presents as a nonoliguric ATN, as observed in K.S., whose urine output is more than 400 mL/day. It is also differentiated from other forms of ATN in that the FE_{Na} is usually less than 1% (vs. the typical >2%). The degree of creatinine rise and the presence of oliguria are widely variable. Because of the lack of an accepted CIN definition and differences in both clinical trial design and populations studied, estimating the true prevalence of CIN is daunting. Nevertheless, patients without risk factors have a relatively minute risk of developing CIN; for those with recognized risk factors, prevalence may approach 50%.[60]

The mechanisms by which radiocontrast media induce AKI are complex. Initially, the radiocontrast medium produces renal vasodilation and an osmotic diuresis. This, however, is followed by intense vasoconstriction in the medullary portion of the kidney, which has been demonstrated by significant decreases in medullary Po_2 after contrast administration.[61] The ischemia is compounded by the increased medullary oxygen consumption because of the osmotic diuresis. Consequently, disequilibrium exists between oxygen supply and demand, creating ischemic ATN. Various vasoactive substances are suspected of decreasing medullary blood flow, including oxygen free radicals, prostaglandins, endothelin, nitric oxide, angiotensin II, and adenosine. Endothelin and adenosine are potent vasoconstrictors that are directly released from endothelial cells on exposure to radiocontrast media.

CASE 29-5, QUESTION 2: What risk factors did K.S. have for developing CIN?

The documented risk factors for CIN are listed in Table 29-5. Any condition that decreases renal blood flow increases the risk of nephropathy. At-risk patient populations include individuals with underlying diabetic nephropathy or eGFR <60 mL/minute/1.72 m^2, heart failure, or volume depletion, or those receiving aggressive diuretic regimens. Contrast volume administered during the imaging procedure as well as type of contrast remain additional risk factors.[62] The use of the ionic high-osmolar or ionic low-osmolar

Table 29-5
Proven Risk Factors for Developing Radiocontrast Media–Induced Acute Tubular Necrosis

Diabetic nephropathy
Chronic kidney disease
Severe heart failure
Diabetes and multiple myeloma
Volume depletion and hypotension
Dosage and frequency of contrast administration
Ionic radiocontrast agents

contrast products increases the risk of nephropathy, as well as the previously discussed medications that markedly reduce renal perfusion (e.g., diuretics, NSAIDs, COX-2 inhibitors, ACE inhibitors, and ARBs). However, newer nonionic low-osmolar agents may be less nephrotoxic than older agents, but still can cause nephrotoxicity in patients at risk. Nonionic iso-osmolar contrast appears to be better tolerated.[63]

On the basis of the published literature, gadolinium-based contrast (GBC) agents are less nephrotoxic than iodinated radiocontrast; however, when GBC agents are used in high dosage with arterial injection in patients with advanced kidney disease, AKI can occur. More concerning is the development of debilitating nephrogenic systemic fibrosis (NSF), which is sometimes fatal. There is no cure for NSF. Patients with AKI or CKD with GFR <30 mL/minute, who have had imaging studies (e.g., magnetic resonance angiography) with GBC agents are at high risk for developing NSF. The U.S. Food and Drug Administration (FDA) has issued an advisory Black Box Warning to avoid using these currently approved GBC agents (Ablavar, Doterem, Eovist, Magnevist, Multihance, Omniscan, Optimark, Prohance) in AKI and stage 4 and 5 CKD.[64–66]

K.S. is at high risk for developing radiocontrast-induced ATN. He is volume depleted, as evidenced by his admission BUN:SCr ratio, which is greater than 20:1. Second, it is very likely that K.S. has underlying diabetic nephropathy, as evidenced by his elevated admission SCr. The presence of retinopathy, coronary artery disease, and peripheral vascular disease suggest long-term uncontrolled diabetes mellitus, a risk factor for nephropathy.

PREVENTION

Case 29-5, Question 3: What strategies could have been performed in K.S. to prevent the occurrence of CIN?

Attempts have been made to minimize or prevent CIN using a variety of approaches. Decreasing contact time and the concentration of contrast media within the kidney tubule lumen may reduce its direct toxic effects. A higher urine output is associated with a lower incidence of CIN in high-risk patients.[67,68] Volume expansion is a rational approach to prevent renal dysfunction in this population because human and animal data have revealed dehydration as a major risk factor for developing CIN. Intravenous hydration with normal saline, hypotonic saline (0.45% sodium chloride), and sodium bicarbonate in dextrose 5% and water have all shown benefits in preventing CIN in high-risk patients. Infusion rates usually start at 1 mL/kg/hour to maintain a goal urine output of 150 mL/hour.

Sodium bicarbonate may be of value, but larger multicenter studies are needed to determine its true effectiveness.[68] Notably, sodium bicarbonate may be more beneficial in decreasing the incidence of radiocontrast nephropathy relative to other fluids because it reduces oxygen free radicals in the renal medulla and, therefore, increases the medullary pH. However, sodium overload is problematic and sodium bicarbonate should be avoided in compromised cardiac states.

Data suggest normal saline should be infused at least 6 hours before and 12 hours after the imaging study to adequately reduce the risk of developing nephropathy. In contrast, sodium bicarbonate should be infused 1 hour before and 6 hours after the imaging study. The antioxidant *N*-acetylcysteine (NAC) has also been used for its renal-sparing effects relative to radiocontrast media, but its role in preventing CIN remains unclear.[69] NAC is believed to work by protecting renal tubule cells from apoptosis related to the reactive oxygen species.[70] Although much data have been generated with NAC, many of these studies have significant pitfalls, including relatively small sample size; single-center design; heterogeneity of patient populations; differing doses, dosage forms, and schedules of NAC therapy; and differing hydration regimens. Therefore, trying to delineate meaningful conclusions from this body of literature is daunting. Given the safety profile and minimal cost impact as well as the significant morbidity associated with CIN in high-risk patients, its continued use is not inappropriate. At this time, recommending a specific dose of NAC is difficult. The commonly accepted regimens at many institutions is 600 or 1,200 mg orally twice daily the day before and the same day of the contrast procedure for a total of four doses along with concomitant intravenous hydration therapy.[71] Higher doses (total of 6,000 mg over 48 hours) may be required for high-risk patients (those with CKD or HF) and needs further investigation.[72]

Currently, a large randomized, double-blind, multicenter trial ongoing trial, The Prevention of Serious Adverse Events following Angiography (PRESERVE),[73] will compare the effectiveness of intravenous bicarbonate versus intravenous normal saline and oral NAC versus oral placebo for prevention of contrast-induced AKI. The trial (ClinicalTrials.gov NCT01467466) will enroll 8,680 high-risk patients undergoing coronary or noncoronary angiography.

Another important point is that the administration of diuretics such as mannitol and furosemide should be avoided.[74] These diuretics result in volume depletion and increase oxygen demand in the medullary portion of the kidney when diuresis occurs, thereby counteracting the benefits of hydration.

Other therapeutic modalities for the prevention of CIN have been studied. A systematic review and meta-analysis of aminophylline and theophylline have affirmed a renoprotective effect in patients who have underlying CKD; however, large-scale clinical trials are lacking.[75] Although the use of calcium-channel blockers theoretically seems rational to prevent contrast-induced ATN, limited clinical data exist. HMG CoA reductase inhibitors have been proposed for prevention of CIN given their antioxidant and anti-inflammatory properties; however, recent studies have not shown a benefit.[76,77] Limited data suggest that ascorbic acid before and after the procedure may be beneficial in preventing contrast nephropathy given its antioxidant effects[78]; however, a recent published report comparing ascorbic acid to NAC showed a greater benefit of high-dose NAC than ascorbic acid in preventing CIN in patients at risk.[79] High doses and long-term use of ascorbic acid should be avoided because of the risk of hyperoxalurea, oxalate-containing urinary stones, and renal damage.

When possible, alternative imaging studies that do not require radiocontrast should be attempted. If this is not practical, the lowest effective dose of nonionic low-osmolar or iso-osmolar radiocontrast media should be used. Concomitant drug therapy that can impair renal perfusion, such as diuretics, NSAIDs, COX-2 inhibitors, ACE inhibitors, and ARBs, should be discontinued 1 day before and 1 day after radiocontrast administration. Metformin is also a risk factor. It is not a nephrotoxin; however, its use has been associated with the development of AKI, systemic complications, and death in rare cases. Metformin should also be discontinued 1 day before giving radiocontrast media and held for at least 2 days after the imaging study because it may cause lactic acidosis if patients experience AKI. If patients are receiving calcium-channel blockers for underlying cardiovascular disease, no change in therapy is warranted. All patients should be well hydrated with normal saline or sodium bicarbonate fluids before and after radiocontrast administration to prevent CIN. The addition of NAC is optional.

CASE 29-5, QUESTION 4: What treatment options are available for established radiocontrast-induced ATN?

Few data exist regarding treatment of existing radiocontrast-induced ATN. The acute management largely involves supportive care that includes strict fluid and electrolyte management to prevent undue sequelae. Approximately 25% of patients will require temporary dialysis therapy; patients who are oliguric generally require long-term dialysis therapy. As already noted, attempts to convert oliguria to nonoliguria with furosemide and mannitol have been largely unsuccessful.

Aminoglycoside-Induced Acute Tubular Necrosis

CASE 29-6

QUESTION 1: T.G. is a 81-year-old, 80 kg white male (height 5 feet, 10 inches) being treated for *Streptococcus bovis* prosthetic valve endocarditis. T.G. is known to have systolic congestive heart failure with an ejection fraction of 25%. T.G. has a low BP at 90/50 mm Hg, pulse 110 beats/minute. Since admission, T.G. has received ceftriaxone 2 g IV daily, and gentamicin 80 mg IV q8 hours. Today, (hospital day 7), significant laboratory values are as follows:

BUN, 67 mg/dL
SCr, 5.4 mg/dL (baseline 0.9 mg/dL)
WBC count, 16,700 cells/μL with continued left shift
FE_{Na} 3%

During the last 2 days, T.G.'s urine output has steadily declined, and today it is 700 mL/24 hours. A urinalysis revealed many WBCs, 3% RBC casts, brush-border cells, and granular casts with an osmolality of 250 mOsm/kg. A serum trough gentamicin concentration obtained with the last dose is 6 mg/L (target, <1.0 mg/L). Given the history and laboratory data, what is the likely source of T.G.'s AKI?

The source of AKI in this situation is likely multifactorial (Table 29-2). Low renal perfusion secondary to low ejection fraction can result in prolonged renal ischemia. Second, T.G. has received 1 week of gentamicin, a well-known nephrotoxic antibiotic. The risk factors for developing aminoglycoside nephrotoxicity are listed in Table 29-6. The latest gentamicin trough concentration of 6 mg/L is far higher than the target value of less than 1 mg/L for a traditional 3-times-daily dosing regimen used for synergy for bacterial endocarditis.[80] Given the laboratory data (Table 29-3) and the clinical course of prolonged hypotension, vasopressor, and aminoglycoside administration, nonoliguric ATN is the most likely diagnosis.

PRESENTATION

CASE 29-6, QUESTION 2: How does aminoglycoside-induced ATN present, and what are the mechanisms of toxicity?

Table 29-6
Risk Factors for Developing Aminoglycoside Nephrotoxicity

Patient Factors
Elderly
Underlying renal disease
Dehydration
Hypotension and shock syndromes
Hepatorenal syndrome
Aminoglycoside Factors
Aminoglycoside choice: gentamicin > tobramycin > amikacin
Therapy >3 days
Multiple daily dosing
Serum trough >2 mg/L
Recent aminoglycoside therapy
Concomitant Drug Therapy
Amphotericin B
Cisplatin
Cyclosporine
Foscarnet
Furosemide
Radiocontrast media
Vancomycin

T.G. illustrates the typical presentation of aminoglycoside-induced nephrotoxicity. Generally, the onset occurs after 5 to 7 days of treatment and presents as a hypo-osmolar, nonoliguric renal failure with a slow rise in SCr.[81] Because of the tubular necrosis that occurs, the urinalysis is often positive for low-molecular-weight proteins, tubular cellular casts, epithelial cells, WBCs, and brush-border cells.[82] T.G.'s plasma and urinary laboratory indices are consistent with those listed for ATN in Table 29-3.

The mechanism of aminoglycoside-induced ATN is complex. Approximately 5% of filtered aminoglycoside is actively reabsorbed by the proximal tubule cells. These agents are polycationic and bind to the negatively charged brush-border cells within the tubule lumen. Once attached, these agents undergo pinocytosis and enter the intracellular space, setting off complex biochemical events that result in the formation of myeloid bodies. With continued formation of myeloid bodies, the brush-border cells swell and burst, releasing large concentrations of aminoglycoside and lysosomal enzymes into the tubule lumen, thereby beginning a cascade of further tubular destruction.[81,83] The following rank order of nephrotoxicity has been collated from human and animal data: neomycin > gentamicin > tobramycin > amikacin > netilmicin > streptomycin.[82]

EXTENDED-INTERVAL DOSING

CASE 29-6, QUESTION 3: Is "extended-interval" aminoglycoside dosing less nephrotoxic than multiple daily dosing regimens?

Extended-interval aminoglycoside dosing entails the administration of one large daily aminoglycoside dose instead of multiple daily dosing. This dosing scheme takes advantage of the concentration-dependent killing activity and post-antibiotic effect observed with aminoglycosides while minimizing time-dependent toxicity.

The net effect of this dosing scheme, purportedly, is greater efficacy with reduced toxicity. Aminoglycoside nephrotoxicity is a function of drug exposure, and it might be minimized with extended-interval dosing because of saturable uptake kinetics in the proximal tubule. That is, only a maximal amount of aminoglycoside is transported into the tubule cell, no matter how much aminoglycoside is present in the tubule. Consequently, once saturation occurs, the remaining aminoglycoside concentration passes through the proximal tubule without being absorbed, and is excreted in the urine. Accumulation is therefore averted.[84] This concept is supported by studies demonstrating that continuous-rate gentamicin infusions, which produce sustained low plasma concentrations, result in greater proximal tubule uptake and nephrotoxicity than extended-interval regimens. This is probably because the achieved drug concentrations are well below those required to saturate the uptake mechanism. Extended-interval dosing results in very high peak concentrations to improve efficacy and generally undetectable trough concentrations before the next dose, thus minimizing accumulation. Numerous clinical trials and meta-analyses have compared the efficacy and toxicity of extended-interval aminoglycoside dosing with conventional multiple daily dosing regimens. For endocarditis, aminoglycosides, such as gentamicin 1 mg/kg q8 hours or 3 mg/kg once daily, adjusted for renal function are recommended by the American Heart Association for the management of selected cases of bacterial endocarditis for their synergistical activity with the β-lactams. The extended interval dosing is less well studied for endocarditis.[80] In summary, extended-interval aminoglycoside dosing appears to result in similar or greater efficacy, with similar or reduced toxicity. This dosing schedule is also less costly when considering therapeutic drug monitoring, preparation, and administration costs. Although the typical extended interval in patients with normal renal function is dosing every 24 hours, the interval may have to be prolonged to several days in patients with renal failure.

Drug-Induced Acute Interstitial Nephritis

Drug-induced AIN accounts for approximately 1% to 3% of all AKI cases.[85–89] A variety of antibiotics, such as penicillins, cephalosporins, quinolones, particularly ciprofloxacin, sulfonamides, and rifampin, as well as NSAIDs, loop diuretics, thiazide-like diuretics, and proton pump inhibitors, have been implicated as common drug causes of AIN. The pathophysiology of this reaction is not well understood; it is suspected that either humoral or cell-mediated immune mechanisms or both are involved.[90] Humoral immune reactions occur within minutes to hours of drug exposure and involve the drug or its metabolite acting as a hapten that binds to host proteins, making them antigenic. The drug–protein antigens become lodged in the renal tubules, which initiate the inflammatory cascade. Cell-mediated injury can occur days to weeks after drug exposure and is identified by the presence of mononuclear inflammation and the lack of detectable immune complexes. This suggests a delayed hypersensitivity rather than a direct cytotoxic effect from a given drug. Both immune mechanisms probably contribute to the development of drug-induced AIN.

PENICILLIN-INDUCED ACUTE INTERSTITIAL NEPHRITIS

CASE 29-7

QUESTION 1: J.S. is a 50-year-old Hispanic woman (height = 5 feet, 3 inches; weight = 160 pounds), who exhibited cellulitis 3 days after a car door was closed on her right hand. She was admitted to the hospital, where blood and wound cultures were found to be positive for methicillin-sensitive *Staphylococcus aureus*. She received 2 full days of nafcillin 2 g IV every 4 hours before being discharged to complete a 14-day course with dicloxacillin 500 mg PO 4 times daily (QID). Ten days after discharge, J.S. returned to the emergency department complaining of malaise, fever, diffuse rash, hematuria, and reduced urine output. The following laboratory values were significant:

BUN, 39 mg/dL
SCr, 2.3 mg/dL
WBC count, 18,500 cells/μL with 18% eosinophils

The urinalysis was positive for elevated specific gravity, WBC, RBC, eosinophiluria, and a FE_{Na} of 3%. What objective data suggest drug-induced AIN?

J.S.'s onset of symptoms suggests antibiotic-induced AIN. As illustrated by this case, the median onset of penicillin-induced AIN generally occurs 6 to 10 days after drug exposure. Hallmark symptoms of antibiotic-associated AIN include fever, macular rash, and malaise. Fever is present in nearly all patients with antibiotic-induced AIN, and rash occurs in 25% to 50% of patients. In contrast, NSAIDs, proton pump inhibitors, and rifampin are less commonly associated with rash, fever, eosinophilia, and the onset of AIN may occur several weeks to months or longer following drug exposure.[89,90] J.S.'s objective laboratory data that suggest AIN include azotemia, elevated SCr, proteinuria, cellular urinary sediment, eosinophilia, and eosinophiluria. Her FE_{Na} of 3% suggests intrinsic renal disease, and her eosinophiluria and eosinophilia indicate an immune-mediated allergic reaction. Drug-induced AIN is generally nonoliguric, but oliguria can develop in severe cases of AIN.

CASE 29-7, QUESTION 2: How should J.S.'s penicillin-induced AIN be treated?

The dicloxacillin should be stopped immediately because most patients recover normal kidney function once the offending agent is discontinued. Clindamycin or doxycycline may be chosen to finish the course of treatment for cellulitis. However, J.S. has completed 12 out of 14 days of antibiotic therapy and alternate agents would be optional. General supportive measures that maintain fluid and electrolyte balance are necessary. Renal recovery may take weeks to months. Corticosteroids have been used with variable results to shorten the duration of AKI, but no clinical guidelines have been developed to delineate when to administer them and for how long. Some clinicians prefer to administer prednisone 1 mg/kg for 7 days and then gradually taper the dose during the next several weeks. The response to corticosteroids may be delayed or absent in some patients. Dialysis may be needed in patients who are oliguric, but it is usually not required for those who are nonoliguric. The clinician should document J.S.'s allergic reaction to penicillins in her medical record, and not rechallenge the patient to antibiotics with similar chemical structures because repeated exposure is likely to result in similar reactions.

POSTRENAL ACUTE KIDNEY INJURY

Any condition that results in the obstruction of urine flow at any level of the urinary tract is termed postrenal AKI. Common causes of postrenal AKI are nephrolithiasis (stone formation), crystal formation, underlying malignancies of the prostate or cervix, prostatic hypertrophy, or bilateral ureter strictures. Conditions that result in bladder outlet obstruction (e.g., prostatic

Table 29-7
Risk Factors for Nephrolithiasis

Low urine volume
Hypercalciuria
Hyperoxaluria
Hyperuricosuria
Hypercitruria
Chronically low or high urinary pH

hypertrophy) are the most common causes of postrenal AKI. The onset of signs and symptoms is generally gradual; it often presents as decreased force of urine stream, dribbling, or polyuria. Drugs can also result in insoluble crystal formation in the urine and should be included in the differential diagnosis.

Nephrolithiasis

Kidney stones generally consist of uric acid, cystine, struvite (also called magnesium ammonium phosphate or triple phosphate nephrolithiasis), and calcium salts. Of these, calcium stones are by far the most prevalent.[91]

Calcium nephrolithiasis constitutes approximately 70% to 80% of all kidney stones,[92] with calcium oxalate and calcium phosphate stones making up most of these. Genetic factors appear to play an important role in the development of calcium nephrolithiasis; the stereotypical patient is a man in his third to fifth decade of life. Other risk factors for developing calcium nephrolithiasis are low urine output, inadequate hydration (e.g., living in a hot climate and not drinking adequate fluids), hypercalciuria, hyperoxaluria, hypocitraturia, hyperuricosuria, and distal renal tubular acidosis (Table 29-7). Generally, more than one of these conditions are present simultaneously. The diagnosis and management of kidney stones are beyond the scope of discussion in this chapter. However, pharmacists can be instrumental in providing proper counseling on hydration and preventive measures.

CRYSTAL FORMATION

Crystal-induced AKI most commonly occurs as a result of acute uric acid nephropathy and following the administration of drugs or toxins that are poorly soluble or have metabolites that are poorly soluble in urine. Other drugs or toxins (e.g., ascorbic acid, ethylene glycol) may be metabolized to insoluble products such as oxalate, which are associated with precipitation of calcium oxalate crystals in the urine within the tubular lumen resulting in kidney injury.[92,93]

PRESENTATION AND TREATMENT

CASE 29-8

QUESTION 1: T.C., a 25-year-old male with a past medical history of schizophrenia, was seen in an outpatient clinic 4 days prior to admission where he was started on oral acyclovir 800 mg 5 times a day for a diagnosis of herpes zoster. He presents to the emergency department complaining of sharp flank pain, gross hematuria, and dysuria. Serum chemistries are ordered and are significant only for a BUN of 34 mg/dL and a SCr of 1.5 mg/dL, which are up from his baseline values of 7 and 0.9 mg/dL, respectively. A urine sample was obtained and visualized with microscopy. Birefringent needle-shaped crystals were seen on polarizing light microscopy. It was consistent with acyclovir-induced nephropathy. On questioning, he admits that he has not been drinking much fluid during the past week owing to a busy work schedule, and his urine volume has been markedly lower than usual. Which drugs can crystallize in the urine and cause AKI?

Table 29-8
Commonly Used Drugs that Cause Crystal-Induced Acute Kidney Injury

Acyclovir
Ciprofloxacin
Indinavir
Methotrexate
Sulfonamide antibiotics
Orlistat
Triamterene

Many commonly prescribed drugs are insoluble in urine and crystallize in the distal tubule (Table 29-8). Risk factors that predispose patients to crystalluria include severe volume contraction, underlying renal dysfunction, or acidotic or alkalotic urinary pH. In conditions of renal hypoperfusion, high concentrations of drug become stagnant in the tubule lumen. Drugs that are weak acids (e.g., methotrexate, sulfonamide antibiotics) precipitate in acidic urine; drugs that are weak bases (e.g., ciprofloxacin, indinavir, and other protease inhibitors) precipitate in alkaline urine. Patients with drug-related crystal-induced AKI are usually asymptomatic, and kidney injury is detected by an increased SCr. Occasionally, like T.C., patients present within 1 to 7 days after initiation of the offending drug with renal colic symptoms such as flank or abdominal pain, nausea, or vomiting. Urinalysis often reveals hematuria, pyuria, and crystalluria. The diagnosis is suggested by the appearance of crystals in the urine, the morphology of which depends upon the specific causative drug. Prevention of crystal-induced AKI is targeted at dosage adjustment for patients with underlying renal dysfunction, volume expansion to increase urinary output, and urine alkalization to enhance renal elimination of drugs that are weak acids or urine acidification to enhance renal elimination of drugs that are weak bases. Dialysis may be necessary in a small percentage of patients. With appropriate pharmacotherapy, crystal-induced AKI is usually reversible without long-term complications.[94]

SUPPORTIVE MANAGEMENT OF ACUTE KIDNEY INJURY

CASE 29-9

QUESTION 1: J.W. is a 75-year-old Native American man (height = 6 feet, 2 inches; weight = 200 pounds), who presents to the emergency room with shortness of breath and progressive worsening edema in both lower extremities. His medical history includes nephrotic syndrome secondary to diabetic nephrosclerosis, type 1 diabetes, hypertension, and chronic obstructive pulmonary disease. His surgical history includes a right-sided nephrectomy many years ago. His chronic medications are furosemide 80 mg PO twice a day, metolazone 10 mg PO once a day, lisinopril 5 mg PO once a day, diltiazem extended-release 120 mg PO once a day, albuterol, inhaler as needed, and subcutaneous 20 units insulin glargine at bedtime, and insulin aspart before meals. Vital signs are temperature 36.3°C, pulse 77 beats/minute, respirations 16 breaths/minute, and BP 179/86 mm Hg. Physical examination reveals periorbital edema, jugular venous distension at a 45-degree angle to the jaw, dullness to percussion halfway up the lungs bilaterally, and 4+ pitting edema in the extremities. Admitting laboratory tests reveal the following:

Sodium, 140 mEq/L
Potassium, 5.5 mEq/L

Chloride, 103 mEq/L
Bicarbonate, 19 mEq/L
Glucose, 249 mg/dL
BUN, 67 mg/dL
SCr, 5.2 mg/dL
Serum albumin, 2.0 g/dL
Spot urine albumin:creatinine ratio, 350 mg/g

Baseline renal function tests 1 month ago are BUN 45 mg/dL and SCr 3.0 mg/dL. J.W. is oliguric with a urine output of 10 mL/hour. The nephrologist wants to use supportive management of AKI by first optimizing diuretic therapy. If no increase in urine output occurs during the next several hours, then the patient will undergo RRT. What is the supportive management of AKI?

Despite years of study, no pharmacologic "cure" for AKI exists. Supportive management is therefore directed at preventing its morbidity and mortality. This is achieved by close patient monitoring; strict fluid, electrolyte, and nutritional management; treatment of life-threatening conditions such as pulmonary edema, hyperkalemia, and metabolic acidosis; avoidance of nephrotoxic drugs; and the initiation of dialysis or CRRT.

An assessment of volume status should be performed in all patients who present with AKI, since correction of volume depletion or volume overload may reverse or ameliorate AKI. The underlying cause dictates management of AKI. Treating the underlying cause is of extremely important. For example, prerenal AKI because of volume-depleted states, such as septic shock, requires administration of fluids and vasopressors to restore renal perfusion and increase urine output. On the other hand, diuretic administration for preload reduction to increase cardiac output would be required for prerenal AKI because of volume-overload states as in congestive heart failure.

As discussed earlier, diuretics currently have no role in preventing AKI progression or reducing mortality, but they can prevent complications, such as pulmonary edema. For edema, intravenous furosemide (e.g., 80–120 mg) is preferred because of its potency and pulmonary vasodilation properties. Oral furosemide therapy should be avoided because gut edema may limit its bioavailability. Torsemide and bumetanide are two other loop diuretics that have excellent oral bioavailability and are unaffected by gut edema. The dosage of diuretic needed is highly patient specific, especially in those with frank proteinuria, glomerulonephritis, or the nephrotic syndrome. Low serum albumin limits drug transport to the kidneys and thus limits diuretic effectiveness. In addition, furosemide is highly protein bound, and thus binds to filtered protein, which negates its pharmacologic effect on the kidneys. Combinations of loop and thiazide diuretics may be needed in patients with AKI if they become diuretic resistant. This combination acts synergistically to block sodium and water reabsorption in both Henle's loop and the distal convoluted tubule. Other alternatives include continuous loop diuretic infusions, such as furosemide 1 mg/kg/hour. The infusion rate should not exceed 4 mg/minute because these rates are associated with ototoxicity, especially when given in combination with aminoglycoside antibiotics. Close monitoring of serum bicarbonate, potassium, magnesium, and calcium is necessary when giving large doses of loop diuretics. Diuresis should aim for a weight loss of 0.5 to 1.0 kg/day. If diuretics fail to achieve the desired fluid overload reduction, dialysis or CRRT can be considered.

Hyperkalemia commonly occurs in patients with AKI because the kidneys regulate potassium homeostasis. It can be life threatening. It is prevalent in oliguric patients who are catabolic or have evidence of active cellular breakdown, such as rhabdomyolysis and tumor lysis syndrome. J.W. is mildly hyperkalemic, but his serum potassium may decrease after furosemide therapy. Management of hyperkalemia is discussed in Chapter 27, Fluid and Electrolyte Disorders. In cases of severe hyperkalemia in which conventional pharmacologic treatment is not feasible, or not working, emergency hemodialysis should be performed. Medications that can cause hyperkalemia such ACE-inhibitors, ARBs, or trimethoprim should be avoided.

Metabolic acidosis is a common manifestation of AKI because the kidneys are responsible for excreting organic acids. Other factors also contribute to severe acidosis among patients with AKI, who are often critically ill. For example, patients with AKI because of septic shock, trauma, and multi-organ failure often have increased production of lactic acid or ketoacids. J.W.'s serum bicarbonate concentration reveals slight acidemia that does not require correction at this time. Commonly used treatments for metabolic acidosis include bicarbonate administration and dialysis. Bicarbonate therapy may be administered as first corrective therapy, in non–life-threatening and non–fluid-overloaded metabolic acidosis. Severe metabolic acidosis ($pH < 7.1$) in the presence of anuria or oliguria and a fluid overload state should be corrected with dialysis, since worsening volume overload can occur with the administration of sodium bicarbonate therapy.

Uremia can interfere with platelet aggregation resulting in hemorrhagic diathesis. Uremic patients display increased bleeding sensitivity to aspirin compared to normal patients taking aspirin. Patients with uremia and major hemorrhagic bleed may benefit from using desmopressin (dDAVP) 0.3 mcg/kg intravenously or subcutaneously for one or two doses. Desmopressin produces a dose-related increase in von Willebrand factor VII and t-PA levels; this shortens activated antithromboplastin time (aPTT) as well as bleeding time. The improvement in bleeding time typically begins within about 1 hour to 4 to 8 hours. Tachyphylaxis typically develops after the second dose. Other modalities that can improve platelet function and reduce bleeding in an AKI patient include dialysis, conjugated estrogens, and cryoprecipitate.[95]

Clinicians should closely monitor the patient's vital signs (e.g., weight, temperature, BP, pulse, and respirations) several times per day. The patient's volume status should be assessed daily, and all fluids should be adjusted based on laboratory chemistries to detect fluid and electrolyte abnormalities, urine output, and gastrointestinal and insensible losses. Pharmacists should pay attention to nutritional support for patients with AKI to provide adequate amounts of energy, protein, and nutrients, while being sensitive to the electrolytes, acidosis, and volume balance issues. The patient's medication profile should be reviewed daily to assess for appropriate dosage adjustment in renal dysfunction. Because estimation of ClCr is difficult in patients with changing renal function, therapeutic drug monitoring should be performed when using drugs with narrow therapeutic indices. When possible, nephrotoxic drugs should be avoided, but this may be difficult in patients who are septic or hypotensive and require nephrotoxic antibiotics and vasopressors. Preventive measures to reduce the likelihood of AKI should be used, such as monitoring volume status to ensure adequate renal perfusion, using dosing strategies or products that are associated with less nephrotoxicity, and avoiding drug therapy combinations that enhance nephrotoxicity (e.g., NSAID, aminoglycosides).

Extracorporeal Continuous Renal Replacement Therapy

RRT is not always indicated in AKI. The A-E-I-O-U mnemonic is used to help remember the indications for RRT, where 'A' stands for intractable refractory acidosis, 'E' refers to electrolyte abnormalities, specifically potassium with EKG changes, 'I' refers to ingestion of toxins such as salicylates and ethylene glycol, 'O' stands for fluid overload causing pulmonary edema, and 'U' refers to symptomatic uremia with confusion, platelet dysfunction and severe bleed, and seizures.

The risks associated with RRT are hypotension, arrhythmias, vascular access placement complications, and increased risk of ESRD. Hence, the decision to initiate RRT has to be carefully discussed. The timing of optimal initiation of RRT is also lacking. Early initiation may decrease mortality in critically ill patients and the need for permanent RRT at discharge.[96]

RRT can be divided into intermittent hemodialysis or CRRT, such as continuous peritoneal dialysis or extracorporeal CRRT. The decision to use one versus the other is most often decided by the nephrologist's experience and comfort level. CRRT may be preferred in patients who are hemodynamically unstable or requiring vasopressor support. Extracorporeal CRRT differs from peritoneal and hemodialysis in its mechanism of solute removal; dialysis modalities rely primarily on solute diffusion across a semipermeable membrane, whereas CRRT relies primarily on convective ultrafiltrate production. This discussion will be limited to extracorporeal (hemofilter membrane is outside of the body) CRRT therapies (see Chapter 30, Renal Dialysis, for a complete overview of peritoneal and hemodialysis).

Not all extracorporeal CRRT is alike[97]; many variations exist and include modalities such as continuous arteriovenous hemofiltration (now obsolete), continuous venovenous hemofiltration (CVVH), continuous venovenous hemodialysis (CVVHD), and continuous venovenous hemodiafiltration (CVVHDF; Fig. 29-5). Differences among these modalities are illustrated in Table 29-9. Drug dosing can be difficult in patients receiving these therapies, especially in those who are undergoing both dialysis and hemofiltration modalities (i.e., CVVHDF).

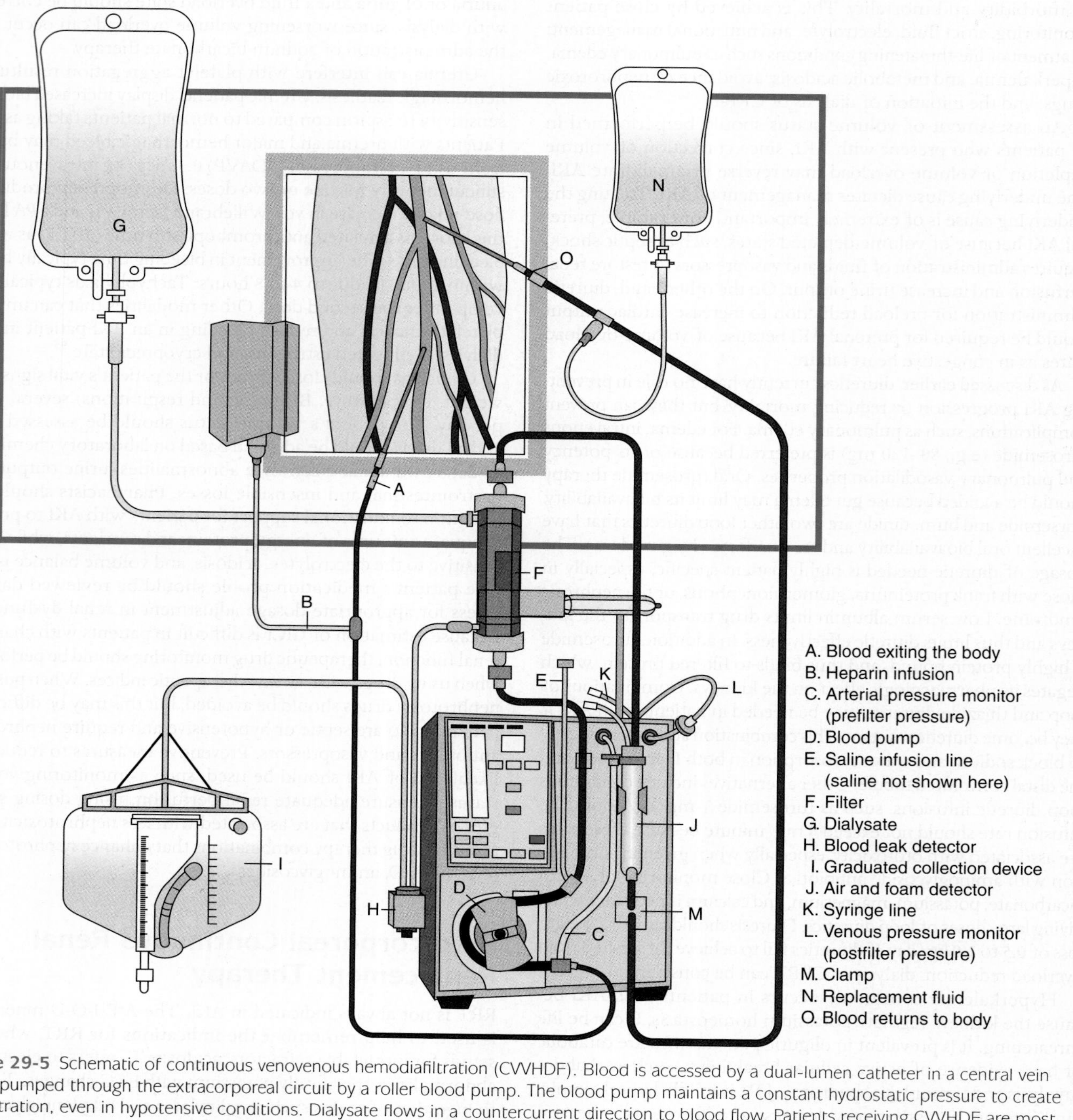

Figure 29-5 Schematic of continuous venovenous hemodiafiltration (CVVHDF). Blood is accessed by a dual-lumen catheter in a central vein and is pumped through the extracorporeal circuit by a roller blood pump. The blood pump maintains a constant hydrostatic pressure to create ultrafiltration, even in hypotensive conditions. Dialysate flows in a countercurrent direction to blood flow. Patients receiving CVVHDF are most often in the intensive care unit and often receive concomitant parenteral nutrition.

Table 29-9
Comparison of Extracorporeal Continuous Renal Replacement Therapies

Parameter	Continuous Venovenous Hemofiltration (CVVH)	Continuous Arteriovenous Hemofiltration (CAVH)	Continuous Venovenous Hemodialysis (CVVHD)	Continuous Venovenous Hemodiafiltration (CVVHDF)
Volume control in hypotensive patients	Good	Variable	Good	Good
Solute control in highly catabolic patients	Adequate	Inadequate	Adequate	Adequate
Blood flow rates in hypotensive patients	Adequate	Poor	Adequate	Adequate
Ease of drug dosing	Published recommendations	Difficult	Difficult	Difficult
Dialytic solute clearance	None	None	Moderate	Moderate
Convective solute clearance	Good	Good	Minimal	Moderate
Corresponding GFR (mL/minute)	15–17	10–15	17–21	25–26
Blood pump required	Yes	No	Yes	Yes
Replacement fluid required	Yes	Yes	Yes	Yes
Pharmacy expense	High	High	High	High

GFR, glomerular filtration rate.

Estimating Drug Removal

Case 29-9, Question 2: Are there ways to calculate drug removal in extracorporeal CRRT modalities?

Recent reviews provide an excellent background on dosing drugs in patients receiving CRRT.[9,32,98–100] The principles for drug removal in hemofiltration are basically identical with those for removal in hemodialysis. Drug removal during CRRT may occur by convection, diffusion, and adsorption. Convection and diffusion have the greatest influence on drug removal. Drug removal is inversely proportional to the percentage of drug that is protein bound. If a drug is >80% plasma protein bound, little will be removed. This principle holds true for convection and diffusion. Ultrafiltration and dialysis flow rates (UFR/DFR) also affect drug clearance. Because CRRT uses highly permeable membranes, the molecular weight (MW) of most drugs has little impact on overall clearance. During convection, clearance of an unbound drug can be dramatic since CVVH can remove easily compounds with MW <15,000 Da. The impact of MW on drug removal during CVVHD is greater than the impact seen during CVVH. Solute clearance during CVVHD is dependent on diffusion and given that diffusion is inversely proportional to MW, the greatest impact is seen with drugs having a low MW <500 Da. Many drugs have low MW and hence CVVHD can impact their removal significantly. Clearance during CVVH is accomplished through the process of convection. The ultrafiltrate produced is replaced either in part or completely. Clearance of unbound drugs during CVVH can be dramatic and dose adjustments are required to prevent underdosing.

The sieving coefficient (SC) of a drug is the non–protein-bound fraction of the drug that is in plasma. SC ranges from 0 to 1 (zero representing no convective clearance). For example, a SC of 0.8 means that 80% of the drug is unbound in plasma. Drug SC can be obtained from the literature or by measuring concentrations simultaneously in the prefilter blood and ultrafiltrate. The ratio of the ultrafiltrate concentration to plasma concentration is the SC. Drug clearance can be calculated by multiplying the SC by the ultrafiltration rate. For example, if a patient is receiving CVVH at an ultrafiltration rate of 1 L/hour, and he or she is receiving vancomycin (which has an SC of 0.8) 1 g/day, the vancomycin clearance while receiving CVVH is $0.8 \times 1{,}000$ mL/hour = 800 mL/hour or 13 mL/minute.

Calculating drug clearance is much more difficult in hemodiafiltration modalities (CVVHDF) because both convection and diffusion account for drug clearance, and it is difficult to predict drug clearance precisely. The use of SC can be useful for small-molecular-weight drugs, but the accuracy declines with larger drug molecules, such as vancomycin. When possible, therapeutic drug monitoring should be performed to maintain therapeutic concentrations and to maximize drug therapy.

Drug references such as Drug Prescribing in Renal Failure provide useful guidelines in a concise tabular format.[101]

KEY REFERENCES AND WEBSITES

A full list of references for this chapter can be found at http://thepoint.lww.com/AT11e. Below are the key references for this chapter, with the corresponding reference number in this chapter found in parentheses after the reference.

Key References

Bellomo R et al. Acute kidney injury. *Lancet*. 2012;380:756. (1)

Churchwell MD et al. Drug dosing during continuous renal replacement therapy. *Semin Dial*. 2009;22:185. (98)

González PM. Acute interstitial nephritis. *Kidney Int*. 2010;77:956. (85)

Heintz BH et al. Antimicrobial dosing concepts and recommendations for critically ill adult patients receiving continuous renal replacement therapy or intermittent hemodialysis. *Pharmacotherapy*. 2009;29:562. (99)

Kidney Disease: Improving Global Outcomes (KDIGO) Acute Kidney Injury Work Group. KDIGO Clinical Practice Guideline for Acute Kidney Injury. *Kidney Int Suppl*. 2012;2:1. (9)

Lapi F et al. Concurrent use of diuretics, angiotensin converting enzyme inhibitors, and angiotensin receptor blockers with nonsteroidal anti-inflammatory drugs and risk of acute kidney injury: nested case control study. *BMJ*. 2013;346:e8525. (39)

Massicotte A. Contrast medium-induced nephropathy: strategies for prevention. *Pharmacotherapy*. 2008;28:1140. (68)

Matzke GR et al. Drug dosing consideration in patients with acute and chronic kidney disease—a clinical update from Kidney Disease: Improving Global Outcomes (KDIGO). *Kidney Int*. 2011;80:1122. (32)

Rahman M. Acute kidney injury: a guide to diagnosis and management. *Am Fam Physician*. 2012;86:631. (22)

Thomas ME et al. The definition of acute kidney injury and its use in practice. *Kidney Int*. 2015;87:62. (3)

Key Website

KDIGO Clinical Practice Guideline for Acute Kidney Injury. http://www.kidney-international.org.

30 Renal Dialysis

Myrna Y. Munar

CORE PRINCIPLES

	CORE PRINCIPLES	CHAPTER CASES
1	End-stage renal disease (ESRD) occurs when there is progressive loss of kidney function over a period of months to years to the point where the kidneys can no longer remove wastes; concentrate urine; maintain acid–base homeostasis; and regulate fluid, electrolytes, and other important body functions.	**Case 30-1 (Question 1)**
2	Dialysis is a process that facilitates the removal of excess water and solutes from the body, both of which accumulate as a result of inadequate kidney function. Solutes from the blood are removed through diffusion and convection. Accumulated water is removed by ultrafiltration.	**Case 30-1 (Question 1), Figure 30-1**
3	The ability of a dialyzer to remove solutes and water is determined by its composition, pore size, surface area, and configuration.	**Case 30-1 (Question 1), Figure 30-1**
4	Dialysate is an electrolyte solution that simulates plasma. The concentration of electrolytes in dialysate can be manipulated to control the diffusion of electrolytes from the blood into dialysate to maintain homeostasis. Metabolic acidosis is controlled with the addition of bicarbonate to dialysate.	**Case 30-1 (Question 1), Figure 30-1**
5	Different types of vascular access are available: arteriovenous (AV) fistula, AV graft, and double-lumen or tunneled catheters. An AV fistula is preferred because of its longer survival rates and low rates of complications.	**Case 30-1 (Question 2)**
6	Anticoagulation is necessary during hemodialysis (HD) to prevent blood from clotting in the extracorporeal circuit. Several methods have been used to provide adequate anticoagulation without increasing the risk of bleeding.	**Case 30-1 (Questions 3–5)**
7	Complications can arise during HD. The most common complications are hypotension and muscle cramps. Graft thrombosis and graft infection are common chronic complications.	**Case 30-1 (Questions 6–9), Case 30-2 (Questions 1–2)**
8	Continuous ambulatory peritoneal dialysis is performed by instilling sterile dialysate into the peritoneal cavity through a surgically placed resident catheter. The solution dwells within the cavity for 4 to 8 hours, and then it is drained and replaced with a fresh solution. This process of fill, dwell, and drain is performed 3 to 4 times during the day, with a longer dwell overnight.	**Case 30-3 (Question 1), Figure 30-2**
9	The process of peritoneal dialysis (PD) is similar to HD; in this process, however, the peritoneal membrane covering the abdominal contents serves as an endogenous dialysis membrane, and the vasculature embedded in the peritoneum serves as the blood supply. Fluid is removed by manipulating the dextrose concentration in dialysate to control the osmotic pressure gradient for fluid removal.	**Case 30-3 (Question 1), Figure 30-2**
10	The most significant complication among patients having PD is peritonitis. Empiric antibiotics can be administered by the intraperitoneal (IP) route and must cover both gram-positive and gram-negative organisms.	**Case 30-3 (Questions 2, 4)**

Continued

		CHAPTER CASES
11	Other medications can be administered IP. Heparin can be added to dialysate to prevent fibrin clots from forming and obstructing outflow from the peritoneal cavity. Regular insulin can be administered IP to patients with diabetes.	Case 30-3 (Questions 3, 7)
12	Prevention of catheter exit-site infections (and thus peritonitis) is the primary goal of exit-site care. Routine care consists of hand cleansing with antiseptics or antibacterial soap before touching the exit site, washing the exit site daily with antibacterial soap, and use of antimicrobial creams around the exit site.	Case 30-3 (Questions 5, 6)

End-stage renal disease (ESRD) occurs when there is progressive loss of kidney function over a period of months to years to the point where the kidneys can no longer remove wastes, concentrate urine, maintain acid–base homeostasis, and regulate fluid and electrolytes and other important body functions. ESRD is classified under stage 5 chronic kidney disease (CKD), which refers to patients with an estimated glomerular filtration rate (eGFR) less than 15 mL/minute/1.73 m^2, or those requiring dialysis or transplantation.[1,2] Demographic characteristics of ESRD population are based primarily on data from the Centers for Medicare and Medicaid Services, because patients with ESRD are eligible for Medicare benefits. Coverage for ESRD began in 1972, when Congress enacted the End-Stage Renal Disease Program as an amendment to Medicare. Data from the ESRD program are reported annually by the United States Renal Data System. According to the 2014 Annual Report, diabetes and hypertension continue to be leading causes of ESRD.[3] Patients aged 45 years and older account for the largest segment of the ESRD population. Racial differences in the prevalence of ESRD persist. While prevalence of ESRD in Native Americans has declined since 2000, prevalence rates remain much higher in Blacks/African Americans than in other racial groups, at nearly twofold higher than Native Americans, 2.5-fold higher than Asians, and fourfold higher than Whites.[3]

In 2012 there were 636,905 prevalent cases of ESRD in the United States, an increase of 3.7% from the previous year. Of these, 402,514 patients were treated by hemodialysis (HD), 40,605 were on peritoneal dialysis (PD), and 17,305 kidney transplantations were performed.[3] The number of kidney transplants has remained stable since 2005. Recipients living with a functioning graft continue to grow, reaching 186,303 in 2012 reflecting a 3.6% increase from 2011. However, the shortage of donor kidneys and the existence of patients with ESRD, who are unacceptable transplant recipients, sustain the demand for dialysis. Kidney transplantation is further discussed in Chapter 34, Kidney and Liver Transplantation.

The two primary modes of dialysis therapy are HD and PD. Both HD and PD were developed as methods for the removal of metabolic waste products across a semipermeable membrane.

HD is an extracorporeal (dialysis membrane is outside of the body) process, whereas PD uses the patient's peritoneal membrane for the clearance of water and solutes. Variations of PD include continuous ambulatory peritoneal dialysis (CAPD) and automated peritoneal dialysis (APD), an increasingly common modality that permits greater patient flexibility with dialysis at home. Among the 443,119 dialysis patients in the United States, 91% undergo HD.[3] Most of these patients receive dialysis 3 times a week in a center designed primarily for stable, ambulatory patients at either a hospital-based or a free-standing dialysis facility. Home HD accounts for less than 1% of dialysis patients. Patients having PD are also managed through dialysis centers for routine care, although less often than patients on HD. The most frequent form of dialysis in children is APD. Several factors are considered in the selection of the type of dialysis for each patient. Often, the overriding consideration is the suitability of the procedure for the patient's lifestyle. A patient who needs flexibility and freedom from a rigid schedule may prefer PD versus HD to avoid the necessity of being at a dialysis center 3 times weekly for a 3- to 4-hour dialysis treatment. Other considerations include the availability of a vascular access site for HD, a patient's ability to perform self-care for dialysate exchanges with PD, or the capability of the patient, parent, or caregiver to carry out APD at home.

Without dialysis or transplantation, patients with ESRD will die from the metabolic complications of their renal failure. Survival on dialysis has improved over the years. Since 1993, mortality rates have fallen across all renal replacement modalities with a 28% reduction for HD patients, 47% reduction for PD patients, and 51% reduction for transplant patients.[3] While these rates are encouraging, only 54% of HD patients and 65% of PD patients survive beyond 3 years after ESRD onset. All-cause mortality rates are 6.1 to 7.8 times higher for dialysis patients compared to the general population, and highest in the second and third months of dialysis. Dialysis patients are expected to live one-third as long as people of the same age in the general population. Transplant patients live longer with an estimated lifetime that is 83% to 87% of the general population.

The rapid growth of the number of patients having dialysis calls attention to the need for practitioners who understand the processes and therapies for these patients. This chapter addresses the fundamental clinical aspects of both HD and PD, including principles, complications, and management. Throughout the chapter, reference will be made, when appropriate, to the Kidney Disease Outcomes Quality Initiative (K/DOQI) clinical practice guidelines developed by the National Kidney Foundation.[4–6]

HEMODIALYSIS

Principles and Transport Processes

Dialysis is a process that facilitates the removal of excess water and toxins from the body, both of which accumulate as a result of inadequate kidney function. During HD, a patient's anticoagulated blood (circulated to the dialyzer from a vein in the arm) and an electrolyte solution that simulates plasma (dialysate) are simultaneously perfused through a dialyzer (artificial kidney) on opposite sides of a semipermeable membrane. Solutes (e.g., metabolic waste products, toxins, potassium, and other electrolytes) are removed from the patient's blood by diffusing across concentration gradients into the dialysate. The rate of removal of various solutes from the blood is a function of blood and dialysate flow rates through the dialyzer, relative concentration of each solute in the blood and dialysis solution (thus determining

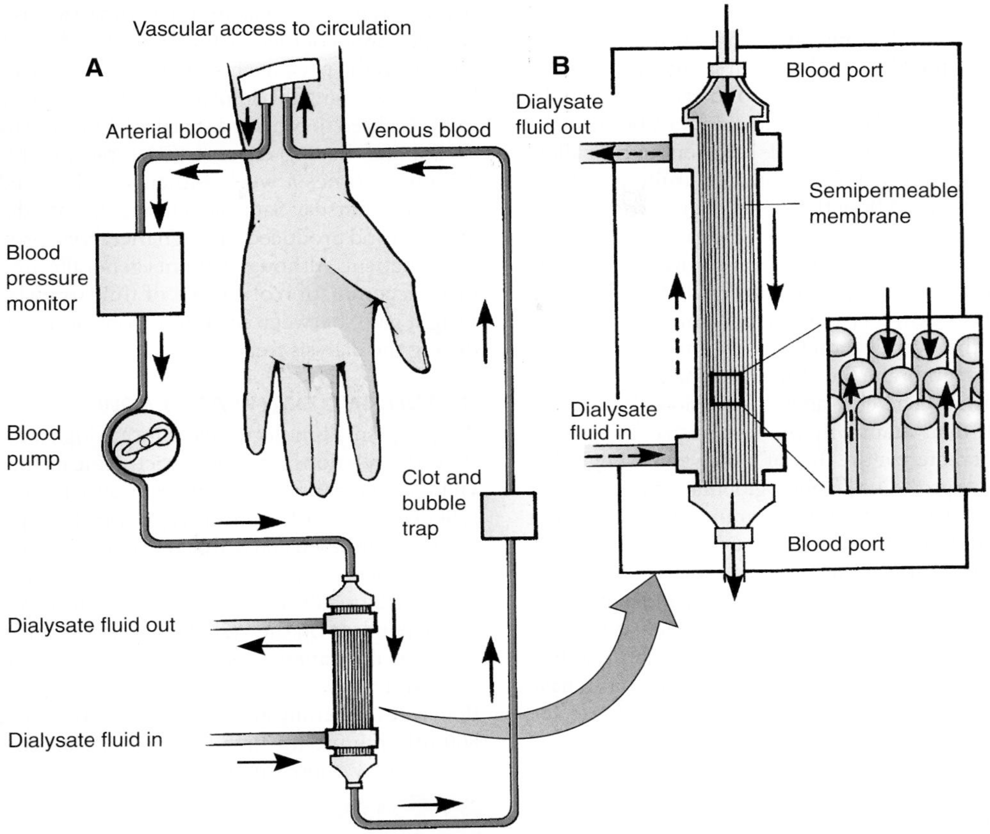

Figure 30-1 Hemodialysis system. **(A)** Blood from an artery is pumped into **(B)**, a dialyzer where it flows through the cellophane tubes, which act as the semipermeable membrane (*inset*). The dialysate, which has the same chemical composition as the blood except for urea and waste products, flows in around the tubules. The waste products in the blood diffuse through the semipermeable membrane into the dialysate. Adapted with permission from Smeltzer SC, Bare BG. *Textbook of Medical-Surgical Nursing*. 9th ed. Philadelphia, PA: Lippincott Williams & Wilkins; 2000.

their concentration gradients across the membrane), physical characteristics of the dialysis membrane (e.g., total available surface area, thickness, and pore size), and properties of the solute being removed (e.g., molecular size in daltons, molecular weight, volume of distribution, and protein binding). Because blood and dialysate flow in opposite directions through the dialyzer, the concentration gradient for each solute across the membrane is amplified (Fig. 30-1). This principle is defined in greater detail in the Dialyzer Characteristics section.

Solutes from the blood are removed through diffusion and convection. Diffusion is the process whereby the molecule moves across its concentration gradient by passing through pores in the dialysis membrane.[7] Once the concentration of a solute reaches equilibrium on both sides of the membrane, the net movement is zero because the rate of movement from the blood to dialysate compartment is equal to the rate from the dialysate to the blood compartment. For most substances, equilibrium is not achieved, either because the blood and dialysate flow rates are too rapid or the molecule is too large to easily move through the pores.

Accumulated water is removed by the process of ultrafiltration. A controlled pressure difference across the semipermeable membrane permits water movement through the membrane pores, carrying solute into the dialysate, thereby further enhancing solute removal. Flux is the rate of water transfer across the dialyzer. Convection is the process that removes toxins and other dissolved solutes during dialysis through the ultrafiltration of plasma water from the blood compartment. The removal of solutes by convection during ultrafiltration generally is small relative to their elimination through diffusion.

DIALYZER CHARACTERISTICS

Dialyzers are characterized by many factors, such as membrane composition, size, and ability to clear solutes. Their primary component is the dialysis membrane, which is made of cellulose (e.g., cuprammonium cellulose), substituted cellulose (e.g., cellulose acetate, cellulose triacetate), cellulosynthetic, or synthetic polymer (e.g., polysulfone, polyacrylonitrile, and polymethylmethacrylate).[8] Membranes differ not only by composition but also by surface area, thickness, and configuration within the dialyzer. The most common configuration is the hollow fiber dialyzer, whereby the membrane is formed as thousands of hollow fibers that run the length of the dialyzer. Blood flows through the fibers and the dialysate flows in the space surrounding the fibers within the dialyzer cartridge. The result is an extremely large surface area for diffusion, which is functionally increased further by the movement of blood and dialysate in opposite directions, so that equilibrium is never fully achieved. Another, less common design is the parallel-plate configuration, whereby blood and dialysate flow between alternating sheets of the membrane.

Functionally, dialysis filters can be differentiated based on their ability to remove solutes and water. The flux of water across the dialyzer is correlated with the clearance of middle molecular weight molecules. Thus, dialyzers are characterized as low-flux or high-flux based on pore size and ability to remove small versus large molecules. One method of categorizing and comparing efficiency (flux) of dialyzer units is to compare the relative in vitro and in vivo clearance rates of marker solutes of varying molecular size. This information is usually printed on the outside of the dialyzer or in the package insert (specification chart) for the dialyzer. For example, urea (molecular size, 60 Da) is a marker of small-molecule transport across the dialysis membrane. Urea (found in the blood as blood urea nitrogen [BUN]) distributes freely throughout body water and is cleared rapidly by HD, even when using standard low-flux dialyzers. Because the pore size of most dialyzer membranes is large enough to allow this small molecule to freely diffuse, the rate-limiting step for the removal of urea is blood flow through the dialyzer. A larger molecule, vitamin B_{12} (molecular size, 1,355 Da), has also been used as a measure of dialysis efficiency. Because vitamin B_{12} is too large to easily cross through the pores of conventional dialysis membranes, its dialysis clearance is less dependent on blood flow than urea. Instead, the overall removal of vitamin B_{12} depends more on the type of membrane (i.e., thickness and pore size) and the duration of dialysis. The clearance of β_2-microglobulin, an even larger molecule than vitamin B_{12} (molecular size, 11,800 Da), has been used to characterize the flux of a dialyzer.[4,8] High-flux dialyzers are defined as providing β_2-microglobulin clearances of at least 20 mL/minute.[4] β_2-microglobulin clearance, however, is not consistently reported in all dialyzer specification charts. High-flux membranes have larger pores and are able to clear larger molecules (e.g., middle molecules such as β_2-microglobulin and leptin) and drugs (e.g., vancomycin or vitamin B_{12}, with molecular weights in the range of 1,000–5,000 Da) more effectively than low-flux membranes with smaller pores. High-flux membranes also have a greater permeability to water, as reflected in a KUf value (to be defined later) of more than 10 mL/hour/mm Hg.

Similarly, molecular weight of drugs is a predictor of dialysis clearance. At a molecular weight of less than 500 Da (e.g., aminoglycosides and theophylline), dialyzability is expected to be high. For these drugs, the actual amount dialyzed will vary based on protein binding (i.e., amount of unbound drug available to cross the dialysis membrane), volume of distribution (Vd) (i.e., a large Vd indicates a relatively small amount of drug will be available in the blood for dialysis), blood flow rate through the dialyzer, dialysis flow rate, and dialyzer surface area. Drugs with a molecular weight between 500 and 1,000 Da (e.g., morphine and digoxin) are less well dialyzed. For digoxin, a greater problem is its large Vd and relatively low serum concentrations. Even if the drug in the blood is effectively removed, tissue-bound drug will quickly redistribute back into the blood as soon as dialysis is completed, a phenomenon known as rebound. Finally, large molecular weight drugs, such as vancomycin, are poorly dialyzed by conventional dialyzers, but they may be removed using high-flux techniques described later in this chapter.

The efficiency of a dialyzer is also a function of its surface area. High-efficiency membranes generally have a large surface area and are able to clear large quantities of small molecules, such as urea. High-efficiency dialyzers can also have small or large pores, resulting in low or high clearance of larger molecular weight solutes. Membranes also differ in their degree of biocompatibility. When free hydroxyl radicals on the surface of cellulose membranes come in contact with blood, the complement pathway is activated and proinflammatory cytokines are produced, which can lead to hypotension, fever, and platelet activation in patients.[9] Use of these membranes has declined. The free hydroxyl groups can be substituted with other chemical structures, such as acetate, to improve biocompatibility. Complement activation and cytokine release occur to a much lesser extent with substituted cellulose or cellulosynthetic membranes, and least of all with synthetic membranes made from plastics.

A typical package insert for a dialyzer will provide information on the clearance of various molecules (e.g., urea, creatinine, phosphate, and vitamin B_{12}). Urea clearance has become a common measure of comparison for membranes; however, clearance also depends on other factors, such as blood and dialysate flow rates. A more standard measure for comparison is KoA_{urea}, the mass transfer area coefficient for urea. Based on the urea clearance data from the package insert, KoA_{urea} can be estimated based on blood flow. Using this information, the dialysis prescription can be individualized to provide a specified dose of dialysis for the patient.

Patients having chronic HD typically are dialyzed for 3 to 4 hours, 3 times a week, either Monday-Wednesday-Friday or Tuesday-Thursday-Saturday. During the interdialytic period, fluids ingested and produced through metabolic processes are retained in the patient. Although patients generally are on fluid-restricted diets, accumulation of 1 to 5 L of fluid (translating into 1- to 5-kg weight gain) between sessions is common and must be removed during the dialysis treatment.

BLOOD AND DIALYSATE FLOW

Although small-molecule clearance is highly dependent on blood flow, the relationship is not strictly linear. Increased blood flow yields a less than proportional response in urea clearance.[10] This is likely because of an insufficient time for equilibration to occur between the blood and dialysate compartments as well as a greater membrane resistance to diffusion from an increased stagnant layer. A typical blood flow rate for dialysis is 400 to 500 mL/minute, but it is dependent on the vascular access site and the cardiovascular status of the patient. Some patients are not able to tolerate this rate, and a lower blood flow rate may be necessary. Dialysate flow rates generally are 500 mL/minute and can be increased to 800 mL/minute for high-flux dialysis, which will increase urea clearance by approximately 10%.[11]

CASE 30-1

QUESTION 1: R.W., a 55-year-old man with stage 4 CKD as a result of poorly controlled hypertension, presents to the renal clinic for reassessment of his kidney function. He is 70 inches tall and weighs 70 kg. Since his last visit 3 months ago, his creatinine clearance (ClCr) has decreased from 22 to 12 mL/minute and the BUN has increased to 89 mg/dL. The serum potassium (K) is 4.8 mEq/L and HCO_3 is 17 mEq/L. He has selected HD as his form of therapy until a suitable donor kidney is available and is expected to begin dialysis within the next 1 to 3 months. When he begins dialysis, he will be dialyzed 3 times a week for 4 hours each treatment, using a Fresenius F-160 dialyzer, with blood and dialysate flows of 400 and 500 mL/minute, respectively, and bicarbonate-containing dialysate. What characteristics of the Fresenius F-160 dialyzer make it a good choice for R.W.? What determines the composition of the dialysate?

The Fresenius dialyzer is a high-flux dialyzer as described previously. This polysulfone membrane is a synthetic membrane with larger pore sizes than conventional cellulose membranes. The F-160 has a KUf (the ultrafiltration coefficient [volume of water removed/mm Hg across the membrane per hour of dialysis]) of 45 mL/mm Hg/hour, indicating a high ultrafiltration capability; an in vitro KoA_{urea} of 1,064, a measure of dialyzer efficiency for urea removal; urea clearance of 266 mL/minute at a blood flow of 300 mL/minute; and a surface area of 1.5 m^2.[8] This information can be located in the product literature from the manufacturer or summary tables from common dialysis references.[8] These data are used to individualize the dialysis prescription for a patient.

DIALYSATE COMPOSITION

Dialysate composition usually is standardized within certain limits of electrolyte content, yet allows for individualization as necessary. Water is obtained through the public water system, which then undergoes treatment by reverse osmosis, followed by ion exchange with activated charcoal to remove contaminants, such as aluminum, copper, and chloramines, as well as bacteria and

Table 30-1
Electrolyte Composition of Hemodialysis and CAPD Dialysate Solutions

Solute	Hemodialysis (mEq/L)	CAPD (mEq/L)
Sodium	135–145	132
Potassium	0–4	0
Calcium	2.5–3.5	3.5
Magnesium	0.5–1.0	1.5
Chloride	100–124	102
Bicarbonate	30–38	
Lactate		35
pH	7.1–7.3	5.5

CAPD, continuous ambulatory peritoneal dialysis.

endotoxins.[12] The dialysate solution does not require sterilization because the dialysis membrane separates the blood and dialysate compartments. Nevertheless, pyrogen reactions may occur, and a greater risk may exist with high-flux membranes because of the increased pore size.

The final dialysate solution is prepared in the dialysis machine by proportioning a dialysate concentrate with the purified water, resulting in a final product, which typically contains those elements listed in Table 30-1. By adjusting electrolyte concentration in the dialysate, the efficiency of dialysis for particular chemicals can be manipulated. For example, if the patient is hyperkalemic, the dialysate contains a low concentration of potassium for diffusion of potassium from blood into dialysate. On the other hand, if the patient is normokalemic at the start of dialysis, the potassium concentration of the dialysate is set at a normal physiologic concentration to minimize flux of this electrolyte across the membrane. If the concentration of a solute is higher in the dialysate than in the blood, the net movement will be into the blood, not out. Metabolic acidosis, which is associated with ESRD because of an inability to excrete the daily obligatory load of acid, is controlled with the addition of bicarbonate buffer to the dialysate solution. Before delivery, dialysate is heated to 37°C to maintain body temperature and avoid hemolysis, which can occur with excessive heating. Dialysate is also deaerated under vacuum to remove dissolved air from the solution.

Vascular Access

CASE 30-1, QUESTION 2: To achieve a sufficient blood flow for dialysis, R.W. must have a vascular site for chronic access. What are the options for chronic vascular access in R.W.?

A permanent vascular access site provides easy access to high blood flow, which cannot be achieved through routine venipuncture of superficial veins. Different types of vascular access are available: arteriovenous (AV) fistula made by joining an artery and vein in the arm, AV graft, a soft tube made of polytetrafluoroethylene to join an artery and vein in the arm, and a double-lumen or tunneled, cuffed catheter placed in a large vein usually in the neck. AV fistulas and grafts are placed in the nondominant arm. Ideal vascular access delivers blood flow rates necessary for chronic HD, has a long period of use, and has a low rate of complications (e.g., infection, stenosis, thrombosis, aneurysm, and limb ischemia).

An AV fistula is created surgically by subcutaneous anastomosis of an artery to an adjacent vein. The AV fistula may not be suitable for patients with poor vasculature, such as elderly patients or those with diabetes, atherosclerosis, or small vessels. The K/DOQI guidelines for vascular access advocate placement of a fistula at the location of the wrist (radial-cephalic), or secondarily the elbow (brachial-cephalic), as the preferred vascular access sites. Once created, vascular access requires time to mature before it can be used for HD. The fistula should preferably be created 3 to 4 months before its intended use to allow the vein to mature. The graft can be used soon after insertion, although 2 weeks will allow for healing at the anastomosis sites and may prolong patency. AV fistulas fail to mature at a higher rate than grafts; however, grafts require fourfold higher interventions per year (elective angioplasty, thrombectomy, or surgical revision) to maintain long-term patency for HD.[13] Central venous catheters are discouraged for chronic vascular access because of high rates of infection and occlusion.

During the dialysis procedure, one needle or catheter is placed into the fistula site to deliver blood to the dialyzer. This is often referred to as the "arterial line" to the dialyzer. Blood exiting the dialyzer is returned back to the patient's fistula site through a second catheter and needle, referred to as the "venous line" from the dialyzer.

If R.W. has adequate vasculature, a fistula should be created for chronic access. Vascular access is critical for chronic HD and often has been labeled the Achilles' heel of dialysis therapy. Complications associated with vascular access are a significant problem in patients having chronic HD. The most common is thrombosis, usually the result of venous stenosis.[6] If not treated, thromboses will result in loss of the access. Access-related complications are a major cause of hospitalization and, therefore, attention to these problems is important both clinically and economically.

ANTICOAGULATION

CASE 30-1, QUESTION 3: Recommend a reasonable anticoagulation regimen for R.W. with the initiation of his HD. What are alternatives for patients at high risk for bleeding?

Most patients undergoing HD are anticoagulated with IV heparin during the dialysis treatment. Anticoagulation is necessary to prevent blood from clotting in the extracorporeal circuit. Several methods have been used in an attempt to provide adequate anticoagulation without increasing the risk of bleeding. Approaches include the administration of heparin in adequate quantities to anticoagulate the patient during the dialysis procedure by either intermittent bolus injections or an initial bolus followed by a continuous infusion.[14] Modern HD delivery systems have incorporated heparin infusion devices that can be programmed to provide the desired infusion rate during dialysis.

With no evidence of a bleeding disorder, recent surgery, or other risk factors for heparin anticoagulation, therapy should be initiated with a 2,000-unit bolus of IV heparin 3 to 5 minutes before initiation of dialysis, followed by an infusion of 1,200 units/hour.[14] The target activated clotting time (ACT) is 40% to 80% above the average baseline for the dialysis unit (e.g., 200–250 seconds, for normal values of 120–150 seconds). The clinician should monitor for signs of bleeding and measure the ACT at 1-hour intervals during dialysis. Heparin should be discontinued 1 hour before the end of dialysis to prevent excessive bleeding after dialysis. Using these standard doses, the estimated elimination half-life for heparin is approximately 50 minutes, and it should have a linear dose–response relationship within the target ACT.[14]

Patients at increased risk of bleeding include those who have had recent surgery, retinopathy, gastrointestinal bleeding, and cerebrovascular bleeding. For these patients, the goal is to prevent clot formation within the dialysis circuit as well as to minimize the risk of active bleeding. This may be accomplished by using "minimal-dose" heparin (tight ACT control), or even heparin-free anticoagulation. The minimal-dose heparin approach individualizes therapy to achieve ACT values 40% above baseline after an initial bolus of 750 units.[14] The ACT is measured 3 minutes after the bolus dose, which should allow for vascular distribution of the heparin to be complete. If the goal ACT level is not achieved, repeat bolus doses of heparin can be administered at a dose that is adjusted based on the expectation of a linear response. For example, if the first dose of 750 units reaches 75% of the ACT goal, an additional 250 units would be appropriate for the second dose. Similarly, the initial heparin maintenance infusion rate of 600 units/hour can be modified by monitoring the ACT at 30-minute intervals. Adjustments in the infusion rate should be proportionate to the bolus dose needed to maintain the ACT at 40% above baseline. Samples collected for determination of ACT should be obtained from the arterial line into the dialyzer, before the infusion of heparin, to reflect systemic anticoagulation effects.

Heparin-free dialysis is an alternative to heparinization for hemodialysis patients who are at a moderate-to-high risk of bleeding or who are actively bleeding.[14] This approach requires priming the hemodialysis circuit and dialyzer with heparin 3,000 units/L in normal saline to coat the extracorporeal surfaces. The heparin-containing priming fluid is allowed to drain by filling the circuit with either the patient's blood or normal saline alone at the outset of dialysis. Next, hemodialysis is set at a high blood flow rate of 300 to 400 mL/minute, if tolerated. During dialysis, the dialyzer is flushed with normal saline every 15 to 30 minutes to rinse away microclots that may have formed. The incidence of clotting with this approach is approximately 5%.

The regional administration of trisodium citrate through the arterial line is an alternative to systemic anticoagulation. It binds free calcium, which is necessary for the coagulation process. The calcium citrate complex is removed by the dialysate and, based on plasma calcium values, calcium chloride is administered on the venous side to replace the citrate-bound calcium to prevent hypocalcemia or hypercalcemia. Some of the administered citrate is returned to the patient and is metabolized to bicarbonate, leading to metabolic alkalosis in some cases. Trisodium citrate may lead to hypernatremia. Regional citrate anticoagulation is reserved for patients who are at risk for bleeding and requires additional monitoring to adjust the dual infusions.[14] In a prospective study of 1,009 consecutive high-flux dialysis procedures in 59 patients, long-term citrate anticoagulation achieved excellent anticoagulation (99.6%) with rare (0.2%) adverse effects on ionized calcium levels, electrolytes, and acid–base balance.[15]

CASE 30-1, QUESTION 4: Can low-molecular-weight heparins (LMWH) be used for hemodialysis?

Enoxaparin, dalteparin, and tinzaparin are LMWH that are commercially available but not yet approved by the US Food and Drug Administration (FDA) for hemodialysis. In a meta-analysis of 11 randomized trials, LMWH was compared with unfractionated heparin in ESRD patients undergoing either hemodialysis or hemofiltration. LMWH did not significantly affect the number of bleeding events (relative risk [RR], 0.96; 95% confidence interval [CI], 0.27–3.43) or extracorporeal circuit thrombosis (RR, 1.15; 95% CI, 0.70–1.91) compared with unfractionated heparin.[16] In a randomized, crossover study comparing the safety and efficacy of enoxaparin with standard heparin, a dose of 1.0 mg/kg body weight of enoxaparin produced less minor fibrin or clot formation in the dialyzer but more frequent minor hemorrhage between dialyses. Dosage reduction of enoxaparin to 0.7 mg/kg body weight resulted in similar efficacy and eliminated the minor hemorrhage.[17] Dalteparin administered as a single bolus dose of 60 high-flux was effective in preventing clotting of the hemodialysis circuit with no reports of bleeding.[18] Tinzaparin has also been shown to be effective as an anticoagulant during HD, using a weight-based IV dose of 75 international units/kg or a fixed IV dose of 2,500 international units just before dialysis.[19,20]

Although LMWH can be used to prevent clotting during HD, several factors need to be taken into account when considering LMWH for prevention and treatment of venous thromboembolism in HD patients. Because LMWH undergoes renal elimination, dose adjustments are necessary in patients with ESRD, accompanied by careful patient monitoring. Although LMWH inhibits factor X_a, factor XII_a, and kallikrein, measurement of antifactor X_a activity is the only available laboratory monitoring parameter for these factors; because active heparin metabolites that are not detected by the factor X_a assay can accumulate in dialysis patients, the clinical utility of this test is unclear.[21–23]

Another concern with LMWH is that patients on dialysis exhibit greater sensitivity to its effect than healthy volunteers.[23] Furthermore, LMWH administered at fixed-weight doses and without monitoring shows unpredictable anticoagulant effects in patients with stage 4 and 5 CKD. In a case series of patients on HD treated with LMWH for acute coronary syndrome, two patients who received as few as two to three doses of LMWH exhibited dialysis–access site bleeding, hematuria, and massive melena. Another subject who received 10 doses experienced hemorrhagic pericardial effusion, resulting in death. Only one patient in the series, who received a total of five doses, did not have hemorrhagic complications.[24] Based on these findings, it is recommended that unfractionated heparin, rather than LMWH, be used in patients on dialysis for prophylaxis and treatment of thromboembolic disease.[25,26]

CASE 30-1, QUESTION 5: Which agents can be used for anticoagulation during hemodialysis in patients with heparin-induced thrombocytopenia (HIT)?

HIT is reported to occur in 0% to 12% of patients on HD receiving heparin for anticoagulation. All forms of heparin, including "heparin-free" dialysis and LMWH must be stopped in patients with HIT. Another class of agents with potential use in patients requiring anticoagulation during HD is the direct thrombin inhibitors, argatroban and lepirudin. The place in therapy for these agents is in individuals who experience HIT. Argatroban is a synthetic derivative of L-arginine, which is approved by the FDA for use in patients susceptible to thrombosis who also have a history of HIT. Most dosage regimens for argatroban consist of an initial bolus dose at the start of HD followed by a continuous infusion during dialysis.[27] Because it is eliminated by non-renal routes, argatroban dosing in patients with renal failure is the same as for patients with normal kidney function.[28] However, dose adjustments are required in hepatic impairment. Murray et al.[29] evaluated three argatroban regimens in patients having high-flux hemodialysis. Anticoagulation was more consistently achieved (ACT > 140% of baseline) when a continuous infusion of 2 mcg/kg/minute with or without a bolus of 250 mcg/kg was used. The infusion was discontinued 1 hour before the end of the HD session. Approximately 20% of argatroban was removed during HD. Argatroban therapy provided adequate, safe anticoagulation throughout HD. No thrombosis, bleeding, or other serious adverse events occurred.[29]

Another antithrombin product, lepirudin, is produced through recombinant DNA technology. It is biologically similar to hirudin, which is isolated from the saliva of leeches. Unlike argatroban, lepirudin is significantly cleared by the kidneys and by most high-flux dialyzers.[30] The loading dose for intermittent hemodialysis in patients with HIT, who need anticoagulation to prevent clotting during dialysis, is 0.2 to 0.5 mg/kg (5–30 mg) with individualized dosage adjustment based on residual renal function.[14,31] An activated partial thromboplastin time ratio (APTTr) measured prior to the next dialysis session targeting an APTTr < 1.5 and, where available, a lepirudan assay targeting a therapeutic range of 0.5 to 0.8 mcg/mL are used to guide dose adjustments.[14] An antidote is not available; however, fresh frozen plasma or factor VIIa concentrates can be used if major bleeding occurs. Bivalirudin is a potential alternative for anticoagulation in patients with HIT, who are at risk for major bleeding. Among the direct thrombin inhibitors, it has the shortest half-life of 25 minutes (in patients without renal dysfunction). Dosing is still being elucidated. A retrospective cohort study of 24 ICU patients undergoing intermittent hemodialysis found that an average dose of 0.07 mg/kg/hour achieved an APTT goal of 1.5 to 2.5 times baseline values,[32] while bivaluridin infused at a lower rate 1.0 to 2.5 mg/hour (0.009–0.023 mg/kg/hour) targeting an APTTr of approximately 1.5 was reported for patency of the hemodialysis circuitry.[33]

Two heparinoids, danaparoid and fondaparinux, have been evaluated for anticoagulation in hemodialysis patients with HIT; however, danaparoid was withdrawn from the United States, and fondaparinux is currently not approved for hemodialysis. A preliminary study found that fondaparinux can be used as an anticoagulant only in patients using low-flux polysulfone dialyzers.[34] An increased risk of thrombosis occurred with high-flux dialyzers attributed to increased removal of fondaparinux, resulting in inadequate anticoagulation. Further studies are necessary to define the role of this agent in patients on chronic HD.

Complications

HYPOTENSION

CASE 30-1, QUESTION 6: The dry weight for R.W. is 69.1 kg. During his most recent dialysis session, he complained of nausea and light-headedness 3 hours into the procedure. His diastolic pressure had dropped from 85 to 60 mm Hg. Ultrafiltration was discontinued, and he recovered without further event. His post-dialysis weight was 69.9 kg. What are the possible etiologies for his hypotension?

In addition to solute removal, the artificial kidney must be used to maintain fluid balance in the patient without renal function. Most patients will become anuric once stabilized on HD, requiring control of ingested fluids between treatment sessions. Fluid removal during dialysis is then necessary to achieve the "dry weight," or weight below which the patient could become symptomatic from volume depletion. Achieving the dry weight is accomplished by ultrafiltration, through adjustment of the transmembrane pressure. The dry weight for R.W. has been set at 69.1 kg. Below this weight, R.W. exhibited symptoms of orthostasis.

Intradialytic hypotension (IDH) can produce a variety of clinical signs and symptoms, including nausea and vomiting, dizziness, muscle cramps, and headache. The reported incidence of hypotension is 10% to 30%, and even higher in patients with specific risk factors, such as autonomic dysfunction associated with diabetes and cardiac disease. It primarily is caused by excessive fluid removal from the vascular compartment at a rate exceeding mobilization of fluid from the interstitial space. As a consequence, patients with an inadequate hemodynamic response to intravascular volume depletion will exhibit a decrease in blood pressure and other symptoms. An ultrafiltration rate greater than 10 mL/hour/kg was found to be associated with higher odds of IDH (odds ratio = 1.30; $p = 0.045$) and a higher risk of mortality (RR, 1.02; $p = 0.02$).[35] It may be necessary to adjust the dry weight upward if the patient is volume-depleted and symptomatic after dialysis.

Other causes of hypotension relate to rises in core body temperature. Sympathetic nervous system activity increases in response to ultrafiltration, leading to vasoconstriction of the dermal circulation and impaired heat dissipation. Increased central heat production can occur during the dialysis procedure. The increase in core body temperature can overcome peripheral vasoconstriction, resulting in hypotension. Excessive heating of dialysate can also produce vasodilation. Cooling of the dialysate to slightly below body temperature may correct this problem, although many patients are uncomfortable and do not tolerate the cooling effect. Eating during dialysis can also cause a fall in blood pressure because of vasodilation of the splanchnic vessels. While food is usually prohibited during dialysis, patients prone to IDH should avoid eating just before dialysis. Antihypertensive therapy before dialysis may exacerbate hypotensive episodes as well; in some patients, these drugs may need to be withheld until after the dialysis session has ended. Immediate treatment of the hypotensive episode can be accomplished by reclining the patient, administering a small (100 mL) bolus of normal saline into the venous blood line, and reducing the ultrafiltration rate.

Several pharmacologic agents have been proposed for the management of IDH, including ephedrine, fludrocortisone, caffeine, vasopressin, L-carnitine, sertraline, and midodrine. Perazella[36] reviewed these agents for their potential use in the treatment of IDH and concluded that only midodrine, sertraline, and L-carnitine show potential benefit in patients. Midodrine is an oral prodrug that is converted to desglymidodrine, a selective α_1-agonist. Doses of 10 to 20 mg, 30 minutes before dialysis are effective for most patients, but the presence of active myocardial ischemia is a major contraindication.[36] Sertraline is a selective serotonin reuptake inhibitor that has shown promise in IDH at daily doses of 50 to 100 mg/day. The mechanism is proposed to be improvement of autonomic function. However, neither midodrine or sertraline have shown additive effects to that of using cool dialysate.[37,38] L-Carnitine has also been tried for treatment of IDH with IV doses of 20 mg/kg at dialysis. Its mechanism of action is not known, but it may be related to improvements in vascular smooth muscle and cardiac functioning.[36] However, a meta-analysis of five studies examining the role of L-carnitine supplementation for IDH failed to confirm a benefit.[39]

An accurate assessment of R.W.'s dry weight is essential. R.W. reports gaining a few extra pounds. If weight gain is related to increased volume, then sodium restriction is needed to minimize weight gain because of fluid retention between dialysis sessions. Another consideration is a change in his lean mass. When questioned about his diet, R.W. reports an improvement in his appetite. It is important to consider "real" weight changes when assessing the dry weight and volume status. Without appropriately increasing the dry weight goal to compensate for his real weight gain, R.W. became volume depleted and hypotensive. His dry weight should be adjusted upward to the point at which he no longer is symptomatic (to approximately 70 kg).

CASE 30-1, QUESTION 7: What other hemodialysis-related complications must be watched for and how can they be treated?

MUSCLE CRAMPS

Perhaps also related to fluid shifts, muscle cramps experienced during dialysis may be induced by excessive ultrafiltration, resulting in altered perfusion of the affected tissues. Several treatments have been attempted, including reduced ultrafiltration, and infusion of hypertonic saline or glucose (in nondiabetic patients) for cramps occurring near the end of dialysis.[40] Exercise and stretching of the affected limbs may also be beneficial. Short-term daily administration of vitamin E 400 IU alone or in combination with vitamin C has been found to reduce episodes of cramping.[41,42]

Vitamin E can cause bleeding and potentiate bleeding with warfarin. Vitamin C therapy is known to produce hyperoxaluria, oxalate-containing urinary stones, and renal damage; therefore, vitamin C supplementation is limited to 60 to 100 mg daily. The long-term effects of vitamin E and vitamin C administration in hemodialysis patients are unknown.

DIALYSIS DISEQUILIBRIUM

Dialysis disequilibrium is a syndrome that has been recognized since the initiation of HD more than 30 years ago. Its etiology is related to cerebral edema, and patients new to HD are at a greater risk because of the accumulation of urea.[43] Rapid removal of urea from the extracellular space lowers plasma osmolality, thereby leading to a shift of free water into the brain. Lowering of intracellular pH, as can occur during dialysis, has also been suggested as a cause. Clinical manifestations occur during or shortly after dialysis and include central nervous system effects, such as headache, nausea, altered vision, and in some cases, seizures and coma. Treatment is aimed at prevention by initiating dialysis gradually by using shorter treatment times at lower blood flow rates in new patients. Direct therapy can be provided in the form of IV hypertonic saline or mannitol.[43]

THROMBOSIS

Dialysis access loss is most often the result of thrombosis, which is usually a consequence of venous stenosis. Prospective monitoring of access function (e.g., intra-access flow; static or dynamic venous pressures; measurement of access recirculation; and physical findings, such as swelling of the arm, clotting of the graft, prolonged bleeding after needle removal, or altered character of the pulse or thrill) is paramount to the prevention of thrombosis. Fistula patency generally is much greater than synthetic graft patency, although thrombosis and loss of function may occur in both.[6] The stenosis may be corrected by percutaneous transluminal angioplasty or, if necessary, surgical revision of the access site. Successful correction is effective as a means to prevent thrombosis. Once it occurs, thrombosis is managed by surgical or mechanical thrombectomy, or use of thrombolytic agents. Alteplase, reteplase, and tenecteplase appear to be effective for thrombolysis of the vascular access site.[44–46] Thrombolytic therapy should be avoided in those patients with an increased risk of bleeding.

For patients who have tunneled, cuffed hemodialysis catheters for hemodialysis, the success rates for clearing occlusions was greatest with reteplase at 88% ± 4%, then alteplase at 81% ± 37%, and tenecteplase at 41% ± 5% with no serious adverse bleeding events reported for thrombolytic therapy.[47] Catheter-locking regimens of heparin 3 times per week or recombinant tissue plasminogen activator instead of heparin at the midweek hemodialysis session was found to reduce the incidence of catheter malfunction and bacteremia.[48]

CASE 30-1, QUESTION 8: Do oral anticoagulants or antiplatelet agents have a role in preventing clots in R.W.'s HD access site?

Anticoagulants and antiplatelet agents have been evaluated in the prevention of graft thrombosis. A large, multicenter, randomized, placebo-controlled trial found a modest effect of extended-release dipyridamole and low-dose aspirin in reducing HD graft stenosis during the period immediately after graft placement, and improving patency duration by 6 weeks.[49] However, approximately three-fourths of patients had loss of graft patency at 1 year. Bleeding occurred at a similar rate (12%) in the treatment and placebo groups. In a cost–utility analysis, aspirin alone was found to be the most cost effective approach,[50] but no prospective studies have evaluated aspirin alone in preventing graft thrombosis. In two separate randomized, placebo-controlled trials, therapy with low-dose warfarin to achieve a target international normalized ratio of 1.4 to 1.9 or combination therapy with clopidogrel and aspirin in patients with polytetrafluoroethylene grafts showed no benefit in the prevention of thrombosis or prolongation of graft survival.[51,52] In both studies, patients receiving active treatment experienced a significantly increased risk of bleeding. A small single-center, randomized, placebo-controlled clinical trial found that fish oil reduced graft thrombosis[52]; however, this benefit was not borne out in a larger, multicenter, randomized, controlled trial.[53]

Based on these studies, oral anticoagulants or antiplatelet agents have no defined role for prophylaxis of graft thrombosis.

INFECTION

CASE 30-1, QUESTION 9: Assessment of the hemodialysis access site is performed at every treatment to identify any signs and symptoms of an access infection. Should R.W. be given prophylactic antibiotics (e.g., cefazolin with each dialysis) to avoid infection of his hemodialysis access site? Explain your rationale.

Access infections, usually involving grafts to a greater extent than a native fistula, are predominantly caused by *Staphylococcus aureus* or *Staphylococcus epidermidis*. Infections with gram-negative organisms as well as *Enterococcus* species occur with a lower frequency.[6] Access infections can lead to bacteremia and sepsis with or without local signs of infection.

There is no evidence that prophylactic antibiotics are of value; to the contrary, indiscriminate use of antibiotics could lead to colonization with resistant organisms. Thus, R.W. should not receive a prophylactic antibiotic. However, if evidence of infection is present, a prompt response is important. K/DOQI clinical practice guidelines for vascular access also advocate surgical incision and resection of infected grafts. Fistula infections are rare and should be treated as subacute bacterial endocarditis with 6 weeks of antibiotic therapy.[6]

CASE 30-2

QUESTION 1: D.B. a 56-year-old, 75 kg woman who undergoes high-flux hemodialysis 3 times a week develops fever, chills, and leukocytosis. What are your recommendations for empiric antibiotic therapy for suspected hemodialysis catheter-related infection?

Antibiotics that permit dosing during or after each dialysis session or antibiotics whose pharmacokinetics are unaffected by dialysis should be chosen. Treatment usually is initiated with vancomycin 20 mg/kg loading dose infused during the last 60 to 90 minutes of dialysis, and then 500 mg during the last 30 minutes of each subsequent dialysis session, depending on the type of dialysis being used.[54] High-flux dialysis results in greater removal of vancomycin than conventional dialysis. Intradialytic dosing of vancomycin is a convenient mode of drug administration in patients receiving high-flux dialysis. It avoids the need for additional intravenous access, longer stays in the hemodialysis unit, or home antibiotic administration. Cefazolin 20 mg/kg after each dialysis session can be used instead of vancomycin in dialysis units with a low prevalence of methicillin-resistant staphylococci.[54] Empiric antibiotic therapy should also include coverage for gram-negative bacilli, with antibiotic selection based on the local antibiogram. For example, gentamicin (or tobramycin) 1 mg/kg, not to exceed 100 mg infused after each dialysis session can be used for empiric gram-negative coverage with appropriate serum concentration monitoring.[54]

CASE 30-2, QUESTION 2: What are your dosing recommendations for intravenous vancomycin and gentamicin therapy for D.B., and how are the infusions prepared?

D.B. weighs 75 kg, therefore she should receive a vancomycin loading dose of 1,500 mg. Parenteral vancomycin is prepared by reconstituting 10 g of sterile vancomycin powder with 96 mL of Sterile Water for Injection for a concentration of 100 mg/mL. Fifteen mL of the vancomycin 100 mg/mL solution is further diluted in 500 mL of 5% dextrose or 0.9% sodium chloride injection, and infused during the last 90 minutes of hemodialysis. For the maintenance dose, vancomycin 500 mg IV (premixed bag) is infused during the last 30 minutes of each subsequent dialysis session. D.B. should receive gentamicin 75 mg infused over 30 minutes after dialysis. Parenteral gentamicin is prepared by diluting the 75 mg dose with 50 to 100 mL of 5% dextrose or 0.9% sodium chloride injection. Vancomycin and gentamicin doses are adjusted according to serum concentrations measured before the next hemodialysis session targeting predialysis concentrations of approximately 20 mg/mL for vancomycin and 3 mg/mL for gentamicin. Subsequent antibiotic therapy should be tailored based on culture and sensitivity results. Antibiotic therapy is continued until blood cultures are negative, no other source of infection is identified, and signs and symptoms of infection have resolved (e.g., resolution of fever and leukocystosis).

Other long-term complications associated with HD include aluminum toxicity, amyloidosis, and malnutrition.

ALUMINUM TOXICITY

Aluminum accumulation in patients undergoing HD was a significant problem before water sources were adequately treated to remove aluminum. Major complications of aluminum toxicity include dementia, aluminum bone disease, and anemia. Aluminum accumulation still occurs in patients treated with aluminum-containing phosphate binders, although not to the degree associated with water supplies. (See Chapter 28, Chronic Kidney Disease, for further discussion.)

AMYLOIDOSIS

Amyloidosis is a painful complication of ESRD caused by the deposition of β_2-microglobulin–containing amyloid in joints and soft tissues over time. Carpal tunnel syndrome, manifested as weakness and soreness in the thumb from pressure on the median nerve, is the most common symptom. Bone cysts also appear along with joint deposition of amyloid, which can lead to chronic arthralgias, joint immobility, bone fractures, and substantial disability. The incidence of amyloidosis is approximately 50% after 12 years of dialysis and nearly 100% after 20 years. β_2-microglobulin (molecular weight, 11,800 Da) is normally eliminated by filtration and tubular catabolism in the intact nephron. Renal failure leads to reduced elimination and accumulation of this substance even during dialysis. High-flux membranes are more effective than conventional membranes for the removal of β_2-microglobulin. Unfortunately, β_2-microglobulin production can exceed its elimination even by high-flux membranes. Initial treatment of carpal tunnel syndrome includes splinting of the wrists and analgesics for pain relief. Newer generations of dialysis membranes may hold some promise in reducing the development of amyloidosis.

MALNUTRITION

Chronic kidney disease produces a catabolic state in patients and, along with the multifactorial complications of ESRD, leads to malnutrition. Serum albumin concentrations less than 3.0 g/dL are associated with an increased mortality rate compared with higher values. Inadequate dietary intake and losses of amino acids by dialysis contribute to protein malnutrition, which in turn can lead to additional complications, such as impaired wound healing, susceptibility to infection, and others. (See Chapter 28, Chronic Kidney Disease, for further discussion.)

L-Carnitine

L-Carnitine supplementation has been used in patients with ESRD to relieve intradialytic symptoms. It is a metabolic cofactor that facilitates transport of long-chain fatty acids into the mitochondria for energy production. This cofactor is found in both plasma and tissue as free carnitine, the active component, or bound to fatty acids as acylcarnitine. The primary source of carnitine is dietary intake, primarily from red meat and dairy products. Carnitine is a small water-soluble molecule that is freely dialyzed, thus its levels are reduced in hemodialysis. The potential benefits of correcting this relative carnitine deficiency have been primarily studied in patients having chronic HD. Although some have suggested that carnitine supplementation benefits muscle cramps and hypotension during dialysis (as well as minimizing fatigue, skeletal muscle weakness, cardiomyopathy, and anemia resistant to large doses of erythropoietic therapy), no evidence supports its routine use in patients undergoing chronic HD.[55]

PERITONEAL DIALYSIS

Peritoneal dialysis is performed using several different modalities, including the most common, CAPD. Development of specialized devices to facilitate the exchange process and improve patient convenience has led to processes referred to as APD, including continuous cycling peritoneal dialysis (CCPD) and nocturnal intermittent dialysis (NIPD). CAPD is the most common method for chronic PD, but the APD methods have grown in popularity, especially among the pediatric population. Although lower rates of peritonitis are observed in APD compared with CAPD,[56] other outcomes measures, such as need for transition to HD and mortality, are similar between the two modalities.[57]

Principles and Transport Processes

Continuous ambulatory peritoneal dialysis is performed by the instillation of 2 to 3 L of sterile dialysate solution into the peritoneal cavity through a surgically placed resident catheter. The solution dwells within the cavity for 4 to 8 hours, and then it is drained and replaced with a fresh solution. This process of fill, dwell, and drain is performed 3 to 4 times during the day, with an overnight dwell by the patient in his or her normal home or work environment (Fig. 30-2). Conceptually, the process is similar to HD in that uremic toxins are removed by diffusion down a concentration gradient across a membrane into the dialysate solution. In this case, the peritoneal membrane covering the abdominal contents serves as an endogenous dialysis membrane, and the vasculature embedded in the peritoneum serves as the blood supply to equilibrate with the dialysate. A primary difference is that because the dialysate solution is resident, the result is a very slow dialysate flow rate of approximately 7 mL/minute when 10 L of fluid is drained per day. Solute loss occurs by diffusion for small molecules, and through convection for larger, middle molecules.

BLOOD AND DIALYSATE FLOW

Hemodialysis provides constant perfusion of fresh dialysate, thereby maintaining a large concentration gradient across the dialysis membrane throughout the dialysis treatment. Unlike hemodialysis, during a typical dwell period for CAPD, urea and other substances increase in the dialysate relative to unbound plasma concentrations. For a daytime dwell period of 4 hours, urea achieves nearly equal concentrations with plasma; therefore, the rate of elimination can become very small. Instillation of fresh dialysate solution will reestablish the diffusion gradient, leading to an increased rate of urea removal. For a patient making four exchanges of 2 L each per day, assuming the urea

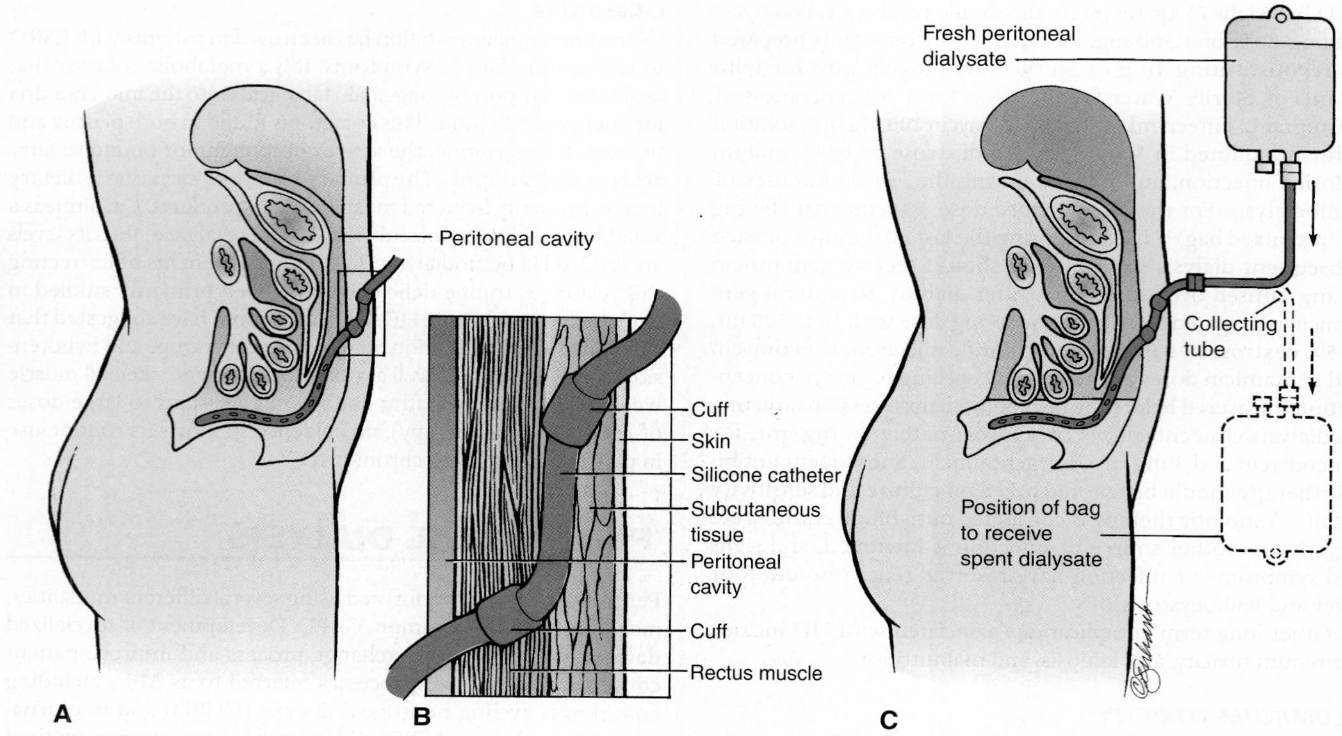

Figure 30-2 Continuous ambulatory peritoneal dialysis. **(A)** The peritoneal catheter is implanted through the abdominal wall. **(B)** Dacron cuffs and a subcutaneous tunnel provide protection against bacterial infection. **(C)** Dialysate flows by gravity through the peritoneal catheter into the peritoneal cavity. After a prescribed period of time, the fluid is drained by gravity and discarded. New solution is then infused into the peritoneal cavity until the next drainage period. Dialysis thus continues on a 24-hour-a-day basis during which the patient is free to move around and engage in his or her usual activities. Adapted with permission from Smeltzer SC, Bare BG. *Textbook of Medical-Surgical Nursing*. 9th ed. Philadelphia, PA: Lippincott Williams & Wilkins; 2000.

dialysate concentration equals the plasma concentration, and 2 L are removed by ultrafiltration, the urea clearance would be approximately 7 mL/minute. This is substantially lower than urea clearances achieved with HD; therefore, CAPD must be performed continually (daily) throughout the week to achieve adequate urea removal. Clearance depends on blood flow; dialysate flow; and peritoneal membrane characteristics such as size, permeability, and thickness. Dialysate flow, the only easily adjusted variable to alter clearance, has been used effectively in acute PD to achieve relatively high clearances with 30- to 60-minute dwell periods in a cycling system. CCPD uses this concept of shorter dwell periods during the sleeping hours with automatic fill, dwell, and drain periods, leaving a high-dextrose dialysate in the peritoneal cavity throughout the day until the next cycling session. NIPD is similar, with nightly exchanges, but the peritoneum is left unfilled, or dry, during the daytime. As a result, urea clearance is lower with NIPD, but it may be suitable for many patients, and preferable to the volume load in the peritoneal cavity throughout the day with CCPD.[58] Electrolyte concentrations in the dialysate solution are near physiologic concentrations to prevent substantial shifts in serum electrolyte levels (Table 30-1). A potential advantage of PD compared with HD is the continuous dialysis of larger, middle molecules that have been implicated as a possible source of toxic effects. These molecules are cleared through convection and follow water as it is removed through ultrafiltration. Clearance of these molecules depends less on flow and more on duration of dialysis. The continuous process of PD, although associated with low clearance values, provides for a more physiologic condition in patients, rather than the intermittent treatment provided with HD.

FLUID REMOVAL

Fluid is removed by ultrafiltration through adjustment of the transmembrane pressure during HD. Because this pressure is not easily adjusted in PD, fluid is removed by altering the osmotic pressure within the dialysate. This is accomplished by the addition of dextrose (glucose monohydrate) to the dialysate in varying concentrations, depending on the degree of fluid removal necessary in the patient. Concentrations of dextrose in commercially available solutions include 1.5%, 2.5%, and 4.25%, with net fluid losses during a 4-hour dwell period of 200 mL and 400 mL for the 1.5% and 2.5% solutions, respectively, and approximately 700 mL for the 4.25% solution after an overnight dwell.[59] As the dwell time persists, the dextrose is absorbed and is diluted by the movement of fluid from the vascular space, so that most ultrafiltration occurs early during the dwell period.

Bicarbonate is not compatible with the calcium and magnesium in the dialysate and can lead to precipitation; therefore, lactate is used in the dialysate. Acid–base balance is achieved through the absorption of lactate from the dialysate, which subsequently is metabolized to bicarbonate in vivo.

Access

Delivery of dialysate into the peritoneal cavity is accomplished through an indwelling catheter inserted through the abdominal wall. The most common design is the Tenckhoff catheter, made of silicone rubber or polyurethane; it consists of a tube, straight or curled, with many holes in the distal end for fluid inflow and outflow. The catheter also has a single or double cuff, which serves to anchor it to the internal and external attachment sites by promoting fibrous tissue growth; this also serves as a barrier to bacterial migration. Several modifications to the original catheter have appeared on the market, mostly in an attempt to overcome problems related to outflow of dialysate. Maintaining an unobstructed outlet port is essential for successful PD.

Delivery of dialysate through the catheter is accomplished using Y sets and double-bag systems. The Y transfer set uses three limbs of tubing, with fresh dialysate attached to the upper arm of the Y, an empty bag to the lower arm, and the stem connected to the catheter. Clamping the inflow arm and opening the stem and outflow arm allow dialysate to drain from the peritoneum into the empty bag. Reversing the clamps then permits infusion of the fresh dialysate solution after a small rinse of the line is performed with the fresh solution. Clamping of the catheter allows removal of the Y transfer set and bags from the patient. The double-bag system uses pre-attached bags to both limbs and the patient and makes only a single connection to the catheter. Use of the Y transfer set has reduced episodes of peritonitis from approximately one for every 9 to 12 patient-months to one for every 24 to 36 patient-months.[60] PD performed with the cycler involves only two disconnections of the system, compared with four for CAPD.

Dialysis Prescription

CASE 30-3

QUESTION 1: M.J., a 27-year-old woman, has a 14-year history of type 1 diabetes mellitus. She is 5 feet, 5 inches tall and weighs 65 kg. One complication of her diabetes is ESRD necessitating dialysis. She has been undergoing CAPD for 1 year and, until now, has done well without any complications. Her dialysis prescription consists of three exchanges with 1.5% dextrose during the day and a fourth, overnight exchange with 4.25% dextrose. She has a double-cuff Tenckhoff catheter and uses a Y transfer set for her exchanges. Her blood pressure is controlled and she shows no evidence of edema. She has no residual renal function. What is the purpose of the addition of 1.5% dextrose to M.J.'s dialysate? Why would the concentration of dextrose be increased to as high as 4.25% in some situations?

The initial CAPD prescription for most patients consists of three exchanges during the day with 1.5% dextrose and a fourth, overnight, exchange with 4.25% dextrose. This would be expected to achieve fluid removal of approximately 1,300 mL, based on 200 mL from each daytime exchange and 700 mL overnight. Based on the assessment of the patient's fluid status, it may be necessary to increase or decrease the dialysate prescription to achieve fluid balance. Fluid retention is solved by increasing the dextrose content of the daytime exchanges, beginning with 2.5% in place of one of the 1.5% solutions. This is expected to result in an additional removal of 200 mL, and therapy can be further adjusted as necessary. For patients with excessive fluid removal, it may be possible to decrease the number of exchanges per day as long as adequate solute removal is present. If four exchanges are needed, the fluid intake can be liberalized to maintain adequate hydration.

Dextrose is the dextrorotatory form of glucose. Glucose is a small molecule that rapidly diffuses across the peritoneal membrane. As glucose is absorbed, the osmotic gradient of the dwell progressively dissipates, reducing ultrafiltration. Toward the end of the long dwell, more dialysate fluid may be absorbed than ultrafiltered, resulting in a negative net ultrafiltration volume where the drained volume is less than the infused volume. A negative net ultrafiltration volume is undesirable. Greater ultrafiltration and fluid management are predictors of survival.[61]

An alternative to dextrose as the osmotic agent in the dialysate solution is icodextrin, a starch-derived, water-soluble, non-dextrose polymer that is approximately 40% absorbed and subsequently metabolized to maltose oligosaccharides. Icodextrin is approved for use in the United States in patients having CAPD or APD during the long-dwell period. Unlike glucose, icodextrin does not readily diffuse across the peritoneal membrane, but it is slowly removed from the peritoneal cavity via convective uptake into the peritoneal lymphatics.[62] It is superior to dextrose solutions for ultrafiltration.[63] Icodextrin has been shown to have less glucose absorption, carbohydrate exposure, fat accumulation, and weight gain than glucose-containing PD fluids.[64]

A number of factors need to be considered when icodextrin is used. Insulin requirements may decrease when icodextrin is substituted for dextrose solutions during the long dwell. On the other hand, a more worrisome concern is that icodextrin can cause false elevations in glucose concentrations with certain glucose-monitoring devices unable to distinguish glucose from maltose.[65] In this situation, insulin and other medications used to manage hyperglycemia may be increased unnecessarily, resulting in iatrogenic hypoglycemia. A pharmacovigilance report identified three cases of iatrogenic hypoglycemia in patients undergoing peritoneal dialysis with icodextrin, with two of these patients in the ICU for severe hypoglycemia.[66] Other undesirable effects of icodextrin include skin rash, mild hyponatremia, sterile peritonitis, and false reductions of serum amylase concentrations which can complicate the diagnosis of pancreatits.[65]

PERITONITIS

CASE 30-3, QUESTION 2: M.J. now presents to the dialysis clinic with complaints of abdominal tenderness and cloudy effluent. Examination of the dialysate reveals a white blood cell (WBC) count of 330 cells/μL with 62% neutrophils. Gram stain is positive for gram-positive cocci. Her diabetes has been controlled by the addition of 10 units of regular insulin to each daytime bag and 15 units to the overnight bag. While awaiting cultures, dual therapy with cefazolin and ceftazidime is ordered. Is this treatment coverage appropriate? Provide the dosages and administration for M.J.'s infection.

The most significant complication among patients undergoing PD is peritonitis. The patient usually presents with abdominal pain, nausea and vomiting, and fever with or without a cloudy effluent. The effluent should be inspected and sent to the laboratory for cell count with differential, Gram stain, and culture, with antibiotic therapy initiated in the interim. Bacterial peritonitis generally is accompanied by an elevated dialysate WBC count greater than 100/μL with greater than 50% neutrophils. Specific consensus recommendations of the International Society for Peritoneal Dialysis Ad Hoc Advisory Committee on Peritoneal Dialysis-Related Infections are located at http://www.ispd.org.[67]

Empiric antibiotics must cover both gram-positive and gram-negative organisms.[67] The increasing prevalence of vancomycin-resistant organisms has resulted in a shift in empiric therapy away from vancomycin, toward first-generation cephalosporins (cefazolin or cephalothin). Without a Gram stain, therapy should be initiated with a combination of cefazolin or cephalothin (to cover gram-positive organisms) and ceftazidime (to cover gram-negative organisms), coadministered by the intraperitoneal route (IP) in the same dialysate solution at a dose of 15 mg/kg (rounded to the nearest 500 mg) for both drugs, once daily.[67] M.J. weighs 65 kg, therefore a 1 g dose cefazolin and ceftazidime IP is appropriate. Both antibiotics are available as 1 g vials. To prepare the doses for IP administration, each sterile antibiotic powder is reconstituted with 3 to 10 mL of Sterile Water for Injection and shaken well. The contents are withdrawn into separate syringes and injected into the peritoneal dialysis bag. Separate syringes must be used to add the antibiotics to dialysis solutions. An aminoglycoside can be used in place of ceftazidime. While aminoglycosides were not found to adversely affect residual renal function,[68] high systemic absorption and prolonged half-life of gentamicin was found in patients with peritonitis, which can lead to drug accumulation.[69] Short-term use appears to be safe and effective, but there is a potential risk of toxicity, such as oto- and/or vestibular toxicity, with prolonged therapy. Gentamicin, tobramycin, or netilmicin are given at doses of 0.6 mg/kg/bag, once daily, and for amikacin, 2 mg/kg/bag once daily. Antibiotics should be allowed to dwell for at least 6 hours, and the minimum duration of therapy is 2 weeks.[67] M.J. should receive the antibiotics in the overnight bag, since it has the longest dwell time. Subsequent antibiotic therapy should be based on culture and sensitivity results, incorporating specific dosage regimens based on the treatment guidelines.

This is M.J.'s first episode of peritonitis. The most likely pathogen, a *Staphylococcus* species, is consistent with the positive Gram stain. Her treatment should consist of monotherapy with cefazolin (or cephalothin) 15 mg/kg IP daily as ordered. Ceftazadime should be discontinued. Vancomycin should not be used for empiric therapy. Instead, it should be reserved for methicillin-resistant *S. aureus* infections or methicillin-resistant *S. epidermidis* if M.J. does not respond to empiric therapy.

CASE 30-3, QUESTION 3: A new order is written to add heparin to M.J.'s dialysate fluid. What is the reason for this? She is also receiving insulin intraperitoneally. Is this appropriate or should she be switched to subcutaneous insulin?

In addition to antibiotics, heparin 500 units/L should be added to each exchange to prevent fibrin clots from forming, obstructing outflow from the peritoneal cavity, and occluding the catheter.[67] M.J.'s blood glucose should be monitored, because infection causes insulin resistance and peritonitis will increase glucose and insulin absorption. Inability to control the blood glucose concentration may require temporary discontinuation of the intraperitoneal (IP) insulin and administration by another route. Also see Case 30-2, Question 7, for other considerations regarding insulin dosing.

CASE 30-3, QUESTION 4: If M.J. was receiving APD instead of CAPD, would the treatment of her infection be different?

Cycler machines automatically cycle dialysate into and out of the peritoneal cavity in APD. Patients having CCPD will generally need three to five exchanges, each lasting approximately 2 hours, using a cycler while the patient sleeps. During the daytime hours, the patient maintains a reservoir of dialysate in the peritoneal cavity, resulting in a long dwell. The cycler process repeats at night. Six to eight exchanges are performed every night for patients having NIPD. The peritoneum is left dry, and patients do not continue dialysis during the day. Nightly dwell times are generally 1 to 2 hours for each exchange, resulting in a higher clearance for small molecules because of the increased dialysate flow rate.[58]

For patients having APD, the choice of first-line antibiotics is the same as for CAPD because the likely organisms are similar. Drug dosage regimens, however, can differ because patients having CCPD or NIPD undergo PD only during the nighttime hours, and those having NIPD do not have residual peritoneal fluid during the day. The rapid exchanges in APD may lead to inadequate time to achieve therapeutic drug concentrations. The dose of cefazolin in APD is 20 mg/kg (rounded to the nearest 500 mg) every day, in the long day dwell.[67] M.J. should receive cefazolin 1,500 mg IP in the long day dwell. A concern is that patients given a single dose of a cephalosporin during the long day dwell may have IP levels at night that are below the MIC of most organisms allowing biofilm-associated organisms to survive, resulting in relapsing peritonitis.[67] A safer approach would be to add the cephalosporin to each exchange in APD. Because of the lack of clinical trials with other antibiotics in patients having APD, extrapolation from the CAPD literature may be necessary. A review addresses the current knowledge and issues surrounding the pharmacokinetics of antibiotics in patients with peritonitis undergoing APD.[70]

EXIT-SITE INFECTION: PROPHYLAXIS

CASE 30-3, QUESTION 5: Catheter exit-site infections are a significant risk factor for developing peritonitis. What information should be provided to educate M.J. in daily catheter care? Recommend an appropriate antimicrobial cream for M.J. to administer around the catheter exit site.

Prevention of catheter exit-site infections (and thus peritonitis) is the primary goal of exit-site care. Several preventative measures are important: adequate catheter placement, dedicated postoperative catheter care, and routine daily care of the exit site. Dressing changes of a newly placed catheter are done by a dialysis nurse using sterile technique until the exit site is well healed, which can take up to 2 weeks. Once the exit site is well healed, M.J. can be educated and trained to do routine exit-site care, including thorough hand cleansing before touching the exit site by rubbing both hands for at least 15 seconds using antiseptics that contain at least 70% alcohol or antibacterial soap.[71] The exit site is then washed daily with antibacterial soap, although use of an antiseptic (e.g., povidone iodine or chlorhexidine) is a reasonable option as long as concentrations are non-cytotoxic.[72] Hydrogen peroxide should be avoided as a routine antiseptic because it causes drying. After daily cleansing, M.J. can be instructed to apply antimicrobial creams (e.g., mupirocin, gentamicin) around the catheter exit site using a cotton swab. Mupirocin ointment, not the cream, can cause structural damage to polyurethane catheters and should be avoided in patients with these catheters.[72]

Catheter exit-site infections are most often caused by *S. aureus* and *Pseudomonas* species.[67] In a randomized, double-blind trial, gentamicin sulfate 0.1% cream was found to be as effective as mupirocin 2% cream in preventing *S. aureus* infections.[73] Gentamicin cream was also highly effective in reducing *Pseudomonas aeruginosa* and other gram-negative catheter infections, whereas mupirocin cream was not. A longer time to first catheter infection and a reduction in peritonitis, particularly gram-negative organisms, was also seen with gentamicin use. For these reasons, daily gentamicin cream at the exit site is considered to be the prophylaxis of choice in patients having PD and would be the preferred treatment for M.J. Finally, the catheter should be immobilized with a small gauze dressing and tape to prevent pulling and trauma to the exit site, which may lead to infection.

EXIT-SITE INFECTION: TREATMENT

CASE 30-3, QUESTION 6: If M.J. were to exhibit an exit-site infection despite appropriate catheter care, could oral therapy be used or is intraperitoneal therapy required?

Empiric therapy for exit-site infections may be started immediately and should always cover *S. aureus*. Oral antibiotic therapy has been shown to be as effective as IP therapy with the exception of methicillin-resistant *S. aureus* infections.[67] Local erythema alone can be treated with topical agents, whereas purulent drainage indicates more significant infection and the need for systemic antibiotics. Gram-positive organisms are treated with first-generation oral cephalosporins, or with oral penicillinase-resistant penicillins. Rifampin may be added at 600 mg/day orally (in single or split dose) for slowly resolving infections. It should not be used as monotherapy, or in areas where tuberculosis is endemic. Rifampin is an inducer of drug-metabolizing enzymes and concurrent medications should be evaluated for potential drug interactions.

Oral quinolone antibiotics are recommended as first-line agents in the treatment of *P. aeruginosa* exit-site infections. Monotherapy is not recommended because resistance develops rapidly, and *P. aeruginosa* infections are difficult to treat often requiring prolonged therapy with two antibiotics. If the infection is slow to resolve or if in cases of a recurrence, a second antipseudomonal drug can be added (e.g., ceftazidime IP). Gram-negative organisms can be treated with ciprofloxacin 500 mg orally twice daily.[74] Scheduling of the quinolone dose is important, so that coadministration with foods or other drug therapies that may chelate the quinolone in the gut is avoided. Potentially chelating agents include calcium products, iron, multivitamins, antacids, zinc, sucralfate, and dairy products. Antibiotic therapy should be continued for a minimum of 2 weeks until the exit site appears entirely normal.

WEIGHT GAIN

CASE 30-3, QUESTION 7: M.J. is noted to have gained weight since starting peritoneal dialysis. Besides fluid retention, what other possible cause is there for the weight gain? How might this affect her insulin requirements?

Dextrose is present in dialysate solutions primarily to serve as an osmotic agent for the removal of fluid during each exchange. Higher concentrations are expected to result in greater fluid removal. Approximately 500 to 1,000 kcal/day are absorbed as glucose from PD solutions, which can lead to weight gain in patients. Some patients may require modification of oral caloric intake to avoid excessive weight gain. Insulin requirements generally are increased in patients with diabetes as a result of the additional calories and, when administered IP, usually are 2 to 3 times the normal subcutaneous dose because of their reduced bioavailability of 20% to 50% by this route. Also see Case 30-3, Question 3, for other considerations regarding insulin dosing.

KEY REFERENCES AND WEBSITES

A full list of references for this chapter can be found at http://thepoint.lww.com/AT11e. Below are the key references and websites for this chapter, with the corresponding reference number in this chapter found in parentheses after the reference.

Key References

Ahmad S et al. Hemodialysis apparatus. In: Daugirdas JT et al., eds. *Handbook of Dialysis*. Philadelphia, PA: Wolters Kluwer Health; 2015:59. (8)

Andrassy KM. KDIGO clinical practice guideline for the evaluation and management of chronic kidney disease. *Kidney Int Suppl*. 2013;3(1):1. (2)

Blake PG. Adequacy of peritoneal dialysis and chronic peritoneal dialysis prescription. In: Daugirdas JT et al, eds. *Handbook of Dialysis*. Philadelphia, PA: Wolters Kluwer Health; 2015:464. (59)

Davenport A et al. Anticoagulation. In: Daugirdas JT et al, eds. *Handbook of Dialysis*. Philadelphia, PA: Wolters Kluwer Health; 2015:252. (14)

Li PK et al. ISPD guidelines/recommendations. Peritoneal dialysis-related infections recommendations: 2010 update. *Perit Dial Int*. 2010;30(4):393. (67)

The National Kidney Foundation–Kidney Disease Outcomes Quality Initiative. NKF-K/DOQI clinical practice guidelines for chronic kidney disease: evaluation, classification, and stratification. *Am J Kidney Dis*. 2002;39:S1. (1)

The National Kidney Foundation–Kidney Disease Outcomes Quality Initiative. NKF-K/DOQI clinical practice guidelines for hemodialysis adequacy: update 2006. *Am J Kidney Dis*. 2006;48(Suppl 1):S2. (4)

The National Kidney Foundation–Kidney Disease Outcomes Quality Initiative. NKF-K/DOQI clinical practice guidelines for peritoneal dialysis adequacy: update 2006. *Am J Kidney Dis*. 2006;48(Suppl 1):S91. (5)

The National Kidney Foundation–Kidney Disease Outcomes Quality Initiative. NKF-K/DOQI clinical practice guidelines for vascular access. *Am J Kidney Dis*. 2006;48(Suppl 1):S176. (6)

Ward RA et al. Dialysis water and dialysate. In: Daugirdas JT et al, eds. *Handbook of Dialysis*. Philadelphia, PA: Wolters Kluwer Health; 2015:89. (12)

Key Websites

NFK KDOQI Guidelines. https://www.kidney.org/professionals/guidelines/guidelines_commentaries.

31 Dosing of Drugs in Renal Failure

David J. Quan

CORE PRINCIPLES

		CHAPTER CASES
1	The pharmacokinetics and pharmacodynamics of many drugs are altered in patients with impaired renal function (e.g., declining glomerular filtration rate) or who are on renal replacement therapy.	**Case 31-1 (Questions 1, 2), Case 31-2 (Question 1), Case 31-3 (Questions 1, 3), Case 31-4 (Questions 1, 2), Case 31-5 (Questions 1, 4), Case 31-8 (Questions 1–3)**
2	Clinicians should be aware of drugs that require dosage adjustment in the setting of renal dysfunction to avoid adverse drug events and poor patient outcomes.	**Case 31-1 (Questions 1, 2), Case 31-3 (Questions 1, 3), Case 31-4 (Question 1, 2), Case 31-5 (Questions 1, 4)**
3	Dosages of drugs that are cleared by the kidneys should be adjusted according to the patient's renal function (e.g., creatinine clearance). The initial dose can be determined using the manufacturer's prescribing information, published guidelines, or published literature.	**Case 31-1 (Questions 1, 4), Case 31-3 (Question 3), Case 31-4 (Question 1), Case 31-5 (Questions 1, 4, 5)**
4	Many drugs have a narrow therapeutic window (range of drug concentrations that will achieve the desired effect), for which there may be lack of efficacy with subtherapeutic levels and adverse events associated with elevated levels. Therapeutic drug concentration monitoring should be performed to achieve the desired target concentration.	**Case 31-1 (Questions 2, 3), Case 31-5 (Question 2), Case 31-7 (Question 1), Case 31-8 (Question 3)**
5	Renal replacement therapy (e.g., hemodialysis, continuous venovenous hemofiltration) can have a significant influence on the extracorporeal removal of drug. Clinicians should be aware of the method of renal replacement therapy and its impact on drug dosing.	**Case 31-1 (Questions 5–8), Case 31-2 (Questions 1, 2), Case 31-3 (Questions 1, 4), Case 31-5 (Questions 3, 4), Case 31-6 (Question 1)**
6	Biotransformation of drugs may be altered in patients with renal failure. Active or toxic metabolites may accumulate in patients with renal failure, leading to adverse effects. Excipients such as diluents can also accumulate in the setting of renal failure, resulting in toxicity.	**Case 31-3 (Question 2), Case 31-8 (Questions 1, 2)**

BASIC PRINCIPLES

The kidneys play an important role in the disposition of many drugs. It is important to design specific pharmacotherapeutic regimens for patients with renal impairment. Without careful dosing and therapeutic drug monitoring for select medications in these patients, accumulation of drugs or toxic metabolites can occur, resulting in serious adverse effects. Many patients are treated with multiple medications, which may require even greater attention to dosage adjustment.

In addition to altered drug elimination, numerous other factors associated with kidney disease predispose patients to potential drug toxicity by altering the pharmacokinetic disposition and the pharmacodynamic effects of drugs. For example, the physiologic changes associated with uremia can change drug absorption, protein binding, distribution, or elimination. These physiologic effects can alter drug concentrations in the plasma or blood, and at the targeted tissue site of activity, thereby affecting drug efficacy and toxicity.

Less is known about the effect of renal disease on drug pharmacodynamics, i.e., the pharmacologic or toxicologic effects produced relative to the drug concentration. Patients with renal disease can be more sensitive to some drugs, and experience an increased frequency of adverse drug reactions.

Effect of Renal Failure on Drug Disposition

BIOAVAILABILITY

Although several factors can potentially affect drug absorption in patients with kidney disease, limited data are available describing altered bioavailability. For example, drug absorption could be impaired in uremia by nausea, vomiting, diarrhea, gastritis, and edema of the gastrointestinal (GI) tract, the latter condition being a complication of nephrotic syndrome. Gastric and intestinal motility, as well as gastric emptying time, can be altered by the neuropathy associated with uremia. Uremia also can increase gastric ammonia, leading to an increased gastric pH, which may affect the bioavailability of drugs that require an acidic environment for absorption such as ferrous sulfate.[1] Similarly, calcium-containing antacids used by patients with renal failure for GI symptoms and hyperphosphatemia neutralize hydrochloric acid in the stomach and increase gastric pH. Patients with end-stage renal disease (ESRD) often take oral phosphate binders, such as sevelamer and lanthanum carbonate, which can impair the absorption of other medications.[2,3]

The bioavailability of orally administered drugs also depends on the extent to which the drug is eliminated by first-pass (presystemic) metabolism. The first-pass hepatic metabolism of oral propranolol was found to be reduced in patients with renal disease, leading to increased bioavailability.[4] Subsequent studies, however, attributed the observed increased concentrations of propranolol in renal failure to a significant increase in the blood to plasma ratio.[5] Intestinal P-glycoprotein activity may be decreased as well.[6] Other drugs exhibiting increased bioavailability in renal disease include cloxacillin, propoxyphene, dihydrocodeine, encainide, and zidovudine (AZT). For example, the area under the concentration–time curve of dihydrocodeine is increased by 70% in those patients with impaired renal function.[7]

PROTEIN BINDING AND VOLUME OF DISTRIBUTION

The extent to which a drug exerts its pharmacologic effects is related to the amount of free or unbound drug available for distribution to target tissues. Patients with renal failure often have alterations in plasma protein binding, which can increase the amount of unbound drug.[8] Clinically, this is most important for highly protein-bound acidic drugs (>80%), whereas the binding of basic drugs is usually unchanged or possibly decreased in renal disease. Decreased protein binding of affected drugs results in increases in the free fraction of drug, an increase in the apparent volume of distribution (Vd), and higher plasma clearance (Cl) for drugs with a low-extraction ratio. However, the simultaneous increase in both the Vd and clearance results in little or no change in the elimination half-life ($t_{1/2}$) of these drugs. Alternatively, the Vd of high-extraction ratio drugs can increase without a concomitant change in clearance. In this situation, the $t_{1/2}$ would increase, based on the following relationships, where Kd is the elimination rate constant of the drug:

$$\text{Kd} = \text{Cl}/\text{Vd} \qquad \text{(Eq. 31-1)}$$

$$t_{1/2} = 0.693 \times \text{Vd}/\text{Cl} \qquad \text{(Eq. 31-2)}$$

In patients with renal failure, the accumulation of uremic toxins may also alter protein binding. When the free fraction of drugs that are highly protein bound changes, the interpretation of the total drug concentration must also be considered. That is, with an increase in the free fraction, the total drug concentration necessary to exert the desired pharmacologic effect is lower than that needed under normal conditions.

Table 31-1
Plasma Protein Binding (%) of Acidic Drugs in Renal Failure

Drug	Normal	Renal Failure
Cefazolin	85	69
Cefoxitin	73	25
Clofibrate	97	91
Diazoxide	94	84
Furosemide	96	94
Pentobarbital	66	59
Phenytoin	88–93	74–84
Salicylate	87–97	74–84
Sulfamethoxazole	66	42
Valproic acid	92	77
Warfarin	99	98

Hypoalbuminemia is a common complication of renal failure. Because acidic rather than basic drugs are bound to albumin, their protein binding tends to be altered in patients with renal failure (Table 31-1).[9] Patients with uremia accumulate acidic by-products that may inhibit binding or displace acidic drugs from albumin binding sites. This is supported by the observed improvement in protein binding after removal of uremic by-products by hemodialysis. Finally, the structural conformation of albumin is altered in renal disease, which may reduce the number or affinity of binding sites for drugs. Studies have demonstrated differences in the amino acid composition of albumin between healthy people and patients with uremia.[10] The anticonvulsant, phenytoin, is a classic example of a drug whose protein binding is altered in renal disease.[11] This is discussed in more detail later in this chapter.

Renal disease can change the Vd of various drugs. The Vd or "apparent volume of distribution" is the "volume" or size of a compartment necessary to account for the total amount of drug in the body if it were present throughout the body at the same concentration as that found in plasma. A decrease in the plasma protein binding of highly protein-bound drugs, such as phenytoin, leads to an increase in the apparent Vd.

Drugs that are not highly protein bound (e.g., gentamicin, isoniazid) have little change in their Vd in renal disease. Digoxin is a unique exception in that its Vd is decreased in renal disease. This is attributed to a decrease in myocardial tissue uptake of digoxin, leading to a decrease in the myocardial or tissue to serum concentration ratio.[12]

ELIMINATION

The extent to which renal disease affects the elimination of a drug depends on the amount of drug normally excreted unchanged in the urine and the degree of renal impairment. As kidney disease progresses, the kidney's ability to excrete uremic toxins diminishes. Consequently, the ability to eliminate certain drugs that are renally excreted also decreases. If the dose of these drugs is not modified for the patient's degree of renal dysfunction, these drugs will accumulate, potentially leading to an increase in the pharmacologic effect and toxicity.

The kidney eliminates drugs primarily by filtration or active secretion. Characteristics of a drug that determine its ability to be filtered include its affinity for protein binding and its molecular weight (MW). Drugs with low protein binding or those that are displaced from proteins in the setting of renal disease are filtered more readily. Molecules with a high MW (>20,000 Da) are not readily filtered because of their large size. The reasons for how renal disease selectively alters the process of glomerular filtration or tubular secretion of specific drugs are not well understood. The elimination of drugs by the kidneys in patients with renal disease usually can be estimated by measuring the ability of the kidney to eliminate substances such as creatinine (i.e., creatinine clearance [CrCl]) (see Chapter 29, Acute Kidney Injury).

Organic anion transporters (OATs) are predominantly found in the basolateral membrane of the renal tubules. OATs facilitate the uptake of small organic anions into renal tubular cells. Decreased OAT activity as a result of acute kidney injury can decrease the renal secretion of various drugs such as methotrexate, nonsteroidal antiinflammatory drugs, and acetylsalicylic acid.[13]

Renal disease can also have an important impact on the elimination of drugs that are primarily metabolized by the liver.[14] Metabolic processes, such as hydroxylation and glucuronidation, often produce inactive, more polar compounds that can be eliminated by the kidney. The metabolites of some drugs (e.g., meperidine, morphine, procainamide) are pharmacologically active or toxic. In patients with renal disease, these metabolites may accumulate, leading to an increase in pharmacologic activity and adverse effects.[15,16] For example, the central nervous system (CNS) toxicity observed in renal disease has been attributed to accumulation of the morphine metabolite, morphine-6-glucuronide. Therefore, careful dosing modifications or avoidance of these drugs is warranted in patients with renal impairment. Metabolic enzymes have been found within renal tissue, and may play a role in the metabolism of some drugs.[17,18] For example, the nonrenal clearance of drugs (e.g., acyclovir) decreases in patients with renal impairment, and is believed to be caused by a decrease in "renal" metabolism.[19]

Excipients used to formulate medications should also be considered. For example, the pharmacokinetics of itraconazole and voriconazole are not significantly altered in the setting of renal dysfunction. However, the parenteral formulations of itraconazole, posaconazole, and voriconazole contain the solubilizing agent, β-cyclodextrin, which is normally rapidly eliminated by glomerular filtration but can accumulate in patients with renal impairment, causing GI disturbances.[20]

Drug Removal by Dialysis

The effect of dialysis on the removal of a specific drug must be considered when using medications in patients undergoing dialysis. Patients may need supplemental doses of a medication after a dialysis session or alteration in their dosage to maintain therapeutic drug concentrations. Dialysis also can be initiated to hasten drug removal from the body in some cases of drug overdose.

When using dialysis to manage a drug overdose, patients may respond clinically to factors unrelated to dialysis of the drug. For example, declining plasma concentrations may be caused by concurrent drug elimination by hepatic metabolism or renal excretion, which is independent of the dialysis procedure itself. Furthermore, clinical improvement may result from removal of active metabolites by dialysis rather than the parent compound.

The primary literature should be used to determine whether any information is available about the ability of dialysis to remove the drug. The application of data from the literature to a specific clinical situation often is difficult, however, and information pertaining to the dialysis of a specific drug may be limited.

When applying information from the primary literature to a specific patient, the specifics of the dialyzer (e.g., type of machine, membrane surface area, pore size, and blood and dialysis flow rates) must be considered (see Chapter 30, Renal Dialysis). Furthermore, patient-specific information (e.g., time of drug ingestion, liver and renal function) from case reports in the literature also should be evaluated appropriately. The method used to calculate dialysis clearance also should be considered. In addition, clinical investigators often use predialysis and postdialysis serum drug concentrations for estimating drug dialyzability without considering the contributing effects of drug metabolism and excretion on drug elimination.

DRUG-SPECIFIC PROPERTIES

The physical and chemical characteristics of drugs can be used to predict the effectiveness of dialysis on drug removal.[21–23] Low MW compounds are more readily dialyzed by conventional hemodialysis procedures because they can pass with greater ease across the dialysis membrane. Using cuprophane dialysis membranes, compounds with an MW of 500 or less are more likely to be significantly dialyzed than compounds with a high MW (e.g., vancomycin, MW approximately 1,400). Newer high-flux dialyzers using polysulfone membranes more effectively remove large chemical compounds (see High-Flux Hemodialysis Section, and Chapter 30, Renal Dialysis). In addition, water-soluble drugs (e.g., aminoglycosides, lithium) are removed more readily by dialysis than are lipid-soluble compounds (e.g., diazepam) or those that partition into red blood cells (e.g., tacrolimus).

Pharmacokinetic characteristics (e.g., Vd, protein binding) also can affect drug dialyzability. A drug with a large Vd that distributes widely into the peripheral tissues resides minimally in the plasma and, therefore, is not substantially removed by dialysis. This is particularly true for highly lipid-soluble drugs such as digoxin (Vd = 300–500 L) and amiodarone (Vd = 60 L/kg). In addition, drugs that are highly protein bound, such as warfarin (99%) and ceftriaxone (83%–96%), are not significantly removed by dialysis because the large protein–drug complex is unable to pass through the dialysis membrane.

Because clearance values are additive, the hepatic and other nonrenal plasma clearance of a drug should be considered in relation to the dialysis clearance. Only when dialysis clearance contributes a substantially additive effect to the patient's own clearance is drug elimination enhanced. For example, AZT has a large nonrenal plasma clearance in patients with severe renal disease (approximately 1,200 mL/minute). Therefore, despite a hemodialysis clearance of 63 mL/minute, the contribution of dialysis to total AZT removal is negligible.

HIGH-FLUX HEMODIALYSIS

High-flux hemodialysis uses higher blood and dialysate flow rates compared with conventional methods. The enhanced efficiency of high-flux dialysis and the larger pore size of the polysulfone membranes allow for small- and mid-MW compounds (e.g., vancomycin) to be partially removed. Drugs such as gentamicin and foscarnet, which are removed by conventional dialysis, are also efficiently removed by high-flux hemodialysis.[24,25] In many cases, the net amount of drug removed during a high-flux dialysis session is greater than the amount removed during conventional dialysis because of the use of higher blood flow rates. The principal difference is the greater efficiency and the ability to clear drugs of larger MW compared with conventional dialysis.

CONTINUOUS AMBULATORY PERITONEAL DIALYSIS

Continuous ambulatory peritoneal dialysis (CAPD) uses the patient's peritoneum as the dialysis membrane. Patients maintained with CAPD undergo infusion of a dialysate solution via a catheter inserted into the peritoneal cavity; the solution is allowed to dwell in the cavity for several hours. The accumulated fluid and uremic by-products diffuse from the blood into the dialysate solution, which is exchanged every 4 to 8 hours (see Chapter 30, Renal Dialysis).

Some drugs, such as antibiotics, can be administered intraperitoneally (IP) in patients on CAPD by directly adding them to the dialysate solution. This is particularly useful for patients with peritonitis who require high intraperitoneal concentrations of antimicrobial agents to treat this infection. After intraperitoneal administration of drugs, such as the aminoglycosides, plasma and intraperitoneal drug concentrations will eventually reach equilibrium. Despite systemic absorption of these drugs from the peritoneal fluid, peritoneal dialysis (PD) usually is inefficient at removing drugs from the plasma.[26] Because CAPD contributes little to the overall elimination of most drugs, dosage modifications are not always necessary in patients having this procedure.

Continuous venovenous hemofiltration (CVVH) is a form of continuous renal replacement therapy (CRRT) used in the critically ill patient with renal failure. CRRT is typically reserved for patients who are unable to tolerate hemodialysis because of hemodynamic instability. As with hemodialysis, this procedure removes fluid, electrolytes, and low- and mid-MW molecules from the blood. Using a hollow fiber that is made of a semipermeable membrane, water and solutes are filtered by hydrostatic pressure. A countercurrent dialysate can be added to the circuit to improve solute removal (continuous venovenous hemodialysis with filtration).

Limited data are available on the effect of CVVH on the removal of drugs. Drugs that have a high sieving coefficient (permeability of a drug through a semipermeable membrane), such as the aminoglycosides, ceftazidime, vancomycin, and procainamide, are readily removed by CVVH.[27–29] Data concerning the removal of drugs by hemodialysis cannot be extrapolated to CVVH because of differences in the membranes used, blood flow rates, ultrafiltration rate, dialysate flow rate, and the continuous nature of the procedure compared with intermittent hemodialysis. CVVH clearance can be estimated to determine the appropriate dosage regimen based on the pharmacologic characteristics of a specific drug (see Case 31-1, Question 8).

HEMOPERFUSION

Hemoperfusion is another method of drug removal that may be used to facilitate the elimination of a drug in the setting of an overdose.[30,31] During the hemoperfusion procedure, blood is passed through a column of adsorbent material (e.g., activated charcoal or resin) to bind toxins and drugs. Hemoperfusion can be particularly useful for removing large MW compounds or highly protein-bound drugs that are not removed efficiently by hemodialysis. Large compounds and drug–protein complexes are adsorbed onto the high-surface-area resin as blood passes through the adsorbent column. Hemoperfusion can also be used to remove lipid-soluble drugs not easily removed by hemodialysis. Lipid-soluble drugs often have a large Vd. Removal of drugs by hemoperfusion is of limited value because a significant amount of these lipophilic compounds resides in peripheral tissues.

Pharmacodynamics and Renal Disease

Few studies have investigated the pharmacodynamics of drugs in patients with renal disease. Clinical observations report that patients with renal disease are more sensitive to various drugs. For example, morphine has been associated with increased neurologic depression in patients with renal failure.[32,33] The ability of morphine to potentiate the CNS-depressant effects of uremia may result from an alteration in the permeability of the blood–brain barrier that results in higher CNS levels of morphine and morphine-6-glucuronide.

Another example of altered drug response in uremia is that of nifedipine, which at similar unbound plasma concentrations has an increased antihypertensive effect in patients with renal disease.[34] The mean maximal effect change in diastolic blood pressure values in the control group and in patients with severe renal failure were 12% and 29%, respectively. Therefore, the dose of nifedipine may need to be adjusted in patients with renal disease because of changes in drug effects rather than pharmacokinetic alterations.

The pharmacokinetics of warfarin is not significantly altered in renal failure. However, patients with renal failure who are prescribed warfarin have a higher incidence of hemorrhagic complications, likely because of platelet dysfunction from uremia, and drug–drug interactions from concomitant medications.[35,36]

PHARMACOKINETICS AND PHARMACODYNAMICS OF SPECIFIC DRUGS IN RENAL FAILURE

Ceftazidime

DOSAGE MODIFICATION: FACTORS TO CONSIDER

CASE 31-1

QUESTION 1: G.G., a 31-year-old, 70-kg woman with a 3-year history of systemic lupus erythematosus, presents to the emergency department (ED) with a 5-day history of fatigue, weakness, and nausea as well, as worsening of her facial rash and a fever of 40°C. Her systemic lupus erythematosus had been moderately controlled until this acute flare. Her admission laboratory workup now reveals the following pertinent values:

Potassium (K), 6.0 mEq/L
Sodium (Na), 142 mEq/L
Serum creatinine (SCr), 3.4 mg/dL
Blood urea nitrogen (BUN), 38 mg/dL

Complete blood count reveals a hematocrit of 32% and a hemoglobin of 9.2 g/dL. The platelet count is 50,000/μL, and her erythrocyte sedimentation rate is 35 mm/hour. Physical examination is significant for a blood pressure of 136/92 mm Hg and 2+ pedal edema. Prednisone is started at a dose of 1.5 mg/kg/day.

During her hospital course, G.G.'s condition worsens and signs of sepsis develop. *Pseudomonas aeruginosa* is cultured from her urine. Therapy with ceftazidime is initiated at a dose of 2 g every 8 hours, a dose commonly used for patients with normal renal function. Considering that G.G.'s renal function has remained stable and that she has an estimated CrCl of 27 mL/minute, what factors should be considered before modifying her dose? What would be an appropriate dose of ceftazidime for G.G.?

Before modifying the dose of any drug, its route of elimination should be established. As a general rule, the degree to which renal impairment affects elimination depends on the percentage of unchanged drug that is excreted by the kidney. Thus, the elimination of most drugs that are primarily cleared by the kidneys will be decreased in the setting of renal impairment. For many drugs dependent on the kidney for elimination, relationships between some measurement of renal function (e.g., CrCl) and some parameter of drug elimination (e.g., plasma clearance or half-life) have been established to help clinicians determine the appropriate dosing modifications in patients with renal disease.

In contrast, the clearance of drugs that are eliminated primarily by nonrenal mechanisms (e.g., hepatic metabolism) is not altered significantly in patients with renal disease. However, some drugs have water-soluble metabolites that have either pharmacologic activity or potential toxicity and that may accumulate with renal dysfunction, warranting dosage adjustment or avoidance of the drug entirely (e.g., meperidine; see Case 31-8, Question 1).

Enzymes with metabolic capacity have also been found within renal tissue, which can result in the kidneys playing a limited role in the metabolism of certain drugs (see Case 31-3, Question 2). The clinical importance of this elimination pathway is unclear.

Another important factor to consider is the "therapeutic window" for a given drug, i.e., the range of drug concentrations thought to be most effective. Drug concentrations below this range are usually subtherapeutic, whereas concentrations above this range can lead to a greater incidence of adverse effects. For drugs with a wide therapeutic window, the difference between toxic and therapeutic concentrations is large. Although many drugs that are cleared primarily by the kidney may require dosing modifications in patients with renal dysfunction, aggressive dose reduction may not be necessary for drugs with a large therapeutic window, particularly if the adverse effects of the drug (e.g., fluconazole) are relatively mild. This is in contrast to drugs (e.g., aminoglycosides, vancomycin, or foscarnet) that are eliminated primarily by the kidney and have narrow therapeutic windows. For these drugs, the toxic plasma concentrations are very close to the therapeutic drug concentrations, with little room for dosing error.

Ceftazidime is a cephalosporin that has excellent activity against most strains of *Pseudomonas* species. As with most cephalosporins, ceftazidime primarily is cleared by the kidneys, with little nonrenal or hepatic elimination. The correlation between the clearance of ceftazidime and CrCl in mL/minute is represented by the following equation[37]:

$$Cl_{ceftaz}(\text{mL/minute}) = (0.95)(\text{CrCl}) + 6.59 \qquad \text{(Eq. 31-3)}$$

Using Equation 31-3, the clearance of ceftazidime in G.G. is estimated to be 32 mL/minute compared with an average normal clearance of approximately 100 mL/minute. Because her drug clearance is approximately one-third of normal, she would require about one-third of the normal daily dose (i.e., 2 g every 24 hours). As with other cephalosporins, ceftazidime has a large therapeutic window.[38] Failure to reduce the dose from a normal dose of 2 g every 8 hours, although likely safe, might lead to accumulation of ceftazidime, predisposing G.G. to seizures and other adverse effects associated with toxic β-lactam antibiotic plasma levels.[39,40] This is in contrast to the aminoglycosides, which must be dosed based on specific pharmacokinetic calculations. Therefore, more generalized or empirical dosage modifications can be made with ceftazidime.

Aminoglycosides

Case 31-1, Question 2: G.G.'s medical team decides that the addition of an aminoglycoside antibiotic is necessary to treat her infection. Considering that her renal function has remained stable, how should gentamicin be dosed in G.G.? Is it best to alter the dose or the dosing interval for this drug?

ALTERATION OF DOSE VERSUS DOSING INTERVAL

The aminoglycosides (e.g., tobramycin, gentamicin, amikacin) are effective in the treatment of serious systemic infections caused by gram-negative organisms such as *Pseudomonas* species. Unlike the cephalosporins and penicillins, however, the aminoglycosides have a relatively narrow therapeutic window. Using pharmacokinetic principles, a dose regimen can be designed to produce specific peak and trough serum concentrations. Peak serum concentrations (Cp_{peak}) (e.g., gentamicin or tobramycin 5–8 mg/L) correlate best with therapeutic efficacy, whereas toxicity tends to correlate with elevated trough levels (Cp_{trough}), which reflects prolonged exposure to high drug concentrations. To minimize the risk of toxicity, trough levels of less than 2 mg/L should be maintained. In patients with normal renal function, these target serum aminoglycoside concentrations are usually obtained after standard doses (e.g., 1.5 mg/kg) administered every 8 hours. Peak and trough levels are typically measured once steady state is achieved, which is typically within 24 hours.[41–44]

Many clinicians now use once-daily dosing of the aminoglycosides (e.g., 5 mg/kg every 24 hours) for patients with normal renal function in an attempt to minimize aminoglycoside accumulation and nephrotoxicity. The rationale for this regimen is based on the aminoglycosides' concentration-dependent killing and postantibiotic effect. This approach is not recommended for patients with advanced renal impairment, however. When once-daily dosing is used, peak concentrations are less helpful; however, trough concentrations should be monitored with a target of being below the limit of analytic detection (<1 mg/L). The discussion regarding aminoglycoside dosing in renal impairment that follows is based on the traditional every 8 hours dosing regimen.

Aminoglycosides are almost completely eliminated by the kidneys; thus, the clearance of these drugs essentially is equal to the glomerular filtration rate (GFR). The pharmacokinetic properties of gentamicin and tobramycin are similar. A close correlation also exists between CrCl (a surrogate for GFR) and gentamicin total body clearance. As renal function deteriorates, aminoglycoside doses must be modified to achieve the desired peak and trough plasma concentrations. Failure to appropriately adjust the dosage of aminoglycosides in renal insufficiency can lead to high drug plasma levels that can result in ototoxicity and nephrotoxicity.

In many cases, the aminoglycoside dose can be modified by extending the dosing interval rather than simply reducing the dose. This permits maintenance of adequate peak plasma concentrations to ensure efficacy, while allowing for sufficient elimination between doses to produce trough levels less than 2 mg/L. The advantages and disadvantages of adjusting the dosing interval versus reducing the dose are summarized in Table 31-2.

Figure 31-1 illustrates the effect of increasing the dosing interval in a patient such as G.G. with renal function that is 30% of normal. Although this is the preferred method for adjusting the dose of aminoglycosides, for many other drugs requiring dose adjustments in renal disease, simple dosage reduction is sufficient. Commonly used drug references such as Facts and Comparisons can be used for dosing guidelines for drugs used in patients with renal failure.[45]

DETERMINATION OF APPROPRIATE DOSE

A number of methods have been developed to determine the appropriate aminoglycoside dose for patients.[46] One method is Bayesian forecasting, in which pharmacokinetic data obtained in the individual patient are integrated with population parameters. Initially, a dose is used that is based on population parameter values adjusted for characteristics such as increased SCr. Drug concentrations for the individual patient are measured at specific times (e.g., peak and trough measurements), and these are compared with the expected values from the population data. Individualized pharmacokinetic parameter estimates are subsequently derived using Bayes' theorem to calculate a more patient-specific dosing regimen.[47]

Because of the wide interpatient variability in aminoglycoside pharmacokinetic parameters and the narrow therapeutic index for these drugs, doses should be adjusted based on pharmacokinetic principles (e.g., Bayesian calculations or methods described later in this chapter) and plasma concentrations that are specific for this patient.

Table 31-2
Advantages and Disadvantages of General Approaches to Dosing Adjustments in Renal Disease

Method	Advantages	Disadvantages
Variable Frequency		
Use the same dose but ↑ the dosing interval	Same Cp_{ave}, Cp_{max}, Cp_{min} Normal dose	Levels may remain subtherapeutic for prolonged periods in patients requiring dosing intervals >24 hours
Variable Dose With Fixed Cp_{ave}		
↓ Dose to maintain a target Cp_{ave}; keep the dosing interval the same	Same Cp_{ave} Normal dosing interval	↓ Peak levels, which may be subtherapeutic; ↑ trough levels, which may ↑ potential for toxicity

Cp_{ave}, average plasma concentration; Cp_{max}, maximum plasma concentration; Cp_{min}, minimum plasma concentration.

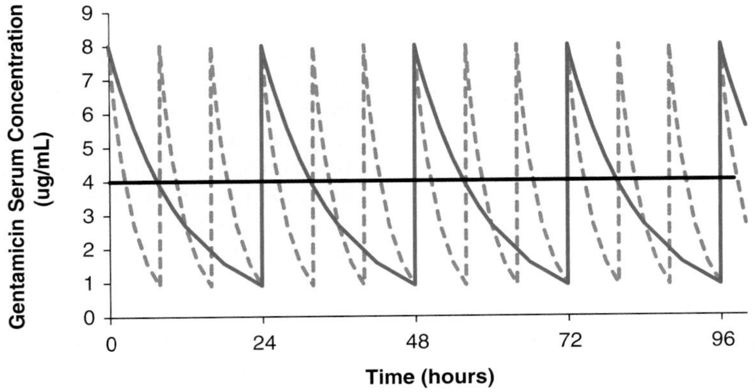

Figure 31-1 Serum concentration versus time profile for a patient with normal renal function (*dotted line*), and for patient G.G. (Case 31-1) whose estimated creatinine clearance is 27 mL/minute (*solid lines*).

Patient-Specific Methods

Sawchuk et al. developed a method to derive patient-specific estimates of Vd and clearance based on the patient's size and estimated CrCl.[43] These parameters can be used to calculate a specific dose for G.G. that will produce the desired gentamicin peak and trough concentrations. If steady-state serum concentrations of gentamicin are known, they can be used to calculate even more specific parameters. To initiate gentamicin therapy, pharmacokinetic parameters should first be estimated from population values.

The clearance of gentamicin (Cl_{gent}) can be calculated based on G.G.'s CrCl. Using the Cockcroft–Gault equation,[48] the CrCl can be estimated as follows:

$$\text{CrCl (males)} = \frac{(140 - \text{age})(\text{IBW})}{(\text{SCr})(72)} \qquad \text{(Eq. 31-4)}$$

$$\text{CrCl (females)} = \frac{(140 - \text{age})(\text{IBW})}{(\text{SCr})(72)}(0.85) \qquad \text{(Eq. 31-5)}$$

where IBW is ideal body weight in kilograms, age is measured in years, and SCr is serum creatinine in mg/dL.

With a SCr of 3.4 mg/dL, an ideal body weight of 70 kg, and an age of 31 years, G.G.'s estimated CrCl, is 27 mL/minute.

For practical purposes, Cl_{gent} is usually considered equivalent to CrCl. Therefore, Cl_{gent} also is approximately 27 mL/minute or 1.6 L/hour. The Vd of gentamicin (Vd_{gent}) is approximately 0.25 L/kg in patients with normal or impaired renal function.[43,48,49]

The Vd_{gent} will be different in obese patients or those who have fluid overload. Although G.G. does have some fluid retention, this is minimal and should not affect her Vd_{gent} significantly. Therefore, the Vd_{gent} for G.G. is as follows:

$$\begin{aligned} Vd_{gent} &= (0.25\ \text{L/kg})(\text{body weight}) \\ &= (0.25\ \text{L/kg})(70\ \text{kg}) \qquad \text{(Eq. 31-6)} \\ &= 17.5\ \text{L} \end{aligned}$$

The loading dose of gentamicin (LD_{gent}) can be determined using the following equation:

$$LD_{gent} = (Vd_{gent})(\text{desired } Cp_{peak}) \qquad \text{(Eq. 31-7)}$$

For treatment of infections caused by *Pseudomonas* species, a peak level of approximately 6 to 8 mg/L is desired:

$$\begin{aligned} LD_{gent} &= (17.5\ \text{L})(7\ \text{mg/L}) \\ &= 122.5\ \text{mg or round off to 120 mg} \end{aligned} \qquad \text{(Eq. 31-8)}$$

Using Cl_{gent} and Vd_{gent}, the elimination rate constant (Kd) and half-life for gentamicin can be estimated as follows:

$$\begin{aligned} Kd &= \frac{Cl_{gent}}{Vd_{gent}} \\ &= \frac{1.6\ \text{L/hour}}{17.5\ \text{L}} \qquad \text{(Eq. 31-9)} \\ &= 0.091\ \text{hour}^{-1} \end{aligned}$$

$$\begin{aligned} t_{1/2} &= \frac{0.693}{Kd} \\ &= \frac{0.693}{0.091\ \text{hour}^{-1}} \qquad \text{(Eq. 31-10)} \\ &= 7.6\ \text{hours} \end{aligned}$$

For the aminoglycosides, the dosing interval (τ) is determined by doubling the half-life because by the end of two half-lives, 75% of the drug will have been eliminated. This will usually lead to a desired trough level of less than 2 mg/L. Therefore, gentamicin should be administered at least every 16 hours. For convenience, an interval of 24 hours can be used, which also will achieve the desired trough concentration.

Gentamicin is usually infused over 30 minutes. To determine the peak gentamicin concentration, serum samples are drawn 30 minutes after the infusion has been completed. Because the estimated elimination half-life of gentamicin in G.G. (7.6 hours) is much longer than the infusion time (0.5 hours), the intravenous (IV) bolus model can be used to calculate an appropriate maintenance dose.

To achieve the peak concentration of 7 mg/L, the following equation can be used:

$$\text{Dose} = \frac{(Cp_{peak})(1 - e^{-Kd\tau})(Vd_{gent})}{(e^{-Kdt_{sample}})}$$

$$= \frac{(7\ \text{mg/L})(1 - e^{-(0.091\ \text{hour}^{-1})(24\ \text{hour})})(17.5\ \text{L})}{(e^{-(0.091\ \text{hour}^{-1})(1\ \text{hour})})} \quad \text{(Eq. 31-11)}$$

$$= 119.2\ \text{mg}$$

$$= \text{or round off to } 120\ \text{mg}$$

where t_{sample} usually equals 1 hour (30 minutes after a 30-minute infusion).

The expected trough level in G.G. can now be estimated by the following equation:

$$Cp_{trough} = (Cp_{peak})(e^{-Kd\tau_{sample}})$$

$$= (7\ \text{mg/L})(e^{-(0.091\ \text{hour}^{-1})(24\ \text{hours})}) \quad \text{(Eq. 31-12)}$$

$$= 0.8\ \text{mg/L}$$

Although not the case for G.G., patients with normal renal function may eliminate a significant amount of gentamicin during the 30-minute infusion. In these patients, the intermittent infusion model should be used to account for this loss of drug, where t_{in} is the duration of the infusion:

$$\text{Dose} = \frac{(Cl_{gent})(Cp_{peak})(1 - e^{-Kd\tau})(t_{in})}{(1 - e^{-Kd\tau_{in}})(e^{-Kd\tau})} \quad \text{(Eq. 31-13)}$$

REVISED PARAMETERS

CASE 31-1, QUESTION 3: After 72 hours of gentamicin therapy, G.G.'s peak and trough levels are 7.6 and 2.6 mg/L, respectively. Her physician attributes this to a gradual decline in renal function. (Her most recent SCr is 4.8 mg/dL.) How would you revise G.G.'s dosing regimen based on these levels?

A gentamicin trough level of more than 2 mg/L suggests that G.G.'s dosing interval is too short. Although her peak concentration is within the normal range of 5 to 8 mg/L, her trough concentration indicates that she is at a potentially toxic level. Her pharmacokinetic parameters can be revised based on these values, and a new Kd can be estimated from the following equation:

$$Kd = \frac{\ln\left(\frac{CP_1}{CP_2}\right)}{\Delta t} = \frac{\ln\left(\frac{7.6\ \text{mg/L}}{2.6\ \text{mg/L}}\right)}{23\ \text{hours}} = 0.047\ \text{hour}^{-1} \quad \text{(Eq. 31-14)}$$

Because little change in G.G.'s Vd_{gent} is expected, a new Cl_{gent} ($Cl_{revised}$) can be estimated from her revised elimination constant (if necessary, a revised Vd_{gent} could be calculated, keeping Cl_{gent} constant, although the clearance is more likely to change than the volume of distribution):

$$Cl_{revised} = (Vd_{gent})(Kd)$$

$$= (17.5\ \text{L})(0.047\ \text{hour}^{-1}) \quad \text{(Eq. 31-15)}$$

$$= 0.82\ \text{L/hour}$$

These revised values for Kd and Cl can now be used to calculate a revised maintenance dose to maintain the Cp_{trough} at less than 2 mg/L using Equation 31-11:

$$\text{Dose} = \frac{(7\ \text{mg/L})(1 - e^{-(0.047\ \text{hour}^{-1})(48\ \text{hours})})(17.5\ \text{L})}{e^{-(0.047\ \text{hour}^{-1})(1\ \text{hour})}}$$

$$= 115\ \text{mg} \quad \text{(Eq. 31-16)}$$

$$Cp_{trough} = (7\ \text{mg/L})(e^{-(0.047\ \text{hour}^{-1})(48\ \text{hours})})$$

$$= 0.73\ \text{mg/L}$$

The revised dose is now 115 mg (or ~110 mg) every 48 hours.

CASE 31-1, QUESTION 4: What are some limitations in calculating G.G.'s CrCl based on her SCr? Can this estimate safely be used to predict gentamicin clearance?

See Chapter 28, Chronic Kidney Disease, for information about equations used to calculate CrCl and estimate GFR. For patients with stable renal function, CrCl can be estimated from SCr using the Cockcroft–Gault equation (see Eqs. 31-4 and 31-5). In a patient such as G.G., however, whose renal function continues to decline during the hospital course, estimation of renal function based on her increasing SCr becomes more difficult. Because her SCr does not reflect a steady-state level, the previous equations can no longer be used to accurately estimate her renal function. Because G.G.'s SCr has increased rapidly from 3.4 to 4.8 mg/dL during the past few days, her CrCl is probably much lower than that estimated using the Cockcroft–Gault method. A rising SCr may represent a decline in renal function manifesting as an accumulation of creatinine.

Although prediction equations such as the Modification of Diet in Renal Disease (MDRD) equations are a good measure of GFR,[50] they were developed in patients with chronic kidney disease, therefore limiting its use in healthy patients. In addition, the MDRD equation has not been validated for the dosing of most drugs in the setting of renal dysfunction.[51,52] There can be significant differences in drug dosing regimens when the MDRD and Cockcroft–Gault methods are used to estimate renal function.[53,54] In 1998, the FDA recommended using the Cockcroft–Gault equation to estimate kidney function when designing pharmacokinetic clinical trials and drug dosing regimens. The Cockcroft–Gault equation has been the standard method to estimate renal function to determine if drug dosage adjustments are necessary. In 2010, the FDA released a draft guidance that included both the Cockcroft–Gault and MDRD equations to determine renal function. It also should be noted that the units for the Cockcroft–Gault equation for CrCl is mL/minute, while the units for the MDRD equation for eGFR is mL/minute/1.73m^2. The manufacturer's prescribing information and available literature should be evaluated to determine the appropriate dosage regimen based on the patient's renal function.

Effect of Hemodialysis

CONVENTIONAL DIALYSIS

Gentamicin

CASE 31-1, QUESTION 5: G.G.'s renal function continues to deteriorate to the extent that she requires hemodialysis. What additional alterations in her gentamicin dosing regimen are necessary when she is having dialysis?

Gentamicin has a MW of about 500 and a relatively low Vd (averaging 0.25 L/kg), and is about 10% bound to proteins, all favoring effective removal by conventional hemodialysis.[44] For a given patient, the observed dialysis clearance of gentamicin using conventional methods also depends on factors such as the physical properties of the dialysis filter, the blood and dialysate flow rates, and the length of dialysis. Studies indicate that dialysis clearance of gentamicin averages 45 mL/minute compared with an average plasma clearance of 5 mL/minute in patients with ESRD.[55,56] Therefore, G.G.'s gentamicin dose must be adjusted to compensate for the amount of drug that will be removed by dialysis. Because drug removal represents a combination of drug elimination by the body and dialysis, the following equation can be used:

$$Cl_{total} = Cl_{dial} + Cl \qquad \text{(Eq. 31-17)}$$

where Cl_{total} is the total clearance of the drug during dialysis, Cl_{dial} is the clearance by dialysis, and Cl is plasma clearance. If dialysis clearance is high relative to plasma clearance, drug removal will be enhanced by the dialysis procedure. The total clearance of gentamicin in a patient with severe renal dysfunction during dialysis is 50 mL/minute (45 mL/minute + 5 mL/minute) or 10 times the clearance while off dialysis. Plasma clearance and dialysis clearance are related to the elimination half-life by the following equation:

$$t_{1/2} = \frac{(0.693)(Vd)}{Cl_{dial} + Cl} \qquad \text{(Eq. 31-18)}$$

Thus, assuming a constant Vd of 17.5 L (i.e., 0.25 L/kg × 70 kg), the elimination half-life on dialysis is approximately 4 hours compared with 40 hours off dialysis. In addition, the extent (fraction) of drug removal (FD) during a timed dialysis run can be predicted from the following equation:

$$FD = 1 - e^{-(Cl + Cl_{dial})(t/Vd)} \qquad \text{(Eq. 31-19)}$$

where t is the duration of dialysis. Therefore, the fraction of gentamicin removed (FD) during a 4-hour conventional dialysis procedure is approximately 50%. If specific data are not available for dialysis and plasma clearance, the following equation will predict fraction removed using the elimination half-life data alone obtained during dialysis:

$$FD = 1 - e^{-(0.693/t_{1/2on})(t)} \qquad \text{(Eq. 31-20)}$$

The estimated value of 50% removal is consistent with literature values indicating that 50% to 70% of a dose of gentamicin is removed during a 4-hour dialysis procedure. A limitation of this equation, however, is that it does not consider the redistribution of drug from the tissues back into the plasma after the dialysis procedure.

It generally is difficult to calculate an appropriate maintenance dose for patients having hemodialysis that will maintain peak and trough concentrations similar to patients with normal renal function, in part because of the large variability found in aminoglycoside pharmacokinetic parameters.[56,57] Sustained plasma concentrations greater than 2 mg/L can increase the risk of toxicity; however, dosing gentamicin to achieve trough concentrations of less than 2 mg/L may lead to prolonged periods of subtherapeutic peak concentrations because one would have to use smaller doses with lower peak concentrations to allow the troughs to decrease before the next dose. Another practical consideration is that unless one expects the patient to recover renal function in the future, renal toxicity of the drug is less of a concern. As a compromise in patients receiving hemodialysis, gentamicin doses are given to achieve a predialysis trough concentration of approximately 3 mg/L. This can generally be achieved with a loading dose of 2 mg/kg, followed by a maintenance dose of 1 mg/kg after each dialysis session.

Ceftazidime

CASE 31-1, QUESTION 6: Why does the dose of ceftazidime in G.G. have to be adjusted because of her hemodialysis when this drug has such a large therapeutic window?

Because only 21% of ceftazidime is protein bound and its Vd is 0.2 L/kg, it should be readily removed by hemodialysis. The mean dialysis clearance of ceftazidime is 55 mL/minute, with 55% of the drug removed during 4 hours of conventional hemodialysis.[58] A supplemental dose of ceftazidime should be given to G.G. after each hemodialysis session to maintain a therapeutic concentration. Half of the daily ceftazidime dose should be administered after each dialysis session.

HIGH-FLUX HEMODIALYSIS

CASE 31-1, QUESTION 7: G.G.'s physician is considering changing her from a conventional dialysis system to a high-flux system that uses high-efficiency polysulfone membranes. How does the dialyzability of gentamicin and ceftazidime differ with high-flux hemodialysis compared with conventional hemodialysis?

High-flux hemodialysis is more effective than conventional dialysis at removing certain pharmacologic agents (see Chapter 30, Renal Dialysis) because the membranes are more efficient and the blood flow through the dialyzer is increased. Although limited data are available, a greater fraction of drugs, such as aminoglycosides, ceftazidime, and vancomycin, are removed by high-flux versus conventional hemodialysis.[59,60] Approximately 50% to 70% of gentamicin is removed during a 2.5-hour, high-flux dialysis session.[24] The clearance of ceftazidime by high-flux dialysis is 75 to 240 mL/minute compared with 55 mL/minute for conventional hemodialysis.[59] Thus, further dosage adjustments for gentamicin and ceftazidime may be necessary if G.G. is converted from conventional hemodialysis to high-flux hemodialysis.

CONTINUOUS VENOVENOUS HEMOFILTRATION

CASE 31-1, QUESTION 8: What changes would be necessary in G.G.'s gentamicin dosing if she were to start a CRRT such as CVVH?

Because of the continuous nature of CVVH, the extent of drug eliminated by CRRTs will differ from intermittent modes such as hemodialysis. The clearance of a drug in a patient receiving CVVH can be described in a fashion similar to Equation 31-17, where Cl_{dial} is replaced with Cl_{cvvh}.

$$Cl_{total} = Cl + Cl_{cvvh} \qquad \text{(Eq. 31-21)}$$

In G.G., the $Cl_{revised}$ from Equation 31-15 can be used for the plasma clearance (Cl). The clearance by CVVH can be described by the following equation:

$$Cl_{cvvh} = Fu \times UFR \qquad \text{(Eq. 31-22)}$$

where Fu is the fraction of drug unbound and UFR is the ultrafiltration rate. Gentamicin exhibits low plasma protein binding (Fu = 0.95). Typical ultrafiltration rates for CVVH are approximately 1 L/hour, but can vary.

$$\begin{aligned} Cl_{cvvh} &= Fu \times UFR \\ &= 0.95 \times 1\ L/hour \\ &= 0.95\ L/hour \end{aligned} \qquad \text{(Eq. 31-23)}$$

$$\begin{aligned} Cl_{total} &= Cl_{revised} + Cl_{cvvh} \\ &= 0.82\ L/hour + 0.95\ L/hour \\ &= 1.77\ L/hour \\ &= 29.5\ mL/minute \end{aligned} \qquad \text{(Eq. 31-24)}$$

Because the clearance of gentamicin approximates that of CrCl, G.G.'s total clearance is approximately one-third the normal clearance of 100 mL/minute. Therefore, the gentamicin dose should be approximately one-third of the normal dose. G.G. should be given 1.5 mg/kg/day or 100 mg of gentamicin as a single daily dose (normal dose is approximately 5 mg/kg/day). Gentamicin trough concentrations should be monitored, and her dose adjusted to maintain a trough concentration of less than 2 mg/L.

CONTINUOUS AMBULATORY PERITONEAL DIALYSIS

CASE 31-2

QUESTION 1: J.J., a 24-year-old man with ESRD, is maintained with CAPD. He presents to the ED with a fever of 38.2°C and complains of severe abdominal pain. He also reports that his peritoneal dialysate has become cloudy in the past few days. All these symptoms are consistent with peritonitis, a frequent complication of CAPD. His culture results reveal *Escherichia coli*, sensitive to gentamicin. How should gentamicin be dosed in this patient?

Management of dialysis-related peritonitis can vary from one institution to another. Antibiotics often are administered IP with or without systemic antibiotic therapy. For less severe cases, IP administration is often considered sufficient. With IP administration, the goal is to deliver a concentration of drug similar to the desired plasma concentration for the treatment of systemic infections. Therefore, 8 mg of gentamicin into each liter of dialysate (or 16 mg into a 2-L bag of dialysate) is recommended. Once equilibrium or steady state is achieved, the dialysate concentration will be comparable to the concentration of gentamicin in the plasma. Despite a more rapid transfer of drug into the plasma because of increased permeability of the peritoneal membrane in patients with peritonitis, there will still be a substantial lag time before steady state is reached. For more serious cases of peritonitis, concomitant systemic antibiotics should be given.

CASE 31-2, QUESTION 2: Is gentamicin eliminated by CAPD?

In general, most drugs are not well removed via CAPD. This is particularly true for drugs that are highly protein bound or for drugs with a large Vd. Gentamicin and other aminoglycosides, on the other hand, are effectively removed by CAPD because they have low protein binding and a small Vd. It is estimated that 10% to 50% of gentamicin is removed by CAPD.[61]

Acyclovir

RENAL CLEARANCE

CASE 31-3

QUESTION 1: D.M., a 28-year-old man with acquired immune deficiency syndrome, presents with a severe herpetic infection requiring IV acyclovir. Because of other complications associated with his human immunodeficiency virus (HIV) infection, D.M. has developed renal insufficiency during his hospital course. His SCr is 4.5 mg/dL, and his CrCl is 20 mL/minute. What are important considerations for dosing acyclovir in D.M. now, and also if he requires dialysis?

Acyclovir is used to prevent or treat a variety of viral infections, such as those caused by herpes simplex and varicella zoster viruses.[62] It is cleared primarily by the kidneys, with approximately 70% to 80% excreted unchanged in the urine. Dosage adjustment is necessary in patients with renal disease.[19,63] Renal tubular secretion in addition to filtration contributes to the elimination of acyclovir, which explains why the renal clearance of acyclovir is about 3 times greater than the estimated CrCl.

Acyclovir also can precipitate in the renal tubules and exacerbate D.M.'s renal failure. This is more likely to occur when high doses are infused too rapidly to patients with renal dysfunction.[63] To minimize nephrotoxicity, the patient should be adequately hydrated to maintain good urine flow, and the acyclovir dose should be infused over the course of 1 hour. Nephrotoxicity is usually reversible on discontinuation of the drug or reduction of the dose. In addition, acyclovir-associated neurotoxicity correlates with elevated plasma concentrations, and further underscores the need for adequate dosage adjustments in patients with renal dysfunction.[64]

The clearance of acyclovir correlates with the CrCl according to the following relationship:

$$Cl_{acyclovir} \text{ in mL/minute/1.73 m}^2 = (3.4)(\text{CrCl in mL/minute/1.73 m}^2) + 28.7 \quad \text{(Eq. 31-25)}$$

In patients with normal renal function, the clearance of acyclovir ranges from 210 to 330 mL/minute; in patients with ESRD, the clearance is 29 to 34 mL/minute.[19,63,65] Although this change in clearance primarily results from decreased renal clearance of the drug, nonrenal clearance of acyclovir also decreases in these patients.[19,65] As a result, the elimination half-life increases significantly from approximately 3 hours in patients with normal kidney function to 20 hours in patients with ESRD. Therefore, doses should be reduced proportionately from a normal daily dose of 15 mg/kg body weight (5 mg/kg given every 8 hours) for serious herpes simplex infections to doses as low as 2.5 mg/kg/day (given as a single daily dose) in patients with ESRD.[66] Because D.M. has a CrCl of 20 mL/minute and an estimated $Cl_{acyclovir}$ of 97 mL/minute (approximately one-third of normal), a single daily dose of 5 mg/kg (one-third of normal) would be appropriate to treat this infection.

DIALYSIS

Acyclovir is moderately removed by conventional hemodialysis, with plasma concentrations decreasing by 60% after 6 hours of dialysis.[67] The elimination half-life on and off dialysis is 6 and 20 hours, respectively, whereas the dialysis clearance averages 80 mL/minute. Therefore, a supplemental dose of 2.5 mg/kg after dialysis is recommended to replace the amount of drug removed by hemodialysis. No data are available on the removal of acyclovir by high-flux hemodialysis.

EFFECT OF RENAL DYSFUNCTION ON METABOLISM

CASE 31-3, QUESTION 2: Does D.M.'s renal dysfunction affect the metabolism of acyclovir? Are there other drugs that are affected similarly?

Approximately 20% of acyclovir is cleared by nonrenal mechanisms.[19,65] The only significant metabolite that has been isolated is 9-carboxymethoxymethylguanine, which accounts for 9% to 14% of an administered dose. It is believed that this metabolite is a product of hepatic metabolism; however, the kidney may also play an important role.[19] Whether renal dysfunction alters hepatic metabolism or metabolic enzymes are present within the kidney is unclear. Renal tissue contains many of the same metabolic enzymes found in the liver. Mixed-function oxidases have been found in segments of the proximal tubule, whereas other metabolic processes, such as glucuronidation, acetylation, and hydrolysis, also occur within the kidney.[17,18,68]

Renal failure can affect hepatic metabolic enzyme activity and drug transporter function.[69,70] Most of these investigations were carried out in animals that had diminished microsomal, mitochondrial, and cytosolic enzyme activities. Renal dysfunction substantially alters the nonrenal clearance of certain antibiotics, such as ceftizoxime, cefotaxime, and imipenem,[71–74] as well as the benzodiazepines, diazepam and desmethyldiazepam.[75,76]

Tenofovir

CASE 31-3, QUESTION 3: D.M. also is being treated with tenofovir as part of antiretroviral regimen for his HIV disease. Will his tenofovir doses need to be adjusted?

DOSAGE ADJUSTMENT

Tenofovir is a nucleotide analog of adenosine monophosphate. Tenofovir undergoes activation by phosphorylation to the active form, tenofovir diphosphate. Tenofovir diphosphate inactivates HIV reverse transcriptase and HBV DNA polymerase by causing chain termination.[77] It is used as part of an antiretroviral regimen in the treatment of HIV infection and can also be used for the treatment of chronic hepatitis B infection.[78] Approximately 70% to 80% of tenofovir is excreted unchanged in the urine. The elimination half-life is approximately 17 hours, and the clearance is significantly reduced in the setting of renal dysfunction. Nephrotoxicity, including cases of acute renal failure and Fanconi syndrome (renal tubular injury and hypophosphatemia) have been reported. Organic transporters in the proximal tubule are believed to mediate nephrotoxicity.[79] The dose of tenofovir must be adjusted in the setting of kidney dysfunction to prevent accumulation, and the potential to worsen renal dysfunction. Tenofovir is also available in combination with other antiretrovirals in a single dose formulation for the treatment of HIV infection. The specific dosing recommendation should be consulted in the setting of renal dysfunction for tenofovir or the combination products.

HEMODIALYSIS

CASE 31-3, QUESTION 4: Is tenofovir significantly removed by dialysis?

Tenofovir is effectively removed by hemodialysis, with an extraction coefficient of approximately 54%. Approximately 10% of a 300 mg tenofovir dose is removed after 4 hours of hemodialysis. The recommended dose of tenofovir is 300 mg orally every 7 days (after approximately 12 hours of hemodialysis or three 4-hour dialysis sessions).[78,80]

Penicillin

DOSAGE ADJUSTMENT

CASE 31-4

QUESTION 1: T.H., a 57-year-old, 85-kg man with chronic kidney disease secondary to poorly controlled hypertension, presents to the ED with a 24-hour history of fever (39°C), altered mental status, nausea, and vomiting. On physical examination he is found to have nuchal rigidity and a positive Brudziński sign. Laboratory analysis reveals the following:

WBC count, 22,000/μL with 89% neutrophils
BUN, 45 mg/dL
SCr, 4.4 mg/dL

A lumbar puncture yields cerebrospinal fluid (CSF) with a WBC count of 2,000/μL (90% polymorphonuclear neutrophils), a glucose concentration of 36 mg/dL, and a protein concentration of 280 mg/dL. Gram-positive diplococci are seen on CSF smear. A diagnosis of meningococcal meningitis is made, and potassium penicillin G is ordered. What dose should be used?

Meningococcal meningitis can be treated with 20 to 24 million units of IV penicillin G in patients with normal renal function. As with many β-lactam antibiotics, penicillin is primarily excreted unchanged in the urine with little or no hepatic metabolism. Thus, the elimination half-life, which averages less than 1 hour in patients with normal kidney function, increases to 4 to 10 hours in patients with ESRD.[81–83]

Methods to modify the dose of penicillin in renal insufficiency have been developed by numerous investigators. The clearance of penicillin correlates closely with CrCl according to the following equation[83]:

$$Cl_{pen} \text{ in mL/minute} = 35.5 + 3.35 \text{ CrCl in mL/minute} \qquad \text{(Eq. 31-26)}$$

This correlation is based on data from patients with varying degrees of renal impairment.

An equation to estimate the total daily dose for patients with renal failure to achieve serum levels similar to those produced by high-dose penicillin (20–24 million units/day) in patients with normal renal function has been developed for patients with an estimated CrCl of less than 40 mL/minute. The dose for T.H. should be given in equal divided doses at 6- or 8-hour intervals:

$$Dose_{pen} \text{ in million units/day} = 3.2 + (\text{CrCl}/7) \qquad \text{(Eq. 31-27)}$$

Using the Cockcroft–Gault method, T.H.'s CrCl is approximately 20 mL/minute. Therefore, his daily dose of penicillin should be 6 million units. A dose of 1 million units every 4 hours would be appropriate for T.H. Penicillin G is often given as the potassium salt (penicillin G potassium), which contains approximately 1.7 mEq of potassium per 1 million units of penicillin. Accumulation of potassium due to renal impairment may lead to hyperkalemia. Penicillin G sodium is an alternative formulation that would be appropriate.

As is true for many agents, these dosing recommendations are empiric and based on pharmacokinetic principles for patients in renal failure. These recommendations have not been subjected to carefully designed clinical trials that establish therapeutic efficacy. Therefore, other factors that can influence host response also should be considered when designing an individualized therapeutic regimen. These include the host's immune status, the presence of other medical conditions, microbial sensitivity patterns, and changes in pharmacokinetic disposition (e.g., concomitant liver disease, fluid overload, dehydration).

PENICILLIN-INDUCED NEUROTOXICITY

CASE 31-4, QUESTION 2: The prescriber fails to consider T.H.'s renal dysfunction when he orders penicillin, and begins a dose of 4 million units every 4 hours. Four days later, T.H. is encephalopathic (confused, disoriented, and difficult to arouse), with some twitching noted on the right side of his face. Are these toxic symptoms associated with high-dose penicillin? What predisposing factors may contribute to this neurotoxicity?

T.H. is experiencing signs of neurotoxicity that are consistent with elevated penicillin concentrations in the plasma and CSF. Penicillin usually produces few serious adverse effects. When large doses are used in patients with renal impairment, toxic symptoms such as those exhibited by T.H. can result. Signs and symptoms of penicillin-induced CNS toxicity include myoclonus, complex or generalized seizure activity, and encephalopathy progressing to coma.[39,40]

Predisposing Factors

T.H.'s renal dysfunction predisposes him to penicillin-induced neurotoxicity. In a review of 46 cases of penicillin-associated neurotoxicity, decreased renal function was present in 35 patients.[40] Several possible explanations for this observation exist. Penicillin accumulates in patients with renal failure. The binding of acidic drugs (such as penicillin) to albumin is decreased, resulting in an increased fraction of free or active drug that can pass into the CSF. Alterations in the blood–brain barrier have been observed in uremic patients, which can lead to further increases in CSF drug levels.[39] High plasma concentrations of penicillin per se may contribute to changes in the blood–brain barrier permeability of this drug.[39] All these factors, together with the increased sensitivity of patients with renal failure to centrally acting agents, make CNS toxicity more likely. Previous neurotrauma, history of seizures, elderly age, and concurrent drugs that lower the seizure threshold can also contribute to neurotoxicity. As with penicillin, the carbapenem antibiotic combination, imipenem–cilastatin, is associated with a higher incidence of seizures in patients with renal dysfunction.[84,85] Other β-lactam antibiotics such as ceftazidime, cefepime, and piperacillin/tazobactam have also been associated with seizures.[86,87]

Antipseudomonal Penicillins

PIPERACILLIN

CASE 31-5

QUESTION 1: M.H., a 44-year-old, 70-kg woman with acute nonlymphocytic leukemia, was admitted to the oncology ward for placement of a Hickman catheter for her chemotherapy. Seven days after treatment with cytarabine and daunorubicin, her temperature spiked to 39.4°C. Other physical findings consistent with sepsis included a blood pressure of 102/68 mm Hg, pulse rate of 112 beats/minute, and a respiratory rate of 27 breaths/minute. M.H. is neutropenic with a WBC count of 1,400/μL (3% polymorphonuclear leukocytes, 70% lymphocytes, and 22% monocytes). Her platelet count is 16,000/μL. M.H. also has renal dysfunction as reflected by an SCr and BUN of 2.6 and 38 mg/dL, respectively. Empiric therapy for sepsis is started with tobramycin, piperacillin/tazobactam, and vancomycin. How should piperacillin/tazobactam be dosed in M.H.?

Piperacillin is an antipseudomonal penicillin that is often used with an aminoglycoside to treat serious infections caused by gram-negative organisms.[88] Piperacillin is commonly given as a combination with tazobactam, a β-lactamase inhibitor.[89] In patients with normal renal function, piperacillin is primarily excreted unchanged by the kidney with a clearance of 2.6 mL/minute/kg, and a half-life of approximately 1 hour.[90,91] Doses of piperacillin/tazobactam can be as high as 4.5 g every 6 hours for the treatment of serious *Pseudomonas* species infections. In patients with ESRD, mean piperacillin clearance and half-life values are 0.7 mL/minute/kg and 3.3 hours, respectively.[90–92] Although these parameters are significantly different, they are less than those expected for a drug primarily cleared by the kidneys, suggesting that some other compensatory mechanism for elimination must be present. Piperacillin is partially cleared by biliary excretion, a route of elimination that is increased in patients with renal failure.[92,93] Therefore, aggressive dosage reductions in M.H. are unnecessary. An appropriate dose of piperacillin/tazobactam for M.H. would be 3.375 g every 8 hours. Widely used drug references such as Facts and Comparisons can be used for dosing guidelines for drugs commonly used in patients with renal failure.[45]

Vancomycin

PHARMACOKINETIC DOSAGE CALCULATIONS

CASE 31-5, QUESTION 2: In addition to the aforementioned regimen for M.H., vancomycin therapy is initiated at 500 mg every 24 hours to cover the possibility of an infection resistant to antistaphylococcal penicillins, such as nafcillin. Is this an appropriate dosing regimen for M.H.?

Vancomycin is a bactericidal antibiotic with excellent activity against most gram-positive organisms such as methicillin-resistant *Staphylococcus aureus* and *Streptococcus* species, including some isolates of *Enterococcus* species. It is used empirically in febrile neutropenic patients because the incidence of infection secondary to resistant organisms is much greater in this patient population. However, cases of vancomycin-resistant enterococci have emerged at rates as high as 50%, raising concern and reducing its empiric use.[94]

Vancomycin is poorly absorbed by the oral route and must be administered IV when used to treat systemic infections. As with many other antibiotics, vancomycin primarily is cleared by the kidneys.[95] Significant toxicities have been associated with elevated serum concentrations, making careful dosing modification in renal failure necessary.[96]

As with the aminoglycosides, pharmacokinetic calculations can be used to individualize a dosing regimen to produce the desired peak and trough plasma levels. Unlike the aminoglycosides, the therapeutic range for vancomycin is less clear. Normally, doses are designed to achieve peak levels of 25 to 40 mg/L and trough levels of 10 to 15 mg/L.[97,98] The correlation between vancomycin toxicity (e.g., ototoxicity) and plasma levels is not well defined. Some clinicians have suggested, however, that plasma levels of 80 mg/L or more may correlate with auditory dysfunction.

Vancomycin has an elimination half-life of 3 to 9 hours in patients with normal renal function.[99] This increases to 129 to 189 hours in patients with ESRD.[100–102] Using pharmacokinetic principles and considering that the plasma clearance of vancomycin is approximately 60% to 70% of CrCl[97] and the Vd averages 0.7 L/kg,[97,99,103] the estimated Vd_{vanco} and Cl_{vanco} can be calculated using the following equation:

$$Cr_{Cl} = 30.5 \text{ mL/minute (calculated from Eq. 31-5)}$$

$$\begin{aligned} Cl_{vanco} &= (0.65)(\text{CrCl}) \\ &= (0.65)(30.5 \text{ mL/minute}) \\ &= 19.8 \text{ mL/minute or rounded off to } 1.2 \text{ L/hour} \end{aligned} \quad \text{(Eq. 31-28)}$$

$$\begin{aligned} Vd_{vanco} &= (0.7 \text{ L/kg})(\text{body weight}) \\ &= (0.7 \text{ L/kg})(70 \text{ kg}) \\ &= 49 \text{ L} \end{aligned} \quad \text{(Eq. 31-29)}$$

Based on estimated values for Cl_{vanco} and Vd_{vanco}, the elimination rate constant can be calculated using the following equation:

$$\begin{aligned} Kd &= \frac{Cl_{vanco}}{Vd_{vanco}} \\ &= \frac{1.2 \text{ L/hour}}{49 \text{ L}} \\ &= 0.024 \text{ hour}^{-1} \end{aligned} \quad \text{(Eq. 31-30)}$$

$$Cp = \frac{\frac{Dose}{Vd_{vanco}}}{1 - e^{-Kdt}}$$

$$= \frac{\frac{500\ mg}{49\ L}}{1 - e^{-(0.024\ hour^{-1})(24\ hours)}} \quad (Eq.\ 31\text{-}31)$$

$$= 23\ mg/L$$

$$Cp_{trough} = Cp_{peak}(e^{-Kdt})$$

$$= 23\ mg/L\,(e^{-(0.024/hour^{-1})(24\ hours)}) \quad (Eq.\ 31\text{-}32)$$

$$= 13\ mg/L$$

Because M.H.'s estimated peak concentration is less than 40 mg/L and her trough falls within the range of 10 to 15 mg/L, the starting dose of 500 mg every 24 hours is appropriate for M.H.

Routine monitoring of plasma vancomycin concentrations in patients with normal renal function is controversial because the likelihood that toxicity will develop in this group is relatively low. However, in patients with renal failure, such as M.H., it is advisable to measure vancomycin levels several days after initiation of therapy to ensure that they are within an acceptable range.[99,101,102,104] This is prudent if an extended course of therapy is anticipated. Vancomycin is usually infused over the course of 60 minutes.

HEMODIALYSIS OF VANCOMYCIN

CASE 31-5, QUESTION 3: M.H.'s renal function begins to deteriorate to the point where she requires hemodialysis. How should her regimen now be altered?

Patients with ESRD may have measurable vancomycin levels for up to 3 weeks after a single dose despite conventional hemodialysis.[102] This suggests that the ability of these patients to eliminate vancomycin is minimal and that little of the drug is removed by conventional hemodialysis. The elimination half-life for vancomycin in these individuals averages 5 to 7 days, which is consistent with a residual vancomycin clearance of 3 to 4 mL/minute.[100–102] Only about 5% of vancomycin is metabolized hepatically in patients with normal renal function.

Conventional hemodialysis removes about 7% of vancomycin during a typical 4-hour dialysis run.[105] The elimination half-life on and off dialysis and plasma levels of the drug before and after hemodialysis do not differ significantly. The poor removal of vancomycin by conventional hemodialysis is attributable to its large MW of 1,400.

Patients receiving conventional hemodialysis are typically given a single, 1-g dose every 7 to 10 days.[99,102,104] Based on M.H.'s estimated Vd of 49 L, this dose will produce an initial peak plasma level of approximately 20 mg/L. If vancomycin is administered weekly, steady-state peak and trough levels of 40 and 16 mg/L, respectively, would be predicted.

Vancomycin is removed to a greater extent by high-flux hemodialysis than by conventional hemodialysis. As a result, more frequent dosing is necessary to maintain therapeutic vancomycin concentrations. High-flux dialysis clearance of vancomycin using the Fresenius polysulfone dialyzer is 45 to 160 mL/minute and varies with membrane surface area.[60,106] Up to 50% of a dose of vancomycin is removed in 4 hours by high-flux hemodialysis compared with 6.9% using conventional dialysis. A rebound phenomenon after dialysis suggests that the total amount of drug removed may be less than initially reported.[107,108] In any case, the efficiency of high-flux procedures in removing vancomycin is greater than that of conventional dialysis. Therefore, plasma levels should be monitored carefully in these patients, and the necessity for postdialysis replacement doses of around 500 mg (~10–15 mg/kg) should be anticipated.

Caspofungin

DOSING

CASE 31-5, QUESTION 4: M.H. continues to be febrile despite her triple antimicrobial regimen. Caspofungin is started empirically for potential fungal infections. In addition, pentamidine is begun to cover *Pneumocystis jirovecii* pneumonia. How should caspofungin be administered in patients such as M.H. with renal dysfunction?

HEMODIALYSIS OF CASPOFUNGIN

Caspofungin is an echinocandin antifungal agent that is slowly metabolized by hydrolysis and N-acetylation, with little being excreted unchanged in the urine.[109] Caspofungin is not removed significantly by hemodialysis or continuous hemofiltration. No dosage adjustment is necessary in patients with renal failure or on renal replacement therapy.[110] The maintenance dose needs to be reduced in the setting of moderate liver failure however.

CASE 31-5, QUESTION 5: What factors need to be considered when other antifungal agents are used in patients with kidney disease?

Amphotericin B is a polyene antifungal agent that has activity against a wide variety of fungi. Amphotericin B is extensively distributed into the peripheral tissue, and has a long elimination half-life of approximately 15 days.[111,112] There is no significant change in the disposition of amphotericin B in patients with liver or kidney disease. The utility of amphotericin B has been limited due to its nephrotoxicity.[113] Lipid-based formulations are associated with a lower incidence of nephrotoxicity and other systemic side effects.[114] Triazole antifungal agents (e.g., fluconazole, posaconazole, voriconazole) or an echinocandin class (e.g., anidulafungin, caspofungin, micafungin) are alternative choices that are not potentially nephrotoxic, nor do they need to be dose adjusted in the setting of renal dysfunction (with the exception of fluconazole). The oral as opposed to the IV formulation of voriconazole and posaconazole should be used in the setting of renal dysfunction or for patients with a CrCl of less than 50 mL/minute to prevent accumulation of sulfobutyl ether β-cyclodextrin, the solvent vehicle found in the IV formulation.[115]

Cefazolin

PERITONEAL DIALYSIS

CASE 31-6

QUESTION 1: M.J. is a 65-year-old woman with chronic kidney disease awaiting a kidney transplant. She has been managed with PD for the past 8 years. She presents with a cloudy effluent and abdominal pain. Analysis of the effluent reveals a WBC count of 323/μL and gram-positive cocci and clusters on Gram stain. The patient has a history of *S. aureus* peritonitis that was readily treated with cefazolin previously. The patient has no allergies, and weighs 52 kg. How should M.J.'s PD-related infection be managed?

Gram-positive cocci such as *S. aureus* are common causes of PD-related infections. The selection of empiric antibiotics should be made based on the patient's and program's history of microorganisms and sensitivities. A first-generation cephalosporin such as cefazolin would be a reasonable choice for M.J. Programs with a high rate of methicillin-resistant organisms should use vancomycin.

IP antibiotics can be given with each exchange (continuous dosing). In this situation, a single 500-mg/L loading dose of cefazolin is given followed by a maintenance dose of 125 mg/L with subsequent exchanges. Antibiotics can also be given intermittently (once daily per exchange). With intermittent dosing, the antibiotic-containing dialysis solution should dwell for at least 6 hours to allow for adequate absorption. Cefazolin 15 mg/kg (rounded off to 750 mg) is typically given in one exchange. For patients on automated PD, the dose of cefazolin is 20 mg/kg every day in a long-day dwell. For patients with residual renal function (e.g., >100 mL/day of urine output), empirically, the dose is increased by 25%. The management of PD-related infections and dosing of various antibiotics is discussed in the International Society for Peritoneal Dialysis guidelines.[116]

Phenytoin

PROTEIN BINDING

CASE 31-7

QUESTION 1: R.S., a 24-year-old man with ESRD from rapidly progressive glomerulonephritis, is treated by hemodialysis 3 times weekly. He has a 7-year history of generalized tonic–clonic seizures and has been treated with phenytoin. He presents to the ED after having had a seizure lasting about 5 minutes. His mother states that he ran out of phenytoin 4 weeks ago. Because his plasma phenytoin concentration on admission was less than 2.5 mg/L, R.S. is given an IV loading dose of fosphenytoin: 15 mg/kg in 30 minutes. Additional admission laboratory work includes the following:

SCr, 8.6 mg/dL
BUN, 110 mg/dL
Potassium, 5.4 mEq/L
Calcium, 9 mg/dL
Albumin, 2.9 g/dL

Eight hours after administration, his phenytoin level is 5 mg/L. Is this level subtherapeutic?

R.S. has severe renal disease, which will affect the total (bound plus free) phenytoin concentration achieved and how this concentration is interpreted. Decreased plasma protein binding will result in lower measured total phenytoin concentrations, and the calculated apparent Vd may increase. In patients with normal renal function, approximately 90% of the measured phenytoin is bound to albumin, and 10% is free. The free fraction of phenytoin is increased to about 20% to 25% in patients with uremia.[11,117–121] Because the free fraction for phenytoin is increased in patients with uremia, lower plasma concentrations will produce therapeutic effects that will be equivalent to those produced by higher phenytoin concentrations in patients with normal renal function.[8,122] Phenytoin is an acidic drug that is bound primarily to albumin. A number of mechanisms have been proposed that account for the decreased binding, including (a) decreased albumin concentration, (b) accumulation of uremic by-products that displace acidic drugs from their binding sites, and (c) alteration in the conformation or structure of albumin in uremic patients, resulting in a reduced number of binding sites or decreased affinity for drugs (see Chapter 60, Seizure Disorders). Other acidic drugs with altered protein binding in renal disease are listed in Table 31-1.

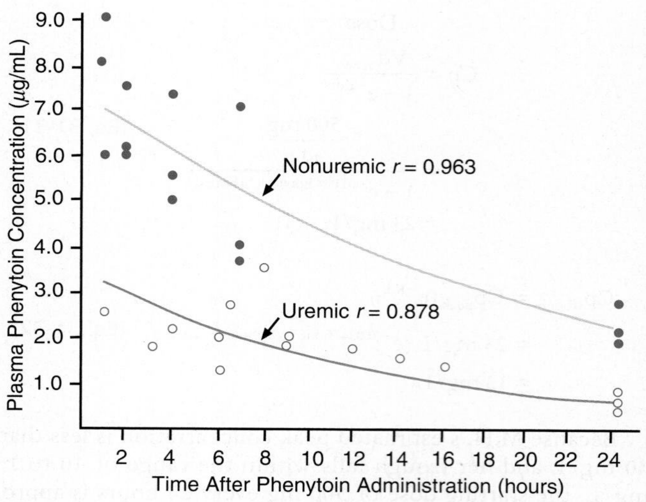

Figure 31-2 Plasma phenytoin concentrations in uremic (∘) and nonuremic (•) patients after 250 mg of intravenous (IV) phenytoin. (Reprinted with permission from Letteri JM et al. Diphenylhydantoin metabolism in uremia. *N Engl J Med*. 1971;285:648. Copyright © 2001 Massachusetts Medical Society. All rights reserved.)

Figure 31-2 illustrates changes in phenytoin levels when uremic and nonuremic patients are given equivalent doses.[123]

The following equation should be used to correct for R.S.'s altered binding owing to his renal dysfunction and hypoalbuminemia[120]:

$$Cp_{\text{Normal Binding}} = \frac{Cp'}{(0.48)(1-\alpha)\left(\frac{P'}{P_{NL}}\right)+\alpha} \qquad \text{(Eq. 31-33)}$$

where Cp′ is the measured plasma concentration reported by the laboratory, and $Cp_{\text{Normal Binding}}$ is the corrected plasma concentration that would be seen if the patient had normal renal function and normal albumin. Alpha (α) is the normal free fraction (0.1), P′ is the patient's serum albumin, and P_{NL} is normal albumin (4.4 g/dL). The factor 0.48 was derived from patients on hemodialysis and represents the decreased affinity of phenytoin for albumin.

For R.S., a total plasma phenytoin concentration of 5 mg/L is comparable to 13 mg/L in a patient without renal failure. Because this falls within the phenytoin's therapeutic range of 10 to 20 mg/L, his measured level is not subtherapeutic.

The factor 0.48 should be used only to estimate changes in protein binding for patients with ESRD receiving hemodialysis. Data for patients with moderate renal disease are limited, and it is unclear what changes exist in the binding of phenytoin to albumin.[118] For patients with normal or moderate renal impairment, the following equation should be used only if the serum albumin is low; the factor 0.48 should be omitted:

$$Cp_{\text{Normal Binding}} = \frac{Cp'}{(1-\alpha)\left(\frac{P'}{P_{NL}}\right)+\alpha} \qquad \text{(Eq. 31-34)}$$

Fosphenytoin, a prodrug of phenytoin, does not need to be dissolved in propylene glycol, and therefore can be administered more quickly. This offers an important advantage for seizures that must be controlled quickly. In patients with renal failure, the conversion of fosphenytoin to phenytoin was equally efficient in patients with renal disease and healthy subjects.[124] Once fosphenytoin is converted to phenytoin, the impact of renal disease on protein binding is expected to be similar to that seen with phenytoin and thus the same considerations should be made for patients with renal failure.

EFFECT OF RENAL FAILURE ON METABOLIZED DRUGS

Meperidine

CASE 31-8

QUESTION 1: F.G., a 56-year-old woman, is admitted for a cervical laminectomy. She has a history of chronic kidney disease (CrCl 20 mL/minute) and arrhythmias that are treated with amiodarone. Her admission laboratory values are as follows:

SCr, 4.4 mg/dL
BUN, 66 mg/dL
Hematocrit, 34%
Hemoglobin, 12.6 g/dL

After surgery, she complains of severe pain and is treated with meperidine 50 to 100 mg intramuscularly every 3 to 4 hours. Three days postoperatively, F.G. experiences a generalized tonic–clonic seizure. She has no history of seizures. What might be responsible for this sudden event?

Meperidine is a narcotic analgesic commonly used to control acute pain. It is metabolized hepatically via *N*-demethylation to normeperidine, a metabolite known to accumulate in renal insufficiency.[15,125] Although meperidine has both CNS excitatory and depressant properties, normeperidine is a very potent CNS stimulant that can cause seizures in patients with renal failure who are receiving multiple doses of the parent drug.[126] Patients with renal dysfunction given merperidine experience more neurologic effects.[126] Because the renal clearance of normeperidine correlates significantly with CrCl, renal dysfunction can lead to its accumulation, resulting in neurologic toxicity. The normeperidine to meperidine plasma concentration ratio was consistently higher in patients with renal failure, averaging 2.0 compared with a mean of 0.6 for patients with good renal function.[126] Table 31-3 lists examples of additional drugs that have active or toxic metabolites that may accumulate in renal disease.

Table 31-3
Drugs with Active or Toxic Metabolites Excreted by the Kidney

Drug	Metabolite
Acetohexamide	Hydroxyhexamide
Allopurinol	Oxypurinol
Bupropion	Threo/erythro-hydrobupropion
Cefotaxime	Desacetylcefotaxime
Chlorpropamide	Hydroxy metabolites
Clofibrate	Chlorphenoxyisobutyrate
Cyclophosphamide	4-Ketocyclophosphamide
Daunorubicin	Daunorubicinol
Meperidine	Normeperidine
Methyldopa	Methyl-*O*-sulfate-α-methyldopamine
Midazolam	α-Hydroxymidazolam
Morphine	Morphine-3-glucuronide
	Morphine-6-glucuronide
Phenylbutazone	Oxyphenbutazone
Primidone	Phenobarbital
Procainamide	*N*-acetylprocainamide (NAPA)
Propoxyphene	Norpropoxyphene
Rifampicin	Deacetylated metabolites
Sodium nitroprusside	Thiocyanate
Sulfonamides	Acetylated metabolites
Tramadol	*O*-Demethyl-*N*-demethyltramadol

Narcotic Analgesics

CASE 31-8, QUESTION 2: Are the pharmacokinetics or pharmacodynamics of other narcotic analgesics altered in patients with renal insufficiency?

MORPHINE

The pharmacokinetic disposition of morphine does not appear to be altered in patients with renal failure[127]; however, its active metabolite, morphine-6-glucuronide, as well as its principal metabolite, morphine-3-glucuronide, do accumulate in renal disease. The elimination half-life of morphine-6-glucuronide increases from 3 to 4 hours in normal subjects to 89 to 136 hours in subjects with renal failure.[128] This metabolite penetrates the blood–brain barrier more readily, has a greater affinity for CNS receptors, and has analgesic activity that is 3.7 times greater than morphine.[129] Therefore, accumulation of morphine-6-glucuronide may be responsible for the morphine-induced narcosis reported in patients with severe renal disease.[32,33]

CODEINE

Other analgesics that have been associated with CNS toxicity in patients with renal failure include codeine, propoxyphene, and dihydrocodeine.[125] The disposition of orally administered codeine does not appear to be altered in renal failure; however, there have been case reports of codeine-induced narcosis.[130] Although the dose of codeine did not exceed 120 mg/day, CNS and respiratory depression persisted for up to 4 days after discontinuing codeine and initiating naloxone administration. The elimination half-life of codeine is prolonged in patients on chronic hemodialysis. Although the Vd of codeine was twice as large, the total clearance was not significantly decreased.[131] A lower initial dose should be used because codeine is metabolized to morphine.

HYDROMORPHONE

Hydromorphone is metabolized in the liver to hydromorphone-3-glucuronide, dihydroisomorphone, dihydromorphine, and small amounts of hydromorphone-3-sulfate, norhydromorphone, and nordihydroisomorphone.[132] All metabolites that are eliminated are excreted by the kidneys. Hydromorphone can be used in patients with renal failure; however, smaller initial doses may be warranted.[131]

Enoxaparin

CASE 31-8, QUESTION 3: Because F.G. is not ambulating well after her surgery, her physician would like to initiate deep vein thrombosis prophylaxis with enoxaparin. Are there any dosing considerations for enoxaparin in this patient?

Enoxaparin is a low MW heparin that is used to prevent and treat various thromboembolic disorders, such as deep venous thrombosis, unstable angina, and non–Q wave myocardial infarction. The kidneys play a major role in the clearance of enoxaparin,[133] and a higher incidence of bleeding complications is associated with the use of enoxaparin in patients with renal dysfunction.[134] The elimination half-life of enoxaparin is prolonged in patients with ESRD, although the other pharmacokinetic parameters are similar to those in healthy subjects.[135,136] The increased incidence of bleeding complications cannot be completely attributed to pharmacokinetic changes, but may also be related to the effects of enoxaparin on antifactor IIa and antithrombin III, as well as the effects of uremia on hemostasis.[137]

Enoxaparin should be used cautiously in patients with a CrCl less than 30 mL/minute, with a recommended lower dosage of 30 mg subcutaneously daily. Although monitoring of the anticoagulant effect by anti-Xa activity is not necessary in clinically stable patients, it may be warranted in patients with renal dysfunction as well as in those who have other factors that may increase the risk of bleeding complications.

ASSESSING RENAL FUNCTION IN THE ELDERLY

Renal function declines physiologically with advancing age and as the result of comorbidities such as hypertension and diabetes.[138] This decrease in renal function can have significant consequences on drug excretion, metabolism, and the potential for adverse drug reactions, particularly in the elderly population that is often prescribed multiple medications.[139] Antithrombotic and antidiabetic drugs are high-risk medications that are often implicated as a cause for hospitalizations due to adverse drug events in elderly patients.[140] Sulfonylurea antidiabetic agents such as glyburide that are eliminated primarily by the kidneys can lead to prolonged hypoglycemia in patients with decreased renal function.[141] In addition, metformin should be used with caution in patients with kidney dysfunction due to the increased risk for lactic acidosis.

Formulas that estimate renal function use the serum creatinine. In elderly adults, a low serum creatinine may not always be indicative of normal renal function. Older adults tend to have lower muscle mass than younger people, and a low serum creatinine may not be indicative of normal renal function, but rather reduced muscle mass. Differences in the estimated GFR between the MDRD and Cockcroft–Gault formulas may result in discordant dosing recommendations in an elderly population.[142]

This highlights the importance of obtaining a comprehensive medication history, assessment of the patient's renal function, and evaluation of the available drug-information resources for appropriate dosing recommendations for each patient.

SUMMARY

The kidneys play a vital role in maintaining homeostasis by regulating the excretion of water, electrolytes, and metabolic by-products. In addition, the kidneys are the primary route of elimination for many drugs. Pharmacokinetic changes, such as altered bioavailability, protein binding, drug distribution, and elimination, can occur with many drugs in patients with renal failure. Pharmacodynamic changes, such as altered sensitivity or response to medications, can also occur in this patient population. Renal replacement therapies, such as hemodialysis, CAPD, and CVVH, will aid in the removal of fluid, electrolytes, and metabolic by-products in drugs as well. Data from clinical trials provide valuable information about the disposition of drugs in patients with renal failure. Pharmacokinetic principles should be applied when appropriate to determine the optimal dose of drugs for patients with renal failure.

KEY REFERENCES AND WEBSITES

A full list of references for this chapter can be found at http://thepoint.lww.com/AT11e. Below are the key references and websites for this chapter, with the corresponding reference number in this chapter found in parentheses after the reference.

Key References

Aronoff GR et al. *Drug Prescribing in Renal Failure: Dosing Guidelines for Adults and Children*. 5th ed. Philadelphia, PA: American College of Physicians; 2007. (49)

Daugirdas JT et al. *Handbook of Dialysis*. 5th ed. Philadelphia, PA: Wolters Kluwer; 2015.

Guidance for industry. Pharmacokinetics in patients with impaired renal function-Study design, data analysis, and impact on dosing and labeling. http://www.fda.gov/downloads/Drugs/Guidances/UCM204959.pdf.

Winter ME. Basic Clinical Pharmacokinetics. 5th ed. Baltimore, MD: Lippincott Williams & Wilkins; 2010.

Key Websites

Cockroft-Gault Calculator. http://www.nephron.com/cgi-bin/CGSI.cgi.
MDRD calculator. http://touchcalc.com/e_gfr.
National Kidney Disease Education Program. http://nkdep.nih.gov/.
2014 Dialysis of Drugs. http://www.renalpharmacyconsultants.com/publications/.

Section Editor: Steven Gabardi

32 Drug Hypersensitivity Reactions

Greene Shepherd and Justinne Guyton

CORE PRINCIPLES

		CHAPTER CASES
1	Drug allergies are a subset of adverse drug reactions that are usually mediated by the immune system. Although typically unpredictable, there are several factors known to influence the frequency of allergic reactions including age, sex, genetics, prior drug exposure, and drug dose and route. A detailed drug history is key to assisting in the diagnosis of a drug allergy.	**Case 32-1 (Questions 1, 2)** **Table 32-1**
2	Skin testing for allergy to penicillin is an important diagnostic tool that assists in determining whether or not a patient is truly allergic to this class of drug. Patients presenting with a history of penicillin allergy but who have a negative penicillin scratch test and a negative intradermal test can be safely given β-lactam antibiotics.	**Case 32-1 (Question 3)** **Table 32-4**
3	There are varying degrees of cross-reactivity between various β-lactam antibiotics. Understanding the frequency of cross-reactivity is important in making treatment decisions if skin testing is not available. The frequency of cross-reaction between penicillins and cephalosporins has been reported to be 5% to 15%, but it is likely much lower. The risk of a cephalosporin reaction in a patient with a penicillin allergy decreases with increasing cephalosporin generation, being lowest with the third- and fourth-generation drugs. The frequency of cross-reaction between penicillins and carbapenems or monobactams appears to be very low (approximately 1%).	**Case 32-1 (Question 4)**
	ANAPHYLAXIS	
1	Anaphylaxis is a serious allergic reaction that has a rapid onset and might cause death. It is caused by the rapid release of immune mediators from tissue mast cells and peripheral blood basophils. Symptoms such as pruritus of the hands, feet, and groin; flushing; light-headedness; hypotension; tachycardia; and difficulty breathing can begin within minutes of exposure to the precipitating agent, which is most commonly foods, insect stings, and drugs. Prompt recognition and treatment are critical to ensure a favorable outcome.	**Case 32-2 (Questions 1, 2)** **Table 32-2**
2	Epinephrine is the drug of choice for treatment of anaphylaxis and should be given immediately upon suspicion of an anaphylactic reaction. Epinephrine should be given intramuscularly into the lateral thigh as often as every 5 minutes to treat symptoms. Intramuscular injection is preferred over the subcutaneous and intravenous (IV) routes because of rapid absorption and ease of administration. The patient should be placed in the Trendelenburg position and second-line treatments including oxygen, IV fluids, and a nebulized β-agonist initiated as needed. Antihistamines and corticosteroids are also commonly used to treat anaphylaxis although there are no data showing an impact on outcome from these therapies.	**Case 32-2 (Question 3)** **Table 32-5**

Continued

	CHAPTER CASES
GENERALIZED REACTIONS	
1 Generalized hypersensitivity reactions can manifest in a number of ways including drug fever, serum sickness, hemolytic anemia, vasculitis, and autoimmune disorders. Specific organ systems such as the lungs, liver, kidneys, and hematopoietic system can also be the target of allergic drug reactions.	**Case 32-3 (Question 1), Case 32-4 (Questions 1, 2), Case 32-5 (Questions 1, 2) Tables 32-6, 32-7, 32-8**
PSEUDOALLERGIC REACTIONS	
1 Pseudoallergic reactions are drug reactions that exhibit clinical signs and symptoms of an allergic response but are not immunologically mediated. Pseudoallergic reactions can be relatively benign (such as red man syndrome from vancomycin) or potentially life-threatening, clinically resembling immune-mediated anaphylaxis as from radiocontrast media. Several drugs are associated with pseudoallergic reactions including aspirin and nonsteroidal anti-inflammatory drugs, opiates, angiotensin-converting enzyme inhibitors, and injectable iron products.	**Case 32-6 (Questions 1, 2, 5), Case 32-7 (Question 1) Tables 32-9**
2 The management of pseudoallergic reactions is the same as for true allergic reactions.	**Case 32-6 (Questions 3, 4), Case 32-7 (Question 2)**
PREVENTION AND MANAGEMENT OF ALLERGIC REACTIONS	
1 The keys to preventing an allergic reaction in a patient with history of allergy are a good description of the reaction and its causes, distinguishing between drug allergy and drug intolerance, and good documentation and communication of the reaction.	**Case 32-1 (Questions 1, 2), Case 32-8 (Question 1)**
2 In some cases, it is necessary to treat a patient with a drug to which they have a significant allergic reaction. To accomplish this, the process of tolerance induction (or desensitization) may be used. Tolerance induction starts with administration of a sub-allergenic dose of the drug to which a patient is allergic and the progressive administration of larger doses with the goal of modifying the patient's response. Once tolerance has been successfully induced, the patient must remain on the drug to maintain the state of tolerance. Tolerance induction should not be used in patients with a history of a severe non–IgE-mediated reaction such as hepatitis, hemolytic anemia, Stevens–Johnson syndrome, or toxic epidermal necrolysis.	**Case 32-9 (Questions 1, 2, 4)**
3 The oral route of tolerance induction is preferred over the IV route. Patients may experience a mild reaction during desensitization, although severe reactions are rare. Even after successful desensitization, patients may experience an allergic reaction during full dose therapy.	**Case 32-9 (Questions 2, 3)**
4 A graded drug challenge (also called test dosing) is a process of giving subtherapeutic doses of a drug to a patient to determine if they are allergic. A graded drug challenge generally uses larger starting doses than tolerance induction and involves fewer steps. Graded drug challenge may be appropriate in patients with a distant or unclear history of drug allergy, when the reaction seems minor or when diagnostic testing is unavailable, or in cases where cross-reactivity is expected to be low. Graded challenge should not be used in patients with a history of a severe non-IgE–mediated reaction such as hepatitis, hemolytic anemia, Stevens–Johnson syndrome, or toxic epidermal necrolysis.	**Case 32-9 (Question 1)**

Adverse drug reactions occur in up to 20% of hospitalized patients and up to 25% of ambulatory patients. Studies have found that up to 6% of all hospitalizations are caused by an adverse drug event. Immunologically mediated adverse drug reactions (also commonly referred to as drug allergy or hypersensitivity) account for about one-third of all adverse drug reactions and may affect 10% to 15% of hospitalized patients.[1–4] In one study of more than 36,000 hospitalized patients, 731 adverse events were identified, with 1% being severe, life-threatening, allergic reactions.[5] The potential morbidity and mortality associated with allergic drug reactions can be significant.

DEFINITION

Adverse drug reactions resembling an immune response are called drug hypersensitivity reactions (DHRs). True drug allergies show evidence of either drug-specific antibodies or T-cells.[1] Clinically, DHRs are commonly classified as immediate or delayed depending on their onset during treatment. Immediate reactions occur within a few hours of exposure and usually are mediated by IgE. Delayed reactions will occur a few days after starting therapy and are typically mediated by T-cells. See Table 32-1.

Chapter 32

Table 32-1
Immunologic Classification of Allergic Drug Reactions

Type	Type of Immune Response	Pathophysiology	Clinical Symptoms	Typical Chronology of the Reaction
I	IgE	Mast cell and basophil degranulation	Anaphylactic shock Angioedema Urticaria Bronchospasm	Within 1–6 hours after the last intake of the drug
II	IgG and complement	IgG and complement-dependent cytotoxicity	Cytopenia	5–15 days after the start of the eliciting drug
III	IgM or IgG and complement or FcR	Deposition of immune complexes	Serum sickness Urticaria Vasculitis	7–8 days for serum sickness/urticaria 7–21 days after the start of the eliciting drug for vasculitis
IVa	Th1 (IFN-γ)	Monocytic inflammation	Eczema	1–21 days after the start of the eliciting drug
IVb	Th2 (IL-4 and IL-5)	Eosinophilic inflammation	Maculopapular exanthema, DRESS	1 to several days after the start of the eliciting drug for MPE 2–6 weeks after the start of the eliciting drug for DRESS
IVc	Cytotoxic T-cells (perforin, granzyme B FasL)	Keratinocyte death mediated by CD4 or CD8	Maculopapular exanthema, pustular exanthema, Stevens-Johnson Syndrome (SJS)/TEN	1–2 days after the start of the eliciting drug for fixed drug eruption 4–28 days after the start of the eliciting drug for SJS/TEN
IVd	T-cells (IL-8/CXCL8)	Neutrophilic inflammation	Acute generalized exanthematous pustulosis	Typically 1–2 days after the start of the eliciting drug (but could be longer)

Source: Demoly P et al. International consensus on drug allergy. *Allergy*. 2014;69:420.

PATHOGENESIS

DHRs cannot be attributed to a single immunopathologic mechanism. Traditionally, an allergic drug reaction was thought to occur in two phases, initial sensitization and subsequent elicitation.[6] Most drugs are small molecules (<1,000 Da) and are unable to stimulate an immune response. Sensitization occurs as a result of covalent binding of a drug or a metabolite to a carrier protein in a process referred to as haptenation.[1,7] This drug–protein (or drug metabolite–protein) complex is sufficiently large to induce the production of drug-specific T- or B-lymphocytes and IgM, IgG, and IgE. On reexposure to the drug, the patient is likely to present with allergic symptoms.[7] Allergic reactions to β-lactam antibiotics occur by this mechanism. This theory, however, cannot explain several allergic phenomena. For instance, some chemically inert drugs (i.e., drugs that cannot form stable covalent bonds and do not have reactive metabolites) can still elicit an allergic response. Lidocaine and mepivacaine are examples. Furthermore, some patients have a strong allergic reaction to a drug on initial exposure, and some allergic reactions rapidly occur after drug exposure, a time period shorter than expected for the development of new antibodies. To account for some of these observations, other models for explaining allergic reactions have been proposed. The direct pharmacologic interaction concept offers one explanation for these observations. This model suggests that some drugs are able to bind directly to T-cell receptors in a reversible, non-covalent manner.[8] The drug–T-cell receptor complex interacts with Major Histocompatibility Complex (MHC) molecules, leading to activation and expansion of T-cells that are directed against the drug.[9]

Recent studies have demonstrated an additional mechanism whereby abacavir and carbamazepine can alter the shape and chemistry of the antigen-binding cleft via non-covalent interactions in patents with specific HLA variants. These alterations cause endogenous peptide to be viewed as foreign and lead to the activation of T-cells. This process is referred to as the altered repertoire model.[10,11] Undoubtedly, the processes involved in allergic reactions are complex and might include some combination of each theory. The three models of hapten sensitization, direct pharmacologic interaction, and altered repertoire are not mutually exclusive. Interested readers are referred to more in-depth reviews.[12]

PREDISPOSING FACTORS

Factors known to affect the incidence of allergic reactions can be categorized as being drug-related or patient-related.[3] Patients with histories of allergic rhinitis, asthma, or atopic dermatitis who experience a systemic drug reaction tend to react more severely than others.[3,13,14]

Age and Sex

Children are less likely to become sensitized than adults, presumably because children typically have less cumulative drug exposure.[1,13] More female than male patients experience allergic reactions (up to 2.3:1), although this may vary by type of reaction, drug, patient age, and setting.[3,14]

Genetic Factors

Familial occurrences of allergic reactions, although rare, have been reported.[15] A patient's ability to metabolize a drug is influenced by his or her genetic makeup and may affect the incidence of DHRs.[12,16–18] In humans the major histocompatibility complex is encoded by a group of genes on chromosome 6 called the human leucocyte antigen (HLA) system. Variations in HLA is probably the most important genetic determinant of drug allergies.[12]

Genetic differences in drug metabolizing enzymes can explain the predisposition to drug allergy and hypersensitivity of some individuals.[12] Examples of the phenotypic expression of these polymorphisms include poor metabolizers (who possess nonfunctional alleles and have reduced metabolic activity) and ultrarapid metabolizers (who have multiple copies of functional genes and have enhanced metabolic activity).[18,19]

Slow acetylators are at risk for sulfonamide hypersensitivity and are also more likely to develop antinuclear antibodies (ANA) and symptoms of systemic lupus erythematosus (SLE) when treated with procainamide or hydralazine.[20] Anticonvulsant hypersensitivity syndrome, characterized by fever, generalized rash, lymphadenopathy, and internal organ involvement, is most associated with aromatic anticonvulsants (e.g., phenytoin, phenobarbital, and carbamazepine). Oxidation of these compounds by cytochrome P-450 enzymes results in arene oxides that are antigenic. Patients with a heritable deficiency in epoxide hydrolase cannot clear the formed antigen and are at increased risk of a drug sensitivity syndrome also known as DRESS (drug rash with eosinophilia and systemic symptoms).[21] A polymorphism might also be responsible for a serum sickness–like reaction to cefaclor.[19]

While polymorphism in drug metabolizing enzymes is responsible for some allergic reactions, variation in MHC appears to be more important.[12,16] HLA polymorphisms mostly map to the antigen-binding cleft, thereby diversifying the repertoire of peptide antigens selected by different HLA allotypes. Several important DHRs reactions are associated with specific HLA alleles.[12] For example, HLA-B*1502 is associated with increased risk (OR 17.6) of SJS with Carbamazepine (CBZ), phenytoin, and lamotrigine.[16] HLA-B*1502 occurs in 10% to 15% of individuals from southern China, Thailand, Malaysia, Indonesia, the Philippines, and Taiwan and has a prevalence rate of 2% to 4%, or higher, in other southern Asian groups, including Indians. It is uncommon in Japan and Korea (<1%) and in European Caucasians (0%–0.1%).[17]

The potentially life-threatening hypersensitivity syndrome seen with abacavir is strongly associated with the HLA-B*5701 haplotype.[12,22–25] HLA-B*5701 in patients predicted abacavir hypersensitivity 100% of the time, and its absence had a 97% negative predictive value.[25] This haplotype appears more commonly in white patients than in other ethnic groups and explains the predisposition of white patients to this severe reaction. Genetic screening of patients for this haplotype before initiating abacavir therapy has significantly reduced the occurrence of hypersensitivity reactions.[25] In the future, it is hoped that screening tests for HLA haplotypes associated with a variety of allergic reactions will become widely available.

A more comprehensive and up-to-date listing of alleles associated with immunologically mediated adverse drug reactions can be found at https://www.pharmgkb.org/.

Associated Illness

Although genes clearly play a role in hypersensitivity reactions, environmental factors (e.g., concomitant illness) also are implicated. For example, the incidence of maculopapular rash with ampicillin therapy is significantly higher in patients with Epstein–Barr virus infections (e.g., infectious mononucleosis), lymphocytic leukemia, or gout.[26] Infection with herpes virus or Epstein–Barr virus has also been linked to DRESS syndrome,[26] and the occurrence of reactions to trimethoprim–sulfamethoxazole in patients who are HIV-positive is about 10-fold higher than in the HIV-negative population.[22] Liver or kidney disease may alter the metabolism or elimination of reactive drug metabolites, increasing the risk of an allergic response.

Previous Drug Administration

A history of an allergic reaction to a drug being considered for treatment, or one that is immunochemically similar, is the most reliable risk factor for development of a subsequent allergic reaction.[1,26] A commonly encountered example is the patient with a history of a severe allergic reaction to penicillin, in whom all structurally related penicillin compounds should be avoided, and in whom the possibility of a hypersensitivity reaction should be considered when using other β-lactam antibiotics.[1,26]

Drug-Related Factors

The dose, frequency of exposure, and route of administration can influence the incidence of drug allergy. For example, penicillin-induced hemolytic anemia requires high and sustained drug concentrations.[27] In β-lactam antibiotic IgE sensitivity, frequent intermittent courses, rather than continuous therapy, are more likely to result in drug sensitization.[21] The route of administration is important in terms of the risk of both sensitization and allergic reaction in a previously sensitized person. Topical administration carries the greatest risk of sensitization, followed by subcutaneous, intramuscular (IM), and oral routes. The intravenous (IV) route is the least sensitizing route of administration.[28] However, in a patient who is already sensitized to a specific medication, the risk of an allergic reaction to that medication is greatest when it is given IV and least when given orally. This is thought to be a function of the rate of drug delivery.[28] Multiple drug therapy is associated with a greater risk of allergic reactions. This may be related to increased demands on metabolic pathways from multiple drugs, leading to the accumulation of reactive metabolites.[28]

Drugs as Allergens and Immunologic Classification

Although there are proposed changes to the nomenclature and classification of drug allergies,[29] the Gel and Coombs classification is the most common. In this system, allergic drug reactions can be classified into one of four types (Table 32-1).[1]

TYPE I: IMMEDIATE HYPERSENSITIVITY REACTIONS

Type I reactions are typically mediated by the immune globulin IgE. Initial exposure to an antigen results in production of specific IgE antibodies that are expressed on the surface of mast cells in the tissue and basophils in the blood. On reexposure, the antigen cross-links with two or more surface-bound IgE antibodies causing the release of several chemical mediators including histamine, tryptase, leukotrienes, prostaglandins, and cyotkines.[28]

A period of several weeks is required after initial exposure and sensitization before a type I reaction can be elicited; once sensitized, however, a type I response can be elicited within minutes as a result of existing antibodies. In addition, a type I reaction can occur on reexposure to small amounts of drug administered by any route.[28,30] Immune-mediated anaphylaxis is the classic example of a type I reaction. Reactions that clinically resemble anaphylaxis, but do not involve immunologic mediators (antibodies), are termed anaphylactoid or pseudoallergic reactions (see Case 32-6, Question 1).

TYPE II: CYTOTOXIC REACTIONS

Cytotoxic reactions involve the interaction of IgG or IgM and can occur by three different mechanisms (Table 32-1). Common clinical manifestations of cytotoxic reactions include hemolytic anemia, thrombocytopenia, and granulocytopenia. Penicillin-induced hemolytic anemia is the best-known example of a cytotoxic drug reaction. This reaction typically appears after 7 days of high-dose therapy.[27]

TYPE III: IMMUNE COMPLEX–MEDIATED REACTIONS

Immune complex–mediated reactions result from the formation of drug–antibody complexes in serum, which often deposit in blood vessel walls, resulting in activation of complement and endothelial cell injury.[30] Also referred to as serum sickness, these reactions typically manifest as fever, urticaria, arthralgia, and lymphadenopathy 7 to 21 days after exposure.[26,30]

TYPE IV: CELL-MEDIATED (DELAYED) REACTIONS

In cell-mediated (delayed) reactions, an antigen binds with sensitized T-cells. Contact dermatitis is the most common manifestation of cell-mediated reactions, although systemic reactions can occur. The variety of clinical manifestations of delayed hypersensitivity has been attributed to distinct patterns of cytokine release and effector-cell recruitment, based on the type of T-cells stimulated. Each pattern of cytokine release recruits specific effector cells, such as macrophages, neutrophils, or other T-cells, and is responsible for the unique clinical manifestations of the reaction. Based on this understanding, type IV reactions have been further subclassified as type IVa, type IVb, type IVc, and type IVd, corresponding to four unique patterns of T-cell and effector-cell involvement.[31]

An understanding of the immunologic mechanism can be helpful in the diagnosis and treatment of an allergic reaction; however, the exact immunologic mechanism is unknown for many allergic reactions to drugs.[26] In addition, patients often present with several symptoms characteristic of more than one of the reactions described herein. The use of many drugs concurrently also makes it difficult to identify the drug responsible for the reaction. Therefore, a careful drug history and diagnostic tests are often necessary for an appropriate diagnosis and treatment of a patient.

DIAGNOSIS

Distinctive Features of Allergic Reactions

The first step in the diagnosis of an allergic drug reaction is to recognize and differentiate it from other adverse drug reactions. This can be accomplished by having a good understanding of the distinctive features of allergic drug reactions (Table 32-2).[26]

CASE 32-1

QUESTION 1: J.A., a 73-year-old woman, is admitted with an infected decubitus ulcer. Cultures reveal *Staphylococcus aureus*, which is sensitive to oxacillin, cefazolin, and vancomycin. On questioning, J.A. reports having experienced a rash to penicillin in the past. Her current medications include oral docusate 100 mg twice daily, oral enalapril 5 mg every morning, oral prednisone 20 mg daily, and oral ibuprofen 800 mg 3 times daily. What information should be obtained to determine whether J.A.'s rash represents an allergic drug reaction?

The single most informative diagnostic procedure for allergic drug reactions is a detailed drug history (Table 32-3), which is helpful in obtaining the information necessary to determine whether a reaction represents a drug allergy and in identifying the culprit drug. In inquiring about prior allergic and medication encounters, it is important to document the drugs to which the patient has or has not previously reacted. This can alert the clinician about certain types of compounds to which the patient is likely to react. The acquired information allows the clinician to characterize the drug reaction and to appreciate how such a reaction might be manifested in the patient on exposure to the same, or an immunologically similar, compound in the future.

The temporal relationship between drugs and reactions is often the strongest piece of evidence implicating an allergic reaction to a particular agent. Drugs that the patient has received for long continuous periods before the onset of a reaction are less likely to be implicated than drugs that have been recently initiated or restarted.[26] Equally important is to determine when an adverse reaction has occurred. Many compounds have been reformulated over the years, resulting in removal of sensitizing

Table 32-2
Clinical Features of Allergic Drug Reactions

- Are unpredictable
- Occur only in susceptible individuals
- Have no correlation with known pharmacologic properties of the drug
- Require an induction period on primary exposure but not on readministration
- Can occur with doses far below therapeutic range
- Can affect most organs, but commonly involves the skin
- Most commonly manifests as an erythematous or maculopapular rash, but includes angioedema, serum sickness syndrome, anaphylaxis, and asthma
- Occur in a small proportion of the population (10%–15%)
- Disappear on cessation of therapy and reappear after readministration of a small dose of the suspected drug(s) of similar chemical structure
- Desensitization may be possible

Source: Schnyder B. Approach to the patient with drug allergy. *Immunol Allergy Clin North Am*. 2009;29:405; Demoly P et al. International consensus on drug allergy. *Allergy*. 2014;69:420.

Table 32-3
Detailed Drug History

- Name of the medication
- Route of administration
- Reason medication was prescribed
- Nature and severity of reaction
- Temporal relationships between drugs and reaction (dose, date initiated, duration, when during the course of treatment did the reaction occur)
- Prior allergy history
- When did the reaction occur (days to weeks vs. months to years)
- Similar reactions in family members
- Prior exposure to the same or structurally related medications
- Concurrent medications
- Management of the reaction (effect of drug discontinuation; therapies required to treat the reaction)
- Response to treatment
- Prior diagnostic testing or rechallenge
- Other medical problems (if any)

Source: Khan DA, Solensky R. Drug allergy. *J Allergy Clin Immunol*. 2010;125 (2 Suppl 2):S126; Celik G. Drug allergy. In: Adkinson NF, ed. *Middleton's Allergy: Principles and Practice*. 7th ed. St. Louis, MO: Mosby; 2008:1205.

impurities (e.g., penicillin and vancomycin). Therefore, it is possible that reexposure to the agent will not result in an adverse event. Inquiring about whether the patient has received the drug since the first episode by asking the patient about other brands or names of other drugs in the same class (e.g., amoxicillin and ampicillin) will assist in determining whether the patient is likely to react to the drug on reexposure. It is usually helpful to chart all the drugs the patient is currently taking, their dose, and start and stop dates of use. This can be compared with the onset and disappearance of the reaction.

CASE 32-1, QUESTION 2: On further questioning, J.A. reports having experienced an urticarial rash in the past when given ampicillin for a kidney infection approximately 2 years ago. The rash developed over her entire body less than a day after starting the antibiotic and disappeared 2 days after discontinuation. Her treatment course was completed with ciprofloxacin. She denies having had a viral infection at the time of the rash to ampicillin. She does not recall having experienced any adverse effects when she received penicillin before this reaction. No other recent changes in her treatment regimen were made before the occurrence of the rash. Why is it likely that J.A. is allergic to penicillin?

Several pieces of information in the drug history obtained from J.A. can be used to determine the likelihood of an allergic reaction to penicillin. J.A.'s rash appeared less than a day after initiation of ampicillin and other drugs had not been added; therefore, the rash probably was caused by ampicillin.

Another important method of identifying a potential drug-induced allergic reaction is to examine the patient's medication list to determine whether the patient is receiving an agent that commonly is implicated in causing the exhibited allergic manifestation. For example, amoxicillin and ampicillin are two of the top three drugs implicated in drug-induced rash.[27]

J.A. received penicillin previously without experiencing any adverse effects until an urticarial rash (a relatively common allergic manifestation) developed on subsequent exposure. This sequence of events follows the typical pattern of an allergic reaction. Allergic reactions commonly require an induction period to sensitize the person to the antigen; however, once sensitized, allergic symptoms typically occur immediately on reexposure.[26] Therefore, a prior exposure to the same or structurally related compounds needs to be documented.

Finally, it is important to evaluate other medical problems that can elicit or mimic a reaction resembling drug allergy (see the "Associated Illness" section). Rashes to ampicillin commonly occur in patients with concurrent Epstein–Barr virus infection.[32] J.A. denies having a viral infection at the time of her rash, thereby strengthening the case that the rash was likely a manifestation of an allergic reaction.

Skin Testing

CASE 32-1, QUESTION 3: Would skin testing for penicillin allergy be appropriate for J.A.?

Although J.A.'s medication history strongly suggests that she is allergic to penicillin, a skin test and a drug rechallenge would more firmly establish her drug allergy. Penicillin degrades to major determinants (95%) and minor determinants (5%). Penicilloyl, the primary metabolite of penicillin, is referred to as the major determinant. The other derivatives are referred to as minor determinants. Of these, the parent compound (penicillin), penicilloate, and penilloate are the minor determinants most associated with allergic reactions. The terms major determinant and minor determinant refer to the frequency of antibody formation to these antigenic penicillin metabolite–protein complexes. These terms do not describe the severity of the allergic reaction. Indeed, the major determinant is thought to be responsible for accelerated reactions, but not anaphylaxis. The minor determinants are responsible for anaphylaxis and immediate systemic reactions.

Skin testing with these determinants is used to identify which patients have IgE antibodies to penicillin and which do not. The skin-testing antigen for the major determinant of penicillin is commercially available as penicilloyl polylysine (PPL; Pre-Pen), which was recently reintroduced into the United States after several years of absence.[33] Skin testing using Pre-Pen is a safe and effective procedure (Table 32-4), with less than 1% of positive responders developing systemic reactions.[34] In those in whom a false-negative response occurred, reactions were mild after penicillin administration and, in most cases, did not require drug discontinuation.[26,34] Skin testing with PPL identifies 80% of patients allergic to penicillin. When PPL is supplemented with skin tests for the minor determinants of penicillin, 99.5% of penicillin-allergic patients can be identified.[26] Of the minor determinants, only penicillin G is available in the United States, although a minor determinant mixture is marketed in Europe and Australia.[35]

The negative predictive value of skin testing was demonstrated when 34 purportedly "penicillin-allergic patients" needed β-lactam antibiotics during hospitalization. Each subsequently tested negative to penicillin skin-testing and no allergic drug reactions occurred.[36]

Penicillin and its metabolites become antigenic when combined with proteins and can precipitate a hypersensitivity reaction in a patient on reexposure. In patients with a history of penicillin hypersensitivity, skin test reactivity is affected by the length of time since the allergic reaction and by the nature of the past reaction. Skin test positivity is greatest 6 to 12 months after a reaction and decreases with time. Skin test positivity in one study was found to be only 40% of patients with a history of anaphylaxis, 17% with urticaria, and 7% for maculopapular rashes.[37] Skin testing should not be performed in patients receiving antihistamines because they block the response to the antigen and can result in misinterpretation. In patients receiving antihistamines (i.e., H_1- or H_2-receptor antagonists) or when skin testing is not possible because of severe skin disease, in vitro assays to detect drug-specific IgE antibodies have been developed for the major and minor determinants of penicillin.

To determine whether skin testing is appropriate for J.A., the risks and benefits must be weighed. Because the time of the last reaction was approximately 2 years ago, J.A. may still retain some skin-test positivity if the previous reaction was truly an allergic response to ampicillin. Testing with PPL (major determinant) and penicillin G (minor determinant) could be useful in determining whether J.A. is likely to experience an urticarial or anaphylactic reaction to penicillin or its derivatives. That J.A. is currently receiving prednisone should not alter the interpretation of the skin test results because the corticosteroids minimally affect the IgE-mediated immediate hypersensitivity reactions. The risks of developing serious systemic reactions to penicillin skin testing are minimal.

The most practical approach to penicillin-allergic patients is simply to avoid the drug. In the unlikely situation in which treatment with a penicillin is essential, penicillin skin testing would be useful.

Cross-reactivity

CASE 32-1, QUESTION 4: J.A. received a scratch test with PPL, which was negative; however, an intradermal test was positive. What treatment options are available to J.A. for her infection?

Table 32-4
Penicillin Skin Testing Procedure

Agent	Procedure	Interpretation
Penicilloyl polylysine (Pre-Pen)	Puncture (scratch) test one drop of full-strength solution (6×10^{-5} mol/L)[a]	*No wheal or erythema or wheal <5 mm in diameter after 15 minutes:* proceed with intradermal test.
Major determinant		*Wheal or erythema of 5 to 15 mm in diameter or more within 15 minutes:* choose alternative agent, consider desensitization if no other alternatives exist.
PPL	Intradermal test: inject sufficient volume PPL to raise an intradermal bleb of 3 mm in diameter[a] Saline: negative control Histamine: positive control (optional; useful if it is suspected that patient may be anergic)	Read at 20 minutes. Negative response: no increase in size of original bleb and no greater than reaction at control site. Positive response: itching and increase in size of original bleb to at least 5 mm and greater than saline control: choose alternative agent; consider desensitization if no other alternatives exist.
Penicillin G potassium (>1 week old) most important of the minor determinants	Scratch test one drop of 10,000 unit/mL solution	Same as scratch test with PPL (see above).
Penicillin G potassium	Intradermal test: 0.002 mL of 10,000 unit/mL solution	Same as intradermal test with PPL (see above).
	Serial testing with 10, 100, or 1,000 unit/mL solutions can be performed in those with strong history or serious reactions	

[a]PPL is administered initially as a scratch test. If no wheal or erythema develops, then intradermal testing is performed.
PPL, penicilloyl polylysine.
Source: *Pre-Pen benzylpenicilloyl polylysine injection solution [package insert]*. Round Rock, TX: ALK-Abelló, Inc; 2015. **http://penallergytest.com/app/uploads/sites/2/Pre-Pen-Package-Insert.pdf** Accessed July 20, 2017.

All penicillin derivatives should be avoided because J.A. had a positive skin-test reaction. Skin tests are not commercially available for cephalosporins and other β-lactam antibiotics. Although cephalosporin-skin testing (i.e., prick followed by intradermal instillation) has been proposed, no prospective studies have evaluated this approach and this practice is not without risk.[38,39] Therefore, clinicians must rely on cross-reactivity data to determine whether a non-penicillin β-lactam antibiotic (e.g., a cephalosporin) can be used in a penicillin-allergic patient.

Cross-reactivity (i.e., cross-antigenicity) between penicillin and cephalosporins has been reported in 5% to 15% of patients[34,37]; however, the true incidence of cross-reactivity is considerably less because these initial percentages were based on the recollection of patients of an allergic history rather than by objective skin tests.

The risk of a cephalosporin reaction in a patient with a penicillin allergy decreases with increasing cephalosporin generation: 5% to 16.5% for first-generation, 4% for second-generation, and 1% to 3% for third-generation and fourth-generation cephalosporins.[40] The risk of a serious allergic reaction with the use of an advanced-generation cephalosporin in a penicillin-allergic patient might be no greater than the risk of any alternative antibiotic.[41] The cross-reactivity between penicillins and cephalosporins formerly was attributed primarily to their common β-lactam chemical-ring structure; however, side-chain–specific reactions are now recognized to be responsible for a significant portion of allergic reactions within and between the penicillin and cephalosporins families.[38,41,42] In a study of 30 patients with immediate allergic reactions to cephalosporins, less than 20% reacted to penicillin determinants (i.e., skin test positivity, radioallergosorbent testing positivity, or both).[42] (Radioallergosorbent testing is a radioimmune test to detect IgE antibodies responsible for hypersensitivity.) This cross-reactivity between penicillin and cephalosporins is significantly less than earlier reports (up to 50%); however, the results of this study could be attributable to the greater use of third-generation, rather than the first-generation cephalosporins, which share more chemical structure similarities with the penicillins. Additional support for the importance of side-chain–specific reactions of β-lactams comes from observational data noting that 30% of patients with immediate reactions to penicillins were selective for amoxicillin.[43] In patients with allergy to amoxicillin, studies have found 2% to 38% cross-reactivity with the cephalosporin cefadroxil; both drugs share the same side chain.[30] Patients allergic to ampicillin may also have a greater risk of allergic reaction to cephalosporins that share the same side chain, such as cephalexin, cefaclor, cephradine, and loracarbef. Some patients also have multiple drug allergies and could manifest an allergic reaction to these drugs (and others that are not β-lactams) in a manner similar to their penicillin reaction.[37]

Cross-reactivity between penicillins and carbapenems (imipenem, meropenem, ertapenem, doripenem) and monobactams (e.g., aztreonam) has also been studied. One hundred twelve patients with a history of immediate reactions to a penicillin and a positive skin test to penicillin underwent skin testing with imipenem–cilastatin. One patient (0.9%) had a positive skin test. One hundred ten of the remaining 111 patients received gradually increasing IM doses of imipenem–cilastatin with no reactions observed.[44] Similarly, 108 children with a history of an immediate hypersensitivity reaction to a penicillin and a positive skin test underwent intradermal skin testing to meropenem. One child (0.9%) had a positive skin test. The remaining 107 subjects received increasing doses of IM meropenem with no reactions reported.[45] There also does not appear to be significant cross-reactivity between penicillins and the monobactam aztreonam.[46] Ceftazidime and aztreonam have an identical side-chain, however, and there is evidence of cross-reactivity between these two antibiotics.[47]

Although desensitization with an appropriate cephalosporin is a potential option for J.A. (see Case 32-9, Question 1), her infection is not life-threatening, and the organism is probably sensitive to another antimicrobial agents. In this case, it would be prudent to treat J.A. with a non–β-lactam antibiotic. If J.A.'s skin tests to cephalosporin were undertaken, and had been negative, she could receive a cephalosporin despite her positive history beginning with a cautiously administered small (i.e., "test") initial dose.[37]

GENERALIZED REACTIONS

Drug allergies can be grouped into three categories: generalized reactions, organ-specific reactions, and pseudoallergic reactions. Generalized reactions involve multiple organ systems and variable clinical manifestations. Anaphylactic reactions, serum sickness reactions, drug-induced fever, hypersensitivity vasculitis, drug-induced vasculitis, and autoimmune drug reactions are the generalized drug reactions presented in this chapter.

Anaphylaxis

CASE 32-2

QUESTION 1: L.P., an 85-kg, 29-year-old man, presents to the emergency department with a chief complaint of a cat bite to the forearm 2 days prior. Physical examination reveals a man in moderate distress with multiple puncture wounds on the volar aspect of the right arm. The area surrounding the wounds is swollen, erythematous, and tender to the touch. L.P.'s history is notable for exercise-induced asthma, controlled with an albuterol metered-dose inhaler as needed, and a history of a laparoscopic appendectomy 3 years prior. He has no known allergies. The wound is cleansed with a germicidal soap and 3 g ampicillin/sulbactam is started intravenously. Three minutes after starting the ampicillin/sulbactam, L.P. notes tingling and pruritus of both his hands and feet, and appears flushed. One minute later he complains of light-headedness, difficulty breathing, and a lump in his throat. His vital signs at this time are blood pressure (BP) 100/60 mm Hg (normal, 125/85), heart rate 70 beats/minute (normal, 60), and respiratory rate 27 breaths/minute (normal, 12). Chest auscultation reveals restricted airflow and stridor. Anaphylaxis is the diagnosis and emergency treatment is started. What subjective and objective evidence support the diagnosis of anaphylaxis in L.P.?

Anaphylaxis is a serious allergic reaction that has a rapid onset and can cause death.[48] The diagnosis is considered probable if one of three clinical criteria are met[49]:

1. an acute onset of a reaction (minutes to hours) with involvement of the skin, mucosal tissue, or both, and at least one of the following:
   a. respiratory compromise
   b. reduced blood pressure or symptoms of end-organ dysfunction
2. two or more of the following that occur rapidly after exposure to a likely allergen for that patient:
   a. involvement of the skin/mucosal tissue
   b. respiratory compromise
   c. reduced blood pressure or associated symptoms
   d. persistent gastrointestinal symptoms
3. reduced blood pressure, after exposure to a known allergen

Anaphylaxis results from the rapid release of immunologic mediators from tissue mast cells and peripheral blood basophils.

The symptoms of anaphylaxis vary widely, depending on the route of exposure, rate of exposure, and dose of allergen.[30] Symptoms often begin within minutes of exposure, as in L.P., and most reactions occur within 1 hour. On rare occasions, anaphylaxis can appear several hours after exposure, and late phase or biphasic attacks have occurred 1 to 72 hours after the initial attack (most commonly within 8 hours). In general, the severity of the anaphylaxis is directly proportional to the speed of onset. L.P. displays symptoms in many of the organs commonly involved in anaphylaxis. Although almost any organ system can be affected, the cutaneous, gastrointestinal (GI), respiratory, and cardiovascular systems are involved most frequently, either singly or in combination.[30] These "shock organs" contain the largest number of mast cells and are the most highly affected.

L.P. exhibits erythema (flushed appearance) and complains of pruritus of his hands and feet, both common initial symptoms of anaphylaxis; the groin is also commonly affected. These symptoms can progress to urticaria and angioedema, especially of the palms, soles, periorbital tissue, and mucous membranes. L.P. describes the early manifestations of angioedema (laryngeal edema) with complaints of a lump in his throat (this may also be described as throat tightness or constriction by some patients).

The upper and lower respiratory tracts can also be involved during an anaphylactic event. L.P. exhibits stridor, indicating upper airway involvement. Hoarseness is another sign of upper respiratory tract involvement. In addition, L.P. is tachypneic with poor airflow, suggesting his lower airway also is affected. L.P. does not display wheezing or acute emphysema, which are further clues of lower airway involvement. Respiratory symptoms can lead to suffocation and death. In one autopsy series, laryngeal edema accounted for 25% of the fatalities and acute emphysema for another 25% of the deaths.[50] Cardiovascular symptoms also are ominous. Cardiovascular collapse and hypotensive shock (anaphylactic shock) are caused by peripheral vasodilation, enhanced vascular permeability, leakage of plasma, low cardiac output, and intravascular volume depletion. Thus, hypotension, as seen with L.P., is a common cardiac manifestation. Tachycardia also commonly occurs in patients with cardiac complications of anaphylaxis. L.P. does not show a significant increase in heart rate; however, he is taking the β-blocker atenolol. Other cardiac manifestations of anaphylaxis include a direct cardiodepressant effect and various electrocardiographic changes, including arrhythmias and ischemia.

Although not demonstrated by L.P., common GI manifestations such as abdominal cramping, diarrhea (which can be bloody), nausea, and vomiting are also manifested during an anaphylactic reaction.[30] In summary, L.P.'s rapid onset and progression of symptoms involving multiple organ systems (i.e., cutaneous, respiratory, and cardiovascular systems) are consistent with an anaphylactic reaction. L.P.'s anaphylaxis is a severe reaction given its speed of onset, the number of organ systems involved, and the degree of involvement. In particular, his respiratory and cardiovascular symptoms indicate a potentially life-threatening reaction.

CASE 32-2, QUESTION 2: What is the mechanism behind anaphylaxis and what is the likely cause of L.P.'s anaphylactic event?

Anaphylaxis occurs through one of three mechanisms.[30] In the first type of reaction, exposure to a foreign protein, either in its native state or as a hapten conjugated to a carrier protein, causes IgE-antibody formation. The IgE antibodies then bind to receptors on mast cells and basophils. On reexposure, the antigen stimulates cellular degranulation through both antigen-IgE antibody formation and cross-linking, which result in massive release of preformed immunologic mediators from the mast cells and basophils. Histamine is the major mediator of anaphylaxis and the primary preformed cellular constituent. Histamine has multiple effects and is likely responsible for vasodilation, urticaria, angioedema, hypotension, vomiting, abdominal cramping, and changes in coronary flow.[30] Leukotrienes (e.g., leukotrienes C_4 and D, also known as slow-reacting substance of anaphylaxis), platelet activating factor, and prostaglandins are generated rapidly as a result of cellular degranulation, and other mediators of anaphylaxis (e.g., tryptase, chymase, carboxypeptidase A, tumor necrosis factor, and other cytokines and chemokines) are released as well.[30] Anaphylactic reactions to *Hymenoptera* venom (e.g., bee stings), insulin, streptokinase, penicillins, cephalosporins, local anesthetics, and sulfonamides occur through this IgE-mediated mechanism.

Anaphylaxis also can occur via the formation of immune complexes that activate the complement system and the subsequent formation of anaphylatoxins C3a, C4a, and C5a. Such anaphylatoxins can directly stimulate mast cell and basophil degranulation and mediator release. In 2008, cases resembling anaphylaxis in patients receiving heparin, particularly those also undergoing dialysis, were reported with almost 100 deaths occurring internationally. The culprit was found to be a contaminant (oversulfated chondroitin sulfate) that caused symptoms by this mechanism.[51,52]

The third mechanism by which substances, such as radiocontrast media and other hyperosmolar agents, can cause anaphylaxis is by the direct stimulation of mediator release (primarily histamine). The pathway by which this occurs is as yet unknown, but it is independent of IgE and complement.

Additionally, when no distinct mechanism can be associated with an anaphylactic event, the term idiopathic anaphylaxis is applied.[30]

Foods, insect stings, and drugs are the most common causes of anaphylaxis.[53] Antibiotics (particularly β-lactams and fluoroquinolones), nonsteroidal anti-inflammatory drugs (NSAIDs), neuromuscular blocking agents, radiocontrast media, chemotherapeutic agents, and monoclonal antibodies are the most common causes of drug-induced anaphylaxis. L.P.'s anaphylactic episode most likely is related to the first mechanism (i.e., IgE-antibody formation). L.P. is receiving a drug from a class of antibiotics well known to cause anaphylaxis. Specifically, L.P. may have received a prophylactic β-lactam antibiotic prior to his appendectomy, a standard of practice. Exposure to the antibiotic at that time stimulated IgE-antibody formation. After exposure to the β-lactam ampicillin/sulbactam in the emergency department, antibody–antigen complexes were formed, resulting in cellular degranulation and anaphylaxis. The temporal relationship of L.P.'s anaphylactic reaction to the administration of the antibiotic also strongly implicates ampicillin/sulbactam as the precipitating agent. Furthermore, L.P. was not exposed to agents known to cause anaphylaxis by one of the other known mechanisms. A review of L.P.'s surgical records is necessary to confirm his prior exposure to a sensitizing antibiotic.

CASE 32-2, QUESTION 3: Given L.P.'s signs and symptoms and the presumed cause of his anaphylactic reaction, how should he be treated?

Effective management of anaphylaxis requires quick recognition and aggressive therapeutic intervention because of the immediate life-threatening nature of the reaction, as illustrated by L.P. The severity of the anaphylactic reaction must be assessed quickly, the probable causative agent determined, the administration of the offending substance discontinued, and the absorption of the offending agent minimized if possible. Recent guidelines on the management of anaphylaxis list the following treatments in order of importance: epinephrine, patient position, oxygen, intravenous fluids, nebulized therapy, vasopressors, antihistamines, corticosteroids, and other agents.[49] All of these interventions must be undertaken promptly and the clinical status of the patient closely monitored. Vital signs, cardiac and pulmonary function, oxygenation, cardiac output, and tissue perfusion in particular must be immediately and continuously assessed.[30,49]

Although not definitively known to be the cause, the infusion of ampicillin/sulbactam should be stopped to prevent further exposure to the presumed precipitating agent. Additionally, the forearm wounds should be flushed with normal saline to remove any residual cleansing agent in the event that this is the cause of the reaction.

Pharmacologic treatment of anaphylaxis has traditionally involved several drugs and drug classes such as epinephrine, antihistamines, and corticosteroids aimed at reversing the clinical manifestations of anaphylaxis and interrupting the biological pathways involved. Recent literature reviews, however, failed to find well-designed and well-conducted randomized controlled trials to support the use of these drugs.[54–56] Recommendations for use are based on tradition, case reports, case series, and expert opinion.

L.P. is showing early signs of anaphylactic shock that must be managed immediately. Epinephrine is the drug of choice for the pharmacologic management of anaphylaxis and all national and international anaphylaxis guidelines recommend epinephrine as first-line treatment.[30,49,57] Studies have shown that failure to use epinephrine early in anaphylaxis is a risk factor for a poor outcome. Use of standard order sets and auto-injectors by emergency departments have been shown to increase epinephrine utilization for anaphylactic patients.[58]

The α-adrenergic effects of epinephrine increase systemic vascular resistance and increase blood pressure while decreasing mucosal edema and relieving upper airway obstruction, angioedema, and hives. These actions counter the vasodilating and hypotensive effects of histamine and the other mediators of anaphylaxis. In addition, the β-adrenergic effects of epinephrine promote bronchodilation and increase cardiac rate and contractility. Epinephrine also inhibits the release of mediators from basophils and mast cells.

The route of epinephrine administration is important. Most guidelines recommend IM epinephrine, 0.01 mg/kg of a 1 mg/mL (1:1,000) solution to a maximum dose of 0.5 mg in an adult or 0.3 mg in a child injected into the lateral aspect of the thigh every 5 to 10 minutes as needed.[58,59] Epinephrine doses should be expressed in mass concentration (e.g., 1 mg in 1 mL) instead of ratios such as 1:1,000, which have been confused with epinephrine concentrations used in cardiac arrest (1:10,000) and caused dosing errors.[57] Epinephrine is vasodilatory in skeletal muscle and because skeletal muscle is highly vascular absorption is rapid. While some guidelines propose the subcutaneous route for epinephrine administration, subcutaneous tissue is less vascular than skeletal muscle, thus there is less rapid absorption of epinephrine. Additionally, epinephrine causes vasoconstriction in subcutaneous tissue, therefore slowing its own absorption. Studies have shown that IM epinephrine injections into the thigh achieve higher blood concentrations more rapidly than do subcutaneous or IM injections into the arm in healthy subjects.[49] The rate and extent of absorption from IM and subcutaneous routes of epinephrine administration, however, have not been studied in patients experiencing anaphylaxis, and there is no evidence that epinephrine is ineffective when given IM or subcutaneously into the arm.[49] Epinephrine should be administered via the IV route in cases of anaphylaxis that have not responded to repeated doses of IM epinephrine and/or are progressing to shock, or in cases where cardiorespiratory arrest appears imminent. Low cardiac output and intravascular volume depletion from shock decrease tissue perfusion and possibly the absorption of subcutaneous or IM injections. In animal studies, the benefits of intermittent IV boluses of epinephrine are short lived and a continuous infusion of epinephrine provides optimal results.[59] In L.P.'s case, an initial dose of 0.5 mg of 1 mg/1 mL epinephrine solution should be injected IM into his lateral thigh. This should be repeated every 5 minutes until symptoms improve.

Some evidence suggests poor outcomes in patients who are in an upright position during anaphylactic shock.[60] Placing L.P. in the Trendelenburg position (patient supine, inclined approximately 45 degrees with head at the lower end and legs at the upper end) might improve survival by enhancing perfusion to vital organs. After repositioning, oxygen should be started and normal saline infused at a rate sufficient to maintain perfusion to vital organs. Normal saline is the preferred crystalloid because it stays in the intravascular space longer than does dextrose and does not contain lactate (e.g., Lactated Ringer's solution), which could worsen metabolic acidosis. Circulating blood volume can decrease by as much as 35% in the first 10 minutes of anaphylactic shock because of vasodilation and fluid shifting from the intravascular to the extravascular space.[49] Therefore, vigorous fluid resuscitation might be necessary (e.g., 1–2 L of normal saline at a rate of 5–10 mL/kg in the first 5 minutes). Cerebral perfusion, as evidenced by adequate mentation, must always take precedence over BP readings when managing shock.

The effect of L.P.'s atenolol must also be considered. Patients taking a β-blocker, whether cardioselective or not cardioselective, could experience more severe episodes and more refractory episodes of anaphylaxis than patients not taking a β-blocker. This effect might be caused by a blunted response to epinephrine when given to treat anaphylaxis, resulting in refractory hypotension, bradycardia, and bronchospasm.[49] If L.P.'s BP and heart rate do not substantially improve shortly after initiating epinephrine, IV glucagon, which can stimulate heart rate and cardiac contractility independent of β-adrenergic blockade, should be given (Table 32-5). Airway protection is important because glucagon may cause emesis and there is a risk of aspiration, especially in drowsy or obtunded patients. Methylene blue, through its ability to reduce nitric oxide production (a known potent vasodilator) has been found to be effective in a small number of cases of anaphylaxis with refractory hypotension.[53,60] Other vasopressors such as dopamine (2–20 mcg/kg/minute) may be needed to maintain blood pressure if there is poor response to epinephrine and glucagon. Second-line treatment for anaphylaxis includes inhaled β-agonists, H_1 and H_2 antihistamines, and corticosteroids. In light of L.P.'s severe pulmonary reaction, he should receive a nebulized β-agonist (e.g., albuterol). If L.P.'s respiratory status fails to improve after pharmacologic intervention, intubation must be considered. Atenolol would not be expected to diminish the effect of albuterol because atenolol is a β_1 cardioselective β-blocker and the dose is low. Because histamine is the primary mediator of anaphylaxis, IV administration of an H_1 antihistamine such as diphenhydramine (50 mg every 6 hours until the reaction resolves) should be considered. Similarly, giving an H_2 antihistamine is a common practice. Both therapies present little acute risk to the patient, but as already noted, there are few data supporting their efficacy in treating anaphylaxis.[55]

Lastly, given the severity of his reaction and his pulmonary involvement, L.P. is a candidate for IV corticosteroids. Methylprednisolone, 125 mg every 6 hours for four doses, might be beneficial and is associated with minimal risk. Although commonly used, corticosteroids will not affect the acute course of the reaction because of their delayed onset of action (typically 4–6 hours after administration). Corticosteroids may impact a prolonged episode of anaphylaxis and could prevent or minimize the occurrence of a biphasic reaction, although this has not been proven in well-controlled trials. The effect of methylprednisolone on L.P.'s diabetes is not a factor because his condition is potentially life-threatening. Once stabilized, L.P. should be transferred to a critical care setting and monitored for a minimum of 24 hours because relapses of the anaphylactic reaction can occur.[30,49]

Serum Sickness

Serum sickness is a type III hypersensitivity reaction that results from the production of antibodies directed against heterologous protein or drug haptens with subsequent tissue deposition. The typical presentation of serum sickness includes fever, cutaneous eruptions (95%), lymphadenopathy, and joint symptoms (10%–50%).[61–64] Symptoms usually occur 1 to 2 weeks after exposure, but accelerated reactions can occur within 2 to 4 days in previously sensitized persons. Laboratory data are relatively nonspecific and are of little diagnostic value. For example, the erythrocyte sedimentation rate (ESR) and the serum concentration of circulating immune complexes usually are increased. Complements C3 and C4 are often low, whereas activation products C3a and C3a desarginine are elevated. Urinalysis might reveal proteinuria, hematuria, or an occasional cast.[61–64]

In most cases, serum sickness reactions are mild and self-limiting and resolve within a few days to weeks after withdrawal of the inciting agent. Antihistamines and aspirin can be used to relieve pruritus and arthralgias. In severe cases, corticosteroids might be used and can be tapered during 10 to 14 days.[61–64] At one time, heterologous serum (e.g., anti-thymocyte globulin made from rabbit or equine serum) was a leading cause of serum sickness. With the decline in use of these products, however, the most common causes of serum sickness today are penicillins and cephalosporins, although biological agents such as rituximab, infliximab, and natalizumab are increasingly associated with serum sickness.[65,66]

Drug Fever

CASE 32-3

QUESTION 1: M.M., a 57-year-old ill-appearing woman, is hospitalized with a 3-day history of difficulty breathing, left-sided chest pain on inspiration, fever, chills, and a productive cough. Her medical history is significant only for hypertension, well controlled on hydrochlorothiazide; she has no known drug allergies. M.M.'s physical findings on admission are temperature, 38°C; respirations, 20 breaths/minute; left-sided crackles heard on auscultation; oxygen saturation 85% on room air; and heart rate, 85 beats/minute. A chest radiograph reveals an infiltrate in her left lower lobe. Her white blood cell (WBC) count is 17,500 cells/μL with the following differential:

Polymorphonuclear neutrophil leukocytes (PMN), 83% (normal, 45%–79%)
Bands, 12% (normal, 0%–5%)
Lymphocytes, 10% (normal, 16%–47%)
Basophils, 0% (normal, 0%–1%)
Eosinophils, 1% (normal, 1%–2%)

Community-acquired pneumonia is the diagnosis, and M.M. is empirically started on ceftriaxone 1 g IV daily, azithromycin 500 mg IV daily, and oxygen at 2 L/minute. Other medications include oral acetaminophen 325 mg every 4 to 6 hours as needed for temperature greater than 38°C, oral famotidine 20 mg BID, and oral hydrochlorothiazide 12.5 mg daily. Seventy-two hours later, M.M. is breathing without pain at a respiratory rate of 12 breaths/minute, her lungs are clear to auscultation, and her

Table 32-5
Drug Therapy of Anaphylaxis

Drug	Indication	Adult Dosage	Complications
First-line Therapy			
Epinephrine	Hypotension, bronchospasm, laryngeal edema, urticaria, angioedema	001 mg/kg to a maximum of 0.5 mg of a 1 mg/1 mL solution IM every 5 minutes PRN; if progressing to cardiorespiratory arrest 1–3 mL of 1:10,000 (0.1–0.3 mg) IV for 3 minutes	Arrhythmias, hypertension, nervousness, tremor
		1 mL of 1 mg/mL (1:1,000) in 250 mL of normal saline IV at a rate of 4–10 mcg/minute	
		3–5 mL of 0.1 mg/mL (1:10,000) intratracheally every 10–20 minutes PRN	
Oxygen	Hypoxemia	40%–100%	None
Albuterol		0.5 mL of 0.5% solution in 2.5 mL of saline via nebulizer (i.e., 2.5 mg)	Arrhythmias, hypertension, nervousness, tremor
IV fluids	Hypotension	1 L of normal saline every 20–30 minutes PRN (rates as high as 1–2 mL/kg/minute may be necessary)	Pulmonary edema, CHF
Second-line Therapy			
Antihistamines	Hypotension, urticaria		
H_1 receptor antagonists[a]		Diphenhydramine 25–50 mg IV over 10–15 minutes Oral H_1 antagonists may be used in less severe cases.	Drowsiness, dry mouth, urinary retention; may obscure symptoms of continuing reaction
H_2 receptor antagonists[a]		Ranitidine 50 mg IV over 10–15 minutes or Famotidine 20 mg IV over 10–15 minutes	
Corticosteroids[a]	Bronchospasm; patients undergoing prolonged resuscitation or severe reaction	Hydrocortisone sodium succinate 100 mg IV every 3–6 hours for two to four doses or Methylprednisolone sodium succinate 40–125 mg IV every 6 hours for two to four doses	Hyperglycemia, fluid retention
Dopamine	Hypotension refractory to epinephrine	400 mg in 500 mL dextrose 5% at 2–20 mcg/kg/minute	Hypertension, tachycardia, palpitations, arrhythmias
Norepinephrine	Hypotension refractory to epinephrine	4 mg in 1 L dextrose 5% IV at a rate of 2–12 mcg/minute	Arrhythmias, hypertension, nervousness, tremor
Glucagon[b]	Refractory hypotension	1 mg IV for 5 minutes, followed by 5–15 mcg/minute in fusion	Nausea, vomiting

[a]Agents in these classes may be used as adjuncts to epinephrine. Controlled studies demonstrating a clear benefit in anaphylaxis are lacking. Do not delay the administration of epinephrine, supplemental oxygen, or IV fluid resuscitation by taking time to draw up and administer a second-line medication.
[b]Glucagon may be particularly useful in patients taking β-adrenergic blockers, because it can increase both cardiac rate and contractility regardless of β-adrenergic blockade. Choice of agent and starting doses should be patient-specific, weighing safety and efficacy.
IM, intramuscularly; IV, intravenously; PO, orally; PRN, as needed.

oxygen saturation is 98% on room air. She appears much better and offers no new complaints. Her temperature during the previous 48 hours has ranged from 38.6°C to 40°C, her pulse has ranged from 90 to 100 beats/minute, and her WBC count is 22,000 with the following differential: PMN, 89%; bands, 5%; lymphocytes, 12%; basophils, 0%; and eosinophils, 7%. Drug-induced fever is considered. What evidence supports this diagnosis? What is the mechanism for drug fever?

Drug fever is described as a febrile reaction to a drug without cutaneous symptoms and is estimated to occur in 3% to 5% of inpatients.[67] Drug fever can be challenging to identify and can be misinterpreted as a new infectious process or failure of an existing infection to respond to treatment. Such failure to recognize a drug fever can lead to prolonged hospitalization and unnecessary tests or medications.[68] Table 32-6 lists the characteristics of hypersensitivity drug-induced fever. The most important finding in the case of M.M. is her clinical improvement with respect to her pulmonary status despite a high-grade fever and persistent leukocytosis; she also appears healthier than expected if she had an untreated infection. Whereas a drop in her WBC count would be anticipated given her improving respiratory function, her WBC count remains elevated, consistent with hypersensitivity drug fever. Notably, her eosinophil count is increased, a frequent sign of hypersensitivity reactions. Despite her high-grade fever, she has a relative bradycardia; that is, her heart rate is not as elevated as expected if an infectious process were ongoing. Further, the timing of the symptoms favors a drug-induced fever (i.e., within days of starting a new medication). A definitive diagnosis can be made only by stopping the suspected offending agent, however, because fever generally resolves within 48 to 72 hours if a rash is not present. When a rash is present, on the other hand, the fever may persist for several days after stopping the implicated drug.

Table 32-6
Hypersensitivity Reactions to Drugs: Drug-Induced Fever

Frequency	True frequency is unknown because fever is a common manifestation and almost any drug can cause fever. Estimate is that 3%–5% of hospitalized patients experiencing adverse drug reaction suffer from drug fever alone or as part of multiple symptoms.
Clinical manifestations	Temperatures may be 38°C or higher and do not follow a consistent pattern. Although patients may have high fevers with shaking chills, patients generally have few symptoms or serious systemic illness. Skin rash (18%), eosinophilia (22%), chills (53%), headache (16%), myalgias (25%), and bradycardia (11%) can occur in patients with drug fever. Onset of fever after exposure to the offending agent is highly variable, ranging from an average of 6 days for antineoplastics to 45 days for cardiovascular agents. Occurrence of fever is independent of the dose of the offending agent.
Treatment	Although drug fever can be treated symptomatically (e.g., with antipyretics, cooling blankets), stopping the offending agent is the only therapy that will eliminate fevers. Patients generally defervesce within 48–72 hours of stopping the suspect drug.
Prognosis	Drug fever is usually benign, although one review[57] found a mean increased length of hospitalization of 9 days per episode of drug fever. Rechallenge with the offending drug usually results in rapid return of the fever. Although reexposure to the suspect drug was previously thought to be potentially hazardous, there is little risk of serious sequelae.

Source: Patel RA, Gallagher JC. Drug fever. *Pharmacotherapy*. 2010;30:57; Mackowiak PA, LeMaistre CF. Drug fever: a critical appraisal of conventional concepts. An analysis of 51 episodes in two Dallas hospitals and 97 episodes reported in the English literature. *Ann Intern Med*. 1987;106:728; Cunha BA, Shea KW. Fever in the intensive care unit. *Infect Dis Clin North Am*. 1996;10:185.

Drug fever can be caused by various mechanisms, although it is ascribed most commonly to a hypersensitivity reaction. Other mechanisms include the pharmacologic action of the drug (e.g., cell destruction from antineoplastic agents releases endogenous pyrogens); altered thermoregulatory function (e.g., increased metabolic rate from thyroid hormone); decreased sweating from drugs with anticholinergic properties (e.g., atropine, tricyclic antidepressants, and phenothiazines); drug-administration-related fever (e.g., amphotericin B and bleomycin); and idiosyncratic reactions (e.g., neuroleptic malignant syndrome from haloperidol, malignant hyperthermia from inhaled anesthetics).[67]

Case 32-3, Question 2: What agent is the most likely cause of drug fever in M.M.?

Most of the information available on drug fever is based on case reports or small case series and reviews of the literature.[68,69] Unfortunately, the literature is inconsistent with regard to the frequency of drug fever (e.g., very common, common, uncommon) and such descriptions are not supported by good clinical data. Nevertheless, some drugs are more commonly associated with drug fever than others. These include anti-infectives as a class (especially β-lactam antibiotics), antiepileptics, and antineoplastics. Drug fever has also been reported frequently with amphotericin B, azathioprine, hydroxyurea, methyldopa, procainamide, quinidine, and quinine.[68–70]

In M.M.'s case, ceftriaxone or azithromycin is the most likely cause of her ongoing fever, given the timing of the reaction relative to beginning the antibiotics and the frequency of febrile reactions attributed to them, especially to β-lactam antibiotics. Febrile reactions have not been associated with acetaminophen, and famotidine is rarely a cause of fever without other symptoms of an allergic reaction. Although diuretics such as hydrochlorothiazide can cause fever, M.M. was taking this medication before admission without any ill effects, making this drug an unlikely culprit.

Case 32-3, Question 3: How should M.M.'s drug fever be treated? Can M.M. receive cephalosporins in the future?

Because M.M. has responded clinically, her antibiotics should be discontinued and her fever curve, WBC count, heart rate, and respiratory status followed. An oral antibiotic from another drug class (e.g., a fluoroquinolone) should be started to complete a 7-day to 10-day antibiotic course of therapy. Acetaminophen and other antipyretics should be avoided unless M.M. becomes uncomfortable from the fever because they can mask the response to the discontinuation of her antibiotics.

As with any hypersensitivity reaction, rechallenge with the offending drug can cause a similar, or sometimes greater, response. In M.M.'s case, reexposure to ceftriaxone (or another β-lactam antibiotic) or a macrolide might cause a febrile reaction. It is unclear, however, how large the risk of reexposure truly is. Although drug fever sometimes precedes more serious hypersensitivity reactions, evidence suggests there may be little risk to reexposure. Should M.M. require ceftriaxone (or another β-lactam or macrolide antibiotic) in the future, it would be prudent to administer the drug in a setting where M.M. can be monitored, at least initially, to ensure prompt treatment if an immediate hypersensitivity reaction develops.

Hypersensitivity Vasculitis

CASE 32-4

Question 1: M.G., a 26-year-old woman with cystic fibrosis, is admitted for treatment of pneumonia. Sputum cultures obtained before admission reveal *Alcaligenes xylosoxidans* sensitive only to minocycline and chloramphenicol. M.G. is initiated on appropriate doses of these two antibiotics for a 2-week course. On day 8 of therapy, M.G. begins to complain of a rash on her legs. Physical examination reveals palpable purpura and a maculopapular rash on both lower extremities. Laboratory data reveal an elevated ESR and leukocytosis. What is the likely cause of M.G.'s rash and laboratory abnormalities?

M.G.'s presentation is suggestive of a diagnosis of hypersensitivity vasculitis.

Hypersensitivity vasculitis, also called cutaneous leukocytoclastic angiitis, is characterized by inflammation of the small blood vessel walls. These reactions occur when immune complex deposition within the small veins and arterioles activates complement, causing the release of chemotactic factors. These factors attract polymorphonuclear cells that cause vessel damage.[71–74]

Drug-induced Vasculitis

Approximately 10% of cases of cutaneous vasculitis are believed to be drug-related.[73] Approximately 100 drugs have been identified as causing vasculitis, including β-lactams, fluoroquinolones, NSAIDs, antiepileptics, and tumor necrosis factor blockers.[72–75] Interested readers are referred to more in-depth reviews.[74–76] The diagnosis of hypersensitivity vasculitis is based on five clinical criteria (Table 32-7), three of which must be present.[76] M.G. meets three of the five criteria, including age greater than 16 years, palpable purpura, and a maculopapular rash. In addition, minocycline, a medication that she was taking at the onset of the rash, has been associated with serum sickness and vasculitic-type reactions. Onset of symptoms typically occurs 7 to 10 days after initiation of drug therapy but can occur sooner on reexposure. Purpuric papules and macular eruptions, the most commonly observed findings, are usually symmetric and occur on the extremities (Table 32-8).[71] Hypersensitivity vasculitis can involve multiple organ systems. Renal damage, ranging from microscopic hematuria to nephrotic syndrome and acute renal failure, is common in patients with disseminated disease.[76] An enlarged liver with elevated enzymes is indicative of hepatocellular involvement. Although the lungs and ears can be involved as well, clinical manifestations are usually mild.[71] Arthralgia is also commonly observed. Laboratory examinations usually show nonspecific abnormalities of inflammation such as an elevated ESR and leukocytosis. In patients with cystic fibrosis experiencing acute pneumonia, these laboratory abnormalities could already be present and, therefore, will not be helpful in establishing the diagnosis of hypersensitivity vasculitis in M.G.

Table 32-7
Criteria for the Classification of Hypersensitivity Vasculitis

Development of symptoms after age 16
Medication at disease onset that may have been a precipitating factor
Slightly elevated purpuric (hemorrhagic) rash over one or more areas of the skin that does not blanch with pressure and is not related to thrombocytopenia
Maculopapular rash over one or more areas of the skin
Biopsy showing granulocytes around an arteriole or venule

The diagnosis of hypersensitivity vasculitis can be made if a patient exhibits at least three of these criteria.

Source: Calabrese LH et al. The American College of Rheumatology 1990 criteria for the classification of hypersensitivity vasculitis. *Arthritis Rheum*. 1990;33:1108.

Table 32-8
Hypersensitivity Reactions to Drugs: Clinical Manifestations of Drug-Induced Vasculitis

- Palpable purpura and maculopapular rash occurring symmetrically predominantly on the lower extremities
- Multiple organ systems may be involved:
  Renal: microscopic hematuria to nephrotic syndrome and acute renal failure
  Liver: enlarged liver, elevated enzymes
  Joints: arthritis
  Gastrointestinal: abdominal pain
- Laboratory data usually show nonspecific abnormalities of inflammation: elevated erythrocyte sedimentation rate and leukocytosis. Peripheral eosinophilia may be present and serum complement concentrations can be low. Histologic findings on biopsy reveal small blood vessels with leukocytoclastic or necrotizing vasculitis
- Onset typically 7–21 days after initiation of therapy

Source: Valeyrie-Allanore L et al. Drug-induced skin, nail and hair disorders. *Drug Saf*. 2007;30:1011.

Case 32-4, Question 2: What additional workup could be performed to confirm the diagnosis of drug-induced vasculitis in M.G.?

In addition to the previous workup, other laboratory and diagnostic procedures might demonstrate peripheral eosinophilia and low serum complement concentrations. A biopsy, which typically reveals granulocytes in the wall of a venule or arteriole and eosinophils at any location, would provide more definitive information.

Case 32-4, Question 3: How should M.G.'s hypersensitivity vasculitis be treated?

The first step is to discontinue the minocycline therapy. Drug-induced vasculitic reactions typically resolve on their own without additional interventions. If the reaction is severe, corticosteroids can be used.

Autoimmune Drug Reactions

CASE 32-5

Question 1: R.F., a 24-year-old white male medical student, has been treated for 5 months with isoniazid because of a positive skin test for tuberculosis. He now is in the clinic with complaints of new-onset myalgias and arthralgias. Laboratory values obtained the morning of the visit are within normal limits except for a positive ANA titer and an elevated ESR. What is the likely cause of R.F.'s symptoms and laboratory abnormalities?

Some drugs can induce an autoimmune process characterized by the presence of autoantibodies and, in some instances, clinical features of an autoimmune disorder. A drug-induced syndrome resembling SLE is usually characterized by myalgias, arthralgias, positive ANA titers, and an elevated ESR (see Chapter 33, Systemic Lupus Erythematosus). All of these characteristics are manifested by R.F.

The first case of drug-induced lupus erythematosus (DILE) was recognized more than 60 years ago and was associated with sulfadiazine.[77] Subsequently, more than 80 drugs have been associated with DILE including isoniazid, chlorpromazine, quinidine, methyldopa, and minocycline; however, hydralazine and procainamide are the drugs most frequently associated with this syndrome.[78–80] As with idiopathic SLE, DILE can be separated into systemic, subacute cutaneous, and chronic cutaneous lupus. An exact incidence of DILE is difficult to ascertain because of changing patterns of drug use; however, it is estimated that 10% of SLE cases are drug-induced with 15,000 to 30,000 cases in the United States annually.[73]

Case 32-5, Question 2: How can the diagnosis of drug-induced lupus be differentiated from SLE in R.F.?

In contrast to idiopathic SLE, DILE is less likely to affect women and black patients.[79] On average, patients with DILE are twice as old as those with idiopathic SLE at the time of diagnosis. Individuals with a slow acetylator phenotype have a greater tendency to exhibit DILE; ANA after exposure to lupus-inducing drugs also appear more rapidly.[81] In general, DILE is a milder disease than idiopathic SLE. Many patients with DILE, however, could fulfill the diagnostic criteria for SLE according to the American Rheumatism Association.[81–83] Arthralgias or myalgias accompanied by a positive ANA test can be the only clinical features for some patients with drug-induced lupus. Symptoms usually appear abruptly after several months to years of continuous therapy with the offending drug. Common complaints include fever, malaise, arthralgias, myalgias, pleurisy, and slight weight loss. Mild splenomegaly and lymphadenopathy have been reported occasionally. The skin is affected in about 25% of cases manifesting as photosensitivity on light exposed surfaces. The classic butterfly malar rash, discoid lesions, oral mucosal ulcers, Raynaud's phenomenon, and alopecia are unusual features in DILE in contrast to idiopathic SLE. In addition, the central nervous system and kidneys rarely are affected.[84] Laboratory abnormalities commonly include anemia and an elevated ESR. The evidence supporting a diagnosis of drug-induced lupus in R.F. includes white male predominance, abrupt onset and relatively mild symptomatology, and lack of the classic butterfly malar rash. More definitive tests include determining whether antibodies to single-stranded (indicative of drug-induced lupus) or double-stranded DNA (indicative of SLE) are present.

CASE 32-5, QUESTION 3: Should ANA have been monitored in an effort to detect drug-induced lupus at an earlier stage in this patient?

No. Although all patients with symptomatic drug-induced lupus test positive for ANA (which consist predominantly of single-stranded DNA and antihistone antibodies),[84] many patients taking lupus-inducing drugs become ANA positive without going on to experience lupus. In patients treated with procainamide, about 50% to 75% are positive for ANA after 12 months and 90% after 2 years or more of continuous therapy; only 10% to 20% of those patients actually experience lupus symptoms.[84–86] Similarly, up to 44% of patients are ANA positive after 3 years of hydralazine therapy, but DILE occurs in only 6.7% of patients after 3 years of treatment.[84] It is not necessary to discontinue therapy in asymptomatic patients with positive ANA because most of them will never exhibit clinical symptoms.[79]

CASE 32-5, QUESTION 4: How should R.F.'s drug-induced lupus be treated?

Musculoskeletal complaints can be treated with aspirin or an NSAID. More severe symptoms from pleuropulmonary or pericardial involvement may require the use of corticosteroids. Clinical features of DILE usually subside and disappear in days to weeks with discontinuation of the offending drug. Occasionally, these symptoms linger or recur over a course of several months before eventually disappearing. Serologic tests tend to resolve more slowly: ANA may persist for a year or longer.[79,87] Drug-induced lupus does not predispose patients to the subsequent development of idiopathic SLE.[88] In most instances, lupus-inducing drugs do not increase the risk of exacerbation of idiopathic SLE[89]; however, long-term treatment with isoniazid may worsen preexisting SLE.[90] Since R.F. has not yet completed his 6- to 9-month course of isoniazid therapy, an alternative agent should be prescribed for R.F. with appropriate monitoring (see Chapter 68, Tuberculosis).

ORGAN-SPECIFIC REACTIONS

The drug allergies in this chapter have been grouped into categories of generalized reactions, organ-specific reactions, and pseudoallergic reactions. The generalized reactions have been described first, the organ-specific hypersensitivity drug reactions affecting the blood, liver, lung, kidney, and skin are described next, and pseudoallergic reactions follow.

Blood: Immune Cytopenias

Drug-induced immune cytopenias (e.g., granulocytopenia, thrombocytopenia, and hemolytic anemia) result from type II–mediated allergic reactions (Table 32-1). A drug or drug metabolite binds to the surface of blood elements such as granulocytes, platelets, and red blood cells. IgG or IgM antibodies are formed and are directed against the drug or drug metabolite bound to the cell (i.e., hapten–cell reaction).[27] Typical symptoms associated with immune thrombocytopenia include chills, fever, petechiae, and mucous membrane bleeding. Granulocytopenia generally manifests with chills, fever, arthralgias, and a precipitous drop in the leukocyte count. Symptoms of hemolytic anemia can be subacute or acute and can be sufficiently severe to cause renal failure. The Coombs test is useful in identifying antibodies bound to red cells or circulating immune complexes directed against red cells. Antibiotics are the most commonly implicated class of drugs causing either neutropenia or hemolytic anemia.

Liver

Hypersensitivity reactions involving the liver can be classified as cholestatic or cytotoxic. Jaundice is usually the first sign of a cholestatic reaction, in addition to pruritus, pale stools, and dark urine. Cholestatic reactions usually are reversible on discontinuation of the offending agent. Cytotoxic reactions can involve hepatocellular necrosis or steatosis and can result in irreversible damage if not recognized early.

Lung

Pulmonary manifestations of drug hypersensitivity include asthma and infiltrative reactions. Asthma typically occurs as part of a generalized systemic reaction. Most reactions to drugs that involve asthma alone represent a pharmacologic side effect rather than a true allergic reaction.

Infiltrative reactions typically develop 2 to 10 days after exposure and manifest with cough, dyspnea, fever, chills, and malaise.[26] Infiltrative reactions vary in presentation from eosinophilic pneumonitis to acute pulmonary edema.

Kidney

The most common hypersensitivity reaction involving the kidney is interstitial nephritis. Typical findings include fever, rash, and eosinophilia. Methicillin is the drug most commonly associated with interstitial nephritis, although penicillins, sulfonamides, and cimetidine also have been implicated in renal hypersensitivity reactions.[27] (See Chapter 29, Acute Kidney Injury, for hypersensitivity reactions to specific drugs that adversely affect the kidney.)

Skin

Adverse reactions involving the skin are the most common clinical manifestation of drug allergy. Although several different types of cutaneous reactions are possible, most drug-induced skin eruptions can be classified as erythematous, morbilliform, or maculopapular in appearance.[27] In a surveillance study of drug-induced skin reactions, amoxicillin was the most common cause, followed by trimethoprim–sulfamethoxazole and ampicillin. Overall, allergic skin reactions were identified in 2% of hospitalized patients.[14]

Treatment of skin reactions includes discontinuation of the offending drug and general supportive care (see Chapter 39, Dermatotherapy and Drug-Induced Skin Disorders).

PSEUDOALLERGIC REACTIONS

CASE 32-6

QUESTION 1: C.C., a 37-year-old man with no known allergies, is hospitalized for treatment of methicillin-resistant *S. aureus* (MRSA) bacteremia associated with an infected central line. His medical history is significant for short-bowel syndrome requiring parenteral nutrition and one previous episode of MRSA line infection successfully treated with vancomycin. Similar to his last admission, vancomycin 750 mg IV for 60 minutes every 12 hours is begun. A trough level taken after the fifth dose, however, is 8 mg/L and the vancomycin dose is doubled to 1,500 mg IV every 12 hours, to be administered at the same rate. Fifteen minutes after the new dose of vancomycin is begun, C.C. experienced hypotension (100/70 mm Hg), tachycardia (85 beats/minute), generalized pruritus, and facial flushing. C.C. is diagnosed as having a pseudoallergic reaction to vancomycin. What subjective and objective data in C.C. are important in differentiating vancomycin pseudoallergic reaction from a true allergic reaction?

Pseudoallergic reactions (also called nonallergic hypersensitivity reactions) are drug reactions that exhibit clinical signs and symptoms of an allergic response but are not immunologically mediated.[91] They can manifest as relatively benign symptoms or as severe, life-threatening events indistinguishable from anaphylaxis (Table 32-9).[91] The latter response is described as an anaphylactoid reaction because it resembles true anaphylaxis, but it does not involve IgE-antibody formation.[27,91] The risk of such potentially severe reactions needs to be considered when prescribing agents known to be associated with anaphylactoid reactions. For example, the prophylactic use of antibiotics such as ciprofloxacin to prevent meningococcal infections during an outbreak was associated with a relatively high rate (1:1,000) of serious anaphylactoid reactions.[92] This would be of potentially greater importance in the setting of a mass prophylaxis program to combat exposure to anthrax. Unlike true allergic reactions, which require an induction period during which a patient becomes sensitized to an antigen, pseudoallergic reactions can occur on the first exposure to a drug. The development of pseudoallergic reactions can be dose related, manifesting when large doses of the drug are administered, when the dose is increased, or when the rate of IV administration is increased.[26]

C.C. has experienced a common pseudoallergic reaction to vancomycin, usually referred to as the "red man syndrome" or "red neck syndrome," which primarily occurs when large doses of vancomycin are administered rapidly. Differentiating between a true allergic response and a pseudoallergic response can be difficult because the signs and symptoms can be indistinguishable. For example, each of the symptoms experienced by C.C. (flushing, tachycardia, pruritus, and hypotension) is caused by histamine release and can occur during an anaphylactic episode (see Case 32-2, Question 2). To conclusively determine the cause of the reaction would require immunologic testing for antibodies to the suspect drug or agent, which is not always possible or practical. In this case, C.C. had uneventfully received vancomycin previously and has tolerated five doses during this hospitalization; therefore, it is unlikely that the reaction is immunologically mediated (i.e., a true allergic reaction). Furthermore, the reaction occurred after an increase in his vancomycin dose, which further supports the diagnosis of a pseudoallergic reaction.

CASE 32-6, QUESTION 2: Why did vancomycin cause a pseudoallergic reaction in C.C.?

Pseudoallergic reactions from vancomycin occur because of a drug-induced histamine release that occurs through an as yet unknown pathway. Direct drug-induced release of histamine does not involve complement activation or IgE-antibody formation. Several other drugs (e.g., deferoxamine, opiates, pentamidine, phytonadione protamine, radiocontrast media) are known to directly stimulate histamine release.[13,91]

Some drugs (e.g., radiocontrast media and protamine) cause pseudoallergic reactions via both complement activation and direct-histamine release mechanisms. Furthermore, some drugs (e.g., vancomycin, quaternary ammonium muscle relaxants, and ciprofloxacin) can cause both true allergic reactions and pseudoallergic reactions.[7]

Table 32-9
Hypersensitivity Reactions to Drugs: Pseudoallergic Reactions

Frequency	Highly variable, depending on the agent involved. For example, up to 30% of patients taking aspirin exhibit a cutaneous pseudoallergic response. On the other hand, pseudoallergic reactions to other agents, such as phytonadione and thiamine, are rare.
Clinical manifestations	Range from benign reactions (e.g., pruritus and flushing) to a life-threatening clinical syndrome indistinguishable from anaphylaxis. Commonly require a higher drug dose to elicit the response than a true IgE-mediated reaction. May arise less quickly (>15 minutes after exposure) than true allergic reaction.
Diagnostic workup	Skin tests and identification of specific antibodies are negative.
Treatment	Pseudoallergic reactions are treated the same as true allergic reactions (i.e., according to the clinical presentations of the patient). Thus, some reactions simply may require removal of the suspect agent, whereas some anaphylactoid reactions may require aggressive therapy (e.g., epinephrine, antihistamines, and corticosteroids).
Prognosis	As with true allergic reactions, patients who have experienced a pseudoallergic drug reaction may have a similar reaction on reexposure. The severity of response may lessen, however, with repeated administration. Furthermore, for some drugs, the frequency and severity of the reaction also may be influenced by the dose or rate of intravenous administration. Pretreatment regimens to reduce the frequency and the severity of responses have been developed for some drugs well known to cause pseudoallergic reactions (e.g., radiocontrast media).

Source: Pichler WJ et al. Drug hypersensitivity reactions: pathomechanism and clinical symptoms. *Med Clin North Am*. 2010;94:645; Schnyder B. Approach to the patient with drug allergy. *Immunol Allergy Clin North Am*. 2009;29:405; Sanchez-Borges M. NSAID hypersensitivity (respiratory, cutaneous, and generalized anaphylactic symptoms). *Med Clin North Am*. 2010;94:853.

CASE 32-6, QUESTION 3: How should C.C.'s pseudoallergic reaction be treated? Does treatment of pseudoallergic reactions differ from that of true allergic reactions?

The first step in treating C.C.'s reaction is to eliminate the underlying cause. Thus, his vancomycin infusion should be held until the reaction resolves. Because the reaction is histamine-mediated, administration of an antihistamine such as diphenhydramine 50 mg IV is warranted. Observation of his BP and heart rate is mandatory. Intravenous fluids should be administered if his BP continues to fall or fails to stabilize. Patients with allergic reactions should be treated based on their clinical signs and symptoms, regardless of the mechanism behind the reaction. Thus, for all intents and purposes, pseudoallergic reactions are treated in the same manner as true allergic reactions.

CASE 32-6, QUESTION 4: Can C.C. continue to receive vancomycin? How can future reactions be prevented?

It is not necessary to discontinue vancomycin therapy in C.C. This reaction can be prevented by administering smaller doses of the drug more frequently (e.g., 1,000 mg every 8 hours rather than 1,500 mg every 12 hours) or infusing the dose for a longer interval, typically 2 hours. Alternatively, pretreatment with an antihistamine 1 hour before vancomycin administration is effective. In addition, tachyphylaxis to vancomycin-induced red man syndrome is independent of pretreatment with antihistamine and is another characteristic that differentiates a pseudoallergic reaction from a true allergic reaction. Pretreatment regimens to prevent pseudoallergic reactions to various other drugs (e.g., radiocontrast media) are also well described and can be effective.

CASE 32-6, QUESTION 5: What other drugs are commonly associated with pseudoallergic reactions?

Many other agents have been associated with pseudoallergic reactions.[7] Some of the agents more commonly associated with pseudoallergic reactions are described next.

Aspirin/Nonsteroidal Anti-Inflammatory Drugs

After penicillins, aspirin is the drug most commonly reported as causing "allergic" reactions. Reactions to aspirin can be divided into three broad categories: respiratory reactions, cutaneous manifestations, and anaphylaxis. None of these reactions has been consistently associated with IgE.[26,93]

RESPIRATORY

The prevalence of bronchospasm with rhinoconjunctivitis is 0% to 28% in children with aspirin sensitivity. In adult asthmatics, the prevalence of aspirin sensitivity ranges from 5% to 20%. The prevalence of aspirin sensitivity during aspirin challenge in adult asthmatics with a history of aspirin-induced respiratory reaction ranges from 66% to 97%.[94] Symptoms usually occur within 30 minutes to 3 hours of ingestion. The triad seen in many sensitive patients is aspirin sensitivity, nasal polyps, and asthma. All potent inhibitors of cyclo-oxygenase can cause respiratory symptoms in aspirin-sensitive patients. Thus, patients who react to aspirin should be considered sensitive to NSAIDs, and vice versa. Weak cyclo-oxygenase inhibitors, such as acetaminophen, choline magnesium salicylate, salicylamide, salsalate, and sodium salicylate, are generally well tolerated in patients with aspirin sensitivity.[93]

CUTANEOUS

The prevalence of cutaneous reactions to aspirin depends on the type of reaction and the population studied. For example, urticaria-angioedema occurs in 0.5% of children, 3.8% of the general adult population, and in 21% to 30% of patients with a history of chronic urticaria. Disease activity at the time of aspirin challenge plays an important role in those with a history of chronic urticaria. In one study, 70% of patients whose urticaria was active at the time of challenge reacted to aspirin, compared with only 6.6% of patients whose urticaria was not active at the time of challenge. Furthermore, aspirin or NSAID may aggravate preexisting urticaria.[93–95] Other dermatologic reactions to aspirin occur with less frequency; for example, eczema, purpura, and erythema multiforme occur in 2.4%, 1.5%, and 1% of the population, respectively.

ANAPHYLAXIS

The true prevalence of aspirin-induced or NSAID-induced anaphylaxis is unknown, but it may range from 0.07% of the general population to 10% of patients with anaphylactic symptoms. Although IgE is not consistently associated with aspirin or NSAID-related reactions (including anaphylaxis), aspirin-induced or NSAID-induced anaphylaxis shares three characteristics with immune-mediated anaphylaxis that point to IgE as a cause. First, the reaction occurs after two or more exposures to the offending agent, suggesting that preformed IgE antibodies are responsible. Second, patients do not have underlying nasal polyposis, asthma, or urticaria. Third, the patient who reacts to aspirin or a single NSAID can tolerate a chemically unrelated NSAID, suggesting that a drug-specific IgE antibody has been formed.[93,96]

The NSAIDs that selectively inhibit cyclo-oxygenase-2 (COX-2) while sparing cyclo-oxygenase-1 (COX-1) include celecoxib, rofecoxib, and valdecoxib, among others. Celecoxib is the only COX-2 inhibitor currently marketed in the United States. Selective inhibition of COX-2 provides anti-inflammatory effects while minimizing the renal effects, GI toxicity, and antiplatelet effects seen with inhibition of COX-1. Aspirin and older NSAIDs are nonselective inhibitors of cyclo-oxygenase, inhibiting both COX-1 and COX-2. Anaphylactoid or hypersensitivity reactions have been reported with celecoxib, and it appears that the rate of hypersensitivity is comparable to that of traditional NSAIDs.[96] Notably, celecoxib prescribing information states that, as with any NSAID, use is contraindicated in patients who have experienced asthma, urticaria, or allergic-type reactions after taking aspirin or other NSAIDs. Several reports, however, describe successful administration of celecoxib and other COX-2 selective agents to patients with aspirin-sensitive asthma or a history of hypersensitivity reactions to traditional NSAIDs, and evidence suggests that inhibition of COX-1 rather than COX-2 is key to initiating these events.[97–100] Nevertheless, COX-2 selective agents can still elicit allergic responses by other means (e.g., IgE-mediated hypersensitivity). Thus, appropriate precautions and monitoring should be followed when initiating therapy in any patient with a history of allergic reactions to aspirin or other NSAIDs.

Angiotensin-Converting Enzyme Inhibitors and Angiotensin II–Receptor Blockers

CASE 32-7

QUESTION 1: K.J., a 48-year-old woman, seeks care at an urgent care center. She presents with impaired speech but is able to swallow; she has red and swollen lips and tongue, and puffy eyes. Her medical history includes hypertension, atrial fibrillation, and a new diagnosis of hypercholesterolemia (plasma cholesterol, 290 mg/dL). Although her BP had been well controlled on hydrochlorothiazide, her diuretic was discontinued about 3 weeks ago because of its effect on cholesterol, and enalapril 5 mg daily was started. K.J. also takes a multivitamin (one tablet each day) and warfarin (5 mg daily). Her physical examination shows BP, 130/87 mm Hg; heart rate, 70 beats/minute; lungs clear to auscultation and percussion; respirations, 12 breaths/minute; and skin without rash or urticaria. Her condition is attributed to angioedema induced by enalapril. What is angioedema, and what evidence supports this diagnosis? What is the mechanism behind angioedema?

Angioedema refers to a localized, transient swelling of the deep skin layers or the upper respiratory or gastrointestinal mucosa. Angioedema commonly manifests as localized erythematous edema, involving the tongue, lips, eyelids, and mucous membranes of the mouth, nose, and throat. However, in rare cases it can occur in the lower gastrointestinal tract. Angioedema can be caused by a variety of mechanisms involving complement, histamine, substance P, and bradykinin that can be hereditary, immunologically acquired, or pharmacologic. ACE inhibitors are the most common pharmacologic cause and have been associated with this adverse effect in about 0.1% to 0.7% of individuals treated with this drug class and account for up to 60% of cases of angioedema that present to emergency departments.[101] The reaction is not dose-related and occurs with all ACE inhibitors. ACE inhibition causes accumulation of excess bradykinin leading to capillary leakage. Bradykinin receptor B2 is a G-protein–coupled receptor found in blood vessels and encoded by the *BDKRB2* gene in humans.[102]

K.J. presents with classic symptoms of angioedema and does not have symptoms of a true anaphylactic reaction, further strengthening the diagnosis of drug-induced angioedema. Symptoms of angioedema usually occur within the first week of starting therapy, although they can occur at any time, even years later. Thus, although angioedema developed 3 weeks after K.J. began enalapril, the temporal relationship is reasonable.

Case 32-7, Question 2: How should K.J. be treated? Would an angiotensin receptor blocker (ARB) be an appropriate substitute for her ACE inhibitor?

Although angioedema can be life-threatening, symptoms are usually mild and resolve within hours to days of stopping the offending drug. The most common life-threatening complication of angioedema is airway obstructions. More severe reactions affecting the upper airway must be treated emergently with appropriate measures to maintain airway patency. A small clinical trial of ACE-induced angioedema comparing treatment with corticosteroid and antihistamine (prednisolone 500 mg IV and clemastine 2 mg IV) to treatment with icatibant (30 mg subcutaneous injection) found that the time to initial relief and complete symptom resolution were significantly shorter with icatibant.[102] Additional trials are currently evaluating icatibant and hopefully will help define which patients will be most likely to benefit from this drug.

K.J. does not need to be hospitalized because her respirations are not compromised and she is not experiencing swallowing difficulty; however, she should be kept under observation at the urgent care center to ensure that her angioedema does not worsen. She can be treated with icatibant 30 mg subcutaneously or she can be observed and later sent home with instructions to seek emergent help if her breathing or swallowing becomes difficult. She should be instructed to discontinue her enalapril, follow up with her primary physician as soon as possible, and to request her community pharmacist to record this adverse reaction to enalapril into her drug profile at the pharmacy. Because angioedema occurs with all ACE inhibitors, K.J. must avoid all drugs in this class.

Angioedema with ARBs has also been reported,[103,104] although with less frequency than with ACE inhibitors. Many of the cases of ARB-induced angioedema involved patients with a history of ACE inhibitor–induced angioedema, but this is not consistently the case. Similar to the ACE inhibitors, angioedema to ARBs can occur at any time during treatment. In K.J.'s case, it would be best to avoid ARBs and ACE inhibitors. Instead, other antihypertensive agents that have little effect on cholesterol (e.g., calcium channel blockers) should be used.

Several other drugs have been associated with angioedema including aspirin, NSAIDs, antibiotics, radiocontrast media, and DPP-IV inhibitors (e.g., sitagliptin and saxagliptin).[101] The causes of angioedema with these drugs are less well understood but often occur after having ACE inhibitor–induced angioedema. These drug should be used with caution if KJ needs them in the future.

Case 32-7, Question 3: Are there other pseudoallergic reactions that occur with ACE inhibitors and ARBs?

Besides angioedema, cough is a pseudoallergic reaction caused by ACE inhibitors. It may occur in up to 39% of patients after 1 week to 6 months of therapy. Interestingly, it is more common in nonsmokers than in smokers; the incidence does not increase in patients with chronic airway disease or asthma. Cough is more common in women than men, is not dose-related, and, as with angioedema, occurs with all ACE inhibitors.[93,101,105] Several mechanisms appear to be responsible, including inhibition of the breakdown of bradykinin in the lung and increases in local mediators of inflammation such as prostaglandins and substance P. Although many approaches to the management of ACE-induced cough have been proposed,[105] angiotensin II–receptor blocking agents are the most promising alternative. Cough can occur with an ARB, but the frequency appears to be no more than that of placebo. Furthermore, most direct comparative trials between ARBs and ACE inhibitors demonstrate that the frequency of cough with ARBs is much lower than with ACE inhibitors.[105]

Radiocontrast Media

Radiocontrast media are widely used diagnostic agents, exceeding 75 million administrations annually.[106] Adverse reactions to radiocontrast media can be divided into immediate reactions (occurring within 1 hour of administration and include nausea, flushing, BP changes, bronchospasm, urticaria, angioedema, cardiac arrhythmias, convulsions, angina, and symptoms indistinguishable from true anaphylaxis) and non-immediate reactions (occurring 1 hour to 10 days after administration and include pruritus, maculopapular drug eruption, Stevens–Johnson syndrome, toxic epidermal necrolysis, and vasculitis). The cause of radiocontrast media reactions remains unknown, although histamine release, complement activation, and direct toxic effects on end organs might all play a role. Many of the adverse effects to radiocontrast media have historically been classified as pseudoallergic reactions because evidence did not support IgE mediation of these reactions. Recently, however, skin tests and laboratory evidence suggest an immunologic mechanism for radiocontrast media reactions.[106] The overall incidence of reaction to radiocontrast media is 0.7% to 13%, depending on the type of agent selected and whether the patient was pretreated before administration.[107] Conventional, ionic, high-osmolality contrast media produce reactions in 4% to 13% of recipients, whereas nonionic, low-osmolality agents produce fewer reactions (0.7%–3.1%). The mortality rate from radiocontrast media is 1 to 2 cases per 100,000 procedures and is the same for ionic and non-ionic agents.[108]

Female sex, a history of asthma, and a history of reaction to contrast media are risk factors for reactions to radiocontrast media. Of these, a history of reaction is the most important; 21% to 60% of patients with a history of reaction to radiocontrast media will have a reaction on reexposure.[106] Several pretreatment regimens have been developed to minimize such occurrences. For example, 32 mg of oral methylprednisolone given 12 hours and 2 hours before a procedure involving a high-osmolality contrast medium can reduce the reaction rate by up to 45%.[107] Another pretreatment regimen uses oral prednisone 50 mg taken 13 hours, 7 hours, and 1 hour before the procedure, plus diphenhydramine 50 mg orally or intramuscularly 1 hour before the examination.[109] This latter regimen lowers the occurrence of pseudoallergic reactions to high-osmolality contrast media, even in high-risk patients (i.e., those with a history of severe anaphylactoid reactions). Note that a "seafood allergy" is not a risk factor for a reaction to radiocontrast media. Patients with food allergies do not require special pretreatment prior to procedures involving these agents.[108,110]

Narcotic Analgesics

Some opiates stimulate histamine release and, thereby, cause hypotension, tachycardia, facial flushing, increased sweating, or pruritus. Severe reactions are uncommon, however. In many cases, the opiate can be continued with administration of an antihistamine to treat the symptoms. If the reaction is significant, a non-narcotic alternate analgesic may be considered, or an opiate that does not cause histamine release can be substituted. Morphine and meperidine cause the greatest histamine release in both in vitro and in vivo studies. Codeine, hydromorphone, oxycodone, and butorphanol stimulate histamine release less commonly; and levorphanol, fentanyl, sufentanil, methadone, and oxymorphone have little to no effect on histamine levels. One of the more frequent reactions to epidurally or intrathecally administered opiates is pruritus, which does not appear to be mediated by histamine because narcotics that do not release histamine (e.g., fentanyl and sufentanil) still cause pruritus after spinal administration. Furthermore, the pruritus tends to develop several hours after the opiate has been administered, when serum levels of histamine are insignificant. The cause of pruritus from spinal opiates remains unclear. The reaction can be managed with antihistamines and low-dose naloxone or nalbuphine, while continuing with the spinal narcotic.[91]

Iron-dextran Injection

Parenteral iron is used in the treatment of iron deficiency when oral iron preparations cannot be used or are ineffective. This is most commonly seen in patients with anemia of chronic renal failure, particularly those treated with epoetin alfa or darbepoetin and undergoing hemodialysis (Chapter 28, Chronic Kidney Diseases). Iron preparations are associated with a wide spectrum of adverse events (e.g., chest pain, hypotension, hypertension, abdominal pain, nausea, vomiting, weakness, syncope, backache, arthralgias, myalgias, and hypersensitivity reactions). Hypersensitivity reactions can be manifested as urticaria, sweating, dyspnea, rash, fever, and as anaphylactoid reactions, which can be fatal. Consistent with a nonimmunologic mechanism, hypersensitivity reactions to iron are not dose-related and can occur with the first drug exposure.[111]

Iron preparations differ in regard to the salt or carbohydrate carrier used, molecular weight, and rate of hypersensitivity reactions. The first commonly used iron preparations were iron dextran, available as a high-molecular weight ferric oxyhydroxide and dextran solution (Dexferrum) and later as a low-molecular weight ferric hydroxide and dextran solution (INFeD). Adverse events occur more often with iron dextran preparations compared to non-dextran preparations and are highest with high-molecular weight iron dextran. Data reported to the FDA MedWatch program between 2001 and 2003 was used to determine the odds of adverse events between iron dextran products and two non-dextran products: sodium ferric gluconate and iron sucrose (also known as iron saccharate). Relative to the InFeD brand of iron dextran, patients receiving sodium ferric gluconate or iron sucrose were half as likely to experience an allergic reaction or any adverse reaction. An equal risk existed of experiencing an allergic reaction, or any adverse reaction, between sodium ferric gluconate and iron sucrose. Although sodium ferric gluconate and iron sucrose were safer than iron dextran, at least one death and five life-threatening reactions were reported with each of the four agents studied.[112] Ferumoxytol, an agent approved in 2009, was designed with a modified dextrose shell to reduce hypersensitivity reactions. In a comparison trial, there was a comparable safety profile but did include one anaphylactoid reaction but no deaths compared to iron sucrose.[113] Since approval, post-marketing FDA surveillance has demonstrated several reports of life-threatening and serious anaphylactoid reactions, including six deaths in a 10-month reporting period.[114] The prescribing information has been updated to include a black box warning for fatal and serious hypersensitivity reactions.[115] The newest iron product is ferric carboxymatltose complex, which releases iron from a carbohydrate polymer. Hypersensitivity reactions are expected to be lower as it does not contain an dextran or modified dextran component. In comparison to iron sucrose, no significant difference was found in the rate of hypersensitivity reactions or anaphylactoid reactions.[116,117] Although approval FDA was initially delayed because of a potential safety imbalance in the risk of death, subsequent pooled analysis has not validated the early findings, and the product was approved with only a warning for hypersensitivity reactions.[118,119]

All patients receiving iron dextran should receive a test dose to assess tolerance, the other iron preparations do not require a test dose per their prescribing information. It appears iron dextran–tolerant patients have little risk of experiencing a serious hypersensitivity or anaphylactoid reaction to sodium ferric gluconate or iron sucrose injection and can safely be given one of these products without a prior test dose. Similarly, patients who have never received any parenteral iron product can be administered sodium ferric gluconate or iron sucrose for injection without a prior test dose. Although studies support the safety of both sodium ferric gluconate and iron sucrose for injection in iron dextran–sensitive patients, such patients may be at increased risk for an anaphylactoid reaction or other serious hypersensitivity response, and test dosing in this population may be reasonable. Because of the risks associated with any of the parenteral iron products, close monitoring of the patient for at least 30 minutes after drug administration is necessary and the availability of resuscitative medication and personnel trained to evaluate and address anaphylaxis is prudent.

PREVENTION AND MANAGEMENT OF ALLERGIC REACTIONS

CASE 32-8

QUESTION 1: A.M., a 40-year-old woman, is hospitalized with a diagnosis of community-acquired pneumonia. Her medical history is noncontributory except for an uneventful course of ampicillin 6 months before admission for an ear infection. A.M. is empirically treated with cefuroxime 0.75 g IV every 8 hours. On day 2 of therapy, she develops a raised pruritic maculopapular rash on her back, abdomen, and upper extremities. Antacid, docusate sodium, albuterol by metered-dose inhaler, and multivitamins were initiated on the same day as the cefuroxime. How should A.M.'s allergic reaction be managed? How might her allergic reaction have been prevented?

When examining methods to prevent allergic reactions, three possibilities exist: (a) the patient has unknowingly been sensitized to a drug and experiences an allergic reaction on receiving the same or a similar drug again; (b) the patient has a history of an allergic reaction to a medication and mistakenly receives the same or a similar medication a second time and again develops an allergic reaction; and (c) the patient has a history of an allergic reaction to a medication and intentionally receives the same or similar medication again. As in the first situation, A.M.'s allergic reaction was unpredictable and, therefore, could not be prevented. To prevent future allergic reactions (i.e., the second situation), however, A.M.'s reaction should be well documented in the medical chart and pharmacy records. In addition, all patients should undergo a thorough drug history on hospitalization. Careful attention should be paid to differentiating drug intolerance (e.g., stomach upset) from true allergic reactions, and any allergic reactions elicited during an interview should be documented appropriately. Adequate communication of allergic reactions is the single most important method of preventing their occurrence.

As described earlier, the first step in managing an allergic reaction is to determine its cause. Given A.M.'s history of exposure to ampicillin, the timing of the reaction, and the low frequency of allergic reactions to her other medications, cefuroxime is the most likely candidate. Second, a decision regarding whether to stop the suspect drug should be made. This decision must be based on the severity of the reaction, the condition being treated, and the availability of suitable alternatives. When possible, an equally effective alternative drug should be substituted for the suspect agent, preferably one that is immunologically distinct to avoid cross-sensitivity (see Case 32-1, Question 4, for a discussion of cross-reactivity).[120] If a suitable alternative exists, the offending agent should be stopped and the reaction treated symptomatically if necessary. In the case of A.M., another antimicrobial (e.g., azithromycin, clarithromycin, trimethoprim–sulfamethoxazole) could be substituted for cefuroxime (Chapter 67, Respiratory Tract Infections) and her symptoms treated with an oral or parenteral antihistamine, as well as a low-potency topical corticosteroid if necessary.

Some cases are described by the third situation: a patient develops an allergic reaction (or has a well-documented history of drug allergy), and it is inappropriate or not possible to change to an alternative drug. If the sensitivity reaction is severe or life-threatening, desensitization should be considered (Case 32-9, Questions 1 and 2); premedication to prevent or minimize anaphylaxis is not effective.[29] If the reaction is minor (e.g., pruritus, rash, or gastrointestinal symptoms), premedication or management of the reaction with antiallergy medications (e.g., antihistamines) might be sufficient to allow completion of therapy. It is rare in such cases for the reaction to progress to more serious allergic symptoms such as anaphylaxis[120]; however, suppression of allergic symptoms should be undertaken cautiously because many immunologic reactions are not IgE mediated and may progress to serious reactions, despite treatment. In general, allergy suppression should be reserved for prevention of mild reactions that are known or strongly suspected to be IgE mediated.[7,120]

Desensitization

β-LACTAMS

CASE 32-9

Question 1: K.A. is a 24-year-old primigravida in her eighth week of pregnancy with a history of angioedema secondary to penicillin. Her initial pregnancy screening revealed a positive Venereal Disease Research Laboratory reaction and a fluorescent treponemal antibody absorption titer of 1:64. K.A. denies a history of genital lesions, currently does not exhibit clinical signs or symptoms of syphilis, and denies previous treatment for syphilis. Based on the serologic evidence and her history, a diagnosis of early latent syphilis is made. Current treatment guidelines indicate that penicillin is the drug of choice for K.A. How can a possible reaction to penicillin be prevented in K.A.? Is premedication an alternative to preventing a reaction?

There are situations where a drug is medically necessary in a patient with a known or suspected allergy to the drug, alternative therapy is not available, and diagnostic testing does not exist. In such cases there are two options: induction of tolerance (also called desensitization) or a graded challenge. Desensitization is the process of administering gradually increasing doses of a drug in an effort to modify a patient's response to the drug so that it can then be safely administered.[108] This process has been used successfully to manage both immune-mediated and non–immune-mediated reactions. A graded challenge (also called incremental test dosing) is the process of careful administration of subtherapeutic doses of drug to determine if a patient is truly allergic. Although similar sounding, there are distinct differences between the two processes.[108] For example, unlike induction of tolerance, a graded challenge does not alter a patient's response to the drug. The initial drug doses used for inducing tolerance are sub-allergenic—as low as 1/10,000th of the final dose and the process can take several hours involving multiple doses, each slightly larger than the preceding dose. Starting doses for a graded challenge may be 1/100th of the final dose. The process generally involves fewer steps (as few as two) and can be typically accomplished more rapidly. If the graded challenge is completed and a therapeutic course of drug tolerated, a graded challenge is not required before future courses of the drug. Tolerance induction, on the other hand, is only maintained as long as the patient receives the suspect drug; any interruption of therapy will require the desensitization procedure to be repeated (see Case 32-9, Question 4).

The choice of drug desensitization or using a graded challenge depends on the likelihood of the patient having a true allergic reaction. A graded challenge may be appropriate in patients with a distant or unclear history of drug allergy; when the reaction seems minor or for which diagnostic testing is unavailable; or in cases where cross-reactivity is expected to be low. For example, a patient with a maculopapular rash to ceftriaxone may undergo a graded challenge to imipenem–cilastatin to assess tolerance. On the other hand, a patient with a well-described, severe IgE-mediated reaction to a drug may be better suited for tolerance induction. Importantly, graded challenge or tolerance induction should not be used in patients with a history of a severe non-IgE–mediated reaction such as hepatitis, hemolytic anemia, Stevens–Johnson syndrome, toxic epidermal necrolysis, or DRESS syndrome because of the risk of provoking a potentially life-threatening reaction.[108] Because K.A.'s reaction to penicillin may be potentially severe, premedication is not an option and desensitization to penicillin should be started. (See Chapter 72 Sexually Transmitted Diseases, for alternative therapy.)

CASE 32-9, QUESTION 2: How should K.A. be desensitized? Why should she be skin-tested before desensitization?

If possible before tolerance induction is begun, K.A. should be skin-tested (see Case 32-1, Questions 3 and 4) to confirm her penicillin allergy.[7,34,120] Patients who have a positive history of penicillin allergy, but whose skin tests are negative, can receive full therapeutic doses without desensitization with little risk of developing an allergic reaction. One author, for example, reported only one case of acute anaphylaxis in a skin test–negative patient given full therapeutic doses of penicillin in more than 1,500 skin tests; similar results have been reported by other investigators.[34,120] If skin testing cannot be performed or if K.A.'s skin test is positive, desensitization should be initiated. Acute oral desensitization to penicillin and other β-lactam antibiotics is well established.[121]

The oral route for β-lactam desensitization is preferred to the parenteral route because (a) exposure by the oral route is less likely to cause a systemic allergic reaction than parenteral exposure; (b) fatal anaphylaxis from oral β-lactam drug therapy is rare; (c) preformed polymers and conjugates of penicillin major and minor determinants to *Penicillium* proteins are not well absorbed after oral administration; (d) blood levels rise gradually, favoring univalent haptenation; and (e) fatal or life-endangering reactions have not occurred using current methods. In addition, oral desensitization can be accomplished over several hours.[7] If oral desensitization is not possible (e.g., if oral absorption is questionable), parenteral desensitization can be instituted. Although the subcutaneous and IM routes have been used, the IV route is quicker and allows better control over the rate and concentration of drug administered, and any untoward reaction can be detected promptly and treated rapidly.[7,122] Oral and parenteral desensitization methods have not been compared formally, however. Patients should not be premedicated before desensitization, because this may prevent detection of minor allergic responses that may precede more serious reactions. In addition, only experienced personnel should undertake desensitization in an appropriate setting where emergency resuscitative equipment is readily available because severe reactions can develop.[120] Thus, K.A. should undergo oral desensitization if her skin test is positive or if skin testing cannot be performed.

CASE 32-9, QUESTION 3: Is K.A. at risk for an allergic reaction during tolerance induction? If tolerance induction is successful, is she at risk for a reaction during full-dose penicillin therapy?

Acute β-lactam desensitization, regardless of the route or protocol chosen, is not without risk. Approximately 5% of patients experience mild cutaneous reactions during desensitization, although one study reported reactions in 20% of patients during oral desensitization.[7,123] If a reaction occurs during the desensitization procedure itself, the reaction may be treated and desensitization continued using lower doses, increased intervals between doses, or both, after the reaction has abated. Severe, fatal reactions during desensitization are rare.[122]

Uneventful β-lactam desensitization, however, does not guarantee patients will be without reaction during full-dose therapy. Approximately 25% to 30% of patients experience a mild reaction during therapy, and 5% experience more severe reactions, including drug-induced serum sickness, hemolytic anemia, or urticaria.[7] Reaction rates are no different in severely ill or pregnant patients compared with stable or nonpregnant patients, although those with cystic fibrosis may be more difficult to desensitize because of their high frequency of allergic reactions.[123,124] Despite the occurrence of reactions, full-dose therapy is possible for most tolerance-induction procedures, but suppression of the reaction (e.g., by diphenhydramine) may be required.[122] Tolerance induction is also dose-dependent as allergic symptoms can appear after a substantial increase in the dose after tolerance has been achieved.[7]

CASE 32-9, QUESTION 4: If K.A. requires penicillin at a later date, will she need to undergo desensitization again? What is chronic desensitization?

The desensitized state, once achieved, will persist for approximately 48 hours after the last full dose of antibiotic; after this time, drug sensitivity will return.[7,122] Thus, if K.A. requires future courses of penicillin, she will need to undergo desensitization once again. In some cases, those requiring long-term antibiotic therapy (e.g., for endocarditis), those who may require β-lactams at a future date (e.g., those with cystic fibrosis), or those who have occupational exposure to β-lactams, maintenance of the desensitized state can be considered. Chronic twice daily dosing of oral penicillin has safely resulted in "chronic desensitization." Similar to acute desensitization, once therapy is interrupted, the allergic state returns.[7,27]

OTHER DRUGS

CASE 32-9, QUESTION 5: Have patients allergic to drugs besides β-lactams been desensitized successfully?

Although most experience with desensitization is with penicillin and other β-lactams, desensitization also has been accomplished with numerous other drugs, including allopurinol, vancomycin, antineoplastic agents, aspirin, and monoclonal antibodies.[66,123,124] Interestingly, not all of these cases represent IgE-mediated hypersensitivity reactions. For example, reactions to trimethoprim–sulfamethoxazole commonly occur in patients infected with HIV and may not be IgE mediated. Yet, given its role in treating and preventing *Pneumocystis jiroveci* pneumonia, successful desensitization to trimethoprim–sulfamethoxazole is commonly used.[124]

KEY REFERENCES AND WEBSITES

A full list of references for this chapter can be found at http://thepoint.lww.com/AT11e. Below are the key references and websites for this chapter, with the corresponding reference number in this chapter found in parentheses after the reference.

Key References

Antonov D et al. Drug-induced lupus erythematosus. *Clin Dermatol.* 2004;22:157. (77)

Baile GR. Comparison of rates of reported adverse events associated with IV iron products in the United States. *Am J Health Syst Pharm.* 2012;69:310. (114)

Barbarino J et al. PharmGKB summary: very important pharmacogene information for human leukocyte antigen B. *Pharmacogenet Genomics.* 2015;25:205. (18)

Baş M et al. A randomized trial of icatibant in ACE-inhibitor–induced angioedema. *N Engl J Med.* 2015;372:418. (102)

Dedeoglu F. Drug-induced autoimmunity. *Curr Opin Rheumatol.* 2009;21:547. (73)

Demoly P et al. International consensus on drug allergy. *Allergy.* 2014; 69: 420. (1)

Frumin J, Gallagher JC. Allergic cross-sensitivity between penicillin, carbapenem, and monobactam antibiotics: what are the chances? *Ann Pharmacother.* 2009;43:304. (46)

Kemp SF et al. Epinephrine: the drug of choice for anaphylaxis. A statement of the World Allergy Organization. *Allergy*. 2008;63:1061. (57)
Lieberman P et al. The diagnosis and management of anaphylaxis practice parameter: 2010 update [published correction appears in *J Allergy Clin Immunol*. 2010;126:1104]. *J Allergy Clin Immunol*. 2010;126:477. (49)
Patel RA, Gallagher JC. Drug fever. *Pharmacotherapy*. 2010;30:57. (68)
Sanchez-Borges M. NSAID hypersensitivity (respiratory, cutaneous, and generalized anaphylactic symptoms). *Med Clin North Am*. 2010;94:853. (95)
Schnyder B. Approach to the patient with drug allergy. *Immunol Allergy Clin North Am*. 2009;29:405. (66)
Solensky R. Drug desensitization. *Immunol Allergy Clin North Am*. 2004;24:425. (122)

33 Systemic Lupus Erythematosus

Jerika T. Lam, Ann M. Lynch, and Mary A. Gutierrez

CORE PRINCIPLES

		CHAPTER CASES
1	Systemic lupus erythematosus (SLE) affects multiple organ systems with diagnoses based on clinical findings and objective criteria from the American College of Rheumatology (ACR) and Systemic Lupus Collaborating Clinics (SLICC) guidelines.	**Case 33-1 (Questions 1–4), Case 33-2 (Question 1), Table 33-2, Figure 33-1**
2	Management of SLE is complex and involves many specialists, including cardiologists and rheumatologists.	**Case 33-2 (Question 2)**
3	SLE treatment includes NSAIDs, corticosteroids, antimalarials, and immunosuppressants. The goals of SLE treatment should be considered when devising a treatment plan.	**Case 33-2 (Question 3), Case 33-3 (Questions 1–3, 5–6), Table 33-4**
4	Pregnancy considerations should be applied when selecting drug treatments for female patients with SLE.	**Case 33-3 (Questions 7–8)**
5	Hydroxychloroquine and cyclophosphamide could cause bothersome side effects. Monitoring parameters and management of hydroxychloroquine and cyclophosphamide side effects should be considered for SLE patients.	**Case 33-3 (Questions 4, 9–11), Table 33-4**
6	Belimumab is the first FDA-approved biologic treatment for SLE. The appropriate use and monitoring parameters should be considered to optimize its efficacy.	**Case 33-3 (Questions 12–17), Table 33-3, Table 33-4**
7	There are several drug–drug interactions pertaining to the treatments for SLE. Concomitant use of hydroxychloroquine and antacids could have a potential adverse effect.	**Case 33-4 (Questions 1, 2), Table 33-5**
8	Pharmacists can play an important role in the education of SLE, management of side effects, and monitoring of drug–drug interactions.	**Case 33-3 (Questions 2, 3, 5-9, 13), Case 33-4 (Questions 2–3), Table 33-4, Table 33-5, Table 33-6**

GENERAL PRINCIPLES

Systemic lupus erythematosus (SLE) is a chronic, autoimmune, inflammatory disease that affects multiple organ systems and primarily the connective tissue. Its presentation and disease progression are unpredictable and highly variable. This multi-organ disease is characterized by inflammation, autoantibody production, the deposition of complement-fixing immune complexes, and a clinical pattern alternating between disease flares and periods of remission.[1] In essence, the immune system attacks the body's own cells and tissue, resulting in a continuous inflammatory response and tissue and/or organ damage over time. While SLE can eventually affect any organ such as the lungs, nervous system, and cardiovascular, it mainly affects the skin, joints, and kidneys.[2] The 10-year survival rate is approximately 70% for patients with SLE.[3]

EPIDEMIOLOGY

SLE is more common among women than men (9:1) and generally occurs during childbearing age, with a peak age of onset between 15 and 45 years.[4,5] It is estimated that more than 16,000 new cases of SLE are reported annually in the U.S. with an average prevalence of 1.5 million Americans. Approximately 5 million people are afflicted with SLE globally.[6] Progression of SLE is usually slow. It typically begins as a benign disease without signs or symptoms (preclinical phase) to disease with mild-to-moderate symptoms with exacerbations or flares, resulting in the involvement of additional organs and sustained damage (clinical phase). Over time the disease will progress, continually relapsing and remitting until eventually reaching severe potentially fatal disease (comorbidities phase).[7] Isolated skin and musculoskeletal involvement are associated with a milder course of disease and a higher survival rate over patients with renal and CNS involvement, which indicate more severe and progressive disease conditions.

PATHOPHYSIOLOGY

The specific cause of SLE is unknown. Many genetic, ethnic, environmental, and hormonal factors are identified as potential causative risk factors. As part of the genetic component involved in the development of SLE, there is no clear Mendelian pattern of inheritance. Siblings of patients with SLE have a risk disease of approximately 2%.[8] Identical twins have approximately 10-fold higher risk of SLE than dizygotic twins.[4] First degree relatives of patients with SLE have a 20-fold increased risk of developing SLE when compared to the healthy population.[9,10] The genetic risk for the disease is more likely associated with multiple genes than the deficiency of a single gene. Interestingly, genome-wide association studies have identified risk alleles shared between SLE and other autoimmune disorders such as rheumatoid arthritis, Graves' disease, multiple sclerosis, type 1 diabetes, and psoriasis.[11] SLE is more likely to develop in women of color, at a rate of 2 to 3 times higher than the rate for Caucasian women.[6] Furthermore, the symptoms are found to be more severe in African-American, Asian, Native American, and Hispanic women.[4,12] However, individuals of all ages, genders, and ancestral backgrounds are susceptible to having the disease.

The association of environmental factors to SLE remains unclear. Some of the exposure-related factors that have been implicated for causing SLE include smoking and ultraviolet radiation.[13] The proposed hypothesis behind cigarette smoke is that it is associated with the indirect generation of anti-double stranded-DNA (anti-dsDNA) and related to immunoregulatory effects of tobacco exposure. Thus, in genetically predisposed individuals with a smoking-related decreased ability to clear apoptotic cells, the excess levels of intracellular antigens may lead to the production of autoantibodies such as anti-dsDNA.[14]

UV Radiation

Exposure to sunlight may cause the occurrence of SLE and could exacerbate preexisting symptoms. Ultraviolet radiation has been implicated in cutaneous manifestations of SLE, such as macular, papular or bullous lesions, and erythema.[15] Systemic disease is rarely induced by ultraviolet radiation. Possible mechanisms that may link the pathogenesis of ultraviolet radiation and SLE include circulating antibodies to the Ro/Sjogren's syndrome type A (anti-Ro/SSA) and anti-La Sjogren's syndrome type B (anti-La/SSB) antigen particles that result in an autoimmune response.[2,15] Nevertheless, both anti-Ro/SSA and anti-La/SSB are more commonly associated with Sjogren's syndrome than with SLE.

Viral Infection

It has been considered for many years that viruses, particularly the herpes families and the Epstein–Barr virus (EBV) may trigger SLE via polyclonal immune activation, resulting in an activation of the autoimmune system.[16] EBV may reside in and interact with B cells, promoting interferon alpha production and contributing to the inflammatory process.

Female Hormones

The increased prevalence in the female gender proposes that hormones such as estrogen or progesterone may play a role in aggravating the disease. Both estrogen and progesterone levels are increased during pregnancy and at conception. These hormones can lead to an increase in mature, high-affinity autoreactive B cells, resulting in an autoimmune reaction.[17] Evidence that SLE worsens during pregnancy ironically does not contribute to this theory as levels of estrogen and progesterone are lower in second- and third-trimester pregnant patients with SLE compared to healthy pregnant patients.[17] Interestingly, hormone replacement therapy is linked to worsening SLE symptoms in postmenopausal women.[18] The X chromosome may also independently contribute to the incidence of SLE, where the combination of two X chromosomes increases the severity of SLE over an XY combination.[19] The gene CD40 is located on the X chromosome and has been known to contribute to the pathogenesis of the disease.[13]

Immunologic Abnormalities

SLE is a disease of an overall dysregulated, aberrant immune function, indicated by a large number of autoantibodies involved. Abnormalities of the immune system include immune complexes, T lymphocytes, cytokines, and antibodies.[13] Antigen receptor-mediated activation is changed in T and B cells for patients with SLE. B cells play a pivotal role in the disease. They produce autoantibodies, which amplify inflammation and mediate tissue damage. The autoantibodies are immunoglobulin G (IgG)-mediated, and T lymphocytes help stimulate B cells to produce antibodies. Moreover, B cells process and present antigen and autoantigen to T cells and contribute to disease manifestation.[20] The innate immune system (i.e., toll receptors, plasmacytoid dendritic cells, and interferon alpha) and adaptive immune network also contribute to the production of autoreactive B cells and autoantibodies.[21] Similarly, cellular debris from apoptosis further stimulate activation of the immune system. The decreased clearance of cellular debris may be related to low-complement levels, such as C1q, C2, and C4, which normally function to help phagocytes and macrophages eliminate apoptotic material and self-reactive B cells. As a result, deposits of immune complexes can lead to organ damage, systemic inflammation, and pain.[5,13]

CLASSIFICATION CRITERIA

In 1971, the Diagnostic and Therapeutic Criteria Committee of the American College of Rheumatology (ACR) developed a disease classification criteria system. As there is no single test to diagnose SLE, the classification criteria have been used for the diagnosis of SLE. The original classification was revised in 1982 and again in 1997 to include more organs than just cutaneous involvement (Table 33-1).[22] In 2012, the Systemic Lupus Collaborating Clinics (SLICC) revised and validated the ACR SLE classification criteria in order to improve its clinical relevance and incorporate updated information about immunology in SLE (Table 33-2).[23] Either classification system, ACR 1997 or SLICC 2012, can be used.

CLINICAL PRESENTATION

The clinical features of the disease are diverse and vary among patients. Signs and symptoms may be subtle early in the course of the disease; and the spectrum of mild to severe symptoms may fluctuate, with periods of remission, throughout the disease process.[24] Clinical patterns of the disease can be categorized as constitutional, musculoskeletal, and mucocutaneous.

Constitutional symptoms usually include fatigue, general malaise, fever, and weight loss. These may occur in the early stages of the disease. Fatigue is the most common complaint and can be a debilitating symptom early on.[25,26] Musculoskeletal symptoms include arthritis, arthralgia, and myalgia. Early in the

Table 33-1
American College of Rheumatology Revised Criteria for Classification of Systemic Lupus Erythematosus, 1982 with 1997 Updates[22,46]

Criterion	Definition
1. Malar rash	Fixed erythema, flat or raised, over the malar eminences, tending to spare the nasolabial folds
2. Discoid rash	Erythematous raised patches with adherent keratotic scaling and follicular plugging; atrophic scarring may occur in older lesions
3. Photosensitivity	Skin rash as a result of unusual reaction to sunlight, by patient history or physician observation
4. Oral ulcers	Oral or nasopharyngeal ulceration, usually painless, observed by physician
5. Arthritis, non-erosive	Involving two or more peripheral joints, characterized by tenderness, swelling, or effusion
6. Serositis	Pleuritis—convincing history of pleuritic pain or rubbing heard by a physician or evidence of pleural effusion *Or* Pericarditis—documented by electrocardiogram (ECG) or rub or evidence of pericardial effusion
7. Renal disorder	Persistent proteinuria >0.5 g/day or >3+ if quantitation not performed *Or* Cellular casts—may be red cell, hemoglobin, granular, tubular, or mixed
8. Neurologic disorder	Seizures—in the absence of offending drugs or known metabolic derangements (e.g., uremia, ketoacidosis, or electrolyte imbalance) *Or* Psychosis—in the absence of offending drugs or known metabolic derangements (e.g., uremia, ketoacidosis, or electrolyte imbalance)
9. Hematologic disorder	Hemolytic anemia—with reticulocytosis *Or* Leukopenia—<4,000/mm^3 on ≥2 occasions *Or* Lyphopenia—<1,500/mm^3 on ≥2 occasions *Or* Thrombocytopenia—<100,000/mm^3 in the absence of offending drugs
10. Immunologic disorder	Anti-DNA: antibody to native DNA in abnormal titer *Or* Anti-Sm: presence of antibody to Sm nuclear antigen *Or* Positive finding of antiphospholipid antibodies on ■ an abnormal serum level of IgG or IgM anticardiolipin antibodies, ■ a positive test result for lupus anticoagulant using a standard method, *Or* ■ a false-positive test result for at least 6 months confirmed by *Treponema pallidum* immobilization or fluorescent treponemal antibody absorption test
11. Positive antinuclear antibody	An abnormal titer of antinuclear antibody by immunofluorescence or an equivalent assay at any point in time and in the absence of drugs associated with drug-induced lupus syndrome

Anti-DNA, anti-deoxyribonucleic acid; Anti-Sm, anti-Smith antibodies; IgG and IgM, immunoglobulins G and M.

course of the disease the symptoms may be confused with rheumatoid arthritis, especially with intermittent symmetric arthritic and joint pain. Arthritis associated with SLE is non-erosive and does not damage the joint even though it affects the joints of the hands, wrist, knees, and feet. Myopathy may also be present during periods of active disease, or secondary to treatment of hydroxychloroquine and corticosteroids.[27]

Mucocutaneous manifestations occur frequently in patients with SLE. The malar or butterfly rash across the face is one of the classic cutaneous signs; however, it may not be present in all patients with SLE. It is an erythematous skin rash distributing over the cheeks and the bridge of the nose but spares the nasolabial folds. It can persist for weeks and resolves without scarring. The malar rash should be differentiated from flushing, glucocorticoid-induced dermal atrophy, rosacea, seborrheic, atopic, and contact dermatitis.[2] Other cutaneous signs may include alopecia, discoid lesions, photosensitivity reactions, periungual erythema, nail fold infarcts, and splinter hemorrhages.[28,29] In comparison, mucosal symptoms can include vasculitis and painful, recurrent ulcers in the mouth, nose, and genital cavity.[27] Raynaud's phenomenon may also occur in patients with SLE. It is described as a vasospastic disorder of the extremities, commonly affecting the hands and is characterized by color changes as a result of decreased temperature or intense stress.[18] It can also lead to avascular bone necrosis, which is a major cause of disability in SLE patients.[2]

Additional clinical presentation of SLE may include the development of antiphospholipid antibodies (e.g., lupus anti-*β*2-glycoprotein, IgG and IgM anticardiolipin antibodies, and IgG and IgM anti-*β*2-glycoprotein I) in the blood and places patients with SLE at increased risk for developing blood clots.[30] Livedo reticularis is a common feature of antiphospholipid syndrome (APS), which will be further discussed in the hematologic section. Common symptoms of SLE are described in Figure 33-1. Other major organ systems may also be affected by SLE, including the nervous system, cardiovascular, pulmonary, gastrointestinal (GI), renal, and hematologic.

Table 33-2
Systemic Lupus International Collaborating Clinics Classification Criteria 2012 for Classifying Systemic Lupus Erythematosus[23]

A patient can be classified as having SLE if he/she	■ Satisfies 4 of the criteria listed in Table 33-1 including at least one clinical criterion and one immunologic criterion *Or* ■ Has biopsy-proven nephritis compatible with SLE and with antinuclear antibody (ANA) or anti-dsDNA antibodies
Clinical and Immunologic Criteria Used in the SLICC Classification Criteria[a]	
Clinical Criteria	
1. Acute cutaneous lupus (includes lupus malar rash; do not count if malar discoid) and the following:	■ Bullous lupus ■ Toxic epidermal necrolysis variant of SLE ■ Maculopapular lupus rash ■ Photosensitive lupus rash in the absence of dermatomyositis *Or* ■ Subacute cutaneous lupus ■ Nonindurated psoriaform and/or annular polycyclic lesions that resolve without scarring, although occasionally with post-inflammatory depigmentation or telangiectasia

2. Chronic cutaneous lupus includes the following:	■ Classic discoid rash
	  ■ Localized (above the neck)
	  ■ Generalized (above and below the neck)
	■ Hypertrophic (verrucous) lupus
	■ Lupus panniculitis (profundus)
	■ Mucosal lupus
	■ Lupus erythematosus tumidus
	■ Chilblains lupus
	■ Discoid lupus/lichen planus overlap

3. Oral ulcers include the following: (in the absence of other causes, such as vasculitis, Behcet's disease, infection (herpes virus), inflammatory bowel disease, reactive arthritis, and acidic foods)	■ Palate
	  ■ Buccal
	  ■ Tongue
	Or
	■ Nasal ulcers

4. Non-scarring alopecia (in the absence of other causes such as alopecia areata, drugs, iron deficiency, and androgenic alopecia)	■ Diffuse thinning or hair fragility with visible broken hairs

5. Synovitis	■ Involving two or more joints
	■ Characterized by
	  ■ Swelling or effusion
	Or
	  ■ Tenderness in two or more joints *and* at least 30 minutes of morning stiffness

6. Serositis	■ Typical pleurisy for more than 1 day *Or* ■ Pericardial effusion *Or* ■ Pericardial rub *Or* ■ Pericarditis by electrocardiography
7. Renal (in the absence of other causes, such as infection, uremia, and Dressler's pericarditis)	■ Urine protein-to-creatinine ratio (or 24-hour protein) representing 500 mg of protein/24 hour *Or* ■ Red blood cell casts
8. Neurologic	■ Seizures ■ Psychosis ■ Mononeuritis multiplex in the absence of other known causes, such as primary vasculitis ■ Myelitis ■ Peripheral or cranial neuropathy, in the absence of other known causes, such as primary vasculitis, infection, and diabetes mellitus ■ Acute confusional state, in the absence of other causes, including toxic/metabolic, uremia, drugs

(continued)

Table 33-2
Systemic Lupus International Collaborating Clinics Classification Criteria 2012 for Classifying Systemic Lupus Erythematosus[23] (*continued*)

9. Hemolytic anemia	
10. Leukopenia	■ <4,000/mm^3 at least once (in the absence of other known causes, such as Felty's syndrome, drugs, portal hypertension, and thrombotic thrombocytopenia purpura)
Immunologic Criteria	
1. ANA	■ Level above laboratory reference range
2. Anti-dsDNA	■ Antibody above laboratory reference range (or >2-fold the reference range if tested by ELISA)
3. Anti-Sm	■ Presence of antibody to Sm nuclear antigen
4. Antiphospholipid antibody positivity as determined by any of the following:	■ Positive test result for lupus anticoagulant ■ False-positive test for RPR ■ Medium- or high-titer anti-β2-glycoprotein antibody level (IgA, IgG, or IgM) ■ Positive test result for anti-β2-glycoprotein I (IgA, IgG, or IgM)
5. Low complement	■ Low C3 ■ Low C4 ■ Low CH50
6. Direct Coombs' test	■ In the absence of hemolytic anemia

[a]Criteria are cumulative and need not be present concurrently.
ELISA, enzyme-linked immunosorbent assay; Anti-dsDNA, anti-double stranded deoxyribonucleic acid; Anti-Sm, anti-Smith antibodies; RPR, rapid plasma reagin.

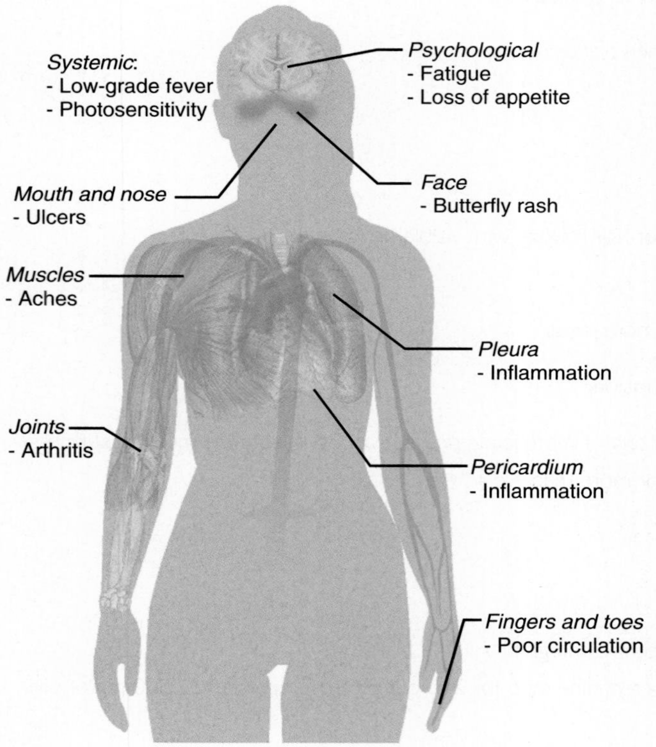

Figure 33-1 Common symptoms of systemic lupus erythematosus. (Source: Haggstrom, Mikael/Wikipedia Commons/ Public Domain. http://www.commons.wikipedia.org/wiki/File:SymptomsofSLE.png. Accessed July 26, 2015.)

Nervous System

SLE affects both the central nervous system (CNS) and peripheral nervous system. The CNS manifestations affect approximately two-thirds of patients with SLE.[30] Collectively, both have been described as neuropsychiatric syndromes. The pathology of the syndromes is not well understood. The syndromes may be ascribed to the autoimmune nature of SLE, where the immune anti-neuronal antibodies attack the neurons causing neuronal damage and leading to cognitive dysfunction, or the production of antiphospholipid antibodies that damage blood vessels and may cause clots in the brain.[28] Neuropsychiatric manifestations are nonspecific and variable. They may occur in less than 40% of patients with SLE, while the remaining events represent complications of the disease, therapies and therapy-related side effects, infections, and metabolic abnormalities.[31] Patients with SLE can present with higher rates of anxiety and depression. Depression is more common in those experiencing changes in appearance and limitations from complications and medication-related side effects.[32] Other manifestations include migraine headaches, memory loss, and seizures. Less common symptoms may also occur, such as psychosis, confusion, peripheral neuropathy, mood disorders, autonomic dysfunction, movement disorders, Guillain–Barre, and cerebrovascular disease.[27] Diagnosis and laboratory tests for neuropsychiatric events related to SLE continue to be challenging, as well as the therapies used for them.[33]

Cardiovascular

Patients with SLE are at increased risk of morbidity and mortality from cardiovascular disease, especially associated with atherosclerosis. Premature atherosclerosis is associated with longer lupus disease duration, more damage, and less aggressive immunosuppressive therapy.[34,35] They are at higher risk for myocardial infarction or stroke compared to the healthy population. In addition, pericarditis and pericardial effusion are the most common cardiac complications associated with SLE, occurring in approximately 45% of patients.[28,29,30,36] They range from mild-to-severe symptomatology. Patients may present with fever, dyspnea, tachycardia, and congestive heart failure. Other clinical features that may occur in more than 80% of patients with SLE include left ventricular dysfunction, segmental wall motion abnormalities, nonspecific ST-T wave changes, and decreased ejection fraction.[2] Valvular abnormalities can also be common and are linked to antiphospholipid antibodies. The most common abnormality is diffuse thickening of the mitral and aortic valves followed by the presence or absence of nonbacterial vegetations (Libman–Sacks), valvular regurgitation, and stenosis.[2] Modifiable risk factors, in addition to comorbid disease screening, include reducing long-term steroid use as it is linked to the development of hypertension, smoking cessation, reducing homocysteine levels with folate supplementation, and preventing thrombosis with aspirin or anticoagulation in patients with APS.[27] These will help to reduce cardiovascular risk and control disease activity by reducing the inflammatory atherogenic effects.

CASE 33-1

QUESTION 1: T.C. is a 45-year-old Hispanic woman with hypertension, hypercholesterolemia, and an 18-year history of SLE. For the first 10 years after the diagnosis of SLE, she had frequent SLE flares and was treated with high-doses of prednisone. As a result, she developed steroid-induced diabetes and osteoporosis. Though her SLE has been relatively stable over the past 2 years, she has not been feeling well 1 month ago. T.C. denies symptoms consistent with her usual SLE flares, but she reports a sharp chest pain that worsens when lying down and improves when leaning forward, significant fatigue and shortness of breath with minor activity. She feels better after resting but has not returned to her previous energy level. She reports good adherence with her medications, which include the following:

Alendronate 70 mg weekly
Hydrochlorothiazide 25 mg every morning
Hydroxychloroquine 400 mg daily
Lisinopril 40 mg daily
Metformin 1,000 mg twice daily
Simvastatin 40 mg daily
Acetaminophen 650 mg prn pain

Findings from an examination of the patient are unremarkable, except for elevated blood pressure. Lupus anticoagulant antibodies are within normal limits. What is the most likely cause of T.C.'s complaints of fatigue and positional chest pain?

Patients with long-standing SLE are at increased risk for cardiovascular disease. Given that T.C.'s SLE is stable, cardiovascular disease is the most likely cause of her current symptoms.

CASE 33-1, QUESTION 2: What tests would best confirm your suspicion?

Electrocardiograms (EKGs), exercise stress tests, and echocardiograms. Cardiac stress test is also considered a best way to determine the presence and extent of her cardiovascular disease, especially for symptomatic patients.

CASE 33-1, QUESTION 3: Along with a referral to a cardiologist, which of the following treatments would you recommend that T.C. initiate at this time?

Aspirin is recommended because her most likely diagnosis is cardiovascular disease. She has no evidence of active SLE, so aspirin would be the most appropriate treatment at this time to prevent risk of thrombosis. Premature atherosclerosis with cardiovascular events tends to manifest as a late complication for patients with SLE. Oral anticoagulants may be considered for T.C. if she has developed antiphospholipid antibodies and APS.

CASE 33-1, QUESTION 4: Late in the disease course of SLE, what is the most common cause of high mortality rates?

Early in the disease course, mortality is primarily from inflammation affecting organ systems. Over time, mortality tends to be mostly from coronary artery disease and complications of chronic steroid therapy and immunosuppression. SLE disease could elevate the LDL and reduce the HDL levels in addition to treatment with systemic steroids that could worsen the cholesterol profile.

Pulmonary

Pulmonary involvement occurs in 30% of patients with SLE.[30] Pleuritis or pleural inflammation is the most common pulmonary manifestation of SLE. It is associated with chest pain, cough, and dyspnea. Pleural effusions are typical findings and are usually linked with antinuclear antibody (ANA)-positive exudates with low complement.[37] Alveolar hemorrhage is a common occurrence in patients with SLE, particularly in those with high titers of anti-dsDNA antibodies and active extrapulmonary disease.[30] Another respiratory complication is identified as the "shrinking lung syndrome," which can occur in 25% of SLE patients.[2] It is characterized as progressive dyspnea (worse in the supine position) and weakness of the diaphragm and respiratory muscles. Acute lupus pneumonitis and pulmonary hypertension, although rare, could also develop as pulmonary complications.

Gastrointestinal

Nonspecific GI symptoms include abdominal pain, nausea, vomiting, diarrhea, and stomach upset. These are reported in 25% to 40% of patients with SLE, which could be disease-related or from medication side effects.[2] Other clinical manifestations include dyspepsia and peptic ulcers.

Renal

Up to 70% of all SLE patients will develop some form of renal complication, which is a poor prognostic indicator. Approximately 60% will have kidney involvement in the first 10 years of the disease.[18] Thirty-five percent of patients will develop nephrotic syndrome or lupus nephritis (LN) by the time of SLE diagnosis.[38] It is a serious kidney complication, which increases the risk of renal failure, cardiovascular disease, and mortality.[39] LN is caused by inflammation and deposits of immune complexes consisting of anti-dsDNA in the glomeruli. It includes proteinuria (>0.5 g/24 hours) and/or hematuria, described as active urinary sediment (>5 RBCs per high-power field, pyuria, or cell casts), in addition to a significant creatinine clearance reduction. For patients with inactive sediment and >500 mg/day of proteinuria, monitoring is recommended with urinalysis every 3 to 6 months for 3 years. More frequent monitoring, such as every 3 months, is preferred for patients with anti-dsDNA antibodies and/or hypocomplementemia.[40]

Aside from performing a urinalysis, a renal biopsy is required in all lupus patients with evidence of kidney involvement to determine the histologic subtype of LN and the extent of disease severity.[41,42] Pathology reports can elucidate the extent of inflammatory (reversible) and chronic (irreversible scarring) changes. LN can be an ongoing disease, with flares often requiring repeat biopsy and repeat treatment (refer to Chapter 28, Chronic Kidney Disease for Lupus Nephritis, Case 28-4).

Hematologic

Hematologic disorders can occur in patients with SLE. The most common hematologic manifestation is normochromic, normocytic anemia, which is often overlooked in young menstruating women. Iron deficiency may also develop. A common cause of anemia is suppressed erythropoiesis from chronic inflammation. Patients may have a positive Coombs test without apparent hemolysis.[42] Leukopenia and thrombocytopenia are also common manifestations that can develop as part of the disease process, or may be a side effect of the pharmacologic treatment for SLE. Oftentimes, leukopenia consists of lymphopenia, not granulocytopenia.[43] Patients with SLE may also develop a thrombotic disorder known as APS. APS is characterized by the development of autoantibodies to phospholipids present in the serum. Antiphospholipid antibodies interfere with the coagulation system, particularly protein C and the function of endothelial cells.[13] APS features are described as venous or arterial thrombosis, miscarriages or spontaneous abortions, and thrombocytopenia from antiphospholipid antibodies.[27] The European League Against Rheumatism (EULAR) recommends low-dose aspirin in individuals with SLE and antiphospholipid antibodies as primary prevention of thrombosis and pregnancy loss.[7] Long-term use of oral anticoagulants is considered as secondary prevention of thrombosis in nonpregnant patients with SLE and thrombosis associated with APS. On the other hand, unfractionated or low-molecular-weight heparin and aspirin should be used in pregnant patients with SLE and APS.

Lymphadenopathy could be a common presentation in SLE, where it may occur in 15% to 26% in patients. Diffuse lymphadenopathy, however, is a very rare occurrence.[44,45] Lymph node biopsy may be considered to exclude alternative diagnoses.

DIAGNOSIS

Diagnosis is based on the presence of 4 or more of the 11 criteria, either serially or simultaneously, of the ACR classification. The revised criteria yields a sensitivity of 83% and a specificity of 96% for SLE diagnosis but are associated with several weaknesses.[22,46] For instance, many patients with biopsy-proven LN do not meet the criteria. Also, there have been numerous advances in imaging, serologic, and cerebrospinal fluid testing that resulted in an outdated CNS definition. The Systemic Lupus International Collaborative Clinics (SLICC) guidelines propose new criteria for the disease.[23] According to the SLICC criteria, a person is diagnosed with SLE when there is presence of at least 4 of the 11 criteria, of which one must be a clinical criterion and one an immunologic criterion.[23] Furthermore, the classification can also be made from a biopsy confirming LN and presence of antinuclear antibodies (ANA), or anti-dsDNA antibodies. Both anti-Smith (anti-Sm) and anti-dsDNA antibodies are highly specific for SLE, but anti-Sm antibodies lack sensitivity.[1] Anti-dsDNA and anti-Sm antibodies are found in approximately 70% and 30% of patients with SLE, respectively.[47] Other markers, such as the lupus anticoagulant and IgG and IgM antibodies to anticardiolipin are specific for APS. Their presence may increase the risk for thrombosis or miscarriages. When compared to the ACR classification, the SLICC criteria have higher sensitivity (97%) but not specificity (84%) (Table 33-2).[18]

The diagnostic workup can be challenging because of the complexity of the disease and overlapping features of many other autoimmune diseases, such as polymyositis, rheumatoid arthritis, and scleroderma. The workup includes an assessment of the clinical presentation, physical examination, diagnostic, and laboratory tests. Approximately 80% of patients have skin involvement manifesting as photosensitivity, alopecia, malar and discoid rash (thick, red, scaly patches on the skin), and ulcers in the oral and nasal cavities or in the vagina, all of which are part of the ACR criteria.[22]

CASE 33-2

QUESTION 1: P.J., a 26-year-old, obese (80 kg, 5-feet tall) African-American woman, presents to the emergency department complaining of chest pain. It is a sharp and substernal pain, but with a component that is diffuse and aggravated by deep aspiration. Two months ago she presented to the emergency department with a 6-week history of fatigue, low-grade fevers, hair loss, joint pain, and oral ulcers. Her laboratory tests showed a positive ANA test result. Blood cultures were negative for infection. The urinalysis was negative for blood, and the urine culture was negative for infection. A chest x-ray showed non-pulmonary infiltrates. Her symptoms improved after a 10-day tapering course of prednisone. Feeling better, P.J. decided not to follow-up with her physician's appointment last week. Today, the medical resident's examination reveals an ill-appearing woman, with a temperature of 100.5°F (38.06°C), oral ulcers, alopecia, and tachycardia with distant heart sounds. What signs and symptoms exhibited by P.J. are consistent with SLE?

According to the "1997 Update of the 1982 American College of Rheumatology Revised Criteria for Classification of Systemic Lupus Erythematosus," the diagnosis of SLE is satisfied when 4 of 11 criteria are present. The criteria contain 4 cutaneous, 4 systemic, and 3 laboratory components (Table 33-1). P.J. meets criteria with the presence of a positive ANA test result, oral ulcers, presumed pericarditis, and presumed arthritis (joint pain). Furthermore, her clinical features are consistent with SLE including fatigue, alopecia, and low-grade fevers (infection ruled out).

CASE 33-2, QUESTION 2: After P.J. has started treatment and further laboratory tests are performed, what other specialists would you involve in her care at this time?

Rheumatologist and cardiologist because of P.J.'s pericarditis. The cardiologist could evaluate the patient's modifiable cardiovascular risk factors, such as hypertension, dyslipidemia, and obesity. Pericarditis with pericardial effusion is most commonly associated with cardiovascular involvement and SLE. Symptoms could include sharp chest pain and fluid around the heart, worsened with deep breathing and certain body positions. Endocarditis, myocarditis, and valvular disease are less common. Over time, other specialists including gastroenterologist, neurologist, pulmonologist, and nephrologist may be considered as part of P.J.'s multidisciplinary team.

PHARMACOLOGIC AND NON-PHARMACOLOGIC TREATMENTS

The management approach for SLE will depend on the severity of the disease and organ involvement. A therapeutic plan is created based on clinical guidelines for the management, treatment, and monitoring of SLE. It should include considerations for pharmacologic and non-pharmacologic approaches with clearly defined goals. Since there is currently no cure for SLE, the goals of therapy are to prevent flares, treat active symptoms of disease, minimize drug toxicity, and reduce risk of complications and organ damage. An effective and successful therapeutic plan is individualized based on the patient's needs, symptoms, lifestyle, and disease complications. Patients should be regularly monitored by their providers every 3 to 6 months.

NSAIDs and COX-2 Inhibitor

Treatment options will differ depending on the level of severity of SLE. For mild disease, nonselective nonsteroidal anti-inflammatory drugs (NSAIDs) and selective cyclooxygenase-2 (COX-2) inhibitor, such as celecoxib, are used. Because of their ability to inhibit the release of prostaglandins and leukotrienes, NSAIDs and the COX-2 inhibitor possess anti-inflammatory, analgesic, and antipyretic properties. They are effective in reducing swelling, relieving muscle and joint pain, fever, as well as pleuritic chest pain.[26,48] Patients with antiphospholipid antibodies and are at increased risk of thrombosis or atherosclerotic disease may benefit from low-dose aspirin for primary prevention, or long-term anticoagulation therapy for secondary prevention.[7] Long-term use of NSAIDs is encumbered with GI, cardiovascular, and renal issues. Common GI side effects include dyspepsia, heartburn, and nausea. More serious GI symptoms such as stomach bleeding and mucosal lesions may occur. Cardiovascular side effects associated with NSAIDs may include hypertension and the risk of myocardial infarction. Fluid retention and acute tubular necrosis with kidney failure may also occur with long-term use, especially in elderly patients.

As a class, NSAIDs work in the same manner; however, not every agent has the same effect on every patient. When a NSAID is used, it needs to be titrated to its maximal dose over 1 to 2 weeks. The agent should not be discontinued until the patient has been on the maximal dose for at least 2 weeks, which is the amount of time NSAIDs reach maximal efficacy.[27] Although all NSAIDs appear to work in the same way, not every agent has the same effect on every person. In addition, patients may do well with one NSAID for a period of time, then may not derive further benefit from it for some unknown reason. Switching the patient to a different NSAID could produce the desired effects. NSAIDs may be appropriate for chronic pain management in aspirin users provided that appropriate GI prophylactic measures are used in high-risk patients. Patients should use only one NSAID at any given time to really know its benefits.

Celecoxib, a COX-2 inhibitor, is more selective in the inhibition of cyclooxygenase, which is involved in the transformation of arachidonic acid to prostaglandin precursors. Celecoxib has the same efficacy as NSAIDs; however, it possesses a milder GI side effect profile. It does not have a direct effect on platelets.[49] Therefore, it is preferred over NSAIDs in patients with thrombocytopenia. There have been many studies and case reports correlating COX-2 inhibitors with cardiovascular risks (e.g., stroke and heart attack), especially with rofecoxib (Vioxx), which was removed from the U.S. market.[49–51]

CASE 33-2, QUESTION 3: Which of the following treatments would P.J. benefit from using at this time?

P.J. could benefit from high-dose NSAIDs. Traditionally, the initial treatment for SLE pericarditis (inflammation of the lining of the heart or pericardium) is high-dose NSAIDs such as ibuprofen. Patients with SLE are at increased risk for coronary heart disease from increased cardiovascular risk factors (i.e., chronic inflammation, dyslipidemia, obesity, and physical inactivity). SLE patients with recurrent pericarditis will need to be on immunosuppressive medications.

Antimalarials

Antimalarials are currently the mainstay therapy for SLE, in particular hydroxychloroquine sulfate (Plaquenil) and chloroquine. They work through immunomodulation by downregulating the production of TNF alpha and other proinflammatory cytokines.[52] Hydroxychloroquine is preferred over chloroquine because it is associated with less corneal deposition (opacities) and retinopathy risks.[33] Ocular side effects occur in a dose-dependent manner where the risk is low when hydroxychloroquine's dose is less than 600 mg daily and less than 6.5 mg/kg/day. It has anti-inflammatory effects and is used to reduce the time to flare-ups, constitutional (i.e., fever and rashes), skin, fatigue, and joint symptoms.[53] Additionally, hydroxychloroquine has antithrombotic and lipid-lowering effects, which can help patients with SLE.[54] Other ocular symptoms may include blurred vision, night blindness, missing or blanched out areas in the central or peripheral fields, light flashes and streaks, and photophobia. Hydroxychloroquine-related side effects may also include a bull's eye appearance in the macular region.[33] The manufacturer recommends eye exams should be performed at baseline and subsequently every 3 months with long-term hydroxychloroquine treatment. In contrast, the American Academy of Opthalmology (AAO) proposes more flexible eye exam criteria. The AAO recommends patients who are at low risk (those taking hydroxychloroquine less than 6.5 mg/kg/day dose for a treatment duration of less than 5 years) be checked at baseline and then, if normal, every 5 years. Patients who are at high risk (those taking hydroxychloroquine more than 6.5 mg/kg/day dose for >5 years, aged more than 60 years old or pediatric patients, or those with existing retinal disease and kidney or liver disease) should be evaluated at baseline and then annually.[55] Patients should be screened for the presence of "premaculopathy" antimalarial retinopathy, or retinal toxicity during scheduled eye exams because it is a reversible stage as long as hydroxychloroquine is discontinued.

Patients may need to take hydroxychloroquine for months to experience the maximal effect. For SLE, the initial oral hydroxychloroquine dose is 400 mg given daily for 3 to 6 months depending on patient response, then tapered to 200 mg daily for maintenance therapy. If the patient does not have any benefit from hydroxychloroquine after 6 months, the drug should be discontinued.

CASE 33-3

QUESTION 1: R.W., a 54-year-old Caucasian woman with a 30-year history of SLE, returns to her rheumatologist for evaluation. She has received prednisone, hydroxychloroquine, and azathioprine in the past. Her SLE has been stable for 2 years. Feeling well, R.W. discontinued all of her medications more than 1 year ago. She recently returns from a family vacation in the Caribbean. Having been out in the sun for a few hours on the first day, she developed an erythematous eruption over photo-exposed areas of her face, ears, and legs despite the application of sunscreen. R.W. returns home, and the lesions are healing. Though she is fatigued, she feels well enough to return to work. You determine that her rash is because of photosensitivity. What would be the best next step in the management of R.W.?

The next appropriate step is to initiate a short-course of low-dose prednisone because it can be used to treat a photosensitive rash from SLE. The rash may occur because with SLE, the body's immune system does not function properly, and the inflammatory response works to damage the patient's own tissues. Prednisone is a corticosteroid that helps to reduce the inflammation and immune response, thereby preventing further damage to the tissues in the body.

CASE 33-3, QUESTION 2: The rash resolves; however, R.W. continues to complain of fatigue and arthralgia. No other clinical signs or symptoms consistent with SLE flare emerge. Laboratory test results reveal continued elevation of anti-dsDNA antibody titers and suppressed complement levels. What is your next step in managing R.W.?

Hydroxychloroquine should be initiated as it is effective for long-term treatment of SLE with rash, fatigue, and arthralgias. Hydroxychloroquine is often prescribed in combination with steroids to reduce the dose required of the steroids. It is prescribed for skin rashes, mouth ulcers, and joint pain. Hydroxychloroquine improves SLE by decreasing autoantibody production, protecting against the damaging effects of ultraviolet light from the sun and other sources, and improving skin lesions. Several studies have reported the benefits of hydroxychloroquine in treating symptoms of SLE, preventing disease flares, and its association with less organ damage.[56]

Case 33-3, Question 3: R.W. is initiated on hydroxychloroquine 400 mg orally daily. How long should she be on the initial treatment dose?

Three to six months of the initial treatment dose of hydroxychloroquine is recommended unless R.W. does not tolerate the side effects or does not benefit from the medication. After R.W. has responded to the initial dose, then hydroxychloroquine can be tapered to 200 mg daily for maintenance therapy.

Case 33-3, Question 4: How often should eye exams be performed for R.W.?

At high doses of hydroxychloroquine and over time, it may damage the retina of the eye (retinal toxicity), causing vision problems. Eye exams should be performed at baseline before initiating hydroxychloroquine and every 3 months based on the manufacturer's recommendation. If based on the AAO, an eye exam should be performed at baseline and then every 5 years. If low doses of hydroxychloroquine are used in the treatment of SLE, the risk of retinal toxicity is low. Long-term users of high-dose hydroxychloroquine will need to monitor their eye health regularly to prevent retinal toxicity.

Case 33-3, Question 5: What are the goals of SLE treatment?

Since there is no cure for SLE, the goals of treatment are to reset the patient's immune system to a state of remission, reduce the incidence of drug toxicity, and prevent multi-organ damage.

Corticosteroids

Corticosteroid treatment is considered for patients with SLE who have not responded to NSAIDs and hydroxychloroquine. Corticosteroids possess anti-inflammatory effects and work by inhibiting T and B cell responses.[57] They provide immediate relief for mild-to-moderate symptoms compared to immunosuppressant treatments. Low-dose corticosteroid, such as prednisone, may be effective for mild-to-moderate symptoms. For instance, low-dose oral prednisone (6–10 mg daily) over a duration of 4 to 6 weeks is recommended for mild disease activity. Short-term use of tapered courses of prednisone will help reduce acute flares with or without systemic symptoms starting at adult doses of 1 mg/kg/day, up to 60 mg daily, and tapered over 8 weeks. Short-term treatment can minimize risks of developing side effects associated with long-term corticosteroid use, such as weight gain, decreased bone mineral density, muscle wasting, hypercholesterolemia, and hyperglycemia. More severe adverse effects associated with long term use of high-dose corticosteroids may include diabetes, osteoporosis, mood changes (e.g., anxiety, insomnia, depression, and delirium), Cushing's syndrome, and risks of cardiovascular events. Topical corticosteroids are recommended for cutaneous SLE manifestations. Adjunctive treatments with NSAIDs or celecoxib may be combined with prednisone to reduce its dose and side effects, or allow it to be administered as an every other day therapy. High-dose oral corticosteroids (e.g., prednisone 40–60 mg daily) or intravenous corticosteroids (e.g., methylprednisolone 0.5–1.0 g daily) are considered for more severe disease.[27]

Case 33-3, Question 6: If R.W. is to be initiated on chronic, high-dose corticosteroid therapy for management of her SLE symptoms, what should she be monitored for?

With the use of high-dose corticosteroids, it important to monitor for weight gain, hyperglycemia, osteoporosis, glaucoma, cataracts, hypercholesterolemia, mood changes, and premature atherosclerosis. Steroid medications can have serious long-term side effects, and the risk of the side effects increases with higher doses and chronic therapy.

Disease-Modifying Antirheumatic Drugs (DMARDs)

Methotrexate (MTX, Rheumatrex, Trexall) is a folate antagonist that inhibits dihydrofolate reductase, an essential enzyme for DNA synthesis. MTX is usually considered for treatment of rheumatoid arthritis, in terms of arthritis and skin manifestations. It is an effective alternative agent to hydroxychloroquine and corticosteroids for SLE patients with arthritis, rash, or serositis.[53,58,59] When used with or without corticosteroids, MTX is dosed between 7.5 mg and 15 mg weekly, orally or subcutaneously, not to exceed 25 mg/week. Subcutaneous injection is recommended for patients who experience drug-induced nausea. Side effects are dose dependent and can range from mild to severe. Mild side effects include gastrointestinal effects (e.g., nausea and vomiting) versus leukopenia or thrombocytopenia which are more severe side effects. Hepatotoxicity could occur from MTX use. Patients should receive baseline liver function tests and periodically throughout therapy. They should also be screened for preexisting liver disease, excessive alcohol use, or diabetes. Patients with liver disease (e.g., hepatitis B or C) should avoid MTX because of liver toxicity risk. Similarly, MTX should be used cautiously in patients with renal disease because of increased risk for renal toxicity. Other adverse effects may include lung toxicities, such as cough, shortness of breath, and pulmonary infiltrates.[53,58] MTX is teratogenic and contraindicated in pregnant women (Pregnancy Category X). Men and women who take MTX should stop 1 to 3 months before trying to conceive. The 3-month period allows the complete elimination of MTX from the body.

Leflunomide (Arava) is a pyrimidine synthesis inhibitor that inhibits the formation of DNA in the cells of the body, particularly the immune cells that contribute to the inflammation, swelling, stiffness, and joint pain. Leflunomide can be used as a steroid-sparing treatment for SLE patients with photosensitive rashes and arthritis. It is also used either as monotherapy or in combination with MTX. Treatment may be initiated with or without a loading dose, depending on the patient's risk for ARAVA-associated hepatotoxicity and ARAVA-associated myelosuppression.[60] Patients who are at a low risk for ARAVA-associated hepatotoxicity and ARAVA-associated myelosuppression, the oral loading dose is 100 mg daily for 3 days, followed by a maintenance oral dose of 20 mg daily. Alternatively, an oral loading dose of 100 mg once a week for 3 weeks, in addition to the maintenance dose have been used to reduce the increased incidence of diarrhea. If diarrhea persists to be a bothersome side effect, in spite of the use of antidiarrheal medication, then the dose can be reduced to 10 mg daily. In contrast, patients who are at a high risk for ARAVA-associated hepatotoxicity (i.e., concomitant MTX use) or ARAVA-associated myelosuppression (i.e., concomitant immunosuppressant use) should receive an oral dose of 20 mg daily without a loading dose.[60] Similar to MTX screening, patients initiated on leflunomide should receive baseline liver function tests and complete blood count tests every 3 to 4 months. Furthermore, they should also be screened for preexisting liver disease and excessive alcohol use. Leflunomide is teratogenic and contraindicated in pregnant women (Pregnancy Category X). Women should use oral contraceptives or other forms of effective birth control methods while taking the drug. More importantly, they should continue to do so until 2 years after discontinuation of leflunomide since its active metabolite, teriflunomide, remains in the plasma. Cholestyramine (Questran) can be used to accelerate the elimination of leflunomide and reduce the plasma levels of teriflunomide.[61]

Immunosuppressants

Azathioprine (Imuran, Azasan), a purine analog, inhibits DNA synthesis and blocks cell proliferation.[58] It is used to treat non-renal SLE manifestations, such as photosensitive rashes. Prior to starting azathioprine treatment, genotyping or phenotyping of the thiopurine S-methyltransferase (TPMT) is strongly recommended.[62] Caution is recommended for patients with reduced thiopurine methyltransferase activity because they may be at increased risk of bone marrow suppression.[57,63] Patients who are homozygous, or carry two nonfunctional TPMT alleles will experience life-threatening myelosuppression when treated with azathioprine because of high concentrations of thioguanine nucelotides. Bone marrow suppression can occur in any patient, is dose-dependent, and is reversible by reducing the dose of azathioprine.[64] Side effects include gastrointestinal (e.g., nausea, vomiting, diarrhea, and stomach pain) and leukopenia. Anemia and thrombocytopenia may result from high doses of azathioprine or from poor metabolizers of the drug.

Mycophenolate mofetil (MMF; CellCept) inhibits inosine monophosphate dehydrogenase, an essential enzyme for DNA synthesis in lymphocytes. Its active metabolite inhibits the proliferation of T and B cells.[57] Similar to methotrexate, MMF treatment could be used to treat SLE patients with arthritis. It is also used for SLE patients with renal symptoms. It has been demonstrated to be superior to azathioprine as maintenance therapy of LN.[65] Patients with SLE and nephritis had a much better response with a 6-month induction trial of mycophenolate versus azathioprine for prolonging time to treatment failure, time to renal flare, and time to rescue therapy. MMF is teratogenic (Pregnancy Category D) and should not be used in pregnant women or who plan to become pregnant. It could cause birth defects and reduces the effectiveness of oral contraceptives. Women who take this drug should wait at least 1 to 3 months after stopping the drug before trying to conceive. Common side effects may include gastrointestinal (e.g., nausea, vomiting, and diarrhea), risk of infection, and decreased white blood cell counts.[53]

CASE 33-3, QUESTION 7: R.W.'s daughter has also been diagnosed with SLE. She is 28 years old and is married. She and her husband want to start a family. R.W. heard about MMF as one of the treatment options for SLE. She asks you if her daughter can benefit from taking MMF.

You explain that MMF is not an option because it is teratogenic and has been associated with infertility even though it is classified as Pregnancy Category D. Furthermore, MMF has been reported to cause risk of birth defects if taken during pregnancy (i.e., cleft lip/palate or ear malformations). Women who take this drug should wait at least 1 to 3 months after stopping the drug before trying to conceive.

Cytotoxic Drug

Cyclophosphamide (Cytoxan) is an alkylating agent. Its active metabolite, aldophosphamide, interferes with DNA links and causes cell death.[52] It is the agent of choice for treatment of LN, severe CNS, lung, or hematologic manifestations.[53,66] It is teratogenic (Pregnancy Category D) and should not be used in pregnant women or who plan to become pregnant. Cyclophosphamide has been reported to cause birth defects, especially if taken during the first trimester. Birth defects may include growth restriction, ear and facial abnormalities, hypoplastic limbs, and absence of digits.[67] Cyclophosphamide has a serious adverse effect profile that includes hemorrhagic cystitis, bacterial and viral (herpes zoster) infections, and infertility. Its metabolite, acrolein, is toxic to the bladder. Hemorrhagic cystitis and bladder cancer risks can be minimized by hydrating the patient (orally and intravenously), frequent bladder emptying, and using mesna as a protectant prior to intravenous use.[53] Mesna (sodium 2-mercaptoethane sulfonate) is a sulfhydryl donor which binds and detoxifies acrolein.[68] Urinalysis testing and monitoring for hematuria should be performed regularly. If patient develops hemorrhagic cystitis, cyclophosphamide therapy should be discontinued. The risk of bladder cancer is increased after receiving a total dose of 30 g.[58]

Because immunosuppressants and cyclophosphamide can increase the prevalence of secondary malignancies, such as cervical cancer in female patients with SLE, the ACR recommends annual Pap exams as part of laboratory monitoring.[53,69] Infertility, from ovarian failure in females or azoospermia in males, can occur in patients with SLE and of childbearing age.[7] Gonadotropin-releasing hormone analogs may preserve gonadal protection and can be considered for patients who are concerned with infertility associated with cyclophosphamide.

CASE 33-3, QUESTION 8: R.W. asks you what other commonly used drugs for SLE treatment should her daughter avoid taking if she wanted to become pregnant.

Other than MMF, her daughter should avoid taking leflunomide (Pregnancy Category X), MTX, (Pregnancy Category X), and cyclophosphamide (Pregnancy Category D) for treatment of her SLE if she plans to get pregnant. Women should use oral contraceptives or other forms of effective birth control methods while taking leflunomide. More importantly, they should continue to do so until 2 years after discontinuation of leflunomide since its active metabolite, teriflunomide, remains in the plasma. Cholestyramine (Questran) can be used to accelerate the elimination of leflunomide and reduce the plasma levels of teriflunomide.[61] Men and women who take MTX should stop 1 to 3 months before trying to conceive. The 3-month period allows the complete elimination of MTX from the body. Cyclophosphamide has been reported to cause birth defects, especially if taken during the first trimester. Birth defects may include growth restriction, ear and facial abnormalities, hypoplastic limbs, and absence of digits.[65]

CASE 33-3, QUESTION 9: Over the next couple of months, R.W. continues to have mild-to-moderate flares of her skin and joints because of SLE, despite hydroxychloroquine therapy. Her primary care physician is considering cyclophosphamide for her. What common toxicity should R.W. be monitored for?

R.W. should be monitored for bladder toxicity. Acrolein, a compound of one of cyclophosphamide's active metabolite aldophosphamide, is toxic to the bladder epithelium and could cause hemorrhagic cystitis.[70] Hemorrhagic cystitis is associated with hematuria and occasional dysuria.

CASE 33-3, QUESTION 10: How is the risk for bladder toxicity reduced?

By administering mesna and plenty of fluids (orally and intravenously) the risk of bladder toxicity is reduced. Mesna (sodium 2-mercaptoethane sulfonate) is a sulfhydryl donor that binds and detoxifies acrolein. Pulsed or intermittent dosing of cyclophosphamide can decrease the cumulative drug dose and reduce bladder exposure to acrolein.

CASE 33-3, QUESTION 11: Considering her present symptoms, should R.W. be initiated on cyclophosphamide?

Because her symptoms are still mild to moderate without signs of CNS, lung, or renal complications, cyclophosphamide is not recommended. Cyclophosphamide is primarily reserved for treatment of LN, severe CNS associated with SLE, lung, or hematologic manifestations.

Biologic Therapy

Belimumab (Benylsta) is the first biologic agent approved for adjunctive treatment of SLE in patients with active, autoantibody-positive SLE. It is a human IgG1 lambda monoclonal antibody that stimulates B-lymphocytes (BLyS). Belimumab is also referred to as a B cell–activating factor (BAFF)-specific inhibitor. B cells have three membrane receptors: B cell–maturation antigen, transmembrane activator and calcium modulator and cyclophilin ligand interactor, and BAFF receptor.[18] BAFF is involved in B cell survival, activation, and differentiation. It is elevated in patients with B cell–mediated autoimmune diseases, such as SLE.[71] Belimumab is hypothesized to decrease the amount of abnormal B cells.

Phase II clinical trials reported that belimumab combined with standard therapy offered better response to patients with active SLE versus standard therapy alone.[71,72] Belimumab's efficacy was further demonstrated in two phase III randomized, placebo-controlled clinical trials (BLISS-52 and BLISS-76). A total of 1,684 patients were randomized to receive either belimumab or placebo in combination with standard therapy.[73,74] The combination of belimumab and standard therapy was found to be superior to placebo plus standard therapy. Furthermore, the combination of belimumab and standard therapy was well tolerated, improved SLE Responder Index response rates, and reduced disease activity and severe flares.[73,74] Belimumab has not been studied in patients with severe active LN or severe active CNS lupus; therefore, it cannot be recommended for use in patients with these symptoms. More importantly, it is not recommended to be administered in combination with other biologics or intravenous cyclophosphamide because it has not been studied in these settings.

Possible side effects (≥5%) of belimumab may include diarrhea, nausea, fever, insomnia, nasopharyngitis, pharyngitis, bronchitis, extremity pain, migraine, and depression.[75,76] More common side effects reported from the belimumab study group were serious infections, primarily upper respiratory tract infections.[75] Therefore, patients being treated for chronic infections should not start belimumab therapy. If an infection develops while receiving belimumab, temporary discontinuation of the drug is recommended. From clinical trials, mortality (resulting from infection, cardiovascular disease, and suicide) was increased in patients receiving belimumab versus those on placebo therapy.[71–74] Hypersensitivity reactions, including infusion reactions and anaphylaxis, may occur. Patients should be closely monitored for potential side effects and reactions.

Belimumab is administered parenterally as an intravenous infusion over 1 hour (Table 33-3). Premedication with an antihistamine for prophylaxis against infusion-related reactions and hypersensitivity reactions is recommended as part of the therapy. There are no dosage adjustments required for patients with hepatic and renal impairment.

Case 33-3, Question 12: Over the next year, R.W. continues to have bothersome symptoms associated with her SLE, despite hydroxychloroquine therapy. She resists the recommendation to use steroids because of risks of weight gain, osteoporosis, and vision problems. She is excited to hear about a recently approved drug for SLE, belimumab. R.W. asks you for the mechanism of action of belimumab.

Belimumab is a monoclonal antibody that inhibits the B cell–survival factor, B-lymphocyte stimulator (BLyS). As a BLyS-specific inhibitor, belimumab blocks the binding of BLyS to receptors on B cells, thus inhibiting the survival of B cells including autoreactive B cells. It also reduces the differentiation of B cells into immunoglobulin-producing plasma cells. Belimumab reduces disease activity and possibly a number of severe flares and steroid use when administered in combination with standard therapy. It is approved for treatment of patients with active, autoantibody-positive lupus in combination with standard therapies (i.e., hydroxychloroquine, azathioprine, and MTX).

Table 33-3
Preparation and Administration Instructions of Belimumab[18,76]

Reconstitution

Remove belimumab vial from refrigerator and allow it to stand for 10 to 15 minutes to reach room temperature. Reconstitute belimumab powder with Sterile Water for Injection, USP, as follows, with reconstituted solution to make a concentration of 80 mg/mL belimumab.

Reconstitute 120 mg vial with 1.5 mL sterile water.

Reconstitute 400 mg vial with 4.8 mL sterile water.

Direct the stream of sterile water to the side of the vial to minimize foaming.

Gently swirl the vial for 60 seconds. Allow vial to sit at room temperature during reconstitution, gently swirling the vial every 5 minutes until powder is dissolved. *Do not shake.* It usually takes 10–15 minutes, but it may take up to 30 minutes. Protect solution from light.

If a mechanical reconstitution device (swirler) is used to reconstitute belimumab, it should not exceed 500 rpm, and the vial should not be swirled for longer than 30 minutes.

Once reconstitution is complete, the solution should be opalescent and colorless to pale yellow and without particles. Small bubbles can occur and are acceptable.

Dilution Instructions

Belimumab should only be diluted with 0.9% sodium chloride injection, USP (normal saline). Dextrose IV solutions are incompatible with belimumab. Dilute the reconstituted product to 250 mL in normal saline for IV infusion. From a 250-mL infusion bag or bottle of normal saline, withdraw and discard a volume equal to the volume of the reconstituted solution of belimumab required for the patient's dose. Then add the required volume of reconstituted solution into the infusion bag or bottle. Discard any unused solution.

Inspect visually for any particular matter and discoloration before administration. Discard if present.

Use reconstituted solution immediately, otherwise it should be stored protected from sunlight and refrigerated at 2°C–8°C (36°F–46°F). Solutions of belimumab diluted in normal saline may be stored at 2°C–8°C (36°F–46°F) or room temperature.

The time from reconstitution to completion of infusion should not exceed 8 hours.

No incompatibilities exist between belimumab and polyvinyl chloride or polyolefin bags.

Administration Instructions

Administer the diluted solution of belimumab by IV infusion only, over a period of 1 hour.

Belimumab should be administered by health care professionals prepared to manage anaphylaxis.

Do not infuse belimumab concomitantly in the same IV line with other agents.

IV, intravenous; USP, US Pharmacopoeia.

Case 33-3, Question 13: How is belimumab dosed and administered?

Belimumab is given at a recommended dose of 10 mg/kg that is administered intravenously as an infusion over 1 hour, 2 weeks apart for the first three doses, and 4 weeks apart thereafter.

Case 33-3, Question 14: What are the necessary precautions taken prior to administration of belimumab?

Antihistamine premedication is recommended as a prophylaxis to prevent infusion reactions and hypersensitivity reactions. Patients should be monitored before and after drug administration. Belimumab should be used with caution in patients with chronic infections. Infections were the most common adverse events associated with belimumab in BLISS-52 and BLISS-76 clinical trials. Upper respiratory tract infections were the most common type, occurring in more than 5% of belimumab patients.

CASE 33-3, QUESTION 15: When is belimumab not recommended for use in patients with SLE?

Belimumab is not recommended in patients with severe active lupus nephritis, or in those with severe active CNS lupus as its efficacy has not been evaluated in these types of patients. Furthermore, depression and suicidality have been reported in clinical trials; therefore, it is not recommended for patients with uncontrolled psychiatric disorders. Belimumab is not recommended in combination with other biologics or IV cyclophosphamide as it has not been studied with these drugs.

CASE 33-3, QUESTION 16: Are there drug–drug interactions between belimumab and other combination treatments for SLE?

There are no clinically significant drug–drug interactions identified with belimumab in the clinical trials. It was administered concomitantly with corticosteroids, antimalarial drugs, statins, NSAIDs, angiotensin-converting enzyme inhibitors, and immunomodulatory and immunosuppressive agents.

CASE 33-3, QUESTION 17: Can R.W. receive immunizations while receiving belimumab treatment?

Live vaccines should not be administered within 30 days before treatment starts or during treatment. Belimumab may interfere with R.W.'s response to immunizations.

Table 33-4 summarizes the current medications used for treating SLE.[53,57,69,75,76] There are drug interactions with the medications used for treating SLE symptoms. Table 33-5 summarizes the possible significant drug–drug interactions.[77,78]

Non-pharmacologic Therapy

Both the ACR and EULAR recommend non-pharmacologic treatments as part of the management of SLE.[22,79] Sunscreens with a sun protective factor of 15 or greater should be used daily. There are patients who are sensitive to UVA light and may require broader-spectrum sunscreens. Patients are advised to apply sunscreen each morning and prior to sun exposure. Wearing protective clothing and/or sun avoidance for patients with SLE is encouraged. Sunbathing and the use of sunbeds in tanning parlors are discouraged. In addition, patients with SLE should be educated about lifestyle modifications, such as smoking cessation, weight control, and regular exercise to reduce comorbidities of atherosclerosis, hypertension, and diabetes.[7] Psychosocial support is also an important aspect of management as the disease and several of the medications may cause depression and anxiety. The medications' side effects can also affect a patient's adherence to treatment and medical office visits.

DRUG-INDUCED LUPUS ERYTHEMATOSUS

Drugs can cause subacute cutaneous lupus erythematosus or drug-induced lupus (DIL) (<1%) by inducing autoantibodies.[4] For as many patients that develop these antibodies, a surprisingly low number of them do not develop signs of an autoantibody-associated condition.[2] Over 38 drugs have been implicated with causing the disease (Table 33-6).[42,80–82] However, most DIL cases have been associated with the following medications: hydralazine, procainamide, and quinidine.

The symptoms of DIL may present as arthralgia or myalgias, fatigue, and the presence of anti-histone antibodies. The symptoms are similar to those of SLE; however, they are generally not as severe. Typically, the symptoms are self-limiting and resolve after discontinuing the offending drug. NSAIDs may be used to help speed up the healing process. Corticosteroids may also be used if more severe symptoms of DIL are present. The development of DIL occurs over long-term and from chronic use of medications that have high risk for causing lupus.

The mechanism by which these drugs exert their effect is not well understood. However, it may be attributed to a patient's genetic predisposition as a slow acetylator, which decreases the metabolism of some drugs such as procainamide and hydralazine. Gene expression is regulated by DNA methylation and histone modifications.[81,82] Procainamide and, particularly, hydralazine are hypothesized to inhibit DNA methylation, which alters gene expression in T lymphocytes. Subsequently, this process induces an over-expression of lymphocyte function-associated antigen 1 (LFA-1 antigen), thus resulting in autoreactivity.[28,80]

INVESTIGATIONAL AGENTS

Aside from the current therapies used for the treatment and management of SLE symptoms, rituximab and abatacept are currently being studied in patients with SLE. Both medications target T and B cells and have already been approved for the treatment of rheumatoid arthritis along with other indications. More recently, investigational biologic agents are being developed and are undergoing Phase I, II, and III clinical trials. These newer biologic agents specifically target different phases of the pathogenesis of SLE, have different mechanisms of action, and possess milder adverse effect profiles. The investigational drug classes include immune cell–targeted therapies, anti-cytokine therapy, therapies targeting costimulatory signaling pathways, and neutralizing monoclonal antibody against interferon alpha.[57]

TREATMENT APPROACHES

The primary goal of treatment for SLE is to control acute flares, and maintenance strategies are used to suppress symptoms and to prevent further organ damage. NSAIDs, hydroxychloroquine, and low-dose corticosteroids are considered maintenance therapy to control mild-to-moderate symptoms of arthritis, dermatitis, and constitutional symptoms. High-dose systemic corticosteroids, DMARDs, immunosuppressants, and belimumab are used for patients with more serious active disease, including those with more life-threatening forms such as LN.[66] Certain DMARDs and immunosuppressants (i.e., leflunomide, MTX, cyclophosphamide, and MMF) should be used with extreme caution in women of childbearing age and in those who are planning to get pregnant because of teratogenic effects.[7] MMF is the preferred maintenance therapy for LN in patients who can tolerate the medication, who are not pregnant, and who respond to it. It can reduce the effectiveness of oral contraceptives and, thus, additional or alternative non-hormonal methods of birth control should be considered. Currently, only hydroxychloroquine and belimumab are FDA-approved for the treatment of SLE. Immunosuppressants and DMARDs (i.e., azathioprine, cyclophosphamide, leflunomide, MTX, and MMF) have been used off-label for managing SLE symptoms for years. Prophylaxis with aspirin or long-term anticoagulation should

Table 33-4
Medications Used for the Treatment of Systemic Lupus Erythematosus[53,57,69,75,76]

Medication	FDA-Approved for SLE	Dose	Side Effects/Toxicities	Monitoring Parameters
Azathioprine	No; off-label	1–3 mg/kg/day	Bone marrow suppression, liver toxicity, elevated lymphocytes	Clinical: symptoms of infection. Laboratory: CBC and platelet count every 1–2 weeks with initiation and dosage changes, then every 1–3 months; monitor LFTs and Scr; Pap test at regular intervals.
Belimumab	Yes	IV: 10 mg/kg every 2 weeks for the first 3 doses and then administer monthly	Serious infusion and anaphylactic reactions; depression with suicidal ideation	Clinical: symptoms of allergic reaction, including hypotension, angioedema, rash, urticarial, pruritus, and difficulty breathing. Symptoms of common infusion reactions, including headache, nausea and skin reactions. Symptoms of infection, including fever, nausea, diarrhea; chest pain or shortness of breath. Laboratory: CBC monthly.
Corticosteroids	No; off-label	Prednisone (or equivalent) 0.125–1 mg/kg/day	Elevated blood pressure, glucose and cholesterol levels; low potassium or reduced potassium levels; reduced bone density; cataracts; weight gain; infections; and fluid retention	Clinical: symptoms of high blood sugar, edema, shortness of breath, high blood pressure, visual changes, bone pain. CNS symptoms of depression, suicidal ideation, insomnia, or other mood changes can occur at higher doses (e.g., prednisone >60 mg). Laboratory: glucose every 3–6 months, cholesterol annually, BP at each visit, bone density.
Cyclophosphamide	No; off-label	IV: 0.5–1 g/m^2 monthly; Oral: 1–2 mg/kg/day	Bone marrow suppression, malignancy, immunosuppression, hemorrhagic cystitis, secondary infertility	Clinical: symptoms of infection and presence of blood in urine. Laboratory: CBC and urinalysis monthly, urine cytology and Pap test annually for life.
Hydroxychloroquine	Yes	200–400 mg twice daily	Ophthalmic damage	Clinical: visual changes. Laboratory: funduscopic and visual field exam, frequency determined by risk.
Leflunomide	No; Off-label	Loading dose: 100 mg daily × 3 days, followed by 20 mg daily; *Or* 100 mg weekly × 3 weeks, then 20 mg daily ARAVA-associated hepatotoxicity or ARAVA-associated myelosuppression: 20 mg daily without a loading dose	Diarrhea, nausea, rash, liver toxicity, myelosuppression	Clinical: frequency and severity of diarrhea. Laboratory: LFTs, CBC
Methotrexate	No; off-label	Oral: 5–15 mg as a single weekly dose, or can be given as 3 divided doses/week given every 12 hours (i.e., 2.5 mg × 3 doses with 12 hours apart)	Bone marrow suppression, lung and liver toxicity, infection	Clinical: symptoms of infection, shortness of breath, nausea, vomiting. Laboratory: initial chest x-ray, CBC and platelet count monthly, LFTs, albumin, Scr every 4–8 weeks.
Mycophenolate mofetil	No; off-label	1,000–3,000 mg daily	Bone marrow suppression, liver toxicity and infection	Clinical: symptoms of infection. Laboratory: CBC and platelet count every 1–2 weeks with initiation and changes in dosage (then every 1–3 months), monitor LFTs and Scr, monitor changes in BP.
NSAIDs	No; off-label[a]	Product dependent	Gastrointestinal bleeding, liver and kidney toxicity, elevated blood pressure	Clinical: dark/black stool, upset stomach, nausea, vomiting, abdominal pain, edema. Laboratory: CBC, LFTs and Scr annually; BP at each visit.

[a]Aspirin is approved for treatment of SLE.
NSAIDs, nonsteroidal anti-inflammatory drugs; BP, blood pressure; CBC, complete blood count; IV, intravenous; LFTs, liver function tests; SCr, serum creatinine.

Table 33-5
Summary of Drug Interactions with Medications for Systemic Lupus Erythematosus[77,78]

Medication	Possible Interaction with Concomitant Drugs
Azathioprine	Allopurinol, cyclosporine, etanercept, infliximab, leflunomide, sirolimus, tacrolimus
Belimumab	Drug interactions have not been formally studied
Corticosteroids	Cimetidine, cisapride, clarithromycin, dihydroergotamine, ergotamine, erythromycin, itraconazole, ketoconazole, lovastatin, mifepristone, quinidine, rifabutin, rifampin, simvastatin, sirolimus, St. John's wort, terfenadine, tofacitinib
Cyclophosphamide	Carbamazepine, etanercept, tofacitinib
Hydroxychloroquine	Antacids, azathioprine, cyclosporine, digoxin, etanercept, infliximab, leflunomide, mycophenolate, sirolimus, tacrolimus
Leflunomide	Azathioprine, cyclosporine, etanercept, infliximab, methotrexate, mycophenolate, sirolimus, tacrolimus
Methotrexate	Celecoxib, diclofenac, etodolac, ketorolac, leflunomide, meloxicam, probenecid, sulfamethoxazole, trimethoprim
Mycophenolate mofetil	Ampicillin, antacids, cholestyramine, colestipol, etanercept, ethinylestradiol, infliximab, leflunomide, nafcillin, quinidine, sirolimus, tacrolimus
NSAIDs	ACE inhibitors, angiotensin receptor blockers, beta blockers, diuretics, other antihypertensives, lithium

be considered for patients with antiphospholipid antibodies and who are at an increased risk of thrombosis.[18] Patients with mild disease require frequent medical evaluations every 3 to 6 months. On the contrary, patients with inactive disease may benefit from being monitored every 6 to 12 months.

ROLE FOR PHARMACISTS

SLE disease is very complex and the symptoms are variable. Successful and effective management of SLE requires the involvement of a multidisciplinary healthcare team comprised of many specialists (e.g., rheumatology, cardiology, nephrology, dermatology, psychology, and ophthalmology) and pharmacists. Pharmacists have an important role in caring for patients with SLE, especially with education, management of their medications, and the monitoring of drug–drug or drug–herbal interactions. As part of the healthcare team, pharmacists can provide drug education and counseling to patients with respect to proper administration of the medications, common side effects, management of the side effects, and reinforcement of adherence to their medications and office visits. Education and counseling of the teratogenic effects of certain DMARDs and immunosuppressants should be offered, as well as the information that the disease should remain inactive for at least 6 months prior to attempting to conceive.[53] More importantly, pharmacists can provide education to help patients with SLE maintain a healthy lifestyle and better quality of life (e.g., regular weight-bearing exercise, sufficient dietary vitamin intake, smoking cessation, and limited alcohol intake to a minimum of two drinks daily).[83,84]

CASE 33-4

QUESTION 1: S.P., a 35-year-old Asian woman with a 10-year history of SLE, sees you for follow-up management of her medications. She currently takes hydroxychloroquine 200 mg PO daily as part of her maintenance regimen. S.P. reports experiencing some heartburn and bloating symptoms over the past several days and purchased an over-the-counter antacid, Tums. Tums helped to alleviate her gastrointestinal symptoms; however, she notices feeling more fatigued lately. What is the potential drug interaction between hydroxychloroquine and Tums?

Antacids that contain calcium carbonate, magnesium, or aluminum (i.e., Tums, Maalox) can interfere with the absorption of hydroxychloroquine and reduce its effectiveness when taken at the same time.

CASE 33-4, QUESTION 2: As her pharmacist, provide advice to S.P. regarding the appropriate administration of hydroxychloroquine and Tums?

Table 33-6
Medications that may Cause Systemic Lupus Erythematosus (DIL)[81–83]

Drug Class	Very Low Risk	Low-to-Moderate Risk	High Risk
Antiarrhythmics	Disopyramide, propafenone	Quinidine	Procainamide
Antimicrobials/antibiotics	Nitrofurantoin	Isoniazid, minocycline	
Anticonvulsants	Phenytoin, primidone, ethosuximide	Carbamazepine	
Antihypertensives	Enalapril, clonidine, atenolol, labetolol, pindolol, minoxidil, prazosin, chlorthalidone, hydrochlorothiazide	Captopril, methyldopa, acebutolol	Hydralazine
Anti-inflammatories	Phenylbutazone	Sulfasalazine, D-penicillamine	
Antipsychotics	Perphenazine, phenelzine, chlorprothixene, lithium	Chlorpromazine	
Anti-thyroids		Propylthiouracil	
Miscellaneous	Lovastatin, levodopa, alpha-interferon, timolol eye drops		

S.P. should be advised to separate the administration of hydroxychloroquine and Tums by at least 4 hours to reduce the risk of a drug interaction. There has been no clinically significant drug–drug interactions reported for concomitant use of hydroxychloroquine and histamine (H_2) receptor antagonists.

CASE 33-4, QUESTION 3: What other counseling points could you offer to S.P. about her health?

S.P. should be advised to incorporate a heart-healthy exercise regimen (low-impact aerobic exercise, such as walking, swimming, or Pilates) and diet (low-sodium, low-fat, and low-carbohydrate) to reduce modifiable cardiovascular risk factors and on approaches to maintain adequate rest. Counseling should also be provided regarding the use of sunscreen, vitamin D supplementation and adequate calcium intake, smoking cessation, maintenance of schedule immunizations, and prompt management of infections.

KEY REFERENCES AND WEBSITES

A full list of references for this chapter can be found at http://thepoint.lww.com/AT11e. Below are the key references and websites for this chapter, with the corresponding reference number in this chapter found in parentheses after the reference.

Key References

Bertsias GK, Tektonidou M, Amoura Z, et al. Joint European League Against Rheumatism and European Renal Association-European Dialysis and Transplant Association (EULAR/ERA-EDTA) recommendations for the management of adult and pediatric lupus nephritis. *Ann Rheum Dis*. 2012;71:1771–1782. (39)

Bertsias G, Cervera R, Boumpas DT. Systemic lupus erythematosus: pathogenesis and clinical features. *EULAR Textbook on Rheumatic Diseases*. 20th ed. Zürich, Switzerland: Eular Fpp. Indd. 2012;476–505. (2)

Krikorian S. Systemic lupus erythematosus. In: Helms RA et al, eds. *Textbook of Therapeutics: Drug and Disease Management*. 8th ed. Philadelphia: Lippincott Williams & Wilkins, 2006:1767–1787. (27)

Petri M, Orbai AM, Alarcon GS, et al. Derivation and validation of the Systemic Lupus International Collaborating Clinics classification criteria for systemic lupus erythematosus. *Arthritis Rheum*. 2012;64:2677–2686. (23)

Tsokos GC. Systemic lupus erythematosus. *N Engl J Med*. 2011;365: 2110–2121. (13)

Key Websites

American College of Rheumatology. 1997 Update of the 1982 American College of Rheumatology Revised Criteria for Classification of Systemic Lupus Erythematosus. Available at http://tinyurl.com/1997SLEcriteria. Accessed July 20, 2015.

American College of Rheumatology (ACR). Position Statement: Screening for hydroxychloroquine retinopathy. ACR website. http://www.rheumatology.org/Portals/0/Files/Screening%20of%20Hydroxychloroquine%20Retinopathy.pdf. Accessed July 15, 2015.

Lupus Foundation of America. What is Lupus? Available at http://www.lupus.org/answers/entry/what-is-lupus. Accessed July 21, 2015.

34 Kidney and Liver Transplantation

David J. Taber and Robert E. Dupuis

CORE PRINCIPLES

	CORE PRINCIPLES	CHAPTER CASES
1	Successful kidney transplantation involves rigorous evaluation of both donor and recipient. This results in immunologic categorization as either a high-risk or low-risk transplant and determines the immunosuppressive regimen an individual recipient should receive. The majority of these patients will receive combination therapy, which includes a calcineurin inhibitor, an antiproliferative agent, and a corticosteroid.	**Case 34-1 (Questions 1, 2), Table 34-1**
2	Induction therapy is used in most kidney transplant cases. Rabbit antithymocyte globulin, alemtuzumab, and basiliximab are common agents. Differences among these agents include dosing regimen and side effect profile. Rabbit antithymocyte globulin and alemtuzumab are often used in high-risk patients, including those with delayed graft function, whereas basiliximab is frequently used in low-risk recipients.	**Case 34-1 (Questions 2–6)**
3	Immunosuppressive combination therapy is directed at prevention of rejection. Acute rejection can be either T-cell-mediated or B-cell-mediated. T-cell-mediated rejection can be successfully treated, whereas B-cell-mediated rejection is much more resistant. Despite success in reducing acute rejections, chronic rejection and chronic graft dysfunction are major causes of graft loss.	**Case 34-1 (Questions 7–9)**
4	Cyclosporine is a calcineurin inhibitor with a complex pharmacokinetic profile associated with multiple adverse effects and requires therapeutic drug monitoring (TDM). Its use has significantly declined since the introduction of tacrolimus.	**Case 34-2 (Questions 1, 2), Case 34-3 (Question 1) Case 34-4 (Question 1)**
5	The mTOR inhibitors, sirolimus and everolimus, have complex pharmacokinetic profiles, significant adverse effects, and require TDM. These agents appear to be most useful in minimizing or avoiding the use of calcineurin inhibitors or other agents.	**Case 34-4 (Question2)**
6	The calcineurin inhibitors cyclosporine and tacrolimus and steroids have significant toxicity profiles, particularly with chronic long-term use. Calcineurin inhibitor-induced nephrotoxicity is a major problem. Steroids have a negative impact on the cardiovascular, bone, and endocrine system. Several strategies have been developed in an attempt to either avoid or minimize these adverse effects.	**Case 34-2 (Questions 1, 2), Case 34-3 (Question 1)**
7	Cardiovascular complications, including hypertension, hyperlipidemia, and diabetes, are prevalent among kidney transplant recipients. These contribute to poor patient survival and graft loss. Other complications such as osteoporosis are frequently observed. Monitoring and treatment of these complications, which may be drug-induced, are an important part of the post-transplant care plan.	**Case 34-5 (Questions 1–4)**
8	BK polyomavirus is almost exclusively seen in kidney transplantation and is associated with graft loss. The best approach to reducing its occurrence is viral surveillance. If it is present, then reduction of immunosuppression appears to be the most effective treatment.	**Case 34-6 (Questions 1–3)**
9	Liver transplantation is considered the treatment of choice for patient with end-stage liver disease. Common early post-transplant complications include surgical (biliary leaks and bleeding), neurologic (continued hepatic encephalopathy, drug toxicity), and infectious (pneumonias, urinary tract infections, and biliary bacteremias).	**Case 34-7 (Questions 1, 2)**

Continued

		CHAPTER CASES
10	Tacrolimus is considered the cornerstone of the immunosuppressant regimen for the vast majority of solid organ transplant recipients. It has complex pharmacokinetics and therefore requires close TDM for optimal use. Tacrolimus is a potent agent that has significantly reduced acute rejection rates; additionally, compared to cyclosporine, tacrolimus has fewer cosmetic side effects (hirsutism, gingival hyperplasia), fewer effects on serum lipoproteins and blood pressure, but has more severe effects on serum glucose levels and more pronounced neurotoxicities.	**Case 34-7 (Questions 3–6)**
11	Acute rejection of the transplanted liver is a common, but usually reversible, consequence after this surgery. It is usually asymptomatic, but can be identified early through serial monitoring of serum transaminases and bilirubin, and definitively diagnosed only through liver biopsy. Treatment usually consists of pulse-dose corticosteroids, followed by a taper, or the use of rabbit antithymocyte globulin for more severe rejections or those refractory to steroid therapy.	**Case 34-7 (Questions 7, 8)**
12	Mycophenolate is considered the adjuvant agent of choice in solid organ transplantation and is used to reduce calcineurin inhibitor exposure or augment immunosuppressant regimen potency. TDM is not common and has yet to prove effective in optimizing therapy. Common side effects with this agent include gastrointestinal issues (nausea, vomiting, and diarrhea) and cytopenias (leukopenia and thrombocytopenia).	**Case 34-7 (Question 9)**
13	Drug interactions with immunosuppressants are numerous and are commonly encountered clinical dilemmas in the transplant recipient. Pharmacists should prospectively screen for these interactions and, depending on their magnitude, may need to prospectively adjust medication regimens. Closer TDM or clinical monitoring is always warranted when adding or removing an interacting medication to a patient on immunosuppression.	**Case 34-8 (Question 1), Table 34-2**
14	Infections, including opportunistic infections, are common complications after transplant. Prophylaxis with antimicrobial agents is critical for the most common and severe pathogens. Hepatitis B and hepatitis C are problematic after liver transplant and require immunoprophylaxis or treatment in certain circumstances.	**Case 34-9 (Question 1), Table 34-3**
15	Cytomegalovirus is the most common and debilitating opportunistic infection after solid organ transplantation. Reactivation or new infection with this virus can lead to severe tissue invasive disease and potentially death. Indirect effects include acute rejection, chronic rejection, graft loss, and potentially, lymphoma. Prophylaxis with potent antivirals (ganciclovir or valganciclovir) is the cornerstone of prevention. Treatment involves a long course of antiviral therapy usually in conjunction with reductions in immunosuppression.	**Case 34-10 (Questions 1–4)**
16	Post-transplant lymphoproliferative disorder (PTLD), which is usually a B-cell lymphoma, is the most common cancer encountered after organ transplant. Early PTLD is generally responsive to reductions in immunosuppression; advanced PTLD is usually not responsive to this nor to traditional chemotherapy. The use of rituximab, a monoclonal antibody directed against B cells, has shown promise for treatment of this disease.	**Case 34-11 (Questions 1, 2)**

INTRODUCTION TO TRANSPLANTATION

Solid organ transplantation, adult and pediatrics, is an established therapeutic option for patients with end-stage kidney, liver, heart, and lung disease. For many of these patients, it is the only option. One-year patient and graft survival for these major organs is between 85% and 98%.[1] Pancreas or combined pancreas–kidney transplantation is available as a treatment for diabetic patients with end-stage renal failure.

Unfortunately, many more patients are in need of transplantation than there are organs available. In 2014, about 30,000 organ transplants were performed, whereas 130,000 people were waiting for all organs and 60,000 for kidneys. Consequently, a significant number of candidates die while on the waiting list.

During the 1960s, azathioprine, prednisone, antilymphocyte serum, and antilymphocyte globulin made the success of kidney transplantation possible. In the 1980s, the introduction of cyclosporine had a remarkable impact on solid organ transplantation, and the first monoclonal antibody approved for human use, OKT3, was introduced, but is no longer available.

Since the 1990s, a number of other agents have been approved. These include tacrolimus, mycophenolate mofetil, mycophenolate sodium, sirolimus (formerly rapamycin), and everolimus; monoclonal antibodies, such as basiliximab; a polyclonal antibody, antithymocyte globulin (rabbit antithymocyte globulin); and belatacept. More recently, several agents, such as alemtuzumab, intravenous immunoglobulins (IVIGs), rituximab, eculizumab, and bortezomib, are incorporated into transplant protocols. Several new agents are undergoing investigation.

Although transplantation has a significant positive impact on the quality of life in most patients, rehospitalizations, retransplantation because of graft failure or disease recurrence, donation source (living-related and unrelated organs), and costs to individuals, insurers, and society are major issues. For example, the average Medicare cost during the first year after kidney transplantation is $83,000 and during the second year is $25,000. After liver transplantation, first-year average Medicare cost is $190,000 and second year $30,000.[2] The ability of transplant recipients to pay for their medications or insurance denial or termination of coverage is another major issue.

The goal of immunosuppressive therapy is to prevent organ rejection, prolong graft and patient survival, and improve quality of life. Short-term (i.e., 1–2 years) survival after transplantation has improved dramatically. Long-term survival also has improved, but not to the same degree.[3] As patients live longer after transplantation, the focus of therapy has shifted to survival and management of long-term complications. Immunosuppressive agents are associated with significant long-term complications. These include nephrotoxicity, hypertension, hyperlipidemia, osteoporosis, diabetes, infection and malignancy, as well as graft loss secondary to, recurrence of primary disease, nonadherence and rejection. Many patients also have several pre- and post-transplant comorbidities and complicated drug regimens, which must be evaluated and managed. Pharmacists play an important role in these patient care activities.[4] Although acute rejection rates are significantly lower, this remains a problem, along with chronic rejection and/or chronic allograft injury and long-term outcomes. The search for safer and more effective immunosuppressive regimens continues, along with a better understanding of optimal long-term immunosuppression.[5] This chapter addresses the immunology of transplantation and rejection, indications for kidney and liver transplantation, appropriate use of immunosuppressive agents, and the management of postoperative and long-term complications in these patients. Many of these issues are similar for the various types of solid organ transplantations, but there can also be significant differences as well. This chapter addresses some of these issues as they relate to kidney and liver transplantation.

TRANSPLANTATION IMMUNOLOGY

Successful organ transplantation has evolved from a greater understanding and application of pharmacology, microbiology, molecular and cellular biochemistry and biology, genetics, and immunology. Suppression of the host's immune system and prevention of rejection are vital for host acceptance of the transplanted organ. The ultimate goal is permanent acceptance or tolerance, a situation in which the new organ is seen as "self" by the host's immune system. In general, the currently used immunosuppressive drugs provide a nonpermanent form of tolerance and lifelong immunosuppression is required. A basic understanding of the immune system and the mechanisms of rejection is key to the effective use of immunosuppressive drugs in organ transplantation.

Major Histocompatibility Complex and Human Leukocyte Antigen

The degree to which allogeneic grafting (e.g., donor and recipient from same species) is successful depends on the genetic similarities or differences between the donor organ and the recipient's immune system. The recipient recognizes the transplanted graft as either self or foreign. This recognition is based on the recipient's reaction to alloantigens or antigens (i.e., substances that initiate an immune response that can lead to rejection of the transplanted organ). These substances, also known as histocompatibility antigens, play a very important role in organ transplantation. The ABO blood group system of red blood cells is also important and, in most cases, the donor and recipient should be ABO compatible; otherwise, immediate graft destruction can occur because of antibodies directed against the ABO antigens.

Histocompatibility antigens are glycoproteins that are located on the surface of cell membranes. These are encoded by the major histocompatibility complex (MHC) genes located on the short arm of chromosome 6. In humans, the MHC is called the human leukocyte antigen (HLA). The gene products encoded on the HLA are divided into classes I, II, and III based on their tissue distribution, antigen structure, and function. Class I antigens (HLA-A, HLA-B, and HLA-C) are present on all nucleated cell surfaces and are the primary targets for cytotoxic T-lymphocyte reactions against transplanted cells and tissues. The three class II antigens (HLA-DR, HLA-DQ, HLA-DP) have a more limited distribution and are found on macrophages, B lymphocytes (B cells), monocytes, activated T lymphocytes (T cells), dendritic cells, and some endothelial cells, all of which can act as antigen-presenting cells (APCs). Individual HLA loci are extensively polymorphic. Each transplant recipient possesses two A, B, and DR antigens, one from each parent. This is called a haplotype. Recognition of these polymorphic loci by recipient T cells appears to account for rejection events. Class III antigens (C4, C2, and Bf) are part of the complement system.

Rejection of a transplanted organ is the outcome of the natural response of the immune system, innate and adaptive immunity, to a foreign substance, or antigen, and is a complex process, the understanding of which continues to evolve. This process involves an array of interactions between antigens, T cells, macrophages, cytokines (soluble mediators secreted by lymphocytes, also called lymphokines [the interleukins]), adhesion molecules (also referred to as costimulatory molecules), and membrane proteins expressed on a wide variety of cells that enhance binding of T- and B cells. This process of organ rejection ultimately can involve all elements of the immune response, but it is predominantly T-cell-mediated. This process can be divided into several important steps, which include antigen presentation, T-cell recognition, activation, proliferation, and differentiation of the various components of the immune response. For foreign antigens to interact with recipient T cells and B cells, they must be prepared for presentation by APCs. These APCs usually are recipient macrophages or dendritic cells (indirect pathway of allorecognition), although initially donor cells—dendritic cells or passenger leukocytes and graft endothelial cells—also can serve as APCs (direct pathway of allorecognition). This phase takes place within the blood, lymph nodes, spleen, and the transplanted organ.

Once antigens are prepared and presented, the next step (signal one) involves T-lymphocyte cell recognition of the antigen presented on the surface of the APC. The primary site for this to occur is at the CD3–T-cell receptor (TCR) complex on recipient T cells. This step involves the binding of the antigen, MHC, and TCR for T-cell activation. These T cells also express other molecules (clusters of differentiation [CD]) on their surfaces that, along with CD3, recognize and respond to different types of antigens. These T cells are known as $CD4^+$ cells (T_H, helper or inducer T cells) and $CD8^+$ cells (T_C, cytotoxic or suppressor T cells). $CD4^+$ cells interact with class II antigens. $CD8^+$ cells interact with class I antigens.

In addition (signal two), proteins known as adhesion molecules or costimulatory molecules promote T-cell signaling and activation. For T-cell activation to occur, binding of these costimulatory molecules as well as binding of the TCR with the presented antigen and MHC is required. Examples of these molecules include intercellular adhesion molecule (ICAM)-1 found on APCs, which bind with lymphocyte function-associated antigen expressed on the surface of T cells; ICAM-1 and ICAM-3 on APCs with CD2 on T cells; B7 (now called CD80 and CD86) on APCs with either CD28 or CTLA4 on T cells; and CD40 on APC with CD40 ligand (now called CD154) on T cells. The binding of costimulatory molecules is critical to T-cell activation. Without this costimulation, T cells undergo abortive activation or programmed T-cell death (apoptosis).

Once recognition and costimulatory binding occurs, T-cell activation and proliferation are initiated. After interacting with class II antigens and stimulation from IL-1 secreted from macrophages, T_H cells produce and secrete cytokines (e.g., interleukin [IL]-2 and interferon [INF]-γ). T_H cells are classified according to their cytokine-secretion pattern into either T_{H1} or T_{H2} cells. T_{H1} cells secrete IL-2, INF, and tumor necrosis factor (TNF), which stimulate cytotoxic T cells (T_C). T_{H2} cells secrete IL-4, IL-5, IL-6, IL-10, and IL-13, which stimulate B-cells. T_H cells, along with T_C cells, are stimulated to express cell-surface IL-2 receptors (IL-2R) and other cytokines. Once the T_C cells express IL-2R, they bind to IL-2 and other cytokines, which leads to signal transduction that results in proliferation, division, and stimulation of T cells (signal 3). These committed T_C cells bind directly to allogeneic cells and produce cell lysis. T_H-secreted cytokines recruit other T cells, which results in further cytotoxicity. During this process, T_H cells also produce cytokines that trigger a cascade of events involving B cells and antibody production, complement fixation, increased macrophage infiltration, neutrophil involvement, fibrin deposition, platelet activation and release, prostaglandin release, and inflammatory response at the graft site. These delayed-type hypersensitivity and humoral responses occur in conjunction with one another and are not mutually exclusive. This results in cellular and tissue injury and graft destruction

The antibodies produced by plasma cells, which are transformed B cells under the influence of cytokines, bind to the target antigenic cells. This leads to local deposition of complement and results in immune complexation and injury to the graft (complement-mediated cell lysis). The newly formed antibodies cause a series of interactions to occur with T cells, which lead to cytotoxicity (antibody-dependent, cell-mediated cytotoxicity). These cell-mediated and humoral immunologic events can impair organ function so significantly that without therapeutic intervention, complete organ graft dysfunction may occur. Under certain circumstances, which are not clear, certain T_C cells, known as suppressor T cells, downregulate the immune response to alloantigen.[6]

Human Leukocyte Antigen Typing

The genetic compatibility between donor and recipient can have a major impact on acute rejection, graft function, graft survival, and patient survival. For example, in kidney transplantation, the closer the HLA matching is between recipient and donor, the better the outcome, particularly over the long term. To determine this compatibility, a number of laboratory tests, including serologic, flow cytometric, genetic-DNA-based, and cellular assessments of donor and recipient serum and lymphocytes, are performed before organ transplantation. This process is referred to as tissue typing. Lymphocytes are typed for HLA-A, HLA-B, and HLA-DR. Typing for HLA is performed using the donor and recipient lymphocytes for serology-based techniques or tissue or fluid containing nucleated cells.[7]

The panel-reactive antibody (PRA) test is commonly used to assess organ compatibility because recipients may have HLA antibodies from previous exposure to antigenic stimuli (e.g., blood transfusions, previous transplantation, and pregnancy). In this test, the recipient's serum is tested against a cell panel of known HLA specificities that are representative of possible donors in the general population. The percentage of cell reactions (recipient with potential donor) determines a recipient's PRA. It is done periodically on patients on the waiting list to determine their immunologic reactivity. The potential recipient with a higher percentage of PRA (>20%–50%) is at higher risk for rejection and will generally a have longer wait time for a kidney than patients with PRA less than 20%. With recent changes (December 2014) to kidney allocation systems, this wait time may change for these patients.

A cytotoxic and/or flow cytometry lymphocyte cross-match is also performed prior to transplantation. In this case, the potential recipient's serum is cross-matched to determine whether preformed antibodies to the donor's lymphocytes are present. A positive cross-match indicates the presence of recipient cytotoxic IgG antibodies to the donor. In kidney transplantation, a positive cross-match is usually considered a contraindication. Recently, a number of transplant programs have utilized desensitization strategies to reduce the level of HLA antibodies present in potential recipients as a mechanism to reduce likelihood of a positive cross-match with either identified living donors or future potential deceased donors. Common strategies to reduce these preformed HLA antibodies include serial delivery of plasmapheresis coupled with IVIG, rituximab, and bortezomib.[8] In liver transplantation, a positive cross-match is not an absolute contraindication because the need is urgent and because the liver appears to be more resistant immunologically to this type of reaction. These liver transplant recipients can, however, experience significant complications and early graft dysfunction. In kidney transplantation, organ allocation and matching now utilize a virtual cross-match in which potential recipients are listed with known unacceptable HLA antigens (those that have been pre-identified in the patient). If a potential donor is identified with a specific HLA antigen that the recipient has known antibodies directed against, they will be skipped on the list.

ABO blood typing is one of the most critical of all evaluations when determining the genetic compatibility for all solid organ transplants. Transplantation of an organ with ABO incompatibility typically results in a hyperacute rejection and destruction of the graft, although in kidney transplant, newer therapeutic approaches to overcome ABO incompatibility have been successful.[7]

IMMUNOSUPPRESSIVE AGENTS

Immunosuppressives, based on an improved understanding of their mechanisms of action and the mechanisms of rejection, have had the most significant impact on patient and graft survival. The currently used immunosuppressives are shown in Table 34-1. These agents can be categorized as induction or maintenance therapy.[9] Sites of action and role of the currently used agents are discussed below.

MAINTENANCE

Azathioprine

Azathioprine is a prodrug of 6-mercaptopurine (6-MP). Azathioprine and 6-MP are purine antagonist antimetabolites. The introduction of cyclosporine, tacrolimus, mycophenolate, and sirolimus has led to a significant reduction of azathioprine use or its elimination altogether in immunosuppressive protocols. It can be useful in some cases, because it is inexpensive, or in patients who cannot tolerate other agents. It continues to be used in other countries.[9]

Table 34-1
Currently Used Immunosuppressive Agents

Drug (Brand Name)	Usual Dose/Route (How Supplied)	Therapeutic Use(s)	Major Adverse Effects
Alemtuzumab (Campath-H1)	IV 0.3 mg/kg or 30 mg × 1 dose (30-mg vial for injection)	Prevention and treatment of acute cellular and antibody-mediated rejection; steroid-free protocols	Lymphopenia, leukopenia, infection
Azathioprine (Imuran)[a]	IV or Oral 1–3 mg/kg/day (50-mg tablet; 100-mg vial for injection)	As maintenance agent to prevent acute rejection	Leukopenia, thrombocytopenia, hepatotoxicity, nausea and vomiting, diarrhea, pancreatitis, infection
Antithymocyte globulin, equine (Atgam)	IV 10–20 mg/kg/day (250 mg/5 mL ampule for injection)	Treat acute rejection (including severe or steroid-resistant forms); as induction agent in high-risk patient to prevent acute rejection	Anemia, leukopenia, thrombocytopenia, arthralgia, myalgias, nausea and vomiting, diarrhea, fevers, chills, hypotension, tachycardia, anaphylaxis, infection
Antithymocyte globulin, rabbit (Thymoglobulin)	IV 1.5 mg/kg/day given daily for 4–10 days (25 mg/5 mL vial for injection)	Treat acute rejection (including severe or steroid-resistant forms); as induction agent in high-risk patient to prevent acute rejection	Fever, chills, nausea and vomiting, hypotension, neutropenia, flushing, rash, itching, joint pain, myalgias, thrombocytopenia, infection
Basiliximab (Simulect)	IV 20 mg × 2 doses 10 mg; 2 doses for children if <35 kg (10- and 20-mg vial for injection)	As induction agent to prevent acute rejection	Abdominal pain, dizziness, insomnia, hypersensitivity reaction (rare)
Belatacept (Nulojix)	IV Initial Maintenance: 10 mg/kg on days 0, 4, 14, 28 and week 8 and12 and monthly thereafter Conversion from CNI: 5 mg/kg q 2 weeks for 5 doses, then every 4 weeks thereafter	As maintenance agent to prevent acute rejection; conversion agent from CNIs in patients with intolerances.	Anemia, neutropenia, diarrhea, UTIs, headaches, peripheral edema, PTLD
Cyclosporine[a] (Sandimmune)	Oral 5–10 mg/kg/dose BID IV 1.5–2.5 mg/kg/dose (100 mg/mL oral solution; 25- and 100-mg capsule; 250 mg/5 mL ampule for injection)	As maintenance agent to prevent acute rejection	Nephrotoxicity, hypertension, neurotoxicity, hair growth, gingival hyperplasia, hyperglycemia, hyperkalemia, dyslipidemia, hypomagnesemia, infection, neoplasm
Cyclosporine (Neoral, Gengraf, various others)[a]	Oral 4–8 mg/kg/day BID (100-mg solution; 25-, 50-, and 100-mg capsule)	As maintenance agent to prevent acute rejection; conversion agent from tacrolimus in patients with intolerance	Same as above
Everolimus (Zortress)	Oral 0.5–1.5 mg BID (0.25-, 0.5-, 0.75-mg tablets	As maintenance agent to prevent acute rejection; conversion agent from CNI in patients with intolerance or poor response	Dyslipidemia, thrombocytopenia, neutropenia, impaired healing, mouth ulcers, proteinuria, pneumonitis (rare)
Methylprednisolone[a] sodium succinate (Solu-Medrol, various others)	10–1,000 mg/dose (40-, 125-, 250-, 500, 1,000-, and 2,000-mg vial for injection)	As induction and maintenance agent to prevent acute rejection; to treat acute rejection	Hyperglycemia, psychosis, euphoria, impaired wound healing, osteoporosis, acne, peptic ulcers, gastritis, fluid, electrolyte disturbances, hypertension, dyslipidemia, leukocytosis, cataracts, cushingoid state, infection, insomnia, irritability
Mycophenolate[a] mofetil (CellCept)	1.5–3.0 g/day BID IV/PO (250-mg capsule; 500-mg tablet; 200 mg/mL oral suspension; 500-mg vial for injection)	As maintenance agent to prevent acute rejection; conversion agent from azathioprine and sirolimus in patients with intolerance or poor response	Diarrhea, nausea and vomiting, neutropenia, dyspepsia, ulcers, infection, thrombocytopenia, anemia
Mycophenolate[a] sodium (Myfortic)	360–720 mg PO BID (180- and 360-mg tablets)	As maintenance agent to prevent acute rejection. Alternative to MMF	Similar side effect profile as MMF

(continued)

Table 34-1
Currently Used Immunosuppressive Agents (*continued*)

Prednisone[a]	Oral 5–20 mg/day (1-, 2.5-, 5-, 10-, 20-, 50-, and 100-mg tablet)	As maintenance agent to prevent acute rejection	See methylprednisolone
Sirolimus[a] (Rapamune)	Oral 2–10 mg/day (0.5-, 1-, and 2-mg tablet; 1 mg/mL oral solution)	As maintenance agent to prevent acute rejection; conversion agent from CNI or mycophenolate or azathioprine in patients with intolerance or poor response	Dyslipidemia, thrombocytopenia, neutropenia, anemia, diarrhea, impaired healing, mouth ulcers, proteinuria, pneumonitis (rare)
Tacrolimus (Prograf, Astagraf XL, Envarsus XR)[a]	Oral 0.15–0.3 mg/kg/day BID IV 0.025–0.05 mg/kg/day as continuous infusion (0.5-mg, 1-mg, and 5-mg capsule; 5 mg/mL ampule for injection) Astagraf XL: Oral 0.1–0.2 mg/kg/day Once daily (0.5-mg, 1-mg, and 5-mg capsules) Envarsus XR: Oral 0.1–0.2 mg/kg/day once daily 80% of total daily dose of tacrolimus when converting from immediate-release formulation (0.75-, 1-, and 4-mg tablets)	As maintenance agent to prevent acute rejection; conversion agent from cyclosporine in patients with intolerance or poor response	Nephrotoxicity, hypertension, neurotoxicity, alopecia, hyperglycemia, hyperkalemia, dyslipidemia, hypomagnesemia, infection, neoplasm
Bortezomib (Velcade)	1.3 mg/m^2 on days 1,4, 8, and 11 IV bolus or sc (3.5 mg single use vial)	Inhibits plasma cells	Bone marrow suppression, thrombocytopenia, neuropathy, hypotension, gastrointestinal
Eculizumab (Soliris)	600–1,200 mg IV infusion (300 mg single use vial [30 mL of 10 mg/mL soln])	Inhibits complement	Infusion reaction, headache, hypertension, leukopenia, infections
Rituximab (Rituxan)	375 mg/m^2 × 1–5 doses or 500 mg/m^2 single-dose IV infusion (100 and 500 mg single use vial, in 10 mg/mL concentration)	Inhibits B-cell production	Infusion reactions (fever, chills, rigors); pain at infusion site, infections
Intravenous Immunoglobulin (Carimune NF, Flebogamma, Gammagard S/D, Gamunex, Iveegam EN, Octagam, Polygam)	100 mg/kg–2 g/kg IV infusion (vial size varies based on manufacturer, ranging from 1, 2.5, 5, 6, 10, 12, 20, 30 and 40 g; usually concentrations are 5% and 10%)	Immunomodulation of T- and B cells and/or immunoglobulin replacement	Infusion reactions (fever, chills, rigors); pain at infusion site, thrombosis, hemolytic anemia, acute renal failure, septic meningitis

[a]Generic products available.
BID, 2 times daily; CNI, calcineurin inhibitor; IV, intravenous; MMF, mycophenolate mofetil; PO, orally.

Azathioprine, a nonspecific antimetabolite immunosuppressive agent, affects both cell-mediated (i.e., T cell) and antibody-mediated (i.e., B cell) immune responses. Because it inhibits the early stages of cell differentiation and proliferation, azathioprine is useful for preventing rejection, but it is ineffective for the treatment of acute rejection. 6-MP, an active metabolite, is incorporated into DNA and RNA, thereby interfering with the intracellular formation of thioguanine nucleotides (TGN). 6-MP is intracellularly converted by hypoxanthine phosphoribosyltransferase to thioinosinic acid and then to thioguanine nucleotides. 6-MP may have two separate immunosuppressive effects: inhibition of cellular proliferation and cytotoxicity. A decrease in the levels of intracellular purine ribonucleotides decreases cellular proliferation, and incorporation of TGN into DNA mediates cytotoxicity.

The major metabolic conversion of azathioprine to 6-MP is via nucleophilic attack by glutathione. The liver and red blood cells are thought to be major tissue sites for this metabolic conversion. The 6-MP formed by this reaction can be metabolized further to thiopurine ribonucleosides and ribonucleotides such as 6-thioguanine nucleotide. These active metabolites, which have longer half-lives, are responsible for immunosuppressive activity. Azathioprine pharmacokinetics are not affected by renal dysfunction, but 6-TGN metabolite concentrations can accumulate in this situation.[1]

The most common adverse effect of azathioprine is bone marrow suppression. Bone marrow suppression may be related to a genetic deficiency of the enzyme, thiopurine methyltransferase. Low activity of this enzyme is rare but in some individuals it leads to greater availability of 6-MP, elevated 6-thioguanine levels, and susceptibility to myelosuppression. Low levels of thiopurine methyltransferase and specific genetic polymorphisms of this enzyme have been associated with severe azathioprine myelotoxicity and reduced efficacy.[10,11] Testing for this polymorphism has been advocated. However, few transplant centers perform genetic testing prior to use.

Mycophenolate Mofetil and Mycophenolate Sodium

As a result of several multicenter comparative registry trials in kidney transplant recipients, mycophenolate mofetil (MMF) has replaced azathioprine in many transplant protocols. MMF is used as adjunctive therapy in combination with cyclosporine or tacrolimus, prednisone, mammalian target of rapamycin (mTOR) inhibitors, and monoclonal and polyclonal antibodies to prevent acute rejection and used for calcineurin inhibitor (CNI) withdrawal and minimization. It is also used as rescue therapy when patients have not responded to, or cannot tolerate, the side effects of other immunosuppressive agents.

MMF is an antiproliferative antimetabolite that inhibits purine synthesis, but in a more selective manner than azathioprine. Unlike azathioprine, MMF interferes with the de novo pathway for purine synthesis. MMF is the morpholinoethyl ester prodrug of mycophenolic acid (MPA), which is the active component. MPA selectively, noncompetitively, and reversibly blocks an enzyme known as inosine monophosphate dehydrogenase (IMPDH) found primarily in actively proliferating T- and B cells. T- and B cells rely on this enzyme and the de novo purine pathway to produce purine nucleotides for DNA and RNA synthesis. Thus, MPA interferes with T-cell and B-cell proliferation. It is more selective than azathioprine. MPA also may affect cytokine production. Other secondary effects include inhibition of B-lymphocyte antibody production, decreased adhesion molecule expression, decreased smooth muscle proliferation and recruitment, and infiltration of neutrophils[12] (MMF pharmacokinetics are complex and discussed in detail in Case 34-7, Question 9).

Another oral formulation of MPA, enteric-coated mycophenolate sodium, is also approved by the US Food and Drug Administration (FDA) to prevent rejection in kidney transplantation, when used in combination with a calcineurin inhibitor (CNI) and corticosteroids. The original purpose of designing the enteric-coated formulation was to reduce or prevent the gastrointestinal (GI) side effects commonly seen with MMF. However, most data suggest that the efficacy rates and side effect profiles of MMF and mycophenolate sodium are nearly identical. These two agents are not bioequivalent.[12] Other aspects of their use, generic products, therapeutic drug monitoring, and adverse effects will be addressed later in this chapter (Case 34-7, Question 9).

Corticosteroids

Prednisone, methylprednisolone, and prednisolone—all synthetic analogs of hydrocortisone—are the primary corticosteroids used to prevent and treat rejection of transplanted organs. These agents usually are given in fixed doses or dosing is based on body weight (mg/kg) despite the pharmacokinetic differences. Although they are an important part of immunosuppression, a goal of most transplantation programs is to minimize, eliminate, or avoid corticosteroid use because of their numerous and significant side effects.

Corticosteroids have multiple effects on most cells and tissues of the body, but it is their anti-inflammatory and, more importantly, their immunosuppressive properties that serve as the basis for their use in organ transplant recipients. The corticosteroids bind with specific intracellular glucocorticoid receptors and interfere with RNA and DNA synthesis as well as transcription of specific genes. Cell function is altered, resulting in suppression or activation of gene transcription. Corticosteroids also affect RNA translation, protein synthesis, cytokine production and secretion, and protein and cytokine receptor expression.

Even after a single dose, corticosteroids cause marked lymphocytopenia by redistribution of circulating lymphocytes to other lymphoid tissues, such as the bone marrow, rather than by cell lysis; however, they also transiently increase the number of peripherally circulating neutrophils. Corticosteroids inhibit IL-1 and IL-6 production from APC, a number of events associated with T-cell activation, and IL-2 and IFN-γ production. They interfere with the action of IL-2 and IL-2R on activated T cells, resulting in the inhibition of T_{H1} function. They can enhance IL-10 regulatory function and enhance T_{H2} cell function. Moderate-dose to high-dose corticosteroids also inhibit cytotoxic T-cell function by inhibiting cytokine production and lysis of T cells. They can inhibit early proliferation of B cells but have a minimal effect on activated B cells and immunoglobulin-secreting plasma cells. The corticosteroids affect most cells and substances associated with acute allograft rejection and inflammatory reactions. They inhibit accumulation of leukocytes at sites of inflammation; inhibit macrophage functions, including migration and phagocytosis; inhibit expression of class II MHC antigens induced by INF-γ; block release of IL-1, IL-6, and TNF; inhibit the upregulation and expression of costimulatory molecules and neutrophil adhesion to endothelial cells; inhibit secretion of complement protein C3; inhibit phospholipase A_2 activity; and decrease production of prostaglandins.[13]

Calcineurin Inhibitors

CYCLOSPORINE

The activity of cyclosporine is mediated through a reversible inhibition of T-cell function, particularly T_H cells. Its major effect is inhibiting the production of IL-2 and other cytokines, including INF-γ. These actions result in an inhibition of the early events of T-cell activation, sensitization, and proliferation. Cyclosporine has little effect on activated mature cytotoxic T cells. Therefore, it has little usefulness in the treatment of acute rejection. Its site of action is within the cytoplasm of T cells after antigenic recognition and signaling occurs. Cyclosporine binds to an intracellular protein (immunophilin) called cyclophilin. Although binding to cyclophilin is required, it alone is not sufficient for immunosuppression. This cyclosporine–cyclophilin complex then binds to a protein phosphatase, calcineurin. This is thought to prevent activation of nuclear factors involved in the gene transcription for IL-2 and other cytokines, including IFN. Also, because of this inhibition, cyclosporine indirectly impairs the activity of other cells, macrophages, monocytes, and B cells in the immune response. Cyclosporine has no effect on hematopoietic cells or neutrophils. Cyclosporine is metabolized extensively in the liver to more than 25 metabolites. Two of these metabolites elicit a lower immunosuppressive effect in vitro. The role of these metabolites in the development of toxicity with cyclosporine is unclear.[14] The pharmacokinetics, dosing, and therapeutic drug monitoring (TDM) of cyclosporine are described in Case 34-3, Question 1 and Case 34-4.

TACROLIMUS

Tacrolimus is a macrolide with a different molecular structure than cyclosporine. Tacrolimus is more effective than cyclosporine in liver and kidney transplant recipients as the primary immunosuppressant in combination with corticosteroids or mycophenolate, azathioprine, mTOR inhibitors, and antibodies. It also is effective in some patients as rescue treatment in liver and kidney recipients experiencing acute or chronic rejection resulting from failure of standard immunosuppressive therapy. Tacrolimus is the preferred CNI over cyclosporine in most transplant centers.[2]

The activity of tacrolimus is similar to that of cyclosporine, but the concentrations of tacrolimus needed to inhibit production of IL-2 are 10 to 100 times lower than those of cyclosporine. Tacrolimus also inhibits production of other cytokines, including IL-3, IL-4, and INF-γ, TNF, and granulocyte-macrophage colony-stimulating factor. It has variable effects on B-cell response and also has anti-inflammatory effects. As with cyclosporine, tacrolimus binds to an intracellular, although different, protein: FK binding protein 12. This protein, which interacts with calcineurin, inhibits gene transcription of cytokines and interferes with T-cell activation.[15] The pharmacokinetics, dosing, and TDM of tacrolimus are described in Case 34-7, Question 3-6.

mTOR Inhibitors

Sirolimus, formerly known as rapamycin, is an FDA-approved agent for prevention of acute rejection and for withdrawal of cyclosporine in kidney transplantation. Positive results for sirolimus also have been observed in other transplant populations; in situations in which it is used in combination with other agents, including antibodies, tacrolimus, mycophenolate and prednisone; and when it has been used for rescue therapy. Its major use is in CNI avoidance, withdrawal, or minimization protocols.

Unlike CNIs, which work earlier in the T-cell activation cycle and inhibit cytokine production, sirolimus is an inhibitor of late T-cell activation. It does not block cytokine production; rather, it inhibits signal transduction, which blocks the response of T cells and B cells to cytokines, such as IL-2. Sirolimus binds to the same immunophilin bound by tacrolimus, FK binding protein. This complex interferes with the action of certain enzymes or proteins involved in cell proliferation signaling. Both cyclosporine and tacrolimus inhibit calcineurin, whereas sirolimus influences a protein called the mammalian target of rapamycin (mTOR). Sirolimus also inhibits an enzyme called P7056 protein kinase, which is involved in microsomal protein synthesis. These effects result in cell-cycle arrest, blockage of messenger RNA production, and blockage of cell proliferation. Sirolimus also inhibits proliferation of smooth muscle cells and may, although it is too early to tell, reduce the development of chronic rejection and, potentially, cancer.

Sirolimus exhibits significant pharmacokinetic variability. Its average bioavailability is 15%; C_{max} and AUC are linear over a wide range of doses. Sirolimus is extensively distributed. It distributes primarily into red blood cells and is highly plasma protein-bound, approximately 92%. It also binds to lipoproteins. Sirolimus is extensively metabolized in the gut and liver by cytochrome P-450 3A4 isoenzymes, and it is a substrate for P-glycoprotein. Its drug interaction profile is similar to that of cyclosporine and tacrolimus. Renal elimination accounts for 2% of a dose. The terminal half-life is approximately 57 to 63 hours and the time to steady state is 10 to 14 days in adults and shorter in children.

Everolimus is the newest FDA-approved mTOR inhibitor for use in both kidney and liver transplantation. Its mechanism of action is similar to sirolimus. Like sirolimus, it is used in CNI avoidance, withdrawal, or minimization protocols.

Everolimus is hepatically metabolized through the cytochrome P-450 3A4 but has a shorter half-life, average 30 hours, and different dose and frequency schedule than sirolimus. Similar to sirolimus, it requires monitoring of trough blood concentrations, although the target range is different from sirolimus. Its role in transplantation is generally similar to sirolimus, but direct comparison to sirolimus is needed.[16] Aspects of its use are discussed in Case 34-4, Question 2.

Belatacept

This agent is the first FDA-approved intravenous (IV) maintenance agent. Belatacept is a CTL4-Ig, which blocks the costimulatory pathway of CD28 or CTL-A4:CD80/CD86 binding interactions. CTLA4-Ig binds to CD80/CD86 to a greater degree than CD28, resulting in inhibition of costimulation and T-cell activation. Belatacept is given once every few weeks in combination with other agents, such as mycophenolate and prednisone, and generally well tolerated. It has been used as initial therapy, or for CNI avoidance or withdrawal (conversion) to reduce development or progression of CNI-induced reduction in renal function. Benefits on renal function have been demonstrated as well as other CNI-associated adverse effects. However, it should be noted that there is an increased risk of acute rejection, when belatacept is used in combination with mycophenolate, as compared to a cyclosporine- and mycophenolate-based regimen. There are no large-scale studies comparing it to tacrolimus-based regimens or in combination with cytolytic induction therapy. In clinical practice, some transplant centers utilize belatacept as a conversion agent in patients that cannot tolerate CNIs. There is an ongoing multicenter study to assess the efficacy of this. Other small studies have been published that utilize belatacept with mTOR therapy. It should be noted that belatacept is contraindicated in patients who are EBV antibody negative, due to risk of post-transplant lymphoproliferative disorder (PTLD). The phase III studies that demonstrated a higher risk of PTLD in those that received belatacept noted this was only the case in EBV-naive recipients, and CNS PTLD was of particular concern. Recent data presented in abstract form, which followed patients from the phase III studies out for greater than 7 years post-transplant, have now demonstrated improved graft survival in the belatacept arm, as compared to the cyclosporine group. Thus, this agent may offer beneficial outcomes for certain low-risk kidney transplant recipients. Use in other organs, particularly liver transplant recipients, is not recommended, due to previous studies demonstrating inferior outcomes, as compared to CNI-based therapy.[17]

INDUCTION

Polyclonal Antibodies

ANTITHYMOCYTE GLOBULINS

Polyclonal antibody products have been used for decades to prevent and treat acute rejection. Polyclonal products used today are administered IV and include equine (lymphoglobulin) and rabbit antithymocyte globulin, which is considered the polyclonal antibody of choice.

Antithymocyte globulin (ATG) preparations have also been made in goats and sheep for investigational study. However, the following discussion is limited to the products produced in horses and rabbits. Regardless of the species from which they are produced, all ATG products have similar pharmacologic effects. Their potency and antibody specificity vary, however, from batch to batch and between products. The production of polyclonal equine or rabbit antibody begins with the injection of homogenized human spleen or thymus preparations into the animals. This injection induces an immune response in the animals directed against human T lymphocytes; serum containing antibodies to T cells is collected from the animals and purified. Other antibodies to human cells are produced as well, however. These antibodies bind to all normal blood mononuclear cells in addition to T lymphocytes and B lymphocytes, resulting in depletion of lymphocytes, platelets, and leukocytes from the peripheral circulation. The mechanism of action of these agents is thought to be linked to lysis of peripheral lymphocytes, uptake of lymphocytes by the reticuloendothelial system, masking of lymphocyte receptors, apoptosis, and immunomodulation. These agents contain antibodies to a number of cell-surface markers on lymphocytes, including CD2, CD3, CD4, CD8, CD11a, CD25, CD44, CD45, HLA-DR, and HLA class I antigens. They also interfere with leukocyte adhesion and trafficking and also have effects against $CD20^+$ B cells. ATG preparations can produce a rapid and profound depletion of circulating T cells, often within 24 hours of the initial dose. The duration of the effect can last several weeks after a course of therapy, particularly with rabbit antithymocyte globulin. Antibodies can be produced to these products as well. This, however, does not appear to influence clinical outcomes (see Case 34-1).[18]

Monoclonal Antibodies

BASILIXIMAB

Basiliximab is an IL-2R antagonist, monoclonal antibody approved for use in combination with other immunosuppressives to prevent acute cellular rejection in kidney transplantation. Basiliximab is a chimeric antibody that contains both murine and human antibody sequences. This agent prevents episodes of acute rejection in kidney transplant recipients. It has been used, although not as frequently, in liver transplants. Comparative studies between basiliximab and other antibodies, such as rabbit antithymocyte globulin, have been conducted. Advantages over these other agents include ease of administration, minimal side effects, low immunogenicity, no greater infections or malignancy rates, and fewer required doses. It is well tolerated, although there are rare reports of anaphylaxis. Basiliximab appears to be most effective in immunologically low-risk patients, whereas in high-risk patients, its use may be limited. It binds to the α-subunit of the IL-2R, also known as CD25 or the TAC subunit, which is expressed only on the surface of activated T cells; this subunit is critical to IL-2 activation of T cells in the acute rejection process. Basiliximab prevents the IL-2R from binding with IL-2, thereby blocking T-cell activation. It does not cause lymphocyte depletion. Basiliximab, with the two-dose IV regimen, on days 0 and 4 post-transplant, saturates the receptor for approximately 30 to 50 days in kidney transplants.[19] See Case 34-1, Question 4.

ALEMTUZUMAB

Alemtuzumab is a humanized monoclonal antibody against CD52 proteins on the surface of T cells and B cells, natural killer cells, macrophages, and granulocytes. Binding of CD52 elicits antibody-dependent lysis of these cells. It is approved for use in certain types of leukemias, but not in organ transplant. Because it causes a profound reduction or depletion in lymphocytes, especially T_H lymphocytes, a number of studies have evaluated its effect as induction therapy to prevent acute rejection after kidney transplant. Several studies have investigated its use in low and high immunologic risk transplants and in steroid avoidance or withdrawal regimens and CNI avoidance or withdrawal regimens. Short-term studies have indicated a role for this agent in these situations. It is rarely used in liver transplantation. Most protocols with this agent give a single IV or subcutaneous (SC) dose in the operating room. With this dose, significant neutropenia and lymphopenia can occur, lasting for months to years in some patients. This single-dose regimen has been successful in reducing the incidence of fungal and viral infections as compared with multiple-dose regimens although infection is still a concern with single dose.[20,21] See Case 34-1, Question 4.

OTHER AGENTS

These agents, although not indicated for kidney transplantation, are being used and studied primarily in kidney transplantation. Intravenous immunoglobulin and rituximab, an anti-B-cell CD20 monoclonal antibody, are being used pre- and post-transplant in order to transplant patients with ABO incompatibility or who are highly sensitized. Eculizumab, a C5 complement inhibitor, and bortezomib, a proteasome inhibitor, are also being used and studied in these situations, as well as for the treatment of antibody-mediated acute cellular rejection.[22,23]

KIDNEY TRANSPLANTATION

Indications and Evaluation

All patients with ESRD are potential candidates for kidney transplantation unless contraindicated. The contraindications (absolute or relative) are determined by the individual transplant center. Absolute contraindications include current malignancy, active infection, active liver disease, HbsAg-positive, severe or symptomatic cardiac or pulmonary disease, specific renal diseases with an accelerated recurrence rate, substance abuse, and abnormal psychosocial and noncompliant behavior. Relative contraindications for the recipient of a kidney transplant include chronic liver disease, active infection, positive for hepatitis C, human immunodeficiency virus (HIV) positive, morbid obesity, current positive cross-match, and age greater than 70 years. The relative contraindication for the elderly with ESRD is controversial because approximately 40% of the ESRD population is older than 65 years and an increasing number of these patients are undergoing kidney transplantation. Patients with ESRD need not wait until they are receiving dialysis before being considered for a kidney transplant because early transplantation is associated with lower cost, better quality of life, and longer survival than patients on dialysis awaiting transplantation. The primary diseases leading to ESRD and transplant are diabetes, hypertension, glomerulonephritis, and polycystic kidney disease.

Diabetes and hypertension are the most likely causes of ESRD. A kidney transplant should return renal function to near normal (i.e., a glomerular filtration rate between 50 and 80 mL/minute), improve quality of life, and correct the complications of ESRD such as anemia, hypocalcemia, and hyperphosphatemia, but not diabetes, hypertension, or hyperlipidemia.

The risk–benefit ratio must be considered when evaluating a patient for any organ transplantation. In general, kidney transplants are performed to improve the quality of life and avoid the complications and outcomes associated with dialysis and renal failure. It is also more cost effective than dialysis. On the other hand, patients who are candidates for liver transplantation will die if the transplanted liver fails. Therefore, the criteria established for organ transplantation must be evaluated carefully before it is offered to any patient.

Donor and Recipient Matching

HLA matching of donor and recipient at the HLA-A, HLA-B, and HLA-DR loci is associated with better graft survival and longer half-lives for both living-related and deceased donor kidney transplants. A six-antigen match is ideal, whereas a zero antigen match is less favorable. The half-life refers to the time it takes for half of the grafts that survive the first year to fail. Organ half-lives are longer with living donors (average 15.9 years) compared with deceased donors (average 11.9 years).[24] For kidney recipients, the 1- and 3-year graft survival for a first deceased donor transplant is greater than 90% and greater than 80%, respectively. These positive factors may be offset, however, by ethnicity. Patient and graft survival after kidney transplantation is reduced in the African-American population compared with others because of immunologic, medical, pharmacologic, pharmacokinetic, pharmacogenomic, and socioeconomic reasons. Along with African-American race, other risk factors associated with decreased survival include advanced donor age, recipient age less than 15 years and greater than 50 years, retransplantation, a high PRA (>20%–50%), and delayed graft function. Recipients who fall into these categories are referred to as high-risk patients.

Because of a limited number of donors, the organ transplant community has devised methods to increase the donor pool by attempting to safely utilize marginal donors. In its most current form, this allocation system has incorporated the use of a predictive tool that determines the degree of marginality, termed the Kidney Donor Profile Index (KDPI). The KDPI uses donor information, including age, height, weight, ethnicity, hypertension, diabetes, cause of death, serum creatinine, hepatitis C status, and circulatory death status to rate kidneys from 0% to 100%. Those in the higher percentile are more likely to fail, as compared to kidneys with lower KDPIs. In the current allocation system, donors with a high KDPI (85% or higher) are reserved for older recipients.[25]

Immunosuppressive Therapy

CASE 34-1

QUESTION 1: G.P. is a 52-year-old, 72-kg African-American man with end-stage renal disease (ESRD) secondary to type 2 diabetes mellitus, hypertension, and hyperlipidemia. He has been undergoing hemodialysis 3 times a week for 4 years. Other medical problems include anemia, hypocalcemia, and hyperphosphatemia. G.P.'s medications include amlodipine 10 mg daily, ramipril 10 mg twice daily (BID), Lipitor 20 mg daily, calcium carbonate two tablets with meals and at bedtime, sevelamer 800 mg with meals, glargine insulin 30 units daily, Novolog 8 units with meals, and erythropoietin 8,000 IU IV 3 times weekly. He has been on the kidney transplant waiting list for 2 years. He is called by the transplant coordinator and admitted for a possible deceased donor (formerly called cadaveric) kidney transplant. G.P. has the same blood type as the donor. His most recent cPRA is 10%. Cross-match is negative, and HLA typing reveals a three-antigen match (A1, A2, and B35) between donor and recipient. On admission to the hospital, his laboratory values are as follows:

Na, 141 mEq/L
Potassium (K), 4.7 mEq/L
Cl, 102 mEq/L
Bicarbonate (HCO_3), 23 mEq/L
Blood urea nitrogen (BUN), 44 mg/dL
Serum creatinine (SCr), 13.9 mg/dL
Calcium (Ca), 7.8 mEq/L
Phosphorus, 6.2 mg/dL
Glucose, 225 mg/dL
Albumin 3.5 g/dl
WBC count, 8.4 cells/μL
Hemoglobin (Hgb), 10.8 g/dL
Hematocrit (Hct), 32%

His serology is negative for HIV, hepatitis B surface antigen (HbsAg), hepatitis C, and cytomegalovirus (CMV), and is positive for antibody to the surface antigen of hepatitis B (anti-Hbs), positive for Epstein–Barr virus (EBV) antibody

Before the transplant procedure, G.P. receives MMF 1 g orally (PO) and cefazolin 1 g IV. During surgery, just before reperfusion of his new kidney, he received methylprednisolone 500 mg IV and rabbit antithymocyte globulin 100 mg IV. He is also given furosemide 100 mg IV after the kidney has been transplanted. Methylprednisolone 250 mg IV is to be given on the day after surgery. The methylprednisolone dose is to be decreased to 100 mg IV on the second postoperative day for one dose. Prednisone 60 mg (1 mg/kg/day) PO is to be given on the subsequent day for one dose and tapered by 0.3 mg/kg/day to 20 mg daily by day 7 after surgery and further tapered to 5 mg daily within a month. Tacrolimus nasogastric (NG) or PO 0.1 mg/kg/day or 3 mg every 12 hours will be started within 12 hours after surgery if renal function improves. The dosage will be adjusted according to tacrolimus whole blood trough concentrations. MMF will be continued at 1 g PO BID. He will also continue with antibody induction with rabbit antithymocyte globulin 100 mg IV on days 1, 2, 3 after surgery. Why is G.P. being treated with this immunosuppressive regimen?

The major goal of immunosuppressive therapy is to prevent rejection and infection with minimal adverse effects and to ensure long-term patient and graft survival as well as improved quality of life. Overall acute rejection rates are <15% during the first year after kidney transplantation. Most of these episodes respond to acute antirejection therapy.

No consensus exists on the best induction and maintenance immunosuppressive regimen, and selection primarily depends on the program and the specific organ to be transplanted. Although studies have evaluated the various regimens, comparisons are influenced by differences in donor selection and condition, organ preservation and procurement, organ ischemic (cold and warm) time, recipient's pretransplant conditions, comorbid and high-risk or low-risk immunologic factors, surgical procedures, postoperative management and monitoring, and length of follow-up. Another important consideration is that many of the these agents show significant effects during the first year, but fail to show a significant impact on long-term effects such as chronic rejection and graft survival[3] The choice of a particular regimen generally depends on the risk factors present at the time of transplantation. During this early time period, because the risk of acute rejection is highest in the first few weeks to months, the number of agents, doses, and target drug concentrations are higher than later on after transplantation.

Most initial combination immunosuppressive drug regimens rely on two to three maintenance agents, although in some cases monotherapy has been used, depending on organ type and risk factors. Common combination regimens include a CNI (tacrolimus and cyclosporine) with MPA or sirolimus/everolimus, and prednisone. The most common regimen is tacrolimus, mycophenolate, and prednisone along with short-term administration of a monoclonal antibody (alemtuzumab, basiliximab) or a polyclonal antibody (rabbit antithymocyte globulin). Regimens that avoid steroids and CNIs, or use a short course, in the early transplantation period, or are withdrawn some time (usually several months) after transplantation in an attempt to avoid the long-term side effects of these agents, are another option. In HLA-identical, living-related kidney transplants, dual therapy (e.g., tacrolimus or mycophenolate and prednisone) gives excellent results; however, acute rejection may still occur, as well as with other regimens. Combination therapy is used to take advantage of different mechanisms of action and to reduce drug toxicity by using sequential therapy and smaller doses of multiple agents rather than larger doses of any agent used alone. These multidrug combinations can lead, however, to increased drug costs, compliance issues, a higher incidence of infection and malignancy, and difficulty in assessing and managing adverse effects.[9]

Because G.P. is receiving a deceased donor transplant and is considered an immunologically high-risk recipient (he is African-American), an antibody plus several maintenance agents would be appropriate. He is started on tacrolimus, mycophenolate, and prednisone. This combination based on the literature is the most effective.[15]

After the first 6 months, drug dosages are reduced over time and maintained at a stable dose for 6 months to 1 year. In G.P., tacrolimus cyclosporine, sirolimus, and everolimus doses are adjusted based on target trough concentration ranges, which are reduced over time as well. MMF may be discontinued later. Although the discontinuation of a drug may reduce adverse effects, it must be counterbalanced against the risk of rejection and potential graft loss. Monotherapy, generally with tacrolimus or cyclosporine, may be achieved in low-risk kidney, liver, transplant recipients at some time after transplantation. Most patients require lifetime immunosuppression.

CASE 34-1, QUESTION 2: What is induction therapy and which is the preferred agent for G.P?

Induction therapy after transplantation refers to the use of an antibody, typically at time of transplant and during the first few days after transplant. rATG, alemtuzumab, and basiliximab are induction agents. Acute rejection and delayed graft function (need for dialysis during first 7 days after transplant) can occur in the early transplant period. Both of these have a negative impact on graft survival. Antibody induction reduces the incidence of early acute rejection, delayed graft function, and has typically been used in immunologically high-risk patients. They allow the use of lower doses, or slower introduction or sequential use of maintenance immunosuppression. They are a major component of early therapy in high-risk patients. Their use in patients at low-to-moderate risk has increased, often as a means of reducing or avoiding the use of CNI and steroids. Currently, approximately 80% of all kidney transplants receive induction therapy, with rabbit antithymocyte globulin making up about 60%.[2,26]

rATG was chosen as induction because G.P. is African-American and is at higher risk for acute rejection. In general, rATG appears to be more effective than ATGAM (horse ATG) and is the antibody of choice. rATG, when used for induction, results in reduced acute rejection, improved survival, and manageable side effect profile. In kidney transplants, this agent is effective in reducing acute rejection and improving short- and long-term graft survival compared to horse ATG and especially in high-risk patients.[26]

Thymoglobulin and Antithymocyte Globulin

DOSING AND ADMINISTRATION

CASE 34-1, QUESTION 3: How would rATG be administered and monitored in G.P.?

Both rATG and horse ATG are effective as induction therapy, although not FDA approved, and as treatment of acute rejection. The dose of rATG ranges from 1 to 6 mg/kg but is typically 1.5 mg/kg/day, and the dose of horse ATG is 10 to 20 mg/kg/day, but is typically 15 mg/kg/day. These drugs can be diluted in 0.9% NaCl for injection and administered for 4 to 6 hours. Both are usually infused into a high-flow central vein to reduce pain, erythema, and phlebitis at the injection site. Peripheral administration has been used successfully with rATG[27] Skin testing is recommended before horse ATG use, but not rabbit-derived rATG. Patients previously sensitized to horse serum are at risk for an anaphylactoid reaction, but the prevalence of anaphylaxis has diminished with improved purification of this product. Patients with a positive pretherapy skin test could undergo desensitization, but alternatives, such as rATG, may be substituted.[18]

DOSE REGIMEN AND DURATION OF THERAPY

The first dose of rATG is usually given intraoperatively. Intraoperative administration of rATG reduces the incidence and severity of delayed graft function as compared with postoperative administration. Duration of therapy with rATG or horse ATG is 3 to 10 days for induction therapy. Protocols used to treat rejection commonly use a 7- to 10-day course of therapy. In patients such as G.P., a four-dose prophylactic regimen has been shown to be as effective as a longer regimen.[18]

ADVERSE EFFECTS

A number of adverse effects have been related to the use of rabbit antithymocyte globulin or ATG. Local phlebitis and pain usually can occur. Anaphylaxis is rare. Chills and fever, erythema, rash, hives, pruritus, headache, leukopenia, and thrombocytopenia are commonly encountered. Fever, chills, hypotension, nausea, and vomiting may be caused by the release of cytokines, such as TNF and IL-6, from lysed lymphocytes. These symptoms can be minimized by premedication with acetaminophen and diphenhydramine before each dose.

Methylprednisolone, up to 500 mg, is given 1 hour before rabbit antithymocyte globulin typically for the first two doses to minimize infusion reactions. Opportunistic viral (cytomegalovirus (CMV) and Epstein–Barr virus [EBV]) and fungal infections are the predominant delayed side effect. Susceptibility to malignancy, such as post-transplantation lymphoproliferative disease (PTLD), is also a concern. Because of the increased risk of CMV infection, patients are often given oral valganciclovir or IV ganciclovir during therapy and then oral valganciclovir, which is continued up to several months after induction.[18]

MONITORING

Vital signs should be monitored hourly during infusion, and WBC and platelet counts should be monitored daily. If the patient's WBC count drops to less than 3,000 cells/μL or if the platelet count drops to less than 100,000 cells/μL, the dose of drug is decreased by 50% or held entirely until the counts return to desired levels. Patients who receive rATG for the treatment of acute rejection may have doses held or decreased based on the degree of leucopenia and thrombocytopenia; however, the need for and response to therapy would be carefully considered in this decision.

Dosages also can be adjusted based on absolute lymphocyte counts or lymphocyte subsets as a way of maximizing efficacy and minimizing infectious complications. For example, the dose can be adjusted by using a target absolute T-lymphocyte count (CD2 or CD3) of less than 25 to 50 cells/μL, particularly if used for treatment of acute rejection. It is less common to adjust doses based on CD2 of CD3 counts when used for induction as in G.P.'s case. Using CD2 and CD3 counts results in a lower dose, less frequent dosing (e.g., every other day instead of daily), lower costs, and a lower rate of viral infection. rATG produces a more profound and longer duration of effect on lymphocytes than horse ATG; however, it does not result in a greater risk for infection and malignancy, although still a concern.[18]

CASE 34-1, QUESTION 4: Could basiliximab or alemtuzumab be used as an alternative to rabbit antithymocyte globulin?

Basiliximab is approved for use as induction therapy in kidney transplantation; however, it is also used in other organ transplant recipients. It is administered in combination with cyclosporine or tacrolimus and steroids with or without MMF or sirolimus. It has a similar safety profile compared to placebo and better safety profile than rATG. It has a limited role in high-risk populations such as G.P., or patients with high PRA or long ischemic times, delayed graft function, or patients who have received a previous transplant. In these patients, induction with polyclonal antibodies is used in most centers. The large initial trials with this IL-2R antibody included very few high-risk patients or excluded them altogether. More potent agents, such as rATG, are still preferred in high-risk patients. A prospective study comparing rATG with basiliximab in high-risk kidney transplants demonstrated that acute rejection rates were lower in patients receiving rATG.[20] Basiliximab is often used for low-risk to intermediate-risk patients and in patients where CNI minimization or steroid avoidance is implemented

Alemtuzumab is another alternative and is used by some centers for low- and intermediate- to high-risk patients. It has been shown to be no less effective than rATG in high-risk patients and more effective in reducing acute rejection than basiliximab in low-risk patients.[28] Adverse effects include frequent and prolonged neutropenia, lymphopenia, thrombocytopenia, anemia, nausea, vomiting, and diarrhea. Infusion reactions can occur although it is given, as a single dose, under anesthesia, in the operating room during the transplant. As with rATG, there is an increased risk of opportunistic infections and malignancy. Rituximab has also been studied as potential induction therapy in nonsensitized or ABO-compatible transplants and found not to be very effective in this population, unlike that in ABO-incompatible recipients.[22]

Postoperative Course and Delayed Graft Function

CASE 34-1, QUESTION 5: G.P. is admitted to the transplant ward for initial post-transplantation management. His urine output during the next 3 hours has decreased from 300 to 40 mL/hour. He is receiving IV fluids at a rate equivalent to his urine output. He received 3 L of fluids in the operating room. His blood pressure is 140/83 mm Hg, heart rate is 87 beats/minute, and temperature is 36.9°C; he has no signs of dehydration. His BUN is 56 mg/dL and his SCr is 12.8 mg/dL. Another dose of furosemide 100 mg IV increased his urine output to 140 mL/hour, but his urine output returned to less than 40 mL/hour in a few hours. Fluids and IV furosemide were given again with similar results. Renal ultrasound indicates no urine leaks, fluid collections, or ureteral obstruction. A diethylenetriamine penta-acetic acid renal scan indicates good perfusion, but decreased accumulation and clearance. During the next 2 days, G.P.'s BP is 150/93 mm Hg, weight is 76 kg (4 kg higher than pretransplantation), urine output has fallen to less than 200 mL/day, and relevant laboratory values are as follows:

BUN, 85 mg/dL
SCr, 13.2 mg/dL
K, 5.8 mEq/L

The decision is made to institute hemodialysis. What has happened to G.P.'s renal function? What is the most likely diagnosis?

The initial renal function after kidney transplantation can reflect excellent, moderate, or delayed graft function. In recipients with excellent function, a good diuresis begins immediately and continues; the serum creatinine rapidly declines to less than 2.5 mg/dL within the first few days after transplantation. Most living-related transplants and between 30% and 50% of deceased donor transplants generally experience this pattern. Kidney transplant recipients with moderate or slow graft function usually experience a slower decline in serum creatinine, which stabilizes within the first week. Recipients with delayed graft function usually have anuria or oliguria, require dialysis in the early period, and take days to weeks to recover. Delayed graft function is most common in recipients of organs from deceased transplant donors, occurring in between 10% and 50% of cases.[29] The diagnosis of delayed graft function is based on clinical, laboratory, and diagnostic criteria that may vary among centers. Traditionally, delayed graft function has been defined as the need for dialysis within the first 7 days post-transplant. Slow graft function is another term that has been used to describe a lag in improvement and does not involve dialysis. Delayed graft function is influenced by the donor (age, condition of organ, prolonged ischemic time), intraoperative conditions (hypotension, fluid imbalance, ischemia or reperfusion injury), and recipient characteristics such as prior transplantation, postoperative hypovolemia or hypotension, and use of nephrotoxic drugs.[29]

In G.P., poor urine output in the first hours after transplantation and subsequent oliguria, the exclusion of other causes of acute tubular necrosis, the results of the renal scan, the lack of improvement in BUN and serum creatinine, and the need for dialysis are indicative of delayed graft function. Delayed graft function reduces kidney long-term graft survival, increases the risk of acute rejection, and influences a patient's early management by requiring dialysis, increasing the length of hospital stay, and increasing the costs of therapy. It also may make the assessment of acute rejection more difficult because the patient already has impaired renal function. In delayed graft function, a renal biopsy may be obtained if no improvement in serum creatinine is seen by day 7.[29]

CASE 34-1, QUESTION 6: What adjustments should be made in G.P.'s immunosuppressive regimen at this time? Are there any therapies that can prevent or treat delayed graft function?

The adverse renal effects of CNIs may contribute to the onset of delayed graft function as well as prolong its duration. Therefore, tacrolimus may be discontinued temporarily or its dose significantly reduced. Because of this effect, some protocols do not include CNIs, use them only in low doses for the first week, or delay their use until kidney function improves. These protocols often include antibodies and provide more intense immunosuppression early after transplantation when the risk of delayed graft function and acute rejection is highest. Rabbit antithymocyte globulin is commonly used in patients with delayed graft function because it may shorten the duration and the need for dialysis when compared with the CNI. Another potential option would be to use basiliximab, which has been shown to reduce acute rejection rates and extend the time to first rejection. One concern with the use of basiliximab is that a CNI may be required sooner than with rabbit antithymocyte globulin because this agent does not provide as long a duration of protection from rejection. One should also confirm that MPA doses be maintained and continue prednisone taper. In G.P., rabbit antithymocyte globulin would be administered for 5 to 10 days, depending on improvement in his SCr and urine output, along with his current regimen of prednisone and mycophenolate. A typical dose would be 1.5 mg/kg/day or every other day, depending on his $CD3^+$ level, and WBC and platelet counts. Tacrolimus will not be started until his SCr decreases.

Recent studies have focused developing therapies that prevent or reverse delayed graft function, with mixed results. There are several therapies being tested within this context, which include therapies to inhibit p53 (I5NP), complement (eculizumab), TLR2 (OPN-305), and hepatocyte growth factor (BB3). Other therapies that have been tested include alteplase, etanercept, ischemic preconditioning, erythropoietin, and dopamine, with the later showing reduced dialysis requirements but none demonstrating improved graft survival. As this is a common and important clinical dilemma, it continues to be a significant area of research and discovery.[29]

Rejection

CASE 34-1, QUESTION 7: G.P. was started on rabbit antithymocyte globulin 1.5 mg/kg as a 6-hour IV infusion on days 0, 1, 2, and 3 for induction, but because of his delayed graft function, he received an additional dose on day 5. He received this along with his prednisone taper and MMF. Tacrolimus PO 3 mg BID was initiated on day 5 after transplant. G.P.'s urine output has increased gradually to 1,600 mL/day after stopping rabbit antithymocyte globulin. His weight has decreased to 73 kg, and the following is recorded:

BP, 142/84 mm Hg
Heart rate, 82 beats/minute
Temperature, 36.7°C
BUN, 23 mg/dL
SCr, 3.2 mg/dL
K, 4.6 mEq/L

Sixty days after stopping rabbit antithymocyte globulin, he is on a regular diet and taking all oral medications. His current medications include MMF 750 mg BID, prednisone 5 mg daily, tacrolimus 5 mg BID, ranitidine 150 mg at bedtime, dioctyl sodium sulfosuccinate 100 mg BID, amlodipine 10 mg daily, metoprolol 50 mg PO BID, glargine insulin 40 IU daily Novolog 10 IU with meals, valganciclovir 450 mg daily, and trimethoprim–sulfamethoxazole (TMP–SMX) double-strength, one tablet on Mondays, Wednesdays, and Fridays. His weight increased to 75.6 kg, and note the following:

BP, 160/94 mm Hg
Heart rate, 98 beats/minute
Temperature, 37.6°C
BUN, 30 mg/dL
SCr, 3.4 mg/dL
K, 4.8 mEq/L
Trough whole blood tacrolimus concentration, 5 ng/mL (target range 8–10 ng/mL)
Urine output decreased during the last 24 hours to 750 mL

He feels tired and has a decreased appetite, but his fluid intake has been adequate during the past day. What evidence is consistent with rejection in G.P.?

Although significant improvements in reduction in acute rejection and improved graft survival have occurred over the past decade, certain types of acute rejection and chronic rejection continue to be a major reason for graft loss in kidney transplants. Rejection episodes can be categorized as cellular and/or antibody mediated, hyperacute, accelerated, acute, or chronic. Kidney biopsy is considered the gold standard for making the diagnosis of rejection after kidney transplant. Approved criteria are used to classify and grade the type and severity of rejection.

HYPERACUTE REJECTION

Hyperacute rejection, which occurs within minutes to hours after transplantation of the allograft, is the result of preformed cytotoxic antibodies against donor-specific class I antigens. This type of rejection is rare because of ABO matching and improved HLA typing before transplant, but it remains associated with a poor prognosis. Clinically, the patient presents with anuria, hyperkalemia, hypertension, metabolic acidosis, pulmonary edema, and, in some cases, disseminated intravascular coagulopathy. A perfusion scan of the kidney would indicate no uptake. If other causes of anuria are excluded and this diagnosis is made, then the transplanted kidney must be removed.

ACCELERATED REJECTION

Accelerated rejection usually occurs within a few days after organ transplantation. This is a result of prior sensitization to antigens that are similar to those of the donor and newly developed donor-specific antibodies to the donor graft. Accelerated rejections of transplanted kidneys occur primarily in recipients who have had prior transplantation, multiple pregnancies, or blood transfusions. These patients usually maintain good renal function for a few days before developing acute renal failure. Accelerated organ rejections generally are more resistant to pharmacologic therapy.

ACUTE REJECTION

Acute rejection is the most common type of kidney rejection in transplant recipients and most episodes respond to therapy. Most episodes of acute rejection are T-cell-mediated (cellular), although some can be B-cell (antibody or humoral)-mediated, and others are a combination of both types. Acute rejection of a transplanted kidney is associated with reduced the half-life and survival of both living-donor and deceased-donor transplants. Acute rejection often occurs in the first week to months after kidney transplantation. The prophylactic use of antibody induction may, however, delay the onset for several weeks, as illustrated by G.P.'s case. If acute rejection occurs, its onset is generally within the first year, with most episodes occurring within the first 60 days after transplantation. Acute rejection can, however, also occur at any time after transplant and can be a result of patient nonadherence (also called noncompliance) to medications and monitoring. The clinical presentation of patients with acute rejection of a kidney ranges from an asymptomatic patient with mild renal dysfunction as indicated by an elevated serum creatinine, which is common, to patients presenting with a flulike illness, hypertension, and acute oliguric renal failure. G.P. presents with subjective complaints of malaise or tiredness and lack of appetite. Such nonspecific complaints occur often in patients with rejection and can be accompanied by myalgias. Objectively, G.P.'s increased weight, hypertension, decreased urine output, and increase in serum creatinine are consistent with acute kidney rejection. In addition, the tacrolimus trough concentration is low, suggesting inadequate immunosuppression. Acute rejection of a transplanted kidney must be distinguished from CNI nephrotoxicity, and infections (e.g., pyelonephritis, CMV, polyomavirus BK) also must be ruled out. Although the clinical evidence in G.P. probably represents an acute cellular rejection, a kidney biopsy is the gold standard for establishing the diagnosis. Biopsy results usually are available within 6 to 8 hours. If there is acute rejection, the biopsy will show an interstitial infiltration of mononuclear cells with tubulitis or intimal arteritis in more severe cases. The severity of acute rejection will be classified and graded according to standardized pathologic criteria and is important in determining treatment. Less severe grades will receive high-dose steroids, whereas more severe grades will often receive raATG.[6]

ANTIBODY-MEDIATED REJECTION

Antibody-mediated (previously called humoral) rejection can be either acute or chronic rejection mediated by antibodies. Over the past several years, there has been an increased recognition of the importance and detrimental impact of this type of rejection on graft outcomes. Antibody-mediated rejection (AMR) is ≤10% of acute rejection episodes but graft loss is near 30%. Histologically, criteria for AMR differ from ACR. Presence of positive staining for the complement component C4d indicates antibody-mediated rejection, although this type of rejection can also occur with negative C4d. Many patients either prior to transplant or after have donor-specific antibodies (DSAs) that can occur hours to years after transplantation. Antibody-mediated rejection often is associated with hemodynamic compromise and is more resistant to drug therapy.[30]

CHRONIC REJECTION

Chronic rejection is a major cause of long-term kidney graft loss after the first year. It can be either cellular- or antibody-mediated.

It occurs slowly in most cases over several years. The characteristic signs of chronic rejection are hypertension, proteinuria, and a progressive decline in renal function leading to renal failure. Because no specific treatment exists, therapy is supportive (e.g., dialysis in the case of kidney transplantation). Ultimately, retransplantation is needed. Some data suggest that some patients may benefit from some of the newer agents, such as mycophenolate and sirolimus, that are considered non-nephrotoxic, but this requires further study. The diagnosis of chronic rejection is determined by clinical signs and biopsy findings indicative of fibrosis of hollow structures and vessels within the graft. The chronic rejection of a kidney must be distinguished from chronic CNI nephrotoxicity, chronic infection, recurrence of the original kidney disease, and other causes of chronic allograft injury and other causes.

CHRONIC ALLOGRAFT INJURY

Chronic allograft injury (CAI) is a term that has been used, generally, as a diagnosis of exclusion that indicates a slow deterioration of renal function over months to years after kidney transplant, where the exact cause is unknown and results in graft loss. Immunologic and nonimmunologic mechanisms play a role in CAI. Immunologic factors that increase the likelihood of CAI include a history of acute rejection, inadequate immunosuppression, nonadherence with immunosuppressive therapy, and previous infection, such as CMV. Nonimmunologic factors are donor-related (age, hypertension, diabetes), increased ischemic times, recipient hypertension, hyperlipidemia, CNI nephrotoxicity, and elevated body mass index. Another term, interstitial fibrosis/tubular atrophy (IF/TA) is another term used to describe this deterioration. It is often considered irreversible and unaffected by increased immunosuppressive therapy.[31]

Acute Rejection Treatment

CASE 34-1, QUESTION 8: A biopsy of G.P.'s transplanted kidney shows grade 1A, moderate acute cellular rejection. G.P. is started on methylprednisolone 500 mg daily IV for three doses. His maintenance oral prednisone is discontinued and will increase MPA and TAC dose. He will be placed on a high-dose oral prednisone tapering regimen after his IV doses. Why is methylprednisolone therapy of G.P.'s first acute episode of rejection appropriate?

High-dose or "pulse" IV methylprednisolone, IV rabbit antithymocyte globulin, IV antithymocyte globulin, and oral prednisone are options to treat acute rejection in all types of solid organ transplants. A high-dose corticosteroid (usually IV methylprednisolone) is considered first-line therapy because it works very quickly in decreasing lymphocyte responsiveness, is easy to administer, and reverses at least 75% of acute rejection episodes. Rabbit antithymocyte globulin is usually reserved for steroid-resistant rejection or more severe grades of rejection. IVIG has also been used as an alternative for resistant rejection. The ideal corticosteroid dosage, route, and regimen are unknown. Corticosteroid protocols vary among transplant programs. IV methylprednisolone and oral prednisone are equally effective in reversing rejection, but oral corticosteroids are given for a longer period and have been associated with a higher incidence of adverse effects. Even though 50 mg of IV methylprednisolone has a similar lymphocyte suppressive effect as a 1-g IV dose, most programs use methylprednisolone 250 to 1,000 mg (most commonly 500 mg) IV every day for three doses and adjust the prerejection oral prednisone regimen accordingly. An example of an oral prednisone regimen is 100 to 200 mg/day tapered for 1 to 3 weeks to baseline maintenance dose. For G.P., IV methylprednisolone is appropriate because corticosteroids are considered first-line therapy for acute rejection of a transplanted kidney, and first rejection episodes (such as G.P.'s) are very responsive. In addition, G.P. has received a prophylactic course of rabbit antithymocyte globulin recently and additional doses should be avoided, if possible. Rabbit antithymocyte globulin is associated with a higher risk of CMV infection and malignancy; it is more difficult to administer, requires more intensive monitoring, is more expensive, and usually is held in reserve for corticosteroid-resistant or more severe forms of rejection.

Nevertheless, high-dose corticosteroids are not without risk. They increase the risk of infection, and long-term therapy can induce ocular, bone, cardiovascular, and endocrine abnormalities. Although G.P. will be receiving high-dose IV methylprednisolone for only 3 days, because he is diabetic, he should be monitored for hyperglycemia, and a change in his insulin requirements should be anticipated because corticosteroids can alter glucose metabolism. Short-course methylprednisolone also can mask signs of infection (e.g., fever, changes in WBC counts, pain associated with inflammation) and delay the diagnosis. Insomnia, nervousness, euphoria, mood shifts, acute psychosis, and mania also can occur with short-term corticosteroid use. If the methylprednisolone regimen is effective in reversing G.P.'s acute rejection, his serum creatinine concentration should decline within 2 to 5 days and his urine output increase.

In addition, it would be appropriate to increase G.P.'s tacrolimus dosage to 7 mg twice a day because the concentration is low (5 ng/mL) and low trough has been associated with a higher risk of acute rejection. Because small changes in tacrolimus dose can increase levels disproportionately, a trough whole blood concentration should be re-evaluated in 2 to 3 days. The mycophenolate dose could be increased to 1 g BID and up to 1.5 g BID, because this dose in combination with a CNI has reduced acute rejection in African-American patients, particularly if the patient was on cyclosporine therapy. There are limited data supporting the increase of the mycophenolate dose beyond 1 g BID with tacrolimus-based regimens.[32,33] If G.P. had been on cyclosporine, another option would be to change cyclosporine to tacrolimus, which has been shown to reduce future episodes of acute rejection. Another important aspect for prevention of future rejection would be to assess G.P.'s adherence with, and understanding of, his medication regimen. Nonadherence is a major cause of acute rejection and graft loss.[34]

CASE 34-1, QUESTION 9: Six months later G.P. is noted to have another elevation in Scr. In addition, donor-specific antibodies are also detected in blood. Did kidney biopsy indicate it as AMR? How would this type of acute rejection be treated?

AMR is more difficult to treat and approaches vary. It may not respond to steroids and thymoglobulin, which is used initially. The most common treatment is plasmapheresis or immunoadsorption. These modalities are used to remove circulating antibodies, and low- or high-dose intravenous immunoglobulin for residual antibody inhibition, given after these procedures. Because of increased recognition and diagnosis, and resistance to treatment, a number of approaches are being used and investigated. Along with plasmapheresis and IVIG, rituximab may be used to treat acute AMR. Other agents, not currently approved for transplantation, are being utilized and studied as treatment, including bortezomib, which causes plasma cell apoptosis/depletion and eculizumab which is an anti C5 antibody. Given the sparsity of large-scale, randomized trials assessing which agents to utilize to treat AMR, there is no consensus regarding which should be considered first-line therapy to treat AMR, although most clinicians do utilize plasmapheresis with IVIG as a starting point, and add on the aforementioned therapies at various stages or severities of AMR.[35]

Calcineurin Inhibitor-Induced Nephrotoxicity

CASE 34-2

QUESTION 1: C.C. is a 60-year-old man who received a deceased-donor kidney transplant 3 years ago. His serum creatinine at 1 year after transplant was 1.5 mg/dL; at 2 years, it was 1.7 mg/dL; now it is 1.9 mg/dL. He says he feels fine. His BP is controlled and urinalysis is negative for protein. A kidney biopsy conducted at this time indicates that he has no signs of acute or chronic rejection, but has evidence of CNI nephrotoxicity. His current regimen is cyclosporine 275 mg BID, MMF 500 mg BID, and prednisone 5 mg daily. His current labs show the following:

Cyclosporine blood trough, 220 ng/mL (target 100–150 ng/mL)
K, 5.5 mEq/mL
Mg, 2.3 mg/dL
Uric acid 8.0 mg/dL
Why does C.C. have CNI nephrotoxicity?

CNI nephrotoxicity is one of the most common adverse effects and occurs to some degree in all patients. The rise in the serum creatinine concentration is more gradual than, and not as high as, that seen with rejection. CNI concentrations may be elevated, although some patients may experience CNI nephrotoxicity even with levels below or within the targeted therapeutic range. Two forms of CNI nephrotoxicity have been identified: functional or acute renal dysfunction and chronic nephrotoxicity.[36]

Acute CNI nephrotoxicity is more likely to occur in the first months after transplantation and associated with high CNI doses and levels. Functional renal dysfunction or acute nephrotoxicity, the most common form of renal dysfunction, is characterized by rapid reversal when the CNI dose is held or reduced. This syndrome typically is not associated with histopathologic abnormalities. Repeated episodes of transient acute renal dysfunction can result in protracted acute renal dysfunction. Recovery of renal function after repeated episodes may not be complete even if the CNI is withdrawn. Protracted acute renal dysfunction can lead to direct tubular toxicity and can be associated with the development of thrombosis of glomerular arterioles or diffuse interstitial fibrosis.

Chronic nephrotoxicity is associated with proteinuria and tubular dysfunction. Renal biopsies in allograft patients with chronic CNI-related nephropathy show tubulointerstitial abnormalities, sometimes with focal glomerular sclerosis. These findings are considered nonspecific. Recently, the role of CNI chronic nephrotoxicity in the development of irreversible chronic renal dysfunction has been challenged and thought to be overdiagnosed in many patients. However, long-term use can result in chronic nephrotoxicity, is usually seen after 6 months of therapy, and may be irreversible. In this situation, renal function progressively declines to a point that dialysis or retransplant is required. The pathophysiology of cyclosporine or tacrolimus-induced transient acute renal failure is not understood completely, but seems to be related to its effects on renal vessels. For example, CNI can induce glomerular hypoperfusion secondary to vasoconstriction of the afferent glomerular arterioles, thereby reducing glomerular filtration. One possible explanation for these effects is that cyclosporine alters the balance of prostacyclin and thromboxane A_2 in renal cortical tissue. Increased thromboxane A_2 results in renal vasoconstriction. Endothelin release from renal vascular cells stimulated by CNI also may contribute to this acute effect through its potent vasoconstrictive properties. Activation of the renin–angiotensin–aldosterone system may also play a significant role. CNI also can cause a reversible decrease in tubular function. The alterations in tubular function reduce magnesium reabsorption and decrease potassium and uric acid secretion. This may be a result of direct tubular toxicity and possibly the result of thromboxane A_2 stimulation of platelet activation and aggregation.

C.C.'s rise in serum creatinine in conjunction with an elevated cyclosporine level suggests acute cyclosporine toxicity as the most likely cause of his findings. In this case, the total cyclosporine dose should be lowered by approximately 25% to 225 mg twice a day, to keep level in target range, and C.C. should be monitored closely for resolution of any symptoms and decrease in serum creatinine or worsening if rejection results from lowering the dose. His elevated potassium and uric acid and low magnesium should correct themselves with this dose reduction if it is acute CNI toxicity. If the nephrotoxicity is caused by cyclosporine, a decrease in the serum creatinine may be evident when the cyclosporine dose is reduced. If no such reduction occurs or if the serum creatinine continues to increase, then other nonimmunologic or immunologic causes should be considered and also need to substitute calcineurin inhibitor with an agent such as sirolimus, everolimus, or belatacept.

Calcineurin Inhibitor Avoidance, Withdrawal/Conversion, or Minimization

CASE 34-2, QUESTION 2: Would it be appropriate to withdraw cyclosporine in C.C.? If attempted, how could this be accomplished?

Cyclosporine and tacrolimus are associated with a number of metabolic, cardiovascular, neurologic, and cosmetic side effects but the most concerning is nephrotoxicity, which is a contributor to graft loss. The potential benefit of withdrawing cyclosporine would be to reduce toxicity, but this has to be weighed against the risk for rejection, graft loss, and toxicities of replacement agents.

Concern for chronic nephrotoxicity, as well as other long-term side effects, has led to the development of cyclosporine or tacrolimus minimization, withdrawal or substitution/conversion protocols, using agents, such as mycophenolate or sirolimus, everolimus, belatacept, or protocols using low doses of cyclosporine or tacrolimus.

Antibody induction, sirolimus, everolimus, mycophenolate, and belatacept, which are not associated with nephrotoxicity, have been evaluated in combination protocols that attempt to avoid, minimize, or withdraw CNI. Protocols completely avoiding CNIs usually contain combinations of these agents. Studies, which were usually done in low-risk populations, observed lower serum creatinine levels and fewer CNI-induced toxicities, but were associated with higher rates of acute rejection, especially when CNI is not used at all. Other trials that compared combinations of rabbit antithymocyte globulin, alemtuzumab, or basiliximab, sirolimus, everolimus, mycophenolate, and steroids with either cyclosporine or tacrolimus withdrawal, or minimization protocols have shown equal effectiveness compared to standard therapy.[37,38]

In the case of early cyclosporine withdrawal, there is a 10% to 20% increased risk of acute rejection, but no change in graft survival. Protocols are used that withdraw the CNI or at least reduce the dose to a minimal level. Many attempts are within the first 3 to 12 months after transplantation in the hope that the nephrotoxic effects can be reversed before significant chronic damage occurs. These approaches add mycophenolate, sirolimus, or both as the CNI is withdrawn or reduced in dose, but they have been primarily tested in low-risk patients. Data with sirolimus suggest that patients without proteinuria and an estimated glomerular filtration rate greater than 40 mL/minute in the first year had better renal function. Whether this applies to other agents remains to be determined. Usually, when sirolimus is added to the CNI regimen, the CNI dose is reduced by 50% initially and in some cases slowly withdrawn altogether during several weeks to months. Improvement in serum creatinine may be seen initially, which may be attributed to the diminution of the CNI vasoconstrictive effects.

CNI minimization or withdrawal may not reverse the nephrotoxicity observed in C.C.'s biopsy, but it may slow the rate of deterioration of his renal function. Because C.C. is currently receiving mycophenolate, one approach would be to continue to reduce his cyclosporine, increase his mycophenolate, and maintain steroids. Another approach would be to replace the mycophenolate with sirolimus/everolimus, because he has no proteinuria and his eGFR is >40 ml/min, maintain steroids, and reduce or withdraw slowly the cyclosporine. Belatacept could also be used as replacement for cyclosporine, while continuing mycophenolate and steroids. Some studies indicate better eGFR, lower incidence of new onset diabetes after transplant, lower blood pressure, lower cholesterol, but no difference in survival compared to CNI.[37] The best regimen for someone such as C.C. has not been established, because the long-term consequences of these changes are not known. If this approach is attempted, C.C. should be watched carefully for acute rejection, and side effects of these agents, which some patients do not tolerate, and infections should be closely monitored. In addition, BP control as well as control of hyperlipidemia and hyperglycemia could improve with reduction or withdrawal of cyclosporine, depending on agent used, and could also be important in minimizing renal injury.

STEROID AVOIDANCE OR WITHDRAWAL

CASE 34-3

Question 1: D.T., a 65-year-old Caucasian woman, will receive a deceased-donor kidney transplant today. She has a negative cross-match to this donor, and her previous cPRA was less than 10%. She will be given alemtuzumab 30 mg IV × 1 and methylprednisolone 500 mg IV × 1, intraoperatively. After transplant, she will be started on tacrolimus 0.05 mg/kg BID, adjusted to trough levels of 8 to 12 ng/mL for the first 3 months, along with MMF 750 mg BID. Methylprednisolone IV will be given as 250 mg IV on postoperative day 1, 125 mg IV on postoperative days 2 and 3, and no maintenance steroids thereafter. Is D.T. a good candidate for steroid avoidance or withdrawal?

Another important issue after kidney transplantation is the role of short-term and long-term steroid use. Most transplant protocols incorporate steroid therapy, although approximately 30% of transplant centers use steroids only in the early postoperative period.[2] The concept of either avoiding or discontinuing corticosteroids is appealing because they cause significant adverse effects such as diabetes, cataracts, infection, hypertension, hyperlipidemia, osteoporosis, avascular necrosis, and psychiatric, neurologic, and cosmetic effects. Steroid withdrawal or avoidance, however, may increase the risk of acute rejection, compromise long-term graft function, and necessitate higher doses of the other immunosuppressives. Steroid avoidance is defined as either no steroid use or steroid use only for the first few days after transplant. Short-term studies, generally in low-risk patients, suggest no adverse impact on short-term graft survival exists and no need is seen for higher doses of other immunosuppressives when corticosteroids are not included in maintenance regimens. These protocols have included regimens such as using induction agents, alemtuzumab, basiliximab, or rabbit antithymocyte globulin along with tacrolimus and cyclosporine, mycophenolate, sirolimus, or everolimus.[39]

Steroid withdrawal is the complete discontinuation of prednisone, typically a few months post-transplant. In the era of cyclosporine (Sandimmune)- and azathioprine-based regimens, withdrawal was associated with a high rate of acute rejection and late graft loss. With the introduction of newer agents, steroid avoidance or withdrawal has been viewed with renewed interest. Steroid withdrawal has been successful in at least 50% of kidney transplant recipients—resulting in reductions in blood pressure and lipid levels. Some protocols withdraw corticosteroids within the first few days to weeks after the initial transplantation period, whereas others withdraw them in 3 to 6 months or later after transplantation. The rate of success depends not only on the immunosuppressives used but on the population (high risk vs. low risk) and timing of withdrawal. Most success takes place in low-risk patients receiving antibody induction, such as rATG, with tacrolimus and mycophenolate with short-term steroids (≤1 week). African-Americans, pediatric patients, patients who have retransplants, highly sensitized patients, patients with a high serum creatinine (>2.5 mg/dL), and those who have had a recent rejection episode are more difficult to withdraw from steroids. This is particularly true early (<3 months) after transplantation. Withdrawal in these cases is associated with a higher rate of rejection. Later withdrawal may be attempted, but the benefits in terms of side effect profile may not be as great. Not all studies have demonstrated significance differences in side effect profiles between steroid withdrawal and continuation. Long-term outcomes are also limited using this approach. Low-risk populations are candidates for steroid avoidance or early withdrawal. First-time transplantation, living-donor, well-matched transplantation, older age, and stable graft function without rejection are factors associated with a positive benefit to steroid withdrawal.[39]

D.T. would be considered a low-risk patient because of her low immunologic activity evidenced by first time transplant, a living donor, low PRA, older age, and ethnicity. Therefore, a steroid avoidance protocol, such as the one indicated here, would be appropriate. As with other transplant recipients, she must be closely monitored for rejection and adverse effects.

Cyclosporine

CASE 34-4

Question 1: B.B. is a 27-year-old, 55-kg African-American man who received a deceased donor kidney transplant. Within 12 hours of the transplantation, his immunosuppression consisted of modified cyclosporine (Neoral) 300 mg PO BID, MMF 1.5 g PO BID, and prednisone. He was taking other medicines for hypertension and infection prophylaxis. What pharmacokinetic and monitoring parameters and adverse effects should be considered with using cyclosporine?

Cyclosporine pharmacokinetic parameters exhibit significant intrapatient and interpatient variability. A number of factors are known to influence its pharmacokinetic behavior and outcomes. These include age, ethnicity, transplant type, underlying disease, time after transplantation, GI metabolism and motility; biliary and liver function; metabolism, body weight, cholesterol, albumin, red blood cell mass; and drug interactions and formulation.[40] For example, children, African-Americans, and patients with cystic fibrosis tend to have reduced absorption, increased clearance of cyclosporine, or both. Patients who are obese or who have decreased liver function will have reduced clearance. Oral absorption of cyclosporine, which has been characterized as slow, incomplete, and highly variable, is the parameter that is most significantly affected. Absorption can depend on the type of transplant, time after transplantation, presence of food and its composition, intestinal function (e.g., diarrhea, ileus), small bowel length, and presence or absence of external bile drainage. Bioavailability ranges from less than 5% to 90%.[41] In most transplant recipients, cyclosporine absorption increases over time.

Because the original cyclosporine (Sandimmune) absorption was so poor and erratic, the IV route was used for the first few days after transplantation, particularly after liver transplantation. Cyclosporine can be given IV as a continuous infusion (2–3 mg/kg/day) or intermittently (2.5 mg/kg/day) over 2 to 6 hours divided into two equal doses. Sandimmune is used in very few patients today.

Neoral and Sandimmune are not bioequivalent and, therefore, not interchangeable. Neoral produces a higher maximum concentration (C_{max}), shorter time to C_{max} (T_{max}), and higher area under the concentration–time curve (AUC) than Sandimmune. It has significantly less intrasubject and intersubject pharmacokinetic variability, and a better correlation exists between single doses and trough concentrations and AUC than Sandimmune. The bioavailability of Neoral is approximately 20% higher than that of Sandimmune. Several other generic capsules and liquid formulations are now available for both.

Cyclosporine is extensively distributed into red blood cells; whereas in plasma it is highly bound to lipoproteins. It is extensively metabolized by both the gut and liver cytochrome P-450 3A4 enzymes and transported by P-glycoprotein. The average half-life is about 15 to 20 hours. Cyclosporine is an inhibitor of CYP3A4 and Pgp, so it can interact with other drugs.[41]

Cyclosporine can cause a number of adverse effects, of which nephrotoxicity is the most frequent and worrisome. Other major effects include hypertension, hyperlipidemia, tremors, headaches, seizures, paresthesias, hypomagnesemia, hypokalemia or hyperkalemia, hyperuricemia, hyperglycemia, gout, gingival hyperplasia, hirsutism, hemolytic–uremic syndrome, and hepatotoxicity. If these occur, they generally respond to a reduction in dose or concentration although some cases require discontinuation of cyclosporine.[42]

Cyclosporine concentrations are monitored to prevent toxicity, optimize efficacy, and assess patient compliance to the prescribed regimen. Most institutions monitor trough cyclosporine levels. During the early postoperative period, cyclosporine levels are often measured daily, keeping in mind that these may not reflect steady-state concentrations, and that dosage changes should be made every few days. The target trough therapeutic concentration of cyclosporine during the first 2 months post-transplant is 150 to 300 ng/mL with most whole blood assays. About 1 to 6 months after transplantation, the cyclosporine trough concentration target is lowered to 150 to 250 ng/mL. After 6 months, the targeted cyclosporine trough concentration is lowered even further to 50 to 150 ng/mL. These ranges differ among institutions and depend on the transplant type, time after transplantation, and other agents used. The range is reduced over time, given that less immunosuppression is required after transplantation and that the pharmacokinetics change over time. A few programs may monitor C2 levels, obtained 2 hours after a dose or determine AUC; however, these are more cumbersome. A number of assay methods are used to measure cyclosporine concentrations, and most institutions use the method that is most familiar to their transplant physicians.[43]

As in all cases, pharmacokinetic and drug level data must be interpreted in conjunction with the patient's clinical condition. In addition, deference always must be given to trends established by multiple cyclosporine levels rather than reacting to a single level. Single levels may be erroneous because of variability in dose administration, incorrect sampling time or techniques, or assay error.

B.B. was started on Neoral 10 mg/kg/day given in two divided doses. Because he is African-American, he may require even higher doses, because the of the increased gut metabolism of cyclosporine in this population. His trough concentration will be monitored closely and adjusted if necessary. Once B.B. is home, cyclosporine monitoring is necessary less frequently and eventually only every 1 to 2 months. He should be watched closely for signs of rejection and toxicity.

CASE 34-4, QUESTION 2: B.B. developed GI intolerance, nausea, vomiting, and diarrhea, to both mycophenolate products (mycophenolate mofetil and mycophenolic acid sodium) and cannot take either one anymore. A decision is made to use an mTOR inhibitor, sirolimus or everolimus instead. What would be important pharmacokinetic considerations, an appropriate regimen, and monitoring parameters for this agent?

mTOR Inhibitors

Sirolimus, and more recently everolimus, could be used as a substitute for other immunosuppressives. Experience and literature is more extensive with sirolimus.[16]. Sirolimus can be used in the immediate post-transplant period although impaired wound healing and lymphocele development in kidney transplantation have limited its use in the early period. In the case of liver transplantation, its use is contraindicated in the early post-transplantation period because of hepatic artery thrombosis. Sirolimus can be added later, as is the practice in many centers, as replacement for or minimization of cyclosporine, tacrolimus, steroids, or mycophenolate. In addition, sirolimus may be used as a substitute for these agents in patients predisposed to or with evidence of malignancy.[44] Early experience advocated an initial loading dose followed by a once-daily maintenance dose; however, because of its adverse effect profile, not all centers use loading doses. The starting maintenance dose is 2 to 5 mg. The typical loading dose is 6 mg followed by 2 mg every day. In high-risk patients, such as African-Americans, a 15-mg loading dose and 5-mg daily dose is recommended along with cyclosporine. Other centers have used loading doses of 10 to 15 mg, followed by 5 to 10 mg/day for the first week with target troughs of 10 to 15 ng/mL for the first month and 5 to 10 ng/mL thereafter when used with tacrolimus. Sirolimus is often given 4 hours after the morning dose of cyclosporine. If administered at the same time as cyclosporine, sirolimus concentrations are on average 40% higher.[45]

As with other immunosuppressives, sirolimus is associated with a number of side effects, including impaired wound healing, lymphedema, oral ulcerations, hypercholesterolemia, hypertriglyceridemia, diarrhea, arthralgias, epistaxis, rash, acne, leukopenia, thrombocytopenia, nausea and vomiting, lymphocele, hypokalemia, anemia, hypertension, pneumonitis, reproductive endocrine disorders, and infection. Dose-related hypertriglyceridemia, as well as hypercholesterolemia, occurs within the first few weeks of therapy and is sufficiently significant to require intervention with lipid-lowering agents, although it may respond to dosage reduction to some degree. Leucopenia and thrombocytopenia are also dose related. Sirolimus is associated with the development of proteinuria in kidney transplant recipients. The exact mechanism is unknown, but many transplant centers are now routinely monitoring for proteinuria in patients on sirolimus therapy and generally avoid its use in patients with preexisting proteinuria. Unfortunately, adverse effects are often the reason for discontinuing this agent in many patients.[46]

Trough blood concentration monitoring plays an important role in the dosing of sirolimus. Trough concentrations correlate well with sirolimus AUC. Because it has a longer half-life than the CNI, concentrations are obtained less frequently and only 5 to 7 days after a dose change. The target trough is usually 5 and 15 ng/mL; however, this continues to be refined with more experience. Early studies achieved concentrations greater than 15 ng/mL, especially when used without a CNI, which were associated with a greater immunosuppression and adverse events. Because sirolimus is synergistic with CNIs, the target concentrations of the CNIs are also reduced when these agents are used together. Target tacrolimus trough targets are 5 to 10 ng/mL, and the cyclosporine trough targets are 75 to 100 ng/mL, and in some patients lower, when used with sirolimus.[46]

B.B. could be started on sirolimus at 2 to 5 mg daily. Sirolimus blood trough concentration should be obtained 5 to 7 days after initiation. B.B.'s cyclosporine may need to be reduced if concentrations exceed 100 ng/mL. Monitoring parameters should include a fasting lipid panel, complete blood count, chemistries, and electrolytes. If everolimus was used, the starting regimen would be 0.5 mg twice daily. Everolimus blood concentrations should be obtained in 3 to 4 days after initiation. Target trough goal would be 3 to 8 μg/mL. Monitoring parameters would be similar to sirolimus.

Post-transplantation Metabolic and Cardiovascular Complications

CASE 34-5

QUESTION 1: J.F. is a 28-year-old African-American man who received a kidney transplant 8 weeks ago secondary to focal segmental glomerulosclerosis. His medical history is significant for hypertension. Before the transplant, he was taking lisinopril 20 mg PO daily and amlodipine 10 mg PO daily. After the transplant, amlodipine 10 mg PO daily was continued. J.F. was started on tacrolimus 8 mg PO BID and MMF 1 g PO BID. He also receives 10 mg prednisone PO twice daily and will be tapered down during the next 6 weeks to 5 mg PO daily. J.F.'s tacrolimus trough concentrations have been between 10 ng/L and 14 ng/L. During the next 12 weeks, he will be maintained on a dose of tacrolimus to achieve trough concentrations between 8 ng/L and 12 ng/L. J.F. currently weighs 95 kg and is 6 feet tall. His body mass index (BMI) is 28.5 kg/m^2. After transplant, he has required a sliding-scale regular insulin regimen to maintain an appropriate blood glucose level and was discharged on an insulin regimen that included lispro and glargine insulin. His BP readings during the past 2 weeks have ranged between 145 and 155/90 and 95. Fasting lipid panel is a total cholesterol, 261 mg/dL; LDL, 161 mg/dL; HDL, 40 mg/dL; and triglycerides, 200 mg/dL.

Why would J.F. have issues with controlling his blood glucose levels, blood pressure, lipid levels, and prevention of bone fractures after transplant?

Post-transplantation diabetes mellitus (PTDM) has also been referred to new onset diabetes after transplant (NODAT) and is another common problem that appears in transplant recipients. Diabetes significantly affects morbidity and mortality in transplant recipients. It is often a preexisting condition in renal transplant recipients and a cause of ESRD. In recipients of other organs, such as livers, diabetes is common as well, both as a preexisting condition and as a post-transplantation complication. The definition of PTDM varies among studies. It has been based on symptoms, plasma glucose and HgbA1c levels, oral glucose challenge results, or the need for insulin or oral antidiabetic drugs after transplantation. Reported rates are 3% to greater than 40%, with most cases of PTDM occurring within the first year after transplantation. Risk factors, besides pretransplantation diabetes, include advanced age, family history, CMV infection, certain HLA phenotypes, race (African-American or Hispanic), increased BMI, and hepatitis C infection in the liver transplant population. One of the most critical factors in the development of PTDM is the immunosuppressive regimen. Cyclosporine, tacrolimus, and prednisone are all associated with PTDM. The CNIs appear to have a direct toxic effect on the pancreatic beta cells leading to decreased insulin synthesis and secretion; this effect seems to be dose-related and generally reversible. Although still debated, the literature suggests that tacrolimus is more likely to cause PTDM than cyclosporine. Additionally, conversion from tacrolimus to cyclosporine has been useful in some patients. Prednisone is a major contributor to PTDM via multiple effects on beta cell sensitivity to glucose and ability to release insulin and insulin resistance in multiple tissues. Sirolimus has also been implicated in development of PTDM, although its role and mechanism is unclear. Other risk factors, such as CNI drug concentrations, steroid doses, transplant type, and time lapsed after transplantation, must also be considered.[47] As with diabetes in the general population, a similar intensive approach in controlling blood glucose should be undertaken. Also, other conditions (e.g., hypertension and hyperlipidemia) should be managed aggressively to reduce cardiovascular and kidney damage. Reducing or withdrawing diabetes-inducing immunosuppression as much as possible without jeopardizing graft function or using agents that are nondiabetogenic (such as mycophenolate) may be beneficial. One important aspect of post-transplant diabetes management is to realize the differences in pharmacologic management in this population, as compared with patients who are not transplant recipients. Often, in the immediate post-transplant period, because of the rapidly changing organ function and the dramatic tapering of corticosteroids, a patient's antidiabetic medicines may need frequent adjustment. During the first several weeks post-transplant, insulin is the agent of choice owing to the ability of the clinician to use sliding scales, the availability of several insulin products, and the ease in changing doses. Once patients are stabilized on their immunosuppressant regimen, and their organ function also, the use of oral antidiabetic agents can be introduced or restarted. Metformin, glitazones, gliptins, and sulfonylureas have been used in kidney transplants, but the use of oral agents is often dictated by renal function. Other considerations would be liver function and weight gain.[48]

J.F. was not diabetic pretransplant but is now requiring insulin. By some clinicians' definitions, he would be classified as having PTDM. Others would wait to see whether J.F. still required insulin after his immunosuppressant regimen was tapered to lower levels. In either regard, because J.F. is African-American, he is considered at high risk for the development of PTDM. At this point, J.F.'s diabetes should continue to be controlled on an insulin regimen. Once J.F.'s immunosuppression regimen is stable, he could be switched to oral antidiabetic agents if needed. J.F. should be counseled on diet and exercise to help control his blood glucose level. Other pharmacologic interventions that may help prevent long-term diabetes in J.F. is changing his tacrolimus to cyclosporine and reducing or withdrawing his prednisone. The risks and benefits of changing immunosuppressant regimens must always be weighed. For instance, changing his tacrolimus to cyclosporine, or reducing or removing J.F.'s steroids, may reduce his blood glucose level and may prevent PTDM, but it also will put J.F. at higher risk of developing acute rejection.

Post-transplant Hypertension

CASE 34-5, QUESTION 2: What pharmacologic options would be used for J.F.'s hypertension?

Cardiovascular disease is very common in patients with ESRD and after kidney transplantation. These patients with prior ESRD can have CAD, LVH and CHF, and arrhythmias and valvular heart disease. Cardiovascular disease after transplant is associated with graft loss and lower patient survival. In those recipients who die with a functioning graft, 40% die secondary to a cardiovascular event. Some immunosuppressives, including cyclosporine, tacrolimus, and steroids, contribute to the development of hypertension. Studies have indicated that blood pressure is higher, with high nighttime systolic blood pressure, and more difficult to manage in patients on cyclosporine compared with tacrolimus.[49] The appropriate blood pressure goals are similar to those in the general population, that is, less than 140/90 mm Hg in patients without proteinuria, as seen in this case. Nonpharmacologic therapies should be implemented; however, in transplant recipients, pharmacologic management is a key, often requiring multiple antihypertensives.

Pharmacologic agents used in transplant recipients are the same as those used in the general population. In the transplant recipient, one must consider the drug interaction profile and comorbidities. For example, nondihydropyridine calcium-channel blockers (CCBs), such as amlodipine, are less likely to interact with CNIs than diltiazem or verapamil. CCBs may also ameliorate some of the vasoconstrictive effects produced by the CNIs. In many programs, CCBs are considered first-line therapy. β-Blockers such as metoprolol are also frequently used in transplant recipients. Many recipients have or are at risk for coronary artery disease, and these agents can be effective in these situations. Angiotensin-converting enzyme (ACE) inhibitors and angiotensin receptor blockers (ARBs) can be used in transplant recipients, those with LVH. Historically, these agents were avoided, because of concern for their association with impaired kidney function. However, these have significant cardiovascular and renal benefits in patients with comorbidities such as diabetes, proteinuria, and congestive heart failure. Their use in transplant recipients has increased and is introduced shortly after transplant to months after transplant when renal function is more stable. Certainly if an ACE inhibitor or ARB is used, SCr and potassium levels must be monitored closely. Diuretics are useful in patients with evidence of fluid overload. In refractory patients, agents such as clonidine, hydralazine, and minoxidil may be required. In J.F.'s case, because he is already on amlodipine, a second agent such as lisinopril or metoprolol would be appropriate at this time with close monitoring and follow-up.

Post-transplant Hyperlipidemia

Case 34-5, Question 3: What would be an appropriate lipid-lowering therapy for J.F.'s hyperlipidemia?

Hyperlipidemia is another cardiovascular issue that must be addressed in transplant recipients. As with hypertension, it is fairly common pretransplant and post-transplant. It is associated with negative cardiac outcomes and reduced graft and patient survival in transplant recipients. Immunosuppressives including cyclosporine, tacrolimus, steroids, sirolimus, and everolimus can cause elevations in total cholesterol, LDL, and triglycerides, and also reduce HDL. Goals of treatment are primarily based on targeting an LDL of less than 100 mg/dL. Treatment involves diet, which alone appears to have minimal effect; therefore, pharmacologic treatment is usually required. Agents utilized in the nontransplant population are effective in reducing lipids in transplant recipients. Considerations in selecting treatments for hyperlipidemia include drug interactions with the immunosuppressives and the side effect profile. Statins are considered first-line treatment and have substantial evidence to support their use. Cyclosporine can increase concentrations of simvastatin and rosuvastatin, therefore limiting their doses and increasing potential for adverse events. Atorvastatin and pravastatin are often used and appear to be safe and effective in this population. Fibrates, ezetimibe, bile acid binders, and niacin are considered second-line agents.[49] In J.F., atorvastatin would be an appropriate choice.

Post-transplant Osteoporosis

Case 34-5, Question 4: Would osteoporosis and bone fractures be a concern and what would be appropriate therapies in this patient?

Rapid bone loss with the subsequent development of osteopenia or osteoporosis is another common post-transplantation disorder. Osteoporosis increases bone fragility and eventually leads to fracture. Studies estimate that osteoporosis occurs in 11% to 56% and fractures 5% to 44%, and increases in time in the transplant population. Osteoporosis risk factors for transplant recipients are similar to those in the general population included. Additional risk factors in kidney transplant include time on hemodialysis before transplant, vitamin D deficiency, pretransplant PTH and FGF-23 levels, diabetes, and steroid dose. Patients with ESRD commonly have at least some evidence of renal osteodystrophy, which includes hyperparathyroidism, osteomalacia, osteosclerosis, and adynamic or aplastic bone disease. Many kidney transplant recipients have already been exposed to medications that can affect bone and mineral metabolism, such as corticosteroids and/or loop diuretics.

Drugs used to prevent organ rejection predispose patients to osteoporosis, especially corticosteroids. The most dramatic reduction in bone loss after transplantation occurs within the first 3 to 6 months, when high doses of steroids are tapered to prednisone doses equivalent to 7.5 to 10 mg every day. As noted, corticosteroid-free or rapid-taper corticosteroid immunosuppressant regimens are being used to minimize or prevent post-transplant bone disease. Most studies suggest a minor effect of CNI on bone. Other currently used agents appear to have little or no effect. Most recommendations are based on the American College of Rheumatology's guidelines for the prevention and treatment of corticosteroid-induced osteoporosis. These recommendations focus on providing calcium and vitamin D (variable dosing depending on kidney and liver functions) to patients who will be receiving continuous corticosteroid therapy. Patients with osteopenia or osteoporosis with bone mineral density scans using dual-energy X-ray absorptiometry (DXA) scans, calcium, and vitamin D analogs are recommended in conjunction with either a bisphosphonate or calcitonin or teriparatide.[50,51]

Clinical trials have demonstrated that bisphosphonates and vitamin D or activated vitamin D analogs are effective in reducing or stabilizing bone loss but fail to show significant improvement in bone fracture rates, bone pain, or immobility owing to bone disease.

Although J.F. is young and likely may not have severe bone disease, a DXA scan should still be performed, as well as FRAX score should be determined. Phosphate, calcium and parathyroid levels, 25OH vitamin D levels, and eGFR should be assessed prior to initiation of any therapy. He could be given calcium and vitamin D because he is receiving steroids, unless he has a contraindication to this therapy. Based on the results of J.F.'s DXA scan, he may need to receive either a bisphosphonate or an activated vitamin D analog, such as calcitriol, vitamin D, and possibly calcium supplementation. A repeat DXA scan should be performed in 1 to 2 years. J.F. should be carefully counseled on how to take his medicine correctly and monitored for adverse effects.

BK Polyomavirus Infection

CASE 34-6

Question 1: K.T., a 45-year-old white man, is now 16 months post-transplant. His post-transplant course has been complicated by two rejection episodes. The first was severe and required rabbit antithymocyte globulin therapy; the second was a mild rejection several weeks later that was adequately treated with three pulse doses of 500 mg IV methylprednisolone. His current immunosuppressant regimen consists of tacrolimus 8 mg PO BID, MMF 1 g PO BID, and prednisone 10 mg PO daily. In addition, he is receiving amlodipine 10 mg PO daily, benazepril 10 mg PO daily, pravastatin 40 mg PO at bedtime, and calcium with vitamin D 500 mg/400 IU PO BID. Today, he is in the transplant clinic for a routine follow-up visit. He has no complaints and says he has been feeling "great," although he has noticed some blood in his urine during the past couple of weeks. Because of this, a urinalysis is ordered in addition to the standard laboratory values. The results are as follows:

Na, 145 mEq/L
K, 4.2 mEq/L
Cl, 104 mEq/L
HCO3, 26 mEq/L
BUN, 32 mg/dL
SCr, 2.7 mg/dL
Ca, 10.1 mEq/L
Phosphorus, 4.5 mg/dL
Glucose, 110 mg/dL
Amylase, 50 IU/L
Lipase, 32 IU/L
WBC count, 7.7 cells/μL
Hgb, 10.4 g/dL
Hct, 31%
Tacrolimus trough, 9 ng/mL
Urinalysis, color yellow
Specific gravity, 1.013
pH, 7.0
Protein, 100 mg/dL
Glucose, negative
Ketones, negative
Bilirubin, negative
Blood, moderate
Nitrite, negative
Leukocyte, negative
Squamous epithelial cells, 3 cells/high-power field
Bacteria, negative

Urinalysis revealed "decoy" cells, and plasma BK virus–PCR was greater than 10^4. Because of an increased serum creatinine, a percutaneous kidney biopsy is performed. The pathologist reviews the histology of the tissue sample and determines that it is consistent with polyoma-associated nephropathy. What is BK polyomavirus? How is it diagnosed and what are its clinical manifestations?

BK virus is a human polyomavirus, first isolated in 1971. Polyomaviruses are small, nonenveloped viruses with a closed, circular, double-stranded DNA sequence. Little is known about the transmission or about the primary infection of BK virus. It is believed that viremia during the initial exposure results in systemic seeding and subsequently becomes a latent infection. The kidney is the main site of BK virus latency in healthy people. More than 50% of the general population express BK virus antibodies by age 3 years. Immunosuppression after transplantation probably leads to the reactivation of the virus, but other factors, such as organ ischemia and coinfection with other pathogens, may contribute to reactivation. Reactivation inevitably leads to viruria or viral shedding into the urine. Asymptomatic viruria occurs in approximately 10% to 45% of kidney transplant recipients.[52]

Diagnosis of polyoma-associated nephropathy is made by careful review of clinical, laboratory, and histologic findings. Patients are often asymptomatic, although hematuria has been noted in some patients. Clinically, BK virus nephritis mimics acute rejection, and increases in serum creatinine often lead to a tissue biopsy. Tissue histology is similar to cases of acute rejection and BK virus nephritis, with mononuclear infiltration as the predominant finding. The abundance of plasma cells, prominent tubular cell apoptosis, collecting duct destruction, and absence of endarteritis are features that may distinguish BK virus nephritis from acute cellular rejection. Although BK virus has been implicated in up to 5% of all cases of interstitial nephritis (of which 30% go on to graft failure), it is still unclear whether asymptomatic biopsy findings in the kidney transplant recipient are a prognostic indicator. Decoy cells in the urine and BK virus–PCR in blood are used as screening tools. Blood or plasma BK virus–PCR is a more sensitive and stable test, and correlates better with renal dysfunction than decoy cells. The American Society of Transplantation recommends screening for BK virus in all kidney transplants, by measuring serial BK PCRs monthly for the first 3 to 6 months post-transplant, then every 3 months until the end of the first year post-transplant, whenever there is an unexplained risk in serum creatinine and after treatment of acute rejection. If the BK–PCR is consistently >10,000 copies/mL, it is recommended to reduce immunosuppression.[53]

Most cases of polyoma-associated nephropathy occur within the first 3 months after transplantation, although a number of cases have been reported as long as 2 years after transplantation. The major risk factor for the development of polyoma-associated nephropathy and subsequent graft dysfunction or loss is the degree of immunosuppression. In addition, accelerated graft loss has been demonstrated in patients who received antilymphocyte antibodies in the presence of polyoma-associated nephropathy misdiagnosed as an acute rejection episode. K.T., like many patients with BK virus, is asymptomatic with an elevated serum creatinine. Because K.T. has received higher doses of immunosuppression recently to treat two acute rejection episodes, he is at higher risk for developing BK virus nephritis.

TREATMENT

CASE 34-6, QUESTION 2: K.T. is told to stop taking MMF and to reduce his tacrolimus dose to 4 mg PO BID with target trough levels less than 6 ng/mL. Why was K.T.'s immunosuppressive regimen significantly reduced?

Because BK virus reactivation and BK nephritis are strongly associated with the degree of immunosuppression, reduction in, or removal of, immunosuppressant agents is considered first-line therapy and most effective approach. Beneficial clinical responses have been demonstrated in some patients when the dose of CNI is reduced and/or other agents removed. Not all patients, however, respond to this maneuver. In addition, reduction in immunosuppression puts patients at higher risk for an acute rejection episode. Close clinical follow-up after reduction of immunosuppression is important to ensure adequate response and to make sure the patient does not experience an acute rejection episode. In K.T.'s case, an improvement of renal function can be expected, as seen by a reduction in serum creatinine over time. Also, monitoring viral loads from both the urine and the serum has been shown to correlate with clinical disease.[54]

CASE 34-6, QUESTION 3: During the next 2 weeks, K.T.'s serum creatinine remains unchanged, and his serum and urine viral loads also remain approximately the same. Are there any additional treatment options for K.T.'s BK nephritis at this time?

ANTIVIRAL THERAPY

Cidofovir, an antiviral agent indicated for the treatment of CMV retinitis, inhibits polyomavirus replication in vitro; however, to date, no well-conducted clinical trials have proved this agent to be effective in treating or preventing polyoma-associated nephropathy in the transplant population. In a small number of case reports and case series, this agent was beneficial, but the appropriate dose and frequency are still undetermined. Most reports have used very small doses (0.25–1.0 mg/kg/dose) to minimize nephrotoxicity. It is given IV either weekly or every other week and usually continued until renal dysfunction is resolved and a decrease in the viral load occurs.

Cidofovir is associated with a high incidence of nephrotoxicity, especially at much higher doses; therefore, patients usually receive predose and postdose hydration with 0.9% NaCl boluses. Close clinical monitoring of the patient is advised if this treatment option is used. Because the doses of cidofovir currently used are approximately 5% to 10% of the standard dose used to treat CMV (5 mg/kg/dose), use of probenecid as a premedication to prevent high-dose cidofovir-induced nephrotoxicity is not advocated. Other therapies that have been tried with mixed success are IVIG and leflunomide in place of the discontinued antimetabolite, such as mycophenolate. Retransplantation has also been conducted with some success.[54]

LIVER TRANSPLANTATION

Indications

CASE 34-7

QUESTION 1: E.P., a 58-year-old, 78-kg man with an 18-year history of chronic liver disease secondary to hepatitis C infection, arrives at the emergency room with a 2-day history of confusion, fever up to 102.2°F, and worsening jaundice, with scleral icterus. Because the patient has severe abdominal distention, a paracentesis is performed, and 7 L of fluid is drained from his peritoneal cavity. A diagnosis of spontaneous bacterial peritonitis is made.

E.P.'s clinical status during the next several days gradually worsens, and he is moved to the intensive care unit for closer monitoring and better supportive care. E.P. continues to be severely jaundiced, with worsening liver function tests (LFTs). He becomes progressively more confused and eventually comatose requiring intubation. Within 3 days of admission into the intensive care unit, a suitable liver donor, matched for size and ABO blood group, is found and E.P. receives an orthotopic liver transplant with a choledocho-choledochostomy (duct-to-duct anastomosis). CMV serology for E.P. is negative, and the donor liver is CMV positive.

After the transplantation, E.P. is started on fluid maintenance with 0.45% normal saline; tacrolimus 2 mg NG/PO BID; and high-dose methylprednisolone with a rapid taper: 50 mg IV every 6 hours for four doses, 40 mg IV every 6 hours for four doses, 30 mg IV every 6 hours for four doses, 20 mg IV every 6 hours for four doses, 20 mg IV every 12 hours for two doses, then 20 mg IV daily; famotidine 20 mg IV every 12 hours; and ganciclovir 150 mg IV daily. Piperacillin–tazobactam 3.5 g IV every 6 hours for 48 hours was begun in the operating room. An order also is written to limit all pain medications and sedatives. E.P. returned from surgery with three abdominal Jackson–Pratt (JP) drains, an NG tube, Foley catheter, and Swan–Ganz central venous catheter. What was the indication for E.P. to receive a liver transplant?

E.P. was diagnosed with end-stage liver failure (cirrhosis) caused by chronic hepatitis C infection. Each center varies with respect to the most causes of cirrhosis leading to liver transplant, but nationwide, hepatitis C and alcohol-induced disease are the number one and two reasons for liver transplantation; however, in recent years, nonalcoholic steatohepatitis (NASH) has been increasing in incidence and is expected to become the most common indication within the next 10 years. Indications for liver transplantation in adults include cholestatic liver disease (e.g., primary biliary cirrhosis and primary sclerosing cholangitis), hepatocellular liver disease (e.g., chronic viral hepatitis B or C, autoimmune, drug-induced, NASH, cryptogenic cirrhosis), vascular disease (e.g., Budd–Chiari), hepatic malignancy, inherited metabolic disorders, and fulminant hepatic failure (e.g., viral hepatitis, Wilson disease, drug-induced or toxin-induced). Controversial indications include alcohol-induced disease and some types of hepatic malignancies. The concern with these indications is either recurrence of disease, as in the case of hepatic malignancies, or recidivism in the case of alcoholics.[55,56]

Contraindications to transplantation have decreased over the past few years. Current contraindications to liver transplantation include malignancy outside the liver, cholangiocarcinoma, active uncontrolled infection outside the biliary system, patients with alcoholic liver disease who continue to abuse alcohol, psychosocial instability and noncompliance, severe neurologic disease, and advanced cardiopulmonary disease. Patients with active infections are considered candidates after the infection has been eradicated.[56] HIV infection is not considered an absolute contraindication to transplantation.[57]

E.P. was within the age limitations for transplantation (in general, up to age 75 years is considered although exceptions are common); he had severe progressive disease and was at risk for death if he had not received a liver transplant. Because he did not have any of the listed contraindications, a liver could be transplanted emergently. His anticipated survival after transplantation at 1 year is greater than 85%; at 5 years, it is greater than 70%.[56]

Patient Monitoring

CASE 34-7, QUESTION 2: How should E.P. be monitored in the initial postoperative period?

Ideally, E.P. should be awake and alert within 12 to 24 hours after the operation, transferred from the intensive care unit to a regular bed in 1 to 2 days, and discharged home within 5 to 10 days. Because function of the transplanted liver is essential for the survival of the patient, extensive clinical, laboratory, and radiologic monitoring are necessary. E.P. has three JP abdominal drains that must be monitored for output production. The serum concentrations of BUN, creatinine, LFTs, potassium, sodium, magnesium, calcium, phosphate, and glucose should be monitored every 6 hours on the first postoperative day.[58] The surgical transplantation of a liver has been associated with coagulopathies and bleeding. Therefore, platelets, prothrombin time, fibrinogen, and factor V levels also should be monitored and deficiencies rapidly corrected when clinically indicated.[58]

Initial LFT results are highly variable; they can either increase for the first day or two after transplantation because of ischemic and reperfusion injury to the allograft, or they can decrease because of initial dilution by high-volume blood replacement. If the liver is functioning well, the LFTs, bilirubin, and prothrombin time all should begin to trend toward normal within a few days after the transplant.

Magnesium, phosphate, and calcium levels may fall in the early postoperative period and should be monitored closely. Ionized calcium serum concentrations are often monitored rather than total calcium because most patients have low serum albumin concentrations. Hypocalcemia can occur because these patients may receive large amounts of citrate through blood transfusions, which can lower serum calcium concentrations. Magnesium deficiency is common in patients with end-stage liver disease and may be exacerbated in the early post-transplantation period by tacrolimus or diuretics. Why patients experience hypophosphatemia is not fully known, but increased demand for phosphate for incorporation into adenosine triphosphate is a possible explanation. Hypokalemia or hyperkalemia can occur, depending on renal function and fluid status. Electrolyte serum concentrations should be followed and electrolytes replaced if needed (see Chapter 27, Fluid and Electrolyte Disorders).

Hyperglycemia, which is a good indication of a properly functioning liver due to its role in glucose homeostasis (gluconeogenesis and glycolysis), may need to be controlled with a continuous IV infusion of insulin initially, and then subcutaneous insulin dosed on the basis of periodic glucose measurements. In contrast, persistent refractory hypoglycemia indicates a poorly functioning liver. Hypertension, which is multifactorial, also is sometimes seen during this time and usually is treated with calcium-channel blockers or β-blockers. Renal dysfunction and neurologic complications also can occur.[58] Neurologic complications, including those that are drug induced, include oversedation, acute psychosis, depression, tremor, headaches, peripheral neuropathy, cortical blindness, paresthesias, paresis, and seizures.[59]

Additional complications that are common within the first 3 days to 3 months after liver transplantation include respiratory distress, intra-abdominal hemorrhage, biliary tract leaks and strictures, hepatic artery thrombosis, and primary graft nonfunction. Because infection is another early postoperative concern, E.P. should be monitored for bacterial, fungal, and viral infections.[58]

Tacrolimus

PHARMACOKINETICS

CASE 34-7, QUESTION 3: Seven days after his liver transplantation, E.P.'s JP abdominal drains, Foley catheter, and NG drain have been removed. Current medications include tacrolimus 4 mg PO every 12 hours; prednisone 20 mg PO daily; TMP–SMX single-strength, one tablet PO daily; and valganciclovir 450 mg PO daily. E.P.'s current laboratory values include the following:

BUN, 27 mg/dL
SCr, 0.9 mg/dL
Aspartate aminotransferase (AST), 170 IU/L
Alanine aminotransferase (ALT), 154 IU/L
γ-Glutamyl transferase (GGT), 320 IU/L
Total bilirubin, 3.4 mg/dL
Tacrolimus 9.4 ng/dL (whole blood by HPLC mass spectrometry)

What important pharmacokinetic factors should be considered when using tacrolimus after transplantation?

Tacrolimus is a highly lipophilic medication that is absorbed rapidly after oral administration; peak blood concentrations are achieved in about 0.5 to 1 hour. Oral bioavailability is usually poor, highly variable, and ranges from 4% to 89% (mean, 25%). Protein binding is approximately 99% and is mainly to erythrocytes and alpha1-acid glycoprotein. Whole blood concentrations are significantly higher than serum concentrations for this reason. Tacrolimus has a large volume of distribution and accumulates in high concentrations in tissues, including the lungs, spleen, heart, kidney, brain, muscles, and liver. Tacrolimus is predominantly metabolized in the liver through the cytochrome P-450 3A4/5 isoenzyme system and is primarily eliminated from the body as several inactive metabolites. Less than 1% of tacrolimus is eliminated as the parent compound in the urine, and renal dysfunction does not alter the pharmacokinetics of this agent. The elimination half-life ranges from 5.5 to 16.6 hours, with a mean of 8.7 hours. Varying degrees of liver dysfunction, including cirrhosis and severe cholestasis, may reduce the metabolism and excretion of tacrolimus. Pediatric patients have a higher clearance, shorter half-life, and larger volume of distribution compared with adults.[60] African-American patients may require higher dosages (0.2–0.4 mg/kg/day orally as opposed to 0.1–0.2 mg/kg/day orally), such as in E.P.[61]

DOSING

CASE 34-7, QUESTION 4: How would you initiate the dosing of tacrolimus for E.P.?

Although tacrolimus can be administered as a continuous IV infusion through a central or peripheral catheter after transplantation (initial dose 0.025–0.05 mg/kg/day), it is preferable to give it via an NG tube or orally because adverse effects, such as headache, nausea, vomiting, neurotoxicity, and nephrotoxicity, occur more commonly with IV administration. If tacrolimus is given IV, patients should be converted as soon as possible to oral therapy (initial doses of 0.1–0.3 mg/kg/day in adults and 0.15–0.3 mg/kg/day in children, divided into 12-hour intervals).[62]

In E.P., the initial starting dose was approximately 0.1 mg/kg/day given orally or through the NG tube every 12 hours. Oral tacrolimus should be administered on an empty stomach or taken consistently in relation to meals. Most institutions extemporaneously prepare an oral solution for NG tube administration because it is not commercially available.[61]

THERAPEUTIC DRUG MONITORING

CASE 34-7, QUESTION 5: E.P.'s tacrolimus concentrations are measured by whole blood HPLC mass spectrometry. Why is it important to monitor E.P.'s tacrolimus concentrations and how should his tacrolimus therapy be monitored?

Because of the large interpatient and intrapatient variability, the narrow therapeutic index, and the large number of potential drug interactions associated with this agent, tacrolimus concentrations should be monitored in patients receiving therapy. Concentrations are monitored to prevent toxicity, optimize efficacy, and assess patient adherence to the prescribed regimen. A relationship exists between concentration, efficacy, and toxicity.[62] The primary monitoring parameter used clinically is the trough concentration because trough concentrations correlate well with overall total body exposure (AUC). The target trough range is 5 to 12 ng/mL for the first 3 months and 4 to 10 ng/mL thereafter, but this can vary with each transplant center's protocols and type of transplant. Most centers are now using mass spectrometry to monitor all immunosuppressant concentrations. HPLC with mass spectrometry is a more reliable method of analysis that does not cross-react with metabolites; therefore, only parent drug is quantitated.[63]

As in all cases, pharmacokinetic data must be interpreted in conjunction with the patient's clinical condition. In addition, deference always must be given to trends established by multiple tacrolimus concentrations over that of a single concentration.

ADVERSE DRUG REACTIONS

CASE 34-7, QUESTION 6: What are the major adverse effects associated with tacrolimus and what clinical parameters should be monitored in E.P.?

Nephrotoxicity, which usually is the limiting adverse effect of tacrolimus, has been reported in more than 50% of patients in some studies.[64] This high incidence may be related to the higher dosages used in earlier trials. Fortunately, dose reduction usually reverses the acute nephrotoxicity. Because IV administration of tacrolimus during the first week has been associated with acute renal failure in 20% of patients, very few centers use this route or rapidly convert to oral therapy. Presumably, liver recipients with poor graft function have a very low tacrolimus clearance and are at a greater risk for acute renal failure.[64] In a multicenter study involving 529 patients, the efficacy and toxicity of tacrolimus was compared with cyclosporine in liver transplant recipients. Both agents increased serum creatinine and decreased glomerular filtration rate comparably.[65] Thus, E.P.'s renal function should be monitored closely.

Major neurologic toxicities (e.g., confusion, seizures, dysarthria, persistent coma) occur in approximately 10% of patients. Minor neurologic toxicities occur in approximately 20% to 60% of patients and include tremors, headache, and sleep disturbances.[65] Hypertension (40%) is another common finding in patients treated with tacrolimus. A greater number of tacrolimus-treated patients, however, are able to discontinue or limit their use of antihypertensives as compared with cyclosporine. Other adverse effects include diarrhea, nausea, vomiting and anorexia, alopecia, hypomagnesemia, hyperkalemia, hemolytic uremic syndrome, alopecia, increased susceptibility to infection and malignancy, and hyperglycemia. Hyperglycemia is reported to occur more often with tacrolimus than cyclosporine. This is most likely to be seen in patients with higher tacrolimus levels, higher steroid doses, and in African-Americans. With reduction in tacrolimus and steroid doses, hyperglycemia may reverse or decrease in severity. Hirsutism and gingival hyperplasia, which occur with cyclosporine, are not seen with tacrolimus use.

Generic Tacrolimus

In August 2009, the FDA approved the first generic tacrolimus. Since that time, there are up to five commercially available generic products. There has been continued controversy and debate regarding the bio- and clinical equivalence of generic tacrolimus products, with studies providing evidence on both sides of this argument. However, recently completed FDA-solicited multicenter crossover studies conducted in organ transplant recipients have demonstrated bioequivalence. The use of generic tacrolimus has become fairly routine across most transplant centers, although clinicians continue to caution against frequent changing of different manufacturers.[66]

Tacrolimus ER

Two new products, which are once-daily extended-release formulations of tacrolimus, have recently been approved for use in the United States (Astragraf XL and Envarsus XR). Studies demonstrate a 1:1 conversion from the normal-release product yields lower peak concentrations, but similar 24 hour AUCs when using Astragraf XL. Randomized clinical trials demonstrate similar rates of acute rejection, graft loss, and death between tacrolimus ER and normal-release formulations; however, specifically within female liver transplant recipients, there was a significant higher rate of death in the ER formulation group, which led the FDA to add a black box warning to the label for Astragraf XL. A number of small follow-up studies have also demonstrated improved adherence to the once-daily formulation, although this is a controversial area of debate amongst clinicians. The conversion from immediate-release tacrolimus to Envarsus XR is 1:0.8; meaning 80% of the preconversion daily dose of tacrolimus of immediate release should be given when using the Envarsus XR formulation.[67,68]

Rejection

Case 34-7, Question 7: E.P. was discharged from the hospital. He went to stay with his brother and was followed up with laboratory tests obtained 3 times a week. The following laboratory values were obtained 2 weeks later:

AST, 36 IU/L
ALT, 52 IU/L
GGT, 65 IU/L
Total/direct (T/D) bilirubin, 1.0/0.3 mg/dL
and another week later:
AST, 158 IU/L
ALT, 322 IU/L
GGT, 321 IU/L
T/D bilirubin, 3.6/3.2 mg/dL

E.P. was readmitted to the transplant center because his LFT rise suggested acute liver dysfunction, and a percutaneous needle liver biopsy was obtained to determine the cause. On admission, he complained of lethargy, severe headaches, a mild tremor, and some pain over the area of the transplanted liver. E.P. also stated that he had not felt like eating for the last 2 to 3 days. The pathologist interpreted the liver biopsy as moderate rejection, and E.P. was given a 500-mg IV bolus of methylprednisolone followed by rapidly tapered doses of IV methylprednisolone: 50 mg every 6 hours for four doses; 40 mg every 6 hours for four doses; 30 mg every 6 hours for four doses; 20 mg every 6 hours for four doses; 20 mg every 12 hours for two doses; then back to the pretaper oral prednisone dose. Three days into the recycle, E.P.'s liver enzyme values had not improved and rabbit antithymocyte globulin therapy was initiated. Laboratory values after 10 days of thymoglobulin IV 1.5 mg/kg/day were as follows:

AST, 35 IU/L
ALT, 108 units/L
GGT, 169 units/L
T/D bilirubin, 1.0/0.6 mg/dL

The 12-hour tacrolimus trough level at the end of the treatment course was 15.2 ng/mL. E.P. was discharged and sent home with the following medications: tacrolimus 5 mg PO BID; prednisone 20 mg PO daily; clonidine 0.3 mg PO BID; felodipine 10 mg PO daily; furosemide 20 mg PO daily; co-trimoxazole one tablet daily Mondays, Wednesdays, and Fridays; and valganciclovir 450 mg PO daily. What subjective and objective evidence of liver rejection is present in E.P.?

Hyperacute rejection rarely occurs with liver transplantation; when this occurs, treatment is supportive and retransplantation is required.[69] Unlike other organs, however, the liver may function adequately, but survival is lower when the organ is transplanted across blood types (ABO incompatible) or in patients that are presensitized to the HLA antigens.[70]

ACUTE LIVER REJECTION

Although acute liver rejection can occur at any time after the transplantation, it is most commonly experienced within the first 3 to 6 months after transplant and in approximately 20% to 50% of patients treated with either cyclosporine or tacrolimus and prednisone.[68] Data in patients treated with tacrolimus, mycophenolate, and prednisone indicate lower rejection rates.[71] Late acute rejections often are a result of either nonadherence, a reduction in dose, or a discontinuation of immunosuppressive agents. These rejection episodes, although somewhat common, rarely lead to graft loss.

E.P. presented with some of the subjective complaints of rejection. Commonly, patients feel poorly and complain of anorexia, abdominal discomfort, and headache. Other symptoms, such as a low-grade fever, back pain, or respiratory distress, may rarely occur. With the use of more potent immunosuppression, symptoms are no longer commonly present with acute rejection and cannot be relied upon for early indication of rejection. Objective evidence for rejection in E.P. included an abrupt rise in transaminases and bilirubin and a liver biopsy that was interpreted as "moderate rejection." These observations led to a diagnosis of rejection. Acute rejection is associated with mononuclear cell infiltration of the graft, edema, and parenchymal necrosis. Rejection should be diagnosed by biopsy using histologic criteria. Areas commonly damaged by rejection are the bile ducts, veins, and arteries, known as portal triaditis.[72]

CHRONIC LIVER REJECTION

Chronic liver rejection, also called ductopenic rejection, usually develops months to years after the transplant in less than 5% of recipients. Characteristics of chronic liver rejection include occlusive arterial lesions, destruction of small intrahepatic bile ducts (often referred to as vanishing bile duct syndrome), intense cholestasis, accumulation of foamy macrophages within the portal sinusoids, and fibrosis, which can lead to the development of cirrhosis.[72] Chronic rejection is almost always irreversible and unaffected by increased immunosuppressive therapy. Retransplantation has been considered the only viable alternative. Some patients with early ductopenic rejection unresponsive to cyclosporine-based therapy have responded to tacrolimus.[73]

Treatment of Rejection

CASE 34-7, QUESTION 8: Was the treatment of E.P.'s rejection of his transplanted liver appropriate?

E.P. was receiving maintenance immunosuppression with tacrolimus and prednisone. Double or triple therapy with tacrolimus and prednisone is commonly used as chronic immunosuppressive therapy. Although E.P.'s tacrolimus concentration appeared adequate, he was treated with a bolus dose of IV methylprednisolone because of clinical evidence that supported a diagnosis of graft rejection. This treatment decision was reasonable because high-dose corticosteroids reverse the majority of acute rejection episodes.[69] The decision to determine E.P.'s response to the initial bolus steroid dosage and the severity of rejection by biopsy also was appropriate before proceeding with further treatment. E.P. had experienced moderate rejection of his transplanted liver, and the subsequent initiation of rabbit antithymocyte globulin was reasonable because he did not adequately respond to the steroid recycle.

Rejection in adult liver transplant recipients is usually treated with 200 to 1,000 mg/day of IV methylprednisolone and tapered rapidly, similar to E.P. When patients fail to respond to recycle corticosteroid therapy, several options are available. E.P. was begun on rabbit antithymocyte globulin therapy; other options include the use of alemtuzumab. Most centers use rabbit antithymocyte globulin as a second-line agent if there is no response to high-dose corticosteroids or first line for severe rejection. The typical dose is 1.5 mg/kg/day given as an infusion for 4 to 6 hours and is continued for 7 to 14 days. Treatment of corticosteroid-resistant rejection with rabbit antithymocyte globulin is effective in about 70% to 80% of liver transplant recipients. Other adjustments in immunosuppression include the addition of mycophenolate or an mTOR inhibitor.[69]

Mycophenolate Mofetil

CASE 34-7, QUESTION 9: After the rejection episode, E.P. is started on MMF. Describe MMF's pharmacokinetic characteristics and adverse effects. How will these characteristics affect the dosing and monitoring of MMF in this patient?

In the vast majority of transplant centers, MMF has replaced azathioprine as the antiproliferative agent used in combination with antibodies, CNI, and prednisone. In E.P., MMF was not initiated immediately after transplant because he has hepatitis C, which can recur after transplant, especially with too much immunosuppression. Therefore, in his case, immunosuppression was initially minimized to limit the chances of severe hepatitis C recurrence.

PHARMACOKINETICS

Mycophenolate mofetil is a prodrug for the active form, MPA. MMF is well absorbed (bioavailability 94%) and is rapidly hydrolyzed to MPA. The C_{max} for MPA occurs between 1 and 3 hours, and it is hepatically and renally glucuronidated to inactive MPAG, which is eliminated by the kidney, but mainly excreted into the bile. Once MPAG is excreted into bile, it then may then undergo enterohepatic recycling in the GI tract, where it is deconjugated to MPA (which is reabsorbed back into the systemic circulation). Because of this recycling, a second peak occurs 6 to 12 hours after dosing. MPA has an elimination half-life of 17 hours on average; the volume of distribution is 4 L/kg, and it is highly protein-bound to albumin (98%). Protein binding correlates well with albumin, and free MPA concentrations somewhat correlate with the immunosuppressive effect. Renal impairment, liver dysfunction, and elevated MPAG concentrations in transplant recipients can reduce protein binding. This may be a function of low albumin concentrations seen in these patients.[12]

ADVERSE EFFECTS

The most commonly reported side effects for MMF are GI (anorexia, nausea, vomiting and diarrhea, gastritis), hematologic (leukopenia, thrombocytopenia, anemia), and infections. GI side effects are common, and all side effects are more common with higher dosages. Patients with GI complaints may respond to administering the dose without other medications, smaller more frequent doses, or lowering of the dose and titrating upward as tolerated.[74] If the WBC count is less than 3,000 or absolute neutrophil count is less than 1,300 cells/μL, the MMF dose should be reduced or discontinued.

DOSING

The usual MMF starting dose in adults is 1 to 1.5 g twice daily PO. Some advocate the higher dosage in high-risk patients (e.g., patients receiving another transplant, patients with a high PRA, African-Americans). The recommended regimen in patients with a glomerular filtration rate less than 25 mL/minute is 1 g twice daily PO. In children, 300 to 600 mg/m^2 or 23 mg/kg/day given 2 times a day PO has been recommended. Due to a drug interaction, doses should be higher when administered with cyclosporine (1 to 1.5 g) compared to tacrolimus (0.75 to 1 g).[12,32]

THERAPEUTIC DRUG MONITORING

Monitoring MPA plasma concentrations is controversial and not generally recommended at this time due to the lack of data demonstrating improved outcomes with TDM. There are a number of studies that have shown some benefit, with others not showing any clinical improvements with MPA TDM. In kidney transplant recipients, low MPA AUCs and troughs have been shown to correlate with acute rejection. In centers routinely performing MPA monitoring, typical AUC_{0-12} targets are 30 to 60 mcg/hour/mL and troughs 1 to 3.5 mcg/mL. MPA monitoring appears to be more beneficial in protocols where CNI sparing, withdrawal, or minimization is used. Once started on MMF, E.P. should be monitored for GI and hematologic side effects, as well as for any signs and symptoms of infection and rejection.[33]

GENERIC MYCOPHENOLATE MOFETIL

In 2009, the FDA approved the use of generic MMF in solid organ transplantation. Currently, there are multiple manufacturers with approved generic formulations of MMF. These products meet FDA standards for bioequivalence and are considered AB-rated to CellCept 250-mg capsules or 500-mg tablets.[75] Currently, there are no studies demonstrating that generic MMF has produced inferior clinical outcomes or increased the risk of medication side effects, and most clinicians are comfortable utilizing the generic formulation of MMF, although frequent changes between manufacturers are not recommended.

Drug Interactions with Immunosuppressives

CASE 34-8

QUESTION 1: C.C. is a 42-year-old woman who underwent a liver transplantation 5 days ago. She was noted to be febrile, with an elevated WBC. Cultures were obtained, and her JP drainage grew *Candida albicans*. C.C. was started on fluconazole 400 mg daily. Her other medications included tacrolimus 3 mg BID, prednisone 20 mg daily, mycophenolate 500 mg BID (low dose due to new onset infection), valganciclovir 450 mg daily, TMP–SMX single-strength tablet daily, and esomeprazole 20 mg every night. The tacrolimus trough level is 11 ng/mL. What drugs interact with immunosuppressive agents? Will the initiation of fluconazole require any adjustments in current medication doses?

Because the immunosuppressants have complex and highly variable pharmacokinetic profiles with relatively narrow therapeutic indexes, drug–drug interactions represent a significant clinical problem. Drug interactions can be separated into two main categories: pharmacokinetic and pharmacodynamic. Pharmacokinetic interactions occur when one medication alters the absorption, distribution, metabolism, or elimination of the immunosuppressant agent.[76,77] Table 34-2 displays the most clinically relevant pharmacokinetic drug interactions that are likely to be encountered in transplant recipients and how to manage these interactions. These include drugs that alter either the absorption or metabolism of the immunosuppressants. Note that this table is not comprehensive.

Pharmacodynamic interactions occur when one medication either potentiates an adverse effect or alters the pharmacologic effects of the immunosuppressant agent.[77] An example is the use of CNI in combination with ACE inhibitors. Because both classes of agents can cause hyperkalemia and potentially decrease renal function, toxicity may be more pronounced when given in combination.[78] Pharmacodynamic drug interactions are usually more difficult to identify and require a thorough knowledge of the pharmacologic effects of the agents. Often, little or no information in the literature on these types of interactions exists to guide the clinician in determining whether this drug interaction will occur. As a general rule, if an agent is known to cause a particular toxicity that is similar to a toxicity associated with the immunosuppressant agent, then there is a high likelihood that a pharmacodynamic interaction will occur. Another example is an interaction between metoclopramide and MMF. Both agents

Table 34-2
Immunosuppressant Drug Interactions

Immunosuppressant	Interacting Drugs	Mechanism	Consequence	Clinical Management
Calcineurin inhibitors (cyclosporine and tacrolimus), sirolimus and everolimus	Clarithromycin,[a] erythromycin,[a] telithromycin,[a] ketoconazole,[a] itraconazole,[a] fluconazole, voriconazole,[a] fluoxetine, fluvoxamine, citalopram, nefazodone,[a] diltiazem,[a] verapamil,[a] delavirdine,[a] ritonavir,[a] cimetidine,[a] grapefruit juice,[a] amiodarone, saquinavir, nelfinavir, indinavir, amprenavir, chloramphenicol[a]	Inhibit CYP 3A isoenzyme in the liver and intestines.	Increase the blood concentration of the IS.	Either prospectively decrease the IS dose or monitor trough concentrations and AUC more closely and adjust doses accordingly.
Calcineurin inhibitors (cyclosporine and tacrolimus), sirolimus and everolimus	Carbamazepine,[a] dexamethasone, phenobarbital,[a] phenytoin,[a] Saint-John's-wort,[a] rifampin,[a] rifabutin,[a] efavirenz,[a] nevirapine,[a] nafcillin, clindamycin	Induce CYP 3A4 isoenzyme in the liver and intestines.	Decrease the blood concentration of the IS.	Either prospectively increase the IS dose or monitor trough concentrations and AUC more closely and adjust doses accordingly.
Calcineurin inhibitors (cyclosporine and tacrolimus), sirolimus, mycophenolate mofetil, and mycophenolate sodium	Cholestyramine, colestipol, probucol, sevelamer, antacids (magnesium and aluminum containing), iron-containing products	Bind to IS and prevent absorption.	Decrease the blood concentration of the IS.	Avoid concomitant administration with IS and monitor trough concentrations.
Azathioprine	Allopurinol	Inhibit metabolism by inhibiting xanthine oxidase.	Increase the blood concentration of azathioprine.	Avoid use together or prospectively reduce azathioprine dose to one-third or one-fourth normal dose and monitor for increased toxicity.

[a]These are considered either potent inhibitors or inducers.
AUC, area under the curve; CYP, cytochrome P-450; IS, immunosuppressant.

are known to cause diarrhea, and a higher incidence or severity of diarrhea likely occurs when these agents are used together.[77]

It is important to be alert for drugs with pharmacologic effects that may alter the efficacy of an immunosuppressant.[77] For example, a drug with immunosuppressant properties, such as cyclophosphamide, could lead to overimmunosuppression of the transplant recipient and a higher incidence or severity of opportunistic infections. Conversely, a drug with immunostimulant properties, such as the herbal medication echinacea, may reduce the efficacy of the immunosuppressant agent and increase the risk of rejection in the transplant recipient.[76,77] Although agents that have pharmacodynamic drug interactions with the immunosuppressants are not absolutely contraindicated, transplant recipients should be closely monitored for either increased risk of drug toxicity or decreased drug efficacy when these agents are used in combination. When a transplant recipient adds any new medication—whether prescription, over-the-counter, or herbal—it should be thoroughly researched to determine whether there is a potential interaction with the immunosuppressant regimen.

In C.C., the addition of fluconazole will lead to a pharmacokinetic drug interaction by inhibiting the cytochrome P-450 3A4 system and may significantly increase tacrolimus concentrations. This interaction is usually evident within 2 to 5 days, and a maximal effect is seen within a week of initiating fluconazole. Therefore, C.C.'s tacrolimus dose should be reduced when fluconazole is started. Tacrolimus blood levels should be monitored, as should signs and symptoms of toxicity. Fluconazole could also influence steroid metabolism, but specific recommendations are not available. In general, drug interactions can be managed and, in some cases, may require only separate administration times. In other cases, an alternative agent can be used within a pharmacologic class that does not interact with these agents.

Infection Prophylaxis

CASE 34-9

QUESTION 1: S.C. is a 20-year-old man who underwent liver transplantation for end-stage liver disease secondary to chronic hepatitis B. Besides his immunosuppressives, he received ampicillin sulbactam 1.5 g every 8 hours for 24 hours perioperatively. After transplantation, he also was started on trimethoprim-sulfamethoxazole (TMP–SMX) double-strength (DS, 800/160 mg) one tablet Mondays, Wednesdays, and Fridays; nystatin 5 mL 3 times a day (TID); lamivudine 100 mg daily; and valganciclovir 900 mg PO daily. Hepatitis B immunoglobulin (HBIG) 10,000 IU was started intraoperatively and given every day for 8 days after transplantation. What is the rationale for the aforementioned agents? Should other measures be considered to prevent infection?

Infection continues to be a major source of morbidity and mortality. Transplant recipients have the same risk of infection from transplant surgery as any other patient having a surgical procedure. The incidence of infections or organ transplant recipients has decreased since the advent of cyclosporine. Infection rates, however, remain high—upwards of 50% in transplant recipients.[79]

Prophylactic antimicrobial therapy decreases the risk of surgical infections; however, prophylactic regimens and antibiotic therapies are highly institution-dependent.[80] Kidney transplant recipients typically receive a first-generation cephalosporin, such as cefazolin, to cover uropathogens and staphylococci. Usually, antibiotic prophylaxis is given preoperatively, prior to skin incision and continued for one to three doses post-transplant. Due to how severely ill a cirrhotic is going into transplant and the fact that the surgery requires multiple anastomoses in an nonsterile environment (the bowel), liver transplantations are associated with the highest rate of life-threatening bacterial infection. Piperacillin–tazobactam commonly is used to cover staphylococci, enterococci, and *Enterobacteriaceae.* Duration of therapy in these patients is individualized, based on the patient's postoperative recovery, but usually lasts from 24 for 96 hours post-transplant.[80] Infections can occur at any time after transplantation, but there are predictable time patterns for certain kinds of infections.[79] The time of highest risk for infection in transplant recipients is during the first 6 months, because they are receiving the highest doses of immunosuppressive agents during this period. Another time of high risk is during and after treatment of acute rejection with high-dose immunosuppression. Patients can acquire new infections (*Pneumocystis jiroveci* pneumonia [PJP], CMV), reactivate old infections (e.g., CMV, BK virus), or experience recurrence of underlying disease (hepatitis B or C). Opportunistic infections are common during this time, as shown in Table 34-3. Because the infections shown in Table 34-3 occur at such a high rate, it is routine to provide specific prophylaxis for many of them. For example, nystatin suspension 500,000 IU by "swish and swallow" 3 to 4 times a day is commonly used for 1 month post-transplant in kidney recipients, and fluconazole 100 mg every day is used to reduce fungal colonization of the GI tract in liver and pancreas transplant recipients; acyclovir, ganciclovir, valacyclovir, valganciclovir, and immunoglobulins can be used for CMV and/or herpes virus infections; and TMP–SMX is used for *Pneumocystis* prophylaxis. For patients with sulfa allergies, alternatives, such as dapsone 50 to 100 mg PO daily, inhaled monthly doses of pentamidine 300 mg and atovaquone are used. These generally are given for the first 3 to 6 months after transplantation and, in some cases, up to 1 year or even for life.[81] S.C. needs prophylaxis with TMP–SMX for PJP prevention; valganciclovir for CMV prevention; and HBIG and lamivudine, adefovir, entecavir, tenofovir, or telbivudine to prevent recurrence of hepatitis B.

Table 34-3
Common Opportunistic Infections After Transplantation

Organisms	Usual Time of Onset After Transplantation
Cytomegalovirus	1–6 months
Herpes simplex virus	2 weeks–2 months
Epstein–Barr virus	2–6 months
Varicella-zoster virus	2–6 months
Fungal	1–6 months
Mycobacterium	1–6 months
Pneumocystis jiroveci pneumonia	1–6 months
Listeria	1 month–indefinitely
Aspergillus	1–4 months
Nocardia	1–4 months
Toxoplasma	1–4 months
Cryptococcus	4 months–indefinitely

Hepatitis B

A major concern for S.C. would be recurrence of hepatitis B in his new liver. If hepatitis B recurs, it is associated with a poorer outcome. Strategies that have been effective are the use of lamivudine, adefovir, entecavir, telbivudine, and tenofovir preoperatively and HBIG, with or without oral antiviral therapy, postoperatively. S.C. was started on lamivudine and HBIG postoperatively because monotherapy with HBIG is associated with recurrence in 10% to 50% patients, whereas HBIG with lamivudine has been associated with a lower incidence of recurrence compared to HBIG monotherapy. Lamivudine resistance rates are reported in 15-30% of patients taking this agent per year. In patients who develop a resistant form of hepatitis B to lamivudine, adefovir, entecavir, telbivudine, and tenofovir have been shown to be effective. After the first week of HBIG, S.C. will continue to receive 10,000 IU IV as a 1-hour to 2-hour infusion weekly for 4 weeks, then 10,000 IU monthly for the first 6 to 12 months after transplantation. During this time, anti-HBs titers are monitored and kept greater than 500 IU/L. Because HBIG is expensive (up to $50,000 per patient per year) and with the newer, more potent, oral antivirals available, more transplant centers now target lower titers (>100 IU/L) and HBIG doses of 1,500 IU intramuscularly every 3 to 4 weeks with lamivudine.[82]

Hepatitis C

Another virus that is a major cause for concern is hepatitis C. Hepatitis C is currently the most common reason for liver transplantation, and recurrence of hepatitis C viral replication after transplantation is universal.[83] Overimmunosuppression can have a significant detrimental effect on this disease after transplantation. Survival rates are significantly lower at 5 years after transplant compared with patients who received liver transplants for non-hepatitis-C causes.[83] Recently, there have been dramatic advances in the treatment of hepatitis C, with the advent of noninterferon-based direct-acting antiviral (DAA) therapies. Preliminary studies have demonstrated sustained virologic response rates of >70%, as compared to rates of 30% to 50% with interferon-based therapies. In addition, the DAA therapies have a much improved tolerability profile, with less cytopenias and limited constitutional symptoms, thus substantially reducing the need to hold or discontinue therapy, as compared to interferon and ribavirin.[84,85]

Cytomegalovirus

CASE 34-10

QUESTION 1: A.A., a 58-year-old, 76-kg man with end-stage liver disease caused by alcoholic cirrhosis, received an orthotopic liver transplant 4 months ago. He presents to the transplantation clinic with a 7-day history of generalized malaise, fatigue, nausea, vomiting, diarrhea, low-grade fevers, and anorexia. At the time of transplantation, the liver he received was positive for CMV antibody, but he had negative CMV serology (CMV naïve). His postoperative immunosuppressant regimen included oral prednisone and tacrolimus 5 mg PO BID, with adjustments made to his dose to maintain a 12-hour trough concentration between 6 and 12 ng/mL. He was also given valganciclovir 450 mg PO daily for 3 months.

His postoperative course was complicated by an acute rejection episode on postoperative day 19, which was treated successfully with a pulse and taper of steroids. At that time, MMF 1 g PO BID was added to his immunosuppressant regimen. He was discharged from the hospital on postoperative day 24, with instructions to return to the transplant clinic in 4 days. Since then, he has done fairly well with no complaints until now, 4 months later. On admission to the hospital, a physical examination was remarkable for an oral temperature of 38.8°C, a BP of 112/79 mm Hg, a heart rate of 104 beats/minute, a respiratory rate of 22 breaths/minute, and a mild tremor. All other findings on his examination were benign. Pertinent laboratory findings include the following:

WBC count, 3,400 cells/μL
Platelet count, 34,000 cells/μL
BUN, 29 mg/dL
SCr, 1.4 mg/dL
Total bilirubin, 2.2 mg/dL
AST, 62 IU/L
ALT, 126 IU/L
CMV PCR 184,000 copies/mL (normal <500 copies/mL)
12-hour tacrolimus concentration, 18.3 ng/dL

His current medications include tacrolimus 6 mg PO BID; MMF 750 mg PO BID; prednisone 10 mg PO daily; TMP–SMX 80 mg PO Mondays, Wednesdays, and Fridays; calcium carbonate 1.25 g PO TID; vitamin D 800 IU PO daily; enteric-coated aspirin 325 mg PO daily; and nizatidine 150 mg PO BID. What is the most likely diagnosis for A.A.?

A major concern in A.A. at this time after transplantation is CMV infection, which is commonly encountered within 1 to 6 months after solid organ and bone marrow transplantation. It is a ubiquitous virus belonging to the herpes virus group. In healthy immunocompetent adults, infection with the virus is usually asymptomatic, whereas in immunocompromised patients, CMV can cause significant morbidity and mortality. CMV can potentiate the risk for developing bacterial and fungal infections and induce chronic injury to the transplanted organ (arteriosclerosis in the heart, obliterative bronchiolitis in the lungs, vanishing bile duct syndrome in the liver, and chronic arteriopathy in the kidneys).[86]

ETIOLOGY

Cytomegalovirus infection in transplant recipients usually occurs when latent viruses from a seropositive donor organ are reactivated owing to immunosuppression. Without prophylaxis, transmission of CMV from a positive donor to a negative recipient leads to an 80% to 100% infection rate and a 40% to 50% disease rate; a positive donor to a positive recipient leads to a 40% to 60% reactivation rate and a 20% to 30% disease rate; and a negative donor to a negative recipient leads to a 0% to 5% infection rate. Transplant recipients at highest risk for developing the disease are (a) those who are or have serologically positive donor and negative recipient (D+/R−) at the time of transplant, (b) elderly, (c) those who received antilymphocyte antibodies, (d) those who received a retransplantation because of acute rejection, and (e) those who received larger amounts of immunosuppressive agents.[86] A.A. is at high risk of CMV infection and disease because his CMV serology is D+/R−, he was treated for rejection, and his immunosuppression regimen is fairly intense for a liver transplant recipient.

DIAGNOSIS

Diagnosis of CMV is based on both clinical and laboratory findings. CMV may be detected by culturing body fluids, such as bronchoalveolar lavage, urine, blood, and tissue biopsies. CMV is contained within the host's leukocytes, which appear to have large intranuclear inclusion bodies. CMV PCR is now readily available with rapid turnaround in most centers for measuring viral loads in the patient's serum. Documented viral shedding alone is not, however, diagnostic for active disease without clinical signs and symptoms.[87] A.A. has laboratory findings consistent with CMV infection: viral shedding, as indicated by the CMV PCR of 184,000 copies/mL, leukopenia, thrombocytopenia, and clinical symptoms consistent with CMV infection, including malaise, fatigue, nausea, vomiting, diarrhea, and anorexia.

CLINICAL MANIFESTATIONS

In healthy immunocompetent adults, the CMV-infected individual is usually asymptomatic but may present with mild complaints of malaise, fever, and myalgias, as well as abnormal liver enzymes and lymphocytosis. More severe reactions are rare.[86,87] CMV may, however, be life-threatening in the immunocompromised. Evidence indicates that CMV infection is associated with graft rejection and that graft rejection in the setting of immunosuppression further exacerbates CMV infection. It often is unclear which comes first. The actual CMV course may be limited to fever and mononucleosis, or it may extend to organs presenting as pneumonitis, hepatitis, gastroenteritis, colitis, disseminated infection, encephalopathy, or leukopenia.

A.A.'s clinical presentation meets the criteria for CMV disease: viremia with clinical signs and symptoms. At this time, it is unclear whether or not A.A. has any end-organ involvement/disease. His liver enzyme concentrations are elevated, and he is having numerous GI symptoms (nausea, vomiting, diarrhea, and anorexia), which may be indicative of CMV hepatitis, CMV gastroenteritis, or CMV colitis, respectively. Alternatively, the increased total bilirubin and serum transaminases may be caused by acute rejection, and his GI problems and leukopenia may be a side effect he is experiencing from his medications (e.g., MMF). To fully differentiate among CMV hepatitis, CMV gastroenteritis, CMV colitis, acute rejection, and medication side effects, tissue biopsies should be obtained.

CASE 34-10, QUESTION 2: What are the treatment options for A.A.'s diagnosed CMV disease? What doses should be used, and how should the effects of these drugs be monitored?

Ganciclovir

Before ganciclovir was available, CMV infection was "treated" by reducing the level of immunosuppression. This may be one of the explanations for an increased prevalence of rejection associated with CMV infections. Graft loss in kidney recipients is undesirable; yet, it is not immediately life-threatening because a patient may return to dialysis. Reducing immunosuppression in liver recipients, however, could result in the patient's death owing to graft loss. Treatment has been largely unsuccessful with acyclovir, adenine arabinoside, and immune globulin. Ganciclovir is the first-line agent for the treatment of CMV disease in solid organ transplant recipients. Although ganciclovir is highly efficacious, there is still a potential 20% relapse rate of CMV after ganciclovir therapy in liver transplant recipients.

Ganciclovir, a virostatic agent, is a nucleoside analog that is phosphorylated in infected cells to its active form and is then incorporated into replicating viral DNA. Although ganciclovir-resistant strains of CMV have been isolated, their occurrence is far more common in patients with HIV; currently, ganciclovir-resistant CMV in solid organ transplantation is not a large concern. A.A. should receive ganciclovir IV, or oral valganciclovir for mild CMV disease; a recent study has demonstrated equivalence between IV ganciclovir and oral valganciclovir. Because relapses of CMV disease after treatment are of concern, some suggest that patients should be placed on maintenance therapy with valganciclovir or oral acyclovir after the IV course is completed.[88]

Dosing

In patients with normal renal function, the usual dose of ganciclovir is 5 mg/kg/dose every 12 hours and the usual dose of valganciclovir is 900 mg PO BID, both for 14 to 21 days. Dosage adjustment is necessary for patients with renal dysfunction with either agent. Because A.A. has an estimated creatinine clearance of 60 mL/minute, he should receive 2.5 mg/kg/dose (190 mg) IV every 12 hours for 2 to 3 weeks, followed by maintenance valganciclovir 450 mg PO daily for 2 to 4 weeks.

The most common adverse effect associated with ganciclovir therapy is neutropenia, occurring in up to 27% of patients.[87] Neutropenia is defined as an absolute neutrophil count of less than 500 to 1,000 cells/μL. The neutropenia usually resolves with a decrease in dosage or discontinuation of the drug, but colony-stimulating factors increase the total white count.[88] Because CMV disease has a propensity to cause neutropenia as well, it is often difficult to distinguish the cause. If laboratory findings and clinical signs and symptoms of CMV disease are resolving and the patient remains neutropenic, the most likely cause is ganciclovir. Thrombocytopenia occurs in approximately 20% of ganciclovir recipients. Patients with initial platelet counts less than 100,000/μL appear to be at greatest risk. Other adverse effects include CNS effects, fever, rash, and abnormal LFT findings.[86,87] A.A.'s WBC with differential and platelet counts should be assessed every 3 to 4 days during therapy, and ganciclovir should be held if neutrophils fall to less than 500/μL or platelets fall to less than 25,000/μL. To monitor either the regression or progression of A.A.'s CMV disease, a weekly serum CMV DNA PCR should be obtained.

Immunoglobulins

The use of immunoglobulins to treat CMV disease in solid organ transplantation is controversial. They are expensive and sometimes in short supply. Immunoglobulins provide passive immunization by potentiating an antibody-dependent, cell-mediated cytotoxic reaction. Basically, the immunoglobulins modify the immunologic response that damages host tissue. Some evidence suggests that immunoglobulins may have synergistic or additive effects with current antiviral drugs in the treatment of CMV disease.[88] Both unselective immunoglobulins and CMV hyperimmune globulin have been studied in combination with ganciclovir. CMV hyperimmune globulin is prepared from high-titer pooled sera that have a fourfold to eightfold enrichment of CMV titers compared with unscreened immunoglobulin.

Cytomegalovirus immunoglobulin may be given as 100 mg/kg/dose every other day for 14 days. This is the dose recommended for treatment of CMV when used in combination with ganciclovir. The most common adverse effects associated with the administration of immunoglobulins are infusion related and include fever, chills, headache, myalgia, light-headedness, and nausea and vomiting.

Foscarnet

Foscarnet is a virostatic pyrophosphate analog that inhibits DNA synthesis; however, unlike ganciclovir, no phosphorylation is required for activation. Because this drug has a high nephrotoxicity propensity and because most transplant recipients are already receiving drugs that are nephrotoxic, experience with the use of foscarnet in solid organ transplantation is limited. In most centers, foscarnet is a second-line or third-line agent to be used only if intolerance or resistance develops with ganciclovir therapy.

The usual dosage of foscarnet is 60 mg/kg/dose every 8 hours for 14 to 21 days. The dosage should be reduced in patients with renal dysfunction. The most serious adverse effect with foscarnet is nephrotoxicity, which occurs in up to 50% of patients and is probably induced by acute tubular necrosis. Therefore, prehydration is suggested to help minimize or avoid nephrotoxicity. GI effects, a decrease in hemoglobin and hematocrit, an increase in LFTs, and alteration of serum electrolyte concentrations are other side effects of foscarnet. All of these appear to be reversible on discontinuation of the drug. SCr should be monitored daily during therapy.[87]

PROPHYLAXIS

CASE 34-10, QUESTION 3: Is there any way to prevent CMV in high-risk patients such as A.A.?

Because of its significant consequences, efforts should be made to prevent CMV disease. Many studies have tried to ascertain the easiest, most cost-effective regimen to prevent CMV disease.

These studies have focused on the combined use of different agents as well as IV followed by oral therapies. Trials have also targeted high-risk patients and assessed the use of CMV PCR monitoring, without the use of universal prophylaxis therapy (preemptive strategy).[88]

Ganciclovir

The use of both the IV and oral formulations of ganciclovir to prevent CMV disease has been studied in liver and kidney recipients.[89] Very few large trials have been conducted, and most of the data in the solid organ transplantation population are from small uncontrolled trials. Another difficulty lies in that large discrepancies exist between the trials with regard to the terminology used to define prophylaxis and high-risk patients. Until the introduction of valganciclovir, ganciclovir was the most widely used prophylactic agent.

In the United States, oral ganciclovir therapy has not been commercially available for a number of years. Thus, most transplant centers are now solely using valganciclovir therapy as their first-line agent. IV ganciclovir is still available and can be used for short periods if the patient is not able to tolerate oral therapy.

Valganciclovir

Valganciclovir was developed because oral ganciclovir has a very low bioavailability (<10%). Valganciclovir is the L-valyl ester of ganciclovir, which is a prodrug that is rapidly and completely converted into ganciclovir by hepatic and intestinal esterases once absorbed across the GI tract. The absolute bioavailability of valganciclovir is approximately 60%, so that a 900-mg single PO dose given with food is an AUC equivalent to a 5 mg/kg IV dose of ganciclovir. This is roughly twice the AUC achieved by 1,000 mg of ganciclovir given orally TID. Valganciclovir is currently FDA-approved for the treatment of HIV-associated CMV retinitis and to prevent CMV disease in heart, kidney, and pancreas transplantation.[90,91] Valganciclovir is not FDA-approved for prevention of CMV disease in liver transplantation, although it is often used in such cases. Several small studies have demonstrated that valganciclovir is effective in treating CMV infection preemptively and potentially preventing CMV disease.[90]

Because valganciclovir is very expensive and has a high potential for causing hematologic toxicities, several studies have been conducted using reduced dosing strategies. Most use half the recommended dose of 900 mg PO daily in patients with good renal function and have shown equivalent clinical outcomes with the potential of reducing cost and toxicities. These studies were conducted in kidney transplant patients, and the dosing of this agent is transplant center-specific based on institutional protocols.[92]

Valacyclovir

One published meta-analysis of 12 trials that included 1,574 patients evaluated valacyclovir as a prophylactic agent in transplant recipients.[93] Valacyclovir was found to be more effective than acyclovir in preventing herpes viruses, including CMV. Most transplantation centers, however, do not use valacyclovir for routine prophylaxis of CMV, and still consider valganciclovir first line.

Cytomegalovirus Hyperimmune Globulin

The role of CMV hyperimmune globulin in preventing CMV disease is controversial. Many studies have combined this agent with either oral acyclovir or ganciclovir, but because of its high cost and IV route, its use as a prophylactic agent has decreased. In addition, in patients who are D+/R−, results have been mixed.[87,94]

Case 34-10, Question 4: Should A.A. have received prophylactic therapy and, if so, which agent should be used?

A.A. has several risk factors that predispose him to developing CMV disease. At the time of transplantation, A.A. was CMV D+/R−, which means that he has about an 80% chance of developing CMV infection and a 40% chance of developing CMV disease. In addition, A.A. had an early acute rejection episode, which means he received higher doses of immunosuppression, also putting him at higher risk for developing CMV disease. Because of these risk factors, A.A. should have (and did) receive CMV prophylaxis for at least 3 months after transplantation. Some centers may extend prophylaxis to 6 months post-transplant in patients like A.A. A.A. developed CMV disease and is being treated with ganciclovir 190 mg every 12 hours IV. Once A.A. is tolerating oral medications, he can start receiving oral valganciclovir at a dose of 900 mg twice daily with food. Because A.A. has renal insufficiency, his oral valganciclovir dose will be adjusted to 450 mg daily.[92]

Cytomegalovirus Resistance to Anti-viral Therapies

Although uncommon, CMV resistance to anti-viral therapies, as defined by continued viral replication despite prolonged treatment, may be present in 5% to 12% of patients that have a high-risk serostatus (D+/R−). There have been two primary gene mutations associated with this resistance, one to the UL97 kinase and the other to the UL54 DNA polymerase gene. The vast majority (90%) of resistant strains to ganciclovir contain mutations to the UL97 gene, which usually does not confer cross-resistance to other anti-viral therapies, including cidofovir or foscarnet.[95]

As illustrated by A.A.'s case, a patient who has received prophylactic therapy does not preclude the development of CMV disease after the prophylaxis is withdrawn or, in rare instances, during prophylactic therapy. The incidence of CMV disease while receiving valganciclovir is significantly lower when compared to oral ganciclovir, probably because drug exposure is approximately 2 times higher.[90–92]

Preemptive Therapy

Because of recent advances in the laboratory tests used to identify and quantify CMV; because prophylactic therapy is not always effective; and because it is often toxic and very expensive, preemptive therapy has also been used to prevent CMV disease. The technique involves withholding prophylactic therapy and monitoring laboratory tests to identify presymptomatic CMV viremia, usually by using serum CMV DNA PCR. Once a patient develops viremia (CMV PCR viral load >2,000 copies/mL), he/she receives treatment with IV ganciclovir or oral valganciclovir. This strategy has been prospectively studied and is as effective as universal prophylaxis, with some potential cost advantages. However, a few recent studies have demonstrated a higher incidence of the indirect effects of CMV in the preemptive group—most-concerning in one study, graft loss. Thus, the preemptive therapy role is controversial, with many centers still using universal CMV prophylaxis in all solid organ transplant recipients.[88]

Post-transplantation Lymphoproliferative Disorder

RISK FACTORS

CASE 34-11

Question 1: A.L., a 16-year-old, 42-kg girl, underwent liver transplant 1 year ago secondary to biliary atresia with a failed Kasai procedure. She now presents with low-grade fever, malaise, pain, and a 1-week history of decreased appetite. She has experienced two episodes of rejection that were treated with 1 to 2 g of methylprednisolone each time, with the last rejection episode requiring rabbit antithymocyte globulin therapy. She received tacrolimus and prednisone after transplantation and had MMF added to her immunosuppressant regimen after the second rejection episode. She has just finished a course of IV ganciclovir (4 weeks) for CMV infection. The donor was CMV-positive, and she is CMV-positive. Her EBV DNA PCR is now 18,000 copies/mL (normal, <500 copies/mL); this value was negative at the time of transplant, but because her last rejection episode has been increasing in value. On physical examination, she was noted to have mediastinal adenopathy. She denies chills, sweats, nausea, vomiting, or diarrhea. A chest computed tomography scan revealed a mediastinal mass. Vital signs and all laboratory tests are within normal limits. Her tacrolimus trough is 9.8 ng/mL. Seven days after admission, a biopsy of this mass shows a thoracic lymphoproliferative lesion identified as a thoracic immunoblastic lymphoma adherent to the right side of the heart. Ten days later, she developed tachy/brady syndrome and a pacemaker was implanted. Given the location of her lymphoma and symptoms, surgery and radiation therapy are not viable options, and chemotherapy is started the next day. What clinical signs and risk factors in A.L. are associated with lymphoma?

A.L. has developed a PTLD, one of many types of malignancies that have been reported after solid organ transplantation. The exact etiology of this condition is unclear and probably multifactorial. The presentation of PTLD varies significantly. Patients can present asymptomatically, with mild mononucleosis-like symptoms or with multiorgan failure. A.L. presents with fever, lymphadenopathy, malaise, and lack of appetite. Although these symptoms are consistent with PTLD, they also are consistent with infection. Because PTLD can involve various organ systems, patients can present with organ-specific symptoms (e.g., acute abdominal pain, perforation, obstruction, bleeding if a tumor is in the GI tract). Depending on its location, a tumor can impinge on the function of other organs, as seen in A.L.[96] Besides immunosuppression, two factors that have been strongly associated with PTLD are the presence of EBV and the age of the patient. Children have a higher incidence of PTLD.[97] A.L. developed EBV DNA viremia, indicating that she had been exposed to this virus at the time of transplantation or afterward. EBV also can be transmitted from the donor liver and/or blood products. Also, EBV-positive recipients at the time of transplantation can experience reactivation of this virus as a result of immunosuppression.

A.L. received a significant amount of immunosuppression. This could lead to an inability to suppress an active viral infection by cytotoxic T cells and result in uncontrolled B-cell proliferation and polyclonal and monoclonal expansion. In addition to this T-cell defect, an imbalance or alteration in cytokine production in response to EBV, which infects B lymphocytes, may contribute to the exaggerated B-cell expansion and transformation; most are classified as non-Hodgkin lymphomas primarily of B-cell origin. Small percentages are of T-cell origin, however, and are harder to treat.[96] The incidence and detection of PTLD has increased. Newer, more potent immunosuppressive agents used in different combinations, increased numbers of transplantation procedures, and closer monitoring contribute to this phenomenon. When cyclosporine-based regimens were compared with azathioprine or cyclophosphamide-based regimens, lymphomas made up 26% and 11% of all cancers, respectively. The lymphomas occurred, on average, within 15 months after transplant in the cyclosporine group versus 48 months in the azathioprine group. One-third of these malignancies occurred in the first 4 months in the cyclosporine group compared with only 11% in the latter group.[96]

The incidence of PTLD increases with rabbit antithymocyte globulin therapy and appears to be related to a cumulative dose and multiple courses. PTLD is not caused by any single agent but probably reflects the intensity of immunosuppression with multiple agents. Chronic antigenic stimulation by foreign antigens, repeated infections, genetic predisposition, and indirect or direct damage to DNA are other variables that might affect the development of PTLD.[98] A.L. had a recent CMV infection, which also could have contributed to this process.

As a percentage of all malignancies, PTLD occurs more commonly in thoracic than in other types of solid organ transplants and is even more common in children. Lymphomas develop in about 1% of kidney transplantations and 2% of liver transplantations. These tumors often appear early and progress rapidly. The overall prevalence of malignancies in the transplantation population averages about 6%, and the risk of cancer increases with time after a transplantation. Major organ transplant recipients are 100 times more likely to have cancer than the general population. Furthermore, the most common types of cancer observed in transplant recipients (e.g., lymphomas, cancer of the skin and lips) are uncommon in the general population. The development of skin and lip cancers in the transplant population has been attributed partially to exposure to sunlight and sensitization of skin to sunlight by an azathioprine metabolite, methylnitrothioimidazole.[96]

TREATMENT AND OUTCOMES

CASE 34-11, QUESTION 2: What are the therapeutic maneuvers and outcomes that would be expected in A.L.?

Treatment of a PTLD depends on timing, presentation, symptoms, extent of involvement, histologic type, and transplant type. Early experiences with PTLD indicated that reduction or discontinuation of immunosuppression led to regression of the cancer. Therefore, the first step in treating PTLD is to consider the discontinuation of all immunosuppressives, with the potential exception of the corticosteroids. This course of action is not feasible for A.L., however, because her transplanted liver is essential for her life. Immunosuppressive drugs can be discontinued in kidney recipients because dialysis can be reinstituted. A.L. will need chemotherapy for her cancer. Therefore, her MMF probably should be discontinued to minimize the potential for severe bone marrow toxicity. Additionally, A.L. will likely have a small reduction in her tacrolimus doses, with the goal of achieving trough concentrations on the lower end of her therapeutic range (4–6 ng/mL); her prednisone should also be reduced to the lowest dose possible. If her immunosuppressive drug therapy is diminished, she should be monitored closely for rejection.[99]

Antiviral therapy with IV acyclovir or ganciclovir has been used to inhibit EBV replication in an effort to treat PTLD. Response is variable and may depend on the type and extent of PTLD. A.L. already has received ganciclovir for 4 weeks during which time she presented with PTLD. Surgery, radiation therapy, and chemotherapy are used to treat PTLD depending on the situation. Interferon and immunoglobulin have been effective in a few cases that appeared unresponsive to other therapies. Monoclonal or immunoblastic, disseminated, rapidly progressive PTLD responds poorly to traditional therapy and has a mortality rate as high as 70%. Rituximab (an anti-B-cell, anti-CD20 antibody) is considered first-line therapy for CD20-postive B-cell PTLD along with reduction or withdrawal of immunosuppression if possible. Patients usually get 375 mg/m^2 weekly for 4 weeks; some groups have used prolonged therapy. Patients may have relapse or disease progression that may respond to chemotherapy regimens such as cyclophosphamide, adriamycin, vincristine, prednisone, or dexamethasone (CHOP); CHOP plus rituximab (CHOP-R); and cyclophosphamide, doxorubicin, etopside, prednisone, cytarabine, bleomycin, vincristine, and methotrexate (PROMACE-cytaBOM).

Transplant recipients have a higher risk of myelotoxic side effects, depending on their maintenance immunosuppression. A.L.'s prognosis is poor given the type and extent of her PTLD, which would have been more responsive to therapy if it had been diagnosed early. Polyclonal PTLD responds well to reduction or discontinuation of immunosuppression and high-dose acyclovir or ganciclovir therapy for several weeks to months. The roles of prophylactic antivirals, immunoglobulins, and EBV PCR monitoring in the prevention of PTLD are currently controversial, with mixed results in current literature.[99]

KEY REFERENCES AND WEBSITES

A full list of references for this chapter can be found at http://thepoint.lww.com/AT11e. Below are the key references and websites for this chapter, with the corresponding reference number in this chapter found in parentheses after the reference.

Key References

Avery RK et al. Update on immunizations in solid organ transplant recipients: what clinicians need to know. *Am J Transpl*. 2008;8:9.

Fishman JA. Infection in solid-organ transplant recipients. *N Engl J Med*. 2007;357:2601. (79)

Kidney Disease: Improving Global Outcomes (KDIGO) Transplant Work Group. KDIGO clinical practice guideline for the care of kidney transplant recipients. *Am J Transplant*. 2009;9(Suppl 3):S44–S46. (56)

Manitpisitkul W et al. Drug interactions in transplant patients: what everyone should know. *Curr Opin Nephrol Hypertens*. 2009;18:404. (77)

Marcen R et al. Immunosuppressive drugs in kidney transplant. Impact on patient survival, and incidence of cardiovascular disease, malignancy, and infection. *Drugs*. 2009;69:2227. (71)

Naesens M et al. Calcineurin inhibitor nephrotoxicity. *Clin J Am Soc Nephrol*. 2009;4:481. (36)

Nankivell BJ, Alexander SI. Rejection of the kidney allograft. *N Engl J Med*. 2010;363:1451. (6)

Marino Z, Londono MC, Forns X. Hepatitis C treatment for patients post liver transplant. *Curr Opin Organ Transplant*. 2015;20:251–258. (84)

Parker A et al. Management of post-transplant lymphoproliferative disorder in adult solid organ transplant recipients—BCSH and BTS Guidelines. *Br J Haematol*. 2010;149:693. (99)

Matas AJ et al. OPTN/SRTR 2011 annual data report: kidney. *Am J Transplant*. 2013;13(Suppl s1):11–46.

Wolfe RA et al. Trends in organ donation and transplantation in the United States, 1999–2008. *Am J Transplant*. 2010;(4, Pt 2):961. (1)

Key Websites

www.ustransplant.org.
www.srtr.org.

Section Editors: R. Rebecca Couris and Susan L. Mayhew

35 Basics of Nutrition and Patient Assessment

Jeff F. Binkley

CORE PRINCIPLES

		CHAPTER CASES
1	A complete nutritional assessment of the patient is imperative before specialized nutrition is initiated. Parameters to be considered are nutrition and weight history, physical examination, anthropometric and biochemical measurements, and malnutrition risk.	**Case 35-1 (Question 1)**
2	The nutritional status of a patient can be assessed using the subjective global assessment (SGA) technique, which has been found to be highly predictive of outcome, because the SGA correlates strongly with other subjective and objective measures of nutrition.	**Case 35-1 (Question 1)**
3	Patients who cannot meet their nutritional needs by consuming food orally should be considered for specialized nutritional support, which is the provision of parenteral or enteral nutrients.	**Case 35-1 (Question 2)**
4	Protein and calorie goals are assessed on the basis of the disease status and body weight of the patient.	**Case 35-1 (Question 3)**
5	Nutritional support regimens should be tailored on the basis of the requirements, response, and tolerance of the patient. Patients with inflammatory bowel disease are particularly at risk for developing vitamin and other micronutrient deficiencies, and therefore, supplementation is warranted.	**Case 35-1 (Question 4)**
6	The fluid needs of a patient are determined by the following steps: (a) need to correct fluid imbalances, (b) maintenance fluid requirements, and (c) replacement of ongoing fluid losses.	**Case 35-1 (Question 5)**
7	Continued success of a nutritional support regimen can be accomplished by appropriate nutritional assessment after the initiation of therapy. The parameters such as patient weight trends, nitrogen balance, and prealbumin are considered when determining the need to adjust therapy.	**Case 35-1 (Question 6)**
8	Overfeeding should be avoided in patients, and a gradual and conservative approach to instituting nutritional support should be used to prevent potential metabolic abnormalities.	**Case 35-1 (Question 7)**

Recognition of the importance of adequate and appropriate nutrition is paramount to the maintenance of optimal health. When an imbalance exists between the supply and the demand for the sources of nutrients and energy by the body, a nutritional disorder can occur. Years of research and clinical experience have led to the creation of various screening tools, assessment techniques, and guidelines to aid practitioners in their quest to delay or prevent patients from developing dangerous sequelae associated with deviations from optimal nutrition.[1] Despite many advances in nutritional science, impaired nutritional status in developing nations continues to be a main cause of morbidity and mortality, especially in young children.

NUTRITION BASICS

Adequate levels of energy sources and essential nutrients are critical for retaining the structural and biochemical integrity of the human body. Energy is provided in the diet by macronutrients such as carbohydrates, protein, and lipid. Essential nutrients, none of which offer any caloric value, are supplied to the body in the form of water, electrolytes, vitamins, and minerals.

Macronutrients

Humans need to consume food to sustain life. The unique structure and function of our cellular architecture allow human beings to convert the chemical free energy contained within the diet into high-energy, biologically active compounds. This transformation of food energy into forms of viable free energy through cellular respiration is an extremely inefficient process. Close examination of the distribution of food energy within the human body reveals that approximately 50% is lost as heat, 45% is available to the body in the form of adenosine triphosphate, and the remaining 5% is thermodynamically required for the conversion to heat because the entropy of the final products is greater than that of the initial substrates. Ultimately, all of the energy derived from food is expended in the form of external work or heat.

In nutritional contexts, the energy available from food is expressed in terms of the calorie. A calorie is technically defined by the amount of heat required to raise the temperature of 1 g of water by 1°C. This unit, however, is too small from a dietary perspective. A food calorie (sometimes written as *Calorie* with a large *C*, although this convention is not strictly followed) is equivalent to 1,000 calories or 1 kilocalorie (kcal). One food calorie is also equal to 4.184 kilojoules.[2] It is not uncommon for a single kilocalorie to be referred to as a calorie when communicating the energy content of food. This ambiguity must be understood by practicing clinicians to communicate properly not only with colleagues but also with patients and the general public who may not have an appreciation for this subtlety and remain confused when reading calories on nutrition labels yet and seeing kilocalories in textbooks, scientific publications, patient records, and Internet.

CARBOHYDRATES

Carbohydrates, also known as saccharides, are organic compounds that are chemically the hydrates of carbon. There are four main types of carbohydrates: monosaccharides, disaccharides, oligosaccharides, and polysaccharides. Dieticians frequently classify carbohydrates as either simple (monosaccharides and disaccharides) or complex (oligosaccharides and polysaccharides); yet, the exact delineation of these categories is often not clear. Although carbohydrates serve as a common source of energy for living organisms, these compounds also function as structural components and building blocks for complex genetic molecules.

Monosaccharides (e.g., glucose) are the simplest of carbohydrates and cannot be hydrolyzed into smaller saccharide molecules. They are the major sources of fuel, because glucose serves as a nearly universal and accessible reservoir of calories. In the context of food science, monosaccharides, collectively along with disaccharides, are commonly referred to as sugars and are found in foods such as candy and desserts. Natural sources of monosaccharides include fruits and vegetables, but these compounds are also found in commercially manufactured products such as high-fructose corn syrup. The latter is a common replacement for table sugar in processed foods composed of a high proportion of fructose relative to glucose.

Oligosaccharides are short chains of monosaccharides typically composed of 3 to 10 molecules linked through glycosidic bonds. These molecules are typically found connected to proteins or lipids functioning as chemical markers for cellular recognition. Their important role in the classification of blood groups is an example. Polymeric carbohydrate structures are referred to as polysaccharides and function either as storage forms of energy, such as glycogen in animals or starch in plants, or as a structural component, such as cellulose in plants. In humans, dietary polysaccharides must be catabolized to their constituent monosaccharides before absorption can occur.[3]

Dietary carbohydrates are composed of approximately 60% polysaccharides, mainly starch, and disaccharides such as sucrose and lactose, which represent 30% and 10%, respectively. All carbohydrates provide 4 kcal of energy/gram. Although the exact amount of dietary carbohydrates sufficient for good health is not known, a mixed-fuel diet in which carbohydrates constitute 45% to 65% of the total energy intake is considered an acceptable distribution range.[4]

PROTEIN

Polypeptides are linear chains of amino acids. These polypeptides can twist and fold alone or together into three-dimensional globular or fibrous structures, generating a biochemical compound known as the protein. Proteins are crucial to all living organisms and participate in a wide spectrum of processes. Many proteins function as enzymes, which serve as catalysts to biochemical reactions and are important for metabolism. Additionally, proteins can play a role in structure and function, such as actin and myosin in muscle—the largest source of protein in higher animals. Some proteins stabilize blood by giving it the appropriate viscosity and osmolarity, and yet, other proteins participate in cell signaling and immune responses.

Protein is the second largest store of energy in the body after adipose tissue.[5] Although protein differs from the other two primary dietary energy sources because of its inclusion of nitrogen, the amino acid residues from proteins can be converted to glucose via gluconeogenesis to supply a continuous source of glucose for the body after the depletion of glycogen. Like carbohydrates, each gram of protein supplies 4 kcal of energy. The loss of more than 30% of body protein, however, can compromise muscle strength, affect respiratory function, and negatively influence the immune system, all of which ultimately lead to organ dysfunction and death. It should be noted that protein and energy requirements of the body are intimately connected. During the times of infection or injury, metabolic rates rise and body protein is suddenly oxidized into amino acids and mobilized for fuel utilization. In most instances, the injuries that patients experience are minimal and self-limiting; however, patients with chronic illnesses or those with complicating factors that result in a long-term hypermetabolic state can subsequently experience a dangerous loss of body nitrogen.

LIPIDS

Lipids comprise a broad spectrum of molecular species ranging from hydrophobic triglycerides and sterol esters to hydrophilic phospholipids and cardiolipins, as well as dietary cholesterol and phytosterols. Biologic lipids function as a form of energy storage, serve as the structural components of cell membranes, and participate as messengers in the vital process of cellular signaling.

In a nutritional context, fats that exist as liquids at room temperature are typically called oils, whereas fats that remain solid at room temperature are labeled as fats. Although the term lipid is frequently used synonymously for fat, fats are actually a subgroup of lipids also known as triglycerides. Triglycerides are synthesized by chemically combining glycerol with three fatty acid molecules. These fatty acids are generally nonbranched hydrocarbons containing an even number of carbon atoms ranging from 4 to 26 carbons. Adipose tissue is composed of fatty acids in varying lengths.

An unsaturated fat is a fatty acid that includes at least one double bond within the fatty acid chain, and therefore, a saturated fat is one that contains no double bonds. Unsaturated fatty acids result in less energy after the oxidation process of cellular metabolism compared with an equivalent amount of saturated fatty acids. Commercial manufacturers of processed food favor saturated fats because they are less vulnerable to rancidity (lipid peroxidation) and remain solid at room temperature. Foods containing unsaturated fats include avocado, nuts, and vegetable oils such as canola and olive oils. Meat products contain both saturated and unsaturated fats.

Importantly, each gram of fat yields 9 kcal of energy, twice that of either carbohydrate or protein. Approximately 35% to 40% of the total daily calories consumed by the average human being are lipids. Higher-fat diets can lead to more rapid weight gain, a positive attribute if the individual is malnourished or underweight, but a negative attribute if the individual is trying to achieve weight loss.[6] Triglycerides make up by far the largest proportion of dietary lipids consumed by humans. Although humans possess the biologic pathways to synthesize lipids, there are two essential lipids that must originate from the diet to prevent essential fatty acid deficiency—linoleic acid and α-linolenic acid.

Essential Nutrients—Water

Water plays a critical role in nearly every biologic function necessary for life. The total body water in an adult male without fluid and electrolyte disorders is approximately 50% to 60% of the lean body weight.[7] Infants and children possess a much higher fractional water content, which then decreases progressively with age. Individuals with a greater percentage of body fat, such as women or obese patients, also tend to have less water for a given weight.

The total aqueous volume in the body can be divided into the intracellular and extracellular compartments. Because the intracellular fluid is the site of major metabolic activity, homeostatic mechanisms are therefore in constant execution to provide an environment of optimal ionic strength. The primary function of the extracellular fluid is to serve as a conduit between cells and between organs. Substantial ionic alterations within extracellular fluid can occur without a clinically significant impact on body function. This extracellular compartment can be further divided into three fractions: the interstitial volume, plasma volume, and transcellular water volume. Interstitial fluid flows around cells, allowing the total surface area of a cell to serve as an area of exchange. Plasma is the route for rapid transit within the body. Transcellular water is the smallest component of extracellular fluid and is the portion of total body water that can be found contained within epithelial-lined spaces. Transcellular water includes the luminal fluid of the gastrointestinal (GI) tract, the fluids of the central nervous system, and the fluid in the eye, as well as the lubricating fluids at serous surfaces.

The basal requirement of water for a given individual is dependent on the sensible (urinary) and insensible losses of water. Urine osmolality and the total amount of solute excreted from the body dictate the volume of water comprising urine. Fever can promote dehydration by increasing one's basal metabolic rate in addition to raising the vapor pressure of expired air and sweat, resulting in higher respiratory and skin water losses, respectively. In the absence of fever and sweating, water loss through the skin is relatively fixed; however, urinary water excretion can vary greatly.

Essential Nutrients—Micronutrients

ELECTROLYTES

A subtle and complex balance of electrolytes exists between the intracellular and extracellular milieu. The precise maintenance of these electrolyte gradients is critical as such gradients regulate hydration and pH and ultimately have an impact on nerve and muscle function. Sodium, chloride, and bicarbonate are the main solutes in the extracellular fluid, whereas potassium, magnesium, phosphate, and proteins are the dominant solutes inside the cell.

Although water can freely travel across the membrane of a cell, the cell membrane itself is only selectively permeable to solutes. Osmotically active solutes are those that are impermeable and thereby exert an osmotic pressure by which the distribution of water between fluid compartments is determined.

Electrolyte balance is traditionally maintained by the oral intake of substances containing electrolytes. Foods such as fruit juices, sports drinks, milk, and many fruits and vegetables are replete with electrolytes. In oral rehydration therapy, electrolyte drinks containing sodium and potassium salts replenish the water and electrolyte levels in the body after dehydration caused by exercise, excessive alcohol consumption, diaphoresis, diarrhea, vomiting, intoxication, or starvation. Hormones, such as antidiuretic hormone, aldosterone, and parathyroid hormone, regulate electrolytes once in the body, and the kidneys function to flush out those excess ions.

VITAMINS

Vitamins are organic compounds that cannot be biologically synthesized in sufficient quantities by human beings and yet remain a vital requirement for the sustainment of life. The biochemical functions of vitamins are diverse. Some vitamins assist in the regulation of electrolyte metabolism, whereas others participate in the control of cell and tissue growth and differentiation. Most vitamins function as cofactors, which are molecules that bind to enzymes to promote their catalytic activities.

Vitamins are classified by their biologic and chemical activity. Vitamins are designated as either water-soluble or fat-soluble. There are four fat-soluble vitamins (A, D, E, and K) and nine water-soluble vitamins (eight B vitamins and vitamin C) in humans. Water-soluble vitamins are used by the body quite rapidly, and amounts in excess are readily excreted from the body in urine. The fat-soluble vitamins are absorbed by the body using processes that closely parallel the absorption of lipids. Fat-soluble vitamins are more likely to lead to toxicity, or hypervitaminosis. Fat-soluble vitamin regulation is also of particular significance in cystic fibrosis.

Vitamins are procured through the diet or supplements. The body can manufacture only three vitamins from nondietary sources: vitamins D and K, and the B vitamin, biotin. Critically ill patients experiencing metabolic stress possess vitamin needs that may increase dramatically. Many disease states such as inflammatory bowel disease, liver and renal disease, short-bowel syndrome, cancer, and acquired immunodeficiency syndrome-associated wasting can also result in a higher demand for vitamins. A parenteral formulation of multivitamins combining both fat- and water-soluble vitamins into an aqueous solution designed for incorporation into intravenous infusions is available for these classes of patients.

TRACE ELEMENTS

Appropriate intake levels of certain dietary minerals have been demonstrated to be required in small amounts to maintain optimal health. These dietary minerals are known as trace elements or ultratrace elements. Iron, zinc, copper, manganese, and fluoride are classified as trace elements. These minerals are required in amounts between 1 and 100 mg/day by adults. Ultratrace elements, or those dietary minerals that are required in quantities less than 1 mg/day, include arsenic, boron, chromium, iodine, selenium, silicon, nickel, and vanadium.

Consuming specific foods rich with the dietary mineral of interest is the recommended method for satisfying these micronutrient requirements. Many trace elements are naturally present in foods; however, some are added to foods to prevent nutrient deficiencies—such as fortifying salt with iodine to prevent development of hypothyroidism and goiter. When dietary intake is insufficient to meet the daily nutrient requirements of an individual or when chronic or acute deficiencies arise from pathology and injury, dietary supplements remain a viable option. Supplements can be formulated to include multiple trace elements, a combination of vitamins, or a single trace element.

MALNUTRITION

Malnutrition may occur when there is any disruption of nutritional status, including disorders resulting from overfeeding or underfeeding or through impaired nutrient metabolism. Clinically, a more useful definition of malnutrition is the state induced by alterations in dietary intake, which results in subcellular, cellular, or organ function changes that expose the individual to increased risks of morbidity and mortality and can be reversed by adequate nutritional intervention.[8] An incidence of malnutrition as high as 30% to 50% has been reported among hospitalized patients.[9,10] In these hospitalized patients, the risk of acute malnutrition development is greater because nutrient intake is often inadequate, nutrient stores can be depleted, or the patients may experience concurrent injury or stress (e.g., trauma, infection, major surgery). The presence of acute stress or injury increases energy requirements to repair tissues. Breakdown of skeletal muscle to release amino acids for energy production by conversion to glucose occurs if exogenous energy is not provided to stressed patients. Even patients who were well nourished before the stressful event may quickly become at risk for this type of iatrogenic malnutrition. Usually conditional, acute malnutrition resolves once the illness or injury improves and normal nutrient intake is resumed.

In stark contrast to stress-induced malnutrition, patients in starvation or semistarvation states slowly adapt to inadequate nutrient intake. In this scenario, endogenous fat stores are used for energy and a slow loss of muscle proteins ensues. Nevertheless, energy and protein stores are not unlimited, and death occurs in previously normal-weight individuals after about 60 to 70 days of starvation.[11,12] Patients with a history of chronic malnutrition who are faced with stress or injury are at the greatest risk of developing malnutrition.

The most common type of nutritional deficiency in hospitalized patients is protein-calorie malnutrition, which includes depletion of both tissue energy stores and body proteins. Complications develop more frequently for hospitalized patients who are malnourished as a result of organ wasting and functional impairments. These complications may include weakness, decreased wound healing, altered hepatic metabolism of drugs, increased respiratory failure, decreased cardiac contractility, and infections such as pneumonia and abscesses. Complications often increase the length of hospital stay and costs of care, and may even ultimately reduce reimbursement for institutions.[13–15]

Malnutrition or its risk may occur in patients with inadequate intake for 7 to 14 days or in patients with an unintentional weight loss of 10% before their illness. For these patients, nutritional intervention is appropriate and should be considered.[16,17] Patients who cannot meet their nutritional needs by consuming enough food orally should be considered for an alternative nutrition mechanism. Specialized nutritional support is the provision of parenteral or enteral nutrients, which are specifically formulated or delivered to maintain or restore nutritional status.[18] For those who cannot eat by mouth but have a functional GI tract, the first line of nutritional intervention to be considered should be enteral feeding through an appropriate access device (see Chapter 37, Adult Enteral Nutrition, and Chapter 38, Adult Parenteral Nutrition).

To mimic the normal physiologic state when possible, the GI tract should be used for providing nutrients. Enteral nutrients may be more beneficial and are generally less costly than those provided by the parenteral route.[19] Enteral nutrients stimulate the intestine, thus maintaining the mucosal barrier structure and function. This has been associated with decreased infectious morbidity in critically ill patients compared with those receiving nutrients parenterally.[20–24] Parenteral nutrition is therefore reserved for patients whose GI tracts are not functional or cannot be accessed, or who do not absorb enough nutrients to maintain adequate nutritional status.[16]

NUTRITION SCREENING

According to The Joint Commission (http://www.jointcommission.org), hospitals are required to screen patients within 24 hours of admission to determine whether they are malnourished or at risk for developing malnutrition. The nutrition screening process identifies needs for further nutritional intervention or monitoring based on nutritional risk. The information collected in the screening process is dependent on the patient population, the healthcare setting, and individual institution policy. A number of screening tools have been described in the literature with varying reliability, specificity, and sensitivity. Some parameters included in nutrition screening may have wider applicability in the outpatient setting than in the inpatient arenas.[1,9]

Patient Assessment

Nutritional assessment of a patient incorporates a collection of historical data, analysis of body composition, evaluation of physiologic function, and complete physical examination. Proper patient assessment should include the examination of multiple factors and should not rely on any one parameter. This assessment serves to identify the presence and severity of malnutrition or the risk of developing malnutrition. A complete patient assessment performed by a trained practitioner can help determine the goals of therapy and specify the need for specialized nutritional support. Goals of therapy may be maintenance of existing nutritional status, repletion of fat and lean body mass, and prevention of complications associated with malnutrition.

NUTRITION HISTORY

A nutrition history is crucial in an effective nutritional assessment. Practitioners may gain valuable information by interviewing the patient or the patient's family and by reviewing the medical record to identify factors that can contribute to malnutrition or increase the risk of developing malnutrition.

Multiple factors can contribute to the development of malnutrition, including the patient's underlying disease states, past medical history, and socioeconomic circumstances. Medications can adversely affect nutritional status by decreasing the synthesis of nutrients, minimizing food intake through alteration of appetite and taste, changing the absorption or metabolism of nutrients, or increasing nutrient requirements. A complete evaluation of present and past body weight habits contributes significantly to an appropriate nutrition history.

The components of a nutrition history are summarized in Table 35-1, some of which are expanded subsequently.

WEIGHT HISTORY

Weight history and influences are important in evaluating nutritional status. Weight loss is a sign of negative energy and negative protein balance and is often associated with poor outcome in hospitalized patients.[9,25] A patient's current weight often is compared

Table 35-1
Components of a Nutrition History

Medical history
Chronic illnesses
Surgical history
Psychosocial history
Socioeconomic status
History of gastrointestinal problems (nausea, vomiting, or diarrhea)
Diet history, including diets for weight gain or loss
Food preferences and intolerances
Medications
Weight history
Increase or decrease
Intentional or unintentional
Time period for weight change
Functional capacity

with a standard for ideal body weight (IBW). Percentage of IBW[9] is determined as shown in Eq. 35-1:

$$\% \text{ IBW} = \text{Current weight (100)/IBW} \quad \text{(Eq. 35-1)}$$

The primary limitation of this method of assessing weight is that the patient's weight is compared with a population standard rather than using the individual as the reference point. For example, a patient who is significantly overweight but has lost large amounts of weight may still be more than 100% of IBW and therefore not considered at risk for developing malnutrition. A more patient-specific method of evaluating weight is to compare current weight with the patient's usual weight. This can be determined using Eq. 35-2:

$$\% \text{ Usual body weight} = \text{Current weight (100)/ Usual body weight} \quad \text{(Eq. 35-2)}$$

Using this method, the obese patient who has lost weight may be determined to be less than 90% of usual weight and therefore nutritionally at risk. It is also important to assess over what time period the change has occurred. Involuntary weight loss is considered severe if loss exceeds 5% of usual weight within 1 month, or 10% of usual weight within 6 months. A nonvolitional weight loss of more than 10% is considered significant for malnutrition.[18] Patterns of weight loss must be evaluated to determine whether the loss is stabilizing or continual, the latter being a more serious concern. Weight gain after a significant weight loss may be considered a positive sign.

PHYSICAL EXAMINATION

Nutritional deficiencies may be identified on physical examination, and these findings may require further evaluation. Muscle and fat wasting (often noticed in the temporal area), loss of subcutaneous fat and muscle in the shoulders, and loss of subcutaneous fat in the interosseous and palmar areas of the hands are readily identifiable. Other physical parameters that may be less obvious are assessment of hair for color changes and sparseness, skin for turgor, pigmentation, and dermatitis, mouth for glossitis, gingivitis, cheilosis, and color of the tongue, nails for friability and lines, and abdomen for signs of ascites or enlarged liver. Additionally, the patient's fluid status must be evaluated as a part of the physical examination.

ANTHROPOMETRICS

Anthropometry is the science of body composition based on measurement of weight, stature, body circumferences, and subcutaneous fat thickness. Physical examination may include measurement of subcutaneous fat and skeletal muscle mass. Assessment of fat stores provides information about fat loss or gain and assumes fat is gained or lost proportionally throughout the entire body. The subcutaneous compartment contains approximately 50% of body fat. Triceps skinfold and subscapular skinfold thickness measurements are methods used to assess subcutaneous fat, allowing associated estimations of total body fat.

Reference standards[26] are used to compare against values obtained in the examination. Somatic protein mass or skeletal muscle mass can be estimated by measuring mid-arm circumference and then calculating arm muscle circumference. These values are also compared with standards, and the amount of muscle mass is then estimated.

Anthropometric measurements accurately reflect total body fat and skeletal muscle mass when used for the long-term comparisons of large, nutritionally stable populations. However, anthropometric measurements of hospitalized patients are of little value. Changes experienced during acute illness and stress may result in errors of interpretation of subcutaneous fat and weight assessments, and peripheral edema can result in inflated values for skinfold thickness and mid-arm circumference.[9,25]

Biochemical Assessment

Biochemical assessment of nutritional status includes the examination of protein status. No single test or group of tests can be recommended as a routine or reliable indicator of protein status. It is a combination of measures—biochemical, anthropometric, dietary, and clinical findings—that produce a more complete picture of protein status.

The protein composition of the human body can be viewed as a two-compartment model—somatic and visceral proteins. Somatic proteins are those constituting skeletal muscle; they account for approximately 75% of total body protein. The remaining 25% of total body protein are visceral proteins, which are found in the internal organs and serum. Albumin, prealbumin, transferrin, and retinol-binding protein are the most common visceral proteins used to assess nutritional status. These proteins are produced by the liver and often reflect hepatic synthetic capability. When hepatic insufficiency develops or when intake of substrates is inadequate for synthesis of proteins, the serum concentration of visceral proteins decreases. During stress or injury, inflammatory cytokines are released and substrates are shunted away from the synthesis of these proteins to synthesize other acute-phase proteins such as C-reactive protein, haptoglobin, fibrinogen, and others.[27] Serum protein concentrations are altered during acute stress or inflammatory states and chronic starvation.[25,27]

Albumin is the classic visceral protein used to evaluate nutritional status and is a prognostic indicator. Serum concentrations of less than 3 g/dL correlate with poor outcome and an increased length of stay of hospitalized patients.[28] Albumin serves as a carrier protein for fatty acids, hormones, minerals, and drugs, and is necessary for maintaining oncotic pressure. Albumin has a large body pool of 3 to 5 g/kg, and 30% to 40% is localized to the intravascular space. The normal hepatic rate of albumin synthesis is 150 to 250 mg/kg/day. Because albumin has a half-life of 18 to 21 days, a decrease in serum albumin concentrations is generally not observed until after several weeks of inadequate nitrogen intake. Serum albumin concentrations decrease rapidly in response to stress (which causes albumin to shift from the intravascular to the extravascular space), burns, nephrotic syndrome, protein-losing enteropathy, overhydration, and decreased synthesis with liver disease.[25,27]

Table 35-2
Visceral Proteins for Nutritional Assessment

Visceral Protein	Half-Life (days)	Normal Serum Concentration
Albumin	18–21	3.5–5 g/dL
Transferrin	8–10	250–300 mg/dL
Transthyretin (prealbumin)	2–3	15–40 mg/dL
Retinol-binding protein	0.5	2.5–7.5 mg/dL

Transferrin, which is involved in the transport of iron, has a half-life of 8 to 10 days and is more sensitive than albumin to acute changes in nutritional status. Normal serum concentrations of transferrin are 250 to 300 mg/dL.

Even more sensitive to changes in energy and protein intake is prealbumin (transthyretin), which has a small body pool (10 mg/kg) and a half-life of 2 to 3 days. Prealbumin transports both retinol and retinol-binding protein. Normal serum prealbumin concentrations are 15 to 40 mg/dL.

Retinol-binding protein has the shortest half-life, 12 hours; normal serum concentrations are 2.5 to 7.5 mg/dL. However, because serum concentrations of retinol-binding protein change rapidly in response to alterations in nutrient intake, monitoring it has limited use in clinical practice. The visceral proteins commonly used for nutritional assessment are summarized in Table 35-2.

Other proteins, such as fibronectin and somatomedin-C (insulin-like growth factor-1), are also used as markers of nutritional status. Fibronectin is a glycoprotein found in blood, lymph, and many cell surfaces. Somatomedin-C is important in regulating growth. Both fibronectin and somatomedin-C have half-lives of less than 1 day and respond to fasting and refeeding. Urinary measurement of 3-methylhistidine, a by-product of muscle metabolism that is excreted unchanged, has been used to estimate skeletal muscle mass. Although these markers have potential use in nutritional assessment, they are used primarily as research tools and are not readily available for routine clinical use.[25]

The interpretation of serum protein concentrations in hospitalized patients may be difficult because other factors more important than hepatic synthesis rate can alter serum concentrations. These factors may include renal, hepatic, or cardiac dysfunction, hydration status, and metabolic stress. Visceral proteins, as with any nutritional assessment parameter, must be used in conjunction with other parameters and comprehensive consideration of the patient's clinical status. Practitioners should evaluate markers of inflammation and stress, such as C-reactive protein, in conjunction with visceral protein markers periodically to ensure that an accurate assessment is made.

Nutritional assessment based on determinations of body composition using anthropometric and biochemical parameters has many limitations. Newer techniques (e.g., bioelectrical impedance, dual-energy X-ray absorptiometry, isotope dilution, neutron activation) are increasingly being used to determine body composition. Other parameters such as hand grip and forearm dynamometry may be used to assess skeletal muscle function, which relates changes in body composition to body function.[1,9,25]

Another nutritional assessment method, subjective global assessment (SGA), combines objective parameters and physiologic function.[29] This easy-to-use tool for diagnosing malnutrition is based on a history of weight change, dietary intake, presence of significant GI symptoms, functional capacity, and physical examination to assess edema and the loss of subcutaneous fat and muscle. Using the SGA system, patients are rated as well nourished, moderately malnourished, or severely malnourished.

Classification of Malnutrition

Malnutrition is categorized through a variety of descriptive terms, each with varying characteristics. Three classic categories include marasmus, kwashiorkor, and mixed protein-calorie malnutrition. A chronic deprivation of energy (calories), or partial starvation, leads to marasmus, which means a "dying away state." For patients with marasmus, physical examination reveals severe cachexia with loss of both fat and muscle mass; however, visceral protein production is preserved, and serum levels may remain at or near the normal range. Patients with chronic wasting diseases such as cancer or anorexia are likely to present with marasmus malnutrition.

Classic kwashiorkor malnutrition results from diets devoid of adequate protein, but with adequate caloric intake. Kwashiorkor-like malnutrition in hospitalized patients often refers to patients who are extremely catabolic from their medical complication (e.g., sepsis) or injury (e.g., trauma, thermal injury). Carbohydrate metabolism involves endogenous production of insulin, which in turn prevents lipolysis and promotes the movement of amino acids into muscle. To meet increased protein demands, protein can be mobilized from internal organs and circulating visceral proteins. Consequently, an individual with kwashiorkor-like malnutrition may have adequate fat and muscle mass, but may demonstrate depleted serum proteins.

Hospitalized patients commonly exhibit components of both marasmus and kwashiorkor-like malnutrition and are classified as having mixed protein-calorie malnutrition. This mixed condition occurs when an acute injury or stress compounds chronic starvation or semistarvation, resulting in wasting of fat and muscle mass, as well as depletion of serum proteins.

Estimation of Energy Expenditure

Estimating energy expenditure constitutes an important aspect of patient evaluation. The most common approach used to determine energy requirements is based on body weight in kilograms. Energy requirements are standardized and are determined by the metabolic condition of the patient.

Many predictive equations for estimating expenditure have been described in the literature.[30,31] The traditional method of assessing energy expenditure is the basal energy expenditure (BEE): the amount of energy (kilocalories) needed to support basic metabolic functions in a state of complete rest, shortly after awakening, and after a 12-hour fast. BEE is most commonly calculated using the Harris–Benedict equations (see Table 35-3). Alternatively, BEE can be estimated at 20 to 25 kcal/kg/day.

Basal metabolic rate (BMR) is the energy expended in the postabsorptive state, approximately 2 hours after a meal. BMR is approximately 10% greater than BEE. Calculations of BEE or BMR do not include additional energy required as a result of stress or activity. The Harris–Benedict equations can be modified to include stress and physical activity factors, or these variables are estimated at 20 to 35 kcal/kg/day for moderate-to-severe stress (Table 35-3).

Indirect calorimetry determines energy expenditure using a machine known as a metabolic cart that measures the patient's breathing or respiratory gas exchange. The cart measures oxygen consumption and carbon dioxide production when standard testing conditions are maintained. The amount of oxygen consumed and carbon dioxide produced for carbohydrate, fat, and protein is constant and known. Energy expenditure, including that caused by stress, is measured for a defined time, and the information is

Table 35-3
Estimation of Energy Expenditure

Basal Energy Expenditure (BEE)	
Harris–Benedict equations	
BEE_{men} (kcal/day) = 66.47 + 13.75 W + 5.0 H − 6.76 A	
BEE_{women} (kcal/day) = 655.10 + 9.56 W + 1.85 H − 4.68 A	
Or	
20–25 kcal/kg/day	
Energy Requirements	
Hospitalized patient, mild stress	20–25 kcal/kg/day
Moderate stress, malnourished	25–30 kcal/kg/day
Severe stress, critically ill	30–35 kcal/kg/day

A, age in years; BEE, basal energy expenditure; H, height in cm; kcal, kilocalories; W, weight in kg.

then subjected to a series of equations to extrapolate the estimated 24-hour energy expenditure.[17,25] This is the measured energy expenditure (MEE). Because the measurement is usually conducted while the patient is at rest, activity is not included in MEE.

Indirect calorimetry is available to many clinicians and is considered the gold standard for energy expenditure determination. Its usefulness is particularly valuable in the energy assessment of critically ill or obese patients. In 2016, the Society of Critical Care Medicine (SCCM) and American Society for Parenteral and Enteral Nutrition (ASPEN) published guidelines for the provision and assessment of nutritional support therapy for the adult critically ill patient.[32] Based on expert consensus, the guidelines suggest that determination of nutritional risk be performed on all ICU patients for whom volitional intake is anticipated to be insufficient. High-risk patients would likely benefit from early enteral nutritional therapy. Additionally, the guidelines suggest that the nutritional assessment should include evaluation of comorbid conditions, function of the gastrointestinal tract, and risk of aspiration. Traditional nutrition indicators or surrogate markers should likely not be used to assess nutritional status in critically ill patients because they have not been validated in the critically ill patient population.

Estimation of Protein Goals

Estimation of protein needs is necessary in nutritional assessment. Protein needs are calculated based on body weight, degree of stress, and disease state. The initial estimation is often made with a degree of subjectivity and clinical judgment, with adjustments made based on patient response. The US-recommended dietary allowance is 0.8 g of protein/kg/day. Well-nourished, hospitalized patients with minimal stress need 1 to 1.2 g of protein/kg/day to maintain lean body mass. The requirement for protein intake may be as high as 2 g/kg/day for a patient in a hypermetabolic, hypercatabolic state secondary to trauma or burns. In addition, protein provision may need to be adjusted and reduced in patients with renal or hepatic dysfunction as a result of altered metabolism. Guidelines for protein needs are summarized in Table 35-4.

Micronutrients

Micronutrients are the electrolytes, vitamins, and trace minerals needed for metabolism. A complete assessment will include identification of risks for deficiencies or toxicities with micronutrients based on the patient's specific nutritional status and concurrent disease processes. These nutrients are available enterally and parenterally from various manufacturers as either single entities or in combinations. It is important to be aware of the specific products available in each institution to avoid providing inadequate or excessive amounts of various micronutrients.

Table 35-4
Estimation of Protein Requirements

US-recommended dietary allowance	0.8 g/kg/day
Hospitalized patient, minor stress	1–1.2 g/kg/day
Moderate stress	1.2–1.5 g/kg/day
Severe stress	1.5–2 g/kg/day

PATIENT ASSESSMENT: WOMAN WITH CROHN'S DISEASE

CASE 35-1

QUESTION 1: S.P., a 34-year-old cachectic woman, is admitted to the hospital with abdominal pain, nausea, vomiting, and diarrhea. She has a history of moderate Crohn's disease diagnosed 4 years ago. She has had extensive treatment with medical therapy, but has not required surgical intervention since her diagnosis. She has experienced extraintestinal symptoms including skin lesions and joint pain. She presents to the hospital with increasing weight loss in the past 3 months, accompanied by regurgitation, vomiting, and poor appetite. Approximately 6 months ago, S.P. weighed 120 lb. Her weight on admission is 92 lb; height is 60 inches. Past medical history is also significant for peptic ulcer disease and occasional bouts of depression. Physical examination reveals a thin woman with wasting of subcutaneous fat in the temporal area and square shoulders. She reports noticing recent hair loss. Attempts at increasing her oral intake with enteral supplements have not been successful owing to self-reported retching.

Admission laboratory values are as follows:
Sodium, 135 mEq/L
Potassium, 4.0 mEq/L
Chloride, 100 mEq/L
Bicarbonate, 25 mEq/L
Blood urea nitrogen, 4 mg/dL
Creatinine, 0.6 mg/dL
Glucose, 87 mg/dL
Calcium, 8.2 mg/dL
Magnesium, 1.7 mg/dL
Phosphorus, 2.8 mg/dL
Total protein, 6.0 g/dL
Albumin, 3.5 g/dL
Prealbumin, 14 mg/dL

Her white blood cell count is 12,600/μL. Based on history and physical findings, S.P.'s working diagnosis includes Crohn's disease exacerbation with cutaneous, joint, and GI involvement. What is her current nutritional status?

To develop an accurate nutritional assessment of any patient, it is important to elicit a thorough history and conduct an appropriate physical examination. Although history and physical examination are of paramount importance, laboratory studies are also integral components to the assessment of S.P.'s nutritional status. S.P.'s nutrition history indicates that she is unable to eat because of vomiting, and the Crohn's diagnosis raises the question of nutrient malabsorption. Most striking about S.P.'s history is her weight loss of 28 lb in 6 months. She is now 76% of her usual weight (Eq. 35-2). Another way of analyzing this is that she has lost 25% of her original weight, which is characterized as severe weight loss. The physical findings of cachectic appearance, temporal wasting, and loss of subcutaneous fat and muscle in her shoulders are significant. No anthropometric measurements are available. S.P.'s visceral proteins are also in low–normal ranges, indicating both short-term (prealbumin) and long-term (albumin) malnutrition. Consideration of these factors leads one to conclude that S.P. is severely malnourished. This assessment can be further validated by using other tools such as the SGA.[29]

Because nutritional assessment can often be difficult, a clinician may choose to use the SGA to appropriately categorize their patients. Application of the SGA technique classifies patients into three areas: class A (the well-nourished patient), with less than 5% weight loss or more than 5% total weight loss but recent gains and improvements in appetite; class B (moderately malnourished), identified by those patients with 5% to 10% weight loss without recent stabilization or gain, poor dietary intake, and mild loss of subcutaneous tissue; and class C (severely malnourished), with an ongoing weight loss of more than 10% with severe subcutaneous tissue loss and muscle wasting, often with edema. The utility of the SGA is its simplicity for implementation and strong correlation with other subjective and objective measures of nutrition.

Clinicians place patients into one of the three categories on the basis of their subjective rating of two broad factors: history and physical examination. There are four elements to the history: (a) weight loss in the 6 months before the examination, expressed as a proportionate loss from previous weight, (b) dietary intake in relation to the patient's usual pattern, (c) presence of significant GI symptoms, and (d) functional capacity or energy of the patient, ranging from full capacity to bedridden. Applying these four elements to S.P., one first finds that S.P. is reporting a 25% weight loss during the past 6 months. It is also important to recognize the pattern of weight loss. Querying a patient regarding recent weight loss (in conjunction with the weight change in 6 months), often in the past 2 weeks, can help establish a pattern of chronic weight loss. In S.P.'s case, she reports increasing weight loss in the past 3 months, which confirms a progression. It is also recommended that clinicians explore weight history by asking for the patient's maximal weight at specific times, such as 1 year ago, 6 months ago, 1 month ago, and at the present time. Confirmation of weight history can be conducted by having the patient to discuss about his/her change in clothing size or how his/her clothes fit.

With respect to the second element regarding dietary intake, S.P. says she has a poor appetite, and attempts to consume supplements have been unsuccessful. Using the SGA, patients are classified as having either normal or abnormal intake in the weeks to months before the examination. In this case, S.P. is clearly experiencing abnormal intake; however, one can also ask S.P. certain questions such as "How has the amount of food you have consumed over the past several weeks to months changed?" or "Are there certain kinds of foods that you no longer can eat?" and "Give me an example of a typical meal" to establish eating patterns. It is also important to determine why a patient is eating less—intentional reduction or unintentional reduction. S.P. is not communicating any intention of wanting to lose weight, and her change in consumption is related to her chronic pathology.

In terms of the third element of the history, significant GI symptoms are those that have persisted on virtually a daily basis for a period longer than 2 weeks. Given the presentation of S.P. to the hospital with her history of 3 months of vomiting, it is highly likely that she satisfies the definition for possessing significant GI symptoms. However, a clinician can always clarify this by asking S.P. more specific questions.

The final element of S.P.'s history, functional capacity, is one that should be explored further; yet, it is not likely to have an impact on the final nutritional assessment given the prior objective findings of the patient. Patients who cannot eat will often complain of weakness and fatigue—many times to the point of which they are bedridden. Observation of the activity levels of patients, their overall mood, skeletal muscle function, and their respiratory movements can all provide clues to the clinician regarding functional impairment. Given the joint pain and squared-off appearance of her shoulders from the combination of muscle and subcutaneous tissue loss, functional capacity of S.P. is likely to be diminished.

Having completed the history component of the SGA, the clinician moves to the second component of the SGA, or the physical. This section of the SGA essentially asks the clinician to look for physical signs of malnutrition such as loss of subcutaneous fat in the triceps and chest region, muscle wasting in areas like the quadriceps and deltoids, presence of ankle or sacral edema, and finally any presence of ascites. For each of the traits, the clinician should consider the severity, if anything present. In the case of S.P., there is definite muscle wasting. Given the history and physical components of the SGA, S.P. would be classified as severely malnourished (class C) as there are obvious signs of malnutrition such as subcutaneous tissue loss and muscle wasting in the presence of a clear and convincing pattern of ongoing weight loss greater than 10%.

CASE 35-1, QUESTION 2: Is S.P. a candidate for specialized nutritional support therapy?

The fundamental goal of specialized nutritional support therapy is to meet the energy requirements of metabolic processes, to support the hypermetabolism associated with critical illness, and to minimize protein catabolism. Crohn's disease is a form of inflammatory bowel disease that is associated with potentially great nutritional insult. Nutritional abnormalities can arise in Crohn's disease patients from malabsorption, decreased food intake, medications, and intestinal losses. Disease location along the GI tract, symptomatology, and dietary restrictions all contribute to the development of protein energy malnutrition with specific nutritional deficiencies. S.P. is admitted to the hospital for tests to evaluate her Crohn's disease, weight loss, and associated symptoms. The subjective and objective evidence points to a nonfunctioning GI tract. If the diagnosis of advanced Crohn's exacerbation is accurate, S.P. may require parenteral nutritional therapy until enteral therapy can be established (see Chapter 38, Adult Parenteral Nutrition). In addition, previous attempts at enteral nutrition were unsuccessful with continued increased retching and vomiting, indicating decreased GI motility. With her malnourished state, continued inadequate nutrition in the hospital will result in further deterioration of her nutritional status. Specialized nutritional support intervention should be implemented.

Goals of Therapy

CASE 35-1, QUESTION 3: Calculate calorie and protein goals for S.P.

Nutritional support begins with an estimation of the patient's caloric requirements.[30,31] Accurate determination of caloric needs is essential to obtain the full benefits of nutritional therapy and aids in preventing the problems associated with underfeeding as well as overfeeding. The Harris–Benedict equation is one of the most commonly used methods for estimating caloric needs or BEE; however, there is still controversy regarding the best method to accurately estimate the caloric needs of a patient. The Harris–Benedict equation may overestimate or underestimate resting energy expenditure in certain critically ill patients, particularly when clinical conditions are changing and when body weight fluctuates because of changes in fluid status. The most common approach is based on body weight in kilograms. The energy requirements are standardized and are determined by the metabolic condition of the patient. S.P.'s initial calorie goals are to meet her current energy expenditure needed for basal metabolism and activity of ambulating. S.P. would fall into the category of "moderate stress, malnourished" requiring 25 to 30 kcal/kg/day. For this calculation, S.P.'s actual weight of 92 lb (41.8 kg) should be used because her metabolism and current energy expenditure reflect this decrease in body mass. Using usual weight or IBW in patients who have severe weight loss may result in overfeeding. For S.P., the caloric goal should be from 1,045 to 1,255 kcal/day.

Protein is the building block of life. Once hepatic glycogen stores are depleted, muscle protein is degraded to provide three-carbon backbones for hepatic gluconeogenesis. Initially, protein catabolism is resistant to the administration of exogenous amino acids, and it can sometimes take weeks until a patient is found to be in a state of positive nitrogen balance. In addition to protein catabolism, exogenous protein is required for wound healing and to replace protein lost in wounds and fistulae. Protein goals are estimated based on weight, degree of stress, and disease state. The goal is to minimize the loss of lean body mass, and as a general rule this requires anywhere from 1.0 to 1.5 g/kg/day of protein depending on the degree of illness and injury. Because S.P. has not had surgery and her stress is minimal, her protein goal should be based on the desire to maintain her current protein status. Using the guidelines provided in Table 35-4, S.P.'s protein dose is 1.2 to 1.5 g/kg/day, or 50 to 63 g/day. As with energy expenditure, calculations of protein needs are only estimates; the patient's clinical course should be monitored, and the protein dose should be adjusted accordingly. If S.P. requires surgery, her energy or calorie goals should be reassessed to include an additional stress factor.

Micronutrients

CASE 35-1, QUESTION 4: What vitamin and mineral deficiencies would you expect to find in S.P.? What options are available to the clinician to address them?

The therapeutic effects of specialized nutritional support accrue through the combined provision of macronutrients and micronutrients. These elements support vital cellular and organ functions, immunity, tissue repair, protein synthesis, and capacity of skeletal, cardiac, and respiratory muscles. As with any medical therapy, a nutritional support regimen should be adjusted based on the requirements, response, and tolerance of the patient. Patients who have inflammatory bowel disease are particularly at risk for developing altered levels of vitamins and other micronutrients. The etiology of these micronutrient losses is multifactorial and encompasses decreased oral intake, increased losses secondary to diarrhea, and malabsorption. In particular, deficiencies in vitamin D, folate, vitamin B_{12}, calcium, magnesium, and zinc are common to this patient population.

Given the prevalence of these deficiencies, S.P. should be prescribed a daily multivitamin and mineral supplement. If it is determined that S.P. has significant fat malabsorption, a water-miscible fat-soluble vitamin formulation can be considered. There is an increased incidence of osteoporosis in patients with Crohn's disease (with or without corticosteroid use), and therefore, S.P. should be assessed to ensure that her calcium and vitamin D intake is normal. Recommended daily oral calcium requirements are from 800 to 1,500 mg/day, but increase from 1,500 to 2,000 mg/day when replacement is needed for a deficiency. S.P. should be consuming a daily amount of 400 international units of vitamin D orally; however, if serum 25-hydroxyvitamin D levels are subtherapeutic, greater amounts will be required and also doses based on the specific disease progression and functionality of S.P.'s GI tract.

Medications such as methotrexate (a folate antagonist) and sulfasalazine (which blocks folate absorption) can be used to treat inflammatory bowel disease and, therefore, increase folate requirements for patients. Daily folate supplementation at a dose of 1 mg orally can be beneficial to S.P. if she is prescribed either of these medications.

Patients with surgical resection of the stomach or terminal ileum are at risk of developing vitamin B_{12} deficiency given the locations of intrinsic factor production and site of absorption, respectively. Given that S.P. has had no surgical intervention to date, it is wise to monitor her vitamin B_{12} status and look for signs of deficiency (i.e., megaloblastic anemia) before instituting aggressive supplementation.

Magnesium deficiency can be a concern in patients with increased intestinal losses, as is the case with many individuals who have inflammatory bowel disease. When considering enteral magnesium supplementation, the change in pH along the GI tract, GI transit time, and fat content of a meal can all affect magnesium absorption. Large doses of enteral magnesium can result in diarrhea; therefore, administering smaller doses throughout the day can lead to improved tolerance and therapeutic efficacy. Choosing a magnesium supplement that can deliver 150 mg of elemental magnesium and dosing it 4 times a day is the recommended oral replacement regimen for patients.

Inflammatory bowel disease patients can experience excessive stool losses resulting in a zinc deficiency. S.P. should receive an oral zinc supplement that delivers 50 mg of elemental zinc daily.

Maintenance Fluids

CASE 35-1, QUESTION 5: Determine the daily fluid requirements for S.P. while she receives specialized nutritional support.

When determining the fluid needs of a patient, the clinician should consider the following steps: (a) correction of fluid imbalances, (b) maintenance fluid requirements, and (c) replacement of ongoing fluid losses.

The extended periods of diarrhea, vomiting, or both that occur with inflammatory bowel disease may lead to dehydration. Dehydration results in a loss of body weight, decreased urine output, dry mouth, and progressive thirst. Hypotension, tachycardia, and poor skin turgor are all clinical signs of dehydration. Apathy, stupor, coma, and death will follow if fluid replacement is not undertaken. Fluid deficits should be estimated from the clinical appearance of the patient, recent weight loss, and serum sodium and blood urea nitrogen concentrations, and replaced by giving half the estimated deficit intravenously over the course of 8 hours. After 8 hours, a new assessment of fluid status should be made, and half of the new estimated deficit should be replaced during the next 8 hours. This process should be repeated until normal hydration is achieved (see Chapter 10, Fluid and Electrolyte Disorders).

Maintenance fluid is that volume of daily fluid intake that replaces the insensible losses and at the same time allows excretion of the daily production of excess solute load in a volume of urine that is of an osmolarity similar to plasma. Maintenance fluid needs can be estimated using several methods. The simplest method uses 30 to 35 mL/kg/day as the basis. Another method is to provide 1,500 mL for the first 20 kg of body weight plus an additional 20 mL/kg for actual weight beyond the initial 20 kg.

Both methods provide estimates of fluid needs for basic maintenance. S.P.'s fluid needs are estimated as follows:

$$\begin{aligned} \text{mL/day} &= 1{,}500\text{ mL} + ([20\text{ mL/kg}][41.8\text{ kg} - 20\text{ kg}]) \\ &= 1{,}500\text{ mL} + (20\text{ mL/kg})(21.8\text{ kg}) \\ &= 1{,}500\text{ mL} + 436\text{ mL} \\ &= 1{,}936\text{ mL} \end{aligned} \quad \text{(Eq. 35-3)}$$

If S.P. experiences vomiting, nasogastric tube output, diarrhea, or other significant fluid losses, additional fluid must be provided. Some losses are measurable and can be directly replaced milliliter for milliliter on a regular basis. Others, however, are not measurable and can only be estimated. The electrolyte composition of the lost fluid is an important consideration for the clinician and dictates the ultimate choice of the replacement fluid.

Evaluating Specialized Nutritional Support Effectiveness

CASE 35-1, QUESTION 6: What parameters should be examined to determine the effectiveness of S.P.'s nutritional support regimen?

Implementing a successful nutritional support regimen begins with proper nutritional assessment of the patient. Nutritional goals that identify macronutrient, micronutrient, and fluid requirements are then established. Follow-up support and monitoring of the patient once nutritional support has been instituted is important to maintain the integrity and efficacy of the therapy.

To minimize the risk of refeeding syndrome in S.P. (a metabolic and electrolyte disturbance that occurs as a result of supplying nutrition to patients who are severely malnourished), all electrolyte abnormalities must be corrected before any nutrition is initiated. Because S.P.'s electrolytes are within normal ranges, no adjustments are necessary. Nutrition should then be implemented slowly, and vitamins administered routinely. Electrolytes, including phosphorus, potassium, magnesium, and glucose, should be monitored at least daily during the first week. Although electrolyte and mineral abnormalities may not be avoided, careful recognition of and close monitoring for refeeding syndrome will prevent serious complications.[33,34]

Although it can sometimes be difficult to obtain a reliable weight for a patient, weight can be an important parameter to help assess not only fluid balance but also the long-term appropriateness of caloric intake. Most patients should gain or lose no more than 1 kg/week when receiving nutritional support (assuming normal fluid status). However, clinicians must be aware of the impact that fluids have on the weight of a patient. Large intake or loss of fluids can influence weight measurements and mask the trends of body mass. Having S.P. record of daily weights, in addition to fluid intake and output, and monitoring trends can serve as one, but not the only, key in determining the effectiveness of her regimen.

Nitrogen balance is another parameter that can help determine the degree of catabolism and protein requirements in a patient. Nitrogen balance is the difference between nitrogen intake and nitrogen excretion. It is estimated by the nitrogen intake along with collecting a 24-hour urine urea nitrogen sample from the patient. Positive nitrogen balance is a reasonable goal during nutritional support therapy for recovery of a patient, but may also require increasing caloric loads on a periodic basis. If a nitrogen balance study is ordered for S.P., increasing protein intake should be considered if results indicate a negative nitrogen balance; however, a negative nitrogen balance may be unavoidable during high-stress states, regardless of the amount of nutrients provided.

Finally, prealbumin levels for S.P. should also be monitored once a week as a marker for short-term gross adequacy of calorie and protein intake. A lack of prealbumin increase is an indicator of poor patient outcomes. With adequate feeding, prealbumin can increase more than 4 mg/dL/week. It should be noted that in the case of S.P. who is suffering from Crohn's disease and may likely be receiving either oral or parenteral corticosteroids as treatment, administration of corticosteroids can falsely elevate prealbumin levels, making S.P. appear to be at a lower nutritional risk.

CASE 35-1, QUESTION 7: Members of the medical team are anxious to have S.P. gain weight and are concerned by her malnourished appearance. Therefore, there is a desire to increase the calories provided to S.P. What potential complications could result from overfeeding S.P.?

Overfeeding should be avoided in all patients because of a plethora of potential complications, especially those with respiratory concerns.[35] Although restoration and maintenance of body cell mass is the goal of nutritional support therapy, a gradual and conservative approach yields fewer metabolic abnormalities. Supplying an abundance of calories to a patient in need of nutritional support increases the metabolic rate, which in turn places greater demands for cardiopulmonary effort and oxygenation. Overfeeding with carbohydrates is particularly detrimental because of the amount of carbon dioxide produced relative to the amount of oxygen consumed. This results in carbon dioxide retention that may lead to acid–base disturbances. Hyperglycemia is also a common metabolic abnormality secondary to excessive carbohydrate administration that can lead to osmotic diuresis and immune dysfunction.

KEY REFERENCES AND WEBSITES

A full list of references for this chapter can be found at http://thepoint.lww.com/AT11e. Below are the key references and websites for this chapter, with the corresponding reference number in this chapter found in parentheses after the reference.

Key References

ASPEN Board of Directors and the Clinical Guidelines Task Force. Guidelines for the use of parenteral and enteral nutrition in adult and pediatric patients [published correction appears in *J Parenter Enteral Nutr.* 2002;26:144]. *J Parenter Enteral Nutr.* 2002;26(1 Suppl):1SA. (16)

Brooks MJ, Melnik G. The refeeding syndrome: an approach to understanding its complications and preventing its occurrence. *Pharmacotherapy.* 1995;15:713. (34)

McClave SA et al. Society of Critical Care Medicine (SCCM) and American Society for Parenteral and Enteral Nutrition (A.S.P.E.N.). *J Parenter Enteral Nutr.* 2016;40(2)159–211. (32)

Mueller C et al. A.S.P.E.N. Clinical guidelines: nutrition screening, assessment, and intervention in adults. *J Parenter Enteral Nutr.* 2011;35:16. (1)

Key Websites

American Society for Parenteral and Enteral Nutrition. http://www.nutritioncare.org.

USDA Food and Nutrition Information Center. http://fnic.nal.usda.gov.

36 Obesity

Dhiren K. Patel and Kaelen C. Dunican

CORE PRINCIPLES

#	Core Principle	CHAPTER CASES
1	Body mass index (BMI) should be measured at each patient encounter and patients should be assessed for overweight and obesity and the risk for related comorbid conditions.	**Case 36-1 (Questions 1, 3)**
2	An understanding of body composition is essential when evaluating the health status of a patient with regard to body fat.	**Case 36-1 (Question 1)**
3	The medication lists of patients with increased body weight should be evaluated for drugs associated with weight gain and alternative agents that are weight neutral or associated with weight loss should be considered.	**Case 36-1 (Question 1)**
4	Obesity is a chronic disease and therapeutic interventions must be long term.	**Case 36-1 (Questions 2, 7)**
5	An appropriate weight loss goal is 5% to 10% of baseline body weight in 6 months.	**Case 36-1 (Question 4)**
6	Management and treatment of overweight and obesity should include a combination of diet and increased physical activity along with behavioral modifications.	**Case 36-1 (Questions 4, 5)**
7	Medication to treat obesity should be considered for patients with a body mass index greater than 30 kg/m^2 without risk factors or greater than 27 kg/m^2 with an obesity-related risk factor such as hypertension, dyslipidemia, sleep apnea, cardiovascular disease, and type 2 diabetes	**Case 36-1 (Questions 6, 7, 9)**
8	Short-term weight loss drugs are unlikely to be clinically useful and should not be recommended.	**Case 36-1 (Question 6)**
9	Medication for chronic weight management includes orlistat, phentermine/topiramate, lorcaserin, naltrexone/bupropion, and liraglutide.	**Case 36-1 (Question 7)**
10	The use of dietary supplements for weight loss is not supported by clinical literature and should be avoided due to safety concerns and lack of regulation.	**Case 36-1 (Question 8)**
11	Bariatric surgery may be considered for patients with a BMI >40 or BMI >35 with obesity-related comorbid conditions.	**Case 36-1 (Question 10)**
12	Alteration of gastrointestinal tract and stomach size after bariatric surgery can alter drug pharmacokinetics and place patients at risk for adverse events associated with some medications.	**Case 36-1 (Question 10)**

Obesity is a chronic disease that is characterized by excess body fat accumulation which may impair health.[1,2] The prevalence of obesity has become an epidemic. More than two-thirds of the US adult population is overweight with more than one-third considered obese.[3] And more than one-third of the worldwide population is overweight.[4] It is recognized by the World Health Organization (WHO) and US Federal Government as a growing problem that is burdening our healthcare organizations and economy. Analyses estimate the total annual US economic costs associated with obesity are in excess of $215 billion.[5]

DEFINITIONS

Overweight and obesity are defined by body mass index (BMI), a measure of weight in relation to height. BMI is calculated as weight (in kg) divided by height (in meters) squared. Normal weight is defined as BMI of 18.5 to less than 25 kg/m^2; overweight is defined as BMI greater than or equal to 25 to less than 30 kg/m^2; and obesity is defined as BMI greater than or equal to 30 kg/m^2 (Table 36-1).[6,7] Obesity is further divided into class I (BMI ⩾30–35 kg/m^2), class II (BMI ⩾35–40 kg/m^2), and class III (BMI ⩾40 kg/m^2). Class III obesity is also referred to as extreme or severe obesity and was formerly known as morbid obesity. Obesity is a chronic metabolic disorder that is determined by multiple biologic and environmental factors, an obesogenic lifestyle, and a genetic predisposition. The increase in the prevalence of obesity and negative health outcomes are major public health problems throughout the world.[1,8]

Body mass index (BMI) is widely accepted as the standard to classify weight. However, a major limitation of BMI is that it does not consider body composition. According to BMI, a person may be classified as "overweight" if their muscle mass is great enough to significantly contribute to total weight. On the other hand, a patient may be considered "normal weight" while having excess fat accumulation and decreased muscle mass. The use of BMI to assess body fat and risk of morbidity and mortality is particularly problematic in certain ethnic groups because BMI does not account for differences in distribution of body fat. For example, research suggests that in the Asian population, BMI underestimates body fat.[9]

Fat distribution in the abdominal region has been linked to many of the metabolic consequences of obesity.[10] Measurement of waist circumference (WC) is used to assess for increased abdominal fat accumulation and to determine health risk. Waist circumference measurements greater than 102 cm (40 inches) in men and 88 cm (35 inches) in women are associated with increased risk of metabolic diseases.[10] Increased WC has been shown to predict obesity-related diseases such as diabetes, hypertension, dyslipidemia, and cardiovascular disease.[10–12] The waist-to-hip ratio (WHtR) also provides an assessment of regional fat distribution. A waist-to-hip ratio >1 in men and >0.8 in women indicates high intra-abdominal fat. Some research suggests that WHtR is superior to both WC and BMI in determining obesity-related cardiometabolic risk. Independent of BMI classification, higher waist circumference is correlated with increased mortality.[13] Therefore, measurement of WC and the WHtR are useful in identifying individuals that are normal weight or overweight with health risk due to increased abdominal fat accumulation.

Table 36-1
BMI and Guidelines for Weight Classes

Weight Status	BMI[a]	Obesity Class
Underweight	<18.5	
Normal	≥18.5–25	
Overweight	≥25–30	
Obesity	≥30–35	I
	≥35–40	II
Extreme or severe obesity	≥40	III

[a]Metric conversion formula using kilograms and meters: BMI = Weight in kg/height in m^2. Nonmetric conversion formula using pounds and inches: BMI = weight in lb/height in inches^2 × 703.

BMI, body mass index.

Source: Jensen, Michael D et al. 2013 AHA/ACC/TOS guideline for the management of overweight and obesity in adults: a report of the American College of Cardiology/American Heart Association Task Force on Practice Guidelines and The Obesity Society. *J Am Coll Cardiol*. 2014;63:2985–3023.

EPIDEMIOLOGY

Obesity is a major public health concern worldwide and is a leading cause of numerous medical conditions (e.g., cardiovascular disease, hypertension, dyslipidemia, diabetes, sleep apnea) and premature death[10,13] (Table 36-2). According to the WHO, there were approximately 1.9 billion overweight and 600 million obese adults globally in 2014.[1] In the United States, the prevalence of

Table 36-2
Obesity-Related Health Conditions

Cardiovascular	Dermatologic
Hypertension	Striae distensae (stretch marks)
Heart failure	Skin tags
Coronary artery disease	Acanthosis nigricans
Stroke	Intertrigo
Pulmonary	**Gastrointestinal**
Obstructive sleep apnea	Gallstones
Asthma	Gastroesophageal reflux disease (GERD)
Metabolic	**Psychological**
Dyslipidemias	Eating disorders
Diabetes mellitus	Depression
Hyperinsulinemia	Social stigma
Cancer	**Gynecologic and Obstetric Complications**
Esophageal	Gestational diabetes
Colon	Preeclampsia
Liver	Infertility
Prostate	**Musculoskeletal**
Uterine	Osteoarthritis
Breast	**Other**
Ovarian	Nonalcoholic fatty liver disease (NAFLD)
Gallbladder	Impotence
Kidney	
Cervix	

Sources: Hildago LG. Dermatologic complications of obesity. *Am J Clin Dermatol*. 2002;3:497–506; Malnick SD, Knobler H. The medical complications of obesity. *Q J Med*. 2006;99:565–579.

obesity has been examined as part of the National Health and Nutrition Examination Survey (NHANES). The NHANES data from 2011 to 2012 showed that 68.5% of US adults were overweight or obese and 34.9% were obese and 6.4% were extremely obese.[3] Adult obesity usually results from a steady weight gain from the mid-20s to between ages 40 and 59, when the prevalence of obesity peaks.[3] Severe obesity is more common in women.[3] The most recent NHANES data report overweight, obesity, and extreme obesity were more prevalent among non-Hispanic black women.[3] Despite the striking increases in obesity prevalence in the 1980s and 1990s, current NHANES data suggest that the prevalence of obesity may be stabilizing, showing nonsignificant increases compared with the 2003 to 2004 NHANES data.[3]

Obesity is also a significant problem among children and adolescents, with alarmingly high prevalence rates. Overweight and obesity in children and adolescents (age 2–19 years) are based on the Centers for Disease Control (CDC) growth charts; overweight is defined as BMI in the 85th to 95th percentile and obese is defined as BMI greater than the 95th percentile.[7] The WHO estimates that greater than 42 million children under age 5 are overweight.[1] NHANES data from 2011 to 2012 reported that 31.8% of children and adolescents (age 2–19 years) were either overweight or obese and 16.9% were obese.[3] Non-Hispanic white youth show lower prevalence of obesity as compared to non-Hispanic black and Hispanic youth. As with adults, the prevalence has stabilized, with no significant change compared with the 1999 to 2000 NHANES data.[3] However, because this prevalence rate has remained alarmingly high, childhood obesity must be addressed because of the health consequences the obese child takes on into adulthood. Childhood and adolescent obesity shows an increased risk for adult overweight and obesity.[14] Also, studies have shown that overweight and obesity in childhood and adolescence are correlated with an increased risk of adult diabetes, hypertension, ischemic heart disease and stroke physical morbidity, and premature mortality.[15]

ETIOLOGY AND PATHOPHYSIOLOGY

Simply stated, obesity results from an imbalance of energy intake and energy expenditure. Body fat accumulation will occur when an individual consumes more calories than are burned. However, the exact cause of obesity is difficult to identify and is likely a mixture of genetic, environmental, behavioral, and neurohormonal factors. Investigators have tried to understand the origin of this disease by studying the influences of society, culture, socioeconomic status, medical conditions, medications that stimulate appetite, parental weight, and hereditary traits on dietary habits and physical activity.[16] Each potential cause of obesity continues to be investigated as a possible target for treatment and prevention of this chronic disease.

There have been several association studies linking short sleep duration and metabolic changes such as obesity, insulin resistance, and diabetes.[17,18] One study showed that children aged 30 months and younger who lacked sleep were at risk of exhibiting obesity at 7 years.[19] Another trial in adults found that sleep duration was negatively correlated with BMI.[20] Alteration of the hypothalamic regulation of appetite and energy expenditure owing to sleep loss is one possible explanation. Normally, when a person has eaten an adequate amount of food, neurotransmitters or peptides in the brain signal the satiety centers in the hypothalamus and there is a reduced desire to eat. Sleep loss has also been shown to be associated with low leptin levels and high ghrelin levels; both factors contribute to signaling of energy deficit and hunger, which may contribute to overeating and obesity.[21]

Recently, research has begun to investigate the role of that gut microbiota in body composition. Data suggest that interventions that negatively impact the biodiversity of the gut microbiota such as Cesarean delivery (vs. vaginal delivery), maternal prepregnancy BMI, and early antibiotic use may increase the risk of obesity.[22] A large cohort trial found that the repeated use of broad-spectrum antibiotics during the first 2 years of life has been associated with early childhood obesity.[23]

Genetic Features

There is a clear link between genetics and obesity, both in childhood and adulthood, shown mostly through twin and adoption studies.[24–29] One study by Wardle et al.[26] demonstrated a heritability estimate of 77% for BMI and 76% for waist circumference. Genetic studies have identified genes that may be associated with weight.[24,30] There is also evidence that body fat distribution is controlled by genetic factors with waist-to-hip ratio showing heritability of up to 60%.[31]

HYPOTHALAMUS DYSREGULATION

The hypothalamus plays a key role in body weight regulation by controlling satiety (the feeling of fullness), hunger, and in turn food intake. Neurobiologic theories of eating disorders have focused on dysregulation of the hypothalamic–pituitary–adrenal, hypothalamic–pituitary–gonadal, and hypothalamic–pituitary–thyroid axes as well as dysregulation of neurotransmitters, neuropeptides, endogenous opioids, growth hormone, insulin, and leptin.[32] Alterations in hypothalamic functioning are associated with appetite changes, mood disorders, and neuroendocrine disturbances.[33] The hypothalamus is the major appetite and eating control center in the brain and is sensitive to a variety of facilitatory and inhibitory neurotransmitters and polypeptide neurohormones from the brain and gastrointestinal (GI) tract. The hypothalamus receives input from peripheral satiety sites (e.g., gastric and pancreatic peptides released secondary to food passing through the GI tract), from leptin that is produced by fat cells, and from the catecholamine neurotransmitter system in the brain.[33,34]

NEUROTRANSMITTER DYSREGULATION

Serotonin

Serotonin plays an important role in postprandial satiety, anxiety, sleep, mood, obsessive–compulsive, and impulse control disorders. Serotonin has an inhibitory effect on appetite and is responsible for satiety or the feeling of fullness after food intake.[35,36] Diminished serotonin activity can contribute to increased food intake and carbohydrate craving.[35] The reduction in serotonin activity may upregulate the appetite or satiety centers in the brain, thereby increasing the amount of food a person wants to eat. Agents that block postsynaptic serotonin activity (e.g., clozapine, mirtazapine, and atypical antipsychotics) can stimulate appetite and may cause weight gain.

Dopamine

Agents that increase dopamine activity (e.g., apomorphine, a dopamine agonist; levodopa, a metabolic precursor of dopamine; and amphetamine, a stimulator of release of dopamine from presynaptic stores) have been shown to have anorexic effects.[37] Dopamine agonists increase dopaminergic transmission and motor activity, which causes loss of appetite and hyperactivity. The central nervous system (CNS) effects of dopaminergic agents occur in the cerebral cortex, in the reticular activating system, and in the hypothalamic feeding center. The mesolimbic–mesocortical dopaminergic circuits are important for behavior reward and reinforcement, and are involved with "addictive" behaviors.[37] Dopamine-augmenting agents such as amphetamines were once used for the treatment of exogenous obesity and produced tolerance, dependence, and withdrawal reactions. Conversely, dopamine receptor antagonists such as chlorpromazine and clozapine may cause dysphoria and are often associated with weight gain.

Norepinephrine

The hypothalamus is innervated by noradrenergic pathways; thus, norepinephrine is involved in the regulation of eating behavior, the hypothalamic control of thyrotropin-releasing hormone secretion, corticotropin-releasing hormone (CRH) release, and gonadotropin secretion.[37] D-Amphetamine, which inhibits the reuptake of norepinephrine, decreases hunger sensations and food intake. Abnormalities in leptin and β_3-adrenergic activity have been associated with obesity and diabetes.[38] The β_3-adrenoceptor is involved in a feedback loop with leptin to regulate energy balance, lipolysis in adipocytes, serum insulin levels, and food intake.[39] People with hereditary obesity or type 2 diabetes mellitus may have abnormalities in the β_3-adrenoceptor or in leptin activity, signaling, or receptors.[38] A genetic variant of the β_3-adrenoceptor in humans has been associated with severe obesity and type 2 diabetes. It is possible that some cases of obesity may be secondary to failure of the β_3-adrenoreceptor on brown adipocytes to respond appropriately to leptin-induced sympathetic activity. β_3-Adrenergic receptor agonists are being studied to induce thermogenic activity and promote weight loss when combined with a calorie-restricted diet.[39]

NEUROPEPTIDE AND LEPTIN DYSREGULATION

Leptin

Leptin is a protein synthesized by adipocytes, gastric chief cells, skeletal muscle, and other organs. It acts on receptors of the hypothalamus to act as an afferent satiety signal in the brain to regulate body fat mass.[33,40,41] Leptin reduces food intake, decreases serum glucose and insulin levels, increases metabolic rate, and reduces body fat mass and weight by reducing neuropeptide Y (NPY) activity (a potent feeding stimulant secreted by the hypothalamus and cells in the gut).[40,42] Leptin serum levels are highly correlated with BMI and body fat and its secretion has a circadian rhythm and an oscillatory pattern similar to other hormones.[38,41,43]

Leptin is supposed to signal the brain to reduce the desire to eat, but this does not occur in patients with obesity.[40] It has been postulated that some individuals with obesity may have partially resistant hypothalamic receptors or that there is a defect in the blood–brain barrier transport system for bringing leptin into the brain.[33,40,43,44] Cerebrospinal fluid leptin levels in some patients with obesity have been found to be much lower than expected compared with serum leptin levels, which suggests that the uptake of leptin into the brain may be defective.[33] Other studies suggest that obese individuals may have a dysregulation of leptin in response to overfeeding, with a lack of serum increase. Compared with lean individuals, this may indicate that the patients with obesity lack a protective mechanism of increase in serum leptin levels in response to increased caloric intake to prevent weight gain.[45] It has been demonstrated that elevated baseline serum leptin levels are associated with inability to maintain weight loss.[46] Another potential mechanism may be reduced leptin receptor protein expression found in skeletal muscle of patients with obesity that could lead to leptin resistance in the presence of elevated leptin serum levels.[47] Leptin and leptin-like products have been investigated for promotion of weight loss, but leptin resistance impedes its clinical utility.[40,48]

Neuropeptides and Neurohormones

Appetite is regulated in part via orexigenic neuropeptides which signal hunger and anorexigenic neuropeptides which signal satiety within the hypothalmus. Neuropeptide Y (NPY) and agouti-related peptide (AgRP) are found in the central nervous system and are potent stimulators of appetite.[49,50] POMC (pro-opiomelanocortin) is a precursor protein to α-melanocyte-stimulating hormone (α-MSH) and binds to melanocortin-3 receptors (MC3R) and melanocortin-4 receptors (MC4R) to suppress food intake.[34,49] Research on MC4R analogs is ongoing, but trials with selective MC3R agonist failed to suppress feeding.[34,49]

Several other neurohormonal signals and peptides play a role in appetite regulation. Ghrelin is a hormone that is released from the stomach before meals and acts to increase appetite via stimulation of NPY and AgRP.[49] There is a negative correlation between ghrelin levels and BMI where patients with obesity have increased ghrelin and levels remain elevated even after weight loss.[49] Peptide tyrosine tyrosine (peptide YY or PYY) and pancreatic polypeptide (PP) are pancreatic are chemically related to NPY but work as appetite suppressants.[49,50] Early studies of experimental PYY administration have found an intranasal formulation to be ineffective for weight reduction and poorly tolerated in obese patients.[51] A small dose escalation study of subcutaneous injections of two forms of PYY, PYY_{1-36}, and PYY_{3-36}, found some positive results on inducing lower subjective hunger and thirst ratings and higher satiety ratings with PPY_{3-36} administration.[52] Amylin is a pancreatic hormone that is released in response to eating and functions as an anorectic hormone.[49] Administration of amylin has been shown to result in reduced food intake and weight loss.[53] Glucagon-like peptide-1 (GLP-1) is secreted from the gut in response to food intake and works to reduce food intake, suppress glucagon secretion, and delay gastric emptying.[49] Cholecystokinin (CCK) is a hormone that is released from the small intestines in response to food intake and works to suppress further food intake.[49]

Environmental Influences and Behavioral Factors

Despite the known genetic influences predisposing certain individuals to obesity, environmental influences play a role by providing exposure to a lifestyle promoting energy imbalance and may influence epigenetic factors. Modern society provides an overabundance of inexpensive, readily accessible calorie-dense food. Decreased energy expenditure due to a sedentary lifestyle has become common, further exacerbating an obesogenic lifestyle. A review of twin and adoption studies by Silventoinen et al.[25] clearly demonstrated that environmental factors affect BMI variation in childhood, but the effect of common environment disappears in adolescence. These results portray a stronger influence of genetics in the incidence of obesity in adulthood.

Medical Conditions and Medications

Although less common, certain medical conditions may cause overweight and obesity.[6] Genetic syndromes may be the primary cause of obesity such as Prader–Willi, Bardet–Biedl, Cohen, Alström, and Froehlich syndromes. Other primary causes of obesity include monogenic disorders such as melanocortin-4 receptor mutation, leptin deficiency, and POMC deficiency. Secondary causes of obesity include neurologic issues such as brain injury, brain tumors, and hypothalamic injury. Endocrine disorders may also be a secondary cause of overweight and obesity such as polycystic ovarian syndrome, Cushing syndrome, and growth hormone deficiency. Hypothyroidism is often cited as a secondary cause of obesity because elevated TSH is correlated with obesity.[54] But the relationship between hypothyroidism and obesity is complex; because leptin and melanocortin influence the release of TSH, causality has yet to be established.[54–56] Psychological causes of obesity include eating disorders and depression when associated

Table 36-3
Common Drugs and Their Effect on Weight

	Associated with Weight Loss	Associated with Minimal Weight Gain or Weight Neutral	Associated with Weight Gain
Antidepressants	Bupropion	Fluoxetine, imipramine	TCAs, MAOIs, paroxetine, fluvoxamine, venlafaxine, duloxetine, mirtazapine
Antipsychotics		Aripiprazole, quetiapine, ziprasidone	Clozapine, olanzapine, risperidone
Neurologic	Topiramate, zonisamide, felbamate	Lamotrigine	Valproic acid, gabapentin, pregabalin, carbamazepine, vigabatrin, lithium
Glucose-lowering	GLP-1 agonists, metformin, pramlintide, SGLT-2 inhibitors	DPP-4 inhibitors, α-glucosidase inhibitors	Insulin, sulfonylureas (especially glyburide), meglitinides, thiazolidinediones
Antihypertensives		ACEIs, ARBs, CCBs, doxazosin	β-adrenergic blockers, (especially propranolol), α-adrenergic blockers (prazosin, terazosin)
Contraceptives		Barrier methods, Oral contraceptives	Injectables (especially medroxyprogesterone)
Antihistamines		Second generation	First generation
Anti-inflammatory		NSAIDs, DMARDs	Corticosteroids

ACEI, angiotensin converting enzyme inhibitor; ARB, angiotensin receptor blocker; CCB, calcium channel blocker; DMARD, disease-modifying antirheumatic drug; DPP-4, dipeptidyl peptidase-4; GLP-1, glucagon-like peptide-1; MAOI, monoamine oxidase inhibitor; NSAID, nonsteroidal anti-inflammatory drug; SGLT-2, sodium-glucose-linked transporter-2; TCA, tricyclic antidepressant.

with overeating or binging. Several medications are associated with weight gain. These include antipsychotics, steroids, insulin, sulfonylureas, thiazolidinediones, some antidepressants, and some anticonvulsants.[57] When treating overweight and obesity, if medications associated with weight gain are identified, substitution with possible alternatives should be attempted. Table 36-3 provides a list of medications that may cause weight gain along with potential alternatives.

CLINICAL FEATURES

CASE 36-1

QUESTION 1: S.B. is a 48-year-old woman with a past medical history of hypertension, sleep apnea, osteoarthritis, and depression. She states that she has been overweight since she was a toddler. She reports having tried multiple diets during the past 30 years, but has had little success with weight loss and always regains any weight she manages to lose. Her height is 168 cm, current weight is 91 kg, and WC is 96 cm. She presents to her primary physician for a routine physical examination. She complains of dissatisfaction with her weight. She reports having tried multiple diets during the past 20 years, but has had little success with weight loss and always regains any weight she manages to lose. S.B. expresses a desire to attempt medication therapy for weight loss. Her current medications include hydrochlorothiazide, metoprolol, naproxen, and paroxetine. Her blood pressure is currently 162/98 mm Hg and she is complaining of daytime fatigue due to sleep apnea. How is obesity defined and assessed in a patient like S.B.?

Initial Assessment

Current guidelines suggest that weight status should be assessed in all patients.[6,7] Initial assessment involves a physical exam and patient interview to classify the presence of overweight or obesity and any obesity-related comorbidities. The preferred method to classify overweight or obesity is to measure the BMI. Measurement of WC will also aid in determining risk of obesity comorbidities. However, measurement of waist circumference in patients with BMI greater than 35 kg/m^2 is not necessary because it will likely be elevated and will add no additional risk information.[7,12] BMI, WC, and obesity-related comorbidities are used to determine the need to initiate treatment. S.B.'s BMI is 32.2 (91 $kg/[1.68\ m]^2$), which is in obesity class I. Her waist circumference is greater than 88 cm, indicating abdominal obesity that puts her at additional risk for increased morbidity and mortality. S.B. also has hypertension, sleep apnea, and osteoarthritis, which are likely related to obesity and will need to be considered in her overall care plan.

During the patient interview, information should be obtained regarding the patient's eating habits and physical activity. It is important to establish baseline data so that response to changes in diet and exercise is noted throughout treatment. Successful weight loss involves a change in energy balance through reduced caloric intake or increased energy expenditure. In S.B.'s case, it will be beneficial to evaluate her current diet and physical activities to determine the most appropriate lifestyle recommendations. It is also important to evaluate a patient's "weight loss readiness" or self-motivation before initiation of therapy. A patient's motivation to lose weight is a significant predictor of success or failure in the weight management program. S.B.'s desire and willingness to make significant lifestyle changes in order to achieve this should be evaluated.

Patients should also be screened for medical conditions or medications that can increase the risk for obesity, and these underlying factors should be corrected before recommending treatment. S.B.'s past medical history does not indicate any overt medical causes of obesity, but it would be appropriate to rule out whether she is overeating due to her depression and to check thyroid function to rule out hypothyroidism. Even though causality between obesity and thyroid dysfunction has yet to be firmly established, hypothyroidism is a common condition in women and may be associated with weight gain or inability to lose weight. S.B. is currently taking paroxetine for depression which has been associated with weight gain.[6,58] S.B.'s prescriber may want to consider switching to fluoxetine which is the SSRI that is associated with the least amount of weight gain or bupropion which is associated with weight loss (Table 36-3).[6,57,58]

Course and Prognosis

CASE 36-1, QUESTION 2: S.B. states that she has struggled with her weight her whole life. She has progressively gained approximately 2 kg/year since her 20s.What is the typical course and prognosis of obesity?

Obesity is a chronic disease that often begins in childhood or adolescence and can be characterized by a slow and steady increase in body weight during adult life. Most patients with obesity battle with weight loss and regain throughout their entire lives. The biologic response to weight loss favors regain with increased ghrelin and reductions in GLP-1, CCK, leptin, and PYY resulting in increased hunger.[6,59] Maintaining weight loss is key to long-term management of obesity. S.B. should be assured that her struggle is common and that she will need to commit to long-term lifestyle changes to manage her obesity.

Medical Complications

CASE 36-1, QUESTION 3: S.B. understands that she already has hypertension, sleep apnea, and osteoarthritis, which are comorbidities that are related to her obesity and increase her risk of morbidity and mortality. She is also at risk for experiencing additional obesity-associated medical comorbidities if she does not lose or continues to gain weight. What are the other common medical conditions associated with obesity? What impact will weight loss have on comorbid conditions?

Obesity is associated with an increased risk of morbidity and mortality. Some obesity-associated diseases that are generally not life-threatening include dermatologic complications, osteoarthritis, reproductive complications, gallstones and their complications, and stress incontinence. Other obesity-related conditions have a tremendous impact on physiologic functioning and medical illnesses. Obesity is linked to many significant health conditions such as type 2 diabetes mellitus, respiratory conditions, gallbladder disease, cancers, osteoarthritis, cardiac disease (hypertension, stroke, congestive heart failure, and coronary heart disease), dyslipidemia and dermatologic problems (intertrigo and stretching of skin), and gynecologic and obstetric complications (Table 36-2).[60,61] Weight loss helps to control diseases associated with obesity and may even help prevent development of these diseases.

Health benefits have been shown with modest sustained weight loss. Weight loss of 2% to 5% is associated with reducing hemoglobin A1C by 0.2% to 0.3% in patients with type 2 with overweight or obesity and weight loss of 5% to 10% is associated with up to 1% reduction in A1C.[7] Five percent weight loss is associated with reducing systolic blood pressure by 3 mm Hg and diastolic blood pressure by 2 mm Hg. Weight loss of 5 to 8 kg has been shown to reduce low-density lipoprotein cholesterol (LDL-C) by approximately 5 mg/dL and increase high-density lipoprotein cholesterol (HDL) by 2 to 3 mg/dL and triglycerides are lowered by 15 mg/dL with just 3 kg weight loss.[7] In S.B.'s case, weight loss could help her decrease or eliminate medications needed to control her hypertension, alleviate pain associated with osteoarthritis, decrease symptoms of sleep apnea, and reduce her BMI and WC, therefore improving her morbidity and mortality risk. In the meantime, her hypertension is currently uncontrolled and should be aggressively managed per the current guidelines.

MANAGEMENT AND TREATMENT

Obesity is a chronic disease that requires lifelong effort for successful treatment.[6,7] Treatment may involve a multidisciplinary approach including the expertise of a general practitioner, dietician or nutrition specialist, pharmacist, psychiatrist, or surgeon depending on the specific needs of the individual. The general goals of weight loss and management are to prevent weight gain, reduce body weight, and maintain weight loss over a long period.

Medical Management

CASE 36-1, QUESTION 4: S.B. reports that she has never received dietary counseling from a medical professional and has always dieted on her own by restricting fat intake. S.B. expresses a desire for weight loss therapy. What are appropriate goals for S.B.'s weight loss? What should the initial treatment plan include?

Weight loss is recommended for patients who have obesity (BMI ≥30) or those who are overweight, who have obesity-related comorbidities or increased waist circumference.[7] An appropriate initial goal for weight loss is 5% to 10% of baseline weight within 6 months.[7] Setting appropriate achievable weight loss goals is important to success; unrealistic expectations for more dramatic weight loss may lead to disappointment and ultimately cause patients to stop any efforts toward weight loss. An appropriate goal for S.B. is 4.55 to 9.1 kg within 6 months. Treatment options to facilitate weight loss include lifestyle interventions and anti-obesity medications. S.B. questioned her physician about weight loss medications, but she has never made an effort to lose weight through a structured weight loss program. The initial treatment plan must always include a reduced calorie diet, increased physical activity, and behavioral modifications. These measures must be attempted and maintained for at least 6 months before considering pharmacotherapy.[7]

Nonpharmacologic Therapy

CASE 36-1, QUESTION 5: S.B. reports that she has never received dietary counseling from a medical professional and has always dieted on her own by restricting fat intake. Although she has not attempted to lose weight recently, S.B. expresses desire to try a program for weight loss and start an exercise regimen. What types of nonpharmacologic therapies are available for weight reduction and relapse prevention?

Comprehensive lifestyle interventions including a calorie-restricted diet, increased physical activity, and behavioral modifications are the foundation of weight loss therapy.

DIET

Diets for weight loss promote caloric restriction. Caloric recommendations for women seeking to lose weight are 1,200 to 1,500 kcal/day and 1,500 to 1,800 kcal/day for men; alternatively, a deficit of 500 to 750 kcal/day is associated with weight loss.[7] Because of the high demand by consumers, there are numerous types of weight loss programs, diets, and products that may or may not be effective for each individual patient. A variety of dietary interventions have been proven successful in weight loss including low-fat diets, higher protein diets, low carbohydrate diets, restricted carbohydrate diets, meal replacement and liquid diets, dietary pattern such as the Mediterranean diet.[7] Research suggests clinically meaningful weight loss is achieved through a reduced calorie diet regardless of the composition of dietary macronutrients.[62]

EXERCISE

Increased physical activity will contribute to the negative energy balance that is required for weight loss. Increased physical activity is essential in preventing weight gain. Overweight children and adults should have at least 30 minutes of moderate-intensity physical exercise daily (with a gradual increment of increasing exercise by several minutes each day up to 30 minutes/day). It has been shown that moderate exercise (e.g., 4 kcal/g/week) can improve physiologic variables.[63,64]

BEHAVIOR THERAPY

The most effective lifestyle intervention includes frequent counseling (>14) group or individual sessions per month with a trained interventionist (registered dietician, nutrition counselor, psychologist, exercise specialist, health counselor, or other trained professional).

Individuals who want to lose weight frequently seek out popular structured programs (e.g., Jenny Craig, Weight Watchers) and these programs have also been proven successful in producing weight loss. Clinical trials that compared dietary interventions conclude that the most effective diet is one that the patient is able to comply with long term.[62,65]

Overall, a combination of a reduced-calorie diet and increased physical activity with support of a trained interventionist is the most effective for reducing and maintaining weight loss. Given that obesity is a chronic condition, S.B. must select a comprehensive lifestyle intervention that is most appealing to her so that she will be able to comply with it long term.

Pharmacologic Therapy

CASE 36-1, QUESTION 6: S.B. returns to her physician for follow-up 6 months later. She has managed to lose 7 kg and is at a weight of 84 kg. Based on her BMI of 29.8 kg/m^2, her weight is classified as overweight. Her depression, osteoarthritis, sleep apnea, and hypertension have improved (current blood pressure is 142/88 mm Hg). Her current medication profile includes bupropion, hydrochlorothiazide, metoprolol, and acetaminophen as needed. Although she has achieved her goal with 7.7% weight loss and is now considered overweight and not obese, S.B. is disappointed that her weight loss has plateaued. She still wants to lose additional weight. She again asks the physician about short-term anti-obesity medications that can help accelerate her weight loss. Would a short-term agent be appropriate for S.B.? What are the mechanisms of action, efficacy, and potential adverse effects of the short-term anti-obesity medications?

As previously stated, a comprehensive lifestyle intervention is the foundation of weight loss management. Although weight loss is possible for most patients, it is not sustainable and regain is common.[66] Obesity is a chronic, lifelong illness that may require long-term medication therapy. Medication should be considered only for patients with a BMI ≥30 kg/m^2 without risk factors or BMI ≥27 kg/m^2 with an obesity-related comorbid medical condition such as hypertension, dyslipidemia, type 2 diabetes, and obstructive sleep apnea (Table 36-2).[6] Medications should not be considered a replacement for diet, behavioral modification, and exercise, but rather as adjunctive therapy. Currently, marketed anti-obesity drugs cause weight loss by suppressing the appetite or decreasing the absorption of fat.[67]

S.B. is a candidate for pharmacotherapy even though her BMI is currently considered overweight at 29.8 kg/m^2, her obesity-related comorbidities of hypertension and sleep apnea qualify her for medication therapy. The most appropriate medication for S.B. must be based on her current medication profile and her comorbid health conditions.

SHORT-TERM THERAPY

Obesity is a chronic disease state; therefore, the clinical usefulness of short-term therapy is unlikely to have a meaningful impact. The FDA has approved several weight loss drugs for short-term use defined as <12 weeks, and these include phentermine, diethylpropion, phendimetrazine, and benzphetamine. All are sympathomimetic agents that function as appetite suppressants.[68,69] Of these drugs, phentermine is the most commonly prescribed and is frequently prescribed, off-label, for long-term therapy.[68]

Phentermine is approved for adjunctive therapy in patients older than 16 years of age, at a dosage of 18.75 to 37.5 mg taken 2 hours after breakfast. Dosing may also be divided into two 18.75 mg doses.[70] The most common adverse effects associated with phentermine therapy are insomnia and dry mouth.[68] Phentermine has also been associated with cardiovascular effects, including case reports of pulmonary hypertension, and as such is contraindicated in patients with cardiovascular disease and hypertension.[71,72] Phentermine also has abuse potential and is considered a controlled substance (schedule IV drug), which further limits its use as a weight loss agent.[69]

Diethylpropion, phendimetrazine, and benzphetamine exhibit appetite suppressive actions similar to phentermine, but are less widely prescribed.[68] They also share adverse effects and contraindications similar to phentermine.[68,69] The abuse potential with these drugs is high, with diethylpropion classified as a schedule IV drug and benzphetamine and phendimetrazine classified as schedule III drugs.[69] Based on their approval for short-term use, adverse effects and abuse potential, none of these agents should be recommended for weight loss therapy.

S.B.'s physician should not prescribe short-term weight loss medications to S.B. Short-term agents for obesity may increase S.B.'s blood pressure. Also short-term agents will not provide the necessary long-term treatment for S.B.'s chronic condition.

CASE 36-1, QUESTION 7: S.B. realizes that her obesity is a chronic condition and inquires about long-term medications for weight loss. What agents are available for the long-term treatment of obesity? (see Table 36-4)

LONG-TERM THERAPY

Orlistat (Xenical, Alli)

Orlistat is FDA-approved for long-term obesity management as an adjunct to lifestyle modification.[73] Orlistat 120 mg was originally marketed under the trade name Xenical. Then, in February 2007, the FDA approved the OTC marketing of orlistat, under the trade name Alli, at a 60 mg dose.[74] Orlistat works to reduce dietary fat absorption by inhibiting GI (stomach and pancreatic) lipase activity.[75,76] Gastric and pancreatic lipase are enzymes that play a pivotal role in the digestion of dietary fat (triglycerides). By inhibiting these lipase enzymes, orlistat prevents the hydrolysis and absorption of triglycerides.[73,77] This results in the excretion of approximately 30% of ingested fat in the feces.[68] Orlistat does not exert appetite suppressant effects, has no CNS effects, and has no systemic absorption.[76] The therapeutic activity of orlistat takes place in the stomach and small intestine and effects are seen as soon as 24 to 48 hours after dosing.

In a meta-analysis, orlistat was shown to produce average weight loss of 2.9 kg or 2.9% greater than placebo.[78] Additionally, a 4-year prospective, double-blind, randomized study, XENDOS, found that orlistat plus lifestyle changes was associated with a 37.3% risk reduction of type 2 diabetes in greater than 3,300 high-risk obese patients.[79] Use of orlistat has also been associated with improvements in blood pressure, as well as improvement in metabolic parameters such as fasting serum lipid profiles and C-reactive protein.[78,80,81]

Table 36-4
Medications for the Treatment of Obesity

Generic Name	Trade Name	Dosing
Orlistat	Xenical	120 mg PO TID
	Alli	60 mg PO TID
Phentermine/topiramate	Qsymia	3.75/23 mg PO QAM × 14 days; then 7.5/46 mg QAM for 12 weeks then evaluate weight loss, if less than 3%, dose may be titrated to 11.25/69 mg QAM × 14 days then 15/92 mg QAM
Lorcaserin	Belviq	10 mg PO BID
Naltrexone/bupropion	Contrave	8/90 mg PO QAM × 1 week then 8/90 mg BID ×1 week then 16/180 mg QAM and 8/90 mg QPM then 16/180 mg BID
Liraglutide	Saxenda	0.6 mg SC daily × 1 week increase dose by 0.6 mg weekly until therapeutic dose of 3 mg daily
Phentermine hydrochloride[a]	Adipex-P	TID; 30–37.5 mg QAM

[a]Not recommended for routine or long-term use.
BID, 2 times a day; OTC, over the counter; PO, by mouth; QAM, every morning; QPM, every evening; SC, subcutaneously; TID, 3 times a day.

The most common adverse effects associated with orlistat include GI problems (loose stools, oily spotting, flatus with discharge, fecal urgency, fatty or oily stools, increased defecation, fecal incontinence, bloating, and cramping).[82] The most common non-GI adverse effect was headache (6%). Side effects usually develop early in treatment and persist for 1 to 4 weeks, but occasionally last longer than 6 months. Because GI adverse effects are worse with a high-fat diet, orlistat may enhance dietary compliance with a low-fat diet. Side effects that continue to be problematic have been associated with nonadherence to orlistat therapy and therefore variability in patient outcomes. Rare cases of oxalate-induced acute kidney injury and liver injury have been reported with use of orlistat.[83,84]

Orlistat may reduce the absorption of fat-soluble vitamins (A, D, E, and K) and patients should take a multivitamin supplement that contains these vitamins.[82] The supplement should be taken once a day at least 2 hours before or after the administration of orlistat, such as at bedtime. Reduced absorption of vitamin K may potentiate the bleeding effects of warfarin. Reduced absorption of vitamin D may lead to metabolic bone disease; supplementation with higher doses of vitamin D may be required.[85] Orlistat may also reduce the absorption of lipophilic drugs including amiodarone, cyclosporine, lamotrigine, and valproic acid.[76,86] Orlistat is contraindicated in pregnancy and in patients with chronic malabsorption syndrome, or cholestasis.[73]

Phentermine/Topiramate ER (Qsymia)

Phentermine/topiramate ER is a combination drug that has been approved by the FDA for long-term obesity management as an adjunct to lifestyle modification.[87] Phentermine is a sympathomimetic agent that functions as an appetite suppressant by increasing the concentration of norepinephrine in the central nervous system.[88] Topiramate is a second-generation antiepileptic agent also approved for the treatment of migraines, which acts as an agonist at γaminobutyric acid ($GABA_A$) receptors and as an antagonist at non-*N*-methyl-D-aspartic acid (NMDA) glutamate receptors.[89] The mechanism by which weight loss occurs with topiramate is unclear, but may be related to a direct action on adipose tissue.[90]

Therapy is initiated at a dose of phentermine 3.75 mg/topiramate 23 mg daily for 14 days, after which the dose is increased to phentermine 7.5 mg/topiramate 46 mg daily. If the patient has not experienced ≥3% weight loss after 12 weeks of therapy at the maintenance dose, the drug should either be discontinued or the dose escalated to phentermine 15 mg/topiramate 92 mg daily. After an additional 12 weeks of therapy, if the patient has not experienced ≥5% weight loss, the drug should be discontinued.[87]

The efficacy of phentermine/topiramate ER has been demonstrated in two phase 3 clinical trials and one expansion trial: CONQUER, EQUIP, and SEQUEL (an extension of the CONQUER trial).[91,92] Phentermine/topiramate ER 7.5/46 mg was shown to produce average weight loss of 7.8% of initial body weight after 1 year and 9.3% after 2 years.[91,93] Phentermine/topiramate ER 15/92 mg was shown to produce average weight loss of 9.8% of initial body weight after 1 year and 10.5% after 2 years.[91,93] Use of phentermine/topiramate ER has also been associated with improvements in cardiometabolic parameters at the 15/92 mg dose.[91,92] Patients taking phentermine/topiramate ER at doses ≥7.5/46 mg also showed reduced progression to type 2 diabetes.[93]

The most common adverse effects associated with phentermine/topiramate ER include paresthesia, dizziness, dysgeusia, insomnia, constipation, and dry mouth.[87] Topiramate has been associated with birth defects, specifically oral clefts when taken during the first trimester, which led the FDA to approve phentermine/topiramate ER with a risk evaluation and mitigation strategy (REMS). This REMS is designed to inform practitioners and patients about the risk of birth defects, the importance of contraceptive use, and the need to immediately discontinue the drug if the patient becomes pregnant.[94] Phentermine/topiramate ER is contraindicated in pregnancy and in patients with glaucoma, hyperthyroidism, MAOI use within the past 14 days, and hypersensitivity to sympathomimetic amines.[87]

Lorcaserin (Belviq)

Lorcaserin is FDA-approved for long-term obesity management as an adjunct to lifestyle modification.[95] It is a selective serotonin 2C ($5\text{-}HT_{2C}$) receptor agonist. It is thought that lorcaserin promotes feelings of satiety by activating $5\text{-}HT_{2C}$ receptors in the hypothalamus.[96,97] It is available as 10 mg tablets and is dosed at 10 mg twice daily. If the patient has not experienced ≥5% weight loss after 12 weeks of therapy at the maintenance dose, the drug should be discontinued.[95]

The efficacy of lorcaserin has been demonstrated in three phase 3 clinical trials: BLOOM, BLOSSOM, and BLOOM-DM.[98–100] Lorcaserin was shown to produce average weight loss of 5.8% of initial body weight after 1 year and 7.2% after 2 years.[98,99] Use of lorcaserin has been associated with significant improvements in lipid profiles and glycemic parameters, including reductions in fasting plasma glucose and HbA1c.[98,100]

The most common adverse effects associated with lorcaserin include headache, dizziness, fatigue, nausea, dry mouth, and constipation in patients without diabetes. In patients with diabetes, the most common adverse effects are hypoglycemia, headache, back pain, cough, and fatigue.[95] In the past, nonselective serotonin agonists (fenfluramine and dexfenfluramine) were withdrawn from the market due to adverse cardiac events, most significantly valvulopathy.[98,101] Based on this, the FDA required data on the rates of valvulopathy with lorcaserin; a pooled analysis of the three previously mentioned phase 3 clinical trials found that the rates of echocardiographic valvulopathy were similar in both the lorcaserin and placebo groups.[102] Rarely reported side effects include priapism, hyperprolactinemia, cognitive impairment, hallucinations, and dissociation.[95]

Based on the serotonergic activity of lorcaserin, it is advised to avoid it with other serotonergic drugs such as SSRIs, SNRIs, MAOIs, and triptans.[95] Lorcaserin is an inhibitor of CYP 2D6; caution should be used when co-administering lorcaserin with drugs metabolized by this enzyme. The use of dextromethorphan is of particular concern because it is metabolized by CYP 2D6 and may have serotonergic effects. Lorcaserin is contraindicated in pregnancy.[97]

Naltrexone/Bupropion (Contrave)

Naltrexone/bupropion is a combination drug that has been approved by the FDA for long-term obesity management as an adjunct to lifestyle modification.[103] Bupropion, an antidepressant that inhibits dopamine and norepinephrine reuptake, has a known side effect of weight loss when used for the treatment of depression and smoking cessation.[104] This weight loss effect is thought to be the result of appetite suppression induced by the stimulation of pro-opiomelanocortin neurons in the hypothalamus.[105] Naltrexone, an opioid receptor antagonist, is believed to enhance this appetite suppression by blocking opioid receptors on these same pro-opiomelanocortin neurons.[104] Naltrexone/bupropion is available as combination 8/90 mg tablets. Patients initiate treatment at a dose of one tablet every morning. This dose is titrated up over the course of 4 weeks to a dose of two tablets twice daily, for a total daily dose of 32/360 mg.[21] If the patient has not experienced ≥5% weight loss after 12 weeks of therapy at the maintenance dose, the drug should be discontinued.[103]

The efficacy of naltrexone/bupropion has been demonstrated in four 1-year, placebo-controlled, phase 3 clinical trials: COR-I, COR-II, COR-BMOD, and COR-Diabetes.[103] Naltrexone/bupropion 32/360 mg was shown to produce average weight loss of 6.1% to 6.4% of initial body weight.[106,107] When coupled with intensive behavior modification, patients taking naltrexone/bupropion 32/360 mg experienced an average weight reduction of 9.3% of initial body weight.[104] Use of naltrexone/bupropion has also been associated with improvements in cardiometabolic parameters, including HbA1c reduction.[104,107,108]

The most common adverse effects associated with naltrexone/bupropion include nausea, constipation, headache, vomiting, dizziness, insomnia, dry mouth, and diarrhea.[103] Slight increases in blood pressure and heart rate have been seen in phase 3 clinical trials; thus, these parameters should be monitored during therapy.[103,109] Contrave has a black box warning for suicidal thoughts and behavior, although increased rates have not been seen in phase 3 clinical trials.[103,109] Bupropion is an inhibitor of CYP 2D6; caution should be used when co-administering naltrexone/bupropion with drugs metabolized by this enzyme.[103] Naltrexone/bupropion is contraindicated in pregnancy and in patients with uncontrolled hypertension; seizure disorders; anorexia nervosa or bulimia; sudden discontinuation of alcohol, benzodiazepines, barbiturates, or antiepileptic drugs; chronic use of opioids; use of MAOIs within the past 14 days; and in patients currently taking other bupropion-containing products.[103]

Liraglutide (Saxenda)

Liraglutide, marketed as Saxenda, is an injectable medication, FDA-approved for long-term obesity management as an adjunct to lifestyle modification.[110] When used for obesity, the dose is titrated to 3 mg daily. It is also marketed under the brand name Victoza at a dose of 1.8 mg daily for the treatment of type 2 diabetes.[111,112] Liraglutide is a glucagon-like peptide-1 (GLP-1) receptor agonist. Activation of this receptor acts via the central nervous system to promote feelings of satiety, thereby reducing food intake.[110,113] If the patient has not experienced ≥4% weight loss by 16 weeks after initiating therapy, the drug should be discontinued.[110]

The efficacy of liraglutide for weight loss has been demonstrated in three phase 3 clinical trials: SCALE Maintenance, SCALE Obesity and Pre-Diabetes, and SCALE Diabetes.[114–116] The results have not yet been published for the SCALE Diabetes trial. The results of the SCALE Maintenance trial indicate that by 12 weeks, liraglutide produces an average weight loss of 6.0% greater than placebo.[114] The results of the SCALE Obesity and Pre-Diabetes trial and the data released thus far for the SCALE Diabetes trial indicate that by the end of 56 weeks of treatment, liraglutide produces an average weight loss of 3.9% to 5.4% greater than placebo.[115,116] Use of liraglutide has also been associated with significant improvements in HbA1c, fasting plasma glucose, and fasting insulin.[110,115]

The most common adverse effects associated with liraglutide include nausea, hypoglycemia, diarrhea, constipation, vomiting, headache, decreased appetite, dyspepsia, fatigue, dizziness, abdominal pain, and increased lipase. In order to reduce the incidence of gastrointestinal side effects, liraglutide is initiated at a dose of 0.6 mg daily and titrated up to the effective dose of 3 mg daily over a 5-week-period.[110] Liraglutide has been associated with an increased risk of medullary thyroid carcinoma and acute pancreatitis. As a result, liraglutide is part of a REMS program to ensure practitioners are informed of these risks.[117] Liraglutide is contraindicated in pregnancy and in patients with hypersensitivity to liraglutide or any of its product components, a personal or family history of medullary thyroid carcinoma, or a personal or family history of multiple endocrine neoplasia syndrome type 2.[110]

Investigational Agents

Several recent investigational agents have shown promise in weight loss pharmacotherapy. In a 24-week phase IIb clinical trial, bupropion/zonisamide ER was shown to produce weight loss of 9.9% of initial body weight, as compared to 1.7% weight loss with placebo.[118] Much like naltrexone/bupropion, this combination drug works through a dual mechanism: Bupropion stimulates pro-opiomelanocortin neurons in the hypothalamus, and zonisamide acts synergistically by suppressing an appetite-stimulating neural pathway.[118] The most common adverse events were headache, insomnia, and nausea.[118]

Cetilistat is a lipase enzyme inhibitor, which acts similarly to orlistat, with a more tolerable side effect profile.[119,120] In a 12-week phase II clinical trial, cetilistat produced a mean weight loss of 4.32 kg when taken at a dose of 120 mg 3 times daily by obese patients with diabetes.[120] The most common adverse events were mild-to-moderate GI effects.[54,120]

Tesofensine, an inhibitor of noradrenalin, dopamine, and serotonin reuptake, was initially developed to treat neurodegenerative disease and found to produce weight loss in obese patients with Parkinson's or Alzheimer's disease.[121,122] Early results evaluating this agent for weight loss in combination with caloric restriction have shown dose-dependent reductions in weight up to 10.6% of baseline body weight after 24 weeks of therapy. Adverse reactions associated with tesofensine included nausea, constipation, diarrhea, insomnia, and dry mouth.[125]

Tauroursodeoxycholic acid has also been proposed as a weight loss agent. It is thought to induce weight loss by increasing sensitivity to leptin, a hormone that acts to suppress appetite.[57,123] However, clinical data are lacking at this time.

The most appropriate pharmacotherapeutic option for weight loss depends on patient-specific parameters including other disease states, concomitant medication use, adverse effects, patient preference, and cost. S.B. should avoid agents that will exacerbate her hypertension; therefore, S.B. should not be prescribed phentermine/topiramate and naltrexone/bupropion. Also, S.B. is currently taking bupropion which would duplicate with naltrexone/bupropion and may cause serotonin syndrome with lorcaserin. Orlistat and liraglutide are the only pharmacotherapeutic options for S.B. that can be safely administered with her hypertension and concomitant medication (bupropion). S.B. should chose the most appropriate agent based on her personal preference including her lifestyle (many gastrointestinal side effects and restricted fat intake and multiple daily doses with orlistat) or the subcutaneous route of administration with the liraglutide.

CASE 36-1, QUESTION 8: S.B. began therapy with orlistat 120 mg and lost an additional 8 kg in 6 months. After 6 months, S.B.'s weight loss began to taper and she regained 2 kg such that 1 year later her total net loss is 6 kg. S.B.'s current weight is 78 kg and her BMI is down to 27.6 kg/m^2 but she is disappointed that she has regained weight and inquires about dietary supplements for weight loss. How would you advise SB with regard to dietary supplements? (Table 36-5)

Table 36-5
Dietary Supplements for weight loss

Supplement	Proposed Mechanism	Clinical Data	Adverse Effects and Safety Concerns
Chitosan	A cellulose-type polysaccharide, reported to bind dietary fat and prevent absorption	Meta-analysis (14 trials) demonstrated average placebo-subtracted weight loss of 1.7 kg; average weight loss 0.8 kg in trials lasting longer than 4 weeks	GI effects common (constipation, diarrhea, flatulence, bloating, nausea, heartburn) Avoid in patients with a shellfish allergy
Caffeine	Increased thermogenesis by inhibiting the breakdown of cAMP	Several clinical trials demonstrate short-term weight loss when used in combination with ephedra (no longer available)	Common adverse effects: insomnia, irritability, tachycardia, anxiety
Green tea	Polyphenols and caffeine act synergistically to decrease fat absorption, reduce lipogenesis, and cause thermogenesis	Several clinical trials demonstrate potential weight loss of up to 2 kg	See caffeine Reports of hepatotoxicity
Guarana (Brazilian cocoa, *Paullinia cupana*)	See caffeine (seed contains 2.5%–7% caffeine)	See caffeine	See caffeine
Yerba mata (Yerba mate, *ilex paraguariensis*)	See caffeine	See caffeine	See caffeine Hot drinks may increase risk of esophageal cancer
Citrus aurantium (bitter orange, Seville orange, sour orange)	Contains synephrine (structurally similar to epinephrine)	No evidence of efficacy when used alone; limited data suggest minimal weight loss when used in combination with caffeine and Saint-John's-wort (less than 1 kg weight loss)	Cardiovascular effects (increase heart rate, blood pressure) Reports of angina, increased QT-interval, seizures, and ischemic colitis Potential drug interactions because of inhibition of intestinal CYP 3A4
Hydroxycitric acid (garcinia, *Garcinia cambogia*)	Theorized to inhibit production of lipids	No evidence of weight loss	Reports of hepatotoxicity, rhabdomyolysis (avoid with statins) May inhibit platelet aggregation
Glucomannan (Konjac)	Fibrous polysaccharide may work similar to fiber (promote/prolong satiety)	Limited data suggest minimal weight loss (1–2 kg)	GI adverse effects (nausea, bloating, flatulence)
Hoodia	Unknown, reported to be an appetite suppressant	No clinical trials to support use	Unknown

cAMP, cyclic adenosine monophosphate; GI, gastrointestinal.
Reprinted with permission from Dunican KC, Jarvis C. Overweight and Obesity. In: Murphy JE, Lee MW, eds. *Pharmacotherapy Self-Assessment Program*. 2014 Book 2 (Chronic Illnesses). Lenexa, KS: American College of Clinical Pharmacy, 2014;59:69.

Numerous dietary supplements are marketed for weight loss. Reliable evidence of efficacy for these agents is limited and safety data are lacking. Clinical data do not support the use of these agents and S.B. should be advised not to use dietary supplement for weight loss.

CASE 36-1, QUESTION 9: S.B.'s health insurance changed and she was no longer able to continue orlistat and she slowly regained the lost weight. Two years after discontinuing orlistat, SB has regained 7 kg. Her current weight is 85 kg and her BMI is 30.1 kg/m². She is frustrated that she has regained weight despite compliance with comprehensive lifestyle interventions. She asks whether her results are usual and inquires about additional options for weight loss.

S.B.'s regain after discontinuing orlistat is typical. Trials with a crossover design have shown that the weight loss achieved with anti-obesity agents is unlikely to be sustained after discontinuation.[6] Weight regain is to be expected after discontinuing anti-obesity agents because the underlying pathology of obesity is not changed.

Medical Devices for Obesity Treatment

A device called the vBloc Maestro Rechargeable System has been recently approved by the FDA as a treatment option for patients with extreme obesity (BMI ≥40 or ≥35 kg/m² with comorbid conditions) who have failed at least one supervised weight management program within the past 5 years.[124] The device is surgically implanted into the abdomen where it emits intermittent electrical pulses to block signaling by the vagus nerve.[124,125] In a recent randomized, double-blind, sham-controlled clinical trial, the vBloc system produced weight loss of 9.2% of initial body weight, compared to weight loss of 6.0% of initial body weight with the sham technology.[126] The most common adverse events were heartburn, dyspepsia, and abdominal pain.[126]

S.B.'s current BMI is 30.1 kg/m² which is below the threshold for use of vBloc; therefore, she is not a candidate for a medical device at this time. In order to sustain weight loss, long-term treatment must continue.

CASE 36-1, QUESTION 10: S.B. returns to her physician 3 years later. She has gained an additional 16 kg and her BMI is now 35.4 kg/m². She reports inability to maintain her weight with diet and exercise therapy after completion of the behavioral modification program in which she was participating. Laboratory tests provide the following results:

Blood pressure, 154/92 mm Hg
Fasting blood glucose, 162 mg/dL
TG, 354 mg/dL
Total cholesterol, 227 mg/dL
HDL, 35 mg/dL
LDL, 182 mg/dL

S.B. requests a referral to a bariatric clinic for evaluation for surgical intervention for weight loss. Is S.B. a candidate for bariatric surgery? How could a bariatric surgical procedure affect medication administration in S.B. postoperatively?

Surgery

Surgery may be an option for individuals with extreme obesity (BMI ≥40 or ≥35 kg/m² with comorbid conditions) who have not responded to lifestyle changes with or without adjunctive pharmacotherapy.[7,127] For severely obese patients (>100% more than normal weight), the most effective treatment is a surgical procedure to reduce the size of the stomach. Bariatric surgical procedures either reduce the absorptive surface of the GI tract resulting in malabsorption, or reduce the stomach volume so that the person feels full after a smaller meal. Procedures include gastric banding, vertical banded gastroplasty, Roux-en-Y gastric bypass, and biliopancreatic diversion; all have demonstrated efficacy, although the degree of weight loss and complications may differ.[128] Gastric bypass has been shown to produce a greater weight loss compared with gastroplasty procedures.[129] In addition, laparoscopic (vs. open surgical) approaches may be preferred for reducing postoperative complications and hospital stay.[128]

The mortality rate from bariatric surgery is estimated to be 0.3% to 1.9% and literature has shown that centers that perform surgeries at high volume have better outcomes.[67] Some of the complications of bariatric surgery include nausea, stomach ulceration, stenosis, anemia, and cholelithiasis. Postsurgical precautions include careful evaluation of meal sizes and timing along with meal content, especially immediately after surgery. Patients should be aware that they will not be able to resume their normal eating habits, and they should be properly educated on lifestyle modifications for maintenance of weight loss. In addition, medications and adequate intake of necessary nutrients are important considerations after surgery. Medications such as nonsteroidal anti-inflammatory drugs, salicylates, and bisphosphonates may cause ulcerations, and medications that are delayed release or extended release may not be absorbed owing to changes in gastric size.[130] Medications may need to be administered using liquid formulation and other dosage routes. Transdermal formulations need to be carefully dosed to account for changes in body surface area postsurgically.[130]

Although S.B. is a candidate for bariatric surgery based on her BMI of 35.4 kg/m² and her comorbid conditions (hypertension and sleep apnea), she may also consider alternative pharmacotherapeutic options. S.B.'s fasting blood glucose indicates that she may have type 2 diabetes. Liraglutide is an option that will lower her blood glucose as well as result in clinically significant weight reduction.

KEY REFERENCES AND WEBSITES

A full list of references for this chapter can be found at **http://thepoint.lww.com/AT11e**. Below are the key references and websites for this chapter, with the corresponding reference number in this chapter found in parentheses after the reference.

Key References

Apovian CM et al. Pharmacological management of obesity: an endocrine society clinical practice guideline. *J Clin Endocrinol Metab.* 2015;100(2):342–362. (6)

Domecq JP et al. Drugs commonly associated with weight change: a systematic review and meta-analysis. *J Clin Endocrinol Metab.* 2015;100(2):363–370. (57)

Garvey WT et al. Two-year sustained weight loss and metabolic benefits with controlled-release phentermine/topiramate in obese and overweight adults (SEQUEL): a randomized, placebo-controlled, phase 3 extension study. *Am J Clin Nutr.* 2012;95(2):297–308. (93)

Jensen MD et al. 2013 AHA/ACC/TOS guideline for the management of overweight and obesity in adults: a report of the American college of cardiology/American heart association task force on practice guidelines and the obesity society. *J Am Coll Cardiol.* 2014;63(25_PA):2985–3023. (7)

Pi-Sunyer X et al. A randomized, controlled trial of 3.0 mg of liraglutide in weight management. *N Engl J Med.* 2015;373(1):11–22. (115)

Rucker D et al. Long term pharmacotherapy for obesity and overweight: updated meta-analysis. *BMJ.* 2007;335(7631):1194–1199. (77)

Smith SR et al. Multicenter, placebo-controlled trial of lorcaserin for weight management. *N Engl J Med*. 2010;363(3):245–256. (98)

Snow V et al. Pharmacologic and surgical management of obesity in primary care: a clinical practice guideline from the American College of Physicians. *Ann Intern Med*. 2005;142(7):525–531. (66)

Torgerson JS et al. XENical in the prevention of diabetes in obese subjects (XENDOS) study: A randomized study of orlistat as an adjunct to lifestyle changes for the prevention of type 2 diabetes in obese patients. *Diabetes Care*. 2004;27(1):155–161. (78)

Yanovski SZ, Yanovski JA. Long-term drug treatment for obesity: a systematic and clinical review. *JAMA*. 2014;311(1):74–86. (67)

Key Websites

Obesity Action Coalition. http://www.obesityaction.org/.

CDC. http://www.cdc.gov/obesity/.

NIH. http://www.nhlbi.nih.gov/health/educational/wecan/healthy-weight-basics/obesity.htm.

37 Adult Enteral Nutrition

Carol J. Rollins and Jennifer H. Baggs

CORE PRINCIPLES

	Core Principle	Chapter Cases
1	Patients should be assessed for the appropriate timing and route for nutrition support.	**Case 37-1 (Questions 1, 2)**
2	The type of tube placement and site of formula delivery are determined by several factors.	**Case 37-2 (Question 1)**
3	Formula selection is based on nutrient requirements, fluid restrictions, and the extent of impaired digestion and absorption.	**Case 37-2 (Questions 2–5)**
4	The administration regimen for feeding is influenced by the feeding route, formula selected, and duration of feeding.	**Case 37-2 (Questions 6–8)**
5	Although the preferred route for nutrition intervention in critical illness is enteral, the ideal formula composition remains unresolved.	**Case 37-3 (Questions 1–4)**
6	Macronutrient content should be considered when selecting an enteral formula for patients with diabetes.	**Case 37-4 (Question 1)**
7	Appropriate monitoring is essential to recognize and prevent complications associated with enteral nutrition.	**Case 37-4 (Question 2)**
8	Medication administration through a feeding tube requires selection of appropriate dosage forms and proper preparation.	**Case 37-4 (Question 3)**
9	Feeding tube occlusion is a common problem influenced by medication-related and nonmedication-related factors.	**Case 37-4 (Question 4)**
10	Patients must meet strict criteria for Medicare coverage of home enteral nutrition.	**Case 37-5 (Question 1)**
11	Diarrhea in patients receiving enteral nutrition is multifactorial, including both tube-feeding-related and nontube-feeding-related causes.	**Case 37-6 (Question 1)**

Enteral nutrition refers to nutrition provided via the gastrointestinal (GI) tract. However, because the term is commonly used, enteral nutrition (EN) is synonymous with delivery of nutrients into the GI tract by tube (e.g., nasogastric or jejunostomy feeding). Tube feeding allows continued use of the GI tract when one or more steps in the normal process of obtaining nutrients from oral intake are disrupted. Table 37-1 lists functional anatomic units of the GI tract along with major steps occurring in preparing nutrients for absorption and examples of conditions potentially impairing each region. Chewing or swallowing may be completely disrupted, but some digestive and absorptive function must remain for tube feeding to be a viable option.

PATIENT SELECTION AND ROUTE OF FEEDING

CASE 37-1

QUESTION 1: G.W., a 59-year-old woman, 5 feet 2 inches tall, 88 kg, was brought to the emergency department (ED) last night complaining of severe left-sided upper abdominal pain. Tests performed in the ED were consistent with acute pancreatitis. G.W. was admitted to the hospital and has "nothing by mouth" (NPO)

Table 37-1
Functional Units of the Gastrointestinal Tract

Functional Unit	Major Steps	Conditions/Diseases Disrupting Function
Mouth and oropharynx	Chew and lubricate food; swallow; taste	Amyotrophic lateral sclerosis, muscular dystrophy, severe RA, CVA, end-stage Parkinson disease, paralysis, coma. Anorexia due to other disease: cardiac or cancer cachexia, renal failure and uremia, liver failure, neurologic disease.
Esophagus	Transport food to the stomach	Esophageal ulcer, cancer, obstruction, or fistula; esophagectomy; CVA.
Stomach	Hold food for mixing and grinding; add acid and enzymes; release chyme to small bowel; osmoregulation	Severe gastritis or ulceration, gastroparesis, gastric outlet obstruction, gastric cancer, severe gastroesophageal reflux.
Duodenum	Osmoregulation; neutralize stomach acid	Severe duodenal ulcer or fistula; cancer: gastric or pancreatic; surgical resection or bypass of the duodenum: Whipple-type procedures.
Small bowel: jejunum and ileum	Digestion; absorption	Enterocutaneous fistula, severe enteric infection, malnutrition, malabsorption, Crohn disease, celiac disease, ileus and dysmotility syndrome.
Pancreas	Secretion of digestive enzymes	Pancreatitis, pancreatic cancer, pancreatic injury, pancreatic fistula.
Colon	Absorb fluid; ferment soluble fiber and unabsorbed carbohydrate; absorb water	Ulcerative colitis, Crohn disease, colon cancer, colocutaneous fistula, colovaginal fistula, diverticulitis, colitis of any etiology, colon surgery.

CVA, cerebrovascular accident; RA, rheumatoid arthritis.

orders in her chart. The gastroenterology service has seen her and scheduled an endoscopic retrograde cholangiopancreatography (ERCP) for tomorrow. A nutrition support consult was ordered. G.W. is currently receiving intravenous (IV) 5% dextrose/0.9% sodium chloride with KCl 20 mEq/L at 125 mL/hour. She is also receiving hydromorphone via a patient-controlled analgesia (PCA) pump.

G.W. has been experiencing crampy upper right quadrant pain on and off for about 3 weeks and saw her primary care physician a week ago. She is allergic (rash) to sulfa. She was told that her symptoms are consistent with gallbladder inflammation; surgery will be necessary if her symptoms continue or the pain worsens. In addition, her doctor said blood pressure and glucose control "needed improvement" and mentioned it might be because her weight was up 8 pounds. She quit smoking 6 months ago; she frequently drinks one glass of wine with dinner.

Laboratory values this morning are as follows:
Sodium, 139 mEq/L
Potassium, 3.8 mEq/L
Blood urea nitrogen (BUN), 10 mg/dL
Serum creatinine (SCr), 0.8 mg/dL
Glucose, 175 mg/dL
Albumin, 3.4 g/dL
Amylase, 705 units/L (down from 1,200 units/L in the ED)
Lipase, 698 units/L (down from 1,198 in the ED)
Triglycerides, 185 mg/dL
White blood cells (WBC), 12.7 × $10^3/\mu L$
Hemoglobin (Hgb), 12.4 g/dL
Hematocrit (Hct), 37.3%
C-reactive protein (CRP), 2.2 mg/dL

Does G.W. require nutritional intervention at this time? When should nutrition intervention be considered for G.W.?

Patients generally are considered at risk for nutrient depletion and associated increased morbidity and mortality when intake is less than 50% to 75% of requirements for 5 to 7 days acutely or when weight loss exceeds 5% or more in 1 month, 7.5% or more in 3 months, or 10% or more of pre-illness weight within a 6-month period.[1,2] For adequately nourished patients, specialized nutrition support is generally not warranted when support will be needed for fewer than 7 to 10 days.[3] Undernourished patients require nutritional intervention sooner. See Chapter 35, Basics of Nutrition and Patient Assessment, for further information on malnutrition. G.W. was adequately nourished before admission based on her weight for height and serum albumin. She has weight gain per the clinic visit, although edema should be ruled out as a cause, and has been NPO for less than 24 hours. Nutrition support is not warranted at this time. However, once the ERCP has been completed, the need for nutrition intervention should be reassessed. If G.W. must remain NPO for a week or more, nutritional intervention would be warranted. Obesity does not preclude the need for nutritional intervention.

CASE 37-1, QUESTION 2: What route of nutrition intervention would be most appropriate for G.W. if she cannot restart her diet in a timely manner?

Routes of nutrition intervention may include modified oral diet, including oral supplements or altered consistency diets (e.g., thickened liquids, pureed foods), EN by tube, or parenteral nutrition (PN). Tube feeding is considered the route of choice in patients with a functional GI tract in whom oral nutrient intake is contraindicated or is insufficient to meet estimated needs.[3] Other than potential "gallstone" pancreatitis, G.W. is expected to have a functional GI tract. The ERCP and pain symptoms will help determine whether G.W. will remain NPO or have a diet started. It appears her pancreatitis is improving based on decreasing amylase and lipase values. For patients with severe acute pancreatitis, Society of Critical Care Medicine (SCCM) and American Society for Parenteral and Enteral Nutrition (ASPEN) Critical Care (SACC) guidelines recommend initiation of EN as soon as volume resuscitation is complete.[4] For patients such as G.W. with mild-to-moderate acute pancreatitis, symptoms typically resolve before nutrition intervention is necessary. When symptoms are prolonged and nutrition support is required, EN is the preferred route of nutrition support because EN may reduce the inflammatory response and decrease complications.[4–6]

EN may be appropriate for patients with the disorders listed in Table 37-1, depending on the extent to which normal intake, transport, digestion, and absorption of nutrients are impaired. Clinical circumstances, not specific diagnoses, should be the determining factor for initiating tube feeding. EN should be used with caution in patients with severe necrotizing or hemorrhagic pancreatitis, distal high-output enterocutaneous fistulae, hypotension with significant inotropic support, GI ischemia, and partial bowel obstruction.[3,4] Contraindications to EN generally include diffuse peritonitis, complete bowel obstruction, severe paralytic ileus, intractable vomiting or diarrhea, severe malabsorption, severe GI bleed, inability to access the GI tract, and when aggressive intervention is not warranted or desired. Frequent reassessment is recommended because patients may become candidates for EN as the condition improves or resolves.

FEEDING TUBE PLACEMENT AND SITE OF FORMULA DELIVERY

CASE 37-2

QUESTION 1: D.S., an 80-year-old man, was hospitalized 7 days ago after collapsing while grocery shopping. He was diagnosed with ischemic stroke, and his condition has changed little since admission. D.S. is estimated to be 5 feet 10 inches tall; his weight is 62 kg; clinic notes from 6 months ago show his weight at 69.3 kg. He appears thin with mild wasting of arm and leg muscles. His maintenance IV drip is 5% dextrose/0.45% sodium chloride with KCl 10 mEq/L at 80 mL/hour. Laboratory evaluation today shows the following:

Sodium, 141 mEq/L
Potassium, 3.7 mEq/L
Chloride, 106 mEq/L
Glucose, 88 mg/dL
SCr, 0.9 mg/dL
Serum albumin, 3.2 g/dL

D.S. failed his swallow study today and will remain NPO for 7 weeks prior to a repeat swallow study, which he must pass before an oral diet is initiated. Nutrition support via tube feeding is ordered.

What is the most appropriate type of feeding tube placement and site for formula delivery?

The type of tube placement and site of formula delivery for EN are determined by the anticipated duration of tube feeding, disrupted region or process in the GI tract, and the risk of aspiration. Figure 37-1 illustrates the two basic types of tube placement—nasal versus ostomy—and the sites available for formula delivery (i.e., gastric, duodenal, or jejunal). The name of the feeding route usually includes both the type of tube placement and the site of formula delivery. For example, nasogastric (NG) indicates nasal placement with gastric delivery of formula, whereas gastrostomy indicates ostomy placement with gastric delivery of formula.

Nasal tube placement is preferred for short-term use in patients expected to resume oral feeding and without obstruction of nasal, pharyngeal, or esophageal passages. The tube is secured to the nose or cheek after placement to prevent the tube from being displaced.

Clinically evident injury from nasal intubation is very low, but patients may suffer mucosal trauma in the nasopharynx.[7–9] Pharyngitis, sinusitis, otitis media, and incompetence of the lower esophageal sphincter are associated with nasal tubes, especially large-bore tubes. The incidence of inadvertent pulmonary placement of small-bore feeding tubes is 4% or less.[7] Radiographic confirmation of tube placement is mandatory to rule out pleural perforation and pulmonary intubation in unconscious patients and remains the standard to ensure correct tube placement in all patients. Tube displacement is a potential complication occurring in 25% to 41% of cases.[7]

Feeding ostomies (tube enterostomies) generally are reserved for long-term EN, interpreted as anywhere from 4 weeks to 6 months, depending on clinical circumstances and the type of tube enterostomy placed. Access for enterostomies can be achieved through open surgery, laparoscopy, or via percutaneous access. Percutaneous access is usually performed under local anesthesia or conscious sedation by endoscope (percutaneous endoscopic gastrostomy [PEG] or jejunostomy [PEJ]) or by radiography (percutaneous radiologic gastrostomy [PRG] or jejunostomy), including fluoroscopy, ultrasound, or computed tomography.[7,10,11] The major advantage of radiologic compared with endoscopic placement is reduced contamination of the puncture site by oral pharyngeal microorganisms, which are implicated in the 5.4% to 30% incidence of site infections.[9] Most patients requiring long-term EN receive either a PEG or a PRG. Less than 5% receive a combined gastric and jejunal access (PEGJ or G-J) tube.[12]

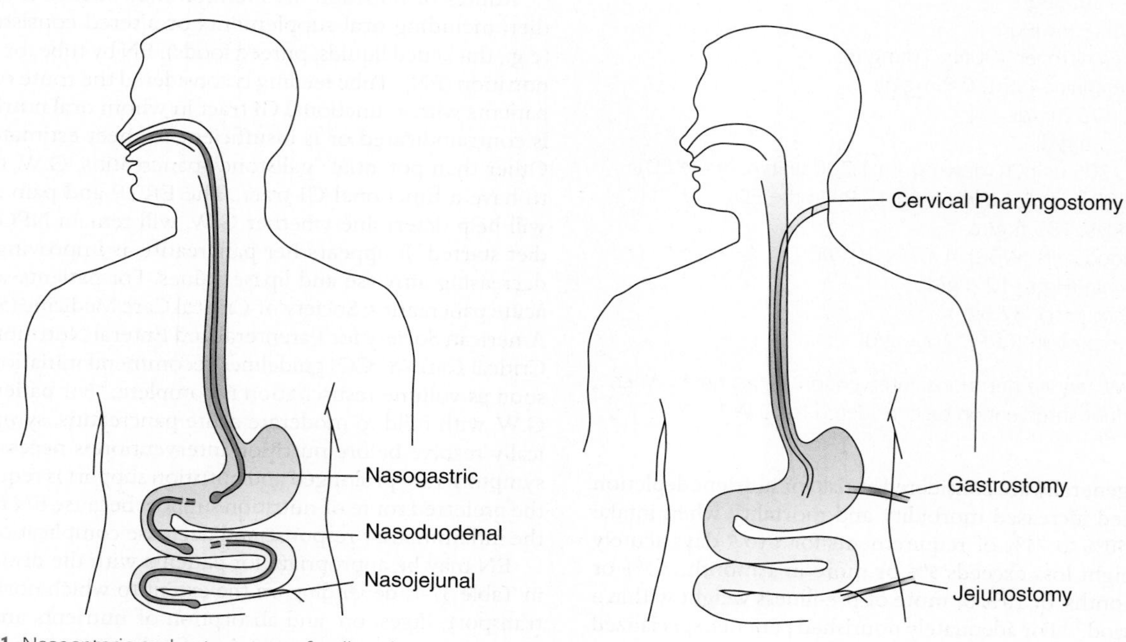

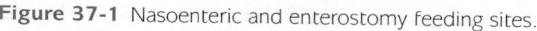

Figure 37-1 Nasoenteric and enterostomy feeding sites.

Endoscopic placement is contraindicated when obstruction prevents passage of the endoscope, but radiographic placement may be possible in such cases. Relative contraindications to percutaneous feeding tube placement include inability to see the endoscopic light through the abdominal wall (e.g., morbid obesity, massive ascites), peritoneal dialysis, coagulopathy, gastric varices, portal hypertension, hepatomegaly, and neoplastic or infiltrative disease of the gastric or jejunal wall.[7–11,13] Prior total or subtotal gastrectomy, including Roux-en-Y gastric bypass and gastric sleeve for obesity reduction, prevents percutaneous gastrostomy placement, but percutaneous jejunostomy may be possible. Major advantages of percutaneous access are shorter procedure time and lower cost; morbidity and mortality appear to be similar to surgical feeding tube access.[13] Major complications, such as aspiration, peritonitis, hemorrhage, gastrocutaneous fistula formation, necrotizing fasciitis, gastric perforation, and migration of the tube through the gastric wall, are generally low but have been reported in up to 2.5% of patients.[7]

Formula delivery into the stomach is preferred because it is the most physiologically normal feeding site. Stimulation of normal digestive processes and hormonal responses associated with eating occur. The stomach serves as a reservoir, typically allowing tolerance of bolus, and intermittent or continuous feeding. Gastric feeding requires adequate gastric motility to prevent accumulation of formula in the stomach. Patients with gastric outlet obstruction, gastroparesis, gastric distension, or gastroesophageal reflux are poor candidates for gastric feeding.

Postpyloric feeding into the duodenum or jejunum may be appropriate when gastric dysfunction or disease is present, for early postoperative feeding when gastric emptying may be impaired, when pancreatic stimulation is to be minimized, or when risk of aspiration is high. Critically ill patients are at risk for aspiration and ventilator-associated pneumonia, with a 25% to 40% incidence of aspiration in patients with long-term nasoenteric feeding.[14] Evidence of reduced aspiration and improved outcomes with postpyloric feeding remains controversial.[4] A study in 428 patients using pepsin as a marker of aspiration showed steady decline in the pepsin positive samples moving from stomach (34.4%) to proximal, mid-, and distal duodenum (20.8%, 17%, and 7.6%, respectively).[15] Conversely, a meta-analysis of 17 randomized, controlled trials failed to find a benefit of postpyloric feeding on aspiration risk and ventilator-associated pneumonia.[16] Poor differentiation between aspiration of oral secretions and aspiration from the GI tract occurs in many studies; however, this is avoided by using pepsin as a marker. Tube placement beyond the ligament of Treitz (into the jejunum) may be best for patients at risk of tube migration and aspiration; however, studies are not conclusive, and either gastric or small bowel feeding is considered acceptable in the intensive care unit (ICU) setting.

D.S. will require EN for at least 7 weeks and may require longer-term EN depending on repeat swallow study results. A feeding ostomy is appropriate for him. Because there does not appear to be a contraindication to feeding into the stomach, a gastrostomy is appropriate. He will likely have a PEG or PRG placed to avoid the need for surgery.

FORMULA SELECTION

CASE 37-2, QUESTION 2: What factors should be considered in selecting an enteral formula for D.S.?

Enteral formula selection is based on nutrient requirements, fluid restrictions, and the extent of impaired digestion and absorption. Many enteral formulas are available, but because of similarities between products, institutional formularies are generally limited but still provide an adequate selection to meet a variety of patient needs. Categorizing formulas as listed in Table 37-2 simplifies the formula selection process. There are three major categories of enteral formulas: (a) polymeric formulas, (b) oligomeric formulas, and (c) specialized formulas.

Polymeric Formulas

Polymeric formulas are designed for patients with full digestive capability and are used most often. Osmolality is decreased and palatability increased in these formulas by the use of relatively intact nutrients, including whole (i.e., intact) proteins. Administration of approximately 1.5 to 2 L of most polymeric formulas provides 100% of dietary reference intakes (DRI) for vitamins and minerals; thus, these formulas sometimes are called "complete" formulas.[17] As indicated in Table 37-2, the relative cost for polymeric formulas tends to be less than that of oligomeric or specialized formulas, although prices can vary considerably based on specific nutrient content (e.g., omega-3 fatty acids [ω-3FAs], antioxidants).

Oligomeric Formulas

Oligomeric formulas, also called predigested, monomeric, or chemically defined formulas, are designed for patients with reduced digestive function. Pancreatic enzyme activity is required for digestion of oligosaccharides (carbohydrates) and fats. Brush-border disaccharidase activity also is required. Minimal digestion is required, however, for the hydrolyzed protein and medium-chain triglyceride (MCT) components. These formulas can be used for patients with pancreatic insufficiency, reduced mucosal absorption, or reduced hydrolytic capability. Although the Canadian Clinical Practice (CCP) guidelines noted patients with GI complications, such as short bowel syndrome and pancreatitis, may benefit from oligomeric formulas, insufficient data were available to make recommendations regarding use of such formulas.[18–20] Pancreatic enzyme supplementation combined with polymeric formulas may be tried before oligomeric formulas for some patients with pancreatic insufficiency (e.g., cystic fibrosis, chronic pancreatitis).

Two subgroups of oligomeric formulas can be differentiated based on the protein source. True "elemental" formulas contain free amino acids, whereas "peptide-based" formulas contain oligopeptides plus dipeptides, tripeptides, and free amino acids from hydrolysis of protein. Amino acids require no digestion, but the sodium-dependent active transport mechanism is somewhat slow and inefficient with only about one-third of dietary protein absorbed as free amino acids; the remaining two-thirds are absorbed as dipeptides and tripeptides.[21,22] Specific carriers for dipeptide and tripeptide absorption, located in small bowel mucosa, do not compete with the free amino acid transport system. Peptides longer than three amino acids require further hydrolysis within the lumen of the small bowel before they are absorbed. Most peptide-based formulas contain a significant portion of peptides requiring hydrolysis before absorption. No well-designed, randomized, controlled trials have clearly delineated clinical differences in elemental (free amino acid) versus peptide-based formulas. Elemental formulas generally have the lowest-fat content (10% or less of calories from fat). Peptide formulas typically contain one-fourth to one-third of calories from fat, but provide 20% to 70% of the fat as MCT to minimize the risk of malabsorption.

Oligomeric formulas are typically hypertonic owing to their partially digested nature; peptide-containing formulas are

Table 37-2
Generic Groups and Subgroups of Enteral Formulas with Relative Costs

Type of Formula	Relative Cost[a,b]	Examples
Polymeric Formulas[c]		
Standard Caloric Density, Standard (or High Nitrogen) Content with Varied Fiber Content		
Fiber free for oral supplement or tube feeding	$	Ensure; Nutren 1.0
Low fiber (from 1– g/1,000 kcal)	$	Nutren Probalance[d]
Moderate fiber (>9–<14 g/1,000 kcal)	$	Ensure with fiber; Fibersource HN[d]
High fiber (≥14 g/1,000 kcal)	$	Glucerna; Jevity 1.2 Cal[d]; Nutren 1.0 with fiber
Standard-Nitrogen Content, Fiber-Free (or Low Fiber) with Varied Caloric Density		
Standard caloric density (1–1.2 kcal/mL)	$	Ensure; Nutren 1.0
Moderate density (1.5 kcal/mL)	$	Boost Plus; Ensure Plus; Isosource 1.5 Cal[e]; Nutren 1.5
Calorically dense (1.8–2 kcal/mL)	$	Nutren 2.0
Standard Caloric Density, Fiber-Free with Varied Nitrogen (Protein) Content		
Low nitrogen (6%–10% of kcal as protein)	$	Resource Breeze
Standard nitrogen (11%–16% of kcal as protein)	$	Ensure; Nutren 1.0
High nitrogen (17%–20% of kcal as protein)	$	Isosource HN; Osmolite 1.2 Cal
Very high nitrogen (>20% of kcal as protein)	$$	Boost High Protein; Promote; Replete
Oligomeric Formulas		
Elemental (free amino acids)[f]	&&	f.a.a.; Tolerex; Vivonex T.E.N.
Peptide Based		
Standard protein	&	Peptamen; Peptamen with Prebio
High protein	&	Peptamen 1.5
Very high protein (NPC:N <100:1; >20% calories as protein)	&&	Crucial; Peptamen AF
Specialized Formulas		
Renal Failure		
Essential amino acid enriched[f]	&&&&	Renalcal
Polymeric, low electrolyte (less than standard potassium, phosphorus, and magnesium)	$$$$	
■ Low nitrogen		Suplena
■ Standard nitrogen		Novasource Renal
■ High nitrogen (for dialysis)		Nepro
Hepatic failure (high BCAA, low AAA[f])	&&&&	Nutrihep
Stress or Critically Ill		
Branched-chain enriched	&&&	
High nitrogen plus conditionally essential nutrients	$$	
Immune modulating	&&	Oxepa
Pulmonary disease (standard; not IMP)	$$	Nutren Pulmonary; Pulmocare
Glucose control	$$$	Diabetisource AC; Glucerna; Nutren Glytrol

[a]Based on average cost per 1,000 calories for equivalent formulas on a University Health System contract from 2010 to 2013.
[b]Index product is a standard caloric density, standard-nitrogen content, fiber-free formula. Cost is indicated relative to an index product given a value of 1:
$ = same cost as index product, up to 1.5 times that cost per 1,000 calories.
$$ = cost is 1.6 to 2.5 times the cost of the index product per 1,000 calories.
$$$ = cost is 2.6 to 3.5 times the cost of the index product per 1,000 calories.
$$$$ = cost is 3.6 to 4.5 times the cost of the index product per 1,000 calories.
& = cost is 11 to 15 times the cost of the index product per 1,000 calories.
&& = cost is 16 to 20 times the cost of the index product per 1,000 calories.
&&& = cost is 20 to 24 times the cost of the index product per 1,000 calories.
&&&& = cost is 25 to 30 times the cost of the index product per 1,000 calories.
[c]All products listed in the table are lactose-free.
[d]High nitrogen.
[e]Low fiber.
[f]Special order, not on formulary used for price calculations.
AAAs, aromatic amino acids; BCAAs, branched-chain amino acids; IMP, immune-modulating pulmonary; NPC:N, nonprotein calorie to nitrogen ratio.

typically less hypertonic than free amino acid products. Osmotic diarrhea can occur because of the hyperosmolality; however, the CCP guidelines meta-analysis found no difference in diarrhea occurrence between patients receiving intact protein and those receiving peptide-rich formulas.[18] Taste and cost are disadvantages of oligomeric formulas. Flavoring packets are available and newer formulas may be better accepted, but patients commonly complain of a bitter taste when these formulas are taken orally. In general, patients do not tolerate adequate oral consumption of an oligomeric formula. As shown in Table 37-2, the cost of oligomeric formulas tends to be greater than 10 times the cost of polymeric formulas.

Specialized Formulas

Specialized formulas are designed for specific disease states or conditions; however, clinical benefits are often controversial. Formulas generally have a good theoretic basis for use, yet many lack conclusive clinical evidence of improved efficacy compared with standard formulas. Well-designed studies showing a difference in outcome between specialized and standard enteral formulas providing equal nitrogen and equal calories are limited for most types of specialized formulas. As shown in Table 37-2, there are several different types of specialized formulas; costs and evidence for use vary greatly among them.

D.S. requires EN because he cannot adequately protect his airway when swallowing. There is no evidence presented to suggest he has problems with digestion or absorption. One of the polymeric formulas on the hospital EN formulary should be selected for D.S. The choice of polymeric formula can be narrowed by several factors, including requirements for calories, protein, fluid and fiber, as well as potential nutrient intolerances.

CASE 37-2, QUESTION 3: What are D.S.'s requirements for calories, protein, and fluid? Does he have any special nutrient requirements?

D.S.'s nutrient requirements must be assessed before proceeding in the selection of enteral formula. Based on his weight–height ratio, 10% weight loss over 6 months, slightly elevated CRP, and mild muscle wasting D.S. has moderate malnutrition in the context of chronic illness. Low serum albumin is a risk factor for morbidity and mortality, but is not a reliable indicator of nutritional status.[2] Weight loss to 85% of ideal body weight ([IBW], 73 kg) most likely is due to chronic deficiency in total energy intake, but may also be associated with significant loss of lean mass, especially in older men.[23]

Because D.S. has an IBW less than the ideal for his height, his actual weight should be used to estimate energy and protein requirements. Use of IBW to estimate requirements for undernourished patients may result in fluid and electrolyte imbalance. Once the patient is stabilized on nutrition support, calories can be increased, if necessary, to achieve weight gain.

D.S.'s level of metabolic stress is relatively low. He has no surgical wounds, fractures or skeletal trauma, burns, or major infections, although CRP indicates mild inflammation. Caloric requirements are only slightly higher than basal needs. Although the term calorie is used interchangeably with kilocalorie (kcal) in nutrition literature, the large "Calorie" or kilocalorie technically is correct and energy requirements generally are listed as kcal/day or kcal/kg body weight when specific numbers are given for a patient. See Chapter 35, Basics of Nutrition and Patient Assessment, for methods of determining nutrient requirements. An estimation of 20 to 25 kcal/kg actual weight can be used based on D.S.'s low level of metabolic stress, but higher caloric intake (25–30 kcal/kg/day) may be needed for weight gain after he is stable.

Protein requirements for healthy elderly people are controversial but estimated to be 1 to 1.2 g/kg/day, which is higher than the DRI of 0.8 g/kg/day.[24] D.S.'s protein needs are estimated to 1 to 1.2 g/kg actual weight per day, minimum, based on inflammation and chronic malnutrition. Renal function appears adequate for D.S. to tolerate 1.2 g/kg/day without experiencing azotemia. SCr, however, may provide a poor estimate of renal function in underweight patients owing to less-than-normal muscle mass.

Daily fluid requirements for geriatric patients can be estimated at 30 mL/kg or 1 mL/kcal ingested, with a minimum of 1,500 mL daily, plus replacement of excess losses from hyperthermia, vomiting, or diarrhea.[24] Baseline requirements of 1,500 mL for the first 20 kg plus 20 mL per each additional kilogram of body weight also can be used to estimate fluid requirements. D.S. does not appear to have any excess fluid losses at this time; therefore, calculation of baseline fluid requirements should provide adequate fluids.

D.S.'s estimated daily requirements are approximately 1,240 to 1,550 total calories, 62 to 74 g protein, and about 1,860 mL of fluid. These are estimated requirements that should be adjusted based on frequent reassessment of D.S.'s response to therapy and changes in his clinical situation. Additional calories and protein may be needed for repletion of weight and protein status.

D.S.'s apparently suboptimal nutrition before hospitalization increases his risk for vitamin deficiencies (see Chapter 35, Basics of Nutrition and Patient Assessment). Medical, medication, and dietary histories should be evaluated to determine nutritional risks associated with specific conditions. D.S.'s age, along with his acute illness and chronic malnutrition, increases his risk of vitamin deficiencies, and he may have at least some subclinical deficiencies. He should receive 100% of the DRI, minimum, for vitamins and minerals daily.[17] If actual deficiencies are identified, D.S. will require higher, therapeutic doses for the specific vitamins that are deficient.

D.S. may be at risk of refeeding syndrome. His weight is low (85% of IBW), although his body mass index is acceptable at 19.5 kg/m^2. Chronic malnutrition can lead to intracellular depletion of potassium, phosphorus, and magnesium, whereas serum concentrations are maintained. When specialized nutrition support begins, refeeding syndrome may develop as these electrolytes move from the extracellular space into the cells, causing a decrease in serum concentrations during the first few days of feeding.[25] Failure to monitor the patient and replace electrolytes as necessary can result in serious electrolyte abnormalities. Knowing D.S.'s weight history, particularly recent weight loss, and his diet history could help assess his potential for clinically significant electrolyte and fluid abnormalities associated with refeeding syndrome.

CASE 37-2, QUESTION 4: Which category of polymeric formulas would be most appropriate for D.S. based on his estimated nutritional requirements?

Polymeric formulas can be divided into several categories based on nutrient sources, caloric density, and protein content. Each category should be evaluated because formula characteristics overlap between the categories.

NUTRIENT SOURCE

Polymeric formulas can be subdivided based on lactose content. Hospitalized patients are presumed to be lactose intolerant due to reduced disaccharidase production during fasting, malnutrition, and various GI tract diseases.[26,27] In addition, most ethnic groups, except northern Europeans, have reduced lactase production in adulthood, leading to lactose intolerance. Lactose ingestion can cause bloating, flatulence, abdominal cramps, and watery diarrhea in patients with permanent or transient lactose intolerance. Lactose-free formulas are the standard for tube-fed adults. Most enteral products are lactose-free, except the powdered products

Table 37-3
General Descriptions of Macronutrient Quantity in Enteral Formulas

	Low	Standard	Moderate	High	Very High
Caloric density (kcal/mL)	<1	1–1.2	1.5	1.8–2	>2
Free water (%)	65%–75%	80%–85%	75%–80%	>85%	
Nitrogen (protein) content: % kcal as protein	6%–10%	11%–16%		17%–20%	>20%
Nitrogen (protein) content: NPC:N	>200:1	200:1–130:1		125:1–100:1	<100:1
Fiber content (g/1,000 kcal)	1–9	None	>9–<14	≥14	

NPC:N, nonprotein calorie to nitrogen ratio.

reconstituted with milk and generally intended for oral consumption. Proteins, even those derived from milk, do not contribute to lactose content because lactose is a carbohydrate. The majority of enteral formulas are also gluten-free to avoid GI symptoms associated with celiac disease.

CALORIC DENSITY

Caloric density influences the volume of formula needed to meet nutrient requirements. Standard caloric density is 1 to 1.2 kcal/mL. Table 37-3 lists the general descriptions for caloric density and macronutrient quantities in enteral formulas. Increased caloric density increases formula osmolality. Gastric emptying can be reduced when osmolality exceeds 800 mOsm/kg and this may result in feeding intolerance.[28] GI intolerance (e.g., nausea, flatulence, abdominal discomfort) also can occur if the capacity of intestinal enzymes is overwhelmed by infusion of a calorically dense formula.

Caloric density reflects the free-water content of EN formulas. Risk of dehydration increases with increasing caloric density; however, standard caloric density formulas can result in fluid overload in patients with congestive heart failure, renal failure, or other fluid-sensitive conditions. Calculation of water provided by EN helps determine the volume of additional fluid needed to meet daily fluid requirements. Free-water content is generally 80% to 85% (800–850 mL/L of formula) for formulas with 1 to 1.2 kcal/mL. Table 37-3 lists free-water content associated with other caloric densities. The available history for D.S. does not suggest a need for fluid restriction; therefore, it would be reasonable to initiate feedings with a standard caloric density product (1–1.2 kcal/mL).

PROTEIN CONTENT

Protein needs increase disproportionately to caloric needs during injury and critical illness, whereas protein tolerance may limit protein provision in other conditions. To meet the need for varying ratios between calories and protein, polymeric formulas are available with a range from low- to very high protein content. Either percentage of calories from protein or nonprotein calories to nitrogen (NPC:N) ratio can be used to define protein content. Table 37-3 lists general descriptions for protein content. High-nitrogen enteral formulas are designed for patients with an increased protein requirement without a proportional increase in caloric needs. Very high nitrogen formulas are generally intended for critically ill patients or those with large wounds to heal. Low-nitrogen formulas are available for patients requiring protein restriction. Some low-nitrogen formulas are designed for patients with reduced renal function and can be classified as specialized formulas.

D.S. could obtain adequate protein from a formula with standard protein content. A formula with slightly higher-protein content (17%–18% of calories) would also be acceptable. A high-nitrogen formula that meets D.S.'s calorie needs will provide protein at the upper end of the estimated requirement (1.2 g/kg/day), whereas a standard-nitrogen formula will provide between 0.8 and 1 g/kg/day. A high-nitrogen formula may replete D.S.'s somatic and visceral protein status sooner but it may not provide adequate calories for weight gain. The decision to use a high-nitrogen versus standard-nitrogen formula depends on the exact nutrient composition of products on the EN formulary.

CASE 37-2, QUESTION 5: Should the EN product selected for D.S. contain fiber and if so, what type and amount?

Fiber has potential physiologic benefits, including increased fecal bulk, decreased bowel transit time in patients susceptible to constipation, increased transit time in patients with diarrhea, reduction of serum cholesterol, and improved glycemic control in patients with diabetes. Recommended daily fiber intake for healthy Americans is 21 to 25 g for women and 30 to 38 g for men, with the lower end of these amounts for people 51 years of age or older.[29] Adequate intake is determined by calorie intake and fiber intake observed to protect against coronary artery disease (14 g/1,000 calories). Optimal fiber intake for ill persons has not been determined. Fiber-supplemented formulas vary considerably in fiber content. There is no standardized terminology for low-fiber, moderate-fiber, and high-fiber content; however, the amounts listed in Table 37-3 can serve as a general guideline.

Enteral formulas may contain either insoluble or soluble fiber, or both. Insoluble fiber is associated with changes in fecal bulk and transit time, whereas soluble fiber tends to be responsible for effects on cholesterol and glycemic control. Soluble fibers, such as pectin, psyllium, and certain gums, tend to form gels and are used as a single fiber source only for low-fiber formulas. Fructooligosaccharides (FOS) are naturally occurring sugars that are added to some enteral formulas for soluble fiber benefits with better formulation characteristics (i.e., less gelling). Soluble fibers and FOS can be fermented to short-chain fatty acids by *Bifidobacterium* in the colon.[30,31] Short-chain fatty acids stimulate colonic blood flow, enhance fluid and electrolyte absorption, and provide a trophic effect in the colon.

The most common fiber source for enteral formulas is soy polysaccharide, or soy fiber. Although soy polysaccharide demonstrates beneficial effects associated with both soluble and insoluble fibers in healthy subjects and non-critically ill patients, studies do not provide clear evidence of improved bowel function in critically ill patients.[31] Routine use of fiber is not supported by available data in critically ill patients.[18–20] Given available data, stable patients on long-term EN appear most likely to benefit from fiber-supplemented formulas. Some patients on short-term EN without GI pathology who experience altered stool consistency may benefit from fiber supplementation.

Addition of fiber to enteral formulas creates some potential problems. Fiber increases viscosity and fiber-containing formulas often require a pump for administration through feeding tubes. GI symptoms from fiber can include increased gas production and abdominal discomfort.[27,31] Improvement in constipation has been noted with FOS administration; however, intake of greater than 45 g/day may cause diarrhea.[32] Flatulence and bloating can limit tolerance to FOS for some patients. Gradual introduction of fiber may help reduce these symptoms. Bezoar formation also has been reported in a patient receiving fiber-containing tube feedings and medications that suppressed GI motility.[31] Caution is advised for the use of fiber-containing formulas in patients with poor GI motility and underlying GI dysfunction. Insoluble fiber should be avoided in critically ill patients, and patients at high risk of bowel ischemia or severe dysmotility should not receive either soluble or insoluble fiber.[4] Inadequate fluid intake may also contribute to the risk of bezoar formation and intestinal blockage with fiber.

D.S. is not critically ill and does not appear to have bowel pathology precluding use of a fiber-containing formula. He will require EN for a moderate duration of time and potentially long term. It would be reasonable to provide a formula with at least moderate fiber content. However, D.S. could experience GI symptoms from the fiber, especially if his diet has previously been of low-fiber content. If necessary, a low-fiber formula could be used initially and then transitioned to higher fiber once symptoms of bloating and gas improve.

CASE 37-2, QUESTION 6: What is an appropriate administration regimen for D.S.'s tube feeding?

The feeding route, formula selected, and anticipated duration of feeding influence the administration regimen. Patient location (e.g., hospital, nursing facility, home) and cost also are considered when developing the regimen, including the rate for initiating and advancing feedings, and the administration method (i.e., syringe, gravity drip, pump).

Limited scientific data exist regarding EN administration regimens; thus, expert opinion plays an important role and different regimens can be used in various settings, all of which appear to meet the needs of the patients and personnel. The administration regimen should be adjusted as necessary for feeding intolerance. Four basic schedules for formula delivery are available: (a) continuous infusion, (b) cyclic infusion, (c) intermittent infusion, and (d) bolus delivery of formula.

Continuous Infusion

Continuous infusion provides formula at a continuous rate for 24 hours/day and can be used with any route of feeding. Intragastric continuous infusion is most commonly used for hospitalized patients, although small bowel feeding may be more appropriate in certain settings (e.g., ICU).[18–20] Risks of gastric distension and aspiration may decrease with continuous infusion compared with intermittent gastric infusion.[14] In addition, the slower infusion rate associated with continuous infusion may be better tolerated as judged by stool frequency and time to attain full nutrition support, especially in the elderly and in metabolically unstable patients.[33–35] However, data were insufficient to include a recommendation for continuous infusion versus other administration methods for critically ill patients in the CCP guidelines.[18–20] Feeding into the duodenum or jejunum is best initiated with continuous infusion because rapid infusion of large formula volumes into the small bowel can result in symptoms of dumping syndrome, including sweating, lightheadedness, abdominal distension, cramping, hyperperistalsis, and watery diarrhea. With time, the jejunum may adapt to larger volumes over a shorter time allowing cyclic or longer intermittent infusions.

Cyclic Feeding

Cyclic feeding provides formula at a continuous rate for less than 24 hours daily. This method is most commonly used for patients who need supplemental nutrition because of an inability to consume adequate oral nutrients, during transition to an oral diet, and for long-term home EN patients. Infusions are typically given at night for 8 to 12 hours to minimize interference with oral intake and normal activities during the day, although cycles can be as long as 20 hours. Most patients do not start on a cyclic regimen; rather, they transition from continuous feeding. Formula volume and osmolality can limit tolerance to cyclic feedings, especially jejunal feedings, and transition from continuous to cyclic infusion may require several days to weeks depending on patient tolerance. For gastric feeding, the transition usually takes only a few days.

Intermittent and Bolus Feedings

Formula is provided in three to eight gastric feedings daily for intermittent and bolus administration. Intermittent infusion occurs for 30 to 60 minutes using a feeding container or bag, with or without an enteral pump, and bolus feedings are for about 15 minutes using gravity administration via a syringe.[34–37] The stomach's reservoir capacity allows administration of relatively large volumes on an intermittent or bolus schedule. This is more physiologic than continuous feeding and more convenient for patients in nursing facilities and ambulatory patients at home on EN.

INITIATION OF FEEDINGS

The regimen for initiating EN primarily depends on the site of feeding and condition of the patient's GI tract. Use of full-strength (i.e., undiluted) formula is recommended for initiation of feedings.[34–37] Dilution delays delivery of adequate nutrients without significantly affecting the incidence of GI intolerance. Hypertonic formulas are diluted rapidly in the GI tract, reaching isotonicity before or shortly beyond the ligament of Treitz (distal end of duodenum). Continuous feedings are commonly initiated at a rate of 10 to 50 mL/hour with advancement by 10 to 25 mL/hour every 4 to 24 hours as tolerated, although stable patients may tolerate initiation of EN at goal rate.[3,34,35] For critically ill patients, those with abnormal GI function, patients without use of the GI tract for a prolonged time, those at risk of refeeding syndrome, and when calorically dense or high-osmolality formulas are used, starting at the lower rate and advancing slowly (i.e., start at 10–20 mL/hour and advance by 10–15 mL/hour every 12 or 24 hours) may be preferable, although this is based on consensus rather than evidence from well-designed studies.[25,33–36]

Patients are typically started on continuous infusion feedings, then transition to intermittent infusions, and eventually to bolus feedings, if desired. Bolus feedings are administered for about 15 minutes to avoid bloating, cramping, nausea, and diarrhea. A rate of less than 60 mL/minute is suggested to minimize GI intolerance with bolus feedings.[36,37] For intermittent feeding, rates of 200 to 300 mL every 4 to 6 hours are generally tolerated; volumes up to 750 mL may be tolerated.[33,36,37] Initiation of feedings at goal rate may be tolerated by some patients, although starting slower is appropriate for most patients.

D.S. receives gastric feeds; therefore, continuous infusion, intermittent infusion, or bolus feedings could all be used. Continuous infusion most commonly is used for hospitalized patients despite no clearly established difference in tolerance compared with intermittent infusion. Full-strength formula should be used to initiate feedings. The goal volume of enteral nutrition for D.S. is 1,440 mL/day of a standard caloric density formula (1.06 kcal/mL,

0.44 g protein/mL, 83.5% free water), or 60 mL/hour continuous infusion. The infusion could be started at 30 mL/hour (half goal rate); however, given D.S.'s risk for refeeding syndrome, it is preferable to start slower. Starting at 15 mL/hour for 12 hours, then increasing by 15 mL/hour every 12 hours would achieve the goal rate of 60 mL/hour within 48 hours. If D.S. experiences diarrhea or abdominal distension, the feeding may be held at 15 mL/hour for 24 hours, then increased by only 10 mL/hour every 12 to 24 hour as tolerated. Extra care is required to ensure he receives an adequate fluid intake until the formula is at goal rate.

Continuous infusion enteral feeding can be administered by gravity drip or by enteral pump. With gravity drip, the infusion rate must be adjusted frequently to maintain a consistent flow rate, and formula flow must be checked regularly to ensure that the flow has not stopped. Gravity infusion has no alarms to alert nurses to kinked tubing or empty delivery containers. Enteral pumps provide a consistent flow rate and alarms for problems with the infusion, but they are more expensive than gravity drips. Pumps often are used for hospitalized patients to help maintain delivery of the prescribed volume of enteral formula. Either gravity drip or an enteral pump could be used for D.S., depending on the hospital's protocol for enteral feeding.

To prevent potentially fatal inadvertent IV infusion of non-IV products, new non-Luer compatible global design standards for small-bore liquid and gas medical device tubing connectors, including enteral feeding connectors, are being introduced under the "Stay Connected" initiative.[38] The connection between the enteral formula bag and the tubing going into the bag changed in 2012. Transition to the new ENFit connector between the administration tubing and feeding tube itself is expected to be completed by 2016. Oral syringes will not fit the new ENFit connectors; therefore, ENFit compatible syringes are required for medication administration, tube flushes, and bolus feeding via syringe.

TRANSITION FROM CONTINUOUS TO INTERMITTENT/BOLUS FEEDING

CASE 37-2, QUESTION 7: D.S. has received EN for 10 days. He has tolerated his continuous tube feeding without problems and has not required electrolyte replacements for the past 4 days. The plan is to transfer D.S. to a skilled nursing facility (SNF) in the next few days. The SNF requests D.S. be on an intermittent/bolus feeding regimen before transfer to the SNF. How should D.S. be changed from continuous infusion to intermittent or bolus feeding?

Many nursing facilities do not routinely use enteral pumps because of increased cost. Without a pump, delivery of the prescribed volume of formula at a consistent rate may not be reliable and increased nursing time may be required to prevent tube occlusion and ensure adequate volume of formula is delivered. D.S. is currently receiving continuous infusion feedings. The transition to intermittent delivery of formula can be accomplished by various methods. An overlapping regimen of gradually decreasing the continuous infusion rate and increasing the intermittent volume appears to be an economical and efficient method of changing the feeding regimen.[33] For D.S., decrease the continuous rate from 60 mL/hour down to 40 mL/hour and add four intermittent feedings of 120 mL over 60 minutes every 6 hours initially. If tolerated, decrease continuous infusion to 20 mL/hour and increase intermittent feeding to 240 mL. Finally, stop the continuous feeding and increase intermittent feedings to 360 mL, or add a fifth feeding to keep the intermittent volume at 285 to 300 mL. To keep the feeding volume in a more convenient increment of 120 mL (half of an 8-ounce can), D.S. could receive two feedings of 360 mL and three feedings of 240 mL if five daily feedings are needed.

Another transition method is to stop continuous feedings and restart feedings with a regimen for initiating intermittent feedings. Starting volume is typically 60 to 120 mL for the first two or three feedings, and feeding intervals are often every 4 hours. Volume is increased by 60 to 120 mL every 8 to 12 hours, as tolerated, until goal is reached.[35] Feeding intervals can be increased once goal volume is reached. D.S. could start with 120 mL over 60 minutes every 4 hours for two feedings, then advance to 240 mL per feeding. If tolerated, the volume per feeding could increase to 360 mL to allow feedings every 6 hours. Once at the desired number of feedings per day, the infusion time could be decreased based on tolerance. If feeding for 30 minutes is well tolerated, D.S. could be changed to bolus administration for 15 to 20 minutes.

The discharge EN prescription should state clearly the desired caloric density, protein content, fiber content per 1,000 kcal, and formula volume, or the daily calories, protein, fiber, and fluid goals. The brand name may be included, but the SNF may not carry the same brand of formula. Any special considerations for the feeding schedule also should be communicated (e.g., D.S. does not tolerate feeding after 9 PM; raise the head of the bed to 45 degrees for 3 hours after the last daily feeding to avoid regurgitation).

FLUID PROVISION

CASE 37-2, QUESTION 8: How much additional fluid must be included in the feeding regimen to meet D.S.'s estimated daily fluid requirements?

The free-water content of EN must be calculated to determine the volume of additional fluid that must be provided. As noted previously, standard caloric density formulas generally contain 80% to 85% free water. The formula selected for D.S. contains 83.5% free water; therefore, at his goal volume of 1,440 mL/day (six cans), the formula provides approximately 1,200 mL of free water daily. Using 1,860 mL daily (30 mL/kg/day $\times$ 62 kg) as D.S.'s fluid requirement (see Case 37-2, Question 5), he will need 660 mL/day in addition to the enteral formula. If D.S. had additional losses from vomiting, diarrhea, or other sources, this volume would be added to the 660 mL to determine total volume in addition to enteral formula. The additional fluid is typically provided with medications and tube irrigation (flushes). Feeding tubes should be irrigated with 30 mL of fluid every 4 hours during continuous feeding, or before and after each intermittent or bolus feeding.[34,35] The tube should be flushed with a minimum of 15 mL of water before and after medication administration through the tube, as well as with 15 mL between each medication.[34–37] Fluid also is required for diluting medications before administration through the tube. The flush volume and/or number of flushes will need to be increased to provide D.S. with adequate fluid because 30 mL every 4 hours plus fluid for medication administration will not provide the 660 mL of fluid needed in addition to his EN. Because D.S. is receiving gastric feedings, hypotonic fluid is of less concern than in the jejunum.[39] Increasing flush volumes to between 100 and 150 mL should meet D.S.'s daily fluid requirement, depending on the amount needed for medication administration. Diluting the formula itself to increase fluid provision is not recommended because this increases the risk of error and contamination.

NUTRITION IN CRITICAL ILLNESS

Nutrition support is an important component of care in critical illness where patients are typically in a catabolic stress state and metabolism may be altered. Multiorgan dysfunction, as well as fluid and electrolyte imbalances, adds to the complexity of this population and confounds attempts to provide proper nutrition. The preferred route for nutrition support is generally EN, although the ideal formula composition remains unresolved. Guidelines are periodically updated. The most recently published guidelines should be consulted to determine current recommendations, especially regarding specialized components discussed in this section.

CASE 37-3

QUESTION 1: J.B., a 68-year-old man with a past medical history of hypertension, presents to the ED with complaints of shortness of breath, productive cough, wheezing, and fever. J.B. subsequently requires intubation and is transferred to the ICU with a diagnosis of pneumonia. During the next 24 hours, his respiratory status further declines, and he is diagnosed with acute respiratory distress syndrome (ARDS). In anticipation of a prolonged course of mechanical ventilation, a feeding tube is placed into the small bowel. The chart indicates a height of 70 inches and an admission weight of 75 kg.

Laboratory evaluation today includes the following:
Sodium, 140 mEq/L
Potassium, 3.9 mEq/L
Chloride, 109 mEq/L
Carbon dioxide content, 22 mM
BUN, 18 mg/dL
SCr, 0.8 mg/dL
Glucose, 118 mg/dL
Albumin, 3.6 g/dL
Aspartate aminotransferase, 32 international units/L
Alanine aminotransferase, 37 international units/L
Alkaline phosphatase, 64 international units/L
Total bilirubin, 0.7 mg/dL
WBC, $15.3 \times 10^3/\mu L$
Hgb, 13.4 g/dL
Hct, 39.9%

Should a specialized critical care formula be used for initiation of EN in J.B.?

J.B. is critically ill and several types of EN formulas have been developed for critically ill patients. However, the role of specialized EN formulas, and certain components in particular, remains controversial in critical illness. Table 37-4 shows a few formulas marketed for critical illness and lists the components which are altered compared to standard polymeric formulas. Due to the catabolic nature of critical illness, formulas are generally high protein, many with an NPC:N ratio less than 100:1 (i.e., high or very high protein content). Other formulas containing slightly lower-protein content (i.e., NPC:N ratio between 100:1 and 125:1) target the inflammatory element of critical illness with addition of components designed to mitigate the inflammatory response. Formulas designed for critical illness are typically fiber-free, although a few formulas include small amounts of soluble fiber. Supplementation of specific amino acids, including branched-chain amino acids (BCAAs), glutamine, and arginine, in EN for critical illness remains an unsettled issue.

Enhanced Branched-Chain Amino Acid Content

Standard EN formulas contain 15% to 20% of protein as BCAAs; enhanced BCAA formulas for critical care contain over 35%, and hepatic failure formulas contain 45% to 50%. High-BCAA stress/critical care formulas are not therapeutically interchangeable with hepatic formulas due to the lower-than-normal concentrations of aromatic amino acids (AAAs), especially phenylalanine, in hepatic formulas.

Guidelines from SCCM–ASPEN recommend a standard enteral formula for patients with acute or chronic liver disease in the ICU.[4] High–very high protein is currently emphasized over BCAA content for critically ill patients.

Glutamine

The proposed role of glutamine in critical illness is enhanced neutrophil function and maintenance of intestinal barrier function, thereby preventing translocation of bacteria and endotoxins from the GI tract into systemic circulation and reducing bacteremia.[40] Glutamine is considered a nonessential amino acid, as it is synthesized in sufficient quantities for its roles in transamination, as an intermediate in numerous metabolic pathways, such as gluconeogenesis and renal ammoniagenesis, as a fuel source for rapidly dividing lymphocytes and enterocytes, and in the synthesis of glutathione. However, during periods of metabolic stress, endogenous synthesis may become inadequate.

Study results are conflicting regarding effects of glutamine supplementation in the critically ill population. Past studies have indicated numerous clinical benefits from glutamine supplementation; however, two recent studies (REDOXs, METAPLEX) suggest increased mortality in critically ill patients receiving parenteral and/or enteral glutamine.[41–44] The CCP guidelines now recommend against the use of enteral glutamine in critically ill patients.[19] Glutamine supplementation should also be avoided in patients with total bilirubin greater than 10 mg/dL or creatinine clearance less than 30 mL/minute because ammonia excretion could be impared.[45] Monitoring for potential complications is essential when glutamine supplementation is used.

Protein-bound glutamine is present in all enteral formulas. Free glutamine is unstable in ready-to-use formulas and, due to poor stability, is not commercially available in an intravenous form. However, glutamine is available as a modular supplement, which can be administered separately from the EN formula. Glutamate is stable in water and functions in many roles attributed to glutamine. Additional research is needed to determine whether physiologic effects are equivalent for glutamate, protein-bound glutamine, and free glutamine.

Arginine

Arginine is a nonessential amino acid synthesized by the urea cycle during detoxification of ammonia and is normally available in sufficient quantities for growth and tissue repair. In times of metabolic stress, however, endogenous synthesis may become inadequate, making arginine conditionally essential. The postulated benefit of arginine in critical illness is related to enhanced protein synthesis, cellular growth, and immune system support. In contrast, several mechanisms have been proposed that suggest potential adverse effects with arginine supplementation, including one in which arginine is used as a substrate in the synthesis of nitric oxide (NO), a potent vasodilating agent, which may also have implications in mitochondria damage, organ dysfunction, and increased gut barrier permeability.[46] Although synthesis of NO increases during sepsis (thereby creating a negative arginine balance), the exact role of this effector molecule remains controversial. Many believe that excess NO is part of an adaptive response directed toward limiting infection, ischemia, coagulation, inflammation, and tissue injury.

Conflicting study results leave considerable uncertainty regarding use of arginine supplemented EN in critically ill patients.[4,18–20,47] Guidelines, consensus statements, and recommendations have been developed to help the clinician provide evidence-based nutrition therapy; however, many barriers to implementation exist.[4,18–20,48,49] Use of arginine-containing, immune-enhancing

Table 37-4
Selected High-Protein Enteral Formulas with Altered Protein or Fat Sources

Formula[a,b,c]	kcal/mL (mOsm/kg)	Free Water (%)	Protein g/L (% kcal)	NPC:N	Protein Source	ARG g/L[d]	GLN g/L[d]	Fat g/L (% kcal)	Fat Sources	Fat kcal as MCT (%)	Ratio of ω-6FA to ω-3FA[d]	Fiber g/L[d]
Crucial[c]	1.5 (490)	77	94 (25)	67:1	Hydrolyzed casein; L-arginine	15	–	67.6 (39)	MCT oil; fish oil (<2%); soybean oil; lecithin	50	1.5:1	–
f.a.a[c]	1.0 (850)	85	50 (20)	100:1	Crystalline amino acids	–	–	11.2 (10)	Soybean oil; MCT	25	–	–
Impact with Fiber[c]	1.0 (375)	87	56 (22)	71:1	Sodium and calcium caseinates; L-arginine	12.5	–	28 (25)	Palm kernel oil; menhaden oil	–	1.4:1	10
Impact 1.5[c]	1.5 (550)	78	84 (22)	71:1	Sodium and calcium caseinates; L-arginine	18.7	–	69 (40)	MCT; palm kernel oil; menhaden oil	33	1.4:1	–
Impact Glutamine[c]	1.3 (630)	81	78 (24)	62:1	Whey protein hydrolysate; free amino acids; sodium caseinates; L-arginine	16.3	15	43 (30)	Palm kernel oil; menhaden oil	–	1.4:1	10
Optimental[b]	1.0 (540)	83.2	51 (20.5)	97:1	Soy protein hydrolysate; partially hydrolyzed sodium caseinate; L-arginine	5.5	–	28.4 (25)	Structured lipid (interesterified sardine oil [EPA, DHA] and MCT); canola oil; soy oil	NA	–	5 FOS
Osmolite 1.2 Cal[b]	1.2 (360)	82	55.5 (18.5)	110:1	Sodium and calcium caseinate	–	–	39 (29)	High-oleic safflower oil; canola oil; MCT oil; lecithin	20	–	–
Oxepa[b]	1.5 (535)	78.5	62.5 (16.7)	125:1	Sodium and calcium caseinates	–	–	93.8 (55)	Canola oil; MCT oil; sardine oil; borage oil	25	–	–
Peptamen AF[c]	1.2 (390)	81	75.6 (21)	76:1	Hydrolyzed whey protein	–	–	54.8 (39)	MCT oil; soybean oil (<2%); fish oil (<2%); lecithin	50	1.8:1	5.2 (FOS and other fibers)
Pivot 1.5 Cal[b]	1.5 (595)	75.9	93.8 (25)	75:1	Partially hydrolyzed sodium caseinate; whey protein hydrolysate	13	6.5	50.8 (30)	Structured lipid (interesterified sardine oil [EPA, DHA] and MCT); soy oil; canola oil	20	–	7.5 FOS

[a]Changes periodically occur in nutrient sources and content; use this table as a general reference only and not for specific patient care issues.
[b]Abbott (Ross) product.
[c]Nestle product.
[d]None or unknown indicated by "–."
AF, advanced formula; ARG, arginine; DHA, docosahexaenoic acid; EPA, eicosapentaenoic acid; FOS, fructooligosaccharides; GLN, glutamine; MCT, medium-chain triglycerides; NPC:N, nonprotein calorie to nitrogen; ω-3FA, ω-3 fatty acids; ω-6FA, ω-6 fatty acids.

diets is not recommended for critically ill patients in the CCP guidelines because higher-quality studies indicated no effect on mortality with these formulas and increased mortality was reported for septic patients in some studies.[18–20]

IMMUNE-MODULATING FORMULAS

Formulas included in Table 37-4 have an NPC:N ratio less than or equal to 125:1 and also contain supplemental arginine, glutamine, or nucleic acids, or a modified fat component. Such formulas are often referred to as "immune-modulating" formulas based on their proposed beneficial modulation of biologic responses to stress. Study formulas frequently contain varying portions of two or more potentially immune-modifying components, making it difficult to determine the effect of any given component. The subset of immune-modulating formulas intended for patients with acute respiratory distress syndrome (ARDS) and acute lung injury (ALI) is distinct from other formulas and is discussed in more detail under pulmonary disease.

The results of clinical trials examining the effects of immune-modulating enteral formulations on mortality, hospital length of stay (LOS), ICU days, incidence of nosocomial infection, duration of mechanical ventilation, and GI complications are conflicting.[4,18–20,40–47] Several meta-analyses have shown benefit on clinical outcomes (e.g., infectious complications, ventilator days, LOS); however, no mortality benefit has ever been found in critically ill patients receiving immunonutrition versus standard EN.[4,18–20,48]

The population which appears to have better outcomes with immune-modulating EN is patients undergoing major elective surgery, particularly surgery for upper GI malignancy. Reduced infection risk and shorter LOS in high-risk elective surgery patients, mostly patients with upper GI malignancy, receiving immunonutrition with EN supplemented with both arginine and fish oil was shown in a meta-analysis.[47] Joint guidelines from SCCM–ASPEN gave the highest recommendation for use of an immune-modulating EN formula in patients undergoing major elective surgery, trauma, burns, and head and neck cancer; the recommendation was slightly lower for critically ill, mechanically ventilated, nonsurgical medical ICU patients.[4] Conversely, CCP guidelines advise against use of formulas with "arginine and other nutrients" in critically ill patients based on failure to show an infectious or mortality benefit and potential for harm in septic patients.[18–20] Neither the CCP guidelines nor the SCC-ASPEN guidelines recommend use of an arginine-supplemented immune-modulating formula for patients with severe sepsis.[4,18–20] Additional studies with well-defined patient populations are necessary to determine the effects of combinations of immune-modulating components (arginine, glutamine, nucleic acids, ω-3FAs), optimal component and dose combinations, and the most beneficial timing for administration of immune-modulating components.

Altered Fat Components

Stress or critical care and immune-modulating formulas contain different sources of fat to alter the type of fatty acids provided. Fat sources commonly include MCTs, along with predominantly canola oil, high-oleic oils, or fish oils. Absorption of MCTs is relatively independent of pancreatic enzymes and bile salts, and is carnitine-independent; thus, they can be absorbed in patients experiencing malabsorption of the long-chain triglycerides. Formulas containing a relatively large percentage of fat calories as MCTs are frequently marketed for critically ill patients with malabsorption.

Canola oil and high-oleic oils have high monounsaturated fatty acid (MUFA) content. MUFAs have been popularized by reports of low cardiovascular disease in populations using olive oil, but further research is needed to determine the role of these fatty acids in ill patients. Usual polyunsaturated vegetable oils (i.e., corn, soy, and safflower oils) are avoided or provided in relatively small quantities in critical care formulas to limit omega-6 fatty acids (ω-6FAs), which are precursors to inflammatory, vasoconstrictive, and platelet-aggregating agents.[50,51] Some ω-6FAs may, however, be converted to γ-linolenic acid (GLA), then to dihomo-GLA, and subsequently to arachidonic acid.[52] Dihomo-GLA competes with arachidonic acid in the pathways for prostaglandin synthesis resulting "1" series prostaglandins with lower proinflammatory effects, similar to "3" series prostaglandins from ω-3FA. Small amounts of ω-6FAs are required in the diet to prevent deficiency of linoleic acid, an essential fatty acid not provided by MCT and fish oils.

Fish oils, including menhaden oil, provide fatty acids primarily from the ω-3 family, with the very long-chain fatty acids eicosapentaenoic acid (EPA) and docosahexaenoic acid (DHA) predominating. The proposed role of ω-3FAs in critical illness is to reduce infectious complications and death in selected patient populations. The ω-3FAs are precursors to less inflammatory and more vasodilatory eicosanoids than those from ω-6FA.[50–52]

Few data are available evaluating effects of only fat modification in EN for critical illness, and combinations of immune-modulating components may produce different effects than single nutrients. Improved clinical outcomes for postsurgical and critically ill patients have been associated with EN-containing ω-3FAs, usually in conjunction with other immune-modulating components, although the effects remain controversial.[4,18,26] Some studies suggest data are inadequate to support routine use of fish oil, whereas others indicate the potential for arginine to counteract the benefit of fish oil in EN containing combinations of immune-modulating components.[53,54]

Studies suggest a minimum of 5 to 7 days of supplementation with immune-modulating components, including ω-3FAs, is necessary to see beneficial effects on postoperative outcomes.[49–51] Incorporation of ω-3FAs into cell membranes may be required to see benefits; this has been demonstrated in humans with supplementation for 5 days.[55] Fat modification to provide high-ω-3FA content also has been studied in ARDS and acute lung injury (as discussed in the Pulmonary Disease section).

The question of whether to initiate EN in J.B. with an immune-modulating formula does not have a clear-cut answer. The data provided for J.B. do not indicate sepsis; thus, he would be a candidate for an immune-modulating formula using the SCCM–ASPEN guidelines.[4] The more conservative CCP guidelines would not recommend an arginine-containing immune-modulating formula.[18–20] The decision of whether to use the immune-modulating formula would likely depend on practices within the hospital and the immune-modulating formulas available. Because J.B. was admitted with pneumonia and now has ARDS, the other consideration would be whether a specialized pulmonary formula would be more appropriate for his EN.

PULMONARY DISEASE

CASE 37-3, QUESTION 2: How do pulmonary formulas differ from standard polymeric formulas? If J.B. receives a specialized pulmonary formula, what nutrient modifications should the formula contain?

There are two types of EN formulas intended for patients with pulmonary conditions. Both have a moderate caloric density (1.5 kcal/mL) and the percentage of calories from fat is relatively high (40%–55%), although the types of fats differ. The premise for higher fat content is that fat metabolism produces less carbon dioxide (CO_2) than carbohydrate metabolism, thereby reducing the work load of the lungs. Early studies comparing isocaloric, high-fat, low-carbohydrate diets with higher-carbohydrate diets showed improved respiratory parameters in ambulatory patients with chronic obstructive pulmonary disease (COPD) as well as reduced time on the ventilator and decreased arterial CO_2 concentrations in mechanically ventilated patients.[26,56,57] Caloric intake in these studies ranged from 1.7 to 2.25 times the measured energy expenditure, which is excessive by current standards. Excess calories contribute to higher CO_2 production; thus, the early studies are of questionable relevance, and in practice, preventing overfeeding is as important for control of CO_2 as high-fat, low-carbohydrate diets.[26,27] In addition, improved respiratory parameters with a high-fat EN product are unlikely in patients without excess CO_2 production or retention. Data from 60 malnourished, underweight patients with COPD do suggest respiratory status in this population is more likely to benefit from a high-fat, low-carbohydrate (28% of calories) formula compared with a high-carbohydrate (60%–70% of calories) formula.[58] Although the percent of calories from fat (55%) in the high-fat formula was similar to traditional pulmonary formulas, fat distribution was considerably different with 20% of fat as MCTs and a predominance of MUFAs. Currently marketed pulmonary formulas contain 20% to 40% of fat calories as MCTs and fat sources providing higher MUFAs. During a period of overfeeding for weight gain, pulmonary formulas may be reasonable; however, they are not warranted for routine use in most patients.

The second type of pulmonary EN formula is an immune-modulating pulmonary (IMP) formula with an anti-inflammatory lipid profile (fish oils rich in ω-3FAs, borage oil rich in GLAs), antioxidants (vitamins C and E, βcarotene), and no supplemental glutamine or arginine, which has been studied in patients with ARDS and ALI.[4,18–20] Three studies comparing this formula with a typical high-fat pulmonary formula with elevated ω-6FA content were included in a meta-analysis by Pontes-Arruda et al.[59] and showed a significant reduction in new organ failures, time receiving mechanical ventilation, ICU LOS, and mortality.

Based on the one study available when the initial CCP guidelines were published, the committee recommended use of IMP formulas with a combination of fish oils, borage oil, and antioxidants in patients with ARDS.[18] The SCCM–ASPEN and updated 2009 CCP guidelines evaluated additional studies and both recommended patients with ARDS or ALI be placed on an IMP formula.[4,20] However, the choice of control formula in these otherwise high-quality studies has been questioned because there is some evidence of harmful effects from administration of ω-6FA-rich fats in critically ill patients.[18]

The study by Grau-Carmona et al.[60] compared an IMP formula to standard EN rather than a high-fat pulmonary formula. In 132 septic patients with ARDS or ALI, no difference was found in gas exchange, ventilator days, or infection rate, although ICU LOS was less with the IMP. Based on inclusion of this study and one other with those available from previous CCP evaluations, the 2013 CCP guidelines downgraded their recommendation to consider use of a IMP formula in patients with ARDS or ALI.[20] An additional study using an IMP formula preemptively in severe trauma patients was included in the 2015 CCP guidelines.[19] No difference was found in the level of oxygenation, development of ALI or ARDS, ventilator days, ICU LOS or mortality; however, more patients in the study group developed bacteremia.[61] The 2015 CCP guidelines remained the same as in 2013.[19]

J.B. was diagnosed with ARDS; therefore, an IMP formula could be considered based on the CCP and SCCM–ASPEN guidelines.[4,19,20] The formula should contain fish oils to provide a high-ω-3FA content, borage oil to provide GLA, and increased antioxidant vitamin content. Delayed gastric emptying is associated with high-fat diets and must be considered when evaluating possible benefits and adverse effects of high-fat EN. This applies to both IMP and routine pulmonary formulas. Abdominal distension, increased gastric residuals, nausea, and vomiting can result from delayed gastric emptying. J.B. has his feeding tube placed in the small bowel, so delayed gastric emptying is not a concern. However, the potential to overwhelm pancreatic lipase activity resulting in fat malabsorption should be considered when a high-fat load, especially long-chain triglycerides, is delivered into the small bowel. Continuous infusion is more likely to be tolerated than other, more rapid delivery methods in most patients. As shown in Table 37-2, the cost of routine pulmonary formulas is slightly higher than for standard polymeric formulas and IMP formulas are significantly more expensive.

RENAL FAILURE

CASE 37-3, QUESTION 3: J.B. has been in the ICU for 10 days. His ARDS has improved; however, he now has acute kidney injury and hemodialysis will start today. Morning laboratory results include the following:

Sodium, 131 mEq/L
Potassium, 5.7 mEq/L
BUN, 80 mg/dL
SCr, 3.8 mg/dL
Glucose, 100 mg/dL on an insulin drip
Magnesium, 2.9 mg/dL
Phosphorus, 5.6 mg/dL
WBC, 9.7 × $10^3/\mu L$
Hgb, 11.4 g/dL
Hct, 34.3%

An EN formula for renal failure is ordered. How do the nutrient components in renal formulas differ from standard polymeric EN formulas? Is a renal formula appropriate for J.B.?

Two types of EN formulas for renal disease/injury are available and both are calorically dense (1.8–2 kcal/mL) to limit fluid provision. Highly specialized formulas with enriched essential amino acid content are based on the theory that recycling of urea nitrogen for nonessential amino acid synthesis reduces the accumulation of BUN.[26,56,57] Clinically significant recycling of nitrogen and incorporation into nonessential amino acids does not appear to occur, however. Essential amino acid formulas may be appropriate for patients with chronic renal failure with glomerular filtration rates less than 25 mL/minute/1.73 m^2 who are receiving very low-protein diets and for whom dialysis is not an option.[56] Use should be limited to no more than 2 to 3 weeks, because hyperammonemia and metabolic encephalopathy have been associated with longer use. These formulas are not appropriate for patients with acute kidney injury, such as J.B., or for those receiving dialysis. The NPC:N ratio is approximately 300:1 in these formulas. Water-soluble vitamins are typically included in currently available high essential amino acid formulas; however, vitamin content should be reviewed as some essential amino acid formulas do not contain vitamins. Renalcal contains higher-than-normal essential amino acids with about two-thirds essential combined with one-third nonessential amino acids.

Polymeric enteral formulas designed for renal failure or renal insufficiency are the standard for hospitalized patients with impaired renal function. These formulas contain a balanced amino acid profile and are not enriched with essential amino acids. The NPC:N ratio varies from about 130:1 (for patients with increased nitrogen losses from dialysis) to 230:1 (typically used for nondialyzed patients).

Lower-than-normal concentrations of potassium, phosphorus, and magnesium are used in these formulas to minimize electrolyte problems. Many critically ill patients receiving dialysis for acute kidney injury tolerate a nonrenal formula; however, those with elevated potassium, phosphorus, or magnesium generally require a renal formula to control electrolyte levels. Based on his electrolytes, J.B. will require a renal formula. A polymeric formula with a lower NPC:N ration (i.e., 140:1; moderate protein content) would be appropriate given the plan for dialysis. Polymeric renal formulas meet 100% of the DRI with less than 2,000 mL/day.

Modular Components

CASE 37-3, QUESTION 4: After several days on the renal formula (NPC:N ratio, 140:1), there are indications that J.B.'s protein intake should be higher. Serum electrolytes today include the following:

Sodium, 137 mEq/L
Potassium, 5.1 mEq/L
Phosphorus, 4.5 mg/dL
Magnesium, 2.6 mg/dL

What are the options for increasing protein provision?

J.B. is receiving a renal formula with moderately high-protein content based on the NPC:N ratio of 140:1. There are no very high protein formulas with low potassium, phosphorus, and magnesium on the market; therefore, a very high protein formula will provide significantly more of these electrolytes than J.B. currently receives. His current serum levels of the renally eliminated electrolytes are near the upper end of normal and would likely rise above the normal range if the EN is changed to a nonrenal formula. Using a lower potassium concentration in the dialysis bath might keep serum potassium within normal range. Addition of a phosphate binder to the medication regimen could be considered; however, the risk of tube occlusion may be increased with a phosphate binder. A better option is to provide additional protein from a modular protein component, although this can also increase the risk of tube occlusion if not administered properly.

Modular components are individual nutrient substrates, or combinations of two substrates, designed for addition to oral diets or enteral formula regimens. They provide only the macronutrient(s) without electrolytes or vitamins, and should only be used to supplement a diet or EN, not as a sole source of nutrition. Protein modules are powders containing 3 to 5 g protein/tablespoon. Most protein modules are intact protein. Arginine and glutamine are available as individual packets to allow supplementation as a single amino acid. Glucose polymers are used to supplement calories as carbohydrate. They do not increase osmolality or alter food or formula flavor. Powdered carbohydrate modules contain 20 to 30 kcal/tablespoon, whereas liquids contain 2 kcal/mL. Protein and carbohydrate modular components typically are mixed with water and administered through the feeding tube rather than being mixed directly into the formula. Additional fat can be provided as 50% safflower oil emulsion (Microlipid) or as MCT oil. A combination carbohydrate and fat modular product is available if both sources of calories are appropriate. A modular fiber product containing soluble fiber in the form of partially hydrolyzed guar gum is also available.

Glucose Control Formulas

CASE 37-4

QUESTION 1: M.P., a 59-year-old man, is admitted to the hospital secondary to dehydration and for a GI workup related to a 35-pound unintentional weight loss during the past 3 months. He states he has been unable to eat for a week due to continual nausea, although he reports no vomiting. M.P. received IV fluids in the ED and currently has 0.9% sodium chloride infusing at 125 mL/hour. Past medical history includes hypertension, hyperlipidemia, gastric reflux, and diabetes mellitus type 2. M.P. is 5 feet 11 inches tall and his admit weight is 130 kg. Laboratory values from this morning show the following results:

Glucose, 230 mg/dL
BUN, 20 mg/dL, down from 31 mg/dL in the ED
SCr, 1.2 mg/dL, down from 2.3 mg/dL in the ED
Sodium, 141 mEq/L
Potassium, 4.3 mEq/L
Chloride, 105 mEq/L

His small bowel follow-through study indicates severely delayed gastric emptying. A feeding tube is to be placed into the small bowel for a trial of enteral feeding.

Should a "glucose control" or "diabetic" formula be used for initiating tube feedings in M.P.? How do formulas for glucose control differ from standard polymeric EN formulas?

No ideal macronutrient distribution has been identified for meals intended for patients with diabetes mellitus and general dietary guidelines for healthy eating are considered appropriate.[62] However, formulas for hyperglycemic patients, known as diabetic formulas, do not necessarily follow this recommendation. Diabetic formulas have caloric distributions of 31% to 40% carbohydrate, 42% to 49% fat, and 16% to 20% protein. The carbohydrate content is lower, and fat content is higher than in most standard polymeric formulas. High MUFA sources predominate to provide greater than 60% of fat as MUFAs. The source and type of carbohydrates in diabetic formulas varies, with a predominance of more complex carbohydrates (i.e., oligosaccharides, cornstarch, fiber) and insulin-independent sugars (i.e., fructose). Fiber sources associated with improved glycemic control, mainly soluble fibers but also soy polysaccharide, are included in these formulas to help minimize postprandial hyperglycemia. Fiber content ranges from 14 to 21 g/L and formulas are 1 kcal/mL; thus, the recommended fiber intake of 25 to 38 g daily generally can be achieved with less than 2,000 kcal/day.[29]

Multiple studies comparing diabetic formulas to standard EN formulas providing equal calories and protein have been conducted. Results of a large meta-analysis including 23 studies, 19 being randomized controlled trials, favor the diabetic formulas for glucose control.[63] Postprandial increases in glucose, glucose area under the curve, and peak blood glucose concentrations were significantly reduced with the diabetic formulas. However, there were no significant effects on total cholesterol, high-density lipoprotein, or triglyceride concentrations, or on overall complication rates. Also, mortality differences were not found in the single 2-week trial reporting mortality for critically ill patients. Ability to utilize results of this meta-analysis in practice is limited by many studies of low methodologic quality, inclusion of single-meal trials, and use of oral supplements in healthy volunteers. For hospitalized patients with hyperglycemia, no well-designed clinical trials of adequate size were found to make a recommendation regarding use of diabetic formulas in the ASPEN guidelines regarding adults with hyperglycemia.[64]

M.P. could receive either a diabetic formula or a standard formula. The meta-analysis discussed previously would suggest glucose control may be better with a diabetic formula; however, the ASPEN guidelines found inadequate data to make a recommendation regarding use of diabetic formulas in hospitalized patients with hyperglycemia and the Academy of Nutrition and

Dietetics suggests following a general pattern of healthy eating for patients with diabetes.[62–64] Either a diabetic or standard formula would be acceptable for M.P. based on available data. Problems with delayed gastric emptying or fat malabsorption must be weighed against possible benefits of improved glucose control with diabetic formulas. These problems are of minimal concern for M.P. as he is being fed into the small bowel and his history does not suggest fat malabsorption. Treatment goals for EN in patients with diabetes mellitus should include individualization of macronutrient composition, avoidance of excess calories, and maintenance of euglycemia.[62–64] M.P. may benefit from a treatment plan that includes gradual weight loss and this may influence the decision of whether to use a diabetic formula or a very high protein formula that would permit lower total calories while still providing adequate protein.

MONITORING ENTERAL NUTRITION SUPPORT

CASE 37-4, QUESTION 2: What types of complications can occur with tube feeding? What steps can be taken to prevent complications in M.P., and how should he be monitored for complications?

Appropriate monitoring of patients receiving EN is essential to recognize and prevent complications. Complications can be divided into three groups: mechanical, metabolic, and GI (Table 37-5).

Mechanical Complications

The major mechanical complications are tube occlusion and aspiration. Mechanical complications often can be avoided with good nursing technique and careful observation of feeding tolerance. Adequate tube flushing is essential to prevent tube occlusion. Flushing with 30 mL of water every 4 hours during continuous feeding or before and after intermittent feedings is recommended.[34,35] Flushing must also occur before and after medication administration and after withdrawal of gastric contents. M.P.'s tube should be flushed using these guidelines. Frequent assessment of tube placement by auscultation, location of markings on the tube, and withdrawal of gastric contents is important to prevent pulmonary aspiration of the formula secondary to displacement of the tube into the esophagus or pharynx. Tube placement should be evaluated every 4 to 6 hours with continuous feeding, or before each intermittent or bolus feeding.[34,36,37,39,57]

Withdrawal of gastric contents through a gastric tube using a syringe allows evaluation of volume in the stomach (gastric residual volume [GRV]). Endogenous secretions from saliva and gastric fluids, about 4,500 mL/day in normal adults receiving food, contribute to GRV when gastric emptying is impaired. Variations in GRV also occur based on the volume and timing of previous feeds, especially for intermittent or bolus feeds, feeding tube characteristics, and patient position and activity.[36,37] Gastrostomy tubes may yield less volume than NG tubes because of their more anterior position in the stomach. Soft, small-bore feeding tubes may collapse when GRV is checked, resulting in falsely low GRV. GRV is not usually checked through tubes placed in the postpyloric region because (a) problems with tube collapse have been reported and (b) the small bowel does not serve as a reservoir for residuals. M.P. has a jejunal feeding tube; thus, GRV is not reliable when checked through his feeding tube. If M.P. has an NG tube in addition to a small bowel feeding tube, GRV can be checked through the NG tube to assess whether formula is "backing-up" or refluxing into the stomach. Previously, methylene blue or blue food coloring was added to the formula to evaluate reflux; however, reports of mortality associated with this practice resulted in its abandonment.[4,14,34,35] The use of glucose oxidase test strips to detect the presence of enteral formula in tracheobronchial secretions lacks sensitivity and specificity, and the results have not been shown to correlate with aspiration; thus, it is not a recommended practice.[33,34,35,36] Current practice recommendations vary on the GRV volume for to holding feeding; CCP guidelines recommend holding at somewhere from 250 to 500 mL whereas SCCM–ASPEN recommendation holds for GRV greater than 500 mL and consider jejunal placement of the feeding tube when GRV is consistently greater than 500 mL.[4,19,20,35] In addition, use of a promotility agent, preferably metoclopramide, should be considered when GRV is greater than 250 mL after a second check.[19,20] These agents may improve feeding tolerance and formula delivery, and the risk of aspiration may be decreased, although the benefit of these agents has been questioned. If the feeding is held because of a high GRV, hourly evaluation of the GRV is recommended until the volume is less than 200 to 250 mL and the feeding is restarted. The fluid withdrawn for GRV assessment may be infused through the tube back into the stomach to minimize electrolyte imbalances; however, CCP guidelines suggest either discarding GRV or feeding back up to 250 mL may be acceptable.[19,20] Elevating the head of the bed to 30 to 45 degrees, with 45 degrees preferred in critically ill patients, during and after feedings also is recommended to reduce the risk of aspiration.[19,35,39]

Metabolic Complications

Major metabolic complications of EN include hyperglycemia, electrolyte abnormalities, and fluid imbalance. Although rigorous studies evaluating monitoring frequency are lacking, regular biochemical determinations similar to those used for PN are recommended to identify and correct metabolic abnormalities before severe abnormalities occur. Baseline values for serum glucose, SCr, BUN, and electrolytes should be available to guide selection of the enteral formula. The few baseline laboratory results available for M.P. may be adequate as a baseline, but additional laboratory parameters will be necessary as part of the monitoring regimen once EN starts.

Capillary glucose measurements every 6 hours or an insulin protocol is recommended before EN starts in diabetic or hyperglycemic patients or if hyperglycemia is anticipated. Given M.P.'s history of diabetes and a baseline glucose greater than 200 mg/dL, diligent monitoring and treatment of his hyperglycemia is warranted even before EN starts. M.P. will require long-term glucose monitoring; however, routine glucose monitoring in nondiabetic patients can be stopped once a stable euglycemic state is established with EN at the goal volume and infusion regimen.

A basic metabolic panel ([BMP]; serum glucose, sodium, potassium, chloride, bicarbonate, calcium, BUN, and SCr) is generally checked daily after feeding starts in critically ill patients and those at risk of electrolyte abnormalities or renal dysfunction. More stable patients may have serum glucose and electrolytes (sodium, potassium, chloride, bicarbonate) monitored rather than a BMP. During the first week of EN, whether initiated in the hospital or alternate site (SNF or at home), a BMP, phosphorus, and magnesium should be monitored a minimum of 2 to 3 times weekly in patients with weight loss; once or twice weekly may be adequate if there is no weight loss. Monitoring frequency can be reduced once tolerance to tube feeding is established and there are no metabolic abnormalities. Daily BMP for a minimum of 4 to 5 days is probably best for M.P. considering his recent dehydration. Daily phosphorus and magnesium also should be considered for a few days in M.P. because of his significant weight loss and risk of refeeding syndrome (see chapter 38 for a more detailed discussion of refeeding syndrome). Despite being obese, M.P. is at risk of electrolyte abnormalities associated with refeeding syndrome.[25]

Table 37-5
Complications of Tube Feeding

Complication	Cause/Contributing Factor	Treatment/Prevention
Mechanical Complications		
Aspiration	Deflated tracheostomy cuff	Inflate tracheostomy cuff before feeding; keep inflated 1 hour after feeding; consider small-bore feeding tube placed past the ligament of Treitz
	Displaced feeding tube	Reinsert tube, check placement; consider hand restraints or feeding tube bridle
	Reduced gastric emptying	Check residuals every 4–6 hours for gastric tube; raise head of bed 30–45 degrees; use lower-fat formula; use prokinetic medication; use small bowel feeding tube
	Lack of gag reflex; coma	Place feeding tube into jejunum; keep head of bed elevated to 45 degrees; provide continuous feeding
Nasal or pharyngeal irritation or necrosis; esophageal erosion; otitis media	Large-bore, polyvinyl chloride tube for long periods of time	Reposition tube daily, change tape; use smaller-bore tube; position tube to avoid pressure on tissues; moisten mouth and nose several times daily
Tube obstruction	Poorly crushed medications	Crush medications thoroughly, dissolve in water; use liquid medications whenever possible; check compatibility of medication with tube and formula
	Inadequate flushing after medications or thick formula	Flush tube with 50- to 150-mL water after medications or thick formula and every 4–6 hours with 30 mL minimum
	Poorly dissolved or mixed formula	Use blender to mix powdered formula (check manufacturer's mixing guidelines); use ready-to-use formula
	Formula mixed with low-pH substance	Avoid checking gastric residuals when safe to do so; use larger-diameter tubes when checking residuals; avoid administering acidic medications through small-diameter tubes; consider a nonacidic therapeutic alternative; flush with a minimum of 30-mL water before and immediately after medication administration
Gastrointestinal Complications		
Nausea, vomiting, distension, cramping	Too rapid administration	Slow administration rate; change bolus to intermittent infusion
	Osmolarity too high; intolerance to volume of formula	Use isotonic formula; increase the number of bolus or intermittent feedings so the volume per feeding is reduced, or change to continuous infusion; change to a more calorically dense formula if volume is the major problem (osmolarity will likely increase with higher caloric density)
	Gastric retention; poor GI motility	Place feeding tube distal to the pylorus; consider a promotility agent, such as metoclopramide; evaluate medications and change those possibly contributing to gastric dysmotility, if possible
Dumping syndrome (weakness, diaphoresis, palpitations)	Hyperosmolar load bolused or infused rapidly into the small bowel	Do not bolus into the small bowel; temporarily decrease continuous infusion rate and gradually increase rate after symptoms subside; use an isotonic formula
	Rate or volume of feeding increased too fast	Temporarily decrease continuous infusion rate or volume of intermittent or bolus feeding, and gradually increase rate after symptoms subside
Diarrhea	Atrophy of microvilli; malabsorption related to a disease process (e.g., pancreatitis, short bowel syndrome, Crohn disease)	Use a oligomeric formula until absorption improves; use a relatively isotonic and advance slowly; use a formula low in long-chain fatty acids when fat is malabsorbed and/or consider pancreatic enzymes
	Hypertonic formula	Change to a lower-osmolarity formula
	Dumping syndrome	See dumping syndrome entry in this table
	Rapid advancement of formula volume	Temporarily reduce rate or volume, then advance slowly; consider enteral pump for better control of administration rate
	Lactose intolerance	Change to lactose-free formula if previously using lactose-containing formula; evaluate lactose content of medications and supplemental foods, if patient is not strict NPO
	Contaminated formula	Hang fresh formula every 4 to 6 hours when using an open administration system; do not add fresh formula to volume remaining in the feeding container; change the formula container and tubing daily; follow clean/aseptic technique when working with the formula or feeding tube; minimize manipulation of the feeding tube; consider changing to a closed enteral system; avoid powdered formulas requiring reconstitution

(continued)

Table 37-5
Complications of Tube Feeding (*continued*)

Gastrointestinal Complications		
	Medications; antibiotics; magnesium-containing antacid; high-osmolarity liquid dosage forms	Check stool for *C. difficile* and treat if present; consider probiotic agent; administer antidiarrheal if not contraindicated; consider alternate therapy such as histamine-2 blocking agent or proton pump inhibitor; use calcium-based antacid; reduce dose or divide dose into 3–4/day, when feasible to do so; dilute medication with water before administrations; consider alternate dosage form (transdermal, IV); change to crushed tablet and use appropriate precautions to avoid tube occlusion
Constipation	Inadequate fluid or free-water intake	Increase volume and/or frequency of tube flushes to increase fluid intake; change to a formula with lower caloric density, if possible
	Inadequate fiber intake	Change to a formula with fiber or with a higher-fiber content; administer fruit juice or bulk-forming laxative (e.g., psyllium) using caution to prevent tube occlusion
	Fecal impaction	Administer stool softener daily using caution to prevent tube occlusion if administered via the tube
	Poor gastric/GI motility	Encourage ambulation; consider promotility agent
	Medications, especially narcotics and anticholinergics	Use lowest effective dose of medication and transition to an alternate medication with fewer constipating effects, if possible
Metabolic Complications		
Hyperglycemia, glycosuria (can lead to dehydration, coma, or death)	Stress response; diabetes mellitus	Monitor fingerstick glucose every 6 hours, use sliding scale insulin plus appropriate routine insulin (e.g., insulin drip in critically ill)
	High-carbohydrate formula	Change formula
	Drug therapy (steroids)	Monitor intake and output accurately
Excess CO_2 production (high RQ)	High percentage of carbohydrate calories or excess calories from any source	Reduce total calories to avoid overfeeding; consider formula with higher-fat calories
Hyponatremia	Dilutional (fluid excess, SIADH); inadequate sodium intake; excess GI losses	Use full-strength formula or change to 1.5–2 kcal/mL formula; add salt to tube feeding (1 tsp = 2 g Na = 90 mEq); use diuretics if appropriate; replace GI losses
Hypernatremia	Inadequate free-water intake	Use 1 kcal/mL formula; monitor intake and output accurately; temperature and weight daily; increase flush volume
	Excess water losses (diabetes insipidus, osmotic diuresis from hyperglycemia, fever)	Correct hyperglycemia and the cause of fever or diabetes insipidus
Hypokalemia	Medications (diuretics, antipseudomonal penicillins, amphotericin B)	Monitor serum potassium; give PO or IV potassium replacement PRN
	Intracellular or extracellular shifts (insulin therapy, acidosis)	Correct underlying problem
	Excess GI losses (NG suction, small bowel fistula, diarrhea)	Routinely provide potassium in replacement fluid
Hyperkalemia	Potassium-sparing medications (triamterene, amiloride, spironolactone, ACE inhibitors); potassium-containing medications (penicillin G potassium)	Monitor serum potassium; change to medications without potassium-sparing effect or without potassium salts
	Renal failure	Monitor renal function; change to formula with lower potassium content
Hypercoagulability	Warfarin antagonism due to formula	Hold formula 1–2 hours before and after warfarin dose; monitor coagulation status; check vitamin K content and change to lower vitamin K, if appropriate (most EN formulas are not high in vitamin K)

ACE, angiotensin-converting enzyme; EN, enteral nutrition; GI, gastrointestinal; IV, intravenous; NG, nasogastric; NPO, nothing by mouth; PO, oral; PRN, as needed; RQ, respiratory quotient; SIADH, syndrome of inappropriate antidiuretic hormone secretion.

Failure to monitor M.P. and replace electrolytes as necessary could result in serious electrolyte abnormalities. Once M.P.'s BMP, phosphorus, and magnesium are stable, the frequency of monitoring could be reduced to once or twice weekly. Critically ill patients generally require daily or every other day monitoring while in the ICU. For patients receiving long-term EN, the frequency of laboratory monitoring gradually is decreased. Laboratory monitoring should be done once or twice yearly in stable patients without significant medical problems. Patients who have medical problems that can affect nutrient, electrolyte, or trace element requirements or tolerances should be monitored as appropriate to the medical condition.

Weight and fluid status are important parameters to monitor throughout EN therapy, especially in patients with unusual losses, an inability to recognize thirst, or inability to voluntarily adjust their oral fluid intake. For hospitalized patients, weight is primarily a reflection of fluid status and increasing weight for 3 or 4 consecutive days may be an indication fluid intake needs to be reduced, whereas decreasing weight may indicate a need for increased fluid unless the patient had been fluid overloaded. Generally, total fluid can be adjusted by the number of times the feeding tube is flushed daily and the volume of each flush. In long-term patients, fluid is an important parameter for adequacy of caloric intake. Consistent increases or decreases from the required enteral formula volume can have significant effects on weight. For example, a weight loss of 12.5 pounds over the course of a year can be expected if the daily intake of a 1-kcal/mL formula is 120 mL less than required. Changing caloric density of the formula may be a potential option to help manage fluid when altering the number or volume of flushes is not adequate for fluid control. For patients with a stable fluid status, the week-to-week weight change can be used as an indicator of appropriate caloric intake. An upward trend in weight (e.g., ≥3 consecutive weeks with an increase) may indicate a need for fewer calories unless weight gain is a goal. A downward trend may indicate a need to increase caloric intake, unless weight loss is desired. A plan that includes gradual weight loss is appropriate for M.P. based on his obesity.

Respiratory status should be evaluated every 8 hours in hospitalized patients, to help recognize pulmonary edema and pulmonary aspiration. Auscultation with a stethoscope should be conducted at least 2 times per week, but simple observation of the patient's breathing pattern is adequate at other times unless altered respirations are noted. Coughing or respiratory distress may be indications of aspiration or other developing respiratory problems. Vital signs also may provide clues to aspiration or other problems, such as dehydration, fluid overload, or infection.

In addition to monitoring for complications, monitoring for response to EN and changes in nutritional status is recommended. This should occur routinely in patients receiving either short-term or long-term EN. Chapter 35, Basic Nutrition and Patient Assessment, discusses parameters used for nutrition assessment and ongoing monitoring of nutritional status.

Gastrointestinal Complications

Assessment of GI symptoms is important for determining EN tolerance because GI complications are frequently associated with tube feeding. Abdominal distension and bloating should be evaluated at least every 8 hours while M.P. is hospitalized. Abdominal distension may be an indication of accumulating formula. The possibility of falsely low GRV due to malposition or collapse of the tube during withdrawal of gastric fluid should be considered if abdominal distension occurs when GRV is low. Gas formation secondary to lactose intolerance or rapid increases in fiber intake, and poor gastric emptying secondary to a high-fat formula, medications, recent surgery, critical illness, or an underlying disease such as diabetes are among the conditions associated with distension. When considerable distension is present, the formula should be held temporarily, and the patient evaluated further to rule out a contraindication to EN.

Nausea, vomiting, abdominal cramping, diarrhea, and constipation are other GI symptoms monitored as indicators of EN tolerance. M.P. has some of these symptoms associated with his gastroparesis, and disease-associated symptoms should not be confused with feeding intolerance. Vomiting creates the most immediate concern because tube displacement and pulmonary aspiration can occur. Nausea and vomiting commonly occur with a high GRV, severe gastric distension, poor gastric emptying during gastric feeding, GI tract obstruction, or poor GI motility. Diarrhea occurs in 2% to 70% of patients, depending on the definition used, and is one of the most difficult problems for patients and caregivers to address.[34–37] Predisposing illnesses, including diabetes mellitus, GI infections, pancreatic insufficiency, and malabsorption syndromes, are more likely to cause diarrhea in patients receiving EN than the formula itself.[30,33,36] M.P. has type 2 diabetes; however, at this time, diarrhea has not been reported as a problem.

Formula-related GI infections could occur from contamination of an opened can or package. Sources of contamination include the water used for reconstitution or dilution, transfer to the delivery bag, formula kept in the delivery bag for a prolonged period, and poorly cleaned feeding bags or administration sets. Water used to flush the tube can also be a source of contamination; therefore, current practice recommendations are to use sterile water as the flush solution for immunocompromised patients.[35] Closed enteral feeding systems using ready-to-hang bags of formula decrease contamination by reducing manipulation of the bag and formula, and are commonly used in the hospital setting. Concurrent drug therapy (e.g., antibiotics) is another major contributor to diarrhea in tube-fed patients, potentially accounting for 61% of diarrhea cases.[30,36]

Bolus feeding into the jejunum can lead to diarrhea and abdominal cramping, as well as nausea and vomiting. Because M.P. is being fed into the jejunum, he should remain on a continuous infusion protocol. Initiation of EN with a hypertonic formula, a rapid rate of infusion or a large volume, and use of formula at refrigerator temperature are other factors often cited as causing GI symptoms. Although controlled studies have not supported these factors as significant contributors to GI intolerance, subjective evidence suggests they are important. Constipation is most likely to occur with long-term tube feeding in nonambulatory patients. Inadequate fluid intake and lack of fiber may be factors associated with constipation. Diabetic EN formulas contain fiber. However, if the decision is to use a very high protein formula for M.P., a fiber-containing formula would be reasonable to use based on his known history.

MEDICATIONS AND ENTERAL NUTRITION BY TUBE

Patients receiving EN often receive medications through the same tube. Feeding tube occlusion, adverse effects caused by changes in pharmaceutical dosage forms, and alteration of medication pharmacokinetics and pharmacodynamics are among the potential problems.[65–68] Interactions related to pharmacologic or physiologic effects of medications or enteral nutrients also may occur. For this reason, oral medication administration should be considered unless a strict NPO status is required. M.P. has severe gastroparesis, a diagnosis not requiring a strict NPO status; however, the medical team is concerned that medications administered by mouth may have erratic absorption and poor efficacy due to delayed gastric emptying. Medications are ordered to be administered through M.P.'s feeding tube.

CASE 37-4, QUESTION 3: M.P. has been receiving EN for 5 days and has been at goal rate for 2 days. Laboratory evaluation today shows the following:

Sodium, 137 mEq/L
Potassium, 2.8 mEq/L (decreased from 3.7 mEq/L yesterday, 4.1 mEq/L the previous day, and 4.8 mEq/L when tube feeding started)
Chloride, 97 mEq/L
Calcium, 7.8 mg/dL
Magnesium, 1.3 mEq/L (decreased from 2.5 mEq/L 2 days ago)
Phosphorus, 2.5 mg/dL (decreased from 4.7 mg/dL 2 days ago)
Albumin, 2.4 g/dL

Micro-K (8 mEq KCl/capsule) has been ordered as six capsules via feeding tube along with calcium carbonate (260-mg elemental calcium/tablet) as two tablets twice daily via feeding tube. Orders were also placed in the chart for warfarin. He was placed on a heparin drip yesterday for a newly diagnosed deep vein thrombosis (DVT) in his left leg, despite prophylactic heparin therapy since admission. Home medications are to be restarted, including enteric-coated aspirin, 81 mg daily; famotidine tablet, 20 mg twice daily; simvastatin tablet, 20 mg daily; metoprolol succinate tablet, 95 mg daily; and verapamil capsule, 240 mg daily. How should M.P.'s medications be administered when he is receiving EN?

Medication Selection

Solid dosage forms are a challenge to administer by feeding tube. Crushing a medication and mixing the powder in water results in an altered pharmaceutical dosage form, and this may affect its efficacy or patient tolerance. Liquid dosage forms are generally recommended for administration through a feeding tube, but they are not without problems, and a liquid dosage form may not always be the best choice. Liquids should be diluted at a minimum of 1:1 with water before administration to avoid coating the tube interior. High-viscosity liquids, such as suspensions, should be diluted 3:1 with water. Pharmaceutical syrups with a pH of 4 or less must be used with caution because immediate clumping and tackiness of formulas mixed with the syrups have been reported.[65,66] For medications not available in liquid form, a therapeutically equivalent medication in a liquid form can be considered. Extemporaneous preparation of a liquid also may be considered, but can increase cost significantly. Medications in a soft gelatin capsule are best avoided for administration through a feeding tube. If there is no alternative, the capsule can be dissolved in warm water. Undissolved gelatin should not be administered, because this may occlude the tube. The safety and efficacy of simple compressed tablets are not affected by crushing and dissolving in water immediately before use. Simple compressed tablets can be crushed to a fine powder, then dissolved or suspended in water for administration. Powder in hard gelatin capsules can be poured into water and mixed thoroughly before administration through a feeding tube. Failure to adequately suspend or thoroughly dissolve any of these dosage forms in water before administration through the tube can result in occlusion. Some medications appear to be particularly troublesome for administration through a feeding tube. Calcium salts, iron salts, lansoprazole, omeprazole, multivitamins, pentoxifylline, potassium chloride, phenytoin, protein supplements, sucralfate, and zinc salts were identified by nurses as the products most frequently contributing to feeding tube occlusion.[67,68] M.P. has both calcium and potassium ordered today.

Calcium carbonate is a simple compressed tablet that can be crushed, suspended in 30 mL of water, and administered through the feeding tube. Risk of tube occlusion from an inadequately crushed tablet may be decreased by use of calcium carbonate suspension (500-mg calcium/5 mL), if available. Administration of either crushed and suspended tablets or commercial suspension requires flushing the tube with 15 mL of water before and after medication administration.[35] Diluting the suspension at least 1:1 with water, preferably 3:1, and flushing with 75 to 100 mL may be advisable because suspensions may otherwise coat the tube. The appropriateness of calcium supplementation should be questioned, however, because M.P.'s serum calcium concentration is within normal limits after correction for his low serum albumin concentration, and the ionized calcium concentration would likely be within normal limits. Administering any medication via the feeding tube may occlude the tube; therefore, administering an unneeded medication through the feeding tube is an unwarranted risk. For calcium, and for electrolytes in general, only oral and IV dosage forms are available, so the easiest and most cost effective route is an oral dosage form via feeding tube if M.P. cannot take oral medications.

Potassium supplementation is ordered today for M.P.'s low serum potassium. Potassium should have been considered yesterday because the serum level has been decreasing since tube feeding began. The selected potassium supplement is inappropriate for administration by tube because Micro-K is a slow-release product. Crushing any type of slow-release or sustained-release product destroys slow-release mechanisms, resulting in the immediate release of several hours worth of the medication at one time. An exaggerated therapeutic response may be seen initially, followed by a loss of response part way through the dosing interval. Deaths have occurred when sustained-release or long-acting products are crushed before administrations; therefore, these dosage forms should not be crushed.[69] Instead, an immediate-release dosage form should be used, with appropriate adjustment of dose and dosing interval, or an alternate administration route (e.g., intravenous, suppository, transdermal patch) may be available. Potassium chloride powder for solution (three packets with 15 mEq KCl/packet) or liquid (10% KCl 35 mL, 15% KCl 25 mL, or 20% KCl 15–20 mL) should be ordered rather than the slow-release product. Dividing the potassium dose into two or three smaller doses and diluting each dose with 60 mL of water may be better tolerated. Giving 45 to 50 mEq of potassium as a single dose may cause nausea, vomiting, abdominal discomfort, or diarrhea. These symptoms might be mistaken as intolerance to EN, resulting in the tube feeding being stopped temporarily. The larger fluid volume for administration also may help reduce the GI irritation associated with potassium doses.

Potassium supplementation could also be partially accomplished by changing part of the potassium ordered to potassium phosphate, which is available as a 250-mg capsule that provides 8.1 mmol of phosphate and 14.2 mEq of potassium. M.P. appears to have a mild refeeding syndrome, with phosphorus and magnesium slightly less than the normal range and having decreased significantly during the past 2 days.[25] Supplements should be started today so that smaller daily quantities can be used before electrolytes are critically low. This may decrease the risk of diarrhea and GI upset caused by the administration of oral phosphate or magnesium. Contents of each potassium phosphate capsule are designed to be dissolved in 75 mL of water for administration, so dissolution is not a concern. One potassium phosphate capsule twice a day plus KCl liquid to provide 20 mEq potassium is the same potassium dose as is ordered currently. The liquid KCl dose should be separated from the potassium phosphate to minimize GI effects.

Magnesium supplementation could be accomplished with a magnesium oxide tablet (400 or 500 mg) administered 2 to 4 times daily. These are simple compressed tablets that can be crushed and suspended for administration via feeding tube. An alternative would be magnesium hydroxide suspension 5 mL 2 to 4 times daily. Magnesium doses are distributed through the day to reduce the risk of diarrhea. The feeding tube must be flushed adequately before and after each dose of electrolyte replacement. The flush volume should be a minimum of 15 mL, although 75 to 100 mL after the magnesium dose may be better to ensure the electrolyte preparation is out of the tube. The volume of other tube flushes can be adjusted to limit the total fluid intake to the estimated requirements. It can be difficult to provide large quantities of potassium, phosphate, and magnesium via feeding tube secondary to the GI intolerance they cause. Therefore, IV electrolyte replacement may be necessary if intracellular depletion is extensive and M.P. does not tolerate oral electrolyte replacement.

Famotidine is a simple compressed tablet that can be crushed. However, both the verapamil and metoprolol dosage forms ordered for M.P. contain multiple doses intended to be slowly released. The once-daily dosing schedule helps identify these two medications as slow-release products and, for metoprolol, the succinate salt is also a clue as this is different than other dosage forms of metoprolol. Both verapamil and metoprolol should be changed to immediate-release dosage forms if M.P. cannot take them by mouth. The dose and frequency of dosing will need to be adjusted to reflect the immediate release dosage form.

Enteric-coated tablets are designed to release medication in the small bowel because the medication is either acid labile or irritates the stomach. Protection for the medication or stomach is lost when enteric-coated tablets are crushed and delivered via feeding tube into the stomach, resulting in decreased efficacy of the medication or increased gastric irritation. When an irritating medication must be given by tube into the stomach, diluting the medication in at least 60 mL of water is recommended.[65] M.P. has enteric-coated aspirin ordered for administration into a jejunal feeding tube. The enteric coating is designed to dissolve in the small bowel and could be dissolved with bicarbonate solution before administration into the small bowel. However, it would be better to use a noncoated tablet for his aspirin dose. If enteric-coated beads, such as those found in several proton pump inhibitor dosage forms, are to be administered through a feeding tube, use of an acidic liquid (e.g., fruit juice) helps prevent the enteric coating from becoming sticky and adhering to the inside of the feeding tube. This should only be considered for a large-bore feeding tube, such as a gastrostomy, or the beads will occlude the tube. Film-coated tablets also cause problems when crushed because the coating does not crush well and becomes sticky in water. M.P.'s simvastatin has a film coating and may be a problem to crush and administer through the feeding tube.

Administering buccal or sublingual dosage forms via feeding tube may result in altered absorption or destruction of the medication by stomach acid. Therefore, therapeutically equivalent medications (e.g., isosorbide dinitrate rather than sublingual nitroglycerin) or an alternate route of administration (e.g., nitroglycerin ointment or transdermal system rather than sublingual nitroglycerin) should be used. A listing of medications that should not be crushed is available at **http://www.ismp.org/Tools/DoNotCrush.pdf**.[70] Carcinogens, teratogens, or cytotoxic agents that should not be crushed are included in the list.

Pharmacokinetic parameters can be altered when medications are administered by feeding tube. M.P. has a jejunal tube and delivering medication into the jejunum could affect bioavailability, although few studies address this issue. Medications taken orally are delivered to the stomach, where dissolution occurs for most dosage forms and hydrolysis of some medications may occur. Delivery into the small bowel may alter these processes, thereby affecting bioavailability. For instance, recovery of digoxin from intrajejunal dosing is higher than with oral administration, primarily because of reduced intragastric hydrolysis.[28,65] Bioavailability of medications also can be affected by the presence of enteral formula in the GI tract. Medications affected by the presence of food are expected to be affected in a similar manner by the presence of formula.[66,68] For example, administration of tetracycline with formula present is expected to reduce tetracycline bioavailability because of interactions with divalent cations. A similar interaction is expected between ciprofloxacin and enteral formula, although some evidence suggests a mechanism other than binding with divalent cations is responsible for reduced ciprofloxacin concentrations with enteral feeding.[28]

Phenytoin is particularly troublesome to manage in patients receiving EN, with reduced phenytoin concentrations reported in numerous case reports and small studies. Methods suggested for management include using a meat-based formula, administering phenytoin capsules rather than the suspension, and stopping formula delivery for 1 to 2 hours before and after the phenytoin dose.[65,71] Holding formula administration before and after phenytoin dosing is often recommended, although others claim that adequate dilution will reduce loss of the medication. None of these methods, however, clearly prevents low phenytoin concentrations; thus, monitoring of serum concentrations is important whenever EN is started or altered. Large-scale, controlled trials are needed to determine the most appropriate method for managing the phenytoin–EN interaction.

Warfarin can also be troublesome to manage in patients with a feeding tube, and M.P. is to start warfarin for a newly diagnosed DVT. Reversal of warfarin anticoagulation by vitamin K included in enteral formulas is an important pharmacologic interaction.[28] The vitamin K content of most enteral formulas today is about the same as found in a mixed diet and is unlikely to interfere with anticoagulation, but should be evaluated if adequate anticoagulation is difficult to achieve. In addition, binding of warfarin to a component of enteral formulas, likely protein, has been proposed to explain warfarin resistance with formulas containing low vitamin K content; others suggest binding to the feeding tube itself may occur.[28,66] Stopping formula administration for an hour before and after warfarin administration appears to prevent this type of interaction. Unfortunately, rigorous, randomized studies to provide evidenced based guidance for the management of this potential interaction are lacking.

Liquid dosage forms are often hypertonic. Diarrhea is a potential problem related to physiologic effects of hypertonic medications. Diluting hypertonic medications (e.g., potassium chloride) with 30 to 60 mL of water before administration is suggested. Dividing the medication dose and separating doses by about 2 hours also decrease GI effects of hypertonic medications. In addition, selection of brands and dosage forms with minimal sorbitol can reduce the risk of diarrhea. Sorbitol is a nonabsorbed sugar alcohol found in many liquid dosage forms. Cumulative sorbitol doses greater than 5 g can cause bloating and flatulence, whereas larger doses may act as a cathartic.[35,65,66]

Tube Occlusion

CASE 37-4, QUESTION 4: M.P.'s feeding tube has occluded (clogged). What are the causes of feeding tube occlusion and how can occlusions be managed? What can be done to avoid occluding M.P.'s tube in the future?

The incidence of feeding tube occlusion is 1.6% to 66%.[9,34,35,67] Pump malfunction, lack of periodic tube flushing, formula characteristics, and tube characteristics are nonmedication-related factors affecting tube occlusion. Important tube characteristics include the inner diameter (bore size), tube material, and the arrangement and number of delivery holes (ports) at the distal end. The most important formula characteristic appears to be the protein source. In vitro studies suggest formulas with intact protein, particularly caseinates or soy, coagulate and clump when exposed to an acidic pH, whereas formulas with hydrolyzed protein do not.[28,65]

Medication-related factors influencing feeding tube occlusion include the administration method, dosage form, pH, and viscosity. Medications must be crushed to a fine powder, mixed with water to form a smooth slurry, and adequately diluted before administration. Medications admixed with formula have the greatest potential for occluding tubes owing to alteration of the texture, viscosity, or physical form of the medication or formula. Therefore, medications should not be admixed directly with formula. The enteral formula infusion should be stopped, and the tube flushed with a minimum of 15-mL water before and after medication administration and with 15 mL between each medication.[34,35,36,39,65] Contact between medications and formula within the tube lumen should be limited to decrease the risk of occlusion. Each medication should be administered separately to reduce the risk of interactions.

When a feeding tube occludes, it must be replaced unless patency can be restored. Frequent tube replacement disrupts nutrient delivery and increases patient discomfort as well as the cost of care. The initial treatment for tube occlusion is to flush the tube with warm water using a large syringe, at least 20 mL but preferably 50 mL, to avoid generation of excessive pressure that could rupture the tube. When a specific cause for occlusion can be identified (e.g., a specific medication) and physiochemical characteristics of the responsible product are known (e.g., solubility, pH), it may be possible to select a more appropriate flush preparation than water. In most cases, however, use of an acidic or basic flush preparation could worsen the occlusion. Acidic liquids (e.g., cranberry juice, diet soda, regular soda) may perpetuate or extend the occlusion, especially when coagulated proteins are the cause.[65,66] When water fails to restore patency, activated pancreatic enzymes may be effective. Previously, one crushed pancrelipase tablet and one sodium bicarbonate tablet (324 mg) were dissolved in 5 mL of warm water just before instillation into the occluded tube.[36,65] A product containing multiple enzymes, buffers, and antibacterial agents in a powder form (Clog Zapper) is commercially available. Adherence to flush protocols and proper medication administration techniques are essential to maintain patency once tube patency is restored.

Transfer to Home on Enteral Nutrition

CASE 37-5

QUESTION 1: D.S., an 80-year-old man, was admitted 2 days ago from an SNF for evaluation of large bruises on his right arm and shoulder and possible collarbone fracture due to a fall. He receives intermittent feedings through his PEG. The volume is 1,680 mL (seven cans) daily. D.S.'s history indicates he was hospitalized approximately 7 weeks ago with an ischemic stroke and was discharged to an SNF (see Case 37-2). D.S.'s tube-feeding volume has increased from 1,440 mL on discharge, but the formula remains the same (1.06 kcal/mL, 0.044 g protein/mL, 15 g fiber/1,000 kcal polymeric formula). His weight has increased 2 kg since hospital discharge, and his overall status has improved. Bone fracture is ruled out and D.S. is able to participate in physical therapy (PT). The PT consult indicates D.S. can ambulate safely with a walker and is able to transfer from bed to chair and to the bedside commode with minimal assistance. He is deemed appropriate for outpatient PT after hospital discharge. The swallow study performed this morning indicates D.S. must continue NPO for at least another 4 months when the swallow study will be repeated again. D.S.'s daughter has made arrangements for him to move in with her family. She is concerned about insurance coverage for the EN therapy and states D.S. has Medicare insurance, including a Part D prescription plan. Will Medicare cover EN?

Before addressing the coverage of EN therapy in the home, it should be determined whether D.S. is an appropriate candidate for home versus return to the SNF. Based on the PT assessment, it is likely D.S. is appropriate for discharge home, providing he will have some supervision and assistance available. Typically, a case manager or social worker is involved in arranging appropriate discharge facilities; however, the healthcare professional managing nutrition support in the hospital setting should facilitate the nutrition support portion of discharge, as necessary. The pharmacist should review the medication regimen to assure it is appropriate for administration through the feeding tube.

Strict guidelines exist for home EN coverage. Medicare Part B (not Part D) will cover 80% of the cost if criteria are met.[72–74] EN must be medically necessary to "maintain weight and strength commensurate with overall health status" and there must be a functional disability of the GI tract (e.g., dysphagia, swallowing disorder) that is expected to be "permanent." The formula must be delivered by feeding tube (i.e., not oral supplements) and must provide most of the patient's nutritional requirements (i.e., not supplemental nutrition). Approval is on an individual basis, requires a physician's written order, and sufficient documentation must be available to support the need for EN. Calories less than 20 kcal/kg/day or greater than 35 kcal/kg/day require additional documentation. The duration of therapy must be 90 days or more to meet the test of permanence. D.S.'s therapy falls within these guidelines. In addition, the formula D.S. receives is in a category that does not require him to meet additional eligibility criteria related to the formula itself. Additional documentation would be needed to justify a pump if D.S. was receiving EN via pump.

Enteral formulas are divided into five categories for reimbursement purposes by Medicare Part B (Table 37-6). Formula manufacturers typically list the Medicare category on the product label. Most polymeric formulas containing intact (whole) protein and 1 to 1.2 kcal/mL are in category I. These products do not require documentation of medical necessity for the specific formula itself, but still require documentation of the need for EN. Clear documentation of medical need for formulas in specific categories (e.g., categories III and IV) is required for their higher reimbursement rates. Appropriate forms available from the Centers for Medicare and Medicaid must be completed for Medicare reimbursement of any EN therapy.[75]

Evaluation of Tube Feeding Intolerance

CASE 37-6

QUESTION 1: J.N., a 30-year-old man, was admitted to the hospital 70 days ago after a motor vehicle crash. He sustained multiple traumatic injuries and exhibited multiple complications requiring several exploratory laparotomies. He has been treated for multiple infections, including pneumonia, sepsis, and wound infection. Treatment for *Clostridium difficile* diarrhea was completed 3 weeks ago and he has not had diarrhea since then. Lysis of adhesions, closure of an enterocutaneous fistula, and placement of a feeding jejunostomy tube (J tube) were done during the last laparotomy

9 days ago. Enteral feedings were started through his J tube 4 days ago and advanced to the goal rate of 90 mL/hour within 24 hours. The EN lactose-free and fiber-free, 460 mOsm/kg, contains 15% of calories from a 50% MCT–50% long-chain triglycerides fat mix, and provides 35 kcal/kg/day and 1.6 g protein/kg/day, which is less than his protein goal. The product is ready-to-use in a closed-system bag. J.N. has received PN for nutrition during most of his hospitalization and the PN rate was decreased as EN increased. J.N. now has diarrhea, which started approximately 12 hours after his EN was increased to goal rate. What is the likely cause of diarrhea? What other information related to the EN regimen would be helpful to determine whether the EN should be stopped and the PN formulation restarted?

Diarrhea develops in 12% to 32% of hospitalized patients, and in up to 80% of high-risk patients; a point preference of 12.4% has been reported.[76] In patients receiving EN, 15% to 40% develop diarrhea, which is multifactorial. Factors associated with diarrhea, but not related to EN, include medications, partial small bowel obstruction or fecal impaction, bile salt malabsorption, intestinal atrophy, hypoalbuminemia, malnutrition, infections such as *C. difficile*, and underlying conditions affecting the GI tract.[4,30,36,37,39,65,66,76–78] The LOS, particularly over 3 weeks, and EN over 11 days have also been associated with developing diarrhea.[77,79] Tube feeding-related causes of diarrhea include high-fat content, lactose content, and bacterial contamination. Formula temperature, caloric density, osmolality, formula strength, lack of fiber content, and method of delivery have been associated with diarrhea, although these factors are not shown to affect diarrhea in some studies, making a cause-and-effect relationship unclear.[78,79]

J.N.'s hospitalization has been unusually long and complicated. Many factors could contribute to diarrhea; however, the diarrhea coincides relatively closely with initiation and advancement of tube feeding. He may have intestinal atrophy and impaired absorptive function because of his prolonged period without GI tract stimulation. He has had multiple surgeries, including GI surgeries, and may have reduced absorptive capacity, bile salt malabsorption, dumping syndrome, or reduced pancreatic enzyme availability related to his complications and surgeries. At least theoretically, an oligomeric formula would be better absorbed if any of these conditions exist. The SCCM–ASPEN guidelines recommend a standard formulation for those not meeting guidelines for an immune-modulating product.[4] The CCP guidelines were downgraded in 2013 from recommending use of a polymeric formula to consider use of a polymeric formula, although clinical outcomes do not appear to differ between the types of formula.[18–20] However, studies have not evaluated patients without use of the GI tract for weeks before EN initiation. Formula selection is often determined by physician preference and the calorie, protein, and fat content of formulas on the institution's formulary. Because J.N. had been more than 2 months without significant use of the GI tract, he was started on an oligomeric formula.

The EN formula selected for J.N. is only slightly more than isotonic. Risk of diarrhea from fat malabsorption should be minimal with the low-fat content and MCT mix. Increasing EN to goal rate within 24 hours may have contributed to diarrhea. Initiation at 10 to 20 mL/hour and advancement by 10 mL every 8 to 12 hours to reach goal in 48 to 72 hours would have been appropriate for J.N. because he had not used his GI tract for over 2 months.[33–37] The jejunum adapts slowly to changes in volume or concentration, and formula volume was increased less than

Table 37-6
Medicare Categories for Enteral Formulas

Category and Code[a]	Description	Examples (Partial Listing)
Category I B4150	Semisynthetic intact protein or protein isolates (general purpose formulas)	Boost, Isosource HN, Jevity 1.0 Cal, Nutren1.0 Fiber, Osmolite 1.2 Cal
Category II B4152	Intact protein or protein isolates; calorically dense	Boost Plus, Ensure Plus HN, Isosource 1.5 Cal, Jevity 1.5 Cal, Nutren 2.0, Resource 2.0
Category III[b] B4153	Hydrolyzed protein or amino acids	Optimental, Peptamen 1.5, Peptamen AF, Perative, Vital HN Documentation that may provide justification for use: dumping syndrome, uncontrolled diarrhea, evidence of malabsorption on appropriate semisynthetic formulas (e.g., isotonic, low long-chain fat content, lactose-free) that resolves with an oligomeric formula or documentation of the disease process causing malabsorption
Category IV[b] B4154	Defined formula for special metabolic need (i.e., disease-specific formulas)	Advera, Alitraq, Glucerna 1.0, Glucerna 1.5, NutriHep, Nepro with Carb Steady, Nutren Renal, Oxepa, Peptamen, Pulmocare, Renalcal, Suplena with Carb Steady Documentation that may provide justification for use: evidence of inability to meet nutritional goals with category I or II products without compromising patient safety and documentation of the specific diagnosis for which a formula is intended
Category V[b] B4155	Modular components for protein, fat, and carbohydrate	*Protein:* Complete amino acid mix, ProMod Liquid Protein Carbohydrate: Moducal, Polycal, Polycose Carbohydrate and Fat: Duocal Fat: MCT oil Documentation that may provide justification for use: inability to meet specific nutrient requirements (i.e., protein, carbohydrate, or fat) with a commercially available formula

[a]Code refers to the Health Care Procedure Code System (HCPCS) billing code used by providers billing the Center for Medicare and Medicaid.
[b]Failure to provide adequate documentation of medical necessity for the specific formula will likely result in denial of claim or payment at the lower category I rate for Medicare Part B insurance coverage.
MCT, medium-chain triglyceride.

24 hours before diarrhea started. Also, an enteral infusion pump should be used to maintain consistent flow. Changing to a lower volume should decrease stool output within 24 hours if the volume change was responsible. If J.N. does not respond to decreasing formula volume, the formula may be held for 24 hours to assess whether diarrhea decreases or stops. Diarrhea related directly to EN usually is an osmotic diarrhea that stops within 24 hours of stopping the formula.[39] A more objective approach than stopping the formula is to measure stool osmolality. Enteral-formula-induced diarrhea is associated with a large osmotic gap, whereas secretory diarrhea (e.g., infectious diarrhea) is associated with a low or negative osmotic gap.[39]

The selected oligomeric formula is ready-to-use and in a closed-system bag; therefore, bacterial contamination from mixing technique is not of concern. Cleanliness during formula transfer to the delivery bag, the period of time formula is in the bag, and methods of cleaning the delivery bag may contribute to bacterial contamination of formula. J.N. is receiving formula from a closed enteral system (i.e., ready-to-hang formula-filled containers), and this virtually eliminates transfer-related contamination when proper technique is used. Any addition (e.g., medication, carbohydrate, fat or protein module, MCT oil) to the prefilled container before hanging can contaminate the system, and guidelines (e.g., hang-time, set changes) for an open enteral system then apply. Even when administered separately from the formula, modular components are a potential contributor to diarrhea due to their osmolarity and potential contamination during preparation and administration. The selected formula does not meet J.N.'s protein requirement; therefore, a modular protein is needed to supplement the enteral formula. The nutrition plan includes addition of a modular protein component; however, on review of the medication administration record, this has been started.

Medications are a major contributor to diarrhea in tube-fed patients.[30,36,77–79] J.N. currently receives antibiotics and has for some time. However, the prevalence of diarrhea with antibiotic therapy is difficult to determine due to failure to report stool frequency and consistency as well as lack of a clear definition of diarrhea. *C. difficile* may have relapsed after his previous treatment. Stool specimens should be sent for culture and/or *C. difficile* toxin. Evaluation of J.N.'s medications may reveal medications associated with diarrhea (e.g., sorbitol-containing products, antacids, oral magnesium, potassium chloride, phosphate supplements, H_2 receptor antagonists) for which therapeutic alternatives or different routes of administration could be considered.[28,36] High-osmolality liquid medications should be diluted before administration to reduce GI side effects.[34,35,65,66]

J.N.'s GI tract should continue to be used to the extent possible. EN appears to be better than PN for maintaining the GI tract barrier and host immunologic function.[4,18–20,49,55] Both the CCP and SCCM–ASPEN guidelines recommend use of EN over PN in critically ill patients.[4,18–20] Both guidelines also recognize the need for PN at some point when EN cannot meet the patient's nutritional requirements; however, neither guideline addresses patients with long-term, chronic critical illness such as J.N. The risk of sepsis increases without enteral stimulation of the GI tract. Whether this occurs through bacterial translocation, an unproved process in humans in which enteric bacteria or endotoxin crosses the GI mucosa into mesenteric lymph nodes and portal circulation, or through another mechanism is unclear. In addition, the GI tract serves an immune function, especially with respect to IgA secretion. Respiratory tract infections, such as pneumonia, may increase without proper stimulation of the GI tract, owing to less-effective protection from IgA. Compared with PN, EN attenuates catabolism in highly stressed patients, although initiation of feedings soon after the stressing event may be required to obtain this response. Before a decision is made to stop J.N.'s EN, all possible causes of diarrhea should be investigated. Possible benefits of improved fluid and electrolyte balance from stopping EN should be weighed against the potential benefits of reduced infections from continued use of the GI tract. Combined EN plus PN can also be considered, especially if J.N. tolerates partial EN but cannot advance to goal rate. Full PN should be provided if EN is stopped for more than 1 or 2 days.

KEY REFERENCES AND WEBSITES

A full list of references for this chapter can be found at http://thepoint.lww.com/AT11e. Below are the key references and websites for this chapter, with the corresponding reference number in this chapter found in parentheses after the reference.

Key References

Bankhead R et al. Enteral nutrition practice recommendations. *JPEN J Parenter Enteral Nutr*. 2009;33:122. (35)

Mueller C et al, eds. The A.S.P.E.N. *Adult Nutrition Support Core Curriculum*. 2nd ed. Silver Spring, MD: American Society for Parenteral and Enteral Nutrition; 2012. (2, 3, 7, 21, 26, 37, 52, 65)

McClave SA et al. Guidelines for the Provision and Assessment of Nutrition Support Therapy in the Adult Critically Ill Patient: Society of Critical Care Medicine (SCCM) and American Society for Parenteral and Enteral Nutrition (A.S.P.E.N.). *JPEN J Parenter Enteral Nutr*. 2016;40(2):159-211. (4)

Dhaliwal R et al. The Canadian Critical Care Nutrition Guidelines in 2013: an update on current recommendations and implementation strategies. *Nutr Clin Pract*. 2014;29(1):29. (20)

Kraft MD et al. Review of the refeeding syndrome. *Nutr Clin Pract*. 2005;20:625. (25)

Key Websites

American Society for Parenteral and Enteral Nutrition. http://www.nutritioncare.org and http://www.nutritioncare.org/Guidelines_and_Clinical_Resources/Clinical_Guidelines/. To access content for:

- McClave SA et al. Guidelines for the Provision and Assessment of Nutrition Support Therapy in the Adult Critically Ill Patient: Society of Critical Care Medicine (SCCM) and American Society for Parenteral and Enteral Nutrition (A.S.P.E.N.). *JPEN J Parenter Enteral Nutr*. 2016;40(2):159-211. (4)
- McMahon MM et al. A.S.P.E.N. clinical guidelines: nutrition support of adult patients with hyperglycemia. *Nutr Clin Pract*. 2013;37910:23. (64)
- Bankhead R et al. Enteral Nutrition Practice Recommendations—[Endorsed by the American Dietetic Association (ADA), the American Society of Health-System Pharmacists (ASHP) and the Institute for Safe Medication Practices (ISMP)]. *J Parenter Enteral Nutr*. 2009;33:122. (35)

Heyland DK et al. Canadian Clinical Practice Guidelines. Summary of topics and recommendations. Critical Care Nutrition. *J Parenter Enteral Nutr*. 2003;27:355. http://www.criticalcarenutrition.com/index.php?option=com_content&review=article&id=18&Itemid=10. Accessed August 20, 2015. (19)

Global Enteral Device Supplier Association (GEDSA). Stay Connected initiative. Enhancing patient safety. http://www.StayConnected2015.org. (38)

Dhaliwal R et al. The Canadian critical care nutrition guidelines in 2013: an update on current recommendations and implementation strategies. *Nutr Clin Pract*. 2014;29(1):29-43. www.criticalcarenutrition.com/cpgs/2013.

Institute for Safe Medication Practices (ISMP). Oral dosage forms that should not be crushed. http://www.ismp.org/Tools/DoNotCrush.pdf. Accessed July 21, 2015. (70)

38 Adult Parenteral Nutrition

Susan L. Mayhew and Richard S. Nicholas

CORE PRINCIPLES

	CORE PRINCIPLES	CHAPTER CASES
1	Parenteral nutrition (PN) formulations are complex intravenous (IV) admixtures that require strict adherence to safe compounding practices.	**Case 38-2 (Questions 5-8), Case 38-3 (Question 8), Case 38-4 (Question 7), Tables 38-1, 38-2 and 38-4**
2	Parenteral nutrition (PN) is indicated in patients with a nonfunctioning gastrointestinal tract. Patients should be assessed for appropriate indications of the use of PN.	**Case 38-2 (Question 1), Table 38-3**
3	Calories, protein, fluid, electrolytes, vitamins and minerals are based on the patient's individual needs and are determined by baseline nutritional status, medical history, clinical presentation and IV access.	**Case 38-1 (Questions 1-6), Case 38-2 (Question 4), Case 38-3 (Questions 1, 4, 5 and 9), Case 38-4 (Question 1, 2, 4 and 5), Tables 38-6–38-8**
4	Before PN is initiated, the practitioner must be aware of potential metabolic and respiratory complications, including refeeding syndrome, increased carbon dioxide production, and hyperglycemia. Appropriate fluid, macronutrient, and micronutrient adjustments to specialized nutrition support must be implemented to avoid or diminish the expected complications.	**Case 38-2 (Questions 3 and 9), Case 38-3 (Questions 2, 3, and 6, 7), Case 38-4 (Question 3)**
5	Appropriate monitoring of the patient's vital signs, body weight, temperature, serum chemistries, hematologic indices, nutrition intake, and fluid intake and output are essential to determine the success of PN therapy and to make changes in therapy.	**Case 38-2 (Question 9), Case 38-3 (Question 7), Table 38-5**
6	Advancements in the delivery of home PN have increased patients' acceptance and empowered engagement in self-care. An understanding of the patient's fluid and nutrient needs is essential for optimal delivery of home PN, to help ensure positive outcomes and the best quality of life for the patient.	**Case 38-4 (Questions 5 and 6)**
7	Practitioners should be aware of the additional complications associated with home (or long-term) delivery of PN including hepatobiliary complications, metabolic bone disease, and catheter-related complications.	**Case 38-4 (Questions 7–9)**
8	Fluid requirements, macronutrient selections, electrolyte quantities, and vitamin and mineral alterations may be warranted in patients presenting with hepatic or renal failure, short bowel syndrome, obesity, diabetes, pancreatitis, and respiratory failure.	**Case 38-1 (Question 2), Case 38-3 (Questions 1-3), Case 38-4 (Questions 3 and 5)**

It has long been established that a patient's nutritional status directly impacts recovery from illness or injury. Malnutrition is associated with multiple complications including poor wound healing, infection, prolonged hospital stays, and increased mortality.[1] The preferred method of providing nutritional support is through the gastrointestinal (GI) tract. If using the GI tract is not feasible, intravenous feeding is an option. For centuries clinicians attempted intravenous feeding using crude intravenous cannulas and nutritional substances ranging from olive oil to cow's milk. Unfortunately, historical attempts at using the vascular system for nutritional support were fraught with challenges. Clinicians were limited by the amount of calories administered, lack of reliable intravenous (IV) access, and risk of infection because of a lack of sterility.[2]

The advent of central venous catheters (CVCs) in the 1960s ushered in the contemporary practice of intravenous feeding—parenteral nutrition (PN) therapy. CVCs allow the administration of concentrated nutritional admixtures that are rapidly diluted in the systemic circulation. Prior to the development of central catheters, peripheral catheters were used which limited the amount of calories and nutrients that could be safely administered.[3]

VENOUS ACCESS SITES

PN formulations are administered through peripheral or central veins. The type of venous access utilized primarily depends on the anticipated duration of therapy and nutrient requirements of the patient.[1]

Peripheral Venous Access

Peripheral venous access is generally the route of choice when PN is expected to be utilized for less than 10 days and when energy and protein requirements are low to moderate. Patients requiring peripheral parenteral nutrition (PPN) must have good peripheral venous access and must be able to tolerate large volumes of fluids, because of the low concentrations of dextrose and amino acids used in PPN formulations.[4]

PN formulations are hypertonic and irritating to peripheral veins. In adults, the osmolarity of PPN formulations should be maintained below 900 mOsm/L (normal serum osmolality 280–300 mOsm/L) to minimize vein irritation and patient discomfort. With peripheral venous access, low final concentrations of dextrose (5%–10%) and amino acids (3%–5%) are necessary and frequent venous access site rotation (every 48–72 hours) is required. Several liters of PPN may be needed daily to meet energy and protein needs of the patient because of the dilute nature of the peripheral admixture. Caloric density of peripheral formulations is less than 1 kcal/mL and can be increased by administering intravenous lipids concurrently or by adding lipids to the dextrose and amino acid mixture. Lipids may protect the vein against irritation through dilution and by a buffering effect.[5,6]

Central Venous Access

Central venous access is the preferred route of administration of PN formulations for patients who have a nonfunctional GI tract, require bowel rest for more than 7 days, have limited peripheral venous access, or have energy and protein needs that cannot be met with peripheral nutrient formulations.[1,4,7]

Traditionally, the CVC is percutaneously inserted into the subclavian vein and threaded through the vein so the tip rests in the upper portion of the superior vena cava (SVC) just above the right atrium. A newer catheter technique involves the use of a peripherally inserted central catheter (PICC) that is inserted in the antecubital vein and advanced until the end of the catheter reaches the upper SVC.[7–9] The internal and external jugular veins may also be used to thread a catheter into the SVC; however, maintaining a sterile dressing on these sites is more difficult than with the subclavian or PICC approach. The SVC is an area of rapid blood flow, which quickly dilutes concentrated parenteral nutrient formulations, thereby minimizing phlebitis or thrombosis. Some patients are not candidates for placement of catheters in the SVC and require a femoral vein insertion with the tip of the catheter in the inferior vena cava. There may be a greater risk for infection with catheters placed using this technique.[6,7]

Differing from PPN, parenteral nutrient formulations designed for administration through central veins often contain relatively high concentrations of dextrose (20%–35%) and amino acids (5%–10%), plus lipids. The central PN formulation typically provides a caloric density greater than 1 kcal/mL and an osmolarity greater than 2,000 mOsm/L. Central PN formulations are often termed total PN because complete nutrient needs of the patient may be delivered by this route.

COMPONENTS OF PARENTERAL NUTRIENT FORMULATIONS

PN formulations are complex mixtures containing up to 40 different nutrient components, including energy substrates such as carbohydrate (dextrose), protein (amino acids), and fat (lipid or IV fat emulsion), along with water, electrolytes, vitamins, and trace minerals. Various combinations of these components are prepared under aseptic conditions based upon individual patient needs.[10,11] The three macronutrients used in PN formulations are available in various concentrations from manufacturers. Sterile water for injection is used to dilute the macronutrients to achieve the prescribed final concentrations of dextrose, amino acids, and lipids, as well as the final volume of the PN formulation.

PN formulations may be prepared in one of two ways, a dextrose–amino acid (2-in-1) mixture in which IV fat emulsion (IVFE) is administered separately as a piggybacked infusion or a total nutrient admixture (TNA or 3-in-1) in which the dextrose, amino acids, and IVFE are combined in solution in the same bag. Premixed PN solutions are also available commercially in different percentages of dextrose and amino acid preparations. Premixed PN solutions are sterile products that have a longer shelf life; however, these formulations limit the ability to customize the final product to meet individual patient needs.

Errors have occurred in preparing and managing this complex therapy, resulting in patient harm and death. A responsibility of the pharmacist is to ensure safe, accurate, and sterile preparation of the PN formulation. Guidelines for safe practices have been developed for situations in which inconsistent practices have the potential to cause harm. Pharmaceutical problem areas that are addressed in the Safe Practices for Parenteral Nutrition Formulations are compounding, formulas, labeling, stability, and filtering of PN formulations.[12]

PN is a costly therapy. Costs associated with PN therapy include not only the admixture but also the expense of obtaining venous access, laboratory monitoring, and treatment of complications of therapy. Because of the cost and complexity of PN therapy, its use should be scrutinized and reserved for patients who will benefit from it.

Carbohydrate

Dextrose in water is the most common carbohydrate for IV use. It is available commercially in concentrations ranging from 2.5% to 70%. Dextrose solutions are mixed with other components of the PN formulation and diluted to various final concentrations with sterile water for injection. Dextrose in its hydrated form provides 3.4 kcal/g, compared with dietary carbohydrate which provides 4 kcal/g.

Another carbohydrate energy substrate is glycerol, a sugar alcohol with a caloric density of 4.3 kcal/g. It is available as a premixed PN formulation (3% glycerol with 3% AAs) for administration as PPN. Because of the dilute concentrations of this premixed formulation, large volumes are generally necessary to meet caloric requirements.

Lipid

Lipid or intravenous fat emulsion (IVFE) is the most calorically dense macronutrient for infusion and a source of essential fatty acids (FA). The optimal composition of IVFE has been a focus of clinical debate because of the potential to influence immune function, inflammatory response, and liver function. This has prompted research into the development of new lipid formulations (structured lipids) in which part of the n-6 polyunsaturated fatty acids (PUFA) has been replaced by less bioactive FAs, such as coconut oil (rich in medium chain saturated FA), olive oil (rich in n-9 monounsaturated FA oleic acid), or fish oil (rich in n-3 polyunsaturated FA)—challenging the traditional soybean oil and soybean/safflower oil emulsions (n-6 FA).[13] While structured IVFEs have been used for years outside of the United States, the US Food and Drug Administration has recently approved an IVFE formulated with a 4:1 combination of olive oil and soybean oil[14] and another IVFE formulation containing soybean oil, medium-chain triglycerides (MCT), olive oil and fish oil.[13,14]

The traditional IVFEs are available commercially as 10% (1.1 kcal/mL), 20% (2.0 kcal/mL), and 30% (3.0 kcal/mL) concentrations. While each gram of fat provides 9 kcal, the caloric density of the IVFE is increased slightly because of the glycerol within the IVFE such that each milliliter of 10% IVFE provides 1.1 kcals, and each milliliter of 20% and 30% IVFE provides 2.0 kcal/mL and 3.0 kcal/mL respectively. Other components of the IVFE include glycerol to make the formulation isotonic, egg phospholipid as an emulsifier, vitamin K, and sodium hydroxide to adjust the final pH. The 10% and 20% IVFEs may be administered concurrently (IV piggyback) with dextrose/amino acid solutions or mixed with dextrose and amino acids within the PN formulation. The 30% IVFE is used exclusively for compounding formulations that combine dextrose, amino acids, and lipid in the same container.[15]

Amino Acids

Synthetic crystalline amino acids serve as the source of protein and nitrogen (6.25 g protein = 1 g nitrogen). Nitrogen is the building block of cell structure and is used to produce enzymes, peptide hormones, as well as structural and serum proteins. When oxidized for energy protein yields 4 kcal/g. Protein calories have not always been included in the calculation of energy needs for patients receiving PN formulations. Ideally, amino acids are used to stimulate protein synthesis and tissue repair and are not oxidized for energy; however, the human body cannot compartmentalize energy metabolism in such a manner. Today, conventional wisdom is to include protein calories in the total calorie calculations. Table 38-1 summarizes available nutrients and their caloric density.

Amino acid concentrations of 3.5% to 20% are available commercially and vary slightly from one product to another in specific amounts of each amino acid, electrolyte content, and pH. Generally, amino acid (AA) products are characterized as standard mixtures or specialty mixtures. Standard AA products provide a balanced mix of essential, nonessential, and semi-essential amino acids, whereas specialty AA products are modified for specific disease states.

Specialty AA mixtures are available for neonatal patients and for adult patients with hepatic encephalopathy, renal failure, or critical illness. Specialty AA formulations designed for patients with hepatic failure contain increased amounts of branched-chain amino acids (BCAA) and decreased amounts of aromatic amino acids (AAA) compared to standard AA products. These formulations are thought to counter the imbalance between AAA and BCAA that can occur in hepatic failure. Elevations in AAA may lead to altered mental status. There is no evidence to suggest that formulations enriched with BCAA improve patient outcomes compared with standard formulas.[16–18] Formulas enriched with BCAA should be reserved for patients with hepatic encephalopathy refractory to standard treatment with luminal acting antibiotics and lactulose.[16] Specialty amino acid products used in renal failure are predominantly comprised of essential amino acids.[19] Their use is based upon the theory that nonessential amino acids can be recycled from urea and essential amino acids. Indications for renal amino acid formulations are limited.[20] Standard amino acids should be used in acute kidney injury.

Modified amino acid formulations are also available for critically ill patients with hypercatabolic conditions such as trauma or thermal injury. These formulations contain increased amounts of the BCAAs (leucine, isoleucine, and valine) to address the increased skeletal muscle catabolism that can be seen in severe metabolic stress. While these BCAA enriched products may slightly improve nitrogen balance, improved patient outcomes have not been demonstrated.[21,22] For a summary of the various amino acid formulas, see Table 38-2.

Table 38-1
Caloric Density of Intravenous Nutrients

Nutrient	kcal/g	kcal/mL
Amino acids	4	
Amino acids 5%		0.2
Amino acids 10%		0.4
Dextrose	3.4	
Dextrose 10%		0.34
Dextrose 50%		1.7
Dextrose 70%		2.38
Fat	10	
Fat emulsion 10%		1.1
Fat emulsion 20%		2
Fat emulsion 30%		3
Glycerol	4.3	
Glycerol 3%		0.129
Medium-Chain Triglycerides	8.3	

Micronutrients

Micronutrients are electrolytes, vitamins, and trace minerals needed for metabolism. These nutrients are available from various manufacturers as either single entities or in combinations. For example, the trace element zinc is available commercially as a single trace element product or as a combination product with copper, chromium, manganese, and selenium. Likewise, electrolytes are available as individual salts or as a combination product to facilitate admixing. Commercially available vitamins for PN formulations are generally prescribed as a combination multivitamin regimen, although some vitamins are available as single additives. It is important to be aware of the specific products available in each institution to avoid providing inadequate or excessive amounts of various micronutrients.

PARENTERAL NUTRITION

Patient Assessment: Population-Based Formulation

CASE 38-1

QUESTION 1: A.A. is an 70 year-old man brought to the emergency department who is unable to speak, has a left-sided facial palsy, and left-sided muscle weakness in his upper and lower extremities. He is admitted to the hospital with a diagnosis of ischemic stroke. Evaluation of swallowing with modified barium swallow shows A.A. is at increased risk of aspiration. Enteral tube feedings are started to prevent aspiration. A.A. develops abdominal pain and bloating while receiving enteral feedings. Other enteral formulas and regimens are tried with the same results. Enteral feedings are stopped at this time and a short-term peripheral PN formulation is to be started. His weight today is 186 lbs; his height is 70 inches.

Nutrition laboratory panel values are as follows:

Sodium (Na), 142 mEq/L
Potassium (K), 4.1 mEq/L
Chloride (Cl), 100 mEq/L
Bicarbonate (HCO_3^-), 25 mEq/L
Blood urea nitrogen (BUN), 10 mg/dL
Creatinine, 1.0 mg/dL
Glucose, 91 mg/dL
Calcium (Ca), 9.4 mg/dL
Magnesium (Mg), 2.1 mg/dL
Phosphorus (P), 3.4 mg/dL
Total protein, 6.0 g/dL
Albumin, 3.6 g/dL
Prealbumin, 18 mg/dL
White blood cell (WBC) count, 8,800/μL

Assess his nutrition status.

A.A. is a well-developed, well-nourished man prior to admission. However, A.A.'s visceral proteins are in low-normal range, indicating he may be at increased risk for malnutrition. See Chapter 35, Basics of Nutrition and Patient Assessment, for a more detailed description of evaluation of patients with nutritional deficiencies. The principles from Chapter 35 will be applied to this and all others cases throughout this chapter. He has a minimal stress level and his baseline electrolytes are within normal limits.

CASE 38-1, QUESTION 2: Calculate calorie and protein goals for A.A. using population estimations.

A.A.'s initial calorie goals are to meet his current energy expenditure needed for basal metabolism and account for mild stress associated with stroke recovery. A.A. would fall into the category of "hospitalized patient, mild stress" requiring 20 to 25 kcal/kg/day (see Table 35-3 in Chapter 35, Basics of Nutrition and Patient Assessment). For this calculation, A.A.'s actual weight of 186 lbs (84.5 kg) should be used because his metabolism and current energy expenditure have caused a decrease in body mass. Using usual weight or ideal body weight in patients who have severe weight loss may result in overfeeding. For A.A., the caloric goal should be 1,690 to 2,113 kcal/day.

Protein goals are estimated based on weight, degree of stress, and disease state. Because A.A. has had a stroke and his metabolic stress is mild his protein goal should be based on the desire to maintain his current protein status. Using the guidelines provided in Table 35-4 (Chapter 35, Basics of Nutrition and Patient Assessment), A.A.'s protein dose is 1.0 g/kg/day (range 1.0–1.2), or 85 g/day. As with energy expenditure, calculations of protein needs are only estimates; the patient's clinical course should be monitored and the protein dose adjusted accordingly. The protein source for PN is synthetic amino acids. Generally, 1 g of protein is equivalent to 1 g of amino acids. A.A. will need 85 to 101 g/day of amino acids.

In patients with chronic kidney disease, protein intake should be adjusted according to catabolic rate, renal function, and possible protein losses from dialysis.[23–25] Patients with compromised renal function may require protein restriction to delay the progression of renal disease. Protein intake for patients receiving continuous renal replacement therapy should range between 1.8 and 2.5 g/kg/day.[23–25] Patients with acute kidney injury who receive hemodialysis may demonstrate positive nitrogen balance with protein dose of 1.5 g/kg/day.[26] The recommended protein intake for patients who receive maintenance hemodialysis is 1.2 g/kg/day,[27,28]

Table 38-2
Amino Acid Product Comparison

Description	Product Name	Available Concentrations (%)
Standard Formulations		
Contain essential[a] and nonessential[b] amino acids, some available with electrolytes[c]	Aminosyn, Aminosyn II	3.5,[c] 5, 7,[c] 8.5,[c] 10,[c] 15
	FreAmine III	3, 8.5, 10
	Novamine	15
	ProSol	20
	Travasol	3.5,[c] 5.5,[c] 8.5,[c] 10
Hepatic Failure Formulations		
Contain essential and nonessential amino acids with a proportion of branched-chain amino acids (leucine, isoleucine, valine)	HepatAmine	8
	HepAtasol	8
Renal Failure Formulations		
Contain primarily essential amino acids; RenAmin also contains a complement of nonessential amino acids	Aminess	5.2
	Aminosyn-RF	5.2
	NephrAmine	5.4
	RenAmin	6.5
Stress Formulations		
Contain percentages of leucine, isoleucine, and valine, as well as all essential and nonessential amino acids	Aminosyn HBC	7
	FreAmine HBC	6.9
Supplements		
Contain only branched-chain amino acids (isoleucine, leucine, valine); must be used with a general formulation	BranchAmin	4

[a]Essential amino acids: isoleucine, leucine, lysine, methionine, phenylalanine, threonine, tryptophan, valine, histidine.
[b]Nonessential amino acids: cysteine, arginine, alanine, proline, glycine, glutamine, aspartate, serine, tyrosine.
[c]These concentrations are available with or without electrolytes.

Source: Zerr KJ et al. Glucose control lowers the risk of wound infection in diabetics after open heart operations. *Ann Thorac Surg*. 1997;63:356; Rose BD. *Clinical Physiology of Acid–Base and Electrolyte Disorders*. 4th ed. New York, NY: McGraw-Hill; 1994:891.

while patients who receive chronic ambulatory peritoneal dialysis should receive 1.3 g/kg/day.[29]

CASE 38-1, QUESTION 3: A.A. has a peripheral IV catheter, and his peripheral access appears to be adequate. Is he a candidate for using a peripheral PPN formulation?

With good peripheral access, A.A. meets one of the criteria for PPN. Furthermore, he should be able to tolerate the volume of a PPN formulation necessary to meet his goals. A common complication (up to 70%) of PPN is thrombophlebitis, which generally occurs within 72 hours.[5,30] Phlebitis is usually attributed to the acidic pH or hyperosmolarity of the PN formulation. The osmolarity of typical peripheral parenteral feedings ranges from 600 to 900 mOsm/L compared with an osmolarity of 280 to 300 mOsm/L of plasma. Osmolarity of a dextrose–amino acid formulation can be approximated quickly by multiplying the percent dextrose concentration by 50 and the percent amino acid concentration by 100. Approximately 150 to 200 mOsm/L should be added to account for the contribution of electrolytes, vitamins, and trace elements. Although the concurrent administration of fat emulsions decreases osmolarity, buffers the pH, and improves peripheral vein tolerance, it does not eliminate the risk of thrombophlebitis.[31] If PN is anticipated to be a long-term therapy for A.A., central venous access should be obtained.

CASE 38-1, QUESTION 4: Design a parenteral nutrient base formulation and determine the amounts of each macronutrient stock solution needed to compound the PN formula for A.A. based on the caloric and protein goals determined previously.

A.A.'s caloric and protein goals are determined to be approximately 1,900 kcal/day and 85 g protein/day. Giving 85 g of protein per day will provide 340 kcal/day (1 g protein = 4 kcal). Subtracting these protein calories from total desired calories results in the amount of nonprotein calories needed (to be provided by carbohydrates and fat). For A.A., this would be 1,900 total calories minus 340 protein calories, or 1,560 nonprotein calories needed. Typically, dextrose should account for 60% to 70% of nonprotein calories, and lipids would account for the remaining 30% to 40% of nonprotein calories. Providing A.A. with 1,092 kcal of dextrose (approximately 321 g of dextrose; 1 g dextrose = 3.4 kcal) will supply 70% of nonprotein calories as dextrose. The remaining 30% of nonprotein calories will be provided by lipids at 468 kcal (46.8 g of lipids; 1 g of IV lipids = 10 kcal).

For dextrose, a 70% stock solution provides 70 g of dextrose/100 mL. To obtain 321 g of dextrose, 459 mL of the stock solution is needed:

$$\begin{aligned}\text{Dextrose Volume mL} &= 321\text{ g dextrose} \times 100\text{ mL}/70\text{ g dextrose}\\ &= 459\text{ mL}\end{aligned} \qquad \text{(Eq. 38-1)}$$

Similarly, the volume necessary to provide 85 g of amino acids with a 10% stock AA solution is 850 mL. IV lipids at 20% provide 2 kcal/mL or 20 g/100 mL. Using this stock solution, 234 mL would provide 46.8 g of lipids. The total volume of the dextrose, AA, and fat solution would be 1,543 mL/day. Additional volume will be required as electrolytes, vitamins, trace elements, and water are included in the final formulation.

CASE 38-1, QUESTION 5: The institution administers PPN using a 3-in-1 system at 100 mL/hr (2,400 mL/day). This PPN regimen will meet the majority of nutrient goals. Will this meet A.A.'s maintenance fluid requirements?

Maintenance fluid needs can be estimated using several methods. The simplest method uses 30 to 35 mL/kg/day as the basis. Another method is to provide 1,500 mL for the first 20 kg body weight plus an additional 20 mL/kg for actual weight beyond the initial 20 kg. Both methods provide estimates of fluid needs for basic maintenance, and additional fluid must be provided for increased losses such as vomiting, nasogastric (NG) tube output, diarrhea, or large open wounds. A.A.'s fluid needs are estimated as follows:

$$\begin{aligned}\text{mL/day} &= 1{,}500\text{ mL} + ([20\text{ mL/kg}][84.5\text{ kg} - 20\text{ kg}])\\ &= 1{,}500\text{ mL} + (20\text{ mL/kg})\,(54.5\text{ kg})\\ &= 1{,}500\text{ mL} + 1090\text{ mL} = 2{,}590\text{ mL}\end{aligned} \qquad \text{(Eq. 38-2)}$$

The PPN formulation is slightly less than A.A.'s needs of 2,590 mL/day. The PPN can be increased to 2,600 mL/day to better meet fluid needs. This will also slightly increase his calorie and protein intake bringing him closer to his goal requirements. Another option would be to provide any additional fluids via a separate IV line. It is important to not supply fluids in excess. The extra fluid intake may put patients at risk for becoming fluid overloaded. Therefore, A.A. should be monitored for signs of fluid overload, including peripheral edema, shortness of breath, daily intake exceeding daily output, hyponatremia, and rapidly increasing weight.

CASE 38-1, QUESTION 6: What are the benefits of using a mixed-fuel system, combining dextrose and fat to meet energy needs?

Providing a portion of calories as fat may reduce the metabolic consequences of excessive dextrose administration. The maximal rate of dextrose metabolism in adults is 5 to 7 mg/kg/minute, or approximately 7 g/kg/day. In doses greater than 7 g/kg/day, dextrose is used inefficiently and converted to fat.[32] The conversion to fat may be associated with respiratory compromise and hepatic dysfunction.[33–35] Hyperglycemia, another complication of excessive dextrose infusion, is associated with electrolyte and acid–base disturbances, osmotic diuresis, increased risk of infections, and altered phagocyte and complement function. Furthermore, using a mixed-fuel system allows the administration of a small amount of IVFE daily and avoids the need for larger boluses of lipid twice weekly to prevent essential fatty acid deficiency (EFAD). Rapid administration of IVFE has been associated with alterations in the reticuloendothelial system that are not observed with continuous administration of small doses.[36] IVFE should be infused at a rate of less than 0.11 g/kg/hour to prevent adverse effects, which include impaired hepatic, pulmonary, immune, and platelet function.[11] Administration of essential fatty acids as 1% to 4% of total caloric intake (e.g., 250 mL of 20% lipid twice a week) is necessary to prevent EFAD.

The essential fatty acids, linoleic acid and α-linolenic acid, are those that cannot be synthesized by humans. Of these, linoleic acid appears to be the only one required by adults. Clinical symptoms of EFAD are dry, thickened, scaly skin, hair loss, poor wound healing, and thrombocytopenia, which may be observed after a few weeks to months of lipid-free parenteral feedings.[29] Biochemical evidence of EFAD, determined by a triene to tetraene ratio of greater than 0.4, may be seen after 1 week of lipid-free parenteral feedings. The continuous infusion of hypertonic dextrose from the PN is associated with high circulating concentrations of insulin. Because insulin promotes lipogenesis rather than lipolysis, linoleic acid cannot be released from adipose tissue.[34]

Patient Assessment: Moderate Stress

CASE 38-2

QUESTION 1: B.B. is a 64-year-old woman who was diagnosed with ovarian cancer 4 years ago. The cancer was treated with a combination of chemotherapy and external beam radiation therapy. B.B. subsequently developed chronic radiation enteritis. She is admitted to the hospital for a complaint of increasing abdominal pain with eating for 7 days, and no stool output for 5 days. Questioning reveals that over the past week she has been drinking only liquids secondary to nausea and vomiting, and her weight has decreased 6 lbs during that time. Review of systems is positive for abdominal pain. On physical examination, B.B. appears thin, and her abdomen is distended. Vital signs are notable for a temperature of 38.5°C, heart rate of 88 beats/minute, and a blood pressure of 102/68 mm/Hg. She is 5 feet 6 inches tall and weighs 110 lbs (50 kg). Her medical record indicates that 1 month ago she weighed 116 lbs (52.7 kg), and 6 months ago her weight was 122 lbs (55.4 kg).

Admission laboratory values are as follows:

Na, 133 mEq/L
K, 4.5 mEq/L
Cl, 100 mEq/L
HCO_3^-, 25 mEq/L
BUN, 15 mg/dL
Creatinine, 0.7 mg/dL
Glucose, 103 mg/dL
Ca, 9.3 mg/dL
Mg, 2.2 mg/dL
P, 4.5 mg/dL
Albumin, 3.1 g/dL
WBC count, 11,800/μL
Hematocrit, 46%
Alanine aminotransferase, 31 units/L
Aspartate aminotransferase, 27 units/L
Alkaline phosphatase, 65 units/L
Total bilirubin, 0.6 mg/dL

Evaluation of B.B. with an abdominal CT scan shows bowel obstruction with a stricture distal to the obstruction and signs of chronic inflammation. B.B. is admitted with complications from chronic radiation enteritis. Why is B.B. a candidate for PN?

PN should be considered when the patient's nutrient intake has been inadequate for 7 days or longer and the GI tract is not functioning. B.B. has eaten little in the past week, and her 5% decrease in weight is a concern. Furthermore, her weight has decreased by more than 10% during the past 6 months, which is considered a severe weight loss. B.B. is not expected to resume oral intake because her radiation enteritis is being managed conservatively with bowel rest.

Assessment of weight loss should include evaluation of hydration status, especially because B.B.'s vomiting and minimal oral intake for the past week place her at risk of dehydration. Loss of lean body mass is probably less than that reflected by the decrease in weight. In addition, B.B.'s admission serum albumin concentration is low at 3.1 g/dL. Her hydration status should be considered when evaluating this visceral protein, since B.B.'s serum albumin concentration will probably decrease further after she is rehydrated. Because B.B.'s GI tract is not functioning, PN is indicated. For a list of the most common primary diagnoses for the use of PN in hospitalized patients, see Table 38-3.

CASE 38-2, QUESTION 2: What type of malnutrition does B.B. have?

B.B. exhibits some loss of fat and muscle, as well as depletion of visceral proteins. She has components of both marasmus and kwashiorkor malnutrition; therefore, she would be considered to have mixed protein-calorie malnutrition (see Chapter 35, Basics of Nutrition and Patient Assessment).

Table 38-3
Most Common Primary Diagnoses for TPN in Adult Hospitalized Patients

Top 10 Primary Diagnoses TPN
Intestinal or peritoneal adhesions with obstruction
Acute pancreatitis
Septicemia
Diverticulitis
Acute respiratory failure
Intestinal obstruction
Aspiration pneumonitis
Gastrointestinal complication
Coronary atherosclerosis
Pneumonia

Source: Wischmeyer PE et al. Characteristics and current practice of parenteral nutrition in hospitalized patients. *JPEN J Parenter Enteral Nutr*. 2013;37:56–67.

CASE 38-2, QUESTION 3: Members of the medical team are anxious to have B.B. gain weight and are concerned by her malnourished appearance. What potential complications could result from aggressively feeding B.B.?

B.B. may be at risk of *refeeding syndrome*. Chronic malnutrition may lead to intracellular depletion of phosphorus, potassium, and magnesium that may not be evident when measuring serum electrolyte concentrations. Refeeding syndrome may occur as phosphorus, potassium, and magnesium shift from the extracellular space into the cells upon consumption of concentrated sources of calories. Carbohydrate calories are converted to glucose which triggers the secretion of insulin, which in turn, facilitates the uptake of glucose, water, phosphorus, and other intracellular electrolytes. This phenomenon was first reported in World War II when chronically malnourished survivors were given normal food and liquid diets. Complications coinciding with refeeding these individuals included hypertension, cardiac insufficiency, seizures, coma, and death. These complications were reported later in the 1970s and 1980s, with the introduction of PN in chronically ill, essentially starved hospitalized patients. Knowing a patient's history of weight loss and diet will help to assess the risk of refeeding syndrome. Specialized nutrition support should be initiated and advanced slowly for "at risk" patients, along with close monitoring to avoid serious electrolyte abnormalities and the cardiovascular consequences thereof.

To minimize the risk of refeeding syndrome in B.B., all electrolyte abnormalities must be corrected before nutrition support is initiated. Because B.B.'s electrolytes are within normal range, no baseline adjustments are necessary. Nutrition should then be implemented slowly and vitamins administered routinely. Laboratory values including phosphorus, potassium, magnesium, and glucose should be monitored at least daily for the first week.[38,39]

Overfeeding should be avoided in all patients, especially those with respiratory concerns (i.e., mechanically ventilated, chronic obstructive airway disease). Overfeeding with carbohydrates is particularly detrimental because of the amount of carbon dioxide produced relative to the amount of oxygen consumed. This results in carbon dioxide retention that may lead to alterations in acid–base balance. Complete oxidation of carbohydrate is demonstrated at dextrose infusions of 4 to 5 mg/kg/minute (20–25 kcal/kg/day). Infusions exceeding this rate increase carbon dioxide production and may cause respiratory distress. In designing a PN formulation for B.B., it is important to provide a moderate calorie dose and to limit her dextrose dose to less than 4 mg/kg/minute.[40,41] For adults, the daily lipid intake should not exceed 2.5 g/kg/day. However, current literature supports a maximum of 1 g/kg/day. It is also important to monitor serum triglyceride levels to assess tolerance to this dose of IVFE. If the blood sample is obtained while the triglycerides are infusing, as with the TNA formulation, a serum triglyceride concentration of 400 mg/dL, although elevated, is acceptable.[42] Hypertriglyceridemia can sometimes be noted quickly by gross observation of turbidity in the blood sample.

CASE 38-2, QUESTION 4: After hydration with IV fluids, B.B.'s weight is 51.5 kg. PN therapy was delayed because within 24 hours after admission, B.B. experienced severe abdominal pain and distension and required surgery. An exploratory laparotomy was performed, and 25 cm of ileum was resected to remove an area of bowel with severe disease and a stricture that was causing the obstruction. Bowel sounds are absent. She has a right Port-A-Cath CVC and PN is to begin on postoperative day 1. Calculate energy and protein goals for B.B.

Energy requirements may be estimated with predictive equations, simplistic formulas (25–30 kcal/kg/day) or measured by indirect calorimetry, the most accurate method. Over 200 predictive equations have been published in the literature, including the Harris–Benedict equation. Using the Harris–Benedict equation for women (see Table 35-3 in Chapter 35, Basics of Nutrition and Patient Assessment) and her current weight of 51.5 kg, height of 167.6 cm, and age of 64 years, B.B.'s basal energy expenditure (BEE) is 1,158 kcal/day. To estimate her total energy expenditure, the BEE should be modified with an activity factor of 1.2 for being confined to bed and a stress factor of 1.2 for surgery. These modifications result in an estimated energy expenditure of 44% greater than her BEE, or 1,668 kcal/day. Therefore, an energy goal of 1,600 kcal/day is reasonable. In a similar manner, her protein goal (see Table 35-4 in Chapter 35, Basics of Nutrition and Patient Assessment) for moderate stress is 62 to 77 g/day of protein (1.2–1.5 g/kg/day).

CASE 38-2, QUESTION 5: Design a TNA parenteral nutrient formulation as a single daily PN bag for B.B. that provides 1,600 kcal and 70 g of amino acids with a non-protein calorie distribution of 75% carbohydrate and 25% lipid. The macronutrients available on the formulary for compounding the parenteral nutrient formulations are 70% dextrose, 30% lipid emulsion, and 10% amino acids.

1. Amino acids calculation

$$\begin{aligned}\text{Calories from amino acids (protein)} &= 70\text{ g} \times 4.0\text{ kcal/g}\\ &= 280\text{ kcal}\\ \text{mL of 10\% amino acids} &= 70\text{ g}/0.1\text{ g/mL}\\ &= 700\text{ mL} \quad \text{(Eq. 38-3)}\end{aligned}$$

2. Dextrose calculation

$$\begin{aligned}\text{Calories from dextrose} &= (1{,}600 - 280)\,(0.75)\\ &= 990\text{ kcal}\\ \text{g of dextrose} &= 990\text{ kcal}/3.4\text{ kcal/g}\\ &= 291\text{ g/mL of 70\% dextrose}\\ &= 291\text{ g}/0.7\text{ g/mL}\\ &= 416\text{ mL} \quad \text{(Eq. 38-4)}\end{aligned}$$

3. Lipid emulsion calculation

$$\begin{aligned}\text{Calories from lipid} &= (1{,}600 - 280)\,(0.25)\text{ or}\\ &\quad (1{,}320 - 990)\\ &= 330\text{ kcal/mL of 30\% lipid emulsion}\\ &= 330\text{ kcal}/3.0\text{ kcal/mL}\\ &= 110\text{ mL} \quad \text{(Eq. 38-5)}\end{aligned}$$

4. Calculation of final volume of energy substrates

$$\begin{aligned}&700\text{ mL amino acids 10\%} +\\ &416\text{ mL dextrose 70\%} + 110\text{ mL lipid emulsion 30\%}\\ &= 1{,}226\text{ mL total volume} \quad \text{(Eq. 38-6)}\end{aligned}$$

B.B.'s goal PN formulation will provide 291 g of dextrose and approximately 33 g of lipids daily. If the PN is infused continuously over 24 hours, B.B. will receive 3.9 mg/kg/minute of dextrose and 0.6 g/kg/day of lipids. Both dextrose and lipid doses comply with the limitations recommended in question 3. Other additives such as electrolytes, vitamins, and trace elements are included in the parenteral nutrient formulation and slightly increase the final volume to 1,680 mL/day. The infusion rate for this formulation can be calculated as follows:

$$\begin{aligned}\text{Hourly infusion rate (mL/hour)} &= \frac{1{,}680\text{ mL/day}}{24\text{ hours/day}}\\ &= 70\text{ mL/hr} \quad \text{(Eq. 38-7)}\end{aligned}$$

B.B.'s parenteral nutrient formulation of 1,680 mL/day will not meet her maintenance fluid needs of 2,130 mL/day (see Case 38-1, Question 5). She will require extra fluid to meet the remainder of her basic fluid needs. These additional fluids should be provided through another IV or added as sterile water to the TNA solution.

CASE 38-2, QUESTION 6: What are the advantages and disadvantages of combining the dextrose, fat, and amino acids in one container?

PN formulations may be prepared in one of two ways: a dextrose–amino acid (2-in-1) mixture in which IVFE is administered separately as a piggybacked infusion or a total nutrient admixture (TNA or 3-in-1) in which the dextrose, amino acids, and IVFE are combined in solution in the same bag.[43]

While the use of TNAs have been widely embraced by home care providers and many institutions for convenience and cost advantages, the addition of IVFE to the traditional mixture of dextrose and amino acids converts the mixture into a complex emulsion with physiologic differences that alter the stability of the product.[44] The differences between these two methods of compounding PN formulations must be considered. Specific advantages and disadvantages of each are summarized in Table 38-4.

CASE 38-2, QUESTION 7: How stable are the TNA parenteral feeding formulations compared to 2-in-1 formulations? Why is an infusion filter necessary?

IVFE gradually deteriorates over time because of increased formation of free fatty acids and a resultant decrease in pH. When lipids are mixed with dextrose and amino acids, this process is accelerated. IVFE consists of an interior oil phase dispersed within an external water phase. Stability of the IVFE is maintained by polar and nonpolar regions on the same fat droplet. The surface of the polar region of the fat droplet is negatively charged and repels other lipid droplets of the same charge. When the surface loses its negativity, fat droplets aggregate into larger globules and the emulsion becomes unstable and unsafe for use, risking occlusion of pulmonary vasculature. Commercially available IVFEs in the United States use an anionic egg yolk phosphatide emulsifier to stabilize the lipid droplets and maintain dispersion. Destabilization of the emulsion occurs in phases that begin with creaming and ends with the coalescence of the lipid particles, or "cracking" of the emulsion. A decrease in pH and the addition of divalent cations (Mg^{2+}, Ca^{2+}) alter the electrical charge on the fat droplet surface and pose a risk to the integrity of the emulsion. Although dextrose decreases the pH, the addition of amino acids provides an adequate buffer for this variable. The amount of

Table 38-4
Advantages and Disadvantages of 2-in-1 and 3-in-1 Parenteral Nutrition

	2-in-1	3-in-1
Advantages	■ Improved overall stability ■ Increased flexibility in concentrating dextrose and amino acids ■ Allows more flexibility to add higher concentrations of electrolytes ■ Better medication compatibility ■ Reduced risk of bacterial growth because of high osmolarity and acidic pH ■ Better visualization of precipitant of particulate matter. Enables the use of bacterial retention filter (0.22-micron) ■ Lower risk of catheter occlusion if IVFE is not used daily	■ All components are aseptically compounded by the pharmacy ■ Simplified regimen for the patient especially at home ■ Less supply and equipment costs ■ Less nursing time needed for administration ■ Decreased preparation cost ■ Decreased risk of contamination ■ Inhibited bacterial growth versus separate IVFE ■ Minimize infusion-related reactions from IVFE because of slower infusion rate ■ May improve lipid clearance because of slower infusion rate ■ Decreased risk of phlebitis with PPN
Disadvantages	■ Increased administration costs and time when lipids are infused separately ■ Increased risk of touch contamination ■ Increased risk of phlebitis, particularly if PPN is not co-infused with IV lipid emulsion ■ IVFE given in a piggyback manner is limited to a maximum hang time of 12 hours.[45]	■ Impaired visualization of particulate matter or precipitate because of opacity of IVFE admixture ■ IVFE is less stable—more prone to lipid separation. Admixture is less stable with concentrated electrolyte additives ■ Larger particle size of IVFE admixture. Must use 1.2-micron. Cannot use 0.22-micron bacterial retention filter. ■ Limited compatibility with medications ■ Containers with diethylhexyl phthalate should be avoided because this toxic material may be extracted by the lipid and may harm patients.

divalent cations added to TNAs should be limited to minimize the risk of emulsion instability. Trivalent cations such as iron should never be added to a TNA parenteral nutrient formulation. PN formulations containing lipid must be assessed visually for signs of phase separation, in which the instability of the emulsion is manifested by "oiling out," indicated by a continuous layer of oil or individual fat droplets. Fat emulsion particles have an average size of 0.5 μm. A destabilized emulsion is not visibly apparent until the lipid particles are 40 to 50 μm. Fat particles as small as 5 μm may occlude pulmonary capillaries.[43,44] Therefore, the use of a 1.2-μm filter is recommended to protect against the infusion of enlarged lipid particles.[12,43]

Using dual-chamber bags may extend the shelf life of TNAs because they allow the lipid to be physically separated from the dextrose, amino acids, and other additives until it is time to administer the feeding. The use of dual-chamber bags has the greatest advantage for home care settings, where up to a week's supply of parenteral feedings are prepared at one time.[43]

After preparation, TNAs should be refrigerated (4°C) to preserve stability. Once the bag is removed from the refrigerator, it may be warmed to room temperature and the contents mixed well before administration. Mixing is best accomplished by gently inverting the container up and down to ensure top-to-bottom transfer of the fluid. Vigorous shaking should be avoided because it introduces air, which can destabilize the emulsion.[43,44]

Case 38-2, Question 8: How does microbial growth differ between 2-in-1 and TNA (3-in-1) formulations?

Dextrose–amino acid PN formulations are not conducive to growth of most organisms because of their high osmolarity (>2,000 mOsm/L) and acidic pH. Lipid emulsions alone, however, are isotonic and have a physiologic pH, providing an optimal growth medium. Combining these three substrates in a TNA provides a formulation with a microbial growth potential that is intermediate between the two.[43,44] The number of CVC violations or manipulations correlates strongly with the incidence of catheter-related infections. From an infection-control perspective, the use of a single daily bag of PN formulation limits the number of manipulations of the CVC to one per day, thereby minimizing touch contamination. The Centers for Disease Control and Prevention guidelines allow TNA formulations to hang for up to 24 hours. However, because of concerns about the potential of lipid emulsions to support microbial growth, the hang time for IVFE when administered alone in a piggyback manner with 2-in-1 PN formulations is 12 hours.[43]

Case 38-2, Question 9: Design a plan to monitor the adequacy of B.B.'s specialized nutrition support and to identify and prevent adverse complications.

Routine monitoring and evaluation of nutritional status and the metabolic effects of therapy are required for patients receiving PN therapy. Nutritional goals established in the patient care plan are estimates of a patient's nutritional requirements and must be evaluated regularly to assess adequacy of therapy. Daily monitoring parameters include vital signs, body weight, temperature, serum chemistries, hematologic indices, nutrition intake, and fluid intake and output.

The adequacy of nutrition therapy should be assessed weekly. This may be accomplished through measuring serum concentrations of visceral proteins (see Table 35-2 in Chapter 35, Basics of Nutrition and Patient Assessment) such as prealbumin and albumin. Because prealbumin has a half-life of only 2 to 3 days, serum concentrations of this protein should increase weekly with adequate nutrition and improving clinical status. Albumin has a much longer half-life of 14 to 20 days that renders it less useful in reflecting an anabolic response to PN therapy. It is, however, a good indicator for morbidity and mortality.[46] Indirect calorimetry, if performed correctly, is the most accurate way to reassess energy expenditure. A method to assess adequacy of protein intake is to evaluate nitrogen balance which compares the amount

Table 38-5
Routine Monitoring Parameters for Parenteral Nutrition

	Suggested Schedule for TPN Monitoring					
Parameter	**Initial**	**Daily (Critically Ill)**	**2-3 × Weekly (Stable)**	**Weekly**	**Monthly (Home Health)**	**As Indicated**
Weight	X	X	X			
BUN, Creatinine, Glucose	X	X	X			
Na, K, Cl, HCO_3^-, Ca, P, Mg	X	X	X			
Albumin, AST, ALT, LDH, Alk Phos, Total Bili, Conj Bili	X			X		X
Prealbumin	X			X		X
Triglycerides	X			X		X
RBC count, Hgb, Hct, WBC count, Platelets	X			X		X

of nitrogen administered to the amount of nitrogen excreted (amount "in" vs. amount "out"). The nitrogen "in" is provided by the AA component of the PN formulation. Each commercially available amino acid formulation has a slightly different amount of nitrogen per gram of amino, so the manufacturer's product information should be consulted to obtain this value. On average about 16% of amino acid is nitrogen or 1 g of nitrogen for every 6.25 g of protein. Most of the nitrogen is excreted in the urine as urea, a byproduct of protein breakdown for energy. Renal excretion of urea nitrogen increases with increasing stress. To determine the nitrogen balance, urine must be collected for 24 hours and the amount of urine urea nitrogen (UUN) measured. Some laboratories have the capability of measuring total urine nitrogen, which measures all nitrogen entities in the urine. In addition, some nitrogen lost via skin, respiration, and stool is not measurable but is estimated to be between 2 and 4 g/day.

$$\begin{aligned}\text{Nitrogen balance} &= \text{Nitrogen in} - \text{Nitrogen out}\\ &= \text{AA (g)}/6.25 - (\text{UUN [g]} + 3\text{ g})\\ &= \text{g} \end{aligned} \quad \text{(Eq. 38-8)}$$

Achieving a positive nitrogen balance is difficult, if not impossible, in critically ill patients; therefore, the calculation may result in a negative number or zero. For convalescing patients, a nitrogen balance of plus 2 to 4 g is acceptable. A negative nitrogen balance prompts a reevaluation of the amount of protein and energy a patient is receiving. For patients with a negative nitrogen balance, it may be helpful to increase intake of both calories and protein.

As with all tests, assessment should include monitoring several parameters, including the patient's clinical status. Most important is the identification of trends that may alert clinicians to impending complications. A suggested schedule for monitoring is provided in Table 38-5.

CASE 38-3

Question 1: C.C., a 56-year-old man, is admitted to the hospital complaining of increasing abdominal pain and vomiting. He is diagnosed with acute pancreatitis. This is his third admission for pancreatitis during the past year. His past medical history is significant for ethanol abuse, chronic obstructive pulmonary disease, and type II diabetes. His social history is significant for 2 packs/day smoking history. A NG tube is inserted, and he is to receive nothing by mouth (NPO). IV fluids are begun for hydration. During the next 5 days, C.C.'s abdominal pain subsides, his pancreatitis resolves, and he is started on an oral diet. Two days after beginning an oral diet, C.C. complains of severe abdominal pain and is vomiting. He is febrile, his WBC count has increased to 21,000/μL, and he is hypotensive, requiring large volumes of IV fluids. Furthermore, he experiences respiratory distress and requires endotracheal intubation and mechanical ventilation. His most recent arterial blood gas (ABG) is notable for pH, 7.44; Pco_2, 40 mm Hg; Po_2, 88 mm Hg; and HCO_3^-, 28 mEq/L. C.C.'s clinical presentation is consistent with severe pancreatic necrosis. A small-bore nasojejunal feeding tube is placed, and enteral nutrition therapy is begun. However, C.C. experiences severe abdominal pain and distension, and bowel sounds are absent, so the enteral feeding is discontinued. The decision is made to begin PN because C.C. is not expected to have a functional GI tract in the near future and his nutrient intake has been inadequate during his hospitalization. C.C. is 5 feet 8 inches tall, and his usual weight is 215 lb.

What adjustments should be made in determining C.C.'s energy goals?

First, C.C. is considered obese, and an adjusted body weight should be calculated and used in nutrition calculations. Obesity is defined as weight exceeding 120% of ideal body weight or a body mass index (BMI) of greater than 30 kg/m^2. C.C. weighs 215 lb, or 98 kg, which is 142% of his ideal body weight of 69 kg. BMI is determined as shown by Equation 38-9.

$$\begin{aligned}\text{BMI} &= \text{W (kg)}/\text{Height (m)}^2\\ &= 98\text{ kg}/(1.73\text{ m})^2\\ &= 32.7\text{ kg/m}^2\end{aligned} \quad \text{(Eq. 38-9)}$$

Obese patients should have their weight adjusted because adipose tissue is not metabolically active. However, about one-fourth of the adipose tissue is composed of some supporting tissue that is metabolically active. Adjusted weight for obesity is calculated using Equation 38-10.[47]

$$\begin{aligned}\text{Adjusted weight} &= (0.25)(\text{Actual weight} - \text{IBW}) + \text{IBW}\\ &= (0.25)(98 - 69) + 69\\ &= 76\text{ kg}\end{aligned} \quad \text{(Eq. 38-10)}$$

Using an adjusted weight will decrease the risk of overfeeding, which can further increase adipose tissue and complicate glucose management, especially in a patient with a history of diabetes mellitus. Another approach is to use the Ireton-Jones predictive equation that includes a factor for obesity. Using indirect calorimetry to obtain a measured energy expenditure may more accurately assess energy expenditure and avoid overfeeding.

C.C. is considered to be a critically ill patient. Guidelines from the American Society for Parenteral and Enteral Nutrition (A.S.P.E.N.) support permissive underfeeding (80% of estimated energy requirements) for critically ill patients to minimize the risk of insulin resistance, infectious morbidity, and prolonged mechanical ventilation. As the patient stabilizes, the PN regimen may be increased to meet a 100% of estimated energy requirments.[21] For critically ill obese patients, the A.S.P.E.N. guidelines go a step further to support that if BMI is in excess of 30, goal caloric intake should not exceed 60% to 70% of target energy requirements or 11 to 14 kcal/kg actual body weight per day (or 22–25 kcal/kg ideal body weight per day). Protein should be provided at >2.0 g/kg IBW for BMI classes I and II and at >2.5 g/kg IBW for BMI class III.[21,48] In the case of C.C., his BMI is 32.7 (BMI Class I) so his energy goal is estimated at 22 kcal/kg of ideal body weight or approximately 1,500 kcal/day.

CASE 38-3, QUESTION 2: Is the use of lipid emulsion contraindicated in patients with pancreatitis?

Several observations have raised concern about the use of IVFE in patients with pancreatitis. The oral ingestion of fats may stimulate pancreatic exocrine function and should be restricted in patients with pancreatitis. Although hyperlipidemia has been well described in patients with alcohol-induced pancreatitis, it is unlikely that it is primarily responsible for initiating the pancreatitis. Acute pancreatitis associated with hypertriglyceridemia is most often seen in patients with hereditary or acquired defects in lipid metabolism. Furthermore, pancreatitis alone may be associated with hypertriglyceridemia.[49]

Several investigators have evaluated the effects of PN formulations containing IVFE's in patients with acute pancreatitis and have found no stimulation of pancreatic exocrine function. Furthermore, IVFE did not result in abdominal pain or relapse in patients with a history of pancreatitis. Available data suggest that IVFE are a safe and efficacious form of calories for patients with pancreatitis.[49]

While consensus has not been reached regarding the optimal composition of lipid emulsions, recent guidelines from the Society of Critical Care Medicine (S.C.C.M.) and the A.S.P.E.N. recommend that during the first week of stay within an intensive care unit, patients should receive PN formulations that do not contain soy-based lipids.[49] The addition of n-3 fatty acids, eicosapentaenoic acid and docosahexaenoic acid, to lipid emulsions is recommended because of positive effects on cell membranes and inflammatory processes.[50]

Monitoring serum triglyceride concentrations should be part of routine management for patients with pancreatitis and those receiving parenteral nutrient formulations containing lipids. Serum triglyceride concentrations should be maintained at less than 400 mg/dL with a continuous infusion of lipids and less than 250 mg/dL when checked 4 hours after the infusion for patients receiving intermittent IVFE infusions.[1,42,49] If serum concentrations exceed these parameters, consideration must be given to decreasing or eliminating the IVFE from the parenteral nutrient regimen.

CASE 38-3, QUESTION 3: What are other considerations regarding PN therapy initiation and formulation design for C.C.?

Patients with mild-to-moderate pancreatitis do not generally require nutrition support therapy. Patients with severe acute pancreatitis should have a nasoenteric tube placed and feedings initiated as soon as the volume resuscitation is complete. If tube feeding is not feasible, PN therapy should be considered and initiated after the first 5 days of hospitalization (after the peak of the inflammatory response).[21] Acute pancreatitis is a complex condition and its severity is highly variable. Severe acute pancreatitis can cause systemic inflammatory response syndrome affecting multiple organ systems often times resulting in organ failure. Compromised or failing organs may necessitate macronutrient and micronutrient adjustments in the PN formula.

Hyperglycemia is the most common complication associated with PN therapy and can be caused by a variety of factors. Patients without a history of diabetes mellitus may exhibit hyperglycemia under conditions of stress. Even greater alterations in glucose metabolism may be observed in patients with diabetes mellitus during critical illness. Stress-induced hyperglycemia may develop as a result of insulin resistance, suppressed insulin secretion, and increased gluconeogenesis and glycogenolysis.[51] Dextrose should be limited to 150 g during the first 24 hours of therapy, the amount of dextrose should not be increased until serum glucose concentrations are consistently less than 180 mg/dL, and capillary blood glucose concentrations should be monitored frequently. With a history of diabetes, coupled with acute pancreatitis, it is anticipated that C.C. will need supplemental insulin when his parenteral nutrient regimen is infused. Insulin therapy may be administered subcutaneously, intravenously with an insulin infusion, or directly in the PN formulation.[52,53] Regular insulin may be added to the PN formulation at a dose of 0.1 units per gram of dextrose as a reasonable starting point and should be adjusted to achieve serum glucose levels between 140 and 180 mg/dL.[54] Alternatively, a separate insulin infusion may be used for more aggressive glucose control. Capillary glucose monitoring is required during PN therapy at least every 6 hours and more frequently in hyperglycemic patients, and it may be necessary to provide additional subcutaneous insulin.[53,55,56]

CASE 38-3, QUESTION 4: C.C.'s current laboratory values are as follows:

Na, 137 mEq/L
K, 4.5 mEq/L
Cl, 102 mEq/L
HCO_3^-, 26 mEq/L
BUN, 9 mg/dL
Creatinine, 0.8 mg/dL
Glucose, 148 mg/dL
Ca, 8.9 mg/dL
Mg, 1.9 mg/dL
P, 2.8 mg/dL
Albumin, 3.0 mg/dL

Which electrolytes should be included in C.C.'s parenteral nutrient formulation?

Once macronutrient goals are achieved and tolerance is established, the daily management of PN therapy revolves around maintaining the patient's fluid and electrolyte needs. All concurrently administered IV fluids and medications must be considered and accurate records of volume intake and output reviewed. Electrolytes added to PN formulations are sodium, potassium, chloride, acetate (which is metabolized to bicarbonate), magnesium, calcium, and phosphate. Electrolyte requirements can vary widely and should be added to the PN formulation based on individual patient needs. However, patients without significant fluid and electrolyte losses, hepatic or renal dysfunction, or acid–base disturbances do well with standard maintenance doses of electrolytes. Electrolytes may be added individually or as commercially available combination products for maintenance doses. General guidelines for electrolyte requirements for parenteral feedings are included in Table 38-6.

CASE 38-3, QUESTION 5: What doses of multiple vitamins and trace elements should C.C. receive in his parenteral nutrient formulation?

Vitamins and trace elements should be included in PN regimens and are essential for normal metabolism and effective nutrient utilization. Guidelines for the 13 essential vitamins have been established by the Nutrition Advisory Group of the American Medical Association[57] (Table 38-7).

Table 38-6
Guidelines for Daily Electrolyte Requirements

Electrolyte	Amount
Sodium	80–100 mEq
Potassium	60–80 mEq
Chloride	50–100 mEq[a]
Acetate	50–100 mEq[a]
Magnesium	8–20 mEq
Calcium	10–15 mEq
Phosphorus (phosphate)	20–40 mmol

[a]As needed to maintain acid–base balance.

Table 38-7
Recommended Adult Daily Doses of Parenteral Vitamins

Vitamins	Dose
Fat-Soluble Vitamins	
A	3,300 IU (990 retinol equivalents)
D	200 IU (5 mg cholecalciferol)
E	10 IU (6.7 mg/dL-α-tocopherol)
K	150 mcg
Water-Soluble Vitamins	
Thiamine (B_1)	6 mg
Riboflavin (B_2)	3.6 mg
Niacin (B_3)	40 mg
Pyridoxine (B_6)	6 mg
Cyanocobalamin (B_{12})	5 mcg
Folic acid	600 mg
Pantothenic acid	15 mg
Biotin	60 mcg
Ascorbic acid (C)	200 mg

Guidelines for daily doses of the trace elements, such as chromium, copper, manganese, and zinc, have also been developed.[58] In addition to these trace elements, many practitioners provide selenium on a daily basis. Recommended doses of the trace elements are listed in Table 38-8. As with vitamins, trace elements are available as single entities or combination products. Molybdenum and iodine are also available commercially.

Case 38-3, Question 6: C.C.'s initial PN infusion is started at a rate of 40 mL/hour. Why is this slow infusion rate selected?

Standard practice for administering PN formulations containing hypertonic dextrose is to begin at a slow infusion rate of less than 250 g of dextrose during the first 24 hours for most patients and less than 150 g of dextrose for patients with known diabetes mellitus or hyperglycemia. The infusion is increased slowly during the next 24 to 48 hours to the goal infusion rate as of 1,800 mL/day as tolerated. This initial period allows the clinician to assess tolerance to the nutrient formulation components and to avoid metabolic complications, primarily hyperglycemia.[37] If C.C.'s serum glucose level consistently remains less than 180 mg/dL, the PN formulation infusion rate can be increased to his goal rate.

Case 38-3, Question 7: During the next 24 hours, a comparison of his intake and output reveals an overall negative fluid balance

Table 38-8
Recommended Daily Adult Doses of Parenteral Trace Elements

Trace Element	Dose
Chromium	10–15 mcg
Copper	0.3–0.5 mg
Manganese	60–100 mcg
Selenium	20–60 mcg
Zinc	2.5–5 mg

because a high volume of gastric fluid is being removed via the NG tube. Laboratory values at this time are the following:

Na, 138 mEq/L
K, 3.1 mEq/L
Cl, 91 mEq/L
HCO_3^-, 33 mEq/L
BUN, 28 mg/dL
Creatinine, 0.9 mg/dL
Glucose, 279 mg/dL
Ca, 7.8 mg/dL
Mg, 1.4 mg/dL
P, 1.8 mg/dL
Albumin, 2.8 g/dL

Arterial blood gas (ABG) results are pH, 7.46; PO_2, 98 mm Hg; PCO_2, 47 mm Hg; and HCO_3^-, 31 mEq/L. What factors contribute to these metabolic abnormalities?

PN therapy may be associated with multiple metabolic complications. The most common abnormalities are hypokalemia, hypomagnesemia, hypophosphatemia, and hyperglycemia. The plan for PN therapy should include routine monitoring of these serum chemistries to identify complications early and institute methods to manage or prevent complications.

Hypokalemia

Hypokalemia, a common metabolic abnormality associated with the initiation of PN, usually occurs within the first 24 to 48 hours. Potassium moves, along with dextrose, from the extracellular to the intracellular space. Furthermore, building lean body mass (i.e., anabolism) requires approximately 3 mEq of potassium per gram of nitrogen provided by the amino acids. Administering dextrose promotes repletion of glycogen stores, which also requires potassium.[37,39,59]

C.C.'s decreased serum potassium concentration is compounded by metabolic alkalosis. With metabolic alkalosis, the renal excretion of potassium is increased. Additional potassium should be administered and can be provided in C.C.'s parenteral feeding or through another IV.

Hypomagnesemia

Magnesium, like potassium, is primarily an intracellular cation and is considered an anabolic electrolyte. It is common to observe decreases in magnesium serum concentrations during the administration of parenteral nutrient formulations. Synthesis of lean tissue requires 0.5 mEq of magnesium per gram of nitrogen.[37,39,59] Additional magnesium can be added to the PN formulation. However, when a TNA formulation is used, the amount of magnesium must stay within the guidelines for the cation content to maintain the stability of the lipid emulsion.

Hypophosphatemia

Hypophosphatemia occurs when phosphorus moves into the cells for the synthesis of adenosine triphosphate (ATP), an important energy carrier. Phosphorus is depleted quickly with the administration of hypertonic dextrose, especially in malnourished patients (see Case 38-2, Question 3, for discussion of refeeding syndrome). Phosphorus is used for ATP synthesis, primarily in the liver and skeletal muscle. Alkalosis also decreases phosphate stores by stimulating the phosphorylation of carbohydrates. As a component of 2,3-diphosphoglycerate, found in red blood cells (RBCs), phosphorus is necessary for the disassociation of oxygen from hemoglobin.[59]

Clinical signs and symptoms of hypophosphatemia usually occur when serum concentrations fall to less than 1.0 mg/dL. They include lethargy, muscle weakness, impaired WBC function, glucose intolerance, rhabdomyolysis, seizures, hemolytic anemia, reduced diaphragmatic contractility, and death. Moderate to severe, complicated hypophosphatemia can be managed by administering up to 0.625 mmol/kg of phosphate IV.[39,59–61] Although C.C.'s serum phosphorus is not less than 1.0 mg/dL, it is low (1.8 mg/dL), and he should receive 15 to 30 mmol of phosphate in the parenteral nutrient formulation per day. Additional supplements may be necessary to replete his phosphorus stores.[60]

Metabolic Alkalosis

C.C. has evidence of a metabolic alkalosis based on his ABG results, hypochloremia, and elevated bicarbonate level. The continued loss of fluid and hydrochloric acid from the NG tube is the most probable cause of his metabolic alkalosis. Management of this type of metabolic alkalosis is to replace the fluid and chloride through another IV. Because acetate is converted to bicarbonate and can further contribute to the alkalosis, the acetate salts in the parenteral nutrient formulation can be changed to chloride salts.[59] Nevertheless, the PN formulation generally is not the primary vehicle for adjusting and supplementing electrolytes and fluids. Instead, the fluid and electrolyte balance may be adjusted with maintenance IV fluid and electrolyte supplements.

Hyperglycemia

Hyperglycemia is the most common metabolic complication of PN therapy, especially in stressed patients. Metabolic stress increases gluconeogenesis and glycogenolysis. This increase in endogenous glucose production coupled with the administration of hypertonic dextrose in PN formulations increases the potential for hyperglycemia.[62] C.C. is at particular risk for hyperglycemia because he is diabetic, experiencing pancreatitis, and recovering from the stress of surgery.

Persistent hyperglycemia may lead to glucosuria and osmotic diuresis, resulting in dehydration and electrolyte abnormalities. Hyperglycemia compromises the immune response altering chemotaxis and phagocytosis and impairing complement function, thereby increasing risk of infection. In extreme cases, hyperglycemia progresses to hyperosmolar, non-ketotic acidosis and coma, a condition associated with 40% mortality.

Hyperglycemia can be minimized by limiting the dextrose infusion rate to less than 4 mg/kg/minute (20 kcal/kg/day).[63] Clinical evidence suggests that treatment of hyperglycemia and maintenance of euglycemia may reduce morbidity and mortality, length of stay, and hospital costs.[53,55,64–66]

CASE 38-3, QUESTION 8: In response to these serum chemistries, the electrolytes in C.C.'s parenteral nutrient formulation are changed to the following per liter: NaCl, 160 mEq; KCl, 140 mEq; phosphate as K salt, 60 mmol; $MgSO_4$, 54 mEq; and calcium gluconate, 30 mEq. How do the doses of calcium and phosphate compare with maintenance doses? What calcium and phosphate incompatibilities should be anticipated? Will the calcium and magnesium content alter the lipid stability?

Calcium and phosphate solubility is a safety concern with PN formulations. The dose of calcium ordered for C.C. is more than 3 times the usual maintenance dose (Table 38-6). This amount of calcium is not necessary because the observed hypocalcemia merely reflects C.C.'s low serum albumin concentration; therefore, less calcium is bound to albumin. C.C. probably does not have true hypocalcemia because his free (or ionized) calcium, which is critical for physiologic function, has not changed. If available, obtaining an ionized calcium concentration is advised. However, some laboratories do not have this test available. In this situation, a "corrected" calcium formulation may be used. For every 1-g/dL decrease in serum albumin concentration, there will be about a 0.8-mg/dL reduction in the serum calcium concentration.[67] For C.C., a serum calcium of 7.8 mg/dL will correct to a serum concentration of 8.8 mg/dL ([4.0–2.8 g/dL albumin][0.8] + 7.8 mg/dL calcium).

The amount of phosphate prescribed for C.C. at this time exceeds the usual recommended dose of 20 to 40 mmol/day (Table 38-7). Although C.C. has a low serum phosphorus concentration and needs additional phosphate, increasing the dosage in the parenteral nutrient formulation to 60 mmol/day may be incompatible with the calcium content, resulting in calcium–phosphate precipitation.

Numerous factors affect calcium–phosphate solubility, and caution is warranted when preparing PN formulations to ensure that solubility limits are not exceeded. If solubility is compromised, microprecipitates can occur and may cause diffuse pulmonary emboli, resulting in respiratory distress or death. Calcium and phosphate precipitation curves have been developed to assist practitioners in safe compounding practices. These guidelines help predict the points at which calcium–phosphate precipitation is likely to occur. The solubility of calcium and phosphate must be determined based on the volume of the formulation at the time the calcium and phosphate are mixed together, not the final volume. For example, if the electrolytes including calcium and phosphate are added to 1,000 mL of a dextrose–amino acid mixture and then 300 mL of IV fat is added, the calcium–phosphate solubility is based on the 1,000 mL, not the final 1,300 mL volume. In addition, some amino acid products contain phosphate ions, and these should be considered when determining calcium–phosphate solubility.[12,68]

The in vitro precipitation of calcium–phosphate depends on the type of calcium salt used in compounding, concentrations of calcium and phosphate, amino acid concentration, temperature, pH of the formulation, and infusion time. Calcium gluconate rather than the chloride salt offers enhanced calcium phosphate solubility. In solution at equimolar concentrations, calcium chloride dissociates more than calcium gluconate, thereby increasing the yield of free calcium available for binding with phosphate. Calcium and phosphate should not be added to the PN formulation in close sequence. It is recommended to add phosphate first and calcium last, thereby taking advantage of the maximal parenteral volume. The PN formulation should be agitated periodically during preparation and inspected for precipitates.[69] Other guidelines for improving the solubility of calcium are a final amino acid concentration of greater than 2.5% and a pH less than 6. An increase in the ambient temperature, such as that found in the heated isolettes within neonatal intensive care units, can facilitate the precipitation of calcium–phosphate. PN formulations should be infused within 24 hours after compounding if stored at room temperature; if refrigerated, it should be infused within 24 hours after rewarming. Increasing temperature and slow infusions may result in calcium–phosphate precipitation in the IV catheter, even if precipitation has not occurred in the infusion container.[12]

The amount of divalent cations, calcium (20 mEq) and magnesium (30 mEq), exceeds the general guidelines for maximal amounts that can be added safely to a TNA without disrupting the stability of the lipid emulsion. A limit of 20 divalent cations per liter is a general guideline. The amount prescribed for C.C.'s regimen is excessive because it provides 50 divalent cations in 1.8 L (28 divalent cations/L) and may result in a potentially unstable admixture.

Last, a 1.2-μm air-eliminating filter should be used when infusing TNA PN formulations, and a 0.22-μm air-eliminating filter should be used for non–lipid-containing admixtures.[12]

CASE 38-3, QUESTION 9: C.C. is recovering from his pancreatitis, and a small-bore nasojejunal enteral feeding tube is reinserted. Tube feeding is considered because he cannot eat by mouth because of the endotracheal tube and mechanical ventilation. How should he be transitioned from parenteral to enteral feedings?

Tube feedings can begin with a full-strength isotonic enteral feeding formulation at a slow continuous infusion rate (10-50 mL/hr and advanced by 10-25 mL/hr every 4 to 24 hours) (see Chapter 37, Adult Enteral Nutrition). Concurrently, the PN formulation should be decreased to avoid fluid overload and to keep the calorie and protein intake constant. It can be anticipated that C.C. can transition from parenteral to enteral feedings in 24 to 48 hours.

CASE 38-4

QUESTION 1: D.D., is a 43-year-old man with a 17-year history of Crohn's disease (CD). He has had several hospital admissions over the past 2 years with exacerbations of Crohn's Disease. D.D. has experienced an unintentional weight loss of 12% over the past year. He is admitted to the hospital for increasing abdominal pain, nausea, and vomiting for 9 days, and no stool output. Prior to admission D.D.'s condition was managed with mesalamine 1 gm QID and prednisone 10 mg QD. On physical examination, D.D. appears thin and his abdomen is distended. Baseline labs are as follows:

Na, 142 mEq/L
K, 4.2 mEq/L
Cl, 99 mEq/L
HCO_3^-, 15 mEq/L
BUN, 12 mg/dL
Creatinine, 0.9 mg/dL
Glucose, 114 mg/dL
Ca, 9.1 mg/dL
Mg, 1.9 mg/dL
P, 5.8 mg/dL
Albumin, 2.8 g/dL
Prealbumin, 28 g/dL

Interpret D.D.'s prealbumin level.

Although D.D.'s prealbumin level indicates his nutritional status is adequate, caution must be exercised with its interpretation. In the 1960s it was shown that prednisone administration may elevate prealbumin levels.[70] Despite his prealbumin level, D.D. has other indicators of chronic malnutrition. His albumin level is low at 2.8 g/dL. He has experienced an unintentional weight loss of 12 lbs over the past year and appears thin. Corticosteroid therapy is fairly common in patients likely to use PN solutions. These patients include patients with inflammatory bowel disease, patients being treated for cancer, and respiratory patients.

CASE 38-4, QUESTION 2: D.D. has a prolonged hospital course complicated by intra-abdominal abscesses, poor wound healing, and necrotic bowel, requiring removal of all but 82 cm of his small intestine but leaving his ileocecal valve and colon intact. D.D. is given a diagnosis of short bowel syndrome (SBS). What is the clinical significance of the presence of D.D.'s ileocecal valve and colon?

The presence of the terminal ileum and colon following small bowel resection is critical in nutritional and hydrational management as the patient may be able to tolerate a very short small intestine without TPN support. The presence of the ileocecal valve is thought to prolong intestinal transit time and serve as a barrier to bacterial reflux into the small intestine. Deficiencies of electrolytes, trace elements, and vitamins are common in Crohn's disease and influenced by the presence of the terminal ileum and colon. Deficiencies are often reflective of chronic blood loss (e.g., iron deficiency), chronic diarrhea (e.g., magnesium, selenium, zinc deficiencies), or loss of specific absorptive sites (e.g., vitamin B_{12}). There is a high prevalence of vitamin D deficiency in patients with Crohn's disease.

CASE 38-4, QUESTION 3: What issues should be addressed in the nutrition and metabolic management of this patient?

SBS occurs from extensive intestinal resection that results in inadequate bowel function to support nutrient and fluid requirements. SBS becomes clinically apparent when about 75% of the small bowel is removed. Recent studies suggest that the average length of the small intestine may be shorter than previously thought (approximately 11 feet), so SBS is best defined using a patient's symptoms and findings rather than solely on remaining length of small bowel.[71] SBS patients frequently experience diarrhea, dehydration, and nutritional deficiencies of minerals, trace elements, and vitamins (see Chapter 28, Lower Gastrointestinal Disorders). In adults, this syndrome is commonly seen in Crohn's disease, radiation enteritis, mesenteric artery infarction, adhesive obstruction, and trauma.[72] Severe malnutrition will develop without adequate nutrition support.

To maintain adequate nutrition status, D.D. will require PN until his remaining intestine begins to adapt. This adaptive period may take several weeks to months to years, with the majority of intestinal adaptation occurring within the first 2 years following massive bowel resection. Gut adaptation is enhanced by stimulation of the enterocytes with nutrients, which is best provided by small, frequent oral meals or tube feeding.[1,73,74] Sometimes the remaining intestine may never adapt, and SBS may necessitate lifelong PN therapy for survival.

A potential complication of SBS is hypersecretion of gastric fluids. The volume and acid content of gastric secretions is directly proportional to the amount of bowel resected.[79–81] The patient can experience symptoms of reflux similar to a Zollinger–Ellison syndrome with epigastric pain and burning. Medications that decrease GI tract motility (antidiarrheals) and secretions (H_2 blockers and proton pump inhibitors) are frequently necessary to reduce the volume of gastric secretions and minimize the damaging effects of hypersecretion of gastric acid. These agents are also important in the management of fluid and electrolyte imbalances because of excessive GI fluid losses. Patients with extensive small bowel resection and an intact colon, such as D.D., may experience diarrhea as a result of bile salt depletion.[1,73,74]

Octreotide may help in decreasing diarrhea in patients with SBS. Octreotide reduces a variety of GI secretions and slows jejunal transit, but the effects are often short-lasting and have not shown improved nutrient absorption.[82] It is important to be mindful that most oral medications are absorbed within the first 50 cm of the jejunum. Delayed-release medications should be avoided.

Patients with SBS are at risk for having vitamin and mineral deficiencies, especially folate, vitamin B_{12}, vitamin D, selenium, and zinc. These patients should receive supplemental vitamin B_{12} and IV parenteral or oral liquid multivitamin supplements. GI losses of trace minerals, particularly zinc and selenium, are increased in SBS, and these minerals should be supplemented.[73,74]

D.D. should be continued on PN support and will most likely need PN therapy at home to sustain his nutrient and fluid requirements. Since oral ranitidine in not an option, the treatment team orders ranitidine 150 mg to be added to D.D.'s PN formula to manage hypersecretion of gastric fluids and diarrhea. D.D.'s fluid status must be monitored and evaluated daily for clinical signs of dehydration or fluid overload. Electrolyte abnormalities, including hyponatremia, hypokalemia, hypomagnesemia, hypocalcemia, and metabolic acidosis, should be anticipated.[74]

CASE 38-4, QUESTION 4: On hospital day 10, he presents with a fever and green, purulent fluid draining from his abdominal incision site. He is diagnosed with an enterocutaneous fistula. The fluid loss from D.D.'s fistula is about 600 mL/day. How will losses from D.D.'s fistula affect his PN?

Enterocutaneous (EC) fistulas are an abnormal communication between the intestine and the skin. Most EC fistulas occur 7 to 10 days following surgery and are classified by site of origin, output volume, etiology, and number of fistulas. Fluid, electrolyte, and trace element losses from the EC fistula will vary depending on the origin of the fistula. Losses must be accounted for and incorporated into the PN formulation or replaced through a separate IV fluid infusion.

CASE 38-4, QUESTION 5: D.D. has stabilized and his physician would like to discharge him home in a few days with the plan to continue TPN at home. D.D. is 5 feet 8 inches tall and weighs 141 lbs at discharge. Design an appropriate PN therapy for home infusion.

Home TPN has allowed patients, such as D.D., to be discharged from the hospital sooner. Candidates for home therapy must be physically and medically stable, have a strong support network in the home setting to assist with care, and have an appropriate home environment. They must be educated regarding the prescribed therapy.[75]

The first step in designing a PN regimen is to estimate energy and protein needs (see Chapter 35, Basics of Nutrition and Patient Assessment). D.D. is 10 days out from surgery, and his estimated requirements are 25 to 30 kcal/kg/day or approximately 1,600 to 1,920 kcal/day. Protein goals must include adequate nitrogen (protein) for wound healing and replacement for losses from the enterocutaneous fistula. A goal of 1.5 to 1.8 g/kg/day (96–115 g) is reasonable. Long-term systemic corticosteroid therapy is commonly seen in Crohn's patients and may cause muscle wasting. Losses of lean body mass from corticosteroids may increase amino acid requirements.

To simplify his nutrition and fluid regimen, all of D.D.'s fluids, including parenteral nutrients, electrolytes, vitamins, trace minerals, and water, should be provided in one TNA container per day. D.D.'s home PN formulation can be provided in 3,000 mL/day to meet maintenance requirements (see Case 38-1, Question 5) and to replace losses from his enterocutaneous fistula (600 mL/day). Nutrients provided include 100 g of amino acids (400 kcal); 264 g of dextrose (884 kcal); 50 g of lipid (500 kcal); and electrolytes, vitamins, and minerals to maintain normal serum chemistries. Initially, daily intake and output must be monitored; therapy should be adjusted based on this information and D.D.'s clinical status.

Adjustments in fluids and electrolytes may be needed. The fluids secreted by the GI tract are rich in electrolytes, including sodium, potassium, chloride, and bicarbonate. Measurement of the electrolyte content of the fistula fluid will determine those that must be replaced, and in what quantities. Both fluid and electrolytes should be replaced to prevent dehydration and electrolyte and acid–base imbalances.

In addition to losses of fluids and electrolytes, the trace element zinc is lost in fluid from the small intestine. Approximately 12 mg of zinc is lost in each liter of small bowel fluid, and should be replaced to prevent zinc deficiency. Furthermore, zinc may play a role in wound healing.[76] Management of enterocutaneous fistulas may include octreotide 50 to 100 mg given subcutaneously 2 or 3 times daily or added to the parenteral nutrient formulation to decrease fistula output.[77]

A home infusion pharmacy will be responsible for preparing D.D.'s PN formulations. Typically, a seven day supply of PN therapy (7 bags) is prepared and delivered to the patient's home. These formulations must be refrigerated until administration; however, formulations should be warmed to room temperature and visually inspected for particulate matter before being administered. Because some additives such as multivitamins are not stable for long periods, the patient or caregiver must add these to the PN formulation just before administration.

Patients and caregivers preparing for home PN therapy must be taught how to manage home therapy. This includes assessment of fluid status, care of a CVC, infection, and the technical aspects of administering parenteral feeding formulations.[75] Preparation for home PN includes placement of a central venous access device for long-term TPN therapy.[7,8]

CASE 38-4, QUESTION 6: What other measures can be used to simplify D.D.'s parenteral feeding regimen and encourage ambulation?

Transitioning D.D. from a 24-hour continuous PN infusion to a cyclic infusion must be considered. After D.D.'s PN regimen is formulated to meet his entire daily nutrient and fluid needs and he is stable on that regimen, his PN regimen can then be cycled. *Cycling* means that the PN formulation is infused for less than 24 hours per day, so that there is time free from PN therapy each day. Cycling is usually done gradually, prior to hospital discharge, and depends on the patient's ability to tolerate the changes in fluid and dextrose intake that occur when the TPN is started and stopped each day. For example, the 24-hour PN infusion is decreased to a 20-hour infusion (e.g., 8:00 PM to 4:00 PM) on cyclic PN day 1 and then the next day is decreased to a 16-hour infusion (e.g., 8:00 PM to 12:00 noon), and the next day a 12-hour infusion (e.g., 8:00 PM to 8:00 AM). With each incremental decrease in time, the infusion rate should be increased such that the total PN volume is infused each day. The infusion rate of the PN regimen is generally tapered up over 1 to 2 hours upon PN initiation to avoid hyperglycemia and tapered down over 1 to 2 hours upon PN discontinuation each day to avoid hypoglycemia. For example, a 16-hour cyclic PN infusion with a 1-hour taper up and down can be calculated by taking the total TNA volume divided by the infusion time minus 1 hour, to estimate the goal infusion rate. The goal infusion rate is then divided by 2 to get the 1 hour taper up and taper down rate. For D.D.'s 3,000 mL TNA, the regimen would start at 8:00 PM at 100 mL/hour for 1 hour, then at 9:00 PM the rate would increase 200 mL/hour for 14 hours. At 11:00 AM the following day the TNA rate would taper back down to 100 mL/hour and then at noon it would stop. Most infusion pumps used at home can automatically make these adjustments in the infusion rate. Eventually, the nutrient formulation can be infused for 10 to 12 hours during the night, leaving D.D. free from his PN infusion during the day.

Vital signs, fluid intake and output, serum electrolytes, and glucose concentrations should continue to be monitored. The serum glucose concentration should be evaluated 30 minutes to 1 hour after the PN infusion is completed to be sure that hypoglycemia does not occur.

CASE 38-4, QUESTION 7: In addition to his PN formula and ranitidine 150 mg IV, D.D. is receiving hydrocortisone 100 mg IV every 8 hours, and he now needs insulin. Can these medications or any other medications be mixed with his PN formula to simplify his medication regimen?

Patients receiving PN therapy often require concomitant drug therapy. Most patients have adequate venous access or have multiple-lumen CVCs, so that mixing medications with the parenteral nutrient formulation is not an issue. However, for some patients with limited venous access, directly added medications or piggybacking medications via a secondary infusion may be considered.

Although regular insulin, histamine type 2 (H_2)-receptor antagonists, and heparin can be added to PN formulations in some circumstances, the routine addition of medications to parenteral nutrient formulations is discouraged. Often times there are requests to add other medications to a PN admixture. Specific criteria for drug admixture with PN are listed below.[83]

1. Stability and compatibility of the drug with the specific parenteral admixture over a 24-hour period must be determined before adding the medication.
2. The medication must have appropriate pharmacokinetics and proven efficacy for continuous infusion.
3. The medication dose must have remained constant throughout the previous 24-hour period before admixture in PN.
4. There should be a stable PN infusion rate for at least 24 hours before the medication is added.
5. PN should include appropriate labeling to avoid pharmacotherapeutic problems associated with abrupt discontinuation of PN.

CASE 38-4, QUESTION 8: After receiving home PN for 3 weeks, D.D.'s liver function tests are found to be elevated. Current values are as follows:

Bilirubin, 0.8 mg/dL
Aspartate aminotransferase, 70 units/L
Alanine aminotransferase, 90 units/L
Alkaline phosphatase, 100 units/L
Could his PN be contributing to these abnormalities?

Elevations in liver function tests are common in adults receiving long-term PN therapy and may be noted as early as 2 to 3 weeks after beginning therapy. The abnormalities are usually mild and transient and do not progress to significant liver dysfunction in adults. The predominant type of hepatobiliary dysfunction is steatosis (fatty liver), whereas other patients develop cholestasis or cholelithiasis (biliary obstruction). Liver-associated enzyme elevations usually resolve when PN therapy is discontinued. Rarely does this dysfunction proceed to hepatic failure.[35,78]

Other than avoiding overfeeding with carbohydrate and lipid, there are few options to prevent or manage PN-associated liver abnormalities. Potential management options include metronidazole and supplements of ursodeoxycholic acid, choline, and carnitine. Transitioning to a lipid emulsion containing n-3 fatty acids should also be considered. Patients with progressive liver disease may be candidates for liver and small bowel transplantation.[78]

The elevations in D.D.'s liver enzymes are not of concern at this time because they are less than 3 times normal. However, since D.D. has been on home PN for 3 weks and his wounds have healed, it is time to decrease his energy and protein intake to maintenance requirements (20-25 kcal/kg/day and 0.8-1.0 g/kg/day of protein). Liver enzymes should be monitored weekly. Because he may not need lifelong PN therapy, the mild elevations are likely to resolve.

It is important to keep in mind that the liver is the primary organ involved with digestion, metabolism, and storage of nutrients. When the functional capacity of the liver is compromised (e.g., cirrhosis), macronutrient intolerance and imbalances may occur. The patient may experience hyperglycemia, hypoglycemia, variations in blood lipid levels, and accumulation of amino acid metabolites (ammonia).

CASE 38-4, QUESTION 9: After 10 months of receiving home TPN, D.D. suffers a fall and fractures his wrist. Fracture of the wrist from a fall raises suspicions of compromised bone density. Subsequent DEXA scan reveals a bone density T-Score of −3.1. Can these results be caused by long-term PN? What are other complications of long-term parenteral therapy?

Long-term complications of PN are adverse effects associated with PN lasting greater than 3 months. The most common complications include central catheter complications (infection or occlusion), metabolic bone disease, and hepatobiliary disease.[84]

The exact cause of metabolic bone disease in long-term PN is unknown; however, its origins appear to be multifactorial. The predominant risks factors for metabolic bone disease in D.D. include Crohn's disease, the medications used to manage it (e.g., corticosteroids) coupled with the use of long-term PN therapy.[85] Both osteoporosis and osteomalacia have been associated with long-term PN use. Osteoporosis is the most common form of metabolic bone disease and is because of loss of bone mass. Osteomalacia is the softening of bones and generally occurs as the result of vitamin D deficiency. A combination of both osteoporosis and osteomalacia may occur. Deficiencies in micronutrients such as calcium, magnesium, and vitamin D are risk factors. Historically, bone abnormalities were thought to be caused by aluminum toxicity. However, as aluminum has been nearly eliminated from TPNs, metabolic bone disease remains an issue. High amino acid concentrations and TPN cycling cause increased renal calcium excretion. Other factors include abnormalities in the handling of calcium, phosphorus, and vitamins D and K.

Central catheter–related complications can vary from occlusion to central catheter–related sepsis. Both of these complications are related to CVC care and are a surrogate measure of overall catheter care.[86] Occlusion develops from fibrin and/or lipid deposits. The consequences of catheter occlusion range from diminished flow to complete occlusion necessitating removal of the catheter. Central catheter infections are associated with the amount of times the catheter is accessed for PN administration and blood sample removal. Patients with CVC infections usually present with symptoms and signs such as pyrexia and tachycardia during PN infusion. The causes of central catheter infections are bacterial and are usually because of skin flora, *Staphylococcus epidermis* and *Staphylococcus aureus*. If CVC-related sepsis is suspected, then the CVC being used should be discontinued and peripheral and central cultures taken, while antimicrobial therapy is started pending culture results.[85]

The incidence of hepatobiliary complications associated with long-term PN ranges from 19% to 75%. These complications are variable, with patients experiencing chronic elevations in liver enzymes to advanced liver disease (fibrosis and cirrhosis). Liver disease associated with PN is termed intestinal failure–associated liver disease (IFALD). IFALD is divided into nonnutrient and nutrient-related causes. Nonnutrient causes of IFALD can include medications, biliary obstruction, bacterial overgrowth, and intrinsic liver disease. Nutrient-related IFALD can be caused by overfeeding, nutrient toxicities, and deficiencies. Nutrient toxicities associated with IFALD include manganese, aluminum, and soybean oil. Some nutrient deficiencies associated with IFALD are taurine, choline, carnitine, and essential fatty acids. The most common histological finding in IFALD is steatosis followed by cholestatic stasis, fibrosis, and finally cirrhosis. Hepatic steatosis is associated with both under and overfeeding, so the importance of ensuring the correct amount of calories is of utmost importance.[84]

KEY REFERENCES AND WEBSITES

A full list of references for this chapter can be found at http://thepoint.lww.com/AT11e. Below are the key references and websites for this chapter, with the corresponding reference number in this chapter found in parentheses after the reference.

Key References

Driscoll DF. Intravenous lipid emulsions: 2001. *Nutr Clin Pract.* 2001; 16:215. (15)

Krzywda EA et al. Parenteral access devices. In: Gottschlich MM et al, ed. *The Science And Practice Of Nutrition Support: A Case-Based Core Curriculum.* Dubuque, IA: Kendall/Hunt Publishing; 2001. (4, 37, 43, 49, 74, 75)

Kearns LR et al. Update on parenteral amino acids. *Nutr Clin Pract.* 2001;16:219. (19)

Mirtallo J et al. Safe practices for parenteral nutrition [published correction appears in *J Parenter Enteral Nutr.* 2006;30:177]. *J Parenter Enteral Nutr.* 2004;28:S39. (12)

Key Websites

American Society for Parenteral and Enteral Nutrition. http://www.nutritioncare.org. http://www.nutritioncare.org/Library.aspx to access content for:

ASPEN Board of Directors and the Clinical Guidelines Task Force. Guidelines for the use of parenteral and enteral nutrition in adult and pediatric patients. *JPEN J Parent Enteral Nutr.* 2002;26(Suppl 1):1SA.

McClave SA et al. Guidelines for the provision and assessment of nutrition support therapy in the adult critically ill patient: Society of Critical Care Medicine (SCCM) and American Society for Parenteral and Enteral Nutrition (A.S.P.E.N.). *JPEN J Parent Enteral Nutr.* 2009;33:277.

Section Editor: Timothy J. Ives

39 Dermatotherapy and Drug-Induced Skin Disorders

Richard N. Herrier and Daniel R. Malcom

CORE PRINCIPLES		CHAPTER CASES
1	The accurate assessment of dermatologic conditions is primarily based on the appearance and location of the skin lesion, plus age, sex, symptoms, and current and past personal and family history.	**Case 39-1 (Question 1)** **Figure 39-1** **Tables 39-3, 39-4, 39-5**
2	Dry skin (xerosis) is a common condition that may occur alone or with a variety of dermatologic disorders and requires appropriate treatment depending on geographic location.	**Case 39-2 (Question 1)** **Table 39-6**
3	The selection of topical corticosteroid is based on the nature of the lesion (wet vs. dry), the concentration of the corticosteroid, the nature of the vehicle, the corticosteroid potency, the location of the lesion, and the thickness of the epidermis.	**Case 39-3 (Questions 1, 2)** **Figure 39-1, Tables 39-1, 39-2, 39-3, 39-4, 39-5, 39-7**
4	Topical corticosteroids can cause a variety of adverse effects and adverse reactions that may require adjustment of therapy including changing products or discontinuing their use.	**Case 39-4 (Questions 1–3)** **Tables 39-7, 39-8, 39-9**
5	Atopic dermatitis is a common dermatologic condition characterized by eczematous lesions, dry skin, and intense pruritus. Most patients have a family or personal history of other atopic diseases such as asthma and allergic rhinitis. Atopic dermatitis is primarily treated with topical corticosteroids and emollients.	**Case 39-5 (Questions 1–5)** **Tables 39-3, 39-5, 39-6, 39-7, 39-10**
6	Allergic contact dermatitis is one of the most common dermatologic conditions seen by pharmacists. Drugs (neomycin), plants (*Rhus*), chemicals, detergents, metals (nickel), and organic products (latex) are common causes. Treatment consists of removal of the antigen and use of topical or systemic corticosteroids.	**Case 39-6 (Question 1)** **Case 39-7 (Questions 1, 2)** **Tables 39-3, 39-5, 39-7, 39-10, 39-11**
7	Medications are a common cause of a variety of dermatologic disorders. Timing relative to medication ingestion and principles of dermatologic assessment are important to identify potential life-threatening adverse reactions.	**Case 39-8 (Question 1)** **Tables 39-8, 39-11**

ANATOMY AND PHYSIOLOGY OF THE SKIN

The skin is the largest organ in the body and constitutes, on average, 17% of a person's body weight. The skin's thickness ranges from 3 to 5 mm. Figure 39-1 shows a cross section of the anatomy of human skin. Physiologically, the major function of skin is to protect underlying structures from trauma, temperature variations, mechanical penetrations, moisture, humidity, radiation, and invasion of microorganisms. There are three layers of skin: epidermis, dermis, and subcutaneous tissue.[1–5]

Epidermis

The major function of the epidermis is to serve as a barrier. The epidermis keeps chemicals and other substances from penetrating into the body and prevents the loss of water from the skin and underlying tissues.

The *stratum corneum*, which is composed of dead cells, provides the greatest resistance to the percutaneous absorption of chemicals and drugs. It behaves as a semipermeable membrane through which drugs are absorbed by passive diffusion. Factors that can enhance drug absorption are hydration of the skin and damage to the stratum corneum. In general, the greater the

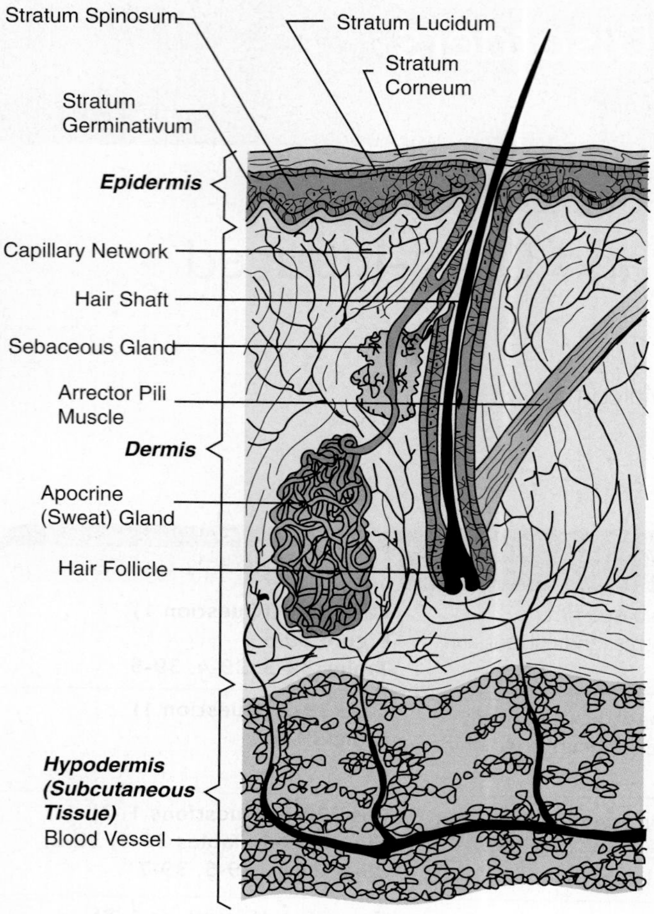

Figure 39-1 Cross section of the anatomy of human skin.

damage to the stratum corneum, the greater is the absorption of topically applied drugs. Skin diseases affecting only the epidermis heal without scarring.[1–5]

Dermis

The dermis is composed of collagen fibers and ranges in thickness from 1 to 4 mm. The major function of the dermis is to protect the body from mechanical injury and to support the dermal appendages (i.e., sweat and sebaceous glands, hair follicles) and the epidermis. It also provides capillary, lymphatic, and nerve supply to the skin and its appendages. The dermis contains large amounts of water, thus serving as a water storage organ as well. Importantly, all but the most superficial injuries to the dermis generally result in scarring as the wound heals.[1–5]

Drugs passing through the epidermis penetrate directly into the dermis and may be absorbed into the general circulation through the capillary network. Only small amounts of topically applied drugs enter the dermis via the sweat glands or the pilosebaceous units.

Subcutaneous Layer

The subcutaneous layer supports the dermis and epidermis and serves as a fat storage area. This layer helps regulate temperature, provide nutritional support, and cushion the outer skin layers.[1–5]

INFLAMMATORY LESIONS

One of the dermatologic axioms regarding therapy is particularly useful in selecting dosage forms: "If it is wet, dry it; if it is dry, wet it." Paradoxically, wet dressings (e.g., Burow solution) are most useful in drying acute, inflamed lesions because they draw out fluid as they evaporate. Ointment-type bases increase hydration to an affected area by slowing water evaporation from the skin and are most useful for chronic, lichenified, scaling lesions. The choice of vehicle for chronic lesions is often based on what the patient has found to work best or is willing to use. Frequently, patients with chronic dermatologic conditions use multiple types of vehicles concomitantly (e.g., cream bases, which are drying because they are oil in water emulsions) during the day, because they are cosmetically acceptable, and ointment bases at night (greasy, but better emollients).

Acute Lesions

Acute inflammatory lesions can be characterized by vesiculation, erythema, swelling, warmth, pruritus, oozing, or weeping. Generally, depending on the part of the body involved, the more severe the dermatitis, the milder is the initial topical therapy would be. For instance, cool water in the form of a wet dressing, soak, or bath is more effective as the initial therapeutic agent than a potent topical corticosteroid applied to a warm, erythematous, weeping dermatitis.[1–6]

Subacute and Chronic Lesions

Subacute lesions are characterized by decreasing vesiculation and are often covered with crusts. They still require cleaning and drying with aqueous preparations, but for a shorter duration than with acute lesions. Chronic inflammatory lesions are characterized by erythema, scaling, lichenification, dryness, and pruritus. There are no absolute rules for treating chronic lesions. If the lesion is dry, an oleaginous or occlusive base should be used.

DERMATOLOGIC DRUG DELIVERY SYSTEMS

Dermatologic formulations are available in a variety of forms: solutions, suspensions or shake lotions, powders, lotions, emulsions, gels, creams, ointments, and aerosols. Each dermatologic delivery vehicle has specific characteristics and uses based on the type, relative acuteness, and location of the lesion.

Solutions

Solutions provide evaporative cooling and vasoconstriction, with resultant mild antipruritic effects. They soothe and cool inflamed skin, dry oozing lesions, soften crusts, aid in cleaning wounds, and assist in the drainage of purulent wounds. Aqueous solutions are most useful for acutely inflamed, oozing lesions; erosions, and ulcers, and are often applied as wet dressings. In most instances, solutions should be the sole therapy until the oozing or weeping subsides. If other topical medications are applied, they will be washed away and will not provide the desired effect. The most commonly used solutions are normal saline (0.9% NaCl) and aluminum acetate 5% solution (Burow solution) diluted 1:10 to 1:40.

The most important component of a solution is water. Although active or inert substances may be added to solutions, the cleansing, drying, and cooling effect of water provides the major therapeutic benefit. Some of the products (e.g., Burow solution) also have *astringent* properties that alter the skin surface and interstitial spaces to cause contraction and wrinkling. Water penetration is reduced to minimize edema, inflammation, and exudation. Table 39-1 lists the most commonly used solutions.

Table 39-1
Solutions for Wet Dressings or Drying Weeping Lesions

Agent[a]	Strength	Preparation (H_2O)	Germicidal Activity	Astringent Activity	Comments
Normal saline	0.9% NaCl	1 tsp NaCl per pint H_2O	None	None	Inexpensive; easy to prepare
Aluminum acetate	5%	Dilute to 1:10–1:40 (0.5%–0.125%)			
(Burow solution) (Domeboro packets/tablets)		One packet or tablet to a pint of water yields a 1:40 solution; two packets or tablets yield a 1:20 solution	Mild	+	
Potassium permanganate	65- and 330-mg tablets	Dilute to 1:4,000–1:16,000; 65-mg tablet to 250–1,000 mL; 330-mg tablet to 1,500–5,000 mL	Moderate	None	Stains skin, clothing
Silver nitrate	0.1%–0.5%	1 tsp of 50% stock solution to 1,000 mL will yield a 0.25% solution	Good	+	Stains; can cause pain
Acetic acid[b]	1%	Dilute 1 pint of standard 5% household vinegar with 5 parts H_2O	Good	+	Unpleasant odor; can be irritating

[a]Although many substances are added to wet dressings, the cleansing and drying effect of the water is the major benefit.
[b]Used primarily for *Pseudomonas aeruginosa* infections.
Source: Arndt KA, Hsu JHS, eds. *Manual of Dermatologic Therapies: With Essentials of Diagnosis*. 8th ed. Philadelphia, PA: Lippincott Williams & Wilkins; 2014.

Boric acid should not be used as a topical agent because it can be absorbed through the skin, causing systemic toxicity.[6]

Depending on the affected area and its size, a patient may soak the affected area directly in the solution for 15 to 30 minutes 3 to 6 times per day. If larger areas are involved or if the affected area cannot be easily soaked (e.g., a shoulder), a clean towel or cloth soaked in the solution (lightly wrung out) is directly applied to the lesion(s) as a wet dressing. The soaked cloth should be left in place for 5 to 10 minutes and then resoaked in the solution and reapplied. The patient may repeat this procedure for 15 to 30 minutes 3 times daily. Solutions applied with a cloth should have the cloth material wrapped around the lesions several times, if possible. If large areas are involved, the patient may draw a bath, add appropriate amounts of medications found in Table 39-1, and soak for 15 to 30 minutes 3 to 6 times/day. In general, no more than one-third of the body should be soaked in this manner at any time. Evaporation can concentrate solutions, potentially making them too irritating to use. Small volumes of a 1:40 concentration of Burow solution left standing open at room temperature after 30 to 60 minutes may yield a 1:10 solution. For this reason, wet dressings should always be freshly prepared (i.e., within 24 hours), kept in closed containers, and never reused. When drying the affected area after a wet dressing has been used, care must be taken not to irritate the inflamed skin by rubbing it with a towel; rather, the area should be patted dry gently with a soft, clean towel.[6]

Baths

In addition to wet dressings and soaks, topical solutions can be applied to large areas of the body through bathing. In using this type of treatment, the bath should be about half full. Soothing and antipruritic colloidal bath additives may be used to treat widespread eruptions. Colloidal oatmeal, in the form of 1 cup of oatmeal (e.g., Aveeno) mixed with 2 cups of cold tap water and poured into 6 inches of a lukewarm bath, produces a pleasing and soothing bath. Alternatively, a starch bath using two cups of hydrolyzed starch (e.g., Linit, a mixture of equal parts baking soda and hydrolyzed starch) may also be used. Epsom salt baths, made by dissolving three cups of magnesium sulfate in 6 inches of lukewarm water in a tub, are useful in treating pyodermas, furuncles, and necrotic acne (especially when the back, shoulders, and buttocks are affected).

Many different bath oils are available: Alpha-Keri, Domol, Lubriderm, and Nutraderm. Adding the oil directly to the bath is not recommended because it makes the tub slippery and potentially dangerous. The concentration of the oil in the water becomes almost insignificant anyway (5–10 mL in 20–40 gallons). Approximately 5 to 10 mL of bath oil may be applied directly to wet skin on leaving a bath and patted dry with a towel for a more significant effect. This is most useful in preventing and treating mild cases of xerosis (dry skin). With moderate-to-severe cases of xerosis, additional topical oleaginous products are generally required to improve the condition.

Powders

Powders are drying and cooling, absorbing moisture and creating more surface area for evaporation. They are used mainly in intertriginous areas (e.g., groin, under the breasts, or in skin folds) to decrease friction, which can cause mechanical irritation. The liberal use of powders on bedridden patients helps prevent pressure ulcers (bedsores). They also are useful in the treatment of chafing, tinea pedis (athlete's foot), tinea cruris (jock itch), and diaper dermatitis (diaper rash).

Powders can be applied with a cotton puff or shaker. Care should be taken to minimize breathing the powder because this can lead to respiratory tract irritation, particularly in infants. Powders that contain starch or cellulose (which are hygroscopic) should be washed off before reapplication, because continued buildup can produce mechanical irritation. Corn starch-containing powders should not be used for intertrigo (inflammation of body folds—thighs, armpits, under breasts, or enlarged abdomen; aggravated by heat, moisture, and maceration) because starch can serve as a substrate for *Candida albicans*. Powders should not be applied to oozing lesions because they tend to cake into hard granules, making them difficult and painful to remove, and promoting maceration. The most commonly used powder is talc.

Lotions

Lotions are suspensions or solutions of powder in a water vehicle. They are usually cooling and drying, but may provide some lubrication, depending on the formulation. Lotions are used to treat superficial dermatoses, especially if there is slight oozing. They are useful if large or intertriginous areas are affected, and they are especially advantageous in the treatment of conditions characterized by significant inflammation and tenderness. In these situations, creams or ointments may cause pain on application. Lotions are also useful for hairy areas of the body and scalp. Generally, lotions not containing corticosteroids are applied 3 or 4 times daily, with each fresh application placed over previous application, unless there is significant oozing present, which could promote caking of dried solid ingredients. If this is the case, the area should be cleansed before repeat application. Because many lotions are suspensions, it is advisable to shake the lotion well before application. Generally, 6 ounces of lotion covers the entire body of an average adult.[6]

Liquid Emulsions

Liquid emulsions can be divided into two classes: *oil-in-water* (o/w) and *water-in-oil* (w/o) emulsions. Creams are generally oil-in-water emulsions, whereas ointments are water-in-oil emulsions. Because the fraction of oil increases, the viscosity of the emulsion will also increase.

The indications for liquid oil-in-water emulsions (e.g., Keri Lotion, Cetaphil) are similar to those for lotions and creams, except that this dosage form provides greater occlusion and is more useful in conditions in which dry skin predominates. Liquid water-in-oil emulsions (e.g., Nivea, Eucerin, or Lubriderm) have similar indications to ointments, except they can be applied more easily than ointments. Water-in-oil emulsions are most useful in conditions in which dry skin predominates; application to hairy or intertriginous areas should be avoided. As with lotions, 6 ounces of a liquid emulsion will cover all exposed skin on an average adult.[7]

Gels

Gels are a form of ointment (semisolid emulsion) that contain propylene glycol and carboxypolymethylene. They are clear, nongreasy, nonstaining, nonocclusive, and quick drying. They are thixotropic (i.e., become thinner with rubbing and may sting on application). Gels are most useful when applied to hairy areas or other areas such as the face or scalp, where it is considered cosmetically unacceptable to have the residue of a vehicle remain on the skin. Because of their ingredients, gels tend to be more drying.

Creams

Creams are the most commonly used vehicle in dermatology. Most are oil-in-water emulsions and are intended to be rubbed in well until they vanish (vanishing creams). Because creams are drying and do not provide much occlusiveness, they are most often recommended for subacute lesions and occasionally for chronic lesions without significant lichenification. The most common mistake made by patients when applying creams is that they use too much or do not rub them in fully. Generally, if the cream can be seen on the skin after application, the patient has made one or both of these application mistakes and the preparation is wasted or the patient is not getting the full therapeutic benefits.

Ointments

Ointments are made of inert bases such as petrolatum or may consist of droplets of water suspended in a continuous phase of oleaginous material (i.e., water-in-oil emulsions such as Aquaphor or Polysorb). Ointments are most useful on chronic lesions, relieving dryness, brittleness, and protecting fissures owing to their occlusive properties. They should not be used on acutely inflamed lesions. Ointments should not be applied to intertriginous, burns, or hairy areas because they tend to trap heat and promote maceration. Ointments are greasy and may be cosmetically unacceptable.

Table 39-2
Appropriate Dermatologic Vehicle Selection Across the Range of Dermatologic Lesions

Range of Lesions	Range of Vehicles
Acute inflammation: Oozing, weeping, vesication, edema, pruritus	Aqueous vehicles and water, and then powder solutions, lotions, sprays, and aerosols
↓	↓
Subacute inflammation: Crusting, less oozing, pruritus	Creams, gels
↓	↓
Chronic inflammation: Lichenification, dryness, erythema, pruritus, scaling	Ointments

Aerosols

Aerosols are the most expensive and inefficient way to apply dermatologic medications. Their only advantage over other dosage forms is that they do not require direct mechanical contact with the skin and may be useful if application causes intolerable pain for the patient. If an aerosol is used, it should be shaken well before use, and the patient should be cautioned not to spray the product around the face where it could get into the eyes or nose or be inhaled. Generally, aerosols should be sprayed from approximately 6 inches above the skin in bursts of 1 to 3 seconds. Aerosols are also useful for application to hairy areas if a special application nozzle is used. Aerosols have a drying effect and should not be used for a long period.

Selection of a Delivery System

Dermatologic vehicles should be matched to the type of lesion for which they will be used. Acute lesions require aqueous vehicles until the lesions become dry. Subacute lesions also benefit from aqueous vehicles, but for shorter periods before switching to creams or gels. Chronic lesions usually require ointments because of their dry, lichenified characteristics. Although there are exceptions, usually due to patient preferences, these principles are depicted in Table 39-2.

ASSESSING THE DERMATOLOGIC PATIENT

CASE 39-1

QUESTION 1: C.B., a 23-year-old, 66-kg woman, complains of a rash. What types of questions should C.B. be asked to help determine the appropriate diagnosis and treatment?

The diagnosis of dermatologic conditions can be simplified by considering six primary factors: appearance (what the lesions look like, pattern of the lesions); location or distribution of the lesions on the body; symptoms, both local and systemic; history of the present condition as well as related conditions; age of the patient; and patient sex. Direct observation of the skin lesion,

Table 39-3
Dermatologic Lesions, Definitions, and Clinical Examples

Name	Definition	Examples
Primary Lesions		
Macule	Nonpalpable, flat, change in color, <1 cm	Freckles, flat moles
Patch	Nonpalpable, flat, change in color, >1 cm	Vitiligo, "café au lait" spots, chloasma
Papule	Palpable, solid mass, may have change in color, <1 cm	Verrucae, noninflammatory acne (comedone), raised nevus
Nodule	Palpable, solid mass, most often below the plane of the skin, 1–2 cm	Erythema nodosum, severe acne
Tumor	Palpable, solid mass, >2 cm, most often above and below the plane of the skin	Neoplasms
Plaque	Flat, elevated, superficial papule with surface area greater than height, >1 cm	Psoriasis, seborrheic keratosis
Wheal	Superficial area of cutaneous edema, fluid not confined to cavity	Urticaria (hives), insect bite
Vesicle	Palpable, fluid-filled cavity, <1 cm, filled with serous fluid (blister)	Herpes simples, herpes zoster, contact dermatitis
Bulla	Palpable, fluid-filled cavity, >1 cm, filled with serous fluid (blister)	Pemphigus vulgaris, second-degree burn
Pustule	Similar to vesicle, but filled with purulent fluid	Acne, impetigo, folliculitis
Special Primary Lesions		
Comedone	Plugged opening of sebaceous gland	Acne, blackhead, whitehead
Cyst	Palpable lesion filled with semiliquid material or fluid	Sebaceous cyst
Abscess	Accumulation of purulent material in dermis or subcutaneous layers of skin; purulent material not visible on surface of skin	
Furuncle	Inflammatory nodule involving a hair follicle, following an episode of folliculitis	Small boil
Carbuncle	A coalescence of several furuncles	Large boil
Secondary Lesions		
Erosion	Loss of part or all the epidermis	Ecthyma
Ulcer	Loss of epidermis and dermis	Stasis ulcer
Fissure	Linear crack from epidermis into dermis	Tinea pedis
Excoriation	Self-induced linear, traumatized area caused by intense scratching	Atopic dermatitis, extreme pruritus
Atrophy	Thinning of skin with loss of dermal tissue	Striae
Crusts	Dried residue of pus, serum, or blood from a wound, pustule, or vesicle	Impetigo, scabs
Lichenification	Thickening of epidermis, accentuated skin markings, usually induced by scratching or chronic inflammation	Atopic dermatitis, allergic contact dermatitis

plus C.B.'s responses to questions about these factors, will allow an appropriate diagnosis and treatment plan.

Appearance (morphology)

Table 39-3 provides a listing of common dermatologic lesions, their respective definitions, and some well-known clinical examples. Lesions may also be classified as either primary or secondary. Primary lesions are lesions because they first appear on the skin, whereas secondary lesions develop from primary lesions. The ability to recognize and describe specific lesions is critical to a successful diagnosis and communication regarding response to therapy.

In addition, many lesions present in a particular distribution or pattern. Poison ivy lesions are commonly distributed linearly. Herpetic lesions are so typical that the term herpetiform is used for lesions caused by other conditions that have a herpes-like distribution. The specific size of the lesion is also important in assessing a patient's condition. Dermatologic terms related to lesion distribution or pattern are shown in Table 39-4. The lesion's consistency (firm vs. soft), borders, and color are also important diagnostic considerations.

Location

Certain lesions or conditions usually occur in specific body locations, usually due to physiologic reasons. Table 39-5 provides a list of anatomic sites with common dermatoses occurring in those locations. For example, diseases of the sebaceous glands (e.g., acne, seborrheic dermatitis, rosacea) occur only in sites with high concentrations of sebaceous glands, such as the scalp, head, neck, chest, and umbilicus. Atopic dermatitis shows a predilection for the flexor surfaces of the body (i.e., antecubital and popliteal fossae).

Symptoms

Most skin conditions have only localized symptoms with the most common symptom being pruritus. Occasionally, localized burning or pain is the predominant symptom.

Table 39-4
Descriptive Dermatologic Terms

Term	Characteristics	Examples
Annular	Ring shaped	Tinea
Acneiform	Acne-like	Acne vulgaris
Arcuate	Shaped like an arc	Syphilis
Circinate	Circular	Tinea
Confluent	Lesions run together	Psoriasis, tinea
Discrete	Lesions remain separate	Psoriasis, tinea
Eczematous	General term for dry, red flaky, or lichenified skin without clear border	Chronic allergic contact dermatitis, atopic dermatitis
Geographic	Shaped like islands or continents; map-like	Generalized psoriasis
Grouped	Lesions clustered together	Herpes
Herpetiform	Appears like herpes simplex	Herpes simplex
Intertrigo	Irritant dermatitis in skin folds	Diaper dermatitis
Iris	Looks like a bull's-eye, lesion within a lesion, target lesion	Erythema multiforme
Keratotic	Horny thickening	Psoriasis, corn, callus
Linear	Shaped in lines	Poison ivy
Multiform	More than one type or shape of lesion	Erythema multiforme
Papulosquamous	Papules with desquamation	Psoriasis
Serpiginous	Snake-like lesions	Cutaneous larva migrans
Zosteriform	Appears like herpes zoster	Herpes zoster

Table 39-5
Common Skin Diseases by Body Location

Location	Skin Diseases
Scalp	Seborrheic dermatitis, dandruff
Face	Acne, rosacea, seborrheic dermatitis, perioral dermatitis, impetigo, herpes simplex, atopic dermatitis
Ears	Seborrheic dermatitis
Chest or abdomen	Tinea versicolor, tinea corporis, pityriasis rosea, acne, herpes zoster
Back	Tinea versicolor, tinea corporis, pityriasis rosea
Genital area	Tinea cruris, scabies, pediculosis, condyloma acuminate (venereal warts)
Extremities	Atopic dermatitis (cubital and popliteal fossa)
Hands	Tinea manuum, scabies, primary irritant contact dermatitis, warts
Feet	Tinea pedis, contact dermatitis, onychomycosis
Generalized or localized	Primary irritant or contact dermatitis, photodermatitis

History

Although a diagnosis may often be made from morphology, location, and symptoms, the patient history provides useful diagnostic and therapeutic information. Similar to the historical information obtained for any acute medical problem, the following questions should always be asked:

1. When and how did the problem start?
2. How has it progressed or changed since its onset? How have the lesions changed in size, color, appearance, or severity?
3. What is the patient's past and current medical history? What other symptoms might indicate that this is a dermatologic manifestation of a systemic disease?
4. What are the patient's other symptoms?
5. What kind of allergies does the patient have?
6. What makes the condition worse or better?
7. What events or happenings have occurred with the onset or worsening of the condition (e.g., increased stress, exposure to new products, recent travel, and changes in climate)?
8. What have you used to treat the condition, and how have the treatments worked?
9. How did the patient use any previous therapy, and for how long did they use it?

Age

Many conditions occur predominantly in certain age groups, such as acne in neonates and those ages 11 to 20 years, seborrheic dermatitis in neonates and those ages 11 to 12 years, rosacea in those older than 30 years, and atopic dermatitis primarily in children younger than 6 years. In fact, atopic dermatitis begins and ends before 6 years of age in 95% of patients. It is equally important to realize that many conditions, such as primary irritant and allergic contact dermatitis, occur independent of age. In addition, the skin of children and patients older than 65 years is more penetrable, thus more responsive and more susceptible to adverse effects from therapy with topical agents. Topical therapeutic agent potency and delivery systems must be carefully evaluated before usage.

Sex

Although most dermatologic conditions occur in both sexes, sometimes frequency and severity are sex dependent. Rosacea occurs more frequently in women, but is often more serious in men.

XEROSIS

CASE 39-2

QUESTION 1: C.R., a 64-year-old woman, requests something for dry skin on her shoulders and back. She has had this problem for a number of years. It is generally not a problem in the summer, with most symptoms troubling her in the winter. She denies any visible rash. When asked what makes it better, she tells you bathing provides some temporary relief. She has no other medical conditions and only takes an occasional aspirin for "arthritis." How would you advise C.R. to manage this condition?

C.R.'s complaints represent a common problem of the elderly, xerosis (dry skin). The seasonal cycle described is frequently called "winter itch." Most cases of dry skin are caused by dehydration of the stratum corneum.[7,8] Cold temperatures decrease the indoor humidity because of increased use of central heating, or living in a low humidity climate, such as in Arizona, dry out the outer layers of the skin. Given fact that bathing (moisture) provides temporary relief points to xerosis as the most likely cause.[7,8] The location of the itching, the lack of a visible rash, the relief with bathing, and no chronic diseases rule out most other causes of xerosis (e.g., atopic dermatitis, diabetes mellitus). However, given her age and sex, hypothyroidism remains a possibility. Table 39-6 gives general recommendations for the treatment of dry skin.

Table 39-6
General Recommendations for Treatment of Dry Skin

1. Use room humidifiers.
2. Keep room temperature as low as comfortable to prevent sweating and water loss from the skin.
3. Keep bathing to a minimum (every 1–2 days) with warm, but not hot, water. After bathing, the patient should immediately apply an emollient. When the skin is soaked for 5 to 10 minutes, the stratum corneum can absorb as much as 6 times its weight in water. Application of an emollient immediately after bathing will trap the water in the skin and reduce dryness.
4. Eliminate exposure to solvents, drying chemicals, harsh soaps, and cleaners. These substances remove oils from the skin and reduce its barrier function. Because the barrier function is lost, water loss from the skin is increased up to 75 times higher than normal. Exposure to cold, dry winds will also enhance water loss.
5. Apply emollients 3 to 6 times a day, especially after bathing to help retain moisture in the skin from bathing.
6. The selection of emollients depends on the atmospheric moisture content of the region. In dry parts of the western United States where humidity is very low, water-in-oil emollients such as Lubriderm, Eucerin, or Nivea are preferred because the high oil content prevents the loss of moisture from the skin. In those areas, a general rule is to avoid products in which glycerin is one of the top four ingredients on the label because glycerin is hygroscopic and in low humidity will pull moisture out of the dermis, leading to drier, cracked skin. In areas with higher humidity such as the eastern United States, glycerin in both types of emollients pulls moisture from the atmosphere into the skin. Regardless of region, if application of an emollient appears to be ineffective, switching to a product with less glycerin and more oil may resolve the dryness.
7. If scaling is a problem, a keratolytic (Lac-Hydrin, AmLactin) or a higher-strength, urea-containing preparation (20%) may be useful.

TOPICAL CORTICOSTEROIDS

Table 39-7 lists the most common topical corticosteroid preparations by their degree of potency according to the Stoughton–Cornell classification system.

Indications

A topical corticosteroid is often the drug of choice for many inflammatory and pruritic eruptions. In addition, topical corticosteroids are useful with hyperplastic and infiltrative disorders. The following conditions generally respond well to topical corticosteroids: allergic contact dermatitis, atopic dermatitis, psoriasis, and seborrheic dermatitis.

Contraindications

The following conditions (predominantly infectious etiologies) are worsened by topical corticosteroids: acne vulgaris, ulcers, scabies, warts, molluscum contagiosum, fungal infections, and viral infections.

CASE 39-3

QUESTION 1: AJ is a 54-year-old male who has suffered intermittently from plaque psoriasis for almost 20 years. Most lesions have been coin-sized in various locations (mostly elbows and knees). Normally, gentle removal of the scales and application of 1% hydrocortisone ointment has been effective over several weeks during which it disappears. He has averaged less than a lesion a year. He saw a dermatologist once 18 years ago. Six weeks ago a much larger hand-sized lesion developed on his elbow. The usual treatment has been ineffective. What are the relevant biopharmaceutic considerations for selecting a topical corticosteroid for A. J.?

Topical corticosteroids are classified into potency categories (Table 39-7). The relative potency assigned to a topical corticosteroid is determined by the ability of the preparation to penetrate the skin after release from the vehicle, the intrinsic activity of the corticosteroid at the receptor, and the rate of clearance from the receptor.[10] Activity of corticosteroids may be enhanced by the use of a more occlusive vehicle, the addition of penetration-enhancing substances (i.e., petrolatum, propylene glycol), and modifications of the steroid molecule. Hydrocortisone has been modified in several ways to enhance potency. The addition of a fluorine atom at the 6, 9, and 21 positions protects the steroid ring from metabolic conversion, resulting in more potent activity. The addition of a double bond between the first and second carbon atoms slows metabolism, increasing duration of action. The introduction of an acetonide bond or lipophilic ester groups increases skin penetration. Many newer topical corticosteroids have incorporated one or more of these molecular changes, resulting in increased-potency agents and a growing armamentarium of agents.[9–13]

Topical corticosteroids penetrate into the stratum corneum by passive diffusion, which varies considerably, depending on thickness of the stratum corneum over the part of the body to which the preparation is applied. When a standard hydrocortisone preparation was applied to various parts of the body, absorption was found to be 0.14% on the plantar surface of the foot, 1% on the forearm, 4% on the scalp, 7% on the forehead, 13% on the cheeks, and 36% on the scrotum. Because penetration is high in

Table 39-7
Topical Corticosteroid Preparations by Stoughton–Cornell Classification of Potency

Corticosteroid	Example Brand Name(s)	Vehicle
1 (Most Potent) no more than 2 weeks' use		
Betamethasone dipropionate	Diprolene 0.05%	Ointment, optimized vehicle
Clobetasol propionate	Temovate 0.05%	Cream, ointment, optimized vehicle
Diflorasone diacetate	Psorcon 0.05%	Ointment
Halobetasol propionate	Ultravate 0.05%	Cream, ointment
2		
Amcinonide	Cyclocort 0.1%	Cream, lotion, ointment
Betamethasone dipropionate	Diprolene AF 0.05%	Cream
Betamethasone dipropionate	Diprosone 0.05%	Ointment
Desoximetasone	Topicort 0.25%	Cream, ointment
Desoximetasone	Topicort 0.05%	Gel
Diflorasone diacetate	Florone, Maxiflor 0.05%	Ointment
Fluocinonide	Lidex 0.05%	Cream, ointment, gel
Halcinonide	Halog 0.1%	Cream
Mometasone furoate[a]	Elocon 0.1%	Ointment
Triamcinolone acetonide	Kenalog 0.5%	Cream, ointment
3		
Amcinonide	Cyclocort 0.1%	Cream, lotion
Betamethasone	Benisone, Uticort 0.025%	Gel
Betamethasone benzoate	Topicort LP 0.05%	Cream (emollient)
Betamethasone dipropionate	Diprosone 0.05%	Cream
Betamethasone valerate	Valisone 0.1%	Ointment
Diflorasone diacetate	Florone, Maxiflor 0.05%	Cream
Fluocinonide	Cutivate 0.005%	Ointment
Fluticasone propionate	Lidex E 0.05%	Cream
Halcinonide	Halog 0.1%	Ointment
Triamcinolone acetate	Aristocort A 0.1%	Ointment
Triamcinolone acetate	Aristocort HP 0.5%	Cream
4		
Betamethasone benzoate	Benisone, Uticort 0.025%	Ointment
Betamethasone valerate	Valisone 0.1%	Lotion
Desoximetasone	Topicort-LP 0.05%	Cream
Fluocinolone acetonide	Synalar-HP 0.2%	Cream
Fluocinolone acetonide	Synalar 0.025%	Ointment
Flurandrenolide	Cordran 0.05%	Ointment
Halcinonide	Halog 0.25%	Cream
Hydrocortisone valerate[a]	Westcort 0.2%	Ointment
Mometasone furoate[a]	Elocon 0.1%	Cream
Triamcinolone acetonide	Aristocort, Kenalog 0.1%	Ointment
5		
Betamethasone benzoate	Benisone, Uticort 0.025%	Cream
Betamethasone dipropionate	Diprosone 0.02%	Lotion
Betamethasone valerate	Valisone 0.1%	Cream
Clocortolone	Cloderm 0.1%	Cream
Fluocinolone acetonide	Synalar 0.025%	Cream
Flurandrenolide	Cordran 0.05%	Cream

Table 39-7
Topical Corticosteroid Preparations by Stoughton–Cornell Classification of Potency (*continued*)

Corticosteroid	Example Brand Name(s)	Vehicle
Fluticasone propionate	Cutivate 0.05%	Cream
Hydrocortisone butyrate[a]	Locoid 0.1%	Cream
Hydrocortisone valerate[a]	Westcort 0.2%	Cream
Prednicarbate	Dermatop 0.1%	Cream
Triamcinolone acetonide	Aristocort 0.25%	Cream
6		
Alclometasone dipropionate	Aclovate 0.05%	Ointment
Betamethasone valerate	Valisone 0.1%	Lotion
Desonide[a]	Tridesilon 0.05%	Cream
Fluocinolone acetonide	Synalar 0.01%	Solution
Triamcinolone acetonide	Kenalog 0.1%	Cream, lotion
7 (Least Potent)		
Hydrocortisone[a]	Generic 0.5%, 1.0%, 2.5%	Cream, ointment
Dexamethasone	Decadron 0.1%	Cream

[a]Nonfluorinated corticosteroid.

the groin, axillae, and face, lower-potency nonfluorinated topical preparations such as hydrocortisone 0.5% to 1% should be used on these areas.[9–13] In areas where penetration is poor, owing to thicker stratum corneum, such as the elbows, knees, palms, or soles, higher-potency preparations should be used.[9–13]

The stratum corneum acts as a reservoir, precluding the need for more than twice daily application. In low-potency preparations, this reservoir effect persists for several days, and with the most potent preparations under occlusion, the effects may persist for up to 14 days.[9–13] The clinical implication of this reservoir effect on chronic conditions is a cumulative effect with repeated application of topical corticosteroids. As a result, the number of applications per day can be reduced, and less potent preparations can be used after the acute inflammatory process has been brought under control. It also allows less frequent administration to maintain remission.

For A.J, a high-potency cream (class 2 or 3 as listed by Stoughton–Cornell class of corticosteroid potency in Table 39-7) should be used because the thicker stratum corneum over the elbow, the presence of scales and a raised plaque decreases penetration.

When equal amounts of a corticosteroid are incorporated into ointments, gels, creams, and lotion bases, the gel and ointment preparations are generally more active than creams and lotions.[9–13] However, with the increased use of optimized vehicles, that rule is not as true as in the past. The addition of certain substances enhances penetration and potency. Using these principles, pharmaceutical manufacturers have increasingly developed optimized vehicles that maximize diffusion of individual corticosteroids into the stratum corneum. Unfortunately, these optimized bases may be labeled as ointments, creams, or gels. Therefore, for new products, the only reliable way to ascertain potency is to consult the manufacturer's literature for its Stoughton–Cornell classification. Increasing the concentration of a corticosteroid in a preparation also increases its potency, but not in a linear fashion.

CASE 39-3, QUESTION 2: Given A.J.'s larger lesion and the failure of his usual therapy should occlusive therapy be used? What complications could develop from occlusion? How should the use of occlusion be explained to A.J.?

Occlusion

Occlusion increases the hydration of the skin and resultant absorption of corticosteroid preparations, thus producing a heightened therapeutic effect. Generally, occlusion can be accomplished by the following: (a) selecting an ointment-based corticosteroid, (b) applying a nonmedicated ointment base over a corticosteroid preparation (gel, cream, lotion, or aerosol), 30 minutes after applying the corticosteroid, or (c) by enveloping the medicated area with plastic (e.g., plastic wrap, gloves, or plastic suit). Occlusion is best used for chronic lesions that are thick and scaly, in which drug absorption is impaired, such as psoriasis. Increasing the hydration of the skin (with a shower or bath) also increases the effects of medications immediately applied after the bath or shower. An appropriate recommendation for A.J. would be fluocinonide ointment 0.05% applied twice daily to only the psoriatic plaques.[4,6,9–13] For other conditions, for example, atopic dermatitis, several hours of occlusion are all that are necessary to increase potency, these relatively short periods of occlusion can be clinically useful. Occlusion can be uncomfortable and can lead to sweat retention and an increased risk of bacterial and fungal infections. To reduce these problems and the chances of systemic adverse effects, occlusion should not be maintained for more than 12 hours in a 24-hour period. Occlusion should not be used for acute lesions, which already have increased absorptive capability and need the vasoconstrictive effects of cooling first.

Pharmacists and practitioners tend to underappreciate that both cloth and disposable diapers are powerful occlusive devices. Therefore, only low-potency nonfluorinated topical corticosteroids should be used in the diaper area for no more than 24 to 48 hours in the rare instances of severe diaper dermatitis not responding to conservative treatment. Use of topical corticosteroids to enhance the effectiveness of antifungals in the face of diaper dermatitis complicated by fungal infection is only theoretic and does not enhance the efficacy of anticandidal antifungals, but does increase the risk of local, potentially irreversible disfiguring local adverse effects of topical corticosteroids.

Adverse Drug Effects

Although relatively infrequent, both localized (i.e., at the application site) and systemic adverse effects (from percutaneous absorption) can be caused by topical corticosteroids. The risks for adverse reactions are influenced by the potency of preparation used, frequency of application, duration of use, anatomic site of application, and individual patient factors. Any of the previously discussed factors that increase potency, such as inflammation and occlusion, increase the chances of adverse effects.[9]

CASE 39-4

QUESTION 1: K.L. is 54-year-old male, recently diagnosed with mild Parkinson disease, presents severe case of seborrheic dermatitis involving the ears, scalp line, forehead, and nasal labial folds. The areas are quite inflamed and red with yellow greasy scales. K.L. is upset with the way it looks. Because suppressing the cause of the disease, the yeast, *malassezia furfur*, will take some time, it is decided to initially use a topical corticosteroid to reduce the redness and improve K.L.'s appearance. What would be an appropriate choice of topical corticosteroid for K.L.?

The biggest concern in K.L. is the potential for epidermal and dermal atrophy (thinning of the skin), telangiectasia (small red or purple clusters of dilated capillaries), localized fine hair growth, bruising, hypopigmentation, and striae. These local complications can result from repeated application of topical corticosteroids.[12] Epidermal changes consisting of a reduction in cell size may begin within several days of therapy and are generally reversible after therapy is stopped.[10] Exposed areas (face) and thin-skinned areas (groin) are most vulnerable to dermal and epidermal atrophy.

Dermal atrophy generally takes several weeks to occur and can be reversed in some cases, depending on how long the patient has used the corticosteroid, and on individual host factors such as skin age. Dermal atrophy can be reversible within 2 months after stopping the corticosteroid.[12]

Telangiectasia, which occurs most often on the face, neck, groin, and upper chest, may not be reversible after stopping corticosteroid therapy. Striae, which occur most commonly in the cubital and popliteal fossa, groin, axillary, and inner thigh areas, are usually permanent.[12] Fine hair growth may be particularly bothersome to female patients using corticosteroid preparations on the face. This problem is generally reversible after stopping therapy. Hypopigmentation, predominantly a problem of dark-skinned patients, is generally reversible after therapy is discontinued.[12]

Especially in thin-skinned areas such as the face, fluorinated corticosteroids are more likely to cause these localized reactions because of their increased-potency than nonfluorinated corticosteroids. Therefore, whenever possible only nonfluorinated topical corticosteroids should be used in thin-skinned areas for the shortest possible time. Because the use of corticosteroids is expected to last less than a week, the risk of developing local complications is minimal with a nonfluorinated product.

Because the lesions are on the face, a nonfluorinated corticosteroid such as hydrocortisone valerate or mometasone should be used to minimize the potential for adverse effects in this thin-skinned area. Although there is minimal oozing and weeping, his sensitivity to appearance would indicate a cream might be more appropriate.

CASE 39-4, QUESTION 2: K.L. calls the next day and complains of a burning sensation lasting for about 30 minutes after each application. He wants to know whether this is potentially an allergic reaction.

Because of the time course of the burning sensation in L.K. (starting the first day and lasting only 30 minutes), it is doubtful that he is actually allergic to this product and points to the cream being the cause. To remedy this situation, L.K. should continue to apply it and if it continues for the next 24 hours to call again. Creams applied to inflamed areas can cause burning initially. Because the inflammation lessens, the burning generally subsides. If the burning persists, an ointment can be substituted, or the cream. If the reaction continues with a new product, an allergy workup may be necessary and patch testing could be considered.

Cortisol is endogenously secreted by the adrenal gland and is essential to life. As a result, allergic reactions to topical corticosteroid preparations are rare. When allergic symptoms do occur, they are generally not caused by the corticosteroid, but rather the preservatives (e.g., paraben) or other ingredients in the formulation or the base (e.g., lanolin). Allergic sensitization can occur within 2 weeks of therapy, but may be difficult to diagnose because the corticosteroid can modify the allergic reaction.[14] One should suspect an allergic reaction if lesions change appearance after starting therapy, if healing does not occur within the expected time, or if the condition improves and then abruptly gets worse. In atopic dermatitis, most case reports of allergic reactions (dryness, itching, burning, or irritation) to topical corticosteroids are nonspecific reaction.[14] The use of creams or gels may cause excessive dryness, burning, and irritation. Switching to an ointment can alleviate those symptoms. Allergic individuals are more likely to react to the vehicle base than the active corticosteroid ingredient.

ACNE

CASE 39-4, QUESTION 3: After several weeks of continuous corticosteroid and adjuvant therapy, K.L.'s seborrheic dermatitis has disappeared, but he has developed four pustules and two closed comedones on his forehead and multiple pustules on his nasal labial folds. What problems from the use of topical corticosteroid therapy on the face does this represent?

The face is particularly vulnerable to corticosteroid adverse effects because of enhanced penetration.[12] Acne, acne rosacea, and perioral dermatitis can develop after several weeks to months of application. Corticosteroid-induced conditions can generally be distinguished from naturally occurring disorders because lesions are uniformly at the same level of development throughout the affected area and are present only in areas treated with the corticosteroid. Generally, steroid acne and perioral dermatitis resolve after discontinuing the drug. Application of corticosteroid preparations (particularly the potent preparations) to areas around the eye can lead to increased intraocular pressure, glaucoma, cataracts, increased risk of ocular mycotic infections, and exacerbation of preexisting herpes simplex infections.[12]

Because K.L.'s original disorder was also treated with topical selenium sulfide shampoo to the face and the scalp to suppress the cause of his seborrheic dermatitis, the corticosteroid can be discontinued.

ADRENAL AXIS SUPPRESSION AND RISK OF INFECTION

Systemic adrenal axis suppression from topically applied corticosteroids appears to be more of a theoretic risk than a practical one in adults, except when the highest-potency preparations are used,[15] or other risk factors are present (Table 39-8). Although suppression has been reported with use of mild to moderately potent agents, these cases can be attributed to excessive use or to application of corticosteroids over large areas of the body for prolonged periods under occlusion. If suppression does occur, it reverses within 2 to 4 weeks after application is stopped. Patients using more than 45 g/week of a high-potency corticosteroid are at risk for adrenal axis suppression.[15] Therefore, the use of preparations such as clobetasol should be limited to no more than 45 g/week for 2 weeks or less. In addition, these preparations

Table 39-8
Risk Factors for Systemic Adverse Effects from Topical Corticosteroids

Duration of application
Prolonged application (>3–4 weeks)
Potency of corticosteroid
Weak or moderately strong, 100 g/week without occlusion
Very potent, >45 g/week without occlusion
Application location
Thin stratum corneum results in easier penetration (eyelids, forehead, cheeks, armpits, groin, and genitals)
Age of patient
Very young children and elderly people have very thin epidermis
Manner of application
Occlusion
Presence of penetration-enhancing substances
Propylene glycol
Salicylic acid
Urea
Condition of the skin
General factors
Compromised liver function
Uremia

should not be used under occlusion and should be reserved for dermatoses that are unresponsive to less potent preparations.

Because young children absorb corticosteroids to a greater extent than adults, they have a greater risk of developing adrenal axis suppression and other systemic adverse effects.[15] To reduce this risk, low-potency topical preparations should be used in children, and their use should be limited to short periods. Patients whose corticosteroid clearance is impaired (e.g., liver failure) should also use hydrocortisone and be monitored closely for signs of systemic toxicity.[12]

The risk of developing an Addisonian crisis during surgery or at other times of stress secondary to adrenal suppression from topical steroids is extremely low. Patients who have used potent topical corticosteroids over large areas of their bodies (>30%) or those who have used occlusion are at greater risk (see previous discussion) and are often given systemic hydrocortisone prophylactically before surgery.[15]

PROPER APPLICATION OF TOPICAL CORTICOSTEROIDS

Because overuse of topical corticosteroids leads to local and/or systemic effects and underuse results in suboptimal treatment, the amount of corticosteroid required to treat certain anatomic areas of the body has long been an issue of debate and discussion.[16,17] To prevent overuse in clinical practice, patients are typically given subjective instructions to apply topical products "sparingly" or "in a thin layer or coat" and left up to the patient or caregiver's interpretation.

The fingertip unit (FTU) was devised as a means of standardizing the way practitioners and pharmacists alike thought about how to prescribe topical corticosteroids and counsel patients on appropriate use. One FTU is defined as the amount of ointment (or other semisolid topical formulation) squeezed from a tube with a 5-mm diameter nozzle (standard in manufacturing), applied from the first distal skin crease to the tip of the index finger of an adult.[18–20] This amount is roughly equivalent to 500 mg of medication. The FTU can serve as a helpful starting point for how much product is used. Because lesions rarely conform to the exact anatomic areas in Table 39-9, adjustments need to be made based on the specific area involved. For example, in an adult with atopic dermatitis on the cubital fossa of both arms, the table does not provide that exact measurement. Because one FTU covers both sides of a hand and the cubital fossa is approximately hand-sized, the patient should be instructed to apply 0.5 FTU to each cubital fossa once or twice daily depending on the specific preparation. Although use of the FTU concept is not a panacea, it does provide

Table 39-9
Fingertip Unit Charts for Adults and Children

Fingertip unit measures for use in adults[3]				
Area of body			**FTU per dose**	
Face and neck			2.5	
Torso and abdomen (front of trunk)			7	
Back and buttocks (back of trunk)			7	
One arm (front and back)			3	
One hand			1	
One leg (front and back)			6	
One foot			2	
Adult fingertip unit measures for use in children (by age of child)[4,5]				
	3–6 months	**1–2 years**	**3–5 years**	**6–10 years**
Face and neck	1	1.5	1.5	2
Arm and hand	1	1.5	1	2.5
Leg and foot	1.5	2	3	4.5
Trunk (front)	1	2	3	3.5
Trunk (back including buttocks)	1.5	3	3.5	5

a more objective benchmark to help patients more consistently apply the correct amount of product and avoid overuse. Use of the FTU concept must be accompanied by counseling and reinforcement based on the individual medication received, size and location of the lesion, and the desired goals of therapy. In addition, the FTU concept can be used to determine the amount to be dispensed to cover a treatment period.

Summary of Principles of Topical Corticosteroid Therapy

The following principles are used to guide the choice of agent and application technique (Table 39-7 and Table 39-9):

- Due to the reservoir effect of the stratum corneum, topical corticosteroids should be applied no more than twice daily. Increasing the application from twice daily to 4 times daily does not produce superior responses, is more expensive, and may lead to increased frequency of topical and systemic adverse effects.[10]
- Preparations should be rubbed thoroughly and, when possible, applied while the skin contains optimal moisture (e.g., after bathing and drying off).[6] Hydration of the skin increases percutaneous absorption and the resultant therapeutic effect of topical corticosteroids.
- Appropriate-strength preparations should be used to control the condition. For maintenance, most dermatologic conditions requiring topical corticosteroids can be managed with medium- or low-potency corticosteroid preparations (i.e., 1% hydrocortisone or a low-strength fluorinated corticosteroid such as triamcinolone acetonide 0.025%).[10,11]
- Occluded areas and certain, thin-skinned areas of the body, such as the face and flexures, are more prone to the development of adverse effects.[9,11] If corticosteroids must be used on the face flexures or other thin-skinned areas, hydrocortisone or other nonfluorinated topical corticosteroids should be used to reduce the probability of adverse effects. These nonfluorinated corticosteroid products are highlighted in Table 39-6.
- Children, elderly patients, and patients with liver failure are at risk for systemic corticosteroid toxicities. In addition, patients who use the highest-potency preparations for longer than 2 weeks are susceptible to percutaneous absorption and systemic toxicity including Addison syndrome upon sudden discontinuation.[9–14]
- With chronic conditions such as atopic eczema or allergic contact dermatitis, it is best to discontinue therapy gradually. This reduces the potential for rebound flares of topical lesions.[6]

Atopic Dermatitis

CASE 39-5

QUESTION 1: P.K., a 17-year-old boy, presents to a dermatology clinic with 5% of his body covered with a pruritic, eczematous rash. There is extensive involvement of popliteal and cubital fossae bilaterally. There is evidence of excoriation with cosmetic disfigurement in the cubital fossae, and on his cheeks, with a history or frequent bouts of impetigo. P.K.'s mother and aunt have asthma. One sister (L.K.), age 15, has seasonal allergic rhinitis and eczema. His father and younger brother, age 11, appear to have no atopic manifestations. A rash was first noted 1 month after birth. The cheeks of the face were the only area affected, and the rash continued with varying degrees of severity until the age of 2 years, when it spontaneously resolved. A similar rash reappeared at age 12, was diagnosed as atopic dermatitis, and has not disappeared since that time. P.K. experienced seasonal allergic rhinitis beginning at age 6 years. He has had a difficult time trying to follow provided nondrug recommendations for eczema. He has used over-the-counter topical hydrocortisone cream to treat flare-ups during the years.

On physical examination, P.K. is a well-nourished, well-developed, adolescent boy with no abnormal physical findings other than marked allergic shiners, pale boggy nasal mucosa, and Dennie–Morgan folds noted near the eyes, plus extensive skin lesions. Oozing, crusted, excoriated areas caused by scratching, with erythematous, eczematous, lichenified eruptions, are his face and the flexor aspects of both arms and legs. There is some evidence of a secondary bacterial infection in both cubital fossae and on portions of the left leg. The presenting history, symptoms, and signs are characteristics of atopic dermatitis (eczema). Describe characteristics of atopic dermatitis and explain the significance of P.K.'s family and medical history because it relates to this disorder.

Atopic dermatitis, a form of eczema, can be acute or subacute, but is more commonly a chronic pruritic inflammation of the epidermis and dermis. Approximately two-thirds of the patients have a personal or family history of allergic rhinitis, eczema, or asthma. Sixty percent of patients are affected within the first year of life, 30% by 5 years of age, with the remaining 10% experiencing atopic dermatitis between 6 and 20 years of age. Atopic dermatitis in infants may be a prelude to the development of other atopic disorders later in life (i.e., allergic rhinitis or asthma). Presence of these disorders many times is the key to differential diagnosis. About 80% of patients with atopic dermatitis have a type I (immunoglobulin E [IgE]-mediated) hypersensitivity reaction occurring because of the release of vasoactive substances from both mast cells and basophils that have been sensitized by the interaction of the antigen with IgE. An allergy workup is rarely helpful in determining the allergen. The disorder affects 0.5% to 1.0% of the general population, although its prevalence in children is 5% to 10%. In infants and young children, the dermatitis often occurs on the face and sternal area of the chest. In older children and adults, it tends to localize to the flexural areas, especially the cubital and popliteal fossae with the neck and face involved in more severe cases.[21]

Pruritus is the hallmark of atopic dermatitis. Atopic dermatitis has been described as "the itch that rashes, rather than the rash that itches." In other words, the itching precedes the rash. The constant scratching leads to a vicious cycle of itch-scratch-rash-itch, with bacterial colonization and infections intertwined. Chronically, untreated atopic dermatitis leads to lichenification of the affected areas. Wool, detergents, soaps, a change in room temperature, and mental or physical stress can precipitate itching. Patients tend to have dry skin (xerosis) all over the body. This is attributable to a reduced water-binding capacity and a higher transdermal water loss. Xerosis is worsened during periods of low humidity, such as winter in northern latitudes. Treating the xerosis can prevent or control the disease in mild or episodic cases.[21,22]

P.K.'s family and medical history are classic for atopic dermatitis. His family history is significant for asthma, allergic rhinitis, and atopic dermatitis. He had his initial outbreak at the age of 1 month and then experienced seasonal allergic rhinitis after his dermatitis went into remission. His skin examination reveals findings of both acute and chronic atopic dermatitis, with typical lesion location and description.

Product Selection

CASE 39-5, QUESTION 2: P.K. received a prescription for halcinonide 0.25% cream, 30 g, to be applied at bedtime to nonfacial areas and mometasone furoate cream 0.1%, 30 g, twice daily to the facial lesions. Based on pertinent biopharmaceutic considerations, why is this prescription appropriate for P.K.?

Results from P.K.'s treatment regimen might be improved by providing more frequent (twice daily) application or a more potent preparation to control inflamed lesions. Once any weeping is stopped, a less potent preparation in the ointment form should be used for maintenance and the number of applications may be reduced. Because of the reservoir effect, control can be maintained in many cases with intermittent regimens such as once daily, every other day, or every third day use of topical corticosteroids. In addition, intermittent regimens can involve alternating corticosteroids and agents such as topical pimecrolimus or tacrolimus to maintain control and minimize adverse effects of either agent.

Because the calcineurin inhibitors are as potent as mid-potency topical corticosteroids without causing atrophy, telangiectasias, or striae, many dermatologists would use either tacrolimus or pimecrolimus on the face in preference to mometasone.[22]

Topical Antibiotics with Corticosteroids

CASE 39-5, QUESTION 3: P.K.'s atopic dermatitis presentation is complicated with areas of erythematous, honey-colored, crusted lesions on his arm, and leg. Can a corticosteroid and an antibiotic preparation be used together? What are the risks associated with topical antibiotics?

It is determined that P.K. has impetigo superimposed on his atopic dermatitis. Because impetigo can be treated with topical antibiotics such as mupirocin, combination therapy with a corticosteroid–antibiotic preparation would appear to be a logical choice. Although mupirocin may be an appropriate alternative for some topical dermatologic infections, the current over-the-counter topical antibiotics (bacitracin, neomycin, and polymyxin) are ineffective for most dermatologic infections and are indicated only for the prophylaxis of skin infections. In addition, because staphylococcal toxins act as superantigens, eliciting the production of IgE, thus worsening the atopic dermatitis, almost all clinicians treat atopic dermatitis-associated impetigo with oral antibiotics such as dicloxacillin, macrolides, or cephalexin, in combination with topical corticosteroids for the atopic dermatitis.[22] Oral antibiotics reduce the bacterial counts faster and have a lower incidence of recurrent impetigo compared with topical agents. In areas in which community methicillin-resistant *Staphylococcus aureus* rates are high, more effective antibiotic therapy might be indicated as an alternative. P.K. would most likely benefit from a treatment course of an oral antibiotic plus a topical corticosteroid preparation.

P.K. is prone to repeated infections and atopic dermatitis flares because his skin is colonized with staphylococci. Many dermatologists upon clearance of the impetigo would initiate dilute bleach baths. These consist of 5- to 10-minute baths twice a week, made by adding 120 cc (1/2 cup) of household bleach (6%) to a full bathtub (approximately 40 gallons) to create a 0.005% solution. Because of the variety of tub sizes, the amount of bleach should be adjusted to the size of the bathtub and the amount of water in the tub.[23]

Pruritus

CASE 39-5, QUESTION 4: As stated in Case 39-5, Question 1, one of P.K.'s complaints is pruritus. What could you recommend for relief of pruritus?

As previously noted, pruritus (itching) is the most common cutaneous symptom in atopic dermatitis.[21] Scratching, which can damage or fatigue receptor nerve endings, is the most common method of relieving pruritus. Topically applied local anesthetics or antihistamines could also be effective in dulling the sensation. However, this approach is often disappointing, probably because the intact epidermis poorly absorbs the salt forms of these drugs. In addition, low concentrations are used in many over-the-counter preparations. If adequate concentrations of local anesthetics are used (lidocaine 3%–4%), pruritus or pain may be reduced for up to 45 minutes. These agents are most useful for relieving pruritus or pain for short periods (e.g., when trying to go to sleep at night).[21] A serious drawback to the use of topical benzocaine and antihistamine preparations is their propensity to induce allergic contact dermatitis.[24]

P.K. could also try cold water or ice cubes, which effectively relieve pruritus via vasoconstriction, as do products containing aluminum acetate (Burow solution), tannic acid, or calamine. A cool bath may be useful for the relief of pruritus from dermatologic lesions if they are widespread.

Moisturizing mixtures such as Eucerin, Nivea, Lubriderm, or even simply mineral or baby oil are useful in the treatment of pruritus caused by dry skin in patients with atopic dermatitis. Bathing should be restricted to avoid washing away normal body oils, the drying effect of water, the irritant effect of alkaline soaps, and the trauma of toweling.[6]

Topical corticosteroid applications can be very effective if dermatologic lesions exist. They reduce inflammation, which helps soothe the affected area.

Systemic antihistamines are effective antipruritic agents, although their major beneficial effect may be attributable to sedation. The newer, nonsedating antihistamines are notably ineffective at relieving itch, with the exception of cetirizine.[25] There is disagreement over which antihistamine or antiserotonin agents are most effective for treatment of pruritus.[21,25,26] Oral hydroxyzine is a commonly used antihistamine; doses of 10 to 25 mg 3 to 4 times a day are commonly used. Oral cyproheptadine is another option. There is little evidence that antihistamines are effective in treating non–histamine-mediated pruritus, except that their inherent sedative effect may be somewhat beneficial in all pruritic conditions. Doxepin, a tricyclic antidepressant with potent H_1-blocking properties, is valuable as a second-line antihistamine topically or systemically if others fail.[27] Because P.K.'s pruritus is worse at night, as is typical with atopic dermatitis, the use of any of the three H_1-blockers mentioned at bedtime would be appropriate.[22]

Nondrug Recommendations for Atopic Dermatitis

CASE 39-5, QUESTION 5: In addition to prescriptions for topical corticosteroids, a systemic antibiotic (cephalexin 500 mg 4 times daily for 10 days), and an oral antihistamine (hydroxyzine 25 mg, one to two tablets by mouth at bedtime as needed), what nondrug interventions should be suggested for P.K.?

The general goals of therapy for atopic dermatitis are to decrease pruritus, suppress inflammation, and moisturize the skin. The nondrug recommendations shown in Table 39-10 are

Table 39-10
Nondrug Recommendations for Patients with Atopic Dermatitis or Other Irritant Dermatoses[28]

- Clothing should be soft and light. Cotton or corduroy is preferred. Wools and coarse, heavy synthetics should be avoided.
- Heat should be avoided because it often makes eczema worse. The environment should be well ventilated, cool, and low in humidity (30%–50%). Rapid changes in ambient temperature should be avoided.
- Bathing should be kept to a minimum (no longer than 5 minutes), and the patient should use a nonirritating soap (e.g., Basis soap). A colloid bath or the use of appropriate amounts of bath oil may be useful.
- The skin should be kept moist with frequent applications of emollients (e.g., Lubriderm, Nivea, Aquaphor, Eucerin, or petrolatum).
- Primary irritants such as paints, cleansers, solvents, and chemical sprays should be avoided.

useful adjuncts and mainstays for use between disease flares for patients such as P.K. with atopic dermatitis or any other irritant dermatitis. Often careful attention to nonpharmacologic measures can markedly reduce the incidence of disease flare. Because even nonlesional skin in patients with atopic dermatitis has reduced moisture, the use of emollients should include all skin surfaces.[28]

P.K. should be warned to avoid people with active herpes simplex infections because severe disseminated infections can occur.

Tachyphylaxis and Calcineurin Inhibitors

Clinicians commonly misdiagnose tachyphylaxis due to corticosteroids. Failure of topical corticosteroids to clear difficult atopic dermatitis after an initial improvement may give the false impression of tachyphylaxis, when the actual problem is a primary failure of the treatment.[29] This could be caused by either inappropriate application technique by the patient or the choice of a product with inadequate potency. Tachyphylaxis can occur within 1 week of therapy, but generally takes several weeks to a month to occur.[29] To treat this problem, patients should discontinue the corticosteroid for a week and restart at an appropriate dose. Alternatively, patients may be switched to topical tacrolimus or pimecrolimus.

Topical tacrolimus or pimecrolimus is an effective alternative to moderate-potency topical corticosteroids and is safe for use in children.[22,23,27] In addition to inhibitory effect on cytokine production, calcineurin inhibitors result in decreased immunologic response to antigens. Transient burning, erythema, and pruritus are the most common adverse effects. Neither pimecrolimus nor tacrolimus causes skin atrophy, making them attractive alternatives for patients with lesions on the face and the neck. Issues regarding the long-term safety of these products have led the U.S. Food and Drug Administration to place a black-box warning in the manufacturer's literature regarding a potential increased cancer risk.[22]

ALLERGIC CONTACT DERMATITIS: POISON IVY, POISON OAK, OR POISON SUMAC

Contact dermatitis is an inflammation of the skin that occurs when a substance comes in direct contact with the epidermal surface. The most common form is irritant contact dermatitis caused solvents or other chemicals that irritate the skin resulting red, painful lesions, for example, dish pan hands, diaper dermatitis. Allergic contact dermatitis is a type IV delayed hypersensitivity reaction controlled by allergen-specific T cells. The resulting dermatitis is pruritic and many times vesicular in nature.[1–6]

Poison ivy (*Rhus*) dermatitis is a major cause of allergic contact dermatitis in the United States, exceeding all other causes combined. Other allergens include latex, leather, nickel, and laundry detergents. It is estimated that 50% to 95% of the population is sensitive to the plants to some degree. The severity of the condition varies from mild discomfort to an extremely painful, debilitating condition. *Rhus* dermatitis is caused by sensitization to an allergic substance in the leaves, stems, and roots of poison ivy, poison oak, and poison sumac plants. All three plants contain the same sensitizing oleoresin, urushiol oil, which contains pentadecacatechol, the actual sensitizing agent. Therefore, the dermatitis caused by the three different plants is identical.

Direct contact with the plant is unnecessary for the rash to occur. Highly sensitive persons may develop severe dermatitis merely from exposure to *Rhus* oleoresin carried by pollen or by smoke from burning leaves. The oleoresin may remain active for months on clothing, shoes, tools, and sporting equipment. Once the toxic substance is exposed to the skin, it can be spread by the hands to other areas of the body (e.g., genitals or eyes) or to people who may come into close contact with the exposed person. Although washing with soap and water may not prevent the dermatitis, even if it is done within 15 minutes of exposure, it will prevent spread of the oleoresin to other parts of the body.

Sensitive individuals should be instructed to avoid contact with the offending plant. If contact is inevitable, every effort should be made to shield exposed areas of the skin with appropriate clothing.

Exposed individuals should bathe or shower as soon as they come in from outdoors and should wash their clothes. Nonprescription topical cleansers (Tecnu, Zanfel, Mean Green Hand Scrub) claim to remove urushiol oil embedded in the skin through the action of microfine scrubbing beads and surfactants, thus possibly preventing the rash or limiting spread. They are applied to exposed areas of the skin, followed by vigorous scrubbing, and rinsed off after application.

After an initial incubation period of 5 to 21 days, a patient would be expected to react to the oleoresin in 12 to 48 hours after re-exposure. A mild exposure to these plants in a sensitized person results in a typical erythematous, vesicular, linear, and sometimes, oozing rash after 2 to 3 days; complete clearing occurs in 1 to 3 weeks.

If a large area is exposed, lesions appear within 6 to 12 hours and may appear blistered and eroded; in some cases, ulcers may appear. Healing occurs more slowly, often requiring 2 to 3 weeks for complete resolution. The following factors contribute to the development of poison ivy, poison oak, or poison sumac dermatitis: the concentration of the oleoresin to which the skin is exposed, area of exposure (i.e., the thickness of the stratum corneum), duration of exposure, site of exposure, genetic factors, and immune tolerance. It is important to determine the areas of the body that are affected. If the eyes, genital areas, mouth, respiratory tract, or more than 15% of the body is affected, the patient should receive a course of systemic corticosteroids. See Case 39-6 below.

Treatment

CASE 39-6

QUESTION 1: K.P., a 27-year-old woman, has recently returned from an outing in the woods. She now has vesicular eruptions that appear in a linear pattern on one arm and hand. She believes that she has had a poison oak reaction and requests therapy. What should be recommended at this point? What should be recommended if the condition becomes more severe?

Weeping lesions should be treated with aqueous vehicles (e.g., Burow solution or saline) as outlined in the beginning of this chapter. Lesions that are not wet or weeping should be treated with calamine lotion applied 2 to 4 times daily. The zinc oxide in calamine lotion may act as a mild astringent, although some people find this preparation to be unacceptable because of its pink color, which can stain clothes. Alternatively, a topical corticosteroid appropriate for the body part affected could be used. If K.P.'s poison oak reaction becomes more severe, additional treatment with prednisone 1 mg/kg/day for at least 2 or 3 weeks will be required; such therapy should be withdrawn slowly (1–2 weeks) to prevent recurrence of the lesions.

SYSTEMIC THERAPY

CASE 39-7

QUESTION 1: Z.T., a 19-year-old man, has just returned from a fishing trip and now has an erythematous, linear, dry eruption on his leg and arm, and a generalized eruption on his hands and face. He has been in areas that have dense poison ivy growth, and he may have burned some in the campfire. Z.T. has washed himself and his clothes thoroughly. How should he be treated?

The fact that Z.T.'s facial rash is not linear (as one would expect if he had just contacted the plant) suggests that he may have contacted the smoke of a burning poison ivy plant. This can be quite serious because the oleoresin can be carried in smoke and, if inhaled, can cause vesiculation of lung tissue leading to severe respiratory problems. Z.T. should be observed for signs of respiratory difficulties and should be treated with a course of systemic corticosteroids.

RELAPSE

CASE 39-7, QUESTION 2: Z.T.'s physician prescribed oral prednisone for his rash. He was instructed to take 80 mg/day for 14 days and to decrease the dose by 5 mg/day each day thereafter. Calamine lotion (3 times daily to affected areas) also was prescribed. After 12 days, Z.T. complains that the lesions seem to be getting worse. The lesions had cleared after 8 days of treatment, and he began rapidly tapering the prednisone at that time. Why is he experiencing a relapse?

Two weeks is the minimum course of treatment when systemic corticosteroids are used for severe cases of poison ivy, poison oak, or poison sumac. The oleoresin remains fixed in the skin, and if the systemic corticosteroid is withdrawn too soon, the lesions return. This is probably the most common reason for treatment failure with systemic corticosteroids. Alternatively, systemic corticosteroids can be discontinued before 2 weeks of treatment and a moderate-potency topical corticosteroid preparation can be started 24 hours before discontinuation of systemic corticosteroids and continued for 7 to 10 days to prevent relapse.

DRUG ERUPTIONS

Clinically recognizable adverse drug reactions are manifested on the skin more often than any other organ or organ system.[30–33] An estimated 1% to 5% of hospitalized patients experience a drug eruption.[31] Outpatient statistics are more difficult to obtain, but are probably within the same range.

Many of the common dermatologic reactions that can be induced by drugs have other causes as well, so a complete workup must include other nondrug etiologies. Viral, fungal, and bacterial infections, as well as certain systemic diseases and foods, have been identified as causes for common reactions such as urticaria, erythema multiforme, and erythema nodosum. The diagnosis of drug eruptions is best made by identifying the type of lesions observed and associating the lesions with specific drug therapy. The most important diagnostic criterion is an accurate assessment of the skin lesions. With this critical information, the clinician can then refer to a drug information source to associate any current or past drug therapy with the specific lesions observed (see Chapter 32, Drug Hypersensitivity Reactions).

Acneiform Eruptions

Acneiform eruptions appear very much like common acne. They may be distinguished from acne by their sudden occurrence, the absence of comedones, uniform appearance (i.e., all at the same stage of development), and the fact that they may occur on any part of the body. Cysts and scarring are rarely associated with drug-induced acne. Eruptions can also occur during any period of the patient's life; thus, drug-induced acne should be suspected when the lesions appear in persons outside the typical age bracket for acne. Drugs implicated include adrenocorticotropic hormone, anabolic steroids, azathioprine, danazol, glucocorticoids, iodides, bromides, lithium, gefitinib, erlotinib. lapatinib, and oral contraceptives. For patients with acne vulgaris, these drugs may worsen existing lesions (see Chapter 40, Acne).

Photosensitivity Reactions

Photosensitivity eruptions require the presence of both a drug (or chemical) and a light source of appropriate wavelength. These eruptions are divided into two subtypes: phototoxic and photoallergic. *Phototoxic* reactions, the most common drug-induced photodermatosis, manifest themselves as an exaggerated sunburn or increased sensitivity to sunburn. The ultraviolet A (UVA) light source alters the drug to a toxic form, resulting in tissue damage independent of any allergic response, and occurs in everyone who gets high enough skin levels of the offending drug. This eruption can occur on first exposure to a drug, is dose-related, and will continue as long as the skin concentration of the drug exceeds the threshold level for the reaction to occur. *Photoallergic* reactions, which are very uncommon, may appear as a variety of lesions, including urticaria, bullae, and eczema. UVA light alters the drug so it becomes an antigen or acts as a hapten. Photoallergic eruptions require previous contact with the offending drug, are not dose related, exhibit cross-sensitivity with chemically related compounds, and are secondary to the use of topical agents. Unfortunately, outside light through a window and fluorescent lighting permit passage of or can emit UVA light. In addition, until recently there were inadequate topical preparations that provide protection against UVA light. Avobenzone, although covering much of the UVA spectrum, is photolabile, losing 60% of its effectiveness in less than 1 hour. However, many products now solve that problem by adding agents such as octocrylene, which stabilize avobenzone's photolability, and are usually labeled "stabilized UVA protection." New products containing ecamsule appear to offer an advance in protection against lower spectrum UVA rays. Most phototoxic and photoallergic reactions occur fairly soon after exposure to light. Implicated drugs are numerous, including among others, antibiotics (tetracyclines, fluoroquinolones, and sulfonamides), antidepressants (tricyclics), antihypertensives (hydrochlorothiazide, β-blockers), hypoglycemics (sulfonylureas), nonsteroidal anti-inflammatory drugs, sunscreens (*p*-aminobenzoic acid [PABA]), oral contraceptives, and antipsychotics (phenothiazines) (see Chapter 42, Photosensitivity, Photoaging, and Burns Injuries).

Allergic Contact Dermatitis

Topical administration of a sensitizing agent produces localized papulovesicular lesions. These lesions are limited only to areas that are exposed to the topical product. Neomycin, benzocaine, and diphenhydramine are well-known topical sensitizers (Table 39-11).[34-36] Systemic administration of a drug to a patient previously sensitized to the drug by topical application can provoke widespread dermatitis. Implicated systemically or topically administered drugs that reactivate allergic contact dermatitis include procaine or benzocaine, radiographic contrast media or iodine, and streptomycin and gentamicin or neomycin, among others.

Erythema Multiforme

As the name implies, erythema multiforme (EM) eruptions take on a varied spectrum of morphologic forms, ranging from the mildest with tiny maculovesicular lesions to more severe forms such as SJS and toxic epidermal necrolysis syndrome (TENS) with extensive bullous lesions and routine involvement of mucous membranes. Although all forms have been reported to have oral lesions, they are much more severe in SJS and TENS, in which genital, nasal, and ocular mucosae can also be involved. Target lesions are usually present in all forms of the disorder, which characteristically are erythematous, iris-shaped papules, and vesiculobullous lesions typically involving the extremities, especially the palms and soles in EM and the torso in SJS and TENS. The lesions take on the appearance of a circular target with a bull's-eye in the middle, thus the term target lesion. Questions have recently been raised about the shared pathologic nature of these forms of EM.[37] EM in its mildest forms, EM minor and EM major, is more common in children and young adults, and is self-limited in nature with only transient hypopigmentation or hyperpigmentation as complications. Sometimes malaise, a low-grade fever, and itching or burning may accompany this type of eruption. Etiologic factors associated with EM include drugs, mycoplasma and herpes infections, radiation therapy, foods, and sometimes neoplasms. Allopurinol, barbiturates, phenothiazine, and sulfonamides are the drugs most often implicated in EM eruptions.

Table 39-11
Frequent Contact Sensitizers

Substance	Found In
Ammonia	Soaps, chemicals, hair dyes
Antihistamines	Topical anti-itch creams and ointments
Balsam of Peru	Cosmetics
Benzyl alcohol	Medications, cosmetics
"Caine" anesthetics	Medications (e.g., over-the-counter benzocaine products)
Carba	Rubber
Chromium	Jewelry
Epoxy resin	Glue
Ethylenediamine	Stabilizer in topical products (e.g., aminophylline)
Formaldehyde	Shoes, clothing, soaps, insulations
Mercaptobenzothiazole	Rubber
Naphthyl	Rubber
Neomycin	Topical medications (e.g., Neosporin)
Nickel sulfate	Jewelry, fasteners
Paraben	Preservative in many topical products
Paraphenylenediamine	Hair dyes, leather
Potassium dichromate	Shoes, leather
Thiomersal	Preservatives, contact lens products
Thiram	Rubber products
Turpentine	Paint products
Wool alcohols	Lanolin-containing products, clothes

Stevens–Johnson Syndrome

SJS is probably the most common type of severe drug eruption. The syndrome is usually a moderate mucocutaneous and systemic reaction. Blisters and atypical target lesions involve less than 10% of body surface area, with some epidermal detachment, which can cause scarring in some cases.

With more extensive involvement, clinical findings are almost indistinguishable from TENS. The skin can become hemorrhagic, and pneumonia and joint pains may occur. Serious ocular involvement is common and can culminate in partial or complete blindness. Besides drugs, this syndrome has been associated with infections, pregnancy, foods, deep radiographic therapy, and neoplasms. Mortality is estimated to be in the range of 5% to 18%. The duration of the syndrome is usually 4 to 6 weeks. The long-acting sulfonamides are most often implicated. Allopurinol, carbamazepine, fluoroquinolones, hydantoin, phenylbutazone, piroxicam, and other sulfa derivatives such as sulfonylureas are also possible causative agents.

Toxic Epidermal Necrolysis Syndrome

Epidermal necrolysis, a severe, life-threatening mucocutaneous and systemic reaction, may be preceded by a prodrome characterized by malaise, lethargy, fever, and occasionally throat or mucous membrane soreness. Epidermal changes follow and consist of erythema and massive bullae formations that easily rupture and peel, giving the skin a scalded appearance.

Hairy parts of the body are usually not affected, but mucous membrane involvement is common. Blisters cover more than 30% of body surface area, with extensive epidermal detachment that can result in scarring. Mortality in TENS patients is roughly 30%, often within 8 days after bullae appear. The usual cause of death is infection complicated by massive fluid and electrolyte loss, similar to patients with extensive burns. Although the skin takes on a grave appearance, healing occurs within 2 weeks in approximately 70% of patients, with some potential for scarring. In addition to drugs, certain bacterial infections and foods are believed to cause this type of eruption. Most causes of TENS in children are owing to infection (e.g., *S. aureus*). A higher incidence of this type of drug eruption appears to occur in HIV-positive patients. Drugs most frequently implicated include allopurinol, aminopenicillins, carbamazepine, hydantoin, phenylbutazone, piroxicam, and sulfa drugs.

Erythema Nodosum

Erythema nodosum eruptions appear as red, indurated, inflammatory nodules on the shins and knees.v

In addition to the unusual distribution, the lesions are tender when palpated. Occasionally, these lesions are accompanied by mild constitutional symptoms, but there is usually no mucous membrane involvement. Etiologic factors associated with the development of erythema nodosum include drugs, female sex, rheumatic fever, sarcoidosis, leprosy, certain bacterial infections (e.g., tuberculosis), and systemic fungal infections such as coccidioidomycosis. Usually, the lesions heal slowly over the course of several weeks after the offending agent is removed. Oral contraceptives are the most frequently implicated drug with this type of eruption. Other implicated drugs include sulfonamides and penicillin.

Drug Hypersensitivity Syndrome

This severe systemic reaction is also known as anticonvulsant hypersensitivity syndrome and as a drug reaction with eosinophilia and systemic symptoms (DRESS). Symptoms begin with a high fever followed by widespread maculopapular–pustular rash on the trunk, arms, and legs that may lead to exfoliative dermatitis with large areas of skin sloughing. Hair and nails are sometimes lost. Eosinophilia occurs in greater than 50% of cases, 30% have abnormal lymphocytosis, and 20% have lymphadenopathy. Internal organ damage appears late in the syndrome with elevations of liver function or renal function laboratory values. These may be accompanied by other general systemic symptoms such as headache and malaise. Secondary bacterial infections can occur. Approximately 10% of patients die, many because of infection. If exfoliative dermatitis occurs, it can take weeks or months to resolve, even after withdrawal of the offending agent. The most commonly implicated drugs are sulfonamides, antimalarials, anticonvulsants, and penicillin. Although rarely reported in the literature, its broad range of symptoms, confusing nomenclature, and symptom overlap with other drug-related adverse effects may lead to underdiagnosis and reporting.

Maculopapular Eruptions

Maculopapular eruptions are subdivided into two groups: scarlatiniform and morbilliform. Most drug eruptions fall within one of these two groups. *Scarlatiniform* eruptions are erythematous and usually involve extensive areas of the body. They are differentiated from streptococcal-induced scarlet fever by the lack of other diagnostic signs and laboratory studies. *Morbilliform* eruptions usually begin as discrete, reddish-brown maculae that may coalesce to form a diffuse rash. These eruptions are differentiated from measles by the lack of fever and other typical clinical signs. In either type of maculopapular eruption, pruritus may or may not be present. Generally, this type of eruption appears within 1 week after the causative drug (2 or more weeks with penicillins) has been started and completely clears within 7 to 14 days after stopping it. Morbilliform eruptions commonly are caused by ampicillin, amoxicillin, and allopurinol.

Urticaria

Urticarial eruptions are immediate hypersensitivity reactions (IgE-mediated) and usually appear as sharply circumscribed (raised), edematous, and erythematous lesions (wheals) with an abrupt onset.

In most cases, individual lesions disappear within 24 hours. These are replaced with new lesions elsewhere until the offending allergen is cleared from the body. Urticarial lesions are associated with an intense itching, stinging, or prickling sensation. Commonly called *hives,* urticarial eruptions are frequently associated with certain drugs, foods, psychic upsets, and serum sickness. The most frequently implicated drugs with this type of reaction are aspirin, penicillin, and blood products. Patients who exhibit urticaria attributable to a drug are at increased risk of anaphylaxis if re-exposed to the same medication in the future.

Angioneurotic Edema

Angioneurotic edema (also called angioedema) is a more severe form of urticaria in which giant hives penetrate more deeply into surrounding tissues.

Lips, mouth, tongue, and eyelids are common locations. Extensive involvement of the tongue, throat, or larynx can be fatal.

Angiotensin-converting enzyme inhibitors (ACEIs) are the most common drug cause of angioedema. Patients taking ACEIs should be warned to look out for any unusual swelling in the facial or oral area and, if present, should go immediately to the nearest emergency room for treatment. Although it usually occurs within the first several months of treatment, cases have been reported up to as long as 3 years after initiation of ACEI therapy (see Chapter 14, Heart Failure and Chapter 32, Drug Hypersensitivity Reactions).

CASE 39-8

QUESTION 1: D.Z., a 42-year-old man with a chronic seizure disorder and long-standing anxiety, was recently given a prescription for penicillin V 250 mg 4 times daily for a group A, α-hemolytic streptococcal-positive pharyngitis. Chronic medications include carbamazepine 200 mg 3 times daily and clonazepam 2 mg 2 times daily. One week later, D.Z. presents with urticarial lesions on his chest and arms. Is this a typical time of onset for a drug-induced dermatologic reaction? How should the drug eruption in D.Z. be managed?

Although most drug eruptions occur within 1 to 2 weeks after starting therapy, it may take 3 to 4 weeks after an initial exposure to a medication for the reaction to occur. Repeated exposure to the same offending agent can reduce the time of onset of the reaction to a few days or even within hours of ingestion. Because D.Z. has been taking clonazepam and carbamazepine chronically and penicillin for only 8 days, the temporal relationship would logically lead to the conclusion that penicillin is a highly probable cause. Almost all cases of urticaria are associated with extensive eosinophilia; however, it is not specific for any particular antigen. However, before labeling penicillin as the cause of his drug eruption, a thorough history to rule out other common nondrug causes should be taken.

For D.Z., a different antibiotic (macrolide) should be substituted for penicillin (to complete the 10-day course of therapy). The individual lesions should begin to clear in 24 hours of eruption (if the penicillin is the cause of the urticaria). If the urticaria does not begin to clear in a few days, another cause should be investigated.

Treatment is primarily supportive, and use of an oral antihistamine (e.g., diphenhydramine 25–50 mg 4 times daily) for several days would be recommended. If the reaction is severe, a 1- to 2-week course of prednisone 40 to 60 mg/day will control most symptoms within 48 hours.

KEY REFERENCES AND WEBSITES

A full list of references for this chapter can be found at http://thepoint.lww.com/AT11e. Below are the key references and websites for this chapter, with the corresponding reference number in this chapter found in parentheses after the reference.

Key References

Arndt KA, Hsu JH. *Manual of Dermatologic Therapies: With Essentials of Diagnosis*. 8th ed. Philadelphia, PA: Lippincott Williams & Wilkins; 2014. (6)

Buddenkotte J, Steinhoff M. Pathophysiology and therapy of pruritus in allergic and atopic diseases. *Allergy*. 2010;65:805.

Carbone A, et al. Pediatric atopic dermatitis: a review of the medical literature. *Ann Pharmacother*. 2010;44:1448.

Eichenfeld LF et al. Guidelines for the diagnosis and management of atopic dermatitis: Section 1, Diagnosis and assessment of atopic dermatitis. *J Am Acad Dermatol*. 2014;70:338. (21)

Eichenfeld LF et.al. Guidelines for the diagnosis and management of atopic dermatitis: section 2, management and treatment of atopic dermatitis with topical therapies. *J Am Acad Dermatol*. 2014;71:116. (22)

Freedberg IM et al, eds. *Fitzpatrick's Dermatology in General Medicine*. 8th ed. New York, NY: McGraw-Hill; 2012. (4)

Lee NP, Arriola ER. Topical corticosteroids: back to basics. *West J Med*. 1999;171:351. (10)

James WD et al, eds. *Andrews' Diseases of the Skin: Clinical Dermatology*. 11th ed. Philadelphia, PA: WB Saunders; 2015. (2)

Pracash AV, Davis MDP. Contact dermatitis in older adults: a review of the literature. *Am J Clin Dermatol*. 2010;11:373.

Tadicherla S et al. Topical corticosteroids in dermatology. *J Drugs Dermatol*. 2009;8:1093. (13)

Key Websites

American Academy of Dermatology Atopic Dermatitis Clinical Guidelines. https://www.aad.org/education/clinical-guidelines/atopic-dermatitis-guideline.

National Eczema Association. https://nationaleczema.org/.

40 Acne

Jamie J. Cavanaugh and Kelly A. Mullican

CORE PRINCIPLES

	CORE PRINCIPLES	CHAPTER CASES
1	Acne is a condition in which the pilosebaceous units of the skin become plugged and distended, presenting as comedones, papules, pustules, or nodules.	**Case 40-1 (Questions 1, 2), Case 40-3 (Question 1), Case 40-4 (Question 1), Case 40-5(Question 1)**
2	Drug therapies work by reducing sebum production, normalizing keratinization in the pilosebaceous units, reducing *Propionibacterium acnes*, or reducing inflammation.	**Case 40-1 (Questions 1, 2), Case 40-3 (Question 1), Case 40-4 (Question 1), Case 40-5(Question 1)**
3	Patients must be counseled that pharmacotherapy works best to prevent future lesions, not to resolve current ones. Therefore, topical therapies should be applied regularly to the entire acne-prone area(s), not just to lesions. Full treatment effect takes time from weeks to months for most treatment options.	**Case 40-1 (Question 3), Case 40-2 (Question 1)**
4	Appropriate choice of vehicle ensures efficacy and tolerability of topical therapy. Gels should be used in patients with normal to oily skin, and lotions and creams should be reserved for those with dryer skin types.	**Case 40-1 (Question 4), Case 40-3 (Question 2)**
5	Topical retinoids are first-line monotherapy for comedonal acne. They are also key components of combination therapies in maculopustular acne and preferred agents to continue for maintenance therapy once acne is under control. If comedonal acne cannot be controlled with topical retinoids alone, then salicylic acid or azelaic acid may be used as adjunctive therapy.	**Case 40-1 (Questions 2, 3), Case 40-2 (Question 1), Table 40-1**
6	Initial treatment for maculopustular acne is a topical retinoid in combination with topical or oral antibiotics. If treatment with topical antibiotics is selected, the regimen should also include topical benzoyl peroxide to reduce the development of antibiotic resistance. Antibiotic duration should be limited to the period needed to obtain control of acne; then the retinoid, with or without benzoyl peroxide, should be continued as maintenance therapy.	**Case 40-3 (Questions 1, 2), Table 40-1**
7	Antiandrogenic therapies, such as combined oral contraceptives or spironolactone, are useful alternative treatment options for maculopustular acne in nonpregnant women.	**Case 40-4 (Question 1), Table 40-1**
8	Oral isotretinoin monotherapy should be used to treat nodular acne. Isotretinoin is extremely effective and can induce a lengthy remission of acne, but the adverse effect profile and the need for laboratory monitoring preclude use in comedonal or maculopustular acne. The iPLEDGE risk management program controls isotretinoin distribution to prevent accidental prescription of this severe teratogen to pregnant women.	**Case 40-5 (Questions 1–6), Table 40-1**

DEFINITION AND EPIDEMIOLOGY

Zits, pimples, whiteheads, and blackheads are all terms commonly used for acne vulgaris, or simply acne. Acne is a condition in which the pilosebaceous units of the skin become plugged and distended, presenting as comedones, papules, pustules, or nodules. Unless otherwise stated, all references to acne in this chapter refer to acne vulgaris.

Acne affects an estimated 9.4% of the world population, including greater than 90% of all adolescents in the United States.[1,2] While teenagers and young adults are typically afflicted by acne, it can occur at any age. Acne often begins when sebaceous gland activity increases in association with puberty. Because the onset of puberty has decreased in recent years, so has the age of acne onset. Acne is now seen as early as 8 to 9 years of age, with peak onset occurring between 16 and 20 years.[3,4] Acne tends to dissipate in most patients by their 30s; however, up to 20% of the patients have acne persisting into adulthood.[5] There is no known cure for acne, but treatment can reduce its severity and minimize scarring.

PATHOPHYSIOLOGY

There are four primary mechanisms responsible for acne: (1) increased sebum production, (2) hyperkeratinization, (3) colonization of *Propionibacterium acnes (P. acnes)*, and (4) release of inflammatory mediators to the skin. Acne begins with the overproduction of sebum, often secondary to an increase in androgen levels.

Androgens such as dehydroepiandrosterone sulfate (DHEAS) are metabolized to dihydrotestosterone (DHT) in the skin, which in turn stimulates sebum biosynthesis. DHEAS levels rise before puberty and begin to decline in early adulthood.[6] An increase in sebum production triggers keratinization which is the proliferation of keratinocytes in the follicular epithelial lining. Keratinization increases cell-to-cell adhesion, interfering with normal desquamation. The cellular debris from keratinization, in addition to excess sebum accumulation, causes sebaceous follicles to plug and form undetectable microcomedones. If the superficial portion of the follicular opening dilates from the pressure of the impaction, an open comedo (blackhead) forms. The dark color of open comedones is caused by light refraction, not by dirt; comedo contents are white when expressed.[7] Such lesions rarely become further inflamed, because as pressure builds from further sebum production and cellular accumulation, follicular contents can escape to the skin surface.[8] If the follicular opening remains narrow and a closed comedo (whitehead) forms, increased pressure can rupture the follicular wall, with infiltration of foreign matter into the dermis inciting a marked local inflammatory response. The depth and extent of this occurrence determine whether a papule, pustule, or nodule results.[9]

Distension in the follicle and increased sebum production allow the gram-positive anaerobe, *P. acnes*, to colonize and proliferate. The occupation of *P. acnes* in the follicle stimulates the upregulation of cytokines and releases proteases, hyaluronidases, lipases, and chemotactic factors that attract neutrophils, T cells, and macrophages.[10] Hydrolytic enzymes released by macrophages may contribute to weakening of the follicular wall, hastening rupture, and resulting progression of comedo to inflammatory lesion.[8] Inflammatory mediators traverse the follicular wall into the dermis and intensify the inflammatory process even before wall rupture.[7]

CLINICAL PRESENTATION

Acne presents as comedones or inflammatory papules, pustules, or nodules. (See Chapter 39, Dermatotherapy and Drug-Induced Skin Disorders.) In severe cases (acne conglobata), multiple lesions coalesce into abscesses with draining sinus tracts. Acne lesions generally appear in areas with the highest density of pilosebaceous units including the face, neck, upper chest, shoulders, and back.[11]

Sunlight and diet may be risk factors for worsening acne, but are controversial.[11] Ultraviolet light may make sebum more comedogenic, but some of the visible wavelengths may reduce the follicular bacterial population.[12] As for diet, studies have investigated lower-milk-intake and lower-glycemic-load diets for potential benefit in acne,[13] but research on dietary modifications is not yet sufficiently robust to alter routine patient care.

Risk factors for acne include a family history and increased body mass index. Worsening of acne has been associated with times of increased stress.[11]

DIAGNOSIS

The differential diagnosis of acneiform eruptions includes (a) acne vulgaris, (b) rosacea, (c) folliculitis caused by gram-negative bacteria, *Pityrosporum*, or mechanical irritation, (d) drug-induced acne (acne medicamentosa) such as that caused by topical or systemic corticosteroids, or by anabolic steroids, and (e) perioral dermatitis.[9,14] Detailed discussions of severe acne variants, such as acne conglobata and acne fulminans, are beyond the scope of this chapter. In addition, acne may be secondary to systemic diseases, such as SAPHO (synovitis, acne, pustulosis, hyperostosis, osteitis) and Apert syndromes.[15]

There is no standard for the grading of acne severity. Initial treatment should be selected based on patient-specific factors including the presence of comedonal, maculopustular and nodular acne, which are used in order to guide treatment decisions. Clinicians may choose to adopt an acne severity scale to assist in the assessment of therapy.[16]

OVERVIEW OF THERAPY

Treatment is individualized and depends on the clinical presentation of the patient. The goals of the treatment are to relieve discomfort, improve skin appearance, prevent scarring, and minimize the psychosocial impact of the condition.

Treatment is largely preventive because little can be done for existing lesions. Slow improvement over the course of weeks to months is expected for all treatments. Therefore, treatment regimens should not be modified more often than every 6 to 8 weeks. Although some acne may resolve without residual changes, it is important to counsel patients that inflammatory acne may result in scaring or hyperpigmentation, which, while reversible, may take several months to fully resolve. Recognition of the duration of improvement of these secondary symptoms is important when considering the efficacy of a medication because patients may not recognize the improvement.[17] Patients should be counseled on the basic pathophysiology of acne, proper drug administration or application technique, delay in onset of therapeutic effect, potential adverse effects of any recommended therapy, and steps to take if adverse effects occur. Clinical practice guidelines are available. Table 40-1 outlines a general approach to the treatment of acne.[10,16,18]

Nonpharmacologic Therapy

Nonpharmacologic therapy plays a minimal role in the management of acne. There is no good evidence to support that acne

Table 40-1
Treatment Selection by Acne Type

Type	Treatment Options
Comedonal acne	Topical retinoid, azelaic acid *Or* Salicylic acid
Maculopapular acne	Topical retinoid + topical antimicrobial (antibiotic or benzoyl peroxide) *Or* Topical retinoid + oral antibiotic + benzoyl peroxide *Or (additional options for female patients)* Combination oral contraceptive Androgen receptor antagonist
Nodular acne	Isotretinoin

can be caused or cured by poor hygiene. Twice-daily washing with warm water and mild facial cleanser may suffice; however, excessive washing and scrubbing should be avoided. Using harsh cleaners disrupts the skin barrier encouraging bacterial colonization and the removal of oil from the skin, which further stimulates its production.[17] To minimize scarring, patients must resist squeezing or picking at acne lesions. Drugs known to cause acne, such as corticosteroids, androgens, and anabolic steroids, should be avoided when possible.[19] In addition, oil-based cosmetics and other known precipitants should be avoided. Oil-free, noncomedogenic moisturizers formulated for facial skin can improve the penetration and tolerability of many topical acne drugs by improving the skin's hydration, especially in patients with sensitive skin.

Dermatologists may use procedures such as surgical comedo extraction, chemical peels, and microdermabrasion as adjunct therapy to improve cosmetic appearance. Current guidelines prefer drug therapy to light and laser therapies because there are less stringent clinical testing for devices versus drugs, concern about long-term effects of therapies aimed at sebaceous gland function, and the inadequate research done on light and laser therapies to date.[10] Acne scarring is treated with various microsurgical techniques such as dermabrasion, laser therapy, chemical peels, and tissue augmentation.[20]

Pharmacotherapy

Available drug therapies exhibit one or more of the following mechanisms: (a) normalizing follicular keratinization (e.g., retinoids, benzoyl peroxide to some degree, azelaic acid); (b) decreasing sebum production (e.g., isotretinoin, hormonal therapies); (c) suppressing *P. acnes* (e.g., antibiotics, benzoyl peroxide, azelaic acid, systemic isotretinoin); and (d) reducing inflammation (e.g., antibiotics, retinoids).

COMEDONAL ACNE CASE

CASE 40-1

QUESTION 1: L.Y. is a 15-year-old female who presents to the pharmacy asking for the best way to treat her "zits." The problem started earlier this year around the same time that she joined the track team. Upon examination, you can see several closed comedones on her nose and chin and open comedones dispersed across her forehead covered by makeup. Her skin is slightly oily, and you can see that she is wearing a sweatband around her head. She would like to know what you recommend to get rid of her "zits." What factors could be contributing to her acne?

There are several factors that may be contributing to L.Y.'s acne. Mechanical irritation caused by the sweatband may cause acne mechanica. Increased sweat and humid conditions encountered while running track can lead to favorable conditions for the colonization of *P. acnes*. Finally, it is important to ask L.Y. whether her makeup is oil based, because oil-based products can be comedogenic.

Pharmacotherapy

CASE 40-1, QUESTION 2: What are the treatment options for L.Y.'s acne?

Topical therapies are the most appropriate first-line treatment for comedonal acne. Options include retinoids, azelaic acid, and salicylic acid.

TOPICAL RETINOIDS

Retinoids, analogs of vitamin A, normalize keratinization by decreasing horny cell cohesiveness and stimulating epidermal cell turnover. These actions combine to unplug follicles and prevent microcomedo formation. Retinoids reduce inflammation by inhibiting the production of inflammatory mediators. It is important to note that topical retinoids have no antibacterial properties.[21]

As the most potent comedolytic agents, topical retinoids are preferred therapy in comedonal acne.[18] They are also a core component of combination therapies for maculopapular/pustule acne and a first-line treatment to maintain remission of acne once it is controlled. Tretinoin, all-*trans*-retinoic acid, is the naturally occurring form of vitamin A acid and is a first-generation topical retinoid. It is generally well tolerated, although it can cause retinoid dermatitis leading to further hyperpigmentation if used too aggressively in patients with darker skin tones. Starting at a low dose or using creams over gels can minimize the risk of worsening hyperpigmentation.[22] Alternatively, adapalene, a retinoid-like product, that binds to specific retinoic acid nuclear receptors can be used. It is generally well tolerated and, in addition to decreasing risk for hyperpigmentation, has a greater anti-inflammatory effect than tretinoin. Tazarotene is a second-generation topical retinoid available and, although effective, is the least tolerated agent in this class.[23]

Topical retinoids and retinoid-like products should be applied once daily at bedtime to avoid degradation in ultraviolet light.[24] Common adverse effects of this class include skin irritation, peeling, erythema, and dryness.[23] The irritation potential depends on the drug concentration and vehicle used. Patients should be counseled to apply daily sunscreen and gentle moisturizing cream while using these agents.[24] Patients should be aware that acne might initially worsen during treatment because pustular flares can occur.

AZELAIC ACID

Azelaic acid is a dicarboxylic acid that works to normalize keratinization and indirectly reduces inflammation through suppression of *P. acnes*.[25] Formulations in the 20% strength are indicated for the treatment of acne, whereas the 15% gel, Finacea, is indicated for rosacea. Although azelaic acid hits several of the pathways leading to acne formation, the evidence for use is not as robust as other topical agents.[21] It is applied twice daily to the skin and could be an option for patients who are unable to tolerate other topical therapies.

SALICYLIC ACID

Topical salicylic acid works as a concentration-dependent keratolytic agent. It is commonly reserved for patients with comedonal acne who cannot tolerate other comedolytic therapies or as augmentation to other therapies as studies have demonstrated that their effectiveness is less than either topical retinoids or benzoyl peroxide.[26] It is typically applied twice daily and is not effective if soly used as needed. Patients should be cautioned regarding chronic use over large body surfaces because it increases the risk of percutaneous absorption that could lead to systemic salicylate toxicity.[27]

CASE 40-1, QUESTION 3: What treatment option is most appropriate for L.Y.?

Topical retinoids are first-line agents for her type of acne. Selection of the specific topical retinoid is provider-specific and generally depends on what is most affordable for the patient. Adapalene should be considered for patients with darker skin tones secondary to the reduced risk for hyperpigmentation. She should be instructed to apply the product to her entire face every other day for the first 2 weeks and then advance to daily as tolerated. It is important to let L.Y. know that this is for routine and not as needed use in order to be effective and that she will need to wait several weeks before judging its effectiveness. She should apply the product at bedtime, ideally 30 minutes after washing her face with a mild cleanser, and wash it off in the morning (or after several hours, if excessive skin dryness or peeling occurs).

CASE 40-1, QUESTION 4: What vehicle would you recommend for L.Y.?

L.Y. has slightly oily skin. Therefore using a gel is the vehicle of choice because it has more drying effects compared to lotions of creams.

CASE 40-2

QUESTION 1: M.G. is a 27-year-old female who presents to the dermatology clinic with open and closed comedones spread across her cheeks and forehead. She was recently prescribed adapalene 0.1% lotion, which she has been applying daily for the last 6 months without much success. She is not sure what else she can do to manage her acne. What would you recommend M.G. to better manage her acne?

Although topical retinoids are first-line treatment for comedonal acne, some patients require additional agents to achieve satisfactory results. M.G. should be instructed to continue adapalene and initiate salicylic acid wash daily. This wash should be used on her entire face, not just areas with active breakouts, twice daily. It is important to remind her that it may take several weeks before she sees an effect.

MACULOPAPULAR ACNE

Pharmacotherapy

ANTIBIOTICS

Although *P. acnes* is part of the skin's normal flora, under the conditions leading to acne, it helps transform comedones into inflammatory pustules or papules. Antibiotics do not resolve existing lesions, but they can prevent future lesions by decreasing both *P. acnes* colonization and inflammation. The antibiotics that are most effective in acne have antioxidant properties. In addition, antibiotics inhibit the release of reactive oxygen species by *P. acnes*, which in turn reduces leukocyte recruitment.[10] Due to this multifactorial mechanism of action, clinical efficacy does not correlate perfectly with reductions in bacterial load; successful antibiotic courses do not necessarily eradicate *P. acnes*.[28]

Topical Antibiotics

Topically applied antibiotics avoid systemic exposure and achieve high follicular concentrations. They can augment topical retinoids when initiating therapy for comedonal and papular acne cases involving inflammatory lesions, or they can be added to regimens for patients failing monotherapy. Topical antibiotics alone in acne treatment should be avoided due to concerns for bacterial resistance.[21]

Topical antibiotics are usually applied once or twice daily for 3 months. Although rare reports of systemic adverse effects exist, topical effects, such as stinging and tingling, are the most common adverse effects, and even these occur less frequently with topical antibiotics compared to other topical therapies.

Doxycycline is most convenient and effective; tetracycline is an alternative.[29] Tetracyclines should not be prescribed for children younger than 9 years of age because of potential impairment of bone growth and discoloration of forming teeth. Pregnant women must avoid tetracyclines because of bone growth effects on the fetus. Minocycline is sometimes tried if other tetracyclines fail, but is more expensive and not clearly better in efficacy, even in resistant acne. It is also associated with a higher rate of serious adverse effects than other tetracycline antibiotics.[30]

Trimethoprim/sulfamethoxazole is also effective, but has a less favorable adverse effect profile when compared to tetracycline. It is reserved for situations when other antibiotics are unable to be used.[16] In patients who are unable to take oral antibiotics mentioned above (including pregnant patients), erythromycin may be an option despite association with higher rates of resistance.

Most oral antibiotics are given twice daily for a 3-month course, followed by continuation of a topical retinoid for maintenance therapy.[23]

Oral Antibiotics

Oral antibiotics should not be used as monotherapy. Benzoyl peroxide may be added for patients with maculopustular or nodule acne. If lesions are widespread or difficult to reach, oral antibiotics are generally preferred over topical agents. They are also used as a step-up therapy when topical antibiotic regimens fail to suppress acne.

Antibiotic Resistance

Antibiotic resistance of *P. acnes* is increasing and correlates with prescribing patterns. Erythromycin has the highest rate of resistance. Resistance to tetracyclines is less common and is increasing at a slower rate than resistance to other antibiotics. In an effort to minimize resistance, guidelines increasingly emphasize that antibiotics should be reserved for acne of at least maculopapular subtype. Antibiotics should be used with drugs exerting additional mechanisms of action, ideally topical retinoids, rather than used as monotherapy, and should be used for the shortest effective duration to obtain acne control (trials to stop antibiotics every 3 months). Antibiotics should not be used for maintenance of control (rather, the retinoid should be continued for maintenance). Including benzoyl peroxide in regimens containing antibiotics reduces the development of resistance, and it is particularly recommended if antibiotic therapy needs to be continued beyond 3 months to maintain control.[21] If adherence to therapy with an antibiotic and both topical retinoid and leave-on benzoyl peroxide formulations is challenging, even a benzoyl peroxide wash product can be helpful.[31,32] Dual antibiotic use is inappropriate because it increases the risk of bacterial resistance without offering therapeutic gain, as bacterial eradication is not a therapeutic goal.

BENZOYL PEROXIDE

Benzoyl peroxide is another effective agent for those with maculopustular acne. It works through three mechanisms: antimicrobial, anti-inflammatory, and keratolytic effects. It is important to note that there is no reported resistance of *P. acnes* to benzoyl peroxide. Benzoyl peroxide is available over-the-counter and by prescription in a variety of dosage forms. It is important to be aware that benzoyl peroxide inactivates some formulations of tretinoin, so they should not be used together, or should at least be applied at different times (morning and evening, respectively).[33] However, benzoyl peroxide can be used in combination with either adapalene or tazarotene to provide additive benefit. Benzoyl peroxide is usually applied to the affected area once or twice daily. The most common adverse effects of benzoyl peroxide include contact dermatitis (occurs in up to 2.5% of patients), erythema, peeling, and skin drying.[27] Those who develop contact dermatitis should be instructed to stop. Patients should be counseled to be careful when applying this medication because it can bleach hair and dyed fabrics.

CASE 40-3

QUESTION 1: R.P. is an 18-year-old male who has had acne since his early teens. He started out with comedonal acne alone, but now has a number of inflammatory pustules across his forehead and nose. Upon further examination, you can also see that he has dry skin with numerous comedones on his chin. R.P. was prescribed tretinoin 0.1% gel in the past, but he stopped this due to skin irritation and dryness. He has been using salicylic acid washes daily, without success. What changes to R.P.'s medication regimen do you recommend?

Guidelines currently recommend topical retinoids as a cornerstone of therapy for patients with comedonal and inflammatory acne. Although R.P. had been unable to tolerate tretinoin gel in the past, it may have been secondary to the vehicle and strength of the medication that he was prescribed. Gels tend to dry out the skin and are not the preferred vehicle for patients like R.P. who have dry skin. Recommend that R.P. restarts a topical retinoid with a cream or lotion formulation. You could also recommend that he starts with a lower strength tretinoin for tolerability (available in strengths as low as 0.02%). Because R.P. also presents with pustules, he could also start on a topical antimicrobial agent such as a topical antibiotic or benzoyl peroxide.

CASE 40-3, QUESTION 2: One year later, R.P. returns to the pharmacy and reports that his acne therapy is "not working." He saw his dermatologist and has been using clindamycin lotion 1% every morning, adapalene cream 0.1% every night, and benzoyl peroxide lotion 4% daily for the past year. Upon examination, you can notice that he continues to have maculopapular acne in addition to a few nodules. What changes do you recommend to his treatment regimen?

R.P. should stop his topical antibiotic and start an oral antibiotic, such as doxycycline. If he is able to tolerate doxycycline, he should continue this medication for 6 to 8 weeks, at which point changes should be made if there is no improvement.[34,35] If the response is adequate, R.P. should try to stop doxycycline after 3 months. Topical retinoid therapy and benzoyl peroxide should be continued during doxycycline therapy and then after the antibiotic course to maintain treatment benefit. If R.P. were to experience a treatment relapse in the future, after successful use of an oral antibiotic, another course of the same antibiotic should be used; switching antibiotics offers no therapeutic benefit and can promote multidrug resistance.[31] With only a few nodules present, it is not appropriate to initiate oral isotretinoin without adequate trials of other treatment options.

CASE 40-4

QUESTION 1: M.J. is a 24-year-old female who presents to the clinic with maculopapular acne. She reports that her acne typically worsens 1 week before her menstrual cycle and improves once menses begins. She says that she is tired of applying all of these creams and is looking for an alternative way to manage her acne. What treatment options would you recommend for her?

HORMONAL THERAPIES

Hormonal therapies with antiandrogenic effects, such as androgen receptor antagonists and combination oral contraceptives, are the only treatments besides oral isotretinoin to attack acne by reducing sebum production. Hormonal therapies may be helpful in patients with normal serum androgen levels, as well as in patients with elevated serum androgen levels, because hypersensitivity to androgens sometimes occurs at the follicular level despite normal circulating androgen levels.[32] These treatments are good options for women with acne who are not pregnant, for those who desire contraception, and for women with polycystic ovary syndrome or other hyperandrogenic conditions or symptoms.[32] Systemic effects of hormonal therapy generally preclude their use in male patients. Response to hormonal therapies can take 3 to 6 months because their mechanism of action, reducing sebum production, is an early step in the cascade of acne pathology.[36]

Androgen Receptor Antagonists

Spironolactone at doses of 25 to 100 mg/day reduces acne because it is an androgen receptor antagonist and inhibits 5-α-reductase. Tolerability and serum potassium should be monitored every 3 weeks until maximum tolerated dose or 100 mg/day is achieved, titrating in 25-mg increments. Spironolactone is generally well tolerated, although gynecomastia, menstrual irregularities, and hyperkalemia are possible.[32] Female patients should use contraception because of the potential for antiandrogen exposure to impair the sexual development of male fetuses. Spironolactone should be used with caution in male patients given the risk for gynecomastia and possibly lower efficacy when compared to female patients.[37]

Combination Oral Contraceptives

Estrogen, usually administered as ethinyl estradiol in a combination oral contraceptive, improves acne in females by reducing ovarian androgen production and by increasing sex hormone-binding globulin concentrations in the serum, thereby lowering free testosterone levels. The manufacturers of Ortho Tri-Cyclen, Gianvi, Loryna, Nikki, Vestura, Estrostep, and Yaz specifically sought and obtained FDA approval for acne indications. Studies of combination oral contraceptives containing levonorgestrel, norethindrone acetate, drospirenone, dienogest, nomegestrol, cyproterone acetate, desogestrel, or gestodene (not available in the United States) have demonstrated efficacy in acne.[38] Comparative trials have not yet clearly established clinically significant superiority of one product over another.[38] In individual patients, products containing progestins with androgenic effects (e.g., norgestrel, levonorgestrel) may override the effect of ethinyl estradiol and worsen acne. Conversely, patients already on a combination oral contraceptive may improve when switched to a formulation with a less androgenic progestin (norgestimate, desogestrel).[39] Other estrogen-containing contraceptives (transdermal patches, vaginal rings) may have similar beneficial effects to combination oral contraceptives, but studies have not been conducted.

If M.J. is not interested in becoming pregnant in the near future, hormonal therapy may be a good option for treatment of her acne. Because the onset of hormonal therapy is delayed, she should be counseled to continue using her current treatments for at least 3 months. At that time, she may try stopping her topical treatments and continuing hormonal therapy as an acne monotherapy.

NODULAR ACNE CASE

CASE 40-5

QUESTION 1: K.S. is a 24-year-old female who first noticed acne when she was 10 years old. As a teen, she used topical benzoyl peroxide, topical adapalene, and systemic erythromycin with limited success. Two years ago, she was diagnosed with polycystic ovary syndrome and began taking Ortho Tri-Cyclen along with her maintenance adapalene treatment, after which her acne improved, but was not eradicated. Ten months ago, she also began taking minocycline 100 mg orally twice daily. After a few months, she experienced significant improvement, but she has not been able to stop antibiotics because of recurrent flare-ups. She now has at least a dozen nodules widely distributed among multiple papules and pustules on her face and back. What pharmacologic therapy would you recommend for K.S.?

Pharmacotherapy

ORAL ISOTRETINOIN

Isotretinoin (Absorica, Amnesteem, Claravis, Myorisan, Zenatane) is the only agent effective for the treatment of nodular acne largely in part due to its mechanism of action. It exhibits all four of the mechanisms of action currently used to attack acne, making it a uniquely effective monotherapy. It is administered by mouth as 10-, 20-, 30-, and 40-mg capsules. In most cases, one or two 5-month-long courses of therapy will induce a remission lasting for several months or even years after the drug is stopped. Although this medication is very effective in the suppression of acne, it is not utilized in more mild cases of acne due to its adverse effect profile. It should be reserved as a last-line therapy for patients with nodular acne and those variants of acne that are prone to scaring.

The most effective medication for K.S. will be oral isotretinoin at an initial dose of 20 mg twice daily (targeting 0.5 mg/kg/day). The dosage should be increased to 40 mg twice daily (1 mg/kg/day) as tolerated after 1 month. The dose should be divided twice daily and given with food. For best results and minimal risk of relapse, treatment should be continued until a cumulative dose of approximately 120 mg/kg is reached, usually about 5 months.[33] Higher dosages are associated with an increased risk of adverse effects. K.S. should stop taking minocycline when isotretinoin therapy begins because isotretinoin is effective monotherapy, and coadministration of isotretinoin and tetracyclines increases the risk of intracranial hypertension.[34] Adapalene is also unnecessary once isotretinoin begins. Her acne should significantly improve within the first month of therapy and gradually resolve by the third or fourth month. A second course of therapy is usually not necessary.

CASE 40-5, QUESTION 2: K.S.'s prescriber discusses enrolling her in iPLEDGE. What is the iPLEDGE program? What should K.S. know about avoiding pregnancy while taking isotretinoin?

Isotretinoin is severely teratogenic.[40] A Food and Drug Administration-mandated Risk Evaluation Mitigation Strategy (REMS) strict risk management program called iPLEDGE regulates the prescription and distribution of isotretinoin in the United States.[41] The program requires all patients, prescribers, pharmacies, and even drug wholesalers involved in distribution and use of the drug to register with a national database. Proper patient monitoring and education, including negative pregnancy tests in female patients of childbearing potential, must be documented in the database each month before initial or refill medication can be dispensed to a patient. Because of the teratogenicity or oral isotretinoin, patients (both male and female) should also be counseled not to donate blood during therapy and for at least a month after therapy, to ensure no pregnant woman receives isotretinoin-contaminated blood products.

Female patients of childbearing potential must use two forms of contraception for at least a month before, during, and a month after isotretinoin therapy. At least one contraception method must be a "primary" method. K.S. is already using an approved primary method with Ortho Tri-Cyclen; approved primary methods also include bilateral tubal ligation, partner's vasectomy, some intrauterine devices, or hormonal methods (other than progestin-only minipills). However, she must also begin using a backup method, such as condoms. The program requires that all female patients of childbearing potential must have two negative pregnancy tests before initiating isotretinoin therapy, one at the time of screening and then another, from an appropriately certified laboratory, after 1 month of using their chosen contraception regimen. The program also requires a negative pregnancy test before each monthly refill is prescribed, immediately after therapy, and a month after therapy. K.S. and her prescriber will both have to verify with the program on a monthly basis that she has been counseled again regarding contraception.

CASE 40-5, QUESTION 3: How should K.S. be counseled with regard to adverse effects of isotretinoin?

In addition to its teratogenic effects, oral isotretinoin can also cause numerous dermatologic effects including dryness, erythema, peeling and photosensitivity.[40] To minimize this, patients should be instructed to use daily moisturizers, sunscreen and protective clothing if going out into the sun. K.S. should also be counseled to avoid waxing, dermabrasions and any other dermatologic procedures during and up to 6 months after the completion of treatment. Other common side effects that K.S. should be cognizant of include hair dryness, hair thinning and nail fragility.

CASE 40-5, QUESTION 4: What laboratory testing should be performed prior to the initiation of oral isotretinoin?

Before beginning isotretinoin therapy, all patients, both male and female, should have the following baseline laboratory tests: a fasting lipid panel; a liver function panel, including both serum transaminases and bilirubin; and a complete blood count, including platelets.[40] For accurate triglyceride results, the blood sample should be collected at least 36 hours after alcohol consumption and 10 hours after having food. A lipid panel should be redrawn 4 and 8 weeks into isotretinoin therapy to document the effect of the drug because 20% of patients develop significant triglyceride elevations.[9,42] Triglyceride levels greater than 400 mg/dL should be treated with diet and reduced alcohol intake; monthly monitoring should continue throughout isotretinoin therapy. In the unusual event that triglyceride levels exceed from 700 to 800 mg/dL, isotretinoin should be discontinued, or continued at a reduced dosage with concomitant gemfibrozil therapy to reduce the risk of pancreatitis.[9] If pancreatitis develops, isotretinoin must be discontinued. Liver function tests and blood counts only need to be redrawn during therapy if symptoms suggestive of hepatitis or blood dyscrasias appear.[9,16]

CASE 40-5, QUESTION 5: K.S. has never had problems with depression, but her prescriber completed a psychiatric history and assessment of current symptoms, and her iPLEDGE patient education materials warn against possible drug-induced depression. The thought of suddenly becoming violent or suicidal concerns her. How significant is this risk?

Isotretinoin product labeling includes a warning that isotretinoin may cause depression, including suicide attempts, psychosis, and violent behavior. Case reports suggest that isotretinoin causes psychiatric symptoms in some patients. Prospective trials and literature reviews have not established a causal relationship between isotretinoin and depressive symptoms.[43] Although the absolute risk is low, drug-induced depression is a possible idiosyncratic reaction to isotretinoin in individual patients. In any case, all patients with severe acne, whether receiving isotretinoin or not, should be monitored for the development or worsening of depression.[16] K.S. should be reassured that the risk of drug-induced psychiatric symptoms is low. If she does notice any of the psychiatric symptoms listed in her medication guide, she should contact her prescriber immediately and stop isotretinoin.

CASE 40-5, QUESTION 6: After 3 weeks of therapy, K.S. complains of dry eyes, dry skin, and cracks with bleeding at the corners of her mouth. What do you recommend to manage these adverse effects?

K.S. should use artificial tears to relieve the discomfort of her dry eyes; if she is still uncomfortable after several days, she can also apply lubricating ophthalmic ointment at bedtime. She should liberally apply moisturizer to dry skin, particularly after bathing (see Chapter 39, Dermatotherapy and Drug-Induced Skin Disorders). Frequent application of a lip balm or emollient, ideally one containing sunscreen, will treat cheilitis. If the symptoms become intolerable, a small reduction in the isotretinoin dose (e.g., reduction of 10–20 mg/day) usually decreases the intensity of skin and mucous membrane reactions. Drug discontinuation is rarely necessary.[40]

KEY REFERENCES AND WEBSITES

A full list of references for this chapter can be found at http://thepoint.lww.com/AT11e. Below are the key references and websites for this chapter, with the corresponding reference number in this chapter found in parentheses after the reference.

Key Reference

Zaenglen AL et al. Guidelines of care for the management of acne vulgaris. *J Am Acad Dermatol*. 2016; 74: 945–973.(16)

Key Websites

American Academy of Dermatology Clinical Guidelines. https://www.aad.org/education/clinical-guidelines.

iPLEDGE Program. https://www.ipledgeprogram.com/.

41 Psoriasis

Jill A. Morgan, Rachel C. Long, and Timothy J. Ives

CORE PRINCIPLES

		CHAPTER CASES
1	Psoriasis is a chronic, proliferative skin disease that is characterized by well-delineated, thickened erythematous skin plaques and is both topical and systemic in nature. It is immune-mediated with both vascular and inflammatory changes, which precede epidermal changes.	**Case 41-1 (Question 1)**
2	Precipitating factors for psoriasis include cold weather, anxiety and stress, viral or bacterial infections, epidermal trauma, or drugs.	**Case 41-1 (Questions 2,4)**
3	Topical corticosteroids are first-line treatment for mild psoriasis because of their prompt relief, convenience, and anti-inflammatory, immunosuppressant, and antipruritic properties.	**Case 41-1 (Question 5)**
4	Alternative topical treatments for mild psoriasis—coal tar, anthralin, calcipotriene, calcitriol, and tazarotene—and phototherapy are not as convenient as topical corticosteroids, but have well-established efficacy for initial management.	**Case 41-1 (Question 6)**
5	Treatment goals for severe psoriasis include both safe and effective resolution of the disease and long-term maintenance using agents to induce immunosuppressive or remittive cellular changes.	**Case 41-2 (Questions 1,2)**
6	Psoriatic arthritis can occur in up to 40% of patients with psoriasis, and mild disease is treated first with nonsteroidal anti-inflammatory drugs and second with an immunosuppressive agent, methotrexate.	**Case 41-3 (Question 1)**
7	Use of immunosuppressive agents can be limited as a result of adverse effects, monitoring requirements, or toxicity. There is also a lack of evidence to support that they modify the long-term disease process. Immunomodulatory therapy, including T-cell agents and TNF-α inhibitors, is thought to target the immune-mediated mechanism of psoriasis.	**Case 41-3 (Question 2)**

EPIDEMIOLOGY

Psoriasis, a chronic, proliferative skin disease, is one of the most common immune-mediated disorders, occurring in 1.5% to 3% of the population worldwide, with northern Europeans and Scandinavians affected most.[1–4] It is characterized by well-delineated, thickened erythematous epidermis or dermal plaques covered with a distinctive silvery scale. Of patients, 75% present with symptoms of psoriasis before the age of 46 years.[2] A family history of psoriasis is found in nearly half of patients. At least 36 chromosomal loci have been identified that increase psoriasis susceptibility.[5–7] Modifiable triggers, such as tobacco and alcohol use, stress, obesity, skin injury, and hormone changes, also play a major role in disease expression.[3,8]

Pathogenesis

Innate and adaptive immunity are both involved in the initiation and maintenance of psoriatic plaques. Because the epidermis is the body's main barrier to environmental insult, epidermal hyperplasia forms a key component of the innate immune response. Natural killer cells and natural killer T cells are part of the cutaneous inflammation in psoriasis.[3,9]

Because $CD4^+$ and $CD8^+$ T-lymphocytic cells constitute most of the leukocyte infiltrates found in plaques early in the development of lesions, current evidence supports an autoimmune mechanism for psoriasis. Cytokines such as interferon-α_2 or interleukin-2 are also found in psoriatic plaques.[10] T cells in the cutaneous infiltrate are positive for cutaneous lymphocyte–associated antigen, a marker for skin-homing leukocytes. Pathogenesis also involves vascular and inflammatory changes, which precede epidermal changes.[11] Alterations in the dermal vasculature also appear to be a result of angiogenesis, the development of new blood vessels, similar to a number of other disease processes, including tumor growth. Many commonly used therapeutic agents for psoriasis have antiangiogenic activity.[1]

The epidermal changes of psoriasis are based on the time required for affected epidermal cells to travel to the surface and be cast off, which is markedly reduced (3–4 vs. 26–28 days in normal cells).[12] This sixfold to ninefold transit time decrease does not allow the normal events of cell maturation and keratinization to take place and is reflected clinically as diffuse scaling. T cells contribute to this keratinocyte hyperproliferation through the secretion of various growth factors.[13,14] Memory T lymphocytes marked with cutaneous lymphocyte–associated antigen, to remember the anatomic site where they first encountered antigen, migrate to the (epi)dermis by a number of immunologic and inflammatory triggering mechanisms released from keratinocytes after minor trauma. On entry into the skin, these T cells complex with epidermal self-antigens presented by major histocompatibility complex molecules that confer the risk of psoriasis. The subsequent release of T-cell cytokines results in further inflammation, the recruitment of additional marked (i.e., with cutaneous lymphocyte–associated antigen) T cells, and, ultimately, the development of psoriatic lesions in susceptible persons.[13,14]

Prognosis

Similar to those with diabetes, cancer, or heart disease, patients with psoriasis experience a reduced quality of life related to an impairment of social, psychological, and physical functioning.[15–17] Although psoriasis is a treatable disease, there is no known cure. Optimism and encouragement are justified and make it easier for patients to conscientiously apply sometimes awkward and messy topical treatments or take medications that have significant adverse effects. The goal of therapy should be to achieve complete clearing of psoriatic lesions, particularly during emotionally critical times, such as the commencement of school, puberty, and the summer months.

Clinical Presentation of Psoriasis

CASE 41-1

QUESTION 1: M.M., a 35-year-old man, presents with complaints of several thick, well-defined erythematous areas on both his elbows and knees that have silvery scales on them. He complains of itching in these areas and that the areas bleed when he removes the scales. M.M. states that he has had these lesions for some time; however, he has used over-the-counter hydrocortisone and some of his friend's triamcinolone 0.025% cream on them for the itching. He feels that the lesions have gotten worse since he went on vacation in the Dominican Republic and got "a pretty bad sunburn." His medical history is noncontributory. His only medications, besides topical corticosteroids, include a recent course of chloroquine for malaria prophylaxis during his recent travel. On physical examination, M.M. is also found to have a few scattered, circumscribed, erythematous, scaly plaques on the flexural surfaces of both arms and legs and a dense scale on his forehead and scalp. Approximately 4% of his body surface area (BSA) is estimated to be affected with psoriasis. The rest of M.M.'s physical examination and laboratory results are within normal limits.

Laboratory values and vital signs include the following:
BP, 132/78 mm Hg
HR, 64 beats/minute
Sodium, 140 mEq/L
Potassium, 4.3 mEq/L
Blood Urea Nitrogen (BUN), 13 mg/dL
Creatinine, 0.9 mg/dL

What classic signs and symptoms suggestive of psoriasis are demonstrated by M.M.?

Most psoriatic lesions are asymptomatic, but not always. Pruritus, for example, is noted in 50% of patients, and it can be severe.[18] Patients also report stinging or burning sensations.[19] The primary psoriatic lesion is a relapsing eruption of scaling papules that rapidly coalesce or enlarge to form circumscribed, erythematous, scaly plaques. The scale is adherent and silvery white and may reveal bleeding points when removed, called the *Auspitz sign*. Scales can become extremely dense on the scalp or macerated and dispersed in intertriginous areas.

The development of lesions of active psoriasis at the site of epidermal trauma is known as the *Koebner phenomenon*. Scratch marks, sunburn, or surgical wounds may heal, leaving psoriatic lesions in their place. The elbows, knees, scalp, gluteal cleft, fingernails, and toenails are favored areas of involvement. Extensor surfaces are affected more than the flexor surfaces, but the disease usually spares the palms, soles, and face. Nail beds may show punctate pitting, profuse collections of keratotic material, yellow-brown discoloration ("oil spot"), or onycholysis (nail plate separation) in approximately 50% of patients.[20] Psoriatic arthritis is a seronegative inflammatory arthritis that occurs in approximately 25% of all patients with psoriasis, with combined features of both rheumatoid arthritis and the seronegative spondyloarthropathies.[2,18]

Most patients (90%) have chronic localized disease (plaque type or *psoriasis vulgaris*), but several other presentations exist.[3] The most severe form of the disease is *erythrodermic psoriasis*, a condition of acute inflammatory erythema and scales involving greater than 90% of the BSA. *Pustular psoriasis* is generally localized to palms and soles, but there is also a generalized version. Both generalized pustular psoriasis and erythrodermic psoriasis can be accompanied by systemic symptoms (i.e., hyperthermia, tachycardia, edema, dehydration, shortness of breath) and can have life-threatening consequences (i.e., hypovolemia, electrolyte imbalance, septicemia) if not promptly treated.[21] Lesions of *Guttate psoriasis* are small, fine, erythematous scales, usually found on the trunk, arms, or legs, classically after β-hemolytic streptococcal pharyngitis. *Flexural* or *inverse psoriasis* is shiny and red, and typically lacks scales and looks more like intertrigo.[2] Of interest, psoriatic skin is rarely secondarily infected, because of the overexpression of the endogenous peptides cathelicidins and β-defensins.[20]

Systemic disorders that can have a causative association with psoriasis include type 2 diabetes mellitus, Chron's disease, metabolic syndrome, depression, and cardiovascular disease.[2,15–17] This increased risk is thought to be caused by the presence of endothelial activation, proinflammatory cytokines, and hyperlipidemia.[2,17,21] Disease severity is also thought to be a factor, because psoriatic patients with more severe conditions have an increased risk of metabolic, coronary heart disease or stroke compared with those with milder forms of psoriasis.[15]

M.M. presents with many classic signs of psoriasis, including symmetric, distinctive, chronic, and erythematous plaques covered with silvery scales on the extensor surfaces of the elbows and knees as well as the flexural surface of his arms and legs. He also shows scalp involvement, but does not appear to have plaques on his trunk or nail or systemic involvement. He exhibits the Auspitz sign and evidence of the Koebner phenomenon because his lesions worsened after skin trauma from the sunburn. His report of pruritus is consistent with the presentation in 50% of patients.

CASE 41-1, QUESTION 2: What are the factors that can precipitate or aggravate psoriasis? What are the potential causes of M.M.'s psoriatic exacerbation?

A thorough medical history may reveal a cause of exacerbations of psoriatic lesions. Most patients report that hot weather, sunlight, and humidity help clear psoriasis, whereas cold weather has an adverse effect on its course. Anxiety or psychological stress is believed to contribute adversely. Viral or bacterial infections, especially streptococcal pharyngitis, may precipitate the onset or flare-up of psoriasis. Cuts, burns, abrasions, injections, and other trauma can also elicit the development of lesions. Any drug that causes a skin eruption to develop can exacerbate psoriasis via this response.

Drug-Induced Psoriasis

A number of drugs have been reported to exacerbate preexisting psoriasis, induce psoriatic lesions on apparently normal skin in patients with psoriasis, or precipitate psoriasis in persons with or without a family history of psoriasis (Table 41-1).[23] Antimalarial agents, such as chloroquine (taken by M.M.), may have an adverse effect on the course of psoriasis and can cause exfoliative erythroderma.[24] Hydroxychloroquine, however, has not shared this association (except for one case report) and usually induces a beneficial response in 75% of patients with psoriatic arthritis.[24] It is preferred over chloroquine in patients with psoriasis who need prophylactic treatment for malaria when both are effective against the particular plasmodium species in the area (see Chapter 81, Parasitic Infections).[24]

Lithium also can precipitate psoriasis and contribute to resistance to treatment through its effects on cell kinetics (increase in circulating neutrophils, accelerated neutrophil turnover, increased epidermal cell proliferation).[22] Psoriasis is not a general contraindication, however, to lithium therapy. More intensive psoriasis treatment can be used if these reactions occur, and lithium must be continued.[22]

β-Blockers and some nonsteroidal anti-inflammatory drugs (NSAIDs) also can precipitate a psoriasiform state.[22] Because both lithium and propranolol inhibit cyclic adenosine monophosphate (cAMP), cyclic nucleosides may play a role in the onset and clinical course of psoriasis. Chemotactic substances, including 12-hydroxyeicosatetraenoic acid and leukotrienes, may accumulate in the epidermis of some patients taking indomethacin, thereby precipitating psoriasis.[22]

When compared with other NSAIDs, indomethacin may selectively inhibit cyclooxygenase more than lipoxygenase pathways of arachidonic acid metabolism. As a result, indomethacin may have a more significant adverse psoriatic effect than other NSAIDs that have been reported to ameliorate psoriasis.[22]

Flare-ups of pustular psoriasis also can be precipitated by withdrawal from systemic corticosteroids or withdrawal from high-potency topical corticosteroids that are applied under occlusion to large areas.[25] Because of this problem and because fatalities have been associated with systemic corticosteroid use and withdrawal, systemic corticosteroids are not routinely used to treat psoriasis.

Chloroquine prophylaxis, a Caribbean sunburn, and triamcinolone tachyphylaxis probably all contributed to the exacerbation of M.M.'s psoriasis.

Categorization of Psoriasis

CASE 41-1, QUESTION 3: How would you categorize M.M.'s psoriasis?

The Self-Administered Psoriasis Area and Severity Index (SAPASI) is a validated, structured instrument that can be used for patient assessment of psoriasis severity and the response to therapy. It closely correlates with the standard clinician assessment instrument, Psoriasis Area and Severity Index (PASI), which includes quantification of the percentage of body involvement

Table 41-1
Drugs Reported to Induce Psoriasis

Anesthetics	Procaine
Antimicrobial agents	Amoxicillin, ampicillin, imiquimod, penicillins, sulfonamides, terbinafine, tetracyclines, vancomycin, voriconazole
Anti-inflammatory drugs	Corticosteroids (after withdrawal), NSAIDs (indomethacin, salicylates), mesalamine
Antimalarial agents	Chloroquine, hydroxychloroquine
Cardiovascular drugs	Acetazolamide, amiodarone, angiotensin-converting enzyme inhibitors (enalapril, lisinopril), β-blockers (atenolol, metoprolol, propranolol, timolol), calcium channel blockers (dihydropyridines, diltiazem, verapamil), clonidine, digoxin, gemfibrozil, quinidine
H_2-antagonists	Cimetidine, ranitidine
Hormones	Oxandrolone, progesterone
Opioid analgesics	Morphine
Psychotropics and neurologic agents	Lithium carbonate, venlafaxine, fluoxetine, carbamazepine, olanzapine, gabapentin, oxcarbazepine, tigabine, valproic acid, zaleplon
Miscellaneous	Potassium iodide, mercury, α-interferon, β-interferons, granulocyte-macrophage colony-stimulating factor (GM-CSF)

NSAIDs, nonsteroidal anti-inflammatory drugs.
Source: Kim GK, Del Rosso JQ. Drug-provoked psoriasis: is it drug induced or drug aggravated? *J Clin Aesthet Dermatol*. 2010;3:32–38; Basavaraj KH et al. The role of drugs in the induction and/or exacerbation of psoriasis. *Int J Dermatol*. 2010;49:1351; Facts & Comparisons eAnswers. Accessed August 21, 2015, with permission.

and severity of lesions.[26,27] A PASI of 75 (a ≥75% decrease in PASI score) at 3 months from baseline has become the most prominent marker to assess systemic agent efficacy (see http://escholarship.org/uc/item/18w9j736, which is *Dermatol Online J.* 2004;10(2):7, for a good reference to teach someone the PASI and SAPASI).[28]

The National Psoriasis Foundation has released a clinical consensus statement on the classification of severity of disease. Rather than using a mild (less than 5% BSA affected) to moderate (5%–10%) to severe (greater than 10% BSA affected) classification system, the statement recommends two categories for patients: those who are candidates for topical therapy (less than 5% of BSA affected) and those who are candidates for systemic or phototherapy (more than 5% of BSA affected).[27,28]

M.M. would be categorized as having mild psoriasis and is a candidate for topical therapy because less than 5% of his BSA is currently affected by psoriasis.

TREATMENT OF MILD PSORIASIS

Many topical and systemic therapeutic agents are available, varying from simple topical emollients to systemic, highly potent immunosuppressant drugs for more recalcitrant conditions. Often, treatment modalities are chosen on the basis of disease severity, cost, convenience, and patient response. Patients with mild disease can generally be treated with topical therapy (Table 41-2). Patients with psoriasis covering more than 5% of the body require more specialized systemic or phototherapy treatment programs (Table 41-3). Nonpharmacologic treatment is also very important and can range from spa therapy to support groups.

Initial Therapy

NONPHARMACOLOGIC MODALITIES

CASE 41-1, QUESTION 4: What role can emotional support play in the comprehensive management of M.M.'s psoriasis?

Psoriasis is often more emotionally or psychologically disturbing than is recognized, and it may cause a reluctance from patients to participate in sports and other outdoor activities that may expose their skin to sunlight. Although exposure to sunlight helps most patients with psoriasis, there is an unwillingness to sunbathe if the lesions can be seen. Furthermore, if the psoriatic lesions become pruritic and are scratched, there can be further deterioration at the site. Many patients alter their lifestyles or use nontraditional medications and modalities, often in desperation.

Emotional support should begin with explanation of the psoriatic condition. M.M. needs to be reassured that many other people have the same condition, that the disorder is not

Table 41-2
Topical Agents for the Treatment of Psoriasis (Mild to Moderate; <5% Body Surface Area Involvement)

Treatment Modality	Advantages	Disadvantages
Emollients	Basic adjunct for all treatments; safe, inexpensive, reduces scaling, itching, and related discomfort	Provide minimal relief alone
Keratolytics (salicylic acid, urea, α-hydroxy acids [i.e., glycolic and lactic acids])	Reduce hyperkeratosis; enable other topical modalities to better penetrate; inexpensive	Provide minimal relief individually; nonspecific; salicylism (tinnitus, nausea, vomiting) with salicylic acid if applied extensively
Topical corticosteroids	Rapid response; control inflammation and itching; best for intertriginous areas and face; convenient, not messy; mainstay topical treatment modality for psoriasis	Temporary relief; less effective with continued use (tachyphylaxis occurs); withdrawal can produce flare-ups; atrophy, telangiectasia, and striae with continued use after skin returns to normalized state; expensive; adrenal suppression possible
Coal tar	Particularly effective for "flaky" scalp lesions; newer preparations are more cosmetically appealing; efficacy enhanced in combination with UVB (i.e., Goeckerman regimen)	Effective only for mild psoriasis or scalp psoriasis; inconvenient with difficult application; stains clothing and bedding, not skin; strong smelling; folliculitis and contact allergy (bronchospasm in atopic patient with asthma after inhalation of vapor); carcinogenicity in animals
Anthralin	Effective for widespread, refractory plaques; produces long remissions; short, concentrated programs preferred; enhanced efficacy in combination with UVB (i.e., Ingram regimen)	Purple-brown staining (skin, clothing, and bath fixtures); irritating to normal skin and flexures; careful application is required; can precipitate generalized psoriasis
Calcipotriene and calcitriol	As effective as topical corticosteroids, although slower onset, without long-term corticosteroid adverse effects; convenient, well tolerated	Slow onset; expensive; potential effects on bone metabolism (hypercalcemia); irritant dermatitis on face and intertriginous areas; contraindicated during pregnancy
Tazarotene	Extended response; convenient (applied once daily, in gel formulation); maintenance therapy; effective on scalp and face; used in combination with topical corticosteroids	Slow onset; local irritation and pruritus; teratogenic (adequate contraception is required)
Ultraviolet B (UVB)	Effective as maintenance therapy; eliminates problems of topical corticosteroids	Expensive; office-based therapy; sunburn (exacerbates psoriasis); photoaging; skin cancers

Table 41-3
Agents for the Treatment of Severe Psoriasis (>5% Body Surface Area Involvement)

Treatment Modality	Advantages	Disadvantages
Psoralens plus UVA (PUVA)	80% efficacy; "suntan" effect is cosmetically desirable	Time-consuming; expensive, office-based therapy (restrictive); sunburn (exacerbates psoriasis); photoaging; both nonmelanoma skin cancer and melanoma; contraindicated during pregnancy and lactation
Acitretin	Not as effective as other systemic agents; efficacy enhanced if given with PUVA or UVB (i.e., RePUVA or ReUVB); less hepatotoxic than methotrexate	Teratogenic (contraception required); contraindicated with liver or renal dysfunction, drug or alcohol abuse, hypertriglyceridemia, hypervitaminosis A
Methotrexate	Effective for both skin lesions and arthritis, as well as psoriatic nail disease	Hepatotoxicity (liver biopsy may be indicated); bone marrow toxicity; folic acid protects against stomatitis (but not against hepatic or pulmonary toxicity); drug interactions; contraindicated during pregnancy and lactation, drug or alcohol abuse; use with caution during acute infections
Cyclosporine	Toxicities and short-lived remissions; used in patients with extensive disease who are unresponsive to other agents; however, given changing pathophysiology and increasing experience at lower dosages, increasing role in rotational therapy to induce remissions	Renal impairment; suppressive therapy (relapse occurs when discontinued); increased risk of skin cancer, lymphomas, and solid tumors; phototoxic; contraindicated during pregnancy and lactation, and with hypertension, hyperuricemia, hyperkalemia, acute infections
Immunomodulators (etanercept, infliximab, adalimumab, golimumab, secukinumab, ixekizumab)	Specific, targeted therapy; effective for both moderate-to-severe skin lesions and arthritis; maintains remission	Expensive; parenteral therapy (often administered in an office-based practice); long-term safety unknown; increased risk of serious infections

PUVA, psoralens plus ultraviolet A light; RePUVA, retinoid-PUVA; UVA, ultraviolet A; UVB, ultraviolet B.

contagious or fatal, and that it can be controlled, although no cure exists.[29] Patients usually are comforted in the knowledge that a wide range of treatments are available. Psychological encouragement and support are justified and make it easier for the patient to conscientiously apply messy topical treatments or to take toxic medications.

TOPICAL CORTICOSTEROIDS

CASE 41-1, QUESTION 5: What topical corticosteroid therapy is appropriate for M.M.?

Topical corticosteroids, the most widely prescribed treatment for psoriasis, are effective in the treatment of psoriasis because of their anti-inflammatory, antimitotic, immunosuppressant, and antipruritic properties.[25,30,31] These properties are explained by a reduction in phospholipase A_2, DNA synthesis, and epidermal mitotic activity, as well as their vasoconstrictive actions. They provide prompt relief, and patients find them convenient and acceptable. Mild-strength topical products or intermediate-strength products, for limited periods, can be used on facial lesions or intertriginous areas, or for maintenance therapy.[32] However, topical corticosteroids can, in a process called tachyphylaxis, also become less effective with continued use, and long-term use after the skin has returned to a normalized state leads to typical corticosteroid adverse effects (atrophy, telangiectasia, and striae). Thin-skinned areas (i.e., facial and intertriginous) are particularly susceptible.[33]

Psoriasis is generally a relatively corticosteroid-resistant disease; therefore, the more potent corticosteroids are frequently necessary, often with occlusion (e.g., plastic food wrap on top of the topical corticosteroid-treated area) (see Table 39-8 in Chapter 39, Dermatotherapy and Drug-Induced Skin Disorders, for a listing of topical corticosteroids by potency). Less-potent agents are more appropriate in intertriginous areas, on the face, and for maintenance. Potent fluorinated corticosteroid preparations should be used cautiously and only for short periods on the face and flexures, if at all. Potent topical corticosteroids may clear psoriasis in 25% of patients in 3 to 4 weeks, with 75% clearing in 50% of treated patients.[34]

Intermittent dosing or "pulse therapy" with several weeks between successive courses appears to yield the best long-term results and minimizes tachyphylaxis and adverse effects. An additional drawback of chronic corticosteroid therapy is an associated acute flare-up of psoriasis when corticosteroid therapy is terminated.[35] Continuous application for more than 3 to 4 weeks should be discouraged in patients with psoriasis, and systemic corticosteroids have no place in therapy.[33,34] Topical corticosteroids occasionally can cause a reversible suppression of the hypothalamic–pituitary–adrenal (HPA) axis, as indicated by a decrease in the morning plasma cortisol level.[33] For anything more extensive than mild disease and short duration of therapy, topical corticosteroids are best used in an adjunctive role. During a flare-up, corticosteroids help reduce inflammation, redness, and irritation and prepare the involved area for initiation of other potentially irritating, but more appropriate, maintenance topical treatments (e.g., coal tar, anthralin, calcipotriene, or tazarotene).

A short course of a potent topical corticosteroid is appropriate for this flare-up of erythematous plaque psoriasis in M.M. This will help reduce inflammation, redness, and irritation before possible initiation of more appropriate chronic topical treatments, such as calcipotriene, coal tar, or anthralin with ultraviolet B (UVB). Topical corticosteroids also may continue to be useful for M.M.

on the face and flexures, where the alternative topical agents are poorly tolerated. His scalp psoriasis can be treated with corticosteroid preparations in gels, lotions, or aerosol sprays. This will allow for a more effective treatment of scaling and pruritus using an agent such as coal tar shampoo lathered into the scalp for 5 to 10 minutes, then rinsed out.

The response to once- or twice-daily corticosteroid application is as effective as or better than that observed with more frequent regimens (owing to a corticosteroid reservoir effect) and is much less expensive. M.M. should apply a topical corticosteroid preparation after a bath, at bedtime with occlusion, and possibly again during the day without occlusion. As the lesions subside, occlusion should be decreased or omitted, emollient use should increase, and the corticosteroid potency should decrease. After lesions have flattened, the topical corticosteroid products can be continued intermittently (e.g., 1–2 weeks on, 1–2 weeks off; or on alternate days [e.g., days 1, 3, 5, and 7]).

ALTERNATIVE TOPICAL TREATMENTS

CASE 41-1, QUESTION 6: M.M.'s acute psoriasis flare-up has responded well to a short course of topical corticosteroid. What alternative topical therapeutic regimens are available for patients such as M.M. who have localized or mild disease?

Effective alternative topical therapies available for patients with localized, mild psoriasis include crude coal tar, anthralin, calcipotriene, calcitriol, and tazarotene.[31] Although anthralin has irritating properties and both coal tar and anthralin generally stain clothing and skin and are somewhat inconvenient to apply, their efficacy is well established and may be an option to consider for initial management. Tachyphylaxis does not occur with chronic use of any of these alternative agents. Once the inflammation and erythema have lessened with corticosteroid use or when a twice-daily, high-potency corticosteroid regimen along with bedtime application of coal tar is ineffective, calcipotriene ointment applied twice daily or tazarotene gel applied once daily is effective in treating flare-ups and maintaining remission. Ointment vehicles are favored because they help moisturize the plaques (in contrast to creams, which dry the plaques further). Also, moisturizers or emollients are often helpful for psoriasis.[31]

Coal Tar

Crude coal tar is a complex mixture of thousands of hydrocarbon compounds.[31,36] It is a time-honored modality for treating psoriasis. It affects psoriasis by enzyme inhibition and antimitotic action (antiproliferative and anti-inflammatory).[36] The efficacy of the combination of tar and UVB light (i.e., Goeckerman regimen) led to its increased popularity beginning in the 1920s. Tar preparations of 2% to 10% are processed as creams, ointments, lotions, gels, oils, shampoos, and coal tar solution. Newer purified preparations, using refined coal tar, are less messy and more cosmetically acceptable, but perhaps not as effective.[36] Tar may be helpful for patients with mild-to-moderate disease, and tar shampoos are useful for psoriasis of the scalp. The potential severity of adverse drug effects from topical tar products is less than that from anthralin and much less than that from topical corticosteroids. Because tar, in every form, is messy, stains the skin, has an odor, and is low potency compared with anthralin, it has been relegated to second-line therapy for most patients, despite its moderate price and newer, more cosmetically appealing formulations.[33,37]

Tar preparations generally are used once or twice daily, and a bedtime application (as a shampoo or cream overnight) is particularly useful in psoriasis of the scalp. Patients should be warned about the staining properties of tar on clothing and bedding. Other adverse effects include photosensitivity, acneiform eruptions, folliculitis, and irritation dermatitis. Care should be taken to avoid use of tar on the face, flexures, and genitalia and with inflammatory psoriasis because of tar's irritant properties.

The polyaromatic hydrocarbons contained in coal tar may be metabolized to active carcinogens by epidermal microsomal enzymes. The incidence of hyperkeratotic lesions, including squamous cell carcinoma, is increased after prolonged industrial exposure to tar; however, extensive reviews of patients who have used tar preparations in psoriasis have not revealed an increased risk of carcinoma.[38]

Anthralin

Anthralin (dithranol in the United Kingdom) is a hydroxyanthrone derivative that inhibits DNA synthesis, mitotic activity, and a variety of enzymes crucial to reducing cell proliferation.[31,34] It is effective for treatment of widespread, discrete psoriatic plaques, but its use has declined in recent years with the availability of more cosmetically appealing preparations. Traditionally, it was applied as a stiff paste overnight and used in conjunction with coal tar baths and UVB light (i.e., Ingram regimen). Most cases of chronic plaque psoriasis clear in 3 weeks. The primary disadvantages of anthralin are its irritant nature and property of staining skin and clothing. Anthralin also can precipitate generalized psoriasis if applied to unstable psoriasis (i.e., plaque transformation to pustular form).

When used, the most current anthralin regimen is a once-daily application of a 1% or 1.2% cream (Dritho-Crème HP and Zithranol-RR, respectively) for a short-contact anthralin therapy (SCAT; apply for 20–30 minutes, then wash off). One factor that limits its use is the brown-to-purple staining of the skin, hair, clothing, furniture, and bedding that occurs immediately with use. Plastic gloves should be used, as well as old bed linens and clothing for sleep. If possible, contact with the face, eyes, mucous membranes, and nonpsoriatic skin should be avoided because of irritant properties. Irritation is a problem and should be evaluated every 48 hours. Patients can apply petroleum jelly around lesions to avoid anthralin contact with unaffected skin. Anthralin is used daily for clearing of psoriasis, then once or twice weekly for maintenance therapy, after a response is seen at 2 to 3 weeks. Short-course regimens clear 32% of lesions and produce greater than 75% improvement in half of patients after 5 weeks. These regimens are comparable in effectiveness to the Ingram regimen and topical corticosteroids, and are associated with fewer adverse drug events.[33,39]

Calcipotriene

Calcipotriene (calcipotriol in Europe) is a topical vitamin D_3 analog that suppresses keratinocyte proliferation and has anti-inflammatory effects.[31,40] It can be applied twice daily as a cream, ointment, foam, or solution. Although systemic absorption is slight and the vitamin D effects of calcipotriene on calcium and bone metabolism are about 100 to 200 times less than those of 1,25-dihydroxyvitamin D_3, serum calcium levels and urinary calcium excretion should be monitored to prevent serious adverse effects. A 100-g/week limit should be enforced; exceeding this limit results in negative effects on calcium and bone metabolism. Other adverse effects of calcipotriene, such as lesional and perilesional irritation, burning, stinging, pruritus, erythema, and scaling, occur in about 30% of patients and preclude use on the face or in intertriginous areas. When used concurrently with topical salicylic acid, calcipotriene will be chemically inactivated.[41]

Calcipotriene may be the topical maintenance treatment of choice in patients with generalized mild-to-moderate psoriasis. The drug is usually effective, relatively easy to apply, odorless, and nonstaining (cream, ointment, or scalp solution). Most patients see improvement, although not clearing, of psoriatic plaques at 2 weeks when treated with calcipotriene, often in combination with potent topical corticosteroids.[42] A maximal response is usually seen at 6 to 8 weeks. Of treated patients, 57% experience greater than 75% clearance of psoriatic plaques, which is comparable to that achieved with corticosteroids, albeit slower in onset and associated with more skin irritation.[30,39] Tachyphylaxis has not been a problem.[42]

Calcitriol

Calcitriol is an active form of vitamin D_3 that blocks keratinocyte proliferation. The ointment should be applied twice a day, while avoiding the face, eyes, and lips. Use should not exceed 200 g/week. Hypercalcemia has occurred in about 25% of patients, and calcitriol should be held until calcium levels return to normal. Nephrolithiasis, hypercalciuria, and irritation of the skin have been reported with calcitriol use. Skin irritation, however, is less than with the use of calcipotriene. Caution should be exercised when combining calcitriol with phototherapy because it is inactivated by ultraviolet light and its vehicle blocks ultraviolet light.[43] Therefore, patients should apply calcitriol after phototherapy. Calcitriol effects are seen as early as 2 weeks, peak in about 8 weeks, and equal calcipotriene efficacy. Approximately 65% of patients continued to show improvement at 52 weeks of therapy.[44]

Tazarotene

Tazarotene is a topical synthetic retinoid that is rapidly converted to its biologically active metabolite, tazarotenic acid.[31,45] By interacting with the predominant retinoid receptors on the skin surface regulating gene transcription, retinoic acids normalize abnormal keratinocyte differentiation, reduce hyperproliferation, and decrease inflammation associated with psoriasis.[45] Treatment success rates compare favorably with corticosteroids (52% clearing of all lesions; 70% clearing of trunk and limb lesions). The antipsoriatic effects of tazarotene are sustained for a longer period after treatment compared with corticosteroids.[34,46] Because local skin irritation and pruritus are common adverse effects of tazarotene use, combination therapy with corticosteroids not only provides additive antipsoriatic effects, but also reduces retinoid-induced irritation.[47] Because oral retinoids are known teratogens, tazarotene is a category X drug and is contraindicated during pregnancy. Women should be warned of the potential risk and the need to use adequate contraception while using these preparations.[45,46]

Similar to calcipotriene, tazarotene works slowly. It is available as a gel, which many patients find more cosmetically appealing than an ointment. It is also effective in a once-daily regimen, which might help to improve compliance.

PHOTOTHERAPY

Phototherapy with ultraviolet (UV) light has a long history of use in the treatment of psoriasis. Unlike immunosuppressive agents, phototherapy is thought to target effector immune cells and upregulate regulatory T cells. Phototherapy also reverses epidermal barrier abnormalities, thus restoring cutaneous homeostasis.[48] If available locally, UV light can be used as an outpatient modality, and newer options for home treatments have become commonplace.[49] This modality produces comparatively long-lasting remissions and is pleasant to use with relatively low toxicity at a reasonable cost when compared with biologic agents.[50] Different protocols require daily exposure or multiple times per week for varied lengths of time, depending on patient variables. The optimal effect of UVB on psoriasis is a dose that produces minimal erythema at 24 hours. The usual time to induce clearing of psoriasis is approximately 4 to 6 weeks.

Ultraviolet B

Ultraviolet B light, sunburn spectrum 290 to 320 nm, induces pyrimidine dimers, inhibits DNA synthesis, and depletes intraepidermal T cells found in psoriatic epidermis (i.e., UVB has antiproliferative and local immunologic effects).[25] UVB light, unlike ultraviolet A (UVA) light, is effective without additional sensitizers (i.e., psoralens). UVB therapy is generally considered pleasant to use and relatively nontoxic. Typically, 60% of patients with chronic plaque psoriasis experience clearing, and an additional 34% achieve a 75% clearance with UVB treatment for 7 to 8 weeks.[35] Humidity and heat from sunlight provide additional positive effects. Narrowband UVB (NB-UVB) phototherapy, having sunburn spectrum of 311 nm, has been found to be more effective than broadband UVB (BB-UVB)[51]; however, it has not demonstrated superiority to psoralens plus ultraviolet A (PUVA) light therapy in terms of clearing psoriatic lesions.[52] In a literature review comparing PUVA with NB-UVB, PUVA tends to clear psoriatic lesions more reliably, with fewer sessions, and with longer-lasting clearance; however, this must be balanced with the increased risk of PUVA in causing skin cancers.[53] In another literature review, NB-UVB was found to be more effective than BB-UVB and was also safer than PUVA.[54]

The greater efficacy of PUVA, however, may be offset by the short-term adverse effects of psoralens (e.g., nausea, headaches), the greater incidence of phototoxic reactions (erythema), and the inconvenience of wearing photoprotective eyewear after treatments. At present, NB-UVB may be preferred because the available data suggest no or minimal risk of carcinogenesis compared with PUVA, it is safer to use in children and pregnant patients, it is devoid of drug-related (psoralen) adverse drug events, and there is no requirement for the use of posttreatment photoprotective eyewear. Although not definitively proven, it is hypothesized that NB-UVB will produce less long-term photodamage and fewer skin cancers than PUVA.

Ultraviolet B treatments are administered 3 times weekly. The use of pretreatment emollients (e.g., petrolatum, mineral or "baby" oil, Eucerin) applied before UVB exposure, long thought to improve results by aiding in descaling or by enhancing UVB penetration, actually inhibits its penetration and should not be used.[55] After the skin clears, therapy is discontinued gradually over the course of 2 to 4 months to prolong remission. The risks of UVB radiation and sunlight are similar: sunburn, photoaging, and skin cancer.

Regimens combining UVB with anthralin (Ingram regimen) or tar (Goeckerman regimen) have been used for years, theoretically taking advantage of the photosensitizing properties of tar and anthralin. The Goeckerman regimen, which consists of use of UVB light and 1% to 10% crude coal tar, involves daily application of coal tar for at least 4 hours, along with UVB exposure. Crude coal tar has been shown to be superior to cleaner tar preparations and other tar derivatives, using a 2-hour application before broadband UVB exposure. A petrolatum base, with a greasy sensation, was not superior to hydrophilic ointment, which has better cosmetic appeal and is easier to apply.[56]

The Ingram regimen combines daily application of anthralin plus coal tar baths with exposure to UVB light, with combination results superior to UVB monotherapy. These two regimens are reported to clear plaques in 75% of patients treated for 6 weeks for chronic plaque psoriasis (vs. 56% with UVB alone). The total number of treatments and the total UVB dose required for clearing are less in the combination groups.[57] Methods of classical treatments are not standardized, and different protocols in different treatment settings are used. Combinations of anthralin with superpotent corticosteroids or with coal tar may be preferred if systemic therapies are not effective or contraindicated.[58] Both the Goeckerman and Ingram regimens can decrease the severity of widespread psoriasis in 3 to 4 weeks, induce remissions that last for weeks to months, and may reduce the long-term adverse effects of UVB exposure.[57] A newer interest is the use of the Goeckerman regimen in those patients who are refractory to biologic agents.[59]

In summary, the first step in the treatment of M.M. would be a high-potency corticosteroid ointment twice daily, along with a coal tar ointment at night. If this is ineffective, either calcipotriene ointment can be added twice daily or tazarotene gel can be used once a day for 8 weeks. Once control is achieved, M.M. may use calcipotriene or tazarotene without topical corticosteroids; these products do not cause corticosteroid atrophy and do not have the potential for systemic adverse effects associated with topical corticosteroids. Topical anthralin, with or without UVB, can be used for resistant cases.

TREATMENT OF SEVERE PSORIASIS

CASE 41-2

QUESTION 1: G.L., a 42-year-old man with a several-year history of psoriasis (fairly localized), presents with diffuse, erythematous plaque-like lesions now extending over 80% of his body. The areas have become inflamed, and application of his maintenance topical medication (anthralin) causes pain and irritation. He expresses frustration with the messiness of the current topical regimen. He has reinstituted topical corticosteroids, which helped the redness and itching but are too expensive to use long term. He is free of cardiovascular, renal, or hepatic disease and takes no systemic medications. He is self-employed as a business consultant. Which "systemic" therapy would be most appropriate for G.L.'s psoriasis at this point?

Systemic therapies for psoriasis include PUVA, acitretin (the systemic retinoid), methotrexate; cyclosporine; and apremilast. Biologic agents, including the tumor necrosis factor (TNF)-α inhibitors (infliximab, etanercept, adalimumab, golimumab, ustekinumab, and secukinumab), have also been used for psoriatic lesions.[60]

Although PUVA and methotrexate are commonly used, cyclosporine and the immunomodulatory agents are being used increasingly more as experience is gained with them for treatment of severe psoriasis.[25,61] The choice of agents depends on patient and drug characteristics. Because patients with psoriasis generally have the disease for the rest of their lives, the goal of treatment is not just safe and effective resolution of lesions at a specific point in time, but also maintenance therapy. Long-term maintenance therapy for psoriasis can generally be achieved even with a weaning or discontinuation of UVB, PUVA, and methotrexate. From a histologic perspective, these drugs have been shown to induce remittive cellular changes. In contrast, partial-to-full doses of acitretin or cyclosporine are necessary to maintain therapeutic effects, because they induce suppressive rather than remittive histopathologic changes. For example, relapse will occur in most patients in a predictable manner 2 to 4 months after cyclosporine is discontinued.[62] Similarly, biologic therapy has demonstrated a very satisfactory antipsoriatic effect; however, the loss of the therapeutic response over time has been reported. Of interest, the addition of NB-UVB to the use of immunomodulatory agents that have lost this response in the control of moderate-to-severe cases in adults has been demonstrated to recover the initial response.[63]

Photochemotherapy

Photochemotherapy combines psoralens with UVA light in the 320- to 400-nm spectrum. The psoralens (methoxsalen, 8-methoxypsoralen, and trioxsalen) are a group of photoactive compounds that, on absorption of UV light, are both antiproliferative and immunomodulatory. When photoactivated by UVA, psoralens form monofunctional adducts and cross-links with pyrimidine bases. PUVA also inhibits cytokine release and depletes both epidermal and dermal T cells. As measured by extent of T-cell depletion and decreases in delayed hypersensitivity, PUVA has greater immunomodulatory effects in the skin than UVB. Use of PUVA for scalp or nail involvement is limited, however, because of lower exposure.[64] Remissions are longer in duration than with UVB. Psoralens are not active without UVA.

Photochemotherapy is used to control severe, recalcitrant, disabling plaque psoriasis. After 10 to 20 treatments over the course of 4 to 8 weeks, more than 80% of patients experience clearing of symptoms, which can be maintained with periodic (twice monthly) treatments.[64] UVA penetrates the skin more deeply than UVB and may have marked effects on the dermis. The use of PUVA requires careful consideration and adherence to strict photoprotective measures. Patients unwilling to adhere to PUVA-related precautions may prefer UVB treatment because it is much less restrictive.

The peak range for UVA light's therapeutic action is between 320 and 335 nm. The most widely used agent, 8-methoxypsoralen, at an oral dosage of 0.6 to 0.8 mg/kg of body weight rounded to the nearest 10 mg, is taken approximately 1.5 hours before exposure to UVA light.[52] The initial dose is selected on the basis of the patient's skin type (i.e., ease of sunburn and inherent skin color). Other options for combination therapy with UVA include calcipotriol-PUVA (D-PUVA) and retinoid-PUVA (RePUVA). Both of these modalities have been shown to have greater efficacy as compared with PUVA alone.[51]

Acute adverse phototoxic effects, such as partial-thickness burns, erythema, and blistering, are dose-related and, therefore, are a serious yet preventable complication of PUVA photochemotherapy.[65] Other acute adverse drug effects include nausea, lethargy, headaches, pruritus, and hyperpigmentation. Topical corticosteroid therapy should be continued until the psoriasis is brought under control. If topical corticosteroids are discontinued at the start of PUVA, an exacerbation of psoriasis usually occurs. Patients should wear protective clothing (with long sleeves and high necklines), use sunscreens that filter out both UVA and UVB, and wear sunglasses that block UVA after PUVA (see Chapter 42, Photosensitivity, Photoaging, and Burns). Because methoxsalen has a short half-life and 80% is eliminated within 6 to 8 hours, physical barriers are most important during the 8 hours immediately after PUVA therapy.

Of greater concern are the potential long-term adverse effects: mutagenicity, carcinogenicity, and cataract formation. A review of studies demonstrated an increased risk of nonmelanoma skin cancers following PUVA.[66] Squamous cell carcinoma has been associated with cumulative PUVA treatments (11-fold increase in patients who receive more than 260 treatments compared with patients who received fewer than 160 treatments).[67] Male patients have an increased risk of having genital squamous cell carcinoma. A relationship exists between the exposure to PUVA and the risk of malignant melanoma. At present, there appears to be a dose-dependent increase in the risk of melanoma associated with high-dose exposure to PUVA. The risk is first manifested at least 15 years after initial exposure to PUVA.[67–69] A cohort study evaluated over 13,000 patients for cancer risk by treatment modality. Patients treated with coal tar did not have increased risk of malignancies, both dermatologic and nondermatologic, and it is considered a safe option for treatment.[70] Long-term maintenance and high cumulative dosages should be avoided. Shielding the face and genitalia during treatment and performing annual examinations to detect skin cancer at an early stage may lessen the risk of long-term adverse effects of photochemotherapy.

Topical psoralens are extremely photosensitizing and hence difficult to administer. Application of methoxsalen 0.1% followed by small UVA doses (i.e., ≤20% of the level of usual doses for oral PUVA) has been used, however, to treat localized areas and to prevent adverse gastrointestinal effects.[64]

SYSTEMIC PHARMACOTHERAPY

Acitretin

Second-generation systemic retinoids are effective for treatment of recalcitrant psoriatic disease. Antipsoriatic effects stem from the drug's ability to modulate epidermal differentiation and immunologic function in addition to an anti-inflammatory action.[71] This latter effect may alleviate the arthritis that accompanies psoriasis.[25,64] Acitretin, a systemic second-line therapy for severe psoriasis, is the principal metabolite of etretinate. It is 50 times less lipophilic than etretinate and has a considerably shorter elimination half-life; however, patients taking any retinoid product should still be monitored closely. It is indicated for patients who have received extensive radiation with PUVA, as a pretreatment for PUVA (1–3 weeks) to accelerate the response rate, for patients who fail to respond to UVB with anthralin or tar, or for patients who are not candidates for methotrexate.[72] Most patients require maintenance or intermittent therapy to prevent relapses.[73] Response to acitretin should be assessed at 4-week intervals with dose titrations to reach therapeutic effect with minimal adverse events.[74]

Numerous other adverse effects are associated with acitretin use, including hypervitaminosis A syndrome (i.e., dry skin, skin thinning and fragility, chapped lips, dry nasal mucosa, skin peeling, alopecia, and nail dystrophy), retinoid rash, extraspinal tendon and ligament calcification and bone changes in children, hyperlipidemia with elevated levels of serum triglycerides and cholesterol, and liver enzyme alteration and hepatitis.[75] Many patients find the adverse effects of the retinoids intolerable and discontinue treatment. Topical corticosteroids can reduce some of the cutaneous retinoid adverse effects.

Acitretin is teratogenic and accumulates in fatty tissues, where it is slowly released into the bloodstream for up to 1 year after final administration.[71] Therefore, strict contraception during treatment and for 2 to 3 years afterward is recommended in women of childbearing age.[69,76] Patients also need to be advised not to donate blood while taking acitretin and up to 1 year after the end of treatment.[71]

Immunosuppressive Agents

METHOTREXATE

Methotrexate, a folic acid analog, inhibits dihydrofolate reductase needed for synthesis of several amino acids, pyrimidines, purines, and, subsequently, DNA, RNA, and protein synthesis. Methotrexate therapy greatly suppresses rapidly proliferating cells, such as those in psoriatic skin. Antipsoriatic mechanisms of methotrexate action include inhibition of keratinocyte differentiation and immunomodulation by destruction of lymphoid cells.[25,77]

Unlike other cytotoxic drugs, methotrexate produces antipsoriatic effects at dosages that are much lower than those used in cancer chemotherapy. Methotrexate is relatively safe and well tolerated, yet the long-term concerns for myelosuppression and hepatotoxicity (fibrosis and cirrhosis) and the need for periodic liver biopsies can discourage many patients and physicians from using it.[78,79] Alcohol and methotrexate are a particularly potent hepatotoxic combination. Patients with psoriasis receiving methotrexate have a 2.5- to 5-fold higher incidence of advanced liver changes than patients with rheumatoid arthritis receiving comparable regimens.[80] Methotrexate hepatotoxicity may be related to both cumulative doses and constant blood levels. Daily administration has been replaced by weekly dosage schedules for this reason. Liver chemistry tests (i.e., serum alanine aminotransferase, serum aspartate aminotransferase, serum albumin, and bilirubin) can be within normal limits, even in the presence of methotrexate-induced liver disease.[77] Therefore, consensus guidelines call for risk stratification for liver biopsies in all patients with psoriasis at baseline, and at intervals of approximately 1 to 1.5 g of cumulative methotrexate dose. Liver function tests, bilirubin, and albumin should be monitored monthly for the first 6 months, and then every 1 to 2 months thereafter.[77]

Bone marrow depression, nausea, diarrhea, and stomatitis are other adverse effects associated with methotrexate. Pneumonitis can occur early in the course of treatment, particularly when methotrexate is given at higher dosages similar to those used in cancer chemotherapy regimens. Folic acid, 1 mg daily, may prevent some of these adverse events, but not hepatitis or pulmonary toxicities. Teratogenesis and miscarriages have occurred, and methotrexate may cause reversible oligospermia. A number of clinically significant drug interactions may enhance the toxicity of methotrexate. Drug interactions are most likely to be clinically relevant problems in patients with decreased renal function.[77]

Relative contraindications to treatment with methotrexate include decreased renal function, significant abnormalities in liver function (i.e., fibrosis, cirrhosis, hepatitis), pregnancy or breast-feeding, anemia, leukopenia, thrombocytopenia, active peptic ulcer disease or infectious disease (tuberculosis, pyelonephritis), alcohol abuse, and patient unreliability.[77] Conception must be avoided during methotrexate therapy and for at least 3 months after cessation of methotrexate in men or one full ovulatory cycle in women.[77] Monthly monitoring of complete blood count with differential and a platelet count should be performed 7 to 14 days after starting therapy, and every 2 to 4 weeks for the first few months, then every 1 to 3 months. Renal function tests (i.e., serum creatinine, BUN) should be obtained at 2- to 3-month intervals.

CYCLOSPORINE

The positive dermatologic effects of cyclosporine highlight the importance of immune alterations in the pathogenesis of psoriasis. The toxicity and the short duration of remissions induced by cyclosporine and tacrolimus limit their usefulness. Cyclosporine is generally reserved for patients with extensive psoriasis who have not responded adequately to topical agents, UVB, PUVA, and other systemic agents.

In psoriasis, cyclosporine primarily acts by inhibition of calcineurin, which is necessary for interleukin-2 (IL-2) production. Interleukin-2 amplifies helper T cells and cytotoxic lymphocytes. Decreased IL-2 production leads to a decline in activated CD4 and CD8 cells in the epidermis. Cyclosporine also inhibits TNF-α and interferon-α_2, both of which are involved in the chemotaxis of inflammatory cells; it inhibits release of cytokines and the growth of keratinocytes.[81]

Cyclosporine is used at relatively low dosages for the treatment of psoriasis. In general, 2.5 to 6 mg/kg of cyclosporine, in one or two divided doses, is recommended for the initiation of psoriasis treatment. Rapid improvement of plaque psoriasis is expected, with 30% of patients experiencing clearing of psoriatic plaques and 50% achieving greater than 75% clearing of lesions within 10 weeks at a dose of 2 to 3 mg/kg/day. Many people relapse 2 to 4 months after the discontinuation of cyclosporine therapy.[82] Cyclosporine showed comparable efficacy to methotrexate in patients with psoriasis with average doses of 4.5 mg/kg/day and 20.6 mg/week, respectively.[78]

Drug-induced renal impairment is common with cyclosporine use, but usually reversible. Hypertension, secondary to vasoconstrictive effects on the smooth muscle of renal blood vessels or drug-induced arteriolar hyalinosis, is dose dependent and gradual in onset. Blood pressure and serum creatinine should be monitored closely in patients receiving cyclosporine.[79] Hypokalemia, hypomagnesemia, hyperuricemia, gingival hyperplasia, hypercholesterolemia, hypertriglyceridemia, adverse gastrointestinal effects, hypertrichosis, fatigue, myalgia, and arthralgia also have been attributed to cyclosporine therapy.[80] The risk of skin cancer, lymphomas, and solid tumors can also increase.[81,82] Patients should be cautioned about excessive sun exposure and should not receive concurrent UVB or PUVA treatment during cyclosporine therapy because of an increased risk of nonmelanoma skin cancers.[83]

PUVA is effective in 80% to 90% of patients, and G.L.'s severe, extensive, plaque psoriasis should be expected to respond accordingly. The systemic drugs (e.g., methotrexate, cyclosporine) may be preferred if G.L. had systemic symptoms (e.g., psoriatic arthritis). Although 3 times weekly PUVA treatments can be disruptive to work schedules, G.L. is self-employed and presumably has some flexibility in his working hours, and this would be a good option for him.

Phosphodiesterase 4 (PDE4) Inhibitors

Apremilast is an oral PDE4 inhibitor with efficacy in the treatment of moderate-to-severe plaque psoriasis and reduces immune responses by increasing intracellular cAMP in T cells. This results in decreased expression of cytokines and other proinflammatory mediators, but increased expression of anti-inflammatory mediators.[84] Mesenchymal cells, which express PDE4, are found in keratinocytes within the dermis, smooth muscle, and vascular endothelium.[85] Two phase IIb studies demonstrated that patients randomized to apremilast 20 mg twice daily achieved 24% and 29% PASI-75 at weeks 12 and 16, compared to 10.3% and 6% of those in placebo groups.[86,87] Of note, all patients enrolled had previously failed other therapy or were receiving concurrent therapy for psoriasis. Therefore, apremilast should not be considered a first-line agent in the treatment of plaque psoriasis.[86]

The recommended dose for apremilast is a 5-day titration up to 30 mg twice daily. The most common adverse effects with apremilast include gastrointestinal (i.e., diarrhea and nausea) and headache. Other adverse effects included upper respiratory infections and rebound psoriasis in 0.3% of patients after discontinuation of therapy. Apremilast is metabolized via the CYP 3A4 pathway and therefore should be evaluated for any drug–drug interactions prior to starting therapy. The dose of apremilast should be reduced when used in patients with impaired renal function (e.g., creatinine clearance less than 30 mL/minute).[85–87]

ROTATIONAL THERAPY

CASE 41-2, QUESTION 2: Does G.L. have options to decrease adverse effects and cost of his PUVA therapy?

No form of therapy used in psoriasis today is without toxicity. Rotational therapy involves the use of alternating monotherapies, which allows the patient to experience extended intervals of a particular treatment.[88] When used in long-term maintenance, rotational therapy limits adverse effects associated with either long-term use of one specific agent or the additive or synergistic interactions when multiple therapies are used concurrently. As discussed, the relative risk of skin cancer associated with PUVA increases after 160 treatments. If a patient in remission is rotated off PUVA to another treatment after 100 exposures, the skin has time to recuperate from the light therapy, and PUVA can eventually be reinstated presumably with lesser risk. Rotational therapy assumes that the patient can tolerate three to four alternative treatments with unrelated toxicity profiles.[88] By rotating each treatment after 12 to 18 months of cumulative use, the potential for long-term toxicity associated with any single treatment is minimized. With this theoretic rationale, cyclosporine could be used for a limit of possibly 3 to 6 months, thus inducing a remission. The patient could then be rotated to another treatment (e.g., methotrexate or PUVA) for maintenance.

Psoralens and UVA irradiation become noticeably effective in 80% to 90% of patients in 6 to 8 weeks.[25] The regimen is time consuming because UV radiation treatments must be administered at least 3 times a week. Methoxypsoralen (8-MOP) is administered (0.6–0.8 mg/kg of body weight), followed by UVA (dose selected based on skin type, ease of sunburn, and inherent skin color) about 75 to 90 minutes later when psoralen blood levels peak. PUVA-induced erythema generally appears later than with UVB therapy, reaching a peak by 48 hours. Consequently, treatment should not be administered more frequently than every second day. The time to produce clearing of psoriatic plaques with PUVA takes longer than with UVB therapy (average 10 weeks compared with ≤3 weeks for UVB).[64] PUVA treatment must be decreased slowly once plaques have been cleared (frequency of treatment is reduced during 2–3 months) to prevent recurrence of psoriatic plaques. In contrast, UVB therapy can be ceased abruptly.

Taking time off from work 3 times weekly for photochemotherapy can be disruptive to some patients' work or school schedules. Technologic advances in home phototherapy equipment have provided patients with choices for therapy in settings that are familiar and comfortable, in addition to continued improvements in efficacy and safety.[41] Advantages of home phototherapy include improved quality of life, greater convenience, lower cost, and less time lost from work and social activities.

Psoralens and UVA should be avoided in patients with a history of skin cancer, in children, during pregnancy, in patients who are immunosuppressed, and in those who have light-colored skin that burns rather than tans. Absolute contraindications to treatment with PUVA include a history of photosensitivity diseases (i.e., lupus erythematosus, porphyria), idiosyncratic or allergic reactions to psoralens, arsenic intake, and exposure to ionizing radiation, skin cancer (relative contraindication), pregnancy, and lactation. Techniques to minimize cumulative dosage of radiation and reduce the risk of long-term adverse effects of photochemotherapy include use of sunscreen, protective clothing, and sunglasses, and use of combination therapy (RePUVA). Other photosensitizing drugs (e.g., fluoroquinolones, phenothiazines, sulfonamides, sulfonylureas, tetracyclines, and thiazides) should be avoided in patients receiving PUVA.

Rotational therapy could be considered at a later time, depending on G.L.'s response and tolerance of PUVA.

PSORIATIC ARTHRITIS

CASE 41-3

QUESTION 1: R.T. is a 46-year-old male aerospace machinist with psoriasis and increasing joint complaints. He describes a flare-up during the last month involving predominantly the middle finger of his right hand. He also has arthralgias of the shoulders, knees, and the rest of his hands. Concomitantly, his skin disease has once again become active, despite nightly betamethasone dipropionate administration. He has a history of chronic depression and alcoholism, although he is currently sober and not being treated with antidepressant medications. Physical examination reveals a significant amount of tenderness of the right third metacarpophalangeal joint, without a great deal of active synovitis. He also has a moderate effusion of his right knee, but the rest of the joint examination is otherwise benign. Active psoriatic lesions are noted on his feet, knees, and elbows, and he has characteristic psoriatic nail changes. An erythrocyte sedimentation rate is mildly elevated. Which systemic therapy would be most appropriate to treat both R.T.'s skin and joint complaints?

Psoriatic arthritis (PsA) is a distinct form of inflammatory arthritis that is usually seronegative for rheumatoid factor. In various reports, 6% to 39% of patients with psoriasis experience PsA, and the prevalence is increased among patients with severe cutaneous disease.[18] Nail involvement occurs in greater than 80% of patients with PsA, as compared with 30% of patients with only cutaneous psoriasis.[18,89] Five clinical subsets of PsA have been identified: distal interphalangeal arthritis (classic; 5%–10%, often accompanied by nail changes), arthritis mutilans (5%, starts in early age, accompanied by osteolysis with severe deformities of fingers and toes), symmetric polyarthritis (rheumatoid-like; <25% incidence, milder course), asymmetric oligoarthritis (most prevalent; 70%, proximal and distal interphalangeal joints, metacarpophalangeal joints, knee, and hip), and spondylitis (5%–40%, often asymptomatic).[90]

The presentation of R.T. is representative of asymmetric oligoarthritis. Traditionally, treatment of this form of PsA consists of an NSAID, local corticosteroid injections, and immunosuppressive agents, including TNF inhibitors. Despite scant clinical evidence of efficacy, NSAIDs are commonly used to suppress the musculoskeletal symptoms of PsA, but do not induce remissions.[89] Systemic corticosteroids are avoided because they destabilize psoriasis (transformation to pustular forms), induce resistance to other effective therapies, and re-exacerbate the skin disease during withdrawal.[91] PUVA and acitretin have negligible anti-arthritic efficacy.

Methotrexate

Methotrexate is one of the most common agents used to produce symptomatic benefits (approximately 30%) in patients with PsA, but data on its efficacy to inhibit articular damage are limited.[91,92] TNF-α inhibitors have also been demonstrated to slow down or halt radiographic progression.[93] For mild joint disease, NSAIDs and intra-articular glucocorticoid injections may be adequate, whereas moderate-to-severe joint disease optimally will be treated with systemic oral disease-modifying antirheumatic drugs or biologics. After a sufficient trial of an NSAID, initiation of a second-line agent such as methotrexate before progression to a biologic intervention is a reasonable approach to manage R.T.'s arthralgias in his shoulders, knees, and hands, as well as his active skin disease.

After obtaining the history and physical examination, baseline laboratory tests should be obtained, which include a complete blood count, platelets, renal function tests (serum creatinine, BUN), liver function tests (LFTs: alanine aminotransferase, aspartate aminotransferase, alkaline phosphatase, and bilirubin), HIV antibody determination, and a purified protein derivative (PPD). Although standard in the past for all patients about to receive methotrexate therapy, a baseline aspiration needle biopsy of the liver, not an innocuous procedure, is obtained currently only in those patients with preexisting severe liver disease.[77] Patients with one or more risk factors for hepatic fibrosis (e.g., persistent abnormal liver chemistries, previous exposure to hepatotoxic agents, obesity, hyperlipidemia, diabetes mellitus, and family history of inheritable liver disease) should receive a baseline liver biopsy and a biopsy every 2 to 6 months until the drug's efficacy and a lack of toxicity have been established. A repeat liver biopsy after 1.0 to 1.5 g of methotrexate has been received is appropriate because it is rare for life-threatening liver disease to develop at this lower cumulative dose.[94]

Therapy with methotrexate usually is initiated with a 2.5- to 5-mg test dose.[77] If no idiosyncratic reaction occurs, doses are gradually increased to a maintenance dose of 10 to 25 mg/week. Methotrexate is best given in a single weekly oral dose or in three 2.5- to 7.5-mg doses at 12-hour intervals during a 24-hour period (e.g., 8 AM, 8 PM, and again at 8 AM). With the introduction of biologic agents in the management of psoriasis and its associated conditions, an increased level of monitoring has developed. Hepatotoxicity, however, may not be apparent on routine laboratory evaluation. Every 4 to 12 weeks, LFTs should be obtained, preferably at least 1 week after the last methotrexate dose because these values are often elevated 1 to 2 days after therapy. If a significant abnormality in the LFTs is noted, therapy should be withheld for 1 to 2 weeks, and the LFT testing should be repeated. LFT values should return to normal in 1 to 2 weeks. If significantly abnormal LFTs persist for 2 to 3 months, a liver biopsy should be considered. As noted previously, a liver biopsy is recommended when the cumulative dosage level reaches 1.0 to 1.5 g, as well as after each subsequent 1.5-g increase in the cumulative dose. Liver function abnormalities may improve after cessation of methotrexate therapy for 6 months.

Immunomodulatory Therapy

CASE 41-3, QUESTION 2: During a follow-up visit to his family physician several months later, R.T. had several somatic complaints that led to a diagnosis of recurrent depression. Subsequent history reveals that he also has resumed use of alcohol. He tends to drink four to five beers a night on weekends or when he is feeling low, although he does admit that his level of alcohol use is sometimes higher. His skin lesions are relatively well controlled, but joint complaints have persisted. What additional options now exist for R.T.?

Methotrexate should be discontinued because the risks probably now exceed the benefits, particularly because rheumatic complaints have not been controlled and alcohol consumption has resumed. Agents such as methotrexate and cyclosporine may reduce inflammatory joint activity in the short term, but evidence of their ability to modify the long-term disease process remains elusive. Close monitoring of the effects of these agents is also required because the toxicities often limit long-term use. R.T. should be referred for physical and occupational therapy, encouraged to exercise regularly, and, if needed, referred for orthotics. An NSAID can be given for symptomatic relief. Sulfasalazine and hydroxychloroquine might be beneficial for mild joint symptoms alone, but the cutaneous manifestations may be controlled with topical agents. Other alternative second-line agents include immunomodulatory agents, anticytokines, TNF-α inhibitors, infliximab, and etanercept. In the case of R.T., it is clear that better therapies for PsA are necessary.

Immunomodulatory Agents

With advances in biotechnology immunomodulatory therapy, important treatment alternatives are becoming available for moderate-to-severe plaque psoriasis and PsA that is resistant to other systemic therapies. These agents are thought to target the immune-mediated and elevated levels of TNF found in psoriasis.

MONOCLONAL ANTIBODIES AND TNF-α INHIBITORS: INFLIXIMAB, ETANERCEPT, ADALIMUMAB, GOLIMUMAB, USTEKINUMAB, SECUKINUMAB, AND IXEKIZUMAB

As a potent cytokine, TNF-α is involved in inflammation and joint damage. Inhibition of TNF-α reduces direct actions as well as the action of other proinflammatory cytokines. The TNF-α inhibitors, infliximab, etanercept, and adalimumab, are FDA approved for the treatment of both plaque and PsA. Golimumab is approved only for PsA. Ustekinumab is approved for both psoriasis and PsA, whereas secukinumab is currently approved only for plaque psoriasis. The mechanism of action of these agents is through blocking the interaction of TNF-α with cell-surface TNF receptors.[95] Ustekinumab is a specific inhibitor of interleukin-12 (IL-12) and anti-interleukin-23 (IL-23).[95] Secukinumab and ixekizumab inhibit interleukin-17A. Dosing is either subcutaneous injection or intravenous infusion (infliximab), on a biweekly, weekly, every other week, or monthly schedule during the initiation phase.

In a 24-week trial to assess the efficacy and safety of etanercept 50 mg administered once weekly in patients with moderate-to-severe plaque psoriasis, at week 12, 37.5% of patients achieved a PASI 75 response, with 71.1% achieving PASI 75 at week 24. No deaths, serious infections, opportunistic infections, demyelinating disorders, or malignancies were reported.[96] Antibody production has been reported in up to 18% of patients; however, they do not impact the efficacy of etanercept.[97]

Infliximab is a human/mouse chimeric anti-TNF-α antibody. One hundred eighty-six patients were given infliximab for moderate-to-severe plaque and nail psoriasis for 46 weeks. A PASI of 75 was demonstrated in 74.6% of patients, and a PASI of 90 was demonstrated in 54.1% at week 50.[98] In spite of clinically significant improvements, induction of antinuclear antibodies and anti–double-stranded DNA antibodies is frequently observed in patients receiving infliximab. To investigate the development of autoimmunity in patients receiving infliximab for severe, recalcitrant forms of psoriasis, 28 patients with psoriasis refractory to three or more systemic treatments were given infliximab 5 mg/kg for 22 weeks.[99] Detection of antinuclear antibodies and of IgM and IgG anti–double-stranded DNA antibodies was performed at baseline and at week 22. The prevalence of positive detection of antinuclear antibodies increased from 12% at baseline to 72% at week 22 and was also observed for IgM anti–double-stranded DNA antibodies. Three patients exhibited nonerosive polyarthritis, without any other criteria for systemic lupus. This study suggests that the incidence of biologic autoimmunity is high in patients with refractory psoriasis receiving infliximab.[99]

In a 52-week trial to assess the efficacy and safety of adalimumab 80 mg load followed by 40 mg administered every other week in patients with psoriasis, at week 16, 71% achieved an improved PASI score. Only 5% of patients continued on adalimumab until week 52 lost response to adalimumab.[100] Antibody formation for adalimumab, a human monoclonal antibody, occurs in up to 50% of patients, which may reduce the efficacy of this medication.[97]

In phase 3 trials, ixekizumab was superior to etanercept for mild-to-moderate psoriasis. By 12 weeks of ixekizumab dosed every other week, 90% of patients achieved a PASI of 75% versus 48% with etanercept. The most common adverse reactions were infection (26%) and injection site reactions (10%).[101]

Pharmacotherapy with TNF-α inhibitors has the best ratio of number-needed-to-treat-to-benefit (NNTB) to number-needed-to-harm (NNTH) of all disease-modifying antirheumatic drugs (DMARDs) in psoriatic arthritis, and is able to induce clinical remission in at least 30% of patients. Of interest, however, is that in many of these clinical studies, the NNTB presented comparisons with placebo. Many studies of TNF-α inhibitor therapies have allowed inclusion of patients who had not received other systemic therapies beyond topical therapies alone.[102] When interpreting the NNTB for TNF-α inhibitors, it is important to compare them with the NNTB for other systemic therapies. Also, having a comparable outcome measure (e.g., PASI 75) is necessary, especially because most established treatments have not been compared with placebo.[103] To determine which TNF-α inhibitor to use in a patient, consider the results from three meta-analyses. Infliximab was most likely to achieve a PASI of 75. Also, ustekinumab and adalimumab achieve significantly higher PASI 75 scores than etanercept. It is important to note this evaluation was based on 16 weeks of therapy.[104–106]

For a patient like R.T., whose disease cannot be treated successfully or safely with methotrexate, proceeding with a TNF-α inhibitor remains an option. These agents produce rapid, well-tolerated, beneficial responses compared with placebo. Benefit is seen anywhere from 2 to 12 weeks, with a PASI 75 being obtained in at least 80% of patients after 10 weeks of infliximab, at least 50% after 12 weeks of etanercept, and at least 50% after 48 weeks of adalimumab treatment.[107,108] R.T. does not have any contraindications to therapy, such as active infection or New York Heart Association (NYHA) class III or IV heart failure. If available, etanercept (25–50 mg subcutaneously twice weekly [3 or 4 days apart] for the first 3 months, followed by 50 mg once a week) may be preferred for convenience; however, in a recent comparative trial of ustekinumab (administered at weeks 0 and 4) and etanercept (administered twice weekly for 12 weeks), ustekinumab patients experienced a superior improvement in PASI 75 scores.[109]

Screening for tuberculosis before beginning therapy with anti-TNF agents is prudent, and those with evidence of prior tuberculous chest infection or with a positive skin test for tuberculosis should be offered prophylactic antitubercular therapy.

Phosphodiesterase 4 (PDE4) Inhibitors

Apremilast was recently approved by the FDA for the treatment of active PsA because clinical trials demonstrated moderate efficacy in the reduction of symptoms of PsA, including tender and swollen joints. Results from both phase II and phase III clinical trials demonstrated improvement in symptoms, quality of life, and pain in patients randomized to apremilast compared with placebo.[110] Of the patients enrolled in the phase III clinical studies, over half received concomitant therapy with DMARDS (e.g., methotrexate) and 10% to 15% had failed therapy with TNF-α inhibitors.[111]

Dosing is similar to that of plaque psoriasis, a titration up to 30 mg twice daily. The most common adverse effects reported in the clinical trials were gastrointestinal (i.e., diarrhea, nausea), fatigue, headache, and nasopharyngitis. The gastrointestinal adverse events were transient in nature and often occurred early on in therapy.[85]

Combination Therapy

The National Psoriasis Foundation recommendations for combination treatments include methotrexate and a TNF-α inhibitor (etanercept or infliximab), acitretin and infliximab, then a TNF-α inhibitor (etanercept or adalimumab) and phototherapy.[112] There is no evidence as yet to support using two biologics or a biologic with cyclosporine.[112]

KEY REFERENCES AND WEBSITES

A full list of references for this chapter can be found at http://thepoint.lww.com/AT11e. Below are the key references and websites for this chapter, with the corresponding reference number in this chapter found in parentheses after the reference.

Key References

Anderson KL, Feldman SR. A guide to prescribing home phototherapy for patients with psoriasis: the appropriate patient, the type of unit, the treatment regimen, and the potential obstacles. *J Am Acad Dermatol.* 2015;72:868–878. (49)

Armstrong AW et al. Combining biologic therapies with other systemic treatments in psoriasis. *JAMA Dermatol.* 2015;151:432–438. (109)

Brezinski EA, Armstrong AW. An evidence-based review of the mechanism of action, efficacy, and safety of biologic therapies in the treatment of psoriasis and psoriatic arthritis. *Curr Med Chem.* 2015;22:1930–1942. (60)

Gladman DD et al. Psoriatic arthritis: epidemiology, clinical features, course, and outcome. *Ann Rheum Dis.* 2005;64(Suppl 2):ii–14. (18)

Jabbar-Lopez ZK, Reynolds NJ. Newer agents for psoriasis in adults. *BMJ.* 2014;349:g4026. (61)

Menter A et al. Guidelines of care for the management of psoriasis and psoriatic arthritis: section 5. Guidelines of care for the treatment of psoriasis with phototherapy and photochemotherapy. *J Am Acad Dermatol.* 2010;62:114. (57)

Naldi L. Scoring and monitoring the severity of psoriasis. What is the preferred method? What is the ideal method? Is PASI passé? Facts and controversies. *Clin Dermatol.* 2010;28:67. (26)

Pariser DM et al. National Psoriasis Foundation clinical consensus on disease severity. *Arch Dermatol.* 2007;143:239. (28)

Key Websites

American Academy of Dermatology Current Psoriasis Guidelines. https://www.aad.org/education/clinical-guidelines.

American Academy of Dermatology Current Psoriasis Pharmacotherapy Reviews. https://www.aad.org/dermatology-a-to-z/diseases-and-treatments/m---p/psoriasis.

Arthritis Foundation (psoriatic arthritis). http://www.arthritis.org/about-arthritis/types/psoriatic-arthritis/.

National Psoriasis Foundation. http://www.psoriasis.org.

42 Photosensitivity, Photoaging, and Burn Injuries

Katherine G. Moore, Molly E. Howard, and Timothy J. Ives

CORE PRINCIPLES

	CHAPTER CASES
PHOTOSENSITIVITY	
1 Ultraviolet radiation (UVR) exposure has been linked to many adverse effects, including malignant melanoma.	**Case 42-1 (Questions 1, 2)**
2 Photoprotection encompasses all methods of UVR blocking, including sunscreens, protective clothing, and sunglasses. Sunscreens are widely used to prevent sunburn and reduce the incidence of premature aging and carcinogenesis, although clothing and avoiding direct sunlight offer greater protection.	**Case 42-1 (Questions 3–9)**
3 The use of tanning beds that use artificial ultraviolet A (UVA) has not been shown to reduce long-term damage to the skin or to provide protection from natural UVR. The use of tanning beds should be minimized, and adherence to Food and Drug Administration (FDA) recommendations on length of exposure should be encouraged.	**Case 42-2 (Questions 1, 2)**
4 Sunburn is a self-limiting condition, which is generally managed with symptomatic treatment including oral analgesics, topical analgesics, and topical anesthetics. Treatment beyond self-management is necessary if the sunburn is accompanied by constitutional symptoms, involves second- or third-degree burns, or is infected.	**Case 42-3 (Question 1)**
5 Phototoxicity and photoallergy are often drug- or chemical-induced reactions to UVR exposure and account for up to 8% of adverse drug reactions.	**Case 42-4 (Questions 1–3)**
PHOTOAGING	
1 Photodamaged skin is characterized as being wrinkled, yellowed, and sagging.	**Case 42-5 (Question 1)**
2 Topical retinoid therapy is most effective for patients of 50 to 70 years of age with moderate-to-severe photoaging and for prophylactic use in patients undergoing the initial changes of photoaging.	**Case 42-5 (Questions 2–5)**
BURN INJURIES	
1 Most burn injuries are minor and can be managed in ambulatory settings.	**Case 42-6 (Question 1)**
2 Major second- or third-degree burns should be immediately triaged to a health system with a multidisciplinary team that can adequately manage all of the potential complications.	**Case 42-6 (Question 1)**
3 Synthetic dressings and skin substitutes have expanded the options and the desired outcomes for recovery.	**Case 42-6 (Question 2)**

ULTRAVIOLET RADIATION (UVR) EXPOSURE

Incidence, Prevalence, and Epidemiology

Changing lifestyles have considerably increased human exposure to sunlight: more outdoor recreational activities, more emphasis on tanning, longer life spans, seasonal population shifts to the Sunbelt, and an emphasis on improving vitamin D deficiency. Epidemiologic evidence clearly implicates sunlight as a causative factor in many skin diseases, and public attitudes toward tanning and sun exposure have slowly begun to change. Skin cancer is the most common of all cancers and yet also one of the most preventable. Squamous cell carcinoma (SCC) and basal cell carcinoma (BCC), which together account for more than half of all malignancies in the United States, are linked closely to exposure to ultraviolet radiation (UVR).[1] Melanoma incidence rates have doubled from 1982 to 2011 in the United States, with 65,647 cases in 2011 and 9,128 deaths. Without intervention, the annual cost of treating newly diagnosed melanomas is projected to triple by 2030, but the CDC estimates that a comprehensive national skin cancer prevention program could potentially avert 230,000 melanoma cases.[2] In July 2014, the acting Surgeon General delivered "The Surgeon General's Call to Action to Prevent Skin Cancer." The purpose of the call was to unite various sectors of the nation to address skin cancer as a major public health problem, increase awareness of skin cancer, and call for action to reduce risk.[3]

Sunburn, photoaging, immunologic changes in the skin, cataracts, photodermatoses, phototoxicity, and photoallergy are other commonly encountered photosensitivity reactions that occur after UVR exposure. Phototoxicity and photoallergy are often drug- or chemical-induced reactions to UVR exposure and account for up to 8% of adverse drug reactions.[4] The appropriate use of sunscreens or other photoprotective behaviors can help mitigate the incidence of the adverse effects of UVR. Despite this fact, sunscreen use remains low, with recent survey-based estimates showing that fewer than 15% of men and 30% of women use sunscreen on both the face and the exposed skin as recommended. Forty-two percent of men reported never using sunscreen at all.[5]

Etiology

ULTRAVIOLET RADIATION SPECTRUM

Ultraviolet radiation, the primary inducer of photosensitivity reactions in humans, is divided into ranges according to the effects of four primary wavelengths: UVA1 (340–400 nm), UVA2 (320–340 nm), UVB (290–320 nm), and UVC (200–290 nm) (Fig. 42-1; Table 42-1). UVA, with a wavelength of 320 to 400 nm, is closest in wavelength to visible light.[6] UVA radiation levels have small fluctuations during the day and are present from sunrise to sunset every day, all year round, even in the winter and on cloudy days. UVA is considerably less likely than a comparable dose of UVB to cause a similar degree of erythema.[7,8] In contrast to UVB, UVA penetrates into the dermal layer and may cause harmful effects not caused by UVB.[5] About 10 to 100 times more UVA reaches the earth's surface than UVB. Consequently, UVA may contribute up to 15% of the erythemal response at midday.[6,9] UVB is the most erythemogenic and melanogenic of the three UVR bands.[6,10] Up to 90% of UVB is blocked by the earth's stratospheric ozone layer, and it is absorbed completely by the epidermal layer of the skin.[11,12] In addition, UVB radiation can alter the immune system,[12] thereby increasing the incidence of certain cancers, including skin cancers. The only known beneficial effect of UVR in humans is exposure to small amounts of UVB, most commonly through sunlight, which converts 7-dehydrocholesterol to cholecalciferol (vitamin D_3). Vitamin D enhances calcium homeostasis and has direct and indirect effects on cells involved with bone remodeling. As a result, vitamin D can decrease the risk of rickets in childhood and fractures and osteomalacia in adults.[13]

The UVC wavelengths are absorbed completely by the earth's stratospheric ozone layer. Artificial sources of UVC have been used in the sterilization and preservation of food and in minimizing bacterial growth in laboratories and hospital operating rooms by germicidal lamps, which can cause erythema or cataracts if mishandled.[6,10]

ENVIRONMENTAL EFFECTS ON UVR

Ozone and Chlorofluorocarbons

The amount of UVR that reaches the earth's surface is influenced by many factors. Concern has been focused on the implications of depletion of the ozone layer caused by

Figure 42-1 Ultraviolet radiation (UVR) spectrum. *Erythrogenic and melanogenic bands of UVR.

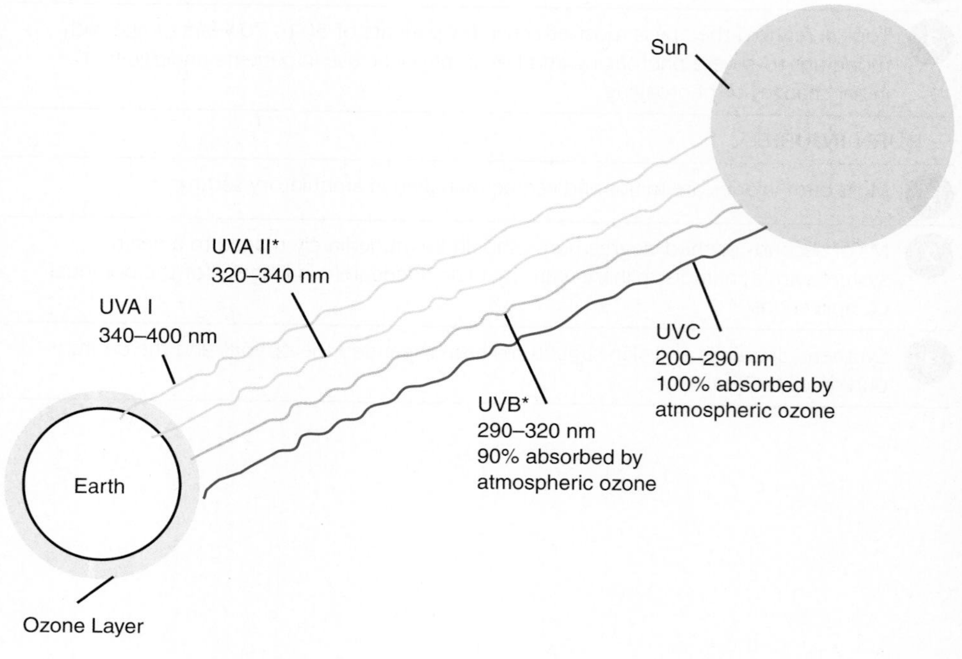

Table 42-1
Types of Ultraviolet Radiation and Characteristics

Radiation	Wavelength (nm)	Characteristics
UVA1 (long UVA; long-wave radiation)	340–400	Not absorbed by the ozone layer Passes through glass Produces some tanning, photoaging, and skin cancers Lower carcinogenic potential than UVA2, but harmful over long-term exposure Levels remain relatively constant throughout the day
UVA2 (short UVA)	320–340	Similar characteristics to UVA1, but greater carcinogenic potential with erythema production similar to UVB
UVB (sunburn range of radiation)	290–320	Partially absorbed by the ozone layer before reaching earth Does not pass through glass Causes erythema, sunburn, tanning, wrinkling, photoaging, skin cancers Daily and seasonal variation, with highest intensity at noon

man-made pollutants such as chlorofluorocarbons (CFCs), nitrous oxide, and other greenhouse gases (GHGs).[9,14] In the decade after this effect was first detected in 1983, ozone levels above the Antarctic had fallen to 50% of normal.[14] In the early 1990s, worldwide estimates from the Environmental Protection Agency (EPA) predicted that for every 1% decrease in ozone, UVB radiation reaching the earth's surface would increase by 2% per year, possibly resulting in a 1% to 3% increase per year in nonmelanoma skin cancer.[15] However, further research is needed to determine whether this prediction has been realized.[16] As GHGs contribute to ozone depletion, and because UVA is only slightly filtered by the ozone layer, any decrease in the ozone layer would result in a disproportionate increase in UVB reaching the earth.

Time of Day, Cloud Cover, and Surface Reflection

The time of day influences the amount of UVR reaching the earth's surface; 20% to 30% of the total daily UVR is received from 11 AM to 1 PM, with 75% between 9 AM and 3 PM. Cloud cover can decrease UV intensity by 10% to 80% and decreases infrared radiation to an even greater extent. This greater attenuation of infrared radiation by cloud cover can lead to an increased risk of UVR overexposure because less infrared radiation will be absorbed by the body and transformed into heat, resulting in less warning of overexposure to UVR. In general, whenever someone's shadow is shorter than his or her height, care should be taken; the shorter the shadow, the more likely a sunburn will occur. Reflection of UVR by substances (e.g., sand, water, snow) also may be important. For example, sand reflects about 25% of incident UVB radiation; therefore, sitting under an umbrella at the beach may not offer adequate protection. Fresh snow can reflect 50% to 95% of incident sunlight. Water reflects approximately 5% of erythemal UVR, whereas 75% of the radiation is transmitted through 2 m of water, offering swimmers little protection.[6] Seasonal changes, geographic latitude, and altitude also influence the amount of UVR reaching the earth's surface.

UV Index

The UV Index/Global UV Index (http://www.epa.gov/sunwise/uvindex.html), developed by the EPA, the National Weather Service, and the Centers for Disease Control and Prevention, is a public health education service that is calculated on a next-day basis for every ZIP code across the United States, and worldwide.[17] This index, with a scale from 1 (low exposure) to 11+ (extremely high exposure), forecasts the probable intensity of skin-damaging UVR expected to reach the surface during the noon hour when the sun is highest in the sky. Theoretically, the UV Index can range from 0 (e.g., during the night) to 15 or 16 (in the tropics at high elevations under clear skies). The higher the UV Index, the greater the dose received of skin- and eye-damaging UVR, and the less time it takes before skin damage occurs.

The amount of UVR exposure needed to damage an individual's skin is affected by the elevation of the sun in the sky, the amount of ozone in the stratosphere, and the amount of clouds present. Clear skies transmit 100% of UVR to the earth's surface, with scattered clouds transmitting 89%, broken clouds, 73%, and overcast clouds, 32%. The darker an individual's skin tone, the longer (or the more UVR) it takes to cause erythema.

Pathophysiology

ERYTHEMA, SUNBURN, AND TANNING

Erythema and Oxygen Free Radicals

Excessive exposure of the epidermal and dermal layers of the skin to UVR can result in an inflammatory erythematous reaction. Excess UVA and UVB cause the release of vasodilatory mediators (e.g., histamine, prostaglandins, cytokines), resulting in increased blood flow, erythema, tissue exudates, swelling, increased sensation of warmth, and a characteristic sunburn.[6,10] Severe UVR exposure, primarily UVB, can cause blister formation, desquamation, fever, chills, weakness, and shock. Erythema caused by UVB begins within 3 to 5 hours after exposure, is maximal after 12 to 24 hours, and usually resolves during the ensuing 3 days.[10] In contrast, erythema caused by UVA begins immediately, plateaus between 6 and 12 hours, and remains for 24 hours. UVA-induced changes in the dermis are characterized by greater damage to the vasculature and dense cellular infiltrates that penetrate to deeper levels of the skin.[10] The dermis also may be damaged when endogenous components of the skin absorb UVR energy and subsequently interact with oxygen to form tissue-damaging oxygen free radicals.[11]

Histology of Sunburn

The skin undergoes adaptive changes in response to UVR exposure.

When keratinocytes in the epidermis are damaged and lose their typical organization, both the epidermis and the stratum corneum thicken and attempt to serve as a barrier to UVR, particularly to UVB.[9] The skin's normal protective immune response, however, is altered with exposure to UVR. Metalloproteinase proteins act as proteolytic enzymes that are produced from low-dose UVR exposure, causing degradation of collagen and elastin in the dermal matrix.[18] Langerhans cells (i.e., antigen-presenting cells in the skin) are decreased in number and function even after small doses of UVB.[18] These cells abnormally activate suppressor T lymphocytes and lose their ability to activate normal effector pathways of the immune system.[19]

Immediate Pigment Darkening and Delayed Tanning

Tanning is an adaptive mechanism of the skin to UVR. Tanning occurs by two different mechanisms: immediate pigment darkening (Meirowsky phenomenon) and delayed tanning. The primary cell involved in tanning is the melanocyte, which produces the radiation-absorbing protein melanin.[6,9] Immediate pigment darkening begins during the actual exposure to UVA and certain bands of visible light,[6,9] and the oxidation of existing melanin in the epidermis transiently turns the skin grayish brown. The degree of immediate pigment darkening depends on the duration and intensity of exposure, the extent of previous tanning (or amount of preexisting melanin), and the skin type of the individual.[5] Immediate pigment darkening is not protective against UVB erythema.[9]

Delayed tanning occurs 48 to 72 hours after exposure to either UVA or UVB. It is most intense 7 to 10 days after UV exposure and can last for weeks to months.[6] Delayed tanning is the result of increased production of melanin, an increase in the size of dendritic processes, increased melanization of melanosomes, and an increase in the rate of transfer of melanosomes (particulate bodies of melanin) to keratinocytes.[6,9] The keratinocyte, now pigmented with melanosomes, migrates to the epidermis, producing the characteristic suntan. Delayed tanning caused by UVA is less protective against sunburn than delayed tanning caused by UVB, because epidermal thickening is not induced by UVA.[6]

PHOTOCARCINOGENESIS

Squamous Cell and Basal Cell Carcinoma

The association between skin cancer in humans and UVR exposure is based primarily on clinical and epidemiologic evidence. Nonmelanoma skin cancers, such as SCC and BCC, occur most commonly on areas that are maximally exposed to sunlight (e.g., the face, neck, arms, back of the forearms, and hands).[6] The prevalence of nonmelanoma skin cancers is inversely related to geographic distance from the equator and to the melanin content of the skin, with SCC more strongly linked than BCC to UVR.[6,20] Persons of skin types most sensitive to sunlight, as well as persons working outdoors, have higher incidences of nonmelanoma skin cancers.[6] A family history of SCC and BCC increases the risk at least twofold, depending on the histology, number of lesions, and degree of invasiveness.[21] Albinism, a genetic disease characterized by partial or total absence of pigment in the skin, hair, and eyes, is associated with increased and premature development of skin cancers.[6]

Cutaneous Malignant Melanoma

The development of cutaneous malignant melanoma (CMM) also may be linked to UVR exposure, specifically exposures that induce sunburn. A history of five or more severe sunburns during adolescence more than doubles the risk of CMM.[20] Similar to nonmelanoma skin cancers, CMM demonstrates an inverse relationship to geographic distance from the equator and melanin content of the skin.[6] Unlike nonmelanoma skin cancers, however, CMM does not demonstrate a clear relationship to the cumulative dose of UVR, and it occurs on areas of the body exposed to the sun intermittently (e.g., on the back in men and the lower legs in women). In addition, it occurs most commonly in the middle-aged population and in individuals who work indoors, as well as in those whose sun exposure is limited to weekends and vacations.[20] A family history of melanoma is a strong risk factor, as 8% to 12% of melanoma patients display a familial propensity for the disease.[22]

Mechanisms of Carcinogenesis

Mechanisms of carcinogenesis may include damage to DNA and alterations in immunologic status. Epidermal and dermal DNA can absorb UVR, which can contribute to abnormal formation of pyrimidine dimers. Under normal circumstances, these dimers are excised and repaired; however, if left uncorrected, these DNA lesions, as well as an inactivity of p53 tumor suppressor gene activity, can lead to interruption of transcription, with possible mutagenesis and malignancy.[23]

PHOTOEFFECTS ON THE EYE

Exposure to UV radiation can cause many types of ocular adverse effects including cataracts, conjunctival degeneration and proliferation, as well as squamous cell carcinoma of the cornea and conjunctiva.[24] Age-related opacification of the ocular lens, or senescent cataracts, has been attributed to a lifetime of exposure to sunlight. The incidence of cataracts increases steadily after age 50, reaching nearly 30% in individuals older than 74.[25] UVB is absorbed by the cornea and lens, which slowly results in protein oxidation and precipitation within the lens. UVA penetrates the ocular lens and can cause cumulative damage to deeper structures of the eye. Decreased transmittance and increased scattering of light by the opacified lens eventually result in blurred vision, rings or halos around lights, changes in color perception, and blindness.[24] In advanced cases, the only treatment is surgical removal of the cataract.

High exposure of the eye to UVR (which can range from a few seconds of exposure to arc welding, a few minutes of exposure to a UVC-emitting germicidal lamp, commercial tanning, or UVR reflection by snow or sand) can cause conjunctivitis or photokeratitis, a painful inflammation of the cornea. Photokeratitis usually begins 30 minutes to 24 hours after the exposure, and time to onset depends on the intensity of the exposure.[26] Conjunctivitis commonly accompanies photokeratitis and is characterized by the sensation of a foreign body or grit in the eyes. Varying degrees of photophobia, lacrimation, and blepharospasm also may accompany photokeratitis.[26] Because the corneal epithelium has a great regenerative capacity, photokeratitis tends to be transient, with regression in 24 to 48 hours. Treatment consists of cool, wet compresses and mild anti-inflammatory analgesics, such as ibuprofen, aspirin, or naproxen sodium.

PHOTOTOXICITY AND PHOTOALLERGY

The most common type of drug-induced photosensitivity reaction is phototoxicity, which is an immediate or delayed inflammatory reaction that occurs when a compound with photosensitizing ability absorbs a sufficient concentration of UVR in or on the skin, and when the skin is exposed simultaneously to a specific wavelength of light.[27,28] When the offending agent is deposited on the skin surface, it is thought to act as a chromophore, absorbing UVR. When the chromophore reaches a sufficient concentration in or on the skin, and when the skin is exposed to the appropriate wavelength of UVR, energy is emitted and transferred to the surrounding molecules, which damages the adjacent tissue to cause a phototoxic reaction. The wavelength of radiation necessary to produce such a reaction depends on the absorption spectrum of the offending agent.[29]

Photoallergy results from a similar mechanism to phototoxicity, except that the immune system is involved. Most commonly, it is caused by polycyclic photosensitizers that react with UVA to form antigenic macromolecules, evoking a delayed hypersensitivity response. In photoallergic photosensitivity reactions, the suspected medication or chemical agent is altered in the presence of UVR to become antigenic or to become a hapten (i.e., an incomplete antigen), which can combine with a tissue antigen. These antigen–antibody or immune-mediated processes differentiate photoallergic from phototoxic reactions. Photoallergic reactions do not occur on first exposure to the medication, but as with other allergic reactions, they require prior or prolonged exposure (sensitization period) to the offending agent.[27,28] Once sensitization has occurred, subsequent exposure to even small amounts of the offending product will produce a photoallergic reaction.

Photoprotection

Photoprotection encompasses all methods of UVR blocking, including sunscreens, protective clothing, and sunglasses. Sunscreens are widely used to prevent sunburn and reduce the incidence of premature aging and carcinogenesis,[30–32] although clothing and avoiding direct sunlight offer greater protection. Sunburn preventive agents are those active ingredients that absorb greater than 95% of UVB radiation, and have the potential to prevent sunburn. Suntanning agents are those with active ingredients that absorb 85% to 95% of UVB radiation, thereby allowing suntanning without significant sunburn in the average individual. Chemical sunscreens include both of the aforementioned designations. Opaque sunblocks, or physical sunscreens, are those active ingredients that reflect or scatter all UVA, UVB, and visible light, thereby preventing or minimizing sunburn and suntanning.[33] The original formulations were developed to protect against the effects of UVB radiation before adverse effects of UVA were recognized. Because UVA plays a significant role in many of the adverse effects associated with UVR exposure, broad-spectrum sunscreen products with absorption spectra in the UVA range have become commercially available, in combination with UVB absorbers. These broad-spectrum products provide additional benefit for patients with photosensitivity reactions caused by wavelengths not covered by single-ingredient sunscreens. Table 42-2 lists the available sunscreen chemicals that have been judged to be both safe and effective.

There is a clear association between UV exposure and the development of BCC and SCC,[34] and limiting UV exposure by starting sunscreen use during childhood is a key to reduce the lifetime risk of nonmelanoma skin cancers; however, some investigators have suggested that sunscreen use, through increased UV exposure, may actually cause melanoma, perhaps because its use allows for a longer exposure to the sun,[35,36] and because historically there was a lack of UVA protection in most products.[37] Sunscreen use has been thought to be associated with the occurrence of nevi (pigmented moles), an important risk factor for melanoma development[38]; however, epidemiologic analyses have refuted this proposed association, largely on the basis of a longer exposure to UVR and less protective clothing in individuals who developed nevi.[39,40]

Table 42-2
Sunscreens and UVR Absorption

Sunscreen	Absorption
Anthranilates	
Meradimate (menthyl anthranilate)	260–380
Benzophenones	
Dioxybenzone	250–390
Oxybenzone (benzophenone-3)	270–350
Sulisobenzone (Eusolex 4360)	260–375
Cinnamates	
Cinoxate (diethanolamine *p*-methoxycinnamate)	280–310
Octocrylene	250–360
Octinoxate (octyl methoxycinnamate, Parsol MCX)	290–320
Dibenzoylmethanes	
Avobenzone (butyl methoxydibenzoylmethane, Parsol 1789)	320–400
Aminobenzoic Acid and Ester Derivatives	
Para-aminobenzoic acid (PABA)	260–313
Padimate O (octyl dimethyl PABA)	290–315
Salicylates	
Homosalate	295–315
Octisalate (octyl salicylate)	280–320
Trolamine salicylate	260–320
Camphor Derivatives	
Ecamsule (terephthalylidene dicamphor sulfonic acid; Mexoryl)	290–400
Others	
Ensulizole (phenylbenzimidazole sulfonic acid)	290–340
Physical Sunscreens	
Titanium dioxide	290–700
Zinc oxide	290–700

UVR, ultraviolet radiation.

Clinical Application of Photosensitivity

SKIN TYPES

CASE 42-1

QUESTION 1: R.J., a 26-year-old woman, and her husband J.J., 28 years old, are spending a week in August vacationing on the Outer Banks of North Carolina with their two children, P.J., a 6-month-old girl, and L.J., an 18-month-old boy. They have plans for time at the beach, bicycling, and sailing. They come to your pharmacy to inquire about sunscreens for the trip. R.J. has a light brown complexion with brown hair and brown eyes, and J.J. has fair complexion with blonde hair and blue eyes. On first exposure to the sun with about an hour of intense midday sunlight, J.J. almost always develops a deep red, painful sunburn, with only minimal subsequent tanning. He freckles easily when exposed to sunlight and remembers being severely sunburned on several occasions as a child. When R.J. is first exposed to the sun in the summer, she usually develops mild erythema, followed by moderate tanning. She cannot recall being severely sunburned as a child, but does recall becoming moderately tanned each summer as a child and adolescent. R.J. is employed as a receptionist for an accounting firm, and J.J. is a lawyer for a local law firm. Both spend considerable amounts of time participating in outdoor activities. Using subjective and objective data in this history, determine the skin types of R.J. and J.J. to guide you to a recommendation of a sunscreen product.

One of the most important pieces of information to include in the patient history is the patient's skin type.[41] Patients can be classified into six sun-reactive skin types based on their response to initial sun exposure, skin color, tendency to sunburn, ability to tan, and personal history of sunburn (Table 42-3). This skin typing system is used by the US Food and Drug Administration (FDA) in its guidelines for sunscreen agents. J.J.'s fair complexion, propensity to sunburn, and minimal tanning classify him as skin type II. R.J.'s light brown complexion, minimal sunburn reaction, and moderate tanning classify her as skin type IV.

Hair and eye colors also provide an indication to skin reactiveness to sunlight. People who have blonde, red, or light brown hair or blue or green eyes tend to have greater skin reactivity to sunlight than people with dark-colored hair or eyes. A history of severe sunburn also can be associated with skin reactivity to sunlight, although self-reported patient histories of sunburn or tanning may not be consistently reliable and personal interviews may be a better indicator. J.J.'s propensity to freckle and his history of severe sunburns as a child may give an indication as to his skin's sun reactiveness. Other important information to consider in the patient before recommending a certain product is medication history, history of sun-reactive dermatoses, history of allergies (particularly contact hypersensitivities to cosmetics or other topical agents), and the intended activities during sunscreen use.

RISK FACTORS

CASE 42-1, QUESTION 2: R.J. and J.J. exhibit several risk factors that place them at risk for the long-term adverse effects of UVR. What are the risk factors for these long-term adverse effects of UVR?

The long-term effects of UVR include photocarcinogenesis and premature aging of the skin (photoaging). The associated risks for the development of these long-term effects are directly related to the congenital pigmentation of an individual (which includes skin type and hair and eye color) and intensity, duration, and frequency of exposure to UVR. With skin type II, J.J. is at high risk for carcinogenesis and photoaging, whereas R.J., with skin type IV, may be at a lower risk. Excessive sun exposure, especially during early childhood, increases the risk of nonmelanoma and melanoma skin cancers. During the first 18 years of life, the average child receives 3 times the dose of UVB of the average adult; consequently, most sun exposure occurs during childhood.[23,42,43] A history of frequent sunburn or intermittent high-intensity exposures to UVR may be associated with the occurrence of malignant melanoma, whereas large cumulative doses of UVR during a lifetime may contribute to the incidence of nonmelanoma skin cancers. J.J.'s history of several severe sunburns as a child may more than double his risk of CMM.[42,43] Cumulative doses of UVR received unintentionally from working outdoors or from participating in outdoor recreational activities also can contribute significantly to the risk of photocarcinogenesis and photoaging.[7] A large number of moles, congenital moles more than 1.5 cm wide, and abnormal moles also appear to be a risk factor for malignant melanoma.[20] Risk for skin cancer is increased among first-degree relatives of patients with skin cancer[44] because frequent sunburns, suboptimal sunscreen use, and high rates of tanning bed use are common among children with a personal or family history of skin cancer.[45]

Photoprotection

Sun Protection Factor

CASE 42-1, QUESTION 3: Before deciding on the exact product for R.J., J.J., and their children, R.J. and J.J. want to know how to differentiate among products and how to interpret the SPF of a product. How will you explain this to them?

The effectiveness of a sunscreen formulation is based on its SPF and its substantivity.[46] SPF is a measure of how much solar energy (UV radiation) is required to produce sunburn on protected skin (i.e., in the presence of sunscreen) relative to the amount of solar energy required to produce sunburn on unprotected skin. Because the SPF value increases, sunburn protection increases. It is defined as the ratio of the minimal dose of UVR required to produce an erythemal response in sunscreen-protected skin compared with unprotected skin.[30] The SPF is based on tests of volunteers with skin types I through III, using either natural sunlight or a solar simulator that generates both UVB and UVA.[30,46] Because the SPF can be influenced by the composition, chemical properties, emollient properties, and pH of the vehicle, sunscreen formulations must be evaluated on an individual basis.[46] The concept of a SPF is commonly misunderstood and is also influenced by a variety of factors including the amount applied to the skin, the time of initial application before UVR exposure, the frequency of application, and environmental factors, such as photodegradation during UVR exposure; therefore, the SPF achieved during actual use can be significantly less than indicated on the label.[47–51] Consumers have been shown to routinely apply only one-fourth to one-half thickness of the layer of sunscreen used to determine the SPF before marketing.[52–55]

A popular misconception is that SPF relates to time of solar exposure. For example, many people believe that if they normally get sunburn in 1 hour, then an SPF 15 sunscreen allows them to stay in the sun for 15 hours (i.e., 15 times longer) without getting

Table 42-3
Suggested SPF for Various Skin Types

Complexion	Skin Type	Skin Characteristics	Suggested Product SPF
Very fair	I	Always burns easily; never tans	20–30
Fair	II	Always burns easily; tans minimally	15–20
Light	III	Burns moderately; tans gradually	10–15
Medium	IV	Burns minimally; always tans well	8–10
Dark	V	Rarely burns; tans profusely	8
Very dark	VI	Never burns; deeply pigmented	8

SPF, sun protection factor.

sunburn. This is untrue because SPF is not directly related to time of solar exposure, but to the amount of solar exposure. Although solar energy amount is related to solar exposure time, other factors have an impact on the amount of solar energy. For example, the intensity of the solar energy has an impact on the amount. Generally, it takes less time to be exposed to the same amount of solar energy at midday compared with early morning or late evening because the sun is more intense at midday relative to other times. The following exposures may result in the same amount of solar energy: one hour at 9 AM versus 15 minutes at 1 PM. Solar intensity is also related to geographic location, with greater solar intensity occurring at lower latitudes. Also, because clouds absorb solar energy, solar intensity is generally greater on clear days than on cloudy days.

In 1978, the FDA Over-the-Counter (OTC) Review Panel on sunscreens reclassified sunscreens from cosmetics to drugs intended to protect the structure and function of the human integument against actinic damage. In 1999, the FDA finalized its original regulations for OTC sunscreens (available at: **http://www.fda.gov/downloads/Drugs/DevelopmentApprovalProcess/DevelopmentResources/Over-the-CounterOTCDrugs/StatusofOTCRulemakings/ucm090244.pdf**). The 1999 regulations listed the active ingredients that can be used in sunscreens as well as labeling and testing requirements. They also provide for uniform, streamlined labeling for all OTC products intended for use as sunscreens to assist consumers in making decisions on sun protection.

Additionally, cosmetic regulations required tanning preparations that do not contain a sunscreen ingredient to display the following warning: "Warning—this product does not contain a sunscreen and does not protect against sunburn. Repeated exposure of unprotected skin while tanning may increase the risk of skin aging, skin cancer, and other harmful effects to the skin even if you do not burn."

In 2006, the FDA introduced further regulations on sunscreen labeling. The term *sunscreen* was redefined: "A product with active ingredients to affect the structure or function of the body by absorbing, reflecting, or scattering the harmful, burning rays of the sun, thereby altering the normal physiological response to solar radiation." These ingredients also help to prevent diseases such as sunburn and may reduce the chance of premature skin aging, skin cancer, and other harmful effects attributable to the sun when used in conjunction with limiting sun exposure and wearing protective clothing. Sunscreen ingredients may also be used in some products for nontherapeutic, nonphysiologic uses (e.g., as a color additive or to protect the color of the product).

In 2007, the FDA proposed a new amendment to its original regulations, which sets standards for formulating, testing, and labeling sunscreen products.[56] The final rule, which did not take effect until June of 2012, limited the maximum SPF value on sunscreen labeling to "SPF 50+," as well as establishing that claims of water resistance must tell how much time a user can expect to receive the stated level of SPF protection while sweating or swimming, based on standard testing.[57] Claims of products being "waterproof" or "sweatproof" are no longer allowed, nor can products be identified as "sunblocks." Qualifications for products to be labeled as "broad spectrum" were standardized and must provide protection against both UVA and UVB radiation. Additional warnings about skin cancer and skin aging were added to products that were not broad spectrum or have low SPF ratings <15. The SPF maximum of 50+ resulted due to the lack of data that SPF levels higher than 50 provide any additional benefit.[57] Despite this new regulation, products listed with SPF >50 are still available for purchase.

In November 2014, the Sunscreen Innovation Act (SIA) was enacted, which provided a new process for the FDA review of the efficacy and safety of nonprescription sunscreen active ingredients.[58] The act amended the Food, Drug, and Cosmetic Act to provide specific timelines and deadlines requiring FDA review of time and extent applications (TEAs) for sunscreen ingredients. This helps to ensure that timely decisions are made on ingredients that had been pending review.[58,59] In response to the SIA in early 2015, the FDA made tentative determinations on eight ingredients that had been pending review, including bemotrizinol, bisoctrizole, drometrizole trisiloxane, octyl triazone, amiloxate, diethylhexylbutamido triazone, ecamsule, and enzacamene. These ingredients were found to have insufficient evidence of safety and effectiveness at the concentrations in question and are in need of more data to determine whether they are generally recognized as safe and effective (GRASE) for use in over-the-counter sunscreen products.[60]

Evaluation of Sunscreens

Substantivity is a measure of the sunscreen formulation's effectiveness. The substantivity of a sunscreen formulation is its ability to be absorbed by, or adhere to, the skin while swimming or perspiring. The substantivity of a product largely depends on the vehicle, as well as the active ingredient.[61] The affinity of a sunscreen to the keratinaceous layer of the stratum corneum is directly related to the keratin or vehicle partition coefficient. The saturation of the active agent in keratin depends on the drug's lipophilicity, whereas its substantivity is independent of its lipophilicity. Sunscreen compounds with a high solubility in the product's vehicle penetrate the skin most easily. Classically, vehicles such as water-in-oil emulsions or ointments tend to have a higher degree of substantivity. Some of the newer products have improved substantivity with the addition of a polymer, such as polyacrylamide, to the formulation.

Molar Absorptivity, Absorption Spectrum, and Photostability

The molar absorptivity and absorption spectrum determine the effectiveness of an individual sunscreen agent, mostly by its chemical structure. *Molar absorptivity* is a measure of the amount of UVR absorbed by a particular sunscreen, and it depends on the concentration of the sunscreen in the product and the amount applied to the skin. Sunscreens with an absorption spectrum in the UVB range, with a maximal absorption between 310 and 320 nm, are the most effective in preventing a sunburn.[46] Sunscreens with absorption spectra in the UVB range are *para*-aminobenzoic acid (PABA) and its esters, cinnamates, and the salicylates. Sunscreens with absorption spectra that extend into the UVA range are the anthranilates (e.g., meradimate), dibenzoylmethanes (e.g., azobenzene), and benzophenones (e.g., oxybenzone). *Photostability* means the ability to stabilize under sunlight. The process of photostability is a key factor in sunscreen protection efficacy. High photostability means the sunscreen will maintain a higher UVA protective barrier longer and not degrade as quickly as other UVA filters when exposed to the sun.

Table 42-2 shows the 17 ingredients that act as sunscreens currently approved in the United States, along with their FDA-allowable maximal concentration and absorption spectrum.

CHEMICAL ORGANIC SUNSCREENS

Chemical organic sunscreens are compounds capable of absorbing UVR, thereby protecting the skin structures from the adverse effects of the selective wavelengths absorbed.[30] After application to the skin, these aromatic compounds convert the high UVR energy into harmless longer-wave radiation, which may or may not be perceived as warmth.[30] Chemical organic sunscreens usually are nonopaque because they do not absorb the wavelengths of visible light.

UVB Filters

Aminobenzoates

Commonly used in the past and the first widely used UV filter, PABA absorbs UVR in the UVB range from 260 to 313 nm, with maximal absorption around 290 nm; its molar absorptivity is considered to be high.[46] PABA readily penetrates and binds to the stratum corneum and, after several days of application, may remain in the skin and provide protection even after swimming, perspiration, and bathing, making it an ideal candidate for water-resistant sunscreens.[46] It is commonly formulated as an alcoholic mixture, which can cause stinging, dryness, or tightness, particularly when applied to the face. Its major disadvantage is the potential to cause contact or photocontact dermatitis, which has been reported to happen in approximately 4% of the population.[62] Responsible for more sensitivity reactions than any other sunscreen,[49] PABA can also cause cross-sensitivity reactions with benzocaine, thiazides, sulfonamides, paraphenylenediamine (a common ingredient in hair dyes), and other PABA derivatives. It can cause discoloration of clothes as well. The use of PABA in commercial sunscreens has decreased to the point where many of the newer sunscreens are promoted as being PABA-free.

The PABA esters include octyldimethyl PABA (Padimate O) and glyceryl PABA. These esters are incorporated easily into formulations, demonstrate good substantivity, and do not discolor clothing. Their absorption spectra are similar to those of PABA (Table 42-2). With a maximal absorption of 311 nm, Padimate O has the lowest likelihood of any PABA ester to cause cross-sensitivity reactions or contact and photocontact dermatitis.[63]

Cinnamates

Octinoxate (octyl methoxycinnamate), which has high molar absorptivity and a maximal absorption of 305 nm, is the most commonly used cinnamate and most potent UVB filter.[64] Cinnamates are related chemically to balsam of Peru, balsam of Tolu, coca leaves, cinnamic acid, cinnamic aldehyde, and cinnamic oil, ingredients that are used in perfumes, topical medications, cosmetics, and flavorings.[65] These agents do not bind well to the stratum corneum, leading to poor substantivity. Cinnamate-based sunscreens tend to be comedogenic because the vehicle may contain other occlusive ingredients that are added to improve the substantivity. Cinnamates are often used in combination with benzophenones, appear to be nonstaining, and rarely cause contact dermatitis.[64]

Salicylates

Salicylates are weak UVB absorbers often found in PABA-free products. Topical salicylates are considered among the safest sunscreens, even though they must be used in high concentrations to meet the SPF requirement.[66] Salicylates have low molar absorptivities, are incorporated easily into formulations, and are used to boost the SPF of combination products, particularly oxybenzone and avobenzone.[67] Octisalate and homosalate are water insoluble, which leads to high substantivity. Sensitization to the salicylates is rare[66]; however, it has been reported with the use of octisalate.[68]

Octocrylene

Octocrylene has a absorption profile similar to the salicylates and cinnamates, with a peak absorption at 307 nm. It has low irritation potential and low substantivity; however, it has become increasingly popular because of its ability to photostabilize avobenzone.[69]

UVA Filters

Benzophenones

Benzophenones, such as oxybenzone and dioxybenzone, are UVB-absorbing sunscreens that have absorption spectra extending into the UVA range.[70] Benzophenones are also found in shampoos, soaps, hair sprays and dyes, paints, varnishes, and lacquers. The maximal absorption for each is about 290 nm, but both are limited because of poor substantivity and sensitization.[70] Photocontact dermatitis with oxybenzone and contact dermatitis with dioxybenzone occur commonly, with the latter usually occurring as a contact urticaria.[71] Systemic absorption has also been noted with oxybenzone, and it can be detected in the urine and bloodstream.[72]

Anthranilates

Anthranilates, such as meradimate (menthyl anthranilate), are weak UVB-absorbing sunscreens with an absorption spectrum extending into the UVA range. As with the salicylates, they have low molar absorptivity, with a maximal absorption of approximately 336 nm.[46] Meradimate has a low risk of sensitization and a desirable absorption spectrum, especially when it is used in combination with other sunscreens to give broad-spectrum protection.

Dibenzoylmethanes

As a prototype of the dibenzoylmethane class, avobenzone (butyl methoxydibenzoylmethane) has high molar absorptivity and absorption spectra exclusively in the UVA range, with maximal absorption at approximately 360 nm.[73] It is commonly formulated with UVB sunscreens to broaden UVR coverage. Avobenzone loses approximately 35% of its absorption capacity about 15 minutes after UVR exposure, because of the photoinstability of the compound, thereby reducing its UVA protection efficacy.[74] One molecule of avobenzone can absorb UVA radiation only once, making it inactive from that time forward as opposed to zinc oxide or titanium dioxide, which can reflect UVA radiation over and over again with minimal decay. All of the avobenzone applied to the skin is virtually rendered inactive after 5 hours of UVA exposure. Avobenzone is also not compatible with octinoxate, the most powerful UVB filter.[75] Photostability of avobenzone can be increased with the use of UV absorbers, as well as non-UV filters. Neutrogena has marketed this technology under the name of Helioplex, which initially stabilized avobenzone using oxybenzone and diethylhexyl 2,6-naphthalate (DEHN), but has now broadened to include additional technologies and ingredients.

Ecamsule

Ecamsule is a camphor derivative that protects against short UVA rays and is photostable and water resistant, and has low systemic absorption.[76] The FDA has only approved ecamsule for use in certain formulations such as the combination of 2% ecamsule / 2% avobenzone / 10% octocrylene cream (Anthelios SX, L'Oreal USA). This OTC product is only available in the United States as a moisturizing cream with an SPF rating of 15, with the FDA determining that more research was needed to evaluate the safety and efficacy of ecamsule in other concentrations.[60] This combination provides continuous protection across most of the UV spectrum (290–400 nm range), with ecamsule providing protection within the short UVA range (320–340 nm), filling the gap between octocrylene and avobenzone capabilities (210–290 nm, and 340–400 nm, respectively). The photostability of the ecamsule and octocrylene–avobenzone combination provides residual protection at 1 and 5 hours (1 hour, 100% UVB protection and 97% UVA protection; 5 hours, 90% UVB protection and 80% UVA protection). Adverse events associated with its use are infrequent and include acne, dermatitis, xerosis, eczema, erythema, pruritus, skin discomfort, and sunburn.

There are two additional formulations of ecamsule. Mexoryl SX is a water-soluble form suitable for daytime sunscreens, including sunscreen-containing moisturizers and facial foundations. Mexoryl XL, an oil-soluble formulation, is suitable for water-resistant sunscreen formulations, including those worn on the beach and during vigorous physical exercise.

INORGANIC SUNSCREENS

Inorganic sunscreens are opaque formulations made of particulate insoluble compounds, incorporated into a vehicle, which scatter and absorb UV rays. Both size of the particles and thickness of the film determine the degree of protection.[77] Currently, there are only two inorganic sunscreens approved by the FDA: titanium dioxide and zinc oxide.[77,78] Other inorganic sunscreens include magnesium oxide, red veterinarian petrolatum, iron oxides, kaolin, ichthammol, and talc. Iron oxides and talc continue to be found in commercially available sunscreen products and cosmetics, whereas kaolin and ichthammol may be found in products such as cleansers, moisturizers, and ointments. These compounds are often used in conjunction with chemical sunscreens to formulate products of higher SPF and as single-ingredient products. When used alone, they are usually placed in an ointment base designed specifically for vulnerable parts of the body, such as the nose, cheeks, lips, ears, and shoulders.[33] Inorganic sunscreens are important in individuals who are unusually sensitive to UVA and visible light, such as those with vitiligo, a skin condition with amelanotic lesions (white patches) surrounded by areas of normally pigmented skin. Appropriately colored formulations can be used to camouflage and protect these vulnerable amelanotic lesions.[33] Inorganic sunscreen agents are preferred for persons who need absolute UVR and visible light protection (e.g., young children, persons with skin types I through IV who receive constant exposure, and persons with drug photosensitivity reactions, xeroderma pigmentosa, lupus erythematosus, and other photosensitive skin reactions).[33]

Despite some advantages, inorganic sunscreens are not widely accepted because they are visible to others, messy, and occlusive when applied to the skin. They have a higher substantivity, but may melt in the heat of the sun, limiting their protection to a few hours. Physical sunscreen products tend to be so occlusive that they may cause or worsen acne or obstruct sweat glands.[33] Substantial effort has been made to improve the shortcomings of these products by reducing the particle size to improve the cosmetic appearance. This has created a growing trend toward incorporating nanoparticles of titanium dioxide and zinc oxide, which have been shown to have superior UV protection while maintaining cosmetic elegance. Concern about toxicity of these agents has been raised because of the potential for increased skin penetration and interaction with lower portions of the epidermis; however, this has been disproved in both in vivo and in vitro studies.[79–83] No current regulation in the United States exists regarding the testing and labeling of nanosized titanium or zinc oxides.

Antioxidants

The addition of botanical antioxidants and vitamins C and E to a broad-spectrum sunscreen may further decrease UV-induced damage compared with sunscreen alone due to neutralization of free radicals.[78,84] Antioxidants have received increased attention for use as photoprotective agents, particularly because of the observation that vitamin C levels in the skin can be severely depleted after UVR exposure.[85] Vitamins C and E, either taken orally or applied topically (incorporated into a commercially available sunscreen product), may provide additive protection against both UVA- and UVB-induced photodamage.[85,86] Topically applied antioxidants do not have adequate diffusion into the epidermal layer, however, and are susceptible to chemical instability.[67] If recommended, they should only be used in conjunction with adequate sunscreen. Commercially available products can be found with combinations of antioxidants and broad-spectrum sunscreens, specifically those formulated for facial use.

Given their plans for the week of vacation and amount of UV exposure likely, R.J. and J.J. should consider a broad-spectrum product with high substantivity and a high degree of water resistance to offer the best protection.

CROSS-SENSITIVITY

CASE 42-1, QUESTION 4: According to your assessment of R.J. and J.J., you determine that they have type IV skin and type II skin, respectively. On further inquiry, you learn that R.J. has no medication allergies; however, she has a history of contact dermatitis on her scalp and around her hairline on several occasions after dyeing her hair and using certain shampoos. As a teenager, J.J. suffered from frequent sinus infections and often was treated with trimethoprim–sulfamethoxazole (TMP-SMX) because of an allergy to penicillin. He remembers developing a severe sunburn after minimal exposure to the sun while taking the sulfa-containing antibiotic. He recently has been started on hydrochlorothiazide (HCTZ), 12.5 mg PO daily, for hypertension. What considerations are important in recommending sunscreens for R.J. and J.J.?

The first consideration for recommending an appropriate sunscreen to R.J. and J.J. is their skin type. R.J. has skin type IV, suggesting that a sunscreen with an SPF of at least 15 would provide adequate protection for her (Table 42-3). J.J. has skin type II, suggesting that a sunscreen with an SPF of 30 to 50 would be required to provide adequate protection for him. Furthermore, the history of contact dermatitis and photosensitivity reaction exhibited by R.J. and J.J., respectively, is important when recommending use of a sunscreen.[87] The contact dermatitis that R.J. experienced from hair dyes and shampoos may have been caused by paraphenylenediamine, an ingredient of hair dyes,[88] or a benzophenone, which sometimes is included in products such as hair dyes and shampoos.[70]

Because cross-reactivity between paraphenylenediamine and PABA or its derivatives is possible, a sunscreen for R.J. that does not contain PABA or a benzophenone should be recommended. Cinnamates and anthralates rarely cause contact dermatoses, which would be ideal for R.J.

Because both contain sulfa moieties, the photosensitivity reaction that J.J. experienced while taking TMP-SMX may indicate that he might be susceptible to a cross-sensitivity reaction with PABA or its derivatives. This reaction to TMP-SMX also indicates that J.J. may be susceptible to a photosensitivity reaction with HCTZ. If a photosensitivity reaction is likely, it is advisable to recommend an SPF of 30 or more. Because drug-induced photosensitivity reactions are caused by UVA, a PABA-free, broad-spectrum sunscreen that absorbs UVA as well as UVB would be necessary to provide J.J. with adequate protection. Broad-spectrum chemical sunscreens commonly contain a benzophenone and a cinnamate. A broad-spectrum sunscreen containing both of these chemical classes would be an acceptable broad-spectrum product. Alternatively, because Padimate O is the least likely of the PABA ester derivatives to cause photocontact dermatitis,[63] a broad-spectrum combination product that contains Padimate O could be recommended for J.J. If the photosensitivity reaction is caused by visible light, it would also be necessary to recommend an inorganic physical sunscreen to block all sunlight or complete avoidance of the sun.[50] With all of these issues considered, it may be preferable to recommend an alternative antihypertensive medication for J.J. that would not place him at risk for a photosensitivity reaction.

PHOTOPROTECTION FOR CHILDREN

CASE 42-1, QUESTION 5: What photoprotective measures should be provided for P.J. and L.J.?

Sun protection during childhood is very important, considering that most of a person's lifetime of sun exposure occurs in childhood and that the harmful effects of UVR are cumulative.[38] However, infants and toddlers are at increased risk of over exposure to topical sunscreen products because of an increased body-surface-area to body-weight ratio compared to adults and a lower ability to metabolize absorbed drug.[89,90] It is therefore recommended that sunscreen should not be used for children younger than 6 months of age.[91] P.J. needs to be kept out of direct sunlight and, when outside, must be protected with proper clothing and shading.[91–95]

L.J. should be protected with a PABA-free, inorganic UV filter sunscreen such as zinc oxide with an SPF of at least 15. Inorganic UV filters are preferred for children between 6 months and 2 years due to lack of systemic absorption.[89,90] Regular use of a sunscreen with an SPF of at least 15 for the first 18 years of life can reduce the lifetime incidence of nonmelanoma skin cancers by about three-fourths.[95] If L.J. is in the sun during 6 hours of maximal exposure (i.e., 10 AM–4 PM), or otherwise for an extended period, he should wear protective clothing, covering as much of his body as possible.[94] Tightly woven clothing, long sleeves, and pants protect the skin from almost all UVR, whereas loosely woven clothing or wet T-shirts can allow up to 30% of UVR to pass through to the skin. Although not complete, water is thought to reduce UVR scattering, thus decreasing its transmission. An average-weight cotton T-shirt provides only an SPF of 7 or 8.[94]

The transmission of UVR through a fabric is measured using a spectrophotometer or spectroradiometer. The ultraviolet protection factor (UPF), rather than SPF, has been recommended as a measure of the sun-protective properties of fabrics.[96,97] It is calculated using a formula based on UV transmission through the fabric and the erythema responsible for human skin. For example, if a fabric has a UPF of 20, then only one-twentieth of the UVR at the surface of the fabric actually passes through it. Certain synthetic fabrics have UPF values that exceed 500, making them vastly superior to sunscreens.[94] Table 42-4 compares the UPF with the amount of effective UVR transmitted and absorbed.

No woven fabric provides complete coverage because the holes between the threads permit UVR transmission. A baseball cap shields little more than the upper central forehead. Broad-brimmed hats can protect the ears, neck, nose, and cheeks, but may provide inadequate protection against SCC of the head or neck.[98] The use of an ultraviolet-absorbing ingredient for fabric softeners (e.g., bisoctrizole, Tinosorb M, BASF) is promoted to reduce transmission of excessive UVA and UVB radiation through fabrics to the skin, through absorption of UV radiation without impairing whiteness. This chemical absorption process has a high affinity for cotton fibers at various washing temperatures. Available as a laundry additive (e.g., Sun Guard, Phoenix Brands), it works by binding to laundered fibers, and through accumulation, it increases the UV protection up to UPF 30 through up to 20 wash and rinse cycles.[99,100]

Product Selection

Two types of sunscreens are appropriate for use in children. A lotion is preferred for total body application versus an alcoholic lotion or gel because alcoholic preparations can cause stinging, burning, and irritation of the skin and eyes. Physical sunscreens (e.g., zinc oxide) are available in bright colors and are recommended for selected body areas, such as the nose, cheeks, and shoulders. PABA and its derivatives are considered potentially harmful to a child's tender skin. For adolescents with acne vulgaris, the use of an oil-free, noncomedogenic sunscreen formulation (e.g., Neutrogena Clear Face Break-Out Free Liquid-Lotion Sunscreen) and a lip balm that contains a sunscreen of at least SPF 15 (e.g., Blistex or ChapStick Sunblock [SPF 30]) would be appropriate.

Application

CASE 42-1, QUESTION 6: What instructions should you provide R.J. and J.J. on how to apply the sunscreen that you have chosen for each of their family members?

Because R.J. and J.J. are planning to be active on the beach, sunscreens that are water resistant are recommended. Before complete application of the sunscreen to the body, because of the risk of cross-sensitivity reactions, patients can perform a patch test by applying a small quantity of the sunscreen to the inner aspect of the forearm and covering with a small bandage overnight.

Most persons apply 20% to 60% of the required amount of sunscreen needed to achieve the SPF of their product.[48,51–54] Because of this, a method has been developed to determine an approximate volume of sunscreen product needed for adequate protection.[101] This rule states that you should use more than half a teaspoon on each of your head and neck area and arms, and more than a teaspoonful on each of your anterior and posterior torso and your legs. This application size was determined based on the dose used in FDA sunscreen testing (2 mg/m^2). Studies of sunscreen application techniques have demonstrated inadequate application at all body sites.[52–54,102] The worst protected areas were the ears and top of the feet, and the back was poorly protected if sunscreen was self-applied. Patients should be reminded to apply sunscreen on those often forgotten areas, such as the hands, cheeks, neck, ears, and dorsum of the feet. It is best to reapply the sunscreen every 1 to 2 hours or after sweating, swimming, or toweling off. There is evidence that early reapplication within 20 to 30 minutes be able to partly compensate for initial underapplication.[47,103–105]

CASE 42-1, QUESTION 7: How long might J.J. expect to be protected with the sunscreen properly applied?

If J.J. (skin type II) normally burns after 30 minutes of exposure to the sun, a sunscreen with an SPF of 15 to 30 may provide up to 7.5 hours (0.5 hours × 15 [SPF 15]) of photoprotection from UVB. However, a high SPF product may provide only partial protection against UVA, with little or no protection from infrared radiation.[46] Because of this, sun exposure should be limited to 90 to 120 minutes for each outing after appropriate sunscreen application. Further, environmental factors, such as elevated atmospheric humidity, and inadequate application techniques, may reduce photoprotection by as much as half.

Table 42-4
Relative Ultraviolet Protection Factor (UPF) by Ultraviolet Ray (UVR) Transmission and Absorption

UVR Transmitted (%)	UVR Absorbed (%)	UPF	Protection Category
10	90.0	10	Moderate protection
5	95.0	20	High protection
3.3	96.7	30	Very high protection
2.5	97.5	40	Extremely high protection
<2.0	>98.0	50	Maximal protection

Sunscreen formulations with SPF as high as 50 can be made using combinations of chemical and physical sunscreen agents.[6] Individuals who are extremely sensitive to the sun may benefit from formulations with higher SPF, but the average fair-skinned person gains adequate protection for sunbathing or for average daily exposure from a product with an SPF of 30.[48]

CASE 42-1, QUESTION 8: Would J.J. gain additional benefit from a product with an SPF greater than 50?

Protection from sunburn increases with higher SPF; however, it is important to remind J.J. that this protection does not correlate to the extent of skin damage from UVA rays. One study reported less sunburn in patients who applied SPF 85 compared with those who applied SPF 50 and spent a similar amount of time in direct sunlight.[106] In the FDA amendment that went into effect in 2012, SPF ratings were limited to a maximum of 50+ due to lack of evidence for greater efficacy at higher SPF ratings.[57] J.J. should also be reminded that the SPF is only accurate if he correctly applies the sunscreen in the adequate amount.

PROTECTIVE EYEWEAR

CASE 42-1, QUESTION 9: Recommend appropriate protective eyewear for R.J. and J.J.'s family while they are on vacation.

R.J. and J.J. should wear sunglasses when outdoors to decrease their lifelong exposure to solar radiation and while at the beach to prevent high exposure of UVR and possible photokeratitis or conjunctivitis. Many manufacturers of sunglasses label their products according to three categories: cosmetic, general purpose, and special purpose. Cosmetic sunglasses block at least 70% of UVB, at least 20% of UVA, and less than 60% of visible light and are appropriate for casual wear when high exposure to UVR is unlikely. General-purpose sunglasses block at least 95% of UVB, at least 60% of UVA, and 60% to 92% of visible light and are appropriate for most activities in sunny environments.[107] Special-purpose sunglasses block at least 99% of UVB, at least 60% of UVA, and at least 97% of visible light and are appropriate for very bright environments, such as ski slopes or tropical beaches.[107] Special- or general-purpose sunglasses are appropriate recommendations for R.J., J.J, and their children to wear while on vacation.

Tanning Booths

CASE 42-2

QUESTION 1: B.P., a 32-year-old woman, is preparing for a business trip to Cancun. She is seeking advice about the use of a tanning bed to stimulate melanin for the prevention of sunburn while on her trip. B.P. has skin type III and light brown hair and green eyes. She recently heard, however, that a tan produced by artificial sunlight may not protect against sunburn and may even cause skin cancer. What advice will you offer her?

Most tanning beds, booths, or salons use an artificial light source that emits about 95% UVA with minimal (i.e., 1%–5%) UVB.[108,109] It was originally thought that UVA is much less likely to produce photoaging and photocarcinogenic changes of the skin than UVB; however, UVA has now been found to cause many of the same effects on the skin as UVB, including immunologic, degenerative, and neoplastic changes, as well as damage to DNA and the formation of reactive oxygen species.[110] UVA also contributes to cataract formation and the activation of herpetic lesions.[25] The high doses of UVA received during a tanning session, as well as increasing cumulative UVA doses over time, raise great concern about the long-term effects of UVA.[111] In addition, UVA may augment the photocarcinogenic effect of UVB,[74] and extensive evidence indicates a relationship between indoor tanning and melanoma.[112] Tanning bed use dramatically increased from less than 1% of Americans in 1988 to 27% of Americans in 2007.[113] However, results from the National Health Interview Survey noted a decrease in adults who frequented tanning salons from 5.5% in 2010 to just over 4.2% in 2013. The decrease is hypothesized to be due to increased awareness regarding the harms of tanning. Concern still exists about the number of Americans choosing to tan, especially within the adolescent population.[114] Participants of the 2013 Youth Risk Behavior Survey conducted by the CDC reported that about 13% of high school students, including 20% of high school girls, had used an indoor tanning device one or more times during the last year.[115] This issue is compounded by evidence that suggests that excessive UV exposure, particularly tanning beds, may have a behavioral component similar to other substance-related disorders, which may be related to an endogenous release of opioids secondary to exposure to UV light.[116] As many as 10% to 53% of young adults meet the criteria for having an addictive component to indoor tanning behavior.[117–121] In an attempt to combat the epidemic of use in young people, the FDA reclassified ultraviolet lamps to be class II medical devices in 2014 and include a black box warning indicating that they should not be used by minors 18 years old or younger.[122] Although this act placed more regulation on tanning booths, concern has been raised that regulating tanning equipment as medical devices implies that they offer a therapeutic benefit, and is not commensurate with other products that are known carcinogens with very little to no offered benefit.[123]

With a skin type III, B.P. may be able gradually to achieve a moderate tan with minimal burning, thus providing some protection from UVR because of increased melanization of the skin. This UVA-induced tan, however, may not be as protective as a tan achieved under normal sunlight conditions because UVA does not thicken the stratum corneum.[118] An artificially produced tan plus subsequent sun exposure has not been found to provide any net reduction in long-term damage to the skin when compared with the same amount of tan obtained by sunbathing alone.[118] For these reasons, B.P. should not use the tanning booth to obtain a protective tan, and she should use appropriate photoprotective measures during her trip.

CASE 42-2, QUESTION 2: What precautions would you recommend if she decides to visit a tanning salon?

If B.P. decides to artificially tan despite your recommendation, she should undertake some precautions. The FDA has recommended exposure schedules for first-time users based on skin type, which determines a person's minimal erythemal dose (MED) of UV radiation. The MED is determined by the amount of UV exposure necessary to produce any visible reddening of the skin 24 hours after exposure. This policy suggests that exposure be limited to no more than 0.75 MED 3 times the first week, followed by a gradual increase to maintenance doses of a maximum of 4.0 MED delivered weekly or biweekly.[124] It is important to remember that MED is specific to an individual, and therefore will be different depending on his or her skin type. Correlating the FDA's policy into time limits for an individual is therefore dependent on skin type as well as the amount of UV exposure provided by the tanning apparatus the individual will use. To minimize cataract development, B.P. should always wear protective eye wear that absorbs all UVA, UVB, and visible light up to 500 nm; simply closing her eyes or wearing regular sunglasses provides no protective effect against eye damage.

CASE 42-2, QUESTION 3: B.P. decides to accept your recommendations to avoid tanning beds; however, she would still like to have a tan before going to Cancun. Will the use of sunless tanning agents confer any photoprotection for B.P. against sunburn?

Sunless tanner is a commercial term that denotes a product that provides a tanned appearance without exposure to the sun or other sources of UVR. One commonly used ingredient in these products is dihydroxyacetone (DHA), a color additive that darkens the skin to orange brown by reacting with amino acids in the stratum corneum. The term *bronzer* is used to describe a variety of products intended to achieve a temporary tanned appearance. For example, among the products marketed as bronzers are tinted moisturizers and brush-on powders. These produce a temporary effect, similar to other types of makeup, and wash off over time. Some products are marketed with other ingredients in addition to DHA to provide a tanned appearance. Generally, neither sunless tanners nor bronzers provide any protective activity to UV exposure by themselves, unless specifically listed with a SPF rating[125] As previously described, the FDA now requires that all suntanning preparations that do not contain sunscreen ingredients are required to carry a warning statement on the label that they do not protect against sunburn.

Tanning pills are promoted for tinting the skin by ingesting massive doses of color additives, usually canthaxanthin. At large doses, canthaxanthin is deposited in various organs, including skin, imparting an orange-bronze color. This color varies from individual to individual. This colorization is not the result of an increase in the skin's supply of melanin. Although canthaxanthin is approved by the FDA for use as a color additive in foods, in which it is used in small amounts, its use in these so-called tanning pills is not approved. Reported adverse events include drug-induced retinopathy, nausea, gastrointestinal cramping, diarrhea, pruritus, and urticaria. None of the above noted unapproved agents should be recommended for use.

Treatment of Sunburn

CASE 42-3

QUESTION 1: G.B., a 31-year-old man with skin type IV, returned a few hours ago from an afternoon of activity in the sun. His shoulders, back, neck, and arms are bright red and are beginning to feel hot, stretched, and painful. G.B. has been otherwise healthy, has no significant medical history, and has no known allergies to medications. What treatment recommendations would you give G.B. for his sunburn?

Sunburn is a self-limiting condition, and treatment is usually symptomatic.[126] Suggested treatments that G.B. can try for his first-degree burn are oral (e.g., ibuprofen, aspirin) or topical (e.g., camphor, menthol) analgesics, topical anti-inflammatory agents (e.g., hydrocortisone cream or aloe vera gel), cooling compresses (tap water, saline, or aluminum acetate solution [Burow solution]) applied to the skin, or cool protectant baths (e.g., colloidal oatmeal). Nonsteroidal anti-inflammatory drugs (NSAIDs), such as aspirin or ibuprofen, may be preferred over acetaminophen because of blockade of the inflammatory prostaglandin-mediated sunburn process; however, although offering symptomatic relief, corticosteroids, NSAIDs, antioxidants, antihistamines, or emollients offer only mild improvement at decreasing the time to recovery.[126]

Topical anesthetics, such as benzocaine or lidocaine, provide only transient analgesia for up to 15 to 45 minutes. These topical agents should not be used in large quantities or applied more than 3 or 4 times a day. In addition, they should not be used on raw, blistered, or abraded skin. Benzocaine has minimal systemic toxicities, but is commonly associated with contact sensitization.[127] In contrast, lidocaine is associated with a low incidence of contact sensitization.[128] Topical corticosteroids have been shown to provide minimal clinical benefit when applied after UV exposure.[129] If G.B. wants to try a topical agent, application or administration is recommended when the pain is particularly bothersome, such as at bedtime. Oral antihistamines may help control pruritus associated with sunburn, as well as aid with sleep, if taken at bedtime; however, no definitive studies have shown benefit in reducing symptoms or benefit of one agent over another.

Treatment beyond self-management is generally unnecessary unless the sunburn is extensive with constitutional symptoms (i.e., fever, chills, nausea, vomiting), involves second- or third-degree burns (particularly if on the eyes or genitalia), or becomes infected. In such cases, referral of the patient to his or her healthcare provider is indicated as a short course (i.e., up to 3 days) of an oral corticosteroid may need to be given (e.g., 1 mg/kg of prednisone or equivalent, given once daily).

Clinical Application of Phototoxicity or Photoallergy

Phototoxic photosensitivity reactions are dose dependent and occur in almost any person who takes or applies an adequate amount of the offending agent. The dose necessary to produce such a reaction varies from person to person and depends on such factors as complexion, hair and eye color, usual ability to tan, and type and amount of UVR exposure. Phototoxic photosensitivity reactions are not immunologically mediated or true allergic reactions; they can occur on first exposure to the agent and generally show no cross-sensitivity to chemically related agents.

A phototoxic reaction usually has a rapid onset, often within several hours after UVR exposure, and presents as an exaggerated or intensified sunburn with erythema, pain, and prickling or burning. Blistering, desquamation, and hyperpigmentation can occur in severe cases.[27,28] Symptoms generally peak 24 to 48 hours after the initial exposure and are usually limited to the areas of UVR-exposed skin. Because phototoxicity reactions do not involve the immune system, prior exposure to the photosensitizer is unnecessary for this reaction to occur. Common drug classes known to be phototoxic include fluoroquinolone, tetracycline, and sulfonamide antibiotics, diuretics, sulfonylureas, nonsteroidal anti-inflammatory agents.

Clinically, photoallergy differs from phototoxicity in that it produces an intensely pruritic, eczematous form of dermatitis.[28] The rash is preceded by pruritus and may subside within an hour. In 5% to 10% of cases, persistent hypersensitivity to light occurs, even after the offending chemical has been eliminated.[27] Photoallergic reactions are not dose-related, and eruptions can also be caused by chemically related agents via cross-sensitivity or cross-allergenicity. As a type of delayed hypersensitivity reaction, time is required to develop an immune response, and the onset of a photoallergic reaction is often delayed for 1 to 3 days. These reactions can present as macular, bullous, or purpuric lesions. Acute urticaria can occur within minutes after UVR exposure. Recovery is slower than from a phototoxic reaction, and it can persist after the offending product has been removed. These reactions may present with erythema and possible edema secondary to the inflammation, but are most commonly found to be eczematous, characterized by erythema; pruritus (possible severe); and papules, vesicles, or both, with weeping, oozing, and crusting. Scaling, lichenification, and pigmentation may occur later.

CASE 42-4

QUESTION 1: D.L., a 16-year-old, blond-haired, blue-eyed teenager with skin type II, presents with a severe sunburn. He states that he started a new summer job 2 days ago with typical sun exposure. He is surprised at the severity of this sunburn, which is worse than normal for the same amount of sun exposure. What further information do you need to know before making treatment recommendations?

Because D.L. is reporting symptoms that differ from previous sun exposures, further questions should be asked regarding the history of the current scenario. Information that may be important in the history of the condition include the temporal relationship between sun exposure and onset of symptoms; the nature and duration of symptoms; recent ingestion or topical application of medications; possible exposure to photosensitizers, chemical irritants, or plants that can cause allergic contact dermatitis (e.g., poison ivy); and the potential for arthropod bites. Information that may be important from the physical examination includes the distribution and morphology of the reaction, as well as areas of the body spared of the reaction.

A drug-induced photosensitivity reaction most commonly appears as a sunburn of greater severity than would normally be expected or as a rash in areas exposed to the sun or tanning apparatus. These reactions can be secondary to oral medications; however, it is important to remember that chemicals with photosensitization potential are found in cosmetics, shampoos, moisturizing lotions, hair dyes or tints, soaps, and other topically applied medications and agents.

Drug-induced photosensitivity reactions can be subdivided into phototoxic and photoallergic reactions. The same medication or agent may produce both phototoxic and photoallergic reactions, and it may at times be difficult to differentiate clinically between the two types of reactions.

CASE 42-4, QUESTION 2: On further questioning, you discover that D.L. first experienced painful erythema of the extensor surface of his hands and forearms, the anterior aspect of his neck, and parts of his face within hours of starting his new job at an outdoor garden and greenhouse. Besides painful erythema, the symptoms also included an immediate prickling and burning sensation. The symptoms continued to worsen until the following morning, about 24 hours after initial exposure to the sun. D.L. does not recall orally ingesting or topically applying any medication or other preparation to his skin, nor does he recall exposure to any chemical irritants, or poison ivy or oak. The morphology of the skin lesions is that of an exaggerated sunburn. The skin lesions are patchy in distribution with greater density on his forearms and hands than on his neck and face. The posterior aspect of his neck and covered areas of his body was spared completely. What are some possible causes of his exaggerated sunburn reaction?

The most likely explanation for D.L.'s exaggerated sunburn reaction is *phototoxicity,* secondary to contact with psoralen-like chemicals from the plants at his job at the outdoor garden and greenhouse. Photoallergy is another possible cause of D.L.'s symptoms. Although much less common than phototoxicity, photoallergy requires prior or prolonged exposure to the photosensitizing compound.

Presumably, D.L. came into contact with psoralen-containing plants and simultaneous exposure to sunlight. With an unusual distribution of lesions on his hands, forearms, neck, and face and the lack of lesions on areas not contacted by the plants or sunlight, the temporal relationship between the exposure and onset of symptoms places phototoxicity higher in the differential diagnosis. D.L. is unlikely to have a photoallergic reaction because of the lack of a delayed temporal relationship between the onset of symptoms and combined exposure to a psoralen-containing plant and sunlight. Unlike phototoxicity reactions, photoallergic reactions can spread to areas that have not been exposed to sunlight; however, D.L.'s lesions were limited to areas of skin exposed to sunlight.

CASE 42-4, QUESTION 3: What nonprescription remedies might you recommend for D.L. at this time?

General recommendations for the management of phototoxicity and photoallergy reactions are focused on the removal of exposure to the potential photosensitizer and reduced exposure to the sun. Patients should be counseled not to take any medications, orally or topically, without first consulting with their healthcare provider to minimize exposure to other photosensitizers. D.L. should try wearing long-sleeved shirts, pants, and gloves when working to limit exposure to plant photosensitizers. He also may try applying a broad-spectrum sunscreen to protect his skin from UVB and UVA radiation. If these measures do not prevent further photosensitivity reactions, D.L. should consider a different type of employment. His presenting symptoms should be managed in a manner similar to that for an exaggerated sunburn.

PHOTOAGING

Incidence, Prevalence, and Epidemiology

Photoaging, or premature aging of the skin, involves skin changes that differ from those associated with normal chronologic aging.[130,131] Aside from advancing age, risk factors that have been associated with photoaging include fair skin, male gender, high sun exposure, and smoking.[115,132] Because recognizing photoaging and photodamage may prevent the progression or development of skin cancer, it is important that they are recognized as real medical problems, not just cosmetic or aesthetic concerns.

Etiology

Normal aging of the skin involves fine wrinkling of the skin, atrophy of the dermis, and a decrease in the amount of subcutaneous adipose tissue, all of which lead to a state of hypocellularity of the skin.[131] Photoaging involves a chronic inflammatory state induced by long-term exposure to UVA radiation from reactive oxygen species (ROS), leading to a hypermetabolic state of the skin.[133] Photodamaged skin is characterized histologically by an accumulation of excessive quantities of thickened, degenerated elastic connective tissue fibers (elastosis).[131] Type I collagen predominates in normal skin, but in photodamaged skin, type III collagen increases about fourfold, and the mature matrix of type I collagen slightly decreases.[110] These degenerative changes in connective tissue may be caused by hyperactive fibroblasts or by enzymatic degradation via cellular infiltrates in inflamed skin.[6] The elastic connective tissue then replaces the collagen in the upper parts of the dermis.[133] The ground substance, composed of proteoglycans and glycosaminoglycans, also is increased considerably in photoaged skin.[6] Capillaries in the dermis become dilated and tortuous, resulting in telangiectasias, ecchymosis, and purpura.[131] The epidermis thickens, and epidermal cells become hyperplastic and possibly neoplastic. Large cumulative doses of UVA, UVB, and possibly infrared radiation during the course of a lifetime are strongly implicated as the cause of these changes in photoaged skin.[6]

Photodamaged skin is characterized as being wrinkled, yellowed, and sagging. Mildly affected skin becomes irregularly pigmented, rough, and dry, with mild wrinkles. Moderately affected skin becomes deeply wrinkled, sagging, thickened, and leathery, with vascular lesions.[131] Largely irreversible, severely affected skin can become deeply furrowed and permanently (and irregularly) pigmented, and may manifest premalignant and malignant lesions.[131] Areas of the body most commonly affected are the face, back of the neck, back of the arms and hands, the V-line of the neck of women, and balding areas of the head of men.

Clinical Application of Photoaging

CASE 42-5

QUESTION 1: P.B. is a 38-year-old woman who has enjoyed many outdoor activities over the years. She lives in a moderate climate, with hot, sunny summers and cold winters. She feels that she appears older than other women her age because of wrinkling and color changes of her skin. Her facial color is somewhat yellowish in appearance, and the fine wrinkles at the corners of her eyes and mouth have become more obvious. She has noticed the formation of small brown spots mottling parts of her face, hands, and forearms. P.B. has skin type III, a clear complexion, and skin that is sensitive to soaps, heavy cosmetics, and perfumes. What nonprescription recommendations can you provide P.B. for treatment of her photoaged skin?

Many nonprescription agents known as cosmeceuticals, products marketed as cosmetic products that contain biologically active ingredients, are targeted at reducing visible signs of aged skin. These products include α-hydroxy acids, retinol, ascorbic acid, hyaluronic acid, and lipoic acid. One particular product class widely used is α-hydroxy acids and polyhydroxy acids. In normal concentrations (5%–17%), they are included in many products to lessen the appearance of damage; however, in high concentrations, they are used as facial skin peels because of their keratolytic properties. They have been shown in studies to reduce skin roughness and sallowness; however, minimal impact was seen on wrinkles.[131,134] Topical ascorbic acid and lipoic acid have also been shown to improve skin texture and wrinkles,[135–137] whereas a co-enzyme Q_{10} derivative (idebenone) may reduce skin roughness and fine lines while increasing skin hydration.[138] In patients who choose to use these products, it should be strongly recommended that they wear at least SPF 15 to 30 because they allow for greater absorption of UVR. These agents are not regulated by the FDA and therefore do not have substantial evidence supporting their effectiveness and can be very costly. Emphasis should be placed on protection from the sun, using photoprotective strategies previously discussed.

CASE 42-5, QUESTION 2: Are there any prescription products that you would recommend to P.B. to discuss with her physician?

There are several topical retinoids currently available that are derivatives of vitamin A and are effective for the signs of photoaging (see Chapter 41, Psoriasis). Tretinoin (all-trans-retinoic acid) is available as a cream (0.02%, 0.025%, 0.0375%, 0.05%, and 0.1%) or gel (0.01%, 0.025%, 0.04% [in microspheres], 0.08% [in microspheres], 0.1% [in microspheres]) and tazarotene (available as a 0.05 or 0.1% cream, 0.1% foam, and a 0.05% or 0.1% gel) are the only two topical retinoids FDA approved for the treatment of photoaging. These agents are effective in partially reversing some of the clinical and histologic changes of photoaging by lessening fine wrinkles, mottled pigmentation, and the tactile roughness associated with photoaged skin through mechanisms such as inhibition of metalloproteinase expression.[139–142] Additional benefits of retinoid therapy include the formation of new dermal collagen and vessels, reduction in the number and melanization of freckles, resorption of degenerated connective tissue fibers, and treatment of premalignant and malignant skin lesions.[143] In one of the initial trials, all subjects treated (100%) demonstrated global improvement in the signs of photoaging, with 53% showing moderate changes and the remainder having at least slight improvement. Of the clinical parameters assessed, the most impressive improvements were found with facial skin sallowness, with respondents developing a healthy, rosy glow.[140] These agents are more potent than the retinoids found in over-the-counter products such as retinyl esters, retinol, and retinaldehyde and therefore produce more profound results.

CASE 42-5, QUESTION 3: Would P.B. be an appropriate candidate for therapy with a topical retinoid product (e.g., tretinoin)?

Topical retinoid therapy is most effective for patients 50 to 70 years of age with moderate-to-severe photoaging and for prophylactic use in patients undergoing the initial changes of photoaging.[139] Recently, P.B. has noticed some of the skin changes consistent with early photoaging and would be a good candidate for prophylactic therapy with topical tretinoin. Treatment may improve her sallow skin color and lessen the mottling on her face and forearms and fine wrinkles at the corners of her eyes and mouth, as well as prevent worsening of the photoaging process that she is experiencing.

CASE 42-5, QUESTION 4: P.B.'s physician calls you asking for dosing recommendations for tretinoin. What advice do you provide?

Because both the beneficial and adverse effects of topical retinoid therapy are dose dependent, the underlying goal is to provide the maximal benefit by using the highest concentration that causes minimal skin irritation. Considering P.B.'s skin sensitivity to soaps, cosmetics, and perfumes, her skin is likely to be irritated easily by topical therapy; therefore, it would be best to initiate therapy with the lowest strength (e.g., tretinoin 0.025% cream or tazarotene 0.05% cream). These agents are usually applied every night at bedtime, but in some instances, they are applied initially on an every-other-night basis until the skin accommodates to the irritant effects. The likelihood of irritation depends on the type of vehicle more than the concentration of the agent.[143] The cream or the microsphere gel formulations cause the least skin irritation and would be preferred for initiating therapy for P.B. The microsphere gel formulation is preferred for patients with persistent acne or for those with focal actinic lesions. Younger patients often prefer the gel because it leaves no residue and is compatible with most cosmetics. The solution and gel may be better tolerated in older patients with oily, thick, pigmented skin.

CASE 42-5, QUESTION 5: You are now dispensing tretinoin cream 0.025% to P.B. What patient counseling should P.B. be given?

Before applying the cream to her face at bedtime, P.B. should wash her face gently, using her fingertips and mild soap, then pat her skin dry with a towel. If gentle washing with her fingers does not remove the dry, peeling skin, a washcloth can be used gently on the face. The treated stratum corneum is fragile, and erosions could occur if P.B. is not careful when washing. After waiting about 15 minutes, she should apply a pea-sized amount of cream to her forehead and spread the cream evenly over her entire face. Care should be exercised while applying the cream to the areas adjacent to the eyes and mouth because tretinoin can cause irritation and burning of mucous membranes.

Skin irritation can be expected to start in the first 3 to 5 days of therapy and, hopefully, will subside in 1 to 3 months. Irritation can manifest as erythema, peeling, burning, and stinging. If P.B. experiences excessive irritation, she can reinitiate the regimen on a slower timeline by applying the cream on an every-other-night or every-third-night basis for the first 2 weeks to reduce skin irritation, or she can also apply a topical corticosteroid product such as hydrocortisone 1% cream. Once she begins to tolerate the therapy, her frequency of applications and strength of cream should be titrated to cause mild scaling with only occasional mild erythema. A thicker film of cream can be applied to photodamaged areas. After 9 to 12 months of therapy, she can begin maintenance therapy, which consists of application two or three nights a week indefinitely.

Because these agents can dry the skin, P.B. should be counseled to use moisturizers during the day to help decrease the dryness and irritation of the skin. Nighttime application of moisturizers should be discouraged when topical tretinoin is being used because the moisturizers can cause a pH incompatibility with the cream and possibly dilute the concentration of tretinoin. With a thinning of the stratum corneum, P.B.'s skin may be more susceptible to the effects of UVR. For this reason, as well as to prevent further actinic damage, P.B. should begin prophylactic daytime application of a sunscreen. Considering her skin type (III) and early photoaging changes, a sunscreen with an SPF of at least 30 would be appropriate. P.B. should be counseled not to become discouraged by any apparent lack of response; her skin damage is mild, her response to therapy will be gradual, and part of the goal of therapy is to prevent further damage. Her wrinkles may actually appear to worsen early in therapy owing to an initial buildup of the stratum corneum. P.B. should avoid facial saunas and irritating soaps and cosmetics. Retinoids are recognized as being teratogenic, and although risk is more highly associated with oral forms more commonly used for acne, use should generally be avoided in any patients who are pregnant or planning to become pregnant.[144]

BURN INJURIES

Incidence, Prevalence, and Epidemiology

Approximately 486,000 Americans are treated for burns annually.[145] Although admission for and mortality from burn injuries continues to decline, the total number of emergency department visits remains elevated, with over 40,000 individuals requiring hospitalization; burns cause an overall yearly mortality of over 3,200.[146] With the development of multidisciplinary burn centers and a better understanding of the pathophysiology of the burn wound, survival of patients with second- and third-degree burns has improved by 5 to 6 times during the last three decades.[147] Data from the 2015 National Burn Repository Annual Report reviewed the combined data set of acute burn admissions for the time period between 2005 and 2014.[147] Key findings included the following:

- Over 68% of the burn patients were men. The mean age for all cases was 32 years old. Children under the age of 5 years accounted for 19% of the cases, whereas patients age 60 or older represented 13% of the cases.
- The two most commonly reported etiologies were fire/flame and scalds, and accounted for almost 8 out of 10 reported. Scald injuries were most prevalent in children under 5, whereas fire/flame injuries dominated the remaining age categories.
- More than 75% of the reported total burn sizes were less than 10% of total body surface area (TBSA), with a mortality rate of 0.6%. The mortality rate for all cases was 3.2% and 5.7% for fire/flame injuries.
- Seventy-three percent of the burn injuries, with known places of occurrence, were reported to have occurred in the home. Seventy-two percent of cases with known circumstances of injury were identified as accident, nonwork-related.

Burn injuries range from relatively minor, superficial injuries to severe, extensive skin loss resulting from contact with hot solids and liquids, steam, chemical agents, electricity, or other physical agents, such as UVR or infrared radiation. Burn injuries occur in 8 to 12% of all reported abuse cases involving children who come to the attention of healthcare professionals.[148] Teenagers and adults between 17 and 30 years of age most commonly are involved in accidents with flammable liquids, but the mortality associated with clothing ignition continues to decrease as a result of the use of flame-retardant forms of fabric in clothing. Both income and income disparity by country are associated with higher rates of burn-related deaths.[149]

Complications such as fluid and electrolyte imbalances, metabolic derangements, respiratory failure, sepsis, scarring, and functional impairment are the primary causes of hospitalization for these cases. Most burns, however, are minor and can be managed in an ambulatory environment, provided the burned patient is evaluated carefully, the severity of the burn is assessed accurately, and proper and continuous follow-up care is ensured.

The number of serious burns is decreasing in the United States because of better prevention (smoke detectors, water temperature regulations, and decreased smoking), and the advances in acute burn wound management have contributed to this decline as well, including its pharmacotherapy, with topical antimicrobial therapy, early excision or enzymatic debridement of devitalized tissue, and skin grafting or substitutes.[150,151]

Etiology

ZONES OF INJURY

The skin functions as a protective barrier of the underlying organ systems from trauma, temperature variations, harmful penetrations, moisture, humidity, radiation, and invasion by microorganisms (see Fig. 39-1 in Chapter 39, Dermatology and Drug-Induced Skin Disorders). It also is involved with carbohydrate, protein, fat, and vitamin D metabolism, produces secretions that lubricate the skin, is involved with the immune response, and provides the body with the sense of touch.

Burn wounds caused by thermal injury can be described by varying zones of injury.[152] The most peripheral area of injury is the *zone of hyperemia*. The tissue in this area is characterized by inflammatory changes with minimal tissue damage. The *zone of stasis* is the next area of injury, extending inward from the zone of hyperemia. This area involves ischemic, damaged tissue, with blood vessels only partially thrombosed. The damaged endothelial linings of blood vessels within this zone of injury may trigger further thrombosis, resulting in further ischemia, cell death, and deepening of the burn wound. This process of further injury can occur 24 to 48 hours after the initial injury. Drying of the burn wound or infection can cause deepening of the burn wound by preventing re-establishment of circulation to injured tissue. The central-most area, or the *zone of coagulation*, is characterized by thrombotic vessels and necrotic tissue. This area absorbs the most thermal energy, resulting in the greatest tissue damage. Minor burns may involve only the most peripheral zones of injury, whereas severe burns encompass all three zones of injury.

EXTENT OF INJURY

Rule of Nines

Total body surface area (TBSA) is used to assess the size of burns of the skin. The burned surface area is calculated as a percentage of TBSA to determine burn size. In adults, the rule of nines is used to approximate the percentage of burned surface area. Burn severity is proportional to the percent of TBSA involvement and depth of the wound. The percent of TBSA for adults can be estimated by using the "rule of nines," in which each arm constitutes 9% of the TBSA, the head 9%, each leg 18%, the front and back of the torso 18% each, and the genitalia 1%.[153] For children younger than 10 years of age, the percent TBSA must be adjusted because their bodies have different proportions. Variations of the Lund and Browder chart have been used for this purpose.[154] At birth, the infant's head constitutes about 19% of the TBSA. For each additional year of age, the head decreases by about 1%, and the BSA of the legs increases by about 1% of the patient's TBSA, so a quick estimation of the size of a burn can be made.

Classification of Wounds

Burn wounds also are classified according to the depth of tissue damage. Determining the depth of the burn wound can be difficult during the first 24 to 48 hours because of the presence of edema and continued tissue ischemia and infection, both of which can cause deepening of the wound. In addition, the depth of destruction can vary within the same burn, and skin surface characteristics may not match underlying tissue damage, making assessment of the burn wound difficult.[152]

First-Degree Burns (Superficial-Thickness Burn)

First-degree burns result from injury to the superficial cells of the epidermis; a common example is a mild sunburn. The burned skin does not form blisters, but it does become erythematous and mildly painful. This superficial-thickness burn heals within 3 to 4 days without scarring.

Second-Degree Burns (Partial-Thickness to Superficial Burn)

Second-degree burns may be superficial or deep, depending on the depth of dermal involvement. Superficial second-degree burns involve the epidermis and the upper layer of the dermis. The burn surface often is erythematous, blistered, weeping, painful, and very sensitive to stimuli. The erythema blanches with pressure, and the hair follicles, sweat, and sebaceous glands are spared. Superficial second-degree burns heal spontaneously within 3 weeks with little, if any, scarring. Deep second-degree burns involve the deeper elements of the dermis and may be difficult to distinguish from third-degree burns. The burn surface is pale, feels indurated or boggy, and does not blanch with pressure. This wound is less painful than more superficial wounds; some areas may be insensitive to stimuli. Healing occurs slowly over the course of about 35 days with eschar formation and possible severe scarring and permanent loss of hair follicles and sweat and sebaceous glands.

Third-Degree Burns (Partial-Thickness to Deep Burn)

Third-degree burns entail complete destruction of the full thickness of the skin, including all skin elements. The wound may appear pearly white, gray, or brown and is dry and inelastic. Pain is sensed only when deep pressure is applied. If the wound is small, healing over the course of several months can occur by epithelial migration from the margins of the injury, with scar and contracture formation. Third-degree burns are repaired by excision and grafting, or excision and primary closure to prevent contractures of the skin.[155]

Fourth-Degree Burns (Full-Thickness Burn)

Fourth-degree burns are similar to third-degree burns except that devitalized tissue extends into the subcutaneous tissue, fascia, and bone. These burns are blackened in appearance; they are dry and generally painless because of destruction of nerve endings and are at great risk for infection.

COMPLICATIONS OF SEVERE BURN WOUNDS

Fluid Loss

In severe burns, release of vasoactive mediators and capillary injury cause sequestration of large amounts of body fluid, plasma, and electrolytes in extravascular compartments, resulting in edema both locally and throughout the entire body. This redistribution of fluid is compounded by the loss of large amounts of fluid, electrolytes, and protein into the open wound. The cumulative effect is a marked decrease in blood volume, a fall in cardiac output, and decreased tissue and organ perfusion. During the first 24 to 48 hours after a severe burn injury, adequate fluid must be given to replace fluid lost from the vascular space to prevent shock and, possibly, multiple-organ failure and death.[156]

Infection

The most important threat to survival of the fully resuscitated patient is infection, with burn wound sepsis and pneumonia being the leading causes of death.[156] The local mechanical defenses of the skin and respiratory tract often are damaged in burn victims, making these common foci for fatal infections. Loss of circulation to the burn wound margins does not allow proper functioning of cellular and humoral defense mechanisms, which increases susceptibility to infection. Devitalized tissue and tissue exudates provide an ideal environment for the proliferation of bacteria. Colonization of gram-positive bacteria occurs if topical antimicrobial therapy is not initiated promptly, and gram-negative bacteria may predominate by the fifth day after injury.[156] Systemic antibiotics are of limited benefit in full-thickness burns and are used only to treat infections documented by wound biopsy, which reveal in excess of 10^5 bacteria per gram of burn tissue.[157] Topical antimicrobials, local wound care, and strict infection control practices are the mainstays of controlling burn wound infections. Devitalized tissue initiates and perpetuates a sepsis-like state in the absence of an identifiable focus of infection.[156] For this reason, as well as for infection control, early excision of devitalized tissue and closure of the burn wound by skin grafting or substitutes have been adopted by many burn centers.

Inhalation Injury

Burn injuries complicated by inhalation injury are associated with greatly increased mortality rates. Injury to the tracheobronchial mucosa is caused by inhalation of smoke or flames and may result in bronchospasm, ulceration of the mucous membranes, damage to cell membranes, edema, and impairment of bacterial ciliary clearance. Even patients with minor burns can have inhalation injury and require hospital admission. The early symptoms of pulmonary injury (hoarseness, dyspnea, tachypnea, and wheezing) may not be evident for 24 to 48 hours, so patients with suspected inhalation injury (i.e., facial burns or entrapment in a closed space) must be examined carefully. Singed nasal hair, a soot-coated tongue or oropharynx, and upper airway edema are indications of inhalation injury. The diagnosis is established by bronchoscopy, and management may include endotracheal intubation and mechanical ventilation. Maintenance of the patient's fluid status is essential. Corticosteroids do not influence survival rates and should not be routinely administered to patients with inhalation injury. They can also increase morbidity and mortality associated with burns and inhalation injury by increasing the risk of infection.[156]

Clinical Management of Minor Burns

TRIAGE

CASE 42-6

QUESTION 1: S.T., a 17-year-old, nonobese boy, has just burned the calf of his right leg on the muffler of his motorcycle. Immediately after being burned, S.T. was able to rinse his leg with cool water from a garden hose. The burn on his leg is about twice the size of the palm of his hand and appears erythematous and weeping. He sustained no other injury, but now he is in considerable pain. S.T. has no significant medical history. Should S.T. be referred to a healthcare provider or can he safely self-treat his burn? What patient information is necessary to consider in making this decision?

Before recommending treatment for a patient with a minor burn, it is important to accurately assess the patient to determine whether he or she can self-treat safely or whether referral or hospitalization is necessary. The location and severity of the burn, the patient's age and state of health, and the cause of the burn injury all must be considered.

American Burn Association Treatment Categories

Three treatment categories for burn injuries are recommended by the American Burn Association: major burn injuries; moderate, uncomplicated burn injuries; and minor burn injuries.[158]

- *Major burn injuries* are second-degree burns with greater than 25% TBSA involvement in adults (20% in children); all third-degree burns with 10% TBSA involvement; all burns involving the hands, face, eyes, ears, feet, and perineum that may result in functional or cosmetic impairment; high-voltage electrical injury; and burns complicated by inhalation injury, major trauma, or poor-risk patients (elderly patients and those with debilitating disease).
- *Moderate, uncomplicated burns* are second-degree burns with 15% to 25% TBSA involvement in adults (10%–20% in children); third-degree burns with 2% to 10% TBSA involvement; and burns not involving risk to areas of specialized function, such as the eyes, ears, face, hands, feet, or perineum.
- *Minor burn injuries* include second-degree burns with less than 15% TBSA involvement in adults (10% in children), third-degree burns with less than 2% TBSA, and burns not involving functional or cosmetic risk to areas of specialized function.

Patients with minor burn injuries may be treated on an outpatient basis if no other trauma is present; if circumferential burns of the neck, trunk, arms, or legs are not present; and if the patient is able to comply with therapy. After initial evaluation by a healthcare provider, patients may self-treat a second- or third-degree burn only if less than 1% BSA is involved.

Major or moderate, uncomplicated burns necessitate hospital admission, and surgical referral is recommended for patients of all ages who have deep second- or third-degree burns covering 3% of the TBSA.

Both the American Burn Association and the American College of Surgeons recommend transfer to a burn center for all acutely burned patients who meet any of the following criteria[159]:

- Partial-thickness burns of at least 20% TBSA in patients aged 10 to 50 years
- Partial-thickness burns of at least 10% TBSA in children younger than 10 or adults older than 50 years
- Full-thickness burns of at least 5% TBSA in patients of any age
- Patients with partial- or full-thickness burns of the hands, feet, face, eyes, ears, perineum, or major joints
- Patients with high-voltage electrical injuries, including lightning injuries
- Patients with significant burns from caustic chemicals
- Patients with burns complicated by multiple trauma in which the burn injury poses the greatest risk of morbidity or mortality (in such cases, if the trauma poses the greater immediate risk, the patient may be treated initially in a trauma center until stable before being transferred to a burn center)
- Patients with burns who suffer an inhalation injury
- Patients with significant ongoing medical disorders that could complicate management, prolong recovery, or affect mortality
- Patients who were taken to hospitals without qualified personnel or equipment for the care of children
- Burn injury in patients who will require special social, emotional, or long-term rehabilitative support, including cases involving suspected child abuse or substance abuse

Age- and Disease-Related Recommendations

Children younger than 2 years of age and elderly patients with a burn injury should be referred for evaluation because these patients may not tolerate any trauma associated with the burn. In addition to medical issues, children with burns that result from suspected child abuse should be hospitalized for legal, psychosocial, and protective reasons. Burn patients with any other medical condition, such as diabetes mellitus, cardiovascular disease, immunodeficiency disorders (e.g., human immunodeficiency virus [HIV]-associated disease, patients receiving cancer chemotherapy), renal disease, obesity, or alcoholism, may be more susceptible to complications from the burn and may have compromised wound healing.

ETIOLOGY

The etiology of a burn should always be considered because this may provide some insight into the burn presentation and its management. Electrical burns can appear to be superficial because external injury may occur at only the entrance and exit sites of the current. These burns, however, can cause extensive damage to underlying nerve and muscle tissue that is not initially evident. Except for very minor electrical burns, these patients should be referred for further evaluation. S.T. has sustained a superficial second-degree burn over about 2% of his TBSA. Even though the burn wound on his leg was caused by thermal injury and is relatively minor, S.T. should be referred for further evaluation and treatment.

TREATMENT

CASE 42-6, QUESTION 2: How should S.T.'s burn be treated? What treatment alternatives may be used for S.T.? What immunization should S.T. be questioned about?

Goals of Treatment and Immediate Care

Treatment goals for first- and second-degree burns are to relieve the pain associated with the burn; to prevent desiccation and deepening of the wound and infection; and to provide a protective environment for healing. Immediate care of the wound should be application of cold, wet compresses or immersion in cool water.

S.T. may have prevented extension of the burn to deeper layers of tissue and alleviated some of his pain from the burn by immediately irrigating the wound with cool water. Next, the area should be cleansed with a mild hypoallergenic soap (e.g., Basis, Purpose) and water. The sterile, nonadherent, fine-mesh gauze dressing impregnated with hydrophilic petrolatum (e.g., Xeroflo, Kendall; 3% bismuth tribromophenate) should be placed over the wound. This type of dressing offers bacteriostatic activity and prevents the gauze from adhering to the wound and allows the burn exudate to flow freely through the dressing, thus preventing maceration.

A second layer of absorbent gauze should be placed over the petrolatum gauze, and a supportive layer of rolled gauze can be used to keep the dressing in place. The outer layer must not be too constricting, and the dressing should be replaced every 48 hours after recleaning the area and inspecting for signs of infection. If S.T.'s wound continues to weep, it may be beneficial to soak his wound or apply a towel saturated with water, normal saline, or Burow solution (diluted 1:20 or 1:40) for 15 to 30 minutes at least 4 times daily (see Chapter 39, Dermatotherapy and Drug-Induced Skin Disorders). The use of butter, grease, or similar home remedies should be avoided in the treatment of burns because these measures tend to retain the thermal energy sustained in the burn and may increase the area of thermal injury. Because burn patients are susceptible to secondary tetanus infections, S.T. should receive a tetanus toxoid booster if he has not been immunized within the previous 10 years.

Skin Substitutes and Synthetic Dressings

Advances in the development of skin substitutes are being used to achieve the elusive goal of finding a skin replacement to mimic completely the interaction and functions of dermis and epidermis. Although this goal has yet to be achieved, a growing number of synthetic and biologic products are available that can serve important roles in caring for burn patients.[159] Examples of some of the current modalities are as follows:

Human Cadaver Skin

Fresh human cadaver skin (allograft) is considered the sine qua non for temporary closure of burn wounds. It adheres well to a healthy wound bed, resulting in reduced contamination and reduced protein, heat, and water loss. With improved stabilization techniques, rejection and disease transmission (e.g., hepatitis) can be delayed for 3 to 5 weeks, and the risk of infection transmission (e.g., hepatitis) is minimized.

Epidermal Substitute: Cultured Epithelial Allografts

Deep injuries (i.e., third-degree or deep dermal burns) lead to dermal damage that impairs the ability of the skin to heal and regenerate on its own. Skin autografting after burn excision is considered the current gold standard of care, but lack of patient's own donor skin or unsuitability of the wound for autografting may require the temporary use of dressings or skin substitutes to promote wound healing, reduce pain, and prevent infection and abnormal scarring. These alternatives include deceased donor skin allograft, xenograft, cultured epithelial cells, and biosynthetic skin substitutes.

Allotransplantation is the transplantation of cells, tissues, or organs, sourced from a genetically nonidentical member of the same species as the recipient. Human deceased donor skin allografts represent a suitable and much used temporizing option for skin cover after burn injury. The main advantages for their use include dermoprotection and promotion of re-epithelialization of the wound and their ability to act as a skin cover until autografting is possible or reharvesting of donor sites becomes available. Disadvantages of its use include the limited abundance and availability of donors, possible transmission of disease, the eventual rejection by the host, and its handling, storing, transporting, and associated costs of provision. The technique of culturing autologous human epidermal cells grown from a single full-thickness skin biopsy into confluent keratinizing sheets suitable for grafting has been available for more than two decades and is especially useful for patients with large wounds.[160] A lack of mechanical stability of cultured epithelium, causing an imperfect cover, remains a major concern; therefore, the development of a dermal substitute (or a vascularized remnant of allogeneic dermis), in combination with cultured epithelial allografts to increase mechanical stability and decrease wound contracture, or a laboratory-derived autologous composite continues to receive scientific investigation.[161]

Animal Substitute: Porcine Skin

Xenografts derived from porcine skin has gained acceptance as a temporary dressing alternative to allograft because of its lower cost and greater availability.[161] At 0°C, frozen porcine skin has a storage life of 6 to 18 months from the date of manufacture. As with an allograft, it has the desirable properties of being able to adhere initially to a clean wound; to cover nerve endings to decrease pain; to function as an autograft test graft; and to diminish heat, protein, and electrolyte loss. Use of porcine xenografts is a cost-effective alternative to allografts in the treatment of burn wounds, especially for partial-thickness skin losses, temporary coverage prior to autograft and to protect meshed autografts. Although porcine skin shares many physical properties with human skin, it is susceptible to hyperacute rejection due to preformed antibodies. A porcine-derived xenograft in a premeshed, de-epithelialized, collagen matrix that can be stored at room temperature (EZ Derm, Mölnlycke Health Care) is thought to be more resistant to bacterial degradation.

Dermal Analogs: Allodermal Grafts

Unlike the epidermis, the dermis can be rendered acellular and still perform its basic protective and supportive functions. With removal of the dermal cells, the antigenic elements are also eliminated; therefore, alloplastic transplantation can occur without rejection. The principle of allodermal grafting is that an ultrathin (0.01 cm) meshed autograft laid on top of the allodermis provides skin quality that is comparable to that obtained from thick partial-thickness skin grafts.

As one example, AlloDerm (LifeCell) is a shelf-stored, freeze-dried, acellular human cadaveric dermal matrix. Integra (Integra LifeSciences) is a porous matrix of cross-linked bovine tendon collagen and glycosaminoglycan and a semi-permeable polysiloxane (silicone) layer. The inner layer of this material is a 2-mm-thick combination of collagen fibers isolated from bovine tissue and the glycosaminoglycan chondroitin-6-sulfate that has a 70- to 200-μm pore size to facilitate host fibrovascular ingrowth. The outer layer is a 0.009-inch polysiloxane polymer with vapor transmission characteristics that simulate normal epithelium. This meshed bilayer allows drainage of wound exudate and provides a flexible adherent covering for the wound surface. The collagen-glycosaminoglycan biodegradable matrix provides a scaffold for cellular invasion and capillary growth.[161]

Semisynthetic or Biosynthetic Dressings

Biobrane (Smith & Nephew), a nylon–collagen mesh, is used commonly for partial-thickness burns.[162,163] It is a bilaminar, semisynthetic, temporary skin substitute made of a silicone film that is bonded to nylon mesh. Once applied to the burn site, blood or sera clot in the nylon matrix to adhere the mesh to the wound until epithelialization occurs. Its adherence is facilitated by collagen peptides bonded to the nylon underlayer. This substitute has been shown to be as effective as frozen human allograft for the temporary coverage of freshly excised full-thickness burn wounds before autografting.[163] Other available biosynthetic dressings are AWBAT (Aubrey) and AWBAT Plus (Aubrey), which contain a silicone–nylon–collagen membrane. Silon TSR (BioMed Sciences) is a synthetic copolymer that serves as a temporary skin replacement, with elasticity, permeability to water vapor and impermeability to bacteria. These agents peel off within approximately 2 weeks as re-epithelialization of the wound bed progresses.[162]

For superficial- to partial-thickness burns, numerous agents are available over-the-counter. Duoderm (ConvaTec) is a hydrocolloid dressing, whereas OpSite (Smith & Nephew) and Tegaderm (3M) are elastomeric polyurethane films. Comfeel (Coloplast) is a semipermeable polyurethane film coated with a flexible, cross-linked adhesive mass containing sodium carboxy-methylcellulose (NaCMC) as the principal absorbent and gel-forming agent. This product is permeable to water vapor, but impermeable to exudates and microorganisms. In the presence of an exudate, NaCMC absorbs fluids and swells to form a cohesive gel that does not disintegrate or leave residues in the wound bed.

Hyaluronic Acid

Produced by fibroblasts, this group of dermal matrices has a demonstrated positive impact on scar-free fetal wound healing and is also used commercially as a dermal filler. It can be obtained from *Streptococcus* fermentation or extracted from rooster combs. It is available as a scaffold for keratinocytes (Laserskin), an acellular dermal matrix (Hyalomatrix), and as a cellular dermal matrix (Hyalograft-3D).[164]

Alternatives in treating S.T.'s second-degree burn include the use of synthetic dressings and topical antimicrobial agents. Synthetic dressings serve as skin substitutes that are applied to fresh, clean, and moist burns. They are trimmed to about the size of the burn and left in place until the burn is healed or the dressing separates from the wound spontaneously. Indicated for superficial second-degree burns, biosynthetic dressings keep the wound warm and moist, allowing for a faster rate of healing. These dressings offer a significantly lower rate of infection, less frequent dressing changes, with less pain and electrolyte and albumin loss.

Tissue-Engineered Biologic Dressings

Tissue-engineered biologic dressings (examples: Dermagraft, Organogenesis; OASIS Wound Matrix, Smith & Nephew) have been used in the treatment of burns, chronic ulcers, surgical wounds, and other desquamating dermatologic conditions.[165,166] Using an appropriate biologically active matrix to accelerate wound healing and achieving skin reconstruction is well established. Cellular components migrate to the wound from preexisting cell populations in adjacent tissue. Both circulating marrow-derived stem cells and preexisting organ-specific stem cells can contribute to tissue regeneration.[165]

Topical Antimicrobial Agents

Silver Sulfadiazine

Silver sulfadiazine 1% cream (Silvadene, generic; Aquacel Ag [hydrofiber dressing with silver]; ConvaTec) is the usual agent of choice because it has broad-spectrum gram-positive and gram-negative antibacterial activity, provides reasonable eschar penetration, and is easy and painless to apply and wash off. The cream is a 1% suspension of silver sulfadiazine in a water-miscible base. As a consequence of poor water solubility, the active agent shows only limited diffusion into the eschar. Silver sulfadiazine cream is most effective when applied to burn wounds immediately after thermal injury to prevent bacterial colonization of the burn wound surface as a prelude to intraeschar proliferation. This agent has the advantages of being painless when applied to the wound and being free from acid–base and electrolyte disturbances. The limitations of silver sulfadiazine cream include the potential for allergic reactions owing to its sulfadiazine moiety, silver staining of the treated burn wound, hyperosmolality, methemoglobinemia, and hemolysis as a result of a congenital lack of glucose-6-phospate dehydrogenase.[167] Leukopenia, previously considered to be an adverse drug event associated with use of silver sulfadiazine, occurs when using other topical agents during burn care.[167] An evidence-based review of use of silver sulfadiazine in burns suggested that whereas there is evidence of antibacterial activity, no direct evidence is seen of improved healing or reduced infection compared with normal dressings.[168] In partial-thickness burns, use of Aquacel Ag offers less treatment to re-epithelialize burns 100% with less pain, as compared with silver sulfadiazine.[169] This agent should not be applied around the eyes or mouth in patients with hypersensitivity to sulfonamides or in pregnant or breast-feeding women.

Mafenide Acetate

Mafenide acetate (Sulfamylon) is an 11.1% cream formulation of mafenide acetate in a water-dispersible base, or a 5% powder for topical solution. A recent investigation in a pediatric burn population demonstrated the effectiveness of a 2.5% solution, without a change in the incidence of bacteremia or wound infection, and without experiencing adverse drug events.[170] As a water-soluble agent, mafenide diffuses freely to establish an effective antibacterial concentration throughout the eschar and at the interface of viable–nonviable tissue, where bacteria characteristically proliferate before invasion. Because of this characteristic, mafenide is the best agent for use if the patient to be treated has heavily contaminated burn wounds, if treatment is delayed for several days after the burn occurred, or if a dense bacterial population already exists on and within the eschar. Adverse effects include hypersensitivity reactions in 7% of patients (usually responsive to antihistamines), pain or discomfort for 20 to 30 minutes when applied to partial-thickness burns (seldom a cause for discontinuation), and inhibition of carbonic anhydrase. The inhibition of carbonic anhydrase can produce both an early bicarbonate diuresis and an accentuation of postburn hyperventilation. The resulting overall reduction of serum bicarbonate levels renders such patients liable to a rapid shift from an alkalotic to an acidotic state. If acidosis should develop during use of mafenide, the frequency of application should be reduced to once daily, or it should be omitted for 24 to 48 hours, with buffering used as necessary and with efforts made to improve pulmonary function.

Either topical silver sulfadiazine or mafenide should be applied in a one-eighth-inch-thick layer to the entire burn wound with a sterile gloved hand immediately after initial debridement and wound care. Twelve hours later, to ensure continuous topical treatment, a one-eighth-inch coat of cream should be reapplied to those areas of the burn wound from which it has been abraded by clothing. The topical cream should be cleansed gently once each day from all of the burn wound, and the wound should be inspected. Daily debridement should be carried out to a point of bleeding or pain without the use of general anesthesia. After debridement, the wound should be covered again by the topical cream.

In S.T.'s case, silver sulfadiazine cream could be chosen to treat his burn on an outpatient basis if an assessment determines that he is at particular risk for infection. The cream would be applied in a thin layer over the wound and covered with absorbent gauze and wrapped with rolled gauze. The dressing must be changed twice daily to maintain an application of cream that is biologically active. Topical bacitracin and the combination of polymyxin B and bacitracin are transparent formulations that also can be used, but, because of limited efficacy, may be desirable for use only on small, second-degree burns on the face.

Oral Analgesics and Topical Protectants

S.T.'s burn pain can be treated with oral OTC analgesics, aspirin, acetaminophen, or ibuprofen. If these analgesics do not provide adequate relief, oxycodone or acetaminophen (or equivalent) may be of additional benefit.[171] Topical protectants, such as allantoin, calamine, white petrolatum, or zinc oxide, are safe and effective in treating first-degree and minor second-degree burns. These agents protect the burn from mechanical irritation caused by friction and rubbing and prevent drying of the stratum corneum.

Postwound Care

Postwound care is an essential part of total burn management to ensure adequate follow-up subsequent to wound healing, including psychological support. Good burn care that helps to alleviate physical discomfort, pain, and scarring and that promotes good wound healing will also provide psychological benefits for the patient. Healed wounds should be moisturized on a regular basis. Pruritus can be a major problem after burn injury. To reduce itching, moisturizers can be applied, and oral antihistamines may be necessary.[172] Protection from the sun will help to prevent further thermal damage or pigmentation changes to the affected area. Patients in this population should avoid the sun after a burn injury whenever possible, with use of a sunscreen with an SPF of at least 50 recommended.[173] If surface changes occur (e.g., skin becomes hypertrophic, or blisters or new wounds appear), the patient should be advised to return for evaluation.

KEY REFERENCES AND WEBSITES

A full list of references for this chapter can be found at http://thepoint.lww.com/AT11e. Below are the key references and websites for this chapter, with the corresponding reference number in this chapter found in parentheses after the reference.

Key References

Brusselaers N et al. Skin replacement in burn wounds. *J Trauma.* 2010;68(2):490.

Bylaite M et al. Photodermatoses: classification, evaluation and management. *Br J Dermatol.* 2009;161(Suppl 3):61. (4)

Department of Health and Human Services. *The Surgeon General's Call to Action to Prevent Skin Cancer.* Washington, DC: U.S. Department of Health and Human Services, Office of the Surgeon General; 2014. www.surgeongeneral.gov/library/calls/prevent-skincancer/call-to-action-to-prevent-skin-cancer.pdf. Accessed May 15, 2015. (3)

Department of Health and Human Services: Food and Drug Administration. Sunscreen drug products for over-the-counter human use; final rules and proposed rules. *Fed Regist.* 2011;76(117):35620–35665. Accessed May 10, 2015. (57)

Moyal DD, Fourtanier AM. Broad-spectrum sunscreens provide better protection from solar ultraviolet-simulated radiation and natural sunlight-induced immunosuppression in human beings. *J Am Acad Dermatol.* 2008;58(5, Suppl 2):S149. (30)

Rigel DS. Cutaneous ultraviolet exposure and its relationship to the development of skin cancers. *J Am Acad Dermatol.* 2008; 58(5, Suppl 2):S129. (1)

Spanholtz TA et al. Severe burn injuries: acute and long-term treatment. *Dtsch Arztebl Int.* 2009;106(38):607. (156)

US Congress Senate. Health, Education, Labor, and Pensions. 2014. *Sunscreen Innovation Act.* 113th Congress. S2141. (58)

Wang SQ et al. Photoprotection: a review of the current and future technologies. *Dermatol Ther.* 2010;23(1):31. (8)

Key Websites

American Academy of Dermatology, Sun Safety. http://www.aad.org/public/sun/smart.html.

Centers for Disease Control and Prevention, Skin Cancer Prevention. http://www.cdc.gov/cancer/skin/basic_info/prevention.htm.

Skin Cancer Organization. http://www.skincancer.org/.

Section Editor: Kamala M. Nola

43 Osteoarthritis

Dominick P. Trombetta and Christopher M. Herndon

CORE PRINCIPLES

	CORE PRINCIPLES	CHAPTER CASES
1	Osteoarthritis (OA) is a chronic, progressive condition, primarily affecting women, that causes loss of articular cartilage in hands, knees, hips, and cervical and lumbar spine. OA causes significant pain and functional disability, and increases costs to our healthcare systems.	**Case 43-1 (Question 1)**
2	The evolving role of cytokines and the resultant imbalance between cartilage maintenance and destruction contribute to the pathophysiology of OA. There are no current disease-mitigating therapies.	**Case 43-1 (Questions 2, 3), Figure 43-1**
3	The typical presentation includes stiffness and pain unilaterally in one or more joints lasting less than 30 minutes after a period of immobility. This causes significant limitations in activities of daily living as well as overall quality of life.	**Case 43-1 (Questions 1, 2)**
4	Conservative treatment strategies include weight loss, self-management, aerobic exercise, strength training, and physical and occupational therapies to best maintain optimal functional status.	**Case 43-1 (Question 4)**
5	Initial trials of routine dosing of acetaminophen, topical agents, nonsteroidal anti-inflammatory drugs (NSAIDs), and intra-articular glucocorticoid injections represent initial pharmacologic interventions of osteoarthritis.	**Case 43-1 (Questions 5, 6), Case 43-2 (Questions 1–4), Tables 43-1–43-3, Figure 43-2**
6	Intra-articular hyaluronan, tramadol, and duloxetine may be considered in those patients with insufficient relief in symptoms and worsening function after initial pharmacologic strategies have been attempted.	**Case 43-2 (Questions 1–6)**
7	A consistent and systematic approach to the management of chronic pain caused by OA can help identify patients with limitations in activities of daily living (ADLs) and prevent further disability. Then, the effectiveness of current therapies can be more appropriately evaluated, and the treatment plan can be updated.	**Case 43-1 (Questions 5, 7), Case 43-2 (Questions 1–6), Case 43-3 (Questions 1, 2)**

INCIDENCE, PREVALENCE, AND EPIDEMIOLOGY

Osteoarthritis (OA) is a chronic, progressive disorder characterized by the changes to articular cartilage and bone primarily in hands, knees, hips, and spine. Incidence rates for OA of the hand have been estimated to be 100 per 100,000 person-years, hip OA, 88 per 100,000 person-years, and knee OA, 240 per 100,000 person-years. Incidence rates increase with advancing age until the 8th decade of life. The Centers for Disease Control and Prevention (CDC) reported in 2005 that approximately 26.9 million people older than 65 years of age are affected, particularly after the age of 50.[1] Women seem to be affected by more severe OA of the knees than men, particularly after the age of 50.[2] Additionally, women experience more severe disease radiographically; however, severity of radiologic disease may not predict severity of subjective symptoms of pain or disability. Men have a lower incidence of knee and hip OA than women.[1] More recently, in 2013, it had been reported that arthritis was the most common cause of disability in U.S. adults, and was noted to co-occur in persons with multiple chronic conditions such as heart disease and diabetes mellitus. This report illustrated that 52.5 million (22.7%) of adults older than 18 years had self-reported provider-diagnosed arthritis, and 22.7 million (9.8% of all adults, 43.2 with arthritis) reported arthritis-attributable activity limitations.[3] Arthritis contributes significant costs to the healthcare system through hospitalizations, joint-related surgeries, and inability to work. An estimated 200 billion US dollars is attributed to OA annually as either direct medical costs or lost productivity.[4]

Arthritis patients perceive lower health-related quality of life. The physical limitations in arthritis-related activities and the subsequent effects on the comorbidities related to obesity are current areas of research.[3] Considering the morbidity and mortality associated with type 2 diabetes mellitus and coronary artery disease is significant. The development of disease-mitigating interventions may benefit not only those with OA but also in cases where inactivity contributes to or worsens obesity-related conditions and complications.

ETIOLOGY

Osteoarthritis has been previously described as disease of cartilage that has undergone significant wear and tear. It is now known to be a more complex and dynamic process. Primary OA cannot be traced to any particular identifiable cause. In secondary OA, a known etiology or cause has been determined. We know osteoarthritis affects not only articular cartilage but also periarticular muscles, subchondral bone and ligaments, synovial membranes, and the entire joint capsule. The interplay of cellular, biochemical, and mechanical processes underlies the disease. Various risk factors have been identified and can be classified as modifiable and nonmodifiable. Modifiable risk factors of OA include obesity and joint trauma. Increased body weight has been correlated with increased risk of OA of the knee, but not the hip. Excess weight contributes to the biomechanical forces and stresses on the knee joints. The cascade of increased pain leading to decreased function and further worsening of obesity can be a difficult cycle to break. Weight loss and moderate amounts of activity improve symptoms of OA of the knee and improve overall health. Nonmodifiable risk factors are advancing age, sex, genetics, and joint location. Typically, the development of symptomatic OA occurs with increased age predominantly in the weight-bearing joints, although many women are affected by localized inflammation of the proximal and distal interphalangeal joints known as Bouchard and Heberden nodes, respectively. Approximately 80% of patients older than 75 years are affected by OA.

Epidemiologic studies provide support for a genetic component to the development of OA as well as the characteristic Heberden and Bouchard nodes. Studies in twins have also supported the influence of genetics and the development of OA. Multiple genes have been identified that are associated with increased risk for OA as well as some genetic mutations associated with OA of early onset. With the increasing development of isolating specific genotypes and pharmacogenomics, more targeted interventions could be implemented to arrest disease progression. OA is particularly more common in the hips and knees than in the ankle joint. Joint trauma can result in the evolution of OA. Biochemical and mechanical changes can occur, resulting in the characteristic joint pain and stiffness. The consequences are articular cartilage with less functionality and resultant characteristics of cartilage, joint capsule, and subchondral bone that are distinctively different from those of normal bone. Regular exercise and physical activity do not increase the risk of OA in normal joints and are necessary to maintain cartilage.[5]

The development of radiologic evidence of OA precedes the clinical symptoms; thus, the initial presentation may not always correlate with disease prognosis. Diminished ability of chondrocytes to maintain and repair articular cartilage has been correlated

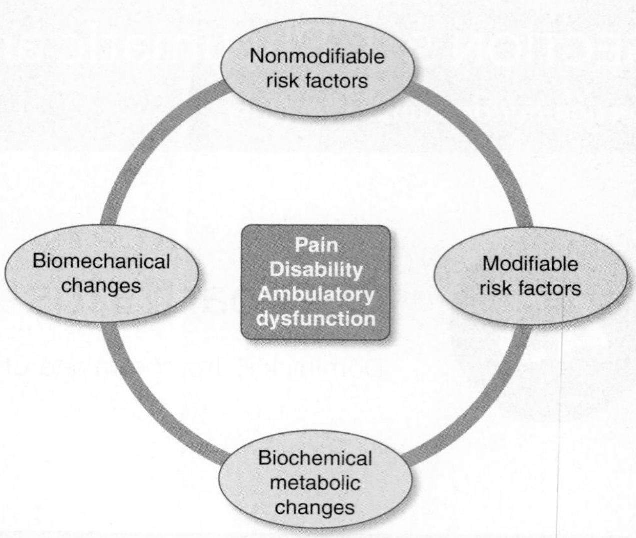

Figure 43-1 Schematic representation of the convergence of modifiable, nonmodifiable risk factors, and morphologic changes associated with osteoarthritis.

with resultant cartilage degradation. These age-related changes in chondrocyte function are associated with a decreased response to anabolic stimuli such as insulin-like growth factor-1 (IGF-1). Thus, the biochemical signal to spur production of proteoglycans and collagen that maintain the strength of cartilage decreases and results in an imbalance between breakdown and repair. The effect of age on chondrocyte apoptosis seems to be strongly related. Perhaps, because of occupational or recreational injury, men tend to have more OA before the age of 50.[5]

PATHOGENESIS

In the early stages of OA, changes occur that appear to begin the complex abnormalities seen in the joint capsule, subchondral bone and ligaments, periarticular muscles, and synovial membranes. Initial insult to the articular cartilage can result from repetitive damage with time. Alternatively, another theory has been proposed that examines articular damage after superficial or deep penetration injury. Either repetitive or traumatic injury to articular surfaces initiates the cascade leading to release of inflammatory cytokines (tumor necrosis factor [TNF], IL-1), nitric oxide, and enzymes that break down the extracellular matrix. The breakdown of extracellular matrix results in cartilage that is less elastic and less able to support joint loads, and stiffening of subchondral bone. The cartilage is less able to support forces, with diminished efficacy for providing joint lubrication and weight distribution across the joint. Cartilage is avascular, however, and contains chondrocytes that under normal conditions are responsible for cartilage breakdown and repair. In early osteoarthritis, chondrocytes attempt to repair joint damage by forming osteophytes, which try to stabilize the joint or alter the biochemical properties of cartilage. The formation of osteophytes may provide an increased surface area over which to distribute the forces across the joint. Cyst formation likely arises via synovial fluid pressure exerted on the fissures or other structural defects in subchondral bone.[5]

Early in the disease process, the water content of the cartilage is increased. However, this less viscous cartilage is structurally weaker than normal cartilage. There are many structural alterations that contribute to the weakened collagen network. One of the early changes is a smaller diameter of type II collagen, in comparison with that in the more structurally intact disease-free joint. With disease progression, the proteoglycan concentrations diminish with shorter glycosaminoglycan side chains resulting in decreases of net aggregate proteins. Type I collagen within the extracellular matrix increases, and keratin sulfate concentrations decrease. Some of the biochemical changes are reflective of those produced in culture by immature tissue. The deposition of calcium crystals represents a curious finding. It is unknown whether calcium deposition has a direct involvement or is reflective of increased chondrocyte activity. Eventually, the initial water swelling of the cartilage is replaced by cartilage with reduced propensity to allow bone to distribute the force and slide on bone.[5] Distinct alterations in cartilage matrix metabolism favor catabolism. Chondrocytes are unable to maintain production of essential macromolecules necessary for healthy cartilage. However, the syntheses of those enzymes that break down the matrix are increased by the same chondrocytes. The enzymes that degrade proteoglycans and collagen are called aggrecanases and collagenases, respectively. The control of these enzymes is complicated by enzymatic activation of latent proteins and inactivation by proteinase inhibitors. In OA, the expression and production of proteinases is increased. Collagen is typically cleaved by matrix metalloproteinases (MMPs), MMP-1, MMP-8, and MMP-13. Most recently, the role of inflammation and inflammatory mediators produced by cartilage is being more closely investigated. Upregulated by IL-1 and TNF, MMPs cleave collagen and break down other important elements of the extracellular matrix. Ultimately, the imbalance between cartilage maintenance and degradation leads to erosion and eventual cartilage destruction.[5]

OVERVIEW OF DRUG THERAPY

The current treatment of OA is to provide analgesia allowing performance of activities of daily living (ADLs), facilitate participation in physical or occupational therapies, and recommend appropriate self-managed exercise programs. There are no disease-mitigating strategies that have demonstrated acceptable safety and efficacy in the treatment of OA. The initial treatment for OA pain and stiffness is acetaminophen given on a routine basis for a 2- to 3-week trial in doses typically less than 4 g/day or less than 3 g/day in patients older than 65 years, unless clinically contraindicated. Acetaminophen offers a considerable degree of safety over nonsteroidal anti-inflammatory drugs (NSAIDs) for mild-to-moderate OA disease. However, many clinical trials have demonstrated significantly better efficacy of NSAIDs as compared with acetaminophen in selected patients, such as those who present with both pain and inflammation, because acetaminophen lacks significant anti-inflammatory effects.[6–8] These patients are more likely to exhibit more moderate-to-severe disease.[5,9,10] Unintentional liver injury may result from overuse of acetaminophen above recommended doses, in combination with over-the-counter acetaminophen containing products, or the opioid–acetaminophen products available by prescription. A trial of a selective or nonselective NSAID would be a reasonable consideration in patients with inadequate response to acetaminophen or presenting with pain and inflammation. A careful risk and benefit analysis must be individualized for each patient starting an NSAID. Adverse events of GI bleeding, diminishing renal function, liver toxicity, and cardiovascular risk of the specific medication considered need to be carefully assessed and a plan for therapeutic monitoring implemented. Additionally, consideration of drug–drug interactions or drug–disease interactions is also warranted. Topical therapies may be therapeutic for selected patients unable to tolerate oral NSAIDs and are becoming more widely recommended by professional practice guidelines.[11,12] Topical therapies include capsaicin creams, capsaicin gels, capsaicin liquids, capsaicin lotions, capsaicin topical patches, lidocaine topical patch, lidocaine topical creams, ointments, and gels, diclofenac topical gel, diclofenac topical patch, and diclofenac topical solution. In patients presenting with effusions of the knee, aspiration of the affected joint and intra-articular injections of corticosteroids may be therapeutic once infectious etiologies have been ruled out. In patients with inadequate relief in symptoms and worsening functions, there are few alternatives outside of surgical interventions. Intra-articular injections of hyaluronic acid derivatives are the last of the conservative strategies before surgical interventions are considered. Tramadol may represent a useful option for many patients unless precluded due to seizures or misuse history or drug–drug interaction potential. There are currently no recommendations for the use of oral glucocorticoids in the treatment of OA. A trial of 6 months of glucosamine and chondroitin can be discussed with those patients interested in pursuing this type of therapy. The use of oral or transdermal opioids or opioid/acetaminophen combinations for pain management should be discouraged because of the limited evidence demonstrating benefit and the high potential for adverse drug reactions.

CLINICAL MANIFESTATIONS

Clinical Presentation of Osteoarthritis

CASE 43-1

QUESTION 1: R.T., a 64-year-old nonsmoking woman, presents to her primary-care physician reporting pain and stiffness in her right knee. The pain is usually worse in the morning and lasts for about 15 to 20 minutes and then subsides throughout the day. She reports some increased difficulty taking care of her grandchildren while her daughter is working. Her medical history is significant for hypothyroidism, hypertension, and hyperlipidemia. Social history is negative for tobacco and alcohol use. R.T. currently takes amlodipine 5 mg daily, levothyroxine 88 mcg daily, and simvastatin 40 mg daily. On physical examination, there is a varus misalignment of the knees. The right knee has no swelling or synovial effusions, and crepitus is noted on examination of passive motion. A radiograph shows right knee joint space narrowing with osteophyte formation at the joint margins.

Laboratory values and vital signs obtained at this visit include the following:

Blood pressure (BP), 135/78 mm Hg
Heart rate (HR), 80 beats/minute
Height, 64 inches
Weight, 205 pounds
BMI, 35.2 kg/m^2
Sodium, 140 mEq/L
Potassium, 4.5 mEq/L
Blood urea nitrogen (BUN), 10 mg/dL
Creatinine, 0.9 mg/dL
Estimated glomerular filtration rate (eGFR), 63 mL/minute
Thyrotropin (TSH), 3.08 mIU/mL
White blood cells (WBC), $5 \times 10^3/\mu L$
Red blood cells (RBC), $4.7 \times 10^6/\mu L$
Hemoglobin, 12.7 g/dL
Hematocrit, 38.2%
Uric acid, 5 mg/dL
C-reactive protein (CRP), 0.9 mg/dL
Erythrocyte sedimentation rate (ESR), 18 mm/hour
Anti-CCP antibodies, negative
Total cholesterol, 160 mg/dL
High-density lipoprotein (HDL), 45 mg/dL

What signs and symptoms suggestive of OA are present in R.T.?

CASE 43-1, QUESTION 2: How do the subjective and objective findings of OA correlate with disease pathogenesis in R.T.?

R.T. presents with unilateral right knee pain that is worse in the morning and subsides throughout the day. The OA diagnosis can be made by a good history and physical examination. Laboratory studies are not needed to confirm the diagnosis of OA, but a normal ESR rules out inflammatory conditions such as gout or septic arthritis. Radiographs demonstrate joint space narrowing that is consistent with OA. However, radiographs do not reliably assess disease severity.

The characteristic joint space narrowing as seen on radiograph without joint destruction is characteristic for OA. Osteophyte formation and bone rubbing against bone are most likely responsible for the pain, stiffness, and crepitus demonstrated on physical examination. Crepitus is an audible "crackling" sound that can be heard with passive or active movement of the joint. Instead of the opposing joint surfaces gliding past each other, the movement of the joint now creates the characteristic crunching or crackling sounds. Additionally, the varus misalignment contributes to the stress on the knee joint and some of the functional impairments R.T. reported to her primary-care physician. A varus misalignment is described as the patient in a standing position with his/her knees appearing further apart (bow-legged), and valgus is when the knees are closer together. Both of these deformities can affect a patient's function and quality of life.

The clinical presentation of OA is usually unilateral pain and stiffness of the knee, hip, or cervical or lumbar spine; the distal interphalangeal joints generally are not painful. More often than not, OA tends to affect more than one joint. There are some distribution associations described between knee and hand OA and knee and hip OA. Elbows, wrists, and shoulders tend not to be affected by OA. Diagnostic criteria from the American College of Rheumatology (ACR) hip criteria have a sensitivity and a specificity of 91% and 89%, respectively, and a sensitivity of 91% and specificity of 86% for knee OA.[3] These criteria usually are not used in clinical practice outside of research studies. Clinical trials typically provide outcome data based on assessment tools such as the Western Ontario and McMaster Universities (WOMAC), predominantly used for knee OA. A WOMAC functional subscale exists to assess for functional disability.[13] Patients usually present to their primary-care provider with complaints of increased pain or stiffness lasting less than 30 minutes, usually in the morning or after periods of prolonged immobility. They usually will report decreases in their ADL, functional status, and overall health-related quality of life. Typically, household activities such as kneeling, stair climbing, and walking tend to be limited. The associated decrease in activities, range of motion, and overall physical activity contribute to muscle weakness and unsteadiness.

Problems with sleep and depression can occur, compromising attempts to lose weight, increase activity, and participate in physical or occupational therapy or in Tai Chi. Joint involvement can be characterized with swelling, easily recognized in the fingers and knees. Joints usually are tender when examined during active motion or application of pressure. Bursitis, tendonitis, muscle spasms, and torn meniscus can cause limitations in range of motion and need to be ruled out. Synovial effusions can be chronic but can also present during times of disease exacerbations. The patellar tap test or the wave test can elucidate joint effusions. Patients with advanced disease may present with the expected loss of cartilage, but also deformities in surrounding bone and soft tissue affecting the ligaments. Joint misalignment is common and contributes to joint unsteadiness. Fingers of patients with the characteristic Bouchard and Heberden nodes are misaligned. Muscle atrophy is demonstrated by simply measuring the circumference of the quadriceps muscles. The use of radiographs is usually not necessary for the diagnosis of OA, but rather is used to rule out conditions such as avascular necrosis, Paget disease of the bone, rheumatoid arthritis, or gouty arthropathies. However, radiographs can be useful to establish disease severity or monitor for disease progression. The clinical features described on radiographs that are characteristic of OA are joint space narrowing, osteophytes at the joint margins, and sclerosis of subchondral bone. As demonstrated in the above case study, R.T.'s knee radiograph revealed joint space narrowing with osteophyte formation.

An ultrasound can be useful for detecting or confirming joint effusion, popliteal cysts, or other erosive inflammatory conditions. Laboratory assessments are usually unnecessary, because the ESR and CRP are typically within reference ranges. Serum uric acid can help differentiate between similar inflammatory presentations. Synovial fluid aspiration is appropriate if septic or inflammatory arthritis is suspected. In the patient with OA, the WBC count is less than 2,000 μL, synovial fluid is clear, and crystals are absent. There are no relevant biomarkers of bone or cartilage remodeling that are used in the routine care of patients with OA. Magnetic resonance imaging (MRI) scans represent an exciting area of research for assessing cartilage, synovium, and bone, but are not routinely used in the diagnosis of OA.

CASE 43-1, QUESTION 3: Cytokines are involved in the pathophysiology of OA. Is it possible to modulate these cytokines and thereby slow or delay the disease process to benefit R.T. before her condition worsens?

The role of IL-1 and TNF in rheumatoid arthritis pathogenesis represented exciting discoveries that have led to highly effective disease remissions. However, in OA, the role of these cytokines in upregulating MMP and the exact mechanism that they play in the disease process have not been clearly elucidated and have not resulted in any disease-mitigating therapies.

TREATMENT OF OSTEOARTHRITIS

CASE 43-1, QUESTION 4: What nonpharmacologic therapies should be recommended in R.T.?

Nonpharmacologic Management of OA

Nonpharmacologic modalities are a primary strategy for OA treatment. As previously discussed, there are no interventions that effectively attenuate the disease process. Pharmacologic strategies have significant untoward effects and modest efficacy in the management of OA pain and disability. Patients typically have difficulty adhering to self-management, aerobic, or strength-training programs. Many times, nonpharmacologic strategies are not even attempted until pharmacologic interventions have failed or side effects necessitate discontinuation of the offending agent.

The ACR outlines a variety of patient education, self-management, weight loss, aerobic, and physical and occupational therapies.[14] A study in middle-aged patients with knee OA has demonstrated equivocal efficacy in comparing self-management with strength training and the combination of both programs. Outcomes assessed were pain, disability, and physical conditioning during the 2 years of the trial.[13] One clinical trial examined the comparison of NSAID therapy with quadriceps home exercise. Quality-of-life surveys and pain scores were not different between the groups reviewed in this small trial.[15] In older patients, Tai Chi has established efficacy through randomized controlled trials in the treatment of knee OA. Wang et al.[16] demonstrated the beneficial effects of Tai Chi not only in improving physical function and lessening pain in patients with OA, but also in having a positive effect on their mental health and overall quality of life. Trial limitations included a small sample size (40 patients) and 3-month study duration. It is unknown whether those demonstrated benefits were sustained. Patients can be referred to the Arthritis Foundation website (http://www.arthritis.org) for further information on various programs or activities in their areas. The Osteoarthritis Research Society International (OARSI) reiterates the effectiveness of nonpharmacologic interventions of self-management, weight loss, exercise, referral to physical therapy, and effective use of bracing for varus or valgus misalignments.[11,12] Nonpharmacologic interventions remain the most effective, yet underutilized, interventions for the treatment of OA.[11,17]

R.T. should be encouraged to lose weight and participate in either self-management or a structured exercise program that includes aerobic and strength-training exercises. Additionally, R.T. should be encouraged to participate in local Tai Chi classes. Weight loss should be the primary goal in obese patients with OA of the knee. Exercise improves muscle strength and helps prevent falls. The use of knee bracing may offer some degree of support in patients with misalignments of the knee joints.

CASE 43-1, QUESTION 5: What is the initial pharmacologic treatment recommendation for R.T.?

Pharmacologic Management of Osteoarthritis

A trial of acetaminophen 1,000 mg PO 3 to 4 times a day should be attempted for 2 to 3 weeks. More aggressive medications are usually reserved for those patients who have failed acetaminophen. Medications such as NSAIDs can increase blood pressure, cause GI ulceration, inhibit renal prostaglandins that are vasodilatory and, therefore, diminish renal function, and potentially increase cardiovascular risks. Given R.T.'s past medical history of peptic ulcer disease and lack of knee inflammation on physical examination, the initial trial of acetaminophen is warranted.

ACETAMINOPHEN

Acetaminophen remains the first choice for the treatment of mild-to-moderate OA of the hands and knees. Clinical practice guidelines from the American College of Rheumatology (ACR), the American Academy of Orthopedic Surgery (AAOS), the European League Against Rheumatism (EULAR), and the Osteoarthritis Research Society International (OARSI) differ in their strength of recommendation, dosing, and length of therapy for acetaminophen.[11,14,18,19]

Chronic acetaminophen use in patients who consume more than three alcoholic drinks per day can increase risk of GI bleeding and elevations of liver enzymes.[20] A 12-week randomized, controlled trial reported in 2007 that extended-release acetaminophen 3,900 mg/day was safe, well tolerated, and more effective than 1,950 mg/day in patients with hip and knee OA.[21] More recently, it has been suggested that select patients presenting with both pain and inflammation without contraindications begin an initial trial with an NSAID instead of acetaminophen.[12]

CASE 43-1, QUESTION 6: What is the role of topical agents in the treatment plan for R.T.?

TOPICAL THERAPY

There are numerous prescription and nonprescription topical analgesics available, containing capsaicin, diclofenac, lidocaine, or methyl salicylate. Both the ACR and OARSI practice guidelines conditionally recommend topical NSAID therapy as a potential first-line therapy for joint-specific OA.[11,14] Topical capsaicin cream is applied to the hands or knees 3 to 4 times daily. If used, R.T. should be counseled regarding proper application, initial burning and sensitivity reactions, and expectations of benefits that may take up to a few weeks. There are no systemic effects or drug interactions with topical capsaicin cream.[11]

Currently, three topical diclofenac products are commercially available in the United States, including a 1% gel, a 1.5% solution, and a 1.3% patch. Topical diclofenac 1% gel, alone or in combination with oral acetaminophen, represents another therapeutic option. Topical diclofenac 1% gel is indicated in the treatment of OA of the upper extremities such as the hands, elbows, and wrists, and the lower extremities such as ankles, feet, and knees. The gel is applied according to "dosing cards" in either 2-g or 4-g measurements. The dose for the upper extremities is 2 g 4 times a day and 4 g 4 times daily to the lower extremities.[22]

Diclofenac topical solution 1.5% w/w in dimethyl sulfoxide, USP (DMSO) 45.5% w/w represent another treatment option for the signs and symptoms of OA of the knee. In two, 12-week, randomized, placebo-controlled trials, oral and topical diclofenac solution was equivocal for the outcome measures of pain and physical function.[23,24] Patients receiving the topical solution reported minor skin irritation, but fewer GI symptoms and abnormal liver function tests than those patients receiving oral diclofenac.

The diclofenac 1.3% patch, although available, is indicated only for the treatment of acute pain due to musculoskeletal sprains and strains.

CASE 43-1, QUESTION 7: What monitoring parameters would be appropriate for R.T.?

Although improved tolerability and decreased toxicity profiles appear promising for topical NSAIDs, the warnings about typical NSAID-related adverse effects are similar for oral and topical agents.[25] Data are lacking for true upper gastrointestinal bleed or cardiovascular event risk with topical versus oral administration. Outside of short-term efficacy trials, the risk for systemic complications with chronic therapy has not been investigated. Additionally, limited comparative efficacy data exist comparing topical diclofenac with other oral NSAIDs or topical capsaicin. Oral and topical NSAIDs should not be used concomitantly unless potential benefit greatly outweighs the risk due to reports of increased incidence of rectal bleeding and abnormal laboratory findings when used together.[26] The combination of acetaminophen and topical diclofenac may be therapeutic for some patients while avoiding other combinations with a higher degree of untoward effects. This combination, however, has yet to be evaluated in the rigor of randomized trials. The risk of significant GI bleeding would be theoretically less with topical preparations as a result of less systemic absorption.[12,23,24,27] In a 2010 systematic review, oral and topical NSAIDs were noted to have similar rates for discontinuation because of a high incidence of topical reactions with the latter.[28] It is unclear whether these skin reactions are caused by the type of formulation, vehicle, or other ingredients in the preparation.

R.T. does not have a history of liver disease or hepatitis C, so a short trial of acetaminophen does not require any monitoring for medication safety. However, it would be important to ask her to keep a daily pain log and complete a comfort assessment on her next visit. These tools are freely available online from multiple sources. This will engage the patient in her own care as well as provide the clinician with information regarding baseline data, medication efficacy, and the impact of medication on functional impairment. Additionally, limitations or improvements in ADLs and instrumental activities of daily living (IADLs) can provide useful information in helping the clinician determine whether any changes in the plan of care need to occur.

CASE 43-2

QUESTION 1: S.L., a 67-year-old woman, presents to her primary-care physician with increased pain and stiffness in her left knee. S.L. reports her left knee as "weak," and she has difficulty getting out of bed in the morning and after sitting on the recliner for some time. She has tried acetaminophen 1,000 mg 4 times daily for 1 month without adequate relief. She also takes metoprolol succinate 50 mg daily, lisinopril 20 mg daily, ranitidine 150 mg twice daily, and citalopram 20 mg daily. Her medical history includes hypertension, osteopenia, depression, gastroesophageal reflux disease, osteoarthritis, and a right knee replacement 2 years ago. Her recent laboratory values and vital signs include the following:

BP, 160/78 mm Hg
HR, 76 beats/minute
Height, 66 inches
Weight, 190 pounds
BMI, 30.7 kg/m^2
Sodium, 145 mEq/L
Potassium, 4.8 mEq/L
BUN, 16 mg/dL
Creatinine, 1.2 mg/dL
eGFR, 48 mL/minute
WBC, 4.5 × 10^3/μL
RBC, 4.2 × 10^6/μL
Hemoglobin, 12.1 g/dL
Hematocrit, 36.6%

Select and recommend a medication to provide adequate pain relief for S.L.

In this patient who has failed an adequate trial of acetaminophen, therapeutic options include celecoxib, a nonselective NSAID, tramadol, or an opioid analgesic. There are no data to suggest any particular NSAID is more effective than another.[29] S.L. does not have any known history of coronary heart disease or peptic ulcer disease. On the basis of the risk factors identified in Table 43-1, S.L. has one risk factor of age, placing her at moderate risk for GI ulceration. Data suggest appropriate treatment of *Helicobacter pylori*, if present, reduces the risk of GI ulceration in patients taking NSAIDs chronically.[30] Therefore, if the decision is made to recommend a nonselective NSAID, then ranitidine would need to be discontinued because of a lack of protection against gastric ulcers, and a proton-pump inhibitor (PPI) such as omeprazole should be initiated to prevent GI bleeding. Either option would represent a reasonable therapeutic recommendation.

Table 43-1
Recommendations for NSAID Selection Based on Gastrointestinal and Cardiovascular Risks[30]

Risk Category	Low GI Risk	Moderate GI Risk	High GI Risk
	0 risk factors	1–2 risk factors	Multiple risk factors, history of previous ulcer events, or continued use of corticosteroids or anticoagulants
Low CV risk	NSAID alone	NSAID + PPI/ misoprostol	Alternative therapy or COX-2 + PPI/misoprostol
High CV risk (low-dose aspirin required)	Naproxen + PPI/ misopr-ostol	Naproxen + PPI/ misoprostol	Alternative therapy recommended

COX-2, cyclooxygenase-2 inhibitor; CV, cardiovascular; NSAID, nonsteroidal anti-inflammatory drug; PPI, proton-pump inhibitor.

Table 43-2
Relative Selectivity of Cyclooxygenase Inhibitors[67]

5- to 50-fold COX-2 Preferential	<5-fold COX-2 Preferential	COX-1 Preferential
Etodolac	Diclofenac	Fenoprofen
Meloxicam	Sulindac	Ibuprofen
Celecoxib	Meclofenamate	Tolmetin
	Piroxicam	Naproxen
	Diflunisal	Aspirin
		Indomethacin
		Ketoprofen
		Flurbiprofen
		Ketorolac

Based on log IC_{80} inhibition ratios COX-2/COX-1.

For those patients with insufficient pain relief from acetaminophen or topical agents, an oral NSAID should be considered. As with any decision regarding pharmacotherapy, the safety and efficacy of the chosen therapy needs to be evaluated in the context of a patient's specific case. The historical perspective and the knowledge of increased cardiovascular risk versus GI safety with COX-2 agents have had a tremendous impact on the use of these agents in clinical practice. Currently available NSAIDs have comparatively unique characteristics in terms of their ability to inhibit COX-1 (constitutive) and COX-2 (inducible). See Table 43-2 for selectivity of COX-2 inhibition.

Patients at increased risk for cardiovascular disease include those with unstable angina, a history of myocardial infarction, coronary artery bypass surgery, ischemic stroke, or a high Framingham risk score.[31] Some clinicians have recommended the addition of low-dose aspirin 81 mg to attenuate the increased risk of cardiovascular disease; however, this practice has not been the primary focus of vigorous clinical trials. The addition of aspirin can potentially increase the risk of GI ulceration and compromise cardioprotection.[32] Additionally, randomized controlled studies have not clearly demonstrated the efficacy and safety of this approach.[31,33]

In a 52-week double-blind study comparing the cardiovascular outcomes of patients with OA exposed to ibuprofen, naproxen, or lumiracoxib, several key findings emerged. First, ibuprofen users taking aspirin had the highest risk of cardiovascular outcomes and heart failure in comparison with lumiracoxib. This supports concerns that ibuprofen can competitively interfere with the ability of aspirin to inhibit platelet aggregation.[34] Second, patients taking naproxen without aspirin had the best safety profile with regard to cardiovascular outcomes. Whether or not naproxen has the lowest risk for cardiovascular side effects has not been clearly elucidated. In fact, recent analysis from the Women's Health Initiative suggests naproxen, in addition to NSAIDs with cyclooxygenase-2 preferential inhibition, exhibits increased risk for cardiovascular events.[35] Conflicting data regarding dose, duration of therapy, and methodological differences in trials have not yet produced clear and concise evidence.[36] Lastly, heart failure was observed more frequently in patients taking ibuprofen than in patients receiving lumiracoxib or naproxen.[37] In a recent AHRQ report, celecoxib has been reported to increase the risk for myocardial infarction,

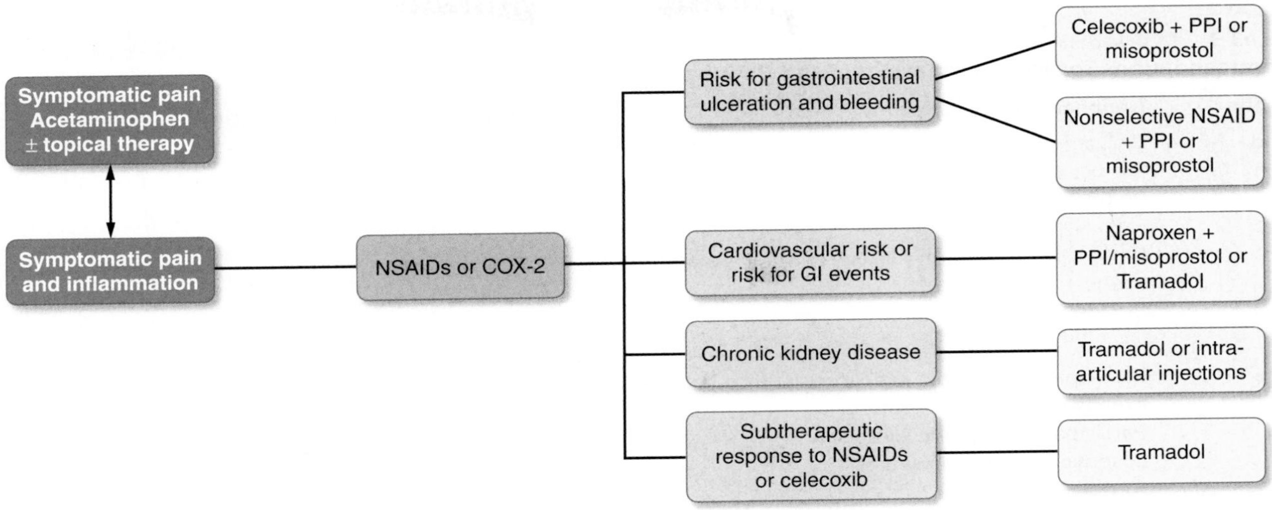

Figure 43-2 Overview of pharmacologic therapy for treatment of osteoarthritis. (Adapted from multiple references.)[11,12,14,18,30]

particularly at higher doses.[27] Other studies have failed to exhibit this finding.[38] In summary, for patients with low cardiovascular risk and moderate-to-higher risk for GI bleeding, a recommendation can be made for once-daily celecoxib or NSAID plus PPI or misoprostol. However, in patients with a higher risk for cardiovascular disease, consider the use of tramadol or naproxen, or nonacetylated salicylates (e.g., diflunisal or salsalate) with careful monitoring of blood pressure and renal function (use of aspirin concurrently with naproxen may need further assessment for clinical need).[39,40]

Case 43-2, Question 2: What monitoring parameters would be appropriate for this pharmacologic treatment recommendation for S.L.?

Many clinicians recommend checking a basic metabolic panel and complete blood count with differential 2 to 4 weeks after starting NSAIDs in older patients. Depending on the initial laboratory results, testing can occur every 3 to 4 months, thereafter for the next year. The risk for GI adverse events decreases after 1 month, but is always present. Liver function should be checked regularly during the first year of treatment and periodically thereafter. Patients with significant comorbidities may need more stringent follow-up and monitoring. Analgesic efficacy is best evaluated using a consistent systematic assessment approach. If S.L. is to remain on chronic NSAID therapy, then monitoring her liver and renal function every 3 months for the first year would be reasonable.

Case 43-2, Question 3: One week later after starting naproxen 500 mg twice daily, S.L. has been adherent with therapy and had a basic metabolic panel completed before this office visit. S.L. reported a decrease in pain since she had been started on naproxen. Laboratory values and vital signs obtained at this visit include the following:

BP, 155/78 mm Hg
HR, 88 beats/minute
Height, 66 inches
Weight, 194 pounds
BMI, 30.7 kg/m^2
Sodium, 135 mEq/L
Potassium, 5.5 mEq/L
BUN, 40 mg/dL
Creatinine, 2.2 mg/dL
RBC, 4.7 × 10^6/μL
Hemoglobin, 10.3 g/dL
Hematocrit, 33.8%

What changes, if any, need to be made with her OA therapy?

Gastrointestinal ulceration and bleeding remain a cardinal concern when evaluating patients for treatment of chronic pain in OA. The addition of a PPI to a nonselective NSAID has been proposed as a less expensive alternative to the more expensive COX-2 inhibitor agent, celecoxib. Older patients with OA have comorbidities requiring aspirin in addition to a COX-2 or NSAID. Goldstein et al.[41] compared celecoxib and aspirin with naproxen, lansoprazole, and aspirin with endoscopically diagnosed ulcers after 12 weeks of therapy. Gastrointestinal ulceration rates were found to be statistically insignificant among groups. In contrast, another randomized controlled trial compared celecoxib with diclofenac and omeprazole in patients with OA and rheumatoid arthritis for 6 months. The risk for GI bleeding was evaluated across the small bowel.[42]

There were less lower and upper gastrointestinal events in the celecoxib treatment group. Consideration of clinically significant anemia not responsive to acid-suppressive interventions (PPIs) distal to the duodenum may provide the clinician with more evidence in patients at increased risk for GI ulceration and bleeding. The results are suggestive of better clinical outcomes with celecoxib versus diclofenac and omeprazole.[42] These results are interesting because they contrast with results found in previous studies. Additionally, it is unknown whether the results found with diclofenac can be extrapolated to naproxen or other NSAIDs. Clearly, further investigation is warranted before changes in practice are suggested. A meta-analysis based on epidemiologic studies illustrates the safety of celecoxib with regard to risk for GI ulceration and bleeding. Additionally, NSAIDs with long half-lives and slow-release formulations were found to demonstrate higher risks for GI events. Higher relative risk (RR) for GI bleeding (>5) was associated with naproxen, indomethacin, ketoprofen, ketorolac, and piroxicam, whereas a lower RR (<5) was found for ibuprofen, diclofenac, celecoxib, meloxicam, rofecoxib, and aceclofenac.[43]

The most frequent reason for withdrawal from this year-long trial was GI adverse events for both medications; however, abnormal liver function tests caused more patients taking diclofenac to withdraw from the study.[42] Diclofenac is associated with elevations in alanine aminotransferase and aspartate aminotransferase levels; however, increases in aminotransferase levels alone are not predictive of liver injury. The FDA recognizes increases in both bilirubin and aminotransferase levels as surrogate markers for drug-induced liver disease. In a study completed by Laine et al.,[44] the risk of hospitalization associated with diclofenac therapy is described as relatively rare (0.023% per 100,000 patient-years). The low rate of hospitalization may be secondary to clinical

Table 43-3
Recommendations for Nonpharmacologic and Pharmacologic Treatments by OA Site[14]

OA Site	Nonpharmacologic Recommendations	Pharmacologic Recommendations
Hand	Evaluate ability to perform ADLs Instruct in joint protection techniques Provide assistance devices, as needed, to help patients perform ADLs Instruct in use of thermal agents for relief of pain and stiffness Provide splints for patients with trapeziometacarpal joint OA	Topical capsaicin Topical/oral NSAIDs, including trolamine salicylate and COX-2 selective inhibitors (patients ≥75 years should use topical NSAIDs) Tramadol **Discourage** Intra-articular therapies (corticosteroids, hyaluronates) Opioid analgesics
Knee	**Participate in aerobic and/or resistance land-based exercise** **Participate in aquatic exercise** **Lose weight (if overweight)** Participate in self-management programs ± psychosocial interventions Use thermal agents and manual therapy in combination with PT-supervised exercise Use medially directed patellar taping Participate in tai chi programs Receive walking aids, as needed If lateral compartment OA, wear medially wedged insoles If medial compartment OA, wear laterally wedged subtalar strapped insoles Some moderate–severe pain patients are candidates for acupuncture or TENS	Acetaminophen Oral/topical NSAIDs Patients ≥75 years should use topical NSAIDs Patients with h/o upper GI ulcer should use COX-2 selective inhibitor or nonselective NSAID + PPI Patients with upper GI bleed ≤1 year ago should use COX-2 selective inhibitor + PPI Tramadol Intra-articular corticosteroid injections Opioids or duloxetine for patients who failed all other therapies and are not candidates for total joint arthroplasty **Discourage** Chondroitin sulfate Glucosamine Topical capsaicin
Hip	**Participate in cardiovascular and/or resistance land-based exercise** **Participate in aquatic exercise** **Lose weight (if overweight)** Participate in self-management programs ± psychosocial interventions Use thermal agents and manual therapy in combination with PT-supervised exercise Receive walking aids, as needed	Acetaminophen Oral NSAIDs Tramadol Intra-articular corticosteroid injections Opioids for patients who failed all other therapies and are not candidates for total joint arthroplasty **Discourage** Chondroitin sulfate Glucosamine

vigilance. This study also found elevations in liver function test concentrations to occur in the initial 4 to 6 months of therapy and does not necessarily parallel clinical significant liver injury.

TRAMADOL AND OPIOIDS

In the week that has passed, there has been an increase in potassium, serum creatinine, and BUN. COX-2 preferential and nonselective inhibitors have the same potential to cause adverse renal effects. Naproxen should be discontinued, and additional monitoring should be ordered to ensure laboratory values return to baseline. The drop in hemoglobin may also be concerning, and appropriate follow-up with either endoscopy or stool occult blood testing should be considered.

CASE 43-2, QUESTION 4: S.L. has seen commercials on television advertising "knee injections." Describe the available therapeutic options.

In many patients with contraindications or subtherapeutic response to acetaminophen, NSAIDs, or COX-2 inhibitors, a trial of tramadol should be considered. Therapeutic alternatives for analgesia are now limited to opioids or tramadol for S.L. Tramadol is a centrally acting analgesic that binds to the mu-opioid receptor and also inhibits the uptake of norepinephrine and serotonin.[45] The ACR recommends tramadol in those patients who have failed or have contraindications to NSAIDs.[14] Tramadol should not be used in patients with a history of seizures or receiving medications with serotonergic activity and requires dose adjustment with diminished renal function.[45,46] Tramadol can be used with acetaminophen, and the combination can be therapeutic.[47] However, she is taking citalopram for depression, and there is a potential drug interaction with tramadol; therefore, this combination should be judiciously considered. Opioid/acetaminophen combinations may be a short-term option in the interim while S.L. is being evaluated for intra-articular injection of either corticosteroid or viscosupplementation (hyaluronic acid injection) by her physician.

In patients in whom the use of tramadol is ineffective or contraindicated, the use of an opioid or opioid/acetaminophen combination can be considered.[48] Side effects from opioids include constipation, confusion, hallucinations, respiratory depression, tolerance, and addiction. A recent Cochrane review evaluated the use of oral and transdermal nontramadol opioids in the treatment of OA of the hip and knee.[49] Although the findings did conclude opioids are effective, their modest benefits are outweighed by their side effect profiles and should thus be avoided. Randomized, placebo-controlled studies have pointed to the efficacy and tolerability of transdermal buprenorphine with or without concurrent acetaminophen in the treatment of hip or knee OA, although long-term safety cannot be concluded at this time.[50,51]

DULOXETINE

Duloxetine, a serotonin and norepinephrine reuptake inhibitor, has been approved for the treatment of chronic musculoskeletal pain, in addition to several other indications. In a 13-week randomized, double-blind, placebo-controlled trial involving 231 patients, duloxetine demonstrated statistically significant reductions in osteoarthritic pain of the knee.[52] The magnitude of difference in average pain between duloxetine and placebo in the reported mean end points and the mean change from baseline was modest, yet the tolerability and adverse effect profile of this medication are preferable to other potential treatment modalities. S.L. is currently receiving citalopram for the treatment of major depressive disorder. The risk-to-benefit analysis of switching citalopram to duloxetine has many considerations. The treatment of the depression and the significant medical history of the patient need to be carefully assessed. S.L. has a past medical history of recurrent depression resistant to several different medications and has been stable for the last year on citalopram. Next, tolerability and cost need to be evaluated because duloxetine may have a higher copay than citalopram, despite both agents' availability as a nonbranded product. Should S.L. be switched to duloxetine for treatment of OA-related pain and depression, she should be counseled on the risk for transient headaches, nausea, and less frequently diarrhea. Liver transaminases are also recommended for periodic monitoring. Specific education regarding expected treatment results should also be provided because the onset of analgesia with duloxetine may be delayed following initiation. Given her concurrent diagnosis of depression, her mood should be reassessed frequently during the transition.

Intra-Articular Therapy

Ultimately, many patients fail oral or topical therapies, and intra-articular (IA) injections represent the last conservative efforts before surgical intervention for OA of the knee. Aspiration of synovial fluid and injections of glucocorticoids or viscosupplementation of hyaluronic acid are strategies that have been offered to patients with severe knee OA. Injections of triamcinolone or methylprednisolone with lidocaine 1% have been shown to be effective for approximately 4 to 8 weeks. Typically, IA glucocorticoids are given no more frequently than every 3 months. Side effects include a paradoxical localized inflammatory reaction.[53]

In a small multicenter, randomized trial, the safety and efficacy of IA treatment with hyaluronic acid in OA of the knee was demonstrated. However, there was a rather large placebo response and a small effect size with treatment in this trial.[54] In a 2005 meta-analysis, intra-articular hyaluronic acid supplementation did not demonstrate clinical efficacy in OA of the knee.[55] In contrast, a more recent Cochrane review found intra-articular injection of hyaluronic acid products to be effective and provide more sustained clinical effects than intra-articular injections of glucocorticoids. The authors acknowledged considerable product variability and corresponding times to clinical response.[56] A 2009 multicenter, randomized, placebo-controlled trial did not find any efficacy of hyaluronic acid in hip OA.[57] A meta-analysis reviewed studies of both intra-articular corticosteroids and hyaluronic acid in the treatment of OA of the knee. Seven studies including 606 subjects were included. Results suggest IA corticosteroids are comparatively more effective from baseline to week 4, after which IA hyaluronic acid appears to have greater durability of effect.[58]

CASE 43-2, QUESTION 5: Two years have passed, and S.L. has now failed all conservative strategies including intra-articular injections into her knee. After discussing all of her options with her physician, S.L. is referred to an orthopedic surgeon for elective left total knee replacement. She is awaiting discharge from the acute care hospital, pending transfer to a short-term rehabilitation facility to facilitate her return to home, and resumption of her previous level of function. S.L.'s current medications are metoprolol succinate 50 mg daily, lisinopril 20 mg daily, citalopram 20 mg daily, enoxaparin 30 mg subcutaneously twice daily, oxycodone CR 10 mg every 12 hours, senna/docusate one tablet twice daily, and oxycodone/acetaminophen 5 mg/325 mg one tablet every 4 hours as needed for moderate pain and two tablets every 4 hours as needed for severe pain. S.L. asks you, as the counseling pharmacist, why she still needs "shots in the belly?"

The American College of Chest Physicians (ACCP)' highest level of evidence for elective knee arthroplasty recommends low-molecular-weight heparin, fondaparinux, dabigatran, apixaban, rivaroxaban or warfarin (international normalized ratio [INR] goal of 2.5) for patients in whom a risk for significant bleeding does not exist. A minimal duration of therapy is for 10 days after surgery and up to 35 days for some patients.[59] It is important to educate S.L. with this information, providing the reason for enoxaparin is to prevent blood clots in her legs or lungs. In cases in which the creatinine clearance is less than 30 mL/minute, the appropriate dosage of enoxaparin would be 30 mg subcutaneously once daily.[60]

CASE 43-2, QUESTION 6: How long will S.L. need oxycodone CR and oxycodone/acetaminophen therapy?

Patients typically need the sustained-release dosing of their opioid analgesic given on a routine schedule only while undergoing aggressive physical and occupational therapy immediately after orthopedic surgery. By the time most patients return to their home environments, the use of as-needed dosing of opioid/acetaminophen combinations may be necessary for the completion of the short-term rehabilitation process. However, the long-term use of opioids in the treatment of chronic pain should be discouraged unless the benefits greatly outweigh the risks.

Comorbid Conditions in the Elderly

CASE 43-3

QUESTION 1: L.P. is a 76-year-old woman who was recently admitted to the hospital for elective right total hip replacement. She had failed all previous conservative interventions. Her medical history is significant for type 2 diabetes, hypertension, dyslipidemia, OA left knee and right hip, a right knee replacement 2 years ago, coronary artery disease, and history of myocardial infarction 1 year ago. Medications include glipizide 10 mg daily in the morning before breakfast, metformin 850 mg twice daily, lisinopril 20 mg daily, atorvastatin 40 mg daily, metoprolol succinate 100 mg daily, rivaroxaban 10 mg once daily with dinner, aspirin 81 mg once daily, celecoxib 200 mg once daily, and oxycodone/acetaminophen 5 mg/325 mg one tablet every 4 hours as needed for right hip pain. Identify L.P.'s risks associated with COX-2 inhibitor use.

The risks associated with nonselective NSAID or COX-2 inhibitor use in older adults with comorbid coronary artery disease include increased blood pressure, heart failure, and worse cardiovascular outcomes. Additionally, diminished renal function and gastrointestinal bleeding risks are relevant and require careful follow-up and monitoring. The lowest effective nonselective NSAID or COX-2 inhibitor dose for the shortest duration would possibly be recommended in situations where continued therapy is clinically indicated.

CASE 43-3, QUESTION 2: Identify any drug–drug interactions that would be clinically significant relative to L.P.'s prophylaxis for deep vein thrombosis after hip replacement surgery.

Caution is encouraged when combining medications to rivaroxaban that may increase the risk of bleeding.[61] In this case, LP requires aspirin for cardiovascular protection after the myocardial infarction. Additionally, celecoxib was added for pain management following hip replacement surgery. The addition of antiplatelet agents and NSAIDs to oral anticoagulant therapy increases the risk for bleeding. A careful evaluation of the risks and benefits of combination therapy would suggest discontinuation of the COX-2 inhibitor.

Dietary Supplements

Dietary supplements offer patients an alternative to prescription medications. Some patients often either fail multiple prescription drugs or have intolerable side effects. Others confuse dietary supplements with natural products and consider them safer than traditional medications. In the case of OA, the role of glucosamine, chondroitin, and the combination products has represented such an alternative to many patients. As with any OTC dietary supplement, the vigor of product consistency and standardization are not equal to FDA requirements for legend drugs. Researchers have found in evaluating the use of glucosamine, chondroitin, and the combinations in OA of the knee that they were all ineffective in reducing pain. However, it is worth noting that treatment effects were more pronounced in the subgroup of patients with moderate-to-severe reports of pain. Also, this trial included a celecoxib treatment group that also did not reach statistical significance with regard to primary outcomes measured.[62] Similar findings were published, concluding the lack of efficacy with glucosamine in treatment of OA of the hip as well as degenerative lumbar OA.[63–65] More recently, in a double-blind, multicenter trial, the combination of glucosamine and chondroitin was compared with celecoxib in patients with osteoarthritis of the knee.[66] The results of this trial in approximately 600 patients demonstrated noninferiority of the glucosamine with chondroitin compared to celecoxib after 6 months for the primary outcome of reduced pain.

Nontraditional alternatives for the pain, stiffness, and discomfort of OA are few and certainly lack the vigor of large-scale, long-term, clinical trials. However, in selected patients who wish to try glucosamine/chondroitin, a time-limited trial can be considered in patients who fail or refuse more traditional approaches to pharmacologic management. However, a general recommendation cannot be made for all patients.

KEY REFERENCES AND WEBSITES

A full list of references for this chapter can be found at http://thepoint.lww.com/AT11e. Below are the key references and websites for this chapter, with the corresponding reference number in this chapter found in parentheses after the reference.

Key References

Fernandes L et al. EULAR recommendations for the non-pharmacological core management of hip and knee osteoarthritis. *Ann Rheum Dis*. 2013;72(7):1125–1135. (17)

Lanza FL et al. Guidelines for prevention of NSAID-related ulcer complications. *Am J Gastroenterol*. 2009;104:728. (30)

McAlindon TE et al. OARSI guidelines for the non-surgical management of knee osteoarthritis. *Osteoarthritis Cartilage*. 2014;22(3):363–388. (11)

Hochberg MC et al. American College of Rheumatology 2012 recommendations for the use of nonpharmacologic and pharmacologic therapies in osteoarthritis of the hand, hip, and knee. *Arthritis Care Res (Hoboken)*. 2012;64(4):465–474. (14)

Key Website

Centers for Disease Control and Prevention. Osteoarthritis. http://www.cdc.gov/arthritis/basics/osteoarthritis.htm. Accessed May 18, 2015. (1)

44 Rheumatoid Arthritis

Steven W. Chen, Rory E. Kim, and Candace Tan

CORE PRINCIPLES

		CHAPTER CASES
1	Rheumatoid arthritis (RA) is a chronic systemic inflammatory disorder characterized by potentially deforming polyarthritis and a wide spectrum of extra-articular manifestations. Diagnosis of RA is based on joint involvement, serology, acute-phase reactants, and symptom duration.	**Case 44-1 (Questions 1, 2)**
2	Treatments for RA include nonpharmacologic (heat or cold therapy, range-of-motion [ROM] exercises, physical therapy, and occupational therapy) and pharmacologic options (nonsteroidal anti-inflammatory drugs [NSAIDs], synthetic [conventional and targeted] and biologic disease-modifying antirheumatic drugs [DMARDs], and corticosteroids). NSAIDs are for symptom management only and must be used cautiously, if at all, because of serious health risks, including gastrointestinal complications and thromboembolic cardiovascular events.	**Case 44-1 (Questions 3–5)** **Case 44-2 (Question 1)** **Case 44-3 (Questions 1, 2)** **Case 44-4 (Question 1)** **Case 44-5 (Questions 1–3)**
3	Owing to the destructive nature of the disease, DMARDs should be initiated as soon as possible once diagnosis has been established. Methotrexate is the most common selection because of efficacy, safety, rapid onset, and cost-effectiveness. Other traditional DMARDs and combinations of traditional DMARDs are selected based on disease severity, disease duration, and the presence of poor prognostic indicators. Regardless of the DMARD chosen, all require diligent monitoring.	**Case 44-5 (Questions 4–7)** **Case 44-6 (Questions 1–7)** **Case 44-7 (Questions 1–5)**
4	Patients with RA, who experience an inadequate response to traditional DMARD monotherapy or intolerable adverse effects, should consider the addition of or switching to a biologic DMARD. Diligent monitoring is also critical with biologic agents owing to the risk of serious adverse effects such as infections and lymphoma.	**Case 44-7 (Questions 6–8)** **Case 44-8 (Question 1)** **Case 44-9 (Question 1)**
5	Corticosteroids when used judiciously at the lowest effective doses and for limited duration, are very effective at quickly controlling inflammation while awaiting onset of DMARD therapy. Although systemic corticosteroids can be prescribed for short-term flares of RA disease activity, intra-articular corticosteroid injections are very effective at managing flares that are limited to a few joints and are not associated with the adverse effects of systemic therapy.	**Case 44-10 (Questions 1, 2)**
6	Juvenile idiopathic arthritis (JIA) describes an assortment of arthritis conditions affecting children and adolescents. Symptoms of JIA, such as joint inflammation and ROM limitation, are present before 16 years of age. As in RA, the diagnosis of JIA is based on clinical manifestations, and all infectious, traumatic, and other etiologies must be ruled out.	**Case 44-11 (Questions 1, 2)**
7	Many nonpharmacologic treatment options are also available to supplement JIA pharmacologic therapy, including exercise, massage, and physical and occupational therapies.	**Case 44-11 (Question 3)**
8	Pharmacologic treatment options for JIA include NSAIDs, traditional and biologic DMARDs, and corticosteroids.	**Case 44-11 (Questions 4–9)** **Case 44-12 (Question 1)** **Case 44-13 (Questions 1, 2)**

EPIDEMIOLOGY

Arthritis refers to more than 100 different joint diseases causing swelling, pain and damage to joints and connective tissue.[1] Rheumatoid arthritis (RA) is the most common chronic inflammatory arthritis and is characterized by potentially deforming polyarthritis and a wide spectrum of extra-articular manifestations resulting from abnormal systemic immune response. It has an estimated worldwide prevalence of 0.5 to 1%, although rates vary between geographic regions.[2,3] In the United States alone, RA afflicts 1.3 million adults, occurring 2 to 3 times more often in women than in men.[3,4] RA prevalence increases with age, with the average age increasing from 63.3 years in 1965 to 66.8 years in 1995. These patterns predict that RA-associated morbidity, mortality, and disability will rise in future years, especially as the United States' baby boomer generation ages.[4]

ETIOLOGY

The exact etiology of RA is unknown, but like many autoimmune diseases it involves interplay among multiple factors including genetic susceptibility, environmental influences, and effects of advancing age on somatic changes in the musculoskeletal and immune system.[3] The onset of RA likely starts years before clinical symptoms develop with activation of specific genes, resulting in innate immunity activity leading the cascade of events.[3] It is suspected that genetics contribute 50% to 60% of the risk of developing RA. The genes with the strongest implication include the *HLA-DRB1* gene of the major histocompatibility complex (MHC) and chromosome 1's *PTPN22* gene. Cigarette smoking increases the production of rheumatoid factor (RF) and anti–cyclic citrullinated peptide antibody (anti-CCP), clinical markers associated with RA, and has been shown to double the risk of developing RA.[5,6] Female sex hormones may also play a role in RA development. In women, peak incidence occurs at the fifth decade, a time when many enter menopause or perimenopause. Estrogen is known to stimulate the immune system; pregnant patients often experience a remission of RA symptoms, and women who take oral contraceptives appear to be somewhat protected against the development of RA.[2,5] Diets rich in fish, olive oil, and other omega-3 fatty acid sources are associated with a lower risk of developing RA.[5]

PATHOPHYSIOLOGY

Pharmacologic therapy for RA targets components of the inflammatory cascade which lead to persistent inflammation of the synovial lining and ultimately cause joint destruction.[7] This normally thin membrane proliferates and transforms into the synovial pannus. The pannus, a highly erosive enzyme-laden inflammatory exudate, invades articular cartilage (leading to narrowing of joint spaces), erodes bone (resulting in osteoporosis), and destroys periarticular structures (ligaments, tendons), resulting in joint deformities (Fig. 44-1).[7,8]

Under normal circumstances, the body can distinguish between self (i.e., proteins found within the body) and nonself (i.e., foreign substances such as bacteria and viruses). On occasion, immune cells (T or B lymphocytes) can react to a self-protein while developing in the thymus or bone marrow. These developing cells are usually killed or inactivated before release from their place of formation; sometimes, however, a self-targeted immune cell can escape destruction and become activated years later to initiate an autoimmune response. Some experts believe the activation of RA is initiated by bacteria (possibly Streptococcus) or a virus containing a protein with an amino acid sequence similar to tissue protein, but this assertion remains disputable.[5] When the activation source (i.e., the self-targeted immune cell) reaches the joint, complex cell–cell interactions take place, leading to the pathology associated with RA.

The initiating interaction for an autoimmune response takes place between antigen-presenting cells (APC), which display complexes of class II MHC molecules, and CD4-lineage T cell lymphocytes (Fig. 44-2). In addition, B cells (previously thought to have little to do with the inflammatory response) can become activated, leading to antibody formation (including RF and anti-CCP), proinflammatory cytokine production, and accumulation of polymorphonuclear leukocytes that release cytotoxins and other substances destructive to the synovium and joint structures. B cells also act as APCs, leading to T cell activation and acceleration of the inflammatory process.[7,8] T cell activation requires two signals: (1) an antigen-specific signal occurring when a class II MHC antigen molecule on an APC binds to a T cell receptor and (2) binding of CD39 on the T cell to either CD80 or CD86 on the APC. T cell activation leads to activation of macrophages and secretion of cytokines, polypeptides that serve as important mediators of inflammation, and cytotoxins, which can directly destroy cells and tissues. Proinflammatory cytokines, such as interleukin (IL) 1 and TNF-α, stimulate both synovial fibroblasts

Figure 44-1 Overview of joint changes in rheumatoid arthritis.

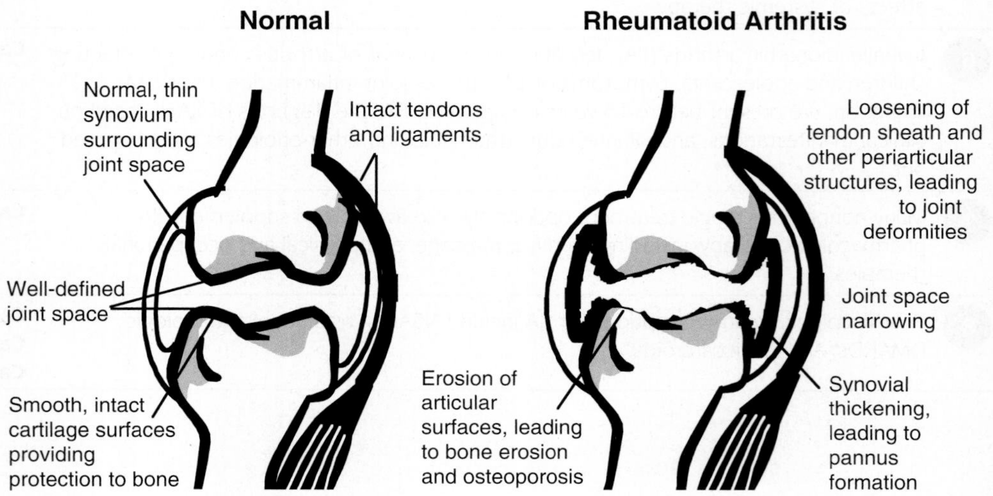

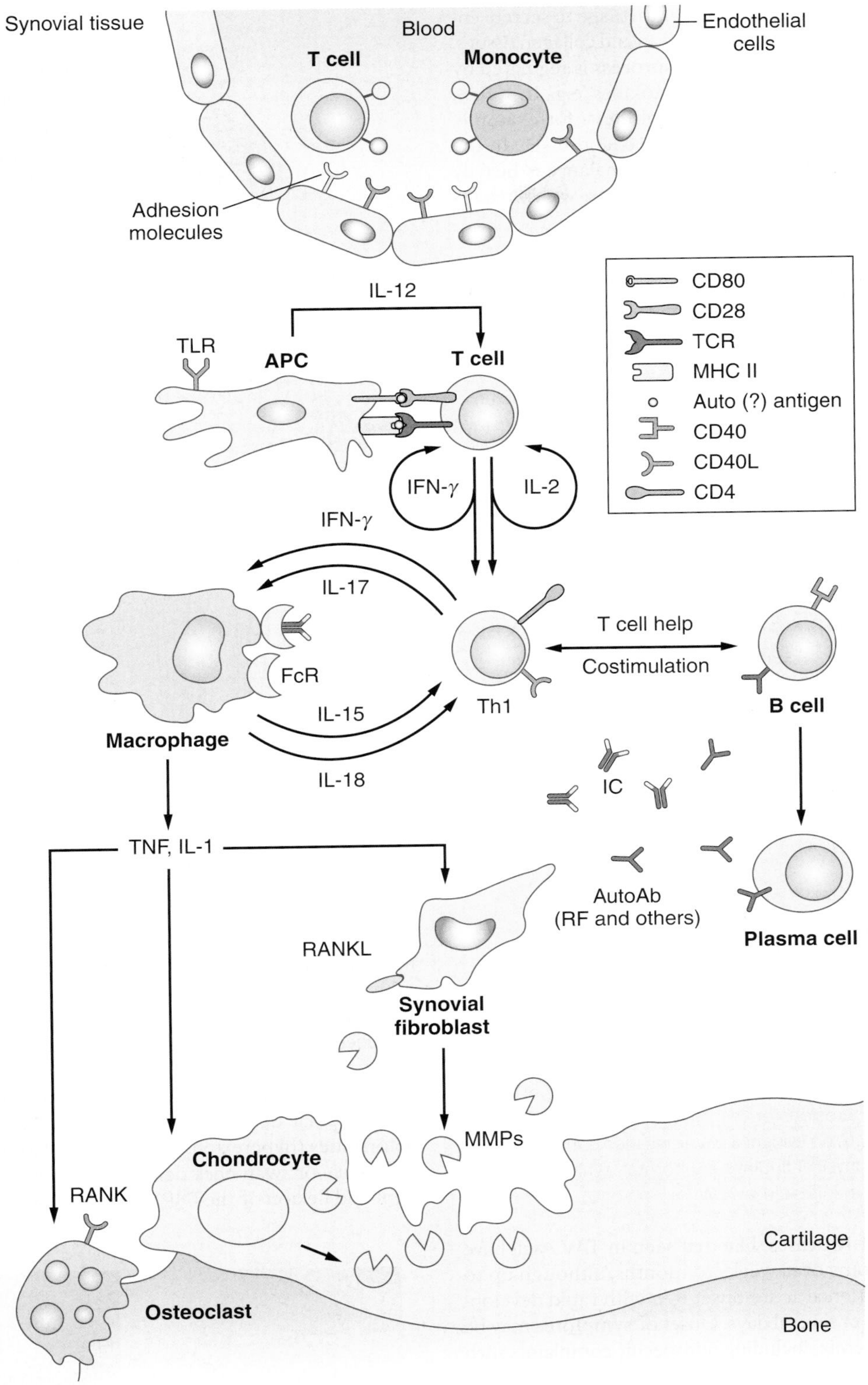

Figure 44-2 Schematic representation of events occurring in rheumatoid arthritis. T cells invading the synovial membrane are primarily CD4+ memory cells, which produce interleukin-2 (IL-2) and interferon-γ (IFN-γ) to a similar extent as antigen-triggered T cells, and which are either already preactivated or become (further) activated by antigen-presenting cells (APCs) in conjunction with arthrogenic (auto) antigen(s) and appropriate major histocompatibility complex (MHC) class II molecules, costimulation (mainly through CD80, CD81, and CD28) and certain cytokines (IL-1, IL-15, IL-18). Through cell–cell contact (e.g., through CD11- and CD69-mediation) and through different cytokines, such as IFN-γ, tumor necrosis factor-α (TNF-α), and IL-17, these T cells activate monocytes, macrophages, and synovial fibroblasts. The latter then overproduce proinflammatory cytokines, mainly TNF-α, IL-1, and IL-6, which seems to constitute the pivotal event leading to chronic inflammation. Through complex signal transduction cascades, these cytokines activate a variety of genes characteristic of inflammatory responses, including genes coding for various cytokines and matrix metalloproteinases (MMPs) involved in tissue degradation. Tumor necrosis factor-α and IL-1 also induce RANK expression on macrophages, which when interfering with RANKL on stromal cells or T cells, differentiate into osteoclasts that resorb and destroy bone. In addition, chondrocytes also become activated, leading to the release of MMPs. Initial events might also involve activation of APCs through Toll-like receptors (TLRs) before T cell engagement. RANK, receptor activator of nuclear factor-κB; RANKL, RANK ligand; RF, rheumatoid factor; TCR, T cell receptor. Reprinted with permission from Smolen JS, Steiner G. Therapeutic strategies for rheumatoid arthritis. *Nat Rev Drug Discov*. 2003;2:473.

and chondrocytes in neighboring articular cartilage to secrete enzymes that cause degradation of proteoglycan and collagen tissues. In healthy individuals, the inflammatory process is regulated by balancing the ratios of proinflammatory cytokines (e.g., IL-1, IL-6, and TNF-α) with anti-inflammatory cytokines—for example, IL-1 receptor antagonist (IL-1Ra), IL-4, IL-10, and IL-11. In the synovium of patients with RA, however, this balance is heavily weighted toward the proinflammatory cytokines, which results in sustained inflammation and tissue destruction.

Clinical Presentation, Diagnosis, and Disease Course

CASE 44-1

QUESTION 1: T.W., a previously healthy 42-year-old, 60-kg woman, has been suffering from morning stiffness that persists for several hours, fatigue, and generalized muscle and joint pain for the past 4 months. In addition, she reports that her eyes seem red most of the time and are unusually dry. Her symptoms have been much worse during the past month and a half, causing her to limit her physical activities somewhat. She also can no longer wear her wedding ring because of swelling of her hand. Physical examination reveals bilaterally symmetrical swelling, tenderness, and warmth of the metacarpophalangeal (MCP) and proximal interphalangeal (PIP) joints of the hands and the metatarsophalangeal (MTP) joints of the feet.

Pertinent laboratory findings include the following:

ESR, 52 mm/hour (reference range: males 0 to 15 mm/hour, females 0 to 20 mm/hour)[9]
CRP, 2.1 mg/dL (reference range: 0 to 0.5 mg/dL)
Hemoglobin, 10.6 g/dL
Hematocrit, 33%
Platelets, 480,000/μL
Albumin, 3.8 g/dL
Serum iron, 40 mcg/dL
Total iron-binding capacity, 275 mg/dL
Positive anti-CCP at 82 units (reference range: <20 units/mL)
Positive RF performed by latex fixation method in a dilution of 1:320 (reference range: <1:80)

Tests for antinuclear antibodies (ANA) and tuberculin sensitivity are negative. Her uric acid level is normal. Radiographic films of the hands and feet show soft tissue swelling, narrowing of joint spaces, and marginal erosions of the second and third MCP and PIP joints bilaterally with no evidence of calcification. Other routine laboratory data and physical findings are normal. What signs and symptoms of RA are manifested by T.W.?

More than 50% of RA cases, like that seen in T.W., will have slow onset of symptoms over weeks to months, although up to 15% of patients experience acute-onset RA, with rapid development of symptoms over several days. Onset of symptoms may be either articular or systemic, including nonspecific complaints such as fatigue, weakness, muscle pains, weight loss, and low-grade fever. Joint involvement is characterized by soft tissue swelling and warmth, decreased range-of-motion (ROM), and sometimes muscle atrophy around affected joints. Most common complaints include pain and stiffness in multiple joints. Classically, as illustrated by T.W., presentation is symmetrical involving wrists, proximal interphalangeal joints, and metacarpophalangeal joints, although asymmetrical joint involvement also occurs with symmetry developing later in the disease course. The peripheral joints of the hands, wrists, and feet are usually involved first. Reflective of joint inflammation, patients usually experience prolonged morning stiffness on awakening lasting at least 30 to 45 minutes, but it can be present all day with decreasing intensity after arising.[10,11]

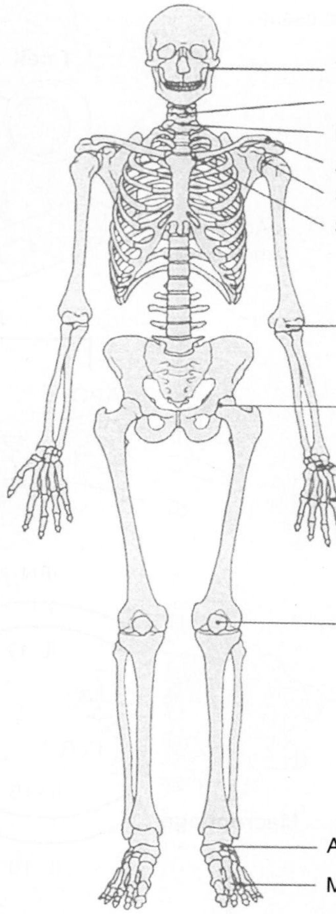

Figure 44-3 Frequency of involvement of different joint sites in established rheumatoid arthritis. MCPs, metacarpophalangeal joints; MTPs, metatarsophalangeal joints; PIPs, proximal interphalangeal joints.

Morning stiffness lasting for more than 1 hour rarely occurs in other diseases outside of RA.[12]

Ultimately, any or all of the diarthrodial joints (elbows, knees, shoulders, ankles, hips, temporomandibular joints, sternoclavicular joints, and glenohumeral joints) can be involved (Fig. 44-3). Progressive disease is characterized by irreversible joint deformities, such as ulnar deviation of the fingers (Fig. 44-4), boutonniere deformities (hyperextension of the DIP joint and flexion of the PIP joint), or swan neck deformities (hyperextension of the PIP joint and flexion of the DIP joint) (Fig. 44-5). Similar irreversible

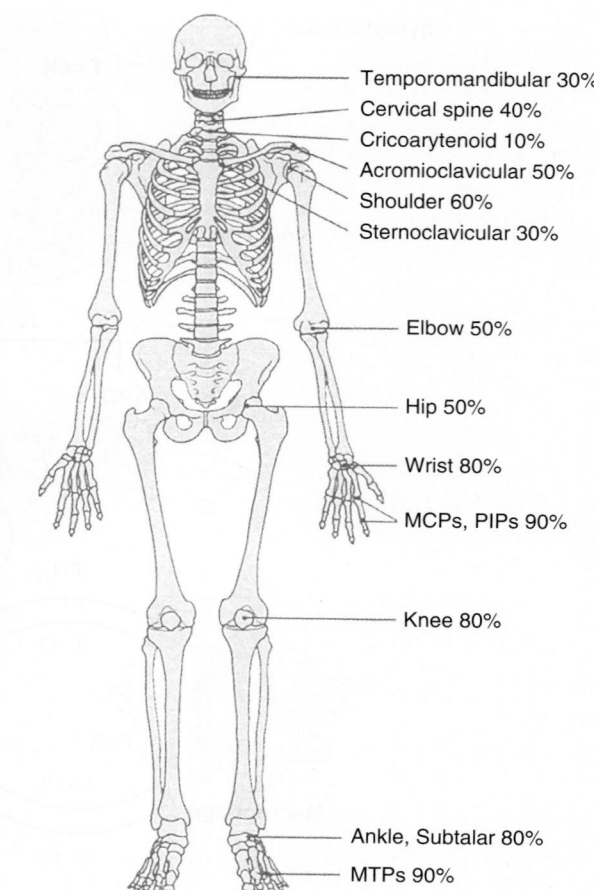

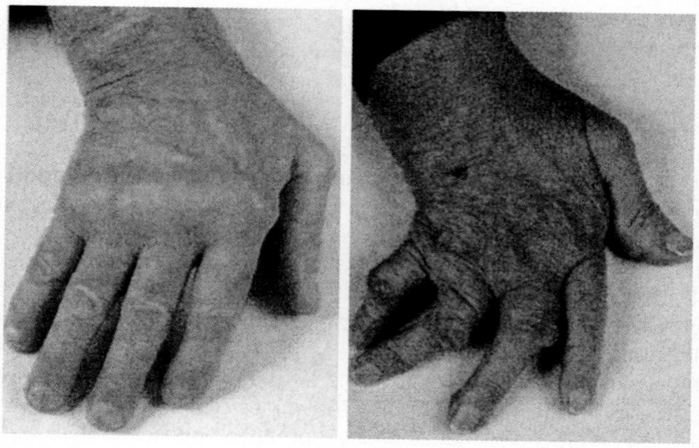

Figure 44-4 Ulnar deviation and metacarpophalangeal synovitis (left). This may progress to more marked lateral deviation with subluxation of the extensor tendons (right finger; right).

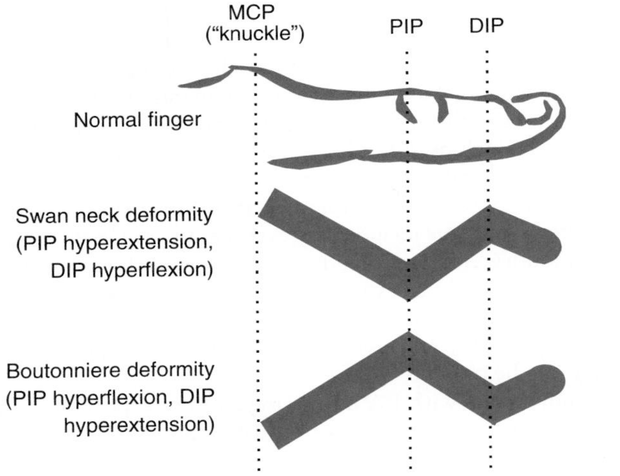

Figure 44-5 Characteristic finger deformities in rheumatoid arthritis. DIP, distal interphalangeal joint; MCP, metacarpophalangeal joint; PIP, proximal interphalangeal joint.

Table 44-1
Criteria for Diagnosis of Rheumatoid Arthritis

Criteria	Score[a]
Joint Involvement	
1 large joint[b]	0
2–10 large joints	1
1–3 small joints[c]	2
4–10 small joints	3
>10 small joints	5
Serology[d] (≥1 result needed)	
Negative RF and negative anti-CCP	0
Low-positive RF or low-positive anti-CCP	2
High-positive RF or high-positive anti-CCP	3
Acute-Phase Reactants	
Normal CRP and normal ESR	0
Abnormal CRP or abnormal ESR	1
Duration of symptoms	
<6 weeks	0
≥6 weeks	1

[a]Score-based algorithm: add score of all categories; score of ≥6/10 needed to classify patient as having definite RA.
[b]Shoulders, elbows, hips, knees, and ankles.
[c]metacarpophalangeal, proximal interphalangeal, second through fifth metatarsophalangeal, thumb interphalangeal joints and wrists.
[d]negative, IU ≤ upper limit of normal (ULN); low-positive, IU higher than ULN but ≤3 times ULN; high-positive, >3 times ULN; if RF assay only available as positive or negative, positive RF interpreted as low-positive.
Source: Aletaha D et al. 2010 rheumatoid arthritis classification criteria: an American College of Rheumatology/European League Against Rheumatism collaborative initiative [published correction appears in *Ann Rheum Dis*. 2010;69:1892]. *Ann Rheum Dis*. 2010;69:1580.
anti-CCP, anti–cyclic citrullinated peptide; CRP, C-reactive protein; ESR, erythrocyte sedimentation rate; RA, rheumatoid arthritis; RF, rheumatoid factor.

deformities can also involve the feet. Patients with more aggressive disease (multiple joint involvement, positive RF) have a greater than 70% probability of developing joint damage or erosions within 2 years of disease onset.[13]

Case 44-1, Question 2: Which laboratory values in T.W. could be used to monitor her RA disease progression?

Physical assessment of an RA patient is fundamental to monitoring and evaluating patient course. For instructions on how to perform a basic musculoskeletal examination, go to http://meded.ucsd.edu/clinicalmed/joints.htm and scroll to select either knee, shoulder, hand, hip, or lower back examinations.

In 2010, the American College of Rheumatology (ACR) and European League Against Rheumatism (EULAR) developed new classification criteria for RA. In comparison to criteria previously outlined in 1987, the intent of the new classification was to identify patients early in disease development so that therapeutic intervention can be initiated as soon as possible, ultimately decreasing disease progression and improving clinical outcomes.[14]

Because no single chemical or laboratory finding is specific for the disease, the diagnosis of RA is based on multiple clinical criteria (Table 44-1). Individuals presenting with clinical synovitis (swelling) not explained by other differential diagnoses such as systemic lupus erythematosus, psoriatic arthritis, or gout, among others, should be tested for RA. RA criteria in the new classification system include quantifying joint involvement and symptom duration as well as detecting presence of autoantibodies and acute-phase reactants.[11,14–16] Using a score-based algorithm based on these four categories, a summative score of 6 or more out of a total possible score of 10, as seen in T.W., suggests RA.[14]

Individually, each of the laboratory findings is characteristic for chronic systemic inflammatory disease with no test being specific for RA, although rheumatoid factor (RF) and anti–citrullinated peptide (anti-CCP) are more definitive than erythrocyte sedimentation rate (ESR) or C-reactive protein (CRP).[9] Specifically, autoimmune diseases are frequently characterized by autoantibodies, with 50% to 80% of RA individuals having RF, anti-CCP, or both.[11,15,16]

RF, an IgM or IgG autoantibody, abnormally reacts with the Fc portion of IgG to form an immune complex. It is found in 75% to 80% of patients with RA. It may also present in up to 5% of healthy individuals and in patients with diseases other than RA, including almost any condition associated with either immune complex formation or with hypergammaglobulinemia (e.g., chronic infections, lymphoproliferative and hepatic diseases, systemic lupus erythmatosus, and Sjogren's syndrome). An RF titer of at least 1:160 is considered a positive test and most patients with RA, such as T.W., typically have titers of at least 1:320.[9,17] Overall, RF is neither sensitive nor specific enough to independently diagnose RA, but it is found in the majority of patients and a higher titer early in disease generally correlates with increased disease severity and progression.[18]

Citrulline, a nonstandard amino acid, is also established as a key component of RA antigenicity and is more specific for RA than RF. Citrullinated proteins and anti-CCP antibodies are abundant in inflamed RA synovium. Anti-CCP antibodies can be detected in 50% to 60% of early RA patients, and the specificity of anti-CCP is very high at 90% to 95%.[9] Anti-CCP is present as early as 1.5 to 9 years before symptom presentation, suggesting a pathogenic role for these antibodies in RA.[19,20] A positive anti-CCP also correlates with an increased likelihood of a more erosive course of RA than either a negative anti-CCP or a positive RF. In summary, a positive anti-CCP antibody test is highly specific for RA, predictive of the development of RA, is a marker for an erosive disease course, and in combination with positive RF also correlates with 99.5% specificity for RA, making the likelihood of T.W. not having RA very minimal.[9,21]

The nonspecific markers for inflammation include ESR and CRP, but unfortunately these acute-phase responses are also not disease-specific. T.W.'s hematologic findings are consistent with a mild anemia of chronic inflammation. Although her serum iron concentration is decreased, her normal iron-binding capacity makes a diagnosis of iron-deficiency anemia unlikely. Her anemia probably results from a failure of iron release from the reticuloendothelial tissues and would not be expected to respond to iron therapy. The mild thrombocytosis is additional evidence of a systemic inflammatory response. The laboratory manifestations of inflammation should improve with effective drug therapy and, along with many of the clinical features of RA, are useful parameters for monitoring disease activity and response to therapy.

Finally, the test for ANA rules out systemic lupus erythematosus in T.W. The ANA, however, can be positive in 10% to 70% patients with RA.[14]

EXTRA-ARTICULAR MANIFESTATIONS AND COMPLICATIONS

The classic RA presentation involves joint findings; however, RA is a systemic disease reflected by accompanying extra-articular and organ system manifestations that, chronically, can occur in up to 46% of patients. These manifestations are also associated with higher disease activity,[22] and those with systemic involvement have higher mortality rates than those without, suggesting that early treatment may lower both the risk and severity of RA complications.[22,23]

Rheumatoid nodules occur in 15% to 20% of patients and are typically found on extensor surfaces, pressure points, and tendons. Pleuropulmonary manifestations include pulmonary nodules, fibrosis, and pleuritis; interstitial pneumonitis and arteritis of the pulmonary vasculature, although rare, can be potentially life-threatening. Vasculitis occurs infrequently, is more common in patients with long-standing and often severe disease. Complications include skin ulceration, peripheral neuropathy, and arteritis of organs.[10]

Some extra-articular manifestations occur as syndromes. Sjögren syndrome includes dry eyes (keratoconjunctivitis sicca), dry mouth (xerostomia), and connective tissue disease. T.W.'s eye complaints may be an extra-articular manifestation of her RA. Felty syndrome is characterized by chronic arthritis, splenomegaly, and neutropenia; thrombocytopenia, anemia, and lymphadenopathy may also be present.[10]

Individuals with RA have a median life expectancy that is 3 to 10 years shorter than non-RA populations, with lower life expectancy associated with more severe disease.[5,24] The excess mortality has been attributed primarily to accelerated cardiovascular disease, responsible for one-third to one-half of deaths among adults compared with one-fourth to one-fifth of deaths among adults without RA. RA is associated with a twofold to threefold increased rate of myocardial infarction (MI), as well as lower MI survival. Management of cardiovascular risk include annual cardiovascular risk evaluations for all patients, multiplying risk scores by 1.5 for patients with more than one marker of severe disease activity, use of statins and cardiovascular medications known to reduce cardiovascular risk, caution when prescribing nonsteroidal anti-inflammatory drugs (NSAIDs) owing to associated cardiovascular risk, and smoking cessation (Table 44-2).[25] Finally, pericarditis and myocarditis, while rare, may also occur.

Table 44-2

Recommendations for Reducing Cardiovascular Risk[a] in Patients with Rheumatoid Arthritis (Evidence/Strength Rating)[b]

1. Rheumatoid arthritis should be considered as a disease in which cardiovascular risk is elevated, because of both an increased prevalence of traditional cardiovascular risk factors and the inflammatory burden. Although the evidence base is less, this may also apply to ankylosing spondylitis and psoriatic arthritis (2b–3/B).
2. To lower cardiovascular risk, adequate control of arthritis disease activity is necessary (2b–3/B).
3. All patients with rheumatoid arthritis should undergo annual cardiovascular risk evaluation with use of national guidelines. This should also be considered for all patients with ankylosing spondylitis and psoriatic arthritis. When antirheumatic treatment has been changed, risk assessments should be repeated (3–4/C).
4. For patients with rheumatoid arthritis, risk score models should be adapted by introducing a 1.5 multiplication factor when the patient meets two of the following three criteria: disease duration of more than 10 years, rheumatoid factor or anti–cyclic citrullinated peptide positivity, and the presence of certain extra-articular manifestations (3–4/C).
5. When using the Systematic Coronary Risk Evaluation model for determination of cardiovascular risk, triglyceride to high-density lipoprotein cholesterol ratio should be used (3/C).
6. Intervention for cardiovascular risk factor management should be performed according to national guidelines (3/C).
7. Preferred treatment options are statins, angiotensin-converting enzyme inhibitors, or angiotensin II blockers (2a–3/C–D).
8. The effect of cyclo-oxygenase-2 inhibitors and most nonsteroidal anti-inflammatory drugs on cardiovascular risk is not completely determined and should be studied further. Clinicians should therefore be very cautious in prescribing these drugs, especially to patients with cardiovascular risk factors or with documented cardiovascular disease (2a–3/C).
9. When corticosteroids are prescribed, this should be at the lowest possible dose (3/C).
10. Patients should be actively encouraged to stop smoking (3/C).

[a]Cardioprotective treatment is recommended when 10-year cardiovascular risk is above the threshold of "moderate" that is established for each country (i.e., either 10% or 20%).

[b]Level of Evidence: Category 1A, from meta-analysis of randomized, controlled trials; 1B, from at least one randomized, controlled trial; 2A, from at least one controlled study without randomization; 2B, from at least one type of quasi-experimental study; 3, from descriptive studies, such as comparative studies, correlation studies, or case-control studies; 4, from expert committee reports or opinions or from clinical experience of respected authorities; Strength of recommendation directly based on A, category 1 evidence; B, category 2 evidence or extrapolated recommendations from category 1 evidence; C, category 3 evidence or extrapolated recommendations from category 1 or 2 evidence; D, category 4 evidence or extrapolated recommendations from category 2 or 3 evidence.

Source: Peters MJ et al. EULAR evidence-based recommendations for cardiovascular risk management in patients with rheumatoid arthritis and other forms of inflammatory arthritis. *Ann Rheum Dis*. 2010;69:325.

Treatment

The treatment goals of RA are to maximize functional status through maintenance or improvement of symptoms (e.g., joint pain and swelling), preserve joint function, and prevent deformity to ultimately improve quality of life and delay disability. Treatment to achieve remission or lowest possible disease activity involves a combination of interventions. Early initiation of pharmacologic therapy starting at the point of diagnosis is critical to quality RA care.[26–28] Other supportive interventions include rest, exercise and physical therapy, occupational therapy, and emotional support.

CASE 44-1, QUESTION 3: What nonpharmacologic therapy should be included in the management of T.W.'s RA?

Systemic and articular rest (achieved by splinting the affected joints) can reduce inflammation significantly. Restful and adequate sleep are particularly important in chronic, fatigue-inducing diseases such as RA. Therefore, T.W. should rest often especially when experiencing acute inflammation, but daytime rest periods should be limited to 30 to 60 minutes each as prolonged rest can also induce rapid losses in strength and endurance. Splinting of joints is typically prescribed throughout the day and night during periods of active inflammation, then only at night for several weeks after cessation of inflammation.[29]

Passive ROM exercises should be prescribed for T.W. because they minimize muscle atrophy and flexion contractures and maintain joint function without increasing inflammation or radiographic progression of disease.[29,30] Regular aerobic exercises, such as cycling, swimming, or walking, enhance muscle function and joint function as well.[31] Overall, physical and occupational therapies can provide valuable assistance to patients with compromised activities of daily living to maximize the potential for self-sufficiency. Some orthoses—medical devices secured to any part of a patient's body designed to support, immobilize, align, correct, or prevent deformity, or improve functioning—can reduce pain and inflammation or improve joint function in targeted joints for RA patients.[32]

Finally, emotional support should be provided to all patients including T.W. As with all chronic debilitating diseases, the potential loss of independence, self-esteem, and employment, as well as altered interpersonal relationships with friends and family, can result in a twofold to threefold increase in depression.[33,34]

The expertise of different health care disciplines (e.g., physical therapists, social workers, health educators, psychiatrists, clinical psychologists, podiatrists, vocational rehabilitation therapists, and pharmacists) should be consulted depending on T.W.'s needs. Pharmacists in outpatient clinical practices can monitor RA drug therapy for therapeutic and adverse effects under collaborative practice agreements with other practitioners and can counsel patients on proper medication use and clarify expectations.[35]

Insufficient literature evidence is available to support the use of spa therapy and thermotherapies such as ultrasound, electrotherapies (e.g., transcutaneous nerve stimulation and electrostimulation of muscles), and laser therapy in the treatment of RA. Heat treatments in general should be avoided during periods of active joint inflammation because heat can further exacerbate pain and swelling.[36]

While symptoms of RA may be controlled by conservative management, more aggressive therapy is needed to prevent disease progression and disability. Nonsteroidal anti-inflammatory drugs (NSAIDs) are often used to provide rapid anti-inflammatory and analgesic effects. However, they do not prevent or slow joint destruction as compared to the disease-modifying antirheumatic drugs (DMARDs) and should be reserved for rapid symptomatic relief while awaiting DMARD onset of action. DMARDs do alter long-term disease course. As such they are the mainstay of pharmacologic care and should be initiated in all patients as soon as they are diagnosed with RA.[26–28] Specific choice of treatment is individualized based on joint function, degree of disease activity, patient age, sex, occupation, family responsibilities, drug costs, and results of previous therapy. The two classes of DMARDs are synthetic chemical compounds (sDMARDs) and biologic agents (bDMARDs). With the recent advent of tofacitinib, EULAR has further subdivided sDMARDs into the conventional sDMARDs (csDMARDs) and targeted sDMARD (tsDMARD).[26,27]

csDMARDs (e.g., hydroxychloroquine [HCQ], sulfasalazine [SSZ], methotrexate [MTX], and leflunomide [LEF]) have demonstrated the ability to slow disease progression. These agents, alone or in combination, are considered as initial therapy for most patients and in the absence of contraindication, MTX is the treatment of choice because of its strong efficacy and favorable safety profile. Other csDMARDs such as azathioprine [AZA], gold, and D-penicillamine are rarely used because of slow onset of action and toxicity profile.[26,27] The first and only tsDMARD, tofacitinib, is considered in those with moderate-to-severe disease who have failed treatment with or are intolerant to methotrexate.[37]

The bDMARDs, also referred to as anticytokines, biologics, biologic modifiers, or biologic response modifiers, target the physiologic proinflammatory and joint-damaging effects of inflammatory mediators, including TNF-α, IL-1, IL-6, T cell, and B cells. Agents in this class include the TNF-α inhibitors (adalimumab [ADA], certolizumab pegol [CZP], etanercept [ETA], golimumab [GLM], and infliximab [IFX]), anti-IL-1 receptor antagonist (anakinra), anti-B cell therapy (rituximab [RXB]), IL-6 receptor antagonist (tocilizumab [TCZ]), and the T cell modulator (abatacept [ABT]). The bDMARDs are typically reserved for patients who fail to achieve an adequate response with csDMARD monotherapy.[28]

Corticosteroids are also potent anti-inflammatory agents that slow the progression of joint damage in RA. However, long-term systemic use should be avoided because of serious adverse effects associated with chronic therapy. Short-term oral therapy may be reserved as bridge therapy in early RA with moderate-to-high disease activity while awaiting onset of DMARD activity, brief periods of active disease, or with therapy failure.[28] Local intra-articular injections may be used for isolated joints experiencing disease flares.

NONSTEROIDAL ANTI-INFLAMMATORY DRUGS

NSAIDs have a long history of use in RA treatment. They are effective for providing short-term pain and inflammation control but do not alter disease course.[38] In addition, NSAIDs are associated with side effects related to COX inhibition such as GI intolerance, nephrotoxicity, and increased risk of bleeding and cardiovascular events. The cardiovascular risk associated with some agents is particularly concerning since RA patients are at higher cardiovascular mortality risk. Therefore, given both the safety profile and the lack of long-term disease-modifying efficacy, NSAID use should be judicious and reserved only as an adjunct to DMARD therapy.[38,39]

Although NSAIDs differ in chemical structure, they generally have similar pharmacologic properties (e.g., antipyresis, analgesia, anti-inflammatory activity, and inhibition of prostaglandin synthesis), mechanisms of action (i.e., inhibition of COX activity), pharmacokinetic properties (e.g., highly protein bound and extensively metabolized to renally cleared inactive metabolites), and side effect profile.[40] Aspirin, an acetylated salicylate, is the standard against which the effectiveness of all other NSAIDs are measured. Other NSAIDs are available, including nonacetylated salicylates (e.g., salsalate, choline salicylate, and magnesium salicylate) and nonsalicylate or nonaspirin NSAIDs (e.g., ibuprofen, naproxen, and cyclo-oxygenase [COX] inhibitors). (Note: For simplicity and clarity, the term NSAID is used henceforth to describe NSAIDs other than acetylated [i.e., aspirin] and nonacetylated salicylates.)[38–40] Choice of particular NSAID has traditionally been based on cost, duration of action, and patient preference because of interpatient variability in response. Courses of several different NSAIDs, even those within the same chemical class, may be necessary to determine the best choice for an individual patient.

CONVENTIONAL SYNTHETIC DISEASE-MODIFYING ANTIRHEUMATIC DRUGS (csDMARDs)

With rare exception, every patient should receive csDMARD therapy soon after diagnosis to minimize loss of joint integrity, function, and risk of cardiovascular disease related to RA.[26,28] Although csDMARDs have the potential to cause serious toxicity, they can substantially reduce joint inflammation, reduce or prevent joint damage, maintain joint function and integrity, and ultimately reduce health care costs and allow patients to remain productive.[26,27] The onset of action of most csDMARDs is slow over 3 to 6 months; however, SSZ, MTX, and LEF can be beneficial within 1 to 2 months.[38] Several factors must be considered when selecting a csDMARD, including convenience of administration, monitoring requirements, medication and monitoring costs, time to therapeutic onset, and frequency and severity of adverse reactions.

MTX, a folate antimetabolite with immunosuppressive and anti-inflammatory properties, remains the mainstay first-line DMARD because of its relatively rapid onset of action and excellent history of efficacy and safety.[26,28] LEF and SSZ are recommended if a contraindication to MTX is present, or if intolerance to MTX occurs. The primary metabolite of LEF, A77 1726 (M1), is responsible for nearly all of its pharmacologic activity. Although the exact mechanism of M1 is not completely understood, it is known that M1 inhibits dihydro-orotate dehydrogenase, an enzyme in cell mitochondria responsible for catalyzing an important step in de novo pyrimidine synthesis; this is believed to be its main mechanism of action. SSZ appears to induce anti-inflammatory effects through one of its active metabolites, mesalamine, which is believed to inhibit both COX and lipooxygenase. HCQ as monotherapy or in combination may be used for relatively mild cases of RA.[26] The mechanism of anti-inflammatory effect of HCQ may be attributable to inhibition of migration of neutrophils and eosinophils, histamine and serotonin blockade, or inhibition of prostaglandin synthesis. Older csDMARDs such as azathioprine, cyclosporine, minocycline, and gold are no longer recommended because of the superior risk–benefit ratio of other csDMARDs, bDMARDs, and tofacitinib.[28]

TARGETED SYNTHETIC DMARD (tsDMARD)

Tofacitinib was recently placed in its own medication subcategory by ACR and EULAR since the janus kinase (JAK) inhibitor, a targeted molecule involved with inhibition of signal transduction pathways, is mechanistically different from the csDMARDs. Tofacitinib inhibits JAKs, enzymes that stimulate inflammatory cytokines; therefore, inhibition modulates leukocyte function and immune response. It is indicated for individuals with moderate-to-high disease activity who have failed csDMARD monotherapy.[26,28]

BIOLOGIC DMARDS (bDMARDs)

In general, the bDMARDs are reserved for patients who have failed to respond to one or more csDMARDs alone or in combination. The ACR and EULAR guidelines recommend the use of bDMARDs in patients with established RA who experience moderate or high disease activity despite csDMARD monotherapy.[26,28] The ACR guidelines also recommend the use of bDMARDs in early RA (<6 months) in patients with moderate-to-high disease activity despite csDMARD monotherapy.[28] Since the late 1990s a total of nine biologic agents have been approved for RA treatment. The earliest biologic agents targeted proinflammatory cytokines, such as TNF-α and IL-1, which play key roles in the immunopathogenesis of RA.[41] These cytokines are abundant in rheumatoid synovial tissues and fluid. Most cytokines can independently induce expression of the others, and IL-1 is capable of upregulating its own expression.[42] Excessive macrophage-produced cytokines (e.g., TNF-α, IL-1, IL-6, and IL-8) correlate closely with RA disease activity and severity. Most importantly, RA improves when the physiologic action of TNF-α or several different ILs are suppressed. In more recent years, new agents have been developed to target additional key processes in RA, including T cell costimulation, the depletion of CD20+ B cells, and the inhibition of IL-6.[39]

The proinflammatory cytokine TNF-α is produced by activated macrophages and T cells in RA-affected joints. It also plays a role in keeping infections localized by increasing platelet activation and adhesion, resulting in local blood vessel occlusion and containment of infection. This action of TNF-α is responsible for its tumor necrosis properties, thus leading to the name. TNF-α exerts its physiologic effects by binding to two different cell-surface receptors known as p55 (i.e., 55 kDa) and p75 (i.e., 75 kDa) on inflammatory cells.[41] These receptors, with portions extending from within the cell cytoplasm to the cell exterior, are capable of binding TNF-α to the domains extending above the cell surface. Soluble forms of these receptors can be found in the serum and synovial fluid and seem to play a role in regulating TNF-α.

Two approaches have targeted the action of TNF-α: (1) the use of soluble TNF receptors with high TNF-binding affinity (i.e., etanercept) and (2) antibodies against TNF-α (i.e., infliximab, adalimumab, golimumab, and certolizumab pegol).[39] Etanercept is a recombinant TNF-receptor Fc fusion protein with the extracellular portion of two p75 receptors fused to the Fc portion of human immunoglobulin G1 (IgG1).[43,44] Infliximab is a chimeric IgG monoclonal antibody directed against TNF-α, and adalimumab is a genetically engineered human IgG1 monoclonal antibody.[45,46] Certolizumab pegol is a polyethylene glycolated (PEG) Fab fragment of a humanized anti-TNF monoclonal antibody. Golimumab is a fully human anti-TNF-α IgG1 monoclonal antibody that targets and neutralizes both soluble and membrane-bound forms of TNF-α.[48,49] All five TNF-α inhibitors render TNF biologically unavailable and are highly effective in reducing RA disease activity. Currently, there is no conclusive evidence from well-controlled comparative trials that any one TNF-α inhibitor is superior to another with regard to efficacy and safety.[50] Comparative efficacy and safety will be discussed further in the section "Pharmacologic Treatment." TNF-α inhibitor selection may be driven by cost, insurance coverage, provider preference, and patient-specific factors.

There are also three non-TNF biologic agents recommended for RA patients who have not responded to at least one csDMARD, which include abatacept, rituximab, and tocilizumab.[28] Each of these agents possesses a novel mechanism of action targeting either T cells, B cells, or IL-6. Abatacept and tocilizumab may be considered as first-line biologic DMARDs along with the TNF-α inhibitors. However, rituximab should only be considered as a first-line bDMARD in the presence of certain contraindications (i.e., recent history of lymphoma, latent TB with contraindications to treatment, or history of demyelinating disease) to the other bDMARDs.[26] There is also one final bDMARD, anakinra, which is seldom used because of lack of comparative efficacy. Anakinra is a recombinant human interleukin-1 (IL-1) receptor antagonist, which inhibits the binding of cytokines IL-1a and IL-1b to their receptor.[39] In healthy individuals, IL-1 overexpression is prevented by naturally occurring IL-1Ra.[41,51] Consequently, inadequate production of IL-1Ra, relative to IL-1, is hypothesized to be an important contributor to active RA. In addition to proinflammatory properties, IL-1 augments cartilage damage and inhibits bone formation. Anakinra has not shown comparable efficacy against other bDMARDs in meta-analyses and is infrequently used, although some individuals may still respond to this agent.[26,27] Anakinra was not included in the most recent ACR 2015 guidelines owing to lack of any new data since 2012 and infrequent use in RA.[28]

Abatacept is a selective costimulation modulator that inhibits T cell activation.[52] For T cells to be fully activated, a CD80/CD86:CD28 costimulatory signal is required.[53] This costimulation is blocked by cytotoxic T-lymphocyte–associated antigen 4. Abatacept, a soluble fusion protein consisting of extracellular cytotoxic T-lymphocyte–associated antigen 4 attached to the Fc portion of IgG1, which inhibits T cell activation by preventing the binding of CD80 and CD86 ligands on the surface of APCs to the CD28 receptor on the T cell.[53]

Rituximab, is a chimeric monoclonal antibody, binds to the CD20 antigen on the surface of pre-B cells and mature B cells, resulting in the depletion of B cells from peripheral blood, lymph nodes, and bone marrow.[54] Stem cells, pro-B cells, and antibody-producing plasma cells do not express CD20 and are not affected by RXB. The exact role of B cells in RA pathogenesis is not known. However, studies have shown that B cells may contribute to the autoimmune and inflammatory processes by producing RF, acting as APCs, activating T cells, and producing proinflammatory cytokines.[54] Owing to its chimeric composition, RXB must be administered with MTX to reduce the risk of human antichimeric antibody (HACA) formation.[55,56] Inhibition of T cell activation and depletion of proinflammatory B cells result in significant reductions in RA-related inflammation and joint destruction.

Tocilizumab is a humanized anti–IL-6 receptor antibody. The pleiotropic proinflammatory cytokine IL-6 is produced by a variety of cell types including lymphocytes, monocytes, and fibroblasts and is involved in multiple immunologic processes, including T cell activation and B-cell proliferation.[57] When bound to the soluble IL-6 receptor, IL-6 activates chemokine production and upregulates expression of adhesion molecules. This leads to the recruitment of leukocytes at inflammatory sites, thus implicating IL-6 as an important factor in RA.[58,59] High levels of IL-6 have been found in the serum and joints of patients with RA. Additionally, IL-6 has been shown to induce proliferation of osteoclasts, which may be a component of the bone degradation seen in RA.[58,59] TCZ is a humanized, monoclonal antibody that can bind to both membranous and soluble IL-6 receptors. This blockade prevents the interaction of IL-6 with the IL-6 receptor, thus interrupting the inflammatory pathways that contribute to the disease processes in RA.[58,59]

Owing to their immunosuppressive nature, all bDMARDs should be avoided in patients with serious infections until the infection has been controlled. All five of the TNF-α inhibitors as well as tocilizumab carry boxed warnings for serious infections. Although these infections occurred primarily among patients with significant risk factors for infection (e.g., poorly controlled diabetes, concurrent corticosteroid use, or concomitant csDMARD therapy), biologic agents should not be given to patients with active infection, history of recurring infections, or medical conditions predisposing them to infection. There has been some debate regarding whether or not bDMARDs are associated with an increased risk of serious infections when compared to csDMARDs. A recent meta-analysis including all currently available bDMARDs concluded that standard and high-dose biologic DMARDs are associated with an increase in risk of serious infections compared to csDMARDs. Risk was increased whether or not the patient was using csDMARDs concomitantly. However, low-dose bDMARDs were not associated with increased risk.[60] It is recommended that all patients be screened for latent tuberculosis infection (LTBI) prior to initiation of a bDMARD or tofacitinib. If LTBI is identified, patients should receive at least 1 month of treatment prior to starting a bDMARD or tofacitinib. Patients with active TB should complete treatment prior to initiation of a bDMARD or tofacitinib. Patients should be monitored for active TB during treatment.[28]

It is recommended that patients receive the following vaccinations prior to the initiation of csDMARD or bDMARD therapy: pneumococcal, influenza, hepatitis B, human papillomavirus, and herpes zoster. However, if not completed prior to the initiation of therapy, these vaccinations, with the exception of herpes zoster, may be given following the initiation of csDMARDs or bDMARDs. Herpes zoster, as well as any other live vaccines, should not be administered in patients receiving bDMARDs.[28]

CORTICOSTEROIDS

Corticosteroids (i.e., low oral doses for multiple joint involvement or injections into isolated joints) can be used as needed at disease onset while awaiting response to DMARD therapy and intermittently during disease flare-ups or following failure of optimized treatment to control symptoms of pain and swelling. Corticosteroids have a long history of use in RA because of their potent anti-inflammatory and immunosuppressive effects and have been shown to enhance the clinical, functional, and structural efficacy of baseline csDMARD or combination csDMARD and bDMARD therapies.[26] Corticosteroids administered orally at low dosages or through local injections are effective in rapidly reducing disease activity and relieving RA symptoms.

Corticosteroids are particularly beneficial when patients are awaiting the onset of DMARD action (known as "bridge therapy") or during flares of active RA involving a small number of joints.[28,61] Oral corticosteroids seem to slow the rate of disease progression and have been shown to reduce radiographic changes for 1 to 2 years.[36,61,62] Use of corticosteroids in combination with DMARD therapy appears to improve clinical outcomes (signs and symptoms, functionality, radiologic damage) for patients with RA above the benefit of a DMARD used alone.[36,61,62] In addition, newer modified-release corticosteroids targeting nocturnal increases in inflammatory mediators, IL-6 and cortisol, have demonstrated a reduction in morning stiffness compared with older, standard immediate release agents.[63–65] Long-term use of corticosteroids, however, is associated with many serious adverse effects (e.g., osteoporosis, weight gain, diabetes, cataract formation, adrenal suppression, hypertension, infections, and impaired wound healing).[66] As a result, oral corticosteroid dosing should be limited to daily doses of $\leq$10 mg of prednisone (or equivalent) and should be administered for as short a time as possible.[28] Frequent corticosteroid injections for an extended period have the potential to accelerate bone and cartilage deterioration; therefore, the same joint should not be injected more than once every 3 months.[66]

SELDOM-USED DISEASE MODIFYING ANTIRHEUMATIC DRUGS AND OTHER THERAPIES

Several DMARDs, including gold, azathioprine, cyclosporine, minocycline, and anakinra, are no longer included in EULAR and ACR treatment recommendations because of infrequent use and lack of any new data supporting clinical benefit, especially in light of other widely available agents with more favorable benefit-to-risk profiles.[26–28]

Two classes of NSAIDs in development may provide GI protection without COX-2 specificity. The first class, nitric oxide NSAIDs, also known as COX-inhibiting nitric oxide donors, are standard NSAIDs structurally linked to a nitric oxide moiety. By donating nitric oxide to the gastric mucosa, nitric oxide NSAIDs produce the same gastroprotective effect as prostaglandins and have a lower rate of gastrointestinal ulceration compared to classic agents.[67] The other class, so-called dual-inhibitor NSAIDs, blocks both enzymatic pathways of arachidonic acid metabolism (i.e., both COX and 5-lipoxygenase) and further broadens the pharmacologic effects of currently available NSAIDs. Although COX inhibition is clearly associated with GI toxicity, inhibition of both enzymatic pathways of arachidonic acid metabolism has been GI sparing in animal and initial human safety studies.[68,69]

RA vaccines are also in development.[70] Only phase II studies have been completed, but a recent trial demonstrated clinical improvement in the majority of RA patients receiving T cell immunotherapy.[71] This RA vaccine induces a specific immune response against T cells that are reactive to joint antigens.[70] Another trial using immune-modulatory therapy targeted toward anti-CCP autoantibodies also demonstrated clinical improvement in patients with active RA.[72]

CLINICAL USE OF DISEASE-MODIFYING ANTIRHEUMATIC DRUGS

Both ACR[27,28] (Fig. 44-6) and EULAR[27] have developed evidence-based recommendations for the use of DMARDs in RA, last updated in 2015 and 2013, respectively. The two sets of guidelines have more similarities than differences. Ultimately, choice of treatment modality will be based on efficacy and safety data as well as on patient-specific parameters.

DMARD treatment should be started as soon as possible following RA diagnosis. MTX remains the gold standard because of high response rate, mild side effect profile, low cost, and long sustained efficacy not just as monotherapy but also in combination with glucocorticoids, other csDMARDs, and bDMARDs.[26,28] Furthermore, MTX therapy is associated with a reduction in cardiovascular morbidity and mortality in patients with RA, important given the strong association between RA and cardiovascular disease.[25] Optimization of MTX therapy also involves appropriate dose titration, adequate trial duration, and folate supplementation. Regardless of disease duration, ACR recommends that in the setting of low, moderate, or high disease activity, a trial of MTX as monotherapy may be started initially, with success predicted in 25% to 50% of individuals within 1 year.[28]

In the setting of moderate or high disease activity unresponsive to csDMARD monotherapy, EULAR recommends use of csDMARD combination therapy. csDMARD combination therapy with MTX may also be considered in the setting of moderate or high disease activity with poor prognostic features (i.e., functional limitation, extra-articular disease, positive RF or anti-CCP, and bony erosions). The most common combination is MTX, SSZ, and HCQ, which has been shown to attain treatment goals faster and with less therapy intensification than MTX monotherapy.[73] Culmination of current data suggests that combination csDMARD therapy may be superior to MTX monotherapy, but results remain controversial because of limitations of the studies themselves. Ultimately, MTX as monotherapy or in combination with other csDMARDs are both appropriate as first-line therapy and selection is determined by patient-specific factors.[26] In the setting of MTX contraindication or intolerance, LEF or SSZ, alone or in combination, may be considered as first-line csDMARDs instead. Both agents have demonstrated similar efficacy compared to MTX.[74,75] In addition to combination csDMARD therapy, ACR also considers addition of a bDMARD (either TNF inhibitor or non-TNF bDMARD) as a viable treatment strategy in the setting of csDMARD monotherapy failure in either early (disease duration <6 months) or established (disease duration ≥6 months) RA. The addition of tofacitinib may also be considered for patients with established RA and moderate-to-high disease activity.[28]

If desired response is not achieved with optimized dosing of the first-line treatment approach within the desired time frame, step-up therapy is warranted. If poor prognostic factors are not present, EULAR recommends the patient trial another csDMARD(s) (i.e., LEF, SSZ, and/or MTX as mono- or combination therapy). If prognosis is poor, then addition of a bDMARD to current csDMARD therapy is warranted. Ultimately, for patients on csDMARD therapy who remain unresponsive, bDMARDs should be initiated as add-on therapy to the csDMARD.

For choice of initial bDMARD, EULAR recommends TNF inhibitors, abatacept or tocilizumab, and in certain clinical scenarios, rituximab, as add-on therapy.[26] While TNF inhibitors have a larger evidence base and extended history of use compared to the non-TNF agents, more recent trial data have not triggered safety concerns for the newer agents.[76–79] Rituximab may be considered as a first-line bDMARD in patients having certain contraindications to other bDMARDs such as recent lymphoma, since this agent is not associated with malignancy.[80–82] ACR gives no preference to any bDMARD over another. Anakinra, the IL-1 inhibitor, is not included in either ACR or EULAR recommendations given lack of efficacy when compared to other bDMARDs and its minimal use in clinical practice.[26,28]

Triple csDMARD therapy has been shown to be non-inferior to combination MTX and TNF inhibitor therapy. There is a lack of trial data comparing csDMARDs to other non-TNF bDMARD agents.[82] It is preferred that the bDMARDs be used in combination with either MTX or other csDMARDs rather than as monotherapy.[28] Furthermore, even if clinical response is achieved with combination therapy, the csDMARD(s) should not be discontinued. If a patient truly cannot be treated with csDMARDs, consideration may be given to monotherapy with etanercept, adalimumab, certolizumab pegol, abatacept or tocilizumab.

If a patient has an inadequate response to the initial bDMARD trial, another bDMARD trial is warranted. There is no preferred step-up bDMARD and choice is dependent on patient-specific factors. However, if a TNF inhibitor was initially chosen, or if a patient has failed successive TNF inhibitor trials, changing to a non-TNF bDMARD is recommended. If a non-TNF bDMARD was initially chosen, switching to another non-TNF bDMARD is preferred. Finally, while indicated for individuals with moderate-to-severe RA who have failed MTX therapy, given the lack of clinical experience and safety data compared to bDMARDs, tofacitinib may be considered following multiple bDMARD treatment failures (i.e., at least one TNF inhibitor and two non-TNF bDMARDs).[26,28]

QUANTIFYING RESPONSE TO DRUG THERAPY

RA disease remission is the highest aim of therapy and has become more realistic as medications capable of halting or slowing disease progression are now widely available and commonly used in clinical practice. The ACR and EULAR consider patients with RA in clinical trials to have achieved remission if either of the following occurs: (1) tender joint count, swollen joint count (of 28 joints), C-reactive protein in mg/dL, and patient global assessment scores (scale of 0–10) are all less than 1 or (2) Simplified Disease

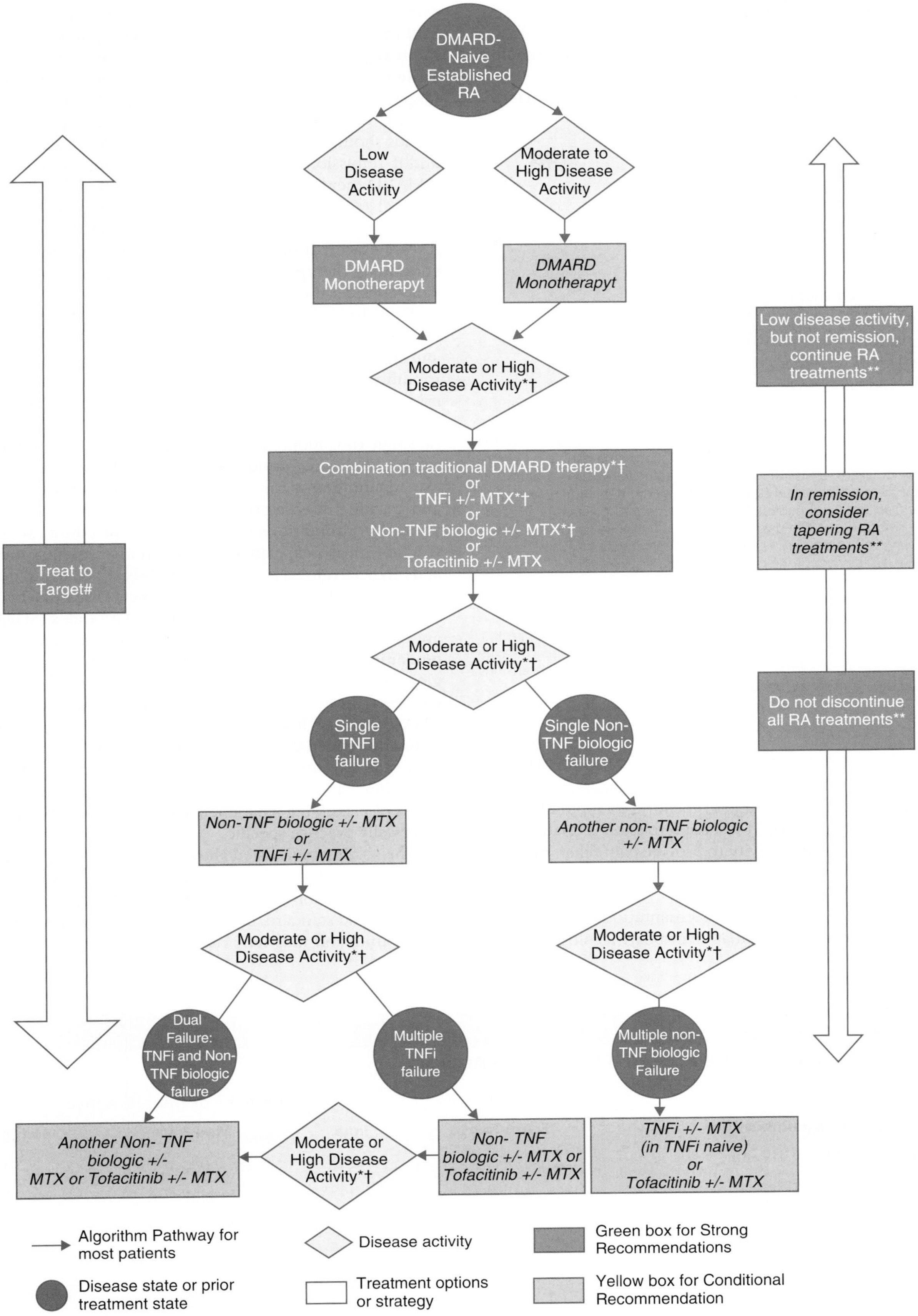

Figure 44-6 2015 American College of Rheumatology recommendations for the treatment of established rheumatoid arthritis. (Redrawn from Singh JA et al. 2015 American College of Rheumatology guideline for the treatment of rheumatoid arthritis. *Arthritis Rheumatol*. 2016;68(1):12.)

Table 44-3

Provisional Criteria for Rheumatoid Arthritis Remission in Clinical Trials from the American College of Rheumatology/European League Against Rheumatism

A patient with rheumatoid arthritis is considered to be "in remission" if either of the following applies:

1. Boolean-based definition
   At any time, patient must satisfy ALL of the following:
   Tender joint count ≤1[a]
   Swollen joint count ≤1[a]
   C-reactive protein ≤1 mg/dL
   Patient global assessment ≤1 (on a 0–10 scale)[b]
2. Index-based definition
   At any time, patient must have a Simplified Disease Activity Index score of ≤3.3[c]

[a]For tender and swollen joint counts, use of a 28-joint count may miss actively involved joints, especially in the feet and ankles, and it is preferable to include feet and ankles also when evaluating remission.
[b]For the assessment of remission, the following format and wording is suggested for the global assessment questions. Format: a horizontal 10-cm visual analog or Likert scale with the best anchor and lowest score on the left side and the worst anchor and highest score on the right side. Wording of question and anchors: For patient global assessment, "Considering all of the ways your arthritis has affected you, how do you feel your arthritis is today?" (anchors: very well–very poor). For physician or assessor global assessment, "What is your assessment of the patient's current disease activity?" (anchors: none–extremely active).
[c]Defined as the simple sum of the tender joint count (using 28 joints), swollen joint count (using 28 joints), patient global assessment (0–10 scale), physician global assessment (0–10 scale), and C-reactive protein level (mg/dL).
Source: Felson DT et al. American College of Rheumatology/European League Against Rheumatism provisional definition of remission in rheumatoid arthritis for clinical trials. *Arthritis Rheum Dis*. 2011;70:404–413.

Activity Index is less than 3.3.37 (Table 44-3). The proportion of patients able to achieve remission with this validated clinical assessment tool is adequate enough to encourage adoption of these criteria in standard practice. If disease remission is unattainable, then minimizing disease activity to provide pain relief, maintain activities of daily living, maximize quality of life, and slow joint damage become primary targets.

In active disease, successful implementation of the treat to target approach requires reevaluation of pharmacologic therapy every 1 to 3 months. Therapy adjustment no later than 3 months into the treatment course is warranted because if there is no improvement by this time then it is unlikely that continuing the same course will achieve satisfactory results. Once treatment targets have been achieved, monitoring may occur less frequently every 6 to 12 months. In patients with good response, glucocorticoids should be the first medications tapered and withdrawn, and if remission is sustained then tapering and discontinuing DMARD therapy (all types) may be considered.[28] This is a conditional ACR recommendation; while the quality of evidence supporting this recommendation is low in terms of the risk of disease exacerbation/recurrence, the long-term risk and cost of continuing therapy that is potentially unnecessary makes this a valid consideration.

Evaluating treatment response using validated clinical assessment tools yield a more accurate assessment of disease activity and improve the likelihood of attaining disease remission through modifications of drug therapy.[87,88] ACR has defined response criteria; however, these are designed for clinical research and may not be practical for clinical practice.[89] Although there is no single tool adopted as the standard of practice in the clinical setting, there are various other validated assessment tools that are advantageous for objectively evaluating disease activity and tracking disease progression (Table 44-4). These tools use various combinations of 28-tender joint count, acute phase reactant measures, pain and function assessments, and patient and physician global assessments of disease activity to determine disease activity. For example, The Clinical Disease Activity Index (CDAI) and the Simplified Disease Activity Index (SDAI) scores are determined through a simple sum of swollen joint count, tender joint count, patient global disease activity, and evaluator global disease activity (both measured by a visual analog scale). However, the SDAI includes CRP in the summation, whereas the CDAI does not.[90] It is important to note that all of these tools have distinctly defined threshold scores corresponding to high disease activity, low-to-moderate disease activity, low disease activity, and remission, although there is little agreement among the tools in terms of classifying a patient's RA activity level. Choice of tool is typically practice-specific.

The scoring tools listed above should be used in conjunction with radiographic evaluation to determine RA course and treatment strategy. Conventional radiography was previously considered the gold standard, but imaging via computed tomography, ultrasound, and magnetic resonance imaging is now available

Table 44-4

Tools Used to Measure Disease Activity in Rheumatoid Arthritis

Measurement Tool	Score Range	Thresholds of Disease Activity		
		Low	Moderate	High
Disease Activity Score in 28 joints	0–9.4	≤3.2	>3.2 and ≤5.1	>5.1
Simplified Disease Activity Index	0.1–86.0	≤11	>11 and ≤26	>26
Clinical Disease Activity Index	0–76.0	≤10	>10 and ≤22	>22
Rheumatoid Arthritis Disease Activity Index	0–10	≤2.2	>2.2 and ≤4.9	>4.9
Patient Activity Scale (PAS) or PASII	0–10	≤1.9	>1.9 and ≤5.3	>5.3
Routine Assessment Patient Index Data	0–30	≤6	>6 and ≤12	>12

Tools incorporate multiple variables such as number of swollen joints and tender joints, erythrocyte sedimentation rate, and measures of general health or global disease activity.
Source: Saag KG et al. American College of Rheumatology 2008 recommendations for the use of nonbiologic and biologic disease-modifying antirheumatic drugs in rheumatoid arthritis. *Arthritis Rheum*. 2008;59:762.

and may offer some benefit in improved resolution compared with standard radiograph technology.[91] Radiographic changes occur in more than half of patients categorized in remission and tracking these can help clinicians objectively evaluate arthritis-related joint damage.[92]

Pharmacologic Treatment

NONSTEROIDAL ANTI-INFLAMMATORY DRUG THERAPY

CASE 44-1, QUESTION 4: T.W. will be treated with a DMARD and concurrent NSAID therapy initially to rapidly control inflammation and swelling. What is the role of NSAIDs in the treatment of T.W.'s RA and which is the NSAID of choice?

T.W.'s clinical presentation clearly warrants DMARD therapy (see Case 44-5, Question 4, and Clinical Use of Disease-Modifying Agents section). The purpose of NSAID therapy, which has no disease-modifying activity, is to provide rapid pain relief and reduction of joint inflammation primarily as bridge therapy while awaiting onset of DMARD activity, which could take weeks to months.[39] In general, there is no NSAID of choice for treatment of RA.[13,93] There is no significant difference among the NSAIDs in efficacy, and it is difficult to predict a given patient's response to a particular agent. The selection of an NSAID is based primarily on patient preference, convenience, cost, and safety.[39,40] A 1- to 2-week trial of any NSAID (Table 44-5) at a moderate-to-high dose on a scheduled basis (i.e., not as needed) is the best method of determining anti-inflammatory efficacy. The analgesic and antipyretic effects are relatively prompt in onset.

Although aspirin at high doses is just as effective as other NSAIDs, it is seldom used today because of well-documented gastrointestinal (GI) toxicity and the availability of other safer and more convenient NSAIDs.[39,40,94] Serum salicylate levels correlate well with both efficacy and toxicity.[93] Anti-inflammatory effects of aspirin can be achieved with dosages sufficient to provide serum salicylate concentrations of 15 to 30 mg/dL. Typically, 5 to 7 days of therapy are needed before steady-state serum concentrations of salicylate are attained. A reasonable initial aspirin dose is 45 mg/kg/day divided into 4- or 6-hour intervals; however, the anti-inflammatory dose of aspirin varies widely because of interindividual variations in metabolism. Nonacetylated salicylates are weak inhibitors of COX in vitro and have less GI toxicity than aspirin, but the risks of GI and renal toxicity are similar to nonselective NSAIDs.[40,94]

The nonaspirin NSAIDs have important differentiating properties, and individualizing selection based on these characteristics is warranted in all patients such as T.W.[93] For example, several NSAIDs increase the risk of MI, with diclofenac, meloxicam, and indomethacin showing the highest risk of thrombosis, although celecoxib and ibuprofen at high doses also carry relatively high cardiovascular risk. Naproxen appears to have the best cardiovascular safety profile.[95,96]

Longer-acting NSAIDs such as piroxicam and ketorolac have been associated with a higher frequency of peptic ulcer disease and GI bleeding, and should be avoided. Other NSAIDs, depending on their COX-2 selectivity, have varying GI toxicity profiles with naproxen conferring moderate risk and ibuprofen lower risk.[97,98] The selective COX-2 inhibitor celecoxib, at least with short-term use, is associated with a 20% lower risk of GI bleeding than traditional NSAIDs.[99] Because this agent does not interfere with COX-1—the isozyme responsible for production of the stomach's mucous lining and for reduced acid secretion—in theory COX-2 inhibitors reduce inflammation as effectively as nonselective NSAIDs while reducing the risk of GI toxicity. However, concurrent daily low-dose aspirin use appears to negate any benefit of COX-2 inhibitor therapy on lowering ulcer risk.[100]

Indomethacin penetrates the blood–brain barrier better than any other NSAID, achieving levels in the cerebrospinal fluid of up to 50% of serum levels. As a result, the incidence of central nervous system side effects of indomethacin such as dizziness often precludes the use of optimal anti-inflammatory doses, particularly in the elderly.[101]

A low-cost NSAID (e.g., naproxen and ibuprofen) with a good safety profile is a good choice for T.W. because she is relatively young and does not have any concomitant illnesses. If convenience of administration is a more important consideration, a longer-acting NSAID (e.g., naproxen) would be preferable. If the first agent chosen is ineffective or not well tolerated, other NSAIDs can be tried to identify the optimal one for this patient.

CASE 44-1, QUESTION 5: Naproxen 500 mg twice daily has been prescribed for T.W. If T.W. were to experience dyspepsia during therapy, should she be given antiulcer prophylaxis or a COX-2 selective NSAID at this time? What is the correlation between dyspepsia and gastroduodenal mucosal injury? What instructions regarding NSAID therapy should be provided to T.W., especially with regard to GI problems?

Patients should be informed that NSAID therapy is being prescribed to provide relief of pain and inflammation associated with RA, but that it will not slow or stop the progression of the disease. It should be explained that the latter can only be accomplished by DMARD therapy. Patients should also understand that moderate-to-high daily doses of NSAIDs are required for anti-inflammatory activity, as opposed to analgesic and antipyretic effects which can be achieved with single and low doses.

About 5% to 15% of patients with RA discontinue NSAID therapy because of dyspepsia, and about 1.3% of patients taking NSAIDs for RA experience a serious GI complication. As expected, the rate is somewhat lower for patients using NSAIDs for osteoarthritis (0.7%) because these patients generally use analgesics only on an as-needed basis. Serious NSAID-induced GI complications account for about 103,000 hospitalizations annually in the United States and approximately 16,500 NSAID-related deaths each year.[98,102] Although these figures warrant concern, most patients who experience NSAID-induced dyspepsia suffer only superficial and self-limiting injury. Nevertheless, prevention of NSAID-induced GI bleeding should be an important focus, particularly in high-risk patients.

Patients should be taught to recognize the signs and symptoms of GI bleeding (e.g., nausea, vomiting, anorexia and gastric pain) including melena (described to the patient as "dark, tarry stool") and emesis of coagulated blood (described to the patient as "coughing or vomiting up what seems to be coffee grounds"). It should be emphasized that GI bleeding can occur without gastric pain. The patient should be instructed to contact their health care provider immediately for further instructions if any of these signs or symptoms occurs.

Gastroduodenal mucosal damage induced by NSAIDs primarily results from inhibition of COX-1 in the mucosal lining.[102] This inhibition of COX-1 decreases bicarbonate secretion, mucosal blood flow, formation of protective mucus, proliferation of gastric epithelium, and the ability of the mucosa to resist injury. Topical damage to the GI mucosa can occur from NSAIDs, but direct injury

Table 44-5
Some Nonsteroidal Anti-Inflammatory Drugs

NSAID Generic Name (Brand Name)	Product Availability	Usual Dosing Interval	Maximum Daily Dose (mg)
Salicylates (Acetylated and Nonacetylated)[a]			
Aspirin, enteric-coated[b]	Tablets: 325 mg; 325, 500, 800, 975 mg SR	QID	4,000
Salsalate (Disalcid)[b]	Tablets: 500, 750 mg	BID–TID	4,800
Magnesium choline salicylate (Trilisate)[c]	Tablets: 500, 750, 1,000 mg	Daily–TID	4,800
	Liquid: 500 mg/5 mL		
Propionic Acid Derivatives			
Fenoprofen (Nalfon)[b]	Capsules: 200, 300 mg	TID–QID	3,200
Flurbiprofen (Ansaid)[b]	Tablets: 50, 100 mg	BID–QID	300
Ibuprofen (Motrin)[b]	Tablets: 200, 400, 600, 800 mg	TID–QID	3,200
	Suspension: 100 mg/5 mL		
Naproxen (Naprosyn)[b]	Tablets: 250, 375, 500 mg; 375, 500 mg SR	BID	1,500
	Suspension: 125 mg/5 mL		
Naproxen sodium (Anaprox)[b]	Tablets: 275, 550 mg	BID	1,375
Oxaprozin (Daypro)[b]	Tablet or capsule: 600 mg	Daily	1,800
Acetic Acid Derivatives			
Diclofenac (Voltaren XR)[b]	Tablets: 25, 50, 75 mg DR; 100 mg XR	BID–TID	200
Etodolac (Lodine, Lodine XL)[b]	Capsules: 200, 300 mg	BID–TID	1,200
	Tablets: 400, 500 mg; 400, 500, 600 mg XL	XL: Daily	XL: 1,000
Indomethacin (Indocin, Indocin SR)[c]	Suppository: 50 mg	TID	
	Suspension: 25 mg/5 mL	TID–QID	200
	Capsules: 25, 50 mg; 75 mg SR	SR: Daily–BID	SR: 150
Ketorolac (Toradol)[b]	Tablet: 10 mg	QID	40
Nabumetone (Relafen)[b]	Tablet: 500, 750 mg	Daily	2,000
Sulindac (Clinoril)[b]	Tablets: 150, 200 mg	BID	400
Tolmetin (Tolectin)[b]	Tablets: 200, 600 mg		
	Capsules: 400 mg	TID–QID	1,800
Oxicam Derivatives			
Piroxicam (Feldene)[b]	Capsule: 10, 20 mg	Daily	20
Meloxicam (Mobic)[b]	Tablets: 7.5, 15 mg	Daily	15
COX-2 inhibitors			
Celecoxib (Celebrex)	Capsules: 50, 100, 200, 400 mg	BID	400

[a]Highly variable half-life; anti-inflammatory doses associated with salicylate serum concentrations from 15 to 30 mg/dL.
[b]Generic version available.
Source: MedicalLetter.org. Drugs for rheumatoid arthritis. *Treat Guidel Med Lett*. 2009;7:37.
BID, 2 times a day; COX-2, cyclo-oxygenase-2; DR, delayed release; NSAID, nonsteroidal anti-inflammatory drug; QID, 4 times a day; SR, sustained release; TID, 3 times a day; XL/XR, extended release.

plays a smaller role than COX-1 inhibition. Table 44-6 provides a comparison of COX-1 and COX-2 isoforms.

Dyspepsia can be managed by ingesting the NSAID with meals or a large glass of water; however, these measures usually are ineffective in preventing GI ulcers. In addition, dyspepsia correlates poorly with endoscopically confirmed mucosal injury.[102–104] Histamine type 2 (H_2) receptor antagonists (e.g., ranitidine, famotidine) significantly reduce dyspepsia among NSAID users; however, NSAID users with RA who take an H_2-receptor antagonist as needed might have a higher risk of developing serious GI complications compared with those who do not take these medications (odds ratio, 2.14; 95% confidence interval, 1.06–4.32).[105] The suppression of dyspepsia symptoms can give a false sense of security to the patient and physician, leading to higher doses of NSAIDs and increased risk of major gastropathy. Also, routine use of H_2-receptor antagonists is associated with tachyphylaxis.[106] Therefore, H_2-receptor antagonists are not recommended for routine use in asymptomatic patients receiving NSAIDs. Proton-pump inhibitors (PPIs; e.g., lansoprazole, omeprazole) relieve dyspepsia better than H_2-receptor antagonists and prevent the development

Table 44-6
Comparison of Cyclo-Oxygenase-1 and Cyclo-Oxygenase-2 Isoforms

	COX-1	COX-2
Expression: continuous or induced	Primarily continuous, although some evidence of induction	Primarily induced, but present continuously in several organs
Common organs/tissues	Nearly all organs, including stomach, kidneys, platelets, vasculature	Induced at sites of inflammation and neoplasms
		Continuously active in kidneys, small intestine, pancreas, brain, ovaries, uterus
Primary role	Housekeeping/maintenance	Inflammation, repair, neoplasia
	May be important when induced in response to inflammation	May be important in housekeeping/maintenance of organs that continuously express COX-2

COX, cyclo-oxygenase.
Source: Hawkey CJ. COX-2 inhibitors. *Lancet*. 1999;353:307.

of NSAID-induced gastroduodenal ulcers.[105,107] They are safe and effective for the treatment of NSAID-induced dyspepsia and should be considered if symptoms develop in T.W.

Effective prevention options for reducing the risk of NSAID-induced ulcers and related complications include a PPI, double the maximal dose of H_2-receptor antagonists, and misoprostol. PPIs are the most efficacious and best tolerated cotherapies with NSAIDs to reduce the risk of peptic ulcers and ulcer complications. Double maximal doses of H_2-receptor antagonists have demonstrated a reduction in NSAID-induced endoscopic peptic ulcers; however, no study has demonstrated that double-dose H_2-receptor antagonists prevent ulcer complications and PPIs remain significantly more effective. Misoprostol, a prostaglandin E_1 analog, is most effective when given at the full dose of 200 mcg 4 times daily; however, intolerable GI upset, particularly diarrhea and abdominal cramping, frequently leads to discontinuation of therapy at this dose. Lower doses are usually prescribed (200 mcg 2 or 3 times daily) with better tolerance but lower efficacy. Sucralfate or antacids are not effective in preventing NSAID-related GI injury.[107]

Routine concomitant antiulcer prophylactic therapy is not warranted for all patients taking NSAIDs; rather the risk for GI ulcer development must be assessed to determine the need for preventive measures. Established risk factors for NSAID-induced GI bleeding include advanced age (>65 years), history of ulcers (a history of complicated ulcers, particularly recent, puts patient at high risk), concurrent use of other ulcer-promoting medications (e.g., corticosteroids, aspirin and anticoagulants), and high-dose NSAID therapy. Patients can be grouped into high, moderate, or low risk of NSAID-induced GI toxicity based on these risk factors. High-risk patients (>2 risk factors) should avoid NSAID therapy or take a COX-2 inhibitor instead along with either a PPI or a misoprostol. Moderate-risk patients (one or two risk factors) should take a PPI or misoprostol with an NSAID; naproxen is the preferred NSAID for high–cardiovascular-risk patients. Low-risk patients (no risk factors) do not need concurrent GI protective therapy and should receive a relatively less GI toxic NSAID at the lowest effective dose.[107] Without risk factors other than NSAID use, T.W. does not need concurrent ulcer prophylaxis or a COX-2 selective NSAID at this time, although a less toxic agent such as naproxen or ibuprofen should be chosen.

Helicobacter pylori infection increases the risk of peptic ulcers in individuals taking NSAIDs.[107] A meta-analysis demonstrated that *H. pylori* eradication significantly reduced the risk of endoscopic ulcers among patients who had not started NSAID therapy; however, eradication did not lower risk among patients who were already receiving NSAIDs.[108] Therefore, *H. pylori* testing, and treatment if positive, should be considered for all patients prior to starting chronic NSAID therapy.[107]

Active NSAID-induced gastroduodenal ulcers are best treated by discontinuing the NSAID and initiating a PPI. PPIs are preferred over H_2-receptor antagonists because of greater efficacy, rapid healing rates, and a shorter duration of treatment (4–8 weeks).[109] If discontinuation of the NSAID is not feasible, ulcer healing can still be accomplished with a PPI but requires a longer duration of therapy (8–12 weeks).[109,110] Patients who test positive for *H. pylori* should undergo *H. pylori* eradication therapy. Other GI treatments, such as misoprostol and antacids, are ineffective for managing active NSAID-induced ulcers.

CASE 44-2

QUESTION 1: C.S., a patient who was hospitalized for evaluation and treatment of his RA, has a history of aspirin allergy. Are other NSAIDs contraindicated for this patient?

C.S. should be asked to describe his reaction to aspirin to determine whether his symptoms are consistent with a hypersensitivity reaction or with a less serious intolerance issue. Many patients who claim to be allergic to aspirin merely experience GI distress. Aspirin is not contraindicated in these patients and tolerance may be improved if the medication is administered with food or as an enteric-coated preparation.

True aspirin hypersensitivity, especially in association with asthma, is a cause for serious concern because exposure can precipitate an acute, life-threatening, bronchospastic reaction.[111] Between 6% and 15% of asthmatics have a history of aspirin-induced bronchospasm; it occurs more often among women than men and rarely in children. The prevalence of aspirin-induced asthma increases with the presence of nasal polyps. Aspirin-sensitive patients can experience a high degree of cross-reactivity to all nonselective NSAIDs; therefore, these agents should be avoided especially in patients who have a history of aspirin-induced asthma.

On the other hand, COX-2 inhibitors have been used safely in aspirin-sensitive asthmatics.[112–114] In theory, COX-2 inhibitors might be safer because they allow COX-1 to continue producing prostaglandin E_2. Prostaglandin E_2 is an important mediator of multiple physiologic processes, including reduction of leukotriene synthesis, suppression of the release of inflammatory mediators from mast cells, and prevention of aspirin-induced bronchoconstriction.

Aspirin desensitization, which is followed by daily aspirin therapy, is an effective treatment option for most patients with aspirin-induced asthma.[111] Patients who appear to benefit the most include those who rely heavily on systemic corticosteroids or with recurrent nasal polyps.

CASE 44-3

QUESTION 1: A.L., a 53-year-old woman with RA, recalls receiving aspirin long ago, but discontinued it because of "ringing in my ears all the time!" Is this a symptom related to aspirin?

Aspirin-induced tinnitus (i.e., a ringing or high-pitched buzzing sensation in the head) is noticeable to most patients with normal hearing when aspirin serum levels reach 10 to 30 mg/dL; however, in some patients tinnitus might not be encountered until serum levels exceed 25 mg/dL.[93] Serum salicylate concentrations are usually within therapeutic range when tinnitus is apparent. As a result, tinnitus has been used to titrate patients on aspirin to therapeutic doses. It is important to note that patients with preexisting hearing loss might not experience tinnitus despite potentially toxic concentrations.[115]

CASE 44-3, QUESTION 2: A.L. is scheduled to have dental surgery. She states that she is currently taking an aspirin-like product for arthritis pain. Why is it important to know the specific NSAID she is taking?

Aspirin, nonacetylated salicylates, nonaspirin NSAIDs, and COX-2 inhibitors have differing effects on platelet function. Nonaspirin NSAIDs can prolong bleeding times by inhibiting platelet aggregation, but these drugs bind reversibly to COX, resulting in transient platelet inhibition.[93] As a result, if A.L. is taking a nonaspirin NSAID, it should be discontinued approximately 5 half-lives before surgical procedures. For most NSAIDs, the impairment of platelet aggregation is reversed within 2 days after the discontinuation.

Nonacetylated salicylates have minimal effects on COX and platelet function and are of little concern in presurgical patients. Likewise, COX-2 inhibitors are not expected to alter platelet function because COX-2 is not found in platelets.[116]

Aspirin is an irreversible inhibitor of COX and impairs platelet aggregation throughout the life of the platelet. It can prolong bleeding time for several days, which may not normalize until new, unbound platelets are released into circulation. This process may take 3 to 6 days after discontinuation of aspirin; however, this does not always necessitate holding aspirin prior to every procedure. If A.L. is also taking low-dose aspirin chronically, whether or not aspirin may be continued prior to surgery depends on the indication for aspirin and type of surgery. For minor dental procedures, low-dose aspirin can usually be continued.[117,118]

CASE 44-4

QUESTION 1: R.Z. is a 28-year-old woman who is planning a pregnancy and is concerned about the possible effects of NSAIDs on her baby. What are the risks to the fetus with uninterrupted consumption of NSAIDs? What are maternal- and lactation-related effects of these medications?

Although NSAIDs, including aspirin, are not teratogenic, they must be used cautiously in women who are pregnant and who plan to breast-feed infants.[119] Fetal effects of NSAIDs include possible premature ductus arteriosus closure, increased cutaneous and intracranial bleeding, transient renal impairment, and a reduction in urine output. High doses of aspirin (greater than 3 g/day) and NSAIDs can inhibit uterine contractions, resulting in prolonged labor. The use of NSAIDs can also increase peripartum blood loss and anemia. Aspirin and nonaspirin NSAIDs should be used sparingly and at the lowest effective doses during pregnancy and discontinued at least 6 to 8 weeks before delivery to minimize adverse fetal and maternal effects.

Aspirin generally should be avoided for women who plan to nurse their baby because salicylate serum concentrations in breast-fed neonates raise concerns about the potential for metabolic acidosis, bleeding, and Reye syndrome. Nonaspirin NSAIDs are generally compatible with breast-feeding, with the best evidence supporting the use of ibuprofen, indomethacin, and naproxen.[120,121]

CASE 44-5

QUESTION 1: T.Z., a 68-year-old man with heart failure previously managed with furosemide 40 mg/day, digoxin 0.125 mg/day, metoprolol 50 mg twice daily, and lisinopril 40 mg/day, returns for a prescription refill of ibuprofen 600 mg 3 times daily, which he takes for his RA. During the past 2 weeks, he has noted increased leg swelling, a weight gain of several pounds, exacerbated shortness of breath, and easy fatigability. Why might these signs and symptoms be associated with ibuprofen use?

Mild fluid retention occurs in approximately 5% of NSAID users, and NSAID-induced kidney disease occurs in less than 1% of patients.[120,121] NSAID therapy should be avoided, if possible, in patients with preexisting heart failure, kidney disease, or cirrhosis.[122] If a patient with these conditions requires NSAID therapy, or patients are taking angiotensin-converting enzyme inhibitors and angiotensin receptor blockers, serum creatinine should be checked soon after NSAID initiation. Inhibition of COX by NSAIDs within the kidney reduces prostaglandin concentrations and unopposed vasoconstriction. Consequently, urine output declines, serum blood urea nitrogen and serum creatinine levels rise, and fluid is retained. In addition, ibuprofen at higher doses is associated with an increased risk of MI, a concern for T.Z. because of his risk of thrombotic cardiovascular events.[95] The provider of T.Z.'s cardiovascular care should be informed of his symptoms of fluid overload, and an alternative to NSAID therapy should be pursued.

CASE 44-5, QUESTION 2: If NSAID therapy is discontinued, what analgesic or anti-inflammatory alternatives are there for T.Z.? What other renal syndromes are associated with NSAID use?

In several studies, sulindac has been associated with fewer adverse effects on the kidney than other NSAIDs.[123] The reasons for this are unclear, but one explanation is that the active sulfide metabolite undergoes renal metabolism and, therefore, might not achieve tissue concentrations within the kidney sufficient to reduce prostaglandin production.[124] Unfortunately, patients do not seem to benefit from sulindac as much as from other NSAIDs, and the evidence overall supporting the safety of sulindac in renal impairment is weak. COX-2 inhibitors do not appear to offer an advantage for renally impaired patients.[123] Although celecoxib has been associated with a slightly lower risk of death and heart failure exacerbation when compared with traditional NSAIDs, it is not a reasonable initial option for T.Z. because celecoxib is also associated with an increased risk of MI and it may contribute to worsening of heart failure.[125]

NSAIDs should be used at their lowest effective doses for minimal periods for T.Z. High-dose NSAIDs should be avoided owing to increased MI risk. Although acetaminophen is not an anti-inflammatory agent, it can provide analgesic relief. Intra-articular corticosteroid injections can be useful if inflamed joints are limited in number, or a short course of oral corticosteroids can provide rapid control of inflammation while reducing the need for longer courses of anti-inflammatory therapy. If T.Z. is not yet being treated with a DMARD, initiation should be considered immediately because disease-modifying therapy can eventually preclude T.Z.'s need for an NSAID. In the meantime, if an NSAID or short course of systemic corticosteroid is used, close monitoring of renal function and fluid retention status is warranted.

In addition to acute renal failure, NSAIDs can induce various adverse renal effects (e.g., nephrotic syndrome, interstitial nephritis, hyponatremia, abnormalities of water metabolism, and hyperkalemia).[126] The nephrotic syndrome, unlike NSAID-induced acute renal failure, can appear anytime (i.e., from days to years) after initiation of therapy and can resolve as quickly as 1 month, or as long as 1 year, after discontinuation of the NSAID. Hematuria, pyuria, and proteinuria without prior renal disease differentiates nephrotic syndrome from other NSAID-induced renal problems. Histologically, NSAID-induced nephrotic syndrome is characterized by interstitial lymphocytic infiltrates, vacuolar degeneration of proximal and distal tubules, and fusion of epithelial foot processes of glomeruli.

Prostaglandin-mediated inhibition of active chloride transport, regulation of medullary blood flow within the kidney, and antagonism of antidiuretic hormone can be suppressed by NSAIDs. As a result, urine is maximally concentrated, free water clearance is limited, and water retention that is disproportionate to sodium retention can occur. The resulting hyponatremia can be severe and could be potentiated by thiazide diuretics.[126] Local prostaglandin synthesis can also stimulate renin production within the kidney. NSAID therapy can critically attenuate this regulatory mechanism in some situations, resulting in reduced aldosterone-mediated potassium excretion and hyperkalemia.

Although the mechanism is poorly understood, some NSAIDs have been associated with sustained mean arterial pressure increases of 5 to 6 mm Hg,[123,127] presumably the result of COX-2 inhibition and sodium and water retention. Several studies suggest that only patients taking antihypertensive medications experienced NSAID-induced mean arterial pressure elevations, but it is now clear that even normotensive individuals can experience elevations in blood pressure from NSAID use.

CASE 44-5, QUESTION 3: How frequently should T.Z.'s renal and liver function be tested during his NSAID therapy?

Patients at high risk for NSAID-induced renal disease, like T.Z. (see Case 44-5, Questions 1 and 2), should have their serum creatinine levels checked regularly (e.g., weekly) for several weeks after initiation of NSAID therapy because renal insufficiency more commonly occurs early in the course of therapy rather than later.[128] NSAID-induced nephrotic syndrome and allergic interstitial nephritis occur, on average, about 6.6 months and 15 days after NSAID initiation, respectively.[126]

In most cases, liver function testing (LFT) is unnecessary.[128] Although NSAIDs can elevate liver enzymes, severe hepatotoxicity is rare. Abnormal LFTs without clinical symptoms have no impact on patient outcome and have not been associated with severe hepatotoxicity. Patients who seem to be at greatest risk for hepatotoxicity are those with established or suspected intrinsic liver disease and those taking diclofenac. These patients should have LFTs performed no later than 8 weeks after initiation of therapy because liver toxicity manifests early in therapy, if at all.

TRADITIONAL DISEASE-MODIFYING ANTIRHEUMATIC DRUGS

CASE 44-5, QUESTION 4: T.Z. was diagnosed with RA 18 months ago, shortly after symptoms began to manifest. He exhibits no features of a poor prognosis and has low disease activity. Which traditional DMARD (csDMARD) therapies are most appropriate for him?

According to ACR, regardless of disease duration, every RA patient should receive DMARD therapy. Monotherapy with MTX is considered the preferred initial treatment for most RA patients. A high and rapid response rate for all levels of RA severity, relatively low cost and toxicity, and radiographic evidence of slowing joint erosion (which is most rapid during the first several years of active disease) are reasons why MTX is preferred[28] (Fig. 44-6). Other csDMARDs to consider are HCQ, SSZ, and LEF. Although most DMARDs are associated with potentially serious adverse effects, these generally are reversible and seldom lead to serious complications if the patient is monitored appropriately.

In addition, low-dose oral corticosteroids or NSAIDs are often prescribed on an as-needed basis for brief periods of severe disease activity or while awaiting the onset of DMARD action. During periods of disease remission, corticosteroid or NSAID therapy can be discontinued. Safety and efficacy data, which reflect several years of DMARD therapy combined with biologic agents, have been excellent, and the combination is now commonly prescribed for patients who fail MTX monotherapy (see Case 44-7, Questions 9-11).[28] Guidelines for DMARD selection were discussed previously (see Treatment section). Combination DMARD therapy is indicated for more severe or more advanced RA patients (see Case 44-7, Question 8).

Antimalarial Drug Dosing

CASE 44-5, QUESTION 5: Although MTX is considered the initial DMARD of choice for newly diagnosed RA, treatment was initiated with HCQ. What dosages would be appropriate, and when should clinical improvement be expected?

Although the manufacturer's literature recommends an initial HCQ adult dose of 400 to 600 mg/day (310–465 mg of base), dosages for HCQ generally range from 2 to 6.5 mg/kg/day.[28] If the patient responds well, the maintenance dose can be reduced by 50% and the medication continued at a dose of 200 to 400 mg/day (155–310 mg of base). About two-thirds of patients who tolerate HCQ respond favorably. Benefits usually are apparent within 2 to 4 months of therapy, but it can vary between 1 and 6 months. About 37% of patients discontinued HCQ within a year and 54% within 2 years, primarily owing to lack of efficacy.[128]

Risk of Retinopathy

CASE 44-5, QUESTION 6: When being counseled regarding HCQ, T.Z. was told that the drug can cause vision problems. How great is the risk of retinopathy from antimalarials when used for the treatment of RA? What monitoring parameters are appropriate?

HCQ is usually well tolerated. The most serious toxicity, retinal damage and subsequent visual impairment, is rare.[28,128] Risk of retinopathy is increased with high cumulative doses ($>$800 g), increased age ($>$60 years), liver disease, and retinal disease. The increased risk of retinopathy in the elderly seems to be related to the increased prevalence of macular disease in this age group. Daily HCQ doses $<$5 mg/kg for the first 5 years are very rarely associated with increased risk of retinal damage, particularly in patients without renal or hepatic dysfunction. HCQ should not be used for patients with significant renal impairment.

Patients should be instructed to stop therapy immediately and undergo an ophthalmologic evaluation if they are experiencing symptoms of antimalarial-associated retinopathy (e.g., difficulty seeing faces or entire words, glare intolerance, poor night vision, and loss of peripheral vision).[129] The fully developed lesion of antimalarial retinopathy is seen on ophthalmoscopy as a pigmentary disturbance with a characteristic bull's-eye appearance in the macular region. The 4-amino-quinolines bind to melanin, and as a result, concentrate in the uveal tract and retinal pigment epithelium. The retinopathy can be progressive even after discontinuation of the drug.

A baseline eye examination is recommended prior to starting HCQ therapy, then annually after 5 years of treatment.[130] More frequent testing is recommended for patients:

- Taking more than 6.5 mg/kg daily
- Who have received a cumulative dose of >200 mg
- With renal dysfunction
- Who are elderly
- With existing poor visual acuity

Sulfasalazine

CASE 44-5, QUESTION 7: If SSZ were chosen as initial therapy for T.Z., when should therapeutic effects become apparent, and what adverse effects might be anticipated?

The onset of SSZ effect is generally more rapid than that of HCQ, usually providing benefits within 2 to 3 months.[130] Overall, SSZ adverse effects are relatively mild, although SSZ is considered to be slightly more toxic than HCQ. Adverse effects include nausea, abdominal discomfort, heartburn, dizziness, headaches, skin rashes, and, rarely, hematologic effects such as leukopenia (1%–3%) or thrombocytopenia. A complete blood count (CBC) is recommended every 2 to 4 weeks for the first 3 months of therapy, then every 3 months thereafter. Leukopenia, agranulocytosis, or hepatitis are rare, but serious side effects of SSZ usually manifest within the first 2 to 3 months of therapy. To minimize GI-related adverse effects, SSZ is initiated at 500 mg/day or 1 g/day, and the dosage is increased at weekly intervals by 500 mg until 1,000 mg 2 or 3 times daily is reached.

Methotrexate

CASE 44-6

QUESTION 1: S.S., a 41-year-old Asian woman diagnosed with RA, presents with inflammation in both hands (MCP and PIP joints), wrists, elbows, shoulders, knees, hips, ankles, and MTP joints. Objective test results include radiographic evidence of joint erosion in both hands and elbows, positive RF (dilution of 1:1,280), positive anti-CCP at 102 units, and ESR of 78 mm/hour. Her SDAI score is 30. When she initially developed symptoms a year ago, she self-treated with ibuprofen 800 mg 3 times daily; however, pain and inflammation have progressively worsened. ROM testing reveals deficits in wrist flexion and extension (20 degrees bilaterally for both motions; normal, 90 and 70 degrees, respectively), elbow flexion (90 degrees bilaterally with flexion contracture; normal, 160 degrees), shoulder abduction (70 degrees right, 90 degrees left; normal, 180 degrees), and plantar flexion of both ankles (20 degrees bilaterally; normal, 45 degrees). Three firm, pea-sized, nontender moveable subcutaneous nodules are found on both elbows at the ulnar border, two on the right and one on the left. A decision is made to treat S.S. with MTX. Why is MTX a good selection for her?

MTX is recommended as initial DMARD therapy for all patients with RA.[28] S.S. has many indicators of severe disease (e.g., an SDAI score indicating high disease activity [see Table 44-7], multiple joint involvement, extra-articular manifestations [i.e., subcutaneous nodules], radiographic evidence of erosions, elevated ESR, positive anti-CCP, positive RF with a high titer of 1:1,280 [high titers correlate with greater disease severity]). MTX is ideal because it has a rapid onset (usually 1–2 months before a plateau of effectiveness), a high efficacy rate at managing symptoms and slowing disease progression, low toxicity, and a long history of successful use.[28]

Dosing

CASE 44-6, QUESTION 2: How should MTX be dosed and administered to S.S.?

In general, MTX is administered orally at an initial dose of 7.5 mg once a week, usually in a single weekly dose. The dose can also be divided into three equal parts (e.g., starting dose of 2.5 mg every 12 hours for a total of three doses) for patients who are unable to tolerate adverse effects, particularly hepatotoxicity.[40] If S.S.'s RA shows no objective response in 1 to 2 months, the dose is increased to 15 mg/week (or 5 mg every 12 hours for three doses) for at least 12 additional weeks. If no response is seen at this time, then (a) the dose can be increased to the maximum of 25 mg/week, (b) the dose can be administered as a subcutaneous or IM injection to address bioavailability concerns, (c) the same dose can be continued for a longer time, or (d) another DMARD can be added to MTX or MTX can be substituted.[131]

When subcutaneous MTX was compared with oral MTX in a 6-month randomized, controlled trial of 384 MTX-naïve patients with active RA,[132] 78% of patients treated with subcutaneous MTX achieved an ACR-20 response, and only 70% of those treated with oral MTX achieved a similar response. At week 16 of this study, patients treated with oral MTX, who failed to attain an ACR-20 response, were switched to subcutaneous MTX; patients treated with subcutaneous MTX who failed to attain an ACR-20 response were given a larger MTX dose (20 mg) subcutaneously. The patients who were converted from oral dosing to subcutaneous dosing and the patients who were given a larger subcutaneous dose had a 30% and 23% ACR response rate at week 24, respectively. As a result, subcutaneous MTX seems to be more effective than oral MTX and not associated with a higher incidence of adverse effects.

Adverse Effects

CASE 44-6, QUESTION 3: What subjective and objective data should be evaluated for evidence of MTX adverse effects in S.S.?

S.S. should be monitored for nausea and other GI distress, malaise, dizziness, mucositis, and mild alopecia, which are commonly encountered adverse effects associated with low-dose MTX therapy.[128] More serious, but less common, adverse effects include myelosuppression, pneumonitis, and hepatic fibrosis and cirrhosis. A CBC, LFTs, and a serum creatinine concentration should be obtained for her at baseline, monthly for the first 6 months of therapy, and then every 4 to 8 weeks during MTX therapy. Renal dysfunction can result in accumulation of MTX and higher risk of myelosuppression. Interstitial pneumonitis, occurring in <1% of patients, has no known risk factors for development, although it may be more common in patients with a history of lung disease.[130] In addition, interstitial pneumonitis can occur at any time during therapy and at any MTX dosage. A baseline chest radiograph is recommended within the year before MTX initiation. If the patient is found to have preexisting lung disease, MTX treatment should be reconsidered because further pulmonary damage could be devastating to the patient. S.S. also should be monitored carefully for cough, dyspnea on exertion, and shortness of breath at each clinic visit.

MTX-induced liver disease is rare, but increased age, long duration of therapy, obesity, diabetes mellitus, ethanol consumption, and a history of hepatitis B or C increase the risk of hepatotoxicity.[131] MTX should be prescribed with great caution, if at all, in patients with preexisting liver disease. The serum concentrations of liver enzymes commonly are modestly increased after administration for 1 to 2 days. However, MTX should be withheld if liver enzymes increase to 3 times the baseline value or if the liver enzyme serum concentrations remain elevated for sustained periods during therapy. Patients taking MTX should avoid alcohol and be instructed to report symptoms of jaundice or dark urine to their primary care provider. Routine liver biopsies to monitor for MTX-induced hepatotoxicity are unnecessary (see Case 44-6, Question 4).

Liver Biopsy and Methotrexate

CASE 44-6, QUESTION 4: The following laboratory test results were obtained for S.S. before starting MTX:

ALT, 28 IU/L
Aspartate aminotransferase (AST), 30 IU/L
Alkaline phosphatase, 100 IU/L
Albumin, 4.5 g/dL
Total bilirubin, 0.8 mg/dL

Should a baseline liver biopsy be performed before S.S. starts MTX?

Liver biopsy is only recommended at baseline for MTX patients who have a history of heavy alcohol consumption, persistently elevated liver function tests (defined as elevations above the upper limit of normal [ULN] in AST for 5 of 9 tests within a 12-month period [or 6 of 12 if tests are performed every month] or a reduction in serum albumin below normal range), or chronic hepatitis B or C. During therapy, patients with persistently elevated liver functions tests or serum albumin below normal range should have a repeat liver biopsy. Otherwise, routine liver biopsy is unnecessary and not cost-effective.[131] Diligent liver function testing has proven to be highly effective at preventing liver injury.[133] When initiating or escalating methotrexate dosing, ALT with or without AST, creatinine and CBC should be checked every 4 to 6 weeks until stable dosing is achieved, then testing should be repeated every 1 to 3 months thereafter along with screening for adverse effects and hepatotoxicity risk factors at every visit.

Because S.S.'s LFTs are normal and there is not a history of liver disease noted, there is no reason to consider a baseline liver biopsy.

Methotrexate and Folate or Folinic Acid

CASE 44-6, QUESTION 5: When should folate (or folinic acid) be administered to reduce the risk of MTX-related toxicity in S.S.?

Folate supplementation appears to reduce the incidence of several MTX-related adverse effects including GI disturbances, mucositis (mouth or GI ulcerations), and LFT elevations.[133] The current consensus and evidence-based recommendation is >5 mg folic acid daily. Although daily doses of folic acid as low as 1 mg are associated with protection against liver toxicity, GI disturbances are best prevented at doses above 5 mg daily. Although folinic acid has also proven to be effective at lowering GI and hepatotoxicity, doses above 5 mg/week are associated with worsening of arthritis symptoms, consistent with the fact that MTX is a folate antagonist, and folic acid supplementation could adversely impact efficacy.[130,133]

Methotrexate-Related Pulmonary Disorders

CASE 44-6, QUESTION 6: S.S. is treated with MTX 7.5 mg and with folic acid 7 mg orally once a week. Nine weeks later, she returns to the clinic with subjective and objective improvement in morning stiffness, fatigability, and joint tenderness and swelling. However, she has noted increased shortness of breath and dyspnea in the past week. Why might these symptoms be related to MTX?

Pneumonitis, a rare complication of MTX therapy, is characterized by a nonproductive cough, malaise, and fever, progressing to severe dyspnea.[134] Risk factors include older age (over 60 years), previous use of DMARDs, low albumin, and diabetes. Recognition of this unusual reaction is important to ensure that MTX is discontinued before the pneumonitis progresses to respiratory failure. After discontinuation of MTX, pulmonary function improves. Corticosteroids can accelerate improvement in pulmonary symptoms associated with pneumonitis. S.S.'s dyspnea and shortness of breath might be related to MTX. If appropriate tests rule out other causes for her pulmonary complaints, MTX-induced pulmonary toxicity should be considered and MTX treatment discontinued.

Methotrexate Interactions

CASE 44-6, QUESTION 7: What major MTX food and drug interactions need to be discussed with S.S. by her providers?

NSAIDs increase MTX serum concentrations and increase the risk of toxicity.[131] MTX doses should be adjusted cautiously if S.S. is taking NSAIDs concurrently to manage her RA pain. Trimethoprim, frequently used as part of the treatment for urinary tract infections, can increase the risk of MTX-induced bone marrow suppression. The concurrent use of MTX and LEF has been associated with major liver damage, including fatalities; as a result, this combination should be avoided. The inorganic acids in cola drinks appear to delay MTX elimination and can increase risk of toxicity, including renal toxicity; as a result, cola drinks should be avoided with MTX therapy.[135] Because MTX is protein bound and renally excreted, other drugs (e.g., salicylates, probenecid, penicillin, and ciprofloxacin) also might interact with MTX.

Leflunomide: Place in Therapy

CASE 44-7

QUESTION 1: B.W., a 36-year-old woman, has severe, progressive RA and is not responding sufficiently to MTX therapy. Would LEF be a reasonable consideration for her?

LEF, an oral csDMARD, seems to be similar in efficacy to MTX with regard to ACR-20, radiographic response, and work productivity.[28] The onset of benefit (as early as 4 weeks) and the percentage of patients who discontinue LEF therapy because of either lack of efficacy or toxicity are similar for LEF, MTX, and SSZ. The preferred initial csDMARD is MTX because of a long history of safety and efficacy, but LEF is a reasonable consideration as a replacement for MTX-intolerant patients, along with bDMARDs.

Dosing and Monitoring

CASE 44-7, QUESTION 2: How should therapy with LEF be initiated in B.W. and how would you monitor B.W. for adverse effects?

The active metabolite of LEF, A77 1726 or M1, is responsible for virtually all the pharmacologic activity of LEF.[131] The serum half-life of the M1 metabolite is approximately 2 weeks. As a result, LEF should be initiated with a loading dose of 100 mg orally once daily for 3 days to reduce time to steady state, followed by 20 mg once daily. If this dose is not tolerated, the dose should be reduced to 10 mg once daily.

Monitoring for Adverse Effects

Diarrhea (20%–30%), rash (10%), alopecia (10%–17%), and reversible liver enzyme elevations more than 3 times the ULN (2%–4%) are common adverse effects of LEF.[131] Routine laboratory testing includes a baseline ALT followed by monthly ALT testing for several months. When it is evident that ALT results are stable and within normal limits, testing can be performed less often according to the clinician's judgment. Because of the risk of liver toxicity and the need for activation by the liver to the M1 active metabolite, LEF is not recommended in patients with preexisting liver disease, including hepatitis B or C.

Potential hepatotoxicity is the greatest concern with LEF; however, the rate of LEF-induced liver enzyme elevation is not significantly different than MTX. Guidelines for managing potential hepatotoxicity include dosage reduction from 20 to 10 mg/day if ALT increases more than 2 times the ULN.[131] If ALT elevations remain steady between 2 and 3 times the ULN and treatment continuation is desired, a liver biopsy is recommended. If ALT elevations are persistently more than 3 times the ULN despite dosage reduction and cholestyramine administration to enhance elimination (see Case 44-7, Question 3), then the drug should be discontinued and another course of cholestyramine elimination therapy should be given.

Enhancement of Elimination with Cholestyramine

CASE 44-7, QUESTION 3: After 2 months of therapy, B.W. does not respond to LEF and the treatment was discontinued, especially because she is beginning to consider starting a family. What precautions must be taken when discontinuing LEF?

LEF (pregnancy category X) has not been tested in pregnant women, but it greatly increases the risk of fetal death or teratogenicity in animals receiving as little as 1% of human equivalent doses.[131] After discontinuation of therapy, however, up to 2 years may be needed to elapse before plasma M1 metabolite levels of LEF are undetectable. As a result, cholestyramine is recommended for all women who discontinue LEF and who are hoping to become pregnant. After stopping the medication, cholestyramine 8 g 3 times daily is administered for 11 days (which need not be consecutive). Plasma levels of the M1 metabolite are reduced by 40% to 65% in 24 to 48 hours and should become undetectable (<0.02 mg/L) at the end of therapy. B.W.'s blood should be tested at least 14 days apart to verify the absence of the metabolite. If plasma M1 levels remain greater than 0.02 mg/L, more cholestyramine should be administered. Cholestyramine also can be used to enhance elimination of LEF in patients who experience hepatotoxicity or who overdose with this drug. Activated charcoal also can reduce plasma M1 levels by 50% after 48 hours and can be an effective alternative to cholestyramine when LEF overdosages need to be managed.

Hydroxychloroquine and Sulfasalazine

CASE 44-7, QUESTION 4: Would it be reasonable to switch B.W. from MTX to either HCQ or SSZ?

Although both HCQ and SSZ are recommended first-line DMARDs for patients with mild-to-moderate RA, it is more common to add either or both of these to the regimen of patients who are not achieving adequate RA control from MTX.[28] HCQ, usually dosed at 200 to 400 mg daily, is a very well-tolerated DMARD. The greatest adverse effect of concern, retinal damage, is rare and easily prevented with diligent monitoring and dose limitations. SSZ, dosed at 2 to 3 g/day divided into two or three doses, is also well tolerated, although toxicity in general is greater than that with HCQ. GI distress (nausea, anorexia) and rash are common. Although leukopenia, agranulocytosis, and hepatitis are serious side effects, they are rare and, if they do occur, normally manifest in the first 2 to 3 months of therapy. As a result, CBC, LFTs, and renal function testing is recommended more frequently early in the course of therapy. Both HCQ and SSZ appear to be safe in pregnancy.

Although B.W. has failed to respond to MTX and LEF, combinations of csDMARDs and bDMARDs offer greater efficacy with lower toxicity and are therefore preferable.[28]

Traditional Disease-Modifying Antirheumatic Drug Combination Therapy

CASE 44-7, QUESTION 5: Is there evidence to support the early and safe use of DMARDs in combination for B.W.?

Because most RA patients develop joint erosions within the first 2 years of disease, the initiation of disease-modifying agents early in the course of therapy, and using them in combination, has been associated with improved patient outcomes. The rationale for combination therapy is based on the premise that a combination of drugs might improve outcomes because of different pharmacologic mechanisms of action or different sites of actions. A combination of drugs also may allow the use of lower doses of individual drugs, thereby reducing the risk of toxicity while maintaining or possibly increasing efficacy. The early use of combinations of potent disease-modifying agents also can expose the patient to increased risks of drug adverse effects.

Current ACR guidelines support csDMARD combinations as an alternative for patients who fail to reach treatment goals on a single csDMARD but give equal weight to considering other treatment options such as bDMARDs with or without MTX and tofacitinib.[28] Few studies have compared csDMARD combinations with bDMARD therapy. However, one study that randomized patients who failed MTX to receive either MTX + SSZ + HCQ or MTX + infliximab found no difference in clinical measures and serious adverse effects between the two groups after 24 months, although radiographic evidence of disease progression was slightly but not significantly greater in patients receiving MTX + SSZ + HCQ.[136]

In summary, every RA patient, including B.W., should receive csDMARD therapy at or shortly after diagnosis, with MTX monotherapy as preferred initial treatment. Patients who experience loss of efficacy or intolerable adverse effects from MTX can add one or two csDMARDs, or add or substitute a bDMARD or tofacitinib which will be discussed in ensuing sections.

Biologic DMARD Drug Therapy

CASE 44-7, QUESTION 6: After 6 months of treatment with csDMARDs (MTX with LEF, then MTX with HCQ), B.W.'s response is inadequate, her RA remains highly active and she has signs of early joint damage. B.W.'s physician would like to try a TNF-α inhibitor. Is a TNF-α inhibitor an appropriate treatment option for B.W.?

According to the EULAR guidelines, biologic DMARDs should be considered for patients with moderate-to-high disease activity with poor prognostic factors, who do not reach treatment targets with the first csDMARD strategy (MTX alone or in combination with another csDMARD) within 6 months or without poor prognostic factors, who fail a second csDMARD strategy.[28] The ACR guidelines recommend the use of bDMARDs for patients with moderate or high disease activity despite trial with csDMARD monotherapy.[28] There are five TNF-α inhibitors available for the treatment of RA including etanercept, adalimumab, infliximab, certolizumab pegol, and golimumab. Given that B.W. has tried two different csDMARD combinations and continues to have highly active RA with poor prognostic factors, it is time to consider a bDMARD. In fact, patients who fail to respond to csDMARD or bDMARD therapy within 3 months should receive consideration for an alternative treatment. A TNF-α inhibitor, adalimumab, or tocilizumab would all be appropriate choices for a first-line bDMARD according to the EULAR guidelines. However, TNF inhibitors have been available on the market for longer and thus have more robust long-term safety data, which may influence prescribers' confidence in these agents. A TNF-α inhibitor would be an appropriate choice in therapy for B.W. Her MTX therapy should be continued with the selected anti-TNF agent.

CASE 44-7, QUESTION 7: Which TNF-α inhibitor should be started in patient B.W.?

There are five TNF-α inhibitors available for the treatment of RA including etanercept, adalimumab, infliximab, certolizumab pegol, and golimumab. While there are multiple studies describing the efficacy and safety of these agents, there is no consensus on the preferred initial TNF-α inhibitor. The use of each of these medications as well as comparisons between them will be explored here.

TNF-α Inhibitors: Place in Therapy and Dosing

Etanercept (ETA) is the first biologic response modifier to be approved by the FDA for reducing the signs and symptoms of moderate to severe active RA, either alone or in combination with MTX.[44] ETA is a soluble TNF receptor that competitively binds two TNF molecules, rendering both molecules inactive. It is self-administered once weekly by subcutaneous injection at a dose of 50 mg.[44] ETA provides rapid and significant improvement in subjective and objective measures of RA, either alone or in combination with MTX.[43,137] The addition of ETA to MTX therapy has shown greater clinical efficacy when compared with MTX monotherapy.[138] ETA has also been shown to be superior to MTX as monotherapy in the reduction of RA symptoms and disease activity.[139,140] ETA has demonstrated decreased radiographic progression of RA as well as long-term safety and efficacy.[141,142] Etanercept is a reasonable choice for B.W. and should be used in combination with MTX for best results.

Adalimumab (ADA) is a genetically engineered, fully humanized IgG1 monoclonal antibody that has been shown to inhibit the structural damage of RA while reducing clinical signs and symptoms. The recommended dose is 40 mg administered by subcutaneous injection every other week. It is recommended to give ADA in combination with MTX.[45] Patients who cannot or choose not to take MTX may benefit from weekly dosing.[45] When ADA 40 mg every other week was added to the treatment regimen of RA patients receiving stable MTX doses, significantly more ADA-treated patients (67%) achieved an ACR-20 response than those receiving only MTX (14.5%, $p < 0.001$) after 24 weeks.[143] Combination therapy with ADA and MTX was shown to be superior to either MTX or ADA monotherapy for RA symptoms and disease progression.[144] In radiographic data reflecting 1 or 2 years of treatment, ADA has been shown to slow the progression of joint damage. Data also support the long-term efficacy and safety of ADA for more than 8 years.[145] ADA would also be an appropriate choice for B.W. and would require less frequent injections than ETA.

Infliximab (IFX) is a chimeric (mouse–human) IgG antibody directed against TNF. Specifically, IFX is approved in combination with MTX for the treatment of moderate to severe active RA. The recommended dose is 3 mg/kg via intravenous infusion at weeks 0, 2, and 6, then every 8 weeks thereafter. Some patients may benefit from an increase in dose up to 10 mg/kg or a decrease in treatment interval to as often as every 4 weeks.[46] IFX should be given with MTX therapy to prevent the formation of antibodies to infliximab. In a randomized, double-blind, multicenter, placebo-controlled trial of active RA patients who failed to respond adequately to at least 12.5 mg/week of MTX, IFX 3 or 10 mg/kg or placebo was administered every 4 or 8 weeks along with MTX therapy. The signs and symptoms of RA were improved in the IFX groups versus MTX alone. This study was unblinded after 1 year because of radiographic evidence of disease modification in patients receiving IFX. Analysis of radiographic results after 2 years demonstrated that IFX significantly protected against joint erosion.[146] IFX would also be an appropriate bDMARD for B.W., particularly if she prefers less frequent intravenous infusions to self-administration of subcutaneous injections. Patient preferences are an important factor to consider when choosing between the anti-TNF agents.

Certolizumab pegol (CZP) consists of a Fab attached to a 40-kDa PEG moiety. The attachment to the PEG moiety increases the half-life of CZP to approximately 2 weeks, which allows dosing every 2 to 4 weeks.[147] The recommended dosing regimen is 400 mg initially and at weeks 2 and 4 followed by 200 mg every other week or 400 mg every 4 weeks by subcutaneous injection.[47] CZP's unique structure lacks an Fc region, so it may not induce complement- or antibody-dependent cell-mediated cytotoxicity, which has been observed in vitro with adalimumab, etanercept, and infliximab.[148] The efficacy of CZP has been demonstrated in patients with moderate to severe active RA in combination with MTX and as monotherapy.[149–151] In a randomized, double-blind, placebo-controlled study in 619 patients with active RA, significantly more patients met ACR response rates with CZP plus MTX than patients treated with placebo plus MTX ($p < 0.001$).[150] Physical function, as evidenced by the mean change in the HAQ disability index (DI) score, DAS28 remission, and radiographic progression of RA were all improved in the CZP plus MTX group.[150] CZP has shown sustained efficacy and safety over 5 years in patients with active RA.[152] Patient B.W. would also be a candidate for CZP. As with ETA and ADA, CZP is self-administered by subcutaneous injection.

Golimumab (GLM) is a human IgG1 monoclonal antibody specific for human TNF-α. It was created using genetically engineered mice immunized with human TNF. GLM binds to both the soluble and the transmembrane bioactive forms of human TNF. This binding prevents the binding of TNF-α to its receptors, thus inhibiting the biologic activity of TNF-α.[49] GLM shares common characteristics with both adalimumab and infliximab. Similar to adalimumab, GLM is a fully humanized bivalent immunoglobulin monoclonal antibody.[153] GLM is made up of light and heavy chains, which are identical to infliximab, but whereas infliximab is derived from both mice and humans, GLM is completely humanized. GLM is approved for the treatment of moderate-to-severe active RA in combination with MTX.[49] It can be administered by subcutaneous injection or intravenous infusion. The subcutaneous injection is a 50 mg injection dosed every 4 weeks.[49] The dose of the intravenous infusion is 2 mg/kg over 30 minutes as weeks 0 and 4, then every 8 weeks thereafter.[154] Clinical trials have demonstrated GLM efficacy in patients with no previous MTX use and in patients with an inadequate response to MTX or a TNF-α inhibitor.[155–157] A randomized, placebo-controlled trial conducted in 444 patients examined the efficacy of GLM in patients with active RA despite concomitant MTX use.[158] Significantly, more patients in the combined GLM plus MTX group achieved an ACR-20 response compared with the MTX plus placebo group (55.6% vs. 33.1%, respectively, $p < 0.001$), and these results were sustained at 52 weeks.[158] In another study assessing the long-term safety and efficacy of GLM in RA patients who discontinued previous TNF-α inhibitors, GLM treatment resulted in sustained efficacy and safety through 5 years.[158] Given this information, GLM would also be an appropriate treatment option for B.W., and she would have the option of choosing between intravenous or subcutaneous dosing.

There are currently no definitive guidelines recommending one TNF-α inhibitor over another. Direct head-to-head comparisons

Table 44-7

Biologic Disease-Modifying Antirheumatic Drug Dosing Information

Generic (Brand)	Mechanism of Action	Dosage Range	Administration Schedule	Routes of Administration	Can Be Self-Administered?
Infliximab (Remicade)	TNF-α inhibitor	3 mg/kg[a]	Weeks 0, 2, and 6 and then every 8 weeks	IV	No
Etanercept (Enbrel)	TNF-α inhibitor	50 mg	Weekly	SC	Yes
Adalimumab (Humira)	TNF-α inhibitor	40 mg	Every 14 days	SC	Yes
Certolizumab pegol (Cimzia)	TNF-α inhibitor	Initial: 400 mg SC on weeks 0, 2, 4 Subsequent: 200 mg every 2 weeks or 400 mg every 4 weeks	Weeks 0, 2, and 4, then every 2 or 4 weeks	SC	Yes
Golimumab (Simponi)	TNF-α inhibitor	50 mg	Every 4 weeks	SC	Yes
Golimumab (Simponi Aria)	TNF-α inhibitor	2 mg/kg infusion over 30 minutes	Weeks 0 and 4, then every 8 weeks	IV	No
Abatacept (Orencia)	Costimulation modulator, T cell activation inhibitor	Weight based: <60 kg = 500 mg 60–100 kg = 750 mg >100 kg = 1,000 mg	Weeks 0, 2, and 4 and then every 4 weeks	IV	No
		Or			
		125 mg	Once weekly (may be initiated with or without IV loading dose)	SC	Yes
Rituximab (Rituxan)	CD20+ B-cell inhibitor	1,000 mg IV infusion: Initial: 50 mg/hour, may increase every 30 minutes to a maximum rate of 400 mg/hour Subsequent: 100 mg/hour, may increase every 30 minutes to maximum rate of 400 mg/hour[b]	Repeat in 14 days, then discontinue	IV	No
Tocilizumab (Actemra)	IL-6 inhibitor	Initial: 4 mg/kg every 4 weeks Subsequent: Titrate to 8 mg/kg based on clinical response Max: 800 mg/dose (8 mg/kg)	Every 4 weeks	IV	No
		Or			
		Weight based SC dosing: <100 kg= 162 mg every other week, followed by an increase to every week based on clinic response ≥100 kg = 162 mg every week		SC	Yes
Anakinra (Kineret)	IL-1 inhibitor	100 mg	Once daily	SC	Yes

[a]For incomplete response, may increase dose to 10 mg/kg or decrease dosing interval to every 4 weeks.
[b]Premedicate with corticosteroid, acetaminophen, and an antihistamine before each dose.
Source: Drug Facts and Comparisons. Facts & Comparisons eAnswers [database online]. St. Louis, MO: Wolters Kluwer Health, Inc. Updated periodically. Accessed August 4, 2015.
IL, interleukin; IV, intravenous; SC, subcutaneous; TNF, tumor necrosis factor.

between the anti-TNF agents are lacking; therefore, prescribers must depend on surveillance data, systematic reviews, and meta-analyses to make clinical decisions regarding comparative efficacy and safety.

In a mixed treatment comparison of the anti-TNF agents, all of the agents demonstrated significant improvement in clinical response across all outcome measures. However, etanercept and certolizumab demonstrated improved outcomes compared to infliximab, adalimumab, and golimumab. All anti-TNF agents were found to be superior to infliximab.[160] Evidence from national registries have also provided insight into the differences among TNF-α inhibitors in clinical practice. Patients in the Czech National Registry had higher survival rates when treated with adalimumab and etanercept compared to infliximab.[161] Data from the Danish and Swedish national registries have shown the drug continuation rates were significantly higher with etanercept and adalimumab than with infliximab.[145,162,163] In a meta-analysis of Cochrane reviews of six biologics for RA (abatacept, adalimumab, anakinra, etanercept, infliximab, and rituximab), it was found that etanercept was associated with lower rates of withdrawal because of adverse events than either adalimumab or infliximab, and the survival rates with adalimumab and etanercept were better than with infliximab.[164] Given this data, etanercept would be an appropriate choice for B.W. as initial therapy with a bDMARD. Systematic reviews seem to demonstrate that etanercept is well-tolerated in comparison to other bDMARDs and has been associated with superior efficacy. Given no other patient specific factors to guide therapy toward another agent, etanercept would be an appropriate option. (Dosing information for the TNF-α inhibitors can be found in Table 44-7.)

CASE 44-7, QUESTION 8: What side effects will need to be monitored when starting B.W. on etanercept?

TNF-α Inhibitors: Side Effects and Monitoring

The greatest concern with etanercept therapy is the risk of immunosuppression and subsequent serious infections, including sepsis. TNF-α is a key mediator of inflammation and plays a major role in immune system regulation. Post-marketing reports of infections, such as TB, mycobacterial infections, and fungal infections, further reinforce the strong recommendation against the initiation of etanercept therapy in patients with sepsis or any chronic or localized active infection.[44] Mycobacterium tuberculosis skin testing and a baseline chest radiograph should be undertaken before initiation of anti-TNF therapy. Therapy should be postponed for patients identified as having latent TB until appropriate antituberculosis therapy has been completed.[28] Clinicians also must be cautious when prescribing etanercept (or any bDMARD) to patients with a history of recurring infection or with underlying illnesses that predispose them to infection (i.e., diabetes). B.W. should receive a TB skin test, undergo a chest radiograph, and be warned of the potential adverse effects of etanercept, particularly the risk of immunosuppression and subsequent infection. Any sign of infection must be reported immediately to her health care provider.

TNF-α has been implicated in the pathophysiology of heart failure, and increased serum levels of TNF-α seem to be associated with worsening heart failure.[165] Proposed mechanisms contributing to the onset or worsening of heart failure include accelerated left ventricular remodeling, negative inotropic effects, and increased apoptosis of myocytes and endothelial cells. However, despite the association between TNF-α and worsening of heart failure, clinical trials with anti-TNF therapy (which have included etanercept and infliximab) have not reduced mortality and heart failure–related hospitalizations. Furthermore, some trials have shown increased cardiovascular risk.[165] As a result, anti-TNF therapy is not recommended for RA patients with moderate-to-severe (New York Heart Association [NYHA] class III and IV) heart failure. Anti-TNF therapy can be used with caution in patients with mild (NYHA class I and II) heart failure, but patients should be closely monitored for cardiac decompensation.[26,28]

Included in the labeling for all anti-TNF bDMARDs is a warning for increased risk of lymphoma. An increased incidence of lymphoma has been observed among patients with RA receiving any of the available anti-TNF agents; however, causation has not been established because both RA and MTX are associated with an increased rate of lymphoma. In an observational study assessing the risk of lymphoma in patients treated with csDMARDs compared to patients treated with anti-TNF agents, there was no evidence of an increased risk in the anti-TNF cohort.[166] A meta-analysis of patients receiving anti-TNF agents suggested a possible increase in incidence of lymphoma; however, given the low incidence of lymphoma overall, this failed to reach statistical significance.[167] Additionally, the FDA has issued a warning following reports of hepatosplenic T-cell lymphoma, a rare cancer of the white blood cells, in patients being treated with TNF blockers, AZA, or mercaptopurine.[168] The majority of these cases were found in adolescents and young adults with Crohn's disease or ulcerative colitis. Incidence was also more common in patients on a combination of immunosuppressive agents. Although it is difficult to measure the added risk associated with anti-TNF agents, caution and monitoring is advised.[168] Other adverse effects, in order of decreasing frequency, include headache, rhinitis, dizziness, pharyngitis, cough, asthenia, abdominal pain, and rash.

CASE 44-8

QUESTION 1: S.K., a 71-year-old woman, was diagnosed with RA approximately 15 years ago. Her initial drug therapy included MTX, followed by the addition of SSZ and HCQ, which seemed to keep her RA in near-remission for 5 years. She then began etanercept along with MTX (without SSZ and HCQ) with good results until 1 year ago. In response to declining disease control, infliximab was substituted for etanercept with excellent results. Then last month, she experienced a flare in RA activity. At that time, her CRP was 5.1 mg/dL, ESR was 90 mm/hour, and anti-CCP was positive at 112 units. She also experienced morning stiffness lasting several hours and multiple joints with swelling (n = 26) and tenderness (n = 38). Of note, S.K. has a history of treated skin melanoma 2 years ago. What are the reasonable treatment options for S.K. at this stage of her disease?

Clinical studies have consistently demonstrated that bDMARDs improve the signs and symptoms of RA as well as slow the progression of structural damage. TNF-α inhibitors have long been considered first-line bDMARDs given the availability of long-term data and clinical experience compared to the non-TNF bDMARDs. However, ongoing registry and trial data suggests that the safety profiles of the non-TNF bDMARDs, abatacept, rituximab, and tocilizumab, are consistent with clinical trial results.[26] Some trials have shown superiority of some of these agents over TNF-α inhibitors. TNF-α inhibitors also fail to produce an ACR-20 response in approximately 30% of patients, which is known as primary failure. Even more patients experience acquired resistance to treatment, known as secondary failure, which is defined as a loss of response with time and is illustrated by S.K.[169] Many patients who lose responsiveness to an initial trial of anti-TNF therapy can be successfully treated with an alternative anti-TNF agent.[170] However, studies have also shown that response rates with sequential anti-TNF therapy may be lower and the reasons for initial anti-TNF failure (inefficacy or adverse effects) may be recurrent.[170,171] Therefore, it is important to consider alternative options for the treatment of patients like S.K. with anti-TNF treatment failure.[170,171]

Abatacept (inhibitor of T-cell activation), rituximab (selective depletor of CD20+ B cells), and tocilizumab (anti-IL-6 receptor antibody) have demonstrated excellent efficacy in patients with inadequate response to csDMARDs (e.g., MTX) as well as to anti-TNF therapy.[26,28] Owing to their differing mechanisms of action, each of these agents possesses unique qualities with regard to efficacy and safety. (Detailed dosing information for the bDMARDs can be found in Table 44-7.)

Abatacept

Abatacept (ABT) is a selective costimulation inhibitor of T-cell activation indicated for the treatment of moderate to severe active RA.[52] ABT may be prescribed as monotherapy or in combination with csDMARDs. It can be administered intravenously or subcutaneously. ABT intravenous dosing is based on body weight (500 mg for patients <60 kg, 750 mg for patients 60–100 kg, and 1,000 mg for patients >100 kg) and should be infused over 30 minutes at weeks 2 and 4 after the first dose, then every 4 weeks thereafter.[52] The dose for the subcutaneous injection is 125 mg weekly. The efficacy and safety profiles have been shown to be comparable between the two preparations.[172]

Abatacept has demonstrated efficacy in patients with an inadequate response to MTX as well as in patients with an inadequate response or adverse reactions to TNF-α inhibitors.[52] In a study comparing ABT plus MTX to placebo plus MTX, significantly more patients in the ABT plus MTX group attained ACR-20 response when compared with the ABT plus placebo group (73.1% vs. 39.7%, respectively, $p < 0.001$) and had significant slowing of structural damage progression compared to the patients treated with placebo at 12-month follow-up.[53] ABT efficacy was maintained in the 5-year open-label extension of this trial. Structural damage progression was reduced by 50% in the second year relative to the first year, with approximately half of the patients who completed all 5 years of ABT treatment exhibiting no structural damage progression.[173] Efficacy and safety data from 7 years of ABT therapy indicate that ABT maintains sustained improvements in disease activity and ACR-70 scores during this period, with no change in safety profile.[174] ABT has also demonstrated efficacy in patients with an inadequate response to one or more TNF-α inhibitors, such as S.K.[175,176]

Finally, ABT has also been compared head-to-head with the TNF-α inhibitor adalimumab. In a 2-year study in RA patients with an inadequate response to MTX, ABT and ADA were found to be similar in both efficacy and safety. Overall, patients experienced similar improvement in clinical markers of disease control and progression. While rates of adverse events in both groups were similar, there were more discontinuations because of adverse events in the ADA group (9.5%) compared to the ABT group (3.8%) (95% CI −9.5 to −1.9).[177]

The side effects of greatest concern with ABT include infections such as pneumonia, cellulitis, urinary tract infection, bronchitis, diverticulitis, and acute pyelonephritis. Infections are significantly more common when ABT is combined with anti-TNF therapy; thus, this combination is not recommended.[52] A few case reports of malignancy have been associated with ABT, and patients with chronic obstructive pulmonary disease are noted to suffer from more respiratory-related and nonrespiratory-related adverse effects than patients with chronic obstructive pulmonary disease treated with placebo.[52]

Rituximab

Rituximab (RXB) is a chimeric monoclonal antibody that binds to the antigen CD20 on B cells. It is approved in combination with MTX for the treatment of moderate to severe active RA in patients who have had an inadequate response to one or more TNF antagonist medications.[54] However, according to the EULAR guidelines, rituximab may be considered as a first-line bDMARD in patients with contraindications to other bDMARDs, such as recent history of lymphoma, latent TB with contraindications to chemoprophylaxis, living in a TB-endemic areas or a previous history of demyelinating disease.[26] RXB, provided in 100- and 500-mg single-use vials at a concentration of 10 mg/mL, is administered as two 1,000-mg IV infusions separated by 2 weeks.[54] RXB must be diluted to a final concentration of 1 to 4 mg/mL with either 0.9% sodium chloride or 5% dextrose in water. To reduce the incidence and severity of infusion-related adverse effects, premedication with IV methylprednisolone 100 mg, or its equivalent, 30 minutes before each infusion is strongly recommended; other premedications (e.g., acetaminophen and antihistamine) may also be beneficial. Antihypertensive medications should be discontinued 12 hours before RXB administration to avoid transient hypotension, which has been reported during RXB infusions. RXB must be given with MTX for maximal efficacy based on clinical trials and to help reduce the risk of developing HACA, which occurs in approximately 9% of patients receiving RXB. It is recommended that subsequent courses of RXB be given every 24 weeks. The dosing interval may be decreased on the basis of clinical evaluation, but must be no less than every 16 weeks.[54]

Rituximab has been shown to be effective in patients who have responded inadequately to MTX therapy as well as in patients who have responded inadequately to anti-TNF medications.[178] The REFLEX (Randomized Evaluation of Long-Term Efficacy of Rituximab in RA) trial evaluated the use of RXB plus MTX versus placebo plus MTX in 499 patients with active, long-standing RA who responded inadequately to one or more anti-TNF medications, such as S.K.[179] At 24-week follow-up, significantly more patients in the RXB group demonstrated an ACR-20 response than those in the placebo group (51% vs. 18%, respectively). And in a 56-week follow-up report of the REFLEX trial, RXB significantly inhibited radiographic progression of joint damage.[180] In the 2-year extension of this trial, RXB showed significant and sustained inhibition of joint damage. These findings support the efficacy and appropriateness of RXB for RA patients, such as S.K., who are refractory to anti-TNF therapy.

In the case of failure with one TNF-α inhibitor, patients may be switched to another anti-TNF agent or to a non-TNF agent. While there are no randomized controlled trials providing head-to-head comparisons between switching to rituximab versus a second anti-TNF agent, there are some observational studies to guide therapy. In the SWITCH-RA trial, a global, observational, comparative effectiveness study, rituximab was compared to an alternative TNF inhibitor in patients with RA with a previous inadequate response to one TNF inhibitor. It was found that the change in DAS28-3-ESR at 6 months was significantly greater in the rituximab patients versus the second TNF inhibitor patients (−1.5 vs. −1.1; $p = 0.007$). However, this difference only remained significant for the patients who discontinued the initial TNF inhibitor because of inefficacy, but not in those who discontinued because of intolerance.[181] Similar results have been found in other observational studies of initial TNF nonresponders.[182] Clinicians should consider reasons for treatment failure, potential side effects, route of administration, ease of use, cost and patient specific factors when choosing an appropriate therapeutic regimen. There is currently no definitive investigation or recommendation for sequencing of bDMARDs. There is a randomized controlled trial underway comparing ABT, RXB, and other anti-TNF therapy following anti-TNF failure, which is expected to provide further insight upon completion.[183]

Infusion reactions, including severe reactions, can be caused by RXB. Severe reactions typically occur with the first infusion; thus, careful monitoring is warranted and premedication with methylprednisolone 100 mg or its equivalent is recommended 30 minutes prior to each infusion. RXB should be discontinued if a serious reaction occurs. Severe mucocutaneous reactions may also occur in patients receiving RXB. Finally, hepatitis B (HBV) reactivation may occur in patients receiving RXB. Therefore, all patients should be screened for HBV infection prior to initiation. The most common adverse reactions in RA patients receiving RXB include upper respiratory tract infections, nasopharyngitis, urinary tract infections, and bronchitis.[54] RXB has not been associated with any increase in malignancy; therefore, it is preferred over anti-TNF agents in patients with a recent history of cancer.[26]

Since S.K. failed two TNF- inhibitors because of inefficacy, either ABT or RXB would be an appropriate choice. Given S.K.'s history of skin melanoma 2 years ago, RXB would be the preferred agent over ABT in this patient.

CASE 44-9

QUESTION 1: Q.O. is a 55-year-old woman with highly active RA for the past year who cannot tolerate MTX therapy. Her doctor would like to start a bDMARD as monotherapy and would like to know which medication would be best?

Tocilizumab

Tocilizumab is a humanized anti-IL-6 receptor antibody indicated for the treatment of adult patients with moderate to severe active RA, who have had an inadequate response to one or more csDMARDs.[57] TCZ may be administered intravenously or subcutaneously. For the intravenous infusion, the recommended dosage is 4 mg/kg, infused IV every 4 weeks with an increase to 8 mg/kg as needed based on clinical response. The dosing for the subcutaneous formulation is 162 mg per injection either weekly or every other week depending on patient weight and response.[57] The safety and efficacy of the intravenous and subcutaneous formulations have been studied and appear to be comparable. However, an increase in injection site reactions in the subcutaneous TCZ group has been seen.[184] TCZ should not be initiated in patients with an absolute neutrophil count less than 2,000 cells/μL, platelet count less than 100,000 platelets/μL, or in patients who have an ALT or AST value greater than 1.5 times the ULN.[57] TCZ treatment should be interrupted if a patient experiences a serious infection; therapy may be resumed once the infection is controlled.[57]

TCZ has demonstrated efficacy in the treatment of RA as monotherapy, in combination with csDMARDs, and in patients who are refractory to anti-TNF medications.[185,186] In a systematic review of eight RCTS, TCZ at a dose of 8 mg/kg in combination with MTX was shown to statistically significantly decrease disease activity and improve physical function when compared to MTX plus placebo.[187] TCZ has also shown decreased radiographic progression of RA compared to csDMARDs.[185,188] In the RADIATE trial, patients with an inadequate response to one or more TNF-α inhibitors were randomly assigned to receive 8 or 4 mg/kg of TCZ or placebo every 4 weeks for 24 weeks.[186] An ACR-20 response was achieved at 24 weeks by 50.0%, 30.4%, and 10.1% of patients in the TCZ 8 mg/kg, 4 mg/kg, and placebo arms, respectively ($p < 0.001$).[186] Given this information, TCZ would also be a reasonable option for patients who have failed one or more TNF inhibitors, like S.K. from Case 44-8.

Tocilizumab is also approved as monotherapy for RA. In the AMBITION trial, TCZ monotherapy compared to MTX monotherapy and TCZ therapy was found to have a superior ACR 20 response (69.9% vs. 52.5%; $p < 0.001$) and DAS28 <2.6 rate (33.6 vs. 12.1%) at week 24.84. In a study comparing TCZ 8 mg/kg plus MTX, TCZ 4 mg/kg plus MTX, TCZ 8 mg/kg monotherapy, and MTX monotherapy, all groups containing TCZ showed superior DAS28 remission compared to MTX alone. However, only the TCZ 8 mg/kg plus MTX group had consistent superiority in clinical, functional, and radiographic outcomes.[85]

According to the ACR and EULAR treatment guidelines, the standard of care indicates that patients should maintain MTX or csDMARD therapy when a bDMARD is added.[26,28] However, for up to 40% of patients, MTX therapy is discontinued because of intolerance or patient preference and as many as one-third of patients may be taking bDMARDs as monotherapy.[86] Three of the TNF inhibitors (etanercept, adalimumab, and certolizumab pegol) and two of the non-TNF bDMARDs (abatacept and tocilizumab) are approved as monotherapy. In a study comparing ADA and TCZ monotherapy in patients who were either intolerant to MTX or MTX was not an appropriate treatment option, patients in the TCZ group were found to have significantly greater improvement in DAS28 as well as most clinical endpoints when compared to the ADA group.[86] Therefore, TCZ is a reasonable therapeutic option for Q.O. as monotherapy for RA and has demonstrated superiority over at least one anti-TNF agent.[186,188]

When starting TCZ, Q.O. should be monitored for potential side effects. The most serious side effects associated with TCZ therapy include severe infections, GI perforation, and laboratory abnormalities. As with the TNF-α inhibitors, TCZ has a boxed warning for increased risk of developing serious infections, especially those caused by opportunistic pathogens. The risk for infection is increased when TCZ is taken in combination with other immunosuppressant agents (e.g., MTX and corticosteroids). As with the anti-TNF agents, a TB skin test result and chest radiograph must be obtained before initiating treatment. In clinical studies the overall rate of fatal serious infections was low at 0.13/100 patient-years.[57]

TCZ has also been associated with a number of blood chemistry changes including neutropenia, thrombocytopenia, elevated LFTs, and lipid changes. Increases in lipids (total cholesterol, low-density lipoprotein, high-density lipoprotein, and triglycerides) have been shown in clinical trials. Increase in lipids may be caused in part by the decrease in inflammatory activity with TCZ use. Lipid elevations respond to lipid-lowering agents. While clinical trials do not indicate an increase in cardiovascular risk, further studies are necessary to assess the effects of TCZ on cardiovascular risk factors.[189,190]

CORTICOSTEROIDS

CASE 44-10

QUESTION 1: W.M., a 57-year-old man, has progressive RA that has not been responsive to SSZ. He is having difficulty working a full day and is seeking an alternative medication. After a discussion of therapeutic options, W.M. declines MTX therapy and asks to start HCQ. Would it be appropriate to initiate corticosteroids concurrently? And if so, at what dose?

Despite the potential for serious adverse effects with long-term therapy, the judicious use of low-dose corticosteroids represents an important component of treatment during the course of unremitting disease. In addition, low-dose corticosteroids may offer some disease-modifying properties, although this is controversial because of the long-term negative effects of corticosteroid use.[65] The benefit of low-dose glucocorticoid therapy is favorable as long as the course of therapy is short.[28] Considering that W.M.'s RA is sufficiently active to compromise his ability to earn an income, MTX is a much better DMARD selection. Regardless, concurrent initiation of a DMARD and an intermediate-acting corticosteroid (e.g., prednisone in a daily or divided dose of 5–10 mg) is justified.[191] A Cochrane review showed that corticosteroid doses equivalent to ≤15 mg of prednisolone were superior to placebo and NSAIDS for joint tenderness and pain in RA.[192] In large cohort studies, prednisone doses greater than 7.5 mg/day have been associated with a greater than twofold increased risk of cardiovascular events (MI, stroke, and heart failure), as well as the risk of developing hypertension with long-term use (at least 6–12 months).[193,194] Therefore, the lowest effective corticosteroid dose is preferred for the shortest duration of time possible.[28] The onset of action of corticosteroids is relatively rapid, and their immediate benefits will allow W.M. to maintain his current employment and continue taking care of responsibilities at home. The corticosteroid dose can be decreased gradually and eventually discontinued as W.M. begins to respond to HCQ therapy. An important goal of low-dose corticosteroid treatment is to provide bridge therapy until the DMARD therapy becomes effective, in hopes of then being able to taper and discontinue the corticosteroid.

CASE 44-10, QUESTION 2: Would intra-articular corticosteroid injections be a safe and effective treatment option for W.M.?

Intra-Articular Corticosteroids

Intra-articular corticosteroid injections are safe and effective for pain relief in patients with RA. This strategy is most sensible when flaring occurs in one or a few joints.[195] Systemic side effects are minimal when compared with oral corticosteroid therapy. Although onset of action is virtually immediate, effects are often short-lived. W.M. could benefit from the use of intermittent intra-articular corticosteroid injections for the treatment of RA flares.

JUVENILE IDIOPATHIC ARTHRITIS

Juvenile idiopathic arthritis is a heterogenous group of chronic arthritic conditions of unknown etiology, occurring before 16 years of age. It is the most common chronic rheumatic disorder in childhood, afflicting approximately 300,000 children in the United States, affecting all races equally with peak age of onset between two and four. However, new cases are seen throughout childhood and often continue into adulthood, causing significant morbidity and physical disability.[196–198]

Clinical Presentation and Classification

By definition, symptoms of JIA (joint inflammation involving swelling, pain, limited ROM, warmth, and erythema) present before the age of 16 and must last for at least 6 weeks in at least one joint.[199] Similar to other rheumatologic disease classifications, the diagnosis of JIA is a diagnosis of exclusion; infectious, traumatic, and other etiologies must be ruled out first.[200]

As with adult RA, JIA begins with synovial inflammation. Because children often cannot articulate complaints, morning stiffness and joint pain may manifest as increased irritability, guarding of involved joints, or refusal to walk. Fatigue and low-grade fever, anorexia, weight loss, and failure to grow are other symptoms. Patients with JIA are categorized as having one of the following seven types of disease as established by the International League of Associations for Rheumatology (ILAR): (1) systemic, (2) oligoarthritis, (3) polyarthritis RF+, (4) polyarthritis RF−, (5) psoriatic, (6) enthesitis-related, and (7) undifferentiated (patients who do not fulfill criteria of other JIA subsets).[201] For a catalog of JIA images, including radiography and ophthalmologic photographs, please go to http://images.rheumatology.org/search.php?searchField=ALL&searchstring=JIA.

The most common type of JIA is oligoarthritis, which comprises about 50% to 60% of all JIA cases. This type of JIA typically presents before the age of 6 years, with 80% cases afflicting girls. Oligoarthritis patients present with four or fewer affected joints, most commonly in the ankles. Those who do not progress beyond four joints are categorized with persistent oligoarthritis, but 50% may eventually develop arthritis in additional joints requiring a change in disease classification to extended oligoarthritis.[198,201]

JIA is classified as a polyarthritis when the disease involves five or more joints during the first 6 months of the disease with few or no systemic manifestations of disease.[201] Polyarthritis may be RF+ or RF− and accounts for up to 40% of all JIA disease, the majority of which is RF−.[202] Both types affect girls more often than boys. Disease onset is typically seen at age 8 or older, and most often in adolescents. RF+ polyarthritis presents very similarly to adult-onset RA, involving aggressive, erosive, and symmetric joint inflammation which may lead to general growth retardation, as well as fatigue, morning stiffness, and elevated inflammatory markers.[196,198]

Psoriatic JIA accounts for a small number of all JIA cases (about 5%) and is diagnosed if chronic arthritis and psoriasis are both evident. Children may also be diagnosed with psoriatic JIA if any two of the following are present: dactylitis (finger or toe inflammation), onycholysis or nail pitting, or family history of psoriasis.[196,201]

Enthesitis-related JIA is manifested as inflammation of the enthesis (the site of attachment of tendon to bone) along with arthritis, typically in the lower limbs, in boys older than 6 years old. Children with enthesitis-related JIA have at least two of the following in addition to arthritis or enthesitis: inflammatory lumbosacral or sacroiliac joint pain, HLA-B27 positivity, symptomatic anterior uveitis, or a family history of enthesitis-related JIA or ankylosing spondylitis (first-degree relative).[201,203]

CASE 44-11

QUESTION 1: J.R., a 4-year-old girl, is brought to the hospital for high fever and arthritis. Several weeks before admission, J.R. had a daily fever ranging from 103°F to 106°F. One week before admission, her knees became painful and swollen. J.R. is listless and irritable during her physical examination, and her rectal temperature measures 102.4°F. She refuses to walk. The right hip is tender, and the right wrist and both knees are warm, red, and swollen. Minimal generalized lymphadenopathy and splenomegaly are present. The Westergren ESR is 82 mm/hour, the white blood cell count is 37,000 cells/μL with a mild left shift, and hematocrit is 33%. Cultures of the throat, urine, stool, and blood are negative. MD global assessment is 4. An intermediate-strength purified-protein derivative, antistreptolysin-O titer, ANA titer, and RF titer are normal, as are radiographs of the chest and involved joints. An electrocardiogram reveals only tachycardia. After withholding aspirin, an evanescent rash becomes apparent in conjunction with fever spikes. What signs and symptoms of JIA does J.R. manifest?

The last category of JIA is systemic JIA, which is distinguished from other forms of the disease by the presence of hallmark systemic features including rash, lymphadenopathy, hepatomegaly or splenomegaly, serositis and cyclical high-spiking fever. J.R. exhibits these distinguishing symptoms and, in addition she also experiences joint pain in her knees, with other commonly afflicted joints including the wrists and ankles. The pain often worsens when fever is elevated, but may not be clinically evident at disease onset. Systemic JIA occurs equally in girls and boys and comprises approximately 15% of all JIA cases. Children presenting with this subtype of JIA may also have a normocytic, hypochromic anemia, elevated ESR, and thrombocytosis. Leukocytosis is common, and a white blood cell count of 30,000 to 50,000 cells/μL is seen occasionally. A positive RF titer is uncommon in JIA and is present in only 5% to 10% of all cases.[197,198]

Prognosis

CASE 44-11, QUESTION 2: What is the expected prognosis for J.R.?

Features of poor prognosis for patients with JIA generally include arthritides that involve cervical spine or hip joints, involvement of the ankle or wrist coupled with significant or prolonged elevation of ESR or other inflammatory markers, and radiographic damage.[199] Disease remission is qualified by lack of active arthritis in joints, absence of systemic symptoms (rash, fever, lymphadenopathy, etc.), symptomatic uveitis not present, normal ESR or CRP, and no disease activity measured on a physician's global assessment scale. While only 5% of patients achieve true remission, sustained periods of good control is becoming more common with treatment advances, and up to 35% to 50% of patients achieve clinical remission on medication therapy. Despite improvements in care, complete remission is still uncommon, and up to one-third of patients with JIA do experience long-term disability and decreased quality of life. Preservation of joint function is least promising in children with RF+ polyarthritis.[204–206] Although J.R. is exhibiting some poor prognostic indicators (hip and wrist involvement, elevated ESR), it is unclear whether these are long-term manifestations. Normal ANA and RF titers and the absence of radiographic damage are favorable for J.R.

Treatment

The goals of JIA treatment are to minimize joint inflammation and its destructive effects, control pain, preserve or restore ROM, facilitate an acceptable quality of life, and achieve long-term disease remission. Choice of medication therapy requires consideration of type of JIA, current treatment, degree of disease progression, level of disease activity, and prognosis.[199]

NONPHARMACOLOGIC THERAPY

In addition to treatment with medication, many patients with JIA can benefit from nonpharmacologic efforts to help preserve joint flexibility, maintain ROM, and prevent disability in adulthood. Patients with JIA are often less physically active and more easily fatigued than their disease-free peers, and they may meet developmental milestones later than children of the same age.[207] Children with JIA are also more prone to decreased bone mineral density than their peers.

CASE 44-11, QUESTION 3: J.R.'s parents understand the need for medication therapy but also want to encourage lifestyle interventions as a way to promote health and combat disease complications. What recommendation can the physician give to J.R. and her family once her acute symptoms are stabilized?

Heat and cold therapy, massage, and regular physical activity can all help reach disease treatment goals of minimizing joint inflammation, controlling pain, and improving quality of life. Regular physical activities, including muscle-strengthening, ROM activities, stretching, and endurance training, are safe and do not worsen arthritis. Weight-bearing exercise can help prevent bone loss, but it should be avoided when joints are acutely inflamed. At these times, low-impact sports such as swimming or bicycling can be enjoyed. Physical therapy and occupational therapy can also help pediatric patients hone gross and fine motor skills, balance, and coordination.[207,208] Once J.R.'s status improves, she should be encouraged to participate in regular exercise and organized therapy sessions to improve exercise capacity and preserve joint functioning.

PHARMACOLOGIC THERAPY AND TREATMENT CONSIDERATIONS

While ILAR differentiates JIA into seven disease types, the ACR treatment recommendations classify treatment groups by a different system, since there is little evidence to support pharmacologic decisions based on disease categorization itself. The five treatment groups consist of (1) history of arthritis in four or fewer joints, (2) history of arthritis in five or more joints, (3) active sacroiliac arthritis, (4) systemic arthritis without active arthritis, and (5) systemic arthritis without active arthritis.[199] However, the 2013 ACR update on systemic arthritis subdivides this treatment category into three distinct clinical phenotypes: (1) with active systemic features and varying degrees of synovitis, (2) without active systemic features and with varying degrees of active synovitis, and (3) features concerning for macrophage activation syndrome (MAS).

The history of arthritis of four or fewer joints treatment group includes ILAR disease-classified patients with extended oligoarthritis, RF− polyarthritis, RF+ polyarthritis, psoriatic arthritis, enthesitis-related arthritis, and undifferentiated arthritis, all have had no more than four affected joints in their disease course. NSAIDs as monotherapy may be initially considered for those with low disease activity; however, step-up therapy includes intra-articular glucocorticoid injections followed by methotrexate, and finally TNF-α inhibitors in those with poor response. NSAIDs can always be used as adjunctive therapy for any patient with JIA; however, it should never exceed 2 months as monotherapy without addition of other treatment. Triamcinolone hexacetonide is the intra-articular glucocorticoid of choice and can provide clinical improvement for a minimum of 4 months; step-up to csDMARD therapy may be warranted if symptoms are not controlled within this period.[209,210] MTX may be initiated in those who either fail initial therapy with NSAIDs and intra-articular injections or in those who have high disease activity and poor prognosis. In those with enthesitis-related JIA specifically, SSZ is the initial csDMARD over MTX because of evidence of improved clinical symptoms and long-term outcomes.[203] Finally, in those who still lack response after 3 to 6 months of optimized MTX therapy, TNF-α inhibitors may be initiated. Since publication of the ACR treatment recommendations, tocilizumab has been approved for polyarticular JIA. While place in therapy is not specified except for systemic JIA, it may be alone or in combination with methotrexate as step-up from initial therapy.[57]

Patients who experience arthritis of five or more joints in the duration of disease course should have MTX considered as first-line therapy. The role of NSAIDs is de-emphasized in this treatment group; patients may undergo a short 1- to 2-month course, but quick escalation to DMARD therapy is cornerstone in order to slow disease progression. Because of extensive experience with LEF, this agent may be considered as an alternative to MTX or in those with high disease activity and poor prognosis. For those who fail DMARD therapy after 3 to 6 months, a TNF-α inhibitor may be initiated, followed by switch to another TNF-α inhibitor or abatacept if response remains poor after 4 months of initial bDMARD therapy. For those who fail both TNF-α inhibitor and abatacept, rituximab is the last-line bDMARD agent.

Patients with active sacroiliac arthritis may include individuals from any of the JIA disease categories, but the treatment group must be defined by both clinical and imaging evidence of the disease. Step-up therapy quickly intensifies to TNF-α inhibitors following failed trials of optimized NSAID or csDMARD (MTX or SSZ).[199]

Systemic JIA is subdivided into three treatment categories based on clinical phenotype. In those without active systemic features, NSAIDs can be used as monotherapy initially but should be reserved for those with low disease activity and should not be continued as sole therapy for longer than 2 months. If four or fewer joints are involved, injectable glucocorticoids may be considered concurrently, but if five or more joints are impacted, favor should be placed on either MTX or LEF over injectable glucocorticoid. Following treatment failure of csDMARD, several bDMARDs including abatacept, anakinra, and tocilizumab may be considered.

About 10% of pediatric patients with JIA develop MAS, a life-threatening complication characterized by fever, pancytopenia, liver insufficiency, and coagulopathy among others and if hospitalized, it is associated with a 6% mortality rate. In these patients, anakinra, calcineurin inhibitors, and systemic glucocorticoid therapy should be considered.[197]

CASE 44-11, QUESTION 4: Are NSAIDS an appropriate choice for initial drug therapy for the treatment of systemic JIA in patient J.R.?

NSAID therapy may be considered as first-line treatment for 1 to 2 months in most cases of oligoarticular and polyarticular JIA.[199] However, the use of NSAIDs as monotherapy beyond 2 months in patients with active arthritis is not recommended, regardless of the presence of poor prognostics features.[199] In the case of systemic JIA, as with patient J.R., NSAIDs may be considered as monotherapy in patients with JIA with an MD global <5 and any level of joint involvement. However, therapy should be stepped up in patients with continued disease activity after 1 month on NSAID monotherapy.[197] NSAIDs are useful in systemic JIA as they target joint inflammation as well as the febrile episodes common in systemic JIA.[198,211] These medications work to control pain, fever, and inflammation by inhibiting prostaglandin synthesis and are usually fairly well tolerated by children. Analgesic effects usually occur first, and with continued use NSAIDs' anti-inflammatory effects will begin within a few weeks.

Many of the traditional NSAIDS as well as celecoxib have been used to treat JIA. The most commonly prescribed NSAIDs for JIA are naproxen and ibuprofen. Naproxen is approved for the treatment of JIA in patients ≥2 years old at a dose of 5 mg/kg by mouth twice daily and is advantageous in school-age children because of the convenient dosing interval and availability in liquid or tablet formulations.[211] Ibuprofen is indicated for the treatment of JIA in patients aged ≥1 years old. For patients from 1 to 12 years, ibuprofen is recommended at a dose of 30 to 40 mg/kg/day given in three or four divided doses. Ibuprofen is also available in tablet and liquid formulations.[212]

In most cases, at least two different NSAIDs should be tried before ruling out this group of medications owing to lack of efficacy or tolerability.[213] Failure to respond to an NSAID in a particular chemical class does not rule out the efficacy of others in the same class. As with adults, it is not possible to predict a pediatric patient's response to any one NSAID.

Given the presence of active systemic features (fever, lymphadenopathy, splenomegaly, and evanescent rash) along with an MD global of <5 and AJC of 4 (right hip, left and right knees, right wrist), either an NSAID or anakinra would be the appropriate first-line agents for J.R.[197] Either ibuprofen or naproxen would be sensible first choices. Ibuprofen is available over-the-counter in liquid and chewable forms, which is an important consideration for a 4-year-old. Naproxen is also available in an oral liquid suspension by prescription and can also be considered as initial therapy.

CORTICOSTEROIDS

CASE 44-11, QUESTION 5: J.R., who weighs 33 lb, was prescribed Naproxen 125 mg/5mL oral suspension at a dose of 75 mg BID. Her parents have given her the medication twice daily as directed for the past 4 weeks, but she continues to have disease activity with persistent fever. What should the next step in therapy be for J.R.?

It is inappropriate to continue NSAID monotherapy in a patient who continues to have disease activity after 1 month of treatment. Therefore, alternate treatment options should be explored. The ACR guidelines recommend the use of systemic glucocorticoid therapy in patients with systemic JIA, but not in patients with nonsystemic JIA.[199]

Despite the potential for serious adverse effects associated with high-dose or long-term therapy, the use of low-dose corticosteroids is sometimes necessary to control disease flares or provide therapeutic relief during initiation of DMARDs with slow onsets of action. Systemic glucocorticoids may be considered as adjunctive therapy for systemic JIA at any point in treatment.[197]

It is preferable that patients take the lowest effective corticosteroid dose for the shortest duration possible to avoid long-term side effects such as hypertension and osteoporosis. Oral corticosteroids are typically dosed once daily in the morning to best mimic physiologic cortisol release and minimize suppression of the hypothalamic–pituitary–adrenal axis. For J.R., systemic glucocorticoids are an appropriate next step in therapy and may be considered as adjunctive therapy, if necessary, throughout the course of her disease.

CASE 44-11, QUESTION 6: What corticosteroid side effects should J.R. be counseled about?

Common side effects of steroids include GI upset and damage to the GI mucosa, mood changes including depression or hyperactivity, and increases in blood pressure and blood sugar.[212] Corticosteroids may also cause impaired skin healing, osteoporosis (especially with long-term use), and vision problems such as cataracts and glaucoma. J.R.'s parents should be counseled about receiving vaccinations during corticosteroid therapy because immunosuppression may attenuate an appropriate immune response. Inactivated vaccines are safe for use in immunocompromised patients and should be administered if indicated.[212] Immunocompromised patients typically have a weaker immune response to vaccines when compared with healthy patients; therefore, higher doses or more frequent revaccinations may be necessary.

Greater caution must be taken with live-virus vaccines in immunosuppressed patients. The risk of immunosuppression in patients receiving corticosteroids is dependent on corticosteroid dose, duration, and route of administration; local corticosteroid treatments (e.g., topical, inhalation, and intra-articular) do not put patients at risk.[214] Patients receiving short-term corticosteroid therapy (i.e., <2 weeks), every-other-day dosing with a short-acting corticosteroid, or doses of no more than moderate range can usually receive live-virus vaccines. Corticosteroid dosing that is considered high risk for immunosuppression is the equivalent of at least prednisone 2 mg/kg/day or 20 mg/day; patients receiving corticosteroid dose equivalents in this range should not receive live-virus vaccines. Patients receiving high-dose corticosteroids systemically for 2 or more weeks should wait at least 3 months before receiving a live-virus vaccine.[214]

Intra-Articular Corticosteroid Therapy

CASE 44-11, QUESTION 7: J.R.'s pain in both knees has continued to limit to her willingness to walk. Her parents are concerned about her lack of activity and would like to know if there are any options for relieving her pain more quickly. Would intrarticular glucocorticoid therapy be an appropriate option for reducing knee pain in J.R.?

Intra-articular corticosteroid therapy seems to be highly effective in JIA. Injections are typically reserved for patients who have not responded to conventional NSAID therapy or who present with monoarthritis or oligoarthritis, and current guidelines suggest they are recommended for all patients with JIA having active disease in four or fewer joints, regardless of activity level, prognosis, or joint deformity.[199] Intra-articular steroid injections are also recommended as adjunct therapy in other forms of JIA, including patients with active disease in five or more joints and those with systemic JIA. Compared with NSAIDs, steroid injections are much better able to reduce duration of joint pain.[213] Full disease remission of injected joints lasting longer than 6 months can be expected in more than 80% of patients with JIA, and 60% of patients may be able to discontinue all oral medications with lasting disease remission in treated joints.[215] In one study, after an average of 30 months of follow-up, long-term negative effects of corticosteroid therapy (e.g., joint stability, osteonecrosis, and soft tissue atrophy) were not encountered. As a result, intra-articular corticosteroid therapy seems to be a safe and effective option for JIA, particularly in oligoarticular disease limited to a few joints.[198]

Intra-articular steroid injections would be appropriate adjunctive treatment for J.R. Her parents should be advised to limit her activity for a couple of days after the injection, but she should be encouraged to resume normal activity and physical therapy to maintain joint flexibility and ROM soon after the treatment.[213] Repeated intra-articular injections are usually given several months apart. Side effects include local lipoatrophy or articular calcification, both of which do not present many issues clinically.

DISEASE-MODIFYING ANTIRHEUMATIC DRUGS

CASE 44-11, QUESTION 8: After 2 weeks of glucocorticoid monotherapy, J.R. continues to have moderate disease activity. Her doctor would like to start DMARD therapy, but it is uncertain whether a csDMARD or bDMARD would be preferred. What would you recommend?

Early csDMARD therapy should be considered for patients with history of arthritis of four or fewer joints (e.g., persistent oligoarthritis) as well as patients with history of arthritis of five or more joints (e.g., extended oligoarthritis and polyarthritis [RF positive and RF negative]).[199] MTX is the DMARD of choice for these forms of JIA. For systemic JIA, MTX or leflunomide should be considered first-line in patients without systemic features and AJC $>$ 4 and as second-line therapy and beyond for any number of active joints. MTX or leflunomide may also be considered for systemic JIA as second-line therapy and beyond for patients with systemic features. However, csDMARDs have not been shown to be as effective against systemic JIA as compared to other forms of JIA.[216,217] For a patient like J.R. with systemic JIA with active systemic features, MTX or lefluonomide could be considered, but given relative lack of efficacy, other options, including several of the bDMARDs, are preferred.

Biologic Agents

CASE 44-11, QUESTION 9: Given that csDMARDs would not be an optimal treatment option for J.R., which of the bDMARDs would be most appropriate for treating systemic JIA in J.R.?

There are currently four FDA-approved biologic agents available to treat forms of JIA: etanercept, adalimumab, and abatacept for JIA and canakinumab for systemic JIA. There are also several bDMARDs which are not FDA-approved for the treatment of JIA but are recommended in the ACR guidelines including anakinra, rilonacept, rituximab, the TNF-α inhibitors as a class, and tocilizumab.[197] While the TNF-α inhibitors have demonstrated excellent efficacy in the treatment of adult RA as well as polyarticular JIA, they have not shown similar efficacy in the treatment of systemic JIA. The exact pathophysiology of systemic JIA remains unclear, but the pro-inflammatory cytokines IL-1 and IL-6 have been identified as targets of pharmacotherapy.[197,217–219] Thus, IL-1 inhibitors anakinra, canakinumab, and rilonacept as well as IL-6 inhibitor, tocilizumab, have demonstrated efficacy in the treatment of systemic JIA, and their use is addressed in the ACR treatment guidelines.[197]

IL-1 inhibitors, anakinra and canakinumab, are recommended for the treatment of systemic JIA, while rilonacept's place in therapy remains unclear. Anakinra blocks the action of IL-1α and IL-1β by inhibiting IL-1 binding to the interleukin-1 type receptor (IL-1R1). While anakinra has shown suboptimal efficacy in the treatment of adult RA, patients with systemic JIA have responded well to anakinra treatment. Case reports of good response to anakinra in patients who were refractory to other treatments for systemic JIA led to increased use of anakinra in patients with systemic JIA.[217,217,220] In a small randomized, controlled trial in patients with systemic JIA, 8 out of 12 patients in the anakinra group achieved the primary outcome (30% improvement in clinical status, resolution of fever, and 50% decrease or normalization of both CRP and ESR) versus 1 out of 12 patients in the control group. Furthermore, 10 of the patients in the control group were switched to anakinra after 1 month and nine of these patients also responded to anakinra treatment.[220] While anakinra is not FDA-approved for JIA, the dose that has been used in clinical trials is 2 mg/kg subcutaneously daily, with a maximum daily dose of 100 mg.[220] As with all of the bDMARDs, patients should be monitored for increased risk of infection when taking anakinra. Anakinra would be an appropriate treatment for J.R. following lack of response to NSAID and glucocorticoid monotherapies.

Canakinumab is a human monoclonal antibody, which binds IL-1β and blocks its interaction with IL-1 receptors. It is FDA-approved for the treatment of systemic JIA at a dose of 4 mg/kg subcutaneously every 4 weeks for patients with a body weight of $\geq$7.5 kg (maximum dose 300 mg).[221] In a randomized, placebo-controlled trial evaluating canakinumab for the treatment of systemic JIA, 84% of subjects experienced a 30% clinical response in the canakinumab group compared to only 10% in the placebo group ($p < 0.001$) 15 days after one dose of canakinumab.[222] In another trial in patients receiving open-label canakinumab for 32 weeks, there was a significantly lower risk of flares in the canakinumab patients and the average glucocorticoid dose was reduced in the canakinumab group.[222] Canakinumab, like other bDMARDs, has been associated with increased risk of infections. It has also been associated with MAS. This association may be attributed to the severity of the disease in patients treated with canakinumab and a causal relationship has not been established.[222] Canakinumab would also be an appropriate treatment option for J.R. The monthly dosing may be preferred over the daily dosing required with anakinra.

Rilonacept is an interleukin 1 inhibitor that binds IL-1β as well as IL-1α and IL-1 receptor antagonist with lesser affinity.[223] While rilonacept has demonstrated efficacy for the treatment of systemic JIA, its place in therapy remains unclear.[224] It should not be used as first-line therapy, and its use for continued disease activity was considered uncertain according to the ACR guidelines.[197]

Tocilizumab is a monoclonal antibody against the IL-6 receptor. It is recommended for patients with systemic JIA with active systemic disease and continued disease activity following a trial of glucocorticoid monotherapy, csDMARD, or anakinra.[197] It is also recommended in systemic JIA patients without systemic features who have an AJC $>$ 0 following treatment with anakinra or a csDMARD.[197] The TCZ dose used in clinic trials for systemic JIA is 8 mg/kg for weight $\geq$30 kg or 12 mg/kg for weight $<$30 kg given intravenously every 2 weeks.[225] In a randomized trial of tocilizumab for systemic JIA, 71% of children who received TCZ experienced a 70% improvement in clinic status, compared to 8%

of patients who received placebo.[227] Like canakinumab, there has been an association between TCZ and MAS, while anakinra has been shown to be effective in the treatment of MAS.[217]

Patient J.R. has tried an NSAID and systemic glucocorticoid, but she continues to have active systemic RA. Anakinra, canakinumab, and tocilizumab would all be appropriate treatment options for J.R. Canakinumab is FDA-approved for systemic JIA and has the most convenient dosing regimen of these three options. Therefore, canakinumab would be the best option for J.R.

CASE 44-12

QUESTION 1: Seven-year-old C.E. has polyarthritis that consistently has not responded to NSAID or MTX therapy. Given the many potential side effects, C.E.'s parents are concerned about her taking steroids and refuse to let their daughter take them. They are worried about permanent joint damage and wish to try a biologic agent in hopes of finally suppressing disease activity. They have heard that biologic drugs are "safer than steroids" and want to know which agents are available to treat JIA in C.E.

There are three FDA-approved biologic agents available to treat JIA: etanercept, adalimumab, and abatacept. As discussed in the previous section, canakinumab is approved for the treatment of systemic JIA.

Etanercept is a recombinant TNF-receptor Fc fusion protein indicated for patients 2 years of age with polyarticular JIA. ETA is recommended for patients with oligoarticular or polyarticular JIA, who continue to have active RA despite 3 months of treatment with MTX at the maximum tolerated dosage.[199] The recommended dose is 0.8 mg/kg (maximum 50 mg) subcutaneously weekly.[44] The safety of etanercept in children is comparable to adults with the exception of significantly more abdominal pain (17% of patients with JIA vs. 5% of adult patients with RA) and vomiting (14.5% of patients with JIA vs. <3% of adult patients with RA). Patients with JIA should be up-to-date on their immunizations before initiation of etanercept therapy because the effect of etanercept on vaccine response is unknown. Safety and efficacy data reflecting up to 10 years of treatment support the long-term use of etanercept for JIA.[226]

Adalimumab is a human monoclonal TNF-α antibody approved for use in patients aged 2 years of age and older with moderately to severely active polyarticular JIA.[45] It is a weight-based dose (10 mg for patients 10 to <15 kg, 20 mg for patients 15 to <30 kg, 40 mg for patients ≥30 kg) given as a subcutaneous injection every other week.[45] In a study involving 171 patients on adalimumab monotherapy and in combination with MTX, children taking combination therapy showed better disease improvement than patients on adalimumab monotherapy.[45] Concomitant steroids, salicylates, NSAIDs, or other analgesic agents may also be continued during adalimumab use.

Abatacept is an injectable biologic agent that inhibits T-cell activation. This drug received approval for JIA in 2008 and is indicated for use in patients 6 years and older with moderate to severe active polyarticular juvenile idiopathic arthritis. Patients weighing less than 75 kg receive a dose of 10 mg/kg via IV infusion for 30 minutes, while patients weighing 75 kg or more should receive the adult intravenous regimen, with a maximum dose of 1,000 mg.[52] All patients receive doses at 2 and 4 weeks after the first infusion and then every 4 weeks thereafter.[52] Unlike TNF-α agents, abatacept does not have an immediate onset and seems to exert its effect best after repeated doses over the course of several months.[213]

Other biologic agents, including the other TNF-α inhibitors, are not FDA-approved for JIA but have been studied. Available data from clinical trials suggest that all of these treatments may be safe and effective for JIA with no evidence of significant risk for serious adverse reactions. Owing to their mechanisms of action, all biologic agents share the side effect of lowered infection resistance, and patients must be monitored for signs of infection during treatment.

Of all FDA-approved bDMARDs, C.E. is a candidate for etanercept, adalimumab, or abatacept therapy. Given that abatacept does not have an immediate onset, etanercept or adalimumab may be preferred. Adalimumab with its biweekly dosing schedule may be preferred compared to weekly dosing with etanercept. C.E. will also be able to continue her concurrent NSAID and MTX therapies during adalimumab treatment, because it is possible she will experience enhanced clinical improvement on combination therapy versus adalimumab alone.

CASE 44-13

QUESTION 1: T.T. presents to rheumatology clinic on referral from her primary-care provider. She is 9 years old and has been complaining at home of her shoes hurting her feet and not being able to run with her classmates at school. On physical examination it is noted she has multiple swollen, erythematous joints (tarsometatarsal and metatarsocuneiform joints bilaterally on the feet, ankles bilaterally, knees bilaterally). Her CBC values are all normal, her ESR is normal, and her RF is positive. In addition to NSAID and steroid therapy, the rheumatologist would like to start a DMARD agent. What DMARD options are available to treat T.T.'s JIA?

Patients with both RF+ polyarthritis and early-onset JIA have poor prognosis in terms of long-term joint function and should receive early consideration for DMARD therapy. MTX is the DMARD of choice for polyarthritic JIA.[227] T.T. is showing classic signs of RF+ polyarthritis and it would be appropriate to choose MTX as a first-line agent for her therapy. The recommended dose of MTX for JIA treatment is 10 mg/m^2 orally or subcutaneously each week. Food reduces the bioavailability of MTX, so MTX should be administered on an empty stomach. Radiologic evidence of improvement or slowing of joint damage has been demonstrated in patients with JIA who responded to MTX therapy during a 2-year period.[228] Other DMARD options for JIA include leflunomide, sulfasalazine, or hydroxychloroquine. MTX is favored over these alternate csDMARDs and leflonomide is the preferred second-line csDMARD.[199]

CASE 44-13, QUESTION 2: What is the expected response to MTX treatment for T.T.?

The likelihood of long-term or permanent JIA-related joint damage is less than that associated with adult RA; therefore, discontinuation of MTX should be attempted when disease remission is apparent. The optimal time to discontinue MTX therapy remains unknown; however, it probably should not be stopped sooner than 1 year after disease remission, with slower withdrawal in patients at high risk for relapse.[229,230] Young age at diagnosis (<4.5 years) and oligoarthritis that progresses to polyarthritis seem to be the greatest risk factors for relapse.[229,231]

Children tolerate MTX therapy well and generally experience few serious or troublesome adverse effects (e.g., transient liver enzyme elevations, nausea, vomiting, and oral ulcerations).[230] These adverse effects are reduced with daily folic acid therapy (1 mg) or weekly folinic acid (the day after MTX dosing). Liver toxicity monitoring in JIA is the same as the guidelines recommend for MTX therapy in adult RA, including biopsy recommendations. The combination therapy of MTX and other DMARDs has not been fully evaluated in pediatric patients.

KEY REFERENCES AND WEBSITES

A full list of references for this chapter can be found at http://thepoint.lww.com/AT11e. Below are the key references and websites for this chapter, with the corresponding reference number in this chapter found in parentheses after the reference.

Key References

Aletaha D et al. 2010 Rheumatoid arthritis classification criteria: an American College of Rheumatology/European League Against Rheumatism collaborative initiative. *Arthritis Rheum*. 2010;62(9):2569–2581. (14)

Beukelman T et al. 2011 American College of Rheumatology recommendations for the treatment of juvenile idiopathic arthritis: initiation and safety monitoring of therapeutic agents for the treatment of arthritis and systemic features. *Arthritis Care Res (Hoboken)*. 2011;63(4):465–482. (199)

Ringold S et al. 2013 update of the 2011 American College of Rheumatology recommendations for the treatment of juvenile idiopathic arthritis: recommendations for the medical therapy of children with systemic juvenile idiopathic arthritis and tuberculosis screening among children receiving biologic medications. *Arthritis Rheum*. 2013;65(10):2499–2512. (197)

Singh JA et al. 2015 American College of Rheumatology Guideline for the Treatment of Rheumatoid Arthritis. *Arthritis Rheumatol*. 2016;68(1):1–26. (28)

Smolen JS et al. EULAR recommendations for the management of rheumatoid arthritis with synthetic and biological disease-modifying antirheumatic drugs: 2013 update. *Ann Rheum Dis*. 2014;73(3):492–509. (26)

Key Websites

The American College of Rheumatology. Rheumatology image bank. http://images.rheumatology.org/. Accessed March 30, 2016.

Arthritis Foundation. What is arthritis? http://www.arthritis.org/about-arthritis/understanding-arthritis/. Accessed July 25, 2015. (1)

45 Gout and Hyperuricemia

Kimberly Ference and KarenBeth H. Bohan

CORE PRINCIPLES

		CHAPTER CASES
1	Gout is a disease that causes acute joint inflammation and pain secondary to the deposition of monosodium urate (MSU) crystals within the synovial fluid and lining. Clinically, acute gout presents as monoarticular inflammation in 85% to 90% of patients with the first metatarsophalangeal joint (great toe) typically affected; this is called podagra. Patients presenting with acute gout may or may not have hyperuricemia.	**Case 45-1 (Question 1), Table 45-1**
2	A definitive diagnosis of gout can be made if MSU crystals are present in a synovial fluid sample. However, this is rarely done in clinical practice, and other diagnostic criteria are available.	**Case 45-2 (Questions 1–3), Table 45-1**
3	The primary goal of treating acute gout attacks is the relief of pain and inflammation. It is not necessary to lower the serum uric acid (SUA) immediately.	**Case 45-2 (Question 3), Table 45-3**
4	Acute episodes of gout are primarily treated with nonsteroidal anti-inflammatory drugs (NSAIDs), colchicine, or corticosteroids.	**Case 45-2 (Questions 4, 5), Case 45-3 (Question 1), Table 45-3**
5	Low-dose oral colchicine is as effective as and safer than traditional high-dose regimens, which are dosed to toxicity (diarrhea); Avoid potential colchicine drug–drug interactions.	**Case 45-2 (Questions 4, 5), Case 45-3 (Questions 1, 5), Table 45-3**
6	Nonpharmacologic therapy for acute and chronic gout includes limiting daily alcoholic beverages, purine-rich meats, and fructose-containing beverages/foods. Specifically, beer and, to a smaller extent, spirits are associated with increased gout attacks; wine is less likely to be a risk factor. Increasing low-fat dairy protein has a favorable effect on SUA.	**Case 45-1 (Question 3), Case 45-2 (Question 6), Table 45-3**
7	Urate-lowering therapy (ULT) should not be initiated or discontinued during treatment for an acute gout attack. Chronic ULT should be started only if the patient has two or more gout episodes in 1 year or the patient has comorbidities such as renal failure, uric acid stones, or urate tophi.	**Case 45-3 (Questions 2, 3), Table 45-3**
8	Patients should be evaluated for drug-induced hyperuricemia before treatment.	**Case 45-3 (Question 3), Table 45-3**
9	The goal of ULT is to lower the SUA to less than 6 mg/dL. If this goal is achieved, most patients can be "cured" of acute gout attacks.	**Case 45-3 (Questions 3–5), Table 45-3**
10	The preferred first-line treatment of gout and hyperuricemia is xanthine oxidase (XO) inhibitors. Monitor for drug–drug interactions.	**Case 45-3 (Questions 4, 5), Tables 45-3**
11	Initiation of ULT can precipitate acute gout attacks, so prophylaxis with either colchicine or NSAIDs is recommended and should be continued for 6 months.	**Case 45-3 (Question 5), Table 45-3**

PATHOPHYSIOLOGY

Gout is a disease that most commonly manifests as recurrent episodes of acute joint pain and inflammation secondary to the deposition of monosodium urate (MSU) crystals in the synovial fluid and lining. MSU deposition in the urinary tract can cause urolithiasis and urinary obstruction.[1] Patients with gout cycle between flares of acute joint pain and inflammation and intercritical gout (i.e., periods of quiescence with no symptoms of the disease). In addition, they can also exhibit chronic tophaceous gout and hyperuricemia.

Tophi are hard nodules of MSU crystals that have deposited in soft tissues and are most commonly found in the toes, fingers, and elbows. Although gout is often associated with hyperuricemia (defined as a serum urate level of greater than or equal to 6.8 mg per deciliter)[2], elevated serum uric acid (SUA) is not a prerequisite for this painful condition.[3] In a retrospective review of two studies on gout, 14% of patients presenting with acute symptoms had a normal SUA concentration less than 6 mg/dL and 32% had an SUA concentration less than 8 mg/dL.[4] Hence, *gout* should be considered a clinical diagnosis and *hyperuricemia* a biochemical one. These two terms are not synonymous and are not interchangeable.

Uric Acid Disposition

Uric acid serves no biologic function; it is merely the end product of purine metabolism. Unlike animals, humans lack the enzyme uricase, which degrades uric acid into more soluble products for excretion. As a consequence, uric acid is not metabolized in humans and is primarily excreted renally, although up to one-third of the daily uric acid produced can be eliminated through the gastrointestinal (GI) tract.[5,6] Therefore, increased SUA concentrations arise from an increase in production or a decrease in renal excretion of uric acid, or a combination of the two.

OVERPRODUCTION

Overproduction of uric acid accounts for approximately 10% of gout cases[5,6] and can result from excessive de novo purine synthesis, which is primarily associated with rare genetic enzyme mutation defects, some neoplastic diseases, aggressive cytotoxic chemotherapy (causing tumor lysis syndrome), and certain myeloproliferative disorders. Overproduction of uric acid can also be the result of excessive intake of dietary purines from meat, seafood, dried peas and beans, certain vegetables (e.g., mushrooms, spinach, asparagus), beer, and other alcoholic beverages.[7,8] Fructose consumption (especially soft drinks) has also been linked with increased uric acid levels.[9] Many patients attempt to avoid intake of these foods; however, dietary restrictions are seldom of much benefit (with the exception of avoiding excessive alcohol, yeast, or liver supplements), and patients should feel comfortable in eating modest quantities of meats, seafood, and vegetables.

UNDEREXCRETION

A defect in the renal clearance of uric acid is the main cause of hyperuricemia and gout in about 90% of patients. Uric acid is filtered in the renal glomerulus and is almost completely (98%–100%) reabsorbed in the proximal tubule. Uric acid is then secreted distal to the proximal tubular reabsorption site, and most is reabsorbed again.[3,6] In normal patients, homeostasis between reabsorption and secretion of urate is maintained. However, many factors (e.g., renal impairment, certain drugs, alcohol excess, metabolic syndrome, hypertension [HTN], coronary heart disease [CHD]) can cause this balance to fail, resulting in excess serum concentrations of uric acid and tissue deposition.[5,10]

ACUTE GOUT

Epidemiology

Classically, gout presents during middle age. The onset of gout is uncommon in prepubertal children, premenopausal women, and men younger than 30 years of age. The appearance of gout in these populations should alert the clinician to the possibility of renal parenchymal disease. The risk of gouty arthritis is approximately the same for both men and women at any given SUA concentration; however, many more men are hyperuricemic. For example, men are six times more likely than women to have SUA concentrations greater than 7 mg/dL. Overall, gout occurs as often in postmenopausal elderly women as in men.[11] Emerging evidence suggests the incidence of gout in increasing in the black population.[12]

Clinical Features

CASE 45-1

QUESTION 1: M.D. is an obese 60-year-old woman who has been referred to a medication management clinic by her primary-care physician. She states that her past medical history includes HTN, type 2 diabetes, hyperlipidemia, and gout. M.D. states she was diagnosed with gout 3 months ago when she had a really painful and swollen right big toe. When asked about that episode, M.D. related the following story: "One morning I just woke up and my big toe was swollen, red, and very painful. I couldn't even put weight on it. I had gone to my husband's 50th high school reunion the night before and it was fine then, because we danced all night. I did have a little too much to drink, though, so I thought maybe I had stubbed my toe without realizing it and broke it." What signs and symptoms did M.D. exhibit that are typical of acute gout?

M.D.'s symptoms of severe, acute pain and an obviously inflamed joint are consistent with the usual presentation of gout. Also, M.D.'s age is consistent with the epidemiologic data that are commonly associated with gout.

PAIN

The pain of gout rapidly reaches its maximum within 6 to 12 hours of onset and is usually accompanied by erythema.[13] It is often so severe that patients cannot even tolerate a sheet lying on top of the affected area.

NUMBER AND TYPE OF JOINTS

M.D.'s report of a very painful big toe is typical, because acute gout attacks affect a single joint 85% to 90% of the time, and most often affect a joint of the lower extremity.[6] The first metatarsophalangeal joint (the great toe) is the most commonly affected joint, and the term *podagra* specifically refers to gout in this joint.

Although initial gout attacks are primarily monoarticular, as many as 39% of the patients in one study experienced polyarticular involvement as their first manifestation of gout.[14] Generally, recurrent attacks are of longer duration than initial attacks, more likely to be polyarticular, and more smoldering in onset.[15]

NOCTURNAL OCCURRENCE

Acute gouty arthritis commonly begins at night. According to the Simkin hypothesis,[16] small amounts of effusion fluid gravitationally enter into degenerative joints of the feet (or other joints) during the day, when most people are busily walking around, and are reabsorbed during the night when the lower extremities are elevated. Thus, the onset of pain in M.D. during the night is typical of gout.

PHYSICAL STRESS

Gout attacks also seem to be more common during episodes of increased physical exercise. Long walks, hikes, golf games, or tight new shoes have historically been associated with the subsequent onset of podagra.[16] The acute episode of toe pain experienced by M.D. after a night of dancing is consistent with the appearance of gout after increased physical exercise.

Risk Factors

CASE 45-1, QUESTION 2: What findings in M.D. place her at risk for gout?

The diagnoses of HTN, type 2 diabetes, hyperlipidemia, and obesity in M.D. have been associated with an increased risk of gout and hyperuricemia.

Common risk factors include alcohol consumption, the use of urate elevating drugs, and certain comorbidities. Conditions associated with an increased risk of hyperuricemia and gout include insulin resistance, obesity, metabolic syndrome, chronic kidney disease, heart failure, organ transplant, history of urolithiasis, and lead intoxication.[2,17]

CORONARY HEART DISEASE

Hyperuricemia is noted to be an independent risk factor for CHD, although it is unlikely to be a primary cause of disease. Several observational studies have shown a link between hyperuricemia and an increase in CHD (e.g., HTN, stroke, heart failure, and ischemic heart disease).[18-21] Researchers continue to study the causality and note that despite the apparent strong relationship, the subject remains controversial. Impaired glucose utilization also has a relationship with hyperuricemia. Because of these close linkages, patients who present with gout and/or hyperuricemia should be monitored closely for the development of CHD and diabetes.

RENAL DYSFUNCTION

Uric acid excretion is decreased in patients with renal dysfunction owing to decreased glomerular filtration, and as a consequence, hyperuricemia is a common finding. The use of xanthine oxidase (XO) in patients with hyperuricemia and chronic kidney disease has been examined in low-quality studies with mixed results. Currently, treating hyperuricemia in patients with renal dysfunction is not recommended unless patients manifest gouty arthritis.[19,22] Appropriate monitoring of renal function in M.D. by obtaining blood urea nitrogen (BUN), serum creatinine (SCr), and electrolytes is important for evaluating her risk factors as well as determining drug doses for treating gout.

CASE 45-1, QUESTION 3: During the medication management clinic visit, M.D. mentions that her doctor said her gout attack could have been caused by drinking too much beer, and she asks you whether this is really true.

ETHANOL CONSUMPTION

Overindulgence of alcohol has been linked to acute gout attacks. Alcohol intake was examined in a prospective cohort of men with new diagnoses of gout from the Health Professionals Follow-Up Study and found that the risk of gout is 2.5-fold in patients who drink two or more beers/day.[23] Ethanol-induced gout or hyperuricemia has been attributed to several mechanisms. M.D.'s episode of overindulgence of beer, possible dehydration from vigorous exercise, and lactic acidemia from muscle energy expenditure made the diagnosis of an acute gout attack the most likely cause of her toe pain and inflammation.

Diagnosis

CASE 45-2

QUESTION 1: E.J., a 52-year-old male school bus driver, reports to the emergency department with the primary complaint of extreme pain in his right elbow. He admits to playing several games of basketball yesterday followed by a few beers with friends. He awoke in the early hours of the morning with a sore and stiff elbow, which he self-medicated with acetaminophen before trying to get back to sleep. He sought medical attention when his pain escalated to the point where he was unable to apply pressure to the area and struggled to move his arm. Pertinent medical history includes the recent diagnosis of HTN and obesity. At visit with his primary-care physician 1 month ago, E.J. was prescribed hydrochlorothiazide 12.5 mg once daily, which is his only medication. He was also encouraged to go on a diet and to increase his exercise. He states that he has no drug or food allergies and is tolerating the antihypertensive well. On physical examination, the right elbow is exquisitely tender and erythematous, and his vital signs are all within normal limits. The elbow is warm to the touch and has moderate swelling. What objective data would be of value in assisting in the diagnosis of E.J.'s elbow pain and inflammation?

JOINT FLUID ASPIRATION

A definitive diagnosis of gout can be established by finding MSU crystals in the aspirated synovial fluid of the affected joint. The absence of MSU crystals in the synovial fluid, however, does not rule out the diagnosis of gout. Although joint fluid aspiration is considered the gold standard for diagnosis of acute gout, it is rarely done in clinical practice. If synovial fluid is aspirated from an inflamed joint, it should also be analyzed for bacteria and a WBC count should be obtained. In gouty arthritis, the WBC count is likely to range from 5,000 to 50,000/L.[3] In septic arthritis, the WBC count of the synovial fluid is usually greater than 50,000/L. E.J.'s physician may consider fluid joint aspiration as a diagnostic measure if E.J. is agreeable and the physician is equipped to conduct the procedure.

LABORATORY TESTS

Because uric acid primarily is excreted renally and renal impairment is a risk factor for gout, the serum concentrations of E.J.'s BUN and SCr should be measured along with an SUA concentration, especially in light of his history of HTN and hydrochlorothiazide therapy. Although infection, in particular *septic arthritis,* could also present as sudden onset of joint pain and inflammation, it is not likely in this case. An elevated systemic white blood cell (WBC) count may be consistent with infection or gout. If joint infection is of genuine concern, synovial fluid aspiration could differentiate between infection and gout.

RADIOGRAPHY

Radiographic findings of the affected joint are nonspecific and generally characterized by asymmetric soft tissue swelling overlying the involved joint. When gout has been long-standing, bony changes can be noticed on a radiograph, along with calcium deposition and increased density in the areas of soft tissue swelling.[24] Ultrasound and computed tomography are also used for diagnosis with the latter showing early changes compared to a traditional radiography. (See http://www.healthinplainenglish.com/health/musculoskeletal/gout/for examples.) A radiograph of E.J.'s elbow should be obtained if other *musculoskeletal disorders* (e.g., bone fracture) are being considered.

PSEUDOGOUT

Deposition of microcrystals (i.e., calcium pyrophosphate, calcium oxalate, calcium hydroxyapatite) into joints can cause acute or chronic arthritis in a manner similar to that caused by MSU deposition.[25] The role of these microcrystals in causing acute synovitis has been greater than previously expected because improved crystallographic technology (e.g., electron microscopy, radiograph diffraction) can differentiate these diagnoses from that of acute gout. Crystal-induced diseases tend to occur in older patients as a result of prior joint disease, especially osteoarthritis (which is generally a disease of the elderly), predisposing them to crystal deposition and acute episodes of joint inflammation. Older adults are also more prone to microcrystal-induced arthritis because these crystals generally accumulate for a long period and must attain a sufficient concentration and size before they precipitate into the synovial fluid and cause inflammation.[26]

CRITERIA FOR DIAGNOSIS

The American College of Rheumatology (ACR) first suggested classification criteria for gout in 1977, which until recently have been commonly used for diagnosis.[27] In 2015, new criteria for the classification of gout were published via a collaboration between ACR and European League Against Rheumatism (EULAR).[28] The new criteria represent the best available evidence and incorporate a multifaceted, objective approach to making a diagnosis. The ACR/EULAR criteria are streamlined into 3 steps. The updated criteria now separate individuals with symptoms of gout undergoing evaluation of joint fluid aspiration from those not undergoing this procedure (Table 45-1).

In order for gout to be considered, a patient must meet the entry criterion (Step 1), which is described as one or more episodes of pain, swelling, or tenderness in a peripheral joint or bursa. If the entry criterion is met, the clinician moves to Step 2. The sufficient criterion described in Step 2 evaluates the presence of MSU crystals from fluid aspiration of the symptomatic joint, bursa, or tophus. If the patient meets the criteria described in Steps 1 and 2, a diagnosis of gout is made. If fluid aspiration is not performed or the results are negative, the clinician moves to the next step. Step 3 examines three different areas consistent with gout: clinical characteristics (i.e., symptoms, timing, clinical evidence of disease), laboratory findings (i.e., SU synovial fluid analysis), and imaging findings (i.e., results consistent with urate disposition, evidence of joint damage). Step 3 utilizes a scoring method for the different characteristics associated with gout, and a diagnosis is made with a score of 8 or greater. A classification calculator can be found at: http://goutclassificationcalculator.auckland.ac.nz/

Case 45-2, Question 2: Laboratory tests were ordered for E.J., and the results are as follows:

SUA, 10.1 mg/dL
BUN, 10 mg/dL
SCr, 1.0 mg/dL
WBC count, 10.2 × $10^3/\mu L$

A radiograph of his elbow shows soft tissue swelling with no evidence of tophi. Does E.J. have gout?

Additionally, Table 45-2 discusses the EULAR propositions for the diagnosis of gout.[13]

E.J.'s objective and clinical presentation fulfills the ACR/EULAR criteria for diagnosis, highlighted in Table 45-1. He presents with symptoms meeting the entry criterion, however, and does not meet the sufficient criterion because he did not undergo joint aspiration. When using the classification calculator, the final criteria score is 8 [e.g., pattern of joint involvement (1), characteristics of symptoms (3), and serum urate (4)]. A score of 8 is consistent with a gout classification.

Management Guidelines

Gout is one of few rheumatologic diseases that can be treated successfully and even cured in many patients.[29] However, despite the availability of adequate pharmacologic interventions, a survey of rheumatologists and internists in the United States (US) found that drug therapy is often not used based on scientific evidence for both acute and chronic gout.[30] Another survey of US primary-care physicians found that evidence-based treatment recommendations were made in only 52.8% of cases of acute gout and 16.7% of cases of chronic gout.[31] Because these common practices are contrary to current scientific data, the ACR Guidelines for Management of Gout were developed to provide evidence-based recommendations for treatment.[32] Other European guidelines include EULAR and British Society of Rheumatology and British Health Professionals in Rheumatology (BSR/BHPR) Guidelines for the Management of Gout.[33,34] A comparison of recommendations from these guidelines is found in Table 45-3.

Treatment of Acute Gout

GOALS OF THERAPY

Case 45-2, Question 3: What is the primary goal in the treatment of E.J.'s acute gout attack?

The primary goal in the treatment of an acute attack of gout for E.J. is to relieve his pain and inflammation. Treatment within 24 hours of symptom onset is recommended to rapidly improve patient symptoms. The immediate goal of therapy should not be aimed at decreasing the SUA concentration with urate-lowering therapy (ULT). Gout sufferers are most likely to have been hyperuricemic for several months or years, and it is not necessary to treat the hyperuricemia immediately. Furthermore, a decrease in the SUA concentration at this time might mobilize urate stores and precipitate yet another acute gout attack. However, if the patient is already receiving ULT, it is not necessary to discontinue therapy during an acute attack.[32–34]

DRUG THERAPY OVERVIEW

Case 45-2, Question 4: What are the pharmacologic options for the treatment of E.J.'s acute pain?

Acute gouty arthritis can be effectively treated in most instances by using monotherapy with one of the following: nonsteroidal anti-inflammatory drug (NSAID), colchicine, or corticosteroids.[32–34] Each therapy has been proven efficacious when compared to placebo; however, to date, there are limited head-to-head comparisons between agents. Treatment should be based on patient preference, previous response or experience with an agent, and patient-specific factors (e.g., comorbidities, current medications, renal or hepatic impairment). Switching to an alternative agent or add-on therapy may be considered in refractory cases. Combination therapy is recommended in severe cases especially those involving multiple joints. Treatment should be continued until patient is asymptomatic (usually 7–10 days).

Nonsteroidal Anti-Inflammatory Drugs

NSAIDs are the preferred first-line therapy for the treatment of acute gout according to the ACR, EULAR, and BSR/BHPR guidelines because of their effectiveness and tolerability.[32–34] Although only a few NSAIDs (i.e., naproxen, indomethacin, sulindac) are US Food and Drug Administration (FDA)-approved for the treatment of pain associated with acute gout attacks, most have been studied and experts consider them equally efficacious.[32,34] The

Table 45-1
The ACR/EULAR Gout Classification Criteria

	Categories	Score
Step 1: Entry criterion (only apply criteria below to those meeting this entry criterion)	At least 1 episode of swelling, pain, or tenderness in a peripheral joint or bursa	
Step 2: Sufficient criterion (if met, can classify as gout without applying criteria below)	Presence of MSU crystals in a symptomatic joint or bursa (i.e., in synovial fluid) or tophus	
Step 3: Criteria (to be used if sufficient criterion not met)		
Clinical		
Pattern of joint/bursa involvement during symptomatic episode(s) ever[a]	Ankle *or* mid-foot (as part of monoarticular or oligoarticular episode without involvement of the first metatarsophalangeal joint)	1
	Involvement of the first metatarsophalangeal joint (as part of monoarticular or oligoarticular episode)	2
Characteristics of symptomatic episode(s) ever		
■ Erythema overlying affected joint (patient-reported or physician-observed)	One characteristic	1
■ Can't bear touch or pressure to affected joint	Two characteristics	2
■ Great difficulty with walking or inability to use affected joint	Three characteristics	3
Time course of episode(s) ever		
Presence (ever) of ≥2, irrespective of anti-inflammatory treatment:		
■ Time to maximal pain <24 hours	One typical episode	1
■ Resolution of symptoms in ≤14 days	Recurrent typical episodes	2
■ Complete resolution (to baseline level) between symptomatic episodes		
Clinical evidence of tophus		
Draining or chalklike subcutaneous nodule under transparent skin, often with overlying vascularity, located in typical locations: joints, ears, olecranon bursae, finger pads, tendons (e.g., Achilles)	Present	4
Laboratory		
Serum urate: measured by uricase method		
Ideally should be scored at a time when the patient was not receiving urate-lowering treatment, and it was >4 weeks from the start of an episode (i.e., during intercritical period); *if* practicable, retest under those conditions	<4 mg/dL (<0.24 mmol/L)[b]	−4
	6−8 mg/dL (0.36−<0.48 mmol/L)	2
	8−<10 mg/dL (0.48−<0.60 mmol/L)	3
	≥10 mg/dL (≥0.60 mmol/L)	4
The highest value irrespective of timing should be scored		
Synovial fluid analysis of a symptomatic (ever) joint or bursa (should be assessed by a trained observer)[c]	MSU negative	−2

Table 45-1
The ACR/EULAR Gout Classification Criteria (*continued*)

	Categories	Score
Imaging[d]		
Imaging evidence of urate deposition in symptomatic (ever) joint or bursa: ultrasound evidence of double-contour sign[e] *or* DECT demonstrating urate deposition[f]	Present (either modality)	4
Imaging evidence of gout-related joint damage: conventional radiography of the hands and/or feet demonstrates at least 1 erosion[g]	Present	4

A web-based calculator can be accessed at: http://goutclassificationcalculator.auckland.ac.nz, and through the American College of Rheumatology (ACR) and European League Against Rheumatism (EULAR) websites.
[a]Symptomatic episodes are periods of symptoms that include any swelling, pain, and/or tenderness in a peripheral joint or bursa.
[b]If serum urate level is <4 mg/dL (<0.24 mmol/L), *subtract 4 points*; if serum urate level is ≥4–<6 mg/dL (≥0.24–<0.36 mmol/L), score this item as 0.
[c]If polarizing microscopy of synovial fluid from a symptomatic (ever) joint or bursa by a trained examiner fails to show MSU monohydrate crystals, *subtract 2 points*. If synovial fluid was not assessed, score this item as 0.
[d]If imaging is not available, score these items as 0.
[e]Hyperechoic irregular enhancement over the surface of the hyaline cartilage that is independent of the insonation angle of the ultrasound beam (note: false-positive double-contour sign [artifact] may appear at the cartilage surface but should disappear with a change in the insonation angle of the probe).[31,32]
[f]Presence of color-coded urate at articular or periarticular sites. Images should be acquired using a dual-energy computed tomography (DECT) scanner, with data acquired at 80 kV and 140 kV and analyzed using gout-specific software with a 2-material decomposition algorithm that color-codes urate (33). A positive scan is defined as the presence of color-coded urate at articular or periarticular sites. Nail bed, submillimeter, skin, motion, beam hardening, and vascular artifacts should not be interpreted as DECT evidence of urate deposition (34).
[g]Erosion is defined as a cortical break with sclerotic margin and overhanging edge, excluding distal interphalangeal joints and gull wing appearance.
Reprinted from Neogi T. 2015 Gout Classification Criteria. *Arthritis Rheum.* 2015;67(10):2564, with permission.

Table 45-2
EULAR Propositions for Diagnosis of Gout 2006

Proposition		A + B (%)[a]
1	In acute attacks, the rapid development of acute pain, swelling, and tenderness that reaches peak intensity within 6–12 hours, especially with overlying erythema, highly suggests crystal inflammation (although not specific for gout).	93
2	For typical presentations of gout (e.g., recurrent podagra with hyperuricemia), a clinical diagnosis alone is reasonably accurate, but not definitive without crystal confirmation.	100
3	Demonstration of MSU crystals in synovial fluid or a tophus permits a definitive diagnosis of gout.	100
4	A routine search for MSU crystals is recommended in all synovial fluid samples obtained from undiagnosed joints.	87
5	Identification of MSU crystals from asymptomatic joints may allow for definite diagnosis in intercritical gout.	93
6	Gout and sepsis can coexist. When septic arthritis is suspected, synovial fluid should be Gram stained and cultured for bacteria even if MSU crystals are identified.	93
7	Serum uric acid concentrations, although the most important risk factor for gout, do not confirm or exclude gout. Many with hyperuricemia do not develop gout, and SUA concentrations during acute attacks can be normal.	93
8	Renal uric acid excretion should be assessed in selected gout patients, especially those with a family history of young-onset gout, onset of gout at younger than 25 years, or those with renal calculi.	60
9	Although radiographs can be useful for differential diagnosis and can show typical features of chronic gout, they are not useful in confirming the diagnosis of early or acute gout.	93
10	Risk factors for gout and comorbidity should be assessed, including features of the metabolic syndrome (obesity, hyperglycemia, hyperlipidemia, hypertension).	100

[a]A + B (%) is the percentage of fully (A) and strongly (B) recommended, based on EULAR ordinal scale.
EULAR, European League Against Rheumatism; MSU, monosodium urate; SUA, serum uric acid.
Adapted with permission from Zhang W et al. EULAR evidence-based recommendations for gout. Part I: Diagnosis. Report of a task force of the Standing Committee for International Clinical Studies Including Therapeutics (ESCISIT). *Ann Rheum Dis*. 2006;65:1301.

Table 45-3
Comparison of ACR, EULAR, and BSR/BHPR Guidelines for Gout

ACR Management of Gout Part 1[17] and Part 2[32]	EULAR Propositions for Gout Management[33]	BSR/BHPR Guidelines for Management of Gout[34]: Summary of Selected Recommendations
Treatment of Acute Gout		
Treat an acute attack within 24 hours of attack with any of the following: oral NSAIDs, colchicine	Treat as soon as possible with oral NSAIDs or colchicine. In the absence of contraindications, an NSAID is a convenient and well-accepted treatment	Treat acute gout with an NSAID, colchicine, or corticosteroid and continue until attack is terminated (1–2 weeks)
NSAIDs or COX-2 is effective at FDA-approved doses for 1 week	NSAIDs are effective at maximum doses	NSAIDs are drug of choice provided no contraindications for use
Use colchicine 1.2 mg, then 0.6 mg 1 hour later. The 0.6 mg once to twice daily until attack subsides	High doses of colchicine cause side effects, and low doses (e.g., 0.5 mg TID) can be sufficient	Use colchicine in doses of 0.5 mg 2–4 times daily
Recommend prednisone 0.5 mg/kg per day for 5–10 days. Intra-articular recommended for acute gout of 1–2 joints	Intra-articular aspiration and injection of a long-acting steroid are effective and safe treatments for an acute attack	Corticosteroids are effective for acute gout in patients who cannot tolerate NSAIDs or are refractory to other therapy: may use intramuscularly, intravenously, or intra-articularly; the latter is highly effective in monoarticular gout
Treatment of Hyperuricemia to Prevent Recurrent Gout		
ULT is indicated in patients with established gouty arthritis and >2 acute attacks per year, tophi, a history of urolithiasis, and CKD (Stage 2 and higher)	ULT is indicated in patients with recurrent acute attacks, arthropathy, tophi, or radiographic changes of gout	Start long-term ULT in uncomplicated gout only if two or more attacks occur per year
Treat to a minimum SUA of <6 mg/dL, may consider a goal of <5 mg/dL in patients without symptomatic relief at <6 mg/dL. Begin ULT once attack is controlled	The therapeutic goal of ULT (i.e., SUA less than or equal to the saturation point for MSU of 6 mg/dL) is to promote crystal dissolution and prevent crystal formation	Plasma urate goal is <300 mmol/L (<5 mg/dL). Start ULT 1–2 weeks after inflammation has resolved
Recommend ULT with a XO inhibitor (allopurinol or febuxostat). Allopurinol should be initiated at 100 mg/d and titrated every 2–5 weeks until target dose reached. May use doses of >300 mg in renal impairment if it is proper education and monitoring	Allopurinol, an appropriate long-term urate-lowering agent, should be initiated at 100 mg/d and increased by 100 mg every 2–4 weeks, if required. The dose must be adjusted in patients with renal impairment. If toxicity occurs, options include other xanthine oxidase (XO) inhibitors, a uricosuric agent, or allopurinol desensitization (if mild rash)	Initial ULT should be allopurinol starting with 50–100 mg/d and increasing by 50–100 mg every few weeks until therapeutic goal of SUA <300 mmol/L to a maximum of 900 mg/d allopurinol (adjust as necessary for renal dysfunction)
Probenecid may be used as a first-line alternative in patients unable to use or intolerant to at least 1 XO inhibitor. Avoid use in patients with a CrCl <50 mL/min	Probenecid can be an alternative to allopurinol in patients with normal renal function, but is relatively contraindicated in patients with urolithiasis	Uricosuric agents should be used only as a second-line drug in those underexcreting urate and in those resistant to or intolerant of allopurinol
Prophylaxis for acute gout is recommended for 6 months. The first-line agent for prophylaxis against acute gout is colchicine or low-dose NSAIDs. Oral corticosteroids are recommended as a second-line agent	Prophylaxis against acute attacks for up to 6 months of initiation of ULT with colchicine (0.5–1 mg/d) or NSAID (with gastroprotection, if indicated)	Prevent gout attacks by giving colchicine 0.5 mg twice daily for up to 6 months; if patient cannot tolerate colchicine, NSAIDs or COX-2 inhibitors can be substituted but limited to 6 weeks
Adjunctive Therapy to Prevent Recurrent Gout		
Patient education on general health, diet, and lifestyle modifications includes limiting daily alcoholic beverages, purine-rich meats, and fructose-containing beverages/foods. Specifically, beer and, to a smaller extent, spirits are associated with increased gout attacks; wine is less likely to be a risk factor. Increasing low-fat dairy protein has a favorable effect on SUA	Optimal treatment of gout requires nonpharmacologic and pharmacologic modalities tailored to specific risk factors (SUA levels, prior attacks); clinical phase of gout; and general risk factors (age, comorbidity, drug interactions) Patient education and lifestyle modifications (e.g., weight loss if obese, reduced beer, and other alcohol consumption) are important	Dietary management: includes skim milk and yogurt; favors soybeans and vegetable proteins; restricts intake of high-purine food (<200 mg/d); avoids liver, kidneys, shellfish, and yeast extracts; reduces intake of red meat; favors cherries, fresh or preserved Alcohol consumption[a]: restrict to <21 units/wk (men) and <14 units/week (women); two 125-mL glasses of wine per day are usually safe; two 25-mL glasses of spirits per day are safer than 1/2 pint of many beers

[a]1 unit equals 10 mL of pure alcohol, so the number of units per drink depends on its alcohol content; generally, 6 ounces of wine is about 2 units, a 12-ounce beer is 1.5 units, and a 2-ounce shot is about 1.2 units.

BSR/BHPR, British Society for Rheumatology/British Health Professionals in Rheumatology; COX-2, cyclooxygenase-2; CrCl, creatinine clearance; EULAR, European League Against Rheumatism; GI, gastrointestinal; HTN, hypertension; MSU, monosodium urate; NSAID, nonsteroidal anti-inflammatory drug; SUA, serum uric acid; TID, three times daily; ULT, urate-lowering therapy.

choice of NSAID should be determined based on patient-specific factors, and dosing should be consistent with the FDA-approved recommendations for the treatment of acute pain and/or acute gout. GI bleeding or ulceration and inhibition of platelet aggregation are two of the most common serious adverse effects of nonselective NSAIDs. Both compound the risk of bleeding when given concomitantly with anticoagulants (e.g., warfarin). Among the nonselective NSAIDs, ibuprofen is the least likely to cause GI adverse effects and is perhaps the safest nonselective NSAID for use in patients at risk for GI bleeding, whereas piroxicam and indomethacin are among the worst offenders.[35] The selective cyclooxygenase-2 (COX-2) inhibitor NSAIDs are another option in patients at risk for GI bleeding or when taking chronic anticoagulants because they do not inhibit platelets at normal doses. Published data to support efficacy in acute gouty arthritis exist for etoricoxib and lumiracoxib (withdrawn in most countries due to hepatotoxicity), but these drugs are not available in the United States. Despite limited evidence for use, celecoxib and meloxicam are available in the United States with FDA-approved indications for the treatment of acute gout. A Cochrane systematic review compared nonselective NSAIDs to COX-2 inhibitors for the treatment of acute gout pain and found no significant differences in efficacy. However, the review demonstrated increased cardiovascular risk and GI adverse effects with nonselective NSAID use.[36]

The potential adverse cardiovascular effects of NSAIDs are of concern.

Cardiovascular risk associated with NSAID therapy has been known for some time (e.g., myocardial infarction, stroke); however, newer literature highlights the significance of this risk. Two separate cohort trials indicate increased risk of cardiovascular morbidity and mortality in patients using NSAIDs after an acute myocardial infarction. This risk was increased in patients receiving antithrombotic therapy and was observed even with short-term use (0–3 days).[37] In patients with a history of myocardial infarction, proceed with caution when considering NSAID use. NSAIDs can also aggravate HTN, cause renal failure, inhibit diuretic-induced increases in renal sodium excretion,[38–41] and decrease the hypotensive effect of diuretics and other antihypertensive drugs.[42,43] Patients with CHD and renal insufficiency can be treated for a short duration with nonselective NSAIDs, albeit with much caution. The nonselective NSAIDs are safe for patients with stable, controlled HTN when given for only a few days and with close monitoring of blood pressure.

Colchicine

Colchicine has been successfully used to treat acute gout for more than 2,000 years despite little published research supporting its efficacy.[44] By inhibiting microtubule polymerization, it decreases the action of inflammatory mediators such as cytokines and chemokines. Traditionally, colchicine has been dosed as one or two 0.5- to 0.6-mg tablets initially followed by 0.5 to 0.6 mg hourly or every other hour, until joint pain was relieved or GI effects (i.e., diarrhea, nausea, vomiting) intervened. To minimize these significant adverse effects, the EULAR and BSR/BHPR guidelines[33,34] recommend lower doses of 0.5 mg twice to four times daily. However, the AGREE trial[45] compared a lower-dose regimen (1.2 mg to start followed by 0.6 mg in 1 hour) with the traditional dosing and found significantly fewer adverse effects with the lower-dose regimen and similar efficacy. A 2014 systematic review, combining the AGREE trial with a separate randomized trial, found similar results.[46] Although colchicine has been marketed in the United States since 1961, it was never approved by the FDA as safe and effective. The AGREE trial was the basis of the FDA approval of a new registered colchicine product in the United States. The FDA granted brand exclusivity to this product. Consequently, there are no approved generic alternatives available in the United States.[47,48] The approved dosage is 1.2 mg to start followed by 0.6 mg in 1 hour for the treatment of acute gout and 0.6 mg once to twice daily for gout prophylaxis with a maximal dose of 1.2 mg per day for chronic dosing, which is also consistent with the ACR recommendations. Colchicine should be used cautiously in patients with creatinine clearance (CrCl) less than 30 mL/minute and with hepatic impairment.[32] Colchicine has a number of significant drug interactions that inhibit either cytochrome P-450 (CYP) 3A4 or P-glycoprotein.[49] A thorough medication history is essential to assure safe prescribing. Some common medications that interact with colchicine include digoxin, fibric acids, statins, nondihydropyridine calcium channel blockers, erythromycin, and antifungals. A table detailing significant colchicine drug interactions can be found online in Table 45-4. Common adverse effects include nausea, vomiting, and diarrhea.

Corticosteroids

Historically, corticosteroids have been considered second-line therapy due to the potential for serious adverse effects and adrenal suppression when used long-term as well as the risk of rebound pain when abruptly discontinued.[3,50] However, a recent systematic review found prednisolone to be as effective as NSAIDs for reducing pain from acute gout, and no differences in serious adverse events were observed.[36,51] Corticosteroids may be particularly useful for elderly patients or those with renal disease or CHD who cannot tolerate NSAIDs.[3,34,50,51] Corticosteroid adverse effects (e.g., osteoporosis, myopathy, peptic ulcer disease, central nervous system effects, HTN, predisposition to infections) are not likely with short courses of treatment for gout attacks. Glucose intolerance, however, can occur with short-term therapy. If the acute gout episode involves only one or two large joints, intra-articular corticosteroid administration is recommended by the ACR[32], EULAR[33], and BSR/BHPR[34] guidelines, despite limited evidence. There is also evidence to support the use of intramuscular corticosteroids especially for patients unable to take oral medications.[32]

Analgesics

When an occasional patient requires more pain control, a dose or two of nonopioid or opioid analgesics can be a reasonable adjunctive therapy to blunt the pain of acute gouty arthritis while awaiting the apparent benefits of NSAIDs, colchicine, or corticosteroids.[6] Most patients, however, generally experience benefits from NSAIDs, colchicine, and corticosteroids soon after a dose is administered.

Other Agents

Alternative regimens include the use of adrenocorticotropic hormone (ACTH) and interleukin-1 inhibitors (IL-1). The ACR guidelines recommend the use of ACTH drugs, such as corticotropin, as an alternative to IM/IV corticosteroids in patients unable to take oral medications; however, the significant expense may outweigh the benefits of this medication.[32] Interlukin-1 agents (e.g., anakinra, rilonacept, canakinumab) have not been approved by the FDA for the treatment of acute gout. A systematic review comparing canakinumab to intramuscular triamcinolone indicated that canakinumab was more effective in pain reduction during an acute flare; however, it had significantly higher serious and nonserious adverse effects.[52] The ACR guidelines recommend reserving these agents for situations where traditional medications are contraindicated to ineffective until there is a clearer idea of the risk and benefit profile.[32] As with the ACTH medications, the cost of IL-agents may prohibit use.

CHOICE OF AGENT

CASE 45-2, QUESTION 5: What therapeutic intervention would be most appropriate for E.J. at this time?

Table 45-4
Colchicine Drug Interaction

Interacting Drugs	Description
Cobicistat	May increase the return concentration of colchicine. Management: Colchicine is contraindicated in patients with impaired renal or hepatic function who are also receiving a strong CYP3A4 inhibiter like cobicistat. In those with normal renal and hepatic function, reduce colchicine dose as directed. Consider therapy modification.
Conivaptan	May increase the serum concentration of CYP3A4 substrates. Avoid combination.
Cyanocobalamin	Colchicine may decrease the serum concentration of cyanocobalamin. Monitor therapy.
CYP3A4 inhibitors (moderate)	May increase the serum concentration of colchicine. Management: Reduce colchicine dose as directed when using with a moderate CYP3A4 inhibitor, and increase monitoring for colchicine-related iconicity. Use extra caution in patients with impaired renal and/or hepatic function. Consider therapy modification.
CYP3A4 inhibitors (strong)	May increase the serum concentration of colchicine. Management: Colchicine is contraindicated in patients with impaired renal or hepatic function who are also receiving a strong CYP3A4 inhibitor. In those with normal renal and hepatic function, reduce colchicine dose as directed. Consider therapy modification.
Dasatinib	May increase the serum concentration of CYP3A4 substrates. Monitor therapy.
Digoxin	May increase the serum concentration of colchicine. Monitor therapy.
Fibric acid derivatives	May enhance the myopathic (rhabdomyolysis) effect of colchicine. Monitor therapy.
Fosamprenavir	May increase the serum concentration of colchicine. Management: Colchicine is contraindicated in patients with impaired renal or hepatic function who are receiving ritonavir-boosted fosamprenavir. In those with normal renal and hepatic function, reduce colchicine dose as directed. Consider therapy modification.
Fusidic acid (systemic)	May increase the serum concentration of CYP3A4 substrates. Avoid combination.
HMG-CoA reductase inhibitors	Colchicine may enhance the myopathic (rhabdomyolysis) effect of HMG-CoA reductase inhibitors. Colchicine may increase the serum concentration of HMG-CoA reductase inhibitors. Consider therapy modification.
Idelalisib	May increase the serum concentration of CYP3A4 substrates. Avoid combination.
Luliconazole	May increase the serum concentration of CYP3A4 substrates. Monitor therapy.
Mifepristone	May increase the serum concentration of CYP3A4 substrates. Management: Minimize doses of CYP3A4 substrates, and monitor for increased concentrations/toxicity during and 2 weeks following treatment with mifepristone. Avoid cyclosporine, dihydroergotamine, ergotamine, fentanyl, pinacide, quinidine, sirolimus, and tacrolimus. Consider therapy modification.
Multivitamins/fluoride (with ADE)	Colchicine may decrease the serum concentration of multivitamins/fluoride (with ADE). Specifically, colchicine may decrease absorption of cyanocobalamin (vitamin B12). Monitor therapy.
Multivitamins/minerals (with ADEK, folate, iron)	Colchicine may decrease the serum concentration of multivitamins/minerals (with ADEK, folate, iron). Specifically, colchicine may decrease the serum concentration of cyanocobalamin. Monitor therapy.
Multivitamins/minerals (with AE, no iron)	Colchicine may decrease the serum concentration of multivitamins/minerals (with AE, no iron). Specifically, colchicine may decrease absorption of cyanocobalamin (vitamin B12). Monitor therapy.
P-glycoprotein/ABCBI inducers	May decrease the serum concentration of P-glycoprotein/ABCBI substrates. P-glycoprotein inducers may also further limit the distribution of P-glycoprotein substrates to specific cells/issues/organs where P-glycoprotein is present in large amounts (e.g., brain, T-lymphocytes, testes). Monitor therapy.
P-glycoprotein/ABCBI inhibitors	May increase the serum concentration of colchicine. Colchicine distribution into certain issues (e.g., brain) may also be increased. Management: Colchicine is contraindicated in patients with impaired renal or hepatic function who are also receiving a P-glycoprotein inhibitor. In those with normal renal and hepatic function, reduce colchicine dose as directed. Consider therapy modification.
Stiripentol	May increase the serum concentration of CYP3A4 substrates. Management: Use of stiripentol with CYP3A4 substrates that are considered to have a narrow therapeutic index should be avoided because of the increased risk for adverse effects and toxicity. Any CYP3A4 substrate used with stiripentol requires closer monitoring. Consider therapy modification.
Telaprevir	May increase the serum concentration of colchicine. Management: Colchicine should not be used with telaprevir in patients with impaired renal or hepatic function. In those with normal renal and hepatic function, reduced colchicine doses (as directed) are required if used with telaprevir. Consider therapy modification.
Tipranavir	May increase the serum concentration of colchicine. Management: Colchicine should not be used with tipranavir in patients with impaired renal or hepatic function. In those with normal renal and hepatic function, reduced colchicine doses (as directed) are required if used with tipranavir. Consider therapy modification.

Source: Facts & Comparisons eAnswers; **http://online.factsandcomparisons.com/MonoDisp.aspx?monoID=fandc-**

An NSAID would be an appropriate first-line therapy for the acute treatment of gout in E.J. because his renal function is normal. Assuming his blood pressure is adequately controlled, a short course of ibuprofen 800 mg now and every 8 hours until resolution of symptoms (usually 7–10 days) is appropriate. The ibuprofen should be prescribed on a scheduled basis rather than "as needed" to reduce inflammation and prevent breakthrough pain. The dose of 2,400 mg/day does not exceed the maximum recommended dose of 3,200 mg/day.

NONPHARMACOLOGIC INTERVENTIONS

Case 45-2, Question 6: What adjunctive therapies would be beneficial for E.J.?

The use of ice, reduction of alcohol consumption, and minor diet modification may be effective and can be considered for E.J.

Ice

The benefit of ice application to the affected joint in acute gouty arthritis should not be overlooked. Evidence from a systematic review indicates the application of ice to an affected joint for 30 minutes four times daily for 1 week reduced the pain of a gout attack when used in conjunction with oral steroids or colchicine.[53]

Alcohol Consumption

Excessive alcohol intake is known to be a risk factor for acute gout episodes. Beer was believed to be more problematic for gout than other alcoholic beverages because of its high purine content. The Health Professionals Follow-Up study[23] examined a cohort of patients with new diagnoses of gout over a 12-year time frame and found that when beer, spirits, and wine intake were examined, the greatest risk was with beer with a significant, but lesser, risk with spirits. Interestingly, wine, even more than two drinks/day, was not associated with an increased risk of gout. A smaller, independent study found that the quantity of alcohol consumed in the 24 hours before an acute attack is more important than the type of beverage consumed.[54] The current ACR,[17] EULAR,[33] and BSR/BHPR[34] guidelines recommend avoiding overuse by advocating moderation in alcohol consumption. The ACR recommends no more than two servings per day for males and one serving per day for women. Despite lack of evidence, the ACR also recommends avoiding alcohol use during an acute attack and frequent, poorly controlled gout attacks.[32] E.J. should avoid alcohol or at least limit his alcohol intake to no more than 2 servings per day.

Diet Modification

Diet has a twofold effect on the epidemiology of gout. First, obese patients are at a greater risk of developing elevated SUA levels, and gout might, in part, be related to insulin resistance of obesity.[7] In a prospective, longitudinal study of male health professionals, weight gain was strongly associated with an increased risk of gout, and weight loss was associated with a decreased risk.[55]

Second, much of the uric acid produced daily comes from metabolism of food. The excessive dietary intake of purine-rich foods, without a concomitant increase in urinary excretion, can lead to elevated SUA concentrations.[7,8] However, the type of protein and purine-rich foods that are detrimental and the true impact of these foods on the incidence of increased SUA and gout episodes are controversial issues due to the quality of evidence available.[56,57] Despite the lack of strong evidence, it is reasonable for clinicians to recommend patients limit certain foods (e.g., organ meats, beef, lamb, pork shellfish, products containing high-fructose corn syrup). Interestingly, low-fat or nonfat dairy products and coffee consumption have been associated with a decreased incidence of gout.[7,58] E.J. should be encouraged to limit or avoid purine-rich meats and fructose-containing beverages/foods and encouraged to increase consumption of low-fat dairy products.

Case 45-3

Question 1: V.D. is a 72-year-old woman who was brought to the emergency department complaining of shortness of breath and dizziness. On arrival, she is noted to have new-onset atrial fibrillation with a heart rate of 130 beats/minute and 2+ peripheral edema bilaterally to her knees. The latter is likely secondary to exacerbation of congestive heart failure caused by her rapid ventricular rate. In addition to administering diltiazem to control her heart rate, V.D. is given 40 mg of IV furosemide every 12 hours for three doses. The following day she complains of severe pain in her left great toe, and it is noted on examination to be erythematous and swollen. V.D.'s CrCl is 70 mL/minute, her SUA concentration is 7.5 mg/dL, and her blood pressure is 160/96 mm Hg. What therapeutic option would be appropriate for V.D.?

The combination of V.D.'s advanced age, acute exacerbation of heart failure, and renal dysfunction is patient-specific parameters that are relative contraindications or precautions for the use of NSAIDs for the treatment of acute gout. Therefore, alternative treatments should be considered. Colchicine is the next drug to consider, but because she is now receiving diltiazem (a moderate CYP3A4 inhibitor) the dose of colchicine would need to be reduced. Because V.D.'s pain is monoarticular, intra-articular or oral corticosteroids could be administered, but the latter would need to be tapered over the course of 10 to 21 days to avoid rebound gout symptoms. It is decided to give V.D. 1.2 mg of colchicine for one dose only, which is appropriate to avoid the diltiazem drug interaction.[47]

HYPERURICEMIA

Chronic Gout

Case 45-3, Question 2: V.D. is ready to be discharged 3 days later. Her toe is no longer inflamed, and her pain is gone. Should ULT be prescribed at discharge to prevent another gout attack?

ULT should be initiated only when patients with gout have recurrent acute attacks (at least two attacks per year), urate tophi, uric acid stones, or chronic kidney disease (Stage 2 and up) with prior gout attack and current hyperuricemia.[17,34] If these indications are absent, ULT should not be prescribed. Long-term ULT should not be started for V.D. at this time because criteria for therapy (see ACR, EULAR, and BSR/BHPR guidelines in Table 45-3)[17,33,34] are not met, and initiation of ULT during an acute episode can mobilize urate from tissues, compounding the problem.

DRUG-INDUCED HYPERURICEMIA

A patient's complete medication list should be reviewed to rule out drug-induced hyperuricemia before adding a medication to decrease SUA concentration. Perhaps, the only treatment needed would be to discontinue the offending agent. Common medications known to increase SUA include thiazide and loop diuretics, niacin, calcineurin inhibitors (e.g., cyclosporine and tacrolimus), and aspirin.[17] The authors of the ACR guidelines recommend continuing low-dose aspirin (used for cardioprotection) in patients with hyperuricemia unless with benefits of discontinuation (i.e., reduction in risk of a gout attack) outweigh the risks.[17]

The association between hyperuricemia and diuretics is well known and is dose related[59]; however, the clinical importance of diuretic-induced gout attacks is now somewhat controversial. Clinicians often discontinue the diuretic, irrespective of possible ancillary benefits of diuretics (especially in HTN and CHF). A 2012 systematic review showed a trend toward increased risk for acute gout with thiazide and loop diuretics; however, the extent of the risk and its clinical significance is still unknown. Therefore, the authors state there is not enough evidence to support discontinuation of these agents in populations that have shown benefit for other comorbidities.[60] In certain cases where diuretics are thought to be a contributing factor to the precipitation of a gout attack, discontinuation of diuretic therapy may be reasonable, particularly if alternatives are available and appropriate for a patient.

GOAL OF URATE-LOWERING THERAPY

CASE 45-3, QUESTION 3: V.D. experienced another episode of acute gout 2 months later, which was treated successfully with colchicine. She is now on chronic warfarin to prevent stroke secondary to her atrial fibrillation and remains on diltiazem for heart rate control. Her blood pressure is 130/70 mm Hg, renal function is stable with a CrCl of 70 mL/minutes, and SUA is 7.2 mg/dL. Would it be appropriate to initiate ULT at this time? If so, when would you initiate treatment?

The general goals for lowering SUA concentrations are the elimination of acute gout attacks and the mobilization of urate crystals from soft tissue. The SUA concentration in a patient who has clinical gout should be decreased to 6 mg/dL or less,[17,34] which is below the saturation point for MSU. However, because some patients may experience continued gouty arthritis attacks even when the SUA is < 6 mg/dL, the ACR and BSR/BHPR guidelines recommend a goal of less than 5 mg/dL in these individuals.[17,34] The BSR/BHPR guidelines recommend as standard of care waiting 1 to 2 weeks after an acute attack to begin ULT due to risk of a recurrent attack.[34] A small, short trial studied the effect of starting allopurinol during an acute flare and was found not to worsen pain or risk of a recurrent flare. V.D. fits the criteria for initiating ULT (2 attacks in less than 1 year); however, this should be preceded by a consideration of whether drug-induced hyperuricemia could be a contributing factor. V.D.'s initial episode of gout after aggressive diuresis with IV furosemide was likely the cause of her first gout attack, but she is not currently on any drugs that cause hyperuricemia.

DRUG THERAPY OF HYPERURICEMIA

Xanthine Oxidase Inhibitors

Allopurinol

Clinical practice guidelines recommend allopurinol as a first-line agent for gout prevention.[17,33,34] It inhibits the production of uric acid and thereby decreases SUA concentrations. A 2014 systematic review of 2 clinical trials, with methodological limitations, shows that when compared to placebo allopurinol was superior at achieving target SUA concentrations, but failed to significantly reduce the frequency of acute gout attacks.[61] The ability of allopurinol to lower SUA concentrations is dose related. An allopurinol dose of 300 mg/day is typical maintenance dose, despite evidence to support that more than 50% of patients are unable to achieve target SUA at this dose or lower.[62, 63] Larger doses up to 800 to 900 mg/day may be needed for those with more severe disease.[34]

The recommended initial dose of allopurinol is 50 to 100 mg once daily and then increased in 50- to 100-mg/day increments every 2 to 5 weeks until the SUA concentration is at the desired goal of less than 6 mg/dL or until patient intolerance.[17,33,34] Starting at a low dose and titrating slowly hypothetically can reduce the risk for hypersensitivity reactions and improve tolerance in renal impairment.

Allopurinol has been associated with a life-threatening hypersensitivity syndrome that may include a desquamative, erythematous rash, fever, elevated liver function tests, and renal failure. Although hypersensitivity reactions are rare (1:1,000 in US), they are very serious.[17] If allopurinol hypersensitivity occurs, the drug should be stopped immediately because this can lead to skin necrosis, exfoliative dermatitis, Stevens–Johnson syndrome, toxic epidermal necrolysis, and even death.[64] Patients who recover should avoid future use of allopurinol, although some have been able to be desensitized and tolerate low doses.[65]

These adverse effects are more common in patients with concomitant diuretic use and preexisting renal insufficiency; therefore, dose adjustment in patients with renal impairment is recommended.[66] In the past, a nomogram based on CrCl has been used to reduce the risk of these adverse effects in renal impairment, but a subsequent study[67] challenged its efficacy and the ACR guidelines[17] recommend against this method. ACR guidelines state that doses of greater than 300 mg may be used in patients with renal impairment (Stage 4 or greater) with slow titration, close monitoring, and patient education.[17] A table detailing significant allopurinol drug interactions can be found online in Table 45-5.

Febuxostat

Febuxostat, a nonpurine XO inhibitor, was approved by the FDA in February 2009 for chronic management of hyperuricemia in patients with gout.[68] Febuxostat is more selective than allopurinol for XO and does not inhibit other enzymes involved in purine and pyrimidine metabolism. A 2012 Cochrane systematic review, with methodological limitations, evaluated six trials comparing febuxostat to allopurinol for clinical SUA-lowering effect, and found febuxostat more effective than allopurinol 300 mg in achieving SUA of less than 6 mg/dL. An important consideration in evaluating the evidence is that although the studies allowed upward titration of febuxostat to achieve maximal SUA lowering, the allopurinol dosage was not titrated to greater than 300 mg daily.[69] Because the urate-lowering effect with allopurinol is known to be dose-related, and some patients have required up to 900 mg/day to achieve a SUA less than 6 mg/dL, these results may not have allowed for an adequate comparison of efficacy between the two drugs. The same review revealed that compared to standard doses of allopurinol higher doses of febuxostat, 120 mg and 240 mg daily, increased the risk of gout flares; however, long-term follow-up studies did not detect an increased risk of flares. The FDA-approved dose in the United States is 80 mg daily; however, doses of up to 240 mg daily are approved in other countries.

In addition, adverse effects were shown to be minor and similar between both drugs in comparative studies with increases in liver function tests, nausea, diarrhea, arthralgias, and rash being the most common adverse effects with greater than 1% incidence.[62,68,70,71] Because febuxostat is more widely used, the clinician should note that thromboembolic cardiovascular events have been reported to the FDA adverse event reporting system. There are two ongoing clinical trials evaluating cardiovascular risk in both allopurinol and febuxostat.[72,73]

The starting dose of febuxostat is 40 mg once daily with a recommended dose increase to 80 mg once daily if SUA concentration is not less than 6 mg/dL by 2 weeks of therapy. It does not require dose adjustments for CrCl greater than 30 mL/minute, and the labeling provides no recommendations for use in patients with more severe renal impairment.[68] A table detailing significant febuxostat drug interactions can be found online in Table 45-6.

CHOICE OF AGENT

CASE 45-3, QUESTION 4: Because a XO inhibitor is first-line therapy to lower SUA concentration, which product should be chosen for V.D.?

Table 45-5

Allopurinol Drug Interactions

Precipitant Drug	Object Drug[a]		Description
Allopurinol	Ampicillin, amoxicillin	↑	The rate of skin appears much higher with allopurinol coadministration than with either drug alone.
Allopurinol	Anticoagulants, oral	↑	Data are conflicting. The anticoagulant action of some agents may be enhanced, but probably not that of warfarin.
Allopurinol	Cyclophosphamide	↑	Myelosuppressive effects of cyclophosphamide may be enhanced increasing the risk of bleeding or infection.
Allopurinol	Theophyllines	↑	Theophylline clearance may be decreased with large allopurinol doses (600 mg/day) leading to increased plasma theophylline levels and possible toxicity.
Allopurinol	Thiopurines	↑	Clinically significant increases in pharmacologic and effects of oral thiopurines have occurred.
ACE inhibitors	Allopurinol	↑	There is possibly a higher risk of hypersensitivity reaction when these agents are coadministered than when each drug is administered alone.
Aluminum salts	Allopurinol	↓	Pharmacologic effects of allopurinol may be decreased.
Thiazide diuretics	Allopurinol	↑	Coadministration may increase the incidence of hypersensitivity reactions to allopurinol.
Uricosuric agents	Allopurinol	↓	Uricosuric agents that increase the excretion of urate are also likely to increase the excretion of oxipurinol and thus lower the degree of inhibition of xanthine of xanthine oxidase.

[a]↑ = object drug increased; ↓ = object drug decreased.
Source: Facts & Comparisons eAnswers; **http://online.factsandcomparisons.com/MonoDisp.aspx?monoID=fandc-hcp13090&quick=176221%7c5&search=176221%7c5&isstemmed=True&NDCmapping=-1&fromTop=true#firstMatch**. Accessed June 18, 2015.

Although febuxostat is clearly efficacious in lowering SUA concentrations, allopurinol is also effective when the dose is appropriately titrated to response and goal SUA concentration. The ACR guidelines[17] do not recommend one over another for first-line treatment. The clinician should keep in mind the significantly higher out-of-pocket cost for febuxostat and consider patient affordability when choosing drug therapy. A 2015 cost-effectiveness analysis (from a US payer perspective) found febuxostat to be a cost-effective option compared to allopurinol at achieving a SUA level < 6 mg/dL despite the fact that the total cost of allopurinol treatment over 5 years was less ($1,882 difference between medications).[74] The National Institute for Health and Clinical Excellence (NICE), an organization that provides medical guidance to healthcare practitioners of the public health system in the United Kingdom, issued a document in 2008 that recommends febuxostat be used only in patients who are intolerant of or have contraindications to allopurinol therapy or for those who cannot achieve adequate SUA concentration lowering on allopurinol therapy.[75] V.D. does not have any contraindications to allopurinol therapy. She is on chronic warfarin, which may interact with allopurinol.[76] This warrants monitoring her international normalized ratio 5 to 7 days after allopurinol therapy is initiated and with any allopurinol dosage adjustments.

Uricosuric Agents

Probenecid is the only uricosuric agent available in the United States. Clinical practice guidelines recommend it as an second-line therapy to XO inhibitors for patients who are unable to take at least one XO inhibitor due to tolerability, contraindications, or significant drug interactions.[17] The clinical evidence for the class of uricosurics is limited to comparisons of benzbromarone, which is not available in the Unites states, to allopurinol. A 2014 Cochrane review concluded that there were no differences between these agents in the number of acute gout attacks prevented or the number of patients who discontinued therapy due to side effects.[77] However, due to the lack of head-to-head comparisons, clinicians must be cautious in extrapolating these results to probenecid. Uricosurics should not be administered to patients with impaired renal function or urolithiasis. It is well absorbed orally, and plasma concentrations peak within 2 to 4 hours. Its biologic half-life is 6 to 12 hours, and its active metabolites extend the duration of action. The usual initial dose of probenecid (250 mg twice daily for the first week of therapy) can be increased to 500 mg twice a day. If necessary, the dose can be increased further to 2 to 3 g/day. Uricosuric therapy should begin with small doses because the excretion of large amounts of uric acid increases the risk of urate stone formation in the kidney. High fluid intake to maintain urine flow of at least 2 L/day also minimizes renal stone formation. This gradual approach to the initiation of ULT also decreases the likelihood of precipitating an acute attack of gout. Common adverse effects include headache and GI upset.

Probenecid inhibits secretion of penicillins into the renal tubule, and thereby prolongs the serum half-life of penicillin and increases penicillin serum concentrations. Probenecid can also compete with salicylates for renal tubular transport, but its interactions with salicylates involve several mechanisms.[78] Low-dose aspirin for cardioprotection is unlikely to interfere with probenecid therapy. Interestingly, high-dose aspirin (e.g., greater than 1 g) has uricosuric activity of its own.[79]

Recombinant Urate Oxidase Drugs (Uricase)

Uricase, an enzyme endogenous in many animal species other than humans, converts uric acid to allantoin, which is much more soluble than uric acid and, therefore, more readily excreted into urine. Recently, two recombinant urate oxidase drugs have been developed for the treatment of hyperuricemia and gout. However, the high-incidence serious adverse reactions (23%–24%) as well as cost prohibit routine use. Rather, they should be considered as alternatives when all other ULTs have failed.[80]

Table 45-6
Febuxostat Drug Interactions

Precipitant Drug	Object Drug[a]		Description
Antacids (e.g., aluminum, magnesium)	Febuxostat	↓	Concomitant ingestion of an antacid containing magnesium hydroxide and aluminum hydroxide with an 80-mg single dose of febuxostat has been shown to delay absorption of febuxostat (approximately 1 hour) and to cause a 31% decrease in C_{max} and 15% decrease in AUC. Because AUC rather than C_{max} was related to drug effect, change observed in AUC was not considered clinically significant. Therefore, febuxostat may be taken without regard to antacid use.
Febuxostat	Didanosine	↑	Systemic exposures of didanosine are increased during coadministration. Concurrent use is contraindicated.
Febuxostat	Xanthine oxidase substrate drugs (e.g., azathioprine, mercaptopurine, theophylline)	↑	Febuxostat is a xanthine oxidase inhibitor. Inhibition of xanthine oxidase by febuxostat may cause increased plasma concentration of these drugs, leading to toxicity. Concurrent use with azathioprine or mercaptopurine is contraindicated. Use with caution when administering with theophylline.

[a]↑ = object drug increased; ↓ = object drug decreased.

Rasburicase

Rasburicase was initially approved by the FDA for the management of hyperuricemia in children who are receiving cytotoxic chemotherapy likely to result in tumor lysis syndrome, and later received approval for the same indication in adults. Rasburicase is administered as a short IV infusion of 0.2 mg/kg daily for up to 5 days.[81] A comparative short-term study in patients with renal impairment found rasburicase was significantly more effective than allopurinol in lowering SUA concentrations at the end of 7 days of therapy.[82] Although lower-quality studies show significant reductions in SUA, rasburicase is not indicated for the treatment of hyperuricemia in patients with gout, due to its short half-life and immunogenicity. Until further studies confirm safety and longer-term efficacy in nonchemotherapy-related hyperuricemia, rasburicase should be reserved for patients with hyperuricemia who are at risk for tumor lysis syndrome.

Pegloticase

Pegloticase, the other available recombinant uricase drug available, has been shown to be effective in reducing SUA concentrations in patients who were refractory to conventional treatment in a few small randomized controlled trials.[83] It received FDA approval in 2010 for treatment in this limited population. Pegloticase is administered IV for 2 hours as a dose of 8 mg every 2 weeks.[84] It has a significant risk of anaphylaxis[85] and infusion site reactions, so each dose must be preceded by prophylaxis with an antihistamine and corticosteroid. It is contraindicated in patients with glucose-6-phosphate dehydrogenase deficiency, and the usual gout flare prophylaxis is recommended for the first 6 months after initiation. Finally, antipegloticase antibodies occurred in the majority of patients studied, and this can ameliorate the SUA-lowering effects by decreasing the half-life of pegloticase. The full implication of this is unknown.

Other Agents

Some medications (e.g., ascorbic acid, antihypertensive agents, and fenofibrate) used to treat conditions commonly seen in conjunction with gout have been proven to have uricosuric properties. However, the currently available trials evaluating these agents have significant limitations and uric acid lowering is minimal. It is also important to note that to date no trials evaluating their effectiveness on clinically relevant outcomes (e.g., gout attacks) have been published. If future randomized trials show promise, some patients with hyperuricemia might be managed better by selecting drugs to manage comorbid conditions rather than requiring the use of the more traditional ULT.

Ascorbic Acid

Vitamin C has a urate-lowering effect that is believed to be mediated by competition with urate for renal tubular reabsorption.[86] However, clinical practice guidelines do not address its place in therapy, and there is a lack of high-quality evidence to support routine use for the prevention of gout attacks.[87,88]

Antihypertensive Agents

In a case–control study, calcium channel blockers and losartan have been shown to decrease the risk of incidence gout.[89] Other antihypertensive agents (e.g., β-blockers, diuretics, angiotensin-converting enzyme inhibitors, and nonlosartan angiotensin II receptor blockers) were also studied and were found to have increased risk of gout. When used with diuretics, losartan appears to mitigate the hyperuricemic effect of the diuretic.[86] It does not seem to be a class effect for the class of angiotensin II receptor blockers because, in a study, patients on losartan achieved significantly lower SUA concentrations than an irbesartan-treated group.[90] In patients with hyperuricemia and HTN, losartan and calcium channel blockers may be a viable option depending on individual patient variables.

Fenofibrate

Fenofibrate has been shown to decrease SUA concentrations by increasing renal urate excretion.[86] In addition to therapeutic lifestyle changes, fibrates (i.e., gemfibrozil, fenofibrate) or niacin is commonly used for the treatment of hypertriglyceridemia. However, with a history of gout and hyperuricemia, a fibrate would be preferred over niacin because niacin can induce hyperuricemia. Fenofibrate is a reasonable option for patients requiring a decrease in triglycerides and a history of gout; however, the selection of a medication to manage this comorbid condition also involves other clinical variables that might be equally applicable.[33,91,92]

FLARE PROPHYLAXIS DURING INITIATION OF ULT

CASE 45-3, QUESTION 5: V.D. is started on allopurinol 100 mg orally once daily for initial ULT. Her SUA concentration will be checked, and her allopurinol will be increased by 50 to 100 mg/day in 2 to 4 weeks if needed until she reaches the goal of less than or equal to 6 mg/dL. What other drug therapy should also be considered when starting ULT?

Paradoxically, initiation of ULT can precipitate acute gout attacks. Guidelines recommend prophylaxis with anti-inflammatory agents for all patients when ULT is initiated.[32–34] The following anti-inflammatory agents should be considered, in order of preference: colchicine, low-dose NSAIDs, and oral corticosteroids.[32] However, when choosing prophylactic therapy, one should also consider patient comorbidities, potential drug–drug interactions, and tolerance issues. Upon initiation of ULT, anti-inflammatory therapy should be continued for at least 6 months. A shorter duration of 3 months may be reasonable in patients without evidence of tophi who achieve SUA target concentrations. V.D. would be a candidate for flare prophylaxis. As stated above, V.D.'s advanced age, acute exacerbation of heart failure, and renal dysfunction are patient-specific parameters that are relative contraindications or precautions for the use of long-term NSAID therapy for flare prophylaxis. Colchicine would be a reasonable option because it is considered first line and she tolerated colchicine during acute attacks. The colchicine dose for flare prophylaxis is 0.6 mg once or twice daily for 6 weeks. V.D. should be monitored for adverse drug reactions.

MONITORING AND FOLLOW-UP

In addition to monitoring for subjective and objective evidence of drug-related adverse effects, SUA concentrations should be monitored monthly until at goal, then every 6 to 12 months, thereafter. The optimal duration of ULT is unclear. Patients with mild gout may go years without experiencing repeat attacks after discontinuation of ULT. Lower SUA concentrations during treatment correlate with a longer interval between acute attacks or before tophi reappear. The majority of patients on long-term ULT are likely to experience recurrent acute attacks, tophi, or both if treatment is stopped.[93] The decision when to discontinue ULT should be made based primarily on patient preference after a shared-informed discussion.

Asymptomatic Hyperuricemia

CASE 45-4

QUESTION 1: T.M., a 50-year-old man, is seen by his physician for a routine evaluation. His physical examination is unremarkable, and his laboratory evaluations are all within normal limits except for a SUA concentration of 9.5 mg/dL. Should his hyperuricemia be treated?

Individuals with high SUA concentrations are more likely to develop acute gouty arthritis than normouricemic individuals. A large percentage of hyperuricemic patients may never experience an acute attack of gout.[2] Therefore, it would be excessive to treat all hyperuricemic individuals with uric acid-lowering medications for lifetime solely to prevent acute attacks of gouty arthritis. If an attack should occur, it can be treated quickly and easily, and if the patient has at least two attacks in a year, ULT can be considered. The ACR guidelines chose not to address this condition due to lack of quality evidence.[17]

The key issue in the treatment of hyperuricemia concerns the effect of uric acid on renal function. Renal disease was commonly associated with gout, and renal failure was believed to be the eventual cause of death in as many as 25% of gouty patients. However, the coexistence of gout and renal insufficiency without HTN is rare.[94] Therefore, the consensus now seems to be that hyperuricemia by itself has no deleterious effect on renal function.[95,96]

PHARMACIST'S ROLE

The pharmacist has an important role in the education and management of gout. As noted several times in this chapter, there are significant drug–drug interactions associated with a majority of the medications used to treat both acute and chronic gout. A 2008 retrospective cohort study showed that 28% of patients did not meet with a provider prior to initiation of ULT and 56% of patients were nonadherent with ULT.[97] Patient education about the role of the medication, including the importance of adherence and how to monitor for and manage adverse drug reactions in the treatment of gout, is an essential part of therapy. In the cases where a provider visit did not occur prior to starting ULT, a pharmacist could have been a resource for education. Pharmacists are equipped with the knowledge and skills to monitor for drug–drug interactions, monitor and educate about medication adherence, and provide general education about gout and lifestyle recommendations. Also, open communication with the patient's primary-care provider has the potential to improve the patient experience related to this condition.

KEY REFERENCES AND WEBSITES

A full list of references for this chapter can be found at http://thepoint.lww.com/AT11e. Below are the key references and websites for this chapter, with the corresponding reference number in this chapter found in parentheses after the reference.

Key References

Choi HK et al. Intake of purine-rich foods, protein, and dairy products and relationship to serum levels of uric acid: the Third National Health and Nutrition Examination Survey. *Arthritis Rheum*. 2005;52:283. (56)

Choi HK et al. Obesity, weight change, hypertension, diuretic use, and risk of gout in men: the health professionals follow-up study. *Arch Int Med*. 2005;165:742. (55)

Hueskes BA et al. Use of diuretics and the risk of gouty arthritis: a systematic review. *Semin Arthritis Rheum*. 2012;41(6):879. (60)

Jordan KM et al. British Society for Rheumatology and British Health Professionals in Rheumatology guideline for the management of gout. *Rheumatology (Oxford)*. 2007;46:1372. (34)

Khanna D et al. American College of Rheumatology guidelines for management of gout. Part 1: systematic nonpharmacologic and pharmacologic therapeutic approaches to hyperuricemia. *Arthritis Care Res*. 2012;64(10):1431. (17)

Khanna D et al. American College of Rheumatology guidelines for management of gout. Part 2: therapy and anti-inflammatory prophylaxis of acute gouty arthritis. *Arthritis Care Res*. 2012;64(10):1447. (32)

Neogi T et al. 2015 Gout Classification Criteria. *Arthritis Rheum*. 2015;67(10):2557.

Neogi T. Clinical practice. Gout. *N Engl J Med*. 2011;364(5):443. (2)

Seth R et al. Allopurinol for chronic gout. Cochrane Database of Systematic Reviews 2014, Issue 10. Art. No.: CD006077. DOI: 10.1002/14651858.CD006077.pub3. (61)

Tayar JH et al. Febuxostat for treating chronic gout. Cochrane Database of Systematic Reviews 2012, Issue 11. Art. No.: CD008653. DOI: 10.1002/14651858.CD008653.pub2. (69)

Terkeltaub RA et al. High versus low dosing of oral colchicine for early acute gout flare: twenty-four-hour outcome of the first multicenter, randomized, double-blind, placebo-controlled, parallel-group, dose-comparison colchicine study. *Arthritis Rheum*. 2010;62:1060. (45)

van Durme CMPG et al. Non-steroidal anti-inflammatory drugs for acute gout. Cochrane Database of Systematic Reviews 2014, Issue 9. Art. No.: CD010120. DOI: 10.1002/14651858.CD010120.pub2. (36)

van Echteld I et al. Colchicine for acute gout. Cochrane Database of Systematic Reviews 2014, Issue 8. Art. No.: CD006190. DOI: 10.1002/14651858.CD006190.pub2. (46)

Wallace SL et al. Preliminary criteria for the classification of the acute arthritis of primary gout. *Arthritis Rheum*. 1977; 20:895. (27)

White WB et al. Cardiovascular safety of febuxostat and allopurinol in patients with gout and cardiovascular comorbidities. *Am Heart J.* 2012;164(1):14. (72)

Zhang W et al. EULAR evidence based recommendations for gout. Part II: Management. Report of a task force of the EULAR Standing Committee for International Clinical Studies Including Therapeutics (ESCISIT). *Ann Rheum Dis.* 2006;65:1312. (33)

Key Websites

American College of Rheumatology. http://www.rheumatology.org/. Accessed June 1, 2015.

Gout and Uric Acid Education Society. http://gouteducation.org/. Accessed June 1, 2015.

MedlinePlus. http://www.nlm.nih.gov/medlineplus/gout.html. Accessed June 1, 2015.

National Health Service. National Institute for Health and Clinical Excellence. Febuxostat for the management of hyperuricaemia in people with gout. 2008. http://www.nice.org.uk/nicemedia/live/12101/42738/42738.pdf. Accessed May 28, 2015. (72)

46 Connective Tissue Disorders

Julie L. Olenak and Jonathan D. Ference

CORE PRINCIPLES		CHAPTER CASES
1	Ninety percent of patients who are affected by systemic sclerosis also have signs and symptoms consistent with Raynaud phenomenon.	**Case 46-1 (Questions 1, 2), Table 46-1**
2	Nifedipine, prazosin, and losartan may decrease severity and frequency of symptoms of Raynaud syndrome.	**Case 46-1 (Question 3), Table 46-3**
3	Many authorities believe polymyalgia rheumatica and temporal arteritis are manifestations of the same underlying process occurring at different times during the clinical course. However, they each have characteristic symptoms and are treated differently.	**Case 46-2 (Questions 1–3), Table 46-4**
4	Reactive arthritis is secondary to certain genitourinary, gastrointestinal, or respiratory infections. Patients with the HLA-B27 gene are more susceptible to spondyloarthritis.	**Case 46-3 (Question 1), Table 46-5**
5	Patients with documented active infections, and their partners when caused by a sexually transmitted disease, should be offered antibiotics. However, efficacy of prolonged antibiotics as a treatment of reactive arthritis is conflicting.	**Case 46-3 (Question 2)**
6	Nonsteroidal anti-inflammatories are appropriate initial therapy for reactive arthritis to control pain and inflammation.	**Case 46-3 (Question 2)**
7	In severe or prolonged cases of reactive arthritis, steroids, DMARDs, and biologicals may be considered.	**Case 46-3 (Question 3)**
8	Polymyositis and dermatomyositis should initially be treated with high-dose corticosteroids. Immunosuppressive agents are recommended if the disease is not controlled with corticosteroids alone, if the response is positive but steroid sparing effects are desired, or if the condition presents initially with extramuscular complications.	**Case 46-4 (Questions 1, 2)**

INTRODUCTION

Despite new knowledge in the immunology and the pathogenesis of the different connective tissue diseases (CTDs), the etiology of these conditions remains unclear.[1] Diagnosing CTDs can be difficult because of the complexity of the diseases and the varying presentation of symptoms. The patient's reported history of symptoms, results of the physical examination, and laboratory testing help guide the diagnosis of a CTD.[1] It has been reported that as many as half of patients who have a diagnosed CTD had been identified as having undifferentiated connective tissue disease.[2] It can take years for a patient to be diagnosed and meet classification criteria. Diffuse CTDs include systemic lupus erythematosus (SLE), scleroderma, polymyositis, dermatomyositis, rheumatoid arthritis, and Sjögren syndrome. Patients may present with findings consistent with more than one CTD, and symptoms generally do not all appear simultaneously. Mixed CTD is an overlap of autoimmune disease features that can include myositis, scleroderma, and lupus.[1,2]

GENERAL SIGNS AND SYMPTOMS

Many patients such as those with SLE can have arthralgias and arthritis as part of the inflammatory disease associated with their CTD. Inflammatory disease is suggested by morning stiffness of greater than 1 hour (a similar problem occurs with sitting or resting), swelling, fever, weakness, and systemic fatigue. In some patients, activities of daily living and function may be excellent despite pain and deformity; in others, because of psychologic and systemic disease, there may be poor function with minimal articular involvement. Other psychosocial aspects of their life, including sexuality, may be affected by many of the inflammatory disorders.

Dermatologic changes are often associated with a particular rheumatic disease. Examples include alopecia with SLE, onycholysis and keratoderma blennorrhagica with reactive arthritis, buccal or genital ulcers with SLE or Reiter syndrome, Raynaud phenomenon with SLE or systemic sclerosis, calcinosis and rash over the knuckles (Gottron papule) with dermatomyositis, and sun sensitivity malar rash with SLE. The presence of nodules, tophi, telangiectasia, or vasculitic changes also may be detected, helping the clinician differentiate which inflammatory disease is present and what management is necessary.

The CTDs are commonly associated with musculoskeletal changes. Joints may display warmth, redness and effusion, synovial thickening, deformities, decreased range of motion, pain on motion, tenderness on palpation, and decreased function. Often, a patient's hand and arm function, as well as gait, may be altered. In addition to the signs and symptoms used to differentiate various rheumatic diseases, laboratory evaluation of patients with rheumatic complaints can often define the extent of disease or detect other organ systems that may be involved.

SELECTED CONNECTIVE TISSUE DISEASES

CTDs and rheumatic diseases encompass a wide range of disorders that are inflammatory in nature and related to the immune system. The following are some of the conditions that are encountered in clinical practice and will be discussed in this chapter: scleroderma, polymyalgia rheumatica, temporal arteritis, reactive arthritis, polymyositis, and dermatomyositis. The reader is also referred to Chapter 33, which covers SLE.

Systemic Sclerosis (Scleroderma)

Systemic sclerosis, or systemic scleroderma, is a CTD associated with autoimmunity characterized by excessive extracellular matrix deposition and vascular injury to the skin and other visceral organs.[3] Systemic sclerosis can be classified into distinct clinical subsets based on the patterns of skin and internal organ involvement, autoantibody production, and patient survival.[3] The most common subsets include limited cutaneous (approximately 60% of patients) and diffuse cutaneous (approximately 35% of patients).[3] The term overlap syndrome may be applied to patients when features common in one or more of the other CTDs are present and affect approximately 11% of patients diagnosed with systemic sclerosis. The limited cutaneous subset is diagnosed when skin thickening is limited to the areas distal to the elbows and knees. A constellation of dysfunctions known as CREST (calcinosis cutis, Raynaud phenomenon, esophageal dysfunction, sclerodactyly, telangiectasia) syndrome is a variant of limited cutaneous systemic sclerosis.[3]

More women than men suffer from systemic sclerosis (female-to-male ratio, 4.6:1), although the mean age at diagnosis does not differ between men and women.[4] Onset of systemic sclerosis generally begins in adults between 30 and 50 years of age and is rare in children and seniors older than 80 years of age.[5] The prevalence is estimated at 276 cases/million adults in the United States.[5] African-American patients are twice as likely as non–African-American patients to have diffuse disease, with the annual incidence in African-American women being twice that of Caucasian women.[4,6] Likely and possible risk factors for the disease include environmental exposure to silica dust (e.g., coal miners) and the presence of a connective tissue growth factor polymorphism, respectively.[7] At this time, there is no conclusive evidence to support an association between silicone breast implants and systemic sclerosis, or any other CTD.[7] Cigarette smoking is not associated with an increased risk of systemic sclerosis.[8]

The underlying pathophysiologic changes that lead to systemic scleroderma remain unknown, but many believe that it results from a lymphocyte-mediated autoimmune reaction with endothelial cells, activated immune cells, and fibroblasts playing a key role in the process. It is hypothesized that the process is initiated by an immune attack on the endothelium leading to endothelial cell activation or injury. This is followed by activation of the fibroblasts, resulting in subendothelial connective tissue proliferation, narrowing of the vascular lumen, and Raynaud phenomenon. T cells are then selectively activated and populate the affected areas such as the dermis and lung tissue. These cells produce cytokines that stimulate resident fibroblasts to produce excessive amounts of procollagen, which is then converted extracellularly to mature collagen. Later, when the inflammatory process subsides, the fibroblasts revert back to normal. The most common, and serious, complications of systemic scleroderma involve the pulmonary system and may include fibrosis or interstitial lung disease as well as pulmonary vascular disease leading to pulmonary arterial hypertension. It is estimated that pulmonary involvement occurs in 40% of individuals and contributes from 13% to 17% of deaths from systemic scleroderma.[7] Other complications include, but are not limited to, poor wound healing, arrhythmia, heart failure, renal failure, and esophageal strictures.[7]

CASE 46-1

QUESTION 1: T.P., a 58-year-old African-American woman with known limited cutaneous scleroderma, presents to your outpatient clinic complaining of pain and discoloration of the fingers on both hands. She describes discoloration as an intermittent loss of color from normal to a pale appearance, and the pain as intermittent numbness and tingling accompanying the loss of color. T.P. states the symptoms only appear when she is exposed to a cold environment. These symptoms are interfering with her quality of life and activities of daily living. In terms of other symptoms, T.P. also experiences intermittent development of thickened, pitted, rough skin patches located distal to her elbows bilaterally. She has no other significant past medical history, nor takes any medications on a regular basis. The physical examination findings revealed patches of skin thickening and nonpitting induration on upper torso. Telangiectasias are also noted in this area. Laboratory samples drawn last week show her ANA is negative and the basic metabolic panel, complete blood count, and liver function tests are all normal. What subjective and objective data present in T.P.'s case are consistent with limited cutaneous scleroderma?

T.P. is complaining of classic symptoms of Raynaud syndrome, which is a common clinical feature of limited cutaneous scleroderma, present in over 95% of cases. In addition, skin fibrosis that is present distal to the elbow or knees, and telangiectasias are suggestive of limited cutaneous scleroderma as opposed to diffuse cutaneous scleroderma. Because ANAs may be present in unaffected patients and absent in afflicted patients, ANA test results must be interpreted within the clinical context and should not be relied on as a sole diagnostic marker.[9]

CASE 46-1, QUESTION 2: Based on these signs and symptoms, which variant(s) of limited cutaneous scleroderma is likely present?

Over 95% of patients who are affected by systemic sclerosis also have signs and symptoms consistent with Raynaud phenomenon, as it is seen with T.P. Patients will typically complain of recurrent,

Table 46-1
Common Clinical Features of Systemic Sclerosis

Subset	Skin Fibrosis	Lung Involvement	Visceral Organ Involvement	Physical Examination Findings
Limited cutaneous	Areas distal to the elbows and knees[a]	Pulmonary arterial hypertension	Severe GERD and Raynaud phenomenon	Telangiectasia, calcinosis cutis, sclerodactyly, digital ischemic complications
Diffuse cutaneous	Areas proximal or distal to the elbows and knees[a]	Interstitial lung disease	Scleroderma renal crisis	Tendon friction rubs, pigment changes

[a]May affect the face.
GERD, gastroesophageal reflux disease.
Adapted with permission from Hinchcliff M, Varga J. Systemic sclerosis/scleroderma: a treatable multisystem disease. *Am Fam Physician*. 2008;78:961.

intermittent vasospastic episodes resulting in a color change in the fingers or toes after being exposed to cold temperatures. Vasoconstriction may lead to local cyanosis and accompanying pain and numbness, with flushing noted on rewarming. Other parts of the body may also be affected, such as the nose, ears, tongue, and nipples.

Common clinical features can be used to distinguish between limited and diffuse cutaneous systemic sclerosis subsets (Table 46-1).[3] In addition, variants of the condition may exist within each subset based on the presence of other symptoms. Manifestations of systemic sclerosis differ based on the organ system(s) involved (Table 46-2).[3] Other disorders that may have similar clinical characteristics, such as amyloidosis and mixed CTD, should be considered and ruled out before the diagnosis of systemic sclerosis. The ACR/EULAR criteria for the diagnosis of systemic sclerosis require the presence of one lone major criterion (skin thickening of fingers of both hands extending proximal to metacarpophalangeal joints) or two minor criteria (skin thickening of fingers, fingertip lesions, telangiectasia, abnormal nailfold capillaries, pulmonary arterial hypertension and/or interstitial lung disease, Raynaud phenomenon, or presence of any of systemic sclerosis-related autoantibodies).[10] Skin biopsy is recommended to confirm scleroderma if the clinical picture is unclear. Separate criteria exist for the diagnosis of juvenile systemic sclerosis.[10] The overall course of systemic sclerosis is highly variable and unpredictable. However, after a remission occurs, relapse is uncommon.

Table 46-2
Manifestations of Systemic Sclerosis

Organ System	Manifestations
Cardiovascular	Abnormal cardiac conduction, congestive heart failure, pericardial effusion, digital ischemic changes, Raynaud phenomenon
Gastrointestinal	Barrett esophagitis or strictures, gastroesophageal reflux disease, dysphagia, halitosis, chronic cough, dental erosions
Genitourinary	Sexual dysfunction, dyspareunia, impotence
Musculoskeletal	Flexion contractures, muscle atrophy, puffy hands, inability to make a tight fist, weakness
Pulmonary	Interstitial lung disease, pulmonary arterial hypertension, basilar and course crackles, dyspnea on exertion
Renal	Renal crisis
Skin	Calcinosis, pruritus, thickened skin, tight skin, excoriations, scabbing, loss of pigmentation

Adapted with permission from Hinchcliff M, Varga J. Systemic sclerosis/scleroderma: a treatable multisystem disease. *Am Fam Physician*. 2008;78:961.

CASE 46-1, QUESTION 3: At this time, which therapeutic agent(s) is recommended to treat T.P.'s manifestations and symptoms of systemic sclerosis?

Clinical practice guidelines exist, which may assist the clinician when determining treatment for systemic sclerosis.[12] However, there is not a specific therapy for systemic sclerosis. Rather, treatment is mainly supportive and symptomatic in nature, targeting the specific organ(s) affected (Table 46-3).[13] Therefore, the primary goals of therapy are to improve the quality of life and minimize the risk of complications. Based on T.P.'s current symptoms, initiating therapy with the dihydropyridine calcium-channel blocker nifedipine is an appropriate option to achieve symptom control. Compared with placebo, nifedipine and prazosin modestly reduced the severity and frequency of Raynaud ischemic attacks.[14,15] However, when losartan was compared with low-dose nifedipine in a nonblinded, randomized, controlled trial (RCT), losartan users experienced

Table 46-3
Treatment Options for Manifestations of Systemic Sclerosis

Manifestation	Treatment Options
Raynaud phenomenon	Nifedipine, verapamil, losartan, prazosin, iloprost, calcium-channel blocker + tadalafil
Pulmonary hypertension	Bosentan, sildenafil, enalapril, iloprost
Interstitial lung disease	Cyclophosphamide, prednisone
Renal crisis	Angiotensin-converting enzyme inhibitors, dialysis, or kidney transplant
Skin fibrosis	Methotrexate, cyclosporine, D-penicillamine
Arthralgias	Acetaminophen and NSAIDs
GERD	Proton pump inhibitors, H2 antagonists, prokinetic agents
Pruritus	Antihistamines, low-dose topical steroids

GERD, gastroesophageal reflux disease; NSAID, nonsteroidal anti-inflammatory drug; H2, type 2 histamine receptor.
Adapted with permission from Usatine RP, Diaz L. Scleroderma (progressive systemic sclerosis). In: Ebell MH et al. *Database Online*. October 15, 2009. Hoboken, NJ: John Wiley & Sons. Accessed March 18, 2011.

a decrease in severity and frequency of Raynaud symptoms in a 12-week period.[16] This should not be considered as definitive evidence that losartan is superior as the lack of blinding may have resulted in an overestimation of losartan's benefit. Although tadalafil monotherapy does not appear effective for Raynaud phenomenon due to systemic sclerosis, when added to a calcium-channel blocker the combination appears to improve symptoms and reduce digital ulcers compared to calcium-channel blocker alone.[17,18] Bosentan (which is restricted in the United States and approved for the treatment of symptomatic pulmonary hypertension) has been shown to decrease the occurrence of digital ulcers caused by Raynaud phenomenon.[19] Compared to placebo, atorvastatin 40 mg daily reduced the number of new digital ulcers in patients with Raynaud phenomenon and systemic sclerosis during a four-month randomized trial: mean number of new digital ulcers per patient 1.6 versus 2.5 comparing atorvastatin versus placebo, respectively.[20] Patients who develop pulmonary artery hypertension early the treatment with an angiotensin-converting enzyme inhibitor may improve prognosis in scleroderma renal crisis.[12,21] For patients who develop pulmonary hypertension, treatment with bosentan, ambrisentan, sildenafil, epoprostenol infusion, or other prostanoids (treprostinil, iloprost) may be considered because they have all been shown to improve functional capacity.[7] The effects of cyclophosphamide, an antineoplastic agent, demonstrated in clinical trials are conflicting. In an RCT comparing cyclophosphamide with placebo in patients with scleroderma lung disease, use of this agent modestly reduced dyspnea and disability while improving lung function.[22] However, a meta-analysis of three RCTs and six cohort studies concluded that cyclophosphamide does not result in significant clinical improvement of pulmonary function.[23] Because this is a potentially toxic drug, patients who take it require close monitoring.

Polymyalgia Rheumatica and Temporal Arteritis (Giant Cell Arteritis)

Polymyalgia rheumatica (PMR) and temporal arteritis, also known as giant cell arteritis (GCA), are closely related clinical syndromes that usually affect the elderly and frequently occur together. Many authorities believe them to be different phases of the same underlying disease process. Polymyalgia rheumatica is 2 to 3 times more common than GCA. However, about 27% to 53% of persons with GCA also have PMR, and 18% to 26% of those with PMR also have GCA.[24] PMR can occur before, with, or after the development of GCA. Inflammation is the hallmark of both conditions. PMR is characterized by aching and morning stiffness in the cervical region and shoulder and pelvic girdles, and may result in disability.[25] Inflammation as a result of GCA most commonly involves the temporal artery, but arteries in other parts of the body can also be affected.[26] Despite certain similarities, PMR and GCA have distinct symptoms, corticosteroid requirements for treatment, and prognoses.

The incidence of PMR and GCA increases in patients after the age of 50 and peaks in those 70 to 80 years of age.[25] GCA is the most common vasculitis among the elderly and can lead to blindness if not diagnosed and treated in a timely manner. Likewise, without treatment, PMR can lead to significant morbidity and disability. Patients with PMR are also at an increased risk of peripheral arterial disease. The primary risk factor for both conditions is age, and both occur more frequently in women than in men. PMR is seen mainly in people of north European ancestry and generally affects whites more commonly than African-Americans, Hispanics, Asians, and Native Americans.[26] The incidence of PMR is 5.9/10,000 patients/year in the United States, with an overall prevalence in the United States of about 740/100,000: 532 for men and 925 for women.[27] The incidence of GCA is 0.17 new cases annually per 1,000 persons older than 50 years of age with a prevalence of 2/1,000 persons.[28]

Although the exact pathogeneses of PMR and GCA are yet to be determined, they are both thought to arise from an autoimmune or inflammatory dysfunction involving similar cellular immune responses from T cells, antigen-presenting cells, macrophage-derived inflammatory cytokines, genetic human leukocyte antigen molecules, and macrophages. A viral cause has been suspected but not confirmed for both PMR and GCA, and some studies demonstrate a cyclic pattern in PMR incidence pointing to environmental infectious triggers (e.g., parvovirus B19, *Mycoplasma pneumoniae*, and *Chlamydia pneumoniae*) as potential causes.[25,29] Branches of the internal and external carotid arteries are most commonly affected in those with GCA, and biopsies often reveal inflammatory changes that lead to a narrowing or occlusion of the vessel and ischemia distal to the lesion.[26] Systemic inflammation is the most prominent feature in PMR, but inflammation of the blood vessels is often clinically undetectable.[26]

CASE 46-2

QUESTION 1: D.C. is an 85-year-old white man presenting to the emergency department complaining of new-onset morning aching pain and stiffness in his shoulders and upper arms. He states his symptoms developed 3 weeks ago and have progressed to the point where his pain and limited range of motion are keeping him from performing activities of daily living. D.C. denies headaches or vision disturbances, but is complaining of overall malaise, fatigue, and anorexia. He has a past medical history significant for hyperlipidemia, type 2 diabetes mellitus, and hypertension. He has been taking his current medications for the past 2 years, which are adequately controlling his hyperlipidemia, diabetes, and hypertension. His current medications include simvastatin 40 mg daily, metformin 1,000 mg twice daily, lisinopril/hydrochlorothiazide 40/25 mg daily, and aspirin 81 mg daily. His physical examination was negative for decreased muscle strength. Limited range of shoulder and upper arm motion is noted along with tenderness of these areas on palpation. Routine baseline laboratory values are within normal limits, with an ESR of 75 mm/hour. D.C. was admitted to a general medical ward with a diagnosis of PMR and was started on prednisone. What signs and symptoms present in this case differentiate PMR from GCA?

No conclusive laboratory test for PMR or GCA exists, and nonspecific clinical features and the absence of physical signs often complicate diagnosis. Appropriate diagnosis requires a thorough history and physical examination. Distinguishing between the two disorders is of importance, as GCA can lead to blindness and requires higher doses of treatment medications. The typical onset of PMR is acute in nature. However, as is the case with D.C., most who present for a medical evaluation describe their symptoms as occurring for 1 month or longer.[26] D.C. is also exhibiting common complaints associated with PMR, which include aching pain and morning stiffness in the shoulders and upper arms, hips and thighs, or neck and torso. The shoulders are affected in 95% of cases. New-onset GCA often manifests as a new headache or a headache that is described as different from previous headaches and has been occurring for 2 to 3 months. Constitutional symptoms such as fatigue, anorexia, and weight loss in an older patient often accompany headaches seen in GCA.[24] The absence of headache in D.C. further supports the diagnosis of PMR. Common findings associated with both conditions are presented in Table 46-4.[26] The most useful laboratory test for diagnosing PMR is the ESR. Patients with GCA usually have an ESR greater than 40 to 50 mm/hour; rates of greater than 100 mm/hour are common. A normal ESR is very helpful in ruling

Table 46-4
Common Findings Associated with Polymyalgia Rheumatica and Giant Cell Arteritis (GCA)

Polymyalgia Rheumatica	Giant Cell Arteritis
Age ≥50 years	Age ≥50 years
ESR >50 mm/hour	ESR >50 mm/hour
Anemia (mild, normochromic, normocytic)	Anemia
Aching, pain, and morning stiffness in the shoulders and upper arms, hips and thighs, or neck and torso	Headache: temporal with temporal artery involvement, or occipital with occipital artery involvement
Symptoms of systemic inflammation	Visual symptoms or jaw claudication
	Fever, weight loss, depression, fatigue
	Arthralgias

ESR, erythrocyte sedimentation rate.
Adapted with permission from Unwin B et al. Polymyalgia rheumatica and giant cell arteritis. *Am Fam Physician*. 2006;74:1547.

out GCA in corticosteroid-naïve patients; however, an elevated ESR (>100 mm/hour) is only minimally helpful in ruling out GCA.[30] Three or more of the following criteria that are present are 93% sensitive and 91% specific for GCA: age of onset of disease greater than or equal to 50 years, new headache, temporal artery abnormality, ESR greater than or equal to 50 mm/hour, or abnormal findings on biopsy of the temporal artery.[31] The BSR/BHPR guidelines recommend biopsy of the temporal artery for the diagnosis of GCA.[32] An abnormal biopsy in the context of positive clinical findings described in Table 46-4 as well as an elevated ESR is strongly predictive of neuro-ophthalmic complications. However, a negative biopsy result does not preclude the diagnosis of GCA if there is strong clinical suspicion.

CASE 46-2, QUESTION 2: What other inflammatory conditions should be considered and excluded before making the diagnosis of PMR or GCA in D.C.?

Other inflammatory or autoimmune disorders, such as fibromyalgia, myalgias from statin therapy, osteoarthritis, polymyositis, and rheumatoid arthritis, should be considered and excluded before the diagnosis of PMR or GCA.[26] Specific alternatives that should be included in the differential diagnosis of PMR include hyperparathyroidism, Parkinson disease, thyroid disorders, adhesive capsulitis, pseudogout, cervical spondylosis, SLE, or multiple myeloma.[24] Other vasculitides (Wegener granulomatosis, polyarteritis nodosa, microscopic polyangiitis), Takayasu arteritis, malignancies, herpes zoster, and migraines (or other causes of headaches) should be included in the differential diagnosis of GCA.[33]

CASE 46-2, QUESTION 3: What is the preferred initial treatment approach for PMR in D.C.? Explain the difference(s) in this approach as compared with those for GCA.

Owing to its anti-inflammatory properties, corticosteroids are considered first-line therapy for either PMR or GCA. Early visual loss may occur in up to 20% of patients and rarely improves once present. Therefore, initiation of corticosteroid treatment should not be delayed pending temporal artery biopsy results.[24] When PMR and GCA occur simultaneously, higher corticosteroid doses (indicated for the treatment of CGA) are required to prevent significant complications. For the treatment of PMR, the British Society for Rheumatology (BSR) and the British Health Professionals in Rheumatology (BHPR) recommend standard initial treatment with oral prednisone 15 mg/day for 3 weeks, 12.5 mg/day for 3 weeks, and 10 mg/day for 4 to 6 weeks, then decrease by 1 mg every 4 to 8 weeks.[29] An alternative treatment regimen includes intramuscular methylprednisolone 120 mg every 3 to 4 weeks, decreased by 20 mg every 2 to 3 months. Beginning low-dose prednisone may improve D.C.'s PMR symptoms within days, but some optimal results could take several weeks to achieve and most patients can expect to receive therapy for 1 to 2 years. Treatment should be tailored to patient symptoms, and inflammatory markers should be followed. Attempts to taper the dose to avoid long-term adverse drug events (e.g., osteoporosis, hypothalamus–pituitary–adrenal axis suppression) should be made once acute relief has been achieved. Tapering the dose (e.g., 1 mg/day/week) should be individualized and based on symptom response because it may take years owing to symptom flares. The Polymyalgia Rheumatica Activity Scale, a disease activity assessment, may be used to monitor and adjust therapy and patient response.[26]

As opposed to PMR, treatment for uncomplicated (no jaw or tongue claudication or visual changes) GCA should begin with high-dose prednisolone (40–60 mg/day).[29] Complicated GCA (evolving visual loss or history of amaurosis fugax) should be treated with IV, methylprednisolone 500 mg to 1 g/day for 3 days, followed by oral prednisolone 60 mg/day.[29] A corticosteroid taper can be initiated after 4 weeks of treatment and resolution of symptoms and normalization of ESR/CRP. It is recommended to decrease the prednisolone dose by 10 mg every 2 weeks until 20 mg is reached, then decrease by 2.5 mg every 2 to 4 weeks until 10 mg is reached, and then decrease by 1 mg every 1 to 2 months.[29] Most will achieve a dose of 7.5 to 10 mg/day after 6 months of therapy, but relapses are common and are managed by restarting steroid therapy or increasing the dose to previous beneficial amounts.[25] The use of low-dose aspirin may reduce the incidence of cranial ischemic complications.

The use of methotrexate as adjuvant therapy for PMR and GCA is not routinely recommended, and its evidence of symptom relief benefit is conflicting.[26] However, a single RCT demonstrated that the use of methotrexate 10 mg once weekly in addition to prednisone in those with GCA resulted in an overall decrease in the amount of prednisone required and in relapse rates.[35] Relapses are common in both PMR and GCA and may be managed by restarting steroid therapy or increasing the dose to previous levels that controlled symptoms, if already receiving steroids. All patients on long-term corticosteroids should be offered calcium (1,200 mg/day) and vitamin D (800 international units/day) for prevention of osteoporosis and be monitored for other complications of steroid therapy. Patients at risk for gastritis should receive prophylactic protection with a proton pump inhibitor.

Patients being treated for PMR or GCA should be monitored closely in response to treatment and disease progression. It is recommended that the first follow-up visit should take place 1 to 3 weeks after the start of corticosteroids.[29] Subsequent visits should occur at 6 weeks as well as 3, 6, 9, and 12 months, or on an as-needed basis if relapses or adverse events occur. At each visit, patients should be assessed for specific symptom improvement and routine blood work should include ESR, CRP, CBC, and CMP. Bone mineral density testing every 2 years may be considered in patients receiving long-term corticosteroids. Professional guidelines recommend a chest X-ray every 2 years to assess for aortic aneurysm in patients diagnosed with GCA.[29] However, a systematic review of imaging studies found limited evidence to guide screening recommendations for thoracic aortic aneurysm/dilation because a chest X-ray may not be sensitive enough to detect thoracic aortic aneurysms.[34]

Reactive Arthritis

Reactive arthritis is defined as peripheral arthritis often accompanied by one or more extra-articular manifestations that appear after certain infections of the genitourinary, gastrointestinal, or respiratory infection. Table 46-5 lists bacterial pathogens associated with the development of reactive arthritis.[36–39] In addition, it shares features with other forms of spondyloarthropathies, which is the grouping it falls under. Reiter syndrome was previously used to describe this condition, but the term reactive arthritis has become the preferred term. The term classic "Reiter triad" associated with this condition was used to describe the specific combination of arthritis, urethritis, and conjunctivitis.[37] The presentation of arthritis is usually a large joint monoarthritis or oligoarthritis usually in the lower extremities, and/or enthesitis which is the inflammation of the entheses. This is the site where the tendon or ligament enters the bone.[36] Typically, the inflammatory disorder would occur 1 to 6 weeks after the infection.[37] The clinical course of reactive arthritis is variable and usually runs a self-limited course of 3 to 12 months.[36] Mortality from reactive arthritis is not common and results from cardiac complications such as aortitis. Approximately 10% to 20% of patients may continue to have chronic, destructive, and disabling arthritis or enthesitis within 2 years after the onset of symptoms. Ten to fifteen percent may progress to ankylosing spondylitis.[39]

The annual incidence reported varies between 9 and 27 for reactive arthritis/100,000/year. Patients with an acute Chlamydia infection develop reactive arthritis. Reactive arthritis most frequently occurs in patients between 20 and 40 years of age, but it can occur at any age. In general, it occurs more frequently in men than in women following genitourinary infection, which is most commonly a sexually transmitted disease. Following bowel infections, the prevalence is equal between men and women.[37]

Reactive arthritis is considered a sterile inflammatory response to a remote infection. Reactive arthritis usually occurs after an infection in a genetically susceptible person, which has been identified as a likely risk factor. Genetics may play a role in pathogenesis of spondyloarthropathies; 30% to 50% of patients are surface antigen HLA-B27 positive, which presents antigenic peptides to T cells. These patients are susceptible to a more severe and prolonged disease.[37] The HLA-B27 gene has a higher prevalence in the Caucasian population.[39]

Onset of symptoms typically occurs 1 to 3 weeks later and may present in an insidious or acute manner. Patients usually present with a chief complaint of mucocutaneous lesions, joint stiffness, myalgia, and low back pain that is worse with rest. Table 46-6 describes the clinical manifestations of reactive arthritis. It may present as arthritic in nature or as dysfunctions of the ocular, skin, genitourinary, or cardiac systems. Urethritis, mild dysuria, and a mucopurulent urethra are the most common symptoms that occur in men. Women may have dysuria, vaginal discharge, and purulent cervicitis or vaginitis. Arthritic complaints are usually asymmetrical, involving the lower extremities, and are associated with the appearance of a "sausage finger" digit.[36]

Table 46-5
Examples of Bacterial Pathogens Associated with the Development of Reactive Arthritis

Gastrointestinal
Salmonella enteritidis and typhimurium
Shigella flexneri
Yersinia enterocolitica and pseudotuberculosis
Campylobacter jejuni
Escherichia coli
Clostridium difficile
Genitourinary
Chlamydia trachomatis
Neisseria gonorrhoeae
Respiratory
Chlamydia pneumoniae
Group A β-hemolytic streptococcus

Source: Hill Gaston JS. Reactive arthritis and undifferentiated spondyloarthritis. In: Firestein G et al, eds. *Kelley's Textbook of Rheumatology*. 9th ed. Philadelphia, PA: Saunders Elsevier; 2013:1221; Reactive arthritis. In DynaMed [Internet]. Ipswich (MA): EBSCO Information Services. 1995 – [cited 2010 March 23]. **http://www.dynamed.com**. Registration and login required. Accessed July 8, 2015; Hannu T. Reactive arthritis. *Best Pract Res Clin Rheumatol*. 2011;25:347; Selmi C, Gershwin ME. Diagnosis and classification of reactive arthritis. *Autoimmun Rev*. 2014;13:546.

CASE 46-3

Question 1: T.K. is a 37-year-old man who presented to the outpatient primary-care clinic 2 weeks after the onset of a low-grade fever associated with pain and stiffness in his left knee and right ankle, pain on urination, and red, irritated eyes. He reports no recent injuries. The patient reports that the last time he engaged in unprotected sex was 3 weeks ago. T.K. denies experiencing chest pain, skin rash, photosensitivity, genital lesions, or urethral discharge and hematuria. Swelling, erythema, and tenderness of the left knee joint, as well as signs of conjunctivitis, were the only findings noted on physical examination. A urine Chlamydia rapid test with first void was positive.

He reports no current medical conditions and a family history of psoriatic arthritis.

Based on the history of symptoms present in this case, what supports a diagnosis of reactive arthritis?

T.K. presents with multiple symptoms following a confirmed infection with Chlamydia trachomatis. He is presenting with an inflamed joint in the lower extremity and also conjunctivitis. Urethritis can be a symptom associated with reactive arthritis but in this case overlaps as a potential symptom of an active Chlamydia infection. A family history of psoriatic arthritis, which is also under the classification as a spondyloarthropathy, may indicate a risk factor for severe or chronicity if T.K. has the HLA-B27 gene. Laboratory testing for the gene is not required for diagnosis.[36,37]

Table 46-6
Clinical Signs of Reactive Arthritis

Musculoskeletal System
Arthritis affecting 1–4 joints
Entheses
Extra-articular disease
Skin Manifestations
Keratoderma blennorrhagica on soles and/or palms
Circinate balanitis on penile gland
Ocular Manifestations
Mucosal ulcers
Conjunctivitis
Uveitis

Source: Hill Gaston JS. Reactive arthritis and undifferentiated spondyloarthritis. In: Firestein G et al, eds. *Kelley's Textbook of Rheumatology*. 9th ed. Philadelphia, PA: Saunders Elsevier; 2013:1221.

CASE 46-3, QUESTION 2: What is an appropriate initial treatment strategy for T.K.?

Empiric antibiotic therapy does not reduce the risk of recurrence of reactive, and antibiotics are therefore not routinely recommended for uncomplicated cases. As is the case with T.K., an active documented infection such as Chlamydia in the urine or bacteria in the stool in gastrointestinal infections should receive treatment. It is possible that by the time arthritis presents stool cultures would be negative following a gastrointestinal foodborne illness. Those with documented *Chlamydia trachomatis* infection and their partners should be offered antibiotics (azithromycin 1 g orally as a single dose or doxycycline 100 mg twice/day for 7 days).[37,38] Further information on appropriate antibiotic therapy for the infections that can cause reactive arthritis can be found in the chapters in Section 14: Infectious Disease. Although some studies have reported success of prolonged use of combination antibiotics specifically in reactive arthritis following Chylmadia,[37,40] a meta-analysis evaluating the efficacy of antibiotics in the routine treatment of reactive arthritis concluded that they did not induce remission, but this issue remains uncertain due to heterogeneity of the studies.[41] Antibiotic use was associated with a 97% increase in gastrointestinal side effects.[41]

Oral nonsteroidal anti-inflammatory drugs may be useful for pain control and inflammation, but there is no evidence that they affect arthritis itself or shorten the clinical course.[37]

CASE 46-3, QUESTION 3: Three weeks later, T.K. reports that he has had resolution of the low-grade fever and any pain on urination but that he is not receiving adequate pain relief in his knee. He complains that it is limiting his activities. What additional therapies can be considered?

Because T.K. is still experiencing pain in his left knee, an intra-articular corticosteroid injection, or oral corticosteroids if more joints are affected, may be considered. Intra-articular corticosteroid injections do not have as dramatic or as sustained a response as in those with rheumatoid arthritis. However, they may be helpful for the treatment of pain and swelling. For those who suffer from a persistence of reactive arthritis, a disease-modifying antirheumatic drug such as sulfasalazine is well tolerated and possibly effective at a dose of 1 g 2 or 3 times daily. Consideration may be given to start DMARD therapy earlier in the course of the disease if a patient is having a recurrence of reactive arthritis or is HLA-B27 positive.[36] Aggressive and unremitting reactive arthritis may be treated with immunosuppressants, if it is confirmed the initial infection is cleared. In severe cases, where patients fail to achieve adequate relief with prior therapies, antitumor necrosis factor (TNF)-α treatment may be considered. Limited evidence is available and is discussed in the literature primarily through case reports. Physical therapy modalities may be an integral part of management to improve mobility and strength and to prevent stiffness and deformities if needed.[36–38]

Polymyositis and Dermatomyositis

Polymyositis (PM) and dermatomyositis (DM) are idiopathic autoimmune and inflammatory disorders of unknown etiology involving a number of voluntary skeletal muscles simultaneously. PM and DM are characterized by the presence of inflammatory myopathies. In addition, DM involves specific skin manifestations, whereas PM does not.[42,43] Dermatomyositis is also associated with an increased risk of malignancies. Fifteen percent of patients over 40 years of age have a preexisting malignancy or will develop one in the future.[44] Therapy is aimed at reducing the risk of respiratory failure, renal failure, and cardiomyopathy as potential complications of either disorder. A proportion of patients (approximately 11%– 40% of those with DM) will meet the diagnostic criteria for other CTDs. This overlap syndrome is thought to occur more frequently in men than in women (9:1 ratio). Patients with myositis are likely, reported in 11% to 40%, to have another connective tissue disease (e.g., scleroderma, SLE, rheumatoid arthritis, and sarcoidosis).[45]

PM typically presents between the ages of 50 and 60 years and is rarely seen in children. DM exhibits a bimodal distribution and affects adults between the ages of 45 and 65 years, as well as a peak in children aged 5 to 15. African-Americans are at an increased risk for these disorders, and both women and men (2:1) are affected.[45] For dermatomyositis, the prevalence in the United States is 5.8 cases/100,000 individuals. In the United Kingdom, the prevalence among children was reported as 3.2/million. Polymyositis is reported in the United States at a prevalence of 9.7/100,000, but it should be noted that polymyositis is a diagnosis that is more difficult to make due to overlap of symptoms with other myopathies.[46] The prevalence is thought to lie between 50 and 100 cases/million for idiopathic inflammatory myopathies.[42]

There is no clear cause of either disorder, and both are thought to involve immune-mediated processes triggered by environmental factors (autoimmune or viral) in genetically susceptible individuals. DM is thought to be a complement-mediated microangiopathy in which inflammatory infiltrates arise owing to ischemic phenomena. In patients with PM, muscle fibers may be damaged by cytotoxic CD8 T lymphocytes. Infectious agents implicated as causative factors include coxsackievirus, influenza virus, retroviruses, cytomegalovirus, and Epstein–Barr virus. Various autoantibodies are found in up to 60% of patients. Expression of a genetic-specific HLA subtype (HLA DRB1-03 in whites and HLA DRB1-14 in Koreans) places individuals from certain ethnic groups at an increased risk. Exposure to UV radiation also increases the risk of developing DM.[45]

Symptom onset for both PM and DM is insidious, and patients initially complain of muscle weakness of the trunk, shoulders, hip girdles, upper arms, thighs, neck, and pharynx. These patients usually report increasing difficulties in everyday tasks requiring the use of proximal muscles such as getting up from a chair, climbing stairs, stepping onto a curb, lifting objects, and combing hair. Frequent falls, fatigue, malaise, weight loss, shortness of breath, and low-grade fever are also often present. Classification of PM and DM can be accomplished by assessing the presence or absence of certain characteristics unique to the condition. Polymyositis rarely affects children as compared to dermatomyositis that occurs more frequently. Specifically, they are largely separated by the involvement of cutaneous changes and calcinosis in dermatomyositis. Specific manifestations seen in DM are described in Table 46-7.[47] At present, no diagnostic criteria for PM and DM have been clearly defined and validated. After other conditions (e.g., human immunodeficiency virus (HIV) infection, lichen planus, SLE, psoriasis, or drug-induced causes) have been considered and ruled out, diagnosis may be confirmed by generally accepted criteria including the presence of proximal muscle weakness, elevated serum concentrations of skeletal muscle enzymes (e.g., creatine kinase, lactate dehydrogenase), myopathic changes on electromyography, evidence of inflammation on muscle biopsy, and skin rash (for DM only).[45,47,48]

CASE 46-4

QUESTION 1: J.A. is a 45-year-old white woman with a history of PM. She was initially diagnosed 1 year ago and was treated with high-dose oral prednisone for 3 months, at which time an attempt to taper the corticosteroid to the lowest effective dose was initiated. Since that time, J.A. has not been able to completely stop corticosteroid therapy without the recurrence of muscle weakness, which affects her ability to perform activities of daily living. In the past 3 months, her symptoms have progressed to the point where she was titrated back to his initial high-dose prednisone regimen in an attempt to gain adequate relief. At this point, J.A. and her primary-care physician are considering alternative options for symptom control. What is a reasonable pharmacotherapeutic option to recommend that may provide J.A. with symptom relief?

The initial and long-term goals of therapy are to improve muscle weakness, thereby improving the activities of daily living. The clinical course of both PM and DM varies in severity from mild to more severe progressive disease. Those with mild forms of the disease usually have a rapid response to therapy, whereas those with more severe or slowly progressive forms of the disease are more likely to not respond to treatment; this is a marker for a poor prognosis. As demonstrated in J.A.'s case, initial therapy with high-dose corticosteroids (e.g., 1 mg/kg) is used, followed by slow taper depending on response to therapy. The approach may include a switch to alternate day dosing during the taper or a 10% reduction in dose every 2 weeks.[45–49] In severe cases, it may be preferred to begin with intravenous corticosteroid therapy with methylprednisolone for 3 to 5 days at a dose of 1,000 mg. Patients who respond early to high-dose corticosteroids typically respond better to corticosteroid-sparing agents (e.g., methotrexate, azathioprine) in the future. J.A.'s failure to respond to corticosteroids should prompt further investigation for other possible pathologic processes including muscular dystrophy, hypothyroidism, or malignancy-associated myopathy. Should those investigations yield no conclusive results, J.A. may be offered methotrexate, azathioprine, mycophenolate mofetil, or cyclosporine as recommended immunosuppressants and steroid-sparing agents if the disease is not controlled with corticosteroids alone, is rapidly progressive, or presents with extramuscular involvement. If the complication of interstitial lung disease is present, cyclophosphamide or tacrolimus may be considered. If a patient does not have a sufficient response to corticosteroids, then intravenous immune globulin can be given over 2 to 5 days.[42,45,49] Ongoing trials will evaluate the potential use of other immune-modulating therapies.

CASE 46-4, QUESTION 2: What preventive health measures may be offered to J.A. to augment her pharmacotherapeutic treatment regimen?

Supportive therapies such as bed rest, physiotherapy, warm baths, and moist heat applications to the affected areas can improve muscle stiffness. If oral lesions are present, irrigation of these lesions with warm saline solution is helpful. Preventive health measures for those experiencing either disorder include application of sunscreen, osteoporosis prevention, minimizing aspiration risk in patients with esophageal dysmotility, and physical therapy or customized exercise in patients with muscle weakness.[45] Although there has been previous concern to not further damage muscle, appropriate exercises including passive range of motion exercises and aerobic and resistance exercises have shown benefit.[44] Female patients placed on teratogenic immunosuppressants should discuss contraception, when appropriate.

Table 46-7
Cutaneous Manifestations of Dermatomyositis

Pathognomonic Skin Lesions of DM
1. Gottron papules: papules having a violaceous hue overlying the dorsal lateral aspect of interphalangeal and/or metacarpophalangeal joints. When fully formed, these papules become slightly depressed at the center which can assume a white, anthropic appearance. Associated telangiectasia can be present.
2. Gottron signs: symmetric macular violaceous erythema with or without edema overlying the dorsal aspect of the interphalangeal/metacarpophalangeal joints, olecranon processes, patellae, and medial malleoli.
Highly Characteristic Skin Lesions of DM
1. Periorbital violaceous (heliotrope) erythema with or without associated edema of the eyelids and periorbital tissue.
2. Grossly visible periungual telangiectasia with or without dystrophic cuticles.
3. Symmetric macular violaceous erythema overlying the dorsal aspect of the hands and fingers (where it can track the extensor tendon sheaths), extensor aspects of the arms and forearms, deltoids, posterior shoulders and neck (the shawl sign), V-area of anterior neck and upper chest, central aspect of the face and forehead.
Compatible Skin Lesions of DM
1. Poikiloderma vasculare atrophicans (poikilodermatomyositis) circumscribed violaceous erythema with associated telangiectasia, hypopigmentation, hyperpigmentation, and superficial atrophy most commonly found over the posterior shoulders, back, buttocks, and V-area of the anterior neck and chest.
2. Calcinosis cuts.

Reprinted with permission from Iaccarino L et al. The clinical features, diagnosis and classification of dermatomyositis. *J Autoimmun*. 2014;48:122–127.

KEY REFERENCES AND WEBSITES

A full list of references for this chapter can be found at http://thepoint.lww.com/AT11e. Below are the key references and websites for this chapter, with the corresponding reference number in this chapter found in parentheses after the reference.

Key References

Barber C et al. Antibiotics for treatment of reactive arthritis: a systemic review and metaanalysis. *J Rheumatol*. 2013;40:916. (40)

Carsten P, Schmidt J. Diagnosis, pathogenesis and treat of myositis: recent advances. *Clin Exp Immunol*. 2014:175:425. (45)

Dasgupta B et al. BSR and BHPR guidelines for the management of polymyalgia rheumatica. *Rheumatology (Oxford)*. 2010;49:186. (29)

Findlay A et al. An overview of polymyositis and dermatomyositis. *Muscle Nerve*. 2015;51:638. (43)

Hill Gaston JS. Reactive arthritis and undifferentiated spondyloarthritis. In: Firestein G et al, eds. *Kelley's Textbook of Rheumatology*. 9th ed. Philadelphia, PA: Saunders Elsevier; 2013:1221. (36)

Hinchcliff M, Varga J. Systemic sclerosis/scleroderma: a treatable multisystem disease. *Am Fam Physician*. 2008;78:961. (3)

Kowal-Bielecka O et al. EULAR recommendations for the treatment of systemic sclerosis: a report from the EULAR Scleroderma Trials and Research group (EUSTAR). *Ann Rheum Dis*. 2009;68(5):620. (12)

Key Websites

Arthritis Foundation. Reactive Arthritis. http://www.arthritis.org/about-arthritis/types/reactive-arthritis/symptoms.php. Accessed June 25, 2015.

Inflammatory myopathies. American College of Rheumatology. http://www.rheumatology.org/I-Am-A/Patient-Caregiver/Diseases-Conditions/Inflammatory-Myopathies. Accessed August 16, 2015.

The Myositis Foundation. http://www.myositis.org/. Accessed August 16, 2015.

Section Editor: Trisha LaPointe

47 Contraception

Shareen Y. El-Ibiary

CORE PRINCIPLES

		CHAPTER CASES
1	Contraceptive choice is based on several factors that include formulation, hormone content, effectiveness, side effect profile, cost, accessibility, past medical history, medication use, privacy of use, prevention of sexually transmitted infections (STIs), and return to fertility time.	**Case 47-1 (Question 1)**
2	Combined hormonal contraceptive (CHC) agents are a combination of estrogen and progestin. They are available in a variety of formulations that include a combination of estrogen and progestin (oral tablet, vaginal ring, and transdermal patch). CHCs may be classified by estrogen content into high dose (50 mcg of ethinyl estradiol), low dose (30–35 mcg of ethinyl estradiol), and very low dose (10–25 mcg of ethinyl estradiol), and can vary in cycle length (e.g., 21, 24, or 84 days of active hormone). Combined oral contraceptives (COCs) can be further classified by hormone content into monophasic, biphasic, triphasic, and quadriphasic.	**Case 47-1 (Questions 3–5, 7), Table 47-3**
3	CHCs have benefits aside from pregnancy prevention that include treatment of acne, hirsutism, premenstrual syndrome (PMS) and premenstrual dysphoric disorder (PMDD), and endometrial cancer; menstrual cycle regulation; and prevention of ovarian cancer and functional ovarian cysts.	**Case 47-2 (Questions 1–3)**
4	Breakthrough bleeding, nausea, acne, and weight gain are among the most commonly reported side effects in women taking hormonal contraceptives. Risks and side effects may be linked to estrogenic, progestogenic, or androgenic properties of hormonal contraceptives.	**Case 47-2 (Questions 4–8), Case 47-3 (Question 1), Table 47-4**
5	There are risks associated with CHCs and contraindications for use in some women. Estrogen-containing contraceptives should be avoided in women who are 35 years or older and smoke more than 15 cigarettes/day, and should have uncontrolled hypertension, history of gallbladder disease, stroke, migraines with aura, cardiovascular disease, and history of thromboembolic events.	**Case 47-1 (Question 2)**
6	Progestin-only contraceptives are alternative agents for women with contraindications to CHCs. Progestin-only contraceptives vary in formulations that include oral tablet, depot and subcutaneous injection, and subdermal implant. Common side effects include weight gain, acne, mood changes, and irregular menses.	**Case 47-3 (Questions 2–6)**
7	Effectiveness of hormonal contraceptives is in part based on proper use and counseling. Patients need to understand how to use the contraceptive, what to do for mishaps (e.g., missed dose, vaginal ring falls out, transdermal patch falls off), and when to use a backup method. Directions for missed doses of progestin-only contraceptives vary from those for COCs.	**Case 47-1 (Question 6, 7), Case 47-3 (Questions 2–6)**

Continued

		CHAPTER CASES
8	Concomitant use of certain drugs may increase or decrease the levels of hormonal contraceptive agents. In particular, antibiotics and hepatic inducers may decrease the effectiveness of CHCs. Progestin-only contraceptives or nonhormonal contraceptives including backup methods may be alternatives in these cases.	**Case 47-1 (Question 8), Table 47-5**
9	Intrauterine devices (IUDs) or intrauterine systems (IUSs) are available in two formulations (copper IUD and levonorgestrel IUS) and are best for long-term pregnancy prevention. To avoid the risk of pelvic inflammatory disease, the products should be used in women involved in a monogamous relationship.	**Case 47-3 (Question 7)**
10	Some nonhormonal contraceptives include diaphragms, condoms, and spermicides. Male and female condoms are the only contraceptive products that also provide protection against STIs.	**Case 47-4 (Questions 1, 2)**
11	Timing is a key for emergency contraception (EC) to be effective. It is best taken as soon as possible after unprotected sexual intercourse but may be effective up to 120 hours after coitus. Emergency contraception can be in the form of high-dose progestin pills, high-dose estrogen and progestin pills (known as Yuzpe method), selective progesterone receptor modulator (SPRM), or copper IUD.	**Case 47-4 (Question 3)**
12	Medical abortion generally consists of mifepristone or methotrexate (to stop development of the pregnancy), or both, in combination with misoprostol (to induce uterine contractions and expel the pregnancy).	**Case 47-4 (Question 4)**

EPIDEMIOLOGY

The world population is greater than 7.3 billion people.[1] In the United States, there are approximately 325 million people, and there is one birth every 8 seconds and 1 death every 12 seconds. This results in an increase in one person every 13 seconds.[1]

Contraception is currently an issue worldwide. Preventing unintended pregnancy is an important goal of contraceptive use, particularly in countries where population control is a goal. Economic implications play a role as well. Data from 2008 to 2011 show an estimated 45% of pregnancies in the United States were unintended, and of these, 42% resulted in abortions.[2] Proper use and understanding of contraceptives is important for preventing unintended pregnancies.

HORMONAL CONTRACEPTION BACKGROUND AND PHARMACOLOGY

Hormonal contraceptives include combinations of estrogens and progestins known as combination hormonal contraceptives (CHCs) or progestin-only contraceptives. Estrogens prevent the development of the dominant follicle by suppressing follicle-stimulating hormone (FSH) secretion and stabilize the endometrial lining to minimize breakthrough bleeding (see Chapter 50, Disorders Related to the Menstrual Cycle, for more information about the menstrual cycle).[3] Progestins prevent ovulation by suppressing luteinizing hormone (LH) secretion. They may work in combination with estrogen in CHCs such as combination oral contraceptives (COCs), the contraceptive patch, and the contraceptive ring, or alone in formulations such as the progestin-only pill (POP), depot intramuscular or subcutaneous injection, subdermal implant, and as part of intrauterine systems. Progestin-only contraceptives hamper the transport of sperm through the cervical canal by thickening cervical mucus and causing alterations in the endometrial lining (so that it is not favorable for implantation) and in the fallopian tubes (affecting ovum transport).

COMBINATION HORMONAL CONTRACEPTIVES

Patient Evaluation

CASE 47-1

QUESTION 1: S.F., a healthy 33-year-old woman, presents to the clinic stating she is getting married soon and would like birth control pills as a method of contraception. She does not have children but would like to start a family in a year or two. Her past medical history is noncontributory other than occasional headaches for which she takes ibuprofen 200 mg by mouth (PO) as needed.

Vital signs: weight, 128 lb; height, 5 feet 4 inches
Blood pressure, 122/72 mm Hg
Heart rate, 85 beats/minute
Temperature, 98.6°F
Social history: smokes one pack/day, denies alcohol
Family history: sister gestational diabetes, mother hypertension, father unknown
Which factors are important in the selection of a contraceptive agent for S.F.?

There are several factors that affect selection of a contraceptive. Among them is effectiveness in preventing pregnancy. It is important to determine the importance of pregnancy prevention for S.F. and choose a method based on this information. For example, patients taking teratogenic medications or those with underlying medical conditions in which pregnancy may not be desired will require a highly effective birth control method or multiple methods. Others may not desire a pregnancy, but for a variety of reasons an unintended pregnancy may be more acceptable.

The effectiveness of contraceptive methods depends on the mechanism of action, availability (e.g., prescription required), patients' concurrent medications, past medical history, and acceptability (e.g., side effects, ease of use, adherence, cost, and religious and social beliefs). Any or all of these factors can account for the discrepancy between the lowest failure rate observed for 1 year in clinical trials (perfect-use failure rate) and the actual failure rate in users (typical-use failure rate) and should be taken into account when selecting a method of contraception (Table 47-1).[3] Return to fertility time is also an important factor to consider. Some contraceptive methods allow a woman to conceive shortly after discontinuation, whereas others may delay fertility longer. S.F. indicated she would like to have children in the near future. Given her age of 33 (fertility decreases more rapidly after age 30) and desire for future pregnancy, it would be best to select a product with a faster return to fertility.[4] However, other factors to consider when selecting a contraceptive agent for S.F. include contraindications and risks for her that may indicate one method over another. A combined hormonal contraceptive (CHC) is used commonly in women and may be appropriate for S.F. once all factors are considered.

Contraindications to Combined Hormonal Contraceptive Use

CASE 47-1, QUESTION 2: Are CHCs an appropriate form of contraception for S.F.? What contraindications to CHC therapy must be considered?

To determine whether any contraindications or precautions exist, the clinician should first obtain baseline health information from S.F. such as past medical history, social history, and family history (Fig. 47-1).[5] The World Health Organization has developed medical eligibility criteria to identify appropriate contraception for patients with specific conditions. In 2010, the Centers for Disease Control and Prevention adopted those guidelines for

Table 47-1
Percentage of Women Experiencing an Unintended Pregnancy During the First Year of Typical Use and the First Year of Perfect Use of Contraception and the Percentage Continuing Use at the End of the First Year: United States

	% of Women Experiencing an Unintended Pregnancy Within the First Year of Use			
Method	Typical Use[a]	Perfect Use[b]	% of Women Continuing Use at 1 Year[c]	Relative Cost[k]
Chance[d]	85	85	—	
Fertility awareness-based methods	24	—	47	None
Standard Days method[e]		5		
TwoDay method[e]	—	4	—	
Ovulation method[e]	—	3	—	
Symptothermal[e]	—	0.4	—	
Withdrawal	22	4	46	
Spermicides[f]	28	18	42	$-$$
Barrier methods				
Sponge				$$
Parous women	24	20	42	
Nulliparous women	12	9	57	
Diaphragm[g]	12	6	57	$$$
Condom[h]				$
Female (Reality)	21	5	41	
Male	18	2	43	
Hormonal contraceptives				
Injectable MPA	6	0.2	56	$$$[l]
Pill				
Progestin only	9	0.3	67	$$-$$$
Combined	9	0.3	67	$$-$$$
Transdermal patch	9	0.3	67	$$-$$$
Vaginal ring	9	0.3	67	$$-$$$
IUD/IUS	—	—	—	$$$$[l]
Copper	0.8	0.6	78	
Levonorgestrel	0.2	0.2	80	
Female sterilization	0.5	0.5	100	$$$$[m]
Male sterilization	0.15	0.10	100	$$$$[m]

(continued)

Table 47-1

Percentage of Women Experiencing an Unintended Pregnancy During the First Year of Typical Use and the First Year of Perfect Use of Contraception and the Percentage Continuing Use at the End of the First Year: United States (*continued*)

Method	% of Women Experiencing an Unintended Pregnancy Within the First Year of Use		% of Women Continuing Use at 1 Year[c]	Relative Cost[k]
	Typical Use[a]	Perfect Use[b]		
Emergency contraceptive pills				$$$
Treatment initiated within 72 hours after unprotected intercourse reduces the risk of pregnancy by at least 75%.[i]				
Lactational amenorrhea method				None
LAM is a highly effective, temporary method of contraception.[j]				

[a]Among *typical* couples who initiate use of a method (not necessarily for the first time), the percentage who experience an accidental pregnancy during the first year if they do not stop use for any other reason. Estimates of the probability of pregnancy during the first year of typical use for spermicides, withdrawal, fertility awareness-based methods, the diaphragm, the male condom, the oral contraceptive pill, and Depo-Provera are taken from the 1995 National Survey of Family Growth corrected for underreporting of abortion; see the source for the derivation of estimates for the other methods.
[b]Among couples who initiate use of a method (not necessarily for the first time) and who use it *perfectly* (both consistently and correctly), the percentage who experience an accidental pregnancy during the first year if they do not stop use for any other reason. See the table source for the derivation of estimates for the other methods.
[c]Among couples attempting to avoid pregnancy, the percentage who continue to use a method for 1 year.
[d]The percentages becoming pregnant in first year are based on data from populations in which contraception is not used and from women who cease using contraception to become pregnant. Among such populations, about 89% become pregnant within 1 year. This estimate was lowered slightly (to 85%) to represent the percentages who would become pregnant within 1 year among women now relying on reversible methods of contraception if they abandoned contraception altogether.
[e]The ovulation and TwoDay methods are based on evaluation of cervical mucus. The Standard Days method avoids intercourse on cycle days 8 through 19. The Symptothermal method is a double-check method based on evaluation of cervical mucus to determine the first fertile day and evaluation of cervical mucus and temperature to determine the last fertile day.
[f]Foams, creams, gels, vaginal suppositories, and vaginal film.
[g]With spermicidal cream or jelly.
[h]Without spermicides.
[i]*ella (ulipristal) is labeled for 120 hours after unprotected intercourse. Plan B One-Step, Next Choice One Dose, MyWay, Take Action, Aftera, EContra Ez, and After Pill are levonorgestrel products specifically marketed for emergency contraception. The labeling for these products says to take the pill within 72 hours after unprotected intercourse. Research has shown that all of the brands listed here are effective when used within 120 hours after unprotected sex.* Research has shown that both pills can be taken at the same time with no decrease in efficacy or increase in side effects and that they are effective when used within 120 hours after unprotected sex. The Food and Drug Administration has in addition declared the following 19 brands of oral contraceptives to be safe and effective for emergency contraception: Ogestrel (one dose is two white pills), Nordette (one dose is four light-orange pills), Cryselle, Levora, Low-Ogestrel, Lo/Ovral, or Quasence (one dose is four white pills), Jolessa, Portia, Seasonale or Trivora (one dose is four pink pills), Seasonique (one dose is four light-blue-green pills), Enpresse (one dose is four orange pills), Lessina (one dose is five pink pills), Aviane or LoSeasonique (one dose is five orange pills), Lutera or Sronyx (one dose is five white pills), and Lybrel (one dose is six yellow pills).
[j]However, to maintain effective protection against pregnancy, another method of contraception must be used as soon as menstruation resumes, the frequency or duration of breast-feeding is reduced, bottle feeds are introduced, or the baby reaches 6 months of age.
[k]$ up to $10/item, $$ up to $50/unit, $$$ up to $80/unit, $$$$ more than $80/unit (These are approximate costs and may vary based on location of purchase and patient insurance.).
[l]Administration or clinic costs not included. Initial cost of product reported but over time similar to $$ cost (e.g., injectable MPA 150 mg/mL suspension one syringe approximately $95, but works for 3 months making its monthly cost similar to COCs or POPs which range from $20 to $45/pack generic, and copper IUD and levonorgestrel IUS may cost more initially but will work for up to 10 years and 5 years, respectively).
[m]Initial cost for procedure but over time may be more cost-effective than other products used frequently (e.g., monthly contraceptives, condoms, or spermicides).
IUD, intrauterine device; IUS, intrauterine system; LAM, lactational amenorrhea method; MPA, medroxyprogesterone acetate.
Source: Hatcher RA et al. *Contraceptive Technology*. 20th ed. New York, NY: Ardent Media; 2011:24, Table 3-2; includes additional information from **www.goodrx.com**. Accessed August 25, 2017; **http://americanpregnancy.org/preventing-pregnancy/diaphragm/**. Accessed June 11, 2017; **https://www.plannedparenthood.org/learn/birth-control/cervical-cap**. Accessed June 11, 2017.

recommendations in the United States and updated them in 2016 (See **http://who.int/reproductivehealth/publications/family_planning/MEC-5/en/**. Accessed June 11, 2017) html for the WHO Medical Eligibility Criteria and CDC link).[6,7] Most data regarding contraindications are based on COCs, but the conclusions are applied to all CHCs (e.g., vaginal ring and transdermal patch).

CIGARETTE SMOKING AND USE OF CHCS

S.F. should be strongly encouraged to stop smoking (see Chapter 91, Tobacco Use and Dependence). Women who are 35 years of age or older and smoke 15 or more cigarettes/day should not use CHCs as a method of contraception. Although S.F. is not yet 35, she is smoking one pack/day (20 cigarettes). In her case, many clinicians would not prescribe CHCs. Although S.F. currently does not have any medical problems that would preclude her from using CHCs, she should be informed that CHCs should not be prescribed for her in 2 years if she continues to smoke. In addition, S.F. should be informed that smoking may decrease fertility and has adverse effects on birth outcomes, which is important given her plans to start a family in the near future.

CARDIOVASCULAR DISEASE

An increased risk of cardiovascular death in women who use COCs has been reported in several studies.[8–11] One study reported that in women who do not smoke or use COCs, the risk of cardiovascular death is 0.59/100,000 women younger than 35 years and 3.18/100,000 women at least 35 years of age. Among nonsmokers, using COCs increased the risk to 0.65/100,000 and 6.21/100,000 women younger than 35 years or at least 35 years of age, respectively. For COC users who smoke, the risk is 3.3/100,000

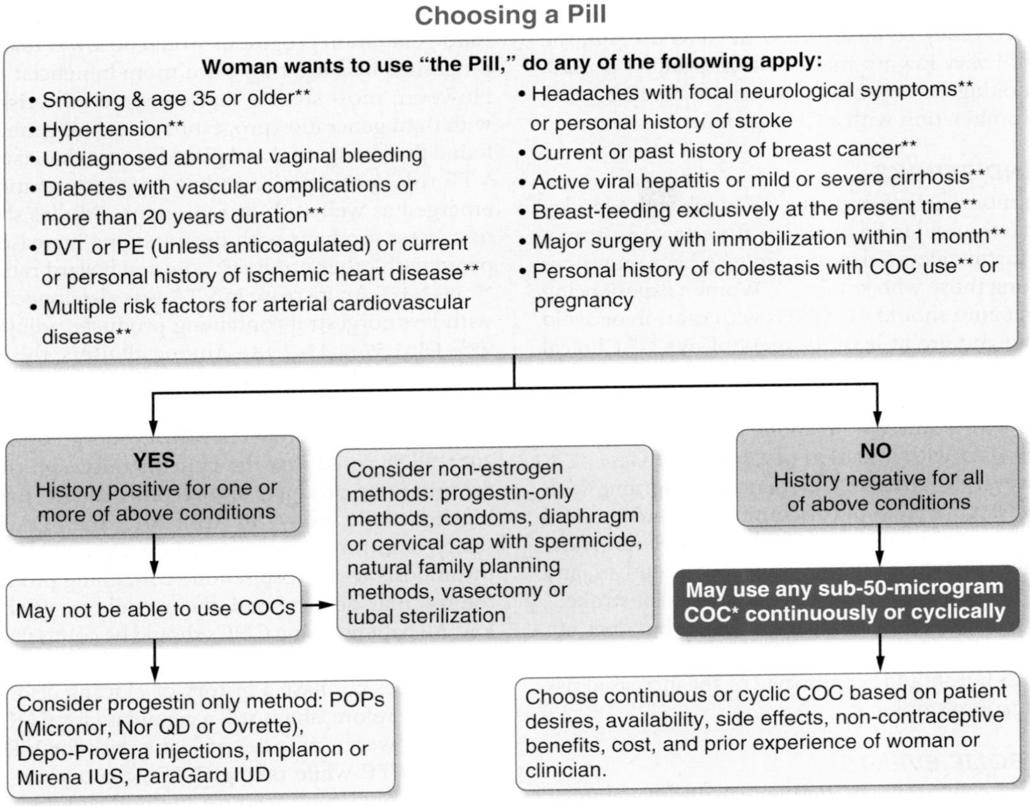

- The World Health Organization and the Food and Drug Administration both recommend using the lowest dose pill that is effective. All combined pills with less than 50 mcg of estrogen are considered "low-dose" and are effective and safe.

- There are no studies demonstrating a decreased risk for deep vein thrombosis (DVT) in women on 20-mcg pills. Data on higher dose pills have demonstrated that the less the estrogen dose, the lower the risk for DVT.

- All COCs lower free testosterone. Class labeling in Canada for all combined pills states that use of pills may improve acne.

- To minimize discontinuation due to spotting and breakthrough bleeding, warn women in advance, reassure that spotting and breakthrough bleeding become better over time.

*The package insert for women on Yasmin and Yaz states [Berlex-2001]: "Yasmin is different from other birth control pills because it contains the progestin drospirenone. Drospirenone may increase potassium. Therefore, you should not take Yasmin if you have kidney, liver or adrenal disease, because this could cause serious heart and health problems. Other drugs may also increase potassium. If you are currently on daily, long-term treatment for a chronic condition with any of the medications below, you should consult your healthcare provider about whether Yasmin is right for you, and during the first month that you take Yasmin, you should have a blood test to check your potassium level: NSAIDs (ibuprofen [Motrin®, Advil®], naproxen [Naprosyn®, Aleve®, and others] when taken long-term and daily for treatment of arthritis or other problems]; potassium-sparing diuretics (sprironolactone and others); potassium supplementation; ACE inhibitors (Capoten®, Vasotec®, Zestril® and others); Angiotensin-II receptor antagonists (Cozaar®, Diovan®, Avapro® and others); heparin."

**These are conditions that receive a WHO:3 or a WHO:4 (based on WHO Medical Eligibility Criteria for Contraceptive Use, 5th ed. 2015, Category 3—A condition in which theoretical or proven risks usually outweigh the benefit of contraceptive method use, Category 4—A condition that represents an unacceptable health risk if contraceptive method is used).

Figure 47-1 Choosing a pill. ACE, angiotensin-converting enzyme; COC, combined oral contraceptive; DVT, deep venous thrombosis; IUD, intrauterine device; IUS, intrauterine system; NSAIDs, nonsteroidal anti-inflammatory drugs; PE, pulmonary embolism; POP, progestin-only pill. (Adapted with permission from Zieman M, Hatcher RA. *Managing Contraception*. Tiger, GA: Bridging the Gap Communications; 2012: Figure 23.1.)

women younger than 35 years and 29.4/100,000 women at least 35 years of age.[12] The increase in mortality is concentrated in smokers of 35 years and older.

Several studies have focused on the effect of COCs on serum lipoprotein concentrations because of the association between lipoproteins and atherosclerotic cardiovascular disease.[13–15] High levels of total cholesterol (TC), triglycerides (TG), low-density lipoprotein (LDL) cholesterol, and very low density lipoprotein (VLDL) cholesterol serum concentrations are associated with the risk of developing atherosclerotic circulatory diseases, whereas high-density lipoprotein (HDL) cholesterol has an inverse relationship. Apolipoprotein levels also affect atherosclerotic risk (e.g., elevations in apolipoprotein increase risk).

Patients taking COCs may be more likely to experience a myocardial infarction (MI) than nonusers.[16] The risk is higher with higher doses of estrogen and especially if the patient is a smoker or has hypertension. It is not clear whether certain types of progestin are more likely to cause MI than others.[10,17] Combined oral contraceptive users may also be at a slightly higher risk of stroke, but some data are conflicting.[16] Those at highest risk of stroke are smokers, patients with hypertension, and patients older than 35 years.

S.F. and her fiance should understand that the risk of adverse cardiovascular effects may be increased with CHC use, but the absolute risk is still very low no matter which product is used. S.F.'s cigarette smoking, however, is a much more significant risk factor for MI in combination with a CHC product.

MIGRAINES AND STROKE

Ischemic stroke is more likely to occur in CHC users with a history of migraines and is thought to be caused by the estrogen component. The risk is further elevated in women who have migraines with aura or among those who smoke.[3,18] Women experiencing migraines without aura should use CHCs with caution or avoid use if they smoke and are at least 35 years of age.[7,19] Clinical experience indicates that women who have increasing migraine attacks with CHCs are not likely to improve when the product is changed to one with a different hormone balance. Headaches or migraines may start with initiation of CHCs (see Case 47-2, Question 6); however, if a patient experiences a migraine with aura while taking CHCs, she should discontinue the product and switch to a nonestrogen method.[18,19] Evidence does not show an increased stroke risk with progestin-only contraceptives, and these agents may be used in women with risk factors for stroke.[19]

S.F. does have a history of occasional headaches but does not have a history of migraines with aura. Therefore, she is still a candidate for CHCs but should be informed of the increased risk of stroke from cigarette smoking.

THROMBOEMBOLIC EVENTS

Combined hormonal contraceptives contribute to thromboembolic events by several mechanisms. Estrogens increase coagulability and thereby increase the possibility of clot formation. Although they have been shown to significantly increase some clotting factors, other studies have shown no changes or decreases in prothrombotic factors.[13,15] Long-term COC use is associated with an increased platelet count and increased platelet aggregation similar to that seen late in pregnancy; this is generally thought to be caused by the estrogen component. More recent data showing increased thrombosis rates in users of third-generation progestins (desogestrel and gestodene [not available in the United States]) suggest that progestin may also have a role in thromboembolism risk.[20]

The baseline risk of venous thromboembolism (VTE) in women is low, at 1 case/10,000 person-years, but increases from 3 to 4 cases with COC use.[21] The best studies looking at thromboembolism in COC users found that most users have a twofold-to-sixfold increased risk of having superficial or deep venous thrombosis or pulmonary embolism (PE).[20] Patients requiring emergency major surgery while taking COCs are more prone to VTE than nonusers. The risk of venous thrombosis does not seem to be associated with duration of COC use or past COC use. A greater risk is associated with ethinyl estradiol (EE) doses greater than 35 mcg.[20]

Women with a mutation in clotting factor V (also called factor V Leiden) or a deficiency in protein C, protein S, or antithrombin are more likely to experience a VTE with COCs than women without a hereditary prothrombotic defect.[22] Women with factor V Leiden using COCs have a 30-fold increase in VTE compared with women without the mutation.[22]

The minimal risk of thrombosis associated with CHCs in the general population does not justify the cost of routine screening for deficiencies and mutations in the coagulation system; however, if a patient has a family history of thrombosis, then measurement of antithrombin III, protein C, activated protein C resistance ratio, protein S, anticardiolipin antibodies, prothrombin G mutation, factor V Leiden, and homocysteine levels should be considered.[5]

Whether third-generation progestins (desogestrel, gestodene) are associated with a higher risk of VTE relative to other progestins is controversial.[20] It was believed that the risk of thrombosis with third-generation progestins would be lower than that with other progestins because they have more beneficial effects on HDL. However, most studies that compared the risk of thrombosis with third-generation progestins to second-generation progestins found that desogestrel and gestodene are associated with a greater VTE risk. A concern regarding fourth-generation progestin has emerged as well with drospirenone. Studies show that among new users products with drospirenone increase VTE risk compared with other products; adjusted hazard ratio 95% CI is 1.77 (1.33–2.35). An increase in VTE was also found when compared with levonorgestrel-containing products; adjusted hazard ratio 95% CI: 1.57 (1.13–2.18). Among all users, the risk of VTE was also increased with drospirenone use; adjusted hazard ratio 95% CI is 1.74 (1.42–2.14), and adjusted hazard ratio 95% CI is 1.45 (1.15–1.83) when compared with levonorgestrel.[23,24] In December 2011, FDA voted that the benefits outweigh the risks of using drospirenone products and recommended labeling changes to highlight VTE risks.[24] In April 2012, the FDA also published a safety communication regarding a possible increased risk of thrombosis with drospirenone-containing products.[25] Although the risk may be increased, the overall rate of thrombosis is still low. All patients using CHCs should be counseled about the VTE warning signs (Table 47-2).[5]

S.F. does not have a history of clotting disorders or previous clots. Therefore, she is still a candidate for CHCs. Her smoking status, however, puts her at higher risk for VTE. If she experiences a VTE while taking CHCs, a progestin-only method or nonhormonal contraceptive method should be recommended and the CHC discontinued.

HYPERTENSION

Combined hormonal contraceptives appear to increase blood pressure. Small studies have found systolic blood pressure to increase by 7 to 8 mm Hg and diastolic blood pressure to increase by 6 mm Hg in normotensive or mildly hypertensive women, and these women may have poorer blood pressure control.[26,27] Other studies have shown differing results on whether women with hypertension who use COCs are more likely to suffer an MI than nonusers.[6,28] A small study of adolescent women showed similar systolic and diastolic blood pressures in users versus nonusers.[29]

The underlying mechanisms for CHC-induced hypertension may be sodium and water retention and increased renin activity.[30,31] Hypertension secondary to COCs may develop slowly during 3 to 36 months and may not decline for 3 to 6 months after COC discontinuation.[32] Women with controlled hypertension may attempt a trial of CHCs with blood pressure monitoring;

Table 47-2
Pill Early Danger Signs (ACHES)[3]

Signals	Possible Problem
Abdominal pain (severe)	Gallbladder disease, hepatic adenoma, blood clot, pancreatitis
Chest pain (severe), shortness of breath, or coughing up blood	Blood clot in lungs or myocardial infarction
Headaches (severe)	Stroke, hypertension, or migraine headache
Eye problems: blurred vision, flashing lights, or blindness	Stroke, hypertension, or temporary vascular problem
Severe leg pain (calf or thigh)	Blood clot in legs

however, progestin-only contraceptives have not been shown to increase blood pressure and may be preferable for women with uncontrolled hypertension.[26]

S.F.'s blood pressure is not elevated at 122/72 mm Hg. Therefore, she is still a candidate for CHCs. If her blood pressure were greater than 140/90 mm Hg, a nonhormonal method or a progestin-only contraceptive would be a preferred form of contraception.

HEPATOTOXICITY

Combined oral contraceptives have been associated with benign liver tumors, hepatic adenomas, and liver cancer.[3,33] The risk of liver cancer is low, and COCs are thought to cause only a modest increase in risk.[33,34] A European study found a small, statistically significant increase in the risk of liver cancer in women without cirrhosis and without hepatitis B or C, which are the types of women that usually use COCs. In this study, COC use in these women increased the risk of liver cancer by 1 case/1.5 million woman-years.[34] S.F. should be reassured that it is very unlikely for her to develop benign or malignant liver tumors associated with COC use.

DIABETES

Generally, low-dose COCs do not alter glucose tolerance.[15,35] Women with a history of gestational diabetes like S.F's sister and those with a strong family history of diabetes in parents or siblings are at greater risk for COC-induced glucose intolerance.[26] Combined oral contraceptives have complex effects on carbohydrate metabolism. Progestins decrease and estrogens increase the number of insulin receptors on the cell membrane. Progestins also may alter insulin receptor affinity. The different progestins in CHCs have different propensities to induce glucose intolerance. Desogestrel seems to have the best glucose values compared with other progestins, but insulin results are not consistent.[35]

Results of one controlled, randomized, prospective study showed no adverse effect on carbohydrate or lipid metabolism in women with a history of gestational diabetes after 6 to 13 months of low-dose CHC use.[36] Both the users and nonusers showed a significant and similar deterioration in glucose tolerance with an overall prevalence of 14% impaired glucose tolerance and 17% diabetes mellitus. The authors concluded that low-dose COCs could be prescribed safely and that serum lipids and glucose tolerance should be monitored closely, regardless of contraceptive choice.

For women with diabetes, the World Health Organization recommends avoiding COCs if they have been diabetic for more than 20 years or they have end-organ damage such as retinopathy, neuropathy, or nephropathy.[6] For women without diabetes, CHC use may protect against developing diabetes. One large prospective, observational study found that women who used COCs had lower fasting glucose levels and lower odds of developing diabetes.[37]

S.F.'s sister having a history of gestational diabetes does not preclude S.F. from using a CHC at this time. Preferably, S.F. should start on a low-dose CHC.

GALLBLADDER DISEASE

The incidence of gallstones has been reported to increase with COC use; however, conflicting data exist. Estrogens and progestins may contribute to bile stasis and gallstones by reducing cholesterol clearance and altering bile acid composition.[38] The incidence of gallbladder disease has been reported to increase during the first year of use but then to decline steadily to a rate lower than that of control women.[39] Conversely, in another large study, long-term COC users experienced slightly lower rates of gallbladder disease than nonusers.[40] In addition, another study found that women who had ever used COCs were not more likely to have symptomatic gallstones, but current and long-term users were. An analysis of 482 women with benign gallbladder disease from the Oxford/Family Planning Association contraception study concluded that it is unlikely that COCs cause gallbladder disease.[41]

The newer COCs with lower progestin and estrogen concentrations should have little effect, if any, on gallstone formation in normal patients. Women who are obese, young, or long-term users of COCs may be the most likely to develop gallstones. At this time, this is not a concern of S.F. in starting COCs.

Combined Oral Contraceptives

CASE 47-1, QUESTION 3: S.F. has decided to quit smoking. Based on her past medical history, she is a candidate for CHCs and indicates she wants to start a COC. Which COC should be selected for her?

Selecting a COC for S.F. can be confusing because of the multitude of products available, the lack of studies directly comparing products, and health insurance medication formulary restrictions. The failure rate of COCs ranges from 0.3% with perfect use to 9% with typical use (Table 47-1).[3]

The COCs are available in varying strengths of estrogens and progestins. Table 47-3[42–51] lists the brand name and generic COCs in the United States. Almost all COCs available in the United States contain the synthetic estrogen, EE. Doses of EE generally range from 10 to 50 mcg with 10- to 25-mcg formulations considered very low dose, 30- to 35-mcg formulations, low dose, and 50-mcg formulations, high dose. Mestranol, another estrogen available in the United States and used internationally, is an inactive prodrug that is hepatically metabolized to EE. Mestranol 50 mcg has approximately the same activity as EE 35 mcg.[3] Estradiol valerate is a third estrogen available in one oral formulation. The formulation of estradiol valerate 2 to 3 mg with 2 to 3 mg of dienogest was compared against EE 20 mcg with levonorgestrel 100 mcg in clinical trials.[47,52]

The COCs also contain one of the following progestins: ethynodiol diacetate, desogestrel, dienogest, drospirenone, levonorgestrel, norethindrone, norethindrone acetate, norgestimate, and norgestrel (a mixture of dextronorgestrel and levonorgestrel; dextronorgestrel appears to be progestationally inert compared with levonorgestrel).[3] Progestins differ significantly in their progestational potency and in the extent of their metabolism to estrogenic substances. Progestins have both estrogenic and antiestrogenic effects. Because the progestins have a chemical structure similar to that of testosterone, they also have varying degrees of androgenic activity (Table 47-3).[53] Minor structural changes in all of the progestins may lead to significant changes in their progestational, estrogenic, antiestrogenic, and androgenic activities, which may affect patients differently (Table 47-4).[3] Drospirenone is a unique progestin because it has antiandrogenic and antimineralocorticoid properties. Drospirenone is chemically similar to the potassium-sparing diuretic spironolactone, and therefore, may increase potassium levels. Drospirenone should be used with caution in patients using medications that can increase potassium levels (e.g., high-dose nonsteroidal anti-inflammatory drugs [NSAIDs], angiotensin-converting enzyme [ACE] inhibitors, heparin, potassium-sparing diuretics, aldosterone antagonists, and angiotensin II blockers).[43]

Because no COC has been shown to be superior to the others, any COC with less than 50 mcg of EE can be used for patients who are COC candidates.[54] The information in Figure 47-1 may be used to select an initial COC for most patients and to change formulations when side effects necessitate an alternative choice.[6] Increased body weight (>70.5 kg) has been associated with increased COC failure.[55] If S.F. were heavier, a COC with a higher dose of EE (e.g., 35 mcg) would be a better option. Any pill containing less than 50 mcg EE can be used for S.F. because she is a healthy woman without medical complications or active medications.

Table 47-3
Oral Contraceptives and Relative Progestin, Estrogen, and Androgen Activities[42–51,53]

Ingredients	Brand Name Examples	Progestin Activity	Estrogen Activity	Androgen Activity	Unique Properties
Monophasic Formulations					
Levonorgestrel 0.1 mg/EE 20 mcg	Amethia Lo, Aubra, Aviane, Camrese Lo, Delyla, FaLessa, Falmina, Lessina, Levlite, LoSeasonique, Lutera, Orsythia, Sronyx	Low	Low	Low	Amethia Lo, Camrese Lo, and LoSeasonique contain 84 active pills and contain 7 pills of EE 10 mcg instead of placebos
Levonorgestrel 0.09 mg/EE 20 mcg	Amethyst	Low	Low	Low	Amethyst is a 1-year continuous formulation available in packs of 28 active pills
Norgestimate 0.25 mg/EE 35 mcg	Estarylla, Mono-Linyah, MonoNessa, Ortho-Cyclen, Previfem, Sprintec	Low	Intermediate	Low	
Norethindrone 0.5 mg/EE 35 mcg	Brevicon, Modicon, Necon 0.5/35, Nortrel 0.5/35, Wera	Low	High	Low	
Norethindrone 0.4 mg/EE 35 mcg	Blaziva, Femcon Fe, Gildagia, Ovcon-35, Philith, Vyfemla, Wymzya FE, Zenchent, Zenchent FE	Low	High	Low	Femcon Fe, Wymza FE, and Zenchant FE are chewable formulations and contain 7 pills of 75 mg ferrous fumarate instead of placebos
Levonorgestrel 0.15 mg/EE 30 mcg	Altavera, Amethia, Ashlyna, Camrese, Daysee, Chateal, Kurvelo, Levora, Introvale, Jolessa, Marlissa, Nordette-28, Portia, Quasence	Intermediate	Low	Intermediate	Introvale, Jolessa, and Quasense contain 84 active pills and 7 placebo pills. Amethia, Ashlyna, Camrese, and Daysee contain 84 active pills and 7 pills of EE 10 mcg instead of placebos
Norgestrel 0.3 mg/EE 30 mcg	Cryselle, Elinest, Low-Ogestrel	Intermediate	Low	Intermediate	
Norethindrone 1 mg/mestranol 50 mcg	Necon 1/50, Norinyl 1+50	Intermediate	Intermediate	Intermediate	
Norethindrone 1 mg/EE 35 mcg	Alyacen 1/35, Cyclafem 1/35, Dasetta 1/35, Necon 1/35, Norethin 1/35, Norinyl 1+35, Nortrel 1/35, Ortho-Novum 1/35, Pirmella 1/35	Intermediate	High	Intermediate	
Norethindrone acetate 1 mg/EE 20 mcg	Gildess 24 FE, Gildess 1/20, Gildess FE 1/20, Junel Fe 1/20, Junel 21 Day 1/20, Junel FE 24, Larin 24 FE, Larin 1/20, Larin FE 1/20, Loestrin 21 1/20, Loestrin Fe 1/20, Lomedia 24 FE, Microgestin Fe 1/20, Minastrin 24 FE, Tarina Fe 1/20	High	Low	Intermediate	"Fe" or "FE" contains 75 mg ferrous fumarate instead of placebos, and Gildess 24 FE, Junel FE 24, Larin FE 24, Lomedia FE 24, and Minastrin 24 FE have 24 active tablets
Norethindrone acetate 1.5 mg/EE 30 mcg	Gildess 1.5/30, Gildess FE 1.5/30, Junel 1.5/30, Larin 1.5/30, Larin FE 1.5/30, Loestrin 21 1.5/30, Loestrin Fe 1.5/30, Microgestin Fe 1.5/30	High	Low	High	"Fe" contains 75 mg ferrous fumarate instead of placebos
Ethynodiol diacetate 1 mg/35 mcg EE	Kelnor 1/35, Zovia 1/35E	High	Low	Low	
Desogestrel 0.15 mg/EE 20 mcg	Azurette, Kariva, Kimidess, Pimtrea, Mircette, Viorele	High	Low	Low	Only 2 days of placebos, other 5 days contain EE 10 mcg

Table 47-3
Oral Contraceptives and Relative Progestin, Estrogen, and Androgen Activities[42–51,53] (*continued*)

Ingredients	Brand Name Examples	Progestin Activity	Estrogen Activity	Androgen Activity	Unique Properties
Desogestrel 0.15 mg/EE 30 mcg	Apri, Desogen, Emoquette, Enskyce, Ortho-Cept, Reclipsen, Solia	High	Intermediate	Low	
Ethynodiol diacetate 1 mg/EE 50 mcg	Zovia 1/50E	High	Intermediate	Low	
Norgestrel 0.5 mg/EE 50 mcg	Ogestrel	High	High	High	
Norethindrone 0.8 mg/EE 25 mcg	Generess Fe, Layolis Fe	No data	No data	No data	"Fe" contains 75 mg ferrous fumarate instead of placebos, and Generess Fe and Layolis Fe contain 24 active pills and 4 pills of ferrous fumarate, chewable formulation
Norethindrone 1 mg/EE 10 mcg	Lo Loestrin Fe, Lo Minastrin Fe	No data	No data	No data	Lo Loestrin Fe and Lo Minastrin Fe contain 24 active pills, 2 pills of 10 mcg EE, and 2 pills of 75 mg ferrous fumarate
Drospirenone 3 mg/EE 20 mcg levomefolate calcium 0.451 mg	Beyaz	No data	No data	None[a]	Provides folate supplementation, FDA-approved use for treatment of acne and PMDD, 24 active pills and 4 days of 0.451 mg of levomefolate calcium instead of placebos
Drospirenone 3 mg/EE 20 mcg	Gianvi, Loryna, Nikki, Vestura, YAZ	No data	No data	None[a]	Antimineralocorticoid properties, FDA-approved use for treatment of acne and PMDD, only 4 days of placebos
Drospirenone 3 mg/EE 30 mcg/levomefolate calcium 0.451 mg	Safyral	No data	Intermediate	None[a]	Provides folate supplementation, 21 active pills, and 7 days of 0.451 mg of levomefolate calcium instead of placebos
Drospirenone 3 mg/EE 30 mcg	Ocella, Syeda, Yasmin, Zarah	No data	Intermediate	None[a]	Antimineralocorticoid properties
Biphasic Formulations					
Norethindrone 0.5, 1 mg/EE 35 mcg	Necon 10/11	Intermediate	High	Low	
Triphasic Formulations					
Norgestimate 0.18, 0.215, 0.25 mg/EE 25 mcg	Ortho Tri-Cyclen Lo	Low	Low	Low	
Norgestimate 0.18, 0.215, 0.25 mg/EE 35 mcg	Ortho Tri-Cyclen, Tri-Estarylla, Tri-Linyah, TriNessa, Tri-Previfem, Tri-Sprintec	Low	Intermediate	Low	FDA-approved use for treatment of acne
Levonorgestrel 0.05, 0.075, 0.125 mg/EE 30, 40, 30 mcg	Enpresse, Levonest, Myzilra, Trivora	Low	Intermediate	Low	
Norethindrone 0.5, 1, 0.5 mg/EE 35 mcg	Aranelle, Leena, Tri-Norinyl	Low	High	Low	
Norethindrone 0.5, 0.75, 1 mg/EE 35 mcg	Alyacen7/7/7, Cyclafem 7/7/7, Dasetta 7/7/7, Necon 7/7/7, Nortel 7/7/7, Ortho-Novum 7/7/7, Pirmella 7/7/7	Intermediate	High	Low	

(continued)

Table 47-3
Oral Contraceptives and Relative Progestin, Estrogen, and Androgen Activities[42–51,53] *(continued)*

Ingredients	Brand Name Examples	Progestin Activity	Estrogen Activity	Androgen Activity	Unique Properties
Norethindrone 1 mg/ EE 20, 30, 35 mcg	Tilia Fe, Tri- Legest 21, Tri-Legest Fe 28	High	Low	Intermediate	Estrophasic (estrogen content changes), FDA-approved use for treatment of acne, "Fe" contains 75 mg ferrous fumarate instead of placebos
Desogestrel 0.1, 0.125, 0.15 mg/EE 25 mcg	Caziant, Cesia, Cyclessa, Velivet	High	Low	Low	
Quadriphasic Formulation					
Dienogest 0, 2, 3, 0 mg/estradiol valerate 3, 2, 2, 1 mg	Natazia	No data	Low	No data	Has 2 placebo pills, 2 pills with 3 mg of estradiol valerate only, 5 pills with 2 mg of dienogest and 2 mg of estradiol valerate, 17 pills with 3 mg of dienogest and 2 mg of estradiol valerate and 2 pills of 1 mg estradiol valerate
Levonorgestrel 0.15, 0.15, 0.15, 0 mg/EE 20, 25, 30, 10 mcg	Quartette	Intermediate	Low	Intermediate	Has 91 pills, 42 contain 0.15 mg of levonorgestrel with 20 mcg of ethinyl estradiol, 21 pills contain 0.15 mg of levonorgestrel with 25 mcg of ethinyl estradiol, 21 pills contain 0.15 mg of levonorgestrel with 30 mcg of ethinyl estradiol, 7 pills contain 10 mcg of ethinyl estradiol
Progestin Only					
Norethindrone 0.35 mg	Camila, Errin, Jolivette, Micronor, Nor-QD, Nora-BE, Deblitane, Heather, Jencycla, Norlyroc, Sharobel	Low	None	Low	No placebos, 28 days of active pills

[a]Preclinical studies have shown that drospirenone has no androgenic, estrogenic, glucocorticoid, antiglucocorticoid, or antiandrogenic activity.
EE, ethinyl estradiol; FDA, US Food and Drug Administration; PMDD, premenstrual dysphoric disorder.
Source: Facts and Comparisons eAnswers. http://online.factsandcomparisons.com/index.aspx. Dickey RP. *Managing Contraceptive Pill Patients*. 15th ed. Dallas, TX: Essential Medical Information Systems; 2014.

Table 47-4
Estrogenic, Progestogenic, and Combined Effects of Oral Contraceptive Pills

Achieving Proper Hormonal Balance in an Oral Contraceptive			
Estrogen		Progestin	
Excess	Deficiency	Excess	Deficiency
Nausea, bloating Cervical mucorrhea, polyposis Melasma Hypertension Migraine headache Breast fullness or tenderness Edema	Early- or mid-cycle breakthrough bleeding Increased spotting Hypomenorrhea	Increased appetite Weight gain Tiredness, fatigue Hypomenorrhea Acne, oily scalpa Hair loss, hirsutism[a] Depression Monilial vaginitis Breast regression	Late breakthrough bleeding Amenorrhea Hypermenorrhea

[a]Result of androgenic activity of progestins.
Source: Facts and Comparisons eAnswers. http://online.factsandcomparisons.com/index.aspx.

LENGTH OF ACTIVE HORMONE: 21-, 24-, OR 28 DAY

The COCs are available in a variety of cycle lengths. The most common is the 28-day pack that contains 21 days of active pills (pills that contain estrogen and progestin) followed by 7 days of placebo pills. Some newer products contain 24 days of active pills followed by 4 days of placebo. Combined hormonal contraceptives with 4 days of placebo may shorten menses and minimize the hormonal withdrawal side effects (e.g., headaches, mood changes) that some women experience during the placebo week.[56]

It is also possible that efficacy is improved; however, this has not been proven in clinical trials.

The 21-day pill packs contain only the active pills. Most patients are instructed to take one pill daily for 21 days and then take nothing for 1 week. Many clinicians prefer the use of 28-day pill packs to minimize confusion; the patient takes one pill daily regardless of whether it is an active or placebo pill. After taking the last pill of a 28-day pack, the patient should begin a new pack the next day. However, when continuous ovarian suppression is indicated to treat estrogen-dependent disorders such as endometriosis, the 21-day cycle products are preferred to facilitate taking active pills continuously. Alternatively, the placebo pills could be removed from 28-day cycle packs. S.F. will not be taking COCs continuously, so a 24- or 28-day pack is recommended.

MULTIPHASIC ORAL CONTRACEPTIVES

CASE 47-1, QUESTION 4: Should S.F. start a monophasic or multiphasic COC? What are the advantages and disadvantages of the monophasic versus multiphasic COC?

COCs have varying amounts of hormones in the active pills, which can be divided in phases that include monophasic, biphasic, triphasic, or quadriphasic (Table 47-3).

Monophasic COCs contain the same dose of estrogen and progestin in each active pill throughout the pill pack, whereas multiphasic COCs have varying amounts of hormones. Because of metabolic and physiologic effects related to the progestin component of COCs, multiphasic products were initially formulated to contain less progestin overall. Some products, however, are now marketed with varying amounts of estrogen to reduce the overall exposure to estrogen or to minimize estrogen withdrawal side effects (e.g., norethindrone/EE [Tri-Legest 21 and Tri-Legest Fe 28]).

A biphasic formulation usually contains a certain amount of progestin and estrogen for the first half of the cycle, then a different amount for the second half, and then a week of placebos. Triphasic formulations have a different amount of hormones for each of the 3 weeks of active pills. No studies, however, show a superiority of one triphasic over another or compared with monophasics. The reduced progestin content is desirable for women with complaints of progestin-associated side effects (e.g., increased appetite, acne, weight gain) or women with cardiovascular disease or metabolic abnormalities.[3] Women with side effects related to progestin deficiency (e.g., late-cycle bleeding) or conditions necessitating progestin dominance (e.g., benign breast disease) may do better with monophasics. Recently, a quadriphasic COC (Natazia) became available, and it contains four different amounts of hormones throughout the pill pack.[47] Advantages of the product remain to be seen, but it may help decrease hormone withdrawal side effects and intermenstrual bleeding.

One drawback associated with triphasic and quadriphasic COC use is the confusion caused by the different-colored pills in each of the three different phases, making the missed-dose instructions more complicated. Monophasics are preferred for women who will be taking COCs continuously (i.e., skipping the placebo pills) because of the same weekly hormone content.

Other unique formulations include Mircette (see Table 47-3 for generic names), which is classified more appropriately as monophasic because the hormone content is consistent throughout the 21-day cycle like other monophasic formulations, but sometimes referred to as biphasic because it does not contain 7 days of placebos. It provides a unique regimen containing 21 days of 0.15 mg of desogestrel plus 20 mcg of EE, then only 2 days of placebo, followed by 5 days of 10 mcg of EE alone.[50] The patient does not need to take missed 10-mcg EE doses or use a backup method when those specific pills are missed. Adding low-dose estrogen for 5 days during the typical placebo week helps minimize breakthrough bleeding with this product and may be useful for patients who have estrogen-deficiency symptoms such as headaches during the hormone-free week. Because S.F. has not been on a CHC before and does not have a history of side effects associated with COCs, she may be started on any of the COC formulations.

EXTENDED CYCLE

CASE 47-1, QUESTION 5: S.F. has heard that she can skip the placebos from her pill pack to have fewer menses each year. She is interested in this approach. Is this a reasonable option for S.F.?

Continuous- or extended-cycle COC regimens (i.e., skipping the placebo pills and taking no break between pill packs, thus having no menses) are often prescribed in women with underlying conditions including anemia, dysmenorrhea (less cramps with fewer menstrual cycles), menorrhagia (heavy menstrual bleeding), and endometriosis (to decrease hormone fluctuations that affect endometrial tissues).[5] In addition, for convenience and lifestyle reasons, many women prefer to take COCs continuously to minimize the number of menstrual periods. Regardless of the reason, any woman who is a candidate for CHCs can use them continuously.

Any CHC (e.g., pill, patch, vaginal ring) may be used continuously; however, from the COCs, monophasic pills are recommended because of the consistent hormone content throughout the cycle. Any duration of continuous pill use is acceptable, but many providers recommend that patients take the active pills for 3 to 4 months (3–4 pill packs) and then stop COCs for 2 to 7 days. Alternatively, providers may prescribe COCs that are specifically packaged for continuous use (e.g., Amethyst, Camrese Lo). Patients should be informed that continuous COC use usually results in more breakthrough bleeding or spotting than traditional COC dosing regimens, with up to 41% of women experiencing some form of irregular bleeding in the first few months of the one-year regimen.[51]

Concerns raised with extended-use regimens include harmful effects on the endometrium; however, one study showed no harmful changes to the endometrium with extended cycles.[57] Long-term side effects of the extended regimens are still being studied. If breakthrough bleeding continues beyond 6 months of continuous COC use, a pelvic examination may be considered. If S.F. is willing to tolerate more irregular bleeding during the first 6 months of continuous COC use, then the extended-cycle regimen may work for her.

Patient Instructions

CASE 47-1, QUESTION 6: What instructions should be given to S.F. about her COC?

WHEN TO START ORAL CONTRACEPTIVES

S.F. should start the first cycle of COCs according to the manufacturer's package instructions or according to one of the following recommendations:[3]

1. Quick start: Take the first COC tablet as soon as possible regardless of cycle day.[58]
2. Day 1 start: Take the first tablet in the COC pack on the first day of menses.
3. Sunday start: Take the first tablet in the COC pack on the first Sunday after the beginning of menstruation. If menses begins on Sunday, start that day.

The quick start method is not described in COC package inserts; however, this method is used by family planning providers.[58,59] The quick start method can minimize the confusion that many patients have about when to start their first pack and can increase adherence. Also, the quick start method provides contraceptive protection sooner and would, therefore, likely lower the risk of unintended pregnancy. More research on and awareness about this method are needed for it to be used routinely by all health-care providers.

WHEN TO USE A BACKUP METHOD OF CONTRACEPTION

Some clinicians recommend that a woman use an alternative method of contraception for the entire first COC cycle. Others believe that alternative methods of contraception are unnecessary if the COC is started on or before the fifth day of the menstrual cycle. Most COC package inserts with the exception of Natazia (estradiol valerate/dienogest) state that a backup method of contraception (e.g., male or female condoms, spermicides, diaphragms) is not necessary if patients use the day 1 start method.[4] If patients use the Sunday or quick start methods, backup contraception should be used for the first week of the COC cycle. A backup method is also recommended when doses are missed, as described in the following section. S.F. has decided to use the quick start method, so she will need to use another method of contraception for her first week of COC use.

COC ADMINISTRATION AND MISSED DOSE INSTRUCTIONS

S.F. should take her COC at the same time each day. Nausea may be prevented or alleviated by taking the dose at bedtime or with food. The best time to take COCs depends on the patient. The optimal time for S.F. is the time when she will have the fewest problems remembering to take her pill each day.

If a woman forgets to take one pill, she must take it as soon as she remembers and refer to the patient instructions in the package insert for further information.[3] Some unique formulations such as estradiol valerate/dienogest (Natazia) have more specific recommendations based on the cycle day missed. If she is taking Natazia, she should be referred to the package insert for information (see **http://www.natazia.com**), as the advice varies from that listed below.

For the majority of COCs, most manufacturers recommend that if she forgets to take one pill, she should take two pills on the day she remembers (e.g., if she forgets her pill on Monday, she should take two pills on Tuesday). Then she should take the remaining pills as usual. A backup method of contraception is not necessary. If she misses two pills in a row in week 1 or 2 of her pack, she must take two pills on the day she remembers and two pills the next day. She should use an alternative method of contraception for 7 days after missing the pills and may consider emergency contraception.

If a woman misses two pills in a row during the third week (for day 1 starters), she must discard the rest of the pack, start a new pack on that same day, and use an alternative contraceptive method for 7 days. For Sunday starters, she should keep taking one pill every day until Sunday, then start a new pack on Sunday. She must use an alternative method of contraception for 7 days after missing the pills and may consider emergency contraception. She may miss her menstrual period this month.

If a woman misses three or more pills in a row during the first 3 weeks (for day 1 starters), she must discard the rest of her pack, start a new pack that same day, and use an alternative method of contraception for 7 days; Sunday starters should keep taking one pill every day until Sunday, start a new pack on Sunday, and use an alternative method of contraception for 7 days after missing the pills, and they may consider emergency contraception. Women may not have a menstrual period this month. If two pills are missed from a low-dose COC (less than EE 30 mcg), some references suggest following the instructions as if three pills were missed.[3] Other references and organizations may cite different recommendations. The recommendations described here are recommended by manufacturers.

CONTRACEPTIVE PATCH AND RING

CASE 47-1, QUESTION 7: S.F. returns to the clinic 3 months later and is very concerned about getting pregnant because she has trouble remembering to take her pill each day. She wants an effective contraceptive method but is wondering whether other dosage formulations are available. She also indicates concern about high doses of estrogen because she has heard high doses of estrogen can lead to blood clots. She wants the lowest possible dose. What do you tell her?

Contraceptive Patch

The contraceptive patch has an estimated failure rate of 0.3% with perfect use and 9% with typical use (Table 47-1). The contraceptive patch (Ortho Evra, Xulane) contains 6 mg of norelgestromin and 750 mcg of EE. It was originally formulated to transdermally deliver 150 mcg of norelgestromin and 20 mcg of EE daily into the systemic circulation; however, higher doses of ethinyl estradiol are now thought to be delivered (see below).[60] The patch is a 1.75-inch square with rounded corners and is beige and thin. One patch is applied each week for three consecutive weeks for a total of three patches used, followed by 1 week with no patch. The day of the week the patch is applied is called the patch change day. Then this cycle is repeated. Menses should begin during the patch-free week. If a woman wants to avoid menses, the patch-free week may be skipped by applying a new patch on week 4 for an extended-use regimen.

The contraceptive patch may be worn on the buttock, abdomen, upper torso, or upper outer arm.[60] The patch should not be applied to the breasts to prevent direct administration of estradiol to the breast tissue. To minimize irritation from the adhesive, S.F. should rotate the patch application sites and not apply the patch to the same location within each month. When applying the patch, S.F. should select the application site and be sure it is clean and dry. She should press firmly on the patch for 10 seconds and trace her finger around the edge of the patch to be sure it adheres securely to the skin. The patch should stay attached during usual activities, including exercising, swimming, and bathing. If the patch falls off and is off less than 24 hours, she should reapply it or apply a new one as soon as possible, and her patch change day will stay the same. No backup contraception is needed. If the patch is off for more than 24 hours, she should start a new cycle of patches, and she will have a new patch change day. She should use backup contraception for 1 week.

The patch may be started using the quick, Sunday, or day 1 start method, and the recommendations for backup contraception are the same as described earlier with CHCs.[60] If S.F. forgets to start the first patch of a new cycle, she should apply it as soon as she remembers. This day will become her new patch change day, and she should use backup contraception for 1 week. If she forgets to change the patch for 1 or 2 days during week 2 or 3, she should apply a new patch as soon as she remembers. This becomes her new patch change day. No backup contraception is needed. If she forgets to wear the patch for more than 2 days, she should start a new cycle as soon as she remembers. She will need to use backup contraception for 1 week and will have a new patch change day.

The effectiveness of the patch is reduced in patients weighing more than 90 kg and should not be used alone for prevention of pregnancy in these women.[60] S.F. does not weigh more than 90 kg, which does not preclude her from using this method.

The most common side effects reported with the patch are breast tenderness, headache, application site reaction, and nausea. Most risks and benefits with the contraceptive patch are thought to be similar to COCs. One notable difference is the rate of VTE. A small pharmacokinetic trial found that overall monthly serum levels of EE are significantly higher in patch users compared with ring or COC users.[61] With the patch, the peak levels of estrogen are lower, but the steady-state concentrations are higher. It has been noted that the patch provides 60% more ethinyl estradiol than an oral 35-mcg tablet.[60] This raised concern that the patch may have a higher incidence of VTE than the other methods; however, it is controversial. One study found no difference in the rate of nonfatal VTE in patch versus COC users, whereas another study found a doubling of VTE risk in patch users compared with COC users.[62–65] The package insert for the transdermal patch was modified to include this new information.[63] Future studies may find that there are other differences in certain risks or benefits between the patch and pill. Given the higher amounts of EE and controversy surrounding VTE with the transdermal patch, this may not be the most appropriate method for S.F. based on her concerns of VTE associated with COC use.

Contraceptive Ring

The failure rate for the contraceptive ring is also 0.3% with perfect use and 9% with typical use (Table 47-1).[3] The contraceptive ring (NuvaRing) delivers 120 mcg of etonogestrel and 15 mcg of EE daily through the vaginal mucosa.[66] The ring is flexible, transparent, and has a diameter of just over 2 inches. The ring is inserted vaginally and kept in place for 3 weeks in a row. After 3 weeks, the ring is removed for 1 week, and then a new ring is inserted (see http://www.spfiles.com/pinuvaring.pdf). For extended use, the ring-free week may be skipped by inserting a new ring on week 4.

The ring may be placed anywhere in the vagina, so S.F. does not need to worry about its exact position.[66] To insert the ring, she should compress it so the opposite sides of the ring are touching, and gently insert it into the vagina.

If she feels discomfort with the ring, it has probably not been inserted into the vagina far enough. Most women do not feel the ring once it is in place. To remove the ring, S.F. should grasp the ring between two fingers or hook one finger inside the ring and pull it out. Menses will usually begin within 3 days of removing the ring. If the ring slips out, it should be rinsed with lukewarm water and reinserted. If the ring is out for less than 3 hours, backup contraception is not needed. If the ring is out for more than 3 hours, backup contraception should be used for 1 week. According to the manufacturer, if the ring has been left in the vagina for longer than 3 weeks but no more than 4 weeks, S.F. should remove it, wait 1 week, then reinsert a new ring. The ring is formulated to contain approximately 35 days of medication but should not be promoted for use beyond 21 days.[66] If it has been in place for more than 4 weeks, she should remove it, confirm that she is not pregnant, reinsert a new one, and use backup contraception for 1 week.

The contraceptive vaginal ring should be inserted anytime during the first 5 days of the menstrual cycle or inserted using the quick start method.[3,66] Backup contraception should be used for the first week. When changing from the COC, S.F. should insert the ring within 7 days of the last active pill and no backup contraception is needed.

The ring is believed to have the same contraindications and precautions as COCs. The most common side effects with the ring are vaginal infections, irritation, and discharge; headache; weight gain; and nausea. Unlike the patch, the ring has not been shown to increase VTE risk or has reduced efficacy in obese women.[66] A study of 1,950 women using the contraceptive ring for 13 months found a high degree of patient satisfaction and adherence to the contraceptive method.[67] The ring provides the least amount of EE exposure when compared with other CHCs.[61] However, despite the lower levels of EE provided, one study has shown an increased risk of VTE with the use of the contraceptive vaginal ring when compared with levonorgestrel-containing contraceptives.[68] Though this study indicated a possible increase in VTE with the vaginal ring, the FDA has not required any labeling changes or communicated any safety issues with the vaginal ring. Given the good adherence rates and lower EE levels, the vaginal ring may be appropriate for S.F. if she is comfortable with the dosage form.

Drug Interactions

CASE 47-1, QUESTION 8: S.F. returns to the clinic 2 months later for a sore throat. She indicates that she is using the contraceptive vaginal ring.

Current vitals at clinic: weight, 132 lb; height, 5′4″
Blood pressure, 125/78 mm Hg
Heart rate, 97 beats/minute
Respiratory rate, 16 breaths/minute
Temperature, 101.1°F
Physical examination: head, eyes, ear, nose, and throat: tonsils 2+, bright red, soft palate erythematous
Laboratory test results: rapid streptococcal antigen test, positive

S.F.'s primary-care physician prescribes Augmentin 875 mg/125 mg (amoxicillin/clavulanate) twice daily by mouth for 10 days. Could this medication affect her contraception? What advice should be provided to S.F.? What other drug interactions are of concern with CHCs?

A variety of drugs may alter the levels of CHCs and in turn affect their efficacy (Table 47-5).[7,69–72] Currently, most data available regarding drug interactions are with COCs. However, as a precaution the potential drug–drug interactions observed with COCs are also applied to the other CHC dosage formulations (e.g., vaginal ring and transdermal patch).

ANTIBACTERIALS

The antibacterials rifampin and griseofulvin are known to cause contraceptive failure, as these products increase the metabolism of estrogen. For other antibacterials, the possible interaction is more complicated.

EE is conjugated in the liver, excreted in the bile, hydrolyzed by intestinal bacteria, and reabsorbed as active drug.[72] Antibacterials, by reducing the population of intestinal bacteria, interrupt the enterohepatic circulation of the estrogen, resulting in a decreased concentration of circulating estrogen. Theoretically, any antimicrobial with significant effects on intestinal bacterial flora could affect COC efficacy. Numerous reports of changes in bleeding patterns and contraceptive failure have been documented.[72] Cases of pregnancy in COC users taking antibiotics have been reported.[72–74] About 30 case reports of contraceptive failure with concomitant COC and antibiotic use have been published.[72] The antibacterials in the case reports include rifampin, ampicillin, penicillin G, tetracycline, and minocycline. In addition, surveys conducted on patients in clinics have revealed about 20 other cases of COC failure.[72] A major limitation of survey data is that it relies on patient reporting, which is often unreliable. Some believe that the probability of a clinically significant drug interaction between COCs and antibacterials is low and the CDC

Table 47-5
Common Combined Oral Contraceptive (COC) Drug[a] Interactions[42,69–71]

Drugs That Increase Effect of CHCs or Side Effects of CHCs	Drugs/Herbals That Decrease the Effect of CHCs	Drugs That May Decrease the Effect of CHCs (controversial)	Metabolism or Clearance Altered by CHCs (levels of drug listed may either increase or decrease depending on patient)
Acetaminophen	Amprenavir	Amoxicillin	Acetaminophen
Ascorbic acid	Aprepitant	Ampicillin	Amprenavir
Atazanavir	Barbiturates	Ciprofloxacin	Antidepressants, tricyclic
Atorvastatin	Bexarotene	Clarithromycin	Benzodiazepines
Ginseng	Bosentan	Colesevelam	β-blockers
Indinavir	Carbamazepine	Doxycycline	Caffeine
Red clover[b]	Darunavir	Erythromycin	Clofibric acid
Rosuvastatin	Efavirez	Fluconazole	Corticosteroids
Tranexamic acid	Felbamate	Itraconazole	Cyclosporine
Voriconazole	Griseofulvin	Ketoconazole	Lamotrigine
	Isotretinoin	Metronidazole	Levothyroxine
	Lopinavir	Minocycline	Morphine
	Modafinil	Penicillins	Paclitaxel
	Mycophenolate mofetil	Phenylbutazone	Salicylic acid
	Nelfinavir	Ofloxacin	Selegiline
	Nevirapine	Tetracyclines	Tacrine
	Oxcarbazepine	Topiramate	Tacrolimus
	Phenobarbital		Theophyllines
	Phenytoin/Fosphenytoin		Tizanidine
	Pioglitazone		Valproic acid
	Primidone		Voriconazole
	Red clover[b]		Warfarin[c]
	Rifamycins		
	Ritonavir		
	Rufinamide		
	Saquinavir		
	St. John's wort		
	Tipranavir		

[a]Drug list is not all inclusive. Some drug interactions may exist that are not cited in this table.
[b]Indicates drug may have variable effect on CHC either increasing or decreasing effect.
[c]May decrease anticoagulant effect of warfarin, not warfarin drug levels.
CHC, combined hormonal contraceptive.
Source: Borgelt L et al., eds. *Women's Health Across the Lifespan: A Pharmacotherapeutic Approach*. Washington DC: American Society of Health Systems Pharmacists; 2010.

US Medical Eligibility Criteria does not recommend a need for alternative birth control methods while taking broad-spectrum antibiotics that do not affect hepatic enzymes.[7,74,75]

Numerous factors may affect the likelihood of an interaction: the hormonal content of the COC relative to the patient's requirements, the dosage and duration of use of the interacting drug, variation in the patient's response to bacterial flora alteration, and the fertility of the couple.[72] The number and complexity of these variables make prediction of outcome in a specific patient exceedingly difficult. Even if a drug produces a several-fold increase in unintended pregnancies in women taking COCs, the likelihood of pregnancy in a given patient still will be low. For patients who require long-term, low-dose tetracycline use for acne therapy (e.g., tetracycline 250 mg by mouth daily), it is unlikely to interfere with COC efficacy.[74] Alternatively, topical antibacterials often can control acne and are viable alternatives to oral medications.

A practical approach to managing patients taking COCs and antibacterials is to educate patients about the available data. To be conservative, S.F. should be advised to use backup contraception while taking the amoxicillin/clavulanate and to continue the backup method until her next menses occurs though this is controversial and the CDC Medical Eligibility Criteria does not call for it.[7] For other antibiotics that affect hepatic enzymes such as rifampin, isoniazid, and griseofulvin, backup contraception should be used while taking the medication and for 4 weeks after discontinuation of the antibiotics.[7]

HEPATIC ENZYME INDUCTION

Ethinyl estradiol is a substrate of cytochrome P-450 3A4 (CYP3A4), so drugs that induce CYP3A4 activity may decrease COC efficacy. In earlier years, COC efficacy was not decreased significantly by other drugs because of their high hormone content. Because the estrogen and progestin concentrations of COCs have gradually been decreasing, reports of menstrual irregularities (e.g., spotting) and unintended pregnancies attributable to drug interactions have been increasing.

Anticonvulsants such as carbamazepine, oxcarbazepine, phenytoin, phenobarbital, primidone, and topiramate are CYP3A4 inducers and are known to cause increased metabolism of COCs (see Chapter 60, Seizure Disorders).[76] Some studies have shown that another inducer of COC metabolism is St. John's-wort.[77,78] Although drugs can influence COC efficacy, COCs also can affect the activity of other drugs. For example, COCs have been reported to decrease serum levels of lamotrigine and can affect seizure control; as well increased levels of lamotrigine have been reported after COC discontinuation.[79] Other drugs may increase the hormone levels of COCs (Table 47-5), increasing the risk of COC side effects (Table 47-4).

Unlike many drug classes that are carefully dosed to maintain a therapeutic range of monitored blood levels, contraceptive estrogen and progestin blood levels are obtained only in clinical drug studies. Therefore, patients are managed by monitoring side effects and by changes in menstrual patterns. Some prescribers suggest using a 50-mcg EE COC in patients taking interacting drugs, although others might recommend using an alternative method of contraception if drug interactions are an issue.

Noncontraceptive Benefits of Combined Hormonal Contraceptives

ACNE

CASE 47-2

QUESTION 1: D.S., a 20-year-old woman, presents to her primary-care physician for a yearly pelvic examination and also complains of moderate acne flares. She has tried a variety of treatments without resolution and is currently using only topical medications. She heard birth control pills can help acne, especially if it occurs right before her period. She also complains of fatigue most days of the month and mood changes, cravings, cramps, and bloating near the time of her period.

Vitals: weight, 118 lb; height, 5′3″
Blood pressure, 118/75 mm Hg
Heart rate, 86 beats/minute
Respiratory rate, 13 breaths/minute
Temperature, 98.6°F
Past medical history: acne (since age 16)
Social history: denies tobacco and alcohol use, not sexually active
Family history: older sister cervical dysplasia grade 2 (age 26), maternal grandmother breast (age 61) and ovarian cancer (age 68)
Allergies: no known drug allergies
Current medications: benzoyl peroxide 5% cream, apply topically twice daily
Benzoyl peroxide 2.5% wash, wash affected area twice daily
Retin-A micro 0.1%, apply topically twice a week as tolerated
Multivitamin with iron by mouth daily
Past medications: doxycycline 100 mg by mouth twice daily for acne, stopped because of vaginal yeast infections
Physical examination: unremarkable with the exception of moderate facial acne
Laboratory test results: white blood cells, $6.0 \times 10^3/\mu L$
Red blood cells, $3.9 \times 10^6/\mu L$
Hemoglobin, 10.8 g/dL
Hematocrit, 32%
Mean cell volume, 79 μL
Mean corpuscular hemoglobin concentration, 31 g/dL
Red blood cell diameter width, 15%

What effect, if any, would CHCs have on her acne? Does D.S. qualify for CHC treatment of acne, and if so, which COC would you recommend for D.S.?

Depending on the patient, a CHC may cause acne to appear, disappear, or significantly improve.[4] D.S. is interested in COCs. Four COC products (norethindrone acetate/EE [Tri-Legest 21 and Tri-Legest Fe 28], norgestimate/EE [Ortho Tri-Cyclen], and drospirenone/EE [YAZ, Beyaz]) are US Food and Drug Administration (FDA)-approved for the treatment of moderate acne vulgaris in women at least 15 years old (at least 14 years old for Beyaz and YAZ), who have no known contraindications to CHCs, reached menarche, desire contraception, and have failed topical acne treatments (Tri-Legest 21, Tri-Legest Fe 28, and Ortho Tri-Cyclen). Most CHCs, however, improve acne mainly as a result of the estrogen component. Higher doses of estrogen may decrease acne by suppressing the activity of sebaceous glands, decreasing the production of androgens, and increasing the synthesis of sex hormone-binding globulin (SHBG). The SHBG binds androgens and thereby diminishes their effects.[80] Progestins with higher androgenic activity may be more likely to increase acne because they stimulate sebaceous glands to produce more sebum. Both desogestrel- and norgestimate-containing oral contraceptives are less androgenic, whereas drospirenone has antiandrogenic properties, thereby decreasing acne associated with androgenic activity.[81] D.S. is 20 years old, has reached menarche, and has not responded to different acne treatments, and she therefore is a candidate for COC therapy. Her acne appears to be hormonally mediated, particularly because it appears around the time of her menses. It is likely that D.S.'s acne should improve with COC use, particularly if she uses a formulation with higher estrogenic activity and low androgenic activity (e.g., Beyaz, Safyral YAZ, Yasmin, Ortho Tri-Cyclen, Ortho Tri-Cyclen Lo, Mircette, Tri-Legest 21; see Table 47-3).

MENSTRUAL CYCLE BENEFITS

CASE 47-2, QUESTION 2: D.S. has iron-deficiency anemia, likely attributed to heavy menses. Will a COC help reduce her menstrual bleeding or menstrual cramps?

COCs help regulate menstrual cycles and reduce monthly blood loss.[28] This may reflect the progressive thinning of the endometrium of COC users and the lack of irregular bleeding. Bleeding may be decreased the most by COCs that have a high ratio of progestin to estrogen because endometrial thinning is maximized.[53] Some COCs have iron pills instead of placebos, often denoted with "Fe" in the name (e.g., Tri-Legest Fe 28, Femcon Fe, Loestrin Fe, Lo Loestrin Fe). Others have folic acid (e.g., Beyaz, Safyral) but D.S. would likely benefit more from the formulations with iron. Another option would be to have D.S. take COCs continuously so she has fewer menses.

Dysmenorrhea, or painful menstruation, may be of unknown origin or may be attributable to endometriosis or uterine fibroids. Data suggest menstrual pain might decrease by 60% after the initiation of a COC.[3] A COC with decreased estrogenic and increased progestational activity may be the best at relieving dysmenorrhea (see Chapter 50, Disorders Related to the Menstrual Cycle).

PREMENSTRUAL SYNDROME AND PREMENSTRUAL DYSPHORIC DISORDER

CASE 47-2, QUESTION 3: D.S. also complains of PMS symptoms such as bloating and mood changes. What treatment approaches are appropriate? What other noncontraceptive benefits do CHCs have?

Premenstrual syndrome (PMS) is a cyclic occurrence of one or more symptoms before the onset of menses. Most women complain of at least one PMS symptom, which includes irritability, bloating, and depressed mood.[82] Premenstrual dysphoric disorder (PMDD) is a more severe form of PMS and has diagnostic criteria by the American Psychiatric Association. Premenstrual tension has been reported to be reduced in COC users, and other premenstrual symptoms seem to improve as well. Nevertheless, the effect of COCs on PMS symptoms is inconsistent and unpredictable, probably because PMS symptoms are neither consistent nor predictable.[83]

There may be augmentation of depression and mood swings by the progestational component, although the probability of this effect is low with a low-dose product (see Chapter 50, Disorders Related to the Menstrual Cycle, for further discussion of PMS). Some patients may also notice depressed mood during the hormone-free period, in which case a continuous-use COC may be helpful.

Two products, drospirenone/EE (YAZ, Beyaz), have the FDA-approved indication for treatment of symptoms of PMDD. Drospirenone/EE has been studied most extensively in patients with PMDD.[42] D.S. may try any CHC to help with her PMS symptoms; however, because YAZ and Beyaz have more data to show that they are effective for PMDD and acne, one of them may be the preferred initial product for her. In addition, both products are 24-day formulations, which may help minimize her menstrual bleeding and help her iron-deficiency anemia.

ENDOMETRIAL CANCER

Clinical data suggest that COCs protect against endometrial cancer. This effect continues for 20 years after the last pill.[83] The protection is directly related to duration of use and may persist for many years after discontinuation of the COC.[4] A meta-analysis of 11 studies showed a 56%, 67%, and 72% reduction in endometrial cancer risk after 4, 8, and 12 years of COC use, respectively.[84]

OVARIAN CANCER AND FUNCTIONAL OVARIAN CYSTS

The risk of developing functional ovarian cysts is decreased, preexisting cysts are more rapidly resolved, and surgery rates for ovarian masses are reduced in women taking COCs.[85,86] This is likely attributable to reducing ovulation, suppressing androgen production, or increasing progesterone levels.

Each year of COC use decreases the relative risk of developing ovarian cancer by 7% to 9%.[86] The risk reduction continues to be seen in women using COCs for more than 15 years and persists after discontinuation.[83] D.S. should be reassured that COC use may decrease her risk of ovarian cancer given that she has a positive family history.

Combined Hormonal Contraceptive Risks and Adverse Effects

Some patients may not be candidates for CHCs because of the risks and adverse effects associated with their use. Other patients may experience minor side effects with CHCs that may be managed by changing to a CHC with different types or doses of estrogen or progestin. All patients should be counseled on the most serious side effects, which include pulmonary embolism or VTE, hepatotoxicity, or visual disturbances (could be a sign of retinal and corneal changes in the eye) and stroke. A helpful acronym to remember when counseling is "ACHES" (Table 47-2),[3] which can be used to increase a patient's awareness of serious potential adverse effects that warrant immediate medical attention.

Other less severe adverse effects are listed in Table 47-4.[53] Most side effects resolve within 3 months of use. If a patient experiences adverse effects other than those described in "ACHES," (Table 47-2) she should be encouraged to continue the CHC for at least 3 months before switching to a different contraceptive.

BREAKTHROUGH BLEEDING, SPOTTING, AND AMENORRHEA

CASE 47-2, QUESTION 4: D.S. comes to the family planning clinic after taking EE 20 mcg/drospirenone 3 mg (YAZ) for 2 months. She had been started on YAZ to help with her acne. She feels her acne has improved but reports irregular menstrual bleeding during her last two menstrual cycles which occurs around the third week of the pill pack and requires a pad. What action should be taken to correct D.S.'s bleeding pattern?

Intermenstrual bleeding is a bleeding that occurs at times other than the regular menses timing. Intermenstrual bleeding that requires a pad or tampon is designated breakthrough bleeding, whereas a lesser amount of intermenstrual bleeding is called spotting. Intermenstrual bleeding is experienced by many women in the first months of starting COCs (30%–50%).[3] Intermenstrual bleeding may also occur if a patient is not adherent to her COCs or taking medications that decrease COC effectiveness (Table 47-5).

Most clinicians will recommend that patients continue the same COC for at least 3 months if breakthrough bleeding or spotting is the only complaint, because this complication usually resolves within 3 months.[3] Early-cycle intermenstrual bleeding, which usually starts before the 14th day of the menstrual cycle (or never ceases completely after menses), is usually caused by insufficient estrogen. Late-cycle intermenstrual bleeding, occurring after day 14, is usually attributable to insufficient progestational support of the endometrium. Another cause of intermenstrual bleeding is drug interactions (see Case 47-1, Question 8, for more information about drug interactions).

The balance between estrogen and progestin components in COCs determines its endometrial activity and, therefore, the likelihood of intermenstrual bleeding problems. It may be helpful to envision the estrogen component as the basic building blocks or "bricks" of the endometrium and the progestational component providing the mortar that holds the bricks together. The estrogenic activity of the progestin component increases the number of bricks, whereas its antiestrogenic activity decreases their numbers. If there are not enough bricks or mortar or if they are present in the wrong proportions, the wall will crumble and bleeding will occur (Table 47-3).

If D.S.'s intermenstrual bleeding continues late in her cycle after 3 months, another COC with the same estrogen activity, more progestin activity, and low androgen activity should be prescribed. Desogestrel 0.15 mg/EE 30 mcg (e.g., Apri, Reclipsen) would be a good choice because progestational activity would be increased and estrogenic activity would be maintained with minimal androgenic liability (Table 47-3). If D.S. had experienced intermenstrual bleeding early in the cycle after several months of use, she should be changed to a formulation with a higher ratio of estrogen to progestin such as norethindrone 0.4 mg/EE 35 mcg (e.g.,Ovcon-35, Femcon Fe, Balziva, Zenchent). For D.S., products with low androgenic activity should be selected because of her acne.

Intermenstrual bleeding may also be the sign of other health conditions such as cervical or uterine cancer. If a patient presents with intermenstrual bleeding and has not had a recent pelvic examination, a healthcare provider may perform an examination to rule out other possible causes of intermenstrual bleeding. D.S. recently had a normal pelvic examination 2 months ago. Given the timing of when she began her COCs, it is likely her intermenstrual bleeding is caused by her COCs.

Some patients experience amenorrhea (no menstrual bleeding) with CHCs. If this occurs, pregnancy should first be ruled out. If the patient is not pregnant and amenorrhea is acceptable to the patient, then the CHC need not be changed. But this does make it difficult for the patient to recognize whether she may become pregnant in the future.

NAUSEA

CASE 47-2, QUESTION 5: D.S. continues to have intermenstrual bleeding late in her cycle after 3 months of use and is placed on a new COC. Five days after starting norethindrone 0.4 mg/EE 35 mcg (e.g., Ovcon-35), D.S. calls with complaints of nausea. What counseling should the clinician provide to D.S.?

Nausea from COCs can generally be attributed to the estrogen component. To help alleviate nausea, D.S. can take her pill at bedtime rather than in the morning. Another alternative may be to take it with food or to try another COC with a lower estrogen strength or property. Ovcon-35 has a higher amount of EE as compared with YAZ (35 mcg of EE vs. 20 mcg of EE), which may be causing nausea to D.S. D.S. should be advised that nausea generally resolves within 3 months of use.

HEADACHE

CASE 47-2, QUESTION 6: Three months later, D.S. returns to the clinic for follow-up and states that she has daily headaches during her placebo week but not when she is taking active pills. How should she be managed?

Headache is a common complaint in women taking CHCs or COCs, as is the case with D.S. Women may notice headaches while taking active pills, which may be related to sensitivity of estrogen. Others may experience headaches during the placebo week as a result of the withdrawal of estrogen.[3] Women with migraines may find that their headaches either improve or worsen when CHCs are initiated.

Mild headaches may improve with time or if the woman is changed to a pill with less estrogen or progestin. Headaches that occur during the placebo week can be managed by trying desogestrel 0.15 mg/EE 10 to 20 mcg (e.g., Mircette, Kariva), which minimizes the estrogen withdrawal by having only 2 days of placebos, or by taking CHCs continuously (i.e., skipping placebo pills or the hormone-free week). Patients with severe headaches should discontinue CHCs and should be evaluated by their healthcare provider (see Contraindications above). D.S. is experiencing headaches during the placebo week, indicating withdrawal of estrogen as the cause. Skipping the placebo pills and using an extended-cycle regimen may help decrease D.S.'s headaches.

WEIGHT GAIN

CASE 47-2, QUESTION 7: During the same visit, D.S. states she is gaining weight and feels "bloated on and off" since starting the new birth control pill. What might be happening, and how should the clinician respond?

Weight gain associated with CHC use is another common concern for women. A Cochrane review of three trials concluded that available evidence was insufficient to determine an association between COCs and weight gain and also stated no large effect was seen.[87] If weight gain is a concern, a low-dose estrogen and low-dose progestin products should be considered. Cyclic weight gain is generally caused by the mineralocorticoid effects of EE-stimulating aldosterone receptors to retain sodium, causing water retention and bloating. Too much progestin may cause an increased appetite and noncyclic weight gain. Drospirenone with antimineralocorticoid properties opposes EE effects, resulting in less water retention and weight gain, and increases in appetite may not be as apparent. D.S. recently increased her estrogen dose, which may be causing the "on and off" bloated feeling and weight gain. She also stopped taking a drospirenone-containing product, which may be why she did not experience the effects of bloating and weight gain with the previous product. The clinician should explain that weight gain is a potential side effect associated with COC use and is likely related to the estrogen component. It is reasonable to consider an alternative COC because she is having estrogen withdrawal headaches and weight gain. Desogestrel 0.15 mg/EE 10 to 20 mcg (e.g., Mircette) has lower estrogen activity than norethindrone 0.4 mg/EE 35 mcg (e.g., Ovcon-35; Table 47-3), which may help to decrease the cyclic weight gain and headaches while still helping to control her acne. In addition, desogestrel 0.15 mg/EE 10 to 20 mcg retains high progestational activity to address D.S.'s previous breakthrough bleeding and has low androgenic activity that will likely help her acne.

BREAST CANCER, CERVICAL DYSPLASIA, AND CERVICAL CANCER

CASE 47-2, QUESTION 8: The medical history and physical examination of D.S. are negative for breast and cervical diseases, except for a history of breast cancer in her maternal grandmother and a history of cervical dysplasia in her sister. D.S. asks how COC use will affect her risk of breast cancer and cervical cancer.

There are conflicting data regarding the association of COC use and breast cancer. The reported overall lifetime risk of breast cancer in American women is 12% to 13%.[88] Older studies have indicated a possible link between COC use and breast cancer.[89–92] More recent studies suggest that COC use does not increase breast cancer risk even with long-term use (e.g., 10 years).[93,94] In addition, other studies concluded breast cancer rates in high-risk women with BRCA 1 and 2 mutations or strong family history of breast cancer did not increase with COC use.[95,96] The American Congress of Obstetricians and Gynecologists (ACOG) does not consider a family history of breast cancer (including BRCA 1 and 2) or benign breast disease a contraindication to COC use.[26]

COCs would not be expected to increase the risk of breast cancer in D.S. She should be instructed to perform monthly breast self-examinations and to return annually for a physical examination by her primary-care physician.

With regard to D.S.'s concern of cervical cancer, it is important to educate D.S. about the incidence of cervical cancer and its relation to COC use. The American Cancer Society estimates that more than 12,000 cases of invasive cervical cancer will be diagnosed in 2017 and more than 4,000 women will die of it.[97] Behavior, not genetics, is the usual cause of cervical cancer.

Women at highest risk for cancer are those who are positive for certain subtypes of human papillomavirus (HPV), who have certain sexual behaviors, who are immunosuppressed, or who smoke.[3] Sexual behaviors associated with cervical cancer include beginning sexual activity at a young age, having multiple male sexual partners, and having a male sexual partner who has multiple partners. Women at low risk for cancer are those who have two or fewer partners, whose partners use condoms, and who do not smoke.

Pooled data on cervical cancer risk from eight case–control studies found that oral contraceptive users positive for HPV were more likely to develop cervical cancer.[98] Women who had ever used oral contraceptives and those who had used oral contraceptives for more than 5 years were 1.5 and 3.4 times, respectively, more likely to develop cervical cancer. This is consistent with older studies that suggest that oral contraceptive users have an increased risk of developing or dying of cervical cancer. In contrast, a large cohort study conducted in England found no significant increase in deaths attributable to cervical cancer in women who had ever used COCs.[99]

Epidemiologic comparisons of the prevalence of cervical cancer in oral contraceptive users versus nonusers often are difficult to interpret because yearly medical examinations and regular Pap smears of COC users result in early detection and treatment of precancerous lesions. Three vaccines for HPV are available for women aged 9 to 26 years. Because D.S. is 20 years old, she may be a candidate for the HPV vaccine (see Chapter 64, Vaccinations). D.S. may use COCs, should be encouraged to have regular Pap smears, and should be counseled on the behaviors that put her at risk for cervical cancer and the risks and benefits of the HPV vaccine.

USE DURING PREGNANCY AND BREAST-FEEDING

CASE 47-3

QUESTION 1: P.K., a 35-year-old woman, comes to clinic stating that she recently took a home pregnancy test that reported a positive result. Her last menstrual period (LMP) was 9 weeks ago. She would like to confirm the results and discuss the effects of her current medications on her unborn baby.

Vitals: weight, 143 lb; height, 5′6″
Blood pressure, 128/82 mm Hg
Heart rate, 97 beats/minute
Respiratory rate, 16 breaths/minute
Temperature, 98.6°F
Past medical history: history of abnormal menses, initiated on COC therapy to help regulate
Medications: desogestrel 0.15 mg/EE 30 mcg (Reclipsen)
Laboratory test results: blood test, qualitative human chorionic gonadotropin >25 mIU/mL

P.K. was started on desogestrel 0.15 mg/EE 30 mcg (Reclipsen) extended regimen 3 months ago because of a history of abnormal menstrual periods. Unknowingly, she became pregnant in the first month and continued her COC for two cycles, and is now 8-week pregnant. What can you tell P.K. about the possible effects of CHC use on her unborn child?

The fact that CHCs were classified as pregnancy category X (contraindicated, fetal risks clearly outweigh maternal benefit) is very misleading.[100] Although older, poorly designed studies found an association between COC use and cardiac or limb anomalies, newer data suggest that CHC use does not substantially increase the risk of anomalies over that expected in other uneventful pregnancies.[4]

Although a CHC should not be started in a woman who might possibly be pregnant, P.K. should be instructed to stop using her COC and be reassured that the risks to her fetus from the use [illegible]ose CHC during the first trimester are likely minimal, [illegible]nforming her no drug is without risk and she should [illegible]th her obstetrician.

CASE 47-3, QUESTION 2: P.K. plans to breast-feed her infant and begin some types of contraception after her discharge from the hospital. Her past experience with condoms and concurrent spermicidal foams or gels resulted in itching and burning. She indicates she would like a contraceptive that would be suitable for long-term use while breast-feeding. What contraceptives are best for her while she is breast-feeding?

P.K. may use CHCs 6 weeks after she has her baby even if she is breast-feeding, although it is preferable for her to use a progestin-only method.[26] The ACOG recommends waiting at least 6 weeks before starting any estrogen-containing contraceptive regardless of breast-feeding status. By this time, the increased risk of thrombosis that occurs during pregnancy should be reduced to baseline. For non-breast-feeding women, a progestin-only contraceptive may be used immediately postpartum and 6 weeks postpartum if solely breast-feeding and in some cases 3 weeks postpartum if partially breast-feeding.[26] However, COCs have been reported to decrease milk quantity and quality.[26] Therefore, many providers suggest avoiding CHCs in women who are exclusively breast-feeding. If P.K. is planning to breast-feed, a progestin-only contraceptive is probably best and may be started 6 weeks postpartum to ensure the newborn is able to metabolize and clear the medication because progestins enter breast milk.

PROGESTIN-ONLY CONTRACEPTIVES

Progestin-Only Pill (Minipill)

CASE 47-3, QUESTION 3: What advantages and disadvantages of the minipill should you discuss with P.K.?

ADVANTAGES

The minipill is devoid of some of the nuisance side effects (Table 47-4) caused by estrogen (e.g., headaches, chloasma).[3] More importantly, estrogen-mediated hypertension and clotting factor changes will be avoided. Confusion with pill taking is minimized because there is no placebo week and all 28 pills in each pack are the same. Therefore, the missed-dose directions are the same whenever any pill is missed. Minipills also have noncontraceptive benefits, including decreased dysmenorrhea and bleeding and possible protection against pelvic inflammatory disease (PID) and endometrial cancer.[3] Women may also choose them because they are not estrogen containing and fertility returns rapidly after discontinuation.[3]

Theoretically, progestin use in the early postpartum period may decrease milk production because milk production is triggered by the decline in progesterone that occurs after delivery. However, no data have consistently shown this to be a problem in postpartum women.[26] Once breast-feeding has been established, progestins have not been shown to interfere with the quantity or quality of milk produced by a nursing mother. Thus, a contraceptive method that is nonhormonal or only contains progestin is preferred for a patient who plans to breast-feed her infant.

DISADVANTAGES

The minipill, with a failure rate of 0.3% to 8%, is similarly effective as COCs in preventing pregnancies (Table 47-1).[3] Minipills, however, must be taken even more regularly than COCs, and therefore, are not used often in women who are not breast-feeding (see Patient Instructions below). Some women on minipills ovulate regularly, and some shift back and forth between ovulatory and anovulatory (no ovulation occurring) menstrual cycles. Women who consistently have menses on the minipill may be ovulating and should consider using a backup contraception or changing to a different method.

Irregular menses, decreased duration, and amount of menstrual flow, spotting, or amenorrhea commonly occur in women taking the minipill.[3] Because of this, patients often are concerned that they may be pregnant. Women who are exclusively breast-feeding will usually have amenorrhea. The high incidence of irregular menses associated with the minipill may mask underlying disease such as uterine fibroids or uterine cancer causing irregular bleeding. Other side effects reported with minipills include headaches, breast tenderness, mood changes, and nausea.

Minipills should be avoided if there is a personal history of breast cancer or unexplained vaginal bleeding. Caution should be exercised when using minipills in women with hepatic disease, multiple risk factors for cardiovascular diseases, ischemic heart disease, a current deep venous thrombosis or PE, or complicated diabetes (e.g., diabetes with nephropathy, neuropathy, retinopathy), or those taking medications that may interact with COCs such as hepatic inducers, St. John's-wort, and Bosentan (Table 47-5).[101,102]

PATIENT INSTRUCTIONS FOR THE PROGESTIN-ONLY PILL

CASE 47-3, QUESTION 4: What instructions should P.K. receive regarding the use of a minipill?

P.K. may begin taking the minipill on the first day of her menses.[3] Because she is breast-feeding and recently postpartum, she is less likely to have a menses. She could begin taking minipills immediately postpartum if she were not breast-feeding. Because she is breast-feeding, it is recommended that she has to wait until 3 weeks postpartum if partially breast-feeding and 6 weeks postpartum to begin minipills if solely breast-feeding. If at 6 weeks postpartum, P.K. started her minipills on the first day of her menses, a backup contraception is not needed with the day 1 start. Alternatively, P.K. can use the quick start method, starting any day of her cycle and using a backup method for 48 hours.[3]

P.K. should be instructed to take the pill at the exact same time each day. If she is more than 3 hours late taking a pill, she should take the pill as soon as she remembers and should use backup contraception for 48 hours. This is quite different from the directions for COCs, so this point should be stressed with patients.

Injectable Medroxyprogesterone Acetate

Progestin-only contraceptives are available in two different injectable formulations of medroxyprogesterone acetate (MPA). Depo-Provera is given as a 150-mg intramuscular injection in the deltoid or gluteus maximus every 11 to 13 weeks.[3,103] More recently, depo-subQ provera 104 was approved. This product also contains MPA; however, it is given subcutaneously as a 104-mg dose every 12 to 14 weeks.[104] Injectable MPA inhibits ovulation, thickens the cervical mucus, and suppresses endometrial growth, making it a very effective contraceptive. Package inserts instruct the patient to begin the injectable MPA methods in the first 5 days of her menses and then no backup is required; however, P.K. may also begin any other time and use backup for 1 week.[3,103]

CASE 47-3, QUESTION 5: P.K. is now lactating and returns to the gynecology clinic for her second IM injection of MPA. She was given her first injection 3 months ago, immediately postpartum. She is experiencing prolonged intermenstrual bleeding and a 3- to 5-pound weight gain. Is this to be expected? What are the advantages and disadvantages of injectable MPA? How are the side effects managed?

ADVANTAGES

Injectable MPA is a reasonable contraceptive choice for P.K. because she is breast-feeding and indicated she needed a long-term contraceptive. Among its benefits are a low failure rate of 0.3% to 3% (Table 47-1), ease of use, lack of estrogenic side effects, decreased dysmenorrhea and monthly blood loss, and a reduced risk of endometrial cancer.[3,26] Other noncontraceptive benefits may include a reduction in seizure frequency in epileptic patients and a possible reduction in ovarian cancer.[3,26] Furthermore, contraceptive efficacy is not reduced by the concurrent use of anticonvulsants or certain antibacterials as is seen with COCs.[6,7] Depo-subQ provera 104 is also indicated for pain caused by endometriosis.[104]

DISADVANTAGES

Patients with breast cancer should not use injectable MPA owing to concerns that breast cancers are hormonally sensitive and the prognosis may worsen for some women.[6,7] Injectable MPA should be used with caution in women with unexplained vaginal bleeding (MPA may cause irregular bleeding and may mask conditions resulting in vaginal bleeding such as cervical or uterine cancer), multiple risk factors for cardiovascular diseases, ischemic heart disease or multiple risk factors for cerebrovascular disease, or a current VTE or PE (for medical eligibility, see https://www.cdc.gov/mmwr/volumes/65/rr/rr6503a1.htm?s_cid=rr6503a1_w).[7] Because clotting factors have not been shown to be clinically affected by injectable MPA, some experts disagree with the manufacturer's labeling for the injectable MPA products, which lists a history of prior thromboembolism as a contraindication.[5–7,103,104] Some clinicians also begin injectable MPA immediately postpartum rather than waiting 6 weeks postpartum, as directed by the package insert.[7]

Estrogen production declines in women using injectable MPA, so P.K. should be told that injectable MPA may decrease bone mineral density (BMD).[103] Loss of BMD may be of particular concern in adolescent patients. Numerous studies have found that women receiving injectable MPA have lower BMD compared with nonusers.[105] Although there have been reports of stress fractures in injectable MPA users, no studies to date have documented an increased rate of hip or vertebral fractures in injectable MPA users.[106] Also, BMD has been shown to recover after discontinuation of the injections.[4] The manufacturer of both products recommends that patients do not use injectable MPA longer than 2 years unless they are unwilling or unable to use other methods.[103]

P.K. must understand that injectable MPA frequently causes irregular bleeding or spotting during the first few months or more of use because estrogen is insufficient to maintain the endometrium. After 1 and 2 years of Depo Provera use, 55% and 68% of women experience amenorrhea, respectively.[103] With depo-subQ provera 104, 56.5% of patients experienced amenorrhea after 1 year.[104] In addition, during the postpartum period, irregular bleeding may occur as well. Although not harmful, amenorrhea leads to discontinuation of injectable MPA in 13% of patients.[103] All patients beginning injectable MPA should be informed that during the first year of use they might have menstrual changes. If unusually heavy or continuous bleeding occurs, P.K. should be evaluated. P.K. should be counseled and reassured that her intermenstrual bleeding probably will resolve in the next few months. If the bleeding is bothersome, a 4- to 21-day course of oral estrogen (e.g., conjugated estrogen 0.625–2.5 mg/day) or a COC with 20 mcg of EE will minimize or eliminate the bleeding.[8] However, the bleeding may recur after discontinuation of the estrogen. Low-dose estrogen may be continued if bleeding recurs.

Weight gain is another concern with injectable MPA. The mean weight gain after 1 year of therapy with injectable MPA was about 5 lb in two-thirds of users.[103] Depo-Provera users typically gair total of about 8 lb in 2 years, nearly 14 lb in 4 years, and 16

6 years. Depo-subQ provera users gain a little less weight, 3.5 lb in the first year of use, and 7.5 lb after 2 years.[104] Other side effects include mood changes, hair loss, and headaches. P.K. should be counseled on the weight gain associated with injectable MPA. P.K. has already reported an increase in weight since she gave birth 3 months ago, which may be caused by injectable MPA, or possibly her weight is fluctuating because of her recent delivery.

The long return to fertility time is another disadvantage of injectable MPA. After the last injection of 150 mg of MPA, conception was delayed approximately 10 months in half of users.[96] The remaining users took longer to become pregnant, with nearly all users becoming pregnant by 18 months. There are less data on return of fertility with the 104-mg dose of MPA. A small study showed that the median time to ovulation was 10 months, with most women ovulating within 1 year of their last injection.[104] Because P.K. is 35 years old, she should be counseled on the return to fertility time with injectable MPA use in case she desired to have children in the near future. She has indicated that she is not interested in having any more children; however, the long return to fertility time with injectable MPA should be explained to all women, especially those older than 35 years of age.

Subdermal Implant

CASE 47-3, QUESTION 6: P.K. returns to the clinic 7 months postpartum for her third MPA injection. She started menstruating today after missing two appointments; she is now 1 month late for her MPA dose. She states her busy family life and work schedule make it difficult to attend appointments. She also does not like the weight gain and prolonged intermenstrual bleeding that has occurred during the past few months. She read that an implant is available and she would like to know whether this might be a better option for her. What information should you give P.K.?

The contraceptive implant (Nexplanon) contains 68 mg of etonogestrel in a single, thin, radiopaque, rod.[107] The rod is inserted subdermally in the upper inner arm using a needle and a local anesthetic. Once inserted, the implant is effective for up to 3 years. Nexplanon should be inserted during the first 5 days of menses, and no backup contraception is required. A small incision is required to remove the implant. The etonogestrel implant has the same mechanism of action as injectable MPA. The product was first marketed as Implanon; however, Implanon was not radiopaque and at times difficult to locate for removal. The radiopaque property of Nexplanon is preferred for ease of removal; therefore, Implanon is no longer manufactured.

ADVANTAGES

The contraceptive implant is a relatively new product, so information on its protection against cancers or effects on other diseases such as cardiovascular disease is limited. Women using the implant reported amenorrhea, decreased menstrual cramping, and less anemia than nonusers.[3] Also, decreases in BMD have not been shown with this product. Fertility returns quickly after the removal of the implant, and this will be a benefit to P.K. if she decides to have another child, given her age.

DISADVANTAGES

As with the injectables, irregular bleeding is likely and is the most common cause of discontinuation. Side effects reported with the implant are headaches, mood changes, and acne. Nexplanon is not recommended for patients on medications [illegible]duce hepatic enzymes (e.g., anticonvulsants) as they may [illegible]ntraceptive efficacy. Weight gain is also common, [illegible]ining 2.8 lb after 1 year and 3.7 lb after 2 years.[108] [illegible]ill experience weight gain with this product. The implant is not recommended for patients with a current VTE; however, it may be used in patients with a personal or family history of VTE.[6,7]

INTRAUTERINE DEVICE AND INTRAUTERINE SYSTEM

CASE 47-3, QUESTION 7: P.K. is concerned about weight gain and is not interested in a subdermal implant. What other long-term, reversible contraceptive methods might work for her? Is P.K. a candidate for an intrauterine device (IUD) or intrauterine system (IUS), and if so, what information would you provide her?

Background and Mechanism of Action

Despite concerns (increased risk of PID, tubal scarring, and infertility) with early IUDs, also known as intrauterine contraceptives (IUCs), the current devices offer a safe and effective method of contraception.[110] Currently, there are four products on the market that include the ParaGard T 380A (copper) IUD, Mirena, Skyla, Kyleena, and Liletta (levonorgestrel) IUSs. Although the IUDs and IUSs available today are a safe and effective method of contraception, they are still not as popular in the United States (1%–6% of women are users) as they are worldwide (12% of married women of reproductive age are users).[110–112]

The copper IUD has a polyethylene body that is wound with copper wire. Once inserted, the copper IUD may be left in place for 10 years.[113] The Mirena, Skyla, Kyleena, and Liletta IUSs also have polyethylene bodies, with levonorgestrel reservoirs in the vertical stem of the T that provide levonorgestrel daily. Mirena and Kyleena are effective for 5 years and provide 20 mcg and 17.5 mcg of levonorgestrel daily, respectively.[114,115] Skyla is slightly smaller in size and provides 14 mcg of levonorgestrel daily after 24 days and is effective for up to 3 years.[116] Similarly, Liletta is effective for 3 years and provides levonorgestrel 18.6 mcg daily, decreasing to 16.3 mcg at 1 year, 14.3 mcg at 2 years, and 12.6 mcg at 3 years.[117]

Failure rate of the copper IUD is 0.6% to 0.8% for the first year compared with 0.2% for the levonorgestrel IUS (Table 47-1). Both IUDs and IUSs are inserted by a healthcare provider in the office. The procedure usually takes only a few minutes and does not require sedation. Many providers will recommend that patients take a dose of an NSAID before the insertion visit.

Possible mechanisms of action for copper IUDs include prevention of fertilization and implantation and the copper interfering with sperm transport, viability, or number.[113] The levonorgestrel IUS is believed to work by thickening the cervical mucus, preventing sperm from entering the uterus, altering the endometrial lining, preventing ovulation, and altering sperm activity.[113]

Advantages

Both the copper IUD and the levonorgestrel IUS are very effective, reversible, long-term methods that are easy to comply with.[3] The copper IUD is a particularly beneficial option for women who desire a nonhormonal method of contraception. The levonorgestrel IUS has the advantages of reducing menstrual bleeding and cramping as a result of the progestin.

Although the initial cost of inserting an IUD or IUS is high (around $500 for the device plus insertion costs), there are no ongoing monthly costs to P.K. as there are with other methods. Therefore, the IUD or IUS becomes more cost-effective when used for more than 1 year.

Disadvantages

Menstrual changes are the most common side effect of IUDs and IUSs.[3] Copper IUD users are more likely to have heavier menstrual bleeding and cramping. Levonorgestrel users should expect to have irregular bleeding and spotting during the first 3 months after insertion. After 3 months, however, levonorgestrel IUS users report lighter menses and reduced cramping.

Both IUDs and IUSs are contraindicated in women with certain anatomic abnormalities of the uterus (e.g., distortion of the uterus, cervical stenosis, or cervical lacerations), unexplained vaginal bleeding, cervical cancer, and PID or other active genital infections. They should be used with caution in women who are HIV-positive or are immunosuppressed (for medical eligibility, see https://www.cdc.gov/mmwr/volumes/65/rr/rr6503a1.htm?s_cid=rr6503a1_w).[7] The levonorgestrel IUSs should be used with caution in women with a current VTE or PE. Although the serum levels of levonorgestrel are low, the manufacturers currently do not recommend that women with active or past breast cancer use the device.

Both IUDs and IUSs are preferred for women in monogamous relationships or who are able to have strict use of condoms as IUD users are more likely to experience PID than nonusers. For all patients, the greatest risk of PID occurs shortly after insertion.[118] To prevent this from occurring, all patients should be tested for gonorrhea and chlamydia before IUD or IUS insertion and evaluated for risk factors of contracting STIs (e.g., multiple partners, unprotected intercourse). Women who are positive for an STI should consider an alternative form of contraception until the infection has resolved. Alternatively, once treatment is provided, an IUD or IUS may be initiated and the woman counseled on ways to prevent STIs.[6,7]

If an IUD or IUS user becomes pregnant, the likelihood that the pregnancy is ectopic is higher (i.e., the ratio of ectopic to uterine pregnancies is higher in IUD or IUS users).[113,114] Common complaints of IUD use include excessive uterine bleeding, spotting, or pain. The device may be removed as a result of these issues. Spontaneous expulsion of the IUD occurs in about 2% to 6% of women within the first year.[3] Rarely, an IUD or IUS may become embedded in the endometrium or partially or totally perforate the uterine wall. P.K. should be instructed to look for the warning signs of a possible complication with IUD or IUS use, such as abdominal pain or abnormal vaginal discharge.

OTHER NONHORMONAL CONTRACEPTION

CASE 47-4

QUESTION 1: C.J. is a 22-year-old HIV+ woman presenting to the clinic for routine checkup and depot medroxyprogesterone acetate injection. She is currently using depot medroxyprogesterone acetate IM injection every 12 weeks and taking Atripla (efavirenz 600 mg/tenofovir 300 mg/emtricitabine 200 mg) 1 tablet by mouth daily.

Vitals today: height, 5′6″; weight, 116 lb
Blood pressure, 124/81 mm Hg
Heart rate, 89 beats/minute
Respiratory rate, 12 breaths/minute
Temperature, 96.8°F
Laboratory test results: CD4, 581
HIV-1 RNA, <75 copies/mL (undetectable)

C.J. wants to make sure she does not get pregnant and is recommended to use a barrier method in addition to depot medroxyprogesterone acetate. C.J. mentions that she is concerned about STIs and more specifically transmission of HIV. What barrier methods are available, and which one is best to recommend for C.J.?

Diaphragm and Cervical Cap

The diaphragm is a soft latex or silicone rubber cap with a metal spring reinforcing the rim.[3] The device is inserted vaginally and placed over the cervical os to mechanically block access of sperm to the cervix. The diaphragm is held in place by the spring tension of the rim, vaginal muscle tone, and the pubic bone.

A cervical cap marketed as FemCap is made of silicone.[119] The FemCap is kept in place by suction formed between the cervix and the device. Because all of these devices do not fit tightly enough to be a complete barrier to sperm, spermicidal gel must be applied to each device before it is inserted.

The first-year failure rate with diaphragms is 6% to 16% (Table 47-1).[3] C.J. should be counseled that diaphragms are less effective than other available methods. Because breast-feeding offers some protection against pregnancy, breast-feeding women may be the best candidates for the diaphragm. Failure rates of cervical caps range from 9% to 16% in nulliparous women and 20% to 32% in parous women (Table 47-1).[3] Studies of an earlier version of the FemCap found a failure rate of about 14% and about 8% for the second-generation FemCap.[119]

TYPES AND FITTING

Diaphragms must be properly fitted to be effective. They are available in different sizes (50–95 mm in diameter) and different styles of construction of the circular rim. The goal of fitting a diaphragm is to select the largest rim size that is comfortable for the patient.[3] A diaphragm that is too small may become dislodged during intercourse because vaginal depth increases during sexual arousal. Conversely, a diaphragm that is too large may cause vaginal pressure, abdominal pain or cramping, vaginal ulceration, or recurrent urinary tract infections. Proper size is estimated during bimanual examination, and several diaphragm sizes may need to be tried by the healthcare provider to find the right size for the patient. If C.J. gains or losses 10 to 20 lb, has a pregnancy, or has abdominal or pelvic surgery, the diaphragm would need to be refitted.

The FemCap is shaped like a sailor's hat[119] (see http://www.femcap.com/). It is available in three sizes, and size selection depends on the patient's pregnancy history; the 22-mm FemCap is for patients who have never been pregnant, the 26-mm one is for women who have miscarried or had a cesarean section, and the 30 mm size is for women who have vaginally delivered a full-term baby.

C.J. would likely be able to tolerate the diaphragm or FemCap. Fitting will depend on the device that she selects. These barrier methods, however, do not protect against STIs, which is important to C.J. when selecting her barrier method, and therefore, are not the best choice.

PATIENT INSTRUCTIONS, ADVANTAGES, AND DISADVANTAGES

The diaphragm and FemCap offer pregnancy prevention without the use of hormones, and women only need to use the devices when they are sexually active.[3,119] All of these devices are available only by prescription, should not be used during menstruation, may be difficult to insert and remove for some patients, and are not as effective as the hormonal methods or IUD. All devices should be inspected for holes or puckering (small areas of wrinkle) before use.

The diaphragm should not remain in the vagina for more than 24 hours.[5] Toxic shock syndrome (TSS) has been associated with diaphragm use, and women should be alert to its symptoms, which include fever, diarrhea, vomiting, muscle aches, and a sunburn-like rash. Allergic reactions to the latex or spermicide also have been reported.

The diaphragm should always be inserted before intercourse; it can be inserted as long as 6 hours before intercourse if desired.[3] The diaphragm should not be removed for at least 6 hours after intercourse. One teaspoon of spermicidal gel should be placed into the dome of the diaphragm before insertion. If intercourse is repeated, a new application of spermicide should be inserted vaginally without removal of the diaphragm.

To use the FemCap, first apply about one-fourth teaspoon of spermicide inside the bowl and one-half teaspoon on the other side that will face the vagina (between the brim and the dome).[119] Insert the FemCap with the long brim side first and the dome side up. Push until the cap is in contact with the cervix. More spermicide should be applied if intercourse is repeated. The FemCap should be inserted at least 15 minutes before sexual arousal and can be left in for up to 48 hours. The FemCap must be left in place for a minimum of 6 hours after intercourse.

Both devices should be washed with mild soap and water, rinsed and dried, and stored in the accompanying container. Oil-based products also may decompose the latex of the diaphragm and should not be used. These devices should be replaced every year or sooner if there are signs of wear or holes.

Vaginal Sponge

The vaginal sponge is another barrier method. It was taken off the market in 1995 and re-released in 2003. The sponge contains a polyurethane foam and 1 g of nonoxynol-9 (spermicide). The sponge is inserted into the vagina and placed against the cervix. It may be worn up to 24 hours. After intercourse, the sponge should remain in place for 6 hours. The sponge works in three ways: It acts as a spermicide, is a mechanical barrier, and absorbs semen. The failure rate reported is 18% for nulliparous women and 36% for parous women (Table 47-1).[3] Irritation or ulceration of the cervix and vaginal mucosa may occur. If the sponge is not removed within 24 hours or if particles remain after removal, toxic shock syndrome could be an issue. Because the sponge may cause irritation and does not provide protection against STIs, it may not be best for C.J.

Male Condoms

Male condoms are an effective method of contraception when used properly. The failure rate with condoms is 2% to 18% (Table 47-1).[3] Many different brands of condoms are available in the United States. The brands differ in size, shape, color, material, and the presence or absence of lubricants or spermicide. The chief noncontraceptive benefit of latex condoms is the prevention of STIs (including gonorrhea, chlamydia, and HIV), and they can be used for vaginal, anal, or oral sex.[6] Condoms are readily available without a prescription and do not cause systemic side effects such as the hormonal methods. However, some complain that condoms reduce sensitivity and spontaneity. The most commonly used and least expensive male condom is made of latex.[3] Male condoms made of polyurethane and lambskin are recommended for men or women allergic to latex. Polyurethane condoms are more expensive and sometimes break more easily than latex condoms, but they also conduct heat better than latex.[120] Lambskin condoms also conduct heat well but do not offer the same protection against STIs as latex and polyurethane. Lambskin condoms are not recommended for those who are concerned about STIs.[120]

Because the pre-ejaculatory secretions may contain sperm, ...condom should be applied before vaginal contact.[3] ...g a male condom, the man or his partner should ... of the condom and unroll it down to the base of ...is.[6,120] Most practitioners recommend lubricated condoms with resevoir ends to prevent breakage and collect the ejaculate. Oil-based lubricants can degrade male latex condoms and should be avoided. Oil-based lubricants, however, may be used with polyurethane or lambskin condoms. Condoms should be used only once by their expiration date and stored in a cool, dry place, away from prolonged periods of heat or light.

Latex condoms would be best for C.J. and her partner to prevent the transmission of STIs.

Female Condoms

The female condom is less effective, with a 21% failure rate (Table 47-1).[3] The original female condom known as the FC1 is made of polyurethane. Recently, the second-generation female condom (FC2) has become available replacing the FC1 (see http://www.fc2.us.com/).[121] The FC2 is made of a nitrale sheath or pouch and polyurethane ring at the closed end of the pouch. Both condoms consist of a smaller, circular, inner ring (which secures the device around the cervix like a diaphragm) and a larger ring around the opening of the condom.

The inner ring should be compressed and inserted vaginally as far as it will go, and the larger ring remains outside of the vagina, protecting the external genitalia. Female condoms should also be inserted before sexual contact; they may be inserted up to 8 hours before intercourse. The FC2 contains a silicone-based lubricant inside of the condom but additional lubricant may be used. Oil-based or water-based lubricants can be used with both female condoms. Just like male condoms, they should be used by their expiration date, not reused, and stored in a cool, dry place, away from heat or light.

Disadvantages of female condoms include cost (about $3 each), squeaking noise during use, and insertion difficulty.[3] Condoms may also break, although this is less likely with the female condom. Male and female condoms should not be used together as this may increase the risk of breakage.

An advantage for C.J. to use the female condom is that she has control of her own protection and does not need to rely on her partner to make sure they are both protected. The female condom is a good alternative for C.J.

Vaginal Spermicides

CASE 47-4, QUESTION 2: C.J. would like to use a spermicide along with condoms. What options does she have and how effective are spermicides when used alone? What dosage form should C.J. use? How should she be instructed to use a vaginal spermicide? What side effects can be anticipated?

Vaginal spermicides currently are available as gels (jellies), suppositories, foams, and films.[3,120] Most of these products use a nonionic surfactant, nonoxynol-9, as the spermicide. First-year failure rates with these dosage forms range from 18% to 29% (Table 47-1).

Table 47-6 compares the different spermicidal products.[3,120] The different characteristics of the products can help guide C.J. when selecting a dosage form. Regardless of the dosage form, a new dose of spermicide should be applied before each act of intercourse.

Spermicides may cause genital irritation and in some patients lead to ulceration. Likely for this reason, spermicides have been shown to increase the transmission of STIs, including HIV, gonorrhea, and chlamydia. Spermicides may not be the best choice for C.J. and her partner to prevent the risk of STI transmission.

Table 47-6
Comparison of Vaginal Spermicides[120]

Formulation	Brand Name Examples	How to Use	Onset of Action	Duration of Action
Gel	Conceptrol, Gynol II	Fill applicator, insert applicator vaginally as far as it will comfortably go, press plunger of applicator to deposit spermicide near the cervix.	Immediate	1 hour
Film	VCF	Fold film in half, fold over finger, use finger to insert as far as it will comfortably go.	15 minutes	3 hours
Foam	VCF	Shake foam canister, fill applicator, insert applicator vaginally as far as it will comfortably go, press plunger of applicator to deposit spermicide near the cervix.	Immediate	1 hour
Suppository	Encare	Unwrap, use finger to insert as far as it will comfortably go.	15 minutes	1 hour

EMERGENCY CONTRACEPTION

Case 47-4, Question 3: C.J. presents to a pharmacy 4 months later and says she missed her MPA injection last month. She had intercourse 4 nights ago with a condom and is worried she might become pregnant. She wants to know whether she should use the "morning-after pill." What do you tell C.J. about emergency contraception options? Is C.J. a candidate for emergency contraception?

Emergency contraception (EC), also referred to as the morning-after pill, is postcoital contraception useful for women who did not use a contraceptive (e.g., forgot, were assaulted) or whose method failed (e.g., broken condom, missed pill). Emergency contraception is available in a few methods, which include oral pills or an IUD.

Emergency Contraception Pills

Emergency contraceptive pills (ECPs) are available in a variety of formulations known as progestin-only, Yuzpe, and selective progesterone receptor modulators.

Currently, the one dose progestin-only (levonorgestrel 1.5 mg) ECPs are available over-the-counter to all ages.[122] The one tablet should be taken within 72 hours of unprotected intercourse according the package labeling. Studies, however, have shown that progestin-only ECPs are still effective if taken up to 120 hours (5 days) after unprotected sex.[108,123] Progestin-only ECPs reduce the risk of pregnancy by a few potential mechanisms: preventing ovulation, preventing fertilization, or preventing implantation.[3] They reduce the average risk of pregnancy by 89% after a single act of intercourse when taken within 72 hours. ECPs are most effective when taken as soon as possible after intercourse; therefore, treatment should not be delayed. Progestin-only ECPs may not be as effective in women with a BMI of 26 or greater and should be recommended to use an alternative ECP but treatment should not be denied due to BMI.[122] The most common side effects with ECPs are nausea and vomiting.[3] C.J. should be instructed that if she vomits within 1 hour of taking ECPs, the dose should be repeated. C.J.'s menses may come early or late, but she should take a pregnancy test if her menses does not come within 3 weeks of taking ECPs. This may further be complicated if C.J. gets her next scheduled dose of injectable MPA.

As an alternative to progestin-only ECPs, regular COCs may be used as long as they contain levonorgestrel or norgestrel as the progestin. This is known as the Yuzpe method, which consists of high-dose progestin and high-dose estrogen. There are no marketed formulations of this method. Depending on the brand of COCs used, a differing number of pills are taken within 120 hours of unprotected intercourse as two separate doses 12 hours apart (see Table 47-1 footnote).[3] Compared with progestin-only ECPs, the Yuzpe method is associated with higher incidence of nausea and vomiting, and patients may wish to take an antiemetic before each dose.[108] Because progestin-only ECPs are widely available, easy to use, and more effective and have limited side effects, COCs are being used less often for EC.

A newer ECP classified as an oral selective progesterone receptor modulator (SPRM), ulipristal acetate (ella), was approved for use in the United States.[124] The 30-mg oral tablet should be taken within 120 hours of unprotected intercourse.[125] It is available by prescription only. Its mechanism of action is somewhat different from that of progestin-only ECPs. It has progesterone receptor antagonist and agonist effects; however, its main mechanism is through receptor antagonism at the uterus, cervix, hypothalamus, and ovaries, thus preventing ovulation even after the LH surge, which progestin-only ECPs may not do.[125] The only other SPRM on the market is mifepristone (RU-486), known for medical abortion use. Concerns were raised about the mechanism of ulipristal disrupting an existing pregnancy and leading to abortion. Current pregnancy exposure data do not suggest an increase in miscarriage. Ulipristal has not been shown to be as effective in women with a BMI of greater than 30 and may be ineffective in women with a BMI of 35 or greater but treatment should not be denied due to BMI.[122,124] It is recommended that those women use an alternative emergency contraceptive method.[122,124] Headache, dysmenorrhea, nausea, and abdominal pain were the most reported side effects in clinical trials.[124,125] If vomiting occurs within 3 hours of taking the dose, a repeat dose is recommended.[124]

In C.J.'s case, progestin-only ECPs are the better choice because she is taking medications that interact with COCs. She is within the window of 120 hours postcoitus making over-the-counter progestin-only ECPs an option. Ulipristal is another option and labeled for use 120 hours postcoitus, but would require a prescription and may delay C.J. from receiving timely emergency contraception.

Intrauterine Devices for Emergency Contraception

The copper-T IUD is also an effective method of emergency contraception when inserted within 5 days of unprotected sex.[3,108] There is no evidence that the progestin IUD is effective. An IU must be inserted by a healthcare provider and as such may not be used regularly for emergency contraception. The biggest advantage of using an IUD for emergency contraception is that it provides continued contraception for the patient. In addition, it is effective in women regardless of their BMI. Because C.J. is HIV-positive, an IUD may not be the best choice for her due to infection risk. Also, having to see a provider for an IUD is less convenient and makes ECPs the better choice for accessibility and timing.

MEDICAL ABORTION

CASE 47-4, QUESTION 4: C.J. presents to the clinic 4 weeks later stating that she missed her period and is concerned she may be pregnant. Her human chorionic gonadotropin test is positive, confirming pregnancy. C.J. considers terminating the pregnancy, stating she is not ready to have a child and is concerned about the antiretroviral medication effects on the baby. What options are there for medical abortion?

It is estimated that about one-half of pregnancies are unintended, so it is important for these women to have safe options.[2] C.J. should be counseled extensively about her options, including keeping the baby, adoption, and medical or surgical abortion. Compared with surgical abortion, medical abortion does not require a surgical procedure, so it is less likely to cause infection and is less costly.[3] Thus, some women feel more in control when choosing this option. However, some patients may not prefer medical abortion because it usually requires more medical visits and follow-up, has a slightly lower success rate (94%–97%; failures will need a surgical procedure), and involves more bleeding and cramping that usually lasts for 2 weeks.

There are many variations in how medical abortions are carried out, but the general treatment remains the same.[3] C.J. would first obtain baseline laboratory tests, including blood type and hemoglobin. She would be given either methotrexate, mifepristone, or both the same day to stop development of the pregnancy. In the United States, mifepristone, a progesterone receptor blocker, is more commonly used. Misoprostol is given to induce uterine contractions and expel the pregnancy.

Typically for a gestational age of 63 days or less, C.J. would be given mifepristone 200 mg orally on day 1, then misoprostol 800 mcg vaginally on day 2 or 3 (6–72 hours after the mifepristone dose).[3] Misoprostol may also be given as 400 or 600 mcg orally or buccally with higher doses of mifepristone (600 mg orally).[3,126–128]

If using methotrexate, 50 mg/m^2 is given IM on day 1 followed by misoprostol 800 mcg vaginally 3 to 7 days later.[3] Side effects may include nausea, vomiting, diarrhea, cramping, and vaginal bleeding (heavier than a menses). With either method, patients should follow up with their healthcare provider on about day 15 to make sure the abortion is complete. If complete miscarriage has not occurred, another method may be used, such as aspiration, to remove all pregnancy tissues.

KEY REFERENCES AND WEBSITES

A full list of references for this chapter can be found at http://thepoint.lww.com/AT11e. Below are the key references and websites for this chapter, with the corresponding reference number in this chapter found in parentheses after the reference.

Key References

ACOG Committee on Practice Bulletins-Gynecology. ACOG practice bulletin. No. 73: Use of hormonal contraception in women with coexisting medical conditions. *Obstet Gynecol*. 2006;107:1453–1472. (26)

ACOG Committee on Practice Bulletins-Gynecology. ACOG practice bulletin No. 110: Noncontraceptive uses of hormonal contraceptives. *Obstet Gynecol*. 2010;115:206–218. (83)

American College of Obstetricians and Gynecologists. ACOG Practice Bulletin No. 152: Emergency contraception. *Obstet Gynecol*. 2015;126(3):e1–11. (108)

Dickey RP. *Managing Contraceptive Pill Patients*. 15th ed. Dallas, TX: Essential Medical Information Systems; 2014. (53)

Hatcher RA et al. *Contraceptive Technology*. 20th ed. New York, NY: Ardent Media Inc; 2011. (3)

Zieman M, Hatcher RA. *Managing Contraception*. Tiger, GA: Bridging the Gap Communications; 2012. (5)

Key Websites

Association of Reproductive Health Professionals. http://www.arhp.org/.

Curtis KM, Tepper NK, Jatlaoui TC, et al. U.S. Medical Eligibility Criteria for Contraceptive Use, 2016. *MMWR Recomm Rep*. 2016;65(No. RR-3):1–104. https://www.cdc.gov/mmwr/volumes/65/rr/rr6503a1.htm?s_cid=rr6503a1_w (7)

Guttmacher Institute. http://www.guttmacher.org. (111)

International Consortium for Emergency Contraception. http://www.cecinfo.org/.

Planned Parenthood Federation of America. http://www.plannedparenthood.org/. (109)

The Emergency Contraception Website. http://ec.princeton.edu. (122)

48 Infertility

Erin C. Raney

CORE PRINCIPLES		CHAPTER CASES
1	Infertility is the inability to conceive after 12 months of unprotected intercourse. A major predictor of infertility is the age of the woman. Additional risk factors for both men and women include lifestyle factors, such as tobacco use and obesity, as well as primary and secondary causes of hypogonadism.	**Case 48-1 (Questions 1–3, 6), Case 48-2 (Questions 1, 2)**
2	The evaluation of infertility in women incorporates data from physical examination and laboratory assessments of pituitary and ovarian function. In men, the semen analysis and laboratory assessments of hormone levels provide key information related to gonadal function.	**Case 48-1 (Questions 3–6), Case 48-2 (Questions 1, 2), Figure 48-1 Table 48-2**
3	Unexplained infertility is diagnosed after a thorough evaluation of both the man and woman reveals no identifiable cause. Treatment is empiric and often combines superovulation with intrauterine insemination or in vitro fertilization.	**Case 48-1 (Questions 7–10)**
4	Clomiphene citrate is a selective estrogen receptor modulator that is considered a first-line agent for superovulation in patients with unexplained fertility. Aromatase inhibitors are under investigation as alternative oral agents.	**Case 48-1 (Questions 8–10)**
5	In vitro fertilization is the most commonly used assisted reproductive technology, or procedure that involves manipulation of oocytes and sperm. Medications are used to stimulate multiple follicles for oocyte retrieval and to optimize implantation after embryo transfer.	**Case 48-2 (Questions 3–9), Table 48-4**
6	Controlled ovarian stimulation with gonadotropins is accomplished with follicle-stimulating hormone alone or in combination with luteinizing hormone. A gonadotropin-releasing hormone agonist or antagonist is administered to prevent interruption of the cycle by endogenous hormones. Human chorionic gonadotropin is injected in a single dose to finalize follicular development for oocyte retrieval.	**Case 48-2 (Questions 4–7), Tables 48-3, 48-5, 48-6, 48-7 Figure 48-3**
7	A rare but serious complication of controlled ovarian stimulation is ovarian hyperstimulation syndrome. The risk is minimized by monitoring the development of follicles carefully with sequential transvaginal ultrasounds and serum estradiol levels.	**Case 48-2 (Questions 5, 7)**
8	Multiple gestation pregnancies are associated with maternal and neonatal risks, including preterm birth and extended neonatal intensive care. These risks are considered when determining embryo transfer and cryopreservation plans.	**Case 48-2 (Question 9)**
9	The diagnosis and treatment of infertility affects the couple emotionally, financially, and socially. Psychosocial support is an important aspect of care from the early phases of evaluation and diagnosis through all stages of treatment.	**Case 48-2 (Question 10), Table 48-8**

INTRODUCTION

Infertility is defined as the inability to conceive after 1 year of unprotected intercourse.[1] The definition is based upon the observation that roughly 85% of couples with normal fertility will achieve pregnancy within 1 year.[2] Data from the 2006 to 2010 National Survey of Family Growth revealed that 6% of married women 15 to 44 years old, or 1.53 million, were infertile and approximately 12% of women in this age group had used infertility services.[3,4] Many factors affect infertility rates, but advancing maternal age appears to be a prominent influence. The incidence of infertility in women 15 to 24 years old was 7%, whereas in women 35 to 44 years old, it was 27%.[3] This is accompanied by an age-related increase in chromosomal abnormalities and spontaneous abortion rates.[5] The physiologic factors of reproductive aging are amplified by a trend toward delayed childbearing in the United States. In 1970, 1 out of 100 women had their first child at age 35 or older. In 2006, this increased to 1 out of 12 women.[6] Male fertility is impacted by age as well, with higher infertility rates after age 39.[3] However, determining the exact contribution of male age to infertility is complicated by the influence of female age.

The complex physical, psychological, and social implications have led to a national focus on infertility as a public health priority.[7] Treatment plans vary widely depending on the contributions of both female and male factors. An individualized approach is necessary to balance the risks and benefits of the various therapeutic options and maximize clinical outcomes.

PATHOPHYSIOLOGY AND DIAGNOSIS

CASE 48-1

QUESTION 1: T.R. is a 32-year-old woman who presents to her gynecologist with concerns that she and her husband, age 37, have not conceived despite having unprotected intercourse on average 2 to 3 times/week for the past 14 months. Her prior contraceptive method was a combined oral contraceptive which she used for 12 years and discontinued 2 years ago. At that time, the couple used male condoms until 14 months ago when they stopped using contraception altogether. What is the recommended initial approach to this couple's concern?

Evaluation of infertility generally begins after a couple has attempted to conceive for at least 12 months without success. Evaluation after just 6 months of unsuccessful conception is recommended in women older than age 35 or in those with a history of conditions associated with infertility, such as amenorrhea, endometriosis, or pelvic inflammatory disease.[2]

This couple has failed to conceive after 14 months of regular, unprotected intercourse, which supports an evaluation of both partners at this time. The diagnostic process first involves a thorough assessment of medical conditions, lifestyle parameters, and medication exposures. This is followed by complete physical examinations and laboratory assessments with other diagnostic procedures as warranted.

General Risk Factors

CASE 48-1, QUESTION 2: Additional information is obtained about the couple's social history. T.R. works as a bank teller and her husband is a financial planner. Neither T.R. nor her husband smoke tobacco or use illicit substances. Both drink one to two cups of caffeinated coffee each day and drink alcohol socially, an average of one to three drinks each on weekends. What lifestyle factors may contribute to infertility in this couple?

Lifestyle factors such as tobacco or illicit drug use and caffeine intake are known contributors to infertility. Tobacco use can be linked to 13% of female infertility cases.[8] In addition to the negative effects on fetal development during pregnancy, tobacco use can worsen ovulatory function. It also induces chromosomal changes that alter sperm production and function.[8] Caffeine is associated with decreased fertility with higher levels of intake, but moderate use of one to two cups of coffee or equivalent appears to have minimal impact. Although a link between alcohol use and infertility is not definitive, it is recommended that women limit their use to no more than one drink per day. Complete abstinence from alcohol is recommended once pregnancy is confirmed.[9] Use of illicit substances such as marijuana impairs fertility and decreases the success of fertility treatments.[9,10] Occupational and environmental exposures to pesticides, heavy metals, and toxins such as organic solvents used in dry cleaning and printing are additional contributors.[9]

The couple's lack of tobacco or illicit drug use eliminates these as potential contributors and their occupations do not fit known high-risk exposure profiles. Their pattern of caffeine and alcohol use is not greater than the amount currently documented to affect fertility. Assessment of other causes of infertility is warranted.

Female Factor Infertility

OVULATORY DYSFUNCTION

CASE 48-1, QUESTION 3: T.R.'s medical history is significant for exercise-induced asthma diagnosed at age 10. Her medications include an albuterol inhaler used as needed for shortness of breath. She is 5 feet 5 inches tall and weighs 140 lb. Her reproductive history reveals menarche at age 13, no prior pregnancies, and regular menstrual cycles approximately 25 to 26 days in length since discontinuing the oral contraceptive. She reports the menstrual bleeding phase to be 4 to 5 days in length and does not complain of excessive bleeding. A physical examination is performed along with a pelvic examination with no notable abnormalities. What information does this provide about possible female factors associated with infertility?

An important focus when evaluating causes of infertility is ovulatory function, which is associated with up to 40% of female factor infertility.[2] A thorough reproductive history should document age of menarche, menstrual cycle patterns, premenstrual symptoms, and previous pregnancies. A history of regular menstrual cycles of 21 to 35 days with premenstrual symptoms or dysmenorrhea is considered consistent with ovulatory cycles.[2]

Ovarian function is regulated through complex feedback mechanisms within the hypothalamic–pituitary–ovarian axis (see Chapter 50, Disorders Related to the Menstrual Cycle, Fig. 50-1). This involves release of gonadotropin-releasing hormone (GnRH) from the hypothalamus, follicle-stimulating hormone (FSH) and luteinizing hormone (LH) from the pituitary gland, and estrogen and progesterone from the ovaries. Table 48-1 provides an overview of abbreviations commonly associated with diagnosis and management of infertility for use throughout the chapter.

Conditions such as thyroid dysfunction, hyperprolactinemia, and polycystic ovary syndrome (PCOS) can disrupt these feedback mechanisms and induce anovulation. Signs may be evident upon physical examination, including an enlarged thyroid (thyroid dysfunction), abnormal discharge from the breast (hyperprolactinemia),

Table 48-1
Common Abbreviations Associated with Infertility Diagnosis and Treatment

ART	Assisted reproductive technology
CC	Clomiphene citrate
COS	Controlled ovarian stimulation
FSH	Follicle-stimulating hormone
GnRH	Gonadotropin-releasing hormone
hCG	Human chorionic gonadotropin
HSG	Hysterosalpingogram
hMG	Human menopausal gonadotropin
IUI	Intrauterine insemination
ICSI	Intracytoplasmic sperm injection
IVF	In vitro fertilization
LH	Luteinizing hormone
OHSS	Ovarian hyperstimulation syndrome
OI	Ovulation induction
SO	Superovulation

or signs of hyperandrogenism (PCOS). Obesity is another feature associated with PCOS. Conversely, extremely low body weight and excessive exercise may negatively impact ovulatory function at the hypothalamic level. Weight gain improves menstrual regulation in women with anovulation associated with low body fat. Primary ovarian failure can result from exposure to chemotherapy agents or radiation treatments as well as ovarian surgery. As previously discussed, the aging process itself is characterized by diminished ovarian follicular reserve.[2]

T.R.'s reproductive history is consistent with regular menstrual cycles which are likely ovulatory. It would be helpful to identify whether she reports any symptoms of premenstrual syndrome or dysmenorrhea which are associated with ovulatory cycles. Her physical examination is unremarkable and her medical history does not reveal any conditions associated with anovulation. Her weight is not likely a factor because her body mass index of approximately 23 kg/m^2 is in the normal range. She has no known history of exposure to chemotherapy or ovarian surgery which could directly impact ovarian function. The only parameter consistent with female factor infertility is T.R.'s age. At 32 years old, she may be experiencing an initial age-related decline in ovarian function consistent with infertility.

CASE 48-1, QUESTION 4: T.R. reports using a home ovulation test kit for the last two menstrual cycles which both yielded positive results. She is referred for a series of laboratory tests with the following findings:

Thyroid-stimulating hormone, 3.2 mIU/L
Prolactin, 8.4 ng/mL
Cycle day 3 FSH, 4 mIU/mL
Cycle day 3 estradiol, 38 pg/mL
What additional information about her ovulatory function can be determined from these results?

Several methods are available to further define ovulatory function. Basal body temperature monitoring is accomplished through the measurement of body temperature every morning upon waking with a basal or digital thermometer. Temperature fluctuations typically follow a biphasic pattern during the menstrual cycle, with a sustained rise in basal body temperature of approximately 0.5°F to 1.0°F after ovulation. If this pattern is apparent through daily documentation in a temperature diary, it can be assumed that ovulation occurred during that cycle. The accuracy of this method is complicated by daily temperature fluctuations, inconsistent measurement technique, and illness. It has largely been replaced by the use of home ovulation test kits that detect urinary LH. The patient initiates daily urine tests during the follicular phase, with the initial testing day determined by the length and regularity of her menstrual cycle (Fig. 48-1). A positive test documents the LH surge, signaling that ovulation will occur in an average of 24 hours.[2,11] Home ovulation test kits that detect changes in cervical mucus or saliva samples are not typically used for diagnostic purposes. They are useful, however, for patients who are timing intercourse during their most fertile period around ovulation.[9,11]

Indirect measurements of ovulation are available, but not widely performed. A serum progesterone concentration measured in the mid-luteal phase greater than 3 ng/mL is considered consistent with an ovulatory cycle. Alternatively, an endometrial biopsy performed just prior to menses measures the degree of progesterone-stimulated growth, signifying whether ovulation likely occurred. The invasive nature of this test limits its feasibility in most diagnostic evaluations.[2]

In patients who are anovulatory, additional laboratory assessments of thyroid function and prolactin levels document potential secondary causes. Anovulation associated with hyperprolactinemia is treated with oral dopamine agonists such as cabergoline.[12] Elevated testosterone levels may correspond with physical signs of hyperandrogenism and PCOS. The treatment of PCOS is discussed elsewhere (see Chapter 50, Disorders Related to the Menstrual Cycle).

Assessment of ovarian reserve may be performed in women older than age 35 to help guide fertility treatment choices. There are multiple methods that can be used. One involves the measurement of basal levels of serum FSH with or without estradiol on day 2, 3, or 4 of the menstrual cycle, with day 1 being the first day of menses. Because the number of ovarian follicles declines with age, pituitary release of FSH increases. Therefore, elevated levels of basal FSH (>10–20 IU/L) suggest diminished ovarian function. Unfortunately, the interpretation is complicated by individual variability in FSH levels from cycle to cycle as well as varying laboratory-specific reference ranges. A serum estradiol level of >60 to 80 pg/mL with normal FSH levels is also associated with a poor prognosis for success with infertility treatments.[2,13] Measurement of inhibin B, which is secreted from the ovarian granulosa cells during the follicular phase of the menstrual cycle, is an additional marker. Low levels of inhibin B correlate with elevated FSH levels and a possible decline in ovarian function. However, due to the variability with this measurement, it is not recommended as a routine evaluation of ovarian reserve.[13]

The clomiphene citrate challenge test provides another option for assessing ovarian reserve. This involves the administration of clomiphene citrate (CC), a selective estrogen receptor modulator, at a dose of 100 mg once daily on days 5 through 9 of the menstrual cycle. In addition to the estradiol and FSH measurements on day 3 as described previously, FSH is also measured on day 10. The expected response is suppression of FSH by the developing ovarian follicles. Elevated levels at either day 3 or 10 suggest diminished ovarian reserve. The value of this test as a predictor of response to ovarian stimulation is not clearly supported in the literature.[2,13]

Direct visualization of the ovaries through a transvaginal ultrasound may be used in conjunction with the hormone testing described previously. An assessment of ovarian volume and the

Figure 48-1 The menstrual cycle.

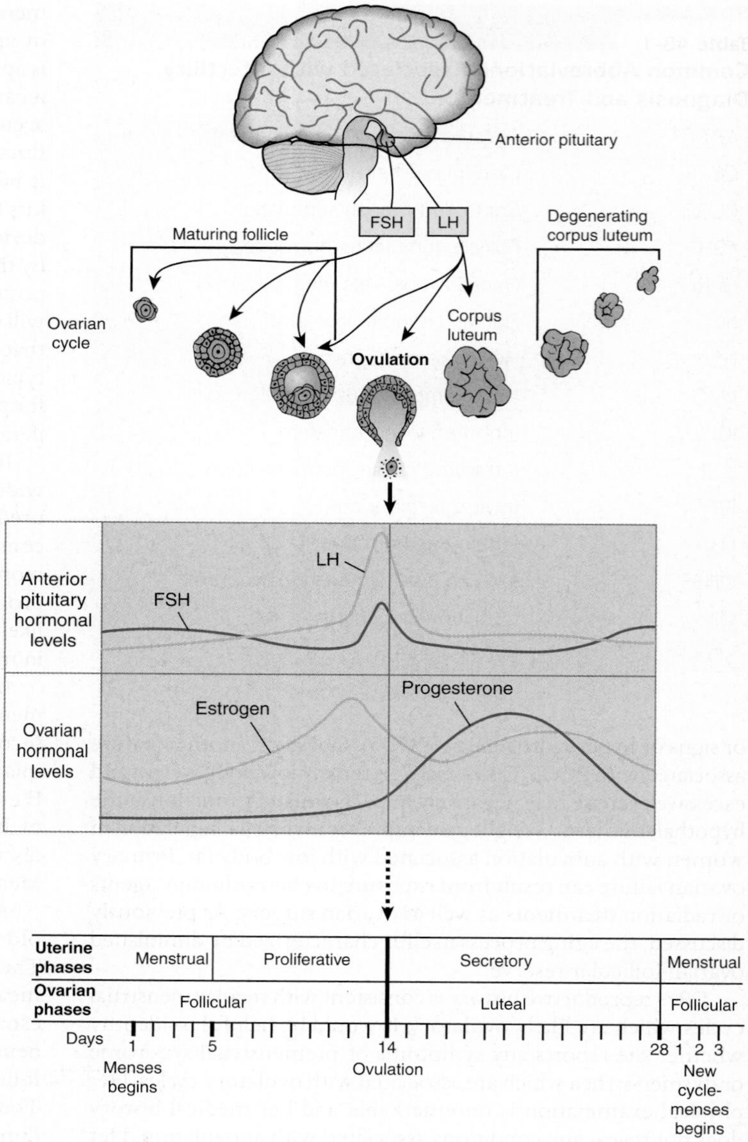

antral follicle count can be made. The antral follicles, or those 2 to 10 mm in diameter, are responsive to FSH in the early follicular phase and decline in number with age. An antral follicle count of 3 to 6 is considered low and predicts poor ovarian response to various infertility treatments.[2,13]

The laboratory assessment of T.R. provides additional data regarding her ovarian function. Ovulatory cycles are supported by the positive urinary LH surge with the home test kit as well as the normal (nonelevated) day 3 FSH and estradiol levels. Her normal thyroid-stimulating hormone and prolactin levels indicate a low probability of secondary causes of anovulation. Because T.R. is younger than 35 and there are no other indicators of ovulatory dysfunction, additional testing of ovarian reserve may not be necessary. The initial findings of T.R.'s infertility assessment show that ovulatory dysfunction is not likely to be a contributor.

STRUCTURAL FACTORS

CASE 48-1, QUESTION 5: Because T.R. has normal ovulatory function, further causes of female factor infertility will be investigated. What testing is recommended to rule out structural causes of infertility?

Structural abnormalities in the uterine cavity or fallopian tubes are additional causes of female factor infertility. These may develop in utero or result from scar tissue or lesions secondary to conditions such as endometriosis. In some cases of endometriosis, surgical interventions improve fertility outcomes, but this is highly dependent on the severity and location of the lesions.[14] Further discussion of the diagnosis and treatment of endometriosis is provided elsewhere (see Chapter 50, Disorders Related to the Menstrual Cycle). Pelvic inflammatory disease from sexually transmitted infections such as chlamydia or gonorrhea is a risk factor for tubal infertility.[2]

The use of invasive procedures to explore structural causes of female infertility is dictated by the reproductive history and findings of the physical examination and laboratory tests. Abnormalities of the ovaries, uterus, and fallopian tubes are evaluated through various procedures. Transvaginal ultrasonography utilizes vaginal insertion of an ultrasound probe to visualize ovarian structure and developing follicles. A hysterosalpingogram (HSG) is performed to confirm normal fallopian tube structure. During this process, dye is injected into the uterus through a catheter and visualized on X-ray to determine any blockages or malformations. Hysteroscopy and laparoscopy are more invasive procedures that allow for direct visualization of the uterus or pelvic anatomy. These are typically reserved for further examination of abnormalities detected by initial testing.[2]

Impaired cervical mucus production and quality are additional structural factors that can impact sperm motility and the fertilization process. Cervical mucus increases in volume and becomes thinner as the follicular phase progresses to facilitate sperm transport at ovulation. The "postcoital test" or microscopic examination of cervical mucus within hours of intercourse can be performed to confirm the presence of motile sperm, but is no longer recommended for routine use.[2]

In the evaluation of this couple, it is important to verify T.R.'s sexual history and any possible exposures to sexually transmitted infections, such as chlamydia. An HSG should be ordered to determine whether she has patent fallopian tubes and to provide basic information about the shape of her uterine cavity. If there are abnormal findings from this test, further hysteroscopic or laparoscopic procedures can be performed. A laparoscopy would be necessary to fully evaluate any peritoneal adhesions from undetected endometriosis, but her medical history does not warrant this invasive procedure at this time.

Male Factor Infertility

CASE 48-1, QUESTION 6: The results of the HSG are normal, so the infertility assessment turns now to the evaluation of T.R.'s husband. He is healthy with no chronic medical conditions or medication use. He denies symptoms of low libido or signs of erectile or ejaculatory dysfunction during intercourse. A complete physical examination, including the genitalia, reveals normal findings. His semen analysis yields the following results:

Semen volume, 5 mL
Sperm number, 400 × 10^6
Sperm concentration, 112 × 10^6/mL
Sperm total motility, 65%
Sperm progressive motility, 61%
Sperm vitality, 80%
Sperm morphology, 30%

A second semen analysis confirms these results. What conclusions about the cause of infertility can be made from these findings?

Infertility is associated with male factors in approximately 20% of cases. Male and female factors contribute to infertility in 30% to 40% of couples.[15] Male factor infertility is often an outcome of impaired sperm production or function, which can originate from a variety of causes. Impaired sperm production may be associated with hypogonadism resulting from testicular trauma, cryptorchidism, radiation, or antiandrogen medications.[15,16] Varicoceles, or dilated scrotal veins, affect testicular function in up to 40% of men with infertility. It appears that the resulting abnormal venous perfusion and elevated testicular temperature impair spermatogenesis.[17] Genetic conditions may disrupt androgen synthesis or cause defects in the LH or FSH receptor. Azoospermia, or no presence of sperm in the ejaculate, is also apparent in certain genetic disorders, such as Klinefelter syndrome. Pituitary tumors can reduce FSH and LH secretion and impair sperm production. Sperm transport defects result from erectile dysfunction, retrograde ejaculation, or obstruction of the vas deferens or epididymis. Medications such as antidepressants or antihypertensives can worsen libido and ejaculatory function.[16]

A complete physical examination of the man is performed to identify signs of androgen deficiency such as small testicular size or an abnormal pattern of male hair growth. In some cases, anatomic defects such as varicoceles can be identified and repaired surgically.[17] However, the primary evaluation tool for male infertility is the semen analysis. Although there are home test kits for male infertility that utilize a semen sample, they are not recommended for diagnostic purposes because a positive result merely confirms that the sperm count is above a predetermined level. There is no quantification of the number of sperm or evaluation of sperm quality, so it does not rule out sperm abnormalities. A detailed semen analysis is required to fully evaluate male factor infertility. The evaluation of two semen analyses on different occasions is recommended.[15] The World Health Organization publishes reference values for semen characteristics (Table 48-2).[18] Results lower than these cut-off values are not definitive for male factor infertility, but do suggest the need to confirm the findings with a second semen analysis.[15]

Table 48-2
Semen Analysis: Lower Reference Limits for Selected Parameters

Parameter	Lower Reference Limit
Semen volume (mL)	1.5
Total sperm number (10^6/ejaculate)	39
Sperm concentration (10^6/mL)	15
Total motility (progressive + nonprogressive, %)	40
Progressive motility (%)	32
Vitality (live spermatozoa, %)	58
Sperm morphology (normal forms, %)	4

Source: World Health Organization, Department of Reproductive Health and Research. *WHO Laboratory Manual for the Examination and Processing of Human Semen*. 5th ed. Geneva, Switzerland: World Health Organization Press; 2010:224.

Abnormal findings on the semen analysis may be suggestive of the underlying cause of infertility. Low semen volume suggests structural causes of ejaculatory dysfunction. Additional hormone testing, including FSH, testosterone, and prolactin levels, may be necessary to distinguish factors associated with a low sperm count or motility. Low FSH and testosterone are consistent with hypogonadotropic hypogonadism.[16] If hyperprolactinemia is evident, any secondary causes such as medications are investigated. Certain antipsychotics, antihypertensives, or antidepressants can increase prolactin levels and should be discontinued and replaced with agents that do not increase prolactin. If the underlying cause cannot be addressed, a dopamine agonist may restore testicular function and sperm production.[12]

T.R.'s husband's medical history does not support an identifiable cause of altered sperm production or function. He does not report any signs of sexual dysfunction or take medications that may negatively affect libido or erectile or ejaculatory function. All components of the semen analysis are above the lower limit defined by the World Health Organization. His normal physical examination and medical history also support a lack of identifiable male causes of infertility. In this case, the extensive testing of both T.R. and her husband has revealed no obvious contributor to infertility.

TREATMENT APPROACHES

CASE 48-1, QUESTION 7: The couple completes their evaluation and is diagnosed with unexplained infertility. What is the initial approach to treatment?

The diagnosis of unexplained infertility, or no identifiable cause after evaluation, accounts for up to 25% of cases.[19] The treatment approach is empiric but typically incorporates medications to stimulate ovulation, often in conjunction with intrauterine insemination or other infertility procedures, which are discussed later in the chapter.

Regardless of the treatment approach, all couples pursuing pregnancy are encouraged to avoid tobacco, alcohol, and illicit substances, and limit caffeine intake.[9] The female partner should take a daily supplement containing 400 to 800 mcg of folic acid to reduce the risk of neural tube defects once pregnancy occurs.[20] Any chronic medications must be evaluated for potential safety issues during pregnancy and discontinued or switched to a safer alternative. Patients are encouraged to achieve and maintain a normal weight.[9] Recommendations pertinent to T.R. include discontinuation of alcohol use, limited caffeine intake, and initiation of a daily multivitamin with 400 to 800 mcg of folic acid. T.R. should also confirm plans for monitoring her asthma symptoms during pregnancy. Albuterol use during pregnancy will be continued, but the frequency of use will be monitored carefully.[21]

Ovarian Stimulation

There are two general treatment approaches to ovarian stimulation: "ovulation induction" (OI) and "superovulation (SO)." The approach depends on a patient's underlying ovulatory function. Ovulation induction is utilized in patients who are not ovulating to promote an ovulatory cycle. This method may be accompanied by timed natural intercourse or the use of insemination procedures to achieve pregnancy. Superovulation, or controlled ovarian stimulation (COS), incorporates many of the same medications, but is appropriate for women who are already having ovulatory cycles but are still experiencing infertility. Additionally, SO is appropriate for infertility procedures where the development of multiple ovarian follicles is desirable (Case 48-2). The general approach to medication use with both strategies is described subsequently.

Anovulatory women with adequate ovarian reserve and no other treatable cause are candidates for OI. This process is designed to mimic the hormonal patterns of the normal menstrual cycle. Follicle-stimulating hormone guides the initial recruitment and development of ovarian follicles early in the menstrual cycle. This is followed by development of a dominant follicle and increased estradiol levels. The elevated estrogen triggers the LH surge and the release of the ovum mid-cycle for fertilization (Fig. 48-1). The goal of OI is the development of a single dominant follicle.[22]

The choice of medications for OI is dictated by hypothalamic–pituitary–ovarian function. With adequate hypothalamic function, an oral regimen of CC, which exhibits estrogen agonist and antagonist activity, is often utilized first line. Clomiphene citrate inhibits estrogen binding in the hypothalamus to stimulate release of GnRH and pituitary gonadotropins and induce ovarian follicular development. Ovulation is successful in approximately 75% of patients using CC.[19] Oral aromatase inhibitors are not approved by the US Food and Drug Administration (FDA) for OI, but also increase release of GnRH and pituitary gonadotropins through an estrogen antagonist effect.[19]

If hypothalamic or pituitary dysfunction is detected or if oral regimens are not successful, injectable gonadotropins are administered. The most common gonadotropin regimens use FSH administered alone or in combination with LH, depending on whether the patient has hypogonadotropic or eugonadotropic hypogonadism (Table 48-3).[23] Injections are initiated at low daily doses until a dominant follicle has matured. Ovulation is then

Table 48-3
Gonadotropins for Ovulation Induction/Superovulation

Ingredient	Product Name	Strength/Dosage Form	Route of Administration
hMG (menotropins)	Menopur	Powder for reconstitution: 75 IU FSH activity and 75 IU LH activity/vial	SC
Urinary FSH (urofollitropin)	Bravelle	Powder for reconstitution: 75 IU FSH activity/vial	IM or SC
Recombinant FSH (follitropin alfa)	Gonal-f multi-dose	Powder for reconstitution: 450 or 1,050 IU FSH activity/vial	SC
	Gonal-f RFF 75 IU	Powder for reconstitution: 75 IU FSH activity/vial	SC
	Gonal-f RFF Rediject	Solution: 300, 450, or 900 IU FSH/pen	SC
Recombinant FSH (follitropin beta)	Follistim AQ Vial	Solution: 75 IU FSH/0.5-mL vial	IM or SC
	Follistim AQ cartridge for Follistim Pen	Solution:300, 600, or 900 IU FSH/cartridge	SC
Urinary hCG	Chorionic gonadotropin (generic)	Powder for reconstitution: 10,000 IU LH activity/vial	IM
	Pregnyl	Powder for reconstitution: 10,000 IU LH activity/vial	IM
	Novarel	Powder for reconstitution: 10,000 IU LH activity/vial	IM
Recombinant chorionic gonadotropin alfa	Ovidrel	Prefilled syringe: 250-mcg r-hCG/0.5 mL	SC

FSH, follicle-stimulating hormone; hCG, human chorionic gonadotropin; hMG, human menopausal gonadotropin; IM, intramuscular; LH, luteinizing hormone; r-hCG, recombinant human chorionic gonadotropin; SC, subcutaneous.
Source: Facts & Comparisons eAnswers. https://fco.factsandcomparisons.com/lco/action/doc/retrieve/docid/fc_dfc/5548530; https://fco.factsandcomparisons.com/lco/action/doc/retrieve/docid/1081/5546104; https://fco.factsandcomparisons.com/lco/action/doc/retrieve/docid/fc_dfc/5548528; https://fco.factsandcomparisons.com/lco/action/doc/retrieve/docid/fc_dfc/5548529; https://fco.factsandcomparisons.com/lco/action/search?q=pregnyl&t=name; https://fco.factsandcomparisons.com/lco/action/search?q=ovidrel&t=name. Accessed June 14, 2017.

triggered with an injection of human chorionic gonadotropin (hCG) to simulate the LH surge that naturally occurs mid-cycle. This is timed with natural intercourse or other infertility procedures to achieve pregnancy.[24]

The oral and injectable medications used for OI are also incorporated into regimens for SO. They are administered in doses and schedules intended to develop multiple ovarian follicles, rather than one dominant follicle. This results in a greater number of oocytes available for fertilization. Because T.R. has ovulatory cycles, but has unexplained infertility, SO is the treatment approach considered most appropriate.

CASE 48-1, QUESTION 8: What medication regimen is recommended for T.R.'s unexplained infertility?

There are multiple methods for ovulation stimulation that utilize oral or injectable medications. Clomiphene citrate is the most common initial choice because of the convenience and low cost of an oral regimen and the widespread experience with its use.

CLOMIPHENE CITRATE

The competitive binding of CC to estrogen receptors in the hypothalamus stimulates release of GnRH. This promotes gonadotropin release from the anterior pituitary, leading to follicular development, increased estradiol production, and ovulation. As previously described, the mechanism of action of CC requires an intact hypothalamic–pituitary–ovarian axis.[25] The typical initial dosing regimen for CC is 50 mg once daily for 5 days starting between days 2 through 5 of the menstrual cycle. Ovulation usually occurs 5 to 12 days after the fifth dose is taken. If ovulation is documented but pregnancy does not occur, the same dose of CC is used in future cycles. If ovulation does not occur, then the dose is increased by 50 mg with each subsequent cycle. Although the product labeling does not recommend doses above 100 mg/day, CC doses as high as 250 mg have been described in the literature.[25]

Superovulation for unexplained infertility with CC is recommended in combination with intrauterine insemination (IUI), because this improves pregnancy and live birth rates over CC alone or no intervention.[25] Intrauterine insemination introduces a processed semen sample directly to the uterus via a catheter placed through the cervix. The procedure is timed with ovulation to maximize sperm exposure for fertilization. This is accomplished by using a urinary ovulation home test kit to identify the natural LH surge or injecting hCG to trigger ovulation and planning the IUI 24 to 36 hours later. Due to the nature of the procedure, patients with bilateral obstruction of the fallopian tubes are not candidates for IUI.[26]

T.R.'s evaluation shows no evidence of hypothalamic or pituitary dysfunction, so she is an appropriate candidate for CC. Once her next cycle begins, she should initiate a 5-day regimen of CC 50 mg once daily starting on the fifth day of menstrual bleeding, with plans for an IUI following documentation of ovulation.

CASE 48-1, QUESTION 9: T.R. begins a regimen of CC and experiences hot flashes and nausea, but chooses to complete the 5-day course. What is the likely cause of her symptoms?

Vasomotor symptoms are a common complaint during a short treatment course of CC, occurring in approximately 10% of users. Additional side effects include headache, breast tenderness, irritability, mood swings, and nausea. Although visual disturbances are reported in less than 2% of patients, symptoms such as blurred vision or light sensitivity should be reported and evaluated to prevent serious complications.[19,25] All medications for SO can result in multiple gestation pregnancies. Clomiphene citrate for unexplained infertility is associated with multiple gestation in approximately 3% to 7% of pregnancies, primarily resulting in twins.[25] Early concerns about increased rates of ovarian cancer in women exposed to more than 12 cycles of CC have been minimized based on recent data.[25]

In this case, T.R. is experiencing side effects commonly associated with CC. They are not treatment limiting, and she is not reporting a change in vision that would require further evaluation. She can safely proceed with treatment by monitoring for an LH surge using a home ovulation test kit and undergoing IUI.

CASE 48-1, QUESTION 10: The pregnancy test after the first cycle of CC and IUI is negative. What other options are available for this couple?

Multiple treatment cycles with the combination of CC and IUI are commonly pursued, but there is little evidence for effectiveness beyond six attempts.[25] In some cases, alternatives to CC for SO may be desirable because of poor tolerability or treatment failure. Aromatase inhibitors or gonadotropins are suitable alternatives to combine with IUI.

AROMATASE INHIBITORS

The aromatase inhibitors letrozole and anastrozole are oral alternatives to CC, although they are not FDA-labeled for OI or SO. Aromatase is an enzyme that converts androstenedione to estrone and testosterone to estradiol. Aromatase inhibitors reduce systemic estrogen levels by blocking this conversion in the ovary, resulting in increased gonadotropin secretion and follicular development. The higher concentration of androgens that remains in the ovary increases follicular sensitivity to FSH and further facilitates development.[27]

The recommended administration schedule is similar to clomiphene: once daily for 5 days beginning on cycle days 3 to 5. Although daily doses of letrozole 2.5 or 5 mg or anastrozole 1 mg have been studied for this purpose, there is more evidence available for letrozole. Pregnancy rates with letrozole appear to be similar to that of CC.[28] Adverse effects experienced with aromatase inhibitors resemble those of CC and include vasomotor symptoms, nausea, and fatigue. The aromatase inhibitors do not affect cervical mucus or endometrial development, but this finding has not translated into improved pregnancy outcomes in clinical studies. Development of fewer follicles may result in a lower risk of multiple gestation pregnancy compared with CC. Initial concerns of the teratogenic potential of aromatase inhibition during fetal development prompted a warning against use in premenopausal women who are or may become pregnant.[27] However, surveillance studies do not demonstrate higher rates of congenital malformations with letrozole as compared to CC.[27,29] The early timing of administration in the cycle reduces the risk of fetal exposure. Continued monitoring of pregnancy outcomes is needed to confirm safety.

GONADOTROPINS

If oral agents are unsuccessful, SO can be attempted with injectable gonadotropins including FSH alone or in combination with LH (Table 48-3).[23] A standard protocol involves daily injections of FSH or a combination of FSH and LH to stimulate follicular development. Human chorionic gonadotropin is commonly administered as a single injection to finalize follicular development and induce ovulation.[19] Dosing recommendations, key differences between formulations, and risks associated with gonadotropin use are reviewed in more detail in Case 48-2.

T.R.'s complaints of vasomotor symptoms are well documented with CC. Although the aromatase inhibitors are another oral option, the likelihood of hot flashes is similar. However, if the couple continues to be unsuccessful with future cycles of CC p

Table 48-4
Description of Select Infertility Procedures

Classification	Procedure	Description
Insemination	Intrauterine, intracervical, intravaginal	Delivery of a prepared semen sample to the intended site (vagina, cervix, uterus) during ovulation
Assisted reproductive technology	Assisted hatching	Mechanical or chemical separation of the blastocyst from the zona pellucida (membrane surrounding the oocyte) during embryonic development in vitro
	Embryo cryopreservation	Freezing and storage of embryos for future ART cycles
	Gamete intrafallopian transfer	Laparoscopic transfer of the unfertilized oocytes and sperm to the fallopian tube for fertilization
	In vitro fertilization—embryo transfer	Transfer of one or more embryos resulting from in vitro fertilization into the uterus through the cervix
	Intracytoplasmic sperm injection	In vitro injection of the sperm into the oocyte
	Preimplantation genetic diagnosis/screening	Examination of oocytes, zygotes, or embryos for specific genetic conditions (diagnosis) or for general genetic alterations (screening)
	Zygote intrafallopian transfer	Laparoscopic transfer of the fertilized oocyte (zygote) into the fallopian tube

ART, assisted reproductive technology.
Source: Zegers-Hochschild F et al. The International Committee for Monitoring Assisted Reproductive Technology (ICMART) and the World Health Organization (WHO) revised glossary on ART terminology, 2009. *Hum Reprod*. 2009;24:2683.

IUI, letrozole can serve as an alternative prior to use of injectable gonadotropins. In vitro fertilization (IVF) is commonly reserved until after multiple IUI procedures are attempted and unsuccessful.

Assisted Reproductive Technology

OVERVIEW AND INDICATIONS

There are a variety of procedures to address infertility factors specific to each couple. Insemination processes (intrauterine, intracervical, and intravaginal) are categorized separately from those using assisted reproductive technology (ART), or the manipulation of oocytes and embryos (Table 48-4).[30] The Centers for Disease Control and Prevention monitors ART in the United States through the National ART Surveillance System. The use of ART is trending upward, with the number of cycles increasing from just over 122,000 in 2003 to more than 157,000 in 2012.[31]

The primary ART is IVF, which involves retrieval of oocytes after SO, fertilization in vitro, and transfer of the embryo(s) directly to the uterus through the cervix, bypassing the fallopian tubes (Fig. 48-2; Table 48-4).[31] Intracytoplasmic sperm injection (ICSI), or the injection of sperm directly into the oocyte during the fertilization process, accompanies IVF if severe sperm dysfunction is evident. A variety of ancillary procedures can be used based upon each couple's history and clinical presentation. These include genetic screening and cryopreservation of embryos. Assisted reproductive technology also allows couples to use donor sperm and/or oocytes to overcome severe sperm or ovarian dysfunction that cannot be addressed through other methods. The option of using donor oocytes uniquely targets infertility due to diminished ovarian reserve.

Figure 48-2 In vitro fertilization process.

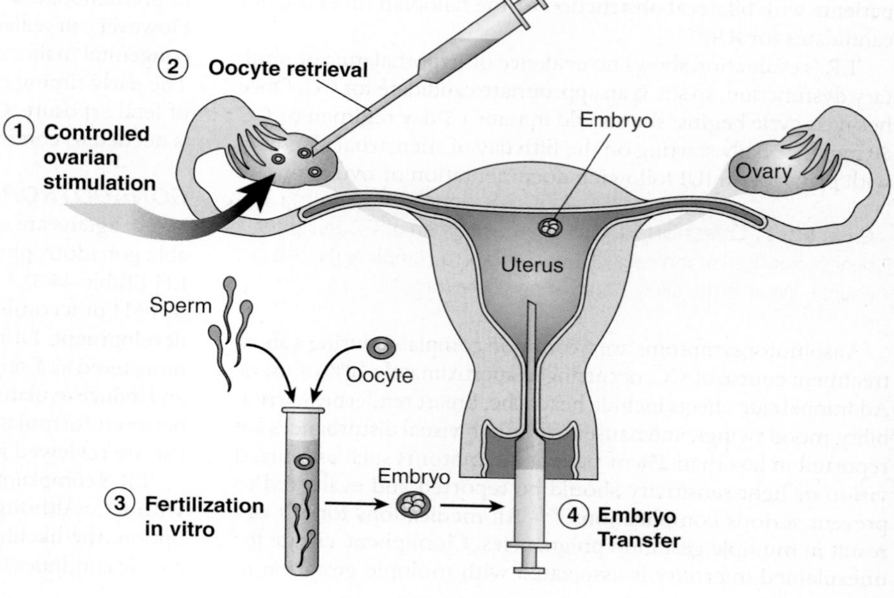

CASE 48-2

QUESTION 1: F.J., a 39-year-old woman, and her 42-year-old husband are a recently married couple undergoing a comprehensive infertility evaluation after 6 months without conceiving. F.J.'s medical history is positive for seasonal allergic rhinitis, dysmenorrhea, and a history of chlamydia at age 21. Her current screen for sexually transmitted infections is negative. F.J.'s reproductive history reveals menarche at age 11, no prior pregnancies, and regular menstrual cycles approximately 30 days in length. Her body mass index is 21 kg/m^2. There are no abnormal findings on her physical examination. She undergoes a CC challenge test and her FSH and estradiol levels on cycle day 3 are 7 mIU/mL and 46 pg/mL, respectively. The day 10 FSH is 6 mIU/mL. Her HSG shows complete occlusion of the left fallopian tube and partial occlusion of the right fallopian tube. What findings support female factor infertility?

This couple is undergoing evaluation of infertility after only 6 months without conceiving because of F.J.'s advanced age (older than 35) and history of chlamydia, which places her at increased risk of complications from pelvic inflammatory disease. The occlusion of her fallopian tubes is most likely from the chlamydial infection at age 21, which may or may not have been detected and treated at that time. Laparoscopy would be necessary to rule out any additional causes such as endometriosis. Further hysteroscopic procedures are warranted to define the location and type of obstruction and to determine whether surgical repair is feasible.[32] Her regular menstrual cycle length and history of dysmenorrhea is supportive of an ovulatory menstrual cycle and her CC challenge test shows adequate ovarian reserve, with normal levels of FSH and estradiol. She is within the normal weight range and has normal findings upon physical examination. However, further laboratory testing may be warranted to confirm normal thyroid and pituitary function and rule out findings associated with PCOS.

CASE 48-2, QUESTION 2: F.J.'s husband has normal findings upon physical examination. His semen analysis yields the following results:

Semen volume, 3 mL
Sperm number, 41 × 10^6
Sperm concentration, 18 × 10^6/mL
Sperm total motility, 35%
Sperm progressive motility, 30%
Sperm vitality, 60%
Sperm morphology, 2%

A repeat analysis produces similar results. Additional laboratory findings include:

Testosterone, 650 ng/dL
FSH, 4 mIU/mL
Prolactin, 14.2 ng/mL

What is the significance of these findings for male factor infertility and the choice of ART for this couple?

The semen analysis is significant for sperm motility and morphology values below the lower reference limit defined by the World Health Organization. The semen volume, sperm number, and vitality measurements are just above the lower reference limit (Table 48-2).[18] Interventions to improve sperm parameters typically target the underlying cause if possible, such as treatment of hyperprolactinemia or supplementation with testosterone. In some cases, sperm production can be stimulated through the use of medications that influence the hypothalamic–pituitary–testicular axis. For example, CC may improve sperm concentrations in men with hypogonadotropic hypogonadism by stimulating hypothalamic release of GnRH. There is no consensus regarding the optimal dosage regimen, which is FDA-labeled for use in women only. Small clinical studies have examined CC in initial daily doses of 12.5 to 25 mg, in addition to alternate-day and cyclic dosing for treatment periods of several months with positive results.[33] Administration of various regimens of injectable gonadotropins (FSH, LH, or hCG) also improves pregnancy rates.[33] Given this patient's normal serum testosterone and FSH, CC or gonadotropins are not recommended therapies. His prolactin is normal as well, ruling out this potential secondary cause. In this case, there is no identifiable cause of the abnormal parameters so it is deemed idiopathic, without a known etiology.

Antioxidants such as vitamin C, vitamin E, folic acid, zinc, selenium, and L-carnitine are reported to counteract negative effects from oxidative stress on sperm. Some small studies have demonstrated improvement in sperm motility, concentration, and morphology. A systematic review documented a possible increase in live birth rates with the use of antioxidants.[34] F.J.'s husband may choose to take a daily antioxidant supplement as they move forward with other treatment modalities.

Insemination procedures are one approach to address abnormal findings on semen analysis. Bypassing the cervix and placing the sperm closer to the fallopian tubes near the time of ovulation can overcome lower sperm counts and motility issues. In regard to this couple, however, F.J. does not have patent fallopian tubes and would not be a candidate for IUI. An ART procedure will be necessary to address both female and male infertility factors.

IVF is more appropriate than gamete intrafallopian transfer and zygote intrafallopian transfer due to F.J.'s tubal findings. Although surgical repair of the obstructed fallopian tubes may be possible in some cases, many couples choose to bypass this option and pursue ART, especially when there are additional male factors.[32] F.J. will need a surgical evaluation to confirm whether this is recommended prior to proceeding to ART. F.J. is ovulatory with adequate ovarian reserve, so the use of donor oocytes is not required. Her husband's abnormal sperm parameters can be addressed through ICSI, with the option of using donor sperm in the future, if necessary.

IN VITRO FERTILIZATION

The basic steps in an IVF protocol include SO/COS, oocyte retrieval, fertilization, embryo culture, and embryo transfer.

CASE 48-2, QUESTION 3: After the completed evaluation, the couple chooses to undergo IVF with intracytoplasmic sperm injection. Although F.J. is very excited to begin the process, she is anxious about administering the multiple injectable medications associated with the procedure. What medication regimen is recommended to initiate the IVF protocol?

Medications are primarily used during three main stages of IVF: COS, oocyte retrieval, and luteal phase support (Table 48-5). (For a step-by-step guide to all the steps in this complex process, go to http://www.sart.org/patients/a-patients-guide-to-assisted-reproductive-technology/general-information/art-step-by-step-guide/) Treatment protocols vary widely in the medications used, dosing regimens, and timing of administration. A sample in vitro fertilization protocol representing F.J.'s experience is provided in Figure 48-3.

Stage One: Controlled Ovarian Stimulation/ Superovulation

The purpose of COS for IVF is the development of multiple follicles for oocyte retrieval. Although oocyte retrieval and fertilization can be performed during a normal ovulatory cycle without stimulation, it is more common and many times necessary to use this process.

Oral Contraceptives

Controlled ovarian stimulation for IVF is designed to manipulate follicular development for oocyte retrieval at the most opti

Table 48-5
Role of Medications in an In Vitro Fertilization Cycle

IVF Stage	Medications[a]	Role
Stage one: controlled ovarian stimulation	Oral contraceptives	Control the onset of menses and the start of controlled ovarian stimulation
	GnRH agonists or GnRH antagonists	Prevent a premature LH surge or disruption of controlled ovarian stimulation
	Gonadotropins (FSH or FSH plus LH)	Stimulate development of multiple ovarian follicles for oocyte retrieval
Stage two: oocyte retrieval	hCG	Induce final follicular maturation to prepare for oocyte retrieval
Stage three: luteal phase support	Progesterone	Maintain the endometrium for embryo transfer and implantation

[a]This list reflects the medications most commonly used during each stage. Alternate regimens vary widely by specialist.
FSH, follicle-stimulating hormone; GnRH, gonadotropin-releasing hormone; hCG, human chorionic gonadotropin; LH, luteinizing hormone.

stage of maturation. Many protocols start with the administration of oral contraceptives for up to 28 days in the preceding menstrual cycle. This serves to control the timing of the onset of the next menses in order to plan for initiating the COS regimen.[35] This is particularly pertinent in women who have irregular or long menstrual cycles, but is also common practice in those with regular menstrual cycles. F.J. has a history of regular menstrual cycles, but is still a candidate for oral contraceptive therapy to conveniently time the remainder of the treatment course.

Gonadotropin-Releasing Hormone Analogs

Once the COS process begins, it can be interrupted by an endogenous surge of LH that triggers ovulation prematurely and threatens the success of the cycle. Most protocols use medications to limit the influence of any endogenous hormone levels as the cycle progresses. Gonadotropin-releasing hormone agonists have been used for this purpose for several decades. Administration of a GnRH agonist initially increases pituitary gonadotropin release, often referred to as a "flare." Continued daily administration leads to receptor downregulation and reduced pituitary secretion of LH and FSH, allowing for direct administration of the gonadotropins by injection.[36]

The most common IVF regimens in the United States use either subcutaneous leuprolide or intranasal nafarelin (Table 48-6).[23] The leuprolide formulation is often dosed in "units" using an insulin syringe to permit measurement of small volumes. Daily doses of 10 to 20 "units" correspond with 0.5 to 1 mg using the 1 mg/0.2 mL product. The depot formulations of leuprolide or goserelin acetate used for endometriosis or hormone-dependent cancers may require higher doses and longer duration of gonadotropin administration for COS.[37] Intranasal nafarelin has been studied in doses of 200 to 400 mcg twice daily.[38] Intranasal absorption can be variable depending on the administration technique, dosage interval, sneezing, or use of nasal decongestants.[39] However, studies indicate that pregnancy rates between the GnRH agonists are similar.[38]

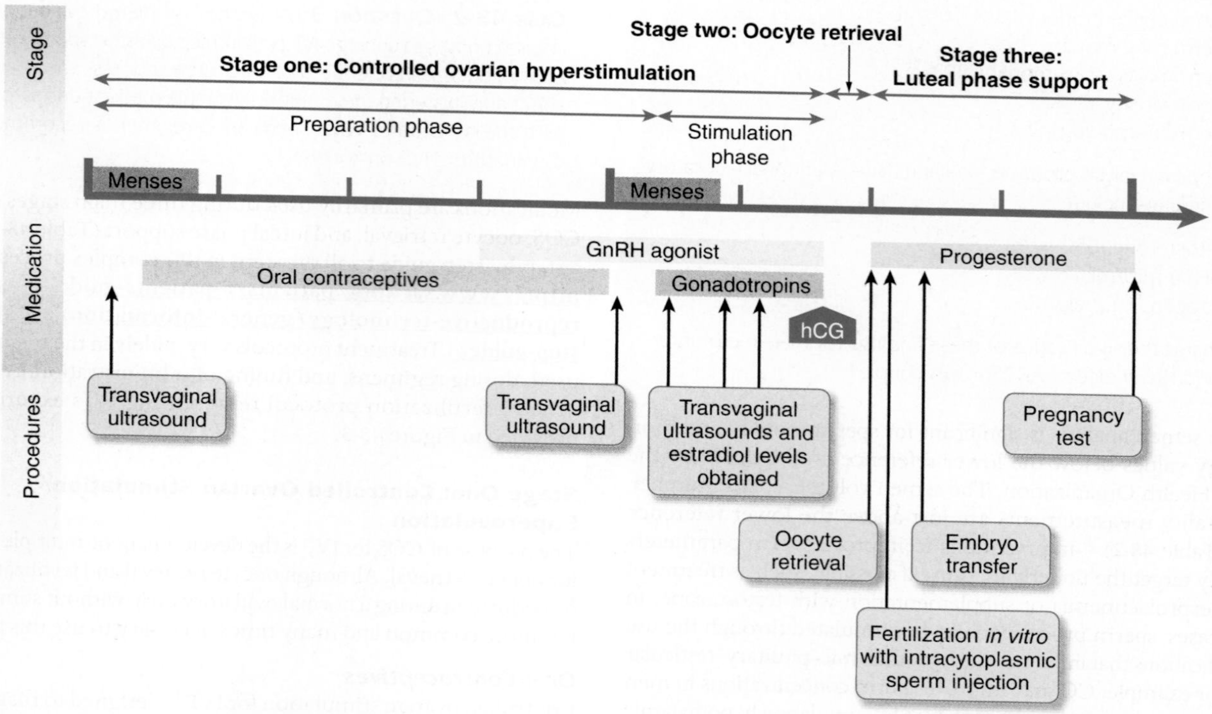

Figure 48-3 Sample in vitro fertilization protocol (Case 48-2).

Table 48-6
Gonadotropin-Releasing Hormone Analogs for In Vitro Fertilization

Analog	Product Name	Strength/Dosage Form	Route of Administration
GnRH agonist	Nafarelin acetate (Synarel)	2 mg/mL solution (200 mcg/spray)	Intranasal
	Leuprolide acetate	1-mg/0.2-mL kit	SC
GnRH antagonist	Cetrorelix acetate[a] (Cetrotide)	0.25-mg kit	SC
	Ganirelix acetate[a]	250-mcg/0.5-mL syringe	SC

[a]FDA-labeled for use with assisted reproductive technology procedures.
Source: Facts & Comparisons eAnswers. https://fco.factsandcomparisons.com/lco/action/doc/retrieve/docid/fc_dfc/5548533; https://fco.factsandcomparisons.com/lco/action/doc/retrieve/docid/fc_dfc/5550316; https://fco.factsandcomparisons.com/lco/action/doc/retrieve/docid/fc_dfc/5548535; https://fco.factsandcomparisons.com/lco/action/doc/retrieve/docid/fc_dfc/5548534; Accessed June 14, 2017. GnRH, gonadotropin-releasing hormone; IM, Intramuscular; SC, subcutaneous.

Treatment protocols are identified by the timing of GnRH agonist administration. In a traditional "long" protocol, a GnRH agonist is initiated during the follicular or luteal phase of the preceding menstrual cycle. Once gonadotropins are initiated, the GnRH agonist is continued at half the daily dose until ovulation is stimulated. If an oral contraceptive is used for pretreatment, the GnRH agonist is often initiated within the last week of the contraceptive regimen. In a "short" protocol, a GnRH agonist is administered in conjunction with the gonadotropins for the stimulation cycle. When used in this manner, the flare, or initial increase in gonadotropin production, aids in the initial recruitment and development of follicles. The continued administration at a lower dose serves to suppress the LH surge. An "ultrashort" protocol reserves the use of the GnRH agonist for just the first 3 days of gonadotropins. The fewer injections in the shorter protocols potentially improves cost and patient convenience. Many other variations of the long and short protocols that adjust the length of GnRH agonist use, dose, and timing of discontinuation are utilized, with wide variability among clinics.[36,40]

Alternatively, the immediate suppression of gonadotropin secretion using GnRH antagonists such as cetrorelix and ganirelix allows for a shorter duration of administration and improved convenience (Table 48-6).[23] Additionally, the lack of FSH and LH flares reduces the incidence of ovarian cysts that can occur with the GnRH agonists. The GnRH antagonists are administered after the gonadotropin-induced follicular development is established, as either a higher-dose single injection or a lower-dose daily injection that is continued until ovulation is triggered.[36,40] Ganirelix is administered as a daily 250-mcg subcutaneous injection and cetrorelix is either a daily subcutaneous injection of 0.25-mg or a single 3-mg dose.[23] The timing of initiation is either "fixed" on a particular day of stimulation or "flexible" based on follicular development.[40] Available data suggest that there is no difference in pregnancy and live birth rates between GnRH agonist and antagonist protocols.[40,41]

In this case, a protocol using a GnRH agonist is chosen for F.J. For the preparation phase, an injectable (such as leuprolide) or intranasal (nafarelin) product can be used. The administration of GnRH analogs in the long protocol is associated with hot flashes, headaches, and sleep disturbances due to hypoestrogenic effects. Concurrent administration of oral contraceptives may help lessen these responses.[42] An intranasal product may appear preferable given F.J.'s concerns about injections. Local reactions at the injection site and nasal and throat irritation are adverse effects expected with the subcutaneous and intranasal routes of administration, respectively.[39,42] However, the symptoms and duration of her seasonal allergic rhinitis should be clarified because the absorption of the intranasal product can be affected by sneezing, congestion, and use of other intranasal medications. Thorough discussion and demonstration of the subcutaneous injection technique can also reduce a patient's fears regarding this route of administration. After discussion, F.J. agrees to administer leuprolide injections. Once she experiences her next menses, she will begin 21 days of an oral contraceptive. On day 16 of this regimen, she will initiate leuprolide 1 mg once daily as a subcutaneous injection in conjunction with the oral contraceptives. A calendar will be provided to help her track the daily doses.

Gonadotropins

Case 48-2, Question 4: F.J. completes the oral contraceptive regimen and starts her menses. A baseline ultrasound rules out ovarian cysts and confirms ovarian suppression. She continues daily injections of leuprolide at a dose of 0.5 mg once daily (half the initial dose) upon initiation of gonadotropins for follicular development. What is the recommended gonadotropin regimen for F.J.?

The exogenous administration of FSH alone or in combination with LH is intended to mimic the natural process of follicular recruitment and maturation. Gonadotropins are available from urinary and recombinant methods (Table 48-3).[23] Human menopausal gonadotropin (hMG) was the first gonadotropin used in the United States as early as the 1950s. The product is extracted from urine of postmenopausal women and standardized to contain 75 IU each of FSH and LH activity. Both LH and hCG are present in the preparation and contribute to the LH activity. Urofollitropin is a urinary FSH that when first marketed in the 1980s retained small amounts of LH and other urinary proteins that were not clinically active. A highly purified urofollitropin is now available that can be injected subcutaneously in place of the earlier intramuscular preparations. The development of the recombinant FSH products (follitropin alfa and follitropin beta) further expanded treatment options in the late 1990s. Although they have unique chemical structures, they result in clinically similar effects.[43]

Women with hypogonadotropic hypogonadism require administration of both FSH and LH because their low endogenous LH levels do not support follicular development. This is achieved through the administration of hMG. Women with normal pituitary function can receive injections of FSH alone, either as urofollitropin or a recombinant product. It is generally demonstrated that urinary hMG and recombinant FSH result in similar pregnancy rates, and there is no consensus recommendation for one preparation over the other.[44]

Dosage regimens for the gonadotropins are intended to promote multiple follicles for oocyte retrieval and vary widely among clinics. A common starting dose in fixed-dose protocols is 150 to 225 IU daily, with further dose adjustments made based on the status of the developing follicles. Treatment may continue for 7 to 12 days, although longer courses may be necessary depending on follicular response. If subsequent cycles are needed, the initial treatment doses are chosen based on the stimulation achieved in the first cycle.[36]

F.J. is undergoing her first cycle of IVF, so there are no data regarding prior gonadotropin response to guide the dose selection. She has no signs of hypothalamic or pituitary dysfunction so she can receive FSH alone or in combination with LH. All of the available highly purified or recombinant products require daily subcutaneous injections. Although this may be a concern for F.J., this is an advantage over earlier formulations that required intramuscular injection. All products require reconstitution of one or more vials of lyophilized powder just prior to injection except certain formulations of the recombinant follitropin alfa and beta. The two recombinant FSH formulations are available in pen injection devices that avoid the need for reconstitution and reduce the complexity of the dose preparation and injection procedure (Table 48-3).[23] Patient education should focus on product-specific instructions for storage, preparation for injection, and the correct subcutaneous injection technique. All products have patient-friendly video demonstrations or handouts available on the Internet to facilitate this process. (For helpful training videos and patient handouts that describe the dose preparation and injection technique, see https://www.ferringfertility.com/products/, and https://fertilitylifelines.com/fertility-treatments/injection-instructional-videos/.) The patient should be instructed to anticipate possible injection-site reactions as well as psychological symptoms of irritability, mood swings, and depression which may increase during this phase.[42]

After consideration of these issues, a recombinant FSH product is chosen for F.J. because of the convenience of the pen device. She will begin a dose of 225 IU of recombinant follitropin alfa injected subcutaneously once daily.

CASE 48-2, QUESTION 5: F.J. begins daily subcutaneous injections of follitropin alfa in addition to her leuprolide injections. What medication monitoring should be provided at this time?

The goal of gonadotropin therapy is to guide the development of multiple follicles for oocyte retrieval without increasing the risk for ovarian hyperstimulation syndrome (OHSS), a rare but serious complication of COS. In its most severe form, this syndrome is characterized by increased systemic vascular permeability that can result in ovarian rupture, thromboembolism, renal failure, and adult respiratory distress syndrome. The risk for this condition correlates most directly with the development of multiple ovarian follicles. Additional risk factors include younger age, low body weight, and history of PCOS. Routine monitoring of ovarian follicular development allows the clinician to maximize efficacy and reduce the risk for overstimulation.[45]

Typical monitoring includes vaginal ultrasounds and serum estradiol measurements performed every 1 to 3 days during the COS phase. The monitoring frequency increases as the follicular development advances, and the gonadotropin doses may be reduced or increased depending on the number and size of the follicles. If hyperresponse is evident, the cycle may be cancelled prior to oocyte retrieval.[45] An alternative to cycle cancellation is "coasting," or discontinuation of gonadotropins until serial estradiol measurements show a plateau or declining trend.[45]

Once F.J. initiates therapy, she is scheduled for serum estradiol and vaginal ultrasound measurements every other day. This increases to daily monitoring on day 7 of the combination of leuprolide and follitropin alfa because the number and size of the follicles continue to increase.

Stage Two: Oocyte Retrieval

Chorionic Gonadotropin

CASE 48-2, QUESTION 6: F.J. presents for her daily monitoring on day 10 and it is determined that she is ready for oocyte retrieval. What medication regimen is recommended at this time?

Chorionic gonadotropin is administered in preparation for oocyte retrieval to simulate the effect of the physiologic LH surge on final oocyte maturation. The oocyte retrieval must be carefully timed to coincide with the completion of the oocyte maturation process, just prior to ovulation. Many clinics schedule oocyte retrieval between 34 and 36 hours after chorionic gonadotropin is injected.

Chorionic gonadotropin is available from urinary or recombinant sources. The urinary hCG product is administered as a single intramuscular injection of 5,000 to 10,000 IU.[23] Doses of 5,000 IU may be administered to patients who are deemed to be at high risk for OHSS.[45] The dose of the recombinant product is 250 mcg injected subcutaneously.[23] A single dose of a GnRH agonist is an alternate method of triggering LH release in IVF protocols that incorporate a GnRH antagonist. This approach appears to reduce the risk for OHSS, but may lower pregnancy rates.[46] F.J. received the GnRH agonist leuprolide in her prestimulation period so she would not be eligible for this approach.

Given F.J.'s concerns regarding injections and the fact that she has been administering the follitropin alfa subcutaneously, it is prudent to continue with this route of administration. F.J. is instructed to inject a single 250-mcg dose of recombinant chorionic gonadotropin subcutaneously. She will discontinue leuprolide and follitropin alfa at this time.

Ovarian Hyperstimulation Syndrome

CASE 48-2, QUESTION 7: F.J. undergoes a transvaginal oocyte retrieval procedure 36 hours after the administration of recombinant chorionic gonadotropin and there are nine oocytes available for fertilization. What additional counseling is recommended for F.J. after the oocyte retrieval?

As previously described, OHSS is a rare complication associated with COS. Careful monitoring of estradiol levels and follicular development on ultrasound limits the incidence. However, if symptoms develop, it is typically within 1 to 2 weeks after oocyte retrieval. It is generally categorized as mild, moderate, or severe, and can occur early (within 9 days after oocyte retrieval) or late (after 10 days, often associated with a pregnancy).[45,47] The clinical signs of OHSS are thought to result from increased capillary permeability due to high levels of vascular endothelial growth factor. However, the specific underlying pathology is poorly understood. A mild presentation of OHSS consists primarily of gastrointestinal symptoms (abdominal pain, nausea, diarrhea, bloating) or weight gain, especially abdominal distension. A patient experiencing these symptoms will be instructed to avoid physical activity, maintain oral fluid intake of at least 1 L/day, and monitor daily weights and urine output. The patient should report any weight gain of 2 lb or more to allow for more intensive outpatient monitoring of liver and renal function, electrolytes, and hematologic parameters. If the condition progresses, the patient may require hospitalization for monitoring and treatment of severe outcomes such as thromboembolism, renal failure, pulmonary distress, or ovarian rupture.[45]

There were no initial indications of hyperstimulation during F.J.'s COS regimen, so she will be instructed to monitor for signs of OHSS during the 2 weeks after oocyte retrieval. She should notify her physician if she experiences gastrointestinal symptoms or weight gain, even if the symptoms are mild. This will facilitate early monitoring to maximize safety during the remainder of the IVF process.

Stage Three: Luteal Phase Support

Progesterone

CASE 48-2, QUESTION 8: After the oocyte retrieval, F.J. is in need of a regimen for luteal phase support. Which agent should be selected?

Supplemental progesterone is administered immediately after oocyte retrieval to provide additional "luteal phase support" during IVF. The luteal phase of the menstrual cycle (Fig. 48-1) is dominated by progesterone released by the corpus luteum that prepares the endometrium for implantation of the fertilized ovum. The disruption of follicles during the oocyte retrieval process delays production of progesterone, necessitating supplementation. Additionally, cycles that utilize a GnRH agonist may be complicated by residual inhibition of pituitary LH secretion and progesterone production into the luteal phase.[48]

Progesterone is available in oral, vaginal, or injectable formulations (Table 48-7).[23] Intramuscular injection of progesterone in oil in a daily dose of 50 mg was the first method used for supplementation and continues to be widely used. However, alternatives to progesterone in oil have been sought due to frequent reports of rash and discomfort at the injection site.[49]

Vaginal progesterone preparations have gained popularity for luteal phase support due to ease of administration and avoidance of injection-site reactions. The 8% progesterone vaginal gel and the 100 mg vaginal insert are the only commercially available FDA-labeled preparations for use in ART procedures. The gel is administered as one 90-mg applicator once or twice daily. The dose of the vaginal insert is 100 mg either twice a day (every 12 hours) or 3 times a day (every 8 hours).[48–50] Patient education should focus on the correct technique for intravaginal administration. Both products utilize a disposable applicator to facilitate correct placement. (Detailed patient instructions are provided by both manufacturers. https://www.ferringfertility.com/products/endometrin/ and https://www.allergan.com/assets/pdf/crinone_pi.)

Table 48-7

Commercially Available Progesterone Products Used in Assisted Reproductive Technology

Product Name	Strength/Dosage Form	Route of Administration
Crinone	8% vaginal gel[a]	Vaginal
Endometrin	100-mg vaginal insert[a]	Vaginal
FIRST-Progesterone VGS	50-, 100-, 200-, 400-mg vaginal suppository (compounding kit)	Vaginal
Progesterone	50 mg/mL (oil)	Intramuscular
Prometrium/micronized progesterone	100-, 200-mg capsule	Oral

[a]FDA-labeled for luteal phase support.

Source: Facts & Comparisons eAnswers. https://fco.factsandcomparisons.com/lco/action/search?q=crinone&t=name; Accessed June 14, 2017.

The vaginal preparations may cause local irritation and vaginal discharge, although the vaginal gel is generally associated with less discharge than the inserts or suppositories. Clinical studies suggest no difference in pregnancy rates between vaginal and intramuscular formulations, so clinician and patient preferences often dictate the selection.[48–50]

Oral formulations are not recommended for the purpose of luteal phase support with ART due to lower absorption and reduced pregnancy rates.[48] Compounded formulations are widely available, including oral micronized progesterone and progesterone vaginal suppositories, gels, and creams. In some cases, patients are instructed to insert oral progesterone formulations intravaginally.

Progesterone is initiated after oocyte retrieval until a pregnancy test is performed and then continued until at least 8- to 10-week gestation.[48] Data suggest that there are no significant risks to the mother or fetus from supplemental progesterone during this time period.[50]

Luteal phase support after oocyte retrieval is important for F.J. because she received a GnRH agonist in her long cycle protocol. Because the efficacy of the parenteral and vaginal formulations is similar, the patient chooses the vaginal route to avoid further injections. She determines that she is most comfortable with 8% progesterone vaginal gel applied once daily and is given instructions regarding the appropriate administration technique.

Embryo Transfer

CASE 48-2, QUESTION 9: The in vitro fertilization process using intracytoplasmic sperm injection yields four cleavage-stage embryos. What considerations are necessary for embryo transfer?

After fertilization, timing of the embryo transfer into the uterus depends on the stage of development. Cleavage-stage embryos are transferred 2 to 3 days postfertilization, whereas embryos in the blastocyst stage are transferred at day 5 or 6.[51] (To reference a tool that gives a representation of the embryo at different stages, see http://visembryo.com/baby/pregnancy1.html.) The number of embryos placed during this process must balance the risks of a multiple gestation pregnancy with the likelihood of successful implantation.

Multiple gestation pregnancies are associated with increased maternal and neonatal morbidity. The mother is at risk for complications such as premature labor, pregnancy-induced hypertension, and gestational diabetes. Preterm labor occurs in approximately 15% of single gestation pregnancies compared with 75% of triplet pregnancies. The neonates are more likely to experience fetal growth restriction and require intensive care for pulmonary, gastrointestinal, and neurologic complications.[22] Additional stressors include the financial and psychosocial implications of raising children with complex medical needs that may persist beyond infancy.[22]

F.J. is 39 years old experiencing her first cycle of IVF. The ASRM has developed embryo transfer recommendations to limit high-order multiple pregnancies (three or more implanted embryos). Based upon her age, if the embryos are judged to have good quality morphology, no more than three cleavage-stage or two blastocysts should be transferred according to ASRM guidelines.[51] A pregnancy test will be performed 9 to 12 days after the embryo transfer to determine the outcome of the cycle.

Long-Term Considerations

Alternate Protocols

CASE 48-2, QUESTION 10: After careful consideration, the couple decides to transfer two cleavage-stage embryos and reserve two for cryopreservation. Unfortunately, the embryo transfer procedure is unsuccessful and the couple plans to pursue a second procedure. What considerations are necessary for future cycles?

Determining an action plan for subsequent procedures requires a thorough evaluation of the response to therapy during the first cycle. If COS is repeated for oocyte retrieval, hormone levels, follicular development, fertilization rates, and numbers of viable embryos are all considered to determine whether dosage adjustments or alternate medication protocols are necessary.

In this case, F.J. experienced adequate follicular development for oocyte retrieval without signs of OHSS. The fertilization procedure was successful and two embryos were cryopreserved for future procedures. The couple can choose to avoid another stimulation process for oocyte removal and move to frozen embryo transfer. Medications remain important for the frozen embryo transfer process, which can occur in a natural cycle or a cycle induced through the use of estrogen and progesterone, with or without GnRH agonists.[52]

Beyond planning the actual protocol, the long-term safety of any repeated medication exposure as well as the psychosocial effects of continuing therapy must be considered. The time needed to gather available information and weigh all considerations will be specific to each couple.

Psychosocial Issues

The financial impact of ART is substantial. The ASRM cites the average cost of an IVF cycle in the United States to be between \$10,000 - \$15,000.[53] Costs vary widely between clinics and many offer financial counseling and payment packages to facilitate treatment. Additionally, the psychological stress of the diagnosis and treatment of infertility must be considered at all stages. There is an observed fluctuation of mood during the course of an IVF cycle, with higher stress points identified at oocyte retrieval and pregnancy testing. This is complicated by potential side effects of medications as well as the baseline mental health of the couple.[54] For couples who undergo successive ART procedures, repeated failures are commonly accompanied by feelings of grief and frustration, and psychological distress is often the reason for discontinuing treatments. Levels of emotional distress, including symptoms of depression and anxiety, can increase with each unsuccessful cycle. This response appears to remit immediately with a successful pregnancy, but in those who continue to be unsuccessful, symptoms can still be significant even 6 months post-treatment.[55]

This couple should be offered individual counseling and social support that extends beyond the initial pretreatment consultation to promote positive outcomes.[56] There are several patient-focused resources for informational fact sheets and videos highlighting the financial, medical, and psychosocial issues of infertility (Table 48-8).

Table 48-8
Patient-Focused Infertility Resources

Sponsor	Website
Path2Parenthood	http://www.path2parenthood.org/
American Society of Reproductive Medicine	http://www.reproductivefacts.org/
Centers for Disease Control and Prevention	http://www.cdc.gov/art/patientresources/preparing.html
Resolve: The National Infertility Association	http://www.resolve.org/
Society for Assisted Reproductive Technology	http://www.sart.org/

KEY REFERENCES AND WEBSITES

A full list of references for this chapter can be found at http://thepoint.lww.com/AT11e. Below are the key references and websites for this chapter, with the corresponding reference number in this chapter found in parentheses after the reference.

Key References

Centers for Disease Control and Prevention, American Society for Reproductive Medicine, Society for Assisted Reproductive Technology. *2012 Assisted Reproductive Technology: National Summary Report*. Atlanta, GA: US Department of Health and Human Services; 2014. (31)

Practice Committee of the American Society for Reproductive Medicine in collaboration with the Society for Reproductive Endocrinology and Infertility. Optimizing natural fertility: a committee opinion. *Fertil Steril*. 2013;100(3):631–637. (9)

Practice Committee of the American Society for Reproductive Medicine. Diagnostic evaluation of the infertile female: a committee opinion. *Fertil Steril*. 2015;103(6):e44–e50. (2)

Practice Committee of the American Society for Reproductive Medicine. Testing and interpreting measures of ovarian reserve: a committee opinion. *Fertil Steril*. 2015;103(3):e9–e17. (13)

Practice Committee of the American Society for Reproductive Medicine. Diagnostic evaluation of the infertile male. *Fertil Steril*. 2015;103(3):e18–e25. (15)

Practice Committee of the American Society for Reproductive Medicine. Use of clomiphene citrate in infertile women. *Fertil Steril*. 2013;100(2):341–348. (25)

Practice Committee of the American Society for Reproductive Medicine. Gonadotropin preparations: past, present, and future perspectives. *Fertil Steril*. 2008;90(Suppl 3):S13–S20. (43)

Practice Committee of the American Society for Reproductive Medicine. Ovarian hyperstimulation syndrome. *Fertil Steril*. 2008;90(Suppl 3):S188–S193. (45)

Practice Committee of the American Society for Reproductive Medicine. Current clinical irrelevance of luteal phase deficiency: a committee opinion. *Fertil Steril*. 2015;103(4):e27–e32. (48)

Practice Committee of the American Society for Reproductive Medicine in collaboration with the Society for Reproductive Endocrinology and Infertility. Progesterone supplementation during the luteal phase and in early pregnancy in the treatment of infertility: an educational bulletin. *Fertil Steril*. 2008;90(Suppl 3):S150–S153. (50)

World Health Organization, Department of Reproductive Health and Research. *WHO Laboratory Manual for the Examination and Processing of Human Semen*. 5th ed. Geneva, Switzerland: World Health Organization Press; 2010:224. (18)

Zegers-Hochschild F et al. The International Committee for Monitoring Assisted Reproductive Technology (ICMART) and the World Health Organization (WHO) revised glossary on ART terminology, 2009. *Hum Reprod*. 2009;24(11):2683–2687. (30)

Key Websites

American Society for Reproductive Medicine. http://www.asrm.org/.
Society for Assisted Reproductive Technology. http://www.sart.org/.

49 Obstetric Drug Therapy

Trisha LaPointe

CORE PRINCIPLES

		CHAPTER CASES
1	The timing and quality of prenatal care can influence an infant's health and survival. Early comprehensive care can promote healthier pregnancies through early detection of risk factors, disease state management, and encouragement of healthy behaviors.	**Case 49-1 (Questions 1, 2)**
2	Important physiologic changes occur in almost all maternal organs during pregnancy to support the growth and development of the fetus.	**Case 49-1 (Question 4)**
3	Drug use during pregnancy presents a significant challenge to clinicians because of the potential adverse effect on the embryo, fetus, and newborn. A thorough assessment, including knowledge of the teratogenic potential of the drug, the critical period of exposure, and magnitude of risk, must be compared with the background risk.	**Case 49-1 (Question 5)**
4	Gastrointestinal (GI) disturbances such as nausea and vomiting and gastric reflux that occur during pregnancy are common. Treatments include intravenous (IV) hydration, pyridoxine (vitamin B_6), antihistamines, and antiemetics for nausea and vomiting. Calcium carbonate, H_2-receptor antagonists, and proton-pump inhibitors may be used for common complaints from reflux.	**Case 49-1 (Questions 6-10)**
5	Urinary tract infections can frequently occur during pregnancy and can easily be treated with nitrofurantoin, cephalexin, or penicillin if cultures are sensitive.	**Case 49-1 (Questions 11)**
6	Diabetes mellitus is the most common maternal medical complication during pregnancy. Tight glycemic control can minimize neonatal and fetal morbidity and mortality associated with diabetic embryopathy.	**Case 49-2 (Questions 1–4), Case 49-3 (Questions 1, 2), Case 49-4 (Questions 1–4)**
7	Women with pregnancy-associated hypertension can be grouped into the following categories: chronic hypertension, preeclampsia–eclampsia, preeclampsia superimposed on chronic hypertension, and gestational hypertension.	**Case 49-5 (Questions 1–13)**
8	The induction of labor involves the artificial stimulation of uterine contractions that lead to labor and delivery.	**Case 49-6 (Questions 1–5)**
9	Premature birth is the leading cause of neonatal mortality (infant death <1 month of age). Tocolytic therapy to stop contractions, corticosteroids for fetal lung maturity, and antibiotics for preterm premature rupture of membranes can help to prolong the pregnancy.	**Case 49-7 (Questions 1–7)**
10	Infectious complications, including bacterial vaginosis and urinary tract infections, can lead to preterm labor. Chorioamnionitis, an infection of the chorion and amnion usually diagnosed during labor with elevations in temperature, should be treated with IV antibiotics until delivery. Human immunodeficiency virus (HIV)-infected mothers should receive IV zidovudine and continue their antiretroviral regimens during labor.	**Case 49-7 (Questions 8–11), Case 49-8 (Questions 1, 2)**
11	Obstetric postpartum hemorrhage is one of the top three causes of maternal mortality in the United States. Pharmacologic therapy for uterine atony includes oxytocin, methylergonovine, carboprost, misoprostol, and dinoprostone.	**Case 49-8 (Questions 3, 4)**

Continued

	CHAPTER CASES
12 Alloimmunization occurs when an Rh D-negative mother becomes immunized after exposure to fetal erythrocytes that carry the D antigen. Rh_o(D) immune globulin should be given to all mothers who are Rh D negative at 28 weeks' gestation.	Case 49-9 (Questions 1–5)
LACTATION AND DRUGS IN BREAST MILK	
1 Breast milk is recognized as the optimal source of nutrition for infants, with documented benefits not only to infants but also to mothers, families, and societies, and breast-feeding should be encouraged if possible.	Case 49-10 (Questions 1, 2), Case 49-11 (Question 1)
2 Most drugs are excreted in the breast milk. The pharmacologic and adverse effects on the infant will be determined by the extent of oral bioavailability, distribution, metabolism, and rate of elimination. A milk-to-plasma ratio can be used to estimate the drug concentration in milk. The relative infant dose (RID) can be calculated to estimate the infant's exposure based on volume of milk ingested.	Case 49-8 (Question 2), Case 49-12 (Question 1), Case 49-13 (Question 1)

PREGNANCY

Definitions

PARITY AND GRAVIDA

Parity and *gravida* are terms used to describe a pregnant woman. Parity is the number of deliveries after 20 weeks' gestation. Parity is independent of the number of fetuses delivered (live or stillborn, single fetus, or twins) or the method of delivery. *Gravida* refers to the number of pregnancies a woman has had regardless of the outcome. For example, a woman who is currently pregnant and has previously delivered one set of twins and had two spontaneous abortions is described as a gravida 4, para 1 (G4, P1).

TRIMESTERS OF PREGNANCY

The average pregnancy is approximately 40 weeks when calculated from the first day of the LMP. Pregnancy is typically divided into three trimesters, approximately 13 to 14 weeks each.[1] The first trimester includes the critical period of organogenesis, the time in which most of the vital organs are developing, which occurs between weeks 5 and 10. The time between the end of the 20th week of gestation and the end of the 28th day after birth is considered the perinatal period.

DELIVERY

Depending on the gestational age at the time of delivery, the result can be an abortion, preterm, term, or post-term birth. An abortion is a delivery before 20 weeks' gestation. A term infant is a fetus delivered between 37 and 42 weeks' gestation. A preterm birth is one occurring between 20 and 37 weeks' gestation, and a post-term (postmaturity) birth occurs after the beginning of 42 weeks' gestation. Parturition refers to labor, and the puerperium is the 6 to 8 weeks after delivery.

Preconceptional Care

CASE 49-1

QUESTION 1: S.C. is a 29-year-old, G1, P1 woman who is interested in becoming pregnant. Her past medical history is significant for hypothyroidism. She currently is taking levothyroxine 88 mcg by mouth daily. Provide appropriate counseling to S.C. with regard to preconceptional care.

It is estimated that 3.9 million live births were registered in the United States in 2013, with an estimated 70.8% of women beginning prenatal care in the first trimester. This can be contributed to several statewide initiatives to increase education and access to prenatal care.[2] Although much improved, prenatal care is still not easily accessible to all women. Early comprehensive care can promote healthier pregnancies through early detection of risk factors, disease state management, and encouragement of healthy behaviors, and will help to ensure normal fetal organogenesis. Appropriate preconception counseling and treatment of women with preexisting high-risk medical conditions, such as diabetes, hypertension, and epilepsy, can greatly improve pregnancy outcomes. In 2013, the mortality rate in the United States (from birth through the first year of life) for infants of mothers beginning prenatal care in the first trimester was 5.96/1,000 live births.[3]

S.C. should see her primary-care provider for regular physical examinations and evaluation of her thyroid function before becoming pregnant. Her first prenatal visit should generally occur by 8 weeks' gestational age when she becomes pregnant.[4]

Vitamins and Mineral Supplementation

CASE 49-1, QUESTION 2: S.C. asks you to recommend vitamin and mineral supplementation and to provide guidance on when should she begin taking these vitamins and minerals.

A balanced diet that provides S.C. with multiple B vitamins, oil-soluble vitamins (A, E, D, and K), folic acid, and minerals (iron, calcium, phosphorus, magnesium, iodine, zinc) should be encouraged. S.C. should be started on a prenatal multivitamin if she has not yet started taking one. Prenatal vitamins should be taken months before conception to ensure that proper nutritional requirements are met during critical periods of organogenesis and fetal growth.

IRON REQUIREMENTS

Iron requirements increase during pregnancy because of maternal blood volume expansion, fetal needs, placenta and cord needs, and blood loss at the time of delivery.[5] Maternal iron deficiency can cause anemia during infancy, spontaneous abortion, premature delivery, and delivery of a low-birth-weight infant, and is associated with low neonatal iron stores.[5,6]

A woman needs about 18 to 21 mg of iron/day during pregnancy; the body compensates by increasing iron absorption from the GI tract by about 15% to 50%.[5] The average diet of women in the United States does not meet these requirements because only about 6 mg of iron is absorbed from 1,000 kcal of food. In addition, some women may already have inadequate body stores of iron before pregnancy. For these reasons, the Centers for Disease Control and Prevention recommends screening for iron deficiency in pregnancy in addition to universal iron supplementation except when genetic conditions such as hemochromatosis are present.[7] Prenatal vitamins usually contain 30 to 60 mg of elemental iron. Women with iron deficiency anemia should be given 60 to 120 mg of elemental iron daily. Iron deficiency anemia during pregnancy generally is associated with a hemoglobin and hematocrit less than 11 mg/dL and less than 33%, respectively, during the first and third trimesters or less than 10.5 mg/dL and less than 32%, respectively, during the second trimester. The classic morphologic changes observed in the erythrocytes in iron deficiency outside of pregnancy, hypochromia, and microcytosis are not prominent in pregnant women. Serum ferritin, however, is low, which has the highest sensitivity and specificity for diagnosing iron deficiency.[6] S.C.'s hemoglobin and hematocrit should be assessed now and again at 26 to 28 weeks' gestation. If her hemoglobin and hematocrit are normal, the amount of iron in her prenatal vitamin should be sufficient.

FOLATE REQUIREMENTS

Folic acid is essential in the synthesis of DNA and RNA. Pregnant women who take 0.4 to 0.8 mg of folic acid daily during the first trimester of pregnancy are significantly less likely to have a child with neural tube defects (NTDs), such as spina bifida and anencephaly.[8,9] NTD can lead to stillbirth, neonatal death, or serious disabilities. Approximately 4,000 pregnancies in the United States are affected by NTD each year.[9]

NTDs develop within the first month of pregnancy at a time when many women are unaware of their pregnancy.[9,10] In 1992, the US Public Health Service recommended that all women with childbearing potential should consume 0.4 mg/day of folic acid to reduce the risk of an NTD-affected pregnancy.[11]

It may be difficult to meet the recommended daily allowance (RDA) for folic acid because foods contain only a small amount of this vitamin; overcooking and high-fiber diets also can reduce the amount of available folic acid from food. Most prenatal vitamins contain 0.8 to 1 mg of folic acid.

Folic acid supplementation is especially important in women with a history of infants born with NTD. Women who have had an NTD-affected pregnancy should receive genetic counseling because they have a 2% to 3% risk of having another such outcome. Women with previous NTD-affected pregnancies who plan another pregnancy should take 4 mg/day of folic acid at least 1 month before conception and through the first 3 months of pregnancy.[11]

Women who require 4 mg/day of folic acid should be prescribed folic acid tablets as an addition to combination prenatal multivitamins (which contain folic acid), rather than just increasing the number of multivitamin tablets. When several fixed-combination multivitamin tablets are taken daily, the mother could be exposed to a potentially teratogenic dose of vitamin A. High doses of folic acid do not prevent NTD better than 0.4 mg/day in women without a previous history of NTD-affected pregnancies and may complicate the diagnosis of a vitamin B_{12} deficiency.[9]

S.C. should be counseled about the risks for NTD, and given she has no history of NTD, she should receive adequate folic acid during the remainder of her pregnancy from a daily prenatal vitamin.

CALCIUM REQUIREMENTS

Calcium is needed during pregnancy for adequate mineralization of the fetal skeleton and teeth, especially during the third trimester when teeth are formed and skeletal growth is greatest. The RDA for calcium during pregnancy is 1,000 mg/day for women of 19 years and older, and 1,300 mg/day for teenagers younger than the age of 19.[12] Large maternal stores can provide calcium if dietary intake is inadequate; however, depleting maternal stores may put S.C. at risk for osteoporosis later in life. Foods rich in calcium (e.g., milk, cheese, yogurt, legumes, nuts, dried fruits) or calcium supplements can be used to meet the calcium RDA.

Commercially Available Home Pregnancy Tests

CASE 49-1, QUESTION 3: S.C starts her prenatal vitamins that contain iron and folic acid immediately. Two months have passed, and now S.C. believes that she may be pregnant because per period is a couple of weeks late. She requests your assistance in selecting an over-the-counter commercially available home pregnancy test. How do these home pregnancy tests work and how should S.C. be counseled?

Commercially available home pregnancy tests are enzyme immunoassays with monoclonal or polyclonal antibodies that bind to hCG in the urine.[13] hCG is detected in the maternal circulation and urine approximately 8 to 10 days after conception.[14] Concentrations in the urine closely parallel those in the maternal blood. The hCG serum concentrations increase rapidly, doubling every 2 days. Peak concentrations are achieved at 60 to 70 days of pregnancy. Thereafter, hCG concentrations decline and reach a low by approximately 120 days, at which point concentrations are maintained for the remainder of the pregnancy.[14]

hCG is composed of an α- and a β-subunit. The α-subunit is identical to the α-subunit of other pituitary hormones (e.g., follicle-stimulating hormone, luteinizing hormone, thyroid-stimulating hormone); however, the β-subunit is specific to hCG. Pregnancy tests specific for this β-subunit are useful diagnostic tests for confirming pregnancy.[1] They can provide accurate results within 1 to 2 weeks after ovulation.[1,13] Several kits are available. The tests can be performed privately and quickly and are easily interpreted. The results are obtained rapidly—within 1 and 5 minutes—and are highly accurate when performed at the start of the first missed menstrual period. Although home pregnancy tests are reportedly 98% to 100% accurate when used correctly, consumer studies have documented accuracy rates as low as 50% to 75% if product directions are not precisely followed.[13] Many home pregnancy tests include a second test, which should be repeated at a specified time after the first negative test result.

S.C. should purchase a product containing two tests and follow the instructions carefully. If the first test result is negative, S.C. should repeat the test in 1 week if she has not started menstruating. False-negative results occur when testing is done before the first day of a missed period or if the urine is not at room temperature.[13] False-negative results can also occur with an ectopic (outside the uterus) pregnancy or in women with ovarian cysts and in those receiving menotropins or chorionic gonadotropin.[13] False-positive pregnancy test results are rare, but can occur with serum testing if the woman has circulating heterophilic antibodies directed against the animal-derived antigen use in pregnancy tests. These antibodies will not interfere with urine assays, however, as they are not present in urine.[15]

S.C.'s home pregnancy test is positive. Because she is pregnant she should be counseled on the possible fetal effects of any medications or herbal products she may be taking and advised to see her primary-care provider as soon as possible.

Pregnancy-Induced Pharmacokinetic Changes

CASE 49-1, QUESTION 4: S.C. is now 6 weeks pregnant. She is concerned about any possible changes that might occur with her medications (levothyroxine 88 mcg orally [PO] daily, prenatal vitamins). Describe pregnancy-induced pharmacokinetic changes that might occur that will affect her medication use and appropriate monitoring.

Important physiologic changes occur in almost all maternal organs during pregnancy to support the growth and development of the fetus. These physiologic changes affect the cardiovascular, respiratory, and GI systems; plasma volume, renal function, and hepatic enzymes can alter the absorption, distribution, metabolism, and elimination of drugs.[16] Alterations in the pharmacokinetics of drugs are influenced by mainly by two factors: (a) maternal physiologic changes and (b) the effects of the placental–fetal compartment.[17]

ABSORPTION

Pregnancy-induced changes affecting drug absorption are (a) a decrease in intestinal motility owing to smooth muscle relaxation by progesterone, resulting in a 30% to 50% increase of gastric and intestinal emptying times; (b) a 40% decrease in gastric acidity, which increases gastric pH; and (c) altered bioavailability or absorption attributable to increased incidence of nausea and vomiting. Bioavailability may be increased for acid-labile drugs and decreased for drugs that require acid medium for stability. Prolonged gastric and intestinal emptying times may decrease the maximum concentration (C_{max}) of a drug and the time to reach C_{max}, whereas the increased intestinal transit time may increase the area under the curve (AUC) and bioavailability of a drug. In contrast, pregnancy-induced vomiting may decrease the amount of drug ingested; it is therefore better to schedule medications during the evening when the incidence of nausea and vomiting is lower, or to use the rectal route for drug administration. In summary, the effect of pregnancy on drug absorption is variable and depends greatly on the physicochemical properties of the drug.[17] Increased blood flow to the maternal skin, which helps dissipate fetal heat production, may also increase the absorption of a topically (transdermal) administered medication.[16]

DISTRIBUTION

Changes in protein binding and increased plasma volume can theoretically increase the apparent volume of distribution (V_d) of drugs during pregnancy. Plasma volume increases by 6 to 8 weeks' gestation and continues to expand to 40% to 50% above pregnancy volumes by 32 to 34 weeks' gestation.[16,17] Plasma volume expands even more with multiple gestations. The total body water (TBW) increases by 8 L; 40% of this increase can be attributable to the mother and 60% to the fetal–placental unit. This increase in TBW necessitates larger loading doses of water-soluble drugs (e.g., aminoglycosides) because of the increase in Vd. A decrease in the C_{max} would be expected.

Plasma albumin concentrations decrease during pregnancy, mostly because of dilution by the increased plasma volume.[16,17] Albumin concentrations may also be decreased as a result of decreased synthesis or increased catabolism.[16] In addition, increased concentrations of steroid and placental hormones may decrease protein-binding sites for drugs.[18] These changes in protein binding generally result in decreased protein binding, increased free fraction (f_u) of drugs, and increased clearance of drugs when clearance is dependent on f_u (e.g., valproic acid, carbamazepine).[18] When both f_u and intrinsic clearance are increased as is the case with increased cytochrome P-450 enzyme activity, both the total and free concentrations are decreased (e.g., phenytoin, phenobarbital).[19] Total protein and α_1-acid glycoprotein concentrations remain fairly unchanged.

METABOLISM

Protein binding, activity of hepatic enzymes, and liver blood flow determine the hepatic clearance of drugs. Increases in estrogen and progesterone during pregnancy affect the hepatic metabolism by stimulating or decreasing different hepatic enzymes of the cytochrome P-450 (CYP) system.[20] CYP3A4 and CYP2D6 activities are increased during pregnancy, which results in increased metabolism of certain drugs such as phenytoin.[17,20] On the other hand, CYP1A2, xanthine oxidase, and *N*-acetyltransferase activity are decreased, resulting in reduced hepatic elimination of drugs such as theophylline and caffeine.[19,21] The clearance of caffeine can be decreased by 70%.[21] Hepatic blood flow as a percentage of the cardiac output is decreased; however, the absolute rate (in L/minute) remains unchanged.[16] The activity of nonhepatic enzymes (e.g., plasma cholinesterase) is also decreased.[19] The extent of the effect on drug therapy of these hepatic physiologic changes during pregnancy is difficult to quantify.

ELIMINATION

The glomerular filtration rate (GFR) begins to rise in the first half of the first trimester and increases by 50% by the beginning of the second trimester.[19] Renal blood flow also increases by 25% to 50% early during gestation. As a result, renal drug excretion (e.g., β-lactams, enoxaparin, digoxin) can increase.[17] This increase in GFR necessitates dosage adjustments up to 20% to 65% for renally excreted drugs throughout pregnancy to maintain therapeutic concentrations.[20] The increased cardiac output and regional blood flow (e.g., renal blood flow) primarily are caused by increased stroke volume and increased heart rate, which can increase drug distribution and drug excretion.

During pregnancy, the serum creatinine concentration is lower because of the increased GFR, resulting in normal serum creatinine values of 0.3 to 0.7 mg/dL in the first and second trimesters.[20] A normal value for serum creatinine in nonpregnant adults is 0.6 to 1.2 mg/dL.[22] Similar changes occur with serum urea nitrogen and uric acid (UA) concentrations. These differences have important implications when assessing renal function during pregnancy. A serum creatinine indicative of normal renal function in a nonpregnant woman may be indicative of renal insufficiency in a woman who is pregnant in her third trimester.

PLACENTAL–FETAL COMPARTMENT EFFECT

Maternal and fetal drug concentrations are dependent on the amount of drug that crosses the placenta, the extent of metabolism by the placenta, and fetal distribution and elimination of drug (Fig. 49-1).[17,20] Diffusion across the placenta is the main mechanism of drug transfer; nonionized lipophilic substances are more readily transferred, whereas less lipid-soluble (e.g., ionized) substances less readily cross the placenta.[17] Highly protein-bound or large-molecular-weight drugs (e.g., heparin and insulin) do not cross the placenta. Both the immature fetal liver and placenta can metabolize drugs. Fetal drug accumulation can be problematic secondary to limited metabolic enzymatic activity along with the concern that approximately half of the blood flow from the umbilical vein bypasses the fetal liver and goes to the cardiac and cerebral circulations.[17] Another mechanism that can also lead to prolonged effects of drugs in the fetal compartment is ion trapping. This phenomenon occurs because the fetal plasma pH is more acidic than the maternal plasma, causing weak bases (e.g., usually nonionized and lipophilic substances) to diffuse across the placental barrier and become ionized in the more acidic fetal blood. The net effect is

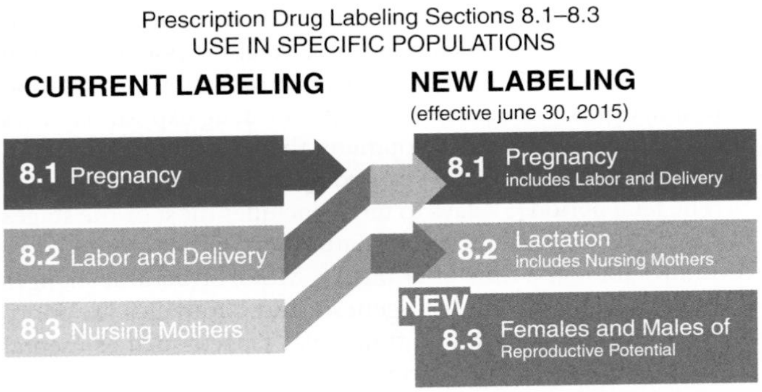

Figure 49-1 FDA Labeling. (Source: http://www.fda.gov/drugs/developmentapprovalprocess/developmentresources/labeling/ucm093307.htm)

movement of drugs from the maternal to fetal compartment. This equilibrium between the maternal and fetal compartments becomes important when therapeutic fetal drug concentrations are desired (e.g., digoxin therapy for intrauterine fetal arrhythmias). Drugs are eliminated by the fetus primarily through diffusion back to the maternal compartment. As the fetal kidney matures, metabolites of drugs are excreted into the amniotic fluid.[17]

S.C.'s thyroid function should be checked regularly to assess the need for an increase in her levothyroxine dosage. During S.C.'s pregnancy, an increase in the Vd of thyroid hormones in the vascular, hepatic, and fetal–placental units, an increase in thyroxine-binding globulin resulting from a rise in estrogen, and an increase in placental transport and maternal metabolism of thyroxine will occur.[22] Most women with hypothyroidism who are taking oral thyroid hormones before pregnancy, similar to S.C., will require an increase in their dosage by about 30% to 50% throughout their pregnancy and then will need decreased dose adjustments postpartum.[22]

TERATOGENICITY

CASE 49-1, QUESTION 5: S.C. is currently 8 weeks pregnant and has become increasingly concerned about her medication use during pregnancy and the risk of birth defects. How should S.C. be counseled regarding the teratogenicity potential of levothyroxine use during pregnancy?

Prevalence of Congenital Malformations

The largest concern with medication use during pregnancy is the risk of congenital malformations, defined as "structural abnormalities of prenatal origin that are present at birth and that seriously interfere with viability or physical well-being."[23] Congenital anomalies or birth defects are estimated to occur in 120,000 babies born per year.[10] Some drug-induced defects relate to changes in functions or conditions that are not structural abnormalities (e.g., mental retardation, central nervous system [CNS] depression, deafness, tumors, or biochemical changes).[24] The broader term *congenital anomalies* include the four major manifestations of abnormal fetal development, which include growth alterations, functional deficits, structural malformations, and fetal death.[25]

The background incidence of birth defects in the general population must be taken into consideration when interpreting the risk of drug-induced birth defects. The prevalence of major congenital malformations discovered at or shortly after birth in the general population is approximately 3%.[25] This number has been derived from large epidemiologic studies completed during the past several decades and depends on how terms are defined (e.g., major versus minor congenital malformations), the thoroughness with which the infant is examined, and how long the exposed person is followed after birth.[25] The collection of malformations data is a complicated task subject to numerous errors and biases. Some studies examined only "significant anomalies," others "major malformations," whereas still others reported only "live births" or "single births" or "birth weights greater than 500 g." Stillbirths and spontaneous abortions, both often associated with congenital malformations, often were excluded from epidemiologic data. Neurodevelopmental delays and growth retardation also are potential long-term effects that will not be diagnosed in the immediate postpartum period. The prevalence of congenital anomalies is likely greater than 3% if minor anomalies and long-term adverse effects are considered.

Despite the significant impact of drug-induced birth defects, it is difficult and unethical to conduct randomized, controlled trials to assess the risk of fetal exposure to drugs in humans. Much of the data available are derived from epidemiologic studies, anecdotal experiences in humans, and animal studies. Because birth defects are species-specific and influenced by many factors including genetic predisposition, the data must be carefully interpreted and the results not overgeneralized.

Causes of Malformations

CLASSIFICATION

Causes of congenital malformations are generally classified into one of five categories: (a) monogenic origin, (b) chromosomal abnormalities, (c) multifactorial inheritance, (d) environmental factors, and (e) unknown.[25] Single gene- and chromosomal-related defects account for approximately 25% of all congenital malformations in live-born infants (monogenetic, 7.5%–20%; chromosomal, 5%–6%).[24–26] *Multifactorial inheritance* refers to defects that are polygenic in origin; it has an environmental component. One surveillance program estimated that this interaction between genetic and environmental factors causes 23% of defects.[26] Congenital dislocation of the hip is an example of a defect in this category: The depths of the acetabular socket and joint laxity are genetically determined, and a frank breech malposition is one of the environmental factors.[27] In most cases, however, the environmental factors in multifactorial inheritance are unknown.

Environmental factors account for approximately 10% of malformations.[28] These include maternal conditions, mechanical effects, chemicals and drugs, and certain infectious agents. Maternal diseases associated with malformations include diabetes, phenylketonuria, virilizing tumors, and maternal hyperthermia. About 9% (range, 6.6%–13.0%) of infants of diabetic mothers develop major congenital defects, primarily consisting of cardiovascular, neural tube, and skeletal malformations.[29] Mechanical effects, such as intrauterine compression and abnormal cord constriction, may result in fetal deformations.[28,29]

Probably, the best known of the teratogenic viruses is rubella, which can cause a fetal rubella syndrome consisting of cataracts, heart disease, and deafness.[30] In utero exposure to rubella in the first trimester can cause defects in up to 85% of fetuses. Cytomegalovirus infection occurs in 0.5% to 1.5% of newborns in the United States, resulting in deafness and mental retardation in 5% to 10% of these infants.[24] Characteristics of cytomegalic inclusion disease, the syndrome produced by cytomegalovirus, include intrauterine growth restriction (IUGR), microcephaly, and at times chorioretinitis, seizures, blindness, and optic atrophy.

Herpes simplex 1 and 2 and varicella are also associated with malformations.[28]

The protozoan generally accepted as a teratogen is *Toxoplasma gondii* which may be present in cat litter.[24] Most infants infected with *T. gondii* show no symptoms and develop normally. When toxicity does occur, the anomalies may consist of hepatosplenomegaly, icterus, maculopapular rash, chorioretinitis, cerebral calcifications, and hydrocephalus or microcephalous.[31] Because of the possible presence of *T. gondii* in cat litter, women should avoid cleaning or touching cat litter while pregnant. *Treponema pallidum* (syphilis) can cross the placenta and cause congenital syphilis as well as other defects, such as hydrocephaly, chorioretinitis, and optic atrophy.[30] In utero exposure to syphilis after the fourth month of pregnancy is associated with higher risk.

The final category, defects of unknown cause, comprises the greatest percentage of congenital malformations, accounting for about 60% to 65% of the total.[26]

Medication Use in Pregnancy and Teratogenicity

The term *teratogen* is used to denote an agent that has the potential under certain exposure conditions to produce abnormal development in the fetus.[25] Many women have the general perception that use of any medication during a pregnancy can harm the developing fetus.[22] This thought may lead to consideration of terminating wanted pregnancies or withholding necessary drug therapy during the course of the pregnancy. The extent to which a drug will affect the development of the fetus depends on the physical and chemical properties of the drug as well as the dose, duration, route, and timing of exposure and the genetic composition and biologic susceptibility of the mother and fetus.[33] Numerous drugs have been associated with congenital anomalies, but only in a few cases has a consensus been reached that a specific agent is teratogenic. Table 49-1[34–36] lists those agents generally considered or suspected to be proven human teratogens. Not all these teratogens will cause developmental toxicity with every exposure, however.

Because every pregnancy has the risk of an abnormal outcome regardless of drug exposure, the objective of evaluating data on drug exposure during pregnancy is to ascertain whether a particular drug increases the risk of developmental toxicity in the fetus beyond the background rate. The following basic principles of teratogenicity should be applied when assessing the potential for teratogenicity of drugs.

CRITICAL STAGE OF EXPOSURE

After fertilization, the development of the embryo and fetus is divided into three main stages: pre-embryonic period, embryonic period, and fetal period.[28] In the first 2 weeks after fertilization or the pre-embryonic period (0–14 days), little is known about the effects of drugs on human development. Exposure to a teratogenic agent during this period usually produces an "all or none" effect on the ovum[31]: The ovum either dies from exposure to a lethal dose of a teratogenic drug or regenerates completely after exposure to a sublethal dose. Some animal studies have suggested, however, that exposure to some drugs during the preimplantation stage can halt growth and development before implantation.[36] Although the damage can be repaired, intrauterine growth may be retarded in the offspring.

During the embryonic period (14–56 days after fertilization), when organogenesis occurs, the embryo is most susceptible to the effects of teratogens or other chemicals.[25,31] Exposure during this sensitive period may produce major morphologic changes (Fig. 49-2). These stages of development differ significantly from other species, and knowledge of these stages is essential for the interpretation of the relationship between congenital malformations and drugs. For example, if a specific drug exposure occurs after the time of organ development, then a structural defect in that organ is less likely to be caused by that specific drug.

The fetal period (57 days to term) includes most of the stages of histogenesis and functional maturation, although the latter continues for some time after birth.[28] Minor structural changes are still possible during histogenesis, but anomalies are more likely to involve growth and functional aspects such as mental development and reproduction.

DOSE–RESPONSE CURVE

All teratogens follow a toxicologic dose–response curve.[25] All teratogens have a threshold dose below which adverse effects will not occur. The threshold dose is the dosage in which the incidence of structural malformations, rate of fetal death, growth restriction, and functional deficits does not exceed the background rate in the general population.[25] Conversely, developmental toxicity may occur when the fetus is exposed to doses above the maximum or threshold dose. There may be an increase in the severity and incidence of malformations when the fetus is exposed to increasingly higher dosages. For example, the risk for major congenital malformations, including NTD and minor anomalies, is increased statistically in patients taking valproic acid dosages greater than 1,000 mg/day during the first trimester.[37]

EXTRAPOLATION FROM ANIMAL STUDIES

In the absence of human trials, data derived from animal studies are used to assess the level of risk of developmental toxicity in humans. Most newly marketed drugs often have to rely on preclinical data to develop an estimation of teratogenic risk based on animal studies until human data become available.[38] The dose used in experimental animal data is expressed as multiples of the human dose using plasma or serum AUC or dose per unit based on body surface area.[39] The drug appears to have a low risk for teratogenicity if the toxic dose in animals (based on AUC or mg/m^2 comparison) is greater than 10 times the anticipated human dose.[40] Risk assessment using animal data is more complicated than just considering the dosage alone. Other major factors, including the effects of metabolism and active metabolites, species differentiation, route of administration, and type of defects, must be considered.[25]

GENETIC VARIABILITY

The most potent teratogenic agent will not produce malformations with every exposure.[25] The teratogenic potential of some drugs is influenced by the genotype of both the mother and fetus. Although the effects of known teratogens can be predictable in the general population, the possibility of individual assessment is difficult. The same dose of a teratogenic agent exposed at the same gestational window will produce variable outcomes in different people. Genetic variability can confer differences in cell sensitivities, placental transport, drug metabolism, enzyme composition, and receptor binding, which may affect how much active drug will reach fetal tissues.[41] One study showed an increased susceptibility to the teratogenic effect of phenytoin, most likely caused by elevated levels of oxidative metabolites (epoxides). These epoxides are normally eliminated from the systemic circulation by enzymes called microsomal epoxide hydrolase. Women who are homozygous for the recessive allele produce low levels of epoxide hydrolase, which may expose the fetus to higher levels of epoxides. These fetuses may be at a higher risk for fetal hydantoin syndrome.[42]

Table 49-1
Drugs with Suspected or Proven Teratogenic Effects in Humans

Alcohol	Growth restriction, mental retardation, mid-facial hypoplasia, renal and cardiac defects
Androgens (testosterone)	Masculinization of female fetus
Angiotensin-converting enzyme inhibitors and angiotensin receptor blockers	Pulmonary hypoplasia, hypocalvaria, oligohydramnios, fetal kidney anuria, and neonatal renal failure
Antithyroid drugs	Fetal and neonatal goiter with iodine use; small risk of aplasia cutis with methimazole
β-Blockers	IUGR and decrease in placental weight in β-blockers with intrinsic sympathomimetic activity if used in second and third trimesters
Carbamazepine	Neural tube defects (NTDs), minor craniofacial defects, fingernail hypoplasia
Cigarette smoking	IUGR, functional and behavioral deficits
Cocaine	Bowel atresias; heart, limbs, face, and genitourinary tract malformations; microcephaly; cerebral infarctions; growth restriction
Corticosteroids (systemic)	Oral cleft lip and palates if used during organogenesis
Cyclophosphamide	Craniofacial, eye, and limb defects; IUGR; neurobehavioral deficits
Diethylstilbestrol	Vaginal carcinoma and other genitourinary defects
Lamotrigine	Oral cleft lip and cleft palate[33]
Lithium	Ebstein anomaly
Methotrexate	CNS and limb malformations
Misoprostol	Möbius sequence (high doses) and spontaneous abortions
Nonsteroidal anti-inflammatory drugs	Constriction of the ductus arteriosus, oral clefts, cardiac defects, and possible spontaneous abortion
Paroxetine	Cardiovascular defects[34]
Phenytoin	Fetal hydantoin syndrome, growth retardation, CNS deficits
Streptomycin and kanamycin	Hearing loss, eighth cranial damage; no ototoxicity reported with gentamicin, tobramycin, amikacin
Systemic retinoids (isotretinoin and etretinate)	CNS, craniofacial, cardiovascular defects
Tetracycline	Permanent discoloration of deciduous teeth
Thalidomide	Limb and skeletal shortening defects, internal organ defects
Topiramate	Cleft lip and cleft palate[35]
Trimethoprim	NTDs and cardiac defects
Vaccines (live)	Live attenuated vaccines can potentially cause fetal infection
Valproic acid	NTDs, developmental delay, and deficits
Vitamin A	Microtia, anotia, thymic aplasia, cardiovascular defects (high dose)
Warfarin	Fetal warfarin syndrome with nasal hypoplasia, stippled epiphyses, and skeletal and CNS defects

Teratogenic effects include the four major manifestations of abnormal fetal development which include growth alterations, functional deficits, structural malformations, and fetal death.
Only drugs that are teratogenic when used at clinically recommended doses are listed. List is not all-inclusive.
CNS, central nervous system; IUGR, intrauterine growth restriction.
Source: Briggs G et al. Drugs in Pregnancy and Lactation: A Reference Guide to Fetal and Neonatal Risk. 11th ed. Philadelphia, PA: Lippincott Williams & Wilkins; 2017; Koren G et al. Drugs in pregnancy. *N Engl J Med*. 1998;338:1128.

PLACENTAL TRANSFER OF DRUGS

At one time, the placenta was thought to present a barrier to the passage of drugs and noxious chemicals to the fetus. It is now known, however, that most medications cross the placenta to the fetus and, in general, what the mother consumes also is consumed by the fetus. Although the placenta acts as a biologic membrane, it initially is composed of four layers effectively separating two distinct individuals.[41] These layers are (a) the endothelial lining of the fetal vessels, (b) the connective tissue in the core of the villus, (c) the cytotrophoblast layer, and (d) the covering syncytium. During gestation, the placenta's surface area increases while its thickness decreases from approximately 25 μm during the first trimester to 2 to 6 μm at term. Both processes tend to favor the transfer of chemicals to the fetus.

Drugs, nutrients, and other substances cross the placenta by five mechanisms: (a) simple diffusion (e.g., most drugs), (b) facilitated diffusion (e.g., glucose), (c) active transport (e.g., some vitamins, amino acids), (d) pinocytosis (e.g., immune antibodies), and (e) breaks between cells (e.g., erythrocytes).[41,42,39] The latter two mechanisms are of no practical importance in the transfer of drugs.

Several factors influence the rate of drug transfer across the placenta, including molecular weight, lipid solubility, ionization, protein binding, uterine and umbilical blood flow, and maternal diseases.[39] Drugs with molecular weights of less than 600 cross

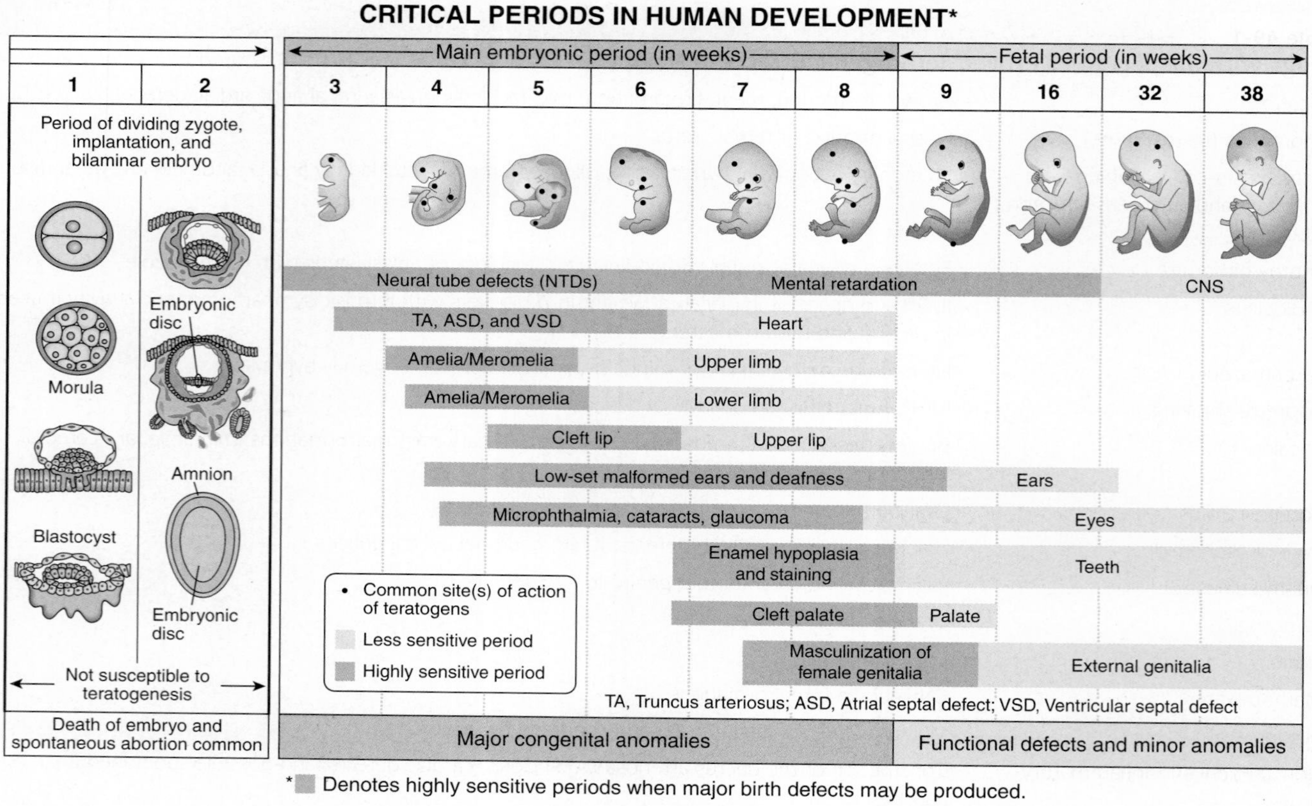

Figure 49-2 Critical stages of human development. (Adapted with permission from Moore KL, Persaud TVN. *The Developing Human: Clinically Oriented Embryology*. 7th ed. Philadelphia, PA: Saunders; 2003.)

easily, whereas those of greater than 1,000 (e.g., heparin) cross with difficulty or not at all. Because most drugs have molecular weights of less than 600, it is safe to assume that most drugs reaching the mother's circulatory system also will reach the fetus. As with other biologic membranes, lipid-soluble substances are transferred rapidly, with the rate of entry primarily governed by the lipid solubility of the nonionized molecule. Conversely, those molecules that are ionized at physiologic pH (e.g., the cholinergic quaternary amines) cross slowly, whereas weak acids and bases with dissociation constant (pK_a) values between 4.3 and 8.5 are transferred rapidly to the fetus. The penetration of highly protein-bound drugs also is inhibited; only the free, unbound drugs cross the placenta.[41,38,39]

Uterine blood flow, a major factor in determining the rate of drug transfer, increases throughout gestation. Several variables can affect uterine blood flow and the rate of drug transfer, including maternal blood pressure (BP), cord compression, and drug therapy. Maternal hypotension reduces uterine blood flow and the rate at which substances are delivered to the membrane. Cord compression reduces the blood flow on the fetal side of the membrane. The use of drugs with α-adrenergic property (e.g., epinephrine) may constrict uterine vessels and thereby reduce blood flow.[27] Maternal diseases, such as pregnancy-induced hypertension, erythroblastosis, and diabetes, change the permeability of the placenta and may reduce or increase transfer.[36]

Food and Drug Administration (FDA) Risk Factors

In 1979, the US FDA introduced a system of rating pregnancy risks associated with pharmacologic agents. This system categorizes all drugs approved after 1983 into one of five pregnancy risk categories, A, B, C, D, and X. It establishes the level of risks to the fetus based on available animal and human data and recommends the degree of caution that should be undertaken with each drug.[38,40–42] This system had many limitations. Effective in June 2015, the FDA introduced pregnancy labeling and category system to include narrative text to provide more clinical management advice that includes consideration of both animal and human data (Fig. 49-1).[43] The structured narratives will include the following sections for each drug: a) pregnancy (including considerations during labor and delivery), b) lactation (includes nursing mother considerations), and c) females and males of reproductive potentionl.[43] For specific information on the FDA pregnancy labeling[43]: **http://www.fda.gov/drugs/developmentapprovalprocess/developmentresources/labeling/ucm093307.htm**

The old FDA pregnancy classification structure states that levothyroxine is a pregnancy category A drug, but does not give any further specific information. The new FDA-structured narrative states "Levothyroxine (T_4) is compatible with all stages of pregnancy. Untreated or undertreated maternal hypothyroidism is associated with low birth weight secondary to medically indicated preterm delivery, preeclampsia or placental abruption, and with lower neuropsychological development of their offspring."[38] S.C. should be counseled that levothyroxine can safely be used during all trimesters of pregnancy including the period of organogenesis, which she is currently in at 8 weeks' gestation. She should not discontinue her levothyroxine. Thyroxine insufficiency has been shown to impair fetal and neonatal development. Levothyroxine therapy has not been observed to increase the risk of congenital malformations beyond the reported background risk of 3%.[38]

MANAGEMENT OF CONDITIONS IN PREGNANCY

Nausea and Vomiting

CASE 49-1, QUESTION 6: S.C. is now 10 weeks pregnant and complains of nausea throughout the day with occasional emesis occurring 2 to 3 times daily. She is able to tolerate at least two meals a day and oral liquids. She reports very little weight gain since she became pregnant. Her current weight is 72 kg. S.C. states that certain smells such as fish, eggs, and beans cause her to gag. How long is her nausea and vomiting likely to last?

According to American College of Obstetricians and Gynecology, nausea and vomiting during pregnancy (NVP) is a common condition occurring in approximately 70% to 85% of pregnancies, during weeks 5 to 12 of gestation.[44] For most women, NVP is a self-limiting condition that usually resolves after the first trimester with no long-term detrimental effect on the fetus.[47] About 91% of cases will resolve by 20 weeks of gestation.[45] The effects of NVP can have an impact on a woman's daily activities, work productivity, and quality of life. Studies estimate $130 million/year is spent on the hospitalization for severe NVP.[46] The cause of NVP is unknown, but is most likely multifactorial including hormonal, psychological, and neurologic factors. Changes in hormonal levels of estrogen, progesterone, and hCG have been implicated as a possible cause of NVP. Mild-to-moderate NVP has been associated with lower rates of miscarriage, preterm delivery, and stillbirth.[47]

NONPHARMACOLOGIC MANAGEMENT FOR NAUSEA AND VOMITING

CASE 49-1, QUESTION 7: What nonpharmacologic approaches should S.C. try for her nausea and vomiting?

Most mild forms of NVP can be managed with psychological support and lifestyle and dietary changes. Advising S.C. to eat smaller frequent meals consisting of a low-fat, bland, and dry diet (e.g., bananas, crackers, rice, toast), to avoid spicy and highly aromatic foods, and to take prenatal vitamins with iron at night may alleviate some of the symptoms. Meals high in protein are more likely to alleviate NVP than carbohydrate-laden or fatty meals. Rest and avoidance of the sensory stimuli occurring from foods, and lotions that may contribute to the effects of NVP can also be helpful.[47] Advise S.C. to avoid the foods (i.e., fish, beans, eggs, spaghetti sauce) that specifically trigger her gag reflex, which may induce emesis.

PHARMACOLOGIC MANAGEMENT FOR NAUSEA AND VOMITING

CASE 49-1, QUESTION 8: S.C. has tried crackers and avoiding the foods that trigger her gag reflex but does not respond to nonpharmacologic treatment of her nausea and vomiting. What pharmacologic agent would be appropriate for her?

Antiemetics are indicated for the treatment of moderate-to-severe nausea and vomiting that fails to respond to nonpharmacologic interventions or when the nausea or vomiting threatens the mother's metabolic or nutritional status (e.g., hyperemesis gravidarum). Traditionally, medications for NVP have been avoided during the first trimester because of fear of the possible teratogenic effects. Most antiemetic therapies (e.g., antihistamines, multivitamins, phenothiazines) can be taken during pregnancy safely. Table 49-2[38,46,48,50,51] shows the most common antiemetics used during pregnancy. The goal of antiemetic therapy is to choose an effective medication to improve a woman's quality of life by maintaining her nutrition and hydration needs, while ensuring fetal safety.

The FDA-recently-approved and prescription delayed-release formulation of 10 mg doxylamine with 10mg of pyridoxine (vitamin B_6) called Diclegis can be considered first-line therapy for the treatment of NVP. Several randomized, controlled trials have demonstrated its effectiveness in reducing NVP. Because of its safety and efficacy profile, doxylamine and pyridoxine are still considered a first-line therapy and are available in combination as prescription or separately as over-the-counter products.[48,52–54]

Other antihistamine H_1 receptor blockers (e.g., diphenhydramine, hydroxyzine, meclizine, dimenhydrinate) have been studied for NVP. The safety of antihistamines was supported in a meta-analysis including more than 200,000 first-trimester exposures, which did not find an increase in teratogenic risk.[49] Sedation is the main side effect that limits the use of this class of antiemetics.

Phenothiazines or metoclopramide is usually prescribed if antihistamines fail.[50,51] Phenothiazines (e.g., promethazine, prochlorperazine) are generally considered safe for both the mother and fetus if used occasionally in low doses. A recent randomized trial compared IV metoclopramide versus IV promethazine in the treatment of hyperemesis gravidarum and found both agents have similar efficacy. However, metoclopramide caused less drowsiness and dizziness.[50] Metoclopramide, a dopaminergic antagonist with prokinetic abilities, can control vomiting and gastric reflux associated with pregnancy. Oral metoclopramide can be added to an antihistamine (e.g., hydroxyzine) or a regimen of doxylamine and pyridoxine.[50,51] A large cohort study of 3,458 women exposed to metoclopramide in the first trimester failed to show an increase in congenital malformations. Metoclopramide issued a black box warning concerning the risk of rare incidences of tardive dyskinesia.[50,51] Risk of tardive dyskinesia increases with longer duration of treatment and total cumulative doses; thus, length of therapy beyond 12 weeks should be avoided.[50,51]

Due to the use of ondansetron, a 5-hydroxytryptamine type 3 antagonist during pregnancy has increased due to more experiences with its use. It is increasingly used for NVP and hyperemesis owing to ease of administration with oral disintegrating tablets and tolerability with minimal sedating side effects or poor fetal outcomes.[46,55] Methylprednisolone is an option for refractory cases; however, its use during the first trimester is associated with a small but significant risk of fetal oral clefts.

Alternative therapies (e.g., vitamin B_6, ginger root, acupuncture, acupressure) have improved NVP in a small number of patients.[38,45] S.C. may be started on doxylamine 10 mg and pyridoxine 10 mg 2 tablets by mouth at bedtime. S.C. may increase to 2 additional tablets in the afternoon if needed to a maximum of 4 tablets per day because of its safety and efficacy profile. Drug selection for S.C. mostly depends on the tolerability of adverse effects. If S.C. continues to have significant nausea and emesis on these antiemetics and fails to tolerate any oral liquids or solids, she should be advised to return to the clinic for evaluation and possibly be admitted for IV hydration and IV antiemetic therapy.

CASE 49-1, QUESTION 9: S.C. returns to the clinic a few weeks later at 12 weeks' gestation stating that she has lost about 4 kg in the past 3 weeks, has been unable to tolerate any liquids or medication for 2 weeks, and feels dehydrated and dizzy. S.C. is referred for admission to the hospital. What recommendations should be given to S.C. to help control her nausea and vomiting?

Severe NVP can persist in less than 1% of pregnancies, leading to a condition called *hyperemesis gravidarum,* which can lead

Table 49-2
Common Antiemetics Used for Nausea and Vomiting During Pregnancy (NVP)

Drug	Dose	Comments
Vitamin B_6 (pyridoxine)	10–25 mg PO TID	First-line therapy[45]; Documented safety in pregnancy
Vitamin B_6 (pyridoxine)–doxylamine combination	Pyridoxine 10–25 mg PO TID–QID; Doxylamine 12.5 mg PO TID–QID Doxylamine 10 mg/ Pyridoxine 10 mg PO QHS, Max 4 tablets/day	First-line therapy; Available OTC; Well-documented safety in pregnancy through large meta-analysis,[54] RX only
Antihistamines		
Diphenhydramine Meclizine Hydroxyzine Dimenhydrinate	25–50 mg PO every 8 hours 25 mg PO every 6 hours 25–50 mg PO every 4–6 hours 50–100 mg PO every 4–6 hours	First-line therapy; Antihistamines have not been shown to be teratogenic[49,50]
Phenothiazines		
Promethazine Prochlorperazine	12.5–25 mg PO, PR every 6 hours 5–10 mg PO every 6–8 hours	Second line of therapy; Available as suppositories; Also suppositories and buccal tablets; Usually add phenothiazine or metoclopramide to therapy if antihistamines fail[45,51]; Can cause EPS
Dopamine Antagonists		
Metoclopramide	10 mg PO every 6 hours	Usually add phenothiazine or metoclopramide to therapy if antihistamines fail[45,51]; Avoid treatment greater than 12 weeks' duration, risk of tardive dyskinesia; Can cause EPS
Droperidol	1.25–2.5 mg IV/IM or Continuous infusion 1 mg/h for treatment of hyperemesis gravidarum[50]	Boxed warning regarding torsades de pointes, may need ECG during administration. Continuous infusion of droperidol requires concomitant diphenhydramine 50 mg IV every 6 hours
5-HT_3 Receptor Antagonists		
Ondansetron	4–8 mg IV/PO every 6–8 hours	Available as ODT tablets; Does not cause sedation; Studies suggest low risk in pregnancy[38,55]
Glucocorticoids		
Methylprednisolone	16 mg PO every 8 hours × 3 days, then taper over 2 weeks	For refractory cases, last line of therapy; Avoid use before 10th week of gestation, associated with oral cleft and palate[38,45]
Ginger extract	125–250 mg PO every 6 hours	Available OTC as food supplement

ECG, electrocardiogram; EPS, extrapyramidal symptoms; IM, intramuscular; IV, intravenous; ODT, oral disintegrating tablet; OTC, over-the-counter; PO, by mouth; QID, 4 times a day; TID, 3 times a day.

Source: Briggs G et al. *Drugs in Pregnancy and Lactation: A Reference Guide to Fetal and Neonatal Risk*. 11th ed. Philadelphia, PA: Lippincott Williams & Wilkins; 2017; Niebyl JR. Clinical practice. Nausea and vomiting in pregnancy. *N Engl J Med*. 2010;363:1544; McKeigue PM et al. Bendectin and birth defects: I. A meta-analysis of the epidemiologic studies. *Teratology*. 1994;50:27; Seto A et al. Pregnancy outcome following first trimester exposure to antihistamines: meta-analysis. *Am J Perinatol*. 1997;14:119.

to detrimental effects on the mother and fetus. Weight loss of more than 5% of prepregnancy weight, ketonuria, and electrolyte abnormalities are associated with this condition. Treatment of hyperemesis gravidarum often requires hospitalization for parental fluid administration, electrolyte replacement, vitamin supplementation, and antiemetic therapy.[47] Metabolic acidosis, ketosis, hypovolemia, electrolyte disturbances, and weight loss may ensue if patients are not treated.[47] Reductions in lower esophageal pressure, gastric peristalsis, and gastric emptying may worsen nausea and vomiting.

In addition to ondansetron as mentioned above used for NVP, droperidol, an IV dopamine antagonist, has been used extensively for many years in the treatment of hyperemesis and the prevention and treatment of postoperative nausea and vomiting.[38] Although the FDA has mandated electrocardiographic monitoring for concern about the risk of prolonged QTc interval, large meta-analysis studies have failed to show an increased risk of arrhythmias when using droperidol at the low doses used for nausea and vomiting.[45] Limited experience with droperidol use in hyperemesis gravidarum has been documented in a small controlled trial.[52] Human and animal data suggest droperidol carries a low risk of teratogenicity to the fetus.[38,50,51]

S.C. should be hydrated with IV fluids with electrolyte replacement therapy and multivitamins including pyridoxine. If hydration with multivitamins does not quell her nausea, IV ondansetron 4 to 8 mg every 4 to 6 hours should be given. IV droperidol therapy should be considered if ondansetron does not work. She should also be evaluated for other causes of nausea and vomiting if her symptoms persist (e.g., gastroenteritis, cholecystitis, pancreatitis, hepatitis, peptic ulcer disease, pyelonephritis, and fatty liver of pregnancy).[47] Enteral nutrition may be needed in the treatment of hyperemesis gravidarum if S.C. cannot tolerate oral liquid and solid intake despite continuous IV antiemetics and hydration. Total parental nutrition should be reserved after multiple antiemetic regimens and enteral therapies have failed because of the substantial risks of catheter sepsis (25%) and thromboembolic clots.[45,46,50]

REFLUX ESOPHAGITIS

CASE 49-1, QUESTION 10: S.C. is now 30 weeks pregnant and no longer complains of nausea or vomiting. However, now she has heartburn that worsens when she lies down. What causes reflux esophagitis in pregnancy, and how should S.C. manage this problem?

Reflux esophagitis or heartburn is a normal occurrence in pregnancy affecting approximately two-thirds of women. The enlarging uterus increases intra-abdominal pressure, and estrogen and progesterone relax the esophageal sphincter. These two factors cause the reflux of stomach acid into the lower esophagus, producing symptoms of substernal burning worsened by eating, lying down, or bending over. Lifestyle and dietary modifications, such as eating smaller meals, avoiding late meals close to bedtime, and elevation of the head of the bed, should be tried first. Avoidance of salicylates, caffeine, alcohol, and nicotine are encouraged to reduce the symptoms of reflux and fetal exposure to these harmful substances.

If these modifications are not successful, S.C. should try a calcium carbonate antacid. Animal studies have not shown antacids to have teratogenic effects.[38] Sodium bicarbonate can cause metabolic alkalosis and fluid overload and should be avoided. Despite evidence of fetal toxicity with aluminum, available data suggest that usual doses of aluminum-containing medications are not harmful to the fetus of a pregnant woman with normal renal function. Sucralfate, which contains aluminum, appears to be safe in pregnancy. The American College of Gastroenterology has classified sucralfate as a medication with benefits that outweigh the risks when used in pregnant women.[38]

H_2-receptor antagonists can be used safely during pregnancy because most studies in animals and humans have not found fetal harm with cimetidine, ranitidine, famotidine, or nizatidine.[38] If H_2-receptor antagonists fail to control symptoms, proton-pump inhibitors (PPIs) should be used as the next treatment option. Recent studies have shown that PPI use during the first trimester and throughout pregnancy is not associated with a significant increase in the risk of congenital anomalies. These studies suggest that PPIs can be safely used at any gestational age.[56,57]

URINARY TRACT INFECTIONS

CASE 49-1, QUESTION 11: S.C. is now 31 weeks pregnant, and a routine urine dip was positive for leukocyte esterase and nitrates. Her urine was sent for urinalysis at her most recent prenatal visit and was positive for 10^5 colony-forming units (CFU) of *Escherichia coli*. She does not complain of any frequency and urgency when urinating and denies any fevers. Her temperature is currently 98.9°F. She denies any allergies to medications. What are the risks of having a urinary tract infection during pregnancy, and how should S.C. be treated?

Pathogenesis

Urinary tract infections are one of the most common complications of pregnancy owing to hormonal and mechanical changes that increase the likelihood of bacteriuria. During pregnancy, increases in progesterone cause relaxation of ureteral smooth muscle, promoting urinary stasis. The enlarging gravid uterus can also mechanically compress the ureters, which may lead to urinary retention. Approximately 90% of pregnant women may exhibit ureteral dilation or hydronephrosis, which can decrease bladder tone and ureteral tone. These physiologic changes along with increases in the GFR, urine alkalization, and glucosuria help to promote bacterial growth.

Asymptomatic Bacteriuria and Acute Cystitis

Urinary tract infections during pregnancy can present as either asymptomatic bacteriuria (ASB) or acute cystitis. ASB is defined as the presence of significant bacteria, greater than 10^5 CFU of bacteria, obtained by two consecutive clean-catch samples in the absence of any urinary symptoms.[58] In contrast, acute cystitis involves an infection of the bladder and manifests with signs and symptoms of frequency, urgency, dysuria, and hematuria without fever or evidence of systemic illness along with significant presence of bacteria of at least 10^5 CFU. Counts of less than 10^5 CFU with two or more organisms likely represent contamination and not true bacteriuria.

ASB is estimated to occur in 2.5% to 15% of pregnant women with about 80,000 to 400,000 cases occurring each year in the United States.[58,59] If ASBs are left untreated, they can lead to complications such as pyelonephritis, low-birth-weight infants, and premature delivery.[60] During pregnancy, treatment of ASB reduces the risk of developing pyelonephritis dramatically down from 20% to 35% to only 1% to 4%.[60] The US Preventive Services Task Force recommends screening for ASB with a urine culture for all pregnant women between 12 and 16 weeks of gestation or at the first prenatal visit if it occurs later.[61] The American College of Obstetrics and Gynecology (ACOG) further recommends repeating a urine culture during the third trimester.[62]

Risk factors for ASB during pregnancy include diabetes, sickle cell disease, immunosuppression, HIV or acquired immunodeficiency syndrome, urinary tract anatomic anomalies, and spinal cord injuries.[63] The primary sources of organisms that cause bacteriuria originate from existing vaginal and perineal flora and migrate up the urethra to cause ASB and cystitis; they include *E. coli* (most common pathogen isolated), *Klebsiella pneumoniae, Proteus mirabilis, Enterobacter* species, *Enterococcus, Staphylococcus saprophyticus,* and group B β-hemolytic *Streptococcus.*[63] Commonly used antibiotics include penicillins, cephalosporins, and nitrofurantoin. Antibiotic selection should be guided by antimicrobial susceptibility testing. For coverage of the most common organism, *E. coli,* oral nitrofurantoin or cephalexin is often used. *E. coli* resistance has been increasing to amoxicillin and trimethoprim-sulfamethoxazole.[63,64] The antibiotic chosen should produce adequate concentration in the urine, have a low resistance rate, and be safe to use during pregnancy. A 7-day regimen of antibiotics should be used whenever possible.[63,64] A recent WHO multicenter, randomized, noninferiority trial found a 7-day regimen with nitrofurantoin was more effective than a 1-day regimen in treating pregnant women with ASB, with bacteriologic cure rates of 86.2% and 75.7%, respectively.[64] Optimal antibiotics and duration of therapy have not been clearly identified and must be individualized for each patient based on cultures and sensitivity results.[60,63] For S.C., who likely has ASB, a 7-day course of nitrofurantoin is reasonable. At this gestation age of 31 weeks, nitrofurantoin can still be used safely. There is a small risk of hemolytic anemia in newborns when nitrofurantoin is used close to delivery.[38]

DIABETES MELLITUS

Diabetes mellitus is the most common maternal medical complications during pregnancy. Diabetes during pregnancy can be detected before or during pregnancy and can be separated into two groups: (a) *pregestational diabetes,* which includes women who have been diagnosed before pregnancy with either diabetes type 1 or diabetes type 2, or (b) *gestational diabetes mellitus* (GDM), defined as carbohydrate intolerance first detected during pregnancy.[65]

More prevalent than pregestational diabetes, GDM accounts for more than 90% of diabetes cases during pregnancy and affects approximately 6% to 7% of live births each year.[66] It is estimated that 50% of women with GDM will go on to develop type 2 diabetes 22 to 28 years postpregnancy.[67,68]

Pregestational diabetes accounts for the remaining 10% of cases. In the United States, more than 8 million women have pregestational diabetes, affecting about 1% of live births each year.[71] Most women with pregestational diabetes have type 2 diabetes characterized by peripheral insulin resistance and relative insulin deficiency.[69] The incidence of type 2 pregestational diabetes has been rapidly rising in the past decade, most likely because of the increasing prevalence of obesity. In contrast to type 2 diabetes, type 1 diabetes is characterized by complete insulin deficiency resulting from autoimmune destruction of pancreatic β-cells.[69] Less than 0.5% of all pregnancies in the United States are complicated by type 1 diabetes.[70]

Fluctuating glucose levels during the first trimester may be the first signs of pregnancy for women with pregestational diabetes owing to increased insulin resistance and reduced sensitivity to insulin action. Placental hormones (e.g., human placental lactogen, progesterone, prolactin, placental growth hormone, and cortisol) are thought to be responsible for the increase in insulin resistance during pregnancy. The ACOG classifies diabetes in pregnancy according to the White classification, modified to include gestational diabetes according to glycemic control. The White classification relies on age at onset, duration of diabetes, and presence of vascular complications for patient classification (Table 49-3).

Preexisting Diabetes Mellitus

FETAL AND INFANT RISKS

CASE 49-2

QUESTION 1: K.H., a 27-year-old, 60-kg woman known to have type 1 diabetes since age 12, has married recently and wishes to have children. She has been conscientious in her diabetes care and self-monitors her blood glucose concentrations two to three times a day (fasting and before meals). During the past month, her fasting blood glucose concentrations have ranged from 90 to 140 mg/dL. Today, her fasting blood glucose and glycosylated hemoglobin (Hgb A_{1c}) laboratory results are 134 mg/dL and 7.8%, respectively. Her BP is 145/94 mm Hg, renal function is normal, serum creatinine is 0.8 mg/dL, and she does not have proteinuria. K.H. reports tingling and pain in her toes. Her current medications include lisinopril 5 mg PO daily, insulin glargine (Lantus) 16 units subcutaneously (SC) every day at bedtime with an insulin lispro (Humalog) sliding-scale of 2 to 10 units before each meal. She reports eating only two meals a day and no snacks in between. How will diabetes affect the health of a child she would like to conceive?

Table 49-3
Modified White Classification of Diabetes During Pregnancy

Class of Diabetes	Age of Onset	Duration	Vascular Complications	Treatment of Choice During Pregnancy
Class A1	First diagnosed during pregnancy	During pregnancy	None	Diet, exercise
Class A2	First diagnosed during pregnancy	During pregnancy	None	Diet, exercise plus oral hypoglycemics or insulin
Class B	Older than 20 years	Less than 10 years	None	Insulin therapy
Class C	Between 10 and 19 years	More than 10 years, less than 19	None	Insulin therapy
Class D	Younger than 10 years	More than 20 years	Background retinopathy Hypertension Microalbuminuria	Insulin therapy
Class F	At any age	Any duration	Nephropathy Macroalbuminuria (>500 mg/day)	Insulin therapy
Class H	At any age	Any duration	Arteriosclerotic heart disease	Insulin therapy
Class R	At any age	Any duration	Proliferative retinopathy Vitreous hemorrhage	Insulin therapy
Class T	At any age	Any duration	Renal transplantation	Insulin therapy

Source: Cunningham FG et al. Diabetes. In: Gary Cunningham F et al, eds. *Williams Obstetrics*. 24th ed. New York, NY: McGraw-Hill; 2014; White P. Classification of obstetric diabetes. *Am J Obstet Gynecol*. 1978;130:228.

Perinatal mortality for infants of diabetic mothers has declined dramatically with strict maternal metabolic control, improved fetal surveillance, and neonatal intensive care.[71] Fetal and neonatal mortality rates are approximately 2% to 4%, and the risk of spontaneous abortion in patients with well-controlled type 1 diabetes is equal to that of women without diabetes.[72] The incidence of stillbirth is greatest after 36 weeks' gestation in women with poor glycemic control, fetal macrosomia (see subsequent discussion), maternal vascular disease, ketoacidosis, or preeclampsia.[65]

The leading cause of perinatal mortality is major congenital anomalies that occur in 9% to 14% of infants born to mothers with diabetes. The major malformations observed include NTDs and other anomalies involving the cardiac, renal, and GI systems, and rarely caudal regression syndrome.[66] Many congenital anomalies occur during organogenesis, before the seventh week of gestation, when women are often unaware that they are pregnant.[73] A direct correlation exists between higher Hgb A_{1c} levels and increased frequency of anomalies.[73] Women with elevated Hgb A_{1c} values during the time of conception have a significantly higher incidence of infants with abomalies compared with women with Hgb A_{1c} closer to the normal range of 4.0% to 5.6%.[74] The risk of fetal anomalies increases dramatically to approximately 20% to 25% when Hgb A_{1c} levels are near 10%.[73] Hgb A_{1c} levels greater than 12% are associated with the same risk of anomalies as infants exposed to known teratogens such as thalidomide, isotretinoin, or alcohol during organogenesis.

Macrosomia, defined as birth weight greater than 4 kg, is thought to be caused in part by fetal hyperglycemia and hyperinsulinemia.[65] Fetal hyperglycemia occurs when glucose crosses the placenta and subsequently stimulates fetal pancreatic β-cells to release excessive insulin. Hyperinsulinemia promotes excessive fetal growth in adipose tissue, causing disproportional fat concentration around the shoulders and chest and doubling the risks of trauma (e.g., shoulder dystocia) during vaginal delivery.

Infants of diabetic mothers also are at increased risk for prolonged hypoglycemia after delivery, respiratory distress syndrome (RDS), hypocalcemia, polycythemia, and hyperbilirubinemia during the neonatal period.[66]

K.H. should be informed that stringent preconception glycemic control is essential for preventing early pregnancy loss and congenital malformations in the infant.[71] Tight glucose control, especially in the months before pregnancy and early in the first trimester, will maximize her chance of having a healthy baby. She should be educated before pregnancy about healthy practices she can institute now to improve a successful pregnancy outcome.

MATERNAL RISKS

CASE 49-2, QUESTION 2: K.H. wants to know what health risks she might incur from becoming pregnant and what measures could minimize these risks?

A prepregnancy assessment, including a history and physical examination, is necessary to determine the risks of or contraindications to pregnancy for K.H. She should be evaluated for ischemic heart disease, neuropathies, or retinopathy, and her renal status must be assessed.[71] Pregnancy can exacerbate the vascular complications of diabetes. For instance, diabetic retinopathy can worsen if strict glycemic control is implemented quickly in pregnant women with proliferative retinopathy; progression to end-stage renal disease can occur in women with mild-to-moderate renal insufficiency (e.g., serum creatinine >1.5 mg/dL or proteinuria >3 g/24 hours).[66,69] The presence of gastroparesis should be noted because it will make controlling her glucose more difficult.[71]

Controlling K.H.'s diabetes before she becomes pregnant may benefit her hypertension and neuropathies and will minimize maternal and fetal problems. Good metabolic control of her diabetes can minimize progression of her diabetes.[73]

PRECONCEPTION MANAGEMENT

CASE 49-2, QUESTION 3: What prepregnancy interventions relative to her general health and diabetes should K.H. undertake before she attempts to become pregnant?

Pregestational care for K.H. should ideally begin 6 months before conception.[71] Recommendations for women with diabetes who want to conceive include suggesting birth control methods until stringent glycemic control can be achieved, consulting a dietitian to develop a patient-specific nutritional diet to attain healthy weight targets, and implementing a self-monitoring blood glucose regimen.[71] Good glycemic control (Hgb A_{1c} levels close to normal) should be achieved months before conception to minimize risks of major congenital anomalies. K.H.'s current regimen may not achieve euglycemia (see Chapter 53, Diabetes Mellitus). Her insulin therapy should be titrated to reduce her average blood glucose range from 90 to 120 mg/dL, targeting an Hgb A_{1c} of less than 6.5% without frequent episodes of hypoglycemia.[71,74] Additionally, K.H. should be started on prenatal vitamins containing at least 400 mcg of folic acid.

Her BP of 145/94 mm Hg is high and should be decreased to a diastolic BP of about 80 mm Hg to minimize risks for preeclampsia (see Case 49-5, Question 6) or exacerbation of her disorder. Many women with pregestational diabetes, such as K.H., are likely on an angiotensin-converting enzyme inhibitor (ACEI) or angiotensin receptor blocker for hypertension treatment or for renal protective effects. Before pregnancy and during preconception planning, K.H. should be switched to another antihypertensive (e.g., methyldopa, labetalol, or calcium-channel blockers) such as methyldopa or labetalol because recent studies have observed possible increased rates of congenital cardiac malformation associated with the use of ACEIs in the first trimester.[75] Further confirmatory studies are needed to define the risk of using ACEIs during the first trimester. However, use of ACEIs is absolutely contraindicated during the second and third trimesters of pregnancy.[38,75]

TYPE 1 DIABETES TREATMENT IN PREGNANCY

CASE 49-2, QUESTION 4: After lowering her BP to 125/80 mm Hg with labetalol 200 mg PO twice daily and her Hgb A_{1c} to 7.3%, K.H. discontinues her oral contraceptive and returns to the clinic 5 months later and is noted to be about 4 weeks pregnant. How should her diabetes be managed at this time?

Goals of Therapy

The overall goals of treatment of K.H.'s diabetes are to reduce the maternal and fetal morbidity and mortality associated with diabetes. Treatment of diabetes (see Chapter 53, Diabetes Mellitus) should include dietary management, appropriate maternal weight gain, insulin therapy to normalize glycemic control, and exercise.

Dietary Management

The goals of dietary management for diabetes during pregnancy are directed at ensuring fetal growth and development, appropriate maternal weight gain, and normalizing maternal glucose concentrations. Patients often benefit from individualized diets developed by a dietitian. Neonatal macrosomia has been associated with high postprandial glucose levels; therefore, a reduction in postprandial hyperglycemia is an important goal.

Blood Glucose and Glycosylated Hemoglobin Monitoring

K.H. should begin to self-monitor her blood sugars more intensively at fasting, before meals, 1 hour postprandially, at bedtime, when she feels symptomatic hypoglycemia, and at 3:00 AM to rule out dawn phenomenon versus Somogyi effect.[76] The goal of therapy is to maintain fasting glucose levels less than 90 mg/dL, premeal values of less than 100 mg/dL, and 1-hour postprandial levels of 100 to 120 mg/dL.[66,69] Tight glycemic control without incidence of hypoglycemic episodes, targeting Hgb A_{1c} levels in the normal range, is the goal. Adjusting therapy based on postprandial glucose levels (as opposed to preprandial levels) can lower Hgb A_{1c} levels and decrease the risk of macrosomia, neonatal hypoglycemia, and cesarean delivery. Hgb A_{1c} levels can be drawn at each trimester to reveal the glycemic control during the previous 3 months.[68,69]

Insulin Therapy

Insulin analogs (e.g., lispro, aspart, glargine) are genetically engineered by recombinant DNA technology and usually differ by a few amino acids from human insulin. Concerns about insulin analog use during pregnancy include placental drug transfer and antibody formation.[77] The use of lispro (Humalog) and aspart (Novolog) insulin during pregnancy is supported by several studies that found minimal passage across the placenta, an absence of antibody formation, and no adverse maternal or fetal effects. Although the rapid onset of insulin lispro and aspart can increase adherence and patient satisfaction, it also may increase the incidence of hypoglycemia. Insulin glargine (Lantus), a long-acting insulin analog, allows for once-daily dosing and produces a peakless basal level of insulin. Only case reports have examined the safety and efficacy of insulin glargine during pregnancy.[38] Glargine is usually reserved for very brittle and sensitive insulin-dependent type 1 diabetes patients. Neutral protamine Hagedorn (NPH) insulin is usually used twice daily during pregnancy in lieu of insulin glargine as a basal insulin because it helps to control fasting blood sugars better than a peakless basal insulin. Newer insulin analogs such as insulin detemir (Levemir) and insulin glulisine (Apidra) have not yet been adequately studied during pregnancy and should not be used until further studies clarify their teratogenicity risk.[39]

Glycemic control is most difficult to establish during the first trimester of pregnancy because of the effect on blood sugars of maternal fluctuating hormones.[66,69] K.H.'s insulin regimen should be optimized by changing from insulin glargine to NPH insulin (with a 1:1 ratio) to help better control her fasting blood sugars and instituting a standard insulin lispro dosage before meals based on her carbohydrate intake. Sliding-scale insulin therapy is rarely used during pregnancy.[66,69] Insulin dosages commonly need to be monitored more strictly (every 2–4 days until glycemic control is achieved) during the first trimester and adjusted usually upward every 2 to 3 weeks during pregnancy.

TYPE 2 DIABETES TREATMENT IN PREGNANCY

CASE 49-3

QUESTION 1: V.W. is a 36-year-old G3, P0 with class B diabetes at 15 weeks' gestation with a history of two spontaneous miscarriages occurring last year. She was diagnosed with diabetes 5 years ago during a routine physical examination. She is morbidly obese with a body mass index (BMI) of 49 kg/m^2, height of 5 feet 5 inches, and weight of 295 pounds. She recently found out that she was pregnant and has not had any prenatal care. Her current medications include metformin 1,000 mg PO twice daily and glipizide 5 mg PO daily. She states she has been noncompliant with checking her blood sugars, maintaining a diabetic diet, and taking her medication. Her last Hgb A_{1c}, which was 8.3%, was 2 months ago. Which medication and treatments should V.W. be started on?

Insulin Therapy

Insulin is the hypoglycemic agent of choice during pregnancy because it does not cross the placenta and has an established safety record for both mother and fetus. The goal with insulin therapy is to imitate the glucose levels of a healthy pregnant woman. Rapid glycemic control is of utmost importance during this critical period of organogenesis when vital organs are developing.[73]

Insulin requirements may vary, depending on the trimester. The first trimester is characterized by unstable diabetes, followed by a stable period.[65] During the first trimester, glucose and gluconeogenic substances in the blood are taken up by the fetus, which can lead to a decrease in maternal insulin requirements and increased episodes of hypoglycemia. On average, insulin dosages range from 0.7 to 0.8 units/kg/day in the first trimester.[66,69] If nausea and vomiting occurs during this time, glycemic control may be unstable and should be monitored closely. At about 24 weeks' gestation, insulin requirements begin to increase from 0.8 to 1 units/kg/day, and insulin doses may need to be adjusted every 5 to 10 days.[66,69] These needs continue to increase during the third trimester from 0.9 to 1.2 units/kg/day, which may be twice as much as the prepregnancy dose, in part because of the placental hormones (i.e., lactogen, prolactin, estrogen, and progesterone), which antagonize the action of insulin. Weight-based dosing may not accurately assess the insulin requirements in all pregnant women, especially in the obese population. Insulin regimens must be individualized for each patient, taking into consideration their educational level, compliance, and schedule constraints. Dosage adjustments must take into account the level of activity, meal plan, and other factors (e.g., steroid use, stress, infections) that may affect glucose control. Some women may be admitted into the hospital in the first trimester to (a) rapidly gain glucose control, (b) accurately assess their insulin requirements, and (c) institute an individualized insulin regimen under careful monitoring of blood sugars.[65]

An insulin regimen with three to four daily injections is most successful at maintaining adequate glucose control. Biosynthetic human insulin (e.g., regular and NPH insulin) is the usual treatment of choice in pregestational diabetes mellitus because of its chemical, biologic, and immunologic equivalency to pancreatic human insulin.[38] These insulins have the most established safety profile during pregnancy, but they require more stringent timing of meals during the day.[38]

V.W. should be switched from her oral hypoglycemic agents to insulin therapy with biosynthetic human regular insulin and NPH insulin. Metformin and glipizide should be discontinued. The total daily insulin dosage can be calculated by taking into account V.W.'s gestational age and actual body weight. Her total daily dose equals 0.8 units/kg $\times$ 134 kg, or 107 units daily. Using three injections per day, her dosage would be 47 units of NPH insulin plus 24 units of regular insulin SC 30 minutes before breakfast, 18 units of regular insulin SC 30 minutes before dinner, and 18 units SC of NPH insulin at bedtime. V.W.'s treatment plan needs to include dietary management; appropriate counseling on maternal weight gain during pregnancy given her morbid obesity; instructions on how to draw up, mix, and inject her insulin therapy to normalize glycemic control; and moderate exercise and walking 20 to 30 minutes after each meal. She should be taught to inject only in the subcutaneous abdomen area where insulin is best absorbed during pregnancy. V.W. should also be given a glucometer and taught how to self-monitor her blood sugars 4 times daily, at fasting and 1 hour postprandially (after the last bite of food from each meal) to target fasting blood glucose levels below 90 mg/dL and 1-hour postprandial levels less than 120 mg/dL.

Oral Hypoglycemic use in Type 2 Diabetes during Pregnancy

Although oral hypoglycemic agents are used commonly to treat type 2 diabetes in nonpregnant women, they are rarely used as monotherapy during pregnancy. A switch to insulin therapy is recommended before conception, if possible, or at the time the pregnancy is confirmed because many patients have inadequate control with oral hypoglycemic agents.[66–69] If insulin is not started before conception, women should be strongly counseled to stay on oral hypoglycemics to adequately control blood glucose until insulin therapy can be implemented. Often, patients will discontinue oral hypoglycemics from fear of taking any medication in pregnancy, resulting in hyperglycemia during the critical period of organogenesis.

The ACOG recommends that the use of oral hypoglycemics for the treatment of type 2 diabetes during pregnancy be individualized until more safety and efficacy data become available.[66–71] There is limited experience with oral hypoglycemic use in type 2 diabetes during pregnancy. Metformin, a biguanide, has been used during pregnancy for hyperinsulinemic insulin resistance or in the treatment of infertility in women with polycystic ovarian syndrome (see Chapter 50, Disorders Related to the Menstrual Cycle). Women taking metformin should be switched to insulin therapy unless specific circumstances (e.g., high insulin requirements during the second or third trimester) warrant its use.[77] Studies have shown the sulfonylureas are inferior to both insulin and metformin and increase risk for neonatal hypoglycemia.[74]

CASE 49-3, QUESTION 2: Should an oral hypoglycemic be added to V.W.'s insulin regimen?

V.W. should remain on insulin therapy with three injections daily. Her insulin regimen should be adjusted every 2 to 3 days until glycemic control is achieved and targeted blood glucose levels are reached without significant hypoglycemia episodes. Metformin should only be added if V.W.'s total daily insulin requirement exceeds 250 to 300 units. If metformin is added, insulin dosages should be decreased to at least half the amount in anticipation of increased insulin sensitivity.

Gestational Diabetes Mellitus

DIAGNOSTIC CRITERIA

CASE 49-4

QUESTION 1: J.B. is a 22-year-old Asian woman in the 24th week of her first pregnancy. She is 5 feet 2 inches, 75 kg (prepregnancy weight), and her BMI is 30 kg/m^2. At her regular prenatal visit, her obstetrician recommends an oral glucose screening test for GDM. Her Hgb A_{1c} was 5.8%. Although her mother has diabetes, J.B. has had no glucosuria during pregnancy. Is J.B. at risk for GDM?

GDM is defined as carbohydrate intolerance that develops or is recognized during pregnancy regardless of severity, necessity for treatment, time of onset, or persistence after pregnancy.[78] GDM occurs in about 7% (range, 1%–14%), and the prevalence varies with the population and methods of detection.[78] Complications noted in the offspring of affected women include macrosomia, hypocalcemia, hypoglycemia, polycythemia, and jaundice. Women with GDM are more likely to experience pregnancy-induced hypertensive disorders or require a cesarean delivery. They also are at risk for type 2 diabetes later, and their children have an increased risk for obesity and diabetes later in life.

Risk factors for GDM include age older than 25 years, obesity (BMI $\geq$25 kg/m^2), family history of diabetes, previous delivery of an infant weighing more than 4 kg, a history of a stillbirth, a history of glucose intolerance, or current glycosuria.[78] African-Americans, Hispanic, Asian, Native American, and Pacific Islander women also are at increased risk for GDM.[66,78]

J.B. is at risk for GDM because she is Asian and obese, and she has a family history of diabetes. Her Hgb A_{1c} at 26 weeks' gestation was normal and ruled her out for overt diabetes. J.B. should undergo the standard screening for gestational diabetes with a 50-g, 1-hour glucose challenge. It is not essential for J.B. to fast before this test. The diagnosis of GDM is important to the mother and the fetus because of the increased risks of fetal hyperinsulinemia and macrosomia.

GESTATIONAL DIABETES MELLITUS TREATMENT

CASE 49-4, QUESTION 2: J.B. is screened with a 50-g, 1-hour glucose challenge resulting at 161 mg/dL. Because her screening test was elevated, a diagnostic 3-hour oral glucose tolerance test (OGTT) was given to her the next day, which required her to be fasting. The results of the 3-hour OGTT showed a fasting plasma glucose of 96 mg/dL, a 1-hour glucose of 183 mg/dL, 2-hour glucose of 140 mg/dL, and 3-hour glucose of 126 mg/dL. These results confirm that J.B. has GDM. How should she be managed?

J.B. requires extensive education about a gestational diabetes diet, use of a glucometer, the signs and symptoms of hyperglycemia and hypoglycemia, and treatment of low blood glucose. She should start to monitor her blood glucose 4 times daily, at fasting and 1 hour after the end of each meal. She should return to the clinic in 1 week for an assessment of her blood sugars to evaluate the need for medication therapy (insulin versus glyburide treatment).

It is suggested that 60% to 85% of patients with GDM can control their glucose with dietary modifications and regular exercise; however, management with medications (insulin vs. oral hypoglycemics) should be initiated if dietary management fails to maintain fasting plasma blood glucose concentrations at 95 mg/dL or less or to achieve a 1-hour postprandial plasma concentration of less than 140 mg/dL.[74] Figure 49-3 outlines recommendations for screening and diagnosis of gestational diabetes.

CASE 49-4, QUESTION 3: J.B. returns to clinic at 30 weeks' gestation with glucometer and logbook for a blood glucose assessment. She has been compliant with her diabetic diet and blood sugar monitoring for the past 4 weeks. She has been able to control her blood sugars with diet and moderate walking after meals. However, she has noticed that her fasting blood glucose has risen in the past week to an average of 98 mg/dL and her dinner postprandial values are averaging 139 mg/dL. How should J.B. be managed at this time?

Treatment of GDM with insulin therapy is implemented similar to the treatment for pregestational diabetes. An optimal insulin regimen for GDM has not been determined. Similar dosing with a weight-based, split-mixed multidose regimen is used. The insulin regimen must be tailored specifically to the needs of the woman to successfully achieve target blood glucose levels.

More recently, the Metformin in Gestational Diabetes trial examined whether metformin treatment could provide equivalent outcomes to insulin treatment. Women with GDM at 20 to 33 weeks' gestation were randomly assigned to open-label treatment with metformin (titrated up to 2,500 mg with the option to add supplemental insulin if glycemic control was not achieved) or to insulin treatment alone.[79] The two groups achieved similar primary outcomes (composite score of neonatal morbidities), but 46% of the group allocated to metformin required supplemental insulin therapy. Those requiring supplemental insulin were more obese and had higher elevations of glycemic values at presentation. The results indicate that metformin can be

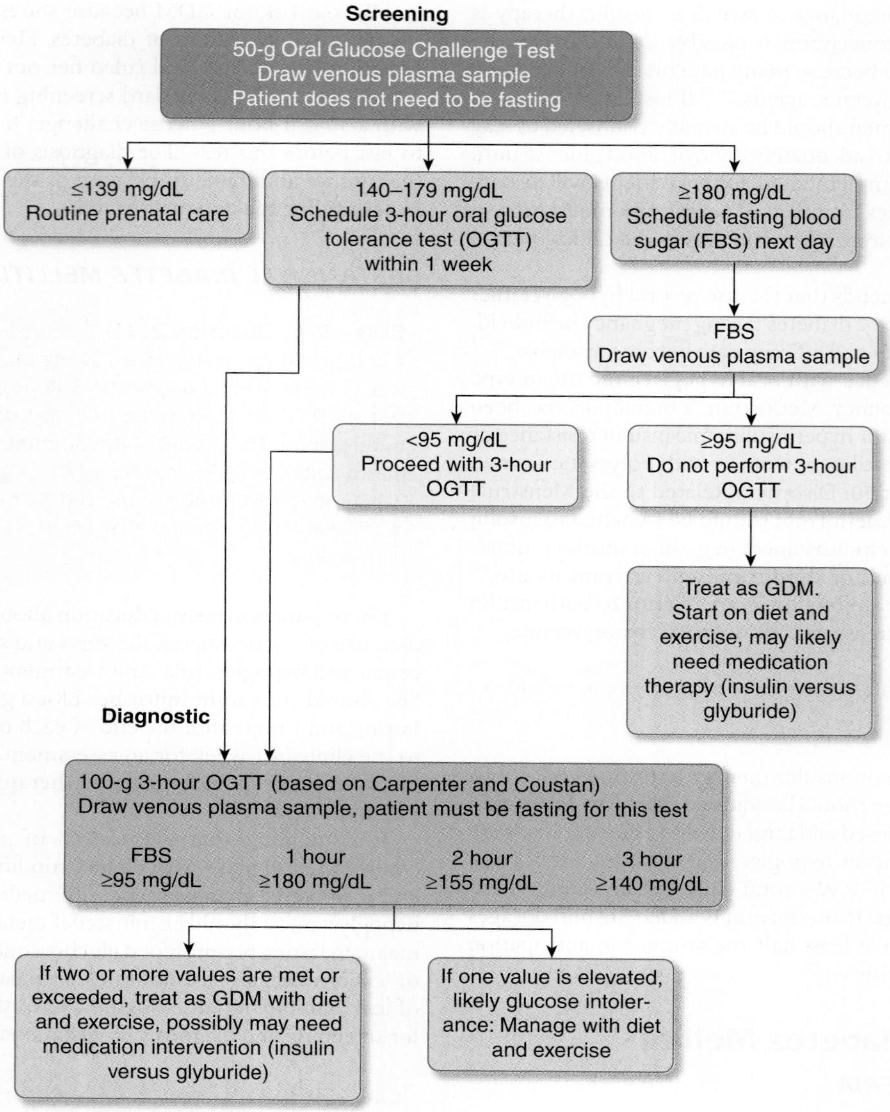

Figure 49-3 Recommendations for screening and diagnosis of gestational diabetes. FBG, fasting blood glucose; GDM, gestational diabetes mellitus; OGTT, oral glucose tolerance test. (Adapted with permission from Screening and diagnosis of gestational diabetes mellitus. Committee Opinion No. 504. American College of Obstetricians and Gynecologists. *Obstet Gynecol*. 2011;118: 751–753.)

used during pregnancy for GDM, but will less likely be successful as monotherapy in women with higher glucose levels.[79] Metformin is usually reserved for patients with high insulin requirements (>300 units daily) in the second and third trimesters.[38] More randomized trials are needed to further determine and to better understand the role of oral hypoglycemic agents in pregnancy.

Other oral hypoglycemics, such as the sulfonylureas, have inferior data and increase risk of adverse effects.[74]

J.B. is a good candidate for insulin therapy because she is greater than 30 weeks' gestation and has a fasting blood sugar level less than 110 mg/dL. Doses should be increased or decreased to achieve glycemic control.

RISK OF DEVELOPING DIABETES MELLITUS

CASE 49-4, QUESTION 4: Why is J.B. at risk for developing diabetes mellitus after delivery?

Glucose tolerance normalizes after delivery for most women. Women with GDM, however, have a 15% to 50% chance of developing nongestational diabetes within 5 to 16 years.[72] The highest risk is in women who are obese or were diagnosed before 24 weeks' gestation or who had marked hyperglycemia during or soon after pregnancy. The risk of developing GDM in a future pregnancy is estimated to be 50% [66,78]

J.B. should try to minimize the potential for development of insulin resistance by exercising and maintaining a normal weight. She should also have her glucose checked with a 2-hour OGTT at her postpartum appointment 6 weeks after delivery and then at least every 1 to 3 years with screening of either fasting blood sugar or HgbA1c. In addition, J.B. should be instructed about the importance of using an effective birth control method to prevent unplanned pregnancies. She also needs to schedule regular appointments with her primary-care clinician.

HYPERTENSION AND PREECLAMPSIA

Chronic Hypertension

CLINICAL PRESENTATION

CASE 49-5

QUESTION 1: T.D., a 37-year-old G1, P0, obese black woman was diagnosed with stage 1 hypertension several months before her pregnancy (BP, 135–145 mm Hg systolic and 90 to 95 mm Hg diastolic). She had no cardiovascular risk factors (i.e., smoking, diabetes mellitus, dyslipidemias) and was prescribed a trial of lifestyle modification (i.e., weight loss and exercise). When she initiated prenatal care at 16 weeks' gestation, her BP ranged from 130 to 135 mm Hg systolic pressure and 82 to 85 mm Hg diastolic pressure. Her BP today at 28 weeks is 142/90 mm Hg. Her serum chemistry values are creatinine (SCr), 0.6 mg/dL, and UA, 4 mg/dL. A random urinalysis did not demonstrate proteinuria. Ultrasound confirms an adequately growing fetus at 28 weeks' gestation. What type of hypertension does T.D. have? What is the likelihood T.D. has preeclampsia?

Hypertensive disease occurs in 5% to 8% of all pregnancies and is a major cause of maternal and perinatal morbidity and mortality.[80] From 15% to 24% of maternal deaths in developed countries are attributed to hypertensive disorders in pregnancy.[81,82] *Hypertension in pregnancy* is defined as a systolic BP of at least 140 mm Hg or a diastolic BP of at least 90 mm Hg on two separate occasions at least 6 hours apart.

Women with pregnancy-associated hypertension can be grouped into the following categories: chronic hypertension, preeclampsia–eclampsia, preeclampsia superimposed on chronic hypertension, and gestational hypertension.[80] After delivery, *gestational hypertension* is ultimately delineated as either (a) transient hypertension of pregnancy if preeclampsia is absent during delivery and BP normalizes by 12 weeks postpartum or (b) chronic hypertension if BP remains elevated.[80]

Chronic hypertension is defined as hypertension diagnosed before conception or before the 20th week of gestation, or hypertension persisting beyond 12 weeks postpartum.[80] Hypertension noted after the 20th week of gestation might be difficult to classify, particularly if a woman has had inadequate prenatal care without appropriate BP monitoring.

Women with chronic hypertension, similar to T.D., commonly have a normal BP during the first half of pregnancy because of the physiologic decline of BP during the second trimester.[83] BP usually returns to the prepregnancy level by the third trimester. T.D.'s diastolic pressure decreased from the prepregnancy levels of 90 to 95 mm Hg to 86 to 90 mm Hg during the second trimester. It is normal for T.D.'s BP to increase during the third trimester. These changes in BP make it difficult to differentiate chronic hypertension from preeclampsia during the second half of pregnancy in women with late prenatal care or inadequate BP monitoring. It is also difficult to diagnose preeclampsia superimposed on existing hypertension using BP measurements alone. A sharp increase in T.D.'s pressure of more than 30 mm Hg systolic or more than 15 mm Hg diastolic could be consistent with preeclampsia. Without coexisting proteinuria ($\geq$0.3 g/24 hours or $\geq$1+ in a random urine sample) or evidence of renal dysfunction, a diagnosis of preeclampsia would be a reach.[83] T.D. has no proteinuria, and a normal SCr and serum UA. T.D has chronic hypertension, but it is unlikely that T.D. has preeclampsia at this time.

RISK FACTORS FOR PREECLAMPSIA

CASE 49-5, QUESTION 2: What risk factors does T.D. have for developing preeclampsia?

Preeclampsia is a pregnancy-specific condition usually occurring after 20 weeks' gestation and consisting of hypertension with proteinuria.[83] Preeclampsia can affect multiple organ systems (e.g., kidney, liver, hematologic, CNS). The signs and symptoms are often unpredictable and can be mistaken for other disorders. Because edema is so common in normal pregnancy and is not specific, it is no longer used as a criterion for the diagnosis of preeclampsia. Preeclampsia is a consequence of progressive placental and maternal endothelial cell dysfunction, increased platelet aggregation, and loss of arterial vasoregulation. A variant of preeclampsia is Hemolysis, elevate Liver enzymes, Low Platelet count (HELLP) syndrome, which consists of hemolysis (H), elevated liver (EL) enzymes, and low platelet (LP) count. HELLP can also be life–threatening and may not always present with proteinuria and increases in BP.[84]

When women with preeclampsia exhibit seizures, the term *eclampsia* is used. Women with preeclampsia may unpredictably progress rapidly from mild-to-severe preeclampsia and to eclampsia within days or even hours. Eclampsia is a potentially preventable complication of preeclampsia. About 20% of women who experience eclampsia have a diastolic BP less than 90 mm Hg or no proteinuria.[85]

The term *gestational hypertension* is used when BP is increased during pregnancy or is increased in the first 24 hours postpartum in a woman without signs or symptoms of preeclampsia and without preexisting hypertension.[80] Women with gestational hypertension are at high risk of recurrence during subsequent pregnancies.

Preeclampsia occurs most commonly during the first pregnancy (two-thirds of cases). Obesity and increasing maternal age are risk factors.[86] Chronic diseases that increase the risk for preeclampsia include diabetes mellitus or insulin resistance and renal disease. Pregnancy-associated risk factors include multifetal gestations, urinary tract infection, certain fetal chromosomal anomalies, and hydatidiform moles. A family history of a sister or mother with preeclampsia significantly increases the risk of developing preeclampsia. Women with previous preeclampsia are at high risk for recurrence in subsequent pregnancies, particularly if it developed before 30 weeks' gestation.[86,87] In addition to her age and obesity, chronic hypertension is the most significant aspect of T.D.'s medical history, which confers a 25% risk of developing superimposed preeclampsia.[87]

Monitoring

CASE 49-5, QUESTION 3: What subjective and objective data should be monitored in T.D. for the development of preeclampsia?

T.D. should have her BP monitored frequently. If protein is detected in a random urinalysis, then a 24-hour urine collection for protein and creatinine can be repeated to determine accurately the degree of proteinuria and severity of disease.[80] Periodic ultrasounds should be obtained to assess fetal growth because IUGR is common in pregnant women with chronic hypertension. T.D. should be taught to recognize and immediately report all signs and symptoms of preeclampsia, such as nondependent edema (i.e., swelling of face or hands), headaches, and visual disturbances. The latter two are signs of severe preeclampsia and may indicate impending eclampsia. Upper abdominal pain also can be a sign of severe preeclampsia, indicating hepatic subcapsular hemorrhage.[86] Because T.D. has chronic hypertension, worsening of hypertension alone may not be a reliable sign of superimposed preeclampsia. Proteinuria is the best indicator of superimposed preeclampsia in a pregnant woman with chronic hypertension and no renal disease.[85]

Antihypertensive Drug Therapy

CASE 49-5, QUESTION 4: Should T.D.'s chronic hypertension be treated with antihypertensive drugs to prevent preeclampsia?

The goal of antihypertensive therapy for women with chronic hypertension during pregnancy is to minimize the risks to the mother of an elevated BP without compromising placental perfusion.[84] The value of treating pregnant women with chronic antihypertension drugs remains an area of ongoing debate. A sustained diastolic BP of more than 100 mm Hg may cause maternal vascular damage, especially if the diastolic pressure is more than 105 to 110 mm Hg.[86] Morbidity is unlikely with a diastolic BP of less than 100 mm Hg. Therefore, many clinicians recommend treatment with antihypertensive drugs to lower diastolic pressures of more than 100 to 110 mm Hg.[80] Treatment of a diastolic BP of less than 100 mm Hg should be reserved for women with chronic hypertension and target organ damage (e.g., left-ventricular hypertrophy) or underlying renal disease because antihypertensive drugs can decrease placental blood flow, which might increase fetal growth restriction.[88,89] Treatment of mild-to-moderate hypertension is associated with a decrease in the risk of developing severe hypertension by approximately 50%, but the overall risk of developing preeclampsia is unchanged.[90] Furthermore, there is no evidence of a reduction in the risk of stillbirth, fetal growth restriction, or preterm birth if women with chronic hypertension with systolic BP of 140 to 169 mm Hg or diastolic BP of 90 to 109 mm Hg are given antihypertensive therapy.[90] Moreover, women treated with antihypertensive therapy were more likely to experience adverse drug effects compared with those who received placebo or were untreated. Antihypertensive therapy, however, is required to reduce the risk of cardiovascular morbidity such as heart or renal failure and acute risk of stroke in pregnant women with severe hypertension (diastolic >110 mm Hg).

T.D. has normal renal function and her BP is less than 100 mm Hg; she does not need antihypertensive drug treatment at this time. If T.D. had been on drug therapy before conception, some experts would have her continue during the pregnancy.[80,85,88] In such cases, however, the doses of the antihypertensive agents often need to be lowered or discontinued altogether to prevent hypotension because the maternal BP naturally decreases during the second trimester. Perinatal outcomes in women with untreated chronic hypertension who do not progress to preeclampsia are similar to those of the general obstetric population.[85] Although chronic hypertension is a major risk factor for preeclampsia, treating T.D.'s uncomplicated mild chronic hypertension is unlikely to prevent the development of preeclampsia.

Methyldopa

CASE 49-5, QUESTION 5: When T.D. returns to the clinic 2 weeks later at 30 weeks' gestation, her BP ranged from 160 to 165 mm Hg systolic pressure and 85 to 92 mm Hg diastolic pressure. Which medication should T.D. be started on?

Methyldopa, a centrally acting α-agonist that decreases sympathetic outflow to decrease BP, is the most commonly used antihypertensive agent for chronic treatment of hypertension in pregnancy in the United States. The usual starting dose of 750 to 1,000 mg/day, to be administered in three to four daily divided doses, can be increased to 2 or 3 g/day if needed. Higher doses may be needed to control BP in pregnancy.[91]

Methyldopa, classified as category B for fetal risk, has the longest and best safety record of all antihypertensive agents during pregnancy. Despite its common use, few adverse effects have been reported in neonates exposed to methyldopa in utero. In addition, no congenital anomalies are associated with methyldopa.[38]

Dizziness and sedation, accompanied by a loss of energy, are among the most common adverse effects reported by pregnant women.[91] Generally, these adverse effects occur early in therapy and tend to subside, but may recur with an increased dosage. Problems with postural hypotension usually do not occur in pregnant women.[91] Patients should be monitored for methyldopa-induced liver damage.[87] Other drugs used to treat hypertension in pregnancy include labetalol and calcium-channel blockers. A review of drug therapies for the treatment of chronic hypertension in pregnancy is listed in Table 49-4.[92–97]

T.D. should be started on methyldopa 500 mg PO 3 times daily. If T.D. cannot tolerate the side effects, she can be switched to labetalol 200 mg PO twice daily. The only antihypertensive drugs absolutely contraindicated during pregnancy are ACEI and angiotensin II receptor blockers because of the association with fetal and newborn morbidity and mortality.[88]

Mild Preeclampsia

CASE 49-5, QUESTION 6: T.D. returns to her obstetrician 1 week later at 31 weeks' gestation complaining of mild hand and leg edema. She has 1+ proteinuria by dipstick, and her BP is 155/102 mm Hg. An ultrasound demonstrates fetal growth restriction. Laboratory results are as follows:

SCr, 0.9 mg/dL
Serum UA, 6.0 mg/dL
Aspartate aminotransferase (AST), 25 units/L
Alanine aminotransferase (ALT), 16 units/L
Platelets, 230,000/μL

She is currently on labetalol 200 mg PO twice daily and has been compliant with her medications. What signs and laboratory evidence are consistent with preeclampsia in T.D.? Does she have mild or severe preeclampsia?

ETIOLOGY AND PATHOGENESIS

The causes of preeclampsia currently remain unknown. Although the pathogenesis begins early in pregnancy, the disease is not clinically evident until the latter half of the pregnancy and persists until the fetus is delivered.[98] Incomplete physiologic placental vascular bed changes and endothelial cell dysfunction are integral to the pathogenesis of preeclampsia.

Placental Ischemia

Early in a normal pregnancy, the trophoblastic migration and invasion of the uterine spiral arteries result in physiologic changes within the placental vascular bed that facilitate maximal intervillous blood flow. The physiologic changes within these spiral arteries are responsible for creating a fixed low-resistance arteriolar circuit, which increases blood supply to the growing fetus. In preeclampsia, these physiologic changes do not occur completely, resulting in decreased perfusion and, consequently, placental ischemia.[98,99]

Endothelial Damage

An intact vascular endothelium assists in preserving the integrity of vasculature, mediating immune and inflammatory responses, preventing intravascular coagulation, and modulating the contractility of the underlying smooth muscle cells.[99]

In normal pregnancy, prostacyclin is increased 8 to 10 times, creating an increased ratio of prostacyclin to thromboxane A_2.[98]

Table 49-4
Drugs for Treatment of Chronic Hypertension in Pregnancy and Lactation

Drug	Dose	Comments
Methyldopa	750–1,000 mg/day start twice a day, increase up to 2–3 g/day, divided in 3–4 doses if needed[99]	Longest safety record in pregnancy. Considered a first-line drug.[88] Dizziness, sedation, and lack of energy are common symptoms, which tend to resolve. Can cause liver toxicity. Low breast milk concentrations, so considered safe in breast-feeding
Labetalol	200–400 mg/day start, increase to up to 2,400 mg/d, divided in 2 or sometimes three doses	Combined α- and β-receptor antagonist properties. Considered a first-line drug.[88] Increasingly preferred to methyldopa owing to fewer side effects. Neonatal effects could include bradycardia and hypotension. Low concentration in breast milk and generally considered safe in breast-feeding[92]
Other β-blockers	Various	Atenolol in particular associated with decreased placental weight and IUGR.[94,95] IUGR thought to be related to β-blocker-induced increased vascular resistance in mother and fetus. Atenolol, acebutolol, metoprolol, nadolol, and sotalol can have high milk-to-plasma ratios and accumulate in breast milk, creating potential risk for neonatal blockade.[96,97] Propanolol found in only small amounts in breast milk and generally considered safe, but infants should be monitored for hypotension, bradycardia, and blood glucose changes
Nifedipine, long-acting	30 mg/day start, increase to up to 120 mg/day, once daily	Limited pregnancy data on nifedipine or other calcium-channel blockers such as verapamil, diltiazem, and amlodipine. Concentrations of nifedipine in breast milk are low and considered compatible with breast-feeding[107,108]
Diuretics	Various	Not first-line agents, although probably safe.[88] Concern regarding potential interference with normal blood volume expansion in pregnancy. Avoid if preeclampsia or IUGR already present. Concentration low in breast milk, but may decrease milk production
ACEI or ARB	Contraindicated	Contraindicated in pregnancy in all trimesters. Fetal renal failure when used after first trimester, resulting in oligohydramnios, limb contractures, pulmonary hypoplasia, skull hypoplasia, and irreversible neonatal renal failure.[38] Increased risk major birth defects with first-trimester ACEI exposure.[75] Minimal amounts of captopril and enalapril in breast milk and both considered compatible with breast-feeding.[229] Minimal amounts of benazepril in breast milk

ACEI, angiotensin-converting enzyme inhibitor; ARB, angiotensin II receptor blocker; IUGR, intrauterine growth restriction.

The biologic dominance of prostacyclin along with nitric oxide plays an important role in maintaining vasodilation throughout pregnancy. Prostacyclin may be responsible for vascular refractoriness to angiotensin II in normal pregnancy. In preeclampsia, the ratio of prostacyclin to thromboxane A_2 is reversed. Thromboxane A_2 is biologically dominant during preeclampsia, leading to increased vascular sensitivity to angiotensin II and norepinephrine.[98] The increased release of thromboxane A_2 is believed to be caused by endothelial cell dysfunction. The end result is vasospasm, which further increases endothelial cell dysfunction and increases BP.[98] Reduced activity of nitric oxide synthase and decreased nitric oxide-dependent or nitric oxide-independent endothelium-derived relaxing factor are believed to increase the vasoconstrictive potential of pressures such as angiotensin II.[80]

Endothelial cell dysfunction in pregnancy is thought to be caused by oxidative stress. Intermittent hypoxic and reperfusion injury that occurs as a consequence of decreased placental perfusion may increase oxidative stress.[98,99] Endothelial damage eventually leads to disruption of the vascular lining, which causes leaking capillary membranes, allowing fluid to leak into the interstitium.[99] In severe preeclampsia, this results in hypovolemia, hemoconcentration, and consequently an increase in hematocrit. The loss of plasma volume, vasospasm, and microthrombi decrease perfusion of the kidney, CNS, liver, and other organs. The loss of intravascular proteins in the urine secondary to renal damage, and through damaged epithelia, decreases plasma oncotic pressure and leads to a rapid onset of nondependent edema. The imbalance of endogenous procoagulants and anticoagulants produces platelet consumption and results in thrombocytopenia and coagulation defects.[99]

T.D.'s diastolic BP is now higher than it was before her pregnancy and has increased by 12 mm Hg in the last 3 weeks. Although an increase in BP by itself is not diagnostic of preeclampsia, the new finding of proteinuria confirms the diagnosis. Other evidence for preeclampsia includes the elevated serum UA concentration, which is a sensitive marker for preeclampsia, and elevated SCr.[86] T.D. denies headaches, visual disturbances, and abdominal pain, which are symptoms of severe preeclampsia. The transaminases and platelet count are normal; therefore, she does not have HELLP syndrome at this time. T.D.'s clinical presentation is consistent with mild preeclampsia; however, a 24-hour urine collection should be obtained to measure protein excretion, quantify the urine output, and further rule out severe preeclampsia.

TREATMENT OF PREECLAMPSIA

General Principles

CASE 49-5, QUESTION 7: T.D. is admitted to the hospital. The 24-hour urine protein is 500 mg/24 hours. Although fetal growth is restricted, all other fetal testing is reassuring. After 24 hours, her BP decreased to 140/95 mm Hg. Her platelet counts remained stable and greater than 200/μL, and transaminases were normal. No other signs and symptoms of preeclampsia were noted. How should T.D.'s mild preeclampsia be managed?

The delivery of the fetus is the only cure for preeclampsia and would be the best treatment option for T.D. if she were at more than 37 weeks' gestation. T.D. has mild disease, however, and is not close to term. Her delivery should be postponed because premature delivery increases neonatal morbidity and mortality. T.D.'s fetus is somewhat growth restricted, which is common in women with chronic hypertension, with or without superimposed preeclampsia. If T.D.'s fetus is severely growth restricted or if subsequent fetal biophysical testing is abnormal, premature delivery would be indicated.[80] Because neither of these is evident in the present circumstances, T.D. should continue her pregnancy under very close medical supervision. It has been suggested that continued hospitalization is appropriate for women with preterm onset of mild preeclampsia, such as T.D.[80] This would allow for rapid intervention in case of rapid progression of disease or associated complications. Probably, a role exists for outpatient monitoring of some select women with very frequent maternal and fetal monitoring, and rehospitalization for worsening disease.[80]

T.D. is also a candidate for administration of glucocorticoids for fetal lung maturation (see Case 49-7, Question 7). Bed rest in the lateral decubitus position is usually suggested and may help reduce BP and promote diuresis by decreasing vasoconstriction and improving renal and uteroplacental perfusion.

T.D. should have her BP measured regularly each day. Liver transaminases, platelets, and creatinine should be measured periodically and whenever her clinical status changes. She also should be assessed for symptoms of severe preeclampsia (e.g., headaches, visual disturbances, epigastric or right upper-quadrant pain). Fetal surveillance is indicated.[80] One approach is to perform a modified biophysical profile, a test performed to ensure fetal well-being using ultrasonography measuring fetal breathing, tone, movement, and amniotic fluid volume with an assessment in fetal heart rate, twice a week and whenever maternal clinical status changes, and an ultrasound for fetal growth every 3 to 4 weeks.

Severe Preeclampsia

CLINICAL PRESENTATION

CASE 49-5, QUESTION 8: T.D.'s BP for about 2 weeks ranged from 140 to 150 mm Hg systolic and 90 to 100 mm Hg diastolic with bed rest. Her proteinuria remained stable at 1+ to 2+ by dipstick. During the past 2 days T.D.'s BP started to increase again, and today her BP is 160/112 mm Hg and her urine dipstick is 3+. She complains of headaches, dizziness, and visual disturbances and has significant edema in her face, hands, legs, and ankles. T.D. is transferred to the Labor and Delivery Unit for delivery. Pertinent laboratory results are as follows:

SCr, 1.3 mg/dL
UA, 6.7 mg/dL
AST, 30 units/L
ALT, 16 units/L
Total bilirubin, 1 mg/dL
Platelets, 95,000/μL
Hematocrit, 38%
Hemoglobin, 13 g/dL
Random urine protein, 4+

Estimated fetal weight by ultrasound is 1,700 g, which is between the 10th and 25th percentile for a gestational age of 34 weeks. What signs, symptoms, and laboratory evidence of severe preeclampsia support this diagnosis in T.D., and what complications may occur?

T.D. has developed severe preeclampsia.[84] Her systolic and diastolic BP are greater than 160 and 112 mm Hg, respectively. She has greater than 3+ protein in a random urine sample, and her SCr is elevated. She complains of headaches and visual disturbances. T.D. is also thrombocytopenic as her platelet count is 95,000/μL. Although her liver transaminases are currently normal, she may be developing HELLP syndrome, a variant of severe preeclampsia associated with a high incidence of maternal and perinatal morbidity and mortality. Therefore, her laboratory values should continue to be monitored even as delivery is being planned.

COMPLICATIONS

T.D. is at risk for cerebral hemorrhage, cerebral edema, encephalopathy, coagulopathies, pulmonary edema, liver failure, renal failure, and eclamptic seizures.[85,86] Severe preeclampsia is dangerous not only to T.D. but also to her fetus because uteroplacental perfusion is compromised. T.D. requires drug treatments to both lower her BP and prevent eclampsia, as well as delivery.

ACUTE TREATMENT OF SEVERE HYPERTENSION

CASE 49-5, QUESTION 9: How should T.D.'s severe hypertension be treated?

The goal of antihypertensive therapy in T.D. is to prevent cerebral complications (e.g., encephalopathy, hemorrhage).[85] Although it is important to reduce the maternal BP, it must be accomplished gradually while the fetus is in utero because a sudden large drop in maternal BP could result in the reduction of uteroplacental perfusion.[86] Because of the potential for fetal bradycardia during or after acute treatment of maternal hypertension, continuous fetal heart rate monitoring should be considered.

Hydralazine

Hydralazine, a direct arterial smooth muscle dilator, has in the past been the drug of choice for the acute treatment of severe hypertension in pregnancy.[85,91] This drug induces a baroreceptor-mediated tachycardia and increases cardiac output, which increases uterine blood flow because the BP is lowered.[86]

The onset of antihypertensive effect for hydralazine ranges from 10 to 20 minutes, and duration of action ranges from 3 to 6 hours after an IV dose.[86,100] Therefore, doses of hydralazine should not be repeated more frequently than every 20 to 30 minutes to prevent drug accumulation.[91] Nausea, vomiting, tachycardia, flushing, headache, and tremors could occur. Some of these hydralazine-induced adverse effects mimic symptoms associated with severe preeclampsia and imminent eclampsia, making it difficult for a clinician to differentiate between drug-associated and disease-related problems.[91] Fetal hydralazine serum concentrations are reportedly the same as or higher than maternal serum concentrations, but drug-associated fetal abnormalities have not been reported.[38]

Labetalol

Labetalol is also a commonly used drug to treat severe hypertension during pregnancy. It should be administered IV in increasing doses of 20, 40, and 80 mg every 10 minutes to a cumulative dose of 300 mg or until the diastolic pressure is less than 100 mm Hg.[101] The onset of action is within 5 minutes, and its effect peaks in 10 to 20 minutes with a duration of action ranging from 45 minutes to 6 hours.

IV labetalol is as effective as IV hydralazine in lowering BP in patients with hypertension during pregnancy, but has fewer reported adverse effects.[91–102] In a meta-analysis of β-blocker trials for the treatment of hypertension in pregnancy, labetalol was associated with less maternal hypotension, fewer cesarean deliveries, and no increase in perinatal mortality.[102] Labetalol also does not appear to decrease uteroplacental blood flow even with a decrease in maternal BP.[91] Labetalol reduces cerebral perfusion pressure, which occurs in up to 43% of women with severe preeclampsia, without negatively affecting cerebral blood flow.[103] Decreased cerebral perfusion pressure may prevent progression to eclampsia. However, it should be avoided in women with asthma and decompensated heart failure.[104,105] Labetalol has also been associated with higher rates of neonatal bradycardia and hypotension than hydralazine, but not higher rates of neonatal intensive care admission.[106,107]

Nifedipine

Nifedipine has been used in doses of 10 mg for acute treatment of severe hypertension during pregnancy because it can be given orally.[91] Nifedipine is effective in decreasing BP without reducing uteroplacental blood flow or decreasing fetal heart rate. Short-acting nifedipine capsules are no longer recommended for the treatment of acute hypertensive urgency, however, because of the risk of stroke or myocardial infarction, and it was never FDA-approved for this indication. Immediate-release nifedipine continues to be used to treat hypertension in pregnancy, however, because this unique patient population may not be at high risk for ischemic events secondary to atherosclerotic disease.[88] Calcium gluconate or calcium chloride should be available for IV administration in the event of sudden hypotension. Caution should be used when giving nifedipine to women concomitantly treated with magnesium sulfate because these drugs have synergistic effects, causing hypotension and neuromuscular blockade.[106]

Several studies comparing immediate-release oral nifedipine with IV labetalol in hypertensive emergencies of pregnancy have found them to be equally effective in lowering BP.[107,108] Nifedipine lowers BP to less than 160 mm Hg systolic and less than 100 mm Hg diastolic earlier than labetalol,[107] but it increases cardiac index[108] (see Chapter 21, Hypertensive Crises). The use of sustained-release nifedipine capsules as an alternative is associated with a delay in BP control to 45 to 90 minutes, which is probably not acceptable.[100]

Hydralazine 5 mg IV for 1 to 2 minutes should be administered to T.D. and repeated in doses of 5 to 10 mg every 20 to 30 minutes to a cumulative dose of 20 mg.[85] T.D. should have repeated measurements of her BP at 15-minute intervals. Because intervillous blood flow depends on maternal perfusion pressure, the goal is to decrease the diastolic pressure to not less than 90 mm Hg.[85,100] Lowering the maternal BP excessively may decrease uteroplacental perfusion and compromise the fetus. A hypotensive overshoot can be observed with hydralazine, particularly in the setting of volume depletion, which is typical of preeclampsia.[100] If one or two doses of hydralazine are not effective in lowering T.D.'s diastolic to less than 100 mm Hg, labetalol 20 mg IV every 10 to 15 minutes can be given.

Eclampsia

MAGNESIUM SULFATE PROPHYLAXIS

CASE 49-5, QUESTION 10: T.D. will undergo an induction of labor for her severe preeclampsia. Which medication should be given to T.D. to prevent seizures?

The precise mechanism of anticonvulsant action of magnesium for the prevention and treatment of eclamptic seizures is unknown. The anticonvulsant activity may be partly mediated through blockade of an excitatory amino acid receptor, *N*-methyl-D-aspartate.[106] Seizures are thought to be caused by decreased cerebral blood flow because of vasospasm. Magnesium sulfate is a potent cerebral vasodilator and increases the synthesis of prostacyclin, an endothelial vasodilator. It also causes a dose-dependent decrease in systemic vascular resistance, which may explain its transient hypotensive effect. Magnesium may also protect against oxidative injury to endothelial cells.[106]

Although termination of the pregnancy is the definitive treatment for severe preeclampsia, the intrapartum and immediate postpartum periods are also the periods of greatest risk for eclampsia.[84] Although the incidence of eclampsia is extremely low, maternal morbidity and mortality are high.[109] In the United States, it has been usual practice to treat all preeclamptic women with magnesium sulfate during labor and for 12 to 24 hours postpartum.[80,85] In the United Kingdom, however, it is common to reserve magnesium sulfate therapy for severe preeclampsia.[110] The evidence for magnesium sulfate prevention of the progression of disease in mildly preeclamptic women had been largely anecdotal in the past. In a large international study of more than 10,000 women, published in 2002, magnesium sulfate clearly decreased the risk of eclampsia in preeclamptic women by 58% compared with placebo.[110] An observational study of nearly 2,500 women with mild preeclampsia (BP of 140/90 mm Hg and 1+ protein) found an incidence of eclampsia of about 1% without the use of seizure prophylaxis.[111]

In a prospective, randomized study, magnesium sulfate was superior to phenytoin for the prevention of eclampsia in hypertensive pregnant women.[109] In addition, magnesium sulfate was more effective than nimodipine for seizure prophylaxis in severely preeclamptic women.[112,113]

A regimen of magnesium sulfate 4 to 6 g IV as a loading dose followed by a continuous infusion of 2 g/hour is the most commonly used regimen in the United States.[115] Lower dosages (e.g., 1 g/hour) have been associated with treatment failures.[116] IV loading doses of 6 g followed by continuous infusions of 2 g/hour maintain therapeutically effective magnesium serum concentrations between 4 and 8 mg/dL.[115] Because magnesium is excreted by the kidneys and will accumulate in cases of renal dysfunction, the continuous infusion rate must be lowered with oliguria or an elevated SCr.

Because of the potential for infusion errors and significant patient morbidity and even mortality with accidental overdoses of magnesium sulfate, the Institute of Medicine has identified magnesium sulfate as a high-risk medication.[116] All infusions of magnesium sulfate must be given through a controlled pump designed to protect against free flow. If such an infusion pump is not available, the intramuscular (IM) route of administration should be used. Dispensing premixed IV bags from the central pharmacy with a standardized concentration of magnesium sulfate and limiting the total grams of magnesium sulfate in each dispensed IV bag also can help guard against inadvertent overdose. Dispensing the loading dose in a separate small bag (e.g., 4 g in 100 mL) from the maintenance bag (e.g., 20 g in 200 mL) also may be helpful.[117]

Magnesium sulfate should be given to T.D. to prevent eclamptic seizures during labor.[80] T.D. should be loaded with magnesium sulfate 4 g IV given for 30 minutes and then started on a continuous infusion of 2 g/hour.

MONITORING MAGNESIUM SULFATE THERAPY

CASE 49-5, QUESTION 11: T.D. has been given magnesium sulfate 4 g IV for 30 minutes and was then started on a continuous infusion of 2 g/hour. What subjective and objective data should be monitored during treatment of T.D. with magnesium?

Deep tendon reflexes (patellar reflex), respiratory rate, and urine output should be monitored periodically during treatment with magnesium sulfate.[109] The loss of patellar reflexes, the first sign of magnesium toxicity, generally occurs at serum concentrations of

8 to 12 mg/dL. The respiratory rate should be monitored hourly and should be greater than 12 breaths/minute. Respiratory arrest can occur with serum concentrations of greater than 13 mg/dL. Urine output should be carefully monitored and should be at least 100 mL every 4 hours (or 25 mL/hour).[109] Magnesium serum concentrations are not routinely measured unless renal dysfunction is evident with oliguria or elevated SCr because magnesium is almost entirely excreted by the kidney.[106,109] Hypocalcemia and hypocalcemic tetany also can occur secondary to elevated magnesium and can be reversed by calcium gluconate 1 g (10 mL of a 10% solution) slow IV push for 3 minutes. Neuromuscular depression can occur in infants whose mothers received magnesium sulfate.[38] Parenteral magnesium sulfate is safe and rarely causes maternal or neonatal toxicity when administered properly but requires stringent, built-in system safeguards to avoid unintended dosing errors.[117]

CASE 49-5, QUESTION 12: How long should magnesium sulfate be continued in T.D.?

Depending on the severity of preeclampsia, magnesium sulfate therapy usually is continued for 24 hours after delivery, which should be the same for T.D.[118] Women with severe preeclampsia or preeclampsia superimposed on chronic hypertension are at greater risk for disease exacerbation when magnesium sulfate is discontinued too soon.

TREATMENT OF ECLAMPSIA

CASE 49-5, QUESTION 13: T.D. delivers vaginally and her magnesium infusion was discontinued by mistake 3 hours postpartum. T.D. experiences an eclamptic seizure 4 hours later when her nurses discover that the magnesium is disconnected. What is appropriate drug therapy for eclampsia?

Lorazepam, diazepam, phenytoin, and magnesium sulfate have all been used to treat eclampsia. The use of magnesium sulfate to treat these seizures results in less maternal morbidity and mortality and less neonatal morbidity.[109,119] Generally, higher serum concentrations of magnesium sulfate are needed to treat than to prevent eclamptic seizures. The same therapeutic range guides both prophylaxis and treatment, however.[114] Seizures unresponsive to magnesium sulfate treatment should prompt an evaluation for other cerebrovascular events (e.g., cerebral hemorrhage or infarction).[115] Lorazepam 2 to 4 mg slow IV push stat should be given for seizure cessation. T.D. should be reloaded with magnesium sulfate and continued on a magnesium infusion for 24 to 48 hours.

DRUG THERAPY MANAGEMENT IN LABOR AND DELIVERY

Induction of Labor

MECHANISMS OF TERM LABOR

In pregnancy, many hormones and peptides, including progesterone, prostacyclin, relaxin, nitric oxide, and parathyroid hormone-related peptide, inhibit uterine smooth muscle contractility. Labor at term occurs because the myometrium is released from its quiescent state.[120] For example, as progesterone concentrations decrease near term gestation, estrogen may stimulate uterine contractility.

Uterine activity is divided into four phases: quiescence (phase 0), activation (phase 1), stimulation (phase 2), and involution (phase 3). Each of these phases is stimulated or inhibited by several factors.[120] During activation, uterotropins such as estrogen, and possibly others, stimulate a complex series of uterine changes (e.g., increased myometrial prostaglandin and oxytocin receptors and myometrial gap junctions), which are important for the coordination of contractions. These changes help prime the myometrium and cervix for stimulation by the uterotonins oxytocin and prostaglandins E_2 and $F_{2\alpha}$. The cervix softens, shortens, and dilates, a process referred to as *cervical ripening*. Uterine stimulation is responsible for the change in myometrial activity from irregular to regular contractions. During phase 3, involution of the uterus occurs after delivery and is mediated mostly by oxytocin.[120]

The exact stimulus of the biochemical scheme leading to labor in humans is unknown. The fetus may help facilitate this process by affecting placental steroid production through mechanical distension of the uterus and by activating the fetal hypothalamic–pituitary–adrenal axis. Ultimately, these lead to increased production of oxytocin and prostaglandins by the fetoplacental unit.

Labor is divided into three stages. Weak, irregular, rhythmic contractions (Braxton-Hicks contractions or "false labor") may happen for weeks before the onset of true labor. The first stage begins with the start of regular uterine contractions and ends with complete cervical dilation. Stage 1 is divided further into the latent phase, active phase, and deceleration phase. During the latent phase, the cervix effaces (thins) but dilates minimally. The contractions become progressively stronger and longer, better coordinated, and more frequent. The duration of the latent phase is the most varied and unpredictable of all aspects of labor, and can continue intermittently for days. During the active phase, contractions are strong and regular, occurring every 2 to 3 minutes. The cervix dilates from 3 to 4 cm to full dilation, usually 10 cm. The second stage starts with complete cervical dilation and ends with the delivery of the fetus. The third stage of labor is the time between the delivery of the fetus and the delivery of the placenta.

INDICATIONS, CONTRAINDICATIONS, AND REQUIREMENTS

CASE 49-6

QUESTION 1: J.T., a 28-year-old primigravida, is admitted to the labor and delivery suite for labor induction. She is at 42 weeks' gestation by dates and ultrasound and has a normal obstetric examination. Cervical examination reveals an unfavorable cervix for labor induction; Bishop score is 4. What are the indications and contraindications for labor induction in J.T.?

The induction of labor involves the artificial stimulation of uterine contractions that lead to labor and delivery. Induction of labor is indicated when the benefits to either the mother or fetus outweigh those of continuing the pregnancy. Examples may include preeclampsia, chorioamnionitis (infection of the fetal membranes, see Case 49-7, Question 11), fetal demise, significant fetal growth restriction, maternal medical problems, and post-term pregnancy.[121] Post-term pregnancy (≥42 weeks' gestation), as in J.T.'s case, is one of the most common indications for induction of labor.[121] Contraindications to labor induction are similar to those for spontaneous labor and vaginal delivery and include, but are not limited to, active genital herpes infection, placenta previa (placenta implanted over the internal cervical opening), prior classic uterine incision, transverse fetal lie (laying longitudinally across the uterus), and prolapsed umbilical cord. Maternal complications that are associated with induction include increased rates of chorioamnionitis and uterine atony (loss of tone in uterine musculature) (see Case 49-8, Question 4) resulting in hemorrhage, as well as a twofold to threefold increased risk of cesarean delivery, particularly in primigravida women.[122]

A complete assessment of both mother and fetus should be performed before inducing labor.[121,123] Gestational age must be assessed accurately before the induction of labor to avoid the inadvertent delivery of a preterm fetus.[121,122] When delivery is necessary before 34 weeks' gestation with intact membranes or before 32 weeks' gestation with ruptured membranes, antenatal corticosteroids should be administered (see Case 49-7, Question 7).[123,124]

The degree of cervical ripeness and readiness for induction of labor should be assessed.[121,125] Success of labor induction is directly related to the favorability of the cervix.[126,127] The Bishop method of evaluating cervical ripeness assigns a score based on the station of the fetal head relative to the maternal ischial spines and the extent of cervical dilation, effacement (thinning of the cervix), consistency, and position.[122,125] Bishop scores of greater than 8 are associated with rates of vaginal delivery similar to those after spontaneous labor.[121] Conversely, Bishop scores of 4 or less, as documented in J.T., are associated with a high likelihood of failed induction and cesarean delivery. As a result, significant research has been directed toward methods of improving the Bishop score and cervix ripeness before stimulation of uterine contractions. However, women with low Bishop scores who undergo cervical ripening before induction of labor still have higher rates of cesarean delivery compared with spontaneous labor.[126] Nevertheless, cervical ripening appears to have some benefit in decreasing time to delivery, shortening labor, and successfully improving Bishop score.[121]

Cervical ripening can be accomplished pharmacologically or mechanically. Pharmacologic methods include the administration of prostaglandins (E_2 and E_1) or low-dose oxytocin. Mechanical methods include membrane sweeping (or membrane stripping), and intracervical balloons.[121,123,125] Osmotic or hygroscopic dilators (e.g., Dilapan, Lamicel) work by absorbing cervical mucus and gradually swelling, thereby dilating the cervical canal.[122,125] In the setting of a favorable Bishop score, labor induction is accomplished most commonly by amniotomy (artificial rupture of the fetal membranes) and oxytocin administration.[121,122]

Although labor induction is medically indicated in J.T. to decrease the risk of an adverse fetal outcome with continuing a post-term pregnancy, such as macrosomia, asphyxia, meconium aspiration, and intrauterine infection, her cervix is unfavorable for induction and she is a candidate for cervix ripening.

CERVICAL RIPENING

CASE 49-6, QUESTION 2: What pharmacologic agents can be used for cervical ripening in J.T.?

Misoprostol (Cytotec)

Prostaglandins induce cervical ripening and enhance myometrial sensitivity to oxytocin by promoting the breakdown of collagen and increasing the submucosal hyaluronic acid and water content.[121,122,125] Misoprostol is a prostaglandin E_1 analog approved for use in the prevention of nonsteroidal anti-inflammatory drug-induced peptic ulcer disease. It also has been used for cervical ripening and the induction of labor in women despite the lack of approval by the FDA for these latter indications.[128,129] In two large meta-analyses, misoprostol was more effective for cervical ripening and labor induction than either placebo or treatment with dinoprostone (prostaglandin E_2).[128,129] In comparisons, intravaginal misoprostol produced labor more often during cervical ripening and resulted in reduced rate of cesarean deliveries, shorter delivery times, and a greater incidence of vaginal delivery within 24 hours but had a higher incidence of uterine contraction abnormalities than either dinoprostone vaginal insert or dinoprostone endocervical gel.[128–132] Uterine tachysystole, excessively frequent uterine contractions, without fetal heart rate abnormalities was more common with misoprostol use. Maternal and neonatal outcomes were similar in both groups. The need for oxytocin is decreased significantly in women treated with misoprostol compared with women treated with dinoprostone.[131]

Oral misoprostol has also been studied for cervical ripening, but comparisons of vaginal and oral misoprostol are complicated by wide variations in dose and dose interval.[132] A meta-analysis of available studies concluded that the only consistent finding was a reduction in low 5-minute Apgar scores with oral misoprostol but no difference in neonatal intensive care unit admissions. When comparing all studies with a wide range of doses, oral misoprostol resulted in similar rates of vaginal delivery not achieved in 24 hours, uterine tachysystole with fetal heart rate changes, and cesarean delivery compared with vaginal misoprostol.[122]

Misoprostol 25 mcg (one-fourth of an unscored 100-mcg tablet) is inserted into the posterior vaginal fornix and repeated as needed every 3 to 6 hours.[130,131] Higher doses of 50 mcg are associated with increased uterine contractile abnormalities.[128,132] Continuous fetal heart rate and uterine monitoring is recommended throughout the administration of misoprostol.[133] If oxytocin is indicated after cervical ripening, administration should be delayed at least 4 hours from the last dose of misoprostol.[121]

Misoprostol should not be used in women with previous uterine scars because of the risk for uterine rupture.[121,130,132] Although misoprostol is a known teratogen in the first trimester of pregnancy, particularly if used in an unsuccessful attempt at medical abortion, there are no such reports with exposure beyond the first trimester.[38,130] Misoprostol's low cost and ease of administration are advantages compared with dinoprostone, and there is extensive clinical experience with this agent; however, its lack of FDA approval for cervical ripening and induction of labor is a disadvantage. Clinical trials of a controlled-release misoprostol vaginal insert are currently ongoing.[133]

Prostaglandin E_2 (Dinoprostone)

There are two FDA-approved forms of dinoprostone available for cervical ripening. Up to half of the women treated with dinoprostone experience labor and deliver within 24 hours, some without oxytocin.[134,136] Dinoprostone cervical gel (Prepidil Gel) contains dinoprostone contains 0.5 mg per 3-g syringe (2.5 mL gel) and is administered endocervically. The dinoprostone cervical gel must be refrigerated, and dinoprostone vaginal inserts must remain frozen until administration. Dinoprostone slow-release insert (Cervidil) contains dinoprostone 10 mg and is inserted vaginally.[137] Post-term women with unfavorable services who receive dinoprostone have shorter durations of labor, and require lower doses of oxytocin, compared with placebo or no therapy.[125,134–136] A large meta-analysis that included more than 10,000 women found that the use of vaginal prostaglandin E_2 compared with no treatment or placebo was associated with increased rates of vaginal delivery within 24 hours, increased rates of cervix ripening, reduced need for oxytocin augmentation, and no difference in cesarean section. The risk of uterine tachysystole with fetal heart rate changes was increased, however.[138]

Both dinoprostone products are effective for cervical ripening, leading to successful induction of labor.[125,134–136] The two dinoprostone formulations differ in dosing and application.[139,141] The dinoprostone 10-mg vaginal insert slowly releases dinoprostone 0.3 mg/hour for a 12-hour period.[137] The insert is contained within a knitted pouch attached to a long tape. Advantages of the vaginal insert include that it is easier for the clinician to place and less uncomfortable for the patient. In addition, the insert can be removed with the onset of active labor or the development of uterine tachysystole with concurrent fetal heart rate tracing abnormalities. It should be removed within 12 hours of placement or after active labor develops, the membranes rupture, or there is evidence of tachysystole with fetal heart rate changes.[141] If dinoprostone cervical gel is used, the dose can be repeated in 6 to 12 hours if there is inadequate change in the cervix and only minimal uterine activity, but no more than three total doses are recommended.[141] The manufacturer of Prepidil recommends a delay in initiation of oxytocin of 6 to 12 hours once the gel has been placed compared with a shorter delay of only 30 to 60 minutes after the vaginal insert has been removed. An initial period of uterine and fetal monitoring of up to 2 hours should occur after placement of the intracervical gel, with continued monitoring thereafter if regular uterine contractions develop and persist.[121]

The most serious side effect associated with dinoprostone administration is uterine hyperstimulation with or without an abnormal fetal heart rate tracing. The incidence of uterine hyperstimulation associated with the use of dinoprostone intravaginal insert is about 5%; the rate of occurrence for dinoprostone endocervical gel is about 1%.[121] Uterine hyperstimulation occurs more frequently if the Bishop score is greater than 4 before administration of dinoprostone and can occur up to 9.5 hours after placement of the intravaginal insert.[121,141] Use of the vaginal insert requires continuous monitoring of fetal heart rate and uterine activity for as long as the insert is in place and for at least 15 minutes after its removal because of possible uterine hyperstimulation anytime during its administration.[135] Most episodes of uterine hyperstimulation with the use of the vaginal insert occur during active labor and resolve within a few minutes after removal of the insert.[136] Uterine contraction abnormalities may be avoided if the insert is promptly removed at the onset of labor.[128] Both dinoprostone formulations are associated with fever, nausea, vomiting, and diarrhea, and neither are associated with adverse neonatal outcomes.[121,137,139]

For J.T., misoprostol 25 mcg should be administered intravaginally every 3 to 6 hours for cervical ripening. Misoprostol is the most cost-effective option for cervical ripening.

OXYTOCIN

Mechanism of Action

CASE 49-6, QUESTION 3: Twelve hours after administration of two 25-mcg doses of misoprostol, J.T.'s cervix has responded and her Bishop score is now 9, but she has not developed a consistent pattern of uterine contractions. What drug therapy should be initiated at this point?

Synthetic oxytocin should be administered to J.T. to stimulate uterine contractions for accomplishing delivery. Oxytocin increases the frequency, force, and duration of uterine contractions.[142] The uterine response to oxytocin increases throughout pregnancy beginning at approximately 20 weeks' gestation and increases considerably at 30 weeks' gestation.[140] Oxytocin is indicated for both the induction and augmentation of labor. A prolonged latent phase or dystocia (difficult labor) caused by uterine hypocontractility in the active phase of labor is the indication for augmentation with oxytocin.[140]

Dosing and Administration

CASE 49-6, QUESTION 4: How should oxytocin be administered to J.T.?

Oxytocin should be administered by continuous IV infusion using a controlled infusion device. The goal of oxytocin administration is to induce uterine contractions that dilate the cervix and aid in the descent of the fetus while avoiding uterine hyperstimulation and fetal distress.[142] There are two opposing views about oxytocin administration for the induction or augmentation of labor. One view is that oxytocin infusions should mimic physiologic doses in the range of 2 to 6 milliunits/minute with the goal being vaginal delivery with as little uterine hyperstimulation and fetal distress as possible.[121] The other view is that oxytocin should be used in pharmacologic doses to cause strong uterine contractions with the goals being shortened labor, timely correction of dysfunctional labor, decreased cesarean deliveries, and reduced maternal morbidity.[121]

Oxytocin plasma concentrations increase linearly with increasing doses, and steady state is reached within 20 to 40 minutes. Oxytocin serum concentrations correlate poorly with uterine activity, however.[143] Factors that may affect response to oxytocin include parity, gestational age, and cervical dilation.[143]

Despite many randomized, controlled trials and much experience with oxytocin, the optimal starting doses, dosage increments, dosing intervals, and maximal doses are different in the various protocols.[140,142,144] Starting doses range from 0.5 to 6 milliunits/minute, and dose increment intervals range from 15 to 60 minutes.[121] Waiting for 30 to 40 minutes between each dosage rate increase allows time to assess the response at steady state. Most low-dose protocols usually start oxytocin 1 to 2 milliunits/minute and increase the rate of infusion by 1 to 2 milliunits/minute every 30 to 40 minutes.[142,145] High-dose protocols start oxytocin at 3 to 6 milliunits/minute with incremental increases of 3 to 6 milliunits/minute every 20 to 40 minutes. The maximal dose of oxytocin has not been established.[121] The ACOG recommends that each hospital's obstetrics departments develop guidelines for the consistent preparation and administration of oxytocin.[121]

Oxytocin protocols using higher doses or shorter dose adjustment intervals (15–20 minutes) for augmentation of labor generally result in fewer cesarean deliveries for labor dystocia, which is an abnormally slow progress of labor.[145–147] The incidence of uterine hyperstimulation during labor induction is higher with high-dose protocols (initial dose of 6 milliunits/minute with incremental increases of 6 milliunits/minute), however, when compared with shorter dosing adjustment intervals of 20 minutes or with longer dose adjustment intervals of 40 minutes.[147] Women undergoing labor induction with high-dose oxytocin have a higher incidence of uterine stimulation and cesarean deliveries for fetal distress, but a reduced incidence of failed inductions and neonatal sepsis compared with women treated with low-dose oxytocin.[147] In general, lower maximal doses are needed for augmentation of labor than for induction of labor.[144,148]

J.T. should be started on an infusion of oxytocin 10 units diluted in 1,000 mL of an isotonic solution (concentration 10 milliunits/mL) at 1 milliunits/minute. She should have continuous uterine and fetal heart rate monitoring throughout the infusion to detect abnormal uterine contraction patterns or fetal heart rate patterns. The goal is to establish a pattern of three to five uterine contractions of 60 to 90 seconds' duration per 10-minute period.[146] The oxytocin infusion should be increased by 1 to 2 milliunits/minute every 30 to 40 minutes as needed for inadequate progression of labor (cervical dilation rate of <1 cm/hour).[121,149] Fluid intake and urine output should be assessed hourly.

Adverse Effects

CASE 49-6, QUESTION 5: What are the adverse effects and complications of oxytocin for which J.T. should be monitored?

Uterine hyperstimulation, usually associated with excessive maternal dosing or increased myometrial sensitivity to oxytocin, may result in uterine rupture, vaginal and cervical lacerations, precipitous delivery, abruptio placentae, emergency cesarean delivery for fetal distress, and postpartum hemorrhage secondary to uterine atony. In general, neonatal outcomes associated with oxytocin use do not differ from those achieved by spontaneous labor.[146] Although oxytocin has only weak antidiuretic properties, water intoxication resulting in seizures, coma, and death has been reported.[121] Oxytocin is structurally and functionally related to vasopressin, also known as antidiuretic hormone. Administration of high concentrations of greater than 40 milliunits/minute and for long periods is associated with hyponatremia, which can lead to lethargy, drowsiness, generalized seizures, and potentially irreversible neurologic injury. IV bolus administration may cause paradoxical relaxation of vascular smooth muscle leading to hypotension and tachycardia. J.T. should be monitored for uterine hyperstimulation with fetal heart rate deceleration because it is the most common adverse effect of oxytocin.[121,142]

Preterm Labor

Preterm delivery occurred in 12.8% of births in the United States in 2006, representing a 20% increase since 1990.[3] Approximately 55% of singleton preterm births follow spontaneous preterm labor, and approximately 8% follow preterm premature rupture of the chorioamniotic membranes.[150] Premature birth is the leading cause of neonatal mortality (infant death <1 month of age), resulting in approximately 70% of deaths.[150] Prematurity is the second leading cause of infant mortality at younger than 1 year of age, and resulted in 17% of such deaths in 2006.[8] However, the more inclusive classification of mortality as being "preterm related" was linked to 36.1% of all infant deaths in 2006.[8]

ETIOLOGY

Spontaneous preterm labor is a heterogeneous syndrome, and several known pathways can lead to preterm birth. These pathways include excessive uterine distension, decidual hemorrhage, activation of the maternal and fetal hypothalamic–pituitary system, and intrauterine infection leading to inflammation. These pathways ultimately lead to a final common response with production of uterine and cervical proteases and uterotonins, which result in progressive cervical ripening and dilation; weakening of the chorioamniotic membranes, which leads to rupture; and uterine contractions. Ultimately, delivery of the infant occurs. Infection, if present, triggers an inflammatory response that results in the release of cytokines, prostaglandins, and proteases, which stimulate uterine activity, induce cervix softening and dilation, and weaken the chorioamniotic membranes.[152] Variations in maternal and fetal genes coding for cytokines have been implicated in the apparent genetic predisposition to preterm birth found in some families and racial groups.[153] Thrombin is another uterotonic agent, which can cause uterine contractions, and has been implicated in causing preterm labor associated with vaginal bleeding caused by placental abruption.[154] Studies have shown a relationship between increasing maternal corticotropin-releasing hormone (CRH) and delivery timing.[155] Maternal and fetal stress can activate the hypothalamic–pituitary system and result in the rapid increase of maternal CRH before premature birth. Infection can also activate the fetal hypothalamic–pituitary system, increasing CRH, cortisol, and, ultimately, prostaglandins.[152,154] Despite some progress in recent years, much remains unknown about the etiology of preterm birth, and little is known about how preterm birth can be prevented.

CLINICAL PRESENTATION AND EVALUATION

CASE 49-7

QUESTION 1: B.B., a 17-year-old white woman, G2, P1, and 29 weeks' gestation, is admitted to the obstetric unit with complaints of backache, cramps, and uterine contractions. She has no symptoms of preterm premature rupture of the membranes (PPROM). She had a previous preterm birth at 32 weeks' gestation. Cervicovaginal secretions are positive for fetal fibronectin. A pelvic examination reveals that her cervix is 2 cm dilated and 80% effaced, which is increased from 1 cm at her prenatal visit last week. Cervical cultures for *Chlamydia trachomatis* and *Neisseria gonorrhoeae* from her previous visit are negative. Vaginal wet-mount preparations are also negative for bacterial vaginosis and *Trichomonas vaginalis*. Vital signs, urinalysis, and complete blood count with differential are normal. Uterine contractions and fetal heart rate are being monitored. Ultrasound reveals a fetus of 30 weeks' gestation size with an estimated weight of 1,200 g. What signs, symptoms, and laboratory evidence support a diagnosis of preterm labor?

B.B. has backache and uterine contractions, which are symptoms of preterm labor. Most women with preterm contractions are not in labor, however, which results in frequent overdiagnosis. In addition, contractions during preterm labor are frequently not painful, are not detected by the woman, and thus are not a sensitive marker for preterm labor. Fibronectin, a protein that serves as an adhesive between the fetal membranes and decidua, normally disappears from the cervical secretions after the first half of pregnancy, reappearing only at term as labor approaches.[156] A negative fibronectin test can exclude imminent preterm delivery in a woman at risk for preterm delivery, between 24 and 34 weeks' gestation with intact amniotic membranes, and with cervical dilatation of less than 3 cm.[157] Because of fibronectin's high negative predictive value of greater than 95% for delivery in the next 1 to 2 weeks, it can be used to avoid overdiagnosis of preterm labor. Although fibronectin testing will yield false-positive results in the presence of blood, vaginal bleeding itself is independently associated with preterm birth. B.B. has the criteria necessary to establish a firm diagnosis of preterm labor. Not only is her fibronectin test positive, but she has persistent contractions with a documented change in cervix dilatation.

RISK FACTORS

CASE 49-7, QUESTION 2: What risk factors does B.B. have for spontaneous preterm labor?

B.B. has several risk factors for preterm delivery. The strongest predictor of preterm birth is prior preterm birth. She has a twofold or higher increased risk of preterm delivery because of one previous preterm delivery.[156] If this pregnancy also ends prematurely, her risk for a third preterm birth in her next pregnancy will be sixfold higher than that in the normal population.[156] Recurrence risk rises as the gestational age of the prior preterm birth decreases, especially for deliveries at less than 32 weeks. Her young age may also be a risk factor. A maternal age younger than 18 or older than 35 years is associated with spontaneous preterm birth, although it is difficult to separate age from the confounding factors associated with age.[156] Her race likely does not contribute to her risk. Black race is an independent risk factor for both preterm labor and lower neonatal birth weight. Other risk factors include low maternal weight before pregnancy, smoking, second- or third-trimester bleeding, multiple gestation, and uterine anomalies, which B.B. does not have.[120,156] Studies of cervix length by transvaginal ultrasound imaging have demonstrated that shorter lengths are associated with greater risk for preterm delivery; however, the positive predictive value varies widely.[156,157] Maternal infections, such as untreated urinary tract infections and pneumonia, are associated with preterm delivery. In addition, genital organisms such as *Gardnerella vaginalis, C. trachomatis, N. gonorrhoeae, Ureaplasma urealyticum,* and *T. vaginalis,* are also associated with preterm births.[142] Although it is important to identify women at risk for spontaneous preterm delivery, only half of all preterm deliveries occur in women with known risk factors.[156]

Goals of Therapy

CASE 49-7, QUESTION 3: What are the goals of tocolysis for B.B.?

Treatment of spontaneous preterm labor primarily has been directed at slowing or stopping contractions (tocolysis), which are the obvious, although likely late, sign of impending preterm birth. It has been presumed that if successful, this should prevent or delay preterm birth. Few placebo-controlled trials have been conducted of agents used to diminish contractions (tocolytics), and most data suggest delay of delivery by at most 1 to 2 days.[158] This might be because of the heterogeneous causes of spontaneous preterm birth and because tocolytic agents may not arrest the underlying process that led to contractions. Most studies have been unable to demonstrate a clear benefit of tocolysis on neonatal morbidity and mortality. Instead, they have evaluated surrogate end points, such as pregnancy prolongation or number of preterm births before various cut-off points.[159] The value of prolonging pregnancy will vary by gestational age, and might be substantial if time is gained to administer glucocorticoids to improve fetal lung maturation and decrease the risk of intraventricular hemorrhage (see Case 49-7, Question 7). All women at risk for preterm birth within 7 days and between 24 and 34 weeks' gestation should be considered for glucocorticoid therapy.[124,159,160] Delay of delivery can also allow transport to a facility best equipped to care for both mother and premature newborn.

Numerous factors affect the decision to treat preterm labor with a tocolytic agent. Fetal factors precluding tocolysis include nonreassuring fetal monitoring, significant IUGR, and lethal congenital anomalies. Maternal factors include evidence of chorioamnionitis, other significant maternal infections or illness, preeclampsia, and advanced labor.[156] Tocolysis is less likely to be effective in women with cervical dilation of greater than 3 cm and is usually unsuccessful if the patient is in advanced labor (cervical dilation >5 cm).[156] Because the etiology of preterm labor is multifactorial, B.B. should be evaluated thoroughly and periodically for potential causes of preterm labor and treated appropriately when diagnosed. For example, urinary tract infections are associated with preterm labor, and they should be diagnosed and treated if present.[156] Additionally, some would also perform amniocentesis to exclude subclinical chorioamnionitis as a cause of preterm labor before initiating or continuing tocolysis, and to evaluate lung maturity at later gestational ages.[160] B.B. has no evidence of overt infection or other complications, and has no contraindications to tocolysis. Prolonging gestation, even for a few days, would be beneficial because B.B. is only at 29 weeks' gestation.

TOCOLYTIC AGENTS

CASE 49-7, QUESTION 4: How should B.B.'s preterm labor be managed? Which tocolytic agent should be used?

Magnesium Sulfate

Magnesium sulfate is the most frequently used parenteral tocolytic agent in the United States and is also prescribed for the prevention and treatment of eclampsia. Magnesium sulfate relaxes uterine smooth muscle at maternal serum levels of 5 to 8 mg/dL.[156] The mechanism by which it exerts this effect is not understood completely, but involves inhibition of myosin light-chain kinase activity by competition with intracellular calcium, reducing myometrial contractility.[159]

Despite its widespread use, the evidence for magnesium's efficacy in prolonging gestation is inadequate. In two published, randomized, placebo-controlled trials, no benefit in mean prolongation of pregnancy or mean neonatal birth weight was demonstrated. In meta-analyses of both placebo-controlled trials of magnesium for tocolysis compared with other active drugs, no prolongation of pregnancy was seen with magnesium.[158,161] Several small randomized, controlled studies have directly compared magnesium with parenteral β-adrenergic agonists, mostly ritodrine.[158] Three of the four showed no differences in birth outcomes. One of the four suggested prolonged pregnancy with magnesium added to ritodrine compared with ritodrine alone. Studies on the efficacy of β-adrenergic agonists (mostly ritodrine) versus placebo have been mixed, but on balance suggest delay of delivery for 48 hours, but not for 7 days. Therefore, because most trials comparing magnesium with β-adrenergic agonists did not show differences, it has been presumed that magnesium is equally effective. Magnesium is better tolerated than the β-adrenergic agonists, with fewer maternal side effects.[158] Magnesium is contraindicated in patients with myasthenia gravis and must be used with caution in renal failure.

β-Adrenergic Agonists

β-Adrenergic agonists are not the first-line choice for preterm labor because of high costs and the significant potential for maternal adverse effects described subseequently.[156,158] Both ritodrine, the only medication approved by the FDA for the treatment of preterm labor, and terbutaline bind to β_2-adrenergic receptors in uterine smooth muscle and ultimately inhibit smooth muscle cell contractility. Results of randomized, controlled trials of ritodrine have been mixed; however, a meta-analysis that included 1,320 women treated with β-agonists demonstrated fewer births at 48 hours but no change in number of births at 7 days. No benefit on neonatal morbidity or mortality was seen; however, the studies are limited by sample size.[162,163] The continued use of β-agonists can result in the development of tachyphylaxis to its effects on the myometrium and may in part explain treatment failures with these drugs.[156,163]

Terbutaline is available for IV, SC, and oral administration. One dose of terbutaline 0.25 mg SC is often administered to women with mild contractions and cervical dilation less than 2 cm. IV β-sympathomimetics are used in cases with more severe and frequent contractions and cervical dilation greater than 2 cm. However, because of potential adverse maternal side effects such as increased heart rate, transient hyperglycemia, hypokalemia, cardiac arrhythmias, pulmonary edema, and myocardial ischemia, the FDA issued a black box warning in 2011 against the use of injectable terbutaline beyond 48 to 72 hours. The FDA also recommended against any use of oral terbutaline for preterm labor owing to both lack of efficacy and the potential for significant maternal side effects.

β-Adrenergic Adverse Effects

β-Adrenergic agonists are not selective for myometrial β_2-adrenergic receptors at pharmacologic doses, and this accounts for their high incidence of adverse effects.[164] Maternal adverse effects such as pulmonary edema, palpitations, tachycardia, myocardial ischemia, hyperglycemia, hypokalemia, and hepatotoxicity result in discontinuation of therapy in up to 10% of patients.[156] Pulmonary edema can occur and, if not recognized promptly, can lead to ARDS and death.[156] β-Sympathomimetics should not be used in women with underlying cardiac disease or arrhythmias, hypertension, diabetes mellitus, severe anemia, or thyrotoxicosis.[156] In addition, these drugs should be avoided if there are signs of chorioamnionitis such as maternal leukocytosis, fetal tachycardia, or maternal fever.[155]

The most commonly reported fetal or neonatal adverse effects associated with β-agonist therapy include tachycardia, hypotension, hypoglycemia, and hypocalcemia, especially if the drug is being administered within hours of delivery.[156,164] Maternal hyperglycemia causing fetal hyperglycemia and hyperinsulinemia can lead to neonatal hypoglycemia if not properly monitored postnatally. Fetal tachycardia rarely leads to fetal myocardial ischemia or hypertrophy.[164] In summary, although β-sympathomimetic drugs have been used commonly in the past, they are now used much less frequently because of side effect profiles and safety concerns.[156]

Indomethacin

Prostaglandins $F_{2\alpha}$ and especially E_2 are important regulators of myometrial contractility and cervical ripening.[120] Prostaglandin synthesis requires cyclooxygenase (COX), also known as prostaglandin synthetase, to convert arachidonic acid to prostaglandin G_2. COX inhibitors such as indomethacin decrease prostaglandin production, which decreases contractions and inhibits cervical change. As with other tocolytics, these drugs have not been adequately studied in multiple randomized controlled trials. A review of available randomized trials of indomethacin compared with placebo found significant reductions in women delivering at less than 37 weeks' gestation, an increase in gestational age at delivery, and a trend toward fewer deliveries at 48 hours and 7 days.[165] In three of eight trials comparing COX inhibitors with other tocolytics, a reduction in both delivery before 37 weeks' gestation and maternal drug reactions was noted. Also, seen in these studies was a trend toward a reduction in delivery within 48 hours.[165] Indomethacin is well tolerated, and GI upset can be mitigated by antacids when it occurs. The available studies are inadequately powered to evaluate neonatal safety and outcomes, however.[165,166]

Although well tolerated by the mother, concerns exist about the fetal and neonatal effects of prostaglandin synthetase inhibition. Indomethacin crosses the placenta rapidly, and fetal levels rapidly approach maternal levels.[164,166] Because indomethacin can decrease fetal urine output leading to oligohydramnios, the amniotic fluid index should be followed and indomethacin discontinued if it falls below 5 cm (normal range, 5–25 cm). Oligohydramnios generally resolves within 48 to 72 hours of the discontinuation of indomethacin. The fetal ductus arteriosus, which is critical to allow blood from the right ventricle to bypass the fluid-filled lungs, constricts in 25% to 50% of fetuses exposed to indomethacin in utero, but generally is reversible.[156] Permanent closure of the ductus arteriosus, however, can lead to fetal right heart failure and even intrauterine demise. The risk for neonatal adverse effects is increased with drug exposure of longer than 48 hours, as well as use after 32 weeks' gestation when premature closure of the ductus occurs more frequently.[156] An increased risk for maternal postpartum hemorrhage has also been reported with indomethacin use but did not reach significance in a meta-analysis.[165] Indomethacin should not be used in the presence of oligohydramnios or suspected fetal renal or cardiac anomaly (see Chapter 105, Neonatal Therapy).

More serious fetal and neonatal effects have been reported in some retrospective and observational studies, including neonatal necrotizing enterocolitis, intraventricular hemorrhage, and renal failure.[166-168] It is difficult, however, to discern whether these complications are causally related to indomethacin or to the use of the drug in cases of refractory preterm labor caused by subclinical intra-amniotic infection.[166,169] An analysis of the risks and benefits of indomethacin suggested its continued use as second-line treatment for preterm labor between 24 and 32 weeks' gestation in women with contraindications to other tocolytics.[166] Typical dosing regimens include a loading dose of 50 to 100 mg either rectally or orally followed by a maintenance dose of 25 mg orally every 4 to 6 hours for 24 to 48 hours.[167]

Calcium-Channel Blockers

The calcium-channel blockers nifedipine and nicardipine inhibit preterm contractions by decreasing calcium influx into uterine smooth muscle and inhibiting myometrial contractions. No placebo-controlled trials have been performed with nifedipine, the most commonly used calcium-channel blocker. A meta-analysis of 12 randomized trials including a total of 1,029 women found that calcium-channel blockers were superior to other tocolytics (mostly β-mimetics) in reducing preterm births within 7 days and before 34 weeks' gestation.[169] A more recent study of 192 women comparing nifedipine with magnesium sulfate for preterm labor found no differences in delivery in 48 hours, gestational age at delivery, or deliveries before 32 or 37 weeks' gestation.[170] Maternal side effects were significantly fewer in patients receiving calcium-channel blockers compared with other tocolytics.[169,170]

Maternal side effects can include tachycardia, headache, flushing, dizziness, nausea, and hypotension in the hypovolemic patient.[164] Nifedipine does not adversely affect uteroplacental blood flow or fetal circulation. Concurrent use with magnesium should be avoided because the combination may potentiate neuromuscular blockade.[106,160,164] The starting dose is usually 10 mg PO with repeated doses of 10 mg every 15 to 20 minutes for persistent contractions, up to a maximum of 40 mg in the first hour.[172,173] Depending on the tocolytic effect, nifedipine is then maintained at 10 to 20 mg PO every 4 to 6 hours.[172] Overall, nifedipine appears to be an attractive alternative for short-term tocolysis because the drug is usually well tolerated.[174]

B.B. should be started on a magnesium sulfate 6-g IV loading dose for 30 minutes followed by 2 g/hour continuous IV infusion through a controlled infusion pump. The hourly rate of magnesium administration for B.B. may be increased until she has one or fewer contractions per 10 minutes or a maximum of 4 g/hour is attained. B.B.'s deep tendon reflexes, respiratory rate, and urine output should be monitored regularly. Close monitoring of fluid balance is important because fluid overload has been associated with pulmonary edema and the drug is renally excreted.[172]

Magnesium serum concentrations are commonly evaluated every 6 to 12 hours in an effort to minimize adverse effects.[175] The patellar reflex disappears with magnesium serum concentrations between 9 and 10 mg/dL, and as long as deep tendon reflexes are present, many practitioners will not measure concentrations. To prevent inadvertent overdoses, a controlled infusion device should always be used to deliver magnesium as a continuous infusion. Hypocalcemia and tetany can occur with hypermagnesemia. Neuromuscular blockade and respiratory arrest develop with magnesium serum concentrations of 15 to 17 mg/dL, and cardiac arrest develops with greater concentrations. The toxic effects of magnesium can be rapidly reversed with 1 g of parenteral calcium gluconate, which should be readily available when patients are receiving magnesium infusion.[164]

The most common side effects of magnesium loading doses are transient hypotension, flushing, a sense of warmth, headache, dizziness, lethargy, nystagmus, and dry mouth.[156,172] Other adverse effects reported with magnesium are hypothermia, paralytic ileus, and pulmonary edema, which may occur in 1% to 2% of patients treated with magnesium sulfate.[172] Pulmonary edema occurs less frequently with magnesium sulfate than with parenteral β-sympathomimetics but is more commonly encountered with prolonged infusions, multifetal pregnancy, and the use of multiple tocolytics.[164] Treatment consists of discontinuing magnesium sulfate and administration of the diuretic furosemide.

Fetal magnesium serum concentrations are similar to maternal concentrations.[172] The most common neonatal adverse effects are hypotonia and sleepiness. Hypotonia may continue for 3 or 4 days in the neonate because of decreased renal elimination of magnesium. Rarely, assisted mechanical ventilation for neuromuscular depression may be needed.[172]

DURATION OF TOCOLYSIS

Acute Therapy

CASE 49-7, QUESTION 5: B.B. has been maintained on magnesium sulfate continuous IV infusion for approximately 48 hours. The dose was increased to 3 g/hour shortly after the start of the infusion. B.B. has had no contractions for the past 24 hours. How long does she need to be treated? Should she be weaned off magnesium sulfate?

B.B.'s contractions have completely stopped for 24 hours. Some protocols maintain magnesium sulfate for 12 to 24 hours after successful tocolysis, or for the time it takes to complete the course of corticosteroids. The weaning of magnesium sulfate is unnecessary, and simple discontinuation of the magnesium infusion is an easier and less costly option.[174]

Chronic Maintenance Therapy

CASE 49-7, QUESTION 6: B.B. heard that preterm labor can return once stopped and asks whether she should stay on medication. Should B.B. be started on chronic maintenance tocolytic therapy?

Maintenance tocolysis has been used in an attempt to prevent recurrence of preterm labor and prolong gestation in women in whom preterm labor was terminated successfully with parenteral tocolytics. β-Adrenergics and oral calcium-channel blockers have been evaluated for maintenance therapy. Results of meta-analysis of trials comparing placebo or no treatment with oral β-adrenergics for maintenance therapy after acute preterm labor showed no benefit in delay of delivery, births at less than 34 or 37 weeks' gestation, or neonatal complications.[181] Moreover, increases in maternal adverse effects occurred, primarily tachycardia, hypotension, and palpitations. Lastly, inadequate data exist to support the use of calcium-channel blockers as maintenance therapy.[160] B.B. should not be started on chronic maintenance tocolysis, because there is not compelling evidence that continued suppression of contractions after acute tocolysis reduces the rate of preterm birth or neonatal morbidities.[155,159]

ANTENATAL GLUCOCORTICOID ADMINISTRATION

CASE 49-7, QUESTION 7: Given B.B. is in preterm labor at 29 weeks' gestation, what medication can be given to help facilitate fetal lung maturation?

B.B. should be given betamethasone 12 mg intramuscularly now and a second dose 24 hours later to facilitate fetal lung maturation by increasing production of fetal lung surfactant, thereby reducing the incidence and severity of RDS.[124] Antenatal corticosteroid administration (betamethasone and dexamethasone) also decreases the incidence of intraventricular hemorrhage, necrotizing enterocolitis, and neonatal death.[124] The greatest reduction in RDS occurs when delivery can be delayed 24 hours up to 7 days after starting treatment. Repeated weekly corticosteroid courses should not be given because of the association with decreased birth weight and head circumference, hypothalamic–pituitary–adrenal axis suppression, deleterious effects on cerebral myelination and lung growth, and neonatal death (particularly in neonates born to mothers who received three or more courses).[125,185] However, a randomized clinical trial has now demonstrated a significant reduction in neonatal respiratory morbidity and composite neonatal morbidity when women with preterm labor and intact membranes who had received an initial course of steroids at less than 30 weeks' gestation were treated again with a single rescue course of steroids (betamethansone 12 mg IM × 2 doses, 24 hours apart) if more than 2 weeks had passed and the gestational age was less than 33 weeks.[186] This rescue course was administered if there was judged to be a recurrent risk of preterm birth. Although long-term outcome data are not yet available, the ACOG now recommends consideration of a single rescue course of steroids under these specific circumstances.[125]

The National Institutes of Health (NIH) Consensus Panel and the ACOG recommend a course of antenatal betamethasone or dexamethasone (dexamethasone 4 mg IM × every 12 hours, for 4 doses) for all women in preterm labor between 24 and 34 weeks' gestation.[124,125] Betamethasone, however, might be the preferred agent because fewer IM injections are needed and because in meta-analysis it was associated with a greater reduction in RDS compared with dexamethasone.[185] That conclusion, however, is not based on direct comparison of betamethasone with dexamethasone and should be interpreted with caution. One study, although limited by its retrospective nature, also suggested an advantage of betamethasone over dexamethasone in the reduction of periventricular leukomalacia, a finding associated with later risks for cerebral palsy.[187] In cases of PPROM, the NIH Consensus Panel recommends that corticosteroids may be given up to 32 weeks' gestation in the absence of chorioamnionitis.[124,125] Recent meta-analysis supports the efficacy of corticosteroids in the reduction of neonatal death, RDS, duration of ventilator use, and intraventricular hemorrhage in infants born after ruptured membranes.[185] Women at more than 32 weeks' gestation can be considered for amniotic fluid testing for the presence of phosphatidylglycerol or a lecithin to sphingomyelin ratio of greater than 2 because these are indicators of fetal lung maturation.[185] Corticosteroids are not recommended for use in pregnant women who are at more than 34 weeks' gestation unless there is an indication of fetal lung immaturity (105, Neonatal Therapy).

Infectious Complications During Pregnancy and Labor

CASE 49-7, QUESTION 8: Preterm labor is often associated with an infectious etiology or source. Does B.B. need to be started on any antibiotic therapy because she is in preterm labor?

PRETERM PREMATURE RUPTURE OF MEMBRANES

Increasing evidence associates preterm labor with intra-amniotic infections.[152,186] Of preterm births, 20% to 40% may be caused by an infectious or inflammatory process.[156] Intrauterine infection is associated with approximately 80% of early preterm deliveries.[154] Most of the bacteria found in amniotic fluid and the placenta are believed to have ascended from the vagina.[156] It has been suggested that the microbes responsible for preterm birth are already present in the endometrium before conception or early in the pregnancy, causing a chronic, subclinical infection weeks to months before eventually causing PPROM or labor.[154,156]

When PPROM has occurred, spontaneous labor and delivery occurs on average within 7 days, although longer intervals from PPROM to delivery occur with earlier gestational ages.[187] The use of a short course of antibiotics has been shown to prolong the period between PPROM and delivery (the latency period) and decrease neonatal morbidity.[187] In the largest and best-designed trial of antibiotic treatment of PPROM, women between 24 and 32 weeks' gestation treated with ampicillin and erythromycin had both prolonged pregnancies and lower rates of chorioamnionitis.[188] Their newborns experienced decreased mortality, as well as decreased morbidity including RDS and necrotizing enterocolitis. These effects were not owing to tocolytics or corticosteroids because these were exclusionary factors. These results were confirmed by the results of a large meta-analysis including more than 6,000 women, although information on the best choice of antibiotics was less clear.[189,190] Therefore, women with PPROM benefit from antibiotic therapy with a broad-spectrum regimen, and IV ampicillin plus erythromycin for 48 hours followed by 5 days of oral amoxicillin plus erythromycin for a total of 7 days treatment is a reasonable choice.[191]

B.B. should not be started on any PPROM antibiotic regimens because her membranes are not ruptured. Antibiotics have not been proved to prevent premature births in the setting of acute preterm labor.[158] There is currently no role for antibiotic use to prolong pregnancy or reduce neonatal morbidity in preterm labor with intact membranes, and it may be associated with long-term harm.[158,192] There may be a role for treatment of bacterial vaginosis antenatally to reduce the risk of preterm birth in women with a past history of spontaneous preterm birth.

BACTERIAL VAGINOSIS

Some, but not all, studies have demonstrated that screening and treating asymptomatic women who are at high risk for preterm delivery for bacterial vaginosis (BV) may reduce the risk of preterm birth.[158,160] A polymicrobial overgrowth of mostly anaerobic bacteria, BV, is one of the most common genital infections in pregnancy, and it is associated with an increased risk of preterm delivery.[193] Treatment of women with BV who had a prior preterm delivery with oral metronidazole in combination with erythromycin decreased the risk of recurrent preterm delivery in one randomized clinical trial, but there was no difference for women without a history of recurrent preterm birth.[197,198] In addition, a meta-analysis including 622 women with prior preterm birth found no reduction in the risk of preterm birth before 37 weeks' gestation after treatment of BV with antibiotics, but did find a reduction in PPROM. In addition, in women with BV who were treated with oral antibiotics before 20 weeks' gestation, there was a reduction in preterm birth at less than 37 weeks.[198] B.B. does not have BV; therefore, treatment with metronidazole is unnecessary.

GROUP B STREPTOCOCCUS INTRAPARTUM PROPHYLAXIS

Antibiotics should be given to women if delivery is anticipated resulting either from preterm labor with intact membranes or after PPROM to prevent group B streptococcal (GBS) infection in the newborn. Other broad-spectrum antibiotic therapy to prevent preterm delivery should not be given routinely to women in preterm labor with intact membranes.

Approximately 10% to 30% of pregnant women are colonized with GBS or *Streptococcus agalactiae* in the vagina or rectum, and 1% to 2% of neonates born to colonized women experience early-onset invasive GBS disease in the absence of IV intrapartum antibiotic prophylaxis.[199] One-fourth of all cases of neonatal GBS infections occur in preterm newborns. B.B.'s fetus, therefore, is at risk for invasive GBS infection from vertical transmission (mother to infant) of bacteria during labor or delivery. The mortality rate for GBS is reported to be between 5% and 20%. Fortunately, the incidence of GBS has declined to a rate of 0.34 to 0.37 cases per 1,000 live births in recent years owing to prevention efforts.[199] During pregnancy, GBS infection can cause maternal urinary tract infection, amnionitis, endometritis, and wound infection. Antibiotics given to the mother during preterm labor and delivery help to prevent neonatal GBS disease, which may lead to sepsis, pneumonia, and meningitis. In the past decade, the routine administration of intrapartum antibiotic prophylaxis to certain subsets of pregnant women has led to a 70% reduction in the overall incidence of GBS disease.[199] The decision to treat women with intrapartum antibiotics has been based on either a positive vaginal and rectal GBS culture routinely obtained at 35 to 37 weeks' gestation or one or more of the following risk factors without culture screening: (a) previous infant with invasive GBS disease; (b) GBS bacteriuria during any trimester of the current pregnancy; (c) unknown GBS status at onset of labor and any of the following: delivery at less than 37 weeks' gestation, amniotic membrane rupture at 18 hours or more, intrapartum temperature of 38°C (100.4°F) or greater.[199]

Vaginal and rectal GBS cultures should be obtained from B.B., and she should be given a loading dose of penicillin G injection 5 million units, followed by 2.5 to 3.0 million units IV every 4 hours until delivery, while awaiting success of tocolysis and culture results. The Centers for Disease Control and Prevention guidelines recommend that the benchmark for optimal prophylaxis should be antibiotics given at least 4 or more hours before delivery. Penicillin G is preferred over ampicillin because it has a narrower spectrum of antimicrobial activity. If B.B. had a severe allergy to penicillin, sensitivities to clindamycin and erythromycin should be requested at the time of culture in the event GBS is found because of increasing resistance to these drugs. If the isolate is susceptible to both clindamycin and erythromycin, then clindamycin 900 mg IV every 8 hours should be used until delivery. Erythromycin is no longer recommended as an option for treatment because it is often associated with inducible resistance to clindamycin. If the isolate is not susceptible to both clindamycin and erythromycin or if sensitivities are not available, penicillin-allergic women at high risk for anaphylaxis should receive vancomycin 1 g IV every 12 hours until delivery. Penicillin-allergic women at low risk for anaphylaxis should receive cefazolin 2 g IV initially, then 1 g IV every 8 hours until delivery.[192,193] Because B.B is only at 29 weeks' gestation and is in preterm labor, she has not yet had her GBS culture obtained, which normally occurs at 35 to 37 weeks. Until the results of her rapid testing for GBS culture returns, she should receive penicillin G, 3 million units IV every 4 hours until delivery to prevent perinatal GBS infection

CASE 49-7, QUESTION 9: B.B.'s culture results are negative for GBS growth. She is still at high risk for imminent delivery. Should penicillin G administration be discontinued?

Penicillin should be discontinued at this time. Vaginal and rectal cultures need not be repeated if B.B. delivers within the next 4 weeks. If tocolysis is successful and delivery is delayed for more than 4 weeks, obtaining cultures and starting penicillin G preemptively should be repeated at that time. Intrapartum prophylaxis is effective only if antibiotics can be given immediately before and during delivery.

CASE 49-7, QUESTION 10: B.B.'s contractions are gone, and her cervical examination remains unchanged for 48 hours. She is able to be discharged home undelivered, but is counseled to stay on bed rest for the duration of the pregnancy. B.B. has a significant history of a prior preterm delivery at 32 weeks' gestation. What medication should be recommended to B.B. now and in her next pregnancy, to decrease her risk and prevent another preterm delivery from occurring?

Recent studies have shown that progesterone supplementation can help to reduce preterm births, but should only be used in women who have had a prior documented history of a spontaneous preterm birth before 37 weeks' gestation.[194] The optimal progesterone product is not known (vaginal suppositories, oral capsules, or IM injectables). Progesterone should be offered to women like B.B. who have had a prior history of spontaneous preterm delivery.[200] A recent randomized, double-blinded, placebo-controlled trial found a significant reduction in the rate of preterm deliveries in these high-risk women with a prior documented history of preterm delivery with the use of 17-α

hydroxyprogesterone (17-OHP).[195] The rate of preterm delivery in the treatment group was 6.3% versus 54.9% in the placebo group.[195] 17-OHP is given as an IM injection prepared as 250 mg/mL once weekly. Therapy should be initiated at 16 to 20 weeks' gestation and continued until 37 weeks' gestation.[195] 17-OHP is widely available from compounding pharmacies, and most recently, a commercially marketed FDA-approved drug called Makena has been released into the market.[196] Although B.B. is already 29 weeks pregnant, she should be started on 17-OHP therapy at 250 mg/mL injected IM once weekly until 37 weeks. She should be counseled that progesterone should be started earlier at 16 weeks in her next pregnancies. The compounded 17-OHP is more affordable, cost-effective, and equally as effective as the marketed Makena product.[196]

Chorioamnionitis

CASE 49-7, QUESTION 11: B.B. returns to labor and delivery at 36 5/7 weeks' gestation with spontaneous rupture of the membranes and is found to be 4 cm dilated and 80% effaced. Her vital signs currently are a BP of 106/79 mm Hg, heart rate of 80 beats/minute, and respiratory rate of 12 breaths/minute with 99% oxygenation on room air. Intrapartum fetal monitoring shows a reassuring reactive fetal heart rate with variability. After being in labor for about 16 hours, her temperature spikes up to 101.1°F. What are the risks of an elevated fever during labor, and how should B.B. be treated?

Chorioamnionitis is an infection of the amniotic fluid, membranes, and placenta occurring before, during, or immediately after birth.[197] Intra-amniotic infections occur in approximately 1% to 5% of term pregnancies and may complicate up to 15% of cases of preterm labor.[204] Maternal fevers are usually the most common clinical presentation in many patients. Diagnosis is based on the presence of fever, defined as 100.4°F (38°C) or greater measured twice at least 4 hours apart, or a temperature of 101°F (38.3°C) measured once. Patients may also present with maternal tachycardia (>100 beats/minute), fetal tachycardia (160 beats/minute), uterine tenderness, foul odor from amniotic fluid, and maternal leukocytosis.[197,198] The exclusion of other sources of infection such as urinary tract infection, viral illness, abscesses, and drug-induced fever (i.e., epidural, misoprostol) must be made. Common organisms ascending from vaginal flora causing polymicrobial intra-amniotic infections include genital mycoplasmas such as *U. urealyticum* and *Mycoplasma hominis,* anaerobes including *G. vaginalis,* enteric gram-negative bacilli, and GBS.[198,199] The two most prominent risk factors of intra-amniotic infections are the number of digital examinations and duration of labor.[197]

Maternal complications from intra-amniotic infections include bacteremia, suboptimal uterine contractility, and risk for postpartum hemorrhage.[198] Increases in rates of neonatal sepsis, pneumonia, meningitis, and mortality have been shown in infants whose mothers had chorioamnionitis.[200] Furthermore, inflammation, intrapartum fever, and infection increase the risk of long-term neurodevelopmental delay and cerebral palsy in these neonates.[201] The risk of cerebral palsy is at least twofold to fourfold higher in infants who were exposed to intra-amniotic infection in utero.[201]

Early administration of broad-spectrum antibiotics immediately after the diagnosis of chorioamnionitis has been shown to have both maternal and neonatal benefit versus postpartum antibiotic administration. A common regimen implemented is ampicillin 2 g IV every 6 hours in addition to gentamicin dosed to a target peak of 8 mcg/mL and trough of 1 mcg/mL.[198] Standard dosing of gentamicin dosed every 8 hours is preferred over once-daily dosing to prevent elevated fetal serum peak levels, although no adverse effects of high-dose therapy were noted.[202] Clindamycin 900 mg IV every 8 hours may be added to the regimen to cover anaerobic organisms. If fevers persist for longer than 24 hours on triple antibiotics with ampicillin, gentamicin, and clindamycin, metronidazole can be substituted for clindamycin to help broaden anaerobic coverage.[198] Other options for antibiotic coverage include extended-spectrum penicillins (i.e., piperacillin–tazobactam, ampicillin–sulbactam) or second-generation cephalosporins (i.e., cefoxitin and cefotetan).[198] Intrapartum antibiotics administered about 1 hour after infusion produce adequate bactericidal concentrations in the fetus and placental membranes.

With a fever of 101.1°F, B.B. meets criteria for a clinical diagnosis of chorioamnionitis. However, she does not exhibit any other symptoms of systemic infection such as tachycardia, uterine tenderness, or fetal tachycardia, which is quite common. Gentamicin and ampicillin should be started promptly after diagnosis to decrease the risk of neonatal sepsis and to avoid possible neurodevelopment sequelae. In addition, clindamycin can be added to cover anaerobic organisms. B.B.'s risk for chorioamnionitis includes multiple digital examinations, preterm labor, spontaneous labor, and long duration of labor. Antibiotics should be continued until B.B. is afebrile for at least 24 to 48 hours or until delivery. Ultimately, immediate antibiotic administration and delivery of the offending source is paramount to ensure fetal health and safety.

Human Immunodeficiency Virus in Labor and Breast-Feeding

CASE 49-8

QUESTION 1: S.L. is a 23-year-old G1, P0 at 38 weeks' gestation and is positive for HIV. She is presenting to labor and delivery with spontaneous rupture of membranes and is having regular contractions every 5 minutes. Her last HIV RNA levels were undetectable, and her CD4 count was 400 cells/μL. Her current combination antiretroviral therapy (cART) consists of zidovudine (AZT), lamivudine, and atazanavir/ritonavir, which was started 2 years ago. What are the risks of HIV perinatal transmission in S.L., and what medications must be started while she is in labor?

Current recommendations state that all HIV-infected pregnant women should receive intrapartum AZT if the HIV RNA level is >1,000 copies/mL, and their infants should receive neonatal AZT immediately after delivery for 6 weeks with a consideration for a 4 week treatment plan if the mother has been maintained on a cART regimen thought out the pregnancy.[203] Many factors must be taken into consideration, including cost, ease of administration for compliance, individual ART resistance patterns, and risks of side effects with the possibility of teratogenicity.[204] Generally, if a woman on cART becomes pregnant, she should continue on therapy throughout the pregnancy, including the first trimester.[203] Women who did not require cART before becoming pregnant should start cART prophylaxis after the first trimester but not later than 28 weeks of gestation.[203] cART is more effective in preventing perinatal HIV transmission if it is started earlier, before 28 weeks' gestation versus 36 weeks' gestation.[203] All HIV-infected women should be counseled and offered cART during pregnancy to prevent perinatal transmission regardless of HIV RNA levels.[203] Avoid the use of stavudine and didanosine entry and fusion inhibitors in women of childbearing age and during the first trimester, if possible due to issues of toxicity and teratogenicity.[203] Efavirenz in the updated guidelines can be continued to be used if the women was on a efavirenz based regimen. A fetal ultra sound is recommended. Further studies are needed to help identify the effectiveness and safety of other cART regimens. Cesarean section delivery is highly recommended.[203]

S.L. should continue on her ART (AZT, lamivudine, and atazanavir/ritonavir) during labor without missing any doses. Prophylactic neonatal AZT should be administered to the infant at a dose of 4 mg/kg (actual weight) PO every 12 hours, within 6 to 12 hours of birth, for a total duration of 6 weeks.[203]

CASE 49-8, QUESTION 2: Should S.L. breast-feed her infant if her HIV RNA levels are undetectable and her CD4 counts are 400 cells/μL?

Although S.L. is currently on effective cART to suppress her HIV RNA levels and maintain her CD4 levels, she should not breast-feed. Breast-feeding is not recommended for HIV-infected women in the United States because of safer and affordable alternatives such as formula. Prophylactic cART in the infant and mother does not entirely eliminate the risk of perinatal transmission through breast milk.[203]

POSTPARTUM HEMORRHAGE

Prevention

CASE 49-8, QUESTION 3: S.L. successfully has a normal spontaneous vaginal delivery with an estimated blood loss of 400 mL. Which medications should be given to S.L. routinely after delivery?

Oxytocin is administered routinely after the delivery of the placenta to promote uterine contraction and vasoconstriction. Meta-analysis of randomized clinical trials demonstrates that the use of oxytocin preventively in the third stage of labor reduces the risk of hemorrhage and need for medical therapy for uterine atony.[205] Uterine atony, the condition in which the uterus fails to contract after delivery of the placenta, is the most common cause of postpartum hemorrhage.[206] Risks for uterine atony include induction and augmentation of labor, prolonged labor, an overdistended uterus such as with twins or polyhydramnios, and previous postpartum hemorrhage.[206] Oxytocin 10 to 20 units IM or diluted in 0.5 to 1 L of parenteral fluid and given as an IV infusion of 200 milliunits/minute until the uterus is firmly contracted reduces the risk for postpartum hemorrhage secondary to uterine atony.[207] Oxytocin should never be administered undiluted as a bolus dose because it can cause severe hypotension and cardiac dysrhythmias.[207]

MISOPROSTOL

Misoprostol 400 to 600 mcg can be administered orally in the third stage of labor to prevent postpartum hemorrhage.[208,209] In a comparison of 600 mcg of oral misoprostol with parenteral oxytocin for prevention of postpartum hemorrhage, oxytocin was marginally but statistically more effective and had fewer side effects.[210] Misoprostol also can be administered rectally. Rectal administration is associated with a lower incidence of fever and shivering, which is common with orally administered misoprostol during the third stage of labor.[210] The rectal route of administration also is associated with lower maximal serum concentrations and lower time to maximal concentrations than when the drug is administered orally. Although not as effective as oxytocin in preventing postpartum hemorrhage, misoprostol, which is inexpensive, stable at room temperature, and not administered parenterally, may be preferred in settings of meager resources for management of the third stage of labor.

S.L. should receive an infusion of oxytocin 20 units in 1 L of lactated Ringer solution at 125 mL/hour.

Treatment

CASE 49-8, QUESTION 4: Within a few hours of delivering her baby, S.L. has visible vaginal bleeding. She has a distended uterus, and the hemorrhage is attributed to uterine atony. Uterine massage, which is standard treatment, does not control the bleeding. What other pharmacologic options are available to treat her postpartum hemorrhage in addition to the infusion of more oxytocin at this time?

ERGOT ALKALOIDS

If the postpartum hemorrhaging does not respond to oxytocin administration, ergonovine maleate (Ergotrate) and its semisynthetic derivative, methylergonovine maleate (Methergine), can be used because of their potent uterotonic effects. IM administration is associated with less frequent adverse effects (nausea, vomiting, hypertension, headache, chest pain, dizziness, tinnitus, diaphoresis) than the IV route.[207] Ergot alkaloids should be avoided in hypertensive and eclamptic patients because of the potential for arrhythmias, seizures, cerebrovascular accidents, and rarely myocardial infarction. The dose of both drugs is 0.2 mg administered IM every 2 hours as needed. This may be followed by 0.2 to 0.4 mg administered PO 2 to 4 times daily for 2 to 7 days to promote involution of the uterus (Table 49-5).[207]

15-METHYL PROSTAGLANDIN $F_{2\alpha}$ (CARBOPROST TROMETHAMINE)

Bleeding caused by uterine atony that is unresponsive to oxytocin can be treated with 15-methyl prostaglandin $F_{2\alpha}$-tromethamine, also known as carboprost tromethamine (Hemabate).[206] Carboprost tromethamine, as with naturally occurring prostaglandins, stimulates uterine contraction and decreases postpartum hemorrhage;

Table 49-5
Uterotonic Medications Used for Postpartum Obstetric Hemorrhage

Drug	Dose	Comments
Oxytocin (Pitocin)	40 IU in 1 L NS or lactated Ringer solution 10 IU IM if no IV site available	Do not give as undiluted IV bolus, can cause hypotension
Methylergonovine maleate (Methergine)	0.2 mg IM every 2–4 hours	Contraindicated in hypertensive patients
Carboprost tromethamine (Hemabate)	0.25 mg IM every 15–90 minutes, not to exceed eight doses	Caution in use with patients with asthma, can cause bronchoconstriction
Misoprostol	1,000 mcg rectally given once	Can be also be given orally or sublingually, but PR is preferred route

IM, intramuscular; IV, intravenous; NS, normal saline; PR, per rectum.
Source: Cunningham FG et al. Obstetrical hemorrhage. In: Gary Cunningham F et al, eds. *Williams Obstetrics*. 24th ed. New York, NY: McGraw-Hill; 2014

it is more potent and has a longer duration of effect than its parent compound, prostaglandin $F_{2\alpha}$.

Carboprost tromethamine is approved for IM use, but also has been also administered through direct myometrial injection.[207,211] Intramyometrial administration has been associated with severe hypotension and pulmonary edema.[212] An initial dose of 0.25 mg IM is given followed by 0.25 mg every 15 to 90 minutes.[207,211] The total cumulative dose should not exceed 2 mg (eight doses maximum).[211] Carboprost tromethamine is effective in treating 60% to 85% of women with uterine atony who have failed standard treatment.[207] Improvement in bleeding typically occurs after one to two injections.

The most common adverse effects of carboprost tromethamine are GI, including nausea, vomiting, and diarrhea. Flushing and fever also occur frequently. Many of the adverse effects are related to the contractile effect of this drug on smooth muscle.[211] Hypertension, although rare, typically occurs in women with preexisting hypertension or preeclampsia. The potent vasoconstricting and bronchoconstricting properties of carboprost can cause uterine rupture, as well as pulmonary and cardiac problems. Carboprost must be used with caution in women with asthma and is relatively contraindicated in the presence of pulmonary, cardiac, renal, or hepatic disease.[206,211]

MISOPROSTOL

Several case series and small randomized trials have reported that misoprostol might be useful in the treatment of postpartum hemorrhage caused by uterine atony. The available data are very limited, however, and large randomized trials are needed to clarify the efficacy of misoprostol compared with standard therapies, as well as the optimal dose and route of administration.[213] A recent double-blind, randomized, placebo-controlled clinical trial was performed to clarify the role of misoprostol for the treatment of postpartum hemorrhage.[214] Treatment was either 800 mcg of sublingual misoprostol or 40 IU of oxytocin in 1 L of IV fluid given for 15 minutes. Resolution of active bleeding occurred within 20 minutes in 89% to 90% of women in each study arm, demonstrating no advantage to misoprostol over standard IV therapy with oxytocin. Furthermore, women who received misoprostol had significantly more shivering and fever greater than 40°C. In areas with meager resources, misoprostol may offer advantages (low cost, prolonged stability, and oral formulation), but the role for misoprostol as an adjunctive therapy when oxytocin is already available remains uncertain.[207]

S.L. does not have any contraindications (i.e., asthma or hypertension) to any of the postpartum hemorrhage medications. She should be given oxytocin 40 IU in 1 L of lactated Ringer solution given for 15 minutes. Methylergonovine maleate 0.2 mg IM and misoprostol 1,000 mcg rectally can be given in succession after oxytocin if bleeding does not subside. Lastly, carboprost tromethamine 0.25 mg IM is an option if those medications fail to control bleeding.

PREVENTION OF RH D ALLOIMMUNIZATION

Maternal–Fetal Rh Incompatibility

CASE 49-9

QUESTION 1: G.G., a 34-year-old primigravida, had her ABO blood group and Rh status determined during her initial prenatal visit. She is found to be type O, Rh negative. Her husband is type O, Rh positive. What are the risks associated with Rh incompatibility that could affect G.G.'s unborn?

Blood group incompatibility between a pregnant woman and her fetus can result in alloimmunization of the mother and hemolytic anemia in the fetus. When a woman is exposed during pregnancy, labor, or delivery to an antigen found on the fetus's red blood cells (i.e., AB, Rh complex) that is not found on her own red blood cells (RBCs), she forms antibodies against fetus's antigen. This is referred to as *alloimmunization*. These antibodies, particularly immunoglobulin (Ig) G antibodies, cross the placenta and can interact with the fetal RBC antigens. The pregnancy in which the alloimmunization has occurred usually results in an unaffected child. The risk is carried on in subsequent pregnancies when maternal antibodies from a tiny amount of blood (less than 0.1 mL) can cross from the mother to child, which can result in the destruction of RBCs and lead to hemolytic disease of the newborn (HDN). Most serious cases of HDN are caused by Rh alloimmunization involving the D antigen. The other four alleles of the Rh gene complex code for the antigens C, c, E, and e. They are also serious, but less common, causes of alloimmunization.[215]

An Rh D-negative mother becomes immunized after exposure to fetal erythrocytes that carry the D antigen. The likelihood of having an Rh D-positive offspring is determined by whether an Rh D-positive father is homozygous or heterozygous for the D antigen. If the father is homozygous for the D antigen, all of his offspring will be D positive (Rh positive). If he is heterozygous for the D antigen, then there is a 50% chance that his offspring will be Rh positive.

Pregnant women can produce detectable IgG antibodies to Rh antigens within 6 weeks to 6 months.[216] These antibodies can cross the placenta during subsequent pregnancies and destroy fetal Rh D-positive RBCs. Of Rh D-negative women who do not receive Rh_o(D) immune globulin during pregnancy, 17% will become alloimmunized during a term pregnancy, with most cases occurring at the time of delivery.[217]

The severity of Rh-associated HDN or erythroblastosis fetalis depends on the concentration of maternal antibodies. The placental transfer of large amounts of antibody can cause substantial RBC destruction. This initially results in anemia and hyperbilirubinemia with compensatory extramedullary erythropoiesis (e.g., liver, spleen). In severe hemolytic diseases, the fetus might develop hepatosplenomegaly, portal hypertension, edema, ascites, and hepatic and cardiac failure. The clinical presentation of profound anemia, anasarca, hepatosplenomegaly, cardiac failure, and circulatory collapse is termed *hydrops fetalis*.[216]

The severity of Rh-associated HDN generally worsens with each pregnancy in the alloimmunized mother if her fetus is Rh positive. Thus, it is important to discuss the consequences of alloimmunization with any woman who is known to be alloimmunized and wishes to have more children in the future.[217]

Rh_o(D) Immunoglobulin

CASE 49-9, QUESTION 2: What interventions should be undertaken to prevent G.G. from becoming alloimmunized?

ANTEPARTUM PROPHYLAXIS

G.G. should have antibody screens at the beginning of each pregnancy and postpartum. Although the American Association of Blood Banks recommends that an antepartum screen should also be obtained at 28 weeks' gestation, the cost-effectiveness of such screening has not been studied, and it is estimated that sensitization before 28 weeks occurs at a rate of less than 0.18%. Therefore, the ACOG has suggested that the decision to obtain a third-trimester antibody screen should be dictated by individual circumstances.[217] As pregnancy progresses, both the incidence and the degree of fetomaternal hemorrhage increase.

Administrating $Rh_o(D)$ immune globulin to G.G. before or shortly after exposure to fetal Rh D-positive RBCs will prevent her from becoming alloimmunized. Giving $Rh_o(D)$ immune globulin at 28 weeks' gestation has been shown to decrease the antepartum sensitization rate from approximately 2% to 0.1%.[217] One mechanism by which $Rh_o(D)$ immune globulin might prevent sensitization is by suppression of the primary immune response to the D antigen.[216] The anti-D immune globulin binds the D antigen, and this complex is filtered by the spleen and lymph nodes whereby it inhibits D antigen-specific B cells from proliferating.

POSTPARTUM PROPHYLAXIS

A second dose of $Rh_o(D)$ immune globulin should be repeated within 72 hours of delivery. A larger dose is needed if a large transplacental bleed occurs at the time of delivery (0.4% of cases). Therefore, all $Rh_o(D)$-negative women who deliver an $Rh_o(D)$-positive newborn should be tested to detect fetal RBCs in maternal blood (e.g., Kleihauer–Betke test) to calculate the correct dose of $Rh_o(D)$ immune globulin. If a woman at risk for sensitization has not been given $Rh_o(D)$ immune globulin within 72 hours, she should still be treated as soon as possible because it has been demonstrated that protection can be seen in some individuals up to 13 days after exposure to Rh-positive RBCs.[217]

ADVERSE EFFECTS OF $RH_O(D)$ IMMUNE GLOBULIN

The plasma from which immune globulin is obtained is tested for viral infections, and the manufacturing process used to produce $Rh_o(D)$ immune globulin inactivates viruses such as HIV, hepatitis B virus, and hepatitis C virus.[218] Adverse reactions associated with the use of anti-D immune globulin are rare. Pain and swelling at the injection site and rash are the most common adverse reactions. Hypersensitivity reactions such as anaphylaxis, although rare, can occur owing to a small amount of IgA in the product. $Rh_o(D)$ immune globulin (RhoGAM) is latex-free and thimerosal-free (contains no mercury).[218]

Prophylaxis for First- and Second-Trimester Events and Procedures

CASE 49-9, QUESTION 3: G.G. will undergo amniocentesis at 16 weeks' gestation. Will she need a dose of $Rh_o(D)$ at that time?

$Rh_o(D)$ immune globulin should be given after all clinical events (e.g., spontaneous abortion) or procedures (e.g., abortion, amniocentesis, fetal blood sampling, or chorionic villus sampling) in which fetomaternal hemorrhage is a risk in an Rh-incompatible pregnancy.[218]Although little evidence supports the need for prophylaxis in the early first trimester, adverse effects are rare and potential benefits are thought by most experts to outweigh the risks.[217,218] Although a 50-mcg dose (MICRhoGAM) is available for first-trimester use (e.g., chorionic villus sampling or abortion), many hospitals do not stock this dose and so a 300-mcg standard dose is often given.

LENGTH OF PROTECTION

CASE 49-9, QUESTION 4: G.G. had an amniocentesis at 16 weeks for which she received $Rh_o(D)$ immune globulin 300 mcg IM. Will she need another dose at 28 weeks' gestation? How long will this dose protect G.G. against alloimmunization?

G.G. will still need a dose of 300 mcg repeated at 28 weeks' gestation and within 72 hours postpartum if her infant is $Rh_o(D)$-positive. The half-life of $Rh_o(D)$ immune globulin is approximately 23 to 26 days.[218] Without a large fetomaternal hemorrhage, a standard dose of 300 mcg will protect against alloimmunization for up to 12 weeks. If more than 12 weeks have lapsed between receipt of anti-D immune globulin and delivery, many practitioners recommend administering another antepartum dose.[217,218]

Failure of Immunoprophylaxis

CASE 49-9, QUESTION 5: What are the most common reasons for Rh D alloimmunization during pregnancy?

The most common reasons for Rh D alloimmunization are (a) failure to give a dose of anti-D immune globulin at 28 weeks' gestation, (b) failure to give $Rh_o(D)$ immune globulin in a timely manner postpartum to women who have delivered an $Rh_o(D)$-positive or untyped fetus, and (c) failure to recognize clinical procedures and situations that increase maternal risk for alloimmunization (i.e., amniocentesis, abortions).[216,217]

Thus, G.G. should be told that with proper prophylaxis with anti-D immune globulin, there is little chance for her to become alloimmunized. She need not worry about her present pregnancy or future pregnancies.

LACTATION

Lactation is controlled primarily by prolactin (PRL), but the entire process is under the intricate control of several hormones. Breast tissue maturation during pregnancy is influenced by many factors, including estrogen, progesterone, PRL, insulin, growth hormone, cortisol, thyroxine, and human placental lactogen.[219] PRL concentrations gradually increase during pregnancy, but high estrogen and progesterone concentrations inhibit milk secretion by blocking PRL's effect on the breast epithelium.[219,220] It is the dramatic decrease in progesterone that triggers lactogenesis or milk secretion for the first 3 days after delivery. Infant suckling at the breast is necessary to maintain an adequate milk supply beyond postpartum day 3 or 4. Nipple stimulation transmits sensory impulses to the hypothalamus to initiate PRL release from the anterior pituitary and oxytocin from the posterior pituitary. PRL stimulates the production and secretion of breast milk, and oxytocin stimulates the contraction of the myoepithelial cells in the breast alveoli and ducts so that milk can be ejected from the breast (milk letdown). Oxytocin also can be secreted through other sensory pathways, which is why women can release milk on hearing, smelling, or even thinking about their infants. PRL, however, is released only in response to nipple stimulation.

PRL synthesis and release depend on the inhibition of hypothalamic prolactin inhibitory factor (PIF) secretion. PRL secretion is regulated primarily by dopamine-releasing neurons. Activating the dopamine receptors on the PRL-secreting cells of the anterior pituitary inhibits the release of PRL. PIF is believed to be closely associated with dopamine.[219,220]

Although PRL controls the volume of milk produced, once lactation is established, milk production is regulated by infant demand. Lactation eventually ceases if milk is not removed from the breast. Absence of suckling stops milk letdown and restores the normal production of PIF. Decreased blood flow to the breast reduces oxytocin delivery to the myoepithelium. Consequently, milk secretion stops within a few days.[219,220]

Stimulation

NONPHARMACOLOGIC MEASURES

CASE 49-10

QUESTION 1: C.C., a 22-year-old woman, vaginally delivered her first child, a healthy term infant. C.C. plans to breast-feed and was educated about breast-feeding during obstetric visits and prenatal classes. After giving birth, C.C. tried to breast-feed in the delivery room with great difficulty. Afterward, she became extremely apprehensive and continued to have trouble breast-feeding. What can be done to encourage C.C. and help her with lactation?

The most effective stimulus for lactation is suckling. Many women nurse in the delivery room after uncomplicated vaginal deliveries because nursing increases maternal–infant bonding and helps establish good milk production. If a mother does not nurse immediately after delivery, she should be encouraged to do so as soon as she is physically able. C.C. did try to nurse after delivery, but experienced problems that may have been related to her emotional or physical state, or to the physical state of her infant. The nursing staff should encourage and support C.C. emotionally to help her relax, be comfortable, and relieve her anxiety about breast-feeding. Healthcare personnel also should emphasize appropriate feeding techniques and proper positioning for breast-feeding. Allowing C.C.'s infant to sleep in her room, rather than the nursery, may help C.C. develop a breast-feeding routine.

Most new mothers who have difficulty breast-feeding initially respond to the emotional and educational support of a good obstetric nursing staff. Few require pharmaceutical intervention.

ENHANCEMENT OF MILK PRODUCTION

CASE 49-10, QUESTION 2: C.C. was successful in establishing breast-feeding. Despite good technique and adequate nutrition, however, she had trouble maintaining adequate milk production after about 2 to 3 weeks and was forced to supplement her infant with formula. How can C.C.'s milk production be enhanced?

Although not an FDA-approved indication, metoclopramide can be used to stimulate lactation in women with decreased or inadequate milk production.[38, 221–223] Metoclopramide, a dopamine antagonist, increases PRL secretion. This is particularly useful in women whose infants do not breast-feed effectively (e.g., preterm infants).[224] Metoclopramide 10 mg PO 3 times daily for 1 to 2 weeks has been shown to help restore milk production.[38,221–223] Improvement in lactation occurs within 2 to 5 days of starting therapy and persists after discontinuing metoclopramide.

The estimated total daily dose of metoclopramide ingested by the nursing infant of a woman on 30 mg/day is 1 to 45 mcg/kg/day.[38] This is below the maximal recommended infant daily dose of 0.5 mg/kg/day. Maternal doses of 30 mg/day do not alter PRL, thyroid-stimulating hormone, or free thyroxin serum concentrations in breast-fed infants.[224] The only adverse effect reported in nursing infants has been intestinal gas.[38,225] The short-term use of metoclopramide for re-establishing lactation appears to be safe, even in preterm infants.[38,221]

Recent randomized control trials have examined the effects of metoclopramide on breast milk volume and duration in women with recent preterm deliveries and found that breast-feeding outcomes were poor despite medication treatment and lactation support.[225,226] In this special population, women likely need lactation support through various resources addressing nutritional, medical, and psychosocial interventions.

Suppression

CASE 49-11

QUESTION 1: After delivery of a nonviable fetus at 24 weeks' gestation, J.G., a 26-year-old G2, P2, informs her obstetrician that she wishes to suppress her lactation. What methods are available to suppress lactation?

Suppression of lactation is indicated for women who do not want to breast-feed, women who have delivered a stillborn infant, and those who have had an abortion. Both drugs and nonpharmacologic methods have been used. In 1988, the FDA, however, recommended against drug-induced suppression of lactation.[227] The only drug therapy that the FDA recommends in women who are not breast-feeding is analgesic for the relief of breast pain. Bromocriptine was approved for the postpartum suppression of lactation; however, the FDA rescinded its approval for that indication because of cardiovascular complications (e.g., stroke, myocardial infarction) associated with its use.[220]

If breast stimulation is avoided (with or without the use of a breast binder), breast milk production will continue, leading to engorgement and distension of breast alveoli. This leads to the termination of lactation after several days. Approximately 40% of women using this method experience breast discomfort and pain; 30% experience milk leakage from their nipples.[227,228] Ice packs may be applied to the breasts for comfort, and a mild analgesic may be used if necessary.

DRUG EXCRETION IN HUMAN MILK

Breast milk is recognized as the optimal source of nutrition for infants, with documented benefits not only to infants, but also to mothers, families, and societies.[229] Evidence indicates that breast-feeding decreases the incidence or severity of many infectious processes (e.g., otitis media, respiratory infections, urinary tract infections) in infants. In children and adults who were breast-fed, the risk of developing certain medical illnesses also may decrease (e.g., obesity, inflammatory bowel disease, celiac disease, childhood leukemia).[230] Breast-feeding may also positively influence cognitive and intellectual development in children and young adults.[231] Numerous benefits to the mother also have been identified, such as decreased postpartum blood loss, more rapid uterine involution, earlier return to prepregnancy weight, and decreased risks of breast cancer, ovarian cancer, and osteoporosis.[229]

The perception that nursing should be discontinued while the mother is medicated persists, although only a finite number of drugs are absolutely contraindicated during lactation.[95] Unlike the use of drugs during pregnancy, drug excretion in breast milk can be approximated to a certain extent. Actual measurements of drug concentrations in milk and clinical observations in breast-fed infants have been published for selected drugs.

Pharmacokinetics

Different pharmacokinetic models of drug excretion in milk have been described.[233] A two-compartment open model presents the maternal fluids as one compartment and breast milk as the other. After ingestion, the drug gets absorbed into the maternal compartment, with a proportion of drug passing into breast milk and the remaining portion distributed in, and eliminated from, the maternal system. Drugs reaching breast milk will ultimately leave this compartment either by diffusing back into maternal fluids or through milk production and nursing.[232] A more popular model describes drug excretion in milk using a three-compartment model that incorporates the pharmacokinetics of the mother, mammary tissues, and infant.[234] The overall risk to the infant depends on the amount of drug bioavailable to the mother, the amount reaching breast milk, and the actual amount of drug ingested and bioavailable to the nursing infant.

Transfer of Drugs From Plasma to Milk

Transfer of drugs from maternal plasma to milk is generally through passive diffusion.[233] Low-molecular-weight, water-soluble substances diffuse through small, water-filled pores, whereas lipid-soluble compounds pass through lipid membranes.[232] Many factors affect the excretion of drugs in breast milk, and they should be carefully assessed before making a recommendation. The extent of drug passage into breast milk is often expressed quantitatively as the milk-to-plasma (M/P) ratio. This ratio should not be used as the sole determinant of whether a drug is safe for use during breast-feeding (see Estimating Infant Exposure section).

Several parameters affect drug excretion into breast milk (Table 49-6). The pK_a of a drug partially determines how much drug can reach the milk, because only the nonionized portion of free drug is transferred. Human milk, with an average pH of 7.1, is slightly more acidic than plasma. In general, drugs that are weak acids (e.g., penicillin) tend to have a higher concentration in plasma than milk (M/P <1). Conversely, the concentration of weak bases (e.g., erythromycin) in milk are more likely to be higher or to reach an equilibrium with that measured in plasma (M/P ≥ 1).[38,219,233] Once in the milk, the proportion of ionized weak base rises in the relatively acidic solution, and thus drug trapping occurs. Drug reabsorption has been found for some agents, and the prevention of passage back into the plasma by trapping may be clinically important. Lipid solubility also is determined to a large extent by the degree of ionization because drugs with relatively high lipid solubility exist in the nonionized form. Diffusion through lipid membranes is probably the most important pathway for drug transfer. Although pH, pK_a, and lipid solubility are important elements, other factors may significantly modify predictions based solely on these chemical characteristics. Two of these other factors are protein binding and molecular weight.[38,233] Drugs with high molecular weights such as insulin (MW $>$6,000) are less likely to transfer into breast milk, whereas those less than 300 transfer more readily.[38] Highly protein-bound drugs such as glyburide (99% protein bound) are less likely to be transferred into breast milk, although infants should still be monitored for signs of hypoglycemia.

Drug transfer also is influenced by the yield of milk, which is related to blood flow and PRL secretion.[233] Lactation is associated with a high blood flow to the breasts, but little is known about this flow during or between feedings. The milk yield (volume) differs slightly depending on the duration of lactation and the time of day. A diurnal pattern has been observed, with highest yields at 6 AM and lowest yields at 6 PM or 10 PM. The mean composition of mature human milk is approximately 87% aqueous solution, 3.5% lipids, 8% carbohydrate (83% of which is lactose), 0.9% protein, and 0.2% nitrogen.[233] The proportions of these components may vary widely from woman to woman and even within the same woman. For example, hind milk (breast milk that is expressed last and contains more fat) contains fourfold to fivefold the fat content of foremilk (breast milk that is expressed first and is high in water content, water-soluble vitamins, carbohydrates, and protein), whereas colostrum (first milk, secreted late in pregnancy and in the first few days after delivery) contains little fat. Fat content also has exhibited a diurnal variation.

After a drug reaches the milk, it equilibrates between the aqueous and lipid phases. The nature of this equilibration can modify how much drug actually reaches the infant. Infant feeding patterns differ significantly from one baby to another. The time spent suckling at each breast, and the volume of milk taken in, also determine the amount of drug ingested, especially if the drug has partitioned into one phase more so than the other. Once the infant ingests the drug via breast milk, the pharmacologic and adverse effects on the infant will be determined by the extent of oral bioavailability, distribution, metabolism, and rate of elimination. These pharmacokinetic parameters differ, depending on the infant's age and whether he or she was born prematurely or at term.

Table 49-6
Factors Affecting the Fate of Drugs in Milk and the Nursing Infant

Maternal Parameters
■ Drug dosage and duration of therapy
■ Route and frequency of administration
■ Metabolism
■ Renal clearance
■ Blood flow to the breasts
■ Milk pH
■ Milk composition
Drug Parameters
■ Oral bioavailability (to mother and infant)
■ Molecular weight
■ pK_a
■ Lipid solubility
■ Protein binding
Infant Parameters
■ Age of the infant
■ Feeding pattern
■ Amount of breast milk consumed
■ Drug absorption, distribution, metabolism, elimination

pK_a, dissociation constant.
Source: Anderson PO. Drugs and breast milk [letter]. *Pediatrics*. 1995;95:957; Dillon AE et al. Drug therapy in the nursing mother. *Obstet Gynecol Clin North Am*. 1997;24:675; Begg EJ et al. Studying drugs in human milk: time to unify the approach. *J Hum Lact*. 2002;18:323; Bennett PN, ed. *Drugs and Human Lactation*. 2nd ed. New York, NY: Elsevier; 1996; Hale TW. *Medications and Mothers' Milk*. 16th ed. Amarillo, TX: Pharmasoft Medical Publishing; 2014.

CASE 49-12

QUESTION 1: H.P. is a 25-year-old woman G3, P3 who recently was diagnosed with a distal deep vein thrombosis (DVT) in her lower left extremity confirmed by a Doppler ultrasound at 5 weeks' gestation. She has a significant history of having multiple DVTs in her prior pregnancies, and her thrombophilia workup was negative. During her pregnancy, she was on therapeutic low-molecular-weight heparin (LMWH) 80 mg (weight, 76 kg) SC every 12 hours. Her dosage was increased to 100 mg SC every 12 hours after subsequent anti-factor Xa levels were subtherapeutic. Her LMWH was discontinued 24 hours before she received an epidural for labor pain. After delivery, H.P. is restarted on LMWH and then changed to warfarin on day 5. H.P. also is breast-feeding. Do either of these drugs present a risk to the nursing infant?

Heparin does not cross into breast milk (see Drug Excretion in Human Milk section) because of its high molecular weight (~12,000) and is therefore safe in breast-feeding. Warfarin is a weakly acidic drug (pK_a 5.05) that is highly ionized at physiologic pH (>99%) in maternal serum.[233] It also is highly protein bound (97%).[38] These pharmacokinetic parameters make warfarin very unlikely to transfer into breast milk. Case reports in lactating mothers confirm that warfarin is not detected in breast milk or infant plasma.[38] The American Academy of Pediatrics (AAP) considers warfarin compatible with breast-feeding,[92] and it is widely considered to be safe in breast-feeding.[92,235] There are no studies to guide duration of anticoagulation in women who have had a DVT associated with pregnancy. However, most recommend anticoagulation for at least 6 weeks postpartum, with total duration of anticoagulation of a minimum of 6 months after the thromboembolic event.[235] H.P. can safely breast-feed her infant while she is on LMWH and warfarin.

Estimating Infant Exposure

The actual amount an infant will ingest is difficult to determine owing to varying maternal, drug, and infant parameters. Available data generally are from single or small numbers of case reports or pharmacokinetic studies involving few mother–infant pairs. An M/P ratio is sometimes used alone as the basis for a recommendation, but this should be avoided because its accuracy can be affected by many factors such as the time of sampling after maternal ingestion (peak versus steady state), dose, length of therapy, route of administration, and milk composition.[233] A RID is sometimes reported in resources or literature, which is expressed as a percentage of the maternal dose.[233] Generally, an RID of less than 10% is interpreted as an acceptable level. This must be interpreted with caution, however, taking into account other variables such as the age and health of the infant and the safety profile of the drug. It is also important to note that these are estimated values, often based on data collected from one or only a few individuals. Applying these equations using measurements specific to a woman and her infant is not clinically practical, however. Compared with the M/P ratio, experts believe that the RID is a better estimate of infant exposure.

Sampling during maternal peak drug concentration attempts to approximate the highest amount of drug that can reach the infant. This assumption is inherently flawed because peak drug concentration in the mother does not necessarily equate with peak drug concentration in milk at that same point in time.[233,236] The amount of drug an infant actually receives also depends on the volume of milk ingested. Even if a drug has a high M/P ratio, the actual amount received by the infant could be low if only a small volume of milk was consumed. Therefore, an M/P ratio describes the likelihood of drug excretion into breast milk, but it does not indicate the level of infant exposure. In general, drugs with lower M/P ratios (<1) are preferred over those with higher M/P ratios (>1) during breast-feeding, but other parameters such as maternal condition and therapeutic efficacy should be considered.

Infant exposure to a drug via ingestion of breast milk can be estimated for some drugs. The M/P ratio is used to estimate the drug concentration in milk (Eq. 49-1) and the dose the infant may ingest (Eq. 49-2).[233,236,237] The variables required to calculate Equation 49-1 can be located in the published literature, but only for some drugs. The actual volume of milk ingested by the infant is difficult to estimate, but the average consumption is approximately 150 mL/kg/day. The estimated infant dose can then be used to calculate an RID, which is expressed as a percentage of the maternal dose.[236]

$$\text{Drug concentration in milk} = \text{Maternal plasma drug concentration} \times M/P \qquad \text{(Eq. 49-1)}$$

$$\text{Infant dose (mg/kg/day)} = \text{Drug concentration in milk} \times \text{milk volume (mL/kg/day)} \qquad \text{(Eq. 49-2)}$$

$$\text{RID \%} = \text{Infant dose (mg/kg/day)/maternal dose (mg/kg/day)} \times 100 \qquad \text{(Eq. 49-3)}$$

CASE 49-13

QUESTION 1: K.J., a breast-feeding, 91-kg woman, is taking hydrochlorothiazide 50 mg PO daily. The drug has a long elimination half-life of about 12 hours. Peak milk levels of the drug occur 5 to 10 hours after a dose. In a recent study, the drug was excreted into milk with a mean concentration of 80 ng/mL. Based only on dose, does this drug represent a significant risk to K.J.'s nursing infant?

The maternal dose is 50 mg/91 kg = 0.55 mg/kg/day. The infant dose is calculated to be 80 ng/mL (1 mcg/1,000 ng) (1 mg/1,000 mcg) (150 mL/kg/day), which equals 0.012 mg/kg/day. The RID equals the actual infant dose (0.012 mg/kg/day) divided by the actual maternal dose (0.55 mg/kg/day) × 100, which equals 2.18%. Therefore, the exposure likely does not represent a risk. K.J. can continue to take hydrochlorothiazide while breast-feeding. The AAP classifies hydrochlorothiazide as compatible with breast-feeding.[38,92]

Reducing Risk of Exposure

If pharmacologic treatment is medically necessary for a nursing mother, every attempt should be made to minimize infant exposure to the drug. Methods of reducing risks have been proposed.[229,233,234] Table 49-7 summarizes critical factors that should

Table 49-7
Reducing Risk of Infant Exposure to Drugs in Breast Milk

A drug should be used only if medically necessary, and treatment cannot be delayed until the infant is ready to be weaned
Drug Selection
Consider whether the drug can be safely given directly to the infant
Select a drug that passes poorly into breast milk with the lowest predicted M/P ratio, and an RID <10%
Avoid long-acting formulations (e.g., sustained release)
Consider possible routes of administration that can reduce drug excretion into milk
Determine length of therapy and if possible avoid long-term use
Feeding Pattern
Avoid nursing during times of peak drug concentration
If possible, plan breast-feeding before administration of the next dose
Other Considerations
Always observe the infant for unusual signs (e.g., sedation, irritability, rash, decreased appetite, failure to thrive)
Discontinue breast-feeding during the course of therapy if the risks to the fetus outweigh the benefits of nursing
Provide adequate patient education to increase understanding of risk factors

M/P, milk-to-plasma ratio; RID, relative infant dose.
Source: Anderson PO. Drugs and breast milk [letter]. Pediatrics. 1995;95:957; Begg EJ et al. Studying drugs in human milk: time to unify the approach. *J Hum Lact*. 2002;18:323; Howard CR, Lawrence RA. Drugs and breastfeeding. *Clin Perinatol*. 1999;26:447.

Table 49-8
Drugs Considered Contraindicated During Lactation

Drug or Drug Class	Effects on Nursing Infants
Amphetamines[a]	Accumulate in breast milk and may cause irritability and poor sleep patterns
Antineoplastics	Potential for immune suppression; cytotoxic effects of drugs on dividing cells in infants unknown[2]
Cocaine[a]	Excreted in milk; contraindicated because of CNS stimulation and intoxication
Ergotamine	Potential for suppressing lactation; vomiting, diarrhea, and convulsions have been reported.[92] Considered contraindicated by some clinicians. AAP recommends using with caution
Heroin[a]	Possible addiction if sufficient amounts ingested
Immunosuppressants	Potential for immune suppression
Lithium	Milk and serum concentrations average 40% of maternal serum levels. Potential for toxicity exists. Considered contraindicated by some clinicians. AAP recommends using with caution
Lysergic acid diethylamide (LSD)[a]	Probably excreted in milk
Marijuana[a]	Excreted in milk
Misoprostol	Excretion in milk has not been studied but contraindicated because of potential for severe diarrhea in infant
Phencyclidine[a]	Potent hallucinogenic properties
Phenidone	Massive scrotal hematoma and wound oozing after herniotomy in one infant; contraindicated
Requiring Temporary Cessation of Breast-Feeding	
Radiopharmaceuticals	Halt breast-feeding temporarily to allow clearance of radioactivity from milk. Suggested times for individual agents are as follows: copper-64 (^{64}Cu) 50 hours; gallium-67 (^{67}Ga) 2 weeks; indium-111 (^{111}In) 20 hours; iodine-123 (^{123}I) 36 hours; iodine-125 (^{125}I) 12 days; iodine-131 (^{131}I) 2–14 days; radioactive sodium 96 hours; technetium-99m (^{99m}Tc) 15 hours–3 days; ($^{99m}TcO_4$) (^{99m}Tc macroaggregates) 15 hours–3 days

This list is not all-inclusive. Selected drugs are listed by drug class and not by individual names.
[a]All drugs of abuse are contraindicated during lactation.
Source: Briggs G et al. *Drugs in Pregnancy and Lactation: A Reference Guide to Fetal and Neonatal Risk*. 11th ed. Philadelphia: Lippincott Williams & Wilkins; 2017; Sachs HC and the American Academy of Pediatrics Committee on Drugs. Transfer of drugs and therapeutics into human milk. *Pediatrics*. 2013;132(3):e796–e809; Hale TW. *Medications and Mothers' Milk*. 16th ed. Amarillo, TX: Pharmasoft Medical Publishing; 2014.

be considered. Except for drugs that are contraindicated during lactation, the decision to continue or discontinue nursing while receiving medication is ultimately the mother's. Therefore, patient education is an integral component in this decision-making process. The mother should be informed of the potential risks, or lack thereof, associated with a drug. She also should be made aware that certain risks may be minimized by altering feeding pattern and drug administration time and by carefully monitoring the infant for early signs of adverse effects.

Resources for Drugs and Lactation

Comprehensive sources reviewing drug use in lactation are available to assist clinicians in weighing the potential risks versus benefits of mothers using medications while breast-feeding. Table 49-8 lists some medications that are contraindicated during lactation. The AAP Committee on Drugs periodically reviews the transfer of drugs and other chemicals into human milk and publishes their findings.[92] The Committee identifies drugs that should be avoided during breast-feeding, drugs that should be used with caution, drugs whose effects on infants are unknown but of concern, and those considered usually compatible with breast-feeding. This rigorous review is an ongoing process, and new guidelines are published every few years; therefore, the reader should locate the latest AAP recommendations available. In addition to the AAP guidelines, several other references also offer comprehensive information and recommendations on drug use in lactation.[38,92,234]

Most drugs are excreted into breast milk to some extent; the reader is referred to specialty sources for an in-depth review of the drug in question. The best sources for information regarding drugs in lactation are (a) *Drugs in Pregnancy and Lactation: A Reference Guide to Fetal and Neonatal Risk* by Briggs, Freeman, and Yaffe[38] and (b) TOXNET, an online lactation database (LactMed) sponsored by the NIH, accessible at http://toxnet.nlm.nih.gov and click on LactMed. These two databases are peer-reviewed and contain referenced sources. Categories assigned to these drugs may change because new data become available for specific drugs.

ACKNOWLEDGMENT

The author acknowledges Kimey D. Ung, Jennifer McNulty, and Gerald G. Briggs, BPharm, for their contributions to this chapter in earlier editions.

KEY REFERENCES AND WEBSITES

A full list of references for this chapter can be found at http://thepoint.lww.com/AT11e. Below are the key references and websites for this chapter, with the corresponding reference number in this chapter found in parentheses after the reference.

MEDICATION USE IN PREGNANCY AND LACTATION

Key References

Briggs G et al. *Drugs in Pregnancy and Lactation: A Reference Guide to Fetal and Neonatal Risk*. 11th ed. Philadelphia, PA: Lippincott Williams & Wilkins; 2017. (38)

Hale TW. *Medications and Mothers' Milk*. 16th ed. Amarillo, TX: Pharmasoft Medical Publishing; 2014.

Ito S. Drug therapy for breast-feeding women [published correction appears in *N Engl J Med*. 2000;343:1348]. *N Engl J Med*. 2000;343:118. (95)

Key Websites

American Congress of Obstetrics and Gynecology. **www.acog.org.**
Motherisk. **www.motherisk.org**.
National Library of Medicine: Drugs and Lactation Database (LACTMED). **http://toxnet.nlm.nih.gov.**
Organization of Teratology Specialists (OTIS). www.otispregnancy.com.
Perinatology. **www.perinatalogy.com/index.html.**
REPROTOX (Reproductive Toxicology). **www.reprotox.org**.

GENERAL INFORMATION

Key References

ACOG Committee on Obstetric Practice. ACOG Committee Opinion No. 475: antenatal corticosteroid therapy for fetal maturation. *Obstet Gynecol*. 2011;117(2, Pt 1):422. (124)

ACOG Committee on Practice Bulletins. ACOG Practice Bulletin. Chronic hypertension in pregnancy. ACOG Committee on Practice Bulletins. *Obstet Gynecol*. 2001;98(1, Suppl): 177. (83)

American College of Obstetricians and Gynecologists. ACOG Practice Bulletin: Clinical Management Guidelines for Obstetrician-Gynecologists Number 76, October 2006: postpartum hemorrhage. *Obstet Gynecol*. 2006;108:1039. (206)

American College of Obstetricians and Gynecologists. Use of progesterone to prevent preterm births. ACOG Committee Opinion No. 419 (Replaces No. 291, November 2003). *Obstet Gynecol*. 2008;112:963. (194)

Bates SM et al. Venous thromboembolism, thrombophilia, antithrombotic therapy, and pregnancy: American College of Chest Physicians Evidence-Based Clinical Practice Guidelines. *Chest*. 2016;149(2): 315–352. (235)

Loebstein R, Koren G. Clinical relevance of therapeutic drug monitoring during pregnancy. *Ther Drug Monit*. 2002;24:15. (16)

Niebyl JR. Clinical practice. Nausea and vomiting in pregnancy. *N Engl J Med*. 2010;363:1544. (46)

Panel on Treatment of HIV-Infected Pregnant Women and Prevention of Perinatal Transmission. Recommendations for Use of Antiretroviral Drugs in Pregnant HIV-1 Infected Women for Maternal Health and Interventions to Reduce Perinatal HIV Transmission in the United State. August 6, 2015. **http://aidsinfo.nih.gov/ContentFiles/PerinatalGL.pdf**. Accessed May 15, 2016

50 Disorders Related to the Menstrual Cycle

Laura M. Borgelt and Karen M. Gunning

CORE PRINCIPLES

	CORE PRINCIPLES	CHAPTER CASES
1	A normal menstrual cycle involves the hypothalamus, anterior pituitary gland, ovaries, and endometrial lining of the uterus to create hormonal release. This process results in follicle development, ovulation, and either pregnancy or menstruation every 28 days (average) during reproductive life.	
2	Polycystic ovary syndrome (PCOS) is a heterogeneous disorder that presents with signs and symptoms of hyperandrogenism (e.g., acne, hirsutism) or ovulatory dysfunction.	**Case 50-1 (Question 1), Figure 50-3**
3	Long-term complications of PCOS may include impaired glucose tolerance, diabetes, metabolic syndrome, infertility, endometrial cancer, and obstructive sleep apnea.	**Case 50-1 (Question 2)**
4	Treatment for PCOS involves nonpharmacologic and pharmacologic management. Pharmacologic management targets the pathophysiologic aspects of the syndrome and individual goals of treatment. Oral contraceptives are preferred when contraception is desired; letrozole or clomiphene citrate is warranted when pregnancy is desired.	**Case 50-1 (Questions 3–7), Table 50-1**
5	Dysmenorrhea, or painful cramping that occurs with the onset and first days of menstruation, can be categorized as either primary (without underlying uterine pathology) or secondary as a result of uterine conditions, including endometriosis, uterine polyps, or fibroids; complications of intrauterine contraceptive device use; or pelvic inflammatory disease. A careful history can distinguish most cases of primary dysmenorrhea that can be effectively treated with over-the-counter medications from secondary dysmenorrhea, which should always be investigated further for its underlying etiology.	**Case 50-2 (Questions 1, 2), Table 50-2**
6	Dysmenorrhea is the single largest cause of lost productivity and school absence among adolescent girls. Healthcare providers can play a significant role in patient education and development of rational evidence-based drug therapy plans that include nonsteroidal anti-inflammatory drugs (NSAIDs) or hormonal contraceptives to decrease symptoms and improve functionality.	**Case 50-2 (Questions 3–8)**
7	Endometriosis is defined as the presence of functional endometrial tissue occurring outside the uterine cavity. It is the most common cause of secondary dysmenorrhea in young women and can result in chronic pelvic pain, infertility, and dyspareunia. A significant delay in diagnosis of endometriosis is common and can result in negative effects on fertility and pain control. Recognition of the potential for a diagnosis of endometriosis, through a careful history and physical examination, is a key for clinicians to provide appropriate care.	**Case 50-3 (Question 1), Table 50-3**
8	Pain control in endometriosis is directed at suppression of endometrial implants that respond to estrogen with bleeding, resulting in subsequent inflammation and pain. Pharmacologic therapy is directed at reducing inflammation (via use of NSAIDs) and reduction in estrogen (through use of hormonal contraception), or the use of gonadotropin-releasing hormone (GnRH) analogs to induce a pseudomenopausal state. A treatment plan should take into account cost, ease of use of therapy, and the patient's desire for future fertility.	**Case 50-3 (Questions 2–4), Case 50-4 (Question 1), Case 50-5 (Question 1), Table 50-4**

Continued

	CHAPTER CASES
9 Endometriosis treatment plans that include GnRH analogs or aromatase inhibitors may also require the use of "add-back" therapy. Add-back therapy is the addition of progestins or estrogens that may be used with GnRH analogs and aromatase inhibitors to decrease menopausal side effects including hot flashes, vaginal dryness, and decreases in bone density.	**Case 50-4 (Question 1), Table 50-4**
10 More than 200 premenstrual symptoms (such as increased energy, libido, ability to relax, abdominal distension, fatigue, headaches, and crying spells) have been described as occurring during the days before menstruation. It is not until the symptoms have a decidedly negative influence on the physical, psychological, or social function of a woman that premenstrual syndrome (PMS) or premenstrual dysphoric disorder (PMDD) exists. Both PMS and PMDD have symptoms that occur in the luteal phase with resolution within a few days of menstruation, lasting across at least two menstrual cycles, and disrupt normal activities.	**Case 50-6 (Questions 1, 3), Tables 50-5 and 50-6**
11 Nonprescription options that have been studied and have shown at least minimal benefit in PMS and PMDD include calcium, magnesium, pyridoxine, chaste tree or chasteberry, and some mind–body approaches.	**Case 50-6 (Question 2)**
12 Treatment for PMS and PMDD includes lifestyle modifications, psychological interventions, selective serotonin reuptake inhibitors (SSRIs), other psychotropic medications, oral contraceptives, GnRH agonists, and danazol. Because serotonin is critical in the pathogenesis of these disorders, SSRIs have become the treatment of choice for PMDD and severe PMS.	**Case 50-6 (Question 4), Table 50-7**

MENSTRUAL CYCLE PHYSIOLOGY

Feedback biologic mechanisms involving the hypothalamus, anterior pituitary gland, ovaries, and endometrial lining of the uterus control the average 28-day menstrual cycle.[1–3] The hypothalamus synthesizes gonadotropin-releasing hormone (GnRH) and secretes the hormone in a pulse-like manner with varying frequencies throughout the menstrual cycle (typically every 60–90 minutes). GnRH stimulates the anterior pituitary to produce and release follicle-stimulating hormone (FSH) and luteinizing hormone (LH). FSH is important for stimulating growth of ovarian follicles, and LH is critical for ovulation and sex steroid production. FSH and LH act on the ovaries to produce estrogen and progesterone. Estrogen in turn acts on the hypothalamus and anterior pituitary, in a negative feedback manner, to stop FSH and LH secretion (Fig. 50-1).

The menstrual cycle can be divided into three phases: the follicular phase, ovulation, and the luteal phase (Fig. 50-2).[1–3] The day bleeding begins is referred to as the first day (or day 1) of the menstrual cycle. Bleeding usually occurs from days 1 to 5 of the cycle, although may be longer in some women. The follicular phase begins at the onset of menstruation and lasts approximately 10 to 14 days (see Fig. 50-2). At the beginning of this phase, several follicles begin to develop within the ovary. In the second half of the follicular phase most of the developing follicles atrophy, while the dominant follicle develops further and produces estrogen in increasing amounts. Elevated estradiol levels during the ovulatory phase lead to a surge in LH and FSH. The LH surge is responsible for final-stage growth and maturation of the follicle, ovulation, and the formation of the corpus luteum. Ovulation usually occurs 14 days before the last day of the cycle and is followed by the luteal phase. The luteal phase is 13 to 15 days in duration and is the least variable part of the human reproductive cycle.[1] During this progesterone-dominant phase, the corpus luteum produces progesterone and estrogen. Progesterone prepares the endometrium for implantation of a fertilized ovum. If implantation does not occur, corpus luteum regression causes a decrease in the levels of estrogen and progesterone. When these hormone levels decrease, the endometrium cannot be maintained and is sloughed off (menstrual phase).

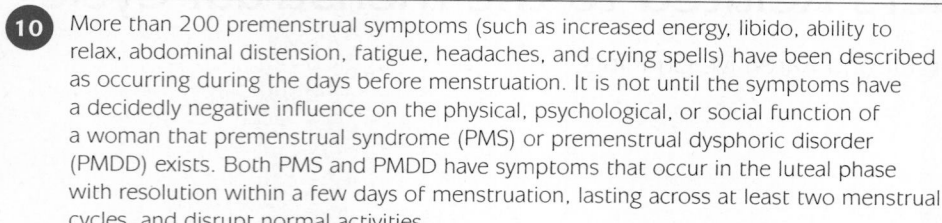

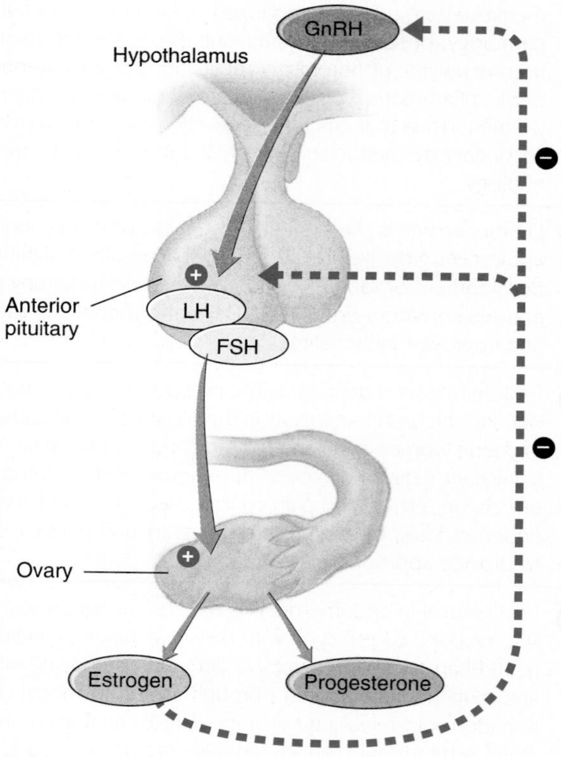

Figure 50-1 Menstrual cycle physiology. FSH, follicle-stimulating hormone; GnRH, gonadotropin-releasing hormone; LH, luteinizing hormone. (Adapted with permission from Premkumar K. *The Massage Connection: Anatomy and Physiology*. Baltimore, MD: Lippincott Williams & Wilkins; 2004.)

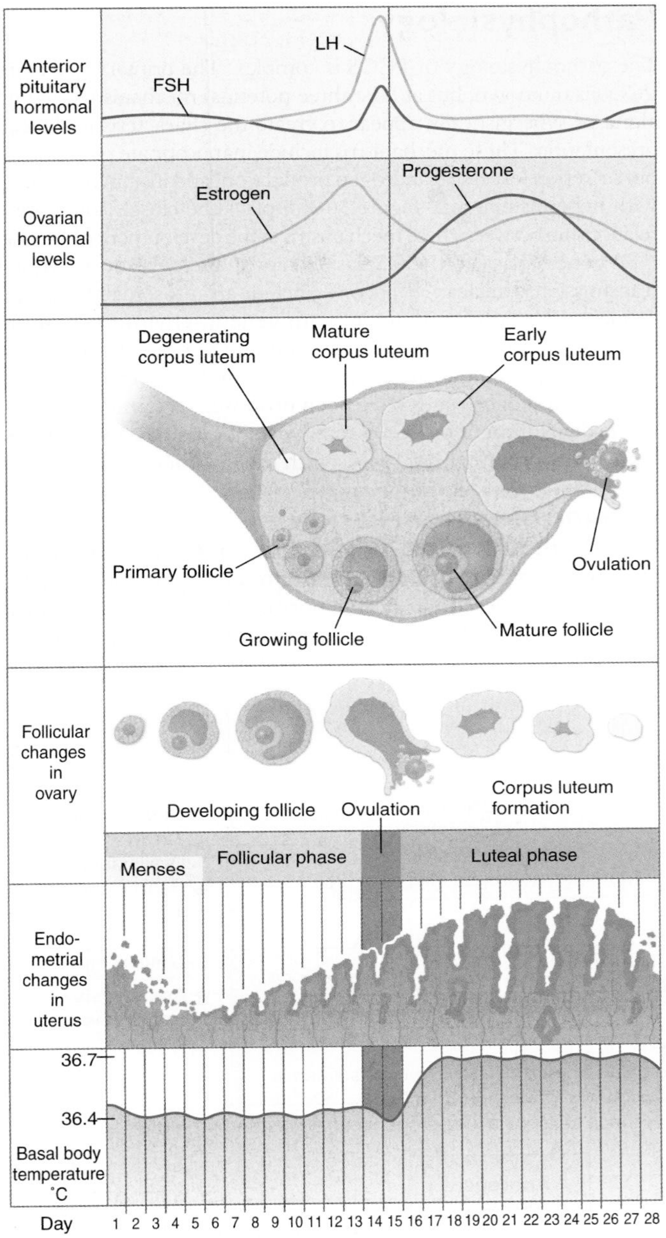

Figure 50-2 The menstrual cycle. FSH, follicle-stimulating hormone; LH, luteinizing hormone. (Adapted with permission from Premkumar K. *The Massage Connection: Anatomy and Physiology*. Baltimore, MD: Lippincott Williams & Wilkins; 2004.)

Using the average 28-day cycle as an example, day 28 is the last day of the cycle and is the day before bleeding begins again for the next menstrual cycle.

POLYCYSTIC OVARY SYNDROME

Polycystic ovary syndrome (PCOS) affects approximately 6% to 15%, or approximately 1 in 10, women of reproductive age, making it the leading cause of anovulatory infertility and the most common endocrine abnormality for this age group.[4] This syndrome, or constellation of symptoms, was first described in 1935 by Stein and Leventhal when they reported infertility and amenorrhea in seven women with enlarged cystic ovaries.[5] Excessive male-patterned hair growth and obesity were added later to the description of this syndrome.[6] PCOS also has been referred to as Stein-Leventhal syndrome, polycystic ovary, polycystic ovarian disease, hyperandrogenic chronic anovulatory syndrome, and functional ovarian hyperandrogenism. The name *polycystic ovary syndrome* has been most widely accepted because "syndrome" best describes the heterogeneous nature of this disorder. However, there have been recommendations to change the name because it focuses on the polycystic ovarian morphology, which is not necessary for diagnosis.[7] It has been suggested that the name should include the complex metabolic, hypothalamic, pituitary, ovarian, and adrenal interactions of the syndrome.

Diagnostic Criteria

The diagnosis of PCOS is complicated by variations among women presenting signs and symptoms of PCOS and because precise and uniform criteria for diagnosis have not been firmly established. Three major diagnostic criteria for PCOS have been proposed by different organizations.

The initial diagnostic criteria were developed in 1990 during an expert conference sponsored by the US National Institutes of Health and US National Institute of Child Health and Human Development. The panel concluded that the major criteria for PCOS should include (in order of importance) the following: (a) hyperandrogenism (clinical signs of hyperandrogenism such as hirsutism) or hyperandrogenemia (biochemical signs of hyperandrogenism such as elevated testosterone levels), (b) oligo-ovulation (infrequent or irregular ovulation with fewer than nine menses/year), and (c) exclusion of other known disorders such as hyperprolactinemia, thyroid abnormalities, and congenital adrenal hyperplasia.[8] The second set of criteria was proposed at an expert conference in Rotterdam sponsored by the European Society for Human Reproduction and Embryology and the American Society for Reproductive Medicine in 2003.[9] They concluded that the presence of two of these three features, after exclusion of related disorders, confirmed diagnosis of PCOS: (a) oligo-ovulation or anovulation, (b) clinical or biochemical signs of hyperandrogenism, or (c) polycystic ovaries. The third set of criteria was developed by a task force of the Androgen Excess Society in 2006 with a complete report including phenotyping in 2009.[10,11] Their criteria include hyperandrogenism (hirsutism or hyperandrogenemia), ovarian dysfunction (oligo-ovulation or polycystic ovaries), and exclusion of other androgen excess or related disorders. Recent practice guidelines support the Rotterdam criteria for diagnosing PCOS.[12]

Criteria for diagnosis of PCOS in adolescence can be difficult to assess due to typical changes during puberty and are different from those used for older women of reproductive age.[4] Specifically, all three Rotterdam criteria should be present or oligomenorrhea or amenorrhea should be present for at least 2 years after menarche (or primary amenorrhea at age 16 years), the diagnosis of polycystic ovaries on ultrasound should include increased ovarian size (>10 cm^3), and hyperandrogenemia rather than just signs of androgen excess should be documented.

Clinical Characteristics

Common clinical signs of hyperandrogenism in PCOS include hirsutism, acne, and alopecia. Hirsutism, the most common of these characteristics, occurs in 60% to 75% of women with PCOS.[4,10–11]

It is defined as an excess of thickly pigmented body hair in a male pattern distribution and commonly found on the upper lip, lower abdomen, and around the nipples. Women seeking treatment for hirsutism may be evaluated for PCOS. Acne affects 15% to 25% of women with PCOS, but this prevalence may not be different from the general population. The prevalence of alopecia occurrence varies widely with reports of 5% to 50% of women with PCOS and presents as scalp hair loss in the crown and vertex areas.[10,13] Although hirsutism is considered a good marker of hyperandrogenism, acne and alopecia should not be regarded as evidence of hyperandrogenism.

Ovulatory dysfunction in PCOS is typically described as oligo-ovulation or anovulation, presenting clinically as a woman with irregular menstrual cycles. Overall, 95% of women with PCOS and oligo-ovulation have menstrual dysfunction, usually oligomenorrhea or amenorrhea.[4] The menstrual disturbances usually begin in the peripubertal years; however, menstrual cycles in women with PCOS become more regular because they approach menopause.[14] Obesity (defined as a body mass index [BMI] $\geq$30 kg/m^2) occurs in approximately 61% to 76% of women with PCOS.[4] Central or abdominal obesity is the typical pattern. Central obesity is a risk factor for the development of diabetes and heart disease and, when present in a woman with PCOS, worsens the clinical features (e.g., insulin resistance) of the syndrome.[4,15] Therefore, lifestyle modification with appropriate diet and exercise is a cornerstone of therapy for many women with PCOS.

Pathophysiology

The pathophysiology of PCOS is complex. The primary defect in PCOS is unknown, but at least three potential mechanisms, acting alone or synergistically, appear to create the characteristic clinical presentation. These mechanisms include inappropriate gonadotropin secretion, excessive androgen production, and insulin resistance with hyperinsulinemia. Figure 50-3 displays the closely integrated relationship between these mechanisms in the development of PCOS.

A genetic basis for PCOS has been postulated, but its mode of transmission is unclear.[7,16] Theories include an autosomal-dominant model and a polygenic model with genetic–environmental interactions. The complex presentation and various mechanisms make it impossible to target just one gene locus; in fact, more than 50 candidate genes have been proposed. A familial pattern to the development of PCOS may exist, because the incidence is higher in women with relatives with the disorder.

GONADOTROPIN SECRETION

In PCOS, there is an increased frequency of GnRH stimulation, leading to an increase in LH pulse frequency and amplitude, whereas FSH secretion remains normal. The development of a dominant follicle does not occur because LH secretion occurs too early in the menstrual cycle. Therefore, a woman is left with

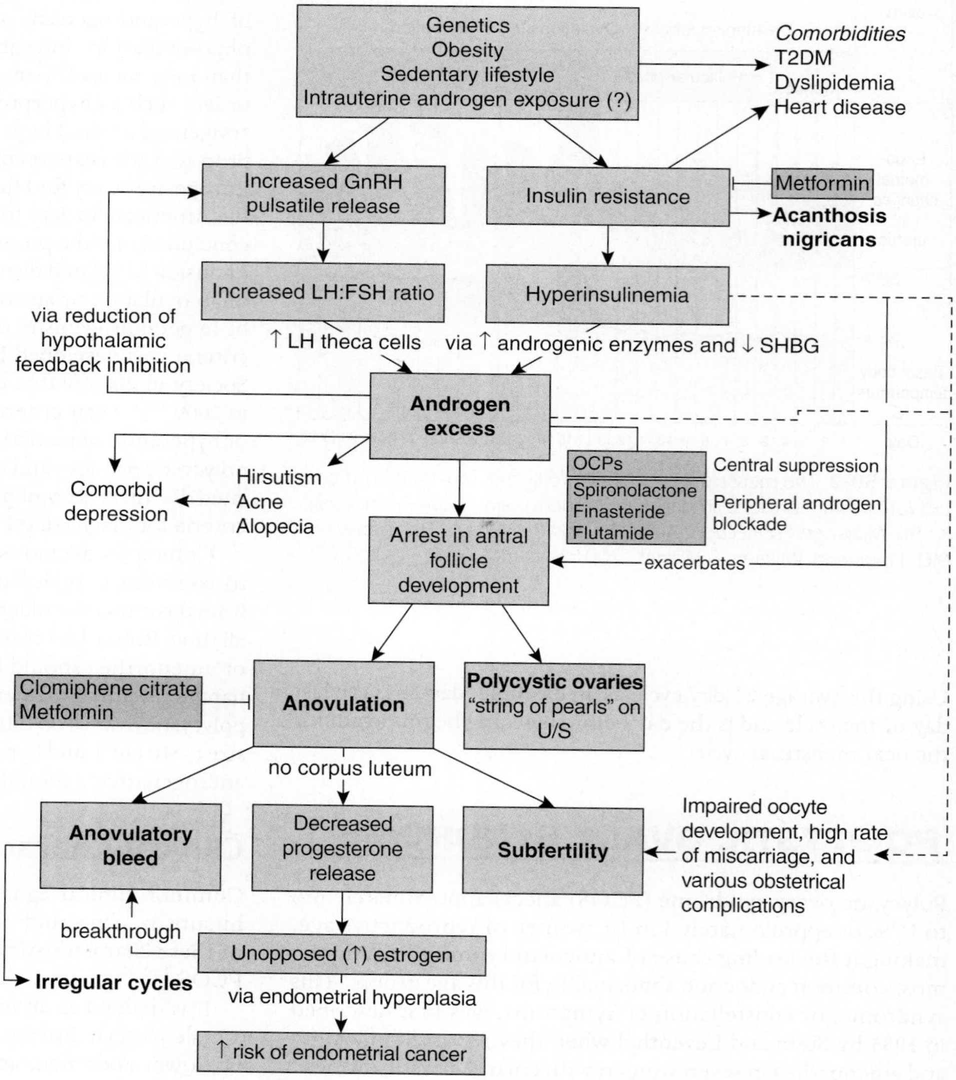

Figure 50-3 Pathophysiology of polycystic ovary syndrome (PCOS). (Redrawn from Wong E. McMaster pathophysiology review. http://www.pathophys.org/pcos/pcos-2/. Accessed March 24, 2016).

several immature follicles and usually will not ovulate. It is not clear whether the abnormal pulse frequency of GnRH is an intrinsic problem in the GnRH pulse generator in the hypothalamus or a result of relatively low progesterone concentrations from infrequent ovulation.[17] A woman with this abnormality does not enter the luteal phase of her menstrual cycle, leaving estrogen unopposed. Unopposed estrogen leads to endometrial hyperplasia and increases the risk for endometrial cancer. Increased LH stimulation also leads to increased steroidogenesis in the ovary, leading to excess androgen production. Amenorrheic women have high antimullerian hormone (AMH) serum concentrations and higher antral follicle counts compared with both oligomenorrheic women and regularly cycling patients with PCOS.[4] Additionally, concentrations of AMH tend to remain persistently elevated over time in women with PCOS.

EXCESS ANDROGEN PRODUCTION

Androgen production occurs in the theca cell of the ovary to facilitate follicular growth and estradiol synthesis in the granulosa cell. In women with PCOS, hypersecretion of LH and insulin increases the production of androgens, causing abnormal sex steroid synthesis, hyperandrogenism, and hyperandrogenemia. The dysregulation in steroid synthesis and metabolism is believed to result primarily from a dysfunction of the cytochrome P-450 (CYP) C17 enzyme in the ovaries, an enzyme with 17-hydroxylase and 17,20-lyase activities that are required to form androstenedione.[17,18] Androstenedione is then converted to testosterone or is aromatized by the aromatase enzyme to form estrone. Theca cells in women with PCOS are more efficient at the conversion to testosterone than normal theca cells.[19] Also, a similar steroid pathway occurs in the adrenal cortex and, when hyperandrogenism or hyperinsulinemic states exist, androgen production is further enhanced.

Elevated androgen levels are seen in approximately 60% to 80% of women with PCOS, mostly as increased free testosterone concentrations.[10,11] Assays for testosterone tend, however, to be highly variable and inaccurate, so measurement of androgen concentrations should be used only as an adjuvant test and never as the sole criterion for diagnosis. Clinical assessment is the primary tool for assessment of excess androgen.

INSULIN

Women with PCOS generally exhibit an increased risk of insulin resistance, yet the cellular and molecular mechanisms for insulin resistance are different from those seen with obesity and type 2 diabetes.[4] Insulin resistance is associated with reproductive and metabolic abnormalities in women with PCOS and can occur in both obese and nonobese women. There are several mechanisms by which this occurs. One proposed mechanism is a postbinding defect in insulin-receptor signaling.[20] Specifically, abnormal receptor autophosphorylation increases serine phosphorylation in targeted cells, which contributes to insulin resistance.[21,22] The insulin resistance in PCOS has been shown to be a selective, tissue-specific process where insulin sensitivity is increased in the ovarian androgenic pathway (causing hyperandrogenism), but insulin resistance is seen in other tissues involved with carbohydrate metabolism, specifically in the fat and muscle. Hyperinsulinemia results because of the compensatory increase in insulin secretion secondary to insulin resistance.

Insulin has both direct and indirect roles in PCOS. In the ovary, insulin acts alone or synergistically with LH to increase androgen production in theca cells. In the liver, insulin inhibits synthesis of sex hormone–binding globulin (SHBG), a key protein that binds to testosterone, and thus increases the free fraction of androgens available for biologic activity. Therefore, hyperinsulinemia is a major contributor to both hyperandrogenism and hyperandrogenemia in PCOS. Treatments targeted to improve insulin resistance in women with PCOS have shown improvements in ovulatory function, hirsutism, androgen levels, and metabolic profiles.[23,24] Indirectly, insulin may enhance the amplitude of LH pulses, further exacerbating the gonadotropin secretion defect in PCOS.[25]

CASE 50-1

Question 1: E.F. is a 27-year-old woman with mild hair growth above her upper lip, mild acne, and a history of irregular menstrual periods. Since age 12, she has had six to nine periods/year at intervals that vary from 30 to 90 days. When she does have a period, she considers them to be "normal" without pain or excessive bleeding. Her irregular periods were not bothersome until recently when she became sexually active and worries about becoming pregnant. She uses condoms for birth control. She reports no other medical conditions. E.F. is 5 feet 7 inches tall and weighs 180 lb (BMI 28.2 kg/m^2). Her vital signs today are blood pressure (BP) 118/84 mm Hg, heart rate (HR) 70 beats/minute, temperature 98.6°F, and respiratory rate (RR) 18 breaths/minute. Her physical examination is normal, with the exception of noted excessive facial hair and mild acne. She takes a multivitamin daily and acetaminophen as needed for headaches. She has no known medication allergies. What signs and symptoms does E.F. have that are consistent with PCOS?

E.F. exhibits several signs and symptoms that would indicate the presence of PCOS. According to the criteria of all organizations, her history of abnormal menstrual periods (oligomenorrhea) and clinical signs of hyperandrogenism, including hirsutism and acne, would indicate PCOS. Furthermore, her combination of hyperandrogenemia and oligomenorrhea signifies the highest metabolic risk among PCOS patients.[4] E.F. is overweight, which is common in women with PCOS but is not considered a criterion for diagnosis. Before a diagnosis of PCOS is made, laboratory testing to exclude other related causes of her symptoms would have to be performed. Studies may include prolactin, thyroid-stimulating hormone, testosterone, and 17-hydroxyprogester-one concentrations to rule out hyperprolactinemia, hypothyroidism, virilizing tumor, and congenital adrenal hyperplasia, respectively. PCOS is primarily diagnosed by clinical assessment; therefore, these tests assist only in confirming or excluding a diagnosis. To determine the presence of polycystic ovaries, defined as more than eight follicles per ovary that are less than 10 mm (usually 2–8 mm) in diameter, a transvaginal ultrasound should be performed.

Long-Term Complications

Case 50-1, Question 2: E.F has a mother with diabetes and hypertension and a father with diabetes, hypertension, and dyslipidemia. Her significant laboratory values include the following:

Fasting glucose, 102 mg/dL
Low-density lipoprotein (LDL), 150 mg/dL
High-density lipoprotein (HDL), 52 mg/dL
Triglycerides, 130 mg/dL
Total cholesterol, 228 mg/dL
What risk does E.F. have for experiencing long-term complications from PCOS?

E.F. has an increased risk for experiencing impaired glucose tolerance, diabetes, and metabolic syndrome, especially considering her family history. Furthermore, the diagnosis of PCOS places her at possible increased risk for sleep apnea and endometrial cancer.

IMPAIRED GLUCOSE TOLERANCE AND DIABETES

Studies have shown that women with PCOS have a higher prevalence of impaired glucose tolerance, gestational diabetes,

diabetes, and insulin resistance compared with women without the syndrome.[4,26,27] A family history increases the risk of these conditions further. In a study of 254 women with PCOS, 38.6% were found to have either impaired glucose tolerance (IGT) or undiagnosed diabetes.[28] Compared with those without PCOS, the prevalence of IGT and diabetes was significantly higher in both obese and nonobese (BMI <27 kg/m^2) women. Waist–hip ratio and BMI appeared to be the most clinically important predictors of glucose intolerance. Women with PCOS who have IGT appear to exhibit type 2 diabetes at higher rates than the general population.[26,27] Therefore, screening and diagnosis of these conditions is important for women with PCOS. E.F. is overweight, and her mildly elevated fasting glucose and overweight suggest that she may be at increased risk for impaired glucose tolerance.

Glucose tolerance should be assessed in all women with PCOS using a fasting and 2-hour oral (75 g) glucose tolerance test.[4,26,29] Routine screening for diabetes with an oral glucose tolerance test should be performed for all women with PCOS by the age of 30 years.[30] The American Diabetes Association or World Health Organization criteria should be used for the appropriate diagnosis of IGT or diabetes. Insulin concentrations are typically not obtained in clinical settings because they are inaccurate.

METABOLIC SYNDROME AND CARDIOVASCULAR RISK

Approximately one-third to one-half of women with PCOS have metabolic syndrome. Using the National Cholesterol Education Panel-Adult Treatment Panel III criteria,[31–34] metabolic syndrome is present when the patient exhibits any three of these symptoms: abdominal obesity (>40 inches in men and >35 inches in women), triglycerides greater than or equal to 150 mg/dL, low HDL cholesterol (<40 mg/dL in men and <50 mg/dL in women), blood pressure greater than or equal to 130/85 mm Hg, and fasting glucose greater than or equal to 110 mg/dL. The incidence of a metabolic syndrome in women with PCOS is significantly higher than the rate for the general US population (45% vs. 6%, ages 20–29 years; 53% vs. 14%, ages 30–39 years) and independent of body weight.[34] It is believed that insulin resistance and hyperandrogenism are contributing factors to metabolic syndrome in women with PCOS.[35] Insulin resistance in the metabolic syndrome has been associated with a twofold increased risk of cardiovascular disease and a fivefold increased risk of type 2 diabetes.[36] Low HDL cholesterol (HDL-C) is seen most frequently in women with PCOS (68%), followed by increased BMI and waist circumference (67%), high blood pressure (45%), hypertriglyceridemia (35%), and elevated fasting glucose (4%).[32] Another group found that elevated fasting insulin concentrations, obesity, and a family history of diabetes conferred higher risk of having the metabolic syndrome in women with PCOS.[33]

Compared with women without PCOS, women with PCOS are reported to have a higher prevalence of cardiovascular risk factors, including hypertension, dyslipidemia, and surrogate markers for early atherosclerosis (e.g., increased C-reactive protein concentrations).[35] With increasing age, and especially as women with PCOS become postmenopausal, the risk of hypertension increases twofold.[37] Dyslipidemia in women with PCOS typically presents as decreased HDL-C (which is a strong predictor of cardiovascular disease in women), elevated triglycerides, elevated LDL cholesterol (LDL-C), and higher LDL–HDL ratios.[38] Women with PCOS are noted to have more atherogenic, small, dense LDL-C compared with controls, and this substantially increases cardiovascular risk.[39] Altered cholesterol levels are more severe in women with hyperandrogenism.[4] Women with PCOS may have other surrogate markers for early atherosclerosis and cardiovascular disease, impaired endothelial dysfunction, and other markers of cardiovascular risk such as coronary artery calcifications and increased carotid intima-media thickness.[35] Women with PCOS are considered to be at risk when any of these risk factors are present: obesity, cigarette smoking, hypertension, dyslipidemia, subclinical vascular disease, IGT, or family history of premature cardiovascular disease.[40] Non-HDL and waist measurement are the best predictors of CVD risk.[4] They are considered to be high risk when they have metabolic syndrome, type 2 diabetes mellitus, or overt vascular or renal disease. Although cardiovascular risk exists, data are inconclusive about whether women with PCOS have increased rates of morbidity and mortality from cardiovascular disease.

OBSTRUCTIVE SLEEP APNEA

Obstructive sleep apnea is cessation of breathing that occurs during sleep. It can disrupt sleep and cause daytime fatigue. Patients may not be aware that they are having the symptoms of sleep apnea, which include snoring and a gasping or snorting when breathing resumes. Studies indicate that the prevalence of obstructive sleep apnea in the PCOS is higher than expected and cannot be explained by obesity alone.[41–43] Insulin resistance appears to be a strong predictor of sleep apnea—more so than age, BMI, or the circulating testosterone concentration.[43] This can be treated with continuous positive airway pressure (CPAP) and may help metabolic dysfunction.[7]

ENDOMETRIAL HYPERPLASIA AND CANCER

Chronic anovulation in women with PCOS results in an endometrium that is exposed to the prolonged effects of estrogen unopposed by progesterone. Therefore, PCOS is a risk factor for endometrial hyperplasia. Women with PCOS have a 2.7-fold (95% CI 1.0–7.3) increased risk for endometrial cancer.[4] It is considered prudent management to induce artificial withdrawal bleeding by administering a course of progestin at least every 3 months to prevent endometrial hyperplasia in women with PCOS who experience either amenorrhea or oligomenorrhea. Alternatively, ultrasound scans can also be used to measure endometrial thickness and morphology every 6 to 12 months.

Treatment Goals

CASE 50-1, QUESTION 3: E.F. worries about becoming pregnant when she does not have regular periods. She also has mild hair growth above her upper lip which is somewhat bothersome. Given these concerns, what are the treatment goals for E.F.?

The primary goals for E.F. are to prevent pregnancy and address her hirsutism. Additionally, treatment goals for E.F. would include maintaining a normal endometrium, blocking the actions of androgens at target tissues, reducing insulin resistance and hyperinsulinemia, reducing weight, and preventing long-term complications. Other goals of treatment in patients with PCOS may include correcting anovulation or oligo-ovulation and improve fertility.

Therapy goals should encompass both long-term and short-term objectives because response to nonpharmacologic and pharmacologic therapy is slow, often requiring 3 to 9 months. Addressing long-term goals can minimize the risk for future complications, and specifying short-term goals can improve motivation and adherence to therapy.

NONPHARMACOLOGIC TREATMENT

CASE 50-1, QUESTION 4: E.F. has indicated that she would like to lose weight. E.F. does not smoke, drinks one to two beers on weekends, and exercises by walking 20 minutes twice weekly. What nonpharmacologic method(s) would be most effective?

Weight reduction programs designed for a modest weight loss (5%–10%) with the incorporation of fitness are effective in reducing metabolic disease, cardiovascular risk, and improving ovulatory potential.[40] A 5% to 10% weight loss in E.F. would be 9 to 18 lb. Diet modification and exercise are the most efficient, cost-effective, and safe ways to produce weight loss and improve the endocrine and metabolic parameters of PCOS.[40,44] Weight reduction should be considered first-line therapy in all overweight or obese women with PCOS, and this should be recommended for E.F.

IMPACT OF WEIGHT LOSS IN POLYCYSTIC OVARY SYNDROME

A minimum 5% weight loss has consistently demonstrated restoration of regular menstrual cycling and ovulation in overweight and obese women with PCOS.[15,45,46] When lifestyle modification is implemented, free testosterone concentrations decrease, but clinical outcomes of acne and hirsutism are not often reported.[15] Obesity in PCOS is associated with a higher risk of developing endometrial cancer, but very limited evidence exists to determine the impact of weight loss on the incidence of endometrial cancer.[15] Studies of weight loss in women without PCOS indicate a 25% to 50% reduced risk of endometrial cancer, so it is logical that addressing weight reduction may lower that risk as well.[47,48] The Diabetes Prevention Program trial demonstrated a 53% prevalence of metabolic syndrome; the incidence of this was reduced 41% in the lifestyle modification group.[49,50] This was significantly better than treatment with metformin. Studies specifically evaluating cardiovascular improvements with weight loss in women with PCOS are limited, but improvements in dyslipidemia and insulin sensitivity have been noted.

DIET COMPOSITION

No single diet has been proven to be ideal for women with PCOS. A diet low in saturated fat and high in fiber from mostly low-glycemic-index carbohydrate foods may, however, be suitable and is recommended.[15,51] Glycemic index is a classification of carbohydrates based on the blood glucose response during 2 hours. Low-glycemic index foods include bran cereals, mixed grain breads, broccoli, peppers, lentils, and soy. High-glycemic index foods, or those that should be minimized, include white rice and bread, potatoes, chips, and foods containing simple sugars (e.g., juice). It has been shown that in women with PCOS, oral glucose intake causes larger fluctuations in plasma glucose, increased hyperinsulinemia, and stimulated adrenal steroid secretion; protein was found to be a preferred nutrient over glucose.[52] The composition of a diet should be individualized to promote adherence and achieve specific goals.

EXERCISE

Exercise is a key component in the attainment and maintenance of weight loss. Exercise with muscle strengthening improves insulin sensitivity.[15] The American Heart Association recommends 150 minutes/week of moderate exercise or 75 minutes/week of vigorous exercise.[53] E.F. should continue to eat a healthy diet. A diet consisting of low saturated fats, high fiber, and foods with a low glycemic index should be encouraged. E.F. should increase her exercise to at least 75 minutes/week for at least 3 days of the week. If she is going to continue walking as her exercise, she should walk at a brisk pace. Titrating her time to a goal of exercising 60 minutes daily will help her lose weight.

Pharmacologic Treatment

CASE 50-1, QUESTION 5: E.F. would like to improve her menstrual irregularity, and be sure that she will not get pregnant. If possible, she would also like to minimize her hirsutism and acne. What options would be appropriate to recommend for E.F.?

Several different pharmacologic options could be recommended to E.F (Table 50-1). A combined oral contraceptive (COC) will address her concerns about irregular menstruation, hyperandrogenism, and pregnancy prevention. An insulin sensitizer would improve her menstrual irregularity and possibly reduce her hirsutism and acne, but it does not address her desire to prevent pregnancy. An antiandrogen, such as spironolactone, would address only hyperandrogenism, and other agents would have to be used concurrently to address pregnancy prevention and other hormonal and metabolic alterations in PCOS.

COMBINED ORAL CONTRACEPTIVES

Estrogen–progestin combination therapy with a COC is the treatment of choice for women seeking regularity in menstrual cycles and relief from hyperandrogenic symptoms (see Chapter 47, Contraception, for a list of possible therapies). The estrogen component suppresses LH, resulting in a reduction of androgen production, and increases hepatic production of SHBG, thereby reducing free testosterone. The progestins in various COCs possess variable androgenic effects, so the choice of the COC may be considered to minimize androgenic exposure. The potential effects of COCs on insulin resistance, glucose tolerance, and lipids have been debated, do not appear to increase metabolic risk, and should be considered when choosing a progestin component.[4,54–56] Caution should be used in those who have insulin resistance, a high propensity to develop type 2 diabetes, or abnormal lipid profiles.

Combined oral contraceptive therapy in PCOS should be initiated with a formulation that contains a low dose or very low dose of estrogen (≤35 mcg of ethinyl estradiol) and a progestin with low androgenic or antiandrogen properties. Most COCs manufactured today have low or very low estrogen doses. Desogestrel and norgestimate are progestins with low androgen potential, and drospirenone is an antiandrogen. A COC containing ethinyl estradiol and desogestrel would prevent pregnancy, improve menstrual cycle regularity, and reduce E.F.'s signs of hyperandrogenism (hirsutism and acne). If E.F. desired monthly cycles, she could take the typical 21/7 regimen (21 days active pill, 7 days inactive pill) or a 24/4 regimen (24 days active pill, 4 days inactive pill). Although not specifically evaluated in women with PCOS, a monophasic regimen may also be prescribed using extended cycles of 84 or even 365 days. Extended regimens reduce the number of cycles/year while providing contraception. Regardless of the COC selected, one of the long-term benefits is that her risk for endometrial cancer would be reduced by 50%, even up to two decades after discontinuation.[57–59] Ideal initial contraceptive options for E.F. include 30 to 35 mcg of ethinyl estradiol and a low-androgenic or nonandrogenic progestin such as drospirenone or desogestrel. If she would like to have her menstrual cycle monthly, she should take 21 active pills followed by 7 inactive pills. If she does not desire to have her menstrual cycle, then taking continuous active pills in an extended (daily) manner is most appropriate. This therapy would address her concerns of menstrual irregularity, contraception, hirsutism, and acne. She should continue therapy for as long as she desires contraception and minimization of the androgenic effects of PCOS.

CASE 50-1, QUESTION 6: Two months later, E.F. reports she is experiencing mood swings and weight gain on her ethinyl estradiol/desogestrel oral contraceptive. She is debating whether she wants to continue with the COC and would like to explore other treatment possibilities. What other therapy options may be beneficial for E.F. if she considers this COC to be intolerable?

Table 50-1
Selected Treatment Options for Polycystic Ovary Syndrome (PCOS)

Drug Class (Example)	Purpose of Therapy	Mechanism of Action	Effective Dose	Side Effects
Combined oral contraceptive (estrogen and progestin)	Menstrual cyclicity, hirsutism, acne	Suppresses LH (and FSH) and thus ovarian androgen production; increases sex hormone–binding globulin, which decreases free testosterone	One tablet orally daily for 21 (or 24) days, then 7-day (or 4-day) pill-free interval	Breast tenderness, breakthrough bleeding, mood swings, libido changes
Progestins (medroxyprogesterone)	Menstrual cyclicity	Creates withdrawal bleeding by transforming proliferative endometrium into secretory endometrium	5–10 mg orally daily for 10–14 days every 1–2 months	Breakthrough bleeding, spotting, mood swings
Biguanide (metformin)	Impaired glucose tolerance, type 2 diabetes	Decreases hepatic glucose production, secondarily reducing insulin levels; may have direct effects on steroidogenesis	1,500 mg orally daily in divided doses (up to 2,550 mg/day)	Gastrointestinal problems, diarrhea, abdominal pain
Antiandrogen (spironolactone)	Hirsutism, acne	Inhibits androgens from binding to androgen receptor	50–100 mg orally twice daily	Hyperkalemia, polymenorrhea, headache, fatigue
Antiestrogen (clomiphene citrate)	Ovulation induction	Increases GnRH secretion, which induces rise in FSH and LH	50 mg orally daily for 5 days; may increase to 150 mg	Vasomotor symptoms, gastrointestinal problems
Aromatase inhibitor (letrozole)	Ovulation induction	Blocks estrogen synthesis to directly affect hypothalamic–pituitary–ovarian function	2.5 mg orally daily for 5 days; may increase to 7.5 mg	

FSH, follicle-stimulating hormone; GnRH, gonadotropin-releasing hormone; LH, luteinizing hormone.

Metformin

Metformin inhibits hepatic glucose output, providing lower insulin concentrations and reducing androgen production in the ovary. Metformin also appears to influence ovarian steroidogenesis directly.[60,61] Metformin is primarily used for IGT or T2D related to PCOS. Metformin has minimal effectiveness for hirsutism or acne and was found to have no benefit improving rate of miscarriage, fertility, or live-birth rates in anovulatory women with PCOS.[4,62–63] Its routine use for treatment of infertility is not recommended.[4] In a Cochrane systematic review comparing COCs and metformin, metformin demonstrated a reduction in fasting insulin and triglyceride levels compared to oral contraceptives, but greater improvement in menstrual pattern and serum androgen levels was observed with COCs.[56]

The most commonly used and most effective dose of metformin in PCOS is 500 mg orally 3 times daily (TID). It should be titrated slowly to this effective dose; doses up to 2,000 mg daily or 2,550 mg daily may be necessary for individual circumstances. The gastrointestinal (GI) side effects of diarrhea, nausea, vomiting, and abdominal bloating are usually transient and dose-related, and can be minimized by taking with food instead. An estimated glomerular filtration rate (eGFR) should be calculated at least annually in women using metformin because it is contraindicated if eGFR is <30 ml/min/1.73 m^2 and not recommended if eGFR is 30–45 ml/min/1.73 m^2.

AGENTS FOR HIRSUTISM

Although frequently used, antiandrogens do not have FDA-approved uses for the treatment of female hirsutism or acne in the United States. Spironolactone is commonly prescribed to women for hirsutism. Drospirenone (a derivative of spironolactone), found in COCs has antiandrogenic properties and has also been evaluated in the long-term treatment of hirsutism.[64] Finasteride has been used for female hirsutism, but its lack of specificity for type I 5α-reductase in the pilosebaceous unit and toxicity may make this a suboptimal treatment choice. Flutamide is effective for hirsutism, but it is not used because of hepatotoxicity. Eflornithine hydrochloride has been approved for topical use in treating facial hirsutism, but has not been well studied in women with PCOS. Electrolysis and laser treatments may be acceptable physical approaches to hair removal for women with PCOS.

Spironolactone

Spironolactone acts by competitively inhibiting dihydrotestosterone (DHT) from interacting with its androgen receptor. This causes a decrease in activity of ovarian-produced testosterone. Spironolactone reduces hair growth by 40% to 88%; however, it takes 6 to 9 months for improvement.[65] Spironolactone may be associated with possible teratogenicity (feminization of the male fetus), so it is prudent to advise women to avoid pregnancy for at least 4 months after the discontinuation of spironolactone. It is recommended that spironolactone be used with a COC to avoid teratogenicity, as well as the side effect of polymenorrhea (more frequent menses) when used as monotherapy. Spironolactone in combination with a COC would also improve hormonal and metabolic manifestations of PCOS as well. The usual effective spironolactone dose is 50 to 100 mg orally twice daily for 6 to 12 months. Serum potassium and renal function should be monitored because this aldosterone antagonist can cause hyperkalemia. Furthermore, spironolactone should not be used with a COC containing drospirenone because of a potential risk for hyperkalemia.

Finasteride

Finasteride is a type II 5α-reductase inhibitor, which decreases the conversion of testosterone to DHT. It provides an approximate

30% reduction from baseline for hirsutism. Compared with spironolactone, finasteride is as or less effective in women with hirsutism.[66] The dose of 5 to 7.5 mg orally daily typically takes 6 months for clinical improvement. It is critical to avoid pregnancy while taking this drug owing to the potential teratogenic effect of abnormal genitalia in the male fetus. Finasteride should not be touched or handled by women who are or may be pregnant. This danger limits the usefulness of finasteride in women with PCOS because most are of childbearing age or desire pregnancy.

E.F. should be encouraged to continue her COC for at least 3 months as most COC side effects resolve within 3 months of use. If E.F. decides that the side effects from the COC are intolerable, an appropriate recommendation for E.F. would be spironolactone 50 mg orally daily. She should continue this therapy for as long as she desires the benefits of this therapy, but it will not provide contraception. E.F. should ensure proper contraception is used while taking spironolactone to avoid teratogenicity.

CASE 50-1, QUESTION 7: E.F. successfully used oral contraceptives for 7 years. After getting married 3 years ago, E.F. and her husband have decided to have children. She lost 30 lb with diet and exercise when she got married and has been able to maintain that weight loss. They have been trying to get pregnant for the last 18 months. The reason for infertility has been identified as oligo-ovulation associated with PCOS. What treatments for ovulation induction should be used in E.F. and why?

Anovulation or oligo-ovulation in women with PCOS is usually first treated with diet, exercise, and weight reduction. Weight loss improves pregnancy rates and reduces miscarriage rates in women with PCOS. E.F. has been successful at losing weight and now must consider agents for ovulation induction.

AGENTS FOR OVULATION INDUCTION

Clomiphene Citrate

Clomiphene citrate induces ovulation via an antiestrogenic effect on the hypothalamus. GnRH secretion is increased, which increases LH and FSH production. The increase in FSH concentrations causes appropriate follicle development and estrogen secretion, which produces a positive feedback on the hypothalamic–pituitary system to create a LH surge for ovulation.

The usual initial dose of clomiphene citrate is 50 mg orally daily for 5 days, started on day 5 after a spontaneous or progestin-induced menses. The clinician must determine whether ovulation occurs with each cycle through laboratory testing, ultrasound monitoring, or both. If ovulation does not occur, the dose can be increased by 50 mg orally daily up to 150 mg orally daily; however, doses greater than 100 mg orally daily for 5 days are not recommended by the manufacturers.[67] A repeat cycle can be administered as early as 30 days after the previous cycle as long as pregnancy has not occurred. If conception does not occur, women can use clomiphene for three to four cycles before considering another regimen. Long-term cyclic therapy is not recommended beyond a total of six cycles because of potential ovarian cancer risk. Most women respond to clomiphene citrate within three to four ovulatory cycles, but 5% to 10% have demonstrated clomiphene resistance and need to consider other options.[67] For women who are clomiphene citrate-resistant, dexamethasone can be used in conjunction with clomiphene or an aromatase inhibitor can be used (e.g., letrozole, anastrozole) as an alternative for infertility in PCOS.[68–71]

Aromatase Inhibitors

Letrozole is an aromatase inhibitor which blocks estrogen synthesis to directly affect hypothalamic–pituitary—ovarian function and increase pregnancy rates. Potential advantages of letrozole over clomiphene citrate include more physiologic hormonal stimulation of the endometrium, a lower multiple-pregnancy rate through single-follicle recruitment, a better side-effect profile with fewer vasomotor and mood symptoms, and more rapid clearance which reduces the chances of periconceptional exposure.[72] In a study of 750 women with PCOS, letrozole or clomiphene was provided for up to five cycles whereas ovulation and pregnancy were evaluated.[73] Women receiving letrozole had more live births compared with those that received clomiphene (27.5% vs. 19.1%; $p = 0.007$) without significant differences in congenital anomalies. The ovulation rate was also higher with letrozole than clomiphene (61.7% vs. 48.3%; $p < 0.001$). Letrozole had a higher incidence of fatigue and dizziness, and clomiphene had a higher incidence of hot flushes. Based on this information and its potential advantages over clomiphene, letrozole may become a first-line agent for ovulation induction in women with PCOS.

Other Agents

If the clomiphene or letrozole is not successful, dexamethasone 0.25 mg at bedtime can be used in combination with clomiphene.[74] Ovarian drilling is the next alternative, followed by administration of gonadotropins or in vitro fertilization. Ovarian drilling is a laproscopic procedure by which a small portion of the ovary is removed via electric current to reduce hyperandrogenemia and improve ovulation. Its effects may only last a few months, and it will not help with clinical signs of hyperandrogenism (e.g., hirsutism, acne). Gonadotropins are effective, but are generally reserved as one of the last options because of ovarian hyperstimulation syndrome. Egg retrieval and in vitro fertilization may be used in conjunction with gonadotropins to increase pregnancy rate and minimize the likelihood of multiple pregnancies by limiting the number of transferred embryos.[67]

Women with PCOS exhibit unique clinical features and have individual concerns that should be addressed when making treatment recommendations. Assessment should include gathering relevant medical information, such as menstrual history, signs and symptoms of hyperandrogenism, time course of symptoms, weight history, previous agents tried, and family history. If PCOS is suspected, laboratory assessments should be performed to rule out any other related disorders. Once a diagnosis has been made, a recommendation about treatment must consider the patient's priorities and motivation. For E.F., letrozole would likely be the pharmacologic agent of choice. Ovulation induction and live birth occur in approximately 48% and 27% of women with PCOS, respectively, using letrozole. The initial dose would be 2.5 mg orally once daily for 5 days, started on day 3 after a spontaneous or progestin-induced menses. If nonresponse occurs, the dose may be increased by 2.5 mg and up to 7.5 mg daily for 5 days on following cycles. Although side effects (e.g., fatigue, dizziness) can occur, the benefit of this therapy outweighs the risk for E.F. Appropriate follow-up for E.F. should include quality-of-life measures, laboratory monitoring when necessary, and medication adherence monitoring. Providers should be educators, facilitators, and empathetic listeners to help women with PCOS become informed and actively engaged in their therapy plan.

DYSMENORRHEA

Dysmenorrhea, or painful cramping that occurs with the onset and first days of menstruation, can be categorized as either primary (without underlying uterine pathology) or secondary (owing to underlying uterine pathology). Secondary dysmenorrhea can result from uterine conditions, including endometriosis, uterine polyps, or fibroids; complications of intrauterine device (IUD) use; or pelvic inflammatory disease.

Up to 93% of adolescents report some pain with menstruation, and up to 15% experience pain that is sufficiently severe and disabling to interfere with activities of daily life.[75] Dysmenorrhea is the single largest cause of lost productivity and school absence among adolescent girls. It most commonly begins within 1 to 2 years after the onset of menses, and up to 91% of adult women report some pain with menses, of which up to 28% experience severe pain and/or limitation of activity.[76]

Clinical Characteristics

CASE 50-2

QUESTION 1: A.B., a 17-year-old girl, presents at the pharmacy with complaints of severe cramping pain associated with her menstrual cycles. The pain predictably begins with the onset of menses and has been occurring for the past 5 years, but is now limiting A.B.'s ability to play sports in high school. A.B. states that she experienced her first menstrual period at age 11. The pain usually is "like a fist, clenching and relaxing," starts in the pelvic area, and radiates to her lower back. She reports no headache, but usually has diarrhea and some nausea, without vomiting. Her symptoms are most severe during the first 12 to 24 hours of her menses, then subside during the next few days. She usually takes two acetaminophen 325-mg tablets when her pain begins and then one tablet every 4 to 6 hours, as needed, with little relief. She has taken no other medications for her symptoms, has no known allergies to medications, and is not taking any other medications. She has no other medical problems. Her social history is significant for occasional social use of less than 10 cigarettes and two to three alcoholic beverages/weekend. A recent physical examination was within normal limits. What clinical manifestations in A.B. are consistent with primary dysmenorrhea?

No specific diagnostic criteria exist for primary dysmenorrhea. Typically, the diagnosis is one of exclusion and is based on response to known effective therapy. Thus, if patients do not respond to therapy, an investigation of pelvic pathology and secondary dysmenorrhea should occur.[77,78] A.B.'s symptoms that are typical of primary dysmenorrhea include cramping pain in the suprapubic area, which may radiate into the back and thighs, nausea, and diarrhea. Some women also experience vomiting, fatigue, headache, lightheadedness, flushing, loss of appetite, irritability, nervousness, and insomnia.[77] Symptom severity seems to correlate with women who have early menarche (onset of menses before age 8) and those with increased duration and quantity of menstrual flow.[79] Risk factors for dysmenorrhea include age younger than 20 years, depression or anxiety, perceived high life or work stress, nulliparity, menorrhagia, and smoking.[76,80]

Primary dysmenorrhea occurs only with ovulatory cycles, which typically begin after the first year following menarche. Dysmenorrhea occurring several years after menarche is most likely secondary dysmenorrhea and should be investigated as such. Because A.B.'s pain began within 1 year of menarche and her physical examination is normal, a trial of therapy can be initiated without further investigation into secondary causes of dysmenorrhea. The typical pattern of dysmenorrhea is to have pain beginning up to 12 hours before menses, increasing in severity for up to 24 hours, and continuing with reduced intensity for 24 to 72 hours.[77] A.B.'s description of pain, as a cramping–relaxing cycle, is typical for dysmenorrhea. Likely, her symptoms will decrease with age, after the onset of sexual activity, as well as after childbirth.[79]

Pathophysiology

CASE 50-2, QUESTION 2: What underlying pathophysiology explains A.B.'s symptoms?

In the normal menstrual cycle, prostaglandins are released by the endometrium in the late luteal phase inducing contraction of the uterine smooth muscle and subsequent sloughing of the endometrium, leading to menstrual flow and the beginning of the follicular phase of the next cycle. Women with primary dysmenorrhea appear to have increased prostaglandin secretion, inducing more intense uterine contractions, leading to decreased uterine blood flow and uterine hypoxia, which results in the cramping and pain that are the hallmarks of dysmenorrhea.[78] The decreasing levels of progesterone in the late luteal phase trigger the release of arachidonic acid from cell membranes, ultimately resulting in the production of prostaglandins and leukotrienes.[78]

The importance of prostaglandin secretion in the pathology of primary dysmenorrhea is confirmed by studies of the exogenous administration of prostaglandin $F_{2\alpha}$ ($PGF_{2\alpha}$), and PGE_2, each of which produce pain and uterine contractions similar to those observed in women with primary dysmenorrhea.[81] These prostaglandins, with potent platelet disaggregation and vasodilatory properties, also induce nausea, vomiting, and diarrhea. Thus, A.B.'s pain, nausea, and diarrhea may be caused by elevated prostaglandin levels. This also explains the rationale for the effectiveness of the two main treatments for primary dysmenorrhea: nonsteroidal anti-inflammatory drugs (NSAIDs), which inhibit prostaglandin synthesis, and hormonal contraceptives, which minimize the progesterone increase typically seen in the luteal phase.

Nearly 85% to 90% of women initially thought to have primary dysmenorrhea respond to NSAIDs with or without oral contraceptive therapy. The remaining women deserve further investigation into potential causes of secondary dysmenorrhea.[82]

Treatment

NONPHARMACOLOGIC TREATMENT

CASE 50-2, QUESTION 3: What nonpharmacologic therapies may be effective for the treatment of A.B.'s symptoms of primary dysmenorrhea?

A.B. should be educated about the causes of primary dysmenorrhea, its associated symptoms, and the rationale behind nonpharmacologic and pharmacologic treatment options. Nonpharmacologic therapies that may have benefit in the relief of A.B.'s symptoms include aerobic exercise, heat therapy, tobacco cessation, omega-3 polyunsaturated fatty acids, and high frequency transcutaneous electrical nerve stimulation.

Exercise, particularly aerobic exercise, has been correlated with decreased menstrual symptoms in observational studies and is, in all patients, associated with positive general health benefits.[83] In addition, specifically yoga exercise, in particular the cobra, cat, and fish poses performed for 20 minutes/day during the luteal phase, was found to reduce pain in adolescent women.[84] The benefit may be due to improved pelvic blood flow and decreased ischemia, or increased release of β-endorphins. Application of local heat to the lower abdomen has been studied in three well-designed clinical trials.[85–87] Heat plus ibuprofen (400 mg orally TID) demonstrated a reduction in the time to pain relief compared with an unheated patch plus ibuprofen in two controlled studies.[85,87] Heat provided better relief than acetaminophen (1,000 mg orally as a single dose).[85] With few adverse effects, heat, in the form of a heating pad or heated patch or wrap device; and exercise (aerobic or yoga) represent reasonable and safe suggestions for women with dysmenorrhea.

Women should be advised and assisted in efforts to stop tobacco use. Although no direct evidence links smoking cessation with improvement in dysmenorrhea, an association exists with increased risk and severity of dysmenorrhea in women who smoke.[79] Increased intake of omega-3 polyunsaturated fatty acids, a low-fat vegetarian diet, or both may decrease the intensity and duration of symptoms.[88,89]

A.B.'s therapy should be based on her specific symptoms, response to previous therapy, and any adverse effects of therapy. The regimen of acetaminophen that A.B. is currently using is not providing relief owing to its relative lack of effect on prostaglandin activity. For A.B., discussion of the nonpharmacologic therapies, particularly continuous low-level heat applied at onset of symptoms, exercise/yoga, and smoking cessation, provides low-risk, potentially beneficial, and low-cost suggestions for pain relief, in addition to drug therapy. A.B should be informed that continuous heat therapy via heat "wraps" or hot water bottle or heating pad should be used cautiously in patients with diabetes and should not be used while sleeping.

CASE 50-2, QUESTION 4: A.B states that her pain is decreased about 50% with the use of a heating pad, but she would rather not be sedentary for hours at a time. She finds the heat wraps uncomfortable and expensive and asks about Pamprin. What are some over-the-counter pharmacologic options for A.B.?

Although nonpharmacologic therapy with heat, exercise, and smoking cessation may have benefit, often the use of pharmacologic therapies is required to significantly improve functionality.

OVER-THE-COUNTER PHARMACOLOGIC THERAPY

Over-the-counter (OTC) pharmacologic therapy for primary dysmenorrhea is focused on reducing prostaglandin activity. Anti-inflammatory drugs act by directly inhibiting prostaglandin synthesis. NSAIDs provide relief from the symptoms of primary dysmenorrhea for most women (See Case 50-2, Question 5, for further information). Naproxen (as the sodium salt) and ibuprofen are approved without a prescription for the treatment of primary dysmenorrhea. Acetaminophen is of limited efficacy in the treatment of dysmenorrhea when compared with NSAIDs or hormonal contraception.[90]

Other therapies, including OTC products marketed for dysmenorrhea and other menstrual disorders (e.g., Pamprin, Midol) (particularly combination products including diuretics), weak muscle relaxants (such as pyrilamine, pamabrom), diuretics (caffeine), and acetaminophen, have limited efficacy for the specific treatment of dysmenorrhea. Because they do not address the underlying pathophysiology of primary dysmenorrhea, combination products, narcotic analgesics, and acetaminophen do not have a role in the treatment of primary dysmenorrhea and may have excessive adverse effects with minimal benefit.

Adolescents with dysmenorrhea frequently use OTC medications to treat primary dysmenorrhea, usually without consultation from a healthcare professional. This lack of professional advice results in the use of lower doses that may not be as effective to treat symptoms. Many women choose ineffective combination medications and/or acetaminophen, indicating patients will benefit from professional advice regarding OTC treatments of dysmenorrhea. Other products include vitamin B_1, vitamin D, magnesium, vitamin B_6, and omega-3 fatty acids, which have all shown some benefit in pain relief compared with placebo, with vitamin D, vitamin B_1, and magnesium showing the most promise.[89,91] Other dietary supplements, including fennel, vitamin E, Neptune Krill Oil, and Toki-shakuyaju-san, have been evaluated in small trials and need further study.[82] At this point, given the limited efficacy of non-NSAID, nonhormonal methods of treatment, they are not an appropriate alternative for A.B. Ibuprofen 200 to 400 mg orally up to TID could be a solid initial plan for A.B.'s menstrual cramps.

Prescription Pharmacologic Agents: Nonsteroidal Anti-inflammatory Drugs

CASE 50-2, QUESTION 5: A.B has tried OTC ibuprofen 400 mg TID starting at onset of her cramping symptoms, but has not had optimal relief. A.B. presents to her family physician for an evaluation. What prescription medications could be recommended for A.B's dysmenorrhea?

The NSAIDs are effective for treatment of dysmenorrhea, but in some cases, OTC doses are not enough and prescription-strength NSAIDs or hormonal contraceptives may be required for adequate relief. Hormonal contraceptives reduce the amount of endometrial proliferation and, as a result, decrease the amount of prostaglandins secreted. By inhibiting ovulation, hormonal contraceptives eliminate the cyclic changes in progesterone that induce prostaglandin release. Choice of therapy depends on the need for contraception, concomitant medical conditions, and patient preference. Treatment efficacy can be monitored by evaluating pain relief, improved functionality, reduced absenteeism, and relief of other symptoms (e.g., diarrhea, nausea) associated with dysmenorrhea. Because A.B. is not sexually active, prescription-strength NSAIDs should be tried for two to three cycles before switching to other agents.

Initial selection of NSAID therapy should be based on effectiveness, incidence of adverse effects, cost, patient history of previous benefit, and availability. In a Cochrane review, 73 trials of NSAIDs for treatment of primary dysmenorrhea were reviewed to assess for any differences in efficacy or safety among the different NSAIDs.[92] When compared with placebo, NSAIDs were significantly more effective (odds ratio [OR], 4.50; 95% confidence interval [CI], 3.85–5.27). When compared with acetaminophen, NSAIDs were, as expected, significantly better at reducing symptoms (OR, 1.90; 95% CI, 1.05–3.44). In limited head-to-head trials comparing NSAIDs, no significant differences in efficacy were seen, with the exception of aspirin being slightly less effective than other NSAIDs when directly compared. Adverse effects seen in these trials were generally mild GI (nausea, upset stomach) and neurologic (sleepiness, dizziness, headache) complaints. When directly compared with each other, no NSAID was found to be better tolerated than another. Naproxen offers the advantage of less frequent dosing compared with ibuprofen.

Some data suggest that an oral loading dose of naproxen sodium (550 mg) might improve pain control in dysmenorrhea. A randomized trial demonstrated increased relief from dysmenorrhea symptoms in adolescents treated with an NSAID regimen that started with a loading dose, versus those who used a flat dosing regimen.[93] Loading doses generally are twice the regular dose. If A.B. experienced adverse effects with the higher loading dose, an alternative strategy is to initiate dosing 24 hours before menses is expected to start, based on the calendar if the patient has predictable cycles, or based on the start of premenstrual syndrome-type symptoms. This prophylactic dosing may be helpful especially for patients who have severe dysmenorrhea with absenteeism and decreased work or school productivity.[78,92] Although no specific evidence supports the use of scheduled NSAID dosing regimens, avoiding as-needed dosing may provide consistent serum levels to maintain reduced prostaglandin levels. As the duration of therapy is typically limited to 2 or 3 days, risk of adverse effects tends to be outweighed by the potential benefit of loading doses, prophylactic dosing, and scheduled versus PRN therapy.

A good recommendation for A.B. could include initiating naproxen sodium 550 mg orally at the beginning of menses, followed by 275 mg every 8 hours thereafter for the 2 to 3 days she experiences dysmenorrhea.

CASE 50-2, QUESTION 6: What adverse effects might A.B. experience from her NSAID?

All NSAIDs have a similar adverse effect profile. Nausea, vomiting, indigestion, anorexia, diarrhea, constipation, abdominal pain, melena, and bloating are common GI complaints.

Careful attention should be given to previous trials of NSAIDs for dysmenorrhea and other conditions, because women may respond favorably to one NSAID over another. If a 2-month or 3-month trial at appropriate doses of one NSAID is unsuccessful for A.B., another agent from a different chemical class may be tried. Because dysmenorrhea is most prevalent in younger women who tend to be healthy, the risk of adverse events may be lower than would be expected in an older population.

Contraindications

CASE 50-2, QUESTION 7: What medical history information is important to avoid serious adverse effects?

A.B should be questioned about medication allergies and any prior history of ulceration or GI bleeding; a history of cardiovascular and renal disease, although uncommon in young women, should be elicited before prescribing therapy. A thorough medication history, including OTC agents and dietary supplements, should be conducted. Particular attention should be paid to any potential therapeutic duplications (e.g., prescription and OTC NSAIDs), drug–drug interaction (e.g., warfarin), and drug–disease (hypertension) interaction.

Women who are allergic to aspirin or have a history of allergic reaction to any NSAID should not use NSAIDs or celecoxib. A.B. has not had a previous allergic reaction to NSAID or aspirin; she is not taking any medications that may interact and does not have any history of medical problems that would prevent her from a trial of NSAID therapy.

Hormonal Contraception

Oral Contraceptives

CASE 50-2, QUESTION 8: After 6 months of treatment, A.B. has some relief of her pain, nausea, and diarrhea with the naproxen sodium, but is unhappy with the amount of time that she is spending at home due to menstrual cramps. She is asking about other treatment options for further pain relief. What other options are available for A.B.?

As mentioned previously, hormonal contraceptives may be an option in A.B. if prescription NSAIDs are not adequate for her symptoms. Oral contraceptives (OCs) suppress ovulation, decrease menstrual fluid volume, and subsequently decrease prostaglandin production and uterine cramping.[75,77] OCs alone, or in combination with an NSAID, are appropriate as first-line treatment in women with or without a need for contraception.[94] OCs relieve dysmenorrhea symptoms in 50% to 80% of women within 3 to 6 months after beginning hormone therapy.[95] A study of healthy adolescent women with primary dysmenorrhea evaluated the effects of a 20 mcg ethinyl estradiol/100 mcg levonorgestrel oral contraceptive pill as compared with placebo during a 3-month period.[96] With OC use, women reported decreased severity of pain and used less pain medication. A Cochrane review of oral contraceptives and primary dysmenorrhea found oral contraceptives containing less than 35 mcg of ethinyl estradiol to be effective at reducing pain, but failed to demonstrate a significant difference between various 35-mcg ethinyl estradiol OC formulations.[95] Selection of an OC should be based on factors presented in Chapter 47, Contraception. A randomized controlled trial has evaluated the use of continuous dosing of oral contraceptives compared to the traditional 21 active days, 7 placebo days regimen, with an initial benefit in favor of decreased pain in the continuous dosing group at 1 and 3 months that was lost after 6 months of use.[97]

Adverse effects and contraindications associated with OC use must be considered (See Chapter 47, Contraception). Although serious complications from OC use are uncommon in young, healthy women, breakthrough bleeding and spotting, nausea, and breast tenderness may occur, especially early in treatment. A.B. may choose to add an OC to her naproxen sodium, with potentially improved pain relief compared with either agent alone. If pain does not respond to either course of therapy, investigation via laparoscopy for causes of secondary dysmenorrhea may be necessary.

Other Hormonal Contraceptive Agents

Other hormonal contraceptive agents that suppress ovulation have also been used in the treatment of primary dysmenorrhea, although none have undergone rigorous trials for this indication.[82] The levonorgestrel intrauterine system (IUS) is associated with amenorrhea and a reduction in dysmenorrhea over time, unlike the copper IUD, which may result in increased pain, cramping, and blood loss. Three years after insertion, fewer women with a levonorgestrel IUS reported menstrual pain (60% baseline, 29% after 3 years), with 47% of women with amenorrhea.[98] In women with primary dysmenorrhea at low risk of sexually transmitted infections, and desiring long-term contraception, the levonorgestrel IUS would be a reasonable option.

Medroxyprogesterone depot injection is another hormonal contraceptive agent that has been used to treat primary dysmenorrhea. Nearly two-thirds of adolescents reported fewer symptoms of dysmenorrhea with injections every 3 months.[77] Negative effects of medroxyprogesterone injections on bone density should be weighed with potential benefit when considering this option (See Chapter 47, Contraception). Given that A.B.'s past history does not include any absolute contraindications to combined oral contraceptives and her dysmenorrhea symptoms have not been well controlled with prescription NSAIDs, she is a candidate for combined hormonal contraception. A trial of combined oral contraceptives would be an appropriate plan for better control of her dysmenorrhea. In addition to smoking cessation, she should be counseled that hormonal contraceptives may require 3 or more months to provide maximal relief of symptoms. The goals of therapy, namely reduction in pain and associated symptoms, as well as improvement in functionality, should be explained to A.B. and reviewed at each contact.

ENDOMETRIOSIS

Endometriosis is defined as the presence of functional endometrial tissue occurring outside the uterine cavity. It is the most common cause of secondary dysmenorrhea in young women and can result in chronic pelvic pain, infertility, and dyspareunia.[77] The ovaries are commonly the site of endometriosis, which can also be found in the pelvic peritoneum, cervix, vagina, vulva, rectosigmoid colon, and appendix.

Less common sites of implantation of endometrial tissue include the umbilicus, scar tissue resulting from surgery, kidneys, lungs, and even arms and legs.[99] Endometriosis is present in up to 45% of women with infertility. Overall, it is difficult to determine the prevalence of endometriosis, because many women do not experience symptoms or seek treatment, and formal diagnostic criteria currently require visual identification of endometrial tissue during surgery. In women who have laparotomies for any reason, endometriosis is identified in 5% to 15%. This increases to 33% in women with chronic pelvic pain.[99] In contrast to primary dysmenorrhea, endometriosis usually occurs in women who have been menstruating for some time; it can provoke pain that is not limited to the time of the menses, but can occur anytime throughout the cycle. Endometriosis is rarely seen in women near the menarche, after menopause, or in amenorrheic women. The average age at diagnosis is 36.4 years, and even before diagnosis, women with endometriosis have higher healthcare costs and utilization, particularly emergency room utilization, than age-matched controls.[100]

Diagnostic Criteria

Diagnosis of endometriosis is difficult, with a delay in diagnosis in the range of 8 to 12 years from initial symptom presentation.[101] Endometriosis, interstitial cystitis, irritable bowel syndrome, and pelvic adhesions represent the four most common causes of chronic pelvic pain (defined as pain not associated with the menses, severe in nature, resulting in functional disability, and lasting at least 6 months).[102] The delay in diagnosis is the unfortunate consequence of the lack of diagnostic laboratory markers and its similarities to these other conditions. The physical examination is often normal, although the most common physical finding is a fixed retroverted uterus, with scarring and tenderness. A definitive diagnosis is only possible with visualization of endometriosis on laparoscopy, although this is not considered as absolutely necessary today as it has been in the past.[103] Although no diagnostic criteria currently exist, endometriosis can be staged at the time of laparoscopy according to the Revised American Fertility Society Classification of Endometriosis.[104] The stages are classified as minimal (stage I), mild (stage II), moderate (stage III), and severe (stage IV), as determined by an accumulated point total, with points based on the location of the endometrial lesions, the size of the lesions, the presence and extent of the adhesions, and the degree of obliteration of the posterior cul-de-sac. The classification system is designed to document the location and extent of endometriosis, does not predict infertility, aid in treatment selection or outcomes, or predict recurrence of disease. Making diagnosis and prognosis more difficult is that the reported severity of pelvic pain and level of functional disability do not seem to be correlated with the stage of endometriosis.[99]

Pathophysiology

Although the first description of endometriosis was made in the 1860s, the precise etiology of endometriosis remains a mystery. Several theories exist regarding the origins of endometriosis, and the exact etiology is probably a complex interplay between physical and individual patient-specific immunologic factors.[99]

The most commonly cited theory is that of retrograde menstruation or the flow of menstrual fluid, endometrial cells, and other debris backward through the fallopian tubes resulting in implantation in the peritoneal cavity. Once endometrial cells reach the peritoneum, stimulated angiogenesis (potentially by estrogen, among other factors) appears to be a determinant of the development and growth of lesions.[105,106] Also at this point, the lesion stimulates an immune response, triggering the activation of macrophages, as well as cytokine and growth factor release. Peritoneal lesions may contribute to more distant disease by spread via hematogenous or lymphatic routes, or even by movement owing to iatrogenic causes, such as cesarean sections and other forms of gynecologic surgery. Although the retrograde menstruation theory makes scientific sense, it has been discovered that retrograde menstruation occurs in nearly all menstruating women (90%) and not all women have endometriosis. This suggests that an additional factor, such as genetic susceptibility or altered immunity, or altered hormone receptor functioning such as progesterone resistance, must be present for the pathogenesis of endometriosis in certain patients.[107]

Another theory for the etiology of endometriosis is the coelomic metaplasia theory. This theory rests on the belief that the coelomic epithelium, the fetal originator tissue for the reproductive tract, retains its ability to differentiate into multiple cell types.[99,107,108] The trigger for differentiation is thought to be, in part, estrogen or environmental factors. This theory would explain the presence of endometriosis in prepubertal girls, in women born without a uterus, and in the rare cases of endometriosis seen in men. Genetics also play a role in the development of endometriosis. For first-degree relatives of women with severe endometriosis, there is a 6 times higher rate of developing endometriosis when compared with women who do not have affected relatives. These woman also have more severe disease and disease that appears earlier in life.[101,109] More than 15 different gene and gene product abnormalities have been documented in women with endometriosis. Environmental factors, as discussed, are intriguing in their role as potential causative factors, but are not definitive.[107,109]

Once endometrial tissue becomes implanted, hormones are necessary for their continued growth. As with intrauterine endometrium, the implants of endometriosis possess estrogen, progesterone, and androgen receptors. The endometrial implants may, however, respond differently to hormonal stimulation than normal endometrium. In general, estrogens stimulate the implants, whereas androgens or lack of estrogen results in implant atrophy. Because of their complex hormonal effects, progestins have variable effects on the implants.[104,107,110] In addition, lesions also show high levels of estrogen biosynthesis, owing to abnormally increased aromatase activity, with a concomitant decrease in the inactivation of estrogen, resulting in high intralesional estrogen concentrations.[107,111] The responsiveness of endometrial implants to ovarian hormones plays a role in the pathology of endometriosis. Withdrawal of estrogen and progesterone causes the endometrial implants to bleed, leading to an inflammatory response in the adjacent tissues. Repetitive cycles of bleeding and inflammation lead to the development of scar tissue and adhesions between adjacent peritoneal tissues. On laparoscopy, these areas of involvement appear as multiple hemorrhagic foci composed of endometrial epithelium, stroma, and glands. Ovarian endometriosis usually involves the formation of endometriomas, blood-filled cysts (chocolate cysts) ranging in size from microscopic to 10 cm. Nodules may form on uterosacral ligaments. Fibrosis usually is present with the endometrial implants, and extensive adhesions may form between pelvic structures.[112]

Clinical Characteristics

CASE 50-3

Question 1: N.H. is a 32-year-old woman who has been married for 6 years and is currently using the vaginal contraceptive ring to prevent pregnancy. She and her spouse have been contemplating the timing of a pregnancy, but have not yet attempted to become pregnant. She presents to her gynecologist to discuss preconceptual planning and reports that she has been having severe lower-abdominal cramps, associated with her menses, occurring on day 1 and lasting until day 4 or 5. This has been occurring for the past 4 years after many years of pain-free cycles and has recently been increasing in severity. The pain is slightly relieved by ibuprofen 400 mg orally TID, and during the past 6 months she has had to work from home at least 1 to 2 days/month owing to pain that has been increasing in frequency. On further questioning, she also reports mild-to-moderate pain that occurs randomly in her cycle, associated with low back pain, constipation with painful defecation, and pain with intercourse. Her menstrual history reveals menarche at age 10 with regular cycles every 26 to 27 days and heavy menses for 6 to 7 days. She reports discussing her symptoms with her mother, who described similar symptoms during her childbearing years.

N.H. is 5 feet 7 inches and weighs 145 lb. She smokes one-half pack of cigarettes/day and does not drink alcohol. She plays recreation league basketball and softball, but does not have a regular exercise regimen. She usually eats five servings of fruits or vegetables per day, but does not like to drink milk. She is concerned about her heart because her father had a cardiac stent placed at age 40, and she has been told she has high cholesterol.

Her physical examination is normal, with the exception of tenderness on palpation of the posterior fornix and a fixed retroverted uterus. A pregnancy test and tests for gonorrhea and chlamydia are negative, and a Pap smear is within normal limits. What subjective and objective data in N.H.'s presentation are compatible with a diagnosis of endometriosis?

A woman presenting with endometriosis may have signs and symptoms that are difficult, initially, to distinguish from primary dysmenorrhea[113] (Table 50-2). N.H.'s symptoms of lower abdominal cramps accompanying her menses are often mistaken for primary dysmenorrhea when other history details are not evaluated in total. N.H.'s age and her nulliparity are consistent with the characteristics of women with endometriosis. Although endometriosis has been diagnosed in women of all ages, it most commonly occurs in women in their late 20s and early 30s who have delayed pregnancy or who have infrequent pregnancies.

N.H.'s menstrual pattern of short cycle length with prolonged flow is characteristic of women with endometriosis. Risk factors for endometriosis are related to exposure to estrogen (i.e., early menarche and late menopause), and shorter menstrual cycle length (<28 days) with longer duration of menstrual flow (≥6 days), as well as having a mother or sister with endometriosis, as may be true with N.H.'s mother.[114] Women who have four or more pregnancies lasting greater than 6 months have a 50% lower risk of being diagnosed with endometriosis, and there is a decrease in risk of endometriosis that is parallel to duration of time spent in breastfeeding.[114] Higher BMI and shorter stature are associated with a lower risk of endometriosis, with a 12% to 14% decreased likelihood of diagnosis for every unit (kg/m^2) increase in BMI.[114] Potential, but not yet confirmed, risk factors that have been identified include higher social class, exposure to dioxins, and intake of caffeine and alcohol.[114] Cigarette smoking appears to reduce the risk for endometriosis, although studies are not conclusive.[108,109] Women with several immune-mediated conditions, including rheumatoid arthritis, systemic lupus erythematosus, hypothyroidism and hyperthyroidism, and multiple sclerosis, also have a higher rate of endometriosis than women without these immune-medicated conditions.[114]

N.H.'s chief complaints center on her progressive pelvic pain occurring throughout the cycle, with worsening during menses, constipation, and pain with intercourse (dyspareunia). Women who report pain during intercourse may have a fixed, retroverted uterus (as N.H. does) or endometriosis located in the posterior fornix of the vagina or along the uterosacral ligaments.[99] This pain may persist for several hours after intercourse. Other symptoms such as the constipation and painful defecation N.H. is experiencing are associated with endometriosis and may (but not always) depend on the organs affected by the location of the endometrial tissue[115,116] (Table 50-3). Depression also is a common symptom in patients with endometriosis, particularly those with chronic

Table 50-3
Location of Endometriosis and Associated Symptoms

Sites	Symptoms
Pelvic	
Cervix	Abnormal uterine bleeding
Ovaries	Dysmenorrhea
Peritoneum	Dyspareunia
Rectovaginal septum	Infertility
Uterosacral ligaments	Pelvic pain
Intestinal	
Abdominal scars	Intestinal obstruction
Sigmoid colon	Mid-abdominal pain
Small intestines	Nausea
	Painful defecation
	Rectal bleeding
Urinary Tract	
Bladder	Cyclic flank pain
Ureter	Hematuria
	Hydronephrosis
	Hydroureter

Source: American College of Obstetricians and Gynecologists. ACOG Practice Bulletin No. 114. Management of endometriosis. *Obstet Gynecol*. 2010;116:223.

Table 50-2
Primary versus Secondary Dysmenorrhea

Characteristic	Primary Dysmenorrhea	Secondary Dysmenorrhea
Onset	Around menarche	Any age (while menstruating)
Timing in menstrual cycle	Worse on day 1, lasts 24–48 hours	Increases in severity, may last days
Change over time	Stable, predictable	Increasing pain with increasing age
Symptoms	Low back pain, premenstrual syndrome, nausea, bloating	Low back pain, dyspareunia, diarrhea or constipation, dysuria, infertility
Signs	Normal pelvic examination	Fixed retroverted uterus, tenderness, but may be completely normal

Source: Reddish S. Dysmenorrhea. *Aust Fam Physician*. 2006;35:82.

pelvic pain, and may express as sadness, somatic complaints, and inability to work or carry on activities of normal living.[117]

Although it is unclear yet whether infertility will be a problem in N.H., endometriosis occurs in up to 45% of women with infertility.[99] The cause of endometriosis-associated infertility is not clear, but is probably caused by a combination of factors, which may include physical distortion of the pelvic architecture, inflammatory factors (including prostanoids, cytokines, and growth factors that may interfere with normal reproductive processes), impaired folliculogenesis (follicle development), or defects in fertilization or implantation.[118,119] Treatment for endometriosis, in inducing a "pseudomenopause," results in impaired fertility while the disease is actively being treated.

N.H.'s limited physical findings are not uncommon in women with endometriosis; physical findings, other than visualization of endometrial tissue during exploratory surgery, may not be present, and outward physical findings may have no correlation with the stage of endometriosis determined with surgery. Many symptoms and physical findings of endometriosis can be associated with other gynecologic conditions or diseases (particularly irritable bowel syndrome), and, if the patient is not responsive to empiric therapy, laparoscopy is indicated to confirm the diagnosis. N.H.'s negative pregnancy, chlamydia, and gonorrhea tests, as well as her normal Pap smear, are reassuring. The CA-125 laboratory test is not sufficiently sensitive or specific enough as a single test to diagnose endometriosis, and while many biomarkers are being studied, none have demonstrated sufficient sensitivity and specificity to be clinically useful.[120]

Treatment

CASE 50-3, QUESTION 2: N.H.'s pain is uncontrolled after trials of three different NSAIDs (ibuprofen, naproxen, and meloxicam), and she would like relief to improve her functionality at work and home. Given the potential mechanisms behind the pathophysiology of endometriosis, what therapeutic approaches are appropriate for the treatment of endometriosis in N.H.?

Therapy for endometriosis should be individualized and should consider N.H.'s desire for future fertility, severity of symptoms, extent of disease, and potential for infertility. This should be done with the knowledge that a high likelihood exists of recurrence and a lack of good prognostic indicators for future severity. The goals of treatment are to relieve symptoms and, if desired, to preserve or improve fertility. Options currently available to treat endometriosis include definitive and conservative surgery, hormonal therapy with estrogen–progestin combinations or progestins alone, danazol, aromatase inhibitors, or the GnRH agonists, and expectant management. Pharmacologic treatment of endometriosis is based on manipulation of this hormonal response: Danazol, GnRH agonists, progestins, aromatase inhibitors, and estrogen–progestin combination all result in endometrial tissue atrophy. No treatment has been shown to provide 100% protection against recurrence when discontinued; even surgical removal of the uterus and ovaries is associated with recurrence rates of up to 10%.[106] Limited evidence-based guidelines for treatment are available and are generally limited by the poor quality of evidence and limited depth of evidence for most treatments, especially those that are emerging.[121]

PAIN MANAGEMENT: PHARMACOLOGIC THERAPY

Nonsteroidal Anti-inflammatory Drugs

NSAIDs, particularly those available as OTC products, are often the first medications that women try for relief of pain from endometriosis, often before they are officially diagnosed. NSAIDs may provide some relief of mild symptoms, particularly in women with endometriosis who have pain associated with the menses (see Dysmenorrhea section), and are an appropriate first choice for women with mild symptoms who do not desire contraception. They should not be the only therapy offered to patients with confirmed endometriosis.[122] Clinicians should be aware of and consider the potential for endometriosis in patients with noncyclic pain, including pain that does not respond to an appropriate trial of an NSAID. N.H. has tried three different NSAIDS with limited relief; a higher dose or trial of another NSAID is not an appropriate strategy at this time. Additional treatment should be considered.

Combined Hormonal Contraceptives

For women who do not receive pain relief from a trial of an NSAID, a reasonable next step for those women desiring contraception is the use of oral contraceptives because they are considerably better tolerated over the long-term versus other hormonal options. They may be used alone or in combination with NSAIDs. OCs improve symptoms of endometriosis by inhibiting ovulation, decreasing hormone levels, and reducing menstrual flow, potentially to the point of amenorrhea. These mechanisms contribute to atrophy of endometrial implants. When used, the most appropriate regimen is continuous OC dosing, so that there is not a "placebo week" that allows for growth of endometrial implants. In a trial of patients who did not respond to cyclic OCs, use of continuous dosing resulted in significant pain reduction.[123,124] A Cochrane review found that the pain reduction seen with OCs (≤35 mcg of ethinyl estradiol) is similar to a GnRH analog (goserelin).[122] After surgery, continuous regimens appear to provide better pain symptom control than cyclic regiments.[125]

Progestins

Similar to oral contraceptives, injectable progestins reduce symptoms of endometriosis by inhibiting ovulation, reducing hormone levels, and inducing endometrial atrophy. They may be particularly useful if estrogen use is contraindicated. Regimens used include oral medroxyprogesterone, depot medroxyprogesterone (see Case 50-3, Question 5), or the levonorgestrel IUS. More recent studies have evaluated the use of the levonorgestrel IUS as a means of providing consistent progestin dosing. The IUS has the advantage of providing longer-term contraception. When compared with leuprolide depot (a GnRH agonist), the levonorgestrel IUS provided similar benefits in reducing pelvic pain, with a decreased potential for hypoestrogenic effects, and an increased potential for early breakthrough bleeding, followed by eventual amenorrhea.[126]

A 3-year direct comparison of the levonorgestrel IUS versus depot medroxyprogesterone was conducted in patients with moderate-to-severe endometriosis for medical control of symptoms after conservative surgery.[127] Although symptoms were improved with both regimens, more IUS patients remained adherent to the regimen, and at 3 years, bone density was increased in the IUS group and decreased in the depot group.

Progestins, despite being as effective as GnRH agonists in the treatment of pain, have increased side effects when compared with OCs, primarily weight gain (particularly with the depot formulation), initial breakthrough bleeding followed by amenorrhea, and, with depot formulations, decreased bone density with prolonged use, placing them after combined hormonal contraception in choice of therapy.[128]

Gonadotropin-Releasing Hormone Agonists

GnRH agonists induce a pseudomenopausal state, resulting in relief of endometriosis symptoms. Because the GnRH agonists have a longer half-life than endogenous GnRH, their binding to GnRH receptors in the pituitary results in downregulation of the hypothalamic–pituitary–ovarian axis, decreasing release of FSH

Table 50-4
Gonadotropin-Releasing Hormone Agonists

GnRH Agonist (Brand Name)	Strength	Dosage Form	Dosage Regimen
Nafarelin (Synarel)	2 mg/mL delivers 200 mcg/spray	Intranasal	200–800 mcg BID
Leuprolide (Lupron)	3.75 mg, 11.25 mg	IM depot	3.75 mg/month or 11.25 mg every 3 months
Goserelin (Zoladex)	3.6 mg, 10.8 mg	SC implant	3.6 mg implant every month or 10.8 mg implant every 3 months

BID, 2 times daily; GnRH, gonadotropin-releasing hormone; IM, intramuscular; SC, subcutaneous.

and LH, leading to low estrogen levels and amenorrhea.[129] GnRH agonists are available in a variety of dosage forms, outlined in Table 50-4. When compared in clinical trials, GnRH agonists have efficacy that is similar to oral contraceptives, progestins, and danazol, but their increased cost and adverse effect profile (including menopausal-type symptoms and decreased bone density) make them second-line agents, after OCs and progestins.[129]

Aromatase Inhibitors

The most recently studied therapy for endometriosis, aromatase inhibitors (AIs), was originally developed for use in patients with breast cancer. Aromatase, the enzyme responsible for the synthesis of estrogens, is required for the conversion of androstenedione and testosterone to estrone and estradiol.[130] Although AIs, OCs, progestins, and GnRH agonists all decrease serum levels of estrogen, only AIs decrease secretion and production of estrogen by endometrial tissue itself. Anastrozole and letrozole are type II AIs, binding reversibly to the enzyme to produce a beneficial effect on endometriosis symptoms.[130] Although AIs effectively decrease estrogen conversion in the periphery, addition of an agent to reduce ovarian estrogen levels is also necessary in premenopausal women; hence, most of the studies in this population have included double therapy with AIs and oral contraceptives or GnRH analog. AIs may be used alone in postmenopausal women.[130]

Although the end result of GnRH agonists and AIs is similar, the adverse effects of the AIs are decreased, with fewer hot flashes, and primarily mild headache, nausea, and diarrhea. Although few long-term trials have been conducted, decreased bone density is suspected with the use of AIs and estrogen add-back therapy is appropriate (described later in this section and Case 50-4, Question 1). All AI studies, although small, have demonstrated reduction in pain and reduced lesion size. The largest study to date used a combination of anastrozole with GnRH agonists compared with GnRH agonists alone in patients after surgery.[131] Although effective at controlling pain, the combination resulted in significantly more bone loss than either regimen alone at 6 months, but no difference was seen at the 2-year follow-up.[131] Further research is needed to determine the role of AIs in the treatment of endometriosis, because currently they do not have an FDA indication for the treatment of endometriosis. Their use should be reserved at this time for those patients with severe endometriosis who have failed other therapies.

Danazol

Danazol, an androgenic drug derived from 17-ethinyl testosterone, also induces a pseudomenopausal state by increasing androgen levels and decreasing estrogen levels. It inhibits the enzymes involved in ovarian steroidogenesis and increases the metabolic clearance of estradiol. By creating a hypoestrogenic, hypoprogestogenic state, danazol causes anovulation, amenorrhea, and atrophy of endometrial implants. Although effective at decreasing pelvic pain, danazol is poorly tolerated because of its significant side effects, which include weight gain, voice changes, edema, acne, hot flashes, vaginal dryness, hirsutism, liver disease, and increased cholesterol; these occur in up to 85% of treated patients.[106] Because of safety concerns, use should be limited to 6 months at a time and should only be initiated in women after all other therapy options have failed.

Emerging Agents

Two new medication classes hold promise for the treatment of endometriosis, with the hope of decreased side effects when compared with current therapy. HMG-CoA reductase inhibitors (Statins) have been studied in one small clinical trial in comparison with a GnRH analog and were found to have similar efficacy in providing pain relief.[132] Further investigation needs to be done with these agents particularly in women who wish to retain the option of fertility.

An additional emerging group of therapeutic agents is the GnRH antagonists, thought to maintain the beneficial effects on pain control in endometriosis, but with decreased side effects. When compared to depot medroxyprogesterone, the first agent in this class studied for endometriosis, elagolix, (a once-daily oral medication) demonstrated noninferiority in its effects on pain control, with little effect on bone density.[133]

PAIN MANAGEMENT: NONPHARMACOLOGIC THERAPY

Definitive Surgery

Definitive surgery, referring to total abdominal hysterectomy, bilateral salpingo-oophorectomy, and removal of all visible endometriosis, theoretically should eliminate the risk of recurrence of the disease. These procedures are not an option for many women with endometriosis who desire pregnancy in the future. It is invasive surgery, reserved for those patients whose pain is unresponsive to other therapies or to conservative surgery. Furthermore, removal of all endometriosis is difficult, and recurring pain is not uncommon. Sinaii et al. surveyed patients with endometriosis regarding treatments and benefits, and found that, of the 1,160 women surveyed, 12% had had definitive surgery, with 40% reporting the surgery was successful, 33% reporting partial benefit, 5.6% reporting no benefit, and 6% of patients actually reported increased pain and symptoms after surgery.[134]

Conservative Surgery

In contrast to definitive surgery, conservative surgery (involving ablation and removal of implants, and lysis of adhesions) preserves fertility and is commonly conducted during the initial diagnostic laparoscopy. In the Sinaii et al. survey, 70% of patients had undergone laparoscopy with removal of lesions, with 30% considering the procedure a success, 50% reporting partial benefit, 15% with no difference in symptoms, and 10% reporting increased symptoms.[134] On average, women reported having three surgical procedures.[134] Drug treatment is used after conservative surgery, because it is not possible to remove all lesions, many of which are difficult to visualize.

Clinical trials in endometriosis have not singled out one treatment as the treatment of choice for all women, with most investigations demonstrating equivalence of the studied therapies. An NSAID and combined hormonal contraception (e.g., N.H.'s contraceptive vaginal ring) are the drugs of choice for initial management, owing to their safety profile and, in this case, the contraceptive agent's dual utility in preventing conception. As a next step, progestins, GnRH agonists, and AIs are options. Because of adverse effects and poor tolerability, danazol should be reserved as an agent of last choice. If N.H. were uninterested in having children in the future, surgical sterilization would be an option. Conservative surgery, including removal of endometriomas and adhesions and ablation of visible lesions, is not curative, but may provide pain relief in 50% to 95% of patients at 1 year.[129] A combination of conservative surgery, followed by postoperative progestin, combined hormonal contraceptive, GnRH agonists, or danazol, has been shown to prolong the duration of pain relief and decrease recurrence after surgery.[129]

Case 50-3, Question 3: N.H. has not had a problem in the past tolerating a variety of contraceptive products, but does have some problems with daily medication adherence, and would like to avoid giving herself injections if possible. How does this information assist in the selection of therapy for her endometriosis?

N.H. is a smoker, with poor calcium intake and some cardiovascular risk factors (family history, high cholesterol), who would rather avoid injectable medication and has trouble with daily medication taking. Danazol, with its ability to increase cardiovascular risk factors and extensive side effects, is not a good option. Although some GnRH analogs are available as nasal sprays or injectable implants, the significant risk of decreased bone density and menopause-like adverse effects place them as a second-line option. Progestins, particularly the long-acting progestins, either in the form of the medroxyprogesterone acetate 3-month depot or subcutaneous injection, or the levonorgestrel IUS, make these appropriate first-line options for N.H., although the risk of diminished bone density with depot formulations remains an issue.

Case 50-3, Question 4: N.H. would like to start the levonorgestrel IUS, but her insurance company will not pay for it to be used in the treatment of endometriosis because of its lack of FDA indication. She decides to start depot medroxyprogesterone acetate. What information can you provide her regarding use, and the benefits and risks of treatment?

Depot medroxyprogesterone acetate (DMPA) is available in two dosage forms: 150 mg to be given intramuscularly (IM) every 3 months and a 104-mg formulation given subcutaneously (SC) every 3 months. Product choice may be based on insurance coverage or potential for the patient to self-administer (the SC product may be more patient-friendly). Because N.H. does not want to self-inject, either choice, administered by her provider's office, or a pharmacist if law allows, would be an appropriate option. Although the DMPA does provide the contraception N.H. desires, she should be informed that it may take longer than usual (up to 1 year) to become pregnant after its use. More than 80% of patients treated with progestins will experience partial or complete pain relief.[123] Although devoid of the menopause-like adverse effects of other medications used to treat endometriosis, DMPA is associated with weight gain (which may be significant in some patients), bloating, and irregular periods or bleeding for several months, with most users eventually experiencing amenorrhea. To reduce bone density loss, which is significant but less than with GnRH agonists, N.H. should be advised to ensure her daily intake by diet or supplementation of calcium is at least 1,000 mg/day and at least 400 to 600 IU of vitamin D/day, receive smoking cessation counseling and pharmacotherapy as appropriate, and start a regular weight-bearing exercise regimen.[135] She should be monitored for pain relief, weight gain, amenorrhea or bleeding changes, and adherence to the quarterly injections. When N.H. desires conception, significant planning is required and she may require a different therapy for her endometriosis because she regains fertility.

GONADOTROPIN-RELEASING HORMONE AGONISTS AND ADD-BACK THERAPY

CASE 50-4

Question 1: M.F., a 24-year-old single woman with a history of moderate-to-severe endometriosis, has been treated with some benefit with NSAIDs (three different NSAIDs at appropriate doses), combined oral contraceptives, and the levonorgestrel IUS. She has no desire for conception and is looking for pain relief. She has also had two conservative laparoscopic surgical procedures, each of which was successful, with pain relief lasting 6 months to 1 year. She recently had her "last ever" (by her description) surgical procedure and is looking to extend the improvement she has seen previously after surgery. She does not mind injections, but has had trouble with adherence in the past. What options are available for the treatment of M.F.'s pain?

M.F. has tried numerous pharmacologic and surgical treatments (NSAIDs, combined oral contraception, and progestin-only contraception) for endometriosis with limited benefit. Given that she does not desire pregnancy at this time, GnRH analogs, aromatase inhibitors, and danazol are other options. Leuprolide, nafarelin, and goserelin are GnRH analogs (agonists) typically used for the treatment of endometriosis (Table 50-4). Although GnRH analogs have not been shown to produce better results than the therapies M.F. has already used, they may provide her with pain relief. Choice of GnRH agonist is driven by patient choice of administration method (nasal twice daily [BID] with nafarelin, monthly SC implant with goserelin, or IM injection either once monthly or once every 3 months with leuprolide). In M.F.'s case, the once every 3 months dosing with leuprolide would be most desirable for her, eliminating the need for daily administration. Efficacy is similar for all the GnRH agonists. Before use of these agents, pregnancy, undiagnosed vaginal bleeding, and breastfeeding should be ruled out. Because M.F. does not desire conception, and use of the GnRH agonists is contraindicated in pregnancy, she should be counseled regarding choices of nonhormonal contraceptive agents.

Onset of response to GnRH therapy depends on the phase in the menstrual cycle during which the agent is initiated. Administration beginning in the luteal phase causes decreased estrogen levels within 2 to 3 weeks, and amenorrhea within 4 to 5 weeks versus the 6 to 8 weeks if started in the follicular phase.[99]

Usual therapy duration is 6 months, although a small pilot study suggested long-term treatment (up to 10 years) with estrogen add-back therapy is without major adverse effects, with continued efficacy.[136] Add-back therapy is based on the concept of an estrogen threshold hypothesis, formulated by Barbieri,[112] which states that there is a critical amount of estrogen that exacerbates endometriosis, and below that level the presence of estrogen serves to decrease adverse effects but does not have an adverse effect on the disease itself. Add-back therapy should be initiated at the beginning of GnRH agonist therapy to try to reduce the occurrence of all hypoestrogenic adverse effects.[136]

Estrogen-containing OCs contain a dose of estrogen that is above the threshold, and they should not be used for add-back therapy. Doses of estrogen equivalent to 0.625 mg of conjugated equine estrogen have been studied in combination with either medroxyprogesterone 2.5 mg daily, or norethindrone 5 mg daily. This dose of norethindrone alone, or a dose of 20 mg of medroxyprogesterone alone, has also demonstrated benefit.[106] To prevent bone loss, a regimen of a progestin plus a bisphosphonate has been studied with positive results. No studies have demonstrated superior efficacy or safety of one regimen over another. Women using add-back therapy should consume in diet or supplement a total of 1,000 mg of calcium daily, and have vitamin D levels in the normal range.[111]

Therapy beyond 3 to 6 months requires the use of add-back therapy to reduce the risk of hypoestrogenic complications. Monitoring for efficacy includes monitoring for amenorrhea, decreases in pain and dyspareunia, and quality of life. After discontinuation of GnRH agonists, menses and ovarian function return to normal in 6 to 12 weeks, although benefits may be maintained for another 6 to 12 months.[99]

Adverse Effects

Adverse effects should be discussed in detail with M.F. because they differ significantly from the other therapies she has tried. Adverse effects are related to the induction of the pseudomenopausal state. Nearly all patients experience hot flashes; vaginal dryness and insomnia also are common. GnRH agonists do not affect SHBG or testosterone levels, so the androgenic side effects of danazol, including changes in lipid profiles, are not experienced with these agents.[99] Significant bone loss can occur, necessitating adequate calcium and vitamin D intake, and estrogen add-back therapy to decrease loss.

A reduction in bone density is a significant concern with GnRH agonists, even at 3 months after the onset of therapy, and is particularly concerning because these agents are being used in young women, many of whom have not reached their peak bone mass. Studies have demonstrated a loss of 3.2% in lumbar spine bone mineral density after 6 months and up to a 6.3% decrease after 12 months of GnRH agonist treatment.[137] It has also been reported that endometriosis itself is also a risk factor for decreased bone density, although a long-term study did not find any association between endometriosis and fracture risk during a 20-year follow-up period.[138] Interestingly, this same study did not find any association between fracture risk and GnRH agonist therapy, although a significant number of women in the study did take add-back therapy.

Monitoring for decreases in bone density should be accomplished via dual-energy X-ray absorptiometry scan every 24 months if GnRH therapy is continued. M.F. should also be counseled regarding adequate calcium and vitamin D intake, smoking cessation, and a regimen of weight-bearing exercise.

M.F should initiate the leuprolide 11.25 mg IM once every 3 months, with add-back therapy consisting of conjugated estrogens 0.625 mg daily with 2.5 mg medroxyprogesterone. A 6-month trial followed by an evaluation of symptom control is reasonable.

MANAGEMENT OF ENDOMETRIOSIS-RELATED INFERTILITY

CASE 50-5

QUESTION 1: K.L. is a 32-year-old woman with a history of stage II endometriosis. She currently is using a levonorgestrel IUS for both contraception and control of her pain, with positive results. She also takes ibuprofen 800 mg TID on a regular basis. She and her spouse would like to have a child. About 6 years ago, they attempted to conceive without success after 24 months. K.L is concerned that she will now have even more difficulty in becoming pregnant, given her advanced age. What are the recommendations for improving fertility in K.L?

Of women presenting to the healthcare system with infertility, 25% to 50% have endometriosis and 30% to 50% of women with endometriosis are infertile.[139] Proposed mechanisms contributing to infertility include adhesions that impair oocyte transport, changes in the peritoneum not compatible with fertility, changes in hormonal function, endocrine or ovulation dysfunction, and disorders of implantation (see Chapter XX, Infertility). No evidence suggests that hormonal therapy, including therapy with GnRH agonists, improves conception rates for women with stage I/II endometriosis, similar to K.L. On the other hand, surgical ablation or resection of visible endometriosis implants is beneficial in improving pregnancy rates in women with stage I/II endometriosis.

For K.L., removal of her IUS, followed by laparoscopic ablation or resection of visible implants, may improve her ability to conceive, barring other factors influencing fertility (e.g., PCOS, male factor infertility, tubal patency).[140] For patients with more advanced disease, or in those patients older than 35 years of age, a more aggressive treatment regimen is appropriate. Options include the use of agents to induce superovulation (clomiphene) and the use of in vitro fertilization techniques with embryo transfer (IVF-ET). In women with endometriosis, the success of IVF-ET is decreased by as much as 20% when compared with women without endometriosis.[99] For women contemplating IVF-ET, three prospective clinical trials have demonstrated a potential benefit in women with stage II–IV endometriosis who were treated for 3 to 6 months or more with GnRH agonists before IVF-ET.[114] The treated subjects had significantly higher pregnancy rates compared with women who did not use GnRH agonists before IVF-ET.[141]

For women who have not yet demonstrated an inability to conceive, a "wait and see" approach, with use of an NSAID for pain, emotional support, and reassurance, for 6 to 12 months is appropriate in women younger than 35 years of age.

PREMENSTRUAL SYNDROME AND PREMENSTRUAL DYSPHORIC DISORDER

Premenstrual symptoms occur in up to 95% of reproductive-age women.[142] Approximately 30% to 40% of these women have more bothersome symptoms of premenstrual syndrome (PMS), and it is estimated that 3% to 8% meet the criteria for premenstrual dysphoric disorder (PMDD), a more severe variant of PMS.[142] More than 200 premenstrual symptoms have been described as occurring during the days before menstruation, including positive symptoms, such as increased energy, libido, and ability to relax, as well as negative symptoms including abdominal distension, fatigue, headaches, and crying spells.[143] It is not until the symptoms have a decidedly negative influence on the physical, psychological, or social function of a woman that PMS or PMDD exists.

Diagnosis

No specific physical findings or laboratory tests can be used to make a diagnosis of PMS. Several different organizations have attempted to provide diagnostic criteria for PMS and PMDD; their criteria are inconsistent and disparate. The International Society for Premenstrual Disorders (ISPMD) published a consensus statement in 2011 that defined core premenstrual disorders as typical, pure, or reference disorders associated with spontaneous ovulatory menstrual cycles and variant premenstrual disorders that are separate from core premenstrual disorders and exist where more complex features are present (e.g., symptoms result from underlying disorder or exogenous progestogen administration).[144] Core premenstrual features (somatic and psychological

Table 50-5

ACOG Diagnostic Criteria for Premenstrual Syndrome

Affective Symptoms	Somatic Symptoms
Depression	Breast tenderness
Angry outbursts	Abdominal bloating
Irritability	Headache
Anxiety	Swelling of extremities
Confusion	
Social withdrawal	

Notes: (1) Diagnosis made if at least one affective or one somatic symptom is reported in the three prior menstrual cycles during the 5 days before the onset of menses. (2) The symptoms must resolve within 4 days of onset of menses and do not recur until after day 12 of the cycle. (3) The symptoms must be present in at least two cycles during prospective recording. (4) The symptoms must adversely affect social or work-related activities.
ACOG, American College of Obstetricians and Gynecologists.
Source: American College of Obstetricians and Gynecologists. ACOG Practice Bulletin. Clinical management guidelines for obstetrician-gynecologists. Premenstrual syndrome. Number 15, April 2000. *Obstet Gynecol*. 2000;95(4); Mishell DR. Premenstrual disorders: epidemiology and disease burden. *Am J Manag Care*. 2005;11:S473.

symptoms) must occur during all or part of the 2-week premenstrual phase and resolve during or shorting after menstruation. A symptom-free interval between the end of menstruation and the time of ovulation must occur. This cyclic pattern must also occur in most (typically two out of three) menstrual cycles. Lastly, the severity of symptoms must (1) affect normal daily functioning; (2) interfere with work, school performance, or interpersonal relationships; or (3) cause significant distress. Core premenstrual disorder is an umbrella term for PMS and PMDD.

The American College of Obstetricians and Gynecologists (ACOG) published a Practice Bulletin in 2000 that defined PMS diagnostic criteria using cyclic patterns of symptoms in women.[145] PMS can be diagnosed if at least one of the affective or one of the somatic symptoms listed in Table 50-5 is reported 5 days before the onset of menses in the three previous cycles. The symptoms must be prospectively recorded in at least two cycles, must cease within 4 days of onset of menses, and must not recur until after day 12 of the menstrual cycle. A key factor that separates PMS from "normal" premenstrual symptoms is that work or social activities are adversely affected in PMS. Other diagnoses that may explain premenstrual symptoms should be excluded, including psychological, thyroid, and gynecologic disorders.[146]

The American Psychiatric Association has developed criteria for PMDD.[147] The criteria for PMDD focus on the mood and mental health symptoms, leading to a higher level of dysfunction compared with PMS. These criteria require prospective documentation of physical and behavioral symptoms (using diaries) being present for most of the preceding year; five or more symptoms present during the week prior to menses, resolving within a few days after menses starts; and PMDD may be superimposed on other psychiatric disorders, provided it is not merely an exacerbation of those disorders. One or more of the following symptoms must be present: mood swings, sudden sadness, or increased sensitivity to rejection; anger, irritability; sense of hopelessness, depressed mood, or self-critical thoughts; and tension, anxiety, or feeling on edge. Additionally, one or more of the following symptoms must be present to reach a total of five symptoms overall: difficulty in concentrating; change in appetite, food cravings, or overeating; diminished interest in usual activities; easy fatigability or decreased energy; feeling overwhelmed or out of control; breast tenderness, bloating, weight gain, or joint/muscles aches; and sleeping too much or not sleeping enough. Symptoms must have been present in most menstrual cycles that occurred the previous year, and the symptoms must be associated with significant distress or interference with usual activities (e.g., work, school, social life).

Although criteria for PMS and PMDD are different, they share three essential characteristics: (a) symptoms must occur in the luteal phase and resolve within a few days of menstruation, (b) symptoms are documented for at least two menstrual cycles and are not better explained by other physical or psychological conditions, and (c) symptoms are sufficiently severe to disrupt normal activities.

The symptoms of PMS and PMDD experienced by women can vary widely. Risk factors for PMS include advancing age (older than 30 years) and genetic factors.[146] Symptoms, however, can begin in adolescents around age 14, or 2 years postmenarche, and persist until menopause.[148] Some studies suggest that women with mothers reporting PMS are more likely to develop PMS than those with unaffected mothers (70% vs. 37%, respectively).[149,150] One article found that traumatic events, such as physical threat, childhood sexual abuse, and severe accidents, increased the risk of developing PMDD.[151]

Pathophysiology

The wide range of symptoms exhibited in patients with PMS or PMDD can be explained by multiple possible mechanisms, probably a result of interactions between sex steroids and central neurotransmitters.[152] Alterations in neurotransmitters, primarily reductions in serotonin, triggered by normal hormonal fluctuations of the menstrual cycle appear to be the most probable factors for the development of PMS or PMDD. Other neurotransmitters, including endorphins and γ-aminobutyric acid (GABA), have also been implicated.[153,154] The levels of estrogen, progesterone, and testosterone are normal in women with PMS, but they may be more vulnerable to normal fluctuations.[154] These potential mechanisms provide a rational basis for the symptoms that appear in PMS and PMDD, but also support the therapeutic benefits of treatments that increase serotonin or GABA levels. Many treatments have limited and variable efficacy, which reinforces the argumentation that PMS or PMDD is a result of multiple factors. Furthermore, placebo responses in trials can be as high as 50% to 80%, which points to an important psychosomatic component and the consideration that PMS or PMDD has relevant biological, psychological, and social factors.[143,155]

CASE 50-6

Question 1: C.P., a 27-year-old woman, presents complaining of significant mood changes that occur the week before her menstrual cycle. She experiences increased irritability and anxiety as well as breast tenderness and abdominal bloating. These symptoms usually subside the first or second day after her menses begin. For 2 to 3 weeks after her menstrual period, C.P. is her "normal, usual self" until the symptoms begin again just before her next menstruation. She has had these symptoms every month for the past several years. She states that she is very uncomfortable when these symptoms occur. Although she is able to work most of the time, she typically avoids going out with her friends when she has these symptoms. Her menstrual cycles are regular, occurring every 28 to 30 days with a light flow lasting 3 to 4 days.

Pelvic, cardiovascular, and neurologic examinations are normal, and all laboratory assessments are within normal limits. Her serum pregnancy test was negative. She is sexually active and uses condoms for contraception. She has no significant past medical history and she does not take any medications. What symptoms does C.P. have that are consistent with a diagnosis of PMS?

C.P. has symptoms that meet the ACOG criteria for PMS. Her affective symptoms include irritability and anxiety, and somatic symptoms include breast tenderness and abdominal bloating. These symptoms occur during the luteal phase of the menstrual cycle, resolve within 4 days of menses, and do not recur until after day 12 of her cycle. C.P.'s symptoms appear to be affecting her social activities. She states that these symptoms have been present for years and that they occur every month, although she has not prospectively recorded this information. C.P. does not meet the criteria for PMDD because her symptoms are not severe or markedly impairing her ability to participate in daily activities.

Treatment: Premenstrual Syndrome

CASE 50-6, QUESTION 2: C.P. asks about nonprescription therapy. Which agents, if any, are appropriate for C.P.?

The management of premenstrual disorders has been outlined by the ISPMD.[155] Treatment may be aimed at symptoms, especially if one particular symptom is dominant. Nonprescription options that have been studied and have demonstrated at least minimal benefit include calcium, magnesium, pyridoxine, chaste tree or chasteberry, and some mind–body approaches. Acetaminophen and NSAIDs may be beneficial for the physical symptoms of PMS, but diuretics found in various OTC products (e.g., ammonium chloride, caffeine, pamabrom) have limited data and unproven efficacy. Given the high placebo response rate in PMS, only agents with clinically proven efficacy should be used.

CALCIUM

Increased estrogen during the middle of a normal menstrual cycle decreases calcium. In women with PMS, intact parathyroid hormone (PTH) increases in response to this change compared with no PTH change in women without PMS.[156] Therefore, women with PMS have mid-cycle elevations of intact PTH with transient, secondary hyperparathyroidism that increases calcium demands. Calcium supplementation may help to normalize these processes and explains why calcium has demonstrated some benefit in women with PMS.

Three calcium trials have shown efficacy of PMS symptoms. A randomized, double-blind crossover trial of 33 women receiving 1,000 mg elemental calcium daily or placebo for 3 months reported a significant overall 50% reduction in PMS symptoms for women taking calcium compared with placebo.[157] In a double-blind study of 10 women assigned to dietary calcium intake, 1,336 mg daily was found to benefit mood, behavior, pain, and water retention symptoms significantly during the menstrual cycle.[158] Perhaps the most convincing evidence comes from a prospective, multicenter, randomized, double-blind, placebo-controlled, parallel-group trial conducted in 466 women with PMS.[159] Elemental calcium 1,200 mg daily (given as 600 mg BID) for three menstrual cycles significantly decreased negative affect, water retention, food cravings, and pain compared with placebo. Overall, the calcium-treated group had a 48% reduction in luteal symptoms compared with a 30% reduction in the placebo group. Because calcium is well tolerated and may provide other benefits (e.g., osteoporosis prevention), calcium supplementation should be recommended to women with symptoms of PMS if inadequate through diet or other supplementation.

MAGNESIUM

Low levels of red cell magnesium have been correlated with women experiencing PMS; therefore, magnesium supplementation has been evaluated for PMS symptoms.[160] A Cochrane review of three small trials comparing magnesium and placebo in women with dysmenorrhea concluded that magnesium was more effective for pain associated with PMS and the need for additional medication was less for those taking magnesium.[89] Magnesium doses that have been studied for PMS vary from 200 to 360 mg orally daily. Trials have reported improvements in fluid retention and negative affect, but findings have not been consistent.[161] The most common side effects affect the gastrointestinal system (e.g., nausea, diarrhea). The conflicting results may be caused by differences in the dosing regimens of the magnesium and differing levels of magnesium stores in the study subjects. Available data support the use of magnesium in PMS, but more research is needed.

PYRIDOXINE (VITAMIN B_6)

Vitamin B_6 has been noted to have positive effects on neurotransmitters, such as serotonin.[162] The most comprehensive information for this nutrient comes from a systematic review of nine trials representing 940 patients with PMS.[163] The overall assessment of the review was that women with PMS are likely to benefit from vitamin B_6 supplementation at a dose of 50 to 100 mg daily. An analysis of four of the trials, which specifically examined depressive symptoms, showed that pyridoxine was more effective than placebo in reducing depressive symptoms (OR, 1.69; 95% CI, 1.39–2.06). Although the conclusions of this review were positive, the authors felt there was insufficient evidence of high quality to recommend vitamin B_6 for PMS. Because neuropathy has been reported with pyridoxine dosages as low as 200 mg/day, patients should be advised to monitor for symptoms, discontinue therapy, and seek medical attention if they occur.[163]

CHASTETREE OR CHASTEBERRY

Chasteberry (Vitex agnus-castus or VAC) is the fruit of the chaste tree, a small shrub-like tree native to Central Asia and the Mediterranean region. Liquid or solid extracts from the dried ripe chasteberry are used to make chasteberry capsules and tablets. The mechanism of action of chasteberry relative to PMS is unclear, but several trials have reported its beneficial effects. In a study of 1,542 women with PMS taking chasteberry extract, 33% of subjects reported total relief of symptoms and an additional 57% reported partial relief after 4 months.[164] Of patients, 2% complained of adverse events including nausea, allergy, diarrhea, weight gain, heartburn, hypermenorrhea, and gastric complaints. A randomized, double-blind, placebo-controlled trial of 170 women taking chasteberry extract 20 mg daily for three menstrual cycles showed a treatment response rate of 52% compared with 24% for placebo ($p < 0.001$).[165] Individual symptoms of irritability, mood alteration, anger, headache, and breast fullness were reduced. Bloating was not significantly altered compared with placebo. The incidence of side effects was low, but long-term safety is unknown. A prospective, randomized, placebo-controlled study in 67 Chinese women showed that one VAC tablet daily containing 40 mg of herbal drug produced an 85% efficacy rate compared with a 56% efficacy rate for placebo on symptom scores after three treatment cycles.[166] In general, data indicate that chasteberry may be effective for PMS, but should probably not be used as routine treatment for PMS.[161]

MIND–BODY APPROACHES

Evidence regarding mind–body approaches for PMS is somewhat limited. Because these modalities are risk-free and they are generally accepted as components of a healthy lifestyle, they are favored in the treatment of PMS. Mind–body approaches that have demonstrated benefit in PMS include relaxation response, cognitive-behavioral therapy, yoga, aerobic exercise, and light therapy.[167] Trials that have evaluated acupuncture have demonstrated benefit to patients with PMS, but there are significant flaws in study designs that prevent it from being recommended as a treatment modality.[168]

NONSTEROIDAL ANTI-INFLAMMATORY DRUGS AND DIURETICS

NSAIDs have been used to relieve the physical symptoms (e.g., headache, joint pain) of PMS, but do not improve the mood symptoms.[146] Regimens have included taking naproxen or mefenamic acid during the luteal phase and stopping therapy after menses begin. Diuretics commonly found in OTC products, such as ammonium chloride, caffeine, and pamabrom, are not effective.

Several OTC options are available to C.P. Trials including calcium, magnesium, pyridoxine, and chasteberry have shown some positive findings, but the evidence is not compelling due to methodological limitations. These treatments should not be recommended for the treatment of PMS, but may already be included in a healthy diet or vitamin regimen. Mind–body approaches, such as yoga and relaxation, are part of a healthy lifestyle and could be recommended to C.P. Because C.P. is having mood symptoms (i.e., anxiety), NSAIDs would not be an effective recommendation.

CASE 50-6, QUESTION 3: C.P. has been taking a multivitamin daily for 3 months with adequate amounts of calcium, magnesium, and vitamin B_6 for PMS relief. She also has been taking naproxen sodium 220 mg orally BID without significant reduction of her symptoms. Her physician requests that she keeps a daily dairy for two consecutive cycles to document her symptoms. What information should be included in this tool?

C.P. should keep a daily diary for two consecutive menstrual cycles to demonstrate a temporal relationship between her symptoms during the luteal phase and to document the severity of these symptoms (Table 50-6). In addition, she should indicate the presence of menstrual flow, weight, and daily basal body temperature readings to help determine when ovulation occurs. The diary establishes a baseline for each patient and documents the most troublesome symptoms. Once therapy is selected for these symptoms, the diary can aid in assessing patient response.

Treatment: Premenstrual Dysphoric Disorder

CASE 50-6, QUESTION 4: C.P. returns to clinic with the diary presented in Table 50-6. The physician determines that C.P. actually has PMDD. What evidence supports this diagnosis and what should be recommended to C.P. for treatment?

C.P. meets the criteria for PMDD as evidenced by her symptoms during the 1 week before her menstrual cycle (luteal phase). Specifically, she has at least five symptoms required for the diagnosis of PMDD: sadness or depression (core symptom), fatigue, irritability, inability to concentrate, breast tenderness, and bloating. She rated several of those symptoms as severe, which indicates the symptoms are disabling and she is unable to meet her daily obligations. There is no reason to suspect any other disorder based on her history. PMDD seems to be the most likely diagnosis for C.P.

Therapy options at this time include lifestyle modifications, psychosocial interventions, and pharmacologic therapy. Psychotropic drugs targeted to her most severe symptoms may include selective serotonin reuptake inhibitors (SSRIs), serotonergic tricyclic antidepressants, and anxiolytics. Oral contraceptives have also been approved for PMDD and could be considered.

SELECTIVE SEROTONIN REUPTAKE INHIBITORS

Serotonin is critical in the pathogenesis of PMDD, and for that reason, SSRIs have become the treatment of choice for PMDD and severe PMS (Table 50-7).[169] SSRIs have demonstrated efficacy in reducing irritability, depressed mood, dysphoria, psychosocial function, and the physical symptoms of PMDD, including bloating, breast tenderness, and appetite changes. Fluoxetine, sertraline, and paroxetine controlled release each have an approved indication for PMDD.

The onset of SSRI effect in women with PMDD or severe PMS is much more rapid than when these agents are used for treatment of major depression or anxiety disorders.[169] Women may experience symptom relief or resolution within the first days of treatment versus 4 to 8 weeks for other psychological disorders.[155] Several different dosing strategies have been studied, including continuous dosing (once daily), intermittent dosing (last 2 weeks of menstrual cycle or luteal phase), and semi-intermittent dosing (continuous administration throughout the cycle with increased doses during luteal phase).[169] Continuous dosing would be reasonable for women with concurrent mood or anxiety disorders or those who may have difficulty in remembering the timing of the intermittent dosing. Intermittent dosing should be considered for patients with regular menstrual cycles who are able to adhere to the regimen, an absence of symptoms during the follicular phase, concerns about long-term effects (e.g., sexual dysfunction) or cost of daily therapy, and few side effects at treatment initiation.[169] Studies evaluating these dosing strategies have reported equal efficacy for continuous or intermittent strategies; treatment should be individualized based on patient history, willingness to adhere to therapy, and drug response.[170]

In a systematic review of 31 randomized controlled trials including fluoxetine, paroxetine, sertraline, escitalopram, and citalopram, SSRIs reduced overall self-rated symptoms significantly more effectively than placebo (end scores for moderate dose SSRIs: SMD −0.65, 95% CI −0.46 to −0.84, nine studies, 1,276 women).[170] Withdrawals due to adverse effects were significantly more likely in the SSRI group (moderate dose: OR 2.55, 95% I 1.84–3.53, 15 studies, 2,447 women) with side effects being dose-dependent and most commonly reported as nausea (NNH = 7), asthenia or decreased energy (NNH = 9), somnolence (NNH = 13), fatigue (NNH = 14), decreased libido (NNH = 14), and sweating (NNH = 14). Overall quality of the evidence was considered to be low to moderate, with poor reporting of methods as the prominent weakness.

OTHER PSYCHOTROPIC AGENTS

Non-SSRI antidepressants that affect serotonin are also beneficial in treating PMS and PMDD (Table 50-7). Venlafaxine, dosed daily, is significantly better than placebo at relieving psychological and physical symptoms of PMDD.[171] Alprazolam is a short-acting benzodiazepine that has been assessed for the treatment of PMS in several studies with differing results.[172] With conflicting data and concerns about dependence, alprazolam should be reserved for women who are unresponsive to other PMS treatments. Luteal-phase dosing may limit the risk of drug dependence of this benzodiazepine, but the dose should be tapered during several days to minimize mild withdrawal symptoms. Buspirone, a partial 5-hydroxytryptamine receptor agonist, demonstrated significant reduction in irritability when given daily, but does not seem to affect the physical symptoms of PMS.[173]

COMBINATION ORAL CONTRACEPTIVES

Two low-dose combination oral contraceptive (COC) formulations containing 20 mcg ethinyl estradiol and 3 mg drospirenone (an antimineralocorticoid spironolactone analog) with a 4-day hormone-free interval have been approved for the treatment of emotional and physical symptoms of PMDD.[174,175] Studies using this agent have shown efficacy for reduced mood, physical, and behavioral symptoms of PMDD, including a 48% improved response with this agent compared with a 36% response using placebo

Table 50-6

Menstrual Cycle Daily Diary Chart

Month 1

Grading Severity of Symptoms:
1 = Mild; general awareness of discomfort but does not interfere with daily activities
2 = Moderate; interferes with activities but not disabling
3 = Severe; symptoms disabling, unable to meet daily social, family, or work obligations
* = Menstrual bleeding
Blank = no symptoms

Each Day
1. List the major symptoms (mood, physical, emotional, behavioral) that you experience during your menstrual cycle
2. Grade the severity of the symptom if present (1–3)
3. Record daily weight
4. Record basal body temperature, which helps determine ovulation date
5. Check the days of the cycle when menstrual flow occurs

Day of month	1	2	3	4	5	6	7	8	9	10	11	12	13	14	15	16	17	18	19	20	21	22	23	24	25	26	27	28	29	30	31
Day of menstrual cycle	18	19	20	21	22	23	24	25	26	27	28	1	2	3	4	5	6	7	8	9	10	11	12	13	14	15	16	17	18	19	20
Menses												*	*	*	*																
Breast tenderness and pain				1	1	1	1	1	1	1	1																				
Sadness or depression				1	2	3	3	3	3	3	3	2	1																		
Fatigue				3	3	3	3	3	3	3	3	2	1																		
Irritability					2	2	3	3	3	3	3																				
Inability to concentrate							2	2	3	3	3																				
Daily weight (lb)	130	130	130	130	130	130	130	130	130	130	130	131	131	131	130	130	130	130	130	130	129	129	129	128	128	129	128	128	128	128	128
Basal body temperature (°F)	98.0	98.2	98.0	98.2	98.0	98.0	98.2	97.8	98.0	97.8	97.6					97.8	97.8	97.6	97.8	97.6	97.8	97.8	97.6	97.4	98.4	98.0	98.4	98.6	98.0	98.2	98.0

Month 2

Day of month	1	2	3	4	5	6	7	8	9	10	11	12	13	14	15	16	17	18	19	20	21	22	23	24	25	26	27	28	29	30
Day of menstrual cycle	21	22	23	24	25	26	27	28	1	2	3	4	5	6	7	8	9	10	11	12	13	14	15	16	17	18	19	20	21	22
Menses									*	*	*	*																		
Breast tenderness and pain				1	1	1	1	1	1		1																			
Sadness/ depression		1	2	3	3	3	3	3	2	2	1																			
Fatigue		2	2	3	3	3	3	3	2	1																				
Irritability	1	2	2	2	3	3	3	3	3	2	2	1																		
Inability to concentrate			1	1	2	2	3	3																						
Daily weight (lb)	128	128	128	128	128	128	128	129	129	129	128	128	128	128	128	128	128	128	128	128	128	128	128	128	128	129	128	128	128	128
Basal body temperature (°F)	98.0	98.2	98.4	98.0	98.2	97.8	98.0	97.4					97.6	97.6	97.8	97.8	97.6	97.8	97.6	97.6	97.6	97.2	97.2	97.0	98.4	98.6	98.0	98.2	98.2	98.0

Table 50-7
Psychotropic Drugs for the Management of Premenstrual Syndrome or Premenstrual Dysphoric Disorder

Drug (Brand Name)	Daily Dosing Regimen (mg)	Intermittent Dosing Regimen (mg)[a]
SSRI		
Citalopram (Celexa)	5–30	10–30
Escitalopram (Lexapro)	10–20	10–20
Fluoxetine (Prozac or Sarafem[b])	20–60	20 or 90 weekly
Fluvoxamine (Luvox)	50–150	NS
Paroxetine (Paxil)	10–30	NS
Paroxetine controlled release (Paxil CR)[b]	12.5–25	12.5–25
Sertraline (Zoloft)[b]	50–150	100
Other Serotonergic Antidepressants		
Nefazodone (Serzone)	200–600	NS
Venlafaxine (Effexor)	50	NS
Anxiolytics		
Alprazolam (Xanax)	NS	1–2[c]
Buspirone (BuSpar)	NS	25–60

[a]Day 14 until onset of menses.
[b]Medication has FDA-approved indication for premenstrual dysphoric disorder.
[c]Dose to be tapered during 2 days after onset of menses to prevent withdrawal symptoms.
NS, not studied; SSRI, selective serotonin reuptake inhibitors.

($p = 0.015$).[176] Side effects occurring in at least 10% of women treated with this medication included intermenstrual bleeding, headache, nausea, breast pain, and upper respiratory infection. Another COC approved for PMDD contains 20 mcg of ethinyl estradiol, 3 mg of drospirenone, and 0.451 mg of levomefolate calcium.[176] In a systematic review of five randomized controlled trials comparing COCs containing drospirenone to placebo or other COCs for effect on premenstrual symptoms, the authors concluded that drospirenone 3 mg plus ethinyl estradiol 20 mcg may help treat PMDD better than placebo.[177] They were unable to determine whether this combination would help women with less severe symptoms or would be more effective than other COCs. For women desiring contraception, these particular agents have only been evaluated for efficacy in PMDD when used for up to three cycles. The effects of other contraceptive agents for PMDD symptoms are currently under investigation.

OTHER AGENTS

Treatment with GnRH agonists has been used for the physical and psychological symptoms of PMS.[178] These agents are not typically used for long periods of time, however, because of vasomotor symptoms and the potential for negative long-term effects on bone. They also have to be administered by injection or nasal spray which may affect adherence. This treatment is reserved for women with very severe PMDD who do not respond to other treatments.

Danazol has been investigated for the treatment of PMS with moderate results. Danazol 200 mg orally BID provides greater symptom relief than placebo for symptoms of severe PMS; however, luteal phase treatment does not appear effective for PMS symptoms.[179] Potential side effects are also a concern with this agent, and therefore, its use in women should be limited to those who have failed other therapies.

C.P. has PMDD and does not need contraception because she uses condoms. Mood symptoms predominate and are impairing her functionality. An SSRI should be started in either a continuous or intermittent manner. C.P. appears to be a good candidate for intermittent therapy because she can adhere to the regimen and does not have a concurrent depression or anxiety disorder. An appropriate initial treatment regimen is fluoxetine 20 mg orally daily for the last 2 weeks of the menstrual cycle. Her response rate should be assessed after three cycles of treatment. An anxiolytic could be tried for symptoms not relieved by the SSRI.

KEY REFERENCES AND WEBSITES

A full list of references for this chapter can be found at http://thepoint.lww.com/AT11e. Below are the key references and websites for this chapter, with the corresponding reference number in this chapter found in parentheses after the reference.

Key References

American College of Obstetricians and Gynecologists. ACOG Practice Bulletin No. 114. Management of endometriosis. *Obstet Gynecol.* 2010;116:223. (116)

Brown J, Farquhar C. Endometriosis: an overview of Cochrane Reviews. *Cochrane Database Syst Rev.* 2014;(3):CD009590. doi:10.1002/14651858.CD009590.pub2.

Legro RS, et al. Diagnosis and treatment of polycystic ovary syndrome: an Endocrine Society clinical practice guideline. *J Clin Endocrinol Metab.* 2013;98:4565–4592.

Nevatte T et al. ISPMD consensus on the management of premenstrual disorders. *Arch Womens Ment Health.* 2013;16:279–291.

O'Brien PMS, Backstrom T, Brown C, et al. Towards a consensus on diagnostic criteria, measurement and trial design of the premenstrual disorders: the ISPMD Montreal consensus. *Arch Womens Ment Health.* 2011;14:13–21

Zahradnik HP et al. Nonsteroidal anti-inflammatory drugs and hormonal contraceptives for pain relief from dysmenorrhea: a review. *Contraception.* 2010;81:185. (99)

Key Websites

Androgen Excess and PCOS Society. http://www.ae-society.org. Accessed June 16, 2017.

Polycystic Ovarian Support Association. http://www.pcosupport.org. Accessed June 16, 2017.

51 The Transition Through Menopause

Louise Parent-Stevens and Trisha LaPointe

CORE PRINCIPLES

		CHAPTER CASES
1	Menopause is the natural progression of reproductive aging in women. It is characterized by declining ovarian function and decreased synthesis of sex hormones.	**Case 51-1 (Question 1), Figure 51-1**
2	Management of women who experience distressing symptoms associated with menopause, including hot flushes and genitourinary atrophy, is targeted at relieving symptoms while minimizing risks.	**Case 51-1 (Questions 1–6), Case 51-2 (Questions 1–2), Figure 51-2**
3	Estrogen therapy (ET), the most effective treatment for menopausal symptoms, is associated with significant risks, including thromboembolic disease and breast and endometrial cancer. Progestogens are added to systemic estrogen therapy (EPT) to provide protection against endometrial hyperplasia and cancer in women with an intact uterus. Women must be adequately counseled so that they can make educated decisions about treatment.	**Case 51-1 (Questions 3, 5), Table 51-1**
4	Hormone therapy (HT), including ET and EPT, can be achieved through a wide variety of dosage formulations and dosing regimens. Based on the current understanding of the risks and benefits of systemic HT, use should be limited to the management of menopausal symptoms at the lowest effective dose for the shortest time possible.	**Case 51-1 (Questions 4, 5), Table 51-2 and 51-3**
5	The optimal time for the use of HT is controversial; some studies suggest decreased cardiovascular risk when HT is initiated soon after menopause, whereas other studies show an increased risk of breast cancer when HT is started shortly after menopause.	**Case 51-1 (Question 3)**
6	Nonhormonal drugs, including serotonergic antidepressants and antiepileptic drugs, are useful alternatives in women who are unable or unwilling to take HT. Although use of herbal medicines for menopausal symptoms is common, efficacy and safety data on these products are limited.	**Case 51-1 (Questions 2, 6), Case 51-2 (Question 2), Table 51-4**
7	As vaginal atrophy does not wane with time after menopause, long-term use of low-dose vaginal estrogen can be recommended.	**Case 51-2 (Questions 1, 2)**

INCIDENCE, PREVALENCE, AND EPIDEMIOLOGY

The perimenopausal or climacteric phase in the female aging process (i.e., the time between the reproductive and nonreproductive years) is distinguished by waning ovarian function and irregular menstrual cycles. Menopause, the last spontaneous episode of physiologic uterine bleeding, is usually identified retrospectively after 12 months of amenorrhea and typically occurs 4 to 5 years after the onset of the perimenopause. If needed, menopause can be confirmed by a follicle-stimulating hormone (FSH) level greater than 40 international units/mL. Postmenopause is characterized by significantly decreased hormone levels that may contribute to an increased risk of disease, including osteoporosis and cardiovascular disease (CVD).[1,2]

The average age of women at menopause has remained relatively constant at 51 years despite a significant increase in life expectancy.[3] Women today may spend one-third of their lives in the postmenopausal state. There are an estimated 40 million postmenopausal women in the United States who are at risk for menopause-related health issues.[3,4] Age at menopause appears to be determined primarily by genetics but may be decreased by low body weight and poor health status. Cigarette smoking decreases age at menopause by 1 to 2 years.[5] Higher socioeconomic status and prior oral contraceptive use may increase age at menopause.[5] Cytotoxic drugs and radiotherapy may induce ovarian failure, and bilateral oophorectomy results in surgically induced menopause. Onset of menopause before age 40 is termed premature ovarian failure.

PATHOPHYSIOLOGY

Perimenopause results from an age-related acceleration in oocyte (immature female egg) degeneration and resistance to gonadotropins. The aging follicles produce less inhibin, which triggers increased production of FSH (Fig. 51-1).[6] Despite this increase in FSH levels, the declining ovary is unable to consistently produce mature follicles, resulting in frequent anovulatory cycles during the years approaching menopause. However, spontaneous ovulation can still occur, and contraception should be used if pregnancy is not desired. When all ovarian follicles have been depleted, menopause occurs. This corresponds with a 10- to 20-fold increase in FSH levels and a threefold increase in luteinizing hormone levels, which peak 1 to 3 years after menopause.[7]

Postmenopausal estrogen production is approximately 10% of premenopausal levels.[7,8] After menopause, circulating estrogen is largely estrone, whereas the more potent estradiol is the primary estrogen during the reproductive years.[7] Unlike the reproductive years, estrogen levels postmenopausally do not vary in a cyclic pattern. The source of postmenopausal estrogen is androstenedione, an androgen converted to estrogen by an aromatase enzyme found predominantly in fat, liver, and skin. Enzyme levels increase with age and body weight, resulting in higher estrogen levels in women with greater body fat.[7,9] The source of progesterone after menopause is the adrenal gland, because the failed ovary no longer produces progesterone. Androgen production declines by approximately 50% with normal aging; however, after menopause, the androgen-to-estrogen ratio increases markedly owing to the greater drop in estrogen levels, often resulting in mild symptoms of androgenism, such as hirsutism.[10]

CLINICAL PRESENTATION

The decrease in estrogen production associated with menopause can result in clinical symptoms, such as hot flushes and genitourinary atrophy. The risk for CVD, the leading cause of death in postmenopausal women, appears to be amplified by estrogen deficiency.[1,2,5,11] Postmenopausal osteoporosis may result from estrogen deficiency (see Chapter 110, Osteoporosis). Loss of estrogen has also been associated with adverse effects on cognition, neurologic functioning, well-being, and sexual health.[2] Other consequences of menopause may not yet be elucidated.

Signs and Symptoms

HOT FLUSHES

CASE 51-1

QUESTION 1: L.K., a 50-year-old woman, is having sudden feelings of warmth over her chest accompanied by flushing of her skin and increased sweating for the past month, especially after drinking coffee or wine or if she is upset. These symptoms often wake her at night. She had a menstrual period 3 weeks ago, but recently her menses have been irregular (five menses in the past 12 months.) Her physical examination is normal for a 50-year-old woman. Her last mammogram 6 months ago was normal. She does not smoke, and her body mass index is 24 kg/m^2. She has hypertension that is controlled with hydrochlorothiazide

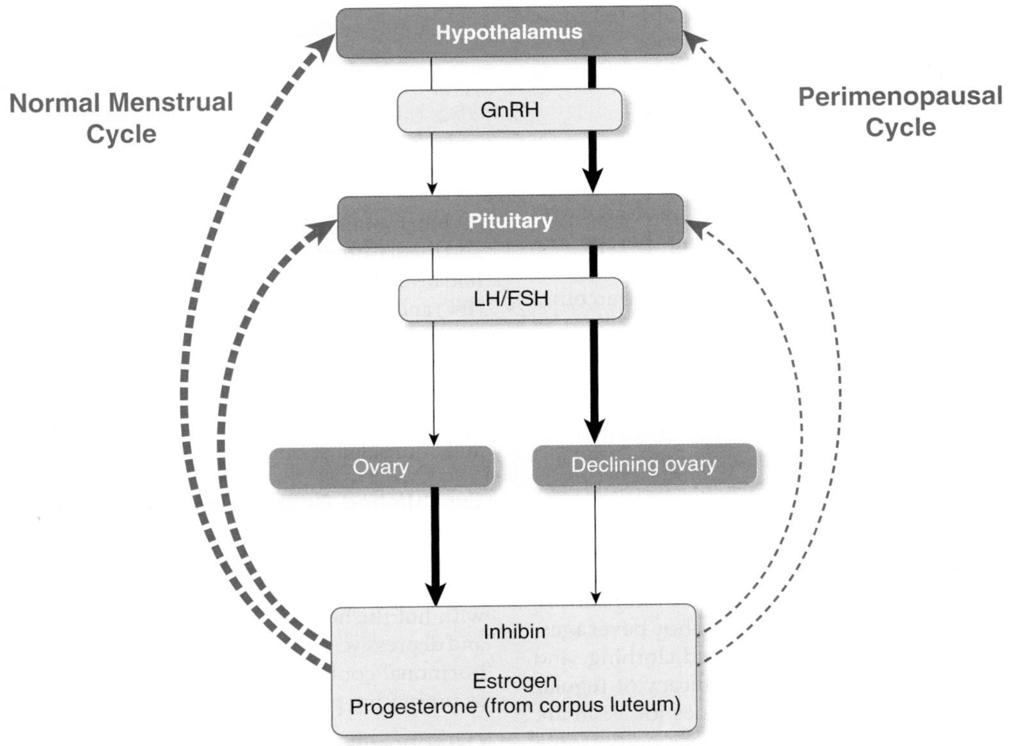

Figure 51-1 Perimenopausal changes in hypothalamus–pituitary–ovary axis. *Dashed line* indicates inhibitory effect, *Solid line* indicates stimulatory effect and *Wider line* indicates more pronounced effect. FSH, follicle-stimulating hormone; GnRH, gonadotropin-releasing hormone; LH, luteinizing hormone.

12.5 mg daily and migraine headaches without aura that she treats with sumatriptan 50 mg orally (PO) as needed. Her family history is positive for osteoporosis, but negative for CVD and breast cancer. Which of L.K.'s current symptoms are consistent with menopause?

It appears that L.K. is having hot flushes, a vasomotor symptom (VMS) experienced by 60% to 80% of women during the menopause transition.[12] The onset of VMS may precede the last menstrual period, but the prevalence peaks 1 year after menopause and declines with time since menopause.[13] Symptoms persist an average of 7 years; up to 30% of women may experience symptoms for longer than 10 years.[14] Obesity and surgically induced menopause are risk factors for more severe hot flushes.[15] Symptoms include a feeling of warmth in the chest, neck, and facial areas that may be accompanied by visible flushing and increased sweating. Nocturnal hot flushes (night sweats) cause nighttime awakening and may lead to insomnia and sleep deprivation. Hot flushes average approximately 4 minutes in duration and are characteristically episodic rather than continuous, but may occur hourly in women with severe symptoms.[10] Increased environmental temperature, ingestion of hot liquids or alcohol, and mental stress may provoke hot flushes.

The specific trigger for hot flushes is unknown, but they are clearly associated with the declining estrogen concentrations that occur during menopause. It is postulated that the drop in estrogen leads to a decrease in serotonin levels and an increase in the levels of norepinephrine and its metabolite, 3-methoxy-4-hydroxyphenylglycol. These hormones are involved in temperature regulation, and their fluctuations trigger an inappropriate activation of the body's heat-release mechanisms, leading to the cutaneous vasodilation and sweating seen with hot flushes.[10,16]

Cognitive and mood changes, including depression, are not uniformly associated with menopause, but are reported more frequently in women during the perimenopausal period.[17] Vaginal atrophy and urinary symptoms are also associated with menopause (see Case 51-2 Question 1).[10,18]

Overview of Therapy

Menopausal symptoms, while distressing, are not associated with increased mortality. Therefore, the goal of drug therapy in a symptomatic woman is to relieve symptoms and improve quality of life without increasing the risk of serious adverse outcomes related to the agents used.

TREATMENT

CASE 51-1, QUESTION 2: L.K. is seeking relief for her hot flushes but is not sure that she wants to use medications for this problem. What nonmedication therapies are appropriate for the management of L.K.'s hot flushes?

Lifestyle Modifications

First-line treatment for hot flushes is lifestyle modification, including avoidance of known triggers (e.g., hot beverages, alcohol, warm environments), wearing layered clothing, and use of personal cooling devices. Data on the efficacy of regular exercise, acupuncture, and relaxation techniques for VMS are limited.[19–21] If the patient continues to experience bothersome symptoms, drug therapy should be considered. It is noteworthy that placebo responses greater than 50% have been seen in clinical trials evaluating interventions for hot flushes.[22]

Black Cohosh

Black cohosh (*Cimicifuga racemosa*), an herbal product derived from a plant in the buttercup family, has a long tradition of use for the management of menopausal symptoms. It does not appear to have estrogenic effects, but may exert a serotonergic effect.[23] The efficacy of black cohosh for hot flushes is controversial; however, good results are reported in trials using a standardized extract containing 1 mg triterpene glycosides/20 mg tablet taken twice daily.[24] Black cohosh is generally well tolerated, but use beyond 12 months has not been evaluated. The most common adverse effects are gastrointestinal upset and rash. There have been case reports of hepatotoxicity which cannot be directly attributed to black cohosh.[23,24]

Phytoestrogens

Phytoestrogens, including isoflavones and lignans, are plant-based substances that exert mild estrogenic effects. Although epidemiologic studies show an association between higher dietary soy intake and fewer menopausal symptoms, meta-analyses of clinical trials of phytoestrogens concluded that they have minimal benefits on VMS.[22] However, several trials of the soy-derived isoflavone, genistein, reported significant improvement in VMS, which warrants further investigation.[22] In general, isoflavones are well tolerated; the most commonly reported side effect is gastrointestinal intolerance. Endometrial stimulation is rare but has been reported in a small number of patients after long-term use.[25,26] Because of their estrogenic effects, phytoestrogens should be avoided or used cautiously in women with a history of estrogen-dependent disease.

L.K. does not have any estrogen-dependent diseases and therefore could try either black cohosh or phytoestrogens for her hot flushes if lifestyle modifications do not provide adequate benefit. She should be counseled that these products have mixed data supporting their benefits and phytoestrogens could potentially have side effects similar to hormone therapy.

Hormone Therapy

CASE 51-1, QUESTION 3: L.K. returns to clinic after 2 months. She initiated lifestyle modifications and tried black cohosh but has noted worsening of her flushes, awakening multiple times nightly from night sweats, which is causing daytime fatigue and irritability. She asks about hormone therapy to control her hot flushes. Is L.K. a candidate for hormone therapy?

Hormone therapy (HT) has received a great deal of scientific and media attention during the past decade. The Women's Health Initiative (WHI), the only large, prospective study of estrogen therapy (ET) and estrogen/progestogen (EPT) therapy in postmenopausal women, and several large cohort studies have provided a great deal of data, some of it conflicting, on the risks and benefits of hormone use after menopause.[27–29] Before selecting a treatment option, women should be evaluated for contraindications to HT and counseled about its possible risks and benefits (Table 51-1).

Established Benefits of Hormone Therapy

Vasomotor Symptoms

Estrogen, with or without a progestogen, is well documented to reduce the frequency and severity of hot flushes. In women with hot flushes, HT has been shown to improve quality of life and depressive symptom.[27] During perimenopause, combination hormonal contraceptives are effective in reducing VMS as well as preventing pregnancy.

Osteoporosis

Estrogen, with or without a progestogen (ET/EPT), is proven to prevent bone loss associated with menopause, reducing the risk of osteoporotic hip and vertebral fractures by approximately 25%.[29]

Table 51-1
Risks and Benefits of Postmenopausal Hormone Therapy

	Evidence	Absolute or Relative Contraindications and Patient Considerations	References
Established Benefits[a]			
VMS	Systemic ET (in women without a uterus) or EPT (in women with a uterus) is most effective therapy for hot flushes. There may be a dose–response relationship. Oral and TD estrogens are equally effective.	This is the primary indication for the use of systemic hormone therapy.	45,79
Osteoporosis	Numerous clinical trials support reduced risk of vertebral and hip fractures with the use of estrogen.	Provides bone protection during use of ET/EPT for menopausal symptoms. May be used in recently menopausal women at risk for osteoporosis if other therapies are not feasible.	30,33,80
Vaginal atrophy	Numerous studies show both local and systemic estrogens reverse the atrophy induced by menopause.	Localized therapy should be used for patients with symptoms related solely to vaginal atrophy.	74,78
Established Risks[a]			
Thromboembolic disease	Increased risk of DVT and PE, greatest within the first year of use, risk with EPT possibly greater than with ET. TD estrogen has lower risk than oral estrogen.	**Absolute contraindication:** current tobacco use, history of thrombosis. **Relative contraindication:** obesity, women 65 years and older. Therapy should be discontinued before surgery or anticipated period of immobilization.	40–43,46
Breast cancer	Risk increased ~25% after 5 years of use, increases with continued use. Greater risk with EPT and shorter exposure gap.	**Absolute contraindication:** personal history of breast cancer. **Relative contraindication:** strong family history of breast cancer.	27,36,37
Cardiovascular disease	Increased risk of MI, when started >10 years after menopause or in women ≥60 years old (see also unconfirmed benefit).	**Relative contraindication:** age 60 years or older, >10 years postmenopause.	27
Endometrial cancer	Risk related to dose and duration of use. Addition of adequate progestogen reduces or eliminates risk.	Rationale for the use of concomitant progestogen in women with uterus. **Absolute contraindication:** undiagnosed postmenopausal vaginal bleeding, prior history of endometrial cancer.	34
Ischemic stroke	30%–50% increased risk for *ischemic* stroke seen. Dose-related risk seen with both ET and EPT, may be less with nonoral route. Risk greater with increasing age (because of underlying age-related risk of stroke). HT does not affect risk of *hemorrhagic* stroke.	**Absolute contraindication:** history of stroke or transient ischemic attacks, current tobacco use. **Relative contraindication:** obesity, uncontrolled hypertension, uncontrolled diabetes.	33,81
Gallbladder disease	~60% increased risk of cholecystitis, cholelithiasis seen with ET and EPT, less risk with nonoral route	**Relative contraindication:** history of gallbladder disease.	29,47
Hypertriglyceridemia	Oral estrogen increases triglycerides. Nonoral route has less effect. EPT may have less effect than ET alone owing to attenuating effect of progestogen.	**Relative contraindication:** hypertriglyceridemia. If estrogen is to be used in woman with elevated TG, select transdermal route and monitor TG levels.	27,82
Unconfirmed Benefits[b]			
Cardiovascular disease	No increased risk or possible decreased risk when initiated prior to age 60 and within 10 years of menopause (see also established risk).	Prevention of CVD is not a primary indication for use; this information can reassure patient needing HT for menopause symptoms or replacement for women with premature ovarian failure.	31,32
Colorectal cancer	Decreased risk is seen with EPT but not with ET.	May be secondary benefit in women using for hot flushes.	83

(continued)

Table 51-1
Risks and Benefits of Postmenopausal Hormone Therapy (*continued*)

	Evidence	Absolute or Relative Contraindications and Patient Considerations	References
Recurrent UTIs	Low-dose localized estrogen treatment can decrease risk for recurrent UTIs.	May be secondary benefit in women using localized therapy for vaginal atrophy.	84
Diabetes mellitus	Decreased incidence of new-onset diabetes in women taking EPT or ET.	This suggests that DM is not a contraindication for women who wish to use EPT/ET.	27
Unconfirmed Risks[b]			
Ovarian cancer	Increased risk seen with ET/EPT, longer durations of treatment	**Relative contraindication:** strong family history of ovarian cancer.	85
Lung cancer	Reports of protective effect but in WHI increased mortality from lung cancer seen in older current/past smokers.	**Absolute contraindication:** current tobacco use (owing to increased risk of TED).	27,28
Urinary incontinence	Systemic estrogen caused or worsened urinary incontinence, not seen with ultralow dose	Avoid systemic estrogen in women with urinary incontinence, monitor for new onset in women taking HT.	48,86
Cognitive effects	Studies report worsening of dementia in women with preexisting dementia; no improvement or protection in older women taking HT.	**Absolute contraindication:** patients with evidence of dementia. Avoid use in women ≥65 years.	87
Migraine headaches	HT may cause worsening of migraine headaches.	**Absolute contraindication:** migraine with aura (increased risk of stroke). **Relative contraindication:** migraine without aura—monitor for changes in HA frequency.	88

[a]Well-documented risk or benefit supported by multiple clinical studies.
[b]Possible risk or benefit shown in limited clinical trials, additional data needed to confirm.
CVD, cardiovascular disease; DM, diabetes mellitus; DVT, deep venous thrombosis; EPT, estrogen and progestogen therapy; ET, estrogen therapy; HA, headache; HT, hormone therapy; MI, myocardial infarction; PE, pulmonary embolism; TD, transdermally; TED, thromboembolic disease; TG, triglycerides; UTI, urinary tract infection; WHI, women's health initiative.

Many estrogen products are US Food and Drug Administration (FDA)-approved for the prevention (but not treatment) of osteoporosis (Table 51-2), and ET or EPT may be used for the prevention of osteoporosis in recently menopausal women, even in the absence of menopausal symptoms, if alternate osteoporosis therapies cannot be used.[27] Systemic ET maintains bone density, but bone loss resumes with estrogen discontinuation. Alternative therapies should be considered in women at risk for osteoporosis who stop ET or avoid its use altogether (see Chapter 110, Osteoporosis).[27,30]

Cardiovascular Disease

The cardiovascular effects of HT are not fully elucidated. Analysis of data from the WHI and other studies found no increased risk of coronary heart disease in women aged 50 to 59 years who began therapy within 10 years of menopause, and a possible reduced risk in women initiating therapy prior to age 55 and within 2 to 3 years of menopause, whereas an increased risk of CVD was seen in women aged 60 years and older who initiated HT more than 10 years after menopause.[31,32] In younger patients such as L.K. who initiate HT for VMS soon after the onset of menopause, the risk of CVD is not significantly increased.

Other Possible Benefits

Other less established benefits of HT (Table 51-1) include effects on urinary tract infections, diabetes mellitus, and colorectal cancer.[33]

Established Risks of Hormone Therapy

Cardiovascular Disease

As noted above, an increased risk of CVD has been noted in women over the age of 60 years who initiated HT more than 10 years postmenopause.[31,32]

Endometrial Cancer

Endometrial proliferation from exogenous estrogen exposure leads to hyperplasia rates of 8% to 62% after 1 to 3 years of use.[34] In a woman with a uterus, use of ET alone increases the risk of endometrial cancer by twofold to 10-fold, with higher estrogen dose and longer duration associated with greater risk.[27] The risk persists for several years after discontinuation of ET.[27] Addition of adequate progestogen significantly attenuates or eliminates the increased risk of endometrial cancer; a progestogen should be added to ET in a woman with an intact uterus (see Case 51-1, Question 4).[27,34]

Breast Cancer

Studies demonstrate a 25% overall increased risk of invasive breast cancer with EPT use, becoming significant 5 years after initiation, increasing with continued use, and returning to baseline approximately 5 years after EPT is stopped.[27,33,35] ET increases this risk less than EPT.[36,37] Risk appears to be similar between oral and transdermal therapies, and no dose–response relationship has been established. Risk may be lower in overweight/obese women.[36] A short time frame between the onset of menopause and initiation of HT appears to significantly increase the risk for breast cancer compared with a longer interval.[27,33,38]

Thromboembolic Disease

HT use increases the overall risk for venous thromboembolic disease (TED), including deep venous thrombosis and pulmonary embolism, twofold.[27] This risk may be mediated by inhibition of hepatic synthesis of anticoagulant factors, including antithrombin, protein S, and protein C.[39] Transdermal estrogen appears to have a significantly lower risk than oral estrogen as it avoids the first-pass metabolic effects of oral therapy.[33,40,41] Observational data suggest that synthetic progesterone derivatives but not bio-identical progesterone further increases risk of TED.[41,42] Women who are older, have a higher body mass index, or have a prothrombotic mutation are at additional increased risk.[43] The

Table 51-2
Agents Labeled for Use in ET and EPT

Drug (Brand Name)	Route, Initial Dosage
Estrogens, Systemic[b]	
Conjugated equine estrogens (Premarin)[a]	PO 0.3 mg
Synthetic conjugated estrogens (Enjuvia)	PO 0.3 mg
Estropipate (piperazine estrone sulfate) (Ortho-Est)[a,c]	PO 0.75 mg
Micronized estradiol (Estrace)[a,c]	PO 0.5 mg
Estradiol transdermal system (various brand name products)[a]	TD 0.014 (ultralow dose)–0.025 mg/24-hour patch applied weekly or twice weekly
Esterified estrogen (Menest)[a]	PO 0.3 mg
Estradiol acetate tablet (Femtrace)[c]	PO 0.45 mg
Estradiol acetate vaginal ring (Femring)[c]	HDV 0.05 mg/24 hour ring inserted vaginally every 90 days
Estradiol topical emulsion/gel/solution (Divigel, Elestrin, Estrogel, Estrasorb, Evamist)[c]	TD 0.0125 mg to 0.75 mg (product dependent)
Progestogens (Minimum Recommended Dose to Prevent Endometrial Hyperplasia)[34]	
Medroxyprogesterone acetate (Provera generic and combo products)	PO 5 mg for sequential regimens; 2.5 mg for continuous regimens
Norethindrone acetate (Aygestin generic and combo products)	PO 2.5 mg for sequential regimens; 1 mg for continuous regimens
Micronized progesterone (Prometrium)[c]	PO 200 mg for sequential regimens; 100 mg for continuous regimens
Progesterone vaginal gel (Prochieve, Crinone)[c] Progesterone vaginal suppository (First Progesterone VGS)	V one full applicator of 4% gel every other day V 200 mg/day for 12 days
Levonorgestrel-releasing IUD (Mirena)	IU 0.02 mg/day
Examples of Estrogen and Progestogen Combination Products	
Prempro[a]	PO 0.3 mg CEE and 1.5 mg MPA
Premphase[a]	PO 0.625 mg CEE for 28 days with 5 mg MPA for last 14 days
Climara Pro[a,c] (estrogen)	TD 0.045 mg estradiol/0.015 mg levonorgestrel/24-hour patch once weekly
Low-dose Vaginal Estrogens (Localized Effect Only)	
Conjugated equine estrogen cream (Premarin)	LDV initial: 0.5–2 g cream (0.3125–1.25 mg CEE) daily Maintenance: 0.5–2 g cream (0.3125–1.25 mg CEE) once/twice weekly based on severity
Estradiol cream (Estrace)[c]	LDV initial: 2–4 g cream (0.2–0.4 mg estradiol) daily Maintenance: 1 g cream (0.1 mg estradiol) twice weekly
Estradiol ring (Estring)[c]	LDV 2-mg ring (0.0075 mg/day) every 90 days
Estradiol hemihydrate tablets (Vagifem and Vagifem LD)	LDV one tablet (0.01 mg) daily for 2 weeks, then one tablet twice weekly

[a]Approved by the US Food and Drug Administration for prevention of osteoporosis.
[b]Requires addition of progestogen in women with a uterus.
[c]FDA-approved bio-identical hormone.
CEE, conjugated equine estrogens; HDV, high-dose vaginal estrogen, sufficient absorption to produce systemic estrogenic effect (i.e., for treatment of hot flushes); IU, intrauterine; IUD, intrauterine device; LDV, low-dose vaginal estrogen, provides localized estrogenic effect (i.e., for vaginal atrophy), owing to low-dose, minimal systemic absorption; MPA, medroxyprogesterone acetate; PO, orally; TD, transdermally; V, vaginal.
Source: Facts & Comparisons eAnswers. **http://online.factsandcomparisons.com/index.aspx**. Accessed June 23, 2015.

risk is greatest within the first year of treatment and decreases upon discontinuation of HT. HT should be avoided in women with a history of or at high risk for TED.[27,43]

Other Possible Risks

Other risks with HT include potential adverse effects on cognition and urinary tract function, an increased risk of stroke and the development of ovarian and lung cancer and gallbladder disease[33] (Table 51-1).

Recommendations

Current guidelines on systemic HT recommend its use only in women with moderate-to-severe hot flushes (Fig. 51-2).[27] For women with premature ovarian failure, it is recommended that HT be given until the typical age of natural menopause to avoid early manifestations of estrogen deficiency.[28,44]

As L.K. continues to experience severe hot flushes that are affecting her quality of life, she is recently postmenopausal, and she has no absolute contraindications to estrogen (such as TED, history of breast or endometrial cancer, uncontrolled hypertension, migraine with aura, tobacco use, obesity), a trial of HT is appropriate.

SELECTION OF THERAPY

CASE 51-1, QUESTION 4: What is an appropriate HT regimen for the management of L.K.'s hot flushes?

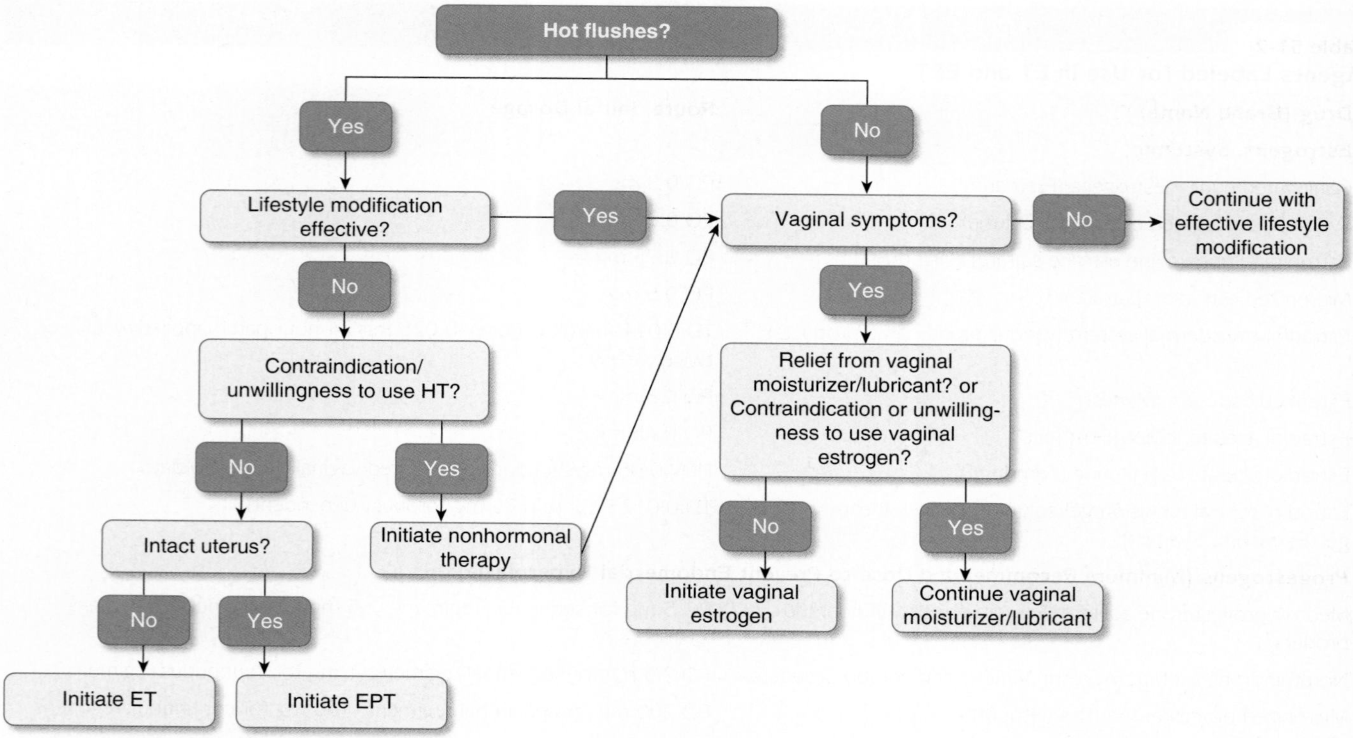

Figure 51-2 Algorithm for the management of symptomatic menopausal women. EPT, estrogen/progestogen therapy; ET, estrogen therapy; HT, hormone therapy.

Estrogens

There are a number of hormonal products currently available for the management of VMS (Table 51-2). Oral and nonoral estrogens appear to be equally efficacious in treating VMS.[27,45] Because it avoids first-pass metabolism, nonoral estrogen is associated with a lower risk for TED, hypertension, and gallbladder disease than oral ET.[42,46,47]

Current recommendations are to initiate estrogen at a low dose (e.g., 0.3 mg of conjugated equine estrogens or 0.025 mg of transdermal estradiol). Ultralow-dose estrogen (TD estradiol 0.014 mg/day) reduces the risk of harm but may not adequately control menopausal symptoms.[48,49] If symptoms persist after 2 to 3 weeks of therapy, the dose of estrogen can be increased to the next available dosage strength for the product being used (Table 51-2).[27]

Bio-identical Hormones

There is strong consumer interest in natural (bio-identical) HT (BHT) as a potentially safer alternative to synthetic estrogens. BHTs are defined as having the same chemical structure as the hormones produced by the human reproductive system and include estradiol, estrone, progesterone, and testosterone. Studies of commercially available BHT products demonstrate a similar efficacy to synthetic hormones; however, clinical evidence to support claims of greater safety is lacking.[50,51] Women desiring to use bio-identical products should be advised of commercially available products (Table 51-2); extemporaneously compounded BHT does not carry FDA-approved warnings and may be of inadequate quality.[51,52]

Progestogens

In women with an intact uterus, such as L.K., a progestogen must be added to the regimen to minimize the risk of endometrial cancer (Table 51-3).[27] Currently, there is no indication for adding a progestogen to ET in women without a uterus. There does not appear to be a difference in the endometrial protective effect between progestogens. Combined continuous regimens may provide better endometrial protection than sequential regimens (Table 51-3). Although not FDA-approved for this indication, progesterone vaginal gel and progestogen-releasing intrauterine systems protect against endometrial hyperplasia from ET.[53–55]

EPT may result in resumption of uterine withdrawal bleeding. The pattern and frequency of bleeding depend on the EPT regimen used (Table 51-3).[56] Lower doses of estrogen are associated with a lower risk of bleeding.[57,58] Patient preference regarding bleeding patterns should be considered when selecting an EPT regimen.

Progestogen monotherapy appears to be similar to estrogen in relieving the symptoms of VMS. Effective regimens include megestrol acetate, 40 mg/day orally, micronized progesterone 300 mg/day orally, and medroxyprogesterone acetate, 10 mg/day orally, 150 mg intramuscularly every 3 months or 400 mg intramuscularly one time.[59–62] Adverse effects of progestogens include vaginal bleeding, fluid retention, increased appetite, breast tenderness, acne, hirsutism, headaches, mood swings, fatigue, and depression. In the absence of ET, progestogens do not appear to increase the risk of TED.[61] However, data on long-term safety, especially in regard to breast cancer, are lacking. Progestogen monotherapy for the treatment of hot flushes is generally reserved for women with contraindications to estrogen use.

DURATION OF HORMONE THERAPY

As some risks of HT increase with longer use, use beyond 5 years has generally not been recommended. However, as many women continue to have VMS beyond this time frame, a thorough risk versus benefit review is needed to determine the appropriate duration for each woman.[63] Because hot flushes are self-limiting, it can be difficult to assess whether symptom relief is related to the treatment or natural resolution of symptoms. Six to 12 months after L.K.'s hot flushes are fully treated, she should attempt discontinuation of EPT. There are no specific guidelines for withdrawing therapy; typical taper regimens involve decreasing the daily estrogen dose to the next available dosage strength or increasing the dosing interval. If symptoms recur during the taper, therapy can be resumed at the lowest effective dose and another taper attempted in 6 months.[64–66]

Table 51-3
ET/EPT Regimens and Expected Vaginal Bleeding Patterns[56,89,90]

Estrogen/Progestogen Dosing	Hormone-Free Interval	Typical Bleeding Pattern
Combined Regimens (EPT) for Patient with Intact Uterus		
Intermittent Sequential		
Estrogen (PO or TD): days 1–25 of each month Progestogen: days 10–25 or 14–25 of each month	3–6 days	Withdrawal bleeding[c] 1–2 days after progestogen dosing ended[a] ~80% experience regular bleeding
Combined Sequential		
Estrogen (PO or TD) and progestogen: days 1–25 of each month	3–6 days	Withdrawal bleeding[c] 1–2 days after progestogen dosing ended[a] Lower incidence than cyclic regimen
Continuous Sequential		
Estrogen (PO or TD): daily Progestogen: 10–14 days every month	None	Withdrawal bleeding[c] 1–2 days after progestogen dosing ended[a] ~80% experience regular bleeding
Long-cycle Sequential		
Estrogen (PO or TD): daily Progestogen: 14 days every third month	None	Withdrawal bleeding[c] 1–2 days after progestogen dosing ended[a] ~70% experience regular bleeding
Continuous Combined		
Estrogen (PO or TD) and progestogen: daily	None	~40% have irregular bleeding for first 6–12 months[b] ~75%–89% become amenorrheic within 12 months
Continuous Pulsed		
Estrogen PO × 3 days then Estrogen + Progestogen PO × 3 days Repeat continuously	None	~70% experience spotting[d] early during treatment ~80% are amenorrheic at the end of 12 months[b]
Estrogen-only Regimens (ET) for Patients Without Uterus		
Continuous Regimen		
Estrogen (PO or TD): daily	None	None

[a]Bleeding earlier than 11 days after beginning of the progestogen suggests need for endometrial evaluation.
[b]Bleeding more than 1 year after initiation of therapy requires endometrial evaluation.
[c]Withdrawal bleeding is vaginal bleeding for multiple days (usually <10 days) that resembles menstrual period and requires use of a tampon or sanitary pad.
[d]Spotting is light bleeding that lasts <1 day.
EPT, estrogen and progestogen therapy; ET, estrogen therapy; PO, orally; TD, transdermally.

ADVERSE EFFECTS

Case 51-1, Question 5: To minimize the risks of TED, L.K. is prescribed a combination estrogen/progestogen patch. How should she be counseled about possible side effects of EPT?

In addition to being counseled about the serious risks of EPT, L.K. should be advised regarding nuisance side effects from HT. These most commonly include resumption of vaginal bleeding and breast tenderness.[27,56] Nausea, weight gain, edema, headache, premenstrual syndrome-like symptoms, and increased vaginal discharge have also been reported. Skin irritation may occur with the use of transdermal products. Frequently, these side effects diminish with time or may respond to a change in dosage or product. Although ET and EPT have not been shown to consistently induce or worsen hypertension, patients with hypertension, such as L.K., should be monitored for increases in blood pressure.[67]

TISSUE-SELECTIVE ESTROGEN COMPLEX

The tissue-selective estrogen complex (TSEC) of conjugated estrogen (CE) and the selective estrogen receptor modulator (SERM), bazedoxifene (BZA), is FDA-approved for the treatment of VMS and the prevention of osteoporosis in postmenopausal women with a uterus. The CE component of this agent reduces VMS and prevents bone loss whereas the estrogen-antagonistic properties of BZA in the breast and uterus mitigate the effects of estrogen on these tissues, eliminating the need for concurrent progestogen.[68] Although not approved for this indication, studies suggest that CE/BZA improves symptoms of vaginal atrophy.[69] Clinical trials have demonstrated that CE/BZA produces fewer bleeding events and breast symptoms than the traditional combination of CE/MPA.[68] This agent is an alternative for women with a uterus who are unable or unwilling to use EPT due to adverse effects.

NONHORMONAL AGENTS

Case 51-1, Question 6: L.K. returns 3 months later. Her hot flushes and night sweats resolved with EPT, but she experienced worsening of her migraine headaches, so she discontinued HT. Her hot flushes recurred soon thereafter. What alternative therapies are available for the management of L.K.'s symptoms?

Table 51-4

Nonhormonal Agents for the Management of Vasomotor Symptoms[70–73,91]

Drug	Recommended Dosage	Adverse Reactions Reported
Serotonergic Antidepressants		
Citalopram (Celexa)	10–30 mg	Dry mouth, ↓ libido, rash/hives, insomnia, somnolence, bladder spasm, palpitations, arthralgias
Desvenlafaxine (Pristiq)	50–100 mg	Asthenia, chills, anorexia, nausea, vomiting, constipation, diarrhea, dizziness, nervousness, mydriasis, dry mouth
Escitalopram (Lexapro)	10–20 mg	Dizziness, lightheadedness, nausea, vivid dreams, increased sweating
Fluoxetine (Prozac)	10–20 mg	Nausea, dry mouth
Paroxetine hydrochloride (Paxil, Paxil CR)	10–20 mg 12.5–25 mg (CR)	Headache, nausea, insomnia, drowsiness
Paroxetine mesylate[a] (Brisdelle)	7.5 mg	
Sertraline (Zoloft)	50 mg	Nausea, fatigue/malaise, diarrhea, anxiety/nervousness
Venlafaxine (Effexor, Effexor XR)	37.5–75 mg 37.5–150 mg XR	Dry mouth, ↓ appetite, nausea, constipation, possible increase in blood pressure at higher doses
Antiseizure Agents		
Gabapentin (Neurontin)	900 mg, possibly up to 2,400 mg	Somnolence, fatigue, dizziness, rash, palpitations, peripheral edema
Pregabalin (Lyrica)	150–300 mg	Dizziness, sleepiness, weight gain, cognitive difficulty
Antihypertensive Agents		
Clonidine	PO: 0.05–0.15 mg TD: 0.1 mg/24 hour	Headache, dry mouth, drowsiness Skin reaction/itching (patch only), risk of rebound HTN if stopped abruptly

[a]FDA-approved for the management of vasomotor symptoms.
HTN, hypertension; PO, orally; TD, transdermally.

Nonhormonal agents, including serotonergic antidepressants and antiepileptic agents, are modestly effective in reducing hot flush frequency and severity. (Table 51-4) Decreased estrogen levels are thought to regulate endorphin concentrations in the hypothalamus thereby affecting serotonin and norepinephrine levels in the thermoregulatory area of the hypothalamus.[70] In clinical trials of serotonergic antidepressants, relief of vasomotor symptoms was seen at lower doses and with a more rapid onset than is seen for their antidepressant effects.[71,72] Venlafaxine and paroxetine, the most studied agents, are considered the drugs of choice; other selective serotonin reuptake inhibitors and serotonin and norepinephrine reuptake inhibitors are considered second-line agents.[72] Low-dose paroxetine mesylate is FDA-approved for the treatment of vasomotor symptoms; the dose of 7.5 mg is lower than that required for the treatment of psychiatric disorders.[70] Studies have shown that paroxetine mesylate is effective in decreasing the severity and frequency of vasomotor symptoms. Dosing should be initiated at the lowest effective dose (Table 51-4); this can be increased after 2 to 3 weeks if the patient has an inadequate response. Patients should be advised not to discontinue therapy abruptly to avoid withdrawal symptoms. Commonly seen side effects of nonhormonal agents are listed in Table 51-4. Of particular concern in postmenopausal women is the risk for anorgasmia and loss of libido; similar sexual dysfunction may also occur as a result of menopause. Patients should be advised to discuss the problem with their care provider if it occurs and is bothersome. The antiepileptic drug gabapentin has been shown in multiple studies to decrease hot flushes through an unidentified mechanism. The therapeutic effect occurs at a dose of 900 mg/day with an onset within 4 weeks of initiation of treatment. To minimize side effects, dosing should be initiated at 300 mg daily and titrated up in 300-mg/day increments as tolerated. Although one study showed benefit with 2,400 mg/day, the optimal dose of gabapentin for hot flushes is unknown.[71,73]

Paroxetine mesylate 7.5 mg daily can be tried in L.K. If her symptoms are not improved after 2 to 3 weeks, the dose can be titrated up to a maximum dose of 25 mg daily.

Genitourinary Atrophy

SIGNS AND SYMPTOMS

CASE 51-2

Question 1: B.L., a 57-year-old woman, presents with a complaint of persistent vaginal dryness and irritation as well as pain associated with intercourse. She has tried vaginal lubricants, which help with intercourse-related pain but do not relieve her daily vaginal symptoms. She experienced menopause at age 50, which was accompanied by moderate hot flushes for 2 to 3 years that have since resolved without intervention. She denies symptoms of urinary incontinence. She does not smoke. On physical examination, her labia minora have a pale, dry appearance, and the labia majora appear flattened. Her vagina is small with a pale, dry epithelium. What is causing B.L.'s condition?

B.L. appears to be experiencing symptoms associated with genitourinary atrophy. Estrogen is the dominant hormone of vaginal physiology. With the postmenopausal loss of estrogen production, the vagina decreases in size and loses its rugal pattern. The mucosa becomes pale, thin, and dry, and vaginal blood flow decreases. A decrease in *Lactobacillus* production of lactic acid leads to an increase in vaginal pH to 5.0 or greater (compared with a premenopausal pH of 3.5–4.5).[18,74,75] These changes make the vagina more susceptible to infection from bacterial colonization and localized trauma secondary to intercourse. Unlike hot flushes, vaginal atrophy does not abate with time since menopause.

Symptoms of atrophic vaginitis include dryness, itching, pain, and dyspareunia (painful coitus). About 10% to 40% of postmenopausal women experience symptoms; however, only 7% of patients report these symptoms to their provider.[74] Postmenopausal women who engage in regular coital activity have less atrophic vaginal changes compared with those of similar age and estrogen levels who do not have regular intercourse.

TREATMENT

CASE 51-2, QUESTION 2: What would be an appropriate regimen for B.L. to decrease her vaginal symptoms?

Nonhormonal Treatment

First-line treatment includes vaginal moisturizers (e.g., Replens), which adhere to the vaginal mucosa, can improve vaginal symptoms but do not reverse atrophy.[75,76] Personal lubricants (e.g., KY jelly or liquid) can be used for women experiencing dyspareunia related to vaginal atrophy. Patients report symptom relief within 3 months of continuous treatment. Nonhormonal treatments used for vasomotor symptoms do not improve vaginal atrophy symptoms.[18,74,75]

Ospemifene (Osphena) is a vaginal tissue-specific estrogen agonist/antagonist. Ospemifene 60 mg once a day has demonstrated significant improvement in dyspareunia and vaginal atrophy. Duration should be restricted to the shortest amount of time possible based on patient's goals. Although ospemifene does not contain estrogen, it does have estrogen agonist effects and postmenopausal women with an intact uterus should be placed on progestin therapy as well. Serious adverse effects include increased risk of endometrial cancer and cardiovascular disorders.[77]

Localized Estrogen Treatment

Estrogen therapy reverses vaginal epithelial thinning, decreases the vaginal pH, and improves the symptoms of vaginal atrophy. Vaginal estrogen therapy has been shown to be more effective than systemic oral estrogen therapy, resulting in 80% to 90% response of vaginal atrophy.[74] For vaginal symptoms alone, low-dose vaginal estrogen is the preferred treatment.[74] The available products (Table 51-2) appear to be equivalent in restoring vaginal cytology and pH and relieving symptoms of vaginal dryness, pruritus, and dyspareunia; product selection should be based on patient preference.[74] Vaginal creams and tablets are initiated with once-daily dosing; after symptoms have resolved, the patient should be switched to maintenance dosing of once- or twice-weekly administration. The low-dose vaginal ring releases a constant dose of estrogen for 90 days.

The most common adverse effects of vaginal estrogens are vaginal irritation and bleeding and breast tenderness. Based on limited studies, the risk of endometrial hyperplasia from low-dose vaginal estrogen is small, and the addition of a progestogen is generally considered unnecessary.[74,78] Women at high risk for endometrial cancer, using higher than usual doses of vaginal estrogen, or experiencing vaginal bleeding during intravaginal ET, should be evaluated for endometrial hyperplasia.[74]

Because B.L. has not had relief with nonhormonal therapy, localized ET such as conjugated estrogen, 1 g of 0.625 mg/g cream, applied vaginally once daily is appropriate. After her symptoms have resolved, the dose can be decreased to a maintenance regimen of twice-weekly administration.

KEY REFERENCES AND WEBSITES

A full list of references for this chapter can be found at http://thepoint.lww.com/AT11e. Below are the key references and websites for this chapter, with the corresponding reference number in this chapter found in parentheses after the reference.

Key References

Carroll DG, Kelley KW. Use of antidepressants for management of hot flashes. *Pharmacotherapy*. 2009;29:1357. (73)

MacBride MB et al. Vulvovaginal atrophy. *Mayo Clin Proc*. 2010;85:87. (75)

McBane SE et al. Use of compounded bioidentical hormone therapy in menopausal women: an opinion statement of the Women's Health Practice and Research Network of the American College of Clinical Pharmacy. *Pharmacotherapy*. 2014;34:410. (51)

Mintziori G et al. EMAS position statement: non-hormonal management of menopausal vasomotor symptoms. *Maturitas*. 2015;81:410. (91)

Mirkin S et al. Conjugated estrogen/bazedoxifene tablets for the treatment of moderate-to-severe vasomotor symptoms associated with menopause. *Womens Health (Lond)*. 2014;10:135. (68)

North American Menopause Society. The 2012 hormone therapy position statement of The North American Menopause Society. *Menopause*. 2012;19:257. (27)

The North American Menopause Society (NAMS) 2013 Symptomatic Vulvavaginal Atrophy Advisory Panel. Management of symptomatic vulvo-vaginal atrophy: 2013 position statement of The North American Menopause Society. *Menopause*. 2013;20(9):888–902. (74)

Santen RJ et al. Executive summary: postmenopausal hormone therapy: an Endocrine Society Scientific Statement. *J Clin Endocrinol Metab*. 2010;95(7, Suppl 1):S1. (33)

Simon JA et al. Low-dose paroxetine 7.5 mg for menopausal vasomotor symptoms: two randomized controlled trails. *Menopause*. 2013;20(10):1027–1035. (70)

Vuvojic S et al. EMAS position statement: managing women with premature ovarian failure. *Maturitas*. 2010;67:91. (44)

Key Websites

European Menopause and Andropause Society. http://www.emas-online.org/home.

NAMS: The North American Menopause Society. http://www.menopause.org.

Women's Health Initiative. https://www.whi.org/SitePages/WHI%20Home.aspx.

SECTION 11 | Endocrine Disorders

Section Editor: Jennifer D. Goldman

52 Thyroid Disorders

Eric F. Schneider and Betty J. Dong

CORE PRINCIPLES

		CHAPTER CASES
1	Thyroid function tests are essential to confirm the presence of thyroid disorders but can be altered by acute and chronic illness and certain drugs. Thyrotropin (TSH) is the most accurate indicator of euthyroidism.	**Case 52-1 (Questions 1, 2), Case 52-2 (Question 1), Case 52-3 (Question 1), Case 52-4 (Question 1), Case 52-5 (Question 5), Case 52-23 (Question 1), Case 52-24 (Question 1), Table 52-1 and 52-7 Figure 52-1 and 52-2**
2	Thyroid hormone deficiency can cause a goiter and hypothyroid symptoms including myxedema coma, heart failure, and hyperlipidemia. The most common cause of hypothyroidism is Hashimoto's thyroiditis.	**Case 52-5 (Question 1), Case 52-8 (Question 2), Case 52-9 (Question 2), Case 52-10 (Question 1), Case 52-11 (Questions 1, 2), Case 52-12 (Question 1), Case 52-13 (Question 1), Case 52-20 (Question 1), Tables 52-2 and 52-3**
3	Generic or branded levothyroxine (L-thyroxine) is the preparation of choice for optimal correction of hypothyroidism. Triiodothyronine (T_3)-containing preparations are not necessary because thyroxine (T_4) is converted to T_3.	**Case 52-5 (Question 2), Case 52-6 (Question 1), Case 52-10 (Question 2), Tables 52-4 and 52-8**
4	The signs and symptoms of hypothyroidism can be corrected by the administration of l-thyroxine on an empty stomach at average oral replacement dosages of 1.6 to 1.7 mcg/kg/day or intravenously. Dosing is altered by weight, comorbidities, and drug interactions.	**Case 52-5 (Questions 3–5), Case 52-7 (Question 1), Case 52-8 (Question 1), Case 52-9 (Question 1), Case 52-10 (Question 2), Case 52-11 (Question 3), Table 52-4, 52-8 and 52-9**
5	The signs and symptoms of hyperthyroidism mimic those of adrenergic excess (e.g., tachycardia, tremors, thyroid storm), but symptoms in the elderly may be absent ("apathetic"). Graves' disease, a common cause of hyperthyroidism, can be complicated by ophthalmopathy.	**Case 52-14 (Questions 1, 2), Case 52-15 (Question 1), Case 52-21 (Questions 1, 2), Case 52-22 (Questions 1, 2), Table 52-5 and 52-6, Figure 52-3**
6	Management of hyperthyroidism includes thioamides, iodides, radioactive iodine, and surgery. β-Blockers can provide symptomatic relief of hyperthyroid symptoms.	**Case 52-15 (Questions 2–9, 12), Case 52-16 (Question 1), Case 52-19 (Questions 1, 2), Case 52-20 (Question 1), Case 52-22 (Question 2), Table 52-10**

Continued

		CHAPTER CASES
7	Methimazole is preferable to propylthiouracil except during the first trimester of pregnancy and during thyroid storm. Thioamide toxicity includes gastrointestinal symptoms, rash, agranulocytosis, and hepatitis.	**Case 52-15 (Questions 4–8, 10, 11), Case 52-18 (Question 1)**
8	Both hypothyroidism and hyperthyroidism can alter metabolism of coadministered medications (e.g., digoxin, warfarin).	**Case 52-14 (Questions 2, 3)**
9	The management of subclinical hypothyroidism and hyperthyroidism should be individualized.	**Case 52-12 (Question 1), Case 52-17 (Question 1)**
10	Certain drugs (e.g., amiodarone, interferon, lithium, tyrosine kinase inhibitors) can cause thyroid disorders.	**Case 52-23 (Question 1), Case 52-24 (Question 1), Table 52-2 and 52-6**

OVERVIEW

Thyroid disease, including hypothyroidism, hyperthyroidism, and nodular disease, is common, affecting 5% to 15% of the general population. Women are affected 3 to 4 times more than men. Triiodothyronine (T_3) and thyroxine (T_4) are the two biologically active thyroid hormones produced by the thyroid gland. The hypothalamic thyrotropin-releasing hormone (TRH) stimulates release of thyrotropin (i.e., thyroid-stimulating hormone [TSH]) from the pituitary in response to low circulating levels of thyroid hormone. TSH in turn promotes hormone synthesis and release by increasing thyroid activity. High circulating thyroid hormone levels block further production by inhibiting TSH release (negative feedback). As the serum concentrations of thyroid hormone decrease, the hypothalamic-pituitary centers again become responsive by releasing TRH and TSH (Fig. 52-1).

T_3 is 4 times more potent than T_4, the major circulating hormone secreted by the thyroid. About 80% of the total daily T_3 production results from the peripheral deiodination of T_4 to T_3 Approximately 35% to 40% of secreted T_4 is converted peripherally to T_3; another 45% of secreted T_4 undergoes peripheral conversion to inactive reverse T_3 (rT_3). Certain drugs and diseases can modify the conversion rate of T_4 to T_3 and reduce the serum T_3 levels (Table 52-1[1,2]; see Case 52-1, Question 2).

T_4 exists in the circulation as 0.03% free (active) and 99.97% protein-bound (inactive), primarily to thyroxine-binding globulin (TBG). This affinity for plasma proteins accounts for T_4's slow metabolic degradation and long half-life ($t_{1/2}$) of 7 days. T_3 is less strongly bound to plasma proteins (99.7%); with about 0.3% free. The lower protein-binding affinity of T_3 accounts for its threefold greater metabolic potency and its shorter $t_{1/2}$ of 1.5 days.

Hypothyroidism is a clinical syndrome that results from a deficiency of thyroid hormone. The prevalence of hypothyroidism is 1.4% to 2% in women and 0.1% to 0.2% in men and is increased in persons older than 60 years, to 6% of women and 2.5% of men. Hypothyroidism can be caused by either primary (thyroid gland) or less commonly, by secondary (hypothalamic-pituitary) malfunction.

Hashimoto's thyroiditis, an autoimmune disorder, is the most common cause of primary hypothyroidism and appears to have a strong genetic predisposition. The pathogenesis of Hashimoto's thyroiditis results from an impaired immune surveillance, causing dysfunction of normal suppressor T lymphocytes and excessive production of thyroid antibodies by plasma cells (differentiated B lymphocytes). The destruction of thyroid cells by circulating thyroid antibodies produces an underlying defect or block in the intrathyroidal, organobinding of iodide. The typical presentation is hypothyroidism and goiter (thyroid gland enlargement), but patients can present with hypothyroidism and no goiter, with euthyroidism and goiter, or rarely (<5%) with hyperthyroidism (Hashitoxicosis).

Other common causes of hypothyroidism, including drug induced, are presented in Table 52-2[3–24]

The clinical presentation, physical findings, and laboratory abnormalities of overt hypothyroidism are summarized in Table 52-3. Myxedema coma is a medical emergency resulting from long-standing, uncorrected hypothyroidism (see Case 52-10). Patients with myxedema coma can present with hypothermia, confusion, coma, carbon dioxide retention, hypoglycemia, hyponatremia, and ileus. Hypothyroid symptoms increase with the severity of the hypothyroidism except in the older patient, who often presents with minimal or atypical symptoms. Patients with subclinical hypothyroidism might have few or no symptoms. Laboratory findings that are diagnostic for overt hypothyroidism include elevated TSH and low free thyroxine (FT_4) levels; for subclinical or early hypothyroidism, the findings are an elevated TSH and normal FT_4 levels.

Levothyroxine (L-thyroxine), at an oral replacement dosage of 1.6 to 1.7 mcg/kg/day administered on an empty stomach, is the

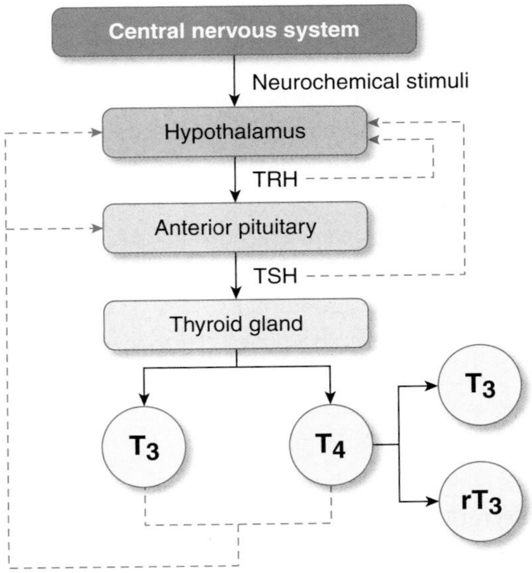

Figure 52-1 Regulation of thyroid hormone secretion. Release of thyroid hormones is controlled by the hypothalamic–pituitary–thyroid axis. Dashed lines represent negative feedback.

rT3, reverse triiodothyronine (inactive); T4, thyroxine; TRH, thyrotropin-releasing hormone; TSH, thyroid-stimulating hormone or thyrotropin; T3, triiodothyronine.

Table 52-1
Factors that can Significantly Alter Thyroid Function Tests in Euthyroid Patients

Factors	Drugs/Situations
$\uparrow$ TBG Binding Capacity	
$\uparrow TT_4$	Estrogens,[1,2] tamoxifen,[55] raloxifene[54]
$\uparrow TT_3$	Oral contraceptives[21]
Normal TSH	Heroin[53]
Normal FT_4I, FT_4	Methadone maintenance[53]
Normal FT_3I, FT_3	Genetic $\uparrow$ in TBG
	Clofibrate
	Active hepatitis[31]
$\downarrow$ TBG Binding Capacity/Displacement T4 from Binding Sites	
$\downarrow TT_4$	Androgens[21]
$\downarrow TT_3$	Salicylates,[21,45,46] disalcid,[46] salsalate[46]
Normal TSH	High-dose furosemide
Normal FT_4I, FT_4	$\downarrow$ TBG synthesis-cirrhosis/hepatic failure
Normal FT_3I, FT_3	Nephrotic syndrome[21,31]
	Danazol[21,31]
	Glucocorticoids[21,31,59]
$\downarrow$ Peripheral T4 $\rightarrow$ T3 Conversion	
$\downarrow TT_3$	PTU
Normal TT_4	Propranolol[200]
Normal FT_4I, FT_4	Glucocorticoids[21,33,59]
Normal TSH	
$\downarrow$ Pituitary and Peripheral T4 $\rightarrow$ T3	
$\downarrow TT_3$	Iodinated contrast media (e.g., ipodate)[249–253]
$\uparrow TT_4$	Amiodarone[3,12,17]
$\uparrow$ TSH (transient)	Non-thyroidal illness[37,39,254]
$\uparrow FT_4I$	
$\uparrow$ T4 Clearance by Enzyme Induction/$\uparrow$ Fecal Loss[a]	
$\downarrow TT_4$	Phenytoin[47,48]
$\downarrow FT_4I$	Phenobarbital[47]
Normal or $\downarrow FT_4$	Carbamazepine[47–52]
Normal or $\downarrow TT_3$	Cholestyramine, colestipol[127]
Normal or $\uparrow$ TSH	Rifampin[47]
	Bexarotene[20]
$\downarrow$ TSH Secretion	
	Dopamine[21,31] dobutamine[255]
	Levodopa[21] cabergoline[256]
	Glucocorticoids[21,33,59]
	Bromocriptine[21,33] Pramipexole[58,59] Ropinirole[58,59]
	Octreotide[32]
	Metformin[60,61]
	Bexarotene[10]
$\uparrow$ TSH Secretion	
	Metoclopramide[21,31,33]
	Domperidone[21,31,33]

[a]Can also cause hypothyroidism in patients receiving levothyroxine therapy.

FT_3, free triiodothyronine; FT_4, free thyroxine; FT_3I, free triiodothyronine index; FT_4I, free thyroxine index; PTU, propylthiouracil; T_3, triiodothyronine; T_4, thyroxine; TBG, thyroxine-binding globulin; TSH, thyroid-stimulating hormone; TT_3, total triiodothyronine; TT_4, total thyroxine.

Table 52-2
Causes of Hypothyroidism

Non-goitrous (No Gland Enlargement)
Primary Hypothyroidism (Dysfunction of the Gland)
Idiopathic atrophy
Iatrogenic destruction of thyroid
Surgery
Radioactive iodine therapy
X-ray therapy
Postinflammatory thyroiditis
Cretinism (congenital hypothyroidism)
Secondary Hypothyroidism
Deficiency of TSH because of pituitary dysfunction
Deficiency of TRH because of hypothalamic dysfunction
Goitrous Hypothyroidism (Enlargement of Thyroid Gland)
Dyshormonogenesis: defect in hormone synthesis, transport, or action
Hashimoto's thyroiditis
Congenital cretinism: maternally induced
Iodide deficiency
Natural goitrogens: rutabagas, turnips, cabbage
Drug-Induced
Aminoglutethimide[21]
Amiodarone[3,12,17]
Bexarotene[10,20]
Ethionamide[18]
Iodides and iodide-containing preparations[16]
Rifampin[22]
Tyrosine kinase inhibitors (e.g., imatinib, sunitinib, sorafenib)[8,9,14,19]
Interleukin[11,23]
Interferon-α[6,7,15,24]
Lithium[4,5,13]
Thiocyanates, phenylbutazone, sulfonylureas[21]

TRH, thyrotropin-releasing hormone; TSH, thyroid-stimulating hormone.

preferred thyroid replacement preparation. Several brand name and less costly generic preparations are interchangeable in most patients. Older patients, and those with severe hypothyroidism, and cardiac disease may require minute T_4 doses initially to avoid cardiac toxicity (Table 52-4); complete reversal of hypothyroidism might not be indicated or possible. In myxedema coma, an intravenous (IV) L-thyroxine (e.g., 400 mcg × 1) loading dose is necessary to reduce the high mortality rate. In subclinical hypothyroidism (see Case 52-12), T_4 replacement therapy is beneficial in those with TSH >10 IU/mL.

The goal of therapy is to reverse the signs and symptoms of hypothyroidism and normalize the TSH and FT_4 levels. Some improvement of hypothyroid symptoms is often evident within 2 to 3 weeks of starting T_4 therapy. Over-replacement of T_4 (i.e., suppressed serum concentrations of TSH) is associated with osteoporosis and cardiac toxicity. The optimal T_4 replacement dosage must be administered for approximately 6 to 8 weeks to achieve steady-state levels. Medications that interfere with T_4 absorption (e.g., iron, aluminum-containing products, some calcium preparations [e.g., carbonate], cholesterol resin phosphate

Table 52-3
Clinical and Laboratory Findings of Primary Hypothyroidism

Symptoms	Physical Findings	Laboratory
General: weakness, tiredness, lethargy, fatigue	Thin brittle nails	↓ TT_4
Cold intolerance	Thinning of skin	↓ FT_4I
Headache	Pallor	↓ FT_4
Loss of taste/smell	Puffiness of face, eyelids	↓ TT_3
Deafness	Yellowing of skin	↓ FT_3I
Hoarseness	Thinning of outer eyebrows	↑ TSH
No sweating	Thickening of tongue	Positive antibodies (in Hashimoto's)
Modest weight gain	Peripheral edema	↑ Cholesterol
Muscle cramps, aches, pains	Pleural/peritoneal/pericardial effusions	↑ CPK
Dyspnea	↓ DTRs	↓ Na
Slow speech	"Myxedema heart"	↑ LDH
Constipation	Bradycardia (↓ HR)	↑ AST
Menorrhagia	Hypertension	↓ Hct/Hgb
Galactorrhea	Goiter (primary hypothyroidism)	

AST, aspartate aminotransferase; CPK, creatinine phosphokinase; DTRs, deep tendon reflexes; Hct, hematocrit; Hgb, hemoglobin; HR, heart rate; LDH, lactate dehydrogenase; Na, sodium; FT_3I, free triiodothyronine index; FT_4I, free thyroxine index; FT_4, free thyroxine; TSH, thyroid-stimulating hormone; TT_3, total triiodothyronine; TT_4, total thyroxine.

Table 52-4
Treatment of Hypothyroidism

Patient Type/ Complications	Dose (L-Thyroxine)	Comment
Uncomplicated adult	1.6–1.7 mcg/kg/day; 100–125 mcg/day average replacement dose; usual increment 25 mcg q6–8wk	2–3 weeks; 4–6 weeks. Reversal of skin and hair changes may take several months. An FT_4 and TSH should be checked 6–8 weeks after initiation of therapy because T_4 has a half-life of 7 days and three to four half-lives are needed to achieve steady state. Levels obtained before steady state can be very misleading. Because 80% is bioavailable, adjust IV doses downward. Small changes can be made by varying dose schedule (e.g., 150 mcg daily except Sunday).
Elderly	≤1.6 mcg/kg/day (50–100 mcg/day)	Initiate T_4 cautiously. Elderly may require less than younger patients. Sensitive to small dose changes. A few patients older than 60 years require ≤50 mcg/day.
Cardiovascular disease (angina, CAD)	Start with 12.5–25 mcg/day. ↑ by 12.5–25 mcg/day q2–6 weeks as tolerated	These patients are very sensitive to cardiovascular effects of T_4. Even subtherapeutic doses can precipitate severe angina, MI, or death. Replace thyroid deficit slowly, cautiously, and sometimes even suboptimally.
Long-standing hypothyroidism (>1 year)	Dose slowly. Start with 25 mcg/day. ↑ by 25 mcg/day q4–6 weeks as tolerated	Sensitive to cardiovascular effects of T_4. Steady state may be delayed because of ↓ clearance of T_4.[a] Correct replacement dose is a compromise between prevention of myxedema and avoidance of cardiac toxicity.
Pregnancy	Most will require 45% ↑ in dose to ensure euthyroidism	Evaluate TSH, TT_4, and FT_4I. normal TSH and TT_4/FT_4I in upper normal range to prevent fetal hypothyroidism. TSH should be no higher than 2.5 microunits/mL during the first trimester and 3.0 microunits/mL in the second and third trimesters
Pediatric (0–3 mo)	10–15 mcg/kg/day	Hypothyroid infants can exhibit skin mottling, lethargy, hoarseness, poor feeding, delayed development, constipation, large tongue, neonatal jaundice, piglike facies, choking, respiratory difficulties, and delayed skeletal maturation (epiphyseal dysgenesis). The serum T_4 should be increased rapidly to minimize impaired cognitive function. In the healthy term infant, 37.5–50 mcg/day of T_4 is appropriate. Dose decreases with age (Table 52-9).

[a]In severely myxedematous patients, steady state may require ≥6 months. In patients who are clinically euthyroid but have ↑ TT_4 and FTI, use TT_3 and TSH as guide to dose adjustments.

CAD, coronary artery disease; FT_4, free thyroxine; FT_4I, free thyroxine index; IV, intravenous; MI, myocardial infarction; q, every; QD, every day; T_4, thyroxine; TSH, thyroid-stimulating hormone; TT_4, total thyroxine.

binders, and raloxifene) should be separated by at least 4 hours from concomitant T_4 administration.

Hyperthyroidism or thyrotoxicosis is the hypermetabolic syndrome that occurs from excessive thyroid hormone production. Hyperthyroidism affects about 2% of women and about 0.1% of men. The prevalence in older patients varies between 0.5% and 2.3% but accounts for 10% to 15% of all thyrotoxic patients.

The classic symptoms of hyperthyroidism are summarized in Table 52-5. The typical symptoms are often absent in the older patient, producing a masked or "apathetic" picture. Because of the atypical presentation in the older patient, occult hyperthyroidism always must be considered, especially in patients with new or worsening cardiac findings (e.g., atrial fibrillation). Untreated hyperthyroidism can progress to thyroid storm, a life-threatening form of hyperthyroidism characterized by exaggerated symptoms of thyrotoxicosis and the acute onset of high fever. The diagnosis of hyperthyroidism is confirmed by high serum concentrations of FT_4 and free T_3 (FT_3) or an undetectable TSH level. Positive thyroid antibodies confirm an autoimmune origin for the hyperthyroidism (e.g., Graves' disease).

Table 52-5
Clinical and Laboratory Findings of Hyperthyroidism

Symptoms
Heat intolerance
Weight loss common, or weight gain caused by ↑ appetite
Palpitations
Pedal edema
Diarrhea/frequent bowel movements
Amenorrhea/light menses
Tremor
Weakness, fatigue
Nervousness, irritability, insomnia
Physical Findings
Thinning of hair (fine)
Proptosis, lid lag, lid retraction, stare, chemosis, conjunctivitis, periorbital edema, loss of extraocular movements
Diffusely enlarged goiter, bruits, thrills
Wide pulse pressure
Pretibial myxedema
Plummer's nails[a]
Flushed, moist skin
Palmar erythema
Brisk DTRs
Laboratory Findings
↑ TT_4
↑ TT_3
↑ FT_4I/FT_4
↑ FT_3I/FT_3
Suppressed TSH
TSI present
TgAb present
TPOAb present
RAIU >50%
↓ Cholesterol
↑ Alkaline phosphatase
↑ Calcium
↑ AST

[a]The fingernail separates from its matrix, but only one or two nails are generally affected.

AST, aspartate aminotransferase; TgAb, thyroglobulin autoantibodies; DTRs, deep tendon reflexes; FT_3, free triiodothyronine; FT_4, free thyroxine; FT_3I, free triiodothyronine index; FT_4I, free thyroxine index; RAIU, radioactive iodine uptake; TPOAb, thyroid peroxidase antibody; TSI, thyroid-stimulating immunoglobulin; TSH, thyroid-stimulating hormone; TT_3, total triiodothyronine; TT_4, total thyroxine.

Graves' disease, an autoimmune disease, is the most common cause of hyperthyroidism. Characteristics include diffuse goiter, ophthalmopathy (exophthalmos), dermopathy (pretibial myxedema), and acropachy (thickening of fingers or toes). The production of excessive thyroid hormone is attributed to a circulating immunoglobulin G or thyroid receptor antibody (TRAb), which has a TSH-like ability to stimulate hormone synthesis. The abnormal production of TRAb by plasma cells (differentiated B lymphocytes) results from a deficiency of suppressor T-cell lymphocytes. Other causes of hyperthyroidism, including iatrogenic, are outlined in Table 52-6.[3,11,12,15,17,21,24–28]

Both Graves' disease and Hashimoto's thyroiditis share similar clinical features and can exist in the same gland: positive antibody titers, goiter with lymphocytic infiltration of the gland, familial tendency, and predilection for women. Thyrotoxicosis can precede the onset of Hashimoto's hypothyroidism, and the end result of Graves' hyperthyroidism is often hypothyroidism.

Effective treatment options for hyperthyroidism include thioamides, radioiodine, and surgery. Therapy selection is influenced by the etiology of the hyperthyroidism, size of the goiter, presence of ophthalmopathy, coexisting conditions (e.g., angina, pregnancy), patient age, patient preference, and physician bias. Radioactive iodine (RAI) is preferred in older patients, those with coexisting cardiac disease, ophthalmopathy, and a toxic multinodular goiter, whereas surgery is appropriate if obstructive symptoms are present or concomitant malignancy is suspected. Pregnant patients can be managed with thioamides or surgery in the second trimester; RAI is absolutely contraindicated.

The thioamides (e.g., methimazole, propylthiouracil) primarily prevent hormone synthesis but do not affect existing stores of thyroid hormone. Therefore, hyperthyroid symptoms will continue for 4 to 6 weeks after beginning thioamide therapy, and initial treatment with β-blockers or iodides is often required for symptomatic relief. Methimazole, given once daily, is considered the thioamide of choice versus propylthiouracil (PTU),

Table 52-6
Causes of Hyperthyroidism

Graves' disease (toxic diffuse goiter); may be caused by polymorphisms in the TSH receptor[27]
Toxic uninodular goiter (Plummer's disease)
Toxic multinodular goiter
Nodular goiter with hyperthyroidism caused by exogenous iodine (Jod-Basedow)
Exogenous thyroid excess through self-administration (factitious hyperthyroidism)
Tumors (thyroid adenoma, follicular carcinoma, thyrotropin-secreting tumor of the pituitary, and hydatidiform mole with secretion of a thyroid-stimulating substance)
Drug induced (iodides,[28] amiodarone,[3,12,17] interleukin,[11,21] interferon-α,[15,24] lithium[25,26])

which requires 2 to 3 times daily dosing and has been associated with severe and fatal hepatitis. PTU should be reserved for use during the first trimester of pregnancy, in thyroid storm, and in those experiencing adverse reactions to methimazole (other than agranulocytosis or hepatitis). The onset of action of PTU is more rapid than methimazole in thyroid storm because PTU can also inhibit the peripheral conversion of T_4 to T_3. PTU is also preferred during the first trimester of pregnancy because congenital defects have been reported with methimazole. Although both drugs are secreted in breast milk, no adverse effects have been reported in the exposed infants. The duration of treatment is empiric, and thioamides typically are prescribed for 12 to 18 months in hopes of long-term spontaneous remission once the drug is discontinued. Although thioamides maintain euthyroidism, they do not change the natural course of the disease, and the likelihood of spontaneous remission, once treatment is discontinued, is about 60%. The combination of thioamide and T_4 therapy to increase the likelihood of remission is not effective nor recommended. Major adverse effects from thioamides include skin rash, gastrointestinal (GI) complaints (e.g., nausea, upset stomach, and metallic taste), agranulocytosis, and hepatitis. Cross-sensitivity between the thioamides is not complete, and the alternative drug can be used if rash or GI complaints do not resolve. This is not true for agranulocytosis and hepatitis, and the alternative agent is not recommended.

Nodular goiters, both multinodular and uninodular, are common thyroid problems that occur in 4% to 5% of the adult population. The nodular goiter is usually found on routine physical examination in asymptomatic and euthyroid patients. A cold nodule is a "hypofunctioning" area of the thyroid that fails to collect radioiodine. Hot nodule is a term used to describe a "hyperfunctioning" or iodine-concentrating area of the thyroid. The hyperfunctioning autonomous nodule typically suppresses activity in the remainder of the gland, but it does not produce clinical or chemical evidence of hyperthyroidism and may remain unchanged for years. Some nodules may develop into toxic goiters, causing overt symptoms of toxicosis. Most hot nodules are benign; malignancies are rarely reported.[29] Treatment options include surgery, RAI, or thyroid replacement therapy if hypothyroid. All goitrogens should be removed if possible. L-Thyroxine suppression therapy is no longer recommended because the dangers from supraphysiologic dosages of T_4 (e.g., osteoporosis and the potential for cardiac arrhythmias) outweigh the benefits. Nontoxic multinodular goiter is a common finding in about 5% of the population.[29] In low-risk patients, long-standing asymptomatic nodules that have not exhibited recent growth are likely to be benign and can be followed or excised surgically for cosmetic reasons. If the patient develops symptoms (swallowing or respiratory difficulty), surgery is the treatment of choice. Observation with close follow-up is the preferred treatment option for most benign multinodular goiters.[29]

Malignancy must be considered if there is recent growth in a "cold" single or dominant nodule, a firm nodule clinically suspicious for cancer on a physical examination, a history of thyroid irradiation, or a strong family history of medullary thyroid carcinoma. Most cold nodules turn out to be benign adenomas rather than cancers. The incidence of malignancy in a cold nodule varies between 10% and 20%.[30] A fine needle aspiration (FNA) of the thyroid nodule can document an underlying malignancy. Surgery is indicated if malignancy is suspected or if any obstructive or respiratory symptoms are present. After a total thyroidectomy for thyroid cancer, RAI ablation is usually given to remove any remaining thyroid tissue. A yearly evaluation for detection of recurrence of some thyroid cancers requires the patient to be off T_4 for 4 to 6 weeks, so that a repeat radioactive uptake and scan can be completed. An elevated TSH level is also necessary to allow thyroglobulin levels, a tumor marker, to rise if any malignant tissue is present. The administration of recombinant human TSH may improve quality of life because comparable elevations in TSH occur without stopping L-thyroxine therapy, reducing the duration of hypothyroidism.

THYROID FUNCTION TESTS

The principal laboratory tests recommended in the initial evaluation of thyroid disorders are the TSH and the FT_4 levels.[31–33] The relationship between laboratory tests and thyroid disorders is summarized in Figure 52-2. The presence of thyroid antibodies indicates an autoimmune thyroid etiology. Adjuncts to the previous tests include the total T_3 (TT_3), free T_3 (FT_3) or FT_3 index (FT_3I), RAIU and scan, TRAb, ultrasound, and FNA biopsy (Table 52-7).

Measurements of Free and Total Serum Hormone Levels

FREE THYROXINE, FREE THYROXINE INDEX, FREE TRIIODOTHYRONINE, AND FREE TRIIODOTHYRONINE INDEX

The free thyroxine (FT_4) and free triiodothyronine (FT_3) are the most reliable tests for the evaluation of hormone concentrations, especially when thyroid hormone–binding abnormalities exist. The FT_3 is most useful in hyperthyroidism but can be normal or low in hypothyroidism. If a direct measure of the free hormone levels is not available, the estimated free hormone indices (FT_4I, FT_3I) can provide comparable information. However, these indices do not correct for changes observed in patients with "euthyroid sick" non-thyroidal illnesses in whom TBG-binding affinity is altered. In these circumstances, the FT_4 and FT_3 are preferable.[34,35]

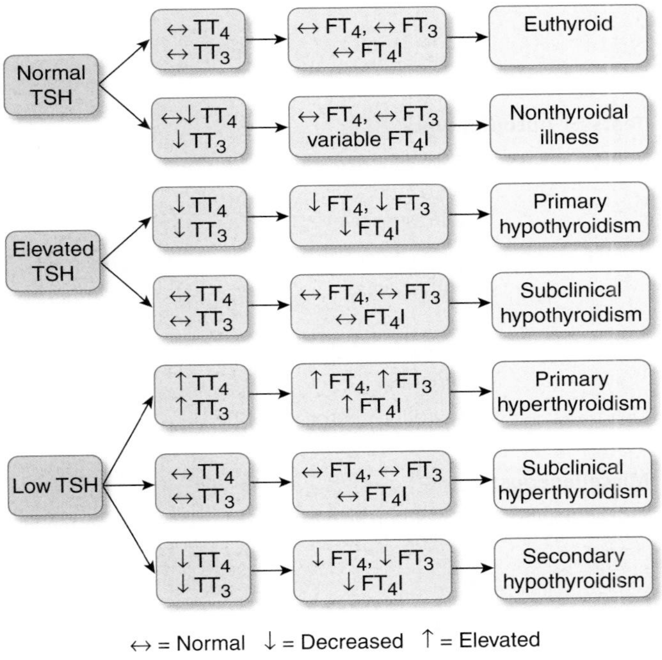

Figure 52-2 Evaluation of thyroid function tests. FT_4, free thyroxine; FT_4I, free thyroxine index; FT_3, free triiodothyronine; TSH, thyrotropin; TT_4, total thyroxine; TT_3, total triiodothyronine.

Table 52-7
Common Thyroid Function Tests

Tests	Measures	Normal[a]	Assay Interference	Comments
Measurement of Circulating Hormone Levels				
FT_4	Direct measurement of free thyroxine	0.8–1.4 ng/dL (10–18 pmol/L)	No interference by alterations in TBG	Most accurate determination of FT_4 levels; might be higher than normal in patients on thyroxine replacement
FT_4I	Calculated free thyroxine index	*T_4 uptake method*: 6.5–12.5 *$TT_4 \times RT_3U$ method*: 1.3–4.2	Non-thyroidal illness (see question 2)	Estimates direct FT_4 measurement; compensates for alterations in TBG
TT_4	Total free and bound T_4	4.8–10.4 mcg/dL (62–134 mmol/L)	Alterations in TBG (Table 52-1)	Specific and sensitive test if no alterations in TBG
TT_3	Total free and bound T_3	58–201 ng/dL (0.9–3.1 nmol/L)	Alterations in TBG levels; T_4 to T_3 (Table 52-1). Non-thyroidal illness (see question 2)	Useful in detecting early, relapsing, and T_3 toxicosis. Not useful in evaluation of hypothyroidism
FT_3	Direct measurement of free T_3	168–370 pg/dL (2.6–5.7 pmol/L)	No interference by alterations in TBG	Most accurate determination of FT_4 levels; might be lower than normal in patients on thyroxine replacement
FT_3I	Calculated free T_3 index	17.5–46	Non-thyroidal illness (see question 2)	Estimates direct FT_3 measurement; compensates for alterations in TBG
Tests of Thyroid Gland Function				
RAIU	Gland's use of iodine after trace dose of either ^{123}I or ^{131}I	5%–35%	False decrease with excess iodide intake; false elevation with iodide deficiency	Useful in hyperthyroidism to determine RAI dose in Graves'; does not provide information regarding hormone synthesis
Scan	Gland size, shape, and tissue activity after ^{123}I or ^{99m}Tc	–	^{154}I scan blocked by antithyroid/thyroid medications	Useful in nodular disease to detect "cold" or "hot" areas
Test of Hypothalamic–Pituitary–Thyroid Axis				
TSH	Pituitary TSH level	0.45–4.1 microunits/mL	Dopamine, glucocorticoids, metoclopramide, thyroid hormone, amiodarone, metformin (Table 52-1)	Most sensitive index for hyperthyroidism, hypothyroidism, and replacement therapy
Tests of Autoimmunity				
TgAb	Thyroglobulin Autoantibodies (ultrasensitive)	<2 IU/mL	Non-thyroidal autoimmune disorders	Present in autoimmune thyroid disease; undetectable during remission
TPOAb	Thyroid peroxidase antibodies	<100 WHO units	Non-thyroidal autoimmune disorders	More sensitive of the two antibodies; titers detectable even after remission
TSI	Thyroid stimulating antibody	<140%		Confirms Graves' disease; detects risk of neonatal Graves'
TRAb	Thyroid receptor antibody	<1.75 IU/L		Confirms Graves' disease; detects risk of neonatal Graves'
Miscellaneous				
Thyroglobulin	Colloid protein of normal thyroid gland	<29.2 μg/L (male) <38.5 μg/L (female)	Goiters; inflammatory thyroid disease	Marker for recurrent thyroid cancer or metastases in thyroidectomized patients

[a]At University of California laboratories.

TgAb, thyroglobulin auto antibodies; FT_3, free triiodothyronine; FT_4, free thyroxine; FT_3I, free triiodothyronine index; FT_4I, free thyroxine index; RAI, radioactive iodine; RAIU, radioactive iodine uptake; T_3, triiodothyronine; T_4, thyroxine; TBG, thyroxine-binding globulin; TPOAb, thyroid peroxidase antibodies; TSI, thyroid receptor–stimulating or thyroid-stimulating antibodies; TRAb, thyroid receptor antibody; TSH, thyroid-stimulating hormone; TT_3, total triiodothyronine; TT_4, total thyroxine; T_3RU, Triiodothyronine resin uptake.

TOTAL THYROXINE AND TOTAL TRIIODOTHYRONINE

The total thyroxine (TT_4) and total triiodothyronine (TT_3) measure both free and bound (total) serum T_4 and T_3. Because the bound fraction is the major fraction measured, situations that change the hormone's affinity for TBG or the TBG level will influence the results. For example, falsely elevated levels of TT_4 and TT_3 are common in the euthyroid pregnant woman (see Case 52-3). In addition, the TT_3 is often low in older patients and in many acute and chronic non-thyroidal illnesses because the peripheral conversion of T_4 to T_3 is decreased (see Case 52-1, Question 2 and Case 52-2). Therefore, careful interpretation of these tests is necessary in situations that alter thyroid hormone binding, TBG levels, or T_4 to T_3 conversion (Table 52-1). The TT_3 (and FT_3) is particularly helpful in detecting early relapse of Graves' disease and in confirming the diagnosis of hyperthyroidism despite normal TT_4 levels. Conversely, TT_3 and FT_3 are not good indicators of hypothyroidism because T_3 levels can be normal. Measurement of only the total hormone levels is less reliable than either the free or estimated free hormone levels when alterations in thyroid-binding globulin or non-thyroidal illnesses exist.[34,35]

Tests of the Hypothalamic–Pituitary–Thyroid Axis

THYROID-STIMULATING HORMONE OR THYROTROPIN

The serum thyroid-stimulating hormone or thyrotropin (TSH) is the most sensitive test to evaluate thyroid function.[31–33] TSH, secreted by the pituitary, is elevated in early or subclinical hypothyroidism (when thyroid hormone levels appear normal) and when thyroid hormone replacement therapy is inadequate. TSH can be abnormal even if the FT_4 remains within the normal range because the TSH is specific for each person's physiologic set point. Polymorphisms in the TSH receptor contribute to this interindividual variability.[27] Consequently, low normal free hormone levels can stimulate the pituitary to synthesize increased amounts of TSH. TSH cannot differentiate between primary hypothyroidism (thyroid failure), which is characterized by elevated TSH levels, and secondary (pituitary or hypothalamus failure) hypothyroidism where TSH levels may be low or normal. The TSH assay can quantitate the upper and lower limits of normal, so that a suppressed TSH level is highly suggestive of hyperthyroidism or exogenous thyroid overreplacement. Of note, TSH is not entirely specific for thyroid disease because abnormal levels are observed in euthyroid patients with non-thyroidal illnesses and in patients receiving drugs that can interfere with TSH secretion. TSH secretion is increased at bedtime and is affected by lack of sleep and exercise.[36] TSH secretion is suppressed physiologically by dopamine, which antagonizes the stimulatory effects of TRH. Therefore, both dopaminergic agonists and antagonists can alter TSH secretion (see Case 52-4). Whether the upper limits of normal for TSH should be lowered to 2.5 microunits/mL is controversial.[27,36]

Tests of Gland Function

RADIOACTIVE IODINE UPTAKE

The radioactive iodine uptake (RAIU), a measure of iodine utilization by the gland, is an indirect measure of hormone synthesis. It is elevated in hyperthyroidism and in early hypothyroidism when the failing gland is trying to increase hormone synthesis. A low or undetectable RAIU occurs in hypothyroidism, thyrotoxicosis factitia, and subacute thyroiditis. Typically, RAIU is used to calculate the dose of RAI therapy for treatment of Graves' disease and to determine the activity of one or several nodules in a gland. The RAIU is not necessary to diagnose classic Graves' disease or hypothyroidism.

A tracer dose of iodine-131 (^{131}I) is administered, and the radioactivity of the gland is measured at 5 and 24 hours after ingestion. It is necessary to measure both the 5- and 24-hour RAIU, so that patients with rapid turnover of iodine will not be missed. In some hyperthyroid patients, the 5-hour uptake is elevated, but the 24-hour uptake can fall to normal or subnormal levels. The normal range of the RAIU (Table 52-7) is affected by any condition that alters iodine intake. Iodine depletion caused by rigorous diuretic therapy or an iodine-deficient diet increases uptake because of replenishment of depleted total iodide pools. Conversely, dilution of ^{131}I with exogenous iodide sources (e.g., contrast dyes) decreases RAIU.

IMAGING STUDIES

Thyroid Scan

A scan of the gland is performed simultaneously with the RAIU or after ingestion of technetium (^{99m}Tc) pertechnetate. The scan provides information concerning gland size and shape, and identifies hypermetabolic ("hot") and hypometabolic ("cold") areas. The possibility of carcinoma must be considered if cold areas are present. A scan is often obtained in the evaluation of a patient with nodular thyroid disease.

Thyroid Ultrasound

A thyroid ultrasound can provide information about gland size and number of clinically palpable or non-palpable nodules or cysts in the thyroid gland.

Tests of Autoimmunity

THYROID PEROXIDASE AND ANTITHYROGLOBULIN ANTIBODIES

Thyroid peroxidase antibodies (TPOAb) and thyroglobulin autoantibodies (TgAb) to the thyroid gland indicate an autoimmune process.[31,33] About 60% to 70% of patients with Graves' disease and 95% of patients with Hashimoto's thyroiditis have positive antibodies to both thyroid antigens. Positive antibodies alone do not indicate thyroid disease because 5% to 10% of asymptomatic patients, as well as patients with other non-thyroidal autoimmune disorders, have positive antibodies.

Clinically, the TPOAb is more specific than TgAb in assessing disease activity. Although both antibodies are elevated during acute flares of the disease, lower titers of TPOAb remain positive during quiescent periods of the disease, while TgAb levels revert to negative.

THYROID RECEPTOR–STIMULATING ANTIBODIES OR THYROID-STIMULATING IMMUNOGLOBULIN

Thyroid receptor–stimulating antibodies (TRAb) or thyroid-stimulating immunoglobulin (TSI) are IgG immunoglobulins that are present in virtually all patients with Graves' disease.[31,33] Like TSH, these immunoglobulins can stimulate the thyroid gland to produce thyroid hormones. High titers of TSI are useful in diagnosing otherwise asymptomatic Graves' disease (i.e., ophthalmopathy), in predicting the risk of relapse of Graves' disease after discontinuing medication, and in predicting the risk of neonatal hyperthyroidism in utero through transplacental passage of TSI from the pregnant mother. Otherwise, TSI measurement is expensive and offers no additional information in the patient with a typical Graves' disease presentation.

EUTHYROIDISM AND NON-THYROIDAL ILLNESS SYNDROME

CASE 52-1

QUESTION 1: R.K., an obese 42-year-old woman, is admitted to the hospital because of increasing fatigue, sluggishness, shortness of breath (SOB), and pitting edema of the legs during the past 3 weeks. Bilateral pleural effusions found on her chest radiograph indicate a worsening of her congestive heart failure (CHF). Her other medical problems include cirrhosis of the liver, type 2 diabetes, and chronic bronchitis, for which she takes glipizide 10 mg every day and an iodine-containing herbal supplement 3 times a day (TID).

Pertinent physical findings include a palpable but normal-size thyroid, bibasilar rales, cardiomegaly, hepatomegaly, 4 + pitting edema, and normal deep tendon reflexes (DTRs). A diagnosis of worsening CHF secondary to hypothyroidism is suspected based on the following laboratory findings:

Cholesterol, 385 mg/dL
RAIU at 24 hours, 13% (normal, 5%–35%[1])
Scan, normal-size gland with homogenous uptake
TT_4, 1.4 mcg/dL (normal, 4.8–10.4 mcg/dL)
TT_3, 22 ng/dL (normal, 58–201 ng/dL)
TSH, 4 microunits/mL (normal, 0.45–4.1 microunits/mL)
FT_4, 1.0 ng/dL (normal, 0.8–1.4 ng/dL)
TPOAb, 30 WHO units (normal, <100 WHO units)
TgAb, 0.3 IU/mL (normal, <2 IU/mL)

Evaluate and explain R.K.'s thyroid status based on her clinical and laboratory findings.

Although low-output failure can be a presenting sign of hypothyroidism, the normal TSH and FT_4 definitely indicates that R.K. is euthyroid, despite the confusing results of her other thyroid function tests. The depressed RAIU is consistent with her history of iodide ingestion and dilution of the ^{131}I. The low TT_4 and TT_3 may be explained by her cirrhosis and non-thyroidal illness syndrome (see Question 2). The negative thyroid antibodies, the normal scan, and normal DTRs further substantiate the diagnosis of euthyroidism. In hypothyroidism, a lower rate of cholesterol degradation can produce an elevated serum cholesterol level. However, because many extrathyroidal factors influence the serum concentration of cholesterol, this test is an imprecise reflection of thyroid status. In this case, the elevated cholesterol level is not related to hypothyroidism.

CASE 52-1, QUESTION 2: Assess the results and explain the significance of R.K.'s TT_4, FT_4I, and TT_3 values.

R.K.'s thyroid function test results are consistent with the non-thyroidal illness syndrome. Abnormal thyroid function tests are commonly found in euthyroid patients with various serious systemic diseases, including starvation, infections, sepsis, acute psychiatric disorders, HIV infection, myocardial infarction (MI), bone marrow transplantation, and severe chronic cardiac, pulmonary, renal, hepatic, and neoplastic diseases.[21,31,33,37–42]

This "euthyroid sick" syndrome occurs in 37% to 70% of chronically ill or hospitalized patients and must be recognized. In general, the sicker the patient, the greater the degree of abnormal thyroid function findings, even though the patient has no thyroid disease.

The most common finding is a low TT_3 (e.g., 15–20 ng/dL) and high inactive reverse T_3 levels (rT_3). Other typical changes include a normal or low TT_4, and a suppressed or normal TSH levels. A borderline-high compensatory TSH occurs as patients recover from illness. In more serious illness, the TT_4, FT_4I, and FT_3 are often low. Free hormone levels (e.g., FT_4, FT_3) are often normal or slightly low. However, these inconsistent findings fuel the controversy over whether thyroid hormone therapy is beneficial or detrimental. These findings are believed to be explained by a central hypothyroidism caused by reduction in hypothalamic TRH because of increased hypothalamic T_3, increased peripheral metabolism of T_3, or by a reduction in serum thyroid hormone–binding proteins.[38] Impaired protein synthesis of thyroid-binding prealbumin (TBPA) and an increase in the proportion of a lower-binding-capacity form of TBG might account for the lower bound hormone levels, but the concomitant increase in the free hormone concentrations would maintain a euthyroid state. Furthermore, circulating substances that inhibit the binding of T_4 and T_3 to the serum-binding proteins might also be present.

Less common changes include a modestly elevated TT_4 and FT_4I in patients with acute viral hepatitis, psychiatric disorders, renal failure, and advanced HIV infection. The TT_3 is usually normal but can be low in critically ill patients. Modest elevations in hormonal binding affinity and increased synthesis of TBG explain these findings.

Several studies have shown a strong inverse correlation between mortality and total serum T_4, T_3, and rT_3 levels.[39–41] Of the 86 hospitalized, intensive care patients, 84% of those with a serum T_4 of <3 mcg/dL died, whereas 85% of those with a serum T_4 of >5 mcg/dL survived.[40] In 331 patients with acute MI, rT_3 levels >0.41 nmol/L were significantly associated with a greater risk of death at 1 year.[41] During recovery, TSH levels increase and hormone levels start to normalize. Therefore, a favorable outcome is associated with reversal of the hormone indices.

Thyroid experts are divided about whether non-thyroidal illness should be treated, and few randomized studies are available to guide therapeutic decisions.[37–42] The few available studies found no survival benefits or favorable clinical outcomes from hormone therapy, although cardiac hemodynamics improved. The benefits of hormone replacement are unproven and might be detrimental. In one trial, the mortality of patients with acute renal failure treated with T_4 was 43% versus 13% in the control group.[42] Other small trials have shown thyroid hormones to be well tolerated and safe.[43] Opponents argue that T_4 therapy, by inhibiting TSH, may interfere with normal thyroid recovery and is preferentially converted to inactive rT3.[43,44] Conversely, proponents argue that there may be cardiovascular benefits and there is no clear evidence that therapy is toxic.[44]

In summary, T_4 and T_3 measurements are not helpful in the diagnosis of thyroid dysfunction in patients with significant non-thyroidal illness. A normal or near-normal TSH is necessary to establish euthyroidism in sick patients with non-thyroidal illness. The available data are not supportive of starting thyroid hormone treatment now. The abnormal laboratory findings should reverse with correction of R.K.'s non-thyroid illness. To confirm euthyroidism, the slightly elevated TSH should be repeated once R.K.'s medical condition improves.

Drug Interference with Thyroid Function Tests

CASE 52-2

QUESTION 1: J.R., a 45-year-old man, complains of fatigue, dry skin, and constipation. His other medical problems include alcoholism for 10 years, cirrhosis, generalized tonic–clonic seizures treated with phenytoin (Dilantin) 300 mg/day and phenobarbital 90 mg

[1]Please note that the normal values used in this chapter are those used at the University of California, San Francisco. Normal values at other locations may differ.

at night, and rheumatoid arthritis for which he takes aspirin 325 mg, 12 tablets/day.

The results of his thyroid function tests are as follows:

TT_4, 4.2 mcg/dL (normal, 4.8–10.4)
FT_4, 0.6 ng/dL (normal, 0.8–1.4)
TSH, 2.5 microunits/mL (normal, 0.45–4.1)

How should these laboratory findings be interpreted? What factors are responsible for the observed changes?

Despite complaints that could be consistent with hypothyroidism (e.g., fatigue, dry skin, constipation) and findings of low serum hormone values, J.R. is euthyroid, as evidenced by the normal TSH level. Secondary hypothyroidism is unlikely at this age without a history of central nervous system (CNS) trauma or tumor. Some non-thyroidal factors could account for J.R.'s low TT_4 and FT_4 values.[21] Anti-inflammatory doses of salicylates >2 g/day and salicylate derivatives (i.e., Disalcid, salsalate) can displace T_4 from both TBG and TBPA, causing these abnormal findings.[21,45,46] Elevation in free T_4 levels and suppression of TSH below normal occur transiently (i.e., no longer than first 3 weeks of administration) but normalize with chronic administration. Cirrhosis, stress, severe infections, and hereditary factors can also decrease TBG and TBPA synthesis to produce similar TT_4 findings. A medication history for drugs such as androgens or glucocorticoids that can lower TBG levels, and therefore TT_4 levels, should be elicited (Table 52-1).[21]

Enzyme inducers, such as rifampin and anticonvulsants (phenytoin, phenobarbital, valproic acid, carbamazepine), can alter serum thyroid hormone levels.[21,47–52] A 40% to 60% reduction in total T_4 serum concentrations results from an increase in the metabolism (non-deiodination) of T_4 and from hormone displacement in patients receiving chronic anticonvulsant therapy. Serum T_3 levels are normal or slightly decreased. In addition, therapeutic levels of phenytoin and carbamazepine interfere with the FT_4 assay, causing a 20% to 40% lower FT_4 than would be expected in euthyroid persons.[48] TSH levels remain normal and patients are euthyroid; however, those who previously required T_4 therapy may need a dosage increase to maintain euthyroidism.[51,52] Valproic acid is reported to have similar but less potent effects on thyroid function.[47,49] Phenobarbital can increase T_4 uptake by the liver and increase the fecal excretion of T_4. Serum binding of thyroid hormones is unaffected by phenobarbital.

In summary, J.R. is taking several drugs that can further compromise the already low serum T_4 levels resulting from his liver disease. FT_4 remains subnormal in euthyroid persons receiving phenytoin. For J.R, the normal TSH confirms euthyroidism, and no thyroid replacement is warranted.

CASE 52-3

QUESTION 1: S.T., a 23-year-old, sexually active woman whose only medication is birth control pills, comes to the clinic complaining of extreme nervousness, diaphoresis, and scanty menstrual periods. Although she appears healthy, the possibility of hyperthyroidism is considered on the basis of the following laboratory values:

TT_4, 16 mcg/dL (normal, 4.8–10.4)
FT_4, 1.2 ng/dL (normal, 0.7–1.9)
TSH, 1.2 microunits/mL (normal, 0.45–4.1)

Based on this information, what would be a reasonable assessment of S.T.'s thyroid status?

The normal FT_4 and TSH confirm that S.T. is not hyperthyroid. The elevated TT_4 is consistent with increased TBG levels observed in patients with acute hepatitis; in pregnancy; and in persons taking estrogens, estrogen-containing contraceptives, tamoxifen, raloxifene, heroin, or methadone.[1,2,21,53–55] Because TBG and therefore bound T_4 levels are increased by estrogens in S.T., total serum T_4 measurements are falsely elevated, but free thyroxine levels remain normal. In patients requiring L-thyroxine, the use of estrogens can increase requirements of hormone replacement because the increased pituitary secretion of TSH cannot increase thyroid production needed to offset the increased binding of T_4.[1] Thyroid function tests should return to normal within 4 weeks after estrogen-containing contraceptives are discontinued. A change to progesterone-only contraceptives that do not affect protein binding, do not alter thyroid function tests, and do not increase thyroid requirements can be considered in S.T.

CASE 52-4

QUESTION 1: J.P., a 55-year-old woman, complains of 3 months of progressive tremors, dizziness, and ataxia. Two months ago, she had a silent MI complicated by malignant ventricular ectopy that was responsive only to amiodarone therapy. Her other medical problems include Parkinsonism, type 2 diabetes, and diabetic gastroparesis. Her current medications include amiodarone, insulin, metformin, metoclopramide, pramipexole, and levodopa/carbidopa. Physical examination of the thyroid was unremarkable. Thyroid function tests yielded the following results:

TT_4, 14.5 mcg/dL (normal, 4.8–10.4)
FT_4, 2.3 ng/dL (normal, 0.8–1.4)
TSH, 3.8 microunits/mL (normal, 0.45–4.1)
TT_3, 40 ng/dL (normal, 58–201)
TPOAb, 40 WHO units (normal, <100)

How should J.P.'s laboratory values be interpreted?

Although the symptoms of tremors, dizziness, and weight loss are suggestive of hyperthyroidism, the low TT_3, negative antibodies, normal TSH, and normal thyroid examination make this diagnosis unlikely. Side effects of amiodarone could be responsible for J.P.'s symptoms. Her drug therapy could also explain her laboratory findings.

Amiodarone produces complex changes in thyroid function tests that are confusing if not properly interpreted.[3,12,56,57] Because amiodarone inhibits both the peripheral and pituitary conversion of T_4 to T_3, FT_4 levels are elevated, and TT_3 levels are subnormal in euthyroid patients. Transient elevations in TSH levels occur (usually <20 microunits/mL) during the first few weeks of therapy but return to normal in approximately 3 months. If TSH levels do not normalize, then amiodarone-induced thyroid disease should be considered. Amiodarone can cause either hypothyroidism or hyperthyroidism in susceptible patients.

The other drugs J.P. is taking—pramipexole, levodopa, metformin, and metoclopramide—also add to the diagnostic confusion. Although these drugs do not affect the actual circulating hormone levels, they affect the dopaminergic system that controls both TSH and TRH secretion.[21,32,33,58] Infusions of dopamine and dobutamine can decrease both TSH secretion and the TSH response to TRH in euthyroid and hypothyroid patients.[21,32,33,59] Therefore, dopamine agonists such as pramipexole, cabergoline, and levodopa can blunt the normal TSH response.[21,32,58,59] In addition, metformin after 1 year of therapy can cause significant TSH suppression without changes in free thyroxine levels by as yet an unknown mechanism of action.[60,61] Conversely, dopamine antagonists such as metoclopramide or domperidone can elevate TSH levels.[21,32] Fortunately, the alterations in TSH caused by these agents are usually not substantial enough to completely obscure the true thyroid abnormality. See Table 52-2 and Cases 52-23 and 52-24 for more information about drug effects on thyroid function.

J.P.'s thyroid tests present a confusing picture; however, the presence of a TSH within the normal range indicates euthyroidism. J.P. should be continued on her current regimen with follow-up monitoring of thyroid tests.

HYPOTHYROIDISM

Clinical Presentation

CASE 52-5

QUESTION 1: M.W., a 70-kg, 23-year-old voice student, thinks that her neck has become "fatter" over the past 3 to 4 months. She has gained 10 kg, feels mentally sluggish, tires easily, and finds that she can no longer hit high notes. Physical examination reveals puffy facies, yellowish skin, delayed DTRs, and a firm, enlarged thyroid gland. Laboratory data include the following results:

FT_4, 0.6 ng/dL (normal, 0.8–1.4)
TSH, 60 microunits/mL (normal, 0.45–4.1)
TPOAb, 136 WHO units (normal, <100)

Assess M.W.'s thyroid status based on her clinical and laboratory findings.

M.W. presents with many of the clinical features of hypothyroidism as presented in Table 52-3. These include weight gain, mental sluggishness, easy fatigability, lowering of the voice pitch, puffy facies, yellowish tint of the skin, delayed DTRs, and enlarged thyroid.[62] The diagnosis of hypothyroidism is confirmed by her laboratory findings of a low FT_4, an elevated TSH value, and positive TPOAb.

A firm goiter, thyroid antibodies, and clinical symptoms of hypothyroidism strongly suggest Hashimoto's thyroiditis. She has no history of prior antithyroid drug use, surgery, or RAI treatment, which are common causes of iatrogenic hypothyroidism. She is also not taking any goitrogens or drugs known to cause hypothyroidism (Table 52-2).

Treatment with Thyroid Hormones

THYROID HORMONE PRODUCTS

CASE 52-5, QUESTION 2: What thyroid preparation should be used to treat M.W.'s hypothyroidism? Are differences, advantages, or disadvantages significant among the various generic and brand name formulations of thyroid hormones?

The principal goals of thyroid hormone therapy are to attain and maintain a euthyroid state. Thyroid preparations (Table 52-8[63–66]) are synthetic (L-thyroxine, L-triiodothyronine, liotrix) or natural (desiccated thyroid). The latter come from animal tissues.

Desiccated Thyroid

Desiccated thyroid is derived from pork thyroid glands, although beef and sheep are also used. Today, starting patients on desiccated thyroid is not justified. The USP requires only that desiccated thyroid contain 0.17% to 0.23% organic iodine by weight. These requirements do not seem stringent enough because potency may vary with changes in the proportion of the two active hormones (T_3 and T_4) or with changes in the amount of organic iodine present.[67,68] This variable potency seems to be particularly true of generic formulations compared with the biologically standardized Armour brand of desiccated thyroid. Inactive desiccated thyroid

Table 52-8
Thyroid Preparations

Drug/Dosage Forms	Composition	Dosage Equivalent	Comments
Thyroid USP (Armour) *Tab:* 0.25, 0.5, 1, 1.5, 2, 3, 4, and 5 gr	Desiccated hog, beef, or sheep thyroid gland Standardized iodine content	1–1.67 gr[a]	Unpredictable T_4:T_3 ratio; supraphysiologic elevations in T_3 levels might produce toxic symptoms; Armour brand preferred
L-Thyroxine (Levoxyl, Levothroid, Synthroid, Unithroid, various) *Tab:* 0.013, 0.025, 0.050, 0.075, 0.088, 0.112, 0.125, 0.137, 0.15, 0.175, 0.2, and 0.3 mg *Inj:* 200 and 500 mcg	Synthetic T_4	60 mcg[a]	Stable, predictable potency; well absorbed; more potent than desiccated thyroid. When changing from >2 gr desiccated thyroid to L-T_4, a lower dosage of L-T_4 might be needed to avoid toxicity. Weight should be considered in dosing (1.6–1.7 mcg/kg/day). L-T_4 absorption can be impaired by iron, aluminum-containing products (e.g., antacids, sucralfate), Kayexalate, calcium preparations, proton pump inhibitors, cholesterol resin and phosphate binders, raloxifene, soy, bran, coffee, fiber enriched foods. L-T_4 metabolism increased by anticonvulsants, rifampin, imatinib, bexarotene, and pregnancy
L-Triiodothyronine (Cytomel) *Tab:* 5, 25, and 50 mcg *Inj:* 10 mcg/mL (Triostat)	Synthetic T_3	25–37.5 mcg	Complete absorption; requires multiple daily dosing; toxicity similar to all T_3-containing products; see desiccated thyroid comments
Liotrix (Thyrolar) *Tab:* 0.25, 0.5, 1, 2, and 3 gr	60 mcg T_4:15 mcg T_3 50 mcg T_4:12.5 mcg T_3	Thyrolar-1	No need for liotrix because T_4 is converted to T_3 peripherally; expensive, stable, and predictable content

[a]Historically, 60 mg (1 gr) of desiccated thyroid = 60 mcg of T_4.[66] This conversion was determined with older TSH assays, without direct measurement of FT_4 and has been challenged. The conversion is now typically reported as 80 mcg[63], 88 mcg,[64] or 100 mcg[65] of T_4 per 60 mg of desiccated thyroid. The T_3 component of desiccated thyroid is an additional factor to consider when converting from one to the other and an exact equivalent dose has not been determined.

gr, grain; Inj, injection; L-T_4, levothyroxine; T_3, triiodothyronine; T_4, thyroxine; Tab, tablet; USP, United States Pharmacopeia.

preparations that contain negligible amounts of T_3 and T_4 or even iodinated casein instead of active hormone have been identified in various brands sold in retail pharmacies and in over-the-counter products found in health food stores.[68–70] Likewise, preparations with greater-than-expected activity caused by an abnormally high T_3 content have resulted in thyrotoxicosis.

Allergic reactions to the animal protein are another concern. In addition, desiccated thyroid suffers from two problems inherent to all T_3-containing preparations. Because T_3 is absorbed more rapidly than T_4, supraphysiologic elevations in plasma T_3 levels occur after oral ingestion, which can produce mild thyrotoxic symptoms in some patients. FT_4 levels are low during T_3 administration and, if misinterpreted, can result in the erroneous administration of more hormone. These problems with T_3 are easily missed unless T_3 levels are routinely monitored. Because significant amounts of T_4 are converted to T_3 peripherally, oral administration of T_3 offers no advantage and is not usually needed (see Triiodothyronine section).

Loss of tablet potency can occur from prolonged storage of desiccated thyroid preparations, but this instability is not as important as once believed. Because the only apparent advantage of desiccated thyroid is its low cost, it should not be considered the drug of choice for replacement therapy. Patients maintained on desiccated thyroid should be encouraged to change to L-thyroxine (T_4). Although 60 mg (1 g) of desiccated thyroid is theoretically equal in potency to 75 to 100 mcg of T_4,[66] this equivalency may not hold true if the desiccated thyroid preparation is less active than its labeled content. The patient's weight should also be considered when switching therapy (see Case 52-5, Question 3).

The synthetic thyroid preparations differ from one another in their relative potency, onset of action, and biological half-life.

Levothyroxine or L-Thyroxine

L-Thyroxine is the thyroid replacement of choice.[35,65,71] Its advantages include stability, uniform potency, relatively low cost, and lack of allergenic foreign protein content. The long half-life of 7 days permits once-a-day dosing and, if necessary, the creation of special convenience schedules, such as the omission of medication on weekends. The mean absorption of a commonly used branded preparation is 81%.[72] Absorption is optimal on an empty stomach.[73] Current guidelines recommend taking L-thyroxine either 60 minutes before breakfast or 3 to 4 hours after the evening meal for consistent absorption.[35,65] Several medications can also impair L-thyroxine absorption (see Case 52-9, Question 1).

Concerns about generic and branded L-thyroxine tablet stability and potency, bioavailability, and product interchangeability existed because L-thyroxine preparations were grandfathered in by the 1938 Food, Drug, and Cosmetic Act. To address these concerns, the U.S. Food and Drug Administration (FDA) required that all manufacturers of L-thyroxine products submit a New Drug Application (NDA) by August 2001 or cease production by 2003 if the NDA was not filed.[74] Several FDA-approved brand and generic (formulations approved under the NDA received AB or BX ratings, indicating interchangeability for some generic and brand preparations. Raising concerns about the methodology the FDA used to determine bioequivalence, the American Thyroid Association, The Endocrine Society, and the American Association of Clinical Endocrinologists issued joint position statements expressing their displeasure with the FDA's conclusions of interchangeability.[75] Abbot Laboratories, the manufacturer of Synthroid, and others also disagreed with the FDA's findings.[76] Although this issue remains controversial, the preponderance of the evidence supports the FDA ratings and suggests that these preparations are likely to be interchangeable in the majority of patients.[35,65,77–80]

Triiodothyronine

T_3 (Cytomel) is not recommended for routine thyroid hormone replacement because of the problems identified earlier with T_3 administration (see Desiccated Thyroid section).[71] Numerous randomized studies now conclude that replacement with combination T_4 and small dosages of T_3 offer no advantage to T_4 alone, despite an initial study showing improved cognitive performance and mood changes[81,82] Furthermore, a prospective study found that T_3 levels post-thyroidectomy in 50 patients receiving only levothyroxine were similar to T_3 levels in these euthyroid patients before surgery confirming that levothyroxine alone is sufficient for replacement.[83] Its use to enhance contractility in coronary bypass surgery is controversial.[84]

Although T_3 is well absorbed, it has a relatively short half-life (1.5 days), necessitating multiple daily dosing to ensure a uniform response. Other disadvantages include higher expense and a greater potential for cardiotoxicity. Its primary use is for patients who require short-term hormone replacement therapy and rarely in those in whom T_4 conversion to T_3 might be impaired. Proponents favoring thyroid treatment of the "euthyroid sick" syndrome identify T_3 as the hormone replacement of choice. T_3 therapy should be monitored using the TSH and TT_3 or FT_3 levels.

Liotrix

Liotrix is a combination of synthetic T_4 and T_3 in a physiologic ratio of 4:1. This preparation is subject to the same disadvantages common to all T_3-containing preparations. It is also stable and potent, but it is more expensive than other thyroid preparations. Because oral administration of T_3 is not needed and there is no advantage of adding T_3 to T_4 therapy, this expensive preparation is not recommended.[81,82] Patients should be changed to an equivalent dosage of L-thyroxine.

THYROXINE

Dosage

CASE 52-5, QUESTION 3: What would you recommend as appropriate starting and maintenance dosages of T_4 for M.W.?

The maintenance dosage for M.W. can be estimated from her weight. Average replacement doses of 1.6 to 1.7 mcg/kg/day (e.g., 100–125 mcg) are sufficient in most patients to normalize the TSH.[62,71] L-Thyroxine dosages that suppress TSH levels to below normal or undetectable levels (subclinical hyperthyroidism) should be avoided to prevent osteoporosis and cardiac toxicity.[71,85–89] Excessive L-thyroxine can cause tachycardia, atrial arrhythmias, impaired ventricular relaxation, reduced exercise performance, and increased risk of cardiac mortality.[85] These considerations are especially important in older patients, who might require less T_4 than their younger counterparts and who are particularly sensitive to minute changes in T_4 doses (see Case 52-6). As patients age, the dosage should be evaluated yearly and decreased if necessary to maintain a normal TSH level.

How rapidly T_4 replacement can proceed depends on the likelihood of invoking cardiac toxicity in susceptible patients. Minute doses of T_4 (e.g., $<$75 mcg) can increase heart rate, stroke volume, oxygen consumption, and cardiac workload before euthyroidism occurs. One double-blind study compared the clinical outcome between starting full replacement doses versus gradual 25-mcg incremental doses in relatively young hypothyroid subjects with asymptomatic cardiac disease and concluded that those receiving full doses normalized thyroid function tests more rapidly (4 weeks) and without any toxicity.[90] Because M.W. has no identifiable risk factors (see Case 52-11, Question 3) for cardiotoxicity that require careful dosage titration (e.g., old age, cardiac disease, long duration of hypothyroidism), she can be started on an estimated full replacement dose of 125 mcg daily of L-thyroxine (70 kg × 1.7 mcg/kg/day = 120 mcg).[35] An alternative conservative approach would be to start with 100 or 112 mcg/day, check the FT_4 or FT_4I and TSH tests after 6 to 8 weeks of therapy, and if the TSH is still elevated without any symptoms of toxicity, increase the dosage to 125 mcg/day. The appropriate replacement dose will produce a TSH of 1 to 2 microunits/mL, normalize FT_4 or FT_4I levels, and reverse clinical symptoms of hypothyroidism. Generally, dosing adjustments should not exceed monthly increments of 12.5 to 25 mcg/day. Even in the absence of overt coronary disease, patients over age 50 to 60 should be started on a lower dose of L-thyroxine (50 mcg/day) and titrated.[35]

Monitoring Therapy

CASE 52-5, QUESTION 4: Ten days after starting L-thyroxine therapy, M.W. continues to complain of tiredness, fatigue, and difficulty singing despite excellent adherence. Thyroid function tests show a TT_4 of 4 mcg/dL (normal, 4.8–10.4), an FT_4 of 0.5 ng/dL (normal, 0.8–1.4), and a TSH of 40 microunits/mL (normal, 0.45–4.1). What therapeutic options are available? How should M.W.'s thyroid function tests be interpreted?

Clinical improvement in the signs and symptoms of hypothyroidism and normalization of laboratory parameters are appropriate therapeutic end points. If the replacement dose is sufficient, some correction of her symptoms should occur after 2 to 3 weeks, but maximal effects will not be evident for 4 to 6 weeks. Typically, improvement of anemia and hair and skin changes is delayed and requires several months of treatment before resolution.[60,66]

In patients with severe myxedema, a transiently elevated T_4 level might occur at 6 weeks because the metabolic clearance of T_4 is decreased by the hypometabolic state associated with hypothyroidism.

FT_4 or FT_4I and TSH should be checked about 6 to 8 weeks after the initiation of therapy because T_4 has a half-life of 7 days, and three to four half-lives are needed to reach steady-state levels. Levels obtained before this time (as in M.W.) may be misleading and should be interpreted cautiously. No change in her L-thyroxine dosage should be attempted at this time.

CASE 52-5, QUESTION 5: Eight weeks later, on a routine follow-up visit, M.W. still feels tired and not back to her normal self. She denies any symptoms of hyperthyroidism. Her thyroid function tests show a TT_4 of 14 mcg/dL (normal, 4.8–10.4), a TT_3 of 100 ng/dL (normal, 58–201), FT_4 of 1.9 ng/dL (normal, 0.7–1.9), and a TSH of 3.5 microunits/mL (normal, 0.45–4.1). How should M.W.'s thyroid function tests be interpreted? What changes, if any, should be recommended in her therapeutic regimen?

Patients treated with L-thyroxine may develop an elevated TT_4 concentration and FT_4 without overt clinical signs of hyperthyroidism.[83,91] Despite these elevated levels, patients are euthyroid, as evidenced by a normal TSH. Because T_3 is not being released from the nonfunctioning thyroid gland, a higher concentration of T_4 is necessary to increase the amount of T_3 obtained from peripheral conversion. Jonklaas et al. reported that the mean FT_4 was significantly higher (1.34 ng/dL) in patients receiving L-thyroxine postoperatively compared to their euthyroid levels before thyroidectomy (FT_4, 1.06 ng/dL).[83] T_3 levels on L-thyroxine replacement were also comparable after surgery to presurgery levels. However, lower T_3 levels were noted only in those in whom TSH levels were greater than 4.5 microunits/mL, indicating that low T_3 levels are likely a result of suboptimal L-thyroxine replacement. Thus, the TSH appears to be the best indicator of euthyroidism in patients treated with L-thyroxine.

Another possibility is that the elevated thyroid levels may only be an artifact of the laboratory collection time. Before any changes in her dosing regimen are made, M.W. should be asked about the time she takes the drug and its relationship to the time of her blood draw. Random sampling of FT_4 and TSH levels can be significantly different when compared with trough levels.[92,93] In one study, the FT_4 level was 12% higher and the TSH level 19% lower when obtained from random samples compared with trough samples.[93] Transient elevations in FT_4 levels were detected for 9 hours after ingestion of the oral L-thyroxine.

The symptoms of fatigue that M.W. is experiencing are likely not because of her hypothyroidism. Patients may continue to have symptoms of hypothyroidism despite normalization of the TSH value. Although some have suggested that the goal TSH be titrated to 1 to 2 microunits/mL or lower for replacement therapy to improve well-being, this is controversial. One study found that changes in T_4 dosing to achieve TSH concentrations of 2 to 4.8 microunits/mL, 0.3 to 1.9 microunits/mL, or <0.3 microunits/mL in hypothyroid patients did not result in improvements in well-being, psychologic, or hypothyroid symptoms, or quality of life.[94] Data justifying the safety of higher T4 replacement doses found that achievement of a low but detectable TSH level (0.04–0.4 microunits/mL) was not associated with an increased risk of cardiovascular disease or fractures compared to those with suppressed (<0.03 microunits/mL) or elevated (>4 microunits/mL) TSH levels.[95]

In conclusion, if an elevated TT_4 and FT_4 are noted without any symptoms of thyrotoxicosis (as in M.W.), the dosage should not be decreased; rather, a trough FT_4 and TSH level should be obtained to eliminate excessive dosing or any laboratory artifacts. Alternatively, obtaining a level at least 9 hours after levothyroxine administration also seems appropriate. Repeat values should be in the normal range if the dosing is correct. An excessively suppressed TSH confirms a dosage that is too high. In M.W., the lack of hyperthyroid symptoms suggests euthyroidism, and no changes in her therapeutic regimen should be attempted until trough levels are available. Evaluation for other causes of fatigue should be explored.

TRIIODOTHYRONINE

CASE 52-6

QUESTION 1: C.B., a 65-year-old woman, complains of fatigue and vague muscle aches and pains, which she attributes to insufficient thyroid medication. On physical examination, the thyroid gland is palpable but not enlarged, and DTRs are 2 plus and brisk. Her dose of T_3 was increased from 25 mcg TID to 50 mcg TID about 2 weeks ago based on the results of a recent FT_4 of 0.5 ng/dL (normal, 0.8–1.4). She denies taking any other medications. Is C.B.'s thyroid hormone replacement appropriate?

As noted previously, T_3 is not the drug of choice for thyroid replacement. The use of L-thyroxine would simplify her dosing regimen and facilitate monitoring.

The low FT_4 did not justify increasing C.B.'s T_3 dose. Because she is receiving T_3, the FT_4, which is a measure of free T_4, will always be low and will never reach normal levels. In fact, her vague complaints may be related to hyperthyroidism because she is receiving the equivalent of 0.2 to 0.3 mg of L-thyroxine daily. TSH and FT_3 levels are most useful in monitoring patients receiving T_3 therapy. A TSH level should be obtained to evaluate her thyroid function. A suppressed TSH and an elevated FT_3 would indicate hyperthyroidism. It is important to remember that in an older patient, hyperthyroidism might not always produce symptoms because of an "apathetic" sympathetic system.

L-Thyroxine should be initiated cautiously in older patients to avoid exacerbating any preexisting arteriosclerotic heart disease that might be masked by the hypothyroidism (see Case 52-11, Questions 2 and 3). In general, older patients require smaller replacement dosages (approximately ≤1.6 mcg/kg/day of T_4) than their younger counterparts.[96–98] Dosages of <50 mcg/day of T_4 are common in patients older than 60 years. However, this lower T_4 dosage is not universal for all older subjects.[98] The reason that older patients need lower dosages is unclear, but it has been suggested that the lower requirements result from an age-related decrease in T_4 degradation rates. Because dosage requirements change with age, patients should be reassessed annually to determine whether the original dosage prescribed is still appropriate.

In C.B., who had been on T_3 without any evidence of cardiac toxicity, a less cautious approach in changing to T_4 can be attempted. An empiric L-thyroxine dosage of 68 mcg/day (40 kg × 1.6 mcg/kg/day) is an approximate dosing end point for C.B. The T_3 should be discontinued and T_4 initiated in a dose of 50 mcg/day; this dosage can be adjusted as needed based on C.B.'s symptoms and thyroid function tests. After T_3 therapy is discontinued, its effects will disappear over 3 to 5 days. In contrast, T_4 levels rise slowly over 4 to 5 days, so no overlap in T_3 administration is necessary to prevent hypothyroidism.

Parenteral Dosing

CASE 52-7

QUESTION 1: G.F., a 70-year-old man with long-standing hypothyroidism, has been receiving L-thyroxine 0.1 mg/day. Currently, he is in the hospital with a stroke and paralysis that prohibits him from swallowing oral medications. His last thyroid function tests were normal. What is a reasonable method of administering thyroid hormone to G.F.?

Because L-thyroxine has a half-life of 7 days, administration can be delayed for up to 1 week, assuming G.F. can resume oral intake at that time. However, if parenteral administration is required, L-thyroxine is available as an intramuscular (IM) or IV injection. The IV route is preferred because IM absorption may be slow and unpredictable, particularly if the circulation is compromised. Because the oral absorption of T_4 is approximately 80%,[72] parenteral doses should be decreased. Once IV L-thyroxine replacement is successful, maintenance with a once-weekly IM injection can be continued if oral ingestion is not feasible.[99]

Hypothyroidism in Pregnancy

CASE 52-8

QUESTION 1: P.K. is a 35-year-old woman with Hashimoto's thyroiditis, who is 6 weeks pregnant. Laboratory test results showed TT_4, 5 mcg/dL (normal, 4.8–10.4) and FT_4, 0.7 ng/dL (normal, 0.8–1.4). She takes her medications in the morning, which include L-thyroxine 0.1 mg/day and a prenatal vitamin enriched with iron and calcium. What dosing adjustments are required because of P.K.'s pregnancy?

Inadequately treated or undiagnosed maternal hypothyroidism can be detrimental to the mother and the developing fetus.[100,101] Miscarriage, spontaneous abortion, hypertension, preeclampsia, and higher rates of cesarean sections and stillbirths have been reported with maternal hypothyroidism. Congenital defects, congenital hypothyroidism (see Case 52-8, Question 2), abnormal fetal development, and impaired cognitive development in the newborn have been attributed to maternal hypothyroidism. The IQ scores of children born to mothers with undiagnosed hypothyroidism during pregnancy averaged 7 points lower than children born to euthyroid mothers.[100] A delay in both mental and motor development was observed in children aged 1 to 2 years old who were born to mothers with hypothyroxinemia but normal TSH levels during the first trimester of pregnancy.[101] Normal maternal thyroid function is essential during early fetal development. Fetal thyroid hormone production begins by the end of the first trimester, with the fetus relying on maternal thyroid hormones until that time. Transfer of maternal thyroid hormones is under the control of the placenta.[102] The risk of congenital hypothyroidism is small if maternal antibodies from Hashimoto's thyroiditis cross the fetal circulation. The infant's cord blood should be assayed at birth to ensure that TSH is normal and that the child is euthyroid.

The majority of women with primary hypothyroidism will require a 30% to 50% increase in the prepregnancy T_4 dosage to maintain euthyroidism during the first trimester of pregnancy.[102–105] The only evidence of increased T_4 demands is an elevated TSH level (e.g., subclinical hypothyroidism) that occurs between weeks 5 (but can be as early as 3) and 16 of gestation. Often, no clinical symptoms of hypothyroidism are evident, and the FT_4 and the index are normal. Because of the adverse consequences associated with maternal hypothyroidism, some have advocated universal TSH screening of all pregnant women[106] as well as empirically increasing the prepregnancy T_4 dosage by 30% (extra 2 pills/week) as soon as pregnancy is confirmed.[104] Because there is a physiologic decrease in TSH during pregnancy caused by the TSH-like activity of human chorionic gonadotropin, the upper limit of the normal TSH range should be adjusted for pregnancy.[102] TSH should be no higher than 2.5 microunits/mL during the first trimester and 3.0 microunits/mL in the second and third trimesters.[105]

Physiologic explanations for the increase in thyroid hormone requirements include the twofold increase in TBPA caused by high estrogen levels, increased volume of distribution of thyroid hormones, as well as maternal transport of T_4.[102,105] Rising HCG concentrations result in increased production of thyroid hormones.[102] Changes in serum proteins cause direct immunoassay of FT_4 to yield incorrect results. A newer assay, measurement of T_4 in the dialysate or ultrafiltrate of serum samples using liquid chromatography or tandem mass spectrometry, has been shown to produce reliable trimester-specific reference ranges for FT_4; however, these assays are not universally available.[107] In the absence of trimester-specific reference ranges for dialysate or ultrafiltrate measured FT_4, the FT_4 index or TT_4 should be used to evaluate thyroxine production.[35] It is important to recognize that coadministration of iron- and calcium-containing prenatal vitamins reduced T_4 absorption (see Case 52-9, Question 1) and that these drug interactions may affect dosage requirements. When prenatal vitamins with iron and calcium were separated by 4 hours from T_4 administration, only 31% of women required an increase in T_4 dose.[108] The increase in thyroid hormone requirements are likely because of a combination of physiologic and drug interaction causes. Women should be followed closely during pregnancy with monthly monitoring during the first half of pregnancy and at least once between gestation weeks 26 and 32. If necessary, the T_4 dosage should be adjusted to maintain a TSH in pregnancy-adjusted ranges and an ultrafiltrate-measured FT_4, FT_4I, or TT_4 in the upper limits of normal based on adjusted normal ranges. When the TT_4 is used, reference ranges should be increased by 50%.[35,107]

P.K.'s low TT_4 and FT_4 are concerning. The TT_4 should be much higher because of pregnancy-associated increases in TBG. The TSH level should be obtained, and the daily dosage of T_4 should be increased to 125 mcg after eliminating the possibility of patient non-adherence and drug interactions. Ingestion of the prenatal vitamins with iron and calcium should be separated by at least 4 hours from T_4. PK could also be instructed to take the T_4 at night for better absorption.[73] The TSH should be repeated in 6 weeks, and the dosage should be adjusted as needed to keep the TSH in the range as above. After delivery, the dosage should be reduced to prepregnancy levels and the FT_4 and TSH rechecked to ensure euthyroidism.

CONGENITAL HYPOTHYROIDISM

CASE 52-8, QUESTION 2: P.K. delivered a healthy baby, T.K., at term without difficulty. T.K.'s postpartum screening serum T_4 level was 5 mcg/dL (normal, 4.8–10.4), and TSH was 35 microunits/mL (normal, 0.45–4.1). At home, T.K. became lethargic, had a weak cry, sucked poorly, and failed to thrive. Assess the situation (including a treatment plan and prognosis). How is mental development affected?

T.K.'s symptoms are suggestive of congenital hypothyroidism, although in most infants the clinical signs and symptoms are so subtle and nonspecific that they are easily missed until the child is several months old. The early clinical findings include prolonged jaundice, skin mottling (cutis marmorata), lethargy, poor feeding, constipation, hypothermia, hoarse cry, large fontanels, distended abdomen, hypotonia, slow reflexes, and piglike facies. Respiratory difficulties, delayed skeletal maturation, and choking (but not palpable goiter) may be present. These infants are also at risk for additional congenital defects or complications.[109] Mass neonatal screening programs have been successful in detecting congenital hypothyroidism within the first few weeks of life before clinical manifestations are apparent and before irreversible changes occur.

The postpartum low serum T_4 concentration and elevated TSH level (>20 microunits/mL) in T.K. are of concern and should be verified. Transient hypothyroidism can result from intrauterine exposure to thioamides or excess iodides, or from transplacental passage of TRAb from the mother. Thyroid function tests often normalize without treatment in 3 to 6 months as the TRAb is cleared by the infant.[109] The diagnosis of hypothyroidism should be confirmed by a low serum T_4, a low FT_4, and an elevated TSH concentration during the next few weeks. Serum T_3 concentrations are often in the normal range and are not helpful. Normal serum T_4 concentrations are higher in the first few weeks of life and gradually return to normal by 2 to 4 months of life. The FT_4I may also be elevated. Because of these confusing changes, thyroid serum levels should be compared with the normal range for the approximate postnatal age.

Thyroid hormones play a critical role in normal growth and development, particularly of the CNS, during the first 3 years of life. If untreated, dwarfism and irreversible mental retardation occur. T.K.'s normal mental (IQ) and physical development will be determined by the age at which treatment is started, the initial dosage of T_4, the serum T_4 level attained during therapy, the adequacy with which treatment is maintained, and the cause and severity of the initial deficiency.[110–116] There is an inverse relationship between the amount of time to reach a euthyroid state and the likelihood of impaired neurologic development.[109]

Sodium L-thyroxine is the preparation of choice for replacement. T_4 tablets can be crushed and mixed with breast milk or formula; suspensions are not stable and should not be used. T_4 tablets should not be mixed with soy-based formulas because decreased absorption and longer time to reach a TSH <10 microunits/mL may occur. If a soy-based formula is required, the dosage of T_4 should be administered halfway between feeds.[109] T_3 is less desirable because its short half-life causes a greater fluctuation in plasma levels (Table 52-8). The initial replacement dose of T_4 should raise the serum T_4 as rapidly as possible to minimize the consequences of hypothyroidism on cognitive function. A delay

Table 52-9
T_4 Recommended Replacement Dose

Age	Daily mcg/kg T_4
3–6 months	10–15
6–12 months	5–7
1–10 years	3–6
>10 years	2–4

T_4, thyroxine.

in starting therapy of even a few days has resulted in a poorer IQ outcome.[111,112,116] A minimum T_4 dosage of 10 to 15 mcg/kg/day is recommended to raise the serum T_4 to >10 mcg/dL (129 nmol/L) by 7 days.[110] However, some suggest that higher than previously recommended dosages of 12 to 17 mcg/kg/day might be more effective, but concern about negative neurologic outcomes exists.[109,111,112] In the full-term healthy infant, full initial replacement T_4 doses are appropriate unless the infant has underlying heart disease or is extremely sensitive to the effects of thyroid hormones. In these infants, reduced doses of T_4 (approximately 25%–33% of the recommended dose) can be started and increased gradually by similar increments until the therapeutic dose is achieved. The recommended replacement dose decreases with age and is shown in Tables 52-4 and 52-9.

Mental development and attainment of normal growth are not severely impaired if adequate T_4 treatment is initiated before 3 months of age to achieve a T_4 level >10 mcg/dL (129 nmol/L).[109–112,114] Children with the most severe congenital hypothyroidism had IQs lower than their siblings.[113] Young adults 20 years after congenital hypothyroidism showed impaired motor and intellectual outcomes after suboptimal T_4 (<7.8 mcg/kg/day) therapy compared to sibling controls.[114] However, those receiving optimal therapy still had some memory, attention, and behavior deficits.[117] Newborns starting L-thyroxine during the first 4 to 6 weeks of life have mean IQs similar to controls. The IQ drops if treatment is delayed until 6 weeks and 3 months (mean IQ, 95), or until 3 and 6 months (mean IQ, 75). When treatment is delayed until 6 months to 1 year of age, normal mental development is impaired despite subsequent treatment. Higher IQs also were found in children who received T_4 dosages >10 mcg/kg/day and achieved a mean T_4 level >14 mcg/dL (181 nmol/L) in the first month of therapy.[109,111,112,116,118] Neurologic deficits were also more likely to occur in infants whose thyroid replacement was delayed or inadequate (T_4 <8 mcg/dL [103 nmol/L] within 30 days of therapy and/or had delayed TSH normalization [18–24 months]). Additional risk factors for low IQs and poor motor and speech skills despite adequate therapy include clinical signs of hypothyroidism during fetal life, T_4 <2 mcg/dL at birth, thyroid aplasia, and retarded bone age.[109,110,112]

The goal of therapy is a T_4 in the upper normal range (e.g., 10–18 mcg/dL and/or an FT_4 of 2 to 5 ng/dL) during the first 2 weeks of therapy, and then a lower target thereafter: a T_4 of 10 to 16 mcg/dL (and/or an FT_4 of 1.6–2.2 ng/dL). IQs are improved if TSH levels are normalized within the first month of therapy but no later than 3 months.[111,112,116,118] Thyroid function tests should be routinely monitored 2 to 4 weeks after starting therapy, then every 1 to 2 months during the first 6 months of life, every 3 to 4 months until age 3, and finally, every 6 to 12 months until growth is complete.[109] Although TSH suppression is the most reliable index of adequate replacement in older children, normalization of the TSH should not be used as the sole monitoring parameter in infants because the TSH may lag behind correction of the T_4 and/or FT_4 levels. Overtreatment should be avoided to prevent brain dysfunction, acceleration of bone age, and craniosynostosis (premature closure of the cranial sutures). Normal growth and development should also be a treatment goal. Other clinical end points include an improvement in activity level, skin color, temperature, facial appearance, and reversal of other symptoms and signs of hypothyroidism. The child will require lifelong replacement therapy.

UNRESPONSIVENESS TO LEVOTHYROXINE AND DRUG–DRUG INTERACTIONS

CASE 52-9

QUESTION 1: R.T., a 45-year-old woman, complains of weight gain, heavy menses, sluggishness, and cold intolerance. Her present medical problems include Hashimoto's thyroiditis, treated with L-thyroxine 150 mcg daily; hypercholesterolemia treated with cholestyramine 4 g 4 times a day (QID); anemia, treated with $FeSO_4$ 325 mg twice a day (BID); dysmenorrhea treated with estrogen-containing birth control pills daily; and a history of peptic ulcer disease, treated with antacids and sucralfate 1 g BID. She was recently started on calcium carbonate 1 g BID and raloxifene 60 mg daily to protect her bones. Her laboratory data include the following findings:

Cholesterol serum concentration, 280 mg/dL
TSH, 21 microunits/mL (normal, 0.45–4.1)
FT_4, 0.6 ng/dL (normal, 0.8–1.4)
Positive TgAb and TPOAb

R.T. admits that she self-increased her L-thyroxine dose because she feels better on the higher dose. Why is R.T. apparently unresponsive to thyroid therapy**?**

R.T.'s complaints and laboratory values confirm inadequate treatment of hypothyroidism despite thyroid therapy. Possible causes of therapeutic failure include non-adherence, error in diagnosis, poor absorption, subpotent medication, rapid metabolism, and tissue resistance.[71,119,120] Thyroid resistance is rare, and non-adherence, error in diagnosis, and rapid metabolism do not appear to be reasonable explanations in R.T.

The most likely explanations are poor bioavailability and/or a subpotent preparation. The timing of T_4 administration with her meals should be ascertained because its bioavailability is improved when it is taken on an empty stomach and at night.[71,73,121,122] Significantly lower TSH levels are achieved when levothyroxine is taken on an empty stomach than with food or at night.[122] Simultaneous coadministration of T_4 with soy proteins, coffee, or high-fiber diets (e.g., oat bran, soybean) should also be avoided because T_4s absorption can be impaired.[123–125] R.T.'s history does not include surgical bowel resection or GI disorders (e.g., steatorrhea, malabsorption). Evidence for incomplete absorption of the hormone can be obtained by comparing R.T.'s response to oral and parenteral T_4.[119]

L-Thyroxine bioavailability can also be compromised by the numerous medications that R.T. is taking. Estrogen therapy can increase T_4 requirements by increasing TBG to increase T_4 binding.[1] Cholestyramine, colestipol, iron sulfate, antacids, sucralfate, calcium preparations, particularly the carbonate salt, and raloxifene can impair thyroid absorption if these medications are administered at the same time.[71,126–133] Cholesterol-lowering agents (e.g., lovastatin) and phosphate binders are also reported to interfere with thyroid absorption.[129,134] R.T. should be questioned about the time she takes her thyroid medication. She should be instructed to take it on an empty stomach or at night,[73] and at least 12 hours apart from the raloxifene and 4 hours apart from the iron, calcium, and cholestyramine.[126–133] Aluminum-containing products (i.e., antacids, sucralfate) should be discontinued because separating the concurrent administration of T_4 and her aluminum-containing preparations does not consistently correct this interaction.[130,131] R.T. should be changed to an aluminum- and calcium-free antacid and, if necessary, an H_2-receptor antagonist. Proton pump inhibitors (e.g., omeprazole) should be avoided because decreased acid secretion may reduce T_4 absorption, although data are conflicting.[135,136] After R.T. has been instructed on the proper times of administration for her medications, the therapeutic response and thyroid function tests should be reevaluated in 6 to 8 weeks before any changes are made.

CASE 52-9, QUESTION 2: Could R.T.'s hypothyroidism be responsible for her hypercholesterolemia?

Type IIa hypercholesterolemia is the most common lipid abnormality observed in patients with primary hypothyroidism.[137] Although the rate of cholesterol synthesis is normal in hypothyroid patients, the rate of cholesterol clearance is decreased. Similarly, slow removal of triglycerides may result in hypertriglyceridemia. Hypercholesterolemia is frequently observed before the appearance of clinical hypothyroidism. Treatment with T_4 alone should lower the cholesterol levels if no other causes are contributing.

Myxedema Coma

CLINICAL PRESENTATION

CASE 52-10

QUESTION 1: R.B., a 65-year-old, agitated woman arrived at the emergency department complaining of chest pain unrelieved by nitroglycerin (NTG). Her medical problems include alcoholic cardiomyopathy, angina, and hypothyroidism. Although she has been advised repeatedly to take her T_4 regularly, she continues to take it sporadically. A FT_4 drawn 4 months ago was 0.5 ng/dL (normal, 0.7–1.9). Haloperidol 2 mg IM and morphine sulfate 10 mg IM were given for the agitation. After the injection, the nurse noticed mental depression, lethargy, and shallow breathing. R.B.'s oral temperature was 34.5°C, and she exhibited chills and shakes. What is your assessment of R.B.'s subjective and objective data?

R.B. has several symptoms consistent with myxedema coma.[138] The classic features are hypothermia, delayed DTRs, and an altered sensorium that ranges from stupor to coma. Other predominant features include hypoxia, carbon dioxide retention, severe hypoglycemia, hyponatremia, and paranoid psychosis. Typical physical findings (Table 52-3) include a puffy face and eyelids, a yellowish discoloration of the skin, and loss of the lateral eyebrows. Pleural and pericardial effusions and cardiomegaly may be present. Because myxedema coma frequently occurs in older women, it is often difficult to distinguish the signs and symptoms from dementia or other disease states, as illustrated by R.B. Precipitating factors include cold weather or hypothermia, stress (e.g., surgery, infection, trauma), coexisting disease states such as MI, diabetes, hypoglycemia, or fluid and electrolyte abnormalities (especially hyponatremia), and medications such as sedatives, narcotic analgesics, antidepressants, and other respiratory depressants and diuretics.

Haloperidol and morphine might be responsible for what appears to be impending myxedema coma in R.B. In severely myxedematous patients, respiratory depressants (anesthetics, narcotic analgesics, phenothiazines, sedative-hypnotics) alone or in combination with the hypothermic effects of the phenothiazines can aggravate the preexisting hypothermia and carbon dioxide retention to precipitate myxedema coma.[138,139] Tranquilizers such as haloperidol should not be given; small doses of less depressive sedative-hypnotics such as the benzodiazepines should be used only when necessary. Myxedematous patients are also inherently sensitive to the respiratory depressant effects of narcotic analgesics, especially morphine. A dose as small as 10 mg may induce coma in a hypothyroid patient or cause death in a patient who is already comatose. If morphine is required, the dose should be decreased to one-third to one-half the usual analgesic dose, and the respiratory rate should be monitored closely.

TREATMENT

CASE 52-10, QUESTION 2: What would be a reasonable therapeutic plan for the management of R.B.'s myxedema coma?

Emergency treatment, usually in the intensive care unit, of myxedema coma is directed toward thyroid replacement, maintenance of vital functions, and elimination of precipitating factors. Despite immediate and aggressive therapy with large replacement doses of thyroid, mortality rates of 60% to 70% are common.[138]

Whether T_4 or T_3 is the drug of choice in myxedema coma is controversial because no comparative trials have been conducted. Although T_3 is potentially more cardiotoxic, it has been recommended because its more rapid onset might reverse coma faster, and the peripheral conversion from T_4 to the biologically active T_3 might be inhibited in severe systemic disease.[139–143] T_4 alone, T_3 alone, and a combination of the two have all been used successfully to treat myxedema coma. However, L-thyroxine is generally regarded as the hormone of choice because of greater clinical experience with T_4 than with T_3. Also, mortality has occurred despite the higher T_3 levels achieved after T_3 administration.[143] T_3 might be considered after failure of T_4 or if concomitant systemic illness (e.g., heart failure) is likely to impair conversion of T_4 to T_3. Supraphysiologic elevations in T_3 levels occur only after oral administration but are not seen after IV T_3 infusion. Factors associated with a higher mortality 1 month after therapy include older age, cardiac complications, and T_4 replacement ≥500 mcg/day or T_3 replacement >75 mcg/day.[139,143]

L-Thyroxine 400 to 500 mcg should be given IV initially in patients <55 years of age without cardiac disease to saturate empty TBG sites and raise the serum T_4 level to 6 to 7 mcg/dL.[138,144] This initial dose can be adjusted based on the patient's weight and other restrictive factors (e.g., age, cardiac disease). The initial T_4 dosage for R.B. should be reduced to 300 mcg/day to avoid worsening her angina. If the proper dosage is given, consciousness, restoration of vital signs, and decreased TSH levels should occur within 24 hours. If T_3 is preferred, the usual dose is 10 to 20 mcg IV, followed by 10 mcg every 4 hours for the first 24 hours, and then 10 mcg every 6 hours for a few days until oral therapy can be started.[138]

Maintenance doses should be titrated to the patient's clinical response. Because myxedema can impair oral absorption, the IV route is preferred to ensure adequate drug concentrations. Oral administration is permitted once GI function returns to normal. The smallest dosage (without untoward effects) administered should be 50 to 100 mcg/day of T_4 or 10 to 15 mcg of T_3 every 12 hours.[138,144]

Supportive measures include assisted ventilation, glucose for hypoglycemia, restriction of fluids for hyponatremia, and the use of blood or plasma expanders to prevent circulatory collapse and to maintain blood pressure. The use of blankets to treat R.B.'s hypothermia is not advised because vasodilation will occur and further compromise the cardiovascular components of shock. Although steroids have not been shown to be clearly beneficial in primary myxedema, they may be lifesaving in patients with hypopituitarism masquerading as myxedema coma. Because it is difficult to distinguish between primary and secondary myxedema, hydrocortisone 50 to 100 mg every 6 hours should be given empirically.[138]

Appropriate measures should be taken to relieve R.B.'s chest pain while ruling out the possibility of an MI. The use of a narcotic antagonist such as naloxone may be beneficial in this instance because it can reverse the effects of the morphine. Naloxone can also arouse comatose patients intoxicated with alcohol.

Hypothyroidism with Congestive Heart Failure

CLINICAL PRESENTATION

CASE 52-11

QUESTION 1: E.B., a 45-year-old woman, is admitted with chest pain, SOB, dyspnea on exertion, and orthopnea suggestive of CHF complicated by an MI. Significant past medical history reveals exertional angina and Graves' disease, treated with RAI ablation 10 years ago. Physical examination reveals cardiomegaly, diastolic hypertension, obesity, facial edema and puffiness, delayed DTRs, and non-pitting pretibial edema. Pertinent laboratory findings include the following results:

FT_4, 0.2 ng/dL (normal, 0.8–1.4)
TSH, 100 microunits/mL (normal, 0.45–4.1)
Creatinine phosphokinase, 300 units/L with negative MB bands
Aspartate aminotransferase (AST), 80 units/L
Lactate dehydrogenase (LDH), 250 units/L
Brain natriuretic peptide, 550 pg/mL
Troponin, 0.3 ng/mL (normal, 0.3–1.5)

A chest radiograph reveals cardiomegaly and pericardial effusions, and an electrocardiogram (ECG) shows bradycardia and flattened T waves with ST depression. Furosemide, nitrates, metropolol, and Lisinopril are started. E.B.'s symptoms improve, but her cardiac abnormalities are not reversed.

Why do these clinical findings suggest hypothyroidism?

E.B.'s abnormal thyroid function tests, symptoms, physical findings, and history of RAI therapy are consistent with severe hypothyroidism. "Myxedema heart" can be confused with low-output CHF because the symptoms are similar: cardiomegaly, dyspnea, edema, pericardial effusions, and abnormal ECG.[85,138] Therefore, hypothyroidism should be ruled out in all patients with new or worsening symptoms of cardiovascular disease (e.g., angina, arrhythmia). Although hypothyroidism alone rarely causes CHF, it can worsen an underlying cardiac condition. Rarely, ventricular arrhythmia, including torsades de pointes, can occur from a prolonged QT interval.

Although E.B.'s enzyme elevations (i.e., AST, CK, LDH, CPK) are suggestive of an MI, they all may be moderately or significantly increased from chronic skeletal or cardiac muscle damage or from decreased enzyme clearance secondary to hypothyroidism. The normal troponin level and negative CPK-MB bands eliminate the likelihood of an MI.

TREATMENT

CASE 52-11, QUESTION 2: What might be the effect of hypothyroidism on the cardiac treatment and status of E.B.?

If E.B.'s cardiac abnormalities are caused by hypothyroidism, adequate doses of T_4 will restore the heart size, normalize the diastolic blood pressure, reverse the ECG findings, and normalize the serum enzyme elevations within 2 to 4 weeks. However, improvement in myocardial function begins only at dosages of 50 to 75 mcg/day of T_4, which may be tolerated poorly by cardiac patients.

The relationship between the altered lipid metabolism of hypothyroidism and increased risk of atherosclerosis is controversial and poorly documented.[137] Angina pectoris and MI are rather uncommon among hypothyroid patients. Theoretically, the hypometabolic state occurring in hypothyroidism may protect the ischemic myocardium by reducing metabolic demands. However, hypothyroidism actually aggravates sub-endocardial ischemia during an acute MI by decreasing erythrocyte production of 2,3-diphosphoglycerate, which shifts the oxyhemoglobin dissociation curve to the left. This effect further diminishes oxygen delivery to already ischemic tissues. Angina or premature beats can develop or worsen with the institution of T_4 therapy,[145–147] so doses should be titrated carefully (see Case 52-11, Question 3). Without organic disease, digitalis is ineffective and may even be harmful. Hypothyroid patients show an increased sensitivity to digitalis, and digitalis toxicity is possible unless the maintenance dose is decreased (see Case 52-14, Question 3).[148,149] Nitrates may precipitate hypotension and/or syncope in hypothyroid patients because these patients have a low circulating blood volume and their response to vasodilation can be exaggerated. Furthermore, if β-blockers are required, the cardioselective β-blockers are preferred. The non-cardioselective β-blockers have produced coronary spasm by exacerbating the compensatory increase in norepinephrine levels and α-adrenergic tone found in hypothyroidism.

Case 52-11, Question 3: How aggressively should thyroid hormone therapy be initiated in a patient like E.B. who has angina? What is the hormone replacement of choice in patients with cardiac disease?

Patients with long-standing hypothyroidism, arteriosclerotic cardiac disease, or advanced age tend to be extremely sensitive to the cardiac effects of thyroid hormone. Initiation of normal or even subtherapeutic doses might produce severe angina, MI, supra- and ventricular premature beats, cardiac failure, or sudden death and underscore the need to replace thyroid cautiously, and sometimes suboptimally, to avoid cardiac toxicity.[145–147,150]

The angina and cardiac status should be controlled before initiating T_4 therapy. In the patient with poorly controlled angina, cardiac catheterization is warranted to assess the coronary artery status before starting hormone therapy. Coronary bypass has been performed safely with minimal complications in the hypothyroid patient to control the angina and may allow institution of full replacement doses without cardiotoxicity.[151]

For E.B., 12.5 to 25 mcg daily of T_4 should be initiated cautiously and increased as tolerated by similar increments of T_4 every 4 to 6 weeks until a therapeutic dosage is reached. The rapidity with which the increments can proceed is determined by how well each increased dose is tolerated. If cardiac toxicity occurs, therapy should be stopped immediately. Once symptoms resolve, therapy can be restarted using smaller dosage increments and longer intervals between dosage adjustments. If cardiac symptoms recur, further T_4 therapy should be stopped pending cardiac evaluation. In patients with severe cardiac sensitivity, complete euthyroidism might never be achieved, and the correct replacement dosage is a compromise between prevention of myxedema and avoidance of cardiac toxicity.[147] E.B.'s clinical status and ECG should be monitored closely during the titration period. T_4 should be discontinued or decreased at the first sign of cardiac deterioration. It is not necessary to monitor thyroid function tests (e.g., TSH or FT_4) during the titration period because the results will remain low until adequate replacement is achieved. Thyroid function tests should be obtained once maximally tolerated or estimated euthyroid dosages are achieved.

Some suggest that T_3 is the agent of choice in patients with cardiac abnormalities because of its shorter duration of action. After therapy is withdrawn, the effects of T_3 dissipate in 3 to 5 days, compared to 7 to 10 for T_4. Thus, if toxicity occurs, the effects of T_3 will disappear rapidly on cessation of therapy, a theoretical advantage in the cardiac patient. Nevertheless, T_3 is not recommended because its greater potency requires finer and more difficult dosage titration to ensure smooth and uniform blood levels. Furthermore, the high serum T_3 levels that occur after oral administration might cause more cardiac toxicity, especially angina.

Subclinical Hypothyroidism

CASE 52-12

Question 1: M.P., a healthy 53-year-old woman, comes in for her regular checkup. She denies any symptoms of hypothyroidism and feels well. She has no other medical problems, takes no medications, and has no known allergies. Her physical examination is within normal limits. Routine screening laboratory tests are normal except for an FT_4 of 1.2 ng/dL (normal, 0.8–1.4) and a TSH of 8 microunits/mL (normal, 0.45–4.1). Does M.P. require thyroid treatment, based on her clinical presentation and laboratory findings?

M.P.'s free thyroid levels are normal, but her TSH level is elevated, indicating subclinical hypothyroidism (SH). The prevalence of SH ranges from 4% to 10% and increases to 26% in the elderly population, particularly women.[87,88] It is unclear whether SH represents the early stages of thyroid failure. The estimated risk of developing overt hypothyroidism after 10 years in untreated patients by Kaplan–Meier curves was 0% for a TSH level of 4 to 6 microunits/mL, 42.8% for a TSH level of 6 to 12 microunits/mL, and 76.9% for a TSH level >12 microunits/mL. This risk increased in patients with positive thyroid antibodies.[152] Because the most common clinical scenarios involve asymptomatic patients with TSH levels <10 microunits/mL, negative thyroid antibodies, and no history of prior thyroid disease, routine thyroid screening has been recommended, particularly in elderly women.[88]

Mild symptoms of hypothyroidism, including psychiatric and cognitive abnormalities, are found in approximately 30% of patients with SH, but the average TSH level usually exceeds 11 microunits/mL. Cardiac dysfunction, including impaired left ventricular diastolic function at rest, systolic dysfunction with exercise, atherosclerosis, CHF, and MI has been reported.[85,88,153–155] Data showing an increased risk of coronary heart disease (CHD) are conflicting and influenced by the severity of SH, study design, and length of follow-up. A meta-analysis noted a 1.6 times increased risk of CHD,[156] a cross-sectional analysis noted an odds ratio of 2.2 only in those with TSH levels of ≥10 microunits/mL, whereas a 20-year longitudinal analysis found a significant risk (hazard ratio (HR) of 1.7) regardless of the degree of TSH elevation.[157] However, a large prospective cohort study found no significant association with atherosclerotic disease or cardiac mortality but observed an increase in all-cause mortality at 10 years of follow-up.[158] Compelling data reported from 11 large prospective cohorts with a median follow-up of 2.5 to 20 years involving 3,450 subjects with subclinical hypothyroidism found an increased risk of CHD (HR 1.89) and mortality (HR 1.5) but not total mortality only in those with TSH level >10 microunits/mL after adjustment for traditional cardiovascular factors. No increased CHD or CHD mortality was noted with more minimal TSH elevations.[159]

Other atypical and nonspecific signs and symptoms reflecting dysfunction of any part of the body may occur, primarily in the elderly. Failure to thrive, mental confusion, weight loss with poor appetite, incontinence, depression, inability to walk, carpal tunnel syndrome, deafness, ileus, anemia, hypercholesterolemia, and hyponatremia have been reported.[87,88,153–155]

Treatment of subclinical hypothyroidism with T_4 is controversial because study results are conflicting. Potential benefits of treatment include (a) preventing progression to hypothyroidism, (b) improving the lipid profile and reducing cardiac risks, and (c) reversing symptoms of hypothyroidism. Patients with higher TSH levels (e.g., >10 microunits/mL), a history of previously diagnosed thyroid disease, elevated lipid levels, or evidence of positive thyroid antibodies gained the most benefit from L-thyroxine therapy.[85,88,152,155,160] L-Thyroxine significantly reduced total cholesterol by 7.9–15.8 mg/dL and low-density cholesterol concentrations by 10 mg/dL; serum HDL cholesterol and triglyceride concentrations remain unchanged.[88,154,155,160] Improvement of elevated intraocular pressures, memory, mood, somatic complaints, and diastolic dysfunction has also been reported after T_4 replacement.[152,154,155,160]

Treatment of older patients requires an assessment of the risks versus benefits of therapy. Thyroid therapy carries the risk of unmasking underlying cardiac disease in older patients. Nevertheless, thyroid replacement appears reasonable in asymptomatic patients with TSH levels >10 microunits/mL and especially those with symptoms of mild hypothyroidism, dyslipidemia, laboratory abnormalities, or end-organ alterations.[87,88,152,154,160] Patients with mild subclinical hypothyroidism (TSH 6–10 microunits/mL) may benefit from therapy with L-thyroxine 25 to 75 mcg/day when there is evidence of cardiovascular risk (e.g., diastolic dysfunction, risk of atherosclerotic disease, diabetes) or clinical indicators suggestive of hypothyroidism (e.g., goiter, antibodies).[88] There is no evidence supporting the treatment of mild subclinical disease in patients over 80 years of age.[88] Conversely, patients with asymptomatic subclinical hypothyroidism and a TSH level <10 microunits/mL do not warrant immediate therapy, but close follow-up is recommended.

Because M.P. is asymptomatic and has a TSH level <10 microunits/mL, it is reasonable to delay therapy and recheck the TSH in a few months.

Hypopituitarism and Thyroxine Replacement with a Normal Thyroid-Stimulating Hormone Level

CASE 52-13

QUESTION 1: J.P. is a 65-year-old woman who complains of fatigue, cold intolerance, dry skin, and weight gain for the past several months. Her thyroid examination and DTRs are within normal limits. A TSH level was 2.5 microunits/mL (normal, 0.45–4.1). She denies taking any other medications. J.P. is started empirically on a 3-month trial of L-thyroxine. How should the TSH level be interpreted? Is T_4 therapy indicated based on her presenting findings?

Despite complaints that could be consistent with hypothyroidism (e.g., fatigue, cold intolerance, dry skin, weight gain), the normal TSH level indicates that J.P. is euthyroid. However, because a diagnosis of hypopituitarism (i.e., TSH level could be normal or low) cannot be ruled out, an FT_4 level should be obtained; a low level would increase the likelihood of hypopituitarism. Some argue that hypopituitarism is underdiagnosed and would advocate adding FT_4 to the primary screening tests.[161]

If the FT_4 level is normal, indicating euthyroidism, then hypopituitarism is unlikely and L-thyroxine therapy is not indicated. A randomized, double-blind, placebo-controlled crossover trial found that T_4 supplementation in patients with hypothyroid symptoms and normal thyroid function tests was not more effective than placebo in improving cognitive function or psychologic well-being despite changes in the TSH and FT_4 levels.[162,163]

In J.P., the T_4 should be discontinued because there is no evidence of its efficacy in euthyroid individuals.

HYPERTHYROIDISM

Clinical Presentation

CASE 52-14

QUESTION 1: S.K., a 48-year-old woman, is admitted to the hospital for a possible MI. Her complaints include chest pain that is unrelieved by NTG, increasing SOB with exercise, nervousness, palpitations, muscle weakness, weight loss despite an increased appetite, and epistaxis; she also bruises easily. She has a history of deep venous thrombosis treated with warfarin 5 mg/day; her last international normalized ratio (INR) was 1.8 (normal, 1; therapeutic, 2–3). She has angina, treated with NTG 0.4 mg, and CHF, treated with digoxin 0.25 mg/day.

Physical examination reveals a thin, flushed, hyperkinetic, nervous woman. Blood pressure (BP) is 180/90 mmHg; pulse is 130 beats/minute, irregularly irregular; respiratory rate is 30 breaths/minute; and temperature is 37.5°C. Other pertinent findings include a lid lag with stare, proptosis with tearing, decreased visual acuity, a diffusely enlarged thyroid gland without nodules, a bruit in the left lobe of the thyroid, positive jugular venous distention (JVD), bibasilar rales, warm moist skin with multiple bruises, new-onset atrial fibrillation (AF), slight diarrhea, hepatomegaly, acropachy, 2+ pitting edema, a fine tremor, proximal muscle weakness, and irregular scant menses.

Laboratory data include the following results:

FT_4, 2.9 ng/dL (normal, 0.8–1.4)
TSH, <0.5 microunits/mL (normal, 0.45–4.1)
RAIU at 24 hours, 80% (normal, 5%–35%)
INR, 4.8 (normal, 1; therapeutic, 2–3)
TPOAb, 200 IU/mL (normal, <0.8)
Alkaline phosphatase, 200 units/L
Total bilirubin, 1.1 mg/dL
AST, 60 units/L
Alanine aminotransferase, 55 units/L

A RAI scan shows a diffusely enlarged gland, 3 to 4 times the normal size. What subjective and objective data are suggestive of hyperthyroidism in S.K.?

S.K. presents with many of the clinical and laboratory features[164] associated with an increased metabolic state resulting from excessive T_4 (Table 52-5). Her ocular symptoms are consistent with Graves' disease and include lid lag (lid falls behind the movement of the eye and a narrow white rim of sclera becomes visible between the upper lid and cornea, producing a "staring" appearance), ophthalmopathy (protrusion of the eyeball), and decreased visual acuity. The thyroid bruit, palpitations, exertional dyspnea, worsening CHF (JVD, bibasilar rales, edema, hepatomegaly), diarrhea, irregular scant menses, nervousness, tremor, muscle weakness, weight loss despite increased appetite, increased perspiration, and flushing of the skin are consistent with a hypermetabolic state. Although sinus tachycardia is the most common arrhythmia in hyperthyroidism, new-onset AF is the presenting symptom in 5% to 20% of patients with hyperthyroidism, particularly in those older than 70 years.[165] Together with S.K.'s symptoms, a diagnosis of Graves' disease is confirmed by an elevated FT_4 level, an undetectable TSH level, an increased RAIU, positive TPOAb, and a diffusely enlarged goiter. Her cardiac status and other medical problems are aggravated by the hyperthyroidism. (Table 52-6 lists the causes of hyperthyroidism.)

Hypoprothrombinemia

CASE 52-14, QUESTION 2: What factors contribute to S.K.'s hypoprothrombinemia? What effect could this have on her subsequent drug treatment?

The hypoprothrombinemia and bleeding observed in S.K. are most likely related to an exaggerated response to warfarin. This may be related to a decrease in the hepatic metabolism of warfarin (secondary to hepatic congestion), but it is more likely that S.K.'s findings are because of the combined effects of hyperthyroidism and warfarin on vitamin K–dependent clotting factors.

WARFARIN METABOLISM

Warfarin metabolism and the metabolism of vitamin K–dependent clotting factors can be altered by thyroid status. Net circulating levels of vitamin K–dependent clotting factors are generally not altered in hyperthyroid patients because both the synthesis and catabolism of these clotting factors are increased. However, an enhanced anticoagulant response occurs when the warfarin-induced decrease in clotting factor synthesis is combined with the hyperthyroidism-induced increase in clotting factor catabolism.[12,166] This may explain S.K.'s elevated INR, bruising, and history of epistaxis.

The opposite occurs in hypothyroidism, in which a decrease in both the metabolism and synthesis of clotting factors occurs. In hypothyroid patients, the response to oral anticoagulants is delayed because the clotting factors are eliminated more slowly.[12,166] Therefore, hyperthyroid patients need less warfarin, whereas hypothyroid patients require more warfarin to achieve the same hypoprothrombinemic response. The anticoagulant response to warfarin should be monitored carefully in patients with thyroid abnormalities, and the dosage adjusted as the thyroid status changes.

THIOAMIDE EFFECTS

Because S.K.'s hyperthyroidism will most likely be treated with a thioamide, caution must be exercised. Treatment of hyperthyroid patients with thioamides, especially PTU, has been associated with hypoprothrombinemia, thrombocytopenia, and bleeding, albeit rarely.[167] These drugs can depress the bone marrow and the synthesis of clotting factors II, III, VII, IX, X, and XIII; vitamin K and prothrombin times may remain depressed for up to 2 months after discontinuation of therapy. These effects may be caused by a subclinical hepatic alteration in synthesis or hepatotoxicity (see Case 52-15, Question 10).[30,168–171] Symptoms occur 2 weeks to 18 months after starting therapy. The bleeding is responsive to vitamin K or blood transfusions. (Also see Case 52-15, Questions 3 and 4 for further discussion of treatment with thioamides.)

Response to Digoxin

CASE 52-14, QUESTION 3: S.K.'s dose of digoxin was increased to 0.5 mg daily because of persistent AF with a rapid ventricular response. Why was such a large dose of digoxin required? What other options can be used to control her ventricular rate?

The AF of hyperthyroidism is often resistant to digitalis. When euthyroid patients with AF were given digitalis before and after exogenous T_3 administration, the daily dose of digoxin required to maintain a ventricular rate of 70 was increased from 0.2 to 0.8 mg after T_3 administration.[172] Higher dosages of digoxin without side effects might be tolerated better by the hyperthyroid patient.[148,149,172] Nevertheless, the goal of digoxin therapy should be a higher target heart rate (i.e., 100 beats/minute) than that achieved with digoxin in the euthyroid patient with AF to minimize cardiac toxicity. If additional rate control is required, β-blockers or calcium channel blockers (e.g., diltiazem or verapamil) can be added. Unless contraindicated by severe bronchospasm, β-blockers rather than calcium channel blockers are preferred because they are more effective in controlling the ventricular rate and are less likely to cause hypotension.

This apparent resistance to digitalis is attributed to intrinsic changes in myocardial function, to an increased volume of distribution for digoxin, and to an increased glomerular filtration of the glycoside.[148,149,172] Conversely, hypothyroid patients are inordinately sensitive to the effects of digitalis and require smaller doses to achieve a therapeutic response. Regardless of the mechanism, one should be aware that higher-than-normal doses might be required in patients with thyrotoxicosis and that the initial dosage should be reduced as the hyperthyroid state resolves.

S.K. should be maintained on warfarin because of a high prevalence of systemic embolization in thyrotoxic patients with AF. Anticoagulation should be started when the AF is first diagnosed and continued until S.K. is euthyroid and in NSR. This is especially true for younger patients at low risk of bleeding with warfarin. The risks versus benefits of anticoagulation should be weighed before therapy (see Chapter 16). Because an increased sensitivity to warfarin is observed, close monitoring is warranted (see Case 52-14, Question 2). Cardioversion, either medical or electrical, should not be attempted if she is still toxic because the success rate is low. If cardioversion is to be used, it should not be attempted until the third or fourth month after achieving euthyroidism.[165]

T_3 Thyrotoxicosis: Clinical Presentation

CASE 52-15

QUESTION 1: C.R., a 27-year-old woman, has a 3-month history of intermittent heat intolerance, sweats, tremor, and severe muscle weakness, which has limited her ability to climb stairs. Her weight has increased because of increased appetite. She is also bothered by the pounding of her heart and some minor difficulty in swallowing. There is a family history of thyroid disease, but she denies taking any thyroid medications or any history of radiation to her neck. C.R. previously received iodide drops with symptomatic improvement, but her disease recurred despite its continued administration. Her other medical problems include type 2 diabetes controlled by diet, and osteoarthritis treated with aspirin 650 mg PO q4h. She has a history of noncompliance with her clinic visits.

Pertinent physical findings include a BP of 180/90 mmHg, a pulse of 110 beats/minute, hyperreflexia, lid lag, and a diffusely enlarged thyroid gland that is about 4 times normal (about 100 g). Laboratory data include the following:

TT_4, 6 mcg/dL (normal, 4.8–10.4)
FT_4, 2 ng/dL (normal, 0.8–1.4)
TSH, <0.01 microunits/mL (normal, 0.45–4.1)
TPOAb, 350 IU/mL (normal, <0.8)
Fasting blood glucose, 350 mg/dL
Assess these subjective and objective data.

C.R.'s laboratory findings of a positive TPOAb and elevated thyroid hormone levels verify an autoimmune hyperthyroid state. However, the serum FT_4 is elevated only slightly and is disproportionately low relative to the severity of her symptoms, the undetectable TSH level, and her other laboratory findings. The low normal TT_4 could be explained by displacement of T_4 from TBG by aspirin (see Case 52-2). The possibility of a variant type of hyperthyroidism known as T_3 toxicosis should be considered. The clinical features include signs and symptoms of thyrotoxicosis, normal or borderline high FT_4, an undetectable TSH level, and elevated T_3 levels. The latter occurs through preferential secretion and peripheral conversion of T_4 to T_3. A T_3 level should be obtained to establish the diagnosis.

Asymptomatic elevations of T_3 levels often precede elevation of T_4 levels and the development of overt hyperthyroidism. T_3 toxicosis probably represents an early stage of classic T_4 toxicosis and is useful for early diagnosis or as an early indicator of relapse after discontinuation of thioamide therapy.

Iodides

CASE 52-15, QUESTION 2: Why were the iodide drops initially effective in improving C.R.'s symptoms and later ineffective? When are iodides indicated? What is their mechanism of action?

Iodides have several effects: They inhibit thyroid hormone release, they block iodotyrosine and iodothyronine synthesis by blocking organification, and they decrease the vascularity of the thyroid gland.[173] However, large doses may accentuate hyperthyroidism because they provide a significant increase in available substrate for hormone synthesis (see Case 52-24).[28,173]

The inhibitory effect of exogenous iodides on the intrathyroidal organification of iodides is known as the Wolff–Chaikoff effect. This is an inherent autoregulatory function of the normal gland to prevent excessive hormone synthesis in the event of a large iodide load. The Wolff–Chaikoff effect occurs when intrathyroidal concentrations of iodides reach a critical level, and this is not overcome by TSH stimulation. However, as illustrated by C.R., the gland can "escape" from this block even with continued iodide use. The gland escapes by decreasing iodide transport or by leaking iodide. Both mechanisms decrease the critical intrathyroidal iodide level, thereby decreasing the block to organification. This effect is illustrated in C.R. Therefore, iodides should not be used as primary therapy for Graves' disease.

Conversely, some patients are responsive to iodide therapy, including (a) patients who already have high intrathyroidal iodine stores (i.e., "hot" nodules, Graves' disease); (b) patients with underlying defects in organic binding mechanisms (i.e., Hashimoto's); (c) patients who develop drug-induced thyroid disorders (see Cases 52-23 and 52-24); and (d) patients with Graves' disease made euthyroid with RAI or surgery and who are receiving no thyroid replacement.

These patients are so sensitive that small doses of iodide can elicit the Wolff–Chaikoff effect, resulting in either amelioration of hyperthyroid symptoms or precipitation of hypothyroidism.[16,28,173] For this reason, patients with recurrent hyperthyroidism after surgery or RAI can often be managed with iodides alone.

The most important pharmacologic effect of iodides is their ability to promptly inhibit thyroid hormone release when dosages of 6 mg/day are given.[16,173] The mechanism is unknown, but it is not related to the Wolff–Chaikoff effect, which may take several weeks to manifest. Unlike the Wolff–Chaikoff effect, this effect can be overcome partially by an increase in TSH secretion. Thus, the normal gland can escape in 7 to 14 days because inhibition of thyroid hormone release stimulates a reflex increase in TSH secretion. Because patients with hyperthyroidism experience an improvement in symptoms within 2 to 7 days of initiation of therapy, inhibition of hormone release must be the predominant mechanism of action for the iodides. This rapid onset is the reason iodides are used in the treatment of thyroid storm and as an ameliorative measure while awaiting the onset of the therapeutic effects of thioamides or RAI.

Large doses of iodides are also used 2 weeks before thyroid surgery to increase the firmness of the thyroid gland by decreasing its size, vascularity, and friability. Iodides facilitate a smoother, less complicated surgery and reduce the risk of postoperative complications by inducing a euthyroid state.[173]

Stable iodine can be administered orally either as an unpleasant-tasting Lugol's solution (5% iodine and 10% potassium iodide), containing 8 mg/drop of iodide, or as the more palatable saturated solution of potassium iodide (SSKI), containing 50 mg/drop of iodide. The minimum effective daily dose is 6 mg,[173] although larger doses (e.g., 5–10 drops QID of SSKI) are often administered.

The advantages of iodide therapy are that it is simple, inexpensive, and relatively nontoxic and involves no glandular destruction. Disadvantages include "escape," accentuation of thyrotoxicosis, allergic reactions, relapse after discontinuation of treatment, and subsequent interference with RAI if used before therapy.

Treatment Modalities

CASE 52-15, QUESTION 3: What are the advantages and disadvantages of the different treatment modalities available for C.R.?

The three major treatment modalities for Graves'-related hyperthyroidism are the thioamides, RAI, and surgery (Table 52-10).[164] In most cases, any of these three modalities can be used, and there is controversy as to which is the most effective therapy. Often the final decision is empiric, depending on the clinician's available resources and the patient's desires. A review of treatment guidelines published by the major endocrine organizations found that RAI is the most common treatment, while surgery is the least common.[174] Patients who are older and those with cardiac disease, concomitant ophthalmopathy, and hyperthyroidism caused by a toxic multinodular goiter are treated best with RAI. Surgery is the preferred therapy for pregnant women who are drug intolerant, when obstructive symptoms are present, or if malignancy is suspected.

THIOAMIDES

The thioamides are the preferred treatment for children, pregnant women, and young adults with uncomplicated Graves' disease.[164,175,176] This is the only treatment that leaves the thyroid gland intact and does not carry the added risk of permanent hypothyroidism often associated with RAI or surgery.

Because the thyrotoxicosis of Graves' disease might be self-limiting, thioamides are used to control the symptoms until spontaneous remission occurs. Thioamides should also be given before treatment with RAI or surgery to deplete the gland of stored thyroid hormone, which prevents subsequent thyroid storm. Although hyperthyroidism from toxic nodules will also respond to thioamides, more definitive therapy (surgery or RAI) is needed because these conditions do not undergo spontaneous remission.

Disadvantages of thioamide therapy include the numerous tablets required, patient adherence, possible drug toxicity, the long duration of treatment, and the low remission rates after discontinuation of therapy (see Case 52-16).

The use of thioamides in C.R. has several potential drawbacks. Her relatively large gland and severe disease make the prognosis for spontaneous remission somewhat less favorable. A delay in the onset of thioamide's effect may be expected if intraglandular stores of thyroid have been increased by her prior iodide therapy. Furthermore, her non-adherence and difficulty swallowing may necessitate another means of treatment. Thioamides may also be prepared for administration by the rectal routes.[177–179]

SURGERY

Surgery is considered the treatment of choice[164,180–182] when (a) malignancy is suspected; (b) esophageal obstruction, evidenced by difficulty swallowing, is present; (c) respiratory difficulties are present; (d) contraindications to the use of thioamides (e.g., allergy) or RAI (e.g., pregnancy) exist; (e) a large goiter that regresses poorly on RAI or thioamide therapy is present; or (f) it is the patient's preference. Some argue that surgery is underused in the treatment of Graves' disease.[180] In a prospective, randomized trial comparing the three treatment modalities, surgery produced euthyroidism more quickly and was associated with a lower relapse rate than either RAI or thioamides.[181] A meta-analysis of 35 studies encompassing 7,241 patients with Graves' disease found that thyroidectomy was successful in 92% of patients with a low recurrence (7.2%) of hyperthyroidism.[183] If C.R.'s minor difficulty

Table 52-10
Treatment for Hyperthyroidism

Modality	Drug/Dosage	Mechanism of Action	Toxicity	Indication
Primary Treatment				
Thioamides				
Methimazole (Tapazole) 5-, 10-mg tablet; rectal suppositories can be made[179]	Methimazole 30–40 mg PO daily or in 2 divided doses (*max:* 60 mg/day) for 6–8 weeks or until euthyroid, then maintenance of 5–10 mg/d PO × 12–18 months	Blocks organification of hormone synthesis, does not block conversion of T_4 to T_3	Skin rashes, GI symptoms, arthralgias, cholestatic jaundice, agranulocytosis, aplasia cutis, and embryopathy syndrome in pregnancy (methimazole only)	DOC in adults/children except in thyroid storm and first trimester of pregnancy (see PTU). Once daily dosing can improve adherence
PTU 50 mg tablet; rectal formulation can be made[177,178]	100–200 mg PO q6–8h (*max:* 1,200 mg/day) for 6–8 weeks or until euthyroid; then maintenance of 50–150 mg daily PO × 12–18 months	Similar to methimazole, and blocks peripheral conversion of T_4 to T_3 (PTU only)	Hepatitis, some fatal. Similar to methimazole	DOC in thyroid storm, first trimester of pregnancy
Surgery				
	Preoperative preparation with iodides, thioamides, or β-blockers before surgery; see specific operative agent	Near total thyroidectomy	Hypothyroidism, cosmetic scarring, hypoparathyroidism, risks of surgery, and anesthesia, vocal cord damage	Obstruction, choking, malignancy, pregnancy in second trimester, contraindication to RAI or thioamides
RAI				
	^{131}I radioactive isotope; 80–100 μCi/g thyroid tissue. Average dose, ≈10 mCi; pretreatment with corticosteroids indicated in patients with ophthalmopathy	Destruction of the gland	Hypothyroidism; worsening of ophthalmopathy; fear of radiation-induced leukemia; genetic damage; malignancy; rarely, radiation sickness	Adults, older patients who are poor surgical risks or have cardiac disease; patients with a history of prior thyroid surgery; contraindications to thioamide usage; increasingly used in kids
Adjuncts to Primary Usage				
Iodides				
Lugol's solution 8 mg/drop (5% iodine, 10% potassium iodide; saturated [SSKI] 50 mg/drop)	5–10 drops TID PO for 10–14 days before surgery; minimum effective dose 6 mg/day	↓ vascularity of gland and ↑ firmness; blocks release of thyroid hormone	Hypersensitivity reactions, skin rashes, mucous membrane ulcers, anaphylaxis, metallic taste, rhinorrhea, parotid and submaxillary swelling; fetal goiters and death	Preoperative preparation before surgery; thyroid storm, provides symptomatic relief of symptoms. *Do not use before RAI or chronically during pregnancy*
β-Blockers				
Propranolol or equivalent β-blocker. *Avoid* those with ISA	Propranolol 10–40 mg PO q6h or PRN to control HR <100 beats/minute; IV 0.5–1 mg slowly	Blocks effects of thyroid hormone peripherally, no effect on underlying disease; blocks T_4 to T_3 conversion	Related to β-blockade; bradycardia, CHF, blocks hyperglycemic response to hypoglycemia, bronchospasm, CNS symptoms at high doses; fetal bradycardia	Symptomatic relief while awaiting onset of thioamides, RAI; preoperative preparation for surgery; thyroid storm
Calcium Channel Blockers				
	Diltiazem 120 mg PO TID–QID or verapamil 80–120 mg PO TID–QID PRN to control HR <100 beats/min	Blocks effects of thyroid hormone peripherally, no effect on underlying disease	Bradycardia, peripheral edema, CHF, headache, flushing, hypotension, dizziness	Alternative for symptomatic relief of hyperthyroid symptoms in patients who cannot tolerate β-blockers
Corticosteroids				
	Prednisone or equivalent corticosteroids 50–140 mg PO daily in divided doses; IV hydrocortisone 50–100 mg q6h or equivalent for thyroid storm	↓ TSI, suppression of inflammatory process; blocks T_4 to T_3 conversion	Complications of steroid therapy	Ophthalmopathy, thyroid storm (use IV steroid), pretibial myxedema, pretreatment before RAI therapy in patients with ophthalmopathy

CHF, congestive heart failure; CNS, central nervous system; DOC, drug of choice; GI, gastrointestinal; HR, heart rate; ISA, intrinsic sympathomimetic activity; IV, intravenous; mCi, millicurie; PO, orally (by mouth); PRN, as needed; PTU, propylthiouracil; q, every; QID, 4 times a day; RAI, radioactive iodine; SSKI, saturated solution of potassium iodide; T_3, triiodothyronine; T_4, thyroxine; TID, 3 times a day; TSI, thyroid receptor–stimulating or thyroid-stimulating immunoglobulin; μCi, microcurie.[87–89] in swallowing persists because of poor regression of goiter size with drug therapy, then surgery is a reasonable alternative. If surgery is contemplated, C.R. must be brought to surgery in a euthyroid state to prevent rapid postoperative rises in T_4 levels and subsequent thyroid storm (see Case 52-22, Question 1). A total or near-total rather than a subtotal thyroidectomy is the procedure of choice when performed by an experienced surgeon.[180,182,183] Although subtotal thyroidectomy theoretically avoids the predictable risk of hypothyroidism from total thyroidectomy, the likelihood of recurrent hyperthyroidism increases in proportion to the amount of residual thyroid tissue remaining.[180,181] Recurrent thyrotoxicosis following a subtotal thyroidectomy should be treated with RAI because the incidence of surgical complications increases with a second surgery.

Surgical complication rates are low when the procedure is performed by a competent surgeon and when the patient is adequately prepared for surgery. The disadvantages of surgery are expense, hospitalization, hypothyroidism, the small risk of postoperative complications, and the patient's fear of surgery (see Case 52-15, Question 12).[180,181,183]

RADIOACTIVE IODINE

RAI, the most common treatment modality in the United States, is the preferred treatment for (a) debilitated, cardiac, or older patients who are poor surgical candidates; (b) patients who fail to respond to drug therapy or who experience adverse drug reactions; and (c) patients who develop recurrent hyperthyroidism after surgery.[164,174,181,184]

Pregnancy is an absolute contraindication to RAI therapy. Previously, the use of RAI was restricted to adults older than an arbitrary age of 20 to 35 years because it was feared that RAI could result in genetic damage or neoplasia. However, its use in adolescents is increasing after more than 50 years of clinical experience with RAI showing that it is safe and effective.[184–187] There is no reported evidence of genetic damage after ^{131}I ingestion, and the dose of radiation to the gonads is <3 rads, which is comparable to other radiographic diagnostic tests (e.g., barium enemas).[188] The incidence of leukemia or malignancy is no higher in recipients of ^{131}I than in thyrotoxic patients treated with drugs or surgery.[185,189] In a retrospective review of 98 adolescents followed for 36 years after receiving ^{131}I, no cancers of the thyroid or leukemia were reported.[187] One interesting finding is that patients receiving RAI should be warned that they can set off radiation detectors at airport screening terminals for up to 12 weeks after RAI and that they should carry documentation of their treatment.[190,191]

RAI is painless, effective, economical, and quick, but unsubstantiated fears about radiation and malignancy, as well as the high incidence of hypothyroidism, may deter its use. RAI could be used safely in this nonpregnant young patient. However, C.R.'s prior use of iodides will dilute the ^{131}I pool. Thus, it will be impossible to achieve therapeutic thyroid concentrations of RAI for as long as 3 to 6 months.

Treatment with Thioamides

PROPYLTHIOURACIL VERSUS METHIMAZOLE

CASE 52-15, QUESTION 4: C.R. is started on PTU 200 mg q8h after baseline FT_4 and TSH levels have been obtained. Three weeks later, she angrily complains that her symptoms are worse and that the medication is not working; however, she reluctantly admits to missing doses because of difficulty swallowing, nausea, vomiting, diarrhea, fatigue, a cough, and a sore throat. What are the advantages of using either PTU or methimazole in the treatment of hyperthyroidism?

Both thioamides are effective in treating hyperthyroidism. The antithyroid effectiveness of the thioamides primarily depends on their ability to block the organification of iodines, thereby inhibiting thyroid hormone synthesis.[175,176] Thyroid autoantibody synthesis may also be suppressed. In most hyperthyroid adults and children, methimazole should be considered the thioamide of choice because of increasing reports of hepatitis, some fatal, from PTU. PTU should be reserved for use in thyroid storm, during the first trimester of pregnancy because of rare teratogenicity from methimazole, and in those allergic to methimazole (except agranulocytosis and hepatitis) who are not candidates for RAI or surgery.[30,169]

Dosing and Administration

Methimazole is effective when administered initially as a single dose compared with the multiple-dose regimen required with PTU to achieve a euthyroid state.[175,176] Although a single-dose regimen of PTU has been tried acutely, it is most effective when given in divided doses. Compared to PTU, methimazole is also less hepatototoxic, less expensive, requires daily ingestion of fewer numbers of tablets, and is not associated with a bitter tablet taste. However, PTU is preferred in thyroid storm because, unlike methimazole, it also blocks the peripheral conversion of T_4 to T_3.[192] Within 24 to 48 hours after PTU administration, a 25% to 40% reduction in peripheral T_3 production is seen, which contributes to PTU's rapid onset. A significantly greater fall in T_3 concentration and the T_3:T_4 ratio can be demonstrated in hyperthyroid patients treated acutely with PTU and iodine than with methimazole and iodides. Lastly, PTU is preferred over methimazole during the first trimester of pregnancy (see Case 52-18).

CASE 52-15, QUESTION 5: Why was the thioamide therapy ineffective in C.R.? Was the dose of PTU appropriate?

The inadequate response in C.R. suggests poor adherence to the thioamide dosing regimen or a delayed response caused by prior iodide loading of the gland.

The onset of action of the thioamides is slow because they block the synthesis rather than the release of thyroid hormone. Therefore, hormone secretion will continue until the glandular stores of hormone are depleted. If adequate doses were given, some improvement of clinical symptoms should be noted after 2 or 3 weeks.[176]

The dosage of PTU is appropriate. Thioamide dosing consists of two phases: initial therapy to achieve euthyroidism and maintenance therapy to achieve remission. Initially, high blocking dosages of PTU (400–800 mg/day, depending on the severity of the toxicosis) should be given in three or four divided doses, as in C.R.[164,175,176] Rarely, dosages of 1,200 mg/day of PTU or its equivalent may be required in patients with severe disease or storm.[192] Equipotent doses of methimazole (which is 10 times more potent than PTU on a mg-per-mg basis) can also be used. However, it is usually unnecessary to use >40 mg/day of methimazole to restore a euthyroid state.[164,175,176] Toxicity is also less common (see Case 52-15, Questions 10 and 11). True resistance to thioamides is rare; thus, most cases of unresponsiveness are caused by poor patient adherence, as in C.R.

C.R.'s adherence is also hindered by the frequency of PTU administration. The serum half-life of PTU is short (1.5 hours), but it is the intrathyroidal drug concentrations that should determine the dosing intervals because they are most clearly related to the drug's antithyroid effects.[176] PTU must be dosed every 6 to 8 hours initially, or as frequently as every 4 hours in cases of severe hyperthyroidism and thyroid storm. In contrast, methimazole has a serum half-life of 6 to 8 hours, remains in the thyroid for 20 hours, and has a duration of activity of up to 40 hours.[176,193]

Poor adherence is often difficult to ascertain and is more likely when multiple daily doses are required. The best option for C.R. is to change to 30 to 40 mg of methimazole, given once daily to improve adherence, or divided into two doses to decrease GI distress. After methimazole is given for 4 to 6 weeks to achieve euthyroidism, the daily dosage can be reduced gradually by 25% to 30% monthly to a dosage that maintains euthyroidism, usually 5 to 10 mg/day of methimazole. If C.R. remains hyperthyroid despite adequate doses of thioamides, then the most likely reason is non-adherence.

Monitoring Therapy

CASE 52-15, QUESTION 6: What additional objective baseline data should be obtained to monitor both the efficacy and toxicity of thioamides?

Before thioamides are administered, a baseline FT_4 and TSH should be obtained. A baseline white blood cell (WBC) count with differential can also help differentiate the leukopenia associated with hyperthyroidism from drug-induced leukopenia and/or agranulocytosis (see Case 52-15, Question 11). Baseline liver function tests can assist in the evaluation of thioamide-induced hepatotoxicity (see Case 52-15, Question 10). A repeat FT_4 and TSH should be obtained after 4 to 6 weeks on therapy and 4 to 6 weeks after any change in the dosing regimen. Once the patient is euthyroid on maintenance dosages, thyroid function tests can be obtained every 3 to 6 months.

Duration of Therapy

CASE 52-15, QUESTION 7: How long should C.R. be continued on thioamide treatment?

Traditionally, thioamide therapy is continued for 1 to 2 years despite the lack of data regarding the optimal treatment period.[164,175,176] The goal of treatment is to control the symptoms of Graves' disease until spontaneous remission occurs. Graves' disease remits spontaneously in about 30% to 50% of patients but relapse is high.[194] Because it is unknown when or if remission will occur, it is understandable why the optimal duration of therapy is unclear. Short-term therapy (i.e., <6 months) has been advocated to save time and money and improve adherence because earlier studies suggested remission rates comparable to a longer course of therapy. However, short-term therapy is not recommended because longer follow-ups of patients receiving short-term therapy have noted poorer remission rates.[175,176]

Most data support a 12- to 18-month course of treatment to achieve remission rates of approximately 60%.[175,176,195,196] Two prospective randomized trials found that extending treatment from 6 to 18 months was beneficial but that 42 months of therapy was not significantly better than 18 months.[195,196] However, one retrospective study of patients treated for >12 months observed remission rates of only 17.5%.[197] These conflicting results underscore the fact that determining the optimal treatment period is confounded by the large variability that exists with regard to spontaneous remission. Nevertheless, treatment periods of 1 to 2 years are justifiable in adherent patients. Therapy can be reinstituted if hyperthyroidism reappears shortly after therapy is discontinued. Methimazole can also be continued indefinitely if there are no side effects, and treatment with either RAI or surgery is not desired. In C.R., this goal might not be achievable, given her history of non-adherence.

PRECAUTIONS

CASE 52-15, QUESTION 8: Can thioamide therapy affect any of C.R.'s preexisting medical conditions?

Thyrotoxicosis can activate or intensify diabetes, primarily by increasing the basal hepatic glucose production and the metabolism of insulin.[198] Therefore, effective therapy with thioamides may restore control of C.R.'s type 2 diabetes.

C.R.'s arthritis should not be affected, although thioamides have been associated with the development of lupus erythematosus (LE), lupus-like syndromes, and vasculitis.[176,199] These adverse drug reactions are rare; the incidence is <0.1%. Lupus-like syndromes include skin ulcers, splenomegaly, migratory polyarthritis, pleuritis and pericarditis, periarteritis, and renal abnormalities. Serologic abnormalities may also occur with these connective tissue disorders and include hyperglobulinemia, positive LE preparations, and positive antinuclear antibodies. Recovery occurs with adequate steroid therapy and withdrawal of the thioamides. Because cross-reaction between methimazole and PTU is likely to occur, patients exhibiting these reactions should be treated with surgery or RAI. C.R.'s treatment should be monitored with this lupus-like adverse effect in mind, but the occurrence of this syndrome is so uncommon that a trouble-free course of therapy can be anticipated.

ADJUNCTIVE THERAPY

CASE 52-15, QUESTION 9: What adjunctive therapy might help alleviate some of C.R.'s symptoms while awaiting the onset of thioamide's effects?

Iodides (see Case 52-15, Question 2), β-adrenergic blocking agents without intrinsic sympathomimetic activity, or calcium channel blockers can be used acutely to ameliorate some of C.R.'s symptoms.[200,201] Because iodides were previously ineffective in C.R., a β-blocker should be tried.

β-Adrenergic blocking agents rapidly decrease the nervousness, palpitations, fatigue, weight loss, diaphoresis, heat intolerance, and tremor associated with thyrotoxicosis, probably because many of the signs and symptoms mimic sympathetic overactivity.[164,200] An increase in the number of β-adrenergic receptors rather than an elevation in catecholamine levels is probably responsible for this overactivity. Because the underlying disease process and thyroid hormone levels are not affected significantly by β-blockers, patients generally remain mildly symptomatic and fail to gain weight. For this reason, they should not be used as the sole treatment for thyrotoxicosis.

All β-blockers without intrinsic sympathetic activity (e.g., atenolol, metoprolol, propranolol) are effective in alleviating the hyperthyroid symptoms, but propranolol is the only β-blocker that significantly inhibits peripheral conversion of T_4 to T_3.[200] Thyroid function tests are generally not affected except for a mild decrease in the T_3 level.

In summary, β-blockers are (a) effective adjuncts in the management of thyroid storm, (b) useful to prepare patients for surgery, and (c) useful in the short-term management of thyrotoxicosis during pregnancy.[180,192,200] Surprisingly, propranolol also improves many of the neuromuscular manifestations of hyperthyroidism, including thyrotoxic periodic paralysis. Current guidelines recommend elderly patients, those with concomitant heart disease, and those with a resting heart rate over 90 beats/minute receive adjunctive therapy with β-blockers.[34]

Diltiazem or verapamil are effective alternatives when β-blockers are contraindicated.[201] Diltiazem 120 mg TID or QID can be tried. The dihydropyridine calcium channel blockers are unlikely to be effective.

Because of C.R.'s history of diabetes, the effects of β-adrenergic blocking drugs on patients with diabetes must be considered (see Chapter 53, Diabetes Mellitus). If β-blockers are instituted, a cardioselective β-blocker would be a better choice for patients on therapy that can cause hypoglycemia. The appropriate dosage should be based on clinical and objective improvement of hyperthyroid symptoms, such as a reduction in heart rate. Metoprolol 25 to 50 mg BID can be started initially and the dosage titrated to maintain the heart rate at <90 beats/minute. Otherwise, diltiazem, verapamil, or a retrial of iodides is warranted.

ADVERSE EFFECTS

CASE 52-15, QUESTION 10: A pruritic area over the pretibial aspects of both legs as well as several maculopapular erythematous patches and abdominal tenderness were noticed during C.R.'s physical examination. Do these reactions require the discontinuation of her PTU?

Thioamide Rash

Although C.R. may be experiencing a drug rash from PTU, pretibial myxedema or the dermopathy of Graves' disease may also be possibilities because of the location of the pruritic area. About 4% of patients with Graves' disease who exhibit infiltrative exophthalmos also have dermatologic changes. The skin is thickened, erythematous, and non-pitting because of mucopolysaccharide infiltration and accentuation of hair follicles. Pruritus or pain may be present. Treatment includes topical corticosteroids, control of the Graves' disease, and reassurance.

Thioamides can produce a maculopapular pruritic rash in 5% to 6% of treated patients.[176] The rash can occur at any time but is more common early in therapy. If the rash is mild, drug therapy can be continued while the patient's symptoms are treated with an antihistamine and a topical steroid; such rashes generally subside spontaneously. Alternatively, another thioamide can be substituted because cross-sensitivity to this side effect is uncommon. Thioamides should be stopped if the rash is urticarial in nature or associated with systemic manifestations (e.g., fever, arthralgias).

Hepatitis

C.R.'s symptoms of nausea, vomiting, diarrhea, fatigue, and abdominal tenderness require further evaluation. Her symptoms could be consistent with mild GI side effects from her PTU therapy, impending thyroid storm from non-adherence (see Case 52-22, Question 1) or more seriously, PTU-induced hepatitis. PTU has been associated with 0.1% severe hepatotoxicity, leading to liver transplants and fatalities primarily in children.[30,169,202,203] Although usually hepatocellular in nature, cholestasis, hepatic necrosis, and fulminant hepatic failures have been reported.[168,170,176] Transient elevations in transaminases occur in approximately 30% of asymptomatic patients within the first 2 months of PTU therapy and may not require drug discontinuation.[168] Liver enzymes usually normalize within 3 months of reducing the PTU to maintenance dosages despite drug continuation. However, PTU should be stopped immediately in patients with clinical symptoms of hepatitis to ensure complete recovery. The mechanism of PTU-induced hepatotoxicity appears to be autoimmune because circulating autoantibodies and in vitro peripheral lymphocyte sensitization to PTU have been detected.[170] Overt hepatitis typically occurs during the first 2 months of PTU therapy and is not dose related. In contrast, methimazole rarely produces a cholestatic jaundice picture that might be more common in older patients and in those receiving higher dosages (i.e., >40 mg/day).[171] In patients with thioamide-induced hepatitis, changing to the alternative thioamide is not recommended because fatalities have been reported on rechallenge. In such patients, either radioactive therapy or surgery should be used.

In C.R., PTU should be stopped while awaiting results of thyroid function tests, transaminases, and bilirubin. Routine monitoring of liver function tests is not recommended during thioamide therapy because patients can be asymptomatic. However, routine monitoring might be reasonable in patients with a history of liver disease and risk factors for hepatitis (e.g., alcohol use). All patients receiving thioamides should be questioned closely during the first 2 months of therapy for symptoms of hepatitis, and hepatic function tests should be obtained if appropriate.

Agranulocytosis

CASE 52-15, QUESTION 11: Assess C.R.'s complaints of sore throat and cough.

C.R.'s complaints should not be dismissed casually because they might indicate PTU-induced agranulocytosis. Agranulocytosis (<500/mm^3 of neutrophils) is the most severe adverse hematologic reaction associated with the thioamides and should be considered strongly in C.R.[176,204] In contrast, drug-induced leukopenia is usually transient, is not associated with impending agranulocytosis, and is not an indication to discontinue thioamide therapy. An accurate history should be obtained from C.R. The clinician should be particularly alert for a temperature of 101°F for 2 or more days, malaise, or other flu-like findings that appeared temporally with her sore throat. If subjective or objective data are consistent with agranulocytosis, the PTU should be discontinued immediately until the results of a repeat WBC count with a differential are obtained. Traditionally, routine serial determinations of WBC counts are not recommended for monitoring the development of agranulocytosis because the onset is so abrupt. Instead, patients should be instructed to immediately report rash, fever, sore throat, or any flu-like symptoms. However, one study suggested that weekly monitoring of the WBC count with a differential during the first 3 months of antithyroid therapy might identify asymptomatic patients with agranulocytosis before infection occurs.[204]

The prevalence of agranulocytosis is about 0.5% but ranges from 0.5% to 6%.[176,204] The risk factors for agranulocytosis are unknown. There is no predilection for either gender, and the reaction may be idiosyncratic or dose related. Some reports suggest that patients older than 40 years or those taking high dosages of methimazole (e.g., >40 mg/day) might be more susceptible than those on any dosage of PTU. Although controversial, patients receiving low dosages of methimazole (e.g., <40 mg/day) might be at less risk than those receiving high or conventional dosages of PTU.[176,204]

Agranulocytosis typically develops within the first 3 months of treatment, although it can occur at any time and as late as 12 months after starting thioamide therapy.[176] A delayed reaction is more common with methimazole therapy than with PTU. In 55 patients who developed agranulocytosis while taking thioamides, the duration of PTU therapy (17.7 ± 9.7 days) was significantly shorter than for methimazole therapy (36.9 ± 14.5 days).[204] The mechanism of thioamide-induced agranulocytosis is unknown. Both allergic- (idiosyncratic) and toxic-type (dose-related) reactions have been suggested. An autoimmune reaction with circulating antineutrophil antibodies and lymphocyte sensitization to antithyroid drugs has been demonstrated.[205] Death usually results from overwhelming infection.

If agranulocytosis is diagnosed, the drug should be discontinued, the patient monitored for signs of infection, and antibiotics instituted if necessary. Granulocyte colony-stimulating factors may shorten the recovery period.[176,206] If the patient recovers, granulocytes begin to reappear in the periphery within a few days to 3 weeks; a normal granulocyte count occurs shortly thereafter.[204,206]

Although some cases of granulocytopenia have resolved with substitution or continuation of thioamides, the risks of drug rechallenge clearly outweigh the benefits, and other treatments should be instituted. Changing to an alternative thioamide should also be avoided because of possible cross-sensitivity between these agents.[176]

In summary, all patients receiving thioamide therapy should be well educated regarding the signs and symptoms of agranulocytosis. If these symptoms develop, they should be advised to contact their physician or pharmacist. If they cannot reach their own physician, patients should inform the emergency physician that they are taking thioamides, and a WBC count with differential should be obtained. Routine monitoring of a WBC and differential is not recommended until further studies justify that it is indicated and cost-effective.

PREOPERATIVE PREPARATION

Case 52-15, Question 12: C.R.'s PTU is discontinued because she developed agranulocytosis and hepatitis, and surgery is scheduled when her granulocyte level returns to normal. What thyroid preparation is needed for C.R. before thyroidectomy? What postoperative complications are associated with thyroidectomy?

C.R. should be in a euthyroid state at the time of surgery to avoid precipitation of thyroid storm and morbidity. Generally, iodides (see Case 52-15, Question 2), thioamides, or propranolol can be used.[173,192,200] The combination of iodides and propranolol is more effective than either used alone. Propranolol used alone has been associated with thyroid crisis postoperatively and may be less effective than iodides in decreasing gland friability and vascularity.[200]

Because C.R. received only 1 week of thioamide therapy, it is likely that her gland still contains large stores of hormone; therefore, pretreatment is necessary.

In addition to the risks of anesthesia and surgery, postoperative complications include hypoparathyroidism, adhesions, laryngeal nerve damage, bleeding, infection, and poor wound healing. However, complications can be minimized if the surgery is performed by experienced surgeons.[180–183,207] Complications are also higher if a total rather than a subtotal thyroidectomy is performed, but there is a lower risk of recurrent hyperthyroidism. Development of hypothyroidism, especially subclinical hypothyroidism, is greatest during the first year after surgery, with an insidious rise in incidence over the next 10 years. The incidence of permanent hypothyroidism varies from 6% to 75% and is related inversely to the amount of remnant tissue left behind.[180–183,207] Thyroid function tests should be monitored annually after surgery. When total thyroidectomy is performed, postoperative L-thyroxine should be initiated at a dose of 1.7 mcg/kg/day.[34] Inadvertent parathyroidectomy can result in life-threatening hypocalcemia. Patients receiving total thyroidectomy should have postoperative measurement of serum calcium and/or intact parathyroid hormone concentrations.[34]

REMISSION RATES WITH THIOAMIDES

CASE 52-16

Question 1: B.D., a 30-year-old woman, has been maintained on methimazole 5 mg daily for >2 years. Her methimazole has been discontinued twice in the past, and each time her hyperthyroidism recurred. She refuses either surgery or RAI therapy. Although she is clinically euthyroid on methimazole, her gland is larger than her usual size and has never decreased with therapy. Recent laboratory tests showed an FT_4 of 1 ng/dL (normal, 0.8–1.4) and a TSH level of 6.5 microunits/mL (normal, 0.45–4.1). What is responsible for the enlarging gland? What subjective or objective data in B.D. would influence her remission rate and justify a longer course of thioamide therapy? Would the addition of T_4 be helpful?

The high TSH level suggests that TSH stimulation caused by excessive suppression of hormone synthesis by methimazole is contributing to the enlarging thyroid gland. The easiest solution to this problem is to decrease the maintenance dose of methimazole to 2.5 mg daily to normalize the TSH value and minimize gland stimulation.

Long-term remission rates achieved with the thioamides are disappointing. Remission rates within 6 years after discontinuing therapy average 50% (range, 14%–75%),[175,176,195–197] although relapse rates are as high as 80%. The rate of permanent remission is usually <25% if the follow-up period is long enough.[175,176,208] Why some patients remain in remission while others relapse once thioamides are discontinued is unclear, although patients who remain euthyroid for >10 to 15 years after discontinuing therapy probably do so because of disease progression to Hashimoto's thyroiditis rather than as a direct result of treatment.[164] In other words, the natural course of Graves' hyperthyroidism might be eventual hypothyroidism regardless of the treatment modality used. Several factors have a limited role in predicting relapse and remission and have been used to guide therapy.

A longer duration of thioamide treatment (see Case 52-15, Question 7) improves the remission rate by changing the basic underlying abnormality of Graves' disease.[175,195–197] Numerous studies show that titers of antithyroid receptor (TSI) and antimicrosomal antibodies fall during thioamide therapy but are unchanged during therapy with placebo or β-blockers.[175,176,196,209] Patients with low or undetectable TSI titers at the end of 12 to 24 months of thioamide therapy had a 45% chance of remission compared to <10% chance of remission for those with higher titers within 1 to 5 years after completing therapy.[208–211] The best response was obtained in those with smaller goiters, less severe disease, and nonsmokers. A higher thioamide dose did not improve the remission rate but resulted in more toxicity, including agranulocytosis, arthralgias, dermatitis, gastritis, and hepatotoxicity.[175,195,208]

Certain clinical features have been associated with a greater chance of disease remission and might help clinicians identify patients who deserve a longer thioamide trial before changing to RAI or surgery. These clinical features include smaller goiter, mild symptoms of short duration, a reduction in goiter size during treatment, nonsmokers, absence of ophthalmopathy, and undetectable or low TSI levels.[176,208,209] Smokers should be advised to discontinue smoking to increase the chance of remission (see Chapter 91, Tobacco Use and Dependence).[212]

In a preliminary study, the addition of L-thyroxine to maintenance doses of thioamides for 1 year, followed by an additional year of L-thyroxine alone, significantly reduced the risk of relapse after stopping thioamides.[211] Those receiving the T_4-methimazole combination experienced significant reductions in TSH receptor antibody titers compared to those taking methimazole alone. At 3 years, the combination-treated patients had a lower rate of recurrence after stopping therapy (1.7%) than those receiving methimazole alone (recurrence rate, 34.7%). Unfortunately, several prospective studies evaluating the addition of T_4 to thioamides have not validated these initial favorable results.[208,210,213,214] Support for this therapeutic approach has waned, and the addition of T_4 to existing thioamide therapy is not recommended.

B.D.'s large goiter reduces her chance of remission with longer therapy. Although thioamide therapy can be continued indefinitely if well tolerated, surgery or RAI therapy should seriously be considered for B.D., who already has received methimazole for >2 years. Alternative therapy is especially crucial if she plans to become pregnant within the next few years (see Case 52-18).

CASE 52-17

QUESTION 1: J.C. is a 68-year-old male who is found to have a TSH level of 0.15 microunits/mL (normal, 0.45–4.1) with normal FT_4 and FT_3 hormone levels on routine blood tests. He is otherwise healthy and denies any symptoms of thyroid dysfunction. On physical exam, his thyroid gland is normal. He denies any family history of thyroid disease and is taking no medications. How should these tests be interpreted? How should J.C. be managed?

J.C.'s laboratory findings of a suppressed TSH value below the limits of normal and normal free thyroid hormone levels are consistent with subclinical hyperthyroidism (SHyper).[87–89] Other unlikely causes of a suppressed TSH in J.C. include medications (e.g., metformin, bexarotene, glucocorticoids) (Table 52-1), pituitary hypothyroidism, and non-thyroidal illness (see Case 52-1, Questions 1 and 2).[10,60] A suppressed TSH may also be a normal finding in healthy elderly patients.

The dangers of SHyper are similar to those of overt hyperthyroidism and include cardiac findings (e.g., atrial and ventricular premature beats, atrial fibrillation [AF], left ventricular hypertrophy, diastolic dysfunction), loss of bone mass, higher fracture rates, especially in postmenopausal women, and if present, subtle symptoms of hyperthyroidism.[85–89] In elderly patients, hyperthyroid symptoms, even if overtly hyperthyroid, may be "apathetic" unapparent because of impaired sympathetic nervous system responsiveness. A significant relationship between atrial fibrillation and degree of SHyper is clear, whereas an association with increased atherosclerotic heart disease or mortality is weak.[158] The relative risk of AF in SHyper may be as high as 5.2 and increased by older age, male gender, higher FT_4 levels, and degree of TSH suppression. In two cohorts followed for 10 to 13 years, the relative risk of atrial fibrillation ranged from 1.6 to 3.1, depending on the degree of TSH suppression.[158,215] The likelihood a patient with endogenous SHyper will progress to overt hyperthyroidism is not clear. Patients may spontaneously revert to euthyroidism, progress to hyperthyroidism or continue with SHyper. Individuals with undetectable TSH concentrations appear most likely to progress, and overall the rate of progression to overt disease is 1% to 5% annually.[88] A study of 2,024 patients with 7-year follow-up of SHyper importantly found 36% reverted back to normal within 7 years, especially those with TSH levels between 0.1 and 0.4 microunits/mL.[216]

The management of subclinical hyperthyroidism is controversial, especially in asymptomatic patients because of limited treatment outcomes evidence.[87–89] Current guidelines recommend treatment of subclinical hyperthyroidism (TSH levels <0.1 microunits/mL) in patients >65 years, postmenopausal woman not taking antiresorptive therapy (see Chapter 110, Osteoporosis), and those with cardiac disease and osteoporosis.[34,87,88] For patients with TSH levels of 0.1 to 0.45 microunits/mL, treatment of patients >65 years of age and those with cardiovascular disease or hyperthyroid symptoms can be considered.[34] A recent review recommends RAI or thioamide therapy only if the TSH level is <0.1 microunits/mL in postmenopausal women, in those 60 years or older, and in patients with a history of heart disease, osteoporosis, or hyperthyroid symptoms.[89] For patients with TSH levels of 0.1 to 0.4 microunits/mL, treatment can be considered if they are in the aforementioned groups; otherwise, therapy is not recommended because TSH normalization may occur.

In J.C., his thyroid function tests should be repeated. An RAIU and scan should be obtained to detect any hyperactive areas or nodules that might be responsible for the suppressed TSH. Because J.C. is generally healthy, treatment can be considered if there are concerns about cardiac disease or bone loss; otherwise, no therapy is reasonable based on the available evidence. Close monitoring of thyroid function tests is recommended every 6 months to 1 year. If hyperthyroid symptoms or changes in cardiac or bone function occur, then RAI therapy is recommended.

HYPERTHYROIDISM IN PREGNANCY

CASE 52-18

QUESTION 1: N.N., a 32-year-old woman who is 3 months pregnant, is referred for management of her Graves' disease. What are the therapeutic ramifications of managing thyrotoxicosis during pregnancy?

Hyperthyroidism develops in 0.02% to 1.4% of pregnant women and often precedes conception.[217] Symptoms of thyrotoxicosis are typically ameliorated during the second and third trimesters and exacerbated early in the postpartum period. Treatment is crucial to prevent damage to the fetus and to maintain the pregnancy. RAI, chronic iodide therapy, and iodine-containing compounds are contraindicated during pregnancy because they will cross the placenta to produce fetal goiter and athyreosis.[217–219] As little as 12 mg/day of iodide has produced neonatal goiter and death. The long-term use of β-adrenergic blockers should also be avoided because it is associated with fetal respiratory depression, a small placenta, intrauterine growth retardation, impaired response to anoxia, and postnatal bradycardia and hypoglycemia.[217,218] However, if rapid control of hyperthyroidism is required, short-term use (<1–4 weeks) of propranolol is safe.[102,105,217–219] Iodide use in pregnancy should be limited to transient preoperative use prior to thyroidectomy or in the management of thyroid storm.[105,220]

Either surgery or thioamide is the treatment of choice for pregnant hyperthyroid patient. Surgery is safe during the second trimester with adequate preoperative preparation. During other trimesters, thioamides are preferred because surgery can precipitate spontaneous abortion. PTU is preferable during the first trimester because of rare reports of teratogenicity from methimazole, but methimazole is preferred thereafter to reduce the risks of PTU-associated hepatitis. Both thioamides are equally effacious,[221] demonstrate similar placental crossing properties,[222] and produce similar thyroid hormone concentrations in fetal umbilical cord blood samples.[223] Methimazole has been associated with anecdotal reports of congenital scalp defects (e.g., aplasia cutis) and an embryopathy syndrome (esophageal and choanal atresia).[224–227] However, the risks of reversible aplasia cutis were not greater in women receiving methimazole (e.g., 2.7%) compared to PTU (e.g., 3%) or hyperthyroid controls (e.g., 6%).[221,224,225] Therefore, methimazole can be considered throughout pregnancy if there is intolerance or non-adherence to PTU[217,218,221] (see Chapter 49, Obstetric Drug Therapy).

Fetal hypothyroidism and goiter can develop when large doses of thioamides are administered to the mother, even if the mother is still hyperthyroid.[217,218] Therefore, to avoid goiter and suppression of the fetal thyroid gland, which begins to function at about 12 to 14 weeks of gestation, the lowest effective thioamide dose should be given. Normal FT_4 levels occur in >90% of neonates when maternal FT_4 is maintained in the upper third of the normal range (1.5–1.9 ng/L).[105,220] Conversely, over 30% of neonates exhibit a low FT_4 when maternal levels are maintained in the lower two-thirds of the normal range.[105] Control of maternal hyperthyroidism increases the risk of fetal hypothyroidism. Start PTU (e.g., maximum of 300 mg/day in three divided doses) or methimazole (e.g., maximum of 20–30 mg given once daily) until control is achieved, then taper PTU to 50–150 mg/day, and after the first trimester, change to 5 to 15 mg/day of methimazole for the remainder of the pregnancy. In many patients, remission of Graves' disease occurs during pregnancy, and some patients can discontinue thioamides in the second half of pregnancy.[217] Measurement of TRAb levels between weeks 22 and 26 of gestation can be useful, because disappearance of TRAb indicates that thioamide therapy may no longer be necessary.[34] Such modest doses of thioamides provide satisfactory control of maternal hyperthyroidism and should not cause clinically evident neonatal thyroid dysfunction. Patients requiring more than the maximum recommended thioamide dosages for control may need to consider the possibility of surgery in the second trimester.

Nevertheless, a small but significant reduction in neonatal serum T_4 occurs even when small (100–200 mg) doses of PTU are administered during pregnancy to mothers with Graves' disease.[217,218,226] It is unclear whether this mild, transient reduction in serum T_4 causes long-term impairment of mental development or is otherwise detrimental to the newborn. To date, no significant differences in intellectual development have been noted between children exposed to PTU or methimazole in utero and their unexposed siblings.[228–230] However, children exposed in utero to >300 mg/day of PTU had lower IQs.[228,229]

Although transient fetal or neonatal hypothyroidism does not appear to be a major threat to the baby, it is advisable to maintain the mother in a mildly hyperthyroid state.[217,218] Mild maternal hyperthyroidism appears to be well tolerated, but maternal hypothyroidism is poorly tolerated by both the mother and the fetus (see Case 52-8, Question 1). T_4 levels should be maintained in the upper third of the normal range to decrease the risk of fetal hypothyroidism because normal thyroid function tests are suggestive of hypothyroidism during pregnancy (high TBG and TBPA levels). The goal of therapy is a suppressed maternal TSH level (0.1–0.4 microunits/mL) because complete correction maternal hyperthyroidism increases the risk of fetal hypothyroidism.[34,102]

It is not rational to add thyroid hormone to the mother's regimen to prevent fetal goiter or hypothyroidism because thyroid hormones do not reach the fetal circulation. Thyroid supplementation only complicates the treatment of maternal hyperthyroidism by increasing thioamide requirements, which can further compromise fetal thyroid hormone production.[217] If the mother has not been thyrotoxic throughout pregnancy, a normal infant can be expected. All pregnant patients with a history of or active Graves' disease should be screened with a TSI during pregnancy to assess the risk of neonatal hyperthyroidism.[217] Neonatal Graves' disease occurs in 1% to 5% of infants born to mothers with the disease; therefore, all newborns should be evaluated for the condition.[105,220] Lastly, both thioamides can be safely used in the lactating mother if the maximal dose of methimazole does not exceed 10 to 20 mg daily or less preferably, if PTU does not exceed 200 mg/day (up to 750 mg/day in one report).[231,232] Propranolol and iodides are secreted in breast milk and should be avoided (see Chapter 49, Obstetric Drug Therapy).

Treatment with Radioactive Iodine

PRETREATMENT

CASE 52-19

QUESTION 1: B.J., a 35-year-old woman, has newly diagnosed Graves' disease complicated by CHF and angina. After a few days of treatment with methimazole 30 mg daily and Lugol's solution, 5 drops/day, B.J. received RAI therapy. Six months later, she is still symptomatic. Evaluate the influence of B.J.'s pretreatment therapy on the efficacy of her RAI therapy.

Older or debilitated patients with severe hyperthyroidism and/or concomitant cardiac disease should receive antithyroid pretreatment before RAI therapy to deplete stored thyroid hormone and minimize post-RAI hyperthyroidism (occurring in the first 10 days after ^{131}I administration) and thyroid storm caused by leakage of hormones from the damaged thyroid gland.[176,192,233] Other hyperthyroid patients can receive RAI safely without pre-therapy.

Lugol's solution or other iodides should not be given before RAI because iodides decrease the gland's uptake of RAI and its effectiveness. This effect of iodides persists for several weeks. Iodides can be given 1 to 7 days after RAI treatment if it is needed to rapidly control symptoms of hyperthyroidism.

Prior to RAI, thioamides achieve a euthyroid state, but pretreatment may lower the cure rate and increase the need for subsequent RAI.[176,184,234] A meta-analysis of 14 trials found that use of thioamides (e.g., PTU, methimazole, carbimazole) before and after RAI was associated with an increased risk of treatment failure (relative risk of 1.28; 95% CI, 1.07–1.52) and a 32% reduced risk of hypothyroidism regardless of the thioamide used.[184] To facilitate optimal uptake and retention of ^{131}RAI by the gland, thioamides should be stopped at least 2 to 3 days, before RAI administration.[234–236] If necessary, thioamides can be restarted 3 to 7 days after RAI administration without impairing its efficacy. β-Adrenergic blocking agents can be used before, during, and after RAI therapy without interfering with its uptake.

B.J. remains symptomatic because methimazole and iodides decreased RAI's efficacy. Propranolol should be given to B.J. before RAI therapy to relieve hyperthyroid symptoms because only a short course of thioamide was given. Iodides might be preferable to propranolol following RAI therapy if B.J.'s CHF worsens. For subsequent RAI doses, methimazole pretreatment should be stopped 2 to 3 days before RAI, thereby allowing a shorter duration of hyperthyroidism.

ONSET OF EFFECTS

CASE 52-19, QUESTION 2: B.J. is still symptomatic 2 weeks after a second dose of RAI. When can she expect to experience the therapeutic effects of RAI therapy? What educational precautions about radiation safety should B.J. receive?

Although some benefits from RAI therapy are evident within 1 month, a period of 6 to 18 weeks is generally required for maximal effects.[164,184,233] Euthyroidism or, more commonly, hypothyroidism occurs in approximately 80% to 90% of patients treated with a single nonablative dose of RAI; the remaining 10% to 20% become euthyroid or hypothyroid after two or more doses. This slow onset is a disadvantage, but symptomatic control can be obtained quickly by administration of a β-adrenergic blocking agent, or iodides starting 1 to 14 days after the ^{131}I dose. Iodides are less preferable if a second dose of RAI is necessary. Thioamides can also be given, although their therapeutic effects are delayed for 3 to 4 weeks.

At least 3 months should elapse before a second dose of RAI is administered, and most recommend waiting 6 months before repeating RAI, unless the patient remains severely thyrotoxic. It is inadvisable to give a second dose before the major effects of the first dose have become apparent. Although the use of iodides before RAI in B.J. may have decreased the amount of ^{131}I retained by her thyroid, it is still advisable to wait at least 3 months before a second dose is given.

Safety precautions are not universal and vary across the United States depending on the dose of RAI administered.[184] B.J. should avoid close contact (e.g. 6 ft) with children for 5 days, with pregnant women for 10 days, and intimate contact with body fluids for 5 days. B.J. should avoid airplane travels, public transportation, and work if contact with others during these activities last more than 2 hours. Other recommendations include sole use of bathroom facilities; sitting while urinating to avoid splashing and to flush the toilet twice with the lid down.

CASE 52-20

QUESTION 1: S.D., a 54-year-old woman, returns to the thyroid clinic after being lost to follow-up for 6 months. She initially received RAI 3 years ago but required a repeat dose of RAI 1 year ago. She has no other medical problems and is not taking any medications. She is a mildly obese, puffy-faced woman wearing several layers of clothing who complains of fatigue and lack of energy. Her reflexes are delayed, and her skin is cool and dry. What is a likely explanation for her symptoms?

S.D.'s clinical presentation and history are compatible with hypothyroidism secondary to RAI therapy. A FT_4 and a TSH level would confirm this diagnosis. Iatrogenic hypothyroidism is the major complication of RAI therapy, although transient hypothyroidism can occur in the first 3 to 6 weeks after therapy.[164] The incidence of iatrogenic myxedema is often reported as 7% to 8%, but it increases at a constant rate of 2.5% per year. The reported prevalence of this complication ranges from 26% to 70% after 1 to 14 years.[233]

The best predictor of eventual hypothyroidism is the total dose of RAI administered. Prevention of iatrogenic hypothyroidism is directed toward calculation of a dose that will produce neither recurrent hyperthyroidism nor hypothyroidism. Unfortunately, when lower doses of RAI were used to avoid hypothyroidism, the cure rate was reduced but the incidence of hypothyroidism was unaffected. Thus, the appearance of iatrogenic hypothyroidism may be inevitable with time. However, hypothyroidism is managed easily and is an acceptable therapeutic end point. Because hypothyroidism after RAI therapy is latent and often insidious, patients should be informed of this and monitored closely at monthly intervals for subsequent hypothyroidism. Awareness of a transient hypothyroidism soon after RAI therapy should minimize the institution of unnecessary hormone replacement.

Ophthalmopathy

CLINICAL PRESENTATION

CASE 52-21

QUESTION 1: H.R., a 50-year-old man, first developed "large eyes with stare" (Figure 52-3), weakness, diaphoresis, and thyroid enlargement when he was diagnosed with Graves' disease. RAI therapy caused some worsening of his eye symptoms. Although he is clinically euthyroid, physical examination reveals severe bilateral conjunctival edema and injection, proptosis of the right eye, incomplete lid closure, and decreased visual acuity. He complains of photophobia, tearing, and extreme irritation, which is worse after smoking cigarettes. His other medical problems include type 2 diabetes treated with metformin and pioglitazone. What is the association of H.R.'s ocular changes with Graves' disease?

H.R. presents with symptoms consistent with the infiltrative ophthalmopathy of Graves' disease.[237–239] The eye signs of Graves' disease are the most striking abnormality of this disorder. Rarely, ophthalmopathy can occur without any evidence of hyperthyroidism. Fortunately, severe ophthalmopathy occurs in only 3% to 5% of patients, while 25% to 50% have some eye findings. Eye disease is more severe in older patients and in men than women. Smokers often have higher levels of TSI and more severe ophthalmopathy.[212,238,240]

It is unknown why the eye and its muscles are attacked in Graves' disease but is likely related to the presence of TSH receptor antibodies found in patients with ophthalmopathy.[239]

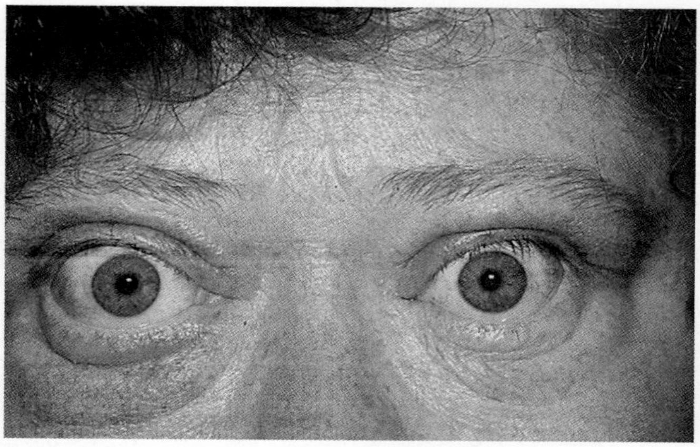

Figure 52-3 Graves' disease ophthalmopathy. (Reprinted with permission from Goodheart HP. *Photoguide of Common Skin Disorders*. 2nd ed. Philadelphia, PA: Lippincott Williams & Wilkins; 2003.)

Histologic examination reveals lymphocytic infiltration, increased mucopolysaccharides, fat (because of increased adipogenesis and glycosaminoglycans), and water in all retrobulbar tissue. Ocular symptoms include edema, chemosis, excessive lacrimation, photophobia, corneal protrusion (proptosis), scarring, ulceration, extraocular muscle paralysis with loss of eye movements, and blindness from retinal and optic nerve damage.

The eye involvement can occur at any time and is usually bilateral. The ocular symptoms usually subside or remain stable once the patient is euthyroid; however, some cases will progress during the euthyroid period or following RAI treatment of the hyperthyroidism (see Case 52-21, Question 2). Pioglitazone has been associated with a 1 to 2 mm increase in eye protrusion by stimulating adipogenesis and increasing retrobulbar fat production.[241] While eye changes were more common in people with a history of thyroid disorders, the overall incidence of eye changes associated with pioglitazone is unknown.[241]

MANAGEMENT OF EYE SYMPTOMS

CASE 52-21, QUESTION 2: Was previous treatment of H.R.'s hyperthyroidism appropriate? How should his current ocular symptoms be managed?

The optimal treatment of hyperthyroidism and its effect on the course of ophthalmopathy remain controversial.[237,238,242] Thioamides might improve eye symptoms through an immunosuppressive mechanism of action and control of the hyperthyroidism or exert a neutral effect.[237] Many clinicians believe that RAI ablation or surgical removal is preferable because it removes the antigen source and prevents progression of the ophthalmopathy.[180,237] However, several studies have confirmed development or worsening of eye symptoms immediately after RAI therapy.[240,242] Concomitant use of 0.4 to 0.5 mg/kg of prednisone begun 1 to 3 days post-RAI continued for one month and tapered over 2 months may be used in patients with mild active eye disease to prevent progression of eye symptoms.[34,240,242] A recent study showed lower dose, shorter duration prednisone therapy (0.2 mg/kg/day for 6 weeks) to conventional doses as effective as conventionally used doses.[243] After 6 months there was no difference in clinical activity score, exophthalmos, or lid retraction. Patients with active moderate-to-severe or sight threatening ophthalmopathy at the time of treatment should be treated with surgery or thioamides instead of RAI.[34] Regardless of the treatment used, control of the hyperthyroidism often improves most eye findings, except for proptosis.

In H.R., prednisone 40 to 60 mg/day should have been started after his RAI treatment and continued for 2 to 3 months until the eye symptoms improved. Because the pathophysiology of the ophthalmopathy is unclear, treatment is limited to symptomatic and empiric measures once the patient is euthyroid.[237,238] H.R. should also be encouraged to stop smoking to prevent progression of the ophthalmopathy.[212] His pioglitazone should be discontinued, in case this is contributing to his ophthalmopathy.

Because periorbital edema and chemosis are worse in the morning after being in the horizontal position, elevating the head of the bed, diuretics, and restricting salt intake may be helpful. Protective glasses can relieve photophobia and external irritation. Topical corticosteroid drops are effective in decreasing local irritation, but they should be used cautiously because they increase the risk of infection. Ocular irritants such as smoke and dust should be avoided. Bothersome symptoms (e.g., dry eye, redness, tearing) caused by eyelid retraction can be relieved by artificial tears and lubricants.[237] Incomplete lid closure predisposes to corneal scarring and ulceration, so lubricant eyedrops should be applied several times daily and at night to keep the bulbs moist. Taping the eyelids shut at night prevents drying and scarring. Lateral surgical closure of the lids (tarsorrhaphy) may be required to improve lid closure.

With severe and progressive ophthalmopathy, an aggressive approach is necessary. Systemic corticosteroids can produce either dramatic or marginal results in the emergency treatment of progressive exophthalmos associated with decreasing visual acuity. Prednisone at dosages of 35 to 80 mg/day is often effective, although dosages as high as 100 to 140 mg/day may be necessary.[237,238] Pain, irritation, tearing, and other subjective complaints often respond within 24 hours of administration. Therapy for about 3 months is necessary to improve eye muscle and optic nerve function disturbances. Initial large doses should be tapered rapidly once the desired response is obtained to minimize adverse effects. Subconjunctival and retrobulbar injections of steroids are not as effective.

Orbital x-ray therapy also relieves congestive and inflammatory symptoms.[237] The combination of orbital irradiation and systemic steroids may be required to achieve maximal benefits. Plasmapheresis and immunosuppressive agents, such as cyclophosphamide, azathioprine, cyclosporine, and methotrexate, combined with steroids have also been used with limited success. Future investigations are focusing on anti-TNF and anti-interleukin receptor antibodies agents that may neutralize some of the inflammatory reactions in the eye.[237,239]

When the previous measures and thyroid ablation fail to arrest the progression of visual loss and exophthalmos, then surgical orbital decompression should be considered.

Thyroid Storm

CLINICAL PRESENTATION

CASE 52-22

QUESTION 1: H.L., a 48-year-old woman, is admitted to the hospital with a 3-week history of fatigue, weakness, dyspnea on exertion, SOB, palpitations, and inability to keep food and liquids down. One year before admission, she began noticing a preference for cold weather and an increase in nervousness and emotional liability. After her husband died a few days ago, she experienced increased nausea and vomiting, irritability, insomnia, tremor, and a 104°F fever, which she attributed to an upper respiratory tract infection. She denies taking any current medications. Her laboratory data obtained on admission included an FT_4 of 4.65 ng/dL (normal, 0.8–1.4) and an undetectable TSH level. Assess H.L.'s subjective and objective data.

The presentation is consistent with thyroid storm, a life-threatening medical emergency that might have been precipitated by the stress associated with the death of her husband. The clinical manifestations of thyroid storm[192] include the acute onset of high fever, tachycardia, and tachypnea, and involvement of the following organ systems: cardiovascular (tachycardia, pulmonary edema, hypertension, shock), CNS (tremor, emotional liability, confusion, psychosis, apathy, stupor, coma), and GI (diarrhea, abdominal pain, nausea and vomiting, liver enlargement, jaundice, nonspecific elevations of bilirubin and prothrombin time). Hyperglycemia is also a common clinical finding in thyroid storm.

Thyroid storm develops in about 2% to 8% of hyperthyroid patients. The pathogenesis of thyroid storm is not well understood, but the condition can be described as an "exaggerated" or decompensated form of thyrotoxicosis. The term *decompensated* implies failure of body systems to adequately resist the effects of thyrotoxicosis. It is not attributed solely to the release of massive quantities of hormones, which can occur after surgery or RAI therapy. Catecholamines also play an important role; the increased quantities of thyroid hormone in conjunction with increased sympathetic and adrenal output contribute to many of the manifestations of thyroid storm. Although thyroid hormones exert an independent effect, many of the symptoms of hyperthyroidism are ameliorated by catecholamine-blocking agents such as β-blockers and calcium channel blockers (e.g., diltiazem, verapamil).

TREATMENT

CASE 52-22, QUESTION 2: What treatment plan (including route of administration) should be initiated promptly in H.L.?

Intensive, continuous, and immediate treatment can significantly reduce the mortality of thyroid storm. Mortality rates in thyroid storm are high, ranging between 20% and 30%.[192] Treatment of thyroid storm should be directed against four major areas discussed in the following sections.[192]

Decrease in Synthesis and Release of Hormones

High dosages of thioamides, preferably PTU 800 to 1,200 mg/day or methimazole 60 to 100 mg/day, should be given orally in four divided doses. If H.L. cannot take oral doses, a rectal formulation of PTU (better bioavailability with enema than suppository) or methimazole, which is as effective as the oral route, can be administered.[177–179] No commercial parenteral preparation is available for either drug, limiting their use by the IV route. PTU is the thioamide of choice because it acts more rapidly than methimazole by blocking the peripheral conversion of T_4 to T_3, a dominant source of the hormone.

Iodides, which rapidly block further release of intraglandular stores of T_4, should be given at least 1 hour after thioamide administration. Given in this way, the substrate for hormone synthesis is not increased, and the therapeutic effect of thioamide is not blocked. The addition of iodides (e.g., Lugol's solution 15 to 30 drops/day orally in divided doses) to the thioamides often ameliorates symptoms within 1 day.

Cholestyramine 4 g orally (PO) QID may assist in lowering hormone levels rapidly but should be administered apart from other agents to prevent inhibiting their absorption.[244] Other effective modalities include plasmapheresis, charcoal hemoperfusion, and plasma exchange.

Reversal of the Peripheral Effects of Hormones and Catecholamines

β-Adrenergic blocking drugs are the preferred agents to decrease the tachycardia, agitation, tremulousness, and other symptoms of excessive adrenergic stimulation seen in thyroid storm. Propranolol is the β-blocker of choice because its clinical efficacy in storm is well documented, and it inhibits the peripheral conversion of T_4 to T_3.[192,200] If rapid effects are necessary, propranolol 1 mg by slow IV push can be given every 5 minutes to lower the heart rate to approximately 90 beats/minute. A 5- to 10-mg/hour IV infusion can maintain the desired heart rate. IV esmolol 50 to 100 mcg/kg/minute can also be given. If perfusion is maintained, oral β-blockers (e.g., propranolol, 40 mg every 6 hours; atenolol, 50–100 mg BID; metoprolol, 50–100 mg daily; nadolol, 40–80 mg daily), titrated to response, can also be given.

Supportive Treatment of Vital Functions

This may include sedation, oxygen, IV glucose, vitamins, treatment of infections with antibiotics, digitalization to maintain the cardiac status, rehydration, and treatment of hyperpyrexia with cooling blankets, sponge baths, and the judicious use of antipyretics. Because hypoadrenalism is often suspected, hydrocortisone 100 to 200 mg should empirically be given IV every 6 hours. Because pharmacologic doses of steroids acutely depress serum T_3 levels, a beneficial effect in storm, their routine use is recommended.

Elimination of Precipitating Causes of Storm

Precipitating causes of thyroid storm include infection (most common), trauma, inadequate preparation before thyroidectomy, surgical operations, stress, diabetic ketoacidosis, pregnancy, emboli, discontinuation or withdrawal of antithyroid medications, drug therapy, and RAI therapy.[192]

DRUG-INDUCED THYROID DISEASE

Lithium

CASE 52-23

QUESTION 1: D.A., a 56-year-old man, complains of sluggishness, cold intolerance, fatigue, and a "rundown" feeling, which doctors attribute to the depressive phase of his bipolar affective illness. He previously had been well controlled with sertraline 100 mg/day, but lithium carbonate 900 mg/day was added 4 months ago because of unreasonable mirthfulness and uncontrollable gift-buying tendencies. Physical examination reveals a puffy face and a large goiter. What is a reasonable assessment of these subjective and objective data?

Thyroid function tests (i.e., TSH, FT_4) and a thyroid ultrasound should be obtained to evaluate the possibility of lithium- and possibly sertraline-induced hypothyroidism and goiter.[4,5,13,245] If the TSH is elevated, T_4 should be initiated and lithium continued if necessary. Although the incidence of goiter and hypothyroidism in the manic-depressive population is unknown, the 10% incidence of baseline-elevated TSH appears higher than in the general population.

The exact mechanism of lithium's antithyroid effect on the gland is unclear, although it is highly concentrated by the gland. Similar to the iodides, chronic lithium therapy inhibits the release of thyroid hormone from the gland. The fall in serum T_4 and T_3 hormone levels leads to a compensatory and transient increase in serum TSH levels until a new steady state is achieved.[4,5,13]

Elevated TSH levels are reported in approximately 19% of patients on chronic lithium therapy.[13] Typically, the serum thyroid hormone levels decrease and the TSH levels increase during the first few months of treatment, returning to pretreatment levels after 1 year. In one study, TSH levels increased within 10 days after starting therapy. Normalization of the TSH level is less likely to occur in patients with preexisting positive thyroid antibodies before lithium therapy. Induction of thyroid antibodies and increases in baseline antibody titers also occur after chronic lithium therapy. Because abnormal thyroid function tests can be transient, a longer period of observation is justified before starting thyroid therapy in patients with subclinical hypothyroidism.

Overt hypothyroidism appears in a small percentage of the population after 5 months to 2 years of therapy; one 15-year study found an incidence of 1.5% but an 8.4 relative risk in females with antibody positivity compared to negative subjects.[4,5,13] Lithium-induced goiter with or without hypothyroidism is common after weeks to months of therapy. Although incidences of less than 6% have been reported, higher rates of 40% to 60% are observed if the goiter is diagnosed using more specific imaging techniques (e.g. ultrasound).[4,5,13] A direct goitrogenic effect of lithium on inducing cell proliferation might explain the occurrence of euthyroid goiter. The goiters respond to discontinuation of lithium or to suppression with thyroid hormone despite continuation of lithium therapy. Surgical removal of the goiter is required if there are local obstructive symptoms. In D.A.'s case, sertraline could be exerting an additive or synergistic antithyroid effect with lithium because antithyroid effects have also been associated with this drug.[245]

Most patients with lithium-induced thyroid abnormalities are women older than 50 years, have a prior history of compromised thyroid function (e.g., Hashimoto's thyroiditis), positive thyroid antibodies before lithium therapy, or a strong family history of thyroid disease.[4,5,13] Therefore, baseline thyroid function tests (i.e., FT_4, TSH), antibodies, and thyroid ultrasound should be obtained before starting lithium therapy, and levels should be checked annually thereafter or more frequently if clinically indicated. Patients should also be questioned about a positive history or family history for thyroid disease and the concurrent use of other, potentially goitrogenic medications (e.g., tricyclic antidepressants, iodides, iodinated expectorants/herbals).

Iodides and Amiodarone

CASE 52-24

QUESTION 1: C.Y., a 54-year-old man with chronic atrial fibrillation presents with a 6-month history of weakness, fatigue, tremor, heat intolerance, and increased palpitations, previously controlled for the last 2 years on amiodarone 200 mg/day. Physical examination reveals a 50-g multinodular gland, which C.Y. says has "been there forever." He denies any family history of thyroid disease or ingestion of any thyroid medication. His current complaints began after a magnetic resonance imaging (MRI) procedure with iodinated radiocontrast media. What might be responsible for C.Y.'s hyperthyroid symptoms?

The iodine load from the MRI or the amiodarone could be responsible for C.Y.'s hyperthyroid symptoms.[3,12,17,28,57,173] Iodide-induced hyperthyroidism, or Jod-Basedow phenomenon, was first described in the 1800s when patients residing in iodide-deficient areas became toxic when given adequate iodide supplementation. Both T_3 toxicosis and classic T_4 toxicosis have been reported following iodide ingestion or injection of roentgenographic contrast media.

Although it is presumed that both iodide deficiency and a multinodular goiter, as in C.Y., are required to invoke the Jod-Basedow phenomenon, iodide-induced disease has been reported in patients residing in iodide-sufficient areas, as well as in euthyroid patients with normal glands and no apparent risk factors (e.g., family history).[28,173]

Amiodarone can cause hypo- or hyperthyroidism in susceptible patients because of its high iodine content.[3,12,16,17,28,57,173] Twelve milligrams (37%) of free iodine is released per 400-mg dose of amiodarone. Patients with multinodular goiters, who lose the ability to turn off iodide organification from increased iodide loads (Wolff–Chaikoff effect), are most likely to develop iodide-induced thyrotoxicosis. Conversely, patients with positive antibodies or with underlying Hashimoto's thyroiditis, who cannot escape from the Wolff–Chaikoff block, are most likely to develop hypothyroidism.

Amiodarone-induced hypothyroidism may occur at any time during therapy and does not appear to be related to the cumulative dose. A low-normal or low FT_4 and a persistently elevated TSH (see Case 52-4) are consistent with amiodarone-induced hypothyroidism, which occurs in 6% to 10% of long-term users. The hypothyroidism responds readily to T_4 therapy, even if the amiodarone is continued.[3,17,57] Amiodarone-induced hypothyroidism typically resolves after stopping the drug, but resolution may be delayed because of its long half-life.

In contrast, amiodarone-induced thyrotoxicosis, which occurs in 1% to 5% of long-term users, occurs early and suddenly during therapy, so that routine monitoring of thyroid function tests is not useful. Elevated hormone levels, an undetectable TSH level, and clinical symptoms consistent with hyperthyroidism are the best indicators of amiodarone-induced thyrotoxicosis. Worsening of tachyarrhythmias may be the first clinical clue to amiodarone-induced thyrotoxicosis.

Amiodarone-induced hyperthyroidism can be classified as either type I or type II.[3,12,55,57] Type I occurs in patients with underlying risk factors for thyroid disease (e.g., multinodular goiter) and is related to the iodine load. The formation of large amounts of preformed hormone from the massive iodine load produces a protracted course of hyperthyroidism, which is challenging to manage. Type II amiodarone-induced hyperthyroidism is because of a destructive thyroiditis, with excessive release of thyroid hormone into the systemic circulation. This occurs most often in patients with normal thyroid glands. Unique laboratory findings include a low RAIU and elevated interleukin-6 levels.

The management of amiodarone-induced thyrotoxicosis is complicated because it is not always possible to identify the type of hyperthyroidism and a mixture of the two types can occur. Stopping amiodarone alone does not immediately improve the hyperthyroidism because of the drug's long half-life (22–55 days) and its sequestration in fat. RAI ablation is never effective because the high iodine load from amiodarone will suppress RAI uptake. The combination of methimazole and potassium perchlorate is the treatment of choice for type I hyperthyroidism.[3,12,17,28,57,173] The addition of corticosteroids to block T_4 to T_3 conversion is less effective because of the already potent inhibitory effects of amiodarone on T_4 to T_3 conversion. However, in patients with type II hyperthyroidism, agents that block T_4 to T_3 conversion (e.g., β-blockers, corticosteroids, and iodinated contrast media if available), rather than the aforementioned agents, are the most appropriate choices.[3,17,28,57,246] A total thyroidectomy can rapidly control the thyrotoxicosis, permitting continued therapy with amiodarone if necessary. Despite underlying cardiac disease in these patients, uneventful surgery and a low complication rate have been observed if patients are treated before surgery with a short course of an oral cholecystographic agent.[246] Changing amiodarone to dronedarone which is devoid of iodine and lacks the undesirable thyroid effects should be strongly considered in C.Y.

Large doses of iodides should be avoided in patients with nontoxic multinodular goiters, who are predisposed to thyrotoxicosis (see Case 52-4 and Case 52-15, Question 2).

Thyrotropin-α and Thyroid Suppression Therapy for Thyroid Cancer

CASE 52-25

QUESTION 1: J.R., a 28-year-old man, had a total thyroidectomy last year for papillary cancer followed by RAI therapy. He is clinically euthyroid on 200 mcg L-thyroxine daily with a TSH level of <0.2 microunits/mL (normal, 0.45–4.1). He is hesitant to discontinue his L-thyroxine, so that an RAIU scan and thyroglobulin testing can be done to evaluate for tumor recurrence. His doctor is concerned about his suppressed TSH level and is also worried about taking J.R. off his L-thyroxine because the patient says he "feels incapacitated" while carrying out these tests. What can you tell his physician about the TSH level and the need to stop L-thyroxine during these tests?

In patients with thyroid cancers, total thyroidectomy, followed by RAI and L-thyroxine therapy to suppress the TSH to subnormal levels, were associated with improved overall survival.[247] The actual degree of thyroid suppression required is complex and depends upon the severity and extent of the thyroid cancer and the likelihood of a disease-free prognosis. The benefits of prolonged thyrotropin suppression to prevent cancer recurrence need to be balanced against the risks and adverse effects (e.g. osteoporosis, cardiac toxicity) of lifelong T_4 suppression. Lifelong TSH suppression to a level of <0.1 microunits/mL is preferred for patients with high-to-intermediate risk of recurrent cancer or metastastes.[29] A low normal TSH of 0.3 to 2 microunits/mL can be considered for disease-free patients. It is important to annually assess recurrence of the malignancy by determining whether any residual cancerous or normal thyroid tissue remains. This is done either by withdrawing suppressive T_4 therapy and allowing endogenous TSH concentrations to rise or by administering recombinant human TSH (thyrotropin-α). If any functioning follicular cells remain, the rise in TSH will cause a rise in thyroglobulin and/or positive RAIU, indicating a need for further RAI therapy. Thyrotropin-α (Thryogen) may be preferred because it allows screening without the troublesome hypothyroid symptoms caused by withdrawal of T_4.[248] Thyrotropin-α failed to detect localized tumor recurrence in 7% of patients compared to 100% detection after hormone withdrawal but detected 100% of patients with metastatic disease.[29,248]

J.R. should be maintained on his current L-thyroxine suppression dosage because his TSH level is appropriately suppressed without hyperthyroidism.

KEY REFERENCES AND WEBSITES

A full list of references for this chapter can be found at http://thepoint.lww.com/AT11e. Below are the key references and websites for this chapter, with the corresponding reference number in this chapter found in parentheses after the reference.

Key References

Bach-Huynh TG et al. Timing of levothyroxine administration affects serum thyrotropin concentration. *J Clin Endocrinol Metab*. 2009;94:3905. (122)

Bahn RS, Burch HB, Cooper DS, et al. Hyperthyroidism and other causes of thyrotoxicosis: management guidelines of the American Thyroid Association and American Association of Clinical Endocrinologists. *Endocr Pract*. 2011;17(3):456–520. (34)

Biondi B, Cooper DS. Benefits of thyrotropin suppression versus the risks of adverse effects in differentiated thyroid cancer. *Thyroid*. 2010;20:135. (247)

Biondi B, Cooper DS. The clinical significance of subclinical thyroid dysfunction. *Endocr Rev*. 2008;29:76. (88)

Brent GA. Clinical practice: Graves' disease. *N Engl J Med*. 2008;358: 2594. (164)

Cohen-Lehman J et al. Effects of amiodarone therapy on thyroid function. *Nat Rev Endocrinol*. 2010;6:34. (57)

Cooper DS. Antithyroid drugs. *N Engl J Med*. 2005;352:905. (176)

Cooper et al. Revised American Thyroid Association management guidelines for patients with thyroid nodules and differentiated thyroid cancer [published correction appears in *Thyroid*. 2010;20:674]. *Thyroid*. 2009;19:1167. (30)

Flynn RW et al. Serum thyroid-stimulating hormone concentration and morbidity from cardiovascular disease and fractures in patients on long-term thyroxine therapy. *J Clin Endocrinol Metab*. 2010;95:186. (95)

Garber JR, Cobin RH, Gharib H, et al. Clinical practice guidelines for hypothyroidism in adults: cosponsored by the American Association of Clinical Endocrinologists and the American Thyroid Association. *Endocr Pract*. 2012;18(6):988–1028. (35)

Grozinsky-Glasberg S et al. Thyroxine-triiodothyronine combination therapy versus thyroxine monotherapy for clinical hypothyroidism: meta-analysis of randomized controlled trials. *J Clin Endocrinol Metab*. 2006;91:2592. (82)

Haugen BR. Drugs that suppress TSH or cause central hypothyroidism. *Best Pract Res Clin Endocrinol Metab*. 2009;23:793. (59)

Jonklaas J, Bianco AC, Bauer AJ, et al. Guidelines for the treatment of hypothyroidism: prepared by the American thyroid association task force on thyroid hormone replacement. *Thyroid*. 2014;24(12):1670–1751. (65)

Jonklaas J et al. Triiodothyronine levels in athyreotic individuals during levothyroxine therapy. *JAMA*. 2008;299:769. (83)

Ross DS. Radioiodine therapy for hyperthyroidism. *N Engl J Med*. 2011;364:542. (184)

Stagnaro-Green A, Abalovich M, Alexander E, et al. Guidelines of the American Thyroid Association for the diagnosis and management of thyroid disease during pregnancy and postpartum. *Thyroid*. 2011;21(10):1081–1125. (107)

Toft A. Which thyroxine? *Thyroid*. 2005;15:124. (77)

Key Websites

American Thyroid Association. ATA Frequently Asked Questions (FAQS). http://www.thyroid.org/patients/faqs.html.

American Thyroid Association. ATA Patient Education Web Brochures. http://www.thyroid.org/patients/brochures.html.

American Thyroid Association. The Professional Community. http://www.thyroid.org/professionals/.

Graves' Disease Foundation. http://www.ngdf.org/.

National Cancer Institute. Thyroid Cancer. http://www.cancer.gov/cancertopics/types/thyroid.

ThyCa: Thyroid Cancer Survivors' Association. http://www.thyca.org/.

53 Diabetes Mellitus

Jennifer D. Goldman, Dhiren K. Patel, and David Schnee

CORE PRINCIPLES

	CORE PRINCIPLES	CHAPTER CASES
1	A glycosylated hemoglobin (A1C) level can be used to diagnose diabetes, in addition to a fasting plasma glucose (FPG) or oral glucose tolerance test (OGTT). Each test must be confirmed on a subsequent day.	**Case 53-2 (Question 1), Case 53-11 (Question 1)**
2	The primary metabolic goals for diabetes are an A1C less than 7%, a systolic blood pressure less than 140 mm Hg, and statin therapy for most patients over the age of 40. Management of cholesterol should include a statin drug, and management of hypertension should include an angiotensin-converting enzyme inhibitor or angiotensin II receptor blocker.	**Case 53-2 (Question 2), Case 53-11 (Question 2)**
3	Glycemic treatment goals should be individualized. For patients with a short duration of diabetes, long life expectancy, and no significant vascular disease, more stringent goals can be considered, if it can be achieved without increasing hypoglycemia. For patients with existing vascular disease, other significant macrovascular or microvascular disease, a history of hypoglycemia, or limited life expectancy, or for those with long-standing diabetes who have difficulty lowering their A1C, a less stringent A1C goal should be considered.	**Case 53-2 (Question 2), Case 53-4 (Question 2), Case 53-11 (Question 2), Case 53-18 (Question 3)**
4	Medical nutrition therapy (MNT) and physical activity are cornerstones to the treatment of diabetes.	**Case 53-2 (Questions 11, 12), Case 53-11 (Question 3), Case 53-18 (Question 4)**
5	Self-monitoring of blood glucose (SMBG) should be performed by all patients with Type 1 diabetes and most patients with Type 2 diabetes, particularly those on antidiabetic therapy that can cause hypoglycemia or those engaged in self-management. The key to SMBG is to educate patients on how to respond to their blood glucose (BG) levels.	**Case 53-2 (Questions 9–11), Case 53-4 (Question 5), Case 53-11 (Question 6)**
6	Basal-bolus insulin regimens should be used for patients with Type 1 diabetes. These can be administered either by multiple daily injections or by an insulin pump. Basal-bolus insulin regimens are also effective for patients with Type 2 diabetes who no longer are able to achieve A1C goals with noninsulin therapies.	**Case 53-2 (Questions 3–6), Case 53-4 (Question 3), Case 53-13 (Question 6)**
7	Metformin is the first-line therapy for Type 2 diabetes unless a patient has a contraindication to its use or is unable to tolerate this agent. It should be added at diagnosis along with lifestyle changes.	**Case 53-11 (Questions 3–5)**
8	After monotherapy, a second antidiabetic agent should be added to the regimen. Factors to consider include the patient's A1C goal, the amount of reduction in A1C required, the patient's kidney and liver function, medication side effects, and cost of therapy.	**Case 53-11 (Question 7), Case 53-12 (Question 1), Case 53-13 (Questions 2–4)**
9	In Type 2 diabetes, insulin therapy should be considered any time the patient's A1C is severely uncontrolled (e.g., A1C >10%) and also when the A1C is more than 8.5% to 9%, and a patient is already on combination oral therapy. It should be considered whether a patient is symptomatic.	**Case 53-11 (Question 7), Case 53-12 (Question 1), Case 53-13 (Question 5)**

Continued

	CHAPTER CASES
10 Owing to concerns about the effects of hypoglycemia and new trials indicating a lack of benefit of very tight glucose control in acutely ill patients, the current-recommended goal BG in hospitalized patients is 140 to 180 mg/dL.	Case 53-7 (Question 1)
11 Although acute hyperglycemic crises can occur in patients with diabetes, most morbidity and mortality occurs over the course of years and can be classified as either microvascular (nephropathy, neuropathy, and retinopathy) or macrovascular (coronary heart disease (CHD), stroke, and peripheral vascular disease).	Case 53-19 (Questions 1–5), Case 53-20 (Questions 1–3)
12 Patients with established vascular disease should remain on lifelong aspirin therapy, whereas patients without established vascular disease need to be carefully considered to determine the appropriateness of antiplatelet therapy.	Case 53-19 (Question 6)
13 The incidence and severity of microvascular complications has a strong correlation with long-term glycemic control as measured by A1C. Macrovascular complications are influenced by glycemic control, but are more dependent on multiple etiologic factors including dyslipidemia, hypertension, and smoking.	Case 53-11 (Question 2)

An estimated 29.1 million people, or 9.3% of the US population, currently have diabetes.[1] Of these, 8.1 million or about one-third are undiagnosed. In 2012 alone, more than 1.7 million new cases in adults were diagnosed. Globally, the prevalence of diabetes for all ages is estimated to be 2.8% in 2000 and projected to increase to 4.4% by 2030.[2] The incidence of Type 2 diabetes is now epidemic, with alarming increases in prevalence in both adults and children. Estimates by the Centers for Disease Control and Prevention indicate that new cases of diabetes annually will increase from 8/1,000 people to about 15/1,000 in 2050, with as many as 1 in 3 Americans having diabetes in 2050.[3] The dramatic increase in Type 2 diabetes in the population is related to obesity and decreased physical activity levels, and also the fact that people with diabetes are living longer. Additional individual factors include a genetic predisposition for increased insulin resistance and progressive β-cell failure. Clinical studies have affirmed that Type 2 diabetes can be delayed or prevented in high-risk populations and that good glycemic control and other interventions can slow its devastating complications.[4]

DEFINITION, CLASSIFICATION, AND EPIDEMIOLOGY

Diabetes is a chronic condition caused by an absolute lack of insulin or relative lack of insulin as a result of impaired insulin secretion and action. Its hallmark clinical characteristics are symptomatic glucose intolerance resulting in hyperglycemia and alterations in lipid and protein metabolism. In the long term, these metabolic abnormalities contribute to the development of complications such as cardiovascular disease (CVD), retinopathy, nephropathy, and neuropathy and a higher risk of cancer.[5,6]

Genetically, etiologically, and clinically, diabetes is a heterogeneous group of disorders. Nevertheless, most cases of diabetes mellitus can be assigned to Type 1 or Type 2 diabetes (Table 53-1). The term gestational diabetes mellitus (GDM) is used to describe glucose intolerance that has its onset during pregnancy. Glucose intolerance that cannot be ascribed to causes consistent with these three classifications includes specific genetic defects in β-cell function or insulin action (usually genetically defective insulin receptors); diseases of the exocrine pancreas; endocrinopathies; drug- or chemical-induced; infections; and other genetic syndromes. Early glucose intolerance or "prediabetes" is identified as impaired fasting glucose (IFG) or impaired glucose tolerance (IGT), and they are considered risk factors for the future development of diabetes and are associated with obesity, hypertriglyceridemia, and/or low high-density lipoprotein (HDL) cholesterol and hypertension.[7]

Approximately 5% to 10% of the diagnosed diabetic population has Type 1 diabetes, which usually results from autoimmune destruction of the pancreatic β-cells. At clinical presentation, these patients have little or no pancreatic reserve, have a tendency to develop ketoacidosis, and require exogenous insulin to sustain life. The incidence of autoimmune-mediated Type 1 diabetes peaks during childhood and adolescence, but it can occur at any age. A minority of patients diagnosed with Type 1 diabetes, mostly of African or Asian ancestry, can have no evidence of autoimmunity; the etiology is, therefore, unknown. In these individuals, the rate of pancreatic destruction seems to occur more slowly, leading to a later onset and less acute presentation.[7]

Most people with diabetes have Type 2 diabetes, a heterogeneous disorder that is characterized by obesity, β-cell dysfunction, resistance to insulin action, and increased hepatic glucose production. Both the incidence and prevalence of diabetes increase dramatically with age, obesity, and lack of physical activity.[7] In the United States, the percentage of patients with diagnosed or undiagnosed diabetes in those 20 to 44 years of age is 4.1%. This increases to 25.9% in those 65 and older.[1] The prevalence of Type 2 diabetes also differs among ethnic populations. Relative to non-Hispanic whites (7.6%), the prevalence of diagnosed diabetes is higher in Asian-Americans (9%), Hispanics (12.8%), African-Americans (13.2%), and American Indians and Alaskan Natives (15.9%).[1] Diabetes is a serious condition that places people at risk for greater morbidity and mortality relative to the nondiabetic population. Diabetes is the seventh leading cause of death in the United States, although deaths attributed to diabetes and its complications are likely to be underreported. Compared with the general population, the mortality rate for people with diabetes is about twice that for people without diabetes.[1]

Medical management of people with diabetes is costly. In 2012, the total cost of diabetes in the United States was estimated to be $245 billion, with 1 of 5 healthcare dollars being spent on people with diabetes.[8] The average healthcare expenditures for people with diabetes were approximately 2.3 times higher than those for individuals without diabetes. The majority (56%) of all healthcare expenditures attributed to diabetes are used by people aged 65 years and older. Hospital inpatient costs, nursing facility resources, home care, physician visits, and medications (not just diabetes agents) made up the majority of these expenditures. Because many expenditures are related to treatment of long-term complications, considerable effort has been directed toward early diagnosis and metabolic control of patients with diabetes.[8]

Table 53-1
Type 1 and Type 2 Diabetes

Characteristics	Type 1	Type 2
Other names	Previously, type I; insulin-dependent diabetes mellitus (IDDM); juvenile-onset diabetes mellitus	Previously, type II; non-insulin-dependent diabetes mellitus (NIDDM); adult-onset diabetes mellitus
Percentage of diabetic population	5%–10%	90%
Age at onset	Usually <30 years; peaks at 12–14 years; rare before 6 months; some adults develop type 1 during the fifth decade	Usually >40 years, but increasing prevalence among obese children
Pancreatic function	Usually none, although some residual C-peptide can sometimes be detected at diagnosis, especially in adults	Insulin present in low, "normal," or high amounts
Pathogenesis	Associated with certain HLA types; presence of islet cell antibodies suggests autoimmune process	Defect in insulin secretion; tissue resistance to insulin; ↑ hepatic glucose output
Family history	Generally not strong	Strong
Obesity	Uncommon unless "overinsulinized" with exogenous insulin	Common (60%–90%)
History of ketoacidosis	Often present	Rare, except in circumstances of unusual stress (e.g., infection)
Clinical presentation	Moderate-to-severe symptoms that generally progress relatively rapidly (days to weeks): polyuria, polydipsia, fatigue, weight loss, ketoacidosis	Mild polyuria, fatigue; often diagnosed on routine physical or dental examination
Treatment	MNT Physical activity Insulin Amylin mimetic (pramlintide)	MNT Physical activity Antidiabetic agents (biguanides, glinides, sulfonylureas, thiazolidinediones, α-glucosidase inhibitors, incretin mimetics/analogs, DPP-4 inhibitors, SGLT-2 inhibitors) Insulin Amylin mimetic (pramlintide)

DPP-4, dipeptidyl peptidase-4; HLA, human leukocyte antigen; MNT, medical nutrition therapy.

CARBOHYDRATE METABOLISM

An understanding of the signs and symptoms associated with diabetes is based on a knowledge of glucose metabolism and the metabolic effects of insulin in nondiabetic and diabetic subjects during the fed (postprandial) and fasting (postabsorptive) states.[9] Homeostatic mechanisms maintain plasma glucose concentrations between 55 and 140 mg/dL. A minimum concentration of 40 to 60 mg/dL is required to provide adequate fuel for the central nervous system, which uses glucose as its primary energy source and is independent of insulin for glucose utilization. When BG concentrations exceed the reabsorptive capacity of the proximal tubule in the kidneys (~180 mg/dL), glucose spills into the urine (glucosuria), resulting in a loss of calories and water. Muscle and fat, which use glucose as a major source of energy, require insulin for glucose uptake. If glucose is unavailable, these tissues are able to use other substrates such as amino acids and fatty acids for fuel.[9]

Postprandial Glucose and Lipid Metabolism in the Nondiabetic Individual

After food is ingested, BG concentrations rise and stimulate insulin release. Insulin is the key to efficient glucose utilization. It promotes the uptake of glucose, fatty acids, and amino acids, and their conversion to storage forms in most tissues. Insulin also inhibits hepatic glucose production by suppressing glucagon and its effects. In muscle, insulin promotes the uptake of glucose and its storage as glycogen. It also stimulates the uptake of amino acids and their conversion to protein. In adipose tissue, glucose is converted to free fatty acids and stored as triglycerides. Insulin also prevents a breakdown of these triglycerides to free fatty acids, a form that may be transported to other tissues for utilization. The liver does not require insulin for glucose transport, but insulin facilitates the conversion of glucose to glycogen and free fatty acids.[9,10]

Free fatty acids are esterified to triglycerides, which are transported by very-low-density lipoproteins (VLDLs) to adipose and muscle tissue. Normal insulin signaling suppresses VLDL secretion by reducing the production of fatty acids in the liver.[10] Once secreted by the liver, VLDL is acted on primarily by hepatic lipase in the liver and by lipoprotein lipase on endothelial cells.[10] Acting through apolipoprotein (apo) CII on the surface of the VLDL particle, these lipases remove free fatty acids from the lipoprotein and convert VLDL to intermediate-density lipoprotein (IDL) and then IDL to low-density lipoprotein (LDL). Insulin plays a role in stimulating apoCII expression, which partly explains the hypertriglyceridemia that occurs in Type 2 diabetes.[10]

Fasting Glucose Metabolism in the Nondiabetic Individual

As BG concentrations drop toward normal during the fasting state, insulin release is inhibited. Simultaneously, a number of counter-regulatory hormones that oppose the effect of insulin and promote an increase in blood sugar are released (e.g., glucagon, epinephrine, growth hormone, cortisol). As a result, several processes maintain a minimum BG concentration for the central nervous system. Glycogen in the liver is broken down into glucose (glycogenolysis). Amino acids are transported from muscle to liver, where they are converted to glucose through gluconeogenesis. Uptake of glucose by insulin-dependent tissues is diminished to conserve glucose for the brain. Finally, triglycerides are broken down into free fatty acids, which are used as alternative fuel sources.[9,10]

TYPE 1 DIABETES

Pathogenesis

The loss of insulin secretion in Type 1 diabetes mellitus results from autoimmune destruction of the insulin-producing β-cells in the pancreas, which is thought to be triggered by environmental factors, such as viruses or toxins, in genetically susceptible individuals.[7,11] This form of diabetes is associated closely with histocompatibility antigens (human leukocyte antigen [HLA]-DR3 or HLA-DR4) and the presence of circulating antibodies, including insulin autoantibodies, glutamic acid decarboxylase autoantibodies (GAD65), islet cell autoantibodies (ICA), and autoantibodies to tyrosine phosphatases (e.g., islet cell antibody 512). The capacity of normal pancreatic β-cells to secrete insulin far exceeds the normal amounts needed to control carbohydrate, fat, and protein metabolism. As a result, the clinical onset of Type 1 diabetes is preceded by an extensive asymptomatic period during which β-cells are destroyed (Fig. 53-1).

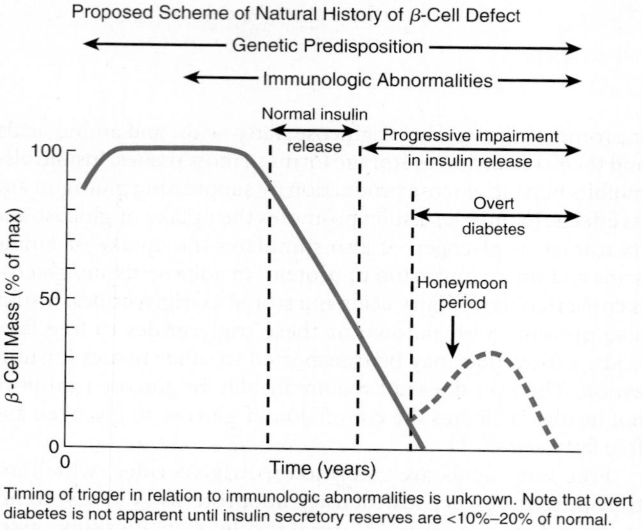

Figure 53-1 Pathogenesis of type 1 diabetes. In an individual with a genetic predisposition, an event (such as a virus or toxin) triggers autoimmune destruction of the pancreatic β-cells, probably during a period of several years. When the number of β-cells diminishes to approximately 250,000, the pancreas is unable to secrete sufficient insulin and intolerance to glucose ensues. At this point, a stressful event, such as a viral infection, can produce acute symptoms of hyperglycemia and ketoacidosis. Once the acute event has passed, the pancreas temporarily recovers, leading to a remission (honeymoon period). Continued destruction of the β-cell ultimately leads to an insulin-dependent state.

β-cell destruction may occur rapidly, but is more likely to take place over a period of weeks, months, or even years. The earliest detectable abnormality in insulin secretion is a progressive reduction of immediate or first-phase plasma insulin response. However, this initial impairment has few detrimental effects on overall glucose homeostasis, and plasma glucose concentrations remain normal. Most affected individuals have circulating antibodies to islet cells or to their own insulin at this stage of the disease. These represent markers of an ongoing autoimmune process that culminates in Type 1 diabetes. Fasting hyperglycemia occurs when the β-cell mass is reduced by 80% to 90%. One or more of the above autoantibodies is usually present in 85% to 90% of individuals at this point. Initially, only postprandial hyperglycemia occurs, but as insulin secretion becomes further compromised, progressive fasting hyperglycemia is seen. Within 8 to 10 years of clinical presentation, β-cell loss is complete and insulin deficiency is absolute.[7,11]

Clinical Presentation

Although the onset of Type 1 diabetes seems to be abrupt, evidence now exists for an extended preclinical period that can precede obvious symptoms by several years. Because insulin secretion becomes compromised, progressive fasting hyperglycemia occurs. Glucosuria, which occurs when BG levels exceed the renal threshold, results in an osmotic diuresis, producing the classic symptoms of polyuria with compensatory polydipsia. If symptoms are untreated, weight loss occurs because glucose calories are lost in the urine and body fat and protein stores are broken down owing to increased rates of lipolysis and proteolysis. Muscle begins to metabolize its own glycogen stores and fatty acids for fuel, and the liver begins to metabolize free fatty acids that are released in response to epinephrine and low insulin concentrations. An absolute lack of insulin may cause excessive mobilization of free fatty acids to the liver, where they are metabolized to ketones. This can result in ketonemia, ketonuria, and, ultimately, ketoacidosis. Patients present with complaints of fatigue, significant weight loss, polyuria, and polydipsia. A significant elevation in A1C confirms weeks or months of preceding hyperglycemia.

Because glucose provides an excellent medium for microorganisms, patients may present also with recurrent respiratory, vaginal, and other infections. Patients also may experience blurred vision secondary to osmotically induced changes in the lens of the eye. Treatment with insulin is essential to prevent severe dehydration, ketoacidosis, and death.

Honeymoon Period

Within days or weeks after the initial diagnosis and implementing treatment, many patients with Type 1 diabetes experience an apparent remission, which is reflected by decreased BG concentrations and markedly decreased insulin requirements. This is called the *honeymoon period* because it may last for only a few weeks to months. Once hyperglycemia, metabolic acidosis, and ketosis resolve, endogenous insulin secretion recovers temporarily (Fig. 53-1). Although the honeymoon period may last for up to a year, increasing exogenous insulin requirements are inevitable and should be anticipated. During this time, patients should be maintained on insulin even if the dose is very low, because interrupted treatment is associated with a greater incidence of resistance and allergy to insulin.

TYPE 2 DIABETES

Pathogenesis

Type 2 diabetes is characterized by impaired insulin secretion and resistance to insulin action. In the presence of insulin resistance, glucose utilization by tissues is impaired, hepatic glucose and free fatty acid production is increased, and excess glucose accumulates in the circulation. This hyperglycemia stimulates the pancreas to produce more insulin in an attempt to overcome insulin resistance. The simultaneous elevation of both glucose and insulin levels is strongly suggestive of insulin resistance. Genetic predisposition may play a role in the development of Type 2 diabetes. People with Type 2 diabetes have a stronger family history of diabetes than those with Type 1. There is no association with HLA types, however, and circulating ICAs are absent.[7,12] People with Type 2 diabetes also exhibit varying degrees of tissue resistance to insulin, impaired insulin secretion, and increased basal hepatic glucose production. Finally, environmental factors such as obesity and a sedentary lifestyle also contribute to the development of insulin resistance.

Despite being the most common form of diabetes, the exact pathogenesis of Type 2 is less well understood. Basal insulin levels are typically normal or elevated at diagnosis. First- or early-phase insulin release in response to glucose often is reduced, and pulsatile insulin secretion is absent, resulting in postprandial hyperglycemia. The effects of other insulinotropic substances such as incretin hormones, which contribute to meal-stimulated insulin release, are also altered.[13] With time, β-cells lose their ability to respond to elevated glucose concentrations, leading to increasing loss of glucose control. In patients with severe hyperglycemia, the amount of insulin secreted in response to glucose is diminished and insulin resistance is worsened (glucose toxicity).

Most individuals with Type 2 exhibit decreased tissue responsiveness to insulin.[12] Excess weight or hyperglycemia may contribute to hyperinsulinemia, which in time may lead to a decrease in or downregulation of the number of insulin receptors on the surface of target tissues and organs. Evidence suggests that decreased peripheral glucose uptake and utilization in muscle is the primary site of insulin resistance and results in prolonged postprandial hyperglycemia. Resistance may be secondary to decreased numbers of insulin receptors on the cell surface, decreased affinity of receptors for insulin, or defects in insulin signaling and action that follows receptor binding. Defects in insulin signaling and action are referred to as postreceptor or postbinding defects and are likely to be the primary sites of insulin resistance.

Patients with Type 2 diabetes also exhibit increased hepatic glucose production (glycogenolysis and gluconeogenesis) reflected by an elevated fasting plasma or BG concentration.[12] As noted, hepatic glucose production is the primary source of glucose in the fasting state. In patients with Type 2 diabetes, altered hepatic glucose production may also contribute to or cause postprandial hyperglycemia. Glucagon, produced by the α-cells in the pancreatic islets and secreted in response to low BG, stimulates hepatic glucose production.[14] Its production is inhibited by insulin. Glucagon response to carbohydrate ingestion is altered in patients with Type 2 diabetes who have a defective or absent early insulin response secondary to β-cell dysfunction or failure. For patients with Type 2 diabetes, untreated fasting and postprandial hyperglycemia caused by decreased glucose uptake and increased hepatic glucose production, hyperinsulinemia, and insulin resistance lead to a vicious cycle that inflicts ongoing damage to tissues and organs.

Patients with Type 2 diabetes are often subclassified based on weight. Obese individuals account for more than 80% of patients with Type 2 diabetes.[12] Patients with Type 2 diabetes who are not obese often have increased body fat distributed in the abdominal area. Nonobese individuals account for about 10% of the Type 2 population. Typically, they develop a mild form of diabetes during childhood, adolescence, or as young adults (usually before age 25), and their insulin levels are low in response to a glucose challenge. Included in this group are patients who have maturity-onset diabetes of the young (MODY).[7,12] MODY is associated with a strong family history that suggests an autosomal-dominant transmission. The underlying defect is heterogeneous, and multiple abnormalities at loci on different chromosomes have been discovered. More common defects include those for hepatic transcription factors and glucokinase (the "glucose sensor" in β-cells). Patients with MODY may present with moderate-to-severe symptoms with or without ketosis. Unlike Type 1 diabetes, however, the disease generally is mild and controlled with diet, oral agents, or low doses of insulin. With the increasing prevalence of obesity and Type 2 diabetes in children and adolescents, it is important to distinguish between a youth with Type 2 diabetes and one who really has autoimmune Type 1 diabetes and is also obese.[15]

Type 2 diabetes is associated with a variety of disorders, including dyslipidemia, hypertension, and premature atherosclerosis (Fig. 53-2). Currently termed the metabolic syndrome, this triad of clinical findings (hypertension, elevated fasting glucose, and dyslipidemia) is proposed to derive from insulin resistance itself and the resulting compensatory hyperinsulinemia.[16] The labeling of this triad as a separate "syndrome" remains the subject of considerable debate, partly because it appears to have little diagnostic utility beyond its component parts.[17] Metabolic syndrome is common in the United States, with an estimated prevalence of more than 34% in adults aged 20 and older, peaking among those 60 to 69 years of age.[18] Because it is highly correlated with cardiovascular events, the National Cholesterol Education Program has suggested criteria for the diagnosis of metabolic syndrome.[19]

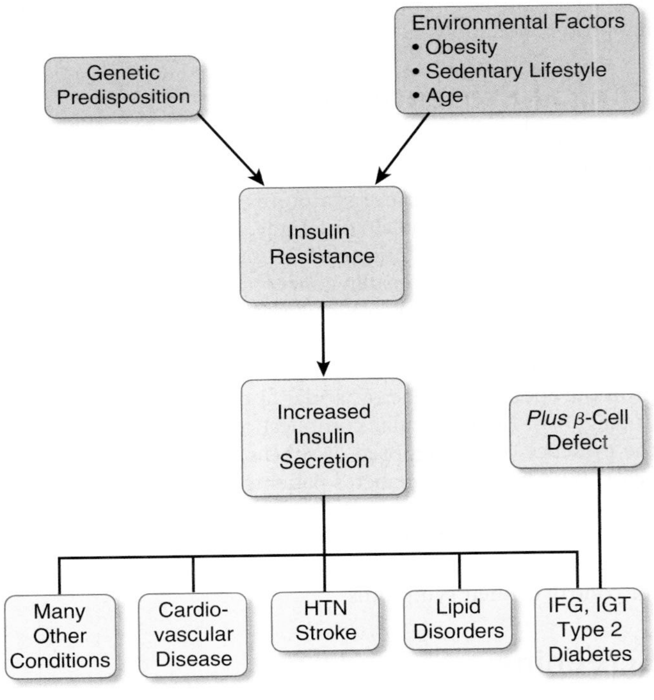

Figure 53-2 Metabolic syndrome. Genetic and environmental factors (visceral obesity, sedentary lifestyle, aging) predispose some individuals to insulin resistance. To overcome the resistance, the pancreas secretes more insulin, leading to hyperinsulinemia. People with insulin resistance and hyperinsulinemia commonly develop a cluster of medical problems and biochemical abnormalities: cardiovascular disease, hypertension, dyslipidemia, hyperuricemia, and type 2 diabetes mellitus. Only those individuals who are further genetically predisposed to β-cell failure go on to develop IGT, IFG, and type 2 diabetes. Many people with type 2 diabetes already have evidence of cardiovascular disease at the time of diabetes diagnosis. The cause-and-effect relationship between insulin resistance or hyperinsulinemia and these clinical conditions has not been clarified. See text for expanded discussion. DM, diabetes mellitus; HTN, hypertension.

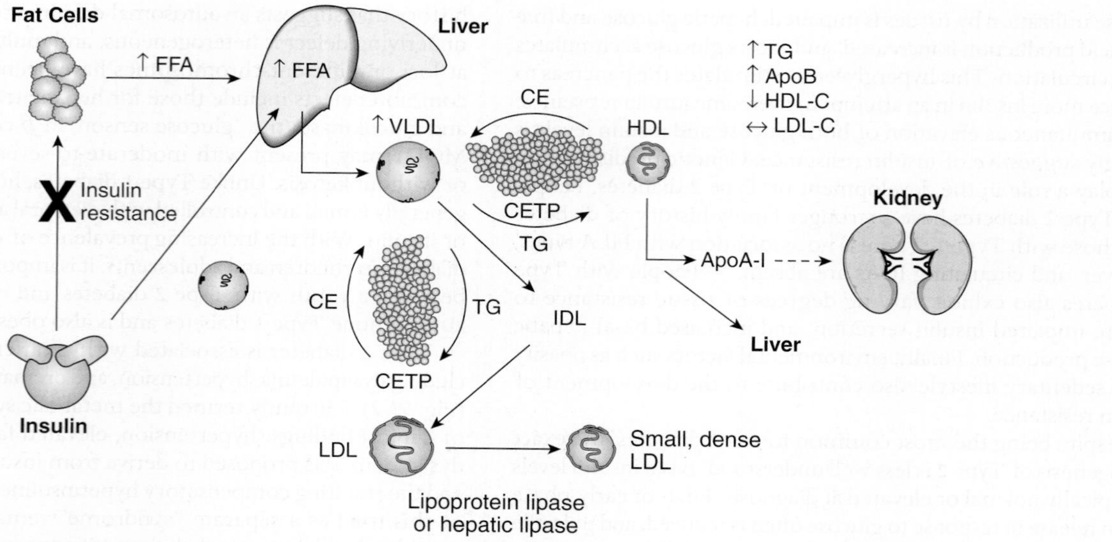

Figure 53-3 Changes in lipoprotein metabolism are a direct consequence of insulin resistance and are present before the onset of overt diabetes.

Not all individuals with the metabolic syndrome progress to IGT or diabetes, but those who do may be genetically predisposed to β-cell dysfunction. Figure 53-3 depicts the typical dyslipidemia pattern seen in diabetes and how insulin resistance affects normal lipoprotein metabolism.

Clinical Presentation

Type 2 diabetes is typically diagnosed incidentally during a routine physical examination or when the patient seeks attention for another complaint. Because symptoms are mild in their onset, patients will rarely complain of fatigue, polyuria, and polydipsia but may admit to them during clinical examination. Because these patients have sufficient insulin concentrations to prevent lipolysis, there is usually no history of ketosis except in situations of unusual stress (e.g., infections, trauma). Weight loss is therefore uncommon because relatively high endogenous insulin levels promote lipogenesis. Macrovascular disease is also often evident at diagnosis. Microvascular complications at diagnosis suggest the presence of undiagnosed or subclinical diabetes for 7 to 10 years. Because Type 2 diabetes patients retain some pancreatic reserve at the time of diagnosis, they generally can be treated with MNT, physical activity, and noninsulin antidiabetic medications for several years. Nevertheless, many eventually require insulin for control of their symptoms.

Screening

The ADA advises that adults without risk factors should be screened starting at age 45.[7] Repeat testing should take place every 3 years if results are normal or yearly if they have prediabetes. Adults may be tested at a younger age and more frequently if they are overweight (body mass index [BMI] ≥25 or 35 kg/m^2 in Asian-Americans) and have one or more of the risk factors listed in Table 53-2. A FPG or A1C is preferred over the OGTT to test for diabetes, because they are much less cumbersome. Asymptomatic children who are age 10 or who experience the onset of puberty before age 10 should be screened every 2 years for Type 2 diabetes if they are overweight (BMI >85th percentile for age and sex; weight for height >85th percentile; or weight >120% of ideal for height) and have two or more of the risk factors listed in Table 53-2.[7]

GESTATIONAL DIABETES MELLITUS

GDM affects about 7% of all pregnancies and is defined as "any carbohydrate intolerance with onset or first recognition during pregnancy."[7,20] The onset of diabetes during pregnancy and its duration affect the prognosis for a good obstetric and perinatal outcome (see Chapter 49, Obstetric Drug Therapy).

Diagnostic Criteria

The categories for normal, increased risk for diabetes, and diabetes for FPG, A1C, and the OGTT are listed in Table 53-3.[7] The Expert Committee of the ADA has established the diagnostic criteria for diabetes for nonpregnant individuals of any age. For these individuals, a diagnosis of diabetes can be made when one of the following is present[7]:

1. An A1C of 6.5% or more. The test must be performed in a laboratory (not with a point-of-care test). It should be performed using a method certified by the National Glycohemoglobin Standardization Program.
2. An FPG of 126 mg/dL or more. *Fasting* means no caloric intake for at least 8 hours.
3. Classic signs and symptoms of diabetes (polyuria, polydipsia, ketonuria, and unexplained weight loss) combined with a random plasma glucose of 200 mg/dL or more.
4. After a standard OGTT (75 g of glucose for an adult or 1.75 g/kg for a child), the venous plasma glucose concentration is 200 mg/dL or more at 2 hours.

The diagnosis must be confirmed by repeating the test, preferably the same test. If two different tests are performed (e.g., FPG and A1C), and both are above the diagnostic threshold, then diabetes is confirmed. If only one test's value is above the diagnostic cut point, the test that is above the diagnostic cut point should be repeated. The diagnosis is made based on the results of the confirmed test.[7]

At times, it may be difficult to classify patients as having Type 1 or Type 2 diabetes mellitus. Type 1 is more likely when a patient is younger than 30 years of age and lean, and has an elevated FPG and signs and symptoms of diabetes. The presence of moderate

Table 53-2

Risk Factors for Type 2 Diabetes Mellitus[7]

Adults	Children[a]
Overweight (≥25 kg/m²) or (≥23 kg/m²) in Asian-Americans	Overweight (BMI >85th percentile for age and sex; or weight >120% of ideal for height)
Family history of diabetes (first-degree relative)	Family history of diabetes (first- or second-degree relative)
Physical inactivity	
Ethnic predisposition[b]	Ethnic predisposition[b]
Previous IFG, IGT, or A1C ≥5.7%	
History of PCOS, GDM, or macrosomia	Maternal history of diabetes (including GDM)
Clinical conditions associated with insulin resistance (e.g., severe obesity and acanthosis nigricans)	Signs of insulin resistance (e.g., acanthosis nigricans)
Hypertension (≥140/90 mm Hg or on antihypertensive therapy)	Conditions associated with insulin resistance (e.g., hypertension, dyslipidemia, or PCOS)
Dyslipidemia	
HDL-C <35 mg/dL (0.90 mmol/L)	
Triglyceride >250 mg/dL (2.82 mmol/L)	
Cardiovascular disease	

[a]Children are younger than 18 years of age.
[b]Ethnic predisposition includes individuals of African-American, Latino, Native American, Asian, or Pacific Islander descent.
A1C, glycosylated hemoglobin; BMI, body mass index; GDM, gestational diabetes mellitus; HDL-C, high-density lipoprotein cholesterol; IFG, impaired fasting glucose; IGT, impaired glucose tolerance; PCOS, polycystic ovarian syndrome.

Table 53-3

Normal and Diabetic Plasma Glucose Levels in mg/dL (mmol/L) and Glycosylated Hemoglobin (A1C) and Normal and Diabetic Plasma Glucose Levels for the Oral Glucose Tolerance Test (OGTT)[7]

	FPG	A1C	OGTT
Normal	<100 (5.6)	≤5.6%	<140 (7.8)
Prediabetes (i.e., impaired fasting glucose (IFG), impaired glucose tolerance (IGT))	100–125 (5.6–6.9)	≥5.7–6.4%	140–199 (7.8–11.0)
Diabetes (nonpregnant adult)	≥126 (7.0)	≥6.5%	≥200 (11.1)

Equivalent venous whole-blood glucose concentrations are approximately 12%–15% lower. Arterial samples are higher than venous samples postprandially because glucose has not yet been removed from peripheral tissues. Capillary whole-blood samples contain a mixture of arterial and venous blood. Fasting levels are equivalent to whole-blood venous samples.
A1C, glycosylated hemoglobin; FPG, fasting plasma glucose; OGTT, oral glucose tolerance test.

ketonuria with hyperglycemia in an otherwise unstressed patient also strongly supports a diagnosis of Type 1 diabetes. Absence of ketonuria, however, is not of diagnostic value. The presence of autoantibodies to insulin or islet cell components may also indicate the need for eventual insulin therapy.[11] Relatively, lean older adults believed to have Type 2 diabetes because they are initially responsive to oral agents or low doses of insulin may be subsequently diagnosed with Type 1 diabetes. In addition, clinicians are beginning to observe more cases of Type 2 diabetes in obese children and adolescents.[21]

Individuals with A1C, FPG, or OGTT values that are intermediate between normal and those considered diagnostic of diabetes are considered to have prediabetes. The terms IFG and IGT should not be used interchangeably because each results from somewhat different physiologic processes. It is important to interpret the categories listed in Table 53-3 as a continuum of increased risk for diabetes, rather than focus on the absolute cutoff points for prediabetes or diabetes.

Many factors can impair glucose tolerance or increase plasma glucose. These must be excluded before a definitive diagnosis is made. For example, an individual who has not fasted for a minimum of 8 hours may have an elevated FPG. Patients who are tested for glucose tolerance during, or very soon after, an acute illness (e.g., a myocardial infarction [MI]) or who are on corticosteroids (e.g., prednisone, dexamethasone) may be misdiagnosed because of the presence of high concentrations of counter-regulatory hormones that increase glucose concentrations. Glucose tolerance often returns to normal in these individuals.

LONG-TERM COMPLICATIONS

Although acute hyperglycemic crises can occur in patients with diabetes, the long-term sequelae of diabetes account for most of the morbidity and mortality in the diabetic population. Complications are typically designated as microvascular or macrovascular in nature. Glucose toxicity contributes most to the development and progression of microvascular complications (retinopathy, nephropathy, and neuropathy) owing to the particular susceptibility of these cell systems to elevated glucose.[22] Diabetes is the leading cause of new cases of adult blindness and kidney failure in the United States.[1] About 60% to 70% of people with diabetes also have some manifestation of peripheral or autonomic neuropathy. Severe peripheral neuropathy coupled with abnormalities in immune function likely contributes to the high rate of lower-extremity amputations among patients with diabetes.[1,23] Finally, poor glucose control promotes development of dental and oral complications and increases the risk of complications during pregnancy for both mother and fetus.[24,25] Macrovascular complications are multifactorial in their etiology and less dependent on hyperglycemia. Diabetes mellitus itself is a well-known risk factor for macrovascular disease (peripheral vascular disease, CVD, stroke). Patients with diabetes have a threefold-to-fourfold elevated risk for MI and cardiovascular death compared with nondiabetic subjects.[26] Insulin resistance and the resultant hyperinsulinemia in Type 2 diabetes mellitus contribute to the development of hypertension, dyslipidemia, and platelet hypersensitivity, all of which then contribute to the increased CVD risk in patients with diabetes.[27] Thus, although tight glycemic control (A1C <7.0%) will dramatically reduce the risk for microvascular disease, its relationship to macrovascular disease is still under intense debate.

RELATIONSHIP OF GLYCEMIC CONTROL TO MICROVASCULAR AND MACROVASCULAR DISEASE

Although epidemiologic studies have shown a general relationship between glucose control and cardiovascular events, recent randomized trials have failed to confirm a benefit of tight glucose control compared with standard control, which highlights the multifactorial nature of macrovascular disease.[28] However, the clear relationship between microvascular events and glycemic control is well established from randomized, clinical trials. The Diabetes Control and Complications Trial (DCCT), and the open-label follow-up trial, DCCT-EDIC (Epidemiology of Diabetes Interventions and Complications), established the benefits of intensive glycemic control on microvascular end points.[29,30] In the DCCT, intensive treatment (A1C 7.1% vs. 9.0%) reduced the risk of clinically meaningful retinopathy, nephropathy, and neuropathy by approximately 60%. The EDIC study was followed as an open-label extension of the DCCT cohorts. Patients originally assigned to the intensive treatment group were shown to have a persistently lower incidence of microvascular complications even after the glucose control reached parity between the two study groups after the end of the randomized portion of the trial.[30,31] The EDIC study also showed a significant reduction in cardiovascular complications among patients previously assigned to the intensive therapy DCCT arm.[32] See Table 53-4 for the glycemic goals of intensive insulin therapy (herein called physiologic or basal-bolus therapy). This persistence of the microvascular benefits of glycemic control has also been demonstrated in patients with Type 2 diabetes in the United Kingdom Prospective Diabetes Study (UKPDS) (see Case 53-11, Question 2).[33]

The relationship between glycemic control and macrovascular disease has always been less clear. Evidence of early atherosclerosis in patients with Type 1 diabetes in whom dyslipidemia and hypertension are typically absent argues strongly for a role of hyperglycemia itself in the development or progression of macrovascular disease.[34] The UKPDS trial was the first to report the benefit of tight BG control on cardiovascular complications in Type 2 diabetes.[35] Although the microvascular benefits were clear, the 21% relative risk reduction for fatal and nonfatal MI and sudden cardiac death failed to reach statistical significance ($p = 0.052$). However, in a planned 10-year follow-up of patients enrolled in the trial, a significant 15% reduction was seen in the risk of MI ($p = 0.01$).[33] A similar finding for macrovascular benefit was reported in a 17-year follow-up of the DCCT-EDIC study.[32] Thus, although glycemic control benefited macrovascular disease, it took more than a decade to see the benefit. Reducing macrovascular risk in patients with diabetes thus takes a more comprehensive approach than just glycemic control. In a trial of multiple risk factor control in Type 2 diabetes, the STENO-2 trial found a significant 53% reduction in macrovascular events with modest control of hypertension, dyslipidemia, and glycemia simultaneously.[36] Control of all major

Table 53-4
Goals of Physiologic (Basal-Bolus) Insulin Therapy

Monitoring Parameter	Adults (mg/dL)	School Age (6–12 years) (mg/dL)	Adolescents and Young Adults (13–29 years) (mg/dL)	Pregnancy (mg/dL)
Premeals	80–130	90–130	90–130	60–99
2-hour postprandial plasma glucose	<180	Not routinely recommended	Not routinely recommended	100–129
Bedtime/overnight (2–4 AM) plasma glucose	>70	90–150	90–150	60–99
A1C[a]	<7.0%[b]	<7.5%[c]	<7.5%[c]	<6%
Urine ketones[d]	Absent to rare	Absent to rare	Absent to rare	Rare

See Case 53-2, Question 2, and Case 53-4, Question 2, for discussion. Basal-bolus insulin therapy is a complete therapeutic program of diabetes management and requires a team approach.
[a]A1C, glycosylated hemoglobin, referenced to a nondiabetic range of 4% to 6% using a Diabetes Control and Complications Trial (DCCT)-based assay.
[b]Acceptable values should be individualized to levels that are attainable without creating undue risk for hypoglycemia. These results are similar to the results achieved in the DCCT trial. The American Diabetes Association recommends consideration for a lower goal (e.g., <6%) in individuals with a short duration of diabetes, long life expectancy, and no significant cardiovascular disease. Less stringent goals may be appropriate for patients with hypoglycemic unawareness, history of severe hypoglycemia, counter-regulatory insufficiency, advanced microvascular or macrovascular complications, or other complicating features (Table 53-10).
[c]A lower goal (<7%) is reasonable if it can be achieved without creating excessive risk for hypoglycemia.
[d]Does not apply to type 2 diabetes patients.
Modified and extrapolated from American Diabetes Association. Standards of medical care in diabetes—2015. *Diabetes Care*. 2015;38(Suppl 1):S5; American Diabetes Association. Preconception care of women with diabetes. *Diabetes Care*. 2004;27(Suppl 1):S76; Kitzmiller JL et al. Managing preexisting diabetes for pregnancy: summary of evidence and consensus recommendations for care. *Diabetes Care*. 2008;31:1060; The Diabetes Control and Complications Trial Research Group. The effect of intensive treatment of diabetes on the development and progression of long-term complications in insulin-dependent diabetes mellitus. *N Engl J Med*. 1993;329:977.

CVD risk factors is highlighted by the ADA for its importance in reducing macrovascular disease risk.[37] See Table 53-5 for the metabolic goals for adults with diabetes.[38,39]

Three trials published in 2008 and 2009 have raised new questions about tight glycemic control in patients with Type 2 diabetes. In the Action to Control Cardiovascular Risk in Diabetes (ACCORD) trial, a higher rate of mortality was seen in the intensive treatment arm, which achieved an A1C of 6.4% compared with the standard arm, which achieved 7.5%.[40] The ACCORD study was a National Heart, Lung, and Blood Institute study of more than 10,000 patients with Type 2 diabetes with known heart disease or multiple cardiovascular risk factors. The intensively treated group had an excess of 3 deaths per 1,000 participants per year compared with the standard group during an average of 4 years on treatment (257 vs. 203 deaths). The higher mortality rate was not attributable to a specific drug therapy or to severe hypoglycemia.[41] A second trial, the Action in Diabetes and Vascular Disease a Controlled Evaluation (ADVANCE), was an even larger study of more than 11,000 patients, which had different findings from ACCORD. In ADVANCE, there was an insignificant trend for reduced cardiovascular mortality and reduced overall mortality with tight glycemic control (A1C of 6.3% compared with 7.0%).[42] Lastly, in the smaller Veterans Affairs Diabetes Trial (VADT), nearly 2,000 patients were studied and found to have an insignificant 12% relative risk reduction in macrovascular end points but a 7% relative increase in overall mortality (95 vs. 102 deaths). Neither finding was statistically significant.[43] After approximately 10-year follow-up to the VADT trial, the study found 1 fewer cardiovascular event/116 person-years without a reduction in mortality. The intensive arm of this study had a mean A1C of 6.9%, not <6.5%.[44]

In the face of these new data, the ADA, along with the American Heart Association (AHA) and the American College of Cardiology (ACC), issued a position statement in 2009.[45] Although acknowledging the findings of the ACCORD trial, the persistent trend for reductions in macrovascular events in all three trials was found to be reassuring. The position of the committee (which continues to be the official position of the ADA in the 2015 guidelines) is that although intensive glycemic control did not improve macrovascular outcomes, a goal of less than 7% is still reasonable based on microvascular benefits and a clear lack of harm across the trials of intensive versus standard glycemic control.[38] However, the ADA does acknowledge that there is room to individualize the A1C goal and that achieving an A1C of less than 7% has limited macrovascular benefit compared with A1C values of 7% to 8%. Patients with Type 2 diabetes and CVD or multiple risk factors for CVD should discuss their treatment goals with their providers. In these patients, a less intensive goal may be appropriate, particularly for patients who have difficulty achieving the goal of less than 7%.[38]

Table 53-5
American Diabetes Association Metabolic Goals for Adults with Diabetes Mellitus[7]

Glycemic goals	
A1C	<7.0% (normal, 4%–6%)[a]
Preprandial plasma glucose	80–130 mg/dL (3.9–7.2 mmol/L)[b]
Postprandial plasma glucose	<180 mg/dL (<10.0 mmol/L)[c]
Blood pressure	<140/90 mm Hg (Refer to Essential Hypertension Chapter 11)
Lipids	Refer to Lipid Chapter 8

Goals must be individualized to the patient. See Case 53-2, Question 2, Case 53-14, Question 2, and Case 53-24, Questions 1–4, for broader discussion.[7]
[a]More stringent goals (i.e., <6%) can be considered for select individuals. American Association of Clinical Endocrinologists/American College of Endocrinology recommends A1C goal of ≤6.5%.[39]
[b]American Association of Clinical Endocrinologists recommends a fasting blood glucose goal of <110 mg/dL (6.1 mmol/L).[39]
[c]American Association of Clinical Endocrinologists/American College of Endocrinology recommends goal of <140 mg/L (7.8 mmol/L).[39]
A1C, glycosylated hemoglobin.

PREVENTION OF TYPE 1 AND TYPE 2 DIABETES MELLITUS

Because the clinical symptoms of Type 1 diabetes mellitus are the overt expression of an insidious pathogenic process that begins years earlier, investigators are focusing attention on strategies that alter the natural history of the disease (Fig. 53-1). First-degree relatives of individuals with Type 1 diabetes mellitus have an increased risk for developing the diabetes and can be identified by the presence of immune markers that may herald the disease by many years.[11] This has led to attempts at immune intervention at the prediabetes stage (primary prevention) or after the development of islet antibodies (secondary prevention). Most immunotherapy trials are tertiary prevention after diagnosis of Type 1 diabetes. Results have not been extraordinary, but will areas of future study. For primary prevention, vaccines, and secondary prevention, immunomodulatory agents will continue to be an area of research.[46] The Diabetes Prevention Program Research Group studied a diverse group of 3,234 individuals at high risk for developing diabetes to determine whether lifestyle interventions or metformin (850 mg by mouth [PO] twice a day [BID]) would prevent or delay the onset of Type 2 diabetes.[47] After 3 years, the incidence of diabetes was reduced by 58% and 31% in the intensive lifestyle and metformin groups, respectively, compared with the control group. Diabetes incidence during 10 years of follow-up was persistently lower in the groups originally treated with lifestyle (34% reduction) and metformin (18% reduction) interventions compared with the control group.[48] Other studies have confirmed the value of lifestyle intervention and other drugs (acarbose, orlistat, and various thiazolidinediones (TZDs)) in the prevention of Type 2 diabetes, but the strongest evidence is with metformin.[49] Lifelong medication therapy, however, is not without its own risks and complications. Current recommendations regarding the treatment for individuals with prediabetes include lifestyle modification (5%–10% weight loss and 150 minutes/week of moderately intense physical activity).[50] Metformin, although less effective than lifestyle changes, can be considered for very high-risk individuals.[49]

CASE 53-1

QUESTION 1: R.P. is a 43-year-old African-American woman visiting a primary-care clinic to obtain a routine physical examination for her new job. Her past medical history is significant for GDM. She was told during her two pregnancies (last child born 3 years ago) that she had "borderline diabetes," which resolved each time after giving birth. Her family history is significant for Type 2 diabetes (mother, maternal grandmother, older first cousin), hypertension, and CVD. She denies tobacco or alcohol use. She states that she tries to walk 15 minutes twice a week. Physical examination is significant for moderate central obesity (5 feet 4 inches; 160 pounds; BMI, 30.2 kg/m^2) and blood pressure (BP) 145/85 mm Hg. R.P. denies any symptoms of polyphagia, polyuria, or lethargy. On checking her electronic medical record, she has documented hypertension and an FPG value of 119 mg/dL, measured 2 months prior. What features of R.P.'s history and examination are consistent with an increased risk of developing Type 2 diabetes?

The features of R.P.'s history that are consistent with an increased risk of developing Type 2 diabetes include her age, ethnicity, weight, family history of diabetes, history of GDM, and a documented IFG. In addition, Type 2 diabetes is also often associated with other disorders such as hypertension. The fact that R.P. has hypertension that is not well controlled and has a family history of hypertension and CVD may indicate that she is predisposed to insulin resistance, further putting her at risk for developing Type 2 diabetes.

CASE 53-1, QUESTION 2: The physician orders an A1C for R.P., which comes back at 6.1%. How should R.P. be managed at this time?

Both the A1C and FPG values are in the prediabetes range. R.P. should be educated about her risk for developing Type 2 diabetes. Working with her healthcare providers, R.P. should be encouraged and educated on how to institute lifestyle modifications (MNT, physical activity) that will help her to lose weight, improve her cardiovascular health, and decrease her risk for developing Type 2 diabetes. A weight-loss goal of 5% to 10% during the next 6 to 12 months should be recommended, and she should increase her level of moderate physical activity to at least 150 minutes/week. Her hypertension should be managed. At this time, the use of pharmacologic agents (i.e., metformin) to prevent the development of Type 2 diabetes is not recommended.

TREATMENT

There are three major components to the treatment of diabetes: diet, drugs (insulin and antidiabetic agents [oral and injectable]), and exercise. Each of these components interacts with the others to the extent that no assessment and modification of one can be made without knowledge of the other two.

Medical Nutrition Therapy

PRINCIPLES

MNT plays a crucial role in the therapy of all individuals with diabetes.[50,51] Unfortunately, patient acceptance and adherence to diet and meal planning are often poor, but revised evidence-based recommendations that are more flexible than previous approaches offer new opportunities to increase the effectiveness of nutrition therapy.

Nutrition therapy is designed to help patients achieve appropriate metabolic and physiologic goals (e.g., glucose, lipids, BP, proteinuria, weight), select healthy foods, and take into consideration personal and cultural preferences. Appropriate levels and types of physical activity to achieve a healthier status are incorporated into the nutrition plan.

NUTRITION THERAPY AND TYPE 1 DIABETES MELLITUS

For patients with Type 1 diabetes taking fixed doses of insulin, a meal plan is designed to provide adequate carbohydrates timed to match the peak action of exogenously administered mealtime insulin. Regularly scheduled meals and snacks should contain consistent carbohydrate amounts, which are required to prevent hypoglycemic reactions. Fortunately, newer insulins and insulin regimens provide much more flexibility in the amount and timing of food intake. Patients who are taught to count carbohydrates can inject rapid- or short-acting insulin doses designed to match their anticipated intake. Integration of food intake, physical activity, and insulin dose is critical and discussed extensively in the cases that follow.

NUTRITION THERAPY AND TYPE 2 DIABETES MELLITUS

For patients with Type 2 diabetes, meal plans emphasize normalizing plasma glucose and lipid levels as well as maintaining a normal BP to prevent or mitigate cardiovascular morbidity. Although weight loss reduces insulin resistance and improves glycemic control, traditional dietary strategies incorporating hypocaloric diets have not been effective in achieving long-term weight loss. A sustainable weight loss can be achieved within structured programs that emphasize lifestyle changes, physical activity, and food intake that modestly reduces caloric and fat intake.[50,51]

SPECIFIC NUTRITION COMPONENTS

MNT is an integral and critical component of diabetes care. For a more extensive discussion of the principles underlying nutrition therapy, the reader is directed to other sources.[51–53] A few key principles are briefly noted below because they are common sources of misunderstanding.

Carbohydrates and Artificial Sweeteners

Carbohydrates include sugar (sucrose), starch, and fiber and are liberally incorporated into the diet of a person with diabetes. In fact, the amount of dietary carbohydrate is the main determinant of insulin demand and is commonly used to determine the premeal insulin dose. Furthermore, patients using fixed doses of insulin or antihyperglycemic medications (e.g., sulfonylureas) must eat meals containing consistent amounts of carbohydrate to avoid hypoglycemia. Because isocaloric amounts of sucrose and starch produce the same degree of glycemia, sucrose can be substituted for a portion of the total carbohydrate intake and should be incorporated into an otherwise healthful diet.

Whole grains, fruits, and vegetables high in fiber are recommended for people with diabetes, because they are for the general population. There is no evidence that larger amounts produce a differential metabolic benefit with regard to plasma glucose and lipid levels. Nonnutritive sweeteners (saccharin, aspartame, neotame, acesulfame potassium, sucralose) and sugar alcohols have been rigorously tested by the US Food and Drug Administration (FDA) for safety in people with diabetes and are safe at approved daily intakes. Fructose and the reduced-calorie sweeteners called sugar alcohols produce lower postprandial glucose responses than sucrose, glucose, and starch. When sugar alcohols (e.g., sorbitol, mannitol, lactitol, xylitol, and maltitol) are consumed, it is recommended to subtract half of their grams from the total carbohydrate amount because their effect on BG is less. Patients should be advised that when these sweeteners are used in foods labeled "dietetic" or "sugar free," they still add to the carbohydrate content and provide substantial calories (2 cal/g). Furthermore, excessive intake of sorbitol-sweetened foods (e.g., 30–50 g/day) can induce an osmotic diarrhea, and excessive amounts of fructose can increase total and LDL cholesterol (LDL-C).

Counting Carbohydrates

When patients are taught to estimate the grams of carbohydrate in a meal, they are given the following guideline: One carbohydrate serving = 1 starch or 1 fruit or 1 cup milk = 15 g carbohydrate. Patients vary with regard to their insulin-to-carbohydrate ratio throughout time and throughout the day; however, a typical starting point is 1 unit/15 g carbohydrate.

Fat

CVD is a major cause of morbidity and mortality in patients with diabetes. Therefore, saturated fats should be limited to less than 7% of calories. The intake of *trans* fat should also be minimized. The recommended cholesterol intake is less than 200 mg/day for patients with diabetes. Two or more servings/week of fish to provide *n*-3 polyunsaturated fatty acids and omega-3 fatty acids are advised.[50,51]

Protein

Data are insufficient to support special dietary protein recommendations for persons with diabetes if kidney function is normal. Generally, 15% to 20% of the daily caloric intake comes from animal and vegetable protein sources in the US diet. This amount may be liberalized in pregnant and lactating women or in elderly people. With the onset of nephropathy, a lower protein intake of 0.8 to 1.0 g/kg/day is considered sufficiently restrictive. For patients in later stages of nephropathy, reduction of protein intake to 0.8 g/kg/day is recommended. High-protein diets are not recommended as a long-term method for weight loss, because the effects on kidney function are not known.[50,51]

Sodium

The ADA recommends a reduced sodium intake of less than 2,300 mg/day in normotensive and hypertensive individuals. For patients with diabetes and symptomatic heart failure (HF), sodium should be further restricted to less than 2,000 mg/day to help reduce symptoms. For all other patients, the ADA has no particular restrictions on sodium intake, but recommends individualizing amounts based on the patient's sensitivity to salt and concurrent conditions such as hypertension or nephropathy.[50,51]

Alcohol

The ADA's recommendation for alcohol is consistent with general recommendations of no more than two alcoholic drinks/day for men or one drink/day for women. A drink is equivalent to 12 ounces of beer, 5 ounces of wine, or 1.5 ounces of distilled spirits (each contains about 15 g of carbohydrate). Nevertheless, its caloric contribution must be considered (1 alcoholic beverage = 2 fat exchanges), and it should always be taken with food to minimize its hypoglycemic effect. In people with diabetes, light-to-moderate alcohol intake (one to two drinks/day) is associated with a decreased risk of CVD. A note of caution: Evening consumption of alcohol may increase the risk of nocturnal and fasting hypoglycemia, particularly in people with Type 1 diabetes.[51]

PHYSICAL ACTIVITY

Physical activity is a key factor in the treatment of diabetes, particularly in Type 2 diabetes, because obesity and inactivity contribute to the development of glucose intolerance in genetically predisposed individuals. Regular exercise reduces cholesterol levels, raises HDL-C, lowers BP, augments weight-reduction diets, reduces the dose requirements or need for insulin or antihyperglycemic agents, enhances insulin sensitivity, and improves psychological well-being by reducing stress. Exercise increases glucose utilization, which is provided initially from the breakdown of muscle glycogen and, subsequently, from hepatic glycogenolysis and gluconeogenesis. These effects are mediated through norepinephrine, epinephrine, growth hormone, cortisol, and glucagon, along with the suppression of insulin secretion. In patients using insulin, hyperglycemia, normoglycemia, or hypoglycemia can occur secondary to exercise depending on the degree of control, recent administration of rapid-acting insulin, and food intake. Exercise in patients taking insulin must be tempered by increased food intake, potential delay in insulin administration, decreased doses of insulin, or a combination of these actions to minimize hypoglycemia.[50,51,54,55]

In patients with Type 2 diabetes, plasma glucose concentrations usually decrease in response to exercise, but symptomatic hypoglycemia is uncommon. The vascular benefits of exercise are particularly helpful in patients with diabetes given their predisposition to CVD. In general, exercise that produces moderate exertion (increase in heart rate of 20%–40% from resting baseline) is recommended with a starting goal of 150 minutes/week. The eventual goal is for patients to be able to achieve 50% to 70% of their age-adjusted maximal heart rate.[50]

Resistance exercise has been shown to improve insulin sensitivity. Therefore, in the absence of any contraindications, people with Type 2 diabetes are encouraged to perform resistance training 3 times/week. Patients with conditions that may preclude certain types of physical activity (e.g., coronary artery disease, uncontrolled hypertension, severe autonomic neuropathy, severe peripheral neuropathy or history of foot lesions, and advanced retinopathy in which retinal detachment may occur) should be carefully evaluated before starting an exercise regimen.

Pharmacologic Treatment

Insulin, along with diet, is crucial to the survival of individuals with Type 1 diabetes and plays a major role in the therapy of people with Type 2 diabetes when their symptoms cannot be controlled with diet or noninsulin antidiabetic agents. Insulin also is used for people with Type 2 diabetes during periods of intercurrent illness or stress (e.g., surgery, pregnancy). The use of antidiabetic agents is primarily reserved for the treatment of patients with Type 2 diabetes whose symptoms cannot be controlled with diet and exercise alone. The clinical use of these agents and the complications associated with their use are discussed later in this chapter.

Overall Goals of Therapy

The overall goal of diabetes management is to prevent acute and chronic complications. Periodic assessments of A1C coupled with regular measurement of fasting, preprandial, and postprandial glucose levels should be used to assess therapy. The following overall goals of therapy are agreed on by most endocrinologists:

1. Landmark randomized, prospective trials of various interventional therapies in patients with both Type 1 and Type 2 diabetes have clearly demonstrated that reductions in hyperglycemia significantly decrease microvascular complications. In both the UKPDS and the DCCT follow-up studies, significant reductions in macrovascular complications were also observed. Target BG goals may need to be adjusted for patients with frequent, severe hypoglycemia or hypoglycemia unawareness (see Case 53-8, Questions 1–3, and Case 53-9), or with CVD. In addition, established renal insufficiency, proliferative retinopathy, severe neuropathy, and other advanced complications are not likely to be improved by tight glucose control. See Table 53-5 for the ADA glycemic goals.[38] The American Association of Clinical Endocrinologists and the American College of Endocrinology established glycemic goals as well (Table 53-5).[39] The ADA guidelines will be discussed throughout this chapter.
2. Try to keep patients free of symptoms associated with hyperglycemia (polyuria, polydipsia, weight loss, fatigue, recurrent infection, ketoacidosis) or hypoglycemia (hunger, anxiety, palpitations, sweatiness).
3. Maintain normal growth and development in children. Intensive therapy is not recommended across any age group with a goal A1C of <7.5%. Goals can be individualized, targeting <7% if can be done so safely with minimum hypoglycemia (see Case 53-4, Questions 2 and 3).
4. Eliminate or minimize all other cardiovascular risk factors (obesity, hypertension, tobacco use, hyperlipidemia; see Table 53-5 for glycemic and blood pressure goals).
5. Try to integrate the patient into the healthcare team through intensive education. The patient's knowledge and understanding of this disease can favorably influence its outcomes (see Table 53-14 later in this chapter).

Methods of Monitoring Glycemic Control

In addition to monitoring signs and symptoms associated with hyperglycemia, hypoglycemia, and the long-term complications of diabetes, an ongoing assessment of metabolic control is an integral component of diabetes management. Ideally, SMBG results combined with laboratory measures of acute and chronic glycemia can be used to evaluate and adjust therapy.[38,56] SMBG and A1C levels continue to be the two primary methods used to access glycemic control. Continuous glucose monitoring (CGM) of interstitial fluid is also available for people with diabetes. CGM is discussed somewhat briefly here because this method is currently recommended for consideration, along with SMBG, for patients with Type 1 diabetes only, especially those with hypoglycemic unawareness.[38,56]

KETONE TESTING

Ketone testing is recommended for patients with gestational and Type 1 diabetes. Urine ketones (acetoacetic acid) should be evaluated when glucose concentrations consistently exceed 300 mg/dL or during acute illness.[56] In addition, a glucose monitor that is able to measure blood β-ketones (e.g., the Precision Xtra has a specific test strip to measure β-hydroxybutyric acid) can be used. Persistently high glucose concentrations of this magnitude signal insulin deficiency that can, in turn, lead to lipolysis and ketoacidosis. A positive test may indicate impending or established ketoacidosis and demands a more extensive diagnostic workup. Testing also is recommended during pregnancy and if the patient has symptoms of ketoacidosis. Although there are generally no ketones in the urine, they may be present in people who are on extremely low-caloric diets and in the first morning sample of women who are pregnant. Also, see discussions of sick day management and ketoacidosis in other sections of this chapter (Cases 53-7 and 53-13).

PLASMA GLUCOSE

FPG concentrations are commonly used to assess glycemic control in the fasting state because this is when glucose concentrations are most reproducible. FPG concentrations generally reflect glucose derived from hepatic glucose production because this is the primary source of glucose in the postabsorptive state. The FPG is the most frequent test performed by patients when self-monitoring. Postprandial glucose concentrations (1–2 hours after the start of the meal) also are used to assess glycemic control when fasting glucose concentrations are within normal limits or when there is a need to assess the effects of food or drugs (e.g., rapid-acting insulins, glinides) on meal-related glycemia. In individuals without diabetes, glucose concentrations generally return to less than 140 mg/dL within 2 hours after a meal. One- to 2-hour postprandial concentrations primarily reflect the efficiency of insulin-mediated glucose uptake by peripheral tissue.

Because glucose concentrations are affected by various factors (e.g., meals, medications, stress), single-time point measurements cannot be used to assess a patient's overall control. Most laboratories measure plasma glucose concentrations rather than whole blood because these values are not subject to changes in the hematocrit. The majority of glucose monitors report plasma-referenced glucose concentrations. Whole BG concentrations are approximately 10% to 15% lower than plasma glucose concentrations because glucose is not distributed into red blood cells.

SELF-MONITORING OF BLOOD GLUCOSE

SMBG has made euglycemia, both preprandially and postprandially, an achievable goal. Patients and their healthcare providers can use SMBG to assess directly the effects of drug dose changes, meals, exercise, and illness on BG concentrations. With improved technology, decreasing costs, and increased coverage by health plans, SMBG is the day-to-day monitoring test of choice for all patients with diabetes. However, SMBG remains expensive for patients without health insurance, is invasive, and can be difficult for some patients to perform depending on their technical ability. Furthermore, to achieve maximal benefit from SMBG, both the clinician and patient must be motivated and willing to spend the time required to interpret the data and modify therapy to improve glycemic control. The frequency and timing of performing SMBG should be dictated by the individual's needs and goals. Selection and use of SMBG testing materials are discussed in Case 53-2, Questions 9 and 10. Patients in whom SMBG is particularly valuable include the following:

- *Patients with Type 1 diabetes:* Frequent BG measurements help the patient to correlate meals, exercise, and insulin dose with BG concentrations. This instant feedback gives the patient an increased sense of control and motivation, leading to improved glucose control.
- *Pregnant patients:* Infant morbidity and mortality are associated with the mother's overall glucose control. Using SMBG, the mother with diabetes who achieves normoglycemia before conception and throughout pregnancy improves her chances of delivering a live, healthy infant.
- *Patients having difficulty recognizing hypoglycemia:* With time, patients with diabetes can develop a sluggish counter-regulatory response to hypoglycemia whereby hypoglycemic symptoms are blunted or even absent. This is often referred to as hypoglycemic unawareness. Routine SMBG to detect asymptomatic hypoglycemia is essential in these individuals. In addition, acute anxiety attacks or signs and symptoms associated with a rapidly falling BG concentration may mimic a true hypoglycemic reaction. This can be evaluated easily by measuring a fingerstick BG concentration.
- *Patients who are using physiologic (e.g., basal-bolus) insulin therapy:* Individuals who are on multiple daily doses of insulin or those using an insulin pump should perform SMBG to evaluate the effectiveness of their insulin regimens and meal plans and to check for hypoglycemic or hyperglycemic reactions (see Case 53-2, Question 10). Knowledge of preprandial, postprandial, bedtime, and nocturnal (e.g., 2 AM) BG concentrations is essential in determining basal and preprandial insulin requirements.
- *Patients with Type 2 diabetes who are on therapy that can cause hypoglycemia:* Individuals taking glinides, a sulfonylurea, or insulin therapy should know how to perform SMBG to detect hypoglycemia when experiencing symptoms consistent with hypoglycemia.
- *Patients with Type 2 diabetes who are engaged in self-management of their diabetes:* Even individuals using noninsulin therapies can benefit from SMBG to evaluate the impact of food, exercise, and antidiabetic medications on their BG.

CONTINUOUS GLUCOSE MONITORING

Like SMBG, CGM provides real-time information on glucose concentrations. However, the difference is that the CMG system automatically detects glucose concentrations (subcutaneous interstitial fluid glucose concentrations) on a continual basis. CGM systems use electrochemical sensors that are inserted into the skin. Sensor probe length varies as does the duration that the sensor can remain in the skin (3–7 days). The sensors transmit a signal to a receiver (wired or wireless), which records and displays the data every 1 to 5 minutes. The sensors require a warm-up or initialization period and have very specific calibration requirements. Calibration is performed by using a BG monitor. Interstitial glucose levels lag behind plasma or BG levels by 8 to 18 minutes, depending on the glucose rate of change.[38,57] Therefore, if a person's glucose is low, or trending downward, SMBG is required. CGM systems have alarms that can go off at certain high and low glucose thresholds. The ability to detect hypoglycemia during the night with these alarms has been a very attractive reason for using CGM. Another key feature is the ability to follow trends and rates of change in BG levels. Any acute treatment changes still require SMBG. Small, short-term studies have demonstrated modest improvements in A1C (0.3%–0.6% reductions) in adults and children with Type 1 diabetes.[38] Just as for SMBG with a glucose meter, use of CGM requires a person to actively assess and react to their readings for this self-management tool to have an impact on A1C.

GLYCOSYLATED HEMOGLOBIN

The glycosylated hemoglobin, or A1C, has become the gold standard for measuring chronic glycemia and is the clinical marker for predicting long-term complications, particularly microvascular complications. A1C is most commonly measured because it comprises the majority of A1C and is the least affected by recent fluctuations in BG. A1C measures the percentage of hemoglobin A that has been irreversibly glycosylated at the *N*-terminal amino group of the β-chain; the plasma glucose level and the life span of a red blood cell (RBC; ~120 days) determine its value. Thus, A1C is an indicator of glycemic control during the preceding 2 to 3 months. In patients without diabetes, A1C comprises approximately 4% to 6% of the total hemoglobin. Values may be 3 times this level in patients with diabetes.[58]

The following formula was developed to convert an A1C into an average glucose: $28.7 \times \text{A1C} - 46.7 = \text{eAG}$ (estimated average glucose). A formula that approximates (not exact) this very closely and is much easier to use in practice is $(\text{A1C} - 2) \times 30$. The ADA now recommends reporting an eAG (units, mg/dL, or mmol/L) along with the A1C. An eAG calculator is available on their website to do this conversion (http://diabetes.org/professional/eAG). The correlation between A1C and eAG is shown in the following table.[59]

A1C (%)	Estimated Average Plasma Glucose (mg/dL)
6	126
7	154
8	183
9	212
10	240
11	269
12	298

Hemoglobinopathies, such as sickle cell trait or chemically modified derivatives of hemoglobin as seen in uremia, in which hemoglobin becomes carbamylated, or acetylated hemoglobin with high-dose aspirin, can affect A1C values (increase or decrease depending on the assay), resulting in inaccurate indications of glycemic control. Alterations in red blood cell survival or turnover, seen in hemolytic anemia and acute blood loss, can falsely lower the A1C. Also a recent blood transfusion or use of intravenous (IV) iron therapy or erythropoietin-stimulating agents in patients with chronic kidney disease can falsely lower A1C values. A glycated serum protein (fructosamine) should be considered for these patients. Antioxidants such as vitamins C and E also may interfere with the glycosylation process.[7,38,60,61]

A1C can be measured without any special patient preparation (e.g., fasting) and generally is not subject to acute changes in insulin dosing, exercise, or diet. A1C values can be used as an adjunct to assess overall glycemic control in patients with diabetes or to diagnose diabetes and prediabetes.[62] Normalization can indicate whether euglycemia has been achieved. However, A1C does not replace the day-to-day monitoring of BG concentrations, which is essential for evaluating acute changes in BG concentrations. These values are needed to adjust the meal plan or medication doses. Sometimes, an A1C is used to verify clinical impressions related to glucose control and patient adherence. It should be measured quarterly in patients who do not meet treatment goals, and at least semiannually in stable patients who are meeting treatment goals.

GLYCATED SERUM PROTEIN, GLYCATED SERUM ALBUMIN, AND FRUCTOSAMINE

Assays for glycated serum proteins reflect the extent of glycosylation of a variety of serum proteins, including glycated serum albumin.[56] The fructosamine assay is one of the most widely used methods to measure glycated proteins (normal, 2–2.8 mmol/L). Because the half-life of albumin is approximately 14 to 20 days, fructosamine provides an indication of glycemic control during a shorter time frame (1–2 weeks) than does the A1C. The ADA does not consider measurement of fructosamine equivalent to that of A1C, although it correlates well with this value. Fructosamine levels may be useful as an adjunct to A1C in determining whether a patient is improving or worsening in the short term (e.g., a patient on insulin therapy undergoing multiple dosage adjustments; for women with Type 2 diabetes during pregnancy or gestational diabetes) or in patients with conditions such as hemolytic anemia in whom the A1C test is inaccurate.

INSULIN

Insulin is a hormone secreted from the pancreatic β-cell in response to glucose and other stimulants (e.g., amino acids, free fatty acids, gastric hormones, parasympathetic stimulation, β-adrenergic stimulation).[63,64] The hormone is made up of two polypeptide chains (a 21-amino acid A chain and a 30-amino acid B chain), which are connected by two disulfide bonds. Proinsulin, the precursor of insulin, is a single-chain, 86-amino acid polypeptide that is processed in the Golgi apparatus of β-cells and then packaged into granules.[63] In the storage granule, the connecting or C-peptide is cleaved from proinsulin to produce equimolar amounts of insulin and C-peptide. Insulin and C-peptide are cosecreted; thus, measurable C-peptide levels indicate the presence of endogenously produced insulin and functioning β-cells. Insulin is crucial to the survival of individuals with Type 1 diabetes, whose β-cells have been destroyed. It also plays a major role in the therapy of many individuals with Type 2 diabetes in combination of antidiabetic agents. Insulin also is used in patients with Type 2 diabetes during pregnancy or periods of illness or stress (e.g., surgery).

Commercially available insulin products differ in their physical and chemical properties as well as in the pharmacokinetics of their action. Prior issues with immunogenicity have been eliminated through modern manufacturing processes and the cessation of use of animal-derived insulin products. Consequently, immunologically mediated sequelae, such as lipodystrophy, hypersensitivity, and insulin resistance caused by "blocking" antibodies, are extremely rare.

Pharmacokinetics: Absorption, Distribution, and Elimination

The route of administration for insulin is primarily via SC injection. Regular insulin, a solution, can be administered by any parenteral route: IV, intramuscularly (IM), or subcutaneously (SC). Most other injectable insulins are only to be used SC with the exception of insulin aspart and insulin lispro which may be used via IV route if they are first diluted. Afrezza (insulin human) is the only insulin currently available as a powder for inhalation. Other routes for insulin administration have been studied, including dermal, nasal, buccal, and oral; however, these formulations are not currently approved for use here in the United States.

After SC injection, insulin is absorbed directly into the bloodstream, bypassing the lymphatic system. The rate-limiting step of insulin activity after SC administration is absorption of insulin from the injection site, which depends on the type of insulin administered, as well as a multitude of other factors. Variations in SC absorption can occur, primarily related to changes in blood flow around the injection site.

Endogenous insulin is secreted directly into the portal circulation and thus is primarily cleared by the liver in nondiabetic individuals (60%), with the kidneys removing only 35% to 40% of it.[63] Exogenous insulin is degraded at both renal and extrarenal (liver and muscle) sites. Degradation also takes place at the cellular level after internalization of the insulin–receptor complex. In contrast to endogenously secreted insulin, up to 60% of exogenous insulin is cleared from the systemic circulation by the kidneys, with the liver accounting for only 30% to 40% of its clearance. Insulin is filtered by glomerular capillaries, but more than 99% is reabsorbed by the proximal tubules. The insulin is then degraded in glomerular capillary cells and postglomerular peritubular cells.[65] See Case 53-6 for changes in insulin requirement in renal dysfunction.

Pharmacodynamics

Clinically, the most important differences among insulin products relate to their onset, peak, and duration of action (not the actual insulin levels, which is pharmacokinetics). Current insulin products can be categorized as rapid-acting, short-acting, intermediate-acting, and long-acting insulin. Products available in the United States are listed in Table 53-6, and the onset of action, peak effect, and durations of action of each insulin category are listed in Table 53-7. However, these data are derived primarily from studies in normal, healthy volunteers in the fasting state or in well-controlled patients with diabetes stabilized in a metabolic ward. In actuality, intersubject and intrasubject variations in response to insulin can

Table 53-6
Insulins Available in the United States

Type/Duration of Action	Brand Name	Manufacturer
Rapid Acting		
Insulin lispro	Humalog	Lilly
Insulin aspart	NovoLog	Novo Nordisk
Insulin glulisine	Apidra	Sanofi Aventis
Short Acting		
Regular	Humulin R[a]	Lilly
	Novolin R	Novo Nordisk
Intermediate Acting		
NPH (isophane insulin suspension)	Humulin N	Lilly
	Novolin N	Novo Nordisk
Long Acting		
Insulin glargine	Lantus	Sanofi Aventis
	Toujeo (U-300)	Sanofi Aventis
Insulin detemir	Levemir	Novo Nordisk
Insulin degludec	Tresiba (U-100 and U-200)	Novo Nordisk
Premixed Insulins		
NPH/regular (70%/30%)	Humulin 70/30	Lilly
	Novolin 70/30	Novo Nordisk
Insulin aspart protamine suspension/insulin aspart (70%/30%)	NovoLog Mix 70/30	Novo Nordisk
Insulin lispro protamine suspension/insulin lispro (75%/25%)	Humalog Mix 75/25	Lilly
Insulin lispro protamine suspension/insulin lispro (50%/50%)	Humalog Mix 50/50	Lilly
Insulin degludec/Insulin aspart (70%/30%)	Ryzodeg 70/30	Novo Nordisk
Inhaled Insulin		
Regular insulin	Afrezza	MannKind

Insulin is made through recombinant DNA technology. Only regular and NPH are human insulin. All other insulins are human insulin analogs. All insulins available in the United States have a concentration of 100 units/mL (U-100), except as noted.
[a]A U-500 concentration is available for use in rare circumstances in patients with severe insulin resistance requiring very large insulin doses.
NPH, neutral protamine Hagedorn, or isophane insulin suspension.

Table 53-7
Insulin Pharmacodynamics

Insulin	Onset (hours)	Peak (hours)	Duration (hours)	Appearance
Rapid-acting (insulin aspart, glulisine, and lispro)	5–15 minutes	30–90 minutes	<5	Clear
Regular	0.5–1	2–4	5–7	Clear
NPH	2–4	4–12	12–18	Cloudy
Insulin glargine U-100	1.5	No pronounced peak	20–24	Clear[a]
Insulin glargine U-300	6	None	24	Clear[a]
Insulin detemir	0.8–2	Relatively flat	5.7–23.2	Clear[a]
Insulin degludec	1	None	42	Clear
Insulin inhalation regular	≤15 minutes	1	3–5	

The onset, peak, and duration of insulin activity may vary considerably from times listed in this table. See text and Table 53-8.
[a]Should not be mixed with other insulins. Some patients require twice-daily dosing.
Source: Levemir [package insert]. Bagsvųrd, Denmark: Novo Nordisk Inc; July 2009; DeWitt DE, Hirsch IB. Outpatient insulin therapy in type 1 and type 2 diabetes mellitus: scientific review. *JAMA*. 2003;289:2254.

be substantial because an individual pattern of response to insulin can be affected by numerous factors (e.g., the formation of insulin hexamers, the presence of insulin-binding antibodies, dose, exercise, site of injection, massage of the injection site, ambient temperature, and interactions between insulins that have been mixed together; see Table 53-8 later in this chapter and Case 53-2, Question 14).[66,67] Nevertheless, knowledge of when one might expect the various insulins to exert their effects is absolutely essential to the rational adjustment of insulin dosages.

RAPID-ACTING INSULIN

Insulin Lispro

Insulin lispro (Humalog) was the first available rapid-acting insulin analog. The natural amino acid sequence of the insulin B chain at positions 28 (proline) and 29 (lysine) is inverted to form lispro. This change results in an insulin molecule that more loosely self-associates into hexamers than does regular human insulin. Consequently, the active monomeric form is more readily available, resulting in an onset of activity (15 minutes), peak action (30–90

Table 53-8
Factors Altering Onset and Duration of Insulin Action

Factor	Comments
Route of administration	Onset of action more rapid and duration of action shorter for IV > IM > SC[87,88]
	Intrapulmonary insulin has onset and duration comparable to SC rapid-acting insulins[89]
Factors altering clearance	
Renal function	Renal failure lowers insulin clearance; may prolong and intensify action of exogenous and endogenous insulin[89]
Insulin antibodies	IgG antibodies bind insulin as it is absorbed and release it slowly, thereby delaying or prolonging its effect[90]
Thyroid function	Hyperthyroidism increases clearance, but also increases insulin action, making control difficult; patients stabilize as they become euthyroid
Factors altering SC absorption	Factors that raise SC blood flow ↑ absorption rates of regular insulin; effect on intermediate- and long-acting insulins is minimal
Site of injection	Rate of absorption is fastest from the abdomen, intermediate from the arm, and slowest from the thigh.[88] Less variation is observed in type 2 diabetes patients; less variation is observed with current rapid-acting and long-acting insulins
	Site — *Half-life absorption (minutes)*
	Abdomen — 87 ± 12
	Arm — 141 ± 23
	Hip — 153 ± 28
	Thigh — 164 ± 15
Exercise of injected area	Strenuous exercise of an injected area within 1 hour of injection can increase absorption rate; rate of absorption of regular insulin is increased, but little effect on intermediate-acting insulin
Ambient temperature	Heat (e.g., hot weather, hot bath, sauna) increases absorption rate; cold has opposite effect

(continued)

Table 53-8
Factors Altering Onset and Duration of Insulin Action (*continued*)

Factor	Comments
Local massage	Massaging injected area for 30 minutes substantially increases absorption rate of regular insulin as well as longer-acting insulins
Smoking	Controversial; vasoconstriction may decrease absorption rate[66]
Jet injectors	Insulin absorption is more rapid, probably secondary to increases in surface area for absorption
Lipohypertrophy	Insulin absorption is delayed from lipohypertrophic sites
Insulin preparation	More soluble forms of insulin are absorbed more rapidly and have shorter durations of action (see Table 53-7 and text); human insulin may have shorter action than animal insulin
Insulin mixtures	The short-acting properties of rapid-acting insulins may be blunted if mixed with NPH insulin (see Case 53-2, Question 15)
Insulin concentration	More dilute solutions (e.g., U-40, U-10) are absorbed more rapidly than more concentrated forms (U-100, U-500)
Insulin dose	Lower doses are absorbed more rapidly and have a shorter duration of action than larger doses

IgG, immunoglobulin G; IM, intramuscular; IV, intravenous; NPH, neutral protamine Hagedorn; SC, subcutaneous.

minutes), and duration (3–4 hours) that more closely simulates physiologic insulin secretion relative to meals. Because it can be injected shortly before eating (0–15 minutes), lispro, and all rapid-acting insulins, provides patients greater flexibility in lifestyle. These insulins lower 2-hour postprandial BG levels and can decrease the risk of late postprandial and nocturnal hypoglycemia compared with regular insulin formulations.[68] Patients who use an insulin pump most often use a rapid-acting insulin instead of regular insulin. One randomized, two-way, crossover, open-label study compared lispro with regular insulin administered for 3 months by continuous SC insulin infusion.[69] Lispro resulted in A1C values that were significantly lower than those produced by regular insulin (7.41% vs. 7.65%). There were no differences in adverse events. Because lispro has a shorter duration of action than regular insulin, hyperglycemia and ketosis may occur more rapidly in patients with Type 1 diabetes if insulin pump delivery is inadvertently interrupted or if the basal insulin dose is missed. Insulin lispro is approved for use in pediatrics (studies included children of age 3 and older), and it is pregnancy category B. Insulin lispro is available in concentrations as both 100 and 200 units/mL. Both formulations are available as an insulin pen (Kwikpen); however, insulin lispro 100 units/mL is available in both vial and insulin pen formulations. The availability of the 200-units/mL formulation allows patients to inject a greater amount of insulin in an overall smaller volume.[70]

Insulin Aspart

Insulin aspart (NovoLog) is a rapid-acting insulin analog that differs from human insulin by substitution of aspartic acid at B28. Insulin aspart is approved for use in pediatric patients, age 2 and older.[71] It is pregnancy category B. Insulin aspart controls postprandial glucose excursions similar to insulin lispro. Insulin aspart is available in both vials and prefilled pen (FlexPen and FlexTouch) formulations.

Insulin Glulisine

Insulin glulisine (Apidra) is a rapid-acting insulin analog that differs from human insulin by substitution of lysine for asparagine at position B3 and glutamic acid for lysine at position B23. Insulin glulisine has been studied in pediatric patients with Type 1 diabetes age 4 and older.[72] It is pregnancy category C. Insulin glulisine lowers postprandial glucose excursions similar to insulin lispro and insulin aspart. Insulin glulisine is available in both vials and prefilled pen (Solostar) formulations.

Inhaled Insulin

Insulin human powder for inhalation (Afrezza) is a rapid-acting insulin indicated for postprandial coverage in patients with Type 1 or Type 2 diabetes.[73] It is produced using recombinant DNA technology and is supplied via inhaler that is breath-activated by the patient. The insulin in the Afrezza inhaler is regular human insulin, and metabolism and elimination are similar to that of regular insulin following pulmonary absorption. The pharmacodynamic profile of inhaled Afrezza is similar to that of rapid-acting insulin. It is pregnancy category C and has not been studied for use in patients less than 18 years old. Insulin human powder for inhalation is available as prefilled inhalers containing 4, 8, or 12 units of rapid-acting insulin to be used at the beginning of a meal. It is contraindicated for use in patients with chronic lung disease such as asthma and chronic obstructive lung disease as well as current smokers.

SHORT-ACTING INSULIN

Regular insulin 100 units/mL (Humulin R and Novolin R) has an onset of action of 30 to 60 minutes, a peak effect at 2 to 4 hours, and a duration of action of 5 to 7 hours. The broad range in peak effect and duration reflects the many variables that affect insulin action (Table 53-7). The 30- to 60-minute onset of action requires proper timing of premeal regular insulin, which is difficult for most patients. Use of regular insulin in patients with both Type 1 and Type 2 diabetes is much less common with the advent of the newer rapid-acting insulins.

Regular insulin U-500 (500 units/mL) is a concentrated insulin that is indicated for SC only. Being 5 times more potent than the 100 units/mL formulation, it is useful in patients who are severely insulin resistant requiring daily insulin doses of greater than 200 units/day because a large insulin dose may be given in a much smaller volume. Its onset of action is approximately 30 minutes and peaks similar to regular insulin U-100. Regular insulin U-500 however has a longer duration of action (up to 24 hours) compared to the U-100 formulation and is therefore recommended to be administered between 2 and 3 times daily.[74] There are no U-500 insulin syringes available; therefore, to avoid confusion, it is recommended to dose U-500 insulin in volume and administer using a tuberculin syringe vs. a typical U-100 insulin syringe. Additionally, the manufacturer of U-500 regular insulin has incorporated multiple differences in packaging between regular insulin U-100 and U-500 to potentially decrease the risk of dispensing errors. Specifically, the regular insulin U-500 vial contains 20 mL compared to the U-100 vial which contains only 10 mL. The U-500 insulin vial is also marked with a band of diagonal brown stripes to distinguish it from the U-100 vial which contains no stripes.[75] The U-500 insulin pen (Humulin R U-500 KwikPen) approved by the FDA in 2016 should eliminate many of these issues.

INTERMEDIATE-ACTING INSULIN (NPH)

Neutral protamine Hagedorn (NPH) or isophane is an intermediate-acting insulin commercially available as Humulin N or Novolin N. Its onset of action is approximately 2 hours (range, 1–3 hours), peak effects occur at approximately 6 to 14 hours, and the duration of action of NPH is approximately 16 to 24 hours. Again, it must be emphasized that this pattern of response is at best a generalization. Patients may have a variable pattern of response to NPH insulin with time, and those on higher doses are likely to have a later peak and a longer duration of action. Up to 80% of these day-to-day fluctuations in BG responses can be accounted for by variation in the absorption of this intermediate-acting insulin.[66] Novolin N is available only in vials, whereas Humulin N is available both in vials and in prefilled pen (KwikPen) formulations.

LONG-ACTING INSULIN

Insulin Glargine

Insulin glargine U-100 (Lantus) is a long-acting insulin that serves to provide a basal level of insulin. It is pregnancy category C.[76] It is approved for once-a-day SC administration for the treatment of adult and pediatric patients (age ≥6 year) with Type 1 diabetes or adult patients with Type 2 diabetes. It can be administered any time during the day, but it is important to take it at the same time each day. It is usually administered at bedtime or, less commonly, in the morning. Insulin glargine is available in both a 10-mL vial and a prefilled pen (Solostar).

Insulin glargine is an insulin analog in which asparagine in position A21 is substituted with glycine and two arginines are added to the C-terminus of the B chain. This change in the amino acid sequence causes a shift in the isoelectric point from pH 5.4 to 6.7, making it more soluble at an acidic pH.[77] Once injected, insulin glargine (which is a clear solution with a pH of 4.0) precipitates at physiologic pH, forming a depot that releases insulin slowly for up to 24 hours. This results in delayed absorption and a less pronounced peak compared with NPH insulin.[78] Zinc is added to further prolong the duration of insulin glargine. In clinical trials of patients with Type 1 and Type 2 diabetes, once-daily injections of insulin glargine were as effective as NPH in lowering A1C values, with less nocturnal hypoglycemia.[79] Insulin glargine is associated with more injection site pain compared with NPH (6.1% vs. 0.3% in one study and 2.7% vs. 0.7% in another), which is likely related to its acidity.[76,80]

Insulin glargine is also available in a concentrated form which is available as 300 units/mL (Toujeo). It is approved for once-daily SC injection in adults with Type 1 or Type 2 diabetes. Toujeo has not been studied for use in the pediatric population. Insulin glargine 300 units/mL is only available in a prefilled pen (Solostar device) which does not require dose calculations or conversions when switching from insulin glargine 100 units/mL.[81]

Insulin Detemir

Insulin detemir (Levemir) is another basal insulin available in the United States and is approved for once- or twice-daily SC administration for the treatment of adult and pediatric patients (age ≥2 years) with Type 1 diabetes or adult patients with Type 2 diabetes. It is pregnancy category B.[82] Unlike other insulin analogs, in which the amino acid sequence is modified, for insulin detemir, a fatty acid moiety is added to the last amino acid on the end of the B chain. Insulin detemir is a neutral, soluble insulin preparation in which the B30 threonine has been removed and the B29 lysine residue has been covalently bound to a 14-carbon fatty acid. The result is an insulin that is more slowly absorbed in the SC tissue because the fatty acid moiety binds to albumin, creating a long-acting insulin.[83] Insulin detemir's kinetics and dynamics are dose-dependent.[84] When used in Type 1 diabetes, two injections daily are usually required to provide adequate basal coverage due to a smaller insulin dose requirement in this patient population. Insulin detemir demonstrates less intrasubject variability than NPH or insulin glargine.[85] The clinical significance and impact of this observation are unclear. Insulin detemir is available in both vial and pen (FlexTouch) formulations.

Insulin Degludec

Insulin degludec (Tresiba) is a long-acting basal human insulin analog approved in the United States in 2015 for once-daily SC administration for the treatment of adults with Type 1 or Type 2 diabetes. It is pregnancy category C and is not indicated for use in the pediatric population. Insulin degludec differs from human insulin in that the amino acid threonine in position B30 has been omitted and a side chain consisting of glutamic acid and a C16 fatty acid has been attached.[86] Insulin degludec has a much longer duration of action (>42 hours) compared to other available basal insulins and is available as a prefilled pen (FlexTouch device) in concentrations of both 100 and 200 units/mL. The FDA has also approved a combination insulin degludec/insulin aspart 70/30 combination (Ryzodeg 70/30) which is intended to be used once to twice daily prior to a main meal.

PREMIXED INSULIN

Products that contain premixed NPH and regular insulin in a fixed ratio of 70:30 are available from Lilly as Humulin 70/30 and from Novo Nordisk as Novolin 70/30. Additional premixed formulations are available in which both insulin lispro and insulin aspart have been cocrystallized with protamine to create an intermediate-acting insulin similar to NPH. Humalog Mix 75/25 and Humalog Mix 50/50 (Lilly) are products with lispro protamine and insulin lispro in a fixed ratio of 75:25 and 50:50, respectively. NovoLog Mix 70/30 (Novo Nordisk) is aspart protamine and insulin aspart in a fixed ratio of 70:30. These premixed insulins are useful for patients who have difficulty measuring and mixing insulins and are dosed twice daily. These insulins are compatible when mixed together and retain their individual pharmacodynamic profiles. Each of these mixed insulin combinations is available as both vials and insulin pens with the exception of Novolin 70/30 which is available in insulin vials only (see Table 53-19 later in this chapter and Case 53-2, Question 15).

TREATMENT OF TYPE 1 DIABETES: CLINICAL USE OF INSULIN

Clinical Presentation of Type 1 Diabetes

CASE 53-2

QUESTION 1: A.H., a slender, 18-year-old woman who was recently discharged from the hospital for severe dehydration and mild ketoacidosis, is referred to the Diabetes Clinic from the University Student Health Service (no records available). A fasting and a random plasma glucose ordered subsequently were 190 and 250 mg/dL. Approximately 4 weeks before she was hospitalized, A.H. had moved across the country to attend college—her first time away from home. In retrospect, she remembers that she had symptoms of polydipsia, nocturia (6 times a night), fatigue, and a 12-lb weight loss during this period, which she attributed to the anxiety associated with her move away from home and adjustment to her new environment. Her medical history is remarkable for recurrent upper respiratory infections and three cases of vaginal moniliasis in the past 6 months. Her family history is negative for diabetes, and she takes no medications.

Physical examination is within normal limits. She weighs 50 kg and is 5 feet 4 inches tall. Laboratory results are as follows: FPG, 280 mg/dL; A1C, 14%; and trace urine ketones as measured by Keto-Diastix. On the basis of her history and laboratory findings, the presumptive diagnosis is Type 1 diabetes. Which findings are consistent with this diagnosis in A.H.?

A.H. meets several of the diagnostic criteria for diabetes. She has classic symptoms of Type 1 diabetes (polyuria, polydipsia, glucosuria, fatigue, recurrent infections), a random plasma glucose greater than 200 mg/dL, and a FPG greater than 126 mg/dL on at least two occasions as well as an A1C greater than 6.5%[7] (Tables 53-1 and 53-3). Features of A.H.'s history that are consistent with Type 1 diabetes, in particular, include the relatively acute onset of symptoms in association with a major life event (moving away from home), recent weight loss, ketones in the urine, negative family history, and a relatively young age at onset.[7]

Treatment Goals

CASE 53-2, QUESTION 2: A.H. will be started on insulin therapy on this visit. What are the goals of therapy? Will normoglycemia prevent the development or progression of long-term complications?

The goal of diabetes management is the prevention of acute and chronic complications. The results of the DCCT and DCCT-EDIC studies convincingly demonstrated that lowering BG concentrations through intensive insulin therapy in persons with Type 1 diabetes slows or prevents the development of microvascular complications.[29,30] The ADA recommends an A1C goal of less than 7% for most patients, and an individual goal as close to normal as possible (<6.5%) if it can be achieved without significant hypoglycemia. For children and adolescents, the ADA recommends an A1C goal of less than 7.5%, and an individualized goal of less than 7% if achievable without significant hypoglycemia.[7]

It is important to understand that physiologic or basal-bolus insulin therapy involves a *complete* program of diabetes management that includes a balanced meal plan, physical activity, frequent SMBG, and insulin adjustments based on these factors (Table 53-4).

In summary, A.H. is a patient newly diagnosed with Type 1 diabetes who has not yet developed any signs or symptoms of long-term complications. Therefore, she is an ideal candidate for basal-bolus insulin therapy, and if she is willing and motivated, normoglycemia with rare hypoglycemic episodes is a reasonable long-term goal. This goal should be achieved gradually over the course of several months with insulin therapy, diet, education, and strong clinical support. A desirable goal is an A1C value as close to the normal range as possible with minimal episodes of hypoglycemia.

Basal-Bolus (Physiological) Insulin Therapy

CASE 53-2, QUESTION 3: What methods of insulin administration are available to achieve optimal glucose control?

A physiologic insulin regimen is designed to mimic normal insulin secretion as closely as possible. Problems with insulin delivery include factors that affect the SC absorption of insulin (Table 53-8).[87,88] Before the development of the rapid-acting insulin analogs and basal insulins, previous insulins lacked pharmacodynamic profiles that allowed one to closely simulate normal pancreatic release of the hormone. In the nondiabetic individual, the pancreas secretes boluses of insulin in response to food. Between meals and throughout the night, the pancreas secretes small amounts of insulin that are sufficient to suppress lipolysis and hepatic glucose output (basal insulin). Clinicians now have more tools to mimic this basal-bolus model. Two methods have been used to achieve this pattern of insulin release: (a) insulin pump therapy (previously referred to as continuous subcutaneous infusion of insulin) and (b) basal-bolus insulin regimens consisting of once- or twice-daily doses of basal insulin coupled with premeal/snackdoses of rapid-acting insulin (see Case 53-2, Questions 3–5).

INSULIN PUMP THERAPY

The use of an insulin pump is currently the most precise way to mimic normal insulin secretion. This consists of a battery-operated pump and a computer that can program the pump to deliver predetermined amounts of insulin (i.e., regular, lispro, aspart, or glulisine) from a reservoir to a SC inserted catheter or needle.[89,90] These systems are portable and designed to deliver various basal amounts of insulin over the course of 24 hours as well as meal-related boluses. Most patients using an insulin pump use a rapid-acting insulin, rather than regular insulin. For meal coverage, the rapid-acting insulin can be given 0 to 15 minutes before eating. The delivery of the bolus can be adjusted depending on the type of food eaten (e.g., piece of cake versus slice of pizza). Caveat: If SC delivery is interrupted, check for rise in glucose and urine ketones after 2 or 3 hours. Because there is no SC pool, effects dissipate quickly.

The preferred meal-planning approach for patients using an insulin pump is carbohydrate counting. The insulin-to-carbohydrate ratio, or how much carbohydrate is covered by 1 unit of insulin, must be determined. One method is to use the "500 Rule." The number 500 (or 450 for regular insulin) is divided by the total daily dose (TDD) of insulin the patient is using to determine the insulin-to-carbohydrate ratio (see Case 53-2, Question 11). Insulin pumps are capable of delivering many basal insulin rates. The basal insulin infusion rate may be adjusted depending on the situation. Many patients find it advantageous to decrease the basal rate during the middle of the night when nocturnal hypoglycemia is most likely to occur. The basal rate also may be increased before awakening to avoid hyperglycemia secondary to the "dawn phenomenon" or adjusted when physically active—adjustments that are not possible using SC basal insulin injections.

Features of the current pump models include the "bolus wizard," which calculates bolus doses based on preset carbohydrate-to-insulin ratios and correction factors, carbohydrate counts for selected foods, and an "insulin-on-board" feature, which helps avoid excessive dosing of insulin by indicating how much insulin from a previously administered dose should still be acting. Most insurance plans provide coverage for insulin pumps for patients with Type 1 diabetes and for some patients with Type 2 diabetes. Factors to consider when choosing a pump include safety features, durability, ability of the manufacturer to provide service, availability of training, clinically desirable features, CGM compatibility, and cosmetic attractiveness for the user.[90,91] The ADA website (www.diabetes.org) contains helpful information about insulin pumps for patients under the Living with Diabetes section.

MULTIPLE DAILY INJECTIONS

CASE 53-2, QUESTION 4: How can insulin be administered to A.H in order to model physiologic release of insulin from the pancreas?

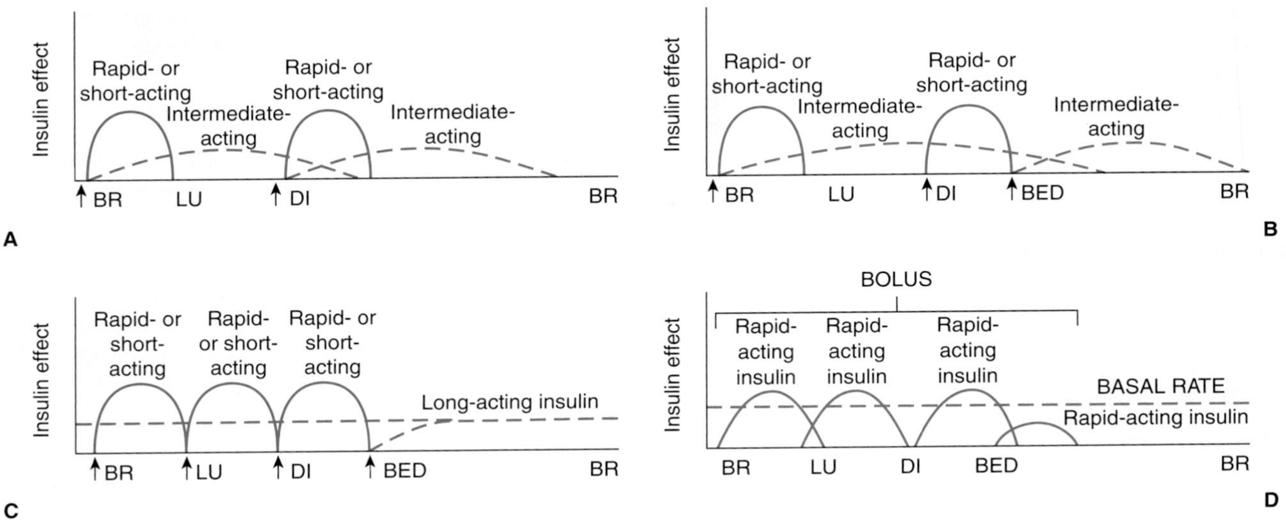

Figure 53-4 Theoretic insulin effect provided by various insulin regimens. **A:** Two daily injections of rapid-acting (insulin aspart, glulisine, or lispro), short-acting (regular), and intermediate-acting insulin (NPH). **B:** Morning injection of rapid-acting or short-acting insulin and intermediate-acting insulin, a predinner injection of rapid-acting or short-acting insulin, and a bedtime injection of intermediate-acting insulin. Suggested for patients with early-morning hypoglycemia, and also those who have early-morning hyperglycemia (owing to rebound phenomenon from hypoglycemia). **C:** Premeal injections of rapid-acting or short-acting insulin and long-acting (e.g., insulin glargine or detemir) or intermediate-acting insulin (NPH) at bedtime. **D:** Continuous subcutaneous insulin infusion, showing an example with bolus given for a bedtime snack. BR, breakfast; Bed, bedtime; LU, lunch; DI, dinner. Arrows indicate time of insulin injection (<15 minutes before meals for rapid-acting insulin and 30 minutes before meals for short-acting insulin).

Endocrinologists have developed a variety of insulin regimens that are intended to mimic the natural release of insulin from the pancreas.[92,93] Examples of these are displayed and illustrated in Figure 53-4. A TDD of insulin is estimated empirically (e.g., 0.3–0.5 units/kg/day for patients with Type 1 diabetes) or according to guidelines listed in Table 53-9. The TDD of insulin then is split into several doses. In general, the basal dose comprises approximately 40% to 50% of the TDD, and the other bolus doses comprise the remaining 50%. If a patient eats three meals/day, the bolus dose would then be divided by three to calculate the number of units of bolus insulin required to cover each meal.

Table 53-9
Empiric Insulin Doses

Estimating Total Daily Insulin Requirements	
These are initial doses only; they must be adjusted using SMBG results. Patients may be particularly resistant to insulin if their blood glucose concentrations are high (glucose toxicity); once glucose concentrations begin to drop, insulin requirements often decrease precipitously. The weight used is actual body weight. Insulin dose requirements can change dramatically with time depending on circumstances (e.g., a growth spurt, modest weight gain or loss, changes in physical activity, stress or illness)	
Type 1 diabetes	
Initial dose	0.3–0.5 units/kg
Honeymoon phase	0.2–0.5 units/kg
With ketosis, during illness, during growth	1.0–1.5 units/kg
Type 2 diabetes	
With insulin resistance	0.7–1.5 units/kg
Estimating Basal Insulin Requirements	
These are empiric doses only and should be adjusted using appropriate SMBG results (fasting or premeal). Basal requirements vary throughout the day, often increasing during the early-morning hours. The basal requirement also is influenced by the presence of endogenous insulin, the degree of insulin resistance, and body weight. Basal requirements are approximately 50% of total daily insulin needs. Thus, basal insulin dose is approximately 50% of TDD. A conservative approach is to reduce the calculated 50% basal dose by 20% to avoid hypoglycemia[93]	
Estimating Premeal Insulin Requirements	
The premeal insulin requirements are approximately 50% of the TDD, usually divided equally into three doses initially, taken with each meal (i.e., breakfast, lunch, and dinner), and then each premeal dose is individually adjusted based on BG readings The "500 rule" estimates the number of grams of carbohydrate that will be covered by 1 unit of rapid-acting insulin. The rule is modified to the "450 rule" if using regular insulin	

(continued)

Table 53-9
Empiric Insulin Doses (*continued*)

500/TDD of insulin = number of grams covered
Example: For a patient using 50 units/d, 500/50 = 10. Therefore, 10 g of carbohydrate would be covered by 1 unit of insulin lispro, glulisine, or aspart. This equation works very well for type 1 diabetes patients in estimating their premeal insulin requirements. Because patients with type 2 diabetes have insulin resistance, the rule may underestimate their insulin requirements
Determining the "Correction Factor"
Supplemental doses of rapid-acting insulin are administered to acutely lower glucose concentrations that exceed the target glucose concentration. These doses must be individualized for each patient and again are based on the degree of sensitivity to insulin action. For example, if the premeal blood glucose target is 120 mg/dL and the patient's value is 190 mg/dL, additional units of rapid-acting insulin could be added to the premeal dose. The correction factor determines how far the blood glucose drops per unit of insulin given and is known as the "1,700 rule." For regular insulin, the rule is modified to the "1,500 rule." The equation is as follows:
1,700/TDD = point drop in blood glucose per unit of insulin
Example: If a patient uses 28 units/day of insulin, their correction factor (or insulin sensitivity) would be 1,700/28 = 60 mg/dL. Therefore, the patient can expect a 60-mg/dL drop for every unit of rapid-acting insulin administered. Patients with a higher-sensitivity factor have lower-insulin requirements. Individuals with a lower-sensitivity factor (higher-insulin requirements) typically achieve a smaller reduction in blood glucose per unit of insulin

SMBG, self-monitored blood glucose; TDD, total daily dose.
Source: DeWitt DE, Hirsch IB. Outpatient insulin therapy in type 1 and type 2 diabetes mellitus: scientific review. *JAMA*. 2003;289:2254; Walsh J, Roberts R. *Pumping Insulin: Everything You Need For Success On A Smart Insulin Pump*. 4th ed. San Diego, CA: Torrey Pines Press; 2006; Walsh J et al. *Using Insulin: Everything You Need for Success With Insulin*. San Diego, CA: Torrey Pine Press; 2003.

A regimen much less commonly used in patients with Type 1 diabetes involves injecting a mixture of intermediate-acting and regular or rapid-acting insulin twice daily, before breakfast and before dinner (Fig. 53-4A). The morning dose of regular or rapid-acting insulin is intended to take care of the breakfast meal; the morning dose of NPH takes care of the noon meal and provides basal insulin throughout the day; the evening dose of regular or rapid-acting insulin takes care of the evening meal; and the evening dose of NPH provides basal insulin levels during the night and takes care of any evening snack that is ingested. Because NPH is an intermediate-acting insulin and has a peak effect, it does not provide true basal insulin coverage. Also, when NPH is injected in the morning, the patient must eat lunch on time because of this peak effect; otherwise, he/she will experience hypoglycemia. Also, when NPH is taken with mealtime insulin before dinner, the patient is at risk for nocturnal hypoglycemia from the peak effect of the evening dose of NPH. The advantage of using a rapid-acting insulin (e.g., insulin lispro, insulin aspart, or insulin glulisine) instead of regular insulin in this regimen is to facilitate the patient being able to take insulin doses immediately before a meal. However, the peak effect of the NPH component in this combined dose still presents the same problems. This type of insulin regimen does not mimic physiologic insulin release.

Figure 53-4B depicts a variation of this method. It is the same except that the evening dose of NPH is given as a third injection at bedtime. This shifts the time of peak effect from approximately 2 to 3 AM to approximately 7 AM. By administering NPH at bedtime, nocturnal hypoglycemia is reduced, and peak insulin activity occurs when the patient is more likely to be awake and ingesting food. This method may be useful for patients in whom nocturnal hypoglycemia and fasting hyperglycemia are particularly troublesome; however, this regimen also does not mimic physiologic insulin release.

The regimen that most closely mimics physiologic insulin release besides the use of an insulin pump is the use of a once-daily basal insulin such as insulin glargine, detemir, or degludec to provide basal insulin levels throughout the day, along with doses of a rapid-acting insulin (preferred) or regular insulin before meals (Fig. 53-4C depicts the long-acting insulin given at bedtime, but it can be given alternatively in the morning). When smaller doses are used, twice-daily insulin detemir and possibly U-100 insulin glargine will be required for 24-hour coverage.[94–96] Insulins U-100 and U-200 degludec and U-300 glargine will last 24 hours with once-daily dosing. This method theoretically provides insulin similar to the insulin pump: constant basal levels plus small boluses for meals and snacks. In doing so, it offers some of the same advantages of the pump in that it permits some degree of flexibility in the patient's lifestyle. For example, if a patient with diabetes chooses to skip a meal, he/she omits a premeal bolus; if the patient chooses to eat a larger meal than usual, he/she increases the premeal bolus. Similar dose adjustments can be made to accommodate snacks, exercise patterns, and acute illnesses. Alternatives to this regimen are depicted in Table 53-4 where the long-acting insulin is replaced with intermediate-acting insulin for basal coverage and or the rapid-acting insulin is replaced with short-acting insulin for bolus coverage. These options however are not preferred because they do not as closely mimic normal physiologic insulin release.

CASE 53-2, QUESTION 5: Should A.H. use an insulin pump or multiple daily insulin injections?

Indications for basal-bolus insulin therapy are listed in Table 53-10. Patients with Type 1 diabetes should be placed on a basal-bolus insulin regimen. A.H. is an ideal candidate to strive for an A1C goal of less than 6.5%. She is newly diagnosed, has not yet developed the long-term complications of diabetes, and should derive the benefits of normoglycemia. Assuming A.H. will be able to manage a basal-bolus insulin regimen, individualized target BG levels that strive for the best level of glucose control possible without placing her at undue risk for hypoglycemia should be prescribed. She must be willing to test her BG concentrations 4 or more times daily and inject herself 4 times daily or learn about the use and care of an insulin pump. She also must be willing to keep detailed BG and food records and participate in an extensive education program that enables her to adjust her insulin doses based on BG concentrations, physical activity, and the carbohydrate content of her snacks and meals.

Transition to an insulin pump is facilitated by patients being able to attain these skills using multiple daily SC insulin injections

Table 53-10
Basal-Bolus (Physiological) Insulin Therapy: Indications and Precautions

Patient Selection Criteria
Type 1 diabetes, otherwise healthy patients (>7 years of age) who are highly motivated, engaged in diabetes self-management and are able to adhere to a complex insulin regimen. Must be willing to test blood glucose concentrations multiple times daily and inject four doses of insulin daily, on average
Women with diabetes who plan to conceive
Pregnant patients with diabetes (preexisting)
Patients poorly controlled on conventional therapy, 2–3 injections daily (includes type 2 diabetes patients)
Technical ability to test blood glucose concentrations
Intellectual ability to interpret blood glucose concentrations and adjust insulin doses appropriately
Access to trained and skilled medical staff to direct treatment program and provide close supervision
Avoid or Use Cautiously in Patients Who Are Predisposed to Severe Hypoglycemic Reactions or in Whom Such Reactions Could Be Fatal
Patients with counter-regulatory insufficiency
β-Adrenergic blocker therapy
Autonomic insufficiency
Adrenal or pituitary insufficiency
Patients with coronary or cerebral vascular disease
(*Note:* Counter-regulatory hormones released in response to hypoglycemia may have adverse effects in these individuals.)
Unreliable, nonadherent individuals, including those who abuse alcohol or drugs and those with psychiatric disorders

before insulin pump initiation. The ADA recommends that the use of insulin pumps be limited to highly motivated individuals under the guidance of a healthcare team trained and knowledgeable in their use. Pumps offer the patient the ability to use multiple basal rates during the 24-hour period and assist with the calculation of bolus and correction insulin doses. Most studies have shown that pump therapy provides equivalent and sometimes better glycemic control than does intensive management with multiple injections.[97,98]

Insulin pumps are particularly useful in patients with frequent, unpredictable hypoglycemia, or marked dawn phenomena (see Case 53-3). Others have described the methods by which insulin doses are established and altered in patients using the insulin pump.[91,99] Because A.H. has just been diagnosed, she should be initiated on a basal-bolus SC insulin therapy. Once she has acquired these skills, she may be considered for pump therapy.

Clinical Use of Insulin

INITIATING INSULIN THERAPY

Case 53-2, Question 6: How should multiple daily insulin injections be initiated in A.H.?

A conservative TDD of insulin is estimated empirically or according to guidelines similar to those listed in Table 53-9 in newly diagnosed patients and will differ in patients with Type 1 and Type 2 diabetes. Many weight-based empiric dose calculations have been proposed as listed in Table 53-9 for patients with both Type 1 and Type 2 diabetes; however, these regimens are mostly beneficial for patients with Type 1 diabetes because these patients are completely insulin deficient. For patients with Type 2 diabetes, initial basal insulin doses that are weight-based or a starting dose of ~10 units daily are appropriate options based on patient-specific information. Insulin doses would then be adjusted based on HBG levels.[100]

For a basal-bolus insulin regimen, insulin glargine, insulin detemir, or insulin degludec could be used as the basal insulin with bolus doses of a rapid- or short-acting insulin (insulin lispro, insulin aspart, insulin glulisine) given at mealtime. During the initial visit, A.H. needs to learn how to inject her insulin (see Case 53-2, Question 8), how to test her BG (Table 53-11), how and when to test for ketones (either urine or blood), and how to recognize and treat hypoglycemia (Table 53-12). She also needs to understand the importance of meal planning and the relationship between carbohydrate intake and insulin action (Table 53-13). It is very important not to overwhelm A.H. with information on the first visit. One should be particularly sensitive to the psychological impact of this diagnosis on A.H., address her major concerns, and provide only the information that is absolutely essential before the next visit. Between visits, she should be assessed and provided information on an as-needed basis by phone. Table 53-14 lists important areas of patient education.

A reasonable first approach for A.H. is to provide a TDD of 24 units of insulin (~0.5 units/kg). Because 50% of the daily dose should be given as basal insulin with the remainder given as rapid-acting insulin divided into three doses, A.H. would take the following: 12 units of insulin glargine once daily (morning or bedtime) with 4 units of insulin aspart or lispro given approximately 5 to 10 minutes before each meal.[71,100] Alternatively, if insulin detemir is used, the dose would generally be split twice daily (6 units BID) as the duration of action of insulin detemir is typically less than 24 hours when given at such a small dose. Caveat: As A.H.'s glucose concentration returns to normal, glucose toxicity will recede and she may require less insulin.

SELECTING AN INSULIN DELIVERY DEVICE

Case 53-2, Question 7: What kind of insulin delivery device should be prescribed for A.H.?

Table 53-11

Self-Monitored Blood Glucose Testing: Areas of Patient Education

When and How Often To Test

Technique

How and when to calibrate the glucose monitor

Review all "buttons" and their purposes. Identify battery type. Review cleaning procedures, if applicable

Preparation

1. Calibrate monitor/set code for batch of test strips, if required
2. Insert test strip to turn machine on (some meters require user to turn machine on)
3. Prepare all materials: tissue, strip, and lancet
4. Remember to close the lid of the strip container immediately. Strips exposed to air and moisture deteriorate rapidly
5. Wash hands with warm water. *Dry thoroughly.* A wet finger causes blood to spread rather than form a drop. Milk the finger from the base to ensure an adequate flow of blood
6. Lance the tip of the finger. Avoid the pads of the finger where nerve endings are concentrated
7. Hold the finger *below* the heart with the lanced area pointing toward the floor
8. Once a sufficient amount of blood is available, *quickly* apply blood to designated area of the test strip. Depending on the strip type, the blood sample is placed in an area on the surface of the strip or it is applied to the side of the strip where it is taken up by capillary action

Record Results in a Log Book and Bring to All Clinician Visits. Include relevant information regarding diet or exercise

How To Use Results To Achieve Glycemic Targets; Educate Patients on What To Do With Their Blood Glucose Readings (e.g., adjust their insulin dose; modify their carbohydrate content)

Table 53-12

Hypoglycemia

Definition

Blood glucose concentration <60 mg/dL: Patient may or may not be symptomatic

Blood glucose <40 mg/dL: Patient is generally symptomatic

Blood glucose <20 mg/dL: Can be associated with seizures and coma

Signs and Symptoms

Blurred vision, sweaty palms, generalized sweating, tremulousness, hunger, confusion, anxiety, circumoral tingling, and numbness. Patients vary with regard to their symptoms. Behavior can be confused with alcohol inebriation. Patients become combative and use poor judgment

Nocturnal hypoglycemia: nightmares, restless sleep, profuse sweating, morning headache, morning "hangover." Not all patients have symptoms during nocturnal hypoglycemia

Clinical Considerations

Irregular eating patterns

↑ Physical exercise

Gastroparesis (delayed gastric emptying)

Defective counter-regulatory responses

Excessive dose of insulin or insulin secretagogues (sulfonylureas, glinides)

Alcohol ingestion

Drugs

Treatment

Ingest 10–20 g of rapidly absorbed carbohydrate. Repeat in 15–20 minutes if glucose concentration remains less than 60 mg/dL or if patient is symptomatic. Follow with complex carbohydrate/protein snack if mealtime is not imminent

The following are examples of food sources that provide 15 g of carbohydrate:

Orange, grapefruit, or apple juice; regular, nondiet soda	1/2 cup
Fat-free milk	1 cup
Grape juice, cranberry juice cocktail	1/3 cup
Sugar	1 tbsp or 3 cubes
Lifesavers	5–6 pieces
Glucose tablets	3–4 tablets

If patient is unconscious, the following measures should be initiated:

Glucagon 1 mg SC, IM, or IV (generally administered IM in outpatient setting; mean response time, 6.5 minutes)

Glucose 25 g IV (dextrose 50%, 50 mL; mean response time, 4 minutes)

IM, intramuscular; IV, intravenous; SC, subcutaneous.

Table 53-13
Interpreting Self-Monitored Blood Glucose Concentrations

Test Time	Target Insulin Dose	Target Meal/Snack
Prebreakfast (fasting)	Predinner/bedtime intermediate-acting or basal insulin	Dinner or bedtime snack
Prelunch	Prebreakfast regular or rapid-acting insulin	Breakfast or mid-morning snack
Predinner	Prebreakfast intermediate-acting insulin or prelunch regular or rapid-acting insulin	Lunch or mid-afternoon snack
Bedtime	Predinner regular or rapid-acting insulin	Dinner
2-hour postprandial	Premeal regular or rapid-acting insulin	Preceding meal or snack
2–3 AM or later	Predinner intermediate-acting insulin or basal insulin if given in AM	Dinner or bedtime snack

Considerations: (a) Assumes a regular meal pattern. For patients who travel, have odd working or sleeping hours, or have irregular meal patterns, these guidelines may not apply. (b) Assumes administration of regular insulin 30 to 60 minutes before meals or rapid-acting insulin 0 to 15 minutes before meals and a normal pattern of insulin response (see Table 53-8 for factors that can alter insulin absorption and response). (c) If prebreakfast concentrations are high, rule out reactive hyperglycemia (Somogyi reaction or posthypoglycemic hyperglycemia). Consider contribution of dawn phenomenon as well. Whenever blood glucose concentrations are high, consider reactive hyperglycemia (excessive insulin doses). (d) Consider accuracy of reported test results: (i) Do they correlate with the glycosylated hemoglobin (A1C) and patient's signs and symptoms? (ii) What is the patient's medication adherence? Could results be fabricated? (iii) Is the patient's technique appropriate? Check timing, adequate blood sample, machine, strips, and calibration (Table 53-11). (iv) Are insulin kinetics altered? (v) What is the carbohydrate content, quality, and regularity of meals?

Table 53-14
Areas of Patient Education

Diabetes: Pathogenesis and the complications
Hyperglycemia: Signs and symptoms
Ketoacidosis: Signs and symptoms (Tables 53-22 and 53-23)
Hypoglycemia: Signs, symptoms, and appropriate treatment (Table 53-12)
Exercise: Effect on blood glucose concentrations and insulin dose (Table 53-19)
Diet: See text. Emphasis placed on carbohydrate counting because the carbohydrate is responsible for 90% of the rise in blood glucose after a meal
Insulins:
Injection technique
Types of insulin
Time action profiles (onset, peak, and duration)
Storage
Stability (look for crystallization and precipitation with NPH insulin)
Therapeutic goals: A1C, fasting, preprandial, and postprandial blood glucose levels, cholesterol, triglyceride, blood pressure (refer to Lipid Chapter 8 and Essential Hypertension Chapter 11)
SMBG testing: Table 53-13
Interpretation of SMBG testing results
Foot care: Inspect feet daily; wear well-fitted shoes; avoid self-care of ingrown toenails, corns, or athlete's foot; see a podiatrist
Sick day management: Table 53-20
Cardiovascular risk factors: Tobacco use, high blood pressure, obesity, elevated cholesterol
Importance of annual ophthalmologic examinations; tests for microalbuminuria; keeping up-to-date with immunizations

A1C, glycosylated hemoglobin; NPH, neutral protamine Hagedorn; SMBG, self-monitored blood glucose.

Insulin delivery is achieved utilizing syringes, prefilled insulin delivery devices (pens), or through oral inhalation. Insulin syringes are plastic, disposable syringes with needles that are extremely fine (typically 30–31 gauge), sharp, and well lubricated to ease insertion. Pen needles and syringes have been improved so that insulin injections are relatively painless if proper technique is used. The lengths of needles are 15/64-inch (6-mm) 5/16-inch (8-mm), or ½-inch (12.7 mm).[100] Research has shown that there is no medical reason why a patient would require use of a needle longer than 4 to 6 mm for insulin administration as skin thickness does not vary between different demographics. Previous thoughts that larger or obese patents require longer needle length for proper insulin administration have been disproven. Manufacturers produce 1-, 0.5-, and 0.3-mL syringes for U-100 insulin. For patients such as A.H., using fewer than 30 units of insulin per injection, the 0.3-mL syringe is preferred for ease of reading the dose markings on the syringe. Insulin syringes are available in 1-unit increments or 0.5-unit increments. One-half-unit increments are useful for pediatric patients and for patients who count carbohydrates, because mealtime insulin doses can be rounded to the 0.5 unit.[101]

Insulin pen devices are also available for injecting insulin. Pen devices are often preferred because they make insulin administration much easier, especially for patients who need to take their insulin doses away from home. They also can increase dosing accuracy. The pens are particularly useful for patients with (a) regimens consisting of multiple daily doses of rapid- or short-acting insulin before meals and snacks (such as A.H.), (b) a fear of needles, (c) impaired visual or dexterity problems, (d) hectic work schedules or lifestyle, or (e) a need to train alternative individuals who administer insulin (e.g., school nurses, siblings). Additionally, studies have shown that use of insulin pen devices vs. vial and syringe insulin administration may result in fewer discontinuations of insulin therapy and improve overall adherence to an insulin regimen.[102,103]

Pens eliminate the need to withdraw insulin, and the insulin dose is dialed up on the device. Pen devices are available as a disposable prefilled pen or a durable pen in which an insulin cartridge is replaced. Most typically used are the prefilled pens which contain a built-in, single-use insulin cartridge. U-100 formulations contain 300 units of insulin, whereas concentrated insulins will contain more units in each device. Pen devices are available to dose insulin in 1-unit (most) and 0.5-unit increments (HumaPen

 Luxura HD). Pen needles are available in 30-, 31-, and 32-gauge needles and 5/32-inch, (4-mm), 3/16-inch (5-mm), 1/4-inch (6-mm), or 5/16-inch (8-mm) lengths, but there is no medical rationale to use needles longer than 6 mm. Patients are advised to use a new disposable needle for each injection. Unfortunately, limited health insurance coverage and higher copays may deter pen use. A detailed review of pen devices (both insulin and noninsulin) was published in 2014.[104]

For insulin delivery using an insulin pump, see Case 53-2, Questions 3 and 5.

If she elected to use a syringe, a 0.3-mL U-100 insulin syringe with a short needle length should be prescribed for A.H. Subjectively, patients can "feel" the difference between different brands, or they may prefer the "ease of bubble removal," physical characteristics, or packaging of one syringe over another. If she elected to use an insulin pen, a prefilled pen for insulin glargine and insulin aspart or insulin lispro are available. The shortest possible needle length (4 mm for pen needles and 6 mm for syringes) should be prescribed for A.H.

MEASURING AND INJECTING INSULIN

CASE 53-2, QUESTION 8: How should A.H. be instructed to administer her insulin injections?

Injection

A.H. should prepare an area for injection. Alcohol swabs may be used to clean the rubber stopper of the insulin vial (or pen device). To inject the insulin SC, A.H. should be instructed to firmly pinch up the area to be injected (this creates a firm surface for the injection) and to quickly insert the needle perpendicularly (90-degree angle) into the center of this area. Note however that if pinching is only necessary then AH is using a syringe that is 6 mm or greater.[101] The syringe should be held toward the middle or back of the barrel, like a pencil. Anxious patients have a tendency to "choke" the hub of the syringe, and this prevents proper needle insertion. A 45-degree angle of injection may be used for infants and very thin individuals who have little SC fat, especially in the thigh area.[101] The site should not be massaged, because this may accelerate the absorption and onset of action of insulin (Table 53-8). When using an insulin pen, the needle should be embedded within the skin for about 5 to 10 seconds after depressing the dosing knob to ensure full delivery of the insulin dose.[101]

Rotating Injection Sites

The primary sites used for injecting insulin are the lateral thigh, abdomen (avoid 2-inch radius around the navel), and upper arm (Fig. 53-5). The ADA recommends that insulin injections be rotated within the same anatomic region to decrease chances of variability in insulin absorption.[101,105] Many practitioners recommend using the abdominal area because absorption from this site is least affected by exercise and is the most predictable. Alternatively, A.H. can be instructed to rotate her morning injection within one region (e.g., the abdomen) and her evening injection in another anatomic region. This minimizes the variables that can alter her response to insulin.

Rotating injection sites also were recommended at one time to avoid the lipodystrophic effect of insulin (lipohypertrophy and lipoatrophy); however, because insulin has been purified, these complications are less common and the importance of rotation is less critical. Nevertheless, repetitive use of the same site of injection may still result in lipohypertrophy, and it does toughen the skin, making needle penetration more difficult. Furthermore, insulin absorption from lipohypertrophic sites can be slowed.[101]

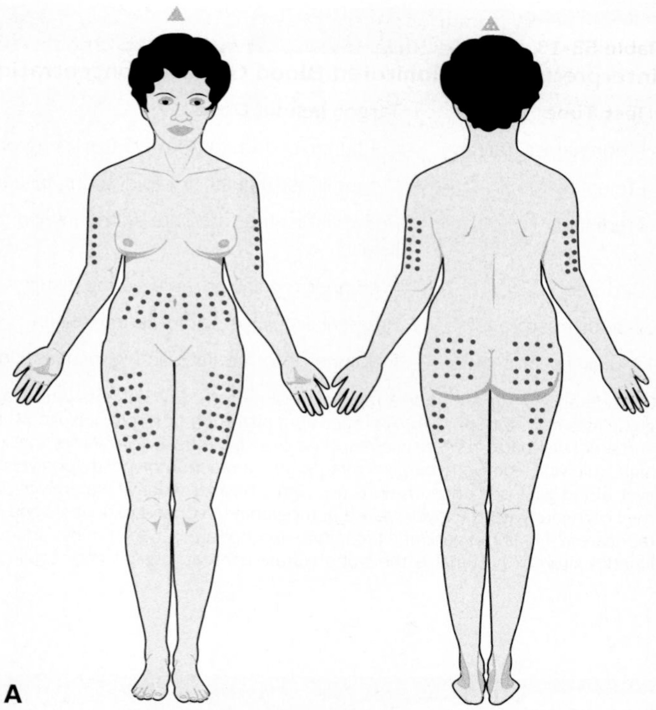
A

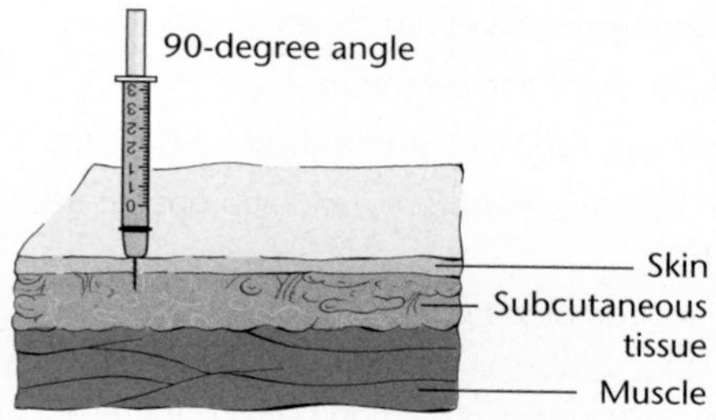

B

Figure 53-5 Selecting insulin injection sites. **A:** Areas of the body most suitable for insulin injections. The actual point of injection should be varied each time within a chosen body area. Give injections at least one inch apart. Patients should consult with their provider or diabetes educator about which area is most appropriate for use. **B:** The site where insulin should be injected. Insulin is injected in the subcutaneous tissue (between the skin and the muscle layer). If the skin is pinched up and the needle is pushed all the way in, the need will reach the proper space under the skin. (**A**, LifeART image © 2011. Lippincott Williams & Wilkins. All rights reserved; **B**, Adapted from Springhouse. Lippincott's Visual Encyclopedia of Clinical Skills. Philadelphia: Wolters Kluwer Health; 2009, with permission.)

Agitation

A.H. does not need to agitate insulin glargine or aspart because these are clear insulins. For NPH insulin, which is a suspension, or a combination/mixed insulin, the vial or pen must be gently agitated before use. The vial should be rolled between the palms of the hands to minimize foaming. A pen device is inverted back and forth to mix the insulin. Agitation is only required for insulin suspensions (i.e., insulin mixtures).

Measurement

First, A.H. should make sure her hands and the injection site are clean. She should withdraw the plunger to the level of insulin she intends to inject (e.g., 12 units for her insulin glargine dose), then she should insert the needle into the vial and inject the air to prevent creation of a vacuum within the vial. The vial then should be inverted with the syringe inserted, and 12 units of insulin glargine should be withdrawn. The bevel of the needle should be well below the surface of the insulin to avoid withdrawing air or bubbles into the syringe. Insulin glargine must not be mixed in the same syringe with her rapid-acting insulin, and it should be injected into a different site if it is injected at the same time as her glargine dose.[101]

The barrel of the syringe should be held at eye level to check for air bubbles and to allow accurate placement of the plunger tip at the 12-unit mark. If bubbles are present, they should be removed by tapping the syringe gently to coax the bubbles to the top of the barrel, where they can be injected back into the insulin vial. To remove air bubbles in an insulin pen, prime the pen with 2 units of insulin before each use (repeat until insulin drop appears at tip of pen needle). Also, remove and discard the pen needle from the device in between uses to prevent air bubbles from accumulating.

SELF-MONITORING OF BLOOD GLUCOSE

CASE 53-2, QUESTION 9: How should A.H. be educated to self-monitor her BG? What types of self-monitoring BG tests are available, and what are the major differences among them? How accurate are results obtained from home BG testing? Should she begin CGM at the same time?

The ADA recommends that most individuals with diabetes should attempt to attain and achieve normoglycemia as safely as possible. SMBG is a tool to allow patients to safely achieve these goals. For patients with Type 1 diabetes, this can be achieved by the routine use of SMBG. SMBG is also important in (a) pregnancy complicated by diabetes, (b) patients with unstable diabetes, (c) patients with a propensity to severe ketosis or hypoglycemia, (d) patients prone to hypoglycemia who may not experience the usual warning symptoms, and (e) patients using an insulin pump. The technology in this area is changing rapidly, with new monitors with advanced features being introduced yearly.[90]

All monitors use test strips and are self-timing, requiring no patient action after the blood is placed on the strip. Several factors should be taken into account when evaluating a monitor and its appropriateness for an individual. The primary considerations are ease of use, accuracy relative to a reference standard, reliability, insurance coverage, and cost.[90] Most monitors no longer require coding for the test strips, which simplifies the process for patients. Convenience factors include meter size, volume of blood required for testing, site to obtain sample (e.g., finger versus alternative site such as forearm), capacity of the meter to store BG values (memory) and data such as comments, required testing time, ability to download BG values, general availability of strips, ability to turn off audible signals, audible readings and instructions for visually impaired, and availability of technical support. Some devices are less reliable for use in anemic patients (e.g., renal transplant patients), and all function most reliably within certain temperature ranges (usually 60°F–95°F) and humidity (generally <90%) conditions. Strips are sensitive to light, moisture, and temperature extremes and must be stored and handled with care.

Patient education regarding any testing procedures, the importance of logging results in a diary, and test times are critical. Ultimately, A.H. should be taught how and when to check her BG levels in order to optimize her insulin regimen (Table 53-15).

Table 53-15
Guidelines for Dosing Insulin

Basic Insulin Doses
First, adjust the basic insulin dose (i.e., the dose that the patient will be instructed to take daily)
Only adjust insulin doses if a *pattern* of response is observed under stable diet and exercise circumstances. That is, the same response to insulin is observed for ≥3 days, particularly for the basal insulin dose. It is important to verify the stability of diet and exercise. Consider adjusting these variables as well
Unless all levels are >200 mg/dL, try to adjust one component of insulin therapy at a time
Start with the insulin component affecting the FBG concentration. This glucose level often is the most difficult to control and often affects all other glucose concentrations measured throughout the day. The basal insulin dose is often what is adjusted to control the FBG. However, if the dinner insulin dose (of rapid-acting or short-acting insulin) is not adequate, this can result in hyperglycemia that can persist into the morning. The basal dose is typically adjusted by 2–4 units, no sooner than every 3–4 days
Prandial/mealtime insulin dose: ■ For patients eating a set amount of carbohydrate at meals: typically adjust the basic insulin dose by 1–2 units at a time. The amount given is based on the individual patient's response to insulin. This can be determined by looking at the patient's total daily dose (TDD) using the "500 rule" (see the following, and Table 53-9) ■ For patients using the insulin-to-carbohydrate method (i.e., 1 unit rapid-acting or short-acting insulin for every *x* g of carbohydrate), adjust the "ratio" based in the patient's response to insulin (e.g., 1:8, 1:10, 1:12, 1:15, 1:18, 1:20)
General Principles
Assumes that diet and physical activity are stable. Set a reasonable goal initially. This may mean the upper limits of the acceptable concentrations may be high initially (e.g., <200 mg/dL). Move toward a more ideal goal slowly.
Supplementary Insulin Doses (with rapid-acting or short-acting insulin)
Once the basic dose of prandial insulin has been established, supplemental doses of rapid- or short-acting insulin can be prescribed to correct *preprandial* hyperglycemia. For example, if the goal is 140 mg/dL and the glucose value is 190 mg/dL, administer one additional unit. Supplemental doses also can be used when the patient is ill (Table 53-15)
Algorithms for correction doses are based on the patient's sensitivity to insulin using the "1,500 or 1,700 rule" (Table 53-9)
If premeal glucose concentrations are <60–70 mg/dL, the dose of aspart, glulisine, lispro, or regular insulin administered before the meal is ↓ by 1–2 units; insulin administration is delayed until just before the meal; the meal should include an extra 15 g of glucose if the value is <50 mg/dL

(continued)

Table 53-15
Guidelines for Dosing Insulin (*continued*)

If supplemental doses before a given meal are required for ≥3 days, the basic insulin dose should be adjusted appropriately. For example, if a patient taking lispro before meals requires an extra 2 units before lunch for ≥3 days, 2 units should be added to the prebreakfast dose, or the insulin-to-carbohydrate ratio at breakfast should be adjusted (e.g., if patient was using a 1:15 ratio, a 1:12 ratio could be used). Rapid-acting insulin doses should be adjusted no more frequently than every 2–3 days
Anticipatory Insulin Doses (with rapid-acting or short-acting insulin)
The basic insulin dose is ↑ or ↓ based on the anticipated effects of diet or physical activity
↑ Aspart/glulisine/lispro or regular insulin by 1 unit for each additional 15 g of carbohydrate ingested (e.g., holiday meal) or ↓ the usual dose by 1–2 units if the meal is smaller than usual (Table 53-9)
See Table 53-19 for recommended insulin adjustments for exercise

FBG, fasting blood glucose.

Used properly, available monitors provide reasonably accurate results that can be used by patients to manage their diabetes. Problems with a monitor can be detected by performing a quality-control test once weekly and with each new vial of strips. Table 53-16 lists factors that can affect results of SMBG test results. Any time SMBG values are inconsistent with the patient's symptoms or A1C values, sources of error should be evaluated. A.H.'s technique should be reviewed periodically, because clinical decisions are often based on the patient's BG testing record.

Because A.H. is just starting insulin therapy and SMBG, it would be reasonable to hold off on considering CGM until she becomes comfortable with these skills. Then, she and her practitioner could assess whether CGM would be useful.

TESTING FREQUENCY

CASE 53-2, QUESTION 10: How often should A.H. test her BG concentrations?

Although the exact frequency and timing of BG tests should be dictated by individualized patient goals, most patients with Type 1 diabetes using basal-bolus insulin regimens should perform SMBG at least 3 times daily or more according to the ADA.[38] Glucose monitoring should also be performed more frequently if needed, such as when therapy is modified, prior to exercise, when the patient suspects hypoglycemia, after treatment of hypoglycemia, or when the patient is performing a critical task such as driving. Because A.H. is being initiated on insulin therapy with the goal of normoglycemia, she should ideally self-monitor her BG 4 times/day (before meals and at bedtime) for 2 weeks until the pattern of blood sugar fluctuation can be assessed and adjustments can be made. Motivated patients may continue this degree of monitoring, but it may be reduced to twice daily for patients on long-term insulin. Varying the time of day in which testing is performed will allow the clinician and patient to make informed decisions on how to make adjustments. For those patients who are not using an intensive insulin regimen, such as patients with Type 2 diabetes using insulin, there is insufficient evidence as to how often a patient should check their BG due to the decreased risk of hypoglycemia. Instead patients along with their providers should determine the appropriate frequency and timing to check BG levels in order to best optimize drug therapy and decrease risk for hypoglycemia.[106]

The objective of ongoing, frequent BG testing is to determine whether normoglycemia is being achieved, assess effectiveness of drug therapy as well as the impact of meals, food, illness, or exercise on BG levels. Typical times to check BG may include: before meals and snacks, 2 hours postprandial, at bedtime and occasionally at 2 to 3 AM. However, it can be challenging for

Table 53-16
Factors that Can Alter Self-Monitored Blood Glucose Test Results: Troubleshooting

Glucose monitor not coded for batch of test strips[a]
An inadequate amount of blood applied to test strip[b]
Improper storage of test strips (temperature and humidity)[a]
Dirty glucose monitor[a]
Low battery[a]
Test performed outside of altitude, temperature, and humidity operating conditions[a]
Low[c] or high[b] hematocrit
Dehydration[b]
Hyperosmolar, nonketotic state[b]
Lipemia[a]
Interfering substances
Nonglucose sugars (e.g., maltose, xylose, galactose) in meters using GDH-PQQ test strips[115]
Large amounts of acetaminophen[c]
Large amounts of ascorbic acid or salicylates (rare)[b]

[a]Effect unpredictable
[b]Values tend to be lower
[c]Values tend to be higher
GDH-PQQ, glucose dehydrogenase pyrroloquinolinequinone.
Source: Heinemann L. Quality of glucose measurement with blood glucose meters at the point-of-care: relevance of interfering factors. *Diabetes Technol Ther*. 2010;12:847.

patients to adhere to such a rigorous regimen. A.H. should set her alarm for 3 AM 2 or 3 times/week and test her BG. BG concentrations measured before meals allow patients and clinicians to determine whether the rapid-acting insulin dose is appropriate for the amount of carbohydrate consumed; FPG levels are used to determine whether the basal insulin dose is adequate; and the 2 to 3 AM BG level is used to identify nocturnal hypoglycemia. For example, the BG measured before dinner reflects the action of A.H.'s prelunch aspart dose on food she has eaten for lunch, as well as hepatic glucose production between meals. Increasingly, patients who use carbohydrate counting with rapid-acting insulins test 2-hour postprandial levels when initiating therapy to enhance proper dosage adjustment (Table 53-13).

The importance of frequent BG testing in patients newly diagnosed with Type 1 diabetes cannot be overemphasized. When BG is tested less frequently than 4 times daily, it becomes difficult to adjust insulin doses based on infrequent readings or to assess patterns in glucose levels (i.e., pattern management). If patients refuse to test 4 times daily, they should be encouraged to test 4 times daily on representative days of the week or to test at different times of the day each day so that a weekly profile can be developed. A.H. also should be encouraged to test her BG concentration any time she is feeling unusual, if she is experiencing hypoglycemic symptoms, or to evaluate the effect of unusual circumstances on her BG concentration (e.g., increased physical exercise, a large holiday meal, final examinations, a family crisis).[38]

USING BLOOD GLUCOSE TEST RESULTS TO EVALUATE INSULIN DOSES

CASE 53-2, QUESTION 11: A.H. was instructed to inject herself with 12 units of insulin glargine each evening and to give 4 units of insulin aspart just before each meal. She was asked to test her BG 4 times daily (before meals and at bedtime), to record her results and other unusual events or symptoms during the day, and to bring her BG logbook to the clinic. A.H. was also instructed to track her food and record the number of carbohydrates she ingested at each meal. The initial goal of therapy is to lower her to eliminate symptoms of hyperglycemia. The ultimate goal is to achieve fasting glucoses of 80 to 130 mg/dL and postprandial values of less than 180 mg/dL. One week later, trends in her BG concentrations were as follows:

Time	Glucose Concentration (mg/dL)
7 AM	160–200
Noon	220–260
5 PM	130–180
11 PM	140–180

Occasional 3 AM tests averaged 160 mg/dL, and A.H.'s urine is negative for ketones. She eats approximately four carbohydrate servings for breakfast (60 g) and two to four carbohydrate servings for lunch and dinner (30–60 g). Subjectively, A.H. feels a bit better, and her weight has stabilized, but she still urinates 2 to 3 times nightly. How would you interpret these results, and how should A.H.'s insulin doses be altered?

Values from SMBG appropriately form the basis for insulin adjustments. Ultimately, the goal is to move motivated patients toward being able to recognize their own glucose trends and make insulin adjustments accordingly based on recommendations between the patient and provider.[56] Before using A.H.'s BG results to adjust her insulin dose, it is important to observe and reassess her testing technique. One also should determine whether there were any unusual circumstances in her life such as acute illness, diet changes, drug therapy changes, or exercise patterns during the past week that may have affected her response to insulin. Once these have been ruled out as confounding factors, one can begin making adjustments in A.H.'s insulin dose, realizing that fine-tuning will be impossible until a consistent diet and exercise pattern have been instituted.

Several principles must be kept in mind whenever BG tests are used to adjust a patient's basic insulin dose (Table 53-17). Because many factors can alter a patient's response to insulin, it is important to review BG concentration *trends* measured for a minimum of 3 days to adjust the basic insulin dose (i.e., the dose the patient will use every day). The only exception to this rule is the use of supplemental insulin doses to correct exceptionally high glucose concentrations after A.H. has acquired sophisticated insulin adjustment skills (see Case 53-2, Question 16). SMBG results should always be evaluated in conjunction with A1C values.

The daily dose of insulin glargine is inadequately controlling A.H.'s FPG and should be increased by 2 to 4 units. A more conservative approach would be to increase the dose to 14 units each evening (or a designated time of day that she will be able to do consistently) and further titrate as needed.[92] She is achieving some response from her lunchtime dose of insulin aspart, but there is room for improvement in her meal insulin coverage overall. The BG concentration of 160 mg/dL at 3 AM indicates that rebound hyperglycemia is an unlikely cause of her high fasting levels (see Case 53-2, Question 13, and Case 53-3). As an initial step toward control, A.H.'s daily dose of insulin glargine should be increased in an attempt to control her fasting hyperglycemia. However, this approach does not address A.H.'s elevated prelunch values. Her intake of carbohydrates also varies from meal to meal. Thus, a more appropriate method would be to calculate the insulin-to-carbohydrate ratio for A.H. and allow her to determine her premeal aspart dose based on the amounts of carbohydrates she will ingest at each meal. A typical starting point for the insulin-to-carbohydrate ratio is 1 unit to every 15 g of carbohydrate ingested. To calculate her insulin-to-carbohydrate ratio, the "500 rule" is used: Divide the number 500 by her TDD of

Table 53-17
Factors that Can Alter Blood Glucose Control

Diet
Insufficient calories (e.g., alcoholism, eating disorders, anorexia, nausea, and vomiting)
Overeating (e.g., during the holidays)
Irregularly spaced, skipped, or delayed meals
Dietary content (e.g., fiber, carbohydrate content)
Physical Activity
See Table 53-19
Stress
Infection
Surgery/trauma
Psychological
Drugs
Certain medications can increase or decrease blood glucose levels. It is important to assess for potential effects on the blood glucose when starting new medications
Hormonal Changes
Menstruation: Glucose concentrations may increase premenstrually and return to normal after menses
Pregnancy
Puberty: hyperglycemia probably related to high growth hormone levels
Gastroparesis
Delays gastric emptying time. Peak insulin action and meal-related glucose excursions may become mismatched
Altered Insulin Pharmacokinetics
See Table 53-8
Insulin Injection Technique
Measuring
Timing
Technique
Inactive Insulin
Outdated insulin
Improperly stored insulin (heat or cold)
Crystallized insulin

 insulin (14 units of insulin glargine plus 12 units of insulin aspart for meal coverage = 26 units):

$$500/26 = 19 \text{ g of carbohydrate covered by 1 unit of insulin} \quad \text{(Eq. 53-1)}$$

Because most single servings of carbohydrate contain 15 g, A.H. decides to start with a ratio of 1 unit for every 15 g or single serving of carbohydrates she consumes at each meal. If A.H. were using regular insulin for meal coverage, she could use the "450 rule": 450 divided by the total daily insulin dose yields grams of carbohydrate covered by 1 unit of insulin.

To evaluate the accuracy of her insulin-to-carbohydrate ratio, A.H. will need to check her BG values 2 hours after each meal (postprandial) to assess the appropriateness of her ratio. She agrees to test her BG level 8 times/day and return in 2 weeks.

CASE 53-2, QUESTION 12: A.H. is getting more comfortable with carbohydrate counting and adjusting her insulin doses accordingly. A review of her food diary reveals that for the most part, she is able to determine the appropriate serving sizes for 15 g of carbohydrate. She admits to difficulty determining carbohydrate amounts when eating out. As a result, A.H. notices that her preprandial BG concentrations exceed her goal of 80 to 130 mg/dL on occasion.[7] Sometimes they are as high as 200 mg/dL. Evaluate A.H.'s BG trends. How should occasional preprandial glucose concentrations that exceed the desired goal of 80 to 130 mg/dL be managed?

Once the basal insulin dose and insulin-to-carbohydrate insulin dose have been established, one can begin to teach A.H. how to use a correction factor to adjust her dose of insulin when preprandial BG concentrations fall above or below the range of BG concentrations that have been established as her goal of therapy (80–130 mg/dL per the ADA; Table 53-15).

A correction insulin dose is used to compensate for unusually high BG concentrations (high-sugar correction). To re-emphasize, this assumes there are no unusual changes in the patient's overall diet or exercise patterns (Table 53-18 explains the effects of exercise on BG). Many clinicians favor rapid-acting insulin versus regular insulin because its action is brief and patients do not have to worry about residual effects 3 to 4 hours after its injection. This is particularly valuable when correctional doses of insulin are needed at bedtime.

The patient's sensitivity to insulin, as reflected by his/her TDD on a unit per kilogram basis, is a major determinant of any algorithm developed. A general approach is to give an additional 1 to 2 units of supplemental rapid-acting insulin for each 30- to 50-mg/dL elevation above the target level.[93] An alternative method of estimating the drop in a person's BG per unit of regular insulin is the "1,500 rule."[99] The derived value is referred to as the "sensitivity factor": The rule was modified to the "1,800 rule" for use with rapid-acting insulin (insulin lispro, aspart, or glulisine). Because these insulins tend to drop the BG level faster and farther, 1,500 turns out to be too aggressive. Others have recommended other numerators such as 1,600, 1,700, 2,000, and 2,200.[107] For this case, the "1,700 rule" will be used. The calculation for A.H. would be as follows:

$$1{,}700/24 = 70 \text{ mg/dL} \quad \text{(Eq. 53-2)}$$

Thus, 1 unit of insulin aspart for A.H. will drop her BG level by about 70 mg/dL. People with a lower-sensitivity factor (higher-insulin requirements) typically achieve a smaller reduction in BG per unit of insulin compared with those with a higher-sensitivity factor (lower-insulin requirement). Thus, an algorithm of 1 unit of insulin aspart for every 70-mg/dL excursion above her goal of 120 mg/dL is a reasonable place to begin. If this dose of insulin is insufficient, one can decrease the BG excursion required per unit of insulin dose (e.g., 50 mg/dL). Correctional insulin doses also are used for sick day management (see Case 53-5). The following is an example of a high-sugar correction algorithm for A.H:

Glucose Concentrations (mg/dL)	Insulin Aspart
<80	1 unit less
80–120	Usual dose
120–190	1 unit extra
191–260	2 units extra
261–330[a]	3 units extra
331–400[a]	4 units extra

[a]Check urine or blood ketone levels. If ketones are positive and BG concentrations remain >300 mg/dL for ≥12 hours, call the physician for directions.

Table 53-18
Exercise in Patients with Diabetes

1. Test blood glucose before, during, and after exercise
2. For moderate exercise (e.g., bicycling or jogging for 30–45 minutes), ↓ the preceding dose of regular or rapid-acting insulin by approximately 30%–50%. If glucose concentration is normal or low before exercise, supplement the diet with a snack containing 10–15 g of carbohydrate
3. To avoid ↑ absorption of regular insulin by exercise, inject into the abdomen or exercise 30–60 minutes after injection. Avoid exercise when rapid-acting insulin is peaking
4. Individuals with low glycogen stores may be predisposed to the hypoglycemic effects of exercise. Examples include alcoholics, fasted individuals, or patients on extremely hypocaloric (<800 calories), low-carbohydrate (<10 g/day) diets
5. Patients taking insulin are more susceptible to hypoglycemia than those taking oral insulin secretagogues (sulfonylureas, glinides). Patients with type 2 diabetes treated with diet are unlikely to develop hypoglycemia
6. Watch for postexercise hypoglycemia. Individuals who have been exercising during the day will likely need to ↑ their carbohydrate intake and should test their blood glucose during the night to detect nocturnal hypoglycemia. Hypoglycemia can occur 8–15 hours after exercise
7. If the glucose concentration is >240–300 mg/dL, the patient should not exercise. This indicates severe insulin deficiency. These patients are predisposed to hyperglycemia secondary to exercise
8. Patients with severe proliferative retinopathy or retinal hemorrhage should avoid jarring exercise or exercise that involves moving the head below the waist

EVALUATING FASTING HYPERGLYCEMIA

CASE 53-2, QUESTION 13: A.H. returns after 1 month. She is currently using 14 units of insulin glargine each evening, 1 unit of insulin aspart for each 15 g of carbohydrate ingested at mealtime, and a high-sugar correction factor of 1 unit of insulin aspart for every 70 mg/dL above 130 mg/dL. Presuming that her diet is consistent, her SMBG results are as follows:

Time	Glucose Concentration mg/dL
7 AM	140–180
Noon	120–150
5 PM	90–130
11 PM	90–120
3 AM	60–90

Overall, A.H. feels her diabetes is in good control. Her energy level has returned to normal, and her nocturia has diminished, but she occasionally gets up 1 or 2 times nightly to urinate. A.H. has also noticed that nightmares or "sweats" sometimes awaken her. When this occurs, she generally has something to eat because she is "famished." She is able to get back to sleep, but wakes up the next morning with a "splitting headache" and a "hungover" feeling. A.H.'s weight remains the same, and she has begun to develop some consistency in her dietary patterns with the help of a dietitian. She has been consistently correcting her prelunch and predinner insulin doses by adding or subtracting 2 units from her premeal insulin doses based on her premeal BG values. The A1C from her last visit is 7.3%. Evaluate A.H.'s BG values. What are possible causes of A.H.'s fasting hyperglycemia?

When evaluating morning hyperglycemia, several causes must be considered:

- An insufficient basal dose of insulin. If the basal dose is insufficient, hepatic glucose output during the fasting state will be excessive, thereby producing hyperglycemia.
- Insufficient dinner coverage with insulin aspart, resulting in hyperglycemia that persists into the morning. This can be distinguished from an insufficient basal insulin by assessing glucose control at bedtime.
- Reactive hyperglycemia in response to a nocturnal hypoglycemic episode (Somogyi effect or rebound hyperglycemia).
- An excessive bedtime snack.
- The dawn phenomenon (see Case 53-3).

The presence of normoglycemia at bedtime, low BG concentrations at 3 AM, and symptoms of nocturnal hypoglycemia (nightmares, sweating, hunger, morning headache) in A.H. are consistent with a rebound hyperglycemic reaction in the morning (i.e., posthypoglycemic hyperglycemia, also referred to as the Somogyi effect).[108]

Theoretically, this effect occurs after any episode of severe hypoglycemia and is secondary to an excessive increase in glucose production by the liver that is activated by insulin counter-regulatory hormones such as cortisol, glucagon, epinephrine, and growth hormone. The waning effects of the basal insulin dose can also be a cause of fasting hyperglycemia because insulin is needed to suppress hepatic glucose output during the fasting state; however, this is not likely in A.H.'s case. Asymptomatic nocturnal hypoglycemia can occur in patients taking more than necessary doses of insulin in the evening and may potentially cause rebound hyperglycemia in the morning. By correcting the nocturnal hypoglycemia, normalization of A.H.'s fasting hyperglycemia also may be achieved. Thus, a decrease in the daily dose of insulin glargine is warranted. A.H. should continue to monitor her BG concentrations at 3 AM to determine whether her BG levels return to normal.

Caveat: If A.H. were using NPH BID to supply her basal insulin, one option would be to shift the evening injection of NPH from before dinner to bedtime. This preferred method effectively shifts the peak action of NPH to the early morning, when she is awake, and decreases the risk of nocturnal hypoglycemia.[93,109,110] This peak action also corresponds to the dawn phenomenon (see Case 53-3) and the breakfast meal.

Another option if a patient is using NPH and experiencing nocturnal hypoglycemia is to change from NPH to either insulin glargine or insulin detemir because these insulins are associated with less nocturnal hypoglycemia.[111,112] When switching from NPH insulin to insulin detemir, a one-to-one dose conversion may be used although higher doses of detemir may be required. In one crossover study of Type 1 diabetes patients, the average detemir basal dose was approximately double that of the NPH basal dose.[113] However, when switching from NPH insulin to insulin glargine, a one-to-one dose conversion is utilized only when a patient is using NPH insulin once daily. If a patient is taking NPH insulin twice daily, then the total daily insulin dose should be decreased by 20% when switching to insulin glargine. In this case of AH, the daily dose of NPH should be decreased by 20% to determine the insulin glargine dose to err on the conservative side.[76]

Although A.H.'s prelunch BG values are above her goal, this may be attributable to the fasting BG being elevated and then continuing to be elevated mid-morning, like a domino effect. It is important to first correct fasting hyperglycemia and generally correct one BG concentration at a time.

MIXING INSULINS

CASE 53-2, QUESTION 14: If A.H. were to use NPH as basal insulin, how should she be instructed to measure and withdraw this insulin mixture?

Although mixing two insulins in the same syringe has become less common with use of basal-bolus therapy (because insulin glargine and detemir cannot be mixed) and the use of rapid-acting insulin pen devices, the procedure used to mix and withdraw NPH and mealtime insulin (regular or rapid-acting insulin) is basically the same as that described in Case 53-2, Question 8. The major difference is that an adequate volume of air must be injected into the NPH vial before the regular or insulin aspart is measured and withdrawn. Also, the mealtime clear insulin is measured and withdrawn into the insulin syringe *first* to avoid contamination of the vial of regular, aspart, lispro, or glulisine insulin with NPH. For example, contamination with NPH ultimately alters the NPH to regular insulin ratio that is administered. When patients withdraw NPH insulin first, the vial of regular insulin eventually becomes cloudy. In contrast, contamination of the NPH insulin with regular insulin is insignificant because the protamine contained in NPH can bind the regular insulin (see Case 53-2, Question 15). The procedure A.H. should use to mix her insulins is described in the following section, using her morning dose as an example.

- After dispersing the NPH insulin suspension, inject 14 units of air into the NPH vial and withdraw the needle.
- Inject 7 units of air into the insulin aspart vial, and withdraw the 7 units of insulin as described in Case 53-2, Question 8.
- Insert the needle into the NPH vial, and pull the plunger down to the 21-unit mark (14 units of NPH plus 7 units of insulin aspart).

STABILITY OF MIXED INSULINS

CASE 53-2, QUESTION 15: Will mixing NPH with a rapid-acting or regular insulin blunt the rapid action of the mealtime insulins? How stable are other insulin mixtures?

Regular insulin and all of the rapid-acting insulin analogs (aspart, lispro, and glulisine) may be mixed with NPH. In general, it is recommended to mix the insulins just before administration. See Table 53-19 for details on compatibility and stability of insulin mixtures. However, with the increased use of insulin pen devices, mixing of insulins in the same syringe has become a less common practice.

PREMEAL HYPERGLYCEMIA

CASE 53-2, QUESTION 16: After reducing the dose of insulin glargine to 14 units each evening, A.H.'s FPG is now 110 to 125 mg/dL. However, her noon BG concentrations remain in the 120- to 150-mg/dL range. Are there any other changes that you would recommend to make at this time?

Table 53-19
Compatibility of Insulin Mixtures[105]

Mixture	Proportion	Comments
Regular + NPH	Any proportion	The pharmacodynamic profiles of regular and NPH insulin are unchanged when premixed and stored in vials or syringes for up to 3 months
Regular + normal saline	Any proportion	Use within 2–3 hours of preparation
Regular + insulin diluting solution	Any proportion	Stable indefinitely
Rapid-acting + NPH[70–72]	Any proportion	The absorption rate and peak action of the rapid-acting insulins are blunted; total bioavailability is unaltered. Rapid-acting insulin and NPH should be mixed just before use (within 15 minutes)
Insulin glargine and detemir[76,82]	Do not mix with other insulins	Pharmacodynamics could be modified

NPH, neutral protamine Hagedorn.

When evaluating mid-morning hyperglycemia, it is important to remember that the FPG concentration can contribute up to 50% of this plasma glucose excursion. Therefore, a key to the control of mid-morning hyperglycemia may be to normalize the fasting glucose concentration. However, for A.H., the reduction in the insulin glargine has now corrected the reactive fasting hyperglycemia.

Hyperglycemia before a meal can be a result of several factors. The following are possible explanations for A.H.'s mid-morning hyperglycemia:

- An insufficient dose of insulin aspart before breakfast. For A.H., this means that her insulin-to-carbohydrate ratio needs to be adjusted.
- Excessive carbohydrate ingestion at breakfast or inaccurate (under) counting of the carbohydrates ingested. Patients having difficulty accurately counting their carbohydrates should meet with a dietitian or diabetes educator for education; this is often necessary periodically throughout their lives as a refresher, just like many other skills require.
- Poor synchrony between meal intake and insulin action. This could be caused by administration of rapid-acting insulin too long before or after the meal (e.g., ≥30 minutes). If regular insulin is used, this could be caused by administering regular insulin just before or after meals.
- An insufficient dose of evening insulin glargine to suppress hepatic glucose production (glycogenolysis and gluconeogenesis) during the fasting state or the dawn phenomenon (see Case 53-3). However, in A.H.'s case, her FBG values are in target, so this is not likely.

The following interventions may be considered:

- Adjust her insulin-to-carbohydrate ratio to increase her insulin aspart dose at breakfast. The ratio should be changed to 1 unit of aspart for every 10 or 12 g (which are typical ratios used) of carbohydrate for the breakfast meal. This assumes a patient is technically able to use a different "ratio" at different mealtimes.
- Alter the carbohydrate content of the meals. This may include decreasing the amount of carbohydrate in the breakfast meal, changing the type of carbohydrate ingested, or adding fiber to that meal to minimize glucose excursions.
- Adjust the high-sugar correction factor if the glucose excursions appear to be caused by reduced insulin sensitivity in the morning. For example, the high-sugar correction can be adjusted to give 1 unit of aspart for every 50 mg/dL above 130 mg/dL.

PREPRANDIAL HYPOGLYCEMIA

CASE 53-2, QUESTION 17: A.H. is now taking insulin glargine 12 units each night and using an insulin-to-carbohydrate ratio of 1:15 (1 unit of insulin aspart for every 15 g of carbohydrate) at lunch and dinner and 1:12 at breakfast. She is continuing with the same high-sugar premeal correction of 1 unit of insulin aspart for every 70 mg/dL more than her premeal BG target of 120 mg/dL. Two weeks later, she brings in her BG records.

Time	Glucose Concentration (mg/dL)
7 AM	110–120
Noon	90–115
5 PM	60–110
11 PM	80–110
3 AM	110–120

A.H. feels that she is now "back to normal." She has no signs or symptoms of hyperglycemia, and her weight has remained stable. Occasionally, she becomes hypoglycemic before dinner, but this most often occurs when her dinner is delayed because of a hectic work schedule. Evaluate A.H.'s BG trends. What could be the cause of her predinner hypoglycemia, and how could she be managed?

A.H.'s BG concentrations indicate that her basic insulin regimen is generally adequate to achieve the overall goal of preprandial BG concentrations of less than 80 to 130 mg/dL.

The hypoglycemia A.H. is experiencing before dinner could be caused by insufficient carbohydrate intake at lunch (inaccurate carbohydrate counting), increased activity during the day, or an excessive dose of insulin aspart (insulin-to-carbohydrate ratio too high). Thus, the problem could be resolved by augmenting A.H.'s lunch meal, adjusting the lunch insulin-to-carbohydrate ratio to 1 unit of insulin aspart for every 18 (or 20) g of carbohydrate, or adding a mid-afternoon snack.

DAWN PHENOMENON

CASE 53-3

QUESTION 1: R.D., a 37-year-old man, has had Type 1 diabetes since age 14. During the past 2 years, he has been very well controlled on the following insulin regimen: insulin glargine 20 units each morning with insulin lispro 3 to 4 units depending on carbohydrate intake before meals. On this regimen, his BG concentrations for the past 2 weeks have been as follows:

Time	Glucose Concentration (mg/dL)
7 AM	140–170
Noon	100–120
5 PM	100–130
11 PM	115–140
3 AM	100–120

What are the likely causes of R.D.'s fasting hyperglycemia?

As discussed in Case 53-2, Question 13, fasting hyperglycemia may be the result of insufficient doses of insulin in the evening and, possibly, reactive hyperglycemia. In R.D.'s case, the dawn phenomenon also must be considered.[98] The *dawn phenomenon* is a rise in the BG concentration that occurs between 4 and 8 AM after a physiologic nadir in the BG concentration that occurs between midnight and 3 AM. This 30- to 40-mg/dL increase in the morning BG concentration cannot be attributed to increases in counter-regulatory hormones secondary to an antecedent hypoglycemic event, but it may be secondary to rising growth hormone levels. This phenomenon is inconsistently observed in individuals with Type 1 and Type 2 diabetes as well as nondiabetic individuals; furthermore, it is inconsistently present from one day to the next.[114]

R.D.'s normal 3 AM BG concentration indicates that posthypoglycemic hyperglycemia is an unlikely cause of his fasting hyperglycemia. Thus, the modest increase in his BG concentration between 3 and 8 AM may be attributed to the waning effects of insulin or the dawn phenomenon. In both cases, an increase in R.D.'s daily dose of insulin glargine would be indicated. Another option would be to switch R.D. to an insulin pump. He has demonstrated a desire and the ability for intensive management with multiple daily injections, frequent SMBG, record-keeping skills, the ability to make appropriate insulin dose adjustments, and accurate carbohydrate counting. The advantage to using a pump is the ability to program an increase in the basal infusion rate in the early-morning hours (e.g., beginning around 2 to 3 AM and continuing until 7 to 9 AM).

Type 1 Diabetes in Children

DIAGNOSIS AND CLINICAL PRESENTATION

CASE 53-4

QUESTION 1: J.C., a 7-year-old, 30-kg (95th percentile), 50 inches tall (90th percentile) girl, was brought to the emergency department by her parents because of nausea, vomiting, and a persistent stomach pain secondary to the flu. For the past week, J.C. had flulike symptoms, resulting in a 6-lb weight loss. Initial laboratory values revealed a BG of 600 mg/dL, serum pH of 6.8 with bicarbonate level of 13 mEq/L, plasma ketone level of 5.2 mmol/L, and positive ketonuria. J.C. was diagnosed with diabetic ketoacidosis (DKA) secondary to new-onset Type 1 diabetes. In retrospect and on further questioning, J.C.'s parents realized that she probably had symptoms as early as 4 weeks before her hospitalization. While on a driving vacation, she drank large quantities of juice and had to stop hourly to urinate. She began experiencing enuresis, which her parents attributed to her increased fluid intake. What signs and symptoms are consistent with the diagnosis of Type 1 diabetes in a child?

The diagnosis of Type 1 diabetes in children is generally straightforward. Presenting symptoms include a several-week history of polyuria, polydipsia, polyphagia, and weight loss, with hyperglycemia, glucosuria, ketonemia, and ketonuria. J.C.'s presentation is typical for a child newly diagnosed with diabetes who is brought in for medical attention because of severe symptoms related to the flu. An acute viral illness can trigger autoimmune destruction of the pancreas and abdominal pain, which may masquerade as gastroenteritis. Abdominal pain is a common presenting symptom of DKA.[115] J.C.'s weight loss probably represents fluid and caloric loss secondary to uncontrolled diabetes as well as decreased caloric intake from the flu. The symptoms of polyuria are less obvious in an infant and are frequently missed until metabolic derangement has occurred. Unlike J.C., infants frequently present with severe dehydration and metabolic acidosis despite a negative history of diarrhea or significant vomiting.

GOALS OF THERAPY

CASE 53-4, QUESTION 2: What are the goals of therapy for J.C.? Do the results of the DCCT apply to children such as J.C.? Are there age-specific goals?

Current ADA guidelines recommend an A1C goal of <7.5% for all pediatric groups and adolescents (<19 years old) such as J.C. with diabetes mellitus. Individualization of goals however is still encouraged.[7]

Additional targets should also be kept in mind, including (a) to achieve normal growth and development, (b) to facilitate positive psychosocial adjustment to diabetes, and (c) to prevent acute and chronic complications. Attainment of these goals requires a tremendous amount of support and education for the parents and can best be provided by a multidisciplinary team of professionals, including a pediatric endocrinologist, nurse educator, pharmacist, dietitian, and mental health professional.[116]

Growth serves as an important clinical indication of overall general health and well-being in children with diabetes. Height and weight should be measured at each visit and plotted on standard growth grids. If, at the time of diagnosis, a child has fallen behind in height or weight, prompt and appropriate treatment should quickly return the child to the appropriate percentile and pattern of growth. An overweight child should be encouraged to achieve a more appropriate percentile of weight gradually, over the course of several months.[117]

Although recommendations for glycemic control are based on data from studies mostly in adult patients with diabetes, achieving the same near-normalization of BG levels in children and adolescents is recommended. However, special consideration must be given to the unique risks and consequences of hypoglycemia in young children. A cohort of adolescents included in the DCCT was analyzed separately.[118] Similar to the adults in the DCCT, adolescents had sustained benefits from intensive management with little further progression to proliferative retinopathy 4 years after the DCCT was terminated.[119] Thus, J.C.'s pediatrician must strive for the best glucose control that she, her family circumstances, and currently available treatment regimens will permit.

The risk of hypoglycemia is of great concern in children younger than 6 years of age as they can have a form of hypoglycemic unawareness that results partly from their reduced capacity to communicate symptoms of hypoglycemia, but may be contributed to by less-developed counter-regulatory mechanisms.[38] In addition, food intake and physical activity are unpredictable in this age group. These factors must be taken into consideration when determining an A1C goal in this patient population where the long-term benefits of achieving a lower A1C need to be weighed against the risk of hypoglycemia.[116] Per the ADA recommendations, the ultimate goal is to achieve the best A1C possible without experiencing symptoms of hypoglycemia. The management of diabetes in children 6 to 12 years of age, such as J.C., is particularly challenging because many children require insulin with lunch or at other times when they are away from home. Administration of insulin at school demands flexibility and close communications between the parents, the healthcare team, and school personnel. (Table 53-4).[38,116,120] The greatest amount of evidence-based data exists for adolescents with diabetes (13–19 years). As mentioned, teenagers included in the DCCT achieved a mean A1C level of 8.06% in an era before the availability of rapid-acting or basal insulins. As stated previously, an A1C goal of less than 7.5% is recommended in this age group.[38,116,120]

INSULIN THERAPY

CASE 53-4, QUESTION 3: How should J.C. be started on insulin? Is the use of an insulin pump appropriate in children such as J.C.?

Generally, rapid-acting and basal insulin analogs are used in children to reduce the risk of hypoglycemia. Insulin requirements are generally based on body weight, age, and pubertal status. Newly diagnosed children with Type 1 diabetes usually require an initial TDD of approximately 0.5 to 1.0 unit/kg.[116] The small insulin requirements of infants and toddlers may be delivered by using diluted insulin (e.g., 10 units/mL, U-10; or 50 units/mL, U-50)[70,71] to measure doses in less than 1-unit increments. Diluents are available for insulin aspart and lispro. Insulin syringes and pens that deliver insulin in 0.5-unit increments are also very useful in pediatric patients. Most children are treated with basal-bolus regimens. These regimens have demonstrated lower FBG levels with less nocturnal hypoglycemia versus regimens using NPH in children and adolescents.[121]

Basal-bolus insulin regimens combined with carbohydrate counting are attractive regimens for middle and high school students. Because children often have erratic eating habits, rapid-acting insulins are advantageous over regular insulin because they can be injected directly before or immediately after a meal, accounting for the portion of the meal a child actually consumed. J.C. should be started on approximately a TDD of 15 units (i.e., 0.5 units/kg/day), such as 3 units of rapid-acting insulin before meals and 7 units of insulin glargine at bedtime.[116,122] In some patients, insulin glargine may not last a full 24 hours; in this case, the dose of insulin glargine should be divided and given twice daily, and then each adjusted based on the BG patterns.[116] Although U-300 glargine or insulin degludec would last 24 hours, they are not FDA-approved in children at this time.

When J.C. and her caregivers become skilled with carbohydrate counting, insulin kinetics, dosing insulin based on her carbohydrate intake, and diabetes management, the use of an insulin pump may be considered. The insulin pump therapy in the pediatric population is increasing rapidly as it provides increased flexibility with meal timing and has been shown to improve glycemic control and quality of life.[123,124] Young children (not just adolescents) are now recommended for consideration of insulin pump therapy.[123] Family and adult support both at home and school is critical for successful pump use until the child is able to manage his/her diabetes independently.

INJECTION SITES

CASE 53-4, QUESTION 4: Where should J.C. administer her insulin? Are the recommended sites of injection different for children? Does the age of the child play a factor?

For infants with abundant SC tissue, injection sites are usually plentiful. For some toddlers who have lost their "baby fat," locating an appropriate site for injection can be difficult. Injecting insulin into the abdomen of children with minimal SC abdominal fat or in very young children may not be advisable. Rotation of injection sites among arms, thighs, and the upper-outer quadrant of the buttock or hip area, as well as the abdominal area in older children, may be beneficial. To achieve consistent absorption, insulin injections can be patterned, for example, using the arms for the morning injection and the thighs for the evening injection. Children and teens should be cautioned to not consistently inject their insulin into a single area, which may be more convenient for them.[125] Fatty deposits and scar tissue can develop secondary to insulin action at the local tissue level. Insulin absorption from these hypertrophied areas is generally poor and unpredictable, resulting in variability in glycemic control. Insulin pen devices are very helpful for use in children because they are easy to use, have the option for an even smaller needle size, and are less intimidating (see Case 53-2, Question 7).

BLOOD GLUCOSE MONITORING

CASE 53-4, QUESTION 5: How often should J.C. monitor her BG?

The eventual goal for children with diabetes is self-management, with insulin dosing decisions based on interpretation of BG results. Self-management skills and basal-bolus insulin regimens rely on frequent SMBG. For children with Type 1 diabetes, four or more BG tests per day are generally necessary. Many home BG meters allow for alternative site testing (arm or thigh), which decreases the discomfort of fingersticks. Enthusiasm for frequent BG testing tends to wane with duration of diabetes. However, families who are instructed on managing diabetes on the basis of test results are better motivated to persevere with SMBG. CGM may also be considered at some point for improved assessment of her metabolic control, particularly to detect nocturnal hypoglycemia. J.C. should test her BG before each meal and at bedtime, at a minimum. Additional tests should be performed whenever J.C. experiences hypoglycemia, ketonuria, or when she becomes acutely ill.

HONEYMOON PERIOD

CASE 53-4, QUESTION 6: During the next 2 months, J.C.'s insulin requirements decreased to a TDD of 10 units (~0.3 unit/kg). Has her diabetes gone into remission?

Approximately 20% to 30% of individuals with Type 1 diabetes go into a remission phase (honeymoon period) within days to weeks of their diagnosis.[116] During this phase, which can last for weeks to months, insulin requirements can fall well below the usual initial dose of 0.5 to 1.0 units/kg/day, and C-peptide can be detected, indicating a return of pancreatic function. A child may require minimal-to-no basal insulin replacement, and mealtime replacement requirements may need to be reduced. As illustrated by J.C., this presents clinically as markedly decreased insulin requirements to maintain normoglycemia. J.C. should continue to perform SMBG and closely monitor for rising BG concentrations, as β-cell destruction continues during the honeymoon phase and she will eventually return to higher-insulin requirements.

HYPOGLYCEMIA

CASE 53-4, QUESTION 7: J.C.'s parents contacted the clinic to report that J.C. is having nightmares and is awakening in the middle of the night complaining of a headache and stomach pain. However, these symptoms resolve by noon the following day. Her current insulin regimen is insulin aspart 2 units before meals and 3 units of insulin glargine twice daily (at breakfast and bedtime). Could J.C. be experiencing nocturnal hypoglycemia? How do the symptoms of hypoglycemia differ in a child compared with an adult? How can the risk of hypoglycemia be minimized for J.C.?

J.C.'s parents are appropriately worried. Hypoglycemia is a serious and often life-threatening complication of diabetes management in children, and the risk of hypoglycemia increases with attempts to maintain meticulous control of BG levels.[116,126] It was previously thought that pediatric patients may be at risk of cognitive impairment following severe episodes of hypoglycemia; however, current literature does not support this finding. Common causes of hypoglycemia include changes in carbohydrate intake, late or skipped meals or snacks, exercise or unusual activity, and administration of excessive insulin. Because very young children may not be able to identify or express symptoms of hypoglycemia, caretakers must observe the child closely and identify symptoms or behaviors associated with a falling BG. Symptoms of hypoglycemia may include crankiness, sudden crying, restless sleep, or nightmares as seen in J.C.

Hypoglycemia is more frequent in children with lower A1C values, a prior history of severe hypoglycemia, larger insulin doses, and younger children.[127] Nocturnal hypoglycemia is reported in 14% to 47% of children with Type 1 diabetes and is thought to be related to impaired counter-regulatory response to hypoglycemia during sleep.[128] Bedtime BG levels are poor predictors of nocturnal hypoglycemia. J.C.'s parents should be instructed to test her BG at 2 AM closely for the next few nights, and then continue to check at least twice weekly. In children, insulin glargine can exhibit a small peak effect during the initial 3 to 5 hours after administration, increasing the risk for nocturnal hypoglycemia.[116] If this is the case, the insulin glargine dose should be moved to dinnertime or in the morning. If this does not correct the nocturnal hypoglycemia, then the dose should be reduced. Use of insulin glargine is associated with less nocturnal hypoglycemia (and asymptomatic nocturnal hypoglycemia) compared with NPH insulin in children and adolescents.[120,121,129] A bedtime snack may also be needed. Treatment of hypoglycemia is addressed in Case 53-8, Question 3.

SICK DAY MANAGEMENT

CASE 53-5

QUESTION 1: G.M., a 32-year-old woman with Type 1 diabetes, has been well controlled on a basal-bolus regimen (four injections daily) for the past 6 months. However, 2 days ago, she began to exhibit signs and symptoms consistent with the flu. This has made her nauseated, and now she has begun to vomit; consequently, her food intake has been minimal. Because R.D. is not eating at this time, should she discontinue her insulin?

Insulin requirements always increase in the presence of an infection or acute illness, even if food intake is diminished. Patients with Type 1 diabetes, such as G.M., commonly decrease or eliminate insulin doses under these circumstances, and it is in just this setting that ketoacidosis may occur.

Therefore, G.M. should be instructed to maintain her usual dose of insulin and test her BG and urine ketones every 3 to 4 hours. If BG concentrations are above the usual range, extra doses of her rapid-acting insulin should be administered according to a prescribed algorithm based on her body's sensitivity to insulin (e.g., 1 unit for each 50 mg/dL above her BG target). People with Type 1 diabetes should be instructed to test for ketones if their BG concentration is 300 mg/dL or higher. G.M. should call her physician if her BG concentration remains more than 240 mg/dL after three corrective insulin doses; if she has moderate-to-large amounts of ketones in her urine or blood (if using a meter that can measure these); if she has been vomiting or having diarrhea for longer than 6 hours; or if she begins to experience signs and symptoms related to ketoacidosis (polyuria, polydipsia, dehydration, ketonuria, and a fruity breath [see Case 53-10]). G.M. also should attempt to maintain her fluid, mineral, and carbohydrate intake with easily digested food and fluids (Table 53-20).[130]

Table 53-20
Sick Day Management[130]

1. Continue taking your basic dose of insulin *even* if you are not eating well or have nausea or vomiting
2. Test your blood glucose more frequently: every 3–4 hours
3. If indicated, give yourself extra doses (high-sugar correction) of lispro, aspart, glulisine, or regular insulin: for example, 1–2 units for every 30–50 mg/dL over an agreed-on target glucose concentration (e.g., 150 mg/dL). Correction doses must be individualized based on the patient's sensitivity to insulin (Table 53-9)
4. Begin testing your ketones (urine or blood) if you have type 1 diabetes. If you have type 2 diabetes, begin testing especially when glucose readings exceed 300 mg/dL
5. Try to drink plenty of fluids (½ cup/hour for adults) and maintain your caloric intake (50 g carbohydrate every 4 hours). Foods such as gelatin, noncarbonated soft drinks, crackers, soup, and soda may be used
6. Call a physician if your blood glucose concentration remains >300 mg/dL, or your urine ketones remain high after two or three supplemental doses of insulin, or your blood glucose level remains >240 mg/dL for more than 24 hours

INSULIN REQUIREMENTS IN RENAL FAILURE

CASE 53-6

QUESTION 1: M.B., a 32-year-old woman, has had Type 1 diabetes for 15 years. During the past 2 years, a gradual deterioration of her renal function—as reflected by increased proteinuria, serum creatinine (SCr), and blood urea nitrogen (BUN) values, and reduced glomerular filtration rate (GFR)—has been observed. What are the anticipated effects of decreased renal function on M.B.'s insulin requirements?

The effects of renal failure on insulin requirements are complex, and under various circumstances, insulin requirements may increase or decrease. The kidney is the most important site of extrahepatic insulin metabolism and excretion. In nondiabetic individuals, the liver extracts approximately 60% of insulin secreted endogenously before it reaches the peripheral circulation.[63] Because exogenous insulin is delivered directly to the periphery, the kidneys play a more important role in its elimination. Insulin is filtered by the glomerulus and reabsorbed in the proximal tubules, where it is destroyed enzymatically. The kidney also clears insulin from the peritubular circulation.[65,131] At that site, insulin can enhance the reabsorption of sodium, which may account for the edema occasionally observed after the initiation of insulin therapy in some individuals.

Diminished renal function can be accompanied by decreased clearance of endogenous and exogenous insulin, resulting in increased plasma concentrations of insulin. Therefore, M.B.'s insulin requirements may diminish as her renal disease progresses. Patients with moderate degrees of renal failure (GFR >22.5 mL/minute) remove 39% of insulin from arterial plasma, similar to normal subjects. In contrast, patients with severe renal insufficiency (GFR <6 mL/minute) have a marked reduction in insulin removal from arterial plasma (9%).[132] Decreased insulin clearance in conjunction with nausea and decreased food intake associated with uremia can lead to hypoglycemia in such individuals. In some patients with diabetes, particularly those with residual endogenous insulin secretion (e.g., Type 2 diabetes), glucose tolerance may normalize as renal function diminishes, eliminating the need for insulin. In contrast, severe uremia is associated with glucose intolerance. This seems to be related to tissue resistance to insulin secondary to an unknown factor that can be removed by dialysis.

As M.B.'s renal function worsens, a reduction in her insulin requirements should be anticipated.

MANAGEMENT OF THE HOSPITALIZED PATIENT

CASE 53-7

QUESTION 1: A.G., a 55-year-old, 60-kg woman with a 35-year history of Type 1 diabetes, was admitted to the critical care unit for an abdominal hysterectomy. Before admission, she was well controlled on 24 units of insulin glargine at bedtime and premeal doses of insulin aspart. How should A.G.'s diabetes be managed while in the critical care unit?

Patients with diabetes account for more than 1 in 5 hospital days in the United States. Of the nearly $176 billion that is spent annually on diabetes, nearly half is spent on inpatient care.[8] A clear, linear relationship exists between hyperglycemia and adverse clinical outcomes in the hospitalized patient.[133] However, this relationship exists regardless of a baseline diagnosis of diabetes at the time of admission, and iatrogenic hyperglycemia in the hospital does not have the same relationship morbidity that spontaneous hyperglycemia does.[133–135] These observations have raised important questions about the relationship between hyperglycemia and morbidity in the hospitalized patient.

Complex responses to acute illness including excess secretion of catecholamines and cortisol result in peripheral insulin resistance and so-called stress hyperglycemia. This makes it difficult to discern whether glycemia is a marker or a mediator of adverse outcomes in the acutely ill patient. Accordingly, historic practice had been to only aim for BG concentrations that prevent glucosuria (<200 mg/dL) and the subsequent risk for dehydration in the hospitalized patient. However, beginning in 2001, a series of randomized trials tested glycemic control in the critically ill patient. Significant changes have subsequently been made to practice recommendations for both the critically and the noncritically ill hospitalized patient.

Although several trials beginning in the 1990s tested intensive insulin regimens in patients with acute MI, they were small, placebo-controlled studies and reached different conclusions that proved difficult to rectify.[136–139] In 2001, the first of the van den Berghe trials tested two different levels of glycemic control in a relatively large number of surgical intensive care unit (ICU) patients with hyperglycemia with or without known diabetes.[140] A liberal glucose control strategy (reduction only if BG rose above 215 mg/dL) was compared with normalization of BG (80–110 mg/dL). Overall, normalization of BG significantly reduced ICU mortality from 8.0% to 4.5%.[140] However, the same researchers were unable to replicate their findings in a subsequent, similarly designed study in medical ICU patients with substantially higher baseline mortality rates.[141] Although a substudy showed that an ICU stay of 3 days or longer was predictive of benefit from tight control, a subsequent and much larger trial not only failed to confirm that finding but found increased mortality from a blood sugar of 80 to 110 mg/dL compared with 140 to 180 mg/dL (27.5%, 829 of 3,010 vs. 24.9%, 751 of 3,012).[142] The incidence of severe hypoglycemia (<40 mg/dL) in the different study groups assigned to tight control was between 7% and 18% and did not explain the different findings between studies. However, several important differences between these trials, which helped to inform current guidelines, should be noted.

The 2001 van den Berghe trial used parenteral nutrition in all patients and allowed for higher glucose values (insulin started if blood sugar exceeded 215 mg/dL) to occur in the conventional glycemia arm.[140] It is therefore possible that the aggressive insulin therapy in the tight control group helped to blunt the excessive glucotoxicity that may have been occurring from the parenteral nutrition. In the second van den Berghe trial as in the NICE-SUGAR study, parenteral nutrition was rarely used and initiation of insulin therapy in the conventional arms began at blood sugar values greater than 180 mg/dL.[141] Additionally, in NICE-SUGAR, a more aggressive target of less than 180 mg/dL was used rather than 180 to 200 mg/dL as in the two van den Berghe studies.[140–142] Table 53-21 summarizes these three trials assessing level of glucose control in critically ill patients.

Overall, numerous individual studies as well as meta-analyses have reached different conclusions regarding whether or not tight control of BG is superior to conventional control in the hospitalized, acutely ill patient.[143,144]

In 2009, the ADA made substantial changes to its 2005 guideline on management of inpatient hyperglycemia. Although existing randomized trials of glycemic control have been performed in critical care settings, the ADA guideline included non-ICU settings. To make recommendations for non-ICU patients, ADA relied on case series and retrospective analyses, which will ultimately need to be subjected to randomized, prospective trials.[145–147] In the meantime, recommendations for both critically ill and noncritically ill hospitalized patients are the same: a premeal or fasting BG target less than 140 mg/dL and random values of less than 180 mg/dL. A tighter goal of 110 to 140 mgl/dl however may be beneficial in specific subgroups of patients, such as open-heart surgery patients.[145–148]

Table 53-21
Summary Data of Three Major Trials of Intensive vs. Conventional Glycemic Control with Insulin in Critically Ill Patients

Trial	N	Glucose Target (mg/dL)		Glucose Achieved (mg/dL)		Primary Outcome	End Point	OR (95% CI)
		Intensive	Conventional	Intensive	Conventional			
van den Berghe et al.[140]	1,548	80–110	180–200	103	153	ICU mortality	4.6% vs. 8%	0.58 (0.38–0.78)
van den Berghe et al.[141]	1,200	80–110	180–200	111	153	Hospital mortality	37.3% vs. 40.0%	0.94 (0.84–1.06)
NICE-SUGAR[142]	6,104	81–108	<180	115	145	90-day mortality	27.5% vs. 24.9%	1.14 (1.02–1.28)

CI, confidence interval; OR, odds ratio.

For perioperative insulin needs, A.G. should receive her usual basal insulin dose (insulin glargine 24 units) on the night before surgery. If the basal insulin is normally administered in the morning, the usual dose can still be given for patients with Type 1 diabetes; for those with Type 2 diabetes, 50% to 100% of the basal insulin is administered the morning of surgery. Correction doses of rapid-acting insulin can be administered the morning of surgery if the BG is more than 180 mg/dL.[149] If a current A1C is not available, it can be measured to assess the patient's glycemic control before admission.

Most insulin infusion protocols include the use of IV regular insulin and maintenance IV fluids, either 5% dextrose in water (D5W) or D5W with 0.45% normal saline (0.45% NaCl). For a patient requiring fluid restriction, 10% dextrose in water (D10W) may be used.[149] The adjustment algorithms are used by nursing to change the rate of infusion (in units/hour) depending on the BG level. Most often, the insulin infusion is prepared in a solution of 1 unit/1 mL normal saline (e.g., 100 units of regular insulin in 100 mL of 0.9% NaCl). A dedicated IV line is used for the insulin infusion to avoid iatrogenic hypoglycemia. The insulin infusion is connected to the maintenance IV containing dextrose (can be Y-connected). Because insulin binds to plastic, the insulin solution should be flushed (e.g., with 20 mL) through the IV tubing before the line is connected to the patient. An IV dextrose infusion is maintained while a patient is on an insulin infusion. Most patients need 5 to 10 g of glucose per hour (or D5W or D5W/0.45% NaCl at 100–200 mL/hour). Additional maintenance fluids (and electrolytes) can be administered via a different port or line. Some protocols include an initial bolus dose of insulin. The initial insulin infusion rate is primarily based on current BG level and BMI; other factors such as body weight, current daily insulin requirements, and renal function should be taken into consideration. An initial rate of 1 unit/hour is common (can range from 0.5 units/hour to ≥2 units/hour). The choice of initial infusion rate is not critical but should be based on patient history. A rate of 0.5 units/hour is appropriate for a patient who has never previously received insulin, whereas 2 units/hour would be appropriate for a patient with known insulin-dependent diabetes. Adjustments in the insulin infusion rate are determined by BG levels every 60 minutes until the BG is stable and close to target. Then, the frequency of BG testing may be reduced to every 2 to 3 hours. Algorithms should consider both the current and previous BG level, the rate of change of the BG level, and the current infusion rate.[38]

Insulin infusion should be started at least 2 to 3 hours before the surgery to titrate to the desired level of glucose control. Examples of protocols are available on the Institute for Healthcare Improvement's website (available at http://www.ihi.org/IHI/Topics/PatientSafety/MedicationSystems/Tools/), and many are published in the medical literature.[150,151]

Thus, A.G.'s usual SC insulin regimen should be discontinued, and she should be initiated on an insulin infusion that is adjusted according to an algorithm. Throughout the perioperative period, she should receive a minimum of 100 g of glucose daily to prevent starvation ketosis.

Assessment of interfering substances with point-of-care BG testing is particularly important for hospitalized patients. Some immunoglobulins and dialysates contain nonglucose sugars (including maltose, xylose, and galactose), which can interfere with glucose measurements with glucose dehydrogenase pyrroloquinolinequinone test strips (will falsely elevate the reading, Table 53-16). BG concentrations should only be performed by the laboratory in these patients.[152]

Adverse Effects of Insulin

HYPOGLYCEMIA

CASE 53-8

Question 1: G.O., a 42-year-old, slightly overweight (5 feet 11 inches, 200 pounds, BMI 27.9 kg/m^2) man, has had a history of Type 1 diabetes mellitus for 17 years. G.O.'s medical care was sporadic until 1 year ago when he referred himself to a diabetes clinic because he was beginning to experience pain and numbness in his feet. At that time, he was poorly controlled on a single daily dose of a premixed NPH and regular insulin mixture (Humulin 70/30), 45 units. He had not been testing his BG concentrations, and his A1C was 13%.

On physical examination, G.O. was found to have an elevated BP (160/94 mm Hg), background retinopathy, and decreased pedal pulses bilaterally. He had decreased sensation to vibration and monofilament testing in both feet. G.O. also complained of impotence and "shooting pains" in both legs. A spot collection for microalbuminuria was 450 mg of albumin/g creatinine (normal, <30 mg/g creatinine).[38]

G.O. was transitioned to a basal-bolus insulin regimen. His physician gave him a premeal BG target of 80 to 130 mg/dL.[38] For the past several months, he has been treated with the following regimen: 14 to 18 units of insulin glulisine before breakfast; 14 to 18 units of insulin glulisine before lunch; 16 to 18 units of insulin glulisine before dinner; and 40 units of insulin glargine at bedtime. If his BG level is high after lunch, he takes additional glulisine (~2 hours after eating). If his BG is high at bedtime (e.g., >150 mg/dL), he takes additional insulin glulisine (7–10 units) because his physician told him his BG level needed to be lowered significantly. BG concentrations have been as follows:

Time	Glucose Concentration (mg/dL)
7 AM	60–320
Noon	140–280
5 PM	40–300

In the past year, G.O.'s A1C has decreased to 7.1%. Currently, he has approximately five hypoglycemic episodes per week, primarily in the late afternoon and early-morning hours. These are characterized by intense hunger, sweating, palpitations, and (according to his wife) a short temper. He has found that he can avoid nocturnal hypoglycemia (night sweats, nightmares, and headaches) by eating a large bedtime snack. During the past 3 months, he has gained 15 lb. Are G.O.'s signs and symptoms consistent with mild, moderate, or severe hypoglycemia? What are the causes?

G.O.'s case illustrates one of the major hazards of aggressive BG targets and intensive insulin therapy: hypoglycemia. Hypoglycemia is a fact of life for patients with Type 1 diabetes, virtually all of whom experience a hypoglycemic episode at one time or another. Nocturnal hypoglycemia is of particular concern. A syndrome called "dead-in-bed" has been described for patients with Type 1 diabetes, who experience repeated hypoglycemia and have an underlying cardiovascular pathology, and die in their sleep.[153]

Hypoglycemia is a BG concentration less than70mg/dL, and its occurrence is potentially fatal if not promptly recognized and treated. However, the exact level at which a patient experiences symptoms is difficult to define. Clinical hypoglycemia is associated with typical autonomic (neurogenic) and neuroglycopenic symptoms relieved by the administration of a quickly absorbed carbohydrate.

Normal brain function depends on glucose, the exclusive fuel for cerebral metabolism. Because the brain is unable to synthesize or store glucose, it must be provided with a constant exogenous quantity via the brain's blood supply. As BG concentrations fall, a series of physiologic responses occur to restore glucose levels. These responses create symptoms warning a patient to take corrective action by consuming carbohydrates. If these counter-regulatory responses fail to alert the patient and BG concentrations fall below a critical level, cognitive function becomes impaired, and confusion and coma may ensue.

In people without diabetes, the peripheral responses to hypoglycemia are so efficient that clinically important hypoglycemia probably never occurs. As glucose levels fall between 50 and 60 mg/dL, a series of neuroendocrine events occur, raising the plasma glucose concentration back toward normal by increasing hepatic glucose output. The major hormone responsible for producing acute recovery from insulin-induced hypoglycemia is glucagon; however, epinephrine alone also can produce near-normal recovery. Rising levels of adrenergic and cholinergic hormones generate warning symptoms of hypoglycemia. When hypoglycemia is prolonged, growth hormone and cortisone play a greater role in producing recovery.

Patients with Type 1 diabetes who maintain insulin depots throughout the day are predisposed to severe hypoglycemic reactions because deficiencies in the normal feedback system occur with time. Glucagon secretion becomes deficient within the first 2 to 5 years after diagnosis, and by 10 years or longer, epinephrine secretion may become impaired. The latter defect leads to asymptomatic hypoglycemia or hypoglycemic unawareness (see Case 53-9).

Certain circumstances predispose patients with Type 1 diabetes to severe hypoglycemia. These include (a) a defective counter-regulatory hormonal response to hypoglycemia (see Case 53-9), which may be further diminished with frequent hypoglycemia, (b) medications such as β-blockers that diminish early warning signs of impending hypoglycemia, (c) intensive insulin therapy that can alter secretion of counter-regulatory hormones, (d) skipped meals or inadequate carbohydrate intake relative to the insulin dose, (e) physical activity, and (e) excessive alcohol intake (Table 53-12).

Symptoms

The signs and symptoms associated with hypoglycemia vary in intensity according to the presence of cognitive deficits and the patient's ability to self-treat the reaction. They vary substantially from one patient to another. Symptoms are conventionally divided into two categories: neurogenic (or autonomic) and neuroglycopenic.[154]

Autonomic symptoms include sweating, intense hunger, palpitations, tremor, tingling, and anxiety. Epinephrine is thought to mediate many of the neurogenic responses to hypoglycemia.

Neuroglycopenic symptoms resulting from neuronal fuel deprivation (glucose) include difficulty concentrating, lethargy, confusion, agitation, weakness, and possibly, slurred speech, dizziness, and fainting. Profound behavioral changes, seizures, and coma are more severe manifestations of neuroglycopenia. Prolonged, severe neuroglycopenia ultimately results in death. Symptoms of mild, moderate, severe, and nocturnal hypoglycemia are as follows:

- *Mild hypoglycemia:* Symptoms include tremor, palpitations, sweating, and intense hunger. Diminished cerebral function is not present, and patients are capable of self-treating.
- *Moderate hypoglycemia:* Moderate hypoglycemic reactions include neuroglycopenic as well as autonomic symptoms: headache, mood changes, irritability, decreased attention, and drowsiness. Patients may require assistance in treating themselves because of the presence of impaired judgment or weakness. Symptoms are more severe, usually last longer, and often require a second dose of a simple carbohydrate.
- *Severe hypoglycemia:* Symptoms of severe hypoglycemia include unresponsiveness, unconsciousness, or convulsions. These reactions require assistance from another individual for appropriate treatment. Approximately 10% of patients treated with insulin experience at least one severe, disabling episode of hypoglycemia per year that requires emergency treatment with parenteral glucagon or IV glucose.[154]
- *Nocturnal hypoglycemia:* Tingling of the lips and tongue is a common complaint of patients who experience nocturnal hypoglycemia. These patients also may complain of headache and difficulty arising in the morning, nightmares, or nocturnal diaphoresis.[154] Family members should be conscious of any unusual sounds or activity while the patient is sleeping.

G.O. has mild-to-moderate hypoglycemic reactions, which he is able to self-treat. These are likely caused by overinsulinization and insulin "stacking" (giving rapid- or short-acting insulin injections too close together, so that the doses "stack" on top of the other) with his rapid-acting insulin.

OVERINSULINIZATION

CASE 53-8, QUESTION 2: Evaluate G.O.'s overall control. What signs and symptoms in G.O. are consistent with overinsulinization and insulin stacking? How should he be managed?

The following is a list of signs and symptoms of overinsulinization in G.O.:

- A total daily insulin dose of more than 1 unit/kg. This dose is unusually high for a patient with Type 1 diabetes, who should not be resistant to the action of insulin.
- Weight gain in the past several months. This is secondary to the anabolic effects of insulin as well as G.O.'s increased carbohydrate intake to match his high insulin doses for treatment of hypoglycemia.
- Frequent hypoglycemic reactions.
- High glycemic variability (i.e., BG concentrations that fluctuate wildly between hypoglycemia and hyperglycemia). In G.O.'s case, high BG concentrations may represent reactive hyperglycemia or overtreatment of hypoglycemic episodes. His low BG level may represent excessive rapid-acting insulin at bedtime and insulin stacking of his rapid-acting insulin after lunch. At lunchtime, he is administering a high-sugar correction dose of insulin glulisine too soon; his mealtime glulisine is still likely at a peak action and working to lower his prandial BG. By administering additional glulisine soon after the meal, the two insulin doses are adding up, or stacking, causing hypoglycemia.
- Near-normal A1C levels indicate mean BG concentrations that must be within the normal range even though the patient has recorded numerous high BG concentrations. Patients treated with intensive insulin therapy in the DCCT experienced hypoglycemic episodes 3 times more often than patients treated with standard insulin therapy.[29] A1C levels were approximately 7.2%.

G.O. should be managed by discontinuing his high-sugar corrections at bedtime and after lunch. He should check his BG premeal, 1 to 2 hours after meals, and at bedtime to obtain a better picture of his glucose patterns and insulin requirements. He should avoid the large bedtime snack because one should not have to add food just to avoid hypoglycemia (i.e., the insulin regimen should be adjusted). He should also begin testing his BG at 2 or 3 AM to assess whether he is still experiencing nocturnal hypoglycemia after stopping the bedtime insulin glulisine. It will be important that he records the actual dose he administers before each meal and brings the record to clinic so that his insulin doses can be fine-tuned. Next, if he is capable, an algorithm for adjusting his preprandial insulin glulisine doses should be provided to minimize hypoglycemic and hyperglycemic reactions (see Case 53-2, Question 12), eventually he can transition to counting carbohydrates (see Case 53-2, Questions 11 and 12).

TREATMENT OF HYPOGLYCEMIA

CASE 53-8, QUESTION 3: How should G.O.'s hypoglycemic episodes be managed?

As G.O. illustrates, many patients with diabetes are frightened of hypoglycemia and have a tendency to over-treat their reactions with, for example, large quantities of juice or regular soda. This should be discouraged because overcorrection together with glucose generated by counter-regulatory hormones ultimately results in hyperglycemia.

The key to successful management of hypoglycemia is recognition and prevention. Because early warning symptoms of hypoglycemia vary from person to person, it is important that G.O. learns to recognize and pay attention to his earliest warning symptoms and treat early. Patients generally can recall prodromal symptoms after recovery from a severe hypoglycemic reaction if they have not developed hypoglycemic unawareness (see Case 53-9). As a caveat, occasionally patients "feel" hypoglycemic after their BG concentrations have been normalized from very high levels with intensive insulin therapy, owing to the amount of BG change. Encourage patients to test their BG level any time they "feel unusual" to verify a low BG concentration before treatment. G.O. should treat his symptoms only if he is truly hypoglycemic.

A second component of prevention is determining its cause and taking preventive or corrective action. This entails assessment of his diet (did he skip or delay a meal or change its content?), exercise pattern, time of insulin administration, insulin dose, and accuracy of carbohydrate counting and dose administered. If hypoglycemic reactions consistently occur at a certain time of day, he should determine whether this corresponds with a mealtime dose of his rapid-acting insulin and reduces that insulin dose by 1 to 2 units. If his FPG is running low, his insulin glargine dose can be reduced.

If a reaction occurs, G.O. should be instructed to treat it as follows (Table 53-12).

Mild Hypoglycemia

Most hypoglycemic reactions are managed readily with the equivalent of 10 to 20 g of glucose (see Table 53-12 for examples of carbohydrate sources containing 15 g of glucose). If the blood concentration remains low after 15 minutes, the patient should ingest another 10 to 20 g of carbohydrate. This quick-acting source of glucose should be followed by a small complex carbohydrate or protein snack (e.g., milk, peanut butter sandwich) to provide a continual source of glucose if a meal is not scheduled within the next 1 to 2 hours. An easy rule of thumb that can be used by patients is "15-15-15": 15 g of glucose followed by a second 15 g if the patient is still symptomatic after 15 minutes.

Glucose tablets are available and have the added benefit of being premeasured to prevent overtreatment of hypoglycemia. Glucose gels, liquid, or small tubes of cake frosting are useful for children or patients who become uncooperative and combative when hypoglycemic.

Moderate-to-Severe Hypoglycemia

Glucagon can be injected by the SC or IM (preferred) route into the deltoid or anterior thigh region. Glucagon is used when a patient is unable to self-treat their hypoglycemia caused by exogenous insulin. The dose of glucagon recommended to treat moderate or severe hypoglycemia for a child younger than 5 years of age is 0.25 to 0.5 mg; for children 5 to 10 years of age, 0.5 to 1 mg; and for patients older than 10 years, 1 mg. Parents, spouses, or other close contacts should be taught how to mix, draw up, and administer glucagon during emergency situations. Kits with prefilled syringes containing 1 mg glucagon are available. Patients who are given glucagon should be positioned so that their face is turned toward the floor to prevent aspiration in the event of vomiting. As soon as the patient awakens (10–25 minutes), he/she should be fed.

Intravenous Glucose

If glucagon is unavailable, the patient should be taken to the hospital's emergency department, where he/she can be treated with IV glucose (~10–25 g administered as 20–50 mL of 50% dextrose for 1–3 minutes) in preference to glucagon. After the bolus injection of glucose, IV glucose (5–10 g/hour) should be continued until the patient has gained consciousness and is able to eat.

HYPOGLYCEMIC UNAWARENESS

CASE 53-9

QUESTION 1: M.M., a 35-year-old, 75-kg, unemployed man, has had Type 1 diabetes since the age of 3. As a consequence of the diabetes, he has developed proliferative retinopathy and progressive diabetic nephropathy (current SCr, 2.2 mg/dL). M.M. has an erratic lifestyle. Because he does not work, he often stays out late at night and sleeps late into the morning. His insulin is injected whenever he awakens, and his meals are irregularly spaced. Each time he comes to the clinic, he brings with him a complete log of glucose concentrations that range from 80 to 140 mg/dL. He has two to three severe hypoglycemic reactions a month that require trips to the emergency department for treatment with IV glucose. On several occasions, his BG concentration has been 30 mg/dL, and he states he may feel a little weak, but otherwise feels "not too bad." M.M.'s last A1C was 10%. He says that he adheres to the following insulin regimen: 18 units NPH/11 units regular insulin before breakfast, 10 units regular insulin before lunch and dinner, and 14 units NPH at bedtime.

At this visit, M.M. comes with his girlfriend. He has a large gash on his nose that occurred 3 days ago when he lost consciousness at approximately 1:30 PM while pushing his stalled car. He was unable to eat lunch at the usual hour because he had problems with his car. Assess M.M.'s hypoglycemic reactions and BG control. Should his current insulin regimen be continued? How should he be managed?

M.M. illustrates a patient with Type 1 diabetes who has defective glucose counter-regulation and, as a result, is unable to counteract a hypoglycemic reaction effectively. He also is an example of a patient who should not have aggressive BG targets because he does not feel the symptoms of a low blood sugar and has already developed end-stage organ damage (proliferative retinopathy and nephropathy). Neither is likely to be reversed with improved glycemic control. In fact, proliferative retinopathy may actually worsen with intensive insulin therapy initially.[38] In the DCCT study, severe hypoglycemic reactions were 3 times more common among patients treated with intensive insulin therapy, and nocturnal hypoglycemia accounted for 41% of the total hypoglycemic episodes.[29] In patients with defective counter-regulation, the risk of severe hypoglycemia may be 25 times higher than in patients with adequate counter-regulatory mechanisms treated with intensive insulin therapy.[154] M.M. is at great risk for death secondary to hypoglycemia.

M.M.'s lifestyle is erratic, he eats irregularly, and his reported BG concentrations (80–140 mg/dL) do not correspond to his elevated A1C value. This may indicate that M.M.'s technique is incorrect or that he simply fills in the log with fictitious numbers before he comes to the clinic. Irregular entries in different colored inks and bloodstains usually indicate authentic records.

As noted, the primary hormones that are secreted in response to a low BG concentration are glucagon and epinephrine. In patients who have had Type 1 diabetes for longer than 2 to 5 years, a deficiency in glucagon secretion is a relatively consistent finding, and these patients must rely on epinephrine to reverse low BG concentrations.[155] Unfortunately, approximately 40% of patients with long-standing Type 1 diabetes (8–15 years) have defective epinephrine secretion as well, and this may be related to the development of autonomic neuropathy. Patients whose diabetes is tightly controlled also have reduced counter-regulatory hormone responses to hypoglycemia. As illustrated by M.M., patients with defective epinephrine secretory responses also lose the warning signs and symptoms of hypoglycemia. These patients are said to have hypoglycemia unawareness because they have no awareness of BG concentrations less than 50 mg/dL. In these individuals, loss of consciousness, seizures, or irrational behavior may be the first objective sign of exceedingly low BG concentrations. The glycemic threshold for symptoms also is lowered in patients on intensive insulin therapy whose glucose concentrations have been lowered to normal or near-normal levels.[154] Consequently, their hypoglycemic reactions may go unnoticed and untreated until they lose consciousness. M.M. should be managed as follows:

- Because his waking, sleeping, and eating patterns are highly irregular, M.M. should be treated with an insulin regimen that addresses his lifestyle. For example, he could be switched to a basal-bolus insulin regimen, in which he can give himself a rapid-acting insulin just before he actually intends to eat. A dose of insulin glargine or detemir could be given before his first meal to supply a basal level of insulin between meals. Additionally, when switching to insulin glargine or detemir MM should be provided this insulin in a pen formulation as to avoid any dosing errors from drawing insulin into a syringe based on MM's current symptoms of visual impairment.
- Because M.M. has no warning symptoms for hypoglycemia, the importance of regular SMBG should be emphasized. When BG testing was reviewed with M.M., it was discovered that his eyesight was so poor that he was unable to distinguish between the right and wrong side of the glucose test strip. Furthermore, because he had lost his depth of field, he was unable to apply the drop of blood into the test strip. To address this situation, M.M.'s girlfriend was taught how to perform BG testing. Also, a glucose monitor that requires a very small blood sample and beeps with an adequate blood sample would be beneficial for him.
- M.M.'s girlfriend also was taught how to recognize and treat symptoms of hypoglycemia and how to administer glucagon. Often, patients ignore early warning symptoms and progress to a point that they lose the judgment needed to treat the condition. If M.M. has not yet become combative, a quick-acting carbohydrate source should be offered. If he has lost consciousness, glucagon should be injected.

All of these maneuvers diminished the frequency of M.M.'s severe hypoglycemic reactions. On the whole, his BG concentrations were maintained below 180 mg/dL, and he remained relatively free of hyperglycemic symptoms. M.M.'s A1C using a basal-bolus insulin regimen was 8.0%.

DIABETIC KETOACIDOSIS

CASE 53-10

QUESTION 1: J.L., a 40-year-old, 60-kg woman with an 8-year history of Type 1 diabetes, is moderately well controlled on 24 units of insulin glargine plus premeal doses of insulin lispro. Her family brings her to the emergency department, where she complains of abdominal tenderness, nausea, and vomiting. According to her family, J.L. was well until 2 days ago when she awoke with nausea, vomiting, diarrhea, and chills. Because she has been unable to eat, she has omitted her usual morning dose of insulin for the past 2 days. Her gastrointestinal (GI) symptoms progressed, and she was brought to the emergency department when she became lethargic.

Physical examination reveals an ill-appearing woman who is lethargic but responsive. Her temperature is 37°C. Skin turgor is poor, mucous membranes are dry, and her eyeballs are shrunken and soft. J.L.'s lungs are clear, but respirations are deep and her breath has a fruity odor. Cardiac examination is within normal limits.

In the supine position, J.L.'s pulse rate is 115 beats/minute and her BP is 105/60 mm Hg. In the upright position, her pulse increased to 140 beats/minute, and her BP dropped to 85/40 mm Hg. There is mild, diffuse tenderness over her abdomen.

Laboratory results on admission disclosed the following:

BG, 450 mg/dL
Sodium (Na), 150 mEq/L
Potassium (K), 5.4 mEq/L
Chloride (Cl), 106 mEq/L
HCO_3, 10 mEq/L
SCr, 2.0 mg/dL
Hemoglobin, 15.7 g/dL
Hematocrit, 49%
White blood cell count, 15,000/μL with 3% bands (normal, 3%–5%), 70% polymorphonuclear neutrophils (normal, 54%–62%), and 27% lymphocytes (normal, 25%–33%)
Serum ketones, moderate at 1:10 dilution (normal, negative)

The urinalysis showed the following:

Glucose, 2+ (normal, 0)
Moderate ketones (normal, 0)
pH, 5.5 (normal, 4.6–8)
Specific gravity, 1.029 (normal, 1.020–1.025)
No white blood cells, red blood cells, bacteria, or casts

Arterial blood gas results were as follows:

pH, 7.05 (normal, 7.36–7.44)
P_{CO_2}, 20 mm Hg (normal, 35–45)
P_{O_2}, 120 mm Hg (normal, 90–100)

What supports the diagnosis of DKA in J.L.?

The fact that J.L. has Type 1 diabetes puts her at risk for developing ketoacidosis. About 80% of DKA cases occur in patients older than 18 years of age with about one-third of those occurring in patients older than 45 years of age.[151] In DKA, an absolute or relative insulin deficiency promotes lipolysis and metabolism of free fatty acids to β-hydroxybutyrate, acetoacetic acid, and acetone in the liver. Excess glucagon enhances gluconeogenesis and impairs peripheral ketone utilization. Physiologic stress contributes to the development of DKA by stimulating release of insulin counter-regulatory hormones including glucagon, catecholamines, glucocorticoids, and growth hormone. Common stress factors include infection, pregnancy, pancreatitis, trauma, hyperthyroidism, and acute MI.

J.L. presented with symptoms of nausea, vomiting, diarrhea, and chills, and these are suggestive of an acute viral gastroenteritis.

Patients such as J.L. commonly discontinue their insulin in this setting, which can rapidly precipitate the development of DKA (see Case 53-5). Table 53-22 lists patient education points with regard to DKA.

As illustrated by J.L., patients with DKA present with moderate-to-high serum glucose concentrations secondary to decreased peripheral utilization and increased hepatic production (Table 53-23). This increases serum osmolality, which initially shifts fluid from the intracellular to the extracellular space. When serum glucose concentrations exceed the renal threshold for reabsorption of about 200 mg/dL, glucose "spills" over into the urine and causes an osmotic diuresis that depletes the total body water and electrolytes. J.L. also has lost fluid and electrolytes from vomiting and diarrhea. Eventually, as losses exceed input, the patient becomes dehydrated (dry mucous membranes; dry skin; soft, shrunken eyeballs; increased hematocrit), and intravascular volume becomes depleted (orthostatic BP and pulse changes).

The finding of hyperkalemia in J.L. is also common in DKA because insulin contributes to the intracellular shift of potassium.[156] The relative deficiency of insulin in DKA results in an extracellular shift of potassium that is worsened by the acidosis that often develops.[157] A finding of hypokalemia in DKA (<3.3 mg/dL) is uncommon and is a marker of more severe disease. In the hypokalemic patient, the combination of the extracellular shift of potassium and polyuria has led to excessive depletion of total body potassium. Care must be used in these patients to replace potassium intravenously before beginning insulin therapy, which will cause further hypokalemia as potassium shifts back into cells.[156]

Table 53-22

Diabetic Ketoacidosis: Patient Education

Definition: DKA occurs when the body has insufficient insulin

Questions to Ask

1. Has insulin use been discontinued or a dose skipped for any reason?
2. If an insulin pump is being used, is the tubing clogged or twisted? Has the catheter become dislodged?
3. Has the insulin being used lost its activity? Is the bottle of rapid-acting/regular or basal insulin cloudy? Does the bottle of NPH look frosty?
4. Have insulin requirements increased owing to illness or other forms of stress (infection, pregnancy, pancreatitis, trauma, hyperthyroidism, or MI)?

What to Look For

1. Signs and symptoms of hyperglycemia: thirst, excessive urination, fatigue, blurred vision, consistently elevated blood glucose concentrations (>300 mg/dL)
2. Signs of acidosis: fruity breath odor, deep and difficult breathing
3. Signs of dehydration: dry mouth; warm, dry skin; fatigue
4. Others: stomach pain, nausea, vomiting, loss of appetite

What to Do

1. Review "sick day management" (Table 53-20)
2. Test blood glucose ≥4 times daily
3. Test urine for ketones when blood glucose concentration is >300 mg/dL
4. Drink plenty of fluids (water, clear soups)
5. Continue taking insulin dose
6. Contact physician immediately

DKA, diabetic ketoacidosis; MI, myocardial infarction; NPH, neutral protamine Hagedorn.

Table 53-23

Common Laboratory Abnormalities in Diabetic Ketoacidosis (DKA)

Glucose	250 mg/dL
Serum osmolarity	Variable, can be >320 mOsm/kg in presence of coma
Sodium	Low, normal, or high[a]
Potassium	Normal or high
Ketones	Present in urine and blood
pH	Mild: 7.25–7.30
	Moderate: 7.00–7.24
	Severe: <7.00
Bicarbonate	Mild: 15–18 mEq/L
	Moderate: 10 to <15 mEq/L
	Severe: <10 mEq/L
WBC count	15,000–40,000 cells/μL even without evidence of infection

[a]Total body sodium is always low.
WBC, white blood cell.

Evidence of excessive ketone production in J.L. includes ketonuria, ketonemia, and the characteristic fruity odor of acetone on the breath. Elevated levels of these organic acids increase the anion gap and decrease the pH and carbonate levels. The respiratory rate is increased to compensate for the metabolic acidosis leading to hypercapnia.[156,158]

Treatment

CASE 53-10, QUESTION 2: How should J.L. be treated?

Treatment of patients with DKA is aimed at expansion of intravascular and extravascular volume, replacement of electrolyte losses, and cessation of ketone production (Table 53-24).

FLUIDS

Rapid correction of fluid loss is most crucial. The usual fluid deficit is difficult to estimate in the absence of overt hypernatremia but approximates 5% to 10% of body weight in most patients depending on the severity of the DKA. In the absence of cardiac compromise, hypernatremia, or significant renal dysfunction, isotonic saline (0.9% NaCl) should be used.[151]

J.L. has evidence of significant dehydration and intravascular volume depletion. Based on body weight, if the patient has the typical 5% to 10% weight loss, that would indicate approximately 3 to 6 L of fluid will be needed to fully replete (10% of 60 kg = 6-kg loss and 1 L = 1 kg). It is recommended that fluids be replaced at the rate of 15 to 20 mL/kg/hour during the first hour (~1 to 1.5 L in the average adult). The subsequent choice for fluid replacement depends on the patient's state of hydration, serum electrolyte levels, and urinary output. If the corrected sodium is normal or elevated, 0.45% NaCl infused at a rate of 4 to 14 mL/kg/hour is appropriate. If the corrected serum sodium is low, 0.9% NaCl is preferred.[156] When serum glucose concentrations approach 200 mg/dL, solutions should be changed to D5W/0.45% NaCl. Glucose is added to allow the continuation of insulin therapy without causing hypoglycemia (see Case 53-10, Question 5).[156]

Table 53-24

Management of Diabetic Ketoacidosis[156]

Fluid Administration	
Start IV fluids using normal saline (0.9% NaCl) unless patient has cardiac compromise	
Rate is 15–20 mL/kg body weight or 1–1.5 L during first hour	
Then, if corrected sodium is normal or elevated, use 0.45% NaCl at a rate of 4–14 mL/kg/h (250–500 mL/hour). Use 0.9% NaCl if corrected sodium is low	
Once serum glucose reaches 200 mg/dL, change to 5% dextrose with 0.45% NaCl at 150–250 mL/hour	
Insulin	
Continuous IV infusion of regular insulin is preferred. Use IM route only if infusion is not available	
Bolus dose: 0.1 units/kg IV	
Maintenance dose: 0.1 units/kg/h IV	
If blood glucose level has not decreased by 50–75 mg/dL after 1 hour, double infusion rate	
Once blood glucose reaches 200 mg/dL, reduce infusion rate to 0.05–0.1 units/kg/hour and change fluid to 5% dextrose with 0.45% NaCl (do not stop insulin infusion)	
When SC insulin can be initiated, administer dose 1–2 hours before discontinuing IV infusion	
For uncomplicated DKA, SC rapid-acting insulin can be considered. A bolus dose of 0.2 units/kg followed by 0.1 units/kg every hour *or* an initial dose of 0.3 units/kg followed by 0.2 units/kg every 2 hours until the blood glucose reaches <250 mg/dL; then the SC insulin dose is decreased by half (to either 0.05 or 0.1 units/kg every 1–2 hours)	
Potassium	
Establish adequate renal function (urine output ~50 mL/hour). If K is <3.3 mEq/L, hold insulin and give 20–40 mEq/hour until K >3.3 mEq/L. If K is >5.5mEq/L, do not give K and check serum K every 2 hours. If K is >3.3 but <5.3 mEq/L, give 20–30 mEq in each liter of IV fluid to maintain K between 4 and 5 mEq/L	
Phosphate	
Initiate if level <1 mg/dL, or in patients with cardiac dysfunction, anemia, or respiratory depression. Use potassium phosphate salt, 20–30 mEq added to replacement fluid. Rarely needed	
Bicarbonate	
Replacement is controversial and may be dangerous	
For adults with pH <6.9, 100 mmol of sodium bicarbonate may be added to 400 mL of sterile water with 20 mEq of KCl; infuse for 2 hours (200 mL/hour). For adults with pH of 6. 9–7.0, 50 mmol of sodium bicarbonate diluted in 200 mL of sterile water with 10 mEq of KCL; infuse for 1 hour (200 mL/hour). No bicarbonate is necessary if pH >7.0	

DKA, diabetic ketoacidosis; IM, intramuscular; IV, intravenous; SC, subcutaneous.

SODIUM

Total body sodium usually is depleted by 7 to 10 mEq/kg of body weight in patients with DKA. In assessing serum sodium in these patients, it is important to remember that falsely low values (i.e., pseudohyponatremia) may be the result of hyperglycemia and hypertriglyceridemia. A corrected sodium value can be estimated by adding 1.6 mEq/L to the observed sodium value for every 100 mg/dL glucose in excess of 100 mg/dL. Sodium is replaced adequately with normal saline, which has a sodium concentration of 154 mEq/L.[156]

POTASSIUM

Potassium balance is altered markedly in patients with DKA because of combined urinary and GI losses. Invariably, total body potassium is at least partly depleted; however, the serum potassium concentration may be high, normal, or low, depending on the degree of acidosis and volume contraction and severity of insulin deficiency. Usual potassium deficits in this situation average 3 to 5 mEq/kg of body weight, although they may be as high as 10 mEq/kg.[156,158]

Thus, J.L. needs approximately 200 to 350 mEq of potassium to replenish her body stores, assuming her normal weight is 70 kg. To prevent hypokalemia, potassium replacement should be started after her serum potassium concentrations decrease to less than 5.3 mEq/L (assuming an adequate urine output of 50 mL/hour). The addition of 20 to 30 mEq/L is usually sufficient to maintain the serum potassium at greater than 4 mEq/L. In cases when serum potassium is low at presentation (<3.3 mEq/L), potassium replacement should be initiated with fluid therapy, and insulin therapy delayed until the potassium level is greater than 3.3 mEq/L to avoid severe hypokalemia and the risk of cardiac arrhythmias and diaphragmatic weakness. In these cases, initial IV solutions should contain 20 to 30 mEq/L of potassium chloride.

PHOSPHATE

Phosphate is lost as the result of increased tissue catabolism, impaired cellular uptake, and enhanced renal excretion. Like other electrolytes, serum levels initially may seem normal, even though body stores are depleted. However, replacement can result in hypocalcemia, and the use of phosphate in DKA has resulted in no clinical benefit to patients.[156] Severe hypophosphatemia (<1.0 mg/dL) can cause cardiac and skeletal muscle weakness as well as respiratory depression. To avoid this, phosphate can be carefully replaced in patients with cardiac dysfunction or respiratory depression when phosphate concentrations are less than 1.0 mg/dL. Potassium phosphate can be added to the replacement fluids in the amount of 20 to 30 mEq/L.

INSULIN

CASE 53-10, QUESTION 3: What is an appropriate insulin dose and route of administration for J.L.?

Insulin therapy is the key to DKA management because it is what stops the production of ketones. As insulin allows glucose metabolism to resume, the counter-regulatory signals for ketone production are turned off. Unless the episode of DKA is mild (pH 7.25–7.30) and uncomplicated, regular insulin by continuous infusion is the treatment of choice. Once hypokalemia (K^+ <3.3 mEq/L) is excluded or treated, an IV bolus of regular insulin at 0.1 units/kg followed by a continuous infusion at a dose of 0.1 units/kg/hour should be administered. This should decrease the plasma glucose by at least 10% in the first hour. If there is not at least a 10% reduction in the first hour, then a second bolus of 0.15 units/kg should be administered. Once the plasma glucose reaches 200 mg/dL, the insulin infusion can be decreased to 0.05 units/kg/hour. Alternatively, insulin can be switched to SC at a dose of 0.1 units/kg every 2 hours. Regardless of the route of insulin therapy, serum glucose should be maintained at less than 200 mg/dL.[156] At this point, the fluid should be changed to D5W with 0.45% NaCl. Thereafter, the rate of insulin administration and the rate of infusion of D5W with 0.45% NaCl are adjusted to maintain the glucose value at around 200 mg/dL until the ketosis is resolved.[156] Resolution of ketosis is marked by a serum bicarbonate level of at least 15 mEq/L, a venous pH greater than 7.3, and a calculated anion gap of 12 mEq/L or less. Once any two of those three findings are present, the patient can be converted to a longer-acting SC regimen.

For mild DKA (serum bicarbonate ≥15 mEq/L, anion gap <15), SC rapid-acting insulin has been used with no differences in patient outcomes. The advantage is that patients can be treated in a non-ICU setting, thus reducing hospital costs. The dosing for rapid-acting insulin is included in Table 53-24.

SODIUM BICARBONATE

CASE 53-10, QUESTION 4: J.L. was treated with fluids, electrolytes, and insulin as discussed in previous questions. Laboratory and clinical data 4 hours after therapy are as follows:

pH, 7.1
BG, 400 mg/dL
K, 3.8 mEq/L
SCr, 3.1 mg/dL
Serum ketones, strongly positive at a 1:40 dilution

Her BP was 120/70 mm Hg with no orthostatic changes. Urine output for the past 3 hours has been 500 mL. Because serum ketones have increased, should J.L. receive more insulin? Should she receive bicarbonate therapy?

The assumption that ketosis is worse in J.L. is incorrect. In DKA, low levels of insulin and elevated glucagon levels promote the metabolism of free fatty acids in the liver to acetoacetate and β-hydroxybutyrate. The standard nitroprusside reaction test for ketones measures only acetoacetate, even though β-hydroxybutyrate is the more important ketone. The conversion of acetoacetic acid to β-hydroxybutyrate is coupled closely with the reduced NADH:NAD ratio. If this ratio is high (as in the presence of alcohol), so much β-hydroxybutyrate may be formed that acetoacetate is virtually undetectable; thus, the absence of ketones in the serum does not rule out ketoacidosis.

Conversely, treatment with insulin begins to suppress lipolysis and fatty acid oxidation; nicotinamide adenine dinucleotide is regenerated, shifting the reaction back in favor of acetoacetate.[156] Thus, even though there seem to be higher concentrations of ketones in the serum, J.L.'s declining BG concentration, improved bicarbonate concentrations, and improved acid–base and cardiovascular responses indicate that she is responding appropriately. Therefore, no change in the insulin dose is indicated. It is important to emphasize that the glucose concentrations normalize before ketones (4–6 hours vs. 6–12 hours) because the latter are metabolized more slowly. For this reason, it is important to continue insulin to maintain suppression of lipolysis until plasma and urine ketones have cleared.

The use of bicarbonate in patients with DKA has been controversial.[151] Most investigators discourage its routine use, reserving it for patients with severe acidemia (pH <6.9) or those in clinical shock. Coma is correlated most closely with BG concentrations (>700 mg/dL) and hyperosmolality (calculated osmolality >340 mOsm/kg).[156] In a small randomized, prospective study, bicarbonate did not affect recovery in patients with severe DKA (arterial pH, 6.9–7.14).[159] Thus, even though J.L.'s acidosis seemed severe on admission (pH, 7.05; bicarbonate, 10 mEq/L; Kussmaul respirations [deep, frequent respirations resulting in blowing off of CO_2]), bicarbonate was not administered. It is apparent that with fluid and insulin therapy alone, her acidosis is beginning to improve.

CASE 53-10, QUESTION 5: What is the expected course of DKA in J.L.?

After 3 L of fluid and a constant insulin infusion of 6 units/hour for 3 hours, J.L.'s glucose concentration had dropped to 400 mg/dL and she had no orthostatic BP changes, reflecting recovery from her volume-depleted status. Potassium (40 mEq/L) was added to her fluids, which were administered at a reduced rate of 300 mL/hour.

Three hours later, the glucose concentration had dropped to 350 mg/dL and her pH had increased to 7.21 with an anion gap of 24 mEq/L. The serum potassium remained low-normal at 3.4 mEq/L, and serum sodium increased to 151 mEq/L. In view of these changes, the IV infusion fluid was changed to half-normal saline with 5% dextrose to which 40 mEq/L of potassium was added. The rate was slowed to 250 mL/hour, and the insulin infusion was continued at 6 units/hour.

Four hours later (10 hours after admission), the BG was 205 mg/dL and the serum potassium was 3.5 mEq/dL. The IV fluids were changed to 5% dextrose with 40 mEq/L of potassium chloride, administered at a rate of 250 mL/hour, and the regular insulin infusion was decreased from 6 to 3 units/hour. J.L. continued to improve during the next 12 hours, and she began taking full oral liquids by the second hospital day. At that time, her IV infusion rate was decreased to 200 mL/hour, but her insulin infusion was continued.

Approximately 24 hours after admission, J.L.'s BG concentration was 175 mg/dL, potassium was 4.6 mEq/L, sodium was 144 mEq/L, and the anion gap had closed down to 16 mEq/L. There were no ketones in the plasma. The urine contained 1% glucose and moderate amounts of ketones. IV fluids were discontinued, and a rapid-acting insulin was administered SC 1 hour before the insulin infusion was discontinued. J.L. continued to receive rapid-acting insulin SC every 4 hours according to a sliding scale (see Case 53-2, Question 12). Thirty-six hours after admission, J.L. was given her usual dose of insulin glargine and insulin lispro and was sent home for follow-up in the clinic.

TREATMENT OF TYPE 2 DIABETES: ANTIDIABETIC AGENTS

Type 2 diabetes must be managed in the context of the metabolic syndrome. At the time of diagnosis, many people with Type 2 diabetes already have evidence of macrovascular and microvascular disease. Every effort to lower glucose concentrations toward normal values and to control BP and lipids is important to delay the onset or slow the progression of these complications, improve the overall quality of the patient's life, and save the healthcare system millions of dollars in hospitalization costs to treat these complications. MNT, physical activity, and SMBG are cornerstones in the treatment of people with Type 2 diabetes. Unfortunately, these measures alone are usually not successful in achieving control for the majority of patients, and drug therapy is eventually required. Because these patients also often require a number of medications to treat related conditions (e.g., hypertension, dyslipidemia, CVD, and depression) and may also be medicating themselves with over-the-counter drugs, herbal products, and nutritional supplements, the aim of therapy for Type 2 diabetes should be the simplest and safest regimen that provides the best glycemic control possible.

Tables 53-25 and 53-26 summarize the comparative pharmacology, pharmacokinetics, and dosing of the noninsulin antidiabetic drugs. The clinical use of these agents in specific situations is illustrated in cases presented later in this chapter.

Biguanides

Metformin belongs to the biguanide class of oral antidiabetic agents. It has been available in the United States since 1995 and became generically available in 2002. Currently, both the immediate-release and the extended-release formulations are available generically. The clinical pharmacology of metformin has been extensively reviewed.[160]

MECHANISM OF ACTION

The biguanides are described more accurately as antihyperglycemic agents. Although they lower BG concentrations in people with Type 2 diabetes, they do not cause hypoglycemia in nondiabetic individuals or individuals with diabetes when used as monotherapy. Partly because of this lack of hypoglycemia, metformin is recommended by the ADA to reduce the risk for developing diabetes in patients at high risk (IGT and IFG) because of its strong evidence base and long-term safety. Metformin is considered first-line therapy for diabetes because it is the only agent with outcome data showing a reduction in all-cause mortality and vascular complications independent of glycemic control.[7,160] Metformin primarily lowers FPG concentrations by decreasing hepatic gluconeogenesis, but it also increases insulin-stimulated glucose uptake by skeletal muscle and adipose tissue and also decreases intestinal absorption of glucose.[160]

Metformin has been shown to activate 5′ adenosine monophosphate-activated protein kinase (AMPK), a major regulator of glucose and lipid metabolism.[161] The primary cellular site of metformin is thought to be complex I in the mitochondria, whose inhibition by metformin leads to the activation of AMPK.[162] Through AMPK activation, acetyl-CoA carboxylase is inactivated, resulting in decreased lipid synthesis and increased fatty acid oxidation. Sterol regulatory element-binding protein-1, a key lipogenic transcription factor, is also suppressed, leading to a reduction in hepatic lipid production. AMPK activation is also thought to play a role in metformin's inhibition of hepatocyte glucose production and induction of muscle glucose uptake.[161,163]

Metformin modestly lowers total cholesterol and triglycerides and may maintain or improve HDL-C levels.[164] The observed effects on lipid metabolism as well as others on clotting factors, platelet function, and vascular function may impart some of metformin's favorable effects on CVD and outcomes (see Case 53-11, Question 3). A key advantage with metformin is that weight loss rather than weight gain is more likely to occur with its use (mean weight loss of 0.5 to 3.8 kg can occur in adults receiving metformin immediate-release tablets as monotherapy and negligible weight loss occurs with extended-release tablets).[164]

PHARMACOKINETICS

Approximately 50% to 60% of metformin is absorbed from the small intestine, and peak plasma concentrations are achieved at approximately 2.5 hours.[164] Approximately 10% of an oral dose is excreted in the feces and about 90% of a dose is excreted through an active tubular process in the kidneys. The rate and extent of absorption are both decreased by food. Metformin has a plasma half-life of 6.2 hours in patients with normal renal function and a whole-blood half-life of 17.6 hours.[164] It is not bound to plasma proteins.

ADVERSE EFFECTS

Gastrointestinal Effects

Transient side effects include diarrhea and other GI disturbances such as nausea, abdominal discomfort, metallic taste, flatulence and anorexia.[164] Relative to placebo, diarrhea is the most common GI complaint with immediate-release tablets (53.2% metformin vs. 11.7% placebo-treated patients) and occurs in roughly 9.6% of patients taking extended-release tablets. Symptoms can be minimized by taking metformin with food and slowly titrating the dose. To enhance adherence to therapy, patients should be informed of the possibility of GI side effects that will likely subside with continued use, and instructed to discuss any suspected side effects with their provider before discontinuing therapy (see Case 53-11, Question 4).

Lactic Acidosis

Much of the perceived risk of lactic acidosis secondary to metformin use is based on historical data for phenformin, a biguanide that was withdrawn from the market in 1977.[165] The risk of lactic acidosis secondary to metformin is 10 to 20 times lower than with phenformin. Unlike phenformin, metformin is not metabolized, does not inhibit peripheral glucose oxidation, and does not enhance peripheral lactate production.[166] However, it may decrease conversion of lactate to glucose (decreased gluconeogenesis) and increase lactate production in the gut and liver.[166,167] Metformin has rarely been associated with lactic acidosis. The few patients in whom this event has been reported had renal, liver, or cardiorespiratory contraindications to the use of biguanides. A Cochrane review including 347 studies compared the risk of lactic acidosis among patients taking metformin, placebo, or other nonbiguanide therapies. The review found no difference between groups in either lactate levels or in the development of lactic acidosis.[157] Despite the rarity of lactic acidosis with metformin therapy, patients should be warned to bring the following symptoms of lactic acidosis to the attention of their physician: weakness, malaise, myalgias, abdominal distress, and heavy, labored breathing (see Case 53-16, Question 2).

CONTRAINDICATIONS AND PRECAUTIONS

Patients with renal impairment, liver disease, or other states predisposing them to hypoxia, acute or chronic metabolic acidosis, DKA, or a history of lactic acidosis should be excluded from therapy.[164] Metformin can accumulate in patients whose renal function is impaired, thereby increasing their risk for lactic acidosis. For this reason, metformin caries a black box warning. Its use is not recommended in patients with a decreased GFR (see Dosage and Clinical Use; see Case 53-16, Question 2, for detailed discussion) or elevated creatinine levels ($\geq$1.4 mg/dL for women or $\geq$1.5 mg/dL for men[164]). Because even a temporary reduction in renal function could cause lactic acidosis in patients taking metformin, the manufacturer recommends withholding it after some radiologic procedures (see Drug Interactions section).

Other predisposing factors for lactic acidosis include the following: excessive alcohol ingestion, dehydration, surgery, decompensated congestive HF, hepatic failure, shock, or sepsis. Because aging is associated with reduced renal function, metformin should be titrated to the minimal effective dose and renal function should be monitored regularly. An estimated GFR (eGFR) or creatinine clearance (ClCr) should be measured in patients older than 80 years of age to ensure adequate renal function prior to metformin use, because these patients are more susceptible to experiencing lactic acidosis.[164]

DRUG INTERACTIONS

- Alcohol potentiates the effect of metformin on lactate metabolism. Patients should be warned against excessive alcohol intake while taking metformin. Metformin should be avoided in patients who are alcoholics.
- Vitamin B_{12} absorption may be decreased in patients taking metformin. Each 1 g/day increment dose of metformin significantly increases the odds of vitamin B_{12} deficiency, as well as taking metformin therapy for more than 3 years.
- Dofetilide should not be administered in patients taking metformin due to the competition for common renal tubular transport systems, which may result in an increase in the plasma concentrations of either drug.
- Topiramate should be avoided in patients on metformin because topiramate may increase the risk of developing lactic acidosis.
- Parenteral contrast studies (e.g., pyelography or angiography) that use iodinated materials can result in acute renal failure and increase the risk of metformin-induced lactic acidosis. For patients requiring such a study, metformin should be withheld at the time of or before and for 48 hours after the procedure. Metformin should be reinstituted only after renal function has been re-evaluated and determined to be normal.

EFFICACY

As monotherapy, metformin can be expected to reduce the A1C by 1.3% to 2.0% and the FPG by 50 to 70 mg/dL.[160] Research suggests that certain genetic variations may impact patient response to metformin therapy. Patients exhibiting reduced function polymorphisms of organic cation transporter 1, which is involved in the hepatic uptake of metformin, may be less responsive to metformin therapy.[168]

DOSAGE AND CLINICAL USE

Metformin is the first line of therapy for Type 2 diabetes.[7,38] The ADA recommends its initiation as monotherapy in combination with lifestyle interventions (e.g., MNT, physical activity, weight-loss education, lifestyle education) on diagnosis. To minimize GI side effects, metformin should be initiated at 500 mg twice a day or 850 mg once a day, to be taken with food, followed by weekly increases in 500 mg increments or 850mg increases every 2 weeks (see Case 53-11, Question 4). Metformin is dosed 2 to 3 times daily (500–1,000 mg/dose; maximal dose 2,550 mg/day or 850 mg PO 3 times a day [TID]), unless an extended-release preparation is prescribed. Using the ER formulation as initial therapy may decrease GI side effects. It should still be initiated at 500 mg daily and titrated similarly. It can, however, be dosed once a day, usually with the evening meal. Clinicians should obtain a SCr/eGFR (using the Modification of Diet in Renal Disease equation) and hepatic function tests at baseline and then annually. A recent review[169] recommends that metformin dose reduction should be considered in patients with an eGFR <45 mL/minute/1.73 m^2 and the TDD should not exceed 1,000 mg/day. Renal function should be closely monitored in these patients every 3 months. Metformin should be discontinued in patients with an eGFR <30 mL/minute/1.73 m^2 or in patients with additional risk factors such as hypotension, hypoxia, sepsis, or an increased risk for acute kidney injury (e.g., use of radiocontrast dye in patients with an eGFR <60 mL/minute/1.73 m^2). Metformin should not be used in patients older than 80 years unless a ClCr/eGFR demonstrates normal renal function.[7] Patients are good candidates for treatment if the ClCr is more than 60 mL/minute (or eGFR >60 mL/minute/1.73 m^2). For patients unable to achieve goals of therapy with metformin alone within 3 months of initiating therapy, addition of insulin or another agent should be considered (also see Case 53-13).

Nonsulfonylurea Insulin Secretagogues (Glinides)

Repaglinide (Prandin) and nateglinide (Starlix) are nonsulfonylurea insulin secretagogues (i.e., they stimulate insulin secretion). They belong to a class of agents referred to as meglitinides and are often called "glinides." Repaglinide was approved by the FDA in December 1997, and nateglinide was approved in December 2000 (Table 53-25).

MECHANISM OF ACTION

These agents close the adenosine triphosphate (ATP)-sensitive potassium channels in the β-cell, which leads to cell membrane depolarization, an influx of calcium, and secretion of insulin. The release of insulin depends on the glucose level and decreases at low concentrations of glucose.[170,171] Unlike the sulfonylureas, they have a rapid onset and shorter duration of action, so they are given with meals to enhance postprandial glucose utilization.

PHARMACOKINETICS

Repaglinide has a bioavailability of 56% and is rapidly absorbed and excreted.[170] Its maximal serum concentration (C_{max}) occurs at approximately 1 hour, and its half-life is 1 hour. Repaglinide is highly (>98%) protein bound (volume of distribution, 31 L). It is completely metabolized (via cytochrome P-450 [CYP] 3A4 and 2C8) by the liver to inactive products, with 90% excreted in the feces and 8% excreted in urine. Nateglinide has a bioavailability of 73%.[171] It is rapidly absorbed, with a C_{max} occurring within 1 hour after dosing and a half-life of 1.5 hours. Nateglinide is metabolized (CYP 2C9, 70%; CYP 3A4, 30%) to less-potent compounds, which are 75% excreted in the urine and 10% in the feces. Sixteen percent is excreted unchanged in the urine. It is highly (98%) protein bound, primarily to albumin, and, to a lesser extent, to α_1-acid glycoprotein.

ADVERSE EFFECTS

Mild hypoglycemia may occur, particularly if patients delay or forget to eat after the dose. A weight gain of 0.9 to 3 kg compared with baseline has been observed.[170,171] Rare side effects include elevated hepatic enzymes and hypersensitivity reactions. There has been at least one case report of repaglinide-induced hepatic toxicity.[172]

CONTRAINDICATIONS AND PRECAUTIONS

Because a functioning pancreas is required, these agents should not be used in people with Type 1 diabetes. They should be used with caution in patients with liver dysfunction. They are contraindicated for use in patients with DKA. Repaglinide clearance is reduced in patients with severe renal insufficiency, but may still be used safely at a reduced dose.[170] The clearance of nateglinide is not affected in patients with moderate-to-severe renal insufficiency.[171]

Table 53-25

Comparative Pharmacology of Antidiabetic Agents

Agent/Generic Name (Brand Name)/ Mechanism	FDA Indications	A1C Efficacy[a]	Adverse Effects	Comments
Insulin Replaces or augments endogenous insulin	Monotherapy; combined with any oral agent	↓ A1C[b] ↓FPG[b] ↓ PPG[b] ↓ TG	Hypoglycemia, weight gain, lipodystrophy, local skin reactions	Offers flexible dosing to match lifestyle and glucose concentrations. Rapid onset. Safe in pregnancy, renal failure, and liver dysfunction. Drug of choice when patients do not respond to other antidiabetic agents
Insulin-Augmenting Agents				
Nonsulfonylurea secretagogues (glinides) Repaglinide (Prandin) Nateglinide (Starlix) Stimulates insulin secretion	Monotherapy; combined with metformin or TZD	Monotherapy: ↓ A1C ~1% (repaglinide) ↓ A1C ~0.5% (nateglinide) Combination: additional 1% ↓ A1C	Hypoglycemia, weight gain	Take only with meals. If a meal is skipped, skip a dose. Flexible dosing with lifestyle. Safe in renal and liver failure. Rapid onset. Useful to lower PPG
Sulfonylureas Various; see Table 53-26. Stimulates insulin secretion. May decrease hepatic glucose output and enhance peripheral glucose utilization	Monotherapy; combined with metformin; combined with insulin (glimepiride)	Monotherapy: ↓ A1C ~1% Combination: additional 1% ↓ in A1C	Hypoglycemia, especially long-acting agents; weight gain (5–10 lb); rash, hepatotoxicity, alcohol intolerance, and hyponatremia rare	Very effective agents. Some can be dosed once daily. Rapid onset of effect (1 week)
Incretin-Based Therapies				
Glucagon-like peptide-1 receptor agonists/incretin mimetic Exenatide (Byetta) Extended-release exenatide (Bydureon) Liraglutide (Victoza) Dulaglutide (Trulicity) Albiglutide (Tanzeum) Stimulates insulin secretion, delays gastric emptying, reduces postprandial glucagon levels, improved satiety	Monotherapy (exenatide only) Combined with metformin, SFU, or TZD; combined with metformin + SFU; combined with metformin + TZD Exenatide and liraglutide can be used in combination with basal insulin	Monotherapy: ↓ A1C 0.8%–0.9% Combination: additional 1% ↓ in A1C	GI: nausea, vomiting, diarrhea; hypoglycemia (with SFUs); weight loss; reports of acute pancreatitis; URTIs	Weight loss. Exenatide: take within 60 minutes before morning and evening meals or before 2 main meals of the day (≥6 hours apart). Liraglutide, extended-release exenatide, dulaglutide, albiglutide: Do not use if personal or family history of medullary thyroid carcinoma (MTC) or in patients with multiple endocrine neoplasia syndrome type 2. Do not use in patients with gastroparesis or severe GI disease. Administered by SC injection; pen device in use does not need to be refrigerated. Rare cases of pancreatitis
DPP-4 inhibitors Sitagliptin (Januvia) Saxagliptin (Onglyza) Linagliptin (Tradjenta) Alogliptin (Nesina) Stimulates insulin secretion and reduces postprandial glucagon levels	Monotherapy; combined with metformin, SFU, or TZD; insulin (sitagliptin, linagliptin, and saxagliptin)	Monotherapy: ↓ A1C 0.5%–0.8% Combination: ↓ A1C 0.5%–0.9%	Headache, nasopharyngitis, hypoglycemia (with SFU), rash (rare)	Dosed once daily. Taken with or without food. No weight gain or nausea. Need to adjust sitagliptin, saxagliptin, and alogliptin dose in renal dysfunction. Reduce dose of SFU when combined. Rare reports of pancreatitis

Table 53-25
Comparative Pharmacology of Antidiabetic Agents (*continued*)

Agent/Generic Name (Brand Name)/ Mechanism	FDA Indications	A1C Efficacy[a]	Adverse Effects	Comments
Amylin Receptor Agonists				
Amylin mimetic Pramlintide (Symlin)	Type 1: Adjunct to mealtime insulin	T1: ↓ A1C 0.33% T2: ↓ A1C 0.40%	GI: nausea, decreased appetite	Take only immediately before meals; administered by SC injection. Do not use in patients with gastroparesis. Reduce dose of mealtime insulin by 50% to avoid hypoglycemia when starting therapy
Stimulates insulin secretion, delays gastric emptying, reduces postprandial glucagon levels, improved satiety	Type 2: Adjunct to mealtime insulin; ± SFU and metformin		Headache; hypoglycemia; weight loss (mild)	
Insulin Sensitizers				
Biguanides Metformin (Glucophage) ↓ Hepatic glucose output; ↑ peripheral glucose uptake	Monotherapy; combined with SFU or TZD; or with insulin	Monotherapy: ↓ A1C ~1% Combination: additional 1% ↓ in A1C	GI: nausea, cramping, diarrhea; lactic acidosis (rare)	Titrate dose slowly to minimize GI effects. No hypoglycemia or weight gain; weight loss possible. Mild reduction in cholesterol. Do not use in patients with renal or severe hepatic dysfunction
Thiazolidinediones Rosiglitazone (Avandia) Pioglitazone (Actos) Enhances insulin action in periphery; increases glucose utilization by muscle and fat tissue; decreases hepatic glucose output	Monotherapy; combined with SFU, TZD, or insulin; combined with SFU + TZD	Monotherapy: ↓ A1C ~1% Combination: additional 1% ↓ in A1C	Mild anemia; fluid retention and edema, weight gain, macular edema, fractures (in women)	Can cause or exacerbate HF; do not use in patients with symptomatic HF or class III or IV HF. Rosiglitazone may increase risk of MI. Increased risk of distal fractures in older women. Pioglitazone may increase risk of bladder cancer when used for >1 year. Slight reduction in TG with pioglitazone; slight increase in LDL-C with rosiglitazone. LFTs must be measured at baseline and periodically thereafter. Slow onset (2–4 weeks)
Glucose Reabsorption Inhibitors				
Sodium–Glucose Cotransporter Type 2 Inhibitors Canagliflozin (Invokana) Dapagliflozin (Farxiga) Empagliflozin (Jardiance) Selectively and reversibly bind to SGLT-2 preventing reabsorption of glucose leading to the excretion of glucose in the urine	May be used as 2nd or 3rd line agent or 1st line in patients who cannot tolerate metformin.	↓A1C 0.7-1.0% ↓FPG ↓PPG May cause weight loss	Genital mycotic infections Urinary tract infections ↓GFR in patients with renal failure	Low risk of hypoglycemia Contraindicated in renal failure GFR<30

(continued)

Table 53-25

Comparative Pharmacology of Antidiabetic Agents (*continued*)

Agent/Generic Name (Brand Name)/ Mechanism	FDA Indications	A1C Efficacy[a]	Adverse Effects	Comments
Delayers of Carbohydrate Absorption				
α-Glucosidase inhibitors Acarbose (Precose) Miglitol (Glyset) Slow absorption of complex carbohydrates	Monotherapy; combined with SFUs, metformin, or insulin	Monotherapy: ↓ A1C ~0.5% Combination: additional ~0.5% ↓ A1C	GI: flatulence, diarrhea. Elevations in LFTs seen in doses >50 mg TID of acarbose	Useful for PPG control (↓ PPG 25–50 mg/dL). LFTs should be monitored every 3 months during the first year of therapy and periodically thereafter. Because miglitol is not metabolized, monitoring of LFTs is not required. Titrate dose slowly to minimize GI effects. No hypoglycemia or weight gain. If used in combination with hypoglycemic agents, advise patients to treat hypoglycemia with glucose tablets because absorption is not inhibited as with sucrose. Avoid use in patients with GI disorders (IBD, Crohn disease, intestinal obstruction)
Bile acid sequestrant Colesevelam (Welchol)	Combined with metformin, SFU, or insulin	↓ A1C 0.3%–0.4%	Constipation, dyspepsia, and nausea; ↑ TG	Added benefit of ↓ LDL-C (by 12%–16%). Administer certain drugs 4 hours before. Take with a meal and liquid
Enhancers of Dopaminergic Tone				
Bromocriptine (Cycloset)	Monotherapy; combined with SFU or metformin in patients with type 2 diabetes	Monotherapy ↓ A1C 0.1%; Combo: ↓ A1C 0.5%	Hypotension, dizziness, syncope, nausea, somnolence, headache, exacerbation of psychotic disorders	Very limited role as a therapeutic agent

[a]Comparative effectiveness data provided for SFUs, glinides, TZDs, and α-glucosidase inhibitors.[256]
Theoretically, unlimited glucose lowering with insulin therapy.
A1C, glycosylated hemoglobin; DPP-4, dipeptidyl peptidase-4; FDA, Food and Drug Administration; FPG, fasting plasma glucose; GI, gastrointestinal; HF, heart failure; LDL-C, low-density lipoprotein cholesterol; LFTs, liver function tests; MI, myocardial infarction; PPG, postprandial glucose; SC, subcutaneously; SFU, sulfonylureas; TG, triglycerides; TID, 3 times a day; T1, type 1 diabetes; T2, type 2 diabetes; TZD, thiazolidinediones.

DRUG INTERACTIONS

Clinically relevant drug interactions include those that occur when these drugs are taken in combination with other glucose-lowering agents or drugs known to induce or inhibit their metabolism.[173] Therefore, BG levels should be closely monitored when either drug is taken in combination with other agents known to lower BG or affect their metabolism. Repaglinide is metabolized by CYP 2C8 and 3A4.[170] Studies have shown that repaglinide has no pharmacokinetic effects on digoxin or warfarin. Gemfibrozil should be avoided in combination with repaglinide owing to the risk of hypoglycemia. The combination of gemfibrozil and itraconazole synergistically inhibits repaglinide metabolism and should be avoided. Concomitant use of clopidogrel may result in increased serum concentrations of repaglinide; therefore, dose reduction of repaglinide may be required. Cyclosporine inhibits the metabolism of repaglinide causing increased serum concentrations of repaglinide; therefore, a dose reduction may be required. Nateglinide is metabolized largely by CYP 2C9 (70%) and to a lesser extent by 3A4 (30%).[171] When evaluated in clinical studies, there were no clinically relevant interactions with nateglinide and glyburide, metformin, digoxin, diclofenac, or warfarin. Concomitant use of oral systemic azole antifungals should be used cautiously due to potential for increased hypoglycemic effects. Fibric acid derivatives including fenofibrate, clofibrate, and gemfibrozil may increase the effects of nateglinide. Concomitant use of either repaglinide or nateglinide with rifampin may lower their efficacy.[173]

EFFICACY

The efficacy of repaglinide is comparable to metformin and the sulfonylureas.[174] When used as monotherapy, the mean decrease in FPG, postprandial glucose, and the A1C values were 61 mg/dL, 104 mg/dL, and 1.7%, respectively, compared with placebo (−31.0

mg/dL, −47.6 mg/dL, and −0.6% compared with baseline).[170] Nateglinide as monotherapy results in a mean decrease in FPG and A1C of 13.6 mg/dL and 0.7%, respectively, compared with placebo (−4.5 mg/dL and −0.5% compared with baseline).[171] In comparison with metformin monotherapy, both drugs produce a similar or slightly smaller reduction in A1C.

DOSAGE AND CLINICAL USE

Repaglinide and nateglinide are approved to treat people with Type 2 diabetes as monotherapy or in combination with metformin or a TZD.[170,171] Because they have the same mechanism of action as the sulfonylureas, combining these agents does not produce any additional benefit. The agents are usually added to therapy for patients with postprandial hyperglycemia, particularly nateglinide. When repaglinide is used as the initial treatment in patients who are naïve to oral antidiabetic therapy or in patients with A1C values less than 8%, the recommended starting dose is 0.5 mg 15 to 30 minutes prior to eating up to 4 times a day. When used in patients who have failed sulfonylureas or in those with A1C values greater than 8%, the initial dose is 1 to 2 mg with each meal up to 4 times a day. Doses can be titrated weekly at a rate of 1 mg/meal to a maximum of 4 mg/dose or 16 mg/day. Repaglinide should be initiated at a 0.5-mg dose in patients with severe renal dysfunction and should be titrated cautiously in patients with liver dysfunction. The recommended starting dose of nateglinide is 120 mg TID 0 to 30 minutes before meals. For patients close to their A1C goal, a dose of 60 mg TID may be used. Doses should be omitted if a meal is skipped and added if an extra meal is ingested (repaglinide only). There are no dosage adjustments required for nateglinide in patients with renal or hepatic insufficiency.[170,171]

Sulfonylureas

Until metformin and other antidiabetic agents became available in the United States, sulfonylureas were the first-line pharmacologic treatment for people with Type 2 diabetes who had failed diet and exercise therapy. Six sulfonylureas are available in the United States. The three first-generation sulfonylureas (chlorpropamide, tolazamide, and tolbutamide) are considered equally effective despite differences in their pharmacokinetic properties and adverse effect profiles (see the following discussion and Tables 53-25 and 53-26).

Glipizide and glyburide, two second-generation sulfonylureas, were first introduced into the United States in May 1984. Glimepiride was approved for use in 1995. Despite being approximately 100 times more potent than the first-generation sulfonylureas on a

Table 53-26
Antidiabetic Pharmacokinetic Data

Drug (Brand Name), Available Tablet Strengths (mg)	Typical Dosing Regimen (mg)	Usual Minimum and Maximum Total Daily Dose (TDD)/ How Divided	Mean Half-Life	Approximate Duration of Activity	Bioavailability, Metabolism, and Excretion	Comments
α-Glucosidase Inhibitors						
Acarbose (Precose) 25, 50, 100 mg	25–100 mg with first bite of each meal Begin with 25 mg; ↑ by 25 mg/meal every 4–8 weeks	Minimum: 25 mg TID Maximum dose is 50 mg TID if ≤60 kg; 100 mg TID if >60 kg	2 hours	Affects absorption of complex carbohydrates in a single meal	*F* = 0.5%–1.7%; extensively metabolized by GI amylases to inactive products; 50% excreted unchanged in the feces	Titrate doses slowly to avoid GI effects
Miglitol (Glyset) 25, 50, 100 mg	25–100 mg with first bite of each meal Begin with 25 mg; ↑ by 25 mg/meal every 4–8 weeks	Minimum: 25 mg TID Maximum: 100 mg TID	2 hours	Affects absorption of complex carbohydrates in a single meal	Dose of 25 mg is completely absorbed; dose of 100 mg 50%–70% absorbed; elimination by renal excretion as unchanged drug	
Biguanides						
Metformin (Glucophage) 500, 850, 1000 mg; 500 mg/mL liquid	Begin with 500 mg daily or BID; ↑ by 500 mg daily every 1–2 weeks	0.5–2.5 g BID or TID	Plasma, 6.2 hours. Whole blood, 17.6 hours	6–12 hours	*F* = 50%–60%; excreted unchanged in urine	Take with food. Avoid in patients with renal dysfunction or those who could be predisposed to lactic acidosis (e.g., alcoholism, severe HF, severe respiratory disorders, liver failure)

(continued)

Table 53-26
Antidiabetic Pharmacokinetic Data (*continued*)

Drug (Brand Name), Available Tablet Strengths (mg)	Typical Dosing Regimen (mg)	Usual Minimum and Maximum Total Daily Dose (TDD)/ How Divided	Mean Half-Life	Approximate Duration of Activity	Bioavailability, Metabolism, and Excretion	Comments
Metformin extended-release (Glucophage XR) 500, 750, 1000 mg	500–1,000 mg daily with evening meal; ↑ by 500 mg every 1–2 weeks	1,500–2,000 mg daily	As for metformin, but active drug is released slowly	24 hours	As for metformin	As for metformin
Nonsulfonylurea Insulin Secretagogues (Glinides)						
Repaglinide (Prandin) 0.5, 1, 2 mg	If A1C is <8% or if this is first drug, begin with 0.5 mg with each meal. For others, begin with 1–2 mg/meal	0.5–4 mg with each meal (16 mg/d) TID or QID	1 hour	C_{max} is at 1 hour; duration is approximately 2–3 hours	*F* = 56%; 92% metabolized to inactive products by the liver; 8% excreted as metabolites unchanged in the urine	Take only with meals. Skip dose if meal is skipped. Maximum dose per meal is 4 mg
Nateglinide (Starlix) 60, 120 mg	120 mg TID 1–30 minutes before meals; 60 mg TID for patients with near-normal A1C at initiation	60 or 120 mg TID	1.5 hours	Onset, 20 minutes; peak, 1 hours; duration, 2–4 hours	*F* = 73%; metabolized to inactive products (predominantly) that are excreted in the urine (83%) and feces (10%)	Skip dose if meal is skipped
First-Generation Sulfonylureas						
Acetohexamide (Dymelor) 250, 500 mg	250 or 500 mg daily; ↑ by 250 mg daily every 1–2 weeks	0. 25–1.5 g daily or BID	5 hours (active metabolite)	12–18 hours	Activity of metabolite greater then parent drug. Metabolite excreted, in part, by kidney	Caution in elderly and patients with renal disease. Significant uricosuric effects
Chlorpropamide (Diabinese) 100, 250 mg	100 or 250 mg daily; ↑ by 100 or 250 mg every 1–2 weeks	0.1–0.5 g daily	≥35 hours	24–72 hours	Inactive and weakly active metabolites; 20% excreted unchanged; varies widely	Caution in elderly and patients with renal impairment. Highest frequency of side effects relative to other sulfonylureas
Tolazamide (Tolinase) 100, 250, 500 mg	100–250 mg daily; ↑ by 100 or 250 mg every 1–2 weeks	0.2–1 g daily or BID	7 hours (4–25)	12–24 hours	Some metabolites with moderate activity excreted via kidney	Active metabolites may accumulate in renal failure
Tolbutamide (Orinase) 250, 500 mg	250 mg BID before meals; ↑ by 250 mg daily every 1–2 weeks	0.5–3 g BID or TID	7 hours	6–12 hours	Metabolized to compounds with negligible activity	No special precautions Shortest-acting sulfonylurea
Second-Generation Sulfonylureas						
Glimepiride (Amaryl) 1, 2, 4 mg	1–2 mg daily initially; usual maintenance dose is 1–4 mg	1–8 mg daily	9 hours	24 hours	*F* = 100% completely metabolized by liver. Principal metabolite is slightly active (30% of parent compound). Excreted by the urine (60%) and feces (40%)	Probably safe in patients with renal failure, but low initial doses recommended for older patients and those with renal insufficiency. Incidence of hypoglycemia may be lower than other long-acting sulfonylureas

Table 53-26
Antidiabetic Pharmacokinetic Data (*continued*)

Drug (Brand Name), Available Tablet Strengths (mg)	Typical Dosing Regimen (mg)	Usual Minimum and Maximum Total Daily Dose (TDD)/ How Divided	Mean Half-Life	Approximate Duration of Activity	Bioavailability, Metabolism, and Excretion	Comments
Glipizide (Glucotrol) 5, 10 mg	2.5 mg daily in elderly, 5 mg daily in others; ↑ by 2.5 or 5 mg every 1–2 weeks	2.5–40 mg daily or BID[a]	2–4 hours	12–24 hours	Metabolized to inactive compounds	No special precautions daily dose >15 mg should be divided. Dose 30 minutes before meals
Glipizide extended-release (Glucotrol XL) 5 mg	5 mg daily; ↑ by 5 mg every 1–2 weeks	5–20 mg daily	4–13 hours	24 hours	Same as glipizide	Use with caution in patients with preexisting GI narrowing owing to possible obstruction
Glyburide (Diabeta, Micronase) 1.25, 2.5, 5 mg	1.25 mg daily in elderly, 2.5 mg daily in others; ↑ by 1.25 or 2.5 mg every 1–2 weeks	1.25–20 mg daily or BID	4–13 hours	12–24 hours	Metabolized to inactive or weakly inactive compounds; 50% excreted in urine and 50% in feces.	Caution in elderly patients with renal failure and others predisposed to hypoglycemia. Daily doses >10 mg should be divided
Micronized glyburide (Glynase PresTab) 1.5, 3 mg	1.5 mg daily; ↑ by 1.5 mg every 1–2 weeks	1.0–12 mg daily	4 hours	24 hours	Metabolized to inactive or weakly inactive compounds; 50% excreted in urine and 50% in feces.	Daily doses >6 mg should be divided. ↑ Bioavailability relative to original formulation. Resulted in reduced dose
Thiazolidinediones						
Rosiglitazone (Avandia) 2, 4, 8 mg	4 mg daily; ↑ to 8 mg daily (or 4 mg BID)	4–8 mg daily in single or divided doses	3–4 hours	Onset and duration poorly correlated with half-life because of mechanism of action. Onset at 3 weeks; max at ≥4 weeks. Offset likely to be similar	F = 99%; extensively metabolized in liver into inactive metabolites; excreted $^2/_3$ in urine and $^1/_3$ in feces.	Food has no effect on absorption. BID dosing may have greater A1C lowering effect. No dose adjustments required in renal failure. Avoid in patients with liver disease and heart failure
Pioglitazone (Actos) 15, 30, 45 mg	15–30 mg daily; ↑ to 45 mg daily. If used with insulin, ↓ insulin dose by 10%–25% once FPG <120 mg/dL	15–45 mg daily	3–7 hours (16–24 hours for all metabolites)	Same as previous	Extensively metabolized in liver; 15%–30% excreted in urine, remainder eliminated in the feces	Food delays absorption but is not clinically significant. No dose adjustments required in renal disease. Avoid in patients with liver disease and heart failure

(*continued*)

Table 53-26
Antidiabetic Pharmacokinetic Data (*continued*)

Drug (Brand Name), Available Tablet Strengths (mg)	Typical Dosing Regimen (mg)	Usual Minimum and Maximum Total Daily Dose (TDD)/ How Divided	Mean Half-Life	Approximate Duration of Activity	Bioavailability, Metabolism, and Excretion	Comments
GLP-1 Receptor Agonists/Incretin Mimetics						
Exenatide (Byetta)	5 mcg SC BID; ↑ to 10 mcg SC BID after 1 month	5–10 mcg BID	2.4 hours	C_{max} is at 2.1 hours; duration 10 hours	Glomerular filtration	Take within 60 minutes before morning and evening meal. Nausea usually subsides with time
Exenatide ER (Bydureon)	2mg SC once weekly	2 mg once weekly	10 weeks	Initial Cmax is at 2 weeks, second peak is at 6 to 7 weeks	Glomerular filtration	Take daily without regard to meals. Nausea usually subsides with time.
Liraglutide (Victoza)	0.6 mg daily for 1 week; ↑ to 1.2 mg daily	0.6–1.8 mg daily	13 hours	24 hours; C_{max} is 8–12 hours after dosing	Metabolized as other large proteins	Take daily without regard to meals. Nausea usually subsides with time
Dulaglutide (Trulicity)	0.75 mg SC once weekly; can ↑ to 1.5 mg once weekly	0.75–1.5 mg weekly	Approximately 5 days	Cmax is at 48 hours	Degraded into amino acids by protein catabolism	Take daily without regard to meals. Nausea usually subsides with time
Albiglutide (Tanzeum)	30 mg SC once weekly; can ↑ to 50 mg once weekly	30–50 mg weekly	Approximately 5 days	Cmax is at 3 to 5 days after administration	Metabolized by ubiquitous proteolytic enzymes into small peptides and amino acids	Take daily without regard to meals. Nausea usually subsides with time
DPP-4 Inhibitors						
Sitagliptin (Januvia)	100 mg daily CrCl ≥30 to <50 mL/minute: 50 mg daily CrCl <30 mL/minute: 25 mg daily	100 mg daily	12.4 hours	24 hours	*F* = 87%; 79% excreted unchanged in urine	Requires dose adjustment in renal insufficiency
Saxagliptin (Onglyza)	5 mg daily CrCl ≤50 mL/min: 2.5 mg daily	2.5–5 mg daily	2.5 hours (3.1 hours for active metabolite)	24 hours	Metabolized by CYP 3A4/5 Excreted by renal and hepatic pathways	Active metabolite is ½ as potent Reduce dose to 2.5 mg with strong CYP 3A4/5 inhibitors
Linagliptin (Tradjenta)	5 mg daily	5 mg daily	12 hours	24 hours	*F* = 30%; 90% excreted unchanged (80% enterohepatic system, 5% urine). Small fraction metabolized to inactive metabolite	No dose adjustment needed in liver or renal disease

Table 53-26
Antidiabetic Pharmacokinetic Data (*continued*)

Drug (Brand Name), Available Tablet Strengths (mg)	Typical Dosing Regimen (mg)	Usual Minimum and Maximum Total Daily Dose (TDD)/ How Divided	Mean Half-Life	Approximate Duration of Activity	Bioavailability, Metabolism, and Excretion	Comments
Alogliptin (Nesina)	25 mg daily CrCl 30 to 59 mL/minute: 12.5 mg daily CrCl <30 mL/minute: 6.25mg daily	25 mg daily	21 hours	24 hours	F=100%, 76% excreted unchanged and 13% eliminated in feces. Small fraction metabolized to inactive metabolite	Requires dose adjustment in renal insufficiency
Amylin Mimetics						
Pramlintide (Symlin)	Type 1 DM: 15 mcg SC before major meals; ↑ by 15-mcg increments after minimum of 3 days Type 2 DM: 60 mcg SC before major meals; ↑ to 120 mcg after 3–7 days	Type 1: 15–60 mcg before major meals Type 2: 60 or 120 mcg before major meals	48 minutes	C_{max} is 20 minutes	*F* = 30%–40%; metabolized by kidneys	Reduce mealtime insulin dose by 50%. Titrate dose if no significant nausea
SGLT-2 Inhibitors						
Canagliflozin (Invokana)	100 mg by mouth before first meal	May increase to 300 mg daily	10.6 hours		*F* = ~65% *Metabolism:* Primarily UGT1A9 and UGT2B4. ~7% Metabolized through CYP3A4	
Dapagliflozin (Farxiga)	5 mg by mouth daily before first meal	May increase to 10 mg daily	12.9 hours		*F* = 78% *Metabolism:* Primarily (UGT) isoenzyme 1A9.	
Empagliflozin (Jardiance)	10 mg by mouth daily before first meal	May increase to 25 mg daily	12.4 Hours		*Metabolism:* Primarily through glucuronidation by UGT2B7, UGT1A3, UGT1A8, UGT1A9	
Bile Acid Sequestrants						
Colesevelam (Welchol)	6 tablets once daily or 3 tablets BID [625 mg tablets]	3.75 g	N/A	N/A	Drug is not absorbed systemically and not metabolized	Take with food and liquid. Do not use if history of bowel obstruction, TG >500 mg/dL, or history of pancreatitis from ↑ TG.

(*continued*)

Table 53-26
Antidiabetic Pharmacokinetic Data (*continued*)

Drug (Brand Name), Available Tablet Strengths (mg)	Typical Dosing Regimen (mg)	Usual Minimum and Maximum Total Daily Dose (TDD)/ How Divided	Mean Half-Life	Approximate Duration of Activity	Bioavailability, Metabolism, and Excretion	Comments
Enhancers of Dopaminergic Tone						
Bromocriptine (Cycloset), 0.8 mg	1.6–4.8 mg once daily in the morning; Begin with 0.8 mg daily and increase by 1 tablet each week until max tolerated dose	1.6–4.8 mg daily	6 hours		*F* = 65%–95% Metabolized extensively by CYP3A4; 93% undergoes first-pass metabolism Excreted primarily in bile; 2%–6% in urine	Take with food to reduce GI side effects. Food increases AUC. Highly protein bound

A1C, glycosylated hemoglobin; BID, 2 times a day; C_{max}, maximal concentration; CrCl, creatinine clearance; CYP, cytochrome P-450; DM, diabetes mellitus; DPP-4, dipeptidyl peptidase-4; F, bioavailability; FPG, fasting plasma glucose; GI, gastrointestinal; GLP-1, glucagon-like peptide-1; HF, heart failure; N/A, not available; QID, 4 times a day; SC, subcutaneously; TG, triglycerides; TID, 3 times a day.

milligram-for-milligram basis, these agents are not more clinically effective. Their duration of activity allows for once- or twice-daily dosing.

MECHANISM OF ACTION

Sulfonylureas stimulate the release of insulin from pancreatic β-cells and enhance β-cell sensitivity to glucose. A specific sulfonylurea receptor closely linked to the ATP-sensitive potassium ion channel exists on the β-cell. Sulfonylureas inhibit this potassium ion channel, thus blocking the efflux of potassium and lowering the membrane potential to cause depolarization. The voltage-dependent calcium channels then open, increasing intracellular calcium concentration. The increased intracellular concentration of calcium ultimately stimulates preformed insulin secretion. Additionally, sulfonylureas can normalize hepatic glucose production and enhance peripheral glucose disposal.[63,175]

PHARMACOKINETICS

The duration of hypoglycemic activity is related to the half-life of these compounds only in very general terms and may correlate poorly in some cases.[176] All sulfonylureas are highly protein bound (90%–100%), mainly to albumin. Binding characteristics, however, vary among individual sulfonylureas. Food does not impair the extent of drug absorption, but may delay the time to peak levels of some agents. The relationship between sulfonylurea doses and their BG-lowering effect remains unclear. Studies of glyburide and glipizide suggest that these agents may operate within a narrow range of plasma concentrations that may be achieved with low (10 mg/day) doses.[177–179] The maximal recommended daily doses of 40 mg for glipizide and 20 mg for glyburide may therefore not be more effective and may decrease β-cell function.[179]

Glipizide is an intermediate-acting second-generation agent with a half-life of 2 to 4 hours, but a duration of action of 12 to 24 hours. Patients receiving less than 20 mg/day may require only once-daily dosing. Food delays its rate of absorption, but not its bioavailability. Glipizide should be taken 30 minutes before meals. The onset of action occurs in 90 minutes, and the maximum decrease in serum glucose occurs within 2 to 3 hours. Glipizide is extensively metabolized by the liver to inactive products that are eliminated primarily by the kidney.[176] An extended-release formulation of glipizide also is available.

Glyburide is a longer-acting second-generation agent similar to glipizide. The half-life is approximately 1.5 to 4 hours after single-dose studies and up to 13.7 hours when chronically administered.[180] Nevertheless, as with glipizide, the duration of action can last for up to 24 hours in many patients, allowing for once-daily dosing with small-to-intermediate doses (<15 mg). Food does not delay the rate or extent of absorption. The onset of action is 2 hours, and the maximum decrease in serum glucose occurs within 3 to 4 hours. Glyburide is metabolized completely by the liver to two weakly active metabolites, half of which are excreted in the urine and feces. A micronized formulation is available (e.g., Glynase PresTab), but it is not bioequivalent to the conventionally formulated tablets. Thus, patients switched between the conventional form and the micronized product must be carefully monitored and the dose titrated again.

Glimepiride is a long-acting second-generation sulfonylurea. Its half-life is 9 hours and its duration of action is 24 hours, allowing for once-daily dosing.[181] The administration of glimepiride with food slightly decreases the AUC and slightly increases the time to peak concentration. Its peak effect on plasma glucose concentrations is observed 2 to 3 hours after each dose. Glimepiride is completely metabolized by the liver, and its principal metabolite has 30% of the activity of the parent drug. Metabolites are excreted in feces and urine. Interestingly, research suggests that the sulfonylureas may close ATP-sensitive potassium channels in cardiac tissue, similar to their action at the β-cell. In the heart, this effect could prevent vasodilation during an ischemic episode (i.e., ischemic preconditioning).[182]

ADVERSE EFFECTS

The primary side effects of the sulfonylureas are hypoglycemia (particularly for those that are long-acting, see Case 53-16, Question 2, and Case 53-18, Question 6) and weight gain (~2 kg).[114] Other adverse effects attributed to the sulfonylureas generally are so infrequent and mild that fewer than 2% of patients discontinue these agents because of them. In general, the type, incidence, and severity of reported side effects are similar for all the sulfonylureas. An important exception is chlorpropamide, which has several unique adverse effects (see following discussion). Adverse reactions to the sulfonylureas include GI symptoms (nausea, fullness, bloating that can be relieved if taken with meals), rare blood dyscrasias, allergic dermatologic reactions and photosensitivity, hepatotoxicity, and hyponatremia (also see Case 53-16).[161]

A disulfiram (Antabuse-like) reaction occurs when patients take certain sulfonylureas (primarily chlorpropamide, occurring in approximately one-third of patients receiving it) and drink ethanol. The flushing reaction is rare with other sulfonylureas.

The syndrome of inappropriate secretion of antidiuretic hormone can occur with chlorpropamide and, to a lesser extent, with tolbutamide, but these agents are rarely used in the United States anymore. If it occurs, the syndrome of inappropriate secretion of antidiuretic hormone is a syndrome of enhanced secretion of vasopressin from the pituitary. This results in an increase in the retention of free water by the kidneys and a dilutional hyponatremia. In the UKPDS study, the increase in BP seen in patients on chlorpropamide was likely attributable to water retention.[35] In contrast to chlorpropamide and tolbutamide, glipizide, glyburide, tolazamide, and acetohexamide have a very mild diuretic effect.

CONTRAINDICATIONS AND PRECAUTIONS

Contraindications to the use of sulfonylureas include the following:

1. Type 1 diabetes;
2. Pregnancy or breast-feeding, because these agents (except glyburide) can cross the placental barrier and can be excreted into breast milk;
3. Documented hypersensitivity to sulfonylureas;
4. Severe hepatic or renal dysfunction;
5. Severe, acute intercurrent illness (e.g., infection, MI), surgery, or other stress that can unduly affect BG control, in which case insulin therapy should be used; and
6. G6PD deficiency—Patients with this deficiency may be at risk for hemolytic anemia if they take chlorpropamide—consider using a nonsulfonylurea medication as an alternative.

DRUG INTERACTIONS

Drug interactions with sulfonylureas have a pharmacodynamic or pharmacokinetic basis. Pharmacodynamic interactions are discussed later in this chapter in sections addressing drug-induced hypoglycemia and hyperglycemia. Most of the reported pharmacokinetic drug interactions with the sulfonylureas involve chlorpropamide and tolbutamide. Because most of the clinically significant interactions occur with drugs that alter liver metabolism or urinary excretion, possible interactions with all of the sulfonylureas must be anticipated, even though the outcomes may be quite different. Glipizide and glyburide also differ from the first-generation agents in that they are highly bound to albumin at nonionic rather than ionic sites.[176] On this basis, these agents are unlikely to interact with other highly protein-bound drugs, such as phenylbutazone, salicylates, or certain sulfonamide antibiotics that have been reported to enhance the effects of the first-generation sulfonylureas. These highly protein-bound drugs, however, seem to interact with the sulfonylureas by altering their hepatic metabolism as well. Therefore, glipizide and glyburide should be used cautiously with drugs reported to interact with first-generation sulfonylureas. Sulfonylureas are CYP 2C9 substrates; therefore, coadministration with a medication that is an inhibitor or inducer of CPY 2C9 will increase or decrease levels of sulfonylurea medications, respectively.[173]

EFFICACY

Like metformin, the sulfonylureas decrease the A1C by 1.5% to 1.7% and the FPG by 50% to 70%. With time and increased duration of Type 2 diabetes, the pancreas may respond less to a sulfonylurea. Whether sulfonylureas actually contribute to β-cell dysfunction and decline remains to be clearly determined.[183]

DOSAGE AND CLINICAL USE

The sulfonylureas are effective, inexpensive, and easy to titrate. Sulfonylureas are generally used as add-on therapy to patients unable to achieve BG goals on metformin monotherapy. Like the other antidiabetic agents discussed here, sulfonylureas may also be considered as monotherapy in patients with contraindications to metformin therapy. The doses of the sulfonylureas are displayed in Table 53-26. As a general rule, one should begin with low doses and titrate upward every 1 to 2 weeks until the desired goal is achieved. Exceeding maximal doses is not likely to produce improvement, but may put the patient at risk for adverse effects (see Case 53-18, Questions 5 and 6).

Thiazolidinediones

MECHANISM OF ACTION

The two available TZDs in the United States, rosiglitazone and pioglitazone, are often referred to as insulin sensitizers. The precise molecular actions of these agents remain to be clarified. TZDs bind to and activate a nuclear receptor (peroxisome proliferator-activated receptor-γ [PPAR-γ]), which is expressed in many insulin-sensitive tissues, including adipose (major site), skeletal muscle, and liver tissue.[184] PPAR-γ regulates transcription of genes that influence glucose and lipid metabolism. For example, PPAR-γ stimulation increases the transcription of GLUT-4, a glucose transporter that stimulates glucose uptake.[185] Reduced expression of GLUT-4 may contribute to the development of insulin resistance. Pioglitazone activates PPAR-α in addition to PPAR-y, which inhibits the transcription of tumor necrosis factor-α-induced vascular cell adhesion molecule (VCAM-1).[185] This duel effect by pioglitazone enables HDL to be raised and triglycerides to be lowered. PPAR-α activation is involved in actions that are anti-inflammatory and the PPAR-y and -α activation can improve insulin sensitivity and lipid profiles.[186]

TZDs either directly or indirectly sensitize adipose tissue to insulin action.[175,184] The effects may include stimulating apoptosis of large adipocytes, increasing the number of small adipose cells, and promoting fatty acid uptake and storage in adipose tissue. The subsequent reduction in free circulating fatty acids may spare other insulin-sensitive tissues (e.g., liver, skeletal muscle, β-cells) from the effects of lipotoxicity. TZDs also lower expression of tumor necrosis factor-α, a cytokine produced by adipose tissue that may contribute to insulin resistance and fatty acid release.[175,184] Other adipokines are likely involved, including adiponectin, resistin, and leptin.[175] TZD interaction with adipocytes may be their primary mechanism of action in sensitizing other tissues to insulin action. As with metformin, TZDs have been shown to directly stimulate the AMPK pathway in liver and adipose tissue, resulting in a lowering of glucose and free fatty acids.[164,184]

Other observed effects of TZDs that may be beneficial in patients with Type 2 diabetes and metabolic syndrome include favorable effects on triglycerides, reduction of inflammatory mediators, inhibition of vascular smooth muscle cell proliferation, improved endothelial function, lowering microalbumin excretion, and enhanced fi brinolysis.[175,184] Despite these apparently favorable effects on surrogate measures of vascular disease, the data regarding TZDs and vascular risk are mixed and controversial. In 2009, the FDA added language to the label for rosiglitazone indicating an increased risk of angina and MI. The Food and Drug Administration and GlaxoSmithKline instituted a Risk Evaluation and Management Strategy (REMS) to restrict the distribution and prescribing of rosiglitazone; however, in May, 2014, the REMS was changed to allow for the prescribing and filling of prescriptions of rosiglitazone.

In summary, the TZDs clinically decrease insulin resistance in muscle and liver, which enhances glucose utilization and decreases hepatic glucose output. They have favorable effects on markers of vascular disease such as triglycerides and inflammatory cytokines.

PHARMACOKINETICS

Rosiglitazone is completely absorbed, with peak plasma concentrations reached in approximately 1 hour.[187] Pioglitazone has a bioavailability of 83%, with peak plasma concentrations reached within 2 hours.[185] Food delays the time to peak concentration, but does not alter the extent of absorption of either drug. Both TZDs are extensively (>99%) protein bound, primarily to albumin. The plasma elimination half-life of rosiglitazone is 3 to 4 hours.[187] Pioglitazone has a serum half-life of 3 to 7 hours, and its metabolites have a serum half-life of 16 to 24 hours.[185] Rosiglitazone is extensively metabolized in the liver by CYP 2C8 and to a much lesser extent by 2C9. Its conjugated metabolites are considerably less potent than the parent drug and are excreted two-thirds in urine and one-third in feces.[187] Pioglitazone is hepatically metabolized, mainly by CYP 2C8 and 3A4, and to a lesser degree by CYP 1A1, to three active metabolites; however, the main metabolites found in serum are M-III and M-IV. Approximately 15% to 30% of the dose is recovered in the urine as metabolites, with the remainder excreted either into the bile as unchanged drug or into the feces as metabolites.[184,185]

Because the action of the TZDs relies on gene transcription and protein production, the onset and duration of action are unrelated to the plasma half-life. The onset of their effect occurs in 1 to 2 weeks, although maximal effects are not usually seen before 8 to 12 weeks. No dose adjustment is necessary in patients with renal impairment. There is no dose adjustment needed for hepatic impairment with pioglitazone; however, rosiglitazone should be avoided in patients with moderate-to-severe hepatic impairment.[185,187]

ADVERSE EFFECTS

Hepatotoxicity

Liver failure has been very rarely reported with either rosiglitazone or pioglitazone, although causality in most cases remains uncertain.[188–190] For both drugs, monitoring of liver function tests (LFTs) is recommended at baseline, and then periodically thereafter (see Contraindications and Precautions section). Many practitioners check the LFTs every 3 to 6 months during the first year of therapy and then every 6 to 12 months thereafter.

Hematologic Effects

TZD therapy may result in small decreases in hemoglobin and hematocrit and, infrequently, anemia.[175,184] These effects may be attributable to dilutional effects (see below).

Weight Gain

Dose-related weight gain (2–3 kg for every 1% decrease in A1C) has been seen with rosiglitazone and pioglitazone.[184] Weight gain is likely caused by fluid retention or fat accumulation. The weight gain seems to be associated with an increase in peripheral adipose tissue along with a reduction in visceral adiposity.[175,184]

Vascular and Cardiovascular Effects

Increases in plasma volume and peripheral edema (4%–6%), possibly caused by increased endothelial cell permeability, occur with the TZDs.[184] The incidence of peripheral edema is greatly increased when TZDs are used in combination with insulin.

The FDA added black box warnings to rosiglitazone and pioglitazone based on the association of their use with an increased risk of developing or exacerbating HF in patients with Type 2 diabetes.[185,187] TZDs are contraindicated for use in patients with NYHA class III or IV HF and are not recommended in patients with acute or systemic HF. Meta-analysis and retrospective observational studies have suggested that rosiglitazone is associated with risk of MI,[191–193] but not for overall cardiovascular or all-cause mortality.[193] Pioglitazone does not appear to increase the risk of MI or mortality.[194–197] TZDs should be used with caution in patients with preexisting edema, which may increase the risk of developing new-onset HF or exacerbating preexisting HF (see Case 53-15).

Other Effects

Hypersensitivity reactions including rash, pruritus, urticaria, angioedema, anaphylactic reaction, and Stevens–Johnson syndrome have been rarely reported with rosiglitazone.[185,187] Macular edema has been rarely reported with TZDs.[185,187,198] Patients experiencing changes or worsening in vision should be referred to an ophthalmologist for follow-up. In some cases, macular edema improved or resolved after discontinuation of TZD therapy.

Pioglitazone has been associated with an increased risk of bladder cancer compared to the general population and is contraindicated in patients with bladder cancer.[199] In patients with previous history of bladder cancer, the need for use of pioglitazone for glycemic control must outweigh the potential recurrence of bladder cancer.[199] The FDA has released a safety communication warning that the use of pioglitazone for longer than 1 year may increase the risk for bladder cancer.[199] Recently analyzed 10-year findings show no statistically significant increase in bladder cancer, but a risk as previously identified cannot be ruled out. This meta-analysis identified a possible increased risk of pancreatic and prostate cancer. Monitoring for causal effect of cancers should be continued.[199]

An increased risk of distal limb bone fractures (e.g., forearm, hand, wrist, foot, and ankle) and bone loss have been observed in women receiving TZDs.[200–203] Men may also be at increased fracture risk, but the evidence is not as strong.[202,203] The mechanism is thought to be reduced osteoblast differentiation as a result of increased adipogenesis in the bone marrow.[204] The potential for fractures in older female patients and patients on chronic steroids should be carefully considered before using a TZD.

CONTRAINDICATIONS AND PRECAUTIONS

- *Type 1 diabetes:* Because insulin is required for their action, TZDs should not be used in people with type 1 diabetes.
- *Patients with type 2 diabetes using insulin:* TZDs should be used with caution because of the increased risk of developing edema.
- *Preexisting hepatic disease:* Pioglitazone and rosiglitazone should not be used in patients whose ALT is more than 2.5 times normal. TZDs should be discontinued if the ALT is more than 3 times normal, if serum bilirubin levels begin to rise, or if the patient complains of any symptoms that could be attributed to hepatitis (e.g., fatigue, nausea, vomiting, abdominal pain, and dark urine).
- *Symptomatic or severe (NYHA classes III and IV) HF:* See previous discussion.
- *Myocardial ischemia* (rosiglitazone only): See previous discussion.
- *Premenopausal anovulatory women:* TZDs may cause resumption of ovulation and menstruation in women with polycystic ovarian syndrome, placing these patients at risk for an unwanted pregnancy.
- *History of hypersensitivity to TZDs.*
- *Patients with osteoporosis or at risk for bone fractures* (e.g., chronic steroid use).
- *Drugs metabolized by CYP 3A4:* See the Drug Interactions section for further details.
- *Patients with a current or previous history of bladder cancer should not use TZDs.*
- *Macular edema:* Patients should receive regular eye examinations to evaluate acute visual changes.

DRUG INTERACTIONS

Coadministration of a TZD with other antidiabetic medications or insulin does not alter the pharmacokinetics of either drug, but may increase the patient's risk for hypoglycemia. Pioglitazone induces CYP 3A4 and may, therefore, decrease effectiveness of other drugs metabolized by this enzyme, such as estrogens, cyclosporine, tacrolimus, and β-hydroxy-β-methylglutaryl-coenzyme A (HMG-CoA) reductase inhibitors. Ketoconazole may significantly inhibit the metabolism of pioglitazone.[185] Patients taking oral contraceptives or estrogen-replacement therapy should be informed of the possible risk of decreased effectiveness of estrogen therapy. Rosiglitazone does not seem to inhibit any of the major CYP enzymes.[187] Rifampin decreases the area under the plasma concentration–time curve (AUC) for both rosiglitazone and pioglitazone, although the clinical significance of this interaction is unknown. Pioglitazone is a substrate of CYP2C8; therefore, interactions may occur when administered with drugs that inhibit or induce CYP2C8.[205] The maximum dose of pioglitazone is 15 mg once a day if given with a strong CYP2C8 inhibitor.[185] Gemfi brozil significantly increases the AUC of both drugs. For patients receiving both a TZD and a gemfi brozil, a dose reduction of the TZD may be warranted.[205]

EFFICACY

The effects of TZDs on A1C and FPG are intermediate between those of acarbose and the sulfonylureas or metformin.[175,184] When combined with other antidiabetic agents in a poorly controlled type 2 diabetes patient, one can expect to see an augmented effect on the A1C (0.9%–1.3% decrease with a sulfonylurea, 0.8%–1.0% decrease with metformin, and 0.7%–1.0% decrease with insulin).[185,187] When added to the therapy of a type 2 diabetes patient taking insulin, rosiglitazone and pioglitazone can enhance glycemic control (approximately 0.6% lower with pioglitazone) while decreasing insulin requirements; however, weight gain (>3 kg) and increased edema will likely occur.[206] Individuals who are minimally responsive or unresponsive to TZD therapy may include those who are not obese and have lower levels of endogenous insulin.

Other potential benefits of the TZDs are their favorable, but variable, effects on lipids.[184,185,187] Pioglitazone and to a lesser extent rosiglitazone may decrease triglycerides. Both drugs may increase HDL-C levels by 10%. Rosiglitazone has been observed to increase LDL-C by 8% to 16%, whereas pioglitazone may not affect LDL-C. As noted, TZD therapy has been associated with weight gain, and this may be substantial when used in combination with sulfonylureas or insulin.

DOSAGE AND CLINICAL USE

Patients who are unable to take or have failed metformin or sulfonylurea monotherapy or who have not responded to combination therapy with other oral antidiabetic agents are usually candidates for TZD therapy. For monotherapy or combination therapy with a sulfonylurea, metformin, or insulin, the starting dose for pioglitazone is 15 or 30 mg once daily with or without food. The dose can be titrated up to a maximum of 45 mg/day.[185] The starting dose for rosiglitazone is 4 mg given once daily or in divided doses. The dose may be increased after 8 to 12 weeks if adequate response is not seen. The maximum daily dose is 8 mg.[187]

Glucosidase Inhibitors

MECHANISM OF ACTION

The α-glucosidase inhibitors, acarbose[207] and miglitol,[208] reversibly inhibit glucosidases present in the brush border of the mucosa of the small intestine. These enzymes break down complex polysaccharides and disaccharides into glucose and other absorbable monosaccharides. Enzyme inhibition delays carbohydrate digestion and subsequent glucose absorption. Postprandial BG concentrations are therefore lowered when these agents are taken with a meal containing complex carbohydrates.

PHARMACOKINETICS

Acarbose is minimally absorbed from the GI tract, with an oral bioavailability of the parent drug of less than 2.0%.[207] It is extensively metabolized by GI amylases to inactive metabolites. The peak plasma concentration occurs in approximately 1 hour and the elimination half-life for acarbose is 2 hours, although there may be a longer terminal half-life. Unlike acarbose, miglitol is absorbed. Absorption of miglitol is saturable at higher doses (>25 mg) and peak concentration occurs in 2 to 3 hours.[208] The drug is primarily distributed in extracellular fluids and is not metabolized. After a 25-mg dose, 95% of the drug is excreted unchanged by the kidneys within 24 hours.

ADVERSE EFFECTS

Flatulence, diarrhea, and abdominal pain are the most frequently reported adverse effects of α-glucosidase inhibitors.[207,208] In placebo-controlled trials of acarbose, these complaints were experienced by 74%, 31%, and 19% of subjects, respectively. GI side effects are attributable to fermentation of unabsorbed carbohydrate in the small intestine and can be minimized by slowly titrating the dose of either agent. GI discomfort usually improves with continued therapy because induction of the α-glucosidase enzymes occurs in the distal jejunum and terminal ileum.

In studies using doses of acarbose 300 mg/day or more, a transient increase in serum hepatic transaminases was reported.[209] The manufacturer recommends monitoring hepatic transaminases every 3 months for the first year of therapy and periodically thereafter. If an elevation of serum transaminases occurs, the dose should be decreased or discontinued if elevations persist. Because miglitol is not metabolized, it does not seem to affect hepatic function.

CONTRAINDICATIONS AND PRECAUTIONS

Acarbose and miglitol are contraindicated with known hypersensitivity to the medications.[207,208] Both medications are contraindicated in patients with DKA and acarbose is contraindicated in patients with cirrhosis.

Gastrointestinal Conditions

Because of their profound GI effects (flatulence, diarrhea), acarbose and miglitol are contraindicated in patients with malabsorption, inflammatory bowel disease, colonic ulceration or other marked disorders of digestion or absorption, or with intestinal obstruction.[207,208]

Renal Impairment

Acarbose has not been studied in patients with severe renal impairment (SCr >2.0 mg/dL) and should not be used in these patients.[209] There is little information with regard to safety of the use of miglitol in patients with a CrCl<25 mL/minute; therefore, its use is contraindicated in these patients.[207,208]

DRUG INTERACTIONS

Patients who use acarbose or miglitol in combination with other antidiabetic agents may experience hypoglycemia. These reactions should be treated with dextrose because acarbose may limit the availability of the disaccharide sucrose (table sugar). Because acarbose and miglitol delay carbohydrate passage through the bowel, they could influence the absorption kinetics of concomitantly administered drugs. Conversely, because their own absorption may be diminished by digestive enzyme preparations and charcoal, they should not be taken concomitantly with these agents.[207–209] The bioavailability of digoxin can be reduced and may require dose adjustment. Miglitol decreases the bioavailability of ranitidine and propranolol by 60% and 40%, respectively.[208]

EFFICACY

By delaying the absorption of glucose after ingestion of complex carbohydrates and disaccharides, the α-glucosidase inhibitors can lower postprandial plasma glucose concentrations in patients with type 2 diabetes by 25 to 50 mg/dL.[207,208] FPG concentrations remain unchanged or are slightly lowered (20–30 mg/dL), but this effect may be related to decreased glucose toxicity, which improves insulin secretion and action. Mean A1C values decline by 0.3% to 0.7%. Acarbose and miglitol have no effect on weight or lipid profiles.[207,208]

DOSAGE AND CLINICAL USE

Because of limited effects on A1C and their side effect profile, α-glucosidase inhibitors are used infrequently and, when used, are usually given as add-on therapy in patients who have failed monotherapy or combination therapy with other oral antidiabetic agents. The recommended initial dose of either drug is up to 25 mg TID, taken at the start of each meal.[207,208] The dosage of acarbose can be gradually increased (e.g., 25 mg/meal) every 4 to 8 weeks to a maximum of 50 mg TID for individuals weighing 60 kg or less, or 100 mg TID for individuals weighing more than 60 kg. The dose for miglitol is titrated up after 4 to 8 weeks to a dose of 50 to 100 mg TID if needed, regardless of a patient's weight. A maximal response is observed at 6 months.

Incretin-Based Therapies

Incretins are insulinotropic hormones secreted from specialized neuroendocrine cells in the small intestinal mucosa in response to carbohydrate ingestion and absorption.[13] The two hormones accounting for most incretin effects are glucose-dependent insulinotropic polypeptide (GIP) and glucagon-like peptide-1 (GLP-1). GIP and GLP-1 stimulate pancreatic β-cells in a glucose-dependent manner, contributing to the early-phase insulin response. GLP-1 also inhibits pancreatic α-cells, thus reducing glucagon secretion and hepatic glucose production. Incretin action is efficient, but short lived. As they enter the blood vessels, incretins undergo rapid metabolism via proteolytic cleavage by dipeptidyl peptidase-4 (DPP-4) to inactive metabolites. Thus, only small amounts are needed to exert their effects on glucose metabolism.

Glucagon-like Peptide-1 Agonists (GLP-1 Mimetics/Analogs)

Exenatide, extended-release exenatide, albiglutide, liraglutide, and dulaglutide are the five available GLP-1 agonists in the United States. The formulations available are a once-daily injection (liraglutide), twice-daily injection (exenatide), and once-weekly injections (extended-release exenatide, albiglutide and dulaglutide).

MECHANISM OF ACTION

GLP-1 mimetics and analogs have stability in the presence of DPP-4, resulting in a longer duration of action than endogenous GLP-1. Exenatide is a synthetic form of exendin-4, a peptide originally discovered from the saliva of the Gila monster.[210] Exendin-4 shares 50% of its amino acid sequence with GLP-1, demonstrating similar affinity for receptor sites but a strong resistance to DPP-4. Liraglutide is a GLP-1 analog that is 97% homologous to human GLP-1, and reversibly binds to plasma albumin owing to the C16 fatty acid side chain, thereby increasing resistance to DPP-4 degradation.[211] Albiglutide has 2 tandem copies of modified human GLP-1 fused to human albumin. The human fragment sequence has been modified to allow for resistance to DPP-IV-mediated proteolysis, and in combination with the human albumin moiety of the fusion protein, the half-life is extended allowing for once-weekly dosing.[212] Dulaglutide is a human GLP-1 receptor agonist that has 90% homology to endogenous human GLP-1.[213] These agents augment early or first-phase insulin response in response to elevated glucose concentrations (i.e., glucose-dependent), moderate glucagon secretion, and decrease hepatic glucose production without impairing the normal glucagon response to hypoglycemia. They slow gastric emptying, thereby reducing the rate at which glucose is absorbed. In addition, they suppress appetite, which may contribute to the prevention of weight gain and the weight loss (1.5–5 kg) observed in patients. A promising action of these agents is their potential to increase β-cell mass and preservation, which has been shown in animal models.

PHARMACOKINETICS

After SC injection, exenatide reaches peak plasma concentrations in 2.1 hours.[214] The injection site (abdomen, thigh, or upper arm) does not significantly alter its kinetics. Both exenatide formulations are eliminated predominantly by glomerular filtration with subsequent proteolytic degradation. The mean terminal half-life of exenatide is 2.4 hours, with levels measurable up to 10 hours, thus allowing for twice-daily dosing. Its metabolism and elimination are dose independent. Extended-release exenatide is released from microspheres over approximately 10 weeks after administration. After discontinuation of therapy, minimal detectable concentrations can be seen in approximately 10 weeks.[215]

Absorption of liraglutide is delayed owing to its self-association in heptameric aggregates within the injection depot that are too large to cross the capillary membranes.[216] On disassociation of the heptamers at the absorption site, liraglutide is absorbed. This delayed absorption is the primary reason for its prolonged action. Liraglutide is highly protein bound (>98%), with a half-life of 13 hours, allowing for once-daily dosing.[211,216] Metabolism of liraglutide occurs endogenously in a manner similar to large proteins and there is no specific organ as its route of elimination.[211,216]

Albiglutide administered SC resulted in maximum concentrations in 3 to 5 days. Steady state is achieved after 4 to 5 weeks of administration. Metabolism to small peptides and amino acids occurs through a metabolic pathway involving proteolytic enzymes in the vascular endothelium. The elimination half-life is approximately 5 days, which allows for once-weekly administration.[212]

Dulaglutide achieves maximum plasma concentration in about 48 hours, and steady state occurs between 2 to 4 weeks with once-weekly administration. There is no statistically significant difference of exposure to dulaglutide between the site of administration in the abdomen, upper arm, or thigh. Metabolism occurs through general protein catabolism pathways into its component amino acids. The elimination half-life is approximately 5 days.[213]

ADVERSE EFFECTS

GI side effects are common and dose-dependent, particularly nausea, vomiting, and diarrhea. Rates vary between agents with albiglutide appearing to have the lowest rates in placebo-controlled trials.[212] These side effects may be lessened by starting patients on lower doses for daily injections, ensuring correct timing and administration of the drug, and titrating the dose slowly. Other reported side effects have included decreased appetite and injection site reactions. Hypoglycemic risk can be increased in patients who are also taking an oral insulin secretagogue (e.g., sulfonylurea) or insulin.[211–215]

These agents have been rarely related to hypersensitivity reactions, acute pancreatitis, and reduced renal function. Patients should be educated about symptoms of acute pancreatitis, including severe abdominal pain accompanied by vomiting, and instructed to report to their practitioner immediately. Patients in whom acute pancreatitis is confirmed with no other probable cause should not be rechallenged with GLP-1 agonists.[211–215]

The development of antibodies against these agents is well established. In general, the presence of antibodies does not appear to significantly affect the A1C reduction seen with GLP-1 agonists, although some patients with high antibody titers may experience reduced efficacy.[211–215,217] Patients who demonstrate adherence to therapy, yet experience no change or worsening in glycemic control, should discontinue therapy and be switched to alternative agents.

CONTRAINDICATIONS AND PRECAUTIONS

GLP-1 agonists are contraindicated in patients with known hypersensitivity. They should not be used in patients with a history of pancreatitis.[211–215] They are not recommended for use in patients with severe GI disease. Exenatide should not be used in severe renal impairment (CrCl <30 mL/minute) or end-stage renal failure, or in those requiring hemodialysis.[215,218] Dulaglutide and albiglutide have limited clinical experience in patients with end-stage renal disease and should be used with caution in these patients. If these patients experience GI adverse effects, renal function should be closely monitored.[212,213]

GLP-1 agonists are contraindicated in patients with a personal or family history of medullary thyroid carcinoma (MTC) or in patients with multiple endocrine neoplasia syndrome type 2 (MEN 2) due to risks in rodents. A causal relationship in humans has not been established.[211–215] Currently, the FDA has required black box warnings on each of the GLP-1 agonists for MTC, MEN 2, and thyroid cancer as well as a REMS program for each medication.

DRUG INTERACTIONS

GLP-1 agonists may increase the risk for hypoglycemia when used with sulfonylureas or insulin. Because of their mechanism of action, they may reduce the rate and extent of absorption of orally administered drugs.[211–215] They should therefore be used with caution in patients taking medications that require rapid GI absorption and are dose-dependent on threshold concentrations for efficacy, such as antibiotics and oral contraceptives. The manufacturers of twice-daily exenatide recommend that patients take the affected medications at least 1 hour before exenatide administration.[214] There have been case reports of an increased international normalized ratio, sometimes associated with bleeding, in patients taking exenatide and warfarin. Patients should be closely monitored, with dose adjustments to warfarin therapy made as needed.[214,215]

EFFICACY

In clinical trials, maximal doses of exenatide combined with a sulfonylurea, metformin, a TZD, or sulfonylurea plus metformin therapy for 30 weeks reduced FBG by 5 to 25 mg/dL, 2-hour postprandial BG by 60 to 70 mg/dL, and A1C by 0.8% to 1.0%.[214,215] Exenatide use for 80 weeks has been reported to reduce body weight by 4 to 5 kg. In a 24-week trial comparing exenatide with extended-release exenatide, the extended-release formulation resulted in a reduction in A1C of 1.6% and a reduction in FBG of 25 mg/dL.[214,215] Clinical trials with liraglutide monotherapy demonstrate decreases in FBG of 15 to 26 mg/dL and A1C of 0.8% to 1.1%, and weight loss of 2.1 to 2.5 kg.[214] When used as combination therapy, additional A1C lowering of 1% to 1.5% can be expected.[219–221]

Albiglutide as monotherapy in a 52-week trial resulted in A1C reduction of 0.7% to 0.9% and reduction in FBG of 16 to 25 mg/dL. When used in combination therapy, albiglutide reduced A1C by 0.6% to 0.8% and reduced FBG by 18 to 23 mg/dL.[212] Dulaglutide monotherapy resulted in a decrease in A1C of 0.7% to 0.8% and a reduction of FBG of 26 to 29 mg/dL, as well as weight loss of 1.4 to 2.3 kg. When dulaglutide is used in combination therapy, it results in an A1C reduction of 0.8% to 1.5%, a reduction in FBG of 16 to 41 mg/dL, and a weight loss of 0.2 to 2.7 kg.[213]

DOSAGE AND CLINICAL USE

Exenatide (not the extended-release formulation) is approved for use as monotherapy, whereas the other GLP-1 agonists are not recommended as monotherapy per the manufacturers.[211–215] GLP-1 agonists are indicated as add-on agents in patients with Type 2 diabetes who have been unable to reach target goals on monotherapy with metformin or in combination therapy. Although not indicated for weight loss, these agents may be helpful in patients with Type 2 diabetes who are obese and struggling with obesity. Albiglutide and exenatide have been studied in patients with Type 2 diabetes already on insulin glargine; albiglutide lowered the A1C by 0.8%, whereas exenatide lowered the A1C by 1.7% and patients required lower doses of insulin glargine compared with the placebo group.[212,214]

The starting dose of exenatide is 5 mcg injected SC into the abdomen, thigh, or arm twice daily within 60 minutes before morning and evening meals. Patients who experience severe GI side effects may try injecting just before meals initially and then move from 30 to 60 minutes before meals. If a patient tolerates the 5-mcg dose, then it can be titrated after 1 month of therapy to the maximal dose of 10 mcg SC twice daily. The dose of extended-release exenatide is 2 mg given SC once weekly without regard to meals at any time of the day. The starting dose of liraglutide is 0.6 mg injected SC into the abdomen, thigh, or arm once daily for 1 week, and then it may be increased to 1.2 mg SC daily. If the A1C goal is not achieved with a 1.2-mg dose, the dose can be further increased to 1.8 mg daily. The starting dose of albiglutide is 30 mg injected SC into the abdomen, thigh, or upper arm once weekly without regard to meals at any time of the day. The dose can be increased to 50 mg once weekly in patients who have not achieved adequate glycemic control. The starting dose of dulaglutide is 0.75 mg injected SC into the abdomen, thigh, or upper arm once weekly given at any time of the day and may be increased to 1.5 mg once weekly if adequate glycemic control is not achieved.[211–215]

When any of these agents are added to the treatment regimen of a patient who is also taking a sulfonylurea or glinide, the insulin secretagogue dose may need to be lowered (by about half) to reduce the risk of hypoglycemia. If used in combination with basal insulin, the insulin dose may need to be decreased.[211–215]

Dipeptidyl Peptidase-4 Inhibitors

Currently, four DPP-4 inhibitors are available in the United States: sitagliptin, saxagliptin, linagliptin, and alogliptin.[218,222–224]

MECHANISM OF ACTION

The DPP-4 inhibitors inhibit the degradation of GIP and GLP-1 on entering the GI vasculature, thus increasing the effects of these endogenous incretins on first-phase insulin secretion and glucagon inhibition.[225] They are all competitive inhibitors of DPP-4. Sitagliptin, at a 100-mg dose, reduces DPP-4 activity by 80% for up to 24 hours,[222] whereas saxagliptin, at a 2.5-mg dose, reduces DPP-4 activity by 50% for up to 24 hours.[223] Alogliptin, at a dose of at least 25 mg, has been shown to reduce DPP-4 activity by more than 80% at a dose of at least 25 mg for at least 24 hours.[224] Linagliptin, at the standard dose of 5 mg, has been shown to reduce DPP-4 activity by more than 80% for up to 24 hours.[218] In contrast to GLP agonists, which increase GLP-1 levels by 6- to 10-fold,[226] these agents only modestly increase GLP-1 levels (2- to 3-fold), but also increase GIP levels. As a result, DPP-4 inhibitors have minimal-to-no effect on satiety and delaying gastric emptying.

PHARMACOKINETICS

Sitagliptin is rapidly absorbed, with an absolute bioavailability of 87%.[222] Absorption is unaffected by food. Peak plasma concentrations occur in 1 to 4 hours, and its terminal half-life is 12.4 hours. Only

38% of sitagliptin is plasma protein bound. Eighty-seven percent of the parent drug is excreted unchanged in the urine, primarily by active renal tubular secretion, and may involve P-glycoprotein and human organic anion transporter-3. Metabolism by CYP 3A4, and to a much lesser extent, CYP2C8, plays a minimal role in the excretion of metabolites in the feces.[227]

Saxagliptin is well absorbed with a bioavailability estimated to be 75%.[223] Although food increases absorption by 27%, it can be administered with or without food. Peak plasma concentrations occur at 2 hours for saxagliptin and 4 hours for the active metabolite. Saxagliptin is metabolized by CYP 3A4/5 to a major metabolite that is one-half as potent.[228] Protein binding of saxagliptin and its active metabolite is negligible. The mean plasma terminal half-lives of saxagliptin and its active metabolite are 2.5 and 3.1 hours, respectively. Saxagliptin is excreted primarily by the kidneys, with 25% excreted unchanged in the urine, and 36% of the active metabolite found in urine. Approximately 22% of drug and metabolite are excreted in feces.[227]

Linagliptin is well absorbed and has a bioavailability of 30%. A high-fat meal can decrease the absorption by 15%; however, this is not clinically significant. Therefore, linagliptin may be administered with or without food. Peak plasma concentrations occur at approximately 1.5 hours after a dose of 5 mg. Linagliptin has a long terminal half-life (>100 hours) due to biphasic decline in plasma concentrations, which is related to the binding of DPP-4. Approximately 90% of linagliptin is excreted unchanged in the urine, and a small percentage is metabolized to an inactive metabolite.[218]

Alogliptin is well absorbed and has a bioavailability of 100%. A high-fat meal results in no significant change in absorption; therefore, it may be administered with or without food. Alogliptin is 20% plasma protein bound, with 60% to 71% of the dose excreted unchanged in urine and 13% excreted in the feces. Limited metabolism occurs via CYP2D6 and CYP3A4. The terminal half-life of alogliptin is approximately 21 hours after the administration of a 25-mg dose.[224]

ADVERSE EFFECTS

Because these agents differ significantly in chemical structure from one another, some adverse events may be unique to the individual agent and may not be indicative of a class wide effect.[225] The most commonly reported side effects with sitagliptin and alogliptin include nasopharyngitis, upper respiratory tract infection, hypoglycemia, and headache.[222,224] Saxagliptin can cause these same adverse effects, as well as urinary tract infection, whereas linagliptin adverse effects can include hypoglycemia, nasopharyngitis, diarrhea, and cough.[218,223] It is possible that DPP-4 inhibitors may have an effect on the immune system, because lymphocytes express DPP-4. These medications have been suggested to increase risk for pancreatitis; however, studies have shown this risk to be low.[229] Additional clinical experience and postmarketing studies are needed to clearly establish the long-term safety of these agents.

CONTRAINDICATIONS AND PRECAUTIONS

All DPP-4 inhibitors should be avoided in patients with a history of serious hypersensitivity reaction to the drug.

DRUG INTERACTIONS

Sitagliptin is not significantly protein bound.[222] It also does not inhibit CYP isoenzymes or induce CYP 3A4; therefore, it is not expected to interact with other drugs that are metabolized by these pathways. Patients taking digoxin, a substrate of P-glycoprotein-like sitagliptin, should be monitored for any signs or symptoms of digoxin toxicity, because a slight increase in the AUC (11%) and C_{max} (18%) has been observed.[222,226]

Saxagliptin does have significant drug interactions because it is metabolized by CYP 3A4/5.[223] Therefore, if used with strong inhibitors of these enzymes (e.g., ketoconazole, itraconazole, clarithromycin, telithromycin, protease inhibitors such as indinavir), the dose of saxagliptin is reduced to 2.5 mg daily.

Linagliptin is a weak-to-moderate inhibitor of CYP3A4 and a P-glycoprotein substrate and inhibits P-glycoprotein-mediated transport of digoxin at high concentrations.[218] Medications that are strong inducers of CYP3A4 or P-glycoprotein, such as rifampin, decrease linagliptin to levels that are subtherapeutic and ineffective; therefore, if treatment with those medications is necessary, an alternative to linagliptin should be used.

Alogliptin is not significantly protein bound, and metabolism through the cytochrome P450 pathway is negligible; therefore, there are no significant drug interactions with alogliptin.[224]

EFFICACY

In monotherapy clinical trials versus placebo, sitagliptin lowers fasting glucose by 12 mg/dL and A1C by 0.5% to 0.6% compared with baseline (0.6%–0.8% compared with placebo)[222]; saxagliptin is comparable, with A1C lowering by 0.5% (0.6% vs. placebo) and FPG by 15 mg/dL.[223] In addition, both agents reduce 2-hour postprandial glucose by approximately 45 mg/dL.[222,223,226] When used as add-on combination therapy, A1C lowering is greater (0.7%–0.9%). Linagliptin, as monotherapy in clinical trials versus placebo, decreased fasting glucose by 13 mg/dL from baseline and decreased A1C by 0.4%.[218] Alogliptin, as monotherapy in clinical trials versus placebo, decreased fasting glucose by 16 mg/dL and A1C by 0.6%.[224] Unlike the GLP-1 mimetics and analogs, DPP-4 inhibitors do not significantly affect body weight, appetite, or satiety, and are considered weight neutral.[226] As is the case for the GLP-1 mimetics and analogs, further studies are needed to more clearly determine the effects of DDP-4 inhibitors on long-term preservation of β-cell function.

DOSAGE AND CLINICAL USE

DPP-4 inhibitors are mainly used as add-on therapy in combination with other agents. However, all are approved for use as monotherapy. Sitagliptin may be initiated at 100 mg taken once daily with or without food.[222] Renal function should be assessed before initiation of this agent. In patients with moderate renal insufficiency (CrCl 30–50 mL/minute), the dose for sitagliptin should be reduced to 50 mg once daily, and in severe renal insufficiency (CrCl <30 mL/minute) or for those in end-stage renal failure requiring dialysis, the sitagliptin dose is 25 mg once daily. Sitagliptin may be administered without regard to the timing of hemodialysis. Only sitagliptin should be used in patients on peritoneal dialysis.

Saxagliptin is dosed at 2.5 to 5 mg once daily with or without food.[223] Renal function should be assessed before initiation of this agent. In patients with moderate or severe renal impairment or end-stage renal disease with a CrCl < 50 mL/minute, the recommended dose is 2.5 mg daily. If patients are taking strong CYP3A4/5 inhibitors, the dose of saxagliptin should be 2.5 mg daily. In hemodialysis patients, the dose is 2.5 mg daily to be administered after hemodialysis.

Linagliptin is dosed at 5 mg once daily with or without food. No dose adjustment is necessary for patients with renal impairment; however, patients with a CrCl <30 mL/minute may be more prone to hypoglycemia; therefore, dosing adjustments of concomitant antidiabetic medications and frequent monitoring may be necessary.[218]

Alogliptin is dosed at 25 mg once daily with or without food. Renal function should be assessed prior to initiation of this medication. In patients with moderate renal impairment with a CrCl of 30 to 60 mL/minute, the recommended dose is 12.5 mg once daily. In patients with severe renal impairment (CrCl <30 mL/minute) or end-stage renal disease, the dose is 6.25 mg once daily. Patients on hemodialysis should be given 6.25 mg once daily and it may be administered without regard to the timing of dialysis.[224]

When any of these agents are added to a patient also on a sulfonylurea or glinide, the insulin secretagogue dose may need to be lowered (by about half) to reduce the risk of hypoglycemia. Similarly, when sitagliptin is added to a patient already on insulin therapy, the dose(s) of insulin may need to be lowered initially and then readjusted depending on the response to sitagliptin.

Amylin Receptor Agonists (Amylinomimetics)

MECHANISM OF ACTION

Amylin is a hormone found in the β-cells where it is comanufactured, stored, and released with insulin in response to food intake.[230] Its actions seem to be centrally mediated and include slowing gastric emptying, suppressing glucagon secretion, and modulating the regulation of appetite. Amylin is absent in patients with Type 1 diabetes. In patients with Type 2 diabetes, its concentrations are altered to mirror those of insulin at different points in the progression of the disease. Pramlintide, a synthetic amylin analog, is available in the United States for the adjunctive treatment of both Type 1 and Type 2 diabetes who use mealtime insulin.

PHARMACOKINETICS

The absolute bioavailability of SC injected pramlintide is 30% to 40%.[231] Subcutaneous injection into the abdomen and thigh allows for more predictable absorption and distribution than when administered into the arm. Approximately 40% of the drug is unbound in plasma. The half-life is about 48 minutes, and time to maximum concentration is approximately 20 minutes. Pramlintide is metabolized by the kidneys to an active metabolite with a half-life similar to the parent drug.

ADVERSE EFFECTS

GI symptoms—including mild-to-moderate nausea (28%–48%), vomiting (8%–11%), and anorexia (9%–17%)—are the most frequently reported adverse reactions associated with therapy.[231] GI symptoms are usually transient, subsiding after 4 to 8 weeks of treatment or with dose reduction and slow dose escalation. Hypoglycemia can occur in up to 16.8% of Type 1 diabetes patients receiving pramlintide and insulin therapy, and in 8.2% of Type 2 diabetes patients receiving pramlintide and insulin.

CONTRAINDICATIONS AND PRECAUTIONS

Pramlintide is contraindicated in patients with known cresol hypersensitivity, hypoglycemic unawareness, and gastroparesis.[231] Severe hypoglycemia can occur when it is used in combination with insulin and medications that can slow gastric emptying. Drugs that can alter glucose metabolism when administered with pramlintide, and therefore cause hypoglycemia, include oral antidiabetics, fibrates, fluoxetine, salicylates, and ACE inhibitors, and should be used with caution if administered concomitantly. Pramlintide has a black box warning for severe hypoglycemia, which can occur within 3 hours following an injection of pramlintide. Caution individuals while driving, those who operate heavy machinery, and those who engage in other high-risk activities due to potential serious injuries that may result during a hypoglycemic episode.

DRUG INTERACTIONS

As noted, severe hypoglycemia can occur in patients who are concurrently taking an oral hypoglycemic agent (e.g., sulfonylurea) or insulin (see Dosage and Clinical Use section).[231] Because pramlintide can delay the absorption of medications that are administered concomitantly, medications that require rapid onset for effectiveness, such as antibiotics, oral contraceptives, and analgesics, should be administered at least 2 hours after or 1 hour prior to the pramlintide injection.

EFFICACY

In clinical studies of patients with Type 2 diabetes with doses up to 150 mcg/day for 52 weeks, pramlintide combined with insulin decreased A1C by 0.3% and weight by 2.57 kg.[231] Clinical studies of patients with Type 1 diabetes taking insulin in combination with pramlintide or placebo demonstrated A1C reductions of 0.2% to 0.4% and weight loss of 0.4 to 1.3 kg.[56]

DOSAGE AND CLINICAL USE

In clinical practice, pramlintide is considered an add-on agent primarily for patients with Type 1 diabetes who have failed to achieve target BG goals on insulin therapy alone. Its practical use is more limited to obese patients with Type 2 diabetes who have failed to achieve target BG levels with a regimen that includes a sulfonylurea or insulin. Pramlintide is available in a pen device (SymlinPen). It cannot be mixed with any type of insulin. The pens (60 pen-injector for 15-, 30-, 45-, or 60-mcg doses and 120 pen-injector for 60- and 120-mcg doses) in use may be stored at room temperature (86°F or 30°C) for up to 30 days.[231]

For patients with Type 1 diabetes, the initial dose is 15 mcg, and for patients with Type 2 diabetes, the initial dose is 60 mcg. Pramlintide is injected SC into the abdomen or thigh immediately before every major meal. A major meal is one that contains 30 g or more of carbohydrate or 250 kcal or more. If a meal is skipped, the pramlintide dose should be skipped. When initiating pramlintide therapy, the dose of premeal insulins must be reduced by at least 50%. Patients should be closely followed and instructed to intensively monitor and record BG (fasting, preprandial, and postprandial) levels and any hypoglycemic episodes until control has stabilized. Pramlintide is titrated based on achieving optimal glucose control with minimal side effects (e.g., nausea). The dose can be increased when no clinically significant nausea has occurred for 3 to 7 days. For patients with Type 1 diabetes, doses may be increased in 15-mcg increments up to a maximum meal dose of 60 mcg. For patients with Type 2 diabetes, the dose may be increased to 120 mcg before every major meal.[231]

Sodium–Glucose Transporter 2 (SGLT2) Inhibitors

SGLT2 inhibitors reduce BG by decreasing tubular reabsorption of glucose in the kidney, thereby increasing the excretion of urinary glucose.[231] These agents are highly selective, reversible inhibitors of SGLT2. Currently, there are three agents in this class: canagliflozin, dapagliflozin, and empagliflozin, which are available as individual agents or in combination with other antidiabetic agents.[232–234] Because their mechanism of action is independent of insulin resistance or β-cell function, these medications can be used in combination with all antidiabetic agent classes, including insulin, for the treatment of Type 2 DM in addition to diet and exercise. These agents have added benefits of weight loss, increase in HDL, and decrease in blood pressure; however, genital and urinary infections may be an adverse effect of these agents.[235]

PHARMACOKINETICS

Canagliflozin has a bioavailability of 65%, and peak plasma concentrations occur within 1 to 2 hours after the dose is administered.[232] There was no effect on absorption when administered with a high-fat meal; therefore, canagliflozin may be administered with or without food. Canagliflozin is 99% protein bound, primarily to albumin. This agent is metabolized primarily by glucuronidation by UGT1A9 and UGT2B4 to two inactive metabolites. Approximately 7% is metabolized by CYP3A4. Approximately 33% of a dose is excreted in the urine as metabolites and <1% is excreted as unchanged canagliflozin in the urine. The terminal half-life is 10.6 hours for a 100-mg dose and 13.1 hours for a 300-mg dose.

Dapagliflozin has a bioavailability of 78% after the administration of a 10-mg dose.[233] The maximal serum concentration (C_{max}) occurs at approximately 2 hours under fasting state. Taking dapagliflozin with a high-fat meal decreases the C_{max} by up to 50%; however, this change is not clinically significant. Therefore, it may be administered with or without food. Dapagliflozin is approximately 91% protein bound and is metabolized primarily by the UGT1A9 pathway and to a small extent by CYP 3A4 to yield inactive metabolites. This agent and the inactive metabolites are excreted 75% in the urine and 21% in the feces, with 15% being excreted as unchanged drug. The terminal half-life is approximately 12.9 hours following a single-dose administration.

Empagliflozin reached peak plasma concentrations at 1.5 hours postoral administration.[234] Plasma concentrations then declined in a biphasic manner with a rapid distribution phase and a slower terminal phase. The C_{max} decreased by 37% after administration with a high-fat meal; however, this was determined to be clinically insignificant. Therefore, empagliflozin may be administered with or without food. Empagliflozin is 86.2% bound to plasma proteins, and the agent is primarily metabolized by glucuronidation by UGT3B7, UGT1A3, UGT1A8, and UGT1A9. No major metabolites were detected in plasma. Approximately 41.2% of the drug was eliminated in feces (unchanged parent drug), whereas 54.4% was eliminated in urine (half is unchanged parent drug). The terminal half-life is approximately 12.4 hours.

ADVERSE EFFECTS

Canagliflozin commonly reported adverse effects include female genital mycotic infections, increased urination, and urinary tract infections.[232] The most common adverse effects associated with dapagliflozin include nasopharyngitis, urinary tract infections, and female genital mycotic infections.[233] The most common adverse effects associated with empagliflozin include female genital mycotic infections and urinary tract infections.[234]

CONTRAINDICATIONS AND PRECAUTIONS

All SGLT2 agents are contraindicated in patients with hypersensitivity reactions to the agents and in patients with severe renal impairment, ESRD, and dialysis.[233–234] Based on the mechanism of action of these agents, they would be ineffective in patients with severe renal impairment and would place these patients at increased risk for renal adverse effects. Renal function should be assessed prior to the initiation of these agents and periodically during treatment. Blood pressure should be assessed in patients prior to initiation with these agents and hypovolemia should be corrected due to the potential of these agents to lower blood pressure, especially in patients already taking antihypertensive medications. Hypoglycemia may occur when SGLT2 agents are used in combination with insulin and secretagogues; therefore, the doses of the concomitant agents may need to be decreased. Renal function may be impaired with use of these agents; therefore, renal function monitoring should occur during therapy. Serum concentrations of LDL may be increased with SGLT2 therapy, which may require medication therapy, and serum LDL concentrations should be monitored. In clinical trials, dapagliflozin has shown an increase in bladder cancer cases as compared to placebo; therefore, patients with previous history of bladder cancer should not take dapagliflozin.[235]

In May 2015, the FDA released a Drug Safety Communication warning that SGLT2 agents may cause ketoacidosis and patients should be warned to seek medical attention if they experience signs and symptoms of ketoacidosis including confusion, fatigue, difficulty breathing, abdominal pain, nausea, or vomiting.[236] The cases were not typical of DKA cases, because blood sugars were not highly elevated. In some of the cases, DKA may have been triggered by major illness. The FDA will monitor the safety of these agents and determine whether prescribing information changes are warranted.

DRUG INTERACTIONS

Canagliflozin weakly inhibits CYP2B6, CYP2C8, CYP2C9, and CYP3A4, is a weak inhibitor of P-gp, and is a substrate of drug transporters P-gp and MRP2.[232] Rifampin decreases the efficacy of canagliflozin; therefore, the dose of canagliflozin may need to be increased. When administered concomitantly with digoxin, there was an increase in the AUC (20%) and C_{max} (36%) of digoxin; therefore, digoxin should be monitored appropriately.

Dapagliflozin does not inhibit CYP enzymes and is a weak substrate of the P-glycoprotein (P-gp) active transporter. The dapagliflozin metabolite is a substrate for the OAT3 active transporter; however, it did not inhibit P-gp, OCT2, OAT1, or OAT3 active transporters with any clinical significance. Therefore, dapagliflozin is unlikely to affect the pharmacokinetics of concurrently administered medications that are substrates of these enzymes. Coadministration of dapagliflozin with rifampin, a nonselective inducer of UGT1A9, may cause a decrease in dapagliflozin serum concentrations, which may lead to a decrease in dapagliflozin efficacy.[233]

Empagliflozin does not induce or inhibit CYP450 enzymes or UGT1A1; therefore, it is not expected to have interactions with concomitantly administered medications that are substrates of the CYP450 pathway or UGT1A1.[234]

EFFICACY

Canagliflozin monotherapy versus placebo decreased A1C by 0.77% to 1.03%, decreased FPG by 27 to 35 mg/dL, and decreased body weight by 2.8% to 3.9%.[232] In a clinical trial comparing dapagliflozin monotherapy to placebo, A1C was decreased by 0.8% to 0.9% and FPG was decreased by 24.1 to 28.8 mg/dL.[233] Empagliflozin monotherapy, in a clinical trial compared to placebo, decreased A1C by 0.7% to 0.8%, decreased FPG by 19 to 25 mg/dL, and decreased body weight by 2.8 to 3.2%.[234]

DOSAGE AND CLINICAL USE

The SGLT2 agents are indicated for use in patients with Type 2 DM as an adjunct to diet and exercise as monotherapy or concomitantly with other antidiabetic agents. The initial dose of canagliflozin is 100 mg once daily taken before the first meal of the day and can be increased to 300 mg once daily in patients who need additional glycemic control and have an eGFR > 60ml/min/1.73 m^2.[237] In patients with an eGFR of 45 to 60 mL/minute/1.73 m^2, the dose is limited to 100 mg once daily and should be discontinued in patients with an eGFR <45 mL/minute/1.73 m^2.[232] Dapagliflozin should be initiated at a dose of 5 mg once daily in the morning, with or without food, and the dose may be increased in patients who need additional glycemic control.[233] Monitor renal function prior to initiation and do not use in patients with an eGFR <60 mL/minute/1.73 m^2. Empagliflozin should be initiated at a dose of 10 mg once daily in the morning, with or without food, and may be increased to 25 mg once daily.[238] Do not initiate empagliflozin therapy in patients with an eGFR <45 mL/minute/1.73 m^2 and discontinue therapy if eGFR persistently falls below 45 mL/minute/1.73 m^2.[234]

Other Agents

COLESEVELAM

In January 2008, the FDA approved a new indication for colesevelam (Welchol), a bile acid sequestrant, to be used as add-on therapy in Type 2 diabetes as an adjunct to diet and exercise.[239]

The mechanism by which colesevelam reduces glucose is not known. It is a hydrophilic, water-insoluble polymer that is not absorbed. Therefore, its distribution is limited to the GI tract.[239–242] The primary side effects of colesevelam are GI (constipation, nausea, and dyspepsia). The following are contraindications for use of colesevelam:

- Patients with triglyceride levels of more than 500 mg/dL
- Patients with a history of bowel obstruction
- Patients with a history of pancreatitis caused by hypertriglyceridemia
- Patients with of Type 1 diabetes or for the treatment of DKA

Because of its constipating effects, it should not be used in patients with gastroparesis, other GI motility disorders, or in those who have had major GI tract surgery and may be at risk for bowel obstruction. The tablets are large and can cause dysphagia or esophageal obstruction; therefore, it should be used with caution in patients with dysphagia or swallowing disorders. It should be used with caution in patients with triglycerides in excess of 300 mg/dL because bile acid sequestrants can cause concentrations of serum triglycerides to increase.[240–242]

Drug interactions are an important consideration for colesevelam because it reduces GI absorption of some drugs. Drugs with a known interaction with colesevelam (e.g., phenytoin, warfarin, levothyroxine, oral contraceptives) should be administered at least 4 hours before colesevelam. The bioavailability of glimepiride, glyburide, and glipizide may be affected by concomitant administration of colesevelam; therefore, these medications should be administered 4 hours prior to colesevelam.[239]

A1C reductions associated with colesevelam are 0.3% to 0.4% compared with baseline (0.5% vs. placebo). Colesevelam also reduces LDL-C by 12% to 16% when used in combination with metformin or a sulfonylurea respectively.[243] Bile acid sequestrants can increase triglycerides by 5% to 22% in patients with Type 2 diabetes, depending on which antidiabetic medications are given concomitantly.[239–242] Colesevelam is approved for use as combination therapy with metformin, a sulfonylurea, and insulin.[239] It has not been studied as monotherapy or in combination with DPP-4 inhibitors. It can provide an added benefit in patients with dyslipidemia. The dose is six (625 mg) tablets once daily or three tablets twice daily taken with a meal and liquid. Alternatively, a 3.75-g packet (powder for oral suspension) once daily or 1.875-g packet twice daily may be used by dissolving each dose in 4 to 8 ounces of water, fruit juice, or diet soda, and administering with a meal. Since its approval, its use for treatment of Type 2 diabetes remains quite limited.

BROMOCRIPTINE

Bromocriptine mesylate, an ergot derivative, is a dopamine-2 receptor agonist that is a quick-release formulation.[244] It was FDA-approved in May 2009 for use in Type 2 diabetes. Bromocriptine has been available since 1978 and was once widely used for Parkinson disease. The mechanism by which bromocriptine improves glycemic control is not known. A normal circadian peak in the central dopaminergic tone occurs in the early morning and has been linked to induction of normal insulin sensitivity and glucose metabolism.[237] It is theorized that taking bromocriptine in the morning will increase central dopaminergic tone and reset the normal circadian rhythm to that of leaner people. The recommended dose of bromocriptine in diabetes is initiation with 0.8 mg daily, increasing by one tablet weekly until the maximum tolerated dose of 1.6 to 4.8 mg is reached. Bromocriptine is administered once daily within 2 hours after waking in the morning.[244] It should be taken with food to help reduce GI side effects such as nausea. Its effect on A1C lowering is very mild: As monotherapy, A1C is lowered by 0.1% compared with baseline (0.4% vs. placebo), and as add-on therapy to a sulfonylurea or metformin, A1C is reduced by 0.5%. Common side effects include hypotension, dizziness, syncope, nausea, somnolence, headache, and exacerbation of psychotic disorders. Bromocriptine is contraindicated in patients with known hypersensitivity to ergot-related drugs, patients with syncopal migraine, and women who are nursing.[244] Bromocriptine is highly protein bound, and when given concomitantly with other drugs that are highly protein bound, such as sulfonamides, salicylates, and probenecid, the unbound fraction of these other drugs may increase, altering their risk of adverse effects or their effectiveness. Bromocriptine is metabolized by CYP3A4; therefore, caution should be used when administering concomitant drugs that are CYP3A4 substrates, inducers or inhibitors. Neuroleptic agents with dopamine receptor agonist properties, such as olanzapine, clozapine, and ziprasidone, may reduce the effectiveness of both bromocriptine and the other drugs; therefore, concomitant use is not recommended. Given the minor A1C lowering, bromocriptine quick release has a very limited role as a therapeutic agent.[244]

TREATMENT OF PATIENTS WITH TYPE 2 DIABETES

Clinical Presentation

CASE 53-11

QUESTION 1: L.H. is a 45-year-old, overweight, Mexican American woman with central obesity (height, 5 feet 5 inches; weight, 165 lb; BMI, 27.5 kg/m^2). Three months ago, she was referred to the diabetes clinic when her gynecologist, who had been treating her for recurrent monilial infections, noted glucosuria on routine urinalysis. Subsequently, on two separate occasions, she was found to have an FPG of 150 and 167 mg/dL; an A1C was also checked and it was 8.2%. L.H. denies any symptoms of polyphagia or polyuria, although lately she has been more thirsty than usual. She does complain of lethargy and takes afternoon naps when she can.

L.H.'s other medical problems include hypertension, which is well controlled on lisinopril 20 mg/day, and recurrent monilial infections, which are treated with fluconazole. She has given birth to four children (birth weights, 7, 8.5, 10, and 11 lb) and was told during her last pregnancy that she had "borderline diabetes." She currently works as a loan officer in a local bank and spends her weekends "catching up on her sleep" and reading. L.H. has been smoking one pack of cigarettes per day for 20 years and drinks an occasional glass of wine. She drinks at least two regular sodas daily and has a "large" glass of orange juice every morning. Her physical activity consists of routine walking during the day (e.g., to her car). Her family history is significant for a sister, aunt, and grandmother with Type 2 diabetes; all have "weight problems." L.H.'s mother is alive and well at age 77; her father died of a heart attack at age 47.

On presentation, fasting laboratory assessment reveals glucose of 147 mg/dL, triglycerides of 400 mg/dL, and an A1C of 8.3% (normal, 4%–6%). All other values (including the complete blood count, electrolytes, LFTs, and renal function tests) are within normal limits. L.H. is given the diagnosis of Type 2 diabetes. What features in L.H.'s history and physical examination are consistent with this diagnosis?

The features of L.H.'s history that are consistent with Type 2 diabetes include an FPG concentration of 126 mg/dL or higher on more than one occasion, a A1C of 6.5% or more, high BMI with central obesity, age older than 40, physical inactivity, family history of diabetes, and Mexican American descent. L.H. also has delivered large babies, which suggests that she may have had undiagnosed gestational diabetes, a condition that places women at high risk for subsequently developing Type 2 diabetes. Diagnosis on routine examination and mild signs and symptoms of hyperglycemia (including increased thirst and lethargy), recurrent monilial infections, hypertriglyceridemia, and indications of CVD (hypertension) also are typical in patients with Type 2 diabetes (see Type 2 Diabetes section and Table 53-1).

Treatment Goals

CASE 53-11, QUESTION 2: What should the goals of therapy be for L.H. and other patients with Type 2 diabetes? Which biochemical indices should be monitored?

The beginning of this chapter discussed general goals of therapy for all people with diabetes, which include eliminating acute symptoms of hyperglycemia, avoiding hypoglycemia, reducing cardiovascular risk factors, and preventing or slowing the progression of both microvascular and macrovascular diabetic complications. The ADA recommends that otherwise healthy patients with Type 2 diabetes strive to achieve the same biochemical goals as those recommended for people with Type 1 diabetes (Tables 53-4 and 53-5).[7] When determining treatment goals for L.H. and others with Type 2 diabetes, the same individual characteristics should be considered as for Type 1 diabetes, such as the patient's capacity to understand and carry out the treatment regimen and the patient's risk for severe hypoglycemia. Given the data from the ACCORD, ADVANCE, and VADT trials, patients with Type 2 diabetes and CVD or multiple CVD risk factors should be carefully assessed when determining their glycemic goals. For example, less aggressive A1C goals should be considered for patients with advanced age (and short life expectancy), longer duration of diabetes (more than 10 years), advanced microvascular complications, or comorbid conditions such as significant cerebrovascular or coronary artery disease because of the serious consequences related to hypoglycemia. Therefore, glycemic goals for patients with Type 2 diabetes must be individualized. Emphasis should be placed on assessment of *all* cardiovascular risk factors, including hypertension, tobacco use, dyslipidemia, and family history.

As presented earlier in the Relationship of Glycemic Control to Microvascular and Macrovascular Disease section, the UKPDS was a landmark study in patients with Type 2 diabetes that conclusively demonstrated that improved BG control reduces the risk of developing retinopathy, nephropathy, and, potentially, neuropathy.[35,44,238] The 10-year follow-up study demonstrated that these outcomes persist even though the conventional group achieved similar glycemic control with time; an overall relative risk reduction in microvascular complications (24%) in the sulfonylurea- or insulin-treated group compared with patients who initially received conventional therapy was seen.[33] The exciting finding was that reductions in macrovascular complications emerged with time, with significant reductions in MI (15%) and death of any cause (13%) in patients initially intensively treated with sulfonylurea or insulin. Metformin appeared to be of particular benefit, with even greater reductions in MI and death of any cause (33% and 27%, respectively).

An additional finding of the UKPDS was that aggressive control of BP also significantly reduced microvascular complications, strokes, diabetes-related deaths, HF, and vision loss; during the 10-year follow-up study, these benefits diminished with time as the BP difference between the two groups was lost (i.e., BP increased in the tight control group and decreased in the conventional group).[245–247] These findings stress the importance of maintaining good BP control to reduce the risk of long-term complications.

Because L.H. is relatively young and has no symptoms of microvascular disease or neuropathy, every effort should be made to normalize her glucose concentrations to prevent these complications. Furthermore, a lipid panel should be ordered, and steps should be taken to achieve normal LDL-C, HDL-C, and triglyceride levels. Often, triglyceride levels improve as BG concentrations decline and the metabolic response to insulin improves. (Management of dyslipidemia is addressed more fully later in this chapter.)

Biochemical indices that should be followed to monitor L.H.'s response to therapy include fasting, postprandial, and preprandial BG concentrations, A1C values, and fasting triglyceride levels, as well as LDL-C and HDL-C concentrations. Based on ADA guidelines initial metabolic goals for L.H. should be an A1C value of less than 7%, an FPG of 80 to 130 mg/dL and postprandial glucose concentrations less than 180 mg/dL.[7]

Treatment

LIFESTYLE INTERVENTIONS AND INITIAL THERAPY WITH METFORMIN

CASE 53-11, QUESTION 3: How should L.H. be managed initially?

Initial therapy of Type 2 diabetes is aimed at lifestyle changes that will minimize insulin resistance and risk for CVD. In L.H.'s case and in the case of other overweight (BMI, 25.0–29.9 kg/m^2) or obese (BMI $\geq$30.0 kg/m^2) Type 2 diabetes individuals, this includes a lower-calorie, low-fat, low-cholesterol diet; regular exercise; smoking cessation (see Chapter 91, Tobacco Use and Dependence); and aggressive management of dyslipidemia and hypertension. Because central obesity is associated with increased insulin resistance, L.H. should be strongly encouraged to decrease her caloric intake, start exercising, and lose weight. Simple changes in her diet (such as cutting out juice and regular soda) and physical activity level can have a large impact on her glucose control. SMBG monitoring should be encouraged, and education that addresses the serious nature of diabetes mellitus and its long-term consequences also should begin. This is discussed in the previous sections, Medical Nutrition Therapy and Physical Activity, under Treatment (See also Table 53-14).

Initial Pharmacologic Therapy with Metformin

The ADA recommends that most patients diagnosed with Type 2 diabetes begin therapy with lifestyle modifications, including those mentioned above. In addition, most patients should begin monotherapy with metformin upon diagnosis. If metformin is contraindicated or poorly tolerated, agent approved for monotherapy may be used.[7] The selection of alternative agents will be discussed later in this chapter.

Although the UKPDS demonstrated that intensive therapy with sulfonylureas, metformin, and insulin reduces glucose with equal effectiveness (TZDs were not studied), metformin is favored as a first-choice agent in Type 2 diabetes, particularly in overweight patients. This is because metformin lowers BG by decreasing hepatic glucose output and insulin resistance (indirectly) without causing weight gain or hypoglycemia. Metformin also has beneficial effects on plasma lipid concentrations as well due to a reduction in LDL as well as fatty acids.[238]

Another reason for metformin being a first choice for initial therapy is not only its proven benefit to reduce risk of microvascular complications, but also macrovascular disease and mortality.[33] Furthermore, in an observational study of patients with Type 2 diabetes, and established coronary artery disease, cerebrovascular disease, or peripheral arterial disease, metformin use was associated with a significant reduction in all-cause mortality (22%) after only 2 years of follow-up.[243] Metformin is also emerging as a therapy that may reduce cancer risk, possibly attributable to its activation of AMPK, which can suppress tumor formation. Data so far have been in animal models and observational studies in humans.[248]

A drawback to immediate-release metformin is that it requires multiple daily dosing and its dose also must be titrated to minimize GI effects. After the dose is established, it is possible to use a long-acting product that can be dosed once daily. Alternatively, extended-release metformin may be initiated at a dose of 500 mg daily and titrated upward as tolerated. Renal function tests should be evaluated before the drug is initiated. L.H. does not have any contraindications (renal or hepatic dysfunction, cardiorespiratory disease, binge alcohol use) to the use of metformin that could predispose her to its most significant side effect, lactic acidosis (see Case 53-16, Question 2). Because L.H. exhibits the typical features of insulin resistance syndrome and has no contraindications for its use, she should be started on metformin. Her A1C goal of less than 7% will require an additional 1.3% lowering in her A1C, which can be achieved with metformin. However, any changes in her lifestyle will further help lower her A1C. L.H. should take metformin 500 mg twice daily with food.

Titrating Metformin Doses

CASE 53-11, QUESTION 4: L.H. is started on metformin 500 mg BID with food and instructed to increase her dosage to 500 mg every morning and 1,000 mg every evening after 1 week. Three days after starting metformin, she phones the clinic complaining of nausea and diarrhea. She admits to taking her doses on an empty stomach. How should L.H.'s symptoms be addressed?

GI disturbances such as diarrhea, bloating, anorexia, abdominal discomfort, nausea, and metallic taste often dissipate with time and can be minimized by initiating metformin in a single 500- or 850-mg dose at breakfast or with the patient's largest meal of the day. Consistently taking metformin with food significantly minimizes the GI side effects. The dosage should be slowly increased (e.g., 500 mg/day every 2 weeks) until the appropriate clinical effect is achieved or the patient is taking the maximal dose (1,000 mg BID or 850 mg TID). Therefore, L.H.'s metformin dose should be reduced to 500 mg daily with her largest meal, and she should be titrated more slowly during a period of several weeks. Metformin is typically dosed 2 to 3 times daily (the long-acting formulation is dosed once daily with dinner). Twice-daily dosing for adherence purposes is preferred if a patient can tolerate a 1,000-mg dose or once daily with the extended-release formulation. If she continues to experience GI symptoms, an alternative approach is to use the extended-release formulation; small studies have demonstrated improved tolerability with the extended-release tablets versus the immediate-release dosage form.[249] A drawback to these tablets is their very large size. Also, patients may complain that metformin has a fishy odor,[250] which seems to be more apparent with certain generic formulations. If this is significant enough to cause a patient to stop taking it, the extended-release formulation can be tried, which may be more tolerable.

Monitoring Metformin Therapy

CASE 53-11, QUESTION 5: How should metformin therapy be monitored in L.H.?

As is standard with other agents, L.H. should be encouraged to perform SMBG (see Case 53-11, Question 6) and have an A1C test performed quarterly until she achieves consistent values less than 7%. Additional evidence of the therapeutic benefits of metformin may include an improved lipid profile and some weight loss. Initially, it is important to monitor GI problems, and although lactic acidosis is unlikely, L.H. should be warned to bring to the attention of her physician any sudden symptoms of shortness of breath, weakness, and malaise. A baseline SCr, LFTs, and complete blood count should be obtained for L.H. and repeated yearly. Metformin can reduce vitamin B_{12} absorption, and it is associated with reductions in vitamin B_{12} levels (19% after 4 years of use in one study) and actual deficiency.[251] Therefore, monitoring of vitamin B_{12} levels every 2 to 3 years should be considered with long-term use.

SELF-MONITORING OF BLOOD GLUCOSE IN TYPE 2 DIABETES

CASE 53-11, QUESTION 6: L.H. is interested in learning how to perform BG testing. What are the advantages and disadvantages of SMBG tests? When and how often should L.H. be instructed to test her BG concentrations?

SMBG is an important self-management tool for patients such as L.H. to assess the efficacy of therapy and guide adjustments in nutrition, exercise, and medications. Disadvantages include cost of testing, inadequate understanding by both healthcare providers and patients regarding the benefits and proper use of SMBG results, patient psychological and minor physical discomfort associated with obtaining a blood sample, and the inconvenience of testing. However, with the current advances in meter technology and proper patient education, most of these potential barriers can be overcome.

The ADA states that SMBG may be a useful guide for patients with Type 2 diabetes treated with MNT or noninsulin therapies, although there is insufficient evidence to determine optimal frequency of testing and demonstrate cost-effectiveness for these patients. Although one meta-analysis of SMBG effects in patients with Type 2 diabetes not on insulin concluded the overall effect on A1C was a 0.4% reduction, others failed to show a benefit.[252,253] SMBG studies in patients with Type 2 diabetes are often limited in that multiple interventions, such as education, diet, and medication adjustments, were used. However, a primary reason studies fail to show a benefit is that patients are not taught what to do with their BG numbers (i.e., how to respond to a low BG reading); the BG values are solely used by the providers to make adjustments to their therapy.[253]

SMBG should be considered for most patients with Type 2 diabetes, particularly those who are learning to adjust their carbohydrate intake and portion sizes and want to measure how well medications and lifestyle changes are working to improve their glucose control. Although not always cost-effective, testing 4 times daily before meals and at bedtime for 1 week is useful, so that the patient can observe his/her glucose profiles. Later, once the desired A1C has been achieved, BG can be tested less frequently. Testing times should vary throughout the day so that fasting as well as postprandial and bedtime values can be assessed. As emphasized by the ADA, intensive patient education regarding testing technique and interpretation are vital to the cost-effective use of this monitoring tool. The patient must learn how to respond to his/her glucose profile and institute lifestyle changes that can have a favorable effect.

Clinical Use of Antidiabetic Agents

CASE 53-11, QUESTION 7: L.H. was quite motivated to improve her glucose control because her grandmother "lost a leg" to diabetes and her aunt is undergoing dialysis because "her kidneys have failed." She is taking metformin 1,000 mg PO BID and tolerating it reasonably well (she occasionally gets some stomach discomfort, but states she is fine with it). She is proud that she remembers to take the metformin every day as instructed. She met with a dietitian who suggested an 1,800-calorie diet and 45-minute walks 3 times weekly. After 3 months, L.H. lost 6 pounds. L.H. stopped drinking regular sodas and juices, but eats either breads or two large tortillas at each meal. She admits to eating only small amounts of "greens" and vegetables. She has not been able to implement her walks 3 times weekly; more often she only walks once a week. Although her FPG fell to 130 mg/dL, a majority of her postprandial BG levels were more than 180 mg/dL. Her A1C is 7.4%, and fasting triglyceride levels are now 260 mg/dL. How should her therapy be adjusted? What factors should be considered when deciding on the next steps for pharmacologic therapy?

L.H.'s A1C has improved by 0.9%. However, she has not fully instituted lifestyle interventions. Although she has cut out juices and regular sodas, she can still further improve her diet and lower her postprandial BG (to <180 mg/dL) by reducing her carbohydrate intake, switching to whole-grain breads, and increasing her vegetable intake. She also can increase her physical activity to at least 3 times weekly. Although the A1C is not less than 7%, a reasonable approach would be to continue metformin at 1,000 mg PO BID and reinforce lifestyle changes at this point before modifying her pharmacologic therapy.

The amount of A1C lowering in response to adding an antidiabetic agent appears to depend on the baseline glycemic level. A meta-regression analysis of 61 clinical trials evaluated the efficacy of the five classes of oral agents (sulfonylureas, glinides, metformin, TZDs, and α-glucosidase inhibitors).[254] Significant correlations were found between the baseline A1C and FPG, and their mean decreases as a result of these agents. Greater reductions in A1C and FPG were observed in groups with higher baseline levels. In addition, a meta-analysis of oral agents found that every 1% higher baseline A1C level predicted a 0.5% greater reduction in the A1C after 6 months of therapy.[255] Overall, on initiation of noninsulin monotherapy, the A1C will typically lower by approximately 1% to 1.25%.[255]

If L.H. is not able to reach an A1C of less than 7% with lifestyle interventions, the next step for her would be to add a second antidiabetic agent. Selecting an antidiabetic agent to treat Type 2 diabetes has become more complex because new agents with unique mechanisms of action have been introduced into the market. Several considerations should be taken into account when choosing initial oral therapy for patients with Type 2 diabetes. As with all therapeutic decisions, clinicians should also blend their knowledge of the drug (e.g., its efficacy, safety, hypoglycemic risk, weight gain, other side effects, route of administration, and cost/hospital formulary) with the unique characteristics of the patient (e.g., level of glycemic control, organ function, other concurrent diseases and medications, ability to adhere to complex medication regimens, health insurance coverage) when making a choice of drug products.[256] The current A1C level and reduction required to reach the A1C goal is a key consideration. It is also important to remember that studies report the glucose-lowering effects of antidiabetic agents by their means; some patients respond more and some respond less than the mean.

Table 53-25 compares and contrasts the efficacy, advantages, and disadvantages of antidiabetic agents used to treat patients with Type 2 diabetes and can be used to help select drugs for a specific patient.

The AACE guidelines recommend consideration of initiating insulin therapy (most often basal insulin) if the A1C is more than 9% with symptoms of hyperglycemia.[39] The ADA guidelines recommend choosing based on patient's level of glycemia and if they are symptomatic.[7] It is an option for dual therapy in all patients, especially if A1C > 9%, but should be strongly considered with an A1C > 10%.[7] Practitioners should attempt to avoid unnecessarily complex therapy that may confuse the patient, increase drug costs, and complicate the clinician's ability to assess each medication's contribution to the overall therapeutic outcome.

The ADA recommends initial therapy with lifestyle changes and metformin monotherapy. If the patient cannot tolerate metformin, any other agent approved for monotherapy may be used. These agents include sulfonylureas, TZDs, DPP-4 inhibitors, SGLT2 inhibitors, GLP-1 receptor agonists, and insulin. Selection of appropriate agents will be discussed later in this chapter. If after 3 months of monotherapy the patient has not achieved their glycemic targets, a second agent may be added. If the patient still has not achieved their glycemic targets after 3 months of dual therapy, a third agent may be added. If glycemic targets still have not been reached after 3 months of triple therapy, different drug classes should be tried and a basal-bolus insulin approach may be considered.[7]

SELECTING AN ALTERNATIVE TO METFORMIN AS MONOTHERAPY

CASE 53-11, QUESTION 8: Which other antidiabetic agents could be considered for L.H. as monotherapy if she cannot tolerate metformin therapy?

Although the ADA recommends the use of metformin, in combination with lifestyle modification, as first-line therapy, other antidiabetic agents are approved for use as monotherapy as well. L.H. is a typical overweight Type 2 diabetes patient with early evidence of CVD (hypertension), but with no evidence of microvascular complications. Her liver, renal, and GI functions are normal. Patients like L.H. have varying degrees of β-cell dysfunction and tissue resistance to insulin. In these individuals, pulsatile insulin secretion and first-phase insulin release are absent, and the pancreas is "blind" or unresponsive to high glucose concentrations (glucotoxicity). Because target tissues are less responsive to insulin, hepatic glucose output typically is increased and higher concentrations of insulin may be needed for peripheral glucose utilization. Insulin causes more weight gain and hypoglycemia than the other antidiabetic agents and is usually reserved for combination therapy unless the initial A1C at diagnosis is very elevated (>10%) or ketonuria is present.[7]

Often, acarbose is eliminated from consideration because slow titration is required to minimize GI effects; anecdotally, however, people of Mexican American origin, such as L.H., seem less susceptible to flatulence and diarrhea. Also, because acarbose has less dramatic effects on the FPG (20–30 mg/dL decrease) and A1C (0.5%–1.0% decrease) than the other agents, biochemical goals are less likely to be achieved in patients whose A1C is 8.5% or higher.

Pioglitazone also can be used as monotherapy, and, like metformin, will not cause hypoglycemia, but weight gain and edema are likely. On the positive side, the TZDs have been shown to have better "glycemic durability" compared with metformin and the sulfonylureas. In a double-blind, randomized, controlled trial of 4,360 patients with Type 2 diabetes, time to monotherapy failure, defined as FPG greater than 180 mg/dL, was assessed for rosiglitazone, metformin, and glyburide (A Diabetes Outcome Progression Trial [ADOPT]).[257] Patients were treated for a median of 4 years. The Kaplan–Meier analysis showed that the cumulative incidence of failure at 5 years was 15% for rosiglitazone, 21% for metformin, and 34% for glyburide ($p < 0.0001$). The suggested explanation for the favorable rosiglitazone results was that it slowed the rate of β-cell function decline. On the negative side, TZDs are associated with many adverse effects including an increase risk in bone fractures and HF.[258] TZDs are associated with an approximately twofold increased risk of HF and thus are contraindicated in NYHA Class III-IV HF.[185,187] In the long-term ADOPT trial, rosiglitazone was associated with a mean weight gain of 4.8 kg, whereas weight decreased by 2.9 kg in the metformin group; glyburide-treated patients had a mean weight gain of 1.6 kg during the first year, and then remained stable.[257] The TZDs also have been found to reduce bone density and increase fracture risk. Given the adverse effects associated with TZDs, and the availability of other agents, their use has fallen out of favor.

Sitagliptin, saxagliptin, and exenatide, which are approved for monotherapy, are often reserved for combination therapy. However, DPP-4 inhibitors may be useful as monotherapy for patients in whom the use of other oral agents is precluded (such as renal dysfunction with metformin or severe HF with pioglitazone). GLP-1RAs may be particularly useful in obese patients.[7,39] It should be noted that AACE recommends GLP-1RAs as first line if metformin can't be initiated first.[39]

Finally, one should not forget that until the newer agents became available, sulfonylureas were used quite successfully to treat obese patients with Type 2 diabetes. Although these agents are relatively effective (average A1C reduction 1%–1.5%), there are still several issues with this class of medications such as unfavorable adverse effects (hypoglycemia and weight gain), durability issues, and may worsen the lipid panel. Although the use of these agents has fallen out of favor due to these effects, they are effective and often utilized when cost is an issue (Table 53-26).

Several products that combine two oral agents into one medication are available. Although many of these products are approved as first-line therapy, thus skipping the monotherapy step, consider reserving them for use in patients who are already established on the two agents or whose medication regimens must be simplified to enhance adherence or decrease cost or are already established on the two agents.

Based on this discussion, metformin is favored as initial therapy in L.H.

CASE 53-12

QUESTION 1: N.H. is a 46-year-old, obese (BMI 33 kg/m^2) man with a history of Type 2 diabetes, and hyperlipidemia. He presents with complaints of fatigue and nocturia. N.H. used to smoke two packs of cigarettes/day for 15 years, but he quit after his diabetes diagnosis. He has a strong family history of CHD. At diagnosis 3 months ago, an elevated A1C was documented (7.6%), confirming the diagnosis of Type 2 diabetes. Tests of liver and renal function are within normal limits. Current medications include lisinopril and atorvastatin. N.H. started metformin but stopped taking it because of GI symptoms (loose stools); he refuses to try this medication again. What is a reasonable next monotherapy option for N.H.?

Unfortunately, N.H. did not tolerate metformin. Although this is less common if patients take metformin with food and the dose is titrated slowly, some do not overcome the GI adverse effects. N.H. is refusing to even consider a retrial. An A1C goal of less than 7% may be appropriate for N.H., although given his young age and long life expectancy, a target of less than 6.5% would be preferred. Therefore, the A1C lowering required to get to goal is only 0.6% to 1.1%.

With a BMI of 33 kg/m^2, hypertension, and dyslipidemia, N.H. has many components of the metabolic syndrome and insulin resistance (see Pathogenesis section). Sulfonylureas or insulin would not be an optimal next choice of drug for N.H. because they do not exert a favorable effect on plasma lipids and generally are associated with weight gain and hypoglycemia. Also, his A1C is not high enough to need insulin therapy yet. However, it must be acknowledged that some sulfonylureas remain the least expensive oral antidiabetic agents, and this may be an important factor in the initial selection of therapy for some patients. Acarbose as monotherapy is not likely to attain near-normal plasma glucose concentrations. Given he is obese, and likely insulin resistant, although pioglitazone improves peripheral target tissue responses to insulin and lipid profiles, avoiding pioglitazone due to adverse effects of weight gain is prudent (see Case 53-11, Question 8, and Case 53-15). A GLP-1 agonist, DPP-4 inhibitor, or SGLT-2 inhibitor are reasonable options for N.H. because they are not associated with weight gain (GLP-1 agonists and SGLT-2 inhibitors may even promote weight loss).

For N.H., initiation of a GLP-1RA, such as liraglutide, is a reasonable option. A GLP-1RA, along with lifestyle changes, should be able to get to his A1C goal. If liraglutide is used, it should be initiated at a dose of 0.6 mg once daily for 1 week and then increased to the therapeutic dose of 1.2 mg once daily thereafter. Some patients may require further titration to 1.8 mg once daily in order to reach their glycemic goals. N.H. should be counseled about the likelihood of GI side effects, which should subside over time, as well as the rare risk of pancreatitis (and to stop taking and notify his provider if he has persistent severe abdominal pain that may radiate to the back and vomiting) and severe allergic reactions.

N.H. was successful in reducing his A1C to 6.4% through a combination of lifestyle modifications and sitagliptin. He was able to lose 10 lb with walking and reduction in fatty food.

N.H. quit smoking 3 months ago. Smoking has been shown to increase the risk of IFG and Type 2 diabetes.[259,260] The mechanism for this is thought to be related to increased insulin resistance and oxidative stress and reduced insulin secretion. Smoking also increases the risk of microvascular and macrovascular disease in people with diabetes.[261] Therefore, N.H. should be congratulated on his cessation, and continued abstinence should be encouraged through follow-up visits (see Chapter 91, Tobacco Use and Dependence).

Failure of Antidiabetic Monotherapy

PATHOGENESIS

CASE 53-13

QUESTION 1: Q.R. is a 68-year-old, 5 feet 1 inch, 155-lb (BMI, 29.3 kg/m^2) woman with an 8-year history of Type 2 diabetes who has been treated with diet, exercise, and metformin. According to clinic records, she was well controlled initially (A1C 6.7%–7.2%) for the first 5 years. When her glycemic control worsened (FPG, 130–160 mg/dL; A1C, 7.5%–8.5%), her metformin dose was increased from an initial dose of 500 mg BID to her current dose of 1,000 mg BID. Recent chart notes indicate that Q.R.'s chief complaints have included loss of appetite and fatigue. Her current A1C is 8.4%. Other medical problems include hypertension managed with hydrochlorothiazide 25 mg daily and mild peripheral neuropathy managed with acetaminophen 500 mg BID. Her eGFR is 70 mL/minute.

At this clinic visit, Q.R., who is well known to you, seems particularly listless and flat in her affect. Her BG records, which are typically meticulous, are incomplete. AM fasting BG values consistently exceed 200 mg/dL and range from 202 to 340 mg/dL. While taking her history, you discover that her husband passed away last year and that one of her adult children has recently been diagnosed with a terminal illness. What factors may be contributing to Q.R.'s poor glucose control?

Several factors may be contributing to Q.R.'s deteriorating BG control and apparent lack of responsiveness to maximal dose of metformin during the past year (as evidenced by her elevated BG and A1C, listlessness, and lack of appetite). Monotherapy failure (also called secondary failure) is characterized by progressively poor glucose control that occurs after a period of good response (months to years). The cause of failure may be related to progressive pancreatic failure; poor adherence to diet, exercise, or medications; and exogenous diabetogenic factors such as increased weight, illness, or drugs that induce hyperglycemia (e.g., atypical antipsychotics or glucocorticoids).

Type 2 diabetes is a progressive condition, which is most likely to require combination drug therapy. The UKPDS confirmed that monotherapy failure represents a natural progression of Type 2 diabetes. In this study, only 16% and 19% of the subjects achieved an FPG less than 108 mg/dL and A1C less than 7%, respectively, after 3 years of dietary therapy alone.[262] By 9 years, only 9% were able to maintain their glycemic goals using just diet therapy. The investigators also found monotherapy failure occurred at the same rate regardless of the initial treatment selected: glyburide, chlorpropamide, metformin, or insulin. In all the monotherapy treatment groups, patients required additional therapies over the course of the study duration.[262] At 3 years, fewer than 55% of patients randomly assigned to single pharmacologic therapy could maintain an A1C less than 7%, and by 9 years this dropped to about 25% of patients. In the ADOPT study, patients were able to maintain A1C levels less than 7% using monotherapy for 60, 45, and 33 months with rosiglitazone, metformin, and glyburide, respectively.[257] The reason for glycemic deterioration is likely owing to the natural progression of Type 2 diabetes in which β-cell function declines with increased duration of disease.

Q.R.'s deteriorating control on a therapeutic dose of metformin after 5 years of reasonable response is consistent with the natural progression of Type 2 diabetes. However, the stress and depression arising out of her life situation have no doubt contributed to her poor control. The latter may have led to a change in her usual adherence to diet, exercise, and medications, and should resolve with time and appropriate management. Women with Type 2 diabetes are at increased risk of depression. Evidence exists for a bidirectional association between diabetes and depression in women.[263] Although hyperglycemia has been attributed to hydrochlorothiazide, the dose prescribed for Q.R. has few adverse metabolic effects.

MANAGING MONOTHERAPY FAILURE

CASE 53-13, QUESTION 2: How should Q.R. be managed? What is an appropriate antidiabetic agent to add?

Q.R. is exhibiting symptoms of depression (e.g., listlessness and flat affect). Her depression likely started after her husband's death. Every effort must be made to address Q.R.'s depression because it is unlikely that she will be able to effectively implement more aggressive treatment of her diabetes until her situation is improved. Resources that may be used include her family, a therapist, and a social worker.

Treatment of monotherapy failure includes identifying and correcting any diabetogenic factors and altering her drug therapy. When failure to any oral agent occurs, one should always add another agent rather than switch to another, unless adverse effects are intolerable or contraindications warrant the discontinuation of the drug. This is supported by a study that evaluated the effect of metformin alone in a population of patients who had failed oral sulfonylureas and the effect of metformin plus the sulfonylureas. Substitution of metformin for glyburide did not produce any significant change in glycemic control, but the addition of metformin to glyburide therapy substantially improved glucose concentrations.[264] Many combinations of antidiabetic agents can be used. The key is that they should have different mechanisms of action. For example, it is not reasonable to combine a sulfonylurea with a glinide (i.e., repaglinide and nateglinide) because they are both insulin secretagogues. Options for Q.R. include adding one of the following to metformin: insulin secretagogue (sulfonylurea or glinide), acarbose, TZD (pioglitazone), DPP-4 inhibitor (sitagliptin, linagliptin, alogliptin or saxagliptin), SGLT-2 inhibitors (canagliflozin, dapagliflozin, empagliflozin), or a GLP-1 agonist (exenatide, exentatide ER, albiglutide, dulaglutide, or liraglutide). SGLT-2 should be used cautiously in this patient because this drug class is associated with genital mycotic infections and urinary tract infections.[228]

Table 53-25 summarizes the FDA-approved combination therapy indications. One also could introduce insulin therapy at this time. However, because Q.R.'s A1C should be effectively lowered to less than 7% with an additional noninsulin agent, two noninsulin antidiabetic agents should be utilized.

In summary, patients such as Q.R. who are unresponsive to the maximally effective dose of metformin should be initiated on combination therapy.

Combination Antidiabetic Therapy

CASE 53-13, QUESTION 3: As anticipated, Q.R. refuses to consider insulin therapy at this time. Which combination of antidiabetic agents is preferred?

When agents from different antidiabetic classes are combined, their effects are essentially additive. With the availability of many antidiabetic agents, there is no one best combination therapy. As discussed, the choice of therapy should take into account the patient's organ function, amount of A1C lowering required to reach an individual's goal, possible adverse effects of a particular drug or drug combination, cost, and patient preference.

A mixed-treatment comparison meta-analysis evaluated the efficacy of second-line antidiabetic therapy added to patients on stable doses of metformin.[265] The risk of weight gain and hypoglycemia was also determined. A total of 27 randomized controlled trials were included in the analysis, with a mean study duration of 32 weeks. Table 53-27 summarizes these findings. In addition, the change in A1C depending on the baseline level of A1C was evaluated and found, as previously discussed (see Case 53-11, Question 7), to be greater when the baseline A1C was 8% or more.

Q.R. is concerned with the costs of her medications, and brand drugs have a higher copay in her insurance plan. Q.R. would like to remain on oral medications if possible. Because she is postmenopausal, avoid a TZD owing to the concerns of increased risk of fractures. Given the significant GI side effects associated with the α-glucosidase inhibitors, their use is often avoided all together. The DPP-4 inhibitors are available by brand only, so initiating a generic is an option. Therefore, she is started on glimepiride 2 mg PO daily.

Combination Antidiabetic Therapy

CASE 53-13, QUESTION 4: Q.R. is titrated to glimepiride 4 mg/day and continued on metformin 1,000 mg BID. This improved her FPG and A1C modestly for approximately 12 months (FPG, 120–150 mg/dL; currently A1C, 7.6%). She remains resistant to starting insulin, despite repeated counseling. She has heard about a new, injectable class of diabetes medications that cause weight loss, and asks whether she is a good candidate to start one. It quickly becomes apparent that Q.R. is referring to the GLP-1 agonists, exenatide, exenatide ER, dulaglutide, albiglutide, and liraglutide; only exenatide is on her health plan's formulary.

Table 53-27
Effects of Adding a Noninsulin Antidiabetic Agent in Patients with Type 2 Diabetes Already on Metformin[265]

	Effects of Adding a Noninsulin Agent Compared with Placebo in Patients Taking Metformin on Change in A1C, Body Weight, and Hypoglycemia					
	% Change in A1C		Change in Body Weight (kg)		Overall Hypoglycemia	
Group vs. Placebo	No. of Trials	WMD (95% CI)	No. of Trials	WMD (95% CI)	No. of Trials	RR (95% CI)
All drugs	20	−0.79 (−0.90 to −0.68)	12	−0.14 (−1.37 to 1.65)	19	1.43 (0.89 to 2.30)
SFUs	3	−0.79 (−1.15 to −0.43)	2	−1.99 (0.86 to 3.12)	3	2.63 (0.76 to 9.13)
Glinides	2	−0.71 (−1.24 to −0.18)	2	−0.91 (0.35 to 1.46)	2	7.92 (1.45 to 43.21)
TZDs	3	−1.00 (−1.62 to −0.38)	1	−2.30 (1.70 to 2.90)	2	2.04 (0.50 to 8.23)
AGIs	2	−0.68 (−1.11 to −0.19)	1	−1.80 (−2.83 to −0.077)	2	0.60 (0.08 to 4.55)
DPP-4 inhibitors	8	−0.79 (−0.94 to −0.63)	4	−0.09 (−0.47 to 0.30)	8	0.67 (0.30 to 1.50)
GLP-1 agonists	2	−0.99 (−1.19 to −0.78)	2	−1.76 (−2.90 to 0.62)	2	0.94 (0.42 to 2.12)

	Effects of Adding a Noninsulin Agent Compared with Placebo in Patients Taking Metformin on Change in A1C, Depending on Baseline A1C	
	Baseline A1C	
Group vs. Placebo	<8% WMD (95% CI)	≥8% WMD (95% CI)
SFUs	−0.57 (−0.75 to −0.39)	−0.97 (−1.35 to −0.62)
Glinides	−0.44 (−0.85 to −0.04)	−0.65 (−1.10 to −0.26)
TZDs	−0.62 (−0.88 to −0.39)	−1.02 (−1.39 to −0.69)
AGIs	NR	−0.65 (−1.07 to −0.24)
DPP-4 inhibitors	−0.51 (−0.69 to −0.34)	−0.89 (−1.11 to −0.68)
GLP-1 agonists	NR	−0.99 (−1.36 to −0.63)

Results are from a subgroup mixed-treatment comparison meta-analysis.
AGIs, α-glucosidase inhibitors; CI, confidence interval; DPP-4, dipeptidyl peptidase-4; GLP-1, glucagon-like peptide-1; NR, not reported; RR, relative risk; SFUs, sulfonylureas; TZDs, thiazolidinediones; WMD, weighted mean difference.

When the A1C is above goal despite the use of a combination of two agents, practitioners often add a third agent before considering insulin. Although this is tempting, depending on a patient's current level of glycemic control, this practice only delays insulin therapy, which is likely to be required to achieve A1C goals. However, because Q.R. is close to an A1C level of less than 7%, it is reasonable to try a third, noninsulin antidiabetic agent. Although glimepiride 8 mg/day is the maximal dose, there is little difference in clinical efficacy compared with 4 mg/day. Therefore, increasing glimepiride to 8 mg/day is not likely to achieve her glycemic goals.[266]

Exenatide is approved for use in patients as monotherapy and also for those taking metformin, sulfonylurea, or a TZD alone, or a combination of metformin plus a TZD or metformin plus a sulfonylurea. When added to patients on a sulfonylurea and metformin, exenatide at 10 mcg BID resulted in a 0.8% A1C reduction compared with baseline.[258] Thus, for Q.R., the addition of exenatide could result in an A1C of less than 7%. The use of exenatide with a sulfonylurea is associated with an increased risk of mild-to-moderate hypoglycemia (28% when used with sulfonylurea and metformin and 36% when used with sulfonylurea alone).[258,267] Most practitioners reduce the dose of the sulfonylurea on initiation of exenatide and then make adjustments based on the patient's response to exenatide.

Q.R. should be started on exenatide 5 mcg SC BID, taken within 60 minutes of the two main meals of the day and at least 6 hours apart. She should be counseled about nausea, which is the most frequent side effect; 44% of patients will experience nausea, but there is only a 3% dropout rate in the clinical trials. The glimepiride should be reduced to 2 (or 3) mg/day to avoid hypoglycemia. After 1 month, if she is tolerating exenatide, the dose should be increased to 10 mcg SC BID. Her A1C should be monitored within 3 months of using the 10-mcg dose. An advantage of exenatide (versus DPP-4 inhibitors) is the potential for weight loss. In a 30-week blinded study of exenatide added onto sulfonylurea and metformin, patients on the 10-mcg dose had an average weight loss of 1.6 kg.[258] In the three open-label, uncontrolled extension trials with exenatide, at 3 years, exenatide progressively reduced (−5.3 kg) and sustained weight loss.[268]

Q.R. should be counseled about the rare risk of pancreatitis. Also, if she finds that nausea is significant enough to reduce her fluid intake, she should contact her provider. The FDA has received case reports of altered renal function and renal failure with exenatide, which are likely owing to dehydration from reduced fluid intake because of the GI side effects (i.e., nausea, vomiting, and diarrhea) caused by exenatide.[214] In patients with significant GI side effects, reduced fluid intake, or preexisting renal dysfunction, the SCr should be monitored more closely. Exenatide should be used cautiously with moderate renal impairment and is not recommended in patients with ClCr of less than 30.[214]

A small proportion of patients will form antiexenatide antibodies. At high titers, these antibodies could result in failure to achieve adequate improvement in glycemic control. If there is worsening glycemic control or failure to achieve targeted glycemic control while on exenatide, the formation of blocking antibodies should be considered as a reason. If this occurs, it may be reasonable to switch over to another GLP-1 analog or exenatide ER. It is important to note that any of the available GLP-1 RAs are options for Q.R. for initial GLP-1 RA therapy. Discussions should be regarding adherence, efficacy, side effects, and cost.

Combination Antidiabetic with Insulin Therapy

Case 53-13, Question 5: If Q.R. were willing to start insulin, why would it be reasonable to use insulin in combination with other antidiabetic agents? How should it be combined with other agents? Is this combination more effective than insulin alone?

Most patients with Type 2 diabetes eventually require insulin. The combined use of insulin with a variety of oral agents has been extensively evaluated, but the studies differ in their interventions. In some studies, single doses of an intermediate- or long-acting insulin or once- or twice-daily doses of premixed insulin are added to a single or combination of oral antidiabetic agents in poorly controlled patients. The primary outcomes that have been evaluated include measures of glycemic control (e.g., A1C, FPG) and the extent to which insulin doses have been decreased. DeWitt and Hirsch published a comprehensive review of these studies, and readers are referred to this article for this evidence.[93] The combined use of insulin and oral agents can be considered based on the ACCE algorithm, particularly when the A1C is higher than approximately 9%.

Before starting insulin, it is important to review the BG profile:

- Fasting hyperglycemia, which may improve or persist throughout the day. This is the more typical glucose profile for patients with Type 2 diabetes, in whom addition of basal insulin at nighttime would be the most appropriate next step.
- Fasting BG is at target, with daytime hyperglycemia. This is less common for people with Type 2 diabetes, in whom addition of prandial insulin would be an appropriate next step for therapy (see Case 53-13, Question 6).

In Q.R.'s case, it makes the most sense to add a single dose of basal insulin to metformin and glimepiride, with the potential to discontinue glimepiride once the insulin dose is optimized. Advantages attributed to adding insulin to an oral agent as the next step after failure, as opposed to using insulin alone, include the following[93]:

- Lower-insulin dosages can be used, and this minimizes weight gain and hypoglycemia.
- Simpler, single-dose insulin regimens are possible (vs. monotherapy with insulin).
- Lowering the fasting glucose concentrations improves glucose control throughout the day because glucose excursions related to meals are layered over lower values. Furthermore, lower glucose values improve β-cell responsiveness to glucose and enhance tissue responsiveness to insulin action.

However, lowering glucose concentrations is the first priority, not attempting to use lower-insulin doses. Q.R. should be started on 10 units or 0.2 unit/kg of NPH, or basal insulin glargine, detemir or degludec. This dose is based on empiric use of insulin in a variety of studies (0.1–0.2 units/kg)[269] and a conservative estimate for basal insulin of approximately 0.5 units/hour (Q.R. weighs 155 lb, or 70.5 kg). The dose also takes into account the possibility that Q.R. is secreting some basal insulin of her own and will have some residual stimulation of insulin secretion by glipizide. The basal dose should be titrated upward based on the FPG for three consecutive days. A common titration method used is the "treat-to-target" schedule.[92,270]

FPG (mg/dL)	Adjustment of Basal Insulin Dose (Units)
≥180	8
160–180	6
140–159	4
120–139	2
100–119	1
80–99	Maintain dose
60–79	−2
<60	−4 or more

Alternatively, the basal insulin dose can be increased by 2 units every 3 days until the FPG is in a target range (80–130 mg/dL); if the FPG is greater than 140 to 180 mg/dL, larger increments can be used (e.g., by 4 units every 3 days).[269] If hypoglycemia occurs or the FPG is less than 70 mg/dL, the dose should be reduced by at least 4 units, or by 10% if the dose is more than 60 units. Of note, U300 glargine and U100 and U200 degludec should not be titrated sooner than every 3 to 4 days. If there is no improvement in glycemic control after 3 months, prandial insulin or a GLP-1RA should be added (see Case 53-13, Questions 6 and 7). At that point, the insulin secretagogue (in Q.R.'s case, glimepiride) is usually discontinued, but metformin should be maintained.

An alternative for Q.R. is to discontinue the sulfonylurea and begin insulin monotherapy using methods similar to those described for Type 1 diabetes patients. This option also is rational based on the observation that patients like Q.R. are likely to require insulin therapy because of progressive β-cell failure. Furthermore, insulin monotherapy may be less expensive and easier to assess than combination oral agents plus insulin therapy. Nevertheless, many clinicians use single doses of basal insulin in combination with oral agents as a bridge to eventual insulin monotherapy, especially for those patients unwilling to adhere to multiple daily insulin injections. In the setting of insulin resistance, such as with Type 2 diabetes, continuing metformin therapy should be a priority if at all possible.

Insulin Monotherapy in Patients with Type 2 Diabetes

INSULIN REGIMENS

Case 53-13, Question 6: Q.R.'s insulin glargine dose was eventually titrated to 25 units at bedtime. In combination with glimepiride 4 mg/day and metformin 1,000 mg BID, her fasting glucose levels fell to the 110s and 120s on most occasions; her A1C dropped to as low as 6.9%. However, after 1 year, she began to note a gradual rise in glucose concentrations throughout the day. This resulted in a further increase in her bedtime insulin glargine to 40 units (0.57 units/kg). Currently, her morning BG levels are 120 to 140 mg/dL, and BG levels before or after meals range between 170 and 200 mg/dL. A recent A1C value was 8.5%. For the past 6 months or so, Q.R. has noted increasing fatigue, bouts of blurred vision, and recurrence of her monilial infections. How should she be managed now?

The next step in managing Q.R.'s diabetes is to institute prandial insulin therapy, which is needed as indicated by her daytime hyperglycemia. Like Type 1 diabetes patients, those with long-standing Type 2 disease may require prandial insulin before meals to minimize postprandial excursions. Insulin lispro has been shown to decrease postprandial glucose concentrations to a greater extent than regular insulin (30% lower at 1 hour and 53% lower at 2 hours) and was associated with a lower rate of hypoglycemia, particularly between midnight and 6 AM (36%). However, A1C levels were not significantly different after 6 months.[271] A similar response with insulin aspart and glulisine would be expected.

Because Q.R. is on insulin glargine, the most appropriate next step is to add prandial insulin using a rapid-acting insulin. Initiation of basal-bolus insulin regimens are discussed in detail in the Type 1 Diabetes Insulin Therapy section (see Case 53-2, Questions 4–6). An easy way to introduce prandial insulin is to initially add only one mealtime dose. The premeal BG levels that are associated with the most hyperglycemia are targeted. For example, if the prelunch BG levels are elevated, a prandial dose at breakfast is added; or if the bedtime BG levels are mainly elevated (owing to large dinners), a prandial dose at dinner is added. Once a patient adjusts to this, prandial insulin is added to the other meals; at that point glimepiride dose should be reduced or discontinued, altogether. Patients with Type 2 diabetes may require large insulin TDDs (>1 unit/kg) to reach A1C targets less than 7%. Although not technically insulin monotherapy, metformin is often continued to assist in reducing insulin resistance and minimizing weight gain with insulin.

PREMIXED INSULINS

CASE 53-13, QUESTION 7: Q.R. has difficulty adhering to a basal-bolus insulin regimen. She is currently taking insulin glargine 38 units at nighttime and approximately 7 units of insulin aspart before each meal (she follows a high-sugar correction scale). What options are available for Q.R.?

Because people with Type 2 diabetes retain some pancreatic function, it often is possible to achieve an acceptable level of control with twice-daily doses of intermediate-acting insulin in combination with rapid- or short-acting insulins, which are available as premixed insulins. These are referred to as split-mixed insulin regimens. Although convenient, they do limit flexibility in dosing, and thus A1C lowering ability without increasing hypoglycemia risk. In the United States, fixed mixtures of NPH and regular insulin in a 70:30 ratio and a 50:50 ratio are available (Table 53-6). Commercial combinations of the rapid-acting insulins plus an intermediate-acting insulin also are available as Humalog Mix 75/25 (a mixture of insulin lispro plus lispro protamine suspension), Humalog Mix 50/50 (a mixture of insulin lispro plus lispro protamine suspension), and NovoLog Mix 70/30 (a mixture of insulin aspart plus aspart protamine suspension). These fixed mixtures are available in prefilled syringes, which can add to their flexibility and convenience for administration.

The Treating to Target in Type 2 Diabetes (4-T) study assessed the efficacy of a basal insulin (detemir), prandial insulin (insulin aspart), and biphasic insulin (NovoLog Mix 70/30) regimen added to patients on metformin and a sulfonylurea.[272] After 3 years, a biphasic-based insulin regimen was found to be less effective in achieving an A1C goal of less than 6.5% compared with prandial and basal insulin regimens (31.9%, 44.7%, and 43.2%, respectively). Despite the findings of this large multicenter study, use of twice-daily, premixed insulin remains a common insulin therapy for patients with Type 2 diabetes.

Q.R. is currently receiving a TDD of insulin of 59 units, or 0.84 units/kg/day. To convert her to a premixed insulin, one could begin with a conservative TDD of 0.5 to 0.6 units/kg/day, split equally before breakfast and dinner. An older method of two-thirds in the morning and one-third in the evening is used less commonly now. When starting an insulin-naïve Type 2 diabetes patient on premixed insulin, doses of 5 to 6 units twice daily (administered before breakfast and dinner) are often used, with the doses being titrated before breakfast (to affect prelunch and predinner glucose levels) and before dinner (to affect the bedtime and fasting glucose levels).[92,273]

If the premixed insulin does not achieve adequate glycemic control, an option is to mix the short- or rapid-acting insulin with NPH in the same syringe. By doing this, each insulin dose can be individually adjusted. A disadvantage to this is the chance for patients to make errors in measuring and mixing insulin, especially in the elderly when they may have vision and/or dexterity issues. Alternatively, a prandial dose of rapid-acting insulin (i.e., a third injection) can be added at lunch; the breakfast dose of premixed insulin should be decreased as well.[93] Another option is to add a third dose of the premixed insulin at lunch (so premix insulin TID); however the lunchtime dose is smaller than the breakfast and dinner dose. An initial premixed insulin lunchtime dose of 2 to 6 units, or 10% of the current TDD of premixed insulin, can be started.[274]

Q.R. should be started on a rapid-acting premixed insulin twice daily, as this has the convenience of being administered right before eating (within 15 minutes). A dose of 20 units SC BID represents a conservative starting dose. She should monitor her fasting and predinner BG levels, at a minimum, to further adjust her insulin doses.

Adding Antidiabetic Agents to a Basal Insulin Therapy-Based Regimen

CASE 53-14

QUESTION 1: M.A., a 62-year-old woman, has had Type 2 diabetes for 11 years. She is currently taking metformin 500 mg PO TID and insulin glargine 47 units at bedtime. Her A1C is 8.2%. She tries to follow a meal plan that a dietitian developed for her, but her BMI remains 31 kg/m^2. Her physical activity is limited because of an arthritic knee, for which she plans to have knee replacement surgery in the future. Other medical problems include hypertension (hydrochlorothiazide 25 mg daily and benazepril 40 mg daily) and dyslipidemia (atorvastatin 40 mg daily), which are both well controlled. Can any antidiabetic agents be added to her current therapy?

The TZDs have been well studied in patients with Type 2 diabetes who are already taking insulin. In a meta-analysis, pioglitazone lowered A1C by 0.58% when added to insulin therapy; unfortunately, it was associated with weight gain (3 kg) and increased peripheral edema and therefore should be avoided.[206]

A GLP-1 agonist would be a logical agent to considering adding in obese patients. Any GLP-1RA would be a good option. The agents should be chosen based on cost, effectiveness, and adherence. For example, exenatide may be the only GLP-1RA on formulary, or perhaps M.A. has trouble remembering to take once-weekly medications, such as dulaglutide, and as such would be more successful with once-daily liraglutide. Adding a DPP-4 inhibitor would be another option. Sitagliptin is FDA-approved for use with insulin; however, the A1C lowering may be less than with a GLP-1 agonist.

Therefore, addition of liraglutide may be a reasonable approach in M.A. Her A1C can reach her target goal of less than 7%, with potential for weight loss and lower-insulin glargine requirements. Liraglutide should be initiated at a dose of 0.6 mg injected SC once daily for 1 week, after which the dose should be increased to 1.2 mg once daily. Some patients may require further titration to a maximum dose of 1.8 mg once daily to reach their glycemic targets.

Use of Antidiabetic Agents in Special Situations

HYPOGLYCEMIA

CASE 53-15

QUESTION 1: C.A. is a 73-year-old woman who has had a 20-year history of Type 2 diabetes and a 5-year history of mild renal dysfunction (SCr, 1.2 mg/dL; eGFR, 47 mL/minute/1.73 m^2; BUN, 22 mg/dL). Her son, who lives with her, quickly called 9-1-1 when he noticed his mother appearing lethargic and sleepy, with her eyes closed, as she was sitting on the couch. He assumed she was having a "low sugar reaction." When the paramedics arrived, her BG concentration was 46 mg/dL. C.A. was able to be aroused, and indicated she could drink something, so 4 ounces of orange juice was administered. After 10 minutes, her BG level was 80 mg/dL, so she was given another 4 ounces of juice. According to her son, C.A.'s diabetes has been well controlled for the past several months with glyburide 10 mg BID and metformin 850 mg TID. For the past 3 days, C.A. has been eating less and vomiting on association, with the "flu." What was the likely cause of her hypoglycemic episode? Were there any predisposing factors?

C.A. has experienced a hypoglycemic episode secondary to glyburide. Hypoglycemia is the most common and potentially severe adverse effect of the sulfonylureas. The incidence and severity of this effect increase with the duration of action and potency of the agents.

Most sulfonylurea-induced hypoglycemia occurs in patients who are predisposed to hypoglycemia in some way, and C.A. is no exception. She is an elderly woman with renal impairment who was on relatively high doses of an agent, a portion of which is excreted unchanged in the urine. Even in the face of decreased carbohydrate intake (reduced appetite and vomiting), she continued to take her usual dose of glyburide. Even though the stress of illness most often raises glucose levels, the decreased food intake resulted in glyburide causing hypoglycemia. Because glyburide has a long duration of action, hypoglycemia may last for several hours.

C.A. and her son should be educated about treatment of hypoglycemia. It is likely that her son did not need to call 9-1-1, and he could have treated the hypoglycemia. Glucagon should not be used to treat hypoglycemia caused by a sulfonylurea, as glucagon can cause a paradoxical fall in the glucose levels.[275]

RENAL DYSFUNCTION

CASE 53-15, QUESTION 2: C.A. has mild renal insufficiency (eGFR, 47 mL/minute/1.73 m^2) and is taking the maximal dose of metformin. What is the risk of lactic acidosis with metformin? How should age and kidney function be taken into account with metformin use? Which agents should be avoided? Which agents could be used?

Sulfonylurea compounds that are metabolized to active products that depend on the kidney for elimination (e.g., acetohexamide, chlorpropamide glyburide, and tolazamide) should be avoided in the elderly and in patients with decreased renal function. Sulfonylureas that are completely metabolized to inactive or weakly active products may be used (i.e., glipizide, glimepiride, or tolbutamide). Although glyburide is unlikely to accumulate in patients with a ClCr greater than 30 mL/minute, it should not be used in C.A because it caused a severe hypoglycemic reaction.[276] C.A. should be instructed to eat regularly because skipped meals may result in recurrent hypoglycemia. Consideration to discontinuing the sulfonylurea and changing adding an agent with a lower incidence of hypoglycemia should be considered.

The most notorious side effect associated with metformin—although extremely rare—is lactic acidosis. The risk of lactic acidosis is increased with renal insufficiency, which can result in accumulation of metformin because it is almost exclusively clear unchanged by the kidneys. Lactic acidosis is a metabolic acidosis characterized by a significant reduction in the arterial pH and an accumulation of serum lactate, a product of anaerobic metabolism. It is a condition that is highly lethal (50% mortality) and resistant to therapy. Lactic acidosis occurs when there is an increased production of or decreased utilization of lactate. Decreased utilization of lactate occurs when tissues are unable to oxidize lactate to pyruvate (these two substances are normally present in the serum in a ratio of 10:1). Metformin might predispose a patient to lactic acidosis by augmenting anaerobic metabolism or by decreasing the kidney's ability to handle an acid load. Other factors that might contribute to lactic acidosis include severe cardiac or pulmonary disease (anoxia, increased lactate production), septic shock, renal dysfunction (retention of metformin and lactate), patients receiving contrast dye, and excessive alcohol intake (increased lactate production and decreased utilization).[165–167]

Signs and symptoms generally are acute in onset and commonly include nausea, vomiting, diarrhea, and hyperventilation. Hypovolemia, hypotension, confusion, and coma also may occur; death is usually secondary to cardiovascular collapse. Typical laboratory findings include a low serum bicarbonate and Pco_2, a low arterial pH, an elevated potassium, a normal or low serum chloride, elevated lactate and pyruvate levels, an increased lactate to pyruvate ratio, and an anion gap of 30 mEq/L or higher.

Although metformin rarely is associated with lactic acidosis, the manufacturer and the FDA have taken extreme measures to prevent its improper use because another biguanide, phenformin, which induced this life-threatening condition, was removed from the market in 1977.[277] The estimated rate of phenformin-induced lactic acidosis was 0.25 to 4 cases per 1,000 users versus 5 to 9 cases per 100,000 users for metformin.[165–167] A group of clinicians from the FDA summarized 47 confirmed cases of metformin-related lactic acidosis (lactate levels ≥5 mmol/L) that had been reported to the FDA between May 1995 and June 1996.[261] Unfortunately, the condition continues to be resistant to treatment; the mortality rate was 43%. Importantly, 43 of the 47 cases (91%) had concurrent conditions that predisposed them to lactic acidosis. These included cardiac disease (64%), decreased renal function (28%), and chronic pulmonary disease (6%). Several patients (17%) were older than 80 years of age and may have had decreased renal function despite normal SCr concentrations. Interestingly, 38% of the patients had HF, and those who died were more likely to be under treatment with digoxin and furosemide. The mean daily dose of metformin was well within the therapeutic range and was not higher in the group that succumbed (1,259 ± 648 mg in the group that died and 1,349 ± 598 mg in the group that survived).

Metformin should be initiated with care in patients older than 80 years of age because of the potential for a low GFR, even when SCr is normal.[164] Because C.A. has moderate renal dysfunction (GFR <60 mL/minute, but >40 mL/minute), lower the dose of metformin to 500 mg BID to minimize the potential for accumulation.

The TZDs are primarily metabolized by the liver and are not contraindicated in patients with mild renal failure. The use of pioglitazone, beginning with low doses, could be considered, as can acarbose, which is poorly absorbed from the GI tract. The DPP-4 inhibitors could also be used, but their doses may require adjustment depending on the degree of renal dysfunction (except for linagliptin). Exenatide can be used in patients with ClCr greater than 30 mL/minute, and the dose does not need to be adjusted.

Liraglutide should be used with caution in renal insufficiency, but does not require dose adjustment. None of these agents cause hypoglycemia when used as monotherapy.

HEPATIC DYSFUNCTION

CASE 53-16

QUESTION 1: B.R., a 60-year-old man with cirrhosis of the liver, is found to have Type 2 diabetes. Glipizide 10 mg/day is initiated. How will B.R.'s liver function affect the disposition of glipizide and his response to this agent?

Most noninsulin antidiabetic agents should be avoided in patients with severe liver disease, and insulin therapy is often the safest option. Because hepatic metabolism is the primary route of elimination for most sulfonylureas, including glipizide, patients with hepatic disease should be expected to have an exaggerated response to those drugs metabolized to less active products. Liver disease can be a separate predisposing factor for severe, prolonged hypoglycemia because glycogenolysis and gluconeogenesis are impaired; thus, sulfonylureas are relatively contraindicated for cirrhotic patients. If they are used, shorter-acting agents are preferred, and small initial doses should be used. For B.R., glipizide could be initiated at a dose no greater than 2.5 mg/day and increased if needed by 2.5-mg increments at no less than weekly intervals. Other options are low doses of repaglinide (0.5 mg) or nateglinide (60 mg) with meals because they are very short acting. Other good options for which severe liver disease is not a specific contraindication include GLP-1RAs, DPP-4 inhibitors, and SGLT2 inhibitors, although there is little data regarding their use in these patients. Basal-bolus or mixed insulin regimens are also good choices.

Diabetes in the Elderly

CLINICAL PRESENTATION

CASE 53-17

QUESTION 1: J.M. is a frail, 82-year-old, unresponsive man who is brought to the emergency department. According to J.M.'s family, he has become increasingly confused, dizzy, and lethargic, with a recent weight loss of 10 lb. J.M. lives by himself and has been generally healthy with the exception of mild-to-moderate chronic obstructive pulmonary disease and arthritis. Fasting serum chemistry reveals the following:

Na, 128 mEq/L
Glucose, 798 mg/dL
Serum osmolality, 374 mOsm/L (normal, 280–295 mOsm/kg H_2O)
Blood pH, 7.5
HCO_3, 22

His serum is negative for ketones. On physical examination, J.M. has poor skin turgor and dry mucous membranes, and is responsive only to deep pain. His BP is 90/60 mm Hg with a pulse of 96 beats/minute. He has rales at the left lower base of his lung, and a chest radiograph confirms pneumonia. Despite aggressive fluid replacement, J.M.'s BG remains consistently greater than 250 mg/dL and his A1C is 11%. J.M. presents with very high glucose concentrations, but has no history of diabetes mellitus. What special factors contribute to a late and atypical presentation of diabetes in the elderly?

Diabetes in the elderly commonly is underdiagnosed and undertreated because it often presents atypically.[278,279] Classic symptoms associated with diabetes mellitus may be masked by other illnesses, entirely absent, or explained away by the normal aging process. For example, polyuria is minimized by higher renal thresholds for glucose, or it may be confounded by urinary incontinence or "prostate problems." Thirst is commonly blunted in elderly persons, increasing their risk of dehydration and electrolyte imbalance. Hunger can be altered by medications or depression. Fatigue often is discounted as "part of getting old," and weight loss, although sometimes profound, may be so gradual that it goes unnoticed for months to years. (See Table 53-28 for a comparison of presenting symptoms for diabetes mellitus in elderly patients compared with younger patients.)

Table 53-28
Presentation of Diabetes Mellitus in Elderly Patients Compared with Younger Patients

Metabolic Abnormality	Symptoms in Young Patients	Symptoms in Elderly Patients
Serum osmolality	Polydipsia	Dehydration, confusion, delirium
Glucosuria	Polyuria	Incontinence
Catabolic state owing to insulin deficiency	Polyphagia	Weight loss, anorexia

HYPEROSMOLAR HYPERGLYCEMIC STATE

CASE 53-17, QUESTION 2: J.M. is diagnosed with hyperosmolar hyperglycemic state (HHS). Why are the elderly predisposed to this condition, and what signs and symptoms are consistent with this diagnosis?

HHS is a condition characterized by extremely elevated plasma glucose concentrations (>600 mg/mL) and high serum osmolality (>320 mOsm/L) without ketoacidosis. Because patients with Type 2 diabetes have some residual insulin production, they are usually protected against excessive lipolysis and ketone production. Patients with Type 2 diabetes may exhibit HHS in later stages of diabetes as loss of β-cells becomes advanced and residual insulin production continues to drop.[156] Measurements of serum ketones and blood pH differentiate this condition from DKA (see Case 53-10). The condition occurs when urinary fluid and electrolyte losses secondary to glucosuria are inadequately replaced by oral fluid intake.[156]

HHS primarily occurs in the elderly because several factors predispose this population to hypodipsia. These include an inability to recognize thirst,[280] an inability to ask for fluids (e.g., dementia, sedation, intubation), and an inability to get fluids on demand (e.g., physical disabilities or restraints). Infections or other acute illnesses (e.g., MI, GI bleeding, pancreatitis) that exacerbate diabetes can interact with the hyperosmolar diuresis and hypodipsia to produce severe dehydration and hyperglycemia. Drugs that increase plasma glucose concentrations (e.g., glucocorticoids), increase diuresis, or decrease mentation also can contribute to this unfortunate situation.

J.M. presents with several symptoms of HHS dehydration, including osmolality greater than 320 mOsm/L, plasma glucose greater than 600 mg/dL, pH > 7.3, elevated bicarbonate, decreased skin turgor, hypotension, and the absence of serum ketones. His pneumonia was probably the precipitating factor. Treatment involves rapid IV hydration. Fluid replacement is provided in the same manner as with DKA. See Case 53-10, Question 2, and Table 53-24 for details.[156] Insulin infusion is given simultaneously. The initiation and rate adjustments are the same as with DKA, except that the plasma glucose cut-off to reduce the insulin infusion rate is 300 mg/dL (not 200 mg/dL as with DKA; see Case 53-10, Question 3, and Table 53-24 for details). Rehydration and insulin administration corrected J.M's metabolic imbalance, allowing his diabetes control to be addressed.

GOALS OF THERAPY

CASE 53-17, QUESTION 3: What are the goals of therapy for J.M.?

It is widely recognized that strict glycemic control is associated with an increased incidence of hypoglycemia.[29] In the elderly patient with age-related autonomic dysfunction and CVD, hypoglycemia may present without the usual premonitory symptoms and can result in severe adverse effects such as angina, seizures, stroke, or MI. Therefore, the general tendency when treating elderly diabetic patients is to aim for slightly less aggressive glycemic goals. Thus, an FBG target of between 100 and 140 mg/dL with postprandial glucose values less than 180 mg/dL and an A1C goal of close to 8%, while avoiding hypoglycemia, is appropriate in this frail patient.[7]

DIET AND EXERCISE

CASE 53-17, QUESTION 4: How should diet and exercise recommendations be modified for elderly diabetic patients such as J.M.?

Nutrition

The ADA recommends individualized MNT for all patients with diabetes mellitus. The Dietary Approaches to Stop Hypertension (DASH) diet and Mediterranean diets have been shown to be effective for glycemic control and lowering CVD risk.[51–53]

Because most elderly patients have Type 2 diabetes, nutrition and exercise programs are the initial steps in therapy. Older people with diabetes, especially those in a long-term care facility, have a tendency to be underweight rather than overweight.[51–53] Therefore, caution should be used when considering a weight-loss diet because this could cause malnutrition or dehydration. For obese individuals, a modest weight loss of 5% to 10% may be indicated. However, an involuntary weight gain or loss of more than 10 lb or 10% of body weight in less than 6 months should be carefully assessed.[51–53]

Several factors can adversely affect proper nutrition in the elderly. They include an impaired ability to shop for and prepare food, limited finances, an age-related decline in taste perceptions, and coexisting illnesses. Ill-fitting dentures, difficulty in chewing and swallowing, and lack of companionship during meals also can contribute to malnutrition as well.

High-fiber diets may lower BG and improve plasma lipids. However, high-fiber diets in frail, elderly patients, particularly those who are bedridden, should be used cautiously because they can be constipating and result in fecal impaction. Ambulatory patients, on the other hand, generally benefit from increased dietary fiber. Because many elderly patients are malnourished, a daily multivitamin preparation containing the recommended daily allowance of each vitamin should be prescribed.[51–53]

Exercise

Exercise in the elderly provides all the benefits derived by younger individuals. It increases well-being and glucose stability, and may decrease a propensity to fall. Exercise also improves BP, the lipid profile, hypercoagulability, and bone density. Physical activity is necessary to minimize any lean body mass loss that can occur with caloric restriction. For patients with arthritis, aquatic exercise may be substituted. Before such an exercise program is initiated, careful evaluation is mandatory to avoid myocardial ischemia or the acceleration of retinopathy.

SELECTING AN ANTIDIABETIC AGENT IN THE ELDERLY

CASE 53-17, QUESTION 5: Why is it important to institute drug therapy to treat J.M.'s diabetes? What considerations should be made in selecting an initial treatment regimen?

As in all patients with diabetes mellitus, poor glycemic control increases the risk of long-term complications. Although it is tempting to minimize the importance of glycemic control because these complications take so long to develop, patients such as J.M. may have had unrecognized hyperglycemia for many years before clinical diagnosis. Thus, many have already begun to develop complications. Furthermore, as life expectancy increases, one can expect that these individuals will live long enough to experience morbidity related to diabetes if they are not treated. Therefore, pharmacologic treatment should be considered in J.M.

The general approach to treating an elderly patient with Type 2 diabetes is basically the same as described in Case 53-11, Questions 3, 7, and 8. The initial choice of an antidiabetic agent should be based on the severity of hyperglycemia. Other considerations include body weight, coexisting diseases, and cost of the agent. Patients with IFG (FPG $>$100, but $<$126 mg/dL) should be treated with diet and exercise tailored to their individual capabilities. For patients with Type 2 diabetes, acarbose, a short-acting insulin secretagogue (e.g., nateglinide or repaglinide), pioglitazone, and a DPP-4 inhibitor are all appropriate options. Sulfonylurea-induced hypoglycemia is a concern in these patients. However, if inability to adhere to the multiple daily regimen is problematic, a short-acting sulfonylurea is an appropriate alternative agent. In J.M.'s case, metformin should probably be used in caution because he has chronic obstructive pulmonary disease increasing the risk of hypoxia. Also, he is older than 80 years of age and requires an assessment of his GFR, which is likely diminished. The favorable effect metformin has on weight is irrelevant in J.M. Thus, although the efficacy of metformin is comparable to that of sulfonylureas, it is not the agent of first choice for elderly patients such as J.M.[281,282] Patients with an FPG greater than 300 mg/dL and no overt stress should be considered insulin deficient and started on insulin therapy.

HYPERTENSION

CASE 53-18

QUESTION 1: L.S. is a 53-year-old, obese man with an 8-year history of Type 2 diabetes. His current problems include a BP of 155/103 mm Hg (documented on two occasions), blurry vision, and impotence, which he now admits has troubled him for the last few years. Physical examination reveals decreased pedal pulses bilaterally, loss of sensation to monofilament testing, and evidence of an amputated toe on the right foot. His laboratory values are as follows:

FPG, 170 mg/dL
A1C, 7.8%
Total cholesterol, 240 mg/dL
Triglycerides, 160 mg/dL

L.S. has normal electrolyte values and albuminuria (180 mg/g creatinine). His only medication is metformin 500 mg PO BID. Describe the pathogenesis of hypertension in patients such as L.S. Why is it so important to treat his hypertension?

Seventy-five percent of adults with diabetes report having a BP of 130/80 mm Hg or more or use medications for hypertension.[1] Hypertension in Type 1 diabetes is usually of renal parenchymal origin and occurs 1 to 2 years after the onset of nephropathy as indicated by albuminuria (see Case 53-19, Question 2).[7] The relationship between Type 2 diabetes and hypertension is more complex and not as closely correlated to nephropathy. In Type 2 diabetes, hypertension is often part of the metabolic syndrome and may be present for years before diabetes is actually detectable.

Patients with diabetes and hypertension have an increased risk for experiencing microvascular complications such as retinopathy and nephropathy. They are also at a twofold increased risk of having CVD.[7] A 5-mm Hg reduction in mean diastolic BP can produce a 37% reduction in microvascular complications, and a 10-mm Hg reduction in mean systolic BP had previously been found to reduce the risk of MI by 11% and death related to diabetes by 15%.[7,245,246] However, because lower BP targets are tested, the benefits are becoming less clear. In the ACCORD blood pressure study, the intensive control arm (achieved systolic BP of 119 mm Hg) did not reduce total cardiovascular events (nonfatal MI, nonfatal stroke or death from cardiovascular causes) compared with standard therapy (achieved systolic BP of <133 mm Hg).[9] However, microvascular benefits were observed, as was a statistically significant reduction in stroke. Therefore, the existing ADA BP goal of less than 140/90 mm Hg is reasonable, and lower goals should not be targeted in practice unless it can be done without adverse effects.[7]

Treatment includes weight management, exercise, sodium restriction (<1,500 mg/day), smoking cessation, and antihypertensive therapy. L.S. should be started on an angiotensin-converting enzyme inhibitor (ACEI). ACEI have traditionally been available as less expensive generics, although angiotensin receptor II blockers (ARB) are also available and appropriate. Many patients require two or three medications to achieve the target BP goal of less than 140/90 mm Hg.[7]

NEPHROPATHY

CASE 53-18, QUESTION 2: What is the significance of the presence of albumin in L.S.'s urine? How should it be managed?

Diabetes is the leading cause of end-stage renal disease and accounted for 44% of new cases of renal failure in 2005.[1,7] Diabetic nephropathy is characterized by nephrotic syndrome and azotemia. It is a major cause of death in patients with Type 1 diabetes and is an increasing source of morbidity in Type 2 diabetic individuals.[283] Thickening of the glomerular capillary basement membranes is the hallmark of diabetic nephropathy.[284] Diffuse deposition of basement membrane-like material expands the mesangium. This process narrows the capillary lumina, impedes blood flow, and thereby reduces the filtering surface area in the glomerulus. Hyperglycemia causes intraglomerular hypertension and renal hyperfiltration. Hyperfiltration is followed by albuminuria with minimal glomerulosclerosis, which still is potentially reversible. If left untreated, overt proteinuria occurs, and the patient usually progresses to nephrotic syndrome. Progression of diabetic renal disease can be accelerated in the presence of hypertension, proteinuria, and diabetic retinopathy. Lipid abnormalities also may contribute to the progression of glomerulosclerosis. Management includes early detection through screening for albuminuria, tight glucose control, use of ACEIs and ARBs for patients with albuminuria (to slow progression), aggressive management of hypertension that includes an ACEI or ARB as first-line therapy,[7] aggressive management of dyslipidemia, and smoking cessation. A thorough discussion on the management of diabetic nephropathy and end-stage renal disease is presented in Chapter 28, Chronic Kidney Diseases, and of hypertension in people with diabetes, in Chapter 9, Essential Hypertension.

Screening for and Confirmation of Albuminuria

The preferred method of screening for albuminuria is measurement of the albumin-to-creatinine ratio in a random spot collection (preferably the first-void or morning sample). Albuminuria is defined as a urinary albumin excretion of 30 mcg or more per milligram of creatinine (or mg albumin/g creatinine) during a spot collection.[7] Because of day-to-day variability in albumin excretion, two of three urine samples collected in a 3- to 6-month period need to be abnormal before a designation is made. Annual screening should be performed in patients with Type 1 diabetes with a duration of at least 5 years and in patients with Type 2 diabetes from the time of diagnosis. More frequent screening is indicated if hypertension, any increase in SCr, or retinopathy develops. Urine albumin concentrations can be falsely elevated over true baseline values by exercise within 24 hours, fever, infection, uncontrolled diabetes, uncontrolled hypertension, and HF.

On the basis of established criteria, L.S. has albuminuria (180 mg albumin/g creatinine). Management includes tight BG control and an ACEI or ARB should be started (L.S. should already be receiving one of these agents to treat his hypertension as noted). After initiation of therapy, continued periodic monitoring of the albuminuria is recommended to assess the response to therapy and progression of disease.[7] Serum potassium and creatinine levels should be followed as well.

CARDIOVASCULAR DISEASE

CASE 53-18, QUESTION 3: L.S. is treated with lisinopril 20 mg/day, which controls his BP and improves his albuminuria. His dose of metformin is titrated to 1,000 mg BID. Recent laboratory values include an FPG of 130 mg/dL, A1C of 6.0%, triglyceride level of 170 mg/dL, total cholesterol of 204 mg/dL, LDL-C of 135 mg/dL, and HDL-C of 35 mg/dL. How does the risk of heart disease for patients such as L.S. compare with that for persons without diabetes? What is the pathogenesis of CHD in persons with diabetes?

CHD is the leading cause of premature death in the Type 2 population and accounts for 50% of the deaths in people with diabetes. Relative to nondiabetic individuals, those with diabetes are 2 to 3 times more likely to develop CHD, and their risk of death after an MI also is 2 to 3 times higher than their nondiabetic counterparts. Women with diabetes, regardless of their age or menopausal status, have equal risk for CHD to that of nondiabetic men. These sobering figures point to the importance of minimizing or eliminating all other preventable risk factors for CVD in patients with diabetes (i.e., tobacco use, hypertension, hypercholesterolemia, obesity) through the prescription of exercise, diet, and appropriate medications.[285]

Pathogenesis

The pathogenesis of CVD in people with diabetes is complex. The metabolic syndrome with its attendant cardiovascular risk factors, dyslipidemia, inflammation, and hemostatic abnormalities are only some of the mechanisms under study.[19,286]

The most common lipid abnormality in Type 2 diabetes is hypertriglyceridemia (>150 mg/dL) with low levels of HDL-C (<40 mg/dL in men or <50 mg/dL in women), similar to the lipid profile seen in L.S. Poor control of Type 1 diabetes also is associated with low levels of HDL-C and a smaller, more-dense LDL particle. These lipid abnormalities, along with a greater prevalence of hypertension, contribute to the risk for CVD.

In patients with diabetes, clinical trials of lipid-lowering therapy (primarily with statins) have demonstrated primary and secondary CHD prevention. Although the evidence for the reduction in "hard" CVD outcomes (e.g., CHD death and nonfatal MI) is stronger in diabetic patients who have a high baseline CVD risk (i.e., known CVD or very high LDL-C levels), the overall benefits of statins in patients with diabetes at moderate or high risk for CVD are convincing. Readers are referred to the ADA Standards of Medical Care for more detailed information on the CVD clinical trials in patients with diabetes.[7]

DYSLIPIDEMIA

CASE 53-18, QUESTION 4: Should L.S. be treated with drug therapy for his dyslipidemia?

The ACC/AHA made important changes in the management of dyslipidemia regarding cholesterol management recommendations. Although the previous ATP III guidelines focused on specific LDL and non-HDL cholesterol target goals, the new guidelines recommend initiating statin therapy based on cardiovascular risk. Cardiovascular risk is determined by age, comorbidities, lipid panel, social, and family history. The ACC/AHA guidelines recommend a moderate-intensity statin for diabetics between the ages of 40 to 75 with LDL between 70 and 189 mg/dL with estimated 10-year ASCVD (atherosclerotic cardiovascular disease) risk <7.5%. A high-intensity statin is recommended for diabetics between the ages of 40 to 75 with LDL between 70 and 189 mg/dL with estimated 10-year ASCVD risk >_7.5%. All patients between the ages of 40 to 75 are recommended a high-intensity statin if they have had a clinical ASCVD, including CHD, MI, unstable/stable angina, stroke, TIA, or peripheral arterial disease. Patients greater than the age of 75 are generally recommended to be initiated on a moderate-intensity statin due to risk of myalgias.[7]

Diet and exercise are cornerstones in the management of dyslipidemia in patients such as L.S. Weight loss is associated with improvements in insulin sensitivity and glucose control, as well as a reduction in triglycerides, total cholesterol, and LDL-C. Physical activity enhances weight loss and increases HDL-C levels. Thus, L.S.'s diet and exercise habits should be reassessed, and instruction in both should be reinforced as appropriate. Because insulin resistance may be the underlying cause of elevated lipids in these patients, efforts should be devoted to reversing insulin resistance as well. Given L.S.'s age and risk factors, a statin is indicated.

For a detailed discussion on statin therapy and other lipid-lowering agents see Chapter 8 (Dyslipidemias, Atherosclerosis, and Coronary Heart Disease chapter).

RETINOPATHY

CASE 53-18, QUESTION 5: L.S. is referred to the ophthalmologist for his persistent complaints of vision problems despite improvement in his glycemic control. He is diagnosed with mild background retinopathy. Should L.S. be concerned?

Ocular disorders related to diabetes are the leading cause of new cases of legal blindness in Americans. Patients with diabetes may experience blurred vision associated with poor glycemic control, but retinopathy, senile-type cataracts, and glaucoma are the complications that threaten sight. Diabetic retinopathy appears as early as 3 years after diagnosis and is evident in 90% of Type 1 diabetic individuals after 15 years. Comparable figures for patients with Type 2 diabetes treated with insulin and for those treated with diet and oral agents are 80% and 55%, respectively. Proliferative retinopathy is less prevalent, but nevertheless is present in 30% of people with Type 1 diabetes and in 10% to 15% of insulin-treated patients with Type 2 diabetes who have had diabetes for 15 years or longer.[287]

Patients with Type 1 diabetes should have a dilated retinal examination within 5 years of diagnosis; evaluation is not necessary before 10 years of age. Patients with Type 2 diabetes should have a comprehensive eye examination soon after diagnosis. The ADA recommends annual comprehensive eye examinations.[7] Less-frequent eye examinations (every 2–3 years) can be considered in patients with normal examinations based on the advice of an ophthalmologist.[287]

Current theories addressing the possible causes of this complication have been thoroughly reviewed.[287] Microvascular disease characterized by thickening of the capillary membrane may be the underlying lesion for two forms of retinopathy. The first and most common presentation is a nonproliferative retinopathy, which is characterized by microaneurysms that may progress to hard, yellow exudates, signifying chronic leakage, retinal edema, and punctate hemorrhage. This form of retinopathy may be associated with loss of central vision, but generally is associated with excellent visual prognosis. Focal laser photocoagulation of the retina in patients with nonproliferative diabetic retinopathy and macular edema decreases the likelihood of visual loss by 50%.[7]

A second, less common presentation is proliferative retinopathy. This form is characterized by neovascularization (presumably owing to retinal hypoxia). Neovascularization ultimately leads to fi brosis, vitreous hemorrhage, and retinal detachment. Photocoagulation therapy may arrest progression and decrease loss of vision associated with neovascularization.[287] Because hypertension, smoking, uremia, and hyperglycemia may lead to more rapid progression of the retinopathy, every effort should be made to eliminate these risk factors for L.S.

The ACCORD study assessed the impact of intensive glycemic, BP, and lipid control on the progression of retinopathy.[268] After 4 years, the rates of progression of diabetic retinopathy were reduced with intensive glycemic control (7.3% vs. 10.4% with standard therapy) and also with fenofi brate (6.5% vs. 10.2% with standard therapy of just a statin alone). Somewhat surprisingly, intensive BP control did not have an effect (10.4% vs. 8.8% with standard therapy). However, on closer interpretation, this finding makes sense as the BP in the standard therapy group achieved excellent control (133.5 mm Hg), so further lowering the BP (119.3 mm Hg in the intensive group) did not provide additional benefit in reducing the rate of retinopathy progression (see Case 53-19, Question 1).

CASE 53-18, QUESTION 6: Should L.S. be started on aspirin therapy?

The issue of aspirin use for primary prevention continues to be debated. The ADA recommends aspirin therapy as secondary prevention in patients with a history of CVD (e.g., MI, vascular bypass procedure, peripheral vascular disease, stroke or transient ischemic attack, claudication, or angina). Primary prevention is indicated in diabetic individuals who have a significant risk of CVD events (10-year risk >10%). Although the ADA lists several risk calculators that can be used in patients with diabetes, the UKPDS calculator can be downloaded and is relatively easy to use (http://www.dtu.ox.ac.uk/riskengine/).[288] In patients with a very low risk (10-year risk <5%), the ADA recommends against aspirin because the risk of significant bleeding outweighs the benefit for vascular event reduction.[288] Because risk calculation in patients with diabetes can be difficult, the ADA also provided more general clinical guidance and recommends that men older than the age of 50 and women older than the age of 60 who have at least one additional major risk factor (a family history of CVD, smoking, hypertension, albuminuria, dyslipidemia) are good candidates for aspirin therapy.[288] In elderly, patients assess the need for aspirin therapy. Clinicians should weigh risks versus benefits for the primary prevention of CVD events in patients >80 years of age. Newer studies have shown antiplatelet therapy renders this patient population to increased incidences of bleeding without significant reduction in CVD events. L.S. has several cardiovascular risk factors (albuminuria, dyslipidemia, hypertension, obesity, and age) and should be started on aspirin therapy as primary prevention. L.S. should take an enteric-coated aspirin, 81 mg daily. Although some authors have suggested that higher doses of aspirin should be used because of the increased platelet reactivity that can be seen in people with diabetes, the clinical literature does not support this approach and the ADA does not recommend doses greater than 162 mg daily.[7,288]

AUTONOMIC NEUROPATHY: GASTROPARESIS

CASE 53-19

QUESTION 1: H.D. is a 36-year-old man with a 20-year history of Type 1 diabetes. He has poor glycemic control (A1C, 12%) and complains of frequent, severe hypoglycemic reactions that "don't make sense." According to H.D., "I have insulin reactions right after I eat, but later on, my glucose concentrations are sky high." H.D. presents to the diabetes clinic with a 2-month history of nausea, postprandial fullness, early satiety, and occasional vomiting, all of which are unrelieved by antacids. H.D. also has peripheral neuropathy involving both his hands and feet and manifestations of autonomic neuropathy (impotence and orthostatic hypotension). An upper GI series was ordered to rule out peptic ulcer disease and gastroesophageal reflux disease, and a solid-meal, gastric emptying study using scintigraphy indicates the diagnosis of diabetic gastroparesis. What is the cause of diabetic gastroparesis? How should H.D. be treated?

Autonomic neuropathy may present as gastroparesis with feelings of bloating and nausea, urinary retention, impotence in men (manifested as retrograde ejaculation or an inability to attain an erection), postural hypotension, tachycardia, and diarrhea with incontinence of stool.[289] The presence of autonomic insufficiency may have profound effects on the patient's response to vasodilating drugs and ability to counteract hypoglycemia.

Poor glycemic control with "unexplained" hypoglycemia may result from the disrupted delivery of food to the intestine; that is, glucose delivery does not correspond with prandial insulin action. As a result, the BG levels can fluctuate greatly. Many patients with diabetic gastroparesis, like H.D., have had diabetes for many years and also have evidence of peripheral and autonomic neuropathies.

Conventional antiemetic therapy is usually not helpful in the treatment of gastroparesis. Prokinetic agents, such as metoclopramide, are considered first-line therapy.[290] Metoclopramide increases gut motility through indirect cholinergic stimulation of the gut muscle. However, symptomatic improvement does not always correlate with improved gastric emptying, which implies that the effectiveness of metoclopramide also is related to its centrally mediated antiemetic activity. A usual starting dose of metoclopramide is 10 mg orally 4 times daily (QID), 30 minutes before meals and at bedtime. Although treatment may not eliminate all symptoms, it should minimize most of the patient's complaints. Patients should be monitored for tardive dyskinesia, a potentially irreversible and disfiguring condition that is characterized by involuntary movements of the tongue, face, or extremities. In 2009, the FDA added tardive dyskinesia as a black box warning for metoclopramide.[291] The risk of tardive dyskinesia increases with the duration of treatment and the total cumulative dose.

Other pharmacotherapeutic interventions include domperidone (not available in the United States), cisapride (withdrawn from the US market), erythromycin, and cholinergic agonists.[290] A key component to treating H.D.'s gastroparesis is improving his glycemic control. Also, H.D. should be advised to try eating smaller, more frequent meals and to chew his food well; this of course will require adjustments to his prandial insulin therapy. Also, eating a low-fiber and low-fat diet may help with his symptoms.[290]

PERIPHERAL NEUROPATHY

CASE 53-19, QUESTION 2: Six months after institution of metoclopramide 10 mg QID and several insulin adjustments, H.D.'s GI symptoms have been alleviated, and his diabetes is now reasonably well controlled as evidenced by elimination of hypoglycemic episodes and a recent A1C of 7.5%. However, H.D. has been complaining of increasing bilateral foot pain, which he describes as a burning, tingling, or prickly sensation. An examination of his feet reveals cool extremities with absent pulses, reduced vibration perception, and loss of 10-g monofilament pressure sensation. What are appropriate steps that can be taken to alleviate H.D.'s peripheral neuropathy?

Diabetic neuropathy may be a consequence of metabolic disturbances in the neurons, microangiopathy affecting the capillary supply to neurons, or an autoimmune process. It affects 60% to 70% of the diabetic population and has a broad spectrum of presentation. Clinically, it most commonly presents as a diffuse symmetric sensorimotor syndrome, as carpal tunnel syndrome, or as autonomic neuropathy (e.g., tachycardia or orthostatic hypotension caused by cardiovascular autonomic neuropathy). Symptomatic diabetic peripheral neuropathy occurs in 25% of patients with diabetes. It is characterized by paresthesia and pain in the lower extremities that may be mild or severe and unrelenting, decreased sensation to monofilament testing, decreased ankle and knee jerks, and decreased nerve conduction velocity. The decreased sensation associated with peripheral neuropathy contributes to the progression of foot injuries and infections that may go unnoticed by the patient until they are severe. The management of diabetic neuropathies has been reviewed.[7,292,293] To view a video of how to perform a complete foot examination, see http://www.medscape.com/viewarticle/708703.

Pharmacologic management consists of symptomatic therapies. Painful neuropathy may respond to simple analgesics (e.g., acetaminophen) or nonsteroidal anti-inflammatory drugs. The analgesic selected should be based on the patient's history of responsiveness to these agents as well as their duration of action and side effect profiles. Side effects include GI upset and bleeding, and renal and hepatic toxicity. Avoid chronic nonsteroidal anti-inflammatory drug use owing to their renal toxicity and development of GI ulcers. Other pharmacologic options include tricyclic antidepressants (TCAs), duloxetine (a serotonin and norepinephrine reuptake inhibitor), gabapentin, pregabalin, and other anticonvulsants (carbamazepine, lamotrigine, topiramate, and oxcarbazepine). Only pregabalin and duloxetine have the FDA indication for the treatment of DPN; others are off label. Efficacy, side effects, drug interactions, renal and hepatic function, and cost should all be considered when an agent is chosen. Often less expensive options are tried first, off label such as gabapentin or a TCA.[294–296]

Topical application of 0.075% capsaicin has been recommended for diabetic neuropathy but may take several weeks to work. Lidocaine 5% patches have also been used. These may be helpful in patients intolerant to oral medications. These may be used in combination with oral medications. Tramadol or opiates may also be used second line.[294–296]

CASE 53-19, QUESTION 3: Can anything be done for H.D.'s peripheral vascular disease?

Peripheral vascular disease or peripheral arterial disease presents as diminished or absent foot pulses, intermittent claudication, skin ulcers, gangrene, or amputation. People with diabetes are 2 to 10 times more likely to experience symptoms of peripheral arterial disease than those without diabetes, and half of all nontraumatic amputations in the United States are performed in patients with diabetes. In one study that followed Type 2 patients for 7 years, 5.5% had an amputation. The prevalence of this condition increases with age, duration of diabetes, and the presence of risk factors such as hypertension or smoking.[293,297]

Signs and symptoms of peripheral arterial disease include leg pain, which is relieved by rest; cold feet; nocturnal leg pain, which is relieved by dangling the feet over the bed or walking; absent pulses; loss of hair on the foot and toes; and gangrene. Treatment of this condition includes elimination and treatment of risk factors such as smoking, dyslipidemia, hypertension, and hyperglycemia; antiplatelet therapy; exercise, which is the mainstay of therapy; and revascularization surgery.[297] H.D. should be thoroughly educated regarding proper foot care, perform daily self-foot examinations, and receive regular care by a podiatrist.[298]

DRUG-INDUCED ALTERATIONS IN GLUCOSE HOMEOSTASIS

Persons with diabetes are likely to take more drugs in their lifetime than any other group of patients. Patients with Type 2 diabetes present with a constellation of chronic conditions, including hypertension, dyslipidemia, and CVD, all of which will likely require drug therapy. Drugs to manage depression, intermittent infections, and neurologic and ophthalmologic conditions also are commonly prescribed. Because we know that the actions of drugs are complex and that for every desired effect there are several other unwanted effects, each time a drug is added to the regimen of someone with diabetes it is important to assess the patient's situation to determine whether a potential exists for a drug–drug or drug–disease interaction or whether the benefit of the newly prescribed drug is likely to outweigh its risks. With the availability of online drug information databases to assist in assessment of drug–drug and drug–disease interactions, a detailed listing of drugs that can exacerbate hyperglycemia and hypoglycemia is not provided. Below, a few case examples are illustrated. Some medications that can have significant hyperglycemic effects include atypical antipsychotics, protease inhibitors, corticosteroids, immunosuppressants (e.g., tacrolimus, cyclosporine), niacin (higher doses), gonadotropin-releasing hormone agonists (used in men for prostate cancer), and pentamidine (can also cause hypoglycemia).[299,300] Patients should be monitored closely for a medication's possible effect on the BG levels.

Drug-Induced Hyperglycemia

CORTICOSTEROIDS

CASE 53-20

QUESTION 1: A.L., a 37-year-old obese woman with systemic lupus erythematosus, has been taking 60 mg/day of prednisone for 6 months. During this period, her weight has increased by 30 lb and she has experienced glycosuria (no ketones). Her primary provider asked her to start SMBG. She was referred to the diabetes clinic, where her predinner and bedtime BG values were found to be 140 to 160 mg/dL and FBG values were 80 to 105 mg/dL. Physical examination shows a 5 feet 2 inch, 150-lb, depressed woman with truncal obesity and an acneiform rash. Her mother and one sister have Type 2 diabetes. How do corticosteroids contribute to diabetes mellitus? How should A.L. be treated?

The term *steroid diabetes* was first used to describe the hyperglycemia and glycosuria seen in patients with Cushing syndrome. Now, it is associated more commonly with exogenously administered glucocorticoids and has been a side effect of parenteral, oral, and even topical therapy. Corticosteroids are one of the most common drug groups that unmask latent diabetes or aggravate preexisting disease, and they may produce hyperglycemia and overt diabetes in individuals who are not otherwise predisposed.

Corticosteroids increase hepatic gluconeogenesis, suppress insulin secretion, and decrease tissue responsiveness to insulin.[300] The primary effect is impaired glucose disposal after meals, resulting in daytime hyperglycemia, and by morning, the glucose levels normalize. Although steroid-induced diabetes generally is mild and rarely associated with ketonemia, a wide spectrum of severity may be encountered—from asymptomatic, abnormal glucose tolerance tests to difficult-to-control, insulin-requiring disease. The onset of glucose tolerance can occur within hours to days or after months to years of chronic therapy. The effect generally is considered dose-dependent and usually is reversible on discontinuation of the drug.

A.L. exhibits many symptoms that can be attributed to supraphysiologic doses of corticosteroids: truncal obesity, depression, acneiform rash, and diabetes. Mildly elevated glucose levels in obese individuals, as in A.L.'s case, sometimes can be controlled by diet, but may require treatment with a short-acting insulin secretagogue or rapid-acting insulin before meals.[300] A person with diabetes whose BG is increased by use of a glucocorticoid should modify treatment appropriately to restore glycemic control. It is important to anticipate the need to modify insulin or other antidiabetic therapy because corticosteroid doses are increased or decreased.

SYMPATHOMIMETICS

CASE 53-21

QUESTION 1: R.C., a 41-year-old man with Type 1 diabetes, is well controlled on a basal-bolus insulin regimen and has been taking pseudoephedrine 30 mg QID for 7 days and Robitussin DM 10 mL QID (which contains 2.92 g of sugar/5 mL) for a cold. Recently, glucose concentrations have been higher than usual. Can pseudoephedrine or the cough preparation be the cause of his poor glycemic control? Discuss the use of sympathomimetics and cough preparations in patients with diabetes.

Over-the-counter drug products, such as decongestants and diet aids, which contain sympathomimetics, carry warning labels that caution against their use in patients with diabetes. Standard sugar- and ethanol-containing cough preparations also carry such warning labels. However, clinically significant drug-induced glucose intolerance probably is very infrequent. It is well established that parenterally administered epinephrine increases BG concentrations secondary to increased glycogenolysis and gluconeogenesis. Other sympathomimetics generally do not have as potent an effect on BG as epinephrine, and their use usually does not pose a practical problem in diabetic patients. Furthermore, the effects of sympathomimetics on BP must be considered in many patients with diabetes. Therefore, antihistamines or occasional use of nasal sprays for severe congestion may be needed.

In summary, pseudoephedrine or the cough preparation may be aggravating R.C.'s glycemic control, although at these low-to-normal therapeutic doses, it is quite unlikely. The stress related to R.C.'s underlying cold is more likely to be impairing his glucose tolerance than these low doses of sympathomimetic agents or the small amounts of sugar contained in the cough syrup.

Drug-Induced Hypoglycemia

ETHANOL

CASE 53-22

QUESTION 1: C.F., a 22-year-old woman with newly diagnosed Type 1 diabetes, enjoys a glass or two of wine with her evening meal. What effect does alcohol have on a patient with diabetes, particularly one using insulin? Is alcohol contraindicated in C.F. or any person with diabetes?

Clinicians often are reluctant to permit the use of alcoholic beverages in patients with diabetes. However, barring contraindications that are similar in the nondiabetic and diabetic patient alike (e.g., alcoholism, hypertriglyceridemia, gastritis, pancreatitis, pregnancy), a person with diabetes can safely enjoy a moderate alcohol intake as long as certain precautions are taken. For an in-depth discussion, the reader is referred to two comprehensive reviews of alcohol and diabetes,[301,302] parts of which are summarized in the following list:

- Drink in moderation. The ADA defines this as a daily intake of one drink for adult women and two drinks for adult men (one drink is defined as 5 ounces of wine, 12 ounces of beer, or 1.5 ounces of distilled liquor). The patient should be aware of his/her own sensitivity to the intoxicating effects of ethanol and adjust consumption downward, if needed. This is particularly important for insulin-dependent patients. When having a drink, be sure to have it with a carbohydrate-containing meal.
- Avoid drinks that contain large amounts of sugar, such as liqueurs, sweet wines, and sugar-containing mixes. Instead, consider dry wines, light beers, and distilled spirits. Not only does the simple sugar content add an additional source of glucose and calories to the diet, but ethanol ingested with simple sugar-containing mixers enhances reactive hyperglycemia.
- Remember to count the calories in alcohol (calories = [0.8] × [proof] × [ounces]); substitute 1 ounce of alcohol for two fat exchanges.
- Be aware that the symptoms of alcohol intoxication and hypoglycemia are similar. If hypoglycemia is mistaken for intoxication by others, appropriate and potentially life-saving treatment can be delayed.
- Be aware of alcohol–sulfonylurea drug interactions, specifically the alcohol-induced enzyme induction of tolbutamide metabolism and the chlorpropamide–alcohol flush reaction.

ACKNOWLEDGMENT

The authors acknowledge Lisa A. Kroon and Craig Williams for their contributions to this chapter in earlier editions.

KEY REFERENCES AND WEBSITES

A full list of references for this chapter can be found at http://thepoint.lww.com/AT11e. Below are the key references and websites for this chapter, with the corresponding reference number in this chapter found in parentheses after the reference.

Key References

ACCORD Study Group et al. Effects of medical therapies on retinopathy progression in type 2 diabetes [published correction appears in *N Engl J Med*. 2011;364:190]. *N Engl J Med*. 2010;363:233. (268)

Action to Control Cardiovascular Risk in Diabetes Study Group et al. Effects of intensive glucose lowering in type 2 diabetes. *N Engl J Med*. 2008;358:2545. (40)

ADVANCE Collaborative Group et al. Intensive blood glucose control and vascular outcomes in patients with type 2 diabetes. *N Engl J Med*. 2008;358:2560. (42)

American Diabetes Association. Standards of medical care in diabetes—2015. *Diabetes Care*. 2015;38(Suppl. 1):S5–S80. (7)

Diabetes Control and Complications Trial Research Group. Effect of intensive diabetes treatment on the development and progression of long-term complications in insulin-dependent diabetes mellitus. Diabetes Control and Complications Trial. *J Pediatr*. 1994;125:177. (118)

Diabetes Prevention Program Research Group et al. 10-year follow-up of diabetes incidence and weight loss in the Diabetes Prevention Program Outcomes Study. *Lancet*. 2009;374:1677. (48)

Duckworth W et al. Glucose control and vascular complications in veterans with type 2 diabetes [published corrections appear in *N Engl J Med*. 2009;361:1028; *N Engl J Med*. 2009;361:1024]. *N Engl J Med*. 2009;360:129. (43)

Handelsman Y et al. American association of clinical endocrinologists and American college of endocrinology—clinical practice guidelines for developing a diabetes mellitus comprehensive care plan—2015. *Endocr Pract*. 2015:21 (Suppl 1);1–87. (39)

Hayward RA et al. Follow-up of glycemic control and cardiovascular outcomes in type 2 diabetes. *N Engl J Med*. 2015;372(23):2197–2206. (44)

Holman RR et al. 10-year follow-up of intensive glucose control in type 2 diabetes. *N Engl J Med*. 2008;359:1577. (33)

Inzucchi S et al. Management of Hyperglycemia in Type 2 Diabetes, 2015: A Patient Centered Approach Update to a Position Statement of the American Diabetes Association and the European Association for the Study of Diabetes. *Diabetes Care*. 2015;38:140–149. (100)

Nathan DM et al. Intensive diabetes treatment and cardiovascular disease in patients with type 1 diabetes. *N Engl J Med*. 2005;353:2643. (32)

Nathan DM et al. Medical management of hyperglycemia in type 2 diabetes: a consensus algorithm for the initiation and adjustment of therapy: a consensus statement of the American Diabetes Association and the European Association for the Study of Diabetes. *Diabetes Care*. 2009;32:193.

NICE-SUGAR Study Investigators et al. Intensive versus conventional glucose control in critically ill patients. *N Engl J Med*. 2009;360:1283. (142)

Riddle MC et al. Epidemiologic relationships between A1C and all-cause mortality during a median 3.4-year follow-up of glycemic treatment in the ACCORD trial. *Diabetes Care*. 2010;33:983. (41)

Skyler JS et al. Intensive glycemic control and the prevention of cardiovascular events: implications of the ACCORD, ADVANCE, and VA diabetes trials: a position statement of the American Diabetes Association and a scientific statement of the American College of Cardiology Foundation and the American Heart Association [published correction appears in *Diabetes Care*. 2009;32:754]. *Diabetes Care*. 2009;32: 187. (45)

Turner R et al. United Kingdom Prospective Diabetes Study 17: a 9-year update of a randomized, controlled trial on the effect of improved metabolic control on complications in non-insulin-dependent diabetes mellitus. Ann Intern Med. 1996;124(1, Pt 2):136. (262)

UK Prospective Diabetes Study Group. Effect of intensive blood-glucose control with metformin on complications in overweight patients with type 2 diabetes (UKPDS 34) [published correction appears in *Lancet*. 1998;352:1558]. *Lancet*. 1998;352:854. (238)

UK Prospective Diabetes Study Group. Intensive blood-glucose control with sulphonylureas or insulin compared with conventional treatment and risk of complications in patients with type 2 diabetes (UKPDS 33) [published correction appears in *Lancet*. 1999;354:602]. *Lancet*. 1998;352:837. (35)

UK Prospective Diabetes Study Group. Efficacy of atenolol and captopril in reducing risk of macrovascular and microvascular complications in type 2 diabetes: UKPDS 39. *BMJ*. 1998;317:713. (245)

UK Prospective Diabetes Study Group. Tight blood pressure control and risk of macrovascular and microvascular complications in type 2 diabetes: UKPDS 38 [published correction appears in *BMJ*. 1999;318:29]. *BMJ*. 1998;317:703. (246)

Key Websites

American Diabetes Association. http://www.diabetes.org.
The American Association of Clinical Endocrinologists. https://www.aace.com/

SECTION 12 | Eye Disorders

Section Editor: Susan Jacobson

54 Eye Disorders

Steven R. Abel and Suellyn J. Sorensen

CORE PRINCIPLES

		CHAPTER CASES
GLAUCOMA		
1	There are different types of glaucoma, including open-angle and angle-closure glaucoma. Angle-closure glaucoma is a medical emergency requiring immediate intervention. Open-angle glaucoma is a chronic condition, which can result in progressive loss of vision leading to blindness if left untreated.	**Case 54-1 (Question 1)**
2	Treatment for open-angle glaucoma is targeted toward reducing intraocular pressure (IOP), a clinical measure of drug efficacy. β-Adrenergic blockers, prostaglandin analogs (PGAs), and α-adrenergic agonists are the mainstay of treatment. Treatment is not curative.	**Case 54-1 (Question 2), Figure 54-1, Table 54-1**
OCULAR AND SYSTEMIC SIDE EFFECTS OF DRUGS		
1	Many widely used medications for various conditions cause ocular side effects. The true incidence is frequently not known, making the reporting of ocular side effects of drugs an important function for any healthcare practitioner.	**Case 54-3 (Question 1), Table 54-3**
2	Conversely, many topically administered ocular medications may cause systemic symptoms.	**Case 54-10 (Question 1)**
COMMON OCULAR DISORDERS		
1	Stye (hordeolum) is a common ocular disorder for which no viable over-the-counter treatment exists.	
2	Conjunctivitis (pinkeye) is frequently related to bacterial or viral infection, or allergy. Viral conjunctivitis is generally self-limiting. Bacterial conjunctivitis should be treated with an appropriate antimicrobial, recognizing that Gram-positive organisms are frequently the cause. A number of agents are available for the treatment of allergic conjunctivitis. Among those, decongestants (e.g., tetrahydrozoline) should be used for no more than 72 hours, because they may mask a more serious condition or result in rebound redness.	**Case 54-5 (Question 1)**
CORTICOSTEROIDS		
1	Topical corticosteroids are used for a variety of ocular inflammatory conditions. The most potent topical corticosteroid is prednisolone acetate 1%.	**Case 54-8 (Question 1), Table 54-4**
2	Topical and oral corticosteroids may be associated with serious side effects such as increases in IOP and cataracts (with long-term use).	**Case 54-8 (Question 1), Table 54-5**
AGE-RELATED MACULAR DEGENERATION		
1	There are two forms, dry (affecting 85% of patients) and the more serious form, wet (affecting 15% of patients).	**Case 54-13 (Question 1)**
2	Wet macular degeneration is associated with abnormal growth of blood vessels behind the retina (choroidal neovascularization) and may be treated by vascular endothelial growth factor (VEGF) inhibitors.	**Case 54-13 (Question 1)**

The eye is a highly complex organ composed of various parts, all of which must function in integration to permit vision. A brief overview of the anatomy and physiology of the eye prefaces the presentation of specific eye disorders. Readers should consult an ophthalmology textbook for an understanding of ocular anatomy, physiology, and general ophthalmology (e.g., *Vaughan and Asbury's General Ophthalmology*).[1]

OCULAR ANATOMY AND PHYSIOLOGY

The eyeball is approximately 1 inch wide and is housed in a cavity (i.e., eye socket) formed by two bony orbits that are lined with fat, which serves to protect the eyeball. Six ocular muscles facilitate movement of the eyeball (Fig. 54-1).

The outer coat of the eye is made up of the sclera, conjunctiva, and cornea. The *sclera* is the white, dense, fibrous protective coating. The episclera, a thin layer of loose connective tissue, contains blood vessels that cover and nourish the sclera. The *conjunctiva* is a mucous membrane that covers the anterior portion of the eye and lines the eyelids. The *cornea* is the transparent, avascular tissue that functions as a refractive and protective window membrane through which light rays pass en route to the retina.

The corneal epithelium and endothelium are lipophilic, and the centrally located stroma is hydrophilic. These three corneal layers are particularly important because they affect drug penetration through the cornea. Ophthalmic medications, which are both fat- and water-soluble, are best able to penetrate through the intact cornea.

The iris, choroid, and ciliary body are known collectively as the uveal tract. The *iris* is a colored, circular membrane suspended between the cornea and the crystalline lens. It controls the amount of light that enters the eye. The *choroid*, located between the sclera and retina, is largely made up of blood vessels, which nourish the retina. The *ciliary body* is adherent to the sclera and contains the ciliary muscle and ciliary processes. The ciliary muscle contracts and relaxes the zonular fibers, which hold the crystalline lens in place. The ciliary processes are responsible for the secretion of aqueous humor, a clear liquid that occupies the anterior chamber. The anterior chamber is bounded anteriorly by the cornea and posteriorly by the iris. The posterior chamber lies between the iris and the crystalline lens.

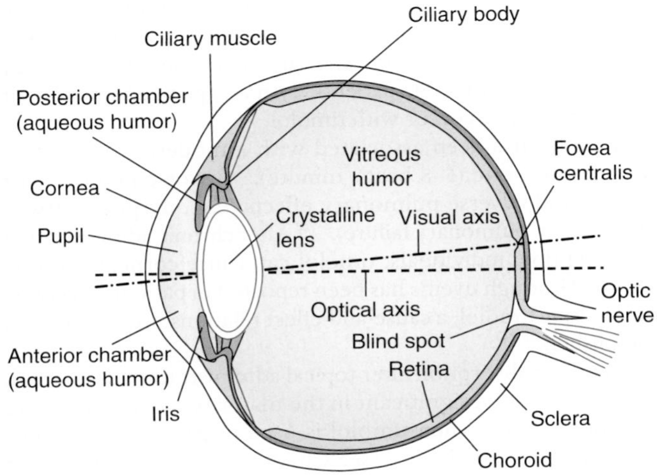

Figure 54-1 Anatomy of the human eye. (Adapted from http://commons.wikimedia.org/wiki/File:Eyesection.svg)

The inner segment of the eye contains the retina with the optic nerve. The *retina*, the light-sensitive tissue at the back of the eye, contains all of the sensory receptors for light transmission. The *optic nerve*, a bundle of more than a million nerve fibers, transmits visual impulses from the retina to the brain.

The crystalline lens, aqueous humor, and vitreous humor assist the cornea with the refraction of light. The *lens*, located behind the iris, functions to focus light onto the retina by changing its shape to accommodate near or distant vision. The innermost part of the lens (i.e., the nucleus) is surrounded by the softer material of the cortex. The *aqueous humor*, the thin watery fluid that fills the anterior chamber (i.e., the space between the cornea and the iris) and posterior chamber of the eye, functions to provide nourishment to the cornea and lens. Disorders involving the aqueous humor are presented in the section on glaucoma. The primary function of the *vitreous humor* (i.e., the jellylike substance between the lens and the retina) is to maintain the shape of the eye and allow the transmission of light to the retina.

The eyelids and eyelashes are the outermost means of protection for the eye. The eyelids contain various sebaceous and sweat glands, which may become infected or inflamed, contributing to many ocular disorders.

The eye is innervated by both the sympathetic and parasympathetic nervous systems. Parasympathetic fibers, originating from the oculomotor nerve in the brain, innervate the ciliary muscle and sphincter pupillae muscle that constrict the pupil. As a result, parasympathomimetic (cholinergic) medications generally are associated with *miosis* (pupillary contraction), and parasympatholytic (anticholinergic) agents with *mydriasis* (pupillary dilation) and *cycloplegia*. The term *cycloplegia* refers to a paralysis of the ciliary muscle and zonules (fibrous strands connecting the ciliary body to the lens) that results in decreased accommodation (adjustment of the lens curvature for various distances) and blurred vision. Tear secretion by the lacrimal glands also is a parasympathetic function.

Sympathetic fibers from the superior cervical ganglion in the spinal cord innervate the dilator pupillae muscle, the blood vessels of the ciliary body, the episclera, and the extraocular muscles. Sympathomimetics cause mydriasis without affecting accommodation.

In this chapter, we will discuss glaucoma, ocular and systemic side effects of drugs, common ocular disorders, ocular inflammatory conditions, and age-related macular degeneration. These are all common conditions that the pharmacist may encounter in all practices of pharmacy. It is important for the pharmacist to be educated on these disorders and their associated treatment so that the pharmacist can evaluate the appropriateness of pharmacotherapy, screen for adverse effects and drug interactions, and counsel patients on their ocular medications.

GLAUCOMA

Glaucoma is a leading cause of irreversible blindness worldwide. The estimated number of suspected cases worldwide is 60 million, increasing to 76 million in 2020 and 111 million in 2040. In the United States, an estimated 3 million Americans are living with glaucoma but only half know they have it. Glaucoma is a nonspecific term used for a group of diseases that can irreversibly damage the optic nerve, resulting in visual field loss. Increased intraocular pressure (IOP) is the most common risk factor for the development of glaucoma; however, even people with "normal"

 IOPs can experience vision loss from glaucoma. Generally, the higher the IOP is, the greater the risk for developing glaucoma. Increasing age, African-American race, family history, thinner central corneas, and larger vertical cup–disc ratios are other risk factors for glaucoma.[1–3]

Intraocular Pressure

The inner pressure of the eye (i.e., IOP) is influenced by the production of aqueous humor by the ciliary processes and the outflow of aqueous humor through the trabecular meshwork. The tonometry test to measure the IOP is based on the pressure required to flatten a small area of the central cornea. Generally, an IOP of 10 to 20 mm Hg is considered normal. An IOP of 22 mm Hg or greater should arouse suspicion of glaucoma, although a more rare form of glaucoma is associated with a low IOP.

Ocular Hypertension

Ocular hypertension has been defined as an IOP exceeding 21 mm Hg, normal visual fields, normal optic discs, open angles, and the absence of any ocular disease contributing to the elevation of IOP. Only a small percentage of patients with ocular hypertension have open-angle glaucoma. An ophthalmoscope can examine the inside of the eye, especially the optic nerve, and a diagnosis of glaucoma can be applied when pathologic cupping of the optic nerve is observed.

Open-Angle Glaucoma

Primary open-angle glaucoma (POAG) occurs in about 1.8% of people older than 40 years of age in the United States; however, glaucoma can affect other age groups, including children.[1–3] In patients with POAG, aqueous humor outflow from the anterior chamber is continuously subnormal primarily because of a degenerative process in the trabecular meshwork. The IOP can vary in the course of a day from normal to significantly high pressures.[1] The decreased outflow appears to be caused by degenerative changes in outflow channels (i.e., the trabecular meshwork and Schlemm canal) and tends to worsen with the passage of time.[1] In rare cases, the outflow is normal even during a phase of elevated IOP, and the elevation appears to be to the result of hypersecretion of aqueous humor.[1]

The onset of POAG usually is gradual and asymptomatic. A defect in the visual field examination may be present in early glaucoma, but loss of peripheral vision usually is not seen until late in the course of the disease. Visual field defects correlate well with changes in the optic disc and help differentiate glaucoma from ocular hypertension in patients with increased IOP. Patients with normal visual fields and an IOP of 24 mm Hg or greater have a 10% likelihood of developing glaucoma in 5 years.[5]

Angle-Closure Glaucoma

Examination of the anterior chamber angle by gonioscopy, using a corneal contact lens, a magnifying device (e.g., a slit-lamp microscope), and a light source, assists in differentiating between open-angle glaucoma and angle-closure glaucoma. Angle-closure glaucoma accounts for approximately 5% to 10% of all primary glaucoma cases. The sole cause of the elevated IOP in angle-closure glaucoma is closure of the anterior chamber angle.[1,5]

Angle-closure glaucoma, which is a medical emergency, usually presents as an acute attack with a rapid increase in IOP, blurring or sudden loss of vision, appearance of haloes around lights, and pain that is often severe. When patients are predisposed to angle-closure glaucoma, their pupils should not be dilated (e.g., during an ophthalmic examination) and they should be taught the signs and symptoms of angle closure. Acute attacks can terminate without treatment, but if the IOP remains high, the optic nerve can be irreparably damaged.[1] Patients with chronic angle-closure generally experience a gradual closure of aqueous humor outflow channels, and patients can be asymptomatic until the glaucoma is in an advanced stage.[1] Permanent medical management of acute or chronic angle-closure glaucoma is difficult: Surgical procedures (e.g., peripheral iridectomies) often are needed.

PRIMARY OPEN-ANGLE GLAUCOMA

Therapeutic Agents for Treatment of Primary Open-Angle Glaucoma

INITIAL THERAPY

Historically, β-adrenergic blockers have been the most commonly prescribed first-line agents for the treatment of POAG. In recent years, prostaglandin analog (PGA) use has reached, if not exceeded, β-adrenergic blocker use. All of the ophthalmic β-blockers currently on the market are available in generic formulation, allowing for cost-effective treatment. Some of the PGAs are available as generic formulations making their cost comparable to β-blockers.

β-Adrenergic Blockers

Ophthalmic β-adrenergic antagonists block the β-adrenergic receptors in the ciliary epithelium of the eye and lower IOP primarily by decreasing aqueous humor production. On average, β-blockers decrease IOP by 20% to 35% depending on the strength used and the frequency of administration.[6–14]

Timolol (Timoptic)

Timolol, a nonselective β_1- and β_2-adrenergic antagonist, is one of the most commonly prescribed glaucoma medications. Because timolol was the first ocular β-adrenergic blocker marketed, subsequently marketed ophthalmic β-blockers usually are compared with timolol for safety and effectiveness. Concentrations or dosages exceeding one drop of timolol 0.5% twice daily (BID) do not produce further significant decreases in IOP.[15] Therapy usually is initiated with a 0.25% solution administered as one drop BID. Monocular administration of timolol has resulted in equal bilateral IOP reduction and can reduce the cost of therapy and side effects for some patients.[16] An escape phenomenon, or tachyphylaxis, can occur with timolol.

Timolol has been associated with a modest reduction of resting pulse rate (5–8 beats/minute),[17,18] worsening of heart failure, and adverse pulmonary effects (e.g., dyspnea, airway obstruction, pulmonary failure).[19,20] After chronic administration in susceptible individuals, timolol can cause corneal anesthesia.[21,22] Although uveitis has been reported in patients receiving ophthalmic timolol, a cause-and-effect relationship has not been established.[23,24]

Systemic absorption after topical administration does occur, but it may not be significant in the majority of patients. Care should be taken when timolol is used in patients with sinus bradycardia, heart failure (see Chapter 14, Heart Failure), or pulmonary disease. Systemic side effects could be exaggerated in elderly patients secondary to inadvertent overdosing associated with poor administration technique (see Case 54-1, Question 3).

Timoptic XE

Timoptic XE, a timolol ophthalmic gel-forming solution, is administered once daily. The ophthalmic vehicle, gellan gum (Gelrite), is a solution that forms a clear gel in the presence of monovalent or divalent cations.[25] This ion-activated gelation prolongs precorneal residence time and increases ocular bioavailability, allowing timolol to be administered once daily.[25] Timoptic XE is comparable to timoptic solution in lowering IOP.[26]

Levobunolol (Betagan)

Levobunolol, a nonselective β-adrenergic antagonist, is approved for either once-daily or BID administration. Levobunolol 0.5% and 1% are comparable to timolol in lowering IOP. The incidence of adverse reactions, including decreases in heart rate, is also comparable to that for timolol.[7,27]

Metipranolol (OptiPranolol)

Another nonselective β-adrenergic blocking agent, metipranolol 0.1% to 0.6%, is comparable to timolol 0.25% to 0.5% in reducing IOP.[8,9] Like timolol, metipranolol produces corneal anesthesia, which occurs within 1 minute of instillation and returns to baseline after 10 minutes.[20] Metipranolol is associated with a greater incidence of stinging or burning on administration and has been associated with granulomatous anterior uveitis.[28,29] As a result of these side effects, the use of metipranolol is limited.

Carteolol (Ocupress)

Carteolol, a nonselective β-adrenergic blocking agent with partial β-adrenergic agonist activity, theoretically should minimize the bronchospastic, bradycardic, and hypotensive effects associated with other ocular β-adrenergic blockers.[30] However, no clinical differences were seen when the cardiovascular and pulmonary function effects of carteolol were compared with those of timolol. Carteolol 1% and timolol 0.25% administered BID are equally effective in reducing IOP.[11–13]

Betaxolol (Betoptic)

In contrast to other β-adrenergic blocking ophthalmic agents, betaxolol is a selective β_1-adrenergic blocker. This cardioselective property may result in less adverse effects on pulmonary function than nonselective β-adrenergic blockers in patients with reactive airway disorders. Betaxolol is slightly less effective than timolol in IOP reduction, and more patients tend to need adjunctive therapy with betaxolol.[14,31–33]

Prostaglandin Analogs

Latanoprost (Xalatan), travoprost (Travatan Z), bimatoprost (Lumigan), and tafluprost (Zioptan) are all PGAs. Latanoprost and travoprost, and tafluprost are analogs of prostaglandin $F_{2\alpha}$, and they lower IOP by serving as selective prostaglandin $F_{2\alpha}$-receptor agonists. Bimatoprost is a synthetic prostamide analog. Tafluprost is a preservative-free formulation supplied in single-use containers.[34]

The prostaglandin analogs increase uveoscleral outflow of aqueous humor and, thereby, decrease IOP.[35] These agents often are prescribed as first-line agents for the treatment of POAG because they are at least as effective as the β-blockers, can be administered once a day, and are associated with minimal systemic adverse effects.

Latanoprost

Latanoprost (Xalatan) is approved for the initial treatment of POAG or ocular hypertension.[36] When administered once daily in the evening, latanoprost is at least as effective as timolol in decreasing IOP. When the effectiveness of latanoprost 0.005% once daily was compared with timolol 0.5% BID, the IOP-lowering effects of latanoprost were superior to those of timolol.[37,38] In addition, the nocturnal control of IOP with latanoprost was superior to that with timolol. Latanoprost 0.005% should be dosed once daily in the evening because the IOP-lowering effects of latanoprost might actually be inferior when administered more frequently.

Systemic side effects are minimal with latanoprost, but local reactions (e.g., iris pigmentation; eyelid skin darkening; eyelash lengthening, thickening, pigmentation, and misdirected growth; conjunctival hyperemia; ocular irritation; superficial punctate keratitis) are relatively common. Latanoprost can gradually increase the amount of brown pigment in the iris by increasing the melanin content in the stromal melanocytes of the iris. This pigment change occurs in 7% to 22% of patients and is most noticeable in those with green-brown, blue/gray-brown, or yellow-brown eyes.[36] The onset of increased iris pigmentation usually is noticeable within the first year of treatment and can be permanent. The nature and severity of adverse events are not affected by the increased pigmentation of the iris.

Latanoprost has additive effects when administered with β-blockers (e.g., timolol), carbonic anhydrase inhibitors (e.g., dorzolamide), and α_2-adrenergic agonists (e.g., brimonidine, apraclonidine). When added to existing therapy, latanoprost decreases IOP an additional 2.9 to 6.1 mm Hg. As a result, latanoprost is a good adjunctive ophthalmic agent for patients who are unable to adequately lower their IOP with single-agent therapy. Although the complementary IOP-lowering effects of latanoprost are comparable to those of brimonidine (at least a 15% reduction in IOP) in patients inadequately controlled on β-adrenergic blocking agents, brimonidine (an α_2-adrenergic agonist) in a comparative study was associated with fewer adverse effects on the quality of life. For example, watery or teary eyes and cold hands and feet were reported more frequently in latanoprost-treated patients.[36] The effectiveness of latanoprost when used once a day alone or as an adjunct to other IOP-lowering drugs and its relative tolerability make it one of the most common if not the most common treatment option for POAG and ocular hypertension.[37–42]

Travoprost

Travoprost (Travatan Z) is US Food and Drug Administration (FDA)-approved for the reduction of elevated IOP and ocular hypertension in patients who are intolerant or who fail to respond to other agents. Travoprost is used as a first-line agent in clinical practice because it is more effective than timolol and at least as effective as latanoprost. The mean IOP reduction with travoprost in African-American patients was 1.8 mm Hg greater than in non–African-American patients. Travoprost, as adjunctive therapy to timolol in patients not responding adequately to timolol alone, reduced IOP an additional 6 to 7 mm Hg. The side effect profile of travoprost is similar to that for latanoprost, including increased iris pigmentation and eyelash changes.[43–45] Local irritation may be less with travoprost because it is free of the preservative benzalkonium chloride (BAK). Rather, travoprost is preserved in the bottle with SofZia, which is a unique ionic buffer containing borate, sorbitol, prophylene glycol, and zinc.

Bimatoprost

Like travoprost, bimatoprost (Lumigan) once daily or BID achieved lower target IOPs than did timolol BID. Bimatoprost BID, however, was less effective than bimatoprost once a day. Iris pigmentation changed in 1.1% of bimatoprost-treated patients. In a 6-month randomized multicenter study, bimatoprost once a day lowered IOP more effectively than latanoprost once a day. Side effects were similar between treatment groups; however, conjunctiva hyperemia was more common ($p < 0.001$) in bimatoprost-treated patients. Overall, the side effect profile of bimatoprost appears to be similar to that for latanoprost and travoprost.[46–48] The local side effects seen with other PGAs also appear to be relatively common with bimatoprost. As a result, the FDA approved the cosmetic use of bimatoprost solution under the trade name Latisse. Latisse solution is applied with an applicator to the base of the upper eyelashes for the treatment of hypotrichosis (inadequate eyelashes). Eyelash lengthening, thickening, and darkening or pigmentation is seen after 8 to 16 weeks of use.[49]

Tafluprost

Tafluprost (Zioptan) is a preservative-free product, US FDA-approved for the reduction of elevated IOP and ocular hypertension. Tafluprost daily in the evening is as effective as latanoprost daily in the evening and timolol 0.5% BID and has demonstrated additive efficacy when administered with timolol. Switch studies evaluating tafluprost in patients receiving BAK containing agents demonstrated some improvement in adverse effects. As a result, tafluprost is an important option for patients with a documented hypersensitivity to BAK or other PGAs. The adverse effect profile is similar to other PGAs.[50–54]

α_2-Adrenergic Agonists

Apraclonidine (Iopidine) and brimonidine (Alphagan) are selective α_2-adrenergic agonists similar to clonidine. Apraclonidine is less lipophilic than clonidine and brimonidine, does not cross the blood–brain barrier as readily, and theoretically has fewer systemic side effects (e.g., hypotension, decreased pulse, dry mouth). Brimonidine is more highly selective for α_2-adrenergic receptors than clonidine or apraclonidine and, theoretically, should be associated with fewer ocular side effects. α_2-Adrenergic agonists appear to lower IOP by decreasing the production of aqueous humor and by increasing uveoscleral outflow.[55]

Brimonidine is an alternative first-line agent in the treatment of POAG. It may also be used as adjunctive therapy in patients not responding to other agents. Apraclonidine 1% is indicated to control or prevent postsurgical elevations in IOP after argon laser trabeculoplasty or iridotomy. The 0.5% apraclonidine solution is indicated for short-term adjunctive therapy in patients on maximally tolerated medical therapy. Long-term IOP control should be monitored closely in patients taking α_2-adrenergic agonists because tachyphylaxis can occur. Common ocular side effects include burning, stinging, blurring, conjunctival follicles, and an allergic-like reaction consisting of hyperemia, pruritus, edema of the lid and conjunctiva, and foreign body sensation. Although ocular side effects are less common with brimonidine than with apraclonidine, systemic side effects (e.g., dry nose and mouth, mild hypotension, decreased pulse, and lethargy) are more common with brimonidine. α_2-Adrenergic agonists should be used with caution in patients with cardiovascular disease, orthostatic hypotension, depression, and renal or hepatic dysfunction.[55,56] Brimonidine (Alphagan P) is available with Purite as a preservative, which facilitates drug delivery into the eye, allowing use of a lower drug concentration.[56]

The IOP-reduction effects (peak and trough) of brimonidine 0.2% BID are 14% to 28%. Although the approved dosing schedule of brimonidine is 3 times a day (TID), brimonidine 0.2% BID lowers IOP comparably to timolol 0.5% BID, and both are slightly better than betaxolol 0.25% BID.[57,58] The IOP-lowering effect of brimonidine also may be comparable to that of latanoprost; however, conflicting efficacy and tolerability results in clinical studies may be related to differences in study design.[59] The combination of brimonidine and timolol is as equally tolerable and effective as the combination of dorzolamide and timolol.[60] The FDA-approved Combigan ophthalmic solution combines an α_2-adrenergic agonist (brimonidine tartrate 0.2%) with a β-adrenergic blocker (timolol maleate 0.5%).

Topical Carbonic Anhydrase Inhibitors

Carbonic anhydrase occurs in high concentrations in the ciliary processes and retina of the eye. Carbonic anhydrase inhibitors (CAIs) lower IOP by decreasing bicarbonate production and, therefore, the flow of bicarbonate, sodium, and water into the posterior chamber of the eye, resulting in a 40% to 60% decrease in aqueous humor secretion.

Although CAIs have been used orally for many years in the treatment of elevated IOPs, they have been replaced by the topical ophthalmic CAIs, dorzolamide (Trusopt) and brinzolamide (Azopt), which are safer and better tolerated. Topical CAIs are excellent alternatives to β-blockers in the initial management of elevated IOPs, and are effective as adjunctive agents. Brinzolamide 1% TID reduces IOP comparably to that achieved with dorzolamide 2% TID and to betaxolol 0.5% BID, but slightly less than timolol 0.5% BID. The IOP-reduction effects (peak and trough) of dorzolamide 2% TID are 16% to 25%. Brinzolamide and dorzolamide are approved for TID dosing; however, BID dosing may be adequate. Dorzolamide provides additional IOP-lowering effects when added to existing β-blocker therapy.[61,62] An ophthalmic solution of dorzolamide hydrochloride and timolol maleate is marketed as Cosopt, and a combination of brinzolamide and brimonidine is marketed as Simbrinza.[63]

The combined use of topical dorzolamide and oral acetazolamide does not result in additive effects and might increase the risk of toxicity. Therefore, the concomitant use of topical and oral CAIs is not advised.[64–66]

The topical CAIs are well tolerated with few systemic side effects. The most common adverse effects reported with dorzolamide are ocular burning, stinging, discomfort and allergic reactions, bitter taste, and superficial punctate keratitis. Brinzolamide causes less burning and stinging of the eyes than dorzolamide, because its pH more closely resembles that of human tears. Dorzolamide and brinzolamide are sulfonamides and may cause the same types of adverse reactions attributable to sulfonamides. These drugs should not be used in patients with renal or hepatic impairment.[64–66]

Pilocarpine

Pilocarpine (Isopto Carpine) historically was an initial treatment of choice, but with the introduction and widespread use of newer agents, pilocarpine has fallen out of favor. Therapy usually is begun using lower concentrations (1%), one drop 4 times a day (QID). Pilocarpine is a direct-acting cholinergic (parasympathomimetic) that causes contraction of ciliary muscle fibers attached to the trabecular meshwork and scleral spur. This opens the trabecular meshwork to enhance aqueous humor outflow. There also may be a direct effect on the trabecular meshwork. Pilocarpine causes miosis by contraction of the iris sphincter muscle, but the miosis is not related to the decrease in IOP.

Carbachol

Carbachol (Isopto Carbachol) is reserved as a third-line agent in patients who are unresponsive or intolerant to initial medications. In addition to having direct cholinergic effects, carbachol is more resistant to cholinesterase than pilocarpine. Added benefits include increased release of acetylcholine from parasympathetic nerve terminals and a weak anticholinesterase effect. Carbachol is administered TID.

Anticholinesterase Agents

If control of IOP is not achieved with optimal use of other topical monotherapy and combination therapy agents, then anticholinesterase agents may be prescribed as a last topical therapy option. Anticholinesterase agents inhibit the enzyme cholinesterase, thereby increasing the amount of acetylcholine and its naturally occurring cholinergic effects.

Echothiophate Iodide

Echothiophate iodide (phospholine iodide), an irreversible cholinesterase inhibitor, primarily inactivates pseudocholinesterase and secondarily inhibits true cholinesterase. Echothiophate iodide may be used if maximal doses of other agents and combination therapy are ineffective. Echothiophate iodide has a long duration of action that affords good control of IOP; however, miosis and myopia are significant side effects. Concentrations higher than 0.06% are associated with a significant increase in subjective complaints (e.g., brow ache).[67]

COMBINATION THERAPY

In general, drugs with different pharmacologic actions have at least partially additive effects in lowering IOP in the treatment of glaucoma. Drugs with similar pharmacologic actions (i.e., from the same pharmacologic class) should not be combined because dose-related adverse effects are more likely and the incremental increase in benefits is likely to be more modest.

Timolol and other β-adrenergic blocking drugs have additive IOP-lowering effects when used in combination with miotic agents, prostaglandin analogs, α_2-agonists, and CAIs. For example, the IOP-lowering effect is greater when timolol is used in combination with pilocarpine, dorzolamide, brimonidine, and travoprost. Likewise, for example, latanoprost has additive effects when administered with timolol, dorzolamide, and α_2-adrenergic agonists.[38–42,68–73] The trend toward the development of fixed-combination products offers many advantages in the treatment of POAG. These advantages include improved adherence because of a reduction in the number of dosages and bottles, eliminating the need to instill two separate drugs 5 to 10 minutes apart to prevent a washout effect from the second medication, improving safety and tolerability by limiting the exposure to the BAK preservative, and a cost savings for the patient by potentially eliminating a copay for one of the medications. There are two β-adrenergic blocker combination products currently on the market, timolol/dorzolamide (Cosopt) and brimonidine/timolol (Combigan). The IOP-lowering effects of timolol/dorzolamide (Cosopt) are comparable to or greater than those of latanoprost monotherapy.[65] Brinzolamide and brimonidine are combined and available as Simbrinza.[63]

Predisposing Factors

CASE 54-1

QUESTION 1: M.H., a 52-year-old African-American woman with brown eyes, presented for routine ophthalmic examination. Visual acuity without correction was 20/40 right eye and 20/80 left eye. Tonometry measured an IOP of 36 mm Hg in both eyes. Ophthalmoscopy revealed physiologic cupping of the optic discs in both eyes, and visual field examination revealed a nerve fiber bundle defect consistent with glaucoma. Pupils were normal in both eyes, and gonioscopy indicated that anterior chamber angles were open in both eyes. There were no signs of cataract formation. M.H. related a positive family history for glaucoma and presently is being treated for hypertension, chronic heart failure (CHF), chronic obstructive pulmonary disease, and asthma. Her medications include the following:

- Amitriptyline, 75 mg at bedtime
- Chlorpheniramine, 4 mg every 6 hours as needed (PRN)
- Lisinopril, 10 mg once daily
- Furosemide, 40 mg BID
- Nitroglycerin, 0.3 mg sublingual PRN
- Fluticasone/salmeterol 250/50 mcg dry powder inhaler, one inhalation twice daily
- Albuterol 90 mcg metered-dose inhaler, 1 to 2 puffs QID PRN
- Tiotropium bromide inhaler, 18 mcg inhaled once daily

Findings on examination indicate that M.H. has POAG. What other factors may predispose M.H. to an increased IOP?

POAG is thought to be determined genetically, and M.H. has a positive family history. The disease is more prevalent and aggressive in African-Americans.[1] In addition, she is taking several medications that have been associated with increases in IOP.

ANTICHOLINERGIC DRUGS

Most reports dealing with drug-induced increases in IOP center around precipitation of angle-closure glaucoma by ophthalmic mydriatic or cycloplegic agents (anticholinergics). In patients with open-angle glaucoma, topical anticholinergics can significantly increase resistance to aqueous humor outflow and elevate IOP while the anterior chamber remains grossly open.[4] As part of any routine ophthalmic examination, the pupils are dilated with a mydriatic or cycloplegic agent (unless otherwise contraindicated). The IOP is always measured before this procedure, so the use of these agents would not have influenced the IOP readings in M.H.

If systemic anticholinergic agents are administered in doses sufficient to cause pupillary dilation, the risk of precipitating angle-closure increases. However, it is unlikely that these agents will aggravate open-angle glaucoma unless the amount reaching the eye is sufficient to cause cycloplegia.[4] Although literature documentation of POAG exacerbation by these agents is scarce, medications with anticholinergic side effects (e.g., antihistamines, benzodiazepines, disopyramide, phenothiazines, tricyclic antidepressants, tiotropium) should be considered. M.H. is receiving chlorpheniramine as needed, amitriptyline at bedtime, and tiotropium bromide once daily, but her pupil examination is normal with no evidence of mydriasis or cycloplegia. Therefore, it is highly unlikely that these medications contributed to her increased IOP.

ADRENERGIC DRUGS

Adrenergic agents, such as central nervous system stimulants, vasoconstrictors, appetite suppressants, and bronchodilators, may produce minimal pupillary dilation. These have no proven adverse influences on IOP in patients with either normal eyes or eyes with open-angle glaucoma. Consequently, the use of salmeterol and albuterol in M.H. is also an unlikely source of the increased IOP.

OTHER DRUGS

Conclusive evidence for the production of angle-closure glaucoma by vasodilators is lacking, although slight increases in IOP have been reported. Use of nitroglycerin as needed in M.H. is not a cause for concern. There have been isolated reports of other medications causing mydriasis in glaucoma patients. These include muscle relaxants (carisoprodol), monoamine oxidase inhibitors, fenfluramine, ganglionic blocking agents, salicylates, and oral contraceptives. Succinylcholine, ketamine, and caffeine have been associated with increases in IOP. Corticosteroid-induced IOP elevation will be addressed in Case 54-8, Question 2. If M.H. requires administration of any other medications associated with increases in IOP, the risk of potential adverse effects can be minimized by routine follow-up.

Initial Therapy

CASE 54-1, QUESTION 2: What is the best initial therapeutic treatment in M.H.?

Topical β-blockers or PGAs are the initial agents of choice in the treatment of POAG (Fig. 54-2). Their efficacy is well documented in numerous studies, and side effects are well characterized. Brimonidine (Alphagan) and topical CAIs are alternative first-line agents. Table 54-1 lists the common topical agents used in the treatment of POAG.

Timolol or other nonselective β-adrenergic blockers should not be initiated for M.H. because of her history of asthma (the

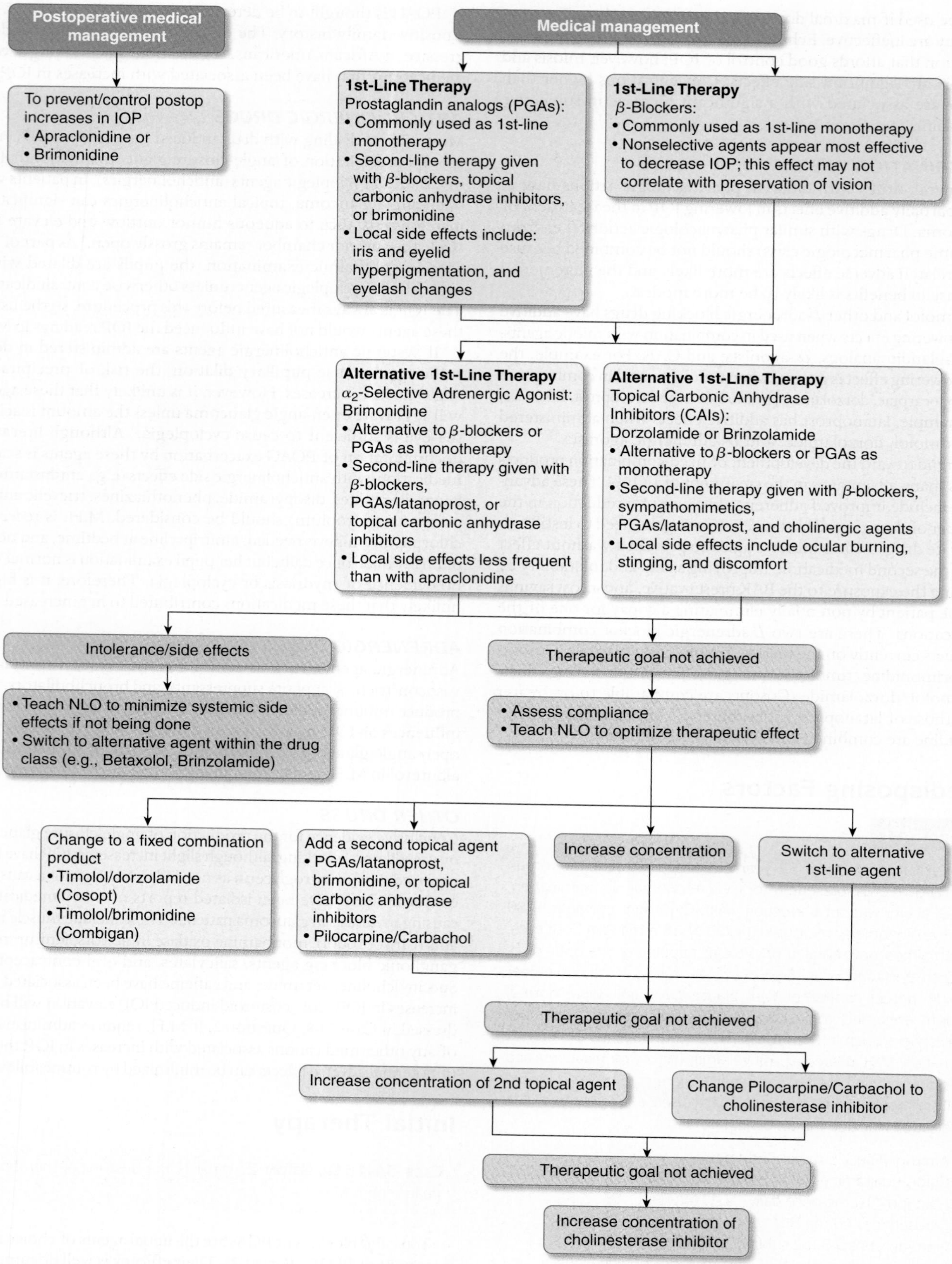

Figure 54-2 Medical management of glaucoma. IOP, intraocular pressure; NLO, nasolacrimal occlusion.

Table 54-1
Common Topical Agents Used in the Treatment of Open-Angle Glaucoma

Generic	Mechanism	Strength	Usual Dosage	Comments
β-Blockers				
Betaxolol (Betoptic [solution], Betoptic S [suspension])	Sympatholytic	0.25% (suspension) 0.5% (solution)	1 drop BID 1 drop BID	Shake suspension well before use. Effective with few associated ocular side effects. BID dosage enhances compliance. Considered β-blocker of choice in patients with preexisting HF or pulmonary disease because of β_1-adrenergic specificity. Patient response may be less than that seen with timolol
Carteolol (Ocupress)	Sympatholytic	1%	1 drop BID	Effective with few associated side effects. BID dosage enhances compliance. Use with caution in patients with preexisting HF or pulmonary disease
Levobunolol (Betagan)	Sympatholytic	0.25%, 0.5%	1 drop daily or BID	Effective with few associated ocular side effects. Daily and BID dosage enhances compliance. Use with caution in patients with preexisting HF or pulmonary disease
Metipranolol (OptiPranolol)	Sympatholytic	0.3%	1 drop BID	Effective with few associated side effects. BID dosage enhances compliance. Use with caution in patients with preexisting HF or pulmonary disease
Timolol (Timoptic) (Betimol) (Istalol)	Sympatholytic	0.25%, 0.5% 0.5% (Istalol) 0.25%, 0.5% preservative-free (Timoptic Ocudose)	1 drop BID 1 drop daily in morning (Istalol)	Effective with few associated ocular side effects. Daily and BID dosage enhances compliance. Use with caution in patients with preexisting HF or pulmonary disease. Proven long-term effectiveness, with well-defined side effect profile
Timolol Gel-Forming Solution (Timoptic XE, Timolol GFS)	Sympatholytic	0.25%, 0.5%	1 drop daily	Once-daily timolol formulation. The ophthalmic vehicle, gellan gum (Gelrite), prolongs precorneal residence time and ↑ ocular bioavailability, allowing once-daily administration
α2-Selective Adrenergic Agonists				
Apraclonidine (Iopidine)	Sympathomimetic	0.5%, 1%	1 drop preoperatively and postoperatively or 1 drop BID to TID	May be used preoperatively and postoperatively for the prevention of ↑ IOP after anterior-segment laser procedures. Use of NLO minimizes systemic side effects and allows for BID dosing. Does not penetrate the blood–brain barrier, therefore negligible systemic hypotension. Local adverse effects fairly common. Tachyphylaxis may be observed
Brimonidine (Alphagan)	Sympathomimetic	0.15%, 0.2%	1 drop BID to TID	Effective long-term monotherapy or adjunctive therapy. Use of NLO minimizes systemic side effects and allows for BID dosing. Penetrates the blood–brain barrier, therefore may cause mild systemic hypotension and lethargy. Local adverse effects less common than with apraclonidine
Brimonidine (Alphagan P)	Sympathomimetic	0.1%, 0.15%	1 drop BID to TID	Contains Purite preservative. Purite preservative and lower concentrations may improve tolerability

(continued)

Table 54-1
Common Topical Agents Used in the Treatment of Open-Angle Glaucoma (*continued*)

Generic	Mechanism	Strength	Usual Dosage	Comments
Topical Carbonic Anhydrase Inhibitors				
Brinzolamide (Azopt)	Decreased aqueous humor production	1%	1 drop TID	Shake suspension well before use. Effective long-term monotherapy or adjunctive therapy. Well tolerated with few systemic side effects. Less burning and stinging compared with dorzolamide
Dorzolamide (Trusopt)	Decreased aqueous humor production	2%	1 drop TID	Effective long-term monotherapy or adjunctive therapy. Well tolerated with few systemic side effects
Prostaglandin Analogs				
Latanoprost (Xalatan)	Prostaglandin $F_2\alpha$ agonist	0.005%	1 drop once a day at bedtime	BID dosing may be less effective than once a day at bedtime dosing. May cause increased pigmentation of the iris and eyelid. Systemic side effects are rare, but may cause muscle, joint, back pain, headaches, migraines, and skin rash. Effective monotherapy or adjunctive therapy. Store unopened bottles in refrigerator. Opened bottles may be stored at room temperature up to 6 weeks
Travoprost (Travatan Z)	Prostaglandin $F_2\alpha$ agonist	0.004%	1 drop once a day at bedtime	BID dosing may be less effective than once a day at bedtime dosing. May cause increased pigmentation of the iris and eyelid. Systemic side effects are rare, but may include colds and upper respiratory tract infections. Effective monotherapy or adjunctive therapy with timolol. May be more effective than timolol and latanoprost and more effective in African-Americans. Does not contain benzalkonium chloride as a preservative. Contains the preservative SofZia that may be better tolerated
Bimatoprost (Lumigan)	Prostamide	0.01%, 0.03%	1 drop once a day at bedtime	BID dosing may be less effective than QHS dosing. May cause increased pigmentation of the iris and eyelid. Systemic side effects are rare but include colds and upper respiratory tract infections and headache. May be more effective than timolol and latanoprost
Tafluprost (Zioptan)	Prostaglandin $F_2\alpha$ agonist	0.0015% preservative-free dropperette	1 drop once a day at bedtime	BID dosing may be less effective than QHS dosing. May cause increased pigmentation of the iris and eyelid. Systemic side effects are rare but include common cold, cough, headache, and urinary tract infections. Store unopened foiled pouches in refrigerator. Single-use container may be stored in the opened foil pouch for 28 days at room temperature
Miotics				
Pilocarpine (Isopto Carpine)	Parasympathomimetic	1%, 2%, 4%	1–2 drops TID or QID	Long-term proven effectiveness. Little rationale for administration more frequently than every 4 hours. Side effects of miosis with decreased vision and brow ache are common sources of patient complaints.
Carbachol (Isopto Carbachol)	Parasympathomimetic	1.5%, 3%	1–2 drops TID or QID	Used in patients allergic to or intolerant of other miotics. May be used as frequently as every 4 hours. Corneal penetration is enhanced by benzalkonium chloride in commercial preparations. Side effects are similar to those of pilocarpine

Table 54-1
Common Topical Agents Used in the Treatment of Open-Angle Glaucoma (*continued*)

Generic	Mechanism	Strength	Usual Dosage	Comments
Echothiophate iodide (phospholine iodide)	Anticholinesterase	0.125%	1 drop BID	Long duration, although usually dosed BID, which enhances compliance. Available as powder + diluent; after reconstitution, stable 30 days at room temperature, 6 months refrigerated. Side effects similar to those of pilocarpine. Increased cataract formation has been associated with its use
Combination Products				
Brimonidine tartrate 0.2%/timolol 0.5% (Combigan)	Sympathomimetic/ sympatholytic	0.2%/0.5%	1 drop BID	Combination products may improve adherence. Eliminates the 5- to 10-minute wait between instillation of drops
Dorzolamide 2%/timolol 0.5% (Cosopt)	Decreased aqueous humor production/ sympatholytic	2%/0.5% 2%/0.5% preservative free (Cosopt PF)	1 drop BID	Combination products may improve adherence. Eliminates the 5- to 10-minute wait between instillation of drops
Brinzolamide 1%/ brimonidine 0.2% (Simbrinza)	Decreased aqueous humor production/ sympathomimetic	1%/0.2%	1 drop TID	Shake suspension well before use. Combination products may improve adherence. Eliminates the 5- to 10-minute wait between instillation of drops

BID, twice daily; HF, heart failure; IOP, intraocular pressure; NLO, nasolacrimal occlusion; QHS, every day at bedtime; GFS, gel-forming solution; QID, 4 times a day; TID, 3 times a day.

indications and use of β-blockers for patients with heart failure are described in Chapter 14, Heart Failure). Betaxolol, a β_1-adrenergic blocker, is better tolerated than the nonselective β-adrenergic blocker, timolol, in patients with reactive airway disease and should be considered when topical β-blocker therapy is indicated in patients such as M.H.[12,31,32,74] Betaxolol 0.25% suspension BID would be reasonable for the initial treatment of M.H.'s glaucoma. Nevertheless, adverse pulmonary and cardiac side effects can occur with betaxolol: M.H. should be followed up closely for these adverse effects. Although ocular burning and stinging have been associated more frequently with betaxolol and metipranolol than with other topical β-blockers, the 0.25% suspension is better tolerated than the 0.5% solution and is as effective.[31] Brimonidine, a topical CAI, and a PGA (e.g., latanoprost) are acceptable alternatives to betaxolol as initial therapy. Although brimonidine, topical CAIs, and latanoprost may not exacerbate her asthma or CHF, they can cause localized side effects and brimonidine can cause systemic hypotension and lethargy.

Patient Education

CASE 54-1, QUESTION 3: Betaxolol 0.25% suspension, one drop in both eyes BID, is ordered for M.H. How should M.H. be instructed regarding the proper use of her betaxolol and expected therapeutic side effects?

M.H. should be instructed to hold the inverted betaxolol bottle between her thumb and middle finger and to rest that hand on her forehead to minimize the risk of inadvertent eye injury caused by sudden unexpected movement of the hand. The index finger is left free to depress the bottom of the container, releasing one drop for the dose. With a little practice, this technique is easy to master. The lower eyelid should be drawn downward with the index finger of the opposite hand or pinched between the thumb and index finger to form a pouch. The patient should look up and administer the drug into the pouch of the eye.

Patients must be encouraged to continue regular use of their medications for effective treatment of glaucoma. Chronic glaucoma is a silent disease and often not associated with symptoms; therefore, the continuation of therapy should be encouraged continuously in patients, especially when side effects to drug therapy can be encountered. Betaxolol is best administered every 12 hours because this schedule of administration is consistent with its duration of action (see Table 54-1).

Systemic side effects (e.g., bradycardia, heart block, CHF, pulmonary distress, central nervous system) are rare with betaxolol, but M.H. should be instructed to report any of these effects to her primary-care provider.

NASOLACRIMAL OCCLUSION

CASE 54-1, QUESTION 4: How much would occlusion of the nasolacrimal ducts (punctal occlusion) by M.H. influence systemic absorption or alter the therapeutic effects of betaxolol?

Nasolacrimal, or punctal, occlusion is a technique that can decrease the amount of drug absorbed systemically.[75] Occlusion of the puncta (through the application of slight pressure with the finger to the inner corner of the eye closest to the nose for 3 to 5 minutes during and after drug instillation) can minimize systemic absorption of ophthalmic medications (e.g., betaxolol), decrease the incidence of side effects, and improve medication effectiveness.[75–77] When a single drop of ophthalmic timolol 0.5% was instilled into the eyes of patients at various times before cataract surgery and the nasolacrimal duct was occluded for 5 minutes, drug levels in the aqueous humor were significantly greater in patients who had their nasolacrimal ducts occluded than those who did not.[76]

Nasolacrimal occlusion is effective and can maximize drug benefits because a lower concentration of an ophthalmic formulation can be used and the dose can be administered less frequently.[69]

Alternative Therapy

CASE 54-1, QUESTION 5: Two weeks after initiation of therapy, M.H. returns to clinic for a follow-up evaluation. Her IOP measures 32 mm Hg in the right eye and 30 mm Hg in the left eye. She denies nonadherence and has no complaints of intolerable side effects. How should therapy be altered? Are there alternative dosage forms or drugs that can be used?

Betaxolol may not be as effective as other ocular β-blockers. Therefore, adjunctive therapy may be required. However, M.H. should be evaluated to determine whether she has been using the technique of nasolacrimal occlusion. If not, M.H. should be again instructed on the technique of nasolacrimal occlusion and the importance of this technique in achieving the maximal therapeutic effect of her therapy (see Case 54-1, Question 4).

After the initiation of therapy, patients should be seen for a follow-up evaluation within about 2 weeks. If M.H. has been adherent to therapy and has been occluding her nasolacrimal ducts, a new course of action is needed because her IOP still is elevated. When the goal of therapy has not been achieved, the drug concentration of the ophthalmic formulation can be increased, adjunctive therapy (e.g., brimonidine, a topical CAI, a PGA) can be initiated, or an alternative first-line agent can be selected. Patients who are experiencing unstable reductions of IOP should be followed up within 4 months.[5] Stable patients usually are evaluated every 6 to 12 months.[5]

Adverse Effects

CASE 54-1, QUESTION 6: Several weeks later, dorzolamide 2% solution, one drop both eyes BID, is added to M.H.'s betaxolol therapy. Two weeks later, M.H. returns for a follow-up evaluation and complains of bilateral stinging and foreign body sensation. Her IOP measures 30 mm Hg in the right eye and 29 mm Hg in the left eye. What are the possible causes of her side effects and poor response to therapy?

The exposure of dorzolamide to the outside environment may result in the aggregation of dry white granules on the tip of the dorzolamide bottle. These granules can drop into a patient's eyes when instilling the medication, leading to local side effects, such as stinging and foreign body sensation. Such foreign bodies may cause enough discomfort to induce nonadherence, resulting in a poor response to therapy. These granules may be rinsed off of the tip with sterile water. M.H. should be questioned about the presence of dry white granules on the tip of her dorzolamide bottle.[78]

These complaints may also be a side effect from the medications, regardless of the granule presence. Ocular burning, stinging, and discomfort were reported in one-third of patients in dorzolamide clinical trials. M.H.'s administration technique should also be assessed to determine whether she is administering the two drugs at least 5 to 10 minutes apart so that the first drug is not washed away by the second drug. This should be a consideration when assessing her response to therapy.[15]

CASE 54-1, QUESTION 7: After further discussions with M.H., it is determined that she has not been adherent to her dorzolamide therapy because of intolerable side effects. The dorzolamide is discontinued and replaced with travoprost 0.004% one drop both eyes once a day at bedtime. Why might this drug selection be especially appropriate for M.H.? What patient education information should be provided to M.H. about travoprost side effects?

Prostaglandin analogs are first-line agents and are appropriate in patients who are not responding to or are having intolerable side effects from other medications. Travoprost is an ideal choice for M.H., because African-Americans respond especially well to travoprost.[43] M.H. still needs to be informed about the PGA-induced potential for hyperpigmentation of the iris, which may be permanent. She also needs to be educated on the possibility of eyelid skin darkening and increased thickness, length, and pigmentation of her eyelashes, which all may or may not be reversible. These side effects might not be as cosmetically concerning to M.H., because she has brown eyes and will be instilling travoprost eyedrops into both eyes.

ANGLE-CLOSURE GLAUCOMA

Treatment

CASE 54-2

QUESTION 1: D.H., a 72-year-old man, presents to the emergency department with an intensely red right eye, a "steamy" appearing cornea, complaints of haloes around lights, and extreme pain. A diagnosis of acute angle-closure glaucoma is made. How should D.H. be managed?

D.H. should be seen by an ophthalmologist because acute angle-closure glaucoma is a medical emergency. Medical treatment usually consists of pilocarpine 2% to 4%, one drop every 5 minutes for 4 to 6 administrations. It is recommended that the puncta be covered during administration to decrease the possibility of systemic absorption. Stronger miotic agents are contraindicated because they may potentiate angle closure. Topical timolol also has been used in acute angle-closure glaucoma, commonly in combination with pilocarpine. However, drugs that decrease aqueous humor production may be ineffective in this situation because they have a decreased ability to reduce aqueous production if the ciliary body is ischemic.[5]

HYPEROSMOTIC AGENTS

Hyperosmotic agents (Table 54-2) act by creating an osmotic gradient between the plasma and ocular fluids.[79] Agents that are confined to the extracellular fluid space (e.g., mannitol) provide a greater effect on blood osmolality at the same dosage than do agents distributed in total body water.[79] Intravenously administered drugs provide a faster, somewhat greater effect than oral agents. Palatability may be a problem with oral agents and can be improved by serving these agents over crushed ice or with lemon juice or cola flavoring.

Orally, 50% glycerin is the usual drug of choice and is administered in dosages of 1 to 1.5 g/kg.[80] Isosorbide is an alternative, especially in diabetic patients because it is not metabolized to provide calories.[81] Parenterally, mannitol is the drug of choice. It is administered in doses of 1 to 2 g/kg, is not metabolized to provide calories, and may be used in patients with renal failure.[82,83]

Primary side effects of hyperosmotic agents include headache, nausea, vomiting, diuresis, and dehydration. It is important that the patient not be allowed to drink because this will counteract the osmotic effects of these agents.

Precipitation of pulmonary edema and CHF has been reported with hyperosmotic agents, and an allergic reaction has been reported with mannitol.[84]

Acetazolamide (Diamox) 500 mg intravenously may be administered in addition to hyperosmotic agents.

Table 54-2
Hyperosmotic Agents

Generic	Mode of Administration	Strength	Onset	Peak	Duration	Dose	Ocular Penetration	Distribution
Mannitol	IV	5%, 10%, 15%, 20%	30–60 minutes	1 hour	6–8 hours	1–2 g/kg	Very poor	E
Glycerin	PO	50%	10–30 minutes	30 minutes	4–5 hours	1–1.5 g/kg	Poor	E
Isosorbide	PO	45%	10–30 minutes	1 hour	5 hours	1.5–2 g/kg	Good	TBW

E, extracellular water; IV, intravenous; PO, orally; TBW, total body water.

OCULAR SIDE EFFECTS OF DRUGS

CASE 54-3

QUESTION 1: B.C., a 64-year-old man, has a history of hypertension managed with hydrochlorothiazide 25 mg/day. He takes amiodarone 800 mg/day for cardiac arrhythmia, and chlorpheniramine 12 mg BID PRN for allergies. Four weeks ago, risperidone 1 mg BID was added to his medication regimen. He also takes sildenafil 100 mg an average of twice weekly. He complains of occasional blurred vision. Could these symptoms be related to his medications?

All the drugs that B.C. is taking have been associated with ocular side effects. Thiazide diuretics have been associated with acute myopia that may last from 24 to 48 hours.[85,86] However, hydrochlorothiazide is an unlikely cause of B.C.'s blurred vision considering its recent onset.

Amiodarone can cause keratopathy, but it is asymptomatic.[87,88] A high percentage of patients who receive this drug exhibit microdeposits within the corneal epithelium that resembles the verticillate keratopathy induced by chloroquine.[85] These corneal deposits are bilateral, dose- and duration-related, reversible, and unassociated with visual symptoms.

Risperidone has been associated with disturbances of accommodation and blurred vision.[89]

B.C. may be in the approximately 1% of the population who experiences blurred vision with chlorpheniramine. This effect has been seen in patients receiving 12 to 14 mg/day.[85] If an antihistamine is indicated, an agent such as cetirizine would be less likely to cause such an effect. Sildenafil has been associated with change in color and light perception as well as blurred vision.[90] These effects generally subside within 4 hours of the dose.

Table 54-3[85–114] outlines some of the more common ocular side effects associated with systemic medications. Each case should be evaluated individually and alternative therapy considered in intolerant patients.

Table 54-3
Ocular Side Effects of Systemic Medications

Drug Class	Effect(s)	Clinical Remarks
Analgesics		
Ibuprofen	Reduced vision	Rare; blurred vision reported in patients taking from four 200-mg tablets/week to six tablets/day; changes in color vision rarely reported[91]
Narcotics, including pentazocine	Miosis	Miosis often with morphine in normal doses; slight with other agents; effect secondary to CNS action on the pupillo-constrictor center[85]
	Tearing Irregular pupils Paresis of accommodation Diplopia	Effects associated with narcotic withdrawal[85]
Antiarrhythmics		
Amiodarone	Keratopathy	Dose and duration related; resembles chloroquine keratopathy. Corneal deposits are bilateral, reversible, and unassociated with visual symptoms. Patients taking 100–200 mg/day have only minimal deposits. Deposits occur in almost 100% of patients receiving 400 mg/day[87,88]
	Cataracts	Previously reported as insignificant, anterior subcapsular lens opacities have been associated with amiodarone therapy. Rarely, such opacities may progress, increasing in density and in the diffuse distribution of the deposits, ultimately covering an area somewhat larger than the undilated pupil's aperture. The mechanism for this effect is unclear, but like chlorpromazine, amiodarone is a photosensitizing agent. Given that the lens changes are limited largely to the pupillary aperture, light exposure may result in the lens changes[85–88]
	Optic neuropathy	Approximately 2% of patients experience optic neuropathy[90]

(continued)

Table 54-3
Ocular Side Effects of Systemic Medications (*continued*)

Drug Class	Effect(s)	Clinical Remarks
Anticholinergics		
Atropine Dicyclomine Glycopyrrolate Propantheline Scopolamine Trihexyphenidyl	Mydriasis Cycloplegia with ↓ accommodation Photophobia	Systemic and transdermal anticholinergic agents may cause mydriasis and, less frequently, cycloplegia. Mydriasis may precipitate angle-closure glaucoma. Photophobia is related to the mydriasis. Accommodation for near objects[85,92]
Anticonvulsants		
Carbamazepine	Diplopia Blurred vision	Ocular adverse reactions when dosage >1–2 g/day; disappear when dosage is reduced[85]
Phenytoin	Nystagmus cataracts	Nystagmus in patients with high blood levels (>20 mcg/mL); rarely occurs with other hydantoins. Cataracts may occur rarely with prolonged therapy[85,93]
Topiramate	Acute myopia, secondary angle-closure glaucoma	Topiramate has been associated with angle-closure glaucoma. Symptoms including ocular pain, headache, nausea, vomiting, hyperemia, visual field defects, and blindness have been reported. This process is usually bilateral, but if symptoms are recognized and the drug is stopped in a timely manner, adverse outcomes may be minimized[90]
Trimethadione	Visual glares	A prolonged glare or dazzle occurs when eyes are exposed to light. The glare is reversible, occurs at the retinal level, and is more common in adolescents and adults; rarely in young children[85]
Vigabatrin	Visual field abnormalities	Visual field abnormalities including bilateral, symmetrical, and irreversible peripheral constriction occur in up to 30% of patients. Most patients are asymptomatic, and <0.1% of patients are clinically affected[90]
Anesthetics		
Propofol	Inability to open eyes	6 of 50 patients undergoing ENT procedures using standardized anesthesia with propofol were unable to open their eyes either spontaneously or in response to verbal commands. This effect lasted from 3 to 20 minutes after the end of anesthetic administration. Two patients showed complete loss of ocular motility. This was a transient, myasthenia-like weakness[94]
Antidepressants		
Tricyclic antidepressants (TCAs)		Mydriasis is the most common ocular side effect of TCAs. Cycloplegia is rare. Reports of precipitation of angle-closure glaucoma.[85]
Fluoxetine	Mydriasis Eye tics	Administration of fluoxetine 20–40 mg/day has been associated with paroxysmal contractions of the muscles around the lateral aspect of the eye. This effect occurred 3–4 weeks after initiation of fluoxetine therapy and resolved within 2 weeks of discontinuation[95]
Antihistamines		
Chlorpheniramine	Blurred vision	Blurred vision occurs rarely (about 1% of patients taking 12–14 mg/day)[85]
	Mydriasis, decreased lacrimal secretions	Rare[85]
Antihypertensives		
Clonidine	Miosis	Miosis is seen in overdose[85]
	Dry itchy eyes	Rare[85]
Diazoxide	Lacrimation	About 20% experience lacrimation, which may continue after drug is discontinued[85]
Guanethidine	Miosis	Sporadically documented. One study reported a 17% incidence of blurred vision in patients taking guanethidine 70 mg/day[85]
	Ptosis	
	Conjunctivitis	
	Blurred vision	
Reserpine	Miosis	Miosis is slight, but can last up to 1 week after a single dose[85]
	Conjunctivitis	Common, secondary to dilation of conjunctival blood vessels[85]

Table 54-3
Ocular Side Effects of Systemic Medications (*continued*)

Drug Class	Effect(s)	Clinical Remarks
Anti-Infectives		
Amantadine	Corneal lesions	Diffuse, white punctate subepithelial corneal opacities have been reported, occasionally associated with superficial punctate keratitis. Onset has been 1–2 weeks after initiation of therapy with dosages of 200–400 mg/day. Resolves with drug discontinuation[96]
Chloramphenicol	Optic neuritis	Rare unless a total dose of 100 g and duration >6 weeks are exceeded. Vision usually improves after the drug is discontinued[85]
Chloroquine	Corneal deposits	Some patients using ordinary doses may develop corneal deposits in a few months. The deposits are visible with use of a biomicroscope and appear as white-yellow in color, but are of no consequence[85]
	Retinopathy (macular degeneration)	Serious retinopathy when total dose >100 g. Usually develops after 1–3 years; can occur in 6 months. Visual loss may be peripheral, with progression to central vision loss and disturbance of color vision. Rarely, effects such as blurred vision are seen earlier when larger doses (500–700 mg/day) are used. Macular changes may progress after drug is discontinued. These agents concentrate in pigmented tissue[85]
Ethambutol	Retrobulbar neuritis	At dosages of 15 mg/kg/day, virtually void of ocular side effects. Such effects are rare at dosages of 25 mg/kg/day for a duration of a few months. Patients treated for prolonged periods should have routine visual examinations including visual fields. Most effects are reversible after the drug is discontinued, but optic neuritis may continue to progress for 1–2 months after the drug has been discontinued[85,90]
Gentamicin	Pseudotumor cerebri	Rare, but has been well documented with secondary papilledema and visual loss[85]
Isoniazid	Optic neuritis	Prevalence not well defined, but appears to be significantly less than peripheral neuritis. Evaluation difficult because most patients are malnourished, chronic alcoholics, or receiving multiple medications. Preexisting eye disease does not appear to be a predisposing factor[85]
Nalidixic acid	Visual sensations	Most common ocular side effect. Main feature is a brightly colored appearance of objects; occurs soon after the drug is taken. Although quinolone antibiotics are nalidixic acid derivatives, they have rarely been associated with these ocular side effects[85]
	Visual loss	Temporary effect (30 minutes–3 days)
	Papilledema	Primarily in infants and young children and secondary to intracranial pressure; reversible on withdrawal of the drug
Sulfonamides	Myopia	Acute and reversible; most common ocular side effect[85]
	Conjunctivitis	Primarily with topical sulfathiazole, 4% incidence between 5 and 9 days of therapy[85]
	Optic neuritis	Even in low dosages. Usually reversible with complete recovery of vision[85]
	Photosensitivity	Associated with use of sulfisoxazole lid margin therapy[97,98]
Tetracyclines	Myopia	Appears to be acute, transient, and rare[85]
	Papilledema	More common in children and infants than adults; rare[85]
Voriconazole	Altered visual perception	May be associated with higher doses or plasma concentrations[99]
	Blurred vision	
Anti-Inflammatory Agents (also see Analgesics; Corticosteroids)		
Cyclooxygenase-2 inhibitors	Blurred vision Conjunctivitis	Discontinuation of therapy leads to resolution without long-term effects[90]
Gold	Corneal Conjunctival deposits	Deposition in the conjunctiva and superficial cornea more common than in the lens or deep cornea. Incidence in cornea of 40%–80% in total doses of 1.5 g; visual acuity is unaffected. One reported case after oral therapy[85]
Indomethacin	Decreased vision	Rare; also changes in color vision have been rarely reported.[85]
Phenylbutazone	Decreased vision	Most common ocular side effect with this drug may be caused by lens hydration.[85]
	Conjunctivitis retinal hemorrhage	Occurs less often than vision. The conjunctivitis may be associated with development of Stevens–Johnson syndrome or an allergic reaction[85]

(*continued*)

Chapter 54

Eye Disorders

Table 54-3
Ocular Side Effects of Systemic Medications (*continued*)

Drug Class	Effect(s)	Clinical Remarks
Antilipemic Agents		
Lovastatin	Cataracts	The crystalline lenses of hypercholesterolemic patients were assessed before and after 48 weeks of treatment with lovastatin 20–80 mg/day. Statistical analyses of the distribution of cortical, nuclear, and subcapsular opacities at 48 weeks showed no significant differences between placebo-treated and lovastatin-treated groups. Visual acuity assessments also were not significantly different among the groups[100]
Antineoplastic Agents		
Busulfan	Cataracts	Reported with high dosages.[85]
Carmustine	Arterial narrowing Nerve fiber layer infarcts Intraretinal hemorrhages	These ocular side effects are not well established. Evidence of delayed bilateral ocular toxicity developed in 2 of 50 patients treated with high-dose IV carmustine (800 mg/m^2). Symptoms of ocular toxicity became evident 4 weeks after IV treatment. Evidence of delayed ocular toxicity (mean onset 6 weeks) ipsilateral to the site of infusion developed in 7 of 10 patients treated with intra-arterial carotid doses of carmustine to a cumulative minimum of 450 mg/m^2 in two treatments[101]
Cytarabine	Keratoconjunctivitis Ocular burning Photophobia Blurred vision	Corneal toxicity and conjunctivitis have been reported with high-dose (3 g/m^2) therapy[102]
Doxorubicin	Conjunctivitis Excessive tearing	May last for several days after treatment[85]
Erlotinib	Trichomegaly and ocular irritation	
Fluorouracil	Ocular irritation Lacrimation	Reversible and seldom interfere with continued therapy[85]
Tamoxifen	Corneal opacities Decreased vision Retinopathy	Generally occurs in patients receiving more than 1 year of treatment when a total dose exceeding 100 g has been taken[85]
Vinca alkaloids (especially vincristine)	Extraocular muscle paresis (EMP) Ptosis	The onset of EMP or paralysis may be seen as early as 2 weeks. Dose related. Most recover fully when drug is discontinued[85]
Barbiturates		
	Miosis Mydriasis Disturbances in ocular movement Ptosis	Most significant ocular side effects occur in chronic users or in toxic states. Pupillary responses are variable; miosis seen most frequently except in toxicity when mydriasis predominates. Nystagmus and weakness in extraocular muscles may be seen. Chronic abusers have a characteristic ptosis[85]
Bisphosphonates (Alendronate, Etidronate, Pamidronate, Risedronate)		
	Blurred vision, pain, photophobia, conjunctivitis, scleritis, uveitis	Adverse events more common with pamidronate. Scleritis and uveitis are of greatest concern. After persistent reduction in vision of sustained ocular pain, refer patient to an ophthalmologist. Ocular NSAID treatment may be of symptomatic benefit[90]
Calcium-Channel Blockers		
	Blurred vision Transient blindness	Primarily blurred vision; transient blindness at peak concentrations has been observed in several patients[103]
Corticosteroids		
	Cataracts	Posterior subcapsular cataracts have been associated with systemic corticosteroids in patients who have received >15 mg/day of prednisone or its equivalent daily for periods >1 year.[103,104] Rare reports of bilateral posterior subcapsular cataracts associated with nasal aerosol or inhalation of beclomethasone dipropionate have been received. Most patients had received therapy for >5 years, often in higher than the recommended dosage. Approximately 40% of patients also were receiving systemic corticosteroids.[106] (Also see Case 54-8, Question 1.)

Table 54-3
Ocular Side Effects of Systemic Medications (*continued*)

Drug Class	Effect(s)	Clinical Remarks
	↑ Intraocular pressure (IOP)	More common with topical corticosteroids than with systemic therapy. Of little consequence in patients without preexisting glaucoma. Glaucoma patients should be monitored routinely if receiving systemic corticosteroids.[85] (See Case 54-8, Question 1.)
	Papilledema	Intracranial hypertension or pseudotumor cerebri from systemic corticosteroids has been well documented. The incidence appears to be greater in children than in adults; primarily associated with chronic therapy
Digitalis		
	Altered color vision, visual acuity	Changes in color vision. A glare phenomenon and a snowy appearance in objects have been associated primarily with digitalis intoxication. In a small number of cases, reversible reduction in visual acuity has been noted. Also associated with changes in the visual fields[85]
	Decreased IOP	Digitalis derivatives can decrease IOP, but clinical use for glaucoma is not practical because the therapeutic systemic dose for this effect is very near the toxic dose[85]
Diuretics		
Carbonic anhydrase inhibitors	Myopia	Acute myopia that may last from 24 to 48 hours. Probably caused by an increase in the anteroposterior diameter of the lens, which may be reversible even if drug use is continued[85]
Thiazides	Myopia	Thiazide diuretics have been associated with acute myopia that may last from 24 to 48 hours.[85,86]
Estrogens		
Clomiphene	Blurred vision Mydriasis Visual field changes Visual sensations	5%–10% experience ocular side effects. Blurred vision is the most common effect, although visual sensations such as flashing lights, distortion of images, and various colored lights (primarily silver) may occur[85]
Oral contraceptives (OCs)	Optic neuritis Pseudotumor cerebri Retrobulbar neuritis	Quite rare. In patients with retinal vascular abnormalities, use of OCs is questionable. Numerous other possible ocular side effects are associated with these agents, and further documentation is required[85]
Hypouricemics		
Allopurinol	Cataracts	Conflicting reports have suggested allopurinol may be associated with anterior and posterior lens capsule changes and with anterior subcapsular vacuoles; 42 cases of cataracts have been reported; these have been observed primarily in age groups in whom normal lens aging changes would not be expected. No cause-and-effect relationship has been proven[85,107]
Immune Modulators		
Imatinib	Visual deficits	Ocular symptoms include blurred vision, conjunctivitis, dry eyes, epiphora, and periorbital edema. The latter occurs in up to 74% of treated patients[108]
Interleukin 2	Visual deficits	Interleukin 2 visual complications have occurred during the first or second treatment cycle, usually within 5–6 days of initiation of therapy. Ocular symptoms included diplopia, binocular negative scotomas (isolated areas of varying size and shape in which vision is absent or depressed; these are not perceived ordinarily, but would be apparent on completion of a visual field examination), and palinopsia (abnormal recurring visual imagery). In most cases, treatment was continued for the entire planned duration of therapy. Symptoms resolved after discontinuation[109]
Phenothiazines		
Chlorpromazine	Deposits on the lens	Rare when total dose <0.5 kg. Visible after a total dose of 1 kg in most cases; incidence may increase to 90% after ≥2.5 kg. Usually, deposits do not affect vision appreciably. The cornea and conjunctiva may be affected after the lens shows pigment changes[85]
	Retinal pigment deposits	The number of reported cases is small; further documentation is necessary[85]
Thioridazine	Pigmentary retinopathy	Primarily associated with maximal daily dosages or average doses >1,000 mg. Daily dosages up to 600 mg are relatively safe; 600–800 mg is uncertain, but rarely suspect. If >800 mg/day is used, periodic ophthalmoscopic examinations may uncover problems before visual acuity is compromised[85]

(continued)

Table 54-3
Ocular Side Effects of Systemic Medications (*continued*)

Drug Class	Effect(s)	Clinical Remarks
Therapy for Erectile Dysfunction		
Sildenafil Tadalafil Vardenafil α-Blockers	Changes in color or light perception, blurred vision, conjunctival hyperemia, ocular pain, photophobia	Color vision alterations are mild to moderate. Blurred vision does not impair visual acuity. Visual alterations usually subside within 4 hours after the dose.[110–112] Ocular adverse effects are uncommon, dose dependent, and fully reversible to date. Incidence is not related to age, but is related to blood concentration. Peak visual effects usually occur within 60 minutes after ingestion[90]
Alfuzosin	Visual defects	Amblyopia, blurred vision, and floppy iris have been reported[113]
Tamsulosin	Floppy iris	Approximately 3% of patients taking tamsulosin for benign prostatic hyperplasia (BPH) experience floppy iris during cataract surgery. Modification of the surgical procedure usually results in successful surgery[114]

CNS, central nervous system; ENT, ear, nose, and throat; NSAID, nonsteroidal anti-inflammatory drug.

OCULAR EMERGENCIES

Chemical Burns

CASE 54-4

QUESTION 1: S.J., a 24-year-old construction worker, has splashed an unidentified chemical in his eyes and runs into a nearby pharmacy complaining of burning in both eyes. Should the pharmacist attempt to treat S.J. or refer him to the emergency department?

Chemical burns require immediate attention. The immediate treatment is copious irrigation using the most accessible source of water (e.g., shower, faucet, drinking fountain, hose, bathtub). After at least 5 minutes of initial irrigation, S.J. should be taken immediately to the emergency department. A water-soaked towel or cloth should be kept on his eyes during transport.

Other Ocular Emergencies

When healthcare professionals are approached by patients with acute ocular emergencies (e.g., chemical burns, corneal trauma, corneal ulcers, acute angle-closure glaucoma), patients require immediate treatment and should be referred to an ophthalmologist if the practitioner has even the slightest doubt about appropriate therapy. It is difficult to effectively evaluate the severity of ocular disorders without the benefit of a thorough ophthalmologic workup and specialized training. In situations of corneal trauma from abrasion or foreign bodies, the patient often complains of a gritty, scratchy feeling and can be aware of a foreign body's presence. The corneal tissue is an excellent culture medium for bacteria (e.g., *Pseudomonas aeruginosa*), and therapy should be initiated as soon as possible to avoid corneal perforation and possible blindness.[1] Signs and symptoms of acute angle-closure glaucoma are reviewed in Case 54-2, Question 1.

Gonococcal conjunctivitis is an ocular emergency, and patients should be referred immediately to an ophthalmologist to minimize the potential of corneal perforation.[1] These patients, who can present with symptoms of red, tender, swollen eyelids with exophthalmos and mild pain, may be suffering from orbital cellulitis or endophthalmitis, which require immediate treatment with systemic antibiotics. Conjunctivitis of other origins (see Acute Bacterial Conjunctivitis [Pinkeye] and Allergic Conjunctivitis sections) generally is not an ocular emergency.

Any loss of vision (whether sudden, complete, or transient), flashes of light, pain, or photophobia can signify potentially damaging ocular disorders (e.g., retinal artery occlusion, optic neuritis, amaurosis fugax, retinal detachment), and an ophthalmologist should evaluate the patient as soon as possible. Referral also is recommended for patients with blurred vision, pupil disorders, diplopia, nystagmus, or ocular hemorrhage.

COMMON OCULAR DISORDERS

Stye (Hordeolum)

Sties are infections of the hair follicles or sebaceous glands of the eyelids. The most common infecting organism is *Staphylococcus aureus*. Treatment consists of hot, moist compresses and topical antibiotics (e.g., sulfacetamide). Over-the-counter products should not be recommended. An ophthalmologist should evaluate sties that do not respond to warm compresses within a few days.

Conjunctivitis

Conjunctivitis, a common external eye problem that involves inflammation of the conjunctiva, usually is associated with symptoms of a diffusely reddened eye with purulent or serous discharge accompanied by itching, smarting, stinging, or a scratching foreign-body sensation. Patients with pain, decreased vision, unequal distribution of redness, irregular pupils, or opacity should be referred immediately to an ophthalmologist because these are signs of more serious eye disease.

Conjunctivitis can be bacterial, fungal, parasitic, viral, or allergic in origin. Most cases of bacterial conjunctivitis are caused by *Staphylococcus. aureus, Streptococcus pneumoniae*, *Haemophilus influenzae* and *Moraxella catarrhalis*, although a number of other organisms may be responsible. The infection usually starts in one eye and is spread to the other by the hands. It also may be spread to other persons. Unlike bacterial conjunctivitis, corneal infections can obliterate vision rapidly; therefore, accurate diagnosis is important.

ACUTE BACTERIAL CONJUNCTIVITIS (PINKEYE)

CASE 54-5

QUESTION 1: L.T. is a 6-year-old boy with diffuse bilateral conjunctival redness that has been present for 2 days. A crusting discharge is deposited on his lashes and the corners of his eyes. His vision is normal, and his pupils are round and equal. The diagnosis of acute bacterial conjunctivitis is made, and sodium sulfacetamide 10% ophthalmic drops, two drops in both eyes every 2 hours while awake, are prescribed. What other measures should be used? What instructions should his caregivers receive?

Although treatment of typical bacterial conjunctivitis such as this is empirical, a culture should be obtained. Other ophthalmic antibiotic drops or ointments, such as neomycin-polymyxin-B-gramicidin combination (Neosporin) or polymyxin-trimethoprim (Polytrim), also are used in these situations. Although other antimicrobials, such as the ocular quinolones, may be used for bacterial conjunctivitis, these agents should be reserved as second-line therapies because of cost and the potential development of resistance. Proper management of this infection also includes mechanical cleaning of the eyelids and hygienic measures that prevent spreading the infection to other children. The deposits should be removed as often as possible with moist cotton swabs or cotton-tipped applicators. A mild baby shampoo can be used to moisten the applicator. Firm adherent crusts may be softened with warm, moist compresses. Because this material is infectious, it should be disposed of in a sanitary fashion. The common use of washcloths by several individuals will spread bacterial conjunctivitis.

ALLERGIC CONJUNCTIVITIS

CASE 54-6

QUESTION 1: N.V., a 10-year-old girl, has experienced redness in both eyes accompanied by "hay fever" for the past 2 months (June and July). There is no crusting on her eyelids, and her vision is normal; she rubs her eyes often because they itch. What treatment is best for N.V.'s allergic conjunctivitis?

Topical vasoconstrictors (e.g., naphazoline, tetrahydrozoline) with or without antihistamines (e.g., antazoline, pheniramine) may be used to treat hyperemia, but they should not be used excessively because rebound congestion can occur. Use of topical vasoconstrictors for longer than 72 hours is not recommended owing to the potential for rebound congestion and masking of more serious ocular inflammatory conditions. Antihistamine tablets or syrup can provide considerable, but temporary, relief. Several ophthalmic histamine H_1-receptor antagonists are effective in the treatment of allergic conjunctivitis. Levocabastine 0.05% is administered BID to QID, olopatadine 0.1% BID (separating doses by 6–8 hours) or 0.2% once daily, emedastine 0.05% QID, ketotifen 0.025% BID to QID, bepotastine 1.5% BID, and alcaftadine 0.25% once daily.[115–117] Ketotifen, olopatadine, azelastine, epinastine, and alcaftadine exhibit both antihistamine and mast cell stabilizing effects. Emedastine was more efficacious than levocabastine when used BID for 6 weeks in adult and pediatric patients with seasonal allergic conjunctivitis.[118] Olopatadine provided superior efficacy and a more rapid resolution of the signs and symptoms of allergic conjunctivitis when compared with ketotifen in a small trial involving adult patients.[119] Azelastine has a slightly quicker onset of therapeutic effect when compared with olopatadine and placebo.[120] Bepotastine 1.5% BID provided better relief of evening ocular and nasal symptoms than olopatadine 0.2% administered once daily for 14 days.[121] Alcaftadine 0.25% and olopatadine 0.2% administered once daily provided relief of ocular itching at 16 and 24 hours postinstallation with alcaftadine also providing significant relief from chemosis.[122] Information to date is insufficient to definitively recommend one of these products as superior to the others. The ideal treatment would be removal of the allergen, but this usually is impossible when the conjunctivitis is secondary to seasonal allergies. Topical corticosteroids provide dramatic relief, but their use must be limited because of potential adverse effects (see Ophthalmic Corticosteroids section).

Cromolyn sodium ophthalmic, a drug that inhibits the release of histamine in response to antigen, may be effective as an alternative for patients who fail to respond to more conservative measures. Lodoxamide, pemirolast, and nedocromil have a similar mechanism of action to cromolyn sodium ophthalmic, but these agents also decrease chemotaxis and activation of eosinophils. In comparative studies, lodoxamide tromethamine 0.1% is at least as effective as cromolyn sodium ophthalmic 2% to 4% in treating allergic ocular disorders, including vernal keratoconjunctivitis.[123,124] Patients in these studies demonstrated more rapid and greater response when treated with lodoxamide, one drop QID. In a 2-week crossover study of nedocromil and olopatadine involving 28 patients of 7 years of age and older, patient acceptance of nedocromil BID was better than for olopatadine BID, but treatment outcomes were essentially equal.[124,125]

Corneal Ulcers

CASE 54-7

QUESTION 1: T.S. presents with a diagnosis of bacterial corneal ulcer in the right eye and prescriptions for "fortified gentamicin" and cefazolin eyedrops, which are not commercially available. What is the rationale for this therapy, and how can the patient obtain it?

The initial choice of therapy for bacterial corneal ulcers commonly is based on a Gram stain and clinical impression of the severity of the ulcer. Single or combination antimicrobial therapy can be prescribed. Although commercial antimicrobial ophthalmic formulations are available, the antimicrobial concentrations in these products might be inadequate to effectively treat bacterial corneal ulcers.[126,127]

Topical antimicrobials for the treatment of bacterial corneal ulcers can be prepared from parenteral antimicrobials or by the addition of parenteral antimicrobials to "fortify" commercially available products. Commonly prescribed products include bacitracin 5,000 to 10,000 units/mL, cefazolin 33 to 100 mg/mL, gentamicin or tobramycin 9.1 to 13.6 mg/mL, and vancomycin 25 to 50 mg/mL. Fortified gentamicin has been prepared by adding 80 mg of parenteral gentamicin to the commercially available gentamicin ophthalmic solution. The final concentration of this solution is 13.6 mg/mL. Cefazolin ophthalmic solution is prepared by reconstituting 500 mg parenteral cefazolin with 2 mL of sterile normal saline. Two milliliters of artificial tears solution are removed from a commercially available 15-mL bottle and replaced with the 2-mL reconstituted cefazolin solution (resulting in a final cefazolin concentration of 33 mg/mL). Therapy initially can be administered as frequently as every 15 to 30 minutes with extension of intervals as the ulcer resolves.[128] The preparation of extemporaneously compounded ophthalmic products must adhere to established federal and state agency guidelines, and must address quality control concerns (e.g., pH, tonicity, sterility, particulate matter). The formulation of sterile products should not be undertaken without due consideration of well-established practice standards. In most situations, these products are prepared within a laminar flow hood.

OPHTHALMIC CORTICOSTEROIDS

Comparison of Preparations and Clinical Use

CASE 54-8

QUESTION 1: S.S. has undergone cataract extraction from his left eye. Prednisolone acetate 1% administered 4 times daily has been prescribed. Is prednisolone acetate an appropriate choice?

The topical ophthalmic corticosteroid preparations are described in Table 54-4. The salt form affects the ability of the preparation to penetrate the cornea. For example, biphasic salts penetrate

Table 54-4
Ophthalmic Corticosteroids

Low Potency	Intermediate Potency	High Potency
Dexamethasone 0.05% (Decadron Phosphate)	Clobetasone 0.1%[a]	Clobetasone 0.5%[a]
Dexamethasone 0.1% (Decadron Phosphate)	Dexamethasone alcohol 0.1% (Maxidex)	Fluorometholone acetate 0.1% (Flarex)
Medrysone 1% (HMS)	Fluorometholone 0.1% (FML) Fluorometholone 0.25% (FML Forte) Loteprednol 0.2% (Lotemax) Loteprednol 0.5% (Alrex) Prednisolone acetate 0.12% (Pred Mild) Prednisolone sodium phosphate 0.125% (Inflamase Mild) Prednisolone sodium phosphate 1% (Inflamase Forte)	Prednisolone acetate 1% (Pred Forte) Rimexolone 1% (Vexol)

[a]Not commercially available in the United States.

the intact cornea better than water-soluble salts. The ability of a formulation to penetrate the cornea, however, does not indicate increased therapeutic effectiveness. Prednisolone acetate 1% and fluorometholone acetate 0.1% have the best anti-inflammatory effects.[129–131] The most commonly prescribed ophthalmic corticosteroid is prednisolone acetate because of its availability in generic form and generally lower cost.

Topical ophthalmic corticosteroids are used for a variety of conditions associated with inflammation of the conjunctiva, cornea, and within the anterior segment of the eye. They are generally contraindicated in individuals with ocular varicella, vaccinia, herpes simplex, and mycobacterial infections.

Adverse Effects

INCREASED INTRAOCULAR PRESSURE

CASE 54-8, QUESTION 2: S.S. continued using topical prednisolone acetate 1%, one drop in the left eye QID for 8 weeks. Before therapy, the IOPs in both eyes were 16 mm Hg, but on the last follow-up visit, his IOP was 16 mm Hg in the right eye and 26 mm Hg in the left eye. Assess these observations.

S.S.'s elevated IOP could be related to topical steroid therapy. In one study, the ophthalmic administration of corticosteroid preparations (Table 54-5) increased IOP in three genetically distinct subgroups.[104,105,132] Fluorometholone acetate increased IOP by more than 10 mm Hg in known steroid responders in 29.5 days (median), whereas dexamethasone did the same in 22.7 days (median).[133] In a retrospective follow-up, 13% of high-corticosteroid responders developed POAG and 63.8% developed ocular hypertension. No low responders developed POAG, and only 2.4% developed ocular hypertension.[133] Although corticosteroid-induced increases in IOP are associated most frequently with topical ophthalmic preparations, systemic corticosteroids may cause a similar response, although the magnitude is somewhat less.[134] The risk for corticosteroid-induced ocular hypertension is greater in patients with high myopia, diabetes mellitus, or connective tissue disease (particularly rheumatoid arthritis).

Topical corticosteroids exert their effects by decreasing aqueous humor outflow, whereas systemic corticosteroids may increase aqueous humor production.[134] The effects on IOP apparently are unrelated to the ability of the corticosteroid to penetrate the cornea. Dexamethasone has been associated with the greatest IOP increase.[135] Fluorometholone, medrysone, rimexolone, and loteprednol have been associated with lower, although sometimes significant, increases in IOP.[136–138] The pressure response often is reversible when the offending agent is discontinued. In subjects with prolonged IOP elevation, glaucomatous field defects are more likely to develop in corticosteroid-responsive patients.[139]

CATARACTS

CASE 54-9

QUESTION 1: G.A., who had asthma, has been taking prednisone 10 mg/day for 1 year. A routine ophthalmic examination revealed early cataract formation. Why could this be related to the prednisone?

Systemic and topical ophthalmic corticosteroids have been associated with the development of cataracts. About 23% of patients treated with 10 to 16 mg/day of prednisone orally (or its equivalent dose) for 1 year or more developed posterior subcapsular cataracts (PSC).[140,141] The estimated occurrence of PSC in patients treated with more than 16 mg/day of prednisone for more than a year increased to more than 70% during the same

Table 54-5
Intraocular Pressure Response to Topical Steroids in Random Populations

Author	Parameter of Response	No. of Subjects	Low	Medium	High	Mean
Armaly[105]	Increase of pressure in eye medicated with 0.1% dexamethasone	80	<5 mm Hg 66%	6–15 mm Hg 29%	16 mm Hg 5%	5.5 mm Hg
Becker et al.[132]	Final pressure in eye medicated for 6 weeks with 0.1% betamethasone	50	<19 mm Hg 70%	20–30 mm Hg 26%	32 mm Hg 4%	17.0 mm Hg
	Time to maximal response		2 weeks	4 weeks	4 weeks	

period. Patients receiving less than 10 mg/day prednisone or its equivalent are unlikely to develop PSC, although some contend that the concept of a "safe" dosage should be abandoned because of variable patient sensitivity to this side effect.[142] As illustrated by G.A., the cataracts cause few subjective complaints and little measurable decrease in visual acuity. Although systemic corticosteroids primarily are implicated, use of topical corticosteroids also has been associated with PSC formation.[143] Patients treated with alternate-day dosing of oral corticosteroids may be at lower risk for PSC formation.[144] Any patient receiving long-term corticosteroids should receive routine ophthalmic follow-up.

SYSTEMIC SIDE EFFECTS FROM OPHTHALMIC MEDICATION

CASE 54-10

QUESTION 1: J.F., a 62-year-old woman, received one drop of phenylephrine 10% in each eye to dilate the pupils. Shortly after administration, her blood pressure increased to 210/130 mm Hg for 5 minutes, and she became confused. How common is this type of reaction in patients receiving topical phenylephrine? What other topical ophthalmic medications have been associated with systemic effects?

In 33 cases, possible adverse effects have been associated with topical phenylephrine 10%.[145] In a double-blind study, no statistically significant differences were observed in blood pressure or pulse rate between experimental and control groups when phenylephrine 10% or tropicamide (Mydriacyl) 1% was administered to 150 patients.[146] Nevertheless, care should be taken when phenylephrine 10% is administered in patients with hypertension or cardiac abnormalities in whom systemic absorption could be hazardous. No similar reports have been associated with topical use of phenylephrine 2.5%.

In addition to the systemic effects from topical administration of cholinergic agents, epinephrine, and timolol that were previously described, topical atropine, cyclopentolate (Cyclogyl), and scopolamine have been associated with psychosis.[147–149] Fatalities have been associated with topical atropine,[150] ataxia has occurred with topical homatropine, and one case of unconsciousness with tropicamide was reported.[151]

Topical chloramphenicol-polymyxin-B sulfate ophthalmic ointment has been associated with bone marrow aplasia after intermittent use for 4 months.[152] A cushingoid reaction has been reported in a 30-month-old baby girl treated with dexamethasone alcohol (Maxidex) 4 times a day in both eyes for 14 months.[153]

The administration of ophthalmic prostaglandins and PGAs are associated with systemic side effects (Table 54-1).

OCULAR NONSTEROIDAL ANTI-INFLAMMATORY DRUGS

CASE 54-11

QUESTION 1: W.A. is scheduled to undergo cataract extraction with implantation of an intraocular lens. Preoperative orders include administration of flurbiprofen 0.03% to inhibit intraoperative miosis. The formulary includes only diclofenac 0.1%. Is this a suitable alternative to flurbiprofen?

Commercially available ophthalmic nonsteroidal anti-inflammatory drugs (e.g., bromfenac, diclofenac, flurbiprofen, ketorolac and nepafenac) share a similar mechanism of action involving inhibition of prostaglandin synthesis and reduction of prostaglandin-mediated ocular effects.[154] Minor clinical differences, which probably are insignificant, exist and approved indications differ (Table 54-6).[155–162] These agents are generally well tolerated, but they can cause transient burning and stinging on instillation. Diclofenac is not approved for prevention of intraoperative miosis, but various dosage regimens have been reported as effective for this use.

OCULAR HERPES SIMPLEX VIRUS INFECTIONS

CASE 54-12

QUESTION 1: P.B., a 34-year-old man, presents with a 2-week history of a red, irritated left eye with watery discharge. Recently, vision in his left eye became blurred, and he complained of light sensitivity. A slit-lamp examination with rose bengal stain revealed a multibranched corneal epithelial defect. This dendritic ulcer is the hallmark of ocular herpes simplex (type 1) infection. What is the therapy of choice for P.B.?

Ocular herpes is common and can be caused by herpes simplex virus or, less commonly, by the varicella-zoster virus (herpes zoster ophthalmicus). Herpes simplex of the eye typically affects the eyelids, conjunctiva, and cornea, and patients often present with symptoms of pain, tearing, eye redness, sensitivity to light, and irritation or a foreign body sensation. When herpes affects the epithelium of the cornea (herpes keratitis), it generally heals without scarring. Occasionally, deeper layers of the cornea are affected (stromal keratitis), and scarring can lead to blindness. Trifluridine is the drug of choice for P.B.

TRIFLURIDINE

In vitro, the mechanism of action of trifluridine is similar to that of idoxuridine (IDU). Trifluridine also inhibits thymidylate synthase, an enzyme required for DNA synthesis.

For the treatment of ocular herpes, one drop of trifluridine 1% ophthalmic solution should be instilled into the affected eye every 2 hours while awake with a maximal daily dose of nine drops. After re-epithelialization, application of trifluridine should be continued for an additional 7 days at a reduced dosage of one drop every 4 hours while awake with a minimum of five drops daily. Continuous administration for periods exceeding 21 days is not recommended because of potential ocular toxicity.

Approximately 96% of treated herpetic corneal ulcers heal within 2 weeks.[163] Therapeutic levels of trifluridine can be found in the aqueous humor after topical administration of a 1% solution, enhancing its possible effectiveness in the treatment of stromal keratitis and uveitis. Trifluridine also is effective in treating herpes simplex virus infections resistant to IDU or vidarabine.

Despite the apparent superiority of trifluridine compared with its antiviral predecessors (IDU, vidarabine), it is not without disadvantages. Trifluridine is activated by uninfected corneal cells and is incorporated into cellular as well as viral DNA. Punctate lesions in the corneal epithelium are clinical manifestations of trifluridine cytotoxicity.[164] However, these effects seem to occur less often with trifluridine than with IDU and vidarabine.

ACYCLOVIR

Acyclovir in in vitro plaque inhibition assays has 5 to 10 times the activity of IDU and trifluridine and more than 100 times

Table 54-6
Ocular Nonsteroidal Anti-Inflammatory Drugs

Indication	Drug/Approval Status for Indication	Dosage(s)
Inhibition of intraoperative miosis	Diclofenac 0.1% (Voltaren, U)[155]	Three reported regimens; 1 drop every 15–30 minutes for four doses; 1 drop TID for 2 preoperative days; 1 drop at 2 hours, 1 hour, and 15 minutes before surgery
	Flurbiprofen 0.03% (Ocufen, A)[156]	One drop every 30 minutes for 2 hours before surgery
	Ketorolac 0.5% (Acular, U)	One drop every 15 minutes beginning 1 hour before surgery
Anti-inflammatory after cataract surgery	Bromfenac 0.09% (Xibrom, A)	One drop BID beginning 24 hours after surgery and continuing through the 2 weeks of the postoperative period
	Diclofenac 0.1% (A)[157] Nepavanac 0.1% (Nevanac, A)	One drop BID to QID, including 24 hours preoperative administration. One drop TID beginning 1 day before cataract surgery, continued on the day of surgery and through the first 2 weeks of the postoperative period (Nevanac prescribing information. Alcon Laboratories, November 2006)
	Ketorolac 0.5% (A)[158]	One drop TID, including 24 hours preoperative administration
Prevention/treatment of cystoid macular edema	Diclofenac 0.1% (U)[159]	Two drops 5 times preoperatively followed by one drop 3–5 times daily
	Ketorolac 0.5% (U)[158,160]	One drop TID or QID, including 24 hours preoperative administration
Ocular inflammatory conditions (iritis, iridocyclitis, episcleritis)	Diclofenac 0.1% (U)	One drop QID
Seasonal allergic/vernal conjunctivitis	Bromfenac 0.1% (U)	One drop BID
	Diclofenac 0.1% (U)	One drop every 2 hours for 48 hours; then QID
	Ketorolac 0.5% (A)[161,162]	One drop QID

A, approved use; BID, twice daily; QID, 4 times a day; TID, 3 times a day; U, unapproved use.

the activity of vidarabine against strains of type 1 and type 2 herpes simplex virus.[165] Acyclovir's apparent superiority lies in its lack of toxicity to normal host cells. In rabbits (rabbit eyes are similar to human eyes), acyclovir 3% ointment healed established herpes simplex epithelial ulcerations at a faster rate and eliminated the virus more effectively than 0.5% IDU and 3% vidarabine ointments.[166] In humans, ulcerative corneal epithelial lesions appear to respond similarly to acyclovir and IDU.[166] In comparison with IDU, the topical application of acyclovir or trifluridine resulted in a greater proportion of subjects healing within 1 week and neither was superior for the treatment of dendritic epithelial keratosis.[167] The dose usually is a 1-cm ribbon of ointment instilled 5 times a day at 4-hour intervals for 14 days or for at least 3 days after healing is completed, whichever is shorter. Detailed dosing instructions are available in product literature of specific manufacturers, and brief reviews of acyclovir and acyclovir resistance are presented in 77, Opportunistic Infections in HIV-Infected Patients, and Chapter 79, Viral Infections.

OTHER DRUGS

Ganciclovir 0.05% and 0.15% gel have been shown to be equivalent to 3% acyclovir ointment in the treatment of superficial herpes simplex keratitis.[168] Cidofovir 1% ointment administered BID was equivalent to trifluridine administered 5 times daily in the rabbit model.[169] Cidofovir was more efficacious than 3% penciclovir ointment administered 2 or 4 times a day.[169]

AGE-RELATED MACULAR DEGENERATION

CASE 54-13

QUESTION 1: E.A., a 77-year-old woman, informs you she read information from the Internet and she thinks her symptoms of blurred vision and the need for a bright light to read are consistent with age-related macular degeneration. She asks which of the available medicines would be best for her.

Age-related macular degeneration is the leading cause of blindness in Americans of European descent who are 55 years of age and older.[170] There are two forms of macular degeneration, wet and dry. The dry form, affecting about 85% of patients, develops as a result of the breakdown of light-sensitive cells in the macula.[171] The most common symptom associated with dry macular degeneration is blurred vision. In this situation, details (e.g., faces, words in a book) are seen less clearly. Wet macular degeneration occurs in 15% of patients and is the more serious form, responsible for the most cases of vision loss. One of the first symptoms of wet macular degeneration is the appearance of straight lines as wavy. Wet macular degeneration is associated with abnormal growth of blood vessels behind the retina, known as choroidal neovascularization. Vascular endothelial growth factor (VEGF) is associated with the pathogenesis of choroidal neovascularization. VEGF may stimulate neovascularization by influencing endothelial cell proliferation, vascular permeability, and ocular inflammation.[172] The correlation between VEGF and wet age-related macular degeneration has led to interest in VEGF inhibitors (pegaptanib, bevacizumab, ranibizumab) as treatment agents.

PEGAPTANIB

Pegaptanib inhibits angiogenesis, decreases permeability of the vascular bed, and decreases inflammation. The efficacy of pegaptanib has been evaluated in two concurrent, prospective, randomized, double-blind trials involving 1,208 patients. A total of 1,190 patients received at least one study treatment, with four subjects being excluded from the efficacy analysis owing to insufficient assessment of visual acuity at baseline. A combined analysis of 1,186 patients at week 54 showed a statistically significant reduction in vision loss associated with pegaptanib, realized as early as week 6 and continued through week 54.[173] The FDA-approved dose of pegaptanib (0.3 mg intravenously every 6 weeks) is no less effective than 1- or 3-mg doses, and the most serious injection-related adverse events were endophthalmitis (12 patients), traumatic injury to the lens (five patients), and retinal detachment (six patients).[173] Patients should be monitored for elevations in IOP after injection; increases in IOP have been seen within 30 minutes of injection and should be monitored within 2 to 7 days after the injection.

BEVACIZUMAB

Bevacizumab is a recombinant humanized monoclonal immunoglobulin G1 antibody approved for intravenous use for first- or second-line treatment of metastatic colorectal cancer. This product has been used off-label via the intravenous and intravitreal routes for the treatment of neovascular ocular disorders in more than 3,500 patients.[172] Intravenous bevacizumab 5 mg/kg was administered every 2 weeks for two or three infusions in 18 patients for whom 12- and 24-week results on subfoveal choroidal neovascularization were published separately. Therapy was associated with improved visual acuity. No serious ocular or systemic adverse effects were noted, although a statistically significant increase in blood pressure was noted at week 3. Nineteen published, uncontrolled case series studies have evaluated the use of intravitreal bevacizumab for the treatment of wet macular degeneration as well as other conditions associated with neovascularization. The most common intravitreal dose was 1.25 mg, usually administered every 4 to 6 weeks. Doses could be repeated if signs of progression occurred. The longest period of study for intravitreal use was 1 year. The majority of patients in these open-label trials were followed up for 3 months. Mean visual acuity improved, and no serious ocular effects were noted.

RANIBIZUMAB

Ranibizumab is a Fab fragment of bevacizumab approved in June 2006 for the intravitreal treatment of wet macular degeneration. Ranibizumab is approximately one-third the size of bevacizumab. Its size may facilitate retinal penetration after intravitreal injection. Ranibizumab has a shorter-systemic half-life and higher VEGF binding affinity than bevacizumab, but bevacizumab has two binding sites per molecule versus one for ranibizumab. The clinical relevance of these pharmacokinetic and pharmacodynamic differences is not known.[172] The recommended dosage of ranibizumab is 0.5 mg via the intravitreal route administered every 4 weeks. This treatment has been associated with maintenance or improvement of vision for 12 to 24 months.[173] The primary ocular side effects associated with ranibizumab administration include conjunctival hemorrhage, eye pain, and increased IOP.

Bevacizumab is significantly less expensive than ranibizumab. Similar efficacy associated with lower cost may lead to increased use for neovascular age-related macular degeneration. The National Eye Institute has initiated the Comparisons of Age-Related Macular Degeneration Treatments Trials, a multicenter, randomized clinical trial of ranibizumab and bevacizumab in the treatment of neovascular age-related macular degeneration.[174]

AFLIBERCEPT

In September 2012, aflibercept became the second VEGF inhibitor approved for treatment of macular edema secondary to choroidal vein retinal occlusion (CRVO). Preliminary results from the ongoing COPERNICUS and GALILEO trials proved the efficacy of this medication in treating macular edema secondary to CRVO. Of the combined 358 patients studied in COPERNICUS and GALILEO, 56% and 60%, respectively, of the patients receiving aflibercept 2 mg monthly achieved at least a 15-letter improvement in best-corrected visual acuity (BCVA) from baseline over 6 months compared with just 12% and 22% in the control group ($p < 0.01$ for both). Additionally, in COPERNICUS and GALILEO, patients achieved a 21.3- and 14.7-letter improvement, respectively, in BCVA compared with placebo ($p < 0.01$ for both).[175]

While efficacy and safety appear similar to other anti-VEGF treatments, the higher potency, binding affinity, and duration of action make aflibercept an appealing new option.

KEY REFERENCES AND WEBSITES

A full list of references for this chapter can be found at http://thepoint.lww.com/AT11e. Below are the key reference and websites for this chapter, with the corresponding reference number in this chapter found in parentheses after the reference.

Key References

Riordan-Eva P, Whitcher JP, eds. *Vaughan and Ashbury's General Ophthalmology*. 18th ed. New York, NY: McGraw-Hill Professional; 2011. (1)

Key Websites

American Academy of Ophthalmology. Primary open-angle glaucoma, preferred practice pattern. San Francisco, CA: American Academy of Ophthalmology; 2010. http://www.aao.org/ppp. Accessed June 2015. (5)

Section Editors: Michele Matthews and Timothy E. Welty

55 Pain and Its Management

Lee A. Kral and Virginia L. Ghafoor

CORE PRINCIPLES

		CHAPTER CASES
1	Perioperative analgesia utilizes nerve blocks via peripheral or spinal local anesthetic delivery. A preoperative pain assessment may identify a history of uncontrolled postsurgical pain, analgesic intolerance or contraindication, risks and benefits of regional anesthesia, and presence of preoperative pain or anxiety.	**Case 55-1 (Questions 1–3)**
2	Multimodal analgesia is a strategy that utilizes a combination of different analgesic modalities to achieve better postoperative pain management and a subsequent reduction in adverse effects. The additive and synergistic effects between different classes of analgesics allow for a reduction in the doses of individual medications while achieving similar or better pain control.	**Case 55-2 (Questions 1–3)**
3	Low back pain is a very common chronic pain condition. It is complex, often involving physical and emotional factors. Patients may have musculoskeletal, neuropathic, and/or central pain that needs to be assessed, as well as comorbidities.	**Case 55-3 (Questions 1, 2)**
4	Chronic pain management requires multimodal therapies, both pharmacologic and nonpharmacologic. Many factors affect analgesic selection, including comorbidities, available routes of administration, and cost.	**Case 55-3 (Questions 3–7)**
5	Neuropathic pain may be caused by injury to peripheral nerves or to the central nervous system. Neuropathic pain is treated with analgesic antidepressants and anticonvulsants. Peripheral or localized nerve pain may be treated with topical agents.	**Case 55-4 (Questions 1, 2)**
6	Elderly patients and patients with multiple comorbidities are at high risk for adverse effects. Pharmacokinetic and pharmacodynamic drug interactions must be considered with the use of anticonvulsants and antidepressants.	**Case 55-4 (Questions 3, 4)**
7	Central neuropathic pain may present with peripheral symptoms that are localized or generalized. Pharmacotherapy provides only modest relief. Central poststroke pain is commonly multifactorial, including neuropathic pain and nociceptive pain. Central pain may respond to traditional neuropathic pain therapies. NSAIDs are ineffective. Comorbidities and drug interactions must be considered.	**Case 55-5 (Questions 1, 2)**
8	Functional pain does not have a clear pathophysiology. Comorbid mental health issues and psychosocial stressors complicate chronic pain management. Analgesic antidepressants and anticonvulsants, in conjunction with cognitive behavioral therapies, are recommended for management of functional pain syndromes (FPSs).	**Case 55-6 (Questions 1, 2)**
9	Opioid therapy requires effective risk assessment to avoid medication abuse, misuse, and diversion. Monitoring recommendations should include use of written opioid agreements, urine drug testing, opioid risk screening tools, and electronic prescription monitoring program records.	**Case 55-7 (Questions 1–6)**
10	Cancer pain may result from one or more causes related to direct tumor involvement, cancer therapy, and psychological factors. Pain management involves assessment of the patient to determine the etiology of pain and development of a care plan to address pain and other symptom management.	**Case 55-8 (Question 1)**

Continued

11	Transdermal fentanyl and methadone are potent opioids commonly used in cancer pain management. Opioid conversion tables for fentanyl and methadone are different due to differences in pharmacokinetics. Supplemental doses of short-acting opioids are recommended for breakthrough pain management.	**Case 55-8 (Questions 2–5)**
12	Opioid adverse effects including sedation, constipation, nausea, vomiting, itching, and respiratory depression should be addressed in the pain management plan. Complementary and alternative medicine therapies are widely used by patients in the management of cancer pain, dyspnea, and nausea and vomiting. Neuraxial opioid administration may be appropriate for patients with intolerable pain who cannot tolerate systemic opioid therapy.	**Case 55-8 (Questions 6–9)**

INCIDENCE, PREVALENCE, AND EPIDEMIOLOGY

Pain is defined as "an unpleasant sensory and emotional experience associated with actual or potential tissue damage or described in terms of such damage."[1] The ability to experience pain is critical for survival because it informs the body of real or potential injury (e.g., touching a hot stove). The body is then able to respond to the threat and protect itself from further injury (e.g., refraining from touching or removing the hand from the hot stove). Pain is a hallmark of many acute and chronic conditions. More than 80% of patients who undergo surgical procedures experience acute pain, 75% of which report the severity as moderate, severe, or extreme.[2,3] Chronic pain affects more than 25% of Americans over the age of 20 years.[4] Many people think that pain is a natural part of growing older, and up to 60% of people believe that pain is just something you have to live with.[5] However, nearly all cases of chronic pain begin as acute pain stemming from surgery, trauma, or illness.[6] The Institute of Medicine in 2011 estimated that $635 billion is spent annually on treatment of chronic pain conditions alone.[7] Back pain and osteoarthritis (OA) are among the top 5 chronic pain conditions associated with high healthcare costs and the prevalence continues to rise with the aging U.S. population. A study of Humana insurance utilization data for Medicare members from 2007 to 2011 found that annual costs were $327 million for OA and $218 million for back pain.[8] There are also gender, racial, and socioeconomic disparities that exist with chronic pain. Chronic pain is reported more often in women than in men, and in non-Hispanic white patients compared with other races and ethnicities.[4] Chronic pain is also more common in those whose income is 2 times less than the level of poverty.

Pain is more complex than just physiology. It is a subjective experience, and sometimes the severity of pain does not appear to equal the extent of tissue damage. A person's perception of pain is affected by environmental, emotional, cultural, spiritual, and cognitive factors. Unrelieved chronic pain affects not only physical well-being but also a person's psychological and social well-being and relationships with loved ones. Recent estimates showed that musculoskeletal-related conditions with low back pain, neck pain, and knee OA ranked within the top 10 noncommunicable diseases for global disability-adjusted life years (i.e., years of life lost and years lived in disability).[9,10]

Factors that increase pain and suffering include sensory factors, cognitive factors, and emotional factors (Fig. 55-1). All are interrelated and illustrate the complex nature of chronic pain.

Pathophysiology

ASCENDING PATHWAY

Nociception, or the sensation of pain, is composed of four basic processes: transduction, transmission, modulation, and perception (Fig. 55-2). *Transduction* is the process by which noxious stimuli are translated into electrical signals at peripheral receptor sites (i.e., free nerve endings located throughout the skin, muscle, joints, fascia, and viscera). Normal sensory stimuli do not activate the pain signal, but if the stimulus is powerful enough to surpass the threshold for innocuous activation, the receptors become *nociceptors* (i.e., pain receptors). These sensory receptors target mechanical (crushing or pressure), chemical (endogenous or exogenous), or thermal (hot or cold) stimuli. Some nociceptors are polymodal, transducing more than one type of stimuli. One of these types of nociceptors is called the transient receptor potential (TRP). This family has a large number of members that are activated by

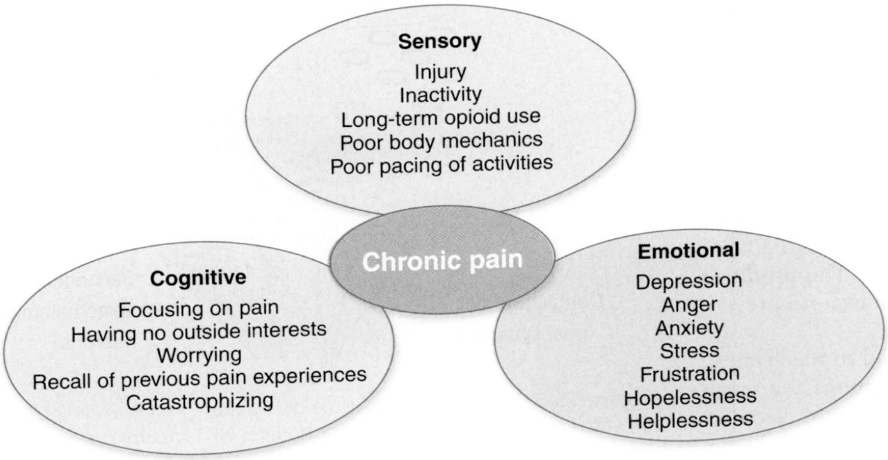

Figure 55-1 Factors affecting chronic pain.

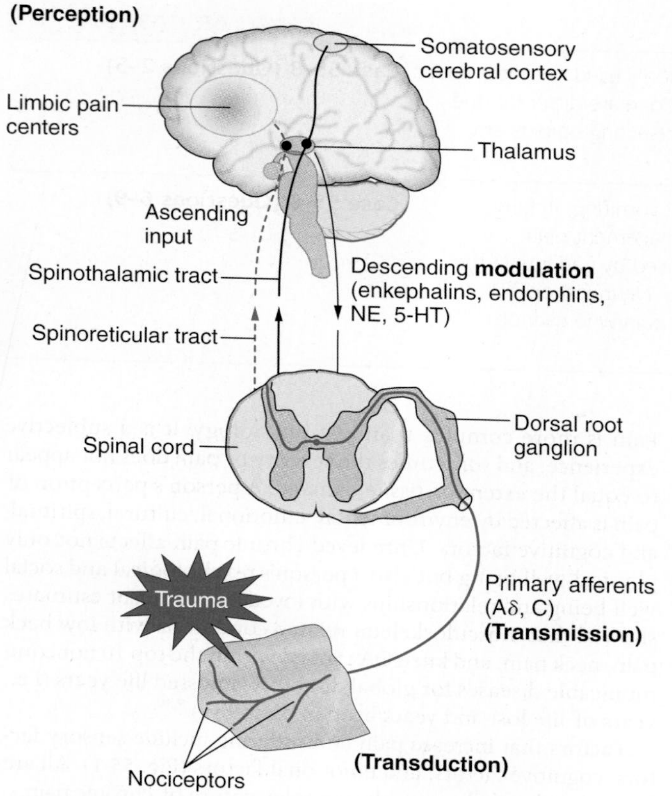

Figure 55-2 Pain pathways. 5-HT, serotonin; NE, norepinephrine.

the whole spectrum of thermal stimuli (very hot to very cold), as well as some mechanical and various chemical stimuli. Other receptors are "silent," but are recruited if the stimulus is more intense or prolonged.

After stimulation of nociceptors, several processes occur. Proinflammatory mediators, including histamine, substance P, prostaglandins, bradykinins, and serotonin are released at the site of injury. Immune mediators are also released, including tumor necrosis factor, nerve growth factors, interleukins, and interferons. These mediators sensitize the nociceptors, lowering the pain threshold in and around the injury (peripheral sensitization). The sensitized nociceptors may fire more frequently and erratically and are stimulated by much weaker stimuli (hyperalgesia). More frequent firing is correlated with an increase in pain intensity.

Transmission is the propagation of the electrical signal along primary afferent nerves, through the dorsal horn of the spinal cord to the central nervous system (CNS). Painful impulses are generated at the nociceptor, with voltage-gated sodium channels initiating the action potentials. Voltage-gated calcium channels are responsible for allowing calcium influx to the presynaptic terminal, causing neurotransmitter release. The message is then transmitted to the spinal cord via two primary afferent nerve types: myelinated A fibers and unmyelinated C fibers. The Aδ fibers are responsible for rapidly conducting impulses associated with thermal and mechanical stimuli. Transmission of signals along Aδ fibers results in sharp or stabbing sensations that alert the patient to an injury (also called "first pain"). This produces reflex signals, such as musculoskeletal withdrawal, to prevent further injury.

The smaller, unmyelinated C fibers respond to mechanical, thermal, and chemical stimuli but conduct impulses at a much slower rate compared with Aδ fibers. Transmission of electrical impulses via C fibers results in pain that is dull, aching, burning, and diffuse (called "second pain"). Prolonged stimulation of C fibers causes an additive effect on the perceived intensity of second pain, called *windup*.

At the level of the dorsal horn of the spinal cord, the primary afferents cause calcium release into the presynaptic terminal. This leads to release of excitatory amino acids (EAAs) like glutamate into the synapse (Fig. 55-3). C fibers also release peptides such as substance P, neurokinins, and calcitonin gene-related peptide (CGRP). The EAAs then stimulate the postsynaptic receptors and the electrical signals stimulate second-order neurons in the CNS. The postsynaptic α-amino-3-hydroxy-5-methyl-4-isoxazoleproprionate (AMPA) receptors are sodium channel-mediated and are responsible for the first pain mentioned previously. *N*-methyl-D-aspartate (NMDA) receptor channels allow both sodium and calcium passage. Usually a magnesium ion holds the channels closed; however, when there is sustained firing from the primary afferents, the magnesium ion is displaced and the NMDA receptor is activated. This sensitizes the second-order neurons that will then discharge at a higher frequency. When sensitization occurs, the firing threshold is reduced, so even slightly painful stimuli (hyperalgesia) and nonpainful stimuli (allodynia) cause sustained activation of second-order neurons. NMDA receptor activation is linked to *windup* and *central sensitization* (i.e., decreased thresholds for response or increased vigor of responses after a sensitizing event) and may contribute to the maintenance of chronic pain conditions with processes occurring both at the dorsal horn level and in the supraspinal areas. Central sensitization may occur with all types of pain when prolonged primary afferent activation causes *plasticity* (adaptation) of the pain sensory thresholds in the CNS.[11]

One of the predominant contributors to pain propagation at the synapse and within the CNS is the glial cell. In the periphery, these are Schwann cells and satellite cells. In the CNS, these include oligodendrocytes, astrocytes, ependymal cells, and microglia. Glial cells account for 70% of the CNS and under normal conditions microglia account for 5% to 20% of glia.[12] The glial cells have historically been seen as support cells for synaptic homeostasis. This is true; however, they also have an important role in the synthesis, release, and uptake of neurotransmitters and serve

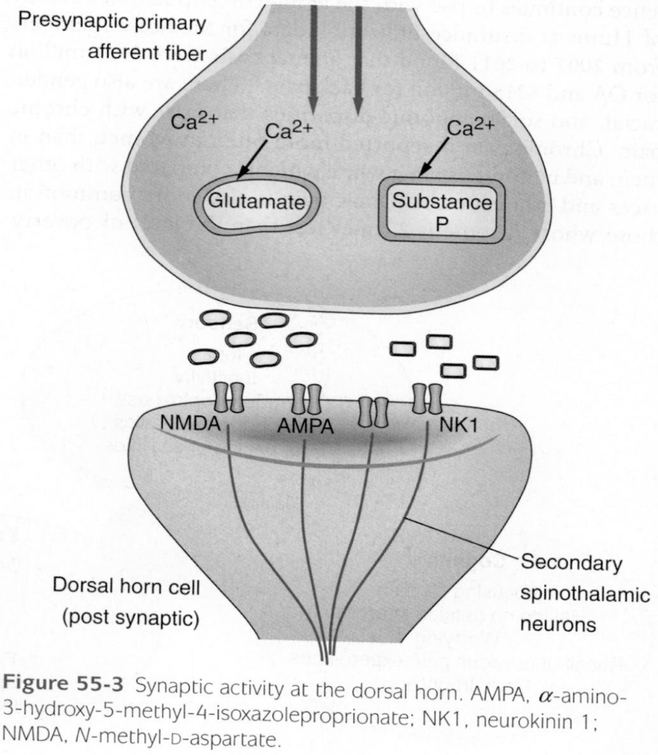

Figure 55-3 Synaptic activity at the dorsal horn. AMPA, α-amino-3-hydroxy-5-methyl-4-isoxazoleproprionate; NK1, neurokinin 1; NMDA, *N*-methyl-D-aspartate.

as a link between the nervous system and the immune system. Nerve damage due to trauma, infection, drugs, or toxins exposes peripheral nerve proteins, and they are seen by the immune system as "nonself," initiating an immune reaction. Glial cells are activated, causing release of cytokines and inflammatory mediators which contribute to peripheral sensitization, increasing nociceptor sensitivity, and lowering of the firing threshold. Continuous nociceptive input results in high levels of glutamate within synapses. In the setting of chronic pain, glial cells swell (called gliosis) and an increase in cell surface markers is seen. The more persistent the stimulus, the more they swell and release inflammatory mediators. This contributes to the development and maintenance of central sensitization.[13] Glial cells and NMDA receptors may also be activated by medications such as opioids. This is thought to contribute to opioid tolerance, dependence, addiction, and a phenomenon called *opioid-induced hyperalgesia* (OIH).[14]

Visceral pain is very complex. It follows somatosensory pathways and also its own systems. Aδ and C fibers have been found in the heart, pleura, abdominal cavity, gallbladder, and testicles. Additionally, the intestinal tract has its own neuronal system called the "brain–gut axis" that operates independently and in conjunction with the rest of the CNS.[15] Like the somatosensory pathways, peripheral and central sensitization occurs with chronic visceral pain. Activation of the autonomic nervous system may also affect visceral sensitivity and the role of emotions in modulating visceral pain. Visceral pain may be referred to areas of the somatosensory system (e.g., myocardial ischemia causes left arm pain), leading to a complex presentation of an individual's pain.[15,16]

SUPRASPINAL MODULATION AND THE DESCENDING PATHWAY

Once nociceptive signals reach the CNS (typically at the spinal cord level), they ascend to the thalamus, primarily via the spinothalamic tract. From the thalamus, tertiary neurons project to many structures in the brain, including the brainstem, diencephalon (includes the thalamus), primary and secondary somatosensory cortices, and frontolimbic area. The somatosensory cortex is where the brain interprets the qualities of pain such as location, duration, and intensity. Tertiary neurons also project to the limbic system, which is involved in the affective or emotional component of pain. *Perception* is when the sensory (physical) and affective (psychological) components of the nociceptive message are integrated into the patient's overall experience. An individual does not experience pain until the brain has processed and interpreted the electrical nociceptive signal.

A second tract, called the spinoreticular tract, ascends to the thalamus, but also branches off at the brainstem to stimulate descending modulation. *Modulation* happens throughout the CNS and results in either an increase or a decrease in transmission. Neurons from the thalamus and brainstem release inhibitory neurotransmitters, such as norepinephrine (NE), serotonin (5-HT), γ-aminobutyric acid (GABA), glycine, endorphins, and enkephalins, which inhibit EAA activity in the ascending pathway. GABA is more active at supraspinal sites, and glycine is more active at spinal sites. The GABA-A receptor is a binding site for benzodiazepines and barbiturates, and the GABA-B receptor is a binding site for baclofen, causing muscle relaxation. Glycine has both pronociceptive and antinociceptive effects, depending on the receptor. Endogenous opioids (endorphins, enkephalins) are the most common group of inhibitory peptides, inhibiting EAA release from the presynaptic terminals and activation of second-order neurons in the postsynaptic terminals. Opioids also enhance the descending pathway via release of NE and 5-HT. In fact, activation of most of the supraspinal structures results in enhancement of NE and 5-HT effects.

Diagnosis and Clinical Presentation

Pain is a symptom and a reactionary response to real or potential bodily harm, but it is not currently defined as a specific disease state. It also cannot be measured objectively. It is a symptom that relies on a patient's subjective report and any physical findings indicative of underlying pathology. Healthcare teams take on the task of identifying the cause of the pain using everything from noninvasive imaging such as magnetic resonance imaging to invasive testing such as electromyelograms and spinal discography.

Pain can be classified in many ways. Some conditions are classified as syndromes because the patient presents with a constellation of symptoms that cannot be attributed to any definitive diagnosis or disease process (e.g., complex regional pain syndrome). Often clinicians simply state the location and type of pain (e.g., neuropathic pain in bilateral lower extremities). Cancer-related pain, whether from the disease process itself or the treatment of the disease (e.g., surgery, chemotherapy, or radiation), presents very much like noncancer pain. One of the most common ways to classify pain is to describe the time course. *Acute pain* is caused by an injury or illness. It alerts an individual to the injury and initiates withdrawal from the noxious stimulus. It typically has an easily identified cause and location. The course is predictable, and the pain is expected to diminish in hours, days, or weeks as the injury heals. It may be associated with an inflammatory response, producing redness and swelling. Inadequately treated acute pain can evoke physiologic hormonal responses that alter circulation and tissue metabolism; these can also produce tachypnea, tachycardia, widening of the pulse pressure, and increased sympathetic nervous system activity. It can also cause emotional distress.

Chronic pain serves no biologic purpose. It is characterized by persistent pain that lasts beyond the length of an illness or the healing of an injury. Sometimes there is no apparent cause. It may be either continuous or recurrent and of sufficient duration and intensity to adversely affect a patient's well-being, level of function, and quality of life. Risk factors for developing chronic pain include individual predisposition (e.g., female sex, increasing age, or a genetic predisposition), environmental factors (e.g., previous painful experiences or abuse), and psychological factors (e.g., anxiety, depression, or catastrophizing).[16]

Chronic pain can be further classified based on mechanism, symptoms, or location of injury. *Musculoskeletal* or *inflammatory pain* is described as constant, aching pain, often mediated by prostaglandins. It is usually caused by injury to the skeletal muscles or joints. Pain may be localized to the joints (as in rheumatoid arthritis and osteoarthritis) or more regional (as with myofascial pain or muscle strain). *Neuropathic pain* is described as tingling, sharp, shooting, stabbing, burning, or other uncomfortable feelings (*dysesthesias*) such as the sensation that there are bugs crawling on the skin. Neuropathic pain may be constant (as in diabetic peripheral neuropathy) or intermittent (as in trigeminal neuralgia). It is typically caused by injury within the nervous system or a nervous system response to persistent pain stimulus from outside the nervous system. *Visceral pain* can have a vague presentation, because the enteric and autonomic nervous systems are involved. Patients may report nausea or generalized abdominal discomfort (as in endometriosis, hepatitis, or pancreatitis). Some people report pain in the absence of physiologic tissue damage; however, their perception of the pain is very real. This is called *dysfunctional pain*. Conditions such as irritable bowel syndrome, fibromyalgia, interstitial cystitis, and some abdominal or pelvic pain fall into this category. In these conditions, pain appears to be generated by an imbalance in pronociceptive signals and antinociceptive signals in the CNS. Patients with dysfunctional pain syndromes are heavily influenced by factors that augment or diminish the CNS pathways (including stress, anxiety, depression, or illness).

Assessment

Pain is very subjective and difficult to measure in quantitative terms. It is essential to obtain a thorough history and examination, both physical and psychological. When obtaining a pain history, clinicians should gather details about the pattern, duration, location, and character of the pain and should additionally determine what makes the pain worse and what makes it better, what medications and nonpharmacologic therapies have been tried in the past, and the result of those therapies (positive or negative outcome) (Table 55-1).

Pain intensity should be measured using an appropriate pain scale according to the patient's ability to communicate (Table 55-2, Fig. 55-4).[17] Single-dimensional pain scales tend to be more accurate in the acute pain setting and not as helpful for chronic pain because they only capture a "snapshot" of what the patient is feeling. Chronic pain symptoms wax and wane over time, so more useful tools are multidimensional pain scales that evaluate function, including sleep, appetite, performance of activities of daily living, work, and social interactions. Examples of multidimensional tools include the McGill Pain Questionnaire and the Brief Pain Inventory.[18,19] Ultimately, the most useful aspect of patient assessment is the information provided by the patient on how pain impacts day-to-day life, such as the number of hours they spend on their hobbies, or how well they can perform activities of daily living. Some of the most difficult patients to assess are young children and patients with cognitive, visual, or hearing impairment. These patients may have difficulty describing and communicating their pain and discomfort. There are multiple assessment tools that are designed and tested in these special populations to increase the accuracy of pain assessment. In addition to physical and functional assessments, psychological evaluations help to identify those patients who may need more psychiatric or psychological therapy to help them cope with their chronic pain. Because controlled substances are used to treat chronic pain, some clinicians advocate for substance abuse screening (see Case 55-7, Question 4).

Table 55-1
Patient Evaluation

General History
Chief complaint
History of present illness (HPI)
Past medical history (PMH)
Family history
Social history
Current medications, including allergies
Pain History
Onset
Duration
Quality
Intensity
Ameliorating factors
Exacerbating factors
Pain rating, if possible
Analgesic History
Current and past analgesics
Dose/route
Duration of use
Effectiveness
Adverse effects
Clinical Examination
Clinician observations of patient behavior (grimacing, withdrawing, guarding)
Physical examination
Functional assessment

Overview of Treatment

Treatment of pain is based on guidelines whenever possible. However, the number of treatment guidelines for pain management is limited. More commonly, clinicians choose a therapy based on the type of pain (e.g., neuropathic, musculoskeletal, visceral, and central). For all types of pain, multimodal therapy including pharmacologic, physical rehabilitation, and cognitive behavioral therapy should be combined. Interventional therapies should be considered if possible.

A treatment plan must always include evaluation of the following factors: age, comorbidities (such as renal and liver disease), route of administration (the oral route may not be suitable), concurrent medications (for duplication or drug–drug interactions), laboratory abnormalities, and financial resources.

Acute pain is usually managed very effectively with nonsteroidal anti-inflammatory drugs (NSAIDs), acetaminophen, and/or opioids, but may include adjunctive therapies as well. Pharmacotherapy for chronic pain is more complex. First-line agents for the treatment of neuropathic pain consist of antidepressants, preferably serotonin and norepinephrine reuptake inhibitors (SNRIs), including tricyclic antidepressants (TCAs). These agents enhance the descending inhibitory pain pathway. Anticonvulsants (e.g., sodium-channel blockers, calcium-channel blockers, or GABA agonists) are also considered first-line therapy for many common types of neuropathic pain. They inhibit activation of sodium and calcium channels, block release of EAAs such as glutamate, or block the postsynaptic receptors. Some anticonvulsants also enhance the inhibitory effects of GABA. If the pain is localized, topical agents may be useful (e.g., capsaicin or local anesthetics). Addition of an opioid may be considered if the former agents fail to provide adequate analgesia. Combination therapy has been shown to be more effective in some cases (TCA–anticonvulsant or opioid–anticonvulsant combinations).[20] Nerve blocks and other interventional therapies may be helpful for short-term relief.[21]

Chronic musculoskeletal pain usually responds to acetaminophen, salicylates, or NSAIDs, in addition to nonpharmacologic therapies such as heat and ice or physical rehabilitation modalities. Localized pain may be amenable to topical therapies (NSAIDs, capsaicin), and trigger points (i.e., taut muscle bands) may be amenable to injections. SNRIs may also be considered for this indication.[22,23]

Visceral pain is complex, and there are no clear treatment guidelines. Because it travels the somatosensory pathways, antidepressants that enhance inhibitory modulation are most commonly used. Additionally, anticonvulsants that reduce central sensitization and hyperalgesia may be helpful.[24]

Trials of any pharmacologic therapy must be monitored for both efficacy and toxicity. Patients must have realistic expectations for any medication trial. Even the most effective analgesics are expected to achieve only about 30% to 50% improvement in chronic pain. This is why multimodal therapy is essential. NSAID therapy should be accompanied by monitoring for dyspepsia, peptic ulcers, and gastrointestinal (GI) bleeding, elevated blood pressure, and declining renal function, at a minimum. Antidepressants do not usually require laboratory monitoring but are known to cause dry mouth, constipation, urinary retention, and drowsiness. Some of the anticonvulsants require laboratory monitoring for liver toxicity, electrolyte imbalance, or bone marrow abnormalities. All anticonvulsants may cause drowsiness, dizziness, and cognitive dysfunction, with short-term memory loss and word-finding difficulty. Opioids

Table 55-2
Pain Assessment Tools for Adults[17]

Tool	Method of Administration	Advantages	Disadvantages
Visual analog scale (VAS)	Verbal, visual	Reliable; sensitive to acute changes in pain	Requires paper/pencil, mechanical skills; decreased reliability with cognitive, visual or auditory impairment; not sensitive to long-term changes in pain
Numerical rating scales (NRS)	Verbal, visual	Reliable; good validity; detects treatment effects acutely	Decreased reliability with extremes of age; requires abstract thought, difficult to use with cognitive, visual, or auditory impairment; not sensitive to long-term changes in pain
Verbal description scales (VDS)	Verbal, visual (4- or 5-point scales)	Reliable; good validity; preferred by older adults; preferred by some over NRS or VAS	Dependent on literacy and language; limited number of response categories, unequal intervals between anchors; not very sensitive to changes in pain
Faces pain scale (FPS)	Visual	Reliable; good validity; good with poor literacy or language barrier; possibly easier than NRS or VDS	Requires abstract thinking; not specific for pain
Brief pain inventory (BPI)	Verbal, written	Reliable; intensity and interference components; sensitive to change in condition over time	Does not assess quality of pain or affective component
McGill Pain Questionnaire (MPQ)	Verbal, written (long form—30 minutes; short form—2–3 minutes)	Reliable; measures sensory and affective components; valid in older patients	Not recommended for illiterate or cognitively impaired patients

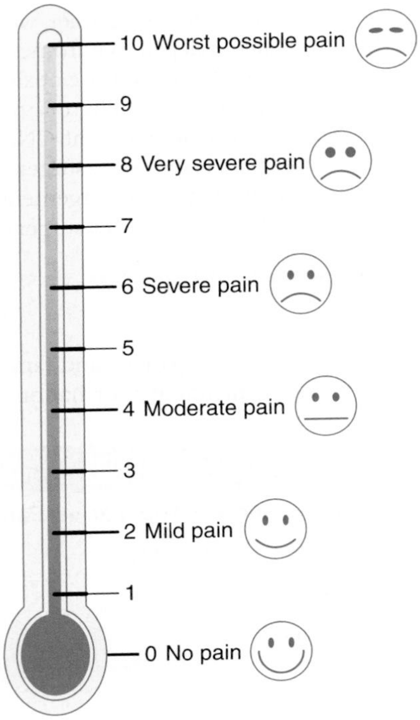

Figure 55-4 Pain assessment scale. (Adapted from Northeast Health Care Quality Foundation [NHCQF], the Medicare Quality Improvement Organization [QIO] for Maine, New Hampshire and Vermont, under contract with the Centers for Medicare & Medicaid Services [CMS], an Agency of the U.S. Department of Health and Human Services.)

require laboratory monitoring for long-term adverse effects such as osteoporosis, hypogonadism, and end-organ impairment, and patients must be routinely screened for sleep apnea, constipation, drowsiness, nausea, and vomiting. Drug interactions, both pharmacokinetic (e.g., hepatic enzyme interactions) and pharmacodynamic (e.g., additive sedation), are common with many of these agents, particularly when used in combination.

Perioperative Pain Management

It is estimated that 25 million inpatient surgeries and 35 million ambulatory surgeries are performed annually in the United States.[25] Greater than 80% of surgical patients experience postoperative pain and of those patients, up to 40% experience "severe" pain.[2] The mismanagement of postoperative pain, whether undertreatment or overtreatment, is associated with negative physiologic consequences such as persistent postoperative pain, impaired rehabilitation, increased hospital length of stay, and adverse events related to excessive analgesic use, including hospital re-admission. Multimodal treatment must be utilized throughout the perioperative continuum to effectively manage pain.

Pain management during the perioperative period can be divided into three phases: pre-, intra-, and postoperative analgesia. Preoperative analgesia is treatment started 1 to 2 hours before surgery, with medications used to decrease peripheral sensitization. Intraoperative analgesia prevents the establishment of central sensitization caused by incisional injury and includes only the intraoperative time period. Postoperative analgesia is aimed at proactively reducing acute pain and preventing central sensitization, thereby avoiding subsequent development of chronic pain.[26]

Table 55-3
Prevalence of Chronic Postsurgical Pain[28]

Type of Surgery	Incidence of Chronic Pain (%)	Clinical Presentation
Limb amputation	30–85	Phantom limb pain
Mastectomy	>50	Scar pain, phantom breast pain, shoulder or arm pain, chest wall pain
Thoracotomy	30–50	Scar pain, chest wall pain
Coronary artery bypass surgery	30–55	Sternal pain, postsaphenectomy pain
Inguinal hernia repair	20–60	Scar pain, ilioinguinal nerve pain, inflammatory pain

Source: Cregg R et al. Persistent postsurgical pain. *Curr Opin Support Palliat Care*. 2013;7:144–152.

Normally, the acute pain trajectory has a rapid decline during the first week after surgery, and most patients fully recover within a few weeks with no residual pain. Although there is no single definition of a time frame for chronic pain, chronic persistent surgical pain (CPSP) is usually regarded as pain of at least 2 months duration and which all other causes have been excluded.[27] The prevalence of CPSP is highest with limb amputation, thoracotomy, mastectomy, hernia repair, and cardiac surgery (Table 55-3).[28] Risk factors for CPSP include history of chronic pain prior to surgery, gender, age, surgical site, invasiveness of surgery, unrelieved postoperative pain, and comorbid anxiety or depression.[29] Genetic factors also account for a significant degree of inter-individual variation in pain sensitivity and treatment response.

CASE 55-1

QUESTION 1: B.B. is a 46-year-old female who sustained a shoulder injury while pulling a cart at work. She will be undergoing shoulder arthroplasty in 2 weeks. She also has fibromyalgia and takes hydrocodone/acetaminophen 5/325 mg 1 to 2 tablets by mouth every 6 hours (usually takes eight tablets daily) as well as duloxetine 30 mg by mouth daily and pregabalin 75 mg by mouth twice daily. She smokes one pack of cigarettes daily and has "a few" glasses of wine nightly to help her pain because she does not think her current analgesic regimen is effective.

What assessment should be done with B.B. prior to surgery? What risk factors does she have for increased pain after surgery?

It is paramount that all patients have a thorough preoperative assessment including review of medical comorbidities, medications, history of chronic pain, and substance abuse, as well as prior postoperative analgesic regimens and responses.[30] This might include evaluating kidney or liver function, pulmonary function, or coagulation status. Pharmacists should also ask about sleep apnea. The presence of central or obstructive sleep apnea is associated with a higher risk for perioperative complications including opioid-induced respiratory depression.[31] If the patient does not have a sleep apnea diagnosis, a screening tool called the STOP-BANG questionnaire can be utilized to assess the risk (Table 55-4).[32] The results of this screening are associated with postoperative critical care admission.[33] As part of a medication review, the pharmacist should consult with the respective state prescription drug monitoring program to determine what controlled substances the patient has been filling. It is expected that patients have only one prescriber of controlled substances so it is helpful to determine whether stated use matches the prescription history. Keeping with The Joint Commission standards, the pharmacist should reconcile outpatient medication profiles, contacting dispensing pharmacies if necessary.[34] Current and past substance use should be addressed in an open and nonjudgmental manner. Some hospitals perform urine drug testing to confirm prescription and/or illicit drug use.

Table 55-4
STOP-BANG Questionnaire[32]

Do you snore loudly?
Do you feel tired, fatigued, sleepy during the day?
Has anyone observed you stop breathing during sleep?
Are you being treated for high blood pressure?
BMI >35 kg/m^2
Age >50 years
Neck circumference >40 cm
Male gender
Yes to 3 or more item = high risk for OSA
Yes to <3 items = low risk of OSA

Patients always bring their past experiences and current fears to surgery. These factors affect how they perceive and cope with acute pain after surgery (Table 55-5). Risk factors for increased pain after surgery in B.B. include female gender, work injury, and chronic opioid therapy. Functional pain syndromes such as fibromyalgia are associated with inefficient diffuse noxious inhibitory control (DNIC). This means that the inhibitory pathway is not effectively blocking pain transmission into the CNS, and she will likely have an exaggerated pain response to surgery. Her chronic opioid use could also complicate pain management because she will likely require higher opioid doses after surgery.

CASE 55-1, QUESTION 2: What should be done to help B.B. prepare for surgery?

Clinicians should provide the patient and family with individually tailored education, including information on treatment

Table 55-5
Risk Factors for Increased Postoperative Pain[29]

Adverse experience with previous surgery
Preexisting pain (moderate–severe >1 month)
Psychological vulnerability
Younger age
Female
Workman's compensation
Inefficient diffuse noxious inhibitory control (DNIC)
Genetic predisposition
Use of chronic opioid therapy

options for management of postoperative pain, making sure to document the plan and goals in the medical record and on paper for the patient to take home.[30] Patient-tailored education has been shown to reduce postoperative opioid consumption, reduce preoperative anxiety, reduce requests for sedatives, and reduce length of stay.[30,35] Education should include changes in analgesics prior to surgery, reporting and assessment of pain and when to report, multimodal pharmacologic and nonpharmacologic options, as well as realistic goals for pain control.[7]

For B.B., there needs to be education about her substance use. Many surgeons require patients to stop smoking prior to surgery to improve healing (see Chapter 91 Tobacco Use and Dependence for smoking cessation strategies). Given her regular intake of alcohol, tapering off this prior to surgery is important, because she may develop alcohol withdrawal after surgery if she continues to consume alcohol. This complicates postoperative care and prevents use of valuable analgesics such as acetaminophen due to additive liver toxicity. Because she is getting little to no benefit from her opioid, it is recommended to discontinue hydrocodone/acetaminophen via taper over the next two weeks to reduce her tolerance and improve her postoperative response to opioid analgesics. Some time needs to be devoted to reducing her anxiety and educating her that she may have an exaggerated pain response. Increasing the dose of pregabalin may help with this as part of a multimodal analgesic regimen, and duloxetine could be continued.

CASE 55-1, QUESTION 3: Based on current guidelines, what postoperative pain management approaches are appropriate for B.B.?

Clinicians should use regional or intraspinal analgesia whenever possible to reduce the neuronal response to surgery. Surgery in the extremities is most often managed with regional nerve blocks, using a local anesthetic such as bupivacaine or ropivacaine. There are both sensory nerves and motor nerves that extend from the spinal cord. The sensory nerves carry pain, temperature, pressure, and chemical messages from the area of injury to the spine and brain for processing. Sensory nerves are small and very sensitive to local anesthetics. Local anesthetics act as sodium-channel blockers and, depending on how concentrated the local anesthetic is (0.05% vs. 0.1%), it is possible to achieve a very dense block and completely stop transmission. Unfortunately, with a really dense block, nerve transmission is retarded or stopped in the larger motor nerves as well, causing loss of motor function. For BB, the anesthesia team will consider a nerve block (likely an interscalene nerve block) either as a one-shot block or a continuous infusion. The one-shot blocks only last a few hours (Table 55-6). Because shoulder surgery is so painful and recovery so long, some hospitals send patients home with a continuous infusion of local anesthetic for pain relief up to 7 days. If they do this for B.B, she will have her arm in a sling because her arm and hand will be numb and not functional while the nerve block is running. This form of longer term acute analgesia has been shown to reduce length of stay as well as provide excellent pain relief.[36] Some surgeons use local anesthetics for localized joint or tissue infiltration in and around the surgical incision to offer short-term analgesia. A liposomal bupivacaine may be used as well. This may offer slightly longer analgesia in the area where administered.

For thoracic and abdominal surgeries, there are several analgesic options to reduce opioid need. Spinals are one-time injections of either opioid and/or local anesthetic into the subarachnoid (intrathecal) space. Because this is not a continuous infusion, the analgesia will wear off according to the half-life of the drug used. Some anesthesiologists use a small amount of epinephrine to cause local vasoconstriction and keep the medication from dispersing through the cerebrospinal fluid (CSF). Common complications with spinal injections include postdural puncture headaches (i.e., CSF can leak after puncture of the subarachnoid dura) and itching (with opioids). More serious complications include delayed respiratory depression (with opioids), hypotension (with local anesthetics), infection, and intraspinal hematomas.

Epidurals offer the convenience of a continuous infusion of opioid and/or local anesthetic. The medication chosen, concentration, and infusion rate all offer different options for a given clinical situation. Morphine, hydromorphone, and an agent from the fentanyl family are the opioids most commonly used. The pKa and lipophilicity help determine the best agent. Morphine and hydromorphone are more hydrophilic so it is more difficult for them to pass through membranes (to get into the CSF or systemic blood) once injected into the epidural space. This is advantageous because they stay in that space, and infusions can be used for up to 7 days. The fentanyl-related agents are highly lipophilic and easily pass through membranes into the systemic circulation and CSF. Typically, they are not used for longer than 24 hours due to this, but are often used for epidurals during labor. All epidural opioids travel cephalad to the brain via the CSF and may cause central respiratory depression. Epidural opioids also cause typical class-related adverse effects such as itching and nausea, and cognitive effects such as sedation or confusion, although these are centrally mediated.

Some clinicians limit opioid use further by only using local anesthetics in epidural infusions. The local anesthetic chosen depends on half-life and toxicity. Lidocaine is used for local infiltration because it has a short onset of action. However, it also has a short half-life so usually bupivacaine or ropivacaine is used for blocks (Table 55-6). Usually these are infused via an epidural

Table 55-6
Local Anesthetics

Agent	Onset (minute)	pKa	Duration (hour)	Maximum dose (mg/kg)
Lidocaine	10–20	7.8	1–2	4.5
Mepivacaine	10–20	7.7	1.5–3	5
Prilocaine (topical)	<60	8.0	1–2	6
Ropivacaine	15–30	8.1	4–8	2.5
Bupivacaine	15–30	8.1	4–8	2.5
Chloroprocaine	10–15	9.1	0.5–1	9
Procaine	2–5	8.9	0.75–1	7
Tetracaine	3–5	8.4	3	1.5
Cocaine (topical)	1	8.7	0.5	0.5

catheter. The catheter tip is placed where the densest block is needed. The greater the concentration, the denser the block. Increasing the infusion rate causes the local anesthetic to spread over more spinal nerve roots. This causes a greater clinical area of anesthesia. For example, if a patient has a total colectomy and the incision area is still painful on the most cephalad part, the infusion rate can be increased so some of the higher nerve roots are covered. Local anesthetics must be monitored not only for pain coverage but also for toxicity. They most commonly cause hypotension, because sympathetic nerves are small. The more cephalad the epidural catheter tip is placed, the more likely that the sympathetic nerves serving the lungs, diaphragm, and heart will be affected. Local anesthetic systemic toxicity (LAST) can be life threatening, causing seizures and cardiac dysrhythmias. The treatment of LAST involves rapid administration of intralipid, which will bind the local anesthetic.[37]

Multimodal Pain Management

CASE 55-2

QUESTION 1: D.K. is a 35-year-old male admitted for elective surgery of an inguinal hernia that has been present for 8 months. The hernia presented as a protruding bulge, 4 cm in diameter, in the lower right abdominal quadrant that was noticeable with standing and retracted inward when lying down. There was no pain initially with the hernia or incarceration of internal structures so conservative management with observation was appropriate until approximately 4 weeks ago when the patient noted the size of the hernia was increasing and experienced pain shooting down the right leg when walking. An ultrasound of the right groin confirmed an inguinal hernia sac, 6 cm in diameter, with no incarceration. The patient was scheduled for an open repair using the Lichtenstein technique with polypropylene mesh reinforcement of the anterior abdominal wall. Prior to admission for the surgery, the patient's medical history included:

Medical conditions:
- Morbid obesity (height 1.8 m, weight 171 kg, BMI 51.5 kg/m^2)
- Type 2 diabetes, noninsulin dependent
- Sleep apnea, uses CPAP at home
- Chronic kidney disease, baseline serum creatinine 1.4 mg/dL
- Hypertension

Medications:
- Glimepiride 8 mg orally once daily
- Lisinopril 20 mg orally once daily
- Ibuprofen 600 mg orally once or twice daily for groin pain

In the postoperative anesthesia care unit (PACU), morphine 2 to 4 mg intravenous every 5 minutes is ordered for severe pain. D.K. received 8 mg of intravenous morphine over 30 minutes then became very drowsy but still reporting severe pain. The nurse is concerned about the level of sedation and does not want to give additional morphine. Is morphine an appropriate opioid for post-operative pain control in D.K.?

After surgery is completed in the operating room, patients are transferred to the PACU for stabilization of respiratory function and pain. Most patients emerging from general anesthesia are still quite sedated when they are transferred to the PACU. When the anesthetic agents begin to wear off, it is very important to achieve rapid control of severe pain so frequent administration of small intravenous opioid doses is common practice in this setting. Currently, there is not a universally accepted standard for titration of intravenous opioids in the PACU. Some institutions will allow use of both intravenous fentanyl to gain fast pain control and morphine for a longer duration of action. Hydromorphone is an acceptable alternative to morphine for patients with renal insufficiency or intolerable side effects to morphine.

Morphine is considered the standard for intravenous opioid administration. The hydrophilic (i.e., water soluble) property of morphine delays penetration across the blood–brain barrier so the relative time to onset is approximately 6 minutes after an intravenous dose. The concentration peak effect (i.e., equilibration time between the plasma and brain) after an intravenous morphine dose is 20 minutes.[38] Major morphine metabolites include morphine-3-glucuronide (M3G) and morphine-6-glucuronide (M6G).[39] The M3G metabolite is inactive but M6G crosses the blood–brain barrier and has potent analgesic activity. Therefore, the analgesic and ventilatory depressant effects of morphine and M6G may not be evident with initial high plasma morphine concentrations.[40] Adverse events may occur 40 to 60 minutes after the last intravenous morphine dose.[40] Patients with renal insufficiency will have M6G metabolite accumulation and be at increased risk for respiratory depression so morphine use is not recommended in this population.[41]

Hydromorphone is commonly used in patients who cannot tolerate morphine or have a history of renal insufficiency.[42,43] Hydromorphone is a hydrogenated ketone analogue of morphine with slightly higher lipid solubility. The concentration peak effect after intravenous hydromorphone administration is between 8 and 20 minutes.[44,45] Hydromorphone has a similar metabolic pathway to morphine producing hydromorphone-3-glucuronide (H3G) and hydromorphone-6-glucuronide (H6G). However, hydromorphone metabolites are devoid of analgesic activity but H3G has been showed to accumulate in animal models leading to dose-dependent myoclonus.[45]

Fentanyl is a synthetic phenylpiperidine compound with high lipid solubility resulting in rapid transfer across the blood–brain barrier. The concentration peak effect after intravenous fentanyl administration can be seen within 4 to 6 minutes.[46] Fentanyl is a good option for rapid pain control but may accumulate in adipose tissue with multiple doses; therefore, it is not the best choice for obese patients.[46]

For management of D.K.'s pain in the PACU, the morphine order should be changed to intravenous hydromorphone at 0.2 to 0.4 mg every 10 minutes for severe pain. Hydromorphone does not have appreciable metabolite accumulation with renal insufficiency and does not distribute into adipose tissue. After D.K.'s pain is stabilized in the PACU, the interval will need to be longer between doses due to the declining acute pain trajectory and addition of other multimodal medications that will decrease the opioid requirements (Table 55-7). In addition to pain management, it is very important to anticipate postoperative nausea and vomiting (PONV) caused by anesthetic agents and opioids. Antiemetics are commonly used for prevention of severe PONV (refer to Chapter 22 for management of PONV).

CASE 55-2, QUESTION 2: Is D.K. an appropriate candidate for intravenous patient-controlled analgesia (PCA)?

For postoperative pain management after discharge from the PACU, the oral route is preferred over intravenous administration unless the patient is unable to use this route or has severe uncontrolled pain.[30] The use of PCA provides a precise and convenient method for intravenous opioid administration that allows the patient to activate the dose for acute pain management. The intravenous PCA route is preferred over nurse-administered intravenous doses because the patient does not have to notify the nurse when more medication is needed, wait until it is given, and then further wait for the peak effect to occur for pain relief. Self-administration of smaller and more frequent intravenous opioid doses reduces the variation between the peak and trough effect of the dosing interval thus better maintenance of the plasma opioid concentration.[47]

Table 55-7

Postoperative Transition of Opioid Doses for Naive Patients >50 Kg[30,42,48]

Postanesthesia Care Unit
Fentanyl intravenous 25–50 mcg every 5 minutes as needed Morphine intravenous 2–4 mg every 5 minutes as needed Hydromorphone intravenous 0.2–0.4 mg every 5 minutes as needed
Medical/Surgical Hospital Floor
Patient-controlled Analgesia (PCA) Starting Dose
Morphine intravenous 1 mg every 10 minutes Hydromorphone intravenous 0.2 mg every 10 minutes Fentanyl intravenous 25 mcg every 10 minutes
Nurse-Administered Opioid Dose for Patients Unable to Use PCA
Morphine intravenous 2–4 mg every 2 hours as needed Hydromorphone intravenous 0.25–0.5 mg every 2 hours as needed
Discharge Planning
Hydromorphone 2–4 mg orally every 4 hours as needed Oxycodone 5–10 mg orally every 4 hours as needed (can be combined with acetaminophen 325 mg) Hydrocodone 5 mg with acetaminophen 325 mg—1 to 2 tablets orally every 4 hours as needed
Important
Long-acting opioid formulations are not recommended for acute postoperative pain management unless the patient was taking opioid therapy for chronic pain prior to surgery.

Evidence-based guidelines on the management of postoperative pain strongly recommend use of PCA for the intravenous route in surgical patients because of ileus, aspiration risk, or inability to take medications orally or enterally.[30]

Patients who are appropriate for PCA must be able to cognitively understand how to use a dose button for opioid self-administration and require intravenous opioid for many hours.[30] The PCA dose button is connected to an infusion pump that will allow the administration of an opioid dose when the button is pushed (i.e., demand). To prevent over dosage by continual demand, all PCA devices use a lockout interval which is the length of time after a successful patient demand during which the device will not administer another dose even if the patient pushes the button.[47] Most patients who start intravenous PCA are opioid-naïve meaning that their opioid use the week prior to surgery was less than 60 mg of oral morphine or its equivalent.[42,48] For this reason, the starting dose for intravenous PCA is standardized for opioid-naïve patients (Table 55-7).

Use of a continuous opioid infusion for postoperative pain management is generally reserved for patients who are opioid-tolerant and were taking opioid medication around-the-clock prior to surgery. The role of the continuous infusion is to provide a steady baseline of opioid medication that mimics the dose taken prior to surgery. Equianalgesic dose calculations are used to determine the dose difference between two opioids to provide the same degree of pain relief. When switching between two opioids, it is recommended to decrease the new calculated dose by 25% to 50% to account for incomplete cross tolerance that may occur.[42] Use of intravenous PCA along with a continuous infusion in opioid-tolerant patients can help fine-tune pain control (refer to Case 55-8 for examples of equianalgesic dose calculations).

Respiratory depression remains the most serious adverse event related to opioid therapy often due to excessive amounts or frequent use of opioid medication beyond what is needed to achieve pain control.[42,47] There are many factors that increase the risk of opioid-induced respiratory depression with intravenous PCA related to comorbid medical conditions. Patients with advanced age >65 years, renal insufficiency, history of sleep apnea, or morbid obesity are at higher risk for developing opioid-induced respiratory depression. To prevent respiratory depression in high-risk patients, the lowest possible starting dose of an opioid should be initiated, and use of a continuous infusion should be avoided. For all patients, avoid administration of more than one drug with sedating properties at the same time with opioids.[30] Medications including antihistamines, benzodiazepines, gabapentin, pregabalin, and skeletal muscle relaxants should be scheduled approximately 2 hours apart to prevent accumulation of sedating side effects.

For hospitalized patients who experience excessive sedation and cannot be aroused with sternal stimulation, or have a significant decline in breathing, naloxone administration may be needed to reverse the opioid CNS effects. Naloxone is a nonselective competitive opioid antagonist of all pharmacologic effects on mu, delta, and kappa receptors. After oral administration, naloxone is extensively metabolized in the liver (i.e., >95% first pass effect) and not effective so intravenous, intramuscular, or subcutaneous administration at a dose of 0.4 mg is required for reversal of life-threatening respiratory depression. The extent and duration of naloxone reversal of opioid-induced respiratory effects is highly variable and is related to many factors, including the specific opioid used, the opioid dose, administration mode, concurrent medication, underlying disease, and pain. Therefore, naloxone administration may need to be repeated every 2 to 3 minutes or given as a continuous infusion until full recovery of respiratory function.[49]

In this case, PCA therapy would be appropriate for D.K. based on the invasive surgery and anticipated severe postoperative pain. Hydromorphone 0.2 mg intravenously with a lockout interval of 10 minutes is recommended because D.K. is at high risk for respiratory depression being opioid-naïve, morbidly obese, and having chronic renal insufficiency. Because D.K. is experiencing sedation due to morphine administration in the PACU, the PCA dose should be started after he is more alert. Other analgesic medications that are not sedating should be used to provide synergistic pain management and can be used throughout the postoperative period.

As soon as DK can tolerate oral medication, the intravenous PCA dose should be discontinued and a short-acting oral opioid such as oxycodone or hydromorphone administered as needed with frequent reassessment of pain. Because DK is opioid-naïve, the lowest starting dose should be prescribed so oxycodone 5 to 10 mg every 4 hours as needed or hydromorphone 2 to 4 mg every 4 hours as needed would be options in this case. Oral short-acting morphine is not recommended due to concern for metabolite accumulation with renal insufficiency. Long-acting oral formulations (i.e., sustained or extended release) should be avoided in opioid-naive patients who cannot tolerate around-the-clock opioid administration for a prolonged period of time. Recent guidelines for postoperative pain do not recommend long-acting oral opioids due to the need for pain titration with short-acting opioid, and studies have not shown that pain control with a long-acting opioid is superior to short-acting opioid administration immediately after surgery.[30]

When DK is ready for discharge, a prescription for a limited supply of short-acting opioid should be written to cover the duration of 3 days.[50] This is particularly important because prescription opioid abuse is a national crisis and prescription opioid overdose is now the leading cause of unintentional deaths in the United

States.[50] It is estimated that 35% to 80% of people addicted to prescription opioids report that they were first exposed to opioids for the legitimate treatment of pain, including postsurgical pain.[6] The use of nonopioid medication can help reduce the need for opioid therapy.

CASE 55-2, QUESTION 3: What other nonopioid medications would be helpful in the management of D.K.'s postoperative pain?

Recent guidelines on postoperative pain management reviewed studies on acetaminophen and NSAIDs in conjunction with opioids and found that the combination of both medications is more effective than either drug alone in reducing pain and opioid consumption.[30] Perioperative oral acetaminophen at a dose of 1,000 mg 3 or 4 times/day for 48 hours after surgery in adults with normal liver function is supported in the literature.[51] After the initial postoperative period, the dose should be reduced to 650 mg and administered on an "as-needed" frequency. To reduce the risk of liver toxicity associated with acetaminophen daily totals exceeding 3,000 mg, patients who will need opioid therapy should not be prescribed combination products containing acetaminophen such as oxycodone/acetaminophen or hydrocodone/acetaminophen. Use of intravenous acetaminophen has generally been reserved for patients who cannot take oral medications after surgery and cannot use NSAIDs due to increased risk of gastrointestinal bleeding or renal insufficiency. Most research indicates that there is no clear difference between intravenous and oral acetaminophen in reducing postoperative pain.[30,52]

Compared with acetaminophen, NSAIDs are more efficacious for reducing postoperative pain due to their anti-inflammatory effects. Most of the oral nonselective NSAIDs are comparable in efficacy so selection may be influenced by other factors such as cost, availability for use over the counter, and lower cardiovascular adverse effects. All NSAIDs are contraindicated for management of perioperative pain in patients who undergo coronary artery bypass graft surgery because of an increased risk of cardiovascular events.[30] Refer to Chapter 43 Osteoarthritis for more detailed information on NSAIDs.

Intravenous ketorolac is a nonselective NSAID and very effective in reducing postoperative pain. The recommended ketorolac dose for adult patients <65 years with normal renal function is 30 mg every 6 hours as needed. For patients over 65 years of age or with mild-to-moderate renal failure, the dose of ketorolac must be reduced to 15 mg every 6 hours as needed. The maximum duration for ketorolac administration is limited to 5 days to prevent adverse events related to gastrointestinal bleeding with prolonged use. It is not recommended to administer ketorolac to patients who are hypovolemic postoperatively due to excessive blood loss or dehydration due to the risk for renal injury.[30]

Gabapentin or pregabalin are neuromodulators that are helpful in reducing postoperative neuropathic pain. The initial dose should be based on the patient's use prior to admission. For patients who were not taking gabapentin or pregabalin for chronic pain prior to surgery, the dose should be titrated up from the lowest dose and adjusted for renal function (Table 55-8). Patients who were taking gabapentin or pregabalin for preexisting neuropathic pain prior to surgery should have their dose and frequency resumed as soon as possible postoperatively to prevent uncontrolled chronic pain.

Table 55-8
Pharmacologic Options for Treatment of Neuropathic Pain

Drug	Dose[a]	Adverse Effects	Monitoring/Comments
Carbamazepine[b]	200 mg TID, titrate to max 400 mg TID	Diplopia, rash, hepatitis, neutropenia, aplastic anemia, dizziness, cognitive effects, hyponatremia	Check LFTs, CBC, sodium at baseline and every 3 months during therapy, periodic serum levels
Oxcarbazepine	75 mg BID, titrate to max 1,200 mg BID	Rash, cognitive effects, hyponatremia, sedation, blurred vision, nausea	Check sodium every 2 weeks for 3 months, then with dose increases
Lamotrigine	25 mg daily, titrate to max 200 mg BID	Desquamating rash, cognitive effects	Requires very slow titration to avoid rash
Topiramate[b]	25 mg BID, titrate to max 200 mg BID	Nausea, anorexia, paresthesias, metabolic acidosis, cognitive effects, nephrolithiasis	Check serum bicarbonate at baseline and every 3 months or with each dose increase
Lacosamide	50 mg BID, titrate to max 200 mg BID	Nausea, vomiting, dizziness, diplopia, ataxia, fatigue, rash, atrial fibrillation/flutter	ECG at baseline and with dose adjustments, especially in patients at risk for cardiac conduction abnormality Reduce dose for renal and liver impairment
Gabapentin[b]	300 mg daily, titrate to max 1,200 mg TID	Somnolence, dizziness, edema, cognitive effects	Reduce dose for renal impairment or elderly patients
Pregabalin[b]	75 mg BID, titrate to max 300 mg BID	Same as gabapentin	Same as gabapentin
Amitriptyline, Nortriptyline	10 mg QHS, titrate to 100 mg QHS	Dry mouth, constipation, urinary retention, orthostatic hypotension, somnolence	Caution in elderly patients
Duloxetine[b]	30 mg daily, titrate to max 60 mg daily	Nausea, dry mouth, headache, diarrhea, fatigue, sweating, anorexia	Contraindicated with liver disease or concurrent alcohol consumption

Section 13 Neurologic Disorders

Table 55-8
Pharmacologic Options for Treatment of Neuropathic Pain (*continued*)

Drug	Dose[a]	Adverse Effects	Monitoring/Comments
Venlafaxine	37.5 mg daily, titrate to max 225 mg daily	Headache, nausea, sweating, sedation, hypertension, seizures, tachycardia	Serotonergic effects <150 mg and noradrenergic effects >150 mg Monitor blood pressure and heart rate
Opioids[b]	10–15 mg morphine every 4 hours or equianalgesic dose of other opioid	Somnolence, respiratory depression, dry mouth, constipation, urinary retention	May cause confusion in elderly patients Use with a bowel regimen Monitor for misuse and abuse
Tramadol[b]	25 mg QID to max 100 mg QID	Somnolence, dry mouth, constipation, Seizures, Serotonin syndrome	Caution with antidepressants
Capsaicin cream[b]	Apply QID	Rash, burning feeling on skin	Avoid contact with mucous membranes, eyes
Capsaicin patch[b]	Apply 1 patch for 1 hour, every 3 months	Skin irritation at application site, burning feeling on skin	Must be applied in medical office
Lidocaine patch[b]	Apply 1–3 patches daily for 12 hours	Skin reaction at site of application	

[a]All oral agents are titrated up to reduce adverse effects and titrated down when discontinuing therapy.
[b]Food and Drug Administration–approved for treating pain conditions.
BID, 2 times a day; CBC, complete blood cell count; ECG, electrocardiogram; LFTs, liver function tests; QHS, every night at bedtime; QID, 4 times a day; TID, 3 times a day.

The use of ketamine is becoming increasingly popular postoperatively in patients with a history of chronic pain that is poorly responsive to traditional analgesic medications including opioids. Ketamine is a NMDA receptor antagonist that is effective in decreasing central sensitization after surgery. There is insufficient evidence in the literature on the optimal ketamine dose and duration of use postoperatively. Doses for postoperative intravenous ketamine bolus dosing or continuous infusion range from 0.1 to 0.5 mg/kg.[30] The main side effect of postoperative ketamine is hallucinations which can be mitigated by keeping the dose low. Ketamine is contraindicated in patients with uncontrolled hypertension.

Intravenous lidocaine has been evaluated as part of multimodal analgesia in patients who underwent open or laparoscopic abdominal procedures. Studies showed that perioperative or intraoperative intravenous lidocaine infusions were associated with shorter duration of ileus and better quality of analgesia compared to placebo.[30] In trials, lidocaine was typically administered as an intravenous bolus (100–150 mg or 1.5–2.0 mg/kg) followed by an infusion of 2 to 3 mg/kg/hour through the end of surgery.[53,54] Topical local anesthetics such as the lidocaine 5% patch may be helpful for incisional pain, but its efficacy is limited due to lack of penetration into deeper tissues.

D.K. should have acetaminophen started at 1,000 mg orally scheduled every 8 hours as soon as he is alert enough to swallow medication without risk of aspiration. NSAIDs should be avoided in the immediate postoperative period until his renal function can be evaluated. If D.K.'s creatinine clearance is >50 mL/minute, ibuprofen 600 mg orally every 6 hours as needed can be used for pain because this was the patient's NSAID choice. Prior to admission, D.K. was reporting pain shooting down the right leg but was not taking medication for neuropathic pain. If the shooting pain persists postoperatively, gabapentin started at a low dose of 100 mg orally scheduled 3 times a day may be helpful. Caution should be used with gabapentin in patients with renal insufficiency which may require a dose adjustment. Intravenous lidocaine is generally not a first-line option for postoperative pain management and should be used only if pain control is suboptimal after maximizing other multimodal medications. Before D.K. is discharged, plans should be made for prescribing the oral multimodal medications for a short duration of time because acute postoperative pain generally abates after one to 2 weeks.

LOW BACK PAIN

Low back pain occurs at a rate of 1.39/1,000 person-years in the United States, including 3.15% of all emergency visits. These are typically injuries occurring in the home.[55] It has been reported that low back pain affects 70% to 85% of adults at some point in their lives, and 12 months after the onset of low back pain, 45% to 75% of people still have pain.[56,57] There is a bimodal distribution with peaks between 25 and 29 years of age (2.58/1,000 person-years) and 95 to 99 years of age (1.47/1,000) without differentiation by underlying etiology.[56] There is an association between psychological factors and the occurrence of low back pain, including anxiety, depression, somatization symptoms, stress, and negative body image. Chronic low back pain patients have higher rates of emotional distress and depression (25%) relative to acute low back pain subjects (2.9%).[58] Socioeconomic risk factors include job dissatisfaction, physical work, psychologically stressful work, low educational achievement, and workers' compensation insurance.[59] Biomechanical and physical work factors such as heavy lifting, repetitive motion, non-neutral body postures, and vibration are established risks for back disorders.[60] Chronic low back pain also creates a large financial burden on the workplace. Low back pain accounts for almost $20 million in lost productivity annually, and patients who have been on disability for more than 1 year rarely return to work.[61]

Low back pain, by definition, affects the lumbosacral spine and associated muscles and nerves. It is multifactorial in nature, either nociceptive (musculoskeletal, myofascial), neuropathic (radicular pain), or has a central sensitization component.[62] In about 85% of cases, no pathophysiologic cause can be found.[63] The functional spinal unit is made up of two vertebral bodies, two zygapophyseal (facet) joints, the intervertebral disc, and the supporting ligamentous structures (Fig. 55-5). The facet joints of the spine form the junction where vertebral bodies meet. The joint space is maintained by cartilage and fluid in the joint. Like

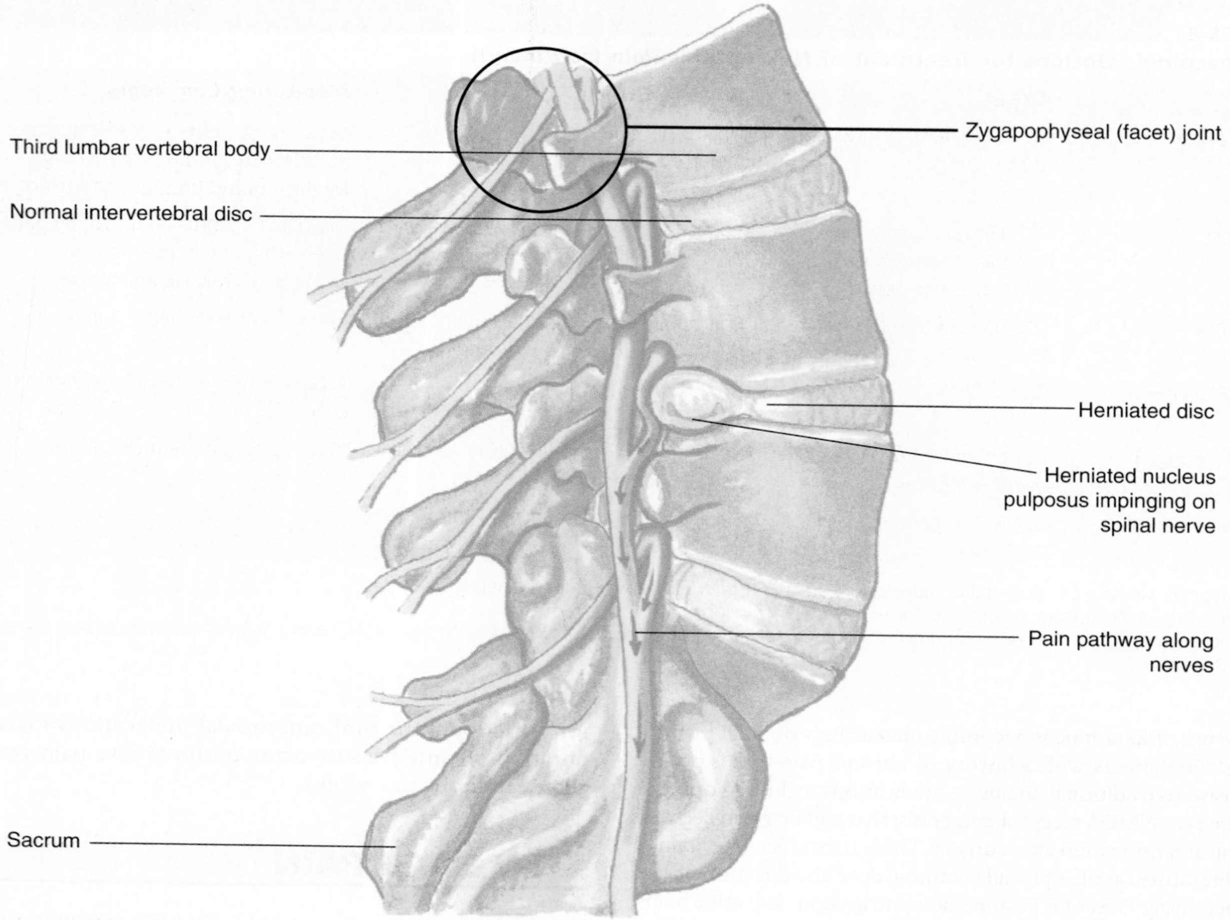

Figure 55-5 Spine anatomy and disc herniation.

all weight-bearing joints of the body, the spine also develops joint space narrowing, bony hypertrophy, and deterioration of cartilage with normal use, resulting in the musculoskeletal pain of OA. If the spine is used more, as with jobs involving heavy lifting and manual labor, the joints deteriorate faster. In addition to deterioration of the facet joint spaces, the intervertebral discs lose water content with time and may become desiccated, reducing the cushion between the vertebral bodies. These discs are fragile and can be torn or damaged and may herniate into the spinal canal foramen (Fig. 55-5). If vertebral bodies shift because of deterioration, spondylolisthesis may occur. This shift, or a herniated disc, may impinge on the spinal nerve root, or cause nerve root irritation, which can produce radicular neuropathic pain. This is sometimes referred to as sciatica. Shifting of the vertebral bodies may also reduce the size of the foramen where the nerves exit the spinal cord (spinal stenosis). If the vertebral bodies shift too far into the central spinal canal, pressure can be exerted on the spinal cord, which may lead to spinal cord injury and subsequent loss of sensory and motor nerve function (paralysis). If the motor nerves are affected (as with lower extremity muscle weakness, bowel or bladder incontinence), a "red flag" is present and surgery may be necessary to preserve function. Table 55-9 lists other serious conditions that call for immediate medical or surgical attention.[64] Sometimes low back pain is more intense than would be expected, or is much more widespread than imaging would predict. These are hallmarks of central sensitization.[62]

Myofascial pain is very common in patients with chronic low back pain. Myofascial pain is localized to specific regions or muscle groups. It affects all age groups and is associated with numerous other pain conditions. It is classically associated with muscle knots called "trigger points." A trigger point is described as a hyperirritable spot in skeletal muscle that is associated with a palpable "taut band" of muscle. Trigger points are hypothesized to evolve from excessive acetylcholine release from the motor endplate, leading to sustained muscle fiber contracture. Development of trigger points is usually associated with mechanical overuse or overload of a muscle group (as with repetitive work). It is also associated with postural problems, prolonged static positions, emotional stress (causing muscles to tense), and nutritional deficiencies (such as vitamins B_1, B_6, B_{12}, and D, iron, magnesium, and zinc) or metabolic problems such as thyroid disease. It is thought that low-intensity exertions related to static posture cause small muscle fibers to be continuously activated, leading to the development of trigger points.[65] Nociceptors are abundant in muscle nerves, and there are a variety of nociceptors that can be stimulated by substances such as prostaglandins, bradykinin, protons, ATP, 5-HT, and glutamate, which are released from damaged tissue. The neuropeptides, substance P and CGRP, are also found in the nociceptor terminals, which stimulate the inflammatory cascade, leading to peripheral sensitization and the clinical manifestation of muscle pain. Continuous activation of muscle nociceptors leads to release of substance P and glutamate from the presynaptic terminal at the dorsal root ganglion. These substances activate postsynaptic AMPA and NMDA receptors, respectively, and subsequently may lead to neuroplasticity (Fig. 55-3).

Table 55-9
Red Flags for Potentially Serious Conditions that Cause Back Pain[64]

Possible Fracture	Possible Tumor or Infection	Possible Cauda Equina Syndrome
Major trauma, such as vehicle accident or fall from height	Age <20 or >50 years	Saddle anesthesia
Minor trauma or strenuous lifting in older or potentially osteoporotic patients	History of cancer	Recent onset of bladder dysfunction (e.g., urinary retention, increased frequency, overflow incontinence)
	Constitutional symptoms (recent fever, chills, unexplained weight loss)	Severe or progressive neurologic deficit in the lower extremities
	Risk factors for spinal infections: Recent bacterial infection IV drug abuse Immune suppression	Unexpected laxity of the anal sphincter
	Pain that worsens when supine	Perianal/perineal sensory loss
	Severe nighttime pain	Major motor weakness: Quadriceps (knee extension weakness) Ankle plantar flexors, evertors, and dorsiflexors (foot drop)

IV, intravenous.

Acetaminophen is considered the safest choice for the management of musculoskeletal pain. Its mechanism of action is not well defined, but it has analgesic activity in the CNS. It has no peripheral clinical effect on prostaglandins, so it lacks typical anti-inflammatory activity. Use of acetaminophen therefore avoids the GI, renal, and cardiovascular toxicities associated with NSAIDs. NSAIDs reduce pain and inflammation by inhibiting cyclooxygenases (COX-1 and COX-2) at the site of injury and along the ascending pain pathway. The NSAIDs are equally effective across the drug class, although some patients may respond to one agent better than another. They are more effective as monotherapy for acute low back pain than in combination with a muscle relaxant or an opioid. A meta-analysis showed that NSAIDs are better than placebo for back pain without neuropathic symptoms, but not for back pain with neuropathic symptoms.[66,67] COX-2 selective inhibitors are as effective as traditional NSAIDs for analgesia but are better tolerated.[67] Celecoxib is the only COX-2 selective inhibitor available in the United States. Acetaminophen may be used in combination with NSAIDs for additive analgesia.

There are several guidelines published for the management of low back pain. Koes et al. reviewed evidence-based management guidelines from 13 different countries and 2 international committees that were published between 2000 and 2008.[65] Table 55-10 presents a summary of common recommendations. All guidelines were in agreement with the use of simple analgesics such as over-the-counter acetaminophen and NSAIDs for first-line therapy for both acute and chronic low back pain. Both of these medication classes are considered effective for short-term use, although their effects are modest. Because the guidelines have been published, a meta-analysis of acetaminophen versus placebo for spinal pain and osteoarthritis found acetaminophen to be ineffective for long-term use in chronic pain.[68] This would make NSAIDs the ideal first-line analgesic, if there are no contraindications.

Most guidelines recommend either muscle relaxants or weak opioids as third-line choices for short-term use in either acute or chronic low back pain. Despite the fact that muscle relaxants are used commonly, there is no evidence that they are effective for chronic low back pain. Agents such as cyclobenzaprine and tizanidine, as well as benzodiazepines such as diazepam, show moderate efficacy in the short-term (<2 weeks) but are associated with a higher incidence of adverse effects than placebo.[69] Weak opioids such as tramadol have also shown modest relief with short-term use (<4 weeks).[70,71] There are several studies showing some efficacy for most long- and short-acting opioids, but they do not show any long-term functional improvement or return to work.[72–74]

A few guidelines, including those from the American Pain Society (APS), recommend use of antidepressants or anticonvulsants for neuropathic pain symptoms.[70] Antidepressants, specifically the TCAs, have shown modest analgesia compared with placebo, but they have not been shown to be effective for acute low back pain, nor have they shown demonstrable improvement in function.[67,68,75,76] Duloxetine, an SNRI, has shown efficacy and

Table 55-10
Summary of Common Recommendations for Treatment of Low Back Pain[65]

Acute or Subacute Pain
Reassure patients that diagnosis is not serious
Advise to stay active
Prescribe medication if necessary
First line: acetaminophen
Second line: NSAIDs
Third line: muscle relaxants, opioids, antidepressants, or anticonvulsants as coanalgesics
Discourage bed rest
Do not recommend supervised exercise program
Chronic Pain
Discourage use of alternative therapies (ultrasound, electrotherapy)
Short-term use of medication/manipulation
Supervised exercise therapy
Cognitive behavioral therapy
Multidisciplinary treatment

NSAIDs, nonsteroidal anti-inflammatory drugs.

safety for the treatment of low back pain.[77] There have been a very small number of trials using the anticonvulsants topiramate and gabapentin for back pain. Anticonvulsants traditionally have been helpful for treating neuropathic pain (e.g., peripheral neuropathies) but produce only small improvements for back pain with radiculopathy.[78–80]

Myofascial pain treatment is aimed at correcting precipitating behaviors including ergonomic factors. Physical rehabilitation is essential for teaching patients appropriate stretching and strengthening exercises, as well as postural support and stabilization. Some clinicians inject the trigger point(s). There are several techniques that are all equally effective, including dry needling, saline injection, local anesthetic injection or botulinum toxin. Several other pharmacologic therapies may be used, but none have more than anecdotal support. General approaches to pain management, including NSAIDs, muscle relaxants, antidepressants, anticonvulsants, and opioids, may be helpful for individual patients. Vitamin D deficiency has been linked to chronic musculoskeletal pain, although this is somewhat controversial.[81,82]

CASE 55-3

QUESTION 1: J.P. is a 48-year-old man who presents with low back and leg pain. He has had chronic back pain for several years, which has progressively worsened during the last several months. He reports an aching pain that is localized to his lumbosacral spine with some radiation into his buttocks and hips. He also describes burning pain into his right leg all the way down to his toes. He rates his pain as 7 out of 10 on the numeric pain scale. On good days, his pain is 5 of 10. He recently did some yard work and had an acute exacerbation of his pain. He reports that this felt like 10 out of 10 on the numeric pain scale, and he was in bed for the following 2 days because of pain. He is usually able to do some chores around the house, but activity makes his pain worse. He sleeps poorly (only about 4–5 hours/night), and he does not go out or socialize very often because he is afraid this will exacerbate his pain. He used to golf and play softball but is not able to participate in these hobbies any more as a result of pain. He smokes two packs of cigarettes daily and drinks about a six-pack of beer each week. He was previously a plumber but had to quit his job earlier this year because of health problems. He denies any lower extremity weakness and also denies loss of bowel or bladder control. He has not found anything that really helps his pain except rest and acetaminophen/codeine that his sister gave him. His past medical history includes hypertension, hyperlipidemia, depression, and morbid obesity. His current medications are lisinopril for hypertension, simvastatin for hyperlipidemia, carisoprodol, cyclobenzaprine as needed, a baby aspirin, and acetaminophen/codeine. He also takes three tablets of over-the-counter strength (200 mg/tablet) ibuprofen and three tablets of extra strength (500 mg/tablet) acetaminophen about four times daily with minimal relief of his pain. Upon physical examination, J.P. has pain with palpation along his lumbar paraspinal muscles with several trigger points noted and marked tenderness at the level of L4–L5. His reflexes are intact, and he has full strength in his lower extremities. The remainder of his physical examination is unremarkable except that general deconditioning is noted. There are no laboratory tests or imaging studies available. He reports that his blood pressure is usually around 150/80 mm Hg with a pulse around 75 beats/minute.

What are the clinically relevant findings (or absence of findings) for J.P.'s pain assessment, and how would you characterize his pain?

The presentation and assessment of back pain can be very complex given its multifactorial nature. Acute low back problems are defined by the Agency for Health Care Policy and Research as "activity intolerance attributable to lower back or back-related leg symptoms of less than 3 months' duration."[64] J.P.'s acute exacerbation would fit this definition. When J.P. has acute exacerbations of his back pain, the numeric pain scale is an accurate assessment tool (Table 55-2, Fig. 55-4). His rating of 10 out of 10 indicates severe acute pain. Clinicians should also consider a patient's vital signs, which may be elevated with acute pain. If a patient is unable to communicate (e.g., on a respirator), changes in vital signs may be the only indicator of discomfort.

J.P.'s chronic back pain assessment must rely heavily on the history he provides, because there is minimal objective evidence to base the assessment on, other than his findings on physical examination or imaging studies. He indicated that his chronic pain is about 7 out of 10 on the numeric pain scale. Even though the numeric pain scale has been validated for chronic pain, it is less useful in this setting because it only gives a snapshot of the whole pain picture. A multidimensional tool, such as the Brief Pain Inventory or the McGill Pain Questionnaire, is more useful to assess chronic pain (Table 55-2).[18,19] Physical activities, sleep, diet, and social interactions may be affected by chronic pain. J.P. notes that his pain is worse with physical activity. He reports sleeping poorly and has limited physical activity and minimal social interaction. All of these factors contribute to a patient's pain experience and must be considered (Fig. 55-1). Assessment of chronic pain is not only more complex, but is more extensive, because the perception and response to chronic pain is widely variable. Each patient experiences pain in his/her own way. A psychological assessment is essential to identify comorbidities such as depression or anxiety and any history of abuse (e.g., physical, verbal, sexual) or previous trauma, as well as to assess a patient's coping ability. It may be helpful to ask J.P. about his spirituality and cultural values, because these may offer unique opportunities (or barriers) to any proposed treatment plan.

If opioids are being considered, many clinicians endorse the use of a substance abuse screening tool such as the Screener and Opioid Assessment of Patients with Pain-Revised (SOAPP-R), Opioid Risk Tool (ORT), or Diagnosis, Intractability, Risk, Efficacy (DIRE) score.[83] J.P. drinks alcohol, smokes tobacco, and has used his sister's acetaminophen/codeine. These factors may warrant use of a screening tool to assess his risk for opioid abuse.

J.P.'s chronic pain has been present for several years and has gradually worsened. Based on his history and current physical examination, he appears to have mechanical musculoskeletal pain. He is a former plumber, which involves bending and lifting, which puts him at risk for facet joint arthritis. He describes the aching, localized pain that is typical of arthritis, either in his spine–hip junction (sacroiliac joint) or his zygapophyseal (facet) joints, which are the most common locations for lumbosacral pain. He demonstrated localized tenderness at the L4–L5 level. This is most consistent with facet joint disease. He also has tenderness along muscles in his low back, reaching into his buttocks, which is very common, because the body attempts to accommodate structural spine abnormalities. Muscular pain may radiate into the mid-back or into the buttocks, but does not travel below the knees. J.P. did not have pain that radiated below the knees. J.P. does not have any motor weakness, past experiences, or comorbidities that would indicate a red flag (Table 55-9). J.P.'s physical examination reveals radicular pain in the L5 dermatome (i.e., an area of the skin supplied by nerves from a single spinal root). Unlike muscular pain, radicular pain travels from the spine past the knee into the distal extremities. J.P. describes burning and shooting pain that radiates from his spine down his right leg to his toes. These are hallmarks of neuropathic pain. J.P. appears to have both musculoskeletal/myofascial and neuropathic pain. This mixed picture is very common with back pain and adds complexity to both diagnosis and treatment plans.

Case 55-3, Question 2: What comorbidities will affect J.P.'s presentation and pain assessment?

J.P. has a concurrent diagnosis of depression, which is quite common in patients with chronic pain. The incidence of depression in chronic pain patients is 2 or 3 times higher than the general population.[84] Depression is often under-recognized in the face of pain as a presenting symptom. Many times healthcare providers investigate for a functional cause of the pain, but overlook the psychosocial aspects of pain. Variables associated with depression in chronic pain are female sex, younger age, lower socioeconomic status, unmarried, Caucasian, and higher pain severity.[85] In fact, because pain severity worsens, depressive symptoms worsen, medical visits become more frequent, and healthcare costs increase.[86] The relative deficiency of NE and 5-HT that occur with depression makes the pain-blocking function of the descending pain pathway less effective. As a result, J.P. may feel more pain physiologically and may also have a greater emotional response to his pain and other stressors. His depression may be contributing to his sleep disturbance and his diminished social interactions. Untreated depression may be detected with a multidimensional pain assessment tool. If identified and treated, his pain may improve concurrently with his depression. Other psychiatric comorbidities that commonly occur with chronic pain include anxiety, personality disorders, and substance abuse.

J.P. also has a diagnosis of hypertension. Although this will not directly contribute to his pain, any acute exacerbations may cause an increase in his pulse and blood pressure. Increases in blood pressure are associated with an increased incidence of stroke. The presence of hypertension is also a factor when developing a treatment plan. He is currently taking ibuprofen for pain, and NSAIDs are known to cause fluid retention, compromise renal function, and diminish the benefits of antihypertensives (such as J.P.'s lisinopril). Corticosteroids, which may be used during an interventional pain procedure, may also increase blood pressure.

Case 55-3, Question 3: How can current low back pain treatment guidelines be applied to J.P.'s pharmacologic regimen?

Acetaminophen is considered first-line therapy for low back pain. J.P. has been using acetaminophen up to 6,000 mg daily, which exceeds the recommended maximum daily dose. He has also been using some acetaminophen/codeine that he obtained from his sister. J.P. is at risk for liver toxicity from high doses of acetaminophen. Additionally, he has not found the acetaminophen to be helpful, so it should be stopped. J.P. is also taking ibuprofen, which is recommended as second-line therapy. He is taking 2,400 mg daily without benefit. His pain relief is unlikely to improve with a dose increase, but he may benefit from rotation to another NSAID with a different chemical structure. Naproxen is an inexpensive agent that is also available over the counter. He does not demonstrate any muscle spasm, so a muscle relaxant is not indicated, nor is it recommended for chronic back pain. He has radicular pain, so a trial of gabapentin may be helpful. He has been using the codeine-containing product and notes that this has been helpful; however, opioids are not recommended for long-term management and have not shown substantial benefit with long-term use. He should be encouraged to reduce or discontinue use of the opioid. Chang et al. recommend a trial of TCAs if NSAIDs and acetaminophen have failed.[87] This may also help his chronic insomnia, but the doses used for analgesia (typically less than 100 mg/day) may not be high enough to have true antidepressant effects. Selective serotonin reuptake inhibitors (SSRIs) may be used to treat depression, but have very little independent analgesic effects. However, if his depression improves, we would expect to see a proportional improvement in his pain. Because SSRIs are better tolerated than TCAs, and TCAs have not demonstrated improvement in function in the long term, J.P. should have a trial of a generic SSRI such as citalopram. SNRI's may also be an effective and well-tolerated option that would treat both his depression and pain.

Case 55-3, Question 4: J.P. has been taking two different muscle relaxants for his back pain. He reports that neither of these is very helpful, and he usually does not have muscle spasms but does have trigger points on physical examination. What would you recommend with regard to continuing these drugs? Would a trial of a different muscle relaxant be appropriate?

Muscle relaxants are commonly used to treat chronic musculoskeletal pain. They are recommended for short-term use for acute low back pain (all are fairly equal).[69] Chou et al. performed a systematic review of trials to compare efficacy and safety of skeletal muscle relaxants.[70] Although the evidence was considered to be of fair quality, they concluded that for the treatment of musculoskeletal pain, tizanidine, orphenadrine, carisoprodol, and cyclobenzaprine were more effective than placebo. There were not sufficient data of good quality to determine whether metaxalone, methocarbamol, chlorzoxazone, baclofen, or dantrolene was better than placebo for this indication. At this time, guidelines do not recommend chronic use of muscle relaxants for musculoskeletal pain. There is a small study that shows improvement in myofascial pain with tizanidine, but there are no data supporting continued use of carisoprodol or cyclobenzaprine.[88] These agents belong to a chemically diverse family, but all work in the CNS, either in the brain or in the spinal cord. They are categorized as either antispasmodics or antispasticity agents. The *antispasmodics* are either benzodiazepines (e.g., diazepam) or nonbenzodiazepines (e.g., cyclobenzaprine) and are used for muscular pain and spasms associated with peripheral musculoskeletal conditions. The *antispasticity* agents reduce spasticity associated with upper motor neuron disorders such as multiple sclerosis (e.g., tizanidine, baclofen) (Table 55-11). Because J.P. has not experienced any improvement in his pain with previous trials of muscle relaxants, switching to another is not likely to yield any improvement in his symptoms, though tizanidine has shown some promise.

Case 55-3, Question 5: J.P. returns after 3 months with a small improvement in his back pain. He is sleeping a bit better (6 hours/night). He is attending physical therapy sessions, although infrequently. He has been taking citalopram 20 mg by mouth daily for his depression and feels that this is somewhat helpful for his mood. He has been taking naproxen 500 mg by mouth 3 times a day and gabapentin 300 mg by mouth 3 times a day for his pain. Neither of these has provided adequate relief. Another provider gave him a prescription for oxycodone 5 mg/acetaminophen 325 mg one to two tablets every 6 hours as needed. J.P. has been taking two tablets every 6 hours on a regular schedule. This helps his pain (30% improvement and he notes that the addition of the opioid has allowed him to start working part time again as a handy man); however, the relief only lasts 3 to 4 hours, and then he is in pain for another 2 to 3 hours before he can take another dose. He also reports a lot of nausea with this regimen. He has heard about "pain patches" and wonders whether these might be an option for him.

J.P. is getting about 30% improvement with oxycodone/acetaminophen, which is a good response for any analgesic, but the duration of relief is short, and he is having nausea after each dose. He has asked about using a pain patch. What therapy might you suggest to optimize J.P.'s analgesia? Is a pain patch a good choice?

Table 55-11
Oral Muscle Relaxants

Drug	Dose	Adverse Effects	Monitoring/Comments
Antispasmodic			
Cyclobenzaprine	5 mg TID, titrate to 10 mg TID	Dry mouth, constipation, urinary retention, somnolence, confusion, blurred vision	Also available in extended-release formulation
Metaxalone	300 mg TID–QID	GI upset, nausea, vomiting, dizziness, headache, somnolence, hemolytic anemia, leucopenia, jaundice	Contraindicated in anemia, liver impairment, renal impairment Monitor liver function, CBC
Methocarbamol	1,500 mg TID, or 1,000 mg QID	Itching, rash, indigestion, nausea, vomiting, dizziness, headache, nystagmus, somnolence, vertigo, blurred vision, arrhythmias, hypotension, leucopenia, urine discoloration	Monitor heart rate, blood pressure
Orphenadrine citrate	100 mg BID	Syncope, nausea, vomiting, dry mouth, dizziness, blurred vision, palpitations	Monitor CBC, liver function
Chlorzoxazone	500–750 mg TID–QID	Lightheadedness, dizziness, somnolence, malaise, liver toxicity	Monitor liver function
Carisoprodol	250–350 mg TID and at bedtime	Dizziness, headache, somnolence, respiratory depression	Monitor for weakness, dizziness, confusion, misuse, or abuse
Antispastic			
Tizanidine	4 mg TID, titrate to max of 12 mg TID	Hypotension, somnolence, muscle weakness	Monitor blood pressure, liver function
Baclofen	10 mg TID, titrate to max of 20 mg QID	Somnolence, muscle weakness, ataxia	
Diazepam	2 mg TID, titrate to max of 10 mg TID	Respiratory depression, somnolence, weakness	Monitor sedation, respiration, misuse, or abuse Risk of physical dependence

BID, 2 times a day; CBC, complete blood cell count; GI, gastrointestinal; QID, 4 times a day; TID, three times a day.

Although opioids are not recommended for chronic low back pain, J.P. has noted an improvement in pain and function.[89] It would be reasonable to consider continuing his analgesic combination. There are several analgesic options available for patients who are unable to tolerate or ingest solid oral dosage forms (tablets and capsules). It is common for patients with feeding tubes and patients who have maxillofacial surgery to use alternative dosage forms such as oral liquids, topicals, or transdermal products (Table 55-12). J.P. has asked about a pain patch. It is likely that he is referring to either a fentanyl transdermal system or a buprenorphine patch. These agents offer extended delivery options, but are often not cost-effective; therefore, a pain patch may not be the best choice for J.P. Because he is able to take oral medications, it would be most reasonable to rotate to an oral opioid that offers a longer duration of action. When considering product rotation for J.P., it is important to consider drug formulation and availability, route of administration, drug interactions, adverse effects, and cost. The oxycodone/acetaminophen product that he is currently using is not providing an adequate duration of analgesia. He may need to use an extended-release/long-acting (ER/LA) opioid to achieve sustained analgesia. There are many ER/LA opioid formulations available including morphine (tablets, capsules), oxycodone (tablets), hydromorphone (capsules), methadone (tablets), oxymorphone (tablets), hydrocodone (capsules, tablets), buprenorphine (patch, buccal film), and fentanyl (patch). Several of these agents are formulated with abuse-deterrent technologies. Because he is getting good pain relief with oxycodone/acetaminophen, converting to a extended-release formulation of oxycodone seems the most logical choice. J.P. is currently taking eight 5-mg tablets of oxycodone daily (40 mg total per day). This may be directly converted to ER oxycodone 20 mg orally twice daily, with elimination of the short-acting product. If he continues to have nausea after his doses of oxycodone, he may need to rotate to another opioid or use a nonoral route of administration, an antiemetic, or a nonopioid analgesic.

J.P. has been using several different analgesics for his pain, including an NSAID, an anticonvulsant, an antidepressant, and an opioid. These agents will offer pharmacologic activity at several points in the pain pathway (Fig. 55-2) and offer additive analgesic effects.[90,91] However, multimodal therapy also carries the risk of additive adverse effects and possible drug interactions. For example, the anticonvulsant and the opioid may cause additive sedation. The balance between adverse effects and analgesia must be considered with any changes in drug therapy. He is also taking lisinopril. Using an NSAID concurrently with an angiotensin-converting enzyme (ACE) inhibitor or an angiotensin receptor blocker may cause hyperkalemia or acute renal blood flow compromise. A nonacetylated salicylate such as salsalate or diflunisal may offer analgesia with a lower risk potential and fewer adverse effects and drug interactions. They have minimal effects on prostaglandin production.

Table 55-12

Analgesics for Patients Who Cannot Take Solid Oral Dosage Forms

Oral Liquids
Acetaminophen (elixir, liquid, solution, suspension, syrup)
Ibuprofen (suspension)
Naproxen (suspension)
Gabapentin (solution)
Pregabalin (solution)
Carbamazepine (suspension)
Oxcarbazepine (suspension)
Nortriptyline (solution)
Oxycodone (solution)
Hydrocodone/acetaminophen (elixir, solution)
Morphine (solution)
Methadone (solution)
Other Oral Products
Lamotrigine (disintegrating tablet)
Fentanyl (mucous membrane lozenge, buccal tablet, buccal film, sublingual)
Buprenorphine (sublingual tablet, buccal film)
Rectal Suppositories
Acetaminophen
Indomethacin
Hydromorphone
Morphine
Topicals
Diclofenac (gel)
Capsaicin (cream)
Local anesthetics (ointment, gel, cream)
Salicylates (gel, cream)
Transdermal Patches
Diclofenac
Lidocaine
Capsaicin
Methyl salicylate
Fentanyl
Buprenorphine

CASE 55-3, QUESTION 6: J.P. returns 6 months later, after seeing a pain specialist and a psychologist. He is now taking gabapentin 1,200 mg by mouth 3 times a day, meloxicam 7.5 mg by mouth once daily, amitriptyline 25 mg by mouth every night at bedtime, and oxycodone controlled-release (CR) 20 mg by mouth twice a day. How should J.P.'s therapy be monitored?

Clinicians must assess each part of J.P.'s care plan, both the positive aspects and the negative aspects. Is J.P. meeting his goals on his personal care plan? Is he getting more sleep? Is he more physically active? Is he managing his stressors better? Is his pain improved? There are several monitoring tools that may be used routinely to record long-term progress. The "5 A's" of monitoring therapy are often used: analgesia, activities of daily living, adverse effects, affect, and potential aberrant drug-related behavior.[92]

In addition to monitoring for efficacy, assessing for adverse effects of his medication is critical. Gabapentin may cause sedation, dizziness, edema, and cognitive impairment of short-term memory, concentration, and word-finding. Meloxicam, an NSAID, may cause GI upset or ulceration, so he should be advised to watch for black, tarry, sticky stools or any sign of internal bleeding. He may experience easy bruising and bleeding related to the platelet inhibitory effects of NSAIDs and should have his serum creatinine and potassium checked regularly to monitor for NSAID-induced renal toxicity. His blood pressure should also be monitored regularly because this has been elevated in the past. Oxycodone may cause constipation, sedation, dry mouth, and urinary retention. If he is using the opioid regularly, he should be advised to also use a bowel regimen with a stool softener, osmotic laxative, or a motility agent. Additionally, if he is using the opioid for an extended period of time, he may need to have his testosterone levels checked and bone density testing done periodically to monitor for hypogonadism and osteoporosis, which are associated with chronic opioid therapy. Amitriptyline may cause additive sedation, constipation, and urinary retention. He is unlikely to have problems with orthostatic hypotension, but this is common in older patients.

CASE 55-3, QUESTION 7: What nonpharmacologic therapies may be beneficial for J.P.'s pain?

Koes et al. found that most guidelines recommend a supervised exercise program, cognitive behavioral therapy, and short-term pharmacologic therapy.[65] The APS recommends that epidural steroid injections and possibly surgery may be considered in patients with persistent radicular low back pain. Because J.P. has radicular pain into his legs and he has tried first-line therapies, he may be a candidate for an epidural steroid injection. This will only offer temporary relief, at best, but may provide him enough relief to participate more in physical rehabilitation. Studies show mixed results with both injections and surgery, so J.P. must be part of the decision-making process.[93]

In the past, patients were advised to use bed rest for acute back pain; it is now recommended that patients remain physically active. This has been shown to improve pain and function at 3 to 4 weeks compared with bed rest.[94] Bed rest is also not recommended for chronic back pain. J.P. still has limited physical activity and was noted to be deconditioned. Inactivity can increase muscular pain. A referral for physical rehabilitation is a key component of management, specifically a supervised exercise regimen. There is no difference in benefit among different forms of exercise, so J.P. and his therapist may build a program that best fits his interests and needs. Physical rehabilitation also may include stretching and strengthening, but these are not effective unless used as part of a comprehensive exercise program. Other modalities such as cold packs to reduce inflammation in the acute phase of an injury and heat to relax muscles may be used, but there is no evidence supporting either of these therapies. Spine manipulation and low back corsets have shown some efficacy, but other physical modalities such as massage, ultrasound, traction, injections, acupuncture, or shoe lifts have not been shown to be effective.[70] J.P. may report that he has more pain after he starts an exercise regimen, because his muscles get reconditioned. J.P. should be encouraged and given assurances that physical activity that is at an appropriate level for his needs may cause him to hurt but will not harm him. He can also learn how to pace his activities so he does not overdo it with yard work as he has done in the past.

Cognitive behavioral therapy (CBT) and mindfulness-based stress reduction (MBSR) have been shown to improve back pain and functional limitations.[95] Mental health care is an essential component of multidisciplinary pain management. CBT works on a patient's perception of pain and expectations, focusing on mood, catastrophizing, negative thinking, and poor coping skills. MBSR focuses on increasing awareness and acceptance of moment-to-moment experiences including physical discomfort and difficult emotions. After J.P.'s depression is addressed, he can work with a therapist on coping skills and how to use self-regulation and manage stressors.

NEUROPATHIC PAIN AND POSTHERPETIC NEURALGIA

Pain may be centrally or peripherally mediated. Peripheral sensory neuropathy usually involves injury or insult to peripheral nerves, like postherpetic neuralgia (PHN), which affects spinal nerve dermatomes. The pain tends to be fairly localized, either regionally or along an associated dermatome. Central pain syndromes originate from injury to the CNS or alteration in central pain processing, as occurs with neuroplasticity. Central pain presents with a larger affected area, up to and including unilateral, head-to-toe pain that may be seen after a stroke.

Herpes zoster occurs in 500,000 Americans each year, and approximately 20% of these patients experience PHN.[96,97] Evidence-based guidelines for treating neuropathic pain have been sponsored by several international organizations in the last several years.[20] Most studies have been conducted in PHN and diabetic peripheral neuropathy (DPN), because these are the most common neuropathic pain conditions. Some types of neuropathic pain (e.g., spinal cord injury and human immunodeficiency virus neuropathy) have been quite resistant to pharmacologic therapy. Studies to date have shown only partial relief of neuropathic pain regardless of pharmacologic treatment. Doses, adverse effects, and monitoring for these agents can be found in Table 55-8.

First-line treatments for neuropathic pain include SNRI antidepressants such as TCAs, venlafaxine, and duloxetine. These antidepressants demonstrate effective pain relief, even in patients without concurrent depression. The TCAs are inexpensive and easily administered once daily; however, they have significant anticholinergic adverse effects, such as dry mouth and constipation that many patients do not tolerate. The secondary amine antidepressants, like nortriptyline, have fewer anticholinergic adverse effects than the parent compound amitriptyline and are similarly effective. TCAs are known to cause orthostatic hypotension and urinary retention in elderly patients and may cause cardiac arrhythmias with higher doses. Venlafaxine functions as an SSRI at low doses and needs to be titrated by 37.5- or 75-mg increments each week to reach a target dose of at least 200 mg daily. At this dose, venlafaxine offers SNRI activity. However, at higher doses (>225 mg/day), increases in blood pressure and heart rate caused by increased NE activity may cause patients to stop therapy. Duloxetine has shown efficacy in treating neuropathic pain with doses of 60 to 120 mg/day.[98] Cardiac rhythm, blood pressure, and pulse rate do not seem to be affected by duloxetine. The most common adverse effect with duloxetine is nausea on initiation and sweating. The dose of duloxetine is titrated up over 2 weeks to minimize the nausea. Duloxetine is contraindicated in patients with liver disease or those who drink alcohol, because there have been reports of liver failure with this medication.[99]

Anticonvulsants that bind to voltage-gated calcium channels are also considered first-line therapies for C fiber-related neuropathic pain (such as DPN and PHN), allodynia, and nonpainful dysesthesias (i.e., abnormal sensations). They have also been very helpful in reducing central sensitization by preventing the release of glutamate and blocking glutamate receptors. Gabapentin and pregabalin (gabapentinoids), both voltage-gated calcium-channel blockers, have shown efficacy and are FDA-approved for treating neuropathic pain, including PHN and DPN.[100–102] These agents must be taken 2 or 3 times daily and may cause dizziness, somnolence, peripheral edema, and cognitive problems. The somnolence is usually managed with a slow titration, but these combined effects may be significant in elderly patients. Although neither agent has many drug interactions, the doses must be reduced for renal insufficiency, because they are mostly renally eliminated.

Anticonvulsants that block sodium channels, such as carbamazepine, oxcarbazepine, and lamotrigine, have been shown to be helpful for A∂ fiber-mediated pain such as trigeminal neuralgia that has sharp, shooting qualities. Carbamazepine is an older agent that requires routine monitoring of complete blood counts (CBCs) for blood dyscrasias, liver transaminases for possible hepatitis, and serum sodium for possible syndrome of inappropriate antidiuretic hormone (SIADH)-induced hyponatremia. It is also a strong cytochrome P-450 enzyme inducer, and there are numerous drug–drug interactions with carbamazepine. Oxcarbazepine has substantially fewer drug interactions and does not require monitoring of CBCs and liver transaminases because it does not form the same 10,11-epoxide metabolite as carbamazepine. It requires monitoring of serum sodium for the first 3 months of therapy and periodically thereafter, because it may cause SIADH and hyponatremia. Lamotrigine has few drug interactions except with valproic acid and does not require any laboratory monitoring. It may, however, cause a desquamating rash (e.g., Stevens–Johnson syndrome) if the dose is escalated too quickly. A newer agent, lacosamide, shows modest efficacy for treating DPN but is not FDA-approved for treating pain.

Topical agents such as local anesthetics and capsaicin are effective for treating localized areas of neuropathic pain, such as PHN. A 5% lidocaine patch is approved by the FDA for the treatment of PHN and is particularly helpful for treating allodynia. It is very well tolerated and easy to apply. It may be cut to the desired shape, and very minimal local anesthetic penetrates the skin, so there is no systemic toxicity with proper administration. Various other topical lidocaine products are available (e.g., ointments and creams), but most do not penetrate the skin deep enough to reach the affected nerve endings. Capsaicin depletes substance P in the periphery and downregulates the transient receptor potential vanilloid 1 (TRPV1) receptors. Because it is derived from chili peppers, it causes a significant amount of burning until the substance P is depleted, and many patients do not tolerate the application of the cream several times daily to accomplish this. Capsaicin cream is available in several strengths, and there is an FDA-approved 8% patch available for medical office use which is applied for an hour under local anesthesia and can be reapplied once every 3 months.[103]

Opioid analgesics have shown moderate efficacy at best in treating neuropathic pain and are not usually considered first-line therapy because of potential long-term effects such as hyperalgesia, tolerance, immunosuppression, and hypogonadism with osteoporosis.[20] Tramadol and tapentadol, atypical opioids, have both opioid activity and SNRI activity and have been shown to be effective in several types of neuropathic pain. Their adverse effects are similar to those of both opioids and SNRIs, including constipation, sedation, and possibly seizures, which are a dose-limiting effect.[20,104]

When compared in a systematic review and meta-analysis, all of the first-line agents and most second-line agents were equally effective with no significant differences in safety.[20]

There are some data that show that a combination of agents, such as an opioid and a gabapentinoid, or a TCA and a gabapentinoid, may offer more analgesia than either agent alone.[90,91] This polypharmacy may offer additive analgesia because different agents act on different parts of the pain-signaling pathways. If more than one agent is used, lower doses of each may reduce adverse effects. However, polypharmacy adds complexity to regimens, which may reduce compliance and cause confusion, particularly in elderly patients.

Postherpetic Neuralgia

CASE 55-4

QUESTION 1: K.J. is a 73-year-old man with a history of Hodgkin lymphoma. He is in remission after chemotherapy and radiation treatment. He is seen in consult for PHN attributable to a case of shingles during chemotherapy. The zoster episode was after his first chemotherapy cycle 2 years ago. The lesions covered an area around his right lower abdomen below the umbilicus in a 10- to 15-cm strip around the lower back and buttock. At rest, his pain is a 1 to 2 out of 10 on the numerical pain scale. At its worst, it is 7 to 8 out of 10. Pain is aggravated by light touch or any jarring motion (such as riding in a car) or rubbing of clothes on the location of the zoster. He has two areas that have greater pain, one located in the lower right aspect of his back and the other in the right lower abdominal quadrant. He describes the pain as a burning sensation. He gets mild relief from topical aquaphilic ointment. If he stays busy, it sometimes takes his mind off the pain. He has not been sleeping well because of the pain. His past medical history includes Hodgkin lymphoma (in remission), low back pain, and benign prostatic hypertrophy (BPH). He currently takes acyclovir 400 mg by mouth once daily, alprazolam 0.25 mg by mouth every night at bedtime as needed for sleep, docusate 100 mg by mouth twice daily as needed for constipation, multivitamin one tablet by mouth once daily, tamsulosin 0.4 mg by mouth every night at bedtime, and zolpidem 5 mg by mouth every night at bedtime. K.J. is married, has never smoked, and denies alcohol and illicit drug use. His physical examination is unremarkable with the exception of scarring noted from the right lower abdomen to the back. Laboratory results and vital signs obtained at this visit are the following:

Serum creatinine, 1.2 mg/dL
Electrolytes, within normal limits
Blood pressure, 137/80 mm Hg
Heart rate, 77 beats/minute
Weight, 80 kg

Which of K.J.'s presenting symptoms are consistent with neuropathic pain and PHN?

K.J. is past the acute phase of his herpes zoster (shingles) pain, but now notices that the pain has a burning quality, localized over the region where his lesions have healed. This is quite typical for a PHN presentation. Another feature that indicates a neuropathic type of pain is his increase in pain with light touch or rubbing of his clothing (allodynia). It is a localized pain that does not radiate past the dermatomal distribution of his zoster infection. Opportunistic infections such as herpes zoster are common in patients who are immunocompromised such as K.J. when he was receiving chemotherapy.

CASE 55-4, QUESTION 2: What factors need to be considered when choosing a medication for K.J.? Which medication is the most appropriate option for treating K.J.'s PHN pain?

POSTHERPETIC NEURALGIA TREATMENT

The American Academy of Neurology (AAN) published PHN treatment guidelines in 2004. Since that time, there have been many more studies published, but there has been very little change in the approach to treating neuropathic pain. The AAN guidelines state that TCAs (e.g., amitriptyline, nortriptyline, and desipramine), gabapentin, pregabalin, opioids, and topical lidocaine patches are effective and should be used in the treatment of PHN.[105] The International Association for the Study of Pain has also published guidelines on the general treatment of neuropathic pain.[20]

Ideally, patients should be treated with the most effective therapy that has the lowest risk of adverse effects. K.J. has peripheral neuropathic pain in a localized area, which is typical of PHN, so a reasonable first-line choice would be a lidocaine patch; however, his pain is in a 10- to 12-cm strip that covers a fairly large surface area from his abdomen to his back. He would need to use at least two patches daily to cover this area, which is fewer than the maximal recommended dose of three patches daily, but it would be an effective barrier against the pain of clothing rubbing against this location. Another localized option would be capsaicin (either as a patch or a cream). Capsaicin cream is available over the counter and is substantially less expensive than lidocaine patches. Insurance plans may require a trial of capsaicin before approving the more expensive lidocaine patch. Unfortunately, many patients cannot tolerate the burning associated with capsaicin.

Another first-line option would be a TCA, which may help him sleep. However, he has BPH, and the anticholinergic effects of a TCA may cause increased urinary retention. These medications also cause orthostatic hypotension and may be a risk for K.J. if he has to get up during the night to use the bathroom (Table 55-8). An SNRI such as duloxetine would have fewer anticholinergic adverse effects but is not FDA-approved for treating PHN.

A calcium-channel blocking anticonvulsant such as gabapentin is also a possibility. The sedating effects of gabapentin may help him sleep if his last dose is given at bedtime, and would not cause the urinary retention, constipation, and orthostatic hypotension associated with TCA use. Given his age, a slow dose escalation starting at 100 mg by mouth 3 times a day would be appropriate. The most important aspect of monitoring for this agent would be for cognitive effects, such as short-term memory problems or difficulty with word-finding.

If the above options do not provide adequate analgesia, addition of an opioid such as morphine or oxycodone may be considered due to the potential for additive analgesia. Initially, a short-acting opioid should be used so that K.J. may be titrated to the optimal analgesic dose. Tramadol is another alternative with some TCA-like activity and mild opioid effects. However, if an opioid is added, it may increase the adverse effects of the above agents, including constipation, sedation, urinary retention, and cognitive effects. Whenever an opioid is added to a medication regimen, a bowel regimen must be implemented as well. A commonly used regimen includes a stool softener such as docusate sodium 100 mg by mouth twice daily or an osmotic agent such as polyethylene glycol 17 g by mouth daily and a mild stimulant laxative such as senna 8.6 mg one to two tablets by mouth once daily.

CASE 55-4, QUESTION 3: K.J. returns after 2 months with complaints that he could not tolerate the burning of the capsaicin cream so discontinued this. He is currently taking gabapentin 1,200 mg by mouth three times daily and tramadol 50 mg one tablet by mouth four times daily. He continues to have 5 of 10 burning pain over his right abdomen and back. He states that he has felt drowsy and has "unclear thoughts" with the gabapentin and does not feel that it has been very effective, despite titrating this to the maximal dose of 3,600 mg daily. His wife reports that he is withdrawing from friends and he does not feel as involved. He is sleeping better, however, and believes that the tramadol is somewhat helpful in "taking the edge off" his pain. Given this information, what would be an appropriate adjustment in his therapy?

MODIFYING THE NEUROPATHIC PAIN REGIMEN

Adverse cognitive effects like K.J. is having are common with anticonvulsants, especially in older patients. Problems with memory, concentration, and word-finding are common. No anticonvulsant is better than any other in this regard; however, some of the adverse effects are dose-related, and patients may exhibit tolerance to some of the effects (like sedation) with time. K.J. is at the maximal recommended daily dose of gabapentin and does not feel that this has been very helpful. At this time, he may need to be tapered off the gabapentin. Sometimes patients do not notice analgesic effects of their medications until they are discontinued. It is a good practice to titrate oral analgesics upward when starting therapy and downward when discontinuing, to avoid a marked increase in pain and withdrawal syndromes that have been reported with both antidepressants and some anticonvulsants. He could reduce his dose by 300 mg every 3 to 5 days until his pain increases or he is off the gabapentin.

A different topical agent would be the lidocaine patch. Because he and his wife are reporting some signs of depression, an antidepressant may be an option. An antidepressant was not chosen previously because of concerns about his BPH symptoms; however, a nontricyclic SNRI agent such as duloxetine may be an effective alternative to treat his depression as well as his pain, although there are no studies reporting its effectiveness for this indication. Another option may be to switch to another anticonvulsant. Pregabalin has very similar pharmacologic activity to gabapentin, so it may not offer any additional analgesia over gabapentin. Possibly, a sodium-channel blocking anticonvulsant such as oxcarbazepine could be used for a trial. However, there are minimal data supporting the sodium-channel blockers for typical C fiber-mediated pain associated with PHN.

CASE 55-4, QUESTION 4: K.J.'s doctor decides to order duloxetine and a lidocaine patch and taper off the gabapentin as tolerated. When the doctor orders K.J.'s new regimen, a drug–drug interaction listed between duloxetine and tramadol is identified. What recommendations are appropriate with regard to the potential drug–drug interactions with analgesics and, in particular, with K.J.'s regimen? What changes to his regimen could be suggested?

ANALGESIC DRUG–DRUG INTERACTIONS

Antidepressants either increase the concentrations of NE or 5-HT or both. Opioids also have serotonergic effects, so it is possible to have a net excess of either of these neurotransmitters, or both. The consequence of an excess of NE is CNS excitation and possible seizures. The consequence of an excess of 5-HT is a possibly life-threatening syndrome called *serotonin syndrome.* Symptoms of serotonin syndrome include muscle rigidity, hyperpyrexia, mental status changes, and possible organ failure. None of these serious adverse effects are very predictable, although they are more likely with higher doses of either agent. If opioids are used with antidepressants, the lowest effective doses should be used, and patients should be counseled to watch for mental status changes.

Pharmacodynamic interactions are more likely to occur with analgesic polypharmacy. Because several analgesics may be used together to decrease the excitatory effects of the pain signal, there is always a risk of additive sedation, dizziness, or even respiratory depression. Several pharmacokinetic drug–drug interactions may occur with analgesics as well. In K.J.'s case, his duloxetine and tramadol are both substrates of cytochrome P-450 2D6 and may compete with each other for this enzyme. This may alter the blood levels and clinical effects of these agents. A table of agents commonly used in pain management, the relevant cytochrome P450 enzyme involved in its metabolism, and potential drug interactions can be found in Table 55-13. K.J. likely needs an antidepressant for his depression symptoms, so alternatives will need to be considered.

Table 55-13
Drug Interactions with Analgesics

CYP1A2	CYP2C9	CYP2C19	CYP2D6	CYP3A4
Substrates				
Amitriptyline	Amitriptyline	Amitriptyline	Amitriptyline, mexiletine	Alprazolam, methadone
Naproxen	Celecoxib	Citalopram	Nortriptyline, morphine	Amitriptyline, prednisone
R-warfarin	Diclofenac	Diazepam	Cyclobenzaprine, codeine	Buspirone, sertraline
Duloxetine	Fluoxetine	Indomethacin	Desipramine, oxycodone	Clonazepam, temazepam
Methadone	Ibuprofen	Topiramate	Doxepin, paroxetine	Codeine, zaleplon
Theophylline	Naproxen		Fluoxetine, sertraline	Cyclobenzaprine, zolpidem
Tizanidine	Piroxicam		Hydrocodone, tramadol	Diazepam, R-warfarin
	S-warfarin		Methadone, venlafaxine	Fentanyl, carbamazepine
	Phenytoin		Fentanyl, duloxetine	Lidocaine, erythromycin
Inducers				
Carbamazepine	Carbamazepine	Carbamazepine	Carbamazepine	Carbamazepine
Phenytoin	Fluoxetine	Phenytoin	Phenytoin	Oxcarbazepine
	Cimetidine			Phenytoin
	Metronidazole			
	Fluconazole			
Inhibitors				
Cimetidine	Carbamazepine	Fluoxetine	Celecoxib	Fluoxetine
Ciprofloxacin	Paroxetine	Indomethacin	Desipramine	Sertraline
	Sertraline	Paroxetine	Fluoxetine	Ketoconazole
	Valproic acid	Topiramate	Methadone	Cyclosporine
	Phenytoin		Paroxetine	
			Sertraline	
			Valproic acid	

CYP, cytochrome P-450.

CENTRAL NEUROPATHIC PAIN: POSTSTROKE PAIN

Pain is one of the most distressing symptoms after a stroke. As mentioned previously, poststroke pain is a central pain syndrome, caused by a lesion in the CNS. Sometimes the cause of central pain syndromes cannot be identified, and even though a stroke presents with a specific lesion, it is still very difficult to treat. There are several different types of pain after a stroke and patients may have more than one type. Nociceptive pain may be related to immobilization, spasticity, and/or muscle contraction in the event of limb paresis. The shoulder is the most common location but musculoskeletal/myofascial pain can occur in the upper back and neck, as well as tension-type headache. The lower extremities may be affected by weakness, muscle spasms, and/or arthralgias from joint disuse. However, by far the most difficult and far-reaching pain is central neuropathic pain generated in the CNS, which is called central poststroke pain (CPSP). CPSP has been reported in as many as 1% to 18% of stroke survivors.[106] The diagnostic criteria for CPSP are as follows: (1) pain within an area of the body corresponding to the lesion of the CNS; (2) history suggestive of stroke and onset of pain at or after stroke onset; (3) confirmation of a CNS lesion by imaging or negative or positive sensory signs confined to the area of the body corresponding to the lesion; and (4) other causes of pain, such as nociceptive or peripheral neuropathic pain, that are excluded or considered highly unlikely.[107] The clinical presentation of CPSP is similar to other neuropathic pain. The onset of pain ranges from immediate to several months after stroke. It may affect a small region of the body or a large area (from head to toe). Central pain after a contralateral stroke is quite common, particularly after thalamic strokes (e.g., patients with a stroke in the left side of the brain will have symptoms on the right side of the body). Because the thalamus is the brain's "relay station," any abnormal signaling may be amplified.[108] Temperature-sensory dysregulation via the spinothalamic tract is common, as well as dysesthesias and allodynia. It is described as "burning," "aching," "squeezing," "pricking," or "cold." These symptoms are frequently aggravated by a cold environment, psychological stress, heat, fatigue, or body movement.

Treatment of CPSP

There are no guidelines for management of CPSP, and few robust studies exist but lack data related to comparative efficacy. Therapy is usually done on a trial and error basis. Current data support use of amitriptyline (with titration from 10 mg/day up to 100 mg/day) as first-line therapy.[109] Nortriptyline may be used as an alternative TCA in patients who do not tolerate amitriptyline. SNRIs have been shown to be beneficial for other types of neuropathic pain but not for CPSP. If pain relief is insufficient, an anticonvulsant may be used. Lamotrigine (titrated to 400 mg/day) may be added or exchanged for the TCA. It has been shown to have some efficacy for CPSP and was fairly well tolerated.[110] Other anticonvulsants that have shown efficacy for both central and peripheral neuropathic pain are listed in Table 55-8.[111] Opioids have been studied in patients with CPSP but were not effective, and there was a high withdrawal rate.[112] Other therapies such as intravenous infusions of lidocaine, morphine, and ketamine are only experimental and are not recommended. It is not unusual to combine agents with different mechanisms of action, though there are no data supporting this for CPSP. Monotherapy should be titrated to the maximum recommended dose.

Nociceptive pain such as shoulder pain related to stroke may be treated with acetaminophen or local/topical agents. NSAIDs are contraindicated due to the increased risk of myocardial infarction and stroke; however, salicylates may be considered. Muscle spasms or spasticity is common after a stroke, and this is usually treated with an antispasticity agent such as baclofen or tizanidine. Skeletal muscle relaxants are generally not effective for long-term use.

Nonpharmacologic therapies for CPSP include deep brain stimulation, motor cortex stimulation, and transcranial magnetic stimulation. Physical rehabilitation (physical and occupational) is essential to help improve function and cognitive behavioral therapy is used to help patients cope with their new circumstances and cognitive or physical limitations.

CASE 55-5

QUESTION 1: W.J. is a 50-year-old man with a history of a right cerebellar ischemic stroke 4 years ago. He initially presented with sudden onset neck pain, nausea, vomiting, and dizziness. Since his stroke, he has had body tingling including all four extremities and his spine. He also has some localized throbbing pain in his neck and headaches. He reports some spontaneous jerking and muscle spasms that affect his extremities (mostly the right side) and sometimes down his back. He notes some right side weakness as well with muscle atrophy. He also describes chronic tinnitus, dizziness, and headache with sharp eye pain (vision is normal per recent eye examination). He has chronic intermittent nystagmus described as eye "throbbing" when looking to the periphery on either side. He has headaches several times a week (frontotemporal and unilateral). Phono- and photophobia are significant when they occur. He has nausea, but rarely emesis. He reports increased pain with cold weather and stress.

He has a past medication history of HTN, type 2 diabetes mellitus, and depression. He takes aspirin 325 mg by mouth daily, insulin glargine 72 units subcutaneously every morning, insulin lispro sliding scale subcutaneously 3 times daily, atorvastatin 20 mg by mouth every night at bedtime, and sertraline 200 mg by mouth once daily. He does not drink alcohol but is a former smoker (quit 5 years ago). He used to work in a factory but had to quit because he fell several times at work. MRI of the neck showed only a mild disc bulge at C5–C6.

He was holding his head in his hands, wincing periodically. Otherwise his physical examination was unremarkable.

He had reduced vibratory sensation in toes and feet to ankles. His neck was tender to palpation and he had some reduced range of motion. His gait was normal but slow but reports being very unsteady on his feet. His vital signs today are as follows:

Blood pressure, 126/75 mm Hg
Heart rate, 72 beats/minute
Respiratory rate, 16 breaths/minute
Weight 149 kg
His pain rating is 9 out of 10.
What symptoms does W.J. have that are consistent with CPSP?

Although W.J. does not have shoulder pain which may be present in CPSP, W.J. has some localized neck pain. He does not have any obvious injury (e.g., from a fall). Because he has not been very active, and he sits with his head in his hands or bowed forward, his neck pain is most likely myofascial. He has frequent headaches that he localizes to his frontotemporal area.

Because W.J.'s stroke was in his cerebellum, he has notable problems with balance and vertigo as well as tinnitus. These are not painful but are disturbing and limit his functionality and predispose him to falling, which may cause injury. He has intermittent nystagmus which he describes as throbbing. His vision and hearing were within normal limits so his symptoms are sensory only.

Since his stroke, W.J. has had body tingling affecting all four extremities. He reports some spontaneous jerking and muscle spasms that affect his extremities (mostly the right side) and right-sided weakness as well, with some muscle atrophy, and he reports that this is his most painful and bothersome symptom; however, on physical examination there is not notable spasticity. He was noted to have decreased vibratory sensation in his feet and ankles bilaterally. The bilateral presentation is more consistent with his diabetes. He describes more pain with changes in the weather and stress, but this is not specific for CPSP.

CASE 55-5, QUESTION 2: Considering W.J.'s comorbidities, what should be recommended for treating his pain?

Treatment goals for W.J. and any stroke patient are to (1) reduce discomfort and suffering, (2) improve or regain as much function as possible, and (3) improve coping. Because there is so little known about what causes CPSP, it is difficult to tailor analgesic therapy. W.J. has diabetes with symptoms suggestive of diabetic neuropathy. Amitriptyline is considered a first-line therapy for CPSP as well as diabetic neuropathy. Tricyclic antidepressants are also used for depression (though at a higher dose) and for headache prophylaxis. It is unknown whether the anticholinergic effects of the TCA will affect his balance issues, because it may cause orthostatic hypotension. Of concern is his current use of a rather high dose of sertraline. SSRIs do not offer any significant analgesia, and the SSRI and TCA combination will provide additive serotonergic effects, putting W.J. at risk for serotonin syndrome (Table 55-13). A discussion with his mental healthcare provider is warranted to review potential analgesic options, including a trial of an SNRI such as duloxetine. Alternatively, the gabapentinoids may be helpful for his diabetic neuropathy, though there is less support for CPSP. Lamotrigine is likely a slightly more effective choice for CPSP, but lacks robust data for use in diabetic neuropathy. There do not appear to be any drug interactions or contraindications for either type of anticonvulsant.

W.J. has some musculoskeletal neck pain and may benefit from a trial of acetaminophen or salicylates or a topical analgesic; however, NSAIDs are contraindicated due to his history of stroke. He also has some intermittent muscle spasms that are quite bothersome for him. Typically, the antispasticity agents are useful so he may benefit from a trial of tizanidine or baclofen (Table 55-11). Nonpharmacologic therapies such as heat, massage, and physical therapy may be most effective.

FUNCTIONAL PAIN SYNDROMES (FPS)

Functional pain syndromes are a cluster of disorders for which the pathophysiologic mechanisms have not been clearly defined to explain the symptoms.[113] FPS includes medically unexplained symptoms for both gastrointestinal and nongastrointestinal disorders such as dyspepsia, irritable bowel syndrome, fibromyalgia, chronic fatigue, and interstitial cystitis. There can be overlap in the syndromes with the presentation of chronic pain and associated psychiatric comorbidities including depression, anxiety, and posttraumatic stress disorder (PTSD).[114,115]

Pain that does not conform to anatomic or neurophysiologic findings is often attributed to psychopathology. Somatic symptom disorder (SSD) is a diagnostic entity in the fifth edition of the Diagnostic and Statistical Manual of Mental Disorders that replaced somatoform disorder terms including pain disorder, somatization disorder, and undifferentiated somatoform.[116] Somatic symptoms associated with significant distress and disruption of daily life are common with FPS. Patients with FPS often have health concerns manifested by disproportionate and persistent thoughts of serious symptoms, a high level of anxiety about symptoms, and excessive time and energy devoted to health concerns.[116,117]

Fibromyalgia is a chronic debilitating condition with the primary symptoms of chronic widespread pain and fatigue. It affects between 3 and 6 million people in the United States, an incidence of 4.9% in women and 2.9% in men.[118] Out of pocket healthcare costs for patients with fibromyalgia is 3 times those without fibromyalgia.[119] It is defined by the American College of Rheumatology (ACR) as pain that is both chronic (lasting longer than 3 months) and widespread (above and below the waist and on both sides of the body). The ACR has published new diagnostic criteria in 2010. They propose using a widespread pain index, in which patients indicate how many areas of their body have pain, and a symptom severity scale, in which patients rate the severity of fatigue, waking unrefreshed, and cognitive and somatic symptoms.[120] Fibromyalgia was previously thought to be peripherally mediated pain related to an inflammatory or muscular disorder, but it has been shown that it may be the manifestation of CNS neurotransmitter dysfunction. Patients with fibromyalgia are more likely to have suffered a traumatic event previously, such as a motor vehicle accident or childhood sexual abuse.[121] Studies have shown an imbalance in neurotransmitters in which excitatory neurotransmitters in the CNS of fibromyalgia patients are increased, including glutamate (a twofold increase) and substance P (a threefold increase), and inhibitory neurotransmitters, NE and 5-HT, are decreased. Patients with fibromyalgia have an enhanced perception of pain at substantially lower forces and at a lower frequency of stimulation than control patients. Pain sensation has a greater amplitude and is more prolonged.[122] Input may be from the periphery or may be triggered by a central stimulus such as a stressor.[123] Heightened sensitivity to lower stimulus seems to contribute to the persistent pain with these patients.[124] This can be widespread and symptoms seem to be largely affected by an exaggerated response to personal stressors, noxious stimuli (hyperalgesia), and non-noxious sensory stimuli (allodynia). Fibromyalgia, as a functional pain syndrome, is associated with other comorbidities that need to be addressed for symptom management, even though treating these symptoms may not directly benefit the hallmark tenderness associated with the syndrome. The assessment tool most often used to assess the impact of fibromyalgia on daily life and function is called the Fibromyalgia Impact Questionnaire (FIQ) (Fig. 55-6).[125]

Fibromyalgia

CASE 55-6

QUESTION 1: G.R. is a 38-year-old woman who presents with chronic widespread muscle pain from her neck down past her buttocks. She also has headaches when her pain is severe. She has had this pain for several years and notes that her pain developed after a car accident in which she sustained a whiplash injury. She describes difficulty sleeping, poor concentration, and fatigue. Her pain rating is 8 out of 10 on most days. She works part time doing some home transcription. She has not identified anything that helps her pain, and physical activity makes the pain worse, so she does not exercise. Her pain is also worse when she is stressed. She was previously told that she has fibromyalgia, and while others have told her that "it's all in her head." Her past medical history includes depression and IBS. She has tried ibuprofen, cyclobenzaprine, carisoprodol, and acetaminophen in the past without relief. She is currently taking tramadol 50 mg by mouth 4 times daily, which provides about 20% pain relief. She is also taking sertraline for depression. G.R. is married and has three children. She smokes one

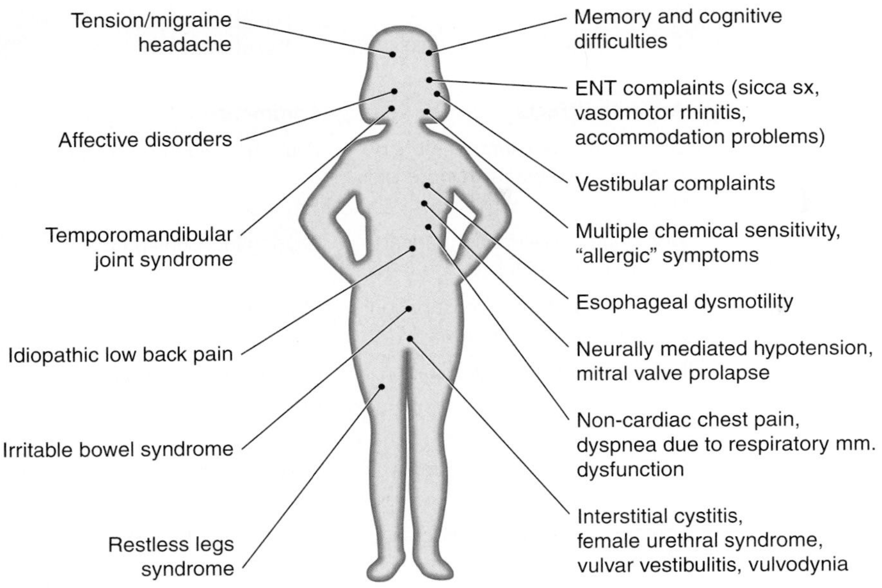

Figure 55-6 Systemic conditions that overlap with fibromyalgia. (Reprinted with permission from Clauw DJ. Fibromyalgia. In: Fishman SM et al, eds. *Bonica's Management of Pain*. 4th ed. Philadelphia, PA: Lippincott Williams & Wilkins; 2010:474.)

pack of cigarettes daily but denies drinking alcohol or using illicit drugs. She reports that her mother and sister have fibromyalgia and depression. She reports diffuse tenderness to palpation along her paraspinal muscles bilaterally, as well as her bilateral trapezius and levator scapulae muscles and her hips bilaterally. Several tender points are elicited. Her only remarkable laboratory result is vitamin D, 24 ng/mL (normal >30 ng/mL).

What part of G.R's presentation supports the presence of a functional pain syndrome?

G.R. likely has fibromyalgia, given her widespread pain that has been present for more than 3 months and was precipitated by a traumatic event (car accident). She reports sleeping poorly, fatigue, and the comorbidities of depression and IBS. On physical examination, she exhibits widespread musculoskeletal tenderness including, but not limited to, several of the identified fibromyalgia tender points, bilaterally, both above and below the waist. Her vitamin D level represents a mild deficiency.

Case 55-6, Question 2: What pharmacologic and nonpharmacologic therapies could be recommended for G.R.?

There have been several evidence-based guidelines published for the treatment of fibromyalgia.[126–130] These guidelines recommended a multidisciplinary approach with pharmacologic and nonpharmacologic therapy. Because evidence indicates a CNS neurotransmitter imbalance, the most effective pharmacologic approaches have targeted these imbalances. Antidepressants have been shown to reduce pain and improve function by increasing levels of 5-HT and NE in the CNS. Historically, the tricyclics (most commonly amitriptyline) have been shown to moderately improve pain, sleep, and to a smaller extent on fatigue and health-related quality of life (HRQOL). SSRIs have also shown some improvement in pain, depression, and HRQOL but the effect sizes were quite small.[131] Duloxetine and milnacipran are both SNRIs that are FDA-approved for fibromyalgia. Milnacipran appears to have more NE activity than duloxetine. This difference does not appear to confer a therapeutic difference. Both of these agents improve average pain scores, FIQ scores, physical functioning, and overall sense of well-being (Table 55-14).[132,133]

Gabapentinoids have been shown to reduce the activity of excitatory neurotransmitters, particularly glutamate. Pregabalin is an anticonvulsant that was approved by the FDA in 2007 for treating fibromyalgia. It targets the increased levels of glutamate in the CNS by binding to the $\alpha_2\delta$ subunit of voltage-gated calcium channels, preventing release of glutamate from presynaptic terminals (Fig. 55-3). This agent has been shown to improve average pain scores and patient perception of improvement, but failed to show improvement in FIQ scores.[134,135] A long-term open-label study found that patients who did well in the short term maintained an improvement in pain for up to 6 months compared with placebo.[136] Gabapentin, a similar compound, has not been formally approved for fibromyalgia but has support for its use. Some insurance companies require a trial with gabapentin before allowing use of pregabalin because of its lower cost.[137] Hauser et al. compared duloxetine, milnacipran, and pregabalin in fibromyalgia and found that duloxetine and pregabalin were better than milnacipran in improving pain and sleep.[138] Duloxetine was better for symptoms of depression, and pregabalin and milnacipran were better for fatigue. Headache and nausea were more common with duloxetine and milnacipran, and diarrhea was more common with duloxetine.

Other drug therapies that have shown some benefit in treating fibromyalgia and its comorbidities include pramipexole, a dopamine agonist, which is beneficial in treating restless legs symptoms, as well as pain and fatigue.[139] NSAIDs, acetaminophen, and opioids are not recommended for treating fibromyalgia pain.[126–130] In fact, Goldenberg, et al. conducted a literature review and found no evidence from clinical trials that opioids are effective for the treatment of FM. The studies reviewed found that patients with FM receiving opioids had poorer outcomes than those receiving nonopioids.[140] More recently, data have been published noting the effectiveness of low-dose naltrexone, an opioid Mu-receptor agonist, in pain reduction, as well as improvement in general satisfaction with life and mood.[141]

An appropriate first step for G.R. is to develop a multidisciplinary approach, including physical rehabilitation, CBT, and pharmacologic therapy adjustments. She is currently taking an antidepressant (sertraline), which may be helpful for her depression but is likely not very helpful for her fibromyalgia. It may be possible to switch her to an SNRI such as duloxetine or milnacipran in consultation with her mental healthcare provider. She is currently taking tramadol with some relief. She has not maximized her dose (maximum daily dose is 400 mg); however, she is also taking an SSRI, which may place her at a higher risk of serotonin syndrome. The risks and benefits of combining antidepressants

Table 55-14
Pharmacologic Treatment of Fibromyalgia

Drug	Oral Dose	Adverse Effects	Comments
Amitriptyline	25–50 mg QHS	Dry mouth, constipation, urinary retention, orthostatic hypotension, somnolence	Caution in elderly patients
Cyclobenzaprine	10–30 mg QHS	Dry mouth, constipation, urinary retention, somnolence	Caution in elderly patients
Duloxetine[a]	30 mg daily × 1 week, then 60 mg daily	Nausea, dry mouth, constipation, fatigue, sweating, anorexia	Monitor liver transaminases
Milnacipran[a]	12.5 mg × 1 day, then 12.5 mg BID × 2 days, then 25 mg BID × 4 days, then 50 mg BID, may titrate to 100 mg BID	Nausea, headache, constipation, insomnia, hot flushes	Monitor blood pressure, heart rate
Pregabalin[a]	75 mg BID, titrate to 150 mg TID	Somnolence, dizziness, edema, cognitive effects	Reduce dose for renal impairment
Gabapentin	300 mg QHS, titrate to 600 mg TID	Somnolence, dizziness, edema, cognitive effects	Reduce dose for renal impairment

[a]Food and Drug Administration–approved to treat fibromyalgia.
BID, 2 times a day; QHS, every night at bedtime; TID, 3 times a day.

with tramadol must be considered on a patient-by-patient basis. Because she is having trouble sleeping, she could be offered a trial of amitriptyline or pregabalin, both of which have sedating side effects (Table 55-7). Pregabalin is a recommended agent and has a different mechanism of action than the medications that she has previously tried. If cost of therapy is a concern, then gabapentin could be tried instead. A vitamin D supplement should also be considered to correct her slightly low vitamin D levels. There is not strong evidence supporting vitamin D supplementation, but there is little harm in correcting her slight deficiency.

Bernardy et al. conducted a systematic review of CBT for fibromyalgia and found that this therapy improves coping with pain and reduces depressed mood and health-care-seeking behavior.[142] Hauser et al. evaluated different regimens of aerobic activity with a meta-analysis and found that land- and water-based aerobic exercise, at a slight to moderate intensity, 2 to 3 times a week for at least 4 weeks resulted in improvement of depressed mood and increased health-related quality of life scores and physical fitness. This was maintained if the patient continued exercise at home.[143] Aquatic training is beneficial for improving wellness, symptoms, and fitness in adults with fibromyalgia.[144] Luciano et al found that CBT is more cost-effective that routine FDA-approved medications for adult FM patients.[145]

Psychological Comorbidity and Opioid Risk Management

CASE 55-7

QUESTION 1: M.T. is a 33-year-old woman with chronic abdominal pain. She first experienced recurrent episodes of abdominal pain at the age of 13 after menarche. At age 21, she was diagnosed with acute pancreatitis secondary to alcohol use. Her pain has persisted despite numerous trials of medications including gabapentin, sertraline, tramadol, and hydrocodone/acetaminophen. She has undergone multiple diagnostic evaluations for the abdominal pain, but all have resulted in negative findings. During the past year, M.T. has had eight visits to the emergency department for severe pain where she usually receives IV hydromorphone and then is discharged with a week's supply of oxycodone/acetaminophen. In addition to the emergency department visits, she has been hospitalized 3 times in the past year for abdominal pain.

Today, M.T. is being seen in the clinic by her primary care physician for continued management of chronic abdominal pain, which she describes as "constantly aching." Over the past 2 years, M.T.'s primary care physician has been prescribing oxycodone in conjunction with an opioid agreement focused on minimizing the use of emergency department visits for pain management. M.T. believes her current management with oxycodone 5 mg by mouth every 4 hours as needed for severe pain is insufficient and would like the 30-day supply limit increased from 180 to 240 tablets.

The primary care physician is concerned about M.T.'s functional status since starting opioid therapy. There has been no noticeable improvement in M.T.'s pain despite three increases in the 30-day oxycodone supply over the past 2 years. During the office visit, M.T. is emotionally labile at times and tearful when discussing her pain but is emphatic that she is not depressed. She states that she drinks one or two "highballs" (whisky and soda) about 2 times a week to help her relax when she is feeling "stressed out." M.T. denies smoking or illicit drug use. She is currently unemployed and seeking permanent disability because the pain interferes with her ability to work. Her physical examination is unremarkable except for diffuse abdominal tenderness.

What is the clinical relevance of M.T.'s self-description of abdominal pain?

Clinical Relevance of Abdominal Pain

M.T.'s self-report of pain is consistent with functional abdominal pain (FAP). FAP is more common in women and peaks around the fourth decade of life. Patients with FAP have high work absenteeism and healthcare utilization.[114,146] Key features in the diagnosis of FAP include abdominal pain that is present for at least 6 months and is not related to gastrointestinal function. The patient will often have a decrease in daily activity with time. The principal criterion differentiating FAP from other gastrointestinal disorders, such as pancreatitis, is constant pain that lacks symptom relationship to food intake or defecation. Psychological

Table 55-15
Symptom-Related Behaviors of Functional Abdominal Pain

Expressing pain of varying intensity through verbal and nonverbal methods
Urgent reporting of intense symptoms disproportionate to available clinical and laboratory data
Minimizing or denying a role for psychosocial contributors, anxiety, depression; attributing symptoms of anxiety or depression to presence of pain
Requesting diagnostic studies or surgery to validate the condition as "organic"
Focusing attention on complete relief of symptoms
Seeking healthcare frequently
Taking limited personal responsibility for self-management
Making requests for narcotic analgesics when other treatment options have been implemented

disturbances are more likely when pain has persisted for a long period and manifests as symptom-related behaviors that dominate a patient's life (Table 55-15).[117,146]

From the physiologic perspective, M.T.'s abdominal pain most likely originated from a combination of somatic and visceral components associated with menses and pancreatitis. When the pain symptoms occur frequently in conjunction with a stressor as in FAP, the main mechanism for altered pain regulation relates to the failure to inhibit the amplification of normal regulatory afferent input from the gut to central mechanisms in the prefrontal, cingulated cortex, and limbic structures (e.g., cognitive and emotions centers of the brain). This impairment in homeostatic inhibition of pain may be related to low levels of 5-HT, NE, endorphin, and other neuropeptides that mediate descending pain transmission in the CNS. Recognition of the brain–gut axis in FAP is essential to understanding its clinical presentation, diagnosis, and therapeutic strategies.[15,113]

FUNCTIONAL ABDOMINAL PAIN TREATMENT

CASE 55-7, QUESTION 2: What are the current recommendations for pharmacologic treatment of FAP? What approaches to the management of FAP are appropriate for M.T.?

Pharmacotherapy for patients with FAP is empirical and not based on results from well-designed clinical trials. Clinical trials have not been targeted to this diagnostic entity, so treatments are typically designed on the basis of data from other chronic pain disorders. The cornerstone to management depends on an effective relationship between the clinician and patient. In this case, the primary care physician needs to listen to M.T.'s concerns but set realistic and consistent limits when ordering tests, medical interventions, and medications. M.T. needs to be an active participant in the pain management plan and take responsibility for self-care.[117,146]

Antidepressants, such as TCAs in low daily dosages, may be useful in treating FAP for both pain and depression owing to their combined noradrenergic and serotonergic effects.[147] In other chronic pain conditions, TCAs generally have been more successful than using SSRIs.[128] Medications with combined 5-HT and NE reuptake activity (e.g., SNRIs such as venlafaxine and duloxetine) have recognized pain-reducing effects with somatic pain conditions and may be useful in FAP. To ensure treatment adherence, M.T. needs affirmation that antidepressant is not prescribed simply to treat depression. It is important that the clinician educate the patient on the role of antidepressants in the treatment of pain. Patient education resources such as diagrams help to show the physiologic basis for treatment of pain and describe descending inhibitory pathways.[117,148]

Gabapentin and pregabalin clinical trials have established their efficacy for neuropathic pain and fibromyalgia, but benefit for visceral or central pain syndromes is not established. NSAIDs offer little benefit because their action is located in the peripheral nervous system. Long-term treatment with benzodiazepines is not recommended because of the abuse potential and tendency to interact with other medications. For patients who are refractory to usual doses of antidepressant medication, referral to psychiatry should be made for treatment with atypical antipsychotic agents such as quetiapine.[117,148]

Risk of Addiction

CASE 55-7, QUESTION 3: There is concern about M.T.'s use of alcohol and escalating use of opioid medication. What is the risk that M.T. will become addicted to opioids?

Opioid use behaviors are stratified based on the risk of aberrant drug use. Aberrant drug use behaviors may occur along a spectrum from those less suggestive of addiction, such as an occasional, sanctioned increase in the opioid dose by a medical provider, to those that may be more suggestive of addiction, such as injecting oral formulations. Table 55-16 provides a list of risk factors for opioid misuse.[148,150] Important but less consistent risk factors include pain-related functional impairment such as sleep disturbance, mental health issues, history of child sexual abuse or neglect, and legal problems.[151,152] With respect to gender, women with chronic pain who report significant emotional issues were at increased risk for opioid misuse.[153]

M.T. has multiple behaviors in which some are more indicative of addiction such as concomitant alcohol use whereas others can be explained given the etiology of FAP. For example, high healthcare utilization for pain validation is common in patients with FAP. Also, aggressive complaining about the need for more opioid medication may be driven by M.T.'s perception that the current dose prescribed by her primary care physician no longer relieves her pain, implying tolerance has developed (Table 55-17).[149,154]

The factor that is most concerning for addiction is M.T.'s continued use of alcohol despite previous pancreatitis and

Table 55-16
Risk Factors for Opioid Addiction[149,150]

Concurrent abuse of alcohol or illicit drugs
Evidence of a deterioration in the ability to function at work, in the family, or socially that appears to be related to drug use
Injecting oral formulations
Multiple dose escalations or other nonadherence with therapy despite warnings
Obtaining prescription drugs from nonmedical sources
Prescription forgery
Repeated resistance to changes in therapy despite clear evidence of physical or psychological effects
Repeatedly seeking prescriptions from other physicians or emergency departments
Selling prescription drugs
Stealing or borrowing drugs from others

Table 55-17
Terms Related to Opioid Use[149,154]

Term	Definition
Misuse	Taking a prescription for a reason or at a dose or frequency other than for which it was prescribed. Use of a medication for a nonmedical use, or for reasons other than prescribed. For example, altering dosing or sharing medicines, which has harmful or potentially harmful consequences.
Abuse	Misuse with consequences involving the use of a substance to modify or control mood or state of mind in a manner that is illegal or harmful to oneself or others. Potentially harmful consequences include accidents, injuries, blackouts, legal problems, and sexual behavior that increases the risk of infectious diseases.
Addiction	A primary, chronic, neurobiologic disease with genetic, psychosocial, and environmental factors influencing its development and manifestations. It is characterized by behaviors that include one or more of the following: impaired control over drug use, compulsive use, continued use despite harm, and craving.
Physical dependence	A state of adaptation manifested by a drug class–specific withdrawal syndrome that can be produced by abrupt cessation, rapid dose reduction, decreasing blood level of the drug, or administration of an antagonist.
Pseudoaddiction	Condition characterized by behaviors that outwardly mimic addiction but are in fact driven by a desire for pain relief (e.g., constantly watching the clock to dose medication "on time" so pain does not become severe).[151]
Tolerance	A state of adaptation in which exposure to a drug induces changes that result in a diminution of one or more opioid effects with time.

misusing it to treat anxiety. There is also a risk of increased opioid side effects, especially sedation and respiratory depression, with concurrent use of alcohol. Multiple literature reports have confirmed there is a strong association between alcohol abuse and opioid addiction.[155,156] Guidelines for chronic opioid therapy strongly recommend clinicians conduct a risk assessment of substance abuse, misuse, or addiction before initiating opioid therapy.[50]

Assessment of Chronic Opioid Therapy

Case 55-7, Question 4: M.T. would like to continue with opioid therapy despite the concerns of her primary care physician. Is M.T. a candidate for chronic opioid therapy?

The Centers for Disease Control released new recommendations for opioid therapy that support the establishment of a treatment plan with the patient before starting opioid therapy that includes realistic goals for pain and function along with consideration of when therapy will be discontinued if benefits do not outweigh risks. Clinicians should continue opioid therapy only if there is clinically meaningful improvement in pain and function that outweighs risks to patient safety.[50] In the case of MT, a pain agreement (e.g., contract) should be established even if the goal is to eventually discontinue opioid therapy. There are multiple sources in the literature for information and guidelines on written agreements between the clinician and patient for chronic opioid therapy (COT).

The written COT agreement should include goals of therapy, how opioids will be prescribed and taken, expectations for follow-up and monitoring, alternatives to COT, expectations regarding use of concomitant therapies, and potential for tapering the regimen and discontinuing.[150] Indications for tapering and/or discontinuation of the opioid include failure to make progress toward therapeutic goals, intolerable adverse effects, or repeated or serious aberrant drug-related behaviors. Patient compliance requirements within the written agreement should include random urine drug screens for illicit substances or opioids obtained from other sources and limited prescribing (e.g., reduced quantities, biweekly prescribing) to help the patient manage use if necessary. In this case, M.T. has not made progress in meeting the goal of decreased emergency department utilization, she continues to use alcohol with her medication, and she has been resistant to trying other therapies despite the ineffectiveness of opioids in treating her pain. These behaviors would indicate M.T. is not a candidate for COT.

Screening tools that assess the potential risks for opioid misuse based on patient characteristics are helpful in determining eligibility for COT. Patient self-report questionnaires for assessing risk of aberrant drug-related behavior include the Screener and Opioid Assessment for Patients with Pain-Revised (SOAPP-R) and the Opioid Risk Tool (ORT).[150,154,157]

The Diagnosis, Intractability, Risk, Efficacy (DIRE) tool is a clinician evaluation instrument designed to assess the potential efficacy of chronic opioid therapy as well as harm.[158] In M.T.'s case, her DIRE score is 10, which would indicate she is not a suitable candidate for long-term opioid therapy. M.T.'s DIRE score and assessment are shown in Table 55-18.

Discontinuing Opioid Therapy

Case 55-7, Question 5: M.T. is going to be discontinued from opioids as part of the pain management plan. What methods are appropriate to safely discontinue opioid therapy in M.T.?

Guidelines strongly recommend that clinicians taper patients from chronic opioids if they have repeated aberrant drug-related behaviors, experience no progress toward meeting therapeutic goals, or experience intolerable adverse effects.[50,150] When tapering patients from long-term opioid therapy, the length of time the patient has been taking opioids needs to be considered. Approaches to opioid tapering range from a slow 10% dose reduction per week to a more rapid 25% reduction every few days. Evidence to guide specific recommendations on the rate of reduction is lacking, although the slower rate may help reduce the unpleasant symptoms of opioid withdrawal.[150,157]

There is insufficient evidence to guide recommendations for the use of short-acting versus long-acting oral opioids, or as-needed versus around-the-clock dosing during taper.[159] In this case, it is recommended that M.T.'s oxycodone dose be

Table 55-18
DIRE Score for Patient M.T.

Score	Factor	Explanation
1	Diagnosis	1 = Benign chronic condition with minimal objective findings or no definite medical diagnosis (e.g., fibromyalgia, migraine headache, nonspecific back pain)
1	Intractability	1 = Few therapies have been tried, and the patient takes a passive role in his/her pain management process
7	Risk	(psychological + chemical health + reliability + social support)
	Psychological	2 = Personality or mental health interferes moderately (e.g., depression or anxiety disorder)
	Chemical Health	1 = Active or very recent use of illicit drugs, excessive alcohol, or prescription drug abuse
	Reliability	2 = Occasional difficulties with compliance, but generally reliable
	Social Support	2 = Reduction in some relationships and life roles
1	Efficacy Score	1 = Poor function or minimal pain relief despite moderate-to-high opioid doses
10	**Total** Score 7–13: not a suitable candidate for long-term opioid therapy Score 14–21: good candidate for long-term opioid therapy	

DIRE, Diagnosis, Intractability, Risk, and Efficacy score.
Adapted with permission from Chou R et al. Clinical guidelines for the use of chronic opioid therapy in chronic noncancer pain. *J Pain*. 2009;10:113.

reduced slowly over 2 months in conjunction with starting psychological therapy for stress management and counseling for alcohol use. M.T. will need to be monitored for signs of withdrawal, which include anxiety, tachycardia, sweating, and other autonomic symptoms. Should withdrawal symptoms occur, they may be lessened by clonidine 0.1 to 0.2 mg orally twice a day.[160]

Cognitive Behavioral Therapies (CBT)

Case 55-7, Question 6: What nonpharmacologic therapies could be offered to M.T. to help with her pain management?

Psychological counseling and CBT are key components to successful management of the patient. The psychological approach to CBT has been shown to be beneficial in the treatment of FAP. CBT typically combines stress management, problem-solving, goal setting, pacing of activities, and assertiveness into a strategy for self-management of pain. Biofeedback, meditation, guided imagery, and hypnosis can all be incorporated within a CBT plan (Table 55-19). The objective is to help patients acquire a sense of hopefulness and resourcefulness, and develop positive coping skills.[161]

Complementary and alternative therapies such as spinal manipulation, massage, and acupuncture are commonly used in patients with chronic pain, but data supporting their use in FAPS are limited. Transcutaneous electrical nerve stimulation has been tried in FAPS patients, but the results are inconclusive.[148,161]

Table 55-19
Cognitive Behavioral Therapy[161]

Meditation—intentional self-regulation of attention using a systematic focus on particular aspects of inner and outer body experience.
Biofeedback—self-regulatory technique that teaches a patient how to exert control over the physiologic processes exacerbating pain. Biofeedback equipment conveys physiologic responses as visual or auditory signals that the patient can observe on a computer monitor. With practice, the patient learns to control and change his/her physiologic responses by manipulating the auditory or visual signals.
Guided imagery—useful method to help patients with pain to relax and achieve a sense of control and distraction. This modality involves the generation of different mental images, evoked either by oneself or with help from the practitioner.
Hypnosis—a state of heightened awareness and focused concentration that can be used to manipulate the perception of pain.

CANCER PAIN AND SYMPTOM MANAGEMENT

Pain is one of the most commonly experienced and feared symptoms of cancer. Cancer pain is defined as pain that results from treatment of the disease or the direct impact of tumor growth. During cancer treatment, 35% to 56% of patients will have pain with up to one-third of those patients having severe pain.[162,163] The type of cancer pain can be classified as somatic, neuropathic, or visceral. Approximately one-half of all cancer pain is somatic, arising from bone, muscle, ligament, subcutaneous tissue, or skin.[164]

Somatic pain is frequent with breast cancer, genitourinary tumors, bone metastasis, and lymphatic malignancies. Neuropathic pain may be caused by surgery, cancer chemotherapy, radiation, herpes zoster (shingles), and tumor progression such as advanced head and neck cancer. Visceral pain often presents with gastrointestinal cancers.[163,164]

Sixty-four percent of patients with advanced cancer report an increased frequency and intensity of pain compared with patients with early-stage cancer.[163] Factors influencing the degree of pain include the primary cancer, stage of disease, location of metastasis, and comorbid medical conditions.[164,165] Each pain complaint must be assessed for time of onset, body location, pattern of progression, impairment of physical function, psychosocial impact, and other associated symptoms such as nausea, fatigue, shortness of breath, constipation, and mental status changes.

The initial treatment of cancer pain is based on the severity as reported by the patient. Factors to consider when starting an analgesic regimen include the pain etiology, patient tolerance (e.g., opioid doses), setting where the medication will be administered, and previous experience with analgesics that were efficacious or produced adverse effects. In general, mild pain (e.g., pain rated ≤4 out of 10 in severity) can be managed with nonopioid or a combination of nonopioid and a low dose of an opioid analgesic. Moderate-to-severe pain (e.g., pain rated >4 out of 10 in severity) usually requires a higher dose of an opioid analgesic. The treatment of neuropathic pain may require the use of anticonvulsant or antidepressant medication. Nerve blocks and invasive surgical procedures are options for pain control that is refractory to conventional medication management.[165]

Presentation and Treatment of Cancer Pain

CANCER PAIN ETIOLOGY

CASE 55-8

QUESTION 1: L.V. is a 58-year-old man who was diagnosed with stage IV squamous cell carcinoma of the subglottis 2 months ago. The cancer is locally advanced with involvement of multiple cervical lymph nodes. He had a modified neck resection to remove the primary tumor and lymph nodes while sparing the larynx. Chemoradiation therapy began 3 weeks after surgery with cisplatin 100 mg/m^2 every 3 weeks (days 1, 22, and 43) and external beam radiation delivering 70 Gy fractionated over the course of 7 weeks. L.V. is now in his fourth week of radiation therapy and continues to have significant neck and shoulder pain described as "sudden shock-like sensations with movement" and rated 6 out of 10 despite a recent increase in his oral ER morphine to 60 mg twice daily with immediate-release morphine 15 mg orally every 4 hours PRN for breakthrough pain. He also reports that his throat is getting so sore that he cannot bear to swallow and rates the pain 10 out of 10. L.V. appears quite fatigued and lethargic during his appointment with the radiation oncologist. The physical examination is remarkable for dry oral mucous membranes, erythema and mild ulceration of the oropharynx, and allodynia with light palpitation of the trapezius and sternocleidomastoid muscles with pain greater on the left side.

The radiation oncologist orders laboratory tests and the results are as follows:

General Chemistry:
Sodium, 132 mEq/L
Potassium, 4.2 mEq/L
Chloride, 101 mEq/L
CO_2, 26 mmol/L
Anion gap, 5 mEq/L
Glucose, random, 70 mg/dL
Urea nitrogen, 28 mg/dL
Creatinine, 1.5 mg/dL
Calcium, total, 9.0 mg/dL

CBC With Differential:
White blood cell count, 7.1 × 10^9/μL
Red blood cell count, 3.25 × 10^6/μL
Hemoglobin, 14 g/dL
Hematocrit, 43%
Mean cell volume, 91 × 10^6/μL
Mean cell hemoglobin, 30 pg/cell
Mean cell hemoglobin concentration, 33 g/dL
Platelet, 369 × 10^3/μL
Absolute neutrophils, 5 × 10^9/L
Absolute lymphocytes, 1.2 × 10^9/L
Absolute monocytes, 0.2 × 10^9/L
Absolute eosinophils, 0 × 10^9/L
Absolute basophils, 0 × 10^9/L

The radiation oncologist decides to admit L.V. to the hospital for dehydration and pain management. What are the possible etiologies of L.V.'s pain?

L.V. is presenting with a new complaint of a severe sore throat and persistent neck and shoulder pain. Laboratory data ruled out infection and myelosuppression. His kidney function may be impaired by dehydration and cisplatin therapy. The most likely causes of L.V.'s pain are the recent surgical neck resection and mucositis from external beam radiation.

L.V. also has postoperative peripheral neuropathy characterized by shock-like sensation in the neck and shoulders after the resection of the tumor. The physical examination of L.V.'s neck and shoulders is remarkable for allodynia, which can be present with neuropathy. The cervical lymph node resection may have caused neuropathy due to nerve damage via crushing, pressure, incision, or inflammation. This results in ectopic firing and changes in the receptive field causing nerve excitability and spontaneous activity (e.g., windup). Neuronal hyperexcitability may be related to overexpression of sodium channels and activation of the NMDA receptor.[166] Cervical plexopathy may also be contributing to the discomfort.

Mucositis occurs in up to 45% of individuals treated for head and neck cancer with the chemoradiation regimen L.V. is receiving.[167,168] Chemotherapy and radiation directly affect the proliferation of epithelial cells and connective tissue, causing damage to and loss of the mucosal barrier. On physical examination, the oropharynx is red and ulcerated, which is indicative of mucositis. Chapter 94, Adverse Effects of Chemotherapy and Targeted Agents provides information on the signs and symptoms of mucositis. Pain associated with mucositis is dependent on the degree of tissue damage, sensitization of nociceptors, and activation of inflammatory and pain mediators. L.V.'s complaint of sore throat pain limiting his ability to swallow is a common presentation of mucositis. In head and neck cancer patients treated with radiation, pain intensity scores directly correspond to mucositis and increase at week 3, often peak at week 5, and persist for weeks after the end of treatment.[166]

In addition, L.V. may have cisplatin-related neurotoxicity. Approximately 30% to 40% of patients may experience sensory loss as a result of direct neuronal DNA damage and apoptotic cell death caused by cisplatin. Neurotoxicity is a dose-limiting side effect for all the platinum agents. Cisplatin peripheral toxicity can occur in patients who receive a cumulative dose of more than 400 to 500 mg/m^2.[169] All sensory modalities are involved, but loss of large fiber function is often prominent. Persistent dysesthetic pain (i.e., an unpleasant abnormal sensation, whether spontaneous or evoked) is a late phenomenon that may continue to progress for several months after cessation of cisplatin.

CASE 55-8, QUESTION 2: L.V. was started on intravenous hydromorphone using patient-controlled analgesia (PCA) with an average usage of 14 mg/day. He now rates his pain as 4 out of 10. Owing to difficulty swallowing secondary to the mucositis and xerostomia, he had a gastric feeding tube placed for nutrition. The plan is to convert the intravenous hydromorphone to a transdermal fentanyl patch. What transdermal fentanyl patch dose should L.V. be started on, and what are the instructions for use?

TRANSDERMAL FENTANYL DOSE CALCULATION

Historically, the World Health Organization (WHO) analgesic ladder has been used to guide cancer pain management.[170] The downside to using this algorithm is that cancer pain rarely progresses in the stepwise fashion that the WHO ladder implies. Therefore, several organizations including the American Pain Society and National Comprehensive Cancer Network have proposed different strategies for managing cancer pain based on the assessment of the patient, development of an individualized care plan for pain, and symptom management.[42,165,171]

Before starting intravenous hydromorphone, L.V. has severe throat pain rated 10 out of 10 and moderate-to-severe neck and shoulder pain rated 6 out of 10. Because of the severity of pain and inability to swallow, intravenous opioid therapy using PCA is appropriate. Hydromorphone is a good choice for intravenous opioid therapy because it does not have active metabolites that could accumulate with renal insufficiency. The transdermal fentanyl patch is an excellent choice for L.V.'s eventual outpatient pain management because it will provide continuous release of opioid and is convenient to use.[172] Kadian, an extended-release morphine capsule, can be administered via a 16 French gastrostomy tube because the capsule can be opened and contents flushed through the feeding tube with water.[173] Limitations to the use of this formulation in L.V. include the need for patient manipulation of the gastric feeding tube with self-administration and the potential for morphine side effects secondary to metabolite accumulation if renal insufficiency persists.

Transdermal fentanyl patches are intended for opioid-tolerant patients with stable chronic pain. Opioid-tolerant patients are those who have been taking daily, for a week or longer, at least 60 mg of oral morphine, 30 mg of oral oxycodone, or at least 8 mg of oral hydromorphone or an equianalgesic dose of another opioid.[174] Respiratory depression associated with opioids is more likely to occur in opioid-naïve patients, patients with postoperative pain, and those with intermittent or mild pain that is managed with PRN opioid administration.[172,174] Before the current hospital admission, L.V. was taking 120 mg of ER morphine per day with additional oral immediate-release morphine for breakthrough pain; therefore, L.V. is a good candidate for a transdermal fentanyl patch.

L.V.'s transdermal fentanyl regimen will need to be determined by converting intravenous hydromorphone using an equianalgesic dose approximation. Doses of two different opioids (or two different routes of administration of the same opioid) are considered to be equianalgesic if they provide the same degree of pain relief. Table 55-20

Table 55-20
Equianalgesic Opioid Dosing[42,179]

	Equianalgesic Dose (mg)			
Opioid	**Oral (PO)**	**Parenteral (IV)**	**Duration (hours)**	**Comments**
Morphine	30	10	IM/IV/SC 3–4 hours	Standard for comparison of opioid analgesics.
			Oral short-acting 3–6 hours	Morphine not recommended in patients with severe renal impairment.
Hydromorphone (Dilaudid, Exalgo)	7.5	1.5	IM/IV/SC 3–4 hours	Exalgo (extended release) dosed every 24 hours.
			Oral short-acting 3–6 hours	Can be used in patients with renal or liver impairment.
Fentanyl[179]		0.05–0.1	IV/SC 1–2 hours	Refer to Figure 55-7 for transdermal fentanyl conversion example. Equianalgesic conversion ratios have not been established for transmucosal and transbuccal fentanyl formulations. Can be used in patients with renal or liver impairment.
Oxycodone	20		Oral short-acting 3–6 hours	OxyContin (controlled release) is dosed every 8 or 12 hours. Can be used in patients with renal impairment.
Buprenorphine (Buprenex, Butrans)[174,175]	0.3 (SL)	0.4		Available as sublingual tablets, sublingual film, transdermal patch, and injection. Suboxone (buprenorphine and naloxone) restricted to treatment of opioid dependence. Partial agonists not recommended for cancer pain management.
Meperidine (Demerol)[42,174]	300	100		Not recommended for routine clinical use by the American Pain Society.[42] Normeperidine is a toxic metabolite that produces anxiety, tremors, myoclonus, and generalized seizures.

SL, sublingual; SC, subcutaneous; PO, oral; IV, intravenous.

provides equianalgesic opioid doses.[42,174] The calculations to convert L.V. from IV hydromorphone to transdermal fentanyl (Duragesic) are shown in Figure 55-7. There are several published tables for converting morphine to transdermal fentanyl that have been developed by researchers and manufacturers of transdermal fentanyl products. They provide slightly different dose conversion recommendations. Duragesic has wide morphine dose ranges, which may result in underdosing the transdermal fentanyl patch in cancer patients.[174,176] Breitbart et al. recommend a 2:1 ratio of oral morphine to transdermal fentanyl (i.e., 2 mg oral morphine/day is equivalent to 1 mcg/hour transdermal fentanyl), resulting in higher transdermal fentanyl doses, which may be excessive for elderly patients.[176] A study by Donner et al. suggested a dose ratio of 60 mg/day oral morphine is equal to 25 mcg/hour transdermal fentanyl, which falls between the manufacturer's table and the study recommendations by Breitbart et al.[176–178] The Donner conversion ratio is used in most references because it is less likely to cause underdosing or overdosing.[178]

L.V.'s transdermal fentanyl patch dose is 116 mcg/hour (Fig. 55-7) using the dose ratio 60 mg/day oral morphine to 25 mcg/hour transdermal fentanyl. Because L.V.'s pain is well controlled based on the intensity rating of 4 out of 10, the dose of transdermal fentanyl should be rounded down to the nearest available patch size, which is 100 mcg/hour.[179] If L.V.'s pain was not controlled, the transdermal patch dose should be rounded up to the nearest available patch size.[174]

Patients who have been on opioid therapy for a prolonged time are likely to exhibit tolerance to the therapeutic effect. However, when switched to a different opioid, the level of tolerance may change (i.e., diminished tolerance to the new opioid) owing to the pharmacokinetic properties of the new opioid. This change in sensitivity to the new opioid is called incomplete cross-tolerance.[174] Most opioid doses need to be reduced by 25% to 50% after the conversion calculation to account for the incomplete cross tolerance.[42] The exception to this is methadone and fentanyl. Conversion ratios for methadone and fentanyl have already accounted for incomplete cross tolerance, so no further reductions are generally needed.[179] Therefore, L.V.'s transdermal fentanyl patch dose should not be reduced for incomplete cross-tolerance.

After the initial transdermal patch is applied, it will take 12 hours to reach the minimal effective blood concentration and up to 36 hours to achieve the maximal concentration. The transdermal fentanyl patch must be changed every 72 hours to maintain the steady-state blood concentration. Elderly, cachectic, or debilitated patients may have altered pharmacokinetics (i.e., more rapid rate of release) as a result of poor subcutaneous fat

Step 1:
Determine the 24-hour total of the opioid that will be converted. For L.V., the 24-hour total of intravenous hydromorphone is 14 mg.

Step 2:
Select the equianalgesic dose ratio that corresponds to the opioid and route that will be converted from Table 55-20. Ratio calculations should be set up to correlate the actual dose with the equianalgesic equivalent as shown below:

$$\frac{\text{"X" mg total daily dose of new opioid}}{\text{mg total daily dose of current opioid}} = \frac{\text{equianalgesic factor of new opioid}}{\text{equianalgesic factor of current opioid}}$$

For conversion of L.V.'s hydromorphone dose, 1.5 mg intravenous hydromorphone is equianalgesic to 30 mg oral morphine:

$$\frac{\text{"X" mg total daily dose of new opioid}}{\text{14 mg intravenous hydromorphone}} = \frac{\text{30 mg oral morphine}}{\text{1.5 mg intravenous hydromorphone}}$$

Step 3:
Cross multiply the ratio to determine the total daily dose of oral morphine.

(1.5)(X) = (14)(30)
1.5X = 420
X = 280 mg of oral morphine

Step 4:
Determine L.V.'s transdermal fentanyl patch dose equivalent to 280 mg oral morphine using the conversion ratio of 60 mg/day oral morphine to 25 mcg/hour transdermal fentanyl will be used for the calculation.

$$\frac{\text{"X" mg total daily dose of new opioid}}{\text{280 mg oral morphine/day}} = \frac{\text{25 mcg/hour transdermal fentanyl}}{\text{60 mg oral morphine/day}}$$

(60)(X) = (280)(25)
X = 116 mcg/hour transdermal fentanyl

Figure 55-7 Conversion of L.V. from intravenous hydromorphone to transdermal fentanyl.

stores, thus requiring the transdermal fentanyl patch be changed every 48 hours.[176]

L.V. should be instructed that the transdermal fentanyl patch should be applied to an intact, nonirritated and nonirradiated flat skin surface such as the chest, back, flank, or upper arm.[174] He should be warned about the risk of elevated body temperature (e.g., 40°C or 104°F) resulting in a faster release of fentanyl from the patch. The increased fentanyl level could cause serious respiratory depression. L.V. should be cautioned about avoiding external heating sources such as electric blankets, heating pads, tanning beds, sunbathing, hot baths, hot tubs, saunas, and heated water beds.[174] Fentanyl transdermal skin patches should not be used if damaged or cut because this may increase the absorption of the medication. L.V. should be told to wash his hands immediately if contact is made with the fentanyl gel that was inside the transdermal patch.

CASE 55-8, QUESTION 3: How should L.V. be transitioned from IV hydromorphone to the transdermal fentanyl patch?

TRANSITION TO TRANSDERMAL FENTANYL

Reducing the intravenous hydromorphone continuous infusion by 50% should occur 6 hours after the initial transdermal fentanyl patch is placed. Discontinuation of the IV hydromorphone continuous infusion and PCA dose should occur 12 hours after the initial transdermal fentanyl patch placement.[174] L.V. may need to use a short-acting (i.e., immediate-release) opioid until the maximal fentanyl blood concentration is achieved. Additional short-acting opioid may be needed for pain that occurs near the end of the 72-hour dose interval.

CASE 55-8, QUESTION 4: What are L.V.'s options for breakthrough pain management?

OPIOID THERAPY FOR BREAKTHROUGH PAIN MANAGEMENT

Breakthrough pain can be classified as spontaneous pain (i.e., frequently idiopathic, occurring with no known stimulus), incident pain (i.e., secondary to a stimulus that the patient may or may not be able to control), or end-of-dose failure (i.e., pain at the end of the dosing interval of the ER/LA opioid).[174] Incident pain can be reduced by instructing the patient to take a dose of short-acting opioid 30 minutes before activity. Spontaneous breakthrough pain should be treated by administering a short-acting opioid as soon as the pain is experienced. For patients on ER/LA opioid formulations experiencing end-of-dose failure, APS guidelines recommend supplementary doses of a short-acting opioid equivalent to 5% to 15% of the total daily dose to be taken every 2 hours as needed.[42] Short-acting opioid/acetaminophen products have a maximal dose to prevent liver toxicity with acetaminophen, thus creating a ceiling limit on the analgesic efficacy. Plain short-acting opioids (e.g., morphine, oxycodone, hydromorphone) should be used for patients requiring large doses for breakthrough pain.

In L.V.'s case, a short-acting opioid solution should be available for breakthrough pain before discontinuation of intravenous hydromorphone. The short-acting opioid can be administered in solution form through the gastric feeding tube or as oral tablets if L.V. can tolerate swallowing. L.V.'s oncologist would like to use oral morphine solution for breakthrough pain management. Because the transdermal fentanyl total daily dose is approximately equal to a total daily dose of 280 mg of oral morphine (Fig. 55-7), 10% of the total daily morphine dose would be 28 mg. The dose should be rounded to the nearest tablet size for a short-acting formulation, which is 30 mg, if L.V. would eventually take morphine tablets.

If more than two supplemental doses of short-acting morphine 30 mg are required daily to keep L.V.'s pain under control, an increase in the transdermal fentanyl patch dose should be considered. Moderate-to-severe pain may require an increase in the opioid total daily dose by 50% to 100%.[179]

Table 55-21
Equianalgesic Doses for Actiq (Transmucosal Fentanyl) and Fentora (Buccal Fentanyl)[180]

Current Actiq Dose (mcg)	Initial Fentora Dose (mcg)
200	100
400	100
600	200
800	200
1,200	400
1,600	400

Fentanyl administration by oral and intranasal transmucosal routes is approved for breakthrough pain management in cancer patients. The dose of both formulations is determined by titration (i.e., starting with the lowest dose and increasing based on pain relief) rather than a percentage of the total daily dose.[179,180] Equianalgesic doses of the transmucosal immediate-release fentanyl products are summarized in Table 55-21. The oral transmucosal route would not be preferred in L.V.'s case due to his dry oral mucous membranes secondary to radiation, which will impact absorption. Xerostomia is a common problem associated with radiation therapy of the head and neck and occurs in 80% of patients by week 7 of treatment. Problems related to xerostomia include difficulty speaking, chewing, swallowing, infections, mouth pain, and dental caries. Reports indicate up to 64% of patients may experience moderate-to-severe xerostomia 3 years after radiation treatment.[169,181] Chapter 94, Adverse Effects of Chemotherapy and Targeted Agents, provides information on topical treatment of mucositis and xerostomia.

CASE 55-8, QUESTION 5: L.V. has now completed chemoradiation therapy, and the mucositis pain has resolved. He continues to have persistent burning neuropathic pain rated 8 of 10 in the neck and shoulders and is using transdermal fentanyl 100 mcg/hour along with five doses of immediate-release oral morphine 30 mg/day. He is also taking gabapentin 900 mg orally 3 times a day and using a lidocaine 5% patch on each shoulder. L.V.'s oncologist wants to switch to oral methadone for neuropathic pain management. What oral methadone dose should L.V. be started on?

METHADONE DOSE CALCULATION

Methadone is an opioid agonist with analgesic activity at mu and delta receptors. Additional mechanisms of action that make it unique from other opioids and a good option for neuropathic pain include 5-HT and NE reuptake inhibition and antagonist effects at the NMDA receptor. Rotation to methadone is recommended when a patient has an inadequate response to other opioids or experiences intolerable side effects such as delirium, myoclonus, or nausea. A trial with methadone is warranted for L.V. because his neuropathic pain is not well controlled with transdermal fentanyl and other coanalgesics, including gabapentin and lidocaine. Refer to Case 55-4 for treatment of neuropathic pain.

Unlike short-acting opioids, methadone has a long half-life that ranges from 15 to 60 hours with a duration of action of 6 to 12 hours.[42] The conversion to methadone is not proportional like other opioid equianalgesic dose calculations. Older opioid dosing tables list a single conversion factor of 20 mg of oral methadone (or 10 mg IV methadone) equianalgesic to 30 mg of oral morphine. The single methadone conversion factor was intended for

Table 55-22
Morphine-to-Methadone Equianalgesic Dose Ratio[182]

Oral morphine dose (mg/day)	<100	101–300	301–600	601–800	801–1000	≥1001
Oral morphine-to-oral methadone ratio	3:1	5:1	10:1	12:1	15:1	20:1

acute pain and does not account for chronic use. The conversion ratios vary with the morphine dose. Contemporary tables contain three or more morphine-to-methadone ratios to adjust for the magnitude of the methadone dose potency with higher morphine daily dose requirements for chronic noncancer and cancer pain. The most commonly used morphine-to-methadone conversions are provided in Table 55-22.[182]

L.V.'s total daily dose of morphine is 390 mg after converting transdermal fentanyl and adding the immediate-release morphine. Figure 55-8 provides the calculation to convert transdermal fentanyl to oral methadone in L.V. The dose of oral morphine falls within the dose range of 301 to 600 mg, which corresponds to a 10:1 oral morphine to oral methadone ratio (Table 55-22). L.V.'s total daily dose of methadone is approximately 39 mg (Figure 55-8). Guidelines recommend when switching to methadone from higher doses of another opioid, start methadone therapy no higher than 30 to 40 mg/day, with initial dose increases of no more than 10 mg/day every 5 to 7 days.[183] For most patients, the recommended methadone dose interval is every 8 hours. Older adults or frail patients may need methadone dosed every 12 hours to reduce the occurrence of side effects such as sedation.[42,174]

L.V.'s total daily dose of methadone should be divided into three doses and administered on an 8-hour interval. However, methadone is available in tablets (5 and 10 mg) or oral solution. The problem with L.V.'s total daily methadone dose is that it does not divide evenly using tablets. Splitting methadone tablets is not recommended because of the inconsistency in the dose with unequal tablet portions. Methadone solution is not convenient to use, and the dose needs to be drawn accurately with an oral syringe to prevent overdosing. L.V. would need approximately 11 to 13 mg of oral methadone solution per dose, which may be difficult to calibrate with the oral syringe. Therefore, L.V.'s methadone dose should be rounded down to the nearest available tablet size (e.g., 10 mg). Using a rapid switch transition from transdermal fentanyl to methadone, L.V. should be instructed to remove the transdermal fentanyl patch and begin methadone 10 mg orally every 8 hours approximately 12 hours after the patch has been removed. L.V. can continue to use morphine sulfate immediate-release 30 mg every 2 hours as needed for breakthrough pain. The immediate-release morphine dose may need to be reduced if L.V. has a good response to methadone.

Because methadone has a long terminal half-life, it will take 4 or more days to achieve steady state. Unless L.V. is experiencing

Step 1:
Determine the 24-hour total of the opioid that will be converted. For L.V., the transdermal fentanyl 100 mcg/hour patch will need to be converted to oral morphine. In addition, L.V. is using 150 mg/day of immediate-release oral morphine.

The conversion ratio of 60 mg/day oral morphine to 25 mcg/hour transdermal fentanyl will be used for the calculation.

$$\frac{\text{"X" mg total daily dose of new opioid}}{\text{100 mcg/hour transdermal fentanyl}} = \frac{\text{60 mg/day oral morphine}}{\text{25 mcg/hour transdermal fentanyl}}$$

(25)(X) = (100)(60)
X = 240 mg oral morphine
Therefore, the total daily dose of oral morphine is 390 mg (240 mg + 150 mg)
The conversion ratio of X = 200 mg/day oral morphine

Step 2:
Select the equianalgesic dose ratio from the methadone table that corresponds to a total daily morphine use of 390 mg using the Donner method in step 1.[161,169]

According to the methadone dose Table 55-22, morphine doses in the range of 301–600 mg correspond to a 10:1 ratio (oral morphine to oral methadone).

$$\frac{\text{"X" mg total daily dose of new opioid}}{\text{390 mg total daily dose oral morphine}} = \frac{\text{1 mg oral methadone}}{\text{10 mg oral morphine}}$$

(10)(X) = (390)(1)
10X = 390
X = 39 mg of oral methadone/day
If the total daily dose of 340 mg oral morphine is used for the calculation, the total daily dose of methadone would be 34 mg.

Figure 55-8 Conversion of L.V. from transdermal fentanyl to oral methadone.

severe pain, the methadone dose should not be increased before 5 days. L.V. should be encouraged to use the immediate-release morphine during the transition period. The methadone dose can be adjusted based on the total daily dose of morphine used for pain control during the transition period.[174]

CASE 55-8, QUESTION 6: What are the signs and symptoms of methadone toxicity that should be communicated to L.V.?

METHADONE TOXICITY SIGNS AND SYMPTOMS

L.V. should be instructed to take methadone exactly as prescribed to prevent serious problems with breathing. He should be told about the signs and symptoms of methadone toxicity including shallow breathing, slowed respirations followed by periods of not breathing, slurred speech or difficulty talking, loud snoring, and inability to walk normally.[174] L.V. should be told to seek medical attention immediately if he experiences any of these signs and symptoms of methadone toxicity. He should also let family members living with him know about the risks of methadone so they can be aware of the signs and symptoms of methadone toxicity. Naloxone nasal spray and injection kits are now available for purchase at pharmacies to prevent fatal respiratory depression caused by opioids. L.V's family members should be counseled that this antidote would be beneficial to keep at home due to the risks associated with methadone.

CASE 55-8, QUESTION 7: What are the recommendations for monitoring cardiac toxicity associated with methadone use in L.V.?

METHADONE TOXICITY MONITORING

Methadone can cause prolongation of the QTc interval and increase the risk for development of torsades de pointes (potentially fatal arrhythmia). Factors associated with QTc prolongation are methadone doses greater than 100 mg/day, hypokalemia, low prothrombin level (suggestive of reduced liver function), and drug interactions involving the cytochrome P-450 3A4 enzyme.[183,184]

Consensus guidelines have been published on cardiac monitoring for patients taking methadone. The guidelines recommend pretreatment screening, electrocardiogram (ECG) evaluation, and risk stratification for QTc intervals exceeding 500 ms. For a QTc interval exceeding 500 ms, the consensus guidelines recommend reducing or discontinuing methadone (Table 55-23).[183,184] L.V. should have an ECG ordered prior to initiation of methadone to check his baseline cardiac function. Periodic ECG monitoring should be done if the dose is increased or L.V. experiences new symptoms such as dizziness or fainting which may signal a change in cardiac function.

CASE 55-8, QUESTION 8: How should opioid-related side effects be managed in L.V.?

OPIOID SIDE EFFECT MANAGEMENT

Appropriate use of opioids requires minimizing the occurrence of side effects including sedation, nausea, vomiting, pruritus, myoclonus, and cognitive impairment.[185] Table 55-24 provides information on the treatment of common opioid-related side effects.[185] In cancer patients, multiple factors may contribute to the emergence of opioid side effects such as renal insufficiency, nausea, and vomiting caused by changes in gut motility or chemotherapy, sedation owing to metabolic disturbances, and concomitant use of other sedatives or antiemetics. Tolerance to most of the opioid side effects develops in 3 to 7 days. If the side effects do not diminish with time, treatment may include switching to a different opioid or adding another medication to counteract the undesired effect.[42]

Respiratory depression is a serious adverse event and often is preceded by sedation. With methadone, the peak respiratory depressant effects typically occur later and persist longer than with other opioids. Naloxone is an opioid receptor antagonist that can be used to reverse respiratory depression caused by opioid medications. Opioid-tolerant patients are exquisitely sensitive to opioid antagonists. If naloxone is necessary, it should be titrated to effect to prevent profound withdrawal, seizures, arrhythmias, and severe pain (e.g., the analgesic effect of opioids is reversed with naloxone).[42] Patients who are overdosed on methadone will require a continuous IV infusion of naloxone for 24 to 36 hours because of the long elimination half-life of methadone.

Table 55-23
Consensus Recommendations for Methadone QTc Prolongation[183,184]

Inform patients of arrhythmia risk before prescribing methadone
Obtain patient history of structural heart disease, arrhythmia, and syncope
Obtain a pretreatment ECG before starting methadone and follow-up 30 days after starting methadone. Annual ECG is recommended. Additional ECG if the methadone dosage exceeds 100 mg/day or patient has unexplained syncope or seizures
Reduce or discontinue methadone if the QTc interval exceeds 500 milliseconds
Screen medication profile use of drugs that also may prolong or slow the elimination of methadone (i.e., SSRIs, antifungal agents, protease inhibitors, phenytoin, rifampin, phenobarbital, droperidol)

ECG, electrocardiogram; SSRIs, selective serotonin reuptake inhibitors.

Table 55-24
Pharmacologic Treatments for Opioid-Related Side Effects[185]

Side Effect	Treatment
Constipation	Stool softener, laxative, methylnaltrexone, oral naloxone, naloxegol
Sedation	Methylphenidate, modafinil
Pruritus	Diphenhydramine, hydroxyzine
Nausea	Prochlorperazine, haloperidol, metoclopramide, ondansetron, antihistamine
Dysphoria	Haloperidol, opioid rotation
Cognitive impairment	Methylphenidate, modafinil, opioid rotation
Myoclonus	Clonazepam, dose reduction, opioid rotation

CASE 55-8, QUESTION 9: What are other options for L.V. if his pain is not controlled with conventional pharmacotherapy?

REFRACTORY CANCER PAIN MANAGEMENT

Neuraxial opioid administration (epidural or intrathecal) can be used to treat cancer pain that is refractory to conventional therapy with opioids and coanalgesic medications. Long-term neuraxial therapy must be administered through an implantable intrathecal pump to avoid infection complications. Indications for use of neuraxial therapy include neuropathic pain and mixed neuropathic–nociceptive pain. Medication selection is based on the patient's allergy history and response to a screening trial. Opioids (e.g., morphine, hydromorphone, fentanyl), local anesthetics (e.g., bupivacaine, ropivacaine), clonidine, ziconotide, and baclofen are commonly used in neuraxial regimens.

Complementary and alternative medicine therapies are widely used by patients in the management of cancer pain, dyspnea, and nausea and vomiting. Auricular acupuncture, therapeutic touch, and hypnosis may help with the management of cancer pain. Music therapy, massage, meditation, and hypnosis may help to reduce anxiety caused by dyspnea. Acupuncture and guided imagery may be beneficial in treating chemotherapy-induced nausea and vomiting.[185]

Oral cannabinoid formulations (dronabinol and nabilone) are approved by the FDA for chemotherapy-induced nausea and vomiting refractory to conventional antiemetic therapy.[186] Several studies of the endogenous cannabinoid receptors (CB_1 and CB_2) have demonstrated efficacy in the management of pain.[187] In the CNS, the CB_1 receptor is expressed in the areas involved in nociceptive processing, including the periaqueductal gray matter and dorsal horn of the spinal cord. The CB_2 receptor is expressed on cells of the immune system and is involved in modulation of inflammation and pain. CB_2 receptor activation has been shown to be analgesic in neuropathic pain models.[188,189] Medical use of cannabinoids has been debated in many states. In October 2009, the Department of Justice issued a memorandum to US Attorneys stating that federal resources should not be used to prosecute persons whose actions comply with their state's laws permitting medical use of cannabis. Currently, 23 states and Washington D.C. allow the use of medical cannabis for various diseases and including cancer pain.[190]

KEY REFERENCES AND WEBSITES

A full list of references for this chapter can be found at http://thepoint.lww.com/AT11e. Below are the key reference and websites for this chapter, with the corresponding reference number in this chapter found in parentheses after the reference.

Key References

Carville SF et al. EULAR evidence-based recommendations for the management of fibromyalgia syndrome. *Ann Rheum Dis*. 2008;67:536. (127)

Chou R et al. Medications for acute and chronic low back pain: a review of the evidence for an American Pain Society/American College of Physicians clinical practice guideline [published correction appears in *Ann Intern Med*. 2008;148:247]. *Ann Intern Med*. 2007;147:505. (70)

Chou R et al. Methadone Safety Guidelines. Methadone safety: a clinical practice guideline from the American Pain Society and College of Problems of Drug Dependence, in collaboration with the Heart Rhythm Society. *Journal of Pain*. 2014; 15(4):321–337 (184)

Chou R et al. Guidelines on the management of postoperative pain. *J Pain*. 2016;17(2):131–157. (30)

Dowell D et al. CDC Guideline for prescribing opioids for chronic pain—United States, 2016. *MMWR Recomm Rep*. 2016;65:1–50. (50)

Dubinsky RM et al. Practice parameter: treatment of postherpetic neuralgia: an evidence-based report of the Quality Standards Subcommittee of the American Academy of Neurology. *Neurology*. 2004;63:959. (105)

Finnerup NB et al. Pharmacotherapy for neuropathic pain in adults: a systematic review and meta-analysis. *Lancet Neurol*. 2015;150:573. (20)

Koes BW et al. An updated overview of clinical guidelines for the management of non-specific low back pain in primary care. *Eur Spine J*. 2010;19:2075. (65)

Manchikanti L et al. American society of interventional pain physicians (ASIPP) guidelines for responsible opioid prescribing in chronic non-cancer pain: part 2 guidance. *Pain Physician*. 2012;15:S67–S116. (151)

McPherson ML. *Demystifying Opioid Conversion Calculations: A Guide for Effective Dosing*. Bethesda, MD: American Society of Health-System Pharmacists; 2010. (174)

Nijs J et al. Low back pain: guidelines for the clinical classification of predominant neuropathic, nociceptive, or central sensitization pain. *Pain Physician*. 2015;18(3):E333–E346. (62)

Substance Abuse and Mental Health Services Administration. *Managing Chronic Pain in Adults With or in Recovery from Substance Use Disorders*. Treatment Improvement Protocol (TIP) Series 54. HHS Publication No. (SMA)12-4671. Rockville, MD: Substance Abuse and Mental Health Services Administration, 2011. (157)

Principles of Analgesic Use. 7th Edition Chicago, IL: *American Pain Society*, 2016. (42)

van Tulder MW et al. Muscle relaxants for non-specific low back pain. *Cochrane Database Syst Rev*. 2003;(2):CD004252. (69)

Key Websites

Centers for Disease Control and Prevention. http://www.cdc.gov/primarycare/materials/opoidabuse/index.html.

National Hospice and Palliative Care Organization. www.nhpco.org.

American Pain Society. http://americanpainsociety.org/.

International Association for the Study of Pain. https://www.iasp-pain.org/.

56 Care of the Critically Ill Adult

Matthew Hafermann, Philip Grgurich, and John Marshall

CORE PRINCIPLES

		CHAPTER CASES
HOME MEDICATIONS IN THE INTENSIVE CARE UNIT		
1	Medications used to treat chronic conditions are often administered in the intensive care unit (ICU) as long as it does not provide harm to the patient. The decision to continue or hold medications that cause bleeding (e.g., warfarin, clopidogrel), have hemodynamic effects (e.g., blood pressure medication), have hypoglycemic effects (e.g., diabetes medications), and/or that can potentially interact with medications administered in the ICU is made on an individual basis based on risk and benefit.	**Case 56-1 (Question 1), Case 56-2 (Question 1)**
PHARMACOKINETICS OVERVIEW AND DRUG SELECTION		
1	Available pharmacokinetic data are often determined in healthy subjects. Critically ill patients may have significant changes in all (ADME) pharmacokinetic parameters. The clinician should be attuned to those disease states most likely to induce alterations and to develop appropriate monitoring and management strategies for specific medications.	**Case 56-3 (Questions 1–8)**
PAIN, AGITATION, AND DELERIUM		
1	Pain, agitation, and delirium commonly occur in critically ill patients for a variety of reasons. Clinicians should vigilantly assess patients for pain and provide adequate analgesia. They should attempt to identify and address underlying conditions leading to agitation and delirium.	**Case 56-4 (Questions 1, 2), Case 56-5 (Question 1), Case 56-6 (Question 1), Table 56-1**
2	Opioids are the most commonly used analgesics in the ICU. Patient-specific characteristics and differences between hydromorphone, fentanyl, and morphine should be considered when designing the optimal analgesic regimen for a patient.	**Case 56-4 (Question 3), Table 56-2**
3	Sedative agents may be utilized in some patients who remain agitated after reversible causes of agitation are thoroughly addressed. Propofol and dexmedetomidine are recommended first-line sedatives in most patients and should be titrated to achieve light sedation.	**Case 56-5 (Question 2), Table 56-3**
4	Clinicians can reduce the incidence of delirium by minimizing patients' exposure to risk factors for delirium and by implementing early mobilization protocols. Limited evidence suggests atypical antipsychotics may help to treat delirium.	**Case 56-6 (Question 2)**
STRESS ULCER PROPHYLAXIS IN THE INTENSIVE CARE UNIT		
1	Stress-related mucosal damage can lead to occult gastrointestinal bleeding in high-risk critically ill patients. All ICU high-risk patients should be evaluated to determine the appropriateness of pharmacologic stress ulcer prophylaxis.	**Case 56-7 (Questions 1–3)**
GLYCEMIC CONTROL IN THE INTENSIVE CARE UNIT		
1	Both hypoglycemia and hyperglycemia result in negative outcomes for critically ill patients. Generally, clinicians should target a blood glucose concentration of <180 mg/dL utilizing insulin to manage hyperglycemia.	**Case 56-8 (Question 1)**

HOME MEDICATIONS IN THE INTENSIVE CARE UNIT

The management of home medications in an intensive care unit (ICU) can be a very challenging aspect of care for the medical team. Medication reconciliation has become an increased priority for hospitals, and pharmacists play a vital role. One study found that 36% of patients admitted to the hospital had at least one medication error, and 85% originated from the patient's medication history.[1] Often the ideal method of obtaining a home medication list is through information obtained in a patient interview. However, this can be difficult in an ICU because of the fact that many patients are intubated, sedated, delirious, and/or unable to participate in a patient interview. Thus, other methods are required, including interviewing family or friends, calling retail pharmacies, locating outside medical records, or looking at previous hospital admissions. Medication reconciliation was shown to decrease discharge medication errors from 57% to 33% on a medical unit and from 80% to 47% on a surgical unit.[2] The importance of restarting home medications in the ICU varies among different agents and medication classes. Multiple types of adult ICUs exist in the United States, including medical, surgical, burn, and neurosurgical. This section will limit discussion to surgical and nonsurgical ICUs and the role of home medications for common situations in these ICUs.

ICU patients can be very complex by definition, and it can be difficult to ensure all important aspects of critical care are addressed daily. To enhance patient care and safety, the medical field has started to incorporate an effective tool borrowed from the airline industry: the checklist. One of the most widely used ICU checklists worldwide is FAST HUG, which stands for **F**eeding, **A**nalgesia, **S**edation, **T**hromboembolic prophylaxis, **H**ead of bed elevation, stress **U**lcer prophylaxis, and **G**lycemic control.[3] These are issues that should be addressed daily because of their impact on morbidity, mortality, and length of ICU stay. Clinical pharmacists working in an ICU have the option to use a personal checklist or other available checklists including a modified version of FAST HUG, FASTHUG-MAIDENS. This acronym stands for **F**eeding, **A**nalgesia, **S**edation, **T**hromboembolic prophylaxis, **H**ypoactive or Hyperactive delirium, **M**edication reconciliation, **A**ntibiotics, **I**ndications for medications, drug **D**osing, **E**lectrolytes, **N**o drug interactions, allergies, duplications, or side effects, and **S**top dates (of medications).[4] These are checklists that could be used in any ICU; however, each pharmacist needs to find what works best for them to ensure optimal medical care for their service and patients.

CASE 56-1

Question 1: S.M. is a 62-year-old male who comes to the ICU with an upper GI bleed. He reports a 2-week history of poor oral intake and weight loss. For the last 2 days he has had several episodes of bloody stools and presented to his local clinic today with the following vitals: 90/51 mm Hg, HR 110 beats/minute, temperature 36.2°C. He is brought immediately to the ED where the following labs are obtained: Hct 17%, WBC 8.2 10^9/L, INR 5.2, Na 128 mEq/L, K 3.1 mEq/L, SCr 1.9 mg/dL. His current home medications are aspirin 81 mg daily, clopidogrel 75 mg daily, atorvastatin 40 mg daily, metoprolol XL 50 mg daily, lisinopril 10 mg daily, and warfarin 7.5 mg daily. The patient is immediately transfused with 2 units of red blood cells and is brought to the ICU. Which of his home medications should be held after he is admitted to the ICU?

Nonsurgical ICU Patients

For the nonsurgical ICU patient, the indication for admission is a major determinant in what medications can be restarted. Often Medical ICU patients come in with hemodynamic instability, reduced left ventricular ejection fraction, and/or alterations in renal or hepatic function, which significantly alter baseline pharmacokinetics. These patients must be evaluated on a case-by-case basis to determine if home medications should be restarted. Patients are admitted to the ICU because they need frequent monitoring and are in constant need of reevaluation. The medical team must consider that withdrawal can manifest from discontinuation of chronic home medications (e.g., β-blockers, baclofen) or from discontinuation of other illicit medications (e.g., heroin, cocaine, methamphetamine). Obtaining thorough patient history helps prevent withdrawal; however, because of the frequent inability to obtain a medical history the ICU team must determine if withdrawal treatment is appropriate based on vital signs and physical exam. This section will discuss home medications and how they should be addressed in common scenarios encountered in ICU patients.

Hemodynamic instability is one of the most common issues encountered in ICUs. Common causes of hypotension include hypovolemia, heart failure, and infection. Knowing the patient's baseline blood pressure can help determine the seriousness of the hypotension. A drop in baseline blood pressure can result in hypoperfusion and in the development of shock. If a patient cannot maintain adequate blood pressure, vasoactive medications (e.g., norepinephrine, epinephrine, phenylephrine, vasopressin) need to be initiated. Common indicators of lack of perfusion are monitored in the ICU, including cool skin, metabolic acidosis, change in mental status, elevated serum lactate levels, and reduced urine output. If a patient comes to the ICU with hypotension and signs of hypoperfusion, home blood pressure medications of all classes are held until there is a resolution of the underlying cause of the hypotension and hypoperfusion. Blood pressure medications should be slowly added back on at reduced doses to the hospital medication regimen.

Severe cases of hypertension in the ICU must be dealt with urgently to prevent stroke and/or end organ damage. Common causes of hypertension in the ICU are missed hemodialysis, medication noncompliance, volume overload, and pain. The differential of high blood pressure is extensive, so determining the cause of the elevated blood pressure will help determine the direction of treatment. Hypertensive emergencies, defined as a large elevation of SBP or DBP ($>$180 or $>$120 mm Hg, respectively), need to be treated immediately because of possible complications, including cerebral infarction, intracranial hemorrhage, aortic dissection, and renal failure.[5] Intravenous medications are often required to control blood pressure in the emergency room or during the early hours of ICU admission. Common medications used are nicardipine, diltiazem, diltiazem, hydralazine, esmolol, labetalol, and enalaprilat. These medications work immediately and can be titrated to lower blood pressures to desired targets. Intravenous medications are used in the short term until chronic antihypertensives can be administered and titrated. Restarting home blood pressure medications in the ICU is important unless there is a contraindication (i.e., new renal dysfunction) or the patient now has a new condition that warrants a change in medication class (i.e., β-blockers and ACEI for new heart failure). This topic is discussed further in Chapter 16, Hypertensive Crisis.

Since renal function is often unpredictable and unstable in the ICU, many classes of medications are withheld in the ICU. Renal function can change very quickly in the ICU and classic indicators of renal function such as SCr, which is used in creatinine clearance equations like Cockcroft and Gault and the Simplified

4-variable MDRD equation, are delayed in acute renal failure or falsely low in the elderly. For this reason, drugs that can be monitored using therapeutic drug monitoring (e.g., vancomycin) should be monitored frequently. Other indicators including urine output, blood pressure, and volume status should be factored into determining an appropriate dosing for medications that are eliminated through the kidney. All medications administered in the hospital setting should be monitored daily and adjusted based on renal function.

Diabetes medications can cause complications in the ICU. Metformin can cause a metabolic acidosis if given to patients with renal dysfunction and is withheld in most ICU patients. Sulfonylureas are also withheld because of the frequent changes in diet in the ICU, which can result in hypoglycemia. As a substitute to prevent hyperglycemia, most patients are converted to a short-acting sliding scale insulin regimen, which accounts for poor oral intake or the withholding of nutrition at certain points in an ICU stay. Sliding scale insulin regimens give varying doses of insulin based on a patient's most recent glucose level. Basal insulin can be considered for known diabetics, who are not receiving adequate control from sliding scale insulin.

Pain and medications used to treat pain are discussed in various chapters in this textbook (see Chapter 55, Pain and Its Management for more details). For a new ICU patient, knowing a patient's home medication pain regimen can be very helpful and often vital to good patient care. A patient on chronic opioids should be continued on a pain regimen, which includes opioids unless there is a contraindication to do so. Often the regimen must be modified to account for renal function and route of administration. For example, many of the long-acting medications cannot be crushed and put down a feeding tube, and a patient with renal dysfunction may need a lower dose or switch to an opioid that is not cleared through the kidney.

The dynamic nature of the ICU can make anticoagulation a very challenging issue in the ICU. Unless the patient will likely be in the ICU for a short period of time, vitamin K antagonists (e.g., warfarin) or the new oral anticoagulants (e.g., dabigatran, rivaroxaban, apixiban) will often be held in the ICU to prevent complications surrounding procedures and the altered pharmacokinetics in ICU patients. A detailed patient history is essential to determine the indication for anticoagulation. This will help the medical team determine if full anticoagulation should be continued. The discussion to continue anticoagulation will be determined on a case-by-case basis after weighing the risks and benefits of anticoagulation and often discussing the issue with consult services such as cardiology, vascular surgery, and the primary care provider. If full anticoagulation is required in the ICU, unfractionated heparin (UFH) may be the best option, because it can be stopped and reversed if needed. Almost all patients in the ICU are at increased risk for a venous thromboembolism (VTE) because of lack of mobility, elderly age (≥70 years), heart failure, respiratory failure, previous VTE, acute infection, obesity, and/or ongoing hormonal treatment. Because of increased risk for VTE, patients should be placed on anticoagulant thromboprophylaxis with low-molecular-weight heparin (LMWH), low-dose unfractionated heparin (LDUH) BID, LDUH TID, or fondaparinux unless a contraindication exists.[6]

One of the biggest complications for a pharmacist in an ICU patient is finding an ideal medication regimen for a patient who cannot take any medications by mouth or that have a feeding tube. For patients who have a feeding tube, medications can be given down the feeding tube in certain circumstances. The pharmacist must determine which home medications can be crushed or come in a solution or liquid form. Often long-acting medications must be converted to immediate release or the medication must be changed so it can be crushed to go down a feeding tube. The ISMP has created a resource for medications that cannot be crushed: http://www.ismp.org/tools/donotcrush.pdf. Certain patients in the ICU will be ordered to not receive anything by mouth including medications. It should always be clarified with the medical teams whether an NPO or "nothing by mouth" order includes medications. Many circumstances allow for the patient to receive oral medications on an NPO order. If medications cannot be given by mouth or there are concerns about absorption in the GI tract, the ICU teams will request that medications be converted from oral to intravenous form. While some medications have intravenous formulations, many do not. A clinical pharmacist can assist with dosage conversions, frequency of administration, and alternative options for medications that do not have intravenous equivalents.

Because of the fact that S.M. is actively bleeding, all anticoagulant and antiplatelet medications should be held. S.M. should have his aspirin, clopidogrel, and warfarin held. Additionally, because he has an elevated INR, he should receive vitamin K to reverse the effect of warfarin. Once his bleeding has stopped the team will have to determine which medications can be restarted and at what time the medications can be restarted.

Surgical Patients

CASE 56-2

QUESTION 1: D.H. is a 68-year-old with a PMH of CAD (drug-eluting stent placed 11 months ago), diabetes, and atrial fibrillation, who will be undergoing a knee replacement procedure in 1 week. His home medications on arrival to the hospital today include aspirin 81 mg daily, clopidogrel 75 mg daily, metoprolol XL 100 mg daily, and metformin 1,000 mg BID. All of his labs are within normal limits on the day of arrival. The surgery team wants your advice on what medications should be continued throughout surgery and what medications should be stopped.

Consequences of stopping a chronic medication before, or failing to restart that medication after surgery, can be significant. For example, abrupt discontinuation of a β-blocker during the perioperative period in a patient who has been on chronic β-blocker therapy can increase the risk of death in the intraoperative and postoperative period. The American College of Cardiology/American Heart Association (ACC/AHA) recommends continuation of β-blocker therapy in patients undergoing surgery who are receiving a β-blocker for treatment of conditions with ACC/AHA Class I guideline indications for the drugs (e.g., angina, symptomatic arrhythmia, post-myocardial infarction).[7] Angiotensin-converting enzyme inhibitors (ACEIs) and angiotensin receptor blockers (ARBs) increase the risk of hypotension after induction of anesthesia when these agents are not withheld 24 hours before surgery.[8] Stopping the ACEI before surgery, however, can result in adverse postoperative effects, such as rebound hypertension and atrial fibrillation. Therefore, the decision to continue or stop the ACEI or ARB before surgery is made on an individual basis, taking into consideration the indication for the ACEI or ARB and the type of surgery. Calcium-channel blockers, clonidine, amiodarone, digoxin, and statins should be continued. Preoperative withdrawal of a statin in a patient undergoing major vascular surgery, for example, increases the risk of myocardial infarction and cardiovascular death after surgery.[9] Diuretics are typically held the morning of surgery to minimize the risk of hypovolemia and electrolyte abnormalities.

Oral antidiabetic agents and noninsulin injectable agents are typically held the morning of surgery and not restarted until normal food intake resumes. In patients with renal dysfunction and those who may receive IV contrast media, metformin should be discontinued 24 to 48 hours before surgery to reduce the risk of perioperative lactic acidosis. For patients on insulin therapy, a portion of the morning dose of intermediate- or long-acting insulin is generally administered on the day of surgery after a check of the patient's blood glucose. Close blood glucose monitoring guides subsequent insulin doses to avoid hypoglycemia.[10]

Antiepileptics, antipsychotics, benzodiazepines, lithium, selective serotonin and norepinephrine reuptake inhibitors (SSRIs and SNRIs), tricyclic antidepressants (TCAs), and carbidopa/levodopa have a greater risk for withdrawal or disease decompensation than for perioperative complications. These medications should therefore be continued up to and including the morning of surgery.

Nonselective nonsteroidal anti-inflammatory drugs (NSAIDs) reversibly inhibit platelet aggregation and are often stopped 1 to 3 days before surgery, depending on the duration of action of the drug. Celecoxib does not affect platelet aggregation and may be continued up to and including the day of surgery. Nonselective NSAIDs and celecoxib should be held if there is a concern for impaired renal function during or after surgery.

For patients on anticoagulant or antiplatelet therapy, the risks for thromboembolism must be balanced with the risk for bleeding during and after the surgical procedure. For patients on warfarin, who are at high risk for perioperative thromboembolism, bridging anticoagulation therapy with IV heparin or LMWH before surgery is recommended. Warfarin may not need to be discontinued if the patient is undergoing minor surgery (e.g., certain ophthalmic, dental, or dermatologic procedures). For patients who have had coronary stents recently placed, discontinuing antiplatelet therapy prematurely can significantly increase the risk of perioperative stent thrombosis and have catastrophic consequences.[11] The 2014 ACC/AHA Guideline on Perioperative Cardiovascular Evaluation and Management of Patients Undergoing Noncardiac Surgery: Executive Summary recommends that patients undergoing urgent noncardiac surgery during the first 4 to 6 weeks after receiving a bare metal stent or drug-eluding stent implantation should continue dual antiplatelet therapy (aspirin plus P2Y12 platelet receptor-inhibitor) unless the relative risk of bleeding outweighs the benefit of the prevention of stent thrombosis. They also recommend that the management of perioperative antiplatelet therapy be determined by a consensus of the surgeon, anesthesiologist, cardiologist, and patient, who should weigh the relative risk of bleeding with those of prevention of stent thrombosis.[12]

Traditionally, it was thought that patients who have been taking long-term corticosteroid therapy before surgery will experience adrenal insufficiency in the perioperative period and should receive a supplemental stress-dose of hydrocortisone or methylprednisolone during and up to 2 to 3 days after surgery.[13] A recent review of the literature, however, found that patients on long-term corticosteroid therapy only require continuation of their normal daily dose of corticosteroid in the perioperative period. These patients are generally able to increase their endogenous adrenal function above their baseline corticosteroid dose to meet the increased demand from surgery; a supplemental stress dose of corticosteroid is not necessary. These patients can be closely monitored, and if hypotension develops, a stress dose of a corticosteroid should be administered at that time. Patients who have a known dysfunctional hypothalamic–pituitary–adrenal axis deficiency (e.g., Addison's disease), on the other hand, will require supplemental corticosteroid doses in the perioperative period as they cannot increase endogenous cortisol production to meet the increased demand from surgery.[14]

Opioid-dependent chronic pain patients who undergo surgery often experience more severe acute pain after surgery. These patients should receive either their chronic opioid medication or a comparable dose of an IV opioid the morning of surgery to meet their daily requirements to avoid uncontrolled pain and opioid-withdrawal symptoms. The use of non-opioid analgesics or analgesic techniques (e.g., acetaminophen, peripheral nerve blockade, epidural analgesia) for perioperative analgesia should be maximized in a postoperative patient.[15] For D.H., since his stent is over 6 weeks old, his clopidogrel should be held 7 days prior to surgery. His warfarin should also be held 5 to 7 days prior to surgery and likely does not need bridging with a UFH or LWMH. His aspirin can be continued through surgery.

PHARMACOKINETIC ALTERATIONS IN THE ICU AND MANAGEMENT STRATEGIES

Pharmacokinetics in the Critically Ill

The dynamic nature of critical illness may cause drastic changes in the pharmacokinetic profile of many medications. Before describing these changes, it is important to first consider where the majority of available pharmacokinetic data is generated.

As a medication makes its way through the discovery process, pharmacokinetic data are obtained in phase I trials and in non-critically ill patients. Phase 1 trials in humans are most commonly done in healthy subjects in highly controlled environments. When pharmacokinetic data are obtained in phase II/III trials, critically ill patients are excluded. As a result, errors may arise in assuming that patients with the disease of interest, and more importantly, critically ill patients have similar pharmacokinetic parameters. While available pharmacokinetic data should always be consulted in formulating a therapeutic regimen, the pharmacist should be attuned to the limitations inherent in the data.

CASE 56-3

QUESTION 1: J.K. is a 67-year-old male who presents to the Intensive Care Unit (ICU) with a 3-day history of cough and shortness of breath. J.K. is diagnosed with severe sepsis due to pneumonia and is intubated on admission to the ICU. J.K. is started on broad spectrum IV antibiotics, including piperacillin–tazobactam and vancomycin. After receiving 6 L of lactated ringers, J.K. remains hypotensive, and a norepinephrine infusion is initiated to maintain his mean arterial pressure >65 mm Hg. J.K. is placed on enoxaparin 40 mg subcutaneously daily and pantoprazole intravenously for DVT and stress ulcer prophylaxis (SUP) respectively. On day 3 of his ICU course, J.K. develops acute kidney injury (AKI) secondary to sepsis/hypoperfusion with his serum creatinine rising from a baseline of 1.1 to 3.4 mg/dL. J.K. has an naso-gastric (NG) tube placed for enteral nutrition. On day 6 of his ICU stay, J.K. develops a severe *Clostridium difficile* colitis for which oral vancomycin is initiated.

What are potential abnormalities of medication absorption in J.K.?

With the exception of intravenous administration, all medications must undergo absorption in order to reach the systemic circulation. Bioavailability (F) is defined as the percentage of the administered dose that reaches the systemic circulation.

Gut function may be altered in J.K. for a variety of reasons including delayed gastric emptying, ischemic bowel, inflammation, and coadministration of interacting substances. Each of these issues may lead to significant delays and/or decreases in the amount of orally/enterally administered medication absorption.

Delayed gastric emptying is a common occurrence in the ICU patient population, occurring in 40% to 60% of patients.[16] It may be caused by many factors including postoperative ileus, trauma, head injury, sepsis, burns, or opioid use.[17] Delayed gastric emptying would be evident in J.K. if he was manifesting high gastric residual volumes or enteral feeding intolerance. Because most medications are absorbed in the small intestine, delayed emptying would most likely affect the rate of absorption, slowing the onset of action of medications in J.K.

Ischemic bowel may also cause J.K. to have alterations in his ability to absorb oral/enteral medications depending on what portion and how much of the bowel is affected. In J.K., ischemic bowel may be caused by vasopressor use and/or the presence of a shock state. Because drug absorption occurs primarily in the small bowel, impaired blood flow to this area would be more likely to decrease the extent of absorption of medications.

Acute gut inflammation may increase the absorption of certain medications in J.K. With the development of severe clostridium colitis on day 6, J.K. may experience increased oral absorption of oral vancomycin. Under normal patient conditions, oral vancomycin is not orally absorbed because of the ionization and large size of the molecule. There have been several reports of therapeutic plasma levels of vancomycin being achieved with oral treatment of severe *C. difficile* infections.[18–21] The postulated mechanism is the severe inflammation in the colon allowing for the passage of larger, charged molecules into the bloodstream.

Oral medications are not the only route that may have altered absorption in the ICU. Subcutaneous absorption has also been shown to be remarkably altered in ICU patients, particularly those on vasoconstrictive (vasopressor) therapy. It is postulated that vasopressor treatment causes a decrease in subcutaneous tissue perfusion, resulting in impaired absorption of subcutaneously administered medications. Studies have shown that patients on LMWH therapy also receiving vasoconstrictive agents have markedly reduced peak and total anti-Xa activity when compared to other hospitalized patients.[22–24]

CASE 56-3, QUESTION 2: How should absorption issues in J.K. be managed?

Generally speaking, when there is a question of gut function in the intensive care unit, intravenous formulations are preferred when available. In cases where a given medication would produce an objective response (antihypertensive, hypoglycemic agents), enteral therapy may be attempted to assess patients' response. As above, the pharmacist should be attuned to the specific pharmacodynamic response of a given medication to assess therapeutic response with oral/enteral dosing.

In the case of J.K., consideration may be given to monitoring anti-factor Xa levels for enoxaparin, while he remains on vasopressor therapy. Trough levels of <0.1 IU/mL have been associated with increased risk of the development of DVT.[25] Additionally, if J.K. is deemed suitable for enteral medication therapy, his proton pump inhibitor therapy could be changed to a dissolvable (solu-tab) formulation, which generally is preferred to crushing and dissolving oral tablets to prevent obstructing tubes and for ease of administration. Consideration could also be given to monitor serum vancomycin concentrations more aggressively, because J.K. may be at risk for significant vancomycin absorption given his severe *C. difficile* infection while also receiving systemic vancomycin therapy.

CASE 56-3, QUESTION 3: What are the potential changes in the distribution of a medication in J.K.?

The distribution of a medication is defined briefly as where the drug goes once it is absorbed into the bloodstream. The extent of distribution of a medication is dependent on both physiochemical drug properties and patient-specific factors. The physiochemical properties of a drug that determine how extensively it distributes to tissues include lipophilicity and protein binding, with high lipophilicity leading to extensive tissue distribution, and lower protein binding contributing to more extensive distribution. Patient-specific factors that determine the distribution of a medication include weight, volume status, and vascular permeability.

J.K. has a multitude of factors that may affect the distribution of hydrophilic (low volume of distribution) medications. These include the presence of sepsis and large-volume crystalloid (normal saline) administration. These conditions result in decreased plasma concentrations of hydrophilic medications, leading to potentially subtherapeutic concentrations.[26]

Patients who have sepsis may possess several factors that would lead to a decreased plasma concentration of hydrophilic medications. These include the presence of capillary leak (third spacing), causing intravascular fluid to distribute to tissues, the administration of large volumes of intravenous crystalloid medications, and reduced tissue perfusion. This is particularly well-documented with antibiotic therapy in this patient population. Most infections occur in the interstitial fluid of tissues, thus interstitial antibiotic concentrations would be most relevant to determine efficacy. Studies have shown that the interstitial fluid concentration and subcutaneous concentration of antibiotics is 5 to 10 times lower and 1 to 5 times lower respectively, in septic patients as compared to normal controls.

Septic ICU patients may also have drastic changes in plasma protein (albumin) concentration because of reduced liver production and third spacing of albumin into tissue sites. Low plasma protein will cause an increase in the unbound fraction of drug, increasing distribution to tissues. Unfortunately, this increased distribution is more than offset by the increase in fluid concentration (secondary to capillary leak and volume administration) of the interstitial tissues, causing low concentrations of antibiotics in interstitial fluid.

Understanding that the distribution of hydrophilic antibiotics in J.K. (piperacillin/tazobactam, vancomycin) is likely increased in J.K., several strategies can be employed to offset these changes. Interventions include giving more frequent doses or continuous infusions with β-lactam therapy, and using large initial doses (30–40 mg/kg/day) of vancomycin in conjunction with targeting trough levels of 15 to 20 mg/L.[26]

CASE 56-3, QUESTION 4: What are the potential alterations in metabolism in J.K.?

Drug metabolism can occur in a variety of body tissues, including the kidneys, GI tract, lung, and liver. The liver is by far and away the predominant metabolizing organ and is the focus of this section. ICU patients may have alterations in hepatic enzyme activity, liver blood flow, and protein binding, all of which may influence the rate at which hepatically metabolized medications are biotransformed.

Liver metabolism is broken into two major categories, phase I and phase II metabolism, both of which transform drugs into more polar substances that are more readily excreted. Phase I metabolism refers to the cytochrome p450 enzyme system that works through oxidation, reduction, and hydrolysis. Phase II metabolism, in contrast, adds large polar molecules to the parent compound, including glucuronidation, sulfation, and acetylation.

There may be significant factors that alter phase I metabolism in J.K. These include kidney injury, inflammation, and hypothermia.

Renal dysfunction can reduce phase I metabolism through reduced hepatic cell uptake of medications and reduced biliary excretion.[27,28] The inflammatory response secondary to trauma has shown variable effects on enzymatic activity, with reduction in CYP 450 3A4, 2C19, and 2E1, with increased 2C9 activity.

Therapeutic hypothermia has been well-documented to reduce cytochrome activity across all isoenzyme families. This is especially well-documented with medications commonly given to these patients, including neuromuscular blockers, fentanyl, phenytoin, and midazolam. It is important to consider that enzyme activity recovers during the rewarming process, necessitating close monitoring and potential dose adjustment.[29]

Hepatic blood flow (perfusion) may also be altered in J.K. Reductions in hepatic blood flow because of hypotension (shock) or shunting (cirrhosis) may have significant effects on prolonging the half-life of medications that are dependent on liver blood flow for metabolism. These medications are defined as having a high hepatic extraction ratio ($E > 0.7$) and would include medications such as midazolam and fentanyl.[17]

Protein-binding alterations may also occur in the critically ill and may subsequently affect the metabolism of select medications. Specifically, albumin concentrations may acutely decrease, thus increasing the free fraction of medications that are normally bound. This is especially relevant for medications that have high extraction ratios, as more medication would be available for removal, causing a net reduction in drug half-life.

CASE 56-3, QUESTION 5: How should metabolism issues be managed in J.K.?

To properly manage metabolism alterations in the ICU, the pharmacist should first be aware of the patient populations who are most likely to have altered metabolic rates/pathways. These include renal dysfunction, burns, therapeutic hypothermia, and decreased hepatic perfusion. In addition to identifying at-risk patients, the pharmacist should be aware of those medications that are most likely to have altered metabolism. These would include medications metabolized through the CYP 450 system as well as those with high extraction ratios ($E > 0.7$). Increased vigilance in monitoring for therapeutic effect/toxicity with these medications in at-risk patients is warranted.[17,29]

CASE 56-3, QUESTION 6: How is elimination altered in J.K.?

Elimination is the process by which a drug or its metabolites are removed from the body. While the kidney is the main organ that eliminates medications, it is important to remember that there are other organs (liver/lung) that also may contribute to elimination.[17] In addition, there exist several therapeutic interventions that occur in the ICU that also contribute to medication elimination, including continuous renal replacement therapy (CRRT) and extracorporeal membrane oxygenation (ECMO).[30]

Glomerular filtration is the primary method of renal clearance of medications, and renal drug removal is usually directly proportional to glomerular filtration rate (GFR). AKI is a common comorbidity in the ICU population, occurring in 1% to 25% of patients, leading directly to reduced medication elimination.[17] Other factors may increase the GFR in ICU patients, including trauma, burns, and use of vasopressors.

Renal function assessment is critical to appropriately dose adjusting renally eliminated medications and proves to be especially difficult in the ICU population. The serum creatinine measurement often lags behind actual GFR, because there exist changes in creatinine production and altered tubular secretion. In addition, most estimates of renal function, including the Cockcroft-Gault (CG) equation and the Modified Diet in Renal Disease (MDRD) equation, were validated only in patients with stable renal function.[31,32] Attempting to apply these equations to a patient with fluctuating serum creatinine measurements will result in inaccurate estimations of renal clearance.

In addition to renal function, there exist other modalities that contribute to drug elimination in specific ICU populations. These include CRRT and ECMO. While a detailed description of these processes is beyond the scope of this chapter, the clinician should remember that both may remove medications in clinically relevant quantities.

It is also important that the pharmacist consider not only the elimination of the parent compound but the presence active/toxic metabolites that require renal elimination. Examples of medications with clinically significant toxic metabolites are nitroprusside and meperidine.[33,34] Renal dysfunction may lead to accumulation of toxic metabolites, causing patient harm. Common medications given in the ICU with active metabolites are midazolam and diazepam. These active metabolites may accumulate in renal insufficiency and cause exaggerated/prolonged sedation/delirium.[35,36]

CASE 56-3, QUESTION 8: How should elimination alterations be managed in J.K.?

Estimation of renal function is critical to appropriately dosing many medications in the ICU. As above, using the usual process of calculating renal function is often inaccurate, and typical equations (CG/MDRD) should only be used in patients with stable creatinine values. In patients with unstable creatinine values, consideration should be given to calculating creatinine clearance using a 24-hour urine collection. Other data points should also be considered when determining an appropriate dose in critical illness and include urine output, trends in serum creatinine, and the specific medication to be dosed. For J.K., this would mean frequent monitoring of Vancomycin serum concentrations, anti-Xa monitoring for enoxaparin, and daily assessment of creatinine and urine output trends. Additionally, medications with active metabolites requiring renal elimination (midazolam) should be avoided if possible.

Pain, Agitation, and Delirium in the ICU

Pain, agitation, and delirium commonly occur in critically ill patients for a variety of reasons. Invasive interventions such as intubation and mechanical ventilation, acute and preexisting disease states, and surgery are just a few of the common causes of pain in critically ill patients.[37] Patients may become agitated and develop delirium because of untreated or inadequately treated pain or because of many other reasons, including drug abuse or withdrawal, adverse effects of medications, sleep deprivation, and the impact of comorbidities or severe illness.[37] Pain, agitation, and delirium are interrelated, and it is often difficult to differentiate these conditions based on symptoms in patients who are severely ill and often unable to communicate. They require prompt and effective interventions because they can lead to patient discomfort, heightened sympathomimetic activity, and negative patient outcomes. Clinicians should judiciously balance management of pain, agitation, and delirium in order to keep patients lucid, calm, interactive, free of pain, and cooperative with their care.[38]

CASE 56-4

QUESTION 1: J.A. is a 28-year-old male who presents to the emergency room after a severe motor vehicle accident. He presents with hemorrhagic shock, multiple rib and leg bone fractures, and a traumatic brain injury. He is immediately intubated and taken to the operating room for control of his bleeding and initial management of his fractures. His past medical history is significant for opioid abuse and bipolar disorder. After the operation, J.A. is transferred to the surgical ICU on mechanical ventilation with multiple chest tubes in place for management of injuries he sustained in the accident.

What causes of pain does J.A. have and what complications might they cause?

Table 56-1
Common Causes of Pain in Critically Ill Patients

Injuries and Diseases	Interventions and Monitoring	Routine Care
Trauma	Endotracheal intubation	Turning
Burns	Endotracheal tube for mechanical ventilation	Suctioning of respiratory secretions
Pancreatitis	Chest tube placement	Physical therapy
Necrotizing fasciitis	Wound care	
Decubitus ulcers	Surgery	
Immobility	Vascular access (arterial catheter)	
Preexisting disease states (e.g., cancer, chronic back pain)		

Up to 77% of patients discharged from ICUs report experiencing moderate or severe pain during their ICU stay.[39,40] This pain occurs during rest and with activity and is the most common memory patients have of their ICU stays.[41] Pain may occur because of injuries or diseases, therapeutic interventions, routine ICU care, or monitoring. Common causes of pain are listed in Table 56-1. Patients consistently report pain as the most traumatic memory from their ICU stay.[42] During the ICU stay, untreated pain can result in increased energy requirements, hyperglycemia, muscle breakdown, immunosuppression, increased risk of wound infection, decreased tissue perfusion, psychological distress, and impaired sleep. Long-term complications of untreated pain include chronic pain syndromes, neuropathy, posttraumatic stress disorder, and a decreased health-related quality of life.[37,43] In light of the acute and long-lasting consequences of pain as well as the prevalence of untreated pain in critically ill patients, it is important to diligently assess patients and utilize appropriate analgesics when indicated.

In J.A., potential causes of pain include trauma, postoperative pain, and the presence of an endotracheal tube and chest tubes. During his ICU stay, he may experience pain from routine care, including turning, suctioning of respiratory secretions, and eventually physical therapy.

CASE 56-4, QUESTION 2: How should J.A. be assessed for pain in the ICU?

Since patient-reported pain assessment is the optimal way to assess pain, whenever possible, clinicians should ask patients to rate their pain on a scale from 0 to 10 with 0 representing no pain and 10 representing the worst pain imaginable. For patients who cannot communicate with caregivers because of mechanical ventilation or other limitations, clinicians should assess patients' pain scores using validated nonverbal pain assessment tools that utilize patients' behaviors as indicators of pain. The two nonverbal pain assessment tools recommended in guidelines are called the Behavioral Pain Scale and the Critical-Care Pain Observation Tool.[37] The maximum score on each tool is 12 and 8, respectively, with higher values indicating more severe pain. Pain assessment should be protocolized such that it routinely occurs throughout each day of the patient's ICU stay. Clinicians should set the goal pain level and utilize analgesics as needed to achieve it while considering potential adverse effects. Generally, hemodynamic parameters such as blood pressure, heart rate, and respiratory rate should not be used to assess pain because they can be affected by other factors and do not correlate with self-reported pain; however, changes in vital signs may be used as a cue to further assess patients.[37]

CASE 56-4, QUESTION 3: How should clinicians manage pain in critically ill patients like J.A.?

Opioids, including fentanyl, hydromorphone, morphine, methadone, and remifentanyl, are the primary analgesics used in the critical care setting. Of these, fentanyl, hydromorphone, and morphine are used most commonly, whereas methadone is mainly used for long-term pain or pain that is refractory to other opioids. Because it is very short acting, very potent, and metabolized in the plasma, remifentanyl is most appropriate for pain that lasts only a short period of time in patients who are mechanically ventilated and in those with severe renal or hepatic dysfunction. Meperidine should not be used because it may cause seizures and other complications.[44] For treatment of acute pain, opioids should be given intravenously since enteral administration may be unreliable in critically ill patients because of incomplete absorption in patients with altered gastrointestinal motility and intramuscular absorption can be erratic.[37] In some cases, it may be impossible to completely alleviate pain because of dose-limiting side effects such as respiratory depression or altered mental status. In these cases, clinicians should attempt to make patients as comfortable as possible without inducing significant adverse effects.

The selection of a specific opioid relates to the pharmacokinetics and pharmacodynamics of the medications and depends on patient-specific characteristics as well as the nature of the pain the patient is experiencing. Table 56-2 lists key considerations for choosing between available opioids. When given as a single intravenous bolus injection, fentanyl has a faster onset and shorter duration of action compared to hydromorphone and morphine. This makes an intravenous injection of fentanyl most appropriate for pain that is short-lived such as procedural pain that might be associated with placement of a chest tube or intravenous catheter. In fact, procedural pain is best treated preemptively through administration of a bolus agent before the procedure.[37] The longer duration of action of hydromorphone and morphine makes these agents better when intravenous treatment of longer lasting pain is indicated. Alternatively, fentanyl, hydromorphone, and morphine may all be administered as continuous intravenous infusions in patients needing ongoing analgesia or those with severe pain.

All opioids can cause constipation, confusion, hallucinations, altered mental status, and respiratory depression when given in high doses. Clinicians should regularly monitor the bowel movements of patients receiving opioid analgesia and a bowel regimen containing both a stimulant laxative and a stool softener should be administered, if indicated. Opioids may all cause a decrease in blood pressure if the patient's blood pressure is increased because of pain and in patients who are hypovolemic. Importantly, morphine is the only opioid that causes histamine release, which can lead to flushing, bronchospasm, and hypotension. These complications underlie the recommendation to avoid morphine in patients who are hemodynamically unstable, at risk for hypotension, or those

Table 56-2
Selected Characteristics of Opioids Used in Critically Ill Patients

	Onset	Duration (IV Bolus Dose)	Active Metabolite	Adverse effects & Other Considerations	Equipotent IV Dose (mg)
Morphine	5–10 minutes	2–4 hours	Yes (cleared renally)	Histamine release (hypotension, bronchospasm, flushing)	10
Hydromorphone	5–15 minutes	2–4 hours	No		1.5
Fentanyl	1–2 minutes	30–60 minutes	No	Accumulates in adipose tissue with prolonged infusion	0.1

with bronchospasm. Morphine has an active metabolite that is cleared by the kidneys, while fentanyl and hydromorphone are metabolized in the liver to inactive metabolites. Thus, hydromorphone and fentanyl are preferred over morphine in patients with renal failure. Another unique side effect relates to QTc prolongation resulting from methadone. Because QTc prolongation can potentially cause cardiac arrest, electrocardiograms should be regularly monitored in patients receiving methadone, especially in patients concurrently receiving other QTc-prolonging agents. Serum concentrations of magnesium and potassium should be monitored, and these electrolytes should be repleted, as needed, to minimize arrhythmias. Because fentanyl is the most lipophilic of the three most commonly used opioid analgesics, prolonged administration via intravenous infusion may lead formation of a depot in adipose tissue. After cessation of the fentanyl infusion, drug may distribute from the fat into the bloodstream and prolong the effects of drug.

In addition to opioids, clinicians may consider adjunctive analgesics in selected patients. For example, nonsteroidal anti-inflammatory agents and acetaminophen may be considered to minimize overall opioid requirements and potentially reduce opioid-related complications. For patients experiencing neuropathic pain, enterally administered gabapentin and carbamazepine can be helpful. Finally, for patients with rib fractures or those who have undergone thoracic or abdominal surgery, thoracic epidural analgesia results in better pain control as compared to opioid monotherapy.[37]

Because J.A. is likely to experience ongoing pain as a result of his trauma, multiple fractures, and surgery, he should be initiated on opioid analgesia. If he remains hypotensive, at risk for hemodynamic compromise, or is in renal failure, morphine should be avoided. Some centers would routinely use fentanyl or hydromorphone in most patients to minimize hemodynamic complications. It would be most appropriate to administer fentanyl as a continuous infusion, while hydromorphone could be given continuously or as repeated intravenous boluses. Because of his rib fractures, J.A. could also be considered for thoracic epidural analgesia with an opioid.

CASE 56-5

QUESTION 1: During his stay in the surgical ICU, J.A. begins to exhibit signs of agitation including diaphoresis, tachycardia, pulling at his endotracheal tube, and even trying to strike his caregivers.

What are some causes of agitation that J.A. might be experiencing and how should he be initially treated?

Agitation is very common in critically ill patients and can lead to adverse consequences arising from sympathomimetic effects.[45] Patient care can be complicated if agitation leads to patient removal of devices, such as endotracheal tubes or intravenous lines, necessary for their care. Patients may exhibit symptoms of agitation for a variety of reasons including pain, delirium, hypoxemia, hypoglycemia, hypotension, or withdrawal from alcohol and other drugs. Given the ubiquity of pain in critically ill patients and the difficulty in assessing patients who cannot communicate, clinicians should always consider pain as a potential cause of agitation and administer analgesics when they suspect pain. In fact, current guidelines recommend analgesia-first sedation strategies that emphasize aggressive use of analgesics before administration of sedative agents.[37] Other general strategies to treat anxiety and agitation in critically ill patients include keeping patients as comfortable as possible, reorienting patients if they misperceive their surroundings or situations, promoting a normal sleep–wake cycle by helping patients to stay awake during the day and minimizing barriers to sleep overnight. Whenever possible, clinicians should attempt to identify and treat the underlying cause of agitation before initiating a sedative agent. For instance, if an agitated patient is found to be hypoglycemic, the hypoglycemia should be corrected, and the patient should be reevaluated before starting a sedative. By identifying and addressing the cause of agitation, clinicians can avoid complications associated with sedative medications, such as over-sedation and delirium.[37]

Clinicians should assess critically ill patients who are agitated using a validated sedation assessment tool.[37] The two most rigorously evaluated tools are the Richmond Agitation-Sedation Scale (RASS) and the Sedation-Agitation Scale (SAS). Both tools effectively discriminate different levels of sedation, have high inter-rater reliability, and have been show to correlate reasonably well with objective measures of brain function.[46–48] Scores on the RASS range from −5 to +4 while the SAS varies from 1 to 7. The lowest numbers of the scales indicate a patient is unarousable, while the highest numbers on the RASS and SAS correspond to combativeness and dangerous agitation, respectively. By quantifying patients' level of sedation using one of these tools, multidisciplinary caregivers can determine the desired level of consciousness and appropriately administer medications to target this level of consciousness while avoiding excessive sedation. Generally, sedatives should be titrated to achieve light levels of sedation, which correspond to RASS scores of −1 to 0 and SAS scores of 3 to 4.[37] Maintaining patients at light levels of sedation instead of deeper levels of sedation, in which they are more difficult to arouse and are less interactive, has been shown to reduce duration of mechanical ventilation and ICU length of stay.[49,50] Sometimes, patients' clinical conditions may necessitate deeper levels of sedation. Some clinical situations in which deeper sedation may be appropriate include active severe alcohol withdrawal, refractory status epilepticus, intracranial hypertension, ventilator dysynchrony, severe lung injury, or paralysis with neuromuscular receptor blocking agents.

J.A. may be agitated because of pain from his traumatic injuries as well as metabolic disturbances or other causes. His level of consciousness should be evaluated using the RASS or SAS. Since he is intubated, J.A. should be assessed for pain using a validated nonverbal pain assessment tool, and his pain should be treated if indicated. His vital signs should be evaluated to identify hypotension or hypoxia, and his blood glucose concentration should be measured. Abnormalities in these values should be corrected as needed. Clinicians should review J.A.'s past medical history, social history, and home medication list to identify any potential that he might be experiencing withdrawal from alcohol, illicit substances, or prescribed medications that he was taking before hospital admission such as benzodiazepines or opioids. If he is unaware of his surroundings or current condition, J.A. should be reoriented. His sleep pattern should be addressed. Finally, the patient's current medication list should be reviewed for medications, such as steroids and anticholinergic drugs, that might cause behavioral changes and these medications should be discontinued if identified. Only after thoroughly assessing the patient for potentially reversible causes of agitation, should the health care team consider initiating a sedative medication with the goal of achieving a light level of sedation in J.A.

CASE 56-5, QUESTION 2: If J.A. requires sedation, which medication would be preferred?

Several agents, including propofol, dexmedetomidine, and benzodiazepines, can be used to treat agitation in critically ill patients. No particular sedative is best for all patients. Although benzodiazepines have been widely used over time, recent guidelines suggest that propofol and dexmedetomidine are preferred in most patients because they may result in decreased ICU length of stay and duration of mechanical ventilation as compared to benzodiazepines.[37,51–53] Decisions about the optimal sedative agent for individual patients depend on the reason for sedation and sedation goals, expected duration of sedation, pharmacology of the medication in the specific patient, and cost-effectiveness.[37] A summary of key clinical considerations relative to commonly used sedatives is provided in Table 56-3.

Propofol is a highly lipophilic sedative that binds to multiple receptors and exerts sedative, hypnotic, anxiolytic, antiemetic, and anticonvulsant properties.[37] Because of its high lipophilicity and formulation in a 10% lipid emulsion, propofol readily crosses the blood–brain barrier and demonstrates a rapid onset of effect and quick offset after short-term use. However, patient awakening after prolonged use can be variable because of its deposition in adipose tissues.[54] Propofol can be rapidly titrated in order to achieve the desired level of sedation. It is suited for regular awakenings that are required for neurologic examinations in patients with brain injuries, and it facilitates daily awakening as part of sedative and ventilator weaning protocols.[53,55] Adverse effects of propofol include respiratory depression, hypotension resulting from vasodilation, bradycardia, hypertriglyceridemia, pancreatitis, myoclonus, and green or white discoloration of the urine.[56,57] Because of the dose-dependent suppression of respiratory drive, continuous infusions of propofol should only be administered to patients who are mechanically ventilated. Patients should be regularly monitored for hypertriglyceridemia when receiving propofol over the course of several days and the drug should be stopped or weaned if significant hypertriglyceridemia develops. Patients with allergies to eggs, soybeans, and sulfites may experience allergic reactions because of components of the lipid emulsion and some generic formulations.[58] In order to reduce burning and stinging associated with administration, propofol should be administered through large-bore intravenous lines whenever possible. Although propofol is formulated with a preservative to prevent bacterial growth, product labeling suggests the bottles and tubing should be changed every 12 hours, and line integrity should be assessed to prevent bacterial contamination. The caloric load of the lipid vehicle should be considered when evaluating nutritional needs in patients receiving propofol.

Propofol may cause a life-threatening syndrome called propofol infusion syndrome (PRIS) in about 1% of patients. PRIS is characterized by metabolic acidosis, hypertriglyceridemia, progressive hypotension, bradyarrythmias, and cardiovascular collapse. Other complications of PRIS may include AKI, hyperkalemia, rhabdomyolysis, and liver failure.[59,60] PRIS has been observed most commonly at doses exceeding 70 mcg/kg/minute and with use beyond 48 hours, but it has been reported at lower infusion rates and with shorter infusions.[61,62] Because PRIS can be difficult to distinguish from other conditions in critically ill patients and because of its high mortality rate, members of the health care team should diligently monitor patients in order to rapidly identify PRIS. When PRIS is suspected, propofol should be discontinued and patients should receive appropriate supportive care.[37]

Dexmedetomidine is a centrally acting α-receptor agonist that is similar to clonidine. It demonstrates greater anxiolytic and fewer sympatholytic properties as compared to clonidine. In addition to anxiolysis, dexmedtomidine also has sedative and opioid-sparing effects. It does not have anticonvulsive characteristics, induce amnesia, or cause respiratory depression.[37] Dexmedetomidine often allows patients to awaken more easily and better interact with caregivers as compared to propofol and benzodiazepines, but it is not appropriate for patients requiring deeper levels of sedation and those paralyzed with neuromuscular receptor antagonists.[63] Dexmedetomidine starts working within approximately

Table 56-3
Clinical Considerations with Sedative Agents

	Receptor Binding Site	Onset (minutes)	Effect of Renal Failure	Effect of Hepatic Failure
Midazolam	$GABA_A$	2–5	Effect prolonged (accumulation of parent drug and active metabolite)	Effect prolonged
Lorazepam	$GABA_A$	15–20	Accumulation of propylene glycol	Effect prolonged
Propofol	$GABA_A$, nicotinic, glycine, muscarinic	1–2	No clinically significant effect	No clinically significant effect
Dexmedetomidine	Central α-2	5–10	No clinically significant effect	Effect may be prolonged in severe hepatic failure

15 minutes after the initiation of an infusion and reaches its peak effect at 1 hour.[64,65] Clinicians may administer a bolus to achieve faster onset, but bolus administration is associated with increased risk of hemodynamic instability, which can manifest as either hypertension or hypotension and bradycardia.[66] Additional adverse effects include nausea, atrial fibrillation, and, rarely, cardiogenic shock.[67] In the United States, dexmedetomidine is approved for use as a continuous infusion at doses up to 0.7 mcg/kg/hour for a maximum of 24 hours, but clinical trials have demonstrated safety and effectiveness at doses up to 1.5 mcg/kg/hour for as much as 28 days.[68–70] Doses may be titrated every 30 minutes. Patients with severe hepatic disease may require lower doses of dexmedetomidine to avoid prolonged offset of effect and excessive hemodynamic effects. Dexmedetomidine-induced hypotension and bradycardia may occur more commonly in patients who are hypovolemic or those who have cardiovascular instability.[71] Importantly, because dexmedetomidine does not cause respiratory depression, it can be continued during and after extubation, unlike propofol.[71,72] When continuing dexmedetomidine in this fashion, clinicians should be aware that it may cause loss of oropharyngeal muscle tone, resulting in airway obstruction. Consequently, patients getting dexmedetomidine without mechanical ventilation must receive continuous respiratory monitoring.

Benzodiazepines are GABA receptor agonists that demonstrate anxiolytic, sedative, hypnotic, and anticonvulsant effects.[73] Current guidelines no longer recommend use of benzodiazepines as first-line sedatives in most critically ill patients, although they remain the mainstay of therapy for management of alcohol withdrawal.[37] Benzodiazepines can potentiate respiratory failure and hypotension, especially when coadministered with opioids.[35] They can also cause mental status changes and are risk factors for development of delirium.[70,74,75] Patients may occasionally experience a paradoxical reaction involving agitation and restlessness. Elderly patients are more likely to experience adverse effects, while patients taking benzodiazepines prior to hospitalization and those on them for long periods of time may demonstrate decreased sensitivity. Usually, benzodiazepines are administered parenterally in the critical care setting and the most commonly used agents are lorazepam and midazolam. Either lorazepam or midazolam may be given via intermittent or by continuous intravenous infusion, but the two drugs have key differences relative to their pharmacokinetic, pharmacodynamic, and adverse effect profiles. Because it is more lipophilic, midazolam has a faster onset and shorter duration of action than lorazepam. However, because midazolam deposits in the adipose tissue, it can lead to variable and prolonged awakening when it is administered continuously over the course of several days.[76] Midazolam undergoes hepatic metabolism to an active metabolite, which is eliminated renally, while lorazepam is inactivated in the liver. Both agents should be used cautiously in renal and hepatic dysfunction because end organ impairment prolongs the elimination half-life of both drugs. Lorazepam is formulated in a propylene glycol vehicle, which can accumulate at doses as low as 1 mg/kg/day and cause metabolic acidosis and AKI.[77,78] When benzodiazepines must be used clinicians should carefully manage the dosing regimen to target the desired level of sedation at the lowest dose possible. Avoiding continuous infusions of benzodiazepines in favor of as needed bolus doses based on symptoms of agitation may result in decreased total benzodiazepine exposure and a lower chance of benzodiazepine-related complications.

After thoroughly assessing J.A. and addressing reversible causes of agitation such as metabolic disorders and withdrawal syndromes, sedation with propofol should be considered if he remains agitated and his hemodynamics are adequate. Propofol and dexmedetomidine are both suggested first-line sedatives according to current guidelines. However, because J.A. may require frequent awakenings for neurologic examinations, the faster offset of effect with propofol may make it more appropriate. J.A.'s blood pressure and heart rate should be monitored when propofol is started, and it should be titrated to a light level of sedation based on the RASS or SAS. His triglyceride concentrations should be evaluated periodically if propofol is administered for several days, and clinicians should be aware of the symptoms of PRIS in order to identify any potential episodes as soon as possible.

CASE 56-6

QUESTION 1: After receiving care in the ICU and remaining intubated and lightly sedated for several days, J.A.'s sedation is lightened, but he does not seem to be himself. He alternates between unresponsiveness and agitation. He is unable to tell caregivers where he is or answer simple questions. Could J.A. be experiencing delirium?

Delirium is a symptom of acute brain dysfunction that involves the following combination of symptoms: acute change or fluctuation from baseline mental status, inattention, and disorganized thinking or altered level of consciousness.[79,80] Patients who are delirious may experience hallucinations, delusions, or hyperactivity, but these symptoms are not present in all delirious patients. In fact, three different forms of delirium have been described based on the symptoms that patients demonstrate. In hyperactive delirium, patients are agitated, while in hypoactive delirium they are calm or lethargic. Patients with mixed delirium fluctuate between these two subtypes.[37]

Delirium occurs at least once during the ICU stay in up to 80% of critically ill patients and is associated with negative patient outcomes, including increased mortality, ICU and hospital-length of stay, long-term cognitive impairment, and health care costs.[81–84] Clinicians are more likely to fail to identify delirium if patients manifest hypoactive delirium rather than hyperactive delirium.[85] In order to identify patients who have delirium, current guidelines recommend that clinicians routinely assess patients several times each day using a validated delirium assessment tool.[37] The two recommended tools for assessing delirium are called the Confusion Assessment Method for the ICU (CAM-ICU) and the Intensive Care Delirium Screening Checklist (ICDSC).

Based on his symptoms, J.A. is likely experiencing delirium. It is clear that his mental status has changed from baseline as "he does not seem to be himself." In addition, the fluctuation between unresponsiveness and agitation combined with the inattention and disorganized thinking he is exhibiting by not being able to answer simple questions fulfill the other criteria of delirium. Clinicians should formally evaluate J.A. for delirium using a validated tool such as the CAM-ICU or the ICDSC.

CASE 56-6, QUESTION 2: How should clinicians work to prevent and treat delirium in critically ill patients like J.A.?

There are a variety of modifiable and non-modifiable risk factors associated with the development of delirium in critically ill patients.[37] Non-modifiable risk factors include baseline dementia, hypertension, alcoholism, and greater severity of illness.[37,75,86] Current evidence suggests that benzodiazepine exposure, very deep sedation, and anticholinergic medications may increase the risk that patients develop delirium. Any association between opioids and propofol and delirium is unclear because of conflicting and limited evidence, respectively.[37]

Evidence suggests delirium may be prevented with early mobilization protocols, in which nurses, physical therapists, and other clinicians assist critically ill patients in getting out of bed and ambulating. Studies of these protocols have demonstrated that they are safe and associated with significant reductions in delirium, hospital and ICU length of stay, and duration of mechanical ventilation when used in critically ill patients.[87,88] No pharmacologic therapy has been shown to prevent delirium in heterogeneous groups of critically ill patients.[37]

Although haloperidol has been used historically to treat delirium in critically ill patients, there is an absence of high-quality published literature in broad groups of critically ill patients. Consequently, current guidelines make no recommendations regarding the use of haloperidol for treatment of delirium. Atypical antipsychotics may be considered to help reduce the duration of delirium; however, published literature supporting their use is very limited.[37,89] Evidence suggests that using dexmedetomidine instead of a benzodiazepine for management of agitation may result in less delirium.[68,70,90]

Delirium can be prevented in patients like J.A. through the use of early mobilization protocols and minimizing risk factors for delirium such as benzodiazepines. No pharmacologic strategy has been convincingly demonstrated to reduce delirium, although evidence suggests that atypical antipsychotics might have some role and could be considered.

Stress Ulcer Prophylaxis in the ICU

The development of stress ulcers in critically ill patients is a common complication of ICU patients. Stress ulcers from critical illness began to be recognized in the 1960s when one study found that 8/150 (5%) of consecutive ICU patients were found to have massive bleeding resulting from stress ulcers.[91] Stress ulcers usually develop in the mucosal layer of the stomach after high stress events and can result in ulceration and progress to clinically significant bleeding.[92] Up to 15% of patients in the ICU will develop an overt gastrointestinal (GI) bleed if not given SUP, which makes it a preventable complication of critical illness.[93] Despite there being a large volume of research in this area, there lacks a consensus on the management and prevention of stress ulcers.

Patients with serious illness or trauma can develop stress ulceration within hours of the inciting event. There are various degrees of stress ulceration and they can develop from hours to weeks after hospital admission. Critical illness often leads to increased vasoconstriction, decreased cardiac output, and a pro-inflammatory state which leads to splanchnic hypoperfusion.[94] The cause of stress ulceration in the ICU evolves from several factors including gastric acid secretion, mucosal ischemia, and upper intestinal reflux. This leads to lack of perfusion and oxygen delivery to intestinal cells, resulting in mucosal damage.

CASE 56-7

QUESTION 1: A.K. is a 76-year-old male admitted to the Medical ICU for likely sepsis from a urinary source. He was acidotic on arrival to the emergency department and intubated. He has a past medical history of hypertension, diabetes, multiple pulmonary embolisms, several urinary tract infections, and reports drinking 10 to 12 beers/day. His home medications include metoprolol XL 100 mg daily, metformin 1,000 mg twice daily, atorvastatin 20 mg daily, lisinopril 20 mg daily, and warfarin 7.5 mg daily. Labs on arrival are Na 131 mEq/L, K 3.2 mEq/L, BUN 33 mg/dL, Scr 2.7 mg/dL, Hct 20%, Plt 47 × $10^3/\mu L$, INR 5.9. What risk factors does A.K. have that would qualify him for SUP?

Several risk factors have been identified to help determine who should get SUP. Cook et al.[95] investigated 2,252 ICU patients and found that there were two major risk factors for clinically important GI bleeding: (1) mechanical ventilation for more than 48 hours (odds ratio, 15.6) and (2) coagulopathy (odds ratio, 4.3) defined as a platelet count of <50,000 mm^3, an International Normalized Ratio of >1.5 or a partial thromboplastin time of >2 times the control value.[95] Other risk factors that have been identified include head injury, burn involving >35% of body surface area, partial hepatectomy, hepatic or renal transplantation, multiple trauma with Injury Severity Score of >16, spinal cord injury, hepatic failure, history of gastric ulceration or bleeding during year before admission, and two or more of the following: sepsis, length of ICU stay >1 week, occult bleeding for at least 6 days, and administration of high dose corticosteroids (>250 mg/day of hydrocortisone or equivalent).[96] Most clinicians will start SUP in patients who have ≥1 major risk factor. For patients who have multiple minor risk factors or patient groups excluded from major trials (spinal cord injury, traumatic brain injury, or thermal injury), SUP is determined by the primary team on a case-by-case basis. A.K. has a major risk factor in that he is likely to be intubated for at least 48 hours. For this reason, he should be started on SUP.

CASE 56-7, QUESTION 2: What medication could be initiated in A.K. to reduce his chance of developing a stress ulcer?

The mechanisms to pharmacologically prevent against stress ulcers are to layer the gastric lining with a protective coating, lowering the gastric pH by neutralizing gastric acid secretions, or by preventing gastric acid secretion. The three classes of medications used for SUP are Histamine 2-receptor antagonists (H_2 blockers), proton-pump inhibitors (PPIs), and protective barrier producing medications. A fourth class of medication, prostaglandin analogs, have been used for SUP in the past, but it has not been shown to be beneficial and will not be discussed in this chapter further.[97]

After deciding to start SUP, the next decision to make is what agent to use. The two most commonly used classes of medications are H_2 blockers and PPIs. H_2 blockers were found to be superior to antacids and sucralfate in two different trials.[98,99] There has been a plethora of research comparing PPIs to H_2 blockers, but there still lacks a consensus on what agent to use based on conflicting data. A recent meta-analysis in over 35,000 ICU patients showed H_2 blockers had a lower risk of GI hemorrhage compared to PPIs (6% vs. 2%; adjusted OR, 2.24; 95% CI, 1.81–2.76).[100] This differed with a previous meta-analysis of 13 randomized trials showing reduced GI bleeding in the PPI prophylaxis group compared to the H_2 blocker group (1.3% vs. 6.6%; OR, 0.30; 95% CI, 0.17–0.54).[101] A meta-analysis of 14 trials and 1,720 patients found that PPIs reduced clinically important upper gastrointestinal bleeding and overt upper gastrointestinal bleeding compared to H_2 blockers.[102] Common agents used for SUP are provided in Table 56-4.

An area of debate is whether a patient who is receiving full caloric supplementation through tube feeds requires pharmacologic SUP. Enteral nutrition has been shown to increase gastric pH to >3.5 more often than H_2 blockers or PPIs.[103] Animal models have shown a protective benefit of alimentation on the gastric mucosa from stress-related damage. The practice of whether to discontinue pharmacologic SUP if enteral nutrition has been started varies among different institutions.

CASE 56-7, QUESTION 3: Are there any adverse effects associated with placing A.K. on SUP?

While pharmacologic SUP has shown to decrease bleeding events, it appears this does not come without risk. Gastric acid plays an important part in sterilizing the upper gastrointestinal tract, and alterations of physiologic pH have shown adverse effects. The higher pH level allows increased colonization of potentially pathogenic bacteria in the gastrointestinal tract.

After the implementation of SUP as a standard of care in ICUs, several studies and meta-analyses identified an increased risk of nosocomial pneumonia and *C. difficile* infections in patients receiving

Table 56-4
Common Agents Used for Stress Ulcer Prophylaxis

Agent	Trade Name	Adult Dosing	Routes	Generic Available
Proton Pump Inhibitors				
Dexlansoprazole[a]	Dexilant	30 or 60 mg	Oral	No
Esomeprazole[a]	Nexium	20–40 mg once daily ≥1 hour prior to a meal	Oral, IV	Yes
Lansoprazole[a]	Prevacid	15 or 30 mg once daily before a meal	Oral	Yes
Omeprazole[a]	Prilosec	20 or 40 mg once daily on an empty stomach ≥1 hour before a meal	Oral, IV	Yes
Pantoprazole[a]	Protonix	40 mg once daily (administer suspension 30 minute prior to a meal)	Oral, IV	Yes
Robeprazole[a]	Aciphex	20–60 mg once daily (administer capsule 30 minutes prior to a meal; if capsule is opened and dispersed on food, administer within 15 minutes of preparation)	Oral	Yes
Histamine H_2 Antagonists				
Famotidine[a]	Pepcid	20 mg twice daily (20 mg daily for CrCl <30 mL/minute)	Oral, IV	Yes
Nizatidine[a]	Axid	150–300 mg daily (150 mg/day for CrCl 20–50 mL/minute; 150 mg every other day for CrCl <20 mL/minute	Oral	Yes
Ranitidine[a]	Zantac	150 mg twice daily (150 mg once daily if CrCl <50 mL/minute)	Oral, IV	Yes
Gastric-Coating Agents				
Sucralfate[a]	Carafate	1 g 4 times daily	Oral	Yes

[a]Off label indication for stress ulcer prophylaxis.
Source: Facts & Comparisons eAnswers. **http://online.factsandcomparisons.com/MonoDisp.aspx?monoid=fandc-hcp14911&book=DFC**. Accessed September 28, 2015.

H_2 blockers or PPIs. The increased pH levels as a result of these medications have been proposed as a mechanism of action. Available data are conflicting on the incidence of nosocomial pneumonia among the agents that alter gastric pH. Two studies showed an increased risk for H_2 blockers compared to those who did not receive acid-suppressive therapy or sucralfate.[99,104] One meta-analysis showed no difference on the incidence of nosocomial pneumonia when comparing PPIs to H_2 blockers.[101] A recent study showed that PPIs had a higher incidence of pneumonia compared to H_2 blockers.[100] Both PPIs and H_2 blockers have been associated with an increased risk of *C. difficile* infection.[105] Most of these studies are observational and did not control for comorbidities, so there is still much debate in the critical care community.

While sucralfate does not alter gastric pH, it can interfere with the absorption of many medications including ciprofloxacin, phenytoin, digoxin, and levothyroxine. To help prevent this, sucralfate should be given 2 hours after these medications. Sucralfate has been shown to bind to tube feeds and cause bezoars and cannot be given through duodenal or jejunostomy feeding tubes. There are several options of SUP for A.K. A PPI or H_2 blocker would be the best choice. Since he is intubated and does not have a feeding tube yet, an IV H_2 blocker such as famotidine (renally dosed) or IV PPI such as pantoprazole would be appropriate.

Glycemic Control in ICU Patients

Critically ill patients may develop hyperglycemia for a variety of reasons, including acute illness, preexisting disease states, and the effects of medications. Glycemic goals and treatments differ for patients managed in the ICU as compared to those treated in other settings, including patients receiving chronic therapy for diabetes as outpatients.

CASE 56-8

Question 1: D.M. is a 74-year-old female admitted to the medical ICU for pneumonia and a COPD exacerbation. Her past medical history includes hypertension, hyperlipidemia, and COPD. On the first day of her ICU stay, she decompensates and develops respiratory failure requiring intubation. Among other laboratory abnormalities, her blood glucose concentration is 212 mg/dL. How should clinicians manage D.M.'s hyperglycemia?

A variety of biochemical mediators, such as cortisol, glucagon, catecholamines, and growth factor, may rise in critical illness and contribute to hyperglycemia by increasing glycogenolysis and decreasing gluconeogenesis.[106] In addition to the effects of critical illness, inadequately treated diabetes, adverse effects of drugs like corticosteroids, and exposure to caloric loads from nutritional regimens or dextrose used as a base for intravenous solutions can contribute to hyperglycemia. Although studies suggest that hyperglycemia of critical illness is associated with poor outcomes, it is not clear whether hyperglycemia leads to worsened outcomes or if it is simply an indicator of disease severity.[107–109] In addition to the magnitude of hyperglycemia, glycemic variability has also been associated with negative outcomes.[110]

The optimal blood glucose range for critically ill patients has not been definitely established.[111] Uncontrolled hyperglycemia has the potential to cause severe effects. Single-center studies of surgical and medical ICU patients treated with intensive insulin therapy to achieve blood glucose concentrations between 80 and 110 mg/dL initially suggested improved outcomes, but these findings have not been replicated in subsequent trials.[112,113] In fact, some studies have suggested that aggressive insulin therapy may increase mortality as compared to liberal blood glucose control typically targeting 140 to 180 mg/dL.[114–117] It has been suggested that the higher rates of hypoglycemia observed in patients receiving intensive insulin may increase mortality by leading to neurologic complications. On the basis of these findings, most clinicians attempt to maintain patients' blood glucose concentrations between 140 and 180 mg/dL. Since parenteral administration of insulin achieves more rapid and reliable results than oral therapy, patients are typically managed with subcutaneous insulin or intravenous insulin infusions while in the ICU. Subcutaneous regimens typically include as-needed sliding scale insulin involving rapid or short-acting formulations. Scheduled long-acting insulin may be combined with sliding scales in some patients; however, clinicians should cautiously dose insulin in order to avoid hypoglycemia. Some patients with significant insulin needs may benefit from a continuous intravenous infusion of regular insulin that is carefully titrated to the blood glucose goal.

Since D.M.'s blood glucose exceeds 180 mg/dL, clinicians should attempt to achieve better glycemic control. First, dextrose-containing fluids should be minimized, and any enteral nutrition she is receiving should be evaluated. Medications, like steroids, that might increase her blood glucose concentrations should be assessed and minimized as possible. If her blood glucose remains high after these measures, it would be appropriate to initially consider sliding scale insulin with regular insulin.

KEY REFERENCES AND WEBSITES

A full list of references for this chapter can be found at http://thepoint.lww.com/AT11e. Below are the key references and websites for this chapter, with the corresponding reference number in this chapter found in parentheses after the reference.

Key References

ASHP Commission on Therapeutics and approved by the ASHP Board of Directors on November 14, 1998. ASHP Therapeutic Guidelines on Stress Ulcer Prophylaxis. *Am J Health Syst Pharm*. 1999;56(4):347–379. (96)

Barr J et al. Clinical practice guidelines for the management of pain, agitation, and delirium in adult patients in the intensive care unit. *Crit Care Med*. 2013;41(1):263–306. (37)

Chanques G et al. A prospective study of pain at rest: incidence and characteristics of an unrecognized symptom in surgical and trauma versus medical intensive care unit patients. *Anesthesiology*. 2007;107(5):858–860. (39)

Guyatt GH et al; American College of Chest Physicians Antithrombotic Therapy and Prevention of Thrombosis Panel. Executive summary: Antithrombotic Therapy and Prevention of Thrombosis, 9th ed: American College of Chest Physicians Evidence-Based Clinical Practice Guidelines. *Chest*. 2012;141(2, Suppl):7S–47S. (6)

Smith BS et al. Introduction to drug pharmacokinetics in the critically ill patient. *Chest*. 2012;141(5):1327–1336. (17)

Varghese JM et al. Antimicrobial pharmacokinetic and pharmacodynamic issues in the critically ill with severe sepsis and septic shock. *Crit Care Clin*. 2011;27(1):19–34. (26)

57 Multiple Sclerosis

Melody Ryan

CORE PRINCIPLES

		CHAPTER CASES
1	Multiple sclerosis (MS) is a chronic inflammatory and degenerative disease of the central nervous system in which demyelination and axonal damage occur. MS can take one of several forms: relapsing-remitting, secondary-progressive, or primary-progressive are the most common forms.	**Case 57-1 (Questions 1, 5), Figure 57-1**
2	The diagnosis of MS is based on clinical symptoms and is supported by magnetic resonance imaging (MRI) and laboratory testing (cerebrospinal fluid oligoclonal bands and immunoglobulin G synthesis rate; evoked potential testing). In an individual patient, dissemination in space and time must be demonstrated before the diagnosis of MS is made.	**Case 57-1 (Questions 1, 5)**
3	Glucocorticoids are the agents of choice for treatment of acute MS relapses.	**Case 57-1 (Question 7)**
4	Clinically isolated syndrome (CIS) is a term used to describe a first demyelinating neurologic event before the diagnosis of MS has been made. When a patient presents with CIS and MRI abnormalities, progression to clinically definite MS is likely, and therapy with interferon β, glatiramer acetate, or teriflunomide helps to prevent this progression.	**Case 57-1 (Questions 1, 2)**
5	Dimethyl fumarate, glatiramer acetate, interferon β-1a, interferon β-1b, and teriflunomide are potential first-line therapies for relapsing forms of MS. The choice of treatment is often based on provider or patient preference.	**Case 57-1 (Questions 3, 5–8)** **Case 57-2 (Question 1), Table 57-3**
6	Adherence to self-injection therapy with interferon β-1a, interferon β-1b, and glatiramer acetate is low.	**Case 57-1 (Question 4), Table 57-7**
7	Alemtuzumab, fingolimod, mitoxantrone, and natalizumab therapy is generally reserved for patients with worsening relapsing forms of MS because of adverse effect concerns.	**Case 57-1 (Question 7)** **Case 57-2 (Question 3)**
8	Patients with MS can experience many symptoms, such as walking problems or impaired ambulation, sexual dysfunction, pain, bladder dysfunction, fatigue, cognitive dysfunction, spasticity, bowel dysfunction, dysphagia or dysarthria, and pseudobulbar affect. These symptoms may require both nonpharmacologic and pharmacologic therapy.	**Case 57-1 (Question 10), Case 57-2 (Question 4), Table 57-2 and 57-4**

EPIDEMIOLOGY, NATURAL COURSE OF THE DISEASE, AND PROGNOSIS

Multiple sclerosis (MS) is a chronic inflammatory and degenerative disease of the central nervous system (CNS) in which demyelination and axonal damage occur.[1] The disease has a mean age at onset of 30 years, with diagnoses typically occurring between the ages of 20 and 50 years.[2,3] Because of the young age at onset, MS has a dramatic effect on employment and, in fact, is the most common cause of disability in young adults.[4] Overall life expectancy is decreased by about 6 years compared with age- and sex-matched control subjects,[5] and patients are three more likely to die than the general population when matched for age and sex.[5] Infection and cardiac causes of death are the most commonly reported, similar to a control population, but occurring in higher frequencies in patients with MS.[5,6] Health-related quality of life is lower in patients with MS than in the general population, and this decrease is related to the severity of MS.[7]

MS affects approximately 0.1% of the US population (400,000 people) and about 2.5 million people worldwide.[3,4] Women are 2 to 3 times more likely to have MS than men.[3] Many environmental and genetic factors have been associated with MS (Table 57-1); however, the causal nature of any of these factors has yet to be established.[8–18] Current thought is that an environmental trigger acting in a genetically susceptible individual is the probable cause of MS.[19]

MS is most frequently encountered between 40 and 60 degrees north or south latitude. Regions with a high prevalence include Western and Northern Europe, Canada, Russia, Israel, Northern United States, New Zealand, and Southeast Australia.[20] Additionally, relapse rates may also vary seasonally with latitude.[21] This finding has spurred many research studies and hypotheses. One hypothesis is that development of MS is related to sunlight exposure or vitamin D. Higher serum concentrations of 25-hydroxyvitamin D (the major circulating form and the one that is measured by clinical laboratory testing) are associated with reduced hazard of an MS relapse, and lower concentrations are associated with higher rates of MS diagnoses.[22,23] Genetically, lack of the vitamin D receptor (VDR) and CYP27B1 (encodes the enzyme responsible for vitamin D activation converting 25-hydroxyl-vitamin D to 1,25-hydroxyl-vitamin D) is associated with impaired immune system.[24] Some investigators have found links between season of birth and development of MS, suggesting that maternal vitamin D status may be important.[24] Relapses also follow a seasonal pattern, with peaks in the early spring and troughs in the autumn in both hemispheres, further suggesting a role of vitamin D in relapses.[21]

Epstein–Barr virus is a ubiquitous infection; however, high EBV titers and a history of infectious mononucleosis both increase risk of developing MS. Smoking is a risk factor, with higher levels of smoking conferring greater risk.[17,24] Dietary salt intake may be associated with higher relapse rates and increased numbers of brain lesions.[18]

There is likely a genetic predisposition to development of MS. First-degree relatives of people with MS have a risk of MS that is 10 to 25 times greater than the general population; the concordance rate in identical twins is 35%.[11,13] There are probably several genetic factors that increase risk for MS, including HLA type and various single-nucleotide polymorphisms that control T-cell receptors, vitamin D receptors, and estrogen receptors.[23,25,26] A specific major histocompatibility complex (MHC) associated with MS is HLA-DRB1*1501 class II, but over 100 different genetic variations have been associated with MS.[24] No genetic association has been found for a particular clinical course or rate of progression.[24]

Although MS is more prevalent in Caucasian populations in the United States, there is evidence that African-American patients may be more likely to have primary-progressive forms and may have a more severe disease course.[27–29]

Table 57-1

Factors Associated with Multiple Sclerosis (MS)

Female sex[3,8]	Low sun exposure[9,10]
Caucasians[11]	Low serum concentrations of vitamin D (25-hydroxyvitamin D)[10]
Higher latitudes of residence[12]	Northern European heritage[13]
High serum antibody titers to the Epstein–Barr virus nuclear antigens[14,15]	Tobacco smoking[14,16]
Infectious mononucleosis[17]	Dietary salt[18]

MS is generally characterized as one of three main types according to the presentation and clinical course of the disease: relapsing-remitting MS, secondary-progressive MS, and primary-progressive MS. These three types of MS are distinguished by their natural histories. Relapsing-remitting MS was named for the relapses (also called *exacerbations* or *attacks*) of clinical disease activity that alternate with periods of symptom remission. Recovery during the remission periods can be complete, or the patient may continue to have some clinical deficits.[30] Between 80% and 90% of patients have relapsing-remitting MS when they are first diagnosed.[1,31] Patient registry data provide insight regarding the prognosis of those with relapsing-remitting MS. Patients diagnosed with relapsing-remitting MS at onset have slower progression to disability than patients with primary-progressive MS; patients having complete or near-complete recovery from the first attack of MS have a longer time to disability compared with those with significant persistent deficits after the first attack.[1,31]

Approximately 80% of patients initially diagnosed with relapsing-remitting MS experience a secondary-progressive form in which fewer relapses occur, but disability continues to progress.[1,2] The cause of the conversion from relapsing-remitting MS to secondary-progressive MS is unknown, but it has been hypothesized that the change occurs when axonal loss in the CNS reaches a critical threshold.[32] The time to development of secondary-progressive MS is quite variable. The usual time to conversion is 20 to 25 years after diagnosis, with a median patient age at the time of conversion of 43 years; however, it may occur much sooner.[1,30,33] It is not known how treatment affects this process. In one study, the number of early relapses (within 2 years of diagnosis) was associated with a shorter time to development of secondary-progressive MS.[34] Therefore, early treatment with a therapy that reduces relapses might be expected to delay development of secondary-progressive MS.

Approximately 10% to 15% of patients have primary-progressive MS.[1,35] This type of MS is progressive from onset with occasional minor improvements or periods of stabilization.[30] Primary-progressive MS is more common in patients who are older than 50 years at diagnosis.[1] Select studies have found this form to be more common in men, but others have found no association with sex.[1,35] Mean time from diagnosis to requiring a cane to walk is approximately 9 years for patients with primary-progressive MS.[36]

In the absence of treatment, patients who initially present with relapsing-remitting MS develop average Expanded Disability Status Scale (EDSS) scores of 4.0 or higher (indicating significant disability) by 7 years after diagnosis.[20] The EDSS is a scale commonly used in MS to measure level of disability and progression of the disease.[37] Some predictors of a more progressive disease course include male gender, multisystem symptoms, incomplete recovery from the initial episode, progressive disease from the time of diagnosis, older age at onset, and abnormal baseline magnetic resonance imaging (MRI) results.[30,38] Although patients present with different types of MS, once progression begins, all forms of progressive MS follow a similar time course for subsequent progression.[30]

A new classification system has been proposed which denotes disease activity and progression.[39] Patients with new, active MRI lesions or with clinical relapses within a specified time frame are classified as active, whereas those without new lesions or relapses are classified as inactive. In a similar way, patients are categorized as progressing if they have steadily increasing objectively documented neurologic dysfunction without recovery or non-progressing. For example, a patient with relapsing-remitting MS who has had a clinical relapse in the last year, but who had full recovery, would be classified as relapsing-remitting MS-active and not progressing.[39] Because MS begins during young-to-middle adulthood, there is a large economic burden associated with the disease. One study in which newly diagnosed patients were matched to healthy control subjects found that patients with MS were 3.5 times as likely to be hospitalized, twice as likely to have at least one emergency department visit, and 2.4 times as likely to have at least one visit for physical, occupational, or speech therapy during the course of a year.[40] These additional services were associated with higher mean annual all-cause healthcare costs ($32,051 vs. $4,732 for MS patients and control subjects, respectively).[41] These estimates do not consider the loss of employment or loss of caregiver employment. When these factors are taken into consideration, the cost of MS is more than $77,938/year.[42]

Ten years after diagnosis, 50% to 80% of patients with MS are unemployed. Surprisingly, only 15% of unemployment is related to physical restrictions.[34] Of the factors most often cited as leading to unemployment, only decreased walking ability relates to physical disability. The other common factors are increased age, decreased verbal fluency, and loss of memory.[34,42]

PATHOPHYSIOLOGY

Many aspects of the pathophysiology of MS remain unclear, although research in this area is progressing rapidly. Foremost in unresolved issues is the identity of the actual initiating factor for the autoimmune and inflammatory processes that characterize MS. Through the years, several dozen triggers have been proposed. Current thinking is that a genetically susceptible individual has an environmental factor which triggers the immune system to cause MS.[44]

There are two pathologic processes that occur during MS. The first is inflammatory. During this process, the body mounts an autoimmune attack on the myelin covering of nerve fibers of the white matter in the CNS. These areas of demyelination are visualized as plaques or lesions and are seen on brain tissue directly (e.g., on autopsy) or on MRI with contrast agents (Fig. 57-1).[25] It is this inflammation that causes the relapses that are seen clinically, and it is the resolution of these relapses that is seen as remission.

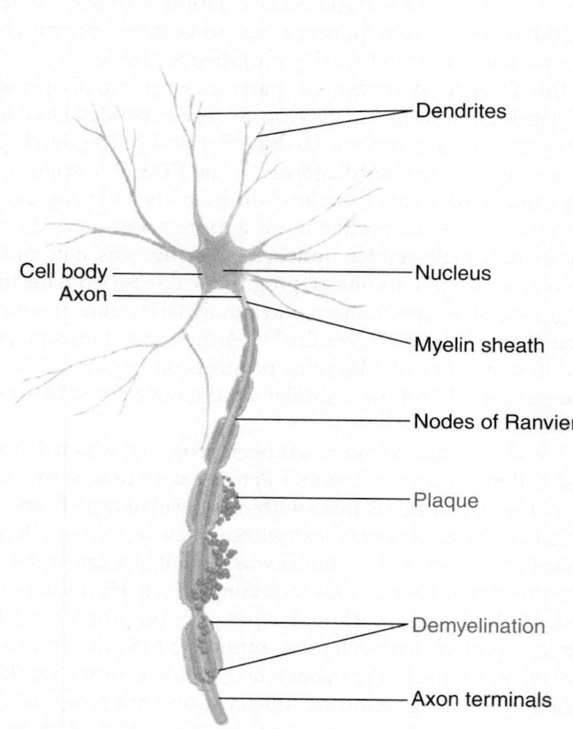

Figure 57-1 Myelin destruction in multiple sclerosis.

The second process is neurodegenerative, during which the axons of nerves in brain white matter are damaged, some irrevocably. This neurodegeneration causes a progressive disability when transmission through the nerve cell is slowed or fails completely. It is cumulative with time and may be irreversible. It is not known whether the inflammatory or neurodegenerative process occurs first in MS or whether they are simultaneous.[19]

Inflammation

The inflammatory cascade in MS is complex. Various types of T cells play a role early in the process.[4] The unknown antigen couples with MHC molecules.[14,44]

These antigen–MHC pairs encounter antigen-presenting cells (APC) such as dendrites, macrophages, and microglia.[9,20] T cells recognize this antigen–MHC–APC complex, become activated, and initiate the immunologic cascade.[4]

Under normal circumstances, regulatory T cells (T_{reg}) monitor for and control autoimmune T-cell formation in the periphery. It has been hypothesized that T_{reg} cells malfunction in people with MS.[19]

The activated T cells then retreat to the lymphatic tissues in the body, such as the spleen and lymph nodes, to expand.[4] At the appropriate time, the T cells exit the lymphatic tissues and rejoin the circulation. Sphingosine-1-phosphate (S1P), a small, circulating lipid molecule, is important in this process. For the T cells to exit the lymphatic tissues, the S1P receptor 1 must be expressed on their surface.[46] The T cells follow an S1P concentration gradient to exit the lymphatic tissues and join the circulation.

The activated T cells must cross the blood–brain barrier to attack myelin in the CNS. An adhesion molecule, $\alpha_4\beta_1$-integrin (VLA4), is found on the surface of T cells.[25] When the T cells approach the blood–brain barrier, they slow and bind to the α_4-integrin and p-selectin glycoprotein ligand 1. This bonding allows the T cells to transmigrate through the endothelial cells of the blood vessel.[46]

Now in the perivascular space, the T cells must be reactivated by new APC.[4] Through the action of matrix metalloproteinases 2 and 9, the activated T cells invade the parenchyma of the brain.[46] Once ensconced in the brain, the T cells begin to secrete various proinflammatory cytokines that further stimulate the inflammatory cascade, including stimulation of microglia.[25,47,48]

The microglia produce proteolytic enzymes, lipolytic enzymes, reactive oxygen species, reactive nitrogen species, excitotoxins, and more proinflammatory cytokines. Activated microglia can also serve as APCs for activation of additional T cells.[47] Nitric oxide, a reactive nitrogen species, is increased during inflammation and can inhibit mitochondrial respiration, inhibit the sodium–potassium adenosine triphosphatase pump, and cause the intracellular release of calcium. The excess calcium leads to degenerative processes within the cell.[4,32]

Although the role of T cells is central to MS pathology, the role of B and NK cells is much less clear. B cells may be involved in antigen presentation and the production of the immunoglobulin found in the CSF of patients with MS.[19] NK cells have been postulated to have both helpful and deleterious effects.[19]

At some point, the resolution of inflammation begins. During the inflammatory cascade, myelin is broken down, and this myelin debris inhibits remyelination. The microglia use phagocytosis to clear myelin structures, axons, apoptotic cells, and myelin debris from the area of inflammation.[47] After this process, the microglia begin to produce immunomodulatory cytokines.[47] Helper T type 2 cells become more prominent and begin secreting immunomodulatory cytokines as well.[47]

Remyelination then begins; however, some evidence suggests that the ability of the body to remyelinate decreases with age.[4]

Microglia produce more cytokines and some growth factors that cause oligodendrocyte progenitor cells to migrate to the area. Remyelination occurs when oligodendrocyte progenitor cells differentiate into new oligodendrocytes.[47] S1P receptors 1 and 5 present on oligodendrocytes appear to help with differentiation.[49] Remyelination may not be complete and, in some cases, does not occur at all. The myelin also may be thinner and shorter than the original myelin.[4]

Neurodegeneration

Axonal injury can occur throughout the course of the disease and may even occur before any clinical symptoms.[3,50] Inside chronic MS lesions, there are 60% to 70% fewer axons compared with other white matter in the same patient.[32] In addition to producing myelin, oligodendrocytes support axons through production of insulin-like growth factor type I and neuregulin; thus, axons can die without the support of the oligodendrocytes. However, axonal loss has been demonstrated at sites separate from MS lesions, particularly the thalamus.[4,32,50] Although oligodendrocytes provide trophic support for the axons, they also inhibit new growth to prevent random neurite sprouting. Three myelin-associated inhibitor factors, myelin-associated glycoprotein, Nogo-A, and oligodendrocyte myelin glycoprotein, lie in the sheath of myelin closest to the axon, where they prevent this sprouting.[3]

Microtubules are also important for neurite growth. The assembly of microtubules is controlled by collapsin response mediator protein 2 (CRMP-2).[3] When CRMP-2 is phosphorylated, neurite growth is inhibited.[3] Ras homolog gene family, member A (RhoA)–guanosine triphosphate (GTP), has action on both the myelin-associated inhibitory factors and CRMP-2. The myelin-associated inhibitory factors signal RhoA–GTP to neurite retraction rather than growth.[3] It also activates Rho kinase, which phosphorylates CRMP-2.[3]

Myelin normally allows saltatory, fast conduction (i.e., conduction via leaps) at the nodes of Ranvier; thus, loss of myelin slows or prevents transmission of nerve impulses.[4]

In the demyelinated state, sodium channels under the myelin sheath may become functional to allow improved nerve conduction.[32] The activation of sodium channels results in sodium entry into the cell. The excess sodium activates the sodium–calcium exchanger to export sodium and import calcium, fueling the degenerative processes within the neuron.[4,32] Additionally, increased numbers of glutamate-regulated α-amino-3-hydroxy-5-methyl-4-isoxazolepropionic acid (AMPA) receptors are seen in demyelinated axons. Activation of these receptors results in increased levels of intracellular sodium and calcium, further contributing to neurodegeneration.[32]

CLINICAL PRESENTATION

Because the demyelination associated with MS can occur in any part of the CNS, many different symptoms are associated with the disease. At first presentation, the most common clinical symptoms are sensory disturbances, particularly of the extremities, partial or complete visual loss, motor dysfunction of the limbs, diplopia, and gait dysfunction.[20] Two demyelinating syndromes are so distinct and they have been recognized, named, and deserve particular mention: optic neuritis and transverse myelitis. Optic neuritis is the acute demyelination of the optic nerve. Symptoms may include ocular pain, blurred vision, or changes in color perception.[51] Transverse myelitis is impairment of motor control or sensory function, or control over bladder, bowel, and sexual functions that are consistent with a lesion at a specific point in the spinal cord, but without a structural cause such as a herniated disc.[51]

Table 57-2
Common Symptoms in Chronic Multiple Sclerosis

Symptom	Prevalence (%)
Sexual dysfunction[57]	85
Walking problems or impaired ambulation[58]	64
Pain[59]	30–90
Bladder dysfunction[60]	75
Fatigue[61]	74
Cognitive dysfunction[62]	70
Spasticity[59]	60
Bowel dysfunction[60]	50
Depression[63]	50
Dysphagia or dysarthria[64]	40
Pseudobulbar affect[65]	10

As concern has developed about neurodegenerative changes that occur early in the course of MS, there has been more interest in very early treatment after the emergence of symptoms to delay or decrease the development of MS. The term clinically isolated syndrome (CIS) describes a first demyelinating neurologic event involving the optic nerve, cerebrum, cerebellum, brainstem, or spinal cord.[51] Up to 85% of people with MS may first present with CIS.[52] Of those who present with CIS, 63% will develop MS during the ensuing 20 years.[52]

Patients younger than 40 years old are more likely to convert from CIS to clinically definite MS than those ≥40 years.[53] Patients with optic neuritis as the presenting diagnosis are less likely than those with other symptoms to develop clinically definite MS. The presence of oligoclonal bands in the CSF, low serum concentrations of vitamin D, and multiple lesions on MRI are associated with a particularly high risk of development of MS.[53,54]

Occasionally, MS-type lesions will be visible on an MRI scan performed for other reasons. If the patient has no other symptoms, this condition is known as *radiologic-isolated syndrome.*[55] About 30% of these patients have a clinical episode within 5 years of the detection of their MRI abnormality.[56] Younger patients, males, and those with lesions on the spinal cord were more likely to develop a CIS.[56] No treatment is suggested for patients with these findings at this time.[56]

With time and with neurodegeneration, many other symptoms can develop in people with MS. The most common symptoms are listed in Table 57-2.[57–65]

DIAGNOSIS

When patients first present for medical care with symptoms of MS, diseases as diverse as infections, cancers, vascular disease, or other inflammatory demyelinating diseases are commonly part of the differential diagnosis. Thus, the addition of MRI and other laboratory findings can help with the diagnosis. At other times, the diagnosis is not apparent until the occurrence of a second attack.[66]

Various diagnostic criteria have been proposed in an effort to standardize diagnoses of MS and to promote earlier treatment. The initial criteria stated that the patient must have experienced at least two demyelination-related episodes separated by time and space (i.e., at least two episodes involving distinct regions of the CNS).[67] Guidelines proposed in 2001 and revised in 2005 and 2010 allow for the use of MRI and CSF findings to fulfill these criteria after an initial clinical attack.[68–70] Primary-progressive MS is diagnosed when there is continuous progression of neurologic symptoms during a 1-year period with characteristic MRI and CSF findings.[70]

OVERVIEW OF TREATMENT

Although the mechanisms of action of MS pharmacotherapies are diverse, they all can be generally categorized as immunomodulating agents. To date, all therapies for MS have targeted the inflammatory response rather than the accompanying neurodegeneration features of the disease.

Treatment of Acute Relapses

Corticosteroids are used in the treatment of MS to control inflammation during acute relapses. Although most patients respond to treatment with corticosteroids, some do not. These agents have several actions that contribute to their acute anti-inflammatory effects. Corticosteroids increase the activity of T_{reg} cells, reduce the activity of T and B cells, reduce adhesion molecule production, and reduce proinflammatory cytokines.[71–73]

Treatment of Relapsing-Remitting Multiple Sclerosis

Most of the therapeutic research conducted in MS has focused on the relapsing-remitting form of the disease. This is the most common form of MS at presentation, and it has an important inflammatory aspect. The agents that are currently US Food and Drug Administration (FDA)-approved for MS include alemtuzumab, beta interferons, dimethyl fumarate, fingolimod, glatiramer acetate, mitoxantrone, natalizumab, and teriflunomide.

ALEMTUZUMAB

Alemtuzumab is a monoclonal antibody aimed at CD52. It reduces the population of circulating B and T cells. The peripheral circulating lymphocytes are undetectable within minutes of infusion.[74] These cells repopulate, but fairly slowly; B cells have a median recovery time of 8 months, $CD8^+$ T cells 20 months, and $CD4^+$ T cells 35 months. However, some patients took as long as 12 years to reach baseline levels.[75] Alemtuzumab reduced relapses and MRI lesions compared to interferon β-1a subcutaneously, but had similar rates of disability progression; 77% of patients taking alemtuzumab were completely relapse-free at 2 years.[76] One long-term study saw benefits sustained from alemtuzumab over 5 years.[77]

BETA INTERFERONS

Beta interferons are thought to work by suppressing T-cell activity, downregulating antigen presentation by MHC class II molecules, decreasing adhesion molecules and matrix metalloproteinase 9, and increasing anti-inflammatory cytokines while decreasing proinflammatory cytokines.[4,47,48,78] There are two types of interferon β (interferon β-1a and interferon β-1b) and a total of four preparations available to treat MS (Table 57-3).[79–82] Placebo-controlled trials of each of the interferon β agents have shown a reduced number of relapses and decreased disease progression measured on the EDSS in patients treated with interferon versus those who were given placebo.[83–85]

Table 57-3
Interferon β Preparations Used in the Treatment of Multiple Sclerosis[79–82]

Interferon Type	Route of Administration	Frequency of Injection
Interferon β-1a	Intramuscular	Weekly
Interferon β-1a	Subcutaneous	3 times weekly
Interferon β-1b	Subcutaneous	Every other day
Peginterferon β-1a	Subcutaneous	Every 2 weeks

Data are available for patients who have been treated with interferon β-1b for up to 16 years. A sustained reduction in relapse rate of 40% was seen in patients who received the drug continuously, an improved response compared with those who received placebo or interferon only for a short time. Patients who received continuous interferon therapy also had slower rates of disease progression.[86,87] Eight-year follow-up data for interferon β-1a given intramuscularly did not show this sustained reduction in relapse rate, but did show that those who began treatment earlier had better long-term outcomes.[86]

DIMETHYL FUMARATE

Dimethyl fumarate is rapidly cleaved in the intestine to form its active form, monomethyl fumarate. The medicine causes a shift in cytokine production from interferon γ and tumor necrosis factor α to interleukin-4 and -5.[88] Dimethyl fumarate also activates the antioxidant effects of nuclear 1 factor (erythroid-related 2)-like 2 (Nrf2) transcriptional pathway which may assist with the neurodegeneration in multiple sclerosis.[88] Dimethyl fumarate reduces the relapse rate by about half and new lesion development on MRI scan compared to placebo.[89]

FINGOLIMOD

Fingolimod is an S1P receptor modulator.[4] It binds to the S1P receptor 1 expressed on T cells.[49] This binding causes the receptor to be internalized in the T cell, where it is unresponsive to the normal signal to exit the lymphoid tissues and recirculate.[49,90] Without the T cells circulating, they are not activated and this disrupts the inflammatory cycle. Fingolimod has been shown to decrease the relapse rate by about half compared with placebo as well as to reduce disability progression.[91,92]

GLATIRAMER ACETATE

Glatiramer acetate decreases type 1 helper T (T_H1) cells while increasing type 2 helper T (T_H2) cells. Additionally, it increases production of nerve growth factors.[4,78] The short-term and long-term efficacy of glatiramer acetate is similar to that of the interferons.[86,93] Regimens of 20 mg subcutaneously daily and 40 mg subcutaneously 3 times weekly are effective compared to placebo.[94]

MITOXANTRONE

Mitoxantrone works as a general immunomodulator. It decreases monocytes and macrophages and inhibits T and B cells.[4] Compared with placebo, mitoxantrone decreased the number of exacerbations and improved MRI in treated patients.[95,96]

NATALIZUMAB

Natalizumab is a humanized monoclonal IgG4 antibody. It blocks T-cell entry into the CNS by binding to $\alpha_4\beta_1$-integrin located on the lymphocyte to keep it from binding to the vascular cell adhesion molecule-1 on the endothelial cell.[4,97,98] In clinical trials, natalizumab was very effective, reducing the 1-year relapse rate by 68%, the risk of progression of disability in 2 years by 42%, and new lesions on MRI by 83%.[99]

TERIFLUNOMIDE

Teriflunomide is the active metabolite of leflunomide. It is thought to act in MS by blocking *de novo* pyrimidine synthesis, inhibiting B- and T-cell division, and blocking the inflammatory pathway prominent in MS.[100] It may also inhibit the pairing of T cells and APC to prevent T-cell activation. Teriflunomide reduces the annualized relapse rate by about 20% to 30% and reduces the risk of new MRI lesions by 60% to 80% compared to placebo in clinical trials.[101,102]

Treatment of Progressive Forms of Multiple Sclerosis

Patients with both secondary-progressive and primary-progressive MS may experience relapses. In these cases, all of the agents used for relapsing-remitting MS may be useful to reduce the number of relapses.[103–106] Some evidence suggests that therapies (specifically, interferon β-1a) are less effective for secondary-progressive MS than for relapsing-remitting MS.[104,106] This finding is consistent with the known mechanisms of action for the currently available agents, which are directed at the inflammatory processes. Treatment of progressive forms of MS is an area in urgent need of scientific investigation. Recently (March 2017), the FDA approved Ocrevus (ocrelizumab), that is the first agent for primary-progressive MS.

Symptom Management

As disability increases, many patients with MS exhibit other associated symptoms that require targeted treatment (Table 57-2).

BLADDER, BOWEL, AND SEXUAL DYSFUNCTION

Bladder, bowel, and sexual dysfunction are very common in patients with MS. Up to 75% of patients have bladder symptoms; constipation or bowel incontinence occur in approximately 50% of patients; and sexual dysfunction occurs in 84% of men and 85% of women.[57,60] It is also known that those patients with more bladder symptoms or sexual dysfunction have lower quality of life compared with patients without these problems.[57,107] The treatment approaches for sexual dysfunction and urinary incontinence in MS are similar to those used when these symptoms occur as part of a primary disorder.

IMPAIRED AMBULATION

In a survey commissioned by the National MS Society, 64% of patients with MS stated that they had some limitation to their walking ability and, therefore, limited activities that involved walking.[58] Physical therapy and conditioning may be of some help for this problem.[59] Another approved treatment option is extended-release dalfampridine. This agent blocks potassium channels and prevents repolarization of the cell, thus prolonging action potentials and nerve impulse transmission in the demyelinated axon.

In clinical studies of extended-release dalfampridine, 57% of treated patients were unable to decrease the amount of time it took them to walk 25 feet. The 43% who did decrease their time were considered responders. On average, they improved their speed to walk 25 feet by 25% (approximately 3 seconds faster).[108] Clinically, it may be difficult to determine which patients respond well to extended-release dalfampridine without conducting timed 25-foot walks.[59]

Adverse effects associated with extended-release dalfampridine include urinary tract infections, insomnia, dizziness, headache, and nausea. Seizures are a less common adverse effect and are related to dose and use of immediate-release dalfampridine. Therefore, this agent is contraindicated in patients with a history of seizures.[109]

PAIN

Between 30% and 90% of patients with MS report experiencing pain.[59] Pain related to MS is of two types: non-neurogenic and neurogenic. Non-neurogenic pain is often related to paralysis, immobility, or spasticity; examples include tension-type headache, low back pain, and limb pain associated with poor mobility or postural changes.[110] Physical therapy, repositioning limbs, and typical analgesics may be effective for treatment of non-neurogenic pain.

A number of painful neurogenic conditions have been described in association with MS (Table 57-4).[111] Patients often describe neurogenic pain as having a burning, aching, pricking, stabbing, or smarting quality.[112] Atypical analgesics are used for neurogenic pain. For trigeminal neuralgia, carbamazepine and oxcarbazepine are first-line treatments.[112] Baclofen, lamotrigine, gabapentin, topiramate, misoprostol, pimozide, or tocainide may be helpful as second-line treatments.[59,112] Surgical options may provide relief if drug treatments are ineffective.[59,112] Antiepileptic medicines and antidepressants are also commonly used for other types of neurogenic pain.

FATIGUE

Often described as the most disabling symptom by patients with MS, 74% experience fatigue.[59,61] The reason that patients exhibit fatigue is not well understood; however, hypotheses include direct effects of cytokines, axonal loss, or cortical disorganization.[63,113] Conduction is impaired in demyelinated axons, and increases in temperature may further worsen conduction.[113] However, fatigue may be caused or worsened by other mechanisms such as sleep dysfunction, depression, or medication adverse effects.[64,114]

Nonpharmacologic approaches are often the mainstay of therapy for fatigue and may include interventions to improve sleep quality, treatment for depression when present, improvements in diet, and increased physical activity.[59] Cognitive behavioral therapy has been helpful for some patients.[63] Cooling therapy with jackets worn over large areas of the body and magnetic therapy have demonstrated benefit in clinical trials.[115–117] Acupressure was shown to help women with fatigue in a small study.[118]

Table 57-4
Types of Neurogenic Pain Associated with Multiple Sclerosis[59,110]

Trigeminal neuralgia—sudden, usually unilateral, severe, brief, stabbing, recurrent episodes of pain in the distribution of one or more branches of the trigeminal nerve.[111]
Lhermitte's phenomenon—sudden onset, brief, electric shock-like sensation traveling rapidly down to the spine or into the arms or legs. Usually caused by flexing the neck. Sometimes occur occasionally for short periods.
Tonic spasms
Burning dysesthesia of the limbs and trunk
Migraine headache

The only pharmacologic therapy for fatigue with proven benefit is amantadine; however, the clinical trials for this agent have included small numbers of patients.[119] Sustained-release fampridine may be helpful in some patients.[120] Modafinil has been used in two placebo-controlled studies, but neither trial showed significant differences in response between modafinil and placebo.[121,122]

COGNITIVE DYSFUNCTION

Cognitive dysfunction may occur early in the course of the disease and has a negative impact on quality of life.[33] Among patients with CIS, 29% had cognitive impairment at the time of presentation. The only predictor of cognitive impairment was the number of lesions on MRI.[123] Between 40% and 70% of MS patients eventually have some cognitive dysfunction.[59] The most common problems are memory impairment, slowed speed of information processing, decreased mental flexibility, and impaired executive functioning.[62] Cognitive dysfunction can also limit the ability of patients with MS to understand discussion of disease and treatments.[124] Breaking down discussions into various components (e.g., intended effects, adverse effects) helps with understanding.[124]

Nonpharmacologic interventions such as cognitive rehabilitation to develop the use of intact cognitive skills to compensate for areas of poor cognitive performance may be beneficial.[125,126] Treatment of MS with immunomodulatory drugs has shown some benefit for cognitive impairments.[127] Additionally, small studies of acetylcholinesterase inhibitors were promising.[128–130] However, trials of memantine, amantadine, pemoline, and gingko biloba have all been negative.[59,130]

SPASTICITY

Spasticity can be defined as an increased resistance of muscle to an externally imposed stretch.[131] Approximately 60% of patients with MS exhibit spasticity, which may worsen with other noxious stimuli such as a full bladder or colon, infection, or MS exacerbations.[59,131] Complications from spasticity may include pain, spasms, reduced mobility, limited range of movement, contractures, fatigue, poor quality of sleep, cardiopulmonary deconditioning, decubitus ulcers, and skin breakdown.[59,131]

Nonpharmacologic therapies, such as repositioning physical therapy, stretching, or splinting, may help with spasticity.[131] These efforts are usually most successful with spasticity that is localized to one area of the body. Injection of intramuscular botulinum toxin can also be beneficial for localized spasticity.[59] Spasticity that is generalized to many areas of the body is best addressed with systemic therapy in addition to nonpharmacologic treatments. Baclofen and tizanidine are first-line therapies for spasticity. Gabapentin, benzodiazepines, and dantrolene are considered second-line agents.[59] In severe cases, intrathecal baclofen can be delivered via infusion pump through a catheter into the intrathecal space.[59] Cannabinoids have been studied with some success for patient-reported improvements in spasticity, but there is little objective evidence for effect.[117,132,133] There is no FDA-approved indication for this use in the US.

PSYCHIATRIC DYSFUNCTION

Psychiatric problems including depression, bipolar disorder, pseudobulbar affect (emotional lability), and psychosis all occur at increased rates in MS patients compared with the general population.[134–136] Depression can affect up to 50% of patients with MS.[63] Several clinical trials of depression treatment have been conducted in patients with MS. In these, cognitive behavioral therapy has been shown to be possibly effective, and fluoxetine and sertraline have been shown to have benefit in some trials.[59,137]

Pseudobulbar affect occurs in approximately 10% of patients with MS and involves frequent and inappropriate episodes of crying, laughing, or both, which may be unrelated to underlying mood. The exact cause of pseudobulbar affect is not known, but it may be caused by disruption of neural pathways from the brainstem and cerebellum. Serotonin, dopamine, and glutamate also appear to be important in the development of pseudobulbar affect. It is not isolated to patients with MS, but may also occur in other neurologic disorders such as stroke. This disorder can be socially stigmatizing and highly disabling.[138–140]

When used together, dextromethorphan and quinidine have shown efficacy for pseudobulbar affect, and a combination product is approved for this indication by the FDA. Dextromethorphan is an agonist at σ-1 receptors, suppressing release of excitatory neurotransmitters, and an antagonist at *N*-methyl-D-aspartate glutamate receptors.[138] Dextromethorphan is metabolized by cytochrome P-450 (CYP) 2D6 to dextrorphan, which does not cross the blood–brain barrier. When a low dose of quinidine, a CYP 2D6 inhibitor, is added, dextromethorphan serum concentrations are increased 20-fold. In a 12-week study of 283 patients, a 49% improvement in inappropriate emotional episodes was demonstrated.[140]

Complementary and Alternative Medicine

Several clinical trials are ongoing to evaluate the therapeutic potential of vitamin D supplementation in patients with MS.[141] In one study, 49 patients with MS were randomly assigned to receive open-label vitamin D or no active treatment (control group). The treatment group was given vitamin D to rapidly raise the serum 25-hydroxyvitamin D concentrations, starting with 4,000 international units/day and increasing to 40,000 international units/day during 28 weeks. In the second phase, subjects were administered 10,000 international units/day for 12 weeks. There was a reduction in annualized relapse rate and a higher proportion of relapse-free patients in the vitamin D group compared with the control group.[141] Another study added 20,000 international units/week of vitamin D or placebo to interferon β-1b. The group given vitamin D had decreased brain lesions on MRI after 1 year of treatment.[143] One study did not find benefits.[144] The results of these trials should be interpreted cautiously, however, because of their small numbers of patients. Vitamin D cannot be taken with impunity, however. An Institute of Medicine reports cautions against intake of more than 10,000 international units daily because of associations with kidney and tissue damage. Elevated serum concentrations of vitamin D have also been associated with hypercalcemia, anorexia, weight loss, polyuria, heart arrhythmias, vascular and tissue calcification, increases in all-cause mortality, some cancers, cardiovascular disease risk, fractures, and falls. Thus, the recommended dietary allowance for adults is 600 IU/day with an upper intake limit of 4,000 IU/day.[145]

CASE 57-1

QUESTION 1: C.B. is a 32-year-old woman of Finnish descent who presents to the neurology clinic with slurred speech and double vision. These symptoms began 2 weeks ago and have not changed. C.B. saw her primary-care physician at that time, who referred her to the neurology clinic. Her past medical history is unremarkable other than a normal gestation and vaginal delivery of a female infant 3 years ago. Today her vital signs are a blood pressure of 126/82 mm Hg, heart rate of 78 beats/minute, respirations at 20 breaths/minute, and a temperature of 37.4°C. Review of systems is negative except as noted above. On neurologic examination, C.B. is alert and her speech is fluent, but slurred. Her cranial nerves examination reveals sixth nerve palsy, and C.B. cannot abduct the right eye on rightward gaze; her visual fields are full. Her tongue and palate are at midline and there is no facial asymmetry. Her motor examination reveals normal tone and strength; her sensory examination is intact to light touch, pinprick, vibration, and position sense. Her finger-to-nose, rapid alternating movements, heel-to-shin, and gait are all normal. On MRI, C.B. has two gadolinium-enhancing lesions in the right mid-pons. Examination of her CSF reveals the following:

Red blood cells, 0
White blood cells, 0
Protein, 24 mg/dL
Glucose, 60 mg/dL

Her CSF is positive for oligoclonal bands, and IgG synthesis rate is 4.3 mg/24 hours (normal less than 3.3 mg/24 hours). Her current medications include a multivitamin one by mouth (PO) every morning, loratadine 10 mg PO every morning, and levonorgestrel-releasing intrauterine system.

What risk factors, signs, and symptoms suggestive of MS are present in C.B.? How do her MRI and CSF findings support or refute a diagnosis of MS?

C.B. has several epidemiologic factors associated with MS (see Table 57-1): She is 32 years old, consistent with onset between the ages of 20 and 50 years; she is female—women are 2 to 3 times more likely to develop MS than men—and she is of northern European ancestry, which also increases her risk of MS. Her symptoms and physical examination findings are consistent with a demyelinating event in the pons area of the brainstem. On MRI, C.B. has two active (gadolinium-enhancing) lesions in this area. This finding on the MRI is abnormal, and gadolinium-enhancing lesions are found commonly in patients with MS. Additionally, her CSF examination on lumbar puncture shows the presence of oligoclonal bands and an increased rate of IgG synthesis. These findings are also consistent with a diagnosis of MS. Although the combined evidence from her history, examination, and CSF and MRI studies make the eventual diagnosis of MS very likely, they do not demonstrate dissemination in space and time. To show dissemination in time, an additional clinical event or another MRI showing a new lesion would be necessary. To show dissemination in space, another clinical event affecting another part of the body or another MRI showing lesions in a different area of the brain would be necessary.[70] At the present time, C.B. would be diagnosed as having CIS.

CASE 57-1, QUESTION 2: Should C.B. begin treatment at this time? If so, what treatment(s) would be appropriate?

Most of the interferon β preparations, glatiramer acetate, and teriflunomide have demonstrated reduced development of MS if taken after the identification of CIS (Table 57-5).[146–150] It should be noted that the subcutaneous administration of interferon β-1a for CIS was less frequent than the usual treatment regimen of 3 times weekly.[149] This may account for the lower response rate seen in the trial with that regimen compared with the other treatments in Table 57-5.[149] C.B. should be educated on the risk of developing clinically definite MS, and she should begin therapy with one of these therapies. There is no evidence on which to base the choice of therapy; commonly the prescriber will have a preference based on discussion with the patient.

CASE 57-1, QUESTION 3: C.B. is started on glatiramer acetate 20 mg subcutaneously daily. How should C.B. be counseled regarding the injection of glatiramer acetate and the potential adverse effects of this treatment? How can she help alleviate or avoid these adverse effects? What monitoring is required?

Glatiramer acetate is supplied as a single-use, prefilled syringe. In general, the recommended administration techniques are similar to those used for other subcutaneously administered products, and the important counseling points are summarized in Table 57-6. The administration technique is slightly different for the intramuscular injection. There are product-specific differences in dose preparation for which it is important to consult the product information. C.B. should be instructed on administration technique, and it is recommended that the first injection be self-administered under the supervision of a healthcare professional.

Glatiramer acetate is initiated at a dose of 20 mg subcutaneously daily. No dosage titration is required. However, for interferon β products, a product-specific titration schedule is recommended to minimize flu-like symptoms.[79–82]

Common adverse effects of glatiramer acetate are injection site reactions and post-injection systemic reactions.[152] Injection site reactions with glatiramer acetate include hemorrhage, hypersensitivity, inflammation, mass, pain, edema, and atrophy at the injection sites. Rarely, necrosis at the injection site can develop. Lipoatrophy may be seen in up to 45% of patients with longer-term use.[153] Acute injection site reactions may be reduced by applying warm compresses or ice to the injection site before injection, warming the medication to room temperature before injection, and ensuring that the needle completely penetrates the skin during injection.[154,155] Symptoms of post-injection systemic reactions include facial flushing, chest tightness, dyspnea,

Table 57-5
Development of Clinically Definite Multiple Sclerosis with Therapy Compared to Placebo

Clinical Study	Treatment	Development of Clinically Definite MS: Active Treatment (%)	Placebo (%)
CHAMPS[146]	Interferon β-1a 30 mcg IM weekly	20	38
ETOMS[147]	Interferon β-1a 22 mcg subcutaneously weekly	34	45
BENEFIT[148]	Interferon β-1b 250 mcg subcutaneously every other day	28	45
PreCISe[149]	Glatiramer acetate 20 mg subcutaneously daily	25	43
TOPIC[150]	Teriflunomide 7 mg PO daily Teriflunomide 14 mg PO daily	19 18	28

IM, intramuscular; MS, multiple sclerosis; PO, orally.

Table 57-6

Patient Counseling Points for Interferon β and Glatiramer Acetate Products[79–82,151]

For all products:
Use clean technique—wash hands with soap and water, clean injection site with an alcohol swab, do not touch site or needle tip to other surfaces or with fingers.
Choose an appropriate site: For subcutaneous injection—fleshy part of upper back, arm, front of thighs, lower abdomen, fleshy area of upper hip. For intramuscular injection—front of thigh, side of thigh, upper arm.
Rotate between injection sites to avoid overuse of any one site.
Examine the reconstituted product for particles, cloudiness, or color changes. The products should be colorless to light yellow.
For subcutaneous injection—pinch up a fold of skin between index finger and thumb for the injection. For intramuscular injection—stretch the skin between index finger and thumb for the injection.
Insert the needle at a 90 degrees angle to the skin.
Release the skin.
Steadily push down on the plunger until all of the medicine is injected.
Pull needle straight out of skin and dispose of it in a hard-walled plastic container.

palpitations, tachycardia, and anxiety.[151] Approximately 16% of patients experience this reaction. When this reaction occurs, its onset is within seconds to minutes after injection, and it may last up to 30 minutes.[152] No specific treatment is recommended for post-injection systemic reactions to glatiramer acetate.

Adverse effects are fairly common with interferon β; they include leukopenia (36%–86%), injection site reaction (6%–92%) and necrosis (3%–6%), flulike symptoms (49%–57%), breakthrough menstrual bleeding (28%), and increased liver function tests (12%–27%).[79–82,156] Depression and suicide are seen in patients treated with the β interferons; however, it is difficult to distinguish the independent contribution of interferon from any possible concomitant effects of MS itself.[157–159]

Flu-like reactions include the symptoms of fever, chills, myalgia, malaise, and sweating, and they occur in about half of patients who are initiated on an interferon β.[78] Symptoms usually begin 3 to 6 hours after administration and last approximately 24 hours. Female patients and those with lower body mass index may have more severe flu-like symptoms.[156] Most patients find that these symptoms decrease with time, with only 10% of patients reporting flu-like symptoms after 1 year of therapy.[78] Helpful tips for patients to reduce flu-like symptoms include administering the injections at night to sleep through the time of peak symptoms, taking ibuprofen or acetaminophen before and every 4 to 6 hours as needed after the injection, and gradual titration to full dose.[156,160]

Injection site reactions vary from 92% with some subcutaneous preparations of interferon β to 6% with the intramuscular preparation.[79–82] These symptoms are similar to those seen with glatiramer acetate except that lipoatrophy is not seen with interferon β. Women appear to be more likely to experience injection site reactions than men.[156] Strategies to reduce injection site reactions include injecting the drug in areas with more subcutaneous fat (abdomen or buttocks), rotating injection sites, using an auto-injection device, icing the site after injection, and using a vitamin K cream on the site.[156,161–164]

Table 57-7

Patient Characteristics and Other Factors Associated with Reduced Adherence to β Interferons or Glatiramer Acetate[166–168]

Secondary-progressive multiple sclerosis	**Younger age**
Female sex	Cognitive impairment
Depression	Perceived lack of efficacy
Unrealistic expectations	Adverse effects
Inconvenience	Needle phobia
Lifestyle or economic instability	Lack of family or other support

General monitoring recommendations for both interferon β and glatiramer acetate include observation of injection sites for infection, necrosis, and atrophy. Specifically for the β interferons, complete blood counts and liver function tests are monitored.[79–82] The frequency of monitoring is not specified in product literature, but a reasonable approach would be at baseline and 1 to 3 months after initiation and then every 6 to 12 months during continuation of therapy. Additionally, patients should be monitored for signs or symptoms of depression. Therefore, the specific counseling and monitoring plan needed for C.B. is instruction in self-injection technique for the subcutaneous injection and discussion of injection site reactions, including their prevention and monitoring, and post-injection systemic reactions. C.B. should also be counseled regarding the value of ongoing clinical monitoring (for efficacy, injection site reactions, and post-injection reactions) during glatiramer acetate therapy.

CASE 57-1, QUESTION 4: Six months later, C.B. returns for an appointment with her neurologist. During the discussion, she states that she is not having any problems with injection technique or adverse effects, but she reveals that she is only using the glatiramer acetate 3 or 4 times a week instead of the daily injection schedule that was prescribed. When questioned, she states, "I just don't know that it's doing anything." How might C.B.'s neurologist deal with this adherence problem?

Adherence is often poor with self-injection of interferons and glatiramer acetate; over 2 to 5 years, only 60% to 76% of patients adhere to therapy.[165] Patient characteristics and other factors that have been associated with poor adherence are listed in Table 57-7.[166–168] In one study, self-efficacy and belief that the medicine would have benefit were strong predictors of adherence, whereas cognitive difficulties, occurrence of adverse effects, depression, more disability, and poor quality of life predicted nonadherence.[169] Adherent patients have a lower risk of relapses, fewer emergency department visits, and fewer hospitalizations.[170]

For C.B., it appears that she has perceived lack of efficacy for the glatiramer acetate; however, other factors associated with nonadherence should be sought and discussed with her. For an individual patient, it is impossible to know what the course of disease would be without treatment; thus, many patients believe that the medicine is not having a positive impact. Particularly for a patient with CIS who does not have ongoing symptoms, embarking on a lifelong therapy can be challenging. Additionally, there is no immediate feedback to the patient that the medication is having an effect, in contrast to some other diseases such as diabetes in which a fingerstick blood glucose measurement provides positive reinforcement.[166] Some evidence suggests that patients would prefer not to take a treatment that causes significant adverse effects until the symptoms experienced from their MS are worse than the perceived adverse effects.[171] Strategies that may improve adherence include establishing a good patient–healthcare provider relationship, patient education and periodic reinforcement, management of adverse effects, involving care partners, and treating depression.[166]

CASE 57-1, QUESTION 5: After re-education and frank discussion, C.B.'s adherence improves, and she does well for a year on glatiramer acetate therapy. However, a routine monitoring MRI scan shows a new gadolinium-enhancing lesion on her right optic nerve. Additionally, a new non-enhancing lesion is apparent on the MRI scan. Does this new information change her diagnosis and treatment?

With these new MRI lesions, the "separation in space and time" criteria for the diagnosis of MS have been met. Thus, C.B. now would be diagnosed with MS. Given her history, it would appear that she has relapsing-remitting MS. To guide the clinician in choosing the most efficacious therapy, there are data from several clinical trials that directly compare first-line therapies (Table 57-8).[76,89,172–177] From the data available, it appears that interferon β-1a intramuscularly once weekly is less effective than the other first-line treatments. Otherwise, the medicines are roughly equivalent for treatment of relapsing-remitting MS. A recently proposed treatment algorithm suggests that patients who present with relapsing-remitting MS should receive dimethyl fumarate, glatiramer acetate, interferon β, or teriflunomide as a first-line therapy. Should disease activity be detected, patients could rotate to another first-line therapy or move to a second-line therapy of natalizumab, fingolimod, or alemtuzumab.[178]

CASE 57-1, QUESTION 6: C.B. admits that she disliked giving herself daily injections and began therapy with dimethyl fumarate delayed-release 120 mg PO twice daily for 7 days, then 240 mg PO twice daily thereafter. What counseling should she receive regarding the adverse effects of this medication?

Table 57-8
Clinical Trials Directly Comparing Active Treatments

Trial	Treatments	Results
First-line Therapies		
INCOMIN[172]	Interferon β-1b 250 mcg subcutaneously every other day vs. interferon β-1a 30 mcg IM weekly	Compared with interferon β-1a-treated patients, more interferon β-1b-treated patients were relapse-free (51% vs. 36%), there were fewer mean relapses (0.38% vs. 0.5%), and fewer patients progressing 1 point on the EDSS (13% vs. 30%) after 2 years.
EVIDENCE[173]	Interferon β-1a subcutaneously 44 mcg 3 times weekly vs. interferon β-1a 30 mcg IM weekly	Compared with interferon β-1a IM-treated patients, interferon β-1a subcutaneously treated patients had fewer mean relapses (0.29% vs. 0.4%) and fewer lesions on MRI after 24 weeks.
REGARD[174]	Interferon β-1a 44 mcg subcutaneously 3 times weekly vs. glatiramer acetate 20 mg subcutaneously daily	No significant differences in time to first relapse or MRI changes.
BEYOND[175]	Interferon β-1b 250 mcg subcutaneous every other day vs. interferon β-1b 500 mcg subcutaneous every other day vs. glatiramer acetate 20 mg subcutaneous daily	No differences in relapse rate, EDSS progression, or MRI lesions.
CONFIRM[89]	Dimethyl fumarate 240 mg PO twice daily vs. dimethyl fumarate 240 mg PO 3 times daily vs. glatiramer acetate 20 mg subcutaneous daily vs. placebo	Compared to placebo, all active therapies reduced annualized relapse rates (0.22, 0.20, 0.29 vs. 0.40), EDSS progression, and MRI lesions. No differences between dimethyl fumarate 240 mg twice daily and glatiramer for any outcome except for one type of MRI lesion.
TENERE[176]	Teriflunomide 7 mg PO daily vs. teriflunomide 14 mg PO daily vs. interferon β-1a 44 mcg subcutaneous 3 times weekly	No differences in relapse rate, treatment failure
Second-line Therapies		
CARE-MS I[76]	Alemtuzumab 12 mg IV daily for 5 days, then 12 mg IV daily for 3 days 12 months later vs. interferon β-1a 44 mcg subcutaneous 3 times weekly	More patients taking alemtuzumab were relapse-free (78%) at 2 years than the interferon group (59%). Fewer patients taking alemtuzumab had disease progression (8% vs. 11%)
CARE-MS II[177]	Alemtuzumab 12 mg IV daily for 5 days, then 12 mg IV daily for 3 days 12 months later vs. interferon β-1a 44 mcg subcutaneous 3 times weekly	More patients taking alemtuzumab were relapse-free (65.4%) at 2 years than the interferon group (46.7%). Fewer patients taking alemtuzumab had disease progression (12.71% vs. 21.13%). Fewer patients taking alemtuzumab had new MRI lesions (9% vs. 23%).

EDSS, Expanded Disability Status Scale; IM, intramuscular; MRI, magnetic resonance imaging; PO, orally; IV, intravenous.

Dimethyl fumarate commonly causes flushing and gastrointestinal (GI) adverse effects; it has been formulated as a delayed-release product to help with these problems. Flushing occurs in about 30% to 38% of patients taking dimethyl fumarate in clinical trials.[89,179] The GI adverse effects include diarrhea 13%, nausea 11%, and upper abdominal pain 10%.[89,179] Taking doses with food helps decrease both of these types of adverse effects. In a small study specifically examining flushing and GI effects, the incidence of flushing was much higher, up to 98% in some groups, but decreased somewhat with continued use. Each event lasted between 1 to 2 hours. Aspirin 325 mg taken 30 minutes prior to the dose decreases the incidence of flushing by about 14%. The subjects also had much higher incidences of GI effects, between 79% and 81%, falling to 53% to 61% during the second month of use. GI event onset was a median time of 2 weeks. Aspirin had no effect on GI symptoms.[180] Metoclopramide, ondansetron, domperidone, antacids, H_2-receptor antagonists, proton pump inhibitors, and antidiarrheals have been recommended to combat the GI symptoms, and antihistamines have been used for flushing but no testing of these approaches has been performed.[181] Lyphopenia occurs in about 2% of patients taking dimethyl fumarate; however, mean lymphocyte count decreases by about 30% in the first year of treatment and then stabilizes. Patients should have a complete blood count at baseline and then annually.[182]

C.B. should be counseled to take her doses with food. Because it is a delayed-release product, she should swallow the capsules whole. If she experiences flushing, aspirin 325 mg PO 30 minutes prior to dosing could be recommended. If she experiences GI problems, those could be treated symptomatically.[182]

CASE 57-1, QUESTION 7: C.B. continued on therapy with dimethyl fumarate. However, 1 year later, she has experienced one relapse and is currently hospitalized with another. She has been adherent to therapy. Her MRI shows several new, gadolinium-enhancing lesions. What therapy should be recommended for acute treatment of C.B.'s current relapse? Would you change her maintenance therapy at this time?

Corticosteroids should be used to decrease the time to recover from acute relapses. The most commonly used regimen is 500 to 1,000 mg intravenous methylprednisolone daily for 3 to 5 days with or without a subsequent regimen of tapering dose oral steroids for 1 to 3 weeks.[183] Comparison of oral and intravenous corticosteroid treatment shows that there are no major differences in clinical outcomes, and both treatments appear to be equally effective and safe.[72] The recommended oral corticosteroid regimen is prednisone 1,250 mg daily every other day for five doses.[184] Some investigators have attempted to use corticosteroids on a chronic basis, giving pulse doses of one or several days monthly; however, this type of regimen does not affect disability progression and should not be recommended.[183,185] Because C.B. is already hospitalized, she should receive methylprednisolone 1,000 mg intravenously daily for 3 days. If she were an outpatient, either intravenous or oral steroid therapy could be recommended, but an oral corticosteroid regimen would be more convenient.

As MS therapies become more effective, tolerance for relapses has decreased. No evidence of disease activity (NEDA) is a composite measure that indicates that there are: (1) no new or enlarging T2-weighted lesions on MRI; (2) no new gadolinium-enhancing lesions on MRI; (3) no relapses; and (4) no progression on EDSS scores over a period of time.[186] An expert panel was convened to help further clarify this classification of NEDA. This group developed a multiple sclerosis decision model (MSDM) which takes into consideration the domains of relapses, progression, neuropsychology factors, and MRI findings.[187] Points are assigned for each of these domains based on assessments, and users are guided to maintain therapy, closely monitor, or change therapy. However, a number of assessments are required to assign the points which may not be practical in many clinic settings. Percentages of patients in clinical trials achieving NEDA status are between 28% and 42% over the first 2 years of therapy; however, this number appears to drop to around 8% after 7 years in one cohort.[188]

It appears that C.B. is failing treatment with dimethyl fumarate because she has experienced two relapses within approximately 1 year and has substantial new lesion formation on MRI; there are several alternatives at this point. C.B. could change to another first-line therapy (βinterferon, or teriflunomide) or she could begin therapy with a second-line agent: mitoxantrone, natalizumab, or fingolimod. There are direct comparator studies of first- and second-line agents (Table 57-8). Additionally, an observational study has addressed the question of the efficacy of the second-line therapies, natalizumab and fingolimod.[189] Patients who had relapse activity on first-line injectable therapies were switched to either natalizumab or fingolimod. The annualized relapse rate for those changed to natalizumab was reduced from 1.5 to 0.2 whereas the rate for those changed to fingolimod was reduced from 1.5 to 0.4 ($p = 0.02$). A careful discussion of the potential risks and benefits of each possible treatment will ensure that the patient is well educated on the options and that an appropriate selection is made.

CASE 57-1, QUESTION 8: After lengthy discussion, C.B. elects to discontinue dimethyl fumarate therapy and start fingolimod 0.5 mg PO daily. How should C.B. be counseled regarding the potential benefits and adverse effects of fingolimod? What monitoring will be necessary?

In studies of fingolimod, 70.4% of patients remained relapse-free for 2 years compared with 45.6% for those treated with placebo. At 1 year, 82.6% of fingolimod-treated patients were relapse-free compared with 69.3% of those treated with interferon β-1a intramuscularly. The annualized relapse rate was 0.16/year for fingolimod, 0.40/year for placebo, and 0.33/year for interferon β-1a intramuscularly.[91,92] C.B. should expect good suppression of her MS with fingolimod treatment.

Because S1P receptors (the targets of fingolimod therapy) are not confined to lymphocytes, adverse effects of fingolimod may affect other body organs and tissues. For example, a transient, dose-dependent reduction in heart rate can occur within 1 hour after the first fingolimod dose (bradycardia in 1.3%); first- and second-degree atrioventricular block can also occur (0.1% and 0.2%, respectively).[91,190] Patients with pre-existing sinus bradycardia or heart block without pacemakers should not be given fingolimod. Other adverse effects include macular edema and a reduction in forced vital capacity.[91] Because the mechanism of action of fingolimod is to prevent lymphocytes from circulating, there is a reduction in peripheral blood lymphocytes and an increase in infections and, possibly, cancers.[91] This reduction in peripheral blood lymphocytes is reversible within 4 to 8 weeks of discontinuation of fingolimod.[49] Fingolimod does not inhibit humoral immunity to infections.[49] Progressive multifocal leukoencephalopathy (PML) has been reported in patients taking fingolimod.[191] PML is caused by JC DNA polyomavirus (JCV) reactivation. JCV then causes an infection of oligodendrocytes that is often fatal or causes permanent disability.[4] Dormant JCV infection is relatively common, with 50% to 86% of adults having antibodies to JCV. When a patient is immunosuppressed, JCV may become reactivated.[192] PML is rapidly progressive and has a mortality rate of approximately 50%.[193] Symptoms of PML include neurobehavioral, motor, language, and cognitive changes; seizures; vision changes; hemiparesis; and tremor.[194,195] Notably, all of these symptoms could be mistaken for an MS relapse.

Table 57-9

Baseline Testing and Monitoring Associated with Fingolimod[196]

Baseline

- Varicella zoster immunity evaluation and vaccination, if needed
- Ophthalmology evaluation for macular edema
- Dermatologic evaluation for melanomas
- Forced expiratory volume in 1 second (FEV_1) or full pulmonary function testing, if patient has history of asthma or chronic obstructive pulmonary disease
- Pulse and blood pressure
- Complete blood count
- Liver function tests

Monitoring

- Observe in clinical area for 6 hours after initial dose with monitoring of blood pressure and pulse
- Ophthalmology evaluation at 4 months and as needed thereafter
- Complete blood count every 6 months
- Liver function tests every 6 months
- Dermatologic evaluation as needed
- FEV_1 as needed

Increases in liver enzymes (transaminase and bilirubin) have also been observed.[91,92] Because fingolimod has a long half-life of 9 to 10 days, its pharmacologic effects will still be present for up to 2 months after therapy is discontinued.[196] Baseline testing and continued monitoring recommended with the use of fingolimod is summarized in Table 57-9. Fingolimod should be given as monotherapy, and the patient should not have had a relapse or have been treated with corticosteroids within 30 days of starting treatment. If patients do not have an existing history of varicella zoster infection or vaccination, vaccination evaluation should be undertaken.[196] Rates of varicella infections are between 7 and 11/1,000 patient-years.[197] C.B. should wait for 30 days after her relapse and any corticosteroid treatment before starting fingolimod. During this time, she can have baseline testing before starting treatment. She should be educated on potential adverse effects and the long-lasting pharmacologic effects of fingolimod that may persist for up to 2 months after therapy is discontinued.

CASE 57-1, QUESTION 9: C.B. is appropriately started on fingolimod and does very well with visits to the neurologist every 6 months. When she is seen 2 years later, she informs her care providers that she is considering having another child. How should C.B. be counseled regarding fingolimod therapy during pregnancy?

It is well documented that the rate of relapses for women with MS decreases during pregnancy, increases in the first 3 months after delivery, then returns to the pre-pregnancy rate.[198] No treatment for MS is recommended for use during pregnancy, and some therapies, such as mitoxantrone, require pregnancy tests before each infusion. However, there are limited data regarding the exposure of fetuses to some of the treatments for MS when given during early pregnancy. No increase in spontaneous abortions or stillbirths was seen with glatiramer acetate or βinterferons.[199–201] However, very few of these exposures were for the full term of pregnancy. A report of 66 pregnancies in women taking fingolimod found fetal abnormalities in 7.6%. In all of these cases, the exposure was in the first trimester.[202] Pregnancy is contraindicated during treatment with teriflunomide, with contraception required for both women and men.[203] Eighty-nine pregnancies (70 in women exposed to teriflunomide and 19 in partners of men exposed to teriflunomide) were reported during clinical trials. Of these, 42 healthy live births, 31 induced abortions, and 14 spontaneous abortions were reported. It should be noted that in almost all cases, teriflunomide was stopped and accelerated elimination procedures were undertaken as soon as the pregnancy was known to minimize fetal exposure.[204] Alemtuzumab is also contraindicated during pregnancy. Women should use adequate contraceptive measures during treatment and for 4 months following treatment. Alemtuzumab can cause thyroid disorders which, during pregnancy, can have serious adverse effects on the fetus.[205]

In general, MS therapy should be discontinued before conception. In the case of C.B., she should be advised that she would need to discontinue fingolimod at least 2 months before conception and stay off the medication while pregnant. It is not known whether fingolimod is excreted into the breast milk of nursing women.[202] Because of the potential adverse effects of fingolimod on an infant's immune system, she should be advised either to not breast-feed or to abstain from taking fingolimod during nursing.

CASE 57-1, QUESTION 10: C.B. discontinued fingolimod, conceived approximately 4 months later, and delivered a healthy male child after a normal gestation and labor. She experienced a relapse of MS 2 months after delivery, discontinued nursing, and was treated with corticosteroids. Two months after the relapse and treatment, she returns to the neurology clinic for a follow-up appointment. She states that she is ready to restart fingolimod therapy at this time. She states that she is often very tired and feels that "she can't continue." However, she admits that this feeling may also be related to being a new mother. She states that her husband and daughter help significantly with care of the infant. She has noticed some jerkiness in her gait, and she states that sometimes her toes will contract toward her head involuntarily. Her neurologic examination shows spasticity in her lower extremities. What treatments would be appropriate for management of C.B.'s spasticity? How should her fatigue be addressed?

Nonpharmacologic therapy such as stretching may help with C.B.'s spasticity. Her symptoms are more generalized (involving the lower extremities) than localized, so systemic therapy may be more beneficial than localized therapy such as splinting or botulinum toxin injections (therapies that might be considered if only her toes were involved).[59,131] Systemic therapies that may relieve spasticity include baclofen and tizanidine; because both agents appear to be equally effective, neither agent is preferred over the other for C.B.

Although fatigue is a common problem when caring for infants, C.B. also may be experiencing fatigue related to her MS. She would likely benefit from nonpharmacologic therapy such as avoiding sleep deprivation to the extent possible and concentrating her infant care during the morning hours, enlisting more assistance in the afternoon and evening. She should also be assessed for any symptoms of depression.[59]

CASE 57-2

QUESTION 1: N.R. is a 47-year-old woman who was diagnosed with relapsing-remitting MS 5 years ago. She has been taking interferon β-1b 250 mcg subcutaneously every other day since diagnosis. For the first 4 years, she did very well with only one relapse. However, in the past year, she has sustained two relapses, and she feels that her treatment is not working as well as it did in the past. Her neurologist sends a blood specimen for neutralizing antibody assay with a result of 160 neutralizing units/mL (reported as high by the laboratory). How might this result assist in the recommendation of future therapy for N.R.?

Neutralizing antibodies develop in many patients given therapy for MS, including β interferons, natalizumab, and alemtuzumab. Neutralizing antibodies are seen in up to 44% of patients given interferon β.[78,93] Fewer patients given interferon β-1a intramuscularly once weekly develop them than those given interferon β-1a subcutaneously 3 times weekly or interferon β-1b subcutaneously every other day.[93] For patients with persistently high antibody titers, their relapse rates are also higher.[93] With time, neutralizing antibodies often disappear.[87]

Despite these observations, the indications for neutralizing antibody testing and the interpretation of test results are areas of ongoing controversy. The Therapeutics and Technology Assessment Subcommittee of the American Academy of Neurology has issued the following statements regarding neutralizing antibodies to interferon β: (a) treatment with interferon β is associated with the production of neutralizing antibodies; (b) it is probable that neutralizing antibodies, especially in persistently high titers, are associated with a reduction in the radiographic and clinical effectiveness of treatment; (c) it is probable that the rate of neutralizing antibody production is less with interferon β-1a compared with interferon β-1b treatment; (d) it is probable that the seroprevalence of neutralizing antibodies is affected by one or more of the following: formulation, dose, route of administration, or frequency of administration of interferon β; and (e) there is insufficient information on the utilization of neutralizing antibody testing to provide specific recommendations regarding the indications for testing or interpretation of antibody titer results.[206]

A panel of MS and neutralizing antibody experts was convened in 2009 to develop practical recommendations. Some of their findings included are as follows: (a) Persistently high titers might provide sufficient guidance to suggest stopping therapy in a patient; however, with low or intermediate titers, additional information might be needed to make a decision regarding therapy continuation; (b) different interferon β products are associated with different rates of antibody formation; chemical formulation, route of administration, and frequency of dosing appear to have an effect; and different formulations of the same molecule may result in different immunogenicity; and (c) to minimize assay variability, antibody measurements should be done in laboratories that have fulfilled the criteria for validation of neutralizing antibody assays, and interferon β-1a should be used in the assays to standardize the assays.[207] Thus, there is continued discussion about the appropriate use of neutralizing antibody assays for β interferons.

Antibodies also form to therapies for MS other than the β interferons. Up to 95% of patients treated with glatiramer acetate have antibodies, but they do not appear to change the efficacy of glatiramer acetate.[152,208] Antibodies may develop to natalizumab and may affect treatment efficacy or increase the likelihood of natalizumab infusion reactions. Many patients who express antibodies to natalizumab do so within the first 6 months of treatment, but these antibodies often disappear with continued treatment. Antibodies to natalizumab are more likely to persist if they develop more than 6 months after treatment initiation.[194] High antibody titers are associated with increased rates of relapse.[209] Neutralizing antibodies have been detected with alemtuzumab, but they do not appear to affect efficacy.[177]

N.R. has a high titer of neutralizing antibodies, and they appear to be associated with a decline in efficacy of her interferon β-1b. Therefore, it would seem appropriate to change therapy at this time. Options would include glatiramer acetate, dimethyl fumarate, teriflunomide, alemtuzumab, mitoxantrone, natalizumab, or fingolimod. Because of the potential for cross-reactivity of the neutralizing antibodies to other β interferons, a change to another β interferon product would not be expected to provide benefit.

CASE 57-2, QUESTION 2: N.R.'s interferon β-1b therapy was discontinued, and she was begun on teriflunomide 14 mg PO daily. What monitoring will be required while taking this medicine?

Elevated ALT, alopecia, and diarrhea were seen in 10% to 20% of patients in clinical trials and more commonly in patients treated with teriflunomide than with placebo.[203] White blood cell counts decrease by about 15% and platelets by about 10% during the first 6 weeks of teriflunomide treatment, and remain low throughout the treatment. A CBC is recommended at baseline.[203] Because of the immunosuppression seen, patients should be monitored for infection, and patients should not receive live virus vaccines while under the effects of teriflunomide.[203] Modest increases in blood pressure were also observed. Other required monitoring includes baseline liver enzymes and bilirubin, blood pressure, and screening for latent tuberculosis infection. The monitoring of ALT should occur monthly for the first 6 months of therapy and periodically thereafter.[203] Teriflunomide rarely causes the serious adverse effects of peripheral neuropathy, acute renal failure, hyperkalemia, and bone marrow suppression.[101] Serious adverse effects are not reported with teriflunomide, but those seen with the parent drug leflunomide are Stevens–Johnson syndrome, interstitial lung disease, and hepatotoxicity.[203] Teriflunomide has a very long half-life of approximately 18 days.[203] Because of this, it can take up to 3 months to achieve steadystate serum concentrations and a proportionally long time to eliminate the medicine (8–24 months). In situations requiring rapid elimination of teriflunomide (e.g., serious adverse effects, desired pregnancy), accelerated elimination procedures are recommended. The recommended accelerated elimination procedures are administration of cholestyramine 8 g every 8 hours for 11 days or administration of activated charcoal powder 50 g every 12 hours for 11 days. Verification of elimination should be undertaken by two teriflunomide serum concentrations of <0.02 mcg/mL taken 2 weeks apart.[203]

Prior to N.R. starting teriflunomide, her immunization status should be carefully checked and she should be screened for tuberculosis. If necessary, her immunizations should be updated and any infectious diseases should be completely treated before starting therapy. She should have a baseline CBC, liver enzymes, bilirubin, and blood pressure. Monthly for the first 6 months, she should have blood drawn for ALT. This would also be an opportune time to check blood pressure and screen for signs of infection.

CASE 57-2, QUESTION 3: N.R. successfully began teriflunomide and continued without adverse effects for 1 year. At her annual MRI visit, however, five new lesions were seen in her brain. She continued for another 6 months and had a follow-up MRI with three additional lesions detected. In discussion with her neurologist, she decided to change therapy. Alemtuzumab, mitoxantrone and natalizumab are considered as therapy alternatives for N.R. How should N.R. be counseled regarding the potential adverse effects and monitoring for these agents?

Common adverse effects of mitoxantrone include nausea, menstrual abnormalities, alopecia, upper respiratory and urinary tract infections, neutropenia, and a temporary change to blue color in the urine and sclera.[210] Dose-related cardiotoxicity occurs with mitoxantrone use, requiring an estimation of left ventricular ejection fraction before each dose.[211] The dose of mitoxantrone for MS is 12 mg/m^2 given as a 5- to 15-minute intravenous infusion every 3 months.[211] Cardiotoxicity limits the lifetime dose of mitoxantrone to 140 mg/m^2 or approximately 3 years of therapy. The most common cardiotoxic effects are cardiomyopathy, decreased left ventricular ejection fraction, and irreversible congestive heart failure.[210] Approximately 12% of

Table 57-10
Monitoring Required for Mitoxantrone Use[211]

Baseline and Before Each Dose
■ Left ventricular ejection fraction
■ Complete blood count
■ Liver function tests
■ Pregnancy test, in women
Ongoing
■ Left ventricular ejection fraction yearly to monitor for late development of cardiotoxicity

Table 57-11
Recommendations for Use of Natalizumab[93,194,215]

Patients Who Should Not Receive Natalizumab
■ Immunocompromised
■ Active viral hepatitis
■ Active malignancy that requires treatment
■ Inability to get MRI
Recommendations for Use
■ Monotherapy with natalizumab only
■ After failure of interferon or glatiramer acetate
■ Therapy-free interval of 14 days after interferon or glatiramer acetate, 3 months after azathioprine, or 6 months after mitoxantrone
Baseline Testing
■ Clinical neurologic examination
■ Human immunodeficiency virus testing
■ Complete blood count
■ Liver function tests
■ MRI with IV contrast
Monitoring
■ Neurologic examination at 3 months, 6 months, and then yearly
■ MRI with IV contrast at 6 months and then yearly

IV, intravenous; MRI, magnetic resonance imaging.

patients experience decreased left ventricular ejection fraction, and 0.4% exhibit congestive heart failure.[212] Treatment-related acute leukemia may occur in 0.81% of mitoxantrone-treated patients. Most cases of leukemia present during the first few years of mitoxantrone therapy, and the development of leukemia may be dose related.[212] It appears that limiting the cumulative dose of mitoxantrone to <60 mg/m^2 may reduce the risk of leukemia.[213] Recommended monitoring for patients taking mitoxantrone is presented in Table 57-10. It should be noted that adherence to mitoxantrone monitoring recommendations is low. In a review of 548 patients, 78% had complete blood counts, 54% had liver function tests, 18% had left ventricular ejection fraction determinations, and 10% of women had pregnancy tests before each infusion.[214] Because of the cardiac and leukemia concerns, mitoxantrone is rarely used for MS.

Adverse effects of natalizumab include fatigue, liver dysfunction, infections, hypersensitivity reactions, and infusion-related reactions.[215] Hypersensitivity reactions are IgE-mediated and occur within 2 hours of the start of the infusion. Patients who exhibit HLA-DRB1*13 or HLA-DRB*14 are more likely to have hypersensitivity reactions.[216] Genotyping may be helpful to identify these patients prior to natalizumab prescribing. Symptoms include urticaria, dyspnea, and circulatory, and vital sign changes. If these symptoms occur, the infusion should be discontinued.[194] Hypersensitivity reactions should be distinguished from infusion-related reactions. These latter reactions are non-allergic and include symptoms of headache, dizziness, fatigue, nausea, sweats, and rigors. If this type of reaction occurs, there is no need to discontinue therapy; the patient can be pretreated with histamine type 1 and 2 receptor antagonists and acetaminophen.[194] Three cases of PML caused the suspension of natalizumab sales shortly after its introduction.[217] Natalizumab was later reintroduced to the market with a limited distribution system and extensive monitoring requirements.

From 2005 to 2009, 28 cases of PML in natalizumab-treated patients were reported in addition to the three cases reported previously. During that period, approximately 65,000 patients with MS were exposed to natalizumab. However, it appears that PML risk is proportional to the duration of natalizumab exposure; one case is reported per 1,000 patients in those who have received 24 or more infusions.[195] Overall, reporting appears to occur at a rate of one or two per month.[195] Of these 28 cases, only eight have been fatal.[195] This may be due to the heightened sensitivity to clinical changes that may suggest PML and aggressive immune reconstitution with either plasma exchange or immunoabsorption if PML is diagnosed. However, this immune reconstitution can lead to immune reconstitution inflammatory syndrome (IRIS), which is itself life-threatening. IRIS usually presents as an acute worsening of MS symptoms and is treated with high-dose corticosteroids.[195] Several groups have developed recommendations for natalizumab use to reduce the risk of PML (Table 57-11).

Several serious adverse effects, infusion reactions, autoimmune conditions, and malignancies, associated with alemtuzumab use have caused the FDA to require a limited distribution program for this agent. Infusion reactions associated with alemtuzumab are triggered by cytokine release, may include rash, fever, headache, itching, nausea, and chills and occur in about 90% of patients; serious reactions occurred in 3% of patients.[74,76,205] Patients should be monitored for 2 hours after each infusion, but reactions may occur later than that time period.[205] Premedication should consist of methylprednisolone 1,000 mg infused immediately before the first infusion and for the first 3 days of each treatment course. Antihistamines and acetaminophen may also be helpful premedications.[205] Autoimmune diseases have been associated with alemtuzumab therapy and may include thyroid disorders (34%), immune thrombocytopenia (2%), and anti-glomerular basement membrane disease (0.3%).[76,177,205] Thyroid disorders have been seen up to 60 months after the initial treatment with alemtuzumab.[177] Of thyroid dysfunction seen, 79% is hyperthyroidism and 21% is hypothyroidism.[218] Patients receiving alemtuzumab had higher rates of some malignancies, including thyroid cancer and melanoma at a rate of 0.3% each.[205] Infections were more common in patients treated with alemtuzumab than those treated with interferon β, including urinary tract infections (17%), herpes virus infections (16%), respiratory infections (16%), and fungal infections (12%).[76,177,205] The herpes virus infections are most common in the month following the infusion and can be significantly reduced by prophylaxis.[74] The recommendation is that patients receive anti-viral prophylaxis for herpetic viral infections starting on the first day of each treatment course and continuing for a minimum of 2 months following treatment or until the $CD4^+$ lymphocyte count is ≥ 200 cells/mcL, whichever occurs later.[205] The dosing of alemtuzumab is unique for MS medicines in that it is a 12 mg/day infusion for 5 days and then an additional 12 mg/day infusion for 3 days 12 months after the first treatment course.[205] No vaccines should be administered during treatment and all should be completed at least 6 weeks prior to treatment,

Table 57-12
Recommended Monitoring for Use of Alemtuzumab[205]

Test	Monitoring Frequency
CBC with differential	Baseline and monthly for 48 months following the last dose
Serum creatinine	Baseline and monthly for 48 months following the last dose
Urinalysis with urine cell counts	Baseline and monthly for 48 months following the last dose
Thyroid-stimulating hormone	Baseline and every 3 months for 48 months following the last dose
Skin examination	Baseline and yearly
Human papilloma virus	Yearly
Tuberculosis	Baseline

including varicella zoster virus vaccine, if patients have not been vaccinated and do not have a history of infection.[205] Monitoring recommendations can be found in Table 57-12.

Of these options, N.R. should probably be started on alemtuzumab or natalizumab. Both of these therapies carry substantial adverse effects about which, she will need to be informed. Additionally, she will need to enroll in the restricted distribution systems for the chosen medicine. Another area that requires consideration is that she may be at higher risk for PML or other opportunistic infections when beginning one of these medicines after taking teriflunomide. Conversely, being completely without medicine allows for return or possible "rebound" of disease activity. Possible strategies include undergoing accelerated elimination procedures for the teriflunomide and then: (1) allowing for a washout period during which the patient receives no treatment, (2) providing a monthly regimen of methylprednisolone while allowing for a washout period, or (3) switching directly to another therapy without a washout period.[219] It is not known which of these options is the best for a patient.

CASE 57-2, QUESTION 4: N.R. experiences another relapse while she is considering which therapy to begin. One month after completing corticosteroid treatment for this relapse, she returns to the neurology clinic for a follow-up appointment. N.R. explains that she has been experiencing episodes of uncontrollable laughing. When these episodes first began, she thought they might be an adverse effect of the corticosteroid treatment for her relapse. However, 1 month after stopping corticosteroid treatment, she is still having these episodes. She states that the episodes are very embarrassing, often occurring at inappropriate times such as in movie theaters, at parent–teacher conferences, and in grocery stores. She is diagnosed with pseudobulbar affect. What treatment is available for pseudobulbar affect, and how should N.R. be counseled regarding this treatment?

Dextromethorphan with quinidine is effective for reducing the rate of pseudobulbar affect episodes and was recently FDA-approved for this indication. It is dosed one capsule (dextromethorphan 20 mg/quinidine 10 mg) orally twice daily.[220] Adverse effects related to the dextromethorphan component may include dizziness and the possibility of serotonin syndrome. Adverse effects associated with quinidine are an immune-mediated thrombocytopenia, lupus-like syndrome, hepatotoxicity, dose-dependent QTc interval prolongation, and anticholinergic effects.[220]

There are several drug interactions associated with dextromethorphan–quinidine.[220] It is contraindicated with monoamine oxidase inhibitors, requiring a 14-day washout before starting therapy. Similarly, caution should be exercised when this therapy is used concomitantly with selective serotonin reuptake inhibitors and tricyclic antidepressants. It is contraindicated with drugs that prolong the QT interval and are metabolized by CYP 2D6. Dextromethorphan–quinidine should be used with caution with drugs that inhibit CYP 3A4. Because quinidine inhibits CYP 2D6, dose adjustments for CYP 2D6 substrates are necessary. Quinidine also inhibits P-glycoprotein, requiring caution and perhaps dose adjustments when this treatment is used in combination with digoxin.

KEY REFERENCES AND WEBSITES

A full list of references for this chapter can be found at http://thepoint.lww.com/AT11e. Below are the key references and websites for this chapter, with the corresponding reference number in this chapter found in parentheses after the reference.

Key References

Aktas O et al. Neuroprotection, regeneration and immunomodulation: broadening the therapeutic repertoire in multiple sclerosis. *Trends Neurosci*. 2010;33:140. (4)

Minden SL et al. Evidence-based guideline: assessment and management of psychiatric disorders in individuals with MS. Report of the Guideline Development Subcommittee of the American Academy of Neurology. *Neurology*. 2014;82:174–181. (136)

Polman CH et al. Diagnostic criteria for multiple sclerosis: 2010 revisions to the McDonald criteria. *Ann Neurol*. 2011;69:292–302. (68)

Thompson AJ et al. Pharmacological management of symptoms in multiple sclerosis: current approaches and future directions. *Lancet Neurol*. 2010;9:1182. (57)

Yadav V et al. Summary of evidence-based guideline: complementary and alternative medicine in multiple sclerosis. Report of the Guideline Development Subcommittee of the American Academy of Neurology. *Neurology*. 2014;82:1083–1092. (117)

Key Websites

National Multiple Sclerosis Society. http://www.nationalmssociety.org.

58 Headache

Steven J. Crosby

CORE PRINCIPLES

	CHAPTER CASES
1 Migraine, tension-type, and cluster headache are classified as primary headache disorders. Subtle differences in symptomatology and the presence of auxiliary symptoms assist in defining headache type.	**Case 58-1 (Questions 1, 2, 3, 6), Case 58-2 (Questions 1, 3), Case 58-4 (Question 1)**
2 Virtually all patients who suffer from migraine, tension-type, and cluster headaches are candidates to receive abortive (or symptomatic) medications during an acute attack. Prophylactic treatment may be considered for all primary headache types and is driven by various factors including headache frequency, the level of disability imparted by the headache, and response to acute treatment modalities.	**Case 58-1 (Questions 4, 7–10, 11, 12), Case 58-2 (Questions 2, 4, 5), Case 58-4 (Questions 2, 3), Case 58-5 (Questions 1, 2)**
3 Triptans are the drugs of choice as migraine-specific treatments for acute episodes. Triptans are effective in managing associated symptoms of migraine (e.g., nausea, photo- and phonophobia). Differences within the class are observed on the basis of pharmacokinetics.	**Case 58-1 (Questions 5, 7, 8), Case 58-2 (Question 4, Table 58-1)**
4 Evidence supports the use of propranolol, amitriptyline, or topiramate as first-line agents for migraine prophylaxis. The decision to initiate prophylaxis takes into account headache frequency, the impact of attacks on patient functioning, and response to acute treatments. Medical history and adverse effect profile are relevant considerations for specific drug selection.	**Case 58-1 (Question 12), Case 58-2 (Question 5)**
5 Overuse of symptomatic or abortive agents (including triptans and over-the-counter, combination, and opioid analgesics) can increase the intensity and chronicity of all headache types. To prevent medication overuse headache, use of these agents should be limited to fewer than 10 days/month.	**Case 58-3 (Question 1)**
6 Cluster headaches are severely painful and short-duration attacks that tend to occur nightly during susceptible periods and then enter remission for a period of months or years. Treatments of choice for abortive treatment must be fast-acting and include subcutaneous sumatriptan, intranasal zolmitriptan, and oxygen inhalation.	**Case 58-4 (Questions 1–3)**
7 Tension-type headaches (previously known as tension or muscle contraction headaches) usually cause mild-to-moderate discomfort. Conventional analgesics are often appropriate for acute management. Some patients with tension-type headache may require prophylactic treatment, for which amitriptyline, mirtazapine, and venlafaxine have demonstrated efficacy.	**Case 58-5 (Question 1, 2)**

EPIDEMIOLOGY AND DESCRIPTION

Prevalence

Previous investigations have determined that migraine prevalence approximates 12%.[1,2] Survey data obtained from the American Migraine Prevalence and Prevention Study (2004) support the same percentage, as applied to meeting International Classification of Headache Disorders-2 criteria.[2] Across ambulatory care settings, migraine accounts for 0.5% of all encounters, with a majority occurring in primary care settings whereas emergency department (ED) visits approximate 3%,[3] being further stratified within the top 10 causes for ED encounters in the U.S.[4] There is demonstrated variability across both gender and age, with a higher incidence in females,[1–3] and a higher prevalence between 30 and 39 years.[1] Such age- and gender-associated prevalence has been further substantiated in surveillance reviews.[4]

Classification

There is inherent difficulty in evaluating and classifying headache, because this symptom may be attributed to either a physiologic, psychological, or pathologic process, or may be an adverse outcome associated with medications. Because the processes contributing to headache are vast, it is imperative to conduct a comprehensive patient assessment. Broadly categorized, headache is defined as primary or secondary, with the latter typically being attributable to an organic cause. Primary headache is inclusive of migraine, tension headache, and trigeminal cephalalgias, of which cluster headache would be one category. Further, headache associated with physical activity, exposure to exogenous stimuli, or those evolving during the sleep cycle would be categorized as primary.[5] Secondary headache may be attributable to, but not limited to, traumatic injury, vascular or nonvascular cranial pathology, tumor formation (neurofibroma), or an infectious process.[5]

The appropriate classification ultimately speaks to the larger issue of optimal management, via either medical procedures or the initiation of medication. Because secondary headache is associated with a causative component, targeting that cause becomes a principle intervention strategy.

PRIMARY HEADACHE DISORDERS

Migraine

The timeline for the evolution of migraine can often be expressed in terms of minutes. The clinical assessment process for differentiating headache type is dependent upon recognizing general characteristics of migraine and further distinguishing such characteristics from other primary headache forms. An assessment of location can be useful but should not be used as a prime differentiator between headache types because migraine location can be unilateral or bilateral in nature. Patient assessment should include an evaluation of both pain intensity and pain quality, because migraines are commonly described as moderate-to-severe pulsating pain.[5] Migraine duration typically ranges from 4 to 72 hours and may be accompanied by auditory (phonophobia) and light (photophobia) sensitivity, as well as nausea and vomiting.[5,6] These auxiliary symptoms are mediated via the hypothalamus and the chemoreceptor trigger zone (CTZ), indicating diffuse neuroanatomic involvement. The aforementioned features have demonstrated reliable predictive value in migraine diagnosis, as defined by the POUND mnemonic (pulsating, 4–72 hour duration, unilateral nature, nausea or vomiting, disabling effect).[7] The presence of 4 out of the 5 criteria indicates high probability of migraine.[7]

Migraine may be preceded by a constellation of optical or sensory features, defined as an aura. The presence or absence of an aura highlights an important differentiator in migraine diagnosis. International Classification of Headache Disorders criteria indicate a disparity in the number of episodes consistent with a diagnosis of migraine without aura (minimum of five episodes) versus migraine with aura (minimum of two episodes).[5] This criterion is not the only parameter considered, because additional criteria pertaining to headache characteristics also need to be met for an appropriate migraine diagnosis. Auras most often affect vision, with either positive (visual feature) or negative (localized blindness) character.[5] Sensory effects can be characterized similarly as positive (pins and needles description) or negative (loss of sensation or numbness).[5] Aura character that extends beyond the visual and sensory, such as motor or speech irregularity, is linked more toward specialized migraine diagnoses.[5] Patients with suspected migraine should be advised to document aura timing and description, because this information can be valuable for accurate diagnosis.

Patient report of pain location in migraine may be widespread due to the branching of the trigeminal nerve, which facilitates sensory effects across facial regions. Anatomically, the trigeminal nerve features branches of V1, V2, and V3.[8] Branch V1 innervates the scalp, orbital region, and meninges, V2 is directed to the top of the jaw and sinus region, and V3 innervates lower mandibular regions.[8] Additionally, patients may report pain referral to the suboccipital region due to the close proximity between occipital nerves and the spinal nucleus.[8]

Cluster Headache

Cluster headache is characterized within the domain of primary headache disorders. Whereas migraine can be unilateral or bilateral, cluster headache is primarily unilateral involving orbital and/or temporal pain, which can persist for up to 3 hours.[5] Independent of duration, such episodes may occur multiple times during the day.[5] Associated symptoms that occur with high prevalence during cluster headache include lacrimation, rhinorrhea, miosis, ptosis, diaphoresis, and flushing.[5] Preferential incidence of cluster headache occurs in males, but there is similarity to migraine on the basis of age prevalence.

Tension-Type Headache

Tension-type headache is of bilateral character and by comparison to migraine, is often associated with less intense pain without a pulsating quality. An individual's subjective description of pain quality and intensity can be useful in differentiation. Patients may use such terminology as "tightening" to characterize symptoms. The *combination* of symptoms of photophobia, phonophobia, and nausea/vomiting is not considered to be consistent with the diagnosis of tension headache; however, the *individual* symptoms of photo- or phonophobia may accompany tension-type headache.[5]

To complete the discussion pertaining to primary headache pathology, the International Headache Society (IHS) defines headache in association with cough, exercise, sexual activity, cold stimuli, and external compression under the umbrella of primary headache disorders.[5]

SECONDARY HEADACHE

Causation is the key principle underlying secondary headache. Such attributable causes include head or neck trauma, cervical vascular dysfunction, nonvascular cranial dysfunction, infection, psychiatric pathology, or substance withdrawal effects.[5] Causation becomes a critically important principle to consider in patient assessment, particularly when headache onset deviates substantially from existing prevalence and epidemiologic data.

Acute Headaches

Acute headaches may be linked to subarachnoid hemorrhage, stroke, meningitis, or intracranial mass (e.g., neurofibroma, abscess, etc.). It is within this clinical context that diagnostic measures of neuroimaging and lumbar puncture are more commonly implemented. Commonalities of headaches associated with such pathology are of severe quality and rapid evolution, perhaps described as the "worst headache" experienced. An increase in intracranial pressure is of particular importance, and recognition of factors that can impact intracranial pressure becomes critical in patient assessment.

Subacute Headaches

Subacute headaches may be a sign of increased intracranial pressure, intracranial mass lesion, temporal arteritis, sinusitis, or trigeminal neuralgia. Trigeminal neuralgia usually occurs after the age of 40 and is more common in women than in men. The pain usually occurs along the second or third divisions of the trigeminal (facial) nerve and lasts only moments. Trigeminal neuralgia is characterized by sudden, intense pain that recurs paroxysmally, often in response to triggers such as talking, chewing, or shaving.

The evaluation of headache pathology should incorporate the consideration of reported prevalence data, patient age, the presence of triggers or aggravating factors, the contribution of past medical history to headache origin, the patient's description and characterization of symptoms and frequency, and any record of self-care interventions employed to manage headache. Evaluating the impact of headache on daily activity and function is a similarly important consideration. A diagnosis may be confirmed on the basis of this information without the need for further laboratory or procedural measures. If objective or subjective information becomes suggestive of a clinical anomaly (e.g., late-age onset of headache, suspected structural anomalies or neural tissue pathology, etc.), a more comprehensive evaluation, inclusive of additional diagnostic measures (e.g., imaging, lumbar puncture), is indicated.

Pathologic Basis

The pathologic picture of headache requires an understanding of vascular physiology and the functions of the trigeminovascular circuit and neuropeptides. Headache involves both peripheral and central pain processing, afferent neuronal excitability, and pain sensitivity of cerebral arteries and venous sinuses.[5,9] The pathology has often been described within the context of interactions between vascular and neurologic systems.[6,10] Muscular tenderness similarly contributes to headache pathology.[9,11] Such an effect is more commonly considered in association with tension headache.

Recent evidence has conferred support for the interplay between vascular and neurologic function. Afferent and efferent fibers of the trigeminovascular circuitry, vasoactive neuropeptides stored within this system, and serotonin (5-HT) maintain significant pathologic importance.[6,12,13] Neuropeptides, such as substance P, neurokinin A, nitric oxide, calcitonin gene-related peptide, and adenylate cyclase-activating peptide, are promoters of neuroinflammation and vessel dilation.[6,13] Recent evidence further suggests an elevation in pro-inflammatory C-reactive protein in migraine sufferers compared to controls.[14] Consequently, therapeutic interventions have focused on modulating the effects of 5-HT with recent efforts directed toward the modulation of neuropeptide function.

Drug Therapy

The primary goal of therapy is the resolution of headache symptoms, most prominently pain, and attenuating disability associated with the headache. Nonpharmacologic recommendations should similarly be paired with therapeutic options. Pharmacologic treatment options can be divided into abortive and prophylactic, the former resolving acute episodes and the latter being administered chronically to reduce the incidence of recurrent headaches. Abortive treatment may sufficiently manage tension-type headache, often negating the need for prophylactic treatment; however, this may be considered when acute treatment is ineffective, overused, or when the headache is chronic or occurring in frequent episodes. Conversely, patients with migraine and cluster headache, while requiring abortive treatment, may commonly also require long-term prophylactic treatment.

Success in managing acute episodes can often be achieved with the use of conventional analgesics or headache-specific medications (e.g., dihydroergotamine, triptans). Medication selection should be based on the patient's prior treatment experience and the level of disability imparted by the headache episode. With regard to prophylactic therapy, evidence supports the use of select antidepressants, anticonvulsants, and antihypertensives. The selection of such agents should be considered within the context of adverse effect profiles and the potential for utility in managing other medical conditions (e.g., prescribing a β-antagonist for migraine prophylaxis in a patient with a history of hypertension). Rational prescribing limits both the potential for polypharmacy and the risk of adverse effects.

MIGRAINE HEADACHE

Migraine is characterized by pain of a throbbing quality with moderate-to-severe intensity and the presence of associated symptoms, including nausea, vomiting, light, and/or auditory sensitivity.[5,6] Migraine can be unilateral or bilateral and can be further classified on the presence of an aura.[5] The occurrence of an aura has diagnostic relevance based upon the number of episodes and can encompass a range of sensory disturbance, not solely limited to visual field effects.[5]

Pathophysiology

Vascular constriction was a prior central focus of migraine pathology, resulting in hypoperfusion and being resolved through compensatory vasodilation.[6,15] Such alterations in blood flow have been observed in neuroimaging of migraine patients.[6,16–18] There are further alterations in neuronal depolarization, termed cortical spreading depression.[6,19,20] There has been further demonstration of causality between cortical spreading depression and the activation of trigeminovascular circuitry.[6,21] Implications of cortical spreading depression include changes in pH, nitric oxide concentration, and the glutamatergic system.[21] The trigeminovascular system consists of afferent fibers with a foundation in trigeminal ganglia, projecting peripherally to intracranial blood vessels and venous sinuses and to extracranial tissues.[6,22] Trigeminal branches innervate the scalp, orbit, meninges, and mandibular regions.[8] Activation of the trigeminovascular system facilitates the release of vasodilatory-promoting neuropeptides (substance P, neurokinin A, calcitonin gene-related peptide, nitric oxide), and subsequent release results in vessel dilation and inflammation.[6,13,23,24] Further effects include the activation of both the superior salivary nucleus and parasympathetic efferent fibers.[20]

Evidence from positron emission tomography scanning (a technique to measure regional cerebral blood flow as an index of neuronal activity) suggests that episodic dysfunction of the brainstem, with corresponding effects on the trigeminal system, is involved.[25] Weiller et al[25] confirmed brainstem activation (periaqueductal gray, dorsal raphe nucleus, and locus coeruleus) at the onset of migraine headaches in a small sample of patients, and this area may represent an endogenous "migraine generator." Whereas the brainstem may be regarded as an anatomic point of initiation, sensory information in migraine is propagated via higher regions of the hypothalamus, thalamus, and cortex. Sporadic dysfunction of the nociceptive system (periaqueductal gray and dorsal raphe nucleus) and the neural control of cerebral blood flow (dorsal raphe nucleus and locus coeruleus) are hypothesized to trigger migraine headache via effects of these brain structures on the trigeminovascular system.

The therapeutic effects of drugs that stimulate 5-HT_1 receptors (e.g., dihydroergotamine, sumatriptan), antagonize 5-HT_2 receptors (e.g., cyproheptadine), prevent 5-HT reuptake (e.g., amitriptyline) or release (e.g., calcium-channel blockers), or inhibit brainstem serotonergic raphe neurons (e.g., valproate) all lend support to the hypothesis that 5-HT is an important mediator of migraine. Furthermore, brainstem nuclei activated during migraine have high densities of serotonergic neurons. Specific 5-HT receptor subtypes, 5-HT_{1B} and 5-HT_{1D}, are largely distributed in blood[26] and nerves,[27] respectively. These same 5-HT receptor subtypes are the targets of antimigraine drugs such as the triptans and ergot alkaloids.

GENETICS

The genetic basis of migraine is perhaps most effectively understood within the context of familial hemiplegic migraine. This subtype has been further categorized into multiple mutation-induced forms with associated genes CACNA1A, ATP1A2, SLC1A3, SLC4A4, and SCN1A.[6,28] Such genes encode α_1 subunits (CACNA1A, SCN1A) and α_2 subunits (ATP1A2), or are linked with glutamate-associated (SLC1A3) and sodium-bicarbonate-associated (SLC4A4) transporters.[6,28] The former α-subunit encoders regulate ion passage through calcium and sodium channels. A further genetic linkage with migraine pathology has been identified in the potassium channel, TRESK.[28] Implications of mutations at this level impact neuronal resting membrane potential, because an identified frameshift mutation negates TRESK action.[28,29] There is further support for the influence of genetics on migraine pathology when considering the disproportionate prevalence across gender. Because prevalence is higher for females, polymorphisms of the estrogen receptor-1 (ESR-1) gene have been associated with increases in migraine risk.[1,30,31] Advances in the understanding of the genetic bases for pathology maintain importance, as such developments impart promise for novel interventional strategies.

Migraine pathology is multifaceted and neuroanatomically diffuse, involving the brainstem trigeminal nuclei, trigeminovascular afferents, thalamus, hypothalamus, CTZ, and cortical regions. Therapeutic strategies target the dysfunction in these regions, the mediation of associated symptomatology, and the modulation of neuropeptides and neurotransmission.

Quantitative Assessment Instruments

Various patient assessment instruments used to evaluate headache impact include the Headache Impact Test (HIT-6), Migraine Disability Assessment (MIDAS), and the Migraine-Specific Quality of Life Questionnaire (MSQ). The HIT-6 utilizes a Likert scale and evaluates pain, social and cognitive function, and psychological impact.[32,33] A higher score on this assessment confers a greater headache impact. Rendas-Baum et al.[33] confirmed validation of this instrument in the context of chronic migraine. The Migraine Disability Assessment (MIDAS) is a self-administered, 7-item questionnaire, assessing headache-induced absenteeism, activity limitations, and headache frequency and intensity. This instrument has demonstrated reliability[34] and validity.[34–36] A regression analysis confirmed a significant, independent association between MIDAS score and pain intensity, headache frequency, and patient age.[34] The MSQ addresses migraine impact across patient social activity, emotional activity, and the capacity of migraine to prevent activity.[33] With established validity and reliability,[37–39] strong correlations between the MSQ and HIT-6 have been confirmed in the context of chronic migraine.[39]

MIGRAINE WITHOUT AURA

CASE 58-1

QUESTION 1: L.P. is a 27-year-old female presenting to her primary care physician (PCP) with a chief complaint of a "severe, throbbing headache." L.P. reports that headaches began 18 months ago, but during the past 3 months, headaches have been occurring with greater frequency, approximating one episode every 2 to 3 weeks. She further describes bilateral headache pain, occurring "without warning," and coinciding symptoms of nausea and vomiting, photophobia, and suboccipital pain. Prior episodes have been self-treated with acetaminophen 500 mg (4–8 tablets/episode as needed) with variable efficacy. Her past medical history is significant for generalized anxiety disorder, gastroesophageal reflux, and seasonal allergies. Current medication usage includes levonorgestrel/ethinyl estradiol 0.10/0.02 mg by mouth daily, venlafaxine XR 75 mg by mouth daily for generalized anxiety disorder (GAD), and omeprazole 20 mg by mouth daily × 2 months for recent-onset gastroesophageal reflux disease symptoms. Social history is negative for both tobacco use and illicit substances. L.P. reports the "occasional" consumption of alcohol, stated as "1 to 2 cocktails after work on Fridays." As headaches have occurred with greater frequency, absenteeism from work has resulted and this issue has prompted a visit with the PCP. Physical and neurologic examinations are unremarkable.

What subjective and objective information is consistent with a migraine diagnosis, and how do these signs/symptoms differ from tension-type headache?

Symptoms reported by L.P. are consistent with migraine. A study by Kelman addressed migraine location, reporting unilateral character in 67% of study subjects and bilateral character in nearly 24%.[40] For L.P., migraine location would not be a differentiating characteristic between migraine and tension headache, because tension headache is more commonly associated with bilateral character.[9] Pain quality, described as "severe" and "throbbing," is consistent with migraine and precipitates interruptions with daily activity (e.g., absenteeism from work) contrasted with tension headache which is associated with sensations of tightness.[9] Similarly, the occurrence of nausea, vomiting, and photophobia more appropriately aligns with migraine.[5]

Migraine prevalence is higher in female patients than in male patients, approximating 17%[2] with a cumulative incidence in females of 43%.[41] Migraine prevalence within the range of 18 to 29 years has been reported as nearly 21%.[2] L.P.'s sex and age would be compatible with prevalence data although it should be noted that a 28% prevalence statistic for females has been reported in the age range of 30 to 39.[2]

CASE 58-1, QUESTION 2: Which characteristics may be classified as precipitating factors, or "triggers," for migraine pathology? What are possible precipitating factors in L.P.?

Factors involved in precipitating migraine should be routinely assessed for all patients. Assessment should address factors within a patient's medical history, medication usage, social history, and environment. L.P.'s medical history is significant for GAD, she denies the usage of tobacco and illicit substances, she does report the occasional use of alcohol. Alterations in neurotrophic factors and an increase in anxiety symptoms have been demonstrated in migraine patients.[42] Such evidence imparts value to assess this aspect of L.P.'s medical history. While the consumption of alcohol should be addressed, the linkage between alcohol consumption and precipitating migraines is less clear.[43,44] The potential provocation of cortical spreading depression, an electrophysiologic factor underlying migraine pathology, in association with alcohol has been suggested.[45] Although not reported by L.P., an evaluation of diet may provide useful information in determining migraine triggers. The evaluation of dietary patterns and quality has yielded disparities, reporting lower-quality dietary intake in migraine patients.[46]

CASE 58-1, QUESTION 3: Are further diagnostic and laboratory tests indicated in the case of L.P.?

The most important diagnostic evaluations of patients presenting with headache should be based on a thorough medical history and physical examination. Imaging (e.g., CT scans, MRI) is generally not required in the context of uncomplicated migraine.[47]

The report of symptoms by L.P. is consistent with migraine and is sufficient for diagnosis. Her symptoms are not associated with a secondary cause, such as trauma or other injury to the head or neck, and her neurologic examination is unremarkable. Similarly, without reason to suspect subarachnoid hemorrhage or symptoms secondary to meningitis, lumbar puncture would not be indicated. Clinical manifestations that may warrant neurologic imaging to identify artifacts or structural anomalies include coordination deficits, localized neurologic pathology, sensory manifestations, an abnormal neurologic examination, or the presence of atypical headache characteristics.[7,47] Further, a change in headache character and headache onset with advanced age warrants neuroimaging.[7]

Case 58-1, Question 4: What are the goals of therapy for the management of headache in L.P.?

The approach to management and the treatment objectives for L.P. include resolving the acute symptoms of pain, nausea, and photosensitivity, educating L.P. on both prescription and self-care treatment, addressing the contribution of past medical history and concurrent medication usage to headache episodes, and identifying potential triggers.

Case 58-1, Question 5: What is the most appropriate recommendation with regard to the use of acetaminophen to treat headache episodes in L.P.?

L.P. has confirmed self-treatment of headaches with acetaminophen, and in such instances, it is critical to not only evaluate each patient's potential for self-care but also determine whether self-care treatment options can effectively and safely manage the diagnosis. Reported efficacy of acetaminophen has been mixed. Evidence does support acetaminophen efficacy in the migraine patient,[48,49] and comparisons of acetaminophen with placebo yielded a nearly 20% difference in headache resolution.[48,49] However, a study evaluating the parenteral administration of acetaminophen for acute management found no significant difference in efficacy versus placebo.[48,50] Considering L.P.'s report of "variable efficacy" and increase in headache frequency, she is not an appropriate self-care candidate and continued, routine use of acetaminophen to manage acute episodes is not recommended.[48]

Case 58-1, Question 6: What drug-related problems associated with the precipitation or worsening of migraine should be addressed in L.P.?

Oral contraceptives may either worsen or precipitate migraine attacks in women without a previous history of this problem.[51] Incidence may be related to estrogen dose[52] and/or duration of oral contraceptive use.[52,53] Alternatively, migraine has been implicated as an effect of estrogen withdrawal.[52,54] Such patients may benefit from use of a continuous combined oral contraceptive product (e.g., one with no hormone-free interval), use of low-dose estrogen supplementation after 21 days of active contraceptives, or the use of a progestin-only oral contraceptive.[51,55,56]

The American Congress of Obstetricians and Gynecologists supports oral contraceptive use in migraine patients, but recommend avoidance in patients with tobacco use, in those 35 years or older, and/or in those with the presence of neurologic signs.[57] None of these factors are present in L.P.; therefore, oral contraceptive use may be continued. However, the implications of oral contraceptive usage and headache should be discussed with L.P. to allow for informed decision-making.

Further, consultation with L.P. should address whether GAD is being optimally managed. The innervation of trigeminovascular circuitry by neurotransmitters (e.g., norepinephrine, 5-HT) linked to affective pathology (e.g., anxiety, depression) has been established[58] and is known to coexist with such patients reporting increased headache frequency.[59] It is prudent to address anxiety management with L.P. and to further assess her response to venlafaxine to determine whether dose adjustments or medication changes are warranted.

Case 58-1, Question 7: Identify treatment strategies and recommend a medication as a first-line treatment option for the management of migraine in L.P.

Treatment should be aimed at rapidly resolving symptoms and the restoration of the patient's routine activity.[47,60] Migraines may be managed via a "step" or "stratified" approach.[60,61] With a "step" care model, conventional analgesics are initiated first with the opportunity to progress to using more targeted therapies as necessary.[60,61] A "stratified" care model is based on the character of the migraine and will further incorporate validated assessment measures into the treatment decision.[60,61] In this model, a more targeted, migraine-specific treatment may be considered first line. A comparison of treatment approaches has favored the "stratified" model.[61] The current treatment approach for L.P. has mimicked a "step" care model, using acetaminophen as a first-line medication.

Triptans (5-$HT_{1B/1D}$ Receptor Agonists)

Triptans, categorized as first (sumatriptan) and second generation (zolmitriptan, naratriptan, rizatriptan, almotriptan, frovatriptan, and eletriptan), are effective and well tolerated in acute migraine management and are considered appropriate for those not responsive to conventional analgesics.

Triptans can be compared on the basis of efficacy, onset, and recurrence potential. Naratriptan and frovatriptan demonstrate lower recurrence potential whereas the remaining agents within the class (sumatriptan, rizatriptan, almotriptan, eletriptan, and zolmitriptan) yield higher efficacy and faster onset.[60] Compared with ergot derivatives, triptans exhibit greater receptor subtype specificity, targeting 5-HT_{1B} and 5-HT_{1D} receptors.[60,62] It is important to note that the specific nature of the effect differs according to receptor subtype. Constriction of the vasculature is mediated via 5-HT_{1B} interaction[60,62,63] whereas interaction via 5-HT_{1D} antagonizes release of neuropeptides.[60,63] Triptans further diminish neuronal excitability within the trigeminovascular circuitry,[64] and there is evidence of impact on nitric oxide-based signal transduction.[63]

Table 58-1 depicts dosing and pharmacokinetic parameters for the triptans.

Sumatriptan

Sumatriptan is the prototype of the triptan class and is available in several formulations, including an oral tablet, nasal spray, and subcutaneous injection (pen devices and a needle-free solution). A recent analysis confirmed efficacy relative to placebo across sumatriptan doses and formulations; however, subcutaneous delivery yielded a more robust analgesic response.[65] Migraine intensity and the character of associated symptoms (e.g., severity of nausea and vomiting, early-onset nausea) impact formulation selection. For patients who are nauseated and prone to vomit during an acute attack, the subcutaneous and intranasal dosage forms are preferred. Both formulations have a rapid onset of effect. Reduction in headache intensity is reported within 10 minutes after subcutaneous injection and within 15 minutes after administration of the nasal spray.[41] Comparisons of orally administered sumatriptan (doses of 25, 50, and 100 mg) have yielded higher efficacy rates relative to placebo in achieving headache relief at 2 hours.[66] Higher sumatriptan doses of 50 and 100 mg were superior to placebo in achieving headache relief at 4 hours.[66]

Comparative efficacy studies with sumatriptan have yielded mixed results. Subcutaneous sumatriptan is more effective and faster acting than dihydroergotamine (DHE) nasal spray.[67] When compared with subcutaneous DHE, subcutaneous sumatriptan is more effective at 1 and 2 hours, but the two treatments are equally effective at 3 and 4 hours.[68] In this trial, headache recurrence rates at 24 hours favored subcutaneous DHE.[68] Intranasal administration of these agents supports efficacy of sumatriptan for both headache relief and the relief of associated symptoms (e.g., nausea) 60 minutes after dosing.[69] Similar efficacy has been reported for comparison with almotriptan[70] and zolmitriptan,[65] with diminished efficacy being reported versus eletriptan[71] and rizatriptan.[65]

Adverse Effects

Although sumatriptan is well tolerated, there is some variability in the adverse effect profile across different formulations. In general, both oral and intranasal sumatriptan formulations are associated with a low incidence of systemic adverse events. Oral administration of sumatriptan has been associated with adverse effects including dizziness, fatigue, nausea, and vomiting,[66,72] whereas intranasal administration may cause abnormal taste and nasal discomfort.[73,74] Parenteral administration is associated with bruising, redness, and discomfort at the injection site.[75] Due to the risk of vasoconstriction associated with triptan use, special attention is required for patients with cardiovascular disease or risk factors. Although the rate of adverse cardiovascular events has been low,[76] sumatriptan should not be used in patients with uncontrolled hypertension, peripheral or cerebral vascular disease, Wolff-Parkinson-White syndrome or arrhythmias associated with other cardiac accessory conduction pathway disorders, coronary artery disease, previous myocardial infarction, Prinzmetal angina, or coronary vasospasm. The provocation of coronary artery spasm secondary to sumatriptan administration has been demonstrated in those with variant angina, an effect likely mediated via the 1B receptor subtype.[77] A baseline electrocardiogram is recommended for patients with potential cardiac risk prior to triptan administration, and such an intervention may be considered for those patients without cardiovascular risk factors experiencing chest tightness following triptan administration.[78] Initial dosing should occur under medical supervision for patients that possess cardiac risk factors but are deemed appropriate treatment candidates.

Drug Interactions

Drug interaction potential associated with sumatriptan centers on the modulation of serotonergic activity, the risk of serotonin syndrome, and the potential for additive vasoconstrictive properties. Serotonin syndrome potential exists with the concomitant use of sumatriptan and ergot derivatives, selective serotonin reuptake inhibitors (SSRIs), lithium, and/or monoamine oxidase inhibitors (MAOIs).[79] A 2006 Food and Drug Administration advisory further underscored the need for caution and consideration of risk versus benefit with combination use of triptans used in combination with SSRIs and serotonin norepinephrine reuptake inhibitors (SNRIs).[80]

The medication profile for L.P. includes venlafaxine, an SNRI, for the management of GAD; however, this does not exclude the possibility of using triptans to manage her migraines. The clinician should evaluate the entire regimen to ensure optimal management of all indications, and if the addition of a triptan is deemed appropriate, L.P. should be educated on the potential for interaction and the clinical implications of the combination. Because L.P. has attempted treatment with conventional analgesics, she would be a candidate for initiating sumatriptan.

Table 58-1

Dosing and Comparative Pharmacokinetic Parameters of Triptans

Pharmacokinetic Parameters of Triptans in Healthy Volunteers and in Patients With Migraine[a, 214-227]

Drug	Dose and Route of Administration	↓ T_{max} (hours)	↓ C_{max} (mcg/L)	↓ Bioavailability (%)	↓ $t_{1/2}$ (hours)	↓ AUC (mcg/L/hour)	↓ Plasma Protein Binding (%)
Almotriptan	↓ 12.5–25 mg orally	1–3	–	≈70	3–4	—	≈35
Eletriptan	↓ 20–40 mg orally	2	–	≈50	≈4	—	≈85
Frovatriptan	↓ 2.5 mg orally	3	4.2/7[b]	29.6	25.7	94	≈15
	↓ 40 mg orally	5	24.7/53.4[b]	17.5	29.7	881	
Naratriptan	↓ 2.5 mg orally	2	12.6	74	5.5	98	≈28
Rizatriptan	↓ 5–10 mg orally	1–1.5, 3.2[c]	–	45	2–3	—	14
Sumatriptan	↓ 6 mg subcutaneously	0.17	72	96	2	90	14–21
	↓ 100 mg orally	1.5	54	14	2	158	—
	↓ 20 mg intranasal	1.5	13	15.8	1.8	48	—
	↓ 6.5 mg/4 hours transdermal	1.1	22	–	3.1	110	14–21
Zolmitriptan	↓ 2.5 mg orally	1.5, 3[c]	3.3/3.8[b]	39	2.3/2.6[b]	18/21[b]	≈25
	↓ 5 mg orally	1.5, 3[c]	10	46	3	42	
	↓ 5 mg intranasal	3	3.93[d]	102[e]	≈3	22.4[d]	

[a]AUC, area under the curve; C_{max}, maximal drug concentration; T_{max}, time to maximal drug concentration; $t_{1/2}$ = terminal half-life.
[b]Value for men and women, respectively.
[c]Orally disintegrating tablets.
[d]Values based on 2.5-mg dose.
[e]Compared with oral tablet.
Source: Facts & Comparisons. eAnswers. http://online.factsandcomparisons.com/MonoDisp.aspx?monoID=fandc-hcp10008#fandc-hcp10008.b11. Accessed June 16, 2015.

Case 58-1, Question 8: During her annual physical examination, L.P. reports success in managing her migraines with sumatriptan but notes that two doses are often required for resolution of symptoms. She inquires as to whether another triptan would be more effective. How do second-generation triptans compare with sumatriptan? Is an alternative triptan appropriate for L.P.?

Second-Generation Triptans

Second-generation triptans include almotriptan, eletriptan, frovatriptan, rizatriptan, naratriptan, and zolmitriptan. All triptans have demonstrated superiority to placebo in terms of efficacy.[62,81] These agents differ based on the pharmacokinetic profile and the capacity for headache recurrence.[60,82] Among the class, zolmitriptan, rizatriptan, eletriptan, and almotriptan are associated with a faster onset and higher likelihood of recurrence compared with naratriptan and frovatriptan, both of which have a slower onset of action with a lower risk of recurrence.[60,82] Naratriptan, in particular, is metabolized by multiple isozymes, without strong enzymatic inhibition or induction potential, creating less potential for CYP-induced interactions[83] whereas frovatriptan is subject to a dual metabolic path via CYP1A2 and renal excretion.[62] Relative to sumatriptan, oral bioavailability of second-generation agents is increased.[83]

Meta-analyses have offered insight into triptan comparisons. For headache response at 2 hours, eletriptan 80 mg and rizatriptan 10 mg elicited higher response rates with sumatriptan 100 mg as the reference whereas eletriptan 20 mg, frovatriptan 2.5 mg, and naratriptan 2.5 mg were inferior to sumatriptan.[83] In assessing sustained freedom from pain, greater efficacy has been observed with rizatriptan 10 mg, eletriptan 80 mg, and almotriptan 12.5 mg.[83] The opposite effect in this efficacy endpoint for almotriptan 12.5 mg has been observed in a parallel-group investigation with sumatriptan 50 mg as a reference.[84] Further comparisons of 74 randomized trials found that among the triptans, eletriptan was associated with the greatest potential of producing a pain-free state at 2 hours and at 24 hours.[85] Favorable efficacy was further observed for rizatriptan (2 hours) and zolmitriptan (24 hours).[85] Comparisons between rizatriptan and frovatriptan have yielded similar pain-free outcomes at 2 hours and have favored frovatriptan for pain-free status at 4 hours.[86] More recently, a therapeutic endpoint of the combination of freedom from pain with no incidence of adverse outcomes has been used in studies involving migraines.[87–90] Using this endpoint as a primary measure of comparison between zolmitriptan (2.5 mg) and almotriptan (12.5 mg) in a multicenter European trial, both treatments were deemed equally efficacious.[87]

Drug Interactions

Striking the balance between theoretic drug interaction risk for triptans and what is observed in clinical practice presents a challenge, especially because it relates to the risk of serotonin syndrome.[80,91,92] For L.P., potential drug interactions exist between triptans and venlafaxine (SNRI) and levonorgestrel/ethinyl estradiol (oral contraceptive). Attributed to metabolism via CYP1A2, a slight increase in frovatriptan AUC has been observed with oral contraceptive administration.[93] Prospective investigations assessing the combination of paroxetine and rizatriptan[91] and fluoxetine and zolmitriptan[91] found no instances of serotonin syndrome. These studies lie in contrast to reports of symptoms of serotonin syndrome with the combination of triptans and SSRIs or SNRIs.[41] The administration of a triptan should not be excluded based on L.P.'s medication profile; however, educating her on the potential for the interaction is warranted.

Increases in rizatriptan and zolmitriptan exposure have been observed secondary to MAO inhibition.[92] Inhibition of CYP3A4 has facilitated increases in eletriptan[92] and almotriptan.[92,94]

L.P. can be considered an appropriate candidate for triptan prescribing. Although associated migraine symptoms are reported, the rapidity of onset for such symptoms (e.g., nausea, vomiting) is less clear and should be a point of discussion with the patient. Such information is important for the optimal formulation selection. A nonoral formulation may be recommended in the context of early-onset vomiting. Although a loss of efficacy is associated with triptan discontinuation,[95] the timeline for triptan use prior to discontinuation has spanned years.[95] Evidence for replacing one triptan with another is mixed. If treatment with one triptan results in suboptimal efficacy, an alternative triptan may be prescribed.[82] However, recent evidence evaluating the impact of such change does not suggest substantial benefit.[96,97]

Case 58-1, Question 9: L.P. has noted that for some migraine episodes, nausea and vomiting has been severe, and asks about the use of DHE and antiemetics. What is the role of ergot alkaloids and/or antiemetics in migraine management?

ERGOT ALKALOIDS

Relative to triptans, ergot alkaloids function as receptor agonists with strong affinity at 5-HT_{1A}, 5-HT_{1B}, and 5-HT_{1D}.[98] In addition, these agents express activity at 5-HT_{1F}, as well as alpha and dopaminergic receptors.[98,99] This pharmacologic profile differs from that of the triptans because the latter exhibit no affinity for dopaminergic or α-receptors.[98] Actions of ergot alkaloids are multifaceted, blocking neuropeptide release, stimulating the ventroposteromedial thalamus, and blocking transmission of afferent signals in trigeminal circuit.[98] Although ergot alkaloids have demonstrated benefit in managing migraine,[82,100,101] the more targeted pharmacologic profile of the triptans has gained preference.

Intranasal administration of dihydroergotamine has yielded significant improvements in both pain reduction and functional status in comparison with placebo.[102] A 2-mg DHE dose achieved headache resolution at 4 hours post administration for 70% of subjects, compared with 28% in the placebo group.[102] This level of efficacy at the 4-hour time point for DHE has been further substantiated in comparison with sumatriptan.[103] Subcutaneous administration of 1 mg DHE or 6 mg sumatriptan resulted in comparable headache resolution.[103] Functional capacity at 1 hour as well as the proportion of patients achieving pain relief at 2 hours postadministration favored sumatriptan.[103] Adverse outcomes of nausea, vomiting, and injection-site pain were more prominent for those administering DHE, whereas incidence of chest pain was more common in the sumatriptan-treated group.[103] Orally inhaled DHE represents a newer, noninvasive delivery (TEMPO inhaler, MAP Pharmaceuticals) system.[104,105] Superiority to placebo has been demonstrated in the FREEDOM-301 Study across endpoints of pain relief and freedom from auditory sensitivity, light sensitivity, and nausea.[104] Associated adverse effects included product taste and nausea, 6% and 4%, respectively.[104] This delivery system is not yet commercially available.

Peripheral and cerebrovascular disease, renal and hepatic disease, sepsis, and cardiac disease qualify as contraindications to the use of ergot alkaloids.[98,100] Further, with the potential to induce uterine contraction and distribute into breast milk, use is contraindicated during pregnancy and lactation.[98,106] In patients with a history of hypertension, it is important to determine whether blood pressure is appropriately controlled before considering the use of these agents in migraine due to the potential for arterial constriction peripherally.[107] Compared with ergotamine, DHE exerts a more variable effect on blood pressure.[107]

Adverse Effects

Nausea is the most prominent adverse outcome with ergot alkaloids.[107] The effect is dose-related and is linked with 5-HT_2 and

$5\text{-}HT_3$ receptor activation.[60] Intranasal DHE and orally inhaled DHE have been associated with prolonged nasal congestion[60] and altered taste.[104] Parenteral administration has been associated with lightheadedness and leg cramping.[107]

Antiemetics

In most patients, triptan agents provide effective relief of migraine-associated nausea. Therefore, specific antiemetic therapy usually is not required. However, as mentioned previously, persistent nausea is more common in patients who use ergotamine for acute migraine therapy. In these patients, and in triptan-treated patients who experience incomplete nausea relief, adjunctive antiemetic therapy should be considered. Results from a more recent comparative trial (prochlorperazine IV 10 mg vs. metoclopramide IV 20 mg) found similar efficacy in managing nausea.[108] Efficacy of metoclopramide has been demonstrated at the lower end of the dosing scale (10 mg), but higher doses (20–40 mg) were not associated with improved outcomes.[109]

Case 58-1, Question 10: In addition to triptans and ergot derivatives, what other abortive agents are available for outpatient treatment of acute migraine?

NONSTEROIDAL ANTI-INFLAMMATORY DRUGS AND COMBINATION ANALGESICS

Many NSAIDs and combination analgesics containing caffeine have been shown to be effective for the acute treatment of migraine headache.[110,111] Significant clinical benefit in double-blind, placebo-controlled trials has been shown for aspirin, ibuprofen, naproxen sodium, and combination analgesics containing acetaminophen, aspirin, and caffeine.[47,111,112] Ketoprofen doses of 75 or 150 mg have demonstrated efficacy relative to placebo in reducing migraine severity.[113]

Case 58-1, Question 11: L.P. reports that her migraines have been successfully managed with naratriptan 2.5 to 5 mg/episode, with most episodes resolving with the lower dose. Naratriptan was selected on the basis of a lower likelihood of recurrence. L.P. has been experiencing a severe migraine for the past few days and has been unsuccessful in treating the episode with naratriptan. She has now sought treatment at a nearby hospital and has been diagnosed with status migrainosus. What is the most appropriate approach to managing status migrainosus in L.P.?

Intractable Migraine

Status migrainosus, or intractable migraine, is characterized by an extended duration of headache, exceeding 72 hours.[5] The typical management strategy usually requires hydration and parenteral therapy with ergot derivatives, sumatriptan, or opioid analgesics.

DIHYDROERGOTAMINE

Dihydroergotamine has demonstrated efficacy in treating intractable migraine by either intermittent or continuous administration.[114] The successful resolution of symptoms by DHE avoids the need for administration of corticosteroids and opioids for the same purpose. Adjunctive antiemetics should be administered for nausea.[114,115]

SUMATRIPTAN

Sumatriptan 6 mg subcutaneously is also effective for the treatment of established migraine.[41] If the first injection does not provide relief at 1 hour, a second injection may be administered. Sumatriptan should not be administered within 24 hours of ergot alkaloids because of the potential for prolonged vasospastic reactions.

PROCHLORPERAZINE

Prochlorperazine has established efficacy in managing migraine-related nausea, with intravenous administration being effective during intractable migraine.[47,114,116] In randomized, controlled trials, prochlorperazine 10 mg IV was more effective than placebo, IV metoclopramide, IV ketorolac, and IV valproate for the treatment of acute migraine in the ED.[116]

CORTICOSTEROIDS

Parenteral dexamethasone may be administered in cases of intractable migraine.[114] Among a subset of patients experiencing migraine symptoms beyond 72 hours, a greater percentage of patients achieved pain-free status following parenteral dexamethasone administration, relative to placebo.[117] Further, lower headache recurrence has been observed in patients receiving dexamethasone after standard abortive treatment.[118]

L.P. may be treated with DHE, sumatriptan, prochlorperazine, or metoclopramide due to demonstrated efficacy and tolerability in comparison with other treatment options.[119]

Case 58-1, Question 12: During a return visit to her PCP, L.P. has reported that most migraine episodes have been successfully managed with naratriptan. Although effective, she expresses concern related to episode frequency noting that in some instances, she is using naratriptan 3 times weekly. Her PCP is considering prophylactic management and wants to prescribe propranolol. Is propranolol an appropriate option for L.P.?

Prophylactic Therapy

CRITERIA FOR USE

The relevance for initiating prophylactic therapy for migraine is not simply defined by one common feature among patients. Rather, the impact of migraine for an individual patient needs to be assessed. Estimates pertaining to prevalence suggest that only a small percentage (around 5%) receive prophylactic management.[120] Targeted outcomes for prophylactic therapy includes a reduction in both migraine frequency and severity, enhancing response to acute management strategies, and a general improvement in daily function.[120] As previous criteria have addressed the frequency of migraine episodes (two or more episodes monthly) as a principle consideration,[120] further guidance on suitability for such treatment should also address disability associated with the episodes, track record of failure with acute treatments or the overuse of acute treatments, adverse effects precipitated by acute treatments, or a more pathologically complex migraine (e.g., basilar or hemiplegic episodes, prolonged auras).[120,121] Optimizing prophylactic treatment may likely require a 2- to 3-month window. This becomes an important consideration to convey to patients with a focus on maintaining adherence. Medications utilized in prophylactic migraine management generally fall into the categories of antihypertensives, antidepressants, or anticonvulsants. A fourth category comprised of nonprescription treatments is considered as well. The evaluation of evidence associated with prophylactic treatments is often challenging due to the lack of studies with comparisons between agents or with crossover design.

An evidence-based guideline for prophylactic treatment of migraine has been created by the US Headache Consortium, published through the American Academy of Neurology.[120] Further evidence has been provided via a combined panel of the American Academy of Neurology and the American Headache Society.[122] Migraine prophylaxis is an area for which the off-label use of medications is a particularly common practical consideration. Only a select number of agents have been approved by the Food and Drug Administration (FDA) for migraine prophylaxis in the

US, including propranolol, timolol, topiramate, valproic acid or divalproex sodium, and botulinum toxin A (onabotulinumtoxinA). The approval of botulinum toxin is within the context of treating chronic migraine. Although triptans are not FDA-approved for migraine prophylaxis, select agents (frovatriptan, naratriptan, and zolmitriptan) are considered off-label for migraine prophylaxis during menstruation.

PROPRANOLOL

Evidence supports propranolol safety and efficacy in migraine prophylaxis.[120–123] Various mechanisms for efficacy may be considered, including the modulation of central catecholamines[124] and interaction with serotonin receptors.[124,125] Propranolol has also demonstrated a suppressive effect on cortical spreading depression in animal models.[124,126] In a small study of migraine patients, propranolol has decreased cerebrovascular reactivity, mediated by action on vascular tone.[127] For L.P., the prescribing of propranolol for migraine prophylaxis could be considered, as there are no contraindications within her profile that would prevent use. A limiting variable to continued use may be the adverse effect profile, including lethargy, fatigue, and sleep disruption.[122,128] As an alternative to propranolol, metoprolol could be considered similarly appropriate for L.P. Comparisons with aspirin[122,129] or propranolol[120] suggest that metoprolol would be appropriately effective. Metoprolol has been further compared with nebivolol.[130] While similarly effective in prophylactic migraine management, better tolerability and ease of titration were associated with nebivolol.[130]

Dosing

Initial dosing for propranolol for prophylaxis of migraine headaches is 20 mg by mouth 2 or 3 times a day with gradual titration (weekly intervals) according to patient tolerability to 80 to 160 mg/day in two to four divided doses.[121] Once the daily dosage of propranolol required to control headaches is established, patient adherence may be improved by changing to a long-acting oral dosage form (e.g., Inderal LA).

Migraine with Aura

CASE 58-2

QUESTION 1: V.M. is a 24-year-old female, reporting to her primary care provider with a 3-month history of "throbbing" headaches. Although V.M. has reported experiencing tension headaches "on and off" in the past, the character of these recent headaches has been different, accompanied by early-onset, severe, nausea and vomiting, and preceded by "flashes of light" and a unilateral facial "numbness." The "numbness" and visual flashes have typically resolved after 30 minutes with headaches developing soon after. She has taken naproxen or ibuprofen for treating recent episodes, but neither has proven effective. The MIDAS score was 11. Medical history includes hypothyroidism, treated with levothyroxine 100 mcg by mouth daily, and a past history of tension headache. Her medication profile also includes an oral contraceptive, norgestimate/ethinyl estradiol, for the past 5 years. She describes herself as an "occasional smoker" and denies a history of alcohol use or illicit substances. Which information is consistent with the diagnosis of migraine with aura in V.M.?

Although both the "throbbing" character of the headache and associated gastrointestinal (GI) symptoms are consistent with migraine, it is the presence of both the visual (light flashes) and sensory (numbness) disturbances correlate with the diagnosis of migraine with aura. Relevant information for confirming this diagnosis would be a minimum of two episodes, the accompaniment of an aura symptom, the duration and unilateral nature of the aura, and the evolution of the headache following the aura.[5]

Propagating glial and neuronal depolarization, characterized as cortical spreading depression, has been implicated in aura.[20,131] It is suggested that the pathologic basis for aura involves gap junction modulation at the neuronal level of the trigeminovascular circuitry.[20] Aura has been associated with migraine in approximately one-third of patients[131] and visual phenomena are typically the most prevalent aura features.[131] It is important to note that visual effects are substantially varied and can include flashing lights, waving lines, or areas of localized blindness (scotoma).[132] Further, a "visual snow" effect has been described in the literature, bearing resemblance to television static.[133] Although visual phenomena are most prevalent, sensory disturbances (e.g., numbness, pins, and needles sensation) may also comprise an aura.[5] In the case of V.M., the aura includes both visual and sensory disturbance, and coupled with the report of additional symptoms (e.g., throbbing headache, n/v), a diagnosis of migraine with aura is appropriate. The temporal relationship between the aura and evolution of the migraine is one of further consideration. Although V.M. reports the evolution of the migraine following the aura, there is evidence to support classical migraine symptoms occurring during the aura phase.[134]

CASE 58-2, QUESTION 2: Should the migraine that V.M. is experiencing be treated according to a stratified-care or step-care model?

In accordance with a step-care model, a conventional analgesic medication would be considered as primary therapy.[61] A stratified-care approach is designed for treatment selection based on patient need.[61] V.M. has reported self-treatment with conventional agents (e.g., naproxen or ibuprofen) without adequate relief. Further considering that V.M.'s MIDAS score corresponds to "moderate" disability and the reported variance of MIDAS score with age,[34] a stratified-care model would be preferable.

CASE 58-2, QUESTION 3: V.M. has been counseled previously regarding the cardiovascular risks associated with oral contraceptives and questions whether she is at greater risk considering her migraine diagnosis. Is an oral contraceptive appropriate for V.M.?

No consistent increased risk for stroke has been found among men, women older than 45 years old, and women who have migraine without aura.[135] Among patients with a diagnosis of migraine with aura, a twofold increase in ischemic stroke risk has been reported.[136] An additional finding in this meta-analysis supported an increased risk among migraine patients using oral contraceptives.[136] The World Health Organization considers migraine with aura in women of any age an absolute contraindication to the use of combined oral contraceptives.[51] The American College of Obstetricians and Gynecologists guidelines permit the use of combined oral contraceptives in women who suffer from migraine with aura as long as they have no focal neurologic signs, do not smoke, and are younger than 35 years of age.[51] V.M. describes herself as an "occasional smoker" so relevant management strategies include discussing other contraceptive options and/or a smoking cessation plan.

CASE 58-2, QUESTION 4: What is the most appropriate recommendation for acute management of V.M.'s migraine?

Given the severity of symptoms and past treatment experience with conventional analgesics, the selection of a migraine-targeted treatment (e.g., ergot alkaloid, triptan) would be preferable. Of similar importance is the presence of severe, early-onset nausea; therefore, a nonoral administration is recommended. Sumatriptan and zolmitriptan are available as nonoral formulations, and either could be considered appropriate for V.M. A limiting factor in the selection of ergot alkaloids as a primary treatment would be the potential for drug-associated nausea.[107]

CASE 58-2, QUESTION 5: V.M. has now returned to her PCP reporting success in managing her migraines with zolmitriptan. The frequency of migraine episodes remains an issue, reporting 4–5 episodes monthly which have caused her to miss work. Her PCP is considering prophylactic treatment but would prefer not to prescribe propranolol. Which medication may be prescribed to prevent migraines in V.M.?

AMITRIPTYLINE

Amitriptyline is an appropriate first-line therapy option for migraine prophylaxis[121,137] with such effects being independent of antidepressant activity.[138–140] Demonstrated blockade of sodium currents in trigeminal neurons and blockade of 5-HT reuptake[141] is the basis for the potential efficacy in managing migraine,[140] although a complete mechanism has not been fully elucidated. Amitriptyline treatment has been associated with significant improvement in MIDAS scores[142] Such an effect has been demonstrated following a 45-day treatment cycle.[142] Particularly applicable to the case of V.M., there is demonstrated benefit for amitriptyline in the treatment of tension-type headache as well,[9] making it a viable option for patients with both headache forms.

Amitriptyline has been compared with propranolol, divalproate, and topiramate in various studies. A randomized trial comparing extended-release divalproate with amitriptyline (150 subjects in each treatment group) yielded similar efficacy, measured by headache frequency at 6 months, while being inferior to divalproate at 3 months.[143] Two separate studies have provided comparison between amitriptyline and topiramate.[144,145] With a primary efficacy measure of monthly migraine episode rate, 100-mg doses of each proved comparable and similarly well tolerated.[144] A smaller study reported similar results; however, the combination treatment of amitriptyline and topiramate was assessed as a separate, third treatment arm.[145] Patient satisfaction among subjects taking the combination was noted to be higher relative to either monotherapy group.[145]

Dosing

The initial dose of amitriptyline is 10 to 25 mg by mouth at bedtime. This nightly dose can be increased at weekly intervals by 10 to 25 mg until the maximal dose of 150 mg/day is reached.

While generally tolerated, common adverse effects attributed to amitriptyline treatment have included drowsiness, anticholinergic effects, and weight increase.[143–145]

TOPIRAMATE

Topiramate is considered a first-line option for migraine prophylaxis.[121,137] In addition to aforementioned comparisons with amitriptyline, prospective studies have reported similar efficacy between topiramate and sodium valproate.[146–148] Three large randomized, placebo-controlled trials have documented the efficacy of this agent for reducing the number of monthly attacks.[149] With initial dosing of 25 mg daily,[144,145,150] target doses of 100 mg daily[144] and 200 mg daily[150] have been assessed. Evidence supports dose titration to 100 mg for optimal outcomes.[148,151] Further titration to 200 mg has not demonstrated significantly better outcomes relative to 100 mg.[148,152]

Paresthesia, fatigue, weight loss, memory, and concentration deficits have been associated with topiramate therapy.[144,145,153]

VALPROATE

Valproate and divalproex sodium are approved for migraine prophylaxis and are viable treatment options for prevention.[121,137] An extended-release divalproex sodium formulation has demonstrated efficacy relative to placebo.[154] Versus active comparators, equivalence in efficacy has been reported for propranolol[155] and topiramate.[147] The selection of valproate as a therapy for women of childbearing age must be evaluated cautiously, in light of potential detrimental effects in cognitive development.[156]

Dosing

Delayed- or extended-release formulations of divalproex sodium (e.g., Depakote or Depakote ER) may be prescribed for prophylaxis with the advantage of the latter formulation being once-daily administration. Initial dosing for the delayed-release formulation is 250 mg by mouth twice daily whereas the extended-release formulation is 500 mg by mouth once daily.

Adverse effects associated with valproate treatment include alopecia, nausea, drowsiness, and weight gain.[147] Potential for hepatotoxicity and pancreatitis[157] limits utility.

GABAPENTIN

Gabapentin possesses a complex mechanism of modulating Ca^{++} channels, increasing GABA concentration centrally, and binding to gabapentin-binding protein.[158] A randomized trial versus placebo demonstrated superiority of gabapentin 2,400 mg/day in reducing migraine rate over 4 weeks.[158] Secondary outcomes related to severity, functional capacity, duration, and aura severity did not yield significant differences between treatment groups.[158]

CANDESARTAN

Candesartan, an angiotensin II type 1 (AT_1) receptor antagonist, has demonstrated efficacy, based on an intention-to-treat analysis of 57 patients, in migraine prophylaxis in a randomized, placebo-controlled, crossover design.[159] Outcomes of migraine frequency (number of days) and duration (number of hours) were favorable with candesartan.[159] Although dizziness was the most frequently reported adverse event associated with treatment, neither this effect nor any other adverse outcome differed significantly from placebo.[159]

TONABERSAT

As both cortical spreading depression and gap junctional modulation have been linked with migraine aura,[20,131] the inhibition of CSD constitutes a potential approach to treatment.[160,161] Tonabersat functions as a gap junction blocker.[161] Comparisons with placebo have been mixed[160,162,163] with efficacy exclusive to migraine with aura.[160] Tonabersat is currently an investigational treatment.

NONSTEROIDAL ANTI-INFLAMMATORY DRUGS

Effectiveness as preventive therapy is considered to be modest compared with the first-line agents.[121] NSAIDs may be effective as short-term therapy for menstruation-associated migraine.[121]

In selecting an alternative prophylactic medication for V.M., evidence supports use of either a selective β-antagonist (e.g., metoprolol), amitriptyline, or topiramate. In all such instances, V.M. should be counseled with regard to dose titrations, adverse effects, and allowing for a sufficient trial duration to adequately determine efficacy.

Medication Overuse

CASE 58-3

QUESTION 1: L.D. is a 39-year-old woman with a 7-year history of migraine (without aura) and tension-type headache who comes to the clinic requesting a refill of her almotriptan. She reports an increase in the frequency of both her "throbbing" and "dull, pressure sensation" headaches during the past year, and lately she has had difficulty distinguishing the two types. In the past 2 months, she has had only 5 days with no headache, and she has been much less productive in her work as a magazine editor. She has reported using 4 to 5 almotriptan tablets weekly with multiple episodes also requiring naproxen sodium, which she has purchased over the counter (OTC). She has requested two refills for her almotriptan during the past 1½ months. What is the role of medication overuse in worsening symptoms, and how should this condition be managed in L.D.?

Medication overuse is defined as the use of triptans, ergot alkaloids, opioid analgesics, or combination analgesics on 10 or more days/month (the criterion for use of simple OTC analgesics is 15 or more days/month)[137] and often occurs in migraine and tension-type headache sufferers.[164] The pathophysiology of medication overuse headache is multidimensional and is related to hypometabolism in neuroanatomic structures,[164,165] neurochemical alterations (e.g., orexinA, corticotropin-releasing factor),[166] and alterations in receptor expression and neuropeptide levels (e.g., increase in CGRP).[167] Chronic daily headaches often have features of both migraine and tension-type headaches.[168] L.D. displays many of the features of medication overuse headache. She reports an increase in the frequency of headaches to a near-daily pattern, and she is no longer able to distinguish between migrainous and tension-type headaches. Laboratory tests should be ordered to assess L.D.'s renal and hepatic function, and she should be questioned regarding the occurrence of GI discomfort, acute bleeding, or a change in her stool color.

In general, patients who receive abortive agents for headache treatment should be counseled to restrict their use of these agents to no more than twice/week.[121] The design of medication withdrawal procedures can be tapered or abrupt, with a tapered withdrawal procedure recommended for opioid, barbiturate, or benzodiazepine overuse.[168] Abrupt discontinuation can be considered suitable for triptans and nonopioid analgesics.[168] For L.D., the discussion of a discontinuation strategy would be recommended. Such an intervention has demonstrated positive outcomes in headache reduction.[169,170] Further, prophylaxis may be considered and topiramate has demonstrated efficacy in this context.[168,171]

CLUSTER HEADACHE

Cluster headache is an uncommon headache disorder (estimated prevalence 0.07%–0.4%) that derives its name from the characteristic pattern of headache recurrence—headaches tend to occur nightly during a relatively short time (e.g., several weeks or months), followed by a long period of complete remission.[172] Cluster headache is more common among males with an average age of onset around 30 years.[173]

Cluster headache is characterized by severe, unilateral pain, potentially described as a pulsating or burning sensation, often involving the orbital, temporal, or maxilla regions.[5,174] In addition to pain, cluster headache typically involves autonomic features (e.g., miosis, nasal congestion, ptosis, lacrimation).[5,174]

Pathophysiology

The pathology surrounding cluster headache includes stimulation of parasympathetic outflow, disturbance at the level of the hypothalamus, and vasodilation.[175,176] Such pathology is also a function of alterations in testosterone levels,[175] melatonin,[175] and diminished response to thyrotropin-releasing hormone.[175] Further assessments of pineal functioning in the context of cluster headache have revealed anomalies in serial plasma melatonin sampling, reflected as diminished peaks.[177] The pathology further includes angiographic changes and the interplay of parasympathetic and sympathetic function at the level of the cavernous sinus.[178]

Signs and Symptoms

CASE 58-4

Question 1: R.H. is a 31-year-old man with a 3-year history of episodic cluster headache. He has been headache-free for the past year, but today states that the headaches are returning in their characteristic fashion. He reports abrupt onset of right-sided retro-orbital pain with occasional superimposed knifelike "jabs" that increase in intensity for several minutes to a severe, unrelenting pain lasting about 90 minutes. The headache then gradually subsides. Associated symptoms include right-sided lacrimation, conjunctival injection, and rhinorrhea. He denies any premonition of ensuing headache or GI upset during the attacks. Physical examination during a cluster headache shows right eyelid droop and pupillary miosis. R.H.'s cluster periods characteristically last about 2 months and usually recur once or twice yearly. The first headache of the current episode awoke him from a short nap. R.H. expects to suffer one or two such headaches daily because this has been the usual pattern during each cluster period. Previous cluster headaches have been symptomatically treated with aspirin and codeine 30 mg. However, R.H. reports only modest relief with this treatment approach.

R.H.'s medical history is unremarkable. He does not use tobacco but admits to occasional social drinking. What subjective and objective evidence in this case is consistent with a diagnosis of cluster headaches?

R.H.'s sex, age of onset, quality and intensity of headache pain, periodicity of headache attacks, and associated symptoms all support the diagnosis of cluster headaches.

An aura may precede a cluster headache episode; however, this effect occurs in a small percentage of patients.[174,179] The episodic timeline of cluster headache is variable, extending from weeks to months, with the potential for extended remission periods.[5] R.H.'s headache quality (severe, unrelenting pain), site (unilateral), evolution and resolution pattern (worsens over several minutes and resolves within 90 minutes), and periodicity of attacks (one or two headaches occurring daily for about 2 months followed by a period of remission that lasts about 1 year) are all compatible with the usual character of cluster headaches.

Associated symptoms reported by R.H. during headache attacks (e.g., lacrimation, rhinorrhea, conjunctival injection) and the absence of GI or neurologic disturbances are also compatible with the diagnosis of cluster headaches.

Case 58-4, Question 2: What abortive measures are available for symptomatic treatment of individual headaches during R.H.'s current cluster period?

Abortive Therapy

The treatments of choice for abortive treatment of cluster headaches are sumatriptan by subcutaneous injection, zolmitriptan nasal spray, and oxygen inhalation.[180,181] Among these agents, subcutaneous sumatriptan is often preferred.[182]

SUMATRIPTAN

Sumatriptan 6 mg administered subcutaneously for cluster headaches reduced severity in 74% of attacks within 15 minutes,

Chapter 58 Headache

compared with 26% of attacks treated with placebo.[182] An additional injection of 6 mg does not appear to give additional headache relief.[182] However, in patients who experience a recurrent headache after initial relief with sumatriptan, a second injection is often useful.[176] Sumatriptan should not be used more often than twice daily during cluster bouts.

A randomized, multicenter trial, assessing intranasal sumatriptan (20 mg) compared with placebo, yielded a significantly better outcome of decreased pain response, 30 minutes following administration.[183] Secondary outcome measures, including resolution of associated symptoms, similarly favored sumatriptan.[183]

OXYGEN

Oxygen may be useful for patients with frequent cluster headaches who would otherwise exceed maximal dosing restrictions of sumatriptan.[172] The mechanism of oxygen's effect is unknown but may be related to a direct vasoconstrictive action.[172] Clinical trial data have been mixed. In a trial of 57 patients with episodic cluster headache, 100% oxygen delivered at 12 L/minute was deemed more effective versus placebo for achieving pain-free status at 15 minutes.[184] A double-blind, placebo-controlled crossover study of hyperbaric oxygen treatment for cluster episodes imparted no significant beneficial effect relative to placebo.[185]

ZOLMITRIPTAN

Two controlled trials have established the effectiveness of intranasal zolmitriptan for the acute treatment of cluster headache attacks. Cluster headache relief rates were 40% and 50% with 5 mg of zolmitriptan, and 62% and 63% with 10 mg of intranasal zolmitriptan in these two studies, respectively.[181,186]

OTHER THERAPEUTIC INTERVENTIONS

The somatostatin analog, octreotide, administered by subcutaneous injection, has demonstrated superiority in efficacy relative to placebo.[187] In addition to headache relief at 30 minutes, octreotide administration yielded improved outcomes for resolving associated cluster headache symptoms.[187] Alternate therapeutic interventions include intranasal capsaicin,[188] local administration of cocaine, and the local administration of lidocaine.[189]

Reasonable options for the acute treatment of R.H.'s acute cluster headaches include subcutaneous sumatriptan, oxygen inhalation, and intranasal zolmitriptan. For many patients, oxygen is a less convenient therapy because the equipment is not easily portable and the patient must sit still during the treatment. The choice can be made on the basis of patient preference or cost.

CASE 58-4, QUESTION 3: What therapeutic agents are available for headache prophylaxis during an active cluster period? Which option is most appropriate for R.H.?

Prophylactic Therapy

Prophylaxis should be considered in the context of chronic cluster headache episodes. An important objective for prophylactic treatment is reducing the risk of overmedication associated with acute treatment.[175]

VERAPAMIL

Evidence supports verapamil efficacy in cluster headache prophylaxis[174,175,190–192] with daily doses in the range of 240 to 320 mg.[175,193,194] Baseline and periodic electrocardiography should be performed for those maintained on verapamil therapy.[174,175] The need for such monitoring is a function of verapamil's electrophysiologic effects on cardiac nodal tissue.

LITHIUM CARBONATE

Where primary treatment is either ineffective or contraindicated, the use of lithium as a second-line option is supported.[191] A double-blind, crossover study found similar efficacy relative to verapamil yet, lithium was inferior to verapamil in tolerability.[195] Lithium serum levels associated with efficacy in cluster headache prophylaxis are usually between 0.4 and 0.8 mEq/L.[182] In addition to assessing serum levels, routine monitoring of electrolytes, hepatic, renal, and thyroid function is required.[191]

SUBOCCIPITAL STEROID INJECTION

One high-quality randomized, controlled trial demonstrated the efficacy of suboccipital steroid injection for the prophylaxis of cluster headache in 26 patients.[196] Injections included 12.46 mg of betamethasone dipropionate and 5.26 mg of betamethasone disodium phosphate mixed with 0.5 mL of 2% lidocaine. Eighty-five percent of patients had relief of headache attacks within 72 hours of injection (compared with none in the placebo group).

TOPIRAMATE

Topiramate has demonstrated efficacy for cluster headache prophylaxis.[191,197–201] In a study of patients with prior prophylactic treatment exposure, topiramate produced favorable outcomes, inducing remission in greater than 50% of treated patients.[197]

Prompt consideration should be given to the aforementioned additional treatments if suppression of headaches during the cluster period is warranted. In general, after response to prophylactic agents such as verapamil and lithium has been established and maintained for at least 2 weeks, attempts can be made to discontinue the drug. Treatment should be reinstituted if headaches recur. With considerations toward patient ease of use and efficacy, treating R.H. with verapamil or topiramate would be rational.

TENSION-TYPE HEADACHE

Prevalence of tension-type headache is variable but has been shown to be as high as 78%.[5,202,203] Women are slightly more affected by tension-type headaches than men, with a ratio of 5:4.[204] Tension-type headache is typically bilateral and is characterized by a milder pain intensity and a tightening quality.[5] Nausea and vomiting are not typical of tension headache presentation but photo- or phonophobia may be present.[5]

Headache frequency is an important determinant for tension headache classification, expressed in terms of headache days/month.[5,202] Episodic tension headache can be either infrequent (<1 day/month) or frequent (1–14 days/month), whereas chronic tension headache is classified with a threshold of 15 headache days/month.[5,202]

Pathophysiology

The pathology of tension headache is theorized to be a function of both peripheral and central pain pathways.[205] Modulation of trigeminal nociceptors and pericranial muscle strain fit within this pathology.[205]

General Management and Abortive Therapy

CASE 58-5

QUESTION 1: K.B., a 27-year-old female financial analyst, presents to her general practitioner with a complaint of recurring headaches that worsened when she started her current job. Before this time, she had experienced infrequent headaches, which she associated with periods of stress. The headaches would occur 3 to 4 times yearly, were of a constant, dull, or "pressing" character, and were present around the entire head. Recently, headaches of similar character have been occurring about 1 to 2 times weekly, usually toward the end of her workday. The pain usually lasts the rest of the day but varies in intensity. Occasionally, a headache is present when she wakes up in the morning as well. K.B. denies GI and aura symptoms associated with her headaches. She has noticed that relaxation and alcohol ingestion seem to relieve these headaches, but aspirin and acetaminophen have been ineffective. Her blood pressure is 120/74 mm Hg; her physical and neurologic examinations are completely normal. What measures should be taken to relieve K.B.'s headaches? What is an appropriate goal for treatment?

K.B. appears to be suffering from frequent episodic tension-type headaches. She reports approximately four to eight headache episodes/month, and these headaches have features that are stereotypical for tension-type headache. As in the treatment of other chronic headache disorders, a cure for recurrent tension-type headache is unlikely. K.B. should clearly understand that the goal of treatment is a reduction in the frequency and severity of headache. Drug therapy and relaxation techniques are the primary means by which tension-type headaches are treated.

ANALGESICS

Conventional analgesics, including NSAIDs, are appropriate first-line treatments for tension headache.[202] A recent meta-analysis of four controlled trials supported the effectiveness of both a combination product (acetaminophen, aspirin, and caffeine) and acetaminophen relative to placebo in achieving pain-free status at 2 hours postadministration for tension headache treatment.[206] Secondary endpoints included pain-free status at 1 hour post, headache response at 2 hours, and level of impact on daily activity, with results being consistent with the primary outcome measure.[206]

An NSAID (e.g., ibuprofen or naproxen) would be an appropriate recommendation for the treatment of K.B.'s tension-type headaches because of her previous inadequate responses to aspirin and acetaminophen.

CASE 58-5, QUESTION 2: K.B. was prescribed ibuprofen 400 mg every 4 to 6 hours as needed for acute relief of recurrent tension-type headaches. At her next scheduled follow-up visit, K.B. reported moderate relief with ibuprofen but complained of GI upset with each dose, even when taken with food. What prophylactic agents are available for continuous suppression of K.B.'s tension-type headaches?

Prophylactic Therapy

Prophylaxis is relevant in the context of both frequent, episodic tension headache and chronic tension headache.[202] Amitriptyline has demonstrated efficacy in managing tension headache.[202,207] A median daily dose of 75 mg yielded a significant improvement in headache index relative to placebo.[207] Mirtazapine and venlafaxine have both demonstrated efficacy in tension headache treatment relative to placebo.[208,209] Superiority for mirtazapine was demonstrated in measures of headache frequency, intensity, and duration for patients with prior treatment experience.[208]

Given K.B.'s increasing frequency of tension-type headache and her intolerance to moderate doses of ibuprofen, prophylactic treatment with amitriptyline would be appropriate. A starting dose of amitriptyline 10 mg nightly, increasing by 10 to 25 mg at 1-week intervals to a maintenance dose of 50 mg/day, should be prescribed, at which time headache response can be assessed and the dose increased or decreased as necessary. If effective, amitriptyline should be continued for 3 to 4 months before gradually decreasing the dose until the drug is completely discontinued. Therapy should be reinstituted if headaches return. Mirtazapine may be initiated as a second-line option for K. B., if amitriptyline is not effective.

Interprofessional Management

Practices in the areas of spiritual meditation,[210] cognitive therapy and stress reduction,[211,212] and acupuncture[213] have been assessed in headache management. A recent study, assessing outcome measures of headache frequency, severity, and medication use, as impacted by either spiritual meditation, secular meditation (internally and externally focused), or muscle relaxation, reported a favorable impact on episode frequency induced by spiritual meditation.[210] A decrease in medication usage was similarly reflected in this cohort; however, neither pain sensitivity or severity differed.[210] Interventions directed toward stress reduction, while deemed feasible, have not met statistical significance for changes in headache severity or frequency.[211] Although stress reduction favorably impacted MIDAS and HIT-6 assessments relative to controls, the study lacked the statistical power to confer significance.[211] Similarly, traditional acupuncture has yielded headache-associated pain relief; however, prospective trials are warranted to better elucidate the therapeutic impact of this practice.[213]

KEY REFERENCES AND WEBSITES

A full list of references for this chapter can be found at http://thepoint.lww.com/AT11e. Below are the key references and websites for this chapter, with the corresponding reference number in this chapter found in parentheses after the reference.

Key References

Bendtsen L et al. EFNS guideline on the treatment of tension-type headache—report of an EFNS task force. *Eur J Neurol*. 2010;17:1318–1325. (202)

Headache Classification Committee of the International Headache Society. The International Classification of Headache Disorders: 3rd edition (beta). *Cephalalgia*. 2013;33(9):629–808. (5)

May A. Cluster headache: pathogenesis, diagnosis, and management. *Lancet*. 2005;366:843–855. (175)

Marmura MJ, Silberstein SD. Current understanding and treatment of headache disorders. *Neurology*. 2011;76(Suppl 2):S31–S36. (28)

Marmura MJ et al. The acute treatment of migraine in adults: The American Headache Society evidence assessment of migraine pharmacotherapies. *Headache*. 2015;55:3–20. (48)

Thorlund K et al. Comparative efficacy of triptans for the abortive treatment of migraine: a multiple treatment comparison meta-analysis. *Cephalalgia*. 2014;34(4):258–267. (85)

Shamliyan TA et al. Preventive pharmacologic treatments for episodic migraine in adults. *J Gen Intern Med*. 2013;28(9):1225–1237. (123)

Tassorelli C et al. A consensus protocol for the management of medication-overuse headache: Evaluation in a multicentric, multinational study. *Cephalalgia*. 2014;34(9):645–655. (169)

Key Websites

American Academy of Neurology. https://www.aan.com/.
American Headache Society. http://www.americanheadachesociety.org/.
American Headache Society (AHS) Committee for Headache Education. http://www.achenet.org/.
International Headache Society. http://www.ihs-headache.org/.

59 Parkinson's Disease and Other Movement Disorders

Kristin M. Zimmerman and Natalie Whitmire

CORE PRINCIPLES

	CHAPTER CASES
1 Parkinson's disease (PD) is a chronic, progressive movement disorder resulting from loss of dopamine from the nigrostriatal tracts in the brain, and is characterized by rigidity, bradykinesia, postural disturbances, and tremor.	**Case 59-1 (Questions 1, 2)**
2 Treatment for PD is aimed at restoring dopamine supply through one, or a combination, of the following methods: exogenous dopamine in the form of a precursor, levodopa; direct stimulation of dopamine receptors via dopamine agonists; and inhibition of metabolic pathways responsible for degradation of levodopa.	**Case 59-1 (Questions 3–17)**
3 Therapy for PD is usually delayed until there is a significant effect on quality of life; generally younger patients start with dopamine agonists or monoamine oxidase type B (MAO-B) inhibitors, whereas older patients may start with levodopa.	**Case 59-1 (Questions 3,4), Figure 59-2**
4 Initial therapy with levodopa-sparing agents is associated with a lower risk of developing motor complications than with levodopa, but all patients will eventually require levodopa.	**Case 59-1 (Questions 4–9), Figure 59-2**
5 Advanced PD is characterized by motor fluctuations including a gradual decline in on-time, and by the development of troubling dopaminergic-induced dyskinesias. Modified carbidopa/levodopa formulations, dopamine agonists, MAO-B inhibitors, and catechol-*O*-methyltransferase (COMT) inhibitors can reduce motor fluctuations; amantadine can improve dyskinesias. Deep brain stimulation of the globus pallidus interna or subthalamic nucleus may benefit patients with advanced PD.	**Case 59-1 (Questions 13–19), Figure 59-4**
6 Antioxidants, dietary supplements, and other investigational therapies have been studied for the management of Parkinson's disease.	**Case 59-2 (Question 1)**
7 Comprehensive therapy for patients should include attention to many progressive complications of PD, including neuropsychiatric disturbances and autonomic dysfunction.	**Case 59-3 (Questions 1, 2)**
RESTLESS LEGS SYNDROME	
1 RLS is a disabling sensorimotor disorder typically marked by irresistible urge to move the legs (akathisia). It is often associated with uncomfortable paresthesias or dysesthesias and often occurs in the evening or night.	**Case 59-4 (Question 1)**
2 Several conditions are associated with or can aggravate RLS. Periodic limb movements of sleep (PLMS) is not the same as RLS but often coexists.	**Case 59-4 (Question 2)**
3 Dopamine agonists are first-line treatments for RLS. They are preferred because they are longer acting than levodopa, and reduce symptoms throughout the entire night. Other effective therapies include carbidopa/levodopa, gabapentin, benzodiazepines, and opiates.	**Case 59-4 (Question 3)**
4 A common problem with long-term use of dopaminergic agents in RLS, particularly levodopa, is an augmentation effect. This refers to a gradual dosage intensification that occurs in response to a progressive worsening of symptoms after an initial period of improvement. Gradual withdrawal of therapy and substitution with other agents should be performed, rather than continued dopaminergic dose escalation.	**Case 59-4 (Question 4)**

Continued

ESSENTIAL TREMOR

1	Essential tremor should be distinguished clinically from tremor associated with PD or other causes.	**Case 59-5 (Question 1)**
2	Treatments of choice for essential tremor include propranolol or primidone. In refractory cases, targeted botulinum toxin A injections can be useful.	**Case 59-5 (Question 2)**

PARKINSON'S DISEASE

Incidence, Prevalence, and Epidemiology

PD is a chronic, progressive movement disorder first described in 1817 by Dr. James Parkinson. Since that time, the term parkinsonism has come to refer to any disorder associated with two or more features of tremor, rigidity, bradykinesia, or postural instability.[1] Most cases of PD are of unknown cause and referred to as idiopathic parkinsonism; however, viral encephalitis, cerebrovascular disease, and hydrocephalus have symptoms similar to PD as part of their clinical presentation.[1] Unless otherwise stated, all references to PD in this chapter refer to the idiopathic type.

The age at onset of PD is variable, usually between 50 and 80 years, with a mean onset of 55 years.[2] Both the incidence and prevalence of PD are age-dependent, with annual incidence estimates ranging from 10 cases/100,000 (age 50–59 years) to 100 cases/100,000 (age 80–89 years) and an estimated prevalence of 1% of the population older than 65 years of age.[3,4] Men are affected slightly more frequently than women.[3] Despite the availability of effective symptomatic treatments to improve both quality of life and life expectancy, no cure exists. The symptoms of PD are progressive, and within 10 to 20 years, significant immobility results for most patients.[5] More rapid rates of symptom progression and motor disability have been observed in patients of older age at disease onset.[6] PD itself does not cause death; however, patients often succumb to complications related to impaired mobility and function (e.g., aspiration pneumonia, thromboembolism) and overall frailty.[5]

Etiology

The etiology of PD is poorly understood. Most evidence suggests it is multifactorial and attributable to a complex interplay between age-related changes in the nigrostriatal tract, underlying genetic risks, and/or environmental triggers. Support for this hypothesis can be found in several historic observations. Notably, the postviral parkinsonian symptoms occurring after epidemics of encephalitis in the early 1900s, and the discovery that ingestion of a meperidine analog, 1-methyl-4-phenyl-1,2,3,6-tetrahydropyridine (MPTP), by heroin addicts in northern California during the early 1980s caused a rapid and irreversible parkinsonism via the oxidation of free radicals during metabolism by the MAO-B enzyme.[7]

For an excellent in-depth discussion of the importance of the MPTP discovery and its influence on PD research, please view the episode "My Father, My Brother, and Me" from the Public Broadcasting System program Frontline at http://www.pbs.org/wgbh/pages/frontline/parkinsons/.

The relative contributions of environment and genetics to the occurrence of PD remain controversial; rural living, pesticide exposure, and consumption of well water have consistently been associated with increased lifetime risk of PD, whereas cigarette smoking and caffeine ingestion appear to be protective.[8] Mutations in several genes, including α-synuclein (SNCA), leucine-rich repeat kinase-2 (LRRK2), parkin, PTEN-induced kinase-1 (PINK1), and DJ-1, have been observed in rare familial inherited cases of PD, but these genes lack typical Mendelian patterns of inheritance, and do not account for the threefold increased risk of developing PD for individuals who have a first-degree relative affected with sporadic PD.[9] Recent advances in molecular genetics and genome-wide association studies have revealed other novel risk genes; however, the exact linkage between genetics, environment, and clinical expression of disease remains uncertain.[10]

Pathophysiology

The salient features of PD result from a loss of dopaminergic neurons in the nigrostriatal tracts of the brain and development of abnormal intraneuronal protein aggregates called Lewy bodies that interfere with neuronal function. The nigrostriatal tracts are neuronal tracts between the substantia nigra and the striatum. They are part of the extrapyramidal system of the brain involving the basal ganglia. This area is involved with maintaining posture and muscle tone by regulating voluntary smooth muscle activity. The pigmented neurons within the basal ganglia have dopaminergic fibers, and in PD, these dopamine-producing neurons are progressively depigmented. The remaining dopaminergic-producing cells have been shown (in postmortem examination) to contain Lewy bodies.[11] Lewy body pathology appears to ascend the brain in a predictable manner in PD, beginning in the medulla oblongata in preclinical stages (which may explain observations of anxiety, depression, and olfactory disturbance), ascending to the midbrain (motor dysfunction), and spreading eventually to the cortex (cognitive and behavioral changes).[12] The loss of dopamine neurons, either from death or from dysfunction, results in loss of dopamine-mediated inhibition of acetylcholine neurons. In PD, the typical balance of dopamine and acetylcholine is lost, resulting in a relative increase in cholinergic activity.

The exact pathologic sequence leading to neurodegeneration is unclear, but free radicals formed as by-products of dopamine auto-oxidation have been implicated. The finding that a critical threshold of neuronal loss (at least 70%–80%) occurs before PD becomes clinically apparent suggests that adaptive mechanisms (e.g., upregulation of dopamine synthesis or downregulation of synaptic dopamine reuptake) may somehow influence disease progression during the preclinical stages.

Clinical Presentation of Parkinson's Disease

CASE 59-1

Question 1: L.M., a 55-year-old, right-handed male artist, presents to the neurology clinic complaining of difficulty painting because of unsteadiness in his right hand. On questioning, he notes that it is becoming increasingly difficult to get out of chairs after sitting for a long period because of tightness in his arms and legs. He also reports having a loss in sense of smell. His medical history is significant for gout (currently requiring no treatment), constipation, benign prostatic hypertrophy, and aortic stenosis. He does not smoke, but usually drinks one alcoholic beverage in the evenings. His only prescription medication is citalopram 10 mg by mouth once daily. On physical examination, L.M. is noted to be a well-developed, well-nourished man who displays a notable lack of normal changes in facial expression and speaks in a soft, monotone voice. Examination of his extremities reveals a slight ratchetlike rigidity in both arms and legs, and a mild resting tremor is present in his right hand. His gait is slow but otherwise normal, with a slightly bent posture. His balance is determined to be normal, with no retropulsion or loss of righting reflexes after physical threat. His genitourinary examination is remarkable only for prostatic enlargement. The remainder of his physical examination is within normal limits. Laboratory values and vital signs obtained at this visit include the following:

Blood pressure, 119/66 mm Hg
Heart rate, 71 beats/minute
Sodium, 132 mEq/L
Potassium, 4.4 mEq/L
Blood urea nitrogen, 19 mg/dL
Creatinine, 1.1 mg/dL
Thyroid stimulating hormone, 3.65 microunits/L
Vitamin B12, 612 pg/mL
Folate, 5.2 ng/mL
White blood cells, 4,400 cells/μL
Red blood cells, $5.9 \times 10^6/\mu$L
Hemoglobin, 13.8 g/dL
Hematocrit, 41%
Uric acid, 6.3 mg/dL

How is PD diagnosed? Is neuroimaging or any other testing helpful in establishing the diagnosis of PD? What signs and symptoms suggestive of PD are present in L.M., and which of these symptoms are among the classic symptoms for diagnosing PD?

The foundation for establishing the diagnosis of PD remains firmly grounded in obtaining a careful history and physical examination.[11] The neurologic examination to assess motor function, along with a positive response to levodopa, is highly diagnostic. The search for biomarkers of premotor PD in blood, cerebrospinal fluid, and urine has not uncovered single, practical candidates that are sensitive and specific.[9] Likewise, although imaging techniques can visualize nigrostriatal nerve terminals of dopamine synthesis and identify presymptomatic pathology, their use remains investigational, and routine use in asymptomatic, at-risk individuals is not yet justified. Other associated premotor symptoms, such as hyposmia (a reduced ability to smell and detect odors), rapid eye movement (REM) sleep disorder, and softening and tonal changes of the voice are among the earliest symptoms to appear; screening for these findings may prove more economically practical in identifying a high risk population worthy of further diagnostic evaluation.[13] With further scientific advancements, the diagnosis of PD may rely on clinical, imaging, genetic, and a panel of laboratory biomarker data. However, by the time patients such as L.M. present with symptoms, a substantial burden of neuropathologic evidence has accumulated, and therefore, a diagnosis can be made clinically, without the need for further laboratory or radiologic testing.

The classic features of PD—tremor, limb rigidity, and bradykinesia—are easily recognized, particularly in advanced stages of disease. Limb rigidity and bradykinesia are direct consequences of dopamine loss; by disinhibiting cholinergic transmission, dopamine loss indirectly causes tremor. It is important to note that not all classic features are required to make the diagnosis of PD. The presence of two or more features indicates clinically probable PD.[14] Tremor, which is most often the first symptom observed in younger patients, is usually unilateral on initial presentation. Frequently, the low-amplitude tremor is of a pill-rolling type involving the thumb and index finger (3–6 Hz); it is present at rest, worsens under fatigue or stress, and is absent with purposeful movement or when asleep.[1] These features help distinguish it from essential tremor, which usually manifests as a symmetric tremor in the hands, often accompanied by head and voice tremor.[11] Approximately 20% of patients with PD do not present with tremor.[11] Muscular rigidity resulting from increased muscle tone often manifests as a cogwheel or ratchet (catch-release) type of motion when an extremity is moved passively.[1] Rigidity may also be experienced as stiffness or vague aching or limb discomfort.[11] Bradykinesia refers to an overall slowness in initiating movement. Early in the disease, patients may describe this as weakness or clumsiness of a hand or leg.[11] Because the disease progresses, difficulty initiating and terminating steps results in a hurried or festinating gait; the posture becomes stooped (simian posture), and postural reflexes are impaired.[1] Symptoms that were unilateral on initial presentation progress asymmetrically and often become bilateral and more severe with disease progression.[1] Patients with PD may develop masked facies, or a blank stare with reduced eye blinking (Figure 59-1).

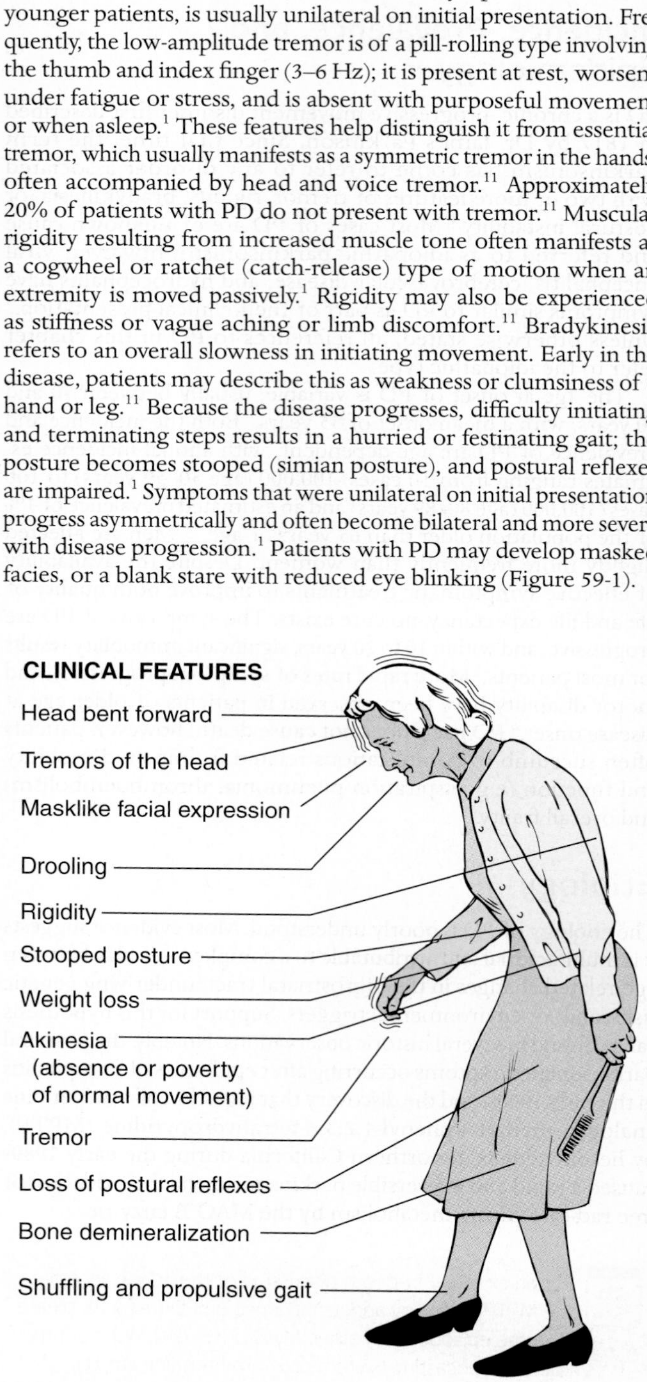

Figure 59-1 Clinical features of Parkinson's disease. (Reprinted with permission from Rosdahl CB. *Book of Basic Nursing*. 7th ed. Philadelphia, PA: Lippincott-Raven; 1999:1063.)

Because the diagnosis of PD is clinical, misdiagnosis can occur, leading to inappropriate, ineffective, or delayed treatment. Several conditions can be mistaken for PD and are important to distinguish from PD because they respond poorly to dopaminergic medications and are associated with worse prognosis.[11] Falls or dementia early in the disease, symmetric parkinsonism, wide-based gait, abnormal eye movements, marked orthostatic hypotension, urinary retention, or marked disability within 5 years after the onset of symptoms suggests alternative diagnoses to PD.[11] Drugs may also mimic idiopathic PD. Drugs that act as antagonists at dopaminergic D_2 receptors (e.g., neuroleptics, prochlorperazine, and metoclopramide), and others such as valproate, amiodarone, phenytoin, and lithium may cause a state of drug-induced parkinsonism. This should be excluded before the diagnosis of PD is established. Although generally reversible, symptoms may persist for weeks or months after discontinuation of the offending agent.[11]

L.M. initially presents with classic premotor features such as his soft, monotone voice and reduced sense of smell, in addition to classic symptoms of PD. A noticeable unilateral resting tremor is present along with decreased manual dexterity, as evidenced by his difficulty handling a paintbrush. Handwriting abnormalities occur frequently, particularly micrographia, a symptom of bradykinesia. Because L.M. is an artist, this abnormality would be particularly troublesome. Rigidity (ratcheting of the arms) and a mask-like facial expression also are present. Although he has a partially stooped posture, it is difficult to attribute this entirely to the disease because postural changes commonly occur with advancing age and, on physical examination, his balance was normal. To confirm the diagnosis of PD, a therapeutic trial of medication (levodopa) may be considered. A positive response to levodopa, as evidenced by an improvement in motor function, suggests the diagnosis of PD. However, patients with the tremor-predominant form of the disease may not respond to levodopa, especially in the early stages of the disease.[11]

Staging of Parkinson's Disease

CASE 59-1, QUESTION 2: What are the stages of PD? In what stage of the disease is L.M.?

To assess the degree of disability and determine the rate of disease progression relative to treatment, various scales have been developed. The most common of these is the Hoehn and Yahr scale (Table 59-1).[2] In general, patients in Hoehn and Yahr[2] stage 1 or 2 of PD have mild disease that does not interfere with activities of daily living (ADLs) or work and usually requires minimal or no treatment. In stage 3 disease, daily activities are restricted and employment may be significantly affected unless effective treatment is initiated. According to the scale, L.M. appears to be in late stage 2, early stage 3 of the disease.

With advanced-stage disease (3, 4), most patients require a double or triple drug therapy strategy. Patients with end-stage disease (stage 5) are severely incapacitated and, because of advanced disease progression, often do not respond well to drug therapy.

Table 59-1
Staging of Disability in Parkinson's Disease (PD)

Stage 1	Unilateral involvement only; minimal or no functional impairment
Stage 2	Bilateral involvement, without impairment of balance
Stage 3	Evidence of postural imbalance; some restriction in activities; capable of leading independent life; mild-to-moderate disability
Stage 4	Severely disabled, cannot walk and stand unassisted; significantly incapacitated
Stage 5	Restricted to bed or wheelchair unless aided

Treatment of Parkinson's Disease

OVERVIEW OF THERAPY

Numerous national and international guidelines exist regarding the management of motor and nonmotor symptoms of PD. These guidelines include the American Academy of Neurology (AAN) Practice Parameters developed in 2002 and 2006,[15,16] the United Kingdom National Institute for Health and Care Excellence (NICE) National Guideline developed in 2006 and revised in July 2017,[17] and the European Federation of Neurological Societies Movement Disorder Society-European Section (EFNS MDS-ES) Guidelines developed in 2013[18]; all are cited throughout the text.

Although most of this chapter is devoted to the drug therapy of PD, the importance of nonpharmacologic, supportive care cannot be overemphasized. Exercise, physical and occupational therapy, and good nutritional support can be beneficial at the earlier stages to improve mobility, increase strength, and enhance well-being and mood.[17] Psychological support is often necessary in dealing with depression and other related problems. Newly diagnosed patients and their family members need to be educated about what to expect from the disease and the various forms of treatment available. The support of family members is vital in establishing an overall effective therapeutic plan.

Nonpharmacologic therapy should continue throughout the course of care; however, due to the progressive nature of PD, pharmacologic therapy is often necessary. Because the salient pathophysiologic feature of PD is the progressive loss of dopamine from the nigrostriatal tracts in the brain, drug therapy for the disease is aimed primarily at replenishing the supply of dopamine. This is accomplished through one, or a combination, of the following methods: (a) administering exogenous dopamine in the form of a precursor, levodopa; (b) stimulating dopamine receptors within the striatum through the use of dopamine agonists (e.g., pramipexole, ropinirole); or (c) inhibiting the major metabolic pathways within the brain that are responsible for the degradation of levodopa and its metabolites. This latter effect is achieved through the use of aromatic L-amino acid decarboxylase (AAD) inhibitors (e.g., carbidopa), COMT inhibitors (e.g., entacapone), or MAO-B inhibitors (e.g., selegiline, rasagiline). Anticholinergics are also used; however, they are solely efficacious for the cholinergic-mediated tremor, and their routine use is limited by central nervous system (CNS) adverse effects, particularly in older patients. A unique agent, amantadine, is also used occasionally and may provide modest benefits via both dopaminergic and nondopaminergic (inhibition of glutamate) mechanisms (Table 59-2). Because PD progresses, additional options, such as surgery, may be appropriate for a subset of patients.

Despite optimization of both pharmacologic and nonpharmacologic therapies in PD, physical disability is progressive and unavoidable. In many instances, adverse effects of the medications themselves can lead to additional problems. These include neuropsychiatric problems (e.g., cognitive impairment and dementia, hallucinations and delirium, depression, agitation, anxiety), autonomic dysfunction (e.g., constipation, urinary problems, sexual problems, orthostasis, thermoregulatory imbalances), falls, sleep

Table 59-2

Medications Used for the Treatment of Parkinson's Disease (PD)

Generic (Trade) Name	Dosage Unit	Titration Schedule	Usual Daily Dose	Adverse Effects
Amantadine (Symmetrel)	100-mg capsule and tablet Liquid: 50 mg/5 mL	100 mg every day; increased by 100 mg every 1–2 weeks	100–300 mg	Orthostatic hypotension, insomnia, depression, hallucinations, livedo reticularis, xerostomia
Anticholinergic Agents				
Benztropine (Cogentin)	0.5-, 1-, and 2-mg tablets Injection: 1 mg/mL	0.5 mg every day increased by 0.5 mg every 5–6 days	1–3 mg given every day to BID	Constipation, xerostomia, dry skin, dysphagia, confusion, memory impairment
Trihexyphenidyl (Artane)	2- and 5-mg tablets Liquid: 2 mg/5 mL	1–2 mg/day increased by 1–2 mg every 3–5 days	6–15 mg divided TID to QID	Constipation, xerostomia, dry skin, dysphagia, confusion, memory impairment
Combination Agents				
Carbidopa–levodopa (immediate release)/entacapone (Stalevo)	12.5-/50-/200-, 18.75-/75-/200-, 25-/100-/200-, 31.25-/125-/200-, 37.5-/150-/200-, 50-/200-/200-mg tablets	Titrate with individual dosage forms (carbidopa/levodopa and entacapone) first, then switch to combination tablet	Varies (see individual drugs)	See individual drugs
Dopamine Replacement				
Carbidopa–levodopa (regular) (Sinemet)	10-/100-, 25-/100-, and 25-/250-mg tablets	25/100 mg BID, increased by 25/100 mg weekly to effect and as tolerated	30/300 to 150/1,500 mg divided TID to QID	Nausea, orthostatic hypotension, confusion, dizziness, hallucinations, dyskinesias, blepharospasm
Carbidopa–levodopa (CR) (Sinemet CR)	25-/100- and 50-/200-mg tablets	25/100 mg BID (spaced at least 6 hours apart), increased every 3–7 days	50/200 to 500/2,000 divided QID	Same as regular Sinemet
Carbidopa–levodopa (ER) (Rytary)	23.75-/95-, 36.25-/145-, 48.75-/195-, 61.25-/245-mg capsules	23.75/95 mg TID; may increase to 36.25/145 mg TID on day 4 and titrate to response	Variable	Same as regular Sinemet
Carbidopa–levodopa (enteral suspension) (Duopa)	4.63-/20-mg/mL in 100-mL cassette	Total daily dose administered over 16 hours	Variable	Same as regular Sinemet
Carbidopa–levodopa ODT (Parcopa)	10-/100-, 25-/100-, and 25-/250-mg tablets	25/100 TID, increased every 1–2 days; if transferring from regular levodopa <1,500 mg/day, start 25/100 mg TID to QID (start 25/250 mg TID to QID if already on >1,500 mg/day of regular levodopa)	25/100 to 200/2,000 divided TID to QID	Same as regular Sinemet; may occur more rapidly than with regular Sinemet
Dopamine Agonists				
Bromocriptine (Parlodel)	2.5-mg tablet, 5-mg capsule	1.25 mg BID, titrate slowly as tolerated (2.5 mg/day every 2-4 weeks)	10–40 mg divided TID; Max 100 mg/day	Orthostatic hypotension, confusion, dizziness, hallucinations, nausea, muscle cramps; retroperitoneal, pleural, pericardial fibrosis; cardiac valve thickening
Pramipexole (Mirapex, Mirapex ER)	Immediate release: 0.125-, 0.25-, 0.50-, 0.75-, 1-, 1.5-mg tablets ER: 0.375-, 0.75-, 1.5-, 2.25-, 3-, 3.75-, 4.5-mg tablets	Immediate release: 0.375 mg divided TID; titrate weekly by 0.125–0.25 mg/dose ER: 0.375 mg once daily; titrate weekly by 0.75 mg/dose	Immediate release: 1.5–4.5 mg divided TID ER: 1.5–4.5 mg once daily	Orthostatic hypotension, confusion, dizziness, hallucinations, nausea, somnolence
Ropinirole (Requip, Requip XL)	0.25-, 0.5-, 1-, 2-, 3-, 4-, 5-mg tablet XL: 2-, 4-, 6-, 8-, 12-mg tablets	0.25 mg TID; titrate weekly by 0.25 mg/dose XL: 2 mg once daily; titrate weekly by 2 mg/day	3–12 mg divided TID XL: 3–12 mg once daily	Orthostatic hypotension, confusion, dizziness, hallucinations, nausea, somnolence

Table 59-2
Medications Used for the Treatment of Parkinson's Disease (PD) (*continued*)

Generic (Trade) Name	Dosage Unit	Titration Schedule	Usual Daily Dose	Adverse Effects
Apomorphine (Apokyn)	10 mg/mL injection	Initial 2-mg subcutaneous test dose; begin with 2 mg; increase by 1 mg every few days	2–6 mg TID	Orthostatic hypotension, drowsiness, yawning, injection site reactions, nausea, vomiting (administer with trimethobenzamide, not 5-hydroxytryptamine-3 [5-HT_3] antagonists)
Rotigotine (Neupro)	1-, 2-, 3-, 4-, 6-, 8-mg/24 hour transdermal delivery system	Early stage: 2 mg/24 hour; Advanced stage: 4 mg/24 hour; titrate weekly by 2 mg/24 hour; Application site should be rotated daily between abdomen, thigh, hip, flank, shoulder, or upper arm and do not use same site within 14 days	4–6 mg/24 hour	Hallucinations, nausea, vomiting, anorexia, somnolence, insomnia, dizziness, hyperhidrosis, visual disturbance, peripheral edema, and application site reactions; avoid in patients with known sulfite sensitivity
COMT Inhibitors				
Entacapone (Comtan)	200-mg tablet	200 mg with each administration of carbidopa/levodopa, up to 8 tablets daily	3–8 tablets daily	Diarrhea, dyskinesias, abdominal pain, urine discoloration
Tolcapone (Tasmar)	100-mg tablet	100 mg TID	300–600 mg divided TID	Diarrhea, dyskinesias, abdominal pain, urine discoloration, hepatotoxicity
Monoamine Oxidase Type B (MAO-B) Inhibitors				
Selegiline (Eldepryl)[a]	5-mg tablet, capsule	5 mg every morning; may increase to 5 mg BID (5 mg with breakfast and 5 mg with lunch)	5–10 mg/day	Insomnia, dizziness, nausea, vomiting, xerostomia, dyskinesias, mood changes; use caution when coadministered with sympathomimetics or serotoninergic agents (increased risk of serotonin syndrome); avoid tyramine-containing foods
Selegiline ODT (Zelapar)	1.25-mg tablet	1.25 mg every day; avoid food or liquids for 5 minutes before and after administration; may increase to 2.5 mg every day after 6 weeks	1.25–2.5 mg every day	Insomnia, dizziness, nausea, vomiting, xerostomia, dyskinesias, mood changes; use caution when coadministered with sympathomimetics or serotoninergic agents (increased risk of serotonin syndrome); avoid tyramine-containing foods
Rasagiline (Azilect)	0.5-, 1-mg tablets	0.5–1 mg once daily	0.5–1 mg/day	Similar to selegiline
Safinamide (Xadago)[b]	50-, 100 mg tablets	50 mg once daily; dose may be increased after two weeks to 100 mg once daily	50-100 mg/day	Similar to selegiline

[a]A transdermal formulation is also available, but not approved for use in PD.
[b]Approved only for use as adjunctive treatment to levodopa/carbidopa in patients experiencing "off" episodes.
BID, twice daily; COMT, catechol-*O*-methyltransferase; MAO-B, monoamine oxidase type B; ODT, orally disintegrating tablet; QID, four times daily; TID, three times daily.

disorders (e.g., insomnia or sleep fragmentation, nightmares, RLS), and motor complications (e.g., disabling periods of either too much [dyskinetic] or too little [akinetic] dopaminergic activity). In general, the more efficacious medications are also those with the greatest risk of serious side effects and motor complications.

Treatment of Early Parkinson's Disease

Case 59-1, Question 3: When should L.M. begin treatment for his PD?

In choosing when to treat the symptoms of PD and which therapy to use, care must be taken to approach each patient individually. Although no consensus has been reached about when to initiate symptomatic treatment, most healthcare professionals agree that treatment should begin when the patient begins to experience functional impairment as defined by (a) threat to employment status, (b) symptoms affecting the dominant side of the body, or (c) bradykinesia or rigidity.[19,20] Individual patient preferences also should be considered. Judging by the symptoms L.M. is displaying, he would likely benefit from immediate treatment. His symptoms are unilateral but are occurring on his dominant side and are interfering with his ability to paint, thus affecting his livelihood. He is also showing signs of rigidity and bradykinesia but can otherwise live independently. An algorithm for the management of patients with early PD is presented in Figure 59-2. The long-term, individualized treatment plan is usually characterized by frequent dosage adjustments because of the chronic and progressive nature of the disease.

CASE 59-1, QUESTION 4: The decision is made to begin drug therapy for L.M. Should therapy be initiated with a levodopa or levodopa-sparing therapy?

Despite advances in pharmacologic treatment options for PD, no therapy has been proven to be disease-modifying or neuroprotective. Therapy continues to be symptomatic, and levodopa remains the most effective antiparkinsonian agent.[11] However, the question of when to begin levodopa in the treatment of PD has been historically debated. With long-term use, the efficacy of levodopa decreases and risk for the development of motor fluctuations and dyskinesias increases. Because escalating doses of levodopa are accompanied by a high frequency of undesirable side effects, other methods of enriching dopamine supply have been developed. Two such methods include the use of dopamine agonists and MAO-B inhibitors. Both of these modalities have proven efficacy early in the disease.[17]

Dopamine agonists, which bind directly to dopamine receptors, do not require metabolic conversion to an active product and therefore act independently of degenerating dopaminergic neurons. In clinical trials comparing dopamine agonists with levodopa, ADLs and motor features are improved to a greater degree with levodopa compared with dopamine agonists.[18] Although they are not as effective as levodopa, the dopamine agonists have potential advantages. Unlike levodopa, circulating plasma amino acids do not compete with dopamine agonists for absorption and transport into the brain, eliminating administration constraints. Dopamine agonists have a longer half-life than levodopa formulations, reducing the need for multiple daily dosing. As a class, dopamine agonists provide adequate control of symptoms when given as monotherapy in up to 80% of patients with early-stage disease.[21]

Short- and long-term comparisons of patients with early disease started on either levodopa or dopamine agonists have varying results. In trials extending 4 to 5 years, therapy with dopamine agonists is associated with fewer motor complications

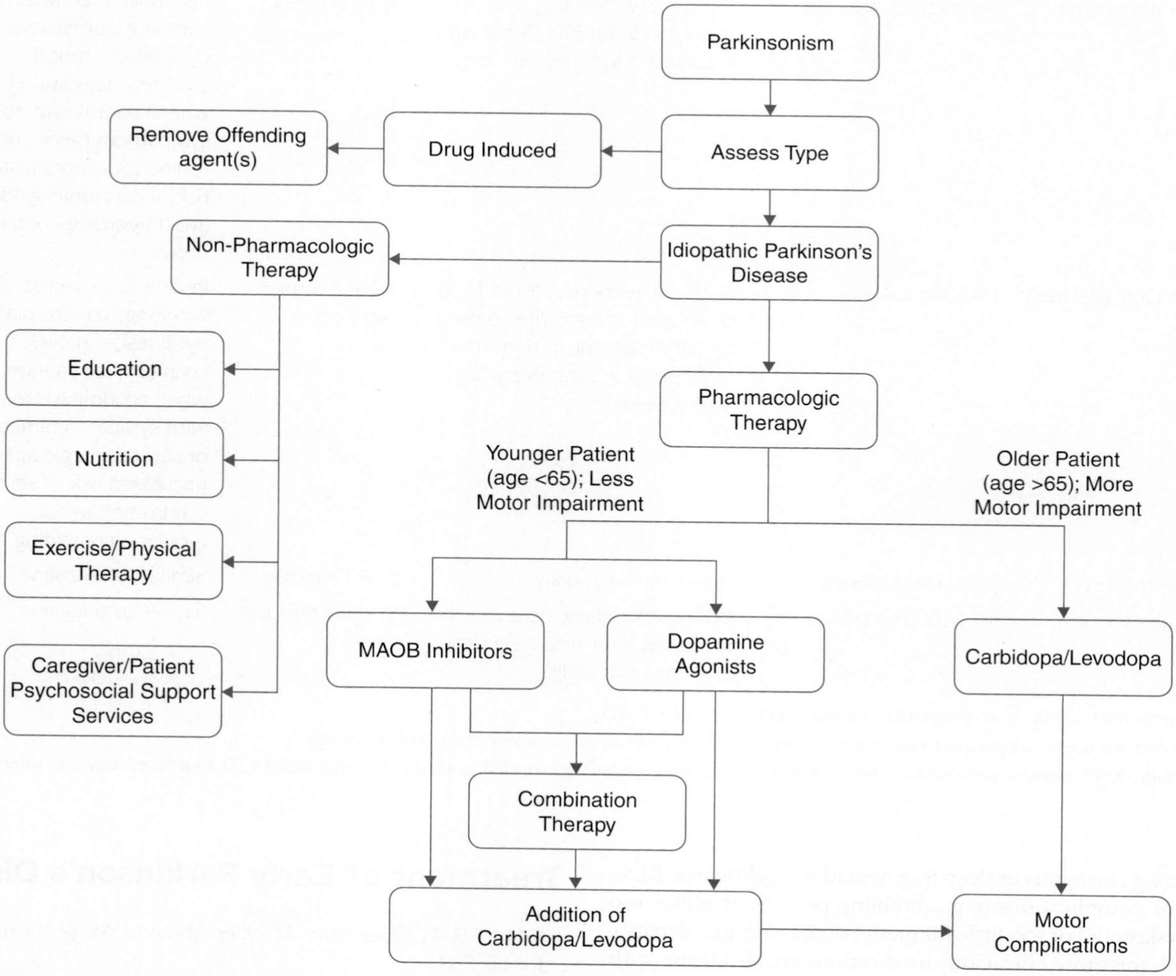

Figure 59-2 Suggested treatment algorithm for the management of early PD.

such as dyskinesias, delayed time to dyskinesias, and delayed need for initiation of dopaminergic therapy.[22–24] Against levodopa as initial therapy, early trials of the dopamine agonists appear to delay the onset of dyskinesias. In a randomized, controlled trial evaluating the development of motor complications with levodopa or the dopamine agonist pramipexole, 301 untreated patients with early PD were randomly assigned to receive either pramipexole 0.5 mg 3 times daily or carbidopa/levodopa 25/100 mg 3 times daily.[24] Patients in both arms could be prescribed open-label levodopa as needed for disability during the maintenance phase of the study. After a mean follow-up of 24 months, fewer pramipexole-treated patients reached the primary endpoint of time to the first occurrence of wearing-off, dyskinesias, or on–off motor fluctuations (28% vs. 51%; $P<0.001$) than the patients initially randomly assigned to levodopa therapy. Additionally, patients in the pramipexole group were receiving lower daily doses of levodopa, theoretically conferring a reduced risk of developing motor complications. Long-term follow-up of this cohort (mean = 6 years) revealed a persistently lower rate of dopaminergic motor complications in the pramipexole-treated patients compared with those receiving levodopa (50% vs. 68.4%, respectively; $P = 0.002$).[25]

Despite the continued increased risk of motor complications in patients started on levodopa, trials extending 10 to 15 years found no significant difference in disease severity rating or rates of disabling dyskinesias.[26,27] Patients treated initially with ropinirole were less likely to experience dyskinesias compared with those treated initially with levodopa at the end of a 5-year evaluation.[22] Patients in the ropinirole group used lower mean daily doses of levodopa (427 mg vs. 753 mg) but were almost twice as likely to need open-label levodopa supplementation (66% vs. 36%). Dyskinesias developed in 20% of the ropinirole-treated patients compared with 45% of the levodopa-treated patients. For ropinirole-treated patients who were able to remain on monotherapy without open-label levodopa supplementation, only 5% experienced dyskinesia, compared with 36% of those receiving levodopa monotherapy. Although the lower incidence of dyskinesias was shown to persist in a long-term open-label follow-up of this study cohort, there was no difference in disease severity between the ropinirole-treated group and the levodopa-treated group at 10 years.[26] There may be additional trends toward better cognitive and health-related quality of life outcomes in the patients started on levodopa.[27] This may be due in part to the fact that although dopamine agonists do delay motor complications, they are not without side effects. Trials have consistently shown higher rates of adverse drug reactions in patients initially started on dopamine agonists.[22,25] One open-label, randomized trial found that 28% of patients discontinued initial therapy with dopamine agonists due to side effects versus only 2% of patients initially given levodopa.[28] Regardless of initial therapy chosen, due to disease progression, levodopa therapy will eventually be required, motor complications will develop, and disability will be present.

MAO-B inhibitors are an alternative method of enriching dopamine supply in early disease. These agents increase nigrostriatal dopamine supply via the irreversible inhibition of MAO-B, a major enzymatic pathway responsible for the metabolism of dopamine in the brain, and require the presence of dopamine for clinical effect.[29] Though MAO-B inhibitors have been shown to delay the need for dopaminergic therapy with levodopa, definitive efficacy comparisons are lacking.[29]

Early guidance from the AAN supported either dopamine agonists or levodopa as initial therapy for PD; more recent NICE and EFNS MDS-ES guidelines additionally support the use of MAO-B inhibitors in initial therapy.[15,17,18] The long-term effectiveness of dopamine agonists and MAO-B inhibitors compared with levodopa as initial treatment for PD (PD MED) trial set out to compare and contrast levodopa versus levodopa-sparing therapies.[28] Patients assigned to monotherapy with MAO-B inhibitors or dopamine agonists were generally younger and healthier than those assigned levodopa as initial therapy. At 7-year follow-up, 72% of patients initially assigned to MAO-B inhibitors withdrew from initial therapy and changed treatment compared to 50% in the dopamine agonist group and 7% in the levodopa group ($P<0.0001$). Among those patients initiated on MOA-B inhibitors, 48% withdrew due to side effects and 36% withdrew due to lack of efficacy, and for patients initiated on dopamine agonists, 82% withdrew due to side effects and 16% withdrew due to lack of efficacy.[28] As shown in prior studies, levodopa improved function and quality of life to a greater degree; however, the primary mobility outcome did not reach the prespecified minimally important difference. Mobility scores were not significantly different between MAO-B inhibitors and dopamine agonists indicating that MAO-B inhibitors are at least as effective as dopamine agonists in early therapy of PD.[28] Additionally, at 7 years, patients on dopamine agonists were on the highest overall amount of medication. The study confirms that initial treatment with a dopamine agonist, MAO-B inhibitor, or levodopa may all be reasonable approaches.

Disease severity, degree of functional impairment, life expectancy, and age guide therapeutic drug selection in early PD. In younger patients (e.g., age <65 years) with milder disease, such as L.M., the initiation of levodopa-sparing therapy with either a dopamine agonist or MAO-B inhibitor would be appropriate. Initiating levodopa therapy later in the course of PD delays the development of motor complications, particularly the troubling peak-dose, levodopa-induced dyskinesias, which eventually develop with advancing PD. Patients with younger age at disease onset, such as L.M., may be at an increased lifetime risk of developing dyskinesias.[19] Although the PD MED trial did conclude that MAO-B inhibitors are at least as effective as dopamine agonists for initial therapy, other meta-analyses show that the degree of symptomatic benefit over placebo is small in comparison with those of dopamine agonists over placebo.[30] Overall, there is a lack of comparative data between MAO-B inhibitors and dopamine agonists. Therefore, use of MAO-B inhibitors in initial therapy is often limited to young patients with more mild functional impairments. In older patients (e.g., age >65 years), those with more significant functional impairments, or those with limited life expectancy, use of levodopa may be warranted, as a result of the large number of symptomatic benefits associated with its use despite the relatively high risk of motor complications and side effects. Additionally, levodopa may be more appropriate initial treatment in older patients, because they may be more likely to experience intolerable CNS side effects from dopamine agonists and less likely to develop motor complications over their lifetime.[19]

In the case of L.M., his relatively young age, mild disease, and moderate functional impairments make him a good candidate for initial therapy with a dopamine agonist. L.M. will require levodopa therapy at a later time, when he reaches more advanced stages of the disease. By initiating therapy first with a dopamine agonist, rescue levodopa therapy can likely be started at smaller doses, and the onset of motor complications that often occur with escalating doses and extended therapy with levodopa may be delayed.

DOPAMINE AGONISTS

CASE 59-1, QUESTION 5: L.M. is to be started on a dopamine agonist. Which agent should be selected?

Table 59-3
Pharmacologic and Pharmacokinetic Properties of Dopamine Agonists

	Bromocriptine	Pramipexole	Ropinirole	Apomorphine	Rotigotine
Type of compound	Ergot derivative	Nonergoline	Nonergoline	Nonergoline	Nonergoline
Receptor specificity	D_2, D_1,[a] α_1, α_2, 5-HT	D_2, D_3, D_4, α_2	D_2, D_3, D_4	D_1, D_2, D_3, D_4, D_5, α_1, α_2, 5-HT_1, 5-HT_2	D_1, D_2, D_3, 5-HT_1
Bioavailability	7% (first-pass metabolism)	90%	55% (first-pass metabolism)	<5% orally; 100% subcutaneous	NA
T_{max} (minutes)	70–100	60–180	90	10–60	15–18 (hours); no characteristic peak observed
Protein binding	90%–96%	15%	10%–40%	>99.9%	89.5%
Elimination route	Hepatic	Renal, 90% unchanged	Hepatic	Hepatic and extrahepatic	Hepatic
Half-life (hours)	2–8	8–12	6	0.5–1	3–7

[a]Antagonist.

5-HT, serotonin; NA, not applicable.

Two generations of dopamine agonists have been used for the treatment of idiopathic PD, in early-stage PD as monotherapy, or as an adjunct to levodopa in patients with advanced disease. The comparative pharmacologic and pharmacokinetic properties of these agents are shown in Table 59-3. The first-generation dopamine agonists, which are derived from ergot alkaloids, include bromocriptine, pergolide, and cabergoline. These older agents are now rarely used because of increased risk of retroperitoneal, pleural, and pericardial fibrosis, as well as a two- to fourfold increased risk for cardiac valve fibrosis when compared with nonergoline dopamine agonists and controls.[31,32] Pergolide was voluntarily withdrawn in the United States (US) in 2007 for this reason, and although cabergoline continues to be used in Europe, it is only indicated in the United States for the treatment of hyperprolactinemia. Pramipexole, ropinirole, apomorphine, and rotigotine are second-generation nonergoline dopamine agonists. Of these agents, pramipexole and ropinirole are commonly prescribed. Apomorphine is available only in injectable form, for use as a rescue agent in the treatment of hypomobility "off" episodes in patients with PD. Rotigotine, a once-daily transdermal formulation, was recently re-introduced to the market.

Dopamine agonists work by directly stimulating postsynaptic dopamine receptors within the striatum. The two families of dopamine receptors are D_1 and D_2. The D_1-like receptor family includes the D_1 and D_5 dopamine subtype receptors and the D_2-like receptor family includes D_2, D_3, and D_4 dopamine subtype receptors. Stimulation of D_2 receptors is largely responsible for reducing rigidity and bradykinesia, whereas the precise role of the D_1 receptors remains uncertain.[33] Pramipexole and ropinirole exhibit selectivity for D_2 receptors without any significant affinity for D_1 receptors whereas rotigotine has activity at all dopamine receptors.[34–36] Although the dopamine agonists differ slightly from each other in terms of their affinities for dopamine receptor subtypes, these agents produce similar clinical effects when used to treat PD, and no compelling evidence favors one agent over another strictly on efficacy measures. Instead, experience with the nonergoline dopamine agonists, specifically pramipexole and ropinirole, makes them currently preferred as initial dopamine agonists. Thus, either agent would be acceptable as initial therapy in L.M.

CASE 59-1, QUESTION 6: The decision is made to begin pramipexole in L.M. How effective is pramipexole in the initial treatment of PD? How does ropinirole compare?

Pramipexole

Pramipexole has been well studied as monotherapy in patients with early-stage PD and as an adjunct to levodopa therapy in advanced-stage disease.[34–36] These trials were multicenter, placebo-controlled, parallel-group studies, and parts of the Unified Parkinson's Disease Rating Scale (UPDRS) were used as the primary outcome measures, specifically improvement in ADLs (Part II) and motor function scores (Part III). Each evaluation on the UPDRS is rated on a scale of 0 (normal) to 4 (can barely perform). Lower scores on the UPDRS after treatment indicate an improvement in overall performance.

To view the UPDRS and other assessment tools for the symptoms of Parkinson's disease, please visit **http://www.movementdisorders.org/MDS/Education/Rating-Scales.htm**.

The evidence for the efficacy of pramipexole in early PD comes from two large-scale, double-blind, placebo-controlled studies that included a total of 599 patients with early-stage PD (mean disease duration of 2 years).[35,36] In the first study, 264 patients were randomly assigned to receive one of four fixed doses (1.5, 3, 4.5, or 6 mg/day) or placebo.[35] The pramipexole-treated patients had a 20% reduction in their total UPDRS scores compared with baseline values, whereas no significant improvement was observed in the placebo-treated patients. A trend toward decreased tolerability was noted because the pramipexole dosage was escalated, especially in the 6 mg/day group. A second study of 335 patients titrated doses up to the maximal tolerated dose (not to exceed 4.5 mg/day) and then followed patients for a 6-month maintenance phase.[36] The mean pramipexole maintenance dosage was 3.8 mg/day. Those treated with pramipexole experienced significant improvements in both the ADL scores (22%–29%; $P<0.0001$) and motor scores (25%–31%; $P<0.0001$), whereas there were no significant changes in the placebo group.

Ropinirole

Similar to pramipexole, ropinirole is a synthetic nonergoline dopamine agonist. Although the drug is pharmacologically similar to pramipexole, it has some distinct pharmacokinetic properties (Table 59-3). Unlike pramipexole, which is primarily eliminated by renal excretion, ropinirole is hepatically metabolized and undergoes significant first-pass hepatic metabolism.[37] Similar to pramipexole, ropinirole is approved for use as monotherapy in early-stage idiopathic PD and as an adjunct to levodopa therapy in patients with advanced-stage disease.

Ropinirole has not been directly compared with pramipexole in randomized, double-blind comparisons, but it appears to have comparable efficacy in indirect comparison. In several randomized, double-blind, multicenter, parallel-group studies comparing ropinirole with placebo, bromocriptine, or levodopa, 6 months of monotherapy with ropinirole in patients with early PD significantly improves UPDRS motor scores by approximately 20% to 30% compared with baseline values.[38–40]

Rotigotine

Rotigotine is a nonergoline dopamine receptor agonist that is formulated in a transdermal patch delivery system designed for once-a-day application. It was voluntarily withdrawn from the U.S. market in 2008 because of problems with crystal formation in the patches; however, the patch was reformulated and re-approved by the Food and Drug Administration (FDA) in April 2012. The original and reformulated patches have demonstrated efficacy as monotherapy in early-stage PD,[41–44] whereas only the original formulation has demonstrated efficacy as adjunctive therapy to levodopa in patients with advanced stages of PD.[45,46] It is, however, used in both situations.

A randomized, controlled trial conducted in Japanese patients with early-stage PD found that the mean improvement in UPDRS Part II and III sum scores was 8.4 in the rotigotine-treated group versus 4.1 in the placebo group ($P = 0.002$; 95% CI, −7.0 to −1.7).[47] The average dose of rotigotine was 12.8 mg/24 hours in this study which exceeds the highest recommended dose for early PD (6 mg/24 hours). Despite clear benefits in improving ADLs and motor function, there is insufficient evidence at this time to support that rotigotine prevents or delays motor fluctuations or dyskinesias.[48]

The transdermal delivery may have several advantages over traditional oral preparations including possible increase in adherence, ease of use in patients with swallowing difficulty, and a more continuous stimulation of dopamine receptors. In theory, these benefits may translate into improved efficacy. In randomized, controlled trials comparing rotigotine to ropinirole as monotherapy or pramipexole as adjunct therapy, rotigotine has been found to be noninferior when typical clinical doses are used.[44,46]

Dosing

CASE 59-1, QUESTION 7: How are pramipexole and ropinirole dosed? What is the appropriate dose of pramipexole for L.M.?

Dopamine agonists should always be initiated at a low dosage and gradually titrated to the maximal effective dose, as tolerated. This approach minimizes adverse effects that may result in nonadherence or discontinuation of the drug. In clinical trials, the maximal effective doses are variable and correlate with disease severity and tolerability. Studies have found no difference in efficacy or safety measures between immediate and long-acting formulations of dopamine agonists.[49] One fixed-dose study of pramipexole in early PD showed that most patients responded maximally at a dosage of 0.5 mg 3 times daily, although it has been shown to be effective and well tolerated in doses as high as 4.5 mg/day (divided).[34]

L.M. has normal renal function; therefore, immediate-release pramipexole should be started at an initial dosage of 0.125 mg 3 times daily for 5 to 7 days. His dosage may be increased weekly by 0.125 to 0.25 mg/dose as tolerated and up to the maximal effective dose, not to exceed the maximum dose of 4.5 mg/day.[34] Patients with a creatinine clearance of less than 50 mL/minute should be dosed less frequently than those with normal renal function.[34] Patients with a creatinine clearance of 30 to 50 mL/minute should receive a starting dose of 0.125 mg twice daily up to a maximal dose of 0.75 mg 3 times daily; patients with a creatinine clearance of 15 to 30 mL/minute should receive a starting dose of 0.125 mg daily up to a maximal dose of 1.5 mg daily. Pramipexole has not been studied in patients with a creatinine clearance of less than 15 mL/minute or those receiving hemodialysis. A once-daily extended-release formulation of pramipexole is also available; patients can be switched overnight from immediate-release pramipexole at the same daily dose. The use of the extended-release formulation is not recommended for patients with a creatinine clearance less than 30 mL/minute or for those receiving hemodialysis.

Ropinirole should be initiated at a dosage of 0.25 mg 3 times daily with gradual titration to clinical response in weekly increments of 0.25 mg/dose over the course of 4 to 6 weeks, not to exceed 24 mg/day.[37] Patients wishing to take the drug less frequently can be switched directly to an extended-release once-daily formulation, selecting the dose that most closely matches the total daily dose of the immediate-release formulation. No dose adjustments for ropinirole are necessary in patients with renal dysfunction and can be used in doses up to 18 mg/day in patients on hemodialysis

Transdermal rotigotine is available in several patch strengths (Table 59-2). For patients with early-stage PD, it is recommended to start rotigotine at 2 mg/24 hours with dose increases of 2 mg/24 hours no sooner than weekly based on clinical response and tolerability.[50] The maximum recommended dose in early PD is 6 mg/24 hours whereas 8 mg/24 hours is recommended in advanced PD. Clinical trials have often used doses up to 16 mg/24 hours.[46,51] The time to reach steady state plasma concentrations of rotigotine is approximately 2 to 3 days after initial patch application.[50] A multinational, open-label study demonstrated that patients with advanced PD taking pramipexole $<$2 mg/day or ropinirole $<$9 mg/day can be safely switched directly to rotigotine with no cross-titration.[52] Rotigotine is metabolized via conjugation and *N*-dealkylation, and the inactive conjugates are excreted in the urine. No adjustments are required for patients with hepatic or renal insufficiency.

Adverse Effects

CASE 59-1, QUESTION 8: What are the adverse effects of pramipexole and ropinirole? How can these be managed?

Because pramipexole, ropinirole, and rotigotine are all approved for use as monotherapy in early-stage disease and as adjunctive therapy in advanced-stage disease, the adverse events of these agents have been evaluated as a function of disease stage. In studies of patients with early-stage disease, the most common side effects were nausea (28%–47%), application site reactions (39%, rotigotine only), dizziness (25%–40%), somnolence (22%–40%), insomnia (17%–19%), constipation (14%), asthenia (14%), hallucinations (9%), and leg edema (5%).[21,34–37,38–40,51] Administration with food may help to relieve nausea and/or vomiting. With continued use, many patients exhibit tolerance to the gastrointestinal side effects. CNS side effects were the most common reason for discontinuation of these agents with older patients particularly susceptible to hallucinations and other CNS side effects. The incidence of orthostatic hypotension was relatively low (1%–9%) and may in part reflect the exclusion of patients with underlying cardiovascular disease in several of the studies.

In advanced-stage disease, the most common adverse events of dopamine agonists were orthostatic hypotension (10%–54%), dyskinesias (26%–47%), application site reactions (46%, rotigotine only, dose related), nausea (25%), insomnia (27%), hallucinations (11%–17%), somnolence (11%), and confusion (10%).[34,37,50,53] The most common reasons for discontinuing these agents are mental disturbances (e.g., nightmares, confusion, hallucinations, insomnia) and orthostatic hypotension. Dyskinesias that are experienced when dopamine agonists are used in combination with levodopa in advanced-stage disease may require lowering the dose of levodopa or, in some cases, the dopamine agonist.

Sudden, excessive daytime somnolence, including while driving, has been reported with dopamine agonists and has resulted in accidents.[34,37,50,54] Affected patients did not always report warning signs before falling asleep and believed they were alert immediately before the event. Labeling for these drugs includes a warning that patients should be alerted to the possibility of falling asleep while engaged in daily activities. Patients should be advised to refrain from driving or other potentially dangerous activities until they have gained sufficient experience with the dopamine agonist to determine whether it will hinder their mental and motor performance. Caution should be advised when patients are taking other sedating medications or alcohol in combination with dopamine agonists. If excessive daytime somnolence does occur, patients should be advised to contact their healthcare practitioner.

Dopamine agonist therapy in patients with PD is associated with 2- to 3.5-fold increased odds of developing an impulse control disorder.[55] The frequency appears similar for both pramipexole and ropinirole whereas it is less clear with rotigotine. In one study, a prevalence of 6.1% was noted for pathologic gambling in patients with PD compared with 0.25% for age- and sex-matched controls.[56] These cases may represent variations of a behavioral syndrome termed dopamine dysregulation syndrome.[57] Other features of the syndrome have been reported, including punding (carrying out repetitive, purposeless motor acts), hypersexuality, walkabout (having the urge to walk great distances during on-times, often with no purpose or destination and abnormalities in time perception), compulsive buying, binge eating, drug hoarding, and social independence or isolation.[57] The syndrome appears to be more common among younger, male patients with early-onset PD, as well as those having novelty-seeking personality traits, depressive symptoms, and current use of alcohol or tobacco.[55,58] Management of impulse control disorders can be challenging, because it often requires modification of dopaminergic therapies, which must be carefully balanced with the accompanying risk of worsening motor function. Underlying depression, if present, should be treated and may improve impulse control. Nonpharmacologic measures (such as limiting access to money or the Internet) may be helpful; in some cases, antipsychotic drugs may be considered, but must also be used carefully to avoid precipitating motor disability.[59]

Although L.M. is younger than 65 years of age, he may be at increased risk for visual hallucinations and cognitive problems from dopamine agonist therapy. He should be monitored closely for occurrence or exacerbation of these side effects. He should also be evaluated for lightheadedness before initiation of pramipexole and counseled to report dizziness or unsteadiness, because this may lead to falls. He should be reassured that if these effects are caused by pramipexole, they should subside with time and that he should not drive or operate complex machinery until he can assess the effect of the drug on his mental status. L.M. should be counseled about the possibility of excessive, and potentially unpredictable, daytime somnolence because pramipexole is introduced. L.M. does not appear to have a problem with excessive alcohol use; however, he and his family should be educated about his increased risk for impulse control disorders and advised to report any new, unusual, or uncharacteristic behaviors or increased use of alcohol.

MONOAMINE OXIDASE-B INHIBITORS

The monoamine oxidase-B inhibitors are irreversible inhibitors of MAO-B, a major enzymatic pathway responsible for the metabolism of dopamine in the brain, and inhibition increases the amount of striatal dopamine.[60] The discovery that ingestion of MPTP causes rapid and irreversible parkinsonism led to the finding that the neurotoxicity associated with MPTP is not directly caused by MPTP itself, but rather the oxidized product, L-methyl-4-phenylpyridinium (MPP).[7] The conversion to MPP is a two-step process mediated in part by MAO-B. Inhibition of MAO-B can inhibit the oxidative conversion of dopamine to potentially reactive peroxides. This finding has led investigators to study whether inhibition of this enzyme is neuroprotective.

Selegiline

In animals, pretreatment with selegiline (also referred to as deprenyl) protects against neuronal damage after the administration of MPTP.[29] The Deprenyl and Tocopherol Antioxidative Therapy of Parkinsonism (DATATOP) study was designed to test the hypothesis that the combined use of selegiline and an antioxidant (α-tocopherol) early in the course of the disease may slow disease progression.[61] The primary outcome was the length of time that patients could be sustained without levodopa therapy (an indication of disease progression). Early treatment with selegiline 10 mg/day delayed the need to start levodopa therapy by approximately 9 months compared with patients given placebo; however, long-term observation showed that the benefits of selegiline were not sustained and diminished with time. In an extension of the study, patients originally assigned to selegiline tended to reach the endpoint of disability after 1 year of observation even more quickly than did those not assigned to receive selegiline.[62] Initial selegiline treatment did not alter the development of levodopa adverse effects such as dyskinesias and wearing-off and on–off phenomena.

Although selegiline did not prove to be neuroprotective, the finding that MAO-B inhibitors can delay the need for dopaminergic therapy by at least several months is clinically relevant and is supported by several randomized, controlled trials.[63,64] Aside from the DATATOP trial, studies of selegiline are limited by relatively small sample sizes. As a result, a large meta-analysis of MAO-B inhibitors in early PD was conducted.[30] When analyzed for selegiline, the levodopa dose necessary to control symptoms was 67 mg (14–119 mg; $P = 0.01$) lower in the selegiline arm. This analysis found that the total, motor, and ADL scores of the UPDRS were significantly improved in the selegiline arm at 3 months. A subsequent Cochrane Review found that the selegiline-treated arms scored 3.79 points better (95% CI: 2.21, 5.3) when looking at the weighted mean difference in motor UPDRS score.[29] Although oral selegiline continues to be FDA-approved only as adjunct treatment to carbidopa/levodopa, the evidence suggests efficacy in monotherapy, and it is used as monotherapy in practice.

Rasagiline

Rasagiline is a second-generation, irreversible selective inhibitor of MAO-B that is FDA-approved as both monotherapy and adjunct therapy in PD. Rasagiline is otherwise differentiated from selegiline primarily in that it is a more potent inhibitor of MAO-B and does not carry the same potential for adverse effects resulting from metabolites.[65] Like selegiline, rasagiline has also been found to protect from MPTP-induced parkinsonism in animal models.[29]

Rasagiline was studied as monotherapy in early PD in a randomized, double-blind, placebo-controlled trial comparing rasagiline 1 or 2 mg daily with placebo ($n = 404$).[66] After 6 months of therapy, the mean adjusted change in UPDRS scores compared with placebo was improved in both the 1- and 2-mg groups ($P<0.001$).[66] These changes are quantitatively similar to those observed with levodopa therapy. This study used a delayed-start design, wherein at the end of the initial 6 months of treatment, patients who received placebo were then switched over to receive active treatment with rasagiline, and the rasagiline-treated patients continued on therapy. After an additional 6 months of study, it was found that patients receiving rasagiline for all 12 months had less functional decline than patients in whom rasagiline was delayed.[67] The mean adjusted difference in total UPDRS scores at 12 months for patients receiving rasagiline 2 mg/day for all 12 months was –2.29 compared with the delayed-start rasagiline 2-mg group ($P = 0.01$). As a result, rasagiline was FDA-approved for use as monotherapy in early PD. These encouraging findings also suggested that neuroprotection might be afforded by rasagiline and prompted a larger, more definitive study.

The Attenuation of Disease Progression with Azilect Given Once-daily (ADIAGO) study was also a randomized, placebo-controlled trial using the delayed-start methodology, but with a much larger sample size (n = 1,176).[68] Patients were randomly assigned to receive rasagiline or placebo for 36 weeks, at which time rasagiline-treated subjects continued therapy, and the placebo group was switched to rasagiline; all patients were then followed for an additional 36 weeks. To prove disease modification attributable to rasagiline with either dose, the early-start treatment group had to meet each of three hierarchic endpoints, based on magnitude and rate of change of UPDRS scores during different periods of the study. At the end of the study, rasagiline failed to meet all of the prespecified endpoints and the authors were unable to confirm any disease-modifying effects.[68]

No direct comparisons of rasagiline and selegiline are available. Existing data were compared in an industry-sponsored, indirect meta-analysis, which found a significant advantage for rasagiline monotherapy on UPDRS scores.[69] Additionally, risk for discontinuation and adverse events favored rasagiline. Rasagiline is primarily metabolized via cytochrome P450 (CYP) 1A2 and *N*-dealkylation, whereas selegiline is metabolized via CYP2B6, CYP2C9, and CYP3A4/5 to amphetamine-like metabolites (L-methamphetamine and L-amphetamine). As a result of their MAO-B inhibition, similar precautions regarding drug interactions exist; caution should be taken when using MAO-B inhibitors with proserotonergic agents such as antidepressants, triptans, and linezolid due to the risk of serotonin syndrome. Although tyramine-challenge studies have not demonstrated any clinically significant reactions with these MAO-B inhibitors, the product labeling still contains a warning that patients should be advised to restrict tyramine intake.[70,71]

Dosing

Selegiline is available in a 5-mg capsule or tablet and as a 1.25-mg orally disintegrating tablet. It is also available in a transdermal patch, but this formulation is not approved for use in PD (approved for treatment of major depressive disorder). The bioavailability of conventional selegiline is low, and it undergoes extensive hepatic first-pass metabolism into amphetamine-based metabolites, which may contribute to neurologic side effects.[60] The usual dosage of conventional selegiline is 10 mg/day administered as 5 mg in the morning and early afternoon. It is not given in the evening because excess stimulation from metabolites (L-methamphetamine and L-amphetamine) can cause insomnia and other psychiatric side effects.[72] The orally disintegrating tablet formulation dissolves in the mouth in contact with saliva and undergoes pregastric absorption. This formulation minimizes the effect of first-pass metabolism in comparison with conventional selegiline, resulting in higher plasma concentrations and reductions in the amphetamine-based metabolites.[60] Selegiline should be used with caution in patients with severe hepatic impairment or with creatinine clearance less than 30 mL/minute.

Rasagiline is available in 0.5- and 1-mg tablets. When used as monotherapy, it is initiated at 1 mg daily. When combined with levodopa, the initial dose is lowered to 0.5 mg daily and can be increased to 1 mg daily based on response. In patients with mild hepatic impairment, the dose should be reduced to 0.5 mg daily, but use should be avoided in those with moderate-to-severe hepatic impairment. Additionally, because rasagiline lacks the amphetamine-like metabolites of selegiline, it also lacks the time-specific dosing constraints.

Adverse Effects

The most common adverse effects of both agents include nausea (6%–20%), dizziness (11%–14%), headache (4%–14%), and dry mouth (4%–6%).[60,70,72] CNS effects such as hallucinations, vivid dreams, and confusion also occur but at a lower rate as compared with dopamine agonists. Although the oral disintegrating tablet reduces the amphetamine-based metabolites, there are higher rates of reported side effects, likely as a result of the higher plasma concentration of selegiline.[60] A large meta-analysis of MAO-B inhibitors in early PD found a higher incidence of reported side effects among the MAO-B inhibitor (all but one study used selegiline) versus non-MAO-B inhibitor groups (OR: 1.36, 1.02–1.8, $P = 0.04$).[30] However, these agents are generally considered well tolerated.[70]

LEVODOPA

CASE 59-1, QUESTION 9: L.M. has responded well to pramipexole 1 mg 3 times daily for the past 18 months, with an increased ability to paint and carry out ADLs. During the past few weeks, however, he has noticed a gradual worsening in his symptoms and once again is having difficulty holding a paintbrush. He currently complains of feeling more "tied up," he has more difficulty getting out of a chair, and his posture is slightly more stooped. He also notes that he feels tired throughout much of the day. He remains able to carry out most of his ADLs without assistance. Should levodopa be considered for the treatment of his PD symptoms at this time?

Dopamine itself does not cross the blood–brain barrier. Levodopa, a dopamine precursor with no known pharmacologic action of its own, crosses the blood–brain barrier, where it is converted by the enzyme aromatic amino acid (dopa) decarboxylase to dopamine. Levodopa has been a mainstay of PD treatment since the 1960s. Nearly all patients will eventually require treatment with the drug, regardless of their initial therapy.

Because significant amounts of levodopa are peripherally (extracerebrally) metabolized to dopamine by dopa decarboxylase, extremely high doses are necessary if administered alone. For this reason, levodopa is always coadministered with a dopa decarboxylase inhibitor. This allows the dose of levodopa to be decreased by 75%.[73] By combining levodopa with a dopa decarboxylase inhibitor that does not penetrate the blood–brain barrier, a decrease in the peripheral conversion of levodopa to dopamine can be achieved, whereas the desired conversion within the striatum remains unaffected. This combination also shortens the time needed to achieve optimal effects by several weeks, because the dopa decarboxylase inhibitor substantially decreases dose-limiting levodopa-induced nausea and vomiting. The two peripheral decarboxylase inhibitors in clinical use are benserazide (unavailable in the US) and carbidopa. A fixed combination of carbidopa and levodopa is available in ratios of 1:4 (carbidopa/levodopa 25/100) and 1:10 (carbidopa/levodopa 10/100 and 25/250). Carbidopa/levodopa is also available as an immediate-release, orally disintegrating tablet and extended-release capsule, both of which may be used in early PD. In addition, controlled-release, extended-release, and intestinal gel formulations are available and are discussed for management of motor complications.

The optimal time to initiate levodopa therapy must be individualized because chronic levodopa use is associated with the development of motor complications and dyskinesias. These observations led to the understanding that chronic levodopa therapy may actually accelerate the neurodegenerative process through formation of free radicals generated by dopamine metabolism.[74] The Earlier versus Later Levodopa Therapy in Parkinson's Disease (ELLDOPA) study was designed to determine whether long-term use of levodopa accelerates neurodegeneration and paradoxically worsens PD.[74] After 42 weeks, the severity of symptoms as measured by changes in the total UPDRS score increased more in the placebo group than in all of the groups receiving levodopa. This validated that levodopa use does not result in accelerated progression of the disease based on clinical evaluations. In untreated individuals, there is little reason to start levodopa until the patient reports worsening of function (socially, vocationally, or otherwise). The need for levodopa therapy may be delayed by initiating therapy first with a dopamine agonist or MAO-B inhibitor. This approach is particularly advantageous in younger patients who will likely live many years with PD and have a high lifetime risk for developing motor complications. In the case of L.M., he is now experiencing bothersome symptoms despite near-maximal dopamine agonist therapy, and it has progressed sufficiently to threaten his job performance. Although the dose of pramipexole could be increased, he may experience more daytime somnolence; thus, levodopa should be added to his regimen.

Dosing

CASE 59-1, QUESTION 10: The decision is made to begin L.M. on carbidopa/levodopa. How should it be dosed?

About 70 to 100 mg/day of carbidopa is necessary to saturate peripheral dopa decarboxylase.[73] It is usually unnecessary and more costly to administer carbidopa in higher amounts. Therapy should be initiated with immediate-release carbidopa/levodopa 25 mg/100 mg 3 times a day. The immediate-release formulation is preferred because it allows for much easier dose adjustment. In the case of L.M., the dose can then be increased by 100 mg of levodopa every day or every other day up to eight tablets (800 mg) or to the maximal effective dose, to individual requirements, or as tolerated.

Troublesome peak-dose dyskinesias may occur as a result of high levels of dopaminergic drug activity. If these occur, the dose or frequency may be adjusted, while giving consideration to balancing the most useful dose (e.g., maximizing the patient's on-time) with that which does not produce unacceptable side effects (e.g., troublesome dyskinesias). Because L.M. is currently being treated with a dopamine agonist, he must be monitored closely for the development of motor complications with the addition of levodopa.

Most patients with early PD will begin therapy on levodopa 300 mg/day and will demonstrate response before reaching 1,000 mg/day.[11,73] When levodopa doses exceed 750 mg/day, patients such as L.M. can be switched from the 1:4 ratio of carbidopa/levodopa to the 1:10 ratio to prevent providing excessive amounts of decarboxylase inhibitor. For example, if L.M. needed 800 mg/day of levodopa, two carbidopa/levodopa 10/100 tablets 4 times daily could be administered. If L.M. had not been initially treated with a dopamine agonist, some clinicians would consider adding a dopamine agonist after the daily levodopa dose has been increased to more than 600 mg because dopamine agonists directly stimulate dopamine receptors, have longer half-lives, and result in a lower incidence of dyskinesias, thus providing a smoother dopaminergic response.

Clinical response to levodopa therapy may be altered by modifying dietary amino acid ingestion.[73] Levodopa is actively transported across the blood–brain barrier by a large neutral amino acid transport system. This transport system also facilitates the blood-to-brain transport of amino acids such as L-leucine, L-isoleucine, L-valine, and L-phenylalanine. Levodopa and these neutral amino acids compete for transport mechanisms, and high plasma concentrations of these amino acids can decrease brain concentrations of levodopa.[75] Patients should be instructed to take immediate-release carbidopa/levodopa 30 minutes before or 60 minutes after meals for optimal efficacy. If nausea develops and administration with food is considered, a low-protein meal should be encouraged.

Adverse Effects

CASE 59-1, QUESTION 11: Since initiating carbidopa/levodopa, L.M. reports feeling restless and agitated at times. To what extent is levodopa contributing to these problems? How should they be managed?

Although levodopa is the most effective agent for PD, it is associated with many undesirable side effects, such as nausea, vomiting, and anorexia (50% of patients); postural hypotension (30% of patients); and cardiac arrhythmias (10% of patients).[11] In addition, mental disturbances are encountered in 15% of patients, and abnormal involuntary movements (dyskinesias) can be seen in up to 55% of patients during the first 6 months of levodopa treatment.[76]

Although more commonly encountered with dopamine agonists, psychiatric side effects are also associated with levodopa therapy and include confusion, depression, psychosis, hypomania, and vivid dreams.[73] Those with underlying or preexisting psychiatric disorders and those receiving high doses of levodopa for prolonged periods are at greatest risk.[77] Concurrent anticholinergics or amantadine therapy can exacerbate these symptoms. Advancement of the PD itself correlates with cognitive decline and greater frequency of CNS findings, possibly mediated through an underlying Lewy body pathology.[17] In some situations, it may be difficult to separate the respective drug from disease effects.

Some patients receiving levodopa experience psychomotor excitation (e.g., overactivity, restlessness, agitation). Similarly, hypomania has been reported in up to 8% of patients and is characterized by grandiose thinking, flight of ideas, tangential thinking, and poor social judgment. Normal sexual activity often is restored with improved motor function; however, hypersexuality and libido are increased in about 1% of levodopa-treated patients.[77]

In general, most of the mental disturbances are dose-related and can be lessened by reducing the dose of the dopaminergic agent. In patients such as L.M. who are concurrently receiving levodopa and a dopamine agonist, the dose reduction should be attempted first with the dopamine agonist. If symptoms do not improve, a reduction in the dose of levodopa may also be warranted. These dose reductions may, however, be impractical for L.M. because a return of parkinsonian symptoms is likely, and the benefits of levodopa therapy may outweigh the risk for mental disturbances.

ANTICHOLINERGICS

CASE 59-1, QUESTION 12: What role do anticholinergic drugs play in the treatment of PD? Should L.M. receive an anticholinergic agent?

Anticholinergic drugs have been used to treat PD since the mid-1800s, when it was discovered that symptoms were reduced by the belladonna derivative hyoscine (scopolamine).[17] Currently, they are used to specifically target tremor. Although tremor may improve with dopaminergic drugs via the restoration of balance between dopamine and acetylcholine, resolution of tremor may be incomplete. Anticholinergic drugs such as benztropine and trihexyphenidyl work by blocking the excitatory neurotransmitter acetylcholine in the striatum, which minimizes the effect of the relative increase in cholinergic sensitivity. Until the late 1960s, when amantadine and levodopa were introduced, anticholinergics were a mainstay of treatment; however, because of their undesirable side effect profile and poor efficacy relative to levodopa in treating bradykinesia and rigidity, anticholinergic agents are no longer used as first-line agents. These drugs produce both peripherally and centrally mediated adverse effects. Peripheral effects, such as dry mouth, blurred vision, constipation, and urinary retention, are common and bothersome.[20] Anticholinergic agents can increase intraocular pressure and should be avoided in patients with angle-closure glaucoma. CNS effects can include confusion, impairment of recent memory, hallucinations, and delusions.[17,20] Patients with PD are often more susceptible to these central effects because of advanced age, intercurrent illnesses, and impaired cognition.[20] Anticholinergics are usually reserved for the treatment of resting tremor early in the disease, particularly in younger patients with preserved cognitive function. Given his history and clinical presentation and based on the absence of tremor, L.M. would not be an appropriate candidate for an anticholinergic drug.

Treatment through the Progression of Parkinson's Disease

LEVODOPA AND ADJUNCTIVE THERAPY

The chronic, progressive nature of PD predicts that patients will develop worsening of motor control through the later stages of the disease; thus, enhanced motor control through the use of levodopa, in conjunction with symptomatic adjunctive agents, will be necessary. Agent selection is guided by efficacy for motor symptom control, adverse effects, and motor complication risk. Agents indicated by the AAN,[16] EFNS/MDS-ES,[18] and NICE[17] guidelines for symptomatic adjunct therapy and management of motor complications in late PD are outlined in Figure 59-3.

MOTOR COMPLICATIONS

CASE 59-1, QUESTION 13: L.M. had a dramatic improvement in all of his parkinsonian symptoms with the initiation of levodopa therapy after being maintained on carbidopa/levodopa 25 mg/250 mg 4 times a day.

After 6 months of treatment, he began to experience dyskinesias occurring 1 to 2 hours after a dose. They manifested as facial grimacing, lip smacking, tongue protrusion, and rocking of the trunk. Decreasing his pramipexole dose to 0.5 mg 3 times daily and gradually decreasing his dosage of carbidopa/levodopa to 25 mg/250 mg 3 times daily lessened the symptoms. After 3 years of levodopa therapy, more serious problems have begun to emerge. In the mornings, L.M. often experiences immobility. Nearly every day, he has periods (lasting for a few minutes) in which he cannot move, followed by a sudden switch to a fluid-like state, often associated with dyskinetic activity. He continues to take carbidopa/levodopa 3 times daily, but gains symptomatic relief for only 3 to 4 hours after a dose. Also, the response to a given dose varies and is often less in the afternoon. At times, he becomes "frozen," particularly when he needs to board an elevator or is required to move quickly. What are possible explanations for these alterations in clinical response?

Though variable, the initial levodopa response period may last up to 5 years. After this initial period of stability, 50% to 90% of patients receiving levodopa for 5 or more years will eventually experience motor complications.[78] Motor complications may present as periods of either too much (dyskinetic) dopaminergic activity, too little (akinetic) dopaminergic activity, or in combination.

In evaluating these motor fluctuations, it is important to ascertain which effects are attributable to the disease and which are

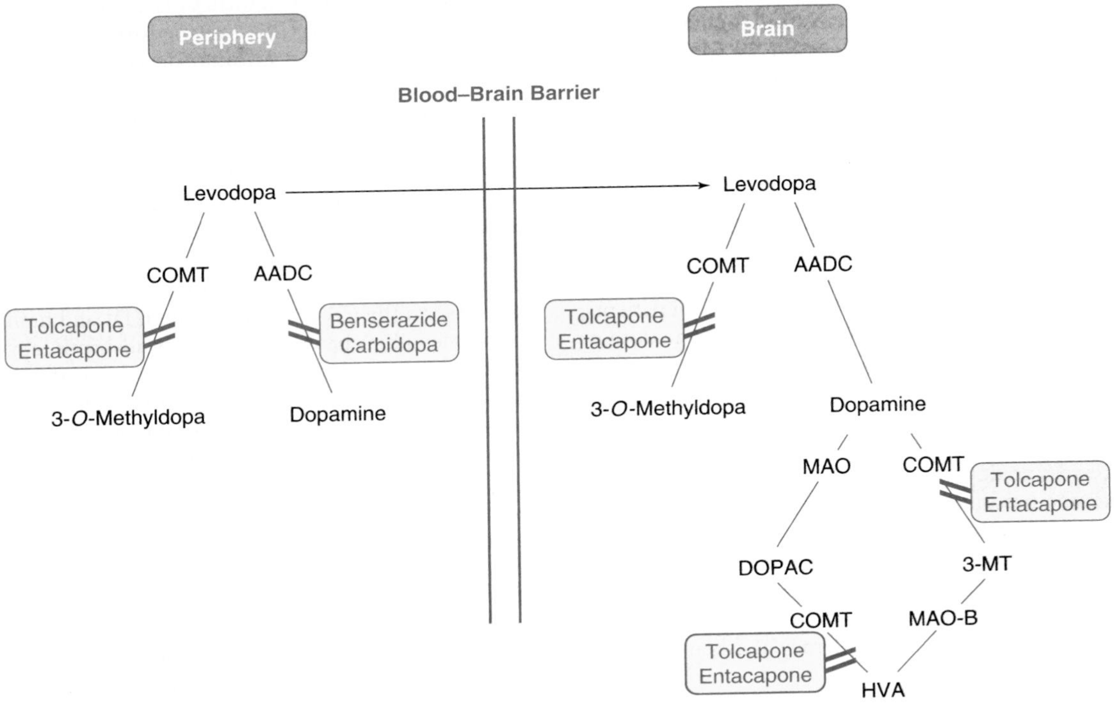

Figure 59-3 Levodopa metabolism in the human body. AADC, aromatic amino acid decarboxylase; COMT, catechol-*O*-methyltransferase; DOPAC, 3,4-dihydroxyphenylacetic acid; MAO, monoamine oxidase; 3-MT, 3-methoxytyramine.

attributable to the drug. For example, levodopa-induced peak-dose dyskinesias often appear concurrently with the development of motor fluctuations.[78,79] Peak-dose choreiform dyskinesias, brief, irregular and jerky movements, are the most common form of dyskinesias that occur with chronic levodopa (and sometimes dopamine agonist) therapy. These symptoms frequently subside at the end of the dosing interval because levodopa levels fall. Their severity is related to levodopa dose, disease duration and stage, and younger age at onset.[79] If peak-dose dyskinesias occur, the following strategies should be considered: The levodopa dose can be lowered but given more frequently; consideration can be given to switching patients to immediate-release tablets if taking modified-release formulations of carbidopa/levodopa (for ease in refining dose adjustments); agents that prolong the half-life of levodopa but do not provide stable levodopa plasma concentrations (e.g., COMT inhibitor, MAO-B inhibitor) can be added; or an antidyskinetic agent such as amantadine can be used. Variations in the rate and extent of levodopa absorption, dietary substrates (e.g., large neutral amino acids) that compete with cerebral transport mechanisms, levodopa drug–drug interactions (Table 59-4), and competition for receptor binding by levodopa metabolites can further explain the variable responses observed to levodopa.

Two of the more common motor complications are the wearing-off effect and the on–off effect. The wearing-off effect is most predictable, occurring in the latter part of the dosing interval after a period of relief. Because levodopa is a short-acting agent with an elimination half-life of about 1.5 hours, much of the effect from the evening dose will dissipate by morning.[73,78] For this reason, it is not surprising that L.M. is experiencing a period of immobility on arising. This is alleviated in most patients shortly after taking the morning dose. Wearing off can be improved by various means such as shortening the dosing interval or with the addition of adjunctive therapy (if not already present) with a dopamine agonist, MAO-B inhibitor or levodopa extender such as a COMT inhibitor. The on–off effect is described as random fluctuations from mobility (often associated with dyskinesias) to the parkinsonian state, which appear suddenly as if a switch has been turned on or off. These fluctuations can last from minutes to hours and increase in frequency and intensity with time. Despite accompanying dyskinesias, most patients prefer to be in an on rather than an off (or akinetic) state; however, for some patients, dyskinesias can be more disabling than parkinsonism.

Early in the course of disease, it is usually possible to control parkinsonian symptoms without inducing dyskinesias via medication adjustments; however, because the disease advances and the therapeutic window narrows, cycling between on periods complicated by dyskinesia and off periods with resulting immobility is common.[78,79] Eventually, despite adjustments in levodopa dose, many patients with advanced PD experience either mobility with severe dyskinesias or complete immobility. In most patients, this effect has no clear relationship to the timing of the dose or levodopa serum levels.[78]

The pathophysiologic basis for motor complications and dyskinesias is not entirely clear, but incomplete delivery of dopamine to central receptors is likely responsible.[78] Because the disease progresses and dopamine terminals are lost, the capacity to store dopamine presynaptically is diminished, impairing the ability to maintain relatively constant striatal dopamine concentrations.[78] As a consequence, dopamine receptors are subject to intermittent, pulsatile stimulation, rather than a more physiologic tonic stimulation. Overactivity of excitatory pathways mediated by neurotransmitters such as glutamate may also be involved.[78]

CASE 59-1, QUESTION 14: What options are available to reduce the motor fluctuations experienced by L.M.?

MODIFIED-RELEASE CARBIDOPA/LEVODOPA FORMULATIONS

A more sustained delivery of levodopa than that achieved with routine oral dosing may theoretically reduce motor complications, by more effectively replicating normal physiology. Three products designed to prolong carbidopa/levodopa delivery include a controlled-release tablet, an extended-release capsule, and an enteral suspension administered as a gastrointestinal infusion. The use of the enteral suspension for gastrointestinal infusion has shown reductions in off-time of 1.91 hours ($P = 0.0018$) and an increase in on-time of 1.86 hours ($P = 0.0059$) in a 12-week study of patients with severe motor fluctuations and hyper/dyskinesias.[80] As a result of its pump administration via a permanent duodenal/upper jejunal tube, this method is typically reserved as last-line therapy for use in specialized centers.

Controlled-Release Carbidopa/Levodopa

A controlled-release (CR) tablet formulation of carbidopa/levodopa is available, containing 25-mg carbidopa and 100-mg levodopa or 50-mg carbidopa and 200 mg levodopa in an erodible polymer matrix that retards gastric dissolution. Although off-time should theoretically be reduced by the slower rate of plasma levodopa decline, clinical study has generally not found a sustained difference in off-time, or a reduction in dyskinesias, with the CR preparation compared with the immediate-release preparation.[17,18] As a result, switching to CR carbidopa/levodopa as a primary strategy to reduce off-time or lessen dyskinesias is not recommended.[17]

A likely reason for the lack of superior effect with CR carbidopa/levodopa as compared with the immediate-release formulation is its variable absorption. Controlled-release carbidopa/levodopa is about 30% less bioavailable than the immediate-release formulation. Patients converted from standard carbidopa/levodopa to the CR formulation should receive a dose that will provide 10% more levodopa, and then the dose should be titrated upward to clinical reponse.[81] Interestingly, administration with food enhances levodopa peak by 25%. Given that there is no obvious advantage to CR carbidopa/levodopa, L.M. should not be switched to this formulation.

Extended-Release Carbidopa/Levodopa

The extended-release (ER) capsule formulation of carbidopa/levodopa contains a combination of both immediate- and extended-release beads designed to circumvent the pharmacokinetic concerns seen with the CR tablet formulation. Although both formulations persist for up to 6 hours, the ER capsule provides a faster time to symptom relief, with a peak that is comparable to the immediate-release formulation (1 hour vs. up to 2 hours for CR).[82] Similar to CR, the ER formulation reduces levodopa bioavailability by approximately 50%.[83] As such, the manufacturer provides specific dose conversions from immediate-release preparations. Converse to the CR preparation, high-fat and high-calorie food reduces levodopa peak and may delay absorption by 2 to 3 hours, and it is recommended that the first dose of the day be given 1 to 2 hours prior to eating. In patients with difficulty swallowing, these capsules may be opened and sprinkled on applesauce, which is an additional advantage to the CR formulation.

The ability of the ER formulation to reduce off-time was evaluated in a placebo-controlled study randomizing 393 patients to immediate or ER formulations over 22 weeks.[84] After being titrated to a stable dose during weeks 1 to 9, patients were followed for an additional 13 weeks. Compared to baseline evaluations, extended-release patients had a reduction in off-time by approximately 1 hour/day ($P<0.0001$) when compared to the IR formulation. This effect was accompanied by an increase in on-time without troubling dyskinesia of approximately 1 hour ($P = 0.0002$). Notably, of patients converted per manufacturer direction, 60% of patients required a further dosage increase and 13% required a dosage decrease.[84]

Table 59-4
Levodopa Drug Interactions

Drug	Interaction	Mechanism	Comments
Anticholinergics	↓ Levodopa effect	↓ Gastric emptying, thus ↑ degradation of levodopa in gut, and ↓ amount absorbed	Watch for ↓ levodopa effect when anticholinergics cause ↓ GI motility. When anticholinergic therapy is discontinued in a patient on levodopa, watch for signs of levodopa toxicity. Theoretic interaction with minor clinical significance
Ferrous sulfate	↓ Levodopa oral absorption by 50%	Formation of chelation complex	Avoid concomitant administration or separate administration by at least 2 hours
Food	↓ Levodopa effect	Large, neutral amino acids compete with levodopa for intestinal absorption	Although levodopa is usually taken with meals to slow absorption and ↓ central emetic effect, high-protein diets should be avoided
MAOI (e.g., phenelzine, tranylcypromine)	Hypertensive crisis	Peripheral dopamine and norepinephrine	Avoid combination use; monoamine oxidase type B (MAO-B) inhibitors such as selegiline can be used, but the dose of levodopa should be reduced after 2–3 days of therapy; carbidopa might minimize hypertensive reaction to levodopa in patients receiving an MAOI.
Methyldopa	↑ or ↓ levodopa effect	Acts as central and peripheral decarboxylase inhibitor	Observe for response; may need to switch to another antihypertensive.
Metoclopramide	↓ Levodopa effect	Central dopamine blockade	Avoid combination use
Neuroleptics (e.g., butyrophenones, phenothiazines)	↓ Levodopa effect	Central blockade of dopamine neurotransmission	Avoid combination use; important interaction
Phenytoin	↓ Levodopa effect	Mechanism unknown	Avoid combination use
Pyridoxine (vitamin B6)	↓ Levodopa effect	Peripheral decarboxylation of levodopa	Not observed when levodopa given with carbidopa; avoid levodopa monotherapy with vitamin B6 supplementation
Tricyclic antidepressants	↓ Levodopa effect	Levodopa degradation in gut because of delayed emptying	Use with caution

GI, gastrointestinal; MAOI, monoamine oxidase inhibitor.

Based upon this evidence, the ER formulation may improve off-time for L.M., but is unlikely to impact his dyskinesias. Therefore, it may not be appropriate to switch therapy. Taking his immediate-release carbidopa/levodopa more frequently while avoiding substantial increases in the total daily dose, which could worsen his dyskinesias, may improve his condition. Taking his morning dose before arising from bed may help with his early-morning problems. If the symptoms that L.M. is experiencing are not improved with these changes, a number of adjunctive agents such as dopamine agonists, apomorphine rescue, amantadine, COMT inhibitors, and MAO-B inhibitors can be considered.

DOPAMINE AGONISTS

The effectiveness of pramipexole added to levodopa therapy in advanced PD was evaluated in a multicenter, placebo-controlled study of 360 patients with a mean disease duration of 9 years.[85] Pramipexole was titrated gradually to the maximal effective dose as tolerated. At the end of a 6-month maintenance period, patients treated with pramipexole had a 22% improvement in their ADLs ($P<0.0001$) and a 25% improvement in their motor scores ($P<0.01$) compared with baseline values. Patients treated with pramipexole also had a 31% improvement in the mean off-time, compared with a 7% improvement in the placebo-treated group ($P<0.0006$). Dyskinesias and hallucinations were more common in pramipexole-treated patients and necessitated levodopa dose reduction in 76% of patients compared with 54% in the placebo group. The total daily levodopa dose was decreased by 27% in those treated with pramipexole compared with 5% in the placebo group.

Ropinirole has been found to improve motor scores when added to levodopa therapy in patients with advanced-stage disease.[53] In a multicenter, double-blind, randomized parallel-group study, patients treated with ropinirole achieved a greater reduction in percent of time spent off during waking hours when compared to placebo (11.7% vs. 5.1%), which was a difference of 0.4 hours. A greater amount of ropinirole-treated patients achieved a significant 20% reduction in time spent off (35% vs. 13%, $P = 0.003$). In those treated with levodopa, the levodopa dose was decreased by an average of 19%.

Long-acting dopamine agonist formulations, including ER ropinirole and rotigotine, have also shown reductions in off-time. In a study of 208 PD patients not optimally controlled with levodopa after up to 3 years of therapy with less than 600 mg/day of levodopa, a prolonged-release, once-daily formulation of ropinirole was found to improve motor scores in a similar fashion to increase the levodopa dose; however, only 3% of ropinirole-treated subjects experienced dyskinesias compared with 17% of levodopa-treated patients ($P<0.001$).[86] In moderate-to-advanced PD, treatment benefits were observed within 2 weeks of initiation.[87] Extended-release ropinirole has been found to reduce off-time more than the immediate-release preparation in advanced PD. A randomized, double-blind trial of 343 patients over 24 weeks found that compared to the immediate-release formulation, significantly more patients given the ER formulation maintained at least a 20% reduction in off-time (adjusted OR: 1.82, 1.16–2.86, $P = 0.009$).[88] These results are confounded by the relatively higher doses of ER ropinirole and greater reductions in levodopa achieved by the ER formulation. Rotigotine has also been evaluated for reduction in off-time in advanced PD patients and has been shown to significantly reduce off-time by approximately 2.5 hours, with benefits seen as early as the first week of therapy.[50]

Because L.M. has advanced disease and is experiencing motor fluctuations despite a treatment regimen that includes a dopamine agonist, further dose adjustments of the dopamine agonist may provide little additional benefit. Any adjustments must be made with consideration of worsening his dyskinesias and the possibility of exacerbating CNS adverse effects.

Apomorphine

Apomorphine is an injectable dopamine agonist that is approved as rescue therapy for treatment of hypomobility or off episodes in patients with PD. In a randomized, double-blind, parallel-group study of 29 patients, rescue treatment with apomorphine resulted in a 34% reduction in off-time, approximately 2 hours, compared with 0% in the placebo group ($P = 0.02$).[89] Mean UPDRS motor scores were reduced by 23.9 points (62%) in those treated with apomorphine, compared with 0.1 (1%) in those receiving placebo ($P<0.001$). Adverse events in the apomorphine group included yawning (40%), dyskinesias (35%), drowsiness or somnolence (35%), nausea or vomiting (30%), and dizziness (20%), although only yawning was statistically different from placebo (40% vs. 0%; $P = 0.03$).

Because nausea and vomiting frequently occur with apomorphine treatment, it should be administered with an antiemetic such as trimethobenzamide. The antiemetic should be started 3 days before initiating apomorphine and continued for the first 2 months of treatment.[89] Apomorphine should not be used with ondansetron and other serotonin antagonists used to treat nausea because the combination may cause severe hypotension. In addition, other antiemetics, such as prochlorperazine and metoclopramide, should not be given concurrently because these dopamine antagonists may decrease the effectiveness of apomorphine.

Doses of apomorphine range from 2 to 6 mg per subcutaneous injection. A 2-mg test dose is recommended while monitoring blood pressure. If tolerated, the recommendation is to start with a dose of 2 mg and increase the dose by 1 mg every few days if needed. Peak plasma levels are observed within 10 to 60 minutes after dosing, so the onset of therapeutic effect is rapid. The test dose and titration are time-consuming and must be done under physician supervision, and patients may require someone else to inject the drug once hypomobility has occurred. In severe cases, subcutaneous infusions have been used, but are limited to research settings and high-level clinical centers. For these reasons, apomorphine is not widely used. Given that L.M. is experiencing motor fluctuations almost daily, long-term frequent apomorphine use would not be a viable solution in his situation.

AMANTADINE

The antiviral agent, amantadine, was serendipitously found to improve PD symptoms when a patient given the drug for influenza experienced a remission in her parkinsonism.[90] Amantadine reduces all the symptoms of parkinsonian disability in about 50% of patients, usually within days after starting therapy; however, early trials indicated that amantadine efficacy might be limited by the development of tachyphylaxis within 1 to 3 months.[91] Although the trials suggested reductions in dyskinesias by up to 40%, previous evaluations of amantadine for the reduction of dyskinesias have been limited by methodological concerns.

The pathophysiologic basis for the efficacy of amantadine in PD is not entirely understood; it may augment dopamine release and possibly inhibit its reuptake.[92] Anticholinergic action has also been suggested. Excess glutamatergic activity has been implicated in the pathophysiology of dopaminergic dyskinesias; amantadine has been found to be an antagonist at *N*-methyl-D-aspartate (NMDA) receptors and to block glutamate transmission.[93] Amantadine has consistently shown approximately 50% reductions in dyskinesia severity and duration, without adversely impacting motor performance.[94–97] Two trials have evaluated long-term efficacy of amantadine in patients with levodopa-induced dyskinesia after treatment for 6 months to 1 year. These trials assessed for change in UPDRS motor examination and motor complication subscores with amantadine washout over 3 weeks to 3 months. Those discontinuing amantadine had deterioration in levodopa-induced dyskinesia compared to the continuing group within a median time of 7 days suggesting the possibility of continued benefit despite the tachyphylaxis suggested in earlier trials.[98,99] Guidance suggests reserving consideration for amantadine use to those in whom dyskinesia is not adequately managed on other therapies.[17]

The decision to use amantadine in L.M. should be based on whether his dyskinesias are deemed more problematic than his duration of off-time. If so, amantadine should be started at 100 mg/day taken at breakfast; an additional 100-mg dose can be taken with lunch 5 to 7 days after initiation. The dose can be increased to a maximum of 300 mg/day; however, doses in excess of 200 mg/day are associated with increased adverse effects and should be used cautiously. Amantadine is renally excreted, and the dose should be reduced in patients with renal impairment.[100] If the dyskinesias that L.M. is experiencing are tolerable but the duration of off-time is more problematic, then selection of another agent such as a COMT inhibitor or MAO-B inhibitor may be more appropriate than the initiation of amantadine at this time.

Side effects of amantadine mainly involve the gastrointestinal (e.g., nausea, vomiting) and CNS (e.g., dizziness, confusion, insomnia, nightmares, and hallucinations). Patients receiving concomitant anticholinergic therapy may experience more prominent CNS side effects.[100] Livedo reticularis, a rose-colored mottling of the skin usually involving the lower extremities, can occur with amantadine as early as 2 weeks after initiating therapy. The consequences of livedo reticularis are entirely cosmetic, and discontinuation of therapy is unnecessary. Ankle edema may be seen in association with livedo reticularis. Elevation of the legs, diuretic therapy, and dosage reduction often alleviate the edema.

CATECHOL-O-METHYLTRANSFERASE INHIBITORS

COMT is an enzyme widely distributed throughout the body that is responsible for the biotransformation of many catechols and hydroxylated metabolites, including levodopa. When carbidopa, an inhibitor of aromatic AAD, is coadministered with levodopa, the peripheral conversion of levodopa to dopamine via this pathway is inhibited; as a consequence, the conversion of levodopa to 3-*O*-methyldopa (3-OMD) by COMT is amplified and becomes the major metabolic pathway for levodopa degradation. The metabolite 3-OMD lacks antiparkinsonian activity and may compete with levodopa for transport into the circulation and brain. By preventing its peripheral degradation, the therapeutic effect of levodopa can be extended via inhibition of COMT.

Entacapone and tolcapone are selective, reversible, and potent COMT inhibitors that increase the amount of levodopa available for transport across the blood–brain barrier (Figure 59-4) to prolong its therapeutic effect. Use of these agents is associated with increased on-time and a decrease in the daily levodopa dose.[101,102] The pharmacologic and pharmacokinetic effects of entacapone and tolcapone are compared in Table 59-5.[101–103] Two uncontrolled trials and one controlled evaluation of patients with motor fluctuations newly placed on entacapone compared switching patients to tolcapone versus continuing the newly started entacapone. These trials alluded to the therapeutic benefits of tolcapone compared to entacapone; however, tolcapone is associated with cases of fatal, acute fulminant liver failure. This has led to stringent liver function monitoring requirements and limited clinical use. If initiated, liver function monitoring should be performed at baseline and every 2 to 4 weeks for the first 6 months, followed periodically thereafter as clinically necessary.[101] Because of the risks for hepatotoxicity associated with tolcapone, entacapone is the preferred COMT inhibitor and would be a good choice for L.M. if he desires an increase in his on-time.

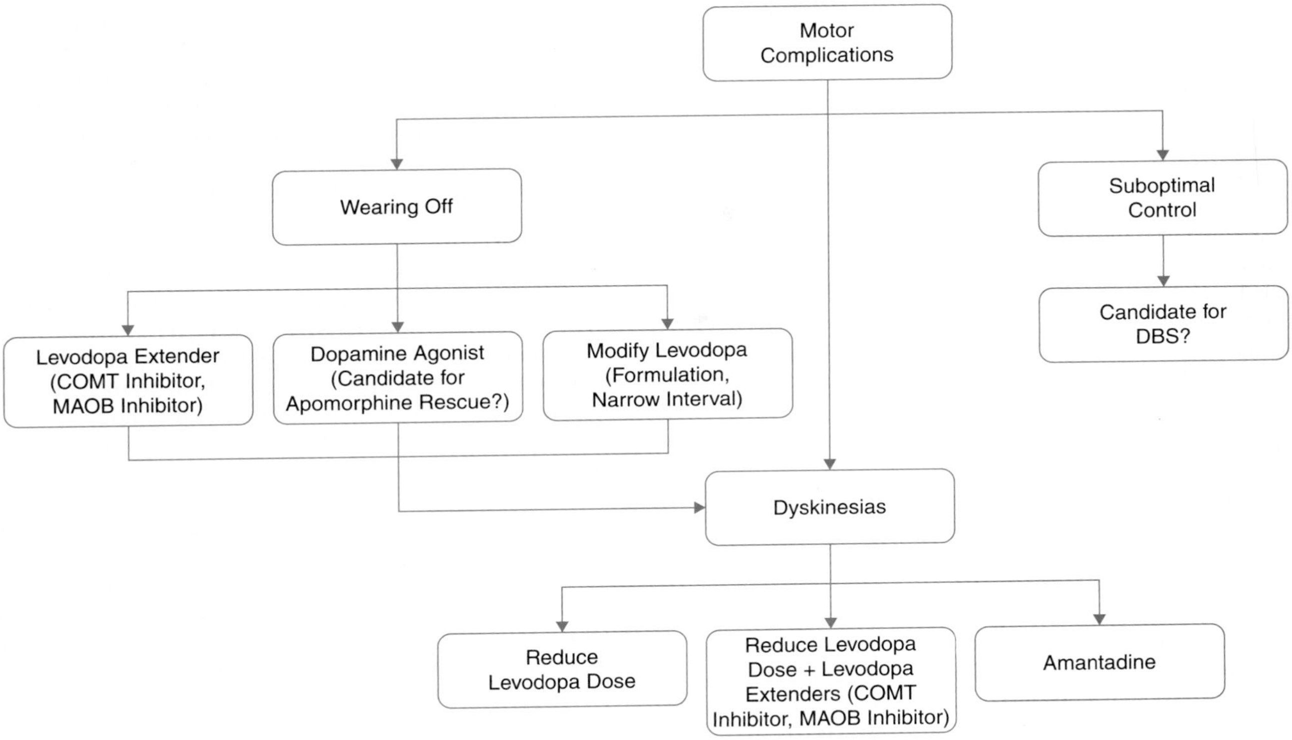

Figure 59-4 Suggested treatment algorithm for the management motor complications in late PD. DBS, deep brain stimulation.

Entacapone

CASE 59-1, QUESTION 15: Six months after adjusting the frequency of his carbidopa/levodopa dose and adding amantadine, L.M. reports that his dyskinesias are not too bothersome, but he is now having increased periods (lasting a few minutes) in which he cannot move. He is currently taking amantadine 100 mg twice daily, pramipexole 0.5 mg 3 times daily, and immediate-release carbidopa/levodopa 25 mg/250 mg 5 times a day, but "even on a good day" gains symptomatic relief for only about 2 to 3 hours after a dose. The decision is made to initiate entacapone therapy and gradually discontinue pramipexole as guided by symptoms or side effects. How effective is entacapone for reducing the symptoms of PD?

Early initiation of a COMT inhibitor at the same time that levodopa is first introduced has been proposed as a way of reducing the development of levodopa-induced motor complications[104]; theoretically, this strategy should provide more stable plasma levels of levodopa and lessen pulsatile stimulation of striatal dopamine receptors normally observed with intermittent levodopa dosing. This strategy was tested in the Stalevo Reduction in Dyskinesia Evaluation in Parkinson's Disease (STRIDE-PD) study, a multicenter, double-blind study that randomly assigned 747 patients to initiate either carbidopa/levodopa or carbidopa/levodopa/entacapone 4 times daily.[104] Surprisingly, patients randomly assigned to receive carbidopa/levodopa/entacapone actually had a shorter time to onset of dyskinesia (hazard ratio: 1.29; $P = 0.04$) and increased dyskinesia frequency at week 134 (42% vs. 32%; $P = 0.02$). These findings may have been confounded by an increased use

Table 59-5
Pharmacologic and Pharmacokinetic Properties of Catechol-*O*-Methyltransferase Inhibitors

	Tolcapone	Entacapone
Bioavailability	65%–68%	35%
T_{max} (hours)	1.7	1
Protein binding	99.9%	98%
Metabolism	Glucuronidation; CYP3A4, CYP2A6 methylated by COMT	Isomerization, glucuronidation
Half-life (hours)	2–3	Biphasic; 0.4–0.7, 2.4
Time to reverse COMT inhibition (hours)	16–24	8
Maximal COMT inhibition at 200-mg dose	>80%	65%
Increase in levodopa AUC	100%	35%
Increase in levodopa half-life	75%	85%
Dosing method	TID, spaced 6 hours apart	With every administration of levodopa

AUC, area under the curve; COMT, catechol-*O*-methyltransferase; CYP, cytochrome P-450; TID, three times daily.

 of dopaminergic therapy in the entacapone group. The findings of the STRIDE-PD study do not support the early administration of entacapone in combination with levodopa to reduce the occurrence of motor complications.

The efficacy and safety of entacapone as an adjunct to levodopa therapy in the presence of motor complications was established in two pivotal multicenter, randomized, double-blind, placebo-controlled trials.[105,106] Subjects for both studies had idiopathic PD with motor fluctuations, including wearing-off phenomena, despite maximal tolerated doses of levodopa. In both trials, patients were randomly assigned to receive either entacapone 200 mg or placebo (up to 10 doses/day) with each dose of carbidopa/levodopa.[105,106] In both trials, significant improvements in off-time (approximately 1 hour), UPDRS scores (10% improvement), and levodopa doses (reductions of approximately 80–100 mg/day) were consistent.

Dosing

CASE 59-1, QUESTION 16: When should entacapone be initiated in L.M., and how should it be dosed?

Entacapone is approved for use as adjunctive therapy to levodopa for the treatment of PD in patients experiencing wearing-off or end-of-dose deterioration. It is given as one 200-mg tablet with each carbidopa/levodopa administration, up to eight tablets/day. It is available in a combination tablet with a 1:4 ratio of immediate-release carbidopa/levodopa that patients can be switched to once they are stabilized on individual formulations of carbidopa/levodopa and entacapone. If dyskinesias occur, it may be necessary to lower the levodopa dose by approximately 10% to 25%, particularly if the patient is receiving more than 800 mg/day of levodopa. Although pramipexole is being discontinued in L.M., he should still be monitored for dyskinesias, especially during the first few weeks of therapy, as it may also be necessary to lower his carbidopa/levodopa dose.

Adverse Effects

CASE 59-1, QUESTION 17: What are the adverse effects of entacapone, and how should they be managed?

Most entacapone-induced adverse effects are consistent with increased levodopa exposure. They include dyskinesias (50%–60%), dizziness (10%–25%), nausea (15%–20%), and hallucinations (1%–14%).[105,106] Reducing the levodopa dosage by 10% to 15% as a strategy for circumventing these effects is successful in about one-third of patients experiencing dyskinesias. Other adverse effects related to entacapone include urine discoloration (11%–40%), diarrhea (10%), and abdominal pain (6%).[105,106] Urine discoloration (brownish orange) is attributed to entacapone and its metabolites and is considered benign, but patients should be counseled regarding this effect. The most common reason for withdrawal from clinical studies and discontinuation of therapy was severe diarrhea (2.5%).[107] Although the results of the STRIDE-PD study indicated that patients taking the combination of carbidopa/levodopa/entacapone may be at an increased risk for cardiovascular events (e.g., heart attack, stroke, and cardiovascular death) compared with those taking carbidopa/levodopa, subsequent FDA analysis has found no increased risk.[108]

MONOAMINE OXIDASE-B INHIBITORS

Selegiline

Selegiline may have a role as a symptomatic adjunct to levodopa in more advanced disease. Studies have found improvement in the wearing-off effect in 50% to 70% of patients and a reduction in as much as 30% in the total daily dose of levodopa without improvements in on-time.[109,110] This improvement has also been shown to arrive with an initial worsening of dyskinesis in 60% of treated patients which may be counteracted with levodopa dose reductions. Selegiline has been shown to reduce off-time by 32% (2.2 hours) compared with 9% (0.6 hours; $P<0.001$) for placebo in a 12-week, randomized, multicenter, parallel-group, double-blind study, but was not reproducible in an identical trial.[111,112] Authors hypothesize that this conflict may be due in part to large and potentially variable placebo effects seen in PD trials. The on–off effect is less responsive to the addition of selegiline.

Rasagiline

Rasagiline has also been studied as an adjunct to levodopa in advanced disease. When added to levodopa therapy, rasagiline can improve motor fluctuations, reducing off-time by 1.4 hours and 1.8 hours (for the 0.5- and 1-mg/day groups, respectively) compared with 0.9 hours for placebo.[113] Patients treated with 0.5 mg/day and 1 mg/day of rasagiline had 0.49 hour (0.08–0.91; $P = 0.02$) and 0.94 hour (1.36–0.51; $P<0.001$) less off-time compared with placebo. Significant improvements were reported in the UPDRS subscores for ADLs in the off state and motor performance in the on state, as well as clinician global assessments. Dyskinesias were slightly worsened in the 1-mg/day group. As adjunctive therapy to levodopa, rasagiline appears to provide similar benefit to entacapone.[16] In the Lasting effect in Adjunct therapy with Rasagiline Given Once daily (LARGO) study, when compared with entacapone 200 mg administered with each levodopa dose, rasagiline 1 mg/day reduced total daily off-time in a similar manner (decrease of 21% or 1.18 hours for rasagiline and 21% or 1.2 hours for entacapone).[114] Reduction of levodopa dose may be necessary if dyskinesias occur when rasagiline is added in combination with levodopa.

Safinamide

Safinamide (Xadago) was approved by the FDA in May 2017 as an adjunct to carbidopa/levodopa for patients experiencing "off" episodes. It is not approved as monotherapy and thus has not been previously discussed. The side effect profile is similar to rasagiline (see Table 59-2). Patients should additionally be monitored for visual changes as retinal detachment and loss of photoreceptor cells were noted in animal studies. The list of contraindicated medications is extensive and should be reviewed prior to starting therapy. Safinamide has a half–life of 20-26 hours, reaches steady state in 5-6 days, and can be taken without regard to meals. It requires hepatic dose adjustment but no renal dose adjustments. The extent of use in clinical practice and eventual place in therapy are unknown at this time.

Surgical Therapies for PD

CASE 59-1, QUESTION 18: L.M. is now classified as Hoehn and Yahr[2] late stage 3. He is now on amantadine 100 mg twice daily, immediate-release carbidopa/levodopa 25 mg/250 mg 5 times daily, and entacapone 200 mg 5 times daily with carbidopa/levodopa administrations. His overall control of his PD has diminished greatly in the last couple of months. His on-time averages around 6 hours/day, with the majority of it accompanied by troublesome dyskinesias. Most days he needs some assistance with ADLs. His cognitive function remains well preserved, and he is not depressed. He has heard about surgical procedures that might benefit patients with PD. Is surgical therapy superior to medical therapy in patients with advanced PD?

Two types of surgical therapies have been used in patients with advanced PD who cannot be adequately controlled with medications. The first involves making an irreversible surgical lesion in a specific location in the brain (e.g., posteroventral pallidotomy or stereotaxic thalamotomy); the second involves

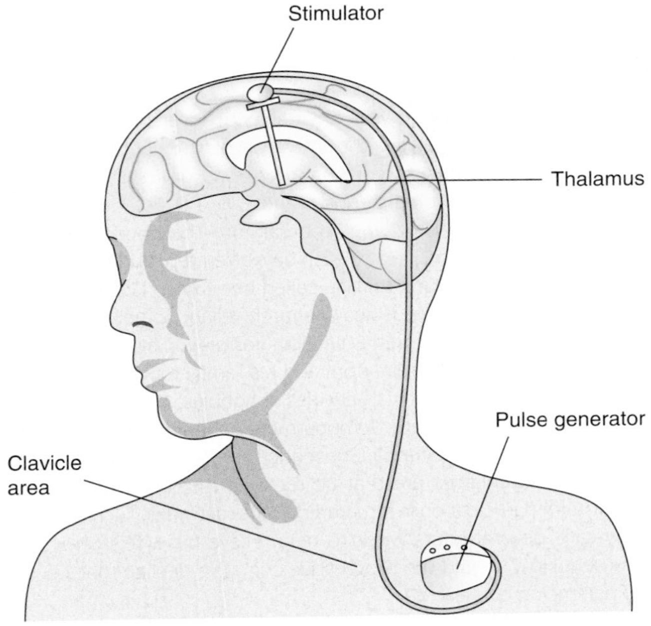

Figure 59-5 Deep brain stimulation. A pulse generator, surgically implanted in a pouch beneath the clavicle, sends high-frequency electrical impulses to the thalamus, thereby blocking the nerve pathways associated with tremors in PD. (Adapted with permission from Smeltzer SC, Bare BG. *Textbook of Medical-Surgical Nursing*. 9th ed. Philadelphia, PA: Lippincott Williams & Wilkins; 2000.)

surgical implantation of a device that sends electrical impulses to specific parts of the brain (e.g., deep brain stimulation [DBS]) (Figure 59-5). Posteroventral pallidotomy has been shown to reduce dyskinesias on the contralateral side and may permit the use of higher dosages of levodopa for managing rigidity and bradykinesia.[115] However, a significant disadvantage is the need to make a lesion near the optic tract, which may risk visual loss. Other possible risks of pallidotomy include weakness, paralysis, and hemorrhage that can cause stroke and speech difficulty. Stereotaxic thalamotomy has been shown to reduce symptoms of debilitating tremor and improve rigidity in patients with PD.[116] This intervention has eliminated contralateral tremor in 80% of patients, and improvement has been sustained for up to 10 years. However, as with pallidotomy, a disadvantage of thalamotomy is the need to make an irreversible lesion in the basal ganglia that may limit the effectiveness of newer procedures because they become available. Thus, DBS is now the preferred surgical method for treating advanced PD that cannot be adequately controlled with medications. DBS uses an implanted electrode in the brain, in either the subthalamic nucleus (STN) or the globus pallidus interna (GPi), which is connected to a subcutaneously implanted pacemaker. This permits delivery of high-frequency stimulation to the desired target. Advantages of DBS include no need for an irreversible brain lesion, and it provides flexibility for altering the target site and program stimulation parameters.

The efficacy of DBS in advanced PD was shown in a two-part study of 255 patients with idiopathic PD responsive to levodopa but with persistent and disabling motor symptoms.[117] Patients were randomly assigned to DBS or best medical therapy and followed for 6 months. Patients receiving DBS gained a mean of 4.6 hours/day of on-time without troubling dyskinesias compared with 0 hours/day for best medical therapy ($P<0.001$). Additionally, 71% of patients receiving DBS experienced clinically meaningful motor function improvements (≥5-point change in UPDRS motor score) compared with only 32% of patients receiving best medical therapy ($P<0.001$).[117]

Case 59-1, Question 19: What surgical therapy would be most appropriate for L.M.?

L.M. appears to be an ideal candidate for DBS. Candidates for DBS should have idiopathic PD and be levodopa-responsive, but continue to experience motor complications or tremor despite optimal pharmacotherapeutic regimens. Ideally, DBS should be avoided in patients with preexisting cognitive or psychiatric problems owing to a slight risk of decline in cognition. No strict age limitation for DBS exists, but patients younger than 70 years of age, such as L.M., appear to recover from surgery more quickly and show greater motor improvements. Deep brain stimulation of the STN consistently demonstrates marked reduction in the need for escalating levodopa dosages compared with DBS of the GPi,[118–121] but data suggest other nonmotor symptoms such as visual processing speed and depression may be affected more favorably when targeting the GPi.[118]

Investigational Pharmacotherapy

CASE 59-2

Question 1: K.B. is a 61-year-old woman who presents to the movement disorders clinic after referral from her family doctor for a presumptive diagnosis of PD. She is Hoehn and Yahr[2] stage 1, with slightly decreased arm swing on the left side and unilateral resting hand tremor. Her past medical history is significant for hypertension and mild renal insufficiency (serum creatinine of 1.4 mg/dL). Since her initial visit with her family physician, she has been researching information about different PD treatments from several PD-related websites. Are there any antioxidants, dietary supplements, or other investigational therapies that may benefit K.B.?

ANTIOXIDANTS

Antioxidants have been hypothesized to benefit patients with PD through their ability to act as free radical scavengers. The most comprehensive evaluation of antioxidant therapy for PD comes from the DATATOP study.[109,122,123] In this study, patients with early PD were assigned to one of four treatment regimens: α-tocopherol (2,000 international units[IU]/day) and selegiline placebo; selegiline 10 mg/day and α-tocopherol placebo; selegiline and α-tocopherol active treatments; or dual placebos. The primary endpoint was time to requirement of levodopa therapy. After approximately 14 months of follow-up, no difference was seen between the α-tocopherol group and placebo group in time to require levodopa.[123] Thus, despite the theoretic benefit, clinical data are lacking to support the routine use of α-tocopherol, and it would not be recommended in K.B.[124]

COENZYME Q10

Coenzyme Q10 (CoQ_{10}) is an antioxidant involved in the mitochondrial electron transport chain and has been shown to be reduced in patients with PD.[125] A futility analysis in untreated PD patients treated with CoQ_{10} failed to show statistical significance but met the threshold for futility. Two subsequent phase III trials of early PD patients failed to show symptomatic or neuroprotective benefits.[125–127] In an evaluation of 600 patients with early PD, subjects were randomized to receive either 1,200 or 2,400 mg of CoQ_{10} daily in addition to 1,200 IU of α-tocopherol. The study was terminated prematurely due to failure to meet prespecified futility endpoints and trend in adverse outcomes compared to placebo.[127] Due to the lack of data supporting CoQ10, K.B. should be counseled to avoid its use.

CREATINE AND MINOCYCLINE

Similar to CoQ_{10}, creatine is thought to play a role in mitochondrial energy production and has been shown to protect from MPTP-induced dopamine depletion in animal models.[128] Minocycline is an anti-infective agent that also displays anti-inflammatory effects and is hypothesized to alter the neuroinflammatory response that occurs because dopaminergic neurons are lost in PD. Minocycline has been shown to be protective in MPTP animal models of PD.[128]

The use of both creatine and minocycline in PD was examined in a futility-design study, in which patients with early PD not requiring therapy were randomly assigned to receive creatine 10 g/day, minocycline 200 mg/day, or placebo.[128] After 12 months, the mean change in the total UPDRS could not be rejected as futile and met criteria for further clinical testing. A long-term follow-up of this trial found that by 18 months, patients requiring symptomatic treatment did not differ but significantly more patients on minocycline discontinued therapy prematurely (23% vs. 9% of creatine and 6% of placebo patients). Given the unresolved issues surrounding the induction of antibiotic resistance with long-term use of an agent such as minocycline and concerns for tolerability, it is generally not recommended. A long-term, randomized, double-blind, placebo-controlled trial of creatine 10 g/day versus placebo in early treated PD was terminated early for futility based upon an interim analysis. The trial concluded that treatment with creatine for at least 5 years does not support its use in PD.[129] Given the lack of data supporting these agents, they should be avoided in K.B.

FUTURE THERAPIES

With developments in PD research and biopharmaceutical technology, new treatment targets and modalities are constantly being investigated. Such targets include transcription factors, proteins, and their mutations. Novel pharmaceutical and biologic technologies under development include small-molecule drug delivery, such as with glial-cell-derived neurotrophic factor, stem cell therapies, and nerve cell grafts.

Nonmotor Symptoms of Parkinson's Disease

Although PD is mostly recognized for its cardinal features of motor dysfunction, nonmotor symptoms are an important part of the disease throughout all stages and are a key determinant of quality of life.[130] More than 98% of patients with PD have at least one nonmotor symptom; the average per patient is nearly eight, with the number and impact increasing with disease duration and severity.[131] Common nonmotor symptoms include autonomic dysfunction (e.g., gastrointestinal disorders, orthostatic hypotension, sexual dysfunction, urinary incontinence, sialorrhea, seborrhea, and constipation), sleep disorders (e.g., RLS, PLMS, excessive daytime somnolence, insomnia, REM sleep behavior disorder), fatigue, and psychiatric disorders (e.g., dementia, depression, and anxiety).[131] In one longitudinal study of patients with PD, the most common nonmotor symptoms were psychiatric symptoms (68%, most commonly anxiety), fatigue (58%), leg pain (38%), insomnia (37%), urinary symptoms (35%), drooling (31%), and difficulty concentrating (31%).[131] Regular screening for these nonmotor symptoms should occur. L.M. has a history of depression treated with citalopram that could be attributable to PD, and his therapy should be periodically evaluated. The forgetfulness and decreased memory described by L.M. could be early signs of cognitive decline and warrant close observation. The management of several commonly encountered nonmotor symptoms is reviewed below.

DEMENTIA

CASE 59-3

QUESTION 1: J.D. is a 74-year-old man with advanced PD, Hoehn and Yahr[2] stage 4. During the last year, his family has noticed that he is increasingly forgetful and anxious. Twice recently, he left home alone for brief periods, and called 9-1-1 because he thought someone was trying to break into the house. He also calls his daughter 2 or 3 times each day, often repeating the same questions and forgetting that he called her earlier. His wife is his primary caregiver, and he is nearly entirely reliant on her for help in performing ADLs. He scored 20 (below normal) on his most recent Mini-Mental Status Examination, and his family reports that he is no longer interested in social activities or hobbies. Neuropsychiatric testing is performed and demonstrates a significant depressive component to his dementia. Subsequent recommendations from the neuropsychiatrist are that he receives 24-hour supervision, along with participation in structured leisure activities, such as adult day care, several hours/week to help relieve his wife's caregiver burden. How should the progressive cognitive decline that J.D. is experiencing be treated?

The prevalence of dementia in patients with PD is high; 48% to 80% of patients may develop dementia during the disease course, at a rate approximately 6 times greater than healthy individuals.[17,132] One longitudinal study of 136 incident cases of PD followed for 20 years found that nearly 100% eventually exhibited dementia.[133] The prevalence of cognitive decline and dementia among patients with PD ranges from 10% to 30% and may be associated with a more rapid progression of disease-related disability.[6] Successful management of cognitive impairment in patients with PD first requires that all potentially reversible causes and underlying contributing factors be addressed. These include treating infections, dehydration, and metabolic abnormalities, as well as eliminating unnecessary medications (particularly anticholinergics, sedatives, and anxiolytics) that can exacerbate dementia or delirium.

Experience with cholinesterase inhibitors for treating cognitive impairment in PD indicates marginal improvements with their use.[134–136] Two randomized, controlled trials of donepezil have failed to show consistent benefit, whereas galantamine has only been evaluated in a single open-label trial.[137,138] Rivastigmine was found to provide clinically meaningful (moderate or marked improvement on the Alzheimer's Disease Cooperative Study–Clinician's Global Impression of Change) benefit to significantly more patients than placebo in a large, randomized, placebo-controlled trial and has demonstrated sustained cognitive benefit for up to 48 weeks.[136,139,140] As a result, rivastigmine was FDA-approved for the management of mild-to-moderate dementia in PD and is therefore the drug of choice. Compared with placebo, the cholinesterase inhibitors often result in statistically significant changes on cognitive scales; though, their impact on function and disposition is unclear.

A cholinesterase inhibitor such as rivastigmine may be considered for patients such as J.D., although he must be monitored closely for signs of deterioration of motor function such as worsening of tremor.[137] Cholinesterase inhibitors are associated with other adverse events that may be overlooked and attributed to the PD itself, including sialorrhea, excessive lacrimation, incontinence, nausea, vomiting, and orthostasis. Perhaps more important than any medication therapy, adequate social support for J.D. should be ensured. Because he becomes further dependent on family members for assistance with ADLs, the increased needs of the caregiver(s) should also be considered. In the case of J.D., attending adult day care several times weekly, if available, would provide a structured, supervised environment for interaction with others, as well as providing a rest period for his caregiver. Dementia is a leading cause of nursing home placement for patients with PD.[137]

DEPRESSION/ANXIETY

CASE 59-3, QUESTION 2: How should anxiety and depression be treated in J.D.?

Despite being one of the strongest predictors of quality of life in PD patients, depression is often poorly recognized and inadequately treated.[137] This is likely because depression and PD share overlapping features that often confound the identification of depression. Withdrawal, lack of motivation, flattened affect, decreased physical activity, and bradyphrenia are examples of overlapping features.[137]

Treatment of depression in PD should first focus on providing adequate treatment of the symptoms of PD by attempting to restore mobility and independence, particularly in patients whose depression can be attributed to lengthy off periods. Antiparkinsonian drugs, such as pramipexole, can be associated with mood-enhancing effects independent of their ability to reduce time in the off state.[137] Small trials and case reports have shown that depression in patients with PD can be successfully treated with antidepressant drugs, including tricyclic agents such as amitriptyline, desipramine, nortriptyline, bupropion, and selective serotonin reuptake inhibitors (SSRIs) such as citalopram and paroxetine.[137] Given the overall lack of high-quality trials, it is difficult to know whether expected benefits reflect class responses or are unique to the individual agents studied. Importantly, the potential for adverse effects should always be considered. For example, some SSRIs, such as fluoxetine, can be activating. Although this may be beneficial in patients who are apathetic or withdrawn, it may worsen symptoms in patients with PD who are agitated. Selective serotonin reuptake inhibitors have additionally been noted to worsen PD tremor in approximately 5% of patients.[141] With tricyclic antidepressants, care must be taken to observe for anticholinergic side effects that may worsen PD symptoms, such as impaired cognition, delayed gastric emptying (which may reduce levodopa effectiveness by increasing levodopa degradation in the gut), urinary problems, orthostatic hypotension, and increased risk of falls. Additionally, consideration should be taken for drug interactions and the risk for serotonin syndrome with concomitant MAO-B inhibitors. Electroconvulsive therapy may be considered in refractory cases, but may adversely affect cognition.

Based on his symptoms, it is reasonable to start J.D. on an antidepressant. Clinical experience suggests a good initial choice for balancing efficacy and safety is an SSRI, such as citalopram. As with other patients with depression, the choice of agent should be individualized based on other pragmatic factors such as cost, potential for adverse effects, and personal or family history of response to prior agents. Regardless of which agent or class of antidepressant is selected, therapy should be started at the lowest dose and gradually titrated to effect. He should be monitored closely for side effects, particularly anticholinergic symptoms with tricyclic antidepressants, and for any adverse effects on mobility. He should be observed carefully for changes in parkinsonian symptoms, including development of extrapyramidal symptoms, as well as any signs of psychomotor agitation. Short-term use of benzodiazepines, such as lorazepam or alprazolam, may also provide relief of anxiety symptoms, but must be used cautiously due to adverse effects on cognition and risk of falling.[142] Generally, anxiety symptoms should improve with treatment of the underlying depression.

PSYCHOSIS

In PD, the incidence of psychotic symptoms increases with age, cognitive impairment, and disease duration.[143] Other risk factors include higher age at PD onset, high doses of dopaminergic drugs, and REM sleep behavior disorder.[144] Symptoms are often more pronounced at night (the "sundowning" effect), and hallucinations are typically visual. As with the management of cognitive impairment, it is important to eliminate or minimize any potential causative factors, particularly anticholinergic medications that could be contributing to the hallucinations or delirium. In some patients, reducing the dose of levodopa improves mental function and also provides satisfactory control of motor features. If it is not possible to achieve a balance between preserving motor control and decreasing neuropsychiatric symptoms through reduction in levodopa dosage, antipsychotics may be considered.

Older antipsychotic medications, such as haloperidol, perphenazine, and chlorpromazine, block striatal dopamine D_2 receptors and may exacerbate parkinsonian symptoms. Therefore, these agents are not recommended. Newer atypical antipsychotics are more selective for limbic and cortical D_3, D_4, and D_5 receptors; they have minimal activity at D_2 receptors and may control symptoms without worsening parkinsonism. Of these agents, clozapine has the best evidence of efficacy in patients with PD without adversely affecting motor function and should be preferentially considered.[137] However, its use is complicated by the need for frequent monitoring of white blood cell counts because of the risk of agranulocytosis. Other newer agents, particularly quetiapine, appear promising and have controlled psychosis without worsening parkinsonism.[17,137] Risperidone and olanzapine have also been studied, but both worsened parkinsonism and were inferior to clozapine in patients with PD.[137,145] Aripiprazole, also a newer atypical antipsychotic, has been associated with worsening motor function in patients with PD, whereas experience with ziprasidone has yielded mixed results.[146]

AUTONOMIC DYSFUNCTION

Patients with PD frequently experience dysautonomia, including orthostasis, erectile dysfunction, constipation, nocturia, sensory disturbances, dysphagia, seborrhea, and thermoregulatory imbalances. Management of these symptoms is generally supportive, and appropriate medical interventions similar to those used in other geriatric patients can be used to treat these symptoms whenever encountered. In some cases, fludrocortisone or midodrine can be considered if orthostatic hypotension is severe, although these drugs have not been well studied in PD patients specifically.[130] Other possibly effective treatments for symptoms of autonomic dysfunction include sildenafil for erectile dysfunction and polyethylene glycol for constipation.[130]

A new atypical antipsychotic, pimavanserin, was FDA-approved in April 2016 based on results from one randomized, placebo-controlled trial. This agent's mechanism of action is unique, acting through serotonin receptors, and as such it avoids interaction with dopamine receptors responsible for the worsening of PD symptoms with other antipsychotics. It is not without its own risks, including cardiovascular and paradoxical worsening of psychosis.[147]

FALLS

Patients with PD and their caregivers should be counseled on the prevention of falls because they can result in serious morbidity and mortality. Falls generally result from one of several factors, including postural instability, freezing and festination, levodopa-induced dyskinesia, symptomatic orthostatic hypotension, coexisting neurologic or other medical disorders, and environmental factors. Prevention remains the best strategy and includes environmental precautions, such as proper lighting, use of handrails, removing tripping hazards, and incorporating physical and occupational therapy. Reversible causes of postural or gait instability should be addressed whenever suspected. Patients with PD are advised to take a vitamin D supplement to reduce their risk of fracture with future falls.[17]

SLEEP DISORDERS

Sleep disorders may occur at any time during the disease course and may even precede motor symptom development.[17] In excessive daytime drowsiness, a common sleep disorder in PD, treatment with modafinil may be considered.[130] Other sleep disorders such as insomnia, sleep fragmentation owing to PD symptoms, RLS, and REM sleep disorder (characterized by vivid dreams that are often acted out, especially if frightening) are common and a source of decreased quality of life. When sleep dysfunction can be directly attributed to PD symptoms, such as akinesia, tremor, dyskinesia, or nightmares, dosage adjustment of dopaminergic medications is indicated. Proper sleep hygiene should be encouraged. Insomnia symptoms unrelated to PD symptoms are treated similar to non-PD patients and can be managed supportively.

Table 59-6
Clinical Features of Restless Legs Syndrome (RLS)

Essential Criteria
Urge to move legs, associated with paresthesias or dysesthesias
Relief of symptoms with movement
Onset or exacerbation of symptoms at rest
Onset or worsening of symptoms during nighttime
Supportive Clinical Features
Accompanying sleep disturbance (sleep-onset insomnia)
Periodic leg movements
Positive response to dopaminergic therapy
Positive family history of RLS
Otherwise normal physical examination

RLS, restless legs syndrome.

RESTLESS LEGS SYNDROME AND PERIODIC LIMB MOVEMENTS OF SLEEP

Clinical Presentation

CASE 59-4

QUESTION 1: J.J., a 47-year-old woman, presents to her family physician complaining of daytime fatigue and difficulty sleeping at night because of "jumpy legs." She reports being able to sleep only 4 to 5 hours/night because of the leg restlessness and feels unrefreshed after sleep. On further questioning, she describes the sensation in her legs as being like "bugs crawling under the skin." The sensation is not painful. She explains that the symptoms worsen in the evening and at night and are partially relieved with walking. She recalls that her mother had similar symptoms. Her spouse notes that she often "kicks" him in her sleep. Review of her medical history shows an otherwise healthy postmenopausal woman. What signs and symptoms are suggestive of RLS in J.J.? What laboratory tests or diagnostic procedures should be performed in J.J. to evaluate her condition?

RLS, also known as Willis–Ekbom disease, is a disabling sensorimotor disorder estimated to affect approximately 2% of the adult population.[148] Although most patients with mild symptoms will not require treatment, RLS can be associated with adverse health outcomes, including sleep-onset insomnia, missed or late work, anxiety, depression, marital discord, and even suicide in severe cases.

Four essential criteria have been established by the International Restless Legs Syndrome Study Group to diagnose RLS (Table 59-6).[149] The pathognomonic trait of RLS is an almost irresistible urge to move the legs (akathisia), often associated with uncomfortable paresthesias or dysesthesias felt deep inside the limbs. Patients describe the sensation as "creepy-crawly" or "like soda water in the veins."[150] The symptoms may occur unilaterally or bilaterally, affecting the ankle, knee, or entire lower limb. With progressive disease, symptoms can begin earlier in the day, and progressive involvement of the arms or trunk may occur. Temporary or partial relief of symptoms can be achieved with movement. If patients attempt to ignore the urge to move the legs, akathisia will progressively intensify until either they move their legs or the legs jerk involuntarily.[150] Symptoms usually manifest in a circadian pattern with onset or worsening during nighttime hours (usually between 6 PM and 4 AM, with peak symptoms between midnight and 4 AM). The circadian pattern persists even in patients with inverted sleep–wake cycles. As a result of their symptoms, patients with RLS become "nightwalkers," spending significant time walking, stretching, or bending the legs in an effort to relieve symptoms.

The symptoms described by J.J. are an example of a classic presentation of RLS. The prevalence of RLS increases with age and appears to be slightly more common in women.[151] She describes "creepy-crawly" sensations that are relieved partially with walking, a core feature of RLS. Her symptoms are worse during the evening hours. J.J. reports that her mother suffered from similar symptoms. The observation of a familial tendency suggests a genetic component, and several chromosomal loci have been linked to the disease.[152] A strong family history of RLS appears to correlate with an early age of onset (<45 years), whereas presentation at a later age is associated with more neuropathy and accelerated disease progression.[150]

Most cases of RLS are considered primary or idiopathic; therefore, the diagnosis does not require elaborate laboratory tests or diagnostic procedures. Several conditions are associated with RLS and include iron deficiency, pregnancy, and end-stage renal disease. Several medications and substances are known aggravators of RLS, including medications with antidopaminergic properties, such as metoclopramide and prochlorperazine. Nicotine, caffeine, and alcohol can aggravate RLS through their own ability to interfere with quality of sleep. Additionally, SSRIs, tricyclic antidepressants, and commonly used over-the-counter antihistamines, such as diphenhydramine, can trigger or worsen RLS symptoms.[152] Hypotensive akathisia, leg cramps, and other conditions such as arthritis, which can cause positional discomfort with extended periods of sitting in one position, can mimic RLS. These conditions are easily distinguished from RLS because they are usually localized to certain joints or muscles, do not have a circadian pattern, and are not associated with an uncontrollable urge to move.

With an otherwise unremarkable physical examination and medical history, specific laboratory tests that should be performed in J.J. are limited to serum ferritin and percent transferrin saturation (total iron-binding capacity) to rule out iron deficiency anemia. Several studies have documented a relationship between low ferritin concentrations and increased symptom severity.[153] J.J. is postmenopausal, so a pregnancy test is not necessary. Polysomnography is not usually indicated unless there is clinical suspicion for sleep apnea or if sleep remains disrupted despite treatment of

RLS. When clinical suspicion from the physical examination or medical history suggests a possible peripheral nerve or radiculopathy cause, a routine neurologic panel should be obtained.[152] In end-stage renal failure, screening for uremia should be considered because this can trigger symptoms.

CASE 59-4, QUESTION 2: What is the difference between RLS and PLMS?

In addition to the presence of RLS, the symptoms reported by the spouse of J.J. are likely related to PLMS. These are also known as nocturnal myoclonus and are best described as involuntary clonic-type movements of the lower extremities while sleeping that usually involve bilateral ankle dorsiflexion, knee flexion, and hip flexion. Approximately 80% of patients with RLS will also have PLMS, but PLMS can occur by itself and is also associated with significant sleep dysfunction. The diagnosis of PLMS usually requires a polysomnogram; the universally accepted criteria for diagnosis are that there should be at least four periodic leg movements (PLMs) in a 90-second period, with contractions typically lasting 0.5 to 5 seconds and recurring every 5 to 90 seconds.[154] A PLM index (PLMI) is calculated by dividing the total number of PLMs by sleep time in hours; an index of more than 5 but less than 25 is considered mild, a PMLI of more than 25 and less than 50 is moderate, and a PLMI of more than 50 is severe. The diagnosis of PLM disorder can be made when patients present with insomnia, tiredness, and daytime sleepiness in the presence of a high PLMI.[155] There is considerable overlap in the treatments of PLMS and RLS. Because J.J. clearly has RLS, there is no need to perform a polysomnogram. The diagnosis of PLMS in her case is incidental and would not alter the clinical management. An exception to this would be whether her medical history revealed the possibility of sleep apnea, because there is a high association between PLMS and upper airway resistance.[156]

Treatment

CASE 59-4, QUESTION 3: The decision is made to initiate drug therapy in J.J. for the management of her symptoms. What pharmacologic therapy should be selected? What nonpharmacologic therapies should be recommended?

It is important to rule out possible reversible causes before treating RLS. Iron supplements can potentially cure RLS symptoms in patients found to be iron deficient.[157,158] If J.J. is iron deficient, she should be prescribed 50 to 65 mg of elemental iron 1 to 3 times daily on an empty stomach with 200 mg of vitamin C to enhance absorption. After ruling out possible reversible causes of RLS, it is important to establish the frequency of her symptoms and to select appropriate therapy.

Several classes of medications are effective for treating RLS.[153,157,158] Dopaminergic therapies are most consistently effective in relieving RLS symptoms, improving sleep, and reducing leg movements. High-quality evidence has found that levodopa/carbidopa improves RLS symptoms.[153,157,158] Dopamine agonists are the preferred dopaminergic class to treat RLS because they are longer acting than levodopa, which allows for more sustained efficacy and control of symptoms throughout the entire night.[153,157,158] J.J. should be started on either ropinirole (0.25 mg initially, up to 0.5–4 mg/day) or pramipexole (0.125 mg initially, up to 0.5 mg/day), because both are FDA-approved for treating RLS. Although rotigotine is approved and supported by guidelines, the transdermal formulation may limit use in the early titration phases of RLS management.[50] Several randomized, controlled clinical trials have documented efficacy of these agents in both objective and subjective ratings of improvement by patients and clinicians with either short- or long-term use.[153,157,158] Ropinirole and pramipexole do not appear to differ with regard to efficacy or adverse effects. When used for RLS, ropinirole and pramipexole should be administered 2 hours before bedtime. Adverse effects are similar to those seen with the use of these agents in PD, and patients should be counseled accordingly.

Other medications may also provide benefit in RLS. Guidelines recommend the use of pregabalin and gabapentin enacarbil.[153,157,158] As a result of their mechanisms of action, these agents may be helpful if JJ had RLS involving neuropathic pain or if she could not tolerate dopaminergic therapy. Though studied, there are inconclusive data to support the use of benzodiazepines, opiates, anticonvulsants, and clonidine.[153,157,158] Opiates may be helpful in patients who experience significant pain related to RLS, but these agents have not proven to conclusively treat RLS symptoms.[153,157,158] Risks associated with the use of opiates, including respiratory depression and addiction, should be reviewed with the patient prior to initiation. Benzodiazepines and opiates should be avoided in concomitant sleep apnea due to their ability to suppress respiratory drive.

In addition to pharmacologic therapy, nonpharmacologic therapies and behavioral techniques should also be recommended for J.J. Most important among these include discontinuing all RLS aggravators and practicing good sleep hygiene. Physical and mental activity (e.g., reading, playing card games, or working on the computer) if patients are unable to sleep can reduce symptoms.[152] Counter stimuli such as massage or hot baths may also be helpful.[152]

CASE 59-4, QUESTION 4: After carefully considering the costs of therapy, J.J. and her physician choose levodopa to treat her RLS instead of a dopamine agonist. She initially responds well to the therapy. One year later, J.J. returns for follow-up. Her dose of carbidopa/levodopa has progressively increased to three 25 mg/100 mg tablets at bedtime. She describes continued worsening of her symptoms that do not seem to be relieved with increasing doses of carbidopa/levodopa. Her symptoms are now starting earlier in the evening, occur almost every night, and are now painful. How should her therapy be further adjusted?

J.J. is likely experiencing augmentation, a common problem with long-term use of dopaminergic drugs, particularly levodopa.[159] Augmentation is described as a progressive worsening of RLS symptoms after an initial improvement and is manifested by gradually intensified symptoms that occur earlier in the evening and spread to other parts of the body.[160] It is the most common side effect occurring with long-term use (>3 months) of dopaminergic agents, and usually occurs 6 to 18 months after therapy is initiated.[152] Doses of dopaminergic agents are often increased in response; however, with each incremental dose increase, symptoms progress more rapidly until they may occur continuously throughout the day.[152] Although augmentation has been clinically recognized for many years, it has not been systematically studied. The exact etiology is uncertain, but it likely relates to the finding that RLS, unlike PD, is actually a hyperdopaminergic condition with an apparent postsynaptic desensitization that overcompensates during the circadian low point of dopaminergic activity in the evening and night. Adding dopamine in the evening initially corrects the symptoms, but ultimately leads to increasing postsynaptic desensitization.

The highest risk for augmentation is with levodopa. An estimated 50% to 85% of patients on levodopa will develop augmentation, compared with only 20% to 30% with dopamine agonists.[161] The primary treatment strategy for the management of augmentation is to withdraw the dopaminergic agent and substitute this with nondopaminergic agents. Given her presentation, J.J. should have her carbidopa/levodopa discontinued. She should be counseled that her symptoms will likely rebound severely for 48 to 72 hours, but approximately 4 to 7 days later her symptoms should gradually return to baseline or pretreatment state.[152]

With the discontinuation of carbidopa/levodopa in J.J., an alternative therapy should be selected. The selection of an alternative agent in cases in which the initial therapy failed or augmentation occurs must be approached on an individual basis. Although a number of agents are available to choose from, clinical experience generally guides the decision because lack of comparative trials precludes development of any formal recommendations. Because J.J. describes increasing pain with her RLS, it would be appropriate to initiate a trial of gabapentin encarbil or pregabalin. If ineffective or not tolerated, J.J. could be prescribed an opiate to manage her pain. Hydrocodone, oxycodone, methadone, codeine, and tramadol have all been evaluated in RLS.[152] Risks associated with opiate use, including respiratory depression and addiction, should be discussed in detail with J.J. prior to initiation. Augmentation does not prevent a future reintroduction of dopaminergic therapy; in the case of J.J., a dopamine agonist could be added after an extended dopaminergic free period if her symptoms are not completely controlled with nondopaminergic agents or if her symptoms were not painful.

ESSENTIAL TREMOR

Clinical Presentation

CASE 59-5

QUESTION 1: K.H. is a 52-year-old white female office manager who was referred to a neurologist for evaluation of bilateral tremor. She is otherwise healthy and reports not taking any regularly prescribed medications. She describes her tremor as being present mainly when she performs voluntary movements. The tremor is not noticeable during rest. She also notices that the tremor seems to disappear in the evening after drinking a couple of glasses of wine. The tremor interferes with several of her ADLs, including writing, eating, drinking from a cup, and inserting her keys into the ignition. She reports mild interference with her job function and some social embarrassment. No bradykinesia or rigidity is elicited on physical examination. A handwriting sample reveals large characters that are difficult to decipher. Family history reveals that her maternal grandmother and mother both had similar symptoms. What signs and symptoms are consistent with essential tremor in K.H.?

Beginning in the mid-20th century, the term essential tremor (ET) has been consistently used to describe a kinetic tremor for which no definite cause has been established. ET is a common neurologic disorder with an estimated incidence of 616 cases/100,000 person-years, and a prevalence of about 0.9% to 4.6%.[162,163] Despite its prevalence, it is underrecognized and undertreated, likely because it has been traditionally viewed as a monosymptomatic disorder of little consequence. More recently, it is recognized to be complex and progressive, resulting in significant disability in ADLs and job performance, and social embarrassment.[162] Both the incidence and prevalence of ET increase with age. In addition, ethnicity and family history of ET are consistently identified risk factors; it is approximately 5 times more common in whites than in blacks, and approximately 50% of patients report a positive family history. The latter finding suggests that genetic predisposition may play a role in ET; however, differences in intrafamilial onset and severity suggest environmental factors may also influence underlying susceptibility to the disease. Several environmental toxins have been proposed as causes of ET, including β-carboline alkaloids (e.g., harmane and harmine) and lead, both of which have been found in elevated concentrations in patients with ET compared with normal control subjects.[165,166]

Because parkinsonian tremor and ET are the most common forms of tremor observed in practice, it is important to distinguish

Table 59-7
Differentiation of Essential Tremor and Parkinson's Disease (PD)

Characteristic	Essential Tremor	Parkinson's Disease
Kinetic tremor in arms, hands, or head	++	++
Hemibody (arm and leg) tremor	0	++
Kinetic tremor > resting tremor	++	+
Resting tremor > kinetic tremor	0	++
Rigidity or bradykinesia	0	++
Postural instability	0	++
Usual age of onset (years)	15–25, 45–55	55–65
Symmetry	Bilateral	Unilateral > bilateral
Family history of tremor	+++	+
Response to alcohol	+++	0
Response to anticholinergics	0	++
Response to levodopa	0	+++
Response to primidone	+++	0
Response to propranolol	+++	+
Handwriting analysis	Large, tremulous script	Micrographia

0, not observed; +, rarely observed; ++, sometimes observed; +++, often observed.

between the two because the treatments differ substantially. Tremor should first be identified as either an action (kinetic, postural, and isometric) or resting tremor. The defining feature of ET is a bilateral, largely symmetrical, 5- to 10-Hz kinetic and postural tremor of the arms. The tremor can also affect the head or voice. The symptoms must be present for greater than 5 years and must not be attributable to other causes such as tremorogenic drugs.[165] Although both kinetic and postural action tremors can be present in ET and PD, the presence of resting tremor is much more common in PD. Lack of resting tremor and absence of bradykinesia or rigidity in K.H. suggest the tremor is not parkinsonian. She describes interference of her tremor occurring with voluntary movement, such as in her ADLs and drinking from a cup. Other signs and symptoms that support a diagnosis of ET include her age, family history, large and tremulous handwriting (as opposed to micrographia in PD), and improvement in tremor with alcohol consumption. Table 59-7 summarizes the similarities and differences of ET and parkinsonian tremor.

Several medications and substances are known to cause tremor, and all patients should have thorough medication history to rule out these causes. Medications commonly implicated include corticosteroids, metoclopramide, valproate, sympathomimetics (e.g., albuterol, amphetamines, pseudoephedrine), SSRIs, tricyclic antidepressants, theophylline, and thyroid preparations.[167,168] In addition, caffeine, tobacco, and chronic alcohol use can cause tremor that resembles ET. K.H. does not report taking any regularly prescribed medications; however, she should be questioned regarding any over-the-counter medication use as well as her alcohol use and caffeine and smoking habits.

The diagnosis of ET is based solely on clinical examination and neurologic history. Neuroimaging is not useful, and there are no available biologic markers or diagnostic tests that are specific to ET. The evaluation of the tremor that K.H. is experiencing should include laboratory analysis to rule out possible medical conditions associated with tremor. Such conditions may include the presence of hyperthyroidism or Wilson disease (particularly in patients younger than 40 years of age).[167,168]

Treatment

CASE 59-5, QUESTION 2: What therapies are effective in treating ET? How should K.H. be treated?

Patients with ET who have mild disability that does not cause functional impairment or social embarrassment can go without treatment. Because K.H. is experiencing tremor that is interfering with her occupation and causing social embarrassment, she should be considered for pharmacotherapy (Table 59-8). It is important to note that although effective treatments exist, tremor is rarely eliminated completely. Factors predicting lack of response have not been readily identified.

Propranolol, a nonselective β-adrenergic receptor blocker, or primidone, an anticonvulsant, is recommended as first-line agent to treat ET.[169,170] Propranolol is typically effective in doses of at

Table 59-8
Pharmacotherapy for Essential Tremor

Drug	Initial Dose	Usual Therapeutic Dose	Adverse Effects
β-Blockers			
Propranolol	10 mg every day to BID	120–320 mg divided every day to BID	Bradycardia, fatigue, hypotension, depression, exercise intolerance
Atenolol	12.5–25 mg every day	50–150 mg every day	Bradycardia, fatigue, hypotension, exercise intolerance
Nadolol	40 mg every day	120–240 mg every day	Bradycardia, fatigue, hypotension, exercise intolerance
Anticonvulsants			
Primidone	12.5 mg every day at bedtime	50–750 mg divided every day to TID	Sedation, fatigue, nausea, vomiting, ataxia, dizziness, confusion, vertigo
Gabapentin	300 mg every day in single or divided doses	1,200–3,600 mg divided TID	Nausea, drowsiness, dizziness, unsteadiness, weight gain, peripheral edema, potential for abuse
Topiramate	25 mg every day	200–400 mg divided BID	Appetite suppression, weight loss, paresthesias, concentration difficulties
Pregabalin	75 mg BID	75–300 mg divided BID	Weight gain, dizziness, drowsiness, potential for abuse
Benzodiazepines			
Alprazolam	0.125 mg every day	0.75–3 mg divided TID	Sedation, fatigue, ataxia, dizziness, potential for abuse
Clonazepam	0.25 mg every day	0.5–6 mg divided every day to BID	Sedation, fatigue, ataxia, dizziness, impaired cognition, potential for abuse
Miscellaneous			
Botulinum toxin A	Varies by injection site: 50–100 units/arm for hand tremor; 40–400 units/neck for head tremor; 0.6–15 units/vocal cords for voice tremor; repeat no sooner than every 3 months (extend as long as possible)		Hand weakness (with wrist injection); dysphagia, hoarseness, breathiness (with neck or vocal cord injection)

BID, 2 times daily; TID, 3 times daily.

least 120 mg/day, with about 50% of patients having long-lasting benefit.[170,171] Long-acting propranolol is as effective as the regular-release formulation. Other beta-1 (β_1)-selective blockers such as atenolol and metoprolol have also been studied, but with mixed findings.[166,170,171] Propranolol has demonstrated greater efficacy than these β_1-selective agents, suggesting that blockade of β_2 receptors is of importance. β-adrenergic receptor blockers with intrinsic sympathomimetic activity, such as pindolol, appear ineffective in ET.[168–170] Caution should be exercised with propranolol in patients with asthma, congestive heart failure, diabetes mellitus, and atrioventricular block.

Several studies have compared propranolol and primidone in ET, and they are considered to have similar efficacy.[169–171] Primidone is metabolized to a phenobarbital-based metabolite; however, phenobarbital is inferior to primidone in treating ET.[171] Acute adverse effects of primidone include nausea, vomiting, and ataxia, which can occur in up to one-fourth of patients, often limiting its use.[169] Primidone should be initiated at 12.5 mg/day and administered at bedtime to reduce the occurrence of acute side effects. It can be titrated gradually as tolerated up to 750 mg/day in divided doses, although side effects become more common at doses greater than 500 mg/day.[169]

Other agents that have demonstrated variable efficacy in ET include gabapentin, pregabalin, topiramate, and benzodiazepines (specifically, alprazolam and clonazepam).[170] They are generally considered to be less-proven, second-line therapies. Adverse effects and potential for abuse should be considered when an agent is selected.

If oral pharmacotherapy options for ET are not beneficial, intramuscular injections of botulinum toxin A or surgical treatments can be used in selected patients.[170] Targeted botulinum toxin A injections can reduce hand, head, and voice tremor; however, they are associated with focal weakness of the adjacent areas.[169] Injections in the wrist can cause hand weakness, and dysphagia, hoarseness, and breathiness can occur with injections into the neck or vocal cords. The use of botulinum toxin injections in the United States is also limited by cost. Treatment should occur with the lowest dose, and the interval should be as long as possible between injections. DBS of the ventral intermediate nucleus of the thalamus or unilateral thalamotomy is possibly efficacious in reducing ET.[170] Greater improvement in self-reported measures of function and fewer adverse events make DBS the preferred surgical option of the two.[170]

Because K.H. is otherwise healthy, she is a good candidate for propranolol therapy. Propranolol can be initiated as needed or on a scheduled basis depending on the degree of impairment and desire of the patient. If the decision is made with K.H. to use propranolol on an as-needed basis, she should begin with one-half of a 20-mg tablet administered 30 minutes to 1 hour before the desired effect. The dose can be increased from one-half to two tablets. An example of a situation in which this may occur is whether she wants to avoid embarrassment with attending a social activity or before certain tasks requiring manual dexterity at work. Given the degree of her impairment, she is probably a better candidate for chronic suppressive therapy with propranolol. In this situation, she can be prescribed 10 mg twice daily, because it can be safely and easily up-titrated every few days to a minimally effective dose, generally not more than 120 to 360 mg/day in divided doses.

KEY REFERENCES AND WEBSITES

A full list of references for this chapter can be found at http://thepoint.lww.com/AT11e. Below are the key references and websites for this chapter, with the corresponding reference number in this chapter found in parentheses after the reference.

Key References

Ferreira JJ et al. Summary of the recommendations of the EFNS/MDS-ES review on therapeutic management of Parkinson's disease. *Eur J Neurol*. 2013;20:5–15. (20)

Fox SH et al. Update on treatments for motor symptom of PD. Update for Website; 2015.

Garcia-Borreguero D et al; European Federation of Neurological Societies; European Neurological Society; European Sleep Research Society. European guidelines on management of restless legs syndrome: report of a joint task force by the European Federation of Neurological Societies, the European Neurological Society and the European Sleep Research Society. *Eur J Neurol*. 2012;19(11):1385–1396. (157)

Garcia-Borreguero D et al. The long-term treatment of restless legs syndrome/Willis-Ekbom disease: evidence-based guidelines and clinical consensus best practice guidance: a report from the International Restless Legs Syndrome Study Group. *Sleep Med*. 2013;14(7):675–684. (156)

Miyasaki JM et al. Practice parameter: initiation of treatment for Parkinson's disease: an evidence-based review: report of the Quality Standards Subcommittee of the American Academy of Neurology. *Neurology*. 2002;58:11. (15)

Miyasaki JM et al. Practice parameter: evaluation and treatment of depression, psychosis, and dementia in Parkinson's disease (an evidence-based review): report of the Quality Standards Subcommittee of the American Academy of Neurology. *Neurology*. 2006;66:996.

National Collaborating Centre for Chronic Conditions. Parkinson's disease: national clinical guideline for diagnosis and management in primary and secondary care. London: Royal College of Physicians; 2006. (17)

Pahwa R et al. Practice parameter: treatment of Parkinson disease with motor fluctuations and dyskinesia (an evidence-based review): report of the Quality Standards Subcommittee of the American Academy of Neurology. *Neurology*. 2006;66:983. (16)

PD Med Collaborative Group, Gray R et al. Long-term effectiveness of dopamine agonists and monoamine oxidase-B inhibitors compared with levodopa as initial treatment for Parkinson's disease (PD MED): a large, open-label, pragmatic randomised trial. *Lancet*. 2014;384(9949):1196–1205. (28)

Zesiewicz TA et al. Practice parameter: treatment of non-motor symptoms of Parkinson disease: report of the Quality Standards Subcommittee of the American Academy of Neurology. *Neurology*. 2010;74:924. (130)

Zesiewicz TA et al. Evidence-based guideline update: treatment of essential tremor: report of the Quality Standards subcommittee of the American Academy of Neurology. *Neurology*. 2011;77(19):1752–1755. (169)

60 Seizure Disorders

James W. McAuley and Brian K. Alldredge

CORE PRINCIPLES

	CORE PRINCIPLES	CHAPTER CASES
1	Epilepsy is a disorder characterized by spontaneously recurring seizures. Seizures can arise from a focal area of the brain (focal or partial seizures) or arise diffusely from both brain hemispheres (primary generalized seizures).	**Case 60-1 (Question 1)**
2	The optimal choice of antiepileptic drug (AED) treatment is based on patient-specific considerations including seizure type (or epilepsy syndrome, if defined), age, sex, concomitant medical conditions and therapies, and AED adverse effects. Monotherapy is preferred; polytherapy should be considered for patients with multiple seizure types and/or when monotherapy (with 2 or 3 agents) fails at maximal tolerated doses.	**Case 60-1 (Questions 2, 3), Case 60-6 (Question 1), Case 60-7 (Questions 1, 3, 4)**
3	Standard AEDs, such as carbamazepine, phenytoin, and valproate, are used commonly for patients with newly diagnosed epilepsy. Newer AEDs (e.g., lacosamide, lamotrigine, levetiracetam, oxcarbazepine, pregabalin, topiramate, zonisamide, ezogabine, perampanel, eslicarbazepine) are often initially approved for add-on therapy in patients with partial-onset seizures who do not respond to other AEDs. Lamotrigine, oxcarbazepine, topiramate, lacosamide, and felbamate are indicated for monotherapy.	**Case 60-1 (Question 3), Case 60-2 (Question 1), Case 60-6 (Question 1)**
4	Enzyme-inducing AEDs (carbamazepine, phenobarbital, phenytoin) increase the metabolism of many other drugs (e.g., warfarin, contraceptive hormones). In addition, carbamazepine induces its own metabolism and levels may decline during the first month of therapy despite excellent adherence.	**Case 60-1 (Question 5), Case 60-11 (Question 1)**
5	Serious idiosyncratic adverse effects have been associated with most standard and new AEDs and include carbamazepine-associated hematologic abnormalities; lamotrigine-associated skin rash; valproate-induced hepatotoxicity; and hypersensitivity syndrome seen with carbamazepine, phenobarbital, and phenytoin. The role of routine laboratory monitoring for detection of these adverse effects is controversial. Patients should know the signs or symptoms that should prompt them to seek medical attention.	**Case 60-1 (Question 4), Case 60-2 (Question 1), Case 60-7 (Questions 8, 9), Case 60-10 (Questions 1, 2)**
6	Unlike other AEDs, phenytoin displays capacity-limited pharmacokinetics at serum concentrations that are clinically useful for epilepsy treatment. As a consequence, phenytoin blood levels often change disproportionately to changes in dosage, and time to steady state varies significantly in individual patients based on the phenytoin concentration.	**Case 60-3 (Questions 2, 3)**
7	Serum concentration monitoring can be useful for selected AEDs when there is a good correlation between concentration and therapeutic or toxic responses. However, clinical criteria (seizure control, medication tolerability) are the primary determinants of the need for dosage adjustments.	**Case 60-7 (Question 7)**
8	The occurrence of seizure clusters (acute repetitive seizures) and status epilepticus (prolonged or repeated seizures without recovery of consciousness) warrants emergent AED therapy. Acute repetitive seizures are often treated by parents or caregivers with rectal diazepam. Status epilepticus is a life-threatening emergency and should be treated with intravenous (IV) lorazepam as initial therapy.	**Case 60-8 (Question 1), Case 60-12 (Questions 1–4)**

Incidence, Prevalence, and Epidemiology

Approximately 10% of the population will experience a seizure at some time in their life. Up to 30% of all seizures are provoked by central nervous system (CNS) disorders or insults (e.g., meningitis, trauma, tumors, and exposure to toxins); these seizures may become recurrent and require chronic treatment with AEDs. Reversible conditions such as alcohol withdrawal, fever, and metabolic disturbances may provoke acute, isolated seizures. These seizures, along with drug-induced seizures, are not considered to be epilepsy and usually do not require long-term AED therapy. Approximately 1% of the general population has epilepsy.[1]

Terminology, Classification, and Diagnosis of Epilepsies

CLASSIFICATION OF SEIZURES AND EPILEPSIES

A seizure is the "transient occurrence of signs and/or symptoms due to abnormal excessive or synchronous neuronal activity in the brain" (p. 471).[2] These signs or symptoms "may include alterations of consciousness, motor, sensory, autonomic, or psychic events" (p. 593).[1] Epilepsy is a "disorder of the brain characterized by an enduring predisposition to generate epileptic seizures and by the neurobiologic, cognitive, psychological and social consequence of this condition" (p. 471).[2] By definition, epilepsy requires the occurrence of two or more seizures that are not acutely provoked by other illnesses or conditions.[3] Guidelines have recently been updated to include a patient who has had one unprovoked seizure and has a high risk (>60%) of a second seizure to be included in the definition of a person with epilepsy.[4] A commonly used classification scheme for epileptic seizures is shown in Table 60-1.[5] Older terms such as "grand mal" and "petit mal" should not be used, because their use may create confusion in the clinical setting. For example, it is common for patients or caregivers to identify any seizure other than a generalized tonic–clonic seizure as a "petit mal" seizure. This labeling may result in the selection of an inappropriate medication.

Generalized tonic–clonic seizures are common. The patient loses consciousness and falls at the onset. Simultaneously, tonic muscle spasms begin and may be accompanied by a cry that results from air being forced through the larynx. Bilateral, repetitive clonic movements follow. After the clonic phase, patients return to consciousness but remain lethargic and may be confused for varying periods of time (postictal state). Urinary incontinence and tongue biting is common. Primary generalized tonic–clonic seizures affect both cerebral hemispheres from the outset. Secondarily generalized tonic–clonic seizures begin as either simple or complex partial seizures. The aura described by some patients before a generalized tonic–clonic seizure represents an initial partial seizure that spreads to become a secondarily generalized seizure. Identification of secondarily generalized tonic–clonic seizures is important because some AEDs are more effective at controlling primary generalized seizures than secondarily generalized seizures. In general, partial seizures are often more difficult to control with AEDs as compared to primary generalized seizures.[3,6,7]

Absence seizures occur primarily in children and often remit during puberty; affected patients may exhibit a second type of seizure. Absence seizures consist of a brief loss of consciousness, usually lasting several seconds. Simple (typical) absence seizures are not accompanied by motor symptoms; automatisms, muscle twitching, myoclonic jerking, or autonomic manifestations may accompany atypical (complex) absence seizures. Although consciousness is lost, muscle tone is maintained and patients do not fall during absence seizures. Patients are unaware of their surroundings and will have no recall of events during the seizure. Consciousness returns immediately when the seizure ends, and postictal confusion does not occur. Differentiation of atypical absence seizures from complex partial seizures may be difficult if only a second-hand account of the episodes is available; identification of a focal abnormality by an electroencephalogram (EEG) often is necessary to identify complex partial seizures. This distinction is important for the proper selection of AED.

Table 60-1
Classification of Epileptic Seizures

Partial Seizure (Focal)
Simple Partial Seizures (Without Impairment of Consciousness)
Motor symptoms
Special sensory or somatosensory symptoms
Autonomic symptoms
Psychic symptoms
Complex Partial Seizures (With Impairment of Consciousness; "dyscognitive features")
Progressing to impairment of consciousness
With no other features
With features as in simple partial seizures
With automatisms
With impaired consciousness at onset
With no other features
With features as in simple partial seizures
With automatisms
Partial Seizures That Evolve to Generalized Seizures
Simple partial seizures evolving to generalized seizures
Complex partial seizures evolving to generalized seizures
Simple partial seizures evolving to complex partial seizures to generalized seizures
Generalized Seizures (Convulsive or Nonconvulsive)
Absence Seizures
Typical seizures (impaired consciousness only)
Atypical absence seizures
Myoclonic Seizures
Clonic Seizures
Tonic Seizures
Tonic–Clonic Seizures
Atonic (Astatic or Akinetic) Seizures
Unclassified Epileptic Seizures
All seizures that cannot be classified because of inadequate or incomplete data and some that cannot be classified in previously described categories

Simple partial (focal motor or sensory) seizures are localized in a single cerebral hemisphere or portion of a hemisphere. Consciousness is not impaired during these events. Various motor, sensory, or psychic manifestations may occur depending on the area of the brain that is affected. A single part of the body may twitch, or the patient may experience only an unusual sensory experience.

Complex partial seizures result from the spread of focal discharges to involve a larger area. Consciousness is impaired and patients may exhibit complex but inappropriate behavior (automatisms) such as lip smacking, picking at clothing, or aimless wandering. A period of brief postictal lethargy or confusion is common.

In 2010, the International League Against Epilepsy recommended modifications to the traditional seizure classification scheme and terminology. Whereas some of the terminology remained unchanged, seizures limited to one hemisphere are now termed "focal seizures" (instead of partial seizures) and the formal distinction between complex partial and simple partial seizures is eliminated.[8] Because most of the existing literature on epilepsy makes use of the traditional seizure terminology, we have retained the use of "partial," "complex partial," and "simple partial" for this chapter.

EPILEPSY SYNDROMES

Epilepsy can be classified based on seizure type as shown in Table 60-1. Epilepsy syndromes can be defined on the basis of seizure type as well as cause (if known), precipitating factors, age of onset, characteristic EEG patterns, severity, chronicity, family history, and prognosis. Accurate diagnosis of epilepsy syndromes may better guide clinicians regarding the need for drug therapy, the choice of appropriate medication, and the likelihood of successful treatment.[1,6,7] Many epilepsy syndromes have been defined; a complete listing is beyond the scope of this chapter. Several are of interest with respect to pharmacotherapy and are described in Table 60-2.[7]

Diagnosis

Optimal treatment of seizure disorders requires accurate classification (diagnosis) of seizure type and appropriate choice and use of medications. Seizure classification may be straightforward if an adequate history and description of the clinical seizure are available. Physicians often do not observe patients' seizures; thus, family members, teachers, nurses, and others who have frequent direct contact with patients should learn to observe accurately and objectively describe and record these events. The onset, duration, and characteristics of a seizure should be described as completely as possible. Several aspects of the events surrounding a seizure may be especially significant: the patient's behavior before the seizure (e.g., Did the patient complain of feeling ill or describe an unusual sensation?), deviation of the eyes or head to one side or localization of convulsive activity to one portion of the body, impaired consciousness, loss of continence, and the patient's behavior after the seizure (e.g., Was there any postictal confusion?). In addition, it is helpful if the observer can record the length of the event and how long it took for the patient to return to baseline. A video of the event could be especially helpful. The patient and caregivers should have a seizure calendar or diary to record events. Many options exist to track seizures including online sites and smart phone applications. Those who observe a seizure should not try to label the seizure but should be encouraged to describe the event fully and objectively.

Accurate seizure diagnosis and identification of the type of epilepsy or epilepsy syndrome also depend on neurologic

Table 60-2
Selected Epilepsy Syndromes

Syndrome	Seizure Patterns and Characteristics	Preferred AED Therapy	Comments
Juvenile myoclonic epilepsy	Myoclonic seizures often precede generalized tonic–clonic seizures. ↓ sleep, fatigue, and alcohol commonly precipitate seizures	Valproate. Levetiracetam FDA-approved as adjunct for myoclonic seizures. Lamotrigine, topiramate, and zonisamide may be effective	5%–10% of all epilepsies; 85%–90% response to valproate. Lifelong therapy usually needed. High relapse rate with attempts to discontinue AED therapy
Lennox–Gastaut syndrome	Generalized seizures: atypical absence, atonic/akinetic, myoclonic, and tonic most common. Abnormal interictal EEG with slow spike-wave pattern. Cognitive dysfunction and mental retardation. Status epilepticus common	Valproate and benzodiazepines may be effective. Lamotrigine, rufinamide, topiramate and clobazam FDA-approved. Felbamate also may be effective, but potential hematologic toxicity limits use. Poorly responsive to AED	Oversedation with aggressive AED trials may ↑ seizure frequency. Tolerance to benzodiazepines limits their usefulness
Childhood absence epilepsy	Typical absences often in clusters of multiple seizures. Tonic–clonic seizures in ~40%. Onset usually between ages 4 and 8 years. Significant genetic component. EEG shows classic 3-Hz spike-and-wave pattern	Ethosuximide or valproate. Lamotrigine less effective	80%–90% response rate to AED therapy. Good prognosis for remission. Tonic–clonic seizures may persist
Mesial temporal lobe epilepsy	Complex partial seizures with automatisms. Simple partial seizures (auras) common; secondary generalized seizures occur in 50%	Carbamazepine, phenytoin, valproate, gabapentin, lamotrigine, topiramate, tiagabine, levetiracetam, oxcarbazepine, zonisamide, pregabalin, lacosamide, perampanel, ezogabine, eslicarbazepine	Often incompletely controlled with current AEDs. Emotional stress may precipitate seizures; surgical resection can be effective when patient is identified as a good surgical candidate

AED, antiepileptic drug; EEG, electroencephalogram; FDA, US Food and Drug Administration.

examination, medical history, and diagnostic techniques, such as EEG, computed tomography (CT), and magnetic resonance imaging (MRI). The EEG often is critical for identifying specific seizure types. CT scanning may help assess newly diagnosed patients, but MRI is preferred. MRI may locate brain lesions or anatomic defects that are missed by conventional radiographs or CT scans.[9]

Treatment

Early control of epileptic seizures is important because it allows normalization of patients' lives and prevents acute physical harm and long-term morbidity associated with recurrent seizures. In addition, early control of tonic–clonic seizures is associated with a reduced likelihood of seizure recurrence. Early control of epileptic seizures also correlates with successful discontinuation of AED treatment after long-term seizure control.[10–12]

NONPHARMACOLOGIC TREATMENT OF EPILEPSY

Alternatives or adjuncts to pharmacotherapy may be helpful in some patients. Surgery is an extremely effective treatment in selected patients. Depending on the epilepsy syndrome and procedure performed, up to 90% of patients treated surgically may improve or become seizure-free. A study of 80 patients with medically refractory temporal lobe epilepsy randomly assigned to either surgery or continued medical treatment showed that after 1 year patients were more likely to be seizure-free after surgery.[13] Surgery is advocated as early therapy for some patients with specific epilepsy syndromes, such as mesial temporal sclerosis. Early surgical intervention may prevent or lessen neurologic deterioration and developmental delay.

Dietary modification may be used for patients who cannot tolerate AEDs or to treat seizures that are not completely responsive to AEDs. In most circumstances, dietary modification consists of a ketogenic diet. This low-carbohydrate, high-fat diet results in persistent ketosis, which is believed to play a major role in the therapeutic effect. Ketogenic diets seem to be most beneficial in children; they are also used as adjuncts to ongoing AED treatment.[14,15]

The vagus nerve stimulator is an implantable device approved for treatment of intractable partial seizures. This device uses electrodes attached around the left branch of the vagus nerve. The electrodes are attached to a programmable stimulator that delivers stimuli on a regular cycling basis; patients can also use "on demand" stimulation at the onset of seizures by swiping the magnet over the subcutaneously implanted stimulator. Approximately 30% to 40% of patients who are so treated have a positive response (50% reduction in seizures).[16] The primary side effect of this device is hoarseness during stimulation; infrequently, this is accompanied by left vocal cord paralysis.

Responsive neurostimulation is a newer non-pharmacologic option for treating intractable partial-onset seizures. Its role in therapy is yet to be determined.

Avoidance of Potential Seizure Precipitants

It is impossible to generalize about environmental and lifestyle precipitants of seizure activity in persons with epilepsy. Individual patients or caregivers may identify specific circumstances such as stress, sleep deprivation, acute illness, or ingestion of excessive amounts of caffeine or alcohol, which may increase the likelihood of a recurrent seizure event. Some women experience an increase in the frequency and/or severity of seizures around the time of menstruation or ovulation. Patients with epilepsy should avoid activities that seem to precipitate seizures; as always, the goal is complete seizure control with as little alteration in quality of life as possible.

ANTIEPILEPTIC DRUG THERAPY

Pharmacotherapy is the mainstay of treatment for epilepsy. Therefore, patient education regarding medications and consultation among health care professionals regarding the optimal use of AEDs are essential to quality patient care. Optimal AED therapy completely controls seizures in approximately two-thirds of patients.[17,18] Optimization of drug therapy depends on several factors, with the choice of appropriate AED, individualization of dosing, and adherence being the most important.

Choice of Antiepileptic Drug

Many AEDs have a relatively narrow spectrum of efficacy against selected seizure types; therefore, choice of appropriate drug therapy for a specific patient depends on an accurate diagnosis of epilepsy. In addition, toxicity must be considered when selecting an AED. Preferred drugs for specific types of seizures and common epileptic syndromes are listed in Tables 60-2 and 60-3. Although certain drugs are preferred, the identification of the most effective drug for a particular patient may be a process of trial and error; several medication trials may be necessary before success is achieved. It is important to keep in mind that certain AEDs can worsen seizures.[19]

The consensus method was used to analyze expert opinion on treatment of three epilepsy syndromes and status epilepticus.[20] The experts recommended monotherapy first, followed by a second monotherapy agent if the first failed. If the second monotherapy failed, the experts were not in agreement on whether to try a third monotherapy agent or to combine two therapies. The experts recommended epilepsy surgery evaluation after the third failed AED for patients with symptomatic localization-related epilepsies.

To assess the evidence on efficacy, tolerability, and safety of many of the new AEDs in treating children and adults with new-onset and refractory partial and generalized epilepsies, a panel evaluated the available evidence.[21,22] They concluded that AED choice depends on seizure and syndrome type; patient age; concomitant medications; and AED tolerability, safety, and efficacy. The results of these two evidence-based assessments provide guidelines for the use of newer AEDs in patients with new-onset and refractory epilepsy.

Therapeutic End Points

The individual patient's response to AED treatment (i.e., seizure frequency and severity, and symptoms of toxicity) must be the major focus for therapy assessment. In general, the goal of AED treatment is administration of sufficient medication to completely prevent seizures without producing significant toxicity.[23] Realistically, this goal may be compromised for many patients; it may not be possible to completely prevent seizures without producing intolerable adverse effects. Thus, the therapeutic end points achieved can vary among patients; optimization of AED therapy for a specific person depends on tailoring therapy to the patient's needs and lifestyle. It is rarely optimal to administer "standard" or "usual" doses of an AED to a patient or to adjust doses to achieve a "therapeutic blood level" without considering the effect of the dose or serum concentration on the patient's condition and quality of life. As with many conditions requiring chronic drug therapy, patient participation in developing and evaluating a therapeutic plan is extremely important. Patients should be educated regarding the expected positive and negative effects of their AED therapy, and they must be encouraged to communicate with their health care provider regarding their responses to prescribed AEDs.

Table 60-3
Antiepileptic Drugs (AEDs) Useful for Various Seizure Types

Primary Generalized Tonic–Clonic	Secondarily Generalized Tonic–Clonic	Simple or Complex Partial (Focal)	Absence	Myoclonic, Atonic/Akinetic
Most Effective With Least Toxicity[a]				
Valproate	Carbamazepine	Carbamazepine	Ethosuximide	Valproate
Levetiracetam	Oxcarbazepine	Oxcarbazepine	Valproate	Clonazepam
Lamotrigine	Levetiracetam	Levetiracetam	Lamotrigine	Rufinamide (Lennox–Gastaut Syndrome)
Levetiracetam	Lamotrigine	Lamotrigine	(Topiramate)[b]	Levetiracetam (Juvenile Myoclonic Epilepsy)
Levetiracetam	Valproate	Valproate		Lamotrigine[b]
Levetiracetam	Gabapentin	Gabapentin		Clobazam (Lennox–Gastaut Syndrome)
(Oxcarbazepine)[b]	Topiramate			(Topiramate)[b]
Perampanel	Tiagabine Zonisamide Levetiracetam Pregabalin Lacosamide Ezogabine Perampanel Eslicarbazepine	Topiramate[b] Tiagabine Pregabalin Zonisamide Lacosamide Ezogabine Perampanel Eslicarbazepine		
Effective, but Often Poorly Tolerated or Cause Unacceptable Toxicity				
Phenobarbital	Phenobarbital	Clorazepate	Clonazepam	(Felbamate)[c]
Primidone	Primidone	Phenobarbital		
(Felbamate)[c]	(Felbamate)[c]	Primidone		
Phenytoin	Phenytoin (Vigabatrin)[d]	(Felbamate)[c] Phenytoin (Vigabatrin)[d]		

[a]Drugs are listed in general order of preference within each category. Recommendations by various authorities may differ. The use of phenobarbital and primidone is discouraged.
[b]The place of some AEDs for select seizure types is yet to be determined. More clinical experience is needed before their roles as possible primary AEDs are clarified.
[c]Felbamate is placed on this table only to indicate the types of seizures for which it appears to be effective. Felbamate has been associated with aplastic anemia and hepatic failure; until a possible causative role is clarified, felbamate cannot be recommended for treatment of epilepsy unless all other, potentially less toxic, treatment options have been exhausted.
[d]Vigabatrin causes progressive and permanent visual field constriction that is related to total dose and duration of exposure. Vigabatrin cannot be recommended for treatment of epilepsy unless other potentially less toxic treatment options have been exhausted.

Serum Drug Concentrations

Relation to Clinical Response

For selected AEDs, proper use and interpretation of serum concentrations are important for optimizing treatment regimens in epilepsy.[24,25] An individual patient's clinical response to AED treatment must be the major focus for therapy assessment. Individual patients often differ dramatically in their response to a particular serum drug concentration; therefore, therapeutic serum concentrations should be considered only as guidelines for treatment. Many patients' condition may be controlled with serum drug concentrations above or below the usual therapeutic range.[26] In these patients, dosage adjustment to get the patient "in range" is not warranted. It is better to "treat the patient, not the level."

Interestingly, a recent Cochrane Review found no evidence that measuring AED concentrations routinely to inform dose adjustments is superior to dose adjustments based on clinical information.[27] However, the authors do state that their review does not exclude the possibility that AED serum concentration might be useful in special situations or in selected patients.

Indications for Use

Measurement of serum drug concentrations may provide clinically useful information in the following situations:

- Uncontrolled seizures despite administration of greater-than-average doses: Serum concentrations of AED may help distinguish drug resistance from subtherapeutic drug concentrations caused by malabsorption, nonadherence, or rapid metabolism.
- Seizure recurrence in a patient whose seizures were previously controlled: This is often owing to nonadherence with the prescribed medication regimen.
- Documentation of intoxication: In patients who exhibit signs or symptoms of dose-related AED toxicity, documentation

of the dose and serum concentration of the responsible drug is helpful.

- Assessment of patient adherence: Although monitoring AED serum concentrations can be used to assess patient adherence with therapy, conclusions must be based on comparisons with previous steady state serum concentrations that reflected reliable intake of a given dose of AED.
- Documentation of desired results from a dose change or other therapeutic maneuver (e.g., administration of a loading dose): When patients are receiving multiple AEDs, it is often appropriate to measure serum concentrations of all drugs after a change in the dose of one agent because changes to one drug frequently affect the pharmacokinetic disposition of other drugs.
- When precise dosage changes are required: On occasion, small changes in the dose of a drug (e.g., phenytoin) can result in large changes in both the serum concentration and clinical response. In addition, cautious titration of dosage and serum concentration may be necessary to avoid intoxication. Knowledge of the serum drug concentration before the dosage change may allow the clinician to select a more appropriate new maintenance dose.
- During pregnancy, AED serum concentrations often decline and dosage adjustments may be warranted to maintain adequate seizure protection. Free (unbound) concentrations should be monitored for highly protein-bound AEDs. AED serum concentrations should be monitored after delivery, particularly when dosage escalations have been made during pregnancy.

Frequent, "routine" determinations of serum AED concentrations are costly and not warranted for patients whose clinical status is stable. Clinicians may tend to focus attention on normal variability in serum concentrations rather than on the patient's clinical status; as a result, unnecessary dosage adjustments may be made to make serum concentrations fit the "normal range." A plan of action for what the clinician is going to do with the information once it is obtained should be in place before obtaining the sample. Therefore, the results of individual serum concentration determinations must be evaluated carefully to decide whether a significant, clinically meaningful change has occurred.[28]

Interpretation of Serum Concentrations

Several factors can alter the relationship between AED serum concentration and the patient's response to the drug. Whenever a change in serum concentration is apparent, pharmacokinetic factors (Table 60-4) should be considered (along with the patient's clinical status) before a decision is made to adjust the AED dosage. Laboratory variability can cause minor fluctuations in reported AED serum concentrations. Under the best conditions, reported values for serum concentrations may be within plus or minus 10% of "true" values.[29,30] Therefore, the magnitude of any apparent change must be considered. Published therapeutic ranges may have been determined in small numbers of patients or may more accurately represent average serum concentrations at usual doses. Inappropriate sample timing can result in inconsistent and clinically meaningless changes in AED serum concentrations.[24] Generally, serum concentrations of AED should not be measured until a minimum of four to five half-lives have elapsed since initiation of therapy or a dosage change. Blood samples should be obtained in the morning, before any doses of the AED have been taken; this practice provides reproducible, postabsorptive (i.e., "trough") serum concentrations. Interindividual variability in response to a given serum concentration of medication is common. Excellent therapeutic response or even symptoms of intoxication may be associated with AED serum concentrations that are classified as "subtherapeutic."[31] Binding to serum proteins is significant for some AEDs (e.g., phenytoin, valproate, tiagabine). Changes in protein binding can result from drug interaction, renal failure, pregnancy, or changes in nutritional status. These changes can alter the usual relationship between the measured total drug concentration (bound and unbound to plasma proteins) and the unbound (pharmacologically active) drug concentration. This change may not be apparent when only total serum concentrations are measured. Determination of serum concentrations of free (i.e., unbound) AEDs is available from many commercial laboratories; these determinations are expensive and results may not be available for several days. If significant changes in protein binding are suspected, measurement of free concentrations of AED may provide additional information useful for adjustment of doses or interpretation of the patient's symptoms.[29,30,32]

Monotherapy Versus Polytherapy

Decades ago, epilepsy was often treated initially with multiple AEDs (polytherapy). A second, third, or even fourth drug was added when seizures were incompletely controlled with a single AED. Evaluation of the effectiveness of polytherapy in subsequent years has shown little advantage for most patients. Use of a single drug at optimal tolerated serum concentrations produces excellent therapeutic results and minimal side effects in most patients. Addition of a second AED significantly improves seizure control in only 10% to 20% of patients.[33,34] Reduction or elimination of existing polytherapy in patients with longstanding seizure disorders often lessens or eliminates cognitive impairment and other side effects; seizure control actually may improve.[33,35–38]

Most experts advocate the use of a single AED (monotherapy) whenever possible. Successful monotherapy may require higher-than-usual AED doses or serum concentrations greater than the upper limit of the usual therapeutic range.[39,40] Addition of a second drug may be necessary in some patients; however, polytherapy should be reserved for patients with multiple seizure types or for patients in whom first-line AEDs have failed to control seizures when titrated to maximal tolerated doses.[20,36,39] When a new AED is added to a patient's regimen with the goal of improving seizure control, the existing AED regimen should be scrutinized for continued value. In some cases, a patient's AED regimen can accumulate drugs that may be unnecessary because they were started and never re-evaluated. Continued vigilance and critical assessment of every drug in a patient's regimen is important.

Use of polytherapy creates several disadvantages that must be weighed against possible benefits. Seizure control may not significantly improve. Health care costs, for medications and for increased laboratory monitoring, may increase significantly with polytherapy. In addition, drug interactions among AEDs can complicate assessment of the patient's response and serum concentrations. Patient adherence often is worsened when multiple medications are prescribed, and adverse effects often increase.

Although AED monotherapy is preferred whenever feasible, the recent introduction of several new AEDs has increased the use of polytherapy.[40] Owing to limitations on the patient populations used for clinical trials of new drugs (i.e., patients with seizure disorders not completely controlled by previous medications), most new AEDs are labeled only for use as add-on therapy. Although reports exist on the efficacy of the new AEDs as monotherapy,[41–44] only felbamate, lacosamide, lamotrigine, oxcarbazepine, and topiramate are US Food and Drug Administration (FDA) approved for monotherapy. More AEDs will undoubtedly follow with monotherapy indications.

Duration of Therapy and Discontinuation of Antiepileptic Drugs

A diagnosis of epilepsy may not necessitate lifelong drug therapy. Several long-term studies have shown that AED therapy may be successfully withdrawn from some patients after a seizure-free

Table 60-4
Pharmacokinetic Properties of Antiepileptic Drugs (AEDs)

Drug	Oral Absorption (%)	Half-Life (hours)	Time to Steady State[a]	Dosage Schedule	Usual Therapeutic Serum Concentration	Plasma Protein Binding (%)	Volume of Distribution (L/kg)
Carbamazepine	90–100	*Chronic*: 5–25	2–4 days	BID to TID	5–12 mcg/mL	75 (50–90)	0.8–1.6
Eslicarbazepine	>90	*Normal renal function*: 13–20	4–5 days	QD	Not determined	<40	0.8
Ethosuximide	90–100	*Pediatric*: 30 *Adult*: 60	5–10 days	Daily (BID)	40–100 mcg/mL	0	0.7
Ezogabine	60	*Normal renal and hepatic function*: 7–11	2–4 days	TID	Not determined	80	2–3
Felbamate	90	12–20	3–4 days	BID to TID	50–110 mcg/mL	24	0.7–0.8
Gabapentin	40–60; ↓ with ↑ dose	*Normal renal function*: 5–9; ↑ with ↓ renal function	*Normal renal function*: 1–1.5 days	TID to QID (every 6–8 hours)	2 mcg/mL (proposed)	0	≈0.8
Lacosamide	100	13 ↑ slightly with renal impairment	2–3 days	BID	Not determined	<15	0.6
Lamotrigine	90–100	*Monotherapy*: 24–29 *Enzyme inducers*: 15 *Enzyme inhibitor (VPA)*: 59	4–9 days	BID	4–18 mcg/mL (proposed)	55	0.9–1.2
Levetiracetam	100	*Normal renal function*: 6–8; ↑ with ↓ renal function	*Normal renal function*: 1–1.5 days	BID	Not determined	<10	≈0.7
Oxcarbazepine	100	8–13	2–3 days	BID to TID	Not determined	40	
Perampanel	100	*Normal hepatic function*: 105	2–3 weeks	QD	Not determined	95	NA
Phenobarbital	90–100	2–4 days	8–16 days	Daily	15–40 mcg/mL	50	0.5–0.6
Phenytoin	90–100	Varies with dose	5–30 days	Daily to BID	10–20 mcg/mL	95	0.5–0.7
Pregabalin	≥90	*Normal renal function*: 6; ↑ with ↓ renal function	24 hours	BID to TID	Not determined	0	0.5
Rufinamide	85	9	1–2 days	BID	Not determined	<35	Dose dependent
Tiagabine	90	*Monotherapy*: 7–9 *Enzyme inducers*: 4–7	1–2 days	BID to QID	Not determined	96	1.1
Topiramate	≥80	12–24	3–4 days	BID	Not determined	10–15	0.7
Valproate	100 (≈80% with divalproex ER)	10–16	2–3 days	BID to QID (daily with divalproex × ER)	50–150 mcg/mL	90+	0.09–0.17
Vigabatrin	80–90	8–12 (not clinically important. Irreversible enzyme inhibitor)	NA	Daily to BID	NA	NA	NA
Zonisamide	≈80	*Monotherapy*: ≈60 *Enzyme inducers*: 27–36	2 weeks	Daily to BID	Not determined	50–60	1.3

[a]Based on four half-lives. This lag time should allow determination of steady state serum concentrations within limits of most assay sensitivities.

BID, twice daily; NA, not available; TID, three times daily; QID, four times daily; VPA, valproic acid.

Table 60-5
Risk Factors Possibly Predicting Seizure Recurrence After Antiepileptic Drug (AED) Withdrawal

- <2 years seizure-free before withdrawal
- Onset of seizures after age 12
- History of atypical febrile seizures
- Family history of seizures
- 2–6 years before seizures controlled
- Large number of seizures (>30) before control or total of >100 seizures
- Partial seizures (simple or complex)
- Abnormal EEG persisting throughout treatment
- Slowing on EEG before medication withdrawal
- Organic neurologic disorder
- Moderate to severe mental retardation

EEG, electroencephalogram.

period of 2 to 5 years.[10–12] Seizures recurred in only 12% to 36% of patients who were followed for up to 23 years after AED withdrawal. Therefore, many patients whose epilepsy is completely controlled with medication can stop therapy after a seizure-free period of at least 2 years.

Discontinuation of medications is advantageous for economic, medical, and psychosocial reasons. Costs associated with health care visits, serum concentration determinations, and the medications themselves are eliminated or reduced. The risk of adverse effects from long-term medication use is eliminated, and patients can expect fewer lifestyle restrictions. Attempts to withdraw AED therapy are associated with risks, however. Primary among them is the reappearance of seizure activity, which can result in status epilepticus, loss of driving privileges, employment difficulties, and/or physical injury.

Risk factors for seizure recurrence after discontinuation of AED have been identified in observational studies; complete agreement, however, is not found among studies regarding the nature and importance of specific risk factors. Opinions and data also differ regarding the optimal duration of the seizure-free period before discontinuation of AED is attempted. Nevertheless, at least some consensus has been reached regarding certain factors that may predict a higher risk of seizure recurrence (Table 60-5).[10–12,45,46]

In nonemergency situations, AED should be withdrawn slowly; if a patient receives multiple drugs, each drug should be withdrawn separately. Too-rapid withdrawal can result in status epilepticus. Clinical studies of AED discontinuation usually used a 2- to 3-month withdrawal schedule for each drug. The optimal rate of withdrawal of AED has not been identified. One study compared withdrawal of individual drugs for a 6-week and a 9-month period and found no difference in seizure recurrence between the groups.[47] Another study compared seizure frequencies in patients withdrawn from carbamazepine rapidly (for 4 days) and in patients withdrawn more slowly (for 10 days).[48] Significantly more generalized tonic–clonic seizures occurred when carbamazepine was withdrawn rapidly; complex partial seizures, however, did not occur at a higher rate with rapid withdrawal. Therefore, withdrawal of each AED for at least 6 weeks would seem to be a safe approach. Gradual withdrawal is recommended even for medications such as phenobarbital that have long half-lives and should theoretically be "self-tapering." In our experience, gradual reduction of medications such as phenobarbital is associated with a significantly higher success rate. If AEDs are withdrawn at an appropriate rate and seizures recur, drug treatment is usually reinstituted. In most patients, good seizure control is regained by restarting therapy. However, approximately 1% of patients had recurrent seizures that could not be controlled again with AEDs.[49] This uncommon, but potentially serious, outcome should be considered when therapy withdrawal is considered.

CLINICAL ASSESSMENT AND TREATMENT OF EPILEPSY

Complex Partial Seizures with Secondary Generalization

DIAGNOSIS

CASE 60-1

QUESTION 1: A.R. is a 14-year-old, 40-kg female high school student. A.R. had three febrile seizures when she was 3 years old. She received phenobarbital prophylaxis "off and on," according to her parents, for about 6 months after her second febrile seizure. Since then, she had no reported seizures until 24 hours before admission. At that time she had a "convulsion" shortly after arriving at school in the morning. A teacher who witnessed the episode describes her as behaving "oddly" before the seizure. She abruptly got up from her desk and began to walk clumsily toward the door; she bumped into several desks and did not respond to the teacher's attempts to redirect her back to her seat. After approximately 1 minute of this behavior, she fell to the floor and experienced an apparent generalized tonic–clonic seizure that lasted approximately 90 seconds. During the episode, she was incontinent of urine and was described as "turning kind of blue." After this episode, A.R. was transported to the hospital.

On arrival at the hospital, A.R. appeared drowsy and confused. Laboratory studies—a complete blood count (CBC), serum glucose, electrolytes, drug and alcohol screen, and lumbar puncture—were normal. Physical examination and a complete neurologic evaluation were normal. An EEG showed diffuse slowing with focal epileptiform discharges in the left temporal area; it was interpreted as abnormal. There was no history of recent illness or injury, although A.R. had stayed up late several nights recently studying for an examination.

A second seizure occurred in the hospital. The nursing staff described an episode similar to the one that occurred at school. After recovery from each episode, A.R. had no memory of events during the seizures; she only remembered a "funny feeling" in her stomach and a "buzzing" in her head before she lost consciousness. She described having these feelings "a couple of times" in the past; she attributed them to "just getting dizzy" and had not reported them to her parents. After these previous episodes, A.R. described feeling "mixed up" and groggy for a few minutes. What subjective and objective features of A.R.'s seizures are consistent with a diagnosis of complex partial seizures with secondary generalization?

A.R.'s clinical pattern of observed seizure activity (an apparent aura preceding her loss of consciousness), her history of apparent complex partial seizures not accompanied by generalized seizures, and the findings of focal abnormal activity on EEG are all concordant with this diagnosis. Postictal confusion and grogginess are common after both generalized tonic–clonic and complex partial seizures. Her unusual or inappropriate behavior represents a complex partial seizure that subsequently generalized. The clinical features, accompanied by her EEG findings, also help rule out possible atypical absence seizures, which can be confused with complex partial epilepsy syndromes based on only clinical presentation. In both syndromes, patients may briefly appear to lose contact with their surroundings and display automatisms and mild clonic movements during seizure activity. In A.R.'s case, the EEG and the generalized tonic–clonic seizures during her episodes would rule out atypical absence as a likely possibility.

DECISION TO USE ANTIEPILEPTIC DRUG THERAPY

CASE 60-1, QUESTION 2: What factors should be considered in a decision to treat A.R.'s seizures with AED therapy?

Once a diagnosis of epilepsy is established, the decision to treat the patient with medication is based on the likelihood of recurrence. The need for AED therapy after a single seizure is controversial, but according to the 2015 evidenced-based guideline on this topic, patients should be informed that their seizure recurrence risk is greatest early within the first 2 years and starting of AED therapy is likely to reduce recurrence risk within the first 2 years.[4]

In A.R.'s case, the potential benefits of immediate introduction of AED therapy appear to outweigh potential risks. She experienced complex partial seizures and some were followed by secondarily generalized tonic–clonic seizures. Recurrence of seizure activity is likely to result in physical injury, social embarrassment, and interference with her participation in activities typical of a person her age. If her seizures are not controlled, she faces future limitation of her driving privileges and may face barriers to employment. Although AED therapy is associated with risks, they probably are outweighed by the potential benefits.

CHOICE OF ANTIEPILEPTIC DRUG

CASE 60-1, QUESTION 3: Which AEDs are commonly used for A.R.'s seizure type? Based on the subjective and objective data available, recommend a first-choice AED for A.R. and a plan for initial dosing of this medication.

Many AEDs would be appropriate choices for A.R.'s complex partial seizures that can secondarily generalize (Table 60-3).[34,50,51] Some AEDs are not FDA-approved as initial monotherapy. Although valproate is effective for treating both generalized and complex partial seizures,[52] it would not be a good initial choice for this patient owing to the increased risks in a woman of childbearing age (see Women's Issues in Epilepsy section).

Eslicarbazepine, ezogabine, felbamate, gabapentin, lacosamide, lamotrigine, levetiracetam, oxcarbazepine, perampanel, pregabalin, tiagabine, topiramate, and zonisamide are effective for control of partial seizures with or without secondary generalization. Most experience with these drugs was obtained when they were used as adjunctive agents when previous AED therapies were unsuccessful. Initial clinical trials with these medications indicate that several of them may be useful as single agents. Felbamate, lacosamide, lamotrigine, oxcarbazepine, and topiramate have monotherapy indications. Most of the more recently approved medications appear to be safe and are usually well tolerated. The usefulness of felbamate is limited, however, owing to its potential for serious hematologic and hepatic toxicity.

Carbamazepine has several advantages that make it a preferred first-choice agent in the opinion of many clinicians. In comparison with phenytoin, carbamazepine is less sedating and is not associated with dysmorphic effects, such as hirsutism, acne, gingival hyperplasia, and coarsening of facial features. Carbamazepine's pharmacokinetic profile also makes dosage adjustment easier. In A.R.'s case, the lack of cosmetic side effects may be especially significant because she may be taking medication for many years. In addition, reduced sedation may be important with respect to her school performance.

CARBAMAZEPINE THERAPY

Initiation and Dosage

Initiation of treatment with full therapeutic maintenance doses of carbamazepine often causes excessive side effects such as nausea, vomiting, diplopia, and significant sedation. Therefore, carbamazepine therapy should be initiated gradually and patients should be allowed time to acclimate to the effects of the drug. Final dosing requirements are difficult to anticipate in individual patients. A reasonable starting dosage of carbamazepine for A.R. would be 100 mg twice a day; her dosage could be increased by 100 to 200 mg/day every 7 to 14 days. The rapidity of increases will depend on A.R.'s tolerance for the drug and the frequency of her seizures.

Hematologic Toxicity

CASE 60-1, QUESTION 4: Carbamazepine has been associated with hematologic and hepatic toxicities. What is the incidence and significance of these toxicities? How should A.R. be monitored for them?

Aplastic anemia and agranulocytosis have occurred in association with carbamazepine therapy.[53] Several cases have been fatal; however, most cases occurred in older patients treated for trigeminal neuralgia. Many patients were receiving other medications, and occasionally the reports were incomplete; thus, assessment of a causal role for carbamazepine is difficult.[54] Severe blood dyscrasias from carbamazepine seem rare (estimated prevalence <1/50,000) and have predominantly occurred in nonepileptic patients. The lack of severe hematologic toxicity in various published series and clinical trials in patients with epilepsy has been notable.[55,56]

Leukopenia is relatively common in patients taking carbamazepine. It is usually mild and often reverses despite continued administration of the drug.[55] Total leukocyte counts may fall to less than 4,000 cells/μL in some patients, but differentials and platelet and erythrocyte counts remain normal. Symptoms (e.g., fever, sore throat) that might suggest early stages of agranulocytosis do not occur. Carbamazepine-associated hematologic disorders are unrelated to drug dosage; thus, these reactions appear to be idiosyncratic.

Routine Hematologic Testing

Laboratory monitoring of A.R.'s hematologic status is recommended during carbamazepine therapy. The likelihood of early detection of aplastic anemia or agranulocytosis through frequent blood counts is low, however, and such monitoring is costly.[55,57] Because hematologic toxicity from carbamazepine primarily occurs early in therapy, a CBC should be obtained before therapy and at monthly intervals during the first 2 to 3 months of therapy; thereafter, a yearly or every-other-year CBC, white blood cell count with differential, and platelet count should be sufficient.

Hepatotoxicity

Carbamazepine-related liver damage is extremely rare despite its being frequently mentioned as a potential problem and strong warnings in the package insert.[58,59] Hepatic adverse reactions are believed to be idiosyncratic or immunologically based. Aggressive laboratory monitoring of liver function tests (LFTs) probably is unnecessary.[57] Alkaline phosphatase and γ-glutamyl-transferase concentrations often are elevated in patients taking carbamazepine (and other AEDs). This is believed to result from hepatic enzyme induction and is not necessarily evidence for hepatic disease.[60]

In summary, hepatic and hematologic toxicities of carbamazepine are rare. Although potentially serious, they are best monitored on clinical grounds rather than by ongoing, intensive laboratory testing. Patients, families, or caregivers should be aware that the appearance of unusual symptoms (e.g., jaundice, abdominal pain, excessive bruising and bleeding, or sudden onset of severe sore throat with fever) should be reported to a health care professional. Baseline (pretreatment) determination of A.R.'s hepatic and hematologic status, possibly with monthly follow-up testing for 2 to 3 months, probably will be sufficient.[56,57] Thereafter, a CBC and a liver function battery should probably be evaluated only every 1 to 2 years, unless signs or symptoms of hepatic or hematologic disorders are observed.

Pharmacokinetics and Autoinduction of Metabolism

CASE 60-1, QUESTION 5: For the subsequent 6 weeks, A.R.'s carbamazepine dosage was gradually increased to 400 mg twice daily (BID) (20 mg/kg/day). Until the last dose increase, she had been experiencing one or two complex partial seizures weekly; she had experienced only one generalized tonic–clonic seizure since her hospitalization. One week after the increase to 20 mg/kg/day, her serum carbamazepine concentration was 9 mcg/mL just before her first dose of the day. No seizures occurred for 4 weeks, and she tolerated the medication well. Subsequent to the 4-week seizure-free period, she again began experiencing one seizure weekly. What factor(s) might be responsible for this reversal of seizure control?

Several factors may account for this change. It is important always to consider the possibility of poor medication adherence when clinical response changes unexpectedly. This should be investigated, and A.R. and her family should be educated regarding the importance of regular medication intake.

The observed changes in A.R.'s seizure control may also be due to unique features of carbamazepine pharmacokinetics. Carbamazepine is a potent inducer of hepatic cytochrome P-450 (CYP3A4). The drug is also a substrate for this enzyme. As a result, carbamazepine not only stimulates the metabolism of other CYP3A4 substrates but also induces its own metabolism by autoinduction. Carbamazepine's half-life after single acute doses is approximately 35 hours; with chronic dosing, its half-life decreases to 15 to 25 hours. This increase in clearance necessitates increased carbamazepine doses, increased frequency of administration, or both. Autoinduction of carbamazepine metabolism appears to be related to dose and serum concentration. Approximately 1 month may be required for the autoinduction process to reach completion after each increase in carbamazepine dose.[61]

Assuming that adherence was not the main problem, A.R.'s carbamazepine dose should be increased. The drug's pharmacokinetics are generally linear with respect to acute dosage changes.[62] A 50% increase in dosage to 1,200 mg/day should re-establish seizure control. Depending on A.R.'s clinical status, further increases in dosage may be necessary.

Bioequivalence of Generic Dosage

CASE 60-1, QUESTION 6: A.R.'s dosage was increased to 600 mg BID. Four weeks later, she was still experiencing approximately one complex partial seizure weekly. A repeat trough serum carbamazepine concentration was 6.5 mcg/mL. On questioning, A.R. denied missing doses of medication, and a tablet count confirmed apparently accurate drug intake. A.R. relates that she experiences some mild nausea after her doses, but she has not vomited. It is noted that her pharmacist has begun substituting a generic carbamazepine tablets for the Tegretol that was previously dispensed. What role, if any, might this change in carbamazepine formulation have played in the failure of A.R.'s serum concentrations to increase as expected? What other factors might be considered in explaining this situation?

Several manufacturers market generic carbamazepine tablets. Bioavailability data supplied by the manufacturers are based on single-dose or short multiple-dose studies in healthy subjects. Therefore, it is impossible to completely predict the results of a change from Tegretol to generic carbamazepine for maintenance therapy in an individual patient.[63] Because of variations in amount of drug available from different products, some patients with epilepsy (aka "generic-brittle") cannot tolerate changes in formulations between brand and generic, generic and generic, or generic and brand.[64] Changes in seizure control from too little drug or toxicity from too much drug have been reported with changes between formulations for several AEDs. On the other hand, two recent in-depth bioequivalence studies have found no evidence to support any pharmacokinetic differences between brand and generic products of lamotrigine in patients with epilepsy.[65,66]

Bioavailability data suggest that the generic carbamazepine preparations currently on the market may be substituted for Tegretol with little need for dosage adjustment. Nonetheless, in A.R.'s case, substitution of generic carbamazepine may be a possible cause for the loss of seizure control. Readjustment of her dose to gain seizure control and consistent use of one manufacturer's product (either brand or generic) might alleviate this problem. Three extended-release forms of carbamazepine (Tegretol XR, Carbatrol, and Equetro) are available and may provide an alternative for A.R. These formulations allow more reliable absorption of drug when administered on a twice-daily dosing schedule. Many patients can better tolerate carbamazepine when these forms are used because large fluctuations in plasma concentrations are avoided. Use of Tegretol XR to avoid 3-times-daily or 4-times-daily dosing schedules has been shown to increase adherence for many patients.[67] It is important to counsel patients on the fact that the empty Oros tablet shell from the Tegretol XR dose does not dissolve as it passes through the gastrointestinal (GI) tract, and it may be visible in the stool. Patients need to understand that the carbamazepine has been absorbed, and that this is an empty shell. Tegretol XR tablets lose their extended-release properties when broken or crushed; Carbatrol beads may be emptied onto food or administered via feeding tube.[68] Equetro is not FDA-approved for epilepsy, it is indicated for the treatment of acute manic and mixed episodes associated with bipolar I disorder.

In conclusion, it may be impossible to identify a single cause for the unexpected change in A.R.'s seizure control. Common reasons for loss of seizure control include sleep deprivation, increased stress, acute illness, and/or medication nonadherence.

TREATMENT FAILURE AND ALTERNATIVE ANTIEPILEPTIC DRUGS

CASE 60-2

QUESTION 1: R.H., a 19-year-old, 64-kg young woman, has experienced simple partial seizures, complex partial seizures, and secondarily generalized tonic–clonic seizures for the past 2 years. She could not tolerate treatment with phenytoin (severe gingival hyperplasia and mental "dullness") or valproate (hair loss, tremor, and a weight gain of 8 kg). In addition, neither phenytoin nor valproate was dramatically effective in reducing her seizures. She currently receives carbamazepine 600 mg 3 times daily (TID). For the past 3 months, while being treated with carbamazepine, she has had approximately five simple partial seizures, three complex partial seizures, and one generalized tonic–clonic seizure. This represents an approximate 30% reduction in her frequency of seizures. She tolerates her present dose of carbamazepine but has experienced significant drowsiness, incoordination, and mental confusion at higher doses. What are possible therapeutic options for R.H.? Evaluate the newer AEDs and their possible usefulness for R.H.

R.H. is exhibiting a partial response to maximally tolerated doses of carbamazepine. An alteration in her current AED regimen is indicated. She has not tolerated other AEDs because of side effects. Although valproate is effective for control of partial seizures, it is not considered an alternative in a woman of childbearing age.

R.H.'s CNS side effects (e.g., persistent drowsiness) with other AEDs would make many clinicians reluctant to consider medications such as phenobarbital or primidone as either alternatives or adjunctive agents to her current carbamazepine regimen. Use of one of the newer AEDs as adjunctive medication may be of value for R.H.

New AEDs marketed in the United States since 1993 for maintenance treatment of epilepsy include the following: eslicarbazepine, ezogabine, felbamate, gabapentin, lacosamide, lamotrigine, levetiracetam, oxcarbazepine, perampanel, pregabalin, tiagabine, topiramate, and zonisamide (Table 60-6). Clinical trials for new AEDs are most often carried out in patients with partial seizures refractory to standard AEDs. Most of these newer or "second-generation" AEDs were initially FDA-approved as "add-on" or adjunctive treatment in patients with partial seizures with or without secondary generalization. Also, consensus is that some of these AEDs may be effective as broad-spectrum agents; for example, lamotrigine appears to be a useful treatment in absence seizures.

Side Effects

Common side effects for the newer AEDs are described in Table 60-6. Most of them are less sedating than older medications such as phenobarbital or phenytoin. The most common side effects seen in the clinical trials with eslicarbazepine were ataxia, blurred and double vision, dizziness, fatigue, headache, nausea, somnolence, tremor, vertigo, and vomiting.[69]

Gabapentin and tiagabine have not been associated with serious side effects; gabapentin can cause weight gain[70] and tiagabine can cause nonspecific dizziness relatively frequently.[71]

Common adverse effects associated with lacosamide include dizziness, headache, diplopia, and nausea. Gradual escalation to the desired dose reduces the adverse event risk.

The most serious adverse effect associated with lamotrigine is skin rash. Rashes occur in approximately 10% of treated patients, usually in the first 8 weeks.[72] Rashes leading to hospitalization occurred in 1 of 300 adults and 1 of 100 children. Widespread, maculopapular rashes usually appear and may progress to erythema multiforme or toxic epidermal necrolysis. Lamotrigine-related rashes may resolve rapidly when lamotrigine is discontinued. Coadministration of valproate with lamotrigine may increase the likelihood of dermatologic reactions; it is partly for this reason that more conservative dosage titration and lower maintenance doses of lamotrigine are recommended for patients receiving concomitant valproate. Higher starting doses and more rapid dose escalation than those recommended by the manufacturer also increase the risk of skin rash.

Levetiracetam is generally well tolerated, with the most common adverse events in clinical trials being asthenia, vertigo, flu syndrome, headache, rhinitis, and somnolence. The most serious adverse effects are behavioral and are more common in patients with a history of behavioral problems.[73] Levetiracetam should be used with caution in patients with a history of suicidal ideations.

Oxcarbazepine, a keto derivative of carbamazepine, is essentially a prodrug for the monohydroxy active metabolite.[74] Oxcarbazepine probably causes less frequent, less severe adverse effects compared with carbamazepine, with the exception of hyponatremia. Hyponatremia is more common with oxcarbazepine than with carbamazepine. Baseline and periodic serum sodium monitoring is indicated during oxcarbazepine therapy. The most commonly reported side effects of oxcarbazepine in clinical trials include ataxia, dizziness, fatigue, nausea, somnolence, and diplopia.

Adverse effects of pregabalin are dose dependent and usually occur within the first 2 weeks of treatment.[75] Somnolence, dizziness, and ataxia are most common. Pregabalin also appears to be associated with a dose-related weight gain.

Topiramate can cause cognitive disturbances, lethargy, and impaired mental concentration when given in large daily doses (especially in combination with other AEDs) or when the dosage is titrated too aggressively.[76] Topiramate has caused nephrolithiasis in approximately 1.5% of treated patients. This adverse effect is believed to be related to inhibition of carbonic anhydrase by topiramate, with resulting increased urinary pH and decreased citrate excretion. Topiramate can also cause acute, secondary angle-closure glaucoma, which presents within the first month of therapy. Topiramate is associated with weight loss.

Zonisamide is a sulfonamide derivative and thus is contraindicated in patients allergic to sulfonamides.[77] The most commonly reported adverse events include ataxia, somnolence, agitation, and anorexia. Kidney stones have developed in 3% to 4% of patients, some of whom had a family history of nephrolithiasis.

Pharmacokinetics

The newer AEDs have somewhat different pharmacokinetic profiles from those of older agents. They also differ in their tendency to interact with other AEDs. Gabapentin is excreted entirely by the kidneys as unchanged drug and is not significantly bound to plasma protein. Gabapentin has a relatively short half-life and should be administered 3 times daily.[78]

Lacosamide is excreted mostly by the kidneys. Dosage reductions are warranted for patients with renal impairment (creatinine clearance <30 mL/minute). It is less than 15% bound to plasma protein, has a 12- to 13-hour half-life, and is administered twice daily.[79]

Lamotrigine is primarily eliminated by hepatic glucuronidation and excretion of metabolites in the urine. Other AEDs, such as carbamazepine and phenytoin, induce the hepatic metabolism of lamotrigine. When lamotrigine is coadministered with enzyme-inducing drugs, its half-life decreases from approximately 24 to 15 hours. Valproate inhibits lamotrigine metabolism, causing increases in half-life and serum concentrations.[80,81] Patients treated with both lamotrigine and carbamazepine may experience more nausea, drowsiness, and ataxia. It appears likely that this interaction represents a pharmacodynamic interaction between lamotrigine and carbamazepine.[82]

Levetiracetam has a short half-life and is eliminated primarily by renal mechanisms. Dosage reductions are warranted for patients with renal impairment (creatinine clearance <80 mL/minute). The drug has a low potential for interactions with other drugs.[83]

Both eslicarbazepine acetate and oxcarbazepine are prodrugs. They cause less hepatic enzyme induction than carbamazepine and may therefore be less likely to interact with other medications. Both, however, increase the metabolism of oral contraceptive hormones.[84,85] Because eslicarbazepine and oxcarbazepine have similar mechanisms of action to that of carbamazepine, it is unlikely that either would offer significant benefits to R.H. because she has not responded to maximal tolerated doses of carbamazepine.[69,74]

Pregabalin is excreted entirely by the kidneys as unchanged drug and is not significantly bound to serum proteins. Unlike gabapentin, which requires more frequent dosing, pregabalin can be administered 2 or 3 times daily.[75]

Tiagabine has a relatively short half-life (4–7 hours). It should be administered at least twice daily.[71] Concurrently administered enzyme-inducing AEDs may reduce the half-life of tiagabine to 2 to 3 hours and necessitate use of larger daily doses and, possibly, shorter dosing intervals. Tiagabine is highly protein-bound (96%), and it is displaced from protein-binding sites by valproate, salicylate, and naproxen. The clinical significance of these protein-binding interactions is unknown.

Topiramate has a half-life of approximately 20 hours, which allows twice-daily administration. It is only partially excreted by hepatic metabolism; approximately 70% of the drug is

Table 60-6

Drugs Used for the Treatment of Partial and Generalized Tonic–Clonic Seizures

AED	Regimen	Adverse Effects	Comments
Carbamazepine (Tegretol, Tegretol XR, Carbatrol, Equetro)	Initial 200 mg BID (adults) or 100 mg BID (children) and weekly until therapeutic response or target serum concentrations. Usual maintenance doses 7–15 mg/kg/day in adults; 10–40 mg/kg/day in children	Sedation, visual disturbance may limit dosage. Severe blood dyscrasias extremely rare. Mild leukopenia more common. Laboratory monitoring of little value. Asian patients positive for HLA-B*1502 are at 10-fold higher risk for Stevens–Johnson syndrome/toxic epidermal necrolysis. Hepatotoxicity rare. May cause hyponatremia. Long-term use may cause osteomalacia	Usually little sedation and minimal interference with cognitive function or behavior. Preferred by most for partial or secondarily generalized seizures. Extended-release products may allow less frequent dosing with fewer peak serum concentration-related side effects. These products may also facilitate adherence
Phenytoin (Dilantin, Phenytek) Fosphenytoin (Cerebyx)	Initiate at maintenance dose of 4–5 mg/kg/day (300–400 mg/day). Titrate on basis of clinical response and target serum concentration. 3–4 weeks between dose ↑ recommended because of potentially slow accumulation	Nystagmus, ataxia, sedation may limit dosage. Gum hyperplasia, hirsutism common. Long-term use may cause osteomalacia. Peripheral neuropathy, hypersensitivity with liver damage rare. Possible increased risk of Stevens–Johnson syndrome/toxic epidermal necrolysis in Asian patients positive for HLA-B*1502	Clearance and half-life change with dose. Small ↑ in dose (30-mg capsule) recommended as plasma concentrations exceed 7–10 mcg/mL. Cautious use of suspension; dose measurement and potential mixing difficulties. IM administration not recommended. Potential precipitation in IV solutions. Fosphenytoin (Cerebyx) recommended for IM and IV use due to faster administration rate, admixture compatibility, and lower rate of injection site complications
Valproate (Depakene, Depakote, Depakote-ER, Depacon)	See Table 60-7	–	–
Phenobarbital	Initial 1 mg/kg/day; titrate to therapeutic response. 2–3 weeks between dose ↑	Sedation (chronic), behavior disturbances common, especially in children. Possibly impairs learning and intellectual performance. Long-term use may cause osteomalacia	Considered outmoded for AED therapy in most patients; adverse effects outweigh benefits. IV use for refractory status epilepticus
Pregabalin (Lyrica)	Initial 50 mg BID then titrate to therapeutic response with maximal daily dose at 600 mg/day in divided doses (BID or TID)	Potential side effects include dizziness, blurred vision and weight gain	No significant interactions with other AEDs. Can be useful for patients with concomitant pain disorders
Gabapentin (Neurontin)	Initial 300 mg/day with titration to 900–1,800 mg/day for 1–2 weeks. Doses of 2,400 mg/day and higher have been well tolerated. Owing to short half-life, TID or QID dosing recommended	Sedation, dizziness, and ataxia relatively common with initiation of therapy. Gabapentin therapy usually not associated with prominent side effects. Commonly associated with weight gain	Excreted unchanged by kidneys. No significant drug–drug interactions. Absorption dose dependent; fraction absorbed ↓ as size of individual dose ↑
Lamotrigine (Lamictal)	*When added to enzyme inducers alone:* Initiate at 50 mg daily HS or 50 mg BID. Daily dose can be ↑ by 50–100 mg every 7–14 days. Usual maintenance doses of 400–500 mg/day. BID dosing may be necessary with enzyme inducer cotherapy. *When added to valproate alone:* Initiate at 25 mg QOD HS. Daily dose can be ↑ by 25 mg every 14 days. Usual maintenance doses of 100–200 mg/day. *For patients not taking valproate or an enzyme inducer:* Initiate at 25 mg QD HS. Daily dose can be ↑ by 25 mg every 14 days. Usual daily doses of 225–375 mg/day	Dizziness, diplopia, sedation, ataxia, and blurred vision can be common with initiation of therapy; limit speed of titration. Incidence of serious rash ranges from 0.8–8.0 per 1,000	Significant ↑ in clearance of lamotrigine when coadministered with enzyme inducers. Significant ↓ in clearance when coadministered with valproate. Slow, gradual titration of dose may reduce risk of skin rash. Estrogen increases clearance

Table 60-6

Drugs Used for the Treatment of Partial and Generalized Tonic–Clonic Seizures (*continued*)

AED	Regimen	Adverse Effects	Comments
Tiagabine (Gabitril)	Initial 4 mg/day. ↑ by 4 mg/day at 7 days. Then ↑ daily dose by 4–8 mg every week. Maximal recommended dose of 32 mg/day in adolescents or 56 mg/day in adults. BID to QID dosing recommended	Drowsiness, nervousness, difficulty with concentration or attention, tremor. Nonspecific dizziness described by some patients	Increased clearance when given with enzyme inducers. TID or QID doses probably needed. Potential for protein-binding displacement interactions with other highly protein-bound drugs (e.g., valproate). Significance of protein-binding displacement not known. Substrate for CYP3A4
Topiramate (Topamax, Trokendi, Qudexy)	Initial 50 mg HS. ↑ daily dose by 50 mg every 7 days. 200–400 mg/day recommended as target dosage range. Larger daily doses associated with increased CNS side effects. BID dosing recommended	Sedation, dizziness, difficulty concentrating, confusion. May be dose related. Possible weight loss. Weak CA inhibitor; may cause or predispose to kidney stones; CA inhibition also possibly related to paresthesias in up to 15%. Risk of hypohidrosis and hyperthermia especially in children. Rarely associated with angle-closure glaucoma	Approximately 70% renal elimination. Phenytoin and carbamazepine may reduce topiramate plasma concentrations and potentially increase dosage requirements. Topiramate may cause small ↑ in phenytoin plasma concentration. Advise patients to drink plenty of fluids. May affect oral contraceptives above 200 mg/day
Levetiracetam (Keppra, Keppra-XR, Spritam)	Initial 250–500 mg BID. ↑ by 500–1,000 mg/day every 2 weeks. Usual maximal dose is 3,000 mg/day. Doses up to 4,000 mg/day have been used. BID dosing recommended	Somnolence, dizziness, asthenia are commonly reported. Behavioral symptoms (agitation, emotional lability, hostility, depression, and depersonalization) reported	No hepatic (CYP450 or UGT) metabolism. 66% excreted unchanged in urine. Less than 10% protein bound. No significant drug interactions reported
Lacosamide (Vimpat)	Initiate at 50 mg BID. Increase weekly by 100 mg/day. Target doses of 200–400 mg/day. Maximum recommended dose is 400 mg/day	Dizziness, ataxia, diplopia, headache, nausea. May slow cardiac conduction. Caution is advised in patients with second-degree AV block. Syncope has been reported	Currently only indicated for treatment of partial seizures in adults. IV form available; currently only approved for short-term replacement of oral therapy. Little evidence of significant risk of drug–drug interactions. Some hepatic metabolism by CYP2C19; significant renal elimination
Oxcarbazepine (Trileptal, Oxtellar)	*Monotherapy:* Initial 300 mg BID. ↑ weekly up to 1,200 mg/day. Can increase to 2,400 mg/day. *Adjunctive therapy:* Initial 300 mg BID. ↑ weekly up to 1,200 mg/day	Dizziness, somnolence, diplopia, nausea, and ataxia are commonly reported. May cause hyponatremia; most cases asymptomatic, more common in elderly. A 25% cross-sensitivity for skin rash reported between oxcarbazepine and carbamazepine	Parent is a prodrug; the MHD is the active component. Readily converted to MHD via omnipresent cytosolic enzymes. Lacks autoinduction properties. In doses >1,200 mg/day, may affect oral contraceptives
Zonisamide (Zonegran)	Initial 100 mg daily. ↑ by 100 mg/day every 2 weeks. Usual maintenance doses of 200–400 mg/day; maximum 600 mg/day	Somnolence, nausea, ataxia, dizziness, headache, and anorexia are common. Weight loss and nephrolithiasis reported. Serious skin eruptions, oligohidrosis, and hyperthermia have also occurred	Broad spectrum, long half-life. 35% of dose is excreted unchanged in the urine. Also a substrate of CYP3A4; enzyme induction may increase clearance. Advise patients to drink plenty of fluids
Ezogabine (Potiga)	Initial 100 mg TID. ↑ by 150 mg/day every week. 600–1,200 mg/day recommended as target dosage range. TID dosing recommended	Dizziness, fatigue and somnolence are commonly reported. Urinary retention, confusion, and hallucinations. Reddish-orange urine discoloration is benign. Prolongs QT interval. Retinal abnormalities and potential vision loss	Phenytoin and carbamazepine reduce ezogabine exposure by 30%–35%. Higher doses may be needed. Monitor vision and eye examination

(*continued*)

Table 60-6

Drugs Used for the Treatment of Partial and Generalized Tonic–Clonic Seizures (*continued*)

AED	Regimen	Adverse Effects	Comments
Perampanel (Fycompa)	Initial 2 mg once daily HS (not on enzyme-inducing AEDs) or 4 mg once daily HS (on enzyme-inducing AEDs). ↑ by 2 mg/day every week. 4–12 mg/day recommended as target dosage range. Once-daily dosing HS recommended	Dizziness, gait disturbance, somnolence and fatigue are commonly reported. Risk of falls in elderly patients. Aggression, hostility, irritability, anger and homicidal ideation. May be worsened by alcohol	Avoidance of alcohol is recommended. Enzyme-inducing AEDs reduce perampanel exposure by 50%–67%. Higher doses may be needed. Perampanel 12 mg/day may reduce effectiveness of hormonal contraceptives containing levonorgestrel
Eslicarbazepine (Aptiom)	Initial 400 mg once daily. ↑ by 400 mg/day after one week. Maximum recommended dose is 1,200 mg/day. Once-daily dosing recommended	Dizziness, somnolence, nausea, and headache	Enzyme-inducing AEDs reduce eslicarbazepine exposure. Higher doses may be needed. May reduce effectiveness of hormonal contraceptives

AED, antiepileptic drugs; AV, atrioventricular; BID, twice daily; CA, carbonic anhydrase; CNS, central nervous system; CYP, cytochrome P-450; GI, gastrointestinal; HS, at bedtime; IM, intramuscular; IV, intravenous; MHD, monohydroxy derivative; PE, phenytoin sodium equivalent; QID, four times daily; QOD, every other day; SIADH, syndrome of inappropriate antidiuretic hormone secretion; TID, three times daily; UGT, uridine diphosphate glucuronosyltransferase; VPA, valproic acid.

excreted unchanged by the kidneys. Topiramate is minimally protein-bound (~10%–15%). When topiramate is coadministered with enzyme-inducing agents, topiramate clearance is increased. This interaction may necessitate titration to somewhat higher doses when topiramate is used with enzyme-inducing drugs.

Zonisamide has a long half-life and low protein binding. It is eliminated by both hepatic metabolism and renal excretion. The average half-life of zonisamide is 63 hours, but there is wide interpatient variation. Serum levels of zonisamide are reduced by enzyme-inducing AEDs but clinical consequences of pharmacokinetic interactions with zonisamide are rare.[77]

On the basis of efficacy and side effect characteristics, gabapentin, lacosamide, lamotrigine, levetiracetam, pregabalin, tiagabine, topiramate, or zonisamide could be considered for use as adjunctive therapy for R.H. In young, active patients such as R.H., sedation might prove to be a problem; however, it is not clear that any of these drugs predictably causes more initial or long-term sedation. The short half-lives of gabapentin and tiagabine and the associated need for R.H. to take several doses during the day might decrease her adherence. Therefore, lacosamide, lamotrigine, levetiracetam, pregabalin, topiramate, or zonisamide would be reasonable choices on the basis of convenience. Because the patient is not tolerating carbamazepine, it does not make sense to switch to either eslicarbazepine or oxcarbazepine.

The reason that ezogabine, felbamate, and perampanel were not discussed in the side effects and pharmacokinetics sections above is that these authors do not believe they are good options for R.H. at this point. Ezogabine and perampanel are very new to the market at the time of this writing and both have FDA boxed warnings (vision problems and behavioral reactions, respectively). Felbamate's usefulness is seriously limited by its association with aplastic anemia and hepatic failure.

Potential Therapies

Other AEDs that may become available in the near future include brivaracetam, ganaxolone, and huperzine A.[86] These drugs may become useful as alternatives or adjuncts to established and newer medications in the future.

With advancing technology and knowledge about genes and brain networks, future treatment strategies should move from controlling symptoms of epilepsy with AEDs to prevention and cure. For AED-resistant epilepsy, much research is examining the role of multidrug transporters (e.g., *P*-glycoprotein) at the blood–brain barrier. These proteins may act as a defense mechanism by limiting the accumulation of AED in the brain.[87] Although it has not yet had much of an impact on the clinical care of patients with epilepsy, pharmacogenetics of AED therapy is continually advancing.[88]

LAMOTRIGINE THERAPY

Initiation and Dosage Titration

CASE 60-2, QUESTION 2: R.H. is to be started on lamotrigine as adjunctive therapy to her carbamazepine. Outline a treatment plan for initiating and monitoring therapy for R.H. What should R.H. and her family be told about this medication and how to use it?

Lamotrigine therapy should be initiated in R.H. with a slow upward dosage titration to minimize early sedative effects and reduce the likelihood of skin rash. An initial dosage of 50 mg/day given at bedtime is recommended; the daily dose can be increased by 50 mg every 1 to 2 weeks. Because R.H. is currently receiving carbamazepine, induction of liver enzymes is likely to increase her dosage requirements for lamotrigine and allow a less conservative dosage titration. A twice-daily schedule is recommended for maintenance therapy. Usual maintenance dosages of lamotrigine are approximately 300 to 500 mg/day. A patient's ability to tolerate this medication ultimately determines dosage limitations. Onset of side effects (e.g., nausea, diplopia, ataxia, and dizziness) may prevent further dosage increases.

R.H. should be told that she may feel drowsy and possibly experience headache and upset stomach, but that these side effects usually disappear with ongoing therapy. She should contact her physician or other health care professional if severe side effects occur that make it difficult to take the medication; this is especially important if she exhibits a rash.

Side Effects and Possible Interaction with Carbamazepine

CASE 60-2, QUESTION 3: Two days after her dosage of lamotrigine was increased to 300 mg/day (12 weeks after beginning therapy), R.H. noticed that her vision was blurring; she also complained of feeling dizzy and having difficulty maintaining her balance. Previously, she had experienced only mild, occasional nausea. She had continued to experience seizures at approximately the same frequency she had before the initiation of lamotrigine. Her physician had encouraged her to continue taking the medication and explained that it would take time to increase the dose to possibly effective levels. Her current carbamazepine serum concentration is essentially unchanged when compared with when she was taking it in monotherapy. Do these new side effects represent treatment failure with lamotrigine? If not, how might these new side effects be managed?

R.H.'s side effects may limit further dosage increases. Her current side effects might represent carbamazepine intoxication, lamotrigine side effects, or an interaction between these two medications. Because R.H. tolerated the same carbamazepine dose previously, carbamazepine "intoxication" seems a less likely cause. Assessing the role of lamotrigine as the only cause is difficult. Obtaining a lamotrigine serum concentration to aid in assessing her adverse effects is not likely to be helpful. A usual "therapeutic range" for lamotrigine serum concentrations has not been established. Clinical studies have failed to demonstrate a significant correlation between lamotrigine serum concentrations and either therapeutic or adverse responses.[89,90] Her symptoms may also be related to an apparent pharmacodynamic interaction between lamotrigine and carbamazepine.[82] The effects experienced by some patients taking both drugs may be relieved by reducing the carbamazepine dosage.

LEVETIRACETAM THERAPY

Initiation and Dosage Titration

CASE 60-2, QUESTION 4: R.H.'s carbamazepine dosage was reduced from 1,800 mg/day to 1,400 mg/day. After 5 days, her side effects persisted and her seizure frequency appeared to be increasing. The clinician decides to abandon lamotrigine therapy and institute treatment with levetiracetam. Recommend a plan for initiating R.H.'s levetiracetam treatment.

R.H. previously tolerated and had a better therapeutic response to a higher carbamazepine dose. Therefore, the dosage of carbamazepine should be returned to 1,800 mg/day before levetiracetam therapy is initiated. Little specific information is available to help determine how lamotrigine can be safely discontinued. As a general rule, rapid discontinuation of AEDs is not recommended in other than emergency situations. Therefore, immediate reduction of R.H.'s lamotrigine dosage to 200 mg/day would seem reasonable. This dosage could then be reduced by 50 to 100 mg every week until lamotrigine is discontinued.

Levetiracetam treatment should be instituted immediately for R.H. because of her continuing seizures. Levetiracetam does not interact with other AEDs. Therefore, discontinuing lamotrigine during initiation of levetiracetam should not create difficulties in assessing R.H.'s response. Levetiracetam should be initiated at a dosage of 250 to 500 mg 2 times daily.[83] Although the manufacturer recommends initiating treatment at 500 mg twice daily, patients may better tolerate lower initial doses and more gradual titration. R.H.'s daily levetiracetam dose can be increased by 500 to 1,000 mg every 2 or 3 weeks, according to her tolerance of side effects and her change in seizure frequency. Although the drug reaches steady state quickly, allowing at least 2 weeks for observation before dosage increases may improve patient tolerability and allow for a more thorough evaluation of therapeutic response. At present, the relationship between serum concentrations of levetiracetam and therapeutic response or symptoms of intoxication is not well defined. Therefore, R.H.'s dose should be titrated to the maximal tolerated amount required to control her seizures. In controlled trials, no clear benefits were apparent at doses greater than 3,000 mg/day.

Patient Education

R.H. should be informed that with levetiracetam she may experience side effects similar to those she had with lamotrigine. R.H.'s mood should be assessed at each visit. Much reassurance and encouragement may need to be given along with this information to help ensure that R.H. adheres to her treatment regimen. Many patients become discouraged when multiple trials of medication are necessary and side effects are prominent. They may express feelings of being "guinea pigs" and may become uncooperative with the therapeutic plan. Given that RH's seizures are still not well controlled, driving restrictions that were likely put into place earlier should be continued. RH should be counseled not to drive until she is seizure-free and her driving privileges have been reinstated according to applicable state law. This restriction can be very hard for some patients to accept because it can significantly decrease their independence.

PHENYTOIN THERAPY

Initiation and Dosage

CASE 60-3

QUESTION 1: J.N., an 18-year-old, 88-kg male college student, was diagnosed with epilepsy. He experiences generalized tonic–clonic seizures that last 2 minutes approximately 3 times monthly. J.N. describes a "churning" feeling in his abdomen before his seizures; this is followed by involuntary right-sided jerking of his upper extremities. An EEG showed diffuse slowing with focal epileptiform discharges in the left temporal area; it was interpreted as abnormal. No correctable cause for his seizure disorder was identified despite a thorough workup. He has no other medical conditions and takes no routine medications. He was treated initially with carbamazepine up to 600 mg/day. He could not tolerate the medication because of nausea and diplopia despite relatively low doses. J.N.'s physician has elected to implement a therapeutic trial of phenytoin. Recommend an initial dosage. What information should be provided to J.N. about his new medication?

Selecting a nontoxic, therapeutic dose of any AED is difficult without having information about the drug's disposition in the individual patient (i.e., prior dosages and clinical response). Although "average" dosages and resulting serum concentrations for phenytoin often are quoted, interpatient variability is significant. An initial phenytoin dosage of 400 mg/day (approximately 4.5 mg/kg/day) would be appropriate for J.N. In most patients, phenytoin therapy is initiated at or near the anticipated maintenance dose (e.g., 300 or 400 mg daily in J.N.). If tolerability problems arise, J.N.'s phenytoin dose could be reduced to 200 mg daily (or 100 mg every 12 hours) and increased by 100 mg/day at weekly intervals until 400 mg/day is reached. Recently, there has been significant interest in using patient-specific genetic information to more accurately dose certain drugs, including phenytoin, with the goals of achieving a therapeutic effect quickly and avoiding dose-related toxicity. Although certain CYP2C9 homozygous allele variants have been shown to confer "slow-metabolizer" status on patients treated with phenytoin,[91] CYP2C9 genotyping of patients is not presently a part of routine clinical practice.

Patient Education

In addition to the name and strength of the medication and instructions for when and how it should be taken, J.N. should be informed that he may experience initial mild sedation from phenytoin. He should be cautioned that symptoms such as blurred or double vision, dysarthria, dizziness, or staggering may indicate that his dosage is too high; he should be instructed to notify his physician, pharmacist, or other health care professional of these symptoms. It is also a good idea to inform patients, at the beginning of therapy, that adjustments of medication dosage may be necessary before the regimen is stabilized. While RH is at relatively low risk for osteomalacia given his age and gender, he should be informed that long-term use of phenytoin (as well as other AEDs; see Table 60-6) is associated with an increased risk of bone mineral loss and that this adverse effect warrants monitoring periodically.

Accumulation Pharmacokinetics

CASE 60-3, QUESTION 2: What are the characteristics of phenytoin accumulation pharmacokinetics?

Phenytoin exhibits dose-dependent (Michaelis–Menten or capacity-limited) pharmacokinetics; therefore, the usual pharmacokinetic concepts of "clearance" and "half-life" are meaningless. The apparent half-life of phenytoin changes with the dose and serum concentration. Thus, the time required to reach a new steady state after dose alteration is difficult to predict because it depends on the dose itself and the patient's pharmacokinetic parameters, V_{max} and K_m.[92] V_{max} is a kinetic constant representing the maximal rate of phenytoin elimination from the body. K_m is the Michaelis constant, the serum concentration at which the rate of elimination is 50% of V_{max}. Values for these parameters vary widely among patients; as a result, patterns of phenytoin accumulation and the time required to achieve steady state also vary.

Many clinicians assume that phenytoin's apparent half-life is approximately 24 hours, and they wait 5 to 7 days before assessing the patient's clinical response and measuring serum phenytoin concentrations. Both clinical studies[93] and model simulations[94] using observed values for K_m and V_{max} have been used to estimate time required for serum concentrations of phenytoin to reach steady state. Up to 30 days may be needed for this to occur either with doses sufficient to produce steady state serum concentrations of 10 to 15 mcg/mL or with doses of 4 mg/kg/day.[92,95] Occasionally, such a dose may exceed a patient's V_{max}; the result is extremely high serum phenytoin concentrations, with probable intoxication. It is important not to assume that steady state has been reached unless widely spaced, serial serum concentrations indicate that accumulation has ceased. Alterations in phenytoin dosage before steady state has been reached can result in significant fluctuations in serum concentrations and the patient's clinical status. Such situations occur frequently and result in unnecessary confusion and expense. As always, serum concentrations in J.N. must be interpreted in the context of his clinical response.

Phenytoin Intoxication

CASE 60-3, QUESTION 3: J.N. was started on phenytoin and is now taking 200 mg every 12 hours. One week after achieving this dose, mild lateral gaze nystagmus was noted, but J.N. had no subjective complaints and was seizure-free. After 3 weeks, J.N. complained of double vision and feeling "drunk" and "unsteady." Significant nystagmus was present. How should J.N.'s phenytoin dosage be altered?

J.N.'s signs and symptoms indicate phenytoin intoxication. Dosage reduction is indicated. Reducing J.N.'s dosage to 360 mg/day (accomplished using both 100-mg and 30-mg phenytoin capsules) would be reasonable. A larger reduction may result in a loss of seizure control. Many clinicians also would have J.N. omit one day's dose of phenytoin before beginning the new maintenance dosage. This would accelerate the decline in phenytoin serum levels. After this dosage change, clinical response should be monitored closely. The new maintenance dose may still be excessive, if J.N.'s V_{max} for phenytoin is low. If this were the case, continued accumulation of drug would occur despite the dosage reduction.[92]

Intramuscular (IM) Phenytoin and Fosphenytoin (Phenytoin Prodrug)

CASE 60-4

QUESTION 1: S.D. is a 24-year-old male institutionalized patient with a history of complex partial and secondarily generalized tonic–clonic seizures. Within the past year, his phenytoin formulation was switched from phenytoin sodium capsules to phenytoin suspension because S.D. was suspected of "cheeking" his medicines and not swallowing the capsules. He has had no seizures in the past 3 months on 275 mg/day of phenytoin suspension. S.D. has now been transferred to the acute medical unit after a 2-day history of anorexia, nausea, occasional vomiting, and abdominal pain accompanied by diarrhea. His chart now states "nothing by mouth." IM fosphenytoin, 275 mg (phenytoin sodium equivalents [PEs]) per day, has been ordered. Discuss the use of IM fosphenytoin, and devise a dosage regimen for S.D.

S.D. is a candidate for parenteral administration of his AED. If placement of an IV line for fluid administration is not planned, then IM administration is an acceptable approach to treatment; however, the type of phenytoin product administered will need to be changed. Phenytoin, itself, should not be administered by IM injection. Injectable phenytoin is highly alkaline (pH 12) and extremely irritating to tissue. After IM injection, the drug may precipitate at the injection site because of the change in pH. As a result, phenytoin crystals form a repository or depot from which the drug is slowly absorbed.[96–98] Often injection site discomfort is noted, although severe muscle damage does not seem to occur.[98]

Fosphenytoin, a phosphate ester prodrug of phenytoin, is highly water-soluble. Its solubility allows this preparation to be administered parenterally without the need for solubilization using propylene glycol or the adjustment of pH to nonphysiologic levels. Therefore, fosphenytoin may be administered either IM or IV with less risk of tissue damage and venous irritation than with parenteral administration of phenytoin.[99–101] (See also subsequent discussion of IV administration of phenytoin and fosphenytoin.) After administration, fosphenytoin is rapidly absorbed and converted to phenytoin by phosphatase enzymes. Ultimately, the bioavailability of phenytoin from IM fosphenytoin administration is 100%.

Fosphenytoin is available as a solution containing 50 mg PE/mL. By labeling fosphenytoin this way, no dosing adjustments are necessary when converting from phenytoin sodium to fosphenytoin or vice versa. Although the prescriber ordered 275 mg PE, S.D. may be underdosed. His oral dosage of phenytoin suspension is providing the equivalent of 300 mg/day of sodium phenytoin. Phenytoin suspension and chewable tablets contain free acid, whereas capsules contain sodium phenytoin. Therefore, phenytoin capsule products contain only 92% of the labeled content as phenytoin acid (i.e., a 100-mg sodium phenytoin capsule contains only 92 mg of phenytoin acid). He should receive a 300-mg dose of fosphenytoin daily to fully replace his current dosage of phenytoin suspension.[101]

Assuming that S.D. will be given 300 mg PE of fosphenytoin daily, he will require a total of 6 mL of this injection given IM. This medication is well tolerated when given IM, and S.D.'s full daily dose can be given in a single injection without causing excessive discomfort. Some clinicians report administering IM injections of fosphenytoin as large as 20 mL in a single site without adverse consequences or serious discomfort.[102] It is also possible to divide his daily dosage into two injections given in two different sites, although many patients prefer to receive fewer injections.

Adverse Effects

CASE 60-5

Question 1: G.R. is a 53-year-old man with partial-onset epilepsy characterized by occasional tonic–clonic seizures. He has taken phenytoin for the past 2 years. His dosage of phenytoin was recently reduced from 400 to 360 mg/day because of symptoms of AED intoxication (mild confusion, occasional diplopia, ataxia, and lateral gaze nystagmus). After the dose reduction, his confusion and diplopia decreased significantly. The neurologic evaluation at the lower dose was within normal limits. No seizures occurred during the subsequent 8 weeks. He continued to complain of being mildly "unsteady" on his feet. He also exhibits mild-to-moderate gingival hyperplasia and significant halitosis. Discuss phenytoin-related gingival hyperplasia and management techniques that may be helpful for G.R. Because G.R.'s seizures are apparently under complete control, is there any problem maintaining him on his current dose of phenytoin?

Gingival Hyperplasia

Gum hyperplasia related to phenytoin is common and troublesome. Prevalence is estimated at 40% to 50% of treated patients.[103] Prevalence and incidence rates, however, are misleading because the occurrence and severity of hyperplasia are related to the dose and serum concentration of phenytoin.[103,104] Gingival hyperplasia is of obvious cosmetic importance. Also, as in G.R., formation of pockets of tissue leads to difficulties with oral hygiene, and halitosis may result.

The mechanism of phenytoin-induced gingival hyperplasia is not well understood. The drug is excreted in saliva and saliva phenytoin concentrations and hyperplasia are correlated; however, this correlation may simply reflect higher serum concentrations producing a greater pharmacologic effect. Phenytoin may stimulate gingival mast cells to release heparin and other mediators that may encourage synthesis of excessive amounts of new connective tissue by fibroblasts. Local irritation caused by dental plaque and food particles may further stimulate this process.[103,104]

Three approaches to the treatment of existing hyperplasia[104] are (a) dosage reduction or replacement of phenytoin with an alternative AED, if possible, which will permit partial or complete reversal of hyperplasia; (b) surgical gingivectomy, which will correct the problem temporarily, but hyperplasia eventually recurs; and (c) periodontal treatment, which will eliminate local irritants and maintains oral hygiene. Treatment for existing hyperplasia and prevention of further tissue enlargement is important. Assuming that phenytoin is producing adequate seizure control, a combination of gingivectomy and follow-up periodontal treatment may be the best approach.

Oral hygiene programs appear to reduce the degree and severity of gingival hyperplasia when they are initiated before phenytoin therapy is started.[104] Patients who are beginning phenytoin therapy should be educated about the role of oral hygiene in diminishing this side effect. The use of dental floss, gum stimulators, and water-flossing appliances may be beneficial adjuncts to other oral hygiene techniques.

Neurotoxicity

Patients chronically maintained on intoxicating doses of phenytoin appear to be at risk for developing irreversible cerebellar damage and/or peripheral neuropathy. Cerebellar degeneration, resulting in symptoms such as dysarthria, ataxic gait, intention tremor, and muscular hypotonia, is of particular concern; this complication has been observed after episodes of acute phenytoin intoxication.[105,106] Generalized seizures also can cause cerebellar degeneration secondary to hypoxia. For this reason, the relative importance of phenytoin in the development of this condition is controversial. Nevertheless, cerebellar degeneration has been reported in several patients without hypoxic seizures.[106,107]

Symptomatic phenytoin-related peripheral neuropathy is rare, although electrophysiologic evidence of impaired neuronal conduction is found in many patients.[105,108] Symptomatic patients may complain of paresthesias, muscle weakness, and occasional muscle wasting. Knee and ankle tendon reflexes are absent in 18% of patients on long-term phenytoin therapy; the upper limbs are rarely affected.[109] Although areflexia may be irreversible,[109] electrophysiologic abnormalities may be closely related to excessive serum phenytoin concentrations and are reversible after dosage reduction or discontinuation.[107]

In G.R., the general discomfort of mild phenytoin intoxication and the potential for producing cerebellar degeneration necessitate a therapy alteration. The phenytoin dose should be reduced to 330 mg/day because it may produce adequate seizure control without toxic symptoms. Should seizures recur at this lower dosage, it may be advisable to consider an alternative AED.

Antiepileptic Drug Impact on Bone

Some AEDs have a negative impact on bone density. People with epilepsy treated with these drugs are at increased risk for bone disorders and fractures.[110] Longer duration of AED therapy and exposure to multiple AEDs are thought to predict bone loss. Enzyme-inducing AEDs (carbamazepine, phenytoin, and phenobarbital) have been associated with bone loss and an increased risk for fracture. Valproate, although not an enzyme inducer, is associated with decreased bone mineral density in children.[111] Less is known about the impact of newer AEDs on bone mineral metabolism.[112] Because of the length of phenytoin use, G.R. is at risk. His bone health should be further evaluated by a DEXA scan to examine his bone mineral density. G.R. should be evaluated for other risk factors of reduced bone health (e.g., immobility, poor diet, family history). Oral calcium and vitamin D supplementation should be implemented. Depending on the outcome of evaluation, a change from phenytoin to an AED with less or no effect on bone should be considered.

New-onset Seizures in the Elderly

CASE 60-6

Question 1: J.R., a 74-year-old man with newly diagnosed partial seizures, is referred to the neurology clinic for evaluation and treatment. The etiology of his new-onset seizures is presumed to be a recent cerebral infarct. His seizures are complex partial seizures (he "blacks out" and loses track of time). He has no history of secondarily generalized tonic–clonic convulsions. He has had three seizures in the last 4 weeks. His last seizure resulted in a fall down a flight of stairs. His wife reports that he is more likely to have a seizure if he gets "overtired" or "stressed-out." He is also being treated for hypertension and diabetes. What options are available for the treatment of J.R.'s epilepsy?

There are relatively few head-to-head comparative studies of AEDs in patients with epilepsy. Even fewer studies address the comparative efficacy of AEDs in elderly patients. Three studies, in particular, are important when discussing AED treatment in elderly persons with epilepsy.

Brodie et al.[113] compared lamotrigine (n = 102) with carbamazepine (n = 48) in elderly patients with newly diagnosed epilepsy via a double-blind, randomized, parallel study. Discontinuation rates because of adverse effects (the primary outcome parameter) were higher for carbamazepine (42%) than for lamotrigine (18%). Using time to first seizure as a measure of efficacy, no differences were found between the two AEDs, and the authors suggested that lamotrigine is "acceptable" as initial treatment in elderly patients with newly diagnosed epilepsy.

Carbamazepine (600 mg/day), gabapentin (1,500 mg/day), and lamotrigine (150 mg/day) were compared for efficacy and tolerability in 593 patients older than 55 years of age (mean age, 72 years) with newly diagnosed epilepsy.[114] Although efficacy was similar in all three groups, study termination for adverse events varied between treatment groups. Carbamazepine had the highest termination rate (31%), followed by gabapentin (21.6%), and then lamotrigine (12.1%) ($P = 0.001$). The authors concluded that lamotrigine and gabapentin should be considered as initial therapy for new-onset seizures in older patients with epilepsy.

Werhahn et al.[115] evaluated carbamazepine (controlled-release), lamotrigine, and levetiracetam in 359 patients 60 years of age and older (mean age, 71.4 years) with newly diagnosed partial epilepsy via a double-blind, randomized, multicenter trial. As with the other two studies, efficacy (as measured by seizure freedom rates), did not differ between the three drugs. But retention rate at week 58 (primary outcome) was significantly higher for levetiracetam (61.5%) than for carbamazepine (45.8%) ($P = 0.02$). The retention rate for lamotrigine (55.6%) was close to that of levetiracetam.

These studies in elderly patients with new-onset epilepsy suggest that gabapentin, lamotrigine or levetiracetam would be good choices for initial treatment of J.R.'s epilepsy. It is noteworthy that none of these AEDs are FDA-approved for newly diagnosed epilepsy.

It is also important to consider drug-interaction profile, dosing frequency, and drug costs when selecting AED therapy. Generally, elderly persons take more medicines than younger individuals. For example, the average number of concomitant medications in the study by Rowan et al.[114] was seven. J.R. is likely to be taking other medicines for diabetes and hypertension. Gabapentin, lamotrigine, nor levetiracetam causes drug–drug interactions, although lamotrigine is influenced more so than gabapentin or levetiracetam by other medicines. Doses of gabapentin and levetiracetam have to be adjusted for renal function.

Adverse Effects

Comparative studies identified minimal differences in efficacy. Newer AEDs, however, showed better tolerability than the older AEDs. In general, elderly patients not only respond to AEDs at lower doses and concentrations but they also exhibit toxicity symptoms at lower doses than do younger patients. Age-related declines in renal and hepatic function may account for those observations. The pharmacokinetics of many AEDs have been studied in the elderly and a decrease in clearance is noted as compared with the young.[116] Decreased clearance of AEDs in the elderly has often been cited as a reason for their increased responsiveness to these drugs.

The impact of AEDs on cognition is an important issue for all patients with epilepsy and perhaps it is an even greater issue in elderly patients.[117–119] As evidenced from the study by Rowan et al.,[114] CNS toxicities such as dizziness, unsteady gait, and ataxia are common adverse effects of AEDs in elderly patients. These symptoms may increase the risk of falls, which are of particular concern in light of the potential negative effects of AEDs on bone mineral density.

J.R. and his family should be informed about the benefits and risks associated with each AED and they should also be incorporated into the decision-making process. AED therapy in the elderly should follow the "start low and go slow" adage, and elderly patients should be monitored for both efficacy (via a seizure calendar) and toxicity (reporting any intolerable side effects).

Absence Seizures

CHOICE OF MEDICATION AND INITIATION OF ETHOSUXIMIDE THERAPY

CASE 60-7

QUESTION 1: T.D., a 7-year-old, 25-kg girl, is reported by her teacher to have three or four episodes of "staring" daily. Each spell lasts 5 to 10 seconds. No convulsive movements occur during the episodes, but her eyelids appear to flutter. She is fully alert afterward. T.D.'s school performance is somewhat below average, despite an intelligence quotient (IQ) of 125. An EEG shows 3-Hertz (Hz) spike-and-wave activity. Typical childhood absence epilepsy is diagnosed. Physical examination and laboratory evaluation findings are normal, and no other positive findings are evident on the neurologic examination. What drug should be prescribed for T.D., and how should therapy with this drug be initiated?

Ethosuximide, valproate, and lamotrigine are commonly used to treat absence epilepsy in the United States. Ethosuximide is a succinimide agent that blocks T-type calcium currents in the thalamus. The drug is effective against absence seizures, but is ineffective against other seizure types. Patients who receive ethosuximide, predominantly children, generally tolerate the drug well and, given its lack of idiosyncratic hepatic toxicity, it has historically been preferred over valproate by many prescribers for the treatment of childhood absence epilepsy. Valproate, a carboxylic acid derivative with broad-spectrum activity against many focal-onset and generalized-onset seizure types, is highly effective but is associated with adverse effects (dose-related, non-dose-related, and severe idiosyncratic) that limits the drug's use among some patient groups. In addition to ethosuximide and valproate, lamotrigine also has been recommended as an initial monotherapy agent for treatment of absence epilepsy, although it is not FDA-approved for this indication[120–122] (Tables 60-2 and 60-6).

Valproate, ethosuximide, and lamotrigine were directly compared for efficacy in the treatment of newly diagnosed childhood absence epilepsy.[123] Efficacy rates for valproate and ethosuximide (based on freedom from treatment failure) were not significantly different, but were significantly higher than for lamotrigine. Attentional dysfunction was significantly more common with valproate than with ethosuximide. Valproate was also more efficacious than lamotrigine for treatment of idiopathic generalized seizures (including absence) in the Standard and New Antiepileptic Drugs (SANAD) trial.[124] Most authorities now consider ethosuximide the drug of first choice for treatment of absence seizures. Valproate is more likely to cause significant nausea and initial drowsiness and it is more likely to interact with other drugs, including AEDs. Valproate usually is reserved for patients whose absence seizures do not respond to ethosuximide.[125] Clonazepam, a benzodiazepine, often is effective for control of absence seizures. Therapy with this drug is limited by prominent CNS side effects (sedation, ataxia, and mood changes) and development of tolerance to its antiepileptic effect after long-term use.[126] Most authorities consider clonazepam a fourth-choice drug for treatment of absence seizures.

T.D. should be started on ethosuximide at a dosage of 15 to 20 mg/kg/day or 250 mg twice daily. The daily dose can be increased by 250 mg every 10 to 14 days as necessary to control seizures. Because the average half-life of ethosuximide in children is ~30 hours, a delay of 10 to 14 days between dosage increments allows ~7 days for achievement of steady state and 7 days for assessment of response.[30]

Patient or Caregiver Education

Educating T.D. and her parents regarding the importance of regular drug administration is extremely helpful in ensuring

Table 60-7
Common Drugs for the Treatment of Absence Seizures

AED	Regimen	Adverse Effects	Comments
Valproate (Depakene, Depakote, Depakote-ER)	Initial 5–10 mg/kg/day (sprinkle caps or syrup); then ↑ by 5–10 mg/kg/day weekly to therapeutic effect or target serum concentration. Manufacturer's recommended usual maximal dose of 60 mg/kg/day often must be exceeded clinically (especially for patients receiving enzyme-inducing AED) to achieve optimal clinical results. Daily dosing recommended for ER product; doses should be 8%–20% higher than non-ER products	GI upset, hair loss, appetite stimulation, and weight gain common. Dose-related tremor and thrombocytopenia may occur. Serious hepatotoxicity extremely rare with monotherapy and in patients younger than 2 years of age	Enteric-coated tablets or capsules or ER tablets may ↓ GI toxicity. Time to peak serum concentrations delayed for 3–8 hours with enteric coating; longer delay if given with food; serum concentrations must be interpreted carefully. Also effective against primarily generalized tonic–clonic seizures. Monitor LFTs and platelet count
Lamotrigine (Lamictal)	See Table 60-6		
Ethosuximide (Zarontin)	Initial 20 mg/kg/day or 250 mg daily or BID; then ↑ by 250 mg/day every 2 weeks to therapeutic effect or target serum concentration	GI upset and sedation common with large single dose, especially on initiation. Daily divided doses may be necessary despite long half-life. Leukopenia (mild, transient) in up to 7%; serious hematologic toxicity extremely rare	Parents/patient should be informed that GI effects and sedation may occur but tolerance usually develops. No good evidence it precipitates tonic–clonic seizures. Up to 50% of patients with absence may exhibit tonic–clonic seizures independent of ethosuximide

AED, antiepileptic drug; BID, 2 times daily; ER, extended release; GI, gastrointestinal.

successful therapy. Nonadherence is common in patients taking AEDs, and rapid discontinuation of these drugs (often secondary to nonadherence) may precipitate status epilepticus. The concept that medication controls rather than cures the seizure disorder should be strongly reinforced. It is also critical to inform both the parents and T.D. that a therapeutic response may not occur immediately and that dosage adjustments may be necessary.

Therapeutic Monitoring

CASE 60-7, QUESTION 2: What subjective or objective clinical data should be monitored in T.D. for evidence of ethosuximide's therapeutic and adverse effects?

T.D.'s seizure frequency and any side effects she experiences are the primary monitoring parameters. If ethosuximide serum concentrations are used to assist in dosing, 40 to 100 mcg/mL is the usual target range; however, a clearly defined toxicity syndrome does not reliably develop when ethosuximide serum concentrations exceed 100 mcg/mL. Gradual and cautious increases in ethosuximide dosage when serum concentrations are beyond the upper limits of the "usual therapeutic range" may improve response in resistant patients. Although ethosuximide traditionally is administered in divided doses, its long half-life allows successful use of single daily doses for many patients. Clinicians should be alert to acute side effects of nausea and vomiting that are associated with large single doses of ethosuximide; should these occur, divided daily doses may be necessary.[30]

Laboratory monitoring for idiosyncratic hematologic toxicity from ethosuximide often is recommended. Ethosuximide causes neutropenia in approximately 7% of patients. Although this reaction often is transient, even if the drug is continued, rare patients may exhibit fatal pancytopenia. Presumably, early detection of neutropenia by means of periodic CBC will allow discontinuation of the drug and potential reversal of this adverse effect.[127] These hematologic reactions, however, can occur unpredictably at any time during therapy and often are missed by routine laboratory monitoring. Patient or caregiver education regarding signs and symptoms associated with leukopenia and pancytopenia (e.g., sudden onset of severe sore throat with oral lesions, easy bruisability, increased bleeding tendency) and instructions to consult the physician if these symptoms occur may be more important than laboratory monitoring.[57]

T.D.'s parents should be informed that nausea or sedation may occur with initiation of ethosuximide. Tolerance to these effects usually develops, although temporary dose reductions may be necessary.

Generalized Tonic–Clonic Seizures Accompanying Absence Seizures

CASE 60-7, QUESTION 3: Three months later, T.D.'s absence seizures have been reduced to a frequency of one every 2 weeks with an ethosuximide dosage of 750 mg/day. Her initial drowsiness has almost disappeared, and nausea was alleviated by administering doses with food. She has, however, experienced two tonic–clonic convulsions in the past month. Both seizures were witnessed by her parents and were well described. No auras or signs of focal seizure activity were apparent, and each episode consisted of typical tonic–clonic activity lasting 1 to 2 minutes. T.D. was incontinent of urine on both occasions, and postictal confusion and drowsiness were significant. Physical examination and laboratory testing showed no abnormalities. A repeat EEG continued to show infrequent 3-Hz spike-and-wave discharges; no abnormal focal discharges were noted. What is the relationship between T.D.'s tonic–clonic seizures and ethosuximide therapy?

It is commonly believed, and often stated in the literature, that ethosuximide may precipitate or worsen tonic–clonic seizures;

however, this effect has not been clearly demonstrated. As many as 50% of patients who initially present with absence seizures also experience tonic–clonic seizures.[128] Historically, it had been common practice to add another AED (e.g., phenobarbital or phenytoin) to ethosuximide therapy to prevent this.[129] However, routine use of drugs for prophylaxis of tonic–clonic seizures may increase the risk of toxicity and potentially reduce adherence with medication regimens. Sedative drugs, especially phenobarbital, actually may aggravate absence seizures in some patients.[130]

In summary, subsequent generalized tonic–clonic seizures are common in patients who initially experience absence spells. It is unlikely that ethosuximide played a causative role for this development in T.D.

ASSESSMENT REGARDING NEED FOR ALTERATION IN ANTIEPILEPTIC DRUG THERAPY AND CHOICE OF ALTERNATIVE ANTIEPILEPTIC DRUG

CASE 60-7, QUESTION 4: What alterations are indicated in T.D.'s drug therapy because of the appearance of generalized tonic–clonic seizures?

Drug therapy for prevention of further tonic–clonic seizures is indicated. Phenytoin, carbamazepine, or valproate might be considered for use in T.D. Owing to her age and sex, many clinicians would avoid using phenytoin because of its dysmorphic and cosmetic side effects. Carbamazepine is widely used for secondarily generalized tonic–clonic seizures and some cases of tonic–clonic seizures in children. It lacks many of the troublesome, common side effects associated with phenytoin. Carbamazepine, however, is not effective for control of absence seizures. Therefore, it is likely that both ethosuximide and carbamazepine would be needed by T.D. Carbamazepine also has been associated with exacerbation of seizures (including atonic, myoclonic, and absence seizures) in children with mixed seizure disorders who exhibit bilaterally synchronous 2.5- to 3-Hz discharges on the EEG.[131,132] The need for polytherapy and the possible risk of seizure exacerbation make carbamazepine a less attractive treatment option for T.D.

Valproate is effective for controlling both absence and primary generalized tonic–clonic seizures.[39,51] T.D. appears to have primary generalized tonic–clonic convulsions; focal signs (e.g., unilateral or single limb involvement) were not observed, and focal discharges (e.g., isolated abnormal electrical activity localized to one portion of the brain) were not found on the EEG. Although neither observation completely rules out secondarily generalized tonic–clonic seizures, the likelihood seems low. Therefore, valproate may offer advantages over carbamazepine in terms of efficacy. In addition, both of T.D.'s seizure types potentially could be controlled with a single medication.

VALPROATE THERAPY

Initiation and Dosage

CASE 60-7, QUESTION 5: T.D.'s physician elects to use valproate. The therapeutic goal is control of her seizures with valproate alone. What procedure should be followed regarding discontinuation of ethosuximide and initiation of valproate?

Techniques used by clinicians to substitute one AED for another depend largely on experience and judgment. Generally, it is best to attain a potentially therapeutic dose of a new medication before attempting to discontinue the previous drug. Serum concentration monitoring may be helpful for some AEDs. Ethosuximide has a relatively long half-life, whereas valproate's half-life is short. Therefore, if necessary, steady state serum concentrations of valproate can be established and evaluated rapidly; evaluation of the effect of decreases in the ethosuximide dosage must await the prolonged elimination of this drug. Once a desired valproate dose or serum concentration has been achieved, the ethosuximide dosage can be reduced gradually by 250 mg/day every 2 to 4 weeks.

Valproate should be initiated at 125 to 250 mg twice daily. Valproic acid syrup or capsules or divalproex sodium can be used. Divalproex often is preferred because it may cause fewer GI side effects than valproic acid. Syrup forms of valproate probably should be avoided unless extremely small doses are required (e.g., infants) or patients cannot swallow. Valproate syrup has an unpleasant taste, and its rapid absorption increases the likelihood of acute, dose-related side effects such as nausea. Lower initial valproate doses are less likely to cause acute side effects (e.g., drowsiness and GI upset). Weekly dosage increases of 5 to 10 mg/kg/day usually are well tolerated and would be appropriate for T.D. More rapid increases may be desirable if tonic–clonic seizures occur frequently. The maximal recommended dosage of valproate is 60 mg/kg/day. Many patients, especially those receiving enzyme-inducing drugs, require higher-than-recommended doses to achieve adequate clinical effect; other patients may respond at much lower doses. Valproate can be titrated in T.D. to produce a "target" serum concentration of approximately 75 mcg/mL. Because ethosuximide is withdrawn, the valproate dose can be further adjusted on the basis of seizure frequency and side effects.

Dosage Forms

CASE 60-7, QUESTION 6: T.D. has been taking valproic acid capsules, 250 mg TID, for 3 weeks. Ethosuximide was discontinued 2 weeks ago; at that time, a valproate serum level just before her morning dose was 68 mcg/mL. She has not experienced generalized tonic–clonic seizures for 6 weeks but continues to have an absence seizure every 2 to 3 weeks. T.D. complains of nausea, epigastric burning pain, and occasional vomiting lasting approximately 1 hour after her doses of valproate. All recent laboratory tests were within normal limits. Administration of the drug with meals is only partially helpful. What alterations can be made in T.D.'s dosing regimen to relieve these symptoms and possibly improve seizure control?

T.D. appears to be a candidate for the use of an enteric-coated valproate preparation or extended-release divalproex. Divalproex tablets are available as an enteric-coated delayed-release preparation, which causes delayed rather than extended absorption of valproate; therefore, these tablets are not a sustained-release product formulation. When patients are switched from nonenteric-coated formulations to divalproex tablets, the frequency of administration should not be decreased. Valproic acid and enteric-coated dosage forms of valproic acid or divalproex are completely absorbed; these can be interconverted at the same total daily dose of medication.[133,134] An extended-release formulation of divalproex sodium is also available that can be administered as a single daily dose. Extended-release divalproex (divalproex ER), however, is not bioequivalent to other dosage forms of valproate.[135] When equal doses are administered, the ER formulation produces serum concentrations that are approximately 89% of those produced by other valproate dosage forms. Accordingly, when patients are converted to divalproex ER from other forms of valproate, the manufacturer recommends an increase of 8% to 20% in the administered dose. T.D.'s valproic acid capsules can be replaced with an equal daily dose of divalproex tablets. Divalproex should be administered on a 3-times-daily dosing schedule. Alternatively, T.D. could be given 1,000 mg of divalproex ER once daily. The results of this change should be apparent within approximately 1 week. By that time, significant relief from GI side effects should have occurred. It may then be possible to increase the dose of divalproex in an effort to improve seizure control.

Capsules containing enteric-coated beads of divalproex also are available; the 125-mg capsule contents can be dispersed in food for administration to children or others who have difficulty swallowing tablets or capsules. In addition, use of the "cap" end of the capsule to measure half of the contents can approximate doses of 62.5 mg.

Pharmacokinetics and Serum Concentration Monitoring

CASE 60-7, QUESTION 7: Two weeks later, T.D. returns for follow-up. Her GI symptoms have resolved. She has been taking divalproex tablets 250 mg with breakfast and lunch and 375 mg with a bedtime snack for the past week. She has had no seizures in the past 2 weeks and complains of no side effects. A valproate serum level before her morning dose today was 117 mcg/mL (considerably higher than her previous valproate level of 68 mcg/mL). The laboratory reports that duplicate determinations of this level agreed within 5 mcg/mL. T.D. denies taking her medication incorrectly; her parents support this, and the tablet count in her prescription bottle is correct. She has taken no other drugs except a multivitamin. How can this disproportionate increase in her valproate serum concentration be explained, and what is its clinical significance? Does valproate exhibit dose-dependent pharmacokinetics?

The observed changes in T.D.'s valproate serum concentrations are probably not the result of dose-dependent metabolism as is seen with phenytoin; instead, these changes are more readily explained by the absorption characteristics of divalproex tablets. Peak serum concentrations of valproate after administration of divalproex may be delayed for 3 to 8 hours, and administration of food may further delay absorption.[136] In addition, diurnal fluctuation in both the rate and extent of absorption of divalproex may be significant. Absorption may be reduced by approximately one-third and peak plasma concentrations may be delayed for up to 12 hours for divalproex doses administered in the evening.[32] Twelve to 15 hours probably elapsed between the administration of T.D.'s last dose and blood sampling; therefore, the currently reported blood level may more closely approximate a peak concentration. Previous blood levels, determined while she was receiving rapidly absorbed valproic acid capsules, are more likely to have been trough concentrations. T.D.'s adherence to her prescribed dosage regimen also may have increased because of the change in dosage form and reduced side effects; her previous serum concentrations may not have reflected administration of the prescribed dose.

Other pharmacokinetic factors may have actually moderated this unusual increase in valproate concentrations. Valproate concentrations may fluctuate throughout the day in a pattern that does not reflect the timing of doses.[137] This fluctuation may be partially related to changes in serum concentrations of endogenous fatty acids that displace valproate from protein-binding sites. Valproate's hepatic clearance is restrictive (i.e., valproate has a low extraction ratio and its clearance is limited by the free fraction of drug in plasma); therefore, when protein-binding displacement occurs, free fraction of drug in plasma and clearance increase. As a result, free serum concentrations of valproate increase only transiently, whereas total serum concentrations decrease persistently. Valproate also exhibits dose dependency in its binding to serum proteins. As concentrations approach 70 to 80 mcg/mL, binding sites on albumin molecules become saturated, and the free fraction of drug in plasma increases.[30,133] This effect also increases valproate clearance and reduces total serum concentrations. Both of these effects may actually "dampen" the apparent increase in plasma concentrations seen in T.D. When also considering the poorly established "therapeutic range" for this drug, it becomes apparent that monitoring serum concentrations is a less useful tool in valproate therapy than with some other AEDs.[133]

The clinical significance of T.D.'s elevated valproate serum concentrations is minimal. She is not experiencing symptoms suggestive of valproate toxicity, and it is too soon after the dosage increase to assess the effect of this change on her seizure frequency. Therefore, alteration in her drug therapy is unnecessary at present and might only confuse evaluation of her response to this drug. She should be observed for an additional 4 to 6 weeks to evaluate seizure frequency before further alterations in her dosing regimen are considered. Further increases in her dosage are not contraindicated as long as she is tolerating the medication and such increases are justified on the basis of seizure frequency.

Hepatotoxicity

CASE 60-7, QUESTION 8: Two months later, T.D. is taking 375 mg of divalproex TID with meals. She has had no absence seizures for 5 weeks and no generalized tonic–clonic seizures for 10 weeks. Yesterday, her valproate plasma concentration was 132 mcg/mL. In addition, her alanine aminotransferase (ALT) was 32 international units/mL and her aspartate aminotransferase (AST) was 41 international units/mL. All other laboratory tests (bilirubin, alkaline phosphatase, lactate dehydrogenase, prothrombin time, and serum albumin) were normal. T.D.'s LFTs have been monitored monthly since she began taking valproate, and they were previously normal. Physical examination was negative for scleral icterus, abdominal pain, or other signs of liver disease. Discuss these laboratory abnormalities and physical findings in relation to possible valproate-induced hepatotoxicity in T.D.

Liver damage related to valproate therapy appears to be caused by accumulation of hepatotoxic metabolites of valproate (probably 4-en-valproate) in certain patients.[138,139] These metabolites may be formed in larger quantities in patients who also receive enzyme-inducing drugs such as phenobarbital. Most cases of fatal hepatotoxicity have occurred in young (<2 years of age) patients with neurologic and metabolic abnormalities who also had severe, difficult-to-control seizures and who were taking multiple AEDs.[138–143] It is important to recognize, however, that severe hepatotoxicity is not limited to this population.[144] Liver damage occurs early in therapy and symptomatically resembles fulminant hepatitis with hepatic failure. Patients may experience vomiting, drowsiness, lethargy, anorexia, edema, and jaundice; these symptoms often precede laboratory evidence of hepatic damage. Liver biopsies in affected patients show evidence of hepatic necrosis and steatosis. Death results from hepatic failure or a Reye-like syndrome.[139,141,145]

Asymptomatic elevations in liver enzymes (such as those found in T.D.) occur commonly during the first 6 months of treatment with valproate and usually are not associated with severe or potentially fatal valproate-induced hepatotoxicity. These changes in aminotransferase usually disappear without alteration in therapy; in some cases, temporary dosage reduction is followed by normalization of laboratory tests within 4 to 6 weeks.[139,141] Without systemic symptoms or other signs of significant liver damage, it is unlikely that the laboratory abnormalities observed in T.D. represent severe liver toxicity from valproate. Because T.D. is responding well to valproate therapy, no change in therapy is warranted at this time. Laboratory testing probably can be repeated in 4 to 6 weeks. T.D. and her family should be educated regarding the possible signs and symptoms of valproate-induced liver damage and instructed to consult their physician if these symptoms are noted.

CASE 60-7, QUESTION 9: What is the usefulness of routinely monitoring LFTs in patients receiving valproate?

Serious hepatotoxicity related to valproate therapy is extremely rare. Historically, the rate of fatal hepatotoxicity decreased significantly (despite substantial increases in the use of valproate) after the use of the drug in high-risk patients (e.g., the very young) decreased and its use as monotherapy increased. Hepatotoxicity is estimated to occur in less than 0.002% of patients treated with valproate.[139,140,142] In children younger than 2 years of age who receive AED polytherapy, the incidence of this complication is 1 in 500 to 1 in 800. Because asymptomatic, apparently benign elevations in liver enzymes are common early in therapy with valproate and symptoms of liver damage often precede laboratory changes, frequent LFTs during early valproate therapy are unlikely to detect serious hepatotoxicity.[57,139–141,146] Education of caregivers or patients regarding potential symptoms of hepatotoxicity, with careful observation and follow-up by health care professionals, is recommended as the most effective method to monitor for this drug-induced illness.

In predisposed patients (i.e., very young children with associated neurologic abnormalities and those receiving polytherapy), significant increases in LFT values that are noted early in therapy may be clinically significant. At the onset of symptoms suggesting this condition, laboratory testing may help confirm its presence.

Acute Repetitive (Cluster) Seizures

RECTAL DIAZEPAM GEL

CASE 60-8

QUESTION 1: B.N., a 7-year-old, 28-kg boy, has had seizures since age 3 months. He suffered anoxia at birth. His seizures usually involve initial confusion and disorientation, shortly followed by generalized tonic–clonic convulsive activity. Despite treatment with carbamazepine at maximal tolerated doses and serum concentrations (300 mg TID; 9–11 mcg/mL), he continues to have approximately two seizures monthly. Recent trials of topiramate and tiagabine as additions to his carbamazepine were unsuccessful and caused intolerable sedation and lethargy. During the past year, he has been admitted to the emergency department (ED) 5 times because of seizure "flurries" consisting of three to six seizures occurring during a period of 12 or fewer hours. Although he regains consciousness between these "flurry" seizures, he remains lethargic. During ED admissions, IV diazepam was administered. This was rapidly successful in terminating seizure activity. B.N.'s mother relates that she usually can identify the onset of seizure flurries; B.N.'s behavior changes and he becomes "clinging" and "whiny" and hyperactive. She also indicates that the initial seizure in a flurry differs from B.N.'s typical episodes. Before the onset of generalized seizure activity, he experiences much briefer periods of confusion. In addition, the generalized seizures are longer and more severe (often with dramatic cyanosis) at the beginning of a "flurry." Why is prophylactic or abortive therapy for B.N.'s seizure flurries indicated? What factors about B.N. predict successful use of such treatment, and how can it be administered?

Frequent ED visits resulting from cluster seizures are expensive and frightening for many patients and their families. B.N. continues to experience seizure flurries despite carbamazepine therapy. He responds well to IV diazepam and has a caregiver who can identify the onset of seizure clusters. His seizure clusters appear to be distinct from the other seizures that he experiences. All of these factors indicate that a trial of caregiver-administered treatment to abort these cluster episodes is likely to be helpful and should be initiated.

Rectal diazepam gel is available for home administration to patients with acute episodes of repetitive seizure activity.[147] When diazepam gel is administered rectally, peak plasma concentrations occur in approximately 1.5 hours,[148] and cluster seizures are often terminated within 15 minutes. Use of diazepam rectal gel is recommended only when caregivers can recognize the onset of cluster seizures, which are different from a patient's usual seizure activity, and when the caregivers can be trained to administer the preparation safely and to monitor the patient's response (e.g., respiratory status) after administration. Caregivers should be informed that this preparation is not for as needed use with every seizure; it should be used only for identifiable cluster seizures or prolonged seizures.

B.N.'s mother should administer rectal diazepam gel at the onset of identifiable cluster seizure activity. A dose of approximately 0.3 mg/kg (10 mg) should be given and repeated, if necessary, within 4 to 12 hours of the first dose. B.N.'s mother should be counseled on the administration of this product and given the patient package insert, which gives complete instructions for the administration of rectal diazepam. After administration, B.N. should be monitored for at least 4 hours to ensure that no respiratory depression or other adverse side effects are occurring and to assess the effect of the medication on his seizures. The most common adverse effect seen with rectal diazepam is somnolence, occasionally accompanied by dizziness and ataxia. Respiratory depression is very uncommon. IM, buccal, and intranasal formulations of benzodiazepines are currently being investigated for their utility in aborting cluster seizures and their use may address some of the barriers associated with rectal drug administration.[149]

Febrile Seizures

INCIDENCE AND CLASSIFICATION

CASE 60-9

QUESTION 1: J.J., a 14-month-old girl, is brought to the ED after having a generalized tonic–clonic convulsion lasting approximately 5 minutes. The episode occurred in association with an upper respiratory infection. On arrival in the ED, her temperature was 39.5°C rectally. She was alert at that time; all laboratory and neurologic findings, including lumbar puncture, were normal. J.J. has no history of neurologic abnormality. Her 7-year-old brother suffers from both absence and generalized tonic–clonic seizures. What is the relationship between febrile seizures and epilepsy? How may J.J.'s convulsion be classified on the basis of the data available?

Up to 8% of children have a febrile seizure between 6 months and 6 years of age.[150,151] Simple febrile seizures occur with a fever of greater than or equal to 38°C in previously normal children younger than 5 years of age. They last less than 15 minutes and have no focal features. The associated seizure does not arise from CNS pathology. Complex febrile seizures show focal characteristics or are prolonged longer than 15 minutes. The child may or may not have previous neurologic abnormalities. The risk of occurrence of unprovoked afebrile seizures after a febrile seizure is 4 times greater than in the general population. A family history of afebrile seizures, complex febrile seizures, and pre-existing neurologic abnormality is a risk factor associated with the later development of chronic epilepsy.[150,151]

J.J.'s seizure appears to be a typical simple febrile seizure that developed in association with her upper respiratory tract infection. The lack of previous neurologic abnormality and normal findings on lumbar puncture and laboratory evaluation help confirm this assessment.

TREATMENT OF ACUTE SEIZURE

Case 60-9, Question 2: How should J.J.'s febrile seizures be treated?

Because J.J. is not having a seizure at present, AED therapy is not required. Measures to reduce her elevated temperature should be initiated; however, these measures may not reduce the risk of further seizures. Acetaminophen and tepid sponge baths usually are helpful.

If patients experience prolonged or repeated febrile seizures, either diazepam or, less commonly, midazolam may be administered.[151–153] Rectal diazepam gel can be used for this purpose.

PROPHYLAXIS AND CHOICE OF ANTIEPILEPTIC DRUG

Case 60-9, Question 3: On the basis of the subjective and objective data available for J.J., is AED therapy indicated on a long-term basis? What are the benefits and risks of AED prophylaxis for febrile seizures?

Long-term treatment or prophylaxis with AED for simple febrile seizures is not recommended. Up to 54% of affected patients will have recurrent febrile seizures, and the risk of recurrence is even greater when the first episode occurs before 13 months of age. Nonetheless, recurrent febrile seizures are not associated with brain damage or development of epilepsy.[150] Although administration of continuous AED treatment may reduce the recurrence rate of febrile seizures, published guidelines recommend against this practice due to the associated adverse effects.[154]

Prophylactic administration of various fast-acting agents, given during fever episodes, has been studied as an alternative to continuous treatment for the prevention of febrile seizures. Agents in both the AED and antipyretic drug classes have been studied in this regard, but no clinically important benefits have been found.[155–159] Thus, AED prophylaxis for febrile seizures is probably not warranted for J.J., even though she is at risk for both development of epilepsy and recurrence of febrile seizures. No evidence supports that medication will significantly affect her later development of epilepsy. Close medical follow-up of J.J. is warranted. Her parents should be counseled to contact a physician if J.J.'s febrile seizure is accompanied by focal features or last longer than 15 minutes; or, if J.J. experiences afebrile seizures. Although antipyretic measures (tepid sponge baths, acetaminophen or ibuprofen) are of questionable benefit, they can be considered at the onset of fever because these interventions are usually safe and well tolerated. Many febrile seizures occur early in the course of an illness before fever is detected[160]; nevertheless, vigilance by her parents and early antipyretic therapy may help prevent further febrile seizures.

Skin Rash: Hypersensitivity Reactions to Antiepileptic Drugs

CASE 60-10

Question 1: R.S., a 34-year-old man, has been taking phenytoin 200 mg BID for the past 7 weeks to control complex partial and secondarily generalized tonic–clonic seizures. Seizures began approximately 4 months ago after surgical evacuation of a subdural hematoma. Today he appears at the walk-in clinic and complains of an "itchy rash" that began 2 days ago. He describes "feeling lousy" for the past week. On examination he is febrile (38.5°C orally). A maculopapular, scaly, erythematous rash covers his upper extremities and torso, and the mucous membranes of his mouth appear to be mildly inflamed. Cervical lymphadenopathy is noted, and the liver is found to be enlarged and tender. R.S. also relates that his urine has become very dark in the past 2 days and that his stools are light colored. What is the significance of R.S.'s skin rash and other signs and symptoms? Are these likely to be related to his phenytoin therapy?

Skin-related adverse reactions (e.g., rash, urticarial) are relatively common (2%–3% of patients) side effects related to AED therapy. Skin rash is most commonly associated with phenytoin, lamotrigine, carbamazepine, and phenobarbital. Most cases are relatively mild, but severely affected patients may exhibit Stevens–Johnson syndrome or a systemic hypersensitivity syndrome accompanied by severe hepatic damage. In R.S.'s case, signs and symptoms suggesting hepatic involvement accompany the skin rash. Fever, lymphadenopathy, and apparent inflammation of mucous membranes also suggest a hypersensitivity reaction to phenytoin with multisystem involvement and the potential for progression to Stevens–Johnson syndrome. Viral infection (e.g., hepatitis, influenza, infectious mononucleosis) should be considered and ruled out as a possible cause of R.S.'s symptoms before they are attributed to phenytoin therapy.[161–164]

DRESS syndrome (which stands for Drug Reaction with Eosinophilia and Systemic Symptoms) is a type of hypersensitivity syndrome that can occur with some drugs, including phenytoin and other AEDs, that is most commonly seen in adults. Typically, patients with this syndrome present with complaints of fever, skin rash, and lymphadenopathy during the first 2 months of AED therapy. Hepatomegaly, splenomegaly, jaundice, or bleeding manifestations may occur. Laboratory manifestations often include leukocytosis with eosinophilia, elevated serum bilirubin, and elevated AST and ALT. When a phenytoin hypersensitivity reaction includes significant hepatotoxicity, fatality may occur in as many as 38% of affected patients.[161]

A high likelihood exists that R.S. has developed a severe reaction to phenytoin; the clinical manifestations and the timing of their appearance are typical of this reaction. Phenytoin should be discontinued immediately pending diagnostic clarification. R.S. should be hospitalized for evaluation of other possible causes of his symptoms such as viral illness and treatment. Treatment of phenytoin-related hypersensitivity and hepatotoxicity is symptomatic and supportive. Intensive therapy with corticosteroids has commonly been used, although little objective evidence exists for beneficial effects of this treatment. Potential complications of this reaction include sepsis and hepatic failure; these conditions should be treated specifically.

Case 60-10, Question 2: R.S. was hospitalized and treated with oral prednisone and topical corticosteroids. Other potential causes for his condition were ruled out, and his signs and symptoms were attributed to cutaneous and systemic phenytoin hypersensitivity. His fever resolved within 5 days; the skin rash became exfoliative but resolved without infectious complications. Laboratory parameters began to normalize after 10 days. While he was hospitalized, R.S. experienced three generalized tonic–clonic seizures that were treated acutely with administration of IV lorazepam. R.S. was afebrile at the time these episodes occurred. What information regarding the pathogenesis of phenytoin hypersensitivity and hepatotoxicity can be used to guide selection of an alternative AED for R.S.?

Further administration of phenytoin to R.S. is contraindicated on the basis of his history of a severe hypersensitivity reaction to this drug. Although the mechanism of this reaction is not fully understood, research implicates reactive arene oxide metabolites of phenytoin (and other chemically similar AEDs) as possible causative agents for hypersensitivity reactions. Affected patients purportedly are predisposed genetically to the development of hypersensitivity, possibly because a relative deficiency of epoxide hydrolase enzymes allows the accumulation of toxic concentrations of reactive epoxide metabolites. These metabolites are believed to exert a direct cytotoxic effect and to interact with cellular macromolecules, thereby functioning as haptens that stimulate an immunologic reaction.[165,166] Carbamazepine, phenytoin, and phenobarbital all are metabolized by similar pathways and converted to reactive arene oxides. It is hypothesized that carbamazepine-induced liver damage also may result from the effects of accumulation of reactive epoxide metabolites; these reactive metabolites differ from the 10,11-epoxide metabolite that accumulates during carbamazepine therapy. For this reason, these drugs potentially cross-react in susceptible patients. Cases of apparent cross-reactivity between phenytoin and phenobarbital or carbamazepine have been documented.[167–169] In addition, both carbamazepine and phenobarbital can produce hypersensitivity reactions similar to those seen with phenytoin. This potential for cross-reactivity should be considered when an alternative AED is selected for R.S. An analysis of cases of AED-related skin rashes found that the most significant nondrug predictor of skin rash was the occurrence of a rash with another AED.[170]

Valproate has been suggested as the preferred alternative AED for patients who have exhibited hypersensitivity reactions to phenytoin.[168] Valproate is not metabolized to arene oxides and also is chemically dissimilar to all other AEDs. Because valproate often shows good efficacy for complex partial seizures with secondary generalization, it would seem to be a safe and potentially effective alternative AED for R.S. Of the newer AEDs, lamotrigine should probably be avoided in R.S. because of its likelihood of causing skin rash and apparent hypersensitivity reactions. Oxcarbazepine is potentially an alternative AED for R.S. because it is not metabolized through the arene oxide pathway. Nevertheless, 25% to 30% of patients who experience a rash in response to carbamazepine will also experience a rash with oxcarbazepine.[171] Therefore, many clinicians would avoid oxcarbazepine. Gabapentin, lacosamide, levetiracetam, pregabalin, tiagabine, topiramate, or zonisamide could be considered as alternative medications for R.S. These medications appear less likely to cause skin rash or hypersensitivity reactions.[170,172]

It is suggested that R.S. be advised to add phenytoin to his list of medication allergies.

Additional recognized genetic risk factors for AED-related hypersensitivity reactions in specific populations are presented in Table 60-6.

WOMEN'S ISSUES IN EPILEPSY

Although epilepsy affects men and women equally, many health issues are of specific importance to women, such as contraceptive interactions with AEDs, teratogenicity, pharmacokinetic changes during pregnancy, breast-feeding, menstrual cycle influences on seizure activity (catamenial epilepsy), AED impact on bone, and sexual dysfunction.[173,174] It is noteworthy that the latter two issues can also occur in men. A great need exists to educate both health care professionals and patients about the many complex issues facing women with epilepsy.[175]

For women of childbearing potential, prepregnancy planning and counseling are important, because significant AED exposure of the fetus often occurs by the time pregnancy is confirmed. This is especially important because of the potential for unplanned pregnancies from the AED–contraceptive drug interactions. Prepregnancy counseling also should include the importance of at least 0.4 mg/day of folic acid supplementation and medication adherence. Patients should be informed about the risk of teratogenicity and the importance of prenatal care.

Although complete seizure control is desirable for all patients with epilepsy, it is especially favorable for a woman's seizures to be well controlled before conception. Monotherapy is preferred whenever possible, because the relative risk of birth defects dramatically increases with AED polytherapy.[160,176] Monotherapy also improves patient adherence. The AED should be given at the lowest effective dose to reduce the possibility of birth defects.[154] Gradual discontinuation of AED before pregnancy may be considered if a woman has been seizure-free for 2 years or longer.

Antiepileptic Drug–Oral Contraceptive Interaction

CASE 60-11

QUESTION 1: P.Z., a 26-year-old woman, experiences complex partial and secondarily generalized tonic–clonic seizures. She is taking phenytoin 400 mg/day and divalproex 2,000 mg/day. She reports having two or three partial seizures and one generalized seizure every 3 to 4 months. Despite taking Lo/Ovral (norgestrel 0.3 mg with ethinylestradiol 30 mcg), she has just learned she is pregnant. Her last menstrual period was 6 weeks ago. What is the relationship between P.Z.'s apparent contraceptive failure and her AED therapy?

There have been several reports of reduced efficacy of oral contraceptives in patients receiving various AEDs.[177,178] These reports describe both breakthrough bleeding and pregnancy. Phenobarbital, phenytoin, carbamazepine, oxcarbazepine, eslicarbazepine, perampanel, and felbamate have been shown to increase the metabolism of ethinylestradiol and progestogens.[179] This effect is not associated with valproate, lamotrigine, gabapentin, tiagabine, zonisamide, levetiracetam, lacosamide, or pregabalin.[179] Topiramate in polytherapy and at high dosages (200–800 mg/day) appears to have a mild, though measurable, effect on oral contraceptive pharmacokinetics; apparent clearance of the estrogen component of combined oral contraceptives is increased in patients taking topiramate.[180] In contrast, topiramate monotherapy in lower dosages (50–200 mg/day) has a lesser impact on the pharmacokinetics of the oral contraceptive.[181]

A lack of contraceptive efficacy may present as irregular or breakthrough menstrual bleeding. Decreased efficacy is not always associated with breakthrough bleeding, however. Oral contraceptive doses can be increased to compensate for the effect of an AED.[182] However, estrogens also may exacerbate seizures in some women.[183] Women older than 35 years of age and those who smoke must consider the risk of thromboembolic complications associated with higher doses of contraceptives. A second contraceptive method (e.g., condoms, intrauterine devices, or spermicide) is recommended to avoid contraceptive failure.[170] Tubal ligation is also an alternative. An additional alternative that could be considered is injectable depot medroxyprogesterone acetate. Although there is a lack of clinical studies substantiating its effectiveness in patients on enzyme-inducing AED, the pharmacokinetic characteristics of this agent suggest that its effect is not reduced by enzyme induction. Medroxyprogesterone is a high-clearance drug; its clearance is directly dependent on hepatic blood flow. Thus, enzyme induction would have little effect on the metabolism of this drug when it is administered by injection. Depot medroxyprogesterone acetate may, however, have other negative effects that would limit its choice as an alternative contraceptive in this situation.[184]

Assuming P.Z. was taking her contraceptive pills on a regular basis, it is possible that her enzyme-inducing AED (phenytoin) is responsible for their failure. Patients receiving enzyme-inducing AED should be prospectively informed that this interaction can occur and advised concerning the use of alternative contraceptives (see Chapter 47, Contraception).

Interestingly, a different drug interaction exists between oral contraceptives and lamotrigine. The estrogen component in oral contraceptives increases the clearance of lamotrigine. Lamotrigine clearance may increase twofold when contraceptive steroids are begun and fall by 50% when contraceptive steroids are discontinued. Changes in lamotrigine levels associated with initiation and discontinuation of contraceptive steroids can result in increased seizure activity in some patients and toxicity in others.[185]

Teratogenicity

CASE 60-11, QUESTION 2: What are the risks of teratogenic effects from P.Z.'s medications? What steps might be taken to minimize these risks?

P.Z.'s child is at risk of congenital malformations because of exposure to several potentially teratogenic drugs: estrogen–progestin combination oral contraceptives, valproate, and phenytoin (also see Chapter 49, Obstetric Drug Therapy).

Many AEDs have teratogenic effects.[186] Animal data regarding the teratogenic potential of the new AEDs are encouraging, but conclusions regarding the teratogenic potential of these AEDs cannot be made because of limited experience in pregnant women. A good resource for clinicians to educate women is the American Epilepsy Society and the American Academy of Neurology series of three Practice Parameter updates on management issues for women with epilepsy focused on pregnancy. They deal with obstetric complications and change in seizure frequency; teratogenesis and perinatal outcomes; and vitamin K, folic acid, blood levels, and breast-feeding.[187–189] The authors evaluated the available evidence based on a structured literature review and provide recommendations.

Most AEDs are believed to exert their teratogenic effects (and possibly other adverse effects such as hepatotoxicity) partly via reactive epoxide metabolites.[160] Enhancement of the formation of these metabolites via hepatic enzyme induction (e.g., by carbamazepine or phenobarbital) or inhibition of their breakdown (e.g., through inhibition of epoxide hydrolase by valproate) would increase the risk of teratogenicity. Combined administration of enzyme inducers and valproate (specifically the combination of carbamazepine, phenobarbital, and valproate with or without phenytoin) is associated with an especially high risk of teratogenicity.[190] In addition, each of the present major AEDs has been associated with congenital malformations when administered alone. Meador et al.[191] provide data from 333 pregnancies in women with epilepsy taking an AED in monotherapy and enrolled in the Neurodevelopmental Effects of Antiepileptic Drugs (NEAD) study. Serious adverse outcomes (major malformations and fetal death) were significantly more likely to occur with exposure to valproate (20.3%) than with carbamazepine (8.2%), phenytoin (10.7%), or lamotrigine (1%). In addition to physical malformations, AED exposure in utero has an adverse effect on neurodevelopment.[192] The NEAD study evaluated age-6 IQ and found that valproate-exposed children had significantly lower scores (mean 97) , even after controlling for the mother's IQ and seizure type.[193] The age-6 IQ scores were significantly lower for children exposed in utero to valproate compared with scores of children exposed to carbamazepine (mean 105), phenytoin (mean 108), and lamotrigine (mean 108) monotherapy. A European task force of epilepsy experts recommends that, where possible, valproate should be avoided in women of childbearing potential.[194]

Several strategies can be used to reduce the potential adverse effects of AEDs on pregnancy outcomes. If feasible, before conception, seizure control should be optimized using the AED of first choice for the prospective mother's seizure type or epilepsy syndrome. Monotherapy at the lowest effective dose is the goal. Maintenance of adequate folic acid stores before conception and during fetal organogenesis is also important. Folic acid supplementation can reduce the risk of congenital neural tube malformations in infants at risk who are born to women without epilepsy, but folate supplementation does not reliably reduce the teratogenic effects of AED. Nevertheless, supplementation of folic acid (and ensuring adequate folate levels) is recommended. Because about half of pregnancies are unplanned and not evident until weeks after conception, folate supplementation should be given routinely to women of childbearing age with epilepsy. No study has been conducted to determine the optimal dose of folic acid supplementation in patients taking AEDs. Clinicians engage in much discussion of this topic, but the current practices are not evidence-based. Even though this is the case, P.Z. should start taking 4 mg of folic acid supplementation each day.

Physiologic changes in pregnant women may affect the pharmacokinetics of AEDs.[171] Absorption can be influenced by nausea and vomiting. Hepatic metabolism and renal function both increase during pregnancy. The binding capacity of albumin is decreased during pregnancy, resulting in decreased protein binding for highly bound drugs. Unbound fractions of phenobarbital, phenytoin, and valproate increase with decreased concentrations of albumin.[195–197] For drugs predominately metabolized by the liver with a restrictive clearance (e.g., carbamazepine and valproate), decreased protein binding without changes in intrinsic clearance should result in a decrease in total drug concentrations; unbound drug concentrations usually remain unchanged. For drugs with both increased hepatic metabolism and decreased protein binding (e.g., phenytoin and phenobarbital), both total and unbound plasma concentrations decrease, but not necessarily proportionately.

The clearance of lamotrigine increases as pregnancy progresses, presumably related to the impact of estrogen on lamotrigine metabolism.[198] This alteration in clearance changes immediately postpartum. Preliminary data suggest that oxcarbazepine concentrations may also decrease as pregnancy progresses.[199]

The effects of changes in renal function during pregnancy on AED concentrations are not well known.[199] Renal blood flow and glomerular filtration rate increase during pregnancy. Thus, the renal clearance of drugs that are predominately excreted through the kidneys, such as gabapentin, levetiracetam, and pregabalin, may increase during pregnancy.

During pregnancy, serum levels of AEDs (including free serum levels for highly protein-bound drugs) can be monitored. In this case, a prepregnancy level would be optimal for comparison. Dosage adjustments may help to prevent the increase in seizure frequency that is seen in approximately 25% of pregnant women with epilepsy. Because falls and anoxia associated with uncontrolled generalized tonic–clonic seizures may increase the risk to the unborn baby, P.Z. should be educated on the value of adherence to her AED regimen.

For P.Z., it can be presumed that significant exposure of the fetus to any teratogenic influence of AED has already occurred. Optimization of seizure control is now the primary concern for her. Any major alterations in P.Z.'s AED regimen should be made cautiously to avoid precipitating seizures. In addition, she should be instructed to contact the AED pregnancy registry at Massachusetts General Hospital (1-888-233-2334 or www.aedpregnancyregistry.org). Information provided to the registry will aid in the ongoing monitoring of outcomes of babies born to mothers taking AEDs. Reports from this registry have provided risk information on many AEDs and regular visits to their website is helpful to learn the latest.

VITAMIN K SUPPLEMENTATION

Babies born to women with epilepsy who are taking enzyme-inducing AED are at risk of hemorrhage owing to decreased vitamin-K-dependent clotting factors. Although some question the evidence, women taking carbamazepine, phenobarbital, primidone, or phenytoin should receive vitamin K 10 mg orally every day from 36 weeks of gestation until delivery, and babies should also receive vitamin K 1 mg IM at birth.[200]

BREAST-FEEDING

In a lactating woman who is taking medications, the risk of drug exposure to the infant needs to be weighed against the benefits of breast-feeding.[201] All drugs transfer into milk to some extent. The extent of protein binding of the drug is the most important predictor of drug passage into milk.[202,203] For the AEDs, a large intersubject variability in the milk/plasma (M/P) ratio exists, presumably owing to a difference in volume and composition of the milk. Thus, the M/P ratio is not useful for predicting infant AED exposure. Reviews on AED and breast-feeding are available.[204] For most first-generation AEDs (carbamazepine, phenytoin, valproic acid), breast-feeding results in negligible AED plasma concentrations in the infants. For the newer AEDs, breast-feeding should be done cautiously and the infant should be monitored for excess AED plasma concentrations and toxicity, if possible. This information should be presented to P.Z. in an appropriate manner. Once she delivers her baby, re-evaluation and optimization of P.Z.'s AED therapy should occur.

STATUS EPILEPTICUS

Characteristics and Pathophysiology

CASE 60-12

QUESTION 1: V.S., a 22-year-old, 85-kg man, was recently diagnosed as having idiopathic epilepsy with generalized tonic–clonic seizures. For the past 3 months, he has been treated with 600 mg/day of carbamazepine, which completely eliminated his seizures. His steady state carbamazepine serum concentration was 10 mcg/mL. While at his parents' home, he had two tonic–clonic seizures, each lasting 3 to 4 minutes. On arrival at the hospital (~30 minutes after the first seizure began), he was noted to be only semiconscious. His blood pressure was 197/104 mm Hg, his pulse was 124 beats/minute, respirations were 23 breaths/minute, and his body temperature was 38°C rectally. Shortly after his arrival, another generalized tonic–clonic seizure began. How does V.S.'s current condition meet accepted diagnostic criteria for status epilepticus? What risks are associated with status epilepticus?

Status epilepticus (SE) is operationally defined as "either continuous seizures lasting at least 5 minutes or 2 or more discrete seizures between which there is incomplete recovery of consciousness."[205] Because V.S. has had three seizures within slightly more than 30 minutes and did not return to his baseline level of consciousness between seizures, his present condition meets this definition. V.S. is experiencing generalized convulsive SE; this is the most common type and it is associated with the greatest risk of systemic and neurologic damage. SE also may be characterized by nonconvulsive seizures that produce a persistent state of impaired consciousness, or by partial seizures (with or without impaired consciousness). These forms of SE are associated with much lower morbidity and mortality than generalized convulsive SE.

Uncontrolled, convulsive SE can cause severe metabolic and hemodynamic alterations. V.S.'s vital signs (tachycardia, elevated blood pressure, increased respiratory rate, and elevated body temperature) are typical for a patient in SE. Prolonged, severe muscle contractions and CNS dysfunction from uncontrolled seizure discharges result in hyperthermia, cardiorespiratory collapse, myoglobinuria, renal failure, and neurologic damage. Even in the absence of convulsive muscle movements, neurologic damage can occur from excessive electrical activity and the resultant alterations in brain metabolism. When seizure activity persists longer than approximately 30 minutes, failure of mechanisms that regulate cerebral blood flow is more likely; this failure accompanies dramatic increases in brain metabolism and demand for glucose and oxygen. Failure to meet the metabolic demands of brain tissue results in accumulation of lactate and cell death. Peripherally, lactate accumulates and serum glucose and electrolytes are altered. After 30 minutes of seizure activity, the body often fails to compensate for increased metabolic demands, and cardiovascular collapse can occur.[206,207] For these reasons, SE is considered a medical emergency that requires immediate treatment to prevent or lessen both systemic and neurologic damage. Mortality in adults with SE is approximately 20%[205]; fatal outcome is often the result of the condition that precipitated SE (e.g., acute symptomatic causes, such as cardiopulmonary arrest, stroke). Long-term neurologic consequences of severe SE may include cognitive impairment, memory loss, and worsening of seizure disorders.

General Treatment Measures and Antiepileptic Drug Therapy

CASE 60-12, QUESTION 2: Describe a general treatment plan for V.S.'s episode of status epilepticus.

The immediate therapeutic concern in V.S. is to ensure ventilation, stabilize vital signs, and terminate current seizure activity. If possible, an airway should be placed for airway protection and if ventilatory support is needed; however, this may not be possible while he is convulsing. Objects (e.g., spoons, tongue blades) should never be placed into the mouth of a patient during a seizure. If airway placement is impossible, V.S. should be positioned on his side to allow drainage of saliva and mucus from the mouth and prevent aspiration. An IV line should be established using normal saline, and blood should be obtained for serum chemistries (especially glucose and electrolytes), AED serum concentrations, and toxicology screens. Glucose, 25 g (50 mL of 50% dextrose solution) by IV push should be administered to correct any hypoglycemia, which may be responsible for SE. Glucose administration should be preceded by IV thiamine 100 mg or vitamin B complex to prevent Wernicke encephalopathy.[208]

IV administration of rapid-acting anticonvulsant medication should begin as soon as possible to terminate V.S.'s seizure activity. Status epilepticus becomes more resistant to treatment the longer the seizure continues; thus, treatment is more likely to stop seizures the sooner it is administered.[205] For in-hospital treatment of SE, IV medication administration is usually preferred.

CASE 60-12, QUESTION 3: Which anticonvulsants are available for IV administration? Evaluate the available drugs and recommend a drug, dosage, and regimen for initial treatment of SE in V.S.

Lorazepam, phenytoin, and fosphenytoin are the agents most commonly used as IV therapy in the initial treatment of SE.[205,209] Phenytoin and fosphenytoin are indicated for treatment of SE, but owing to limitations on their rates of infusion, the onset of their peak effect may be delayed. Therefore, phenytoin or fosphenytoin is usually used after initial treatment with lorazepam.

IV sodium valproate (Depacon) is available, but it is not FDA-approved for the treatment of SE. Although the manufacturer recommends that Depacon be administered slowly (<20 mg/minute), it has been administered safely at high doses and faster infusion rates.[208] There is growing experience with the use of IV valproate for SE that fails to respond to lorazepam and phenytoin, and for patients in whom phenytoin is contraindicated (e.g., phenytoin allergy).[209] An IV form of levetiracetam is available. This drug also is FDA-approved only for patients who cannot receive oral dosage forms of levetiracetam. Rapid IV administration of levetiracetam has been used; however, experience with this agent is limited.[210] Lacosamide is also available in an IV formulation and there are several case reports of its successful use for refractory nonconvulsive SE.[211,212] IV phenobarbital is usually reserved for SE that does not respond to benzodiazepines and phenytoin.[205]

Four IV regimens for generalized convulsive SE were directly compared in one randomized controlled trial.[213] The study evaluated diazepam followed by phenytoin, lorazepam alone, phenobarbital alone, and phenytoin alone. For initial IV treatment of overt generalized SE, lorazepam was more effective than phenytoin alone. Lorazepam was as effective as the other two regimens, and it was easier to use.

IV administration of either diazepam or lorazepam is usually effective for rapid termination of seizure activity in SE.[214] Owing to diazepam's higher lipid solubility, it redistributes from the CNS to peripheral tissues rapidly after administration; this results in a short duration of action (<60 minutes).[215] Lorazepam's lower lipid solubility prevents rapid redistribution and accounts for its longer duration of action.[215] Lorazepam may be effective for up to 72 hours.[216,217] Owing to this longer duration, lorazepam is the preferred benzodiazepine for immediate treatment of SEs.[208,209]

Lorazepam 0.1 mg/kg given intravenously at 2 mg/minute would be appropriate initial therapy for V.S.[208] Lorazepam may cause significant venous irritation, and the manufacturer recommends dilution with an equal volume of normal saline solution or water for injection before IV administration. Lorazepam may be repeated after 5 minutes if seizures continue. The efficacy of lorazepam depends on rapid achievement of high serum and CNS concentrations. Although lorazepam can be administered IM, this route should not be used for treatment of SE because it is unlikely that it would achieve serum concentrations necessary for termination of seizure activity and there is little experience with its use for terminating SE. Midazolam given IM has been shown to quickly and effectively terminate SE when used in out-of-hospital settings. This treatment is an acceptable alternative for in-hospital use when IV access is not feasible.[218,219] The most common adverse effects after IV administration of benzodiazepines are sedation, hypotension, and respiratory arrest.[215] These side effects are usually short-lived and, when adequate facilities are available for assisted ventilation and administration of fluids, they usually can be managed without major risk to the patient. Respiratory depression occurs most commonly in patients who receive multiple IV medications for control of SE.

INTRAVENOUS PHENYTOIN AND FOSPHENYTOIN

CASE 60-12, QUESTION 4: V.S. was given lorazepam 8 mg IV. Seizure activity ceased 2 minutes after the injection was completed. What drug should be administered to V.S. for prolonged control of seizures? Recommend a dose, route, and method of administration.

Continued effective seizure control is important for patients who experience SE. Previously, when diazepam was the benzodiazepine predominantly used for immediate control of SE, a long-acting AED such as phenytoin was routinely administered at the same time to ensure continued suppression of seizure activity. Routine use of phenytoin has been somewhat de-emphasized with increased use of lorazepam[208]; lorazepam's apparent longer duration of effect may make routine use of IV phenytoin less necessary. Nevertheless, many centers still use phenytoin in conjunction with lorazepam.

The availability of fosphenytoin for IV administration has provided an additional option for administration of phenytoin in the treatment of SE, and in most centers, fosphenytoin is preferred over phenytoin. Use of this phenytoin prodrug allows more rapid administration of large IV loading doses of phenytoin with less risk of injection site complications. Fosphenytoin is also better tolerated than phenytoin.[219] Fosphenytoin itself is inactive; the therapeutic effect results from its conversion to phenytoin.[100,101]

In the U.S., phenytoin (administered as either sodium phenytoin injection or as sodium fosphenytoin injection) is considered the long-acting anticonvulsant of choice for most patients with generalized convulsive SE.[209] Phenytoin causes much less sedation and respiratory depression than drugs such as phenobarbital when it is used in conjunction with IV benzodiazepines.[208] V.S.'s maintenance carbamazepine therapy was previously effective. Without obvious precipitating factors such as head trauma, CNS infection, and drug or alcohol abuse, SE, in a patient with a history of epilepsy, most commonly results from poor adherence with maintenance AED medication. Therefore, IV fosphenytoin is a good choice for re-establishing effective AED therapy for V.S. Phenytoin is an acceptable alternative if fosphenytoin is unavailable.

Loading Dose

Whether or not V.S. has a detectable serum concentration of carbamazepine, he should be given an IV loading dose of either fosphenytoin (20 mg/kg PE IV at 150 mg/minute) or phenytoin (20 mg/kg IV at 50 mg/minute). After administration of either of these loading doses, serum phenytoin concentrations should remain greater than 10 mcg/mL for approximately 24 hours; this will allow time for determination of V.S.'s serum carbamazepine concentration and estimation of an appropriate maintenance dose of oral carbamazepine once oral therapy can be restarted. In this setting, the use of IV phenytoin or fosphenytoin is a temporary measure. V.S.'s previous positive response to carbamazepine indicates that he should likely continue to receive this drug as his oral maintenance medication.

IV phenytoin can be administered by direct injection into a running IV line. The rate of administration should be no faster than 50 mg/minute to minimize the risk of hypotension and acute cardiac arrhythmias. Cardiovascular status (blood pressure, electrocardiogram) should be monitored closely during administration. Hypotension or electrocardiographic abnormalities usually reverse if the administration of phenytoin is slowed or stopped temporarily. Fosphenytoin can be given by either direct IV injection or, after dilution in any suitable IV solution, by infusion at up to 150 mg PE/minute.[100] Absence of propylene glycol as a diluent renders fosphenytoin potentially less likely than phenytoin to cause cardiovascular adverse effects, but this advantage is not well supported.[220] Electrocardiographic and blood pressure monitoring is recommended when this drug is given IV. Pruritus and paresthesias, usually localized to the face and groin, are relatively common side effects during IV fosphenytoin administration. These sensations are not allergic reactions to the medication. Their occurrence is related to the administration rate, and they are reversible with temporary discontinuation or slowing of the injection.[100]

Maintenance Therapy

The undetectable serum carbamazepine concentration appears to confirm the role of nonadherence in this episode of SE. Because V.S. was previously well controlled on 600 mg/day, this would be a reasonable target dose. Because V.S. may not tolerate carbamazepine if restarted at the prior maintenance dose, gradually escalating up to this dose should be initiated as soon as V.S. can take oral medication. V.S. should be counseled regarding the importance of taking his medication according to directions and any potential barriers to adherence should be addressed.

Alternative Therapies for Refractory Status Epilepticus

Phenobarbital may be useful for treatment of SE if the patient cannot tolerate phenytoin or when seizures continue after administration of appropriate loading doses of phenytoin. Patients who receive phenobarbital after being treated with IV benzodiazepines should be monitored closely for respiratory depression because this effect may be additive. Equipment and personnel to provide ventilatory assistance should be available.[208]

Status epilepticus that does not respond to lorazepam and a longer-acting agent (e.g., phenytoin/fosphenytoin, valproate, levetiracetam, phenobarbital, or lacosamide) is considered *refractory status epilepticus*. From 20% to 40% of patients with SE will progress to refractory status epilepticus. In such circumstances, an alternative longer-acting agent from those mentioned above may be considered; and, in recent years, the use of such "third-line" agents was a common practice. Recently, it has become a more common practice to escalate therapy to the use of an anesthetic agent after failure of second-line therapy.[209] The most commonly used anesthetic agents for refractory status epilepticus are midazolam and propofol; pentobarbital is also sometimes used. Significant respiratory depression is expected with these therapies; patients require intubation and mechanical ventilation. In addition, vasopressors, such as dopamine or dobutamine, may be required to control hypotension. Constant EEG monitoring also is required to assess the anticonvulsant effect of the drug and to gauge the level of anesthesia.

Midazolam is given as a loading dose of 0.2 mg/kg IV and is followed by an IV infusion of 0.2 to 0.6 mg/kg/hour.[208] Many practitioners adjust the infusion rate to either control electrographic seizures and/or to produce a burst-suppression EEG pattern.[221] Most protocols for anesthetic therapy of refractory SE recommend attempts at gradually reducing the dose of medication after 12 to 24 hours of treatment. If clinical or EEG seizure activity recurs, the dose is increased again to produce the desired EEG pattern. Anesthetic agents may need to be continued for several days or even weeks in some patients.

Continuous IV infusions of propofol or midazolam are also useful for refractory SE. These therapies appear to be less likely than pentobarbital to cause severe hypotension that is refractory to vasopressors.[222–225] Because no direct comparative trials of pentobarbital, propofol, and midazolam have been performed, physician familiarity and preference often guide the choice between these agents for the treatment of refractory SE.

KEY REFERENCES AND WEBSITES

A full list of references for this chapter can be found at http://thepoint.lww.com/AT11e. Below are the key references and websites for this chapter, with the corresponding reference number in this chapter found in parentheses after the reference.

Key References

Bialer M et al. Progress report on new antiepileptic drugs: a summary of the Twelfth Eilat Conference (EILAT XII). *Epilepsy Res*. 2015;111:85. (86)

Werhahn KJ et al. A randomized, double-blind comparison of antiepileptic drug treatment in the elderly with new-onset focal epilepsy. *Epilepsia*. 2015;56:450. (115)

French JA, Pedley TA. Clinical practice. Initial management of epilepsy. *N Engl J Med*. 2008;359:166. (3)

Glauser T et al. Evidence-based guideline: treatment of convulsive status epilepticus in children and adults: report of the Guideline Committee of the American Epilepsy Society. *Epilepsy Curr*. 2016;16:48–61. (225)

Glauser TA et al. Ethosuximide, valproic acid, and lamotrigine in childhood absence epilepsy. *N Engl J Med*. 2010;362:790. (123)

Harden CL et al. Management issues for women with epilepsy-Focus on pregnancy (an evidence-based review): I. Obstetrical complications and change in seizure frequency, II. Teratogenesis and perinatal outcomes, III. Vitamin K, folic acid, blood levels, and breast-feeding. Report of the Quality Standards Subcommittee and Therapeutics and Technology Subcommittee of the American Academy of Neurology and the American Epilepsy Society. *Epilepsia*. 2009;50:1229. (187)

Krumholz A et al. Evidence-based guideline: management of an unprovoked first seizure in adults: report of the Guideline Development Subcommittee of the American Academy of Neurology and the American Epilepsy Society. *Neurology*. 2015;84:1705. (4)

Marson AG et al. The SANAD study of effectiveness of valproate, lamotrigine, or topiramate for generalised and unclassifiable epilepsy: an unblinded randomised controlled trial. *Lancet*. 2007;369:1016. (124)

Meador KJ et al. Fetal antiepileptic drug exposure and cognitive outcomes at age 6 years (NEAD study): a prospective observational study. *Lancet Neurol*. 2013;12:244. (193)

Potschka H. Transporter hypothesis of drug-resistant epilepsy: challenges for pharmacogenetic approaches. *Pharmacogenomics*. 2010;11:1427. (87)

Betjemann JP, Lowenstein DH. Status epilepticus in adults. *Lancet Neurol*. 2015;14:615. (209)

Key Websites

American Epilepsy Society. http://www.aesnet.org.

Epilepsy and Seizure Information for Patients and Health Professionals. http://www.epilepsy.com.

AED Pregnancy Registry. http://www.aedpregnancyregistry.org/.

61 Ischemic and Hemorrhagic Stroke

Oussayma Moukhachen and Philip Grgurich

CORE PRINCIPLES

		CHAPTER CASES
1	Ischemic and hemorrhagic stroke are diseases involving the vascular system of the brain. In the United States, approximately 87% of strokes are ischemic in nature and 13% are hemorrhagic.	**Case 61-1 (Question 1)**
2	Ischemic and hemorrhagic stroke are medical emergencies, requiring prompt medical attention at the first sign of symptoms. Signs and symptoms of cerebrovascular disease usually occur acutely and vary depending on the area of the brain involved. Ischemic and hemorrhagic events have similar symptoms and must be distinguished before initiating treatment.	**Case 61-2 (Question 1)**
3	Primary prevention is vital to reducing the risk of a stroke. Lifestyle modifications and control of risk factors are the mainstay of primary prevention. Important modifiable risk factors include cardiovascular disease, hypertension, obesity, dyslipidemia, diabetes, smoking and physical inactivity. The use of antiplatelet agents is recommended for cardiovascular (including but not specific to stroke) prophylaxis and reasonable for people whose 10-year risk is >10% as estimated by cardiovascular risk calculators (see Core Principle 4).	**Case 61-1 (Questions 1, 2)**
4	Patients with atrial fibrillation and patent foramen ovale require primary prevention pharmacotherapy according to their ischemic stroke risk. Antiplatelet agents or anticoagulants should be used in patients with these conditions, with selection of an agent dependent on patient characteristics.	**Case 61-1 (Question 2)**
5	Secondary prevention of ischemic stroke and transient ischemic attacks involves the use of antiplatelet agents. Selection of an agent is dependent on patient characteristics.	**Case 61-2 (Questions 5,6, 7, 8, 9 , 10)**
6	Acute treatment of ischemic strokes includes the use of alteplase given intravenously. Alteplase should be started after confirming an event is ischemic and not hemorrhagic. The treatment window for use of alteplase is limited to 4.5 hours after the onset of neurologic symptoms. Strict criteria for administration of alteplase must be followed to reduce the risk of intracranial hemorrhage (ICH) and hemorrhagic complications should be carefully monitored.	**Case 61-2 (Questions 2, 3, 4, 5)**
7	The strongest risk factor for hemorrhagic stroke because of non-traumatic intracerebral hemorrhage is uncontrolled hypertension. Intracerebral hemorrhage may also occur as a result of an anatomic abnormality in the brain or a disease process, such as a brain tumor. Bleeding disorders, including those induced by anticoagulant drugs, also predispose patients to intracerebral hemorrhage.	**Case 61-3 (Question 1)**
8	Acute treatment of intracerebral hemorrhage focuses on minimizing hemorrhage expansion through careful blood pressure control and reversal of coagulopathies, when appropriate, as well as prevention and management of elevated intracranial pressure.	**Case 61-3 (Questions 2-6)**
9	Modifiable risk factors for hemorrhagic strokes include blood pressure control, smoking cessation, and avoiding excessive alcohol and cocaine use.	**Case 61-3 (Question 7)**

Continued

10 Rehabilitation after a cerebrovascular event is essential to patient recovery. Common complications encountered in rehabilitation included spasticity, depression, and neurogenic bowel or bladder. Pharmacotherapy interventions should be directed at each of these complications with the goal of improving the patient's quality of life and ability to function independently.

CHAPTER CASES

Case 61-5 (Question 1)

ISCHEMIC STROKE, HEMORRHAGIC STROKE, AND TRANSIENT ISCHEMIC ATTACKS

Ischemic stroke, hemorrhagic stroke, and transient ischemic attacks result from either inadequate blood flow to the brain (i.e., cerebral ischemia) with subsequent infarction of the involved portion of the central nervous system (CNS) or hemorrhages into the parenchyma or surrounding structures of the CNS and subsequent neurologic dysfunction. This group of disorders is the fourth leading cause of deaths among adults in the United States.[1]

Definitions

TRANSIENT ISCHEMIC ATTACK

A transient ischemic attack (TIA) is now defined as transient episode of neurologic dysfunction caused by focal brain, spinal cord, or retinal ischemia not associated with permanent cerebral infarction.[2] It used to be described as the clinical condition in which a patient experiences a temporary (lasting less than 24 hours) focal neurologic deficit such as slurred speech, aphasia, weakness or paralysis of a limb, or blindness. However, the original description is no longer valid because it is implied that TIAs are minor and that symptoms disappeared completely, while recent studies and imaging techniques have shown that TIA can actually lead to brain injury and increased risk of recurrent stroke. Some would argue that TIA term should not be even used at all.

ISCHEMIC STROKE

Ischemic stroke is defined as an infarction of the CNS. Unlike TIAs, ischemic stroke may be either symptomatic or silent.[2] Clinical signs of focal or global cerebral, spinal or retinal dysfunction caused by a CNS infarction are the manifestation of a symptomatic stroke. The two primary causes of infarction and persistent ischemia are atherosclerosis of cerebral blood vessels or an embolus to the cerebral arteries from a distant clot.

INTRACRANIAL HEMORRHAGE

Intracranial hemorrhage involves movement of blood from blood vessels inside the brain into the brain tissue, or parenchyma, and its surrounding structures. Clinical symptoms associated with intracranial hemorrhage are similar to but often more severe than those because of ischemic strokes. These symptoms commonly include neurologic deficits as well as headache, vomiting, and a decreased level of consciousness. Some patients may experience other symptoms including seizures, EKG abnormalities, and a stiff neck. Depending on the type and size of intracranial hemorrhage, symptoms may develop abruptly or worsen slowly over minutes to hours.

The location of the hemorrhage within the intracranial vault determines the type of intracranial hemorrhage. Intracerebral hemorrhages (ICHs) occur when blood moves into the brain parenchyma, whereas other types of hemorrhages develop when blood moves into spaces around the brain tissue.

Epidemiology

Each year an estimated 795,000 individuals in the United States experience a new or recurrent stroke and approximately 610,000 of these are first attacks. It is the fourth most common cause of death in adults after diseases of the heart, cancer, and chronic lower respiratory disease. There is a higher regional incidence and prevalence of stroke and a higher stroke mortality rate in the southern United States than in the rest of the country. Younger men have a higher incidence of stroke than women in the same age group; however, in age group >75 years, women have a higher incidence. Blacks and Hispanics have an increased risk of stroke compared with whites in the United States. The precise reasons for these differences are unclear, but genetic, geographic, dietary, and cultural factors have been considered.[3] In addition, the incidence of risk factors for stroke such as hypertension, diabetes, and hypercholesterolemia differs among racial groups.

In the United States ischemic stroke is the most common type of infarction (Fig. 61-1). Atherothrombotic disease of the large cerebral blood vessels is responsible for the majority of cerebral ischemic events and infarctions. Disease of penetrating arteries that are responsible for oxygenation and nutrition of the CNS, thromboembolic causes (e.g., atrial fibrillation), and other causes such as infection or inflammation of arteries are also responsible for ischemic stroke.

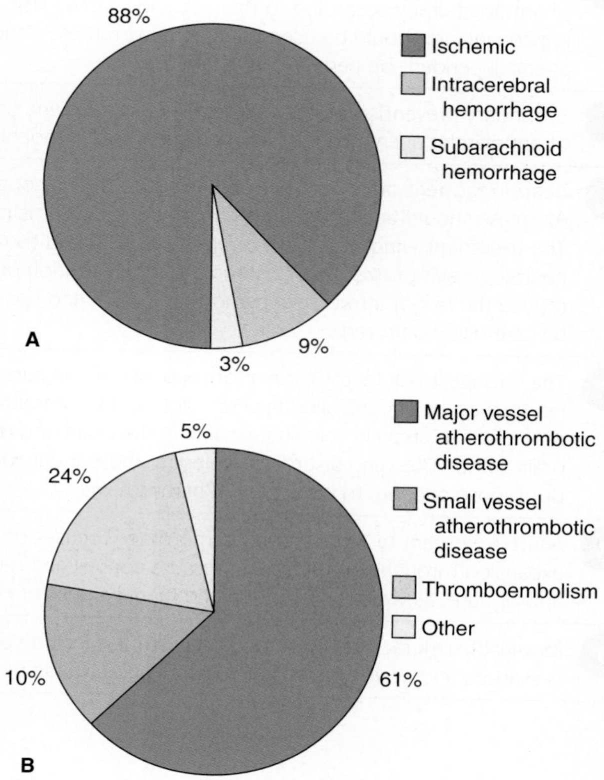

Figure 61-1 Etiology of strokes. Causes of all strokes.

Table 61-1
Risk Factors for Transient Ischemic Attack and Ischemic Stroke

Modifiable	Potentially Modifiable	Non-modifiable
Cardiovascular disease (coronary heart disease, heart failure, peripheral arterial disease) Hypertension Cigarette smoking Diabetes Asymptomatic carotid stenosis Atrial fibrillation Sickle cell disease	Metabolic syndrome Alcohol abuse (≥5 drinks daily) Hyperhomocysteinemia Drug abuse (e.g., cocaine, amphetamine, methamphetamine) Hypercoagulability (e.g., anticardiolipin, factor V Leiden, protein C deficiency, protein S deficiency, antithrombin III deficiency)	Age (doubling each 10 years after age 55) Race (blacks > Hispanics > whites) Sex (men > women) Low birth weight (<2,500 g) Family history of stroke (paternal > maternal)
Dyslipidemia (high total cholesterol, low HDL)	Oral contraceptive use (women 25–44 years old)	
Dietary factors (sodium intake <2,300 mg/day; potassium intake <4,700 mg/day)	Inflammatory processes (e.g., periodontal disease, cytomegalovirus, *Helicobacter pylori* seropositive)	
Obesity Physical inactivity	Acute infection (e.g., respiratory infection, urinary tract infection)	
Postmenopausal hormone therapy (women 50–74 years old)	CD40 ligand >3.71 ng/mL in women free of cardiovascular disease	
	IL-18 upper tertile	
	hs-CRP >3 mg/L in women 45 years or older	
	Migraine headaches	
	High Lp(a)	
	High Lp-PLA_2	
	Sleep-disordered breathing	

HDL, high-density lipoprotein; hs-CRP, high-sensitivity C-reactive protein; IL, interleukin; Lp(a), lipoprotein(a); Lp-LPA_2, lipoprotein-associated phospholipase A_2.
Source: Meschia JF et al. Guidelines for the primary prevention of stroke: a statement for healthcare professionals from the American Heart Association/American Stroke Association. *Stroke*. 2014;45:3754.

There is a strong relationship between the occurrence of TIA and an increased risk for subsequent cerebral infarction.[1,2] The risk of an ischemic stroke is highest in the first 30 days after a TIA, and the risk within 90 days of a TIA is 3% to 17.3%. Additionally, nearly 25% of patients who experience a TIA will die within a year.[2] Risk factors for cerebral infarction are listed in Table 61-1. Risk factors for stroke are classified as either non-modifiable (e.g., age, race, gender) and modifiable if they can be altered (e.g., hypertension, high cholesterol level, smoking). Cerebral infarct prevention efforts will be focused on elimination and control of the modifiable risk factors.[4,5] The control of risk factors is of primary importance in managing a patient with a TIA or cerebral infarction.

Intracerebral hemorrhages account for 10% of all strokes in North America, while subarachnoid hemorrhage, most commonly resulting from cerebral artery aneurysms, comprises 3% of all strokes. Hypertensive hemorrhage is the most common cause of ICH, with 46% of ICHs resulting from hypertension. In fact, hypertension more than doubles the risk of ICH. A number of medications including warfarin and other anticoagulants, such as dabigatran, rivaroxaban, and apixaban, significantly predispose patients to ICH. Less commonly, ICH may occur because of an arteriovenous malformation (AVM), which is a clump of arteries and veins that are intertwined, resulting in weakened blood vessel walls.

Pathophysiology

The neurologic sequelae of cerebral ischemia or infarction directly result from an embolic or thrombotic source. A clot may form in the heart, along the wall of a major blood vessel (e.g., aorta, carotid, or basilar artery), or in small arteries penetrating deep into the brain. If the clot is located near the infarction, it is a thrombus; however, when the clot has migrated to the brain from a distant source, it is an embolus. Either can diminish or block blood flow to the affected area of the brain. Disorders such as atrial fibrillation, mitral or aortic valve disease, patent foramen ovale, or coagulopathies are associated with formation of clots that may embolize to the brain.

Inflammatory mechanisms also contribute to the development of ischemia, especially thrombotic lesions. Substances, such as C-reactive protein, a mediator of inflammation, are elevated in patients with an acute stroke. Inflammation is thought to enhance the development of thrombotic lesions and result in sudden, intermittent occlusion of blood vessels. Disorders such as arteritis (Takayasu, Giant cell), and Moyamoya syndrome are examples of diseases where inflammation plays an important role for the development of brain ischemia.

Cerebral blood flow in the normal adult brain is 30 to 70 mL/100 g of brain tissue/minute. When a thrombotic or embolic clot partially occludes a cerebral artery, causing a reduction in blood flow to less than 20 mL/100 g/minute, various compensatory mechanisms are activated. These include vasodilation and increased oxygen extraction. If the artery is further occluded and cerebral blood flow is reduced to less than 12 mL/100 g/minute, the affected neurons become sufficiently anoxic to die within minutes (Fig. 61-2).[6] Rapid reestablishment of blood flow to the ischemic area can delay, prevent, or limit the onset of infarction, improving the outcome of the acute stroke.

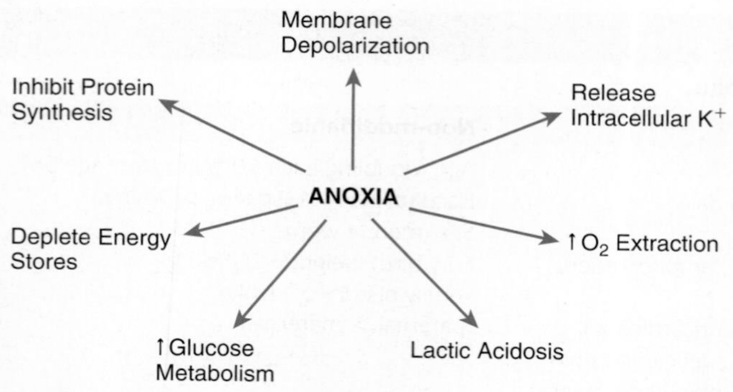

Figure 61-2 Physiologic effects of cerebral anoxia.

Ischemia in the brain usually involves a core or focal region of profound ischemia that results in neuronal death. The extent of this region is dependent on the amount of brain that is perfused directly by the blood vessel that becomes occluded. There is a surrounding area of brain that becomes marginally ischemic with normal function being disrupted. This region of marginal ischemia is frequently called the *ischemic penumbra.* If ischemia continues, neurons in this region will die. However, if normal blood flow is restored quickly, neurons in this area will survive.

When neurons become ischemic, excitatory neurotransmitters are released, causing neurons to rapidly and repeatedly discharge. Increased neuronal activity results in extreme metabolic demands, disrupts neuronal homeostasis, depletes stores of adenosine triphosphate, and synergistically increases the effects of hypoxia. Especially vulnerable to ischemic effects are neurons in the middle layers of the cerebral cortex; portions of the hippocampus (CA1 and subiculum regions), a structure running parallel to the parahippocampal gyrus; and Purkinje cells in the cerebellum.[7] There is also a rapid intracellular influx of calcium. Both voltage-dependent and chemical-dependent calcium channels are unable to act as a gate to prevent the movement of calcium, owing to depletion of cellular energy sources. Intracellular stores of calcium ions also are disrupted, causing release of calcium into the cytoplasm. Increased concentration of calcium ions enhances phospholipase and protease activity and increases reactive metabolites, such as superoxide and hydroxide ions, and nitric oxide. This eventually causes neuronal death.[6,7] In addition, lipolysis of cell membranes occurs in the presence of an accumulation of neurotoxic free radicals.

Immediate therapeutic intervention is needed to limit and prevent permanent neurologic damage from these rapidly occurring events.

INTRACRANIAL HEMORRHAGE

Intracranial hemorrhages occur because of weakened intracranial blood vessels, elevated pressure inside the blood vessels, and anatomical abnormalities. Specific causes include hypertension, cerebral amyloid angiopathy, brain tumors, anatomical derangements such as AVMs, coagulopathies, and trauma. Pathophysiologic mechanisms differ depending on whether the bleeding occurs outside the brain parenchyma in the subarachnoid, epidural, or subdural space or within the intracerebral space.

In subarachnoid hemorrhage, blood moves quickly into the cerebrospinal fluid (CSF), causing an acute elevation of intracranial pressure (ICP). ICP refers to the pressure inside the intracranial vault and may be elevated because of brain tissue swelling, the development of a hematoma (collection of blood) inside the brain, or other conditions. Blood may also migrate into the intraventricular space or into the brain tissue.[8,9] Obstruction of CSF fluid reabsorption and movement out of the brain because of the presence of blood in the brain can result in hydrocephalus, which is the buildup of CSF within the ventricles of the brain. Delayed cerebral ischemia, commonly referred to as "vasospasm" of the cerebral vasculature, may also complicate subarachnoid hemorrhage.

Epidural and subdural hematomas are other types of intracranial hemorrhages that occur outside the brain parenchyma. Depending on their size, epidural and subdural hematomas may significantly compress and displace brain tissue, resulting in elevated ICP and brain herniation because of mass effect. Brain herniation refers to abnormal movement of brain tissue across structures inside the skull that occurs because of elevated pressures within the intracranial vault. This squeezing of brain tissue can significantly compress cerebral blood flow, consequently compromising oxygen delivery to the brain and causing brain cells to die.

Spontaneous intracerebral hemorrhage because of hypertension develops in areas of the brain where smaller blood vessels branch out from large blood vessels at 90 degree angles, exposing the smaller vessels to the higher pressure of the preceding blood vessel and eventually resulting in bleeding of the smaller vessels.[10] In intracerebral hemorrhage, the movement of blood from blood vessels into the brain parenchyma causes local irritation of the brain tissue and edema. In the case of large hemorrhages and significant edema, mass effect can ultimately increase ICP, reducing blood flow to the brain and potentially causing brain tissue herniation.[11] Secondary brain injury occurs in many patients after spontaneous ICH. It is caused by a disrupted blood–brain barrier, release of inflammatory mediators, and progressive edema that may last 7 to 12 days.[12–15]

In spontaneous intracerebral hemorrhage, hematoma enlargement is associated with poor outcomes. Non-modifiable risk factors for hematoma expansion are large hematoma size and contrast extravasation on computed tomography (CT) at the time of presentation, while potentially modifiable risk factors include coagulopathies and ongoing uncontrolled hypertension after hospital admission.[16,17]

General Treatment Principles

Rapid recognition of stroke symptoms and immediate initiation of treatment are essential to the management of ischemic or hemorrhagic stroke. Appropriate pharmacotherapy of stroke requires a precise diagnosis. It is vital to differentiate between an ischemic stroke and a hemorrhagic stroke, because an inaccurate diagnosis can lead to the use of drugs that may cause severe morbidity or mortality. Interventions to prevent and treat ischemic strokes are directed at reducing risk factors, eliminating or modifying the underlying pathologic process, and reducing secondary brain damage. In hemorrhagic stroke, the emphasis of treatment is on preventing hematoma expansion, managing intracranial pressure, and providing supportive therapy to maximize neurologic function and minimize complications. Rehabilitation is a key component of long-term care for many patients, regardless of whether the stroke is ischemic or hemorrhagic.

PRIMARY PREVENTION OF ISCHEMIC STROKE AND TRANSIENT ISCHEMIC ATTACKS

Risk Factors Modification

CASE 61-1

QUESTION 1: R.B. is a 60-year-old, 5 feet 6 inches tall, 85-kg woman who is concerned about having a stroke. Her father died of a stroke, and her 85-year-old mother has had several episodes diagnosed as TIAs. R.B.'s blood pressure is 140 to 150/90 to 100 mm Hg, and she was recently diagnosed with diabetes mellitus. She does not have a history of TIA or stroke. Additionally, she smoked for 25 years but has not used tobacco for the past 10 years. Her current medications include lisinopril, metformin, conjugated estrogen/medroxyprogesterone, and acetaminophen. She approaches her pharmacist because of concerns about having a stroke and being "like her parents." What can R.B. do to reduce her risk of stroke?

Any plan for *primary prevention* (i.e., prevention of a first event) of TIA or stroke must address the control or reduction of risk factors (Table 61-2).The reader is referred to a detailed discussion of treatment of diseases such as hypertension, diabetes, coronary artery disease, chronic kidney disease, etc. in their respective chapters (see Chapters 9, 13, 28, 53) .

For R.B., hypertension is the most important and well-documented risk factor that requires immediate attention.[4] Adequate control of her blood pressure should reduce R.B.'s risk of stroke by 35% to 44%. On the basis of the eighth Report of the Joint National Committee on Prevention, Detection, Evaluation, and Treatment of High Blood Pressure (JNC-8) guidelines, R.B.'s blood pressure goal should be less than 140/90 mm Hg.[18] Antihypertensives that have been associated with a stroke reduction risk are the angiotension converting enzyme inhibitor (ACE-I), hydrochlorothiazide, and calcium-channel blockers.[19] Because she is already receiving lisinopril and her blood pressure is poorly controlled, it is likely that a combination therapy is needed. The addition of hydrochlorothiazide 25 mg/day is advisable to R.B.[4]

Diabetes is another important risk factor for in RB. In older women, diabetes is a more significant risk factor for stroke than it is for men.[20] There is controversy regarding the intensity of glucose control that optimally reduces stroke risk. Clearly, good control of diabetes results in better control of hypertension and other risk factors for stroke.[21] Additionally, use of oral hypoglycemics may reduce the risk of stroke through mechanisms other than glycemic control. However, strict control of blood glucose did not reduce the risk of stroke over the course of 9 years in one study.[21] There is evidence that angiotensin-converting enzyme inhibitors (ACEIs) and angiotensin receptor blockers (ARBs) reduce the risk of stroke in diabetics, with or without hypertension.[22,23] For diabetic patients with at least one additional risk factor for cardiovascular disease, taking a β-hydroxy-β-methylglutaryl-CoA (HMG-CoA) reductase inhibitor appears to reduce the risk of stroke by approximately 24% even in the absence of hypercholesterolemia.[24,25] It is known that HMG-CoA reductase inhibitors have anti-inflammatory activity that may influence the development of atherosclerotic plaques and cerebral ischemic processes.[26–28] Because of these effects of HMG-CoA reductase inhibitors, these drugs should be started for primary prevention of ischemic stroke and TIA even in patients who do not have dyslipidemia if the estimated 10-year risk of cardiovascular events is high, as recommended in the 2013 "ACC/AHA guideline."[4]

Chapter 61
Ischemic and Hemorrhagic Stroke

Table 61-2
Primary Prevention of Ischemic Stroke

Factor	Goal	Recommendation
Hypertension	Blood pressure <140/90 mm Hg	Follow JNC-8 guidelines; after lifestyle modification thiazide-type diuretic, angiotensin-converting enzyme inhibitor, or angiotensin receptor blocker, CCB (full discussion in Chapter 9, Essential Hypertension)
Atrial fibrillation	When warfarin is used, INR 2–3	Aspirin 75–325 mg/day or warfarin, rivaroxaban, dabigatran, apixaban, or edoxaban as determined by the use of the $CHADS_2$ or CHA2DSC2-VASC score (full discussion in Chapter 15, Cardiac Arrhythmias)
Dyslipidemia	National Cholesterol Education Program III goals	Lifestyle modification, HMG-CoA reductase inhibitor (full discussion in Chapter 8, Dyslipidemias)
Women (>65 years, history of hypertension, hyperlipidemia, diabetes, or 10-year cardiovascular risk ≥10%)	Reduce risk without bleeding complications	Aspirin 75–325 mg/day; use the lowest possible dose
Cigarette smoke	Elimination of cigarette smoke	Smoking cessation; avoidance of environmental tobacco smoke
Physical inactivity	≥30 minutes daily of moderate-intensity activity	Establish exercise program of aerobic activity
Excessive alcohol intake	Moderation	≤2 drinks/day for men or ≤1 drink/day for nonpregnant women
Diet and nutrition	≤2.3 g/day of sodium; ≥4.7 g/day of potassium	Institute a diet that is high in fruits and vegetables and low in saturated fats
Elevated lipoprotein(a)	Reduction of lipoprotein(a) by ≥25%	Niacin 2,000 mg/day as tolerated

HMG-CoA, β-hydroxy-β-methylglutaryl-CoA; INR, international normalized ratio; JNC-8, Eighth Report of the Joint National Committee on Prevention, Detection, Evaluation, and Treatment of High Blood Pressure.
Source: Meschia JF, et al. Guidelines for the primary prevention of stroke: a statement for healthcare professionals from the American Heart Association/American Stroke Association. *Stroke*. 2014;45:3754–3832

Niacin, fibric acid derivatives, ezetimibe, or bile acid sequestrants can be considered for patients who do not tolerate HMG-CoA reductase inhibitors or have low high-density lipoprotein cholesterol concentrations; however, their efficacy in preventing a stroke is not established. The benefits of HMG-CoA reductase inhibitors appear to be a class effect, so selection of a specific agent should be based on the individual characteristics of the patient. For R.B., she should maintain tight control of her diabetes, continue her lisinopril, and start an HMG-CoA reductase inhibitor, such as simvastatin or atorvastatin.

The body mass index for R.B. is 30.2 kg/m^2, placing her in the obese category. Multiple large studies have demonstrated a direct relationship between increased body weight and an increased risk of stroke.[29,30] There are no data available to establish the precise effect of weight reduction on reducing the risk of stroke. However, increasing physical activity and proper nutrition are essential to achieve weight loss and improve diabetes and blood pressure control.[31]

A diet high in sodium is associated with an increased risk in stroke, whereas a diet high in potassium appears to reduce the risk of stroke.[32,33] Current recommendations for diet are for sodium intake of 2.3 g/day or less and potassium intake of at least 4.7 g/day.[4] In addition, a DASH-style diet, which emphasizes fruits, vegetables, and low-fat dairy products and reduced saturated fat is recommended to lower blood pressure and thereby reduce the risk of stroke.

Regarding physical activity, several studies have shown an inverse relationship between physical activity and risk of stroke.[34,35] Therefore, at least 40 minutes/day of moderate-intensity exercise is recommended three to four times/week.[4] Cigarette smoking is an independent risk factor for stroke and potentiates other risk factors. In addition to active smoking, passive inhalation of cigarette smoke also appears to be a risk factor for stroke.[36] Smoking cessation does result in a rapid reduction in the risk of stroke, but the risk never returns to levels seen in individuals who have never smoked.[37]

Finally, five studies have specifically investigated the effect of hormone replacement on stroke risk.[38–42] On the basis of the results from these studies, R.B. should discontinue her conjugated estrogen/medroxyprogesterone product unless she is taking this medication for a specific reason other than control of menopausal symptoms or prevention of cardiovascular events. R.B. should be encouraged to avoid passive smoke and to continue avoiding the use of tobacco. R.B. should initiate a weight-reduction program that includes a low-sodium and high-potassium diet with an exercise program.

Pharmacotherapy Primary Prevention of Ischemic Stroke and Transient Ischemic Attacks

CASE 61-1, QUESTION 2: Would R.B. benefit from any antiplatelet or anticoagulation for the primary prevention of ischemic stroke and TIAs?

Aspirin has been carefully investigated for primary prevention of stroke. Although aspirin is recommended in the primary prevention of coronary heart disease, it is not generally recommended for the primary prevention of stroke or TIA in low-risk patients (10-year risk $<$10%).[4] In high-risk patients ($>$10-year risk $>$10%), the use of aspirin for cardiovascular (including but not specific to stroke) prophylaxis is reasonable. A patient's 10-year risk can be calculated using online calculators such as http://my.americanheart.org/cvriskcalculator.

In a study of 22,071 male physicians who took 325 mg of aspirin or placebo every other day for 5 years, stroke incidence was similar between groups. In addition, there was an increased risk of cerebrovascular events caused by hemorrhage in the aspirin group. Chen et al. reported a meta-analysis of 40,000 patients randomly assigned to aspirin and found a reduction from 47% to 45.8% in death and disability attributable to stroke.[44] Another study considered the role of aspirin for primary stroke prevention in women.[45] Women who took one to six tablets of aspirin per week had a slightly reduced risk of stroke and a lower risk of large-artery occlusive disease (relative risk, 59%; 95% confidence level, 0.29–0.85; $p = 0.01$). An increased risk of stroke was seen in women who took more than 7 aspirin weekly, and an excess risk of subarachnoid hemorrhage was seen in those taking more than 15 aspirin a week. The Women's Health Study also investigated the use of 100 mg/day in asymptomatic women and followed them for 10 years, monitoring for nonfatal cardiovascular events including stroke.[46] In this study, there was a 17% reduction in the risk for all strokes and a 24% reduction in the risk for ischemic stroke, whereas there was a nonsignificant increase in the risk for hemorrhage. Women 65 years of age and older at entry into the trial showed the most consistent risk reduction, but hemorrhagic strokes negated some of the benefit. Additionally, women with a history of hypertension, hyperlipidemia, or diabetes, or a 10-year cardiovascular risk of at least 10% had the most benefit. There are very limited data currently available regarding the use of other antiplatelet drugs for primary prevention of stroke except for cilostazol in patients with peripheral artery disease.[4]

Although oral anticoagulants are not generally considered safe for primary prevention of non-cardioembolic, patients with atrial fibrillation are candidates for primary prevention. These individuals are at risk for an embolic event arising from clot formation in the atrium of the heart. The CHADS2 score has been a widely used system of stratifying the risk of thromboembolism in non-valvular atrial fibrillation for a decade. It is generally accepted that low-risk patients (CHADS2 score = 0) should not be treated with anticoagulants but may be considered for antiplatelet therapy, while higher-risk patients (CHADS2 score $\geq$2) should be anticoagulated with oral anticoagulants such as warfarin, dabigatran, apixaban, rivaroxaban, or edoxaban (detailed discussion is available in Chapter 15, Cardiac Arrhythmias). The tool recommended in the new guidelines, called "CHA_2DS_2-VASc," also considers whether a patient has had prior vascular disease, evaluates people at younger ages (between 65–74) and factors in gender.[47] This is important because women face higher stroke risks. CHA_2DS_2-VASC score of $\geq$2 warrant the use of anticoagulants as first-line option. Numerous studies have clearly shown that warfarin prevents embolic cerebrovascular events for patients with valvular and non-valvular atrial fibrillation.[48–51] In these studies, the warfarin dose was adjusted to maintain an international normalized ratio (INR) of 1.5 to 4.5, with most recommendations to adjust the dose for an INR of 2 to 3. The selection of the antithrombotic agent depends on various factors including patient factors (risk of falls and hemorrhagic events), cost, age of the patient, tolerability, patient preference, and potential drug interactions. The Stroke Prevention in Atrial Fibrillation (SPAF) trial included aspirin combined with warfarin in one study arm and indicated that some benefit may be derived by combining antiplatelet agents with anticoagulants.[52] A follow-up study was performed and showed no difference between warfarin and aspirin in preventing stroke in atrial fibrillation.[51] In patients with non-valvular atrial fibrillation, aspirin can be used as an alternative to warfarin in patients with atrial fibrillation, based on the $CHADS_2$ score or CHA_2DS_2-VASC score (Table 61-3).[5,47] Additionally, warfarin may be used in primary prevention of embolic stroke because of a patent foramen ovale.[5]

Table 61-3
$CHADS_2$ and CHA2DS2—VASC Score: Primary Stroke Prevention in Atrial Fibrillation

CHADS2 score	CHAD2DS2—VASC score
Add points for the following items. If score is <2, aspirin can be considered. If score is ≥2, anticoagulants (warfarin, apixaban, rivoraxaban, edoxaban) are recommended.	
Congestive heart failure = 1 point	Congestive heart failure = 1 point
Hypertension = 1 point	Hypertension = 1 point
Age >75 years = 1 point	Age >75 years = 2 points
Diabetes mellitus = 1 point	Diabetes mellitus = 1 point
Prior stroke or TIA = 2 points	Prior stroke or TIA = 2 points
	Vascular disease (e.g., peripheral artery disease, myocardial infarction, aortic plaque) = 1 point
	Age 65–74 years = 1 point
	Sex category (i.e., female) = 1point

TIA, transient ischemic attack.
Source: January C et al. 2014 AHA/ACC/HRS Guideline for the management of patients with atrial fibrillation: a report of the American College of Cardiology/American Heart Association Task Force on practice guidelines and the Heart Rhythm Society. *Circulation*. 2014;130:23.e199–e267.

For R.B., primary prevention of stroke with aspirin 81 mg/day can be considered because of her history of hypertension and diabetes. Given that she has no atrial fibrillation, she is not a candidate for anticoagulation therapy (see Table 61-4).

TREATMENT OF ACUTE ISCHEMIC STROKE AND TIA

Goals of Therapy

The immediate goal is to reestablish adequate blood flow in the diseased cerebral vessels, minimize brain injury, and treat medical complications. Longer-range objectives are to prevent reocclusion and decrease the risk of a future ischemic stroke.

Early Management of Acute Ischemic Stroke

CLINICAL PRESENTATION AND DIAGNOSTIC TESTS

CASE 61-2

QUESTION 1: P.C., a 65-year-old man (100 kg, 5 feet 9 inches), is admitted through the emergency department (ED) with right-sided weakness. As per report the patient was last seen well around 8:30 PM by his wife. Around 9:15 PM, the patient's son heard a bump and went upstairs to find his father on the floor. The patient had a slurred speech and had a right facial droop. At this point 911 was called and patient arrived at 9:45 PM to ED. He regained consciousness by the time he arrived in the ED. Both right extremities are flaccid. He is unable to speak but is capable of understanding instructions (i.e., expressive aphasia). Gross ophthalmologic examination indicates right-sided neglect (inability of his eyes to track to the right or acknowledge the right side of his body). His blood pressure is 165/95 mm Hg; other vital signs are normal. Laboratory studies are all within normal limits. What interventions should have been initiated before arrival in the ED?

Table 61-4
Drugs for Preventing Transient Ischemic Attacks and Ischemic Stroke

Drug	Action	Dose	Adverse Effects
Aspirin	Antiplatelet	50–325 mg/day	Diarrhea, gastric ulcer, GI upset
Dipyridamole	Antiplatelet (use in combination with aspirin)	200 mg sustained-release twice daily With aspirin 50 mg BID	GI upset
Ticlopidine	Antiplatelet	500 mg/day	Diarrhea, neutropenia, rash
Clopidogrel	Antiplatelet	75 mg/day	Thrombocytopenia, neutropenia
Cilostazol	Antiplatelet	100 mg BID	Headache, peripheral edema. Contraindicated in congestive heart failure patients
Warfarin	Anticoagulant (only in patients with cardioembolic cause of stroke/TIA	Titrate to goal INR 2–3 for most patients 2.5–3.5 with mechanical valve	Bleeding, bruising, petechiae
Rivaroxaban	Anticoagulant (only in patients with cardioembolic cause of stroke/TIA	If CrCl >15 mL/minute, 20 mg once daily with evening meal	Bleeding
Apixaban	Anticoagulant (only in patients with cardioembolic cause of stroke/TIA	5 mg BID If Scr ≥1.5 mg/dL, 2.5 mg BID (if age >80 years or weight ≤60 kg)	Bleeding
Edoxaban	Anticoagulant (only in patients with cardioembolic cause of stroke/TIA	60 mg daily If CrCl 15–50 mL/minute 30 mg daily	Do not use if CrCl >95 mL/minute as high risk of ischemic stroke
Dabigatran	Anticoagulant (only in patients with cardioembolic cause of stroke/TIA	150 mg BID If CrCL 15–30 mL/minute: 75 mg BID	GI bleed

GI, gastrointestinal; INR, international normalized ratio; BID, 2 times daily; CrCl, creatinine clearance; TIA, transient ischemic attack; Scr, serum creatinine.

Immediate recognition of, and response to, stroke symptoms are essential to an optimal outcome. As soon as stroke symptoms are recognized, the emergency medical system should be activated. Emergency medical personnel should be trained to gather important historical information, especially when the symptoms started. This is defined as "when the patient was at his or her previous baseline or symptom-free state. For patients unable to provide information or who was awaken with stroke symptoms, the time of onset is defined as when the patient was last awake and symptom-free or known to be normal."[53] Use of a standardized evaluation tool such as the Cincinnati Prehospital Stroke Scale or Los Angeles Prehospital Stroke Screen is useful in distinguishing stroke symptoms from other disorders, such as conversion disorder, hypertensive encephalopathy, hypoglycemia, complicated migraine, or seizures.[53,54]

General supportive care for respiratory and cardiovascular function should be initiated before transporting the patient to the ED. An important key to effectively managing acute stroke patients is to have a well-designed evaluation and treatment algorithm that addresses assessment and care of the patient from initial onset of symptoms through rehabilitation. Patients with suspected cerebral infarction should be transported, if possible, to the closest certified primary care center. A certified primary care center would have a multidisciplinary team and would be activated and notified by the emergency personnel while potential stroke patient is en route (Fig. 61-3).[53] If a primary stroke center is not locally available, patients can be stabilized in community hospital. In these situations, local providers may use practice arrangements with larger centers that allow the provision of advanced care under the supervision of experts at a primary stoke center.

CASE 61-2, QUESTION 2: What diagnostic tests and evaluations will be helpful in guiding P.C.'s therapy?

Basic laboratory and diagnostic tests should be quickly performed to exclude non-cerebrovascular causes of P.C.'s symptoms, such as metabolic or toxicologic derangement or infections. These tests include a routine serum chemistry profile (electrolytes, blood urea nitrogen, serum creatinine, hepatic enzymes, calcium, phosphorus, magnesium, albumin), complete blood count, and toxicology screen. Coagulation studies, including a prothrombin time with INR and partial thromboplastin time, should be performed to provide baseline values for potential anticoagulation or thrombolytic therapy. In addition, a thorough physical, neurologic, cardiovascular, and mental status examination should be performed. The neurologic examination will assist in localization of the lesion in the CNS. The physical examination should include use of the National Institutes of Health Stroke Scale.[54] In addition to providing important information for diagnosis of his neurologic compromise, these tests will provide baseline data for ongoing assessment of P.C.'s progress and recovery.

The etiology of a stroke (ischemic versus hemorrhagic) is difficult to discern based solely on a physical and neurologic examination. As a result, CT or magnetic resonance imaging (MRI) is valuable in the evaluation of these patients. An MRI is preferred to a CT because of its superior tissue contrast, ability to obtain images in multiple planes, absence of artifacts caused by bone, vascular imaging capabilities, absence of ionizing radiation, and safer contrast media. MRI also allows for a magnetic resonance angiogram to be performed, allowing visualization of the cerebro-vasculature and possible identification of the precise location of the thrombus or embolus. Within the first 24 hours of an ischemic stroke, an MRI is clearly more sensitive than a CT. After 48 hours, the MRI and CT are equally effective in detecting ischemic infarcts. The primary disadvantages of the MRI are that it is more sensitive to artifacts, more difficult to perform in unstable patients, and not always available in smaller hospitals or communities. In addition, MRI is also not safe to be done in patients who have metallic implants, or pacemakers.

P.C. must have either a CT or an MRI before initiation of any specific therapy for stroke. A follow-up CT or MRI in 5 to 7 days is useful to determine the extent of neurologic damage resulting from the ischemic stroke.

Angiographic, Doppler, or sonographic examination of the cerebral vasculature may be helpful in identifying the location of the vascular lesion. These tests usually are performed after the patient has been stabilized, unless angioplasty with stents, mechanical retrieval devices, or use of intra-arterial fibrinolytics is anticipated. A lumbar puncture with collection of CSF for evaluation may be helpful in identifying the presence of blood in the CNS. In the presence of suspected increased intracranial pressure, a lumbar puncture must be avoided because of the potential for tentorial herniation.

Treatment

CASE 61-2, QUESTION 3: A head CT revealed left MCA territory infarct with no cerebral hemorrhage or edema. Is PC a candidate for intravenous thrombolysis?

The critical primary event in a thromboembolic stroke is the development of an acute thrombus. Prospective cerebral angiography has demonstrated an arterial occlusion corresponding to the area of acute neurologic deficit in greater than 90% of cases.[55]

Occlusion of cerebral arteries does not cause complete ischemia because collateral circulation from other arterial sources provides unstable and incomplete circulation to the ischemic region of the brain.[56] When blood flow is sustained in the range of 10 to 18 mL/100 g/minute, irreversible cellular damage may occur. Blood flow must be restored quickly after the event. Experimental studies in dogs and cats have shown that when blood flow is restored within 2 to 3 hours, neurologic deficits are prevented.[57,58] Thrombolytic agents can reestablish blood flow to ischemic regions of the brain. The most important factor in successful thrombolytic therapy is early treatment. The selection of appropriate candidates for thrombolysis is extremely important and requires the correct neurologic evaluation by a specialized team. Before the initiation of thrombolytics, patients with high blood pressure should have their blood pressure lowered carefully to systolic BP <185 and diastolic BP <110 mm Hg (see Table 61-5 and the discussion later on blood pressure).

Randomized, controlled-trials have shown that intravenous tissue plasminogen activator (tPA), alteplase, to be beneficial for select patients with acute ischemic stroke who start treatment within 4.5 hours. For eligible patients (Table 61-6), once a CT ruled out a hemorrhage, intravenous tPA should be started within 4.5 hours of clearly defined symptoms. There are specific criteria to select patients for alteplase eligibility if they present within 3 hours of onset of symptoms versus if they present up to 4.5 hours of symptoms (see Table 61-6).

Several thrombolytics (streptokinase, alteplase, tenectaplase, reteplase, urokinase) are available. However, only alteplase trials have shown benefits and improved outcomes.[59–62]

In three studies, streptokinase was used as the thrombolytic, and all of these studies were terminated early owing to high rates of mortality and intracranial hemorrhage associated with streptokinase.[59,60,63] The rates of intracranial hemorrhage ranged

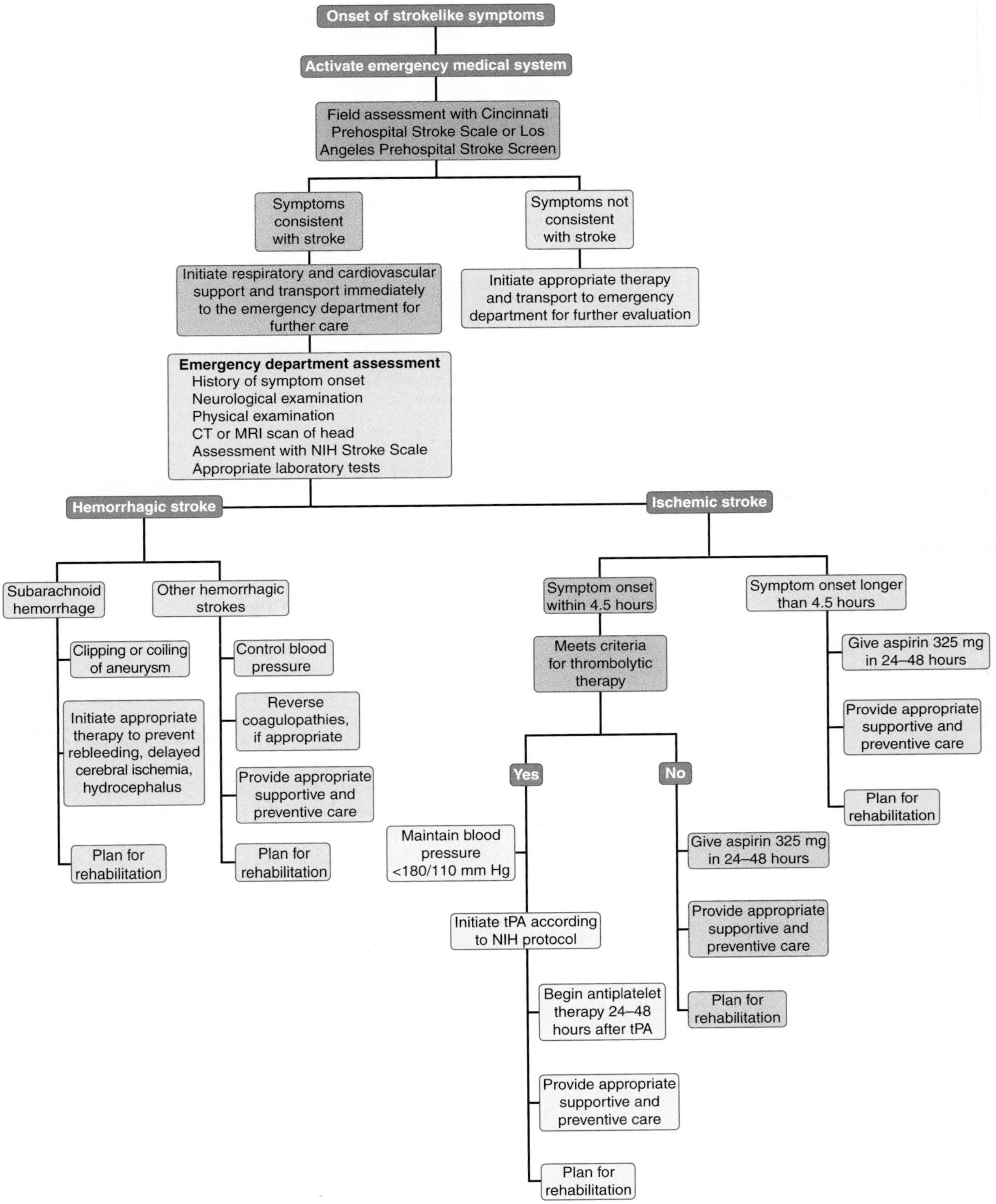

Figure 61-3 Treatment algorithm for management of patient with acute stroke-like symptoms. CT, computed tomography; MRI, magnetic resonance imaging; NIH, National Institutes of Health; t-PA, alteplase. (Source: Adams HP et al. Antifibrinolytic therapy in patients with aneurysmal subarachnoid hemorrhage: a report of the cooperative aneurysmal study. *Arch Neurol*. 1981;38:25.)

from 6% to 17% for patients receiving streptokinase compared with 0.6% to 3% for patients receiving placebo.

The National Institute of Neurological Disorders and Stroke (NINDS) alteplase trial[61] and the European Cooperative Acute Stroke Study (ECASS I)[62] used different doses, inclusion criteria, and treatment protocols. Both trials showed the benefit of alteplase in at least some outcome parameters. In the NINDS alteplase study, patients were enrolled within 3 hours of symptom onset using strict inclusion and exclusion criteria. When enrolled, patients received either alteplase 0.9 mg/kg (maximal dose, 90 mg), with 10% of the dose given as a bolus for 1 minute and the remainder infused for 60 minutes, or placebo. In this study, there were no differences at 24 hours in responses between the placebo group and those who received alteplase. However, at 3 months, patients who received alteplase were 30% more likely to have minimal or no disability. There was an 11% to 13% absolute increase in the number of patients with excellent outcomes and a corresponding decrease in the number of patients with severe neurologic

Table 61-5
Management Guideline for Blood Pressure Treatment in Acute Ischemic Stroke

Treatment	Received Alteplase	Did Not Receive Alteplase
No treatment recommended	If BP is <185/110 mm Hg	If BP <220/120 mm Hg unless there is another specific medical condition
Nicardipine 5 mg/hour, titrate up by 2.5 mg/hour every 5–15 minutes (maximum 15 mg/hour) Labetalol 10–20 mg IV over 1–2 minutes, may repeat to maximum of 300 mg total, or Labetalol 10 mg IV followed by continuous infusion 2–8 mg/minute	If BP >185/110 mm Hg Goal is to lower below 185/105 mm Hg to limit risk of ICH	If systolic BP >220 mm Hg or diastolic 120–140 mm Hg
IV sodium nitroprusside 0.5 mcg/kg/minute	If BP not controlled by above or if diastolic BP is >140 mm Hg	If not controlled or if diastolic BP >140 mm Hg

Source: Jauch EC et al. Guidelines for the early management of patients with acute ischemic stroke: a guideline for healthcare professionals from the American Heart Association/American Stroke Association. *Stroke.* 2013; 44:870–947.

Table 61-6
Criteria for Alteplase Use in Treatment of Acute Stroke

Inclusion Criteria	Exclusion Criteria
18 years of age or older Clinical diagnosis of stroke with clinically meaningful neurologic deficit Clearly defined onset within 180 minutes before treatment Baseline CT with no evidence of intracranial hemorrhage	CT signs of intracranial hemorrhage, or multilobar infarction, or symptoms of subarachnoid hemorrhage Active internal bleeding History of intracranial hemorrhage Stroke or serious head injury within 3 months Current use of direct thrombin inhibitors or direct factor Xa inhibitors with elevated sensitive laboratory test Systolic BP >185 mm Hg, diastolic BP >110 mm Hg Current use of anticoagulant with INR >1.7 Current use if direct thrombin inhibitors with elevated sensitive laboratory tests (such as aPTT, INR, ECT, TT, and factor Xa activity assay) Heparin received in last 48 hours resulting in abnormal elevated aPTT Glucose <50 or 400 mg/dL Symptoms of subarachnoid hemorrhage Platelet count <100,000/mm³ Relative exclusion criteria Only minor or rapidly improving stroke symptoms Pregnancy Seizure at onset with postictal residual neurologic impairments Major surgery or serious trauma within 2 weeks GI or urinary tract hemorrhage within 3 weeks
	Additional Relative Exclusion Criteria for Alteplase Use 3–4.5 hours after Onset of Symptoms
	Age >80 years NIHSS score >25 Taking an oral anticoagulant regardless of INR History of both diabetes and prior ischemic stroke

BP, blood pressure; CT, computed tomography; GI, gastrointestinal; NIHSS, National Institutes of Health Stroke Scale; ECT, ecarin clotting time; aPTT activated partial thromboplastin time; TT, thrombin time.

impairment or death at 3 months. Intracranial hemorrhage occurred more frequently among patients receiving alteplase (6.4%) than in patients receiving placebo (0.6%). Despite the increased incidence of intracranial hemorrhage, outcomes remained better for patients receiving alteplase. For the ECASS I trial, patients were enrolled within 6 hours of the onset of symptoms.[62] The treatment protocol consisted of intravenous alteplase 1.1 mg/kg (maximal, 100 mg) or placebo. There was no difference in the primary outcome measures of functionality at 3 months. However, with target population analysis, there was a significant difference favoring alteplase. Of alteplase-treated patients, 41% had minimal or no disability compared with 29% of placebo-treated patients. A variety of secondary outcome measures favored alteplase. There was no difference in 30-day mortality rates, but 19.8% of alteplase-treated patients had major parenchymal hemorrhages compared with 6.5% of placebo-treated patients.

Since NINDS and ECASS-I, three subsequent trials, the ECASS-II and Alteplase Thrombolysis for Acute Non-Interventional Therapy in Ischemic stroke (ATLANTIS A and B) found largely same effects as NINDS when therapy was initiated in the

≤3-hour time period. The ECASS-II study used an alteplase dose of 0.9 mg/kg and replicated the NINDS trial[64]; however, patients were enrolled up to 6 hours after the onset of stroke symptoms. This study found no difference between alteplase and placebo. Too few patients were enrolled with stroke symptoms within 3 hours to reliably evaluate the influence of this variable on outcome.

Since NINDS, several trials have also investigated the use of intravenous alteplase up to 6 hours after stroke onset. ECASS-I, ECASS-II, ATLANTIS A and B, all enrolled patients with extended window use of alteplase. None of these trials found individually a benefit; however, a pooled analysis suggested improved outcomes.[65] Hence, the ECASS-III study was conducted to evaluate the efficacy and safety of alteplase administered used the NINDS alteplase dose (0.9mg/kg maximum of 90mg), but it focused on the efficacy and safety of alteplase administered 3 to 4.5 hours after the onset of symptoms.[66] A significantly greater number of patients receiving alteplase had favorable outcomes on the mRS global disability scale compared with placebo (odds ratio, 1.34; 95% confidence interval, 1.02–1.76). Although the rate of intracranial hemorrhage was greater with alteplase, mortality and reports of adverse events were similar between the two groups. When considering the use of alteplase in the 3- to 4.5-hour window, the ECASS-III criteria should be followed (Table 61-6). A second large randomized placebo-controlled trial was recently published. In this third International Stroke Trial (IST-3), following NINDS dosing scheme for alteplase, patients enrolled with 6 hours of symptoms onset, there was a significant improvement in functional outcome in the Oxford Handicap score (0 to 2, alive and independent) (OR 1.27; 95% confidence interval 1.10–1.47). There were more deaths at 7 days in the alteplase group though. ITS-3 included patients >80 years of age in comparison to ECASS-III and a broader blood pressure eligibility.[67] Because P.C. presented to the ED within 3 hours of the onset of his stroke symptoms, he is a candidate for alteplase therapy in accordance with the NINDS study protocol making sure the patient has no exclusion criteria based on Table 61-6.

CASE 61-2, QUESTION 4: What general treatment interventions should be made for P.C.?

In addition to the general supportive therapy needed for a hospitalized patient, several issues are important to the proper management of a stroke patient.

Assessing vital signs and ensuring stabilization of airway, breathing and circulation is the initial part of the evaluation. Intubation and mechanical ventilation may be required to ensure adequate ventilation and to protect the airways from aspiration. Careful attention should be given to fluid and electrolyte control. Excessive hydration or inadequate sodium supplementation may result in hyponatremia, potentially causing cerebral edema. This can result in compression and displacement of brain tissue which can disrupt cerebral perfusion. In addition, hyponatremia can produce seizures, which increases the metabolic demand on compromised neurons. Thus, 0.9% saline or lactated Ringer's are the preferred fluids in patients at risk for cerebral edema.[53]

Attention to body temperature needs to be given. Studies have shown that even small increases in temperature are associated with worse outcomes after acute stroke.[68,69] Hypothermia is neuroprotective, and a reduction in body temperature of 0.26°F can be beneficial in stroke patients.[53,70] Use of antipyretics, such as acetaminophen, are advised to maintain normal or slightly subnormal body temperatures.

Another metabolic parameter that must be followed carefully is the serum glucose concentration, because hyperglycemia may adversely affect ischemic infarction outcomes. A review of multiple studies on the effects of hyperglycemia in acute stroke concluded that hyperglycemia results in poor outcomes and increased mortality.[71] If hyperglycemia is detected, appropriate insulin therapy should be initiated to keep the serum glucose concentration less than 140 mg/dL without causing hypoglycemia.[53]

Caution should be exercised in the acute management of P.C.'s blood pressure. Decreasing the blood pressure too rapidly will compromise cerebral blood flow and expand the region of ischemia and infarction, whereas hypertension may place him at a greater risk for cerebral hemorrhage, especially if a thrombolytic agent is used. However, a study comparing treated and untreated patients who were hypertensive in association with an acute stroke failed to demonstrate any difference in outcomes between the groups.[72]

For patients with a systolic blood pressure greater than 185 mm Hg or diastolic blood pressure greater than 110 mm Hg, who are otherwise candidates for intravenous fibrinolytic treatment, labetalol, nitroglycerin paste, or intravenous nicardipine should be used to reduce the blood pressure to these goals before starting alteplase.[53] A reasonable goal is to lower blood pressure by 15% during the first 24-hours after onset of stroke. After administration of alteplase, a systolic blood pressure should be kept less than 180/105 mm Hg to limit the risk of intracranial hemorrhage. Specific blood pressure management recommendations are outlined for the management of acute ischemic stroke patients (Table 61-5). In other patients, the only consensus on blood pressure control is that treatment is required when pressures exceed 220/120 mm Hg. If there is a clinical deterioration of neurologic function associated with the reduction of blood pressure, the infusion rate of the antihypertensive agent should be slowed or the drug discontinued. After the first 24 hours of stroke onset, maintenance antihypertensive therapy can then be initiated using an oral agent, such as a thiazide diuretics, calcium-channel antagonist or ACEI or ARB. The reader is referred to more detailed discussion of hypertension management in Chapter 9.

The general daily needs of the patient should be assessed and provided on an as-needed basis. These include nutrition, urination, defecation, delirium, and prevention of deep venous thrombosis, and decubitus ulcers. Neurologic deficits will compromise the ability of many patients to adequately meet these needs, increasing the necessity for medical assistance.

CASE 61-2, QUESTION 5: Should anticoagulation or antiplatelet agents be used acutely in P.C.?

Several studies have evaluated the use of anticoagulants in the treatment of acute strokes. However, most of these studies are poorly designed or underpowered to determine the efficacy of these agents.

HEPARIN AND HEPARINOIDS

Three studies have evaluated the use of heparin in acute stroke.[73–75] In one double-blind study, heparin doses were adjusted to maintain the partial thromboplastin time (aPTT) at 1.5 to 2 times control and continued for 7 days.[73] There were no significant differences in death at 7 days, no differences in functional ability 1 year after the stroke, and a greater mortality rate at 1 year for heparin-treated patients. Another study compared aspirin, subcutaneous heparin (5,000 international units or 12,500 international units BID), both, and neither treatments for patients with acute ischemic stroke.[74] There was no reduction of mortality or morbidity for patients receiving either dose of heparin. Heparin use has also been studied in progressing stroke (stroke with evolving neurologic symptoms), and no benefit was demonstrated with its use.[75] No studies have demonstrated that heparin is useful in mitigating the neurologic effects of a stroke.

Low-molecular-weight heparins (LMWHs) and heparinoids have been evaluated in several studies for acute stroke. Two doses of nadroparin were compared with placebo in one randomized, double-blind, placebo-controlled trial.[76] There were no differences in death rates or functional ability at 3 months among the three treatment arms. However, at 6 months, patients receiving high-dose nadroparin (i.e., 4,100 anti-Xa international units BID) had improved function. A large randomized, placebo-controlled trial of dose-adjusted danaparoid, a low-molecular-weight heparinoid, did not demonstrate improvement in danaparoid-treated patients.[77] In addition, no improvements were observed in studies of dalteparin and certoparin.[78,79] Similar to heparin, LMWHs and heparinoids are not indicated in the acute treatment of stroke.

Deep vein thrombosis and pulmonary embolism are common complications in patients following a stroke. Intermittent Compression Devices such as Venodynes, which prevent pooling of blood in the lower extremities, should be applied within 24 hours of admission to the hospital unless contraindicated. The incidences of deep vein thrombosis and pulmonary embolism were reduced in most studies in which patients received heparin, LMWHs, or heparinoids.[80]

Unfractionated heparin 5,000 units subcutaneously twice daily or three times daily can be initiated in P.C. for deep venous thrombosis prophylaxis after 24 hours of thrombolytic administration once a repeat head CT ruled out ICH. Heparin is considered a cheap and effective option compared to LMWHs.

ANTIPLATELETS

Aspirin

One study evaluated early administration of aspirin in acute stroke. The Chinese Acute Stroke Trial compared 160 mg/day of aspirin administered within 48 hours of the onset of stroke symptoms with placebo.[81] Patients who received aspirin had reduced early mortality rates, but there was no difference in the primary endpoint of death or dependency at discharge from the hospital. Two other studies did not demonstrate benefit with aspirin.[63,74] When data from these studies are combined, a slight beneficial effect of aspirin is seen with regard to reducing the risk of early stroke recurrence. Current recommendations are for aspirin 325 mg to be administered within 24 to 48 hours of the onset of stroke symptoms, except when alteplase is administered. When alteplase is given aspirin should be given 24 to 48 hours after alteplase administration but still within 48 to 72 hours of onset of stroke symptoms.[53] In our patient, P.C., alteplase was used, aspirin should not be given until 24 to 48 hours after the end of the alteplase infusion and once a repeat 24 hour head CT ruled ICH.

There has been limited published evidence available for the usage of other antiplatelets such as clopidogrel or dipyridamole in the acute treatment of ischemic stroke. Small pilot studies suggested some utility to these antiplatelets without providing solid evidence of a clear benefit of the well-established aspirin in acute ischemic stroke treatment. In the clopidogrel with aspirin in acute minor stroke or TIA (CHANCE), the investigators randomized in a double-blind, placebo-controlled study 5,170 patients within 24 hours after the onset of symptoms of a minor stroke or TIA to an initial loading dose of 300 mg clopidogrel followed by 75 mg/day for 90 days with aspirin at a dose of 75 mg/day for the for the 21 days, or to placebo plus aspirin 75 mg for 90 days. This study conducted in China found that the combination was superior to aspirin in reducing the risk of stroke in the first 90 days. The patients' selection did not include major stroke or patients who received thrombolytics.[82] Given that our patient received thrombolytic, aspirin is the preferred option.

Glycoprotein IIb/IIIa Inhibitors

Platelet glycoprotein IIb/IIIa inhibitors have also been studied in acute stroke. A placebo-controlled phase II trial of abciximab given within 24 hours of acute stroke showed a trend toward improved functionality in abciximab-treated patients, but the study was not powered to show the significance for this outcome.[83]

In another placebo-controlled, phase II study of patients with acute stroke, the direct thrombin inhibitor, argatroban, was associated with statistically significant improvements in neurologic symptoms and daily living activities.[84] The number of patients enrolled in this study was small, but the results show promise. Currently, the use of these agents is limited to clinical trials.

ENDOVASCULAR INTERVENTIONS

CASE 61-2, QUESTION 6: What other non-pharmacological interventions might be also considered for the acute treatment of stroke in P.C.?

A number of endovascular treatment options for ischemic stroke are available and include intra-arterial fibrinolytics, mechanical thrombectomy with coil retrievers such as the Mechanical Clot Retrieval System (Merci) or stent retrievers such as Solitaire FR and Trevo, combination intra-arterial thrombolytics with mechanical thrombectomy, mechanical clot aspiration with the Penumbra system, and acute angioplasty and stenting.[53]

Intra-arterial thrombolytics administration requires an experienced stroke center and careful selection to identify patients who would benefit. As with intravenous fibrinolytics, intra-arterial thrombolytics should be administered within 6 hours of onset of symptoms, in patients with occlusions of the middle cerebral artery who are not a candidates for intravenous alteplase. Urokinase is the only fibrinolytic with randomized trials that has been shown to be effective in clot lysis, resulting in recanalization and restoration of blood flow.[85,86] While intra-arterial thrombolytics can be considered when intravenous fibrinolytics is predicted to fail (large vessel occlusion) or is contraindicated, these therapies, if available to be administered by a skillful interventional neuroradiologist, should be considered. Lack of identification of optimal dose and evidence of effectiveness in occlusions outside of the middle cerebral artery limit the widespread use of intra-arterial thrombolytics.[53] Mechanical removal of the clot has been evaluated alone or in combination with pharmacological fibrinolysis. Four devices are currently available: MERCI, Penumbra, Solitaire FR, and Trevo. The most current guidelines recommend using the stent retrievers (Solitaire or Trevo) over coil retrievers, such as Merci.

The most recent evidence with these devices is promising. In patients with stroke secondary to occlusions in the proximal anterior intracranial circulation, patients who underwent thrombectomy using a stent retriever device (Solitaire) after receiving intravenous alteplase reduced significantly the 90 days disability without increasing risk of ICH or mortality compared to intravenous alteplase monotherapy.[87] Similar results were also found in four other trials comparing endovascular therapy with intravenous thrombolytics to standard therapy with intravenous thrombolytics alone for documented large occlusions in the proximal anterior circulation. Intra-arterial thrombectomy reduced disability and improved outcomes.[88–91] These trials compared to earlier trials required angiographic confirmation by CT of an intracranial occlusion for eligibility, while earlier trials that did not require such confirmation or used older devices (Merci and Penumbra) did not find such benefit.[92–95]

Stroke Education

CASE 61-2, QUESTION 7: What information and instruction should be given to P.C. regarding future stroke symptoms?

Early treatment of acute stroke with available or investigational drugs appears to be the most important factor in determining optimal outcome. Nearly every clinical trial demonstrating some benefit of pharmacotherapy for acute stroke has shown the greatest effect for patients who are treated within a few hours of the onset of stroke symptoms. Immediate detection of stroke symptoms and initiation of treatment are imperative. The primary rate-limiting step in diagnosis and provision of medical care is recognition by the patient of stroke symptoms. Every patient who is at increased risk of stroke should be carefully instructed to seek emergent medical attention if they experience any weakness or paralysis, speech impairment, numbness, blurred vision or sudden loss of vision, or altered level of consciousness. These symptoms should be handled with the same urgency as the symptoms of a myocardial infarction. The pharmacist should ensure that P.C. and his caregivers know the symptoms of stroke and understand what to do if they occur.

Complications

CASE 61-2, QUESTION 8: What complications associated with stroke might P.C. experience?

Agitation, delirium, stupor, coma, cerebral edema, and increased intracranial pressure are other acute symptoms that can be associated with ischemic stroke. These symptoms correlate with the specific blood vessels that are affected, and the development of these complications in P.C. would depend on the progression of his stroke.

Seizures may occur in up to 20% of stroke patients. Pneumonia, pulmonary edema, cardiac arrest, deep vein thrombosis, and arrhythmias are commonly associated with ischemic stroke and should be managed as they occur. In P.C., these may occur soon after his stroke or be related to a rapidly developing neurologic event such as further infarction, hemorrhage, or severe cerebral edema. Pneumonia or deep venous thromboses are related primarily to inactivity, and the risk of these events will increase the longer P.C. remains immobile.

Stroke patients frequently experience psychologic reactions. The most common psychiatric complication is depression, occurring in 30% to 50% of patients.[96]

The severity of depression varies from mild to major depressive episodes. If the depression interferes with recovery and the rehabilitative process, it should be managed with the use of a selective serotonin reuptake inhibitor or other appropriate agent. Severe psychomotor depression may respond to CNS stimulants, such as methylphenidate or dextroamphetamine. Because of P.C.'s hypertension, stimulants should be used only with careful blood pressure monitoring.

Prognosis

CASE 61-2, QUESTION 9: After 4 days in the hospital, P.C.'s neurologic status is stabilized. Will further neurologic improvements be realized?

Neurologic deficits in stroke patients are not considered stable or fixed until at least 8 to 12 months have elapsed. During this time, neurologic function may return but rarely to normal. The prognosis after ischemic stroke depends on a variety of factors including age, hypertension, coma, cardiopulmonary complications, hypoxia, and neurogenic hyperventilation. However, infarction of the middle cerebral artery is associated with a poor chance for recovery. Recently, physical and occupational therapy techniques involving restriction of activity in the unaffected limb or limbs have proven to be effective in patients regaining lost function. Therefore, it is possible that P.C. will experience further neurologic improvement.

SECONDARY PREVENTION AFTER ISCHEMIC STROKE OR TIA

CASE 61-2, QUESTION 10: What antiplatelet or anticoagulation therapy would be recommended for secondary stroke prevention for P.C.?

Antiplatelet Therapy for Secondary Prevention

Because platelets play a key role in the formation of atheromatous clots, various antiplatelet drugs, such as aspirin, combination aspirin/dipyridamole, ticlopidine, clopidogrel, and cilostazol, have been studied for secondary prevention. Cilostazol is the only agent not approved by the Food and Drug Administration (FDA) for secondary prevention of ischemic strokes and TIAs arising from non-cardioembolic origin. These agents generally work by either preventing the formation of TXA_2 or increasing the concentration of prostacyclin. These actions seek to reestablish the proper balance between these two substances, thus preventing the adhesion and aggregation of platelets (Table 61-4). Around 22% relative risk reduction of stroke, myocardial infarction, or death is noted with these agents compared to placebo in patients with prior TIA or stroke.[97] Based on the current guidelines for non-cardioembolic ischemic stroke and TIAs secondary prevention, aspirin, clopidogrel, or combination aspirin/dypiridamole extended release are considered first-line therapy.[5]

ASPIRIN

The effectiveness of aspirin for secondary prevention of non-cardioembolic ischemic stroke and TIA is supported by evidence of high quality. At least 15 randomized trials, with 7 being placebo-controlled, have studied aspirin alone or in combination with other antiplatelet drugs in the prevention of vascular events.[45,98–102]

Patients were enrolled in these studies for as long as 5 years after experiencing a vascular event (i.e., TIA, stroke, unstable angina, or myocardial infarction). Follow-up periods lasted from 1 to 6 years. The incidence of ischemic stroke or TIA ranged from 7% to 23%: the aspirin-treated patients experienced an average 22% decrease in relative risk of a stroke compared with those receiving placebo. In 10 trials that considered only TIA or stroke patients, there was a 24% relative risk reduction in the incidence of nonfatal stroke associated with the use of aspirin. The risk reduction rate is equal for men and women.[98,103]

Dosages of aspirin used in clinical trials have ranged from 30 to 1,500 mg/day. In a meta-analysis of placebo-controlled studies comparing 900 to 1,500 mg/day of aspirin with similar studies of 300 to 325 mg/day, there was a 23% reduction in the risk of cerebrovascular events for patients receiving 900 to 1,500 mg/day and a 24% reduction in risk for patients receiving 300 to 325 mg/day.[97] A prospective comparison of aspirin doses in 3,131 patients showed a 14.7% frequency of nonfatal stroke or nonfatal myocardial infarction in patients receiving 30 mg of aspirin a day and a 15.2% frequency in patients receiving 283 mg of aspirin a day, a nonsignificant difference between these two doses.[104] The Swedish Aspirin Low-Dose Trial showed an 18% reduction in stroke in patients taking 75 mg of aspirin daily compared with placebo.[105] Helgason et al. compared the effects of 325, 650, 975, and 1,300 mg of aspirin a day in stroke patients.[106] Platelet aggregation studies were performed to determine the effects of aspirin. Eighty percent of patients had complete suppression of aggregation at a daily dose of 325 mg, an additional 5% responded at 650 mg/day, only 1% more responded at 975 mg/day, and there was no further response at 1,300 mg. As aspirin doses increase, so does the risk of gastrointestinal (GI) bleeding.[107]

The recommended dose for aspirin is 50 to 325 mg/day. The goal is to use the lowest effective aspirin dosage, thereby limiting the risk of GI adverse effects. In the United States, a dose of 81 mg enteric-coated aspirin is usually started.

TICLOPIDINE

Ticlopidine is an antiplatelet agent approved only for the prevention of TIA and stroke for patients with a prior cerebral thrombotic event. By inhibiting ADP-induced platelet aggregation, its activity differs from that of aspirin. While effective in reducing risk of stroke, its use is limited by serious hematological and GI adverse effects.[108,109]

CLOPIDOGREL

Clopidogrel is chemically related to ticlopidine and works by inhibiting platelet aggregation induced by ADP. A randomized, double-blind, international trial (Clopidogrel vs. Aspirin in Patients at Risk of Ischaemic Events [CAPRIE]) compared clopidogrel 75 mg/day with aspirin 325 mg/day.[110] Patients enrolled in the study had a history of atherosclerotic vascular disease manifested by recent ischemic stroke, myocardial infarction, or symptomatic peripheral vascular disease. Using intention-to-treat analysis, a 5.3% risk of an event in patients receiving clopidogrel and a 5.83% risk in patients receiving aspirin were observed. This represents a statistically significant relative risk reduction of 8.7%, favoring clopidogrel. On-treatment analysis showed a relative risk reduction of 9.4%, again in favor of clopidogrel. For patients whose primary condition for entry into CAPRIE was stroke, the relative risk reduction was 7.3%; however, this difference was not statistically significant. Patients receiving clopidogrel more frequently experienced rash and diarrhea compared with those receiving aspirin. Patients receiving aspirin were more frequently affected by upper GI distress, intracranial hemorrhage, and GI hemorrhage. Significant reductions in neutrophils occurred in 0.10% of patients on clopidogrel and in 0.17% of patients on aspirin. Some cases of thrombocytopenia purpura are reported in the literature.[111]

Clopidogrel is as effective and safe as aspirin. Clopidogrel is an alternative to aspirin in secondary prevention of stroke.[5] Polymorphisms in the hepatic enzymes involved in the metabolism and activation of clopidogrel (CYP 1A2, CYP3A4, CYP2C19) or within the platelet $P2Y_{12}$ receptor may affect clopidogrel's antiplatelet therapy. Similarly, drug interactions affecting the CYP2C19 P450 cytochrome can lead to decreased effectiveness of clopidogrel. Commonly prescribed proton pump inhibitors, such as omperazole, have been suggested to decrease efficacy of clopidogrel. It is suggested to avoid the combination of omeprazole and clopidogrel until more solid evidence is available.[5]

ASPIRIN/DIPYRIDAMOLE

Dipyridamole inhibits phosphodiesterase and augments prostacyclin-related platelet aggregation inhibition. Four large randomized clinical trials have evaluated the secondary prevention effect of aspirin and dipyridamole combination among patients with stroke or TIAs. Two European studies have shown benefit with a combination of aspirin and dipyridamole. In the first study, a combination of aspirin 325 mg/day and immediate release 75 mg dipyridamole three times/day was compared with placebo.[112] Results from this study showed that the combination reduced the combined risk of stroke and death by 33% and the risk of stroke by 38%. The Second European Stroke Prevention Study enrolled patients who had experienced a previous stroke or TIA and found that aspirin combined with dipyridamole was more effective than placebo, dipyridamole alone, and aspirin alone.[113]

A sustained-release formulation of dipyridamole was used for this study. A 37% relative risk reduction was found for the combination treatment, and a 23% relative risk reduction was found for aspirin alone. The dipyridamole dose for this study was 200 mg twice a day (BID), and the aspirin dose was 25 mg BID. Absolute risk reduction was approximately 1.5% annually. Headache occurred more frequently in patients receiving dipyridamole alone or in combination with aspirin. Bleeding complications were less frequent in patients receiving dipyridamole compared with aspirin alone. As a result of these findings, a combination product of aspirin and dipyridamole is available. The combination of sustained-release dipyridamole and aspirin is an acceptable alternative for secondary prevention of stroke when initial secondary prevention has failed.

In the 2006 open label European/Australian Stroke Prevention in Reversible Ischemia Trial (ESPRIT), with a mean follow-up of 3.5 years, the combination aspirin/dipyridamole was associated with an absolute risk reduction of 1%/year for the composite primary outcome of vascular mortality, nonfatal stroke, nonfatal MI, or major bleeding (13% vs. 16%) Bleeding rates were similar between the two groups. Combination aspirin/dipyridamole was discontinued secondary to headaches in 8.8% of patients. Of note, the aspirin dose ranged from 30 to 325 mg, and 83% of the patients took the extended release formulation of dipyridamole.[114]

Clopidogrel was compared with the combination aspirin and extended release dipyridamole in the non-inferiority Prevention Regimen for Effectively Avoiding Second Strokes trial.[115] Among the patients with non-cardioembolic ischemic stroke who were followed for a mean of 2.5 years, there was no difference in stroke rates between the two intervention arms. The risk of gastrointestinal hemorrhage was higher in the aspirin plus extended dipyridamole group compared to clopidogrel (4.1% vs. 3.6%). Clopidogrel was better tolerated with less bleeding and less headaches than the combination.

CILOSTAZOL

Cilostazol is a vasodilator and antiplatelet agent. It has action on intracellular cyclic AMP and is a phosphodiesterase-3 inhibitor that is used mainly for intermittent claudication in patients with peripheral artery disease.[116] In Asian studies, cilostazol 100 mg twice daily was found to equally reduce risk of vascular events compared to aspirin in non-cardioembolic stroke. However, headache, diarrhea, palpitations, dizziness, and tachycardia were more frequent with cilostazol than aspirin, leading to more discontinuation in therapy (20% vs. 12%).[117,118] Given the ventricular tachycardia risk associated with cilostazol, it is contraindicated in patients with heart failure.[116]

WARFARIN AND ORAL ANTICOAGULANTS

Large randomized trials have compared oral anticoagulants with aspirin in the secondary prevention of stroke and TIA. In one study, aspirin 30 mg/day was compared with oral anticoagulants in doses adjusted to maintain an INR between 3.0 and 4.5.[119] This study was terminated early when the mortality rate attributable to major bleeding events in the anticoagulant group was double the rate in the aspirin group. In this study, there was no difference between anticoagulants and aspirin in the frequency of stroke. A second study compared warfarin, dosed to maintain the INR between 1.4 and 2.8, and aspirin 325 mg/day.[120]

Results from this study did not demonstrate a significant difference between aspirin and warfarin with regard to the prevention of stroke or major hemorrhagic events. However, minor hemorrhages were significantly more frequent among patients receiving warfarin. A third study was terminated early because of safety concerns in the warfarin arm of the study.[121] The target INR for this study was 2 to 3 in the warfarin arm compared with aspirin. The study was stopped owing to significantly higher rates of adverse events in individuals receiving warfarin and no difference in the risk of stroke. Events including major hemorrhage, myocardial infarction, or sudden death, and overall death were increased in those receiving warfarin. Warfarin is not generally recommended for secondary prevention of non-cardioembolic stroke. In secondary prevention of cardioembolic stroke originating from atrial fibrillation, warfarin or the newer oral anticoagulants are preferred first-line therapy.[47]

ASPIRIN COMBINED WITH CLOPIDOGREL

A major study has compared clopidogrel 75 mg/day with the combination of clopidogrel 75 mg/day and aspirin 75 mg/day.[122] There was no difference in the risk of recurrent stroke or other cardiovascular outcomes between the groups, but the combination therapy group had a significant increase in life-threatening bleeding. Some individuals may be resistant to aspirin's effects on platelets.[123] Although poorly understood and studied, aspirin resistance may be related to the presence of extra platelet sources of TXA_2 and an interaction with over-the-counter nonsteroidal anti-inflammatory drugs or high levels of circulating 11-dehydro-thromboxane B_2. Cyclooxygenase-2 expression is induced during human megakaryopoiesis and characterizes newly formed platelets.[124–126] There are no data to suggest that increasing the aspirin dose will overcome possible resistance to the antiplatelet effects of aspirin, but it is clear that an increased dose of aspirin increases the risk of major bleeding.

Surgical Interventions for Secondary Prevention

Carotid endarterectomy and carotid artery stenting are available to prevent ischemic stroke or TIAs. These are designed to either remove the source for an embolism or improve circulation to ischemic areas of the brain.

CAROTID ENDARTERECTOMY

Carotid endarterectomy (CEA) is a common surgical procedure for correcting atheromatous lesions responsible for causing a TIA or ischemic stroke. In this procedure, the carotid artery is surgically exposed, and the atheromatous plaque is excised. CEA combined with pharmacotherapy is considered first-line option for patients with a high-grade (>70% angiographic stenosis) atherosclerotic carotid stenosis.[5] Other patients do not benefit as much from such procedure, and the benefit does not outweigh the risk of such procedure. CEA is most effective for patients with an ulcerated lesion or stenotic clot that occludes greater than 70% of blood flow in the ipsilateral carotid artery and who experience symptoms of a TIA or stroke. Use of CEA in these patients may result in a 60% reduction in stroke risk during the subsequent 2 years.[127] Of six to eight patients treated with CEA, one stroke will be prevented within 2 years.[128] The use of CEA in other patient groups must be balanced with the risk of the procedure and life expectancy.[129] CEA is beneficial in patients with 50% to 69% stenosis of the carotid artery.[5] Surgery should be done within 2 weeks of a TIA or stroke. Generally, CEA is not indicated in patients who have permanent neurologic deficits or total occlusion of the carotid artery. CEA should be done by a surgeon with less than 6% morbidity and mortality rates.

Aspirin also has been used for prevention of restenosis after CEA. During the first year after CEA, 25% of patients will redevelop a stenotic lesion, with more than half of these causing a greater than 50% reduction in carotid blood flow.[103]

Stent placement is useful in preventing restenosis. Initial studies indicated that combination therapy with aspirin 325 mg/day and dipyridamole 75 mg three times a day would decrease the rate of restenosis. However, a subsequent randomized, placebo-controlled study using this regimen in post-CEA patients did not substantiate the earlier findings.[130] A combination of clopidogrel with aspirin has been shown to reduce postoperative ischemic events.[131]

Carotid Artery Angioplasty and Stenting

As an alternative to CEA, balloon angioplasty and placement of stents can also improve blood flow through a stenosed artery. This is a less invasive procedure associated with less patient discomfort and a shorter recovery time. During this procedure, a catheter with a small, deflated balloon is placed in the stenosed artery, and the atherosclerotic lesion is pressed into the arterial wall when the balloon is inflated. A small, plastic tube stent is placed in the artery to prevent the vessel from collapsing at the site of the lesion.

Carotid artery angioplasty and stenting (CAS) is another alternative. The initial study of this procedure was halted because of poor outcomes.[132] Subsequently, two studies have shown that CAS is not inferior to CEA, but further study is underway to determine whether CAS is more beneficial than CEA.[133,134] CAS can be used in patients who are not candidates for CEA.

SPONTANEOUS INTRACEREBRAL HEMORRHAGE

Clinical Presentation and Treatment

CASE 61-3

QUESTION 1: S.P. is a 58-year-old man who is sitting at home watching television with his wife when he develops confusion, nausea, severe headache, and right arm weakness. His wife immediately calls for an ambulance and by the time paramedics arrive, S.P. is slumped in his chair and unresponsive. Significant past medical history includes poorly controlled hypertension, atrial fibrillation, and osteoarthritis. He takes lisinopril 10 mg by mouth daily, warfarin 4 mg by mouth daily, and acetaminophen 1,000 mg by mouth three times daily for these conditions. Upon presentation to the ED, his blood pressure is 184/114 mm Hg. A CT scan shows an intracerebral hemorrhage. Key electrolyte concentrations, coagulation studies, and blood counts are within normal limits except for an INR of 4.8 and a blood glucose level of 194 mg/dL.

S.P.'s neurologic symptoms and the appearance of blood on his CT scan are consistent with a diagnosis of intracerebral hemorrhage (ICH).

What risk factors for spontaneous intracerebral hemorrhage does S.P. have?

S.P.'s uncontrolled hypertension and his use of warfarin has increased his risk of ICH.[135] Specifically, use of warfarin increases the risk of ICH by two to five times depending on the degree of anticoagulation.[136,137] Patients, such as S.P., who are taking warfarin before ICH and present with an INR >3 are at greater risk for developing larger hematomas, which are associated with worse outcomes, compared to those taking warfarin and presenting with a lower INR.[138,139] Patients taking oral anticoagulants are also at greater risk of death after ICH versus those not taking anticoagulants.[136] Other drugs that may increase the risk of ICH include target-specific oral anticoagulants, such as dabigatran, rivaroxaban, apixaban, and edoxaban; heparin,

 LMWHs, fondaparinux, and other parenteral anticoagulants; aspirin and other antiplatelet agents; selective serotonin reuptake inhibitors; and sympathomimetics, such as amphetamines, phenylpropanolamine, cocaine, and caffeine-containing medications.[140–144] Additional risk factors for non-traumatic ICH include advanced age, history of stroke, diabetes, smoking, excessive alcohol consumption, African American ethnicity, and low cholesterol levels, especially in the absence of HMG-CoA reductase inhibitor use.[145,146] Genetic predisposition does not play a role in most hemorrhagic strokes except for those caused by AVMs.

CASE 61-3, QUESTION 2: What are the key principles of therapy in patients presenting with spontaneous intracerebral hemorrhage?

Initial management of spontaneous ICH involves (1) preventing hematoma expansion and (2) preventing and managing elevated intracranial pressure.

To minimize hematoma expansion, anticoagulants should be reversed immediately in patients such as S.P., who present with drug-induced coagulopathies, and blood pressure should be carefully managed. Methods for preventing and managing elevated ICP include avoiding hypotonic fluids as well as medical and surgical methods. Ancillary therapies including treatment of fever and avoiding hypoglycemia and hyperglycemia are also suggested.

CASE 61-3, QUESTION 3: What pharmacotherapy should be initiated to reverse S.P.'s anticoagulant-induced coagulopathy?

Up to 20% of patients with ICH present with a drug-induced coagulopathy, like S.P.[147,148] Because hematoma growth within the first 24 hours of ICH is directly associated with worse outcomes and reversal of warfarin-induced coagulopathies within 4 hours of ICH has been shown to limit hematoma expansion, it is important to reverse coagulopathies in a timely manner.[149,150] All anticoagulant and antiplatelet medications should be immediately discontinued, and agents should be administered to remove the anticoagulant medication from the body and reverse its effect.[151] Although S.P. was using warfarin for prevention of ischemic stroke in the setting of atrial fibrillation, because of his acute ICH, the benefit of reversing the warfarin in order to improve neurologic outcome greatly outweighs the short-term risk of ischemic stroke resulting from anticoagulant reversal. If a patient has taken an oral anticoagulant within the last two hours, activated charcoal may be considered to prevent absorption; however, it is important to ensure the patient can tolerate enteral administration. Historically, fresh frozen plasma (FFP) has been used to reverse warfarin-induced coagulopathies in patients such as S.P.; however, prothrombin complex concentrates (PCCs) have recently become the recommended agents to rapidly reverse anticoagulation because of warfarin.[152] FFP contains all the clotting factors depleted by warfarin but can take several hours to thaw and administer and may be associated with pulmonary complications and edema because of the volume required. In contrast, PCCs may reverse the INR within minutes because they can be administered more rapidly. Additionally, PCCs are associated with a lower risk of volume overload and pose a lower risk of infection than FFP. Use of PCCs in this setting has been shown to more effectively limit hematoma expansion compared to FFP, but improvement in clinical outcomes has not been demonstrated to date.[153,154] Three-factor PCCs contain factors II, IX, and X while 4-factor PCCs also includes factor VII. PCC availability may be limited by institutional policies, in part, because of the high cost of treatment relative to other therapeutic options.[155] Because the effect of PCC and FFP is short-lived, patients with warfarin-induced coagulopathy should concomitantly receive 10 mg of IV vitamin K (phytonadione) by slow infusion.[152]

Newer oral anticoagulants indicated for non-valvular atrial fibrillation include dabigatran, rivaroxaban, apixaban, and edoxaban.[156–158] Although data regarding management of ICH patients receiving these agents are limited, some experts suggest using a PCC product. Idarucizumab is a monoclonal antibody that can be used to reverse dabigatran. Agents for reversal of other target-specific anticagulants are under study. Importantly, dabigatran can be removed through hemodialysis. As with warfarin-induced coagulopathies, reversal agents should be administered promptly and activated charcoal should be considered.

Other drug-induced ICHs may occur in patients receiving heparin, LMWHs, the parenteral factor Xa inhibitor fondaparinux, and antiplatelet agents such as aspirin and clopidogrel. Protamine sulfate may be used for the reversal of heparin and LMWH, while fondaparinux activity may be antagonized with PCCs. No intervention has been shown to be clearly beneficial in patients experiencing ICH and taking antiplatelet agents, although studies are ongoing.[151]

To reverse his warfarin-induced coagulopathy, S.P. should receive a weight-based dose of a PCC product and 10 mg IV vitamin K by slow IV infusion.

CASE 61-3, QUESTION 4: How should S.P.'s acute hypertension be managed?

Excessive hypertension may expose patients with ICH to elevated risk of hematoma expansion, neurologic deterioration, and worse outcomes.[159,160] Lower blood pressures have been suggested to potentially worsen prognosis; however, this phenomenon is not as well documented as it is with ischemic stroke.[161,162] Several studies have shown that rapid blood pressure reduction to a SBP of less than 140 mm Hg is safe in patients with ICH presenting with hypertension.[163–166] Additionally, studies suggest that aggressive acute blood pressure control can improve functional outcomes and may be associated with a trend toward a reduction in death.[159,163] It is important to note that patients presenting with SBPs above 220 mm Hg and those with very severe ICHs have not been well represented in studies.

Based on these studies, current guidelines suggest that lowering SBP to less than 140 mm Hg in patients presenting with an SBP 150 to 220 mm Hg and no contraindications to antihypertensive therapy is safe and may improve outcomes. In patients presenting with an SBP >220 mm Hg, it is recommended to initiate aggressive antihypertensive therapy with an IV infusion and to carefully monitor the patient.[151] Nicardipine and labetalol are most commonly used antihypertensive agents in patients with ICH, but hydralazine, nitroprusside, or nitroglycerin may be considered depending on the clinical situation. If labetalol is used to control acute blood pressure, it should be administered as IV boluses, potentially in combination with an IV infusion. Nicardipine is only administered as an IV infusion.

S.P.'s blood pressure exceeds 150 mm Hg, so IV antihypertensive therapy is indicated. It would be appropriate to initiate an IV nicardipine infusion at 5 mg/hour and titrate every 5 minutes to achieve an SBP of less than 140 mm Hg in S.P.

CASE 61-3, QUESTION 5: Hours after admission, S.P.'s mental status worsens, likely because of severely elevated ICPs. What therapy should S.P. receive for his elevated ICP?

Elevated ICP refers to excessive pressure inside the intracranial vault and may occur in patients with severe hemorrhagic and ischemic strokes as well as in those suffering from traumatic brain injury, brain tumors, hydrocephalus, and hepatic encephalopathy. It can lead to brain hypoxemia and cause herniation. S.P.'s worsened mental status may be consistent with elevated ICP. Other symptoms of elevated ICP include headache, vomiting, cranial nerve palsies, and the combination of bradycardia, respiratory depression, and hypertension.

In patients with neurologic emergencies, such as S.P., hypotonic fluids such as dextrose 5% in water should be avoided in favor of isotonic fluids such as 0.9% sodium chloride (normal saline) and Lactated Ringers because hypotonic fluids can exacerbate cerebral edema and worsen ICP.[151] When considering fluids patients are receiving, it is important to evaluate both maintenance fluids patients are getting and the fluids in which IV medications are diluted. In patients with elevated ICPs, IV medications should be diluted in 0.9% sodium chloride rather than dextrose 5% in water or other hypotonic fluids whenever possible.

Treatment of elevated ICP involves patient care measures, pharmacotherapy, and surgical interventions. First, the head of the bed should be elevated to at least 30 degrees once it is clear that S.P. is not hypovolemic in order to minimize blood and fluid accumulation in the brain. Hyperventilation (increasing the patient's respiratory rate and/or the volume of air he breathes with each respiration) with a $PaCO_2$ goal of $<$30 mm Hg may be considered for a very short time in S.P. until other interventions can be implemented. Hyperventilation should not be continued long-term because it can compromise cerebral blood flow.

S.P. should receive aggressive analgesic medications, such as fentanyl and morphine. Sedatives, such as propofol, should also be administered.[151] Hyperosmolar agents, including intravenous mannitol, dosed at 0.25 to 1 g/kg every 4 to 6 hours, or hypertonic sodium chloride may be considered to establish an osmotic gradient that can facilitate the movement of fluid out of the brain, thus reducing ICP.[151,167] Clinicians may place an intracranial pressure monitor or utilize neurologic exams to guide treatment with hyperosmolar agents. If an ICP monitor is used, hyperosmolar therapy would be indicated to maintain an ICP of $<$20 mm Hg while if an ICP monitor is not utilized, a worsening in neurologic exam consistent with elevated ICP would warrant therapy. If S.P. continues to exhibit elevated ICPs after hyperosmolar and aggressive analgesia and sedation, a continuous infusion of a neuromuscular blocking agent should be administered. Last-line measures that may be considered include use of a barbiturate coma.

In patients who develop hydrocephalus because of an ICH or another condition, a ventriculostomy may be employed. A ventriculostomy is a surgically placed drain that resides in the ventricle and is used to drain CSF. Finally, open craniotomy, or removal of a portion of the skull, in the area of edema, may be considered in highly selected situations; however, the efficacy of this approach is questionable in many patients.

CASE 61-3, QUESTION 6: What other ancillary therapies may be appropriate for S.P.?

S.P. may benefit from (1) maintenance of normothermia with acetaminophen if he develops a fever and (2) avoiding hypoglycemia or excessive hyperglycemia.

Although the clinical benefit of antipyretic therapy has not been clearly established in ICH, fever is associated with a worse prognosis.[168] It is recommended that S.P.'s body temperature should be monitored and acetaminophen may be administered to achieve normothermia.[151] Studies evaluating mild hypothermia are ongoing.

Both hypoglycemia and hyperglycemia should be avoided in hemorrhagic stroke. Hypoglycemia can directly lead to neurologic injury while hyperglycemia is associated with worsened neurologic outcome after from stroke. Current guidelines recommend avoiding both hypoglycemia and hyperglycemia but do not suggest a specific blood glucose range.[151] Considering that his blood glucose is markedly elevated, S.P. should be initiated on an insulin regimen in accordance with institutional policies.

Seizures can complicate approximately 16% of all strokes and may be difficult to observe because they are often non-convulsive.[151,169] However, because studies of prophylactic antiepileptic therapy have failed to demonstrate consistent benefit and have sometimes indicated harm,[170] current guidelines do not recommend routine seizure prophylaxis.[151] Antiepileptic therapy should be initiated promptly if a patient develops seizures during or after the development of an ICH.

CASE 61-3, QUESTION 7: What secondary prevention strategies should be recommended for S.P. after he recovers from his ICH?

For S.P. and any patient who has suffered an ICH, key modifiable risk factors that should be addressed upon stabilization include maintaining blood pressure at less than 130/80 mm Hg, smoking cessation, treating sleep apnea, avoiding excessive alcohol use, and abstaining from cocaine and other illicit drugs.[151,169]

REHABILITATION

CASE 61-4

QUESTION 1: Patient J.A. has had a stroke and has received appropriate acute care. He is ready to be discharged from the hospital but still has trouble walking, talking, and performing activities of daily living. For patients who require rehabilitative care after hospital treatment of an ischemic or hemorrhagic stroke, what interventions will aid their recovery?

Patients who have suffered ischemic and hemorrhagic strokes often require long-term rehabilitation after their acute treatment. Rehabilitation is directed at managing daily functions, enhancing existing neurologic function, and attempting to regain lost function. Considerations for daily functions include activities of daily living and bowel and bladder management through balanced pharmacologic interventions. Efforts should be made to allow patients to function independently with activities of daily living and manage the psychologic effects of stroke. Enhancement of current neurologic function and minimizing depression includes elimination of drugs that may compromise patients' memory and mental function. These include benzodiazepines, major tranquilizers, and sedating antiepileptic drugs.

Localized spasticity is a common complication after strokes. Spasticity affecting a single limb frequently responds to regional motor nerve blocks with botulinum toxin. Aggressive physical therapy is also essential to the management of spasticity. Systemic antispasticity agents such as diazepam, baclofen, or dantrolene sodium are not used routinely because of the risk for toxicity. They are used only when spasticity involves multiple parts of the body or is unresponsive to other therapies.

Other less common impediments to patients' recovery after stroke include decubitus ulcers, hypercalcemia, and heterotopic ossification (e.g., the laying down and calcification of a bone matrix in muscle surrounding major joints). Prevention through meticulous skin care is the key to the management of pressure ulcers. Mobilizing patients as soon as possible after stroke can prevent hypercalcemia and heterotopic ossification.

KEY REFERENCES AND WEBSITES

A full list of references for this chapter can be found at http://thepoint.lww.com/AT11e. Below are the key references and websites for this chapter, with the corresponding reference number in this chapter found in parentheses after the reference.

Key References

Easton JD et al. Definition and evaluation of transient ischemic attack. *Stroke*. 2009;40:2276–2293. (2).

Eikelboom J et al. Antiplatelet drugs. Antithrombotic therapy and prevention of thrombosis, 96th ed: American College of Chest Physicians evidence-based clinical practice guidelines. *Chest*. 2012;141(2, Suppl): e89s–e119s. (116).

Hacke W et al. Thrombolysis with alteplase 3 to 4.5 hours after acute ischemic stroke. *N Engl J Med*. 2008;359:1317–1329. (66).

Jauch EC et al. Guidelines for the early management of patients with acute ischemic stroke: a guideline for healthcare professionals from the American Heart Association/American Stroke Association. *Stroke*. 2013;44:870–947. (53).

Kernan WN et al. Guidelines for the prevention of stroke in patients with stroke and transient ischemic attack: a guideline for healthcare professionals from the American Heart Association/American Stroke Association. *Stroke*. 2014;45:2160–2236. (5).

Meschia JF et al. Guidelines for the primary prevention of stroke: a statement for healthcare professionals from the American Heart Association/American Stroke Association. *Stroke*. 2014;45:3754–3832. (4).

Mozaffarian D et al. Heart disease and stroke statistics—2015 update: a report from the American Heart Association. *Circulation*. 2015;131:e29–e322. (1).

Hemphill JC 3rd et al. Guidelines for the Management of Spontaneous Intracerebral Hemorrhage: A Guideline for Healthcare Professionals from the American Heart Association/American Stroke Association. *Stroke*. 2015;46(7):2032–2060. (151).

Key Websites

American Heart Association. http://www.americanheart.org/presenter.jhtml?identifier=4755.

American Stroke Association. http://www.strokeassociation.org/STROKEORG/.

Center for Disease Control and Prevention. http://www.cdc.gov/stroke/.

National Institute of Neurological Disorders and Stroke. http://www.ninds.nih.gov/disorders/stroke/stroke.htm.

Section Editors: Dorothea C. Rudorf, G. Christopher Wood, and Caroline S. Zeind

62 Principles of Infectious Diseases

B. Joseph Guglielmo

CORE PRINCIPLES

	CORE PRINCIPLES	CHAPTER CASES
1	Although acute infection generally is associated with an increased white blood cell count, fever, and localizing signs, these symptoms may be absent in less severe disease. More severe infection, including sepsis, may be associated with hypotension, disseminated intravascular coagulation, and end-organ dysfunction.	**Case 62-1 (Questions 1, 2) Figure 62-1**
2	Other disease states, particularly autoimmune disease and malignancy, may mimic infectious diseases. Although it should be considered a diagnosis of exclusion, drug-induced fever should be ruled out, particularly in patients without other classic signs and symptoms of infection.	**Case 62-1 (Question 3)**
3	Site-specific signs and symptoms and host factors generally predict the most likely pathogens, and empirical antimicrobial therapy should be directed against these organisms. Rapid detection tests improve the efficiency identifying a pathogen; however, they are more costly than traditional methodology.	**Case 62-1 (Questions 4, 5, Tables 62-1, 62-2)**
4	Isolation of an organism may reflect infection; however, colonization and contamination must be ruled out to avoid unnecessary antimicrobial exposure. Once a pathogen is identified, susceptibility tests, particularly disk diffusion or broth dilution, can demonstrate the most active antimicrobial agents.	**Case 62-1 (Questions 6, 7, Tables 62-3 through 62-7)**
5	Once the site of infection is confirmed and the likely pathogens are identified, drug distribution to the site of infection, dosage, route of administration, antimicrobial toxicity, side effects, and costs, must be considered before selection of therapy.	**Case 62-1 (Questions 8–10, Table 62-8)**
6	Antimicrobial dosing should reflect site of infection, route of elimination, and pharmacokinetics and pharmacodynamics.	**Case 62-1 (Questions 11–13, Table 62-9)**
7	Antimicrobial failure may be related to pharmacologic factors (inadequate dosing, insufficient penetration to the site of infection, and inadequate duration) and host factors (presence of prosthetic material, undrained focus of infection, and immune status). Adjunct therapies, including pressors and volume repletion, may improve outcomes in critically ill patients.	**Case 62-1 (Questions 14–17)**

APPROACHING THE PROBLEM

The proper choice, dose, and duration of antimicrobial therapy are based on several factors. Before initiating therapy, it is important first to confirm an infectious versus noninfectious process. Once infection has been documented, the most likely site must be identified, and signs and symptoms (e.g., erythema associated with cellulitis) generally direct the clinician to the likely source. Because certain pathogens are known to be associated with a specific site of infection, empirical therapy often can be directed against these organisms. Additional laboratory tests, including the Gram stain, serologic analysis, and antimicrobial susceptibility testing, generally identify the primary pathogen and active agents. Spectrum of activity, established clinical efficacy, adverse effect profile, pharmacokinetic disposition, and cost considerations ultimately guide the choice of therapy. Once an agent has been selected, the dosage and duration should be based on the size of the patient, site of infection, route of elimination, and other factors.

ESTABLISHING THE PRESENCE OF AN INFECTION

CASE 62-1

QUESTION 1: R.G., a 63-year-old, 70-kg man in the intensive care unit, underwent emergency resection of his large bowel. He has been mechanically ventilated throughout his postoperative course. On day 20 of his hospital stay, R.G. suddenly becomes confused; his blood pressure (BP) drops to 70/30 mm Hg, with a heart rate of 130 beats/minute. His extremities are cold to the touch, and he presents with circumoral pallor. His temperature increases to 40°C (axillary), and his respiratory rate is 24 breaths/minute. Copious amounts of yellow–green secretions are suctioned from his endotracheal tube.

Physical examination reveals sinus tachycardia with no rubs or murmurs. Rhonchi with decreased breath sounds are observed on auscultation. The abdomen is distended, and R.G. complains of new abdominal pain. No bowel sounds can be heard, and the stool is guaiac positive. Urine output from the Foley catheter has been 10 mL/hour for the past 2 hours. Erythema is noted around the central venous catheter.

A chest radiograph demonstrates bilateral lower lobe infiltrates, and urinalysis reveals >50 white blood cells/high-power field (WBC/HPF), few casts, and a specific gravity of 1.015. Blood, endotracheal aspirate, and urine cultures are pending. Other laboratory values include the following:

Sodium (Na), 131 mEq/L (normal, 135–147)
Potassium (K), 4.1 mEq/L (normal, 3.5–5)
Chloride (Cl), 110 mEq/L (normal, 95–105)
CO_2, 16 mEq/L (normal, 20–29 mEq/L)
Blood urea nitrogen (BUN), 58 mg/dL (normal, 8–18)
Serum creatinine (SCr), 3.8 mg/dL (increased from 0.9 mg/dL at admission; normal, 0.6–1.2)
Glucose, 320 mg/dL (normal, 70–110)
Serum albumin, 2.1 g/dL (normal, 4–6)
Hemoglobin (Hgb), 10.3 g/dL (13.5–17.5 g/dL male patients)
Hematocrit (Hct), 33% (normal, 39%–49% [male patients])
WBC count, 15,600/μL (normal, 4,500–10,000/μL) with bands present
Platelets, 40,000/μL (normal, 130,000–400,000)
Prothrombin time (PT), 18 seconds (normal, 10–12)
Erythrocyte sedimentation rate (ESR), 65 mm/hour (normal, 0–20)
Procalcitonin, 1 mcg/L (normal <0.25mcg/L)

Which of R.G.'s signs and symptoms are consistent with infection?

R.G. has numerous signs and symptoms consistent with an infectious process. His WBC count (15,600/μL) is increased, and a "shift to the left" (presence of bands, i.e., immature neutrophils) is observed on the differential. An increased WBC count is commonly observed with infection, particularly with bacterial pathogens. The WBC differential in patients with a bacterial infection often demonstrates a shift to the left owing to the bone marrow response to infection. Although infection is usually associated with an increased WBC, overwhelming sepsis can also be associated with a markedly decreased WBC count. In less acute infection (e.g., uncomplicated urinary tract infection, localized abscess), the WBC count may remain within the normal range because less bone marrow response would be anticipated.

R.G.'s temperature is 40°C by axillary measurement. Fever is a common manifestation of infection, with oral temperatures generally greater than 38°C. Oral and axillary temperatures tend to be approximately 0.4°C lower compared with rectal measurement. As a result, R.G.'s temperature would be expected to be 40.4°C if his temperature had been taken rectally. In general, rectal measurement of temperature is a more reliable determination of fever. Some patients with overwhelming infection, however, may present with hypothermia with temperatures less than 36°C. Furthermore, patients with localized infections (e.g., uncomplicated urinary tract infection, chronic abscesses) may be afebrile.

The bilateral lower lobe infiltrates on R.G.'s chest radiograph, the presence of copious amounts of yellow–green secretions from his endotracheal tube, and the erythema surrounding his central venous catheter is also compatible with one or more infectious processes. Furthermore, R.G. has signs and symptoms consistent with sepsis.

ESTABLISHING THE SEVERITY OF AN INFECTION

CASE 62-1, QUESTION 2: What signs and symptoms manifested by R.G. are consistent with a serious systemic infection?

The term *sepsis*, while a poorly defined syndrome, generally suggests a more systemic infection with the presence of pathogenic microorganisms and/or their toxins in the blood. A uniform system for defining the spectrum of disorders associated with sepsis has been established, but it remains difficult to precisely define.[1]

The pathogenesis of sepsis is complex (Fig. 62-1) and only partially understood.[2,3] Gram-negative aerobes produce endotoxin that results in a cascade of endogenous mediator release, including tumor necrosis factor (TNF), interleukin 1 (IL-1) and interleukin 6 (IL-6), platelet-activating factor (PAF), and various other substances from mononuclear phagocytes and other cells. Although this initial stimulus commonly is associated with gram-negative endotoxin, other substances, including gram-positive exotoxin and fungal cell wall constituents, may also be associated with cytokine release. After release of TNF, IL-1, and PAF, arachidonic acid is metabolized to form leukotrienes, thromboxane A_2, and prostaglandins, particularly prostaglandin E_2 and prostaglandin I_2. IL-1 and IL-6 activate the T cells to produce interferon, IL-2, IL-4, and granulocyte-macrophage colony-stimulating factor (GM-CSF). Increased endothelial permeability ensues. Subsequently, the endothelium releases two hemodynamically active substances: endothelium-derived relaxing factor (EDRF) and endothelin-l. Activation of the complement cascade (fragments C3a and C5a) follows, with additional vascular abnormalities and neutrophil activation. Other potentially important agents in this cascade include adhesion molecules, kinins, thrombin, myocardial depressant substance, endorphins, and heat shock protein. The net result of this cascade involves several hemodynamic, renal, acid–base, and other disorders. Uncontrolled inflammation and coagulation have a particularly important role in this sepsis cascade.[3]

Hemodynamic Changes

Critically ill patients often have central intravenous (IV) lines in place for measuring cardiac output and systemic vascular resistance (SVR). In other words, these lines are placed in the pulmonary artery and allow for more precise measurement of critical hemodynamics. A normal SVR of 800 to 1,200 dyne·s·cm^{-5} may fall to 500 to 600 dyne·s·cm^{-5} in septic shock as a result of extensive vasodilation. In response to vasodilation the heart rate increases leading to increased cardiac output from a normal 4 to 6 L/minute to up to 11 to 12 L/minute in septic patients; stroke volume remains unchanged or decreased. In addition to reflex tachycardia causing a rise in heart rate, stress-induced catecholamine release (norepinephrine, epinephrine) also contributes. The initial increase in cardiac output generally is insufficient to overcome the vasodilatory state, and hypotension ensues. In overwhelming septic shock, myocardial depression may result, resulting

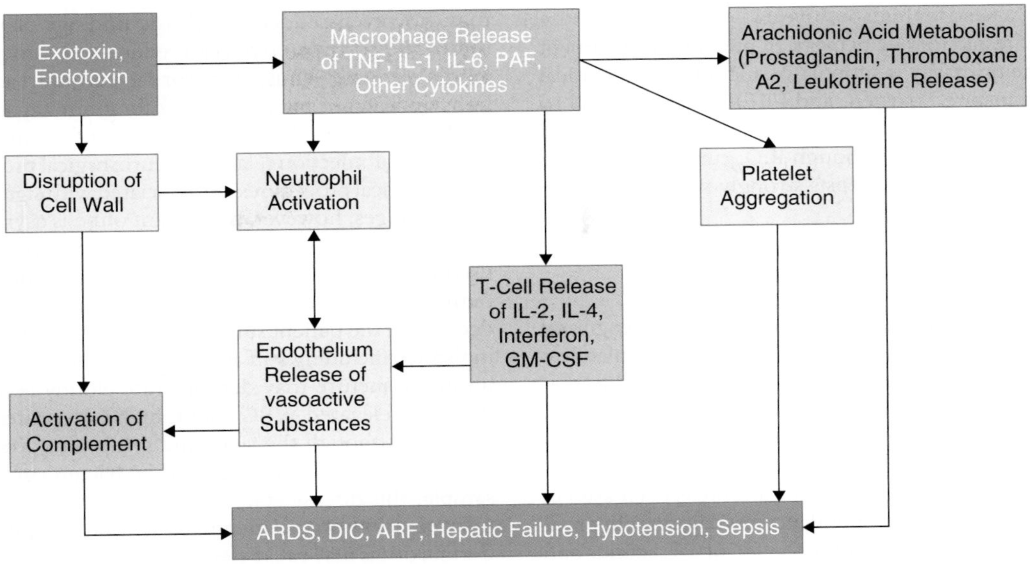

Figure 62-1 The sepsis cascade. ARDS, acute respiratory distress syndrome; ARF, acute renal failure; DIC, disseminated intravascular coagulation; GM-CSF, granulocyte-macrophage colony-stimulating factor; IL-1, interleukin-1; IL-2, interleukin-2; IL-6, interleukin-6; PAF, platelet-activating factor; TNF, tumor necrosis factor.

in a decreased cardiac output. The combination of decreased cardiac output and decreased SVR results in hypotension often unresponsive to pressors and IV fluids. R.G. has hemodynamic evidence of septic shock. He is hypotensive (BP, 70/30 mm Hg) and tachycardic (130 beats/minute), presumably in response to vasodilation and catecholamine release.

Although vasodilation commonly occurs in sepsis, this dilation is unequal and chaotic. Some vascular beds constrict and others dilate, resulting in maldistribution of blood flow. In sepsis, blood generally is shunted away from the kidneys, mesentery, and extremities.

When sepsis has progressed to septic shock, blood flow to most major organs is decreased. Normal urine output of approximately 0.5 to 1.0 mL/kg/hour (30–70 mL/hour for a 70-kg patient) can decrease to less than 20 mL/hour in sepsis. The urine output for R.G. has decreased to 10 mL/hour, consistent with sepsis-induced perfusion abnormalities. Decreased blood flow to the kidney as well as mediator-induced microvascular failure can cause acute-tubular necrosis. R.G.'s uremia (BUN, 58 mg/dL) and increased serum creatinine concentration (3.8 mg/dL) are consistent with decreased renal perfusion secondary to sepsis. Decreased blood flow to the liver may result in "shock liver," in which liver function tests, including alanine aminotransferase (ALT), aspartate aminotransferase (AST), and alkaline phosphatase, become elevated. The liver function tests for R.G. are not available; however, his serum albumin concentration is low (2.1 g/dL) and his PT of 18 seconds is prolonged. Decreased blood flow to the musculature classically is characterized by cool extremities, and decreased blood flow to the brain can result in decreased mentation. R.G. is confused, his extremities are cold, and the area around his mouth appears pale. All these signs and symptoms provide strong evidence that he is in septic shock.

Cellular Changes

The sepsis syndrome is associated with significant abnormalities in cellular metabolism. Glucose intolerance commonly is observed in sepsis, and patients with previously normal blood glucose levels may experience sudden increases in blood sugar. In some cases, a rise in glucose is one of the first signs of an infectious process. R.G.'s increased blood glucose concentration (320 mg/dL) is, therefore, consistent with infection. Other sensitive indicators of sepsis-associated inflammation include the ESR, C-reactive protein, and procalcitonin, nonspecific tests that are commonly elevated in various inflammatory states, including infection. The ESR, C-reactive protein, or procalcitonin can be used to follow the progression of infection; currently, R.G.'s ESR is elevated at 65 mm/hour. With appropriate management of infection, the ESR would be expected to decrease; inadequate treatment would be associated with persistent elevation of the ESR and C-reactive protein. Procalcitonin is a more specific indicator for infection than ESR or C-reactive protein and has been used as a tool to discontinue antibiotics in patients with noninfectious inflammation.[4] At present, R.G.'s procalcitonin is 1.0 mcg/L, which is consistent with infection-associated inflammation.

Respiratory Changes

Production of organic acids, such as lactate, increased glycolysis, decreased fractional extraction of oxygen, and abnormal delivery-dependent oxygen consumption are observed in sepsis.[3] This process leads to metabolic acidosis, with accompanying decreased serum bicarbonate levels. The lungs normally respond to metabolic acidosis in a compensatory manner with an increased respiratory rate (tachypnea), resulting in an increased elimination of arterial carbon dioxide. R.G.'s acid–base status is consistent with sepsis-associated metabolic acidosis (CO_2, 16 mEq/L) and compensatory respiratory alkalosis (respiratory rate, 24 breaths/minute).

A late complication of the above-mentioned sepsis cascade is acute respiratory distress syndrome (ARDS). ARDS initially was described as noncardiogenic pulmonary edema with severe hypoxemia caused by right-to-left intrapulmonary shunting resulting from atelectasis and edema-filled alveoli. The primary pathophysiology of ARDS is a breakdown in the natural integrity of the alveolar capillary network in the lung.[5] In the early phase of ARDS, patients have severe alveolar edema with large numbers of inflammatory cells, primarily neutrophils. The chronic phase of ARDS (10–14 days after development of the syndrome) is associated with significant lung destruction. Emphysema, pulmonary vascular obliteration, and fibrosis commonly are observed. Severe ARDS is associated with ratios of arterial oxygen level to fraction of inspired oxygen (Pao_2/Fio_2) of less than 100, low lung compliance, a need for high positive end-expiratory pressure (PEEP), and other respiratory maneuvers. At present, the treatment for this syndrome primarily is supportive, including mechanical ventilation, high inspired oxygen, and PEEP. If patients fail to show improved gas exchange by day 7, the mortality associated with ARDS is high (>80%).[6] Although R.G. currently does not have ARDS, the severity of his sepsis strongly suggests he may develop this complication.

Hematologic Changes

Disseminated intravascular coagulation (DIC) is a well-recognized sequel of sepsis. Huge quantities of clotting factors and platelets are consumed in DIC as widespread coagulation and inflammation take place throughout the circulatory system.[3] As a result, the ratio of prothrombin time (PT) to international normalized ratio (INR) and the activated partial thromboplastin time (aPTT) are prolonged, and the platelet count commonly is decreased in sepsis. Decreased fibrinogen levels and increased fibrin split products generally are diagnostic for DIC. The PT of 18 seconds and the decreased platelet count of 40,000/μL in R.G. are consistent with sepsis-induced DIC.[3]

Neurologic Changes

Central nervous system (CNS) changes, including lethargy, disorientation, confusion, and psychosis, are commonly observed in septic patients. Altered mental status is a well-recognized symptom associated with CNS infections, such as meningitis and brain abscess. These changes, however, are also commonly observed with other sites of infection. R.G.'s confused state is consistent with that expected with septic shock.[2–3]

PROBLEMS IN THE DIAGNOSIS OF AN INFECTION

CASE 62-1, QUESTION 3: R.G.'s medical history includes temporal arteritis and seizures chronically treated with corticosteroids and phenytoin. Perioperative "stress doses" of hydrocortisone recently were administered because of his surgical procedure. What medications or disease states confuse the diagnosis of infection?

Confabulating Variables

Various factors, including major surgery, acute myocardial infarction, and initiation of corticosteroid therapy, are associated with an increased WBC count. Unlike infection, however, a shift to the left does not occur with these disease states or drugs. In R.G., the stress dose of hydrocortisone and his recent surgical procedure might have contributed to the increased WBC count. The presence of bands in this patient, however, strongly suggests a bone marrow response to an infectious process.

Drug Effects

The ability of corticosteroids to mimic or mask infection is noteworthy. Corticosteroids are associated with an increased WBC count and glucose intolerance with the initiation of therapy or when doses are increased. Furthermore, some patients experience corticosteroid-induced mental status changes that may mimic those associated with sepsis. Although corticosteroids mimic infection, they also have the ability to mask infection. For example, bowel perforation in a patient with ulcerative colitis would result in significant peritoneal contamination. Considering their potent anti-inflammatory effects, concomitant receipt of glucocorticoids may, however, reduce the classic findings of peritonitis. Furthermore, corticosteroids can reduce and sometimes ablate the febrile response. Thus, these corticosteroid-treated patients may be asymptomatic but at great risk for gram-negative septic shock.

Another example of the influence of corticosteroids on the diagnosis of infection relates to neurosurgical procedures. Certain neurosurgical procedures are associated with significant trauma to the meninges; however, the patient often is asymptomatic while receiving high-dose dexamethasone, a corticosteroid commonly used to reduce the inflammation and swelling associated with neurosurgical procedures. When the dexamethasone dose is decreased, the patient subsequently may experience classic meningismus, including stiff neck, photophobia, and headache. The lumbar puncture may demonstrate cloudy cerebrospinal fluid (CSF), an elevated WBC count, high CSF protein, and low CSF glucose. Although the signs and symptoms are consistent with infectious bacterial meningitis, if no bacteria grow from the CSF sample, this disease state represents an aseptic meningitis (i.e., inflammation of the meninges without an infectious origin).[7] Certain drugs may cause aseptic meningitis, including nonsteroidal anti-inflammatory agents, sulfonamides, and certain antiepileptics.[8]

Fever

Fever is also a common finding with autoimmune diseases, such as systemic lupus erythematosus and temporal arteritis, or with sarcoidosis, chronic liver disease, and familial Mediterranean fever.[9,10] Acute myocardial infarction, pulmonary embolism, postoperative pulmonary atelectasis, and certain cancers are also commonly associated with fever. Factitious fever or self-induced disease must be considered in certain patients. More recent evaluations of fever of unknown origin have resulted in an inability to diagnose the etiology of the fever; in many instances, the fever has resulted in the unnecessary use of antibiotics.[10] After infection, autoimmune disease, and malignancy have been ruled out, drug fever should be considered. Drugs, including certain antimicrobials and antiepileptics, have been associated with drug fever. Drug fever generally occurs after 7 to 10 days of therapy and resolves within 48 hours of the drug's discontinuation.[11] Some clinicians claim that patients with drug fever generally feel "well" and are unaware of their fever. A rechallenge with the offending agent usually results in recurrence of fever within hours of administration. Drug fever should be considered a diagnosis of exclusion, however, and should be considered only after eliminating the presence of other disease states.

In summary, R.G. has an autoimmune disease, temporal arteritis, which is known to be associated with fever. Similarly, his corticosteroid administration and phenytoin use may confound the diagnosis of infection. His other signs and symptoms, however, strongly suggest that R.G.'s problems are of an infectious origin.

ESTABLISHING THE SITE OF THE INFECTION

CASE 62-1, QUESTION 4: What are the most likely sources of R.G.'s infection?

Independent of the presumed site of infection, in septic patients a series of blood samples for culture tests must be drawn to demonstrate the presence of bacteremia. After blood culture sampling, a thorough physical examination often documents the source of infection. Urosepsis, the most common cause of nosocomial infection, may be associated with dysuria, flank pain, and abnormal urinalysis.[12] Tachypnea, increased sputum production, altered chest radiograph, and hypoxemia may direct the clinician toward a pulmonary source. Evidence for an infected IV line might include pain, erythema, and purulent discharge around the IV catheter. Other potential sites of infection include the peritoneum, pelvis, bone, and CNS.

R.G. has several possible sites of infection. The copious production of yellow–green sputum, tachypnea, and the altered chest radiograph suggest the presence of pneumonia. The abdominal pain, absent bowel sounds, and recent surgical procedure, however, suggest an intra-abdominal source.[13] Further, the abnormal urinalysis (>50 WBC/HPF) and the erythema around the central venous catheter suggest urinary tract and intravenous catheter infections, respectively.

DETERMINING LIKELY PATHOGENS

CASE 62-1, QUESTION 5: What are the most likely pathogens associated with R.G.'s infection(s)?

R.G. has several possible sources of infection and likely pathogens. Table 62-1 provides a classification of infectious organisms (e.g., gram-positive, gram-negative, aerobic, and anaerobic), and Table 62-2 lists the most likely organisms associated with sites of infection. Bacterial pneumonia is caused by various pathogens, including *Streptococcus pneumoniae*, *Enterobacteriaceae*, and "atypical" pathogens (e.g., *Legionella pneumophila*).[14] However, empirical antimicrobial therapy directed against all the above organisms is not necessary in all patients. Community-acquired pneumonia in normal hosts is generally associated with bacterial, *S. pneumoniae*, *Haemophilus influenzae*, and "atypical" bacterial pathogens.[15] In contrast, nosocomial (acquired in hospital or in other health care facilities, e.g., nursing home) pneumonia is associated with gram-negative bacilli (e.g., *Escherichia coli*, *Klebsiella* species, *Enterobacter* species, and *Pseudomonas aeruginosa*) and *Staphylococcus aureus*. If the pneumonia is a result of a gastric aspiration, empirical antibacterial treatment of mouth anaerobes generally takes place; however, their true pathogenicity in aspiration pneumonia is not clear. For the empirical treatment of hospital-associated pneumonia or ventilator-associated pneumonia, knowledge of a hospital epidemiology is useful. If *P. aeruginosa* or *Enterobacter cloacae* predominate in an institution, then broad-spectrum agents should be used directed against these pathogens. Similarly, prior or concurrent receipt of antimicrobial therapy significantly impacts the choice of empirical therapy. Age is an important determinant in the epidemiology of infection. For example, meningitis in a neonate is commonly caused by group B streptococci, *E. coli*, and *Listeria monocytogenes*, whereas these bacteria are uncommon meningitis pathogens in normal adults. The presence of concomitant diseases, such as chronic obstructive pulmonary disease (COPD) or alcohol and IV drug use, also influences the specific pathogen. As an example, patients with COPD-associated

Table 62-1
Classification of Infectious Organisms

1. Bacteria
   - Aerobic
     - Gram-positive
       - Cocci
         - Streptococci: pneumococcus, viridans streptococci; group A streptococci
         - *Enterococcus*
         - Staphylococci: *Staphylococcus aureus*, *Staphylococcus epidermidis*
       - Rods (bacilli)
         - *Corynebacterium*
         - *Listeria*
     - Gram-negative
       - Cocci
         - *Moraxella*
         - *Neisseria (Neisseria meningitidis, Neisseria gonorrhoeae)*
       - *Rods*
         - Enterobacteriaceae (*Escherichia coli, Klebsiella, Enterobacter, Citrobacter, Proteus, Serratia, Salmonella, Shigella, Morganella, Providencia*)
         - *Campylobacter*
         - *Pseudomonas*
         - *Helicobacter*
         - *Haemophilus* (coccobacilli morphology)
         - *Legionella*
   - Anaerobic
     - Gram-positive
       - Cocci
         - *Peptococcus*
         - *Peptostreptococcus*
       - Rods (bacilli)
         - Clostridia (*Clostridium perfringens, Clostridium tetani, Clostridium difficile*)
         - *Propionibacterium acnes*
     - Gram-negative
       - Cocci
         - None
       - Rods (bacilli)
         - Bacteroides (*Bacteroides fragilis, Bacteroides melaninogenicus*)
         - Fusobacterium
         - Prevotella
2. Fungi
   - *Aspergillus, Candida, Coccidioides, Cryptococcus, Histoplasma, Mucor, Tinea, Trichophyton*
3. Viruses
   - Influenza; hepatitis A, B, C, D, E; human immunodeficiency virus; rubella; herpes; influenza; cytomegalovirus; respiratory syncytial virus; Epstein–Barr virus; severe acute respiratory syndrome (SARS) virus
4. Chlamydiae
   - *Chlamydia trachomatis*
   - *Chlamydia psittaci*
   - *Chlamydophila pneumoniae*
   - Lymphogranuloma venereum (LGV)
5. Rickettsiae
   - Rocky Mountain spotted fever, Q fever
   - Ureaplasma
6. Mycoplasmas
   - *Mycoplasma pneumoniae, Mycoplasma hominis*
7. Spirochetes
   - *Treponema pallidum, Borrelia burgdorferi* (Lyme disease)
8. Mycobacteria
   - *Mycobacterium tuberculosis*
   - *Mycobacterium avium intracellulare*

Table 62-2
Site of Infection: Suspected Organisms

Site/Type of Infection	Suspected Organisms
1. Respiratory	
Pharyngitis	Viral, group A streptococci
Otitis	Viral, *Haemophilus influenzae*, *Streptococcus pneumoniae*, *Moraxella catarrhalis*
Acute sinusitis	Viral, *S. pneumoniae*, *H. influenzae*, *M. catarrhalis*
Chronic sinusitis	Anaerobes, *Staphylococcus aureus* (as well as suspected organisms associated with acute sinusitis)
Epiglottitis	Viral, *H. influenzae*
Pneumonia	
Community-Acquired	
Normal host	*S. pneumoniae*, viral, mycoplasma
Aspiration	Normal aerobic and anaerobic mouth flora
Pediatrics	*S. pneumoniae*, *H. influenzae*
COPD	*S. pneumoniae*, *H. influenzae*, *Legionella*, *Chlamydia*, *Mycoplasma*
Alcoholic	*S. pneumoniae*, *Klebsiella*
Hospital-Acquired	
Aspiration	Mouth anaerobes, aerobic gram-negative rods, *S. aureus*
Neutropenic	Molds, aerobic gram-negative rods, *S. aureus*
HIV	Molds, *Pneumocystis*, *Legionella*, *Nocardia*, *S. pneumoniae*, *Pseudomonas*
2. Urinary Tract	
Community-acquired	*Escherichia coli*, other gram-negative rods, *S. aureus*, *Staphylococcus epidermidis*, enterococci
Hospital-acquired	Resistant aerobic gram-negative rods, enterococci
3. Skin and Soft Tissue	
Cellulitis	Group A streptococci, *S. aureus*
IV catheter infection	*S. aureus*, *S. epidermidis*
Surgical wound	*S. aureus*, gram-negative rods
Diabetic ulcer	*S. aureus*, gram-negative aerobic rods, anaerobes
Furuncle	*S. aureus*
1. Intra-abdominal	*Bacteroides fragilis*, *E. coli*, other aerobic gram-negative rods, enterococci
2. Gastroenteritis	*Salmonella*, *Shigella*, *Helicobacter*, *Campylobacter*, *Clostridium difficile*, amoeba, *Giardia*, viral, enterotoxigenic-hemorrhagic *E. coli*
4. Endocarditis	
Preexisting valvular disease	*Viridans streptococci*
IV drug user	*S. aureus*, aerobic gram-negative rods, enterococci, fungi
Prosthetic valve	*S. epidermidis*, *S. aureus*
5. Osteomyelitis and Septic Arthritis	*S. aureus*, aerobic gram-negative rods
6. Meningitis	
<2 months	*E. coli*, group B streptococci, *Listeria*
2 months–12 years	*S. pneumoniae*, *Neisseria meningitidis*, *H. influenzae*
Adults	*S. pneumoniae*, *N. meningitidis*
Hospital-acquired	*S. pneumoniae*, *N. meningitidis*, aerobic gram-negative rods
Postneurosurgery	*S. aureus*, aerobic gram-negative rods

COPD, chronic obstructive pulmonary disease; IV, intravenous.

pneumonia are more likely to be infected by *S. pneumoniae* and *H. influenzae*, whereas chronic alcoholics are more likely to have *Klebsiella* species as a source of pneumonia.

Immune status is an important predictor of likely pathogens. HIV/AIDS patients or those receiving Atgam, cyclosporine (or tacrolimus), sirolimus, and corticosteroids have lymphocyte deficiency or dysfunction-associated infections, including those caused by cytomegalovirus, *Pneumocystis jiroveci*, atypical mycobacteria, and *Cryptococcus neoformans*. Patients with leukemia and neutropenia are at risk for infection caused by aerobic gram-negative bacilli, including *P. aeruginosa*, *Candida* species, and *Aspergillus* species, as well as the above-mentioned pathogens.

In R.G., the abdomen, respiratory tract, urinary tract, and IV catheter are all potential sites of infection. Intra-abdominal infection is likely caused by aerobic gram-negative enteric bacteria, *Bacteroides fragilis*, and possibly enterococcus; nosocomial urinary tract infection is usually caused by aerobic gram-negative bacteria. R.G.'s pneumonia could be attributable to gram-negative bacilli and staphylococci, as well as other organisms. Furthermore, his long-term use of corticosteroids may predispose him to infection caused by more opportunistic organisms, including *Legionella*, *P. jiroveci*, and fungi. Lastly, his IV catheter infection suggests infection caused by staphylococci, including *Staphylococcus epidermidis* and *Staphylococcus aureus*.

MICROBIOLOGIC TESTS AND SUSCEPTIBILITY OF ORGANISMS

CASE 62-1, QUESTION 6: A Gram stain of R.G.'s tracheal aspirate shows gram-negative bacilli. What tests may assist with the identification of the pathogen(s)?

Once the site of infection has been determined and host defense and other epidemiologic factors have been evaluated, additional tests can be performed to identify the pathogen. The Gram stain uses crystal violet solution and iodine staining bacteria gram positive or gram negative; some organisms are gram variable. In addition, the shape of the organism (cocci, bacilli) is readily apparent with the use of the Gram stain. Streptococci and staphylococci are gram-positive cocci, whereas *E. coli*, *E. cloacae*, and *P. aeruginosa* appear as gram-negative bacilli (Table 62-1).[16] If the Gram stain of the tracheal aspirate demonstrates gram-positive cocci in clusters, empirical antistaphylococcal therapy is indicated. In contrast, if the Gram stain shows gram-negative rods, antimicrobials with activity against these pathogens should be used.

Similar to the Gram stain in bacterial infection, the India ink and potassium hydroxide stains are helpful in the identification of certain fungi. The acid-fast bacilli stain is critical in the diagnosis of infection caused by *Mycobacterium tuberculosis* or atypical mycobacteria.

In R.G.'s case, the Gram stain suggests that antimicrobials active against gram-negative bacilli should be used. Table 62-3 provides a classification of antibacterials (e.g., different generations of cephalosporins). Tables 62-4, 62-5, and 62-6 list in-vitro susceptibilities of aerobic gram-positive, gram-negative, and anaerobic bacteria, respectively.

Culture and Susceptibility Testing

Culture and susceptibility testing provides final identification of the pathogen, as well as information regarding the likely effectiveness of various antimicrobials. Although these tests provide more information than the Gram stain, they generally require 18 to 24 hours to complete. After the pathogen has been identified, Table 62-7 can be used in conjunction with institution-specific susceptibility studies to select the most appropriate antimicrobial.

Table 62-3
Classification of Antibacterials

β-Lactam Antibiotics	
Cephalosporins	Penicillinase-resistant penicillins
First-generation	Isoxazolyl penicillins (dicloxacillin, oxacillin, cloxacillin)
Cefadroxil (Duricef)	Nafcillin (Unipen)
Cefazolin (Ancef)	Combination with β-lactamase inhibitors
Cephalexin (Keflex)	Augmentin (amoxicillin plus clavulanic acid)
Second-generation	Avycaz (ceftazidime plus avibactam)
Cefaclor (Ceclor)	Timentin (ticarcillin plus clavulanic acid)[a]
Cefamandole (Mandol)[a]	Unasyn (ampicillin plus sulbactam)
Cefonicid (Monocid)	Zerbaxa (ceftolozane plus tazobactam)
Ceforanide (Precef)	Zosyn (piperacillin plus tazobactam)
Cefotetan (Cefotan)	Aminoglycosides
Cefoxitin (Mefoxin)	Amikacin (Amikin)
Cefprozil (Cefzil)	Gentamicin (Garamycin)
Cefuroxime (Zinacef)	Neomycin (Mycifradin)
Cefuroxime axetil (Ceftin)	Netilmicin (Netromycin)
Third-generation	Streptomycin
Cefdinir (Omnicef)	Tobramycin (Nebcin)
Cefditoren (Spectracef)	Protein synthesis inhibitors
Cefixime (Suprax)	Azithromycin (Zithromax)
Cefotaxime (Claforan)	Clarithromycin (Biaxin)
Cefpodoxime proxetil (Vantin)	Clindamycin (Cleocin)
Ceftazidime (Fortaz)	Chloramphenicol (Chloromycetin)
Ceftibuten (Cedax)	Dalfopristin/Quinupristin (Synercid)
Ceftizoxime (Cefizox)	Dirithromycin (Dynabac)
Ceftriaxone (Rocephin)	Erythromycin (Erythrocin)
Fourth-generation	Fidaxomicin (Dificid)
Cefepime (Maxipime)	Linezolid (Zyvox)
Fifth-generation	Tedizolid (Sivestro)
Ceftaroline (Teflaro)	Telithromycin (Ketek)
	Tetracyclines (doxycycline, minocycline, tetracycline, tigecycline)

Table 62-3
Classification of Antibacterials (*continued*)

***β*-Lactam Antibiotics**

- Carbacephems
  - Loracarbef (Lorabid)
- Monobactams
  - Aztreonam (Azactam)
- Penems
  - Doripenem (Doribax)
  - Ertapenem (Invanz)
  - Imipenem (Primaxin)
  - Meropenem (Merem)
- Penicillins
  - Natural penicillins
    - Penicillin G
    - Penicillin V
  - Aminopenicillins
    - Ampicillin (Omnipen)
    - Amoxicillin (Amoxil)
    - Bacampicillin (Spectrobid)[a]
- Folate inhibitors
  - Sulfadiazine
  - Sulfadoxine (Fansidar)
  - Trimethoprim (Trimpex)
  - Trimethoprim-sulfamethoxazole (Bactrim, Septra)
- Quinolones
  - Ciprofloxacin (Cipro)
  - Gemifloxacin (Factive)
  - Levofloxacin (Levoquin)
  - Moxifloxacin (Avelox)
  - Norfloxacin (Noroxin)
  - Ofloxacin (Floxin)
- Dalbavancin (Dalvance)
- Daptomycin (Cubicin)
- Oritavancin (Orbactiv)
- Telavancin (Vibativ)
- Vancomycin (Vancocin)
- Metronidazole (Flagyl)

[a]Not on the US market.

Table 62-4
In-Vitro Antimicrobial Susceptibility: Aerobic Gram-Positive Cocci

Drugs	*Staphylococcus aureus*	*Staphylococcus aureus* (MR)	*Staphylococcus epidermidis*	*Staphylococcus epidermidis* (MR)	Streptococci[a]	Enterococci[b]	Pneumococci
Ampicillin	+		+		++++	++	+++
Augmentin	++++	+	++++		++++	++	++++
Aztreonam							
Cefazolin	++++		++++		++++		++
Cefepime	++++		++++		++++		+++
Cefoxitin/ Cefotetan	++		++		++		+
Ceftaroline	++++	++++	++++	++++	++++	+	++++
Cefuroxime	++++		++++		++++		+++
Ciprofloxacin[c]	+++	+	+++	++	+	+	++
Clindamycin	++++	++	++++	+	+++		+++
Cotrimoxazole	++++	+++	++	+	++	+	+
Dalbavancin	++++	++++	++++	++++	++++	++	++++
Daptomycin[f]	++++	++++	++++	++++	++++	++++	++++
Erythromycin (Azithromycin, Clarithromycin)	++		+		+++		++
Imipenem (Doripenem, Ertapenem, Meropenem)	++++		++++		++++	++	+++
Levofloxacin (Gemifloxacin, Moxifloxacin)	++++	++	+++	++	+++	++	++++
Linezolid[f] (Tedizolid)	++++	++++	++++	++++	++++	++++	++++
Nafcillin (Oxacillin)	++++		++++		++++		++
Oritavancin[f]	++++	++++	++++	++++	++++	++++	++++

Table 62-4
In-Vitro Antimicrobial Susceptibility: Aerobic Gram-Positive Cocci (*continued*)

Drugs	*Staphylococcus aureus*	*Staphylococcus aureus* (MR)	*Staphylococcus epidermidis*	*Staphylococcus epidermidis* (MR)	Streptococci[a]	Enterococci[b]	Pneumococci
Penicillin	+		+		++++	++	+++
Quinupristin/dalfopristin[d,f]	++++	++++	++++	++++	++++	++++	++++
TGC[e]	+++		++		++++		+++
Telavancin	++++	++++	++++	++++	++++	++++	++++
Tigecycline[f]	++++	++++	++++	++++	++++	++++	++++
Timentin	++++		++++		++++	+	+
Unasyn	++++		++++		++++	++	+++
Vancomycin	++++	++++	++++	++++	++++	+++	++++
Zosyn	++++		++++		++++	++	+++

[a]Nonpneumococcal streptococci.
[b]Usually requires combination therapy (e.g., ampicillin or ampicillin and ceftriaxone) endocarditis.
[c]Levofloxacin (e.g., gemifloxacin, moxifloxacin) is more active than ciprofloxacin against staphylococci and streptococci.
[d]Active against *Enterococcus faecium* but unpredictable against *E. faecalis*.
[e]Cefotaxime, ceftizoxime, ceftriaxone, cefoperazone. Ceftazidime has comparatively inferior antistaphylococcal and antipneumococcal activity. Cefotaxime, ceftriaxone, and cefepime are the most reliable cephalosporins versus *Streptococcus pneumoniae*.
[f]Active versus vancomycin-resistant *E. faecium*.
MR, methicillin resistant; TGC, third-generation cephalosporin.

Table 62-5
In-Vitro Antimicrobial Susceptibility: Gram-Negative Aerobes

Drugs	*Escherichia coli*	*Klebsiella pneumoniae*	*Enterobacter cloacae*	*Proteus mirabilis*	*Serratia marcescens*	*Pseudomonas aeruginosa*	*Haemophilus influenzae*	*Haemophilus influenzae*[a]
Ampicillin	++			+++			++++	
Amikacin	++++	++++	++++	++++	++++	++++	++	++
Augmentin	+++	++		++++			++++	++++
Aztreonam	++++	++++	+	++++	++++	+++	++++	++++
Cefazolin	+++	+++		++++			+	
Cefepime	++++	++++	+++	++++	++++	+++	++++	++++
Ceftazidime	+++	+++	+	++++	++++	+++	++++	++++
Ceftazidime-avibactam	++++	++++	++++	++++	++++	++++	++++	++++
Ceftolozane-tazobactam	++++	++++	++++	++++	++++	++++	++++	++++
Ceftaroline	++++	++++	+	++++	++	+++	++++	++++
Cefuroxime	+++	+++		++++	+		++++	++++
Cotrimoxazole	++	+++	+++	++++	+++		++++	++++
Ertapenem	++++	++++	++++	++++	++++	+	++++	++++
Gentamicin	++++	++++	++++	++++	++++	+++	++	++
Imipenem/Meropenem/Doripenem	++++	++++	++++	+++	++++	+++	++++	++++
Quinolones	+++	++++	+++	++++	++++	++	++++	++++
TGC[b]	++++	++++	+	++++	++++	+	++++	++++
Tigecycline	++++	++++	++++	++	++++	–	++++	++++
Timentin	+++	++	+	++++	+++	+++	++++	++++
Tobramycin	++++	++++	++++	++++	+++	++++	++	++
Unasyn	+++	+++		++++	++		++++	++++
Zosyn	++++	++++	++	++++	++++	++++	++++	++++

[a]β-Lactamase-producing strains.
[b]Cefotaxime, ceftizoxime, ceftriaxone.
TGC, third-generation cephalosporin.

Table 62-6
Antimicrobial Susceptibility: Anaerobes

Drugs	*Bacteroides fragilis*	Peptococcus	Peptostreptococcus	Clostridia (Non-difficile)
Ampicillin	+	++++	++++	+++
Aztreonam				
Cefazolin		+++	+++	
Cefepime	+	+++	+++	+
Cefotaxime	++	+++	+++	+
Cefoxitin (Cefotetan)	+++	+++	++++	+
Ceftazidime		+	+	+
Ceftizoxime	+++	+++	+++	+
Ciprofloxacin	+	+	+	+
Clindamycin	+++	++++	++++	++
Moxifloxacin	+++	+++	+++	++
Imipenem (Doripenem/Ertapenem/Meropenem)	++++	++++	++++	++
Metronidazole	++++	+++	++	+++
Penicillin	+	++++	++++	++++
Piperacillin-tazobactam (Amoxicillin-clavulanate, Ticarcillin-clavulanate)	++++	++++	+++	+++
Unasyn	++++	++++	++++	++++
Vancomycin		+++	+++	+++

Table 62-7
Antimicrobials of Choice in the Treatment of Bacterial Infection

Organism	Drug of Choice	Alternatives	Comments
Aerobes			
Gram-positive cocci			
Streptococcus pyogenes (group A streptococci)	Penicillin	Clindamycin, macrolide, cephalosporin	Clindamycin is the most reliable alternative for penicillin-allergic patients.
Streptococcus pneumoniae	Ceftriaxone, ampicillin, oral amoxicillin	Macrolide, cephalosporin, doxycycline	Although the incidence of penicillin-nonsusceptible pneumococci is 20%–30%, high-dose penicillin or amoxicillin is active against most of these isolates.
			Penicillin-resistant pneumococci commonly demonstrate resistance to other agents, including erythromycin, tetracyclines, and cephalosporins.
			Antipneumococcal quinolones (gemifloxacin, levofloxacin, moxifloxacin), ceftriaxone, and cefotaxime are options for treatment of high-level penicillin-resistant isolates.
Enterococcus faecalis	Ampicillin ± gentamicin	Piperacillin-tazobactam; vancomycin ± gentamicin; daptomycin, linezolid, tigecycline	Most commonly isolated enterococcus (80%–85%). Most reliable antienterococcal agents are ampicillin (penicillin, piperacillin-tazobactam), vancomycin, and linezolid. Monotherapy generally inhibits but does not kill the enterococcus. Daptomycin is unique in its bactericidal activity against enterococci. Aminoglycosides must be added to ampicillin or vancomycin to provide bactericidal activity. High-level aminoglycoside resistance should be determined for endocarditis.

Table 62-7
Antimicrobials of Choice in the Treatment of Bacterial Infection (*continued*)

Organism	Drug of Choice	Alternatives	Comments
Enterococcus faecium	Vancomycin ± gentamicin	Linezolid, daptomycin, dalfopristin/quinupristin (D/Q), oritavancin, tigecycline	Second most common enterococcal organism (10%–20%) and is more likely than *E. faecalis* to be resistant to multiple antimicrobials. Most reliable agents are daptomycin, D/Q, and linezolid. Monotherapy generally inhibits but does not kill the enterococcus. Aminoglycosides or ceftriaxone must be added to cell wall–active agents to provide bactericidal activity. Ampicillin and vancomycin resistance is common. Daptomycin, D/Q, and linezolid are drugs of choice for vancomycin-resistant isolates.
Staphylococcus aureus (methicillin-resistant)	Nafcillin, oxacillin	Cefazolin, vancomycin, clindamycin, dalbavancin, linezolid, oritavancin	10%–15% of isolates inhibited by penicillin. Most isolates susceptible to nafcillin, cephalosporins, trimethoprim-sulfamethoxazole, and clindamycin. First-generation cephalosporins are equal to nafcillin. Most second- and third-generation cephalosporins adequate in the treatment of infection (exceptions include ceftazidime and cefonicid). Methicillin-resistant *S. aureus* must be treated with vancomycin; however, trimethoprim-sulfamethoxazole, daptomycin, D/Q, linezolid, vancins, doxycycline, or minocycline can be used.
	Vancomycin	Trimethoprim-sulfamethoxazole, minocycline, daptomycin, tigecycline, telavancin, ceftaroline	
Staphylococcus epidermidis (methicillin-resistant)	Nafcillin, oxacillin	Cefazolin, vancomycin, clindamycin	Most isolates are β-lactam-, clindamycin-, and trimethoprim-sulfamethoxazole– resistant. Most reliable agents are vancomycin, daptomycin, D/Q, and linezolid. Rifampin is active and can be used in conjunction with other agents; however, monotherapy with rifampin is associated with development of resistance.
	Vancomycin	Daptomycin, linezolid, D/Q	
Gram-positive Bacilli			
Diphtheroids	Penicillin	Cephalosporin	
Corynebacterium jeikeium	Vancomycin	Erythromycin, quinolone	
Listeria monocytogenes	Ampicillin (±gentamicin)	Trimethoprim-sulfamethoxazole	
Gram-negative Cocci			
Moraxella catarrhalis	Trimethoprim-sulfamethoxazole	Amoxicillin-clavulanic acid, erythromycin, doxycycline, second- or third-generation cephalosporin	
Neisseria gonorrhoeae	Ceftriaxone		
Neisseria meningitidis	Penicillin	Third-generation cephalosporin	
Gram-negative Bacilli			
Campylobacter fetus	Imipenem	Gentamicin	
Campylobacter jejuni	Azithromycin	A tetracycline, amoxicillin-clavulanic acid, quinolone	
Enterobacter	Trimethoprim-sulfamethoxazole	Quinolone, carbapenem, aminoglycoside	Not predictably inhibited by third-generation cephalosporins. Carbapenems, quinolones, trimethoprim-sulfamethoxazole, cefepime, and aminoglycosides are most active agents.
Escherichia coli	Third-generation cephalosporin	First- or second-generation cephalosporin, gentamicin	Extended-spectrum β-lactamase (ESBL) producers should be treated with a carbapenem.
Haemophilus influenzae	Third-generation cephalosporin	β-Lactamase inhibitor combinations, second-generation cephalosporin, trimethoprim-sulfamethoxazole	
Helicobacter pylori	PPI, clarithromycin, and amoxicillin or metronidazole	PPI, bismuth, tetracycline, and a nitroimidazole	

(*continued*)

Table 62-7
Antimicrobials of Choice in the Treatment of Bacterial Infection (*continued*)

Organism	Drug of Choice	Alternatives	Comments
Klebsiella pneumoniae	Third-generation cephalosporin	First- or second-generation cephalosporin, gentamicin, trimethoprim-sulfamethoxazole	ESBL producers should be treated with a carbapenem.
Legionella	Fluoroquinolone	Erythromycin ± rifampin, doxycycline	
Proteus mirabilis	Ampicillin	First-generation cephalosporin, trimethoprim-sulfamethoxazole	
Other *Proteus*	Third-generation cephalosporin	β-Lactamase inhibitor combination, aminoglycoside, trimethoprim-sulfamethoxazole	
Pseudomonas aeruginosa	Antipseudomonal penicillin or antipseudomonal cephalosporin) ± aminoglycoside (or quinolone)	Quinolone or imipenem ± aminoglycoside	Most active agents include aminoglycosides, doripenem, imipenem, meropenem, ceftazidime ceftazidime/avibactam, cefepime, ceftolozane/tazobactam, aztreonam, and the extended-spectrum penicillins. Monotherapy is adequate for most pseudomonal infections.
Salmonella typhi	Quinolone	Ceftriaxone	
Serratia marcescens	Third-generation cephalosporin	Trimethoprim-sulfamethoxazole, aminoglycoside	
Shigella	Quinolone	Trimethoprim-sulfamethoxazole, ampicillin	
Stenotrophomonas maltophilia	Trimethoprim-sulfamethoxazole	Ceftazidime, minocycline, β-lactamase inhibitor combination (Timentin)	
Anaerobes			
Bacteroides fragilis	Metronidazole	β-Lactamase inhibitor combinations, penems	Most active agents (95%–100%) include metronidazole, the β-lactamase inhibitor combinations ampicillin-sulbactam, piperacillin-tazobactam, ticarcillin-clavulanic acid, and penems. Clindamycin, cefoxitin, cefotetan, cefmetazole, ceftizoxime have good activity but not to the degree of metronidazole. Aminoglycosides and aztreonam are inactive.
Clostridia difficile	Metronidazole	Vancomycin Fidaxomicin	Oral vancomycin is the drug of choice for severe infection. Fidaxomicin superior to other agents in the prevention of relapse
Fusobacterium	Penicillin	Metronidazole, clindamycin	
Other Oropharyngeal			
Prevotella	β-Lactamase inhibitor combination	Metronidazole, clindamycin	
Peptostreptococcus	Penicillin	Clindamycin, cephalosporin	Most β-lactams active (exceptions include aztreonam, nafcillin, ceftazidime)
Other			
Actinomyces israelii	Penicillin	Tetracyclines	
Nocardia	Trimethoprim-sulfamethoxazole	Amikacin, minocycline, imipenem	
Chlamydia trachomatis	Doxycycline	Azithromycin	
Chlamydophila pneumoniae	Doxycycline	Azithromycin, clarithromycin	
Mycoplasma pneumoniae	Doxycycline	Azithromycin, clarithromycin	
Borrelia burgdorferi	Doxycycline	Ampicillin, second- or third-generation cephalosporin	
Treponema pallidum	Penicillin	Doxycycline	

DISK DIFFUSION

The most widely used tests for bacterial susceptibility are the disk diffusion and the broth dilution methods. The disk diffusion (Kirby–Bauer) technique uses an agar plate on which an inoculum of the organism is placed. After inoculation, several antimicrobial-laden disks are placed on the plate, and evidence of bacterial growth is observed after 18 to 24 hours. If the antimicrobial is active against the pathogen, a zone of growth inhibition is observed around the disk. Based on guidelines provided by the Clinical and Laboratory Standards Institute (CLSI), the diameter of inhibition is reported as susceptible, intermediate, or resistant. CLSI zones of inhibitions are determined taking into account known achievable antibacterial concentrations. However, broth dilution determination of minimum inhibitory concentration (see the following text) better links with achievable antibacterial concentrations.

BROTH DILUTION

The broth dilution method involves introducing a bacterial inoculum into several tubes or wells filled with broth. Serial dilutions of antimicrobials (e.g., nafcillin 0.5, 1.0, and 2.0 mcg/mL) are placed in the respective wells. After bacteria are allowed to incubate for 18 to 24 hours, the wells are examined for bacterial growth. If the well is cloudy, bacterial growth has occurred, suggesting resistance to the specific antimicrobial at that concentration. As an example, if bacterial growth is observed with *S. aureus* at 0.5 mcg/mL of nafcillin but not at 1.0 mcg/mL, then 1.0 mcg/mL would be considered the minimum inhibitory concentration (MIC) for nafcillin against *S. aureus*.

Similar to the disk diffusion method, the CLSI provides guidelines[17] that also take into account the pharmacokinetic characteristics of an antimicrobial to determine whether the MIC should be reported as susceptible, intermediately susceptible, or resistant. MIC interpretations are both pathogen- and antimicrobial-specific. For example, ciprofloxacin achieves serum concentrations of only 1 to 4 mcg/mL, whereas the fourth-generation cephalosporin, cefepime, achieves peak serum concentrations of 75 to 100 mcg/mL; consequently an MIC of 4.0 mcg/mL for *P. aeruginosa* would be interpreted by CLSI as resistant to ciprofloxacin but susceptible to cefepime.

Although these tests provide an accurate assessment of in-vitro susceptibility, the time delay (18–24 hours) can hinder streamlining of therapy. An alternative efficient, but more expensive, MIC test is the E test, which uses an antibiotic-laden plastic strip with increasing concentrations of a specific antimicrobial from one end to the other. The strip is placed on an agar plate with the actively growing pathogen. Inhibition of growth observed at specific marks on the strip coincides with the MIC of the organism. Numerous studies have confirmed that the E test is as effective as traditional susceptibility testing. Several automated antimicrobial susceptibility systems are available in the United States, including Phoenix (Becton Dickinson, Franklin Lakes, NJ), Vitek (bioMérieux, Durham, NC), MicroScan WalkAway (Siemens Healthcare Diagnostics, Tarrytown, NY), and Sensititre (Trek Diagnostics, Cleveland, OH). These systems generally use a computerized algorithm for interpreting results and determine the antibiotic MIC for the organism by using specialized decision technology. Two major advantages of automated susceptibility methodologies include a reduction in labor and faster reporting of susceptibility results, potentially leading to the earlier initiation of appropriate antibiotic therapy. Although these represent advantages, disadvantages exist, particularly with cystic fibrosis isolates. Most clinical microbiology laboratories use automated susceptibility testing systems. While these automated antimicrobial susceptibility systems are an improvement over traditional broth dilution and disc diffusion methods, other emerging technologies including PCR and other "next generation" systems are likely to result in more rapid identification of pathogens and their associated antimicrobial susceptibility.

Although susceptibility testing is relatively well standardized for aerobic gram-negative and gram-positive organisms, its utility is not as established for anaerobes[18] and fungi.[19] In general, despite improvements in the standardization of testing in anaerobes, institutions do not routinely perform susceptibility testing for these bacteria. In contrast, susceptibility testing is now available for *Candida* species, and these in-vitro data have been demonstrated to predict clinical success in the patient care setting.

The consensus of the CLSI and other experts is that anaerobic isolates from blood, bone and joint sources, brain abscesses, empyemic fluid, and other body fluids that are normally sterile should be considered for susceptibility testing. However, in general, these susceptibilities are rarely performed.[18] Progress has been made in developing a standardized test for determining fungal susceptibility, but the primary emphasis has been on the susceptibility of *Candida* species to azoles in the treatment of candidiasis.[19] Although standardized susceptibility testing for molds is established by the CLSI and other organizations, the correlation with clinical outcome is variable; the best correlation between antifungal susceptibility testing and efficacy lies with the use of azoles in the treatment of disseminated aspergillosis.[20]

DETERMINATION OF ISOLATE PATHOGENICITY

CASE 62-1, QUESTION 7: *Serratia marcescens* grows from a culture of R.G.'s endotracheal aspirate. How can it be determined whether an isolate represents a true bacterial infection versus colonization or contamination?

A positive culture may represent colonization, contamination, or infection. Colonization indicates that bacteria are present at the site; however, they are not actively causing infection. Poor sampling techniques or inappropriate handling of specimens can result in contamination. Contamination differs from colonization in that these isolates are not truly at the site in question. The *S. marcescens* growing from R.G. could represent infection, colonization, or contamination. If a suction catheter was used to sample R.G.'s endotracheal aspirate, the infecting organism likely would be cultured; however, other nonpathogenic flora would also appear in the culture medium (colonization). Furthermore, if the sample is not handled aseptically by the clinician or the microbiology laboratory, bacterial contamination is possible.

In summary, culture results do not solely identify true pathogens. In R.G., the *Serratia* may be a pathogen, contaminant, or colonizer. Nevertheless, considering the severity of R.G.'s illness and his associated respiratory symptoms, treatment directed against this pathogen is necessary.

ANTIMICROBIAL TOXICITIES

CASE 62-1, QUESTION 8: In light of the positive culture for *Serratia*, his increased respiratory secretions, and a worsening chest radiograph, ventilator-associated pneumonia is likely present. Pending susceptibility results, R.G. is empirically started on imipenem and gentamicin. In review of his patient records, R.G. has no known allergies. Are there equally effective, less toxic options for this patient?

Adverse Effects and Toxicities

Before antimicrobial therapy is started, it is important to elicit an accurate drug and allergy history. When "allergy" has been reported by the patient, it is necessary to determine whether the reaction was intolerance, toxicity, or true allergy. For example, gastric intolerance caused by oral doxycycline is common; however, this adverse effect does not represent an allergic manifestation. Although R.G. has no known allergies, neither imipenem nor gentamicin are optimal choices. Imipenem is associated with seizures, particularly in patients with renal failure and in doses in excess of 50 mg/kg/day. Considering R.G.'s acute onset of renal failure and his history of seizures, other carbapenems, such as meropenem or doripenem, or alternative classes of antibacterials would be preferable. Gentamicin similarly may not be a good choice in R.G. His increased age and declining renal function predispose him to aminoglycoside nephrotoxicity and ototoxicity (cochlear and vestibular).[21] A reasonable recommendation pending susceptibility results would be to discontinue imipenem and gentamicin and treat with meropenem or doripenem with or without a fluoroquinolone. Table 62-8 lists common antibiotics adverse effects and toxicities.

Table 62-8
Antibiotic Adverse Effects and Toxicities

Antibiotics	Side Effects	Comments
β-Lactams (penicillin, cephalosporins, monobactams, penems)	*Allergic:* anaphylaxis, urticaria, serum sickness, rash, fever	Many patients will have "ampicillin rash" or "β-lactam rash" with no cross-reactivity with any other penicillins/β-lactams. Most commonly observed in patients with concomitant EBV disease. Likelihood of IgE-mediated cross-reactivity between penicillins and cephalosporins approximately 5%–10%. Most recent data strongly suggest minimal IgE cross-reactivity between penicillins and imipenem/meropenem. No IgE cross-reactivity between aztreonam and penicillins.
	Diarrhea	Particularly common with ampicillin, augmentin, ceftriaxone. Antibiotic-associated colitis can occur with most antimicrobials.
	Hematologic: anemia, thrombocytopenia, antiplatelet activity, hypothrombinemia	Hemolytic anemia more common with higher doses. Antiplatelet activity (inhibition of platelet aggregation) most common with the antipseudomonal penicillins and high serum levels of other β-lactams. Hypothrombinemia more often associated with those cephalosporins with the methyltetrazolethiol side chain (cefamandole, cefotetan). Reaction preventable and reversible with vitamin K.
	Hepatitis or biliary sludging	Hepatitis most common with oxacillin. Biliary sludging and stones reported with ceftriaxone.
	Phlebitis	
	Seizure activity	Associated with high levels of β-lactams, particularly penicillins and imipenem.
	Potassium load	Penicillin G (K^+).
	Nephritis	Occasionally reported for most β-lactams.
	Neutropenia	Nafcillin.
	Disulfiram reaction	Associated with cephalosporins with methyltetrazolethiol side chain (cefamandole, cefotetan).
	Hypotension, nausea	Associated with fast infusion of imipenem.
Aminoglycosides (gentamicin, tobramycin, amikacin, netilmicin)	Nephrotoxicity	Average 10%–15% incidence. Generally reversible, usually occurs after 5–7 days of therapy. *Risk factors:* dehydration, age, dose, duration, concurrent nephrotoxins, liver disease.
	Ototoxicity	1%–5% incidence, often irreversible. Both cochlear and vestibular toxicity occur.
	Neuromuscular paralysis	Rare, most common with large doses administered via intraperitoneal instillation or in patients with myasthenia gravis.
Macrolides (erythromycin, azithromycin, clarithromycin)	Nausea, vomiting, "burning" stomach, cholestatic jaundice, ototoxicity, prolonged QT interval	Oral administration. Azithromycin and clarithromycin associated with less nausea than erythromycin. Cholestatic jaundice reported for all erythromycin salts, most common with estolate. Ototoxicity most common with high doses in patients with renal or hepatic failure. Torsades de Pointes and increased risk of cardiac death associated with increased QT interval.

Table 62-8
Antibiotic Adverse Effects and Toxicities (*continued*)

Antibiotics	Side Effects	Comments
Telithromycin	Hepatotoxicity; upper GI	Severe, sometime fatal hepatotoxicity associated with telithromycin.
Clindamycin	Diarrhea	Most common adverse effect. High association with antibiotic-associated colitis.
Tetracyclines (including tigecycline)	Allergic	
	Photosensitivity	
	Drug Interactions	↓ Oral bioavailability with multivalent cations." similar to that stated in the Quinolones section
	Teeth and bone deposition and discoloration	Avoid in pediatrics (<8 years old), pregnancy, and breast-feeding.
	GI	Upper GI predominates.
	Hepatitis	Primarily in pregnancy or the elderly.
	Renal (azotemia)	Tetracyclines have antianabolic effect and should be avoided in patients with ↓ renal function. Less problematic with doxycycline.
	Vestibular	Associated with minocycline, particularly high doses.
Vancomycin	"Red Man Syndrome": hypotension, flushing	Associated with rapid infusion of vancomycin. More common with increased doses.
	Nephrotoxicity	Reversible nephrotoxicity with high doses or in combination with other nephrotoxins.
	Ototoxicity	Only with receipt of concomitant ototoxins such as aminoglycosides or macrolides.
	Phlebitis	Needs large volume dilution.
Dalfopristin/quinupristin	Phlebitis	Generally requires central line administration.
	Myalgia	Moderate to severe in many patients.
	Increased bilirubin	
Daptomycin	Myalgia	Primarily at high doses and reversible.
Linezolid (Tedizolid)	Thrombocytopenia, neutropenia, anemia, MAO inhibition, neuropathy	Bone marrow suppression and neuropathy duration- and dose-dependent with linezolid. Tedizolid may have less association with bone marrow suppression and neuropathy.
Dalbavancin, Oritavancin, Telavancin	Renal toxicity and prolonged QT with telavancin	
Sulfonamides	GI	Nausea, diarrhea.
	Hepatic	Cholestatic hepatitis, ↑ incidence in HIV.
	Rash	Exfoliative dermatitis, Stevens–Johnson syndrome. More common in HIV.
	Hyperkalemia	Only with trimethoprim (as a component of trimethoprim–sulfamethoxazole).
	Bone marrow	Neutropenia, thrombocytopenia. More common in HIV.
	Kernicterus	Caused by unbound drug in the neonate. Premature liver cannot conjugate bilirubin. Sulfonamide displaces bilirubin from protein, resulting in excessive free bilirubin and kernicterus.
Chloramphenicol	Anemia	Idiosyncratic irreversible aplastic anemia (rare). Reversible dose-related anemia.
	Gray syndrome	Caused by inability of neonates to conjugate chloramphenicol.
Quinolones	GI	Nausea, vomiting, diarrhea.
	Prolonged QT	Moxifloxacin; possibly all quinolones as a class.
	Drug interactions	↓ Oral bioavailability with multivalent cations.
	CNS	Altered mental status, confusion, seizures.
	Cartilage toxicity	Toxic in animal model. Despite this toxicity, appears safe in children including patients with cystic fibrosis.
	Tendonitis or tendon rupture	Common in elderly, renal failure, concomitant glucocorticoids.

(*continued*)

Table 62-8
Antibiotic Adverse Effects and Toxicities (*continued*)

Antibiotics	Side Effects	Comments
Antifungals		
Amphotericin B products	Nephrotoxicity	Common. May depend on patient sodium load. Caution with concomitant nephrotoxins (e.g., aminoglycosides, cyclosporine).
	Hypokalemia	Predictable. Probably caused by renal tubular excretion of potassium. More common in patients receiving concomitant piperacillin–tazobactam.
	Hypomagnesemia	Less commonly observed than hypokalemia.
	Anemia	Long-term adverse effect. Similar to anemia of chronic disease.
Caspofungin, Micafungin, Anidulofungin	Mild LFT increase with concomitant cyclosporine	Anidulofungin is reconstituted with alcohol (about the equivalent of a beer).
Flucytosine	Neutropenia, thrombocytopenia	Secondary to metabolism of flucytosine to fluorouracil. More commonly observed with flucytosine levels >100 mg/mL. More common in patients with HIV.
	Hepatitis	Usually moderate ↑ in LFT. Rarely clinical hepatitis.
Ketoconazole (fluconazole, isavuconazole, itraconazole, posaconazole, voriconazole)	Drug interactions	↓ Oral bioavailability of ketoconazole tablet, and itraconazole capsules with ↑ gastric pH. Azoles are CYP450 substrates and also inhibitors of CYP450 3A4 and other CYP isoenzymes. Voriconazole most likely to be associated with CYP drug interactions
	Hepatitis	Ranges from mild ↑ in LFT to occasional fatal hepatitis.
	Gynecomastia, ↓ libido	More common with high-dose ketoconazole (>400 mg/day). Less common with other azoles.
	Visual disturbance	Unique to voriconazole, particularly first week of therapy.
Antivirals (Excluding Antiretrovirals and Hepatitis Antivirals)		
Acyclovir	Phlebitis	Caused by poor solubility of IV preparation. Reported in 1%–20% of cases.
	Renal failure	Low solubility of acyclovir associated with renal failure. Dehydrated patients, as well as rapid infusions, predispose to toxicity.
	CNS	1% incidence in AIDS. ↑ Incidence with dose in >10 mg/kg/day.
Foscarnet	Nephrotoxicity	Occurs in up to 60% of patients. May be prevented with normal saline bolus before dose. Frequent monitoring of renal function imperative.
	Mineral and electrolyte abnormalities	↑ and ↓ calcium or phosphate may be observed. Hypocalcemia, hypo- and hyperphosphatemia, hypomagnesemia, hypokalemia. ↑ Risk of cardiomyopathy and seizures.
	Anemia	Anemia in 33%; usually manageable with transfusions and discontinuation of foscarnet.
	Nausea, vomiting	
Ganciclovir	Neutropenia, thrombocytopenia	↑ Incidence in AIDS. ↑ Incidence with doses in excess of 10 mg/kg/day.
	Hepatitis	Usually mild to moderate in LFT.
Oseltamavir	Nausea	

AIDS, acquired immunodeficiency syndrome; CNS, central nervous system; EBV, Epstein–Barr virus; GI, gastrointestinal; HIV, human immunodeficiency virus; IV, intravenous; LFT, liver function tests; MAO, monoamine oxidase.

Concomitant Disease States

Concomitant disease states should also be considered in the selection of therapy. As discussed above, older patients with hearing deficits are poor candidates for potentially ototoxic aminoglycoside therapy. Diabetic or kidney transplant patients with candidemia may be better treated with fluconazole or an echinocandin rather than nephrotoxic amphotericin B products. Patients with a preexisting seizure history should not receive imipenem if less toxic therapy can be used. In summary, the toxicologic profile of a drug must be taken into account in the selection of antimicrobial therapy.

ANTIMICROBIAL COSTS OF THERAPY

Case 62-1, Question 9: What factors should be included in calculating the cost of R.G.'s antimicrobial therapy?

The true cost of antimicrobial therapy is difficult to quantify.[22] Although acquisition cost traditionally has been the primary factor in the overall cost of therapy, drug administration labor costs (i.e., nursing and pharmacy) and the use of IV sets, piggyback bags, and infusion control devices must be included in the analysis. As a result, a drug that must be administered several times daily, such as intravenous penicillin, will incur increased administration costs compared with one, such as ceftriaxone, that requires once-a-day dosing.

Some drugs, such as aminoglycosides, are associated with increased laboratory costs (e.g., aminoglycoside serum concentrations, serum creatinine, and audiometry) that are not required for other agents,[23] such as the third-generation cephalosporins and quinolones. Similarly, drugs with a high potential for misuse or toxicity can be associated with increased costs because of monitoring (e.g., medication use evaluation, pharmacokinetic monitoring). If meropenem with or without ciprofloxacin had been selected for R.G., this therapy would be expected to be associated with relatively few laboratory costs. However, the broad spectrum of activity[24] of these agents, potential for misuse, and development of resistance might, however, result in increased monitoring costs and overall cost to society.

Costs that are difficult to quantitate include those associated with failure of antimicrobial therapy and antimicrobial toxicity. Ineffective or toxic therapy can prolong hospitalization and may require expensive interventions, such as hemodialysis,[23] mechanical ventilation, and intensive care unit admission. The net effect of these latter costs can be significantly greater than the acquisition and administration costs of antimicrobial therapy.

In summary, determining the true cost of antimicrobial therapy is complex. Acquisition cost, IV bags, infusion controllers, and labor must be incorporated into the analysis. Although they are difficult to estimate, other costs, including antibiotic toxicity and failure of therapy, should also be included.

ROUTE OF ADMINISTRATION

Case 62-1, Question 10: The *Serratia* was determined to be susceptible to ciprofloxacin. Oral ciprofloxacin was considered for the treatment of R.G.'s presumed *Serratia* pneumonia, but the IV route was prescribed. Why is the oral administration of ciprofloxacin reasonable (or unreasonable) in R.G.?

The proper route of antibiotic administration depends on many factors, including the severity of infection, antimicrobial oral bioavailability, and other patient factors. In patients who appear "septic," blood flow often is shunted away from the mesentery and extremities, resulting in unreliable bioavailability from the gastrointestinal (GI) tract or muscles. Consequently, hemodynamically unstable patients should always receive antimicrobials by the IV route to ensure therapeutic antimicrobial levels. Furthermore, some drug interactions with oral agents can result in subtherapeutic serum concentrations (e.g., reduced bioavailability associated with concomitant quinolone and antacid administration and the decreased absorption of itraconazole with concurrent proton-pump inhibitor [PPI] therapy).

R.G. is clinically septic with a possible *Serratia* pneumonia. Considering his unstable state, the bioavailability of oral ciprofloxacin cannot be guaranteed; thus, he should be treated with IV antimicrobials.

ANTIMICROBIAL DOSING

Case 62-1, Question 11: What dose of IV ciprofloxacin should be given to R.G.? What factors must be taken into account in determining a proper antimicrobial dose?

The choice of dosing regimen is based on many factors. Table 62-9 provides a guide for the dosing of more commonly administered antimicrobials. Selection of the appropriate dosage should be based on evidence confirming the efficacy of the dosage in the treatment of a specific infection. Patient-specific factors, including weight, site of infection, and route of elimination, must also be considered in dosage selection. The patient's weight is important, particularly for agents with a low therapeutic index (e.g., aminoglycosides, imipenem, and flucytosine); these drugs should be dosed on a milligram per kilogram per day basis. Other agents with a more favorable adverse effect profile, such as cephalosporins, are less likely to require weight-specific dosing in most disease states.

Site of Infection

Site of infection results in different dosage requirements. An uncomplicated urinary tract infection requires lower doses considering the high urinary drug concentrations that are achieved with most renally cleared agents. In contrast, a more serious upper urinary tract infection, such as pyelonephritis, requires increased doses to ensure therapeutic drug levels in tissue and in serum.

Anatomic and Physiologic Barriers

Anatomic and physiologic barriers must also be considered in evaluating a dosing regimen. For example, penetration into cerebrospinal fluid requires high doses to ensure adequate antimicrobial concentrations.[25] Vitreous humor[26] and the prostate gland[27] are additional sites in which therapeutic antimicrobial concentrations are more difficult to achieve.

Route of Elimination

Route of elimination must also be considered in the dosage calculation. In general, antimicrobials are eliminated renally or nonrenally (metabolic or biliary). Renal function can be estimated via 24-hour urine collection or with equations, such as the Cockcroft and Gault equation[28]:

$$\text{Creatinine clearance} = ([140 - \text{age}] \times [\text{weight in kg}])/(72 \times \text{SCr}) \quad \text{(Eq. 62-1)}$$

Several anti-infectives are eliminated renally (Table 62-9). Most β-lactams are eliminated by the kidney. In contrast, ceftriaxone and most antistaphylococcal penicillins (e.g., nafcillin, oxacillin, and dicloxacillin) are eliminated both renally and nonrenally. Aminoglycosides, vancomycin, acyclovir, and ganciclovir are cleared primarily by the kidney. Thus, dosage adjustment is recommended for these drugs in patients with renal failure (Table 62-9). Because azithromycin, clindamycin, and metronidazole are primarily eliminated by the liver, no dose reduction is required in renal failure for these agents. Using the Cockcroft and Gault equation, R.G.'s age (63 years), weight (70 kg), and current serum

Table 62-9
Adult Antimicrobial Dosing Guidelines for Hospitalized Patients (Selected Drugs)

Drug	CrCl > 50 mL/minute	CrCl 10–50 mL/minute	CrCl <10 mL/minute (ESRD not on HD)	Dialysis (HD or CRRT)
Acyclovir	*Herpes simplex infections* 5 mg/kg/dose IV every 8 hours	5 mg/kg/dose IV every 12–24 hours	2.5 mg/kg IV every 24 hours	HD: 2.5 mg/kg IV ×1 now then 2.5 mg/kg every evening (give after HD on HD days) CRRT: 5 mg/kg every 24 hours
	HSV encephalitis/Herpes zoster 10 mg/kg/dose IV every 8 hours	10 mg/kg/dose IV every 12–24 hours	5 mg/kg IV every 24 hours	HD: 5 mg/kg IV ×1 now then 5 mg/kg every evening (give after HD on HD days) CRRT: 5–10 mg/kg every 12–24 hours
Ampicillin	*Meningitis or endovascular infection* 2 g IV every 4 hours *Uncomplicated infection* 2 g IV every 6 hours	2 g IV every 6 hours	1 g IV every 8–12 hours	HD: 1–2 g IV every 12 hours CRRT: 1–2 g IV every 6 hours
Ampicillin/sulbactam	3 g IV every 6 hours	1.5 g IV every 6 hours	1.5 g IV every 12 hours	HD: 1.5–3 g IV every 12 hours CRRT: 1.5 g IV every 6 hours
Aztreonam	2 g IV every 8 hours	2 g IV every 12 hours	1 g IV every 12 hours	HD: 1 g IV ×1 now then 1 g every evening (give after HD on HD days) CRRT: 2 g IV every 12 hours
Cefazolin	*Gram negative or complicated Gram positive* 2 g IV every 8 hours *Uncomplicated Gram positive* 1–2 g IV every 8 hours	1–2 g IV every 12 hours	1 g IV every 24 hours	HD: 2 g after HD only CRRT: 2 g IV every 12 hours
Caspofungin Severe hepatic dysfunction: 70 mg LD, then 35 mg IV daily	LD: 70 mg × 1, then 50 mg every 24 hours Increase maintenance dose to 70 mg when given with phenytoin, rifampin, carbamazepine, dexamethasone, nevirapine, efavirenz	No change	No change	No change
Cefepime Less severe infections Febrile neutropenia, meningitis, pseudomonas infections, critically ill patients	>60 mL/minute 2 g IV every 12 hours 2 g IV every 8 hours	**30–60 mL/minute:** 2 g IV every 24 hours; 2 g IV every 12 hours **10–30 mL/minute:** 1 g IV every 24 hours; 2 g IV every 24 hours	<10 mL/minute 500 mg IV every 24 hours 1 g IV every 24 hours	HD: 2 g after HD only CRRT: 2 g IV every 12 hours
Ceftazidime	2 g IV every 8 hours	2 g IV every 12–24 hours	500 mg IV every 24 hours	HD: 1 g after HD only CRRT: 2 g IV every 12 hours
Ceftriaxone Meningitis: 2 g every 12 hours Endocarditis and osteomyelitis: 2 g every 24 hours	1 g IV every 24 hours	No change	No change	No change

Table 62-9
Adult Antimicrobial Dosing Guidelines for Hospitalized Patients (Selected Drugs) (*continued*)

Drug	CrCl > 50 mL/minute	CrCl 10–50 mL/minute		CrCl <10 mL/minute (ESRD not on HD)	Dialysis (HD or CRRT)
Ciprofloxacin[IV-PO] Pseudomonas infections	400 mg IV every 12 hours 500–750 mg PO every 12 hours 400 mg IV every 8 hours 750 mg PO every 12 hours	30–50 mL/minute No change No change	10–30 mL/minute 200–400 mg IV every 12 hours 250–500 mg PO every 12 hours	< 10 mL/minute 200 IV every 12 hours 250 mg PO every 12 hours	HD: 400 mg IV every 24 hours or 500 mg PO every 24 hours (give after HD on HD days) CRRT: 400 mg IV every 12 hours
Clindamycin	600–900 mg IV every 8 hours	No change		No change	No change
Daptomycin Not effective in the treatment of pneumonia	4–10 mg/kg IV every 24 hours Dose depends on indication	<30 mL/minute 4–10 mg/kg IV every 48 hours			HD: 4–10 mg/kg IV every 48 hours CRRT: 4–10 mg/kg IV every 48 hours
Doxycycline[IV-PO]	100 mg IV/PO every 12 hours	No change		No change	No change
Ertapenem	1 g IV every 24 hours	<30 mL/minute 500 mg IV every 24 hours			HD: 500 mg every 24 hours CRRT: 500 mg every 24 hours
Ethambutol	15–20 mg/kg PO every 24 hours	<30 mL/minute 15–25 mg/kg 3 times/week			HD: 15–25 mg/kg 3 times/week (after HD) CRRT: 15–25 mg/kg 3 times/week
Fluconazole[IV-PO]	*Oropharyngeal candidiasis* 100 mg every 24 hours *Esophageal candidiasis* 200 mg every 24 hours *Severe infection* Loading dose of 800 mg then 400 mg every 24 hours	50–200 mg IV/PO every 24 hours		50–100 mg IV/PO every 24 hours	HD: 400 mg after HD only CRRT: 400–800 mg every 24 hours
Flucytosine (5FC)	*Meningitis* 25 mg/kg/dose PO every 6 hours	25–50 mL/minute 25 mg/kg/dose PO every 12 hours	10–25 mL/minute 25 mg/kg/dose PO every 24 hours	12.5 mg/kg/dose PO every 24 hours	HD: 12.5–25 mg/kg PO every 24 hours CRRT: 12.5–37.5 mg/kg/dose PO every 12–24 hours
Ganciclovir	>70 mL/minute 5 mg/kg/dose IV every 12 hours	50–69 mL/minute 2.5 mg/kg/dose IV every 12 hours	25–49 mL/minute 2.5 mg/kg IV every 24 hours	10–24 mL/minute 1.25 mg/kg IV every 24 hours	HD: 1.25 mg/kg after HD only CRRT: 2.5 mg/kg every 24 hours
Gentamicin	See Tobramycin	See Tobramycin	See Tobramycin		See Tobramycin
Imipenem	500 mg IV every 6–8 hours max 50 mg/kg/day	500 mg IV every 8 hours		<20 mL/minute 250–500 mg IV every 12 hours	HD: 250 mg IV every 12 hours CRRT: 500 mg IV every 8 hours
Isoniazid	300 mg PO every 24 hours	No change		No change	No change

(*continued*)

Table 62-9
Adult Antimicrobial Dosing Guidelines for Hospitalized Patients (Selected Drugs) (*continued*)

Drug	CrCl > 50 mL/minute	CrCl 10–50 mL/minute	CrCl <10 mL/minute (ESRD not on HD)	Dialysis (HD or CRRT)
Levofloxacin[IV-PO] Urinary tract infection Pneumonia Pseudomonas infections	250–500 mg IV/PO every 24 hours 750 mg IV/PO every 24 hours	500 mg ×1, then 250 mg IV/PO every 24 hours 750 mg ×1; then 750 IV/PO every 48 hours	500 mg ×1, then 250 mg IV/PO every 48 hours 750 mg ×1, then 500 mg IV/PO every 48 hours	HD: 500 mg ×1, then 250 mg every 48 hours CRRT: 500 mg ×1, then 250–500 mg every 24 hours
Linezolid[IV-PO]	600 mg IV/PO every 12 hours	No change	No change	No change
Meropenem Meningitis, documented or suspected Pseudomonas infections or critically ill	0.5–1 g IV every 8 hours 2 g IV every 8 hours	25–50 mL/minute: 0.5–1 g IV every 12 hours; 2 g IV every 12 hours 10–25 mL/minute: 0.5 g IV every 12 hours; 1 g IV every 12 hours	0.5 g IV every 24 hours 1 g IV every 24 hours	HD: 500 mg IV ×1 now then 500 mg every evening (give after HD on HD days) CRRT: 1 g IV every 12 hours
Metronidazole[IV-PO]	500 mg IV/PO every 8 hours	500 mg IV/PO every 8 hours	500 mg IV/PO every 12 hours ESRD not on HD	500 mg IV/PO every 8 hours
Moxifloxacin[IV-PO]	400 mg IV/PO every 24 hours	No change	No change	No change
Nafcillin Meningitis, osteomyelitis, endovascular infection	1–2 g IV every 4–6 hours 2 g IV every 4 hours	No change	No change	No change
Penicillin G Meningitis, endovascular infection	2–3 MU IV every 4–6 hours 3–4 MU IV every 4–6 hours	1–2 MU IV every 4–6 hours	1 MU IV every 6 hours	HD: 1 MU IV every 6 hours CRRT: 2 MU IV every 4–6 hours
Piperacillin/ tazobactam (Zosyn) Documented/suspected Pseudomonas infections	3.375–4.5 g IV every 6–8 hours 4.5 g every 6 hours for CrCl >20 mL/minute	3.375–4.5 g every 6–8 hours	2.25 g every 8 hours	HD: 2.25 g IV every 8 hours CRRT: 4.5 g IV every 8 hours or 3.375 g IV every 6 hours
Posaconazole Must be administered with high-fat meal or nutritional shake, e.g., Ensure Neutropenia prophylaxis	400 mg PO every 12 hours or 200 mg PO every 6 hours 200 mg PO every 8 hours	No change	No change	No change
Pyrazinamide	20–25 mg/kg/day PO every 24 hours	<30 mL/minute 25–35 mg/kg 3 times/week		HD: 25–35 mg/kg 3 times/week after HD CRRT: 25–35 mg/kg 3 times/week
Rifampin Mycobacterial infection Endocarditis Prosthetic device infection	600 mg PO every 24 hours 300 mg PO every 8 hours 450 mg PO every 12 hours	No change	No change	No change
Tigecycline Severe hepatic disease: 100 mg IV ×1, then 25 mg IV every 12 hours	100 mg IV × 1, then 50 mg IV every 12 hours	No change	No change	No change

Table 62-9
Adult Antimicrobial Dosing Guidelines for Hospitalized Patients (Selected Drugs) (*continued*)

Drug	CrCl > 50 mL/minute	CrCl 10–50 mL/minute	CrCl <10 mL/minute (ESRD not on HD)	Dialysis (HD or CRRT)
Tobramycin (and gentamicin) Gram negative infection Dose is based on ideal body weight (IBW) except in obese patients or those under their IBW. Use actual body weight if patient weight is less than IBW. Use adjusted body weight if patient is obese. (calculations see below)	For CrCl > 60 mL/minute, not morbidly obese or fluid overloaded, give once daily regimen: 7 mg/kg/dose IV every 24 hours. For those patients not qualifying for once daily dosing, see conventional dosing below.			
For conventional dosing peak and trough levels should be monitored.	>60 mL/minute 1.6 mg/kg IV every 8 hours	40–60 mL/minute 1.2–1.5 mg/kg every 12–24 hours	<20 mL/minute 2 mg/kg loading dose, then follow drug levels	HD: 2 mg/kg IV × 1 then 1 mg/kg IV after HD CRRT: 2 mg/kg IV × 1 then 1.5 mg/kg IV every 24 hours
TMP/SMX[IV-PO] When switching to oral therapy, consider that a single-strength tablet has 80 mg of TMP, a double-strength tablet 160 mg of TMP.	*Systemic GNR infections* 10 mg TMP/kg/day IV divided every 6–12 hours *Pneumocystis pneumonia* 15–20 mg TMP/kg/day IV divided every 6–8 hours	5–7.5 mg TMP/kg/day IV divided every 12–24 hours 10–15 mg TMP/kg/day IV divided every 12–24 hours	2.5–5.0 mg TMP/kg IV every 24 hours 5–10 mg TMP/kg IV every 24 hours	HD: 2.5–5 mg TMP/kg/day every 24 hours CRRT: 5–7.5mg TMP/kg/day divided every 12–24 hours
Vancomycin Uncomplicated infections Serious infections	>60 mL/minute 10–15 mg/kg IV every 12 hours[1] 15–20 mg/kg IV every 8–12 hours[2] 40–60 mL/minute 10–15 mg/kg IV every 12–24 hours	20–40 mL/minute 5–10 mg/kg IV every 24 hours 10–20 mL/minute 5–10 mg/kg IV every 24–48 hours	<10 mL/minute 10–15 mg/kg IV loading dose ×1; redose according to serum levels	HD: 15–20 mg/kg load, then 500 mg IV after HD only CRRT: 10–15 mg/kg IV every 24 hours
Round dose to 250 mg, 500 mg, 750 mg, 1 g, 1.25 g, 1.5 g, 1.75 g, or 2 g (maximum 2 g/dose). Trough levels should be obtained within 30 minutes before fourth dose of a new regimen or dosage change. Vancomycin troughs are *not* recommended in patients in whom anticipated duration of therapy is ≤3 days. [1] For patients with uncomplicated infections requiring vancomycin, trough levels of 10–15 mcg/mL are recommended. [2] For patients with serious infections caused by MRSA (central nervous system infections, endocarditis, ventilator-associated pneumonia, bacteremia, or osteomyelitis), trough levels of 15–20 mcg/mL are recommended.				
Voriconazole[IV-PO]	LD = 400 mg every 12 hours × 1 day, then 200 mg every 12 hours (PO)	No change	No change*	No change*
PO should be used when possible, as oral bioavailability >95%. IV dose: LD = 6 mg/kg/dose every 12 hours × 1 day, then 4 mg/kg/dose every 12 hours. *The use of the IV formulation should be avoided in patients with CrCl <50 mL/minute owing to accumulation of IV vehicle and is contraindicated in ESRD and hemodialysis. May require dose adjustment in hepatic dysfunction.				

Doses are those recommended for systemic infections in hospitalized patients commonly treated with these agents for moderate/severe infections. Abstracted in part from doses developed by the UCSF Antibiotic Advisory Subcommittee and the Pharmacy & Therapeutics Committee (updated 6/2015). More mild infection may require decreased doses compared with moderate to severe infection. Dosing guidelines may differ in other institutions.

Estimate of renal function using Cockcroft and Gault equation: CrCl (mL/minute) = (140 – age) × Wt (kg)/72 × SCr (mg/dL) (for females multiply by 0.85).

Ideal body weight equation:

Males: IBW = 50 kg + 2.3 kg for each inch over 5 feet.

Females: IBW = 45.5 kg + 2.3 kg for each inch over 5 feet.

Adjusted body weight: ABW = IBW + 0.4 (actual weight – IBW).

CrCl, creatinine clearance; CRRT, continuous renal replacement therapy (assumes an ultrafiltration rate of 2 L/hour with continuous venovenous hemofiltration and an ultrafiltration rate of 1 L/hour and dialysate flow rate of 1 L/hour with continuous venovenous hemodiafiltration and residual native glomerular filtration rate <10 mL/minute); ESRD, end-stage renal disease; HD, intermittent (high-flux) hemodialysis (when administering a daily dose with HD, the drug should be administered after the HD session); HSV, herpes simplex virus; IV, intravenous; IV-PO, high oral bioavailability (consider initiating with or switching to PO therapy when patient tolerating orals); LD, loading dose; MRSA, methicillin-resistant *Staphylococcus aureus*; PO, by mouth; SCr, serum creatinine.

creatinine (3.8 mg/dL) results in a calculated creatinine clearance of 14 mL/minute. R.G. normally would be given an IV dosage of ciprofloxacin at 400 mg every 12 hours. His increasing creatinine, however, suggests that his dosage should be decreased to 200 to 300 mg every 12 hours.

Although renal function can be approximated with the use of the Cockcroft and Gault equation (or a similar equation), hepatic function is more difficult to evaluate. No standard liver function test (AST, ALT, alkaline phosphatase) has been demonstrated to correlate well with hepatic drug clearance. Some tests, such as PT, INR, and albumin, are markers of hepatic function, but even these tests do not clearly predict drug clearance. Patients receiving hemodialysis or continuous hemofiltration provide additional dosing challenges. Table 62-9 provides dosing recommendations in patients receiving hemodialysis or continuous hemofiltration.

Patient Age

It is important to note that most dosing information is derived from a younger, relatively healthy patient population. It is clear that the very young and the elderly have a decreased ability to clear drugs; thus, dosage requirements for many agents are likely to be decreased in neonatal and geriatric patients.

Fever and Inoculum Effect

The impact of other factors on the selection of an antimicrobial dose is less clear. Fever increases and decreases blood flow to mesenteric, hepatic, and renal organ systems,[29] and it can either increase or decrease drug clearance. Inoculum effect has taken place when higher concentrations of a bacterial inoculum result in an increase in the MIC.[30] As an example, piperacillin may demonstrate an MIC of 8.0 mcg/mL against *P. aeruginosa* at a concentration of 10^5 colony-forming units/mL (CFU/mL); however, at 10^9 CFU/mL, the MIC may increase to 32 to 64 mcg/mL. This phenomenon is well recognized, particularly with β-lactamase–producing bacteria treated with β-lactam antimicrobials. The more stable the antimicrobial is to β-lactamase, the less the influence of the inoculum effect. Aminoglycosides, quinolones, and imipenem appear to be less affected by the inoculum effect than β-lactams. The inoculum effect probably is most relevant in the treatment of a bacterial abscess, in which extremely high concentrations of bacteria would be expected. As a result, antimicrobials that are more susceptible to the inoculum effect may require increased drug dosages for optimal outcome in the treatment of abscesses.

PHARMACOKINETICS AND PHARMACODYNAMICS

CASE 62-1, QUESTION 12: R.G.'s respiratory status remains unchanged; thus, the ciprofloxacin is discontinued and cefepime and gentamicin are started empirically. The use of a prolonged 3 hour IV infusion of cefepime is being considered in R.G. In addition, the use of single daily dosing of gentamicin is being discussed. What is the rationale for these approaches, and would either be advantageous for R.G.?

β-Lactams, such as cefepime, are not associated with increased bacterial killing with increasing drug concentrations. Pharmacodynamic activity with β-lactams best correlates with the duration of time that antimicrobial levels are maintained above the MIC.[31] The animal model suggests that β-lactam antimicrobials should be dosed such that their serum levels exceed the MIC of the pathogen as long as possible.[31] This observation appears to be most important in the neutropenic model, in which the use of a constant infusion more reliably inhibits bacterial growth compared with traditional intermittent dosing. An additional benefit of the use of constant infusions of β-lactams is that smaller daily doses appear to be as effective as higher doses administered intermittently. Other than this latter outcome, it is unclear, however, whether constant infusions have any distinct advantages or disadvantages compared with usual dosing of β-lactams. The efficacy of quinolones, vancomycin, and daptomycin best correlates with the peak plasma concentration to MIC ratio or area under the curve (AUC) to MIC ratio.[31] In light of this pharmacodynamic principle, it is possible that ciprofloxacin was underdosed in this patient, contributing to the therapeutic failure, particularly if the MIC was in the upper range of susceptibility for this agent.

Aminoglycosides traditionally have been administered every 8 to 12 hours to achieve peak serum gentamicin levels of 5 to 8 mcg/mL to ensure efficacy in the treatment of serious gram-negative infection.[32,33] Gentamicin troughs of greater than 2 mcg/mL have been associated with an increased risk for nephrotoxicity.[33,34] These studies attempting to correlate efficacy and toxicity with serum levels and the association of peaks or troughs with clinical outcomes have been questioned.[21] Vancomycin troughs of 5 to 10 mcg/mL have been traditionally recommended[35,36]; however, current recommendations suggest higher troughs (10–20 mcg/mL) depending on the pathogen, site of infection, and severity of illness.[37]

Several antimicrobials (e.g., aminoglycosides) have been associated with a pharmacodynamic phenomenon known as a post-antibiotic effect (PAE). PAE is delayed regrowth of bacteria after exposure to an antibiotic[31,38] (i.e., continued suppression of normal growth in the absence of antibiotic levels above the MIC of the organism). As an example, if *P. aeruginosa* is cultured in broth, it will multiply to a concentration of 10^9 CFU/mL. If piperacillin is added in a concentration above the MIC for the organism, a reduction in the bacterial concentration is observed. As described previously, a β-lactam antibiotic should be present in concentrations above the MIC to optimize its time-dependent killing. When piperacillin is removed from the broth, immediate bacterial growth takes place. If the above experiment is repeated with gentamicin, a reduction in bacterial CFU is observed. In contrast to that observed with β-lactam antibiotics, if the gentamicin is removed from the system, a lag period of 2 to 6 hours takes place before characteristic bacterial growth occurs. This lag period is defined as the PAE. A PAE has also been observed with quinolones and imipenem against gram-negative bacteria. Although most β-lactam antibiotics, such as antipseudomonal penicillins or cephalosporins, do not exhibit PAE with gram-negative organisms, PAE has been demonstrated with β-lactam with gram-positive pathogens such as *S. aureus*.

Once-Daily Dosing of Aminoglycosides

As a result of PAE and other pharmacodynamic factors, certain antimicrobials may be dosed less frequently. The greatest clinical experience has been with the aminoglycosides in the treatment of gram-negative infection.[39,40] Earlier data suggested that the maximal aminoglycoside peak level to MIC ratio correlates well with clinical response. Thus, the higher the achievable peak, the greater likelihood of a favorable outcome. Consequently, greater, less frequent doses of aminoglycosides should work at least as well as the more traditional lower, more frequent doses. Once-daily dosing of aminoglycosides in the treatment of gram-negative infection is as efficacious as traditional multiple daily dosing.[21]

Single daily dosing of aminoglycosides has been investigated primarily in patients with normal renal function, and few critically ill patients have been treated with this nontraditional regimen.

Thus, patients in septic shock are less clear candidates for once-daily dosing. The utility and proper timing of serum aminoglycoside concentrations and association with clinical outcomes are debatable with nontraditional once-daily aminoglycosides.

In summary, the use of a prolonged IV infusion of cefepime is possible in R.G., but the benefit of this mode of administration is not clear. Considering the severity of R.G.'s infection and his elevated serum creatinine level, he is not a candidate for single daily dosing of aminoglycosides (i.e., 5–6 mg/kg every 24 hours). Independent of the aminoglycoside-associated PAE, his current renal function requires a reduced gentamicin dose to treat his infection.

Antimicrobial Protein Binding

CASE 62-1, QUESTION 13: Ceftriaxone (Rocephin), rather than cefepime, is being considered for the treatment of R.G.'s infection. Ceftriaxone is more highly protein bound than cefepime. Why is protein binding important in the selection of therapy?

Free (i.e., unbound) rather than total drug levels are best correlated with antimicrobial activity,[41] and the degree of protein binding may have important clinical consequences in some patients. Chambers et al.[42] reported treatment failures with the highly protein-bound cefonicid (98% protein bound) in patients with endocarditis caused by *S. aureus*. Despite achievable serum drug concentrations well above the MIC of the organism, breakthrough bacteremia occurred in three of four patients. Although total drug concentrations greatly exceeded the MIC of the pathogen, free concentrations were consistently below the level necessary to inhibit bacterial growth. Similar experiences have been reported with daptomycin (90% to 93% protein bound).[43] Thus, clinical cure appears to be more likely if unbound antibiotic concentrations exceed the MIC of the infecting organism. Although ceftriaxone is 85% to 90% protein bound, the free concentrations probably remain far above the MIC of the *Serratia*. Therefore, protein-binding considerations are unlikely to be important in the treatment of R.G.'s infection.

ANTIMICROBIAL FAILURE

Antibiotic-Specific Factors

CASE 62-1, QUESTION 14: Despite "appropriate" treatment, R.G. is unresponsive to antimicrobial therapy. What antibiotic-specific factors may contribute to "antimicrobial failure"?

Antimicrobials may fail for various reasons, including patient-specific host factors, drug or dosage selection, and concomitant disease states. One of the most common reasons for antimicrobial failure is drug resistance.[44–46] Several clinically important pathogens have been associated with emergence of resistance during the past decade, including *M. tuberculosis*,[47] enterococci,[48] gram-negative rods,[44] *S. aureus*,[49] *S. pneumoniae*,[50] and others. Of particular concern is the isolation of glycopeptide-resistant *S. aureus*,[49] and multidrug-resistant *Acinetobacter* and *Pseudomonas*.[51] Development of resistance during therapy, although less common than initial intrinsic resistance, may also account for failure to respond to therapy. Organisms that produce extended-spectrum β-lactamase or amp C β-lactamases may be unresponsive to β-lactam therapy despite associated in-vitro susceptibility.[52]

Superinfection may also play a role in the unsuccessful treatment of infection. Superinfection has taken place when a new pathogen resistant to the current antimicrobial regimen is isolated. If R.G.'s ceftriaxone-treated *Serratia* pneumonia subsequently worsens and a tracheal aspirate returns positive for *P. aeruginosa*, then supercolonization and, perhaps, superinfection have occurred.

Combination Therapy

Most infections can be treated with monotherapy (e.g., an *E. coli* wound infection is treatable with a cephalosporin). Some infections, however, require two-drug therapy, including most cases of enterococcal endocarditis and perhaps certain *P. aeruginosa* infections. Hilf et al.[53] studied 200 consecutive patients with *P. aeruginosa* bacteremia and demonstrated a 47% mortality in those receiving monotherapy (antipseudomonal β-lactam or aminoglycoside) versus 27% in those in whom two-drug therapy was used. Thus, monotherapy appeared to contribute to antimicrobial failure in this specific study.

In contrast to the findings of the previous trial, almost all later investigations do not support the use of two drugs over monotherapy in the treatment of serious gram-negative infection, including *P. aeruginosa*.[54–56] An exception to this rule is bacteremia caused by *P. aeruginosa* in neutropenic patients.

If two antimicrobials are used in the treatment of infection, one of three sequelae will result: indifference, synergism, or antagonism.[57] Indifference occurs when the antimicrobial effect of drug A plus that of drug B equals the anticipated sum activity of the two drugs. Although numerous definitions exist, synergism generally occurs when the addition of drug A to drug B results in a total antibiotic activity greater than the expected sum of the two agents. Antagonism occurs if the addition of drug A to drug B results in a combined activity less than the sum of drug A plus drug B. An example of antagonism is the combination of imipenem with a less β-lactamase–stable β-lactam, such as piperacillin.[58] If *P. aeruginosa* is exposed to imipenem and piperacillin, the imipenem induces the organism to produce increased β-lactamase. Imipenem is remarkably β-lactamase stable and is not degraded by this β-lactamase. In direct contrast, piperacillin is easily degraded by the β-lactamase. Thus, imipenem antagonized the effectiveness of piperacillin. Antagonism is not unique to antibacterials; itraconazole may antagonize amphotericin B in the treatment of certain fungal infections.[59]

Pharmacologic Factors

CASE 62-1, QUESTION 15: What pharmacologic or pharmaceutic factors may be implicated in failure of therapy?

Subtherapeutic dosing regimens are commonplace, particularly for agents with a low therapeutic index, such as the aminoglycosides. For example, a serious gram-negative pneumonia may not respond to aminoglycoside therapy if the achievable peak gentamicin serum levels are only 3 to 4 mcg/mL.[21,32] Considering that only 20% to 30% of the aminoglycoside penetrates from serum into bronchial secretions, only 0.5 to 1.0 mcg/mL may exist at the site of infection,[60] a level that may be inadequate to treat pneumonia. Another example of dosing contributing to antimicrobial failure centers on the use of loading doses. Aminoglycosides or vancomycin should be initiated with a loading dose, particularly in patients with renal failure. If the clinician neglects to use a loading dose, it may take several days before a therapeutic level is achieved. As described previously, yet another reason for subtherapeutic antimicrobial levels and potential drug failure is reduced oral absorption secondary to drug interactions (e.g., concomitant oral ciprofloxacin with antacids or iron).

An emerging problem relates to the use of vancomycin in the treatment of serious methicillin-resistant *S. aureus* (MRSA) infection. By CLSI standards, an isolate of MRSA with an MIC of 2 mcg/mL is considered susceptible. Current vancomycin dosing schemes are designed to achieve an AUC/MIC ratio of ≥400 to ensure maximal efficacy. However, a meta-analysis of patients with *S. aureus* bacteremia demonstrated no differences in the risk of death when comparing patients with *S. aureus* exhibiting high-vancomycin MIC (≥1.5 mg/L) to those with low-vancomycin MIC (<1.5 mg/L).[61] The infection site also potentially contributes to antimicrobial failure. Most antimicrobials concentrate in the urine, resulting in therapeutic levels even with low doses. In some infections, such as meningitis, prostatitis, and endophthalmitis, antimicrobial penetration to the site of infection may be inadequate. Agents that penetrate well into these sites are associated with a more favorable outcome.

Another potential reason for antimicrobial failure is inadequate therapy duration. A woman with a first-time uncomplicated cystitis may respond adequately to a 3-day course of an antibiotic. In contrast, patients with recurrent urinary tract infections are not candidates for this short course of therapy, however, and failure would be expected with only 3 days of therapy.

Host Factors

Case 62-1, Question 16: What host factors may contribute to the failure of antimicrobial therapy?

Several host factors may limit the ability of an antibiotic to cure infection. Infection of prosthetic material (e.g., IV catheters, orthopedic prostheses, mechanical cardiac valves, and vascular grafts) is difficult to eradicate without removal of the hardware. In most cases, surgical intervention is necessary. To treat R.G.'s IV catheter infection adequately, removal of his central intravenous catheter would be optimal. Similar to removal of prostheses, large undrained abscesses are difficult, if not impossible, to treat with antimicrobial therapy. These infections generally require surgical drainage for successful outcome.

Diabetic foot ulcer cellulitis may not respond adequately to antimicrobial therapy. Reasons for antimicrobial failure in patients with diabetes include poor wound healing and reduced delivery of antibiotics to the infection site.

Immune status, particularly neutropenia or lymphocytopenia, also affects the outcome in the treatment of infection. Profoundly, neutropenic patients with disseminated *Aspergillus* infections are unlikely to respond to even the most appropriate antifungal therapy. Similarly, patients with AIDS, who have low CD4 lymphocyte counts, cannot eradicate various infections, including those caused by cytomegalovirus, atypical mycobacteria, and cryptococci.

Once these factors have been eliminated as causes for antimicrobial failure, noninfectious sources must be ruled out. As discussed, malignancy, autoimmune disease, drug fever, and other diseases must be evaluated.

Case 62-1, Question 17: Other than initiation of adequate antimicrobial therapy, what adjunct measures can be considered in this patient with septic shock?

The 2013 Surviving Sepsis Campaign: International Guidelines for Management of Severe Sepsis and Septic Shock consultants developed key recommendations toward the early goal-directed resuscitation of the septic patient.[62] These recommendations include the use of "sepsis bundles", i.e., multiple interventions taking place at the same time. Key recommended adjuncts include administration of broad-spectrum antibiotics within 1 hour of diagnosis of septic shock, administration of either crystalloid or colloid fluid resuscitation, and norepinephrine or dopamine to maintain mean arterial pressure of at least 65 mm Hg. In addition, stress-dose steroid therapy can be given to those patients whose blood pressure is poorly responsive to fluid resuscitation and vasopressors. While one might expect improved survival with adherence to such guidelines, the results have been mixed. A large meta-analysis evaluated the influence of performance improvement programs regarding compliance with sepsis bundles. These programs have been found to be associated with increased adherence to resuscitation and management sepsis bundles and with reduced mortality in patients with sepsis, severe sepsis, or septic shock.[63] In contrast, in patients with septic shock who were identified early and received intravenous antibiotics and adequate fluid resuscitation, hemodynamic management according to a strict early goal-directed therapy protocol did not lead to an improvement in outcome.[64]

KEY REFERENCES AND WEBSITES

A full list of references for this chapter can be found at http://thepoint.lww.com/AT11e. Below are the key references and websites for this chapter, with the corresponding reference number in this chapter found in parentheses after the reference.

Key References

Angus DC, van der Poll T. Severe sepsis and septic shock. *N Engl J Med*. 2013;369(9):840. (3)

Boucher HW et al. Bad bugs, no drugs: No ESKAPE! An update from the Infectious Diseases Society of America. *Clin Infect Dis*. 2009;48(1):1. (44)

Czock D et al. Pharmacokinetics and pharmacodynamics of antimicrobial drugs. *Expert Opin Drug Metab Toxicol*. 2009;5(5):475. (31)

Dellinger RP et al. Surviving sepsis campaign: international guidelines for management of severe sepsis and septic shock. *Intensive Care Med*. 2013;39(2):165. (62)

Hooton TM et al. Diagnosis, prevention, and treatment of catheter-associated urinary tract infection in adults: 2009 International Clinical Practice Guidelines from the Infectious Diseases Society of America. *Clin Infect Dis*. 2010;50(5):625. (12)

Horowitz HW. Fever of unknown origin or fever of too many origins? *N Engl J Med*. 2013;368(3):197. (10)

Kalil AC et al. Association between vancomycin minimum inhibitory concentration and mortality among patients with Staphylococcus aureus bloodstream infections: a systematic review and meta-analysis. *JAMA*. 2014;312(15):1552. (61)

Mandell LA et al. Infectious Diseases Society of America/American Thoracic Society consensus guidelines on the management of community-acquired pneumonia in adults. *Clin Infect Dis*. 2007;44(Suppl 2):S27. (15)

Rybak MJ et al. Vancomycin therapeutic guidelines: a summary of consensus recommendations from the infectious diseases Society of America, the American Society of Health-System Pharmacists, and the Society of Infectious Diseases Pharmacists. *Clin Infect Dis*. 2009;49(3):325. (37)

Solomkin JS et al. Diagnosis and management of complicated intra-abdominal infection in adults and children: guidelines by the Surgical Infection Society and the Infectious Diseases Society of America [published correction appears in *Clin Infect Dis*. 2010;50(12):1695]. *Clin Infect Dis*. 2010;50(2):133. (13)

Vincent JL et al. Evolving concepts in sepsis definitions. *Crit Care Clin*. 2009;25(4):665, vii. (1)

Wacker C et al. Procalcitonin as a diagnostic marker for sepsis: a systematic review and meta-analysis. *Lancet Infect Dis*. 2013;13(5):426. (4)

Weisfelt M et al. Bacterial meningitis: a review of effective pharmacotherapy. *Expert Opin Pharmacother*. 2007;8(10):1493. (25)

63 Antimicrobial Prophylaxis for Surgical Procedures

Daniel J. G. Thirion

CORE PRINCIPLES

		CHAPTER CASES
1	Assessment of the risk of infection is based on patient and procedure risk factors.	**Case 63-1 (Question 1)**
2	Surgical antibiotic prophylaxis is indicated for patients at high risk of infection or in those at high risk of complications from postoperative infection.	**Case 63-2 (Question 1), Case 63-4 (Question 1)**
3	The choice of agent is based on the most likely pathogen associated with surgical site infection. Institutional patterns of pathogens, their resistance profiles, and antibiotic cost impact agent selection.	**Case 63-2 (Question 2), Case 63-6 (Questions 1, 2), Case 63-7 (Question 1), Case 63-8 (Question 1)**
4	To maximize the benefit of prophylaxis, antibiotic administration should be completed within 1 hour before incision to achieve adequate drug levels at the surgical site.	**Case 63-2 (Question 3), Case 63-5 (Question 1)**
5	Intravenous administration is most commonly used. Coadministration of an oral regimen is recommended in colorectal surgery.	
6	Antimicrobials with shorter half-lives may require administration of an additional intraoperative dose in prolonged surgical cases.	**Case 63-2 (Question 4)**
7	Single-dose preoperative prophylaxis is sufficient for most surgical procedures.	**Case 63-3 (Questions 1, 2), Case 63-5 (Question 1)**
8	Continuation of postoperative prophylaxis for up to 24 hours in cardiac surgery has been recommended by some professional organizations.	**Case 63-4 (Question 1)**
9	Continuation of prophylaxis beyond these time frames is not associated with improved outcomes and increases the risk of superinfections, emergence of resistance, adverse effects, and cost.	**Case 63-8 (Question 2)**
10	Surgical site infections are classified as superficial or deep incisional and usually occur within 30 days after the surgical procedure. Deep organ or space infections can occur up to several months after surgery and up to a year after implantation of prosthetic material.	**Case 63-5 (Question 2)**
11	Continuous quality improvement is critical in the prevention of surgical infection and should be overseen by a multidisciplinary team.	**Case 63-9 (Question 1)**

Surgical site infection (SSI) occurs when a pathogenic organism multiplies in a surgical wound, leading to local and sometimes systemic signs and symptoms. Infections complicate surgical procedures in about 2% to 5% of cases but can be as high as 20%, depending on the surgical procedure and the patient.[1–3] Surgical site infections are the most common health-care associated infections.[2] They put patients at risk of death, increase morbidity, extend the duration of hospitalization,[4] and are associated with an annual cost of $3.5 billion to $10 billion in the United States.[5,6]

Prophylactic antibiotics are widely used in surgical procedures and account for substantial antibiotic use in many hospitals.[7] The purpose of surgical antibiotic prophylaxis is to reduce the prevalence of postoperative wound infection. Appropriate use of prophylactic antimicrobial agents results in decreased patient morbidity and hospitalization costs for many surgical procedures.[8] However, the benefits of prophylaxis are questionable for surgical procedures at low risk of infection (e.g., urologic operations in patients with sterile urine).[9] Consequently, inappropriate or indiscriminate use of prophylactic antibiotics can expose the patient to unnecessary risk of drug toxicity and superinfections, promotes the selection of resistant organisms, and increases cost.[10–12]

RISK FACTORS FOR INFECTION

CASE 63-1

QUESTION 1: C.P., a 78-year-old woman with osteoarthritis, is hospitalized for an elective hip surgery. She is 165 cm tall, weighs 90 kg, and is a nonsmoker. The surgery is planned to last within the usual time frame of the operation, which is about 1 to 2 hours. What is the risk of infection following surgery for her?

The likelihood for development of postoperative site infection is related to the degree of bacterial contamination during surgery, the virulence of the infecting organism, and host defenses. Risk factors for postoperative site infection can be classified according to procedure-specific factors and patient characteristics.[13–15] Bacterial contamination can occur from exogenous sources (e.g., the operative team, instruments, airborne organisms) or from endogenous sources (e.g., the patient's microflora of the skin, respiratory, genitourinary, or gastrointestinal [GI] tract).[16] Procedure-specific factors such as the surgeon's experience and technique, the duration of the procedure, and the operating room environment have important influence on SSI rates. Infection control procedures to minimize all sources of bacterial contamination, including patient and surgical team preparation, operative technique, and incision care, are compiled in Centers for Disease Control and Prevention guidelines for surgical site infection.[17]

The risk of postoperative wound infection is influenced by host factors, such as extremes of age, obesity, tobacco use, malnutrition, and comorbid states, including diabetes mellitus, glycemic control in diabetic patients, remote infection, ischemia, oxygenation and body temperature during the procedure, colonization with microorganisms, immune status, and immunosuppressive therapy.[9]

Measuring and predicting risk of infection determines which patients should receive antibiotic prophylaxis. The Centers for Disease Control and Prevention Study on the Efficacy of Nosocomial Infection Control (SENIC) developed an index that included the level of wound contamination and three other criteria based on procedure-related and patient-related factors.[18] Modification of this tool has led to the National Nosocomial Infection Surveillance (NNIS) System risk index that takes into account the patient's preoperative assessment (American Society of Anesthesiologists Assessment),[19] the level of contamination of the procedure, the duration of the procedure, and the use of a laparoscope.[13] This last criterion was added because of the associated decreased incidence of infection with the introduction of laparoscopic procedures. Indexes like these are particularly useful for comparison of performance among institutions and public reporting.

Based on these risk factors for infection, the decision whether a given patient should receive antimicrobial prophylaxis depends on a number of factors. Antimicrobial prophylaxis should be given for surgical procedures (a) with a high rate of infection (i.e., clean-contaminated or contaminated procedures), or (b) involving the implantation of prosthetic materials, or (c) in which an infection would have catastrophic consequences.[9] A widely used surgical wound classification system to assist in this decision-making process follows.

C.P. is at relatively low risk of infection. There is only one point as attributed to the NNIS score because she will undergo a clean surgery within the average time frame. Her American Society of Anesthesiologists score is 2, being known with mild systemic disease (obese, rheumatoid arthritis, age over 60).

CLASSIFICATION OF SURGICAL SITE INFECTIONS

From 1960 to 1964, the National Academy of Sciences National Research Council conducted a landmark study of surgical site infections and formulated a widely used standard classification based on the risk of intraoperative bacterial contamination (Table 63-1).[20] Current recommendations for surgical prophylaxis pertain to clean surgeries at high risk of complications and/or involving implantation of prosthetic material, clean-contaminated surgeries, and select contaminated wounds. Antimicrobial therapy for dirty surgeries in which infection already is established is considered treatment instead of prophylaxis and is not discussed further in this chapter. Table 63-2 lists suspected pathogens and recommendations for

Table 63-1
National Research Council Wound Classification

Classification	Criteria	Infection Rate (%) without Antibiotic Prophylaxis	Infection Rate (%) with Antibiotic Prophylaxis
Clean	No acute inflammation or entry into GI, respiratory, GU, or biliary tracts; no break in aseptic technique occurs; wounds primarily closed	>5	0.8
Clean-contaminated	Elective, controlled opening of GI, respiratory, biliary, or GU tracts without significant spillage; clean wounds with major break in sterile technique	>10	1.3
Contaminated	Penetrating trauma (<4 hours old); major technique break or major spillage from GI tract; acute, nonpurulent inflammation	15–20	10.2
Dirty	Penetrating trauma (>4 hours old); purulence or abscess (active infectious process); preoperative perforation of viscera	30–100	Therapeutic antibiotics

GI, gastrointestinal; GU, genitourinary.
Adapted from Berard F, Gandon J. Postoperative wound infections: the influence of ultraviolet irradiation of the operating room and of various other factors. *Ann Surg*. 1964;160(Suppl 2):1.

Table 63-2
Suggested Prophylactic Antimicrobial Regimens for Surgical Procedures

Procedure	Predominant Organisms	Recommended Agent(s)[a,b]	Alternative Agents[a,b]
Clean			
Neurosurgery	*Staphylococcus aureus*, *Staphylococcus epidermidis*	Cefazolin	Clindamycin, vancomycin
Cardiac (all with sternotomy, cardiopulmonary bypass, pacemaker, and automated defibrillator placement)	*S. aureus*, *S. epidermidis*	Cefazolin	Cefuroxime, clindamycin, vancomycin
Thoracic	*S. aureus*, *S. epidermidis*, gram-negative enterics	Cefazolin	Ampicillin–sulbactam, clindamycin, vancomycin
Vascular (aortic resection, groin incision, prosthesis)	*S. aureus*, *S. epidermidis*, gram-negative enterics	Cefazolin	Clindamycin, vancomycin
Orthopedic (total joint replacement, internal fixation of fractures)	*S. aureus*, *S. epidermidis*	Cefazolin	Clindamycin, vancomycin
Clean-Contaminated			
Head and neck (involving incisions through mucosa)	*S. aureus*, oral anaerobes, streptococci	Cefazolin + metronidazole	Ampicillin–sulbactam, clindamycin
Gastroduodenal (only for procedures entering the stomach)	Gram-negative enterics, *S. aureus*, mouth flora	Cefazolin	Clindamycin or vancomycin + aminoglycoside
Appendectomy (uncomplicated)	Gram-negative enterics, anaerobes (*Bacteroides fragilis*), enterococci	Cefoxitin	Cefazolin + metronidazole, metronidazole + aminoglycoside
Biliary tract (only for high-risk procedures)	Gram-negative enterics, enterococci, Clostridia	Cefazolin	Cefoxitin, ampicillin–sulbactam, clindamycin + aminoglycoside
Colorectal	Gram-negative enterics, anaerobes (*B. fragilis*), enterococci	Cefazolin + metronidazole	Ampicillin–sulbactam, metronidazole + aminoglycoside
Cesarean section	Group B streptococci, enterococci, anaerobes, gram-negative enterics	Cefazolin	Clindamycin + aminoglycoside
Hysterectomy	Group B streptococci, enterococci, anaerobes, gram-negative enterics	Cefazolin	Clindamycin or vancomycin + aminoglycoside
Genitourinary (only for high-risk procedures)	Gram-negative enterics, enterococci	Fluoroquinolone	Aminoglycoside + clindamycin

[a]Dose of antibiotics are ampicillin–sulbactam 3 g, cefazolin 2 g in patients weighing up to 120 kg and 3 g if weighing more than 120 kg, cefuroxime 1.5 g, cefoxitin 2 g, ciprofloxacin 400 mg, clindamycin 900 mg, gentamicin 5 mg/kg based on dosing weight and single dose, levofloxacin 500 mg, metronidazole 500 mg, vancomycin 15 mg/kg.
[b]Vancomycin and ciprofloxacin require longer infusion times and should be administered within 2 hours before surgery.

site-specific prophylactic antimicrobial regimens; a detailed examination of clinical trials supporting these recommendations is presented elsewhere.[9]

PRINCIPLES OF SURGICAL ANTIMICROBIAL PROPHYLAXIS

Decision to Use Antimicrobial Prophylaxis

CASE 63-2

QUESTION 1: M.R., a 72-year-old woman, is admitted to the hospital with severe abdominal pain, nausea and vomiting, and temperature of 39.3°C. A diagnosis of acute cholecystitis is made, and M.R. is scheduled for biliary tract surgery (cholecystectomy). Why is antimicrobial prophylaxis warranted for M.R.?

Biliary tract surgery is considered a clean-contaminated procedure and, therefore, carries a risk of surgical wound infection approaching 10% (Tables 63-1 and 63-2). Prophylaxis for biliary tract surgery is limited to high-risk categories, which include obesity, age older than 70 years, diabetes mellitus, acute cholecystitis, obstructive jaundice, common duct stones, emergency procedures, pregnancy, immunosuppression, nonfunctioning gallbladder, or insertion of prosthetic device.[9] Prophylaxis is not recommended for low-risk procedures such as elective laparoscopic cholecystectomy. Thus, prophylaxis is warranted in M.R., who falls into at least two high-risk categories (age older than 70 years and acute cholecystitis).

CASE 63-2, QUESTION 2: An order for intravenous (IV) cefazolin 2 g on call to the operating room (OR) is written for M.R. Why is this an appropriate (or inappropriate) antibiotic selection?

The selected prophylactic agent should be directed against likely infecting organisms (Table 63-2) but need not eradicate every potential pathogen. In general, pathogens associated with infection originate from the skin or the associated structures contiguous to the regions involved in the surgical procedure. Cefazolin has been proved effective for most surgical procedures, including biliary tract surgery, given that the goal of prophylaxis is to decrease bacterial counts below critical levels necessary to cause infection. Broad-spectrum agents, such as third-generation cephalosporins, should be avoided for prophylaxis because they are no more effective than cefazolin and may alter microbial flora, increasing the emergence of microbial resistance to these otherwise valuable agents. The 2 g cefazolin dose is appropriate for all adults weighing less than 120 kg and should be 3 g for patients over 120 kg.

Timing of Antimicrobial Administration

CASE 63-2, QUESTION 3: Why is the administration time for this antimicrobial appropriate (or inappropriate) for M.R.?

Classic animal studies conducted by Burke[21] and others[22] clearly demonstrated the need for therapeutic antibiotic concentrations in the bloodstream and in vulnerable tissue at the time of wound contamination. Bacteria were most likely to enter the tissue beginning with the initial surgical incision and continuing until the wound was closed; antibiotics administered more than 3 hours after bacterial contamination were ineffective in decreasing the rate of wound infection.[21,22] This 2- to 3-hour period after the surgical incision was deemed the "effective" or "decisive" period for prophylaxis, when the animal's wound was most susceptible to the beneficial effects of the antibiotic. This decisive period for administration of prophylactic antibiotics has been confirmed in humans to be somewhere within 2 hours before incision as compared to earlier administration or anytime after incision.[23–26] The precise window for optimal outcomes is still being investigated.[27]

For maximal efficacy, an antibiotic should be present in therapeutic concentrations at the incision site as early as possible during the decisive period and continuing until the wound is closed. Because an antibiotic administered postoperatively cannot achieve therapeutic concentrations during the decisive period, postoperative administration does not prevent postoperative wound infections, and infection rates are similar to those in patients who receive no antibiotics.[28]

Consequently, prophylactic antibiotics should be administered before the surgical procedure in the operative suite.[9] Prophylactic antibiotics are most effective when given within the 1-hour window before surgical incision; rates of infection increase significantly if antibiotics are administered more than 1 hour before incision or postoperatively.[25,26] Administration of vancomycin and fluoroquinolones should begin within 120 minutes before surgical incision because of the prolonged infusion times required for these drugs. If a tourniquet is required to control blood flow to a limb during surgery, the evidence is insufficient to recommend administering the dose before or after inflation of the tourniquet.[16]

The "on-call" prescribing practice for surgical prophylaxis, as with M.R., has fallen into disfavor because the time between antibiotic administration and the actual incision may exceed 1 hour. This delay may result in subtherapeutic antibiotic concentrations during the decisive period.[9,29] M.R.'s cefazolin should be ordered preoperatively and should be administered in the OR within 1 hour of the surgical incision.

CASE 63-2, QUESTION 4: Will M.R. require a second dose of cefazolin during the surgical procedure?

The duration of the surgical procedure and the half-life of the administered antibiotic should be considered when determining the need for an additional intraoperative dose. The longer the duration of the surgical procedure, particularly with short half-life antibacterials, the greater the incidence of postoperative infection.[24,30,31] Cefazolin, with a half-life of approximately 1.8 hours, is effective in a single preoperative dose for most surgical procedures. For prolonged procedures, or those with major blood loss,[32,33] additional intraoperative doses should be administered every 2 half-lives of the drug.[9] M.R. should require an additional intraoperative cefazolin dose only if the surgical procedure is prolonged (>4 hours).

Route of Administration

CASE 63-3

QUESTION 1: G.B., a 55-year-old woman recently diagnosed with carcinoma of the large bowel, is admitted to the hospital for an elective colorectal surgical resection; the surgery is expected to last 5 hours. Physical examination reveals a cachectic woman with a 9-kg weight loss during the previous 3 months (current weight, 60 kg). Increased frequency of bowel movements and chronic fatigue are noted; all other systems are normal. Laboratory data include the following:

Hemoglobin (Hgb), 10.4 g/dL (normal, 12.1–15.3 g/dL; SI units, 104 g/L)
Hematocrit (Hct), 29.7% (normal, 36%–45%; SI units, 0.297)
Prothrombin time (PT), 15 seconds (normal, 10–13 seconds)

Stool guaiac is positive. Vital signs are within normal limits. G.B. is taking no medications and has no history of drug allergies. The following orders are written to begin at home on the day before surgery: (a) clear liquid diet; (b) mechanical bowel cleansing with polyethylene glycol-electrolyte lavage solution (CoLYTE, GoLYTELY); and (c) neomycin sulfate 1 g and erythromycin 1 g orally (PO) at 1, 2, and 11 pm. Comment on the appropriateness of the oral route of administration of antibiotic prophylaxis for G.B.

In general, oral administration of surgical antimicrobial prophylaxis is not recommended because of unreliable or poor absorption of oral agents in the anesthetized bowel. Oral nonabsorbable agents, however, function effectively as GI decontaminants because high intraluminal drug concentrations are sufficient to decrease bacterial counts.[34] The concentration of bacteria in the colon may approach 10^{16} bacteria/μL, and colorectal procedures, such as the one G.B. will undergo, carry a relatively high risk of postoperative infection. Antimicrobial regimens with activity against aerobic and anaerobic bacterial fecal flora (*Escherichia coli* and other Enterobacteriaceae and *Bacteroides fragilis*) are effective in preventing postoperative wound infections.[34]

A widely used oral antimicrobial regimen is 1 g each of the nonabsorbable antibiotics neomycin sulfate (for gram-negative aerobes) and erythromycin base (for anaerobes), given 1 day before surgery at the times indicated for G.B.[35] Mechanical bowel cleansing, such as with polyethylene glycol-electrolyte or sodium phosphate lavage solution, precede administration of this regimen; the purpose of bowel purging is to evacuate the colonic contents as completely as possible to decrease colonic bacterial counts. Effective oral alternatives to neomycin plus erythromycin include metronidazole with or without neomycin or with kanamycin, or kanamycin plus erythromycin[36,37]; however, clinical situations warranting the use of such alternatives over the well-established neomycin–erythromycin regimen are practically nonexistent. Thus, the regimen selected for G.B. is highly appropriate.

CASE 63-3, QUESTION 2: The surgical resident has canceled the oral neomycin–erythromycin bowel regimen for G.B. Instead, he orders cefoxitin (Mefoxin) 1 g IV preoperatively. Is this change in therapy an effective and rational choice for G.B.?

Numerous parenteral regimens, specifically with agents that possess both aerobic and anaerobic activity, are effective as surgical prophylaxis in colorectal procedures. The second-generation cephalosporins with significant anaerobic activity (e.g., cefoxitin) are superior to first-generation cephalosporins, which lack sufficient anaerobic activity.[38] Mechanical bowel preparation with the combination of oral and intravenous antibiotics is superior to oral or intravenous agents alone.[35]

Also, the cefoxitin order for G.B. would be unacceptable if the surgery lasts longer than 3.5 hours (the relatively short half-life of cefoxitin could be associated with inadequate antibacterial levels and predispose her to infection).[39] For prolonged procedures (>3 hours) such as anticipated for G.B., an alternative agent with a longer half-life, such as ertapenem, or a second dose of cefoxitin should be considered. Ertapenem has been found to be superior to cefotetan in preventing infection after colorectal surgery.[40] This improved efficacy may be because of the long half-life or broader antibacterial activity.[41] Whereas ertapenem may offer certain advantages as a prophylactic antibiotic, its use in this indication is discouraged by most clinicians.[9] Although unproven, the potential impact of widespread ertapenem utilization on subsequent carbapenem resistance is of hypothetical concern.[42] The increased acquisition cost of ertapenem also needs to be considered. Thus, for G.B., the importance of redosing intravenous regimens with short half-lives in prolonged surgery should be stressed to the resident.

CASE 63-3, QUESTION 3: The surgical resident has reconsidered the cefoxitin order and decides to prescribe both the oral and parenteral prophylactic regimens for G.B. Will the combination significantly reduce the rate of postoperative wound infection compared with either regimen administered singly?

Coadministration of an oral regimen followed by a parenteral antibiotic prior to incision is equivalent or superior to administration of either regimen alone in reducing infection rates.[35,43] Oral antibiotics, however, have only been evaluated in combination with mechanical bowel preparation. The optimal agents and regimens as prophylaxis in colorectal surgery remain to be adequately determined. For now, combination of oral and parenteral antimicrobial prophylaxis with mechanical bowel preparation is recommended for colorectal surgery.[9]

Duration of Administration

CASE 63-4

QUESTION 1: L.G., a 28-year-old man with a history of rheumatic heart disease, has a 12-year history of a heart murmur consistent with mild mitral stenosis and mitral regurgitation. During the past 4 months his murmur has become much more prominent. In addition, he has experienced severe dyspnea with light physical activity and 3+ pitting edema over both lower legs. Physical examination is notable for coarse rales and an S_3 gallop. For the past 6 weeks, he has been maintained on digoxin and diuretics without significant relief of his shortness of breath (SOB). The cardiothoracic surgeon recommends mitral valve replacement and orders the following surgical antibiotic prophylaxis regimen: cefazolin 1 g IV preoperatively, then every 8 hours for 24 hours. Is cefazolin the most appropriate antimicrobial for L.G.? Why was prophylaxis ordered for only 24 hours?

Although the incidence of postoperative wound infection for cardiothoracic procedures is low (<5%), the devastating consequences of a postoperative endocarditis (after valve replacement) and mediastinitis or sternal osteomyelitis (after sternotomy) warrant antimicrobial prophylaxis.[44–46] Common pathogens associated with cardiothoracic surgery include *Staphylococcus aureus* and *Staphylococcus epidermidis* (particularly with hardware placement) (Table 63-2); based on these potential pathogens, successful prophylactic regimens include cefazolin and cefuroxime. When cefazolin has been compared with cefuroxime or cefamandole, a statistical trend in favor of the second-generation cephalosporins has been noted, and collective wound infection rates were slightly higher in the cefazolin group.[47–49] In contrast, a comparison of prophylactic cefazolin and cefuroxime in patients having open heart surgery noted a significantly greater incidence of sternal wound infection and mediastinitis in the cefuroxime group.[50] Other studies similarly have not observed improved efficacy with cefuroxime compared with cefazolin.[51,52] In conclusion, cefazolin probably is at least as effective as second-generation cephalosporins; therefore, the choice of agent should be based on an institution's antimicrobial susceptibility and cost data. Hospital-specific antimicrobial resistance patterns are especially important in determining the incidence of methicillin-resistant *S. aureus* (MRSA) or methicillin-resistant *S. epidermidis* (MRSE) surgical site infection rates. Although vancomycin has not been determined to be superior to cefazolin, vancomycin is the drug of choice for prophylaxis in patients colonized with MRSA.[9,53] Patients are at higher risk of MRSA carriage if they are frequently hospitalized or have a prolonged hospital stay, are exposed to broad-spectrum antibiotics, are known for comorbid conditions, or have severe underlying illness. The population to be screened for MRSA carriage and undergo decolonization with mupirocin is still being debated but is mostly considered for patients undergoing an orthopedic or cardiac procedure. Surveillance of susceptibility of *S. aureus* isolated from SSIs should be done if mupirocin is used for decolonization.[54]

Meta-analyses reveal no differences between first- and second-generation cephalosporins or between β-lactams and glycopeptides in the prevention of surgical wound infection.[55,56] Thus, the cefazolin prophylaxis selected for L.G. is acceptable, provided the patient is not colonized with MRSA or MRSE. Additional empiric coverage with an aminoglycoside, a fluoroquinolone, or aztreonam may be considered when gram-negative pathogens are a concern according to local epidemiology and risk factors including hospital admission greater than 48 hours before surgery, diabetes, and ventilator-dependency.[9,57]

With regard to duration, the shortest effective prophylactic course of antibiotics should be used (i.e., single dose preoperatively or not more than 24 hours postoperatively for most procedures).[58] Postoperative doses after wound closure are usually not required and may increase the risk of resistance. Single-dose prophylaxis, a viable option for many surgical procedures (see Case 63-5, Question 1), is still being evaluated for cardiac procedures.[9] In practice, cardiothoracic antimicrobial prophylaxis often is continued up to 24 hours after surgery, as in L.G. No benefit is seen to prolonging prophylaxis to more than 24 hours, and such use should be discouraged. The duration of antimicrobial prophylaxis ordered for L.G. is appropriate.

CASE 63-5

QUESTION 1: G.J., a 27-year-old woman, is admitted to the obstetrics unit at term with her first pregnancy. She is scheduled for a cesarean section because the baby is in a breech presentation. Cefazolin 1 g IV to be administered after the cord is clamped and every 8 hours for 24 hours is ordered. Is this surgical prophylaxis appropriate or inappropriate?

As noted previously, the shortest effective duration of prophylaxis should be used. In the past, 1- to 5-day antimicrobial regimens were commonly used for cesarean section, but single-dose regimens have been proven to be as effective as these longer regimens.[59] Faro et al.[59] demonstrated that a single 2-g dose of cefazolin was superior to either a single 1-g dose or a three-dose, 1-g prophylactic regimen. Others have noted similar results (i.e., a single cefazolin dose administered after the umbilical cord is clamped is sufficient in preventing postoperative wound infections in cesarean section).[60–63] Single-dose prophylaxis is less costly and minimizes the development of bacterial resistance.[12] Antibiotic prophylaxis has traditionally been administered after clamping of the umbilical cord to minimize infant drug exposure. This early exposure could theoretically mask the signs of neonatal sepsis and favor the acquisition of resistant organisms. However, administration before initial incision and cord clamping decreases the incidence of maternal infections without adverse consequences to the child.[63–65] Thus, G.J. should receive a single 2-g dose of cefazolin before incision, without the three additional doses.

Single-dose prophylaxis has been found to be effective in a variety of GI tract, orthopaedic, and gynecologic procedures.[30] A single dose of an antibiotic with a short half-life, however, may provide insufficient antimicrobial coverage during a prolonged surgical procedure. Repeated intraoperative dosing or selection of an agent with a longer half-life is recommended when the duration of surgery is long to maintain adequate tissue concentrations throughout the procedure.[9,31]

Signs of Surgical Site Infection

CASE 63-5, QUESTION 2: G.J. is discharged on the fifth hospital day and instructed to observe her incision site carefully for signs of infection. What are the typical signs of site infection? What is the typical time course for signs of site infection to manifest?

Most surgical site infections involve the incision site and are defined as either *superficial* (involving the skin and subcutaneous fat) or *deep incisional* (involving fascia and muscle). Typically, an infected incision site wound is red, warm, and purulent and sometimes swollen, tender, or painful. Poor wound healing or dehiscence (premature opening of the incision) is highly suggestive of infection. A surgical site infection can also involve any part of the anatomy (e.g., organs or spaces), other than the incision, which was opened or manipulated during an operation.[16] The purulent drainage, if present, should be cultured to identify the causative pathogen and direct antimicrobial therapy. Empiric therapy directed against the most likely pathogens should be instituted while awaiting culture and sensitivity test results. Although most incision site infections are diagnosed shortly after surgery (within 30 days), some deep-seated infections present indolently during weeks to months, for example, abscess formation.[16] Infection of surgically implanted prosthetic hardware may take place up to a year after the surgical procedure.[16]

Selection of an Antimicrobial Agent

CASE 63-6

QUESTION 1: L.T., a 46-year-old woman, has a recent history of abnormal uterine bleeding and vaginal discharge. Endometrial biopsy is positive for squamous cell carcinoma; however, there does not appear to be an invasive disease. The diagnosis is carcinoma in situ, and a vaginal hysterectomy is scheduled. What would be an appropriate surgical prophylaxis antimicrobial regimen for L.T.?

The selection of a prophylactic regimen should be based on the spectrum of activity of the agents and the most likely pathogens associated with the given surgical procedure (Table 63-2), pharmacokinetic characteristics (e.g., half-life), adverse event profile, impact on bacterial resistance selection, and cost.

The usefulness of antimicrobial prophylaxis in vaginal hysterectomies is well established and should be directed against vaginal microflora, including gram-positive and gram-negative aerobes and anaerobes (Table 63-2).[66] The most-effective, yet most narrow-spectrum agent should be selected considering that the goal of prophylaxis is not to eradicate every potential pathogen but to reduce bacterial counts below a critical level necessary to cause infection. Cefazolin has been proven to be as effective a prophylactic agent as ceftriaxone for vaginal hysterectomy.[67] This finding reinforces the fact that a more broad-spectrum agent (e.g., a third-generation cephalosporin) is unwarranted.

Similar to vaginal hysterectomy, cefazolin and numerous agents (cefotetan, cefoxitin, ampicillin–sulbactam, etc.) decrease the incidence of postoperative surgical infection when the abdominal approach is used.[66,68] As with vaginal hysterectomy, most trials have not revealed significant differences between first- and second-generation cephalosporins.[68] In contrast, Hemsell et al.[69] observed a significantly higher incidence of major postoperative surgical infections in patients receiving the first-generation agent cefazolin when compared with the second-generation cephalosporin cefotetan. Cefazolin exhibits a favorable toxicity profile and has a relatively long half-life (~1.8 hours), and a single dose has proven prophylactic efficacy.[67] Cefazolin also is considerably less expensive than broader-spectrum agents and is currently recommended by the American College of Obstetricians and Gynecologists.[70] Although it has a broader spectrum of coverage, a single dose of cefoxitin would also be an appropriate choice for this patient.

CASE 63-6, QUESTION 2: Because cefoxitin has an increased spectrum of activity against the anaerobe *B. fragilis*, it is being considered as an alternative to cefazolin prophylaxis for L.T. Comment on the appropriateness of this proposed change in prophylaxis.

The second- and third-generation cephalosporins and ampicillin–sulbactam generally are not more effective than the first-generation cephalosporins for surgical prophylaxis in vaginal hysterectomy or in gastroduodenal, biliary, and clean surgical procedures.[9] One exception to these findings is in the prevention of infection after colorectal procedures and perhaps hysterectomy. Several investigations have documented the failure of first-generation agents when used as prophylaxis in colorectal procedures, probably a consequence of their weak anaerobic coverage.[71] As stated previously, second- and third-generation agents and ampicillin–sulbactam generally are no more efficacious than cefazolin and should not be used for surgical prophylaxis in most procedures. Cefoxitin, however, would be a reasonable choice in colorectal surgery or hysterectomy. Considering that this patient is having a hysterectomy, either cefazolin or cefoxitin is appropriate.

CASE 63-7

QUESTION 1: S.N., a 57-year-old woman with rheumatoid arthritis and degenerative joint disease, has been admitted for total hip arthroplasty. She states that she had an anaphylactic reaction to penicillin in the past. How does this allergy history impact on the selection of surgical prophylaxis for S.N.?

Cefazolin is the preferred prophylactic agent for most clean procedures, including cardiac, vascular, and orthopedic procedures

(Table 63-2). Although the risk of cefazolin cross-allergenicity to penicillin is relatively low, S.N. experienced a serious, accelerated reaction (hives, SOB) with penicillin; consequently, she should not receive cefazolin. The organisms most likely to cause postoperative infection after total hip replacement are *S. aureus* and *S. epidermidis* (Table 63-2). Nafcillin, cefazolin, and vancomycin possess excellent activity against *S. aureus*; however, the β-lactams have only marginal activity against *S. epidermidis*. Regardless, nafcillin (and cefazolin) should be avoided because of the penicillin allergy, and the preferred agent for S.N. is vancomycin.

Preoperative vancomycin 15 mg/kg should be administered IV slowly, during at least 60 minutes. This slow rate of infusion is necessary to reduce the risk of infusion-related hypotension.[72]

CASE 63-8

QUESTION 1: B.K., an 18-year-old woman, complains of severe acute abdominal pain and nausea; the pain is localized to the periumbilical region. B.K. has a temperature of 39.5°C. After initial examination by her pediatrician, she is admitted to the hospital with presumed appendicitis, and an exploratory laparotomy is scheduled. What surgical antimicrobial prophylaxis should be ordered for B.K.?

As with colorectal surgery, the most likely infecting organisms in appendectomy are *Bacteroides* species and gram-negative enterics (Table 63-2). On surgical inspection, if the appendix appears normal (not inflamed, without perforation), then antimicrobial prophylaxis is unnecessary.[73] If the appendix is inflamed without perforation, a single preoperative antibiotic dose is necessary. If the appendix is perforated or gangrenous (complicated), infection is already established and postoperative treatment is warranted. The status of the appendix, however, cannot be determined before surgery; therefore, all patients should receive at least one preoperative dose of an appropriate antibiotic.[74] After surgical inspection of the appendix, the need for postoperative antibiotic therapy can be determined.

Based on the pathogens likely to be encountered, an antimicrobial agent with both aerobic and anaerobic activity should be used. Consequently, cefoxitin is an acceptable choice for prophylaxis.[75]

Risks of Indiscriminate Antimicrobial Use

CASE 63-8, QUESTION 2: On surgical exploration, B.K. was found to have uncomplicated (non-perforated, non-gangrenous) appendicitis; however, cefoxitin therapy was continued for 3 days. What are the risks of indiscriminate use of antimicrobials for surgical prophylaxis?

The risks of indiscriminate use of antimicrobials include the potential for adverse effects and superinfection. The administration of any β-lactam agent poses the risk of a hypersensitivity reaction, and many antibiotics, including cefoxitin, as is being used in B.K., predispose patients to *Clostridium difficile*–associated disease. The risk of developing this superinfection increases with duration of antibiotic exposure.[11] Avoiding unnecessary initial and prolonged exposure reduces the risk of this superinfection and its associated complications.[76] In addition, prolonged use of antimicrobials increases the selection of resistant organisms in a given patient that could be nosocomially spread to other hospitalized patients.[77]

OPTIMIZING SURGICAL ANTIMICROBIAL PROPHYLAXIS

CASE 63-9

QUESTION 1: As the new infectious disease pharmacist of the institution, you are informed by the infection control team that antibiotic prophylaxis prescribed by the surgeons is not the same as what is indicated in the institution guidelines. Which criteria would you want to measure antibiotic prophylaxis prescription performance? What interventions could improve how antibiotics are used in prophylaxis?

Antibiotic control strategies have improved the appropriate use of antimicrobial agents for surgical prophylaxis. Numerous factors including individual knowledge, attitudes, beliefs, and practice; team communication and allocation of responsibilities; and institutional support for promoting and monitoring practice influence antibiotic prophylaxis measures.[78] Interventions for improvement are focused on education of practitioners, standardization of the ordering, the delivery and the administration processes, and providing feedback on performance as measured by infection rates and compliance with improvements. The Surgical Care Improvement Project (SCIP), a national multidisciplinary initiative developed by the Centers for Medicare and Medicaid Services, aims at improving surgical care. Reducing surgical site infections is among one of the targeted goals of this initiative.[79] Prophylactic antimicrobial received within 1 hour before surgical incision, prophylactic antimicrobial consistent with published guidelines, and prophylactic antimicrobial discontinued within 24 hours of surgery end time are three performance measures included in this quality improvement process. The first two, antibiotic timing of administration and appropriate antibiotic selection, are associated with a decrease in the surgical site infection rate.[8]

Smaller scale projects have also been successful at improving antibiotic use and decreasing infection rates. A multidisciplinary team generated electronic quick orders allowing for a computer-enhanced decision-making process and developed an antibiotic administration protocol. Appropriate selection of antibiotics increased from 78% to 94%, timely administration improved from 51% to 98%, and clean wound infection rate decreased from 2.7% to 1.4%.[80]

In collaboration with other health care providers, pharmacists should be responsible for optimizing the timing, choice, and duration of antimicrobial surgical prophylaxis. Education of surgical, anesthesia, and nursing staff, supported by hospital policy changes initiated by pharmacists, improved appropriate timing from 68% to 97% and resulted in significant cost avoidance.[81] Post-discharge surveillance is also critical in reducing surgical site infections.[82]

KEY REFERENCES AND WEBSITES

A full list of references for this chapter can be found at http://thepoint.lww.com/AT11e. Below are the key references and websites for this chapter, with the corresponding reference number in this chapter found in parentheses after the reference.

Key References

Anderson DJ et al. Strategies to prevent surgical site infections in acute care hospitals. *Infect Control Hosp Epidemiol.* 2008;29(Suppl 1):S51. (17)

Bratzler DW et al. Clinical practice guidelines for antimicrobial prophylaxis in surgery. *Am J Health Syst Pharm.* 2013;70(3):195–283. (9)

Bratzler DW, Hunt DR. The surgical infection prevention and surgical care improvement projects: national initiatives to improve outcomes for patients having surgery. *Clin Infect Dis.* 2006;43:322. (79)

Classen DC et al. The timing of prophylactic administration of antibiotics and the risk of surgical-wound infection. *N Engl J Med.* 1992;326:281. (26)

Key Websites

Centers for Diseases Control and Prevention. Healthcare Associated Infections. Surgical Site Infection (SSI). http://www.cdc.gov/HAI/ssi/ssi.html.

Centers for Diseases Control and Prevention. Healthcare Infection Control Practices Advisory Committee (HICPAC). General Guidelines. https://www.cdc.gov/infectioncontrol/guidelines/index.html.

Centers for Diseases Control and Prevention. National Healthcare Safety Network. Data and Statistics. http://www.cdc.gov/nhsn/datastat.html.

Safer Healthcare Now! Surgical Site Infection (SSI). http://www.patientsafetyinstitute.ca/en/Topic/Pages/Surgical-Site-Infections-(SSI).aspx.

National Institute for Health and Clinical Excellence. Surgical Site Infection. http://www.nice.org.uk/guidance/CG74.

64 Vaccinations

Molly G. Minze and Katherine Dillinger Ellis

CORE PRINCIPLES

	CHAPTER CASES
GENERAL VACCINE PRINCIPLES	
1 **Adverse Effects:** Immunization adverse effects are in part dependent upon the type of vaccine preparation used. Adverse effects from live attenuated vaccines mimic the disease but are less severe and occur 7 to 10 days postvaccination. Inactivated (killed whole virus) vaccination adverse effects include soreness at the site of administration within 24 hours after vaccination. Vaccination adverse effects are significantly less severe than the disease itself.	**Case 64-1 (Question 1)**
2 **Immunization Schedules:** Recommended immunization schedules are designed to optimize immune response, standardize regimens, and enhance immunization rates. Birth to 18 years and adult immunization schedules are reviewed and updated annually.	**Case 64-2 (Question 1)**
3 **Catch-up Immunization Schedules:** To catch up within an immunization series, it is not necessary to restart from the first dose of the schedule. A delay in receiving subsequent doses does not interfere with final immunity gained from the vaccination.	**Case 64-3 (Question 1)**
INACTIVATED VACCINES	
1 **Hepatitis B:** Hepatitis B vaccination is effective for both pre-exposure and postexposure prophylaxis. To prevent vertical transmission to an infant from a mother, it is key to provide vaccination within 12 hours of birth along with hepatitis B immunoglobulin for those mothers who test hepatitis-B–positive.	**Case 64-4 (Question 1)**
2 **Hepatitis B:** The highest incidence of hepatitis B infection occurs in young adults. Hepatitis B vaccination is recommended for adults who participate in high-risk behaviors and those in close contact with the infected persons.	**Case 64-4 (Question 2)**
3 **Hepatitis A:** Hepatitis A immunization is targeted toward toddlers with the aim of preventing transmission to adolescents and adults.	**Case 64-5 (Question 1)**
4 **Diphtheria, tetanus, and acellular pertussis/Pertussis booster:** Waning immunity against pertussis has resulted in outbreaks of pertussis in the United States. Adolescents and adults, particularly those with close contact with young infants, should receive a single dose of pertussis booster vaccine.	**Case 64-6 (Question 1)**
5 ***Haemophilus influenzae* b:** Immunization recommendations for *Haemophilus influenzae* type b is age-dependent. The older an infant is at presentation, the fewer doses needed to elicit a response. A single vaccine dose may be considered in children and adults with underlying diseases that place them a risk for infection.	**Case 64-7 (Question 1)**
6 **Polio:** Inactivated polio vaccine is recommended over the oral attenuated vaccine for polio vaccination in the United States because inactivated vaccine is associated with a lower incidence of vaccine-associated paralytic polio.	**Case 64-8 (Question 1)**
7 **Polio:** Routine vaccination of adults against polio with inactivated poliovirus vaccine is not recommended unless individuals plan travel to endemic areas. Oral polio vaccine may be considered only in unique situations.	**Case 64-9 (Question 1)**

Continued

		CHAPTER CASES
8	**Meningococcal:** Vaccination is recommended within populations at increased for risk for contracting *Neisseria meningitidis*, including travelers to endemic areas, patients with specific immunodeficiencies, functional/anatomic asplenia, lab personnel dealing with meningococcus, and college students.	**Case 64-10 (Question 1)**
9	**Human Papillomavirus:** This three-dose vaccination series is recommended for adolescent females for the prevention of cervical and anogenital cancers, anogenital warts, and recurrent respiratory papillomatosis. It is also recommended for males in the prevention of genital warts.	**Case 64-11 (Question 1)**
10	**Pneumococcus:** *Streptococcus pneumoniae* mostly affects young children and the elderly. The conjugate vaccines protect against 80% (PCV 7) and 90% (PCV 13) of infectious strains that cause disease in children younger than 6 years old.	**Case 64-12 (Question 1)**
11	**Pneumococcus:** The polysaccharide vaccine does not elicit immune response in children younger than 2 years old, and protects against 23 strains of *S. pneumoniae* that typically cause adult disease.	**Case 64-12 (Question 2)**
12	**Influenza:** Vaccination is recommended for anyone older than 6 months of age who does not have a current contraindication. The inactivated vaccine is delivered intramuscularly or intradermally, whereas the live attenuated vaccine is delivered as a nasal spray formulation.	**Case 64-13 (Question 1)**
LIVE ATTENUATED VACCINES		
1	**Rotavirus:** Infants vaccinated with the rotavirus vaccine shed the virus in the feces after immunization; however, the risk of transmission to an immunocompromised contact is relatively low with appropriate precautions.	**Case 64-14 (Question 1)**
2	**Measles/Mumps/Rubella (MMR):** Parents are fearful of the risk of autism which has been falsely associated with the MMR vaccine. Pharmacists must provide counseling to overcome parental fears and ensure protection against measles.	**Case 64-15 (Question 1)**
3	**Varicella:** Postexposure vaccination with the varicella vaccine is recommended within 5 days of exposure for those unvaccinated or who have not received a second dose of vaccine.	**Case 64-16 (Question 1)**
4	**Varicella:** Herpes zoster vaccination is recommended in adults older than 60 years of age to prevent reactivation of previously acquired wild-type varicella zoster infections. It is not recommended for anyone who previously received the varicella zoster vaccine.	**Case 64-16 (Question 2)**
IMMUNIZATION PRACTICES		
1	**Vaccine Administration:** Intramuscular vaccinations are administered at a 90-degree angle into the muscle using a 1-inch needle. Subcutaneous vaccinations are administered at a 45-degree angle into the subcutaneous tissue by pinching this tissue up to prevent insertion into the muscle. When multiple injections are given at the same site, separate each injection by 1 inch.	**Case 64-17 (Question 1)**
2	**Advocacy and Establishing Services:** Pharmacists have an important role as immunization advocates to positively increase immunization rates. Pharmacist immunization training is widespread throughout the United States, but pharmacists must adhere to guidelines and principles established by their state pharmacy practice act when administering immunizations to patients.	**Case 64-18 (Question 1)**

The use of immunizations to control common infectious diseases is a major public health achievement. Children, adolescents, and adults are now routinely immunized against 17 infectious diseases.[1] Immunization rates are high overall and have remained stable in the United States with more than 80% of children 3 years of age receiving all the recommended vaccines.[2] As a result, low levels of vaccine-preventable diseases are occurring. Rates of immunization for adults against influenza and pneumococcus range from 20-43%, with higher coverage for individuals older than 65 years.[3] Unfortunately, despite overall high rates of immunization coverage, disparities still exist in vaccination coverage for the socioeconomically disadvantaged and by ethnicity.[2] Clearly, there is room for improvement and an opportunity for all health professionals to have an impact.

The need for timely immunization administration is key to preventing disease resurgences.[4] As the incidence of vaccine-preventable disease continues to decrease, patients are becoming less aware of the significance and severity of the diseases that could be prevented.[5–8] This, along with parental concerns regarding vaccine safety, may jeopardize previous vaccination achievements.[7] Health care providers play a vital role in clarifying misconceptions and educating parents and other health professionals about the importance of proper and complete immunizations.[7] Any contact with a patient represents an opportunity to promote immunization, and thus every medication history should include a review of immunization status to detect any deficiencies.[8]

VACCINE PRINCIPLES

General Principles

The principle of vaccination against disease is that the introduction of a small amount of the pathogen to the body produces protective immunologic memory (active immunity) and, if the pathogen is reintroduced at a later date, a greater immunologic response is elicited but without inducing disease.[9] The ideal vaccine would present a non-virulent form of a pathogen that produces a strong immunologic response once in the body.[10]

Current vaccine types include live attenuated, killed (inactivated) whole organism, subcellular/subunit, and DNA-based vaccines.[10] (See Table 64-1 for a listing of common vaccines and their formulation type.) Live attenuated vaccines contain weakened or inactivated forms of the pathogen, which causes replication within the host and ultimately elicits antibody and cell-mediated immunity within the body via B-cell and T-cell responses.[10,11] Live vaccine administration produces a mild, typically asymptomatic infection at the time of vaccination followed by long-lived immunity from a single immunization.[12,13]

Killed whole organism and subcellular/subunit vaccines do not replicate within the host, nor can they revert to pathogenicity, but they often require adjuvants and/or multiple doses to increase the duration of immune response to the antigen.[9,10] Because the organisms in whole pathogen vaccines are inactivated (killed), their effectiveness may be impaired by circulating antibodies, maternal antibodies (in infants), or concomitant infections. Toxoids are a specific kind of inactivated vaccine formed by modifying a biological toxin (e.g., diphtheria and tetanus), usually by mixing it with formaldehyde.

Subunit vaccines contain either a protein or polysaccharide antigen within the vaccine and elicit less reaction than whole pathogen vaccines, thus immune responses are weaker and require multiple doses similar to inactivated vaccines.[9] Conjugated subunit vaccines, consisting of a polysaccharide-protein-conjugate where the protein is the antigenic toxin, produce improved immune responses because of B-cell activation by the polysaccharide component and T-cell activation by protein component. Recombinant vaccines available include hepatitis B, human papillomavirus (HPV), recombinant influenza, and live typhoid vaccine.[14]

Adverse Effects

CASE 64-1

QUESTION 1: H.P. is a 38-year-old woman concerned about the side effects of the annual influenza "shot." What information can be provided regarding expected adverse effects for H.P.?

Adverse reactions to inactivated vaccines include pain at the injection site and fever within 48 to 72 hours of administration.[15–17] In contrast, adverse effects from live attenuated vaccines occur 7 to 10 days after immunization, after the virus has replicated and the immune system has responded. Adverse reactions to live attenuated vaccines mimic the symptoms of disease. Transient rash occurs in 5% of patients receiving measles, mumps, rubella (MMR) immunizations, and a mild varicella-like rash (median of five lesions) occurs in fewer than 5% of patients receiving the varicella vaccine. Syncope, usually occurring within 30 minutes of immunization, has been reported, with 70% of syncopal episodes occurring within 15 minutes of immunization, and occurs more commonly in female patients and adolescents.

Although anaphylactic reactions to vaccines are rare, an allergic reaction may occur as a result of specific allergy to the vaccine itself or to trace components in the vaccine (e.g., preservatives, antibiotics).[18] Patients with egg allergy can receive vaccines produced in chick-embryo-fibroblast tissue culture (e.g., MMR) because the risk for serious reaction to these vaccines in egg-allergic individuals is very low.[19–21] MMR should be used cautiously in individuals with a history of a severe reaction to gelatin, which is a stabilizer in the MMR vaccine. Trace amounts of streptomycin, bacitracin, and neomycin are present in oral polio virus vaccine, inactivated polio vaccine, and MMR; therefore, these vaccines should not be administered to individuals with a history of an anaphylactic reaction to these antibiotics.[22]

Overall, vaccinations are safe, especially when compared with the risks of the diseases that these vaccines prevent, and the safety of immunizations are scrutinized continually.[22–24] In response to concerns about vaccine safety, the National Vaccine Injury Compensation Act mandated an ongoing review of evidence regarding the possible adverse effects of vaccines and established a no-fault injury compensation program for selected vaccines.

Contraindications

Misconceptions about contraindications and precautions for immunization often result in missed opportunities to provide needed immunizations.[1,25] Acute, severe febrile illness; history of anaphylaxis to the vaccine or vaccine components; and history of a severe reaction to an immunization are clear contraindications to immunizations. Immunizations, however, should not be delayed in a patient who has a minor illness (e.g., upper respiratory tract infection, otitis media, diarrhea) even in the presence of a low-grade fever. A family history of seizures, allergies, and sudden infant death syndrome are not contraindications for immunizations. Immunization of a patient with a history of anaphylaxis to a vaccine or vaccine component should be withheld until he or she has undergone desensitization. Preterm infants should begin to receive routine immunizations based on their chronological age for all vaccines, although initiation of the hepatitis B series should begin at 1 month of age.

Allergic reaction to previous exposure to vaccine components, immunosuppression (e.g., immunosuppressive therapy, immunodeficiencies), encephalopathy, recent administration of blood products, and pregnancy (although the risk in pregnancy is largely theoretical) are contraindications to live attenuated virus or live bacterial vaccines. Pooled blood products (e.g., immunoglobulins, packed red blood cells, platelet transfusions) can impair the immune response to a live vaccine because these products contain antibodies, which can prevent one's immune system from mounting an adequate response.[1] The impairment of an immune response to an immunization varies, depending on the type and amount of blood product administered, and immunizations may need to be delayed for up to 12 months if pooled blood products have been administered recently.[1] With any question about immune response, antibody titers can be obtained to determine if a patient needs to be re-immunized.

Table 64-1
Vaccine Overview

	Vaccines	Recommended Regimens	Comment
Diphtheria, tetanus, pertussis (inactivated; intramuscular)	DTaP, DT Tdap Td	2, 4, 6, 15–18 months; booster at 4–6 years 11–12 years Every 10 years	Minimum age 6 weeks; fourth dose can be administered at 12 months of age if at least 6 months since third dose Minimum age 10 years (Boostrix) and 11 years (Adacel)
Haemophilus influenzae type b (inactivated; intramuscular)	Hib	2, 4, 6, 12–15 months	Minimum age is 6 weeks If PRP-OMP at 2 and 4 months, no 6-month dose indicated Hiberix should only be used for final dose (12 months–4 years)
Hepatitis B (inactivated; intramuscular)	Hep B	Birth, 1–2 months, 6–15 months	Monovalent vaccine to be administered for any doses before 6 weeks Administer birth dose within 12 hours if HBsAG+ mother Final dose should not be given before 6 months of age
Hepatitis A (inactivated; intramuscular)	HepA	Two doses 6 months apart First dose at 23 months	Minimum age 12 months
Human papillomavirus vaccine (inactivated; intramuscular)	HPV2 HPV9	Three doses 9–26 years Second dose 1–2 months after first Third dose 6 months after first	Administer to females before sexual activity Administer to males to reduce likelihood of genital warts
Influenza (IIV = inactivated; intramuscular) (LAIV 4 = live attenuated; intra-nasal)	IIV, LAIV4	Annually Two doses 4 weeks apart at first annual vaccination	Minimum age IIV 6 months Minimum age LAIV 4 2 years Two doses required for patients aged 2–8 years at first annual vaccination
Measles, mumps, rubella (live attenuated; subcutaneous)	MMR	12–15 months; repeat dose 4–6 years	Minimum age 12 months; second dose may be administered at 4 years as long as 4 weeks from previous dose
Meningococcal (MCV = inactivated; intramuscular) (MPSV = subcutaneous)	MCV4 MPSV4	Two doses 8 weeks apart age 2–10 years One dose age 11–55 years Ages 56 and older	Minimum age 2 years Two doses for patients with immunodeficiency One dose for patients at high risk
Pneumococcal (inactivated polysaccharide; usually intramuscular, but subcutaneous ok)	PCV 13 PPSV 23	2, 4, 6, 12–15 months 1 PCV 13 dose 1 dose ≥65 years 2 doses if <65 at time of first dose	PCV minimum age 6 weeks PPSV minimum age 2 years Administer PCV 13 dose before PPSV 23 Administer second dose of PPSV 5 years after first
Polio (inactivated; usually intramuscular, but subcutaneous ok)	IPV	2, 4, 6–18 months	IPV minimum age 6 weeks If four or more doses given before 4 years of age, repeat booster at 4–6 years Final dose should be after fourth birthday and at least 6 months after previous dose
Rotavirus (live attenuated; oral)	RV1 RV5	2, 4 months 2, 4, 6 months	Initial dose: minimum age 6 weeks, maximum age 14 weeks 6 days Final dose: maximum age 8 months Rotarix (RV1): 6-month dose not indicated
Varicella (live attenuated; subcutaneous)	VZV	12–15 months; repeat dose at 4–6 years	Minimum age 12 months; second dose may be administered at 4 years as long as 3 months from previous dose
Zoster (live attenuated; subcutaneous)	ZV	50 years of age (usually >60)	1 dose

HBsAG+, hepatitis-B–surface antigen positive; PRP-OMP, PedvaxHIB or Comvax (Hep B-Hib).
Sources: National Center for Immunization and Respiratory Diseases. General recommendations on immunizations—recommendations of the Advisory Committee on Immunization Practices (ACIP). *MMWR Recomm Rep*. 2011;60:1; Strikas RA; Advisory Committee on Immunization Practices (ACIP); ACIP Child/Adolescent Immunization Work Group. Advisory Committee on Immunization Practices recommended immunization schedules for persons aged 0 through 18 years—United States, 2015. *MMWR Morb Mortality Wkly Rep*. 2015;64:93–94; Kim DK et al; Advisory Committee on Immunization Practices (ACIP), ACIP Adult Immunization Work Group. Advisory Committee on Immunization Practices Recommended Immunization Schedule for Adults aged 19 years or older—Unites States, 2015. *MMWR Morb Mortality Wkly Rep*. 2015;64:91–92; Kim et al; Advisory Committee on Immunization Practices (ACIP). Advisory Committee on Immunization Practices recommended immunization schedule for adults aged 19 years or older: United States, 2015. *Ann Intern Med*. 2015;162(3):214–223.

GUIDELINES

Schedule for Immunizations

CASE 64-2

QUESTION 1: K.C., a 2-month-old baby girl, is brought to the clinic for a scheduled well-baby visit. K.C.'s mother inquires about immunizations for her daughter. What are the current recommendations for immunizing pediatric patients? When should these immunizations be given to K.C.?

The goal of immunization is to prevent specific infectious diseases and their sequelae. For maximal effectiveness, a vaccine must be administered to the susceptible population before anyone has been exposed to the pathogen. The age at which immunizations are administered to specific individuals depends on several factors (e.g., age-specific risks of the disease, risks of complications, presence of maternal antibodies transferred through the placenta, maturity of the immune system). Usually, immunizations are administered at the youngest age that the child is able to develop an adequate antibody response.

The recommended childhood and adolescent immunization schedules are reviewed annually by the Advisory Committee on Immunization Practice (ACIP) and American Academy of Pediatrics (AAP), and supported by the American Academy of Family Physicians (AAFP), the American College of Obstetricians and Gynecologists (ACOG), and published within the Morbidity and Mortality Weekly Report[26,27] and are available online (**http://www.cdc.gov/schedules**). A partial summary of vaccination schedules is included in Table 64-1, but the reader is referred to the online publication of immunization schedules for a more complete listing of the most current recommendations. The minimal immunization requirements for entry into public schools and day-care centers vary with each state and the departments of health of individual states need to be consulted for these guidelines. The ACIP reviews the adult immunization schedule annually as supported by the American College of Physicians (ACP), American Academy of Family Physicians (AAFP), and the American College of Nurse-Midwives (ACNM) and published within the Annals of Internal Medicine and Morbidity and Mortality Weekly Report[28–30] (available online at **http://www.cdc.gov/schedules**). The respective schedules for children and adults should be reviewed annually, and policies and procedures revised to ensure compliance.

A review of the childhood immunization schedule reveals that the recommended vaccines to be administered at 2 months of age include diphtheria, tetanus, and acellular pertussis (DTaP), inactivated polio (IPV), *Haemophilus influenzae* type b (Hib), conjugated pneumococcal vaccine (PCV13), and rotavirus vaccine. A second dose of the Hepatitis B (Hep B) vaccine should also be administered if the first dose was given at birth. If Hep B vaccine was not given to K.C. at birth, the first dose should be given today, then repeated at 1 to 2 months and again at 6 months (see Case 64-4 Question 1).

CASE 64-3

QUESTION 1: K.C.'s mother also mentions that she personally received two doses of an HPV vaccine series. Her physician asked her to receive a third dose in December, and it is now March. Does K.C.'s mother need to restart the vaccination series for HPV?

Immunization schedules can be adjusted to meet individual needs and may begin at any time of the year. Vaccines should not be administered at time intervals shorter than those recommended to allow for maximal immune responses before the administration of subsequent doses.[1] A "catch-up" schedule for immunizations of children and adolescents who begin their immunizations late or who are more than 1 month behind schedule in their immunizations and recommendations for minimal intervals between doses for the administration of various vaccine can be implemented.[1,26,27] It is not necessary for adults who delay administration of a subsequent dose of an immunization series to restart the vaccination series. An interruption or delay in the recommended schedule does not interfere with the final immunity gained.

Alternative immunization recommendations are available for patients with altered immunocompetence to ensure protection from vaccine associated disease, yet prevent adverse effects or acquiring disease from the vaccine itself in the case of live attenuated vaccines.[1,27,30,31] K.C.'s mother should receive a third dose of HPV vaccine as soon as possible, but she does not need to restart the whole series.

INACTIVATED VACCINES

Hepatitis B

CASE 64-4

QUESTION 1: A.G. is an infant (weight 2,100 g) born to a mother in whom the hepatitis B surface antigen (HBsAg) status is unknown. How should A.G. be managed?

Hepatitis B virus (HBV) can be transmitted via exposure to contaminated blood (e.g., blood products or medical instruments, non-sterilized needles used in intravenous drug abuse, or tattooing), exposure to body fluids (e.g., sexual intercourse), and transplacentally from an HBsAg-positive mother. The prevention of HBV maternal transmission to an infant is essential because acute disease can progress to a chronic carrier state, which can lead to chronic liver disease and primary hepatocellular carcinoma. Children acquiring HBV infection before 5 years of age are at an especially high risk of developing chronic infection.[32] All pregnant women should be tested for HBsAg, and infants born to HBsAg-positive mothers should receive their first vaccine dose in addition to hepatitis B immune globulin (HBIG) within 12 hours of birth to prevent vertical transmission.[33] When combined, HBIG plus HBV vaccine are 99% effective in preventing acute and chronic infection in infants born to HBsAg-positive mothers.[33] If the mother's HBsAg status is unknown, the infant should be also immunized within 12 hours of birth regardless of birth weight. For infants weighing less than 2,000 g, HBIG should also be administered within 12 hours of birth. The mother's HBsAg status should be determined as soon as possible and if the mother is HBsAg-positive, HBIG should be administered to infants weighing >2,000 g as soon as possible, but no later than day 7 of life.[33] Infants weighing >2,000 g born to HBsAg-negative mothers should begin their immunization series within 24 hours of birth. All other infants born to HBsAg-negative mothers should begin their immunization series before hospital discharge. In all situations, subsequent vaccine doses should be administered at age 1 to 2 months and again at age 6 months. All unimmunized children should receive HBV vaccine as soon as they are identified.[33]

AG should receive Hep B vaccine within 12 hours of birth and the mother's status should be determined. If her mother is found to be HBsAg-positive, HBIG should also be administered within 7 days of birth. A.G. can receive her subsequent doses of HBV vaccine according to the childhood immunization schedule. Two Hep B vaccines are currently available for use in the United States. Recombivax-HB and Engerix-B are yeast-derived recombinant vaccines administered as a three-dose series.[33,34] Either formulation can be used because the immune response from an immunization series using different vaccines is comparable to that of a full series using a single vaccine.[1,35]

Case 64-4, Question 2: A.G.'s mother has not been immunized herself against hepatitis B. Should she begin receiving the Hep B series as well?

Despite a decline in hepatitis B infections in the United States after universal childhood immunization, more than a million adults are living with chronic hepatitis B infection. The highest incidence of acute hepatitis B in the United States occurs in adults 25 to 45 years of age, the majority of which occur in individuals with high-risk behaviors including multiple sexual partners, anal intercourse, and injectable drug abuse.[34] Individuals who have close contact with patients infected with hepatitis B, including health care workers, are also at risk of infection.[34] Children and adolescents not vaccinated during infancy should be given a three-dose series of intramuscular injections. Similarly, adults aged 19 to 59 years old with type 2 diabetes are recommended to receive the three-dose series.[36] Other at-risk adult groups who should receive the hepatitis B vaccination include sexually active persons not in a long-term monogamous relationship, persons seeking treatment for a sexually transmitted infection, or men who have sex with men, patients with end-stage renal disease, HIV, who receive hemodialysis or have chronic liver disease, household contacts and sexual partners of hepatitis B surface antigen positive persons, staff of institutions for persons with developmental disabilities, international travelers to areas with high prevalence of hepatitis B, and adults in settings of STD treatment facilities, HIV testing and treatment facilities, or facilities providing care for patients at risk of having hepatitis B.[28–30,34] Antibody screening after immunization is only recommended in high-risk groups in whom future clinical management may depend on knowledge of immune status (e.g., health care workers). Recommendations for serologic testing and revaccination and postexposure prophylaxis for such situations are available.[34] Patients on dialysis and other immunocompromised patients may require a fourth dose if the anti-HBs level is less than 10 MIU/mL 2 months after the third dose.[34]

A.G.'s mother should begin a three-dose series of Hep B vaccine. Monovalent vaccines are preferred for the initial vaccination; however, combination vaccines may be used[1,35] (see Table 64-2). Combination vaccines should not be used for infants younger than 6 weeks of age; therefore, only single antigen doses should be used for birth doses.[33]

Hepatitis A

CASE 64-5

Question 1: A mother presents with her 2-year-old to her pediatrician for a well-child visit. Her pediatrician encourages her to have her child immunized against hepatitis A. What are the differences between hepatitis B and hepatitis A infections, and what are the immunization recommendations?

Hepatitis A infection can present as either an acute or chronic illness, but it is often asymptomatic in infants and young children. However, infections in older children and adults typically present with fever, malaise, anorexia, nausea, abdominal discomfort, and jaundice.[37] Clinical illness usually lasts 1 to 2 months, but it may be relapsing and can last up to 6 months. Approximately one-third of hepatitis A cases occur in children younger than 15 years of age.[38] Among all reported cases, the most common source of infection is household or sexual contact, followed by day-care attendance or employment, international travel, and food or waterborne outbreaks. Asymptomatic children serve as a source of infection, especially for household or other close contacts.[38]

Vaccination programs targeting toddlers and young children are important because children are often asymptomatic and unwittingly transmit the virus to adolescents and adults. In addition, data suggest a "herd effect" when vaccination of children is widespread (i.e., large population immunization programs indirectly protect those who are not immunized because the risk of being exposed to an infected individual is reduced).[39] A program aimed exclusively at toddlers in an endemic area reduced the prevalence

Table 64-2
Combination Vaccines

Combination Vaccine[a]	Antigens[b]	Age Indicated	Regimen
Kinrix	DTaP-IPV	4–6 years	Only for fourth dose IPV and fifth dose DTaP
Quadracel	DTap-IPV	4-6 years	For fourth or fifth dose IPV series and fifth dose DTaP
Pediarix[c]	DTaP-Hep B-IPV	6 weeks–6 years	2, 4, 6 months
Pentacel	DTaP-IPV-Hib	6 weeks–4 years	2, 4, 6, 15–18 months An extra monovalent IPV recommended for IPV at 4–6 years (total, five doses)
ProQuad[d]	MMR-V	12 months–12 years	12–15 months, 4–6 years
Twinrix	HepA-Hep B	18 years+	0, 1, 6 months

[a]Vaccine interchangeability: If combination and single antigen vaccines are used to complete an immunization series, it is preferred to use products from the same manufacturer. Immunogenicity of vaccine antigens between different manufacturers is unknown.
[b]Extra antigens: Administration of extra antigens by using combination vaccines should be avoided. Availability of monovalent vaccines should be provided to avoid giving extra antigens and increase risk of adverse effects, particularly for inactivated vaccines which are reactogenic (e.g., DTaP vaccine).
[c]Hepatitis B: Combination vaccines not recommended for hepatitis B birth doses (<6 weeks).
[d]ProQuad: MMRV may be associated with an increased risk of febrile seizures when used at age 12–47 months. The use of MMR is preferred during this time.
DTaP, diphtheria, tetanus, and acellular pertussis; HepA, hepatitis A; Hep B, hepatitis B; Hib, *Haemophilus influenzae* type b; IPV, inactivated poliovirus vaccine; MMR, measles, mumps, and rubella vaccine; V, varicella vaccine.
Sources: National Center for Immunization and Respiratory Diseases. General recommendations on immunizations—recommendations of the Advisory Committee on Immunization Practices (ACIP). *MMWR Recomm Rep*. 2011;60:1; CDC. Combination vaccines for childhood immunization: recommendations of the Advisory Committee on Immunization Practices (ACIP), the American Academy of Pediatrics (AAP), and the American Academy of Family Practice (AAFP). *Pediatrics*. 1999;103:1064; Marin M et al. Use of combination measles, mumps, rubella and varicella vaccine: recommendations of the Advisory Committee on Immunization Practices (ACIP). *MMWR Recomm Rep*. 2010;59(RR-3):1.

of hepatitis A by more than 90%, not only in the 2- to 4-year-old vaccine recipients but in all age groups.[39]

There are two hepatitis A (Hep A) vaccines on the market, Havrix and Vaqta, each with adult and pediatric formulations. The pediatric formulations of the vaccine are indicated for infants older than 12 months of age and contain half the antigen of the adult formulations.[37] Vaccination involves a two-dose regimen with the second dose to be administered 6 to 18 months after the initial dose, depending on the formulation (see Table 64-1). Two doses of hepatitis A vaccine should be administered at least 6 months apart to previously unvaccinated persons who live in areas where vaccination programs target older children, or who are at increased risk for infection.[27] Adults for whom Hep A vaccination is recommended include those with high-risk behaviors, individuals who work with hepatitis A virus-infected primates or in a hepatitis A research laboratory setting, patients with chronic liver disease or who require clotting factor concentrates, and those traveling to areas where hepatitis A is endemic.[28–30,37] A combination vaccine containing both Hep A and Hep B is available and indicated in individuals older than 18 years of age on a three-dose schedule (see Table 64-2).

Diphtheria/Tetanus/Pertussis Vaccines

CASE 64-6

QUESTION 1: N.R. is a nurse who cares for children in a hospital setting. She calls with confusion regarding the need for her to receive a "pertussis booster." She indicates that she received her DTaP immunization series as recommended during childhood and her last tetanus shot was 3 years ago. Should N.R. receive the pertussis booster (Tdap)?

Pertussis ("whooping cough"), an infectious disease caused by *Bordetella pertussis*, is characterized by a paroxysmal cough with a whoop-like, high-pitched inspiratory noise; vomiting; and lymphocytosis. It is a highly communicable infection, which can affect 90% of infants and young children in nonimmunized households, and can be associated with serious sequelae, particularly in young infants. An estimated 0.3% to 14% of patients with pertussis experience encephalopathy, 0.6% to 2% have permanent neurologic damage, and about 0.1% to 4% die.[40] This serious childhood infection has been mitigated with the availability of an acellular pertussis vaccine (aP), which commonly is administered in combination with diphtheria (D) and tetanus (T) vaccines (DTaP). A primary series of four doses of DTaP is recommended at 2, 4, 6, and 15 to 18 months followed by a booster dose at school entry or 4 to 6 years of age.[27,41] The efficacy of the DTaP vaccines against pertussis after primary immunization (three doses) is greater than 80%.[41] Protection increases to 90% after the last booster (age 4–6 years) and then decreases during the next 12 years, after which protection is minimal.[42,43]

Historically, DTaP vaccines contained whole cell pertussis antigens. However, because of concerns regarding adverse effects, products currently available contain acellular pertussis antigens (see Table 64-1). Despite a more favorable adverse effect profile, the DTaP vaccine is contraindicated in anyone experiencing an anaphylactic reaction or encephalopathy within 7 days of immunization with DTaP when these symptoms cannot be attributed to another cause.[41] In addition, careful consideration of subsequent doses should be given to infants experiencing a temperature of 105°F (not resulting from another cause) or persistent, inconsolable crying lasting more than 3 hours within 48 hours after the administration of a pertussis-containing vaccine.[41] The pertussis component of the DTaP vaccine should be eliminated (i.e., continue vaccination with DT) in any child experiencing collapse or a hypotonic–hyporesponsive episode. If an evolving neurologic disorder is present, pertussis immunization should be deferred until the neurologic problem has been fully evaluated. Preexisting, stable neurologic conditions (e.g., well-controlled seizures) are not contraindications because the benefits of pertussis immunization outweigh the risks. A family history of seizures or other central nervous system (CNS) disorder is not a contraindication for vaccination.[42]

Two DTaP vaccines (Infanrix and Daptacel) are approved for the primary vaccination series. Combination vaccines may also be used; however, their use for primary vaccination is product dependent (Table 64-2).[35] If possible, the same DTaP product should be used for all five doses because the immunity, safety, and efficacy associated with the interchanging of different DTaP vaccines are unknown.[1,27] If the product information is unknown or unavailable from prior vaccinations, however, any licensed DTaP vaccine can be used to complete the vaccination series.[1,27]

Despite the availability of an effective vaccine and a high rate of vaccine coverage, pertussis remains poorly controlled in the United States.[44] Decreased immunity in adolescents and adults is believed to contribute to this problem. About 12% of adult patients with a cough lasting more than 2 weeks have pertussis.[45] Although the illness is typically mild in adults and adolescents, they serve as a source of transmission to unprotected infants. This has led to the development and recommendation of acellular pertussis booster vaccines for adolescents and adults with a tetanus and diphtheria toxoids and acellular pertussis vaccine (Tdap).[1,27,44] (Note the designation as *dap* compared with *DaP* for primary vaccines.) The routine use of a single dose of pertussis booster (Tdap) is recommended for adolescents at 11 to 18 years of age, for adults 19 to 64 years of age, pregnant females during each pregnancy, and for those older than 65 years of age who may be in contact with infants younger than 12 months of age.[27–30,44,46] The pertussis booster (Tdap) may be administered regardless of the time since receipt of a tetanus booster (Td). Two Tdap vaccine formulations (BOOSTRIX and ADACEL) are US Food and Drug Administration (FDA)–approved for use as a booster dose for children 11 to 18 years of age.[44] Recommendations for catch-up immunization of unvaccinated or undervaccinated individuals with DTaP/Tdap are available.[1,27–30] N.R. should receive the Tdap vaccination, particularly because she works in an environment with young children, and she has not received a booster since her childhood DTaP series. She may be given a dose without regard to her prior tetanus booster vaccination.

Diphtheria and tetanus toxoids have been administered in combination with pertussis vaccination in the United States since the 1940s. Both diphtheria and tetanus are rare diseases in the United States as a result of universal childhood immunization. When disease does occur, it does so primarily in the elderly or those who were inadequately vaccinated.[47] For both diseases, it is the toxin-producing strains (toxigenic *Corynebacterium diphtheriae* and *Clostridium tetani*) that result in severe disease and, therefore, the vaccine antigens target the toxoids which they produce. The concentration of diphtheria toxoid in vaccine preparations for adults (designated as *d* as compared with *D* in primary vaccination) is reduced relative to those for children owing to increased reactions with repeated injections and improved response to lower antigen doses.[47] DTaP and diphtheria and tetanus toxoids (DT) are to be used for primary vaccination in children younger than 7 years of age, whereas the tetanus and diphtheria toxoids (Td) are for use in children older than 7 years of age and adults. Booster doses of tetanus (Td) should be administered every 10 years.[47]

Haemophilus Influenzae B

Haemophilus influenzae type b (Hib) was the most common cause of bacterial meningitis and a leading cause of serious, systemic bacterial diseases in children younger than 5 years of age until an effective vaccine was added to the routine immunization schedule.[48–50] The mortality rate associated with Hib meningitis was approximately 5%, with neurologic sequelae observed in 25% to 35% of survivors.[51,52] Epiglottitis, cellulitis, septic arthritis, osteomyelitis, pericarditis, and pneumonia also were commonly caused by *H. influenzae.* Although *H. influenzae* is associated with otitis media and respiratory tract infections, type b strains account for only 5% to 10% of these infections.[53,54]

CASE 64-7

QUESTION 1: P.M. is a 12-month-old child who has not been immunized against Hib. His parents wish to enroll him in day care and are now trying to catch him up on his immunizations. How many doses of vaccine against Hib should he receive?

The Hib vaccine is a conjugate polysaccharide vaccine which is associated with a 95% reduction in the incidence of Hib disease in children younger than 5 years of age.[54] The three currently available monovalent conjugate Hib vaccines are as follows: Hib meningococcal protein conjugate vaccine or PRP-OMP (Pedvax-HIB), Hib tetanus toxoid conjugate vaccine or PRP-T (ActHIB and Hiberix).[56] The immunogenicity of the conjugate vaccines are age-dependent (i.e., older children have an improved immune response).[51,55] The three conjugated vaccines are all approved for use in infants, the group at greatest risk for *H. influenzae* infection; however, they vary in their dosing regimens. The HbCV immunization series requires a priming series followed by a booster dose at 12 to 15 months. PRP-OMP's primary series is administered at 2 and 4 months of age in contrast to a schedule of 2, 4, and 6 months' primary series for the other vaccines.[1,27,56] Ideally, the primary series should be completed with the same HbCV; however, data support the interchangeability of the products for the priming and booster doses.[27,56] If PRP-OMP is used in a priming series with another HbCV, the number of doses necessary to complete the series for the other product should be administered.[56] Combination vaccines may also be used according to indications for each (see Table 64-2).[27,56]

The number of doses of HbCV vaccine needed in previously unimmunized older infants and children depends on their age at presentation. Children who begin HbCV at 7 to 11 months of age should receive a primary series of two doses of a vaccine containing PRP-T, or PRP-OMP followed by a booster dose at 12 to 18 months of age administered at least 2 months after the previous dose.[27,56] Children aged 12 to 15 months should receive a primary series of one dose followed by a booster dose 2 months later. If a child reaches 15 months of age without receiving HbCV, only one dose is necessary.[27,56] HbCV is not routinely recommended in children younger than 5 years of age or adults. Adults who have anatomical or functional asplenia or sickle cell disease, or are undergoing elective splenectomy should receive 1 dose of Hib vaccine if they have not previously received Hib. Adults with a hematopoietic stem cell transplant (HSCT) should receive 3 doses of Hib in at least 4-week intervals 6 to 12 months after transplant regardless of their Hib history. Hib is not routinely recommended for adults with human immunodeficiency virus infection because their risk for *Haemophilus influenzae* type b infection is low.

Polio

Polio, an infectious disease caused by a highly contagious enterovirus, can strike at any age, but primarily affects children younger than 3 years of age (>50% of cases). The three identified serotypes of poliovirus are transmitted person to person by direct fecal–oral contact or indirect exposure to infectious saliva, feces, or contaminated water.[57,58] After household exposure, 90% of susceptible contacts become infected.[57] The poliovirus enters through the mouth and then multiplies in the throat and intestines. Once established in the intestines, poliovirus can enter the bloodstream and invade the CNS, which may result in paralysis.[57–59]

Immunity to polio can be achieved after natural infection with poliovirus; however, infection by one serotype of the poliovirus does not protect an individual against infection from the other two serotypes.[57] Immunity can also be achieved through immunization, and the development of effective vaccines to prevent paralytic polio was one of the major medical breakthroughs of the 20th century. Since the advent of the trivalent oral polio vaccine (OPV) and inactivated polio vaccine (IPV), the incidence of paralytic poliomyelitis has been reduced dramatically.[59]

CASE 64-8

QUESTION 1: H.G. is the mother of a 2-month-old infant who is surprised when the nurse brings in a polio vaccine injection. She remembers that she received an oral form of the vaccine as a child. Why is H.G.'s infant receiving a different form of polio vaccine than she received?

Historically, the live attenuated oral polio vaccine (OPV or Sabin vaccine) was the formulation of choice in the United States. Its advantages include low cost, ease of administration, and induction of lifelong immunity.[57] In addition, OPV provides a high level of gastrointestinal immunity, thus preventing the carrier state. The fecal shedding of the attenuated OPV virus after vaccination is also an effective way to immunize or boost the preexisting immunity in close contacts.[57,59] Despite these benefits, OPV carries the risk of vaccine-associated paralytic polio (VAPP), especially after the first dose in immunocompromised patients such as those with B-lymphocyte disorders (e.g., agammaglobulinemia, hypogammaglobulinemia).[58] In contrast to OPV, the enhanced IPV (IPOL), which is administered intramuscularly, has not been associated with VAPP or other reactions.[58,60] Although IPV provides similar systemic immunity as OPV, it induces less immunity in the gastrointestinal tract.[57,59] The risks of VAPP from OPV, despite its high efficacy, have resulted in the recommendation of IPV as the preferred dosage form for childhood immunization.[1,27,60]

The ACIP and AAP guidelines recommend that all children should receive four doses of IPV at ages 2 months, 4 months, 6 to 18 months, and 4 to 6 years. The first dose of vaccine should be administered no sooner than 6 weeks of life.[60] The last dose of the four-dose series should be administered after 4 years of age and at least 6 months after the previous dose.[27,60] Combination vaccines containing IPV are available and may be used to provide the initial four IPV doses. However, to ensure adequate immunity, it is recommended that an additional IPV booster be administered at 4 to 6 years, for a total of five doses[55] (see Table 64-2).

CASE 64-9

QUESTION 1: L.G. is a 28-year-old graduate student who is planning extensive travels through the African continent and is concerned about polio because she had not been immunized as a child. What would be a prudent immunization schedule for her if her trip includes travel to a polio-endemic area?

Routine poliovirus vaccination of persons older than 18 years of age is not necessary in the United States because US residents are at minimal risk of exposure. Vaccination, however, should be considered for adults at high risk of polio exposure (e.g., travel to an area endemic for polio, close contact with children who will be receiving OPV, close contact with patients who may be excreting wild polioviruses, or work that requires handling poliovirus specimens).[59,60] IPV is the vaccine of choice because adults have a higher incidence of VAPP from OPV than children. Ideally, L.G. should receive two doses of IPV, administered 4 to 8 weeks apart, followed by a third dose 6 to 12 months later. If exposure is likely in less than 8 weeks, two doses of IPV should be administered at least 4 weeks apart.[59] If L.G.'s travel must be undertaken on short notice (<4 weeks) she should receive one dose of IPV with receipt of the remaining doses at a later date according to schedule.[59] Even if L.G. had been immunized as a child, a single dose of IPV may be considered for booster effect.[59]

Currently, OPV is recommended only in special circumstances, such as vaccination to control outbreaks of paralytic polio, unvaccinated infants traveling in less than 4 weeks to areas endemic for polio, and children of parents who reject the number of vaccine injections.[59,60] In parents who are concerned about the number of injections, OPV may be considered for the third and fourth vaccination after receiving systemic protection with IPV for the first two doses.[59] IPV is the only poliovirus vaccine that should be used in patients with an immunodeficiency disorder, those receiving immunosuppressive chemotherapy, or those living with a person who is known or suspected to have these conditions.[59,60]

Meningococcus

CASE 64-10

Question 1: J.C. is a 12-year-old girl who presents for a check-up with her pediatrician. In discussion, it is found that her cousin attends a university where an outbreak of meningococcal disease recently occurred. Should she receive meningococcal vaccine?

After dramatic reductions of *Streptococcus pneumoniae* and *H. influenzae* type b strains of meningitis secondary to conjugate vaccines, *Neisseria meningitidis* has become a more prominent cause of bacterial meningitis. The ACIP recommends routine vaccination of adolescents, with first dose at age 11 to 12 years and a booster at 16 years, persons >2 months of age at increase risk for meningococcal disease, and patients in at-risk groups to control outbreaks.[61] Patients with increased risk for meningococcal disease include those with persistent complement deficiencies, functional or anatomic asplenia, travel to countries where meningococcal disease is hyperendemic or endemic, or who are at risk during an outbreak. Patients aged 2 months to 55 years not previously vaccinated should receive the vaccination if they have persistent complement deficiency, functional or anatomic asplenia, have HIV, are first-year college students in residential housing, travel to countries where meningococcal disease is hyperendemic or endemic, or who are at risk during an outbreak, or are microbiologists who are routinely exposed to *N. meningitides*.[61]

The two available meningococcal vaccine options include two different conjugated vaccines (MCV) covering serotypes A, C, Y, and W-135 of *N. meningitides*. The two conjugate vaccines available (Menactra and Menveo), both MCV4 conjugate vaccines, are indicated for individuals 11 to 55 years of age.[61] The ACIP recommends administration of this vaccine to all persons at 11 to 12 years of age (or at high school entry if there is no history of vaccination) and to unvaccinated college freshmen residing in dormitories. Additionally, as stated earlier, the ACIP recommends a booster dose around the age of 16 years, and a two-dose primary vaccination for patients with reduced response to a single dose.

Adverse effects (e.g., fever, headache, chills, malaise, and arthralgias) from both vaccines are similar and relatively rare; however, the Centers for Disease Control and Prevention (CDC) and FDA issued a warning regarding the potential for increased risk of Guillain–Barré syndrome in patients receiving the Menactra conjugate vaccine.[62] Over the course of a 16-month period beginning in June 2005, 15 cases were reported in the 11- to 19-year age group, and two cases in those older than 20 years of age. All patients recovered. Despite this apparent small increased risk of Guillain–Barré syndrome, current recommendations remain the same, but monitoring of this development will continue. No cases of Guillain–Barré syndrome have been reported with Menveo; however, surveillance is ongoing. At this time, J.C. should receive one of the two MCV4 vaccines and be advised to receive a booster dose at age 16.

Human Papillomavirus

CASE 64-11

Question 1: J.S. is a 12-year-old girl who is healthy and not currently sexually active. Her mother and she would like background information including the role of the human papillomavirus (HPV) vaccine and recommendations for use of the vaccine in J.S.

HPV commonly infects the genital tract and is primarily transmitted by sexual contact. Infection with HPV has been associated with cervical cancer as well as other anogenital cancers (vulvar and vaginal cancers in females and penile cancers in males), anogenital warts, and recurrent respiratory papillomatosis, and it is estimated to be the most common sexually transmitted infection in the United States.[63–65] HPV affects both sexes with similar infection rates, and it is usually asymptomatic, unrecognized, or subclinical.[63,66] Acute HPV infections typically resolve without clinical complications within 1 year; however, 10% to 15% of infections remain persistent and pose a risk of invasive cervical carcinoma and other anogenital carcinomas.[67] Although not all HPV infections cause cervical cancer, almost all (99%) cervical cancer in women is associated with a previous HPV infection.[64,67] The majority of disease associated with HPV is caused by the HPV types 6, 11, 16, and 18, with HPV strains 16 and 18 accounting for 64% of invasive HPV-associated cancers[65] and approximately 50% of cervical cancer precursors.[69,70] In contrast, HPV strains 6 and 11 account for the cause of 90% of genital warts and most cases of recurrent respiratory papillomatosis.[68,71] Infection with one strain of HPV does not prevent infection from other strains; thus, repeated infections can occur through one's lifetime,[67] and those with prior HPV infections benefit from immunization as well.

Three vaccines are available for the prevention of HPV infection: a quadravalent product (Gardasil), a nine-valent product (Gardasil 9), and a bivalent product (Cervarix). The quadravalent product is active against HPV strains 6, 11, 16, and 18; the nine-valent product is active against these strains in addition to 31, 33, 45, 52, and 58. Both of these products are indicated for males and females aged 9 to 26 years.[65] The bivalent product is active against only HPV strains 16 and 18 and is indicated only for females 10 to 25 years old.[71] Gardasil is indicated for males for the purpose of prevention of genital warts and anal cancers.[72]

Routine vaccination with any HPV vaccine is recommended for female patients at 11 to 12 years of age and may begin at 9 years of age.[65] Vaccination at this age attempts to achieve an immune response before the sexual debut[63] and involves a two-dose series administered at intervals of 0 and 6-12 months for patients initiating vaccine before 15 years old.[65] Immunization against HPV is 90% effective in reducing persistent HPV infections and 100% effective in preventing HPV-related diseases such as genital warts or lesions.[68,71] The quadravalent and nine-valent vaccines are recommended for females aged 13 to 26 years, males 13 to 21 years, and it may be given to males 22 through 26 who are men who have sex with men or immunocompromised if they have not been previously vaccinated.[65] The bivalent vaccine is recommended for females aged 13 to 26 years.[65]

The current vaccination rates for HPV vaccination remain below goal for *Healthy People 2020*, despite various strategies to improve rates and reduce the burden of disease and cancer caused by HPV.[64] The CDC recommends immunization for adolescent girls, regardless of current sexual activity, to decrease the lifetime risk of cervical cancer and to protect against infection when the time comes that an individual chooses to become sexually active.[71] Based on the current recommendations, J.S. should receive the HPV vaccine.

Pneumococcus

CASE 64-12

QUESTION 1: M.T. is a 5-year-old boy with a history of asthma. His pediatrician recommends that he receive the pneumonia vaccine. What is the evidence behind this recommendation?

S. pneumoniae (pneumococcus) infection can cause meningitis, pneumonia, sinusitis, and otitis media, and it is a major source of illness and death among children and adults.[73–75] Infants, young children, and older patients are at highest risk for exhibiting pneumococcal infections.[73] The risk for disseminated pneumococcal infections is increased by underlying medical conditions (heart failure, chronic obstructive pulmonary diseases), chronic liver disease (e.g., cirrhosis), functional or anatomic asplenia (e.g., sickle cell disease, splenectomy), and acquired or inherited immunosuppressive conditions (e.g., HIV, cancer, immunosuppressive therapy).

Two pneumococcal vaccines are available: the original polysaccharide vaccine (Pneumovax, PPSV 23) and a conjugate-pneumococcal vaccine (Prevnar, PCV 13).[73,74] Pneumovax contains 23 of the most prevalent or invasive purified capsular-polysaccharide antigens types of *S. pneumoniae*. Antibody response to Pneumovax is inconsistent in children younger than 2 years of age partially because the antigens included in Pneumovax protect against strains that typically cause adult disease, but not childhood disease. In contrast, the conjugate pneumococcal vaccines (Prevnar 13) improve immunogenicity and efficacy in infants and toddlers.[74] The PCV 13 vaccine provides protection against the thirteen pneumococcal strains that cause 90% of all pneumococcal invasive disease in children younger than 6 years of age.[76] ACIP recommends giving the conjugate 13 vaccine (PCV 13) to all children aged 2 to 59 months and children aged 60 to 71 months with underlying medical conditions that place them at high risk for experiencing pneumococcal disease or its complications.[74] Because M.T. has already passed the recommended age for vaccination and has asthma, he should receive the PCV 13 vaccine today.

Immunocompromised patients typically have an unreliable response to vaccines, but because of the potential benefits the pneumococcal vaccines should be administered. PCV 13 and PPSV23 is recommended for children 6 to 18 years old and adult patients >19 years old with immunocompromising conditions, functional or anatomic asplenia, cerebrospinal fluid leaks, or cochlear implants.[75,77] In children, PCV 13 should be administered first, followed by PPSV 23 8 weeks later, and a second PPSV 23 dose 5 years later.[77] Similarly, PCV 13 should be administered first to adults aged 19 to 64 years with immunocompromising conditions, followed by PPSV 23 8 weeks later, with a second PPSV 23 dose 5 years later. Additionally, adults who received PPSV 23 before 65 years old should receive another PPSV 23 dose at 65 years old, or later if it has been 5 years since their last PPSV 23.[75]

CASE 64-12, QUESTION 2: M.T.'s grandfather is a 68 years old who is a previous smoker and has cardiovascular disease. Should M.T.'s grandfather receive pneumococcal vaccine?

In the adult population, PCV 13 and PPSV 23 are recommended for patients over the age of 65 years and older.[78] Since *S. pneumoniae* causes significant morbidity and mortality within the elderly population, the PCV 13 vaccine was studied for efficacy in preventing pneumococcal community acquired pneumonia, non-bacteremic and invasive community acquired pneumonia, and invasive pneumococcal disease.[79] The PCV 13 vaccine was found to prevent pneumococcal, bacteremic, and non-bacteremic community-acquired pneumonia, but it failed to show a prevention of community-acquired pneumonia from any cause. The Centers for Disease Control and Prevention recommend adults >65 years old who have not received a pneumococcal vaccine receive a dose of PCV 13 followed by a dose of PPSV 23 6 to 12 months afterward.[78] The vaccines cannot be coadministered, and the minimum interval between the two vaccines should be at least 8 weeks. For patients >65 years old who have already received a PPSV 23 vaccine should also receive a PCV 13 vaccine >1 year after the most recent PPSV 23. If a second PPSV 23 is indicated, then the PPSV 23 should be administered 6 to 12 months after the PCV 13 or >5 years since the most recent PPSV 23. The 23-valent pneumococcal polysaccharide vaccine (Pneumovax) is also recommended for patients aged 19 to 64 years with certain underlying medical conditions.[73] These underlying medical conditions include immunocompetent patients with chronic heart disease, chronic lung disease, diabetes mellitus, cerebrospinal fluid leaks, cochlear implants, alcoholism, chronic liver disease, functional or anatomic asplenia, cigarette smoking, or who reside in nursing homes or long-term care facilities.[28–30,73] Specifically, adult patients with asthma and those who are cigarette smokers are proven to benefit from the pneumococcal vaccine.[73] A second dose of the vaccine should be administered 5 years after the first dose in patients 19 to 64 years old with functional or anatomic asplenia or who are immunocompromised who received the initial pneumococcal vaccine prior to 65 years of age.[73] If a patient is uncertain as to the accuracy of their vaccination, or when they received it, they should not receive revaccination because of lack of clinical evidence regarding the benefit of revaccination safety and benefit.[73] M.T.'s grandfather (a previously unvaccinated 68-year-old man) should receive one dose of PCV 13, followed by a dose of PPSV 23 6 to 12 months after receiving the PCV 13 vaccine.

Influenza

Annual influenza vaccination is the most effective method for preventing influenza viral infections, complications, and sequelae.[80] Recommendations for influenza vaccination include anyone older than 6 months of age who does not have a contraindication.[81] Routine vaccination has been supported since 2010, and clinical evidence confirms that annual influenza vaccination is a safe and effective preventative health measure with potential benefit for all ages of the population.[81] Vaccination should occur before the onset of influenza virus within the community and patients should receive their dose as soon as available.

Each year, the influenza vaccine is formulated to contain three or four inactivated influenza virus strains (usually, two type A and one or two type B) predicted to be in circulation within the United States during the upcoming flu season.[81] The vaccine is available in intramuscularly administered formulations including the following: inactivated vaccine (IIV) in both trivalent and quadrivalent standard-dose formulations, a trivalent recombinant hemagglutinin influenza vaccine (RIV3), a trivalent cell-cultured based inactivated vaccine (ccIIV3), and a trivalent inactivated high-dose formulation. There is a standard-dose trivalent intradermal inactivated vaccine and a quadrivalent intranasal live attenuated influenza vaccine (LAIV4).[81] Each season the composition of the vaccine is evaluated, and the trivalent formulations contain two influenza type A strains with one type B strain, whereas the quadrivalent formulations contain two type A strains and two type B strains.[80]

The injectable IIV is indicated for use in children at least 6 months old to adults, including those with high-risk conditions.[81] The LAIV4 (intranasal) is indicated for use in healthy nonpregnant patients aged 2 to 49 years old.[81] In patients over 18 years with a history of anaphylactic egg allergy, the trivalent recombinant influenza vaccine (RIV3) and the cell-cultured based inactivated influenza vaccine (ccIIV3) are considered safe for use.[81]

Influenza vaccine should be administered annually for adequate protection. Children younger than 9 years of age require two doses of the vaccine administered 1 month apart to achieve adequate antibody response during the first season they are vaccinated.[81] Influenza vaccine contains a small amount of egg protein, and historically it has been contraindicated in patients with a severe egg allergy.[81] Evidence indicates that even patients with severe egg allergies, including hives, or those who can eat lightly cooked eggs can safely receive the influenza vaccine in the setting of health care personnel in case anaphylactic treatment is necessary. The RIV3 and ccIIV3 are alternatives to patients with egg allergies.

The intradermal IIV is recommended for patients aged 18 to 64 years delivered via a microinjection system into the dermis.[81] Increased injection site reactions occur with this formulation compared to the intramuscular route.[81]

CASE 64-13

QUESTION 1: H.N. is a 72-year-old man inquiring about a new high-dose influenza vaccine. Is this a recommended vaccine for H.N.? Could he be given the LAIV instead?

A high-dose IIV (Fluzone High-Dose) is indicated for patients aged 65 years and older. Standard-dose inactivated trivalent influenza vaccines contain a total of 45 mcg (15 mcg of each of the three recommended strains) of influenza virus hemagglutinin antigen per 0.5-mL dose. In contrast, Fluzone High-Dose has 4 times the activity and is formulated to contain a total of 180 mcg (60 mcg of each strain) of influenza virus hemagglutinin antigen in each 0.5-mL dose. The older than 65 population is targeted to receive the high-dose formulation because older patients respond with a lower antibody titer to the conventional IIV.[82] When antibody titers were measured after patients received the high-dose vaccine, significantly higher antibody titers for all three influenza strains were present.[83–85] In a study to confirm that the high-dose influenza IIV improves protection against laboratory confirmed illness, the high-dose IIV produced higher antibody response and provided improved protection compared to the standard-dose IIV.[86] The high-dose recipients rates for pneumonia, cardiorespiratory conditions, hospitalizations, non-routine medical visits, and medication use were lower than the standard-dose recipients, thus concluding an estimate of improved relative efficacy for the high-dose IIV versus the standard-dose IIV.

The LAIV4 (FluMist) is available for use in healthy, nonpregnant patients 2 to 49 years of age. After administration, recipients become infected with attenuated virus strains, which stimulates both local IgA and circulating IgG antibodies.[87–90] Because live attenuated influenza viral particles are present within the LAIV4, recipients may experience mild signs or symptoms related to influenza infection, such as rhinorrhea, nasal congestion, fever, or sore throat.[91] The LAIV4 is indicated for nonpregnant patients aged 2 to 49 years old without medical conditions that predisposes to complications from the influenza virus. However, the LIAV is not recommended to be preferenced for use over the use of IIV3 at this time.[81] Individuals who should not receive or may not be able to receive the live vaccine include patients[92]:

- with a severe allergy to eggs, or inactive ingredients monosodium glutamate, gelatin, arginine, sucrose, dibasic potassium phosphate, monobasic potassium phosphate, or gentamicin
- with previous life-threatening reactions to previous influenza vaccinations
- currently wheezing or have a history of wheezing if under 5 years of age
- pediatric and adolescent patients currently taking aspirin therapy
- known or suspected immunodeficiency
- history of Guillain–Barré syndrome
- have a history of heart, kidney, or lung disease or diabetes
- are pregnant or nursing

Because of his age, HN should not be given the intranasal vaccine, but he could receive either the standard or high-dose inactivated vaccine.

LIVE ATTENUATED VACCINES

Besides the live attenuated flu vaccine discussed previously, there are several other live attenuated vaccines currently available for use (Table 64-1).

Rotavirus

Rotavirus is a major cause of gastroenteritis and subsequent dehydration in the United States. Almost all children in the United States will experience rotavirus gastroenteritis within the first 5 years of their lives and up to 50% of hospitalizations secondary to gastroenteritis in children are caused by rotavirus infection.[93,94] The AAP and the CDC currently recommend routine immunization of infants with the rotavirus vaccine.[27] There are two oral, live attenuated rotavirus vaccines currently commercially available: Rotateq (RV5), a pentavalent vaccine, and Rotarix (RV1), a monovalent vaccine.[95] Both vaccines are believed to be equally effective despite lack of head-to-head comparison trials. The RV5 vaccine is administered in a three-dose series at 2, 4, and 6 months, whereas the RV1 vaccine follows a two-dose series at 2 and 4 months.[95] Initial vaccination should begin at a minimum of 6 weeks of age and the maximum age at which to administer the last dose is at 8 months of age.[95] It is preferred that all doses be administered with the same product; however, if a combination of RV5 and RV1 is used, a total of three doses should be administered.[95] Although immunization against rotavirus does not prevent all future episodes of rotavirus infection, it can significantly reduce the severity of infections and reduce hospitalization rates.

CASE 64-14

QUESTION 1: J.M., a 24-year-old mother, presents her 2-month-old infant to receive immunizations. She is concerned about the administration of the rotavirus vaccine because the infant's grandmother is undergoing chemotherapy for breast cancer, and she is concerned that the vaccine may put her mother at risk for infection as well as cause "bowel problems" for her baby.

Because the rotavirus vaccine is a live attenuated vaccine and infants can shed the virus after administration, the immunocompromised person (the grandmother) should avoid contact with the infant's feces and adhere to good handwashing procedures, particularly during the first week after vaccine administration.[93–95] Although an immunized infant can spread the rotavirus to an immunocompromised person, the risk is believed to be small relative to the benefits and risks to the immunocompromised individual. For example, if not immunized the infant may become infected with rotavirus and shed much higher amounts of the virus in their stool with a greater potential of spreading the illness to others. Thus, rotavirus immunization of infants under this circumstance still is strongly encouraged.[93]

The immunization of infants who themselves are immunocompromised is more controversial. Rotavirus immunization in this circumstance requires the medical practitioner to discuss risks and benefits with the infant's parents.

Despite being a live attenuated vaccine, the rotavirus vaccine may be administered at any time relative to the administration of blood products and antibody-containing products.[95] There appears to be no interference with the antibody response to the vaccine with the use of these products because much of the immune response is local within the gastrointestinal tract, which leads to protection from gastroenteritis.

Measles/Mumps/Rubella

CASE 64-15

QUESTION 1: J.C. is a 15-month-old girl who is scheduled to receive her MMR vaccination. J.C.'s mother is concerned about the risks of autism and other adverse effects from the vaccine. How should the mother be counseled?

Measles, historically a highly contagious and common disease of childhood, often is associated with symptoms such as high fever, rash, cough, rhinitis, and conjunctivitis.

Complications, although uncommon, include pneumonia and encephalitis. Live attenuated measles virus vaccine produces a benign infection that is thought to produce lifelong immunity. Infections with measles, mumps, or rubella are uncommon in the United States secondary to a significant decrease in the incidence of measles when American children were required to receive the vaccine before entering school.[96,97] During the 1985 to 1988 epidemic, most measles transmission occurred in areas with 95% immunization rates, indicating that some children fail to respond adequately to the initial vaccine dose.[98] In addition, up to 47% of reported cases of measles in the United States result from international importation; the remaining cases result from outbreaks in school-age children who did not receive a second dose of the vaccine.[97,99] Unfortunately, many parents are refusing immunization of their infants with the MMR vaccine because of media reports (now proven unfounded) about the risk of autism.

The concern regarding the risk from autism after vaccination with the MMR vaccine stems from a report by Wakefield et al. published in 1998. This report identified a causal relationship with the administration of the MMR vaccine and the subsequent development of autism in 12 children.[100] The results of this report became highly publicized and sparked fear in parents across the world. Further investigation revealed numerous counts of scientific misconduct for financial gains by Dr. Wakefield, which led to 10 of the 12 coinvestigators retracting their claims. The CDC has coordinated numerous investigations to uncover any relationship between the vaccine and autism, but despite years of research have been unable to find any association. Regrettably, efforts to counter the negative publicity for the MMR vaccine have not had success.

J.C.'s mother should be counseled regarding the lack of an association between autism and the MMR vaccine. If she still decides to refuse vaccination, appropriate forms for documenting such are available through the respective state's Department of Health.

The first dose of the MMR vaccine should be administered to children at 12 to 15 months of age, followed by a second dose at entrance to grade school (age 4 to 6 years).[1,27,97] Studies indicate that infants receiving the vaccine may be at higher risk of exhibiting a febrile seizure during the 2 weeks after vaccination when peak virus replication occurs.[101] The risk appears to be higher with the combination vaccine ProQuad. Because of this concern, the CDC recommends the preferential use of the MMR vaccine in children aged 12 to 47 months. Although studies have not shown a benefit with the use of antipyretics for preventing febrile seizures from the vaccine, it is recommended that caregivers be counseled regarding the management of fever. No increased risk of febrile seizures has been noted with the second dose of the vaccine administered at 4 to 6 years of age, thus the use of the combination vaccine is recommended at this age to reduce the number of injections and enhance compliance.[97]

Adult vaccination with MMR vaccine is also important to protect from epidemics. Adults should receive a second dose of MMR if they were born between 1963 and 1967, previously vaccinated with killed measles vaccine, are students in postsecondary institutions, work in health care facilities, travel internationally, or were recently exposed to a measles outbreak.[97] Persons born after 1957 should receive one dose of a measles-containing vaccine.[28–30,97] Health care workers must show documentation of having receipt of the appropriate number of doses or laboratory evidence of immunity to comply with infection control policies.[102]

Mumps and rubella antigens are combined with measles in the MMR vaccine in the United States. Mumps illness in children rarely produces complications.[97] Meningoencephalitis generally is a benign meningitis, and postinfectious encephalitis, a serious complication, is extremely rare (1 of 6,000). Deafness, commonly considered a risk of mumps, occurs rarely (1 of 15,000) and is usually unilateral. Orchitis, another complication, occurs in approximately 3% to 10% in postpubertal males since the postvaccine era and rarely causes sterility. The most significant consequences of rubella infection occur in pregnant women (e.g., spontaneous abortions, miscarriages, stillbirths, fetal anomalies), especially when infection occurs during the first trimester.[97]

Varicella

CASE 64-16

QUESTION 1: J.T. is a 6-year-old girl who comes home from school with a note from the school nurse indicating that a child in her kindergarten class has been diagnosed with chickenpox. J.T.'s mother is quite concerned because J.T. has not been immunized with the varicella vaccine. She wants to know whether administration of the vaccine at this time will protect J.T. from becoming infected.

Varivax, a live attenuated vaccine against varicella-zoster (chickenpox), is the first herpesvirus vaccine to be widely tested in healthy and high-risk children and adults.[103–105] Chickenpox is a highly contagious, mild childhood disease in healthy children, but it can be severe and even fatal, especially in the immunocompromised patient.

Unusual complications (e.g., severe bacterial superinfections, Reye syndrome, encephalopathies) are markedly reduced with an immunization program.[103] Before the vaccine was available, approximately 4 million cases of chickenpox were reported annually, with 4,000 to 9,000 hospitalizations and 100 deaths.[103] Historically, 55% of varicella-related deaths occurred in adults, many of whom were infected by exposure to unvaccinated preschool-aged children with typical cases of varicella.[106]

Despite high vaccine coverage rates and 85% vaccine efficacy with the previous single dose vaccination, outbreaks of breakthrough varicella continued to occur in the United States.[107] As a result, current guidelines recommend a two-dose series for all children, adolescents, and adults without evidence of immunity.[1,27,107] The first varicella vaccine dose should be administered at 12 to 15 months of age, followed by the second dose at 4 to 6 years of age. For persons 7 to 12 years of age who have not received varicella vaccine, two doses of varicella vaccine should be administered at least 3 months apart. For persons older than 13 years of age, administer two doses of varicella vaccine at least 4 weeks apart.[107]

Postexposure varicella vaccination should be considered for J.T. Chickenpox infection can be prevented or symptoms reduced if varicella vaccine is administered within 3 days of exposure and may provide some protection within 5 days.[105,107] If J.T. also needs MMR vaccination, the quadrivalent combination vaccine ProQuad containing measles, mumps, rubella, and varicella antigens may be considered. A second dose of varicella vaccine in 3 months should be recommended to ensure long-term protection.

The most common adverse effect associated with varicella vaccine administration is rash. Transmission of the virus from the vaccine has been documented in only 3 of 15 million doses administered, all of which occurred in the presence of a vesicular rash after vaccination.[103] Caution should be used when patients exhibit a rash postvaccination to avoid contact with immunocompromised individuals until rash resolution.[107]

Although varicella vaccine might not entirely prevent the occurrence of chickenpox in an immunocompromised patient, it can modify the disease. In the National Institutes of Health's Collaborative Varicella Vaccine Study, a seroconversion rate of only 85% was observed after a single dose in adults, compared with 95% in healthy children and 90% in children with leukemia.[108] Varicella vaccine is generally not recommended in children who have cellular immunodeficiencies, but it can be used in those with impaired humoral immunity.[107] The vaccine should be avoided in children with symptomatic HIV, but it may be considered in asymptomatic or mildly symptomatic patients.[103,107]

CASE 64-16, QUESTION 2: If the varicella vaccine is now universally recommended, what is the role of the herpes zoster vaccine?

After a primary infection with varicella, 15% to 30% of the population experiences a latent infection in the sensory nerve ganglia that reactivates, causing herpes zoster (HZ).[107,109] HZ typically occurs decades after initial varicella infection. This reactivation can result in post-herpetic neuralgia or dissemination which results in skin eruptions ("shingles") and potential CNS, pulmonary, or hepatic complications.[107,109] Although some have theorized that universal varicella vaccination should eventually reduce the incidence of HZ because it prevents primary infection, others debate that the attenuated virus may have greater potential for becoming latent and reactiving.[107,109] Still others argue that with the elimination of wild-type virus in the community, the exposure of individuals with latent wild-type varicella to help boost immunity and prevent HZ is reduced. In this situation, the risk of HZ may be increased.[107,109] Routine varicella immunization began in 1995 and only long-term studies of vaccinated individuals will answer the questions about the impact of the varicella vaccination upon the incidence of HZ. However, currently the majority of adults are not immunized against varicella (unless required as a health care worker) and have previously acquired wild-type varicella infections. Therefore, most adults in the United States are at risk for exhibiting HZ as they age.

The zoster vaccine (Zostavax) is a live attenuated varicella zoster vaccine that uses the same strain and antigens as the varicella vaccines (Varivax and ProQuad); however, it is 14 times more potent and contains additional antigenic components. It was initially recommended for all individuals older than 60 years of age as a single subcutaneous injection to prevent HZ.[28–30,109,110] In 2011, FDA approval was given to use HZ vaccine in individuals 50 years of age or older; however, ACIP recommendations remain for patients 60 years and older.[110] It may be given to patients with a previous history of HZ, but it is not indicated to treat acute zoster or prevent further complications during an acute episode.[109] It is not recommended for routine immunization for anyone who has previously received the varicella vaccine. The zoster vaccine was shown in the Shingles Prevention Study to reduce the incidence of HZ by more than 50% and resulted in reductions in the severity and duration of pain, in addition to preventing the development of post-herpetic neuralgia.[111]

ADMINISTRATION TECHNIQUES

Vaccines or other biological agents are typically administered as either an intramuscular (IM) or subcutaneous injection.

Because appropriate administration by the correct route and technique is critical to the effectiveness of the specified vaccine, it is essential to consult the prescribing and administration information for each specific vaccination administered to a patient (see also Table 64-1). The technique of vaccine administration by either route should include sterilizing the skin surface, drawing up the vaccine from the vial into a syringe using sterile technique, protecting the patient and health care provider regarding biological hazards, performing proper disposal of biohazardous/sharps materials (needles and blood-borne products), observing for adverse effects after administration, and reassuring the patient postvaccine administration. Table 64-3 includes general guidelines for safe and effective parenteral administration.

CASE 64-17

QUESTION 1: B.D., a nurse from a family medicine clinic, frantically calls you because she mistakenly administered a Pneumovax vaccination subcutaneously. How to you respond to B.D.'s call?

The majority of vaccines, including Pneumovax, specify IM administration. This technique involves penetration of the appropriate muscle at a 90-degree angle. For graphical illustration of intramuscular vaccine administration, see **http://www.immunize.org/catg.d/p2020.pdf**. Site of IM injections include the anterolateral thigh muscle in infants and toddlers, and the deltoid (upper arm) muscle for children and adults.[1,112] The typical needle used to administer an IM injection is 1 inch long and 22 to 25 gauge. A shorter needle (e.g., 5/8 inch) may be used for newborns, whereas a 1 to 1/2-inch needle may be

Table 64-3

Subcutaneous and Intramuscular Vaccine Administration Techniques

Patient Age	Site	Injection Area	Typical Needle Length (inch)	Needle Gauge
Birth to 12 months	Subcutaneous	Fatty tissue over the anterolateral thigh muscle	5/8	23–25
12 months and older	Subcutaneous	Fatty tissue over anterolateral thigh or fatty tissue over triceps	5/8	23–25
Newborn (0–28 days)	Intramuscular	Anterolateral thigh muscle	5/8	22–25
Infant (1–12 months)	Intramuscular	Anterolateral thigh muscle	1	22–25
Toddler (1–3 years)	Intramuscular	Anterolateral thigh muscle OR Deltoid muscle of arm if muscle mass is adequate	1–1¼ 5/8–1	22–25
Children (3–18 years)	Intramuscular	Deltoid muscle OR Anterolateral thigh muscle	5/8–1 1–1¼	22–25
Adults ≥19 years	Intramuscular	Deltoid muscle OR Anterolateral thigh muscle	1–1½	22–25

Sources: National Center for Immunization and Respiratory Diseases. General recommendations on immunizations-recommendations of the Advisory Committee on Immunization Practices (ACIP). *MMWR Recomm Rep*. 2011;60:1–61; Immunization Action Coalition. How to Administer Intramuscular (IM) Vaccine Injections. **http://www.immunize.org/catg.d/p2020.pdf**. Accessed May 27 2015; Immunization Action Coalition. Administering Vaccines: Dose, route, site, and needle size. **http://www.immunize.org/catg.d/p3085.pdf**. Accessed May 27 2015.

needed for adults weighing greater than 90 kg for women and 118 kg for men.[112,113] Multiple IM injections given in the same extremity during the same time period should be placed at least 1 inch apart.[1] Although most vaccine products specify the route of administration, Pneumovax may be administered either IM or into subcutaneous tissue.[114] Therefore, B.D. should be reassured that she has administered the Pneumovax correctly because it is acceptable to administer this vaccination by either route.

Subcutaneous vaccinations involve injection of vaccine into fatty subcutaneous tissue between the layer of skin and the layer of muscle.[1,112] Subcutaneous vaccinations are administered with a 5/8-inch needle, 23 to 25 gauge, inserted at a 45-degree angle to the skin, while pinching up on the subcutaneous tissue to prevent injection into the muscle. For graphical illustration of subcutaneous vaccination administration, see **http://www.immunize.org/catg.d/p2020.pdf**. Sites of subcutaneous injections include the fatty tissue over the anterolateral thigh muscle in children newborn to 1 year old, and fatty tissue over the triceps in children 1 year old to adults. Multiple subcutaneous injections given in the same extremity during the same time period should be placed at least 1 inch apart.

Other routes of administration for vaccinations include the oral, intranasal, and intradermal routes. Rotavirus and oral typhoid are the only orally administered vaccines in the United States.[1] Inactivated influenza is the only intranasal vaccine, administered via a nasal sprayer with a dose divider. Intradermal influenza is the only intradermally administered vaccine, and it is administered in the area of the deltoid at a 90-degree angle into the skin.[113]

LEGAL REQUIREMENTS

CASE 64-18

QUESTION 1: What are the requirements necessary to become a pharmacist immunizer? How are pharmacists advocates for improving population immunization rates?

Pharmacists have varying authority to administer vaccinations within the United States based on each state's Pharmacy Practice Act. The rationale for pharmacists to deliver immunizations to the public includes pharmacist accessibility in every community and overall low vaccination rates throughout the population.[115] The Department of Health & Human Services and Centers for Disease Control and Prevention recognized pharmacist's unique position to promote vaccines and also influence vaccination in diverse populations through a letter from the Assistant Surgeon General.[116] This letter also acknowledged pharmacist's contribution to increase immunization awareness in the past, but it also requested continued assistance in this endeavor through the following:

- Increasing vaccine awareness in the adult and adolescent population
- Ensuring patient's vaccine requirements are assessed when they visit pharmacies
- Offering vaccinations to patients with certain medical conditions (high risk)
- Entering adult immunizations into vaccine registries where possible
- Partnering and collaborating with local and state health departments, immunization coalitions, medical providers, and other vaccination outreach programs

The American Pharmacist's Association has developed a national competency-based certificate training program for pharmacists, and most schools of pharmacy across the country contain or provide an opportunity to learn immunization administration within their curriculum.[117] These programs include both didactic and hands-on training and prepare the learners to be public health educators regarding immunizations, to promote vaccinations within their community, and to administer vaccines at their practice sites.

Although each state's requirements regarding necessary training, protocols, and notification systems may differ, there are some standardized requirements a pharmacist immunizer must follow. Current cardiopulmonary resuscitation certification is a common requirement for pharmacist immunizers. Immunization administration curricula typically contain information regarding basic immunology, specifics regarding vaccine information, practice implementation, legal and regulatory issues, and administration techniques.[117] Each state stipulates the statutes on patient age that may receive a pharmacist-administered vaccination; what types of vaccinations pharmacists are able to administer; and the mechanism by which pharmacists are authorized to administer vaccines by physicians, such as through a prescription, collaborative drug therapy management agreement, protocol, or standing order.[118] Some states require continuing-education credit maintenance specific to immunizations or vaccinations for pharmacists who immunize; some states are very specific in their requirements, and others are more general. It is important to check with the state licensing board regarding specific statutes and regulations relating to pharmacist immunization practices. In addition, a growing number of states have passed legislation allowing pharmacy interns with the necessary training to administer immunizations. Currently, 44 states and territories have adopted legislation allowing pharmacy interns to administer vaccines, given the student has completed an immunization certificate program and operates only under supervision of an immunizing pharmacist.[118]

Patient consent forms for immunization and vaccine information sheets are important aspects for patient safety that pharmacists are required to use as part of an approved immunization program. Consent forms should include screening questionnaires specific for each vaccine, should be signed prior to vaccine administration, and should be reviewed by the pharmacist with the patient present. Vaccine information sheets are patient information developed by the CDC providing specific individual vaccine information benefits and risks, and they are required to be distributed to the patient with each vaccine by the National Childhood Vaccine Injury Act of 1986. Resources for pharmacists are available through the CDC, Immunization Action Coalition, and American Pharmacists Association.[119–121]

KEY REFERENCES AND WEBSITES

A full list of references for this chapter can be found at http://thepoint.lww.com/AT11e. Below are the key references and websites for this chapter, with the corresponding reference number in this chapter found in parentheses after the reference.

Key References

Bonten MJM et al. Polysaccharide conjugate vaccine against pneumococcal pneumonia in adults. *N Engl J Med*. 2015;372:1114–1125. (80)

Centers for Disease Control. Prevention and control of influenza with vaccines: recommendations of the Advisory Committee on Immunization Practices (ACIP), 2010 [published corrections appear in *MMWR Recomm Rep*. 2010;59:1147; *MMWR Recomm Rep*. 2010;59:993]. *MMWR Recomm Rep*. 2010;59(RR-8):1. (92)

Centers for Disease Control. Updated recommendations for prevention of invasive pneumococcal disease among adults using the 23-valent pneumococcal polysaccharide vaccine (PPSV23). *MMWR Morb Mortal Wkly Rep*. 2010;59:1102. (74)

Centers for Disease Control and Prevention. Prevention and control of meningococcal disease: recommendations of the Advisory Committee of Immunization Practices (ACIP). *MMWR Morb Mortal Wkly Rep*. 2013;62(RR-2):1-22. (62)

Centers for Disease Control and Prevention. Updated recommendations for use of tetanus toxoid, reduced diphtheria toxoid, and acellular pertussis vaccine (Tdap) in pregnant women: Advisory Committee on Immunization Practices (ACIP). *MMWR Morb Mortal Wkly Rep*. 2013; 62:131–135. (46)

Cortese MM et al. Prevention of rotavirus gastroenteritis among infants and children: recommendations of the Advisory Committee on Immunization Practices (ACIP) [published correction appears in *MMWR Recomm Rep*. 2010;59:1074]. *MMWR Recomm Rep*. 2009;58(RR-2):1. (96)

Harpaz R et al. Prevention of herpes zoster: recommendations of the Advisory Committee on Immunization Practices (ACIP). *MMWR Recomm Rep*. 2008;57(RR-5):1. (110)

Marin M et al. Prevention of varicella: recommendations of the Advisory Committee on Immunization Practices (ACIP). *MMWR Recomm Rep*. 2007;56(RR-4):1. (108)

Marin M et al. Use of combination measles, mumps, rubella and varicella vaccine: recommendations of the Advisory Committee on Immunization Practices (ACIP). *MMWR Recomm Rep*. 2010;59(RR-3):1. (102)

Mast EE et al. A comprehensive immunization strategy to eliminate the transmission of hepatitis B virus infection in the United States: recommendations of the Advisory Committee on Immunization Practices (ACIP) part I: immunization of infants, children, and adolescents [published corrections appear in *MMWR Morb Mortal Wkly Rep*. 2006;55:158; *MMWR Morb Mortal Wkly Rep*. 2007;56:1267]. *MMWR Recomm Rep*. 2005;54(RR-16):1. (33)

Mast EE et al. A comprehensive immunization strategy to eliminate the transmission of hepatitis B virus infection in the United States: recommendations of the Advisory Committee on Immunization Practices (ACIP) part II: immunization of adults [published correction appears in *MMWR Morb Mortal Wkly Rep*. 2007;56:1114]. *MMWR Recomm Rep*. 2006;55(RR-16):1. (34)

National Center for Immunization and Respiratory Diseases. General recommendations on immunizations—recommendations of the Advisory Committee on Immunization Practices (ACIP). *MMWR Recomm Rep*. 2011;60:1. (1)

Nuorti JP et al. Prevention of pneumococcal disease among infants and children—use of 13-valent pneumococcal conjugate vaccine and 23-valent pneumococcal polysaccharide vaccine. Recommendations of the Advisory Committee on Immunization Practices (ACIP). *MMWR Recomm Rep*. 2010;59(RR-11):1. (75)

Petrosky et al. Use of 9-valent human papillomavirus (HPV) vaccine: updated HPV vaccination recommendations of the Advisory Committee on Immunization Practices. *MMWR Morb Motal Wkly Rep*. 2015;64:300–304. (66)

Key Websites

American Pharmacists Association. Immunization Center. http://www.pharmacist.com/immunization-center. Accessed June 1, 2015.

APhA authority to immunize website. http://www.pharmacist.com/sites/default/files/files/Pharmacist_IZ_Authority_1_31_15.pdf. Accessed June 1, 2015.

Centers for Disease Control. Vaccine information statements. http://www.cdc.gov/vaccines/hcp/vis/index.html. Published April 27, 2015. Accessed June 1, 2015.

Centers for Disease Control and Prevention. Immunization schedules: adult immunization schedules, United States, 2017. http://www.cdc.gov/vaccines/schedules/hcp/adult.html. Accessed June 5, 2017.

Centers for Disease Control and Prevention. Immunization schedules: birth-18 years & "catch-up" immunizations schedules, United States, 2017. http://www.cdc.gov/vaccines/schedules/hcp/child-adolescent.html. Accessed June 5, 2017.

Immunization Action Coalition. Administering Vaccines: dose, route, site, and needle size. http://www.immunize.org/catg.d/p3085.pdf. Accessed May 27, 2015.

Immunization Action Coalition. Handouts: clinic resources. http://www.immunize.org/handouts/screening-vaccines.asp. Reviewed March 27, 2015. Accessed June 1, 2015.

Immunization Action Coalition. How to Administer Intramuscular (IM) Vaccine Injections. http://www.immunize.org/catg.d/p2020.pdf. Accessed May 27, 2015.

65 Central Nervous System Infections

Gregory A. Eschenauer, Deanna Buehrle, and Brian A. Potoski

CORE PRINCIPLES

		CHAPTER CASES
1	The most common symptoms of meningitis include the triad of fever, stiff neck, and altered mental status. In neonates and infants, irritability and poor feeding may be reported along with fever. In the elderly, signs may be absent or more subtle.	**Case 65-1 (Question 1)**
2	Adjunctive dexamethasone should be initiated in all patients with suspected bacterial meningitis either before or concomitant with the first dose of antibiotic.	**Case 65-1 (Question 4)**
3	Intraventricular antibiotics should be considered for patients with meningitis who have an external drainage device in place. Such therapy should be used in combination with systemically administered therapy.	**Case 65-4 (Question 4)**
4	Cerebrospinal fluid (CSF) is essential in confirming the diagnosis of meningitis. The CSF typically contains many white blood cells (WBCs) with a predominance of neutrophils. Additionally, CSF protein is typically elevated to greater than 100 mg/dL with a low CSF glucose concentration (either less than 50 mg/dL or less than 50-60% of a simultaneously obtained serum glucose value).	**Case 65-1 (Question 2)**
5	Response to therapy should be monitored by resolution of fever, altered mental status, and stiff neck. A baseline level of mental status should be evaluated for this reason. Delays in response to therapy may require a repeat lumbar puncture to re-examine CSF cultures, which are usually sterile after 18 to 24 hours of therapy. Clinical response should be seen between 24 and 48 hours of initiation of therapy.	**Case 65-1 (Question 6)**
6	The choice of empiric therapy in patients with meningitis is primarily driven by age and the presence of predisposing conditions (postneurosurgical, head trauma, immunocompromised).	**Case 65-1 (Question 3)**
7	Brain abscess is associated with a different spectrum of pathogens, including oral anaerobes, staphylococci, and aerobic gram-negative bacilli, depending on the patient. The barrier from the blood to brain parenchyma differs from that between blood and CSF. Consequently, the choice of antimicrobial for brain abscess may differ from that associated with meningitis.	**Case 65-5 (Questions 1–3)**

The pharmacotherapy of central nervous system (CNS) infections presents numerous challenges. Antibiotic penetration often is limited, and host defenses are absent or inadequate. Thus, morbidity and mortality from infections of the CNS remain high despite the availability of highly potent, bactericidal antibiotics. In a review of 3,155 episodes of bacterial meningitis between 1998 and 2007, the mortality rate was 15%.[1] Although eradication of bacteria is essential, it is only one of the variables that affect mortality from CNS infections. In an attempt to decrease morbidity and mortality, the pathophysiologic mechanisms of CNS infections continue to be studied.[2]

A number of infectious processes can occur within the CNS (e.g., meningitis, encephalitis, meningoencephalitis, brain abscess, subdural empyema, and epidural abscess). In addition, prosthetic devices placed into the CNS (e.g., CSF shunts for management of hydrocephalus) often are complicated by infection. Many etiologic agents are capable of inducing CNS infections, including bacteria, viruses, fungi, and certain parasites. This chapter focuses primarily on bacterial infections of the CNS, with an emphasis on the pharmacotherapy of bacterial meningitis and brain abscess. (Also see Chapter 76, Pharmacotherapy of Human Immunodeficiency Virus Infection, and Chapter 77, Opportunistic Infection in HIV-Infected Patients, for presentations pertaining to CNS infections in these populations).

REVIEW OF CENTRAL NERVOUS SYSTEM

Anatomy and Physiology

MENINGES

Proper therapy of CNS infections requires an understanding of anatomic and physiologic characteristics. The brain and spinal cord are ensheathed by a protective covering known as the meninges and suspended in CSF, which acts as a shock absorber to outside trauma. The meninges consist of three layers of fibrous tissue: the *pia mater*, *arachnoid*, and *dura mater*. The pia mater, the innermost layer of the meninges, is a thin, delicate membrane that closely adheres to the contours of the brain. Separating the pia mater from the more loosely enclosed arachnoid membrane is the subarachnoid space, in which the CSF resides. The pia mater and arachnoid, known collectively as the *leptomeninges*, lie interior to the dura mater, a tough outer membrane that adheres to the periosteum and vertebral column. *Meningitis* is a term describing inflammation (often the result of infection) of the subarachnoid space. Abscesses also can form outside the dural space (epidural abscess), often with devastating consequences.[3]

CEREBROSPINAL FLUID

CSF is produced and secreted by the choroid plexus in the lateral ventricles and, to a lesser extent, by the choroid plexuses within the third and fourth ventricles. CSF flows unidirectionally from the lateral ventricles through the foramina of the third and fourth ventricles into the subarachnoid space, then over the cerebral hemispheres and downward into the spinal canal. CSF is absorbed through villous projections (arachnoid villi) into veins, primarily the cerebral venous sinuses. About 0.35 to 0.4 mL of CSF is secreted per minute, with 50% of the total volume of CSF being replaced every 5 to 6 hours.[4] The flow of CSF is unidirectional from the ventricles to the intralumbar space. Therefore, intrathecal injection of antibiotics results in little, if any, antibiotic reaching the cerebral ventricles.[3] This unidirectional flow of CSF presents a problem because ventriculitis commonly occurs in conjunction with bacterial meningitis. Direct intraventricular instillation of antibiotics, usually by means of a reservoir, is preferable in the setting of ventriculitis (see Case 65-4, Question 4).[5]

In adults, children, and infants, the volume of CSF is approximately 150 mL, 60 to 100 mL, and 40 to 60 mL, respectively.[4,6] Knowledge of approximate CSF volume facilitates estimation of the CSF concentration of a drug subsequent to intrathecal administration. For example, administration of gentamicin 5 mg (5,000 mcg) intrathecally should result in a CSF concentration of approximately 33 mcg/mL in an adult shortly after administration.

The composition of CSF differs from other physiologic fluids. The pH of CSF is slightly acidic (normal pH, 7.3), and with the exception of chloride ion, electrolyte concentrations are slightly less than those in serum.[5] Under normal conditions, the protein concentration in CSF is 15 to 45 mg/dL, CSF glucose values are 50 to 80 mg/dL (approximately 60% those of plasma), and few if any WBCs are present (<5 cells/μL).[3] When the meninges become inflamed (i.e., in meningitis), the composition of the CSF is altered. In particular, the protein concentration in the CSF increases, and the glucose concentration in the CSF usually declines with meningitis. Therefore, careful evaluation of CSF chemistries is useful when establishing a diagnosis of meningitis.

BLOOD–BRAIN BARRIER

The blood–brain barrier plays a crucial role in protecting the brain and maintaining homeostasis within the CNS.[3,4] Actually, two distinct barriers exist within the brain: the blood–CSF barrier and the blood–brain barrier. The blood–CSF barrier is characterized morphologically by porous capillaries (Fig. 65-1). This allows proteins and other molecules (including antibiotics) to pass freely into the immediate interstitial space. Diffusion of substances into the CSF is restricted by tightly fused cells lining the ventricular side of the choroid plexus (Fig. 65-1). Cerebral capillary endothelial cells make up the blood–brain barrier, which separates blood from the interstitial fluid of the brain. Unlike capillaries in other areas of the body, the capillary endothelia of the brain are packed closely together, forming tight junctions that in effect produce a barrier physiologically similar to a continuous lipid bilayer. The surface area of the blood–brain barrier is more than 5,000 times greater than that of the blood–CSF barrier; thus, the blood–brain barrier plays a more important role in protecting the brain and regulating its chemical composition.[7] Many antimicrobials traverse the blood–brain barrier with difficulty (see section on *Antimicrobial Penetration Into the Cerebrospinal Fluid* below).

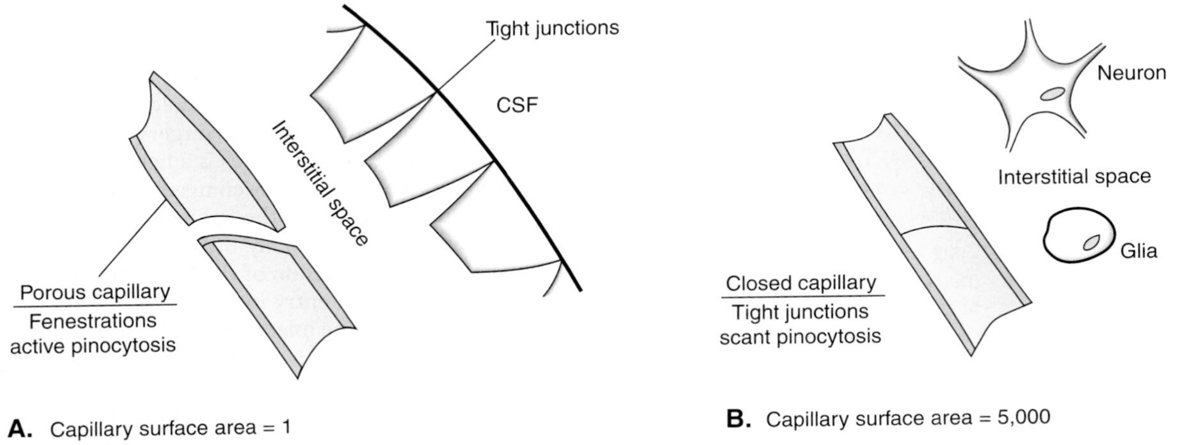

Figure 65-1 The two membrane barrier systems in the central nervous system: the blood–cerebrospinal fluid (CSF) barrier (left) and the blood–brain barrier. Blood–brain barrier: interface between internal medicine and the brain.

MENINGITIS

Meningitis is the most common type of CNS infection. The signs and symptoms associated with bacterial meningitis usually are acute in onset, evolving over the course of a few hours. Prompt recognition and early institution of therapy are essential to ensuring beneficial outcomes.[8] In contrast, a diverse group of infectious (e.g., viruses, fungi, and mycobacteria) and noninfectious (e.g., chemical irritants) agents produce a meningitic picture often of a less acute or chronic nature.[9,10] Drugs that can induce aseptic meningitis include trimethoprim–sulfamethoxazole (TMP-SMX), intravenous (IV) immunoglobulins, OKT3 antibodies, and nonsteroidal anti-inflammatory drugs such as ibuprofen, naproxen, and sulindac.[9]

Microbiology

Generally, meningitis is a disease of the very young and very old: Most cases occur in children younger than 2 years of age and in elderly adults.[1] The bacterial causes of meningitis correlate well with age and underlying conditions (Table 65-1).[11]

Neonates (infants <1 month) are at an especially high risk of experiencing meningitis. Meningitis in preterm neonates is most often caused by *Escherichia coli* whereas meningitis in term neonates is most often caused by group B streptococci (*Streptococcus agalactiae*). These highly virulent pathogens usually are acquired during passage through the birth canal or from the hospital environment and are associated with significant morbidity and mortality, particularly in premature infants.[1,12] Consensus recommendations regarding intra-partum administration of penicillin to women colonized with group B streptococci have led to an 80% decrease in early-onset infection due to this pathogen.[13] *Listeria monocytogenes* is another important and often overlooked pathogen in neonates.[1] Because *L. monocytogenes* is resistant to many antimicrobial agents, including third-generation cephalosporins, selection of initial (empiric) therapy in neonates must be approached with this pathogen in mind.[11]

Infants and children 2 to 23 months old are also at a high risk of meningitis. Historically, in this age group, the disease was caused predominantly by three pathogens: *Haemophilus influenzae*, *Streptococcus pneumoniae*, and *Neisseria meningitidis*. Up to 45% of all cases of meningitis in the United States before 1985 were caused by *H. influenzae* type b (Hib).[14] From 1991 to 1996, however, Hib invasive disease incidence in children <5 years of age decreased by >99%. This reduction in *H. influenzae*-induced meningitis correlates with the widespread vaccination of children against invasive *H. influenzae* disease with the Hib polysaccharide–protein conjugate vaccines.[15]

In adults and children who have received the conjugated Hib vaccine, community-acquired meningitis most often is caused by *S. pneumoniae* (the pneumococcus) and *N. meningitidis* (the meningococcus). Meningococci more commonly are implicated in individuals aged 2 to 34 years, whereas pneumococci are the predominant pathogens in adults older than 34 years of age.[1] The incidence of pneumococcal meningitis has decreased by 26% from 1998 to 2006–2007 with the introduction of pneumococcal conjugate vaccines, with a decrease of 92% if only serotypes contained in the seven-valent conjugate vaccine are considered.[16] Unfortunately, use of the 13-valent conjugate vaccine has not resulted in further decreases in meningitis cases in children, with nonvaccine serotypes replacing those contained in the vaccine.[17] The incidence of meningococcal disease has decreased by 73% from 1996 to 2011. Interestingly, most of this decline in incidence occurred prior to the routine use of meningococcal conjugate vaccines.[18]

Patients of advanced age and those who undergo neurosurgical procedures or experience head trauma are also susceptible to meningitis. The most likely causative pathogens in these patient populations are listed in Table 65-1.

Table 65-1
Microbiology of Bacterial Meningitis

Age Group or Predisposing Condition	Most Likely Organisms[a]
Neonates (<1 month)	Group B streptococcus (*Streptococcus agalactiae*), *Escherichia coli*, *Klebsiella* species, *Listeria monocytogenes*
Infants and children (1–23 months)	*Streptococcus pneumoniae*, *Neisseria meningitidis*, *S. agalactiae*, *Haemophilus influenzae*,[b] *E. coli*
Children and adults (2–50 years)	*N. meningitidis*, *S. pneumoniae*
Adults (>50 years)	*S. pneumoniae*, *N. meningitidis*, *L. monocytogenes*, *E. coli*, *Klebsiella* species, and other aerobic gram-negative bacilli
Postneurosurgical	*Staphylococcus aureus*, aerobic gram-negative bacilli (e.g., *E. coli*, *Klebsiella* species, *Pseudomonas aeruginosa*), *Staphylococcus epidermidis*[c]
Closed head trauma	*S. pneumoniae*, *H. influenzae*, group A β-hemolytic streptococci
Penetrating trauma	*S. aureus*, *S. epidermidis*, aerobic gram-negative bacilli (e.g., *E. coli*, *Klebsiella* species, *P. aeruginosa*)
CSF shunt	Coagulase-negative staphylococci (particularly *S. epidermidis*), *S. aureus*, aerobic gram-negative bacilli (including *P. aeruginosa*), *Propionibacterium acnes*

[a]Organisms listed in descending order of frequency.
[b]Need to consider this pathogen only in children not vaccinated with Hib.
[c]Most commonly seen in association with prosthetic devices (e.g., cerebrospinal fluid shunts).
CSF, cerebrospinal fluid.

Pathogenesis and Pathophysiology

In general, meningitis can develop from *hematogenous* spread of organisms, by *contiguous* spread from a parameningeal focus (e.g., sinusitis or otitis media), or by direct bacterial *inoculation*, as occurs with head trauma or neurosurgery. In contiguous spread, colonization of mucosal surfaces is a necessary first step in the pathogenesis of meningitis. Meningeal pathogens then adhere to, and penetrate through, the epithelial surface and enter the intravascular space. Eventually, organisms multiply to sufficient numbers that allow invasion of the blood–brain barrier.[2,19,20]

Once bacteria gain entry into the CSF, host defenses are inadequate to contain the infection, and bacteria replicate rapidly. Humoral immunity (both complement and immunoglobulin) essentially is absent within the CSF. In addition, opsonic activity in CSF is negligible, and although leukocytosis ensues shortly after bacterial invasion, phagocytosis also is inefficient. Therefore, this relative immunodeficiency state necessitates the initiation of bactericidal therapy.[2,19,20]

Inflammation of the meninges is initiated by contents within the bacterial cell wall. Release of these contents (lipopolysaccharide for gram negatives and teichoic acid for gram positives) induces the production and secretion of inflammatory cytokines, which promote the adherence of leukocytes to cerebral capillary endothelial cells and facilitate the migration of leukocytes into the CSF. This results in the characteristic CSF leukocytosis as well as an eventual increase in blood–brain barrier permeability.[2,19,20]

Inflammation of the blood–brain barrier may lead to brain edema, which, combined with obstruction of CSF outflow, increases intracranial pressure and alters cerebral blood flow. Resultant hyperperfusion or hypoperfusion of the brain may ultimately result in neuronal injury, cerebral ischemia, and irreversible brain damage. The inflammatory response in meningitis also can be aggravated by some antibiotics, notably the penicillins and cephalosporins.[19] When the β-lactam antibiotics lyse bacterial cell walls, large amounts of cell wall products are liberated, and these products amplify the inflammatory response. The long-term benefits of β-lactam therapy far outweigh such detrimental effects, and the use of adjunctive corticosteroids in certain patient populations can substantially reduce inflammation and the subsequent neurologic sequelae of meningitis.[2,19,20]

In a systemic review of approximately three decades of data surrounding neurologic sequelae, the median risk of developing at least one major or minor sequela was 19.9% (12.3%–35.3%).[21] The type and severity of neurologic complications vary with the specific infecting organism, the severity of the infection, and the susceptibility of the host. In a long-term prospective study of 185 children with acute bacterial meningitis, permanent hearing loss occurred in 6%, 10.5%, and 31% of children with meningitis caused by *H. influenzae*, *N. meningitidis*, and *S. pneumoniae*, respectively. Although seizures are fairly common on initial presentation, long-term epilepsy occurs in approximately 7% of patients. Other important long-term complications include spastic paraparesis, behavioral disorders, and learning deficits.[22]

Diagnosis and Clinical Features

CLINICAL AND LABORATORY FEATURES OF BACTERIAL MENINGITIS

CASE 65-1

QUESTION 1: S.C., a 5-year-old boy, is brought to the emergency department (ED) by his mother, who says her son has a temperature of 39°C, is irritable and lethargic, and has a rash. S.C. was in his usual state of good health until last night, when he awoke crying. When she went to investigate, her son began to stiffen up and rock back and forth in his bed. Because he was not arousable, S.C.'s mother rushed him to the hospital. S.C.'s medical history is noncontributory except for an allergy to amoxicillin described as a skin rash. S.C., his mother and father, and his 7-year-old brother recently moved to the United States. S.C.'s vaccination history currently is unknown. S.C. and his brother currently attend a community day-care center.

On physical examination, S.C. was in marked distress, with a temperature of 40°C, blood pressure of 90/60 mm Hg, and a respiratory rate of 32 breaths/minute. His weight on admission was 20 kg. Neurologic examination showed evidence of nuchal rigidity; he was lethargic and difficult to arouse. Brudzinski and Kernig signs were positive. On head, eyes, ears, nose, and throat examination, S.C. demonstrated photophobia (he squinted severely when the examiner shone a light in his eyes), but no evidence was noted of papilledema. A petechial rash was visible on his extremities. The remainder of S.C.'s examination was essentially normal.

Blood drawn for laboratory tests revealed the following results:

Sodium (Na), 128 mEq/L
Potassium (K), 3.2 mEq/L
Chloride (Cl), 100 mEq/L
Bicarbonate (HCO_3), 25 mEq/L
Blood urea nitrogen (BUN), 16 mg/dL
Serum creatinine (SCr), 0.6 mg/dL
Serum glucose, 80 mg/dL

The WBC count was 18,000 cells/μL with 95% polymorphonuclear (PMN) cells; the hemoglobin (Hgb), hematocrit (Hct), and platelet count all were within normal limits. What clinical and laboratory features does S.C. display that are suggestive of meningitis?

Table 65-2
Signs and Symptoms of Acute Bacterial Meningitis

Fever	Anorexia
Nuchal rigidity (stiff neck)	Headache
Altered mental status	Photophobia
Seizures	Nausea and vomiting
Brudzinski sign[a]	Focal neurologic deficits
Kernig sign[a]	Septic shock
Irritability[b]	

[a]See text for description of sign.
[b]Symptoms seen in infants with meningitis.

The clinical features of bacterial meningitis are summarized in Table 65-2. The most common symptoms include the triad of fever, stiff neck (nuchal rigidity), and altered mental status. When all three of these features are present, as is S.C.'s case, meningitis should be strongly suspected. Other less common signs and symptoms include headache, photophobia (unusual intolerance to light), and focal neurologic deficits, including cranial nerve palsies.[23] A positive Brudzinski sign (reflex flexion of the hips and knees produced on flexion of the neck when lying in the recumbent position) and Kernig sign (pain on extension of the hamstrings when lying supine with the thighs perpendicular to the trunk) provide physical evidence of meningeal irritation.[24] Brudzinski and Kernig signs both were positive in S.C. Seizures occur on initial presentation in up to 60% of patients and may be focal or generalized.[23] The presence of seizures or a severely depressed mental status (i.e., obtundation or coma) generally is associated with a poorer prognosis.[25] According to the most recent practice guidelines for the management of bacterial meningitis, a computed tomographic (CT) scan should be obtained before lumbar puncture in patients with specific criteria. These include immunocompromised state, history of CNS disease, new-onset seizure, papilledema, abnormal level of consciousness, and focal neurologic deficit. Although controversial, brain herniation can occur when lumbar puncture is performed in patients with elevated intracranial pressure because of the pressure changes induced within the cranial vault.[11]

S.C. has many of the clinical features associated with acute bacterial meningitis. Furthermore, the low blood pressure (hypotension) and increased respiratory rate are characteristic findings in severe, life-threatening types of bacterial infection (e.g., septic shock, meningitis) and are likely the result of endotoxin release.

The signs and symptoms of meningitis in the very young and very old differ from those in older children and adults. In neonates, signs of meningeal irritation may be absent; fever, irritability, and poor feeding are often the only symptoms manifested.[23] Because S.C. is 5 years of age, accurate assessment of his mental status is challenging. Irritability (crying), as was manifested by S.C., is an important finding that suggests an altered mental status.

In elderly patients, many of the classic signs of meningeal irritation are absent as well, and the disease presentation can be subtler.[23] Therefore, given the grave consequences of a misdiagnosis, clinicians caring for infants and elderly patients must have a particularly high index of suspicion for meningitis.

Laboratory evaluation of meningitis should include serum chemistries and a hemogram as well as a detailed examination of the CSF.[23] The peripheral WBC count often is markedly elevated in acute bacterial meningitis, usually with a left shift evident on the differential. This finding, however, is nonspecific and occurs in many acute inflammatory and infectious diseases. S.C. has a marked leukocytosis with a predominance of PMN cells on the differential.

The abrupt onset of S.C.'s clinical symptoms is consistent with an acute bacterial process rather than a fungal or viral etiology. Given his age (5 years) and the community-acquired nature of the infection, the most likely pathogens for his meningitis are *H. influenzae*, *N. meningitidis*, and *S. pneumoniae*. The presence of maculopapular lesions argues for *N. meningitidis* as the causative pathogen because this is a common finding in cases of meningococcemia or meningococcal meningitis.[20] To make an accurate clinical and microbiologic diagnosis in S.C., it is necessary to obtain CSF for analysis. Thus, a lumbar puncture is required as soon as possible.

CEREBROSPINAL FLUID EXAMINATION

CASE 65-1, QUESTION 2: The resident in the ED performs a lumbar puncture, which yielded the following:

Opening pressure, 300 mm Hg (normal, <20)
CSF glucose, 20 mg/dL (normal, 50-60% of plasma glucose)
Protein, 250 mg/dL (normal, <50 mg/dL)
WBC count, 1,200 cells/μL, with 90% PMN, 4% monohistiocytes, and 6% lymphocytes
The CSF red blood cell (RBC) count was 50/μL. A stat Gram stain of CSF revealed numerous WBCs but no organisms. CSF, blood, and urine cultures are pending. Provide an assessment of the CSF results.

Careful examination of the CSF is essential to confirm the diagnosis of meningitis.[6] Table 65-3 compares the typical findings in CSF obtained from patients with acute bacterial meningitis with those seen with fungal or viral causes.[11,26,27] In acute bacterial meningitis, the CSF is often purulent, containing numerous WBCs with a predominance of PMNs, and often is turbid. CSF protein nearly always is elevated, and the CSF glucose concentration is low.[11] In contrast, CSF obtained in viral and fungal cases of meningitis usually is clear and characterized by a much lower WBC count with a mononuclear or lymphocyte predominance. Although the CSF protein concentration often is elevated, it may be normal. A variable effect is observed with CSF glucose.[11,26,27]

MICROBIOLOGIC EVALUATION

Microbiologic evaluation should include examination of CSF by Gram stain and culture as well as cultures obtained from other potential sites of infection (e.g., blood, sputum, urine). The presence of organisms on smear is indicative of a high bacterial inoculum (i.e., inoculum $>10^5$ colony-forming units/mL) and is associated with more fulminant disease.[22] The absence of organisms on Gram stain by no means rules out infection, but does make selection of empiric therapy more difficult. Although a positive Gram stain should prompt a re-evaluation of empiric therapy to ensure appropriate coverage, Gram stain results should not, by themselves, prompt a narrowing of appropriate empiric therapy.[8]

Table 65-3
Cerebrospinal Fluid (CSF) Findings in Various Types of Meningitis

Microbial Etiology	WBC Count (cells/μL)	Predominant Cell Type	Protein	Glucose
Bacterial	>500	PMN	Elevated	Low
Fungal	10–500	MN	Elevated	Variable
Viral	10–200	PMN or MN	Variable	Normal

MN, mononuclear cells; PMN, polymorphonuclear neutrophils; WBC, white blood cell.

S.C. has a negative Gram stain, which may be the result of previous antibiotic therapy or the early detection of disease. Given the negative CSF Gram stain result, S.C. must receive antibacterial therapy sufficiently broad to cover all pathogens associated with meningitis in his age group until the results from his CSF culture are available (usually within 24–48 hours). The CSF culture nearly always is positive in purulent meningitis, although CSF cultures can be negative in a patient who clearly has meningitis, particularly with antecedent receipt of antibiotic therapy.[6] Finally, results from cultures of other sites, such as the blood, urine, and sputum (when appropriate), can yield useful microbiologic information.

The CSF findings in S.C. also strongly support the diagnosis of bacterial meningitis. He has a markedly elevated opening CSF pressure, CSF leukocytosis (with a predominance of PMNs), an elevated CSF protein concentration, and a depressed CSF glucose value. A few RBCs are present in the CSF, which suggests contamination with peripheral blood caused by the traumatic nature of the lumbar puncture. Precise identification of the offending organism is not possible until CSF culture results are available.

Treatment Principles

Prompt institution of appropriate antimicrobial therapy is essential when treating meningitis. Delay in antibiotic administration is associated with increased morbidity and mortality.[8] When choosing antimicrobial therapy, a number of factors must be considered. First, the antibiotics selected must penetrate adequately into the CSF. In addition, the regimen chosen must have potent activity against known or suspected pathogens and exert a bactericidal effect.[28]

ANTIMICROBIAL PENETRATION INTO THE CEREBROSPINAL FLUID

The ability of antimicrobials to penetrate into CSF is affected by lipid solubility, degree of ionization, molecular weight, protein binding, and susceptibility to active transport systems operative within the choroid plexus. In general, the penetration of most antibiotics into the CSF is increased when the meninges are inflamed. Antimicrobial penetration into CSF is most commonly reported as a ratio of CSF to serum antimicrobial levels. Table 65-4 summarizes the CSF penetration characteristics of various antimicrobials during acute bacterial meningitis.[28,29] Metronidazole, sulfamethoxazole, and trimethoprim are small, highly lipophilic compounds and penetrate into the CSF well, achieving adequate concentrations even when meningeal inflammation is absent. Rifampin is lipophilic but is a larger compound with a high degree of protein binding. Thus, it achieves satisfactory CSF penetration and may be combined with vancomycin to treat coagulase-negative staphylococcal infections in the CNS. Because β-lactams usually are ionized at physiologic pH, they are more polar and do not penetrate into the CSF as well.

Table 65-4
Cerebrospinal Fluid Penetration Characteristics of Various Antimicrobials

Very Good[a]
Commonly recommended: metronidazole (brain abscess), TMP-SMX (2nd line to ampicillin for empiric coverage of *Listeria*) Uncommonly utilized; reserve use for specific scenarios[b]: linezolid, rifampin, fluoroquinolones (ciprofloxacin, moxifloxacin, levofloxacin)
Good[c]
Penicillins: penicillin G, ampicillin, piperacillin, nafcillin
Other β-lactams: aztreonam, clavulanate, imipenem, meropenem, sulbactam, tazobactam
3rd- and 4th-generation cephalosporins[d]: cefotaxime, ceftazidime, ceftriaxone, cefepime
Other agents: vancomycin, doxycycline
Fair to Poor[e]
Aminoglycosides: amikacin, gentamicin, tobramycin *Polymyxins:* colistin, Polymyxin B
1st-generation cephalosporins: Cefazolin *Other agents:* macrolides (azithromycin, clarithromycin, erythromycin), clindamycin, daptomycin

[a]Generally achieve levels ≥20% of serum concentrations; generally penetrate CSF well regardless of meningeal inflammation.
[b]See text for details.
[c]Generally achieve levels 10% to 20% of serum concentrations; adequate CSF penetration achieved when the meninges are inflamed.
[d]Cefuroxime has similar CNS penetration, but is not recommended due to inferior efficacy.
[e]Penetration often inadequate even when the meninges are inflamed.
CSF, cerebrospinal fluid; TMP-SMX, trimethoprim–sulfamethoxazole.

β-Lactams penetrate poorly when the meninges are intact, but when the meninges are inflamed, most penicillins and the third- and fourth-generation cephalosporins achieve CSF concentrations sufficient to treat meningitis (~10%–30% of simultaneously obtained serum concentrations). First- and second-generation cephalosporins are not recommended in the treatment of meningitis due to inadequate penetration and/or inferior efficacy.[30,31] Ceftriaxone achieves sustained, reliable bactericidal activity within the CSF despite its high protein binding and has been used successfully to treat meningitis in both children and adults. An additional factor working against maintenance of therapeutic concentrations of *β*-lactams in the CSF is the active transport system of the choroid plexus, which pumps these organic acids out of the CSF. Meropenem achieves CSF levels 10% to 40% of serum levels.[28,29] At the present time, data are too limited to draw conclusions on the utility of the newer agents ceftaroline, ceftolozane/tazobactam, or doripenem in the treatment of CNS infections.

The aminoglycosides have a low therapeutic index, and adequate CSF concentrations are difficult to achieve with IV dosing alone without risking significant toxicity. Thus, when aminoglycoside therapy is initiated for adults with CNS infections, concomitant intrathecal therapy is usually required. Similarly, the polymyxins are large hydrophilic compounds with substantial toxicity, and thus intrathecal administration is preferred.[28,29]

Vancomycin is a large hydrophilic compound with moderate protein binding (50%) and as such does not diffuse well across the blood–CSF barrier. Therapeutic concentrations in the CSF (up to 30% of serum concentrations) may be attained with systemic vancomycin therapy when the meninges are inflamed. Other studies have found much lower penetration, however, and as such, concomitant intraventricular therapy also may be necessary in selected circumstances.[28,29] Consensus guidelines recommend aggressive dosing (troughs 15–20 μg/mL) when treating meningitis.[32]

Fluoroquinolones are moderately lipophilic, have a molecular weight of ~300 Da, and are not protein bound to a large extent. As would be expected, they penetrate reasonably well into the CSF on a percentage basis (~40%–60% or higher).[28,29] Despite this, clinical data supporting the use of fluoroquinolones for bacterial CNS infections are lacking, although some hypotheses may be made. First, given its potent activity against *S. pneumoniae*, moxifloxacin may be an option for pneumococcal infections with limited therapeutic options, such as infections caused by penicillin- and ceftriaxone-resistant isolates.[33] Second, CSF concentrations attained are likely inadequate for infection caused by bacteria with higher MICs (≥0.125–0.5 mcg/mL, depending on the specific organism and drug).[34] This is especially relevant because concerns regarding CNS toxicity have generally limited the study and practice of nonstandard, increased fluoroquinolone dosages for bacterial CNS infections.[28,29] Finally, given the high rates of gram-negative resistance to fluoroquinolones, these agents should not be considered reliable as empiric therapy options in patients considered at risk for infections caused by such organisms.[35] Taken together, the fluoroquinolones are rarely utilized for the treatment of bacterial CNS infections.

Macrolides such as erythromycin and clarithromycin have a relatively high molecular weight and are substrates for a transporter that is abundant at the blood–brain barrier, *P*-glycoprotein. As such, they do not reach adequate concentrations when meningeal inflammation is lacking, and their lack of bactericidal activity further limits their utility in the treatment of bacterial meningitis. Bacteriostatic activity against *S. pneumoniae* also limits the utility of the tetracyclines and tigecycline. Clindamycin penetrates the CSF poorly and should not be used in the treatment of meningitis. Linezolid is also generally bacteriostatic, but as it often retains activity against multiresistant gram-positive pathogens and achieves CSF levels comparable to those in plasma, it may be considered an option for infections caused by gram-positive infections that are resistant or refractory to frontline options. Daptomycin is generally bactericidal and active against multiresistant gram-positive pathogens, but it is a large, highly protein-bound compound, and thus, CSF penetration is low (≤10% of plasma levels). Use of higher doses and intrathecal administration are being actively explored, but current utility is limited.[28,29]

EMPIRIC THERAPY FOR CHILDHOOD MENINGITIS

CASE 65-1, QUESTION 3: A detailed medication and vaccination history reveals that S.C. and his brother appropriately received vaccination for Hib when they were 2 months of age. What constitutes appropriate empiric therapy for childhood meningitis? Which antibiotic would be appropriate for S.C.? What dose and route of administration should be used?

Because results from culture and sensitivity testing of CSF will not be available for >24 hours, empiric therapy must be instituted promptly. The regimen should take into consideration the patient's age, any predisposing conditions, results from the CSF Gram stain, history of allergy, and the presence of organ dysfunction. Table 65-5 gives recommendations for empiric antimicrobial therapy for acute bacterial meningitis.[11,36]

S.C. is 5 years of age and has a negative CSF Gram stain. Therefore, therapy with a third-generation cephalosporin, such as ceftriaxone or cefotaxime, is preferred. Either of these two agents will provide excellent coverage of the most likely pathogens in this age group (*S. pneumoniae* and *N. meningitidis*).[11,36] Of these two pathogens, S.C.'s

Table 65-5
Empiric Therapy for Bacterial Meningitis

Age Group or Predisposing Condition	Recommended Therapy	Alternative Therapy
Neonates (<1 month)	Ampicillin + cefotaxime	Ampicillin + gentamicin
Infants and children (1–23 months)	Cefotaxime or ceftriaxone + vancomycin	Vancomycin + aztreonam/meropenem
Older children and adults (2–50 years)	Cefotaxime or ceftriaxone + vancomycin	Vancomycin + aztreonam/meropenem
Elderly (>50 years)	Ampicillin, cefotaxime, or ceftriaxone + vancomycin	Vancomycin + TMP-SMX + aztreonam or vancomycin + meropenem
Postneurosurgical	Vancomycin + ceftazidime/cefepime	Vancomycin + meropenem
Closed head trauma	Cefotaxime or ceftriaxone + vancomycin	Vancomycin + aztreonam/meropenem
Penetrating head trauma	Vancomycin + ceftazidime/cefepime	Vancomycin + meropenem
Immunocompromised	Vancomycin + cefepime + ampicillin	Vancomycin + TMP-SMX + aztreonam or vancomycin + meropenem

rash suggests that *N. meningitidis* is likely.[37] *H. influenzae* is not very likely because he was vaccinated against Hib. Thus, initiation of ceftriaxone plus vancomycin would be appropriate for S.C. at this time.

Use of a cephalosporin in this case is appropriate despite the allergic history with amoxicillin (history of skin rash). Patients with a documented penicillin allergy carry a 5% to 11% risk of cross-reactivity when cephalosporins are prescribed, depending upon the agent. In this setting, the type of reaction to penicillin is important to consider. Patients with a history of accelerated hypersensitivity reactions (e.g., hives, shortness of breath [SOB], or anaphylaxis) to penicillins should not be given cephalosporins in most instances. Conversely, a benign skin rash would not contraindicate use of a cephalosporin.[38] If S.C. had experienced an accelerated reaction to penicillin, vancomycin plus aztreonam, or meropenem would be the best alternative choice (Table 65-5).[11]

DOSING CONSIDERATIONS

In general, therapy of meningitis requires the use of high dosages of antimicrobials administered by the IV route. Table 65-6 lists the recommended dosing regimens for the treatment of CNS infections. S.C. should receive ceftriaxone in a dosage of 100 mg/kg/day given in one or two doses. A ceftriaxone regimen of 1,000 mg IV Q 12 hours is reasonable for S.C.

ADJUNCTIVE CORTICOSTEROID THERAPY

CASE 65-1, QUESTION 4: What is the rationale for adjunctive corticosteroid therapy in acute bacterial meningitis, and would it be appropriate for S.C.? How should dexamethasone be dosed and monitored for S.C.?

Corticosteroids, particularly dexamethasone, can reduce cerebral edema and lower intracranial pressure.[39] In addition, corticosteroids reduce the synthesis and release of the proinflammatory cytokines TNF-α and IL-1β from monocytes and astrocytes. These two cytokines play a central role in initiating the cascade of events that lead to neuronal tissue damage and neurologic sequelae.[40] Theoretically, then, inhibition of cytokine synthesis by corticosteroids in meningitis should lead to a decreased risk of hearing loss and other neurologic sequelae. Indeed, a prospective, randomized, double-blind multicenter trial evaluating the use of dexamethasone in adults with acute bacterial meningitis supported this theory.[41] A total of 301 patients were randomized to receive dexamethasone or placebo 15 to 20 minutes before or with the first dose of antibiotic every 6 hours for 4 days. Dexamethasone reduced the risk of unfavorable outcome, defined as a Glasgow Coma Scale score of 1 to 4 at 8 weeks (relative risk, 0.59; $P = 0.03$), and of death (relative risk, 0.48; $P = 0.04$). When the outcomes were analyzed based upon culture results, mortality reduction (14 vs. 34 percent) and all unfavorable outcomes (26 vs. 52 percent) were only seen with dexamethasone therapy in patients with meningitis caused by *Streptococcus pneumoniae*. Outcomes in patients with meningitis caused by organisms other than *S. pneumoniae* were independent of whether they received dexamethasone or not. Neither GI bleeding nor other adverse effects were increased in the dexamethasone group.

In children, several studies have also evaluated the role of adjunctive dexamethasone therapy in bacterial meningitis. Some prospective placebo-controlled, randomized trials have demonstrated that adjunctive dexamethasone therapy significantly reduces audiologic and neurologic sequelae in children >2 months of age. *H. influenzae*, however, was the causative pathogen in most of these meningitis cases, whereas the number of children with streptococcal and meningococcal meningitis in these trials was small.[2,42–46] As previously mentioned, the number of Hib cases has decreased dramatically, making the data from these trials difficult to apply to the present day. More recently, of the 166 patients enrolled in a trial comparing dexamethasone to placebo, 35 and 26 cases were caused by *S. pneumoniae* and *N. meningitides*, respectively, in the treatment arm. Fewer audiologic and neurologic sequelae were observed in the dexamethasone-treated group compared with the placebo group, but the difference did not reach statistical significance.[47]

Most recently, a 2013 Cochrane meta-analysis evaluated data from 25 randomized trials that included over 4,000 children and adults. In the overall population, glucocorticoid administration did not significantly reduce mortality. However, glucocorticoids did reduce mortality in the subgroup of patients with meningitis caused by *S. pneumoniae* (RR, 0.84; 95% CI, 0.72–0.98). In studies conducted in high-income countries, glucocorticoids reduced severe hearing loss (RR, 0.51; 95% CI, 0.35–0.73), any hearing loss (RR, 0.58; 95% CI, 0.45–0.73), and short-term neurologic sequelae (RR, 0.64; 95% CI, 0.48–0.85). In the subgroup of over 2,000 children, the administration of dexamethasone did not affect mortality but did reduce the incidence of severe hearing loss, particularly in those with *H. influenzae* meningitis.[48]

The 2004 IDSA meningitis guidelines recommend that dexamethasone be initiated prior to (or concomitant with the first dose of) antimicrobial therapy in all adult patients with suspected or proven pneumococcal meningitis.[11] Controversy remains over whether dexamethasone should be continued in adults if the causative

Table 65-6
Suggested Antibiotic Dosing Regimens for Treatment of Central Nervous System Infections

	Daily Dose (interval in hours)[a]			
	Neonates			
Antibiotic	**0–7 days old**	**8–28 days old**	**Infants and Children**	**Adults**
Ampicillin	150 mg/kg (8)	200 mg/kg (6–8)	300 mg/kg (6)	12 g (4)
Aztreonam				8 g (6)
Nafcillin	75 mg/kg (8–12)	100–150 mg/kg (6–8)	200 mg/kg (6)	12 g (4)
Penicillin G	0.15 mU/kg (8–12)	0.2 mU/kg (6–8)	0.3 mU/kg (4–6)	24 mU (4)
Meropenem			120 mg/kg (8)	6 g (8)
Cephalosporins				
Cefotaxime	100–150 mg/kg (8–12)	150–200 mg/kg (6–8)	225–300 mg/kg (6–8)	12 g (4)
Ceftriaxone			80–100 mg/kg (12–24)	4 g (12)
Ceftazidime	100–150 mg/kg (8–12)	150 mg/kg (8)	150 mg/kg (8)	6 g (8)
Cefepime			150 mg/kg (8)	6 g (8)
Aminoglycoside[b,c]				
Gentamicin	5 mg/kg (12)	7.5 mg/kg (8)	7.5 mg/kg (8)	5–7 mg/kg (8–24)
Tobramycin	5 mg/kg (12)	7.5 mg/kg (8)	7.5 mg/kg (8)	5–7 mg/kg (8–24)
Amikacin	15–20 mg/kg (12)	30 mg/kg (8)	20–30 mg/kg (8)	15 mg/kg (8–24)
Others				
Moxifloxacin				400 mg (24)
Linezolid				1,200 mg (12)
Rifampin		10–20 mg/kg (12)	10–20 mg/kg (12-24)	600 mg (24)
TMP-SMX[d]			10–20 mg/kg (6–12)	10–20 mg/kg (6–12)
Vancomycin[c,e]	20–30 mg/kg (8–12)	30–45 mg/kg (6–8)	60 mg/kg (6)	30–45 mg/kg (8–12)

[a]Recommended daily dose when renal and hepatic functions are normal.
[b]Concurrent intraventricular doses of 5–10 mg (gentamicin, tobramycin) or 20 mg (amikacin) often required when treating gram-negative bacillary meningitis.
[c]Dose should be individualized based on serum level monitoring.
[d]Dose is based on the trimethoprim component.
[e]Concurrent intraventricular doses of 5–20 mg recommended if response to IV therapy is inadequate.
Source: Tunkel AR et al. Practice guidelines for the management of bacterial meningitis. *Clin Infect Dis*. 2004;39:1267.

agent is found not to be pneumococcus because the number of patients in the studies with meningitis caused by other organisms was small.[49] However, the guidelines do recommend discontinuing dexamethasone if the organism is found to be something other than *S. pneumonia*.[11] Regarding pediatrics, the American Academy of Pediatrics (AAP) Committee on Infectious Diseases suggests that dexamethasone therapy may be beneficial in children with Hib meningitis if given before or at the same time as the first dose of antimicrobial therapy.[50] The AAP Committee on Infectious Diseases also suggests that the decision to use adjunctive dexamethasone therapy should be individualized but considered for infants and children older than 6 weeks with pneumococcal meningitis.[51] At this time, there can be no firm recommendation as to whether steroids should be continued in children if the pathogen is found not to be *H. influenzae* or *S. pneumoniae*.

Thus, S.C. should receive dexamethasone therapy, 0.15 mg/kg/dose given IV Q 6 hours for 2 to 4 days. For S.C., who is 20 kg, this would be 3 mg Q 6 hours, with the first dexamethasone dose given 15 minutes before initiating ceftriaxone therapy.

Potential adverse effects associated with dexamethasone include GI bleeding, mental status changes (e.g., euphoria or encephalopathy), increases in blood glucose, and possibly elevations in blood pressure. For S.C., the complete blood count (CBC), serum chemistries, and stool guaiac should be monitored daily while he is receiving dexamethasone. He also should be questioned about possible GI upset and assessed for changes in mental status (e.g., confusion, combativeness). Given the short duration of corticosteroid therapy, dexamethasone can be discontinued abruptly without tapering.

EFFECT ON CENTRAL NERVOUS SYSTEM PENETRATION OF ANTIBIOTICS

Another important issue to consider is whether dexamethasone, a potent anti-inflammatory agent, reduces the ability of antimicrobials to penetrate across the blood–brain barrier into CSF. Because CSF penetration of the penicillins, cephalosporins, and vancomycin is greatest when the meninges are inflamed, a hypothetical concern is that concomitant dexamethasone may reduce CSF concentrations of these agents, resulting in reduced efficacy. Early animal models suggest that vancomycin penetration into the CSF is reduced in dexamethasone-treated animals compared with animals not treated with steroids.[52] In a rabbit meningitis model, the coadministration of dexamethasone and vancomycin resulted in 29% less penetration of vancomycin into the CSF. By increasing the daily dose of vancomycin in these rabbits, however, therapeutic CSF levels were achieved, suggesting that giving larger daily doses of vancomycin circumvents the steroid effect on CNS penetration.[53] Additionally, current human data suggest that CSF penetration of vancomycin or ceftriaxone is not diminished with concomitant administration of dexamethasone.[54–57] Based on these encouraging findings, it is recommended that dexamethasone be utilized in all patients.[11]

Neisseria meningitidis Meningitis

DEFINITIVE THERAPY

Case 65-1, Question 5: Twenty-four hours after admission, S.C.'s culture results from his blood and CSF samples are available. The CSF culture is growing *N. meningitidis* (penicillin MIC, 0.06 mg/L), and *N. meningitidis* is also growing in both of the two collected blood cultures. What modification in S.C.'s antimicrobial therapy is necessary at this time?

Once culture and sensitivity results become available, definitive therapy can be instituted, often with a single agent (Table 65-7).[11,36] As suspected, S.C.'s CSF culture is positive for *N. meningitidis*. Cefuroxime, a second-generation cephalosporin, has activity against *N. meningitides*; however, it is less effective for meningitis than third-generation cephalosporins and should not be used.[58,59] The reason for the inferiority of cefuroxime relative to ceftriaxone most likely is related to reduced potency.[58]

Because *N. meningitidis* is susceptible to penicillin and ampicillin currently, penicillin is the drug of choice. However, S.C.'s questionable history of amoxicillin rash makes the use of ceftriaxone a reasonable choice (See Table 65-6 for dosing).

MONITORING THERAPY

Case 65-1, Question 6: What subjective and objective data should be monitored to evaluate the efficacy and toxicity of treatment of patients with meningitis, and what specifically should be monitored in S.C.?

Clinical signs and symptoms attributable to the disease, such as fever, altered mental status, and stiff neck, should be checked periodically throughout the day and monitored for resolution. S.C.'s temperature and mental status should be assessed often. Accurate assessment of S.C.'s mental status can be difficult because of his young age. Thus, his baseline level of mental status should be evaluated (e.g., whether he is awake and alert, or lethargic and difficult to arouse). If awake and alert, S.C. should be observed for irritability, because this often is the only sign of altered mentation. Questions can be used to assess his orientation: Does he know where he is? Does he know his name? Can he recognize his mother or other family members? In general, signs of clinical improvement should be evident within 24 to 48 hours for most uncomplicated cases of acute bacterial meningitis, with defervescence of fever achieved in a mean of 3.3 days in one trial of cefotaxime in children.[60]

Laboratory tests should be monitored as well. A CBC with differential, serum electrolytes (e.g., Na, K, Cl, HCO_3), blood glucose, and renal function tests (e.g., BUN, SrCr) should be performed daily. Abnormal electrolyte results may require more frequent monitoring. Laboratory abnormalities, such as leukocytosis and hyponatremia, may take longer to normalize than clinical symptoms. CSF chemistries usually improve within 48 hours of starting therapy, although CSF WBC and protein may remain elevated for a week or more.[61,62] With effective therapy, the CSF culture usually is sterile after about 18 to 24 hours of therapy.[58,60] Delays in CSF sterilization are associated with a higher propensity for neurologic complications.[58] If S.C. responds to therapy in a straightforward manner, he need not to have a repeat lumbar puncture. If the response is inadequate, as evidenced by

Table 65-7
Definitive Therapy for Bacterial Meningitis

Pathogen	Recommended Treatment	Alternative Agents
Haemophilus influenzae		
β-Lactamase negative	Ampicillin	Cefotaxime or ceftriaxone; aztreonam
β-Lactamase positive	Cefotaxime or ceftriaxone	Aztreonam
Neisseria meningitidis	Penicillin MIC < 0.1 mcg/mL: penicillin G or ampicillin	Cefotaxime or ceftriaxone; meropenem
	Penicillin MIC 0.1- 1.0 mcg/mL: cefotaxime or ceftriaxone	
Streptococcus pneumoniae	Penicillin MIC ≤ 0.06 mcg/mL: penicillin G or ampicillin	Cefotaxime or ceftriaxone
	Penicillin MIC ≥ 0.12 mcg/mL: cefotaxime or ceftriaxone if susceptible	Vancomycin or meropenem
	Penicillin and cefotaxime/ceftriaxone nonsusceptible: vancomycin + cefotaxime/ceftriaxone ± rifampin	Vancomycin + moxifloxacin
Streptococcus agalactiae	Penicillin G or ampicillin + gentamicin	Cefotaxime or ceftriaxone
Listeria monocytogenes	Penicillin G or ampicillin ± gentamicin	TMP-SMX or meropenem
Enterobacteriaceae[a]		
Escherichia coli, *Klebsiella* species	Cefotaxime or ceftriaxone	Cefepime; aztreonam; meropenem
Enterobacter, *Serratia* species	Cefepime; meropenem	TMP-SMX; aztreonam
Pseudomonas aeruginosa	Cefepime or ceftazidime; meropenem	Aztreonam
Staphylococcus aureus[a]		
Methicillin-susceptible (MSSA)	Nafcillin or oxacillin	Vancomycin ± rifampin; meropenem
Methicillin-resistant (MRSA)	Vancomycin± rifampin	TMP-SMX; linezolid
Staphylococcus epidermidis[a]	Vancomycin ± rifampin	TMP-SMX; linezolid

[a]Concomitant intrathecal therapy may be required for optimal response (most commonly an intrathecal aminoglycoside for gram-negative or intrathecal vancomycin for gram-positive infections).
MIC, minimum inhibitory concentration; TMP-SMX, trimethoprim–sulfamethoxazole.

persistent fever or deteriorating mental status, S.C. will require a repeat lumbar puncture to re-examine the CSF parameters.[11]

In addition to monitoring the therapeutic response, side effects of the antimicrobial regimen also need to be assessed frequently. Meningitis requires high-dose therapy, making the likelihood of adverse effects much greater. Currently, S.C. is being treated with ceftriaxone. The adverse effects most often associated with ceftriaxone include hypersensitivity reactions, mild pain and phlebitis at the injection site, and GI complaints.[63] S.C. should be observed for the formation of an antibiotic-related skin rash or evidence of an accelerated allergic reaction (e.g., hives, wheezing). The IV catheter site should be observed daily for redness, tenderness, or pain on palpation of the vein. S.C. should be watched closely for loose stools or diarrhea. Although mild diarrhea is a common side effect of most antimicrobials that rarely requires a change in therapy, diarrhea that is severe, persistent, or accompanied by fever, unexplained leukocytosis, or abdominal cramping should prompt testing for *C. difficile* colitis.[59,64]

CEFTRIAXONE-INDUCED BILIARY PSEUDOLITHIASIS

CASE 65-1, QUESTION 7: After 5 days of treatment, the nurse caring for S.C. notes that his appetite is markedly diminished, and he complains of an upset stomach. S.C. was afebrile and alert and oriented, but abdominal examination revealed "guarding," with pain localized in the right upper quadrant area. Laboratory data at this time are as follows:

WBC count, 6,000 cells/μL
Hgb, 12.5 g/dL
Hct, 34%
Platelets, 120,000/μL
Na, 135 mEq/L
K, 3.6 mEq/L
Cl, 98 mEq/L
Aspartate aminotransferase (AST), 35 units/L
Alanine aminotransferase (ALT), 33 units/L
Alkaline phosphatase, 110 MU/dL
Total bilirubin, 1.2 mg/dL
Amylase 70 units/L

A stool guaiac is negative. What are possible causes of S.C.'s abdominal discomfort?

A number of possible causes exist for S.C.'s abdominal discomfort. His corticosteroid therapy may have caused acute GI bleeding; however, the dexamethasone was discontinued 3 days ago and S.C.'s hemoglobin and hematocrit values are in the low-normal range. The negative stool guaiac result also argues strongly against a GI bleed. Acute pancreatitis is unlikely given the normal amylase result. Viral or drug-induced hepatitis is another possibility but also is unlikely given his normal AST, ALT, and bilirubin results. An intra-abdominal infection also is possible, but this is improbable because he is afebrile and has a normal WBC count. Other causes, such as acute cholecystitis or appendicitis, require further diagnostic evaluation.

CASE 65-1, QUESTION 8: An abdominal ultrasound reveals sludge in the gallbladder. What is the significance of this finding in S.C., and how should this abnormality be managed?

The abnormality on S.C.'s abdominal ultrasound explains his right upper quadrant pain. S.C. has what appears to be a condition known as biliary pseudolithiasis (i.e., biliary "sludging"). Biliary sludging can occur in conditions of gallbladder hypomotility (e.g., recent surgery, burns, total parenteral nutrition) and, in some instances, can be drug-induced. S.C. has been receiving ceftriaxone for treatment of his meningitis, and this drug can cause biliary pseudolithiasis.[65]

Antibiotic-associated biliary pseudolithiasis is seen almost exclusively with ceftriaxone. The biliary excretion associated with ceftriaxone results in very high concentrations of the drug in gallbladder bile. In selected circumstances, the biliary concentration of ceftriaxone may exceed solubility limits, resulting in formation of a fine, granular precipitate (i.e., sludge), which differs in composition and ultrasound features from true gallstones. The precipitate is composed of a ceftriaxone–calcium complex, the formation of which is dose dependent. Given the high dosages required for meningitis therapy, it is not surprising that this adverse effect has occurred in S.C.[65] In the comparative randomized trial between ceftriaxone and cefuroxime cited previously, evidence of biliary pseudolithiasis on abdominal ultrasonography was observed in 16 of 35 (46%) patients who received ceftriaxone and in none of 35 patients receiving cefuroxime.[58] Pseudolithiasis usually appears 3 to 10 days following the start of therapy and, in most instances, it is clinically asymptomatic. Symptoms similar to acute cholecystitis are evident in some individuals and include nausea with or without vomiting and abdominal right upper quadrant pain.[65]

Prompt recognition of this adverse effect and discontinuation of ceftriaxone therapy are required to effectively manage biliary pseudolithiasis. Once S.C.'s ceftriaxone is discontinued, the condition should resolve gradually over a period of weeks to months; the clinical symptoms should disappear within a few days.[65] Cefotaxime can be substituted for ceftriaxone; cefotaxime is not associated with biliary complications, and the efficacy of these two agents is equivalent.[63] For S.C., the cefotaxime dosage would be 1,000 mg IV every 6 hours (Table 65-6).

DURATION OF THERAPY

CASE 65-1, QUESTION 9: What is the recommended duration of antimicrobial therapy for S.C.?

The optimal duration of therapy for meningitis is difficult to ascertain because few trials have been designed to address this issue.[66] Although general guidelines exist, the duration should be individualized based on the response to therapy, the presence of complicating factors (e.g., immunosuppression), and the specific causative pathogen. Table 65-8 lists the recommended treatment durations for uncomplicated cases of bacterial meningitis according to the specific pathogen. Patients such as S.C. with meningitis caused by *N. meningitidis* should be treated for 7 days.[11] Complicated cases, such as those with delayed CSF sterilization, require therapy for longer periods (up to 2 weeks or more).

Table 65-8
Duration of Therapy for Bacterial Meningitis

Etiology	Duration of Therapy (days)
Haemophilus influenzae	7
N. meningitidis	7
Streptococcus pneumoniae	10–14
Group B streptococci (*Streptococcus agalactiae*)	14–21
Listeria monocytogenes	≥21
Gram-negative bacilli	21

PREVENTION OF NEISSERIA MENINGITIDIS MENINGITIS

CASE 65-1, QUESTION 10: S.C. is ready to be discharged home. How can the potential spread of meningococcal disease be prevented in persons with whom S.C. has contact?

Despite an excellent response to therapy, S.C. still may harbor *N. meningitidis* in his nasopharynx and could transmit this organism to individuals with whom he has close contact.[18,67,68] Therefore, chemoprophylaxis to prevent secondary cases of *N. meningitidis* is indicated for S.C. and his close contacts. In this context, close contacts include the following: a household member including roommates and young adults in dormitories, child-care center contacts, and any person directly exposed to the patient's oral secretions (e.g., through kissing, mouth-to-mouth resuscitation, or endotracheal intubation) in the 7 days before symptom onset and until 24 hours after initiation of appropriate antibiotics.[67,69] Health-care personnel and any passenger on a flight who had direct contact with respiratory secretions or for anyone seated directly next to an index patient on a prolonged flight (e.g., one lasting ≥8 hours) should also receive chemoprophylaxis.[69]

S.C.'s 7-year-old brother, the children at the day-care center, and close contacts at the hospital who have been caring for S.C. are at risk for invasive *N. meningitidis* disease and should receive chemoprophylaxis. Because the risk of secondary disease is greatest immediately after onset of disease in the index patient, chemoprophylaxis should be instituted as soon as possible and ideally within 24 hours.[67] Administering chemoprophylaxis 14 days or more after identification of the index case is of little value. Regimens to reduce nasopharyngeal carriage of *N. meningitidis* include rifampin, ciprofloxacin, and ceftriaxone. The most frequently used regimen for children ≥1 month is rifampin, given every 12 hours in a dosage of 10 mg/kg/dose for 2 days. For adults, rifampin given every 12 hours in a dosage of 600 mg for 2 days is commonly used. The index patient should also receive prophylaxis if he/she was treated with an agent other than a third-generation cephalosporin as soon as he/she is able to tolerate oral medications and prior to being discharged from the hospital.[69]

Because S.C. is receiving ceftriaxone, he does not need chemoprophylaxis. S.C.'s brother, parents, and day-care contacts should be treated with appropriate doses of rifampin as soon as he is diagnosed. Because rifampin is not recommended for pregnant women, ceftriaxone would be a viable alternative.

Streptococcus pneumoniae Meningitis

CLINICAL FEATURES, PREDISPOSING FACTORS, AND DIAGNOSIS

CASE 65-2

QUESTION 1: A.L., a 58-year-old man with a long history of alcohol abuse, is admitted to the ED febrile and unresponsive. During the past several days, A.L. has experienced intermittent episodes of fever, chills, SOB, and a worsening productive cough. A friend visiting A.L. called 9-1-1 when he could not arouse him. A.L.'s medical records indicate that he has hypertension, adult-onset diabetes mellitus, peptic ulcer disease (PUD), and chronic obstructive pulmonary disease (COPD). A splenectomy was performed 10 years ago after trauma to the abdomen. A.L. is divorced and lives alone in a low-income apartment. He has no known drug allergies. His records show him to be a smoker for more than 30 years. Current medications include hydrochlorothiazide 50 mg every other day, glipizide 5 mg orally (PO) twice daily, famotidine 20 mg PO every bedtime, and doxycycline PO twice daily as needed for cough and increased sputum production.

On admission to the ED, A.L. had a temperature of 40°C, blood pressure of 90/50 mm Hg, and pulse and respiratory rates of 115 beats/minute and 25 breaths/minute, respectively. His weight is 59 kg. A.L. was unresponsive but withdrew all extremities to painful stimuli. His pupils were equal and sluggishly reactive to light; papilledema and evidence of meningismus were present. Wheezes and crackles were heard throughout both lung fields, with dense consolidation noted in the left lower lobe. The remainder of his physical examination was noncontributory.

Stat laboratory tests revealed the following:

WBC count, 18,000 cells/μL, with 80% PMN, 15% bands, 3% lymphocytes, and 2% basophils
Hgb, 10.5 g/dL
Hct, 34%
Platelet count, 250,000/μL
K, 3.0 mEq/L
Glucose, 250 mg/dL
AST, 190 mg/dL
ALT, 140 mg/dL
BUN, 35 mg/dL
SCr, 2.4 mg/dL

The prothrombin time was high normal, and albumin was 3.1 mg/dL. A stat blood alcohol level of 100 mg/dL was reported, and a urine toxicology screen was negative. A.L.'s serum theophylline concentration was 18 mg/dL. Stool guaiac was positive.

A CT scan showed no evidence of mass lesions or cerebral hematoma. Lumbar puncture yielded the following results:

CSF opening pressure, 200 mm Hg
Protein, 120 mg/dL
Glucose, 100 mg/dL
WBC count, 8,500 cells/μL, with 92% PMN, 4% monohistiocytes, and 4% lymphocytes
RBC count, 400/μL

Gram-positive, lancet-shaped diplococci were visible on CSF Gram stain. In addition, a sputum Gram stain revealed numerous WBCs, few epithelial cells, and numerous gram-positive cocci in pairs and in short chains. Blood, CSF, urine, and sputum cultures are pending. What are the clinical and laboratory features of pneumococcal meningitis? What features of pneumococcal meningitis are present in A.L.?

A.L. presents to the ED with many signs and symptoms suggestive of pneumococcal meningitis. He is 56 years of age, and *S. pneumoniae* is the most common bacterial etiology for meningitis in adults >30 years of age (Table 65-1). As is evidenced by A.L.'s presentation, invasive pneumococcal disease often is associated with significant morbidity, and mortality rates remain high.[1] However, likely due to the introduction of conjugate vaccines, the incidence of *S. pneumoniae* meningitis in the United States has significantly decreased, from 0.8 cases per 100,000 people in 1997 to 0.3/100,000 in 2010.[70] Predisposing factors to invasive pneumococcal disease include advanced age, cigarette smoking, alcoholism, diabetes, chronic pulmonary disease, and functional (sickle cell disease) or anatomic (splenectomy) asplenia. In addition, individuals infected with the human immunodeficiency virus (HIV) or with other immunocompromising conditions (such as solid organ or bone marrow transplantation) are at higher risk. Patients with CSF otorrhea or rhinorrhea induced by closed head trauma or neurosurgical procedures are more susceptible to develop pneumococcal meningitis as well.[71]

A.L. has many predisposing factors for pneumococcal meningitis. He smokes, has a long history of alcohol abuse, has had a splenectomy, and has diabetes and COPD. A diagnosis of pneumococcal meningitis in A.L. is supported by the high fever, stiff neck (meningismus), and altered mental status. He is unresponsive, which is a definite negative prognostic factor.[72] Results from CSF chemistries and microbiologic analysis are highly suggestive of pneumococcal meningitis. A.L. has an elevated opening CSF pressure and a markedly elevated CSF protein and WBC count with a predominance of neutrophils on differential examination. The normal CSF glucose level (100 g/dL) is misleading because A.L. is diabetic. The calculated ratio of CSF to serum glucose for A.L. is <50%, which is consistent with acute bacterial meningitis (Table 65-3). The presence of gram-positive, lancet-shaped diplococci in pairs on the CSF Gram stain strongly supports the diagnosis of pneumococcal disease. The signs and symptoms of pneumococcal pneumonia (cough, SOB, increased sputum production, and pulmonary consolidation) as well as the sputum Gram stain result also lend support to a diagnosis of invasive pneumococcal infection.

EMPIRIC THERAPY IN ADULTS

CASE 65-2, QUESTION 2: What would be appropriate therapy for A.L?

Table 65-7 provides therapy recommendations for pneumococcal meningitis based on penicillin and ceftriaxone/cefotaxime susceptibility. Resistance among pneumococci to penicillin G (MIC ≥0.12 mcg/mL) is a significant concern. In a surveillance study from 2006 to 2007, 27.5% of *S. pneumoniae* isolates from patients with meningitis were resistant to penicillin.[73] *S. pneumoniae* strains in CSF with MIC >0.5 mcg/mL to cefotaxime or ceftriaxone are intermediate (1 mcg/mL) or resistant (≥2 mcg/mL). Reduced activity of ceftriaxone and cefotaxime against penicillin-resistant pneumococci affects the therapeutic ratio achieved in CSF and has been associated with clinical failure. Optimal therapy for fully penicillin-resistant pneumococcal meningitis should include vancomycin. The combination of vancomycin and ceftriaxone was superior to either agent given alone in a rabbit model of penicillin-resistant pneumococcal meningitis. Ceftriaxone or vancomycin combined with rifampin also may be superior to either drug given alone.[74] With its potent pneumococcal activity and satisfactory CNS penetration, moxifloxacin may be an option for pneumococcal meningitis caused by penicillin- and ceftriaxone-resistant isolates.[33] However, clinical data supporting the use of moxifloxacin in this scenario are lacking. Thus, until more information is available, the combination of ceftriaxone or cefotaxime with vancomycin represents the most reasonable approach to empiric therapy for potential penicillin-resistant pneumococcal meningitis.

Until culture and susceptibility results are available, the recommended antibiotic in this situation is ceftriaxone 2 g given IV Q 12 hours and vancomycin 30 to 45 mg/kg/day IV divided Q 8 to 12 hours. A.L. weighs 59 kg, and because his renal function is not normal (SrCr, 2.4 mg/dL; creatinine clearance, 30 mL/minute), a dosage adjustment was made.

CORTICOSTEROID THERAPY FOR ADULT MENINGITIS

CASE 65-2, QUESTION 3: Should A.L. receive corticosteroid therapy in addition to his antibiotic therapy?

A.L. presents with profoundly altered mental status, and his signs and symptoms are consistent with a fulminant course of disease. His age, underlying medical problems, likely streptococcal meningitis, and deteriorating clinical status all point to a poor prognosis and argue for the use of adjunctive dexamethasone. On the other hand, A.L. is diabetic and has an elevated glucose concentration. He also has PUD, which may be active given that he is anemic and has a positive stool guaiac result. High-dose dexamethasone therapy may impact upon his mental status, making assessment even more difficult. Although each of these issues is a concern, none is so critical as to preclude the use of corticosteroids. Therefore, dexamethasone given in a dosage of 10 mg IV Q 6 hours could be instituted before starting ceftriaxone therapy provided that the diagnosis of bacterial meningitis is confirmed. Dexamethasone can be continued for up to 4 days if *S. pneumoniae* is found to be the causative pathogen. Dexamethasone may be discontinued if *S. pneumoniae* is not the causative pathogen.[11] To control blood glucose, a sliding-scale dosing schedule of regular insulin is recommended. A.L.'s PUD should be properly worked up and treated if necessary.

TREATMENT OF PENICILLIN-SUSCEPTIBLE PNEUMOCOCCAL MENINGITIS

CASE 65-2, QUESTION 4: Results from A.L.'s CSF, blood, and sputum cultures are available and are positive for *S. pneumoniae* at each site. Sensitivity testing in CSF revealed an MIC of 0.06 mcg/mL to penicillin, 0.25 mcg/mL to cefotaxime and ceftriaxone, and 0.25 mcg/mL to vancomycin. What therapy is indicated for A.L.?

A.L. is infected with a strain of *S. pneumoniae* that is susceptible to penicillin G (Table 65-7).[75] The dosage usually is 24 million units/day in adults with normal renal function (Table 65-6). A.L. has renal impairment, however, which means he should receive a reduced penicillin dosage. For A.L., who has a calculated creatinine clearance of ~28 mL/minute (according to the method of Cockcroft and Gault), the daily dose would be 12 to 16 million units, or 3 to 4 million units Q 6 hours. This revised regimen should provide penicillin serum concentrations similar to those achieved with high-dose therapy when kidney function is normal. Failure to adjust the dosage appropriately is equivalent to providing massive doses of penicillin, and seizures may result.[76] In patients unable to tolerate penicillin G, the best alternatives are ceftriaxone or cefotaxime (Table 65-7).[11,36]

Gram-Negative Bacillary Meningitis

CASE 65-3

QUESTION 1: R.R., a 40-year-old, 80-kg man, is admitted to the hospital for a cervical laminectomy with vertebral fusion. His surgical procedure was complicated by a dural tear. On the third postoperative day, drainage at his surgical excision site was noted, and R.R. was febrile to 38.2°C. A Gram stain of the drainage revealed few gram-positive cocci and moderate gram-negative bacilli. Therapy with IV cefazolin 1 g every 8 hours was begun. The following morning, R.R. was oriented to person, place, and time, but he was slightly obtunded and had a temperature of 40°C. Neck stiffness could not be assessed because of his recent surgery. A magnetic resonance imaging (MRI) scan of the head and neck was negative, and lumbar puncture yielded the following CSF results:

WBC count, 3,000 cells/μL, with 95% PMN
Glucose, 20 mg/dL
Protein, 280 mg/dL

What important clinical and laboratory features of gram-negative bacillary meningitis are manifested in R.R.?

EPIDEMIOLOGY

R.R. has developed gram-negative meningitis as a complication of his recent neurosurgical procedure. Gram-negative organisms are important pathogens particularly after neurosurgical procedures such as craniotomy.[70] Historically, mortality rates from gram-negative bacillary meningitis have been extremely high, ranging from 40% to 70%. With the availability of third-generation cephalosporins, some studies report fatalities have declined to <40%; however, a recent study of 40 adults with spontaneous gram-negative meningitis reported a mortality rate of 53%.[77] Increasing resistance among certain gram-negative bacilli, such as *Enterobacter* species and *P. aeruginosa*, presents a therapeutic dilemma in that mortality associated with these pathogens is high and therapeutic options are fewer.

PREDISPOSING FACTORS

Individuals at greatest risk for gram-negative bacillary meningitis include neonates, the elderly, patients with underlying conditions such as diabetes mellitus or malignancy, patients with open trauma to the head, and individuals such as R.R. undergoing neurosurgical procedures.[78] Although meningitis is a rare complication of clean neurosurgical procedures (e.g., craniotomy, laminectomy), the consequences can be devastating when it does happen.[77]

MICROBIOLOGY

Escherichia coli and *K. pneumoniae* have historically been the most common gram-negative bacteria causing meningitis; however, rates of pseudomonal meningitis appear to be increasing.[77,79] *E. coli* is the most common gram-negative cause of neonatal meningitis, whereas *K. pneumoniae* is isolated more often in the elderly population.[80,81] The remaining cases are generally divided evenly among *Proteus*, *Serratia*, *Enterobacter*, *Citrobacter*, *Pseudomonas*, and other less common bacilli.[77]

CLINICAL FEATURES

In general, clinical laboratory features of gram-negative bacillary meningitis are similar to other types of bacterial meningitis.[1,11] Because of high virulence, gram-negative bacillary meningitis often is a fulminant, rapidly progressive disease. An exception to this rule is meningitis after neurosurgery.[81] As is evidenced by R.R.'s clinical presentation, postneurosurgical gram-negative bacillary meningitis can present in a more subtle fashion. In such patients, many of the symptoms of meningitis (e.g., altered mental status, stiff neck) are masked by underlying neurologic disease. Thus, a high index of suspicion is warranted in the postsurgical setting. In addition to gram-negative bacilli, staphylococci also are associated with postneurosurgical meningitis.[82] The presence of what looks like staphylococci on R.R.'s wound drainage fluid is of concern, but the abundance of gram-negative rods on his CSF Gram stain supports the latter as being the most likely causative pathogen.

TREATMENT OF GRAM-NEGATIVE BACILLARY MENINGITIS

Case 65-2, Question 2: What empiric therapy is appropriate for A.L. at this time?

Fewer choices are available for treatment of gram-negative bacillary meningitis than for other meningitides. Ampicillin is active against only *E. coli*, *P. mirabilis*, and *Salmonella* species, but resistance has essentially eliminated its use. Aminoglycosides are limited by their inability to achieve therapeutic CSF concentrations, as well as reduced activity in the acidic milieu of purulent CSF.[83] Intraventricular administration, which results in therapeutic CSF concentrations, is usually reserved for difficult-to-eradicate shunt infections in combination with IV therapy because of the absence of data supporting their use.[21,43] Unlike intraventricular administration, intralumbar injections will not result in therapeutic CSF concentrations in the ventricle.[43]

Empiric antimicrobial regimens should include an agent with activity against *P. aeruginosa* in patients with penetrating head trauma, a CSF shunt, or in patients who recently underwent a neurosurgical procedure. Because R.R. recently had a neurosurgical procedure, his empiric therapy should include an antipseudomonal agent such as cefepime, ceftazidime, or meropenem (Table 65-5).[11] Cefepime has excellent activity against *E. coli* and *K. pneumoniae* and is active against other enteric gram-negative bacilli as well (Table 65-7).[31] Resistance to third-generation cephalosporins among *Enterobacter*, *Citrobacter*, and *Serratia* is so prevalent that these agents cannot be relied on for the treatment of meningitis caused by these pathogens.[84] With this in mind, therapy of gram-negative meningitis in situations where third-generation cephalosporin resistance is likely (e.g., nosocomial or postneurosurgical meningitis) should result in the use of cefepime or meropenem. If a pathogen is isolated, therapy may be tailored based on culture results, antibiotic sensitivities, and antibiotic penetration into the CNS. For example, success rates exceed 80% with cefotaxime and ceftriaxone for gram-negative bacillary meningitis caused by *E. coli* or *K. pneumoniae*.[85,86] For R.R., cefazolin should be discontinued, and treatment with cefepime adjusted for renal insufficiency (2 g IV Q 8 hours) should be instituted until the return of culture and sensitivities.

TREATMENT OF ENTEROBACTER MENINGITIS

Case 65-3, Question 3: Culture results from R.R.'s wound drainage and CSF both are positive for *Enterobacter cloacae*. Sensitivity data reveal resistance to ceftriaxone, cefepime, ceftazidime, piperacillin–tazobactam, and aztreonam. Drugs to which the isolate is sensitive include imipenem, meropenem, TMP-SMX, gentamicin, tobramycin, and ciprofloxacin. What alteration in antimicrobial therapy is most appropriate for R.R. at this time?

Treatment of meningitis caused by *Enterobacter* and related species (e.g., *Serratia*, *Citrobacter* species) presents a particular challenge.[31,87] Furthermore, some isolates that are sensitive to third-generation cephalosporins can become resistant during therapy by virtue of selecting for derepressed mutants.[88] Thus, in contrast to gram-negative bacillary meningitis caused by *E. coli* and *Klebsiella* species, alternative therapies are needed when treating meningitis caused by *Enterobacter*, *Serratia*, *Citrobacter*, and *Pseudomonas* species. The isolate is sensitive to imipenem, but the higher propensity for seizures compared with other β-lactams (including penicillin G) argues against its use in R.R.[87] Meropenem is not considered to be epileptogenic and should be used preferentially to imipenem for meningitis.[89] Clinical trials have evaluated the efficacy and safety of meropenem versus cefotaxime in the treatment of meningitis in children. Clinical outcomes were similar among the patients randomized to either group, and the incidence of seizures was similar in the treatment groups.[90,91] Thus, after consideration of the aforementioned options, meropenem appears to be the best choice of therapy for R.R and carries FDA (Food and Drug Administration) approval for this indication; however, TMP-SMX, although not FDA-approved, may be an option as well.[92] Cefepime should be discontinued and, if confirmed to be susceptible, therapy started with meropenem 2 g IV every 8 hours adjusted for renal insufficiency.

DURATION OF THERAPY

The optimal duration of therapy for gram-negative bacillary meningitis has not been clearly established. Because of the high mortality and morbidity associated with these pathogens and the reduced susceptibility of enteric pathogens to antimicrobial agents, 21 days has been suggested and should be provided for R.R. (Table 65-8).[11]

Staphylococcus epidermidis Meningitis or Ventriculitis

CLINICAL PRESENTATION OF CEREBROSPINAL FLUID SHUNT INFECTIONS

CASE 65-4

QUESTION 1: T.A., a 21-year-old woman with a history of congenital hydrocephalus, is admitted to the neurosurgery unit for worsening mental status and fever. T.A. has a history of multiple revisions and placements of intraventricular shunts for control of hydrocephalus. Currently, she has a ventriculoperitoneal (VP) shunt, which was placed 1 month ago and previously had been functioning normally. During the past few days, T.A. has exhibited worsening obtundation, stiff neck, and a temperature of 39.5°C. A CT scan performed today reveals enlarged ventricles consistent with acute hydrocephalus.

T.A.'s medical history is noncontributory except for a seizure disorder for which she takes phenytoin 400 mg PO at bedtime. She also takes Lo-Ovral for birth control. T.A. is allergic to sulfa drugs (severe skin rash). Her weight on admission is 60 kg.

Laboratory analysis was significant for the following:

WBC count, 14,000 cells/μL, with a differential of 85% PMNs and 10% lymphocytes
BUN, 19 mg/dL
SCr, 0.9 mg/dL

A tap of T.A.'s shunt was performed, and the ventricular fluid was notable for the following results:

Total protein, 150 mg/dL
Glucose, 40 mg/dL
WBC count, 200 cells/μL, with 85% PMNs and 10% lymphocytes

Gram stain of the ventricular fluid showed numerous gram-positive cocci in clusters. What are the subjective and objective findings of CSF shunt infections, and what manifestations of this type of infection are present in T.A.?

T.A. likely has meningitis with ventriculitis secondary to infection of her VP shunt. The most important way to manage hydrocephalus involves the use of devices that divert (shunt) CSF from the cerebral ventricles to other areas of the body such as the peritoneum (VP shunts) or atrium (ventriculoatrial shunts).[93] This approach alleviates increased CSF pressure and substantially reduces morbidity and mortality.[94] Infection of these devices, however, is a common cause of shunt malfunction, as seen in T.A. The reported incidence of CSF shunt infections in children is approximately 11% in recent studies and varies in adults from 2.5% to 15% depending on patient factors, surgical technique, and the type and duration of the procedure performed (i.e., shunt revision vs. placement of a new device).[95–97] T.A., who has been hydrocephalic since birth and has a history of multiple shunt procedures, is at high risk for such an infection.

Clinical symptoms associated with infected CSF shunts vary widely from asymptomatic colonization to fulminant ventriculitis with meningitis. Fever is common and, in many instances, is the only presenting symptom. CSF findings also are slightly different in shunt infection compared with acute meningitis: The WBC count usually is not as elevated, the decrease in CSF glucose is less pronounced, and the protein value may be normal or slightly elevated. CSF culture is positive in most patients.[98] T.A.'s clinical presentation, CSF findings, and radiographic evidence of hydrocephalus are highly suggestive of a VP shunt infection. She is febrile and has altered mental status. The presence of a stiff neck strongly suggests meningeal involvement. Evaluation of T.A.'s ventricular fluid reveals a slightly elevated WBC count, with a predominance of PMNs, an elevated protein concentration, and a slightly lower-than-normal glucose concentration.

Skin microflora are the most common causes for CSF shunt infections. Coagulase-negative staphylococci (usually *S. epidermidis*) account for roughly 50% of all cases and *Staphylococcus aureus* accounts for roughly one-fourth of all cases. Other less common pathogens include diphtheroids, enterococci, and *Propionibacterium acnes*. Enteric gram-negative bacilli are responsible for a small percentage of cases; these cases usually occur when the distal end of the shunt is inserted improperly into the peritoneal cavity.[98,99] The gram-positive cocci in clusters on Gram stain of T.A.'s CSF strongly suggest a staphylococcal shunt infection. Determining the coagulase status of the isolate will allow differentiation between *S. aureus* and coagulase-negative staphylococci, likely *S. epidermidis*.

TREATMENT OF CEREBROSPINAL FLUID SHUNT INFECTIONS

CASE 65-4, QUESTION 2: Culture and sensitivity tests of T.A.'s ventricular fluid are positive for *S. epidermidis*. The isolate is resistant to nafcillin but sensitive to vancomycin, rifampin, and TMP-SMX. How should T.A.'s CSF shunt infection be treated?

For T.A.'s CSF shunt infection to be optimally treated, a combined medical and surgical approach is required. Studies have demonstrated poorer outcomes for systemic antibiotic therapy alone versus systemic antibiotic therapy plus shunt removal.[100] Because many patients cannot tolerate the complete removal of their shunt for long, externalization of the distal end of the shunt, or shunt removal and placement of an external drainage device, often is necessary during systemic antibiotic therapy. The presence of an externalized device permits sequential sampling of ventricular fluid and also provides a convenient way to administer antibiotic intraventricularly (see the following discussion entitled *Intraventricular Dosing of Vancomycin*).

Glycocalyx

Although *S. epidermidis* is not as virulent a pathogen as *S. aureus*, it is extremely difficult to eradicate this organism from prosthetic devices such as CSF shunts. This is because many strains of *S. epidermidis* produce a mucous film or slime layer known as *glycocalyx*, which allows the staphylococci to adhere tightly to the shunt material, protecting them against phagocytosis.[101] As expected, antibiotic failures are much more likely with slime-producing strains of *S. epidermidis*.

Vancomycin is the drug of choice for treatment of shunt infections caused by *S. epidermidis* and should be instituted immediately in T.A.[11,102] This is because a high percentage (>60%) of coagulase-negative staphylococci are resistant to methicillin (e.g., methicillin-resistant *S. epidermidis* [MRSE]). T.A.'s isolate also is sensitive to TMP-SMX, as is the case with many strains of MRSE (and also methicillin-resistant *S. aureus* [MRSA]), but it must be avoided because T.A. is allergic to this drug combination. Although not considered a first-line therapy, linezolid has been shown to be effective for VP shunt infections in small case series and may be considered in vancomycin-allergic patients.[103,104] Additionally, many staphylococcal isolates (both *S. epidermidis* and *S. aureus*) are susceptible to rifampin, but monotherapy with this drug is not recommended because of rapid emergence of resistance. However, rifampin may be used in addition to an antistaphylococcal agent to enhance bactericidal activity, especially if the prosthesis is retained.[102]

CASE 65-4, QUESTION 3: What would be an appropriate IV dosage for vancomycin in T.A.? What subjective or objective data should be monitored to evaluate the efficacy and toxicity of the treatment?

Vancomycin therapy for T.A.'s CSF shunt infection requires the use of doses similar to those used for bacterial meningitis. For adults such as T.A., vancomycin dosages of 30 to 45 mg/kg/day have been endorsed.[11] For children with meningitis or infected shunts, the recommended dosage of vancomycin is 40 to 60 mg/kg/day, given IV in two to four divided doses (Table 65-6).[105] Targeted serum trough concentrations of vancomycin should be between 15 and 20 mcg/mL.[11,32]

T.A., who weighs 60 kg, should be started on a vancomycin regimen of 1 g IV every 8 to 12 hours because her renal function is normal. In either case, trough serum concentrations should be obtained at steady state to assess whether the initial dosing regimen is adequate. Another consideration for T.A. is the addition of rifampin to her vancomycin regimen. This is based on the excellent staphylococcal activity of rifampin, its moderate CSF penetration, and the potential for synergy between these two agents.[106] Whether rifampin plus vancomycin is superior to vancomycin alone has not been determined. For T.A., it is best to avoid rifampin because evidence supporting its efficacy is weak, and she currently is taking phenytoin and oral contraceptives. Rifampin is a potent inducer of hepatic microsomal enzymes, which can lower serum phenytoin concentrations (possibly resulting in seizure activity) and increase the possibility of an unplanned pregnancy (from reduced effectiveness of the birth control pill).

Intraventricular Dosing of Vancomycin

CASE 65-4, QUESTION 4: Should T.A. receive intraventricular vancomycin? If so, what would be an appropriate dosage?

T.A. should receive IV vancomycin. In addition, T.A. has a long history of hydrocephalus and will require placement of an external drainage device after removal of her VP shunt. The external drainage device allows for intraventricular administration of vancomycin, and such treatment should be instituted promptly. Although dosage recommendations vary from 5 to 20 mg/day, most use 20 mg/day and this dose should be used for T.A. Also, serial (daily) cultures of CSF are recommended to monitor her response to therapy. Therapy should be continued for at least 10 days after sterilization of her ventricular fluid is documented, at which time a new VP shunt can be placed.[11]

In contrast to T.A.'s situation, vancomycin therapy for patients with MRSA meningitis not associated with a CSF shunt or indwelling ventricular catheter is more problematic. The latest MRSA clinical practice guidelines from 2011 endorse a 2-week course of IV vancomycin 15 to 20 mg/kg/dose IV every 8 to 12 hours, with the potential addition of rifampin 600 mg daily, or 300 to 450 mg every 12 hours. Additionally, in seriously ill patients, including those with meningitis, a loading dose of 25 to 30 mg/kg of actual body weight may be considered. Trough concentrations between 15 and 20 mcg/mL are recommended.[32] In the setting of drug allergy, intolerance, or adverse events, alternatives include linezolid 600 mg PO or IV every 12 hours, or TMP-SMX 5 mg/kg/dose IV every 8 to 12 hours.[107]

BRAIN ABSCESS

Epidemiology

Although not nearly as common as meningitis, abscesses of the brain parenchyma (brain abscess) remain an important type of CNS infection. The reported incidence of brain abscess caused by any type of organism ranges from 0.4 to 0.9 cases per 100,000 population.[108,109] On a busy neurosurgical service, 4 to 10 cases a year typically are seen.[110,111] For reasons that are not entirely clear, men are more likely to develop abscesses within the brain than women.[109,110] Brain abscess can occur at any age, but the mean age most recently reported is 34 years of age, with a minority of cases occurring in children.[112]

Despite advances in antimicrobial therapy over the past several decades, mortality rates from brain abscess have remained above 40% until recently. Developments in imaging techniques (e.g., CT and MRI scanning), which allow early recognition of abscesses and the ability to serially monitor the radiographic response to antimicrobial therapy, have had the most profound impact on reducing morbidity and mortality from brain abscess. A recent meta-analysis of 123 studies found case fatality rates declined from 40% to 10% over the decades from 1970 to 2013 whereas the rates of full recovery increased from 33% to 70%. With the combined medical and surgical approach currently recommended, mortality rates continue to average <10%.[112]

Predisposing Factors

Brain abscesses most commonly arise from a contiguous suppurative source of infection (e.g., sinusitis, otitis, mastoiditis, or dental infections).[112] The formation of a single abscess cavity usually is found when infection develops from a contiguous source. In addition, the abscess nearly always is formed in close proximity to the primary focus of infection (Table 65-9). For example, abscesses of sinusitic origin more commonly involve the frontal lobe, whereas otitic infections often lead to temporal lobe abscess formation.[113] Brain abscess also occurs as a consequence of hematogenous spread of organisms from a primary site of infection (e.g., lung abscess, endocarditis, osteomyelitis, pelvic, and intra-abdominal infections). Multiple abscesses suggest a metastatic source of infection. As with meningitis, brain abscess occurs as an infrequent complication of head trauma or neurosurgery.[112] No identifiable source (cryptogenic abscess) is detected in as many as 30% of cases.[113]

Staging

Once an intracranial focus of infection is established, the evolution of brain abscess involves two distinct stages: cerebritis and capsule formation. The cerebritis stage evolves gradually over the first 9 to 10 days of infection and is characterized by an area of marked inflammatory infiltrate that contains a necrotic center surrounded by an area of cerebral edema. Capsule formation occurs about 10 to 14 days after the initiation of infection, and once formed, the capsule continues to thicken over a period of weeks. The stage of abscess development has important implications for therapy. Although it is best to wait until the capsule is fully formed before attempting any type of surgical intervention, antimicrobial therapy alone may resolve the infection if discovered in the early cerebritis stage.[114]

Microbiology

The microbiology of brain abscess is distinctly different from that of meningitis. Streptococci are implicated in 50% to 70% of cases and include anaerobic as well as microaerophilic streptococci of the *S. milleri* group.[112] Other anaerobes, particularly *Bacteroides* species (including *B. fragilis*) and *Prevotella* species, are the second most common cause of brain abscess and are usually in mixed culture.[110,112] These organisms are followed by staphylococci and gram-negative bacteria as other common pathogens.[112] Although

Table 65-9

Predisposing Conditions, Microbiology, and Recommended Therapy for Bacterial Brain Abscess

Predisposing Condition	Usual Location of Abscess	Most Likely Organisms	Recommended Therapy
Contiguous Site			
Otitis media	Temporal lobe or cerebellum	Streptococci (anaerobic and aerobic), *Bacteroides fragilis*, gram-negative bacilli	Ceftriaxone + metronidazole
Sinusitis	Frontal lobe	Streptococci (predominantly), *Bacteroides* species, gram-negative bacilli, *Staphylococcus aureus*, *Haemophilus* species	Vancomycin + ceftriaxone + metronidazole
Dental infection	Frontal lobe	*Fusobacterium* species, *Bacteroides* species, and streptococci	Ceftriaxone + metronidazole
Primary Infection			
Head trauma or neurosurgery	Related to site of wound	Gram-negative bacilli, staphylococci, streptococci, *Clostridium*	Vancomycin + cefepime + metronidazole

somewhat imprecise, a reasonable correlation exists between the various predisposing conditions and the microbiologic etiology of brain abscess (Table 65-9).[113]

In the immunocompromised patient, a diverse group of microorganisms can induce abscesses within the brain. In patients with AIDS, *Toxoplasma gondii* is the most common infectious cause of focal brain lesions.[115] Transplant recipients and those receiving immunosuppressive therapy are susceptible to infection from *Nocardia* species and fungi (e.g., aspergillus or candida species).[116] In Mexico and other Central American countries, cysticercosis remains a common cause of intracerebral infection.[117]

Clinical and Radiologic Features

CASE 65-5

QUESTION 1: L.Y., a 40-year-old man, is brought to the ED by a friend. L.Y. complains of severe headache, fever, weakness in his left arm and leg, and increasing drowsiness. During the past week, L.Y. has suffered from headaches, which have gradually worsened in intensity, and from intermittent episodes of fever. Despite getting plenty of sleep, L.Y. has been feeling increasingly drowsy during the past several days. When he noticed weakness in his left arm and difficulty concentrating this morning, he called a friend and asked to be taken in for evaluation.

L.Y. has a history of chronic sinusitis that has been treated with a variety of oral antibiotics. His last episode of sinusitis, which occurred about 1 month ago, was treated with a 10-day course of cephalexin. He denies any nausea or vomiting and has not experienced any seizures in the recent past. L.Y. was tested for HIV 6 months ago, and the result of his antibody test was negative. He takes no current medications, denies smoking and use of recreational drugs, and drinks alcohol only on social occasions a few times a month. L.Y. has no known drug allergies.

Physical examination reveals L.Y. to be in mild distress, with a temperature of 38.2°C. He is slightly lethargic and is oriented to person and place but not time. The strength in L.Y.'s left arm is 3/5; the strength in his left leg is 4/5. The remainder of his neurologic examination is grossly normal. L.Y. described moderate pain on palpation of his frontal sinuses, and a purulent discharge is noted.

Laboratory evaluation shows the following:

WBC count, 8,000 cells/μL, with 70% PMN, 25% lymphocytes, and 5% monocytes
BUN, 16 mg/dL
SCr, 1.2 mg/dL
Erythrocyte sedimentation rate (ESR), 40 mm/hour
Hgb, Hct, platelets, and serum chemistries are within normal limits.

A CT scan with contrast dye reveals a right frontal ring-enhancing lesion with a small amount of surrounding cerebral edema. L.Y. is admitted to the neurosurgery unit for further evaluation and treatment. What clinical signs and symptoms does L.Y. display that are suggestive of bacterial brain abscess? How can brain abscess be diagnosed in L.Y.?

L.Y. has presented to the ED with many signs and symptoms suggestive of bacterial brain abscess. He is 40 years of age and a man, both of which place him in a group with the highest likelihood of having a brain abscess. In contrast to the diffuse nature of meningitis, brain abscess presents as a focal neurologic process. Notable in L.Y.'s presentation is left-sided (arm and leg) weakness. Symptoms of brain abscess range in severity from indolent to fulminant, and in most patients, the duration of symptoms at the time of presentation is ≤2 weeks.[113] Headache is the most common symptom of brain abscess, occurring in approximately 70% of cases. L.Y.'s clinical manifestations have become gradually worse over the past week, and his worsening headaches, increasing drowsiness, and difficulty in concentrating all are consistent with bacterial brain abscess.

L.Y. presents with the classic triad of fever, headache, and focal neurologic deficits. Although this triad should always be looked for, fewer than half of patients with confirmed bacterial brain abscess present in this manner.[112]

The absence of fever does not rule out infection because fever is found in <50% of patients.[110,113] Focal neurologic deficits are present in approximately 50% of patients and vary in nature and severity in relation to the location and size of the abscess and surrounding cerebral edema. Although L.Y. does not have a history of seizure activity, approximately 25% of patients experience partial seizures that often become generalized. Papilledema and nuchal rigidity occur in ≤25% of cases and often are not useful in confirming the diagnosis. Symptoms associated with a contiguous focus of infection should always be sought, and in some situations, they may dominate the clinical picture.[112] L.Y. has a history of sinus infection, and the pain on palpation of his sinuses coupled with the purulent sinus drainage suggests active infection at this site.

As can be seen from L.Y.'s test results, laboratory evaluation usually is not very helpful when diagnosing brain abscess. L.Y. does not have a peripheral leukocytosis, but he does have an elevated ESR. A normal peripheral WBC count is not unusual in patients with intracranial suppuration. The ESR often is elevated in brain abscess, but this test is nonspecific and only indirectly supports the diagnosis.

L.Y. did not have a lumbar puncture because this procedure is contraindicated for diagnosing brain abscess. The diagnostic yield from CSF is low because chemistries (e.g., protein, glucose, WBC) usually are normal and culture of the CSF in patients with brain abscess is unlikely to yield the causative pathogen. More important, performing a lumbar puncture in patients with space-occupying lesions of the brain can produce cerebral herniation as a consequence of the shifting pressure gradient induced within the cranial vault after insertion of the lumbar puncture needle.[118]

Of paramount importance is the abnormality detected on the CT scan of L.Y.'s brain. When dye is injected before the CT scan, brain abscesses will appear to "ring enhance." Furthermore, cerebral edema can be identified as a variable hypodense region immediately surrounding the abscess cavity. As stated earlier, CT and MRI scanning techniques have revolutionized the diagnosis and treatment of brain abscess.[112,119] In general, a good correlation exists between the clinical and radiologic response to therapy of bacterial brain abscess.

Treatment

CASE 65-5, QUESTION 2: How should L.Y.'s brain abscess be treated?

SURGICAL TECHNIQUES

A combined medical and surgical approach is the best form of therapy for L.Y.'s brain abscess. Response rates to antimicrobial therapy alone have been disappointing, and with a few exceptions, surgical intervention is necessary to ensure optimal results. Modern stereotactic neurosurgical techniques allow almost any brain abscess that is ≥1 cm in diameter to be drained via stereotactic aspiration, regardless of location. Primary medical therapy may be indicated if imaging does not show a central cavity in the abscess or if surgery is withheld for other reasons such as poor health status.[113]

The two types of surgical approaches for brain abscess are (a) stereotactic navigation with needle aspiration and (b) intraoperative ultrasonography through a burr hole or craniotomy for direct abscess drainage.[113] Stereotactic aspiration of abscess is highly effective and is associated with lower morbidity and mortality than craniotomy.[120] Modern medical advances leave total resection with a very limited role unless an abscess is superficial or when there is high suspicion of fungal or tuberculous infection.[113]

ANTIMICROBIAL PENETRATION INTO BRAIN ABSCESS

Antimicrobial therapy is an essential component of brain abscess therapy. Penetration of antibiotics into brain abscess fluid has not been studied as carefully as penetration into CSF, and as discussed earlier, the barrier involved is different (Fig. 65-1).[7] Penicillins and cephalosporins penetrate adequately into abscess fluid, but certain agents (e.g., penicillin G) may be susceptible to degradation by enzymes present within the abscess milieu.[110] Third-generation cephalosporins (e.g., cefotaxime, ceftriaxone) penetrate sufficiently into the abscess and thus are appropriate choices when gram-negative bacteria are present.[110,121] Metronidazole achieves abscess fluid concentrations equal to or in excess of serum levels and is bactericidal against strict anaerobes. The unique mechanism of action of metronidazole makes it particularly useful in the necrotic core of the cavity, where the oxidation-reduction potential is low and bacteria replicate slowly or are dormant. For these reasons, metronidazole is the drug of choice for anaerobic gram-negative bacterial brain abscess.[110] Vancomycin and carbapenems also penetrate sufficiently into brain abscess fluid.[110,122] Although specific abscess-penetration data are unavailable, successful treatment of cerebral nocardiosis with TMP-SMX and CNS toxoplasmosis with clindamycin suggests that these compounds also achieve adequate penetration into cerebral abscess cavities.[123,124]

ANTIBIOTIC THERAPY

When antibiotic therapy should be instituted depends on the status of the patient and the stage of abscess development. For patients diagnosed during the cerebritis stage, before formation of a well-circumscribed capsule, surgery should be delayed and antimicrobial therapy begun in patients with significant symptoms.[110,121] If capsule formation already has taken place and if the patient's clinical status allows, it is reasonable to delay initiation of antibiotics until after surgery if surgery is to be performed within hours to increase the microbiologic yield from tissue and fluid samples. If the disease is fulminant, antibiotics must be instituted promptly and surgical intervention performed as quickly as possible.[113]

L.Y.'s clinical presentation suggests an advanced brain abscess. The presence of ring enhancement on CT and the onset of symptoms over 2 weeks support this conclusion. Because he is not critically ill, antibiotic therapy may be delayed until surgery is performed. Specimens obtained from the surgical procedure should be sent for aerobic and anaerobic culture and an immediate Gram stain.

Initial antibiotic therapy for brain abscess needs to be sufficiently broad to cover the most likely pathogens (Table 65-9). When the implicated source is contiguous such as oral, otogenic, or sinus, metronidazole plus ceftriaxone (with the addition of vancomycin with a sinus source) is recommended.[110,113] Metronidazole will provide coverage for strict anaerobes, including *Bacteroides* and *Prevotella* species. When the implicated source is head trauma with skull fracture or is associated with a neurosurgical procedure, empiric therapy should consist of vancomycin, metronidazole, and a third- or fourth-generation cephalosporin. For hematogenous sources, a third-generation cephalosporin, metronidazole, and vancomycin are recommended.[113] Vancomycin is added to cover staphylococcal infection.

For L.Y., therapy with ceftriaxone 2 grams IV Q 12 hours, vancomycin 1 gram IV Q 8 hours, and metronidazole 500 mg IV Q 8 hours should be started postoperatively (Table 65-6).

ADJUNCTIVE CORTICOSTEROID THERAPY

Adjunctive corticosteroid therapy for bacterial brain abscess is controversial. Steroids can interfere with antibiotic penetration into abscesses and obscure the interpretation of serial CT scans when assessing response to therapy. Therefore, steroids are indicated only if significant cerebral edema is present, particularly if it is accompanied by rapid neurologic deterioration.[110,121] L.Y. should not receive dexamethasone because his mental status is only mildly depressed and the cerebral edema seen on CT scan is not massive.

ADJUNCTIVE ANTICONVULSANT THERAPY

L.Y. has shown no sign of seizure activity thus far and, therefore, does not require anticonvulsant therapy. Anticonvulsants should be used in the acute setting when seizures are present, however.[110,121] Agents with activity against partial and complex partial seizures are preferred (e.g., phenytoin, carbamazepine, and potentially levetiracetam). The long-term use of anticonvulsants depends on whether seizure activity persists. Insufficient information exists regarding how long to continue anticonvulsants in such cases. Therefore, discontinuation of these agents must be individualized.

No formal guidelines are available regarding the optimal duration of therapy for bacterial brain abscess. Given the serious nature of the infection and the difficulty associated with antibiotic penetration, therapy with high-dose IV therapy should continue for at least 6 to 8 weeks.[110,113] The duration of therapy should be evaluated on a case-by-case basis. In an attempt to ensure complete eradication of infection, some experts recommend long-term (2–6 months) oral antibiotics after the IV course, provided agents with good oral absorption and activity against the offending pathogens are available.[110]

MONITORING THERAPY

CASE 65-5, QUESTION 3: How should L.Y. be monitored for therapeutic response and toxicity?

Although L.Y. is on antibiotic therapy, weekly or biweekly CT scans should be obtained to evaluate abscess resolution. His clinical response to therapy also should be assessed daily. If therapy is effective, L.Y.'s mental status should improve gradually (e.g., he will become more alert and oriented) over a period of several days. L.Y.'s headaches and hemiparesis (weakness in his arm and leg) also should resolve eventually. It may take a week or longer, however, to see a complete resolution of symptoms.[110] In general, radiologic improvement (i.e., reduction in abscess size) correlates reasonably well with clinical response, but not always. Persistent symptoms or failure to detect a reduction in abscess size on CT scan or the appearance of new abscesses may indicate improper antimicrobial therapy or the need for more surgery.[110,121] Repeated surgical intervention with appropriate reculturing may be required in some instances to optimize therapy.

Adverse effects associated with the penicillin G therapy that L.Y. is receiving are similar to those of other β-lactam antibiotics. Seizures are a potential complication when high doses of penicillin are used in the presence of a mass lesion in the brain.[125] L.Y. should be observed closely by those providing care and questioned regularly for any evidence of seizure activity. Metronidazole usually is well tolerated, but may also cause neurotoxicity, most commonly peripheral neuropathy. L.Y. should be assessed for the presence of numbness or tingling in his hands or feet. Seizures, although uncommon, occasionally occur with metronidazole. If L.Y. experiences peripheral neuropathy or seizures, a switch to meropenem would be appropriate. Other adverse effects associated with metronidazole include mild nausea, brownish discoloration of the urine, and the potential for a disulfiram-like reaction with concomitant ethanol ingestion.[126] L.Y. should be counseled regarding the possibility of gastric upset and discoloration of the urine, and he should be strongly cautioned to avoid alcoholic beverages while receiving metronidazole. Given his young age, the absence of significant underlying diseases, and the relative early detection of his brain abscess, there is every reason to expect a good response to his treatment and, eventually, a complete resolution of his abscess.

KEY REFERENCES AND WEBSITES

A full list of references for this chapter can be found at http://thepoint.lww.com/AT11e. Below are the key references and website for this chapter, with the corresponding reference number in this chapter found in parentheses after the reference.

Key References

Brouwer MC et al. Corticosteroids for acute bacterial meningitis. *Cochrane Database Syst Rev*. 2013;6:CD004405. (48)

Brouwer MC et al. Brain Abscess. *N Engl J Med*. 2014;371:447–456. (113)

Castelblanco RL et al. Epidemiology of bacterial meningitis in the USA from 1997 to 2010: a population-based observational study. *Lancet Infect Dis*. 2014;14:813–819. (70)

de Gans J et al. Dexamethasone in adults with bacterial meningitis. *N Engl J Med*. 2002;347:1549. (41)

Di Paolo A et al. Clinical pharmacokinetics of antibacterials in cerebrospinal fluid. *Clin Pharmacokin*. 2013;52:511. (28)

Nau R et al. Penetration of Drugs through the Blood-Cerebrospinal Fluid/Blood-Brain Barrier for Treatment of Central Nervous System Infections. *Clin Microbiol Rev*. 2010;23:858. (29)

Thigpen MC et al. Bacterial meningitis in the United States, 1998–2007. *N Engl J Med*. 2011;364:2016–25. (1)

Tunkel AR et al. Practice guidelines for the management of bacterial meningitis. *Clin Infect Dis*. 2004;39:1267. (11)

van de Beek D et al. Clinical features and prognostic factors in adults with bacterial meningitis [published correction appears in *N Engl J Med*. 2005;352:950]. *N Engl J Med*. 2004;351:1849. (72)

66 Endocarditis

Michelle L. Chan and Annie Wong-Beringer

CORE PRINCIPLES

		CHAPTER CASES
1	Infective endocarditis (IE) is a microbial infection of the heart valves or other endocardial tissue, usually associated with an underlying cardiac defect. Disease incidence has remained stable over time accounting for 15,000 to 20,000 new cases per year. *Streptococcus viridans*, *Staphylococcus aureus*, and *Enterococcus* species are common causes of IE. Other rare pathogens affecting special populations include *Staphylococcus epidermidis*, *Pseudomonas aeruginosa*, and *Candida* species.	**Case 66-1 (Question 1), Case 66-2 (Question 1), Case 66-3 (Question 1), Case 66-4 (Question 1), Case 66-5 (Questions 1, 4, 6)**
2	Clinical presentation may be highly variable and characterized by nonspecific symptoms such as fever, weight loss, fatigue, night sweats, and arthralgias. Peripheral manifestations specific to IE include conjunctival petechiae, Janeway lesions, and splinter hemorrhages. Major embolic episodes and infarction involving other organs can develop in up to one-third of cases. Congestive heart failure (CHF) is the most common cause of death in IE, and the most common indication for surgery.	**Case 66-1 (Question 1), Case 66-2 (Question 2), Figures 66-1–66-3**
3	The American Heart Association (AHA) recommends use of the modified Duke criteria as the primary diagnostic schema to evaluate patients suspected of IE. The most important factor confirming IE is positive blood cultures. Transesophageal echocardiogram (TEE) is a valuable tool to strengthen diagnosis and identify patients at risk for complications and need for surgical interventions.	**Case 66-1 (Question 2), Tables 66-1, 66-2**
4	General treatment approach to organism eradication requires the administration of parenteral bactericidal antibiotics at high doses for a prolonged duration of 4 to 6 weeks. Combination therapy may be needed to achieve synergy for some pathogens. Selection of regimen should be based on organism sensitivity, tissue penetration, and host tolerance of the antibiotic agent(s). The AHA treatment guideline by organisms should be followed.	**Case 66-1 (Questions 3, 4), Case 66-2 (Question 3), Case 66-3 (Questions 2–4), Case 66-4 (Questions 1–5), Case 66-5 (Questions 2, 3, 5, 7), Tables 66-3–66-5**
5	Treatment of IE caused by methicillin-resistant *Staphylococcus aureus* (MRSA) and by enterococci presents significant challenges owing to emergence of resistance to standard therapy, vancomycin. Higher doses of vancomycin targeting a trough concentration of 15 to 20 mcg/mL are advocated for treatment of MRSA IE, but may be associated with increased incidence of nephrotoxicity. Alternative agents for treatment of IE caused by vancomycin-resistant enterococci have limited clinical success or lack of clinical evidence.	**Case 66-3 (Questions 3, 4), Case 66-4 (Question 5)**
6	Fungal endocarditis is rare, but carries poor prognosis. It occurs primarily in intravenous (IV) drug users, patients with prosthetic heart valves or IV catheters, and those with a compromised immune system. Management generally requires early valve replacement and combination antifungal therapy.	**Case 66-5 (Questions 1–3)**
7	The AHA recommends the use of antibiotic prophylaxis in select patients with specific cardiac conditions associated with the highest risk of adverse outcomes from endocarditis, who are undergoing dental or respiratory procedures known to cause significant bacteremia. Antimicrobial prophylaxis should be directed against the viridans group of streptococci.	**Case 66-6 (Questions 1, 2), Tables 66-6 and 66-7**

INFECTIVE ENDOCARDITIS

IE is a microbial infection of the heart valves or other endocardial tissue, often associated with an underlying cardiac defect. IE is classified based on the causative organism to provide information on the probable cause and course of the disease (acute or subacute), the likelihood of underlying heart disease, and the appropriate antimicrobial regimens.[1]

Pathogenesis

The pathogenesis of endocarditis involves a complex series of events that ultimately result in the formation of an infected platelet-β-fibrin thrombus on the valve surface.[1,2] This thrombus is called a *vegetation.*

The first step in the formation of the vegetation involves modification of the endocardial surface, which is normally nonthrombogenic.

Valvular insufficiency caused by aortic stenosis or ventricular septal defects can produce regurgitant blood flow, high-pressure gradients, or narrow orifices, resulting in turbulence and endocardial damage.[1,2] In patients with rheumatic heart disease, endocardial injury (e.g., mitral valve stenosis) occurs as a result of immune complex deposition or hemodynamic disturbances.

Once the endocardial surface of the valve is traumatized, small, sterile thrombi consisting of platelets and fibrin are deposited, forming the lesion called nonbacterial thrombotic endocarditis (NBTE).[1,2] NBTE occurs most commonly on the atrial surfaces of the mitral and tricuspid valves and on the ventricular surface of the aortic valve.

NBTE serves as a nidus for microbial colonization during periods of bacteremia (e.g., procedures involving perforation of the oral mucosa, respiratory tract, genitourinary tract, or infected skin). Organisms such as *Streptococcus viridans* group, *Enterococcus* species, *Staphylococcus aureus*, *Staphylococcus epidermidis*, *Pseudomonas aeruginosa*, and *Candida albicans* possess adherence factors that facilitate their pathogenicity. In particular, platelet aggregation has been shown to be an important virulence factor in experimental streptococcal endocarditis potentially leading to larger vegetations and multifocal embolic spread.[3] Once the NBTE lesion becomes colonized by microorganisms, the surface is rapidly covered with a sheath of fibrin and platelets. This avascular encasement provides an environment protected from host defenses and is conducive to further bacterial replication and vegetation growth.[2] The bacterial colony count can be as high as 10^4 to 10^5 bacteria per gram of valvular vegetation.

Endocarditis can result in life-threatening hemodynamic disturbances and embolic episodes affecting many organs. Without antimicrobial therapy and surgical intervention, IE is virtually 100% fatal. Because of bacterial proliferation to high densities in the fibrin mesh protected from normal host defenses, cure of infection requires prolonged therapy of 4 to 6 weeks with relapse not uncommon.

Epidemiology

In 2009, there were 38,976 hospital admissions of endocarditis with an hospital mortality rate of 14% to 20%.[4,5] The overall incidence has been stable; however, health–care-associated IE has emerged as a result of increased use of invasive medical devices and procedures (e.g., IV catheters, total parenteral nutrition [TPN] IV lines, hemodialysis shunts or fistulas, intracardiac prosthesis, central venous pressure monitoring lines).[1] With the exception of IV drug users, the mean patient age has shifted from younger than 30 years in the 1920s to older than 55 years today.[4,6] This increase in age is likely attributable to (a) a decline in the incidence of acute rheumatic fever and rheumatic heart disease counterbalanced by degenerative valvular disease in an increasing elderly population, (b) the increasing longevity of the general population, and (c) increased exposure to more intense and invasive medical procedures in both the overall and the aging populations. Men are infected more often than women (roughly 2:1), and the disease remains uncommon in children, primarily in association with underlying congenital cardiac defect and nosocomial catheter-related bacteremia.[1]

Predisposing Factors

In general, any structural cardiac defect that leads to the turbulence of blood flow predisposes to the development of IE. Rheumatic heart disease was at one time the most common underlying cardiac defect associated with endocarditis; however, the proportion of cases related to rheumatic heart disease have declined to 25% or less in developed countries while remaining the predominant defect in developing countries.[4,5] Mitral valve prolapse with thickened leaflets and valvular redundancy is a recognized predisposing risk to IE, with a documented occurrence rate of 10%. Clinical presentation is often subtle with lower associated mortality in these individuals compared with left-sided IE of other types. In the absence of underlying valvular defects, degenerative cardiac lesions, such as calcified mitral annulus secondary to atherosclerotic cardiovascular disease and postmyocardial infarction thrombus, may be a significant risk factor for the elderly. IV drug users constitute a unique population at greatest risk for recurrent and polymicrobial IE.[4]

Hemodialysis dependency (8%), diabetes mellitus (16%), and congenital heart disease (12%) are the most common demographic characteristics associated with IE.[7] Up to 25% of all cases are acquired in health-care-related settings. Notably, in the United States, health-care-associated IE is more likely compared with community acquisition.

Bacteriology

Streptococci and staphylococci are the cause of 80% to 90% of cases of IE. When comparing epidemiologic studies in the aggregate during the past decades, staphylococci are increasingly prevalent as a cause of IE. *Viridans streptococci* remain the predominant cause of IE in children and in young women with isolated mitral valve involvement.[1]

Staphylococcus aureus is the leading cause of IE.[7,8] Acquisition of IE in nearly half of these cases was likely health-care-related, supporting a low threshold to evaluate underlying IE in the setting of health-care-related *S. aureus* bacteremia. More importantly, methicillin-resistant strains account for up to 40% of IE cases involving *S. aureus*.[4,6]

Endocarditis in IV drug users often is caused by *S. aureus*, whereas prosthetic valve endocarditis (PVE) is more commonly caused by coagulase-negative staphylococci, such as *S. epidermidis*. Gram-negative bacilli and fungi together account for less than 10% of all endocarditis cases, which usually are associated with IV drug use, valvular prostheses, and hospital IV access procedures. Endocarditis caused by anaerobes and other organisms is rare. Polymicrobial IE (caused by at least two organisms), although uncommon in the typical patient, is being recognized more frequently in IV drug users and certain postoperative patients. *Candida* species, *S. aureus*, *P. aeruginosa*, *Serratia marcescens*, and non-β hemolytic group D streptococci are the organisms involved most frequently in these populations.

Site of Involvement

The site of heart valve involvement is determined by the underlying cardiac defect and the infecting organism.[2,4,6,7] The mitral valve is affected in more than 85% of cases caused by *viridans streptococci* with underlying rheumatic heart disease. The tricuspid valve is the common site of involvement in staphylococcal endocarditis associated with IV drug use. Overall, the distribution ranges from 28% to 45% for mitral valve, 5% to 36% for aortic valves, and 0% to 6% for tricuspid valves, and the pulmonary valve is rarely affected.[9] Multiple heart valves may be affected simultaneously. Some studies have shown that aortic valve involvement is increasing in frequency and is associated with higher morbidity and mortality.

STREPTOCOCCUS VIRIDANS GROUP ENDOCARDITIS

Clinical Presentation

CASE 66-1

Question 1: A.G., a 57-year-old, 60-kg man with chief complaints of fatigue, a persistent low-grade fever, night sweats, arthralgias, and a 7-kg unintentional weight loss, is admitted to the hospital for evaluation. Visual inspection reveals a cachectic, ill-appearing man in no acute distress. Physical examination is significant for a grade III/IV diastolic murmur with mitral regurgitation (insufficiency) increased from preexisting murmur, a temperature of 100.5°F, petechial skin lesions, subungual splinter hemorrhages, and Janeway lesions on the soles of both feet (Figs. 66-1, 66-2, and 66-3). Nail clubbing, Roth spots, or Osler nodes are not evident. The remainder of his physical examination is unremarkable. A.G.'s medical history is significant for mitral valve prolapse and, more recently, a dental procedure involving the extraction of four wisdom teeth. The history of his present illness is noteworthy for the development of symptoms 2 weeks after the dental procedure (about 2 months before admission). His only current medication is ibuprofen 600 mg orally 4 times a day (QID).

Relevant laboratory results include the following:

- Hemoglobin (Hgb), 11.4 g/dL (SI units, 114 g/L [normal, 140–180])
- Hematocrit (Hct), 34% (SI units, 0.34 [normal, 0.39–0.49])
- Reticulocyte count, 0.5% (SI units, 0.005 [normal, 0.001–0.024])
- White blood cell (WBC) count, 35,000/μL with 65% polys and 1% bands (SI units, 35 × 10/L with 0.65 polys and 0.01 bands [normal, 3.2–9.8 with 0.54–0.62 polys and 0.03–0.05 bands])
- Blood urea nitrogen (BUN), 21 mg/dL (SI units, 7.5 mmol/L of urea [normal, 2.9–8.9])
- Serum creatinine (SCr), 1.2 mg/dL (SI units, 159 mmol/L [normal, 53–133])

A urinalysis (UA) reveals 2+ proteinuria and 10 to 20 red blood cells (RBCs) per high-power field (HPF). The erythrocyte sedimentation rate (ESR) is elevated at 66 mm/hour (normal, ≤30 mm/minute), and the rheumatoid factor (RF) is positive. Results from a transthoracic echocardiogram (TTE) were unrevealing.

Three blood cultures were obtained during 24 hours, and all cultures obtained on day 1 are growing gram-positive cocci in pairs and chains, presumed α-hemolytic streptococci. Although confirmation and speciation of the organism is being performed, A.G. is started on penicillin G, 2 million units IV every 4 hours (12 million units/day), and IV gentamicin, 120 mg (loading dose) followed by 60 mg every 12 hours. Antimicrobial susceptibility results are pending. What clinical manifestations and laboratory abnormalities in A.G. are consistent with IE?

The clinical presentation of IE is highly variable and can involve almost any organ system.[1] A.G. appears pale and chronically ill, and represents the typical patient with subacute disease (e.g., that caused by *viridans streptococci*). Nonspecific complaints consistent with endocarditis in A.G. include fatigue, weight loss, fever, night sweats, and arthralgias. Fever alone is present in most (90%) patients with endocarditis. The fever is characteristically low grade and remittent, with peaks in the afternoon and evening. Fever may be absent or minimal in patients with CHF, chronic renal and liver failure, prior use of antimicrobial agents, or IE caused by less virulent organisms.[1] Musculoskeletal complaints (e.g., arthralgias, myalgias, and back pain) are common and may mimic rheumatic disease. Other symptoms can include lethargy, anorexia, malaise, nausea, and vomiting.[1] Because signs and symptoms are nonspecific and subtle, diagnosis is often difficult to make. In addition, the time from bacteremia to diagnosis is often prolonged because of the insidious progression of symptoms.[1] Delayed diagnosis occurs more commonly in the elderly. Fever may be absent in 30% to 40% of patients older than 60 years of age, whereas it can be present in more than 90% of patients younger than 40 years of age. Elderly patients are less likely to have new or changed heart murmurs. The most common presenting complaints in the elderly with endocarditis are confusion, anorexia, fatigue, and weakness, which may be readily attributable to stroke, heart failure, or syncope.

The temporal relationship between A.G.'s dental procedure and the onset of symptoms suggests it was the etiology of bacteremia and subsequent endocarditis. Although it is assumed that prophylactic antibiotics were administered before the procedure, endocarditis can develop despite receipt of adequate chemoprophylaxis.[1,7,9]

A.G. has an increase in his preexisting diastolic murmur with mitral insufficiency, a finding consistent with endocarditis. Cardiac murmurs are present in more than 85% of patients with endocarditis. Murmurs frequently are absent in patients with acute disease (e.g., staphylococcal endocarditis), right-sided disease (e.g., endocarditis in IV drug users), or mural infection.[1]

A.G. exhibits several peripheral manifestations of IE, including conjunctival petechiae, Janeway lesions, and splinter hemorrhages. Overall, peripheral manifestations are observed in 10% to 50% of cases, but none of these is pathognomonic for IE.[1] These manifestations are usually a result of septic embolization of vegetations to distal sites, or immune complex deposition. Mucocutaneous petechial lesions of the conjunctiva, mouth, or pharynx are present in 20% to 40% of patients, especially those with long-standing disease.[1] These lesions generally are small, nontender, and hemorrhagic in appearance, and occur as a result of vasculitis or peripheral embolization. Janeway lesions are painless, hemorrhagic, macular plaques most commonly found on the palms and soles (Fig. 66-1). Splinter hemorrhages are nonspecific findings that appear as red to brown linear streaks in the proximal portion of the fingers or toenails (Fig. 66-2). Other findings can include Roth spots (small, flame-shaped retinal hemorrhages with pale white centers found near the optic nerve) and Osler nodes (purplish, nonhemorrhagic, painful nodules that develop on the subcutaneous pads of the fingers and toes or on palms and soles) Clubbing (broadening and thickening) of the nails also may be observed in patients with prolonged disease. Petechial skin lesions also are seen (Fig. 66-3).

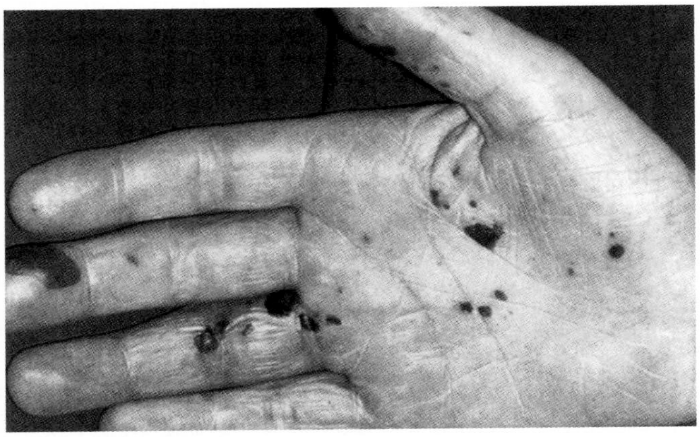

Figure 66-1 Janeway lesions. Extensive ecchymotic embolic lesions in a case of acute bacterial endocarditis.

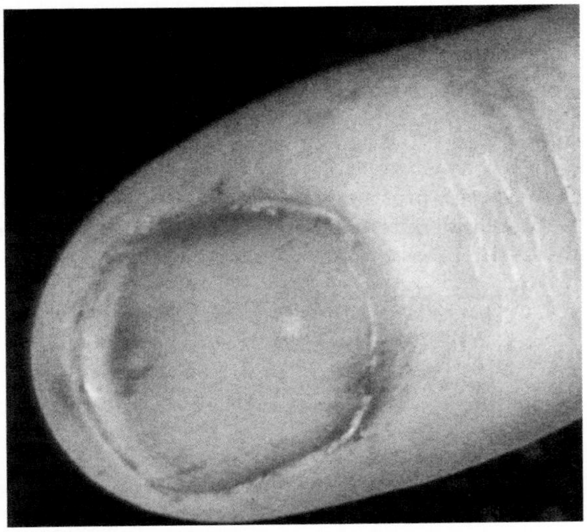

Figure 66-2 Splinter hemorrhages in the nail bed.

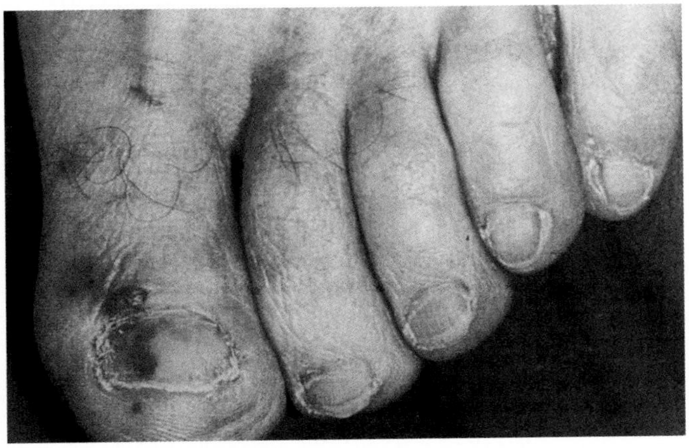

Figure 66-3 Petechial skin lesions in a case of acute staphylococcal endocarditis.

Several laboratory findings are consistent with IE in A.G. A low Hgb and Hct with normal red cell indices suggest anemia of chronic disease. Of patients with subacute disease, 70% to 90% will have a normochromic, normocytic anemia. Leukocytosis with a left shift, although not evident in A.G., commonly is seen in those with acute, fulminant disease such as staphylococcal endocarditis. The ESR nearly always is elevated in IE, but this finding is nonspecific and can be associated with several other disease entities. RF (an immunoglobulin M antiglobulin) and circulating immune complexes can be detected in most patients with long-standing disease, but both are nonspecific findings.[1]

Major embolic episodes and infarction involving the kidney, spleen, lung, and brain may develop as secondary complications in up to one-third of cases.[1] A.G. exhibits some degree of renal damage, as evidenced by moderate hematuria and proteinuria. Alterations in A.G.'s renal function (increased BUN and creatinine) probably are a result of immune complex deposition (diffuse glomerulonephritis) or secondary to renal embolization (focal glomerulonephritis). Erythrocyte and leukocyte cast formation also may be present. Renal impairment usually is reversible with the institution of effective antimicrobial therapy.[1,10]

Cardiac complications occur most frequently. CHF from infection-induced valvular damage is the most common cause of death in IE and is the most common indication for surgery.[1,10] As many as two-thirds of patients with endocarditis develop CHF. Aortic valve infection is more frequently associated with CHF than mitral valve infection. Other manifestations include paravalvular abscesses, pulmonary edema, and pericarditis.[10] Mitral valve injury caused by *viridans streptococci* generally is better tolerated hemodynamically than aortic valve injury caused by staphylococci. Although A.G. has no apparent signs of overt heart failure, he should be monitored closely for the development of hemodynamic instability.

Neurologic complications, most commonly stroke, rank second to cardiac complications in frequency, but they may be the leading cause of death in patients with endocarditis.[10] A stroke syndrome in a patient with underlying valvular abnormalities should prompt the clinician to rule out IE. Other clinical manifestations include headache, mental status change, transient ischemic attack, seizures, brain abscess, or intracranial mycotic aneurysms.[1,10] Neurologic symptoms associated with high mortality can be observed in up to 35% of *S. aureus* endocarditis patients who are not drug addicts.[11]

Metastatic abscesses can develop in virtually any organ secondary to systemic septic embolization. The most commonly involved metastatic foci are the spleen, kidney, liver, and iliac and mesenteric arteries.[10] Splenomegaly, although not part of A.G.'s findings, occurs in 20% to 60% of all cases and is more common in subacute disease.

Diagnosis

Case 66-1, Question 2: How was the diagnosis of IE established in A.G.?

BLOOD CULTURES

Although A.G.'s medical history (mitral valve prolapse, recent dental procedure) and clinical presentation are highly suggestive of IE, blood culture is the single most important diagnostic workup for IE.[1] Bacteremia (when present) secondary to endocarditis is continuous and low grade; more than 50% of the cultures show only 1 to 30 bacteria/mL. Despite the low concentration of organisms, at least one of the first two blood cultures is positive in 95% of cases.[1] In order to achieve a high yield, at least three sets of blood cultures collected by separate venipunctures should be obtained during the first 24 hours of presentation.[1] Administration of antibiotics within the previous 2 weeks may significantly decrease this yield.[12]

It is also important to establish the exact microbiologic cause before initiating antimicrobial therapy. In patients who are acutely ill, empiric therapy should start as soon as the appropriate cultures are obtained to avoid further valvular damage or other complications.[1]

Echocardiography is a valuable tool in establishing early diagnosis (e.g., the presence and size of vegetations), identifying patients at high risk for complications, and optimizing the timing and mode of surgical intervention by detecting and monitoring associated pathologic changes such as valvular abscess.[1,13,14] The transducer may be placed on the chest (transthoracic echocardiogram [TTE]) or in the esophagus (transesophageal echocardiogram [TEE]).[14] TTE is a rapid and noninvasive procedure with 98% specificity for vegetations. Sensitivity for vegetations may be less than 60% to 70%, however, for adult patients with obesity, hyperinflated lungs caused by emphysema, or a prosthetic valve. TEE is more costly and invasive, but is significantly more sensitive in detecting vegetations while maintaining high specificity. All patients with suspected IE should have echocardiography on admission and repeated during their course, to help guide future medical management and timing of intervention.[14] In particular, compared with TTE, TEE is superior in the diagnosis of pacemaker IE and IE in the elderly. A.G. has a negative TTE result on admission. Given the high clinical suspicion for IE in A.G., a follow-up TEE is recommended to rule out a false-negative TTE result.

In summary, IE should be suspected in any patient who has a documented fever and heart murmur and a preceding risk of bacteremia. Prior cardiac disease, peripheral manifestations, splenomegaly, various laboratory abnormalities, and a positive echocardiogram strengthen the diagnosis, but microbiologic documentation is the most important factor in confirming IE. Disease entities with overlapping clinical presentation and laboratory abnormalities should be excluded using the appropriate tests.[1]

Diagnostic criteria for IE which integrate clinical, laboratory, microbiologic, and echocardiographic data are listed in Tables 66-1 and 66-2.[7,15] Based on published evidence involving nearly 2,000 patients, the 2015 AHA guidelines suggest that the modified Duke criteria be used as the primary diagnostic schema to evaluate patients suspected of IE.[7]

A.G. possesses one major criterion (positive blood cultures) and three minor criteria (fever, predisposing heart condition, vascular and immunologic phenomena); therefore, he meets the diagnostic criteria for definite IE.[15]

Table 66-1
Definition of Infective Endocarditis (IE) According to the Modified Duke Criteria

Definite IE[a]
PATHOLOGIC CRITERIA
Microorganisms: demonstrated by culture or histology examination of a vegetation, a vegetation that has embolized, or an intracardiac abscess specimen; *or*
Pathologic lesions: vegetation or intracardiac abscess confirmed by histologic examination showing active endocarditis
CLINICAL CRITERIA
Using specific definitions listed in Table 66-2; two major criteria *or* one major and three minor criteria *or* five minor criteria
Possible IE
One major criterion and one minor criterion; or three minor criteria
Rejected
Firm alternative diagnosis explaining evidence of IE; *or*
Resolution of IE syndrome with antibiotic therapy for <4 days; *or*
No pathologic evidence of IE at surgery or autopsy, with antibiotic therapy for <4 days; or not meet criteria for possible IE as above

[a]Modifications shown in bold.
Reprinted with permission from Li JS et al. Proposed modifications to the Duke criteria for the diagnosis of infective endocarditis. *Clin Infect Dis*. 2000;30:633.

Table 66-2
Definitions of Terminology Used in the Modified Duke Criteria for the Diagnosis of Infective Endocarditis (IE)

Major Criteria[a]

BLOOD CULTURE POSITIVE FOR IE

- Typical microorganisms consistent with IE from two separate blood cultures:
  1. *Viridans streptococci*, *Streptococcus bovis*, HACEK group; *or*
  2. *Staphylococcus aureus* or community-acquired enterococci in the absence of a primary focus; *or*
- Microorganisms consistent with IE from persistently positive blood cultures defined as follows:
  1. At least two positive blood cultures drawn >12 hours apart; *or*
  2. All of three or a majority of four separate cultures of blood (with first and last sample drawn at least 1 hour apart)
- **Single positive blood culture for *Coxiella burnetii* or antiphase 1 IgG antibody titer >1:800**

EVIDENCE OF ENDOCARDIAL INVOLVEMENT

- Echocardiogram positive for IE **(TEE recommended for patients with prosthetic valves, rated at least "possible IE" by clinical criteria or complicated IE [paravalvular abscess]; TEE as first test in other patients)** defined as follows:
  1. Oscillating intracardiac Masson valve or supporting structures, in the path of regurgitant jets, or on implanted material in the absence of an alternative anatomic explanation; *or*
  2. Abscess; *or*
  3. New partial dehiscence of prosthetic valve
- New valvular regurgitation (worsening or changing of preexisting murmur not sufficient)

Minor Criteria

- Predisposition: Predisposing heart condition or IV drug use
- Fever >38°C (100.4°F)
- *Vascular Phenomena*: major arterial emboli, septic pulmonary infarcts, mycotic aneurysm, intracranial hemorrhage, conjunctival hemorrhages, Janeway lesions
- *Immunologic Phenomena*: glomerulonephritis, Osler nodes, Roth spots, RF
- *Microbiologic Evidence*: positive blood culture but not meeting major criterion as noted above[b] or serologic evidence of active infection with organism consistent with IE
- **Echocardiographic minor criteria eliminated**

[a]Modifications shown in bold.
[b]Excludes single positive cultures for coagulase-negative staphylococci and organisms that do not cause endocarditis.
HACEK, *Haemophilus* species, *Actinobacillus actinomycetemcomitans*, *Cardiobacterium hominis*, *Eikenella* species, and *Kingella kingae*; TEE, transesophageal echocardiography.
Reprinted with permission from Li JS et al. Proposed modifications to the Duke criteria for the diagnosis of infective endocarditis. *Clin Infect Dis*. 2000;30:633.

Antimicrobial Therapy

GENERAL PRINCIPLES

CASE 66-1, QUESTION 3: What would be a reasonable duration of antibiotic therapy for A.G.? When is determination of minimum bactericidal concentration (MBC) useful in treating bacterial endocarditis?

The avascular nature of the vegetation results in an environment that is devoid of normal host defenses (e.g., phagocytic cells and complement); this permits uninhibited growth of bacteria.[2] Therefore, to eradicate the causative organism, high doses of an IV bactericidal antibiotic generally are administered for 4 to 6 weeks.[1,7] For some infections, it may be necessary to use two antibiotics to achieve synergistic activity against the organism. Once an organism has been identified, its in vitro susceptibility pattern is determined by the minimum inhibitory concentration (MIC) for various antibiotics. Standard Kirby-Bauer disk diffusion testing is inadequate in the setting of IE to aid in selection of antibiotics without the quantitative information provided by the MIC.[1] In addition, the MBC may be useful in detecting tolerant strains, particularly in the setting of unexplained slow response or treatment failure. Routine MBC determination is not recommended, however.[1] Treatment of endocarditis requires antibiotics with bactericidal activity; therefore, the serum concentration of the antibiotic must greatly exceed the MBC for the particular organism. For endocarditis caused by *viridans streptococci* acquired from the community, this usually is achieved without much difficulty because most isolates are sensitive to penicillin at an MIC of less than 0.12 mcg/mL[7]; corresponding MBCs are, at most, one or two tube dilutions higher.[9] The emergence of strains demonstrating resistance to penicillin and related β-lactams, such as ceftriaxone, is a significant problem, particularly among bloodstream isolates obtained from the nosocomial setting and neutropenic cancer patients.[9,16,17] The increasing prevalence of β-lactam-resistant clinical isolates highlights the importance of determining the MIC and continued close monitoring of the antibiotic susceptibility of *viridans streptococci*. An increasing number of reports have described suboptimal response to vancomycin therapy for the treatment of invasive infection caused by methicillin-resistant *S. aureus* (MRSA) strains showing borderline susceptibility (MIC 2 mcg/mL).[18,19] Many such strains demonstrated tolerance to vancomycin as defined by a high MBC-to-MIC ratio (≥32).[20] Thus, these data support the need to determine MBC, especially in the setting in which the treatment option for IE caused by *S. aureus* is limited to vancomycin and suboptimal response is observed.[20]

REGIMEN SELECTION

CASE 66-1, QUESTION 4: What factors must be considered in selecting a regimen for A.G.? Which regimen should be used for A.G.?

Patients with endocarditis caused by penicillin-sensitive strains of *viridans streptococci* and nonenterococcal group D streptococci (e.g., *Streptococcus gallolyticus*; MIC <0.1 mcg/mL) can be treated with any one of three regimens as outlined in the 2015 AHA treatment guidelines.[7] The suggested regimens (Table 66-3) are associated with cure rates of up to 98% and include (a) high-dose parenteral penicillin for 4 weeks, (b) high-dose parenteral ceftriaxone for 4 weeks, and (c) 2 weeks of combined therapy with high-dose parenteral penicillin and an aminoglycoside.[7,21–27] Ceftriaxone with an aminoglycoside for 2 weeks appears to be equally effective.[28,29]

Table 66-3
Suggested Regimens for Therapy of Native Valve Endocarditis Caused by *Streptococcus viridans* group and *Streptococcus gallolyticus*

Antibiotic	Dose[a,b] and Route	Duration
Penicillin-Susceptible [minimum inhibitory concentration (MIC) ≤0.12 mcg/mL]		
Aqueous crystalline penicillin G[c]	*Adult*: 12–18 million units/24 hour IV either continuously or in four to six equally divided doses	4 weeks
	Pediatric: 200,000 units/kg/24 hour IV (max: 20 million units/24 hour) either continuously or in four to six equally divided doses	
Ceftriaxone sodium[c]	*Adult*: 2 g once daily IV or IM	4 weeks
	Pediatric: 100 mg/kg once daily IV or IM	
Aqueous crystalline penicillin G	See penicillin-susceptible dosing for penicillin above	2 weeks
Ceftriaxone sodium	See penicillin-susceptible dosing for ceftriaxone above	2 weeks
With gentamicin sulfate[d]	*Adult*: 3 mg/kg once daily IV or IM	2 weeks
	Pediatric: 3 mg/kg once daily IV or IM or in three equally divided doses	
Relatively Penicillin G Resistant (MIC >0.12 mcg/mL and <0.5 mcg/mL)		
Aqueous crystalline penicillin G	*Adult*: 24 million units/24 hour IV either continuously or in four to six equally divided doses	4 weeks
	Pediatric: 200,000–300,000 units/kg/24 hour IV (max: 20 million units/24 hour) either continuously or in four to six equally divided doses	
With gentamicin sulfate[d]	*Adult*: 3 mg/kg once daily IV or IM *Pediatric*: 3 mg/kg once daily IV or IM or in three equally divided doses	2 weeks
Ceftriaxone sodium	*Adult*: 2 g once daily IV or IM *Pediatric*: 100 mg/kg once daily IV or IM	4 weeks

(continued)

Table 66-3
Suggested Regimens for Therapy of Native Valve Endocarditis Caused by *Streptococcus viridans* group and *Streptococcus gallolyticus* (continued)

Antibiotic	Dose[a,b] and Route	Duration
β-Lactam Allergic Patients		
Vancomycin hydrochloride[e]	*Adult*: 30 mg/kg/24 hour IV in two equally divided doses (max: 2 g/24 hour unless serum concentrations are monitored)	4 weeks
	Pediatric: 40 mg/kg/24 hour IV in two or three equally divided doses (max: 2 g/24 hour unless serum concentrations are monitored)	

[a]Pediatric doses should not exceed that of a normal adult.
[b]Antibiotic doses for patients with impaired renal function should be modified appropriately.
[c]Preferred in most patients >65 years of age and in those with impairment of the eighth nerve or renal function.
[d]Two-week regimen not intended for patients with known cardiac or extracardiac abscess or for those with creatinine clearance of <20 mL/minute, impaired eighth cranial nerve function or *Abiotrophia*, *Granulicatella*, or *Gemella* infection. Gentamicin nomogram should be used for preferred single daily dosing; when three divided doses are used, dosage should be adjusted to achieve peak serum concentrations of 3–4 mcg/mL and trough serum concentrations of <1 mcg/mL. Other potential nephrotoxic drugs should be used with caution in patients receiving gentamicin therapy.
[e]Vancomycin dosage should be reduced in patients with impaired renal function. Vancomycin given on a milligram per kilogram basis produces higher serum concentrations in obese patients than in lean patients. Therefore, in obese patients, dosing should be based on adjusted body weight. Each dose of vancomycin should be infused for at least 1 hour to reduce the risk of the histamine-release red man syndrome. Trough concentrations should be obtained within half an hour of the next dose and be in the range of 10–15 mcg/mL.
IM, intramuscular; IV, intravenous.
Source: Baddour LM et al. Infective endocarditis in adults: diagnosis, antimicrobial therapy, and management of complications. A Scientific Statement for Healthcare Professionals from the American Heart Association (AHA); on behalf of the AHA Committee on Rheumatic Fever, Endocarditis, and Kawasaki Disease of the Council on Cardiovascular Disease in the Young, Council on Clinical Cardiology, Council on Cardiovascular Surgery and Anesthesia, and Stroke Council: Endorsed by the Infectious Diseases Society of America. *Circulation*. 2015;132:1435–1486.

HIGH-DOSE PENICILLIN FOR 4 WEEKS

Ten to 20 million units/day of IV penicillin G for 4 weeks resulted in a cure rate of 100% for 66 patients with nonenterococcal streptococcal endocarditis.[23] Another study using penicillin monotherapy reported relapse in only 2 of 49 patients; however, both of these patients received less than 4 weeks of therapy.[24] The large range of 12 to 18 million units/day of penicillin is recommended to allow flexibility in dosing based on the patient's renal function and disease severity. Ampicillin 2 g every four hours is a reasonable alternative.

SINGLE DAILY CEFTRIAXONE FOR 4 WEEKS

Ceftriaxone is active against viridans streptococcal strains isolated from patients with endocarditis. In one study, all 49 strains of *viridans streptococci* and 11 strains of *S. bovis* were inhibited at <0.125 mcg/mL of ceftriaxone; one strain of *Streptococcus sanguinis* was inhibited at an MIC of 0.25 mcg/mL.[30] Although no direct comparative trials have been performed evaluating ceftriaxone against high-dose penicillin for the treatment of streptococcal endocarditis, it appears to be comparable to high-dose penicillin when treatment is given for 4 weeks.[31,32] Of the 70 assessable patients who received ceftriaxone 2 g as a single daily dose for 4 weeks, all were cured, except for one patient who had a probable relapse 3 months after completion of therapy. All strains of *viridans streptococci* were inhibited by ceftriaxone at an MIC of 0.25 mcg/mL in both studies. Although the simplicity of single daily treatment with ceftriaxone is attractive for outpatient use, careful patient selection based on microbiologic, clinical, and host factors is critical to the success of treatment and the proper and timely management of potential complications. (See Case 66-6, Question 1, for a detailed discussion of outpatient therapy.)

HIGH-DOSE PENICILLIN OR CEFTRIAXONE PLUS AN AMINOGLYCOSIDE FOR 2 WEEKS

The combination of 2 weeks of streptomycin (or gentamicin) with 4 weeks of penicillin is synergistically bactericidal for most streptococci, including enterococci (see Case 66-4, Question 4).[27,33] This in vitro synergy also has been correlated with a more rapid rate of eradication of *viridans streptococci* from cardiac vegetations in the rabbit model.[25] A shortened combination regimen consisting of high-dose penicillin G and streptomycin for 2 weeks is an effective alternative to the previously described regimens. The reported cure rate in 104 patients treated at the Mayo Clinic with this regimen was 99%.[26,27]

Although clinical experience with combination therapy has been primarily with penicillin and streptomycin, in vitro and animal data support that streptomycin and gentamicin are reasonably interchangeable. Administration of gentamicin once daily versus thrice daily when added to penicillin appears equally effective in the treatment of viridans streptococcal endocarditis.[21]

Combination therapy with ceftriaxone and aminoglycoside for 2 weeks has also been evaluated.[24,28] Clinical cure rates of 87% to 96% were observed in patients infected with penicillin-susceptible streptococci when given once daily ceftriaxone 2 g plus netilmicin or gentamicin at 3 mg/kg. This study excluded patients with suspected or documented cardiac or extracardiac abscesses and those with PVE. Although the aminoglycoside agent (netilmicin or gentamicin) was administered as a single daily dose in both studies, all of the patients had measurable serum trough levels. Therefore, the efficacy of "extended-interval dosing" of aminoglycoside (whereby trough levels are not detectable, allowing a drug-free interval) in short-course combination therapy remains uncertain.

Based on available data, the 2-week regimen of penicillin or ceftriaxone plus an aminoglycoside appears to be efficacious for uncomplicated cases of penicillin-susceptible *viridans streptococci* endocarditis. It is not currently recommended for patients with extracardiac complications or intracardiac abscesses. Patients infected with *Abiotrophia* species (formerly known as nutritionally variant *viridans streptococci*) or *viridans streptococci* with a penicillin MIC greater than 0.1 mcg/mL or patients who have prosthetic valve infections should not receive short-course therapy.[7]

SPECIAL CONSIDERATIONS

The risk of relapse may be higher in patients who have had symptoms for more than 3 months before the initiation of treatment.[1,7,31]

These patients should be treated with 4 to 6 weeks of penicillin combined with an aminoglycoside for the first 2 weeks.[1,7,31]

Nutritionally deficient or variant streptococci (NVS) have been reclassified into a new genus, *Abiotrophia*, which includes *Abiotrophia defectiva*, *Abiotrophia adiacens* (renamed again as *Granulicatella adiacens*), and *Abiotrophia elegans*. *Abiotrophia* species are slow-growing, fastidious organisms that are responsible for approximately 5% of IE cases.[34] Previously, NVS were the cause of most of the cases of endocarditis diagnosed as "culture-negative," initially owing to its requirement for the addition of vitamin B_6 (pyridoxal HCl) to the culture media for laboratory growth. Laboratory identification is no longer a significant problem, however, because of current culture media and laboratory techniques.[9]

NVS are less susceptible to penicillin when compared with other streptococci. Many NVS have a relatively high MIC to penicillin (0.2–2.0 mcg/mL), and some show high-level resistance to penicillin (MIC >4 mcg/mL).[9] In addition, tolerance to penicillin has been described in many strains.[9] An animal model of endocarditis indicates that a penicillin–aminoglycoside (streptomycin or gentamicin) combination is significantly better than penicillin alone in reducing bacterial counts.[35] High rates of bacteriologic failure and relapse may be expected in patients despite completion of the treatment course for strains highly susceptible to penicillin.[9] All patients infected with NVS or *Abiotrophia* should receive 4 to 6 weeks of high-dose penicillin (or ampicillin) in combination with gentamicin.[7] A 6-week course of combination therapy with penicillin and gentamicin is recommended for patients with symptoms longer than 3 months in duration and those with PVE caused by these strains.[7,9] Patients with endocarditis caused by relatively resistant *viridans streptococci* with penicillin MIC of greater than 0.5 mcg/mL or enterococci should receive a similar treatment regimen, as described above.[7]

Patients allergic to β-lactams should receive vancomycin 30 mg/kg/day divided into two doses for 4 to 6 weeks. Although the addition of an aminoglycoside to vancomycin enhances bactericidal activity in vitro, it is unknown whether the addition of an aminoglycoside confers any additional clinical benefit.[7] Assuming the *viridans streptococci* isolated from A.G. are not resistant to penicillin and he has no other complicating factors, any of the suggested regimens would be appropriate. Because no compelling reason exists to use the 4-week regimens, the 2-week penicillin–aminoglycoside regimen could be the optimal choice. Although A.G. has mild renal impairment, this is most likely secondary to the endocarditis and should improve once adequate antimicrobial therapy has been instituted. A.G. was begun on 12 million units/day of penicillin G, which would be reasonable for his age and mild renal impairment. If nephrotoxicity were a major concern in A.G., penicillin or ceftriaxone alone for 4 weeks is reasonable. If gentamicin is used, A.G.'s renal function should be monitored and the dose should be adjusted appropriately if not using a single daily regimen. Multiple aminoglycoside dosing requires frequent monitoring for signs of toxicity by taking periodic peak and trough aminoglycoside concentrations.

STAPHYLOCOCCUS EPIDERMIDIS: PROSTHETIC VALVE ENDOCARDITIS

Etiology

CASE 66-2

QUESTION 1: F.T., a 65-year-old man, presents with chief complaints of anorexia, fever, chills, and weight loss. His medical history is significant for replacement of his mitral and aortic heart valves (both porcine) 1 month ago for aortic stenosis, mitral regurgitation, and mitral stenosis secondary to rheumatic heart disease. Two weeks later he was readmitted with fever, a right pleural effusion, a pericardial friction rub, and pericarditis. The impression at that time was either postpericardiotomy or Dressler syndrome. F.T. was sent home on anti-inflammatory agents but failed to improve. After continued complaints of anorexia, nausea, chills, and fever to 101°F, he returned to the hospital. On readmission, his physical examination was noteworthy for a systolic ejection murmur at the left sternal border and 3+ pedal edema. Blood cultures were obtained, and routine laboratory studies were performed. His history and clinical presentation were strongly suggestive of PVE. What are the most likely organisms responsible for PVE in F.T.?

PVE is a life-threatening infectious complication of artificial heart valve implantation that accounts for 7% to 25% of cases of IE in developed countries.[36,37] The prevalence of complications resulting in death has been as high as 20% to 40%.[37] The risk of PVE after surgery is approximately 1% at 12 months and 2% to 3% at 60 months. PVE is categorized as early or late, depending on the onset of clinical manifestations after cardiac surgery.[36,37] Early PVE occurs within 2 months after surgery and is thought to represent infection acquired during valve placement. It usually is caused by skin organisms that were implanted into the valve annulus (suture site where the valve is attached to cardiac muscle) at the time of surgery.[36,37] The most common organisms cultured from patients such as F.T. with early PVE are coagulase-negative staphylococci (primarily *S. epidermidis* [>30%], most of which are resistant to methicillin), followed by *S. aureus* (20%), and gram-negative bacilli (10%–15%). Miscellaneous organisms, such as diphtheroids and fungi, account for the remainder. In contrast, streptococci are a more common cause of late PVE (>2 months after surgery).[36,37]

Nosocomial bacteremia and fungemia in a patient with prosthetic heart valves contribute to a significant risk for the development of PVE. One study noted that bacteremia caused by staphylococci and gram-negative bacilli resulted in 55% and 33% of subsequent PVE cases, respectively.[38] Another study observed the development of PVE in 25% (11 of 44) of patients after nosocomial candidemia.[39]

Prophylaxis

CASE 66-2, QUESTION 2: What measures can be taken to prevent early PVE?

The overall frequency of early PVE, despite antibiotic prophylaxis, is 1% to 4%.[40] Complications are severe and include valve dehiscence, acute heart failure, arrhythmias, and outflow obstruction. Although antibiotic prophylaxis before valve surgery (a "clean" procedure) has not been proved to reduce the frequency of early PVE, it is indicated nevertheless because the complications of infection are catastrophic. The antimicrobial regimen used most commonly for cardiac surgery prophylaxis (see Chapter 63, Antimicrobial Prophylaxis for Surgical Procedures) consists of an antistaphylococcal cephalosporin, such as cefazolin, given in the operating room at the time of induction of anesthesia or within 60 minutes before the procedure. Vancomycin could be considered the prophylactic agent of choice for cardiovascular procedures, including prosthetic valve replacement and implantation of prosthetic grafts, in the presence of any of the following: (a) documented penicillin allergy, (b) prior receipt of broad-spectrum antimicrobial therapy and high likelihood of being colonized with cephalosporin-resistant staphylococci or enterococci, or (c) performance of the procedure in a center experiencing outbreaks or a high endemic rate of surgical infection with methicillin-resistant staphylococci.[41]

Antimicrobial Therapy

CASE 66-2, QUESTION 3: What are the treatment options for F.T.?

As noted earlier, F.T. most likely is infected with coagulase-negative staphylococci. For those rare coagulase-negative staphylococci that remain sensitive to β-lactams (<20%), a penicillinase-resistant penicillin (nafcillin or oxacillin) is the drug of choice (Table 66-4).[42] For the treatment of PVE caused by methicillin-resistant, coagulase-negative staphylococci, vancomycin should be used.[42] Most staphylococci are sensitive to vancomycin at concentrations of 2 mcg/mL or less; however, strains of staphylococci with intermediate susceptibility to vancomycin have emerged.[43,44] Refer to the IDSA guidelines for vancomycin dosing and drug level monitoring.[19]

The AHA currently recommends the use of triple-drug combination (vancomycin, gentamicin, and rifampin) therapy for the treatment of PVE caused by methicillin-resistant, coagulase-negative staphylococci (MRSE).[7] When isolates of MRSE are resistant to all available aminoglycosides, aminoglycoside treatment should be omitted. A fluoroquinolone active against the isolate may be considered as substitute for the aminoglycoside in the three-drug regimen. In addition to medical therapy, most patients also required valve replacement surgery.[36,37,42]

Table 66-4
Treatment of Staphylococcal Endocarditis

Antibiotic	Dosage and Route	Duration
Without Prosthetic Material[a]		
OXACILLIN/METHICILLIN—SUSCEPTIBLE STAPHYLOCOCCI		
NONPENICILLIN-ALLERGIC PATIENTS		
Nafcillin *or* oxacillin	*Adult*: 2 g IV every 4 hours *Pediatric*: 150–200 mg/kg/24 hour IV (max: 12 g/24 hour) in four to six equally divided doses	6 weeks
PENICILLIN-ALLERGIC PATIENTS		
Cefazolin[d]	*Adult*: 2 g IV every 8 hours *Pediatric*: 100 mg/kg/24 hour IV (max: 6 g/24 hour) in equally divided doses every 8 hours	6 weeks
Vancomycin[b,e,f]	*Adult*: 30 mg/kg/24 hour IV in two or four equally divided doses (max: 2 g/24 hour unless serum levels monitored) *Pediatric*: 40 mg/kg/24 hour IV in two or four equally divided doses (max: 2 g/24 hour unless serum levels monitored)	6 weeks
OXACILLIN/METHICILLIN—RESISTANT STAPHYLOCOCCI		
Vancomycin[b,e,f]	*Adult*: 30 mg/kg/24 hour IV in two or four equally divided doses (max: 2 g/24 hour unless serum levels monitored) *Pediatric*: 40 mg/kg/24 hour IV in two or four equally divided doses (max: 2 g/24 hour unless serum levels monitored)	6 weeks
With Prosthetic Valve or Other Prosthetic Material[g]		
OXACILLIN/METHICILLIN—RESISTANT STAPHYLOCOCCI		
Vancomycin[b,e,g]	*Adult*: 30 mg/kg/24 hour IV in two or four equally divided doses (max: 2 g/24 hour unless serum levels monitored) *Pediatric*: 40 mg/kg/24 h IV in two or four equally divided doses (max: 2 g/24 h unless serum levels monitored)	≥6 weeks
With rifampin[h]	*Adult*: 300 mg IV/PO every 8 hours *Pediatric*: 20 mg/kg/24 hour PO (max: 900 mg/24 hour) in three equally divided doses	≥6 weeks
With gentamicin[b,g,i,j]	*Adult*: 3 mg/kg IV or IM in two or three equally divided doses *Pediatric:* 3 mg/kg IV or IM in three equally divided doses	2 weeks
OXACILLIN/METHICILLIN—SUSCEPTIBLE STAPHYLOCOCCI		
Nafcillin *or* oxacillin[k]	*Adult*: 2 g IV every 4 hours *Pediatric*: 150–200 mg/kg/24 hour IV (max: 12 g/24 hour) in four to six equally divided doses	≥6 weeks

Table 66-4
Treatment of Staphylococcal Endocarditis (*continued*)

Antibiotic	Dosage and Route	Duration
With rifampin[h]	See prosthetic valve dosing for rifampin above	≥6 weeks
With gentamicin[b,g,i,j]	See prosthetic valve dosing for gentamicin above	2 weeks

[a]Antibiotic doses should be modified appropriately for patients with impaired renal function. Shorter antibiotic courses have been effective in some drug addicts with right-sided endocarditis caused by *S. aureus*. (See text for comments on the use of daptomycin and rifampin.)
[b]Dosing of aminoglycosides and vancomycin on a milligram per kilogram basis will give higher serum concentrations in obese than in lean patients.
[c]The benefit of additional aminoglycoside has not been established. The risk of toxic reactions because of these agents is increased in patients >65 years of age or those with renal or eighth nerve impairment.
[d]There is potential cross-allergenicity between penicillins and cephalosporins. Cephalosporins should be avoided in patients with immediate-type hypersensitivity to penicillin.
[e]Trough serum concentrations should be obtained within half an hour prior to the next dose and should be in the range of 10 to 15 mcg/mL. (See text for detailed discussion on the need for high trough target of 15 to 20 mcg/mL for strains with reduced susceptibility to vancomycin. Each vancomycin dose should be infused for 1 hour.)
[f]Vancomycin and gentamicin doses must be modified appropriately in patients with renal failure.
[g]Rifampin is recommended therapy for infections caused by coagulase-negative staphylococci. Its use in coagulase-positive staphylococcal infections is controversial. Rifampin increases the amount of warfarin sodium required for antithrombotic therapy.
[h]Serum concentration of gentamicin should be monitored, and the dose should be adjusted to obtain a peak level of approximately 3 mcg/mL.
[i]Use during initial 2 weeks. (See text on alternative aminoglycoside therapy for organisms resistant to gentamicin.)
[j]First-generation cephalosporins or vancomycin should be used in penicillin-allergic patients. Cephalosporins should be avoided in patients with immediate-type hypersensitivity to penicillin and those infected with oxacillin-resistant staphylococci.
IM, intramuscular; IV, intravenous; PO, orally.
Source: Baddour LM et al. Infective endocarditis in adults: diagnosis, antimicrobial therapy, and management of complications. A Scientific Statement for Healthcare Professionals from the American Heart Association (AHA); on behalf of the AHA Committee on Rheumatic Fever, Endocarditis, and Kawasaki Disease of the Council on Cardiovascular Disease in the Young, Council on Clinical Cardiology, Council on Cardiovascular Surgery and Anesthesia, and Stroke Council: Endorsed by the Infectious Diseases Society of America. *Circulation*. 2015;132:1435–1486.

Although alternative agents such as quinupristin/dalfopristin, linezolid, daptomycin, telavancin, ceftaroline, dalbavancin, and oritavancin have shown potent in vitro activity against coagulase-negative staphylococci, clinical experience in the treatment of IE caused by these strains is lacking.[42,45,46]

STAPHYLOCOCCUS AUREUS ENDOCARDITIS

Intravenous Drug User Versus Nonuser

CASE 66-3

Question 1: T.J., a 36-year-old human immunodeficiency virus (HIV)-seropositive man with a long history of IV drug abuse, was admitted to the hospital 4 months after being released from the state prison. His chief complaints included fever, night sweats, pleuritic chest pain, shortness of breath, dyspnea on exertion, and fatigue. Physical examination was remarkable for a temperature of 101.2°F, splenomegaly, and a pansystolic ejection murmur at the left sternal border, best heard during inspiration. The chest radiograph revealed diffuse nodular infiltrates. TTE was positive for a small vegetation on the tricuspid valve leaflet. Significant laboratory results included the following:

WBC count, 14,000/μL with 65% polys and 5% bands (SI units, 14 × 10/L with 0.65 polys and 0.05 bands [normal, 3.2–9.8 with 0.54–0.62 polys and 0.03–0.05 bands])
CD4 cell count, 350/μL
Hgb, 13.1 g/dL (SI units, 131 g/L [normal, 140–180])
Hct, 39% (SI units, 0.39 [normal, 0.39–0.49])
ESR, 55 mm/hour (Westergren) [normal, ≤30 mm/minute]

IE was suspected. Blood cultures were obtained, and all six samples were positive for coagulase-positive, gram-positive cocci, later identified as methicillin-sensitive *S. aureus* (MSSA). How do the clinical presentation and prognosis of endocarditis in the IV drug user differ from that of the nonuser? What impact does HIV infection have on the risk and outcomes of endocarditis in the IV drug user?

The annual incidence of endocarditis among IV drug users is estimated at 1% to 5%; parenteral cocaine addicts have the highest risk.[47] The presentation, pathophysiology, and prognosis of endocarditis in those who acquire the disease secondary to IV drug use differ from those in nonusers.[1,47,48] *S. aureus* is tenfold more likely than other pathogens to cause infection in this population.[7] *S. aureus* is part of the normal skin flora and is introduced when the illicit drug is injected. The following are differences between addicts and nonaddicts with *S. aureus* endocarditis: Addicts are significantly younger; they have fewer underlying diseases and more right-sided (tricuspid) involvement (in contrast to the predominance of left-sided disease in nonaddicts); they are less likely to have heart failure or central nervous system complications; and they exhibit fewer signs of peripheral involvement and have a lower incidence of death.[48] Among patients without history of IV drug use, MRSA was involved in one-third of a cohort of 424 patients with definite *S. aureus* IE. Clinical features that characterized MRSA IE were persistent bacteremia, chronic immunosuppressive therapy, health-care-associated infection, a presumed intravascular device source, and diabetes mellitus.[6]

The prevalence of HIV seropositivity is 40% to 90% among IV drug users with IE.[47,49] HIV-related immunosuppression may be an independent risk factor for the development of endocarditis.[50]

METHICILLIN-SENSITIVE STAPHYLOCOCCUS AUREUS

CASE 66-3, QUESTION 2: What are the therapeutic options for treating *S. aureus* endocarditis in T.J.?

The susceptibility of *S. aureus* to methicillin is the major determinant of which antibiotic is selected to treat T.J.'s endocarditis. T.J. is infected with MSSA. Therapy of choice for methicillin-sensitive strains is a penicillinase-resistant penicillin, such as nafcillin or oxacillin.[7] (Table 66-4). Penicillin G rarely is appropriate because nearly all isolates of *S. aureus* produce penicillinase. A 6-week course of therapy with high-dose (12 g/day) nafcillin is the therapy of choice.[51,52] Vancomycin may be less efficacious than nafcillin as an antistaphylococcal agent.[7,51] IV drug addicts, for the reasons previously identified, have a higher response rate to appropriate therapy compared with nonaddicts. In one study, 31 addicts were successfully treated with 16 days of parenteral therapy followed by 26 days of oral dicloxacillin.[53]

Addicts with uncomplicated right-sided endocarditis caused by MSSA have been treated successfully with a 2-week course of combination therapy with a penicillinase-resistant penicillin and an aminoglycoside.[54–56] In one study, 47 of 50 patients (94%) were cured after treatment with the combination of IV nafcillin (1.5 g every 4 hours) and tobramycin (1 mg/kg every 8 hours) for a total of 2 weeks. Notably, 2 of 3 patients treated with vancomycin relapsed, resulting in early termination of this arm of study. Thus, vancomycin should not be used to substitute for nafcillin in this regimen. An abbreviated course of treatment can be used in a defined group of IV drug users with right-sided endocarditis. These patients should have the following characteristics: (a) clinical and bacteriologic response within 96 hours of initiation of therapy; (b) no evidence of hemodynamic compromise, metastatic infection, or neurologic or systemic embolic complications at either the initiation or completion of 2 weeks of therapy; (c) no echocardiographically demonstrable vegetations larger than 2 cm^3; (d) not infected with MRSA; and (e) not receiving antibiotics other than penicillinase-resistant penicillins, such as first-generation cephalosporins and glycopeptides.[7,55] HIV-seropositive patients (CD4 counts $>300 \times 10^6$ cells) with tricuspid involvement included in the above studies also responded favorably to these short-course regimens; thus, a short-course regimen is an option for T.J.[55]

Recent studies suggest that the addition of an aminoglycoside to the treatment regimen does not improve overall response for patients who meet the above criteria for short-course therapy and is associated with increased toxicity. Therefore, the AHA guidelines do not favor the antibiotic combination anymore. Also, all patients receiving the short regimen should be carefully evaluated for evidence of continuing infection or complications before discontinuing therapy at the end of the 2-week treatment course; extension of therapy with a β-lactam agent to at least a 4 to 6-week duration is recommended with any evidence of active disease or complications. Although response to antibiotic therapy has been shown to be similar between asymptomatic HIV-seropositive and HIV-seronegative IV drug users, short-course therapy should be avoided in more immunosuppressed individuals (CD4 cell counts $<200\ \mu L$) until more definitive outcome data are available in this subgroup.[47]

Oral Regimen

An oral treatment regimen consisting of ciprofloxacin (750 mg every 12 hours) plus rifampin (300 mg every 12 hours) has also been evaluated in addicts with uncomplicated right-sided endocarditis. In one small, noncomparative study, 10 addicts were successfully treated with the combination of ciprofloxacin and rifampin for 4 weeks.[57,58] Ciprofloxacin was given IV (400 mg every 12 hours) for the first 7 days, followed by oral administration (750 mg every 12 hours) for the remaining 21 days of therapy. Another study prospectively compared the oral regimen with standard parenteral therapy for this subgroup.[58,59] Patients were randomly assigned to receive 28 days of therapy with oral ciprofloxacin plus rifampin or oxacillin (2 g IV every 4 hours) plus gentamicin (2 mg/kg IV every 8 hours). Vancomycin (1 g IV every 12 hours) was substituted for oxacillin in the penicillin-allergic patients. One of 19 patients in the oral group versus 3 of 25 in the IV group failed treatment; however, approximately half of the study patients in either group had possible endocarditis. Given the small number of patients who completed treatment, therapeutic equivalency between the oral and parenteral regimens will need to be confirmed in larger trials. In addition, emerging quinolone resistance in *S. aureus* and the compliance and monitoring required of this regimen when administered in the outpatient setting are of concern. Nonetheless, it appears that a 4-week oral regimen with ciprofloxacin and rifampin may be a useful alternative treatment option in addicts with uncomplicated right-sided endocarditis.

Penicillin-Allergic Patients

Treatment of penicillin-allergic patients with *S. aureus* endocarditis is somewhat controversial. First-generation cephalosporins have been used with some success for the treatment of patients with mild penicillin allergy, but treatment failures with cefazolin are difficult to explain.[60] The stability of cefazolin when exposed to staphylococcal β-lactamase has been proposed as a mechanism for these failures.[61] Notably, staphylococci are capable of producing four penicillinase subtypes, to which the stability of cefazolin varies. These susceptibility differences are apparent on MIC testing only if a larger-than-usual inoculum is used (i.e., $>10^6$ organisms).[61] It is possible that treatment failures with cefazolin may be caused by a combination of the recalcitrant nature of the infection and the instability of cefazolin against a particular subtype of penicillinase produced by the staphylococcal strain, which is not readily detectable via routine MIC testing. For patients with endocarditis caused by *S. aureus* who have immediate-type hypersensitivity to penicillin, vancomycin or daptomycin may be used. Other treatment options include linezolid and quinupristin/dalfopristin.[62] Selection of agent depends on organism susceptibility, potential of drug–drug interactions, and host predisposition for development of adverse effects.

Combination Therapy

An enhanced response to combination therapy in the experimental animal model of MSSA endocarditis has prompted clinical trials to evaluate whether the addition of gentamicin to nafcillin confers any additional benefit. The combination of nafcillin and gentamicin resulted in more rapid clearing of organisms from the blood, but the response rates were similar to patients treated with nafcillin alone.[51] As expected, the group receiving gentamicin had a higher incidence of nephrotoxicity. Thus, for the routine management of endocarditis caused by MSSA, the addition of a second drug does not appear to offer additional benefit when a penicillinase-resistant penicillin is used and is discouraged due to the lack of clearly established efficacy and aminoglycoside toxicity. (see Case 66-3, Question 2, previous discussion). For patients who remain bacteremic or who fail to improve clinically (usually nonaddicts), imaging studies are often performed to identify metastatic sites of infection (i.e., occult abscess) with possible need for surgical intervention.

METHICILLIN-RESISTANT STAPHYLOCOCCUS AUREUS: *VANCOMYCIN*

CASE 66-3, QUESTION 3: How would T.J.'s therapy differ if he were infected with MRSA?

Staphylococcus aureus IE involving methicillin-resistant strains has become increasingly common and accounts for up to 40% of cases.[4,6] MRSA-infected patients have more chronic comorbid conditions (e.g., diabetes mellitus, hemodialysis dependency) and are more likely to have health-care-associated infection (76% vs. 37%) and an indwelling intravascular catheter or hemodialysis fistula as the presumed source of infection (60% vs. 31%) when compared with patients infected with MSSA.[4,6] Persistent bacteremia was more common with MRSA IE, occurring in 43% versus 9% of patients infected with MSSA. Of interest, in this study, patients with *S. aureus* IE from the United States were significantly more likely to be infected with MRSA, to receive vancomycin therapy, and to develop persistent bacteremia.[63]

In 20% of patients with MRSA IE, identifiable health-care contact was absent. MRSA infection is traditionally associated with health-care contact in the nosocomial setting, but is now becoming more prevalent in the community (CA-MRSA).[6] Young and otherwise healthy individuals without the traditional risk factors are infected in the community.[64] CA-MRSA strains are distinct from health-care-associated strains in that most possess a distinct virulence gene encoding for the Panton-Valentine leukocidin (PVL). Expression of this pore-forming toxin that causes severe necrosis in polymorphonuclear neutrophil cells in a rabbit model has been implicated to cause invasive infections, including necrotizing pneumonia and skin abscesses.[65–71] Specifically, CA-MRSA PVL-producing strains causing IE have been reported.[72]

Treatment Options

Vancomycin has been the accepted standard of treatment for MRSA endocarditis. Response to treatment, however, is slower than with semisynthetic penicillins (e.g., nafcillin) for MSSA endocarditis. The mean duration of bacteremia in patients with MSSA endocarditis has been reported to be 3.4 days for nafcillin alone and 2.9 days for the combination of nafcillin and gentamicin.[54] In contrast, the median duration of bacteremia for MRSA endocarditis was 7 days for vancomycin alone. Failure rates of up to 40% have been documented in patients even with right-sided involvement. Of great concern is the emergence of resistant strains of *S. aureus* after repeated and prolonged exposure to vancomycin therapy.[44,73]

Either vancomycin or daptomycin at 8 mg/kg IV once daily (up to 12 mg/kg/day) may be used to treat patients with MRSA endocarditis.[63] The AHA recommends daptomycin 8mg/kg/dose. Vancomycin 30 mg/kg/day in two divided doses for a total of 6 weeks is recommended for adults with normal renal function. Vancomycin peak levels are not recommended. Given the emergence of MRSA strains with reduced susceptibility to vancomycin, published guidelines from the Infectious Diseases Society of America recommend a target trough of 15 to 20 mcg/mL[7,63,74] in an attempt to overcome increasing MIC of clinical strains and limited tissue penetration. Measurement of trough serum vancomycin concentrations is typically 30 minutes prior to the fourth dose for patients receiving a dosing interval of every 12 hours. A dosage regimen of vancomycin aimed to achieve an area under the curve-to-MIC ratio of 400 or an unbound trough at 4 to 5 times MIC of the infected strain has been proposed as the optimal pharmacodynamic target.[75–77]

Persistent Bacteremia

CASE 66-3, QUESTION 4: T.J. has been treated with vancomycin 1 g IV every 12 hours for 5 days for his MRSA endocarditis, but does not seem to be clinically improving. His blood cultures are still positive, and his WBC count remains elevated at 12,500/μL with 55% polys and 7% bands. He continues to have a low-grade fever since starting vancomycin. His vancomycin trough level on the second day of therapy was 17 mcg/mL. The infected MRSA strain had a vancomycin MIC of 1.5 mcg/mL as determined by Epsilometer test (Etest). What factors may be contributing to T.J.'s poor response to treatment? What other therapeutic options are available for T.J.?

In a large multinational study of nearly 1,800 patients with definite IE, persistent bacteremia, receipt of vancomycin, and healthcare contact were significantly more common in patients with MRSA IE from the United States compared with those from other geographic regions.[6] The authors speculated that the higher rates of persistent bacteremia in US patients may be attributable in part to the receipt of vancomycin therapy.

Vancomycin MICs against *S. aureus* have been increasing over the years. At one university medical center, vancomycin MICs were determined by broth microdilution for 6,000 nosocomial MRSA isolates collected during a 5-year period. In the year 2000, 80% of the strains had vancomycin MIC of 0.5 mcg/mL; however, by 2004, 70% of isolates had MICs of 2 mcg/mL.[78] In response to increasing reports of vancomycin failures caused by strains that are in the susceptible range, the vancomycin breakpoint for susceptibility was reduced from 4 to 2 mcg/mL for *S. aureus* in 2005 per the Clinical and Laboratory Standards Institute.[79,80]

Widespread use of vancomycin has led to the emergence of glycopeptide-intermediate S. *aureus* (GISA) or heteroresistant GISA (hGISA) strains.[44] Reduced susceptibility to glycopeptides results from an increase in the production of peptidoglycan precursors leading to a thickened cell wall and decreased penetration of glycopeptides into the bacterial cell membrane.[81] In the absence of vancomycin, hGISA strains may revert to glycopeptide susceptibility, making it difficult to detect these strains in vitro. As such, several investigators have found that hGISA strains have an MIC range that overlaps with the currently defined susceptible range and that the prevalence among hospitalized patients is increasing.[82–84] Routine susceptibility testing methods performed in the clinical laboratory are unreliable in detecting MRSA strains with hGISA phenotype.[85] MIC determined by Etest best predicts treatment outcome with vancomycin.[21,63,86,87]

Experts have recommended a target vancomycin trough concentration of 15 to 20 mcg/mL to overcome increasing MIC when treating pneumonia or endocarditis caused by MRSA.[63,87] A published study of adult infections with MRSA reported that 54% (51 of 95) of clinical isolates had vancomycin MIC of 2 mcg/mL.[20] Notably, invasive infections, such as bacteremia and pneumonia, were linked to higher MIC. Infections caused by those strains were associated with lower end of treatment responses (62% vs. 85%) and increased mortality (24% vs. 10%) compared with strains with MIC of 1 mcg/mL or less, irrespective of attaining a goal trough of 15 to 20 mcg/mL (achieving the goal of 4 to 5 times greater than MIC of an infected strain that has an MIC of 2 mcg/mL). Borderline susceptibility (MIC 2 mcg/mL) and severity of underlying disease were independent predictors of poor treatment response. Many strains demonstrated tolerance to vancomycin as defined by the MBC-to-MIC ratio of 32, and up to 10% exhibited heterogeneous vancomycin-intermediate resistance phenotype (hVISA).[21,88] Vancomycin monotherapy of hVISA was associated with treatment failure, whereas combination therapy responded favorably.[88] Combination regimens included vancomycin plus rifampin, linezolid, or daptomycin. These findings suggest a role for combination therapy or alternative agents when treating invasive infections caused by MRSA strains with borderline susceptibility. However, the above study was not designed to compare the efficacy of vancomycin monotherapy with combination therapy for the treatment of MRSA infections, and the sample size of patients infected with hVISA in this study was small. Therefore, the role of vancomycin as the treatment of choice for MRSA IE will need to be re-evaluated against other available treatment options.

Despite attaining a pharmacodynamic goal of unbound vancomycin trough level of at least 4 times MIC of the infected strain, T.J. fails to clinically improve and has persistent bacteremia. It is possible that T.J. is infected with a hVISA strain; thus, a change in therapy is warranted.

Daptomycin (Cubicin) is a cyclic lipopeptide that has been approved for treatment of *S. aureus* bacteremia and right-sided endocarditis. In vivo, it has a wide spectrum of activity against gram-positive bacteria, including *S. aureus* (including MRSA), *Enterococcus faecalis*, *Enterococcus faecium*, streptococci, and most other species of aerobic and anaerobic gram-positive bacteria. It was approved for the treatment of *S. aureus* bacteremia and endocarditis in a noninferiority study in patients receiving daptomycin or standard therapy consisting of an antistaphylococcal penicillin or vancomycin in addition to low-dose gentamicin.[89] Successful outcome was seen in 46% (41 of 90) of patients who had presumed or definite staphylococcal endocarditis at their baseline diagnosis. Of those, MRSA endocarditis was successfully treated in 42% (15 of 36) of cases. In patients with confirmed uncomplicated and complicated right-sided endocarditis, treatment success was similar between the daptomycin group (8 of 18) and the group receiving standard therapy (7 of 16) at 44%. Microbiologic failure occurred in seven patients in the daptomycin group and in five patients receiving standard therapy. Overall, the most common cause of daptomycin failure was persistent or relapsing infections, accounting for 16% of failures. In contrast, failure of standard therapy was more often the result of treatment-limiting adverse events, accounting for 15% of failures. Increase in the MIC of the infected strain was observed more often in the daptomycin group compared with standard treatment (six in the daptomycin group vs. one patient in the standard therapy group). The use of daptomycin for treatment of left-sided endocarditis is not established because only nine patients were treated and only one had treatment success.

Daptomycin at >8 mg/kg/day for a total duration of 6 weeks should be used for the treatment of endocarditis. Considering its concentration-dependent effects, some recommended higher doses (up to 12 mg/kg/day) which appear to be safe.[63,90] High-dose daptomycin should be considered in patients who have previously failed vancomycin treatment, who are severely ill, or who are infected with an isolate with elevated vancomycin MICs. Daptomycin should be dosed based on total body weight because obese patients have a larger volume of distribution as well as increased clearance compared with the nonobese population.[91] Creatine kinase levels should be obtained at baseline and weekly to monitor for elevations, and more frequently in patients who may be at risk for developing skeletal muscle dysfunction. High-dose daptomycin at 8 to 12 mg/kg daily should be considered as alternative therapy in T.J. Emergence of cross-resistance to daptomycin after vancomycin exposure has been documented.[92,93] Similar to a thickened cell wall contributing to decreased susceptibility to vancomycin, the same mechanism is thought to contribute to daptomycin resistance in *S. aureus*.[94] Therefore, it is important to confirm MRSA susceptibility to daptomycin when used in a patient who had prior vancomycin exposure. Either gentamicin (at 1 mg/kg every 8 hours or 5 mg/kg daily) or rifampin 300 to 450 mg orally (PO) twice daily or both may be used in combination with daptomycin as in vitro synergy has been demonstrated for the combinations.[63] Alternatively, daptomycin 10 mg/kg/dose IV once daily plus linezolid 600 mg PO twice daily may be used, particularly with concomitant pneumonia.[95]

Once daptomycin therapy is initiated, continued monitoring of clinical response and organism susceptibility to daptomycin is warranted because resistance development has been reported during prolonged therapy.[96–99] Daptomycin MIC increase during therapy for *S. aureus* endocarditis was demonstrated in six patients.[97] Baseline MIC increased from 0.25 to 2 mcg/mL in five isolates and from 0.5 to 4 mcg/mL in one isolate. Five of those six isolates were MRSA.

A potential treatment option for T.J., if his infected MRSA strain demonstrates reduced susceptibility to daptomycin, is the addition of an antistaphylococcal β-lactam agent such as nafcillin or oxacillin to daptomycin based on in vitro synergy studies and few case reports.[100,101]

Linezolid (Zyvox), an oxazolidinone, is not approved by the US Food and Drug Administration (FDA) for the treatment of endocarditis, but has been used in cases of treatment failures, intolerability to standard therapy, or in infections with multidrug-resistant gram-positive cocci.[102] In a review article that included 33 case reports of endocarditis treated with linezolid, 63.6% of patients had successful outcomes at the end of the follow-up period.[102] MRSA and vancomycin-intermediate *S. aureus* were the most common pathogens, accounting for 24% and 30% of cases, respectively. Failure with linezolid treatment was documented in seven cases, including four deaths attributed to endocarditis and three owing to persistent positive blood cultures. Thrombocytopenia was the most common adverse effect, occurring in eight of nine patients. In a compassionate-use program, linezolid achieved 50% clinical and microbiologic cure rates at 6-month follow-up in 32 patients with definite IE; MRSA was the causative agent in seven of those patients. The most common adverse events reported in this group were gastrointestinal system effects and thrombocytopenia, each occurring in 15% of patients.[103] The degree of thrombocytopenia associated with linezolid correlates with the extent of drug exposure, as measured by area under the concentration curve and duration of treatment.[104] Of note, treatment failure with linezolid for MRSA endocarditis caused by persistent bacteremia has been described in two patients and in one patient with relapse of infection.[105,106] Thus, additional efficacy data are needed before linezolid can be recommended for the treatment of IE caused by MRSA. Tedizolid (Sivextro), a novel oxazolidinone, was shown to have only moderate bactericidal activity in vivo in a rabbit model of MRSA endocarditis and was less active than either vancomycin or daptomycin.[107] At this time, tedizolid cannot be recommended as a primary agent in treatment of endocarditis.

ENTEROCOCCAL ENDOCARDITIS

Antimicrobial Therapy

ANTIBIOTIC SYNERGY

CASE 66-4

QUESTION 1: G.S., a 35-year-old woman, has been complaining of anorexia, weight loss, and fever for the past 2 months. Her medical history is significant for an aortic aneurysm with insufficiency that resulted in an aortic valve replacement (porcine) 3 years before admission. Approximately 2 months before admission, G.S. had a cesarean section followed by a tubal ligation. She did not receive antibiotic prophylaxis for either procedure. Physical examination revealed a thin woman (5 foot 0 inches, 48 kg) in no acute distress with evidence of a systolic heart murmur, splinter hemorrhages, and petechiae on her soft palate. Her temperature was 100.2°F. Her WBC count was 14,000/μL (SI unit, 14 × 10/L) with a slight left shift; all other laboratory results were within normal limits. She was not taking any medications, and she has a documented allergy to penicillin (rash, urticaria, and wheezing). The working clinical diagnosis was probable bacterial endocarditis, which was confirmed when four sets of blood cultures grew gram-positive cocci. Antibiotic therapy with gentamicin (50 mg IV every 8 hours) and vancomycin (1,000 mg IV every 12 hours) was begun. Biochemical testing subsequently identified the organism as *E. faecalis*, highly resistant to streptomycin (MIC >2,000 mcg/mL). Why were two antibiotics prescribed for the treatment of enterococcal endocarditis in G.S.?

Enterococci, unlike streptococci, are inhibited but not killed by penicillin or vancomycin alone.[108,109] The synergistic combination of penicillin (or ampicillin, piperacillin, or vancomycin) with an aminoglycoside is required to produce the desired bactericidal effect.[108,109] One definition of synergy is when a combination of antibiotics lowers the MIC to at least one-fourth the MIC of either drug alone.[110] The mechanism of synergy against enterococci is explained by an increased cellular uptake of the aminoglycoside with agents that inhibit cell wall synthesis (e.g., β-lactams and vancomycin).[111] Because G.S. is allergic to penicillin, vancomycin was prescribed with an aminoglycoside. Relapse rates are unacceptably high if penicillin is used alone for the treatment of enterococcal endocarditis.[7,108,110,111] Numerous in vivo[110,111] and clinical studies have confirmed the in vitro synergy for penicillin in combination with streptomycin or gentamicin for enterococcal endocarditis.[16]

Streptomycin Resistance

As many as 55% of all enterococcal blood isolates are highly resistant to streptomycin (MIC >2,000 mcg/mL), and the combination of streptomycin with penicillin is not synergistic for those isolates. In contrast, gentamicin in combination with penicillin, ampicillin, or vancomycin is synergistic for most blood isolates of enterococci, regardless of their susceptibility to streptomycin.[1,108,112] In addition, ototoxicity in the form of vestibular dysfunction secondary to streptomycin therapy occurs in nearly 30% of patients in the treatment of enterococcal endocarditis and is most often irreversible. High peak concentrations and prolonged drug therapy have been associated with ototoxicity, but laboratory assays for streptomycin levels are not readily available. For these reasons, gentamicin in combination with penicillin (or ampicillin) or vancomycin is recommended by most authorities for the treatment of aminoglycoside-susceptible and, in particular, streptomycin-resistant enterococcal endocarditis, as it was for G.S.[7] Of note, other aminoglycosides cannot be used to substitute for gentamicin or streptomycin because of the uncertain correlation between in vitro synergy and in vivo efficacy.[7] Table 66-5 lists the suggested regimens for the treatment of enterococcal endocarditis.

Gentamicin Resistance

Of the aminoglycosides, gentamicin and streptomycin are often tested with penicillin (or ampicillin) for synergistic bactericidal activity. About 10% to 25% of the clinical isolates of *E. faecalis*

Table 66-5
Therapy for Endocarditis Caused by Enterococci (or Streptococci viridans with an MIC ≥0.5 mcg/mL)

Antibiotic[a,b]	Dose and Route	Duration
Nonpenicillin-Allergic Patient		
Penicillin G	*Adult*: 18-30 million units/24 hour IV given continuously or in six equally divided doses	4–6 weeks
	Pediatric: 300,000 units/kg/24 hour IV (max: 30 million units/24 hour) given continuously or in four to six equally divided doses	4–6 weeks
With gentamicin[c,d]	*Adult*: 1 mg/kg IM or IV every 8 hours	4–6 weeks
	Pediatric: 1 mg/kg IM or IV every 8 hours	4–6 weeks
Ampicillin	*Adult*: 12 g/24 hour IV given continuously or in six equally divided doses	4–6 weeks
	Pediatric: 300 mg/kg/24 hour IV (max: 12 g/24 hour) in four to six equally divided doses	4–6 weeks
With gentamicin[c,d]	See nonpenicillin-allergic dosing for gentamicin above	4–6 weeks
With ceftriaxone	4 g/24 hour IV in two equally divided doses	6 weeks
Penicillin-Allergic Patients[f]		
Vancomycin[e]	*Adult*: 30 mg/kg/24 hour IV in two equally divided doses (max: 2 g/24 hour unless serum levels monitored)	6 weeks
	Pediatric: 40 mg/kg/24 hour IV in two to three equally divided doses (max: 2 g/24 hour unless serum levels monitored)	6 weeks
With gentamicin[c,d]	*Adult*: 1 mg/kg IM or IV (max: 80 mg) every 8 hours	6 weeks
	Pediatric: 1 mg/kg IM or IV (max: 80 mg) every 8 hours	6 weeks

[a]Antibiotic doses should be modified appropriately in patients with impaired renal function.
[b]Enterococci should be tested for high-level resistance (gentamicin: MIC ≥500 mcg/mL).
[c]Serum concentration of gentamicin should be monitored and dosage adjusted to obtain a peak level of approximately 3 mcg/mL. (For shorter-course gentamicin therapy for enterococcal endocarditis, see comment in text.)
[d]Dosing of aminoglycosides and vancomycin on a mg/kg basis gives higher serum concentrations in obese than in lean patients.
[e]Trough serum concentrations should be obtained within half an hour of the next dose and should be in the range of 10 to 20 mcg/mL. Each dose should be infused over 1 hour; 6 weeks of vancomycin therapy recommended because of decreased activity against enterococci.
[f]Desensitization should be considered; cephalosporins are *not* satisfactory alternatives.
IM, intramuscular; IV, intravenous; MIC, minimum inhibitory concentration.
Source: Baddour LM et al. Infective endocarditis in adults: diagnosis, antimicrobial therapy, and management of complications. A Scientific Statement for Healthcare Professionals from the American Heart Association (AHA); on behalf of the AHA Committee on Rheumatic Fever, Endocarditis, and Kawasaki Disease of the Council on Cardiovascular Disease in the Young, Council on Clinical Cardiology, Council on Cardiovascular Surgery and Anesthesia, and Stroke Council: Endorsed by the Infectious Diseases Society of America. *Circulation*. 2015;132:1435–1486..

and up to 50% of *E. faecium* are resistant to gentamicin.[112,113] Without conclusive data, some groups favor long-term (8–12 weeks) therapy with high-dose penicillin (18–30 million units/day IV in six divided doses) or ampicillin (2–3 g IV every 4 hours) for treatment of resistant enterococci. Ampicillin plus the β-lactamase inhibitor sulbactam (Unasyn) would be substituted for β-lactamase-producing, high-level gentamicin-resistant enterococci. In light of the increasing prevalence of enterococci with high-level aminoglycoside resistance, the potential synergistic interaction between ampicillin or amoxicillin and a third-generation cephalosporin was explored in vitro and in experimental models of IE.[114] A bactericidal synergistic effect was shown between amoxicillin and cefotaxime against 50 strains of *E. faecalis*. Amoxicillin MIC decreased from 0.25 to 1 mcg/mL to 0.01 to 0.25 mcg/mL for 48 of 50 strains tested.[115] Additionally, Brandt et al.[116] demonstrated a synergistic bactericidal effect for amoxicillin in combination with imipenem against vancomycin–aminoglycoside-resistant *E. faecium* strains. The authors speculated that saturation of different penicillin-binding proteins by different β-lactam agents may be the underlying mechanism for the synergy observed. In an observational, nonrandomized multi-center study, 159 patients were treated with ampicillin (2 g IV every 4 hours) and ceftriaxone (2 g IV every 12 hours) and 87 were treated with ampicillin and gentamicin.[23] There were no differences in mortality (while on antibiotics and at 3-month follow-up), treatment failure, and relapses. The 2015 AHA guidelines recommend double β-lactam therapy with ampicillin and ceftriaxone as a reasonable option for infections caused by aminoglycoside-resistant *E. faecalis* strains.

GENTAMICIN

Dosing

CASE 66-4, QUESTION 2: What is the optimal dosage of gentamicin for G.S.?

Because patients with enterococcal endocarditis require prolonged therapy with aminoglycosides, the optimal serum concentration should minimize toxicity without jeopardizing clinical cure. Early in vitro data indicated that the bactericidal activity of gentamicin against enterococci was not significantly different between peak concentrations of 5 and 3 mcg/L; however, the differences between 3 and 1 mcg/mL were significant.[114] Animal models of endocarditis show discordant results in bacterial counts per gram of vegetation in animals on low-dose versus high-dose aminoglycosides.[117,118] In experimental endocarditis, multiple daily dosing is more effective than single daily dosing in reducing bacterial titers in vegetations.[119–121] In contrast, *viridans streptococci* endocarditis can be managed with single daily dosing[28] (see Case 66-1, Question 4). Thus, extended-interval dosing of aminoglycosides cannot be recommended for the treatment of enterococcal endocarditis at this time.

The only study comparing high-dose (>3 mg/kg/day) and low-dose (<3 mg/kg/day) gentamicin with penicillin in humans with enterococcal endocarditis evaluated 56 patients during a 12-year period (36 with streptomycin-susceptible and 20 with streptomycin-resistant infections).[122] The relapse rate of patients infected with streptomycin-resistant organisms (n = 20) was not significantly different between the high- and low-dose treatment groups (n = 10 each). Furthermore, patients who received the higher doses of gentamicin experienced a greater prevalence of nephrotoxicity (10 of 10 vs. 2 of 10; $P<0.001$). Mean peak and trough concentrations of gentamicin in patients who received the high doses were 5 and 2.1 mcg/mL, respectively; corresponding levels for patients receiving the low-dose regimen were 3.1 and 1 mcg/mL.

Given the available data, it would be reasonable to start G.S. on a gentamicin dosage of 1 mg/kg every 8 hours (assuming her renal function is normal) and to maintain peak concentrations of 3 to 5 mcg/mL and trough concentrations of less than 1 mcg/mL.

In Combination with Vancomycin

CASE 66-4, QUESTION 3: Why was vancomycin used in combination with gentamicin in G.S.? Is this combination effective against enterococci?

G.S. has a history of penicillin allergy. Most clinicians favor a combination of vancomycin and gentamicin for penicillin-allergic patients with enterococcal endocarditis, although vancomycin plus streptomycin is a suitable alternative.[7,108,122] The combination of vancomycin and gentamicin demonstrates bactericidal synergy for about 95% of enterococci strains. In contrast, the vancomycin and streptomycin combination demonstrates bactericidal synergy for about 65% of enterococci. Because G.S. has PVE, she should receive approximately 30 mg/kg/day, or roughly 1.5 g/day (750 mg every 12 hours), of vancomycin in combination with gentamicin (3 mg/kg/day). Serum levels of vancomycin and gentamicin should be monitored as previously discussed.

DURATION OF THERAPY

CASE 66-4, QUESTION 4: How long should G.S. be treated?

Historically, enterococcal endocarditis has been treated with penicillin plus an aminoglycoside for 6 weeks; the overall cure rate with this regimen is about 85%.[7] Four weeks of therapy is probably adequate for most patients with enterococcal endocarditis.[7,122,123] One study evaluated the efficacy of a treatment regimen involving shorter-course aminoglycoside therapy (median of 15 days) in combination with a cell wall-active agent for a median of 42 days in patients with PVE and native valve enterococcal endocarditis.[123] Clinical cure was observed in 75 of 93 (81%) patients overall, 78% of patients with PVE, and 82% of patients with native valves. Among those who had a clinical cure, 52% received a β-lactam, 12% received vancomycin, and 36% received a combination of both. Ampicillin was given in 88% of patients receiving a β-lactam. The causative organism was *E. faecalis* in 78 patients and *E. faecium* in five patients. Clinical success was also achieved in all eight patients with native valve IE who received either vancomycin (50%), ampicillin (25%), or combination of both (25%) without synergistic aminoglycoside therapy.[123]

Patients with complicated courses should receive 6 weeks of therapy, including patients infected with streptomycin-resistant organisms (such as G.S.), those who have had symptoms for more than 3 months before the initiation of antibiotics, and patients with PVE (such as G.S.).[7,12] Some clinicians recommend 6 weeks of therapy for all patients in whom the duration of illness cannot be firmly established; this accounts for many patients who present with subacute disease.

CASE 66-4, QUESTION 5: How do enterococci develop resistance to vancomycin? What are the therapeutic implications if G.S. is infected with glycopeptide-resistant enterococci?

GLYCOPEPTIDE RESISTANCE IN ENTEROCOCCI

Vancomycin resistant enterococci (VRE), particularly *E. faecium*, have emerged in the United States since 1987.[124,125] The increased use of vancomycin since the mid-1980s has coincided with the increased resistance to this class of compounds. Between 1989 and 1993, the percentage of nosocomial enterococci reported as resistant to vancomycin in the United States rose more than 20-fold, from

0.3% to 7.9%.[125] Enterococcal isolates from intensive care units increased even more dramatically, from 0.4% to 13.6%, during that time. Data from the Centers for Disease Control and Prevention National Nosocomial Infections Surveillance (NNIS) system indicate that the rate of increase has slowed down from 31% in 2000 to 12% in 2003.[126,127] A 12% increase was found in VRE infections in intensive care units between 2003 and the prior 5-year period (1998–2002). Nonetheless, epidemiologic studies conducted by the NNIS system, as well as others, have shown that VRE bacteremia is associated with significantly increased morbidity and mortality.[126,127]

Although *E. faecalis* is responsible for 80% to 90% of infections caused by enterococci, *E. faecium* is more likely to exhibit resistance to glycopeptides compared with *E. faecalis*; more than 95% of VRE recovered in the United States are *E. faecium*. Glycopeptide-resistant enterococci synthesize abnormal peptidoglycan precursors that lower the binding affinity of glycopeptides to peptidoglycans.[124] VRE can be broadly classified into three separate phenotypes (A, B, and C) based on three structurally different genes and gene products (e.g., altered ligases).[124] Most (approximately 70%) of resistant enterococci are of the VanA phenotype, which are resistant to high levels of vancomycin (MIC >256 mcg/mL). Expression of resistance is inducible, usually plasmid mediated, and transferable to other organisms via conjugation. The VanB strains exhibit moderate vancomycin resistance (MIC 16–64 mcg/mL), and the VanC strains are the least resistant (vancomycin MIC 8–16 mcg/mL, because of chromosomal-mediated constitutive expression (i.e., not inducible as are VanA and VanB); however, VanC isolates usually are associated with the much less common *Enterococcus gallinarum* and *Enterococcus casseliflavus* infections.

Vancomycin, and also extended-spectrum cephalosporins and drugs with potent antianaerobic activity are risk factors for VRE.[124]

Few therapeutic alternatives exist for VRE, and synergistic combinations are required for bactericidal activity and clinical cure in endocarditis. Consequently, the treatment of choice is unknown. As a result, practitioners must make decisions using the available data from in vitro synergy studies, experimental models of endocarditis, and scattered case reports. Of additional concern, glycopeptide-resistant isolates often exhibit concomitant high-level resistance to aminoglycosides and β-lactams (e.g., ampicillin, penicillin) secondary to either β-lactamase production or alteration in the target penicillin-binding proteins.

Several antibiotic combinations appear promising in vitro and in preliminary animal models of endocarditis, but few data are currently available in humans. Those combinations include high-dose ampicillin (20 g/day) or ampicillin/sulbactam plus an aminoglycoside; vancomycin, penicillin or ceftriaxone, and gentamicin; ampicillin and imipenem; ciprofloxacin and ampicillin; and ciprofloxacin, rifampin, and gentamicin.

Streptogramin and Oxazolidinone

Quinupristin/dalfopristin (Synercid) and linezolid (Zyvox) are two agents with activity and proven efficacy against some infections caused by VRE. Quinupristin/dalfopristin received accelerated approval by the FDA in late 1999 specifically for the treatment of vancomycin-resistant *E. faecium* bacteremia. However, in 2010, with other therapies available for the treatment of VRE, this FDA-labeled indication was removed. The fixed product is generally bactericidal against susceptible streptococci and staphylococci (including methicillin-resistant strains), but it is bacteriostatic against *E. faecium*. Specifically, *E. faecalis* is not susceptible to the agent because of the presence of an efflux[128] pump conferring resistance to dalfopristin.

Linezolid has bacteriostatic activity against enterococci, including vancomycin-resistant *E. faecium* and *E. faecalis*. It is also active against other gram-positive cocci, including *Streptococcus pneumoniae* and methicillin-resistant staphylococci.[129] Vancomycin-resistant *E. faecium* isolates resistant to linezolid have been isolated.[130,131] Treatment experience with linezolid under the compassionate-use protocol reported clinical and microbiologic cure rates of 50% at 6-month follow-up for patients with endocarditis. Vancomycin-resistant *E. faecium* was the causative organism for 19 of the 32 patients treated.[103] Common adverse effects associated with linezolid include nausea, headache, diarrhea, rash, and altered taste. Of greater concern is its potential to cause myelosuppression. Thrombocytopenia, leukopenia, anemia, and pancytopenia have all been reported. Up to 30% of patients treated experience thrombocytopenia (platelet counts <100,000 platelets/μL).[129] Linezolid given orally or via enteral feedings is completely bioavailable.[132] A dosage of 600 mg twice daily is recommended for adults.

Daptomycin

Daptomycin is active against enterococci in vitro, with a MIC range of 0.25 to 4 mcg/mL and MIC_{90} of 4 mcg/mL for 219 vancomycin-resistant *E. faecium* isolates from the United States. For 40 vancomycin-resistant *E. faecalis* isolates, the MIC range is 0.015 to 2 mcg/mL, with a MIC_{90} of 2 mcg/mL. Of concern is the emergence of daptomycin resistance during therapy for VRE infections.[133,134] In a case report of a patient with vancomycin-resistant *E. faecium* pyelonephritis, the initial isolate had an MIC of 2 mcg/mL; however, after 17 days of treatment, a blood culture yielded growth of vancomycin-resistant *E. faecium* with an MIC increase to 32 mcg/mL.[135] Clinical experience with daptomycin for vancomycin-resistant *E. faecium* endocarditis is limited, and treatment failure has been reported.[136] If daptomycin therapy is chosen, a dose of 10–12 mg/kg/day is recommended.[7]

FUNGAL ENDOCARDITIS CAUSED BY *CANDIDA ALBICANS*

Prognosis and Treatment

CASE 66-5

QUESTION 1: B.G., a 35-year-old male heroin addict, was admitted to the hospital with chief complaints of pleuritic chest pain and dyspnea on exertion. Physical examination revealed a cachectic man with a temperature of 104°F, a diastolic regurgitant heart murmur heard loudest during inspiration, splenomegaly, and pharyngeal petechiae. Funduscopic examination was noncontributory. On the chest radiograph, several pulmonary infiltrates with cavitation were evident. UA was significant for microscopic hematuria and RBC casts. A TEE demonstrated vegetations on both the tricuspid and aortic heart valves. B.G. had evidence of moderate heart failure, although his hemodynamic status at that time was "stable." Six sets of blood cultures were drawn over the course of 2 days, and broad-spectrum empiric coverage consisting of vancomycin, gentamicin, and ceftazidime was initiated. Two days later, two of the cultures grew *Candida albicans*, and a diagnosis of fungal endocarditis was established. What is B.G.'s prognosis, and how should his fungal endocarditis be treated?

Fungal endocarditis is a rare but life-threatening infection that is difficult to diagnose and even more difficult to treat.[1] Most cases are caused by *Candida* and *Aspergillus* species. Fungal endocarditis occurs primarily in IV drug users, patients with prosthetic heart valves, immunocompromised patients, those with IV catheters, or patients receiving broad-spectrum antibiotics.[137–140]

Management of fungal endocarditis generally requires early valve replacement and aggressive fungicidal therapy with amphotericin deoxycholate B 0.6 to 1 mg/kg/day with or without

 5-flucytosine (5-FC) 25 mg/kg orally QID. If B.G. had poor renal function, liposomal formulations of amphotericin B 3 to 5 mg/kg daily can be used as an alternative.[141]

These antifungal agents should be prescribed for B.G., and his broad-spectrum antibiotic should be discontinued. B.G.'s clinical presentation and chest radiograph indicate that fragments of vegetation have already embolized to his lungs and possibly to other vital organs (e.g., spleen, kidneys). Because of the morbidity and mortality associated with major emboli and valvular insufficiency, B.G. should undergo surgery within 48 to 72 hours after antifungal therapy has been initiated. The prognosis for B.G. is dismal even with proper medical and surgical treatment. In a series analyzing 270 cases of fungal IE occurring during a 30-year period, mortality for those who received combined medical and surgical management was 45%, compared with 64% for those who received antifungal therapy alone.[137] Despite initial response to treatment, the rate of relapse is high (30%–40%), and relapse can occur up to 9 years after the initial episode of infection.[137–140] Most deaths in IV drug users with endocarditis are secondary to heart failure, a finding already evident in B.G.[1] In addition, replacement of a heart valve for fungal endocarditis in a heroin addict carries a significant risk of late morbidity and mortality.[137]

COMBINATION THERAPY WITH 5-FLUCYTOSINE AND AMPHOTERICIN B

CASE 66-5, QUESTION 2: Why is it important to treat B.G.'s fungal endocarditis with the combination of 5-FC and conventional or lipid-based amphotericin B? What is the optimal duration of therapy?

The poor prognosis associated with fungal endocarditis warrants the administration of 5-FC in combination with amphotericin B, despite its potential for causing bone marrow suppression and hepatotoxicity.[137] The vegetations from B.G.'s tricuspid or aortic heart valves already have broken off and caused pulmonary cavitation and possibly splenomegaly. His clinical presentation is consistent with a potentially fatal outcome; therefore, his blood isolates should be tested for in vitro susceptibility to amphotericin, 5-FC, and azoles. Fungi resistant to 5-FC alone may still be susceptible to the synergistic effect of the 5-FC–amphotericin B combination.[142] If the organism is resistant to 5-FC, in vitro synergy between these two antifungals should be performed or therapy with an echinocandin should be considered.

The optimal dose and duration of antifungal therapy for fungal endocarditis have not been determined by clinical studies; however, postoperative treatment with amphotericin B and 5-FC (if it has in vitro activity) for a minimum of 6 weeks (total dose, 1.5–3 g of amphotericin B) is recommended and is supported by the poor penetration of amphotericin B into heart valve tissue.[143] In patients with fungal PVE, some experts advocate secondary prophylaxis for a minimum of 2 years or lifelong suppressive treatment with an oral antifungal agent for nonsurgical candidates in light of the high rates of relapse.[1,137,139,142–145]

Nephrotoxicity caused by amphotericin B is often a serious dose-limiting factor to completion of therapy, particularly in patients who require a prolonged treatment course. Renal dysfunction secondary to the conventional formulation of amphotericin B may stabilize or improve with the switch to lipid-formulated amphotericin B products (i.e., Abelcet, AmBisome).[146] The efficacy of the new formulations in the treatment of endocarditis has been demonstrated only in anecdotal reports.[137,139,142,143,147] Alternative antifungal agents, including echinocandins and azoles, are potential options in patients who experience significant renal toxicities.

ALTERNATIVE ANTIFUNGALS

CASE 66-5, QUESTION 3: If B.G. experiences significant toxicities because of prolonged combination treatment with amphotericin and 5-FC, what alternative antifungal agent(s) can be used to treat his fungal endocarditis?

Fluconazole (Diflucan) is a triazole compound active against *Candida* species, particularly *C. albicans* and *Candida parapsilosis.* It also has a favorable toxicity profile compared with amphotericin and 5-FC.[148]

Successful experience with fluconazole treatment of fungal endocarditis in humans has been described in only a few case reports.[149–152] Patients with various *Candida* species were treated with 200 to 600 mg of fluconazole daily for 45 days to 6 months or until death. Fluconazole therapy reduced or completely removed all cardiac vegetations and resolved clinical symptoms. Because of the lack of adequate clinical experience, however, the use of fluconazole in treating fungal endocarditis cannot be advocated except in patients who require lifelong therapy because of the following situations: (a) The patient is a poor surgical candidate, (b) the patient has relapsed at least once since the initial infection episode, or (c) the patient has PVE.

Another alternative treatment option is the echinocandins which are fungicidal against most *Candida* species, including those in biofilms. A limited but growing body of literature primarily in case reports describes the successful outcomes with use of the echinocandins in *Candida* IE. Echinocandin-based regimens including caspofungin, micafungin, and anidulafungin were found to be as effective and to have similar mortality rate as amphotericin-based therapies based on a subgroup analysis of 25 patients in a prospective international cohort of patients with *Candida* IE.[153]

GRAM-NEGATIVE BACILLARY ENDOCARDITIS CAUSED BY *PSEUDOMONAS AERUGINOSA*

Prevalence

CASE 66-5, QUESTION 4: Fourteen months after completing his course of antifungal therapy, B.G. was readmitted to the hospital with a 48-hour history of fever, shaking chills, rigors, and night sweats. His vital signs at that time were blood pressure, 100/60 mm Hg; pulse, 120 beats/minute; respirations, 24/minute; and temperature, 103.7°F. A new-onset systolic murmur was noted on auscultation. Two-dimensional echocardiography revealed two small vegetations on the prosthetic valve. Empiric therapy consisting of amphotericin B, 5-FC, vancomycin, and gentamicin was initiated. Three blood cultures drawn on the day of admission were positive for *P. aeruginosa* with the following antibiotic susceptibilities: gentamicin (8 mcg/mL), tobramycin (2 mcg/mL), piperacillin–tazobactam (16 mcg/mL), and ceftazidime (2 mcg/mL). A presumptive diagnosis of PVE caused by *P. aeruginosa* was made. Why was the finding of *Pseudomonas* expected in B.G.?

The prevalence of endocarditis caused by gram-negative organisms has increased significantly over the years, especially in IV drug users such as B.G. and patients with prosthetic heart valves. Gram-negative organisms are responsible for about 15% to 20% of endocarditis cases in these populations.[43] Most gram-negative endocarditis cases are caused by *Pseudomonas* species, *S. marcescens*, and *Enterobacter* species, although numerous other gram-negative organisms have been known to cause endocarditis.[43,128,154–157] In narcotic addicts with gram-negative endocarditis, the tricuspid, aortic, and mitral valves are involved in 50%, 45%, and 40% of cases, respectively.[128]

Antimicrobial Therapy

CASE 66-5, QUESTION 5: How should B.G.'s gram-negative endocarditis be treated and monitored?

The previous empirical antimicrobials should be discontinued because *P. aeruginosa* has been cultured from B.G.'s blood. A bactericidal combination of antibiotics usually is required to provide in vivo synergy and to prevent resistant subpopulations from emerging during therapy.[1,158] Endocarditis caused by *P. aeruginosa* (as in B.G.) should be treated for at least 6 weeks with a combination of an aminoglycoside and an antipseudomonal penicillin (piperacillin–tazobactam) or cephalosporin (ceftazidime).[1,156,159–161] The combination of an antipseudomonal penicillin and an aminoglycoside is synergistic in vitro and in the rabbit model of *P. aeruginosa* endocarditis,[160,161] and clinical experience has confirmed this finding in IV drug users. Combination therapy with high dosages of tobramycin or gentamicin (8 mg/kg/day) has been associated with a significantly higher cure rate and lower mortality rate compared with an older, low-dose regimen (2.5–5 mg/kg/day).[43,156,159] B.G., therefore, should be treated with ceftazidime (2 g IV every 8 hours) with concurrent high-dose tobramycin (3 mg/kg IV every 8 hours). Aminoglycosides (tobramycin or gentamicin) should be dosed to produce peak and trough serum concentrations of 15 to 20 mcg/mL and less than 2 mcg/mL, respectively, to ensure maximum efficacy.[1] Finally, the infected valve should be surgically excised for the reasons previously discussed.

Other antibiotics including imipenem, meropenem, aztreonam, cefepime, and ciprofloxacin are active against many of the gram-negative organisms causing endocarditis. Clinical data regarding their use in the treatment of endocarditis are very limited, however.[162–165] Ceftolozane/tazobactam (Zerbaxa) is a novel cephalosporin combination β-lactamase inhibitor with enhanced activity against *Pseudomonas* and may be an alternative for treatment of multi-drug resistant *Pseudomonas* infections. Its efficacy for the treatment of endocarditis is still being investigated.

CULTURE-NEGATIVE ENDOCARDITIS

CASE 66-5, QUESTION 6: B.G.'s history, clinical presentation, and imaging studies are strongly suggestive of IE. If his blood cultures had been negative after 48 hours of incubation, the working diagnosis would have been culture-negative endocarditis. What are the possible reasons for culture-negative endocarditis, and what measures should be taken to establish a microbiologic etiology?

The proportion of patients with culture-negative endocarditis has diminished considerably, presumably as a result of improved microbiologic culture techniques. Negative blood cultures are present in only 5% to 7% of patients who meet strict criteria for the diagnosis of IE and have not recently received antibiotics.[166] The prior administration of antimicrobials is thought to account for most cases of culture-negative endocarditis.[166] B.G.'s blood cultures may remain negative for several days to weeks if he has taken antibiotics recently.

Slow-growing and fastidious organisms, such as gram-negative bacilli in the *Haemophilus–Actinobacillus–Cardiobacterium–Eikenella–Kingella* group (HACEK), *Brucella*, *Coxiella*, chlamydiae, strict anaerobes, and fungi, should be pursued in culture-negative patients. This usually is accomplished by the use of special culture media or by obtaining appropriate serologic acute and convalescent titers. Blood cultures should be saved for at least 3 weeks to detect slow-growing organisms.[166] Of note, previously NVS has been the cause of most of the cases of endocarditis diagnosed as culture-negative, initially because of its requirement for the addition of vitamin B_6 (pyridoxal HCl) to the culture media for laboratory growth; however, laboratory identification is no longer a significant problem with current culture media and laboratory techniques.[9]

Empiric Therapy

CASE 66-5, QUESTION 7: The causative organism remains unidentified. Recommend an antimicrobial regimen for the empiric treatment of B.G.'s presumed culture-negative endocarditis.

In the hemodynamically stable patient, antibiotic therapy should be withheld until positive blood cultures are obtained.[1] Based on B.G.'s clinical presentation and echocardiographic findings, empiric antibiotics should be initiated as soon as necessary cultures have been collected. Because staphylococci (often MRSA) and gram-negative bacilli account for most cases of endocarditis in the narcotic addict with a prosthetic heart valve, B.G. should be started on a four-drug regimen: vancomycin targeting a trough of 15 to 20 mcg/mL, gentamicin targeting a peak of 3 to 4 mcg/mL, cefepime 2 g IV every 8 hours, and rifampin 300 mg IV/PO every 8 hours.[7] Because B.G. may be experiencing a relapse caused by *C. albicans*, the addition of amphotericin B and 5-FC would be appropriate. Depending on the gram-negative pathogens common to the region and their anticipated susceptibilities, a third-generation cephalosporin (ceftriaxone or ceftazidime) or piperacillin–tazobactam could be used. The combination of an aminoglycoside and piperacillin–tazobactam also will provide coverage for enterococci.

B.G.'s clinical status and the positive echocardiogram indicate that early surgical valve excision and replacement are necessary. Cultures obtained from the excised valve may allow for identification of the causative organism and subsequent alteration of his antimicrobial regimen depending on susceptibilities.

PROPHYLACTIC THERAPY

Rationale and Recommendations

CASE 66-6

QUESTION 1: B.B., a 74-year-old man with poor dentition, is scheduled to have all of his remaining teeth extracted for subsequent fitting of dentures. His medical history is significant for numerous infections of the oral cavity and prosthetic valve replacement 2 years ago. His only current medications are oral digoxin (Lanoxin) 0.125 mg/day and furosemide (Lasix) 40 mg every morning. What is the rationale for antibiotic prophylaxis?

Because IE is associated with significant mortality and long-term morbidity, prevention in susceptible patients is of paramount importance.[1] Estimates are, however, that less than 10% of all cases are theoretically preventable.[167] The incidence of endocarditis in patients undergoing procedures known to cause significant bacteremia, even without antibiotic prophylaxis, is low. In addition, endocarditis may develop after the administration of seemingly appropriate chemoprophylaxis. Therefore, it is not surprising that the efficacy of prophylaxis has never been established through placebo-controlled clinical trials. Approximately 6,000 patients would be necessary to demonstrate a statistical difference (if one exists) between untreated controls and a group receiving prophylaxis.[168]

Without conclusive clinical data from prospective trials, recommendations for antibiotic prophylaxis have been based largely on in vitro susceptibility data, evaluation of antibiotic regimens using animal models of endocarditis, and anecdotal experiences.[168]

Prophylactic antibiotics are thought to provide protection by decreasing the number of organisms reaching the damaged heart valve from a primary source. Thus, antibiotics theoretically prevent bacterial multiplication on the valve and interfere with bacterial adherence to the cardiac lesion.[168]

The 2007 AHA recommendations for antibiotic prophylaxis before common medical procedures are outlined in Table 66-6.[168] Compared with the previous (1997) guideline, the current guidelines only recommend the use of prophylaxis in patients with specific cardiac conditions (associated with the highest risk of adverse outcomes from endocarditis) who are undergoing only dental or respiratory tract procedures. The use of prophylaxis for patients undergoing genitourinary or gastrointestinal procedures is not recommended because of a continuing lack of evidence to support efficacy.

DENTAL AND UPPER RESPIRATORY TRACT PROCEDURES

Analysis of published data shows that viridans streptococcal bacteremia can result from any procedure that involves the manipulation of the gingival tissue or the periapical region of the teeth or perforation of the oral mucosa. Placement or removal of prosthodontic or orthodontic appliances, adjustment of orthodontic appliances, taking dental radiographs, bleeding from trauma to the lips or oral mucosa, and instantaneous shedding of deciduous teeth do not require chemoprophylaxis. Endotracheal intubation also does not require prophylactic therapy.

Antimicrobial prophylaxis should be directed against the viridans group of streptococci because these organisms are the most common cause of endocarditis after dental procedures. Invasive surgical procedures involving the upper respiratory tract, such as incision or biopsy of the respiratory mucosa (e.g., tonsillectomy, adenoidectomy), can cause transient bacteremia with organisms that have similar antibiotic susceptibilities to those that occur after dental procedures; therefore, the same regimens are suggested. Prophylaxis is not recommended for bronchoscopies unless the procedure involves incision of the respiratory mucosa. Amoxicillin is currently recommended for oral prophylaxis in susceptible persons having dental or upper respiratory tract surgery. Oral clindamycin, clarithromycin, or azithromycin is recommended for patients with immediate-type hypersensitivity reaction to penicillins. Only patients with outlined cardiac conditions should receive prophylactic antibiotics.

Most cases of endocarditis caused by bacterial flora from the mouth do not follow dental procedures but rather are the result of poor oral hygiene. The cumulative exposure to random bacteremias from daily oral activities is estimated to be 5,730 minutes during a 1-month period compared with only 6 to 30 minutes for a dental procedure. Furthermore, it is estimated that the cumulative exposure to bacteremia from routine daily activities may be up to 5.6 million times greater than a single tooth extraction.[168] Based on the study results, concerns for antimicrobial resistance, and cost, changes to restrict the use of antibiotic prophylaxis before dental procedures to the highest-risk patients may be expected with future guidelines issued by the AHA.

Table 66-6
Cardiac Conditions for Which Prophylaxis is Recommended

Cardiac Conditions
Prophylaxis Recommended
■ Prosthetic cardiac valves
■ Previous bacterial endocarditis
■ Congenital heart disease
■ Unrepaired cyanotic CHD, including palliative shunts and conduits
■ Completely repaired congenital heart defect with prosthetic material device during the first 6 months after the procedure
■ Repaired CHD with residual defects at or adjacent to the site of the prosthetic device or patch
■ Mitral valve prolapse with valvular regurgitation and/or thickened leaflets
■ Cardiac transplantation recipients who develop cardiac valvulopathy

CHD, congenital heart disease.

Source: Wilson W et al. Prevention of infective endocarditis: guidelines from the American Heart Association: a guideline from the American Heart Association Rheumatic Fever, Endocarditis, and Kawasaki Disease Committee, Council on Cardiovascular Disease in the Young, and the Council on Clinical Cardiology, Council on Cardiovascular Surgery and Anesthesia, and the Quality of Care an Outcomes Research Interdisciplinary Working Group. American Heart Association [published correction appears in *Circulation*. 2007;116:e376]. *Circulation*. 2007;116:1736.

Indications and Choice of Agent

Case 66-6, Question 2: Is prophylactic antibiotic therapy indicated for B.B.? If so, which antibiotic(s) should be used?

Based on the current recommendations, B.B. is a candidate for antibiotic prophylaxis. Presence of a prosthetic aortic valve while undergoing multiple tooth extractions places him at risk for experiencing endocarditis. He also is scheduled to have all of his remaining teeth extracted, a procedure likely to result in bacteremia. According to Table 66-7, B.B. should receive a single 2-g oral dose of amoxicillin 1 hour before the procedure.

Table 66-7
Endocarditis Prophylaxis Regimen Indicated for Patients with Cardiac Conditions

Drug[a]	Dose
Dental or upper respiratory tract procedures	Single dose 30–60 minutes before procedure
Standard Regimen	
Amoxicillin	*Adult*: 2 g
	Pediatric: 50 mg/kg
Allergic to Penicillin or Ampicillin	
Clindamycin	*Adult:* 600 mg
	Pediatric: 20 mg/kg
Cephalexin[b,c]	*Adult*: 2 g
	Pediatric: 50 mg/kg
Azithromycin or clarithromycin	*Adult*: 500 mg
	Pediatric: 15 mg/kg
Unable to Take Oral Medications	
Ampicillin	*Adult*: 2 g IM or IV
	Pediatric: 50 mg/kg IM or IV

Table 66-7
Endocarditis Prophylaxis Regimen Indicated for Patients with Cardiac Conditions (*continued*)

Drug[a]	Dose
Allergic to Penicillin or Ampicillin	
Clindamycin	*Adult*: 600 mg IM or IV
	Pediatric: 20 mg/kg IV
Cefazolin[b]	*Adult*: 1 g IM or IV
	Pediatric: 50 mg/kg IM or IV

[a]See Table 66-6.
[b]Cephalosporins should not be used in individuals with immediate-type hypersensitivity reaction (e.g., urticaria, angioedema, or anaphylaxis) to penicillins or ampicillin.
[c]Other first- or second-generation oral cephalosporins in equivalent adult or pediatric dose.
IM, intramuscular; IV, intravenous.
Source: Wilson W et al. Prevention of infective endocarditis: guidelines from the American Heart Association: a guideline from the American Heart Association Rheumatic Fever, Endocarditis, and Kawasaki Disease Committee, Council on Cardiovascular Disease in the Young, and the Council on Clinical Cardiology, Council on Cardiovascular Surgery and Anesthesia, and the Quality of Care an Outcomes Research Interdisciplinary Working Group. American Heart Association [published correction appears in *Circulation*. 2007;116:e376]. *Circulation*. 2007;116:1736.

KEY REFERENCES AND WEBSITES

A full list of references for this chapter can be found at http://thepoint.lww.com/AT11e. Below are the key references and website for this chapter, with the corresponding reference number in this chapter found in parentheses after the reference.

Key References

Baddour LM et al. Infective endocarditis in adults: diagnosis, antimicrobial therapy, and management of complications. A Scientific Statement for Healthcare Professionals from the American Heart Association (AHA); on behalf of the AHA Committee on Rheumatic Fever, Endocarditis, and Kawasaki Disease of the Council on Cardiovascular Disease in the Young, Council on Clinical Cardiology, Council on Cardiovascular Surgery and Anesthesia, and Stroke Council: Endorsed by the Infectious Diseases Society of America. *Circulation*. 2015;132:1435–1486.

Fowler VJ, Jr et al. Endocarditis and intravascular infections. In: Mandell GL et al, eds. *Mandell, Douglas, and Bennett's Principles and Practice of Infectious Diseases*. 8th ed. Philadelphia, PA: Elsevier Saunders; 2015. Chapter 77. (1)

Fowler VG, Jr et al. *Staphylococcus aureus* endocarditis: a consequence of medical progress [published correction appears in *JAMA*. 2005;294:900]. *JAMA*. 2005;293:3012. (6)

Fowler VG, Jr et al. Daptomycin versus standard therapy for bacteremia and endocarditis caused by *Staphylococcus aureus*. *N Engl J Med*. 2006;355:653. (89)

Howden BP et al. Reduced vancomycin susceptibility in *Staphylococcus aureus*, including vancomycin-intermediate and heterogeneous vancomycin-intermediate strains: resistance mechanisms, laboratory detection, and clinical implications. *Clin Microbiol Rev*. 2010;23:99. (44)

Li JS et al. Proposed modifications to the Duke criteria for the diagnosis of infective endocarditis. *Clin Infect Dis*. 2000;30:633. (15)

Le T, Bayer AS. Combination antibiotic therapy for infective endocarditis. *Clin Infect Dis*. 2003;36:615. (16)

Liu C et al. Clinical practice guidelines by the Infectious Diseases Society of America for the treatment of methicillin-resistant *Staphylococcus aureus* infections in adults and children. *Clin Infect Dis*. 2011;52:e18. (63)

Palraj R. Prosthetic valve endocarditis. In: Mandell GL et al., eds. *Mandell, Douglas, and Bennett's Principles and Practice of Infectious Diseases*. 8th ed. Philadelphia, PA: Elsevier Saunders; 2015:1029. Chapter 83. (37)

Pappas PG et al. Clinical practice guidelines for the management of candidiasis: 2009 update by the Infectious Diseases Society of America. *Clin Infect Dis*. 2009;48:503. (141)

Rupp M et al. *Staphylococcus epidermidis* and other coagulase-negative staphylococci. In: Mandell GL et al., ed. *Mandell, Douglas, and Bennett's Principles and Practice of Infectious Diseases*. 8th ed. Philadelphia, PA: Elsevier Saunders; 2015:2272. Chapter 197. (42)

Sexton DJ et al. Ceftriaxone once daily for four weeks compared with ceftriaxone plus gentamicin once daily for two weeks for treatment of endocarditis due to penicillin-susceptible streptococci. Endocarditis Treatment Consortium Group. *Clin Infect Dis*. 1998;27:1470. (30)

Wilson W et al. Prevention of infective endocarditis: guidelines from the American Heart Association: a guideline from the American Heart Association Rheumatic Fever, Endocarditis, and Kawasaki Disease Committee, Council on Cardiovascular Disease in the Young, and the Council on Clinical Cardiology, Council on Cardiovascular Surgery and Anesthesia, and the Quality of Care an Outcomes Research Interdisciplinary Working Group. American Heart Association [published correction appears in *Circulation*. 2007;116:e376]. *Circulation*. 2007;116:1736. (168)

Key Websites

www.clevelandclinicmeded.com/medicalpubs/diseasemanagement/infectious-disease/infective-endocarditis/

67 Respiratory Tract Infections

Jason Cross, Evan Horton, and Dinesh Yogaratnam

CORE PRINCIPLES

CORE PRINCIPLES	CHAPTER CASES
ACUTE BRONCHITIS	
1 Acute bronchitis is a commonly encountered clinical diagnosis exhibited by cough for more than 5 days and generally does not require treatment with antimicrobial agents.	**Case 67-1 (Questions 1 and 3)**
ACUTE EXACERBATION OF CHRONIC OBSTRUCTIVE PULMONARY DISEASE	
1 Antibiotics should be provided to patients with acute exacerbations of chronic obstructive pulmonary disease (AECOPD) if three primary symptoms (increased dyspnea, increased sputum volume, and increased sputum purulence) are present, if two primary symptoms are present and increased sputum purulence is one of the symptoms, or with required mechanical ventilation.	**Case 67-2 (Question 4)**
2 Hospitalized patients with AECOPD should both be optimally treated, and their COPD management be assessed to decrease the likelihood of readmission. Baseline COPD medications should be examined and adjusted based on disease severity. Additionally, an assessment of patients' understanding of the role of medications (maintenance therapy vs. rescue medications), ability to use inhalers correctly, access to prescribed medications, and discussions regarding pulmonary rehabilitation should take place. Consideration for pharmacologic venous thromboembolism prophylaxis should also be made in this high-risk population.	**Case 67-2 (Question 6)**
3 Vaccinations to prevent influenza and *Streptococcus pneumoniae* in patients with COPD or previous pneumonia reduce disease-associated morbidity.	**Case 67-2 (Question 7)**
COMMUNITY-ACQUIRED PNEUMONIA	
1 The first decision after a diagnosis of community-acquired pneumonia (CAP) is to determine the need for hospitalization. Several predictive rules including the pneumonia severity index (PSI) and CURB-65 (confusion, uremia, increased respiratory rate, low blood pressure, and age ≥65 years) have been developed to facilitate site-of-care decision making.	**Case 67-3 (Question 2)**
2 The most frequently isolated bacterial pathogen causing CAP, regardless of epidemiologic factors and severity of illness, is *S. pneumoniae*.	**Case 67-3 (Question 4)**
3 The most important consideration when selecting empiric therapy is to identify patients at risk for infection with drug-resistant *S. pneumoniae* (DRSP).	**Case 67-3 (Question 5)**
4 Patients who continue to have a positive laboratory test result for influenza more than 48 hours after the onset of illness are at high risk of requiring hospitalization, or who are not improving should also be treated.	**Case 67-4 (Question 2)**

Continued

HOSPITAL-ACQUIRED, VENTILATOR-ASSOCIATED, AND HEALTH CARE–ASSOCIATED PNEUMONIA

1	Hospital-acquired pneumonia (HAP) is defined as pneumonia that occurs at least 48 hours after hospital admission. Ventilator-associated pneumonia (VAP) refers to pneumonia that arises 48 to 72 hours after endotracheal intubation. Health care–associated pneumonia (HCAP) is diagnosed in any patient who has been hospitalized in an acute-care hospital for 2 or more days within 90 days of infection; resided in a nursing home or long-term care facility; received intravenous antibiotic therapy, chemotherapy, or wound care within the past 30 days of the current infection; lived in close contact with a person with a multidrug-resistant (MDR) pathogen; or attended a hospital or hemodialysis clinic.	**Case 67-5 (Question 1)**
2	The major difference in the bacteriology between CAP and HAP/HCAP/VAP is a shift to gram-negative pathogens, MDR pathogens, and methicillin-resistant *Staphylococcus aureus* (MRSA) in HAP/HCAP/VAP.	**Case 67-5 (Question 1)**
3	Risk factors for pneumonia caused by MDR pathogens include antimicrobial therapy in the previous 90 days, current hospitalization of 5 days or more, immunosuppressive disease or therapy, or any risk factor for HCAP.	**Case 67-5 (Question 1)**
4	Patients with early-onset pneumonia (<5 days) and no MDR risk factors can be treated with a single agent, including a non-antipseudomonal third-generation cephalosporin or ertapenem, ampicillin/sulbactam, or an antipneumococcal fluoroquinolone. Empiric therapy in those with late-onset pneumonia (≥5 days) or MDR risk factors should include a combination of antibiotics active against *Pseudomonas aeruginosa*. This regimen usually includes an antipseudomonal β-lactam, plus either an aminoglycoside or ciprofloxacin/levofloxacin. Vancomycin or linezolid should be added if MRSA risk factors are present or if there is a high incidence at the health care facility.	**Case 67-6 (Question 2)**

ACUTE BRONCHITIS

Definition and Incidence

Acute bronchitis (AB) is defined as an acute, self-limiting respiratory illness of the upper bronchi accompanied by cough for more than 5 days that can last up to 3 weeks.[1–3] AB may be associated with or without purulent sputum production, and fever is rare.[2] Patients can be diagnosed with AB when there is no evidence of pneumonia and when acute asthma, an acute exacerbation of chronic obstructive pulmonary disease (AECOPD), or the common cold have been ruled out as the cause of cough.[3] While the true incidence of AB is unknown, it is considered to be one of the most common conditions encountered in clinical practice, accounting for more than 6.7 million outpatient visits per year.[4]

Pathophysiology and Epidemiology

AB is characterized by the inflammatory response to infection in the epithelium of the bronchi. Further progression of this inflammation leads to thickening of the tracheal mucosa.[1,2] Sloughing of cells from the tracheobronchial epithelium and inflammatory mediators causes bronchospasm and reduced forced expiratory volume in 1 second (FEV_1) that usually improves after 5 weeks. Spread of pathogen and inflammatory response correlate with patient symptoms. Although bacteria can be isolated from sputum, bacterial invasion of the bronchial tree rarely occurs, and the role of bacterial pathogens in AB is limited.[5] The vast majority of cases of AB are presumed to be caused by viruses.[2,5–7]

Clinical Presentation

Cough lasting for more than 5 days is the hallmark sign of AB. Although the illness is self-limited, cough can last for up to 3 weeks (typical duration 10–20 days). Sputum production occurs in up to 50% of cases, but it does not indicate bacterial infection.[3] Fever is unusual in most cases; when present, it should prompt investigation for influenza (during appropriate seasons) or for pneumonia (if other clinical signs are present).

Overview of Drug Therapy

Antimicrobials do not significantly reduce symptoms of AB, and their use increases the risk of adverse drug events and antimicrobial resistence.[8] Expert guidelines in the United States and abroad recommend against the use of antimicrobial agents for the treatment of AB.[3,6,7,9] Despite the evidence refuting their use, greater than 70% of AB cases are treated with antibiotics in the United States. Furthermore, the agents used for AB are increasingly broad-spectrum drugs, further exacerbating bacterial resistance pressure.[10] Non-antimicrobial treatment considerations include bronchodilators or antitussives depending on symptoms, even though evidence to support the use of many of these modalities is limited.[3,11,12]

Clinical Presentation

CASE 67-1

QUESTION 1: A.R. is a 50-year-old man presenting with a chief complaint of cough. His symptoms have persisted for 8 days, and he now produces yellow sputum with each cough. He has had no recent illnesses; however, his 14-year-old son in high school has experienced recent mild colds. A.R. denies nausea, vomiting, or fever and chills. A review of systems reveals fatigue and difficulty sleeping because of cough. Past medical history includes hypertension managed with lisinopril and hyperlipidemia for which he takes atorvastatin. He also takes low-dose aspirin for stroke prevention. Vital signs indicate a temperature of 37.1°C, heart rate of 70 beats/minute, blood pressure of 130/70 mm Hg, and respiratory rate of 18 breaths/minute with accompanying oxygen saturation of 98% on room air. His physical examination is positive for coarse breath sounds that clear with coughing, but it is otherwise normal. What signs and symptoms in A.R. are consistent with AB?

Persistent cough in the absence of other symptoms including fever or myalgia is typical with AB.[3] Cough can last up to 3 weeks and is usually self-limited. The typical duration of symptoms in AB is 5 to 14 days.[2] Pneumonia must be ruled out; however, normal oxygen saturation and lack of focal signs on pulmonary physical examination makes this diagnosis less likely. Sputum production is common, although not present in all cases of AB. Symptoms can be present at night, contributing to A.R.'s symptoms of fatigue.

Microbiology

Case 67-1, Question 2: What are the most likely causes of A.R.'s case of AB?

The causative agent for AB is identified in a minority of cases; however, when pathogens are isolated, they are usually of viral etiology.[2,5–7] A limited number of bacterial pathogens are associated with AB and should primarily be considered in patients with underlying COPD, mechanical ventilation (tracheobronchitis), or in cases of outbreaks and exposures (e.g., *Bordetella pertussis*). A list of common pathogens with their specific symptoms is included in Table 67-1.[2]

Sick contacts, duration of incubation (2–7 days for viruses vs. weeks for atypical bacteria), and previous exposures should be considered when determining the etiologic agent responsible for AB. Specific symptoms reveal infection caused by specific pathogens, such as an inspiratory whoop and post-tussive emesis (*B. pertussis*), pharyngitis and cough lasting longer than 4 weeks (*Mycoplasma pneumoniae*), hoarseness with low-grade fever (*Chlamydophila pneumoniae*), or cough with fever and myalgias (influenza).[2] Given A.R.'s lack of sick contacts with bacterial infections (his son's recent colds are most likely of viral etiology), time course of present illness, and absence of symptoms suggestive of influenza, a viral etiology (other than influenza) is most likely to be the cause of his symptoms.

Clinical Diagnosis and Treatment

Case 67-1, Question 3: Should A.R. be provided an antimicrobial agent for his AB?

Antibiotics have not been shown to substantially reduce the duration of illness in AB.[8] Thus, guidelines recommend against the routine use of antimicrobial therapy for AB.[3,6,7,9] Despite these recommendations, antimicrobials are frequently prescribed for this condition.[10] Inappropriate use of antimicrobial therapy is a public health concern because it may lead to adverse events and antimicrobial resistance. One exception to avoidance of antimicrobial therapy in AB is if *B. pertussis* infection (whooping cough) is suspected. In these cases, antibiotic therapy with a macrolide antibiotic is recommended, and patients should remain in isolation for the first 5 days of treatment to prevent disease transmission.[3] In A.R.'s case, no antimicrobial agent is warranted.

Case 67-1, Question 4: Should a sputum culture be obtained from A.R.? What other diagnostics should be considered?

Obtaining a sputum sample for culture to determine the presence of the causative agent or diagnostic screening for atypical pathogens is not routinely indicated for AB. The rationale is that most of the identified pathogens have no specific treatment (viral illnesses), and the isolated organisms often are not true pathogens. Diagnostic screening, however, should be performed during influenza season or during outbreaks of *B. pertussis* or other atypical pathogens for infection control purposes. The use of biomarkers for the diagnosis of bacterial infection, such as procalcitonin or C-reactive protein (CRP), may decrease inappropriate antimicrobial use in AB, but their widespread use cannot be recommended at this time.[13,14]

Case 67-1, Question 5: What symptom-guided therapies should be offered to A.R.?

Table 67-1
Causes of Acute Bronchitis

Pathogen	Comments
Viruses	
Influenza	Quick onset with fever, chills, headache, and cough. Myalgias are common and may be accompanied by myopathy.
Parainfluenza	Epidemics in autumn. Outbreaks may occur in nursing homes. Croup in child at home suggests presence of the organism.
Respiratory syncytial virus	About 45% of family members exposed to infant with bronchiolitis become infected. Outbreaks prominent in winter or spring. Twenty percent of adults have ear pain.
Coronavirus	Can cause severe respiratory symptoms in elderly. Epidemics present in military recruits.
Adenovirus	Similar presentation as influenza; abrupt onset of fever.
Rhinovirus	Fever is uncommon and infection generally mild.
Atypical Bacteria	
Bordetella pertussis	Incubation period of 1–3 weeks. Whooping occurs in a minority of patients, and fever is uncommon. Marked leukocytosis with lymphocytic predominance can occur.
Mycoplasma pneumoniae	Incubation period is 2–3 weeks. Outbreaks in military personnel and students have been reported.
Chlamydophila pneumoniae	Incubation period is 3 weeks. Onset of symptoms, which include hoarseness before cough, is gradual. Outbreaks reported in nursing homes, college students, and military personnel.

Source: Wenzel RP, Fowler AA 3rd. Clinical practice. Acute bronchitis. *N Engl J Med*. 2006;355:2125.

Symptom-guided therapies include the use of inhaled β-agonists (albuterol) for shortness of breath, particularly in patients with underlying reactive airway disease; inhaled or systemic steroids for persistent cough; nonsteroidal anti-inflammatory drugs (NSAIDs), aspirin, or acetaminophen to alleviate myalgias or fever; or antihistamines (brompheniramine), antitussives (codeine, dextromethorphan, or benzonatate), or mucolytics (guaifenesin) for cough. These symptom-guided treatments, however, are not backed by strong evidence demonstrating a clear benefit in patients with AB.[1–3,11,12] As such, each of these treatments should be approached with an appropriate consideration of the balance between perceived benefit and risk of adverse events. Given A.R.'s troublesome cough that has kept him up at night, a trial of an antitussive such as dextromethorphan is a reasonable first option. NSAIDs should be avoided given his concurrent aspirin use and lack of clear indication. An inhaled β-agonist or steroid is also not necessary at this time.[12,15]

CASE 67-1, QUESTION 6: Should a chest radiograph be ordered for A.R.? What other illnesses may be considered as the cause of his symptoms?

It is important to distinguish AB from pneumonia with chest radiograph or other imaging tests when fever, tachycardia, tachypnea; physical examination findings such as egophony or rales; or hypoxemia or mental status changes (especially in the elderly) are present.[2,3] Clinical differentiation of AB from AECOPD, postnasal drip, gastroesophageal reflux disorder (GERD), and asthma must also be made (discussed separately in this chapter and in Chapter 23 Upper Gastrointestinal Disorders, and in Chapter 18 Asthma, respectively). In A.R.'s case, no signs of pneumonia are seen on physical examination or on reviewing symptomatology; therefore, no chest radiograph is warranted. Frequent symptoms over time or risk factors for COPD would warrant an investigation for chronic bronchitis. Wheezing or frequent AB outbreaks and GERD symptoms would guide evaluations for asthma or gastrointestinal disorders, respectively.

Patient Education

CASE 67-1, QUESTION 7: What education would you provide to A.R. to dissuade his perceived need for an antibiotic?

An evaluation of A.R.'s expectations for therapy is important to alleviate concerns about the decision to not to prescribe antimicrobials. Overuse of antibiotics in AB is often driven by either prescriber knowledge or patient request. Communication is key with each patient to provide insight into the potential causative agents of AB, the natural course of the disease, the role of symptomatic relief, and reasons for avoiding prescriptions for antibiotics.

ACUTE EXACERBATION OF CHRONIC OBSTRUCTIVE PULMONARY DISEASE

Definition, Incidence, and Epidemiology

According to the Global Initiative for Chronic Obstructive Lung Disease (GOLD), Chronic Obstructive Pulmonary Disease (COPD) is a persistent and progressive reduction in airflow that results from repeated exposure to noxious particles. The chronic inflammation in the lungs results in a narrowing of the small airways, destruction of alveoli, and loss of elastic recoil. Of note, COPD may or may not be accompanied by increased sputum production and chronic cough. This disease is also characterized by acute exacerbations (AECOPD), which is defined as a worsening of symptoms that is more severe than the typical day-to-day variations that patients experience during the stable phase of their disease. Acute exacerbations of COPD typically require a change in medication to relieve symptoms and improve outcomes.[16] Maintenance therapy for COPD (discussed separately in Chapter 19 Chronic Obstructive Pulmonary Disease) is often targeted to reduce the severity and frequency of AECOPD.

COPD is associated with high health care expenditures, decreased quality of life, significant morbidity, and high mortality around the world. AECOPD is responsible for most of this burden. In the United States and Canada, COPD is the third and fourth leading cause of death, respectively. In 2009 in the United States, 1.5 million emergency department visits and 715,000 hospitalizations were attributable to COPD.[17] Direct health care costs associated with COPD in 2010 were estimated to be $29.5 billion in the United States.[17] AECOPD is associated with a decrease in quality-of-life measurements and an increase in the rate of decline in lung function, particularly if not treated early.[16]

The primary precipitating factors for AECOPD are infection of the bronchial tree and air pollution.[16,18–20] As many as one-third of the cases of AECOPD do not have a cause identified.

Pathophysiology

Bacteria, viruses, and pollutants lead to inflammatory responses.[20] Airway inflammation, associated with increases in interleukin-8, tumor necrosis factor-α, and neutrophils, contributes to pulmonary remodeling, decreased ciliary clearance of mucus, worsening airflow obstruction, and the respiratory symptoms associated with AECOPD.

Viruses have been identified as the etiologic cause of AECOPD in up to one-third of the cases, while bacteria have been identified in up to one-half of cases.[20] The micro-organisms most commonly associated with AECOPD include *Haemophilus influenza*, *Streptococcus pneumoniae*, and *Moraxella catarrhalis*. In patients with GOLD 3 (severe) or GOLD 4 (very severe) COPD, *Pseudomonas aeruginosa* is more prevalent.[16] Many patients with COPD are also colonized with bacteria during the stable phase of their illness.[21] Evidence suggests that either an increased burden of the same colonizing microorganism(s) or acquisition of a new bacterial species may be associated with exacerbating COPD symptoms.[16,21] Decreases in adaptive immune responses occur as COPD disease progresses, making patients susceptible to more frequent exacerbations caused by bacterial pathogens. Additionally, pathogens associated with exacerbations tend to increase in virulence and antimicrobial resistance as the underlying disease progresses.[16,19,20,22] A possible mechanism for prolonged infection and colonization in patients with COPD is suggested by interactions between both viruses and bacteria altering immune respone.[20]

Clinical Presentation and Diagnosis

Common features of AECOPD include the following: breathlessness, increased cough, increased sputum volume, and increased sputum purulence. In contrast to AB, purulent sputum in AECOPD is associated with an acute bacterial infection.[22] Other less specific symptoms include insomnia, fatigue, tachycardia, tachypnea, and a decrease in exercise tolerance. Patients often report a decrease in ability to conduct activities of daily living.[16]

Diagnostic considerations in the evaluation of patients with AECOPD include pulse oximetry and arterial blood gases, electrocardiogram, and complete blood count including white blood cell (WBC) differential. Chest radiographs are helpful to rule out pneumonia, pneumothorax, or pleural effusion. An assessment of comorbidities, such as the presence of heart failure or lung diseases (e.g., asthma or lung cancer), should be performed to aid in both prognosis and diagnosis.[16,18] Collection of sputum samples for Gram stain and culture are not generally recommended, but it may be helpful if patients are failing initial therapies.

Overview of Treatment

Pharmacotherapy directed at AECOPD includes bronchodilators and supplemental oxygen, antimicrobial therapy to decrease the burden of microorganisms, and corticosteroids targeting the inflammatory response.[16,18] Methylxanthines (aminophylline or theophylline) are rarely used owing to conflicting and limited evidence of efficacy and concerns about toxicity.[16] Nonpharmacologic AECOPD treatment considerations include decisions regarding the site-of-care and the level of respiratory support. These nondrug considerations are not discussed in detail in this chapter but are available in the GOLD Guidelines.[16]

Disease Severity

CASE 67-2

QUESTION 1: T.H. is an 81-year-old white woman presenting to the emergency department (ED) because she "cannot catch my breath." At baseline she is on 4 L of oxygen continuously via nasal cannula. However, during the last week she has experienced worsening dyspnea necessitating help with daily activities including bathing and feeding. Her daughter had contacted T.H.'s primary-care physician who directed the patient to the ED when T.H. seemed "out of it" and was difficult to arouse. T.H.'s daughter indicates that T.H. has been "having a cold" with increased sputum that is more yellow than in the past with frequent coughing spells. Past medical history is significant for very severe COPD, atrial fibrillation, depression, obstructive sleep apnea, morbid obesity, and a left humerus fracture. No medication allergies are noted. Medications at home include aspirin 81 mg PO daily, citalopram 20 mg PO daily, diltiazem extended-release capsule 240 mg PO daily, salmeterol–fluticasone dry powdered inhaler 50/250 one puff twice daily, and albuterol inhaler four puffs every 6 hours as needed for shortness of breath. Social history is significant for a greater than 80-pack-year history of cigarette smoking, but she quit 4 to 5 years ago. In the ED she was afebrile, heart rate was 96 beats/minute, respiratory rate was 23 breaths/minute, blood pressure was 135/75 mm Hg, and oxygen saturation was 60% on 4 L of oxygen. T.H. is in some distress, alert and oriented times two, and is using accessory muscles for breathing. Initial physical examination was significant for distant breath sounds and decreased air movement bilaterally, a noted absence of lower extremity edema, and an irregularly irregular heartbeat. Laboratory findings are as follows:

Arterial blood gases: pH, 7.34, Pco_2, 60 mm Hg, Po_2, 72 mm Hg
WBC, 9.8 × $10^3/\mu L$ (neutrophils 71%)
Hemoglobin, 12 g/dL
Platelets, 319 × $10^3/\mu L$
Sodium, 135 mmol/L
Potassium, 3.7 mmol/L
Chloride, 91 mmol/L
Bicarbonate, 39 mmol/L
Blood urea nitrogen (BUN), 15 mg/dL
Serum creatinine (SCr), 1.21 mg/dL
Glucose, 104 mg/dL
Brain natriuretic peptide, 66 pg/mL
Troponin, <0.07 ng/mL
Thyrotropin, 1.63 micro-international units/mL

Chest radiograph indicated small pleural effusions, but it was otherwise negative for infiltrates or consolidation. An electrocardiogram indicated the presence of atrial fibrillation. Pulmonary function tests (obtained 1 year ago) indicated an FEV_1 to forced vital capacity ratio of 0.39 and an FEV_1 of 37% predicted. How would you stage the severity of this exacerbation for T.H.?

T.H. has several risk factors for a poor outcome, including the presence of atrial fibrillation and severe COPD defined by her home oxygen requirement and low baseline FEV_1.[16]

Clinical signs and symptoms consistent with a severe exacerbation include the use of accessory respiratory muscles, paradoxical chest wall movements, worsening or new cyanosis, peripheral edema, hemodynamic compromise, signs of right heart failure, and alterations in mental status. T.H. has two of these factors: reduced alertness and use of accessory muscles.[16,18]

Disease Prevention

CASE 67-2, QUESTION 2: Which therapies should be made available to T.H. to alleviate her shortness of breath?

Supplemental oxygen to alleviate hypoxemia is a foundation of treatment for AECOPD. Controlled provision of oxygen should be implemented to provide an oxygen saturation of greater than 90% or a Pao_2 of greater than 60 mm Hg. Hypoxia that is not easily reversible warrants further examination for venous thromboembolism, pneumonia, or other causes. A repeat arterial blood gas should be obtained within 1 hour of initiation of supplemental oxygen to assess for carbon dioxide retention or acidosis.

The use of short-acting bronchodilators should be initiated promptly in all patients with AECOPD. β-Agonists, such as albuterol, with or without an anticholinergic agent (ipratropium), are the preferred agents.[16] If the patient does not respond, a methylxanthine (theophylline or aminophylline) may be considered as second-line therapy. There is no role for long-acting bronchodilators in AECOPD at this time.

CASE 67-2, QUESTION 3: Does T.H. need to be treated with antimicrobial therapy?

The "cardinal" symptoms of AECOPD include increases in sputum purulence, sputum volume, and dyspnea.[23] The use of cardinal symptoms as a method of staging AECOPD severity has been used in several prospective studies and is recommended in the GOLD guidelines.[16,24]

Experts advocate for the use of antibiotics for AECOPD, particularly when two or three cardinal symptoms are present.[16,18] Specifically, the GOLD Guidelines recommend antibiotics for patients with three cardinal symptoms (increased dyspnea, increased sputum volume, and increased sputum purulence); when two cardinal symptoms are present if increased sputum purulence is one of the symptoms; or in all patients requiring mechanical ventilation for their AECOPD.[16]

T.H. is exhibiting all three of the cardinal symptoms and therefore should receive antibiotics. Likely benefits would be enhanced treatment success, prevention of relapse, decreased risk for rehospitalization, improvement in pulmonary function, and reduction of the severity of her exacerbation.

CASE 67-2, QUESTION 4: Which antimicrobial agent should be selected for treating T.H.? What duration of treatment would be recommended?

Given T.H.'s history, diminished mental status, and risk factors for poor outcomes, intravenous (IV) administration seems appropriate for the initial antibiotic administration. Potential risk factors for *P. aeruginosa* should be evaluated. If T.H. demonstrates risk factors for *P. aeruginosa*, an anti-pseudomonal β-lactam, such as cefepime, would be an appropriate initial agent. If no risk factors for *P. aeruginosa* exist, a β-lactam/β-lactamase inhibitor such as ampicillin/sulbactam, a third-generation cephalosporin such as ceftriaxone, or a respiratory fluoroquinolone such as moxifloxacin or levofloxacin should be selected. All these therapies are active against drug-resistant *S. pneumoniae* (DRSP). If T.H. improves on one of these parenteral agents and is ready for discharge, T.H. could transition to an oral respiratory fluoroquinolone or high doses of amoxicillin/clavulanate.

Another important consideration for initial selection of antimicrobials is an evaluation of antibiotic history. Alternative antimicrobials from another class should be considered if patients have been previously treated in the last 3 months.[16] Additionally, if no improvements in symptoms occur within 72 hours, consider obtaining a sputum sample for directed therapy.[16]

The duration of treatment of antibiotics for AECOPD suffers from lack of solid evidence-based recommendation. Given findings from CB investigations, a duration of 5 to 10 days has been suggested, but this is an area in need of further research.[16]

CASE 67-2, QUESTION 5: Should T.H. be treated with corticosteroids? If so, which dose and duration would be selected?

In the setting of AECOPD, systemic corticosteroids help to improve lung function, shorten recovery time, and prevent relapses. Based on available evidence, the GOLD Guidelines recommend a corticosteroid regimen of 40 mg/day of prednisone for 5 days in patients with AECOPD.[16] This regimen would be appropriate for T.H., although an equivalent intravenous regimen could be considered if she was not able to take an oral regimen. Higher doses and longer durations of therapy have not been found to confer a clinical advantage, and intravenous and oral regimens are considered equally effective.[25,26] In those patients receiving more than 3 weeks of steroids or multiple course of steroids in the previous months, tapering the dose should be considered. Although it is more expensive, nebulized budesonide may be considered as an alternative to oral corticosteroids for treatment of AECOPD.[16]

Enhancing Patient Outcomes

CASE 67-2, QUESTION 6: What factors should be assessed for T.H. during her hospitalization, and what follow-up should be planned to help assure she recovers fully and is not readmitted for COPD?

Hospitalized patients with AECOPD should both be optimally treated, and their COPD management be assessed to decrease the likelihood of readmission. T.H.'s baseline COPD medications should be examined and adjusted based on disease severity (see Chapter 19 Chronic Obstructive Pulmonary Disease for details). Additionally, an assessment of her understanding of the role of medications (maintenance therapy vs. rescue medications), ability to use inhalers correctly, access to her prescribed medications, and discussions regarding pulmonary rehabilitation should take place.[16,17] Consideration for pharmacologic venous thromboembolism prophylaxis (see Chapter 11 Thrombosis) should also be made in this high-risk population.[16,27]

PREVENTION OF COMMON RESPIRATORY INFECTIONS BY VACCINATION

CASE 67-2, QUESTION 7: Which vaccines should be considered for T.H. as part of her COPD management?

Vaccination records for influenza and *S. pneumoniae* should be evaluated in T.H. Annual influenza vaccination is recommended for all patients ≥6 months with COPD, and it has been shown to reduce the risk of AECOPD.[16,17] Vaccination against *S. pneumoniae* with the 23-valent polysaccharide vaccine is recommended for patients ≥19 years old with COPD. Unlike the influenza vaccine, however, vaccination against *S. pneumoniae* has not been clearly linked with a reduced risk of AECOPD. The pneumococcal vaccine is recommended by guidelines, however, as part of the overall health plan of the patient.

COMMUNITY-ACQUIRED PNEUMONIA

Definition, Incidence, and Epidemiology

Pneumonia is an infection of the lung parenchyma. Community-acquired pneumonia (CAP) refers to pneumonia acquired in the absence of health care system exposure (i.e., hospital, long-term care, chronic antibiotic exposure). Diagnosis is dependent upon clinical features and radiologic evidence of an infiltrate, but it may be further supported by physical examination and/or hypoxemia.

Current estimates show that CAP accounts for 24.8 cases per 10,000 discharges in the US adult population with the elderly being primarily affected (65–79 years: 63/10,000; ≥80 years: 164.3/10,000).[28] In the pediatric population, CAP accounts for 15.7 cases per 10,000 discharges, with infants and young children showing increased risk (<2 years: 62.2/10,000).[29] The overall mortality rate for patients ≥65 years is 5.6% and is more pronounced in hospitalized patients (8.5%) compared to outpatients (3.8%).[30] Seventeen percent of older patients who develop CAP will suffer cardiac complications.[31]

Pathophysiology

Development of CAP occurs through the inhalation of infectious particles via droplets or aerosols, or the aspiration of oral flora. Rarely, hematogenous spread of bacteria from distant sources into the lungs may occur, as well as direct extension of infection to the lung from contiguous areas, such as the pleural or subdiaphragmatic spaces.

Once bacteria reach the tracheobronchial tree, defects in local pulmonary defenses facilitate infection. Contributing factors include inflammation-mediated injury to bronchial epithelium leading to depressed mucociliary clearance and a blunted cellular and humoral response. Patients with underlying or acquired immunodeficiencies are at an increased risk.

Clinical Presentation and Diagnosis

In the majority of CAP cases, patients present acutely with high fever, chills, tachypnea, tachycardia, and productive cough. Physical examination findings are usually localized to a specific lung zone and can include crackles, rhonchi, bronchial breath sounds, dullness, or egophony. On rare occasions, CAP exhibits a subacute presentation with fever, nonproductive cough, constitutional symptoms, and absent or diffuse findings on lung examination. Children with CAP may present with vomiting.

A chest radiograph or other imaging technique revealing an infiltrate is required for the diagnosis of CAP.[32] Radiographic manifestations of diseases such as congestive heart failure and malignancy can obscure the infiltrate, reinforcing the need to utilize both clinical and chest radiographic findings.

Pretreatment blood cultures and a respiratory sample (expectorated or induced sputum or endotracheal aspirate in intubated patients) should be obtained for culture and Gram stain. Although these cultures are often negative, when they are positive, they allow fine-tuning of the empirical antibiotic selection.

Overview of Drug Therapy

Antibiotic therapy for CAP is empirical in the majority of cases and should always be based on the most likely pathogen(s), underlying patient characteristics, and the severity of disease. Based on these variables, clinicians can triage patients for risk of infection caused by antibiotic-resistant pathogens and appropriately tailor therapy.

CLINICAL PRESENTATION

CASE 67-3

QUESTION 1: J.T. is a 45-year-old woman presenting to the ED with fevers, chills, and chest pain. Her symptoms have persisted for 4 days, and she has a productive cough with rusty-colored sputum and dyspnea on exertion. She has had no recent illnesses and no known sick contacts, but she was recently released from a 2-year period of incarceration. She has tried acetaminophen to alleviate her fever and chest pain. Past medical history is positive for asthma, for which she is prescribed fluticasone and albuterol, and depression, for which she takes paroxetine. Vital signs reveal a temperature of 40.1°C, heart rate of 128 beats/minute, blood pressure of 130/76 mm Hg, and respiratory rate of 32 breaths/minute with accompanying oxygen saturation of 85% on 5 L of oxygen by nasal cannula. The remainder of the physical examination is notable for orientation to person but not place or time and for diffuse crackles bilaterally, which are most apparent on the right side. Laboratory results include the following:

WBC count, 15,500 cells/μL
Hematocrit, 29.3%
Sodium, 133 mmol/L
Potassium, 3.8 mmol/L
BUN, 23 mg/dL
SCr, 0.8 mg/dL
HCO_3, 28 mEq/L
Glucose 148, mg/dL
Arterial blood gases: pH 7.42, Po_2, 61 mm Hg, Pco_2, 46 mm Hg

A test for human immunodeficiency virus is negative. Chest radiograph reveals a right lower lobe infiltrate. What signs, symptoms, and tests are consistent with CAP in J.T.?

In the majority of cases, patients with CAP present with cough with sputum production, dyspnea, and pleuritic chest pain.[33] Patients may show signs of the systemic inflammatory response syndrome, including tachycardia, tachypnea, fever, and an abnormal WBC count.[34] Auscultatory examination often reveals decreased breath sounds, crackles or rhonchi, or egophony in patients with consolidation. Signs and symptoms associated with severe pneumonia are grouped into minor and major criteria defined by the Infectious Disease Society of America (IDSA)/American Thoracic Society (ATS) Guidelines for CAP.[32] Minor criteria include respiratory rate greater than 30 breaths/minute at admission; ratios of the Pao_2 to fraction of inspired oxygen (Fio_2) (Pao_2/Fio_2) less than 250 mm Hg; systolic blood pressure (SBP) less than 90 mm Hg, or diastolic blood pressure (DBP) less than 60 mm Hg; confusion; multilobar infiltrates; SBP less than 90 mm Hg despite aggressive fluid resuscitation; BUN of at least 20 mg/dL; leukopenia; thrombocytopenia; and hypothermia. Major criteria include requirement of mechanical ventilation and requirement of vasopressors for more than 4 hours.[32]

Clinical findings and a positive infiltrate by chest radiograph or other imaging technique is required for the diagnosis of pneumonia.[32] Patients who are hospitalized based on clinical symptoms absent of positive imaging should have repeat imaging performed 24 to 48 hours post-admission.

Disease Severity

CASE 67-3, QUESTION 2: Given the clinical condition of J.T. in the ED, where should her care be continued?

The first decision after a diagnosis of CAP is to determine whether the patient requires hospitalization. Several predictive rules have been developed to facilitate site-of-care decision making. The two best-studied tools that are endorsed by the IDSA/ATS guidelines are the pneumonia severity index (PSI) and the CURB-65 rule.

The PSI uses individually scored demographic characteristics (age, gender, nursing home residence), comorbidities (liver disease, CHF, renal disease, neoplasm), physical examination findings (mental status, RR, SBP, temp, HR), and laboratory data (Na^+, glucose, Hct, BUN); the total PSI score categorizes patients into one of five classes that are associated with an escalating risk of death (Table 67-2).[35] The CURB-65, developed by the British Thoracic Society, is a simple tool that focuses on five assessments: confusion (owing to pneumonia), uremia (BUN >19 mg/dL), respiratory rate of at least 30 breaths/minute, SBP less than 90 mm Hg systolic or DBP less than 60 mm Hg, and age of at least 65 years.[36] Each criteria receives one point, and the cumulative score is associated with a specific (rising with higher score) 30-day mortality risk. Based on the score, subsequent care should be as follows: 0–1 = outpatient; 2 = admission to ward; ≥3 = ICU care. Both scales identify patients at low risk of death, but the CURB-65 has been found to be more discerning of patients who need ICU care and with the highest risk of death.[37] The need for ICU admission can be subjective; however, the IDSA/ATS guidelines recommend that patients with three or more minor criteria, or at least one major criteria for severe CAP, be admitted to the ICU.[32]

CASE 67-3, QUESTION 3: What testing should be performed to obtain a microbiologic diagnosis in J.T.?

Patient J.T. can be assessed as follows using the PSI: 45-year-old woman (35 points [45 for age – 10 for gender female]), respiratory rate greater than 30 breaths/minute (20 points), heart rate greater than 125 beats/minute (20 points), temperature greater than 40°C (15 points), hematocrit less than 30% (10 points), and altered mental status (20 points). A total score of 120 points places J.T. in risk strata IV (30-day mortality risk: 9.3%–27%), and she should be admitted to the hospital, potentially to the ICU. Using the CURB-65, J.T. has a score of 3 (30-day mortality of 9.2%) based on uremia, confusion, and increased respiratory rate, and she should be admitted to the ICU.

Microbiologic testing is optional for outpatients with CAP. However, the IDSA/ATS guidelines recommend attempting to

Table 67-2
Predicted Pneumonia Mortality and Recommended Site of Care

System and Score	Predicted 30-Day Mortality (%)	Recommended Site of Care
PSI strata I–II (≤70)	0.1–0.7	Outpatient
PSI strata III (71–90)	0.9–2.8	Admit to hospital ward
PSI strata IV–V (≥91)	9.3–27	Admit to hospital; consider ICU
CURB-65 score 0–1	0.7–2.1	Outpatient
CURB-65 score 2	9.2	Admit to hospital ward
CURB-65 score ≥3	14.5–57	Admit to ICU

CURB-65, confusion, uremia, increased respiratory rate, low blood pressure, and age ≥65 years; ICU, intensive care unit; PSI, pneumonia severity index.
Source: Fine MJ et al. A prediction rule to identify low-risk patients with community-acquired pneumonia. *N Engl J Med*. 1997;336:243.

make a microbiologic diagnosis in patients with CAP who are hospitalized.[32] Microbiologic diagnosis (via sputum or endotracheal aspirate) can help guide empiric therapy as well as identify rare and usual etiologies and cluster cases.

Urine antigen tests for pneumococcus and *Legionella pneumophila* serogroup 1 are available for patients with severe CAP. Both tests are sensitive (>80%) and specific (>90%), and have the advantage of detecting pathogens after antibiotics have been administered.

The IDSA/ATS guidelines recommend consideration of influenza testing during traditional "flu season" and during times of an outbreak.[32] Detection of influenza should be via reverse transcriptase polymerase chain reaction (RT-PCR), which is the most sensitive and specific method, with a quick turnaround time for results (4–6 hours).[38] Rapid influenza antigen detection tests may be used, but because of lower sensitivity and specificity RT-PCR is recommended to confirm negative test results reported by the rapid antigen test. Viral isolation in standard cell culture should be routinely performed with respiratory specimens during the influenza season.

Microbiology

CASE 67-3, QUESTION 4: What pathogens are most likely in J.T.?

The major pathogens for CAP are summarized in Table 67-3. The most frequently isolated bacterial pathogen, regardless of epidemiologic factors and severity of illness, accounting for approximately 27% of CAP worldwide, is *S. pneumoniae.*[32] Two survival strategies are utilized by *S. pneumoniae.*[39] The first is related to a noninvasive phenotype that uses surface adhesions, immune evasion strategies, and secretory defenses to promote long-term carriage within the nasopharynx. Deficits in host defense, such as an immunocompromised state, allow colonizing strains of low virulence to cause invasive disease. The second survival strategy depends on efficient person-to-person transmission and associated rapid disease induction by an invasive phenotype. Age younger than 2 or older than 64 years, asplenia, alcoholism, diabetes mellitus, antecedent influenza, defects in humoral immunity, and human immunodeficiency virus infection are risk factors for the invasive pneumococcal phenotype.[40] Other risk factors less likely to be associated with invasive disease include poverty and crowding, cigarette smoking, chronic lung disease, severe liver disease, recent exposure to antibiotics, and chronic proton-pump inhibitor use.

Following the introduction of the first pneumococcal conjugate vaccine in 2000 (PCV7) and the expanded PCV13 in 2010, the incidence of invasive disease and all-cause pneumonia have significantly fallen. The advent of these vaccines has not led to a significant pneumonia decline in high-risk pediatric patients, specifically children younger than 5 years with moderate-to-severe asthma, or asthma with one or more of the following comorbid conditions: heart disease, lung disease, diabetes, or neuromuscular disease.[40] The effect of the newly approved pneumococcal polysaccharide vaccine (PPSV23) on the high-risk populations has yet to be realized.

Atypical pathogens, including *L. pneumophila*, *C. pneumoniae*, and *M. pneumoniae*, account for approximately 25% of CAP worldwide.[41] However, atypical pathogens may be present in up to 60% of CAP episodes because of coinfection.[42] Polymicrobial

Table 67-3
Microorganisms Common in Community-Acquired Pneumonia

Ambulatory	Hospitalized, Non-ICU	Hospitalized, ICU
Streptococcus pneumoniae	*S. pneumoniae*	*S. pneumoniae*
Mycoplasma pneumoniae	*M. pneumoniae*	*S. aureus*
Haemophilus influenzae	*C. pneumoniae*	*Legionella* species
Chlamydophila pneumoniae	*Staphylococcus aureus*	Gram-negative bacilli
Respiratory viruses[a]	*H. influenzae*	*H. influenzae*
	Legionella species	
	Respiratory viruses[a]	

[a]Influenza A and B, adenovirus, respiratory syncytial virus, and parainfluenza.
Source: Mandell LA et al. Infectious Diseases Society of America/American Thoracic Society consensus guidelines on the management of community-acquired pneumonia in adults. *Clin Infect Dis*. 2007;44(Suppl 2):S27.

Table 67-4
Community-Acquired Pneumonia: Underlying Conditions and Commonly Encountered Pathogens

Condition	Commonly Encountered Pathogen(s)
Alcoholism	Oral anaerobes, *Klebsiella pneumoniae*, *Acinetobacter* sp., *Mycobacterium tuberculosis*
COPD or smoking	*Pseudomonas aeruginosa*, *Legionella* sp.
Aspiration	Gram-negative enteric pathogens, oral anaerobes
Lung abscess	CA-MRSA, oral anaerobes, endemic fungal pneumonia, *M. tuberculosis*, atypical mycobacteria
Exposure to bat or bird droppings	*Histoplasma capsulatum*
Exposure to birds	*Chlamydophila psittaci* (if poultry: avian influenza)
Exposure to rabbits	*Francisella tularensis*
Exposure to farm animals or parturient cats	*Coxiella burnetii* (Q fever)
HIV infection (early)	*M. tuberculosis*
HIV infection (late)	*M. tuberculosis*, *Pneumocystis jiroveci*, *Cryptococcus* sp., *Histoplasma* sp., *Aspergillus* sp., atypical mycobacteria (especially *Mycobacterium kansasii*), *Pseudomonas aeruginosa*
Hotel or cruise ship stay in previous 2 weeks	*Legionella* sp.
Travel to or residence in southwestern United States	*Coccidioides* sp., hantavirus
Travel to or residence in Southeast and East Asia	*Burkholderia pseudomallei*, avian influenza, SARS
Cough >2 weeks with whoop or post-tussive vomiting	*Bordetella pertussis*
Structural lung disease (e.g., bronchiectasis)	*P. aeruginosa*, *Burkholderia cepacia*, *Staphylococcus aureus*
Injection drug use	*S. aureus*, anaerobes, *M. tuberculosis*
Endobronchial obstruction	Anaerobes, *S. aureus*
In context of bioterrorism	*Bacillus anthracis* (anthrax), *Yersinia pestis* (plague), *F. tularensis* (tularemia)

CA-MRSA, community-acquired methicillin-resistant *Staphylococcus aureus*; COPD, chronic obstructive pulmonary disease; HIV, human immunodeficiency virus; SARS, severe acute respiratory syndrome.
Source: Mandell LA et al. Infectious Diseases Society of America/American Thoracic Society consensus guidelines on the management of community-acquired pneumonia in adults. *Clin Infect Dis*. 2007;44(Suppl 2):S27.

infection including atypical pathogens may lead to a more complicated course with extended lengths of stay. Several studies have shown that antibiotic regimens that include coverage against these pathogens demonstrate a survival benefit over regimens that do not.[43–47] Legionnaires' disease, caused primarily by *L. pneumophila* serogroup 1, accounts for 2% to 7% of CAP.[42] CAP caused by *L. pneumophila* is considered to be more severe among hospitalized patients, and it may present with high fever, nonproductive cough, low serum sodium concentration, high concentration of lactate dehydrogenase, and low platelet counts.[48,49]

Epidemiologic factors may favor the presence of certain bacterial pathogens and are listed in Table 67-4.[32] This highlights the importance of the performance of a thorough patient history to assist in the direction of therapy. Additional factors such as chronic oral steroid use (≥10 mg prednisone / day), immunosuppression, and frequent antibiotic therapy will likely place the patient into the category of health care–associated pneumonia (HCAP), which will require augmented therapy options.[49]

S. aureus is recognized as a major cause of nosocomial pneumonia; however, its significance in CAP is less clear. Traditionally, *S. aureus* has not been considered a common cause of CAP (approximately 2.5% of cases), but it is most likely to occur in association with influenza or in patients with lung abscess.[32,50] Community-associated MRSA (CA-MRSA) is significantly different from the typical hospital-acquired strain. These differences include susceptibility to non–β-lactam antibiotics (e.g., clindamycin and doxycycline) and clinical syndrome (necrotizing radiographic presentation, empyema formation, hemoptysis, and profound hypoxemia) associated with toxins including Panton–Valentine leukocidin.[51] Toxin-producing strains are also part of methicillin-sensitive *S. aureus*'s (MSSA) virulence.[52] The outcomes of patients with MRSA and MSSA CAP are similarly poor with prolonged length of hospital stay and a nearly 25% mortality.[53]

The influenza A H1N1 outbreak in 2009 highlighted the contribution of respiratory viruses as an etiology of CAP. Respiratory virus can be the primary cause of CAP, but it can also be a major contributing factor that predisposes the patient to infection by another pathogen, often bacterial (11%–15%). Using contemporary nucleic acid amplification tests, the incidence of viral CAP ranges from 19% to 32%.[54–56] Respiratory viruses that cause CAP include influenza A and B, respiratory syncytial virus, rhinovirus, parainfluenza, adenovirus, human metapneumovirus, and coronavirus. In patients coinfected with both viral and bacterial pathogens, the most common bacteria are *S. pneumoniae*, *S. aureus*, and atypicals.

Possible microbes causing J.T.'s CAP include *S. pneumoniae*, *M. pneumoniae*, *C. pneumonia*, *S. aureus*, *H. influenzae*, *Legionella* species, and respiratory viruses.

Antibiotic Therapy

CASE 67-3, QUESTION 5: Which antimicrobial agent(s) should be chosen for the initial management of J.T.?

An approach to the patient with CAP, and recommended antibiotic regimens based on the patient's site of care and severity of illness, are provided in Figure 67-1. Delayed antibiotic therapy has been associated with an increased length of hospital stay and decreased survival in CAP; therefore, a rapid and correct diagnosis

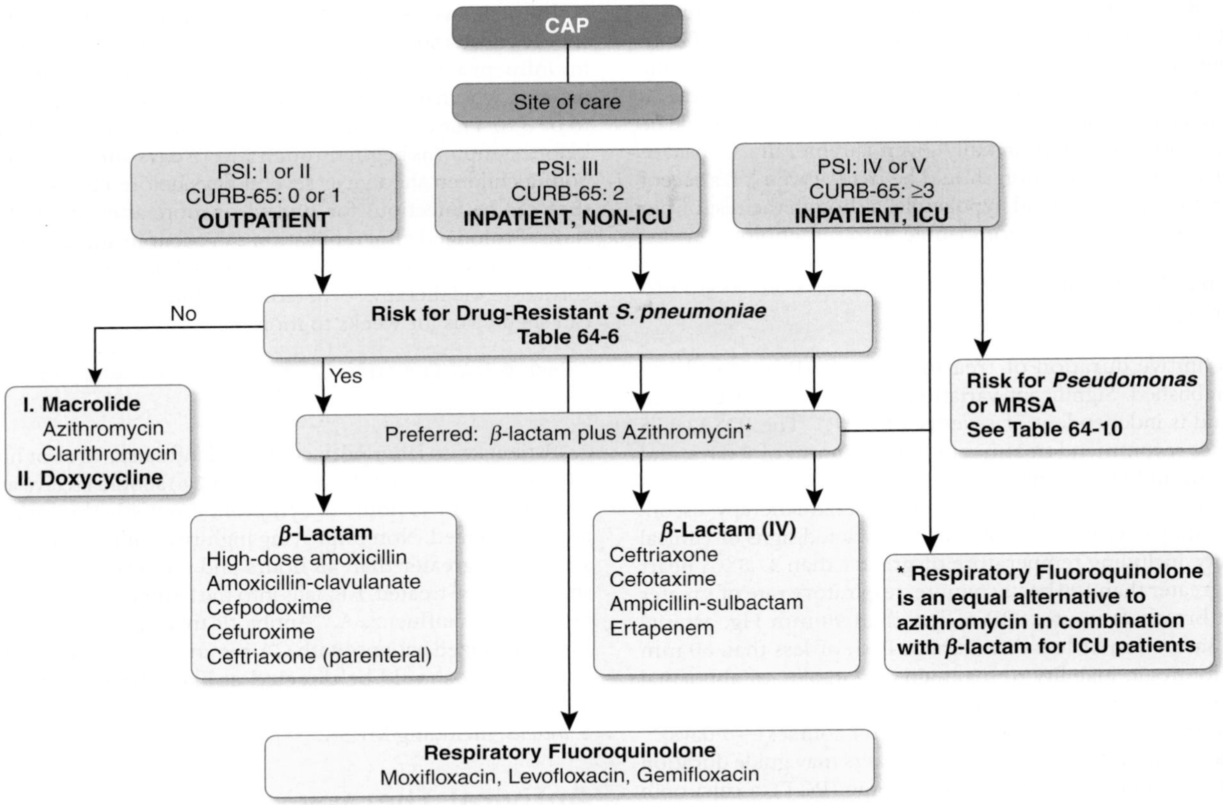

Figure 67-1 Approach to empiric antibiotic therapy in patients with community-acquired pneumonia. CAP, community-acquired pneumonia; CURB-65, confusion, uremia, respiratory rate, blood pressure, and age of at least 65 years; IV, intravenous; MRSA, methicillin-resistant *Staphylococcus aureus*; PSI, pneumonia severity index.

is imperative.[57,58] The most recent IDSA/ATS CAP treatment guidelines recommend the first dose of antibiotic be given in the ED in an effort to avoid treatment delays associated with the hospital admission process.[32]

All patients should be empirically treated for pneumococcus and atypical pathogens. The choice of the initial regimen should be based on medical comorbidities or epidemiologic factors, including the possibility of antibiotic-resistant causative organisms. Factors that increase the risk of DRSP are located in Table 67-5.

Macrolide antibiotics (e.g., azithromycin and clarithromycin) or doxycycline are preferred as monotherapy for noncomplicated outpatient treatment and are used in combination with β-lactams for complicated outpatients and those treated on inpatient wards.[32] Macrolides should not be employed as monotherapy for inpatient care, as nearly 30% of pneumococcal isolates demonstrate resistance.[59] Several mechanisms are responsible for macrolide resistance, including ribosomal modification mediated by *erm* (B), efflux from the bacterial cell controlled by *mef* (A), or a combination of both.

Patients with comorbidities, exposure to antibiotics within the past 3 months, DRSP risk factors, or who live in an area with a high prevalence of DRSP should receive a combination β-lactam and macrolide regimen or a respiratory fluoroquinolone (e.g., levofloxacin, moxifloxacin, and gemifloxacin).[32] Preferred β-lactams include high-dose amoxicillin (1 g PO TID), amoxicillin-clavulanate (2 g PO BID), or ceftriaxone (1–2 g IV daily). β-lactam resistance occurs through alteration of one or more of the penicillin-binding proteins that mediate the bacterial cell wall production.[60] Penicillin-binding protein alterations in resistant strains decrease the affinity to all β-lactams such that higher concentrations are required for binding and inhibition of the enzyme. Thus, appropriate dosing of β-lactams in the treatment of CAP minimizes development of resistance and promotes optimal clinical outcomes.[61,62] Fluoroquinolones are the preferred agents for CAP in penicillin-allergic patients. Fluoroquinolone resistance, mediated by mutations in the DNA gyrase gene *gyrA* and the topoisomerase IV genes *parC* and *parE*, as well as efflux pump–mediated, has increased because of their widespread use; however, overall pneumococcal resistance rates are low.[63] IDSA/ATS guideline-concordant therapy for hospitalized patients has been associated with improved patient outcomes including decreases in time to achieve clinical stability, total duration of parenteral therapy, and hospital length of stay, as well as improved in-hospital survival.[64,65]

Table 67-5
Risk Factors for β-Lactam-Resistant *Streptococcus pneumoniae*

Age <2 or >65 years
β-Lactam therapy within the previous 3 months (also at risk for organisms associated with HCAP)
Alcoholism
Medical comorbidities
Immunosuppressive illness or therapy (also at risk for organisms associated with HCAP)
Exposure to a child in a day-care center

HCAP, health care–associated pneumonia.
Source: Mandell LA et al. Infectious Diseases Society of America/American Thoracic Society consensus guidelines on the management of community-acquired pneumonia in adults. *Clin Infect Dis*. 2007;44(Suppl 2):S27.

J.T.'s treatment should be started in the ED after obtaining a respiratory specimen and pretreatment blood cultures for Gram stain and culture. J.T. does not possess risk factors for specific bacteria, such as *Enterobacteriaceae* or *P. aeruginosa*; therefore, a β-lactam (ceftriaxone) plus a macrolide (azithromycin) should be initiated empirically, both initially given parenterally. Consideration of CA-MRSA infection should be made given J.T.'s recent incarceration and profound hypoxemia, although the rest of her clinical presentation is not compatible with this etiology.

CASE 67-3, QUESTION 6: What is the appropriate length of therapy for J.T.?

A definitive duration of treatment for CAP has not been well established. Significant variation in duration of treatment exists and is independent of severity of CAP.[66] The IDSA/ATS guidelines recommend treatment for a minimum of 5 days, and patients should be afebrile for 48 to 72 hours before therapy is discontinued. In addition, patients should not have therapy discontinued if they have two or more CAP-associated signs of clinical instability, including temperature of greater than 37.8°C, heart rate of greater than 100 beats/minute, respiratory rate of greater than 24 breaths/minute, SBP of less than 90 mm Hg, arterial oxygen saturation of less than 90% or Pao_2 of less than 60 mm Hg on room air, inability to maintain oral intake, or abnormal mental status. Evidence suggests that longer courses of therapy (>7 days) are no more effective than shorter courses (3–7 days).[67]

Serial monitoring of infection biomarkers may guide duration of antibiotic therapy. A fall in procalcitonin (PCT), a calcitonin precursor elevated in infection, trauma, and burns, has been associated with a significant reduction in total duration of antibiotic use compared with standard care and may be a useful indicator of adequate therapy.[68]

CASE 67-4

QUESTION 1: F.E. is a 56-year-old man presenting to the ED with the complaints of fever, chills, nausea, and vomiting for the last 7 days, and more recently, shortness of breath with productive cough with white sputum for the past 4 days. He visited his family approximately 2 days prior to symptoms, where two of his relatives were thought to have an unconfirmed viral illness. Initial assessment reveals the patient to be alert and oriented times three, but falling asleep during assessment, pulses present with brisk capillary refill, decreased lung sounds bilaterally, and no peripheral edema. Past medical history is significant for hypertension and diabetes mellitus. The patient has an allergy to penicillin, with a reported reaction of rash. Medications at home include aspirin 81 mg PO daily, hydrochlorothiazide 25 mg PO daily, lisinopril 20 mg PO daily, and atorvastatin 40 mg PO daily. Social history is significant for smoking one pack of cigarettes per week. In the ED he had a temperature of 38.9°C, heart rate of 112 beats/minute, respiratory rate of 22 breaths/minute, SBP/DBP of 126/80 mm Hg, and oxygen saturation of 93% on 2 L. Laboratory results include the following:

WBC count, 2,900 cells/μL
Hematocrit, 47.1%
Platelets 129,000 cells/μL
Sodium, 127 mmol/L
Potassium, 4.6 mmol/L
BUN, 7 mg/dL
SCr, 0.73 mg/dL
Glucose 117, mg/dL

Chest radiograph showed bilateral interstitial infiltrates; RT-PCR was positive for influenza A. What is the most likely reason for F.E.'s influenza infection?

Influenza viruses spread when an infected person coughs or sneezes near a susceptible person.[69] The usual incubation period for influenza is 1 to 4 days, and the time between onset among patients who have come into contact with one another is likely to be 3 to 4 days.[70] Adults can shed influenza virus from the day before symptoms begin through 5 to 10 days after illness onset.[71] Young children shed virus several days before illness onset, and they can be infectious for 10 days or more after onset of symptoms. Prolonged viral replication can occur in adults with severe disease, including those with comorbidities or those receiving corticosteroid therapy.[72,73] Severely immunocompromised persons can shed virus for weeks to months.[74,75]

CASE 67-4, QUESTION 2: Should F.E. be treated with antiviral agents?

Patients with laboratory-confirmed influenza virus or high-risk patients suspected of infection (Table 67-6) should receive antiviral therapy within 48 hours of symptom onset whether or not they are hospitalized. Non-improving high-risk patients or those with symptoms greater than 48 hours and requiring hospitalization should also be treated. F.E. falls into the latter category and should be treated for influenza A.[38] Antibiotic treatment is recommended for hospitalized patients with CAP, even if influenza is suspected, and therapy should be directed at likely bacterial pathogens associated with influenza such as *S. pneumoniae*, *S. pyogenes*, and *S. aureus*, including MRSA.[32]

Antiviral Therapy

CASE 67-4, QUESTION 3: Which antiviral agent(s) should F.E. be treated with?

Table 67-6
Patients at High Risk of Complications from Influenza

Unvaccinated infants aged 12–24 months
Persons with asthma or other chronic pulmonary diseases (e.g., COPD, cystic fibrosis)
Persons with hemodynamically significant cardiac disease
Persons with immunosuppressive disorders or who are receiving immunosuppressive therapy
HIV-infected persons
Persons with sickle cell anemia and other hemoglobinopathies
Persons with diseases that require long-term, high-dose aspirin therapy, such as rheumatoid arthritis
Persons with chronic renal dysfunction
Persons with cancer
Persons with chronic metabolic disease, such as diabetes mellitus
Persons with central nervous system disorders that may compromise the handling of secretions such as neuromuscular disorders, cerebral vascular accidents, or seizure disorders
Adults aged ≥65 years
Residents of any age of nursing homes or other long-term care institutions

COPD, chronic obstructive pulmonary disease; HIV, human immunodeficiency virus.
Source: Harper SA et al. Seasonal influenza in adults and children: diagnosis, treatment, chemoprophylaxis, and institutional outbreak management: clinical practice guidelines of the Infectious Diseases Society of America. *Clin Infect Dis*. 2009;48:1003.

Table 67-7
Comparison of Current Neuraminidase Inhibitors for Influenza

	Oseltamivir	Zanamivir
Influenza activity	A and B	A and B
Route of administration	Oral	Oral inhalation
Treatment dosage	Adults: 75 mg PO BID Children ≥12 months: ≤15 kg: 30 mg PO BID 15–23 kg: 45 mg PO BID 24–40 kg: 60 mg PO BID ≥60 kg: 75 mg PO BID	Adults: two inhalations (5 mg each) PO BID Children ≥7 years: two inhalations (5 mg each) PO BID
Side effects	Nausea, vomiting, abdominal pain	Nasal and throat discomfort, headache, bronchospasm

BID, two times a day; PO, by mouth.
Source: Harper SA et al. Seasonal influenza in adults and children: diagnosis, treatment, chemoprophylaxis, and institutional outbreak management: clinical practice guidelines of the Infectious Diseases Society of America. *Clin Infect Dis*. 2009;48:1003.

Influenza susceptibility profiles to antiviral agents evolve rapidly, and treating clinicians should be familiar with updated resistance data found at the Centers for Disease Control and Prevention website: www.cdc.gov/flu. Neuraminidase inhibitors including oseltamivir or zanamivir are the primary antiviral agents recommended for the treatment of influenza (Table 67-7).[38] The inhibition of neuraminidase prevents cleavage of sialic acid residues on the cell surface of the virus, thereby preventing the release of virus from infected cells. Considering the high rate of resistance, adamantines (amantadine and rimantadine) are not currently recommended for treatment of influenza. FE should be treated with either oseltamivir 75 mg PO BID or zanamivir 10 mg inhaled every 12 hours. Both medications should be used for a total of 5 days.

Neuraminidase inhibitors should be initiated as soon as possible after illness onset, ideally within 48 hours, as this is when the majority of viral replication occurs. However, treatment of any person with confirmed or suspected influenza requiring hospitalization is recommended for up to 96 hours post-illness onset.[76,77] For patients whose illness is prolonged, treatment regimens may need to be extended beyond 5 days.

Development of resistance to zanamivir or oseltamivir has been identified during treatment of seasonal influenza.[78] Oseltamivir resistance is caused by a specific mutation leading to a histidine to tyrosine substitution (H275Y) in neuraminidase.[79] Oseltamivir resistance, which can occur within one week of treatment initiation, has been reported particularly among immunocompromised patients infected with the 2009 H1N1 virus.[80,81]

HOSPITAL-ACQUIRED PNEUMONIA, AND VENTILATOR-ASSOCIATED PNEUMONIA

Definitions and Incidence

Despite advances in therapy and prevention, hospital-acquired pneumonia (HAP) and ventilator-associated pneumonia (VAP) are associated with significant morbidity and mortality. HAP is defined as pneumonia that occurs at least 48 hours after hospital admission. VAP refers to pneumonia that arises 48 to 72 hours after endotracheal intubation. HCAP occurs within 48 hours of admission in patients with previous risk factors for infection caused by potentially drug-resistant pathogens, including hospitalization in an acute-care hospital for 2 or more days within 90 days of infection; residence in a nursing home or long-term care facility; receipt of recent IV antibiotic therapy, chemotherapy, or wound care within the past 30 days of the current infection; living in close contact with a person with a multidrug-resistant pathogen; or attending a hospital or hemodialysis clinic.[49]

Epidemiology

HAP is the second most common nosocomial infection in the United States, with urinary tract infections as the most common.[49] Based on a prospective cohort study, approximately 7% of ICU patients developed HAP and over 75% of them had VAP.[82] A retrospective cohort study of 4,543 hospitalized patients with culture-positive pneumonia observed that HCAP accounted for 21.7% of the cases, HAP for 18.4%, and VAP for 11%. Mortality rates associated with HAP groups were comparable (19.8% and 18.8%, respectively) and both were significantly lower than those for VAP (29.3%). Mean lengths of stay differed with pneumonia category: HAP patients for 15.2 ± 13.6 days, and VAP patients for 23 ± 20.2 days.[83]

The disease onset is an important epidemiologic variable and risk factor for specific pathogens and outcomes in patients with HAP and VAP. Early-onset HAP and VAP are defined as occurring within the first 4 days of hospitalization, usually carry a better prognosis, and are more likely caused by antibiotic-sensitive bacteria. Late-onset HAP and VAP (occurring after ≥5 days of hospitalization) are more likely to be caused by multidrug-resistant (MDR) pathogens and are associated with increased morbidity and mortality.[49]

Pathogenesis

Microorganisms gain access into the lower respiratory tract via aspiration of oropharyngeal pathogens and leakage of secretions around the endotracheal tube cuff in intubated patients.[84,85] Invasive-care devices, contaminated equipment, and transfer of microorganisms among staff and patients serve as the primary pathogen sources,[86] and although more controversial, the gastrointestinal tract may also play a role in bacterial colonization.[87]

Clinical Presentation and Diagnosis

HAP and VAP are all diagnosed on the basis of radiographic findings, clinical features, and health care setting when there is initial evidence of infection. Patients must demonstrate new or progressive infiltrates on imaging as well as two of three of the following signs: fever greater than 38°C, leukopenia or leukocytosis, and purulent sputum. Patients will often experience declines in oxygen saturation, but this finding is less specific for determining the need for empiric antimicrobial agents.[88]

Respiratory cultures may be taken from endotracheal aspirates, bronchoalveolar lavage, or protected-specimen brush samples. Blood cultures lack sensitivity, and when positive, consideration should also be given to a potential extrapulmonary source.[89]

Overview of Treatment

The IDSA/ATS have published guidelines for the treatment of HAP.[49] The five major principles underlying the management of HAP and VAP include the following: (a) failure to initiate prompt, appropriate therapy is associated with increased mortality; (b) the variability of bacteriology from one institution to another, as well as within specific sites in a hospital, can be significant; (c) the overuse of antibiotics should be avoided by focusing on accurate diagnosis; (d) therapy should be tailored based on lower respiratory tract cultures and the duration of therapy should be shortened; and (e) prevention strategies directed at modifiable risk factors should be applied. The likelihood of an infection with a potential pathogen is based largely on the time to onset of HAP, severity of the condition, and underlying risk factors. In general, patients with early-onset disease who are not severely ill and have no risk factors for MDR organisms can be treated with a single agent including a non-antipseudomonal third-generation cephalosporin or an antipneumococcal fluoroquinolone (Table 67-8). Empiric therapy in those with late-onset or severe disease should include a combination of antibiotics active against *Pseudomonas*. This regimen usually includes an antipseudomonal β-lactam, such as cefepime, imipenem, meropenem, doripenem, or piperacillin-tazobactam, plus either an aminoglycoside or ciprofloxacin/levofloxacin. Vancomycin or linezolid should be added if MRSA risk factors are present or there is a high institutional incidence (Table 67-9).[49]

Microbiology

The major difference in the bacteriology between CAP and HAP, HCAP, or VAP is a shift to gram-negative pathogens, MDR pathogens, and MRSA. Gram-negative bacilli commonly colonize oropharyngeal secretions of patients with moderate-to-severe (acute and chronic) diseases without exposure to broad-spectrum antibiotics.[90] Patients admitted to the hospital with acute illnesses are rapidly colonized with gram-negative organisms. Approximately 20% are colonized on the first hospital day, and this number increases with the duration of hospitalization and severity of illness. Approximately 35% to 45% of hospitalized patients and up to 100% of critically ill patients will be colonized within 3 to 5 days of admission.[90,91]

In the past, gram-negative bacteria accounted for 50% to 70% of all cases of HAP and VAP[49,92–96]; however, gram-positive organisms have become increasingly common, with *S. aureus* responsible for upward of 40% of cases of HAP and VAP. This is in stark contrast to CAP bacteriology, in which *S. aureus* represents 25% or less of cases. *P. aeruginosa* remains the most prevalent gram-negative organism in HAP and VAP, accounting for approximately 20% to 25% of infections.[97] In patients who are ventilator dependent, *Acinetobacter* species is an increasingly common gram-negative pathogen. Other organisms with special risk factors include *Legionella*, which is associated with high-dose corticosteroid use and outbreaks secondary to water supplies and cooling systems,[91,98] and *Aspergillus*, which is associated with neutropenia or organ transplantation.[99]

Risk factors for MDR pathogens include patient-specific factors such as antimicrobial therapy in the previous 90 days, current hospitalization of 5 days or more, and immunosuppressive disease or therapy. Coverage for MDR organisms should also be initiated if there is a high frequency of community, hospital, or health care facility (i.e., nursing home) antibiotic resistance.[100]

CASE 67-5

QUESTION 1: M.L. is a 71-year-old man admitted to the hospital for a deep vein thrombosis. His past medical history is significant for chronic kidney disease (CrCl 40 mL/minute), diabetes mellitus, COPD, GERD, hypertension, and a recent diagnosis of non–small cell lung cancer for which he is not currently receiving chemotherapy. M.L.'s home medications include lisinopril, famotidine, aspirin, insulin glargine, insulin aspart, tiotropium, fluticasone/salmeterol, and as-needed albuterol. What characteristics does M.L. exhibit that place him at risk for HAP?

Table 67-8

Empiric Therapy for Hospital-Acquired Pneumonia and Ventilator-Associated Pneumonia in Patients with No Known Risk Factors for Multidrug Resistant Pathogens and Onset <5 Days

Possible Pathogens	Recommended Therapy	Dosage
Streptococcus pneumoniae[a]	Ceftriaxone	1–2 g IV every 24 hours
Haemophilus influenza	*Or*	
MSSA		
Antibiotic-sensitive enteric GNB	Levofloxacin	750 mg IV every 24 hours
Escherichia coli	*Or*	
Klebsiella pneumonia	Moxifloxacin	400 mg IV every 24 hours
Enterobacter sp.		
Proteus sp.	*Or*	
Serratia marcescens	Ertapenem	1 g IV q24 hours
	Or	
	Ampicillin-sulbactam	3 g IV q6 hours

[a]The frequency of penicillin-resistant *S. pneumoniae and* multidrug-resistant *S. pneumoniae is* increasing; levofloxacin or moxifloxacin are preferred to ciprofloxacin.

GNB, gram-negative bacilli; IV, intravenous; MSSA, methicillin-sensitive *Staphylococcus aureus*.

Source: Management of Adults With Hospital-acquired and Ventilator-associated Pneumonia: 2016 Clinical Practice Guidelines by the Infectious Diseases Society of America and the American Thoracic Society. *Clin Inf Dis*. 2016;63;1–51

Table 67-9

Empiric Therapy for Hospital-Acquired Pneumonia and Ventilator-Associated Pneumonia in Patients with Late-Onset Infection (≥5 days) or Risk Factors for Multidrug Resistant Pathogens

Possible Pathogens	Recommended Combination Therapy	Adult Dosage[a]
MDR pathogens	*Antipseudomonal cephalosporin*	
Pseudomonas aeruginosa	Cefepime	1–2 g IV every 8–12 hours
	Ceftazidime	2 g IV every 8 hours
Klebsiella pneumoniae (ESBL$^+$)[b]	*Or*	
Acinetobacter sp.[b]	*Antipseudomonal carbapenem*	
	Imipenem–cilastatin	500 mg IV every 6 hours or 1 g IV every 8 hours
	Doripenem	500 mg IV every 6–8 hours[c]
	Meropenem	1 g IV every 8 hours
	Or	
	β-Lactam/β-Lactamase inhibitor	
	Piperacillin–tazobactam	3.375–4.5 g IV every 8 hours (infused over 4 hours)
	Plus	
	Antipseudomonal fluoroquinolone[d]	
	Ciprofloxacin	400 mg IV every 8 hours
	Or	
	Levofloxacin	750 mg IV every 24 hours
	Or	
	Aminoglycoside	
	Amikacin	15–20 mg/kg IV every 24 hours[e]
	Gentamicin	5–7 mg/kg IV every 24 hours[e]
	Tobramycin	5–7 mg/kg IV every 24 hours[e]
MRSA[d]	*Plus*	
	Vancomycin	15 mg/kg every 12 hours
	Or	
	Linezolid	600 mg every 12 hours[f]
Legionella pneumophila[g]	Azithromycin	500 mg IV every 24 hours

[a]Dosages are based on normal renal and hepatic function.
[b]If an ESBL$^+$ strain, such as *K. pneumoniae*, or an *Acinetobacter* sp. is suspected, a carbapenem is a reliable choice.
[c]Studied infusion times range from 30 minutes to 4 hours.
[d]If MRSA risk factors are present, or there is a high incidence locally.
[e]Trough levels for gentamicin and tobramycin should be <1 mcg/mL; for amikacin, they should be <4–5 mcg/mL.
[f]Trough levels for vancomycin should be 15–20 mcg/mL.
[g]If *L. pneumophila* is suspected, a combination antibiotic regimen including a macrolide (e.g., azithromycin) or a fluoroquinolone (e.g., ciprofloxacin or levofloxacin) should be used.
ESBL, extended-spectrum β-lactamase; IV, intravenous; MDR, multidrug-resistant; MRSA, methicillin-resistant *Staphylococcus aureus*.
Source: Management of Adults With Hospital-acquired and Ventilator-associated Pneumonia: 2016 Clinical Practice Guidelines by the Infectious Diseases Society of America and the American Thoracic Society. *Clin Inf Dis*. 2016;63;1–51.

Several risk factors for HAP have been identified, including intubation and mechanical ventilation, aspiration, a patient's body position, the administration of enteral feeding, prior use of antibacterial agents, gastrointestinal bleeding prophylaxis (i.e., histamine type 2 antagonists and proton-pump inhibitors), immunosuppressive therapy, and poor nutrition status or glucose control. Other nonmodifiable risk factors associated with developing HAP include age older than 70 years and chronic lung disease.

An important factor in the cause of pneumonia is colonization of the oropharynx, common in alcoholism and with prolonged hospitalization, and previous antimicrobial exposure.[49] Several factors may contribute to the colonization of M.L.'s oropharynx with gram-negative bacteria. In addition to his pulmonary disease, an altered immune response in diabetics and the elderly can predispose M.L. to respiratory infection. The use of drugs that inhibit the production of gastric acid, such as famotidine and omeprazole, increases the possibility of oropharyngeal colonization and pneumonia; yet acid suppressive medications are commonly used to prevent gastric stress ulcers in mechanically ventilated patients.[101–104]

Antibiotic Therapy

Case 67-5, Question 2: Three days after admission, while receiving anticoagulation for the deep vein thrombosis, M.L. exhibits a fever to 39.3°C. Antibiotics were inappropriately delayed, and over the next 24 hours, his respiratory function declined significantly requiring intubation (PaO_2/FIO_2 250). Additionally, objective findings showed elevated WBC count (17,200 cells/μL), left shift (immature leukocytes, bands 18%), and a new infiltrate on his daily chest radiograph. Sputum cultures are sent, and the decision is made to start M.L. on antibiotics. How should antimicrobial therapy be managed for M.L.?

Because delays in the administration of appropriate therapy have been associated with increased hospital mortality from HAP, the prompt administration of empiric therapy is essential. Importantly, changing therapy once culture results are available may not reduce the excess risk of hospital mortality if inappropriate initial therapy is selected.[49] To this end, local bacteriologic patterns and in vitro susceptibility data should be made available and updated as frequently as possible to allow for appropriate selection of initial empirical therapy. In addition to the selection of an appropriate agent, the selection of adequate dosing regimens will optimize the pharmacodynamic properties of the antibacterial agent(s) and improve clinical outcomes and mortality rates.[49]

Resolution of HAP can be defined both clinically and microbiologically. Clinical improvement usually is apparent after the first 48 to 72 hours of therapy. During this time, the selected antibacterial regimen should not be changed unless progressive deterioration takes place or microbiologic studies confirm the pathogen.

If culture results are negative or inconclusive (because of known specimen contamination with mouth flora), the patient's response to the initial antibiotic therapy should be used to evaluate modification of the antibiotic regimen. If the patient responds to the initial regimen, consideration should be given to narrowing coverage to the most likely causative pathogens.

If the patient is not responding to the initial antibiotic therapy, one should consider whether (a) the pathogen is not covered in the initial choice of antibiotic therapy, (b) the dose of antibiotic is insufficient, and (c) any other factors are responsible for the failure to respond to therapy. Such factors include poor pulmonary clearance of necrotic tissue and cellular debris, lung abscesses or empyema, and severely altered host defenses leading to a rapidly fatal underlying disease.

Of note, if one of the following organisms is isolated (*Serratia*, *Pseudomonas*, indole-positive *Proteus*, *Citrobacter*, or *Enterobacter* species), in vitro reports indicating susceptibility should be carefully evaluated, as these organisms often possess an inducible β-lactamase gene (also referred to as a type I β-lactamase enzyme).[105] In vitro testing may demonstrate susceptibility to third-generation cephalosporins and extended-spectrum penicillins, but this may not translate into efficacy in the clinical setting. As a possible scenario of infection with these organisms, after initiation with one of the above agents, the patient may initially respond; however, after approximately 1 week, the patient's condition begins to worsen. Because treatment with the β-lactam agent induces the expression of the type I enzyme, a subsequent sputum specimen sent after approximately 1 week is now likely to demonstrate resistance to the third-generation cephalosporins and extended-spectrum penicillins.[105] Although cefepime is more likely to be active against these isolates, a large inoculum of organisms (e.g., that present in pneumonia) can result in β-lactamase degradation of this agent as well.[106] Considering that this phenomenon will not be identified by using usual in vitro testing, cefepime should be used cautiously in these patients.[107] The preferred therapy in these patients includes trimethoprim–sulfamethoxazole, a fluoroquinolone, or a carbapenem.[105] *Acinetobacter* species are increasingly resistant to many commonly used antibacterial agents. Treatment of this often multiply-resistant pathogen requires the use of very high doses of ampicillin–sulbactam (up to 24 g/day) or colistin.[108,109]

CASE 67-5, QUESTION 3: Seventy-two hours after empiric antibiotics were initiated, the microbiology laboratory reports that greater than 100,000 colonies/mL of MRSA have grown on M.L.'s sputum culture. Antibiotics are de-escalated to vancomycin therapy alone, to which the isolate is susceptible. After a loading dose and aggressive maintenance regimen, vancomycin trough concentrations have been 17 to 22 mcg/mL. However, M.L. remains febrile, demonstrates progression of his infiltrates on chest radiograph, and has acute worsening of renal function requiring dialysis and necessitating vancomycin dose adjustment. Repeat tracheal cultures again grow only *S. aureus* with susceptibility to vancomycin, sulfamethoxazole–trimethoprim, daptomycin, and linezolid. Should M.L.'s antibiotic therapy be modified?

The first IDSA MRSA infection treatment guidelines[110] were published in 2011 and are discussed subsequently in collaboration with the first vancomycin therapeutic monitoring guidelines jointly developed by the American Society of Health-System Pharmacists, the Society of Infectious Diseases Pharmacists, and the IDSA.[111]

For MRSA pneumonia, IV vancomycin, or linezolid 600 mg by mouth (PO) or IV twice daily, or clindamycin 600 mg PO or IV 3 times daily (if the strain is susceptible) is recommended for 7 to 21 days, depending on the extent of infection. Daptomycin should not be used for the treatment of MRSA pneumonia, because its activity is inhibited by pulmonary surfactant, rendering it inactive in the treatment of lung infection.[110]

VANCOMYCIN

The recommended dosing of IV vancomycin is 15 to 20 mg/kg/dose (actual body weight) every 8 to 12 hours, not to exceed 2 g/dose, for patients with normal renal function. A loading dose of 25 to 30 mg/kg (actual body weight) may be considered. Some patients may experience an adverse event during the infusion of vancomycin known as red man syndrome. Extending the infusion time to 2 hours for larger doses or premedicating patients who have experienced this phenomenon with an antihistamine may alleviate this adverse event.[110]

Vancomycin trough concentrations of 15 to 20 mcg/mL are recommended for the treatment of pneumonia[110] as higher trough serum concentrations should increase the likelihood of optimizing the area under the curve (AUC) and minimum inhibitory concentration (MIC) and, therefore, take into account higher vancomycin MIC values appreciated in some isolates. It has also been postulated that targeting higher trough values may help to overcome vancomycin's inherent impaired penetration into epithelial lining fluid and respiratory secretions.[111] Of note, there are no data confirming that achievement of more aggressive trough levels is associated with improvement in clinical cure.[112]

LINEZOLID

Linezolid achieves higher concentrations in lung epithelial fluid than in plasma[113] and serves as an alternative to vancomycin for the treatment of MRSA pneumonia. A retrospective analysis of two prospective trials[114,115] for the treatment of HAP found that patients in the subgroup of MRSA cases randomly assigned to linezolid experienced higher cure rates and lower mortality compared with vancomycin.[116] In contrast, a meta-analysis of eight randomized control trials comparing glycopeptide antibiotics to linezolid for suspected MRSA pneumonia found no evidence to support superiority of linezolid.[117] The ZEPHyR study compared linezolid with vancomycin in patients with proven nosocomial MRSA pneumonia in a randomized, double-blind fashion. This is the largest trial conducted in this population to date, and it showed a statistical improvement with linezolid in clinical outcomes at the end of study; yet the confidence interval was close to no significance and only showed a benefit with linezolid in identified nosocomial MRSA pneumonia.[118] These results make it difficult for initial selection over vancomycin for empiric therapy of MRSA coverage. Therefore, it remains uncertain whether linezolid or vancomycin should be considered superior.

M.L. is at risk for MDR pathogens (current hospitalization of 5 days or more and immunosuppressive diseases) and should be started empirically with an anti-MRSA agent (vancomycin), and double coverage for resistant gram-negative pathogens (cefepime and gentamicin or ciprofloxacin). (Table 67-9) Dosing and frequency of antimicrobial agents will require renal adjustments because of M.L.'s chronic renal issues. When culture results are known, the antibiotic regimen can be modified and individualized. For patients with uncomplicated HAP or VAP, who have received appropriate empiric antibiotics with a satisfactory subsequent clinical response, 7 to 10 days of therapy is recommended.[49] However, patients infected with nonfermenting gram-negative bacilli (i.e., pseudomonas and acinetobacter) may benefit from longer courses (14 days or greater) to prevent recurrence.[119] M.L.'s clinical response should be monitored to determine whether the selected antibiotics are effective in treating this infection. These parameters include the ability to discontinue mechanical intubation and decreases in temperature and WBC count with resolution of the left shift.

Since M.L. remains febrile despite MRSA sensitivities to vancomycin with appropriate trough concentrations, it is appropriate to consider alternative MRSA coverage. Despite MRSA susceptibility to daptomycin, the drug does not penetrate lung surfactant, and therefore it is not appropriate to use in the treatment of pneumonia. Sulfamethoxazole–trimethoprim is a less appealing option owing to the patient's dialysis requirement. M.L. should be switched to linezolid. Linezolid quickly reaches high lung concentrations and is safe to use in the setting of acute renal failure. Linezolid has been associated with thrombocytopenia and neutropenia. Platelet counts and WBC should be monitored at baseline and at least every 7 days during treatment.

ALTERNATIVE AGENTS

Doxycycline, clindamycin, and sulfamethoxazole–trimethoprim are not reliably active against MRSA strains, and recent research has focused on novel agents. Although active against MRSA, tigecycline has been associated with worsened clinical outcomes when used for the treatment of HAP, including MRSA pneumonia.[120] Telavancin has been compared with vancomycin in the treatment of HAP caused by gram-positive pathogens. Treatment with telavancin achieved higher clinical cure rates in patients with monomicrobial *S. aureus* infection and in those with isolates that demonstrated a vancomycin MIC of at least 1 mcg/mL. However, lower cure rates were observed in the telavancin group in those who had mixed infections. Telavancin use was also associated with a higher incidence in serum creatinine elevation; yet the drug was approved by the US Food and Drug Administration in 2013 for HAP when other alternatives are not suitable.[121]

AMINOGLYCOSIDES

Individualization of aminoglycoside dosing is imperative as the therapeutic outcome (efficacy and toxicity) of aminoglycosides correlates with plasma concentrations in patients with gram-negative pneumonia.[122–125] In patients receiving multiple daily doses of gentamicin or tobramycin and achieving a 1-hour postinfusion peak plasma concentration of greater than 7 mcg/mL, a successful outcome occurs more often than in those with lower plasma concentrations.

The aminoglycosides are concentration-dependent killing antibiotics. The rate and extent of killing organisms is maximized by increasing their peak serum concentration relative to the MIC of the pathogen. In addition to maximizing bactericidal activity, in vitro evidence has demonstrated that this concentration goal also minimizes the development of resistance. The use of once-daily dosing strategies to minimize nephrotoxicity of the aminoglycosides has been studied extensively. Single doses of gentamicin and tobramycin (5–7 mg/kg/day) and of amikacin (15–20 mg/kg/day) have been reported to be as effective as standard dosing (smaller single doses given every 8 or every 12 hours) of these agents in controlled clinical trials. However, none of the trials has enrolled a sufficient number of patients required to demonstrate a lower incidence of nephrotoxicity. There are several advantages of once-daily dose aminoglycoside therapy: (a) it is no more nephrotoxic than traditional dosing, (b) clinicians are ensured that a therapeutic peak serum level will be achieved with the first dose, (c) it is the only safe and effective way to achieve serum peak levels of 10 to 20 times the MIC for difficult-to-treat organisms such as *P. aeruginosa*, and (d) it is a more efficient dosing regimen (fewer doses and administration times per day; fewer serum level measurements are required).[49]

Despite the use of individualized aminoglycoside dosing, morbidity and mortality rates attributable to gram-negative pneumonia remain high. This is because the success of antibiotic therapy depends on the ability of the antibiotic to reach the site of infection and remain biologically active.[125] Concentrations of the aminoglycosides in bronchial secretions range from 1 to 5 mcg/mL (30%–40% of serum concentrations) 2 to 4 hours after parenteral administration.[126,127] These concentrations may be insufficient to inhibit the growth of many gram-negative organisms, especially *Pseudomonas*.

Lastly, aminoglycosides bind to purulent exudates and cellular debris and are inactivated by these agents.[128–130] In summary, the aminoglycosides penetrate poorly into bronchial secretions and are less active at the site of infection because of local pH effects and binding to cellular debris. These properties may result in the need for increased dosages, placing patients at increased risk for ototoxicity and nephrotoxicity. Therefore, unless no reasonable alternative exists, aminoglycoside monotherapy for the treatment of pneumonia should be avoided.

INHALED AGENTS FOR MULTIDRUG-RESISTANT PATHOGENS

Because of the growing incidence of pneumonia caused by MDR gram-negative organisms, interest has been renewed in the use of inhaled aminoglycosides and polymyxin products. When given systemically, both classes have been associated with poor pulmonary penetration and with nephrotoxicity, with polymyxin carrying the additional risk of neurotoxicity, and with aminoglycosides ototoxicity. However, the proposed high drug concentrations at the site of pulmonary infection, minimal systemic exposure after nebulized administration, and data showing benefit in both the prevention and treatment of *Pseudomonas* pulmonary infection in cystic fibrosis patients make aerosolized antibiotic therapy an appealing strategy for the treatment of VAP. The IDSA/ATS guidelines state that aerosolized antimicrobials may be considered in patients with MDR organisms not responding well to IV therapy.[49]

The use of adjunctive inhaled antibiotics in VAP has been evaluated in several studies. A systematic review of 16 observational studies and randomized trials without blinding revealed that aerosolized colistin was associated with microbial eradication (OR, 1.61; 95% CI, 1.11–2.35) and improved clinical response (OR, 1.57; 95% CI, 1.14–2.15) but the results were limited by several biases.[131] A systematic review of 12 observational and randomized trials with some blinding showed that nebulized antibiotics in patients with VAP had some benefit in patient outcomes. Nebulized antibiotics were associated with increased rate of clinical cure (RR, 1.23; 95% CI, 1.05–1.43).[132] Neither studies showed an improvement in mortality, duration of mechanical ventilation, or length of stay in the intensive care unit.

ALTERNATIVE DOSING OF ANTIBIOTICS FOR MULTIDRUG-RESISTANT PATHOGENS

Carbapenems, cephalosporins, and extended-spectrum penicillins or β-lactamase inhibitors demonstrate time-dependent killing, and it is known that bactericidal killing for these drug classes is optimized if their free drug concentrations are greater than the MIC (30%–40%, 50%–60%, and 60%–70% of the time, respectively). Prolonged or continuous infusions have been used to increase the time that free drug concentrations are greater than the MIC, theoretically leading to improved patient outcomes.[133]

Continuous infusions were first used in the late 1970s with suggested improvement in clinical cure rates,[134] but until recently they were largely abandoned owing to logistical concerns about medication stability, drug compatibility, and limited IV access. These concerns were lessened by use of contemporary prolonged infusions. This latter strategy is supported primarily by Monte Carlo simulation, a mathematical modeling technique that estimates the probability of pharmacodynamic target attainment at each MIC for a given MIC range.

Patients diagnosed with VAP and treated with cefepime (2 g every 8 hours for 3 hours) have been evaluated using Monte Carlo methodology. Investigators found that at an MIC of 1 mcg/mL, all regimens had a probability of target attainment greater than 90%. However, at an MIC of 8 mcg/mL, when compared with 30-minute intermittent infusions of 1 to 2 g every 8 hours and 2 g every 12 hours, only the prolonged infusion (3 hours) of 2 g every 8 hours maintained 90% probability of target attainment. As one might predict, this phenomenon was only demonstrated in patients with preserved renal function as defined as a creatinine clearance of 50 to 120 mL/minute.[135]

Intermittent and continuous infusion dosing strategies have also been compared when using piperacillin–tazobactam to treat *Pseudomonas* infections. Lodise et al.[136] retrospectively compared intermittent infusions of 3.375 g IV piperacillin–tazobactam (infused over 30 minutes every 6 hours) versus extended infusions of 3.375 g IV piperacillin–tazobactam (infused over 4 hours every 8 hours). Results indicated a shorter length of hospital stay (21 days vs. 38 days; $p = 0.02$) and lower 14 day mortality rate among patients with Acute Physiological and Chronic Health Evaluation-II scores >17 (12.2% vs. 31.6%; $p = 0.04$) in patients receiving extended infusion therapy.[136]

Ventilator-Associated Pneumonia Prophylaxis

The substantial risk of pneumonia in the ICU has prompted aggressive methods to prevent this disease.[137] The most important recommendations include the use of the semi-upright position to reduce the risk of aspiration, infection control (including hand washing) to prevent the spread of pathogens from one patient to the next, and surveillance for ICU infections.[138]

Several strategies for prevention of VAP are controversial, including selective decontamination of the digestive tract (SDD), selective oral decontamination (SOD), and topical antiseptics applied to the oral mucosa. These three strategies address the concept that VAP occurs after colonization of the upper respiratory tract. Because digestive tract flora may play a role in this colonization, the impact of various decontamination approaches has been studied. For SDD a combination therapy including topical tobramycin, polymixin E, and sometimes amphotericin B is administered to the stomach and oropharynx 4 times daily in combination with IV administration of ciprofloxacin or a second-generation cephalosporin. SOD uses a similar antimicrobial strategy to SDD, except that the IV agents are omitted and the combination therapy is applied to the oropharynx.

Historically, SDD and SOD are more widely used in Europe, and most of the literature investigating these techniques in thousands of patients and supporting their use results from outside the United States. In 2009, De Smet et al.[139] performed a large crossover study comparing standard of care ventilation bundles versus SDD versus SOD in mechanically ventilated patients and found a statistically reduced risk of 28-day mortality with an OR of 0.83 (95% CI, 0.72–0.97) for SDD and 0.86 (95% CI, 0.74–0.99) for SOD.[139]

In 2015, Roquilly et al.[140] produced the largest meta-analysis of VAP prevention techniques to decrease mortality. Over 37,000 patients were involved from 157 randomized trials. Although the overall mortality reduction was 5% in the intervention group, in a subgroup analysis, only SDD significantly decreased mortality compared to control with a RR of 0.84 (95% CI, 0.76–0.92).[140] Despite the overwhelming evidence supporting SDD, leading clinicians suggest there are still concerns of North American practitioners who fear that widespread use of antibiotics for SDD will increase antibiotic resistance and *Clostridium difficile* infections, particularly in the United States where drug resistance is more prevalent than in Northern Europe.[141]

KEY REFERENCES AND WEBSITES

A full list of references for this chapter can be found at http://thepoint.lww.com/AT11e. Below are the key references and websites for this chapter, with the corresponding reference number in this chapter found in parentheses after the reference.

Key References

Management of Adults With Hospital-acquired and Ventilator-associated Pneumonia: 2016 Clinical Practice Guidelines by the Infectious Diseases Society of America and the American Thoracic Society. *Clin Inf Dis*. 2016;63;1-51. (49)

Braman SS. Chronic cough due to acute bronchitis: ACCP evidence-based practice guidelines. *Chest*. 2006;129(1, suppl):95S. (3)

CDC. Prevention of pneumococcal disease: recommendations from the Advisory Committee on Immunization Practices (ACIP). *MMWR Recomm Rep*. 1997;46(RR-8):1.

Criner GJ et al. Prevention of acute exacerbation of COPD. American College of Chest Physicians and Canadian Thoracic Society Guideline. *Chest*. 2015;147:883. (17)

Gonzales R et al. Principles of appropriate antibiotic use for treatment of acute respiratory tract infections in adults: background. *Ann Intern Med*. 2001;134:521. (7)

Smith SM et al. Antibiotics for acute bronchitis. *Cochrane Database Syst Rev*. 2014;(3):CD000245. (8)

Quon BS et al. Contemporary management of acute exacerbations of COPD: a systemic review and meta-analysis. *Chest*. 2008;133:756. (18)

Harper SA et al. Seasonal influenza in adults and children: diagnosis, treatment, chemoprophylaxis, and institutional outbreak management: clinical practice guidelines of the Infectious Diseases Society of America. *Clin Infect Dis*. 2009;48:1003. (38)

Mandell LA et al. Infectious Diseases Society of America/American Thoracic Society consensus guidelines on the management of community-acquired pneumonia in adults. *Clin Infect Dis*. 2007;44(Suppl 2):S27. (32)

Key Websites

Centers for Disease Control and Prevention. Seasonal Influenza Vaccination Resources for Health Professionals. http://www.cdc.gov/flu/professionals/vaccination/.

From the Global Strategy for the Diagnosis, Management and Prevention of COPD, Global Initiative for Chronic Lung Disease (GOLD) 2017. Available from: http://goldcopd.org/"http://goldcopd.org. Accessed June 17, 2017. (17)

68 Tuberculosis

Michael B. Kays

CORE PRINCIPLES

		CHAPTER CASES
1	Tuberculosis is an infectious disease caused by *Mycobacterium tuberculosis*, and the most common site of infection is the lungs. Active disease is characterized by fever, chills, cough, night sweats, weight loss, and changes on chest radiography. Several risk factors for tuberculosis have been identified, including immune suppression, exposure to close contacts, and smoking.	**Case 68-1 (Questions 1, 2)**
2	Diagnosis of active disease includes tuberculin skin testing, chest radiography, and sputum collection for acid-fast bacilli stain and culture. Nucleic acid amplification tests and interferon-γ release assays may aid in the diagnosis of tuberculosis. Human immunodeficiency virus (HIV) screening is recommended for all patients with tuberculosis.	**Case 68-1 (Questions 3–7)**
3	The goals of therapy include cure and prevention of transmission of *M. tuberculosis*. Treatment of active pulmonary disease requires administration of multiple-drug therapy for a minimum of 26 weeks. Directly observed therapy is a core management strategy for all patients to ensure adherence to therapy.	**Case 68-1 (Questions 8–13)**
4	Patients should be monitored for resolution of symptoms and questioned about the occurrence of adverse events, especially hepatitis. Sputum smears and cultures should be obtained every 2 to 4 weeks initially and then monthly after cultures become negative. If treatment failure occurs, three new drugs should be added to the treatment regimen.	**Case 68-1 (Questions 14, 15)**
5	Patients with latent tuberculosis infection have a positive tuberculin skin test or interferon-γ release assay but no clinical symptoms or radiographic evidence of active disease. Isoniazid for 6 to 9 months is preferred, and rifampin for 4 months and weekly isoniazid plus rifapentine for 12 weeks are alternatives.	**Case 68-2 (Questions 1, 2)**
6	Adverse events associated with isoniazid include hepatotoxicity and peripheral neuropathy. Rifampin is associated with hepatotoxicity, flu-like syndrome, thrombocytopenia, and discoloration of body fluids. Pyrazinamide can cause hepatotoxicity and increased uric acid, whereas ethambutol can cause optic neuritis.	**Case 68-3 (Questions 1–3), Case 68-4 (Question 1)**
7	The case rate for tuberculosis in the elderly is greater than that in all other age-groups. Principles of treatment of tuberculosis in the elderly are the same as those for other age-groups.	**Case 68-5 (Question 1)**
8	Multidrug-resistant tuberculosis can develop as a result of nonadherence to treatment. Successful treatment of multidrug-resistant tuberculosis is possible depending on the host, adherence to therapy, and the number of drugs to which the organism remains susceptible. Treatment with six to seven drugs may be required in the intensive phase.	**Case 68-6 (Questions 1, 2)**
9	HIV infection is an important risk factor for tuberculosis. The clinical manifestations in HIV-infected persons will vary depending on the severity of immunodeficiency at presentation. Principles and recommendations for treatment of active disease and latent infection in HIV-infected persons are the same as those for HIV-negative persons.	**Case 68-7 (Questions 1–3), Case 68-8 (Question 1)**

Continued

		CHAPTER CASES
10	In antiretroviral-naïve patients, the optimal timing for initiating antiretroviral therapy is dependent on the patient's CD4+ cell count. Antiretroviral therapy may be delayed to decrease the potential for immune reconstitution inflammatory syndrome. If patients are receiving antiretroviral therapy, treatment of tuberculosis should begin immediately with modification of antiviral therapy as needed.	**Case 68-7 (Questions 4, 5)**
11	Treatment of active disease in pregnant women is the same as that for nonpregnant women. Pyrazinamide is not recommended in pregnancy due to insufficient safety data. The minimum duration of therapy is 9 months.	**Case 68-9 (Question 1)**
12	Infants and children have a higher risk of disseminated tuberculosis, and treatment should be initiated promptly. Ethambutol is generally avoided because it is difficult to assess visual acuity in children. Many experts prefer to initiate therapy in children with three drugs and treat for a minimum duration of 6 months.	**Case 68-10 (Question 1)**
13	Extrapulmonary tuberculosis may require longer durations of therapy. Tuberculous meningitis may require 9 to 12 months of therapy, and corticosteroids reduce sequelae and improve survival.	**Case 68-11 (Question 1)**

HISTORY

Tuberculosis (TB) is an ancient disease with evidence of spinal TB in pre-Columbian and early Egyptian remains. TB emerged as a major health problem in the 17th and 18th centuries when crowded living conditions of the industrial revolution contributed to its epidemic spread throughout Europe and the United States. Early physicians referred to TB as *phthisis,* derived from the Greek term for wasting, because its clinical presentation consisted of weight loss, cough, fevers, and hemoptysis. The etiologic agent was identified in 1882 when Robert Koch isolated and cultured *Mycobacterium tuberculosis* and demonstrated its infectious nature. With this knowledge, early treatment in the mid-1800s to the early 1900s consisted of placing patients with TB in a sanatorium for bed rest and fresh air. With the advent of radiographic film, pulmonary cavitary lesions were found to be a pivotal component in the evolution of the disease. Therapy included pneumoperitoneum, thoracoplasty, and plombage to reduce the size of the cavitary lesion, and some of these therapies are still used today for severe and refractory cases.

The modern era of medical TB therapy began in 1944 with the discovery of streptomycin and, shortly thereafter, *p*-aminosalicylic acid. Addition of isoniazid in 1952 and rifampin in the late 1960s greatly increased treatment success and provided hope for the eventual elimination of TB. However, multidrug-resistant TB (MDR-TB) emerged in the 1990s as a threat to the control of TB in the United States and other countries.[1–3] In the subsequent decade, published reports described the worldwide emergence of extensively drug-resistant TB (XDR-TB)[4–6] and, more recently, the emergence of totally drug-resistant (TDR) or super XDR-TB strains.[7] Because TB strains become increasingly resistant to currently available agents, the likelihood of achieving global control and elimination of this disease are diminished. Therefore, a high index of suspicion for TB, rapid pathogen identification, susceptibility testing, patient isolation, and appropriate antimicrobial therapy are critical to prevent further development and spread of drug-resistant TB.

Incidence and Epidemiology

Assuming lifelong infection, approximately 2.0 billion people (30% of the world's population) are infected with *M. tuberculosis.*[8] TB is the second most common causes of death from an infectious disease in the world after human immunodeficiency virus (HIV) and acquired immunodeficiency syndrome (AIDS). Globally, there were an estimated 9 million new cases of TB in 2013; the majority of these new cases were identified in the Southeast Asia, Western Pacific, and the African regions.[9] The countries with the largest number of new cases were India, China, Nigeria, and Pakistan.[9] Approximately 13% of the new TB cases in 2013 were identified in patients infected with HIV, with the African region accounting for 78% of these cases.[9] In 2013, approximately 1.1 million deaths were reported among HIV-negative cases and 0.36 million deaths were reported among HIV-positive cases.[9] These deaths include 510,000 women and 80,000 children.[9]

In the United States, 9,421 cases of TB were reported in 2014, and the incidence rate was 2.96/100,000 population, which represents the lowest recorded rate since national reporting began in 1953.[10] However, the incidence rate remained substantially higher than the national goal for elimination of TB (<1 case per 1,000,000 population).[10] Twenty-one states reported increased numbers of TB cases in 2014, and four states (California, Texas, New York, and Florida) accounted for 51% of all TB cases.[10] The number of TB cases and the incidence rates declined for both foreign-born and US-born persons, but foreign-born and ethnic and racial minorities continue to be disproportionally affected by TB in the United States. In 2014, 66% and 34% of all TB cases were reported in foreign-born and US-born persons, respectively, and the TB rate was 13 times higher in foreign-born persons compared with US-born persons (15.4 vs. 1.2 per 100,000 population).[10] Five countries accounted for more than half of TB cases in foreign-born persons: Mexico (21%), the Philippines (12%), India (8%), Vietnam (8%), and China (7%).[10] TB rates for Hispanics, non-Hispanic blacks, and Asians were 8, 8.5, and 30 times greater than the rate for non-Hispanic Caucasians.[10] Among US-born persons, the greatest number of TB cases was reported in blacks. Among persons with TB whose HIV status was known, 6% of these patients were coinfected with HIV.[10]

In the United States, 9.3% of isolates from patients with no previous history of TB were resistant to isoniazid in 2014; resistance was 7.5% in US-born individuals and 10.2% in foreign-born individuals.[10] Globally, there were approximately 480,000 cases of MDR-TB, defined as resistance to both isoniazid and rifampin, resulting in 210,000 deaths in 2013.[9] The largest number of MDR-TB cases were reported in China, India, the Russian Federation, and South Africa.[9] In the United States, 67 cases of MDR-TB were reported in 2014.[10] The overall proportion of MDR-TB cases in the

Table 68-1

Conditions and Risk Factors for Persons with Increased Risk of Drug-Resistant Tuberculosis

History of treatment for latent tuberculosis infection or active disease
Patients from areas with high prevalence of initial or primary drug resistance (urban population, northeast United States, Florida, California, Texas, United States–Mexico border)
Foreign-born persons from areas with high prevalence of drug-resistant tuberculosis (Southeast Asia, Mexico, South America, Africa)
Contact with persons with active infection caused by drug-resistant *Mycobacterium tuberculosis*
Tuberculosis in persons who are homeless, abusers of intravenous drugs, and HIV infected
Patients with positive sputum smears and cultures after 2 months of treatment

HIV, human immunodeficiency virus.

United States has been stable over the last decade, ranging from 0.9% to 1.3%.[10] Foreign-born persons accounted for 85% of these MDR-TB cases.[10] The percentage of MDR-TB is approximately 7 times higher for persons with a previous history of TB compared with persons with no previous history of TB.[10] Several conditions and risk factors for persons with increased risk of infection with drug-resistant TB are shown in Table 68-1.

In the mid-2000s, XDR-TB emerged as another major threat to global health.[4–6] The definition of XDR-TB is resistance to isoniazid and rifampin among first-line agents, resistance to any fluoroquinolone, and resistance to at least one second-line injectable drug (amikacin, kanamycin, or capreomycin).[11] According to the World Health Organization, XDR-TB strains have been identified in 100 countries worldwide, and an estimated 9% of patients with MDR-TB have XDR-TB.[9] One of the first reports described 53 patients infected with XDR-TB from South Africa.[12] HIV status was known in 44 patients, and all of these patients were HIV positive. Fifty-five percent of the patients had no prior history of TB treatment, and 98% died with a median survival period of only 16 days after collection of the first sputum specimen.[12] In the United States, 49 cases of XDR-TB were identified between 1993 and 2006, and mortality was strongly associated with concomitant HIV infection.[13] Since 2009, 15 cases of XDR-TB have been reported in the United States, and 11 cases were among foreign-born individuals.[10]

Risk factors for XDR-TB include previous treatment for TB, HIV infection, homelessness, and alcohol use.[14] In a retrospective analysis of patients with documented MDR-TB, emergence of XDR-TB was associated with baseline chronic disease and nonadherence to MDR-TB therapy.[15] Treatment success is significantly lower for XDR-TB, and XDR-TB is associated with increased all-cause and TB-related mortality.[16] However, treatment outcomes are significantly improved when later-generation fluoroquinolones are added to the treatment regimen for XDR-TB, even if fluoroquinolone resistance was demonstrated on susceptibility testing.[17]

The evolution of TB resistance continued in 2009 with the identification of strains that were reported to be TDR, which was defined as resistance to all first-line and second-line agents.[7] Fifteen (10.3%) of 146 MDR-TB strains tested were found to be TDR-TB in Iran, and cultures remained positive in these cases after 18 months of treatment with second-line agents.[7] All of these TDR-TB cases were HIV negative. This report illustrates the critical need to develop new and effective agents for the treatment of TB caused by MDR, XDR, and TDR strains.

Etiology

TB is caused by *M. tuberculosis,* an aerobic, non-spore-forming bacillus that resists decolorization by acid alcohol after staining with basic fuchsin. For this reason, the organism is often referred to as an acid-fast bacillus (AFB).

M. tuberculosis is different from other bacteria in that it replicates slowly—once every 24 hours instead of every 20 to 40 minutes as with some other bacteria. The organism thrives in environments in which the oxygen tension is relatively high, such as the apices of the lung, the renal parenchyma, and the growing ends of bones.

Transmission

M. tuberculosis is transmitted through the air by aerosolized droplet nuclei that are produced when a person with pulmonary or laryngeal TB coughs, sneezes, speaks, or sings. Droplet nuclei may also be produced by other methods, such as aerosol treatments, sputum induction, bronchoscopy, endotracheal intubation, suctioning, autopsy, and through manipulation of lesions or processing of secretions in the hospital or laboratory.[18] These droplet nuclei, which contain one to three *M. tuberculosis* organisms, are small enough (1–5 μm) to remain airborne for long periods and reach the alveoli within the lungs when inhaled. Tubercle bacilli are not transmitted on inanimate objects, and organisms deposited on skin or intact mucosa do not invade tissues.

Several factors influence the likelihood of transmission of *M. tuberculosis,* including the number of organisms expelled into the air by the index patient, the concentration of organisms in the air determined by the volume of the space and its ventilation, the length of time an exposed person breathes the contaminated air, location of the exposure (small room vs. outdoors), and the immune status of the exposed individual.[19] Family household contacts, especially children, and persons working or living in an enclosed environment (e.g., hospitals, nursing homes, prisons) with an infected person are at a significantly increased risk for becoming infected. If the index case is smear positive, 50% of household contacts will have a conversion of the tuberculin skin test from negative to positive; however, if the index case is smear negative, only 5% will become infected.[19] Individuals with impaired cell-mediated immunity, such as HIV-infected persons or transplant patients, are more likely to become infected with *M. tuberculosis* after exposure than persons with normal immune function.[19] Travelers to TB-endemic areas with international medical exchange programs are also at risk of TB infection, regardless of involvement in direct patient care activities or duration of stay.[20]

Several techniques are effective in limiting airborne transmission of *M. tuberculosis* by reducing the number of droplet nuclei in a given airspace. Adequate room ventilation with fresh air is very important, especially in the healthcare setting, in which six or more room air exchanges per hour are desirable.[18,21] New construction or renovation of existing facilities should be designed so that airborne infection isolation rooms achieve 12 or more room air exchanges per hour.[21] Ultraviolet irradiation of air in the upper part of the room can also reduce the number of viable airborne tubercle bacilli. All healthcare workers and visitors who enter the room of a patient with TB should wear at least N95 disposable respirators, and the mask should be molded to fit tightly around the nose and mouth.[21] Patients with presumed or confirmed infectious TB should wear a protective mask when being transferred to another area of the institution or after hospital discharge until they are noninfectious.[21] However, the most important means of reducing transmission of *M. tuberculosis* is by treating the infected patient with effective antituberculosis therapy.

Pathogenesis

LATENT INFECTION VERSUS ACTIVE DISEASE

Latent Infection

A clear distinction should be made between latent infection and active disease (tuberculosis). Latent infection occurs when the tubercle bacilli are inhaled into the body. After inhalation, the droplet nuclei containing *M. tuberculosis* settle into the bronchioles and alveoli of the lungs. Development of infection in the lung is dependent on the inoculum of organisms inhaled, the virulence of the organism, and the innate immune response of the host.[22–24] In the nonimmune (susceptible) host, the bacilli initially multiply unopposed by normal host defense mechanisms. The organisms are then phagocytized by alveolar macrophages and resident dendritic cells, but they may remain viable, multiplying within the cells for extended periods.[24] After 14 to 21 days of replication, the tubercle bacilli spread via the lymphatic system to the hilar lymph nodes and through the bloodstream to many other organs of the body.

Fortunately, certain organs and tissues in the body, such as the bone marrow, liver, and spleen, are resistant to subsequent multiplication of these bacilli. Organs with high blood flow and Pao_2, such as the apices of the lungs, kidneys, bones, and brain, are favorable for organism growth and may lead to extrapulmonary disease. Organisms replicate for 2 to 12 weeks until they reach a concentration of 10^3 to 10^4, plateauing coincident with the development of a T-cell-mediated immune response in the host.[24] $CD4^+$ T cells produce interferon-γ, which is an essential cytokine for activation of macrophages and mycobacterial killing, as well as other cytokines.[24] At this point, the patient has developed cell-mediated immunity, which can be detected by a reaction to the tuberculin skin test or interferon-γ release assay (IGRA), and bacterial replication is halted.[24]

In persons with intact cell-mediated immunity, activated T cells and macrophages may result in formation of a granuloma, a hallmark of TB, that is thought to represent a physical and immunologic barrier to control the infection and limit dissemination of the bacilli to the surrounding environment.[24] Cells found within the granuloma include $CD4^+$ and $CD8^+$ T cells, B cells, neutrophils, macrophages, multinucleated giant cells, and fibroblasts.[24] The organisms tend to localize in the center of the granuloma, which is frequently necrotic, and the tubercle bacilli may remain viable indefinitely within the granuloma. In addition, maintenance of the integrity of the granuloma allows for control of bacterial replication and depends on the immune status of the patient.[24] Tumor necrosis factor (TNF) is a key cytokine that is critical for the integrity of the granuloma.[25] Most patients with latent TB infection are asymptomatic with no radiographic evidence of the infection.[22] In some patients, there may be a healed, calcified lesion on chest radiograph, but bacteriologic studies are negative. A positive tuberculin skin test or IGRA is the only indication that the person has been infected with *M. tuberculosis*. Individuals with latent TB infection are not infectious and thus cannot transmit the organism to other individuals.[18]

Active Disease

In the majority of patients, active TB disease results from reactivation of a previously controlled latent infection, termed reactivation TB. It has been estimated that approximately 10% of individuals who acquire TB infection and do not receive therapy for the latent infection will develop active TB disease, and the risk of developing active disease is greatest during the first 2 years after infection.[18,22,23] In a population-based tuberculin skin test survey conducted in Florida between 1997 and 2001, the rate of reactivation with latent TB infection but without HIV coinfection was 0.040 to 0.058 cases per 100 person-years.[26] However, a recent study reported that 1 in 4 cases of active TB in the United States may be caused by recent transmission.[27] The study included patients with culture-positive TB, and the *M. tuberculosis* isolates were fully characterized by genotype. Clusters were defined as cases with *M. tuberculosis* that were an exact match by genotype within specific geospatial zones. Cases that were both genotypically and spatially clustered were considered recent TB transmission, and cases that were not genotypically and spatially clustered were considered reactivation TB. Of the 36,860 cases where genotyping was performed, 8,499 cases (23.1%) met the criteria for recent TB transmission.[27] Groups at greatest risk for recent transmission were HIV-infected individuals, members of a minority group or ethnic race, men, individuals born in the United States, children 4 years of age or younger, substance abusers, and the homeless.[27] These patients may have limited access to health care, resulting in delayed diagnosis and extended periods of infectivity.

Reactivation of TB in persons with latent TB infection is primarily a function of the immune status of the host. The ability of the host to respond to *M. tuberculosis* infection is reduced by certain diseases, such as diabetes mellitus, silicosis, chronic renal failure, and diseases or drugs associated with immunosuppression (e.g., HIV infection, anti-TNF-α agents, organ and hematologic transplantation, corticosteroids, and other immunosuppressive agents). The likelihood of progression from latent infection to active TB disease is greater in persons with these conditions.[22–24] HIV-infected persons, especially those with low $CD4^+$ T-cell counts, develop active TB disease rapidly after becoming infected; up to 50% of these individuals may develop active disease in the first 2 years after infection.[28] In addition, a person with untreated latent TB infection who acquires HIV infection will progress to active TB disease at an approximate rate of 5% to 10% per year.[29,30] The relative risk for progression from latent infection to active disease is 1.6 to 25 times higher in patients treated with anti-TNF-α agents, depending on the clinical setting and the agents used.[31] Physical or emotional stress, gastrectomy, intestinal bypass surgery, alcohol abuse, hematologic disease, reticuloendothelial disease, and intravenous drug use are risk factors for development of active disease. The elderly, adolescents, and children younger than 5 years of age are also at increased risk of developing active disease.[18,22–24,32]

Overview of Drug Therapy

Drug treatment is the cornerstone for management of patients with TB. In a patient with active TB, the overall treatment goals are to cure the individual patient and to minimize transmission of *M. tuberculosis*. The primary goals of chemotherapy are rapid bacterial killing, prevent emergence of drug resistance, and eliminate persistent tubercle bacilli to prevent relapse.[33] To accomplish these goals, treatment must be tailored to each patient's clinical and social circumstances to ensure adherence to and completion of treatment (patient-centered care). Effective TB treatment requires a substantial period of drug therapy, and optimization of the initial treatment phase prevents emergence of resistance and ensures success of TB therapy. Current guidelines recommend four drugs for the initial 8-week treatment phase: isoniazid, rifampin, pyrazinamide, and ethambutol.[33] The drug regimen and duration of the continuation phase depends on patient response, susceptibility of the isolate, host factors, extent of the disease (pulmonary vs. extrapulmonary), and drug tolerability.[33] The shortest duration of therapy is 6 months, but longer durations may be required with drug-resistant strains.[33] Because patients must be treated for months, directly observed therapy (DOT) is the preferred core management strategy to ensure adherence.[33–35]

In patients with latent TB infection, monotherapy with isoniazid for 6 to 9 months remains the preferred regimen although other attractive options are available.

Clinical Presentation of Active Disease

CASE 68-1

QUESTION 1: H.G. is a 35-year-old Hispanic man who presents with a 4-week history of a productive cough. The cough was initially nonproductive but became productive of yellow sputum after 2 weeks. The patient has been self-medicating with over-the-counter antitussives without relief, and he experienced hemoptysis this morning. He complains of subjective fevers, chills, night sweats, dyspnea on exertion, fatigue, and an unintentional 15-lb weight loss during the last 2 months. He immigrated to the United States from Mexico when he was 12 years old, but he has not traveled outside the United States for more than a decade. He currently works as a laborer on new home construction projects, and several of his coworkers, who moved to the United States from Mexico within the past year, have similar respiratory symptoms. He is currently married with three children. The patient has a 20-pack-year smoking history and drinks alcohol on weekends but denies illicit drug use.

On physical examination, H.G. is a thin-appearing man in mild respiratory distress. His heart rate is 94 beats/minute, his respiratory rate is 24 breaths/minute, and his temperature is 38.9°C. Bronchial breath sounds are noted in the right upper lobe on chest auscultation, and chest radiography shows extensive patchy infiltrates in the right upper lobe. Significant laboratory data include the following:

White blood cell count, 13,200/μL (72% polymorphonuclear leukocytes, 3% bands, 12% lymphocytes, 13% monocytes)
Red blood cell count, $3.7 \times 10^6/\mu L$
Hemoglobin, 11.2 g/dL
Hematocrit, 34%
Platelets, $269 \times 10^3/\mu L$
Serum electrolytes, renal function, and hepatic function are within normal limits.

He is 69 inches tall, and his weight is 68 kg. The remainder of his physical examination is unremarkable. What signs and symptoms consistent with active TB disease are present in H.G.?

H.G.'s history of cough (which gradually became productive), fever, night sweats, fatigue, and weight loss are classic symptoms of active TB.[18] Cough may be nonproductive early in the course of the illness, but with subsequent inflammation and tissue necrosis, sputum is usually produced and is key to the diagnostic studies. Sputum may contain blood (hemoptysis) in patients with advanced cavitary disease, which is particularly worrisome because cavitary lesions harbor high concentrations of organisms and the pulmonary location facilitates airborne transmission. Dyspnea is unusual unless there is extensive disease.[18] Other symptoms of TB may include pleuritic chest pain and general malaise.

In pulmonary TB, the chest radiograph usually reveals patchy or nodular infiltrates in the apical or posterior segments of the upper lobes, but changes may be observed in any segment.

The patchy infiltrates on H.G.'s chest radiograph are consistent with pulmonary TB. Cavitary lesions may be seen; however, these were absent in this patient. Moderate elevation of the white blood cell count with increased monocytes and eosinophils and anemia are the most common hematologic manifestations of TB.[18] H.G. had an elevated white blood cell count with increased monocytes, and he was also anemic.

Many patients with active pulmonary TB have no acute symptoms, and a lack of symptoms may hinder diagnosis. In one study, approximately 50% of active TB cases without classic symptoms were misdiagnosed.[36] More than one-third of the patients with active TB had no sweats, chills, or malaise, and fewer than 50% were febrile. Cough was evident in 80% of these patients, and only 25% had hemoptysis. Although dullness over the apices of the lungs and posttussive rales are expected in TB, less than one-third of these patients had any abnormal pulmonary signs. Similar findings were reported in another study.[37] Absence of specific clinical symptoms underscores the importance of skin testing, sputum smears for AFB, and chest radiographs in suspected TB. Lastly, cases of active TB are often found after routine chest radiographs for other illnesses.

Because many of the symptoms of TB also occur in persons with preexisting pulmonary disease or pneumonia, they may be overlooked and not attributed to TB.

CASE 68-1, QUESTION 2: What risk factors for TB are present in H.G.?

The close contact with his coworkers, who have similar respiratory symptoms, and their geographic origin from Mexico are risk factors for TB in H.G. In addition, studies have implicated cigarette smoking as a risk factor for TB.[38–40] In a cohort study conducted in Taiwan, smoking was associated with a twofold increase in the risk of active TB. Furthermore, a significant dose–response relationship was identified for number of cigarettes smoked per day, number of years of smoking, and number of pack-years smoked.[40] Smoking impairs mucociliary clearance, decreases phagocytic pulmonary alveolar macrophage function, decreases intracellular production of tumor necrosis factor-α, and causes iron overload in macrophages.[41–44] These defects in host defense mechanisms increase the risk of active disease after exposure to *M. tuberculosis.*

Diagnosis of Active Tuberculosis

CASE 68-1, QUESTION 3: A tuberculin purified protein derivative (PPD) skin test (5 test units [TU]) is ordered and placed on the volar aspect of his left arm. Sputum is collected and sent for AFB stain, culture, and susceptibility testing. His smear is positive for AFB, and the result of the tuberculin skin test, read at 48 hours, was a palpable induration of 14 mm. What is tuberculin PPD skin testing? How should the result be interpreted in H.G.?

The tuberculin skin test (Mantoux method) has been used as a diagnostic tool for infection with *M. tuberculosis* for decades, but a positive skin test is not necessary for the diagnosis of active TB disease. The test is frequently referred to as the PPD (purified protein derivative) test, which contains a protein prepared from a culture of the tubercle bacilli. Skin testing is performed by injecting 0.1 mL of solution containing 5 TU of PPD *intracutaneously* into the volar or dorsal surface of the forearm.[18,45] The injection is made using a one-quarter to one-half-inch, 27-gauge needle and a tuberculin syringe. The solution should be injected just beneath the surface of the skin, avoiding subcutaneous tissue.[18,46] A discrete, pale elevation of the skin (a wheal) 6 to 10 mm in diameter is produced when the injection is performed correctly. If the first injection was administered improperly, another test dose can be given at once, selecting a site several centimeters away from the original injection site.[18]

If the patient has been infected with *M. tuberculosis,* sensitized T cells are recruited to the skin site where they release cytokines.[47]

These cytokines induce an induration (raised area) through local vasodilatation, edema, fibrin deposition, and recruitment of other inflammatory cells to the area.[18] Typically, the reaction to the tuberculin protein begins 5 to 6 hours after injection with maximal induration observed at 48 to 72 hours. Therefore, the test should be read between 48 and 72 hours after injection because tests read after 72 hours underestimate the actual size of the induration.[18,23] For standardization, the diameter of the induration should be measured transversely to the long axis of the forearm and recorded in millimeters.[18] The diameter of the induration should be measured and not the erythematous zone surrounding the induration.

An induration of at least 5 mm in diameter read 48 to 72 hours after injection is a positive reaction in an individual with a recent history of close contact with a person with active TB, a person with fibrotic changes on chest radiograph consistent with previous TB, organ transplant patients and other immunosuppressed patients (receiving the equivalent of ≥15 mg/day of prednisone for >1 month), or HIV-infected persons.[18,45,48,49]

An induration of at least 10 mm in diameter is a positive reaction with clinical conditions associated with increased risk for TB, such as diabetes mellitus, silicosis, chronic renal failure, malnutrition, leukemia, lymphoma, gastrectomy, jejunoileal bypass, and weight loss of greater than 10% of ideal body weight.[18,45,49] In addition, an induration of at least 10 mm is considered to be positive in recent immigrants (<5 years) from countries with a high prevalence of TB, injection drug users, residents and employees of high-risk congregate settings (e.g., prisons, nursing homes, homeless shelters), healthcare workers, mycobacteriology laboratory personnel, and children younger than 4 years of age or infants, children, and adolescents exposed to adults in high-risk catgories.[18,45,49] The skin test is also considered positive for persons with an increase in induration diameter of at least 10 mm within a 2-year period.[45,49] For individuals with no risk factors for TB, an induration of at least 15 mm is required for a positive reaction.[45,49]

It is very likely that H.G. has been in close contact with persons with active TB, that is, his coworkers, even though they have not yet been diagnosed with active TB. When all factors are considered, the PPD of 14 mm should be considered to be positive in H.G.

CASE 68-1, QUESTION 4: Because H.G.'s PPD skin test is positive, does this confirm his diagnosis of active TB? What other laboratory tests may be performed to aid in the diagnosis of TB in H.G.?

H.G.'s positive reaction to 5 TU of PPD alone does not imply active TB disease. It only confirms that he has previously been infected with *M. tuberculosis.* To confirm the diagnosis of active TB disease in H.G., *M. tuberculosis* must be detected and isolated from sputum, gastric aspirate, spinal fluid, urine, or tissue biopsy, depending on the site of infection.[18] As was performed in H.G., detection of AFB in stained sputum smears examined microscopically should be the first test to confirm the presence of mycobacteria in a clinical specimen. It is the easiest and fastest procedure that can be performed and allows preliminary confirmation of the diagnosis. Sputum samples for AFB stain and culture are best obtained early in the morning on at least three separate days.[34] The cough reflex is usually suppressed at night, and the first early morning expectoration represents secretions accumulated in the chest overnight. The number of organisms in the morning sample is greater, and the diagnostic yield is higher. Smears may be prepared directly from clinical specimens or from concentrated preparations by placing the specimen on a glass slide under a microscope with a Ziehl–Neelsen or fluorochrome stain (not a Gram stain).[18] Sensitivity of sputum smear microscopy is low because 5,000 to 10,000 bacilli/mL of specimen must be present for AFB detection in stained smears.[18,50] Therefore, a negative AFB smear does not rule out active TB disease, and patients with active TB and negative AFB smears may facilitate transmission of *M. tuberculosis.* Additional limitations of the AFB smear are its inability to differentiate among mycobacterial species and between viable and nonviable organisms. In many areas of the United States, *Mycobacterium avium* complex organisms are commonly isolated from the sputum of patients in whom a diagnosis of TB is highly probable, such as the elderly and patients with HIV infection.[51] This finding has resulted in a marked decrease in the specificity and positive predictive value of the sputum smear, in some cases to as low as 50%.[52]

The gold standard for laboratory confirmation of TB is culture.[53] Some patients may have a negative AFB smear, but a sufficient number of organisms may be present to produce a positive culture. Only 10 to 100 organisms are needed for a positive culture.[18] As a result of the limitations of the AFB smear, a positive culture for *M. tuberculosis* is necessary to definitively diagnose TB in H.G. and all patients, even if the AFB smear is positive. In addition, culture allows for genotyping and susceptibility testing of the isolate.[51] Because *M. tuberculosis* grows slowly (i.e., once every 24 hours), it may take several weeks for the cultures to become positive.[18] Broth-based culture systems such as BACTEC, MGIT, MB/BacT, Septi-Check, and ESP, when combined with DNA probes, can result in positive cultures in 2 weeks or less for sputum smear-positive specimens and in 3 weeks or less for smear-negative specimens.[51]

Nucleic acid amplification (NAA) tests are available to enhance and expedite direct identification of *M. tuberculosis* in clinical specimens independent of mycobacterial culture.[54,55] These tests amplify the specific target sequences of nucleic acids in *M. tuberculosis* that can be detected by a nucleic acid probe within 24 to 48 hours. Two NAA tests are approved by the Food and Drug Administration (FDA) for use in the United States. The enhanced amplified *M. tuberculosis* direct test is approved for detection of *M. tuberculosis* in AFB smear-positive and smear-negative respiratory specimens. The sensitivity of this test is greater than 95% for patients with AFB-positive smears and 75% to 90% for patients with AFB-negative smears. The Amplicor *M. tuberculosis* test is approved for detection of *M. tuberculosis* in AFB smear-positive respiratory specimens. Sensitivity of the Amplicor test is greater than 95% for patients with AFB-positive smears and 60% to 70% for patients with AFB-negative smears. Specificity of the NAA tests is greater than 95% for both AFB smear-positive and smear-negative pulmonary specimens.

Compared with AFB smears, additional benefits of NAA testing include the ability to rapidly confirm the presence of *M. tuberculosis* in a majority of patients with AFB-negative smears and the positive predictive value of greater than 95% for AFB-positive specimens in settings where nontuberculous mycobacteria are common.[53] NAA tests are cost-effective because they prioritize contact investigations, improve decision making regarding respiratory isolation, and decrease unnecessary TB treatment.[56,57] Current guidelines recommend NAA testing on at least one respiratory specimen from a patient with signs and symptoms of pulmonary TB for whom a diagnosis has not been established and for whom the test result would alter case management and infection control activities.[53] If the NAA result and the AFB smear result are positive, the patient is presumed to have TB, and drug treatment should be initiated while awaiting culture results.[53] If the NAA result is positive and the AFB smear result is negative, clinical judgment should be exercised regarding initiating drug therapy, and additional diagnostic testing may be needed. If the NAA result is negative and the AFB smear result is positive, a test for inhibitors should be performed and an additional specimen should be tested with NAA. Sputum specimens (3%–7%) might contain inhibitors that prevent or reduce amplification and cause false-negative NAA results.[53] If the NAA result and the AFB smear result are negative, clinical judgment is recommended in the decision to begin drug therapy because NAA tests lack the sensitivity in AFB smear-negative specimens needed to exclude the diagnosis of TB.[53]

CASE 68-1, QUESTION 5: Would a negative tuberculin skin test have eliminated the possibility of infection with *M. tuberculosis* in H.G.?

A negative response to 5 TU of PPD in H.G. would not exclude active infection with *M. tuberculosis*. The PPD skin test has a reported false-negative rate of 25% during the initial evaluation of persons with active tuberculosis.[18] This high false-negative rate is attributable to poor nutrition and general health, overwhelming acute illness, or immunosuppression. False-negative results usually occur in persons who have only recently been infected or are anergic. Anergy, the decreased ability to respond to antigens, may be caused by severe debility, advanced age, immaturity in newborns, high fever, sarcoidosis, corticosteroids, immunosuppressive drugs, hematologic disease, HIV infections, overwhelming TB, recent viral infection, live-virus vaccinations, and malnutrition.[18] If anergy is suspected, control skin tests (*Candida*, mumps, or *Trichophyton*) may be placed in the contralateral arm. If the control test results are positive and the PPD test result is negative, infection with *M. tuberculosis* is less likely. The Centers for Disease Control and Prevention (CDC) changed its recommendations regarding anergy skin testing in HIV-infected patients with a negative PPD. They cite problems with standardization and reproducibility, a low risk for TB associated with a diagnosis of anergy, and the lack of apparent benefit of therapy for latent TB infection in anergic HIV-infected patients. Therefore, the use of anergy testing in conjunction with PPD is no longer routinely recommended in this population or other patients who are immunocompromised.[48,58,59]

CASE 68-1, QUESTION 6: On further questioning, H.G. informs the medical team that he received the BCG vaccine when he was a child in Mexico. What is the BCG vaccine? What effect does the BCG vaccine have on the results of the tuberculin skin test? What other test may be performed in H.G. for detection of *M. tuberculosis* infection?

BCG, or bacille Calmette–Guérin, is a live vaccine derived from an attenuated strain of *Mycobacterium bovis*, and it is used in many foreign countries with a high prevalence of TB to prevent the disease in persons who are tuberculin negative. Many different BCG vaccines are available worldwide, and they differ with respect to immunogenicity, efficacy, and reactogenicity. Additional factors, such as genetic variability in the vaccinated subjects, the nature of the mycobacteria endemic in different parts of the world, and the use of different doses and immunization schedules, may contribute to the varied degrees of protection provided by the vaccine. The protective effect derived from BCG vaccines in case–control studies ranges from 0% to 80%.[60] Two meta-analyses calculated estimates of the protective efficacy of BCG vaccination for preventing TB. Results from the first meta-analysis indicated a 75% to 86% protective effect against meningeal and miliary TB in children.[61] In the second meta-analysis, the overall protective effect of BCG vaccines was approximately 50%.[62] Vaccine efficacy was higher in studies in which persons were vaccinated during childhood in contrast with those vaccinated at older ages.[62] Unfortunately, neither study could confirm vaccine efficacy for preventing pulmonary TB.

Prior vaccination with BCG usually results in a false-positive tuberculin skin test in patients who are not infected with *M. tuberculosis*, but skin test reactivity does not correlate with protection against TB.[18,60] There is no reliable method of distinguishing tuberculin reactions caused by BCG vaccination from those caused by natural mycobacterial infections.[18,60] Therefore, it is prudent to consider "positive" reactions to 5 TU of PPD in BCG-vaccinated persons as indicating infection with *M. tuberculosis*, especially among persons from countries with a high prevalence of TB.[18] Even though H.G. received the BCG vaccine when he was a child, the results of the PPD skin test should still be considered positive, especially in light of his symptoms.

In general, BCG vaccination is not recommended for routine prophylaxis in the United States because the risk of exposure to TB is relatively low. BCG vaccination should be considered only for very select persons who meet specific criteria and in consultation with a TB expert. BCG vaccination should only be considered for infants or children who are PPD negative and are continually exposed to a highly infectious, untreated patient with active TB or a child who is continually exposed to a person with infectious pulmonary TB caused by *M. tuberculosis* strains resistant to isoniazid and rifampin.[60] BCG vaccination of healthcare workers should be considered on an individualized basis in settings in which a high prevalence of patients is infected with MDR-TB, transmission of MDR-TB strains to healthcare workers and subsequent infection are likely, and comprehensive infection control precautions have been unsuccessful.[60] BCG vaccination is contraindicated in pregnancy and in persons who are immunocompromised (e.g., HIV infection) or persons who are likely to become immunocompromised (e.g., organ transplantation).[60] Adverse reactions to the BCG vaccine vary according to the type, dose, and age of the vaccine. Osteitis, prolonged ulceration at the vaccination site, lupoid reactions, regional suppurative lymphadenitis, disseminated BCG infection, and death have been reported.[60]

An interferon-γ release assay (IGRA) is preferred over the tuberculin skin test for persons who have received the BCG vaccine.[63] Two IGRAs are currently approved by the FDA as an aid for diagnosing both latent and active *M. tuberculosis* infection: the QuantiFERON-TB Gold test and the T-SPOT.TB test. These IGRAs assess response to synthetic peptides that represent specific proteins, early secretory antigenic target-6 (ESAT-6) and culture filtrate protein-10 (CFP-10), that are present in all *M. tuberculosis* strains.[63] In sensitized patients, ESAT-6 and CFP-10 are recognized by T cells and stimulate release of interferon-γ. The QuantiFERON-TB Gold test measures the interferon-γ concentrations released using an enzyme-linked immunosorbent assay. The T-SPOT.TB test uses an enzyme-linked immunospot assay (ELISpot) to detect increases in the number of cells that secrete interferon-γ. However, ESAT-6 and CFP-10 are not present in BCG vaccine strains and most nontuberculous mycobacteria; therefore, IGRAs have improved specificity in BCG-vaccinated persons compared with the tuberculin skin test.[63] Results are available within 24 hours compared to 2 to 3 days for tuberculin skin testing.

CASE 68-1, QUESTION 7: Should H.G. be tested for HIV infection?

The CDC recommends HIV screening for all patients with TB as well as those persons suspected of having TB disease and contacts of patients with TB.[64] Therefore, H.G. should be tested for HIV. HIV infection is the most important risk factor for progression of latent TB infection to active disease, and progression is more rapid in HIV-infected persons. Unlike other AIDS-related opportunistic infections, CD4 count is not a reliable predictor of increased risk of TB disease in HIV-infected persons.[65] TB may be the first manifestation of HIV infection because patients can have a relatively high CD4 count when TB disease develops.[65]

TREATMENT OF ACTIVE DISEASE

Initial Therapy

CASE 68-1, QUESTION 8: H.G.'s HIV test is negative. How should treatment be initiated in H.G., pending the results of sputum culture and susceptibility testing? Can he transmit *M. tuberculosis* to others during treatment?

There are four basic regimens recommended for the treatment of adult patients with active TB caused by organisms that are known or presumed to be drug susceptible (Table 68-2).[33] Because H.G. has not been treated previously for TB, he should be started on isoniazid, rifampin, pyrazinamide, and ethambutol. However, he has been in close contact with persons with symptoms resembling TB who are from an area (Mexico) with a high prevalence of drug-resistant TB. Therefore, H.G. must be closely monitored for resolution of symptoms, results of repeated sputum smears, and culture and susceptibility results, regardless of the initial treatment regimen. Previous guidelines recommended the addition of ethambutol only if the local prevalence of isoniazid-resistant *M. tuberculosis* is at least 4%.[34,66] In the United States, 9.3% of *M. tuberculosis* isolates recovered from patients with no previous history of TB were resistant to isoniazid in 2014.[10] The prevalence of isoniazid resistance was higher in foreign-born persons (10.2%) compared with US-born persons (7.5%).[10] In patients with a history of previous of TB, 18.9% of strains were resistant to isoniazid in 2014, with 24.7% resistance in foreign-born persons versus 4.4% resistance in US-born persons.[10] Because of the relatively high likelihood of TB caused by isoniazid-resistant organisms, four drugs are necessary in the initial 8-week treatment phase.[33]

The initial four-drug regimen may be administered daily throughout the 8-week period (regimen 1), daily for the first 2 weeks and then twice weekly for 6 weeks (regimen 2), or thrice weekly throughout (regimen 3).[33] Based on clinical experience, administration of drugs for 5 days/week is considered to be equivalent

Table 68-2

Treatment Regimens for Pulmonary Tuberculosis Caused by Drug-Susceptible Organisms

Initial Phase			Continuation Phase			Rating (Evidence)[a]		
Regimen	Drugs	Interval and Doses (Minimal Duration)	Regimen	Drugs	Interval and Doses (Minimal Duration)[b]	# Total Doses (Minimal Duration)	HIV–	HIV+
1	INH RIF PZA EMB	7 days/week for 56 doses (8 weeks) *OR* 5 days/week for 40 doses (8 weeks)[c]	1a	INH/RIF	7 days/week for 126 doses (18 weeks) *OR* 5 days/week for 90 doses (18 weeks)[c]	182–130 (26 weeks)	A (I)	A (II)
			1b	INH/RIF	Twice weekly for 36 doses (18 weeks)	92–76 (26 weeks)	A (I)	A (II)[d]
			1c[e]	INH/RPT	Once weekly for 18 doses (18 weeks)	74–58 (26 weeks)	B (I)	E (I)
2	INH RIF PZA EMB	7 days/week for 14 doses (2 weeks) *then* twice weekly for 12 doses (6 weeks) *OR* 5 days/week for 10 doses (2 weeks)[c] *then* twice weekly for 12 doses (6 weeks)	2a 2b[e]	INF/RIF INH/RPT	Twice weekly for 36 doses (18 weeks) Once weekly for 18 doses (18 weeks)	62–58 (26 weeks) 44–40 (26 weeks)	A (II) B (I)	B (II)[d] E (I)
3	INH RIF PZA EMB	3 times weekly for 24 doses (8 weeks)	3a	INH/RIF	3 times weekly for 54 doses (18 weeks)	78 (26 weeks)	B (I)	B (II)
4	INH RIF EMB	7 days/week for 56 doses (8 weeks) *Or* 5 days/week for 40 doses (8 weeks)[c]	4a	INH/RIF	7 days/week for 217 doses (31 weeks) *Or* 5 days/week for 155 doses (31 weeks)[c]	273–195 (39 weeks)	C (I)	C (II)
			4b	INH/RIF	Twice weekly for 62 doses (31 weeks)	118–102 (39 weeks)	C (I)	C (II)

[a]Definitions of evidence ratings: A, preferred; B, acceptable alternative; C, offer when A and B cannot be given; E, should never be given; I, randomized clinical trial; II, data from clinical trials that were not randomized or were conducted in other populations; III, expert opinion.
[b]Patients with cavitation on initial chest radiograph and positive cultures at completion of 2 months of therapy should receive a 7-month continuation phase (31 weeks; either 217 doses [daily] or 62 doses [twice weekly]).
[c]Five-day-a-week administration is always given by directly observed therapy (DOT). Rating for 5 days/week regimens is A (III).
[d]Not recommended for HIV-infected patients with $CD4^+$ cell counts <100 cells/μL.
[e]Options 1c and 2b should be used only in HIV-negative patients who have negative sputum smears at the time of completion of 2 months of therapy and who do not have cavitation on the initial chest radiograph.
EMB, ethambutol; INH, isoniazid; PZA, pyrazinamide; RIF, rifampin; RPT, rifapentine.

to 7 days/week administration and either regimen 1 or 2 may be considered "daily." However, 5-day-a-week administration should always be given by DOT.[33] Drug dosages for these recommended regimens are listed in Table 68-3. H.G. should be started on isoniazid 300 mg daily, rifampin 600 mg daily, pyrazinamide 1,500 mg daily, and ethambutol 1,200 mg daily. He should also receive pyridoxine 25 mg/day to minimize the risk for development of isoniazid-induced peripheral neuropathy.

Fixed-dose combinations of drugs have been advocated to improve adherence to the prescribed regimen, especially during the critical initial treatment phase. There are two fixed-dose combination preparations available in the United States: Rifamate, which contains isoniazid 150 mg and rifampin 300 mg/capsule, and Rifater, which contains isoniazid 50 mg, rifampin 120 mg, and pyrazinamide 300 mg/tablet. These formulations are a means of minimizing inadvertent monotherapy, especially when DOT

Table 68-3
Drugs Used in the Treatment of Tuberculosis in Adults and Children

Drug	Dosing (Maximum Dose)	Primary Side Effects	Dose Adjustment in Renal Impairment	Comments
First-Line Agents				
Isoniazid	Adults: 5 mg/kg (300 mg) daily; 15 mg/kg (900 mg) once, twice, or thrice weekly Children: 10–15 mg/kg (300 mg) daily; 20–30 mg/kg (900 mg) twice weekly	Increased aminotransferases (asymptomatic), clinical hepatitis, peripheral neuropathy, CNS effects, lupus-like syndrome, hypersensitivity reactions	No	Peripheral neuropathy preventable with pyridoxine 10–25 mg. Hepatitis more common in older patients and alcoholics. Potent inhibitor of CYP2C9, CYP2C19, CYP2E1. ↑ serum level of phenytoin
Rifampin	Adults: 10 mg/kg (600 mg) once daily, twice weekly, or thrice weekly Children: 10–20 mg/kg (600 mg) once daily or twice weekly	Pruritus, rash, hepatotoxicity, GI (nausea, anorexia, abdominal pain), flu-like syndrome, thrombocytopenia, renal failure	No	Orange-red discoloration of body secretions (sweat, saliva, tears, urine). Potent inducer of CYP3A4, CYP1A2, CYP2A6, CYP2B6, CYP2C8, CYP2C9, CYP2C19, and CYP3A5.
Rifabutin	Adults: 5 mg/kg (300 mg) once daily, twice weekly, or thrice weekly Children: unknown	Neutropenia, uveitis, GI symptoms, polyarthralgias, hepatotoxicity, rash	No	Orange-red discoloration of body secretions (sweat, saliva, tears, urine). Weaker inducer of hepatic microsomal enzymes than rifampin.
Rifapentine	Adults: Active disease, 10 mg/kg (600 mg) once weekly during continuation phase; latent infection, 15 mg/kg (900 mg) once weekly Children 2-11 years: 15 mg/kg (900 mg) once weekly	Similar to rifampin	Unknown	Drug interactions due to induction of hepatic microsomal enzymes (see rifampin).
Pyrazinamide	Adults: 40–55 kg: 1 g daily, 2 g twice weekly, 1.5 g thrice weekly; 56–75 kg: 1.5 g daily, 3 g twice weekly, 2.5 g thrice weekly; 76–90 kg: 2 g daily, 4 g twice weekly, 3 g thrice weekly Children: 15–30 mg/kg (2 g) daily; 50 mg/kg (2 g) twice weekly	Hepatotoxicity, nausea, anorexia, polyarthralgias, rash, hyperuricemia, dermatitis	Yes	Monitor aminotransferases monthly.
Ethambutol	Adults: 40–55 kg: 800 mg daily, 2 g twice weekly, 1.2 g thrice weekly; 56–75 kg: 1.2 g daily, 2.8 g twice weekly, 2 g thrice weekly; 76–90 kg:1.6 g daily, 4 g twice weekly, 2.4 g thrice weekly Children: 15–20 mg/kg (1 g) daily; 50 mg/kg (2.5 g) twice weekly	Optic neuritis, skin rash, drug fever	Yes	Routine vision tests recommended; 50% excreted unchanged in urine.

(continued)

Table 68-3

Drugs Used in the Treatment of Tuberculosis in Adults and Children (*continued*)

Drug	Dosing (Maximum Dose)	Primary Side Effects	Dose Adjustment in Renal Impairment	Comments
Second-Line Agents				
Cycloserine	Adults: 10–15 mg/kg/day (1 g), usually 500–750 mg/day in 2 divided doses Children: 10–15 mg/kg/day (1 g)	CNS toxicity (psychosis, seizures), headache, tremor, fever, skin rashes	Yes	May exacerbate seizure disorders or mental illness. Some toxicity preventable by pyridoxine (100–200 mg/day). Monitor serum concentrations (peak 20–35 mcg/mL desirable).
Ethionamide	Adults: 15–20 mg/kg/day (1 g), usually 500–750 mg/day in one daily dose or 2 divided doses Children: 15–20 mg/kg/day (1 g)	GI effects (metallic taste, nausea, vomiting, anorexia, abdominal pain), hepatotoxicity, neurotoxicity, endocrine effects (alopecia, gynecomastia, impotence, hypothyroidism), difficulty in diabetes management	Yes	Must be given with meals and antacids. Monitor aminotransferases and thyroid-stimulating hormone monthly.
Streptomycin	Adults: 15 mg/kg/day (1 g); ≥60 years, 10 mg/kg/day (750 mg) Children: 20–40 mg/kg/day (1 g)	Vestibular or auditory dysfunction of eighth cranial nerve, renal dysfunction, skin rashes, neuromuscular blockade	Yes	Audiometric and neurologic examinations recommended; 60%–80% excreted unchanged in urine. Monitor renal function.
Amikacin	Adults: 15 mg/kg/day (1 g); ≥60 years, 10 mg/kg/day (750 mg) Children: 15–30 mg/kg/day (1 g)	Ototoxicity, nephrotoxicity	Yes	Less vestibular toxicity than streptomycin. Monitoring similar to streptomycin.
Capreomycin	Adults: 15 mg/kg/day (1 g); ≥60 years, 10 mg/kg/day (750 mg) Children: 15–30 mg/kg/day (1 g) as single dose or twice-weekly dose	Nephrotoxicity, ototoxicity	Yes	Monitoring similar to streptomycin.
p-Aminosalicylic acid (PAS)	Adults: 8–12 g/day in 2–3 doses Children: 200–300 mg/kg/day in 2–4 divided doses	GI intolerance, hepatotoxicity, malabsorption syndrome, hypothyroidism	Yes	Liver enzymes and thyroid function should be monitored.
Levofloxacin	Adults: 500 to 1,000 mg/day	Nausea, diarrhea, abdominal pain, anorexia, headache, dizziness, QT prolongation, tendon pain or rupture	Yes	Do not give with divalent or trivalent cations (aluminum, magnesium, iron, etc.).
Moxifloxacin	Adults: 400 mg/day	Nausea, diarrhea, abdominal pain, anorexia, headache, dizziness, QT prolongation, tendon pain, or rupture	No	See levofloxacin.
Bedaquiline	Adults: 400 mg once daily for 2 weeks, then 200 mg thrice weekly for 22 weeks	Nausea, arthralgias, headache, increased transaminases, hemoptysis, chest pain, anorexia, rash, QT prolongation	No	Take with food. CYP3A4 substrate, avoid concomitant administration with inducers and inhibitors. Increased mortality compared to placebo.

CNS, central nervous system; GI, gastrointestinal.

is not possible, and they may decrease the risk of acquired drug resistance while reducing the number of capsules or tablets that must be ingested each day.[33] Safety and efficacy of a four-drug fixed-dose combination regimen was compared with each drug administered separately in patients with pulmonary TB.[67] The combination tablet contained isoniazid 75 mg, rifampin 150 mg, pyrazinamide 400 mg, and ethambutol 275 mg, and two to five tablets were ingested per day based on body weight. The number of patients who were culture negative at 18 and 24 months was similar between the treatment groups, in addition to the number of treatment failures, relapses, and death. The four-drug fixed-dose combination was noninferior to each drug administered separately.[67] It should be noted that there was no difference in outcomes based on HIV status, but less than 7% of the study subjects were HIV positive.[67]

The high risk of transmission of *M. tuberculosis* to other persons mandates that hospitalized persons with suspected or confirmed infectious TB be placed in respiratory isolation until they are determined not to have TB, they are discharged from the hospital, or they are confirmed to be noninfectious.[34] Based on H.G.'s subjective and objective findings, he should be placed in respiratory isolation. H.G.'s symptoms should improve within the first 4 weeks. He would be considered to be noninfectious when he is receiving effective drug therapy, is improving clinically, and has had negative results for three consecutive sputum AFB smears collected on different days.[34] Patients who have responded clinically may be discharged to home despite positive smears if their household contacts have already been exposed and these contacts are not at increased risk of TB (e.g., infants, HIV-positive and immunosuppressed persons). In addition, patients discharged to home with positive smears must agree not to have contact with other susceptible persons.[34]

Fluoroquinolones as Initial Therapy

Interest in fluoroquinolones for the treatment of TB dates back more than 30 years with a report describing the use of ofloxacin in 19 patients with chronic, drug-resistant TB disease.[68] Several fluoroquinolones possess in vitro activity against *M. tuberculosis*, but moxifloxacin and gatifloxacin are four- to eightfold more potent than levofloxacin.[69] Moxifloxacin was compared with ethambutol in the first 2 months of treatment in adults with smear-positive pulmonary TB.[70] Patients were randomly assigned to receive moxifloxacin 400 mg daily or ethambutol (based on body weight), and all patients received isoniazid, rifampin, and pyrazinamide. Patients receiving moxifloxacin were more likely to have negative sputum cultures at 4 weeks and 6 weeks, but the 2-month conversion rates were equal in each group.[70] In another study, sputum culture conversion at 8 weeks was significantly greater in patients treated with moxifloxacin when compared with ethambutol (80% vs. 63%).[71] Culture conversion rates were also significantly higher in the moxifloxacin group at weeks 1, 2, 3, and 4, and the median time to consistently negative cultures was 35.0 days in the moxifloxacin group and 48.5 days in the ethambutol group.[71]

Moxifloxacin has been compared with isoniazid during the intensive phase of treatment of pulmonary TB.[72] Patients were randomly assigned to receive moxifloxacin 400 mg or isoniazid 300 mg daily, and all patients received rifampin, pyrazinamide, and ethambutol.[72] After 8 weeks, negative sputum cultures were observed in 60.4% of the patients in the moxifloxacin group and 54.9% of patients in the isoniazid group, but this difference was not statistically significant.[72]

Despite the reported efficacy of fluoroquinolones in the treatment of TB, clinicians must be cognizant of the potential development of resistance to this important drug class. Fluoroquinolone resistance in *M. tuberculosis* has been described, occurring more frequently in multidrug-resistant isolates.[73] Fluoroquinolones are the most commonly prescribed antibiotic class in the United States, and outpatient use for infections other than TB could be a potential risk factor for TB resistance in a patient who becomes infected with *M. tuberculosis*. In a study evaluating risk factors for fluoroquinolone-resistant *M. tuberculosis*, investigators identified newly diagnosed patients with culture-confirmed TB in a Medicaid population.[74] Of the 640 patients evaluated, 116 (18%) patients had fluoroquinolone exposure within the 12 months before diagnosis with TB, and 16 (2.5%) patients were infected with *M. tuberculosis* strains that were fluoroquinolone resistant.[74] The study found that receipt of a fluoroquinolone for more than 10 days, occurring more than 60 days before diagnosis of TB, was associated with the highest risk for fluoroquinolone resistance.[74] Therefore, judicious use of fluoroquinolones, especially in patients at risk for TB infection, is mandatory to maintain the utility of fluoroquinolones in the treatment of TB.

Susceptibility Testing

Drug susceptibility testing is essential to ensure proper treatment of patients with active disease and should be performed on the initial isolate of *M. tuberculosis* from all patients.[18] Susceptibility testing should also be performed if cultures remain positive after 3 months of therapy or if negative cultures become positive after a period of time. Traditionally, susceptibility testing is performed by growing the organism on solid or in liquid media containing the drug. The agar proportion method allows for quantitation of the proportion of organisms that are resistant to a given drug, which is expressed as a percentage of the total organism population tested.[18] A drug will not be useful for therapy if 1% or more of the total population are resistant to the drug. Unfortunately, susceptibility results may not be available for several weeks because of the slow growth of the organism and the need to isolate the pathogen before susceptibility testing can be performed.[18]

To expedite susceptibility reporting, molecular drug resistance tests have been developed to detect mutations in the chromosomal sequence encoding for resistance to a specific drug directly on clinical specimens without the need for growth on culture.[54,55] For example, mutations in the *rpoB* gene block the activity of rifampin by preventing the drug from binding to RNA polymerase. Approximately 95% of rifampin-resistant *M. tuberculosis* carry this mutation, and treatment failures have been associated with the presence of *rpoB* mutations.[75,76] The molecular drug resistance test amplifies the target genetic sequence using polymerase chain reaction, and a second assay, such as DNA sequencing and hybridization assays, is used to determine whether the sequence contains a mutation associated with drug resistance. If a mutation is detected, the organism is considered to be drug resistant, but the organism is presumed to be drug susceptible if a mutation is not detected. Molecular tests can reliably detect the presence of known mutations within 1 to 2 days, which may result in earlier initiation of effective therapy, shorter durations of infectivity, and reduced spread of TB. However, these molecular drug resistance tests can only detect a specific set of known mutations and cannot identify novel mutations conferring resistance.[55] Therefore, traditional susceptibility testing continues to play an important role in confirming results of molecular testing.[54]

Kits for detecting mutations associated with rifampin resistance include GenoType MTBDR(*plus*) and INNO-LiPA Rif.TB. Compared with culture-based drug resistance tests, the sensitivity and specificity of the MTBDR(*plus*) line-probe assay were 98% and 99%, respectively, for detecting rifampin resistance in isolates or directly from clinical specimens.[77,78] The sensitivity of the INNO-LiPA Rif.TB assay ranged from 80% to 100% and the specificity was 100% for detecting rifampin resistance directly from clinical specimens.[77,78] Molecular beacons are hybridization probes that use fluorescent-labeled, hairpin-shaped DNA probes with a fluorophore adjacent to a molecule that prevents fluorescence.[35] Using a real-time polymerase chain reaction assay, fluorescence occurs if the amplified PCR products have the wild-type gene sequence, but fluorescence is not detected if mutations are present in the target sequence. These tests have high sensitivity (96%–97%) and specificity (99%–100%) for rifampin resistance in clinical specimens.[79] Molecular drug resistance tests for other antitubercular drugs are not fully developed compared with tests for rifampin resistance. For detecting mutations associated with isoniazid resistance, the specificity of the MTBDR(*plus*) assay was 100%, but the sensitivity ranged from 57% to 100% (pooled sensitivity 85%).[79] However, rifampin resistance is a reliable surrogate for MDR-TB in the United States because isolated rifampin resistance is uncommon.

The Xpert MTB/RIF assay is an automated molecular-based test that uses nested real-time polymerase chain reaction, allowing for simultaneous detection of *M. tuberculosis* and rifampin resistance. The test is approved for diagnostic testing of raw sputum samples, and results are available within 2 hours.[54] Sensitivity is 95% to 98.2% in AFB culture or smear-positive specimens, but performance is correlated with bacterial load because sensitivity is only 55% to 72.5% in smear-negative specimens.[80,81] Sensitivity is also lower in patients with HIV infection. Specificity was 94% to 99.2% in patients with negative cultures.[80,81] The Xpert MTB/RIF test also correctly identified 98.1% of patients with rifampin-susceptible bacilli and 97.6% of patients with rifampin-resistant bacilli.[80]

CASE 68-1, QUESTION 9: Is H.G. a risk to the community and does anyone need to know?

Yes! Each case of active TB disease must be reported to the local, state, or both public health departments.[18,34,82] This not only results in optimal therapy by monitoring adherence to therapy, but it also ensures that contact and source-case investigations will be performed. All individuals who have been in close contact to H.G. should be evaluated for latent TB infection or active disease. Considering their close contact to H.G. and his coworkers, his family members should be evaluated. Reporting of cases also permits record-keeping and surveillance to determine whether public health TB control efforts are achieving their goal of preventing the spread of TB.[34,82]

Continuation Therapy

REGIMENS

CASE 68-1, QUESTION 10: Four weeks later, H.G.'s initial sputum cultures were reported to be positive for *M. tuberculosis*. Drug susceptibility testing to isoniazid and rifampin revealed susceptibility to both agents. What drug regimen should be used for continued treatment of H.G.? How long should treatment be continued?

Successful treatment of uncomplicated TB can be achieved in 6 months (26 weeks) if isoniazid, rifampin, pyrazinamide, and ethambutol are used for the first 2 months (8 weeks) and if patient adherence to the regimen and the organism susceptibility can be assured.[33] Therefore, after 8 weeks of DOT with isoniazid, rifampin, pyrazinamide, and ethambutol, H.G.'s regimen may be streamlined to isoniazid and rifampin daily (5 days or 7 days/week) or 2 to 3 times/week under continued DOT for an additional 18 weeks (Table 68-2). Because H.G. is HIV negative and cavitary lesions were not present on his chest radiograph, he may also be a candidate for once-weekly administration of isoniazid and rifapentine, as long as his sputum AFB smear is negative after completing the initial 8 weeks of therapy.[33]

The effectiveness of a primarily twice-weekly treatment regimen has been demonstrated in both pulmonary and extrapulmonary TB.[83] The regimen consisted of isoniazid 300 mg, rifampin 600 mg, pyrazinamide 1.5 to 2.5 g, and streptomycin 750 to 1,000 mg intramuscularly daily for 2 weeks, followed by the same drugs twice weekly for an additional 6 weeks. The regimen was then reduced to isoniazid and rifampin twice weekly for the remaining 16 weeks (4 months). At 3 months, 75% of patients had negative sputum cultures, and all patients were culture negative at 20 weeks.[83] Relapse occurred in two patients and only minor adverse effects were reported. Another important feature is that this regimen is highly cost-effective. Among the 6- and 9-month regimens, it is the second lowest in cost, primarily because of the least number of patient–healthcare worker encounters (62 directly observed doses).

If pyrazinamide cannot be included in the initial regimen, therapy should be initiated with isoniazid, rifampin, and ethambutol for the first 8 weeks. Therapy should be continued with isoniazid and rifampin for 31 weeks given either daily or twice weekly.[33] If drugs other than isoniazid and rifampin are used in the initial phase, treatment must be continued for 18 to 24 months.[66]

Twice-weekly administration of isoniazid (900 mg) and rifampin (600 mg) is recommended for H.G. because this approach requires fewer doses and should result in substantial cost savings.[33] In addition, the relapse rates for the twice- and thrice-weekly isoniazid and rifampin continuation regimens are significantly lower than the once-weekly regimen of isoniazid and rifapentine 600 mg.[84,85] Five characteristics were associated with increased relapse risk in the isoniazid and rifapentine group: sputum culture positive at 2 months; cavitation on chest radiograph; underweight; bilateral pulmonary involvement; non-Hispanic Caucasian race.[85] A potential explanation for these results is the high protein binding of rifapentine (98%). A study evaluated the safety and tolerability of rifapentine 600, 900, and 1,200 mg once weekly (with isoniazid 15 mg/kg) in 150 HIV-negative patients.[86] A trend toward more adverse events was observed in the 1,200-mg treatment arm ($p = 0.051$), but the 900-mg dose was well tolerated.[86] However, relapse rates for the higher-dose weekly rifapentine regimens with isoniazid are unknown. A subsequent study demonstrated that low plasma concentrations of isoniazid were associated with failure or relapse with once-weekly isoniazid and rifapentine.[87] Two patients who relapsed with *M. tuberculosis* monoresistant to rifamycin had very low isoniazid concentrations. Rapid acetylation status was a risk factor in those patients who failed or relapsed.[87] Rifamycin pharmacokinetics did not influence patient outcomes, however.[87]

Treatment with isoniazid and rifampin should be continued for a minimum total duration of 26 weeks. A full course of therapy can be more accurately determined by the total number of doses ingested, not solely by the duration of therapy.[33] Thus, 26 weeks is the minimum duration of treatment and accurately indicates the amount of time the drugs are given only if there are no interruptions in drug administration.[33] Pyridoxine 10 to 25 mg/day should be continued throughout the treatment period. If H.G. is symptomatic, or smear or culture is positive after 3 months of therapy, he should be re-evaluated for possible nonadherence with his therapy, malabsorption of the drugs, or infection with drug-resistant organisms. Evaluation should include a second culture and a second susceptibility test, consideration of DOT (if not already instituted), and consultation with experts in the treatment of TB.[34]

CASE 68-1, QUESTION 11: H.G. is concerned about the long duration required for treatment of his infection. He asks whether there is any way to shorten the length of treatment. Are there any effective treatment regimens that may be administered for less than 26 weeks?

Treatment of active TB for 26 weeks is a challenge to ensure patients adhere to the prescribed regimen for the total duration of therapy. Shorter-course treatment regimens, if efficacious, could be helpful in improving adherence rates, decreasing treatment costs, and reducing adverse events. Three published studies evaluated the treatment of drug-susceptible TB for a total duration of 4 months using modified regimens that included a fluoroquinolone (moxifloxacin or gatifloxacin).[88–90] The control regimen was the same in each study and consisted of 8 weeks of isoniazid, rifampin, pyrazinamide, and ethambutol followed by isoniazid and rifampin for 18 weeks. In all three studies, unfavorable outcomes and culture-confirmed relapse/recurrence were more common in patients receiving the short-course regimens; therefore, noninferiority was not demonstrated for any of the 4-month regimens.[88–90] Based on these studies, H.G. should receive 26 weeks of therapy, and every effort should be made to ensure adherence to the treatment regimen.

Directly Observed Therapy

CASE 68-1, QUESTION 12: What is directly observed therapy, and why is it important for H.G. to be treated by directly observed therapy?

Directly observed therapy (DOT) is the practice of a healthcare provider or other responsible person observing as the patient ingests and swallows the TB medications. DOT is the preferred core management strategy for *all* patients with TB.[33–35] The purpose of DOT is to ensure adherence to TB therapy. DOT not only ensures completion of therapy, but it may also reduce the risk of developing drug resistance. By improving these two factors, it also reduces the risk of transmission of TB to the community. DOT can be administered with daily or twice- and thrice-weekly regimens. It can be administered to patients in the office or clinic setting, or it can be given at the patient's home, school, or work.[33,66] Often, enablers or incentives, such as food, clothing, or transportation, are used to improve adherence to DOT. A comprehensive review of DOT-related articles found that the completion rate of TB therapy exceeds 90% when DOT is used along with enablers.[35,91] A study found that culture-positive patients treated for active pulmonary TB with DOT had significantly higher cure rates (97.8% vs. 88.6%; $p < 0.002$) and lower TB-related mortality (0% vs. 5.5%; $p = 0.002$) compared with patients treated using self-administered therapy.[92] Although DOT is recommended for all patients, public health departments may not be able to provide DOT for all patients because of the associated costs. The initial cost of DOT is greater than self-administered therapy; however, when costs of relapse and failure are included in a cost-effectiveness analysis, DOT is significantly less expensive than self-administered therapy.[93] When drug resistance develops (in those instances in which DOT is not used), the cost of salvage therapy increases to $180,000.00 per patient.[94] It is, therefore, widely accepted that patients with TB should receive DOT.[93,95]

Multiple-Drug Therapy

CASE 68-1, QUESTION 13: Why are multiple drugs recommended for treatment of active TB disease? What is the role of each drug in the treatment of active TB?

The key to treating active TB disease is multiple-drug therapy for a period sufficient to kill the organisms and to prevent development of resistant strains of *M. tuberculosis*. Most cavitary lesions contain a concentration of 10^9 to 10^{12} organisms, and the frequency of mutations that confer resistance to a single drug is approximately 10^{-6} for isoniazid and streptomycin, 10^{-8} for rifampin, and 10^{-5} for ethambutol.[33] Considering the inoculum of organisms involved, patients with active TB disease likely harbor organisms with random mutations that confer drug resistance to a given drug. If a single drug is given, it would reduce the number of drug-susceptible organisms but allow the drug-resistant organisms to replicate. By using multiple-drug therapy, the likelihood of encountering organisms with mutations to multiple drugs is reduced. For example, the frequency of concurrent mutations to isoniazid and rifampin would be 10^{-14} (10^{-6} for isoniazid and 10^{-8} for rifampin), making simultaneous resistance to both drugs an unlikely event in an untreated patient.[33] Therefore, monotherapy should never be used in the treatment of active TB disease.[33,94]

Multiple-drug therapy also serves to sterilize the sputum and lesions as quickly as possible. The drugs available for the treatment of TB vary in their ability to accomplish this task.[33] Drugs effective against tubercle bacilli can be divided into first-line and second-line agents (Table 68-3). The foundation of treatment should be with first-line agents, such as isoniazid, rifampin, pyrazinamide, and ethambutol. Of the various agents, isoniazid has the most bactericidal activity versus rapidly multiplying *M. tuberculosis* during the initial phase of therapy (early bactericidal activity), followed by ethambutol, rifampin, and streptomycin.[96–98] Drugs that have potent early bactericidal activity more rapidly decrease the infectiousness of the patient and reduce the likelihood of developing resistance.[33] Pyrazinamide has weak early bactericidal activity during the first 2 weeks of therapy and is less effective at preventing emergence of drug resistance than isoniazid, rifampin, and ethambutol.[33,96,99] Therefore, pyrazinamide should not be combined with only one other agent when treating active TB disease. Rifampin also has activity against intracellular organisms that are usually dormant but undergo periods of active growth. This ability to penetrate and destroy the persistent intracellular organisms makes rifampin extremely valuable in short-course chemotherapy regimens.[100]

Pyrazinamide is most effective against tubercle bacilli in the acidic environment within the macrophage or areas of tissue necrosis. In addition, it is most effective in sterilizing lesions when used in the first 2 months of treatment, but it does not offer substantial sterilizing activity after 2 months. Pyrazinamide should be considered an essential component of short-course regimens.[33,66]

Ethambutol is bacteriostatic at low doses, but bactericidal at higher doses. It is moderately effective against the fast-growing bacilli. It has little sterilizing activity and is primarily used to prevent the emergence of drug-resistant organisms.[66]

Streptomycin is bactericidal against rapidly multiplying extracellular organisms and is effective when given daily for 2 months followed by twice- or thrice-weekly administration thereafter. In the past, streptomycin was administered by intramuscular injection, but these intramuscular injections were painful. Therefore, although it is not labeled for intravenous use, streptomycin may be given in 50 to 100 mL of 5% dextrose in water or normal saline and infused for 30 to 60 minutes.[101] Streptomycin can cause ototoxicity and nephrotoxicity, as with other aminoglycosides.

Other drugs used in the treatment of TB (bedaquiline, capreomycin, amikacin, cycloserine, ethionamide, *p*-aminosalicylic acid) are usually reserved for cases involving drug-resistant organisms, treatment failures, drug toxicity, or patient intolerance to the other agents. Their use is discussed later in the chapter.

Monitoring Drug Therapy

CASE 68-1, QUESTION 14: What subjective and objective findings should be followed to ensure therapeutic efficacy and to minimize drug toxicity? Should H.G. be followed closely after completion of his treatment regimen?

H.G. should be questioned about the occurrence of adverse reactions associated with his therapy (Table 68-3). Specifically, he should be asked about anorexia, nausea, vomiting, or abdominal pain, which may be an indication of possible hepatitis secondary to isoniazid, rifampin, or pyrazinamide. He should be questioned about numbness and tingling in his extremities; however, isoniazid-induced peripheral neuropathy should not be a problem in H.G. because he is also taking pyridoxine, which should prevent this adverse effect. H.G. also should be examined for, and questioned about, petechiae or bruises, because thrombocytopenia occurs occasionally with intermittent rifampin therapy. This effect purportedly occurs more frequently with intermittent rifampin therapy, but it is rare at the currently recommended intermittent rifampin dose of 10 mg/kg/day (≈600 mg).[66]

In a study comparing 6- versus 9-month antituberculosis therapies of mostly isoniazid and rifampin, the incidence of side effects was similar between the two groups. Adverse effects occurred in 7.7% of patients in the 6-month arm compared with 6.4% in the 9-month arm, a difference that was not statistically significant.[102] Hepatic abnormalities occurred in 1.6% of patients in the 6-month regimen, a nonsignificant difference from patients in the 9-month regimens (1.2%). Hematologic events were rare at 0.2% and 0.0% in the 6- and 9-month groups, respectively. Other reported effects, gastrointestinal (GI) problems, rash, and arthralgias were minor and infrequent in both regimens.[102]

OBJECTIVE SIGNS

A pretreatment complete blood count, platelet count, blood urea nitrogen, hepatic enzymes (serum aminotransferases), bilirubin, and serum uric acid should be evaluated. Baseline visual examination should also be considered for patients receiving ethambutol. These tests are performed to detect any abnormality that may complicate or necessitate modification of the prescribed regimen. These tests should be repeated if the patient experiences any evidence of drug toxicity or has abnormalities at baseline.[33,66]

H.G. is 35 years of age and at increased risk for development of drug-induced hepatotoxicity. Isoniazid can cause asymptomatic increases in serum transaminases as well as overt hepatitis.[33] Pyrazinamide has also been associated with hepatotoxicity, but the incidence is less common at doses of 25 mg/kg/day or less. Transient asymptomatic hyperbilirubinemia and cholestatic hepatitis can occur in patients receiving rifampin.[33] Therefore, it is important that H.G. be educated about possible symptoms of hepatotoxicity, primarily nausea, vomiting, abdominal pain, anorexia, and jaundice. Monthly serum liver function tests (LFTs) are no longer recommended because they are costly, and transient, asymptomatic elevations in LFTs may occur, which could result in unnecessary discontinuation of optimal therapy. The CDC recommends that medical personnel question patients about symptoms once monthly.[66]

Sputum cultures and smears for AFB should be ordered every 2 to 4 weeks initially and then monthly after the sputum cultures become negative. With appropriate therapy, sputum cultures should become negative in more than 85% of patients after 2 months. Radiologic examination (chest radiographs) is not as important as sputum examination, but it may be useful at the completion of therapy to serve as a comparison for any future films.

Patients who are culture positive at 2 months need to be carefully re-examined. Drug susceptibility testing should be performed to rule out acquired drug resistance, and special attention should be given to drug adherence (i.e., DOT should be used). If drug resistance is demonstrated, the regimen should be modified as needed. Sputum cultures should also be obtained monthly until negativity is achieved.[66]

As was the case for H.G., weight loss and nutritional depletion are common in patients with active TB disease. In a large TB treatment study, 7.1% of patients experienced relapse, with relapse greatest in patients who were underweight at diagnosis or with a body mass index less than 18.5 kg/m^2.[103] In those patients underweight at diagnosis (defined as ≥10% below ideal body weight), weight gain of 5% or less between diagnosis and completion of 2 months of therapy was independently associated with relapse.[103] In addition, the relapse rate was 50.5% in underweight patients with a cavitary lesion on chest radiograph, positive sputum cultures after 2 months of therapy, and a 5% or less weight gain in the first 2 months of therapy.[103] Therefore, it may be prudent to monitor H.G.'s body weight during the initial 2 months of therapy, and he may need to receive more intensive therapy or a longer duration of therapy.

Routine follow-up usually is not required after the successful completion of chemotherapy with isoniazid and rifampin. It may be prudent, however, to re-examine the patient 6 months after completion of therapy or at the first sign of any symptoms suggestive of active TB. This is especially important in patients who were slow to respond to therapy or who have significant radiologic findings at completion of therapy. These recommendations are only for those patients with organisms fully susceptible to the medications being used.[66]

Patients who are culture negative but have radiographic abnormalities consistent with TB should have an induced sputum or bronchoscopy performed to establish a microbiologic diagnosis and monitored radiographically. Patients with extrapulmonary TB should be evaluated according to the site of involvement.[33,66]

Treatment Failure

CASE 68-1, QUESTION 15: If H.G. does not respond to his currently prescribed treatment regimen, should one more drug be added to his regimen?

No! Adding a single drug to a failing regimen is the most common and devastating prescribing error in TB therapy. This practice is essentially monotherapy because the assumption is that the organisms are resistant to the medications currently being used. Resistance to the new drug will eventually develop, further reducing the patient's chance of cure. At least two, and preferably three, new drugs to which susceptibility can be inferred should be added to lessen the probability of further acquired drug resistance. Empiric retreatment regimens may include a fluoroquinolone, bedaquiline, an injectable agent (e.g., streptomycin, amikacin, or capreomycin), and an additional oral agent (e.g., *p*-aminosalicylic acid, cycloserine, or ethionamide).[33] New drug susceptibility testing should be performed and treatment adjusted accordingly.[33,94]

TREATMENT OF LATENT TUBERCULOSIS INFECTION

CASE 68-2

QUESTION 1: J.G., the 32-year-old wife of H.G., and their children are tested to determine whether they have been infected with *M. tuberculosis*. For his wife, the induration from 5 TU of PPD was 12 mm, which is reported as positive. J.G. states that she has never received the BCG vaccine. The PPD results for the children were negative. J.G. does not have any clinical symptoms or radiographic findings suggestive of active TB at this time, and her current weight is 60 kg. Is she at risk of developing active disease? What are the current recommendations for drug therapy for persons with latent TB infection? Should J.G. receive treatment?

Because J.G. is a household contact of a person with active TB disease and has a positive tuberculin skin test, she is at great risk of developing active disease.[22,23,48,49] During the first year after infection from the index case, a household contact's risk of developing active disease is 2% to 4%, and contacts with a positive tuberculin skin test are at the greatest risk.[66] As with active disease, the tuberculin skin test is usually performed to detect the presence of latent TB infection. However, for contact investigation, studies have demonstrated that IGRAs are a more accurate indicator of the presence of latent TB infection than tuberculin skin testing.[104,105]

Therefore, many health departments in the United States have adopted IGRAs as screening tests for contact investigations.[106] The majority of people with a negative IGRA after exposure to a person with active TB disease do not have TB infection; however, the immune reaction to TB can take several weeks to develop so the IGRA should be repeated 8 to 12 weeks after the last exposure to rule out infection.[23,106] Tuberculin skin testing is preferred for screening children younger than 5 years old.[23]

Treatment of latent TB infection is effective in preventing active TB disease in patients with a positive tuberculin skin test or IGRA result and in those at risk for reactivation of active TB; therefore, it is *strongly* recommended.[22,23] Treatment decreases the population of tubercle bacilli and reduces future morbidity from TB in the groups at high risk for developing active disease. Because J.G. is infected with *M. tuberculosis* but does not currently have active TB disease, she should be treated for latent TB infection.

There are four approved regimens for the treatment of latent TB.[22,23] Isoniazid monotherapy prevents active TB in 90% of patients who complete a 9-month regimen compared to 60% to 80% of patients who complete a 6-month regimen.[107] Therefore, isoniazid 300 mg daily or 900 mg twice weekly for 9 months is preferred. The twice-weekly regimen should be administered by DOT to ensure patient adherence.[19] A 6-month regimen is an acceptable alternative in patients who cannot complete 9 months of therapy.[22] The benefits of treating latent TB infection outweigh the risks of isoniazid-induced hepatitis because all persons infected with TB are at risk for developing active disease throughout their lifetime. All patients receiving isoniazid should receive pyridoxine 25 mg/day to minimize the risk of peripheral neuropathy.

Unfortunately, patient adherence to these isoniazid regimens is very poor. In a population of patients beginning isoniazid treatment for latent TB, only 64% of patients completed at least 6 months of therapy.[108] Younger age, Hispanic ethnicity, and non-US country of birth were associated with greater likelihood of completing therapy.[108] Lower completion rates were associated with homelessness, excess alcohol intake, and experiencing an adverse event.[108] In another study, 52.7% of patients receiving treatment for latent TB infection failed to complete the prescribed course of therapy.[109] More than 93% of these patients were receiving isoniazid. Risk factors for failing to complete therapy included receipt of a 9-month isoniazid regimen, residence in a congregate setting (nursing home, shelter, jail), injection drug use, and employment at a healthcare facility.[109] In addition, this study reported that employees at healthcare facilities were more likely to decline treatment for latent TB infection.[109]

Because of concerns for isoniazid toxicity and abysmal adherence rates, shorter rifampin-based regimens may be utilized. Daily isoniazid plus rifampin for 3 months and daily rifampin monotherapy for 4 months are acceptable alternatives to isoniazid therapy.[22,23,107] For the patients randomly assigned to receive daily rifampin for 4 months, 91% took 80% of the doses, and 86% took more than 90% of the doses at 20 weeks.[110] For the patients randomly assigned to receive daily isoniazid for 9 months, 76% took 80% of the doses, and only 62% took more than 90% of the doses at 43 weeks.[110] Discontinuation of therapy due to an adverse events was more common in the isoniazid group (14%) versus the rifampin group (3%).[110] Another study reported significantly fewer grade 3 to 4 adverse events and hepatitis and significantly higher treatment completion rates with 4 months of rifampin compared with 9 months of isoniazid.[111] Rifampin for 4 months is an effective, safe, and cost-effective strategy to consider when treating latent TB infection in selected populations of patients.[110–114]

An attractive alternative for the treatment of latent TB infection is the combination of isoniazid and rifapentine administered once weekly for 12 weeks.[22,23] In one study, patients received either isoniazid 15 to 25 mg/kg (maximal dose 900 mg) plus rifapentine 900 mg (with adjustments for patients weighing less than 50 kg) once weekly for 12 weeks by DOT or isoniazid 5 mg/kg (maximal dose 300 mg) once daily for 9 months.[115] Completion of therapy was significantly higher in the isoniazid/rifapentine group (82% vs. 69%; $p < 0.001$). Overall, TB developed in 7 of 3986 patients receiving isoniazid/rifapentine and 15 of 3,745 patients receiving isoniazid (hazard ratio 0.38 for the combination; 95% CI 0.15–0.99; $p = 0.05$).[115] Hepatotoxicity was higher in the isoniazid group (2.7% vs. 0.4%; $p < 0.001$), whereas hypersensitivity reactions were higher in the combination group (3.8% vs. 0.5%; $p < 0.001$). Permanent drug discontinuation for any reason was higher in the isoniazid group (31.0% vs. 17.9%; $p < 0.001$), but permanent drug discontinuation due to an adverse event was higher in the combination group (4.9% vs. 3.7%; $p = 0.009$).[115] The combination is recommended as an equal alternative to daily isoniazid for 9 months in patient 12 years or older with a greater risk of developing active TB disease.[116] These patients include those with recent exposure to a person with active TB, conversion of the tuberculin skin test or IGRA from negative to positive, or radiographic evidence of healed pulmonary TB. Isoniazid/rifapentine may also be considered in patients unlikely to complete 9 months of isoniazid or in a setting where the combination offers practical advantages (e.g., correctional facilities, homeless shelters). The combination is not recommended in women who are pregnant or who expect to become pregnant during treatment.

J.G. should be placed on isoniazid 300 mg/day or 900 mg twice weekly for at least 6 months and preferably up to 9 months, rifampin 600 mg for 4 months, or isoniazid 900 mg plus rifapentine 900 mg weekly for 12 weeks.[22,23,116] She should be educated and questioned frequently about the clinical symptoms of hepatitis, such as GI complaints. Pretreatment serum aminotransferases and bilirubin should be assessed to rule out preexisting liver disease. The American Thoracic Society and the CDC do not recommend routine monitoring of LFTs unless symptoms suggest hepatotoxicity.[66]

ADVERSE DRUG EVENTS

Isoniazid

HEPATOTOXICITY

CASE 68-2, QUESTION 2: J.G. is started on daily isoniazid. After 2 months of therapy, she presents to the clinic complaining of nausea, vomiting, and abdominal pain. Liver function tests were ordered, and her aspartate aminotransferase (AST) was 150 IU/L. Discuss the presentation, prognosis, and mechanism of isoniazid-induced hepatitis. What are the risk factors for developing hepatitis? Should isoniazid be discontinued to prevent further liver damage?

Approximately 10% to 20% of patients treated with isoniazid alone for latent TB infection will develop elevated serum aminotransferases, which are generally transient and asymptomatic.[33,117] Most patients with mild, subclinical hepatic damage do not progress to overt hepatitis and recover completely even while continuing isoniazid. In contrast, continuation of isoniazid in patients with symptoms of hepatitis increases the risk of mortality compared with immediate discontinuation.[33] The risk of death from TB, however, is estimated to be 11 times higher than the risk of death from isoniazid hepatotoxicity.[118]

Isoniazid-induced hepatotoxicity generally occurs within weeks to months of initiating therapy; 60% of cases occur in the first 3 months and 80% occur in the first 6 months.[117] Constitutional symptoms may be seen early and may last from days to months. Nausea, vomiting, and abdominal pain are seen in 50% to 75% of patients with severe hepatotoxicity.[117] Jaundice, dark urine, and clay-colored stools may also be seen. Recovery may take weeks after discontinuing isoniazid therapy. The development of isoniazid hepatotoxicity has been linked to several factors, including acetylator phenotype, age, daily alcohol consumption, and concurrent rifampin use. Additionally, women may be at higher risk of death, especially during the postpartum period.[118]

The mechanisms responsible for isoniazid hepatotoxicity remain unclear. Previously, it was thought that rapid acetylators had a greater risk for isoniazid hepatotoxicity than slow acetylators. Rapid acetylators of isoniazid form monoacetylhydrazine, a compound that can cause liver damage, more rapidly than slow acetylators.[119] Rapid acetylators, however, would eliminate monoacetylhydrazine at a faster rate, and this should equalize the risk of toxicity between slow and fast acetylators.[120] One study demonstrated a different incidence of hepatitis between Asian men and women. Because both groups were fast acetylators, this study suggests that hepatitis is associated with factors other than acetylator phenotype.[121] Some evidence supports the theory that isoniazid-induced hepatitis is a hypersensitivity reaction; however, many patients tolerate isoniazid on rechallenge, discounting this theory.[122,123]

Age and concurrent daily alcohol ingestion are the most consistent risk factors for isoniazid hepatitis.[66] Progressive liver damage is rare in persons younger than 20 years of age. It occurs in approximately 0.3% of persons between the ages of 20 and 34 years, 1.2% of those between the ages of 35 and 49 years, and 2.3% of persons older than 50 years of age.[66] One prospective cohort study, however, demonstrated a low incidence of isoniazid hepatitis. Of 11,141 patients receiving isoniazid alone for the treatment of latent TB infection, only 11 (0.1% of those starting and 0.15% of those completing therapy) developed clinical hepatitis.[124] Previous studies suggested a higher incidence of clinical hepatitis in patients receiving isoniazid alone, and a meta-analysis of six studies estimated the rate to be 0.6%.[33] However, severe hepatotoxicity may occur with isoniazid treatment of latent TB infection. The CDC reported 17 severe hepatic adverse events with isoniazid in 15 adults and 2 children (ages 11 and 14 years).[125] Five patients, including one child, underwent liver transplantation, and five adults died (including one liver transplant patient).

High-risk patients should be followed with routine monitoring of LFTs. These patients include those who consume alcohol daily, persons older than 35 years of age, those taking other hepatotoxic drugs, those with preexisting liver disease, intravenous drug users, black and Hispanic women, and all postpartum women. In these high-risk patients, isoniazid should be discontinued if the AST level exceeds 3 to 5 times the upper limit of the normal value.[66] Because J.G. is experiencing nausea, vomiting, and abdominal pain and her AST is greater than 3 times the upper range of the normal value, isoniazid should be discontinued temporarily until the AST returns to normal. At that time, isoniazid should be resumed, and her LFTs rechecked. If the AST increases again, the drug should be discontinued, and J.G. should be followed frequently for development of active TB.

CASE 68-3

QUESTION 1: C.M., an 80-kg, 35-year-old woman, is being treated for active TB disease with isoniazid 1,200 mg and rifampin 600 mg twice weekly. Is 1,200 mg of isoniazid twice weekly an appropriate dose for a 80-kg patient? What isoniazid side effects, other than hepatotoxicity, should be anticipated?

The usual twice-weekly isoniazid dose is 15 mg/kg, with a maximal dose of 900 mg. Even though she weighs 80 kg, C.M. should be receiving no more than 900 mg rather than 1,200 mg of isoniazid. Although high doses or increased serum concentrations have not been linked with hepatitis, elevated serum isoniazid concentrations have been associated with increased central nervous system (CNS) events, ranging from somnolence to psychosis and seizure. GI complaints are also more commonly observed at doses greater than 20 mg/kg.

PERIPHERAL NEUROPATHY

Although uncommon at the recommended daily and intermittent doses, isoniazid can cause a peripheral neuropathy by interfering with pyridoxine (vitamin B_6) metabolism.[33,48] As many as 20% of patients may experience this problem with isoniazid doses greater than 6 mg/kg/day. Numbness or tingling in the feet or hands is the most common neuropathic symptom. In patients with medical conditions in which neuropathy is common, including diabetes mellitus, alcoholism, HIV infection, malnutrition, and renal failure, supplemental pyridoxine 25 mg/day should be given with isoniazid.[33,48] Women who are pregnant or breast-feeding and persons with seizure disorders should also receive supplemental pyridoxine with isoniazid.[48]

ALLERGIC AND OTHER REACTIONS

Allergic reactions consisting of arthralgias, skin rash, swelling of the tongue, and fever have also been reported. Isoniazid has been associated with arthritic symptoms and systemic lupus erythematosus; approximately 20% of patients receiving isoniazid develop antinuclear antibodies.[33] Other less common reactions reported with isoniazid are dry mouth, epigastric distress, CNS stimulation and depression, psychoses, hemolytic anemia, pyridoxine-responsive anemia, and agranulocytosis.[122]

DRUG INTERACTIONS

Isoniazid is a relatively potent inhibitor of several cytochrome P450 isoenzymes (CYP2C9, CYP2C19, CYP2E1), but has minimal effects on CYP3A.[33] Isoniazid inhibits the hepatic metabolism of phenytoin and carbamazepine, resulting in increased plasma concentrations of these drugs. Patients receiving either of these two drugs with isoniazid should be observed for signs of phenytoin or carbamazepine toxicity, such as nystagmus, ataxia, headache, nausea, or drowsiness. Plasma phenytoin and carbamazepine concentrations should be monitored periodically so that the doses can be adjusted if necessary. Carbamazepine also may induce isoniazid hepatitis by inducing its metabolism to toxic metabolites.[126] In addition, isoniazid inhibits the metabolism of diazepam and triazolam. It is important to note that rifampin has the exact opposite effect on hepatic metabolism. Rifampin is a stronger inducer than isoniazid is an inhibitor as documented by the fact that isoniazid–rifampin combination therapy induces the metabolism of diazepam, phenytoin, and other agents metabolized by the cytochrome P450 system.[127]

Rifampin

FLU-LIKE SYNDROME

CASE 68-3, QUESTION 2: One month after beginning her twice-weekly DOT regimen, C.M. exhibited symptoms of myalgias, malaise, and anorexia. Laboratory data were normal except for a slightly decreased platelet count. Could C.M.'s symptoms be related to her drug therapy? What adverse reactions other than hepatotoxicity should be anticipated in a patient receiving rifampin?

A flu-like syndrome has been reported in 1% of patients receiving intermittent rifampin administration. This syndrome is rarely seen with usual doses of 600 mg twice weekly, but the incidence increases with twice-weekly doses greater than 900 mg. The incidence also increases if the dosing interval is increased to 1 week or longer.[128,129] Unless the symptoms are severe, discontinuation of the drug is unnecessary. Because C.M. is receiving rifampin 900 mg twice weekly, her dose should be reduced to 600 mg and administered daily until the symptoms subside. Temporary administration of a nonsteroidal anti-inflammatory drug has been used to alleviate the flu-like symptoms. Twice-weekly therapy may then be resumed as long as the dose of rifampin dose does not exceed 600 mg.

HEPATOTOXICITY

Rifampin (rifapentine) is associated with a less than 1% rate of hepatotoxicity. Therefore, the risk of drug-induced hepatotoxicity is greater with isoniazid than with rifampin. On occasion, rifampin can cause hepatocellular injury and potentiate hepatotoxicity of other antituberculosis drugs.[117] Although elevations of liver enzymes may be seen, rifampin is more likely to produce cholestasis, as manifested by increases in alkaline phosphatase and hyperbilirubinemia without hepatocellular injury.[117] Elevations of all liver function tests may be seen transiently during the first month of rifampin therapy, but they are usually benign.[33]

THROMBOCYTOPENIA

Thrombocytopenia is more frequently associated with intermittent or interrupted rifampin administration, likely caused by production of immunoglobulin G and immunoglobulin M antibodies to rifampin. These antibodies likely fix complement onto platelets, resulting in platelet destruction. Hypothetically, intermittent or interrupted rifampin therapy results in increased antibody production. Once thrombocytopenia occurs with rifampin, its subsequent use is contraindicated because the problem will likely recur.[130,131]

MISCELLANEOUS REACTIONS

In addition to the side effects associated with high-dose, intermittent therapy, 3% to 4% of patients taking normal doses of rifampin may experience adverse reactions.[130] The most common of these are nausea, vomiting, fever, and rash. Other reactions to rifampin include the hepatorenal syndrome hemolysis, leukopenia, anemia, and arthralgias as part of a suspected drug-induced lupus syndrome.[33,132] Development of these latter reactions requires discontinuation of the drug.

ACUTE RENAL FAILURE

Acute renal failure has been reported rarely with rifampin.[33] This hypersensitivity reaction may occur with both intermittent and daily administration and may last as long as 12 months.[128] Rifampin should be discontinued, and other drugs (e.g., pyrazinamide and ethambutol) should be given. Doses of ethambutol and pyrazinamide should be adjusted for renal dysfunction, if necessary. Both rifampin and isoniazid may, however, be given in normal dosages to patients with preexisting renal failure.[133,134]

DISCOLORATION OF BODY FLUIDS

Another important characteristic of rifampin relates to its chemical makeup. It is an orange-red crystalline powder that is distributed widely in body fluids. As a result, it can discolor saliva, tears, urine, sweat, and cerebrospinal fluid.[33] Patients using rifampin should be warned of this effect and cautioned not to use soft contact lenses because of possible discoloration. This effect may also be used to monitor adherence to rifampin therapy.

DRUG INTERACTIONS

Rifampin is a very potent inducer of cytochrome P450 CYP3A4 and also induces other cytochrome P450 isoenzymes, including CYP1A2, CYP2A6, CYP2B6, CYP2C8, CYP2C9, CYP2C19, and CYP3A5.[33,135,136] Rifampin induces phase 2 drug-metabolizing enzymes (e.g., UDP-glucuronyltransferases, sulfotransferases) and expression of transporter proteins (e.g., P-glycoprotein, multiple drug resistance protein 2, organic anion-transporting polypeptide).[135] Complete induction of these isoenzymes and transport proteins occurs approximately 1 week after starting rifampin and returns to baseline approximately 2 weeks after discontinuing the drug.[135] Rifamycins differ in their ability to induce cytochrome P450 isoenzymes, in which rifampin is the most potent, rifapentine is intermediate, and rifabutin is the least potent enzyme inducer.[33] Rifampin increases the metabolism of protease inhibitors, certain non-nucleoside reverse transcriptase inhibitors (NNRTIs), macrolide antibiotics, azole antifungal agents, corticosteroids, oral contraceptives, warfarin, cyclosporine, tacrolimus, theophylline, phenytoin, quinidine, diazepam, propranolol, metoprolol, sulfonylureas, verapamil, nifedipine, diltiazem, enalapril, and simvastatin.[33,127] Although the patient is receiving rifampin, it may be necessary to monitor serum concentrations of the aforementioned drugs, when appropriate, or increase their dosages. Also, women who are taking rifampin and oral contraceptives should use an alternative method of birth control. When treating any patient with rifampin, the healthcare professional should carefully evaluate all concomitant medications for the possibility of drug–drug interactions.

Isoniazid–Rifampin

HEPATOTOXICITY

CASE 68-3, QUESTION 3: Will the combination of isoniazid and rifampin increase the risk of hepatotoxicity in C.M. to a greater extent than either drug alone?

Some initial evidence suggested that the concomitant use of isoniazid and rifampin was associated with a greater incidence of hepatotoxicity. The mechanism was thought to be attributable to rifampin induction of the metabolism of isoniazid to either monoacetylhydrazine or to other hepatotoxic products of hydrolysis. Steele et al.[123] performed a meta-analysis reviewing the incidence of hepatitis using regimens that contained isoniazid without rifampin, rifampin without isoniazid, and regimens containing both drugs. They found the incidence of clinical hepatitis was greater in regimens containing both isoniazid and rifampin (2.7%) versus regimens of isoniazid alone (1.6%), but this effect was additive, not synergistic, and therefore expected.[123] The use of the two drugs together, therefore, is not contraindicated, but caution should be used in high-risk groups such as the elderly, alcoholics, those receiving concomitant hepatotoxic agents, and those with preexisting liver disease.[117]

Ethambutol

OPTIC NEURITIS

CASE 68-4

QUESTION 1: S.E., a 65-year-old woman, was placed on isoniazid 300 mg/day, rifampin 600 mg/day, pyrazinamide 1,500 mg/day, and ethambutol 1,200 mg/day for initial treatment of active pulmonary TB. Two months after the initiation of therapy, she began to complain of blurred vision. A routine eye examination and visual field tests yielded a diagnosis of optic neuritis. No evidence was seen of glaucoma, cataracts, or retinal damage. Laboratory tests were within normal limits except for an elevated serum uric acid (9.7 mg/dL) and a slightly elevated serum creatinine (1.6 mg/dL). No symptoms of joint pain were associated with the elevated serum uric acid, and there was no history of gout. Her estimated creatinine clearance based on her weight of 65 kg was 36 mL/minute. Could the visual problem and increased uric acid levels be related to her medications?

S.E.'s decrease in visual acuity is compatible with ethambutol-induced optic neuritis. This condition is characterized by central scotomas, loss of red-green color vision, or less commonly, a peripheral vision defect. The intensity of these ocular effects is related to the duration of continued therapy after decreased visual acuity is first noted. Optic neuritis is related to both dose and duration, and it rarely occurs at doses of 15 mg/kg.[137–139] The incidence is estimated to be 6% for doses of 25 mg/kg and increases to 15% for doses in excess of 35 mg/kg. Recovery, which may take months, is usually, but not always, complete when the drug is discontinued.

Optic neuritis manifested in S.E. is probably caused by the use of an increased ethambutol dose (18.5 mg/kg) in a patient with impaired renal function. Because ethambutol adds no additional benefit to isoniazid and rifampin after the first 2 months for susceptible organisms, it can be discontinued. Ethambutol is excreted by the kidney (50%–80%), and her ethambutol dosing interval should have been increased based on the decline in creatinine clearance.[133] Her visual acuity should be monitored closely through periodic eye examinations, and she should be instructed to contact her physician immediately if she experiences any further visual changes.

S.E.'s elevated serum uric acid also may be attributed to her ethambutol as well as a decline in her renal function, but it is more likely caused by pyrazinamide, which decreases the tubular secretion of urate.[102] Asymptomatic hyperuricemia secondary to drugs usually does not require treatment.

SPECIAL TREATMENT CONSIDERATIONS

The Elderly

INCIDENCE

CASE 68-5

Question 1: G.H., a 75-year-old, 80-kg man who resides in a nursing home, becomes disoriented, refuses to eat, and has a productive cough. Physical examination reveals a thin man with slight difficulty breathing. Laboratory findings are essentially normal with the exception of a slightly elevated blood urea nitrogen of 25 mg/dL and serum creatinine of 1.3 mg/dL. Chest radiography reveals infiltrates in the right lower lobe. He has a history of congestive heart failure, which is well controlled. Blood, urine, and sputum samples are sent for culture and susceptibility testing. The initial Gram stain is negative. Because the nursing home has recently had two cases of active TB, a PPD skin test and sputum smear for AFB are ordered. The PPD skin test induration is 16 mm, and the sputum smear is positive for AFB. G.H.'s admission skin test several months ago was negative. Discuss the presentation of TB in the elderly, and the appropriate treatment of active disease in G.H. Is the incidence of drug side effects higher in the elderly? Should other patients in close contact with G.H. receive isoniazid therapy?

In 2014, the overall case rate of TB in adults 64 years or older was higher than all other age-groups (4.8/100,000 population).[10] Similar to other age-groups, the case rate for persons 64 years or older has declined every year since 1993 when the case rate was 17.7/100,000 population.[10] In 2014, 2.2% of TB cases were reported in residents of long-term care facilities,[10] and the case rate for nursing home residents is 1.8 times higher than that for elderly persons living in the community.[140] Active TB disease in the elderly has been attributed to decreased immune function followed by reactivation of an earlier infection, but active disease is a common, endemic infection in nursing home patients with no previous immunity (negative skin test) to *M. tuberculosis.*[140,141] The incidence of positive tuberculin skin tests increases after patients have been in the nursing home longer than 1 month. Therefore, all patients entering a nursing home should be tested with 5 TU of PPD. If the initial test is negative and a source case is present in the nursing home (as illustrated by this case), this test should be repeated in 1 month. The rate of tuberculin skin test conversion (from negative to positive tests) in this population is approximately 5%. If these recent converters are not treated with isoniazid, approximately 17% will develop progressive pulmonary TB.[142]

DIAGNOSIS

Diagnosis of active TB in elderly patients is difficult because classic symptoms of cough, fever, night sweats, and weight loss are often absent, and elderly patients may describe their symptoms poorly. The chest radiograph and PPD skin test may be the only signs of TB infection.[140,142] Frequently, the chest radiograph is atypical, resembling pneumonia or worsening heart failure. Chest radiographs in the elderly are less likely to reveal upper lobe infiltration; however, more commonly they will show extensive infiltration of both lungs.[143] If the patient's clinical disease is caused by reactivation, the chest radiograph often shows apical infiltrates or nodules. If the disease is progressing from an initial infection, as in the case of G.H., lower lobe infiltrates may be present.[140] TB in this population may present clinically with changes in activities of daily living, chronic fatigue, cognitive impairment, anorexia, or unexplained low-grade fever. Nonspecific signs and symptoms that range in severity from subacute to chronic and that persist for weeks to months must alert clinicians to the possibility that unrecognized TB is present.[144] Sputum examination for *M. tuberculosis,* and AFB smear and culture should be performed in all patients, including the elderly.

TREATMENT OF ACTIVE DISEASE IN THE ELDERLY

The principles of TB treatment are the same for the elderly as for any other age-group.[33,140] Because G.H. has clinical symptoms of a respiratory infection, positive sputum smears for AFB, and a positive tuberculin skin test, he should be treated with a four-drug regimen for active TB disease. Most TB cases in elderly patients are caused by drug-susceptible strains of *M. tuberculosis;* however, notable exceptions would be older patients who are from a country or region where the prevalence of drug-resistant strains is high, persons who have been inadequately treated in the past, or persons who acquired the infection from a recent contact known to be infected with drug-resistant *M. tuberculosis.*[144] G.H.'s drug regimen should include isoniazid 300 mg, rifampin 600 mg, pyrazinamide 2,000 mg, and ethambutol 1,600 mg daily for 8 weeks followed by isoniazid and rifampin daily or 2 to 3 times a week for 16 weeks (DOT). Another option might be isoniazid, rifampin, pyrazinamide, and ethambutol daily for 2 weeks, followed by twice weekly for 6 weeks, then isoniazid and rifampin twice weekly for 16 weeks.[144] Some clinicians prefer treating the elderly with 9-month regimens of isoniazid and rifampin. G.H. should also receive pyridoxine 10 to 50 mg with each dose.[66]

ADVERSE DRUG EFFECTS

Although isoniazid hepatitis is more common in elderly patients, both isoniazid and rifampin are generally well tolerated within this age-group, with major hematologic or hepatic side effects occurring in 3% to 4% of patients.[145] Therefore, serum aminotransferases should be assessed at baseline, and G.H. should be observed monthly for clinical signs of hepatitis. As discussed earlier, routine monitoring of LFTs remains controversial because transient, asymptomatic elevations do occur among the elderly.[145]

Although uncommon at 600 mg, rifampin given twice weekly may cause a greater incidence of flu-like symptoms. Because potential drug interactions with isoniazid and rifampin are possible, any medication added to the patient's regimen should be carefully evaluated. Considering that G.H. has age-related decreased renal function, signs of ethambutol-induced visual dysfunction should be monitoring carefully.

TREATMENT OF LATENT INFECTION IN THE ELDERLY

Treatment of elderly patients with positive tuberculin skin tests but no active TB disease with isoniazid 300 mg daily for 6 to 9 months is essential if a source case is present in the nursing home. Stead et al.[142] reported only one case of active disease in patients receiving therapy for latent TB infection compared with 69 cases in untreated patients. In patients with recently converted skin tests, one patient in the group receiving isoniazid therapy had active disease compared with 45 who received no treatment.[142] Daily rifampin for 4 months or weekly isoniazid plus rifapentine for 12 weeks are also acceptable regimens in the elderly.[116,140]

Multidrug-Resistant Organisms

DEFINITION AND ETIOLOGY

CASE 68-6

QUESTION 1: M.S., an ill-appearing 29-year-old Asian man, is admitted to the hospital with signs and symptoms of pneumonia. He is coughing, and his chest radiograph indicates bilateral infiltrates. He is placed in respiratory isolation pending the results of sputum testing for *M. tuberculosis*. He states that he was diagnosed with TB approximately 3 months ago, and treatment was initiated with isoniazid, rifampin, pyrazinamide, and ethambutol. However, he stopped taking his medication after 1 month. An HIV test was performed 3 months ago, which was negative. What is the likelihood of acquired drug resistance in *M. tuberculosis*?

In the United States, isoniazid resistance was 18.9% and resistance to both isoniazid and rifampin was 7.1% in patients with previous TB in 2014.[10] Resistance in *M. tuberculosis* is either primary or acquired. Primary drug resistance occurs when a patient harbors a resistant strain before any drugs have been administered. Acquired drug resistance occurs when resistant subpopulations are selected as a result of treatment errors, such as addition of a single drug to a failing regimen, inadequate primary regimen, failure to recognize resistance, and, most importantly, nonadherence to the prescribed regimen. Sporadic ingestion, inadequate dosages, or malabsorption of medications can cause susceptible *M. tuberculosis* strains to become resistant to multiple drugs within a few months.[146,147] These resistant organisms can then be transmitted to persons who have never received treatment and lead to primary resistance in those patients.

M.S. is a foreign-born person of Asian ethnicity and may have primary resistance from his country of origin, making a detailed exposure history essential for the treatment of his infection. M.S. is also an example of the problem of treatment failure caused by nonadherence and the potential development of drug-resistant organisms. Homelessness and lack of awareness of the severity of TB have been shown to be significantly associated with interruptions in TB therapy.[148] Therefore, educational efforts to improve a patient's understanding of TB disease are critical for appropriate treatment of the disease.

Many factors can affect the outcome of therapy for MDR-TB, including HIV status, treatment adherence, the number of drugs to which the tubercle bacilli remain susceptible, and the time since the first diagnosis of TB.[149–151] In one study, all 11 patients who were HIV positive died during observation.[150] In another study, 77% of patients with MDR-TB had sputum cultures convert to negative in a median time of 60 days (range, 4–462 days), but 23% of patients never converted to negative cultures.[151] Of the patients who converted, 60% converted after 4 months of therapy.[151] Predictors of a longer time for sputum culture conversion were high initial sputum colony counts, bilateral cavitation on chest radiograph, previous treatment of MDR-TB, and the number of drugs the initial isolate was resistant to at the beginning of therapy.[151]

CASE 68-6, QUESTION 2: Can M.S. be cured by drug therapy, and if so, how should he be treated?

Because his recent HIV test was negative, M.S. has a higher probability of treatment success. In HIV-negative patients, 32 (97%) of 33 patients with MDR-TB were cured, and these patients received an average of five second-line drugs.[150] Only one relapse occurred 5 years after treatment.[150] Therefore, M.S.'s current regimen should be re-evaluated, drug susceptibility testing should be determined, and the patient should be referred to a specialist or consultation at a specialized treatment center.[33] Molecular drug resistance testing should be performed to evaluate resistance to rifampin, which is a reliable surrogate for MDR-TB. Standard susceptibility testing methods should be performed for the other agents, although results may not be available for several weeks. If the rapid molecular test detects the presence of mutations to rifampin, the patient should then begin therapy for MDR-TB. However, there is no standard treatment regimen for MDR-TB. When revising a treatment regimen, at least three previously unused drugs to which the organism is susceptible should be used, and one of these agents should be injectable.[33] A new regimen should contain at least four drugs, possibly more, depending on disease severity and resistance pattern. Treatment should be given by DOT, and the recommended duration is 18 to 24 months.[33,149] However, only 40% of patients with MDR-TB complete a full 18 to 24 months of therapy.[152]

The efficacy of a standardized treatment regimen for a shorter duration of therapy was evaluated in patients with documented MDR-TB.[153] The study population consisted of 427 patients with a mean age of 34 years, 81.5% had bilateral disease on chest radiograph, and patients had exhibited TB for approximately 30 months on average. The mean body mass index was 16.1 kg/m^2, indicating severe emaciation. The intensive phase consisted of three or more months of therapy with six to seven agents, and doses were based on body weight.[153] Daily ofloxacin and gatifloxacin doses were 400, 600, and 800 mg for body weights less than 33 kg, 33 to 50 kg, and greater than 50 kg, respectively.[153] The most effective treatment regimen required a minimum of 9 months of therapy with gatifloxacin, clofazimine, ethambutol, and pyrazinamide throughout the treatment period with the addition of high-dose isoniazid, prothionamide, and kanamycin for a minimum of 4 months during the intensive phase. Among 206 patients receiving this regimen, the relapse-free cure rate was 87.9%. The most common adverse events with this regimen were vomiting (21.4%), diminished hearing acuity (6.3%), dysglycemia (3.9%), and ataxia (3.9%).[153] These results suggest that it may be possible to adequately treat patients with MDR-TB with shorter courses of therapy. However, prothionamide and kanamycin are unavailable in the United States.

Fluoroquinolones are active against mycobacteria, including *M. tuberculosis,* and they penetrate rapidly into macrophages and exhibit intracellular mycobactericidal activity.[149] Fluoroquinolones inhibit DNA gyrase in *M. tuberculosis,* but the other molecular target of these agents, topoisomerase IV, is absent.[149] Ciprofloxacin, ofloxacin, and levofloxacin have been used long term for the treatment of mycobacterial infections and were well tolerated with few serious adverse effects.[154,155] Limited data suggest that moxifloxacin is an acceptable option in the treatment of MDR-TB.[156] Selection of fluoroquinolone resistance has been observed in vivo, and complete cross-resistance within the class is the accepted rule.[149] Other second-line medications used for MDR-TB include *p*-aminosalicylic acid, cycloserine, ethionamide, and capreomycin. These agents are associated with numerous side effects and should not be prescribed without the guidance of an expert in the treatment of MDR-TB.

Bedaquiline was FDA-approved in late 2012 as part of combination therapy with at least three or four other drugs in adults with pulmonary MDR-TB when other alternatives are not available. Bedaquiline is a novel drug that inhibits mycobacterial adenosine 5′-triphosphate synthase, thereby inhibiting energy production in *M. tuberculosis*.[157] The drug is available in 100 mg tablets, and the recommended dosage is 400 mg daily for 2 weeks followed by 200 mg thrice weekly for 22 weeks.[157] Bioavailability of bedaquiline is increased twofold when administered with food, and each dose should be administered by DOT.[157] Bedaquiline is metabolized by CYP3A4, and it is recommended to avoid concomitant administration of bedaquiline with moderate (e.g., efavirenz) and strong (e.g., rifamycins) CYP3A4 inducers. Strong CYP3A4 inhibitors may increase systemic exposure and adverse events of bedaquiline, and use of strong CYP3A4 inhibitors for more than 14 consecutive days should be avoided while the patient is receiving bedaquiline.[157] Bedaquiline can cause QT prolongation, and additive prolongation may occur with other drugs known to prolong the QT interval.

Bedaquiline received accelerated FDA approval based on the surrogate marker of time to sputum culture conversion in phase 2 studies. In the first study, 47 patients with MDR-TB received bedaquiline or placebo added to a preferred background regimen of kanamycin, ofloxacin, ethionamide, pyrazinamide, and cycloserine or terizidone for 8 weeks.[158] After 8 weeks, the background regimen was continued for a total of 96 weeks. Time to sputum culture conversion was significantly reduced in the bedaquiline group, and sputum cultures were negative in 48% of patients in the bedaquiline group compared to 9% in the placebo group at 8 weeks.[158] After 24 weeks, 81% of patients in the bedaquiline group had negative sputum cultures compared to 65.2% in the placebo group.[159] However, after 104 weeks, treatment success was achieved in 52.4% and 47.8% of patients in the bedaquiline and placebo groups, respectively.[159]

In the second study, 160 patients with pulmonary MDR-TB received either placebo or bedaquiline 400 mg daily for 2 weeks followed by 200 mg thrice weekly for 22 weeks with the same background regimen described previously.[160] After 24 weeks, patients continued the background regimen for a total of 18 to 24 months. The median time to sputum culture conversion was 83 days in the bedaquiline group compared to 125 days in the placebo group ($p < 0.001$).[160] Compared to placebo, significantly more patients in the bedaquiline group had negative cultures at 24 weeks (79% vs. 62%, $p = 0.008$) and at 120 weeks (62% vs. 44%, $p = 0.04$).[160] However, mortality was significantly higher in patients receiving bedaquiline (13% vs. 2%, $p = 0.02$).[160]

Human Immunodeficiency Virus Infection

TREATMENT OF ACTIVE DISEASE

CASE 68-7

QUESTION 1: F.R. is a 32-year-old man who presents to the emergency department complaining of mild pleuritic chest pain and a productive cough. He also has experienced weight loss, fatigue, and night sweats for the past 3 weeks. On questioning, F.R. states that he is bisexual and frequently engages in unprotected sex. Chest radiography reveals bilateral interstitial infiltrates. Sputum samples are ordered, and the workup includes AFB smear and culture. A PPD skin test is placed, and an HIV test is ordered. The results of the AFB smear and HIV test are positive, and the induration from the PPD is 6 mm. A $CD4^+$ count is ordered, which is 150 cells/μL. What are the clinical manifestations of active TB in patients infected with HIV? How effective is skin testing in the diagnosis of TB infection in patients infected with HIV? What diagnostic tests should be performed in F.R.?

HIV infection is an important risk factor for active TB disease because HIV infects and destroys $CD4^+$ cells, leading to impaired cell-mediated immunity. The immunodeficiency allows for rapid development of active TB disease in a person who is infected with *M. tuberculosis*. TB is a common opportunistic infection in persons infected with HIV, but unlike other opportunistic infections in this population, $CD4^+$ cell count is not a reliable predictor for risk for TB disease.[65] Active TB disease can occur at any $CD4^+$ cell count, but the risk increases as a patient's immunodeficiency progresses.[161]

Common symptoms of active disease (productive cough, fever, sweats, weight loss, fatigue) may be present in HIV-infected individuals, but the clinical manifestations of TB depend on the severity of the immunodeficiency at the time of presentation. TB in an HIV-infected person will clinically resemble TB in an HIV-uninfected person if the immunodeficiency is less severe ($CD4^+$ count >350 cells/μL).[65,161] The disease will primarily be limited to the lungs in these patients, and upper lobe involvement with or without cavitation will be seen on chest radiography. However, the findings on chest radiography are markedly different in patients with advanced HIV disease. Lower lobe, middle lobe, interstitial, and miliary infiltrates are common, whereas cavitation is seen infrequently.[65,161] In these patients, TB may be difficult to distinguish from other HIV-related pulmonary opportunistic infections (*Pneumocystis jiroveci, M. avium* complex), and TB should be ruled out in any HIV-infected patient with pulmonary symptoms. Patients with advanced HIV disease may also have normal chest radiographs but still have positive sputum smears for AFB and positive cultures for *M. tuberculosis*.[161] Therefore, a normal chest radiograph does not exclude the possibility of active TB disease. Extrapulmonary TB is more common in HIV-infected persons with $CD4^+$ counts less than 200 cells/μL.[65,161] Because of F.R.'s clinical presentation and positive HIV test, a high index of suspicion and diagnostic workup for active TB are appropriate.

A PPD skin test should be placed on HIV-infected patients with suspected TB infection, but sensitivity and specificity of skin testing are poor in patients with HIV infection. Only about 30% to 50% of patients with AIDS and TB will respond to a PPD skin test with an induration greater than 10 mm. Therefore, an induration of 5 mm or more is considered to be a positive reaction in this population.[48,161] F.R.'s reaction of 6 mm to the tuberculin skin test should be considered positive. Theoretically, the sensitivity and specificity of IGRAs are also limited in patients with HIV infection because the tests depend on adequately functioning $CD4^+$ cells. In a study of 294 HIV-infected subjects, indeterminate results were more likely to occur in subjects with a $CD4^+$ count less than 100 cells/μL compared with those with a $CD4^+$ count of 100 cells/μL or more.[162] Additional studies found only 64% sensitivity for detection of active TB disease, and false-negative results occurred in approximately 25% of HIV-infected patients with documented pulmonary TB.[163,164] These studies suggest that IGRAs should not be used alone to exclude active TB in this population.

The diagnostic workup for HIV-infected persons is similar to that for HIV-uninfected persons. Chest radiography and sputum samples for AFB smear and culture of three sputum specimens should be obtained.[161,165] NAA tests can be used to assist in evaluation of HIV-infected persons with positive AFB smears, and a positive NAA result in a patient who is AFB smear positive likely represents active TB.[65,161] Drug susceptibility testing for all first-line agents should be performed on the initial isolate for all patients, and testing should be repeated if sputum cultures remain positive after 4 months of treatment or become positive after at least 1 month of negative cultures.[161] Susceptibility testing of second-line agents should be limited to specimens from patients who have received prior therapy, are contacts of persons with drug-resistant TB disease, have demonstrated resistance to rifampin or other first-line agents, have positive cultures after

3 months of therapy, or are from regions with a high prevalence of MDR-TB or XDR-TB.[166] Molecular drug resistance tests may also be used to yield faster results. Patients with symptoms of extrapulmonary TB should undergo needle aspiration or tissue biopsy of skin lesions, lymph nodes, or pericardial or pleural fluid, and blood cultures for AFB should be obtained.[65]

CASE 68-7, QUESTION 2: What is the preferred treatment regimen for TB in F.R.?

Given his symptoms and positive AFB smear, F.R. should be started on multiple-drug therapy for treatment of active TB disease. DOT is recommended for all patients with HIV-related TB.[33,65,161] F.R.'s treatment plan should be based on completion of the total number of doses ingested rather than the duration of therapy. Principles and recommendations for treatment of TB in HIV-infected adults are similar to those for HIV-uninfected adults, with a notable exception (Table 68-2). The initial 8-week treatment phase in F.R. should include isoniazid, rifampin or rifabutin, pyrazinamide, and ethambutol administered daily by DOT (7 days/week for 56 doses or 5 days/week for 40 doses).[33,65] However, twice- or thrice-weekly dosing regimens during the intensive phase have been associated with increased risk of treatment failure or relapse with acquired rifamycin resistance; therefore, intermittent dosing regimens are no longer recommended during the intensive phase.[161] F.R. should also receive supplemental pyridoxine. After the initial phase, if no drug resistance is evident on susceptibility or molecular testing, F.R. can be treated with isoniazid and rifampin (or rifabutin) daily or 2 to 3 times a week by DOT for a minimum of 26 weeks.[65] Although not applicable to F.R. because his $CD4^+$ cell count is 150 cells/μL, it should be noted that twice-weekly continuation therapy with isoniazid and rifampin or isoniazid and rifabutin is not recommended for HIV-infected patients with a $CD4^+$ count less than 100 cells/μL because of an increased frequency of acquired rifamycin resistance.[33,65,167,168] Twice-weekly administration in the continuation phase may be considered in F.R. because his $CD4^+$ count is greater than 100 cells/μL, but the data supporting this recommendation are limited (Table 68-2).[33,65] In addition, the once-weekly continuation regimen of isoniazid and rifapentine is contraindicated in HIV-infected patients because of a high rate of relapse with organisms that have acquired resistance to the rifamycins.[33,65]

A randomized clinical study evaluated the efficacy of 6 months and 9 months of fully intermittent therapy in HIV-infected patients with TB.[169] All patients received 2 months of isoniazid, rifampin, pyrazinamide, and ethambutol, and then patients were randomly assigned to receive either 4 months ($n = 167$) or 7 months ($n = 160$) of isoniazid and rifampin. Throughout the study duration, doses were administered thrice weekly. The median viral load was 155,000 copies/mL, and the median $CD4^+$ cell count was 160 cells/μL. Favorable clinical response was similar between the two groups; however, bacteriologic recurrence occurred significantly less frequently in the 9-month group compared with the 6-month group (7% vs. 15%; $p < 0.05$).[169] These data may provide support for 9 months of therapy if a fully intermittent regimen is prescribed for TB therapy in HIV-infected patients.

CASE 68-7, QUESTION 3: How should TB therapy be monitored in F.R.?

If F.R. had cavitary disease on chest radiography or if cultures are positive after 2 months of therapy, treatment with isoniazid and rifampin or rifabutin should be continued to complete a total of 9 months of therapy. If F.R. was suspected of having extrapulmonary disease caused by drug-susceptible strains, the recommended treatment is isoniazid, rifampin, pyrazinamide, and ethambutol for 2 months followed by isoniazid and rifampin for 4 to 7 months. However, longer durations of therapy are recommended for extrapulmonary TB involving the CNS (meningitis or tuberculoma) or bone and joints. For these infections, many experts recommend 9 to 12 months of therapy.[65,161]

Baseline and monthly evaluations of hepatic function, renal function, complete blood count, and $CD4^+$ cell count are recommended in all HIV-infected patients with active TB disease.[65] In the absence of symptoms, elevations of AST <3 times the upper limit of normal should not cause a change in therapy.[161] If the AST is >3 times the upper limit of normal in a patient with symptoms, >5 times the upper limit of normal regardless of symptoms, or if a significant increase in alkaline phosphatase and/or bilirubin occurs, hepatotoxic drugs should be stopped and the patient evaluated.[161] For pulmonary TB, at least one sputum specimen should be obtained monthly for AFB smear and culture until two consecutive specimens are culture negative.[65,161] If the AFB smear is positive at the initiation of treatment, AFB smears may be obtained every 2 weeks to provide an early assessment of bacteriologic response to therapy.[33,65] Results of sputum samples obtained after the initial 8-week treatment phase are important because determination of the duration of the continuation phase will be based on these results. Susceptibility testing should be performed on all isolates, and susceptibility testing should be repeated on a newly obtained sputum sample if cultures are positive for *M. tuberculosis* after 3 months of therapy.[65] Patients with positive cultures at or after 4 months of therapy should be considered treatment failures.

At every visit, patients should be questioned about adherence to therapy and possible adverse events to the treatment regimen. If a patient is experiencing adverse events, the first-line drugs should not be discontinued permanently without strong evidence that a specific agent is the cause of the adverse event.[65,161] Drug concentration monitoring may be useful to help guide therapy in patients who respond slowly to the prescribed treatment regimen.[170]

CASE 68-7, QUESTION 4: When should antiretroviral therapy (ART) be initiated in F.R.?

Optimal management of active TB disease in patients infected with HIV requires treatment of both infections. Sequential treatment of TB followed by treatment of HIV is not recommended.[161] In patients with HIV infection, $CD4^+$ cells multiply in response to *M. tuberculosis,* and then HIV replication accelerates within the lymphocytes and macrophages, which leads to progression of HIV disease. Therefore, initiation of ART can prevent progression of HIV disease and reduce morbidity and mortality associated with TB and other opportunistic infections.[65,161] However, this approach may be associated with cumulative drug toxicities, significant drug interactions, a higher pill burden, and the potential for development of immune reconstitution inflammatory syndrome (IRIS).[65,161]

Three studies addressed the optimal timing to initiate ART during the treatment of active TB disease.[171–173] In ART-naïve patients, ART should be initiated within 2 weeks of starting TB therapy in patients with a $CD4^+$ count less than 50 cells/μL. Early initiation of ART significantly reduces mortality in these patients, but the risk of IRIS is increased. In patients with $CD4^+$ counts of 50 cells/μL or greater who present with severe TB disease (low Karnofsky score, low body mass index, low hemoglobin, low albumin, organ system dysfunction, or extensive disease), ART should be initiated within 2 to 4 weeks of starting TB therapy. In patients with $CD4^+$ counts of 50 cells/μL or greater who do not have severe TB disease, ART should be initiated within 8 to 12 weeks of initiating TB therapy.[171–173] If IRIS develops, neither therapy for TB nor HIV should be discontinued. Because F.R. is ART naïve and his $CD4^+$ count is 150 cells/μL, ART should be initiated within 8 to 12 weeks of starting treatment for active TB.

If F.R. was receiving ART when diagnosed with TB, treatment for TB should be started immediately, and ART should be modified to maintain virologic suppression while reducing the risk for drug–drug interactions.[161] ART should not be withheld simply because the patient is being treated for TB, and a rifamycin should not be excluded from the treatment regimen for fear of interactions with certain antiretroviral agents.[33,174] Exclusion of a rifamycin will likely delay sputum conversion, prolong the duration of therapy, and possibly result in a poor outcome.

CASE 68-7, QUESTION 5: Because F.R.'s CD4$^+$ count is 150 cells/μL, the decision is made to begin ART after the initial 8-week intensive phase to decrease the potential for IRIS. What is IRIS? What drug interactions are likely in an HIV-infected patient receiving treatment for TB and HIV?

Immune reconstitution inflammatory syndrome, or IRIS, occurs in approximately 30% of patients who begin therapy for both HIV and TB in close temporal proximity.[161,174] This syndrome is thought to reflect recovery of immune responses to *M. tuberculosis* and usually occurs in the first 1 to 4 weeks after initiation of ART.[161] IRIS lasts for 2 to 3 months on average, but some patients may experience IRIS symptoms for months. The immune response can be an exaggerated inflammatory response during TB therapy in a patient known to have TB infection, or it may unmask a previously undiagnosed TB infection. The risk of IRIS is greater when ART is initiated within the first 2 months of TB therapy and when the CD4$^+$ count is less than 100 cells/μL.[65,161] Symptoms include high fever, malaise, and local reactions in organs, depending on the location of the mycobacterial infection (e.g., lungs, lymph nodes, CNS). IRIS is usually self-limiting, but supportive therapy may be required if symptoms are severe. Moderate IRIS reactions should be treated with nonsteroidal anti-inflammatory drugs without any changes to TB therapy or ART.[65] No specific treatment recommendations are available for severe IRIS; however, prednisone or methylprednisolone at doses of 1 mg/kg body weight and tapered for 1 to 2 weeks has been beneficial.[65]

Simultaneous treatment of TB and HIV can be complicated by drug interactions with the rifamycins and ART.[135,161] Rifampin is a potent inducer of cytochrome P450 isoenzymes, but rifabutin is not a potent inducer.[33,35,65] Rifabutin is highly active against *M. tuberculosis,* and data from clinical trials suggest equal efficacy with rifampin- and rifabutin-based treatment regimens.[33,161] Because of fewer drug interactions and documented efficacy, rifabutin is recommended in place of rifampin for the treatment of active TB in HIV-infected patients receiving certain protease inhibitors or NNRTIs.[33,161] However, some antiretroviral agents may either induce or inhibit cytochrome P450 isoenzymes, depending on the specific drug, and may alter rifabutin serum concentrations.[33,167]

For the NNRTIs, rifampin was shown to decrease efavirenz exposures by 26%, but two additional studies did not show a significant effect of rifampin on efavirenz exposure.[175–177] Therefore, the preferred treatment regimens are rifampin-based TB therapy with an ART regimen consisting of efavirenz plus two nucleoside reverse transcriptase inhibitors.[161] The efavirenz dose should be 600 mg daily.[161] Efavirenz decreases rifabutin exposure by 38%, necessitating a dosage increase for rifabutin to 450 to 600 mg daily.[161] For patients unable to take efavirenz due to early pregnancy or intolerance, nevirapine-based ART can be used, but rifampin significantly decreases nevirapine exposures.[161] If used concomitantly, the nevirapine dose should be 200 mg twice daily.[161] However, rifabutin-based TB therapy may be considered with a nevirapine-based ART regimen because dosage adjustments are not needed for either agent.[161] Concomitant administration of etravirine and rilpivirine with rifampin should be avoided due to significant reduction in exposures of these NNRTIs.[161]

Rifampin should not be used in patients receiving protease inhibitor-based ART, regardless of boosting with ritonavir, because rifampin causes a dramatic decrease in exposures of the protease inhibitors.[65,161] Rifabutin has a negligible effect on ritonavir-boosted lopinavir or atazanavir and only moderate increases in darunavir and fosamprenavir concentrations.[161] For patients unable to tolerate efavirenz or nevirapine or if the HIV strain is resistant to NNRTIs, a rifabutin-based TB regimen is preferred with an ritonavir-boosted protease inhibitor regimen.[161] However, all protease inhibitors markedly increase rifabutin concentrations. If doses of rifabutin are not adjusted, adverse drug events, such as uveitis, neutropenia, arthralgias, skin discoloration, may occur.[65,167] Therefore, the rifabutin dose should be decreased to 150 mg daily when administered with protease inhibitors.[161]

HIV nucleoside and nucleotide reverse transcriptase inhibitors and the fusion inhibitor enfuvirtide are not metabolized by CYP isoenzymes. As a result, these agents can be administered with the rifamycins.[135] Rifampin decreases the concentrations of the integrase inhibitors, raltegravir and elvitegravir. The raltegravir dose should be increased to 800 mg twice daily, but no dosage adjustment is recommended with rifabutin.[161] Co-administration with elvitegravir with rifampin and rifabutin should be avoided.[161] Maraviroc, a CCR5 antagonist, is a substrate for CYP3A and P-glycoprotein, and concomitant administration with rifampin significantly decreases exposures.[135] The maraviroc dose should be increased to 600 mg twice daily, but no dosage adjustment is needed with rifabutin.[161]

TREATMENT OF LATENT TUBERCULOSIS INFECTION IN HUMAN IMMUNODEFICIENCY VIRUS INFECTION

CASE 68-8

QUESTION 1: N.M. is the 32-year-old partner and roommate of F.R. Because of his close contact with F.R., he is evaluated for exposure to TB by an infectious diseases specialist. N.M.'s HIV test is positive, and a tuberculin skin test produces an induration of 8 mm, which is positive. All other studies are negative for active TB. Should N.M. receive treatment for latent TB infection? If so, what therapy should he receive?

The risk of N.M. developing active TB disease is significant; therefore, he should receive treatment for latent TB infection. HIV-infected persons, regardless of age, should be treated for latent TB infection.[65] Pape et al. conducted a randomized, placebo-controlled trial of isoniazid therapy in HIV-infected patients.[178] Patients receiving placebo were 6 times more likely to develop active TB than those receiving isoniazid, and patients receiving isoniazid were also less likely to develop AIDS.[178] The preferred treatment for latent TB infection in N.M. is isoniazid 300 mg daily or twice weekly for 9 months.[65,161] Isoniazid does not increase the risk of hepatitis when used with efavirenz- or nevirapine-based ART regimens.[161] N.M. should also receive pyridoxine 25 mg daily to prevent peripheral neuropathy. Rifampin and rifabutin for 4 months are alternatives to isoniazid, but the potential for drug interactions should be considered. Weekly isoniazid plus rifapentine are not recommended for HIV-infected patients due to the potential for significant drug interactions with rifapentine and ART.[161]

Pregnancy

CASE 68-9

QUESTION 1: E.F. is a 25-year-old Hispanic woman who is being treated with isoniazid 900 mg and rifampin 600 mg twice a week for pulmonary TB. She completed 2 months of therapy with isoniazid, rifampin, pyrazinamide, and ethambutol, and began the new regimen 2 months ago. She recently became pregnant, and her obstetrician is concerned about the possible teratogenic effects of her TB regimen. What are the risks of TB and its treatment to the mother and the fetus? Are these drugs teratogenic?

Although concerns about the use of any medication during pregnancy always exist, it is now recognized that untreated TB represents a far greater risk to a pregnant woman and her fetus than the treatment.[33,66] TB is one of the leading nonobstetric causes of maternal mortality.[179] The World Health Organization recommends that treatment of TB in pregnant women should be the same as that for nonpregnant women, with few exceptions.[179] Isoniazid, rifampin, pyrazinamide, and ethambutol are not teratogenic in humans.[180,181] In the United States, pyrazinamide is not recommended for use during pregnancy because of insufficient safety data.[33] If pyrazinamide is not included in the initial treatment regimen, the minimal duration of therapy is 9 months.[33] All pregnant women receiving isoniazid should also receive pyridoxine 25 mg/day because of the possibility of peripheral neuropathy.

Streptomycin should not be used during pregnancy except as a last alternative because it has been associated with mild-to-severe ototoxicity in the fetus.[179] Ototoxicity can occur throughout the gestational period and is not confined to the first trimester. With the exception of streptomycin ototoxicity, the occurrence of birth defects in women being treated for TB with the above agents is no greater than that of healthy pregnant women.[182,183] Therefore, administration of antituberculosis drugs is not an indication for termination of pregnancy.[33] Because E.F. likely became pregnant after completing the first 2 months of therapy, she should continue her current regimen for a total of 6 months because she received pyrazinamide as part of the initial regimen.

MULTIDRUG-RESISTANT TUBERCULOSIS IN PREGNANCY

Little is known about the efficacy and safety of second-line drugs for the treatment of MDR-TB during pregnancy. Two reports with small numbers of patients have suggested that treatment is effective with no adverse effects to mother or child.[184,185] In a study of seven women treated for MDR-TB during pregnancy, no obstetric complications or perinatal transmission of MDR-TB was observed.[184] Five women were cured, one experienced treatment failure, and one stopped therapy prematurely.[184] No evidence of drug toxicity was seen among their children exposed to second-line drugs in utero, although one child was diagnosed with MDR-TB.[185] There are no well-controlled studies with bedaquiline in pregnancy; therefore, the drug should only be used in pregnancy if clearly needed. More data are needed, but pregnancy should not be a limitation to the treatment of MDR-TB.

LACTATION

When the baby is born, E.F. may breast-feed while continuing her medication. Drug concentrations in breast milk are minimal and do not provide sufficient quantities for the treatment or prevention of TB in the nursing infant.[33,66]

Pediatrics

CASE 68-10

QUESTION 1: A.M., a 3-year-old African American boy, is suspected of having TB. His father has been receiving treatment for TB for the last 2 months. A.M. has a productive cough, fever, and general malaise. His sputum is positive for AFB, and his PPD skin test is positive (10 mm). What is the incidence of TB in children? How should A.M. be treated?

The incidence of TB in children younger than 15 years of age has declined from 1,660 cases (2.9/100,000 population) in 1993 to 460 cases (0.8/100,000 population) in 2014.[10] Children commonly have active TB disease as a complication of the initial infection with *M. tuberculosis,* and the disease is characterized by intrathoracic adenopathy, middle and lower lung lobe infiltrates, and the absence of cavitation on chest radiography.[33,186] Because of the high risk of disseminated TB in infants and children, treatment should be started as soon as the diagnosis of TB is suspected. In general, regimens recommended for adults are also recommended for infants, children, and adolescents, with the exception that ethambutol is not used routinely in children.[33] Ethambutol is often avoided because it is difficult to assess visual acuity in children. A.M. should be started on isoniazid 10 to 15 mg/kg/day, rifampin 10 to 20 mg/kg/day, and pyrazinamide 15 to 30 mg/kg/day.[33,66,186] Many experts prefer to treat children with three drugs (rather than four) in the initial phase because the bacillary population is usually lower than in an adult and it may be difficult for an infant or child to ingest four drugs. If resistance is suspected, ethambutol 15 to 20 mg/kg/day or streptomycin 20 to 40 mg/kg/day should be added to the regimen until susceptibility of the organism to isoniazid, rifampin, and pyrazinamide is known. Pyridoxine is recommended for infants, children, and adolescents who are receiving isoniazid.[33]

If resistance is not suspected and drug susceptibility is confirmed, A.M. should receive the isoniazid, rifampin, and pyrazinamide daily for 8 weeks. He can then continue to take the isoniazid and rifampin daily or 2 to 3 times a week (DOT) for an additional 4 months. The dosage for isoniazid and rifampin in a 2 to 3 times a week regimen would be 20 to 30 mg/kg/dose and 10 to 20 mg/kg/dose, respectively (Table 68-3).

A.M. should be examined routinely for signs and symptoms of hepatitis. Although antituberculosis medications are generally well tolerated in children, LFTs are commonly 2 to 3 times the upper limit of normal during therapy. These are often benign and transient; however, the incidence of hepatitis in children from isoniazid with rifampin may be 4 to 6 times more common than in children receiving isoniazid alone. Most hepatitis occurs within the first 3 months of therapy and generally is associated with higher than recommended doses of isoniazid or rifampin.[123,187]

Children and adolescents should be screened for risk factors for TB using a questionnaire, and they should be skin tested with 5 TU of PPD if one or more risk factors are present.[188] Insufficient data are available to recommend use of IGRAs in children. Isoniazid for 9 months is recommended for treatment of latent TB in this population.[188] Daily rifampin for 6 months is an acceptable alternative, especially in children who cannot tolerate isoniazid or those exposed to a source case whose isolate was isoniazid resistant.[188]

Extrapulmonary Tuberculosis and Tuberculous Meningitis

CASE 68-11

QUESTION 1: R.U. is a 64-year-old, 82-kg man who is brought to the emergency department after a 4-day period during which he became progressively disoriented, febrile to 40.5°C, and obtunded. He also had severe headaches during this time. Physical examination revealed moderate nuchal rigidity and a positive Brudzinski sign (neck resistant to flexion). An initial diagnosis of possible meningitis was made, and a lumbar puncture ordered. The cerebrospinal fluid (CSF) appeared turbid, and laboratory analysis revealed an elevated protein concentration of 200 mg/dL, a decreased glucose concentration of 30 mg/dL, and a white blood cell count of 500/μL (85% lymphocytes). A Gram stain of the spinal fluid and a sputum smear for AFB were negative, but the AFB smear of the CSF was positive. Other laboratory tests were within normal limits. A diagnosis of tuberculous meningitis was made. Discuss the presentation and prognosis of tuberculous meningitis. How should R.U. be treated?

Tuberculous meningitis is only one of the extrapulmonary complications of infection with *M. tuberculosis*.

Successful treatment of extrapulmonary TB can usually be accomplished in 6 to 9 months with an acceptable relapse rate.[33,66,189] Some forms, such as bone or joint TB, miliary TB, or tuberculous meningitis, may require 9 to 12 months of therapy.[33] Because specimens for culture and susceptibility testing may be difficult or impossible to obtain from a site, response to treatment must be based on clinical and radiographic improvement.

Tuberculous meningitis in older persons is usually caused by hematogenous dissemination of the tubercle bacilli from a primary site, most commonly the lungs. In its early stages, tuberculous meningitis often is confused with aseptic meningitis because the Gram stain is negative. The most common symptoms of tuberculous meningitis are headache, fever, restlessness, irritability, nausea, and vomiting. A positive Brudzinski sign and neck stiffness may be present. As illustrated in R.U., the CSF is usually turbid with increased protein and decreased glucose concentrations. There is an increase in the CSF white blood cell count with a predominance of lymphocytes. Culture of the CSF for *M. tuberculosis* may not be helpful because rates of positivity for clinically diagnosed cases range from 25% to 70%.[190] Early recognition and treatment are essential for a favorable outcome. Thus, empirical treatment before receipt of confirmatory culture and susceptibility results is common in suspected tuberculous meningitis. Multiple-drug therapy should be used because irreversible brain damage or death can occur as soon as 2 weeks after the onset of infection (not clinical symptoms).[190]

TREATMENT

Treatment should be initiated in R.U. with daily administration of isoniazid 300 mg, rifampin 600 mg, pyrazinamide 2,000 mg, and ethambutol 1,600 mg for the first 8 weeks.[33] After this initial phase of treatment, R.U. should receive daily isoniazid and rifampin for an additional 7 to 10 months, although the optimal duration of therapy is unknown.[33] In addition, because R.U. is older, pyridoxine 10 to 50 mg/day should be given to prevent the occurrence of peripheral neuropathy from isoniazid. It should be reiterated that rifampin can impart a red to orange color to the CSF.

Isoniazid readily penetrates into the CSF, with CSF concentrations reaching up to 100% of those in the serum. Rifampin is often included in tuberculous meningitis regimens and may be associated with reduced morbidity and mortality; however, even with inflammation, CSF concentrations of rifampin are only 6% to 30% of those found in the serum. Ethambutol should be used in the highest dosage to achieve bactericidal concentrations in the CSF because its CSF concentrations are only 10% to 54% of those in the serum. Streptomycin penetrates into the CSF poorly even with inflamed meninges.[191]

CORTICOSTEROIDS

Corticosteroids in moderate-to-severe tuberculous meningitis appear to reduce sequelae and prolong survival.[192] The mechanism for this benefit is likely owing to reduction of intracranial pressure. Dexamethasone 8 to 12 mg/day (or prednisone equivalent) for 6 to 8 weeks should be used and then tapered slowly after symptoms subside.[192] Corticosteroids are likely indicated for R.U.

THERAPEUTIC DRUG MONITORING

The pharmacokinetics of the drugs used to treat tuberculosis are highly variable and depend on weight, sex, genetic traits, and underlying comorbidities. Subtherapeutic concentrations may be associated with a delayed response to therapy, increased risk of relapse, or acquired drug resistance. Several studies measured drug concentrations in patients with slow clinical response to TB treatment and found subtherapeutic concentrations for isoniazid, rifampin, ethambutol, and rifabutin in a substantial percentage of patients evaluated.[87,193–195] In one study, time to sputum culture conversion was longer in patients with low serum concentrations.[195] In a prospective observational study, 2-hour plasma concentrations were measured in 35 patients, and plasma concentrations were below the normal ranges in 71%, 58%, 46%, and 10% of patients for isoniazid, rifampin, ethambutol, and pyrazinamide, respectively.[196] In addition, 45% of patients had subtherapeutic concentrations for both isoniazid and rifampin. Treatment failure occurred significantly more frequently when concentrations of isoniazid and rifampin were below the normal ranges ($p = 0.013$) and below the median 2-hour drug concentration achieved in the study ($p = 0.005$).[196] In 142 patients with active TB, poor long-term outcomes were predicted by a 24-hour area under the concentration–time curve (AUC) ≤363 mg × hour/L for pyrazinamide, ≤13 mg × hour/L for rifampin, and ≤52 mg × hour/L for isoniazid.[197] Poor outcomes occurred in 32/78 patients with at least one drug with an AUC below these threshold values compared to 3/64 patients without any low AUCs (odds ratio = 14.14; 95% CI 4.08–49.1). Low rifampin and isoniazid peak concentrations and AUCs predicted acquired drug resistance in all cases.[197]

Based on these studies, therapeutic drug monitoring may be useful in patients with poor or slow clinical response to therapy and allow for dosage adjustment to achieve therapeutic drug concentrations. Additional patients who may benefit from therapeutic drug monitoring include those with severe disease, diabetes, HIV infection, renal dysfunction, and hepatic dysfunction.[198] A 2-hour postdose blood sample can be obtained to estimate the peak concentration for most drugs, whereas a 3-hour postdose blood sample would be needed for rifabutin.[198] A second blood sample at 6 hours postdose (7 hours for rifabutin) may also be obtained. Trough concentrations for most agents are below the detection limit of the assays at the end of a dosing interval and are not useful clinically.[198] Blood samples should be collected in red-top test tubes and processed promptly because some drugs are not stable at room temperature in blood or serum. Once the drug concentrations are known, comparisons can be made to the normal ranges for each drug and doses adjusted accordingly. However, normal ranges for drug concentrations have not been studied in regard to clinical outcome, and optimal drug concentrations for clinical and microbiologic efficacy are not known.[196] Although therapeutic drug monitoring may provide useful information, clinicians must remember that serum concentrations are only one factor among multiple factors affecting treatment outcomes.

KEY REFERENCES AND WEBSITES

A full list of references for this chapter can be found at http://thepoint.lww.com/AT11e. Below are the key references and websites for this chapter, with the corresponding reference number in this chapter found in parentheses after the reference.

Key References

Alsultan A, Peloquin CA. Therapeutic drug monitoring in the treatment of tuberculosis: an update. *Drugs*. 2014;74:839. (198)

Baciewicz AM et al. Update on rifampin and rifabutin drug interactions. *Am J Med Sci*. 2008;335:126. (127)

Blumberg HM et al. American Thoracic Society/Centers for Disease Control and Prevention/Infectious Diseases Society of America. Treatment of tuberculosis. *Am J Respir Crit Care Med*. 2003;167:603. (33)

Centers for Disease Control and Prevention. Recommendations for use of an isoniazid-rifapentine regimen with direct observation to treat latent *Mycobacterium tuberculosis* infection. *Morb Mortal Wkly Rep*. 2011;60:1650. (116)

Centers for Disease Control and Prevention. Reported tuberculosis in the United States 2014. http://www.cdc.gov/tb/statistics/reports/2014/pdfs/tb-surveillance-2014-report.pdf. Accessed October 9, 2015. (10)

Diacon AH et al. Multidrug-resistant tuberculosis and culture conversion with bedaquiline. *N Engl J Med*. 2014;371:723. (160)

Getahun H et al. Latent *Mycobacterium tuberculosis* infection. *N Engl J Med*. 2015;372:2127. (22)

Gillespie SH et al. Four-month moxifloxacin-based regimens for drug-sensitive tuberculosis. *N Engl J Med*. 2014;371:1577. (88)

Gordin FM, Masur H. Current approaches to tuberculosis in the United States. *JAMA*. 2012;308:283. (19)

Lin SYG, Desmond EP. Molecular diagnosis of tuberculosis and drug resistance. *Clin Lab Med*. 2014;34:297. (54)

Prahl JB et al. Clinical significance of 2 h plasma concentrations of first-line anti-tuberculosis drugs: a prospective observational study. *J Antimicrob Chemother*. 2014;69:2841. (196)

Sterling TR et al. Three months of rifapentine and isoniazid for latent tuberculosis infection. *N Engl J Med*. 2011;365:2155. (115)

Wlodarsha M et al. A microbiological revolution meets an ancient disease: improving the management of tuberculosis with genomics. *Clin Microbiol Rev*. 2015;28:523. (55)

Worley MV, Estrada SJ. Bedaquiline: a novel antitubercular agent for the treatment of multidrug-resistant tuberculosis. *Pharmacotherapy*. 2014;34:1187. (157)

Key Websites

Centers for Disease Control and Prevention. Tuberculosis (TB). http://www.cdc.gov/tb

World Health Organization. Global tuberculosis report 2014. http://www.who.int/tb/publications/global_report/gtbr14_main_text.pdf. Accessed September 22, 2015. (9)

69 Infectious Diarrhea

Gail S. Itokazu and David T. Bearden

CORE PRINCIPLES

#	CORE PRINCIPLES	CHAPTER CASES
1	The most common complication of any diarrheal illness is loss of fluids and electrolytes, which in extreme cases can lead to hypovolemia, shock, and death. Depending on the degree of dehydration, fluid and electrolyte losses are replaced intravenously or orally.	**Case 69-1 (Questions 1, 2)**
2	Classification of infectious diarrheas as either an inflammatory or noninflammatory diarrheal illness provides a basis for preparing a focused list of suspected pathogens, thus guiding the overall diagnostic and therapeutic plan.	**Case 69-1 (Questions 3–4)**
3	*Vibrio cholerae* 01 and 0139 are toxigenic strains of *Vibrio* species, which cause epidemic cholera; severe dehydration requiring vigorous fluid replacement may be necessary. Non-cholera *Vibrio* species do not possess the virulence factors required to cause epidemic cholera. Antimicrobial treatment differs between toxigenic and non-toxigenic *Vibrio* species.	**Case 69-2 (Questions 1–3), Case 69-3 (Questions 1, 2)**
4	*Salmonella* species are classified as non-typhoidal and typhoidal salmonellae. Non-typhoidal salmonellae may cause the clinical syndromes of gastroenteritis, bacteremia, and localized infection, whereas typhoidal salmonellae may cause typhoid fever and chronic carriage. The role of antimicrobials in the management of salmonellosis is based on the clinical syndrome, its severity, and underlying health problems of infected persons.	**Case 69-7 (Question 1), Case 69-8 (Questions 1, 2), Case 69-9 (Question 1), Case 69-10 (Question 1), Case 69-11 (Questions 1–7)**
5	Severe dysentery caused by *Shigella* species is most commonly caused by *Shigella dysenteriae*, whereas a milder illness is typically caused by *Shigella sonnei*. Antimicrobials alleviate the symptoms of shigellosis, and decrease the period of time that shigellae can be spread by person-to-person contact.	**Case 69-12 (Questions 1–5), Case 69-13 (Question 1)**
6	Fluoroquinolone-resistance in *Campylobacter* species is a common finding in both developed and underdeveloped areas of the world; when indicated, macrolide antimicrobials are recommended.	**Case 69-14 (Questions 1–3)**
7	Travelers to destinations where acquisition of Travelers' diarrhea (TD) is a concern should bring a travel kit including medications (e.g., loperamide and antimicrobials) and instructions for self-treatment at the onset of illness. The selected antimicrobial depends on the area of travel. Long-term postinfectious complications of TD may occur in some returning travelers.	**Case 69-15 (Questions 1–6)**
8	*Escherichia coli* O157:H7 is a specific toxin-producing strain of *E. coli* bacteria that can lead to the severe sequelae of hemolytic uremic syndrome.	**Case 69-16 (Questions 3, 4)**
9	*Clostridium difficile* infection causes a wide range of severity of illness. Mild-to-moderate disease is typically treated with metronidazole as first-line therapy, and oral vancomycin is preferred for severe disease.	**Case 69-17 (Question 6)**
10	Severe *C. difficile* infection can be life-threatening and often necessitates multiple therapeutic interventions.	**Case 69-18 (Questions 4, 5)**

PREVALENCE AND ETIOLOGY

Worldwide, diarrhea accounts for more than 2.5 million deaths annually,[1] mainly affecting infants and children living in poverty.[2] Prolonged episodes of diarrhea lead to malnutrition and in children contribute to impaired growth and developmental delay.[2] In the United States, about 48 million foodborne diarrheal illnesses occur each year, resulting in 128,000 hospitalizations and 3,000 deaths.[3]

Infectious diarrhea is caused by the ingestion of food or water contaminated with pathogenic microorganisms (e.g., bacteria, viruses, protozoa, or fungi) or their toxins (Table 69-1).[2] In the United States, noroviruses account for about 50% of diarrheal outbreaks, while common bacterial pathogens include *Campylobacter*,

Table 69-1
Predisposing Factors, Symptoms, and Therapy of Gastrointestinal Infections

Pathogen	Predisposing Factors	Symptoms	Diagnostic Evaluations	Drug of Choice[a,c]	Alternatives[a,c]
Salmonella (non-typhoidal)[b]	Ingestion of contaminated poultry, raw milk, custards, and cream fillings; foreign travel	Nausea, vomiting, diarrhea, cramps, fever, tenesmus. Incubation: 6–72 hours	Fecal leukocytes, stool culture	Fluoroquinolone, azithromycin, third-generation cephalosporins	Amoxicillin, TMP–SMX
Salmonella (typhoidal)	Ingestion of contaminated food; foreign travel	High fever, abdominal pain, headache, dry cough	Fecal leukocytes, stool culture, blood culture	Fluoroquinolone, azithromycin, third-generation cephalosporins	TMP–SMX, amoxicillin
Shigella	Ingestion of contaminated salad, raw vegetables, swimming in water contaminated with sewage; foreign travel	Fever, dysentery, cramps, tenesmus. Incubation: 24–48 hours	Fecal leukocytes, stool culture	Fluoroquinolone, azithromycin, ceftriaxone	TMP–SMX, ampicillin
Campylobacter	Contaminated eggs, raw milk, or poultry; foreign travel	Mild-to-severe diarrhea; fever, systemic malaise. Incubation: 24–72 hours	Fecal leukocytes, stool culture	Erythromycin, azithromycin	–
Clostridium difficile	Antibiotics, antineoplastics	Mild-to-severe diarrhea, cramps	*C. difficile* toxin, *C. difficile* culture, colonoscopy	Metronidazole	Vancomycin
Staphylococcal food poisoning	Custard-filled bakery products, canned food, processed meat, ice cream	Nausea, vomiting, salivation, cramps, diarrhea; usually resolves in 8 hours. Incubation: 2–6 hours	–	Supportive therapy only	–
Travelers' diarrhea (Enterotoxigenic *Escherichia coli*, *Campylobacter*)	Contaminated food (vegetables and cheese), water; foreign travel	Nausea, vomiting, mild-to-severe diarrhea, cramps	Stool culture	See Table 69-3	–
Shiga toxin–producing *Escherichia coli* (*E. coli* O157:H7)	Beef, raw milk, water	Diarrhea, headache, bloody stools Incubation: 48–96 hours	Stool cultures on MacConkey's sorbitol	Supportive therapy only	–
Cryptosporidiosis	Immunosuppression, day-care centers, contaminated water, animal handlers	Mild-to-severe diarrhea (chronic or self-limited); large fluid volume	Stool screening for oocytes, PCR, ELISA	See Chapter 77, Opportunistic Infections in HIV-Infected Patients	–
Viral gastroenteritis	Community-wide outbreaks, contaminated food	Nausea, diarrhea (self-limited), cramps. Incubation: 16–48 hours	Special viral studies	Supportive therapy only	–

[a]Sources: Navaneethan U, Giannella RA. Mechanisms of infectious diarrhea. *Nat Clin Pract Gastroenterol Hepatol.* 2008;5:637; DuPont HL. Acute infectious diarrhea in immunocompetent adults. *N Engl J Med.* 2014;370:1532. See text for doses and duration of therapy.
[b]Not all cases require antibiotic therapy. See text for details.
[c]If susceptible. See text for details.

ELISA, enzyme-linked immunosorbent assay; PCR, polymerase chain reaction; TMP–SMX, trimethoprim–sulfamethoxazole.

…oidal *Salmonella*, *Shigella*, and Shiga toxin–producing …oli.[3]

…apter focuses on the diagnosis and management of the …on microbial causes of acute infectious diarrhea.

DEFINITIONS

Diarrhea is often defined as three or more episodes of loose stools or any loose stool with blood during a 24-hour period, which may be accompanied by nausea, vomiting, or abdominal cramping.[3] The duration of illness is considered acute if symptoms are present for less than 2 weeks duration, persistent if symptoms last for 14 to 29 days, and chronic if symptoms last ≥30 days.[3] Classifying diarrheal syndromes as either a noninflammatory (watery diarrhea) or an inflammatory (bloody diarrhea) illness provides a basis for predicting the most likely microbial cause for the intestinal illness.[1]

PATHOGENESIS

The pathogenesis of infectious diarrhea involves an interplay among bacterial virulence factors, host factors, and predisposing factors to infection. Diarrhea is more likely to occur in the setting in which an imbalance among these factors favors the enteropathogen.

Bacterial Virulence Factors

Enteropathogens possess virulence factors that contribute to the organism's pathogenicity.[2] Enterotoxins targeting the small bowel cause net movement of fluid into the gut lumen, leading to voluminous watery stools and potentially life-threatening dehydration. Cytotoxins targeting the colon cause direct mucosal damage, leading to fever and bloody diarrhea. Invasive properties of *Shigella* species and invasive strains of *E. coli* allow these bacteria to invade and destroy epithelial cells, causing bloody or mucoid stools. Some enteropathogens induce a vigorous host response through the release of proinflammatory cytokines from intestinal epithelial cells, leading to diarrhea. Finally, adhesions allow enteropathogens to attach to and colonize the gastrointestinal (GI) mucosa, facilitating toxin delivery, invasion, dissemination, or host cell lysis.[2]

Host Defenses

The human GI tract possesses numerous defense mechanisms to protect against enteric infection. Normal bacterial flora compete for space and nutrients with potentially pathogenic organisms, or produce substances, e.g., short-chain fatty acids, that are inhibitory to enteropathogens.[2] Gastric acidity of the stomach prevents acid-susceptible pathogens from passing from the stomach into the intestinal tract, whereas gastrointestinal mucus and mucosal tissue integrity provide physical barriers against infection. Intestinal immunity includes defensins that are bactericidal to some enteropathogens, local production of antibodies, and toll-like receptors that recognize enteropathogens and activate the immune response.[2] Intestinal peristalsis moves bacteria and their toxins along and out of the GI tract. Finally, specific host genetic factors are protective against enteric infection.[3]

Predisposing Factors

Inadequate sanitation facilities increase the risk that local inhabitants and travelers will be exposed to contaminated food and water. Outbreaks of foodborne or waterborne illnesses in both industrialized and developing countries facilitate the spread of infectious organisms. Industrialized countries that rely on imported food items risk the possibility of importation of contaminated food products.[4] Immunocompromised hosts, such as organ transplant recipients and patients receiving immunosuppressive therapies, are more susceptible to intestinal infection. Institutional settings such as day-care centers, hospitals, and extended-care facilities are high-risk settings for dissemination of disease. Finally, poor personal hygiene is a risk for infectious diarrhea.

The use of pharmacologic agents, e.g., drugs that increase gastric pH (Table 69-2), increases the risk for infection with acid-susceptible pathogens such as *Salmonella* species and *Vibrio cholerae*.[5] The use of proton-pump inhibitors predisposes patients to *Clostridium difficile* diarrhea.

Table 69-2
Pharmacologic Agents that May Promote Gastrointestinal Infection

Drug	Mechanism
Antacids, H_2-receptor antagonists, proton-pump inhibitors	Increase of gastric pH; passage of viable pathogens to lower gut
Antibiotics	Alteration of intestinal flora
Cancer chemotherapy	Unclear but may include the antimicrobial activity of chemotherapeutic agents, or chemotherapy-induced intestinal damage and necrosis favoring an anaerobic environment for the growth of *C. difficile*.

Source: DuPont HL. Acute infectious diarrhea in immunocompetent adults. *N Engl J Med*. 2014;370:1532; Cohen SH et al. Clinical practice guidelines for *Clostridium difficile* infection in adults: 2010 update by the Society of Healthcare Epidemiology of America (SHEA) and the Infectious Diseases Society of America (IDSA). *Infect Control Hosp Epidemiol*. 2010;31:431; Anand A, Glatt AE. *Clostridium difficile* infection associated with antineoplastic chemotherapy: a review. *Clin Infect Dis*. 1993;17:109.

MANAGEMENT OVERVIEW

Rehydration Therapy

The most common complication of any diarrheal illness is loss of fluids and electrolytes, which in extreme cases can lead to hypovolemia, shock, and death.[1] Depending on the degree of dehydration, fluid and electrolyte losses are replaced intravenously (IV) or orally. Once replacement of fluid and electrolyte losses is completed, additional laboratory tests and drug therapies can be considered.

Laboratory Tests

Inflammatory diarrheal illnesses are characterized by the presence of bloody or mucoid stools. Therefore, stool specimens with red blood cells (RBCs) or occult blood, or those that contain large numbers of white blood cells, suggest infection attributable to invasive pathogens.[6]

Identification of bacterial toxins in stool specimens is a useful diagnostic tool. For example, because only the toxigenic strains of *C. difficile* are pathogenic, the presence or absence of bacterial toxins in stool specimens is more important than a positive culture for the organism.[7]

In clinical practice, routine microbiologic identification of pathogens utilizes selective media which favors the growth of suspected pathogens.[7] Stool cultures are recommended for patients with one of the following: acute diarrhea that is severe or associated with a temperature >38.5°C; dysentery—which is an inflammatory diarrheal illness characterized by bloody or mucoid stools with abdominal cramps; profuse cholera-like watery diarrhea; dehydration; elderly or immunocompromised patients; nursing home patients; food handlers; and day-care workers.[3] Hospitalized patients should be evaluated for *C. difficile* infection. Culture of specimens from extraintestinal sites of infection (e.g., blood cultures) can be used to identify the microbial etiology.

PCR-based diagnostic tests are widely available in industrialized countries, offering improved sensitivity but focusing on genes versus virulence factors.[3]

Drug Therapy

Drug therapy for infectious diarrhea includes medications to provide symptomatic relief or to eradicate the causative pathogen.

LOPERAMIDE AND DIPHENOXYLATE/ATROPINE

Loperamide and diphenoxylate/atropine reduce the frequency of diarrheal stools by slowing intestinal transit time; additionally, loperamide possesses antisecretory properties.[8] Loperamide is preferred over diphenoxylate/atropine because of its greater efficacy, better tolerance, and over-the-counter availability. Diphenoxylate/atropine causes drowsiness, dizziness, dry mouth, and urinary retention owing to the atropine component, and its use in the elderly is not recommended (see Chapter 107 Geriatric Drug Use).

The use of antimotility drugs is not recommended in persons with fever, bloody diarrhea,[3] or when invasive pathogens are suspected.[1] The primary concern is that prolongation of clearance of pathogens from the intestinal tract could worsen the severity of illness. However, in non-critically ill patients with bacillary dysentery, loperamide was not harmful when administered with antimicrobials to which the infecting pathogen was susceptible.[9]

BISMUTH SUBSALICYLATE (BSS)

Bismuth subsalicylate's antidiarrheal properties are because of its antisecretory, adsorbent, and antimicrobial properties.[10] Problems with BSS include the inconvenience of dosing 4 times per day, and adverse effects such as darkening of the tongue and stools, and tinnitus secondary to salicylate absorption. Each recommended antidiarrheal dose of BSS of 526 mg contains 263 mg of salicylate, and this needs to be considered in patients already taking salicylate products.

CROFELEMER

Crofelemer is a recently U.S. Food and Drug Administration (FDA)–approved non-absorbable agent indicated for the symptomatic treatment of noninfectious diarrhea in HIV-infected persons on antiretroviral therapy.[11] Its antisecretory effect is because of the unique inhibition of two distinct channels responsible for chloride and fluid secretion into the GI tract. Crofelemer improves diarrheal symptoms in patients with noninfectious diarrhea; larger trials are needed to further assess its efficacy and safety in patients with infectious diarrhea. Common side effects of cofelemer include flatulence (7%) and abdominal pain (5%).[11]

PROBIOTICS

Interest in probiotics stems, in part, from their potential to decrease the use of antibiotics. These live microbial mixtures of bacteria and yeasts are used to restore the normal intestinal flora, thereby reducing intestinal colonization with pathogenic organisms. Probiotics also produce pathogen-inhibiting substances, prevent pathogen adhesion to the GI tract, inhibit the action of microbial toxins, and stimulate immune defense mechanisms.[12] Further studies are needed to clarify the role of specific probiotics for the treatment and prevention of acute infectious diarrhea.[12,13]

ANTIMICROBIALS

In selected cases, antimicrobials are prescribed to decrease the duration and the severity of diarrheal illnesses, to prevent the progression to invasive infection, and prevent person-to-person transmission of pathogens. Antimicrobials are generally recommended for the severely ill, for patients with conditions compromising normal enteric defenses, for immunocompromised patients, and for the treatment of extraintestinal infection.[3]

Ongoing surveillance of antimicrobial resistance is important to guide treatment recommendations. Extensively used in the past and resulting in widespread resistance to common enteropathogens, trimethoprim–sulfamethoxazole (TMP–SMX), the aminopenicillins, nalidixic acid, and tetracyclines are unsuitable empiric choices for the treatment of many enteropathogens. Depending on the circumstances surrounding the diarrheal illness, including where the pathogen was acquired (e.g., domestic vs. travel-related), age, and allergy history of the patient, commonly recommended antimicrobials include selected third-generation cephalosporins (e.g., ceftriaxone or cefotaxime), azithromycin, rifaximin, fluoroquinolones, and others.[3]

The fluoroquinolones, although still recommended because of their efficacy against susceptible organisms[3] and their availability as oral formulations, must be used cautiously as common enteropathogens, e.g., *Shigella*, *Salmonella*, and *Campylobacter* species, are frequently fluoroquinolone-resistant.[14] Another consideration with using fluoroquinolones is that they are not FDA-approved for use in children because lesions on cartilage tissue have been reported in juvenile animals. Nevertheless, because of the emergence of multidrug-resistant enteropathogens in some geographic areas, clinical trials using fluoroquinolones in children have been performed,[15] and the available data suggest that a short course of these agents is safe. Finally, antimicrobial use should be limited to instances where their benefits outweigh their risks for adverse effects and resistance.

Prevention

Good personal hygiene along with proper food handling, cooking, and storage are essential to prevent the spread of enteropathogens. When visiting areas with inadequate facilities for the disposal of sewage, travelers should follow the rule, "boil it, cook it, peel it, or forget it." Effective vaccines are available to prevent typhoid fever, rotavirus, and cholera (not available in the United States); studies of vaccines to prevent *Campylobacter*, enterotoxigenic *E. coli*, and *Shigella* infections are ongoing.[1]

EVALUATION AND TREATMENT OF PATIENTS WITH INFECTIOUS DIARRHEA

CASE 69-1

QUESTION 1: B.K. is a 78-year-old man presenting to his physician with a diarrheal illness for 1 day. His illness began with vomiting and was followed by abdominal pain, nausea, and watery, but non-bloody, diarrhea. Despite not feeling well, he is able to drink fruit juices. B.K.'s history of present illness is significant for eating raw oysters at a local seafood restaurant 2 days ago, and he has

…ed that other patrons are experiencing a similar illness. … significant medical history. He denies recent hospital- … contact with small children, recent travel, or recent use of …microbials. On physical examination B.K. is alert and oriented, is not "toxic" appearing, afebrile, and has stable vital signs. The remainder of his examination is significant for decreased skin turgor and dry mucous membranes. What is your general approach to the management of B.K.'s diarrheal illness?

Because infectious diarrhea is typically a self-limiting illness, patients may never seek medical attention, and in many cases, replacement of fluids and electrolytes is all that is required. In general, medical evaluation is warranted for patients with profuse watery diarrhea with dehydration, bloody stools, temperature greater than 101.3°F, or illness of more than 48 hours duration. Other persons requiring medical evaluation include patients older than 50 years of age with severe abdominal pain and immunocompromised patients (e.g., those with acquired immunodeficiency syndrome, organ transplant recipients, or patients being treated with cancer chemotherapies). Noninfectious causes for the illness such as medications, inflammatory bowel disease, consumption of poorly absorbable carbohydrates (e.g., sugarless candies or chewing gum), or malabsorption syndromes should be considered.[6]

CASE 69-1, QUESTION 2: What rehydration plan would you recommend for B.K.?

B.K.'s physical examination is significant for decreased skin turgor and dry mucous membranes, findings consistent with mild-to-moderate volume depletion.[16] Given that B.K. is not "toxic" appearing, with stable vital signs, and is tolerating oral liquids, oral beverages containing glucose (e.g., lemonades, sweet sodas, or fruit juices) or soups rich in electrolytes are appropriate.[17] In developing countries, significant reductions in dehydration-related mortality is attributed to oral replacement therapy solutions containing optimal concentrations of sodium, potassium, chloride, bicarbonate, and glucose; the glucose content of these solutions is responsible for accelerating the absorption of sodium.[5]

Intravenous replacement therapy is warranted for severe dehydration—characterized by lethargy, very sunken and dry eyes, a very dry tongue and mouth, a pulse that is fast, weak or non-palpable, poor urine output, and low blood pressure—or for persons with intestinal ileus or who are unable to drink on their own.[16]

CLINICAL PRESENTATION

CASE 69-1, QUESTION 3: How does B.K.'s clinical presentation as a noninflammatory versus inflammatory diarrheal illness help to guide further treatment?

The clinical presentation (e.g., the specific symptoms, the severity and duration of symptoms), along with the history of present illness (e.g., risk factors for infection), allows for classification of diarrheal syndromes as noninflammatory versus inflammatory illnesses. Such a classification allows the physician to consider a more focused list of potential enteropathogen(s), and based on the list of suspected organisms, a diagnostic and therapeutic plan can be developed.[7]

B.K.'s history of present illness and clinical presentation are consistent with a noninflammatory diarrheal illness. Voluminous, watery, non-bloody diarrhea is characteristic of pathogens targeting the small bowel, which is responsible for absorption of most fluids entering the GI tract.[7] The clinical manifestations of noninflammatory, watery diarrheal illnesses are a consequence of bacterial enterotoxins that promote the secretion of water and electrolytes into the intestinal lumen; or of viruses infecting and damaging the absorptive villus tips, resulting in voluminous watery diarrhea.[7] Like B.K., patients with noninflammatory diarrheal illnesses are not severely ill, are afebrile and without significant abdominal pain[2,7]; most patients require only supportive therapies. Noninflammatory diarrheas are typically caused by viruses (e.g., rotaviruses and noroviruses), bacteria (e.g., *Staphylococcus aureus*, *Bacillus cereus*, and *Clostridium perfringens*), or parasites (e.g., *Cryptosporidium parvum* and *Giardia lamblia*).[1]

In contrast, inflammatory diarrheas are generally a more severe illness characterized by diarrhea with or without dysentery, abdominal pain, and fever.[2] Pathogens targeting the distal small bowel and colon disrupt the epithelial barrier, causing the bloody or mucoid stools.[2] In addition to supportive therapies, selected persons with inflammatory diarrheal illnesses may benefit from antimicrobial therapy directed at the causative pathogen. The clinical manifestations of inflammatory diarrheal illnesses are a consequence of the production of cytotoxins (e.g., as produced by *C. difficile*, Shiga toxin–producing *E. coli* , and enteroaggregative *E. coli*), or of the pathogen's ability to invade the intestinal mucosa (e.g., *Campylobacter jejuni*, *Shigella* species, and *Salmonella* species).[18]

VIRAL GASTROENTERITIS

Clinical Presentation and Treatment

CASE 69-1, QUESTION 4: B.K.'s stool is negative for WBCs and RBCs. With B.K.'s history of dining at the same restaurant as other patrons having a similar illness, the physician calls the Board of Health to find out if similar illnesses are being reported throughout the city. The physician is informed that an outbreak of norovirus (previously called Norwalk-like virus) gastroenteritis was confirmed at the restaurant where B.K. had dined. Why is B.K.'s history of present illness and clinical presentation consistent with the presumptive diagnosis of a viral gastroenteritis, specifically the norovirus? What supportive therapies are recommended?

Noroviruses are responsible for major outbreaks of foodborne viral illnesses in both adults and children, usually in association with restaurants, schools, and day-care centers. The virus is spread by eating inadequately cooked clams and oysters harvested from contaminated waters and other contaminated foods (e.g. salads, sandwiches), by person-to-person contact, or by exposure to contaminated recreational waters. Like B.K., within 12 to 48 hours after exposure to the virus, patients complain of nausea, vomiting, diarrhea, and abdominal cramps. B.K. will likely experience a mild intestinal illness lasting 1 to 3 days. Supportive therapies to correct fluid and electrolyte losses and to replace ongoing losses are the mainstay of treatment for viral gastroenteritis. Preventing future outbreaks will require the restaurant to ensure proper food-handling practices.[19]

Other common causes of viral gastroenteritis are rotaviruses and astroviruses which are responsible for 30% to 60% of all cases of severe, watery diarrhea in children. After an incubation period of 1 to 3 days, patients experience fever, vomiting, and non-bloody, watery diarrhea; otherwise healthy persons are typically ill for 5 to 7 days.

In the United States, two oral rotavirus vaccines are available for the prevention of rotavirus gastroenteritis in infants and children, a pentavalent (three-dose series) and a monovalent (two-dose series). Vaccine effectiveness in high and upper middle income countries ranges from 79% to 100%, with the benefit of vaccination outweighing vaccine risks, e.g., intussusception (when a part of the intestine folds into another adjacent part of the intestine, referred to as "telescoping," which can lead to intestinal obstruction).[20] As rotaviruses are spread by the fecal–oral route, proper hand washing and disposal of contaminated items are essential to limit the spread of infection.

VIBRIO SPECIES

Vibrio species are curved gram-negative rods whose natural habitats are the environmental waters throughout the world. *V. cholerae* 01 and 0139 are noninvasive enteropathogens responsible for epidemic cholera in humans. The ongoing seventh cholera pandemic began in 1961, subsequently spreading through Asia to Africa, Europe, and Latin America.[5] Prevention of cholera relies on the provision of safe drinking water and adequate sanitation. Cholera vaccines are not routinely incorporated into cholera control efforts, in part related to financial and logistical reasons.[5] Non-cholera *Vibrio* species (e.g., *Vibrio parahaemolyticus*) do not possess the virulence factors required to cause epidemic cholera but do cause gastroenteritis, wound infections, and in susceptible hosts, fulminant sepsis.[21]

Vibrio Cholerae

RISK FACTORS AND CLINICAL PRESENTATION

CASE 69-2

QUESTION 1: M.M. is a 50-year-old man hospitalized for severe watery diarrhea, vomiting, muscle cramping with weakness, and confusion, notably unable to recognize his family members. His history of present illness is significant for returning 1 day ago from Haiti where he visited with relatives, several of whom were recovering from diarrheal illnesses caused by *V. cholerae*. Approximately 24 hours before admission, he noted the onset of watery diarrhea and immediately began drinking the oral rehydrating solution remaining from his trip to Haiti. However, over the past several hours he has been unable to drink on his own, and his family noticed "white flecks" in his stools. M.M. lives in Florida, and his past medical history is significant for peptic ulcer disease for which he takes a proton-pump inhibitor.

In the emergency department, M.M.'s vital signs are as follows: afebrile, blood pressure is 70/40 mm Hg, and heart rate is 130 beats/minute. Physical examination reveals a severely ill-appearing man with altered mental status, sunken eyes, poor skin turgor, and dry mucous membranes. The physician's assessment is severe dehydration because of massive diarrhea, most likely caused by *V. cholerae*. What are his risk factors for cholera and why is his clinical presentation consistent with this diagnosis?

Risk Factors

M.M. has two risk factors to explain his presumed diagnosis of cholera. First, he has just returned from Haiti, a county suffering from epidemic cholera following a major earthquake in 2010 that severely damaged public health facilities.[5] In developed countries, cholera has been virtually eliminated because of modern sewage and water treatment systems. However, sporadic cases, like M.M., occur in travelers returning from areas where cholera is epidemic or endemic, or from the consumption of contaminated and undercooked seafood (e.g., improperly preserved fish, raw oysters, and shellfish) from waters off the Gulf Coast States or imported from endemic areas.[22] Second, M.M.'s daily use of a proton-pump inhibitor reduces his stomach's acidity, thus allowing the acid-susceptible *V. cholerae* to pass from the stomach into the small intestine.[5]

Clinical Presentation

Cholera epidemics are caused by toxin-producing strains of *V. cholerae* 01 or 0139.[5] The characteristic voluminous, watery, and colorless stools with "white flecks" of mucus (referred to as rice-water stools because of their similarity to the appearance of water after washing rice) are caused by the cholera toxin which promotes the intestinal secretion of fluids and electrolytes.[5]

The severity of cholera and likelihood of infection is influenced by host factors and the setting in which it occurs.[5] Severe disease is more common in previously unexposed persons like M.M. who are immunologically naïve (e.g. epidemic cholera), while less severe disease occurs in areas where cholera is endemic.[5] Following ingestion of contaminated foods, a watery diarrheal illness begins within 12 hours to 5 days and may progress to life-threatening dehydration.[5]

TREATMENT

CASE 69-2, QUESTION 2: What are the signs and symptoms suggesting M.M. is severely dehydrated, and how should his dehydration be treated?

M.M. is one of the 2% to 5% of persons with *V. cholerae* infection who experience severe dehydration (≥10% dehydration), losing up to 1 L/hour of fluid, and whose condition may, within hours, progress to hypovolemic shock and death.[5] M.M. shows signs of severe dehydration as manifested by his altered mental status, sunken eyes, poor skin turgor, dry mucous membranes, low blood pressure, and increased heart rate.[5] Acidosis may occur as a result of massive bicarbonate losses through diarrheal stools, and it may be exacerbated by lactic acidosis from shock and hypovolemic renal failure.[5] M.M. should receive vigorous IV hydration with Ringer's lactate solution to replace the large quantities of sodium, potassium, and bicarbonate lost through his watery stools; his muscle weakness could be attributed to depletion of electrolytes, specifically potassium and calcium.[5] Monitoring of blood pressure and normalization of heart rate are critical interventions.

Once M.M. is able to drink fluids, oral hydration can be started, even with ongoing IV hydration. Oral replacement solutions containing less than 75 mEq/L of sodium are inappropriate because of the large amounts of sodium lost through cholera stools.[5] Oral rehydration solutions can be made by mixing together one-half teaspoon salt, six teaspoons sugar and 1 liter of safe water.[5]

CASE 69-2, QUESTION 3: Would M.M. benefit from the administration of antimicrobials, and what antimicrobial treatment options are available?

Antimicrobials are recommended for patients with moderate-to-severe dehydration from cholera infection.[5] Effective antimicrobial therapy decreases the volume of diarrheal losses, shortens the duration of illness by up to 50% and reduces the period of shedding infectious organisms from >5 days[23] to 1–2 days.[5] Antimicrobials should be administered after the initial fluid deficit has been corrected and if applicable, after vomiting has resolved.[5]

Antimicrobials

If susceptible, the following single- and multiple-dose regimens are effective treatments for *V. cholerae*; single-dose regimens are preferred because of their ease of administration, and compared to multiple doses of erythromycin, they are better tolerated.[24]

doxycycline 300 mg orally × 1 dose, or azithromycin × 1 dose, or ciprofloxacin 500 mg orally twice a days,[5] or tetracycline 500 mg orally every 6 hours days, or erythromycin 250 mg orally 4 times daily for 3 ays.[5] TMP–SMX resistance precludes its empiric use for the treatment of cholera.[5]

- Children: ciprofloxacin 15 mg/kg/dose orally twice a day × 3 days, or azithromycin 20 mg/kg orally × 1 dose, or erythromycin 12.5 mg/kg/dose orally every 6 hours for 3 days. Pediatric doses should not exceed maximum adult doses.[5]

For M.M., a single 300 mg oral dose of doxycycline is a good empiric choice as the strain of *V. cholerae* circulating in Haiti is currently susceptible to tetracycline (indicative of susceptibility to doxycycline).[23] Empiric ciprofloxacin is not recommended because the circulating strain in Haiti has reduced susceptibility to ciprofloxacin which is associated with lack of clinical and microbiologic improvement.[25] Additionally, until M.M. has recovered from this cholera infection, he should refrain from taking his proton-pump inhibitor which, by reducing his stomach's acidity, allows the acid-susceptible *V. cholerae* to pass from the stomach into the small intestine.

Vibrio Parahaemolyticus

CLINICAL PRESENTATION

CASE 69-3

QUESTION 1: C.T. is a 45-year-old man presenting to his physician with 1 day of non-bloody, watery diarrhea. Two days before his illness, he ate a meal of raw oysters at a restaurant specializing in fresh local seafood. C.T. lives along the coast of Florida and has no significant medical history. His physical examination reveals no evidence of dehydration. Why is C.T.'s history of present illness and clinical presentation consistent with non-cholera *Vibrio* gastroenteritis?

A key piece of information from C.T.'s history of present illness consistent with the presumptive diagnosis of non-cholera *Vibrio* gastroenteritis is consumption of raw oysters harvested from the coastal areas of Florida, where *V. parahaemolyticus* species have been identified. Diarrhea, abdominal cramps, nausea, vomiting, and fever begin after a median incubation period of 17 hours (range, 4–90 hours); bloody diarrhea occurs in 9% to 29% of cases.

TREATMENT

CASE 69-3, QUESTION 2: Should a course of antibiotics be prescribed for C.T.?

In otherwise healthy adults like C.T., *V. parahaemolyticus* gastroenteritis is usually a mild, self-limiting illness lasting for a median of 2 to 6 days.[21] There are no data to support the benefit of antibiotics in this setting, although patients with diarrhea lasting longer than 5 days may benefit from treatment with tetracycline or a fluoroquinolone; minocycline 100 mg orally every 12 hours and cefotaxime 2 g IV every 8 hours have also been recommended.[21]

Individuals with liver disease or alcoholism are at risk for severe *Vibrio* infections including septicemia[21]; such individuals should avoid eating raw or undercooked shellfish, and avoid exposure of open wounds to seawater especially during the warmer months when water temperatures favor the growth of *Vibrio* species.

STAPHYLOCOCCUS AUREUS, BACILLUS CEREUS, AND CLOSTRIDIUM PERFRINGENS

S. aureus, *B. cereus*, and *C. perfringens* are important causes of toxin-mediated foodborne illnesses. Gastrointestinal symptoms typically begin within 24 hours after the ingestion of contaminated foods, which is in contrast to the longer incubation periods for illnesses caused by *Salmonella*, *Shigella*, and *Campylobacter* species. *B. cereus* causes two different intestinal syndromes: the short-incubation disease characterized by vomiting and a long-incubation disease characterized by a diarrheal illness.[1]

Clinical Presentation and Treatment

CASE 69-4

QUESTION 1: S.A. is an otherwise healthy 23-year-old college student, who presents to the Student Health Center with an acute gastrointestinal illness after eating at the school cafeteria. S.A. recalled eating the salad and the cream-filled pastries, and stated that within 3 hours she felt nauseous and began vomiting. Why is S.A.'s history of present illness and clinical presentation consistent with food poisoning caused by *S. aureus* or *B. cereus* (short-incubation)?

Foodborne illnesses are often grouped by their usual incubation period: less than 6 hours, 8 to 16 hours, and greater than 16 hours.[26] The rapid onset (within 6 hours) of S.A.'s intestinal symptoms after eating suggests the illness is caused by preformed toxins, such as those produced by *S. aureus* or *B. cereus* (short-incubation disease, emetic syndrome). Diarrhea and abdominal cramps may also occur. Although cooking kills the toxin-producing bacteria, it does not destroy toxin that has already been produced. Foods implicated in staphylococcal food poisoning include salads, cream-filled pastries, and meats, whereas foods implicated in *B. cereus* food poisoning include fried rice, dried foods, and dairy products.[26]

CASE 69-5

QUESTION 1: C.P. is also an otherwise healthy 23-year-old college student presenting to the same Student Health Center as S.A. (Case 69-4) with an acute gastrointestinal illness. C.P. recalled having lunch at the cafeteria, selecting a fish and poultry meal. Approximately 10 hours after eating she experienced diarrhea and abdominal cramps. Why is C.P.'s history of present illness and clinical presentation consistent with food poisoning caused by *C. perfringens* or *B. cereus* (long-incubation disease)? Should empiric antibiotics be prescribed to either of these students?

In contrast to S.A., the longer incubation period before the onset of symptoms is consistent with illness caused by *C. perfringens* or *B. cereus* (long-incubation disease, diarrheal syndrome). These bacteria are associated with an incubation period of 8 to 16 hours and symptoms of diarrhea and abdominal cramps; vomiting is not a prominent symptom in these illnesses.[26]

C. perfringens or *B. cereus* (long-incubation disease) produce heat-labile toxins after the ingestion of contaminated foods, explaining the longer incubation period compared with illness caused by the ingestion of preformed toxins. Foods implicated in *C. perfringens* food poisoning include improperly stored beef, fish, poultry dishes, pasta salads, and dairy products, whereas foods implicated in long-incubation *B. cereus* food poisoning include meats, vanilla sauce, cream-filled baked goods, and salads.[26]

Foodborne illnesses caused by these toxin-producing bacteria usually resolve within 24 hours; therefore, antibiotic therapy is not indicated for either student.

CRYPTOSPORIDIUM PARVUM

The protozoan parasite *C. parvum* is an important cause of human intestinal illness in both healthy and immunocompromised persons. The role of antiprotozoal agents and the clinical response to antiprotozoal therapy depends on the competence of the host's immune system.

Clinical Presentation

CASE 69-6

QUESTION 1: C.K. is a 35-year-old, previously healthy man presenting to his physician with complaints of 15 days of watery diarrhea and a 5-pound weight loss. He is concerned that his illness is related to the announcement by the Board of Health notifying the community of an outbreak of cryptosporidiosis from contaminated water supplies. Why is C.K.'s history of present illness and clinical presentation consistent with cryptosporidiosis? Should antiprotozoal agents be prescribed to treat cryptosporidiosis in otherwise healthy persons such as C.K.?

A key finding from C.K.'s history is his exposure to water supplies known to be contaminated with cryptosporidium oocysts; other modes of spreading cryptosporidiosis include animal contact (cattle and sheep) and person-to-person contact.[27]

C.K. is presenting with persistent diarrhea, i.e., diarrhea lasting longer than 14 days. Common microbial causes of persistent watery diarrhea include parasites, such as *Isospora belli*, *Microsporidia*, *G. lamblia*, and *C. parvum*. The spectrum of infection with *C. parvum* ranges from asymptomatic carriage to a persistent, noninflammatory diarrheal illness; vomiting, abdominal cramps, weight loss, and fever may also occur.[27] Immunocompetent patients like C.K. can generally expect a self-limiting illness lasting approximately 2 weeks.[27]

In contrast, in immunocompromised patients cryptosporidiosis can be a chronic, debilitating, diarrheal illness associated with malnutrition, increased mortality, and in children, long-term cognitive impairment.[28]

Treatment

For immunocompetent hosts with cryptosporidiosis, other than replacement of fluids and electrolytes no specific therapy directed at the organism is generally required. However, nitazoxanide is an FDA-approved treatment for diarrhea caused by *C. parvum*. A randomized, double-blind, placebo-controlled trial in immunocompetent adults and children found that diarrhea resolved in 80% of those treated with nitazoxanide versus 41% of patients given placebo; oocyst shedding was also significantly reduced in the treatment group. Diarrhea generally resolved within 3 to 4 days of starting treatment.[29] Nitazoxanide 500 mg orally twice daily for 3 to 14 days is recommended for the treatment of cryptosporidiosis.[3]

In contrast, in immunocompromised persons a meta-analysis of treatments for cryptosporidiosis found no evidence to support the role of chemotherapy.[30] These findings are consistent with randomized trials concluding that neither a short, 3-day course of nitazoxanide nor a more intensive regimen of nitazoxanide (200–400 mg orally twice daily for 28 days) provided any benefit to HIV-positive children. For HIV-infected persons, reconstitution of the immune system with effective antiretroviral therapies i the mainstay of treatment for cryptosporidiosis.

SALMONELLA

Salmonellae are enteric gram-negative bacilli belonging to the *Enterobacteriacae* family. Widely found in nature colonizing animal hosts including mammals, reptiles, and birds,[31] they are major causes of foodborne illness as a consequence of consuming contaminated foods including poultry or poultry products and dairy products. Worldwide, the annual incidence of salmonellosis is about 1.3 billion cases, and of the nearly 3 million persons who die,[32] most live in developing areas of the world.

The role of antimicrobials in the management of salmonellosis depends on the clinical syndrome, its severity, and underlying health problems of infected persons. Non-typhoidal salmonellae (e.g., *Salmonella typhimurium*, *Salmonella enteritidis*, *Salmonella choleraesuis*, and many others) cause the clinical syndromes of gastroenteritis, asymptomatic carriage in the stool, bacteremia, and localized infection.[33] Typhoidal salmonellae (*Salmonella typhi* and *Salmonella paratyphi* A, B, and C) cause the syndromes of enteric fever (also referred to as typhoid or paratyphoid fever) and chronic carriage.[31]

Non-typhoidal Salmonellosis

CASE 69-7

QUESTION 1: An outbreak of *Salmonella* gastroenteritis being investigated by the Department of Public Health has traced the source of the outbreak to Restaurant A, specifically the popular turkey dinner special. Anticipating that infected diners with specific clinical syndromes associated with *Salmonella* infection will benefit from antimicrobial treatment, and that antimicrobial resistant *Salmonella* species are increasingly problematic, the Department of Health has asked you to address the following question of what antimicrobials are available for the treatment of non-typhoidal salmonellosis.

CHLORAMPHENICOL, TRIMETHOPRIM–SULFAMETHOXAZOLE (TMP–SMX), OR AMPICILLIN

Until the late 1980s, standard treatments for non-typhoidal *Salmonella* were chloramphenicol, TMP/SMX, or ampicillin. By the early 1990s, widespread multidrug-resistance (MDR) defined as simultaneous resistance to ampicillin, chloramphenicol, streptomycin, tetracyclines, and sulfonamides precluded their use as empiric therapies for the treatment of salmonellosis.[31] Depending on the geographic area, rates of MDR *Salmonella* species are as high as 80% in East Asia and southern Europe and 30% to 40% in the United States.[32] As MDR-resistant *Salmonella* species remained susceptible to the fluoroquinolones, these antimicrobials became the agents of choice for the treatment of salmonellosis. Interestingly, since the early 2000s there has been a decline in the prevalence of MDR-non-typhoidal *Salmonella* in some areas of the world.[32]

FLUOROQUINOLONES

With the advent of MDR-non-typhoidal *Salmonella*, fluoroquinolones were widely prescribed for the empiric treatment of non-typhoidal salmonellosis.[31] During the 1990s, suboptimal clinical responses following treatment with fluoroquinolones were noted when isolates were resistant to nalidixic acid. Both nalidixic acid and the fluoroquinolones are related compounds belonging to the quinolone family of antimicrobials. As these isolates also displayed elevated ciprofloxacin MICs compared to

...cid–susceptible strains (i.e., 0.12–1 mcg/mL vs. ≤0.06 ...hey were referred to as having decreased ciprofloxa- ...bility (DCS).[34] Consequently, nalidixic acid resistance ... a surrogate marker for isolates with DCS, for which ...ofloxacin was not an optimal antimicrobial choice.

In subsequent years, additional fluoroquinolone-resistance mechanisms in *Salmonella* species emerged which were not detected by nalidixic acid screening (i.e., isolates were nalidixic acid susceptible but had elevated ciprofloxacin MICs); thus, nalidixic acid resistance was no longer a reliable surrogate marker to detect *Salmonella* with DCS.[34] Consequently, in 2012 the Clinical Laboratory Standards Institute (CLSI) lowered for *Salmonella* species the breakpoint for susceptibility to ciprofloxacin from <1 to <0.06 mcg/mL, a change which would reliably detect *Salmonella* with DCS. The CLSI also recognized that not all laboratories (e.g., resource-limited settings) would be able to institute these new ciprofloxacin breakpoints, and because nalidixic acid–susceptible isolates with concurrent decreased susceptibility to ciprofloxacin are still uncommon, CLSI allowed for the continued use of nalidixic acid screening,[34] though prescribers should be made aware of its limitations as a marker for isolates with DCS.

Currently, nalidixic acid–resistant non-typhoidal *Salmonella* are prevalent in Asia and increasingly more common in the United States, reportedly 0.4% in 1996 and 2.3% in 2003. Antimicrobial treatment options for nalidixic acid–resistant *Salmonella* include azithromycin and selected third-generation cephalosporins.[34]

β-LACTAMS

Non-typhoidal salmonella resistance to ceftriaxone is currently uncommon, but it has been reported worldwide, including in Africa, Europe, Asia, the Philippines, and the United States[31]; some isolates are also simultaneously resistant to fluoroquinolones.[32,35] Carbapenems[35] have been successfully used for the treatment of invasive infection caused by ceftriaxone- and ciprofloxacin-resistant *Salmonella enterica* serotype choleraesuis,[36] though carbapenem-resistant *Salmonella* have also been reported.[31]

AZITHROMYCIN

Azithromycin displays good in vitro activity against non-typhoidal *S. enterica*[37] and is a recommended treatment for non-typhoidal salmonellosis requiring antimicrobial treatment,[3] including the treatment of nalidixic acid–resistant isolates.

Anticipating the need for recommendations to guide prescribers regarding which diners with salmonellosis should receive antimicrobial therapy, the Department of Health has asked you to address the following question: "Considering a diner's severity of illness and underlying health problems, should antimicrobials be prescribed for diners with the following clinical syndromes: (a) uncomplicated gastroenteritis in the immunocompetent host, (b) asymptomatic stool carriage, or (c) extraintestinal *Salmonella* infection? If appropriate, what specific antimicrobial therapies would you recommend?"

UNCOMPLICATED GASTROENTERITIS IN THE IMMUNOCOMPETENT HOST
Clinical Presentation and Treatment

CASE 69-8

QUESTION 1: B.B., a 35-year-old, otherwise healthy man presents with a 1-day history of fever, abdominal pain, nausea, vomiting, and non-bloody stools. B.B. has no significant medical history. Physical examination is significant for a non-ill appearing, febrile male; his presumptive diagnosis is mild, uncomplicated non-typhoidal *Salmonella* gastroenteritis. Should he receive antimicrobial therapy?

Like B.B., within 6 to 72 hours of ingesting contaminated foods patients begin experiencing the clinical manifestations of *Salmonella* gastroenteritis including acute onset of fever, diarrhea, and abdominal cramping; in more severe illness, bloody diarrhea and dehydration may occur.

In otherwise healthy individuals with uncomplicated non-typhoidal *Salmonella* gastroenteritis, antimicrobials are not recommended as salmonellosis is typically a self-limiting illness lasting for 2 to 5 days. Antimicrobials do not reduce the duration or severity of illness and may be harmful, by placing patients at risk for adverse drug reactions, prolonging the asymptomatic carriage of salmonellae, and promoting the emergence of antimicrobial-resistant bacteria.[33,38] Most individuals like B.B. will only require replacement of lost fluids and electrolytes.

ASYMPTOMATIC STOOL CARRIAGE
Clinical Presentation and Treatment

CASE 69-8, QUESTION 2: Three weeks after resolution of B.B.'s episode of *Salmonella* gastroenteritis, he continues to excrete *Salmonella* bacteria from his stool, despite remaining asymptomatic. Should antimicrobials be prescribed to eliminate B.B.'s intestinal carriage of non-typhoidal *Salmonella*?

Antimicrobials should not be prescribed to eliminate asymptomatic intestinal carriage of non-typhoidal *Salmonella*.[18] A randomized, double-blind trial in healthy, asymptomatic adults from areas where non-typhoidal *Salmonella* infection is endemic found that neither norfloxacin nor azithromycin were better than placebo in eradicating intestinal carriage of *Salmonella* species.[18] The median duration of fecal shedding of non-typhoidal *Salmonella* is about 1 month in adults and 7 weeks in children younger than 5 years of age.[39]

GASTROENTERITIS IN PATIENTS AT RISK FOR EXTRAINTESTINAL SALMONELLA INFECTION
Clinical Presentation and Treatment

CASE 69-9

QUESTION 1: W.M., a 50-year-old male with a past medical history significant for a recently diagnosed malignancy, presents with a 1-day history of fever, severe abdominal pain, nausea, vomiting, and non-bloody stools. One day prior to the onset of these symptoms, he ate cream-filled pastries from a bakery that has since been closed by the Department of Health because of its association with an ongoing outbreak of *Salmonella* gastroenteritis. Should antimicrobials be prescribed for his presumed diagnosis of *Salmonella* gastroenteritis, and if so, what would you recommend?

Antimicrobials are indicated for patients at risk for developing extraintestinal *Salmonella* infection such as persons with malignancy (like W.M.), diabetes, rheumatologic disorders, HIV infection,[32] persons receiving immunosuppressive therapies, very young age, low gastric pH (e.g., as in infancy, pernicious anemia, or medication-induced), severe infection,[33] and persons older than 50 years of age who may have atherosclerotic lesions which could become hematogenously infected.[40] Overall, less than 5% of patients with non-typhoidal *Salmonella* gastroenteritis become bacteremic, though infection with some serotypes, e.g., *S. choleraesuis* and *Salmonella dublin* are more likely to cause bloodstream infection.[33] Once in the bloodstream extraintestinal complications include osteomyelitis, septic arthritis, meningitis, or infectious endarteritis. Lastly, antimicrobials have been used when rapid interruption of fecal excretion of organisms is needed to control outbreaks of salmonellosis in institutionalized persons.[40]

For patients at risk for extraintestinal infection or with severe diarrhea, antimicrobial options include an oral fluoroquinolone (e.g., levofloxacin 500 mg once daily) for 7 to 10 days, azithromycin 500 mg once daily for 7 days, or parenteral ceftriaxone 1 to 2 grams daily for 7 to 10 days (14 days is recommended for patients with immunosuppression).[3] For HIV-infected persons with a CD4 ≥200 cells/μL, the recommended duration of therapy for gastroenteritis without bacteremia is 7 to 14 days, and for patients with a CD4 <200 cells/μL, 2 to 6 weeks is often recommended.[41]

EXTRAINTESTINAL SALMONELLA INFECTION

Clinical Presentation and Treatment

CASE 69-10

QUESTION 1: B.T., an "ill-appearing" 70-year-old man with a history significant for the same cream-filled pastries as B.T. (Case 659-9, Question 1), who is hospitalized for severe abdominal pain, bloody diarrhea, new-onset right hip pain, high fever, and low blood pressure. His past surgical history is significant for a right hip prosthesis. Would B.T. benefit from antibiotic therapy, and if so, what would you recommend?

B.T. is presenting with signs and symptoms of *Salmonella* gastroenteritis, bacteremia (fever, low blood pressure) and possible localized infection of his right hip prosthesis (new onset hip pain).

Treatment of *Salmonella* bacteremia without localized infection is generally successful after 10 to 14 days of antimicrobial therapy.[3,32] For HIV-infected persons, a longer course of therapy (2–6 weeks) is recommended.[35,41] If infection of B.T.'s hip prosthesis is confirmed, surgery may be required to cure his infection.[39] Recommended treatment durations for extraintestinal non-typhoidal salmonellosis are available.[40]

Considering the antimicrobial resistance patterns from where the *Salmonella* infection was acquired (e.g., travel history), prior antimicrobial therapy, and site of infection, until susceptibilities are available empiric therapy options include selected IV third generation cephalosporins (e.g., ceftriaxone 1 g IV q24, cefotaxime 1 g IV q8),[41] an IV or oral fluoroquinolone (e.g., ciprofloxacin 400 mg IV q12h, ciprofloxacin 500–750 mg PO q12h, levofloxacin 750 mg IV or PO q24h), or the combination of a third-generation cephalosporin with a fluoroquinolone.[40] For bacteremic patients, some experts prefer the IV route of administration,[40] particularly until the patient has stabilized,[32] while other experts recommend either the IV or oral route of administration.[41]

Typhoidal Salmonellosis—Typhoid Fever (Enteric Fever)

CLINICAL PRESENTATION

CASE 69-11

QUESTION 1: B.C. is a 49-year-old obese woman, presenting to the emergency department with a 1-week history of fever, confusion and delirium, severe abdominal pain, headache, anorexia, and diarrhea and, for the past 1 day, a red rash on her chest. Her history of present illness is significant for returning 10 days ago from travel to the Indian subcontinent where she stayed with relatives, some of whom were recovering from typhoid fever. B.C.'s medical history is significant for gallstones. She lives in California with her husband. Admission vital signs show a temperature of 101°F, a heart rate of 60 beats/minute and a stable blood pressure. Physical examination is significant for a "toxic appearing" female with a red rash on her chest, splenomegaly, and hepatomegaly. Laboratory tests include the following: WBC is $3.0 \times 10^6/\mu L$, liver function tests are mildly elevated, and the results of two sets of blood cultures are pending. B.C. is given the presumptive diagnosis of severe enteric fever and encephalopathy most likely attributable to *S. typhi*. Why is her history of present illness, clinical presentation, and laboratory results consistent with this diagnosis?

A key piece of information from B.C.'s history of present illness supporting the diagnosis of typhoid fever is her recent travel to the Indian subcontinent where typhoid fever is endemic, and her contact with relatives recovering from this infection. Other developing countries with endemic typhoid fever include Southeast Asia, Africa, and Latin America.[42] In developed countries, enteric fever is a sporadic disease occurring mainly in travelers returning from areas where the disease is endemic; in the United States 85% of cases of typhoid fever are travel-related.[43]

B.C.'s clinical presentation and laboratory findings are classic for enteric fever. During the 7- to 14-day incubation period,[42] salmonellae multiply within macrophages and monocytes, and systemic manifestations of infection appear after the release of bacteria into the bloodstream. Patients usually present with fever, abdominal pain, anorexia, diarrhea or constipation, headache, dry cough, splenomegaly, and hepatomegaly, while severe illness is characterized by concomitant GI bleeding, encephalopathy, and shock. Bacteremia may be followed by localized infection to the liver, spleen, bone marrow, gallbladder, and Peyer's patches of the terminal ileum.[42] Laboratory abnormalities consistent with typhoid fever include B.C.'s low WBC count and mildly elevated liver function tests.[31]

TREATMENT

CASE 69-11, QUESTION 2: Would B.C. benefit from a course of antimicrobials to treat her presumptive diagnosis of typhoid fever? If so, what options are available?

B.C. would benefit from effective antimicrobial treatment for typhoid fever in the following ways: (1) shortening the resolution of fever from 3 to 4 weeks to 3 to 5 days,[44] with clearing of all symptoms within 7 to 10 days,[45] (2) decreasing mortality from usually 5% to 10% to less than 1%,[31] (3) eradicating fecal shedding of *S. typhi*, thereby limiting further spread of infection,[45] and (4) preventing relapse of infection. Most cases of typhoid fever are effectively treated with oral antimicrobials; IV therapy is reserved for severely ill patients or patients with persistent vomiting and severe diarrhea.[42]

Chloramphenicol, TMP–SMX, or Ampicillin

Until the late 1980s, typhoid fever was cured in more than 90% of patients treated with 14 to 21 days of chloramphenicol, TMP–SMX, or ampicillin.[46] By the early 1990s multidrug-resistant (i.e., simultaneous resistance to chloramphenicol, ampicillin, and TMP-SMX) *S. typhi* caused outbreaks of typhoid fever in Asia and Africa. Fortunately, these multidrug-resistant isolates remained susceptible to the fluoroquinolones, which then became the antimicrobials of choice. Interestingly, there has been a reduction in multidrug-resistant *S. typhi* to as low as 12% in some areas of the world.

Fluoroquinolones

Short-treatment courses (less than 5 days) of oral fluoroquinolones were once as effective or better than previously used treatments (e.g., TMP–SMX, ampicillin, or chloramphenicol).[46] By the late 1990s, short-course fluoroquinolone therapies used in parts of Asia were associated with clinical failures in up to 50% of patients.[43] Microbiologic evaluation revealed these isolates were resistant c acid and had higher ciprofloxacin MICs (0.125–1 mpared to *Salmonella* that was fully susceptible to (MICs of <0.03 mcg/mL).[47] Gatifloxacin, a newer on fluoroquinolone (no longer marketed in the United s) with lower MICs compared to ciprofloxacin (0.19 vs. 0.5 cg/mL, respectively) cured greater than 95% of children with typhoid fever, most of whom were infected with nalidixic acid–resistant *S. typhi*.[15] In areas with a high prevalence of nalidixic acid–resistant *S. typhi*, alternatives to fluoroquinolones include azithromycin and selected third-generation cephalosporins.

Azithromycin

Azithromycin is effective for patients with mild-to-moderate typhoid fever.[48] Azithromycin (20 mg/kg/day) for 7 days cured greater than 95% of children with uncomplicated typhoid fever in Vietnam where 96% of *S. typhi* are nalidixic acid–resistant; fever clearance time was 106 hours and there were no relapses.[15] In contrast, lower azithromycin doses (10 mg/kg/day) in the setting of nalidixic acid–resistance are associated with lower cure rates (82%).[49] Concerning is the identification of azithromycin-resistant *S. typhi*[50] and non-response to azithromycin.[51]

β-lactams and Tigecycline

Cefixime, an oral third-generation cephalosporin, is variably effective for the treatment of typhoid fever. Failure rates range from 4% to 27%[50] and some experts do not recommend its use for the treatment of typhoid fever.[43] The lower clinical response to cefixime may be related to the poor intracellular penetration of the β-lactam because the intracellular compartment is the primary site of *S. typhi* colonization.[52]

Ceftriaxone, an intravenous third-generation cephalosporin, is recommended for the treatment of severe typhoid fever[44] with the caveat that longer treatment courses are recommended to prevent relapse of infection. In patients with bacteremia caused by ceftriaxone-susceptible isolates, relapse of infection was higher among patients treated with a 7-day course of ceftriaxone versus azithromycin, 14% versus 0%, respectively.[53] No relapses were reported when a longer course (14 days) of ceftriaxone was used for infection caused by multidrug-resistant *S. typhi*.[54] Patients treated with ceftriaxone may remain febrile for as long as 10 days.[55] Ceftriaxone-resistant *S. typhi* have been reported in India, the Philippines, China, the United States, and elsewhere.[56] Potential alternatives to ceftriaxone include carbapenems (imipenem, meropenem, and ertapenem) and tigecycline, though clinical data are lacking.[48]

TREATMENT—SEVERE VERSUS UNCOMPLICATED TYPHOID FEVER

CASE 69-11, QUESTION 3: What specific empiric antibiotic regimen would you recommend for the treatment of B.C.'s complicated (severe) typhoid fever? How would her treatment differ if she had uncomplicated typhoid fever?

For complicated typhoid fever, empiric therapy with ceftriaxone is recommended.[57] Once susceptibility data are available, treatment options include 10 to 14 days of ceftriaxone (1–2 grams IV once daily) continued for at least 7 days after defervescence to minimize the risk for relapse,[48] or a fluoroquinolone for 10 to 14 days.[44]

Uncomplicated typhoid fever is typically treated in the outpatient setting.[44] Empiric oral regimens include azithromycin 500 mg daily × 5 to 7 days,[44] or a fluoroquinolone (e.g., levofloxacin 500 mg once daily or ciprofloxacin 500 mg twice daily).[3] For children, azithromycin or ceftriaxone is recommended.[3] Interestingly, with the reduction in MDR *S. typhi* in some areas, ampicillin, amoxicillin, TMP–SMX, or chloramphenicol are again options for susceptible isolates.[44]

ADJUNCTIVE TREATMENT

CASE 69-11, QUESTION 4: Besides the administration of antibiotics, what adjunctive therapies could benefit B.C. for the treatment of severe typhoid fever?

Enteric encephalopathy, i.e., altered mental status, is associated with a mortality rate as high as 56% if effective treatment is not promptly administered.[58] In patients with enteric encephalopathy, retrospective data report improved survival when appropriate antimicrobial therapy is combined with high-dose dexamethasone (3 mg/kg IV followed by 1 mg/kg every 6 hours IV for eight doses).[58] The mechanism of action of dexamethasone in enteric encephalopathy is not known.[58]

CASE 69-11, QUESTION 5: Fourteen months after discharge from the hospital, B.C. remains free of symptoms associated with typhoid fever, but follow-up testing reveals she continues to excrete *S. typhi* in her stools. Additionally, their adult son who has dinner with them every Sunday, presents to his clinic doctor with fever, headache and chills, and is confirmed to have uncomplicated typhoid fever. He has no significant past medical history and has no recent travel history. How might her son have acquired typhoid fever? What treatment recommendations can be provided to this family?

Unlike his mother B.C., her son has no travel history to an area where typhoid fever is endemic. Instead, he is likely to have contracted typhoid fever from consuming foods prepared by his mother who is now a chronic carrier of *S. typhi*. Most patients with typhoid fever continue to excrete *S. typhi* in their stools for 3 to 4 weeks after recovery from their illness. However, 1% to 3% of persons like B.C. become chronic carriers who continue to excrete *Salmonella* from stool or urine for more than 1 year after infection and serve as reservoirs for spreading infection. Unlike for non-typhoidal salmonellae, humans are the only natural host and reservoir for *S. typhi*.[55] B.C.'s risk factor for becoming a chronic carrier is her history of gallstones which allows the sequestration of organisms within her abnormal biliary tract.

CHRONIC TYPHOID CARRIERS

Treatment

CASE 69-11, QUESTION 6: What therapeutic options are available to cure B.C.'s chronic carrier state?

Treatment options for chronic *S. typhi* carriers like B.C. include a prolonged course of antibiotics, cholecystectomy, or suppressive antimicrobial therapy.[42] Fifty to ninety percent of chronic carriers may be cured after prolonged courses of antibiotics,[59–62] although efficacy may be lessened when anatomic abnormalities (e.g., cholelithiasis) are present.[59] Relapse is usually detected within the first several months after completing antimicrobial therapy[63] but can occur up to 24 months after completing therapy.[64] For susceptible *S. typhi*, curative oral antimicrobial regimens include amoxicillin 2 g 3 times daily for 28 days,[61] ampicillin 1 g 4 times daily for 90 days,[60] ampicillin 1.5 g 4 times daily plus probenecid for 6 weeks,[59] TMP–SMX 160/800 mg twice a day for 3 months,[62] ciprofloxacin 500 to 750 mg twice a day for 3 to 4 weeks,[65–67] or norfloxacin 400 mg twice daily for 4 weeks.[68]

Prevention

CASE 69-11, QUESTION 7: B.C.'s sister is planning a trip to the Indian subcontinent and is concerned about acquiring typhoid fever. What can she do to reduce her risk for becoming infected?

The U.S. Centers for Disease Control and Prevention recommends vaccination for travel to areas where the risk for *S. tyhi* is increased including many Asian, African, and Latin American countries.[69] In the United States, two licensed vaccines are available to protect against *S. typhi* but not against *S. paratyphi*. The intramuscular vaccine for persons older than 2 years of age is 55% effective in preventing typhoid fever; adverse effects include local pain and swelling, fever, and headache.[69] The oral live-attenuated vaccine Ty21a vaccine (series of 4 doses) for persons older than 6 years of age is well tolerated, and it affords a protective efficacy rate around 55%.[69] Since the oral vaccine is a live-attenuated vaccine, it should not be administered to immunocompromised persons. Additionally, to ensure full vaccine activity, the live-attenuated vaccine should not be given until at least 3 days after the last dose of an antimicrobial, and if possible, antimicrobials should not be initiated within 3 days of the last dose of the oral vaccine; longer intervals should be considered for long-acting agents such as azithromycin.[69]

Finally, because the protective efficacy of available vaccines against *S. typhi* is not 100%, and because neither vaccine is licensed to protect against *S. paratyphi* which in some Asian countries accounts for up to 50% of blood isolates from patients with enteric fever,[70] it is still necessary to reinforce the importance of good hygiene and the avoidance of foods with a high risk for being contaminated with enteropathogens.

SHIGELLA SPECIES

Shigella are gram-negative intracellular bacterial pathogens belonging to the *Enterobacteriacae* family. They are the most frequent cause of dysentery, which is an inflammatory diarrheal illness characterized by bloody or mucoid stools with abdominal cramps. Of the four *Shigella* species, severe dysentery is most commonly caused by *Shigella dysenteriae* followed by *Shigella flexneri*, whereas milder illness characterized by watery diarrhea with or without blood is typically caused by *Shigella sonnei* and *Shigella boydii*.[71]

Shigellosis—Severe Illness

CLINICAL PRESENTATION

CASE 69-12

QUESTION 1: M.T. is a 60-year-old, ill-appearing man hospitalized for bloody diarrhea and fever. Two days before admission he noted the onset of fever, abdominal cramps, and six to seven nonbloody, watery stools. His diarrhea has since worsened to 10 to 12 small-volume stools with blood and mucus, and he now complains of painful straining while passing his stools. His history of present illness is significant for returning 3 days ago from a business trip to Indian subcontinent. During the business portion of the trip, he remained at the hotel where all his meals were prepared by hotel staff well trained in the sanitary preparation of foods. However, on the day of his departure he opted to mingle with local residents to get a first-hand taste of native foods and beverages from street vendors. M.T. lives alone in Florida, has no significant medical history or drug allergies, and takes no medications. On admission, his temperature is 101°F and physical examination reveals a critically ill man with severe abdominal tenderness. Why is M.T.'s history of present illness and clinical presentation consistent with the diagnosis of dysentery, most likely caused by *S. dysenteriae type 1*.

M.T.'s diagnosis of dysentery, likely caused by *S. dysenteriae type 1* is consistent with his recent travel to the Indian subcontinent where *S. dysenteriae type 1* is both epidemic and endemic,[71] primarily as a consequence of inadequate systems for disposal of sewage.[71] M. likely became infected from the consumption of contaminated foods or beverages prepared by local street vendors, by person-to-person contact with symptomatic persons with diarrhea, or from asymptomatic persons continuing to excrete shigellae from their stool.[72] As few as 10 to 100 shigellae can cause illness[71] in healthy hosts, explaining why shigellosis is a very contagious infection.

Once ingested virulence factors allow shigellae to evade detection by the immune system and invade colonic and rectal epithelium. Enterotoxin production causes fluid secretion into the intestinal lumen and cytotoxin production causes cell death; both toxins lead to the severe clinical manifestations of shigellosis.[71]

As with M.T., within 24 to 48 hours after ingestion of *Shigella* bacteria symptoms of dysentery begin and include fever, fatigue, malaise, and anorexia.[72] Watery diarrhea generally precedes dysentery, and frequently is the only manifestation of mild infection.[72] Progression to dysentery may follow within hours to days and is characterized by frequent, small-volume, bloody, and mucoid stools; abdominal cramps; and tenesmus which is described as painful straining when passing stools.[72] Hemolytic uremic syndrome (HUS) is a serious complication of shigellosis, occurring in up to 13% of patients with dysentery caused by *S. dysenteriae type 1*. HUS is a consequence of the production of shiga-toxin 1, most commonly produced by *S. dysenteriae* but also rarely by *S. flexneri*.[71] Longer-term health complications of diarrheal illness caused by invasive pathogens like *Shigella* species, as well as *Salmonella* and *Campylobacter* species, include postinfectious irritable bowel syndrome[73] or reactive arthritis.[74]

TREATMENT

CASE 69-12, QUESTION 2: Would M.T. benefit from antimicrobials to treat the bloody diarrhea and fever (dysentery), presumably caused by *S. dysenteriae type 1*?

For several reasons, M.T. would benefit from antimicrobial therapy for dysentery presumably caused by *S. dysenteriae type 1*. First, effective antimicrobial therapy reduces the average duration of illness from 5 to 7 days to about 3 days[72] and reduces the risk of death and serious infection-related complications. Within 48 hours of starting treatment M.T. should notice a reduction in stool frequency, volume of bloody stools, and fever. Second, effective antimicrobial therapy quickly reduces the carriage and excretion of shigellae, thus limiting the spread of infection. Despite the aforementioned benefits of antimicrobial therapy, there has been concern that antimicrobials could increase the risk for developing HUS. However, Bennish et al.[75] reported that early administration of effective antimicrobials (i.e., within 3–4 days of the onset of dysentery) is associated with a low risk for developing HUS.

CASE 69-12, QUESTION 3: What empiric antimicrobial regimens are available for the treatment of shigellosis?

Shigella species are well known for rapidly developing resistance following exposure to antimicrobials; therefore, selection of empiric therapy should be based on local antimicrobial susceptibility patterns.[71]

Ampicillin, TMP–SMX, and Nalidixic Acid

During the 1960s to 1980s, ampicillin, TMP–SMX, or nalidixic acid were the standard treatments for shigellosis. During the 1990s, multidrug-resistant (i.e., resistance to ampicillin, TMP–SMX, and chloramphenicol) *Shigella* precluded their empiric use for shigellosis, but as these multidrug-resistant isolates remained susceptible to fluoroquinolones, these agents became the drugs of choice for this infection.[71]

...inolones

...l ciprofloxacin 500 mg twice daily for 3 to 5 days is ...inst multidrug-resistant *S. dysenteriae type 1* infection ...tting where all isolates are susceptible to ciprofloxacin ...alidixic acid.[10] With the widespread introduction of fluoroquinolones as the drugs of choice for the treatment of shigellosis, not unexpectedly, quinolone-resistant shigellae have emerged.[76] Ciprofloxacin resistance in *Shigella* species from Asia and Africa has progressively increased from 0.6% prior to 2000 to 29.1% during 2007 to 2009.[77] Although the prevalence of ciprofloxacin-resistant *Shigella* remains low (less than 5%) in Europe and America,[77] international travel is strongly associated with the importation and subsequent circulation, within the United States, of ciprofloxacin-resistant *Shigella sonnei*[78] and other multi-drug resistant *Enterobacteriacae*.[79]

Azithromycin

In the setting of epidemic dysentery caused by *S. dysenteriae type 1*, similar clinical outcomes were observed in adults treated with a single 1 g oral dose of azithromycin or multiple doses of ciprofloxacin (500 mg orally twice daily for 3 days). In this study, the mean number of days until resolution of symptoms after starting therapy was similar (2.5 days for azithromycin vs. 2.3 days of ciprofloxacin) but only 17% of isolates were nalidixic acid–resistant.[80]

In adults with moderate-to-severe shigellosis caused by multidrug-resistant *Shigella* species, clinical efficacy is similar with oral azithromycin (500 mg on day 1, then 250 mg daily for 4 days) or oral ciprofloxacin (500 mg every 12 hours for 5 days), 89% versus 82%, respectively ($P > 0.2$).[81] In a subgroup analysis, a greater proportion of patients infected with *S. dysenteriae type 1* failed therapy with either azithromycin (29%) or ciprofloxacin (17%), compared with patients infected with other *Shigella* species (failure rate of 6% for either antibiotic).[81] Nearly all (97%) of the *S. dysenteriae type 1* isolates were nalidixic acid–resistant (median ciprofloxacin MIC of 0.125 mcg/mL) whereas only 6% of other *Shigella* species were nalidixic acid–resistant (median ciprofloxacin MIC of 0.016 mcg/mL).

Concerning is the intercontinental spread through sexual transmission of azithromycin-resistant shigellosis and treatment failure following azithromycin therapy.[82] *S. sonnei* with reduced susceptibility to azithromycin remains susceptible to ceftriaxone,[83] and ceftriaxone has successfully treated a patient with azithromycin-resistant shigellosis failing azithromycin therapy.[84]

β-lactams

The oral third-generation cephalosporin cefixime is unreliable for the treatment of shigellosis, with failures reported in 11% to 47% of patients.[85] Parenteral ceftriaxone and cefotaxime have excellent in vitro activity against *Shigella* species and have been used alone[39] or with amikacin[46] for patients failing ciprofloxacin therapy. Though uncommon, ceftriaxone-resistant *Shigella* have been reported in Asia.[71] Ongoing surveillance to detect changes in antimicrobial susceptibility among *Shigella* species is needed to direct local empiric treatment recommendations.

CASE 69-12, QUESTION 4: Should loperamide be started in patients with dysentery?

The role of antimotility drugs in patients with dysentery has been debated, the concern being that prolonging the clearance of pathogens from the intestinal tract could worsen the severity of illness. However, loperamide (in combination of ciprofloxacin) has been safely used in non-critically ill adults with bacillary dysentery primarily caused by *Shigella* species, decreasing the number of unformed stools and shortening the duration of diarrhea; fever was not prolonged in these patients.[9] However, the authors stress that all *Shigella* isolates in the study were susceptible to the antimicrobial used (i.e., all isolates were susceptible to ciprofloxacin and nalidixic acid) and none of the patients were critically ill; thus, it would not be prudent to extrapolate the findings from this study to critically ill patients like M.T.[9]

CASE 69-12, QUESTION 5: What empiric antimicrobial regimen could be started in patients like M.T. with severe dysentery, likely caused by *Shigella* species?

Ciprofloxacin, azithromycin, and ceftriaxone are the primary agents used for the treatment of shigellosis,[3,76] though resistance to all of these agents has been reported. In the setting of severe dysentery associated with nausea and vomiting, parenteral ceftriaxone is a reasonable empiric option.[71] Fluoroquinolones are a less desirable option given the widespread prevalence of fluoroquinolone-resistant *Shigella* species in areas including the Indian subcontinent[77] where M.T. likely became infected.

Shigellosis—Mild Illness

CLINICAL PRESENTATION

CASE 69-13

QUESTION 1: F.F. is a 30-year-old, previously healthy woman, presenting to her physician with non-bloody, watery diarrhea of 3 days' duration. Her history of present illness is significant for the following: 2 days before the onset of her gastrointestinal symptoms she visited with her 4-year-old nephew in California who was recovering from an intestinal illness caused by *S. sonnei* acquired at his day-care center. F.F. has no significant medical history. Overall, she feels better compared to the previous day and is afebrile. How does F.F.'s clinical presentation of shigellosis differ from that of M.T. (Case 69-12, Question 1)? Should F.F. be treated with antimicrobials for her presumed, mild case of shigellosis?

TREATMENT

Compared to M.T., F.F. is experiencing a much milder, and likely self-limiting case of shigellosis. In industrialized countries, risk factors for shigellosis include settings where individuals are in close contact such as in child-care centers, military barracks, and institutional housing.[72] International travel[78] and sexual transmission in men who have sex with men[82] are other means of spreading shigellosis. Secondary attack rates as high as 40% occur within 1 to 4 days after exposure to the primary case; infected persons may continue to asymptomatically shed *Shigella* in stool following recovery from their illness.

S. sonnei accounts for 90% of shigellosis in developed countries. As most patients have a mild and self-limiting illness, antimicrobials are not generally required. However, from a public health standpoint they are often prescribed to shorten the duration of illness to reduce the infectious period.[86] On the other hand, with the emergence of multidrug-resistant *Shigella* species, some experts favor reserving antimicrobials for only severely ill persons.[87]

Empiric antimicrobial options include a 3-day course of either ciprofloxacin 500 mg orally twice daily or azithromycin 500 mg orally once daily; ceftriaxone can also be used.[87] Clinical improvement may be evident within 24 hours.[71]

PREVENTION

Prevention of shigellosis requires good hygiene including proper hand washing and reducing fecal–oral exposure during sexual contact.[88] Development of an effective vaccine has been limited by poor vaccine immunogenicity, decreased vaccine protection because of the changing prevalence of infection caused by non-vaccine serotypes and adverse effects.[71]

CAMPYLOBACTER JEJUNI

Clinical Presentation

CASE 69-14

QUESTION 1: M.U. is a 20-year-old, previously healthy woman presenting to the Student Health Center with the following complaints for the past 24 hours: malaise, fever, diarrhea, abdominal pain, and bloody diarrhea. One day before the onset of symptoms, she dined at a restaurant near campus, noting that the chicken she ate was not thoroughly cooked. She has no significant medical history, no recent travel history, and is a full-time student at a university in the United States. On physical examination, M.U. is not ill appearing. The physician tells her that during the past week several students with gastrointestinal symptoms similar to hers have been diagnosed with *C. jejuni* gastroenteritis, and all had recently eaten at the same restaurant. Why is M.U.'s history of present illness and clinical presentation consistent with *Campylobacter* gastroenteritis?

M.U.'s presumptive diagnosis of *Campylobacter* gastroenteritis is consistent with her recent history of eating undercooked chicken at a restaurant associated with an ongoing outbreak of *Campylobacter* gastroenteritis. In industrialized nations, the most important risk factor for acquiring *Campylobacter* infection is the consumption of contaminated undercooked poultry, dairy products, unpasteurized foods, or contaminated water.[89] Prevention of *Campylobacter* infection involves careful food preparation and cooking practices.[90]

Beginning 24 to 72 hours after consumption of contaminated foods, clinical manifestations of *Campylobacter* gastroenteritis typically include diarrhea, fever, and abdominal cramps with either loose and watery or bloody stools.[89] Postinfectious complications of *C. jejuni* gastroenteritis include Guillain–Barré syndrome, reactive arthritis, and postinfectious irritable bowel syndrome; the latter associated with diarrhea lasting more than 7 days.[89]

Treatment

CASE 69-14, QUESTION 2: Would M.U. benefit from antimicrobial therapy to treat her *Campylobacter* gastroenteritis?

Because *C. jejuni* gastroenteritis is typically an acute, self-limiting illness resolving within 3 to 7 days,[91] antibiotic therapy is usually not necessary.[89] Antibiotics are recommended for patients with symptoms lasting longer than 1 week, high fevers, bloody stools, pregnant women, or immunocompromised hosts.[92] As M.U.'s clinical presentation includes fever with bloody stools, antimicrobial therapy is warranted. Effective antimicrobial therapy shortens the duration and the severity of illness by a mean of 1.3 days, and it is most beneficial when started with 3 days of the onset of illness.[89]

CASE 69-14, QUESTION 3: What empiric antimicrobial therapies could be initiated to treat M.U.'s presumed case of *C. jejuni* gastroenteritis?

MACROLIDE/AZALIDE

Macrolides (or an azalide) remain the drugs of choice for the treatment of *Campylobacter* gastroenteritis.[3] Macrolide resistance has remained relatively stable around 5%,[89] but depending on geographic location, higher macrolide resistance has been reported from Eastern Europe and China (5%–11%)[93] and India (22%).[94]

FLUOROQUINOLONES

Once considered the drugs of choice for *Campylobacter* infection, fluoroquinolones are no longer first-line options as a consequence of widespread fluoroquinolone resistance, largely attributed to their use in veterinary medicine and food animals (e.g., poultry); the latter practice has since been banned in the United States.[93] Fluoroquinolone-resistant *C. jejuni* exceeds 80% in Spain, Thailand, and Hong Kong, and it is about 50% in selected European Union States.[95] In the United States, the prevalence of ciprofloxacin-resistant *C. jejuni* remained between 20% and 30% from 2007 to 2011.[89,93,96] However, higher quinolone-resistance among *Campylobacter* isolates in international travelers returning to the United States compared to non-travel-associated isolates (60% vs. 13%)[93] underscores the need to consider local resistance patterns from where infection was acquired, when selecting empiric antimicrobial therapy for returning travelers.

Recommended oral treatments for *C. jejuni* gastroenteritis for adults are azithromycin 500 mg once daily for 3 days or erythromycin 500 mg 4 times daily for 5 days.[3] Children may be treated with azithromycin 10 mg/kg/day once daily for 3 to 5 days or erythromycin 30 mg/kg in two to four divided doses for 3 to 5 days.[3] On the basis of M.U.'s medical history and clinical presentation, empiric therapy with oral azithromycin can be started.

TRAVELERS' DIARRHEA

Of the nearly one billion people traveling each year from industrialized countries to developing areas of the world, approximately 10% to 60% will experience an acute self-limiting episode of travelers' diarrhea (TD).[14,97] Long-term postinfectious complications occur in a small proportion of returning travelers.[14] Experts recommend pretravel education focusing on the prevention of TD and instructions for the self-treatment of TD at the onset of illness.[98]

CASE 69-15

QUESTION 1: W.D. and B.D. are healthy 23-year-old females beginning a 2-week backpacking trip through Latin America. Prior to their departure both travelers attended a travel clinic where they received instructions to minimize their risk for TD, and a travel kit including instructions and medications for the self-treatment of TD. On the day of their arrival, both travelers seek out local street vendors, sampling their fresh fruits, vegetables, prepared foods, and unbottled beverages.

On the second day of their vacation both travelers are not feeling well. W.D. notes only the passing of two to three watery stools without blood, and mild nausea. In contrast, B.D. is feeling much worse noting the passing of six to seven loose, bloody stools, abdominal cramps, and feeling "feverish." Neither traveler feels dizzy or thirsty, and both are able to continue drinking unbottled water and juices. What are their risk factors for TD and why are their clinical presentations consistent with this diagnosis?

Risk Factors

Both travelers have several risk factors for acquiring TD. First, their travel to Latin America, a destination considered "high-risk" for TD (i.e., ≥20% risk within the first 2 weeks of travel); other

1459

…stinations include South Asia and West/Central Africa.[14] …use the highest risk for TD is during the first 2 weeks …ir recent arrival to an at-risk destination increases the …d for infection; the risk for TD lessens during the second …o risk) and third (3.3% risk) weeks of travel.[14] Third is their …avel style of eating foods with a high-risk for contamination with enteropathogens such as foods from local street vendors and drinking unbottled beverages. Additional high-risk foods include ice cubes, raw milk, unpeeled fruits and vegetables, uncooked foods, moist foods; foods remaining at room temperature for prolonged periods of time, allowing bacteria to multiply or release their enterotoxins[99]; use of acid-inhibiting medications allowing acid-susceptible enteropathogens to pass through to the intestines; and genetic predisposition.[14]

Clinical Presentation

TD is defined as three or more loose, unformed stools per day plus at least one symptom of enteric infection such as abdominal cramps, nausea, vomiting, fever, fecal urgency, tenesmus, or the passage of bloody or mucoid stools. Like in these travelers, illness typically begins within 24 to 48 hours after consuming fecally contaminated foods. Left untreated, TD is generally a self-limiting illness lasting 4 to 5 days.[14]

General Management

CASE 69-15, QUESTION 2: What general approach should W.D. and B.D. take to manage their diarrheal illnesses?

Realizing that their symptoms are consistent with TD, both travelers review their pretravel information for the self-management of TD.

Hydration

To replace fluid and electrolyte losses they should continue to drink only bottled or boiled liquids such as tea, broth, carbonated beverages, and fruit juices.[99] Electrolytes can be replaced by eating salted crackers or similar sources of sodium chloride. For travelers able to drink fluids ad libitum, a modified World Health Organization oral rehydration solution offers no additional benefit over the administration of loperamide alone.[100] Neither traveler has symptoms indicative of significant dehydration such as thirst, dizziness, or altered mental status.

SAFE FOODS—"PEEL IT, BOIL IT, OR FORGET IT"

Travelers should avoid consuming foods with a high risk for contamination with enteropathogens such as raw vegetables, fruit they have not peeled themselves, cooked food not served steaming hot, and tap water.[101] Instead, they should only eat fruits that they have peeled themselves or that have been adequately washed, and well-cooked foods served steaming hot. Enteropathogens are killed at 100°C and foods served piping hot at 60°C are generally safe.[14]

Despite adherence to dietary restrictions and precautions, prevention of TD is not always possible, likely reflecting the difficulty with adhering to sanitary standards for the preparation and serving of foods, the lack of facilities for employees to wash their hands after going to the bathroom, or the lack of screens or windows to prevent flies from contaminating foods.[14]

SELF-TREATMENT OF TRAVELERS' DIARRHEA

Antimotility agents alone provide rapid relief of symptoms but do not cure the infection, whereas antimicrobials alone will cure the infection but symptoms may persist for a longer time.[99] In the appropriate setting, antimotility drugs plus antibiotics provide the fastest relief of diarrheal symptoms.[99] Selection of a self-treatment plan is, in part, based on the traveler's severity of illness and manifestations of their diarrheal illness.

Microbial Etiology, Clinical Manifestations, and Treatment Options

CASE 69-15, QUESTION 3: For travelers with the following manifestations of TD, (a) watery diarrhea without blood or fever, or (b) bloody diarrhea or fever, or (c) diarrhea while taking chemoprophylaxis, what are the common microbial etiologies, and what treatment options are available to manage these diarrheal syndromes?

The microbial etiology of TD is recognized in 50% to 94% of patients, with bacteria most commonly identified; viruses and parasites are less frequently isolated.[14] For travelers to developing countries, the most common enteropathogen is enterotoxigenic *E. coli* (ETEC), followed by enteroaggregative *E. coli* (EAEC), diffusely adherent *E. coli*, noroviruses, rotaviruses, *Salmonella* species, *C. jejuni*, and *Shigella* species.[14] The likely enteropathogen afflicting individual travelers can in part be predicted by the clinical manifestations of the diarrheal illness and the travel destination (information which is helpful for selecting an appropriate self-treatment plan).[102]

WATERY DIARRHEA WITHOUT FEVER OR BLOODY DIARRHEA

ETEC is suspected in the setting of acute watery diarrhea, especially in travelers to Latin America and the Caribbean (≥35% of reported pathogens), Africa (25%–35% of reported pathogens), and South Asia (15%–25% of reported pathogens).[14] ETEC produce enterotoxins that stimulate the intestinal mucosa to secrete fluid into the gut lumen, leading to diarrheal stools.

Loperamide, Diphenoxylate/Atropine, Bismuth Preparations

Loperamide alone can be considered in patients with a mild diarrheal illness, e.g., two loose stools and mild symptoms,[103] without fever or bloody stools.[101] Loperamide rapidly relieves diarrheal symptoms, often within <24 hours[101] and is better tolerated than diphenoxylate/atropine. Mild diarrheal illness may be less likely to be infectious in etiology, but instead because of noninfectious causes such as anxiety, diet changes, and stress.[103] Bismuth subsalicylate is moderately effective in improving diarrheal symptoms.[14]

Alternatively, travelers on a short and critical trip (e.g., business) might consider the addition of an antibiotic. However, the potential adverse consequences of antimicrobial therapy such as the risk for adverse drug events, additional cost, and antimicrobial resistance should also be considered. A recent prospective study reported that depending on the travel destination, the risk for a traveler with diarrhea becoming colonized with extended-spectrum beta-lactamase producing *Enterobacteriacae* was greatest (28%–80%) if an antimicrobial was taken versus if no antibiotic was taken (8%–47%).[79] After returning home up to 24% of travelers remain colonized at 6 months and 10% remain colonized at 3 years.[79] Consequently, some experts do not recommend antimicrobials for mild-to-moderate disease nor for the prevention of TD.[79]

Antimicrobials Alone

Rifaximin, ciprofloxacin or levofloxacin, or azithromycin[102] are recommended for travelers with watery diarrhea without fever or dysentery[102] (Table 69-3). For travelers to Mexico[104,105] or Kenya,[106] where ETEC is a frequent cause of TD, a single dose of ciprofloxacin

Table 69-3
Therapy for Travelers' Diarrhea in Adults

Drug	Treatment
Ciprofloxacin	500 mg twice daily for 1–3 days[a]
Levofloxacin	500 mg daily for 1–3 days[a]
Azithromycin	1,000 mg in a single dose or 500 mg once daily × 3 days
Rifaximin	200 mg 3 times daily for 3 days

[a]Single dose may be effective. If diarrhea improves 12–24 hours after the first dose, the antibiotic can be stopped; otherwise, may continue antibiotic for up to 3 days.

Source: Hill DR, Beeching NJ. Travelers' diarrhea. *Curr Opin Infect Dis*. 2010;23:481; DuPont HL et al. Expert review of the evidence base for self-therapy of travelers' diarrhea. *J Travel Med*. 2009;16:161.

500 mg, azithromycin 1 g, or levofloxacin 500 mg decreased the median time to passage of the last unformed stool to 22 to 33 hours versus 54 to 66 hours for travelers given placebo.[107] For travelers to Mexico or India, oral rifaximin 200 mg 3 times daily or ciprofloxacin 500 mg twice daily for 3 days significantly reduced the median time to passage of the last unformed stool to 32 hours and 29 hours, respectively, versus 66 hours for travelers taking placebo.[108] Rifaximin is not systemically absorbed, is well tolerated and has a low potential for the development of antibiotic resistance.[109]

Antimotility Drugs Plus Antimicrobials

The combination of antimotility drugs plus antimicrobials provide the fastest relief of diarrheal symptoms. The antimotility drug quickly acts to reduce the number of stools, whereas the antimicrobial cures the infection.[104] In military personnel stationed in Turkey with TD primarily caused by ETEC, the median time to the passage of the last unformed stool was shortened to as little as 3 hours in recruits taking oral loperamide (4 mg initially, then 2 mg as needed; maximum 16 mg/day) plus either levofloxacin (single 500-mg dose) or azithromycin (single 1-g dose).[110] In otherwise healthy US students at least 18 years old attending school in Mexico, the combination of rifaximin (200 mg orally 3 times daily for 3 days) plus loperamide (4 mg initially, then 2 mg after each unformed stool) relieved diarrheal symptoms faster (27 ± 4.13 hours) than rifaximin alone (32.5 ± 4.14 hours) or loperamide alone (69 ± 4.11 hours).[109]

BLOODY DIARRHEA WITH OR WITHOUT FEVER, OR DIARRHEA WHILE TAKING CHEMOPROPHYLAXIS[102]

Invasive pathogens including *Shigella*, *Campylobacter*, and less commonly *Salmonella*, non-cholera *Vibrios* and *Aeromonas* species are suspected in the setting of acute bloody diarrhea with fever. *Campylobacter* species are frequent causes of TD in travelers to Southeast Asia (25%–35% of reported pathogens) and South Asia (15%–25% of reported pathogens).[14]

Antimicrobials Alone

A comparative study reported the highest cure rate with a single dose of azithromycin 1 g (96%), followed by 3 days of either azithromycin 500 mg daily (85%) or levofloxacin 500 mg daily (71%).[110] The lower cure rate with levofloxacin was because of infection with levofloxacin-resistant *Campylobacter* species. Nausea during the 30 minutes after receipt of the first antimicrobial dose was more common in persons given 1 g of azithromycin versus the other regimens (14% vs. <6%, respectively).[110]

Rifaximin should not be used in patients with diarrhea complicated by fever and bloody stools, being ineffective against invasive enteropathogens, e.g., *Salmonella*, *Shigella*, and *Campylobacter* species.[102]

CASE 69-15, QUESTION 4: Based on the symptoms each traveler is experiencing, what drug therapies are available for W.D. and B.D. that can be considered to reduce the duration and severity of their TD?

For travelers with *mild* watery diarrhea without fever or bloody stools (like W.D.), loperamide can be used, often relieving symptoms in less than 24 hours.[101] If improvement is not evident within 12 hours, an antimicrobial could be started.[103]

For travelers with moderate-to-severe diarrhea with fever or bloody stools (like B.D.), antimicrobial therapy is recommended to shorten the duration and severity of the diarrheal illness.[101] Treatment options include a fluoroquinolone or azithromycin (Table 69-3). Azithromycin is recommended for travelers to areas with a high prevalence of fluoroquinolone-resistant *Campylobacter* species,[101] including Thailand (93%), Nepal (71%), Asia (70%), Latin America (61%), and Africa (31%),[102] or for travelers not responding within 48 hours to a fluoroquinolone.[101] Rifaximin is not effective for TD caused by invasive enteropathogens[14] and not recommended for B.D.

POSTINFECTIOUS COMPLICATIONS OF TD

CASE 69-15, QUESTION 5: Three weeks after returning from their trip, unlike W.D. who is free of intestinal symptoms, B.D. continues to have episodes of loose stools and abdominal discomfort, for which she seeks medical attention. On physical examination her vital signs are stable and she is afebrile. The physician believes her symptoms are consistent with postinfectious irritable bowel syndrome (PI-IBS). What are B.D.'s risk factors for PI-IBS and why is her clinical presentation consistent with this diagnosis? What therapies can be recommended to manage her symptoms?

Clinical Presentation and Risk Factors

Postinfectious complications of TD include reactive arthritis and Guillain–Barré syndrome which are associated with *C. jejuni* infection and PI-IBS which may occur in 3% to 17% of travelers following a diarrheal episode[14] by invasive pathogens including *Campylobacter*, *Salmonella*, and *Shigella* species.[7] Risk factors for PI-IBS include a severe episode of TD (like B.D.), the number of episodes, pretravel diarrhea, pretravel adverse life events, and infection with heat-labile toxin-producing ETEC.[14]

Management

Treatment of PI-IBS is aimed at providing symptomatic relief; antimicrobials have not been proven to be beneficial and may be harmful.[111] Diarrheal symptoms can be managed with loperamide; if postprandial fecal urgency is problematic, taking loperamide 30 minutes before meals is recommended. Bloating and abdominal discomfort can be managed with simethicone or antispasmodic agents[73]; chronic abdominal symptoms can be managed with low doses of amitriptyline and selective serotonin reuptake inhibitors.[111] About 50% of patients with PI-IBS recover within 6 years, although recovery is less likely in the setting of persistent depression or anxiety.[111]

Prevention of PI-IBS with chemoprophylaxis of TD has not been proven. A recent randomized, double-blind, placebo-controlled study evaluating prophylactic rifaximin for the prevention of diarrhea in travelers to South and Southeast Asia did not find rifaximin to reduce the occurrence of new-onset IBS. The absence of a benefit could be attributed to inadequate power of the study to detect a true difference; more studies are needed to address this issue.[112]

...ylaxis

...-15, Question 6: On hearing of the travels of W.D. ...D., friends J.G. and T.M. begin planning a similar vacation to ...entral America, but they want to prevent the occurrence of any diarrheal illness. Neither friend has any significant medical history. Should prophylaxis be recommended for these travelers? What drug therapies can be recommended for the chemoprophylaxis of TD?

CANDIDATES FOR ANTIMICROBIAL PROPHYLAXIS AND SPECIFIC AGENTS

Antimicrobial prophylaxis for TD is recommended when the benefit of prophylaxis outweighs the risks of drug therapy including adverse drug reactions such as photosensitivity with fluoroquinolones, bacterial resistance, and expense.[112] In otherwise healthy persons, TD is typically a self-limiting illness lasting several days, and should it occur, traveler's self-management of TD reduces the time to the last unformed stool to within 24 hours of the onset of illness.[113] For these reasons, routine chemoprophylaxis for TD is not recommended.

Chemoprophylaxis could be considered for travelers at greatest risk for infection or its complications, including persons in whom a short-term illness could ruin the purpose of the trip (e.g., athletes, politicians, lecturers, others); persons in whom a diarrheal illness could complicate an underlying medical problem (e.g., insulin-dependent diabetes mellitus, congestive heart failure, reactive arthritis, inflammatory bowel disease, advanced cancer, or HIV infection); and persons with conditions which increase the risk for enteric infection (e.g., genetic predisposition, gastric disease or surgery, or use of acid-reducing medications).[104] If offered, chemoprophylaxis should not extend beyond 2 to 3 weeks.[14,101] Thus, these travelers are not candidates to receive antimicrobial prophylaxis for TD. Instead, at the onset of illness, they should follow their self-treatment plan for TD they received from their pretravel clinic visit.

For travelers who are candidates for chemoprophylaxis of TD, the following options are available.

Antimicrobials

Chemoprophylaxis with a fluoroquinolone (ciprofloxacin 500 mg or levofloxacin 500 mg given daily during travel but not exceeding 2–3 weeks and for 2 days after return) is recommended to reduce the incidence of diarrheal illness.[14,101] However, the current efficacy of fluoroquinolones should be viewed with caution, given rising fluoroquinolone resistance in common enteropathogens[112] including ETEC and EAEC in India, and *Campylobacter* species in Asia and Latin America.[102] Azithromycin 250 mg daily is an alternative chemoprophylactic agent and preferred for travel to destinations where *Campylobacter* species is a common cause of TD, e.g., South and Southeast Asia.[101]

Rifaximin is not FDA approved for the prophylaxis of TD, but it has been effective for the prevention of TD in students traveling from the United States to Mexico where ETEC is a common enteropathogen.[114] A more recent randomized, double-blind, placebo-controlled study showed only a modest (48% protection) benefit of rifaximin compared to placebo in otherwise healthy travelers to South and Southeast Asia—areas where enteroinvasive pathogens are frequent causes of TD.

Miscellaneous Agents

Bismuth subsalicylate, two tablets (526 mg/dose) 4 times daily for a maximum of 3 weeks has a protective efficacy of 65% against TD.[115] The problems with BSS because of inconvenient dosing, salicylate content, and unpleasant adverse effects as mentioned before need to be considered.

Probiotics have been studied on the basis of their ability to prevent enteropathogen colonization. The effectiveness of probiotics has not been determined and more studies are needed before these agents can be routinely recommended.[102]

ESCHERICHIA COLI O157:H7

Epidemiology

CASE 69-16

Question 1: P.J., a 3-year-old girl, is brought to the ED because of "stomach pains" and non-bloody diarrhea that has progressed to bloody diarrhea over the past 48 hours. Five days before the onset of diarrhea, the family celebrated her birthday at a fast-food restaurant; P.J.'s parents ate fish sandwiches and P.J. ate a hamburger. P.J.'s mother noted that the hamburger was not thoroughly cooked because the juices from the hamburger were still pinkish. P.J. has no significant medical history. During the week, she attended a day-care center.

On physical examination P.J. is afebrile, with signs of mild-to-moderate dehydration. A stool sample is negative for fecal leukocytes. The physician assesses her illness as bloody diarrhea, possibly caused by Shiga toxin–producing *E. coli* (STEC). The plan is to admit P.J. to the hospital for hydration, observation, and further workup. What clinical and laboratory findings and epidemiologic history are consistent with the diagnosis of STEC as the cause of P.J.'s illness?

E. coli O157:H7 is a strain of *E. coli* that produces Shiga toxins as one of its mechanisms of causing GI illness. A second virulence factor of STEC strains is their ability to attach to and damage the intestinal mucosa.[116] These *E. coli* bacteria cause a wide spectrum of illness, including asymptomatic carriage, mild and non-bloody diarrhea, bloody diarrhea (hemorrhagic colitis), HUS, and thrombotic thrombocytopenia purpura.[117]

E. coli O157:H7 should be suspected in the setting of abdominal cramps with non-bloody diarrhea that progresses to bloody diarrhea over 1 to 2 days.[118] Unlike bloody diarrhea associated with *Shigella* species or *Campylobacter* species, fever is often absent or of low grade because this pathogen is not invasive.[119] Patients with severe illness are more likely to have fever, however.[120]

STEC is most commonly spread by consumption of undercooked beef products that are contaminated with *E. coli* O157:H7, although other modes of acquiring this infection have been reported. The incubation period for this infection is usually 3 to 4 days, which is consistent with P.J.'s recent history of eating undercooked hamburger. In most instances, the illness resolves in 5 to 8 days.[121] Fecal leukocytes may or may not be found in stool samples.[122]

Laboratory Diagnosis

Case 69-16, Question 2: How can P.J.'s diagnosis of *E. coli* O157:H7 infection be confirmed?

In the United States, *E. coli* O157:H7 is the most common STEC serotype associated with this infection.[122] Unlike other *E. coli*, O157:H7 does not rapidly ferment sorbitol, thus allowing the use of special culture media (Sorbitol-MacConkey) to help in identifying this organism. P.J.'s stool should be cultured using this media. Because of other sorbitol-fermenting organisms and non-O157 STEC, further testing for Shiga toxins or the genes encoding them is increasingly performed.[121,123]

Hemolytic Uremic Syndrome

CASE 69-16, QUESTION 3: Forty-eight hours after admission to the hospital, P.J. is pale and has developed several "bruises" on her extremities. The nurse recorded only a minimal output of darkened urine during the past 24 hours. New laboratory tests reveal blood urea nitrogen (BUN), 150 mg/dL; serum creatinine (SrCr), 6 mg/dL; serum potassium (K), 6.8 mEq/L; WBC count, 20,000 cells/mm^3; hemoglobin (Hgb), 5 g/dL; platelets, 50,000 cells/mm^3; and urinalysis is positive for blood and protein. The stool specimen sent on admission is positive for *E. coli* O157:H7. What complication of *E. coli* O157:H7 infection does P.J. now display?

The new clinical and laboratory findings support the diagnosis of HUS, a well-known complication of STEC infection. HUS is characterized by the triad of thrombocytopenia, microangiopathic hemolytic anemia, and acute renal failure with oliguria.[124] On physical examination, P.J.'s "bruises" on her extremities are consistent with thrombocytopenia, which is confirmed by the low platelet count. Her pale appearance is consistent with anemia and is confirmed by the low Hgb. The dark urine is caused by the color imparted from bilirubin because of red cell lysis (hemolytic anemia). Finally, P.J.'s decreased urine output and increased serum creatinine and BUN concentrations are consistent with renal failure.[125] P.J. has several risk factors for HUS: her age (i.e., children aged <5–15 years, median age 4–8 years), fever, increased peripheral WBC count, and the season of the year (i.e., summer).[120,124,126–129] Although not present in this case, other possible risk factors for developing HUS are age >65 years[122] and treatment with antimotility or antidiarrheal agents,[130] although this has not been universally confirmed.[120,129] The progression of *E. coli* O157:H7 gastroenteritis to HUS typically becomes apparent about 1 week after the onset of diarrhea.[120,124,126] Of children, 3% to 7%[130] may develop HUS, with a mortality rate ranging from 3% to 5%.

In adults, *E. coli* O157:H7 infection progresses to HUS in as many as 27% of patients, with a higher rate in patients >65 years of age.[120] HUS-related mortality has reached 42% in patients >15 years of age[120]; elderly nursing home patients have a mortality rate of up to 88%.[131]

Treatment

CASE 69-16, QUESTION 4: Would P.J. benefit from drug therapy, including antimicrobial, antimotility, or antidiarrheal agents?

Other than supportive measures to manage the complications associated with illness caused by *E. coli* O157:H7, no specific drug therapy for this infection exists.[118] In retrospective and prospective studies, antibiotics have not influenced the severity of illness, or the duration of diarrhea or other GI symptoms.[132] When TMP–SMX was started a mean of 7 days after the onset of diarrhea, the duration of E. coli O157:H7 excretion was not altered.[133]

The effect of antibiotic administration on the risk of *E. coli* O157:H7 complications (e.g., HUS) remains controversial. A prospective cohort study of 71 children with diarrhea caused by *E. coli* O157:H7 found that antibiotic treatment increased the risk of progression to HUS.[129] Previous publications have supported these findings,[130,133,134] whereas others have reported that antibiotics do not increase the risk of progression to HUS.[120,135] A systematic review of these and other studies revealed no association between antibiotic administration and development of HUS.[136] Antibiotic selection, dosing, timing of administration, small sample sizes, and a lack of placebo use in the selected studies complicate the analysis. Thus, the role of antibiotics in the treatment of *E. coli* O157:H7 infection remains controversial. Currently, clinicians do not recommend antibiotic treatment for STEC, though active US surveillance reports nearly 2/3 of patients with this diagnosis receive antimicrobial therapy, including 29% of patients receiving therapy after confirmed diagnosis.[137] Despite these numbers, P.J. should not receive antibiotic therapy at this time. Clinicians must carefully weigh empiric antibiotic treatment before an organism has been identified.[136]

Antimotility drugs are not recommended for patients with *E. coli* O157:H7 infection because they have been variably associated with an increased risk of progression to HUS,[130,135] although other studies have failed to find an association.[120,129] Despite these concerns, recent reports suggest up to 31% of patients continue to receive antimotility agents for this infection.[137] Although the explanation for the increased risk is unknown, the reduction of bowel motility may decrease the clearance of organisms from the GI tract, thereby increasing the absorption of toxins. Administration of antimotility drugs within the first 3 days of illness has been associated with a longer duration of bloody diarrhea.[138]

Prevention

CASE 69-16, QUESTION 5: P.J.'s family members want to know what they could have done to prevent this infection. On discharge from the hospital, is it safe for P.J. to return to her day-care center?

STEC is often spread to humans by consumption of contaminated beef products that are not thoroughly cooked.[117] Because thorough cooking kills this organism, meat should be well cooked (i.e., juices from meat should be clear, not pink). In addition, this infection can be acquired by consuming other contaminated foods, including water, unpasteurized milk, apple cider, lettuce, and sprouts.[117,118]

Finally, because contact with infected persons commonly results in transmission of this infection to others,[130,131,134] P.J. should not return to day care until at least 48 hours after her diarrhea has ceased.[132]

CLOSTRIDIUM DIFFICILE INFECTION

Mild-to-Moderate Infection

CLINICAL PRESENTATION AND DIAGNOSIS

CASE 69-17

QUESTION 1: B.W., a 35-year-old woman, is admitted to a 10-bed medical ward for the treatment of *Streptococcus pneumoniae* meningitis. On arrival, she is started on ceftriaxone (Rocephin) 2 g IV q12 hours and improves over the next few days. On day 7 of antibiotic therapy, she complains of feeling warm, with cramping abdominal pain and diarrhea. She begins passing mucoid, greenish, foul-smelling watery stools, and has a temperature of 101°F. Microscopic examination of a stool sample is positive for fecal leukocytes. The physician's assessment of B.W.'s clinical and laboratory findings is antibiotic-associated diarrhea (AAD), most likely caused by *C. difficile*. What is the most likely mechanism for this patient's AAD?

ADD is a common complication of antimicrobial therapy.[139] The mechanisms by which antibiotics cause diarrhea include direct allergic and toxic effects on intestinal mucosa, and alterations of GI motility (e.g., erythromycin) and of normal intestinal flora.

the normal bowel flora can lead to changes in carbo- ...e acid metabolism by intestinal bacteria or to over- ...nogenic bacteria, either of which may be followed ...a.[139] Bacteria known to be associated with AAD include ...*ringens*, *S. aureus*, *Klebsiella oxytoca*, *Candida* species, and *C. ...ficile*. *C. difficile* infection (CDI) is the most clinically relevant microbial cause and the focus of this section.

A spore-forming, gram-positive anaerobic bacillus, *C. difficile* can cause a wide spectrum of syndromes, including asymptomatic carriage, diarrhea of varying severity, colitis with or without formation of pseudomembranes, toxic megacolon, colonic perforation, and death.[140]

The pathogenesis of CDI involves disruption of the normal colonic flora, most commonly by antibiotics (Table 69-4). An increasing number of cases in the outpatient setting have been identified without any antibiotic exposure, making additional risk factors difficult to find.[141] Recent data suggest that proton-pump inhibitors may be responsible for CDI.[142,143] Alteration of the colonic microflora is followed by overgrowth of toxin-producing strains of *C. difficile*.[139,140] These toxins, primarily toxins A and B, are responsible for causing colonic inflammation and the clinical manifestations of this infection.[139,140]

A highly pathogenic strain of *C. difficile* has been described in outbreaks in the United States and around the world.[140,144] This strain, labeled BI/NAP1 (or ribotype 027), generally causes more severe disease. Among its increased virulence factors are an increased production of both toxins A and B and a binary toxin. This ribotype has become endemic in some facilities and appears to cause more severe disease even in non-outbreak situations.[145]

Table 69-4
Medications Implicated in Clostridium difficile–Associated Diarrhea

Commonly Implicated
Cephalosporins
Clindamycin
Ampicillin
Fluoroquinolones
Less Commonly Implicated
Erythromycin
Clarithromycin
Azithromycin
Other penicillins
Trimethoprim–sulfamethoxazole
Rarely Implicated
Aminoglycosides
Rifampin
Tetracycline
Vancomycin
Metronidazole
Antineoplastic agents

Source: Owens RC, Jr et al. Antimicrobial-associated risk factors for *Clostridium difficile* infection. *Clin Infect Dis*. 2008;46(Suppl 1):S19; Cohen SH et al. Society for Healthcare Epidemiology of America; Infectious Diseases Society of America. Clinical practice guidelines for *Clostridium difficile* infection in adults: 2010 update by the Society for Healthcare Epidemiology of America (SHEA) and the Infectious Diseases Society of America (IDSA). *Infect Control Hosp Epidemiol*. 2010;31:431.

CASE 69-17, QUESTION 2: Why is B.W.'s history and presentation consistent with AAD caused by *C. difficile*?

B.W.'s major risk factor for acquiring CDI is her receipt of an antibiotic within the last 2 weeks. *C. difficile* is a common cause of nosocomial diarrhea. The clinical and laboratory findings consistent with CDI include mucoid, greenish, foul-smelling watery stools and crampy abdominal pain. Patients usually present with low-grade fevers, but temperature may be >104°F.[146] Peripheral leukocytosis is common with CDI, sometimes with WBC >30,000 cells/mm^3.[146,147] Fecal leukocytes are variably present in CDI and are not clinically useful for diagnosis.[148]

The onset of symptoms of CDI varies widely from a few days after the start of antibiotic therapy to 8 weeks after the agent is discontinued.[146] Other risk factors for acquiring CDI are admission to a hospital in which *C. difficile* is endemic or in which there is an ongoing outbreak of CDI.

CASE 69-17, QUESTION 3: How can B.W.'s diagnosis of CDI be confirmed?

Finding toxins in unformed stool of symptomatic patients is the gold standard for diagnosis. Older enzyme immunoassays detecting toxins A/B have largely been replaced by polymerase chain reaction (PCR) tests, because PCR is much more sensitive.[149] An advanced two-step diagnostic method is increasingly recommended. The two-step test first looks for the presence of glutamate dehydrogenase (GDH) antigen as a quick and inexpensive screening test. GDH is produced by all *C. difficile* strains, so positive GDH tests are then followed by toxin-detecting PCR.[150] Samples negative for GDH are considered negative and not tested further. Culture, though helpful, is complicated by the fact that of the *C. difficile* strains isolated from various populations, 5% to 25% do not produce toxins (non-toxigenic) and do not cause colitis or diarrhea.[146] Routine testing for specific *C. difficile* strains such as ribotype 027 is not typically available in most settings.[149]

Colonoscopy with biopsy is used to make the diagnosis of *C. difficile* colitis rapidly. The characteristic colonic changes are raised, yellowish nodules or plaque-like pseudomembranes, often with skip areas of normal mucosa.[146] Because the characteristic pseudomembranes may be scattered throughout the colon, the diagnosis of pseudomembranous colitis can be missed with colonoscopy.

CASE 69-17, QUESTION 4: How can B.W.'s CDI be differentiated from enigmatic AAD?

Only 10% to 20% of cases of AAD are positive for toxigenic *C. difficile*; the remaining cases have an unknown cause and are referred to as simple, benign, or "nuisance" diarrhea.[139] The clinical resolution of benign diarrhea is a self-limited illness that resolves with nonspecific supportive measures and discontinuation of antibiotics. These clinical entities can be differentiated from one another by several objective measures. In hospitalized patients, watery diarrhea, low functional capacity, acid suppression, low albumin, and a WBC >13,000 cells/mm^3 were significant predictors of CDI.[151] Other clinical features that suggest CDI rather than enigmatic diarrhea are constitutional symptoms, lack of an antibiotic dose relationship to the illness, and hospital-wide epidemics of diarrhea.[152]

TREATMENT

CASE 69-17, QUESTION 5: B.W.'s stool sample is positive for both GDH and *C. difficile* toxin. What is the general plan to treat B.W.'s CDI?

After replacement of fluids and electrolytes, there are several steps to most effectively manage B.W.'s CDI. The first is to discontinue the offending drug (if possible), which in B.W.'s case is probably the antibiotic ceftriaxone. While some data suggest that withdrawal of the precipitating antibiotic and supportive care may be sufficient for mild disease, all available guidelines suggest specific antimicrobial treatment.[150,153]

Because B.W. is being treated for bacterial meningitis, a life-threatening infection, discontinuing antibiotics is not an option. A second option is to change her antimicrobial therapy to an agent less likely to cause CDI. B.W. is taking a cephalosporin, which, as with ampicillin, amoxicillin, and clindamycin, is frequently implicated as a cause of *C. difficile* diarrhea (Table 62-4). In contrast, antibiotics, such as TMP–SMX, and aminoglyclosides, are less commonly associated with CDI.[154–156] None of these antimicrobials, however, is a suitable alternative for treating *S. pneumoniae* meningitis.

B.W. should also receive therapy directed against *C. difficile* while continuing to take ceftriaxone for the treatment of her bacterial meningitis.

Specific *C. difficile*–directed Antimicrobials

CASE 69-17, QUESTION 6: What antibiotic should be selected to treat B.W.'s CDI?

The oral agents most commonly used to treat CDI are metronidazole and vancomycin. The differentiation between these two agents is complex and evolving, but it is guided in part by severity of illness[157–161] (Table 69-5). The most optimal definition of severe disease is not well established, but general markers of instability of vital signs with high white counts and changes in albumin and serum creatinine are suggested.[150,162] In patients categorized as having mild-to-moderate disease severity, metronidazole is generally recommended as the preferred initial agent.[158] In a randomized trial that enrolled patients with CDI and colitis, no significant difference was found in the efficacy of these drugs after 10 days of treatment.[160] Overall, >95% of patients treated for a first episode of CDI with oral metronidazole or vancomycin are expected to respond to therapy.[160,161] Recent reports have shown increases in *C. difficile* resistance to metronidazole and vancomycin, but the clinical significance in treatment selection is unknown.[163] Antibiotic sensitivities, therefore, are not routinely performed on *C. difficile*.

Metronidazole is well absorbed after oral administration and is excreted through the biliary tract before reaching the colon. Common adverse reactions include nausea, vomiting, diarrhea, dizziness, confusion, and an unpleasant metallic taste.[154] A disulfiram-like reaction can occur when alcohol or alcohol-containing medications are taken concurrently with metronidazole.[164] Because metronidazole is a carcinogen and, in some animal species, a mutagen, it should be used in pregnancy only if clearly needed. Similarly, metronidazole's safety in children has not been proved, and many prefer not to use it in this population if other options exist.[154]

Oral vancomycin produces fecal concentrations that are several 100 times the concentration needed to inhibit toxin-producing strains of *C. difficile*.[161] A 10 to 14-day course of oral vancomycin (125–500 mg orally 4 times daily) is recommended for the treatment of CDI, with all dosing regimens equally effective in the patients studied.[154,161,165,166] Because of equal efficacy and high concentrations in the colon with all doses, vancomycin 125 mg is the most commonly prescribed dose. Although oral vancomycin is not well absorbed, measurable serum concentrations have been found in patients with both normal and compromised renal function, though higher and longer dose regimens, severe infection, and renal dysfunction were more associated with serum concentrations.[167]

Fidaxomicin is the newest antimicrobial indicated for the treatment of CDI.[168,169] Fidaxomicin is a macrocyclic antibiotic active against *C. difficile* that is poorly absorbed and achieves high colonic concentrations.[170] It has limited antimicrobial spectrum and largely preserves colonic flora. In the primary clinical trial, patient outcomes on initial infection were similar when compared with vancomycin.[169] This finding, along with a significantly higher cost of therapy, has led many clinicians to suggest fidaxomicin be reserved as second-line therapy.[150,171] However, one potential advantage for fidaxomicin was in recurrence rates, which were

Table 69-5
Clostridium difficile Infection Severity of Disease

	Published guidelines	
Severity	*Am J Gastroenterology 2013*	*SHEA/ISDA 2010*
Mild-to-moderate	Diarrhea plus signs and symptoms that do not meet severe or complicated criteria	White blood count ≤15,000 cells/μL AND Serum creatinine <1.5× baseline
Severe	Serum albumin <3 g/dL PLUS *either* white blood count ≥15,000 cells/μL *or* Abdominal tenderness	White blood count >15,000 cells/μL OR Serum creatinine ≥1.5× baseline
Severe-to-complicated	Admission to intensive care unit Hypotension Fever ≥38.5°C Ileus or significant distension Mental status changes White blood count ≥35,000 or <2,000 cells/μL Serum lactate >2.2 mmol/L End organ failure	Hypotension or shock, ileus, megacolon

Source: Cohen SH et al. Society for Healthcare Epidemiology of America; Infectious Diseases Society of America. Clinical practice guidelines for *Clostridium difficile* infection in adults: 2010 Update by the Society for Healthcare Epidemiology of America (SHEA) and the Infectious Diseases Society of America (IDSA). *Infect Control Hosp Epidemiol*. 2010;31:431; Surawicz CM et al. Guidelines for diagnosis, treatment, and prevention of *Clostridium difficile* infections. *Am J Gastroenterol*. 2013;108:478.

… significantly lower with fidaxomicin compared to … (15.4% vs. 25.3%, $P = 0.005$). While recurrence … CDI treatment, it is not yet clear if it is possible … patients for whom the higher cost would provide an …onal benefit from this effect.

Because B.W. is not critically ill, metronidazole (500 mg orally 3 times daily) for 10 to 14 days is recommended as first-line treatment.[157–159] Oral metronidazole and oral vancomycin are generally considered equally efficacious in mild-to-moderate disease,[158] but vancomycin use should be limited to prevent emergence of vancomycin-resistant organisms.[172] In addition, oral vancomycin capsules are significantly more expensive than a course of oral metronidazole. Some of this cost differential can be offset by using the IV vancomycin preparation to prepare an oral solution which can be flavored and prepared as directed in the package insert.

Once therapy directed against *C. difficile* is initiated, diarrhea or cramping should subside within 2 to 4 days. If B.W.'s symptoms have not resolved, vancomycin can be tried.[152]

ALTERNATIVE THERAPIES

Toxin Binders

Traditional anion-binding resins (e.g., cholestyramine, colestipol) are not as reliable or as rapidly effective as oral metronidazole or vancomycin and are not recommended as routine therapy.[173]

Probiotics

Using probiotics introduces probiotic microorganisms into the normal flora to counteract disturbances and reduce the colonization with pathogenic species.[174] Although orally administered, *Lactobacillus* species and the yeast *Saccharomyces boulardii* have been used to treat CDI, no data support the use of probiotics alone. Adjunctive use has been suggested to prevent CDI and its recurrences. A hospital trial looking at prevention of all ADD with *Lactobacillus* reported positive results for the prevention of CDI.[175] The results of that study, however, are tempered by the methodological exclusion of patients receiving antibiotics with a high risk of causing CDI, making generalization to other patient groups difficult. The exact role of probiotics in treatment or prevention of CDI is not yet known.[150,171] Adding further caution to the widespread use of probiotics, reports of isolated adverse effects, including fungemia, with ingestion of viable *S. boulardii* have been reported.[158,176]

Antidiarrheals

CASE 69-17, QUESTION 7: Should B.W. be given any antidiarrheal agent to relieve her symptoms?

Opiates and other antiperistaltic agents should be avoided in patients with CDI. Although these types of drugs may relieve diarrheal symptoms, they may also delay toxin removal from the GI tract. Evidence supporting these negative effects is minimal as data are scarce,[9] but caution would suggest avoiding any antimotilty agent in B.W.

CASE 69-17, QUESTION 8: Following resolution of B.W.'s CDI, is it necessary to send a follow-up stool sample to determine whether it is negative for *C. difficile* toxin?

After resolution of diarrhea, obtaining a follow-up stool sample to determine whether it is negative for *C. difficile* toxin is not recommended as part of routine practice because most patients with positive tests will not develop a recurrence of their diarrhea.[158] In addition, up to 3% of healthy adults carry small numbers of *C. difficile* in their feces, whereas colonization rates are much higher (31%–37%) in hospitalized patients and infants under 1 month.[177,178]

Transmission

CASE 69-18

QUESTION 1: H.T., a 76-year-old man with multiple medical conditions, is admitted to the same 10-bed hospital ward as B.W. H.T.'s medical history is significant for a stroke that has left him bedridden in a nursing home. His only medications are those used to manage his hypertension. On day 4 of his hospitalization, H.T. complained of severe abdominal pain and watery, loose stools with blood. Physical examination revealed an ill-appearing man with a temperature of 101°F and hypotension. His WBC is 21,000 cells/mL. A stool specimen is positive for *C. difficile* toxin, and colonoscopy reveals pseudomembranes and colitis. A surgical consultant is considering an emergent colectomy because of possible bowel perforation secondary to the CDI. What are H.T.'s risk factors for acquiring *C. difficile*–associated pseudomembranous colitis during his hospitalization?

H.T.'s risk factors for acquiring CDI include his advanced age, bedridden status,[179] underlying diseases,[180] and admission to the hospital. CDI is spread when hospital personnel or equipment contaminated with *C. difficile* spores come into contact with susceptible patients. Physical proximity to an infected patient has been associated with an increased risk of CDI.[181] Therefore, measures to prevent the spread of CDI include hand disinfection before and after contact with infected patients; the use of gloves and gowns; enteric isolation precautions; and proper hand washing with soap and water (to remove any potential spores) after contact with infected patients with CDI. Contaminated equipment should be properly disinfected.[182]

Although *C. difficile* is often thought of as a nosocomial pathogen, it is being increasingly isolated in outpatient settings.[141,183] This changing epidemiology has led to a standard definition of community-associated CDI in patients without any health-care facility exposure within the last 12 weeks.[162] While many community-associated CDI infections appear in patients without antimicrobial exposure, antimicrobial use remains the highest risk factor.[184] Although proton-pump therapy and other acid suppression has been increasingly suspected as a cause of these infections, a meta-analysis of community-associated CDI did not find acid suppression to be a significant risk; however, corticosteroid use was associated with the disease.[184]

CASE 69-18, QUESTION 2: Over the next few days, all 10 patients on the ward with B.W. and H.T. are found to have *C. difficile* toxin in their stools. Five patients have diarrhea and the other five are asymptomatic. What is the role of antibiotic therapy directed at *C. difficile* in controlling this outbreak?

Neither oral metronidazole nor vancomycin is reliably effective in eradicating the carrier state (i.e., asymptomatic fecal excretion), and neither is recommended for use in this situation.[185] The lack of efficacy of these drugs is probably because of the fact that, unlike the vegetative forms of *C. difficile*, the spores of *C. difficile* are resistant to the action of antibiotics.[182] Furthermore, compared with placebo, vancomycin administration is associated with a significantly higher rate of *C. difficile* carriage 2 months after treatment.[185]

Controlling overall antibiotic use in the hospital can be a useful strategy. Antimicrobial stewardship is increasingly seen as a major control mechanism for CDI.[150] Restricting the use of single agents like clindamycin can be an effective component in efforts to control nosocomial epidemics of CDI.[179] With the emergence of the BI/NAP1 strain, control of all antibiotic use, especially fluoroquinolones, may be important in outbreak control.[186]

Finally, the overuse of acid suppressive therapy in the hospital setting, particularly proton-pump inhibitors, has been linked with increases in CDI.[187] Efforts to control use of these drugs have been increasingly recommended.[188]

CASE 69-18, QUESTION 3: What effect will the current CDI outbreak have on the outcomes of the infected patients and on health care costs?

In a prospective study, hospitalized patients who developed CDI had a 3.6-day increase in length of stay.[189] A large retrospective cohort study in the Veterans Affairs Administration reported a 2.3-day increase in hospitalization, with an increase of 4.4 days with severe disease.[190] A review of available economic data suggests additional hospital costs of $8900 to $30,000 for each case of CDI.[191] The current outbreak on the hospital ward is likely to increase both hospital costs and individual lengths of stay.

Severe *C. difficile* Infection

CASE 69-18, QUESTION 4: What treatment is recommended for H.T. who is critically ill from a CDI? What criteria should be used to characterize patients as "critically ill"?

Up to 57% of patients with antibiotic-associated pseudomembranous colitis who require surgical intervention (colectomy) die.[192] Although the precise definition of "critically ill" is not clear, it has variably included patients with pseudomembranes, age over 60, serum albumin <2.5 mg/dL, fever >38.3°C, severe abdominal pain, and marked leukocytosis (greater than 15,000–20,000 cells/mL).[146,193] Recent guidelines from the Society for Healthcare Epidemiology of America and the Infectious Disease Society of America have suggested the definition of severity as presence of any of either of the following two parameters: white blood cell count ≥15,000 cells/mL or serum creatinine 1.5 times baseline[158] (See Table 69-5). Growing evidence suggests that vancomycin 125 mg orally 4 times daily may be more effective than metronidazole in patients with predefined severe disease.[158,193] An additional definition of "severe, complicated" disease has been suggested for patients like H.T., who have hypotension, shock, ileus, or megacolon. The recommended therapy for H.T. would be a combination of vancomycin 500 mg orally 4 times daily and metronidazole 500 mg intravenously every 8 hours.[158] This combination therapy was shown to reduce mortality from 36.4% to 15.9% when compared with monotherapy in a small observational study.[194] The combination of high-dose therapies is theorized to overcome the difficulties for either medication to get to the site of action in the colon.

NON-ORAL TREATMENT

CASE 69-18, QUESTION 5: Three days after oral vancomycin and intravenous metronidazole is initiated, H.T. develops an ileus and cannot take anything by mouth. What therapeutic options are available to treat H.T.'s pseudomembranous colitis?

Adequate antibiotic levels in the colon are necessary to treat *C. difficile*–associated pseudomembranous colitis. If the oral route is not feasible (e.g., patients with an ileus or bowel obstruction), the clinician must choose an agent that is either secreted or excreted into the GI tract in its active form. IV vancomycin is not a desirable agent in this situation because it is not secreted into the GI tract. In contrast, intravenous metronidazole is eliminated by both renal and hepatic routes, and bactericidal concentrations are achieved in both serum and bile.[195]

The literature contains few reports of successful attempts to treat CDI or pseudomembranous colitis with IV metronidazole (500 mg q6–8h) alone.[196–198] Likewise, unsuccessful attempts to treat CDI with IV metronidazole have been reported.[196,199] The clinical response of CDI to PO vancomycin in a patient who did not survive was difficult to ascertain.[161]

In adults, enteral vancomycin 500 mg 4 times daily can be given through an ileostomy or colostomy (if present). Several reports of successful outcomes using intracolonic vancomycin (as an adjunct to oral or IV antibiotics) in patients with CDI have been documented. Rectal doses of vancomycin have varied from 500 mg q4–8h to 1,000 mg/L q8h.[200] Rectal vancomycin administration volumes of 500 mL are suggested to better ensure delivery to the transverse and distal colon.[150] Saline can be used as a carrier, but electrolytes should be monitored because absorption can occur. Lactated Ringer's solution may be preferred if hyperchloremia is present.[150]

Because patients with CDI are at risk for colonic perforation, enteral vancomycin should be administered cautiously.

Relapse

CASE 69-19

QUESTION 1: P.V. is a 57-year-old male who acquired CDI on the same ward as the other infected patients. P.V. was treated with metronidazole 500 mg orally 3 times daily for 10 days while in the hospital. One week after discharge from the hospital, P.V. once again developed abdominal pain and diarrhea. His clinic physician assumed these symptoms could not be related to a relapse of his CDI because he had responded so well to metronidazole. What is the likelihood that CDI has recurred?

Regardless of the antibiotic regimen prescribed for CDI, symptomatic relapse occurs in 5% to 30% of patients who respond to their initial treatment regimen.[155,182] Relapses occur 2 weeks to 2 months (median of 7 days) after treatment has been discontinued.[201] In most instances, relapses are caused by germination of dormant spores that are intrinsically resistant to antibiotics. Reinfection with *C. difficile* from external sources, however, may account for up to half of all second episodes.[202] In rare instances, either vancomycin[203] or metronidazole[204] may have caused CDI.

Risk factors for recurrent CDI include increasing age (≥65 years), use of proton-pump inhibitors, renal insufficiency, continued use of antimicrobials during CDI treatment, and glucocorticoid use.[205,206]

Data suggest that patients with a poor immune response to *C. difficile* toxin A are more likely to have a relapse of CDI.[207] It is not clinically helpful in the case of P.V., because no standard tests are currently available for this immune response. The influence of the immune system, however, has led to the usage of IV immune globulin in refractory or severe cases of CDI.[208,209] The utility of the usage of immune globulins has been debated in small single institution reviews. Immune globulins would not be the considered the next line of therapy for P.V.

CASE 69-19, QUESTION 2: How should P.V.'s CDI relapse be treated?

Most infections resulting from relapse are not related to bacterial resistance and they respond to retreatment with the same antibiotic used for initial treatment of the CDI.[155,210] Thus, an appropriate approach for P.V. is to administer another 10 to 14-day course of oral metronidazole.

For patients with multiple recurrences of CDI, the optimal management plan is unresolved.[182] Different approaches have been tried, including (a) high-dose oral vancomycin (2,000 mg/

a 4- to 6-week course with vancomycin, after which ...ered over a 1- to 2-month period[211,212]; (c) exchange ...ith or without antibacterials; (d) "pulse" dosing of ...cin every 2 to 3 days[211]; or (e) a combination of vanco... and rifampin (600 mg orally twice daily).[215] Tapered and pulse therapy with vancomycin were shown to be most effective in a clinical trial comparing multiple strategies.[211] When combined with standard antibiotic therapy, a clinical trial with the probiotic *S. boulardii* for cases of relapsing CDI noted a 65% response rate versus a 36% response rate for combination therapy with placebo.[216] The relapse rate was reduced to 17% when *S. boulardii* was combined with high-dose vancomycin.[217]

Following treatment with vancomycin, a "chaser" course of rifaximin, a poorly absorbed rifamycin derivative, was successful in separate case series for patients with multiple relapses.[218,219] Concern must be raised that the single failure occurred in concert with emerging rifaximin resistance.[218]

Because of its more minimal impact on fecal flora, fidaxomicin may be recommended for recurrent infections, although there is less evidence for its use in recurrence compared to other recommended agents.[171] Fidaxomicin's inherent advantage in limiting recurrence with initial treatment and treatment of first recurrences may lie in cost savings.[220,221]

Finally, fecal microbiota transplant (FMT) therapy has been more widely investigated in second and third relapses and has shown significant promise.[222] Healthy fecal donors, often family members, are the usual source for fecal microbiota, though frozen "banks" of FMT samples have been increasing.[223] Administration of FMT can be provided through nasogastric or nasojejeunal tubes, colonoscopy, or colonic enemas. Although published data overall remain small, a systematic review of the literature supports the efficacy (85% cure rates) and limited adverse effects of this therapy.[222] Long-term follow-up from a multi-center study of 17 patients found 88% to 94% success rates.[224] A single cost-effectiveness model, using literature-based data, found FMT to be more cost-effective compared to treatment of recurrences with vancomycin.[224]

KEY REFERENCES AND WEBSITES

A full list of references for this chapter can be found at **http://thePoint.lww.com/AT11e.** Below are the key references for this chapter, with the corresponding reference number in this chapter found in parentheses after the reference.

Key References

Cohen SH et al. Clinical Practice Guidelines for *Clostridium difficile* Infection in Adults: 2010 Update by the Society for Healthcare Epidemiology of America (SHEA) and the Infectious Diseases Society of America (IDSA). *Infect Control Hosp Epidemiol.* 2010;31(5):431–455. (162)

Crump JA et al. Epidemiology, clinical presentation, laboratory diagnosis, antimicrobial resistance, and antimicrobial management of invasive salmonella infections. *Clin Microbiol Rev.* 2015;28(4):901–937. (31)

DuPont HL. Acute infectious diarrhea in immunocompetent adults. *N Engl J Med.* 2014;370(16):1532–1540. (3)

Goldstein EJ et al. Pathway to prevention of nosocomial *Clostridium difficile* infection. *Clin Infect Dis.* 2015;60(Suppl 2):S148–S158. (188)

Harris JB et al. Cholera. *Lancet.* 2012;379(9835):2466–2476. (5)

Navaneethan U, Giannella RA. Mechanisms of infectious diarrhea. *Nat Clin Pract Gastroenterol Hepatol.* 2008;5(11):637–647. (2)

Meltzer E, Schwartz E. Enteric fever: a travel medicine oriented view. *Curr Opin Infect Dis.* 2010;23(5):432–437. (55)

Pawlowski SW et al. Diagnosis and treatment of acute or persistent diarrhea. *Gastroenterology.* 2009;136(6):1874–1886. (7)

Surawicz CM et al. Guidelines for diagnosis, treatment, and prevention of *Clostridium difficile* infections. *Am J Gastroenterol.* 2013;108:478–498. (150)

70 Intra-Abdominal Infections

Sheila K. Wang and Carrie A. Sincak

CORE PRINCIPLES

		CHAPTER CASES
1	Acute cholecystitis is the acute inflammation of the gallbladder, presenting with fever, prolonged abdominal pain, and positive Murphy's sign of the right upper quadrant followed by nausea and vomiting. Acute cholangitis is an acute inflammation of the common bile duct with accompanying classic Charcot's triad: fever, jaundice, and right upper quadrant pain.	**Case 70-1 (Question 1)**
2	Empiric therapy for severe biliary tract infections may include combination therapy with either ciprofloxacin, levofloxacin, or cefepime plus metronidazole or monotherapy with piperacillin/tazobactam or an antipseudomonal carbapenem (imipenem/cilastatin, meropenem, doripenem) if multidrug-resistant gram-negative rods are suspected.	**Case 70-1 (Question 3)**
3	Spontaneous bacterial peritonitis (SBP) is largely a monomicrobial infection commonly caused by aerobic enteric gram-negative rods, such as *Escherichia coli* and *Klebsiella pneumoniae*.	**Case 70-2 (Question 1)**
4	Empiric therapy for SBP may include a third-generation cephalosporin such as ceftriaxone or cefotaxime or parenteral fluoroquinolone with activity versus *Streptococcus pneumoniae*. Length of therapy depends on the reduction of polymorphonuclear leukocyte counts (<250 cells/μL) in peritoneal fluid, generally occurring in 5 days or fewer.	**Case 70-2 (Question 2)**
5	For secondary peritonitis, empiric antimicrobial therapy for community-acquired infections is routinely initiated without obtaining Gram stain and culture. Blood cultures may be useful, however, in health care–associated infections for detection of gram-positive cocci, yeast, or multidrug-resistant pathogens.	**Case 70-4 (Question 2)**
6	Therapy for secondary peritonitis should include antimicrobial coverage directed at gram-negative bacteria and anaerobes. Therapy may include (a) certain extended-spectrum β-lactams or β-lactamase inhibitor combinations, (b) carbapenems, or (c) a fluoroquinolone with metronidazole.	**Case 70-4 (Question 3)**
7	Duration of therapy for intra-abdominal infections typically ranges from 4 to 7 days. Clinical response and source control influence duration of therapy.	**Case 70-4 (Question 4)**
8	Acute penetrating abdominal trauma requires a short course (<24 hours) of antimicrobial therapy. Delay of therapy or development of infection necessitates a 5 to 7-day course of therapy.	**Case 70-7 (Question 2)**

INTRODUCTION

Despite the introduction of new antimicrobial agents and improvements in diagnostic and surgical techniques, the treatment of intra-abdominal infections remains a therapeutic challenge. However, advances in radiographic and interventional techniques with timely source control, improved fluid and nutritional management, and the selection of appropriate antimicrobial agents have decreased mortality in intra-abdominal infections.[1]

Intra-abdominal infections are those contained within the peritoneal cavity, which extends from the undersurface of the diaphragm to the floor of the pelvis or the retroperitoneal space. Intra-abdominal infections can present as a localized infection (e.g., appendicitis), a diffuse inflammation throughout the peritoneum (peritonitis), or as abscesses, which can form within the abdomen, between bowel loops, or in such as the liver, biliary tract, spleen, pancreas, or organs.

ic antimicrobial therapy should be initiated as soon as an abdominal infection is suspected. Therapy should be selected the basis of the suspected pathogens; however, antimicrobial therapy alone is insufficient, especially in the setting of diffuse peritonitis. *Source control* is a term used to involve all physical measures needed to eradicate an infection, such as debridement of necrotic tissue or drainage of an abscess or fluid collection. If adequate source control is delayed, bacteremia, multiple organ failure, and mortality are more likely to occur.[2]

Normal Gastrointestinal Flora

The stomach of fasting individuals contains very few bacteria (i.e., <100 colony-forming units [CFU]/mL) as a result of gastric motility and the bactericidal activity of normal acidic gastric fluid.[1] The bacterial population of the stomach can be altered by drugs or diseases that increase gastric pH or decrease gastric motility. Not surprisingly, patients with bleeding or obstructing duodenal ulcers, gastric ulcers, gastric carcinomas, or those receiving proton pump inhibitors or histamine-2 receptor antagonists have an increased number of oral bacteria colonizing the stomach.

The upper small intestine (duodenum and jejunum) usually contains relatively few bacteria and harbors mainly oral flora. The lower small intestine serves as a transitional zone between the sparsely populated stomach and the abundant microbial flora of the colon.[3,4]

In the ileum, facultative gram-negative and gram-positive species, as well as obligate anaerobes, are encountered. As the distal ileum is approached, the quantity and variety of bacteria increase. Substantial numbers of anaerobic bacteria are present, including *Bacteroides* species, as well as *Escherichia coli* and *Enterococcus* species.[1,3]

In the large bowel, anaerobic bacteria, particularly *Bacteroides* species, predominate. In the distal colon, bacterial counts average 10^{10} CFU/mL of feces, with anaerobes outnumbering other organisms by a ratio of 1,000 to 10,000:1.[3] Among the facultative aerobes, *E. coli* is the most frequently isolated species.[1,3] Given these differences in regional microflora populations, it is not surprising that trauma to the colon carries a much higher risk of intra-abdominal infection in comparison with the stomach or jejunum[5] (Fig. 70-1; Table 70-1).

Resistant flora are more common in health care–associated infections, including *Pseudomonas aeruginosa*, *Acinetobacter* species, extended-spectrum β-lactamases (ESBLs) and carbapenemase producing *E. coli* and *Klebsiella* species, methicillin-resistant *Staphylococcus aureus* (MRSA), enterococci, and *Candida* species.[6–10]

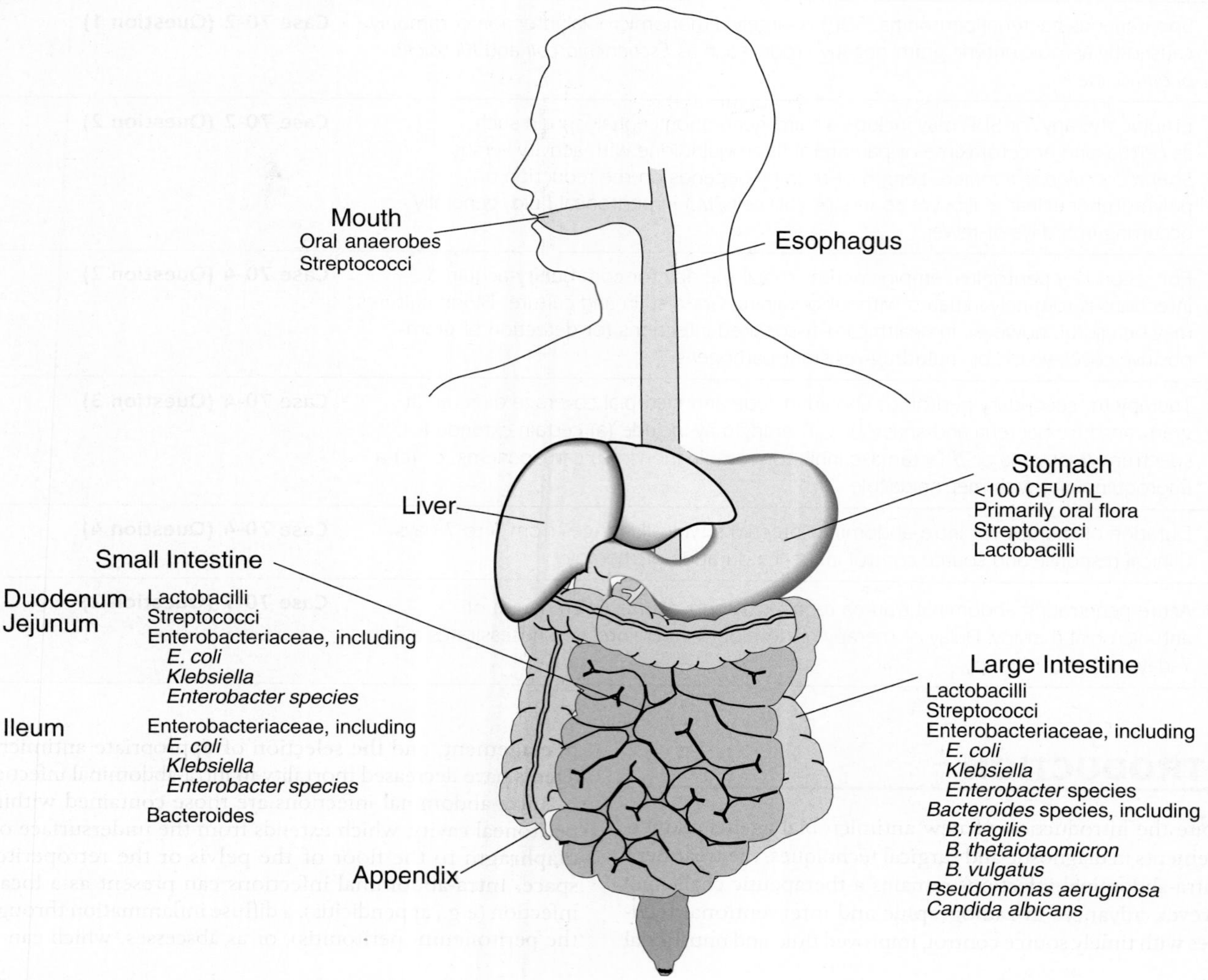

Figure 70-1 Microflora of the gastrointestinal tract.

Table 70-1
Common Pathogens in Intra-Abdominal Infection

Disease	Common Pathogens	Comments
Cholecystitis, cholangitis	*E. coli*, *Klebsiella pneumoniae*, *Enterococcus*, and anaerobes	*Enterococcus* species and anaerobes are less frequently isolated, but they have been associated with nosocomial infections and chronic surgical infections, particularly in patients receiving broad-spectrum antimicrobials.
Primary peritonitis	*E. coli*, *K. pneumoniae*, *Streptococcus pneumoniae*, occasional anaerobes	Also known as spontaneous bacterial peritonitis presented in cirrhotic patients. Often monomicrobial. Anaerobes less likely than aerobes.
Secondary peritonitis	*E. coli*, *Bacteroides fragilis*, *Enterococcus*, and anaerobes	Generally polymicrobial with both aerobic and anaerobic pathogens. *Enterococcus* species should be considered in the setting of health care–associated infections.
Chronic ambulatory peritoneal dialysis	*Staphylococcus epidermidis*, *Staphylococcus aureus*, diphtheroids, gram-negative rods	Dwell time of exchange with intraperitoneal antibiotics must be a minimum of 6 hours.

INFECTIONS OF THE BILIARY TRACT

Cholecystitis and Cholangitis

Cholecystitis and cholangitis originate as inflammatory conditions, usually as a result of obstruction in the gallbladder or common bile duct. The obstruction is typically caused by the presence of stones. The biliary tract is sterile under normal conditions, and the flow of bile, along with its bacteriostatic properties, functions to maintain the sterility. Infection typically occurs as a secondary event to obstruction.[4,5]

Acute cholecystitis is the acute inflammation of the gallbladder. The presence of gallstones in greater than 90% of cases prevents the outflow of gallbladder drainage by obstructing the neck of the gallbladder, Hartmann's pouch, or the cystic duct.[4] The obstruction causes an increase in intraluminal pressure, gallbladder distension, and edema, which triggers an acute inflammatory response. The potential consequences of this obstruction and inflammation include infection, ischemia, perforation, and necrosis.[4,11] The reduction in gallbladder outflow leads to biliary stasis, which provides an ideal environment for bacterial proliferation and subsequent infection (Fig. 70-2).

Acute cholangitis is an acute inflammation of the common bile duct. The most common cause of cholangitis in the United States is common bile duct obstruction as a consequence of choledocholithiasis. Less common causes include neoplastic obstruction, postoperative obstruction after biliary intervention, benign strictures, and primary sclerosing cholangitis.[4] The decrease in biliary outflow results in biliary stasis and bacterial proliferation. Infection results in a rapid rise in biliary pressure, which facilitates the spread of bacteria into lymphatics and the bloodstream via alterations in membrane permeability. In comparison with cholecystitis, acute cholangitis generally carries a poorer prognosis.[4,12]

CLINICAL PRESENTATION AND DIAGNOSIS

CASE 70-1

QUESTION 1: D.S., a 54-year-old man, presents to the hospital with a 1-week history of abdominal pain and tenderness, localized to the right upper quadrant, fever of 38.9°C, and chills. He complains of nausea, with three episodes of emesis occurring in the past 24 hours. D.S. appears jaundiced and reports dark-colored urine. His laboratory values are the following:

White blood cell (WBC) count, $17 \times 10^3/\mu L$
Serum creatinine (SCr), 1.1 mg/dL
Total bilirubin, 6 mg/dL
Alkaline phosphatase, 270 U/L

What evidence of cholangitis exists in D.S.? How does the presentation of cholecystitis differ from cholangitis?

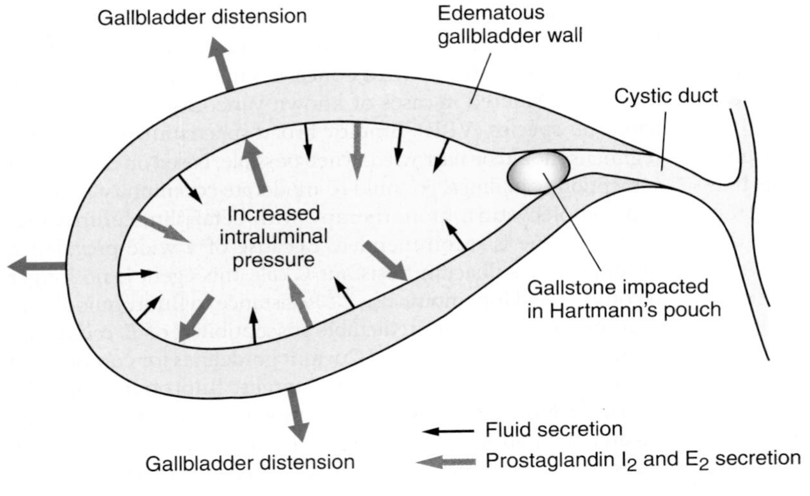

Figure 70-2 Pathogenesis of acute cholecystitis.

The clinical manifestations of acute cholangitis vary, but the classic presentation involves Charcot's triad, which consists of fever, jaundice, and right upper quadrant abdominal pain. Fever is present in 90% of cases, and jaundice and abdominal pain occur in 60% to 70% of cases.[4] A smaller percentage of patients, generally with gram-negative septicemia, may present with changes in mental status and hypotension.[4] Laboratory findings of acute cholangitis include leukocytosis, elevated bilirubin (>2 mg/dL), and alkaline phosphatase, and mildly elevated liver transaminases.[4,13] The clinical signs and symptoms of cholangitis, as exemplified by D.S., include high fevers (38.9°C), chills, jaundice, and right upper quadrant abdominal pain. Laboratory evidence supportive of cholangitis includes leukocytosis with WBC of $17 \times 10^3/\mu L$, increased bilirubin of 6 mg/dL, and elevated alkaline phosphatase of 270 U/L.

The clinical presentation of acute cholecystitis involves fever and prolonged constant abdominal pain typically localized to the right upper quadrant, followed by nausea and vomiting. On physical examination, tenderness in the right upper quadrant and a positive Murphy's sign (inspiration is inhibited by pain on palpation) are often present.[4,11] Laboratory findings include leukocytosis with increased neutrophils (left shift) and mild elevations in transaminases. Jaundice is less common in patients with cholecystitis (bilirubin <4 mg/dL) compared with cholangitis.[4,11]

Diagnostic imaging for acute cholecystitis and cholangitis involves ultrasonography. Findings for acute cholecystitis may reveal pericholecystic fluid, distension of the gallbladder, thickening of the gallbladder wall, stones, and a sonographic Murphy's sign.[14] Ultrasound is less sensitive for choledocholithiasis, but it may reveal biliary dilation with stones. Hepatobiliary scintigraphy is another diagnostic tool used to identify obstruction of the cystic duct. After intravenous injection with technetium hepatobiliary iminodiacetic acid (Tc-HIDA), failure to observe gallbladder filling suggests acute cholecystitis.[6,14] Computed tomography (CT) imaging may be superior in determining the extent of biliary obstruction.[4] Endoscopic retrograde cholangiopancreatography (ERCP) is an alternative mode of imaging for cholangitis.[4,13]

ETIOLOGY

CASE 70-1, QUESTION 2: What are the most likely organisms causing infection in D.S.? What clinical specimens are helpful to identify the causative pathogen(s)?

The most common pathogens associated with acute cholangitis include *E. coli*, *Klebsiella* species, and *Enterobacter* species. However, *P. aeruginosa*, skin flora (*Staphylococcus* species, *Streptococcus* species), and oropharynx bacteria may be implicated. Anaerobic organisms, commonly *Bacteroides* species, are associated with approximately 15% of infections, particularly in elderly patients undergoing biliary tract surgery.[4,15] The etiology of cholecystitis typically involves *E. coli*, *Klebsiella* species, and *Enterococcus* species. Anaerobes are less commonly isolated (Table 70-1).[4,11]

As described above, the stasis of bile flow results in proliferation of bacteria within the gallbladder or common bile duct. Acute cholangitis results in increased pressure within the common bile duct with dissemination of bacteria from the biliary tree to the bloodstream. Blood cultures may be positive in up to 40% of patients with symptomatic acute cholangitis.[4] Acute cholecystitis may reveal positive bile cultures in 20% to 75% of patients with symptomatic disease, but the utility of bile cultures has yet to be determined.[3] In contrast to cholangitis, bacteremia is unlikely with cholecystitis. The choice of antibacterial agents is largely empiric covering the aforementioned common causative pathogens.

TREATMENT

Definitive therapy for both cholangitis and cholecystitis must involve source control, using surgery, percutaneous drainage, or endoscopic intervention. Empiric antibacterial therapy should be added owing to the likelihood of secondary infection and to prevent complications. Supportive measures include fluid and electrolyte supplementation and analgesia.[4,5,11,13]

To decompress or drain the biliary ductal system in cholangitis, ERCP is used with a success rate of greater than 90% in the treatment of cholangitis.[4] Alternatively, percutaneous transhepatic biliary drainage or endoscopic sphincterotomy can be used to drain the contents. Open surgery is a less favored option to decompress the biliary tree as it is associated with increased mortality.[4] Acute symptomatic cholecystitis requires removal of the gallbladder (cholecystectomy). The procedure of choice is laparoscopic cholecystectomy within 48 to 72 hours of onset of symptoms. Early intervention is associated with decreased morbidity and length of hospital stay compared with delayed surgical intervention.[4,11] In high-risk patients, in whom the risks outweigh the benefits of early surgery, percutaneous cholecystostomy can be performed to drain the contents of the gallbladder. The procedure improves the clinical symptoms in 75% to 90% of patients who cannot undergo surgery. Cholecystectomy, however, should take place once the patient is stable enough for surgery.[4]

ETIOLOGY

CASE 70-1, QUESTION 3: Based on the most likely causative pathogen(s), what empiric antimicrobial therapy is recommended for D.S., given a diagnosis of cholangitis?

Empiric antimicrobial therapy for acute cholangitis and cholecystitis should be initiated after blood cultures have been collected. The empiric choice of therapy should cover enteric gram-negative pathogens, particularly *E. coli* (Table 70-2).[5,6] In general, the addition of anaerobic coverage is not mandatory for cholecystitis; however, it should be considered in the setting of severe cases such as acute cholangitis, biliary-enteric anastomosis, or health care–associated infections.[6] Empiric coverage for *Enterococcus* species should be considered for patients at risk for health care–associated infections, such as immunocompromised patients, patients who have required long-term hospitalization, patients who have received broad-spectrum antimicrobial therapy, or patients with valvular heart disease or prosthetic intravascular materials.[6] Antimicrobial therapy must be guided by drug pharmacokinetics and pharmacodynamics, local resistance patterns, and patient factors, such as drug allergies, renal or hepatic dysfunction, and cost.

Considering their activity versus multidrug-resistant gram-negative bacilli, carbapenems generally should be reserved for infection caused by these pathogens. Vancomycin may be added empirically in health care–associated biliary infections in which ampicillin-resistant enterococci and MRSA are of concern. Linezolid or daptomycin may be considered in cases of known vancomycin-resistant *Enterococcus* species (VRE). Empiric broad-spectrum antimicrobial regimens should be narrowed, when possible, based on culture and susceptibility findings. For mild-to-moderate community-acquired acute cholecystitis, monotherapy with cefazolin, cefuroxime, or ceftriaxone is recommended. Because of a wide prevalence of ampicillin–sulbactam resistant *E. coli*, this agent is no longer recommended for empiric use.[6,15] Resistance to fluoroquinolones is problematic with unpredictable susceptibility of *E. coli* to ciprofloxacin and levofloxacin.[16] Current guidelines for complicated intra-abdominal infections (cIAI) suggest fluoroquinolones be considered for therapy when institutional antibiograms indicate greater than 90% susceptibility of *E. coli*.[6] Use of aminoglycosides is not routinely recommended because of the need for

Table 70-2
Treatment Options for Intra-Abdominal Infections[5,6,66,67]

Infection	Agents and Regimens	Agent Dosing[d]
Mild-to-moderate in severity: Community-acquired perforated or abscessed appendicitis *Or* Acute cholecystitis	**Single agent** Cefoxitin Ertapenem Moxifloxacin[a] Tigecycline **Combination** Cefazolin *Or* Ceftriaxone *Or* Cefotaxime *Or* Ciprofloxacin *Or* Levofloxacin[a] + Metronidazole	Cefoxitin 2 g IV every 6 hours Ertapenem 1 g IV every 24 hours Tigecycline 100 mg initially then 50 mg IV every 12 hours Cefazolin 1–2 g IV every 8 hours Ceftriaxone 1–2 g IV every 12–24 hours Cefotaxime 1–2 g IV every 6–8 hours Ciprofloxacin 400 mg IV every 12 hours Levofloxacin 750 mg IV every 24 hours Moxifloxacin 400 mg IV every 24 hours Metronidazole 500 mg IV every 8–12 hours Cefepime 1-2 g IV every 8 hours and Ceftazidime 1-2 g IV every 8-12 hours Piperacillin–tazobactam 3.375 g IV every 4–6 hours or 4.5 g IV every 6 hours[e]
High risk in severity: Community-acquired acute cholecystitis with severe physiologic disturbance, advanced age, or immunocompromised state Or Acute cholangitis associated with biliary-enteric anastomosis Or Health care–associated intra-abdominal infections	**Single agent** Imipenem–cilastatin Meropenem Doripenem Piperacillin–tazobactam **Combination** Cefepime *Or* Ceftazidime *Or* Ciprofloxacin *Or* Levofloxacin[a] + Metronidazole	Imipenem–cilastatin 500 mg IV every 6 hours or 1 g every 8 hours Meropenem 1 g IV every 8 hours Doripenem 500 mg IV every 8 hours Vancomycin[b] 15–20 mg/kg IV every 8–12 hours (normal renal function) Aztreonam[c] 1–2 g IV every 6–8 hours Ceftazidime/avibactam 2.5 g IV every 8 hours or Ceftolozane/tazobactam 1.5 g IV every 8 hours + Metronidazole 500 mg IV every 8–12 hours

[a]Selection of fluoroquinolones should be based on local antibiogram or susceptibility reports.
[b]May be added to each regimen in the setting of health care–associated intra-abdominal infections (e.g., methicillin-resistant *Staphylococcus aureus* or ampicillin-resistant enterococcal infection).
[c]For patients who are intolerant of β-lactams, aztreonam may be considered as an alternative agent for gram-negative coverage.
[d]normal renal function dosing
[e]Extended infusion: 3.375 g IV every 8 hours over 4 hours
IV, intravenous.

therapeutic drug monitoring and potential nephrotoxicity and ototoxicity.[6] Furthermore, in comparison with other regimens, aminoglycoside-based regimens are inferior in the treatment of intra-abdominal infections.[17] However, some argue the decreased efficacy of aminoglycosides has been caused by inadequate dosing. An appropriate empiric regimen for D.S. would be piperacillin–tazobactam 3.375 g intravenously (IV) every 6 hours.

BILIARY CONCENTRATIONS

CASE 70-1, QUESTION 4: The physician caring for D.S. questions the need for an antibiotic that concentrates in the bile. Is there a benefit to using an antibiotic that is extensively excreted into bile?

Common bile duct obstruction prevents the entry of antibiotics into the bile, and the need for high biliary concentrations of antibiotics in the treatment of cholangitis has been debated.[18] Nagar and Berger[19] concluded that a number of antibiotics with excellent in-vitro susceptibility, but poor biliary excretion, are still clinically effective. Biliary antibacterial concentrations do not correlate with an improved clinical outcome.[4] Highly biliary-excreted versus moderately biliary-excreted antibiotics have been compared.[18] Serum concentrations are more important than biliary levels in reducing the septic complications of biliary tract surgery. Furthermore, biliary excretion of any antibiotic is minimal in the presence of obstruction.[18]

The treatment of D.S.'s biliary tract infection must include biliary drainage. Piperacillin–tazobactam should be continued for 4 to 7 days.

PRIMARY PERITONITIS

Peritonitis is inflammation of the peritoneum as a result of infectious or chemical inflammation within the peritoneal cavity.[3,20] Infectious peritonitis can be classified as primary, secondary, or tertiary. Primary peritonitis involves the development of infection in the peritoneal cavity in the absence of intra-abdominal pathology.[20,21] Secondary peritonitis classically results from contamination of the peritoneum with gastrointestinal (GI) or genitourinary microorganisms as a result of the loss of mucosal barrier integrity. Tertiary peritonitis is clinical peritonitis along with signs of sepsis and multi-organ dysfunction persisting or recurring after the treatment of secondary peritonitis.[3,20]

Primary peritonitis is also known as spontaneous bacterial peritonitis (SBP) and is most frequently identified in adults with cirrhosis and ascites. Nearly 10% to 30% of hospitalized patients with cirrhosis and ascites have SBP.[3,21,22] Primary peritonitis is associated with post-necrotic cirrhosis, chronic acute hepatitis, acute viral hepatitis, congestive heart failure, metastatic malignancy, or systemic lupus erythematosus.[3,20]

Spontaneous Bacterial Peritonitis in Cirrhotic Patients

CLINICAL MANIFESTATIONS AND DIAGNOSIS

Patients with SBP may present with fever, signs of peritonitis, including abdominal pain, altered mental status, changes in GI motility, nausea, vomiting, diarrhea, or ileus.[22] Fever is common, occurring in 50% to 80% of patients.[3] Some patients have an atypical presentation or even lack symptoms.[22] The diagnosis of SBP is made on clinical presentation and examination of the peritoneal fluid via paracentesis. The ascitic fluid is tested for cell counts with WBC differential, and the presence of microorganisms is based on Gram stain and culture. Ascitic fluid with an elevated polymorphonuclear (PMN) count ($\geq$250/μL) is diagnostic for SBP.[22]

ETIOLOGY AND PATHOGENESIS

CASE 70-2

QUESTION 1: M.W., a 51-year-old man with alcoholic cirrhosis and significant abdominal ascites, presents with a 4-day history of fever of 38.4°C and abdominal pain. Ascitic fluid obtained by paracentesis was cloudy, and culture of the ascitic fluid is pending. Laboratory values include ascitic fluid PMN count, 450/μL; serum WBC count, 12.2 × 10^3/μL; and total bilirubin, 4.4 mg/dL. What organisms are likely to be cultured from M.W.'s ascitic fluid?

An estimated 70% of cases of SBP are caused by aerobic enteric organisms considered normal flora of the GI tract.[22] *E. coli* is the most common pathogen, followed by *K. pneumoniae*.[3] Other common causes of SBP include *Streptococcus pneumoniae* and other *Streptococcus* species, accounting for 20% of cases. *Enterococcus* species are isolated in approximately 5% of cases.[22] *Staphylococcus* species, anaerobes, and microaerophilic organisms are rarely reported in community-acquired SBP. SBP is largely a monomicrobial infection.

One of the main mechanisms of pathogenesis associated with the development of SBP is bacterial translocation, which is the migration of microorganisms through the GI wall to mesenteric lymph nodes and other structures outside the intestine, including the bloodstream. Bacteria then infect the ascitic fluid by hematogenous or lymphogenous spread.[22,23] Certain characteristics of cirrhotic patients facilitate the pathogenesis of SBP, including bacterial overgrowth, decreased motility, structural intestinal damage, and decreased host-defense mechanisms that normally function to eliminate microorganisms. Bacterial overgrowth in the face of decreased motility and increased gut wall permeability, secondary to structural damage, facilitates subsequent systemic infection. Reduced opsonic activity and phagocytosis allow the microorganisms to escape the hosts' defenses and subsequently infect the ascitic fluid.[23] SBP with underlying cirrhosis was previously associated with a greater than 90% mortality rate, but with the advances in antibacterial therapy the rate has been reduced to approximately 30% to 40%.[3,22] Gram-negative pathogens are associated with increased mortality compared with gram-positive pathogens.[3] Early diagnosis and effective antibacterial treatment of SBP are associated with reduced rates of mortality.[24] Patient characteristics associated with increased mortality include renal insufficiency, hypothermia, hyperbilirubinemia, and hypoalbuminemia. To decrease the rate of renal dysfunction associated with SBP, intravenous albumin at 1.5 g/kg within 6 hours of diagnosis and 1 g/kg on day 3 may be administered. Albumin acts as a volume expander to lessen hemodynamic changes, thereby preserving renal function. Albumin is recommended in patients with a serum creatinine >1 mg/dL, blood urea nitrogen (BUN) >30 mg/dL, or total bilirubin >4 mg/dL.[22]

ANTIMICROBIAL THERAPY

CASE 70-2, QUESTION 2: Pending ascitic fluid culture results, what empiric antimicrobial therapy should be recommended for M.W.? What is an appropriate duration of therapy, and how should the response to therapy be monitored?

Although a positive Gram stain and culture guides antibacterial therapy, nearly 60% of patients with signs and symptoms of SBP have negative cultures.[3,24] Initial antibacterial therapy for patients with a diagnosis of SBP is typically empiric and targeted toward the most likely pathogens as described previously. Ampicillin plus an aminoglycoside was the traditional choice for empiric therapy; however, third-generation cephalosporins (cefotaxime and ceftriaxone) represent safer, more-effective options.[25,26] A fluoroquinolone may be considered an alternative in patients with β-lactam allergies. Levofloxacin and moxifloxacin are preferred over ciprofloxacin, because of their superior activity against *S. pneumoniae*, the most commonly isolated gram-positive bacterial pathogen. Although parenteral therapy is preferred, oral fluoroquinolones may be as effective in patients with uncomplicated SBP.[25] As described earlier, aminoglycosides are not recommended in cirrhotic SBP therapy because of the risk of nephrotoxicity, and the decision whether or not to use fluoroquinolones should be based on institutional antibiogram reports.[22]

Antibiotic therapy is recommended until the PMN count from the ascitic fluid falls below 250 cells/μL, which normally occurs within 5 days.[24] França et al.[27] concluded that a 5-day course of cefotaxime for the treatment of SBP was as effective as a 10-day course.

M.W. should receive empiric therapy with an antimicrobial agent effective against *E. coli* and other common pathogens such as *Klebsiella* species and *S. pneumoniae*. Any of the above-mentioned options would be reasonable empiric choices.

PROPHYLAXIS

CASE 70-2, QUESTION 3: After treatment is completed, should prophylactic antimicrobial therapy be initiated in M.W.?

Recurrence rates for SBP are high. Cirrhotic patients who survive an episode of SBP have a 1-year recurrence rate of nearly 70%. Antibiotic prophylaxis should be administered to the following patients since they are considered high risk for the development of SBP: patients who have had one or more episodes of SBP; cirrhotic patients with gastrointestinal bleeding; cirrhotic patients with ascites, who have impaired renal or liver function; or cirrhotic patients with a low ascitic protein (<1.0 g/dL) or elevated serum bilirubin (>2.5 mg/dL).[22]

Antibiotic prophylaxis in cirrhotic patients is typically initiated to provide selective decontamination of the GI tract. The goal of this therapy is to reduce the burden of bacteria and subsequently prevent bacterial translocation and infection.[22] Prospective, randomized studies in cirrhotic subjects with ascites support the use of oral antibacterial agents to reduce the rate of recurrence. The agents studied include oral norfloxacin,[28] ciprofloxacin,[29] and trimethoprim–sulfamethoxazole.[30] Rifaximin, a nonabsorbable derivative of rifamycin, has also been shown to significantly reduce the occurrence of SBP.[31] Long-term prophylaxis is recommended based on the significant reduction in rates of recurrence in clinical trials. Long-term prophylaxis in patients with low ascitic protein, elevated bilirubin, or both may also be beneficial, but it has not been associated with decreased overall infection or mortality and, therefore, is not uniformly recommended.[22,23,28–30] Clinical trials have provided evidence to support the use of short-course therapy (7 days) of norfloxacin (no longer available in the United States) or ceftriaxone in cirrhotic patients presenting with GI hemorrhage.[23,32] Prophylactic therapy prevents bacterial infection and reduces the risk of rebleeding.[23] Several cost analyses have been performed demonstrating that prophylactic therapy in high-risk groups of cirrhotic patients is cost-effective.[23]

Because rates of fluoroquinolone-resistant and trimethoprim–sulfamethoxazole–resistant organisms are more prevalent in patients who receive long-term prophylactic therapy, its long-term use must be considered when initiating antibacterial therapy for the treatment of new infections in this patient population.[33,34]

M.W. has cirrhosis, a previous episode of SBP, and a high total bilirubin; thus, he is at high risk for recurrence. Prophylactic antimicrobial therapy should be considered and may be a cost-effective measure. M.W. would benefit from ciprofloxacin 500 mg PO daily. The use of trimethoprim–sulfamethoxazole would depend on local resistance patterns.

Continuous Ambulatory Peritoneal Dialysis–Associated Peritonitis

PATHOGENESIS AND CLINICAL PRESENTATION

CASE 70-3

QUESTION 1: H.M., a 33-year-old woman with HIV and end-stage renal disease, has undergone continuous ambulatory peritoneal dialysis (CAPD) daily for the past year. She presents with abdominal pain and a cloudy dialysate fluid. H.M. has negligible residual urine output. What are the most common causative organisms related to CAPD-associated peritonitis? What empiric antimicrobial therapy should be initiated? How should antimicrobial agents be administered?

Following SBP, peritoneal dialysis is another cause of primary peritonitis. An estimated 45% of patients undergoing CAPD will experience at least one episode of peritonitis in the first 6 months of dialysis. Approximately 60% to 70% of patients exhibit peritonitis during the first year of dialysis, and recurrent infection occurs in 20% to 30% of patients.[3] CAPD-associated peritonitis is theorized to originate from contamination of the catheter by organisms of the normal skin flora, contamination of the peritoneum from an exit-site or subcutaneous-tunnel infection, contamination of the dialysate fluid, or bacterial translocation.[3] Alterations in host defenses of the peritoneum may also have a role in the development of CAPD-associated peritonitis.[3]

Clinical manifestations of CAPD-associated peritonitis include abdominal pain and tenderness, which is observed in 60% to 80% of patients. Nausea and vomiting occur in approximately 30% of patients, whereas 10% will have diarrhea and 10% to 20% will present with fever. The diagnosis of peritonitis is made on the basis of clinical signs and symptoms along with examination of the dialysate fluid for cell counts, Gram stain, and culture. Characteristically, the dialysate fluid will be cloudy and have a WBC count greater than 100 cells/μL with a neutrophilic predominance (at least 50%).[35] The Gram stain may be negative in 5% to 10% of cases, and blood cultures are typically negative.[3] In most cases, peritonitis is commonly caused by a single organism.[36]

ETIOLOGY

The most common causative organisms are gram-positive bacteria, accounting for 60% to 80% of isolates. Coagulase-negative *Staphylococcus* species (*S. epidermidis*) are the most common causative organisms, followed by *S. aureus* and *Streptococcus* species. Gram-negative bacilli are isolated in approximately 15% to 30% of cases, with *E. coli* being the most common. Other common gram-negative organisms include *Klebsiella* species, *Enterobacter* species, *Proteus* species, and *P. aeruginosa*. Anaerobes, fungi, and mycobacteria constitute the less commonly encountered pathogens.[3]

ANTIMICROBIAL THERAPY

In general, empiric antibiotic therapy should be directed against the most common causative organisms, both gram-positive and gram-negative, until cultures of peritoneal fluid are available. Intraperitoneal (IP) delivery of antibacterial agents is the preferred route of administration for the treatment of CAPD-associated peritonitis. The IP route provides very high local concentrations of antibacterial agents as well as the ability to avoid a venipuncture and allow the patient to self-administer therapy at home.[35]

Empiric IP administration of antibiotics should be administered when CAPD-associated peritonitis is suspected. When culture and susceptibility results are available, antibacterial therapy should be adjusted as necessary. With appropriate therapy, a clinical response should be expected within the first 48 hours.[35]

Treatment guidelines for CAPD-associated peritonitis provide a systematic approach for antimicrobial selection, dosing guidelines, and duration of therapy. Initial IP therapy recommendations include vancomycin or a first-generation cephalosporin for gram-positive coverage plus an antibacterial agent with antipseudomonal coverage.[35] Because of the increasing rates of MRSA and methicillin-resistant *S. epidermidis*, vancomycin may be the most appropriate initial therapy for gram-positive organisms, although cefazolin remains effective in certain geographical areas.[36–38] Gram-negative therapy options include ceftazidime, cefepime, piperacillin–tazobactam, or a carbapenem.[35,39] For patients who are intolerant of β-lactams, aztreonam may be considered as an alternative agent for gram-negative coverage.[35,39] Fluoroquinolones represent an option for CAPD-associated peritonitis given the extent of distribution into the peritoneal cavity; however, oral therapy should not be used in severe cases of peritonitis. The increasing prevalence of fluoroquinolone-resistant gram-negative *E. coli*, however, is decreasing the utility of these agents.[40,41]

Refractory peritonitis, presence of cloudy effluent after 5 days of IP therapy, may require removal of the catheter, suggesting an exit-site or tunnel infection. Oral antibiotic therapy, or intravenous therapy if severe, may be required for cases involving *S. aureus* or *P. aeruginosa*. When *S. aureus* is isolated, the infection usually necessitates the removal of the dialysis catheter. Vancomycin is recommended for MRSA (with or without rifampin) for 1 week, although monotherapy with vancomycin is adequate, particularly if the infected catheter is removed. Conversely, cefazolin alone is adequate for MSSA. Coagulase-negative *Staphylococcus* species do not require prompt catheter removal as they typically respond well to antimicrobial therapy. Methicillin resistance is common for *S. epidermidis*; thus, vancomycin is normally used. *Enterococcus* species or *Streptococcus* species should be treated with ampicillin if susceptible. Vancomycin should be used for ampicillin-resistant enterococcus; however, VRE require treatment with linezolid, quinupristin–dalfopristin, or daptomycin. In the case of culture-negative peritonitis and clinical improvement after 3 days of empiric coverage, a single agent directed toward gram-positive organisms may be continued for a total of 2 weeks.[35]

When a single gram-negative organism is cultured (e.g., *E. coli*, *Klebsiella* species, or *Proteus* species), therapy can be narrowed based on susceptibility. Isolation of *P. aeruginosa* most often indicates a severe infection, which may also involve the dialysis catheter. Therapy options include an antipseudomonal β-lactam such as ceftazidime, cefepime, or piperacillin–tazobactam with or without a fluoroquinolone or an aminoglycoside. In general, the β-lactam antimicrobials achieve peritoneal fluid concentrations exceeding typical minimum inhibitory concentrations for most commonly encountered facultative gram-negative and anaerobic bacteria.[35,42,43]

Aztreonam can be used in the case of severe immunoglobulin E (IgE)-mediated penicillin allergy. Polymicrobial peritonitis is uncommon and may indicate a more complicated intra-abdominal

Table 70-3
Intraperitoneal Antibiotic Dosing Recommendations for CAPD Patients

		Continuous Dosing[b] (mg/L)	
	Intermittent Dosing[a]	LD	MD
Amikacin	2 mg/kg	25	12
Amoxicillin		250–500	50
Amphotericin			1.5
Ampicillin			125
Ampicillin–sulbactam	2 g every 12 hours	1,000	100
Aztreonam		1,000	250
Cefazolin	15 mg/kg	500	125
Cefepime	1,000 mg	500	125
Ceftazidime	1,000–1,500 mg	500	125
Ceftizoxime	1,000 mg	250	125
Ciprofloxacin		50	25
Daptomycin	40 mg every 4 hours	100	20
Fluconazole	200 mg every 24–28 hours		
Gentamicin	0.6 mg/kg	8	4
Imipenem–cilastatin	1 g twice daily	250	50
Levofloxacin	500 mg PO every 48 hours[c]		
Linezolid	200–300 mg PO daily		
Meropenem	500–1,000 mg daily		
Nafcillin			125
Oxacillin			125
Penicillin G		50,000 units	25,000 units
Polymixin B	150,000 units (IV) every 12 hours		
Quinupristin–dalfopristin	25 mg/L in alternate bags[d]		
Tobramycin	0.6 mg/kg	8	4
Vancomycin	15–30 mg/kg every 5–7 days	1,000	25

Empiric doses for patients with residual renal function (>100 mL/day urine output) should be increased by 25%.
[a]Per exchange, once daily.
[b]All exchanges.
[c]Oral levofloxacin is recommended to be given with weekly IP vancomycin in centers with low fluoroquinolone resistance.
[d]Given in conjunction with 500 mg IV twice daily.
CAPD, continuous ambulatory peritoneal dialysis; LD, loading dose; MD, maintenance dose; IV, intravenous.
Sources: Li PK et al. Peritoneal dialysis-related infections recommendations: 2010 update. *Perit Dial Int.* 2010;30:393.
Gilmore et al. Treatment of enterococcal peritonitis with intraperitoneal daptomycin in a vancomycin-allergic patient and a review of the literature. *Perit Dial Int.* 2013;33(4):353–357.

process. Table 70-3 lists antimicrobial dosing guidelines for the treatment of peritonitis associated with CAPD.[44]

An example of an appropriate regimen for H.M. may include vancomycin plus cefepime or an aminoglycoside given intraperitoneally. The clinician should monitor culture and sensitivity results to adjust therapy based on guidelines, local sensitivity patterns, and therapeutic response.

FUNGAL CAPD-ASSOCIATED PERITONITIS

CASE 70-3, QUESTION 2: Two years later, H.M. presents with abdominal pain and cloudy dialysate fluid. *Candida albicans* is cultured from the dialysate fluid. No other organisms are present. How should H.M. be treated?

Fungal peritonitis is a rare complication of CAPD that is associated with significant morbidity and mortality. The rate of mortality in fungal peritonitis is approximately 25%.[35] Considering the high rate of failure of therapy, CAPD patients with fungal peritonitis should have their catheters removed.[37] Patients who have received prolonged or multiple courses of antibiotics, are on immunosuppressant therapy for a malignancy, transplant, or inflammatory disease, or have a postoperative or recurrent intra-abdominal infection are at increased risk for fungal peritonitis and should be treated with antibiotics.[3,5,45] Most cases are caused by *Candida* species, most commonly *C. albicans*; however, an increase in infection attributable to non-albicans species has emerged in many areas.[45] Empiric antifungal therapy should be broad and include most *Candida* species; echinocandins such as caspofungin, micafungin, or anidulafungin are the empiric drugs of choice. Amphotericin B may be administered intravenously (IV) or IP, but when given IP, conventional amphotericin B is very irritating to the peritoneum.[35] The azole antifungal agents can be administered orally, IV, or IP. Fluconazole is active against *C. albicans*, but it has dose-dependent activity against certain types of non-albicans species, such as *Candida glabrata*. In general, fluconazole is the drug of choice for *C. albicans*; however, other options, such as a polyene or echinocandin, may be needed for azole-resistant *Candida* species. Therapy should continue for a minimum of 2 weeks after catheter removal, and the total duration may be based on severity and clinical response.[35]

H.M.'s treatment should include temporary catheter removal and administration of antifungal agents. Antifungal therapy with oral fluconazole 400 mg daily should be continued for at least 14 days.

SECONDARY PERITONITIS

Pathogenesis and Epidemiology

Secondary peritonitis usually occurs after fecal or urinary contamination of the peritoneal cavity or its surrounding structures.[2] The process leading to an infection commonly includes an acute perforation associated with appendicitis, diverticulitis, the uterus, neoplasm, and inflammatory bowel disease (IBD). Secondary peritonitis can also result from postoperative or posttraumatic perforation of the GI or genitourinary tract related to blunt trauma or ingestion of foreign material.[46,47]

Localization of infection without eradication of bacteria results in intraperitoneal or visceral abscesses. Intraperitoneal abscesses occur most often in the right lower quadrant in association with appendicitis or a perforated peptic ulcer. Other causes can include diverticulitis, pancreatitis, IBD, trauma, and abdominal surgery. Visceral abscesses generally are found in the pancreas but may also occur in the liver, spleen, or kidney.[3]

Mortality with secondary peritonitis can be as high as 68%.[48] Timely source control with surgical intervention is imperative for clinical success of infections resulting from secondary peritonitis. Management with appropriate antimicrobial therapy, intensive care support, and the overall health of the patient are also critical for the outcome.[47]

Clinical Presentation and Diagnosis

CASE 70-4

QUESTION 1: R.C., a 48-year-old man, presents with severe abdominal pain and nausea. He states he has been taking nonsteroidal anti-inflammatory drugs (NSAIDs) for joint pain over the last 2 weeks. An esophagogastroduodenoscopy reveals a perforated peptic ulcer. Vital signs include temperature of 38.7°C and tachycardia (pulse, 105 beats/minute). Bowel sounds are absent. Laboratory values are WBC count, 16.5 × $10^3/\mu L$ and BUN, 34 mg/dL. What signs and symptoms of secondary peritonitis does R.C. display?

Making the diagnosis of a localized intra-abdominal infection may be difficult, despite the presence of signs and symptoms typical of severe infection. Moderate-to-severe abdominal pain with anorexia, nausea, and vomiting are commonly experienced. Fevers with or without chills, tachycardia, sparse urination secondary to fluid loss into the peritoneum, faint or absent bowel sounds, and abdominal distention may accompany primary GI symptoms associated with peritonitis. Inflammation around the intestines and peritoneal cavity results in local paralysis and reflex rigidity of the abdominal wall muscles and the diaphragm, causing rapid and shallow respirations.[3] These signs usually are accompanied by an elevated WBC count with a predominance of neutrophils (left shift). The hematocrit (Hct) and BUN may be elevated as a result of dehydration. Initially, patients are usually alkalotic owing to emesis and hyperventilation, but in the later stages of peritonitis, acidosis usually occurs. Untreated or partially treated peritonitis can result in generalized sepsis and hypovolemic shock, in addition to, a gradual development of intraperitoneal abscesses. Therefore, patients with a sudden turn in disposition after treatment and recovery from peritonitis or abdominal surgery should be assessed for intraperitoneal abscess formation.[2,3]

R.C. is likely to have a community-acquired intra-abdominal infection suggestive of a secondary peritonitis resulting from an acute perforated peptic ulcer after using an NSAID for 2 weeks. His current clinical status is highlighted by complaints of severe abdominal pain and nausea, fever with tachycardia, a significant elevation in WBC, and signs of dehydration with a BUN of 34 mg/dL.

CASE 70-4, QUESTION 2: Given these findings, what are the most likely pathogens for R.C.'s secondary peritonitis?

ETIOLOGY

The normal flora consistent with the perforated segment of the GI tract determines the most likely pathogens, consisting of both aerobes and anaerobes the more distal the source.[49] In general, the stomach and small bowel consist of few microbes, such as *Candida* species, lactobacilli, and oral streptococci, in the fasting state. However, the number and variety of gastric microbiota can increase with meals, achlorhydria (use of histamine [H2] blockers or proton pump inhibitors), obstruction, and presence of blood.[3] The most common facultative bacterium is *E. coli*, which is found in approximately 50% of cultures. A variety of other facultative gram-negative bacteria include *Klebsiella* species, *P. aeruginosa*, *Proteus* species, and *Enterobacter* species (Table 70-4).[2,50–53] The presence of anaerobic bacteria in the culture is indicative of a polymicrobial infection with a predictable group of pathogens.[2,33,50–53] *E. coli*, enterococci, and a predominant presence of obligate anaerobes, including *Bacteroides fragilis*, *P. melaninogenica*, *Peptococcus* species, *Peptostreptococcus* species, and *Fusobacterium* species, are found in the ileum and colon of the large bowel. *B. fragilis* is the most frequently isolated obligate anaerobe after perforation of the colon.[3,54] Anaerobic cocci (*Peptostreptococcus*) and facultative gram-positive cocci, such as streptococci, are also isolated.[3,6,51,54] *Enterococcus* species

Table 70-4
Bacteriology of Intra-Abdominal Infections[1,44–47,49]

Bacteria	Patients (%)
Facultative and aerobic gram-negatives	
Escherichia coli[a]	71
Klebsiella species	14
Pseudomonas aeruginosa	14
Proteus mirabilis	5
Enterobacter species	5
Anaerobes	
Bacteroides fragilis[a]	35
Other *Bacteroides* species	71
Clostridium species	29
Prevotella species	12
Peptostreptococcus species	17
Fusobacterium species	9
Eubacterium species	17
Aerobic gram-positives	
Streptococcus species	38
Enterococcus faecalis	12
Enterococcus faecium	3
Staphylococcus aureus	4

[a]Most common in community-acquired intra-abdominal infections.

 are isolated less frequently.[3,6,51,54] *B. fragilis* and *E. coli* are the most common pathogens found in blood culture samples after bacteremia related to an intra-abdominal infection.[3] Highly antibiotic-resistant strains of *P. aeruginosa*, Enterobacteriaceae producing ESBLs or carbapenemases, *Acinetobacter* species, and *Enterococcus*, as well as *Candida* species, are often isolated from hospitalized patients who experience secondary peritonitis.[3,6]

Gram stain and culture do not need to be routinely obtained in community-acquired intra-abdominal infections before the initiation of antimicrobial therapy. It may be useful in health care–associated infections for detection of gram-positive cocci, yeast or multidrug-resistant pathogens.[3,6] The presence of pleomorphic gram-negative bacilli, a strong odor, or tissue gas is strongly suggestive of infection with anaerobes, particularly *B. fragilis*.

R.C.'s secondary peritonitis is likely because of the presence of a facultative gram-negative bacteria, such as *E. coli*, *Proteus*, *Klebsiella*, or *Enterobacter* or possibly an obligate anaerobe, such as *B. fragilis*. R.C. does not present with a history of hospitalization or recent receipt of broad-spectrum antimicrobials; therefore, an infection caused by more resistant health care–associated pathogens (e.g., *P. aeruginosa*, ESBLs, carbapenemases) is less likely.

CASE 70-4, QUESTION 3: How should R.C. be treated? On the basis of clinical studies, what empiric antimicrobial therapy is appropriate for R.C. at this time?

Antimicrobial Therapy

EMPIRIC THERAPY

Therapy for secondary peritonitis should include early administration of antimicrobial agents directed at facultative gram-negative bacteria and obligate anaerobes, fluid therapy, and support of vital organ function, as well as source control measures. Antibiotics should be administered within 1 hour of presentation of septic shock and within 8 hours after hospital admission in those with stable hemodynamic or organ status.[6] Adequate source control involving surgical debridement and drainage, in conjunction with appropriate antimicrobial therapy, decreases morbidity and mortality.[2,3,55] In general, when an intra-abdominal infection is present, antimicrobial agents should be started immediately after appropriate specimens (e.g., blood, peritoneal fluid) have been obtained and before any surgical procedures are performed.[2,3,6,56] The parenteral route should be used to ensure adequate systemic and tissue concentrations, especially in patients in whom shock or poor perfusion of the muscles or GI tract precludes the use of oral administration. Table 70-2 outlines dosing recommendations for antibiotics commonly used in the treatment of intra-abdominal infections.

For mild-to-moderate community-acquired infections, empiric monotherapy with ertapenem, moxifloxacin, tigecycline, or cefoxitin is recommended. Moxifloxacin has good coverage against gram-positive and gram-negative aerobic organisms (excluding *P. aeruginosa*), in addition to anaerobic organisms, and penetrates well into inflamed GI tissue, peritoneal exudates, and abscesses.[53,57,58] Earlier concerns for resistance among *Bacteroides* species to moxifloxacin were reevaluated in recent studies and found moxifloxacin to be a safe and effective monotherapy option for mild-to-moderate community-acquired cIAI.[6,51,59,60] However, moxifloxacin should be used cautiously in infections with recent fluoroquinolone use. Tigecycline offers added in-vitro activity against resistant pathogens such as MRSA, VRE, and penicillin-resistant *S. pneumoniae*; however, tigecycline lacks activity against *Proteus* species and *P. aeruginosa*. Caution should be practiced when using tigecycline for severe infections, including cIAI, as the US Food and Drug Administration announced a boxed warning of increased risk for mortality and non-cure rates. Therefore, the use of tigecycline should be considered when alternative antibiotic options are not available. Ertapenem is another monotherapy option for mild-to-moderate community-acquired cIAI. In comparative trials of ertapenem versus piperacillin–tazobactam, the two agents were shown to be similar in efficacy and safety.[61–63] Because monotherapy has been shown to be efficacious in numerous trials, combination therapy is now rarely used. Combination therapy with either a cephalosporin or a fluoroquinolone (ciprofloxacin or levofloxacin) plus metronidazole is also reasonable.[6] For severe community-acquired intra-abdominal infections, meropenem, imipenem–cilastatin, doripenem, and piperacillin–tazobactam are empiric monotherapy options that may be used. An antipseudomonal third- or fourth-generation cephalosporin, fluoroquinolone (ciprofloxacin or levofloxacin), or aztreonam in combination with metronidazole represent alternative options for severe infections.[6,61]

Tertiary peritonitis is described as persistent peritonitis with systemic signs of sepsis even after appropriate management of the infection has been initiated.[3] As a health care–associated infection, tertiary peritonitis often presents in critically ill patients and those immunocompromised where adequate source control may be improbable. With tertiary peritonitis, pathogens can vary from those that are less virulent such as enterococci, including VRE, coagulase-negative *Staphylococcal* species, and *Candida* species to the more resistant health care–associated pathogens with little to no antibiotic options. Empiric use of meropenem, imipenem–cilastatin, doripenem, or piperacillin–tazobactam[6] should be reserved for health care–associated infections in cases of sepsis and presumed or documented multidrug-resistant pathogens. Two new combination antibiotics, ceftolozane/tazobactam and ceftazidime/avibactam, both used with metronidazole, were recently approved for cIAI (Table 70-2).[64,65] Ceftolozane/tazobactam and ceftazidime/avibactam offer in-vitro activity against challenging resistant gram-negative pathogens, including ESBLs and AmpC-producing *Enterobacteriaceae* and multi-drug resistant *P. aeruginosa*. Ceftazidime/avibactam also has in-vitro activity against *K. pneumoniae* carbapenemases.[66,67]

Empiric use of ampicillin–sulbactam is no longer recommended for complicated intra-abdominal infections because of increasing rates of *E. coli* resistance.[6,68] Clindamycin and cefotetan are not recommended for community-acquired cIAI because of rising resistance rates from *B. fragilis*. The association of clindamycin with *Clostridium difficile*–associated diarrhea has also resulted in the use of other options.[6,50,61–63,69,70] With the risk of toxicity when using aminoglycosides, safer agents are now considered first-line treatment options. Fluoroquinolone-resistant *E. coli* has become more common in the community. Caution should be taken when using fluorquinolones empirically, particularly if hospital antibiograms indicate <90% susceptibility of *E. coli*.[6] Susceptibility patterns within the community and institutional antibiograms may assist with selection of optimal empiric antimicrobials when managing community-acquired cIAIs.

R.C. should receive antimicrobial therapy with activity against facultative gram-negative bacteria and anaerobes, including *B. fragilis*. Ertapenem 1 g IV every 24 hours would be an appropriate treatment for R.C.'s mild-to-moderate cIAI.

CASE 70-4, QUESTION 4: How long should R.C. receive antimicrobial therapy?

DURATION OF ANTIMICROBIAL THERAPY

Recommendations for the duration of therapy for intra-abdominal infection vary from 4 to 7 days and depend primarily on the patient's clinical response to therapy and need for surgical drainage.[6] In general, antimicrobial therapy should be continued until resolution of signs of infection takes place, including return of WBC count to normal and elimination of fever.

ENTEROCOCCAL INFECTION

CASE 70-5

QUESTION 1: B.B. is a 58-year-old, non-obese woman with gangrene of the bowel from strangulation. One day after undergoing surgical resection of the duodenum, she has a fever of 38.9°C, shaking chills, and abdominal pain. Laboratory values include a WBC count of $18.4 \times 10^3/\mu L$ and creatinine of 1.1 mg/dL. B.B.'s peritoneal fluid cultures grew *E. coli*, *B. fragilis*, *C. albicans*, and *Enterococcus*. Blood cultures are negative. Should she receive additional antimicrobial therapy active against *Enterococcus*?

Although *Enterococcus* is commonly cultured in patients with secondary peritonitis, its pathogenicity has been questioned. *Enterococcus* can cause serious infections (e.g., endocarditis, urinary tract infections), but it is less virulent in the setting of polymicrobial infections such as intra-abdominal infections.

An important issue is whether empiric treatment should include antibiotics with activity against *Enterococcus*. Some investigators believe that *Enterococcus* species are commensal organisms that need not be treated in most clinical settings. They point to clinical studies in which antibiotic regimens lacking in-vitro activity against *Enterococcus* have been successful. The pathogenicity of *Enterococcus* lies in its ability to enhance the formation of abscesses.[2,3] The presence of enterococci suggests active disease; however, use of anti-enterococcal antibiotics has not shown to improve outcomes.[2,71]

In general, coverage is warranted if *Enterococcus* is present in blood cultures or is the sole organism on culture.[3,6] Anti-enteroccocal therapy is recommended in patients with nosocomial or health care–associated infections,[6] particularly those who received antibiotics selecting for *Enterococcus* spp. (e.g., cephalosporins), are immunocompromised, have postoperative infection, or have valvular heart disease or prosthetic intravascular materials.[6] If susceptible, *Enterococcus* species should be treated with ampicillin or piperacillin/tazobactam. Vancomycin should be reserved for ampicillin-resistant enterococcus, whereas VRE can be treated with linezolid or daptomycin. Because B.B.'s blood cultures are negative and ascitic culture has demonstrated mixed pathogens, *Enterooccus* coverage, specifically VRE, may not be necessary. B.B. should be treated with an antimicrobial regimen that has activity against gram-negative `pathogens, anaerobes and susceptible enterococci for a postoperative infection.

CASE 70-5, QUESTION 2: Should B.B.'s antimicrobial therapy include an agent with antifungal activity?

ANTIFUNGAL THERAPY: TREATMENT OF CANDIDA

The need to treat *Candida* species as a solitary isolate or as part of a polymicrobial infection is controversial. Certainly, *Candida* has the potential to cause peritonitis, IP abscesses, and subsequent candidemia. Mortality resulting from *Candida* peritonitis ranges from 25% to 60%.[72] Risk factors for *Candida* peritonitis have included recurrent abdominal surgery, GI tract perforation, particularly in those untreated within the first 24 hours, surgical drains, intravenous and urinary catheters, severe sepsis, and colonization by *Candida* species.[72,73] Significance for intra-abdominal candidiasis worthy of treatment rises when *Candida* species are isolated surgically or directly from an intra-abdominal collection (e.g., within 24 hours of drain placement) in patients with severe community-acquired or health care–associated infections.[6,74] This may include patients who recently received immunosuppressive therapy for neoplasm, has a perforated gastric ulcer while on acid suppression, has malignancy, transplantation or inflammatory disease, or a postoperative or recurrent intra-abdominal infection.

Echinocandins and azoles are initial options for fungal peritonitis.[6,20] Concerns about the toxicity of conventional amphotericin B have limited the use of this agent. To date, no clinical trials have assessed the efficacy and safety of lipid-based amphotericin B, azoles, or echinocandins in the treatment of intra-abdominal fungal infections. Fluconazole is considered an appropriate drug of choice for *C. albicans*.[6] For *C. glabrata* or other fluconazole-resistant species, an echinocandin (caspofungin, micafungin, or anidulafungin) or an amphotericin product is an appropriate option.[6] If critically ill, initial therapy with an echinocandin is recommended.

Therapy with an antifungal agent such as fluconazole 400mg daily is acceptable for B.B and the *C. albicans* isolated.

CASE 70-5, QUESTION 3: The surgical resident initiated piperacillin–tazobactam for the treatment of B.B.'s intra-abdominal infection. Should culture and sensitivity results be used to monitor for anaerobic activity?

ANAEROBIC BACTERIA

With the introduction of broad-spectrum antimicrobial agents with in-vitro activity against *B. fragilis* and a significant problem of increasing resistance, the choice of a specific antianaerobic agent has become more complex. Multiple mechanisms of resistance are encountered, and resistance rates differ among various geographic areas of the United States. Although *Bacteroides* resistance to metronidazole is rare,[20,75] resistance to clindamycin has increased substantially.[20] Although the carbapenems and the β-lactamase inhibitor combinations are exquisitely active against *Bacteroides*, occasional resistance has been reported.

The Clinical and Laboratory Standards Institute has suggested that susceptibility testing be performed only to determine patterns of anaerobic susceptibility to new antimicrobial agents and to monitor susceptibility patterns periodically on a geographic and local basis.[76]

Because most anaerobes are cultured in the setting of mixed flora, isolation of individual components of a complex mixture can be time-consuming. In addition, most anaerobes are very slow growing, and it may take days to weeks for a definitive culture and sensitivity report. If specimens are not collected and transported in optimal media or in a timely manner, inaccurate or misleading results may be reported. The methods for susceptibility testing of anaerobic bacteria are not well standardized, and many hospital laboratories do not have resources to perform extensive culture and sensitivity testing. Routine cultures rarely impact the choice of antibiotic regimen, and thus the empiric choice of therapy usually determines the outcome.[77] Routine susceptibility testing for patient-specific cases is not recommended because of the prolonged time needed to achieve results, but it may be useful when resistant organisms are suspected or high-risk patients have been identified.[78]

Intra-Abdominal Abscess

CASE 70-6

QUESTION 1: R.K. is a 28-year-old woman with a history of diverticulitis, who presents with abdominal pain and distension, fever, and chills. An intra-abdominal abscess is visualized by CT scan. How did this abscess develop? What considerations should be taken into account in the selection of appropriate antimicrobial agents?

Abscesses are collections of necrotic tissue, bacteria, and WBCs that form during a period of days to years. They generally result from chronic inflammation and the body's attempt to localize organisms and toxic substances by formation of an avascular fibrous wall. This process isolates bacteria and the liquid core from opsonins and antimicrobial agents.

Microbiology

Pathogens encountered in intra-abdominal abscesses often include facultative aerobic gram negatives (e.g., *E. coli*) and obligate anaerobes (e.g., *B. fragilis*).[46] Mixed infections involving *E. coli* or enterococci with *B. fragilis* have been associated with a synergistic mechanism responsible for late intraperitoneal abscess development.[79,80]

ANTIMICROBIAL THERAPY

Abscesses pose a therapeutic challenge because they typically contain large bacterial inocula that are likely to include subpopulations of resistant bacteria.[55] Furthermore, the rate of penetration of antibiotics into abscesses is hindered by the low surface-to-volume ratio, low pH, and decreased permeability. Although percutaneous drainage or surgical debridement of R.K.'s abscess is crucial, adjunctive therapy with antimicrobial agents is warranted. The optimal antimicrobial agent should penetrate into the abscess in adequate concentrations and have an adequate spectrum of activity.[20,55] R.K. should be placed on an antimicrobial regimen, such as piperacillin–tazobactam 3.375 g IV every 6 hours, that covers gram-negative bacteria and anaerobes.

INFECTIONS AFTER ABDOMINAL TRAUMA AND POSTOPERATIVE COMPLICATIONS

Risk factors for infection after penetrating abdominal trauma include the number, type, and location of injuries; the presence of hypotension; large transfusion requirements; prolonged operation; advanced age; and the mechanism of injury.[81]

Most investigators stress the importance of instituting antimicrobial therapy as close to the time of trauma as possible. Bozorgzadeh et al.[82] demonstrated a significant reduction in the incidence of postoperative infections when antibiotics were administered before surgical repair of the penetrating abdominal trauma.

Penetrating Trauma

CASE 70-7

QUESTION 1: T.I., a 19-year-old man, is admitted to the emergency department within 1 hour after sustaining a gunshot wound to the stomach and colon. He is to undergo emergency laparotomy. What antimicrobial therapy is appropriate at this time?

As with other types of intra-abdominal infections, antibiotics active against both aerobic and anaerobic pathogens should be used.

Anti-infective therapy has been studied in patients who have sustained penetrating trauma to the abdomen (usually from knife or gunshot wounds). In several comparative trials, single-drug therapy with cefoxitin was as effective as the combination of clindamycin or metronidazole plus an aminoglycoside.[83] In evaluating these studies, however, it is important to note that most patients did not sustain injuries to the colon, where the risk of infection is highest. Although the age of this patient suggests he would tolerate aminoglycoside therapy, monotherapy with cefoxitin or one of the β-lactamase inhibitor combinations would be appropriate.

Consensus guidelines regarding the duration of therapy were published by the Eastern Association for the Surgery of Trauma (EAST) Practice Management Group. These investigators reviewed all literature from 1976 to 1997 regarding the duration of antimicrobial use after penetrating abdominal trauma. They concluded that antimicrobial use should not exceed 24 hours in this patient population.[81]

CASE 70-7, QUESTION 2: How long should antibiotic therapy be administered to T.I.?

The shortest duration of antimicrobial therapy that has been shown to be effective has been 12 hours with the possibility that a short course (<48 hours) is as efficacious as 5-to 7-day course if antimicrobial therapy is promptly instituted.[6] Several other trials have confirmed no additional benefit exists in providing a longer treatment duration.[6,77,81,84–86]

Because antimicrobial therapy carries a risk of adverse reactions, development of resistance, and unnecessary costs, short-term therapy seems warranted as long as it is instituted soon after the injury.[81,87] If the initial dose of antibiotic is administered more than 3 to 4 hours after injury, therapy should be continued for 3 to 7 days because the incidence of infection in this circumstance is high.

Antimicrobial therapy was instituted soon after T.I. sustained the colonic injury; therefore, a short course of antimicrobial therapy is appropriate. Therapy should be continued for 24 hours.

Appendectomy

CASE 70-8

QUESTION 1: S.R. is a 12-year-old girl with a 2-day history of periumbilical pain migrating to the right lower quadrant, abdominal distension, fever of 39°C, diarrhea, and decreased bowel sounds. Her WBC count is $15.8 \times 10^3/\mu L$. A presumptive diagnosis of acute appendicitis is made. What antimicrobial therapy is indicated, and for how long should it be continued?

Clinical manifestations commonly encountered with acute appendicitis include right lower quadrant abdominal pain, rebound tenderness, and low-grade fever complicated by nausea, vomiting, and anorexia.[3,6,35]

A variety of antimicrobial agents are effective in the treatment of acute appendicitis.[88–92] Antimicrobial therapy selection for uncomplicated appendicitis can follow those recommended for community-acquired intra-abdominal infection where therapy for less than 24 hours is sufficient.[6] Patients with gangrenous or perforated appendices are associated with the highest risk of infection. In several well-designed, randomized, placebo-controlled trials, therapy with imipenem–cilastatin, β-lactams, and β-lactamase inhibitor combinations has been found to be as effective as the combination of clindamycin or metronidazole plus an aminoglycoside.[27,89,91] Patients with gangrenous or perforated appendices who were afebrile for 48 hours have been treated for durations ranging from a single dose[92] to 3 to 5 days.[90]

S.R. should receive a preoperative dose of β-lactam antimicrobials with activity against facultative gram-negative and anaerobic bacteria, such as cefoxitin alone or cefazolin plus metronidazole (Table 70-2). Cost, potential side effects, and ease of administration guide selection of a specific agent. If a gangrenous or perforated appendix is found during surgery, antimicrobial therapy should be continued for a minimum of 3 to 5 days or until S.R. has been afebrile for 48 hours.

KEY REFERENCES AND WEBSITES

A full list of references for this chapter can be found at http://thepoint.lww.com/AT11e. Below are the key references and websites for this chapter, with the corresponding reference number in this chapter found in parentheses after the reference.

Key References

Garcia-Tsao G. Current management of the complications of cirrhosis and portal hypertension: variceal hemorrhage, ascites, and spontaneous bacterial peritonitis. *Gastroenterology*. 2001;120:726. (22)

Hoban DJ et al. Susceptibility of gram-negative pathogens isolated from patients with complicated intra-abdominal infections in the United States, 2007–2008: results of the Study for Monitoring Antimicrobial Resistance Trends (SMART). *Antimicrob Agents Chemother*. 2010;54:3031. (16)

Horton JD et al. Gallstone disease and its complications. In: Feldman M et al., eds. *Sleisenger and Fordtran's Gastrointestinal and Liver Disease: Pathophysiology/Diagnosis/Management*. 7th ed. Philadelphia, PA: Saunders; 2002:1065. (12)

Levison ME, Bush LM. Peritonitis and intraperitoneal abscesses. In: Bennett JE et al, eds. *Mandell, Douglas, and Bennett's Principles and Practices of Infectious Diseases*. 8th ed. Philadelphia, PA: Elsevier Saunders; 2015:935–959. (3)

Li PK et al. Peritoneal dialysis-related infections recommendations: 2010 update. *Perit Dial Int*. 2010;30:393. (35)

Luchette FA et al. Practice management guidelines for prophylactic antibiotic use in penetrating abdominal trauma: the EAST Practice Management Guidelines Work Group. *J Trauma*. 2000;48:508. (82)

Sifri CD, Madoff LC. Infections of the liver and biliary system (liver abscess, cholangitis, cholecystitis). In: Bennett JE et al, eds. *Mandell, Douglas, and Bennett's Principles and Practice of Infectious Diseases*. 8th ed. Philadelphia, PA: Elsevier Saunders; 2015:960–968. (5)

Sirinek KR. Diagnosis and treatment of intra-abdominal abscesses. *Surg Infect (Larchmt)*. 2000;1:31. (55)

Solomkin JS et al. Diagnosis and management of complicated intra-abdominal infection in adults and children: guidelines by Surgical Infection Society and the Infectious Diseases Society of America [published correction appears in *Clin Infect Dis*. 2010;50:1695. Dosage error in article text]. *Clin Infect Dis*. 2010;50:133. (6)

71 Urinary Tract Infections

Douglas N. Fish

CORE PRINCIPLES

		CHAPTER CASES
1	Urinary tract infection (UTI) is usually bacterial in etiology, may be either acute or chronic, and may affect any part of the upper or lower urinary system. UTI is often classified as either uncomplicated or complicated based upon patient characteristics and on the clinical setting in which the infection is acquired (e.g., community-acquired vs. health care–acquired).	**Case 71-1 (Questions 1–6), Case 71-2 (Questions 1, 2)**
2	Uncomplicated UTI occurs in women who are otherwise healthy and have normal structure and function of the urinary tract. These infections are primarily caused by *Escherichia coli* (75%–95% of infections) and other gram-negative bacilli, as well as gram-positive organisms such as *Staphylococcus saprophyticus* and *Enterococcus*.	**Case 71-1 (Questions 1–3)**
3	Symptoms commonly associated with lower UTI (e.g., cystitis) include dysuria, frequent urination, suprapubic pain, hematuria, and back pain. Patients with upper tract infection (e.g., acute pyelonephritis) often present with similar findings as well as loin pain, costovertebral angle tenderness, fever, chills, nausea, and vomiting.	**Case 71-1 (Questions 1, 2), Case 71-5 (Questions 1–3)**
4	The cornerstone of effective treatment of UTI is appropriate selection and use of antibiotics. Resistance among *E. coli* and other uropathogens is increasing and is an important consideration in antibiotic selection. Consensus clinical guidelines recommend trimethoprim–sulfamethoxazole (TMP–SMX) for 3 days, nitrofurantoin for 5 days, or a single dose of fosfomycin as preferred first-line antibiotics for treatment of acute uncomplicated cystitis in women.	**Case 71-1 (Questions 1–6), Case 71-2 (Question 1), Tables 71-1, 71-2, 71-3**
5	Fluoroquinolones are commonly used for treatment of UTI and are highly effective. However, growing concerns of increasing resistance and potential adverse effects limit the use of fluoroquinolones in uncomplicated UTI to patients unable to receive other preferred agents because of drug resistance, allergies, or other contraindications. Similar recommendations restrict the use of β-lactam antibiotics for uncomplicated UTI.	**Case 71-1 (Question 3), Case 71-2 (Questions 1, 2), Case 71-3 (Question 1), Tables 71-1, 71-2, 71-3**
6	Complicated UTI is associated with abnormalities of the urinary tract that interfere with normal urine flow or function; men, children, patients with diabetes, pregnant women, and hospitalized patients are examples of commonly affected populations. Complicated infections are frequently caused by drug-resistant gram-negative bacilli or other pathogens with reduced antibiotic susceptibility. Antibiotic selection for complicated UTI should be guided by culture and susceptibility testing, and patients usually require longer durations of antibiotic therapy (7–14 days).	**Case 71-1 (Questions 1–4), Case 71-2 (Question 1), Case 71-4 (Question 1), Case 71-10 (Questions 1, 2), Case 71-11 (Questions 1–3)**
7	Pyelonephritis may be more severe in presentation and is often associated with bacteremia and other complications. However, most cases are uncomplicated and can be treated on an outpatient basis with oral antibiotics such as fluoroquinolones. Patients who cannot take oral antibiotics or who are clinically unstable should be hospitalized for initial treatment with intravenous antibiotics.	**Case 71-5 (Questions 1–5), Tables 71-1, 71-2, 71-5**

Continued

		CHAPTER CASES
8	Recurrent UTI may be caused by either reinfection or relapse because of treatment failure. Relapse usually occurs within two weeks of the original infection and is caused by the same pathogen. Selection of antibiotics for treatment of relapsed UTI should be guided by culture and susceptibility testing, and the duration of antibiotic therapy should be at least 2 weeks in length.	**Case 71-6 (Questions 1–3, 6-8), Case 71-7 (Questions 1, 2)**
9	Recurrent UTI, which occurs more than 2 weeks after the original infection, is treated as a new infection with antibiotic considerations similar to those for the initial infection. Women with frequent infections (3 or more/year) may be considered for chronic prophylaxis therapy. Women with identifiable causes of reinfection (e.g., associated with sexual intercourse) may self-administer prophylactic antibiotics.	**Case 71-6 (Questions 4, 5, 7, 8), Tables 71-3, 71-4**
10	Asymptomatic bacteriuria ($\geq 10^5$ bacteria per milliliter of urine in the absence of clinical signs/symptoms of UTI) is particularly common in children, the elderly, pregnant women, and in patients with diabetes. Treatment of asymptomatic bacteriuria for prevention of subsequent infection and associated complications is routinely recommended in children and pregnant women. However, treatment of the elderly and patients with diabetes has not shown clear benefits and is not currently recommended.	**Case 71-7 (Questions 3, 4), Case 71-8 (Questions 1, 2), Case 71-9 (Questions 1, 2)**
11	Prostatitis is a relatively common infection in men and is caused by bacteria similar to those causing uncomplicated UTI in women. Acute bacterial prostatitis is usually treated with either a fluoroquinolone or TMP–SMX for a period of 2 to 4 weeks. Chronic prostatitis persists in a small percentage of men after acute infection and is usually treated for 4 to 6 weeks, although longer courses may sometimes be required.	**Case 71-12 (Questions 1, 2)**

URINARY TRACT INFECTION

Incidence, Prevalence, and Epidemiology

Urinary tract infection (UTI) is an acute or chronic infection, usually bacterial in origin, that may affect any part of the upper or lower urinary system.

Infections of the bladder are referred to as cystitis, and infections involving the parenchyma of the kidneys are known as pyelonephritis. UTIs occur frequently in both community and hospital environments and are the most common bacterial infections in humans.[1–3] The term UTI encompasses a spectrum of clinical entities ranging in severity from asymptomatic infection to acute pyelonephritis with sepsis.[1–4] Approximately 8 to 9 million cases of acute cystitis and 250,000 cases of acute pyelonephritis occur annually in the United States, resulting in more than 100,000 hospitalizations.[2,5,6] Direct costs associated with the diagnosis and treatment of UTI have been estimated at approximately $3 billion annually in the United States.[3,6,7] UTI is predominantly a disease of females with more than 50% of all women experiencing at least one infection during their lifetime.[2,5] The overall likelihood of developing a UTI is approximately 30 times higher in women than in men.[3,7,8] Women have more UTIs than men, probably because of anatomic and physiologic differences. The female urethra is relatively short and allows bacteria easy access to the bladder. In contrast, males are partly protected because the urethra is longer and antimicrobial substances are secreted by the prostate.[1,3,7,8]

Approximately 1% of boys and 3% to 5% of girls experience at least one UTI during childhood and 30% to 50% of these will have at least one recurrence.[9] The incidence of UTI in neonates is about 1% and is more frequent in male neonates, frequently because of congenital structural abnormalities.[10] The mortality rate among newborns with UTI was earlier reported to be as high as 10%[10]; however, this rate is now much lower because of an increased awareness of the high frequency of UTI in children, improved diagnostic techniques, and more effective management.[10] UTIs in males also occur with increased frequency after age 50, when prostatic obstruction, urethral instrumentation, and surgery influence the infection rate. Infection in younger men is rare and requires careful evaluation for urinary tract pathology.[11,12]

Of women between the ages of 15 and 24 years, 1% to 5% have bacteriuria; the incidence increases 1% to 2% for each decade of life, and approximately 10% to 20% of women are bacteriuric after age 70.[1,8,13,14] In general, 5% to 20% of all elderly living at home have bacteriuria, and this number increases to 20% to 50% in extended care facilities and 30% in hospitals.[3,13,15,16] For those 65 years or older the frequency of UTI continues to rise with increasing age. Most UTI in these patients are asymptomatic, but it may also result in symptomatic infection.[13,15,16] Reasons for higher UTI rates in elderly persons include the high prevalence of prostatic hypertrophy in men, incomplete bladder emptying caused by underlying diseases or medications, dementia, and urinary and fecal incontinence.[8,15–17] Whether bacteriuria in old age is associated with decreased survival is controversial[17,18]; however, the presence of asymptomatic bacteriuria is associated with decreased functional ability of institutionalized persons,[13,15] and symptomatic UTI has been independently associated with a threefold increased risk of vertebral fractures.[19]

Etiology

UNCOMPLICATED VERSUS COMPLICATED INFECTIONS

An important distinction in the characterization and treatment of UTI is that of uncomplicated versus complicated infections. Uncomplicated UTI, either cystitis or pyelonephritis, occurs in women who have normal structure and function of the genitourinary tract and who have no other factors which would put them at risk for more severe or complex infections.[3,5,20] By contrast, complicated infections are those which are associated with conditions that increase the risk for acquiring infection, the potential for serious outcomes, or the risk for therapy failure. Such conditions are often associated with genitourinary tract abnormalities that may interfere with normal urine flow. Infections in men, children, and pregnant women are automatically considered complicated, as are those which are health care–associated in origin. Other examples of complicated infections include those associated with structural and neurologic abnormalities of the urinary tract, metabolic or hormonal abnormalities, impaired host responses, instrumentation and catheterization of the urinary tract, and those caused by unusual pathogens (e.g., yeasts, *Mycoplasma*).[3,5,20] Uncomplicated infections are invariably community-acquired and are caused by the organisms typical to that etiology. Complicated UTI may be caused by pathogens associated with either community-acquired or health care–associated infections, depending on the source of bacterial acquisition and specific underlying patient risk factors. Complicated infections are also more often polymicrobial in etiology, associated with more antibiotic-resistant pathogens, and generally require a longer duration of therapy.

COMMUNITY-ACQUIRED INFECTIONS

Most UTIs are caused by gram-negative aerobic bacilli from the intestinal tract. *Escherichia coli* cause 75% to 95% of community-acquired, uncomplicated UTIs.[1,3,20] Coagulase-negative staphylococci (e.g., *Staphylococcus saprophyticus*) account for another 5% to 20% of UTIs in younger women.[1,3,5] Other Enterobacteriaceae (e.g. *Proteus mirabilis, Klebsiella*) and *Enterococcus faecalis* also are common pathogens.[1,3,20] Uncomplicated infections are nearly always caused by a single pathogen.

HEALTH CARE–ASSOCIATED INFECTIONS

UTIs occur in up to 10% of hospitalized patients and represent 20% to 30% of all nosocomial infections.[21–23] *E. coli* remains the most common pathogen in hospital-acquired or other complicated UTI, but it is responsible for only 20% to 30% of these infections. Other gram-negative organisms, such as *Pseudomonas aeruginosa, Klebsiella, Proteus, Enterobacter,* and *Acinetobacter*, cause significantly more infections (up to 25%) than in the community setting.[5,22,23] *Enterococcus* is also a common pathogen in hospital-acquired UTIs and causes approximately 15% of infections.[22,23] UTIs because of *Staphylococcus aureus* are usually the result of hematogenous spread, although this pathogen is also associated with urinary catheterization.[1,22–24] Finally, *Candida* is a common pathogen in hospital-acquired infections and may be involved in 20% to 30% of cases.[21–23] In contrast to the usually monomicrobial uncomplicated infections, UTIs associated with structural abnormalities or indwelling urinary catheters are often caused by multiple pathogens.[1,21–24]

Pathogenesis and Predisposing Factors

The typical pathway for the spread of bacteria to the urinary tract is the ascending route. A UTI usually begins with heavy and persistent colonization of the introitus (i.e., vaginal vestibule and urethral mucosa) with intestinal bacteria. Colonization of the urethra leads to retrograde infection of the bladder and the development of cystitis.[25,26]

The bladder has defense mechanisms that prevent spread of the infection after urethral colonization has occured.[1,3,22] Urination washes bacteria out of the bladder and is effective if urine flows freely and the bladder is emptied completely. Substances in the urine, including organic acids (which contribute to low pH) and urea (which contributes to high osmolality), are antibacterial. The bladder mucosa also has antibacterial properties.[1,3,22] Lastly, other substances, including immunoglobulin A and glycoproteins (e.g., Tamm–Horsfall protein), are actively secreted into the urine and prevent adherence of bacteria to uroendothelial cells.[22,25,26]

Focal renal involvement leading to pyelonephritis may result from the spread of bacteria via the ureters and may be facilitated by vesicoureteral reflux or decreased ureteral peristalsis. Ureteral peristalsis is decreased in pregnancy, by ureteral obstruction, or by gram-negative bacterial endotoxins.[1,25,26] Reflux can be produced by cystitis alone or by anatomic defects.

A variety of factors contribute to the development of UTI, for example expression of bacterial virulence factors such as specific adhesin molecules, bacterial polysaccharides, and bacterial enzymes. Other factors predisposing to the development of UTI are dependent on the host and may include extremes of age, female sex, sexual activity, use of contraception, pregnancy, urinary tract instrumentation or catheterization, urinary tract obstruction, neurologic dysfunction, renal disease, previous antimicrobial use, and expression of A, B, and H blood group oligosaccharides on the surface of epithelial cells.[1–3,17,25,27]

The incidence of bacteriuria in pregnant women is as high as 17%, which is approximately twice that of similarly aged non-pregnant women.[1,13,28,29] The incidence of acute symptomatic pyelonephritis in pregnant women with untreated bacteriuria also is high and may reach 40%.[3] Many factors contribute to the increased susceptibility of the pregnant female to infection; these include hormonal changes, anatomic changes, progressive urinary stasis, and glucose in the urine.[28,29] Hormonal changes have also been linked to a significantly higher risk of UTI in menopausal women.[3] Estrogen promotes an acidic vaginal pH and proliferation of normal flora such as *Lactobacillus*, both factors which reduce pathogenic colonization of the vagina. Reduction of estrogen production during menopause allows significant colonization of the vaginal tract with *E. coli* and other enteric bacilli, thus predisposing to subsequent infection.[3]

Renal disease increases the susceptibility of the kidney to infection.[1] The incidence of UTI among renal transplant recipients ranges from 35% to 80% without prophylactic antibiotic therapy.[30] Patients with spinal cord injuries, stroke, atherosclerosis, or diabetes may have neurologic dysfunction predisposing to UTI. The neurologic dysfunction can cause urinary retention, requiring catheterization. Furthermore, prolonged immobilization facilitates hypercalciuria and stone formation in some of these patients.[1,5,25]

Previous antimicrobial use (within the previous 15–28 days) for UTI or other infections increases the relative risk for UTI in women threefold to sixfold.[3] The proposed mechanism for this is alteration of normal flora of the urogenital tract and predisposition to colonization with pathogenic bacterial strains.[2,3]

Diabetes mellitus is associated with a higher risk for UTI because of glucose in the urine, promoting bacterial growth and impairing leukocyte function. Anatomic, neurologic, and immunologic abnormalities of the urinary tract in diabetics contribute to the risk of infection, often because of more frequent urinary tract instrumentation.[31,32] Several studies have documented a twofold to threefold increase in UTI in women with diabetes compared to those without; rates of relapses and reinfections, as well as complications such as pyelonephritis, are also higher.[31–33] Autonomic neuropathy associated with diabetes also contributes to increased frequency and severity of UTI.[25,31,32]

Finally, studies have supported an association between sexual intercourse and UTI among otherwise healthy women.[2,3,25,34] Specific contraceptive practices, particularly the use of spermicides, and the use of a diaphragm, cervical cap, or condom in combination with spermicidal jelly increases the risk of UTI compared with the use of the barrier method alone.[2,27,34] Diaphragm users are approximately 3 times more likely to experience a UTI than women using other contraceptive methods, especially when the diaphragm is used in conjunction with spermicidal jelly.[2,27] Oral contraceptive use has also been linked with increased risk of UTI, although this is still unclear.[2,3,27,34] The exact mechanisms of infection related to sexual intercourse and contraceptive methods are unclear but appear to be related to alterations in vaginal flora that allow for bacterial overgrowth and subsequent infection.[1–3]

URINARY CATHETERS

Instrumentation or catheterization of the urinary tract is an important predisposing factor for health care–associated UTI. Catheter-associated UTI, the most common type of hospital-acquired infection, occurs in up to 30% of catheterized patients.[23] Catheterization and other forms of urologic instrumentation are present as risk factors for infection in 65% to 95% of all hospital-acquired UTI.[22] These UTIs also are a major cause of nosocomial gram-negative bacteremia.[21,23] Other urologic procedures, such as cystoscopy, transurethral surgery, prostate biopsy, and upper urinary tract endoscopy, are much less likely to result in infection unless there is preexisting bacteriuria or other contaminated sites (e.g., prostate, renal stones). Any obstruction to the free flow of urine (e.g., urethral stenosis, stones, tumor) or mechanical difficulty in evacuating the bladder (e.g., prostatic hypertrophy, urethral stricture) also predisposes patients to UTI. Furthermore, infections associated with urethral or renal pelvic obstruction can lead to rapid destruction of the kidney and sepsis.[1]

Catheter infection can occur by bacterial entry from several routes. The urethral meatus and the distal third of the urethra normally are colonized by bacteria; therefore, initial catheter insertion can introduce bacteria into the bladder. Bacteria contaminating catheter junctions and the urine collection bag can migrate through the catheter lumen to the bladder, initiating infection.[23] The extraluminal space in the urethra also has been considered a potential route of contamination. The risk of infection is directly related to catheter insertion technique, care of the catheter, duration of catheterization, and the susceptibility of the patient. A diagnostic or single, short-term catheterization is associated with a much lower risk of infection than indwelling, long-term catheterization.[23] Despite careful technique, the risk of contaminating a sterile bladder with urethral bacteria is always present. The incidence of infection after a single catheterization is 1% in healthy young women and 20% in debilitated patients. Each reinsertion of the catheter introduces a risk of infection.[23]

Infections have been reduced dramatically by the closed sterile drainage system, the most common type of catheter currently in use. With this system, the drainage tube leads from the catheter directly to a closed plastic collection bag. The overall incidence of infection from the closed system with careful insertion and maintenance is about 20%; the risk increases to 50% after 14 days of catheterization.[23] Condom catheters are associated with a lower incidence of bacteriuria than indwelling urethral catheters. These catheters avoid problems associated with insertion of a tube directly into the urinary tract; nevertheless, urine within the catheters may have high concentrations of organisms so that colonization of the urethra and subsequent cystitis may develop.[23]

Application of antibacterial substances to the collection bag or the catheter–urethral interface does not decrease the incidence of bacteriuria.[23,35,36] The use of antimicrobial-coated catheters (e.g., silver, rifampin plus minocycline) has been shown in some studies to decrease rates of bacteriuria and UTI.[23,35,36] The overall effects of these catheters on infection rates, patient outcomes, and antibiotic resistance are not known, however. The routine use of antibiotic-coated catheters is not currently recommended.[23,35]

Clinical Presentation

Symptoms commonly associated with lower UTI (e.g., cystitis) include burning on urination (dysuria), frequent urination, suprapubic pain, blood in the urine (hematuria), and back pain. Patients with upper tract infection (e.g., acute pyelonephritis) may also present with loin pain, costovertebral angle (CVA) tenderness, fever, chills, nausea, and vomiting.[1–5,37]

Clinical signs and symptoms correlate poorly with either the presence or the extent of the infection. Symptoms common to lower UTI often are the only positive findings in upper UTI (i.e., subclinical pyelonephritis).[1,4] The probability of true infection in women who present with one or more symptoms of UTI is only about 50%.[38] The presence of dysuria, back pain, pyuria, hematuria, bacteriuria, and a history of previous UTI may enhance the probability of true infection; the absence of dysuria or back pain, and history of vaginal discharge or irritation significantly decrease the likelihood of infection.[38,39] The combination of dysuria plus urgency or frequency in the absence of vaginal discharge or irritation increases the probability of true infection to greater than 90%.[38,39] Fever, chills, flank pain, nausea and vomiting, or CVA tenderness are highly suggestive of acute pyelonephritis rather than cystitis.[4,5,37] Many elderly patients with UTI are asymptomatic without pyuria. Additionally, because many patients have frequency and dysuria, it is difficult to distinguish between noninfectious and infectious causes based on symptoms.[1] Nonspecific symptoms, such as failure to thrive and fever, may be the only manifestations of UTI in neonates and children younger than 2 years of age.[1]

Diagnosis

Diagnosis of UTI based on clinical findings alone is accurate in only approximately 70% of patients.[40] Urinalysis (UA) is a series of laboratory tests commonly performed in patients suspected of having a UTI; in combination with appropriate clinical findings, the UA effectively improves the overall diagnostic accuracy for UTI.[41] A technician first performs a macroscopic analysis by describing the color of the urine; measuring its specific gravity; and estimating the pH and glucose, protein, ketone, blood, and bilirubin contents using a rapid "dipstick" method. Then the urine sediment, obtained by centrifugation, is examined under a microscope for the presence and quantity of leukocytes, erythrocytes, epithelial cells, crystals, casts, and bacteria.

Rapid diagnostic dipstick tests are widely available and easily performed. The nitrite test detects nitrite formation from the reduction of nitrates by bacteria. Although a positive nitrite reading is useful, false-negative results do occur.[40] Dipstick testing can also be used to perform the leukocyte esterase test, which detects the esterase activity of activated leukocytes in the urine. A positive test correlates well with significant pyuria[42]; however, both false-negative and false-positive findings can occur with the leukocyte esterase panel as well.[40] Nitrite and leukocyte esterase tests are useful in ruling out the presence of infection if results of both tests are negative, whereas positive results of both tests in combination are highly suggestive of the presence of infection.[40]

Microscopic examination of urine sediment in patients with documented UTI reveals many bacteria (usually >20 per high-power field [HPF]). Gram staining of uncentrifuged ("unspun") urine shows at least one organism per immersion oil field and usually correlates with a positive urine culture. Pyuria (i.e., ≥8 white blood cells [WBC] per milliliter [mL] of unspun urine or 2–5 WBC/HPF of centrifuged urine) is frequently seen in patients with UTI. WBC casts in the urine strongly suggest acute pyelonephritis.[1,41]

The gold-standard criterion for the diagnosis of UTI is the urine culture with a positive UA.[1–3,37] Proper interpretation of these cultures depends, however, on appropriate urine collection techniques. Urinating into a sterile collection cup using the midstream clean-catch technique is the most practical method of urine collection. This method of urine specimen collection is especially useful for male patients, but it is less useful in female patients because contamination is extremely difficult to avoid.[1] The external urethral area must first be thoroughly cleaned and rinsed, then the urine specimen collected after initiation of the urine stream (hence "midstream").

Urinary catheterization for a urine culture sample yields fairly reliable results if performed carefully. However, infections can result from the procedure itself because organisms might be introduced into the bladder at the time of catheterization. Suprapubic bladder aspiration generally is not painful and is quite reliable. It is not practical for routine office or clinic practice, but it may be useful when voided urine samples repeatedly yield questionable results or when patients have voiding problems. Because contamination is negligible, any number of bacteria found by this method reflects infection.[1–3]

Urine must be plated on culture media within 20 minutes of collection to avoid erroneously high colony counts from bacterial growth in urine at room temperature. Otherwise, urine should be promptly refrigerated until it can be cultured. Colony counts are also affected by the concentration of bladder urine; bacterial counts are higher in first-voided morning urines compared with those obtained from the same patient later in the day.[1,37]

Greater than 10^5 colonies of bacteria/mL cultured from a midstream urine specimen confirms a UTI. A single, carefully collected urine specimen provides 80% reliability, and two consecutive cultures of the same organism are virtually diagnostic.[1–3] It is important to understand that the classic definition of UTI as greater than or equal to 10^5 bacteria/mL is fairly inaccurate in diagnosing patients with UTI. Approximately 30% to 50% of actual cases of acute cystitis have less than 10^5 bacteria/mL.[5,13] In a symptomatic patient, using a definition of greater than or equal to 10^2 bacteria/mL is more accurate and avoids failure to diagnose infection in many patients.[5]

Diagnosis of UTI in men also requires different interpretation of laboratory data. Contamination of urinary specimens is much less likely to occur in men compared with women, and numbers of bacterial colonies in specimens are therefore much lower. Greater than 10^3 bacteria/mL is thus highly suggestive of UTI in men.[11,12] In addition, although a positive nitrite test in a symptomatic man is highly indicative of the presence of an acute UTI, a negative nitrite test does not necessarily exclude infection and should be confirmed with a urine culture.[43]

Diagnosis of UTI in children is particularly problematic because of the difficulties and high contamination rates associated with commonly used methods of urine specimen collection. Suprapubic aspiration is the most accurate method in children, followed by urinary bladder catheterization.[3,37] Although clean-catch and bag methods (i.e., collecting urine into a bag placed around the urogenital area) are most susceptible to contamination and inaccurate results, they are also the most preferred methods for parents and health care personnel because they are simple and noninvasive. The choice of diagnostic tests for children will therefore vary and be based on the experience, skill, and preferences of those involved with the child.[37]

Simplified culture methods such as the filter-paper method (e.g., Testuria-R), dip-slide method (e.g., Uricult), and pad-culture method (Microstix) are as reliable as traditional laboratory methods for bacterial identification and quantification. The filter-paper method is relatively inexpensive but does not differentiate between gram-positive and gram-negative organisms. The dip-slide and pad-culture methods are accurate, differentiate between gram-positive and gram-negative organisms, and are similar in cost. The dip-slide method has the added advantages of ease of storage and a nitrite indicator pad.

Overview of Drug Therapy

The cornerstone of effective treatment of UTI is the appropriate selection and use of antibiotics. Antibiotic treatment of UTI has been well studied and, compared to many other infectious diseases, the choice of specific antibiotic and duration of therapy for acute, uncomplicated infections are reasonably clear. Recently published consensus guidelines from the Infectious Diseases Society of America (IDSA) and the European Society for Microbiology and Infectious Diseases (ESMID) recommend a 5-day course of nitrofurantoin, trimethoprim–sulfamethoxazole (TMP–SMX) for 3 days, or a single dose of fosfomycin trometamol as first-line antibiotics for treatment of acute uncomplicated cystitis in women.[20] Whereas nitrofurantoin and TMP–SMX are familiar agents, fosfomycin is a previously little used antibiotic which has been available for many years. However, it has recently made a resurgence in clinical use because of low rates of resistance among common uropathogens. Fosfomycin also has usefulness against multidrug-resistant pathogens which are becoming more common in certain practice settings; these include methicillin-resistant *S. aureus*, vancomycin-resistant enterococci, and extended spectrum β-lactamase (ESBL)-producing gram-negative bacteria.[20,44] Fluoroquinolones and β-lactam antibiotics, such as amoxicillin–clavulanate or various cephalosporins, are recommended by the IDSA/ESMID guidelines as alternative agents for treating acute uncomplicated cystitis.[20] These same guidelines recommend fluoroquinolones, cephalosporins, aminoglycosides, TMP–SMX, extended-spectrum penicillins (i.e., piperacillin–tazobactam), or a carbapenem for the treatment of acute pyelonephritis in women.[20] The choice of a specific agent for pyelonephritis depends primarily on whether or not the patient is hospitalized or treated as an outpatient, local susceptibility patterns, and whether therapy is empiric or based on known susceptibilities. The duration of therapy for acute pyelonephritis ranges from 5 to 14 days and is dependent on which specific antibiotic is being used.[20] Parameters for monitoring response to treatment of either uncomplicated cystitis or pyelonephritis are primarily resolution of clinical signs and symptoms, and repeat urinary cultures are not usually required. Patients with complicated UTI or recurrent infections may require additional monitoring and long-term follow-up, and antibiotic selection must be guided by culture and susceptibility (C&S) testing. Patient monitoring related to the safety and tolerability of antibiotic therapy is required regardless of type of infection, as is effective patient counseling.

LOWER URINARY TRACT INFECTION

Initial Patient Evaluation and Determining Goals of Therapy

CASE 71-1

QUESTION 1: V.Q., a 20-year-old woman with no previous history of UTI, complains of burning on urination, frequent urination of a small amount, and bladder pain. She has no fever or CVA tenderness. A clean-catch midstream urine sample shows gram-negative rods on Gram stain. A urine sample for culture and susceptibility testing is ordered, and the results of a UA are as follows:

Appearance, straw-colored (normal, straw)
Specific gravity, 1.015 (normal, 1.002–1.028)
pH, 8.0 (normal, 5.5–7.0)
Protein, glucose, ketones, bilirubin, and blood, all negative (normal, all negative)
WBC, 10 to 15 cells/LPF (normal, 0–2 cells/LPF)
Red blood cells (RBC), 0 to 1 cells/LPF (normal, 0–2 cells/LPF)
Bacteria, many (normal, 0 to rare)
Epithelial cells, 3 to 5 cells/LPF (normal, 0 to few cells/LPF)

Based on these findings, V.Q. is presumed to have a lower UTI. What should be the goals of therapy of V.Q.'s infection at this time? What factors should be considered before selecting an antibiotic for V.Q.?

The goals of therapy for treatment of acute cystitis are to effectively eradicate the infection and prevent associated complications, while minimizing adverse effects and costs associated with drug therapy. To accomplish these goals, selection of a specific antimicrobial agent should be made after considering several factors: (a) most likely pathogens, (b) resistance rates within the specific geographic area, (c) desired duration of therapy, (d) clinical efficacy and toxicity profiles of various agents, (e) cost and availability of specific agents, and (f) patient characteristics such as allergies, compliance history, and underlying comorbidities.[20] Because resistance rates among various pathogens vary considerably among geographic areas, clinicians must be familiar with resistance rates prevalent within their specific practice area.[20,45,46]

Drug treatment of a lower UTI often is started before C&S results are known because the most probable infecting organisms and their susceptibility to antibiotics can be predicted reasonably well (Table 71-1). Approximately 75% to 95% of community-acquired infections are caused by Enterobacteriaceae (especially *E. coli*). Although these organisms may be sensitive to ampicillin, amoxicillin, and the sulfonamides (such as TMP–SMX), resistance to these agents is common.[45–49] Ampicillin resistance occurs in 25% to 70% of community-acquired isolates[45–49]; resistance nationwide is currently about 30% to 40%.[1,5,20,45–49] TMP–SMX has been a traditional agent of choice for many years; however, TMP–SMX resistance has significantly increased in recent years and may be as high as 20% to 40% among community-acquired *E. coli* isolates in some geographic areas.[20,45–49] Although traditionally associated with hospital-acquired infections, resistance among *E. coli* and *Klebsiella* caused by production of ESBL enzymes which confer resistance to penicillins and cephalosporins has also been steadily increasing among community-acquired pathogens.[50,51] Another relatively common organism is *S. saprophyticus*. Most strains are susceptible to sulfonamides, TMP–SMX, penicillins, and cephalosporins. Commonly used medications and doses are shown in Table 71-2.

Table 71-1
Overview of Treatment of Urinary Tract Infections

Organisms Commonly Found	Antibacterial of Choice
Uncomplicated UTI	
Escherichia coli	TMP–SMX[a]
Proteus mirabilis	TMP–SMX[a]
Klebsiella pneumoniae	TMP–SMX[a]
Enterococcus faecalis	Ampicillin, amoxicillin
Staphylococcus saprophyticus	First-generation cephalosporin or TMP–SMX
Complicated UTI[b,c]	
E. coli	First-, second-, or third-generation cephalosporin; TMP–SMX[c]
P. mirabilis	First-, second-, or third-generation cephalosporin
K. pneumoniae	First-generation cephalosporin; fluoroquinolone
Enterococcus faecalis	Ampicillin or vancomycin ± aminoglycoside
Pseudomonas aeruginosa	Antipseudomonal penicillin ± aminoglycoside; ceftazidime; cefepime; fluoroquinolone; carbapenem
Enterobacter	Fluoroquinolone; TMP-SMX; carbapenem
Indole-positive *Proteus*	Third-generation cephalosporin; fluoroquinolone
Serratia	Third-generation cephalosporin; fluoroquinolone
Acinetobacter	Carbapenem; TMP-SMX
Staphylococcus aureus	Penicillinase-resistant penicillin; vancomycin

[a]Caution in communities with increased resistance (>10%–20%).
[b]Drug selection based on culture and susceptibility testing when possible.
[c]Oral therapy when appropriate. Nitrofurantoin, fosfomycin, fluoroquinolone, or cephalosporins should be used in areas with increased TMP–SMX resistance.
TMP–SMX, trimethoprim–sulfamethoxazole; UTI, urinary tract infection.

ROLE OF URINE CULTURES

CASE 71-1, QUESTION 2: Is it necessary to order a pretreatment urine C&S test for V.Q.?

Many investigators question the value of pretreatment urine cultures for acute uncomplicated UTI.[1,2,5,20] Women with lower UTI usually have pyuria on UA and respond rapidly to appropriate antimicrobial treatment. Pyuria may be a better predictor of treatable infection than the colony count obtained on urine culture. Furthermore, the urine culture accounts for a large portion of the cost of treating a patient with a UTI.[52] Consequently, in patients such as V.Q. with uncomplicated, acute, lower UTI, it is more cost-effective to order a UA and, if pyuria is present on UA, to forego a urine culture. Instead, the patient should be empirically treated with a conventional course of antibiotic therapy. If V.Q. remains symptomatic 48 hours later, a C&S test can then be ordered. Considerations are quite different in patients with complicated infections. In complicated UTI, predisposing factors that lead to infection and frequent history of previous antibiotic use make both causative pathogens and associated antibiotic susceptibilities much less predictable. Use of C&S testing is therefore commonly recommended for treatment of complicated UTI in order to choose appropriate antibiotics.[1–3,5,20]

INITIAL ANTIBIOTIC SELECTION

CASE 71-1, QUESTION 3: What antibiotics may be appropriate for treatment of V.Q.'s infection?

Table 71-2
Commonly Used Oral Antimicrobial Agents for Acute Urinary Tract Infections[1–3,5,29,47,48,91]

Drug	Usual Dose		Pregnancy[a]	Breast Milk[a]	Comments[b]
	Adult	Pediatric			
Amoxicillin	250 mg every 8 hours or 3 g single dose	20–40 mg/kg/day in 3 doses	Crosses placenta (cord) = 30% (maternal)[c]	Small amount present	High resistance rates, not for empiric use.
Amoxicillin + potassium clavulanate	500 + 125 mg every 12 hours	20 mg/kg/day (amoxicillin content) in 3 doses	Unknown	Unknown	
Ampicillin	250–500 mg every 6 hours	50–100 mg/kg/day in 4 doses	Crosses placenta	Variable amount; milk = 1–30% of serum[c]	High resistance rates, not for empiric use. Should be taken on an empty stomach.
Cephalexin	250–500 mg every 6 hours	15–30 mg/kg/day in 4 doses	Crosses placenta	Enters breast milk	Cephalosporins are alternate choices for patients allergic to penicillins, although cross-hypersensitivity can occur. May be associated with higher failure rates compared to other drug classes.
Cefaclor	250–500 mg every 8 hours	20–40 mg/kg/day in 2–3 doses	Crosses placenta	Small amount present	
Cefpodoxime proxetil	100 mg every 12 hours	10 mg/kg/day in 2 doses	Crosses placenta	Variable amounts; milk = 0–16% of serum	
Cefdinir	300 mg every 12 hours or 600 mg every 24 hours	14 mg/kg/day in 1 or 2 doses	Crosses placenta	Not detectable after single 600 mg dose	
Norfloxacin[d]	400 mg every 12 hours	Avoid	Arthropathy in immature animals	Unknown	*Avoid antacids, divalent and trivalent cations, and sucralfate. Monitor INR in patients on warfarin. May cause dizziness.*[e]
Ciprofloxacin[d]	250–500 mg every 12 hours	Avoid	Arthropathy in immature animals	Unknown	Alternate choice for patients allergic to β-lactams.[e] Useful for pseudomonal infection.
Levofloxacin	250 mg every 24 hours	Avoid	Arthropathy in immature animals	Milk = 100% of serum[c]	
Nitrofurantoin	100 mg every 12 hours (e.g., Macrobid) 50–100 mg every 6 hours (e.g., Macrodantin)	5–7 mg/kg/day in 2–4 doses	Hemolytic anemia in newborn	Variable amounts; not detectable up to 30%; may cause hemolysis in G6PD-deficient baby	Alternate choice. *To be taken with food or milk. May cause brown or rust-yellow discoloration of urine.*
Sulfamethoxazole (SMX)	1 g every 12 hours	60 mg/kg/day in 2 doses	Crosses placenta; displacement of bilirubin may lead to hyperbilirubinemia and kernicterus, avoid after 32 weeks of gestation; teratogenic in some animal studies	Enters breast milk; displacement of bilirubin may lead to neonatal jaundice; may cause hemolysis in G6PD-deficient baby	Alters bowel flora to favor resistant organisms. *To be taken on an empty stomach with a full glass of water. Photosensitivity may occur.*

Table 71-2
Commonly Used Oral Antimicrobial Agents for Acute Urinary Tract Infections (*continued*)

	Usual Dose				
Drug	**Adult**	**Pediatric**	**Pregnancy[a]**	**Breast Milk[a]**	**Comments[b]**
Trimethoprim (TMP)	100 mg every 12 hours		Crosses placenta (cord) = 60%; (maternal) folate antagonism, avoid during first trimester; teratogenic in rats	(milk) >1 (serum)[c]	Alternate choice.
TMP–SMX	160 + 800 mg every 12 hours	10 mg/kg/day (TMP component in 2 doses)	Crosses placenta (cord) = 60%; (maternal) folate antagonism, avoid during first trimester; teratogenic in rats	(milk) >1 (serum)[c]	*To be taken on an empty stomach with a full glass of water. Photosensitivity may occur.* Monitor HIV-infected patients closely for development of adverse hematologic reactions.
					First-line agent for prostatitis.
Fosfomycin	3 g single dose	No data	Crosses placenta	Unknown	Recommended option for uncomplicated cystitis.

[a]Also see Chapter 49, Obstetric Drug Therapy.
[b]Includes unique patient consultation information in italics.
[c]Denotes drug concentration.
[d]May increase theophylline concentrations when given concurrently. Carefully monitor theophylline serum concentrations during quinolone use.
[e]Same comments apply to all fluoroquinolones.
G6PD, glucose-6-phosphate dehydrogenase; HIV, human immunodeficiency virus; TMP–SMX, trimethoprim–sulfamethoxazole.

Updated IDSA/ESMID guidelines for the treatment of acute uncomplicated cystitis and pyelonephritis were published in 2011, and serve as the basis for selection of antibiotics in V.Q. (Table 71-3).[20] The recommended first-line agents for treatment of this patient's uncomplicated cystitis include TMP–SMX, nitrofurantoin, and fosfomycin trometamol; a fourth recommended antibiotic, pivmecillinam, is not commercially available in the United States.

TMP–SMX is effective for therapy of uncomplicated cystitis.[1–3,20,53] Gram-positive and gram-negative organisms, with the notable exceptions of *Enterococcus*, *P. aeruginosa*, and anaerobes, are generally susceptible to TMP–SMX.[20,54] Although TMP–SMX may appear active against enterococci in vitro, clinical efficacy against this pathogen does not always correlate well and is variable. Individually, trimethoprim and sulfamethoxazole are bacteriostatic, but in combination they are bactericidal against most urinary pathogens.[54] Furthermore, this combination is almost uniformly successful in the treatment of uncomplicated UTI, even against organisms that originally were resistant to either agent alone. Although rates of trimethoprim resistance have increased over the past several years,[20,45–49,55] resistance rates remain relatively low in some geographic areas and trimethoprim alone may be effective in managing UTI in many patients.

The ratio of trimethoprim to sulfamethoxazole in the available tablet products is 1:5 (e.g., 80 mg trimethoprim and 400 mg sulfamethoxazole). This combination has been chosen to achieve peak serum concentrations of the two drugs that approximate a 1:20 ratio. This ratio is optimal for synergistic activity against most microorganisms, although the drugs remain synergistic and bactericidal in ratios ranging from 1:5 to 1:40 in vitro.[54,56] Urinary concentrations of trimethoprim and sulfamethoxazole far exceed the minimum inhibitory concentrations (MIC) for most susceptible urinary pathogens. Therefore, good in-vitro activity, excellent clinical success which is similar to that of the fluoroquinolones and other alternative agents in susceptible strains, relatively low resistance rates among common pathogens, and low cost make TMP–SMX a reasonable choice in V.Q.[20] The 2011 IDSA/ESMID guidelines recommend TMP–SMX as an appropriate initial agent of choice in the treatment of acute, uncomplicated lower UTI in geographic areas where the incidence of TMP–SMX resistance among *E. coli* is less than 20%.[20,57]

Nitrofurantoin is also recommended as an appropriate agent for empirical treatment of acute uncomplicated cystitis.[20] Nitrofurantoin is almost completely absorbed after oral administration, but it barely reaches detectable levels in the plasma because it is rapidly eliminated (half-life, 20 minutes) into the urine and bile; the resulting high urine levels are 50 to 250 mg/L and are well in excess of the MIC for most common pathogens causing UTI.[58] Food substantially decreases the rate of absorption, but it increases the total bioavailability of nitrofurantoin from both the macrocrystalline capsules and the microcrystalline tablets by about 40%. This effect lengthens the duration of therapeutic urine concentrations by about 2 hours.[58]

Nitrofurantoin has a spectrum of activity which includes *E. coli*, some strains of *Pseudomonas*, *S. saprophyticus*, streptococci, and enterococci; on the other hand, *Proteus*, *Enterobacter*, and *Klebsiella* are more likely to be resistant (susceptibility <60%).[20,48,59] Nitrofurantoin does not significantly alter the fecal or introital flora, and the development of resistance in previously sensitive strains does not often occur.[20,60] In contrast to ampicillin, TMP–SMX, and other drugs with relatively high resistance rates, nitrofurantoin has maintained excellent activity against most uropathogens; susceptibility rates among *E. coli* currently range from 90% to 99% in most geographic areas.[20,45–49,59] Finally, nitrofurantoin has been shown in comparative clinical studies to be as effective as TMP–SMX, fluoroquinolones, or fosfomycin in the treatment of acute uncomplicated cystitis.[20] Nitrofurantoin is thus recommended in the most recent clinical guidelines as an appropriate choice for treatment of uncomplicated UTI in patients such as V.Q. (Table 71-3).[20]

Most practitioners in the United States have little experience with fosfomycin trometamol, but the drug has, nevertheless, been

Table 71-3
Summary of Evidence-Based Recommendations for Treatment of Acute Uncomplicated Cystitis and Pyelonephritis[20]

Recommendations	Recommendation Grades[a]
Cystitis	
Preferred Agents	
Nitrofurantoin monohydrate/macrocrystals 100 mg PO twice daily × 5 days	A-1
TMP–SMX 160/800 mg (1 double-strength tablet) PO twice daily × 3 days	A-1
Trimethoprim 100 mg PO twice daily × 3 days is considered equivalent to TMP–SMX and is the preferred agent in some regions	A-3
Fosfomycin trometamol 3 g PO × 1 dose	A-1, but appears to have inferior microbiological efficacy compared with standard short-course therapies with agents such as trimethoprim or nitrofurantoin
Pivmecillinam 400 mg PO twice daily × 3–7 days (not commercially available in the United States)	A-1, but may have inferior efficacy compared with other available therapies
Resistance Considerations	
A specific antibiotic is no longer recommended for empirical treatment when the prevalence of resistance is ≥20%	B-3 for TMP–SMX No recommendation for other agents
Alternative agents	
fluoroquinolones	
Fluoroquinolones (ciprofloxacin or levofloxacin) PO × 3 days are highly efficacious for acute cystitis	A-1
Fluoroquinolones should be reserved for other important clinical uses because of propensity for collateral damage	A-3
β-lactams	
β-Lactams (including amoxicillin–clavulanate, cefdinir, cefaclor, and cefpodoxime–proxetil) PO × 3–7 days are appropriate when other recommended agents cannot be used	B-1
Other β-lactams such as cephalexin are less well studied but may also be appropriate in certain settings	B-3
β-Lactams generally have inferior efficacy and more adverse effects compared with other antimicrobials for UTI	B-1
Pyelonephritis	
All Patients	
Urine culture and susceptibility testing should be performed and initial empirical antibiotic therapy tailored appropriately based on results	A-3
Outpatient Treatment	
fluoroquinolones	
Ciprofloxacin 500 mg PO twice daily × 7 days, ± an initial IV dose of ciprofloxacin 400 mg, a long-acting parenteral cephalosporin (e.g., ceftriaxone 1 g) or a consolidated 24-hour dose of an aminoglycoside (e.g., gentamicin 5–7 mg/kg)	A-1
Ciprofloxacin 1,000 mg extended release tablet PO once daily × 7 days, or levofloxacin 750 mg PO once daily × 5 days	B-2
If the local prevalence of fluoroquinolone resistance among uropathogens is >10%, an initial one-time IV dose of a long-acting parenteral cephalosporin or a consolidated 24-hour dose of an aminoglycoside should be administered	B-3
Alternative agents	
TMP–SMX 160/800 mg (1 double-strength tablet) PO twice daily × 14 days	A-1
If TMP–SMX susceptibility is not known, an initial IV dose of a long-acting parenteral cephalosporin or a consolidated 24-hour dose of an aminoglycoside should be administered	B-2 for a cephalosporin B-3 for an aminoglycoside
Oral β-lactams × 10–14 days are less effective than other available agents	B-3
If an oral β-lactam is used, an initial IV dose of a long-acting parenteral cephalosporin or a consolidated 24-hour dose of an aminoglycoside should be administered	B-2 for a cephalosporin B-3 for an aminoglycoside

Table 71-3
Summary of Evidence-Based Recommendations for Treatment of Acute Uncomplicated Cystitis and Pyelonephritis (*continued*)

Recommendations	Recommendation Grades[a]
Hospitalized Patients	
One of the following antibiotic options may be used initially, based on local resistance data and tailored based on susceptibility results: IV fluoroquinolone; IV aminoglycoside ± IV ampicillin; extended-spectrum IV cephalosporin or extended-spectrum IV penicillin ± aminoglycoside; or IV carbapenem.	B-3

[a]Strength of recommendations: A, B, C = good, moderate, and poor evidence to support recommendation for or against use, respectively.
Quality of evidence: 1 = evidence from ≥1 properly randomized, controlled trial; 2 = evidence from ≥1 well-designed clinical trial without randomization, from cohort or case-control analytic studies, from multiple time series, or from dramatic results from uncontrolled experiments; 3 = evidence from opinions of respected authorities, based on clinical experience, descriptive studies, or reports of expert committees.
IV, intravenous; PO, orally; TMP–SMX, trimethoprim–sulfamethoxazole; UTI, urinary tract infection.

used quite successfully in the treatment of UTI in many other parts of the world.[20,44] Fosfomycin is a phosphonic acid derivative which has been shown to irreversibly block bacterial cell wall synthesis through inhibition of early cytoplasmic stages of peptidoglycan synthesis.[44,61] It has bactericidal activity against a broad range of gram-negative and gram-positive organisms including *E. coli* and other Enterobacteriaceae, *Pseudomonas aeruginosa*, and *Enterococcus* as well as many multidrug-resistant pathogens such as methicillin-resistant *S. aureus*, vancomycin-resistant enterococci, and ESBL-producing gram-negative bacilli.[20,44] Fosfomycin is approximately 40% absorbed after oral administration as granules marketed in a sachet form and is rapidly and almost completely excreted unchanged in the urine. Fosfomycin achieves mean urinary concentrations greater than 500 mg/L within 6 to 8 hours after administration and maintains concentrations greater than 100 mg/L for a duration of more than 26 hours after a single oral dose.[44,61] Single 3-g oral doses of fosfomycin are clinically as effective as trimethoprim and nitrofurantoin, although microbiological efficacy may be less.[20] Nevertheless, fosfomycin is currently recommended for treatment of acute uncomplicated cystitis in the 2011 IDSA/ESMID guidelines (Table 71-3).[20] It should be noted that although fosfomycin is commercially available in the United States, it is substantially more expensive than either TMP–SMX or nitrofurantoin.

Alternative agents for the treatment of UTI in V.Q. include the fluoroquinolones and various oral *β*-lactam antibiotics.[20] The fluoroquinolones remain highly effective in the treatment of UTI. However, increasing rates of resistance among common uropathogens and the potential for significant collateral effects on normal flora leading to complications such as *Clostridium difficile* infection have led to recent recommendations that the fluoroquinolones not be routinely used as preferred agents in the treatment of uncomplicated UTI such as that present in V.Q.[20] Further details regarding the use of fluoroquinolones for UTI are discussed in Case 71-2.

Amoxicillin–clavulanate and several oral cephalosporins have been studied for the treatment of uncomplicated UTI; these studies have shown the *β*-lactams to be generally comparable to TMP–SMX, but less clinically or microbiologically effective than the fluoroquinolones.[20] *β*-lactams require longer durations of treatment (see Case 71-1, Question 4), which makes them less attractive from the standpoint of ensuring patient adherence and may also predispose to higher rates of drug-related adverse effects.[20] Finally, these relatively broad-spectrum agents may be associated with more frequent emergence of bacterial resistance, including ESBL-producing gram-negative bacilli.[20] Thus, the *β*-lactam antibiotics (with the exception of pivmecillinam) are currently only recommended for empirical treatment of uncomplicated cystitis when none of the other agents previously discussed can be used (Table 71-3).[20] Of note, ampicillin and amoxicillin are specifically discouraged for empirical treatment of UTI because of the high resistance rates previously noted.[20]

V.Q. could be appropriately treated with either TMP–SMX, nitrofurantoin, or fosfomycin. She has no apparent patient characteristics that would favor the use of one agent over another. In this case, the most important factor to consider would be local antibiotic susceptibilities among community-acquired uropathogens, particularly *E. coli*. Local costs and availability of the different options would also be important to consider in V.Q.

Note that the current IDSA/ESMID guidelines do not apply to the empirical selection of antibiotics for complicated UTI. Complicated infections are often associated with more difficult pathogens (e.g., *P. aeruginosa*) and increased risk of antibiotic resistance; fluoroquinolones are therefore considered preferred agents for initial treatment of complicated UTI with subsequent antibiotic therapy guided by the results of C&S testing.[1–3,5,24]

DURATION OF ANTIBIOTIC THERAPY

CASE 71-1, QUESTION 4: V.Q. is started on TMP–SMX for treatment of her infection. What would be the preferred duration of therapy of antibiotic therapy for V.Q.?

Outpatients with acute, uncomplicated UTI can be treated successfully with a traditional 7- to 14-day course of oral medications, a shorter 3- to 5-day course of therapy, or with single-dose therapy.[1–3,5,20,62] The traditional 7- to 14-day course of antibiotic therapy now is considered excessive for most patients with uncomplicated infections and is seldom used.[1–3,5,20,62] A 3- to 5-day antibiotic treatment regimen is just as effective as a 10-day regimen in achieving clinical cures and eradicating urinary tract organisms, although this is somewhat antibiotic class–specific.[1–3,5,20,62] TMP–SMX is recommended as the preferred agent for 3-day treatment regimens; the fluoroquinolones may also be used in this shorter duration (Table 71-3).[20] A 5-day course of nitrofurantoin is as effective as a 3-day course of TMP–SMX for acute uncomplicated cystitis, and nitrofurantoin is thus currently recommended as a 5-day regimen.[20,63] *β*-Lactam antibiotics are more appropriately reserved for longer treatment courses of 3 to 7 days.[5,20] Longer treatment courses are also used in cases of treatment failure after regimens of shorter duration, as well as in the treatment of complicated UTI where longer courses of therapy (7–14 days) are associated with higher clinical success rates and improved outcomes.[1–3,24]

Even a single dose of an antibiotic may be effective. Bacteria disappear from the urine within hours after antibacterial therapy has been initiated.[20] This, coupled with the urinary bladder's ability to defend itself through micturition, acidification, and inherent antibacterial activity, gives theoretic support to the clinical evidence that a large single dose of an antibiotic can eradicate a UTI. Fosfomycin trometamol is a perfect example of this principle: very high urinary concentrations of this bactericidal agent are maintained for more than 24 hours after a single 3-g oral dose and contribute to the favorable clinical efficacy observed in comparative trials.[20,44,61]

Although not recommended in the current guidelines, single doses of antibiotics other than fosfomycin are also occasionally used in treating acute, lower UTI in young women.[5,8,20] Commonly used regimens are TMP–SMX (two or three double-strength tablets), trimethoprim 400 mg, amoxicillin–clavulanate 500 mg, amoxicillin 3 g, ampicillin 3.5 g, nitrofurantoin 200 mg, ciprofloxacin 500 mg, and norfloxacin 400 mg.[1,20] Again, choice of a specific agent should be based on local susceptibility patterns, patient allergies, and relative drug costs. Female patients with history or clinical presentation suggestive of complicated infection (e.g., systemic manifestations of infection, renal disease, anatomic abnormalities of the urinary tract, diabetes mellitus, pregnancy), a history of antibiotic resistance, or a history of relapse after single-dose therapy should not receive single-dose regimens. Single-dose therapy is also not appropriate for male patients with UTI. Because V.Q. does not have any of these contraindications, she could theoretically receive single-dose therapy with an appropriate agent.

The advantages of single-dose treatment of UTI include improved compliance, reduced cost, proven efficacy in a defined population of patients (i.e., young women with acute, uncomplicated lower UTI), minimal side effects, and a potentially decreased incidence of bacterial resistance associated with antibiotic overuse. However, several concerns also exist regarding single-dose therapy.[5,8,20] First, sample sizes in most comparative studies were relatively small. Consequently, it is difficult to determine whether differences in effectiveness or incidence of side effects between single-dose and multiple-dose therapy are clinically significant. Meta-analysis of studies comparing either single-dose or 3-day regimens with TMP–SMX therapy has demonstrated that single-dose therapy is significantly less effective in eradicating bacteriuria than regimens of $\geq$5 days (83% vs. 93%, respectively, $p < 0.001$) or $\geq$7 days in duration (87% vs. 94%, respectively; $p = 0.014$).[20,53,62] As discussed in Case 71-1, Question 3, reduced microbiological efficacy was also observed with single-dose fosfomycin.[20] Although fewer studies have directly compared single-dose versus 3-day therapies, numerous studies have shown that 3-day courses are as effective as courses of longer duration.[20,62] Finally, single-dose therapies have been associated with higher rates of recurrence compared with therapies of longer duration.[5] A 3-day on 5-day course of therapy is therefore currently recommended by the IDSA/ESMID for uncomplicated cystitis; a large single dose of fosfomycin is the sole single-dose regimen endorsed by the guidelines.[18]

Based on the preceding information, and according to current guidelines, a 3-day course of TMP–SMX, a 5-day course of nitrofurantoin, or a single dose of fosfomycin would be most appropriate for treatment of V.Q.'s infection (Table 71-3).[20]

When using short-course regimens, it is important to counsel the patient that the clinical signs and symptoms of infection may often not be completely resolved for 2 to 3 days after initiation of therapy. Therefore, symptoms that persist for a short while after beginning therapy (or actually completing therapy, in the case of single-dose regimens) are not necessarily indicative of treatment failure.

PHENAZOPYRIDINE

CASE 71-1, QUESTION 5: Along with TMP–SMX, phenazopyridine is also prescribed because of V.Q.'s complaints of significant dysuria. Is phenazopyridine appropriate for this patient?

Phenazopyridine, a urinary tract analgesic, occasionally is prescribed alone or along with an antibacterial agent for the symptomatic relief of dysuria. Although phenazopyridine at a dose of 200 mg orally three times a day may relieve dysuria, it is ineffective in the actual eradication of true UTI. Phenazopyridine plus an antibiotic is not any better than an antibiotic alone; therefore, the drug is not likely of significant value in V.Q. and should not be routinely recommended. However, although most patients have resolution of symptoms within 24 to 48 hours after beginning therapy, certain patients with severe dysuria or delayed response to antibiotic therapy may benefit symptomatically from a short trial (1–2 days) of phenazopyridine.[5] The need for, and duration of, analgesic therapy must be individualized.

Phenazopyridine is an azo dye and may discolor the urine to an orange–red, orange–brown, or red color that can stain clothes. Other adverse effects of phenazopyridine occur after acute overdose, or as a result of accumulation in older patients or in patients with decreased renal function who take the drug chronically. In vivo, about 50% of phenazopyridine is metabolized to aniline, which can cause methemoglobinemia and hemolytic anemia. Hemolytic anemia associated with phenazopyridine occurs primarily in patients with glucose-6-phosphate dehydrogenase (G6PD) deficiency.[64] Cases of reversible acute renal failure and allergic hepatitis have also been rarely reported after brief exposure to phenazopyridine.[64]

INTERPRETATION OF URINE CULTURE AND SUSCEPTIBILITY TEST RESULTS

CASE 71-1, QUESTION 6: Two days after V.Q. begins treatment for her infection with TMP–SMX, results of the C&S studies become available and reveal greater than 10^5 bacteria per milliliter of *P. mirabilis*, which is susceptible to ampicillin, amoxicillin–clavulanate, cephalosporins, and gentamicin. The *Proteus* is intermediately sensitive to nitrofurantoin, and it is resistant to TMP–SMX and ciprofloxacin. V.Q. reports that she is symptomatically better since starting antibiotic therapy and that her dysuria and bladder pain are now almost completely resolved. How should these test results be interpreted? Is a change in V.Q.'s antibiotic therapy necessary?

Most women with either lower or upper UTI have greater than 10^5 bacterial colonies/mL of urine. However, a major revision in the diagnostic criteria for symptomatic UTI has been the abandonment of the absolute requirement for growth of $\geq 10^5$ bacterial colonies/mL of urine. The criterion of greater than or equal to 100 bacteria/mL results in excellent sensitivity and specificity in correctly diagnosing and treating women with symptomatic infection.[13] This same criterion should also be applied to lower UTI when *S. saprophyticus* is isolated, because UTIs caused by this pathogen often are associated with low urine bacterial colony counts, suboptimal growth on commonly used media, and negative findings on nitrite screening.

Mixed flora (more than two organisms) is unusual except in severely debilitated persons and other complicated infections. Thus, mixed flora in the setting of uncomplicated infection frequently suggests contamination, and a repeat specimen should be obtained.

Bacterial susceptibility to different antimicrobial drugs is usually determined by referencing interpretive criteria that correlate with achievable serum concentrations of those drugs. However, drugs useful in the treatment of UTI are excreted primarily by the kidney, and urine concentrations of these drugs may be 20 to 100 times greater than serum concentrations. Therefore, infections caused by organisms that are only intermediately susceptible, or even "resistant" to the tested concentration of antibacterial drug, might still be effectively treated with the high concentration of drug achieved in the urine.

Although in-vitro susceptibility testing is not always predictive of patient response to therapy of UTI, studies clearly show that patients infected with a resistant pathogen are at increased risk of treatment failure.[51,57,65,66] Clinical response to infection occurred in only 24% to 61% of patients with organisms resistant to TMP–SMX compared with 83% to 92% of patients infected with susceptible organisms[51,57,65]; furthermore, patients infected with TMP–SMX-resistant pathogens were 17 times more likely to fail therapy compared with patients with susceptible strains.[67] Patients treated with TMP–SMX, who were infected with drug-resistant organisms, were also found to have longer median times to symptom resolution (14 vs. 7 days, $p = 0.0002$), more frequent return clinic visits within 1 week (36% vs. 6%, $p < 0.0001$), more frequent need for subsequent antibiotic therapy (36% vs. 4%, $p < 0.0001$), and higher rates of significant bacteriuria after 1 month (42% vs. 20%, $p = 0.04$).[65]

Although up to 75% of patients with resistant organisms may experience failure of TMP–SMX therapy, antimicrobial therapy is usually chosen empirically without the benefit of C&S testing results. Appropriateness of antibiotic therapy is, thus, usually judged according to subsequent clinical response. If the infecting organism is susceptible, the urine will usually be sterile for 24 to 48 hours. If a urine specimen collected 48 hours after initiation of therapy is not sterile and the patient has been taking the medication properly, the antibiotic may be inappropriate or the focus of infection may be deeper (e.g., pyelonephritis, abscess, obstruction). If the urine specimen is sterile and the patient is symptomatically improved, the appropriate antimicrobial is being used (regardless of susceptibility studies) and the full course of therapy should be completed. Because V.Q. reports significant improvement in her subjective symptoms, her 3-day course of TMP–SMX should be completed as originally ordered and V.Q. should be closely monitored for any evidence of relapse. A repeat C&S test should be performed in the event that V.Q. reports any new signs or symptoms which are consistent with antibiotic failure and relapse of her infection, and a different antibiotic should be selected for treatment at that time.

FLUOROQUINOLONE THERAPY

CASE 71-2

QUESTION 1: I.B., a 48-year-old woman, presents with a community-acquired UTI. She has a past medical history significant only for several previous episodes of UTI. A UA is ordered with the following results:

- Appearance, straw-colored and turbid (normal, straw-colored and clear)
- Specific gravity, 1.028 (normal, 1.002–1.028)
- pH, 6.3 (normal, 5.5–7.0)
- Glucose, ketones, and bilirubin, all negative (normal, all negative)
- Blood and protein, both trace positive by dipstick (normal, both negative)
- WBC, 10 to 15 cells/LPF (normal, 0–2 cells/LPF)
- RBC, 5 to 10 cells/LPF (normal, 0–2 cells/LPF)
- Bacteria, many (normal, 0 to rare)
- Epithelial cells, 3 to 5 cells/LPF (normal, 0 to few cells/LPF)
- Leukocyte esterase and nitrite tests by dipstick, both positive (normal, both negative)

Of note, I.B. has experienced a rash with TMP–SMX and a type I hypersensitivity reaction to penicillins in the past. What is the role of fluoroquinolones in the treatment of I.B.'s community-acquired UTI?

Several fluoroquinolones are indicated for the treatment of uncomplicated or complicated UTI; these include norfloxacin, ciprofloxacin, and levofloxacin. The fluoroquinolones are usually administered orally in the treatment of UTI and have excellent in-vitro activity against most gram-negative organisms, including *P. aeruginosa*.[68] They are also active in vitro against many gram-positive organisms including *S. saprophyticus*.[68] The activity of many fluoroquinolones in vitro is antagonized by urine (acidic pH, divalent cations); however, this is unlikely to be clinically significant because urine concentrations are several hundred-fold greater than serum levels.[68] A large number of clinical trials have demonstrated that fluoroquinolones are very effective in the treatment of acute uncomplicated UTI with efficacy rates typically greater than 90%.[20,53]

Although the fluoroquinolones are as effective as TMP–SMX, nitrofurantoin, or β-lactams in treatment of uncomplicated UTI, they are no longer recommended as first-line empirical therapy because they are more expensive and provide no additional treatment benefits.[5,8,20,53,68] Concerns also exist regarding the overuse of fluoroquinolones and the promotion of drug resistance among community-acquired uropathogens. Resistance to fluoroquinolones among organisms causing acute uncomplicated UTI is usually less than 1% to 2%.[21] Fluoroquinolone resistance may, however, be more frequent in some geographic areas and in complicated infections[45–49,55]; recent studies have documented resistance to ciprofloxacin in 2% to 10% of acute uncomplicated infections, whereas it is 8% to 60% in complicated UTI.[20,46–49,69] Furthermore, these quinolone-resistant strains often are resistant to multiple other antimicrobials.[46–49,69] Concerns also exist regarding the potential for fluoroquinolones to produce collateral effects on normal flora, these alterations leading to increased risk of infection because of methicillin-resistant *S. aureus* and *C. difficile*.[20]

Fluoroquinolones are recommended as appropriate alternatives for patients with allergies or other contraindications to the use of other first-line agents, or for patients infected with organisms resistant to multiple antibiotics, such as *P. aeruginosa*. Fluoroquinolones are appropriate initial therapy in geographic areas with greater than 20% resistance of *E. coli* to TMP–SMX[20]; however, many patients in such areas may be appropriately treated with nitrofurantoin or some other options (Table 71-3).[20] Finally, the fluoroquinolones are effective in treating patients with structural or functional abnormalities of the urinary tract and other complicated infections.[20,68]

A fluoroquinolone may be considered for I.B. because she has experienced previous adverse reactions to penicillins and sulfonamides. However, nitrofurantoin or fosfomycin should be preferentially considered for I.B. based on current IDSA/ESMID recommendations.[20] If a fluoroquinolone was deemed appropriate for I.B. based on other unspecified factors such as availability, cost, or tolerability issues with other treatment options, the fluoroquinolones are similar in efficacy and the choice would be based on comparative costs and compliance considerations.[20] The duration of fluoroquinolone therapy in I.B. would be 3 days.[20]

NITROFURANTOIN-INDUCED ADVERSE EFFECTS

CASE 71-2, QUESTION 2: The decision is made to begin I.B. on nitrofurantoin rather than a fluoroquinolone. After beginning nitrofurantoin monohydrate 100 mg twice daily, she complains of nausea and gastrointestinal (GI) upset after the ingestion of each dose. I.B. had her nitrofurantoin prescription filled with nitrofurantoin monohydrate because it was the less expensive product at her local pharmacy. How can these GI effects be minimized in I.B.? What other important adverse effects are associated with nitrofurantoin?

Nausea is a common complication of nitrofurantoin therapy, and the patient's adherence with the prescribed regimen may be affected by this side effect. It is not known whether the mechanism by which nitrofurantoin produces nausea is central or local. Taking nitrofurantoin with food may reduce nausea either through serving as a buffer or slowing the rate of absorption and reducing peak concentrations of the drug. Food, however, may also increase the bioavailability of nitrofurantoin. Slowing of absorption is particularly beneficial in decreasing the incidence of nausea and vomiting associated with the microcrystalline product.[59] Use of the macrocrystalline preparation may also reduce adverse effects through slowing rates of dissolution and absorption, and producing lower serum levels. A disadvantage of the macrocrystalline form is the cost, which may be 2 to 10 times that of the microcrystalline form, depending on the product source. Finally, because nausea and vomiting appear to be dose related and occur more frequently in small persons, reducing the daily dose of nitrofurantoin may also improve tolerability.[58,59] However, the best-studied and clinically effective dose of nitrofurantoin is 100 mg twice daily[20], which I.B. is currently receiving. I.B. should remain on her current dose; taking the drug with food and/or switching to a macrocrystalline product should allow her to successfully finish her course of nitrofurantoin at the recommended dose.

Several hundred cases of nitrofurantoin-induced acute, subacute, or chronic pulmonary reactions have been reported.[70] Acute toxicity often manifests within several days of initiating the drug with a sudden flu-like syndrome consisting of fever, dyspnea, and cough; eosinophilia may also be present. The subacute form usually occurs after at least a month of exposure; symptoms include fever and dyspnea. The chronic form tends to be more insidious with milder dyspnea and low-grade fever. In all forms, rales are common and pulmonary infiltrates may be present on chest radiograph.[70] Discontinuation of nitrofurantoin results in complete symptomatic recovery after several weeks; however, permanent fibrotic changes may persist with chronic pulmonary reactions. Rechallenge with oral nitrofurantoin results in rapid reappearance of pulmonary symptoms in those who have had an acute reaction; the drug must therefore be avoided in patients with history of nitrofurantoin-induced pulmonary toxicity.[70]

Peripheral neuropathy may also occur during nitrofurantoin therapy and is characterized by symmetric dysesthesia and paresthesia in the distal extremities, which progresses in a central and ascending fashion.[58,71] Neuropathy usually occurs within the first 60 days of chronic nitrofurantoin treatment and is rarely seen during shorter courses of therapy.[58,71] Symptom severity is not dose-related and is generally reversible, although more severe cases may require up to several months to resolve completely. Renal failure is a risk factor for both neurotoxicity and pulmonary toxicity, but neuropathy has also been reported in patients with normal renal function.[58,71]

FLUOROQUINOLONE USE IN PEDIATRIC INFECTIONS

CASE 71-3

QUESTION 1: C.S. is a 2-year-old girl with a history of multiple recurrent UTIs caused by congenital urinary tract abnormalities that have not been corrected. She has had at least nine UTIs since birth and has received multiple courses of antibiotics, including ampicillin, amoxicillin, amoxicillin–clavulanate, and TMP–SMX. She has also been on chronic low-dose antibiotic prophylaxis with TMP–SMX. C.S. was brought to her pediatrician 48 hours ago with signs and symptoms consistent with a new UTI. Suprapubital aspiration was performed and urine samples sent for C&S testing at that time, and C.S. was empirically begun on amoxicillin–clavulanate pending laboratory test results. C&S results, however, are now available and show $>10^5$ colonies/mL of *P. mirabilis*. The organism is susceptible to ciprofloxacin, gentamicin, and ertapenem and resistant to ampicillin, trimethoprim, TMP–SMX, cephalexin, cefaclor, cefpodoxime, tetracycline, nitrofurantoin, and erythromycin. C.S. has not clinically improved while receiving empiric amoxicillin–clavulanate. What antibiotic therapy would be most appropriate for continued management of this acute infection in C.S.?

This case illustrates the serious dilemmas caused by antibiotic resistance among uropathogens. The pathogen isolated from C.S. is resistant to all commonly used, orally administered antibiotics that have been proved effective in the treatment of UTI in pediatric patients. Penicillins, cephalosporins, nitrofurantoin, and sulfonamides are frequently recommended for treatment of pediatric UTI; however, multiple past treatment regimens and chronic antibiotic prophylaxis make these agents less suitable for treatment of this new infection in C.S. Although in-vitro susceptibility testing does not accurately predict clinical response to therapy in all cases, the risk of treatment failure and poor patient outcome is significantly increased when agents to which isolates are resistant are administered.[57,65] Alternative treatment is required; however, few desirable options exist for C.S.

The recommended duration of antibiotic therapy in C.S. would be at least 2 weeks for the treatment of this complicated and recurrent infection (refer to subsequent sections of this chapter). Although the organism isolated from C.S. is susceptible to gentamicin and this drug would be effective, parenteral (intramuscular or intravenous) administration would be required and the lengthy required treatment duration makes this far from ideal. Use of aminoglycosides would also be less desirable because of toxicity concerns. Although ertapenem would also likely be effective, there is relatively little clinical experience with this agent in the pediatric population and ertapenem would also require parenteral administration for the duration of the treatment regimen.

Fluoroquinolones are contraindicated in children and adolescents younger than 18 years of age because of concerns regarding potential musculoskeletal toxicities in juvenile populations. Although not approved for pediatric use, fluoroquinolones have been formally studied for febrile neutropenia, infectious gastroenteritis, otitis media, bacterial meningitis, and other uses in pediatric patients.[72–74] The use of fluoroquinolones has substantially increased in children and adolescents, most likely owing to resistance to other antimicrobials; approximately 520,000 prescriptions were written for patients younger than 18 years of age during 2002, of which nearly 3,000 prescriptions were for children younger than 2 years.[72] Several reviews summarized data related to the safety of fluoroquinolones in children. Although tendinopathy or other musculoskeletal toxicities have been recorded, these toxicities have been usually mild, reversible, and occurring at rates comparable to that seen in adults.[72–74] Based on currently available information and in consideration of antimicrobial resistance, the American Academy of Pediatrics has published recommendations regarding the use of fluoroquinolones in children and adolescents.[72] These indicate that fluoroquinolones may be considered in special circumstances including (a) infections caused by multidrug-resistant pathogens for which there are no other safe and effective alternatives and (b) times when parenteral therapy is not feasible and no other effective oral agent is available. Treatment of UTI caused by multidrug-resistant, gram-negative pathogens are specifically mentioned as a potentially appropriate use for fluoroquinolones in pediatric patients.[72]

Selection of a specific agent for the treatment of UTI in C.S. should be based on careful consideration of potential risks and benefits of available antibiotic options. The feasibility, risks, expenses, and inconvenience associated with prolonged (≥2 weeks) parenteral administration of an aminoglycoside or carbapenem are problematic; however, the ease of oral fluoroquinolone administration must be carefully balanced against the possible risks of using these agents in C.S. Clearly, no antibiotic of choice exists for treatment of C.S. and both the providers and the child's parents must be involved in development of an acceptable and well-informed treatment plan.

TREATMENT OF LOWER-TRACT INFECTION IN RENAL FAILURE

CASE 71-4

QUESTION 1: K.M., a 55-year-old man with a history of hypertension and chronic renal failure, experiences a UTI. His creatinine clearance, determined from a recent 24-hour urine collection, is 20 mL/minute. What antimicrobial agent should be prescribed?

The major problem in treating UTI in patients with renal failure is how to achieve adequate urine concentrations of the drug without causing systemic toxicity. The ideal drug would be (a) inherently nontoxic, even at high serum concentrations, making dosage adjustments unnecessary; (b) excreted unchanged in the urine (i.e., not metabolized); and (c) eliminated by renal tubular secretion rather than glomerular filtration. Because renal tubular secretion remains active in all but the most severe cases of renal failure, antibiotics eliminated by this mechanism would reach adequate urinary levels; however, no such ideal drug exists.

Nitrofurantoin and many sulfonamides are substantially metabolized by the liver and generally produce low urine levels in uremic patients. The aminoglycosides are eliminated almost exclusively by the kidneys, but uremic patients are at high risk of drug-induced toxicities and alternative agents are usually recommended. Penicillins, cephalosporins, and trimethoprim are partially metabolized by the liver but are also eliminated by the kidney to a significant extent. These agents are suitable for use in renal failure according to the criteria described above. Certain fluoroquinolones, specifically ciprofloxacin and levofloxacin, are highly excreted in the urine through a combination of filtration and tubular secretion and reach extremely high urinary concentrations. These agents are also considered safe and effective in the treatment of UTI in patients with renal failure.

Acute Pyelonephritis

SIGNS AND SYMPTOMS

CASE 71-5

QUESTION 1: L.B., a 45-year-old woman with type 1 diabetes mellitus, comes to the emergency department complaining of severe nausea, frequent vomiting, frequent urination, fever, shaking chills, and flank pain. Positive physical findings include a temperature of 103°F, a pulse of 110 beats/minute, blood pressure of 90/60 mm Hg, and CVA tenderness. A Gram stain of L.B.'s urine reveals gram-negative rods, and a UA demonstrates glucosuria, macroscopic hematuria, 20 to 25 WBC/LPF, numerous bacteria, and WBC casts. She also has a blood sugar level of 400 mg/dL. L.B. is admitted to the hospital with a diagnosis of acute bacterial pyelonephritis, and routine laboratory tests including a blood chemistry profile and complete blood count with differential, and specimens of urine and blood for C&S are ordered. L.B. is started on intravenous (IV) normal saline, ampicillin 1 g IV every 6 hours, and a sliding-scale schedule of regular insulin based on every 6-hour blood sugars. Which signs and symptoms in L.B. are consistent with pyelonephritis?

It is not always possible to differentiate clinically between upper and lower urinary tract infections. Symptoms common in lower UTI often are the only positive findings in upper UTI (i.e., subclinical pyelonephritis).[1–5,75] L.B., however, does manifest signs and symptoms of systemic infection consistent with acute bacterial pyelonephritis, including tachycardia, hypotension, fever, nausea and vomiting, shaking chills, flank pain, CVA tenderness, hematuria, and WBC casts. In addition, her diabetes may predispose her to various renal infections, including pyelonephritis, possibly because diabetic patients have altered antibacterial defense mechanisms.[2–5,75]

Treatment

TRIAGE FOR HOSPITALIZATION

CASE 71-5, QUESTION 2: Why was L.B. hospitalized?

Most patients with clinical pyelonephritis have relatively mild infection and usually can be treated as outpatients. The need for hospitalization often is determined by the patient's social situation and ability to maintain an adequate fluid intake and tolerate oral medications.[2–5,8,20] Patients who experience significant nausea and/or vomiting may not be able to maintain adequate hydration and thus may be at higher risk for cardiovascular complications of infection. Such patients may also require parenteral therapy initially in order to guarantee adequate initial antibiotic therapy. Finally, patients such as L.B. with diabetes should be hospitalized because acute pyelonephritis may predispose her to diabetic ketoacidosis.

Although blood cultures are usually obtained in patients with moderate-to-severe pyelonephritis, one study found that blood cultures were of low yield in the setting of acute uncomplicated pyelonephritis; they rarely provided any additional information not already obtained from the urine culture and were not helpful in the clinical management of such cases.[76] Blood cultures may be positive in up to 25% of patients with severe or complicated pyelonephritis, however, and they are still recommended for hospitalized patients such as L.B.[2–5,75,76]

ANTIMICROBIAL CHOICE FOR PYELONEPHRITIS

CASE 71-5, QUESTION 3: Was ampicillin appropriate treatment for L.B.?

Ampicillin is not an appropriate choice for L.B. because diabetic patients (and patients treated with corticosteroids) are susceptible to colonization with unusual or more resistant organisms. As with lower tract UTI, pyelonephritis is often classified as uncomplicated or complicated. L.B.'s infection would be classified as a complicated infection because of her underlying diabetes.[2–5,8,20,75]

E. coli remains the predominant pathogen in complicated pyelonephritis, but other gram-negative organisms (e.g., *Klebsiella*, *Proteus*, *Pseudomonas*) are found frequently.[2–5,8] Because L.B. is acutely ill and has gram-negative organisms in her urine, she should be treated with an antibiotic that has a better spectrum of activity against gram-negative organisms. Because of high rates of ampicillin resistance among common uropathogens, ampicillin and amoxicillin are inappropriate for the empirical therapy of UTI, including pyelonephritis.[20] Current IDSA/ESMID recommendations for the initial oral management of acute pyelonephritis are shown in Table 71-3. Because L.B. is to be hospitalized, broad-spectrum antibiotics appropriate for initial therapy would include parenteral third-generation cephalosporins (e.g., ceftriaxone), IV fluoroquinolones (e.g., ciprofloxacin, levofloxacin), extended-spectrum penicillins, such as piperacillin–tazobactam, or carbapenems.[2–5,8,20] Aminoglycosides may be used empirically as either monotherapy or in combination with various β-lactams: in combination with ampicillin to provide better activity against suspected enterococci, or together with cephalosporins or piperacillin–tazobactam to provide enhanced gram-negative activity.[20] The choice of a specific regimen is based on local susceptibility patterns and should be tailored as needed on the basis of C&S test results.[20] It is not always necessary to initially treat patients with antipseudomonal therapy; thus, agents such as ceftriaxone with relatively less activity against

Pseudomonas are often appropriate as initial therapy in patients such as L.B.[4,8,20] Because most hospital laboratories can report C&S results within 48 hours, these antibiotics can be replaced with more specific ones if appropriate.

SERUM VERSUS URINE CONCENTRATIONS

CASE 71-5, QUESTION 4: Is it necessary to achieve bactericidal concentrations of antimicrobials in the serum, or are high urinary concentrations adequate for L.B.? How long should she be treated? How should therapeutic success be determined?

In patients with pyelonephritis and infection of the renal parenchyma, adequate tissue concentrations of antimicrobial agents are needed. Therefore, antibiotics that achieve bactericidal concentrations in serum and kidney tissues as well as in the urine should be selected.[20,77] Patients requiring hospitalization should be treated with parenteral antibiotics until fluids can be taken orally and the patient is symptomatically improved and afebrile for 24 to 48 hours.[2–5] This should be followed with a course of oral antibiotics for a total duration of antimicrobial therapy of approximately 14 days; less severe infections not requiring hospitalization are usually treated with 7- to 14-day courses, depending on the specific agent chosen.[20] Although it is customary to observe the patient in the hospital for 24 hours after switching from parenteral to oral antibiotics before discharge, this is probably of limited benefit.[2–5,8] Specimens for C&S testing should be obtained on the second day of therapy (to rule out treatment failure), 2 to 3 weeks after the completion of therapy, and again at 3 months.[1,4]

For patients who have relapsed after 14 days, retreatment for 6 weeks usually is curative. There have been reports of successful retreatment of relapsed infection with only 5 days of treatment[76]; however, longer courses are recommended.[4,8,76]

ORAL THERAPY FOR PYELONEPHRITIS

CASE 71-5, QUESTION 5: Would oral therapy have been appropriate for the initial treatment of acute pyelonephritis in L.B.?

Patients with mild, acute pyelonephritis (no nausea, vomiting, or signs of sepsis) can be treated with oral antibiotics such as fluoroquinolones for 5 to 7 days, or with TMP–SMX for 14 days.[2–5,20] Oral fluoroquinolones are preferred agents for initial empirical therapy of acute pyelonephritis in patients not requiring hospitalization because of lower rates of resistance among common uropathogens compared to TMP–SMX, and higher rates of clinical and microbiological efficacy compared to β-lactams.[20] Fluoroquinolones may be particularly useful for patients potentially infected with resistant organisms because of their excellent in-vitro activity against gram-negative organisms and high kidney tissue concentrations (2-fold to 10-fold greater than serum).[68] However, fluoroquinolone resistance and risk of inappropriate initial therapy may be more common in certain geographic areas. If fluoroquinolone resistance among *E. coli* exceeds 10%, treatment for acute pyelonephritis should be initiated with an intravenous dose of extended-spectrum cephalosporin or an aminoglycoside until C&S test results are known (Table 71-3).[20] Oral agents such as amoxicillin–clavulanate, cefuroxime, cefpodoxime proxetil, or cefdinir also can be used in this setting, but the most recent guidelines suggest that oral β-lactams are less effective than other available options and their use is somewhat discouraged as first-line treatment options.[20]

Patients such as L.B. with evidence of bacteremia (e.g., fever, shaking chills) or sepsis (e.g., hypotension) should be hospitalized and treated with parenteral antibiotics[4,8,20] (see Table 71-4). L.B.'s frequent vomiting and potential inability to be successfully treated with oral antibiotics would also make initial therapy with parenteral antibiotics more favorable. Although L.B. will be initially treated with parenteral antibiotics, early switch to oral therapy after as few as 1 to 4 days of treatment is recommended; clinical outcomes with oral antibiotics are similar to those achieved with continued parenteral therapy (i.e., 5 days or longer).[78]

RECURRENT URINARY TRACT INFECTIONS

Relapse versus Reinfection

CASE 71-6

QUESTION 1: T.W. is a 28-year-old woman with a history of recurrent UTIs who now exhibits a new *E. coli* UTI. Her last episode occurred 5 months previously. Her current infection is treated with TMP–SMX for 10 days. A repeat UA was scheduled for the completion of antibiotic therapy, but she canceled her appointment because she "felt fine." Twelve weeks later, she returns to the clinic with signs and symptoms of another UTI. The only other medication she has taken is an oral contraceptive. Why would C&S testing of a urine sample be especially useful at this time?

Recurrent infections develop in approximately 20% to 30% of women with acute cystitis.[3,5,34,79,80] Repeat C&S data should help determine whether this infection represents a relapse or a reinfection. Relapse refers to a recurrence of bacteriuria caused by the same microorganism that was present before initial therapy. Most relapses occur within 1 to 2 weeks after the completion of therapy and are caused by persistence of the organism in the urinary tract. Relapses often are associated with an inadequately treated upper UTI (e.g. medication non-adherence), structural abnormalities of the urinary tract, or chronic bacterial prostatitis.[1,34,79,80]

Reinfection implies recurrence of bacteriuria with a different organism than was present before therapy. Reinfections can occur at any time during or after the completion of treatment, but most appear several weeks to several months later. Approximately 80% of recurrences are caused by reinfection.[1,34] Reinfection is generally caused by introital colonization with Enterobacteriaceae from the lower intestinal tract[1]; of these, *E. coli* is the most common. Certain *E. coli* strains have been shown to adhere to vaginal epithelial cells and, in women with recurrent UTI, adherence of these organisms to epithelial cells is increased.[26] Considering T.W. was symptom-free for 8 weeks suggests that this is a reinfection, rather than a relapse. Patients with reinfection should be investigated for modifiable predisposing factors such as use of a diaphragm with or without spermicides. Patients with frequent reinfections should also be evaluated for risk factors such as anatomical abnormalities, undiagnosed glucose intolerance or diabetes, or other factors.

Treatment for Reinfection

CASE 71-6, QUESTION 2: Pending the C&S test results, what therapy should be instituted in T.W.?

T.W. has a history of recurrent infections and now probably has a reinfection. Because reinfection is not caused by failure of previous therapy, TMP–SMX may be a reasonable choice once again. The probability that a resistant organism will be responsible for the infection increases when the interval between infectious episodes is short. If several months elapse between each episode of antimicrobial therapy, normal fecal bacterial flora become reestablished and the risk of infection with resistant pathogens is reduced.

Table 71-4
Parenteral Antimicrobial Agents Commonly Used in the Treatment of Urinary Tract Infections

Class	Drug	Average Adult Daily Dose: UTI	Average Adult Daily Dose: Sepsis	Usual Dosage Interval[a]	Comments
Penicillins	Ampicillin	2–4 g	8 g	Every 4–6 hours	Use should be based on local susceptibility patterns.
	Ampicillin–sulbactam	6 g	12 g	Every 6 hours	
	Piperacillin–tazobactam	9 g	18 g	Every 4–6 hours	
First-generation cephalosporins	Cefazolin	1.5–3 g	6 g	Every 8–12 hours	More effective than second- or third-generation cephalosporins against gram-positive organisms.
Second-generation cephalosporins	Cefoxitin	3–4 g	8 g	Every 4–8 hours	Intermediate between first- and third-generation cephalosporins against gram-negative organisms.
	Cefuroxime	2.25 g	4.5 g	Every 8 hours	
Third-generation cephalosporins	Cefotaxime	3–4 g	8 g	Every 6–8 hours	Better coverage than first- and second-generation cephalosporins against gram-negative organisms. Ceftazidime and cefepime are most effective against *Pseudomonas*. All generations of cephalosporins are ineffective against *Enterococcus faecalis* and methicillin-resistant staphylococci.
	Ceftriaxone	1 g	2 g	Every 12–24 hours	
	Ceftazidime	1.5–3 g	6 g	Every 8–12 hours	
Fourth-generation cephalosporins	Cefepime	1–2 g	4 g	Every 12 hours	Ceftaroline has activity against methicillin-resistant staphylococci.
	Ceftaroline	0.6	0.6 g	Every 12 hours	
Carbapenems	Imipenem–cilastatin	1 g	2 g	Every 6 hours	The most broad-spectrum coverage of any antibiotics listed. Ertapenem not active against *Pseudomonas*. Resistance may develop especially with *Pseudomonas*. Toxic in some pregnant animals.
	Meropenem	1.5–3 g	3 g	Every 8 hours	
	Ertapenem	0.5–1 g	1 g	Every 24 hours	
Monobactam	Aztreonam	1–2 g	6–8 g	Every 8–12 hours	Active against gram-negative aerobic pathogens, including *Pseudomonas* sp.
Aminoglycosides	Gentamicin	3 mg/kg	5–7 mg/kg	Every 24 hours	Potent against gram-negative bacteria including *Pseudomonas*. Associated with possible eighth nerve toxicity in the fetus. Amikacin should be reserved for multiresistant bacteria.
	Tobramycin	3 mg/kg	5–7 mg/kg	Every 24 hours	
	Amikacin	7.5 mg/kg	15–20 mg/kg	Every 24 hours	
Quinolones	Ciprofloxacin	400–800 mg	800 mg	Every 12 hours	Use for resistant organisms. Change to oral Therapy when indicated.
	Levofloxacin	250–500 mg	500–750 mg	Every 24 hours	

[a]Assuming normal renal function. Dose adjustments need to be made in patients with compromised renal function (see Chapter 62, Principles of Infectious Diseases)
UTI, urinary tract infection.

The alteration of fecal flora caused by the sulfonamides makes these drugs poor choices for repeated use in cases of frequent reinfection, especially when C&S results are unknown. The development of bacterial resistance also may limit the usefulness of these agents for chronic antimicrobial therapy.[20,34,79,80] However, because her most recent infection was 12 weeks ago and the UTI prior to that was 5 months earlier, TMP–SMX would again be a reasonable choice at this time.

CASE 71-6, QUESTION 3: If T.W. exhibited an adverse reaction to TMP–SMX, what are some other therapeutic alternatives?

Nitrofurantoin is highly effective against *E. coli* with relatively low rates of resistance (<10%) in most geographic areas. It does not significantly alter the fecal or introital flora, and the development of resistance in previously sensitive strains does not often occur.[20,60,81] Therefore, it is generally a useful agent for the treatment of recurrent *E. coli*, *S. saprophyticus*, and *Enterococcus* infections.[20]

The fluoroquinolones also are useful in this setting, especially in geographic areas with high rates of TMP–SMX resistance.[34,78] Their widespread use should not be encouraged for reinfections as in T.W. in light of their high cost and concern regarding selection of resistant organisms.[20,34,80] Cephalosporins (e.g., cefuroxime, cefpodoxime proxetil) and trimethoprim have also been recommended as alternative agents in this setting.[3,79,80]

Antibiotic Selection for Treatment of Relapse

CASE 71-6, QUESTION 4: Greater than 10^5 bacteria per milliliter of *P. mirabilis*, sensitive to ampicillin and TMP–SMX, are cultured from T.W.'s urine. One week after completing her second course of TMP–SMX therapy, signs and symptoms of a UTI again appear. Pending C&S results, TMP–SMX is again prescribed. Is this still a reasonable medication for T.W. at this time?

Because the *P. mirabilis* cultured during the last recurrence was still susceptible to TMP–SMX, this agent would again be a reasonable choice until C&S test results are obtained. Alternatively, use of a different agent (e.g., nitrofurantoin, fluoroquinolone) could be considered because the relapse occurred within 1 week of completing the previous treatment and resistance may have developed.[5,34,80] Additional reasons for treatment failure, including failure to adhere to previously prescribed medication regimens, should also be investigated in patients with apparent recurrent infections.

CASE 71-6, QUESTION 5: How long should antibiotic therapy be continued in T.W. for her relapsed infection?

The duration of therapy for relapsing infections usually is 14 days. In patients who relapse after a second 2-week course of therapy, treatment for 6 weeks should be instituted.[1–3,34] If relapse occurs after a 6-week course, some experts recommend longer courses of 6 months to 1 year.[1–3] These prolonged courses should be reserved for children, adults who have continuous symptoms, or adults who are at high risk for experiencing progressive renal damage. Asymptomatic adults without evidence of obstruction should not receive these longer courses. T.W. should be treated for at least 2 weeks and perhaps as long as 6 weeks.[34,80]

CASE 71-6, QUESTION 6: Although T.W. tolerated TMP–SMX well during her previous treatment, on this occasion she experiences significant nausea and vomiting after taking the medication. Would trimethoprim alone be an appropriate substitute for TMP–SMX in the treatment of T.W.'s infection?

Trimethoprim alone and in combination with sulfamethoxazole is active in vitro against many of the Enterobacteriaceae associated with UTI and is an effective alternative to TMP–SMX in the management of both acute and chronic UTI.[1–3,5] It would be especially appropriate for T.W. because GI intolerance to TMP–SMX is most commonly attributed to the sulfamethoxazole component, and trimethoprim is associated with a lower incidence of side effects. Some concern exists for the potential development of resistant organisms, but studies using trimethoprim alone have failed to demonstrate a significant increase in bacterial resistance.[79,80] Trimethoprim is used for the treatment of acute, uncomplicated UTI in a dosage of 200 mg/day.

Chronic Prophylaxis

CASE 71-6, QUESTION 7: T.W. was treated successfully with trimethoprim for 6 weeks. Is prophylactic antimicrobial therapy indicated? If so, how long should it be continued?

Cases of chronic UTI in adult patients may be managed by treating each recurrent infection with an appropriate antibacterial drug or by administering chronic, low-dose prophylactic therapy. The frequency of urinary infections probably is the main determinant of whether chronic suppressive therapy should be used, because repeated treatment of recurrent infections eventually will result in a decreased incidence of subsequent infections.[1,34,80,82] Long-term prophylactic therapy clearly reduces the frequency of symptomatic infections in nearly all patients.[15,34,80,82]

From a cost-effectiveness standpoint, women having more than one episode of cystitis per year may benefit from antimicrobial prophylaxis.[79] For women with three or more episodes of cystitis per year, prophylaxis clearly is more cost-effective than treating individual infections. Therefore, it is recommended that chronic antimicrobial prophylaxis may be considered in any adult patient with two or more episodes of UTI per year.[2,34,80]

The duration of prophylactic therapy is also determined by the frequency of infection. Women with three or more UTIs in the 12 months before a 6-month course of antimicrobial prophylaxis have a significantly higher recurrence rate (75%) in the 6 months after prophylaxis than women who have had only two infections in the 12 months before prophylaxis (26% recurrence rate).[82] Therefore, prophylaxis should be continued for 6 months in patients with fewer than three UTIs per year and for at least 12 months in adult patients with three or more UTIs per year.

Before chronic antimicrobial suppressive therapy is initiated, active infections must be completely eradicated with a full course of appropriate antibiotic therapy. The low doses of antimicrobials used for chronic prophylaxis suppress bacterial growth but do not eliminate active infection. Furthermore, surgically correctable anatomic abnormalities that predispose the patient to recurrent infections (e.g., obstruction, stones) should be ruled out.[34,79,80] Age also should be considered when contemplating chronic antimicrobial therapy. An asymptomatic, elderly patient taking many other medications is usually not an ideal candidate for chronic prophylactic treatment because of problems of non-adherence, cost, and potential drug interactions or toxicities.[79,80] Younger patients, however, are good candidates for long-term suppressive therapy.[80]

Because T.W., a 28-year-old woman, has had at least three UTIs in the past few months, has undergone extensive evaluation, and has just been successfully treated with a standard course of trimethoprim, a 12-month course of antimicrobial prophylaxis would seem reasonable. She also should be evaluated at regular intervals for recurrent UTI and for the development of resistant organisms.

Although the foregoing discussion applies to antimicrobial prophylaxis in adults, the use of long-term prophylaxis of recurrent UTI in children remains controversial. One study examined risk factors for recurrent UTI and associations with antimicrobial prophylaxis in a prospective cohort study involving nearly 75,000 children 6 years of age or younger.[83] Among the children in this study, antimicrobial prophylaxis was not associated with decreased risk of recurrent UTI; however, prophylaxis was associated with a 7.5 times increased risk of infection caused by resistant bacteria. A second study examined 576 children younger than 18 years of age with a history of one or more microbiologically proven UTIs randomly assigned to receive either placebo or prophylaxis with TMP–SMX for 12 months.[84] Children randomly assigned to receive TMP–SMX experienced a 40% reduction in UTI during the study period; this benefit was independent of underlying risk factors such as history of vesicoureteral reflux. However, other outcomes such as hospitalization, secondary infections, or evidence of parenchymal disease on renal scans were not significantly different between groups; the one exception was that children receiving antibiotics were significantly more likely to experience UTI caused by an organism resistant to TMP–SMX.[84] Finally, a meta-analysis of 11 studies evaluating long-term antibiotic prophylaxis in children found no significant benefits of antibiotic administration overall.[85] Based on the conflicting data in the literature, current recommendations are that long-term antimicrobial prophylaxis should not be routinely recommended for prevention of recurrent UTI in children.[1–3,79,80,85–87]

Case 71-6, Question 8: What drugs could be appropriately used for long-term suppressive therapy in T.W?

Although numerous drugs are used for prophylaxis, TMP–SMX may be the drug of choice for chronic antimicrobial therapy owing to extensive experience, proven efficacy, infrequent toxicities, and low cost.[34,80] TMP–SMX also has the effect of decreasing vaginal colonization with uropathogens.[34,80] TMP–SMX single strength, either one-half or one full tablet daily, is commonly prescribed for chronic UTI prophylaxis and is an effective, well-tolerated, and convenient prophylactic regimen.[34,80]

Successful prophylaxis, however, is significantly decreased in patients with urologic abnormalities or renal dysfunction. Also, infections that are not eradicated by a short-term therapeutic trial of TMP–SMX are not likely to respond to a long-term regimen.[79] Finally, enterococci may colonize introitally in patients taking chronic TMP–SMX.[82]

Fluoroquinolones are effective for chronic suppressive therapy but should be used only when antimicrobial resistance or intolerance to other recommended drugs is present. Cephalosporins also have been recommended, but they are best reserved for patients intolerant to or failing prophylaxis with other agents.[79,80]

When selecting a drug for chronic antimicrobial therapy, it is important to consider efficacy, the likelihood that resistant organisms will develop, long-term toxicity, convenience, and cost to the patient. The most commonly used agents are listed in Table 71-5.

Based on the available information, T.W. could be switched to TMP–SMX. Although she has a history of GI distress because of this drug, this may not be a problem with the lower doses used for prophylaxis. If she is intolerant, trimethoprim alone, nitrofurantoin, or a fluoroquinolone also should be effective.

Cranberries and probiotics have long been of interest for their potentially beneficial effects in preventing UTI. Cranberries contain known compounds (i.e., flavonols, anthocyanidins, proanthocyanidin-tannins) that prevent *E. coli* from adhering to uroepithelial cells in the urinary tract.[88] A wide variety of cranberry products (e.g., juice concentrate, juice cocktail, cranberry extracts in capsules and tablets) and different dosing regimens have been evaluated in the prophylaxis of UTI, but the results are inconclusive overall and there are no formal recommendations regarding cranberry products for prevention of UTI.[88–90] A recent meta-analysis found that cranberry-containing products were effective in prevention of UTIs, with particular benefits seen in women (51% reduction in risk of infections), women with recurrent UTI (47% reduced risk of recurrences) and children (67% reduction in UTI risk).[88] However, this analysis also noted that available studies are quite heterogeneous, and the results of the meta-analysis should be interpreted with caution.[88] Probiotics (particularly *Lactobacillus* strains) may prevent colonization with pathogens associated with UTI.[91] Studies of probiotics for prophylaxis, however, are inconclusive at this time. Lack of standardization of ingredients (i.e. purity, dosage strengths) among available products and paucity of well-designed clinical studies are among the reasons for lack of clear recommendations regarding probiotics for this use. Further research is required to clarify unanswered questions regarding the role of cranberries or probiotics in the prevention of UTI.[88–91]

Urinary Tract Infection and Sexual Intercourse

CASE 71-7

Question 1: On routine screening, asymptomatic bacteriuria is noted in W.W., a 30-year-old pregnant woman in her first trimester. Five years ago, during her first pregnancy, she experienced acute bacterial pyelonephritis, which required hospitalization and treatment with parenteral antibiotics. Since that time, she has had recurrent UTI, apparently related to sexual intercourse. These subsided when she began taking a single dose of nitrofurantoin after coitus, but she discontinued the practice before this pregnancy because she was afraid of the potential effects of this drug on the fetus. What is the association between sexual intercourse and the occurrence of UTI?

Table 71-5
Antimicrobial Agents Commonly Used for Chronic Prophylaxis Against Recurrent UTIs[1–3,5,77–79,82]

Agent	Adult Dose	Comments[a]
Nitrofurantoin	50–100 mg nightly	Contraindicated in infant <1 month of age. *To be taken with food or milk. May cause brown or rust-yellow discoloration of urine.*
Trimethoprim	100 mg nightly	Not recommended in children <12 years of age.
Trimethoprim 80 mg + sulfamethoxazole 400 mg	0.5–1 tablet nightly *Or* 3/week	Not recommended for use in infants <2 months. *To be taken on an empty stomach with a full glass of water. Photosensitivity may occur.*
Norfloxacin	200 mg/day	*Avoid antacids*; monitor theophylline levels.
Cephalexin	125–250 mg/day	
Cefaclor	250 mg/day	
Sulfamethoxazole	500 mg/day	

[a]Includes unique patient consultation information in italics.

Studies strongly support an association between sexual intercourse and UTI.[1–3,27] A direct relationship seems to exist between the number of days with intercourse within the previous week and the risk of developing a UTI.[1–3,27] One study found the relative risk of infection in women with 1, 4, and 7 days of intercourse within the previous week to be 1.4, 3.5, and 9.0, respectively, compared with women who were sexually inactive within the previous week. Another study found that the risk of UTI was doubled in women having intercourse more than 4 times/month compared with those women who did not.[27] Studies also indicate that introital colonization by fecal bacteria has a definite role in recurrent infections related to intercourse. The migration of these colonizing bacteria into the bladder appears to be facilitated during intercourse, but the exact mechanism remains unclear.[1–3] Because UTI are uncommon in men, transmission of an infection from the man is unlikely. Occasionally, bacteria harbored under the foreskin of an uncircumcised man may be transmitted to his partner through intercourse.[25]

CASE 71-7, QUESTION 2: Was it rational to treat W.W.'s repeated infections with a single dose of an antibiotic after intercourse?

Postcoital antibiotic prophylaxis is useful when recurrent UTI results from sexual intercourse. Theoretically, a single dose of an antimicrobial agent produces bactericidal activity in the urine before bacteria have a chance to multiply, and the infection is averted. Patients should be instructed to empty their bladder just after intercourse and before taking the medication to minimize the number of bacteria present in the bladder and to reduce dilution of the drug in the urine. Because most drugs effective for UTI are rapidly excreted by the kidney and quickly reach high urinary concentrations, this regimen is reasonable and decreases the incidence of postcoital infections.[92,93] However, this practice is not recommended in patients with structural abnormalities of the urinary tract or decreased renal function. Symptomatic infection must be completely treated before beginning prophylaxis.

Depending on the frequency of intercourse, postcoital prophylaxis may result in less antibiotic use compared with continuous prophylaxis. TMP–SMX or nitrofurantoin is the most commonly recommended agent; however, other agents such as fluoroquinolones and cephalexin may be used.[77–93]

Urinary Tract Infection and Pregnancy

CASE 71-7, QUESTION 3: Because W.W. is asymptomatic at this time, should treatment be withheld because of her pregnancy?

W.W. should be treated because acute symptomatic lower UTI or pyelonephritis may develop in pregnant women with untreated bacteriuria. In addition, a UTI during pregnancy has been suggested to be associated with increased rates of preterm labor, premature delivery, and lower birth-weight infants.[27] A cause-and-effect relationship between UTI and maternal or infant risk has not been definitely established; in fact, a recent retrospective cohort study in nearly 86,000 mothers with or without UTI during pregnancy found no adverse pregnancy outcomes.[94] Nevertheless, treatment with an appropriate antimicrobial agent is currently recommended for all pregnant patients with significant bacteriuria.[13,28,29]

Nitrofurantoin is often recommended during pregnancy because teratogenic effects have not been observed clinically.[95,96] In vitro and retrospective investigations, however, suggest a slight mutagenic potential.[97,98] During lactation, nitrofurantoin could cause hemolytic anemia in a G6PD-deficient nursing infant; however, only small amounts have been detected in breast milk.[98] The fluoroquinolones are contraindicated in pregnancy because of the arthropathy observed in immature animals.[68]

The penicillins and cephalosporins are safe for use during pregnancy. These drugs, along with the others listed in Tables 71-3 and 71-5, cross the placental barrier; thus, the risk of toxicity or teratogenicity to the fetus must always be considered before deciding to treat a pregnant patient with a UTI.[98]

In this case, a cephalosporin or sulfisoxazole could be safely prescribed for treatment of W.W. Although sulfisoxazole is felt to be safe in the first trimester of pregnancy, trimethoprim and trimethoprim/sulfamethoxazole should be avoided because of the folate antagonist actions of trimethoprim and concerns regarding neural tube and cardiovascular defects potentially associated with maternal folate deficiency during the first trimester. Sulfisoxazole should not be used after 32 weeks of gestation because of concerns regarding neonatal hyperbilirubinemia, jaundice, and kernicterus. W.W. was correct in discontinuing her nitrofurantoin before pregnancy because of the risk to the fetus, although small, tends to offset the advantage of antimicrobial prophylaxis. W.W. must receive proper follow-up care.

CASE 71-7, QUESTION 4: For how long should W.W. be treated?

Few studies have compared single-dose and 3-day therapy with conventional 7-day therapy in pregnant patients. Available trials suggest, however, that cure rates of single-dose therapy were lower than 7- to 10-day therapy.[27,95] Although more recent trials have shown that single-dose therapy effectively eradicates bacteriuria in pregnancy, these studies were conducted in a small number of patients. Therefore, similar to other populations, it is recommended that pregnant patients receive either a 3-day regimen or a 7- to 10-day regimen rather than single-dose therapy.[13,27,95]

Irrespective of the duration of therapy, appropriate follow-up of patients is crucial. Clinicians must document elimination of pathogens 1 to 2 weeks after therapy and follow the patient monthly for the remainder of gestation. If bacteriuria recurs, therapy should be given for relapse or reinfection and the patient evaluated radiologically for structural abnormalities.[1,27]

ASYMPTOMATIC BACTERIURIA

Antibiotic Treatment

CASE 71-8

QUESTION 1: A.K., an asymptomatic 6-year-old girl, is found to have significant bacteriuria on routine screening. Should she be treated with an antimicrobial agent?

The treatment of patients with asymptomatic bacteriuria depends on the clinical setting in which it is found. Asymptomatic bacteriuria occurs in a heterogeneous group of patients with different prognoses and risks. Therefore, recommendations for treatment of asymptomatic patients with significant bacteriuria (two consecutive voided urine specimens showing $\geq 10^5$ bacteria/mL of urine in women, or a single clean-catch voided specimen in men) are based on specific age, sex, and clinical characteristics.[1,10,13,28] These recommendations consider the risk for development of acute UTI and subsequent long-term complications. Generally, patients who benefit most from antibiotic treatment are those with urinary tract structural abnormalities, immunosuppressive therapy, and procedures requiring urinary tract instrumentation or manipulation.[1–3,13] Short-course regimens (i.e., single-dose or 3-day) are usually recommended when treatment is desired,[3] although longer regimens have also been recommended.[13]

Urinary tract infections in infants and preschool children (predominantly girls) occasionally are associated with renal tissue damage, although the incidence of renal damage has been estimated as low as 0.4% in children with previously normal renal function, and the overall risk of UTIs in this regard is now controversial.[9,99] Asymptomatic bacteriuria of childhood is also important because it may be a manifestation of an anatomic or mechanical defect in the urinary tract. Therefore, it should be evaluated fully. Because most cases of renal scarring as a result of bacteriuria occur within the first 5 years of life, it is controversial whether treatment should be limited to infants and preschool children or whether all children should be treated regardless of age. Screening for bacteriuria in children and treating those with positive cultures, regardless of their clinical presentation, seems reasonable and is frequently recommended.[99] Treatment of A.K., although still controversial, seems prudent because any renal damage resulting from asymptomatic bacteriuria generally occurs during childhood. Should the decision be made to treat, principles of therapy are similar to those for symptomatic infections.

Pregnant Patients, the Elderly, and Other Adult Populations

Case 71-8, Question 2: The decision to treat the asymptomatic bacteriuria of A.K. was based primarily on the increased probability of renal damage during childhood. What other population groups should be treated for asymptomatic bacteriuria?

Without urinary tract obstruction, UTI in adults rarely lead to progressive renal damage.[3,5] Therefore, asymptomatic bacteriuria does not require treatment in most adult patients who have no evidence of mechanical obstruction or renal insufficiency. As previously discussed, antimicrobial therapy is appropriate during pregnancy because as many as 40% of pregnant women with asymptomatic bacteriuria later develop symptomatic UTI, particularly pyelonephritis.[13] In addition, studies have confirmed associations between acute pyelonephritis during pregnancy with increased rates of preterm labor, premature delivery, and lower birth-weight infants.[27] The treatment of asymptomatic bacteriuria in pregnancy is therefore justified to decrease the risk of associated complications.[13]

Bacteriuria in the elderly is common; it is estimated that 20% of all women and 10% of all men aged 65 years and older have bacteriuria.[14,15,16] Although bacteriuria in this population often leads to symptomatic infection, clinical studies have consistently documented no beneficial outcomes in treated patients compared with untreated patients.[13,15] Consequently, therapy is not recommended for the asymptomatic older patient because the expense, side effects, and potential complications of drug therapy appear to outweigh the benefits.[13,15] Patients experiencing symptomatic infections should be treated as usual.

The treatment of asymptomatic bacteriuria in women with diabetes does not reduce complications and is not currently recommended.[13,28]

SYMPTOMATIC ABACTERIURIA

Clinical Presentation

CASE 71-9

Question 1: R.D., a 22-year-old woman, complains of urinary frequency and painful urination, which have developed during the past 4 to 5 days. UA reveals 10 to 15 WBC/LPF, but no bacteria are seen on a Gram stain of the urine. What is a reasonable assessment of R.D.'s clinical presentation?

Acute urethral syndrome is defined as symptoms consistent with lower UTI but with no organisms evident on Gram stain or culture. The lack of detectable pathogens may mean that the urine specimen is sterile or that the concentration of the organisms in the urine sample is low. Patients with these symptoms still may have a UTI even though the voided urine is sterile or contains less than 10^5 microorganisms/mL.[100] The causative organisms and the pathogenesis of infection in these cases are the same as for lower UTI. Other organisms that can cause urethritis in this setting, especially in the presence of pyuria, are *Chlamydia trachomatis*, *Neisseria gonorrhoeae*, and *Trichomonas vaginalis*.[100] Conversely, in patients with acute urethral syndrome without pyuria, noninfectious causes of urethritis are common and should be sought. Because R.D. is symptomatic, has 10 to 15 WBC/LPF in her urine, and no bacteria on Gram stain, infection with *C. trachomatis* or some other more atypical pathogen is likely.

Interstitial cystitis, also known as painful bladder syndrome or bladder pain syndrome, is a chronic clinical syndrome characterized by bladder or pelvic pain and urinary frequency or urgency.[101] Although the exact cause of interstitial cystitis is not known, it is apparently not an infection-related disorder and does not respond to antibiotic therapy. The clinical presentation of interstitial cystitis is very similar to that of symptomatic abacteriuria, but absence of pyuria is a key difference. Interstitial cystitis should be suspected in patients with clinical findings suggestive of lower UTI but who do not manifest pyuria and who have not responded to previous empiric antibiotic therapy; no antibiotics should be administered without further diagnostic evaluation.[101]

Antibiotic Treatment

Case 71-9, Question 2: Should R.D. be treated with antibiotics?

A double-blind, placebo-controlled study evaluated the use of doxycycline 100 mg twice a day (BID) in patients with UTI and low bacterial counts. Clinical cure of bacteriuria and pyuria was significantly greater in the doxycycline-treated group, but doxycycline did not reduce symptoms in patients without pyuria.[100] Because *E. coli*, other gram-negative bacteria, and *C. trachomatis* are the usual causes of acute urethral syndrome, an antibiotic such as doxycycline with activity against *Chlamydia* is a reasonable initial treatment for patients such as R.D. presenting with urinary tract symptoms (without bacteriuria) and with pyuria. All tetracyclines and sulfonamides, with or without trimethoprim, also are likely to be effective in such patients, but doxycycline has been best studied to date. Of the fluoroquinolones, newer agents, such as levofloxacin, offer promise as alternatives to doxycycline but have not been well studied in this setting.[100] Azithromycin as a single dose also has a major role in treating chlamydial infections (see Chapter 72, Sexually Transmitted Diseases).

Prolonged therapy of 2 to 4 weeks in duration and treatment of sexual partners may be required to prevent reinfection through intercourse. Prolonged therapy is appropriate if the patient has a history consistent with *Chlamydia* urethritis; a sexual partner with recent urethritis; a recent new sexual partner; a gradual, rather than abrupt, onset of symptoms that has occurred during a period of days (as in R.D.); and no hematuria. Patients without such a history can be treated with a short course of antibiotics as any other patient with a lower UTI.

HOSPITAL-ACQUIRED ACUTE URINARY TRACT INFECTION

CASE 71-10

QUESTION 1: P.M., an alert, 70-year-old woman with chest pain, was hospitalized to rule out acute myocardial infarction. This is her third hospitalization for chest pain in the past 6 months. A urinary catheter was temporarily placed as part of her routine medical care. Two days after admission, she complained of burning on urination and bladder pain. TMP–SMX double-strength, one tablet BID was ordered after microscopic examination of the urine indicated a UTI. Was this empiric therapy appropriate?

Hospital-acquired (or nosocomial) UTIs occur in about one-half million patients per year and most are associated with the use of indwelling bladder catheters. Approximately 10% to 30% of catheterized patients exhibit infection.[23] Complications of catheter-associated UTI are significant. Nosocomial UTIs are the source of up to 15% of all nosocomial bloodstream infections, occurring in about 4% of all catheterized patients[23]; the associated mortality rate is approximately 15%.[23] Nosocomial UTI also prolongs hospitalization by an average of 2.5 days and costs an additional $600 to $700.[23] Prevention is the best way to manage nosocomial UTI, but antibiotic treatment is usually initiated in hospitalized patients who exhibit UTI symptoms.

The susceptibility of hospital-acquired pathogens to antimicrobial agents differs from community-acquired bacteria, and these susceptibilities frequently vary from one hospital to another. Therefore, the microbiology department of a particular hospital should be consulted to determine current trends in the antibiotic susceptibility of bacteria acquired in that setting. In general, *E. coli* is still the predominant urinary tract pathogen. An increased proportion of infections is caused, however, by other gram-negative bacteria such as *Proteus* and *Pseudomonas*, gram-positive pathogens such as *Staphylococcus* and *Enterococcus*, and yeast (e.g., *Candida*).[21,23]

Repeated courses of antibiotic therapy, anatomic defects of the urinary tract, old age, increased length of hospital stay, and repeated hospital admissions are associated with a higher incidence of infection with antibiotic-resistant organisms.[21,23,102] *Pseudomonas, Proteus, Providencia, Morganella, Klebsiella, Enterobacter, Citrobacter,* and *Serratia* are particularly difficult to eradicate because they usually are less susceptible to commonly used antimicrobial agents.

P.M. is elderly, hospitalized, and has been repeatedly exposed to potentially resistant organisms during her previous hospitalizations. Oral fluoroquinolones are most commonly used as empiric therapy in this setting because of their greater activity against potentially resistant pathogens compared to TMP–SMX; however, TMP–SMX is an acceptable empirical therapy in P.M. as long as her clinical and laboratory data are appropriately monitored.[21,23,103] Cultures of P.M.'s urine should be performed and, once C&S test results are known, therapy promptly changed according to susceptibility reports. To achieve the most cost-effective therapy, oral agents should be administered to all patients capable of taking medications by mouth unless the isolated pathogens are resistant to oral medications, or underlying GI dysfunction makes adequate absorption of oral antibiotics questionable.[23,75,103] The recommended duration of antibiotic therapy for patients such as P.M., who present with mild-to-moderate symptoms, is 5 to 7 days; patients who do not respond promptly to treatment may be treated for a total of 10 to 14 days.[23]

CASE 71-10, QUESTION 2: If P.M. had additional symptoms of fever, chills, flank pain, and vomiting, how would her treatment differ?

In seriously ill patients with possible sepsis, broad-spectrum parenteral antibiotics with activity against *P. aeruginosa* are usually preferred as initial therapy (Table 71-4). Suitable antibiotic choices include antipseudomonal cephalosporins (e.g., ceftazidime, cefepime), extended-spectrum penicillins (e.g., piperacillin-tazobactam), carbapenems (imipenem-cilastatin, meropenem), IV fluoroquinolones (e.g., ciprofloxacin, levofloxacin), and aztreonam. These antibiotics are at least as effective as the aminoglycosides and lack the ototoxic and nephrotoxic potential. However, these fluoroquinolone and β-lactam agents are more costly and associated with the emergence of resistant organisms and superinfection.

In general, antipseudomonal β-lactam antibiotics remain the drugs of choice for nosocomial urologic sepsis.[103] Although combination therapy may be useful initially in neutropenic patients with urologic sepsis, it should be narrowed to single-agent therapy once culture results are available.[103] The recommended duration of antibiotic therapy in seriously ill patients is 10 to 14 days.[23]

Urinary Catheters

CASE 71-11

QUESTION 1: J.W., an 18-year-old woman, was hospitalized after a diving accident that resulted in a spinal cord injury with paralysis. Included among several initial interventions was insertion of an indwelling catheter with a closed drainage system because of bladder incontinence. Two weeks after admission to the hospital, J.W. has developed asymptomatic bacteriuria. Should this be treated?

A systemic antibiotic selected specifically for the infecting organism will temporarily result in sterile urine. Reinfection, often by a resistant organism, occurs in 30% to 50% of these cases if closed drainage catheterization is continued during therapy.[1,23] For this reason, it generally is recommended that systemic antimicrobial therapy be initiated after or just before catheter removal.[1,23,104] Because long-term catheterization is necessary in many patients and because bacteriuria is an inevitable consequence, it is often recommended that asymptomatic patients (such as J.W.) be left untreated to avoid the complications of recolonization and potential infection with resistant organisms.[1,13,23,104] Therapy must be started, however, if fever, flank pain, or other symptoms indicative of an actual UTI develop.[1,23]

CASE 71-11, QUESTION 2: Is systemic antimicrobial prophylaxis useful for J.W.?

The benefits of systemic antibiotics in preventing catheter-induced UTI are not clear. Studies using closed drainage systems with diligent catheter care indicate that systemic antibiotics decrease the daily and overall incidence of infection in patients with sterile urines before catheterization.[35,36] The preventive effect of antimicrobials is greatest for short-term catheterizations or during the first 4 to 7 days of long-term catheterization.[35,36] Thereafter, the rate of infection increases. Although the overall infection rate remains lower than in untreated patients, the emergence of resistant organisms is significant. Therefore, in deciding to use systemic antimicrobials, it is important to consider the patient's underlying diseases, risk factors, probable duration of catheterization, and potential complications of drug toxicity or resistant organisms that can result from the chronic use of antimicrobials. Because long-term catheterization is anticipated for J.W., antimicrobial prophylaxis for J.W. is not recommended.[23]

CASE 71-11, QUESTION 3: J.W. eventually recovers urinary continence and the catheter is able to be removed. However, 2 days after removal of the catheter, she still has asymptomatic bacteriuria. How should she be managed?

Because asymptomatic bacteriuria in patients with urinary catheters is very common (approximately 25% with short-term catheterization and virtually 100% long-term) but is associated with few complications, antibiotic therapy for asymptomatic bacteriuria is not recommended as long as the catheter remains in place.[23] However, antibiotic treatment may be considered in asymptomatic women with catheter-acquired bacteriuria that persists >48 hours after catheter removal.[13,23] Such patients may be treated with either a single large dose or a 3-day regimen of TMP–SMX, even if the patient is asymptomatic.[13,23,24] Older women (>65 years) probably should be treated with a 10-day course; however, the optimal duration in this age group is unknown. Whether these same treatment regimens are advisable in male patients requires further study.[23]

PROSTATITIS

Incidence, Prevalence, and Epidemiology

Prostatitis is an acute or chronic inflammatory condition affecting the prostate, approximately 5% of cases being caused by proven bacterial infections.[11,12] Other noninfectious types of prostatitis include chronic calculus prostatitis, nonbacterial prostatitis, and prostatodynia.[11,12] Chronic bacterial prostatitis, defined as prostatitis in which symptoms persist for at least 3 months, is one of the most common causes of recurrent UTI in men. The lifetime probability of a man being diagnosed with prostatitis is greater than 25%; recurrence rates reportedly range from 20% to 50%.[11,12] Approximately 5% of men with acute prostatitis will experience chronic infection.[11]

Etiology, Pathogenesis, and Predisposing Factors

ACUTE BACTERIAL PROSTATITIS

Acute bacterial prostatitis in most patients probably begins as an ascending infection of the urethra. A simple UTI then eventually involves reflux of infected urine into the ejaculatory and prostatic ducts through the prostate gland, where bacteria are difficult to eradicate.[12] Acute prostatitis may also result from urethral stricture or after instrumentation of the urinary tract or prostate biopsy, especially in the presence of bacteriuria at the time of the procedure.[12] Bacterial prostatitis is predominantly caused by aerobic gram-negative bacilli, with *E. coli* causing 50% to 90% of cases. Other Enterobacteriaceae such as *Proteus* and *Klebsiella* account for an additional 10% to 30% of cases, followed by *Enterococcus* (5% to 10%) and *Pseudomonas* (<5%); less common causes include staphylococci, streptococci, and atypical organisms such as *C. trachomatis*, *T. vaginalis*, and *Ureaplasma urealyticum*.[11,12]

CHRONIC BACTERIAL PROSTATITIS

Chronic prostatitis is commonly associated with spinal cord injuries, infectious stones, anatomic or physiologic abnormalities of the urinary tract such as obstruction or voiding dysfunction, and immune dysfunction. However, recurrent infections are also commonly caused by relapses of acute prostatitis caused by persistence of bacteria in the prostate.[11,12] Normally, men secrete a prostatic antibacterial factor; however, this substance is often absent or significantly reduced in men with chronic prostatitis. The most common pathogens isolated from chronic bacterial prostatitis are *E. coli* (>80% of cases) and other gram-negative bacilli, although atypical bacteria have also been more commonly reported in chronic prostatitis compared to acute infections.[11,12]

Clinical Presentation and Diagnosis

ACUTE BACTERIAL PROSTATITIS

Acute bacterial prostatitis is characterized by the sudden onset of chills and fever; perineal and low back pain; urinary urgency and frequency; nocturia, dysuria, and generalized malaise; and prostration. Patients may also complain of myalgias, arthralgias, and symptoms of bladder outlet obstruction. Rectal examination usually discloses an exquisitely tender, swollen prostate that is firm and warm to the touch. The pathogens generally can be identified by culture of the voided urine. In patients with acute bacterial prostatitis, prostatic massage (see following discussion) should be avoided because of patient discomfort and the risk of bacteremia.[11,12] The diagnosis of acute prostatitis is therefore usually based on clinical presentation and physical examination.

CHRONIC BACTERIAL PROSTATITIS

The clinical manifestations of chronic bacterial prostatitis are highly variable and many patients are asymptomatic. The disease usually is suspected when a male patient treated for UTI or acute prostatitis relapses. The diagnosis of chronic prostatitis is confirmed by examination of expressed prostatic secretions.[11,12] To ensure accurate localization (i.e., to distinguish prostatic from urethral bacteria), segmented urine samples are taken. The first 10 mL of voided urine represents the urethral sample, the midstream urine collected represents the bladder sample, and the first 10 mL voided immediately after prostatic massage represents the prostate sample. When the bladder sample is sterile or nearly so, bacterial prostatitis is diagnosed if the bacterial count in the prostate sample is at least one logarithm greater than that in the urethral sample.[11,12]

Overview of Treatment

Treatment of bacterial prostatitis is challenged by poor penetration of many antibiotics across the non-fenestrated prostatic capillaries and through prostatic epithelium into infected tissues and fluids. Fluoroquinolones are often considered the preferred antibiotics for treatment of acute or chronic prostatitis because of good penetration into the prostate (10%–50% of serum concentrations) and good activity against most causative pathogens, although fluoroquinolone resistance has become a growing problem.[11,12] Trimethoprim alone or TMP–SMX are also commonly used agents. β-Lactams, tetracyclines, macrolides, and clindamycin have also been successfully used in the treatment of both acute and chronic infections, but their penetration into the prostatic tissues and fluids may be somewhat less than the fluoroquinolones or TMP–SMX. Also, the antimicrobial activity of these drugs is not necessarily ideal for covering the most common causative pathogens.[11,12] The duration of antibiotic therapy in acute prostatitis is usually 2 to 4 weeks, depending on the severity of the infection and rate of response to treatment.[11,12] Chronic prostatitis is usually treated for 4 to 6 weeks, although longer courses may be required in the presence of prostate stones or other types of genitourinary pathology, and long-term suppressive therapy is sometimes used for patients with a history of rapid and/or multiple recurrences.[11,12] Monitoring parameters consist primarily of clinical signs and symptoms, and the end point of treatment is complete resolution of clinical findings.[11,12] Supportive treatment consists primarily of drugs for symptomatic relief such as acetaminophen or nonsteroidal anti-inflammatory agents; warm compresses to the perineal area are also sometimes recommended, although there are few data to support this practice.[11,12]

CASE 71-12

QUESTION 1: D.G., a 60-year-old man, experienced his first UTI at age 40, with symptoms of frequency, dysuria, nocturia, perineal pain, fever and chills but no flank pain. Acute prostatitis was diagnosed. *E. coli* was cultured from the urine, and treatment with a sulfonamide was successful. After 12 asymptomatic years, acute prostatitis caused by *E. coli* recurred and again responded to sulfonamide therapy. Two more *E. coli* infections that responded to sulfonamide therapy occurred during the next 8 years. Why were sulfonamides appropriate treatment for D.G.'s repeated acute episodes of bacterial prostatitis?

Most antibacterial drugs appropriate for UTI, including sulfonamides, can be used to treat acute bacterial prostatitis because the diffuse, intense inflammation of the prostate gland allows many drugs to readily penetrate into the prostatic fluid and tissues. Antimicrobial therapy should be continued for at least 2 to 4 weeks to prevent the development of chronic prostatitis.[11,12,24]

CASE 71-12, QUESTION 2: Taking into account the pathophysiology of prostatitis, what would be a reasonable choice of therapy for D.G. should he have future recurrences of prostatitis?

In addition to antibiotics, other supportive measures may provide symptomatic relief to patients with acute bacterial prostatitis. These measures include liberal hydration, nonsteroidal anti-inflammatory drugs for pain relief, sitz baths, and stool softeners.

In retrospect, sulfonamides were appropriate for D.G. because they effectively treated his infections. Other options, particularly the fluoroquinolones, would also have been appropriate in the treatment of D.G.'s episodes of acute prostatitis.

Most antibiotics that are acidic do not readily cross the prostatic epithelium into the alkaline prostatic fluid except in the presence of acute inflammation. Theoretically, the high alkalinity of prostatic fluids should impair the diffusion of trimethoprim and enhance the diffusion of tetracyclines, certain sulfonamides, and macrolide antibiotics, such as erythromycin. Nevertheless, TMP–SMX historically has the best documented cure rates in the treatment of acute and chronic bacterial prostatitis. Long-term therapy of chronic bacterial prostatitis with TMP–SMX for 4 to 16 weeks is associated with a cure rate of 32% to 71%, which significantly exceeds the cure rate associated with short-term therapy of 2 or fewer weeks.[11,12]

The fluoroquinolones are alternatives to TMP–SMX and are now considered by many to be the agents of choice for the treatment of prostatitis.[11,12,24] A number of studies have documented bacteriologic cure in 80% to 90% of patients treated with norfloxacin, ciprofloxacin, or levofloxacin for 4 to 12 weeks, rates comparable to or substantially higher than those achieved with TMP–SMX.[11,12] The fluoroquinolones have an important role in the treatment of prostatitis owing to their bactericidal activity against common pathogens and excellent penetration into prostatic tissues and fluid. The fluoroquinolones are often used as initial empiric therapy of prostatitis and are also excellent alternatives to other agents in patients who are unresponsive or intolerant to conventional therapy, or in those infected with resistant organisms.[11,12,24] Fluoroquinolones also have been used for chronic suppressive therapy (one-half normal doses) in patients who relapse after conventional treatment.[1]

D.G. should be treated with TMP–SMX for a minimum of 6 weeks; some authorities recommend a 2- to 3-month total course of therapy. If an adequate trial of TMP–SMX is unsuccessful, fluoroquinolone therapy can be used. Alternatively, a fluoroquinolone could be used as initial therapy for this or future episodes.[11,12,24]

If D.G. continues to experience recurrent infections after a trial of fluoroquinolone therapy, chronic low-dose treatment with TMP–SMX, fluoroquinolones, or nitrofurantoin can alleviate the symptoms of episodic bladder infection associated with chronic bacterial prostatitis. Infections eventually recur with greater frequency in most of these patients. Chronic, low-dose antibacterial therapy sterilizes the bladder, alleviates symptoms, confines bacteria to the prostate, and prevents infection of and damage to the rest of the urinary tract. Chronic bacterial prostatitis is one of the few indications for continuous antibiotic therapy.

KEY REFERENCES AND WEBSITES

A full list of references for this chapter can be found at http://thePoint.lww.com/AT11e. Below are the key references for this chapter, with the corresponding reference number in this chapter found in parentheses after the reference.

Key References

Craig JC et al. Antibiotic prophylaxis and recurrent urinary tract infection in children [published correction appears in *N Engl J Med*. 2010;362:1250]. *N Engl J Med*. 2009;361:1748–1759. (84)

Epp A et al. Recurrent urinary tract infection. *J Obstet Gynaecol Can*. 2010;250:1082–1101. (34)

Gupta K et al. International clinical practice guidelines for the treatment of acute uncomplicated cystitis and pyelonephritis in women: a 2010 update by the Infectious Diseases Society of America and the European Society for Microbiology and Infectious Diseases. *Clin Infect Dis*. 2011;52:e103–e120. (20)

Hooton TM Jr. Uncomplicated urinary tract infection. *N Engl J Med*. 2012;366(11):1028–1037. (2)

Hooton TM et al. Diagnosis, prevention, and treatment of catheter-associated urinary tract infection in adults: 2009 international clinical practice guidelines from the Infectious Diseases Society of America. *Clin Infect Dis*. 2010;50:625–663. (23)

Karlowsky JA et al. Fluoroquinolone-resistant urinary isolates of *Escherichia coli* from outpatients are frequently multidrug resistant: results from the North American Urinary Tract Infection Collaborative Alliance-Quinolone Resistance Study. *Antimicrob Agents Chemother*. 2006;50:2251–2254. (69)

Katsarolis I et al. Acute uncomplicated cystitis: from surveillance data to a rationale for empirical treatment. *Int J Antimicrob Agents*. 2010;35:62–67. (49)

Lipsky BA et al. Treatment of bacterial prostatitis. *Clin Infect Dis*. 2010;50:1641–1652. (11)

Nicolle LE et al. Infectious Diseases Society of America guidelines for the diagnosis and treatment of asymptomatic bacteriuria in adults. *Clin Infect Dis*. 2005;40:643–654. (13)

Nicolle LE. Uncomplicated urinary tract infection in adults including uncomplicated pyelonephritis. *Urol Clin North Am*. 2008;35:1–12. (5)

Popovic M et al. Fosfomycin: an old, new friend? *Eur J Clin Microbiol Infect Dis*. 2010;29:127–142. (44)

Raynor MC et al. Urinary infections in men. *Med Clin North Am*. 2011;95:43–54. (7)

Schito GC et al. The ARESC study: an international survey on the antimicrobial resistance of pathogens involved in uncomplicated urinary tract infections. *Int J Antimicrob Agents*. 2009;34:407–413. (47)

Shuman EK et al. Recognition and prevention of healthcare-associated urinary tract infections in the intensive care unit. *Crit Care Med*. 2010;38(Suppl):S373–S379. (22)

Vouloumanou EK et al. Early switch to oral versus intravenous antimicrobial treatment for hospitalized patients with acute pyelonephritis: a systematic review of randomized controlled trials. *Curr Med Res Opin*. 2008;24:3423–3434. (78)

72 Sexually Transmitted Diseases

Jeffery A. Goad, Karl M. Hess, and Albert T. Bach

CORE PRINCIPLES

		CHAPTER CASES
GROWTH AND DEVELOPMENT		
1	Urethral gonorrhea is initially characterized in males by a purulent discharge associated with dysuria. Discharge may become more profuse and blood tinged as the infection progresses. Some strains of gonorrhea have a propensity to cause asymptomatic or minimally symptomatic infections.	**Case 72-1 (Question 2)**
2	In females, the most common symptom of urethral gonorrhea is vaginal discharge. Many women infected with gonorrhea have abnormalities of the cervix, including purulent or mucopurulent endocervical discharge, erythema, friability, and edema of the zone of ectopy. Pelvic inflammatory disease (PID) is a serious complication and can lead to infertility and chronic pelvic pain.	**Case 72-1 (Question 4)**
3	The standard of treatment for gonorrhea is third-generation cephalosporins, such as ceftriaxone. Fluoroquinolones should not be used owing to high levels of resistance.	**Case 72-1 (Questions 6, 7)**
4	Depending on the site of exposure, gonococcal infections may also cause anorectal and pharyngeal infections. Anorectal infections may cause proctitis with anorectal pain, mucopurulent anorectal discharge, constipation, tenesmus, and anorectal bleeding. Pharyngeal infections may be characterized by sore throat, pharyngeal exudates, or cervical lymphadenitis. The treatment for anorectal or pharyngeal gonorrhea is ceftriaxone.	**Case 72-2 (Questions 2–4)**
5	Disseminated gonococcal infection (DGI) can lead to complicated gonorrhea infections that cause pustular acral skin lesions, tenosynovitis, polyarthralgia, or arthritis. DGI may also lead to rare cases of perihepatitis, endocarditis, or meningitis. Treatment for DGIs requires high-dose ceftriaxone.	**Case 72-4 (Questions 2, 3)**
PELVIC INFLAMMATORY DISEASE		
1	PID may be treated on an inpatient or outpatient basis. Those with mild-to-moderate PID can be admitted and treated with parenteral antibiotics; however, clinical efficacy and overall outcomes are equal between parental and oral therapy.	**Case 72-3 (Question 1)**
NONGONOCOCCAL URETHRITIS		
1	Nongonococcal urethritis (NGU) is a common sexually transmitted disease (STD) in males and is frequently caused by *Chlamydia trachomatis*.	**Case 72-5 (Question 1)**
2	NGU typically produces less severe and less frequent dysuria and less penile discharge as compared with gonococcal urethritis. NGU and gonococcal urethritis cannot be reliably differentiated on the basis of symptoms and signs.	**Case 72-5 (Question 2)**
3	NGU may be treated with either azithromycin or doxycycline; however, azithromycin is superior in its coverage of both *Mycoplasma genitalium* and *Chlamydia*.	**Case 72-5 (Questions 3, 4)**

Continued

		CHAPTER CASES
LYMPHOGRANULOMA VENEREUM		
1	Lymphogranuloma venereum (LGV) is characterized by three stages of infection and may be treated with either doxycycline, erythromycin base, or azithromycin.	**Case 72-6 (Questions 1, 2)**
SYPHILIS		
1	Syphilis is characterized by four stages of infection: primary, secondary, latent, and tertiary. Penicillin G is the drug of choice for all stages of syphilis.	**Case 72-7 (Questions 1, 3, 4), Case 72-8 (Question 1)**
2	The Jarisch–Herxheimer reaction is a benign, self-limited complication of antibiotic therapy that may develop after treatment of primary and secondary syphilis.	**Case 72-8 (Question 2)**
CHANCROID		
1	Uncircumcised males have an increased risk of infection and may not respond to therapy as well as circumcised males. Current treatment options include azithromycin, ceftriaxone, ciprofloxacin, and erythromycin base.	**Case 72-9 (Questions 1, 2)**
VAGINITIS		
1	Common causes of vaginitis include bacterial vaginosis, trichomoniasis, and vulvovaginal candidiasis. General symptoms may include itching, burning, irritation, and abnormal discharge and can be differentiated based on signs, symptoms, and laboratory testing.	**Case 72-10 (Question 1), Case 72-11 (Questions 2–4), Case 72-12 (Question 1)**
2	Vulvovaginal candidiasis may be effectively treated with nonprescription medications; however, patients must be assessed fully before self-treatment is initiated.	**Case 72-11 (Questions 1, 6–9)**
GENITAL HERPES		
1	Genital herpes, transmitted either from symptomatic or asymptomatic individuals, often presents with painful vesicles in those with HSV-2 primary infection, and recurrent infections are common, although the frequency decreases with time.	**Case 72-14 (Questions 1–3)**
2	Genital herpes is best treated with oral antivirals, such as acyclovir or valacyclovir, and prevented with either suppressive or standby antivirals.	**Case 72-14 (Question 5)**
GENITAL WARTS		
1	Genital HPV warts are highly contagious and may now be prevented by vaccination, in addition to condoms.	**Case 72-17 (Question 1)**
2	Genital warts often recur even with treatment, which is primarily local, including antimitotics, immune modulators, chemical and surgical ablation, and cryotherapy.	**Case 72-17 (Question 1)**

Sexually transmitted diseases (STDs) are discussed in the earliest written records. However, only in the last several decades have the common STDs been differentiated from each other; unique STD syndromes continue to be described today. For example, of the common STDs, bacterial vaginosis (BV) was not described clearly as a syndrome (initially called *Haemophilus vaginalis* vaginitis) until the 1950s; herpes simplex virus (HSV) type 2 (the cause of genital herpes) was not differentiated from HSV type 1 until the 1960s; the spectrum of genital chlamydial infections was not defined until the 1970s; and the human immunodeficiency virus (HIV) as an STD was not recognized until the 1980s. Since 1980, eight additional sexually transmitted pathogens have been identified. They include the human papillomaviruses (HPV), human T-lymphotropic virus (HTLV-I and II), *Mycoplasma genitalium*, *Mobiluncus* species, HIV-1 and -2, and the human herpes virus type 8 (associated with Kaposi sarcoma).[1] More recently, the Centers for Disease Control and Prevention (CDC) report while hepatitis C virus (HCV) infection is not efficiently transmitted through sexual contact, men who have sex with men (MSM) coinfected with HIV are more likely to transmit to HCV than through heterosexual contact.[2]

See http://www.cdc.gov/std/training/othertraining.htm for general resources from the Centers for Disease Control and Prevention for various sexually transmitted diseases.

GONORRHEA

Gonorrhea (see http://www.cdc.gov/std/training/clinicalslides/slides-dl.htm for symptoms of this STD) is caused by *Neisseria gonorrhoeae*, a gram-negative diplococcus. Depending on the site of exposure, this disease can cause uncomplicated cervical, urethral, rectal, and oropharyngeal infections in both males and females. *N. gonorrhoeae* infection in women is also a major cause of pelvic inflammatory disease (PID). Disseminated gonococcal infection (DGI), the bactermic spread of *N. gonorrhoeae* to joints and other tissues, can lead to complicated gonorrhea infections that cause pustular acral skin lesions, tenosynovitis, polyarthralgia, or arthritis. DGI may lead to rare cases of perihepatitis, endocarditis, or meningitis. In the 1930s, sulfonamides became the first form of effective antimicrobial therapy for gonorrhea until penicillins and tetracyclines became the mainstays of

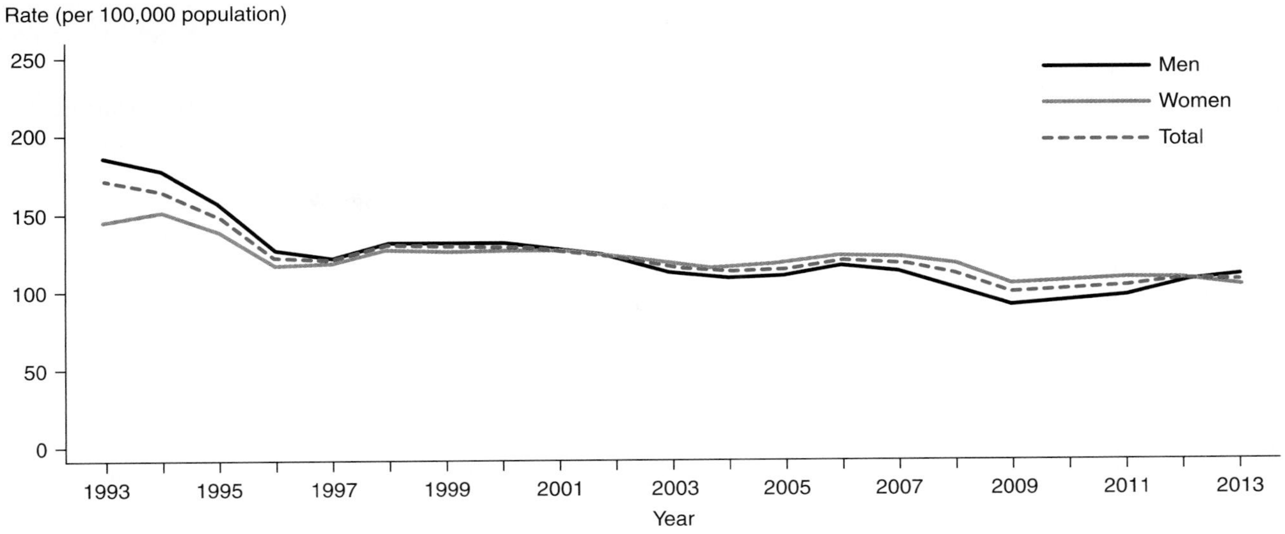

Figure 72-1 Gonorrhea: rates by sex, United States, 1993 to 2013. Note: the Healthy People 2020 target for gonorrhea is 257 new cases per 100,000 for females aged 15 to 44 and 198 new cases per 100,000 for males aged 15 to 44. Source: Centers for Disease Control and Prevention. *Sexually Transmitted Disease Surveillance 2013*. Atlanta, GA: US Dept of Health and Human Services; 2014.

therapy; however, the high levels of resistance to these two antimicrobial agents have eliminated their use in the treatment of this disease state.

In the United States, the incidence of gonorrhea fell 74.3% between 1975 and 1997 after the establishment of national gonorrhea control programs. From 1996 to 2006, the rate fluctuated at around 115 cases per 100,000 individuals, and from 2006 to 2009, the rates declined to a historic low of 98.1 cases per 100,000 individuals in 2009.[3,4] After slight rate increases each year from 2009, the national gonorrhea rate of 106.1 cases per 100,000 individuals in 2013 (representing a total of 333,004 cases) was a decrease from 107.5 in 2012.[4] The current Healthy People 2020 goals for gonorrhea are 257 cases per 100,000 women aged 15 to 44 and 198 cases per 100,000 men aged 15 to 44 (Fig. 72-1).[5] Although there was a decrease of 9.1% in gonorrhea rates among African Americans from 2009 to 2013, rates of gonorrhea remain the highest among African Americans compared to other race and ethnic groups. During this same time period, all other race and ethnic groups saw an increase in gonorrhea rates.[4]

The highest incidence of gonorrhea is in men aged 20 to 24 years and in women aged 15 to 24 years of age. Additional risk factors for women acquiring gonorrhea include a previous gonococcal or other STD infection, new or multiple sex partners, inconsistent condom use, or engaging in commercial sex work or drug use.[6] Although the risk of gonorrhea was greater in homosexual men than in heterosexual men in the past, the incidence dropped in homosexual men during the 1980s AIDS epidemic, because of a reduction in sexual risk behaviors. Currently, the incidence of gonorrhea in MSM continues to rise, from 21.5% in 2006 to 35.1% in 2013.[4]

Uncomplicated Gonorrhea

TRANSMISSION

CASE 72-1

QUESTION 1: D.S., a 23-year-old male naval officer recently stationed in the Philippines, complains of dysuria, meatal pain, and a profuse yellow urethral discharge for 2 days. He admits to extramarital sex with a prostitute during the past week. He is accompanied by his pregnant wife, C.S., who is asymptomatic. D.S. engages in vaginal sex but there is no history of oral or anal sex with either partner. Assuming the prostitute has gonorrhea, what is the likelihood that D.S. and C.S. have been infected?

After one or two episodes of unprotected vaginal intercourse with an asymptomatic infected prostitute, a man has approximately 50% risk of acquiring a urethral infection; the risk increases with repeated exposures and high prevalence among commercial sex workers.[7] The prevalence of infection in women who are secondary sex contacts of infected men is as high as 80% to 90%.[8] Therefore, the likelihood that D.S. and C.S. are infected is high. Because D.S. had sex with a prostitute, both D.S. and C.S. should also be tested for HIV infection.

SIGNS AND SYMPTOMS: MALES

CASE 72-1, QUESTION 2: What signs and symptoms in D.S. are consistent with the diagnosis of gonorrhea? Describe D.S.'s anticipated clinical course if he remains untreated.

In men, gonorrhea usually becomes clinically apparent 1 to 7 days after contact with an infected source. A purulent discharge associated with dysuria is the first sign of infection; D.S. exhibits both. The discharge, which is presumably caused by chemotactic factors such as C5a released when antigonococcal antibody binds complement, may become more profuse and blood tinged as the infection progresses. Some strains of gonorrhea have a propensity to cause asymptomatic or minimally symptomatic infection with negative Gram stain.

Patients with asymptomatic or minimally symptomatic disease may serve as reservoirs for the infection, evading treatment for prolonged periods.[9] At one time, only women were thought to have asymptomatic gonorrhea, but now it is known that men may be asymptomatic carriers as well.[10]

In the area before antimicrobials, gonococci occasionally spread to the epididymis, causing unilateral epididymitis; the prevalence was 5% or more in patients in some studies. Now epididymitis occurs in less than 1% of men with gonorrhea. Urethral stricture after

Table 72-1

CDC Recommendations for Treatment of Uncomplicated Gonorrhea

Presentation	Drugs of Choice (% Cured)	Dosage	Alternative Regimens
Urethritis, cervicitis, rectal[a]	Ceftriaxone (99.2)	250 mg IM once	Cephalosporin single dose regimens[b]
Pharyngeal[a]	Ceftriaxone (98.9)	250 mg IM once	

[a]Because a high percentage of patients with gonorrhea have coexisting *Chlamydia trachomatis* infections, many clinicians recommend treating all patients with gonorrhea with a single-dose azithromycin 1 g orally for treatment of Chlamydia.

[b]Additional cephalosporin regimens include cefixime 400 mg PO, ceftizoxime 500 mg IM, cefoxitin 2 g IM (administered with probenecid 1 g PO), and cefotaxime 500 mg IM.

Adapted from Workowski KA, Bolan GA; Centers for Disease Control and Prevention (CDC). Sexually transmitted diseases treatment guidelines, 2015. *MMWR Recomm Rep*. 2015;64(RR-03):1–137.

repeated attacks and sterility after epididymitis are rare complications of gonococcal infection owing to the effectiveness of antibiotics.

DIAGNOSIS: MALES

CASE 72-1, QUESTION 3: Intracellular gram-negative diplococci were seen on the Gram stain of D.S.'s urethral exudate. Is any further diagnostic testing required?

Demonstration of intracellular gram-negative diplococci in the gram-stained exudate confirms the diagnosis in symptomatic men. Until recently, some experts recommended that cultures be reserved for individuals with negative Gram stain of urethral exudate. However, today cultures are recommended for all patients to permit isolation and testing of the bacteria for antibiotic susceptibility. Cultures usually are performed on Thayer–Martin medium, an enriched chocolate agar to which vancomycin, colistimethate, and nystatin have been added. Cultures from the throat should be obtained if D.S. were exposed by cunnilingus to the prostitute. In D.S.'s case, a urethral culture is indicated.

SIGNS AND SYMPTOMS: FEMALES

CASE 72-1, QUESTION 4: C.S., D.S.'s wife, is asymptomatic. What symptoms would be consistent with gonorrhea in C.S.? Do the symptoms differ because she is pregnant? What is the natural course of gonorrhea in women if left untreated?

Urogenital gonococcal infections in women are commonly asymptomatic. Because the endocervical canal is the primary site of urogenital gonococcal infection in women, the most common symptom is vaginal discharge. Many women infected with gonorrhea have abnormalities of the cervix, including purulent or mucopurulent endocervical discharge, erythema, friability, and edema of the zone of ectopy.[8] The incubation period for urogenital gonorrhea in women is variable.[11] PID is a serious complication in 10% to 20% of women with acute gonococcal infection and can lead to infertility and chronic pelvic pain.[8,12] The assessment of signs and symptoms in women with gonorrhea often is confounded by nonspecific signs and symptoms and a high prevalence of coexisting infection, especially with *Chlamydia trachomatis* or *Trichomonas vaginalis*.

Although lower genital tract symptoms in women may disappear, they remain carriers of *N. gonorrhoeae* and should be treated. Complications of urogenital gonorrhea in pregnancy include spontaneous abortion, premature rupture of the fetal membranes, premature delivery, and acute chorioamnionitis.[12–14] Other complications include gonococcal arthritis (see Case 72-4, Question 1) conjunctivitis, and ophthalmia neonatorum in the newborn.[15] For these reasons, it is critical that C.S. be worked up thoroughly for gonorrhea.

CASE 72-1, QUESTION 5: How should gonorrhea be ruled out in C.S.?

DIAGNOSIS: FEMALES

Nucleic acid amplification tests (NAATs), such as polymerase chain reaction, are recommended for the detection of *N. gonorrhoeae* at urogenital sites in men and women regardless if symptoms are present.[16] Although NAATs are not FDA approved for the detection of *N. gonorrhoeae* at non-urogenital sites, laboratories should meet CLIA requirements and performance specifications for use with rectal and oropharyngeal specimens; NAATs are the recommended detection method for rectal and orophyaryngeal specimens. Although culture for *N. gonorrhoeae* is not ideal for routine diagnosis, cultures should be performed for isolation and identification, antibiotic susceptibility, and resistance surveillance. Cultures should also be performed in cases of suspected treatment failures, defined as those that have received CDC-recommended treatment and subsequently has a positive *N. gonorrhoeae* test result 7 days after treatment and did not engage in sexual activity during those 7 days.[16] In C.S., a NAAT from anal specimen also could be performed because the rectum can serve as a reservoir for gonococci.

TREATMENT

CASE 72-1, QUESTION 6: Compare the various drug regimens used for uncomplicated gonorrhea.

The CDC recommendations are summarized in Table 72-1. Many strains of *N. gonorrhoeae* exhibit plasmid-mediated resistance to penicillin and tetracycline (penicillinase-producing *N. gonorrhoeae* [PPNG] and/or tetracycline-resistant *N. gonorrhoeae* [TRNG], respectively (Fig. 72-2). In addition, significant levels of chromosomally mediated resistance to penicillin, tetracycline, and cefoxitin have been reported.[17] In 2013, all isolates in the Gonococcal Isolate Surveillance Project (GISP) were susceptible to ceftriaxone; therefore, a single dose of intramuscular (IM) ceftriaxone 250 mg is preferred for the treatment of gonorrhea.[18,19] Cefixime 400 mg orally (PO) as a single dose is no longer recommended as a first-line treatment by the CDC but as an alternative option when ceftriaxone cannot be used. Because of the emergence of high levels of quinolone-resistant *N. gonorrhoeae* (QRNG), the CDC no longer recommends the use of fluroquinolones, such as ciprofloxacin and ofloxacin, for the treatment of gonorrhea.[2,20] Because a high percentage of patients with gonorrhea are also coinfected with *C. trachomatis*, a single dose of azithromycin is recommended to be taken concurrently for a presumed infection (see Case 72-1, Question 7).[2,19]

Intramuscular spectinomycin, which traditionally had been used in individuals who could not tolerate fluoroquinolones or cephalosporins, is still unavailable from the manufacturer.[21] Although limited data exists for treatment of gonorrhea in patients

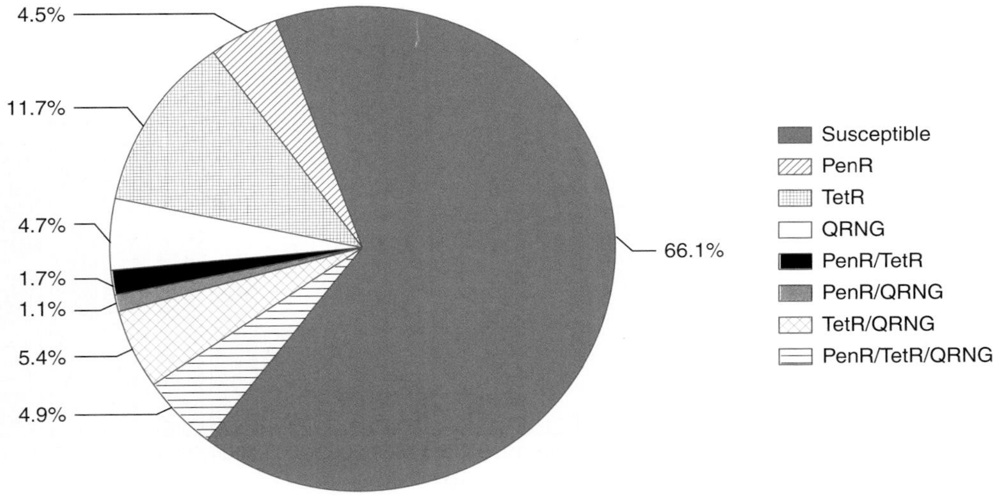

Figure 72-2 *Neisseria gonorrhoeae* Isolates with Penicillin, Tetracycline, and/or Ciprofloxacin Resistance, Gonococcal Isolate Surveillance Project (GISP), 2013. Note: PenR, penicillinase-producing *Neisseria gonorrhoeae* and chromosomally mediated penicillin-resistant *N. gonorrhoeae*; TetR, chromosomally and plasmid-mediated tetracycline-resistant *N. gonorrhoeae*; and QRNG, quinolone-resistant *N. gonorrhoeae*.

Source: Centers for Disease Control and Prevention. *Sexually Transmitted Disease Surveillance 2013*. Atlanta, GA: US Dept of Health and Human Services; 2014.

with cephalosporin or IgE-mediated penicillin allergy, potential alternative treatments are a single dose of gemifloxacin 320 mg PO plus azithromycin 2 g PO, or a single dose of gentamicin 240 mg intramuscularly plus azithromycin 2 g PO.[2,22] Individuals who have either penicillin or cephalosporin allergies should be desensitized to cephalosporins before treatment begins.[23]

Ceftriaxone and Other Cephalosporins

Ceftriaxone, a third-generation cephalosporin, is given as a single, small-volume IM injection that eradicates gonorrhea at all anatomic sites and is also safe in pregnancy (U.S. Food and Drug Administration [FDA] pregnancy category B). Ceftriaxone is ineffective against *C. trachomatis* and in the prevention of postgonococcal urethritis, whereas ofloxacin and levofloxacin for 7 days have similar efficacy to doxycycline.[12] Other injectable cephalosporins (notably ceftizoxime, cefoxitin, and cefotaxime) have been found to be safe and highly effective, but they do not offer any advantage over ceftriaxone for urogenital infections, and their efficacy in pharyngeal infections is not as well-established. A single oral dose of cefixime 400 mg is also effective in curing 92.3% of uncomplicated urogenital and anorectal gonorrhea infections.[2] However, in 2012, the CDC no longer recommended cefixime as a first-line regimen because of concerns about declining cefixime susceptibility among urethral *N. gonorrhoeae* isolates in the United States during 2006 to 2011.[19] Other oral cephalosporins, such as cefpodoxime and cefuroxime, are not recommended because of inferior efficacy and less favorable pharmacodynamics; however, they are FDA approved to treat uncomplicated *N. gonorrhoeae*.

Fluoroquinolones

Fluoroquinolones have been routinely used since the 1990s for the treatment of gonorrhea; however, the GISP has continuously documented fluoroquinolone resistance in *N. gonorrhoeae* isolates, which has necessitated changes in the CDC Sexually Transmitted Disease treatment guidelines (Fig. 72-3). Because of this increased resistance, the CDC no longer recommends ciprofloxacin, levofloxacin, ofloxacin, or other fluoroquinolones for the treatment of gonorrhea. This recommendation also extends to the treatment of gonorrhea-associated conditions, such as PID.[2,20]

Prescribing Patterns

The CDC's 2013 Sexually Transmitted Disease Surveillance Program observed that 96.9% of treated patients received ceftriaxone 250 mg. The number of those treated with cefixime decreased from 5.3% in 2011 to 0.02% in 2013.[4] This decrease in cefixime use was expected as CDC recommendations to avoid use of cefixime at any dose as first-line therapy was issued in 2012. Other most prescribed medications, followed in order by ceftriaxone, azithromycin, "other less frequently used drugs," and cefixime (Fig. 72-4). Dual therapy with azithromycin or doxycycline was prescribed in 95.4% and 4% of those treated with ceftriaxone, respectively.[4]

Case 72-1, Question 7: How should D.S.'s urethritis be treated? Because C.S. is totally asymptomatic and the results of her cultures are pending, should she be treated empirically? If so, what drug(s) would you recommend?

Because D.S. has gonococcal infection limited to the urethra (uncomplicated), a few treatment regimens are possible, as outlined in Case 72-1, Question 6. Ceftriaxone is the preferred treatment, with cefixime as an alternative, only if ceftriaxone is not available. Quinolones should be avoided because of increased resistance in *N. gonorrhoeae* and because D.S.'s infection was likely obtained in the Philippines, where quinolone resistance occurs in more than half of all isolates.[20,24] Patients with gonorrhea may also be coinfected with Chlamydia and therefore presumptive cotreatment with azithromycin 1 g PO as a single dose could be initiated if coinfection is suspected.[19,25] Although single-dose azithromycin 2 g monotherapy has been used to treat concurrent gonorrhea and *Chlamydia*, it is more expensive and poorly tolerated because of increased gastrointestinal (GI) side effects and may lead to macrolide-resistant *N. gonorrhoeae*, or treatment failure.[2]

Sexual Partners

C.S. also should be treated even though she appears asymptomatic. All partners who have had sexual exposure to patients with gonorrhea within 60 days should be treated. If the patient

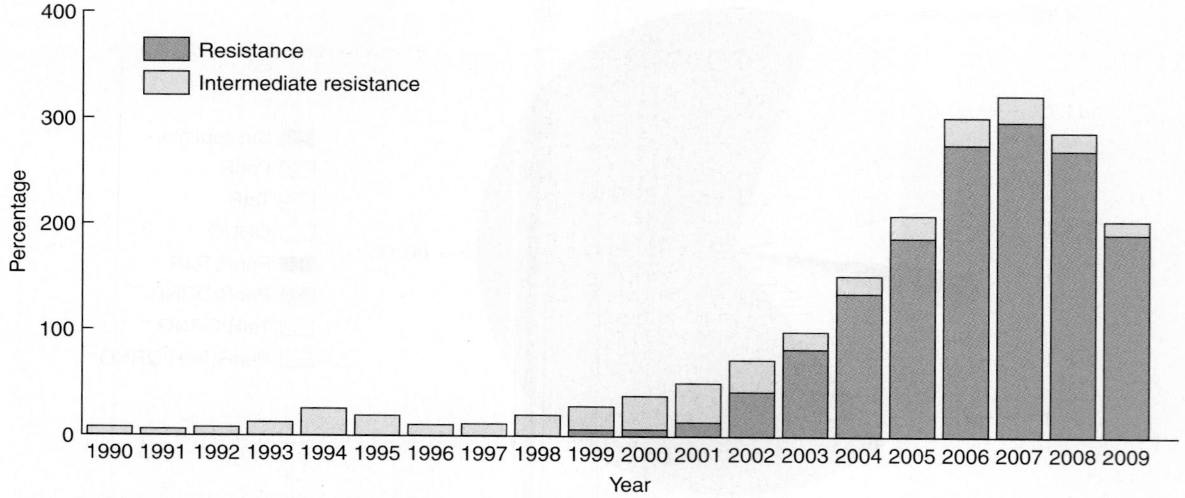

NOTE: Resistant isolates have ciprofloxacin minimum inhibitory concentrations (MICs) ≥1 mcg/mL. Isolates with intermediate resistance have ciprofloxacin MICs of 0.125–0.5 mcg/mL. Susceptibility to ciprofloxacin was first measured in GISP in 1990.

Figure 72-3 Gonococcal Isolate Surveillance Project (GISP)—Percent of *Neisseria gonorrhoeae* isolates with resistance or intermediate resistance to ciprofloxacin, 1990 to 2009. Source: Centers for Disease Control and Prevention. *2009 Sexually Transmitted Disease Surveillance*. Atlanta, GA: US Dept of Health and Human Services; 2010.

has not been sexually active for 60 days, the most recent sexual partner should be treated. This is especially true when the partner is pregnant because gonorrhea during pregnancy is associated with chorioamnionitis and prematurity, as well as neonatal infection. Pregnant women can be treated safely with cephalosporins and azithromycin for gonorrhea and Chlamydia.

Follow-Up

CASE 72-1, QUESTION 8: How does one determine whether the drug therapy of gonorrhea has been effective in D.S. and C.S.?

If recommended therapies are used for treatment of uncomplicated gonorrhea, a test-of-cure is not necessary for either C.S. or D.S. because cure rates are close to 100%.[2] However, a test-of-cure should be done 14 days after treatment in those with pharyngeal infection treated with an alternative treatment regimen.[2] If symptoms persist in D.S., who was treated with ceftriaxone, cultures should be done to determine antibiotic susceptibility, and to rule out other causes of urethritis.

Antibiotic-Resistant *Neisseria gonorrhoeae*

CASE 72-1, QUESTION 9: D.S. states that he was treated with penicillin in the past for a gonococcal infection. Why are penicillins not prescribed routinely today?

Failure of penicillin to eradicate the gonococcus can be the result of plasmid (e.g., PPNG) or chromosomally mediated resistant *Neisseria gonorrhea* (CMRNG) antibiotic resistance. PPNG contain plasmids, which determine the production of lactamase, an enzyme that hydrolyzes the lactam ring of penicillin G or ampicillin. Chromosomally mediated resistance does not involve β-lactamase production and often is associated with increased resistance to other β-lactams. The clinical significance of CMRNG is questionable because serum levels of approved antibiotics are achieved far above the minimum inhibitory concentration, such that treatment failure is unlikely. However, to date, CMRNG remain largely susceptible to ceftriaxone. High-level tetracycline resistance is defined by gonococci that carry plasmid-encoded resistance to 16 g/mL or more of tetracycline. These strains are known as TRNG. Although not of major concern in the United States, development of resistance to alternative therapies is a continuing concern.

The first cases of PPNG infection were reported in the United States in 1976. PPNG are especially prevalent in Southeast Asia, the Far East, and West Africa, where the prevalence often exceeds 50%. In the United States, the percent of PPNG strains reached a peak of about 11% in 1991; since then, cases have steadily declined to 0.4% in 2007, according to the CDC's GISP (Fig. 72-2).[26] Strains of TRNG were first identified in 1985, but fortunately most TRNG isolates still are sensitive to β-lactam antibiotics. The use of tetracycline was officially abandoned by the CDC in 1985 and penicillin was abandoned in 1987. In the late 1990s, the number of TRNG and PPNG plus TRNG cases plateaued at about 5% and 1%, respectively. Therefore, because approximately 21% of gonococcal isolates are resistant to tetracycline and/or penicillin within the United States, it is not acceptable to use these agents in the initial management of uncomplicated genital gonorrhea; IM ceftriaxone remains the drug of choice. Antibiotic susceptibility testing is recommended in cases of persistent infection after treatment.

QRNG was first reported in 1990 and was reported to be 0.2% of isolates in the continental United States.[3,17] In the 2013 GISP report, 11% of isolates from Honolulu, Hawaii, were QRNG, whereas among California sites, 31.8% to 44.4% of isolates were QRNG.[27] *N. gonorrhoeae* resistance to quinolones has increased almost every year since reporting began in 1990 and has become widespread in the United States, resulting in the CDC recommending against using quinolones for the treatment of gonococcal or related conditions (e.g., PID) acquired in the United States.[12,20] In 2013, 16.1% of all isolates collected by the GISP demonstrated resistance to ciprofloxacin.[4] Resistance to fluoroquinolones is associated with mutations of GyrA and is commonly identified in strains that produce β-lactamase and strains exhibiting chromosomally mediated resistance to penicillin and tetracycline.[28] *N. gonorrhoeae* strains may therefore exhibit decreased susceptibility or complete resistance to the recommended dose of quinolones, and the clinical importance of strains with decreased susceptibility is unknown.[29]

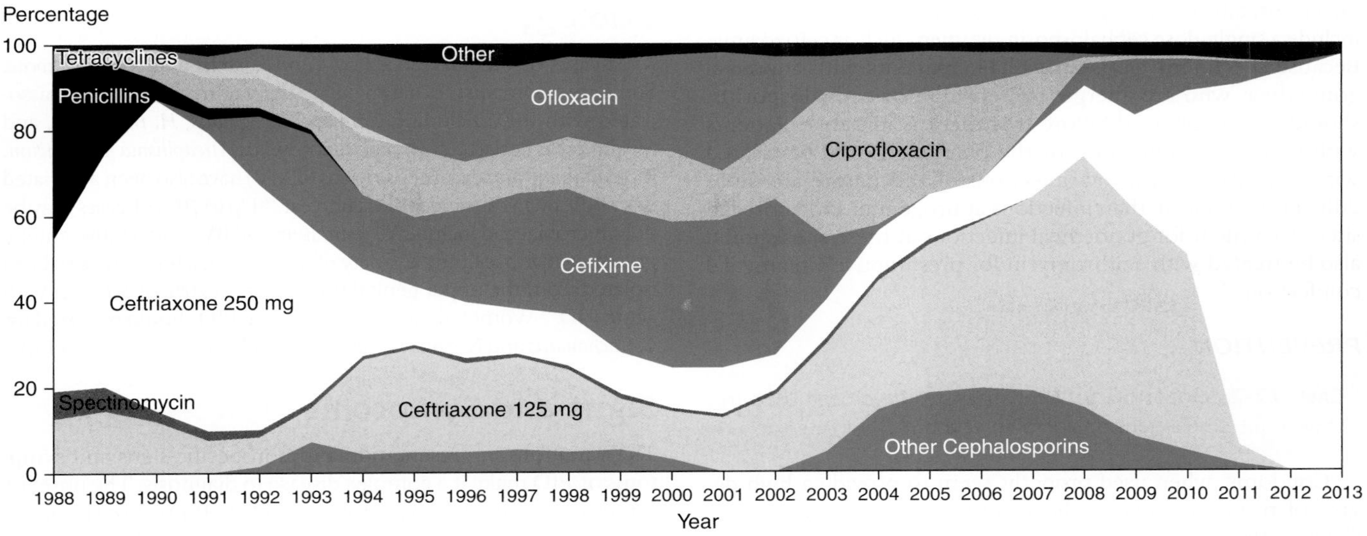

Figure 72-4 Gonococcal Isolate Surveillance Project (GISP)—Drugs used to treat gonorrhea in GISP participants, 1988 to 2013. Note: For 2013, "Other" includes no therapy (0.9%), azithromycin 2 g (1.7%), and other less frequently used drugs (<0.1%).
Source: Centers for Disease Control and Prevention. *Sexually Transmitted Disease Surveillance 2013*. Atlanta, GA: US Dept of Health and Human Services; 2014.

D.S. was likely infected with *N. gonorrhoeae* in the Philippines, and QRNG is highly likely; thus, an appropriate cephalosporin antibiotic such as IM ceftriaxone should be recommended. If he had been initially treated with ceftriaxone, the expectation would be that he would be free of gonococcal infection within 3 days. To date, ceftriaxone-resistant strains of *N. gonorrhoeae* have not been reported in the United States, but GISP data has documented decreased cefixime susceptibility among urethral *N. gonorrhoeae* isolates.[19]

Anorectal and Pharyngeal Gonorrhea

EPIDEMIOLOGY

CASE 72-2

QUESTION 1: M.B. is a 24-year-old, sexually active, homosexual man with a 2-month history of perianal itching, painful defecation, constipation, a bloody mucoid rectal discharge, and a sore throat. Sigmoidoscopy revealed rectal mucosal inflammation but no apparent ulcers or fissures. Stool examination for parasites was negative and a Venereal Disease Research Laboratory (VDRL) test was nonreactive. Both rectal and pharyngeal cultures revealed *N. gonorrhoeae*. How does gonorrhea in homosexual men compare with gonorrhea in heterosexual men?

Rectal infection occurs rarely in strictly heterosexual men, whereas in the male homosexual population, anorectal (25%) and pharyngeal (10%–25%) gonococcal infections occur more often.[8,30] Because pharyngeal[30,31] and anorectal gonococcal infections are often asymptomatic, a large reservoir of carriers in the homosexual male population may exist and annually screening should be done if they have engaged in receptive oral or anal intercourse in the preceding year. By comparison, very few urethral gonococcal infections are asymptomatic. In addition, data indicate that pharyngeal infections may be an important source of urethral gonorrhea in homosexual men, spread by fellatio.[30,32]

SIGNS AND SYMPTOMS

CASE 72-2, QUESTION 2: Are M.B.'s signs and symptoms consistent with gonorrhea?

Rectal gonorrhea produces the syndrome of proctitis with anorectal pain, mucopurulent anorectal discharge, constipation, tenesmus, and anorectal bleeding. The differential diagnosis of proctitis in the homosexual male includes rectal infection with *N. gonorrhoeae*, *C. trachomatis*, HSV, and syphilis. Proctitis, limited to the distal rectum, should be differentiated from proctocolitis, which is often caused by *Shigella* species, *Campylobacter* species, or *Entamoeba histolytica* in homosexual men. The incidence of rectal gonorrhea and Chlamydia has risen dramatically since 1996.[33] Rectal Chlamydia is often asymptomatic and observed more often than gonorrhea, necessitating testing for both pathogens.[34] Although pharyngeal gonorrhea is often asymptomatic, a review of system and physical exam may reveal a sore throat, pharyngeal exudates, or cervical lymphadenitis.

CASE 72-2, QUESTION 3: How should M.B.'s diagnosis be managed?

TREATMENT

The treatment of choice for patients such as M.B. with anorectal or pharyngeal gonorrhea is ceftriaxone 250 mg IM as a single dose (Table 72-1).[12] Azithromycin should also be given to treat possible coexisting rectal chlamydial infection. Patients, such as M.B., with either anorectal or pharyngeal gonorrhea should be advised to avoid further unprotected sexual activity and should be counseled and tested for infection with HIV.

CASE 72-2, QUESTION 4: What are the alternative regimens for patients with isolated anal or pharyngeal gonorrhea?

Patients with anorectal gonorrhea alone should be treated with ceftriaxone. Oral cefixime is a recommended alternative, but it should not be used as a first-line agent. As with urogenital infections, alternative regimens for isolated anorectal infection include a single-dose cephalosporin regimen, such as ceftizoxime. Because spectinomycin is unavailable, patients with anorectal gonorrhea, who are allergic to penicillin or cephalosporins, should be desensitized before treatment is initiated. Patients with gonococcal infections of the pharynx should be treated with ceftriaxone; however, infections of this nature are more difficult to eradicate than infections at urogenital and anorectal sites. Treatment for gonorrheal infections at these sites should also be treated with azithromycin for presumptive Chlamydial coinfection.[19]

PREVENTION

Case 72-2, Question 5: What measures have been used to prevent the sexual transmission of infection?

Condoms, when used properly, seem to provide a high degree of protection against the acquisition and transmission of STDs.[2,35] Previous studies indicated that the use of the spermicide nonoxynol-9 had activity against gonorrhea and Chlamydia; however, in light of recent evidence suggesting that nonoxynol-9 might actually increase the risk of acquiring HIV and other STDs, the FDA currently requires manufacturers of nonoxynol-9 products to include a warning statement on the product's label that it does not protect against HIV or other STDs.[12,36] Topical antibacterial agents, urinating, and washing after intercourse are of little value in preventing the transmission of STDs. Douching may increase the risk of other STDs, such as trichomoniasis.[37]

The prophylactic administration of antibiotics immediately before or soon after sexual intercourse is not recommended owing to increased costs and antimicrobial resistance. Use of rapid, specific tests and empiric symptomatic management enhances detection and treatment of gonorrhea.

PELVIC INFLAMMATORY DISEASE

The term PID refers to a variety of inflammatory disorders of the upper female reproductive tract. This term does not denote the primary infection site (the fallopian tubes) nor the causative microorganisms. PID also has been used to connote an infection that occurs acutely when either vaginal or cervical micro-organisms traverse the sterile endometrium and ascend to the fallopian tubes. Acute salpingitis may also be used to describe an acute infection of the fallopian tubes. Therefore, the terms PID and salpingitis are used interchangeably in this discussion to denote an acute infection involving the fallopian tubes.

PID affects approximately 1 million women annually in the United States.[38] However, the National Disease and Therapeutic Index (NDTI) estimates that from 2002 to 2012, the number of initial visit to physicians for PID for women aged 15 to 44 decreased 39.8%.[4] Many cases of acute PID occur by sexual transmission, especially in young women 16 to 24 years, who are more likely to have multiple sexual partners.[39] Risk factors for the development of PID include unprotected sexual intercourse before age 15, douching, BV, sex while menstruating, and smoking.[40] It is unclear whether an intrauterine device (IUD) increases the risk of PID, but it may be prudent to avoid placement when the patient has chlamydial or gonococcal cervicitis.[41] Two-thirds of PID cases resulting in infertility are asymptomatic, and up to one-third are incorrectly diagnosed owing to low specificity of diagnostic techniques. In the United States, infertility occurs in about 12.1% of women after the first episode of PID.[42] The estimated costs for treatment of PID and its sequelae exceeds $4.2 billion annually.[38]

Etiology

Most cases of PID are caused by *C. trachomatis* and *N. gonorrhoeae*. Some microorganisms that make up the vaginal flora are also associated with PID, including *Gardnerella vaginalis*, *H. influenzae*, and *Streptococcus agalactiae*. *Mycoplasma hominis*, *Ureaplasma urealyticum*, *M. genitalium*, and cytomegalovirus (CMV) have also been associated with PID, but a causative role is unclear.[12] Up to 70% of cases may be polymicrobial and include *M. genitalium* and BV.[43] Facultative enteric gram-negative bacilli and a variety of anaerobic bacteria have also been isolated from the upper genital tract of up to 70% of women with acute PID.[43] Women diagnosed with acute PID should be tested for *C. trachomatis* and *N. gonorrhoeae* using NAAT and screened for HIV.[2]

Signs and Symptoms

The variations in presentation and nonspecific signs and symptoms of PID make it a complex disease to diagnosis. The onset of symptoms of abdominal pain attributable to PID caused by either gonococci or chlamydia often occurs soon after the menstrual period. Symptoms of PID, if present, are often nonspecific, which can create a delay in or failure of diagnosis. Vaginal discharge, menorrhagia, dysuria, and dyspareunia are commonly associated with PID. Pelvic examination findings include cervical motion tenderness, uterine tenderness, or adnexal tenderness. Temperatures greater than 101°F, abnormal cervical or vaginal mucopurulent discharge, white blood cells (WBC) on saline microscopy of vaginal secretions, elevated erythrocyte sedimentation rate, an elevated C-reactive protein, or laboratory documentation of cervical infection with *N. gonorrhoeae or C. trachomatis* support a diagnosis of PID.[2] Clinical diagnosis has sensitivity for PID of about 65% to 90%, whereas laparoscopy and a newer technique, transvaginal Doppler ultrasound, are about 100% specific, resulting in the combination of laparoscopy and clinical impression serving as the gold standard.[2,44,45] Unfortunately, laparoscopy and Doppler ultrasound are costly and often not readily available for acute cases and they are not diagnostic for endometritis; thus, clinical impression is critical. A key to reducing the incidence of PID may be through active screening of *Chlamydia* in young, sexually active women.[46,47]

Clinical Sequelae

An abscess may form in the pelvic or abdominal cavity and in one or both fallopian tubes. Chronic abdominal pain develops in 18% of women with PID and may be the result of pelvic adhesions surrounding the tubes and ovaries. After a single episode of PID, tubal occlusion and fibrosis secondary to fallopian tube inflammation (salpingitis) result in 12% infertility, 25% infertility after two episodes, and 50% infertility after three or more episodes.[42] Other sequelae include ectopic pregnancy (9%) and chronic pelvic pain (18%).[48] The risk of ectopic pregnancy is increased approximately eightfold after one or more episodes of PID.

Diagnosis and Treatment

CASE 72-3

Question 1: H.C., a 19-year-old, sexually active woman, complains of mild dysuria, a purulent vaginal discharge, fever, and moderately severe, bilateral, lower abdominal pain of 3 days duration. Examination confirms uterine and adnexal tenderness, a purulent cervical exudate, and a temperature of 39°C. Laboratory examinations show a nonreactive VDRL and negative urinalysis. A pregnancy test performed was negative. The peripheral WBC count was mildly elevated (11,000/μL) with 70% polymorphonuclear leukocytes. Does H.C. have PID? How should she be treated?

Table 72-2

Antimicrobial Regimens Recommended by the CDC for Treatment of Acute Pelvic Inflammatory Disease

Treatment Setting, Drugs, Schedule	Advantage	Disadvantage	Clinical Considerations
Inpatient (Parenteral) Therapy			
Regimen A			
Cefotetan 2 g IV every 12 hours OR cefoxitin 2 g IV every 6 hours PLUS doxycycline 100 mg IV or PO[a] every 12 hours Continue doxycycline (100 mg PO twice daily) after discharge to complete 14 days of therapy	Optimal coverage of *N. gonorrhoeae* (including resistant strains) and *C. trachomatis*	Possible suboptimal anaerobic coverage	Penicillin-allergic patients may also be allergic to cephalosporins; doxycycline use in pregnant patients may cause reversible inhibition of skeletal growth in the fetus and discoloration of teeth in young children
Regimen B			
Clindamycin 900 mg IV every 8 hours PLUS gentamicin loading dose IV or IM (2 mg/kg) followed by a maintenance dose of 1.5 mg/kg every 8 hours[b]	Optimal coverage of anaerobes and Gram-negative enteric rods	Possible suboptimal coverage of *N. gonorrhoeae* and *C. trachomatis*	Patients with decreased renal function may not be good candidates for aminoglycoside treatment or may need a dosage adjustment
Alternative Regimen			
Ampicillin/sulbactam 3 g IV every 6 hours PLUS doxycycline 100 mg PO or IV every 12 hours	Optimal coverage of *N. gonorrhoeae* and *C. trachomatis*	Inadequate coverage of anaerobes necessitates use of metronidazole or ampicillin/sulbactam	Not appropriate in pregnancy or in young children
Outpatient (Oral) Therapy[c]			
Regimen A			
Ceftriaxone 250 mg IM in a single dose PLUS doxycycline 100 mg PO twice daily for 14 days WITH or WITHOUT metronidazole 500 mg PO twice daily for 14 days OR cefoxitin 2 g IM in a single dose and probenecid, 1 g PO administered concurrently in a single dose PLUS doxycycline 100 mg PO twice daily for 14 days WITH or WITHOUT metronidazole 500 mg PO twice daily for 14 days OR other parenteral third-generation cephalosporins (e.g., ceftizoxime or cefotaxime) PLUS doxycycline 100 mg PO twice daily for 14 days WITH or WITHOUT metronidazole 500 mg PO twice daily for 14 days	Good to excellent coverage of *N. gonorrhoeae* and optimal coverage of *C. trachomatis*	Possible suboptimal anaerobic coverage necessitating the addition of metronidazole	Optimal cephalosporin is unclear; more complicated regimen requiring combination of parenteral and oral therapies

[a]Considering the oral bioavailability of doxycycline, PO therapy should be preferentially used over IV.
[b]Single daily dosing (3–5 mg/kg) may be substituted.
[c]Consider for mild-to-moderate acute PID.

Adapted from Workowski KA, Bolan GA; Centers for Disease Control and Prevention (CDC). Sexually transmitted diseases treatment guidelines, 2015. *MMWR Recomm Rep*. 2015;64(RR-03):1–137.

Although fever and leukocytosis are often absent in mild or subacute PID, these findings in a woman with uterine and adnexal tenderness with cervical exudate increases the likelihood of acute PID. Recommended treatment regimens for PID are listed in Table 72-2 and should be initiated immediately after diagnosis of PID to prevent clinical sequelae; confirmation of the actual pathogen rarely takes place. Patients such as H.C. with mild-to-moderate PID can be hospitalized and treated with parenteral antibiotics; however, clinical efficacy and overall outcomes are equal between parental and oral therapy, and H.C. could also be treated on an outpatient basis. For inpatient treatment, the CDC recommends either intravenous (IV) cefotetan 2 g every 12 hours or IV cefoxitin 2 g every 6 hours for at least 24 hours beyond the first signs of clinical improvement along with doxycycline 100 mg every 12 hours. Once clinical improvement is noted, parenteral therapy may be discontinued and PO doxycycline 100 mg every 12 hours can continue to complete 14 days of therapy. For outpatient treatment, the CDC guidelines recommend either IM ceftriaxone 250 mg as a single dose or IM cefoxitin 2 g as a single dose (with probenecid 1 g PO for one dose) plus PO doxycycline 100 mg twice a day for 14 days with or without PO metronidazole 500 mg twice daily for 14 days.[2] A tetracycline derivative or an alternative agent that is active against *C. trachomatis* should be included in the treatment of PID; however, monotherapy with a tetracycline is not recommended because of the lack of activity against gram-negative aerobic and anaerobic organisms and *N. gonorrhoeae*. The addition of metronidazole, which covers anaerobic bacteria, should also be considered; anaerobes have been isolated from the upper reproductive tract of women with PID and may cause tubal and epithelial destruction.[2,49] Metronidazole is widely used by clinicians, because BV is frequently associated with PID.[2] Fluoroquinolones, such as levofloxacin and ofloxacin, are no longer recommended for the treatment of PID because of the increase in prevalence of QRNG in the United States.[20]

Both oral and IV doxycycline have similar bioavailability; therefore, doxycycline should be given PO whenever possible.[2] Substantial clinical improvement is usually seen within 3 days after initiation of therapy. Clindamycin plus gentamicin can be used alternatively in penicillin-allergic and pregnant women.[2] Because H.C. is sexually active, any sexual partners within the previous 60 days (or if >60 days, then the most recent sexual partner) should be empirically treated because of the risk of gonococcal or chlamydial urethritis as well as to reduce the risk of reinfection.[2]

COMPLICATED GONORRHEA

Disseminated Gonococcal Infection

SIGNS AND SYMPTOMS

CASE 72-4

QUESTION 1: S.P., a 28-year-old, sexually active woman, was seen for stiffness and pain of the right wrist and left ankle and fever (38°C). On physical examination, the knee and wrist joints were found to be hot, red, and swollen; papules and pustular lesions were observed on S.P.'s legs and forearms. A latex fixation test for rheumatoid factor was negative. A tap of the right knee yielded an effusion with a WBC count of 34,000/μL (80% polymorphonuclear leukocytes). Cultures of the skin lesions were negative, but *N. gonorrhoeae* was isolated from the throat, cervix, blood, and synovial fluid. A chest radiograph, echocardiogram, and electrocardiogram all were normal, and no murmur could be appreciated. Assess S.P.'s clinical presentation.

S.P.'s signs, symptoms, and laboratory findings are consistent with gonococcal bacteremia, which today occurs in less than 1% of women and men with gonorrhea. The most common manifestation of gonococcemia is the gonococcal arthritis–dermatitis syndrome or DGI exhibited by S.P. Symptoms include fever, occasional chills, a mild tenosynovitis of the small joints, and skin lesions; the latter primarily involving the distal extremities are petechial, papular, pustular, and hemorrhagic in appearance.[2]

Diagnosis of DGI is made by NAAT or culture of specimen from routine sites of gonococcal infections (e.g., urethra, cervix, pharynx, and rectum), as well as culture from disseminated sites of infection (e.g., synovial fluid, blood, skin, and CNS). However, blood cultures are positive in only 33% of DGI cases, even when culture samples are obtained early in the course of the infection.[12] The low positive yield from blood cultures may be attributable to the low inoculum or intermittent bacteremic period.

TREATMENT

CASE 72-4, QUESTION 2: How should S.P. be managed? How quickly will she respond to therapy?

Patients like S.P. with gonococcal arthritis and bacteremia should be hospitalized for treatment with ceftriaxone 1 g IV or IM daily until substantial clinical improvement is sustained for 24 to 48 hours, at which time therapy may be switched to an oral agent guided by antimicrobial susceptibility for a total treatment course of at least 7 days (Table 72-3).[2] Initiation of treatment should also include azithromycin 1 g PO in a single dose. Symptoms and signs of tenosynovitis should be improved markedly within 48 hours. Septic gonococcal arthritis with purulent synovial fluid may require repeated aspiration and resolves more slowly.

Table 72-3
Treatment of Disseminated Gonococcal Infection

No Penicillin Allergy[a]
Parenteral
Recommended[b]—Ceftriaxone 1 g IV or IM every 24 hours
Alternative[b]—Cefotaxime 1 g IV q8h or ceftizoxime 1 g IV every 8 hours
Oral[c]
Cefixime 400 mg PO twice daily

[a]Parenteral treatment should be continued for 24 to 48 hours beyond clinical improvement.
[b]Treatment should include a single dose of Azithromycin 1 g PO.
[c]Treat for 7 days after switching from parenteral therapy.

Adapted from Workowski KA, Bolan GA; Centers for Disease Control and Prevention (CDC). Sexually transmitted diseases treatment guidelines, 2015. *MMWR Recomm Rep.* 2015;64(RR-03):1–137.

Treatment of Gonococcal Endocarditis and Meningitis

CASE 72-4, QUESTION 3: How should gonococcal endocarditis and meningitis be treated?

Gonococcal endocarditis and meningitis, occurring in only 1% to 3% of DGIs, require high-dose IV therapy, such as ceftriaxone (1–2 g IV every 12–24 hours), for 10 to 14 days in the case of meningitis and for at least 4 weeks in the case of endocarditis.[2] Like other gonococcal infections, a single dose of azithromycin 1 g PO should be given.

Neonatal Disseminated Gonococcal Infection: Treatment

CASE 72-4, QUESTION 4: How should neonatal DGI and meningitis be managed?

Neonatal DGI and meningitis can be treated with either ceftriaxone 25 to 50 mg/kg (IV or IM) daily or cefotaxime 25 mg/kg (IV or IM) every 12 hours. Treatment is for 7 days for DGI; however, meningitis requires 10 to 14 days of treatment.[2] Although ceftriaxone is also effective in the treatment of neonatal DGI and meningitis, cefotaxime is considered a safer choice in the neonatal population.

CHLAMYDIA TRACHOMATIS

The rate of reported *Chlamydia* infections has climbed steadily each year since the 1980s, and it is the most commonly reported STD in the United States. During 1993 to 2012, the reported rate of chlamydial infections increased from 178 to 453.3 cases per 100,000 individuals.[4] This increase may be attributable to the increased development and use of more sensitive screening tests, improved national reporting efforts, or a true increase in the incidence of disease.[12] In 2013, the United States saw the rate of chlamydial infections decrease for the first time to 446.6 cases per 100,000.[4] Women are 3 times more likely than men to be infected with *Chlamydia*—623.1 cases versus 262.6 cases per 100,000 individuals, respectively, in 2013. However, from 2009 to 2013, the infection rate among men increased 21% compared with 6.2% in women. The highest rate of infection is in women 15 to 19 years (3,043.3 cases per 100,000 females) and in men 20 to 24 years (1,325.6 cases per 100,000 males).[4] If left untreated, chlamydial infection in women can lead to serious sequelae, such as PID, ectopic pregnancy, and infertility. Asymptomatic infection is also observed in both men and women; however, routine screening is recommended for sexually active women up to 25 years of age and older women with risk factors for infection (e.g., multiple sexual partners or having a new sexual partner). Screening sexually active men for *C. trachomatis* can be considered in settings or populations with a high prevalence of the infection (e.g., MSM populations).[2]

C. trachomatis, an intracellular obligate organism, can be diagnosed either by culture, direct immunofluorescence assay (DFA), enzyme immunoassay (EIA), or NAAT of endocervical or male urethral swabs.[12] However, *C. trachomatis* is a difficult organism to demonstrate in clinical specimens because cell culture techniques are not readily available to the practitioner. Because few practitioners have access to facilities for isolation of *C. trachomatis*, most chlamydial infections are diagnosed and treated based on clinical impression and laboratory techniques. Nonculture diagnostic tests, such as NAATs, DFAs, and EIAs, are generally sensitive methods for detecting *C. trachomatis.* Ligase chain reaction and PCR are two NAATs with wide commercial availability, are relatively simple to use, can be performed using urine or genital swab specimens, and are more sensitive than non-NAATs.[15] NAATs are approximately 20% to 35% more sensitive than EIAs and DFAs and are the recommended test method for detection of *C. trachomatis* in men and women with and without symptoms.[2,16] A test-of-cure is not necessary unless patient compliance is questionable, symptoms persist, or reinfection is suspected. Repeat testing with NAATs fewer than 3 weeks after initiation of treatment is not recommended because false-negative results may occur as a result of undetectable *C. trachomatis* organisms. Moreover, false positives may occur with repeat NAATs with the continued excretion of dead organisms.

A variety of clinical syndromes are caused by *C. trachomatis*, including cervicitis, urethritis, bartholinitis, endometritis, salpingitis, and perihepatitis in women, and urethritis, epididymitis, prostatitis, proctitis, and Reiter syndrome in men.[12] The spectrum of chlamydial infections closely resembles those caused by the gonococcus, which is why many patients presenting with these syndromes are treated with drugs effective against both organisms.

There is controversy in how *C. trachomatis* is cultured and what the in vitro results mean clinically, especially in the 10% to 15% of cases that fail treatment.[50] The CDC thus uses cure rates instead of microbial susceptibilities to make treatment recommendations. Only azithromycin and doxycycline have 97% and 98% cure rates, respectively.[2,51] Alternatives include erythromycin, ofloxacin, and levofloxacin. Other quinolones should not be used because they have not been evaluated adequately or are not reliably effective.[2]

Nongonococcal Urethritis

ETIOLOGY

CASE 72-5

QUESTION 1: T.K., a 26-year-old, sexually active man, complains of mild dysuria and a mucoid-like urethral discharge beginning 15 days after his last intercourse. He has no fever, lymphadenopathy, penile lesions, or hematuria. A Gram stain smear of an anterior urethral specimen showed 20 polymorphonuclear neutrophilic leukocytes (PMNs) per oil immersion (1,000) field and no gram-negative diplococci. What pathogens are associated with nongonococcal urethritis (NGU)?

In the United States, NGU is the most common STD in men.[52,53] *C. trachomatis* is a frequent cause of NGU, representing 15% to 40% of all cases. Other agents that have been associated with NGU include *M. genitalium*, *T. vaginalis*, *HSV*, and *adenovirus*; however, the cause for the majority of NGU cases is unknown.[12] The variety of pathogens and disparity among identification techniques require sound clinical judgment and an algorithmic laboratory testing approach to accurately identify and treat the cause. A NAAT, if available, should be performed to rule out the presence of *C. trachomatis* and *N. gonorrhoeae*.

SIGNS AND SYMPTOMS

CASE 72-5, QUESTION 2: Describe the clinical presentation of a person with NGU. Is T.K.'s presentation consistent with NGU? How does one differentiate between NGU and gonococcal urethritis?

T.K.'s presentation is typical. Compared with gonococcal urethritis, NGU typically produces less severe and less frequent dysuria and less penile discharge. Chlamydial urethral infection is completely asymptomatic more often than gonococcal urethral infection. The incubation period for gonococcal urethritis is 2 to 7 days, whereas the incubation period for NGU is typically 2 to 3 weeks.

Nonetheless, NGU and gonococcal urethritis cannot be reliably differentiated solely on the basis of symptoms and signs. If there is objective evidence of a urethral discharge (expressed by milking the urethra), a Gram stain with $\geq$2 WBCs per oil immersion field in the urethral secretion, positive leukocyte esterase test demonstrating 10 WBCs per high-power field, the diagnosis of NGU is made by excluding the presence of *N. gonorrhoeae* by Gram stain and/or culture.

TREATMENT

CASE 72-5, QUESTION 3: How should T.K. be treated?

If *C. trachomatis* cannot be ruled out, therapy with azithromycin 1 g PO for one dose or doxycycline 100 mg PO twice daily for 7 days should be ordered. Compared to doxycycline, *M. genitalium* responds better to azithromycin as doxycycline does not effectively eradicate *M. genitalium*.[2] Azithromycin also has the advantage of a single-dose regimen, which may aid in patient compliance. Erythromycin base 500 mg PO 4 times a day or erythromycin ethylsuccinate 800 mg PO 4 times a day for 7 days are alternative CDC-approved regimens. Additionally, ofloxacin 300 mg PO twice daily or levofloxacin 500 mg PO every day for 7 days are other alternatives, but they offer no significant advantages compared with the previously mentioned agents, may not treat *U. urealyticum* adequately, and are significantly more expensive.[2,54] Ciprofloxacin should be avoided because treatment failures have been reported.[55] Patient counseling should emphasize the need for abstinence from sexual intercourse at least until the prescribed course of therapy has been completed (or 7 days after single-dose therapy) by the patient and his sexual partner(s).[2] There is some indication that the proportion of NGU caused by *C. trachomatis* is declining, potentially being replaced by an increased proportion of *U. urealyticum*, which is variably cured at 2 weeks by azithromycin (73%) and doxycycline (65%).[56]

Recurrent Infection

CASE 72-5, QUESTION 4: T.K. was treated with doxycycline 100 mg twice daily for 7 days. He remained asymptomatic for 14 days after completion of his therapy, when he again noticed similar symptoms of dysuria and a mucoid-like urethral discharge. How should T.K.'s recurrent infection be treated?

The major problem encountered in the treatment of NGU is the high rate of recurrent infections. Men receiving treatment should follow-up if symptoms persist or recur after completion of therapy. Approximately 20% to 60% of patients experience recurrent or persistent urethritis within 1 to 2 weeks after treatment.[57] The rate of recurrence is highest in patients with idiopathic urethritis, that is, those not infected with *C. trachomatis* or *U. urealyticum*. Recurrence suggests reexposure to an untreated partner, whereas persistent urethritis (without improvement during therapy) suggests the presence of other organisms, including *M. genitalium*, *U. urealyticum*, or *T. vaginalis*.[2,58,59] NGU that persists or recurs should be retreated with the initial regimen if the patient was not compliant or the sexual partner was not treated. For patients with persistent symptoms, who were compliant with the initial regimen and were not reexposed, the CDC recommends using a single 1 g dose of azithromycin if not used for the initial episode, or moxifloxacin 400 mg PO daily for 7 days if the patient has failed azithromycin.[2]

Men with acute epididymitis often have chlamydial or gonococcal infection, particularly if they are younger than 35 years of age or have a urethral discharge. *Escherichia coli* and *Pseudomonas* species are common pathogens in homosexual men. In older men, sexually transmitted epididymitis is less common and is more commonly caused by urinary tract instrumentation, surgery, systemic disease, or immune suppression.[2] If testicular tenderness is present with urethritis, and the clinical impression is consistent with epididymitis caused by *Chlamydia* or gonorrhea, the CDC recommend a single dose of ceftriaxone 250 mg IM plus doxycycline 100 mg PO twice for 10 days. For acute epididymitis caused by enteric organisms or with a negative gonococcal culture or NAAT, ofloxacin 300 mg PO twice daily or levofloxacin 500 mg PO once daily for 10 days may be used.[2,49] In men who practice insertive anal sex, where the most likely cause of acute epididymitis is caused by *Chlamydia*, gonorrhea, and enteric organisms, the CDC recommends ceftriaxone 250 mg IM in a single dose plus levofloxacin 500 mg PO daily or ofloxacin 300 mg PO BID for 10 days.[2]

SEXUAL PARTNERS

CASE 72-5, QUESTION 5: A.C., T.K.'s girlfriend, comes into the clinic 3 weeks after T.K.'s last visit. She is worried that she may have a similar infection, although she has no signs or symptoms. What clinical manifestations of chlamydial infections are seen in women? Should A.C. be treated for suspected chlamydial infection?

In the absence of cultures for Chlamydia, empirical treatment against chlamydia of women who are sexual partners of men with NGU is recommended. Many partners are asymptomatic but from 30% to 70% are culture positive if tested. A.C. should be examined carefully for mucopurulent cervicitis and salpingitis. Although many women with chlamydial infection of the cervix are asymptomatic, up to one-quarter have evidence of mucopurulent discharge.[60] A Gram stain of appropriately collected mucopurulent endocervical discharge from patients with Chlamydia infection shows many PMNs and no gonococci.

Regardless of findings, treatment should be initiated with the same azithromycin or doxycycline regimen used for NGU. However, if A.C. is pregnant, tetracyclines and fluoroquinolones should be avoided. Azithromycin 1 g PO as a single dose or amoxicillin 500 mg PO 3 times a day for 7 days could be used instead. Alternatively, either erythromycin base 500 mg PO 4 times a day for 7 days, erythromycin base 250 mg PO 4 times a day for 14 days, erythromycin ethylsuccinate 800 mg PO 4 times a day for 7 days, or erythromycin ethylsuccinate 400 mg PO 4 times a day for 14 days can be used.[2] Erythromycin estolate should be avoided in pregnancy because of the increased risk of hepatotoxicity. Azithromycin is safe and effective during pregnancy.[61,62] High rates of GI side effects limit the use of erythromycin. In pregnant women, a repeat NAAT is recommended 3 weeks after completion of therapy to ensure therapeutic cure.[2] Coinfection with *Chlamydia* is common in heterosexual men and women with gonorrhea. Therefore, drug regimens effective against both organisms are recommended in patients with gonorrhea to prevent postgonococcal chlamydial morbidity (epididymitis, mucopurulent cervicitis, salpingitis) and to reduce the genital reservoir of *C. trachomatis.*

Lymphogranuloma Venereum

ETIOLOGY AND SIGNS AND SYMPTOMS

CASE 72-6

QUESTION 1: S.F., a 32-year-old male student who reports having sex with men, presents to the STD clinic with a chief complaint of pain and swelling in the groin. He reports the appearance of a small ulcer on his penis about 2 weeks ago, which resolved rapidly. On examination, he has a bubo (inflammatory swelling of one or more lymph nodes in the groin) with surrounding erythema on his right side. S.F. also has a fever (39°C). Laboratory findings are remarkable for a mild leukocytosis (WBC count, 12,000 cells/μL). What organisms are responsible for lymphogranuloma venereum (LGV)? Describe its clinical course. What subjective and objective manifestations in S.F. are consistent with LGV?

LGV or Nicolas–Favre disease has historically been considered a rare disease in the United States and other developed nations; however, outbreaks have been recently reported in The Netherlands and Great Britain as well as in the United States in New York, Texas, and San Francisco.[63,64] Since 2003, the number of cases of LGV, especially proctocolitis, in MSM in developed countries has been increasing.[65,66] The cause of LGV is usually *C. trachomatis* serovars L1, L2, or L3, which are different from those serovars responsible for chlamydia urethritis.[67] Three stages of LGV infection are recognized in heterosexual men.[68]

Stage I is characterized by a small genital papule or vesicle that appears between 3 and 30 days after exposure. The patient usually is asymptomatic; the ulcer heals rapidly and leaves no scar. This primary lesion is consistent with that reported by S.F. Many patients with LGV recall no primary lesion. Stage II is characterized by acute, painful lymphadenitis with bubo formation (the inguinal syndrome); it is often accompanied by pain and fever, as illustrated by S.F. Without treatment, the buboes may rupture, forming numerous sinus tracts that drain chronically. Adenopathy above and below the inguinal ligament results in the "groove sign." Healing occurs slowly, and most patients suffer no serious sequelae. Patients in this stage may also present with an anogenitorectal syndrome, which is accompanied by proctocolitis and hyperplasia of intestinal and perirectal lymphatic tissue. Stage III is characterized by perirectal abscesses, rectovaginal fistulae (in women), rectal strictures, and genital elephantiasis.[68] Appropriate treatment of stage II LGV usually prevents these late complications.

An acute anorectal syndrome of LGV occurs in homosexual men who acquire the infection through rectal receptive intercourse. In these cases, a primary anal ulcer may be noted with associated inguinal adenopathy (anal lymphatics drain to inguinal nodes). Subsequently, acute hemorrhagic proctocolitis occurs with tenesmus, rectal pain, constipation, and a mucopurulent, bloody rectal discharge. Rectal biopsy may show granulomatous colitis, mimicking Crohn's disease. Perirectal pelvic adenopathy also occurs.

TREATMENT

Case 72-6, Question 2: How should S.F. be treated?

Current CDC recommendations for LGV include doxycycline 100 mg PO twice daily or erythromycin base 500 mg PO 4 times a day for 21 days.[2] Surgical intervention may be needed for later forms of the disease. Azithromycin 1 g weekly for 3 weeks may be effective, as well as fluoroquinolones, but clinical data on its use are lacking.[2]

SYPHILIS

Epidemiology

Syphilis is caused by the spirochete, *Treponema pallidum*. The rates of primary and secondary syphilis in the United States increased in the late 1980s secondary to crack cocaine use (and associated unsafe sex practices), but from 1990 to 2000 the rates have decreased to those reported in 1941 when reporting began, representing a 89.7% decrease since 1990.[4,69,70] However, the number of cases of primary and secondary syphilis have steadily risen since 2000, reaching a high of 17,375 cases in 2013.[4] Another concern is that syphilis facilitates the transmission of HIV, and a high proportion of syphilis is reported in HIV-positive MSM.[4,71] Since 2008, the rates of congenital syphilis have not increased until 2013, when 348 cases were reported to the CDC representing 8.7 cases per 100,000 individuals, a 0.3% increase from 2012 (Fig. 72-5).[3] This increase was attributable to the increase in the rate of primary and secondary syphilis cases in the West among females during 2010 to 2013. The *Healthy People 2020 (HP)* goals for primary and secondary syphilis among women is 1.4 cases per 100,000 individuals and among men it is 6.8 cases per 100,000 individuals (Fig. 72-6).[5]

The clinical manifestations of syphilis have not changed appreciably since their first description. However, early diagnosis, treatment, and greater physician/patient awareness of the disease have reduced the incidence of its severe forms. Penicillin continues to be the mainstay of therapy.

Clinical Stages

CASE 72-7

Question 1: D.M., a 27-year-old homosexual man, presents to the STD clinic with complaints of malaise, headache, and fever of 4 days' duration. He also reveals that he had a sore on his penis about 8 weeks ago, but it has since resolved. Upon examination, he is afebrile and has a widespread maculopapular skin rash that involves the soles of his feet; general lymphadenopathy also is appreciated. Medical history is unremarkable except for one episode of gonorrhea 2 years ago that was treated with procaine penicillin. Laboratory findings include a normal peripheral WBC count, a negative serology for HIV antigen, and a positive rapid plasma reagin (RPR) test and fluorescent treponemal antibody absorption (FTA-ABS) test. Describe the clinical course of syphilis. Are D.M.'s symptoms consistent with this infection?

PRIMARY STAGE

The average incubation period for syphilis is 3 weeks and ranges from 10 to 90 days.[72] During this incubation period, *T. pallidum* can be demonstrated in the lymph and blood. The primary chancre develops at the site of inoculation as a painless papule that becomes ulcerated and indurated. The ulcer is nontender and filled with spirochetes. The chancre usually involves the penis in the heterosexual male; the penis or anus in the homosexual male; and the vulva, perineum, or cervix in the female. Occasionally, the lip or tongue is involved. Regional lymph nodes are enlarged, firm, and nontender. Unfortunately, the typical chancre described earlier often is missed, particularly in women or homosexual men.[73] Without treatment, the primary chancre resolves spontaneously, usually in 2 to 6 weeks. The differential diagnosis of genital ulcers also includes chancroid and genital herpes. Like chancroid, genital herpes produces painful, superficial, nonindurated ulcers with tender inguinal adenopathy. However, unlike chancroid, lesions of genital herpes characteristically proceed through a vesicular state and often are associated with urethritis, cervicitis, and constitutional symptoms, such as fever and chills. Syphilis can be differentiated from herpes by a nonpainful versus painful lesion, a papular

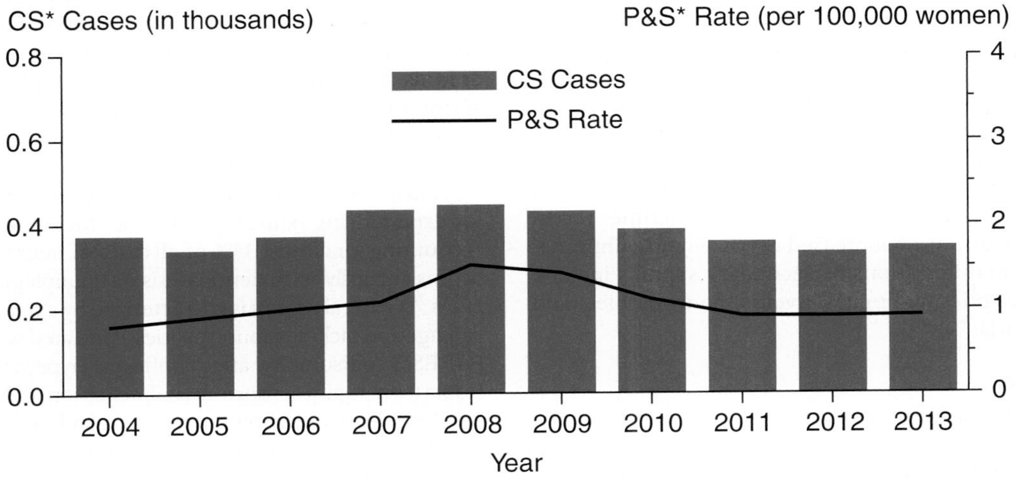

Figure 72-5 Congenital syphilis—Reported cases among infants by year of birth and rates of primary and secondary syphilis among women, 2004 to 2013. Reprinted from Centers for Disease Control and Prevention. *Sexually Transmitted Disease Surveillance 2013*. Atlanta, GA: US Dept of Health and Human Services; 2014.

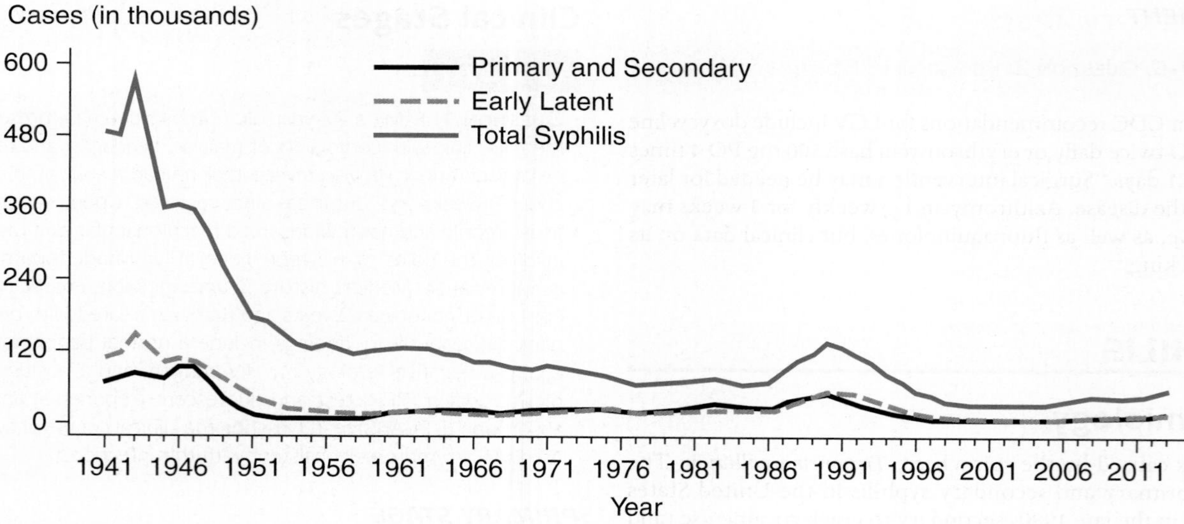

Figure 72-6 Syphilis—Reported Cases by Stage of Infection, United States, 1941 to 2013. Note: the Healthy People 2020 target for primary and secondary syphilis is 1.4 new cases per 100,000 for females and 6.8 new cases per 100,000 for males. Reprinted from Centers for Disease Control and Prevention. *Sexually Transmitted Disease Surveillance 2013*. Atlanta, GA: US Dept of Health and Human Services; 2014.

versus vesicular appearance, and single versus multiple lesions. Chancroid is more difficult to differentiate from syphilis, although chancroid tends to have a more-tender lesion, jagged border, and striking inguinal lymphadenopathy.[72]

SECONDARY STAGE

Approximately 6 weeks after a chancre first appears, the untreated patient manifests signs and symptoms of the secondary stage of syphilis. This stage is currently evidenced by D.M. Skin lesions of secondary syphilis may erupt in a variety of patterns and are usually widespread in distribution. A macular lesion is often the earliest manifestation in this stage. The lesion is round or oval, occurs primarily on the trunk, and is rose or pink in color. As lesions mature, they become papular or nodular with scaling (the so-called papulosquamous rash). The differential diagnosis of diffuse papulosquamous rashes includes psoriasis, pityriasis rosea, and lichen planus. In syphilis, the palms and soles are characteristically involved, and oral lesions (mucous patches) may occur. Generalized lymphadenopathy usually is present, and patchy alopecia may be seen. The most infectious lesion of secondary syphilis is condyloma latum. Condylomata lata are characteristically wet, indurated lesions occurring primarily in the perineum or around the anus as a result of direct spread from the primary lesion. Laboratory studies sometimes reveal anemia, leukocytosis, or an increased erythrocyte sedimentation rate. Other manifestations of secondary syphilis include mild hepatitis, aseptic meningitis, uveitis, neuropathies, and glomerulonephritis.[74]

LATENT STAGE

By definition, untreated, asymptomatic persons with serologic evidence for syphilis have latent syphilis. The latent stage is divided into two phases: the early latent (<1 year's duration) and late latent (>1 year's duration). In the Oslo study of patients with untreated syphilis, 25% experienced secondary relapses, usually within the first year.[75] Patients who relapse to the secondary stage are infectious; those in the late latent stage are not infectious and are immune to reinfection with *T. pallidum*.

TERTIARY STAGE

Serious morbidity and mortality are caused by pathologic progresses involving the skin, bones, central nervous system, and cardiovascular system. Infectious granulomas (gummas), the characteristic lesions of tertiary syphilis, are observed infrequently. Most gummas respond quickly to specific therapy, although if critical organs are involved (heart, brain, liver), they can be fatal.[76] The most common manifestations of syphilitic cardiovascular disease are aortic insufficiency and aortitis, with aneurysm of the ascending aorta.

Neurosyphilis may be classified as asymptomatic early or late, meningeal, parenchymatous, or gummatous. Although neurosyphilis has been a rare complication for more than 40 years because of the widespread of use of penicillin, syphilitic meningitis, an early form of neurosyphilis, may be more common in HIV-positive patients.[72,77] Late neurosyphilis may be asymptomatic or accompanied by a variety of manifestations; the most common syndromes are meningovascular syphilis, general paresis, tabes dorsalis (locomotor ataxia), and optic atrophy. In patients with asymptomatic neurosyphilis, examination of the cerebrospinal fluid (CSF) typically reveals mononuclear pleocytosis, an elevated protein concentration, and a positive VDRL reaction.

Patients with asymptomatic neurosyphilis are at increased risk for experiencing neurologic disease. Meningovascular syphilis, accounting for almost 38% of all cases of neurosyphilis, typically begins abruptly with hemiparesis or hemiplegia, aphasia, or seizures.[78] General paresis is characterized by extensive parenchymal damage and includes abnormalities associated with the mnemonic PARESIS (personality, affect, reflexes [hyperactive], eye [Argyll Robertson pupil], sensorium [hallucination, delusions, illusions], intellect [decreased recent memory, calculations, judgment], and speech). Tabes dorsalis occurs after demyelinization of the spinal cord. Symptoms observed include an ataxic, wide-based gait and foot slap; paresthesias; bladder irregularities; impotence; areflexia; and loss of position, deep pain, and temperature sensation. The Argyll Robertson pupil, seen in both paresis and tabes dorsalis, is a small, irregular pupil that reacts to accommodation but not to light.

Laboratory Tests

Case 72-7, Question 2: Evaluate D.M.'s laboratory findings.

DARK-FIELD EXAMINATION

Exudate expressed from the chancre or from condyloma latum is examined with a dark-field microscope. The diagnosis of syphilis is made if spirochetes with characteristic corkscrew morphology and mobility are present. Dark-field examination is the most specific and sensitive method but only with an experienced microscopist.[79,80] Three dark-field examinations on consecutive days should be performed before considering the test negative in suspected primary syphilis. This technique and other methods, such as DFA and PCR, which detect *T. pallidum* directly from exudate or tissue are definitive diagnostic methods for syphilis.

SEROLOGIC TESTS

Serologic tests become reactive during the primary stage, but they may be negative at the time of presentation with primary syphilis. When the history or examination suggests primary syphilis, a VDRL should be sent to the laboratory, or an RPR test should be performed in the clinic (see discussion on nontreponemal tests, next). If initial serology and dark-field examinations are negative, the serology should be repeated in 1 to 4 weeks to exclude primary syphilis. If the dark-field examination is positive, an RPR may still be ordered to establish a baseline for follow-up after treatment.

Serologic tests are uniformly positive in secondary syphilis.[72] Two types of tests are used for the serodiagnosis of syphilis: nontreponemal tests, which measure serum concentrations of reagin (antibody to cardiolipin), and treponemal tests, which detect the presence of antibodies specific for *T. pallidum*.

Nontreponemal Tests

Nontreponemal tests are not specific for *T. pallidum* but can be quantified. They are inexpensive and useful for screening large numbers of people. The most widely used nontreponemal tests are the VDRL test and the RPR Card Test. The RPR test is the most widely used because it is simpler to perform than the VDRL. Although they are equally valid assays, results of the VDRL and RPR are not interchangeable; thus, the same test should be used throughout the posttreatment monitoring period.[2,81]

The result reported in the quantitative VDRL test is the most dilute serum concentration with a positive reaction. This test may be used to follow the decline in VDRL titer after effective therapy (see Case 72-7, Question 5). In some individuals, a serofast reaction occurs in which nontreponemal antibodies may remain at a low titer for up to their entire lives. When false-positive tests occur, the titer usually is low (e.g., VDRL or RPR titer of 1:8).[82] In secondary syphilis, sensitivity of the RPR and VDRL approach 100% owing to the high antibody concentrations.[83]

Treponemal Tests

Specific treponemal tests, such as FTA-ABS, *T. pallidum* particle agglutination assay (TP-PA), and various EIAs, confirm a positive nontreponemal test. The FTA-ABS test is the most commonly used treponemal test. Because treponemal tests are relatively difficult and expensive to perform, they are not traditionally used for screening.

Treatment

Case 72-7, Question 3: How should D.M. be treated?

The CDC recommends penicillin G for the treatment of all stages of syphilis (Table 72-4).[2] Every effort should be made to rule out penicillin allergy before choosing alternative agents. Considering that penicillin-resistant *T. pallidum* has never been observed, treatment regimens for syphilis have changed relatively little during the years.

As shown in Table 72-4, recommended therapy for primary, secondary, or latent syphilis (with negative findings in the CSF) of less than 1 year's duration is a single, IM 2.4 million-unit dose of benzathine penicillin G. If penicillin is contraindicated, tetracycline 500 mg PO 4 times a day or doxycycline 100 mg PO twice a day for 14 days are the main alternatives. If the patient is allergic to penicillin, is not pregnant, and cannot receive tetracycline or doxycycline, a 10- to 14-day regimen of ceftriaxone 1 g IM or IV every day or a single 2 g dose of azithromycin are options.[2] The use of erythromycin as an alternative is no longer recommended by the CDC because of its poor efficacy. The optimal dose, duration, and efficacy of these alternative regimens are not well-defined, necessitating close follow-up of patients. However, recent studies have shown that azithromycin 2 g PO as a 1-time dose is at least equivalent to benzathine penicillin G.[84,85] Skin testing should be performed for individuals who claim allergy to penicillin. If the patient is truly allergic, he or she should be desensitized.[2] Late latent syphilis (>1 year's duration) and tertiary syphilis (gummas or cardiovascular syphilis) are treated with IM benzathine penicillin G (50,000 units/kg, up to 2.4 million-units) weekly for a total of 3 weeks.[2]

NEUROSYPHILIS

Case 72-7, Question 4: Would D.M.'s treatment differ if his CSF had tested positive for syphilis?

Neurosyphilis can present at any stage of syphilis. When conventional IM doses of benzathine penicillin G are administered, measurable levels of penicillin are not obtainable in the CSF. However, this does not mean that penicillin does not concentrate in meningeal tissue.[86] Treatment failures, as well as late clinical progression to neurosyphilis, can occur after treatment with the recommended IM regimen. After one dose, benzathine penicillin reaches peak plasma concentrations slower (13–24 hours) but with more prolonged treponemicidal plasma concentrations (7–10 days) when compared with procaine penicillin (1–4 hours to peak; 12–24 hour treponemicidal plasma concentrations).[86] Reports of benzathine penicillin failures in the 1970s has resulted in the CDC recommending treatment with aqueous crystalline penicillin G, 3 to 4 million-units IV every 4 hours, or 18 to 24 million-units per day continuous infusion for 10 to 14 days. Alternatively, neurosyphilis can be treated with concurrent procaine penicillin (2.4 million-units IM daily) and probenecid (500 mg PO 4 times a day) for 10 to 14 days. Some experts add benzathine penicillin G (2.4 million-units IM once a week for up to 3 weeks) after the completion of aqueous penicillin G or procaine penicillin.[2] Penicillin-allergic patients should be skin tested to confirm allergy and, if confirmed, the patient should be desensitized and treated with an appropriate penicillin regimen. Some data suggest that ceftriaxone 2 g IM or IV daily for 10 to 14 days can be used as an alternative in patients whose concern for cross-sensitivity between ceftriaxone and penicillin is negligible.[2] Alternatively, the World Health Organization recommends penicillin-allergic nonpregnant patients receive either doxycycline 200 mg PO twice a day or tetracycline 500 mg PO 4 times a day for 30 days.[87]

FOLLOW-UP

Case 72-7, Question 5: D.M. was treated with a single IM dose of benzathine penicillin (2.4 million-units). How should his response to therapy be monitored?

Table 72-4
Treatment Guidelines for Syphilis

Stage	Recommended Regimen	Alternative Regimen
Early (primary, secondary, or early latent)[a]	Benzathine penicillin G 2.4 million-units single dose IM	Doxycycline 100 mg PO BID for 14 days *or* Tetracycline 500 mg PO QID for 14 days *or* Ceftriaxone 1 g IM/IV every day for 8 to 10 days *or* Azithromycin 2 g PO × 1 dose
Late latent or latent syphilis of unknown duration	Lumbar puncture	Lumbar puncture
	If CSF normal: benzathine penicillin G 2.4 million-units/week × 3 weeks IM	If CSF normal: doxycycline 100 mg PO BID for 28 days *or* Tetracycline 500 mg PO QID for 28 days
	If CSF abnormal: Treat as neurosyphilis	If CSF abnormal: treat as neurosyphilis
Neurosyphilis[b] (asymptomatic or symptomatic)	Aqueous crystalline penicillin G 18–24 million-units IV every day × 10–14 days[c]	Procaine penicillin 2.4 million-units IM daily *plus* probenecid 500 mg PO QID, both for 10–14 days
Congenital	Aqueous crystalline penicillin G 100,000–150,000 units/kg/day, administered as 50,000 units/kg/dose IV q12h during the first 7 days of life, and every 8 hours thereafter for a total of 10 days[d]	If CSF normal: benzathine penicillin G 50,000 units/kg/dose IM in a single dose
	Procaine penicillin G 50,000 units/kg/dose IM a day in a single dose for 10 days	
Syphilis in pregnancy	According to stage	According to stage

[a]Some experts recommend repeating this regimen after 7 days for HIV-infected patients.
[b]Because of the shorter duration of therapy as compared with latent syphilis, some experts recommend giving benzathine penicillin G, 2.4 million-units/week for up to 3 weeks, after the completion of these neurosyphilis regimens to provide a comparable total duration of therapy.
[c]Administered as 3–4 million-units IV every 4 hours or continuous infusion.
[d]All infants born to women treated during pregnancy with erythromycin must be treated with penicillin at birth.

Adapted from Workowski KA, Bolan GA; Centers for Disease Control and Prevention (CDC). Sexually transmitted diseases treatment guidelines, 2015. *MMWR Recomm Rep*. 2015;64(RR-03):1–137.

Physical examination and a quantitative VDRL or RPR test for primary and secondary syphilis should be repeated at least 6 and 12 months after therapy.[2] Retreatment should be considered when the RPR or VDRL titer does not decline fourfold in 6 months. Patients with HIV coinfection should receive periodic serologic testing.[72] Patients with latent syphilis should be retested 6, 12, and 24 months after treatment. Close serologic monitoring is necessary if antibiotics other than penicillin are used; CSF examination should be performed in these patients at their last follow-up visit. Patients with neurosyphilis should be monitored serologically every 6 months; CSF examinations should be repeated at 6-month intervals until normal. If still abnormal at 2 years, retreatment should be considered. Return of lesions, a fourfold increase in titer, or a titer of 1:8 that does not fall at least fourfold within 12 months necessitates retreatment. Suspected treatment failures, especially with abnormal CSF, should be treated as described for neurosyphilis. However, false-positive serologic results should be ruled out.

Within 2 years, most patients with early syphilis become seronegative. However, if the disease is treated during the late stages, complete seroreversion may not occur. Patients treated with oral doxycycline or erythromycin are less likely to become seronegative.[88] Therapy is considered adequate in patients who never become seronegative as long as the titer decreases fourfold. Although the disease process may be halted in patients with tertiary syphilis, existing damage to the cardiovascular or nervous systems cannot be reversed.

PREGNANCY

CASE 72-8

Question 1: N.W., a 27-year-old woman in her 19th week of gestation, has a positive VDRL and FTA-ABS. How should N.W. be managed? How would management be altered in the face of penicillin allergy?

Although pregnancy may be associated with false-positive nontreponemal tests,[74] the presence of both a positive treponemal test (e.g., FTA-ABS) and a nontreponemal test (e.g., RPR) virtually excludes a false-positive reaction.[80] The next step is to determine whether N.W. already has been treated adequately. If she has previously received adequate treatment and follow-up and shows no evidence of persistence or recurrence of syphilis, then she requires no further therapy. Pregnancy has no known effect on the clinical course of syphilis.[89] However, her infant should be observed carefully. If N.W. has not been treated previously for syphilis, then she should be treated with penicillin in the same doses recommended for nonpregnant women; some experts recommend a second dose 1 week later of 2.4 million-units of benzathine penicillin.[2]

The goal of therapy should be to treat the mother with syphilis as soon as possible. Syphilis transmission can occur transplacentally as early as 9 to 10 weeks' gestation via direct contact with lesions in the birth canal.[89,90] If the mother is left untreated, 70% to 100% of fetuses born to mothers with primary or 40% with secondary syphilis may be aborted, stillborn, or born with congenital syphilis (see Case 72-8, Question 3).[91,92]

There is no completely satisfactory alternative for the pregnant woman with an accelerated allergic reaction to penicillin. Tetracycline, as well as doxycycline, should be avoided during pregnancy, especially during the second or third trimester, because of tetracycline's known effects on the fetus (tooth staining and inhibition of bone growth).[93] Erythromycin has been used to treat pregnant patients with syphilis; however, the transplacental transfer rate of erythromycin is inadequate,[94] potentially explaining the increased rate of aborted or stillborn infants in erythromycin-treated patients. Erythromycin and azithromycin are not recommended as alternative therapy for syphilis during pregnancy.[2] A woman with a history of allergy to penicillin should be skin tested; if allergy is confirmed, she should be desensitized and treated with penicillin.[2] It is possible that the newer cephalosporins may ultimately prove to be acceptable alternatives to penicillin G in the pregnant woman with syphilis, who is allergic to penicillin, but there is sufficient evidence for the CDC to recommend their use. Adequate treatment with penicillin can prevent up to 98% of fetal infections.[95,96] Serologic titers, at a minimum should be followed up at 28 to 32 weeks' gestation and at delivery. Monthly serologic titers may be considered in women at high risk for reinfection or those in geographical areas of high syphilis rates; thereafter, she should be followed up as any other patient with syphilis.[2]

JARISCH–HERXHEIMER REACTION

CASE 72-8, QUESTION 2: N.W. was treated with an IM injection of 2.4 million-units of benzathine penicillin G. Six hours later, she complained of diffuse myalgias, chills, headache, and an exacerbation of her rash. She was tachypneic, but normotensive. What is this reaction? How should N.W. be managed?

N.W. has developed the Jarisch–Herxheimer reaction (JHR), a usually benign, self-limited complication of antitreponemal antibiotic therapy that develops within hours after treatment of early syphilis.[2] The cause of JHR is not well understood, but it is probably related to the release of cytokines.[97] Clinical manifestations include fever, chills, myalgias, headache, tachycardia, and hypotension. The pathogenesis of the syndrome is uncertain, but the reaction should not be interpreted as an allergic reaction to penicillin. It typically begins within the first 24 hours after antibiotic administration and normally subsides spontaneously, generally subsiding even while antibiotics are continued.[2,98] Notably, JHR can occur after administration of many antimicrobials and is not exclusive to penicillins, nor is it exclusive to syphilis treatment, occurring in other spirochetal diseases, such as Lyme disease and relapsing fever.[99] Usually self-limiting in nonpregnant patients, the primary risk of this reaction in pregnant women is miscarriage, premature labor, or fetal distress.[2,100] Pregnant women should seek medical attention if contractions or a change in fetal movements are noted. Close monitoring of JHR should be observed for patients with ophthalmic or neurologic syphilis. For these patients, prednisolone 10 to 20 mg 3 times a day for 3 days given 24 hours before syphilis treatment may prevent fever, but it will not control local inflammation.[86] Tumor necrosis factor-α has been demonstrated to have some success in the prevention of JHR in spirochete disease.[101] Although there is no proven effective preventive therapy, some experts still recommend antipyretics, hydration, and patient education; antibiotic therapy should not be discontinued.

NEONATAL SYPHILIS

CASE 72-8, QUESTION 3: How should N.W.'s baby be treated if a diagnosis of congenital syphilis is confirmed?

Infants born to mothers who have been treated for syphilis during pregnancy should be carefully examined at birth with a quantitative nontreponemal serologic test. If tests are reactive, the infant should be followed and have serologic testing every 2 to 3 months until nontreponemal tests are nonreactive.[2] Newborn serology is difficult to interpret because of transplacental transfer of nontreponemal and treponemal immunoglobulin G to the infant. Treatment decisions are largely based on evidence of syphilis in the mother, adequacy of maternal treatment, comparison of maternal and neonatal nontreponemal serology, and/or presence of clinical or laboratory evidence of syphilis in the neonate. In addition, infants should be treated at birth, even if they are asymptomatic, when maternal treatment is unknown or inadequate, or when infant follow-up cannot be guaranteed. In most cases, a CSF examination should be performed before treatment is begun to rule out neurosyphilis.

CHANCROID

Chancroid or soft chancre is a painful genital ulcer disease that is often associated with tender inguinal adenopathy. It is caused by *Haemophilus ducreyi*, a gram-negative bacillus. Chancroid is endemic in developing countries, but its incidence in the United States has steadily declined. In 2013, 10 cases of chancroid were reported in the United States, down from 28 cases in 2009.[4] Chancroid and other genital ulcers have also been implicated in the acquisition and transmission of HIV.

Signs and Symptoms

CASE 72-9

QUESTION 1: T.G., a 31-year-old uncircumcised sexually active male, presents to the STD clinic with complaints of tender lesions on the penis and inguinal regions. He noticed the penile lesions on the external surface of the prepuce (foreskin) 2 days before his visit. The lesions were sharply demarcated but were not indurated; the base of the penile ulcer was covered by a yellow–gray purulent exudate. Right inguinal adenitis was present and extremely painful on palpation. A dark-field examination of the purulent exudate was negative. Gram stain revealed a mixture of gram-positive and gram-negative flora. T.G. claims to have an allergy to penicillin, but no other drug allergies are reported. What is the natural course of chancroid? Does T.G. have signs or symptoms consistent with chancroid? What diagnostic procedures are necessary?

Uncircumcised men, as well as circumcised men, may have an increased risk of chancroid infection and may not respond to therapy. In fact, evidence suggests circumcision is protective against nearly all STDs, including HIV, as well as protecting women against *T. vaginalis* and BV.[2] A painful genital ulcer appears 3 to 10 days after exposure and begins as a tender, red papule that becomes pustular and ulcerates within 2 days. Chancroid can be suspected if all of the following criteria are met: (1) one or more painful genital ulcers present, (2) regional lymphadenopathy, (3) no evidence of *T. pallidum* by dark-field examination, and (4) a negative HSV PCR test or HSV culture. As illustrated by T.G., the ulcer may be covered by a grayish or yellow exudate. A Gram stain can be misleading because of the polymicrobic nature of the ulcer and culture and because isolation of *H. ducreyi* is difficult, requiring specialized specimen collection and growth media.[2]

CASE 72-9, QUESTION 2: How should T.G.'s chancroid be treated?

Most strains of *H. ducreyi* produce a TEM-type β-lactamase, and many strains are resistant to the antimicrobials that traditionally were used to treat chancroid, such as sulfonamides and tetracycline.[102,103] Currently recommended CDC treatment regimens include azithromycin 1 g PO for 1 dose, ceftriaxone 250 mg IM once, ciprofloxacin 500 mg PO twice a day for 3 days, or erythromycin base 500 mg PO 3 times a day for 7 days. Ciprofloxacin is contraindicated in pregnant and lactating women. Because T.G. has a history of penicillin hypersensitivity, azithromycin as a single oral dose is a preferred treatment regimen. Treatment may not be as effective for patients who are coinfected with HIV or who are uncircumcised; therefore, HIV testing should occur at the time of chancroid diagnosis and if negative, should be repeated 3 months after the diagnosis. Follow-up should occur 3 to 7 days after treatment is initiated. Depending on the size of the ulcer, the time required until complete recovery will vary; larger ulcers may require longer than 2 weeks. Because T.G. is also sexually active, his sexual partner should be evaluated and treated if they had contact during the 10 days prior to the onset of symptoms.[2]

VAGINITIS

Approximately 10 million physician office visits are made annually in the United States for women seeking evaluation and treatment of vaginitis.[104] The term *vaginitis* refers to such nonspecific vaginal symptoms as itching, burning, irritation, and abnormal discharge that may be caused by infection or other medical conditions. The most common vaginal infections are BV (22%–50% of cases), vulvovaginal candidiasis (VVC; 17%–39% of cases), and trichomoniasis (4%–35% of cases). However, approximately 30% of cases of vaginitis remain undiagnosed.[105]

Bacterial Vaginosis

Bacterial vaginosis (BV) is the most common genital tract infection amongst reproductive aged women.[106] While the exact prevalence of BV varies, one estimate places it at 29.2%. In addition, many sexually active women are infected with *G. vaginalis*, yet as much as 84% are asymptomatic.[107] During an episode of BV, the normal vaginal lactobacillus flora is replaced by *Mobiluncus* species, *Prevotella* species, *Ureaplasma* species, *Mycoplasma* species, and increased numbers of *G. vaginalis* and is associated with an increased, malodorous vaginal discharge.[2]

The evidence for definitive risk factors in BV is inconclusive. Multiple sexual partners, a new sexual partner, douching, lack of condom use, and decreased concentrations of vaginal lactobacilli have been associated with BV. Non-sexually active women are rarely affected.[2] In addition, studies among women who generally have sex with other women show evidence for sexual transmission.[108] The routine treatment of male sexual partners is not recommended because a woman's response to therapy or her likelihood of relapse or recurrence is not impacted by treatment of her sexual partner(s).[2]

SIGNS, SYMPTOMS, AND DIAGNOSIS

CASE 72-10

QUESTION 1: H.H. is a 24-year-old, sexually active woman with a 1-week history of moderate vaginal discharge that has a "fishy" odor, most notable after coitus. She has no complaints of vaginal pruritus or burning. On examination, the discharge appears thin, white, homogeneous, and notably malodorous. A wet mount of the vaginal secretion revealed few leukocytes and numerous "clue cells." The vaginal pH was 4.8, and a characteristic fishy odor was noted when the discharge was mixed with 10% potassium hydroxide (KOH). Does H.H. have signs and symptoms consistent with BV? What diagnostic tests are required?

H.H.'s signs and symptoms are typical of BV. The clinical diagnosis can be confirmed by a vaginal Gram stain that shows overgrowth of the vagina with *G. vaginalis* and other organisms as noted earlier. A 10% KOH solution mixed with the vaginal secretions yields a transient fishy odor because of the increased production of biogenic diamines (positive amine test). A wet preparation of the specimen reveals "clue cells" (exfoliated vaginal epithelial cells sometimes with adherent coccobacillary pathogens), vaginal pH greater than 4.5, and the characteristic KOH "whiff" test.[2,109] If there are many white cells, other infections (e.g., *T. vaginalis*) should be suspected. Self-diagnosis is correct only about 3% to 4% of the time because most women attribute symptoms to poor hygiene.[110]

TREATMENT

CASE 72-10, QUESTION 2: How should H.H. be treated?

Nonpregnant women with symptomatic disease require treatment. CDC-recommended regimens include oral metronidazole 500 mg twice a day for 7 days, metronidazole gel 0.75% intravaginally daily for 5 days, or clindamycin cream 2% intravaginally at bedtime for 7 days.[2] The FDA has approved metronidazole extended release 750 mg once daily for 7 days and a single dose of clindamycin intravaginal cream for the treatment of BV; however, limited data have been published comparing these regimens to established therapies. Alternatively, the CDC recommends either tinidazole 2 g PO every day for 2 days, tinidazole 1 g PO every day for 5 days, clindamycin 300 mg PO 2 times a day for 7 days, or clindamycin ovules 100 mg intravaginally once at bedtime for 3 days.[2] Patients should be instructed to avoid consuming alcohol during treatment with metronidazole and for 72 hours afterward to avoid disulfiram-like reactions. Additionally, clindamycin cream is oil based and may weaken latex condoms or diaphragms. Alternative products include probiotics which have been evaluated in non-pregnant women and have shown to improve cure rates and reduce the reoccurrence of BV, although more studies are needed to establish their role in treatment.[111,112]

BV has been associated with preterm labor and premature delivery and treatment is recommended for all symptomatic women. The CDC recommends metronidazole 250 mg PO 3 times daily for 7 days or 500 mg PO twice a day for 7 days, or clindamycin 300 mg PO twice daily for 7 days. Teratogenic data suggest that metronidazole is not harmful to the fetus. More recent data suggest that the use of intravaginal clindamycin cream is also safe to use for pregnant women.[2]

Vulvovaginal Candidiasis

Candida albicans is the causative organism of VVC in 80% to 92% of cases, with *Candida glabrata* and *Candida tropicalis* accounting for most of the remaining cases.[2,12,113,114] The latter organisms have been identified increasingly as the causative agents of VVC during the past two decades. Approximately 75% of women will experience at least one episode of VVC during their reproductive years and 40% to 45% will have two or more episodes within their lifetime.[105] Less than 5% of women who have VVC have recurrent candidal episodes (defined as four or more episodes of VVC in 1 year). Vulvovaginal candidiasis is not usually described as an STD because celibate women may also experience it; however, the incidence of VVC increases when women become sexually active.[114] Because of this, VVC is often diagnosed during evaluation for a suspected STD when women present with vaginal symptoms.

ASSESSING SELF-TREATMENT

CASE 72-11

QUESTION 1: L.L., a 23-year-old woman, purchases a nonprescription antifungal agent to relieve vaginal symptoms that she believes are caused by a vaginal yeast infection. L.L. asks the pharmacist for assistance in the selection of an antifungal agent. What information should be obtained from L.L. before a medication is recommended?

The pharmacist should ask L.L. if this is her first episode of vaginitis or whether she has experienced similar symptoms previously that have been diagnosed as a vaginal yeast infection and treated by a physician. The nonprescription antifungal agents are indicated for the treatment of VVC in women who previously were diagnosed and treated by their physician. Additional questions that should be asked by the pharmacist include current symptoms, whether they are pregnant or not, other current medical conditions or medications, and allergies. Patients should be referred to a physician if any of the following are present: first episode of VVC, has had more than three episodes of VVC within the past 12 months, last episode was less than 2 months ago, is pregnant, is younger than 12, fever, lower abdominal, back, or shoulder pain, severe symptoms, or has a malodorous vaginal discharge.[115]

SIGNS AND SYMPTOMS

CASE 72-11, QUESTION 2: L.L. has experienced two episodes of vaginal yeast infections, with the most recent case occurring approximately 1 year ago. On both occasions she was diagnosed as having VVC by her physician and responded to antifungal therapy. L.L. currently describes vaginal and vulvar itching, vaginal soreness, and vulvar burning accompanied by a thick, white vaginal discharge that has the consistency of cottage cheese. She has been unable to have sexual intercourse because of pain. These symptoms are similar to those she experienced with her previous vaginal yeast infections. L.L. has no underlying major health problems. Her current medications include oral tetracycline for acne and Ortho Tri-Cyclen for birth control. She has regular menstrual cycles and her last menstrual period ended 4 days ago. What clinical manifestations does L.L. exhibit that are consistent with VVC? What are the other common manifestations?

L.L. exhibits signs and symptoms associated with VVC (i.e., vulvar and vaginal pruritus, vaginal soreness, vulvar burning, dyspareunia, and a thick, white vaginal discharge that appears to be curd-like). Women may also have vaginal discharge which is usually described as nonodorous, highly viscous, and white in color that may vary in consistency from curd-like to watery. Vulvar erythema may also be present.[104]

DIFFERENTIAL DIAGNOSIS

CASE 72-11, QUESTION 3: How can VVC be differentiated from other vaginal infections?

VVC should be differentiated from other vaginal infections because a nonprescription antifungal agent could delay the appropriate treatment of other vaginal infections. The physical appearance of the vaginal discharge may be useful in predicting VVC if it is a viscous, nonodorous, white, curd-like discharge and the patient has a normal vaginal pH (pH <4.5). The quantity of the discharge may be scanty to profuse. Some women with VVC exhibit only vaginal erythema with minimal discharge or an increased amount of normal vaginal secretion. Table 72-5 characterizes the vaginal discharges associated with VVC, BV, and trichomoniasis. The vaginal discharge from a woman with signs and symptoms of VVC should be examined for the microscopic presence of *Candida* using a wet-mount preparation with 10% KOH or a Gram stain of the vaginal discharge. The use of KOH improves the visualization of yeast or pseudohyphae that are seen in approximately 70% of women diagnosed with VVC. If the wet mount is negative, the patient's vaginal discharge should be cultured for *Candida* in an appropriate growth medium. Isolation of *Candida* without signs and symptoms should not result in treatment, because *Candida* is part of normal vaginal flora in approximately 10% to 20% of women. It is the proliferation of *C. albicans* or other yeasts that lead to vulvovaginitis symptoms. Nonprescription home screening tests are also available that measure pH levels within the vaginal epithelium (e.g., Vagisil Screening Kit and Fem-V), which are highly sensitive to pH changes but suffer from low specificity.

Physiologic Vaginal Discharge and Symptomatic Normal pH Vulvovaginitis

CASE 72-11, QUESTION 4: Do women such as L.L., who have an increased vaginal discharge and symptoms consistent with VVC, necessarily have a vaginal infection?

Although the possibility of vaginal infection must be addressed when a woman presents with an increased vaginal discharge with

Table 72-5
Characteristics of Vaginal Discharge

Characteristics	Normal	Candidiasis	Trichomoniasis	Bacterial Vaginosis
Color	White or clear	White	Yellow–green	White to gray
Odor	Nonodorous	Nonodorous	Malodorous	Fishy smell
Consistency	Floccular	Floccular	Homogeneous	Homogeneous
Viscosity	High	High	Low	Low
pH	<4.5	4–4.5	5–6.0	>4.5
Other characteristics		Thick, curd-like	Frothy	Thin

Source: Ries AJ. Treatment of vaginal infections: candidiasis, bacterial vaginosis, and trichomoniasis. *J Am Pharm Assoc (Wash)*. 1997;NS37(5):563–569; Sobel JD. Vaginitis. *N Engl J Med*. 1997;337(26):1896–1903; and Carr PL et al. Evaluation and management of vaginitis. *J Gen Intern Med*. 1998;13(5):335–346.

 or without symptoms, other conditions are associated with an increased discharge. First, a physiologic vaginal discharge must be distinguished from a pathologic discharge. Physiologic discharges (Table 72-5) characteristically are nonodorous, white or clear, highly viscous or floccular, and acidic (pH ~4.5). Physiologic discharge may also become more profuse at midcycle secondary to increased cervical mucus or vaginal epithelial cells. Other conditions resulting in excessive vaginal discharge include retention of foreign bodies (e.g., tampons) and allergic reactions or contact dermatitis secondary to the use of vaginal spermicidal agents, soaps, deodorants, douches, vaginal lubricants, and condoms. Episodes of vulvovaginitis-like symptoms can be associated with frequent use of hot tubs, Jacuzzi baths, or swimming pools that contain chemically treated water with high levels of chlorine.[116]

RISK FACTORS FOR VULVOVAGINAL CANDIDIASIS

Case 72-11, Question 5: What specific groups of women are most susceptible to VVC? Does L.L. fit into any group at high risk for VVC?

C. albicans colonization and symptomatic VVC increases during pregnancy and with use of high-estrogen containing oral contraceptives. Estrogens increase binding affinity of vaginal epithelial cells to *C. albicans*.[117] Women with high glycogen concentrations (e.g., uncontrolled or poorly controlled diabetes mellitus); women with depressed cell-mediated immunity secondary to disease (e.g., cancer, HIV infection); and women receiving broad-spectrum antibiotics or immunosuppressive drugs (e.g., cytotoxic agents, corticosteroids) are also at risk for VVC.[115] Individual cases of VVC, although not related to intercourse, may be related to orogenital sex.

L.L. is taking tetracycline, which may increase her risk for VVC. Antibacterials increase the risk for *C. albicans* overgrowth by suppressing the normal vaginal flora (e.g., lactobacilli), which normally protect against *C. albicans*. L.L. is also taking a low-estrogen–containing oral contraceptive; however, low-dose oral contraceptives have not been consistently associated with an increased risk of VVC. The use of diaphragms, vaginal sponges, and IUDs may also be risk factors for VVC.[115]

Stress-induced VVC and an increased incidence of VVC before menstruation have been described.[117] The cause of both is currently unknown. Although various dietary factors have been postulated as a cause of vaginal yeast overgrowth, the role of diet in the development of VVC remains inconclusive.[117]

TREATMENT OF VULVOVAGINAL CANDIDIASIS

Vaginally Administered Azoles

Case 72-11, Question 6: What vaginally administered therapy is effective for L.L.'s VVC?

L.L. is an appropriate candidate for nonprescription therapy (Table 72-6) because she had previous vaginal yeast infections with symptoms similar to those she currently is experiencing and her VVC is uncomplicated (defined as sporadic disease with mild-to-moderate symptoms in an immunocompetent host). When a patient's VVC appears complicated (defined as a recurrent infection, severe symptoms, non–*C. albicans* infection, presence of uncontrolled diabetes, immunosuppression, and/or pregnancy), she should be referred to her medical practitioner.[2] L.L. should respond well to short-term topical azole therapy. In addition, L.L. should ask her physician whether continuation of antibiotics is truly needed. If L.L. had been evaluated by her physician, a prescription for single-dose oral fluconazole or 3-day intravaginal therapy might have been an option.

The available azole antifungals are equally effective in treating VVC with cure rates between 80% to 90% when a full course of therapy is completed.[2,12,118] All the azole antifungal products listed in Table 72-6 are superior to nystatin, which is no longer recommended by the CDC.[2] The medication used to treat L.L.'s VVC should be selected based on response or failure to previous therapy, convenience, ease of use, length of therapy, dosage form, and cost. L.L. should select a non–oil-based product if a latex condom or a diaphragm is used as a form of contraception (Table 72-6).

Other Treatments for ACUTE Vulvovaginal Candidiasis

Oral lactobacillus and lactobacillus-containing yogurt are advocated for the treatment of VVC; however, evidence in support of this treatment is inconclusive.[119] Boric acid 600 mg capsules inserted in the vagina at bedtime for 14 days is effective for the treatment of recurrent VVC with eradication rates of 70%, but vaginal burning and irritation are common side effects and is poisonous if inadvertently ingested.[2,12,119] Gentian violet preparations also have limited use in the treatment of candidiasis because they stain clothing and bed linens and cause local irritation and edema.

Oral Azoles

Case 72-11, Question 7: How effective are orally administered azoles in the treatment of an acute VVC infection such as the one L.L. is experiencing?

Fluconazole is the only oral antifungal agent currently recommended by the CDC for the treatment of acute VVC. A single 150 mg oral dose of fluconazole is as effective as 3- to 6-day regimen of intravaginal clotrimazole.[120,121] Although some women may prefer an orally administered drug to one that is administered intravaginally, their use for mild-to-moderate VVC is of some concern because of the possibility for systemic adverse effects and drug–drug interactions.

Adverse Effects Associated with Azoles

Case 72-11, Question 8: What adverse effects might L.L. experience from intravaginally or orally administered azoles?

When used intravaginally, azoles are associated with dose-dependent adverse reactions similar to symptoms women report from VVC. Thus, it can be difficult to differentiate disease symptoms from adverse drug reactions. If the vaginal symptoms worsen after therapy is started, the patient should contact her health care provider. In addition, if symptoms have not improved within 3 days after initiation of therapy or continue past 7 days, the patient should contact her physician to rule out more severe disease or treatment of the wrong disease.[117] Topical azole therapy has been associated with a variety of adverse drug reactions, including headaches, allergic contact dermatitis, vulvovaginal pruritus and irritation, dyspareunia, and general burning, soreness, and genital pain. Oral fluconazole has been associated with headaches, nausea, abdominal pain, diarrhea, dyspepsia, dizziness, taste perversion, angioedema, and rare cases of anaphylactic reactions. In addition, intravaginal miconazole has been reported to interact with warfarin, increasing the risk of bleeding and bruising.[122]

PATIENT COUNSELING

Case 72-11, Question 9: How should L.L. be counseled about the use of a nonprescription vaginal antifungal product?

Table 72-6

Recommended Regimens for the Treatment of Candida Vulvovaginitis

Drug	Availability	Trade Names	Dosing Regimens
Nonprescription Products			
Butoconazole	2% vaginal cream[a]	Femstat 3	Nonpregnant women: administer 1 applicatorful intravaginally QHS for 3 consecutive days Pregnant women during second and third trimesters: administer 1 applicatorful intravaginally QHS for 7 consecutive days
Clotrimazole	1% vaginal cream[a]	Gyne-Lotrimin 7; Mycelex-7; Clotrimazole 7; various generics	Administer 1 applicatorful intravaginally QHS for 7 to 14 consecutive days
	2% vaginal cream[a]	Gyne-Lotrimin 3; various generics	Administer 1 applicatorful intravaginally QHS for 3 consecutive days
Miconazole	2% cream[a]	Monistat 7; Femizol-M; various generics	Administer 1 applicatorful intravaginally QHS for 7 consecutive days
	4% cream[a]	Monistat 3; various generics	Administer 1 applicatorful intravaginally QHS for 3 consecutive days
	100-mg vaginal suppositories[a]	Monistat 7	Insert 1 suppository intravaginally QHS for 7 consecutive days
	200-mg vaginal suppositories[a]	Monistat 3	Insert 1 suppository intravaginally QHS for 3 consecutive days
	1,200-mg vaginal suppositories[a]	Monistat 1 daytime Ovule	Insert 1 suppository intravaginally QHS for 1 dose only
Tioconazole	6.5% vaginal ointment	Vagistat-1	Administer 1 applicatorful intravaginally at QHS for 1 dose only
Prescription Products			
Butoconazole	2% vaginal cream[a]	Gynazole 1	Nonpregnant women: administer 1 applicatorful QHS for 1 dose only
Fluconazole	150-mg oral tablet	Diflucan	Take 1 tablet PO for 1 dose only
Terconazole	0.4% vaginal cream[a]	Terazol 7	Administer 1 applicatorful intravaginally QHS for 7 consecutive days
	0.8% vaginal cream[a]	Terazol 3	Administer 1 applicatorful intravaginally QHS for 3 consecutive days
	80-mg vaginal suppositories[a]	Terazol 3	Insert 1 suppository intravaginally QHS for 3 consecutive days

[a]The CDC states that the use of vaginally administered oil-based preparations may weaken latex products such as condoms and diaphragms.

QHS, at bed time.

Adapted from Workowski KA, Berman S; Centers for Disease Control and Prevention (CDC). Sexually transmitted diseases treatment guidelines, 2013. *MMWR Recomm Rep*. 2015;64(RR-03):1–137.

The details of intravaginal administration should be reviewed with L.L., including instructions on how to clean the applicator. To minimize leakage and annoyance, L.L. should apply the product at bedtime to increase retention in the vagina. She should be advised that the nonprescription vaginal antifungal creams and suppositories are oil based and thus may weaken condoms or diaphragms, thereby reducing their effectiveness.

L.L. should be informed about the importance of completing a full course of therapy even if her symptoms subside beforehand and to continue her antifungal treatment through her menstrual period should it occur. In addition, L.L. should be instructed to see her physician if her symptoms persist, if she experiences symptoms that signal a more serious problem (e.g., abdominal pain, fever, a foul-smelling or bloody vaginal discharge), and/or if another yeast infection occurs within 2 months.

L.L. also should be advised to avoid wearing tight-fitting, unventilated underwear (e.g., nylon panties or panty hose) and tight-fitting jeans because a warm, moist environment can facilitate fungal growth. However, a study addressing risk factors for VVC found no relation between type of underwear and the incidence of VVC.[123] In fact, many risk factors for VVC are not consistently associated with this infection.[115] L.L. also could be alerted to the possible relation between candidiasis and swimming in a heavily chlorinated pool or frequent use of a Jacuzzi or hot tub.

Complicated Vulvovaginal Candidiasis

Case 72-11, Question 10: How would management of L.L.'s VVC differ if she had poorly controlled diabetes?

VVC in a woman with uncontrolled diabetes is usually considered to be complicated VVC. A diagnosis of complicated VVC is also warranted when the VVC is severe, recurrent (as defined), caused by non–C. *albicans* species or when VVC occurs in an immunosuppressed, debilitated, or pregnant woman. The treatment of complicated VVC varies depending on the underlying reason for the complication. Severe VVC (e.g., extensive vulvar erythema, edema, excoriation, and fissures) may be treated with either a 7- to 14-day course of topical azoles or two oral doses of fluconazole 150 mg given 72 hours apart. Infection with non–C. *albicans* species should be treated with a 7- to 14-day course of an oral or intravaginal azole; however, the optimal treatment is unknown. Oral fluconazole has poor activity against non–C. *albicans* species and should not be used. Boric acid 600 mg capsules administered intravaginally once daily for 14 days can also be used, which has shown eradication rates of 70%.[2]

Recurrent Vulvovaginal Candidiasis

CASE 72-11, QUESTION 11: L.L. experiences another case of VVC 1 month later. Does she have recurrent VVC? How should she be treated?

Most women have only occasional episodes of VVC, but approximately 5% experience recurrent VVC infections defined as four or more episodes per year. To determine whether L.L. has recurrent VVC, a diagnosis of *Candida* needs to be confirmed by vaginal cultures. Then, underlying risk factors for VVC, such as uncontrolled diabetes mellitus, consumption of excess sugars, IUD placement, and use of antibiotics, must be ruled out.[124] Based on the timing of L.L.'s episodes and the absence of risk factors, L.L. does not meet the definition for recurrent VVC. If a patient meets the criteria for recurrent VVC, an underlying cause of the problem may not be determined. In addition, the role of sexual transmission is not currently well understood.[114] In most patients, the pathogenesis of recurrent VVC cannot be determined.

Treatment of recurrent *C. albicans* vulvovaginitis should include a prolonged (7–14-day) course of topical therapy or a three-dose regimen of oral fluconazole (100, 150, or 200 mg) administered every 3 days. A 6-month maintenance regimen should be initiated after remission has been achieved (Table 72-7). Despite the efficacy of these regimens, discontinuation of therapy after 6 months can result in relapse in 30% to 50% of women.[2] Azole-resistant strains of *C. albicans* are rare; therefore, culture and sensitivity testing is not usually performed to help guide treatment before initiation.

Table 72-7
Maintenance Regimens for Recurrent Vulvovaginal Candidiasis

	Dose	Frequency
Topical agents		
Clotrimazole	200 mg	Intermittently
Clotrimazole vaginal suppositories	500 mg	Intermittently
Oral agents		
Fluconazole tablets	100, 150, or 200 mg	Weekly for 6 months

[a]Given as examples only, CDC does not indicate a preferred regimen.

Adapted from Workowski KA, Bolan GA; Centers for Disease Control and Prevention (CDC). Sexually transmitted diseases treatment guidelines, 2015. 2015;64(RR-03):1–137.

Vulvovaginal Candidiasis During Pregnancy

CASE 72-11, QUESTION 12: What teratogenic risks are associated with the use of azole preparations?

Vaginal colonization with *Candida* and symptomatic VVC are common during pregnancy.[125] Asymptomatic colonization is not associated with increased maternal or fetal risks and need not be treated.[126] However, symptomatic VVC should be treated. Although doses of oral fluconazole used to treat VVC have not been associated with increased fetal defects, higher doses may be teratogenic. Therefore, topical antifungal agents are preferred for treatment of VVC in pregnant women. The CDC currently recommends a 7-day course of topical antifungal therapy for VVC during pregnancy; however, a 3-day regimen with appropriate follow-up to assess efficacy has been shown to be effective in mild-to-moderate cases. Clotrimazole is also classified as a category B drug for fetal risk, and the remaining vaginally administered azoles are designated as category C.[126]

Trichomoniasis

SIGNS AND SYMPTOMS

CASE 72-12

QUESTION 1: N.B. is a 31-year-old woman with a recent history of diffuse vaginal discharge and irritation. A wet-mount examination of vaginal secretions revealed numerous trichomonads. Examination confirms the presence of an increased, yellow–green vaginal discharge. What subjective and objective clinical data support a diagnosis of trichomoniasis?

Trichomoniasis is the most prevalent nonviral STD caused by the protozoan *T. vaginalis*.[2] The overall prevalence is estimated at 3.1% with the highest prevalence among African Americans at 13.3%. Trichomoniasis in women is asymptomatic or with minimal symptoms about 70% to 85% of the time. In men, *T. vaginalis* presumably infects the urethra, although the site of infection (urethra vs. prostate) is uncertain. Classic symptoms of trichomoniasis in women include a diffuse, yellow–green discharge with pruritus, dysuria, and a "strawberry" cervix (cervical microhemorrhages). The latter are typically seen only in 2% to 25% of cases.[127] In almost all cases of trichomoniasis, a vaginal pH greater than 5 is observed.[128] The Papanicolaou smear is associated with a 48.4% error in diagnosis when used alone.[127] Direct microscopic observation of trichomoniasis using a wet mount is inexpensive and yields a high specificity, but it has a low sensitivity.[129] Other testing options include culturing, rapid antigen tests, and NAATs.[130]

TREATMENT

Metronidazole and Tinidazole

CASE 72-12, QUESTION 2: How should N.B.'s trichomoniasis be treated?

The only class of drugs that is effective for the treatment of trichomoniasis is the nitroimidazoles. In the United States, metronidazole and tinidazole are the only available nitroimidazoles and both are CDC-recommended first-line agents given as a single 2 g oral dose. In addition, sexual partners should be simultaneously treated to prevent reinfection. Metronidazole cure rates are reported to be 84% to 98%, whereas tinidazole cure rates are reported to be 92% to 100%; concurrently treating sexual partners might increase these rates. Tinidazole offers other advantages, such as higher serum and genitourinary levels, a longer half-life, and fewer gastrointestinal adverse reactions.[2]

Approximately 4% to 10% of *T. vaginalis* isolates exhibit a low-level resistance to metronidazole therapy and 1% to tinidazole therapy; however, higher-level resistance appears to be rare.[2,131] If metronidazole 2 g PO for one dose fails and reinfection is excluded, metronidazole 500 mg PO twice daily for 7 days can be used. However, if this regimen fails either metronidazole or tinidazole 2 g PO as a single dose for 7 days should be used. In the case of allergy to nitroimidazole compounds, patients should be desensitized to metronidazole and subsequently treated.[2]

Adverse Effects

CASE 72-12, QUESTION 3: N.B. was treated with metronidazole 2 g as a single dose; however, while attending a party, N.B. experienced a severe headache, followed by nausea, sweating, and dizziness. Could N.B.'s symptoms be caused by metronidazole?

Minor side effects associated with metronidazole therapy include nausea, vomiting (especially with single-dose therapy), headache, skin rashes, and alcohol intolerance. The alcohol intolerance may be attributable to a metronidazole-induced inhibition of aldehyde dehydrogenase, which results in the buildup of high serum acetaldehyde levels, although the true risk of this interaction has been debated.[132] According to the manufacturer, patients should be warned about the possibility of nausea, vomiting, flushing, and respiratory distress after alcohol consumption, although reliable evidence is lacking.[123] As a general rule, patients should avoid alcohol ingestion during treatment and for 72 hours after metronidazole or tinidazole therapy. In those patients who cannot otherwise tolerate oral metronidazole or tinidazole, a combination of intravaginal miconazole and metronidazole may be an effective alternative.[133]

PREGNANCY

CASE 72-13

QUESTION 1: S.G., a 31-year-old woman, is in her first trimester of pregnancy and has a history of recurrent trichomoniasis. She now complains of a diffuse, yellow vaginal discharge. The preliminary diagnosis of trichomoniasis is confirmed by a wet-mount examination of vaginal secretions revealing numerous trichomonads. S.G. has read much in the lay press on metronidazole and is concerned about her own safety as well as that of her fetus. Can metronidazole be used for S.G.?

During pregnancy, trichomoniasis is associated with premature rupture of the membranes, preterm delivery, and low birth weight. In one study, rates of preterm delivery appeared to increase in women who received metronidazole, but a definitive causation could not be determined.[134] However, caution should still be exercised if metronidazole must be administered within the first trimester. Metronidazole is mutagenic in facultative bacteria and contains a nitro-reductase enzyme. Long-term, high-dose metronidazole in laboratory mice is associated with the development of pulmonary and hepatic tumors. Midline facial defects have been documented in humans, but two literature reviews indicate that metronidazole is not a teratogen.[135,136] In contrast, the use of metronidazole in asymptomatic women has not been shown to decrease rates of preterm labor despite eliminating the organism from its host.[137]

Treatment

CASE 72-13, QUESTION 2: How should S.G. be treated?

All symptomatic women should be treated with metronidazole 2 g PO as a single dose. Metronidazole is classified as pregnancy category B. Tinidazole 2 g PO as a single dose could be suggested as an alternative regimen; however, it is classified as pregnancy category C.[2]

GENITAL HERPES

The word *herpes* is of Greek origin and means "to creep." HSV is a DNA-containing virus that consists of two antigenically distinct serotypes: HSV-1 and HSV-2. The primary cause of herpes labialis (cold sores), herpes keratitis, and herpetic encephalitis is HSV-1. Genital herpes and neonatal herpes primarily are the result of HSV-2 infections. However, up to 50% of all reported cases of primary genital herpes are caused by HSV-1 infections acquired through oral sex.[138,139]

Etiology

Most people are exposed to HSV-1 early in life with more than half being positive for HSV-1 antibodies before 18 years and more than 90% of the population positive by 70 years of age.[140] The infection is often asymptomatic and generally acquired through primary infection of mucocutaneous surfaces. The initial, primary disease is a gingivostomatitis characterized by vesicles in the oral cavity and occasionally an elevated temperature; life-threatening encephalitis or keratitis may appear during this interval. Usually after primary exposure, HSV-1 enters cells of the trigeminal ganglion, where it may remain latent for the lifetime of the host.[141]

Initial HSV-2 infections usually occur after puberty and coincide with the onset of sexual activity, although transfer to a neonate from an infected mother can occur. After primary infection, the virus enters a state of latency in the sacral dorsal root ganglia in many infected individuals; a high percentage of infected persons may never manifest the disease clinically.[141,142]

In both HSV-1 and HSV-2 infections, the latent virus can reactivate. Recurrent disease may occur even when circulating antibody and sensitized lymphocytes are present. Clinically, the lesions periodically erupt usually at the same location, and the interval between episodes varies widely between individuals.

Epidemiology

Although herpes was recognized several thousand years ago, genital herpes was not described until the 18th century. The seroprevalence of genital herpes (HSV-2) has remained the same in the United States since 1999—at approximately 16.2% overall in 19- to 49-year olds, but 20.9% in women and 39.2% in non-Hispanic blacks—making it still one of the most common STDs in the United States.[143] In 2013, US physicians saw more than 300,000 new patients presenting with genital herpes simplex and nearly 20% of non-Hispanic white females and more than double that in non-Hispanic black females are already seropositive in the United States.[4]

Demographic characteristics obtained at the University of Washington indicate that the mean number of lifetime sexual partners before acquisition of the disease was 8.8 in women compared with 32.8 in men, with the overall chance of acquiring HSV-2 of 5 per 1,000 sex contacts.[144] The range of time from the last sexual exposure to the onset of disease is 5 to 14 days.[142] Whether causal or not, HSV-2 infection increases the risk of HIV acquisition.[145] Of recent concern, the seroprevalence of HSV-1 in 14- to 19-year olds declined by 23% from 1999 while the rate of HSV-2 remained unchanged, indicating that many young adolescents will not have protective HSV-1 antibodies at sexual debut and HSV-2 prevalence may rise.[146]

CASE 72-14

QUESTION 1: B.J., a 28-year-old, sexually active man, complains of painful penile lesions and tender inguinal adenopathy. The lesions are vesicular and limited to the scrotum, glands, and shaft of the penis. The onset of the lesions was preceded by a 1-week period of fever, malaise, headache, and itching. Viral culture of the lesions was positive for HSV infection. Describe the typical course and clinical presentation of herpes genitalis in men and women. What subjective and objective clinical data in B.J. are compatible with herpes genitalis?

Most initial episodes of genital herpes, especially in the male, are symptomatic. As illustrated by B.J., the symptoms usually start about 1 week after the initial exposure with prodromal signs of tingling, itching, paresthesia, or genital burning. The prodromal stage, which can last from a few hours to several days, is followed by the appearance of numerous vesicles. The vesicles eventually erupt, resulting in painful genital ulcers. The pain and edema associated with genital herpetic lesions, especially if they are infected secondarily, can be severe enough to result in dysuria and urinary retention. Bilaterally distributed lesions of the external genitalia are characteristic. The lesions usually are limited to the glands, corona prepuce, and shaft of the penis in males and to the vulva and vagina in females. However, lesions can occur on the buttocks, thighs, and urethra.[142] Asymptomatic or mucopurulent cervicitis occurs in about 15% to 20% of women with primary HSV-2 infections.[147] Rectal and perianal HSV-2 infections are more common in MSM and immunocompromised individuals.[148] Symptoms include anorectal pain and discharge, tenesmus, and constipation.

Prior infection with HSV-1 may ameliorate the severity of the first episode of genital herpes, but it does not impact the rate of recurrence.[149] In primary infections, the local symptoms of pain, itching, and urethral or vaginal discharge last from 11 to 14 days, with a complete disappearance of lesions in 3 to 6 weeks.[142,150] The clinical course of primary herpes is presented in Figure 72-7. Most patients have minor symptoms or are asymptomatic and unaware of their disease; they are most infectious within the first year of acquisition of the virus.[151]

Recurrence

CASE 72-14, QUESTION 2: Is B.J.'s infection likely to recur?

Most first episode HSV-2 symptomatic patients experience a recurrence of their initial infection.[2] The rate of recurrent infections varies among individual patients. Approximately 38% experience at least six episodes, and 20% have more than 10 recurrences.[150] Natural infection with HSV-2 induces type-specific immunity against exogenous reinfection, but it does not affect recurrences.[152] The severity of the primary episode and recurrence appear to be influenced by the host's immune status, especially a depressed T-cell response.[142] Recurrent infections usually appear at or near the site of the initial infection, and prodromal symptoms are reported by about 50% of persons with recurrent infection. Men recur more frequently than women. In contrast with primary infections, there are fewer lesions and they are often unilateral.[142] Constitutional symptoms such as lymphadenopathy, fever, and malaise generally are also milder. Recurrent infections are shorter in duration (average, 1 week); local symptoms such as pain and itching last 4 to 5 days and the lesions themselves last 7 to 10 days.[142] Although there is wide variability, patients may have four to five recurrences during the first year, but reactivation frequency can decline by three reactivations per year during the first 2 years.[153,154] By about 5 years after the initial infection, recurrence rates decrease greatly.[155] Genital infections with HSV-1, however, recur infrequently and decrease by 50% between 1 and 2 years after infection.[156]

Transmission

CASE 72-14, QUESTION 3: B.J. states that this is the first time he has had such lesions and that he has had only one sexual partner for the last 14 months. His sexually active female partner has no history of herpes genitalis or any other STD. The couple is very curious as to how B.J. acquired his infection. How is HSV transmitted?

Transmission of HSV occurs by direct contact with active lesions or from a symptomatic or asymptomatic person shedding virus at a peripheral site, mucosal surface, or secretion.[157] Genital HSV-2 infections usually are acquired through sexual (vaginal or anorectal) intercourse, whereas genital HSV-1 infections are acquired through orogenital sexual practices. Because HSV is inactivated readily by drying and exposure to room temperature, aerosol and fomite spread are unusual means of transmission.[158] Condoms may act as an effective barrier to viral transmission in women, but this method does not offer complete protection for men as women often have perigenital lesions.[159] Evidence suggests

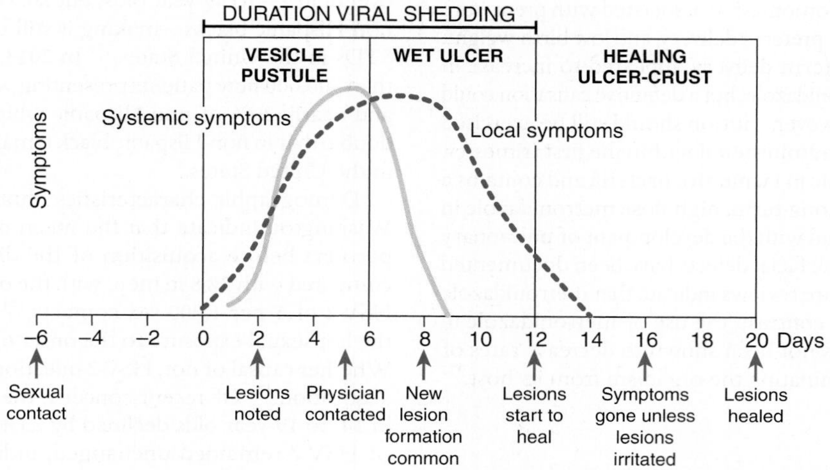

Figure 72-7 The Clinical Time Course of Primary Genital Herpes Infections. (Adapted with permission from Corely L, Wald A. Genital Herpes. In: Holmes K et al., eds. *Sexually Transmitted Diseases*. 4th ed. New York, NY: McGraw-Hill; 2008:399.).

that the frequency of correct condom use is directly proportional to protection against acquisition of HSV-2 and that condoms are more likely to be worn when lesions are present.[160,161]

A patient with genital herpes is contagious only when shedding the virus. The patient begins to shed virus during the prodromal phase, which may be several hours to days before the actual lesions first appear. Patients can, however, be asymptomatically diagnosed by serology and subsequently develop clinical lesions or be symptomatic on diagnosis and have recurrent episodes of clinical lesions. Symptomatic viral shedding occurs twice as often than in asymptomatic HSV-2 seropositive individuals, but subclinical viral shedding (i.e., no lesions present) still occurs approximately 10% of days, regardless of gender.[162] From a public health standpoint, unrecognized subclinical shedding may indicate a greater need for serologic testing to reduce transmission.[163,164] Lesions are most contagious during the ulcerative phase. The median duration of viral shedding as defined from onset to the last positive culture is about 12 days.[142] The mean time from the onset of vesicles to the appearance of the crust stage (~10.5 days) correlates well with the duration of viral shedding. However, there is considerable overlap between the duration of viral shedding and the duration of crusting. Women require a longer healing time than men, 19.5 and 16.5 days, respectively.[142] The mean duration of viral shedding from the cervix is 11.4 days. Therefore, patients should be advised to refrain from sexual activity until the lesions have completely healed; however, subclinical viral shedding may also transmit HSV-2.

A genital herpes infection may be acquired from an individual who has never had symptomatic genital lesions. States of asymptomatic or subclinical viral shedding occur in the majority of women with recurrent genital herpes as a result of reactivation of latent infection. These recurrent infections can have a primary disease presentation, causing the patient to blame the most proximate sexual partner when in actuality the exposure could have occurred in the distant past.[165] Serologic and virologic typing can be used to determine whether this is a true primary infection. Using sensitive detection techniques, such as PCR, women with recurrent HSV infections shed virus up to 28% of the time, but the relationship between a PCR-positive HSV test and true communicability has yet to be determined.[166] In addition, asymptomatic spread can occur from multiple anatomic genital sites and in a bilateral fashion, even with previous outbreaks of unilateral lesions.[167]

Seropositive HSV patients also should be counseled to practice safer sex, using male or female condoms, at all times, not just during symptomatic episodes.[168]

Diagnostic Tests

CASE 72-14, QUESTION 4: Viral culture was negative for B.J., but HSV-2 point-of-care (POC) serology was positive for both B.J. and his sexual partner. How should these laboratory tests to be interpreted?

The accuracy with which herpes genitalis can be diagnosed without the aid of laboratory tests generally is difficult to achieve, especially if the infection is not symptomatic. Thus, because of the potentially severe psychologic and physiologic ramifications of such a diagnosis, either virologic and/or serologic confirmation of the diagnosis may be obtained.

The laboratory diagnosis of HSV-1 or HSV-2 infection depends on isolation of virus using viral culture, while HSV DNA detection by PCR is more expensive than viral culture and not as widely available or HSV antigen detection using EIA or DFA. Both PCR and EIA can differentiate HSV-1 from HSV-2. Currently, HSV DNA PCR is the most sensitive method for detecting mucocutaneous herpes simplex infection rather than simple viral culture in those with genital ulcers and is the preferred method for CSF samples.[142] Tests that measure serologic response, antibody production, are valuable in documenting primary infection, but they are not very useful in recurrent infections or to determine when the initial infection occurred. It is possible to differentiate between antibodies to HSV-1 and HSV-2 by means of type-specific serologic assay. POC devices using HSV-2—specific antibody testing kits offer ease, reduced time, differentiation between HSV-1 and HSV-2, and high sensitivities and specificities.[12,169,170]

Viral culture is more likely to yield false-negative results than other testing methods.[12] A better antigen detection test could have been used, such as an EIA or DFA. The lack of a positive viral culture does not rule out the diagnosis of a primary infection in B.J., especially because the antibody test was positive. The fact that B.J.'s partner's antibody test was positive without a history of symptomatic disease suggests a distant infection with asymptomatic shedding.

Treatment

CASE 72-14, QUESTION 5: How should B.J.'s lesions be managed? Because the likelihood of recurrence of genital herpes is high, what treatment and prevention measures are recommended currently?

A diagnosis of genital herpes is concerning because there is no cure for the condition. Therapies ranging from antiviral agents and photoinactivation to investigational vaccines have been tried. Currently, only acyclovir (ACV), famciclovir (FCV), and valacyclovir (VCV) are useful in the treatment and prevention of genital herpes.

The ideal anti-HSV agent should (a) prevent infection, (b) shorten the clinical course, (c) prevent the development of latency, (d) prevent recurrence in patients with established latency, (e) decrease transmission of disease, and (f) eradicate established latent infection.[142] To date, no agent has been successful in achieving all of these goals.

All three agents, ACV, FCV, and VCV, are effective for the short-term treatment of some HSV infections. ACV, a nucleoside analog, is a substrate for HSV-specific thymidine kinase. Through a series of phosphorylation steps, ACV is transformed to ACV-triphosphate, a competitive inhibitor of viral DNA polymerase. ACV has potent in vitro activity against both HSV-1 and HSV-2 and is far less active against varicella-zoster and CMV.[171] FCV, a prodrug of penciclovir, has increased oral bioavailability compared with acyclovir. Once converted in the intestine and liver to the active form, penciclovir, it is quickly phosphorylated in HSV in a similar manner as ACV. VCV is the L-valyl ester prodrug of ACV. The oral bioavailability of VCV is also significantly better than ACV, producing plasma levels of ACV comparable to those attained with IV administered ACV, often eliminating the need for parenteral therapy.[172] All three antiviral drugs are equally effective for genital herpes infections.

Intravenous ACV (5 mg/kg/dose every 8 hours) significantly reduced the duration of viral shedding in primary genital herpes, decreasing the duration of signs and symptoms of disease by a mean of 5 days, and the time to healing of lesions by a mean of 6 to 12 days compared with placebo-treated patients.[12,173] Similar findings have been shown in the immunocompromised patient population.[174] IV and oral ACV or VCV also prevent HSV reactivation in seropositive immunocompromised patients who are undergoing bone marrow transplantation.[175] For patients with HIV, ACV 400 mg PO 3 times daily, FCV 500 mg twice daily, or VCV 500 mg twice daily for 5 to 10 days have been used for recurrent episodes.[2] Currently, IV therapy is recommended only for patients with severe genital or disseminated infections who cannot take oral medication.

Table 72-8
Antiviral Chemotherapy of Genital HSV-2 Infections

	Acyclovir	Valacyclovir	Famciclovir	Duration	Comments
First clinical episode	400 mg PO TID *or* 200 mg PO 5 per day	1 g PO BID	250 mg PO TID	7–10 days	May extend treatment duration if healing is incomplete
Episodic recurrent infection	400 mg PO TID *or* 800 mg PO BID *or* 800 mg PO TID × 2 days	1 g QD *or* 500 mg PO BID × 3 days	125 mg PO BID *or* 1,000 mg PO BID × 1 day *or* 500 mg PO × 1, then 250 mg BID × 2 days	5 days	Most effective if initiated within the first 24 hours of onset of lesions or during the prodrome
Daily suppressive therapy	400 mg PO BID[a]	500 mg PO QD[b] or 1 g PO QD	250 mg PO BID	Daily	Reduces the frequency of genital herpes recurrences by ≥75% among patients who have frequent recurrences (i.e., ≥6 recurrences per year); use should be reevaluated at 1 year
Severe disseminated	5–10 mg/kg IV q8h	Not indicated	Not indicated	Variable	Hospitalize and treat until clinical resolution of symptoms Follow-up IV therapy with PO ACV to complete 10 days
HIV-infected: episodic	400 mg PO TID *or* 200 mg 5 per day	1 g PO BID[c]	500 mg PO BID	5–10 days	Treat until clinical resolution of lesions
HIV-infected: suppressive	400–800 mg PO BID or TID	500 mg PO BID[d]	500 mg PO BID		

Note: Regimen recommendations derived from 2002 CDC Recommendations.[13]

[a]Safety and efficacy up to 6 years have been documented with the use of acyclovir.

[b]Valacyclovir 500 mg QD seems less effective in patients with >10 episodes per year. Thus, 1 g QD should be used in these patients.

[c]Dosages up to 8 g/day have been used, but an association with a syndrome resembling either hemolytic uremic syndrome or thrombotic thrombocytopenic purpura was observed.

[d]Effective in decreasing both the rate of recurrences and the rate of subclinical shedding among HIV-infected patients.

Topical therapy with ACV ointment (5% in polyethylene glycol) has minimal effect on the duration of viral shedding, symptoms, and lesion healing in first-episode primary genital herpes, and it has no effect on the recurrence rate[175] and is not recommended for primary genital herpes. Penciclovir 1% cream applied every 2 hours while awake is effective for treatment of herpes simplex labialis,[176] but insufficient data exist to recommend its use for genital herpes infections.

Oral antivirals speed the healing and resolution of symptoms of first and recurrent episodes of genital HSV-2 infections.[177] Treatment of primary infection after the first week of infection does change the natural history of recurrent outbreaks; thus, patients should be educated about risk of sexual transmission and prompt recognition of signs and symptoms and the early use of antivirals.[178] The frequency of recurrence decreases with time in most patients. Recurrent episodes of genital HSV-2 infection can be treated with any of the three available oral antivirals (Table 72-8). Rather than having to go into clinic, patients with recurrent infection should have a supply of their antiviral drug with them to allow early initiation of therapy, which may abort or reduce symptoms by 1 to 2 days.[179,180]

Daily suppressive therapy with ACV, FCV, or VCV reduces the frequency of recurrent episodes up to 70% to 80% among patients with frequent (five to eight episodes per year) genital herpes.[2,181] Recurrent outbreaks diminish with time; thus, after each year of continuous suppressive therapy, an effort should be made to discuss discontinuing therapy with the patient. The use of suppressive therapy does not completely eliminate viral transmission. However, a randomized, controlled clinical trial of serodiscordant HSV-2—positive couples demonstrated a statistically significant decrease in the rate of transmission to uninfected partners when infected partners took 500 mg/day of VCV.[154] This 8-month study was restricted to heterosexual partners with fewer than 10 recurrences per year. The CDC recommends various dosing regimens for VCV, but the 500-mg once-daily dose appears to be less effective than the 1-g once-daily dose in patients with frequent recurrent episodes (i.e., >10 episodes per year).[2] However, one meta-analysis showed a consistent prophylactic benefit if VCV was dosed at 250 mg twice daily or 500 mg once daily.[182] Immunocompromised patients may require higher doses or more frequent intervals for suppression.[183] Most cases of ACV-resistant HSV occurs in the immunocompromised host; however, the resistance is less than 5%.[184] All ACV-resistant strains are also resistant to VCV, and most are resistant to FCV as well. Foscarnet 40 to 80 mg/kg IV every 8 hours or cidofovir 5 mg/kg once weekly until clinical resolution may be used for severe ACV-resistant genital HSV infections.[2] Cidofovir 1% gel (not commercially available in the United States but has been compounded by pharmacists) applied once daily for 5 days may be an alternative to IV foscarnet, but more studies are needed.[2,185]

B.J. is not yet a candidate for daily suppressive ACV therapy. A summary of the indications for ACV, FCV, and VCV is outlined in Table 72-8.

ADVERSE EFFECTS

CASE 72-14, QUESTION 6: What adverse effects associated with ACV, FCV, or VCV should be anticipated?

Overall, all forms of ACV, including VCV and FCV, are associated with relatively few adverse reactions largely because of the drugs' affinity for viral thymidine kinase over cellular kinase.

Hematuria and an increase in blood urea nitrogen and serum creatinine may occur, primarily in patients with underlying renal disease or those receiving concomitant nephrotoxic agents. However, this complication is almost entirely associated with the IV route. In addition, severe local reactions are possible with IV administration. In patients with HIV/AIDS, VCV at a dosage of 8 g/day was associated with a hemolytic uremic syndrome or thrombotic thrombocytopenic purpura-like syndrome. However, this complication has not been observed with normal therapeutic doses. As described previously, when given intravenously in high doses or with significant dehydration, ACV crystallizes in the renal collecting tubules of animals, leading to renal insufficiency.[186] ACV should not be rapidly infused or administered at concentrations greater than 10 mg/mL. Dose adjustment is necessary for all three antiviral agents in patients with decreased renal function.

Although neurotoxicity is a rare side effect, case reports of coma and delirium have been reported in patients with renal failure.[187,188]

Intravenous ACV occasionally has been associated with cutaneous irritation and phlebitis, reversible leukopenia,[189] and transient elevations of liver transaminases. Oral ACV and VCV are relatively safe and do not produce any serious side effects at normal doses. Patients receiving oral ACV, VCV, or FCV may complain of nausea, dizziness, diarrhea, and headaches.

Patient Education and Counseling

CASE 72-14, QUESTION 7: What are the roles for education and counseling in patients with genital herpes? Are other forms of local or symptomatic care useful?

Most genital herpes infections are benign, and lesions heal spontaneously unless the patient is immunocompromised or the lesions have become infected secondarily. The patient should be instructed to keep the involved areas clean and dry. To prevent autoinoculation, the patient should be told not to touch the lesions and to wash his hands immediately afterward if he comes in contact with the lesion. Local anesthetics provide relief from the pain of genital lesions, but they should be avoided if possible because they counteract efforts to keep the lesions dry. Local corticosteroid therapy is contraindicated because it may predispose the patient to secondary infections.

Patient counseling should include the source contact and any future partner. Health care practitioners should attempt to relieve patients' feelings of guilt and anxiety; discussion of long-term consequences should take place after the acute symptoms of the infection have resolved.

For individuals with frequent recurrences, efforts should be made to identify and avoid stimulatory factors such as sunlight, trauma, or emotional stress. The limitations of therapy and the decreased severity and frequency of recurrences with time should be explained to the patient. The periods of infectivity and the need to avoid sexual activity even when lesions are not present should be emphasized, indicating the need for continuous barrier protection. Women with herpes genitalis should be scheduled for routine Pap smears and should be instructed to discuss their HSV with their physicians if they become pregnant.

Currently, there is no completely effective way to prevent the transmission of HSV-2 infection. Barrier forms of contraception, in particular condoms, may reduce the transmission of HSV, but this may be limited only to male-to-female transmission owing to the large area that herpes lesions may occupy on the woman.[159] However, greater use of condoms by men can increase protection and is recommended to prevent HSV infections.[160] Nonoxynol-9, a spermicide that has in vitro anti-HSV activity, is ineffective in the prevention of established genital HSV infection and may actually increase the risk of transmission of HSV by causing genital ulceration.[190]

Complications

CASE 72-15

QUESTION 1: M.F. is a 23-year-old, sexually active female student with a history of frequent and severe recurrences of genital herpes since her initial infection 3 years ago. M.F. has tried numerous therapies, including suppressive and episodic antivirals. None of these therapies has provided M.F. with any relief of her symptoms, nor have they decreased the frequency of her recurrences. M.F. has read much in the lay press about herpes and is concerned about the possible complications of the disease, especially cervical cancer. What are the potential complications of herpes genitalis?

Previous research suggested that HSV-2 might be an oncogenic agent responsible for carcinoma of the cervix. However, a large longitudinal nested case-control study using nearly 20 years of seroepidemiologic and epidemiologic data combined with a meta-analysis concluded that it is very unlikely that HSV-2 is associated with the development of invasive cervical carcinoma.[191] Severe complications of herpes genitalis include central nervous system disease, such as meningitis and encephalitis, and disseminated disease.[142]

PREGNANCY

CASE 72-16

QUESTION 1: A.P., a 26-year-old woman in her 32nd week of gestation, was hospitalized with complaints of painful genital lesions, headache, fever, increased vaginal discharge, and dysuria of 1 week's duration. Multiple ulcerative lesions consistent with genital herpes were present on the cervix, vulva, labia minora, and thighs. How should A.P. be treated?

Herpes genitalis seropositivity in pregnant women occurs more frequently than in nonpregnant women, with 20% to 30% of all pregnant women having serologic evidence of HSV-2 infection.[192] When HSV is acquired by the mother near the time of delivery, transmission to the neonate can be 30% to 50% but less than 1% in those who acquired it early in pregnancy or had recurrent infection.[2] Unfortunately, a large proportion of those infections occurring during pregnancy are limited to the cervix and are totally asymptomatic, often eluding diagnosis.

Pregnant patients with a history of recurrent genital herpes should be examined carefully when they present in labor for evidence of active disease. The safety of systemic ACV and VCV in pregnant women has not been established in controlled trials, but the CDC cites the lack of documented fetal harm to assert that ACV can be used safely in all stages of pregnancy.[2] Thus, it is reasonable to recommend ACV to treat HSV in this patient. Some small studies suggest ACV administered for several weeks before delivery may decrease recurrent outbreaks and lessen the need for herpes-related cesarean section,[193] whereas a larger randomized clinical trial did not show a benefit in reducing the need for a cesarean delivery with primary infection.[194] In general, it does seem that patients with symptomatic genital herpes benefit from cesarean section.[195] The manufacturer of Zovirax (ACV) maintains an extensive database of fetal complications related to ACV use. To date, no link between ACV and birth defects has been established.[196] The decision to treat HSV with ACV during pregnancy should depend on the clinical severity of infection. Fetal exposure data to FCV or VCV are limited. If the mother has an active herpes genitalis infection at the time of delivery (either active genital lesions or HSV-2 cervicitis), the baby should be delivered by cesarean section within 4 hours after the membranes have ruptured to prevent exposure of the neonate to the virus.[142] However, if no genital lesions are present at the time of labor, vaginal delivery may be recommended.[12] There is evidence that up to 70% of neonatal herpes cases occur in asymptomatic women, and the use of ACV or VCV after 36 weeks gestation may decrease clinical disease and viral shedding to the fetus.[197]

Neonatal herpes is a devastating systemic infection of the newborn, associated with high morbidity and mortality, especially when infected with HSV-2 versus HSV-1.[198] HSV is usually transmitted to the newborn during passage through an infected birth canal, approximately 300 times greater than when HSV is not present.[195] The risk of transmission to the newborn is greatest in mothers who acquire an initial infection late in the third trimester and lower in mothers with recurrent infection or those who acquire herpes in the first trimester (25%–50% vs. <1% for preexisting infection).[198]

GENITAL WARTS

CASE 72-17

QUESTION 1: S.L., a 19-year-old woman, presents to the women's health clinic for her annual pelvic examination. One week later, her Pap smear is read as showing koilocytosis. A colposcopy is subsequently performed, revealing changes consistent with cervical flat warts. What is the cause of S.L.'s infection? How should she be managed?

Human papiloma virus (HPV) is the cause of genital warts, or condylomata acuminata. Types 6 and 11 account for more than 90% of genital warts.[199] Other types of HPV, including 16 and 18, account for as much as 70% of cervical cancer worldwide.[200,201] They are associated with Pap smear changes, including koilocytosis and cervical dysplasia. In the United States, the seroprevalence of HPV 6, 11, 16, and 18 is 32.5% for women and 12.2% among men aged 14 to 59 years.[202]

Cervical intraepithelial neoplasia (CIN) is a common cervical cancer grading system using histologic changes to classify specimens in three categories: CIN-1, -2, and -3. The higher the number, the greater the chance of progressing to invasive cervical cancer. Most new cases of HPV infection spontaneously regress but with progressive histologic changes, the chance of spontaneously regressing diminishes (CIN1, 60%; CIN2, 30%; CIN3, 10%).[203] Types of HPV are also classified as high risk, or those likely to cause cancer, and low risk, those less likely to cause cancer. HPV types 16, 18, 31, 33, 45, 52, and 58 are considered high risk and types 6 and 11 are low risk, the latter mostly resulting in genital warts. In women, visible warts occur on the labia, introitus, and vagina. Subclinical lesions also commonly occur on these sites and on the cervix, as in S.L.'s case. They are visible only by colposcopy after applying acetic acid. Men can sexually transmit HPV infections to women as well as exhibit genital warts, and anal and penile cancer associated with oncogenic HPV types, especially type 16.[204] The goal of HPV therapy is the removal of symptomatic warts. Several therapeutic options are available and include patient-administered treatments to visible warts, such as podofilox 0.5% solution or gel, imiquimod 3.75% and 5% cream and sinecatechins 15% ointment; provider-administered products include topical treatments (podophyllin 10%–25%, trichloroacetic acid 80%–90%, and cryotherapy), surgery (laser or scalpel), and intralesional interferon.[12] In a recent meta-analysis, locally applied interferon showed a 44% lesion clearance compared with 27.4% for systemic interferon.[205] None of these treatments can eradicate HPV infection or alter the natural history of HPV. It is important to individualize therapy, considering location and number of warts, patient preference, cost, and convenience.

Podophyllin, compounded as a 10% to 25% solution in tincture of benzoin, is applied by the health care provider to visible warts. After application, it is washed off 3 to 4 hours later and then reapplied once or twice a week until the warts have disappeared. Podofilox 0.5% solution or gel, the active component of podophyllin resin, may be applied by the patient with a cotton swab, or podofilox gel with a finger, to visible genital warts twice a day for 3 days, followed by 4 days of no therapy. A total of four cycles, 0.5 mL/day, or application of an area larger than 10 cm^2 should not be exceeded. Podofilox solution is not suitable for use with perianal warts; the gel is more practical for this region. Podophyllin is potentially neurotoxic if absorbed in large amounts. Podofilox has the advantage over podophyllin resin in that it has a longer shelf life, does not need to be washed off, and has less systemic toxicity.[206] Therefore, it should be applied in limited doses and should also be avoided in pregnancy. The rate of wart recurrence after podophyllin therapy is extremely high, probably 50%. With the high cost of clinic care and the high recurrence rate, home treatment of HPV with podofilox solution may be more cost effective and equally efficacious.[207]

Imiquimod induces cytokines and activates the cell-mediated immune system. In initial trials, complete clearance of warts took place in 37% to 50% of immunocompetent patients, but up to 20% experienced recurrence.[208] The 5% cream is optimally applied by finger at bedtime 3 times per week and the 3.5% cream once daily for up to 16 weeks.[209,210] It is usually left on for 6 to 10 hours before it is washed off with soap and water. Imiquimod may take as long as 8 weeks before warts are cleared. Mild-to-moderate local irritation occurs in more than half of the patients who use it, especially when used daily instead of 3 times weekly as directed. The cream may weaken condoms and diaphragms.

Sinecatechins are green-tea extracts that contain active catechins with purported immunostimulatory, antiprofliferative, and antitumor properties. In the United States, a 15% topical ointment is available. There are limited data on this product, but literature suggests it may be more effective than imiquimod or podofilox by clearing up to 55% of external genital warts.[211] It is applied by finger directly to the wart 3 times a day up to 16 weeks with the most common side effects being local erythema, pruritus, burning, and pain.[12]

Cryotherapy by application of liquid nitrogen can be more effective than podophyllin, but it requires special equipment and highly trained personnel. Pain and skin blistering after treatment is common. Cryotherapy is associated with minimal systemic toxicity and is useful against oral, anal, urethral, and vaginal warts.

Trichloroacetic acid (80%–90%) is used topically in the treatment of some genital warts, but its efficacy is uncertain. To date interferons are not recommended because of expense and toxicity. Cases refractory to topical drug therapy should be considered for surgical treatment.

Prevention

In 2006, the first vaccine to prevent HPV types 6, 11, 16, and 18 was approved in the United States. This quadrivalent vaccine was tested in women from 15 to 26 years of age and demonstrated 98% to 100% protection against HPV types contained in the vaccine.[212,213] In males, the quadrivalent vaccine efficacy was 62.1% to 89.4% against genital warts, depending upon previous HPV exposure, leading to its approval for men and boys 9 to 26 years old.[214] Using bridging data, it is estimated that 99% to 100% of 9- to 15-year olds will seroconvert. In 2014, a 9-valent HPV vaccine was approved to replace the quadrivalent vaccine. The extra 5 types (31, 33, 45, 52, and 58) add 15% more cervical cancer coverage protection to the 66% covered by types 16 and 18 in the quadrivalent.[215] This three-dose series can be given as early as 9 years of age, but it is CDC recommended at 11 to 12 years as part of a routine adolescent health care visit and ideally before commencement of sexual activity. Because there are more than 30 types of HPV associated with anogenital disease, a previous HPV infection is not a contraindication to vaccination. It is also important to note that receipt of the HPV vaccine does not change the recommendation for Pap smears. Lastly, it should not be considered a therapeutic vaccine as it has no impact on active HPV infection.

VACCINES

Prevention and control of STDs have largely revolved around education and antimicrobials. Immunization, however, holds the promise of protecting large numbers of people before they are at risk for STDs as well as targeting those who already have the infection. Hepatitis B is an example of an STD with a highly effective vaccine that is now mandatory for school-aged children. The nine-valent HPV vaccine is gaining momentum and a bivalent (HPV 16 and 18) is also approved by the FDA, but the latter is not indicated for prevention of genital warts. Herpes simplex vaccines have been extensively studied, but no candidate vaccine has been submitted for approval.

KEY REFERENCES AND WEBSITES

A full list of references for this chapter can be found at http://thepoint.lww.com/AT11e. Below are the key references and websites for this chapter, with the corresponding reference number in this chapter found in parentheses after the reference.

Key References

CDC. Sexually transmitted diseases treatment guidelines, 2015. *MMWR Recomm Rep*. 2015;64(3):1–138. http://www.cdc.gov/std/tg2015/tg-2015-print.pdf. (2)

CDC. Sexually Transmitted Disease Surveillance 2007 Supplement, Gonococcal Isolate Surveillance Project (GISP) Annual Report 2007. Atlanta, GA: U.S. Department of Health and Human Services, Centers for Disease Control and Prevention, March 2009; 2009. (23).

Key Websites

Centers for Disease Control and Prevention. Sexually Transmitted Disease Surveillance 2014. Atlanta: U.S. Department of Health and Human Services; 2015; http://www.cdc.gov/std/stats. Accessed May 2, 2015.

US Department of Health and Human Services. Healthy People 2020 topics and objectives: sexually transmitted diseases. 2011; http://www.healthypeople.gov/2020/topics-objectives/topic/sexually-transmitted-diseases/objectives. Accessed: May 2, 2015.

73 Osteomyelitis and Septic Arthritis

Jacqueline L. Olin, Linda M. Spooner, and Karyn M. Sullivan

CORE PRINCIPLES

OSTEOMYELITIS	CHAPTER CASES
1 Acute hematogenous osteomyelitis is characterized by the abrupt onset of localized pain and tenderness at a single site, fever, and increased inflammatory markers (erythrocyte sedimentation rate, C-reactive protein). Imaging techniques and blood and bone cultures (if done) may reveal findings consistent with bone changes in osteomyelitis and the responsible pathogen.	**Case 73-1 (Questions 1, 2), Table 73-1**
2 Initial empiric antibiotic therapy for acute hematogenous osteomyelitis should be directed at gram-positive cocci, including methicillin-resistant *Staphylococcus aureus* (MRSA). Protein binding and bone concentrations of antibiotics are not critical factors in predicting successful treatment, as long as the responsible pathogen is susceptible to the chosen therapy, and treatment is given in high doses for long duration.	**Case 73-1 (Question 3), Table 73-2**
3 If blood or bone cultures grow the likely pathogen, then therapy should be de-escalated when possible based on organism susceptibilities. Assuming no allergies, methicillin-sensitive *Staphylococcus aureus* (MSSA) should be treated with oxacillin or nafcillin. The overall duration of therapy (by intravenous [IV] route and possibly orally) should be at least 4 weeks.	**Case 73-1 (Questions 4–6), Tables 73-2, 73-3**
4 Osteomyelitis secondary to a contiguous focus of infection typically occurs after trauma and the consequent orthopedic corrective surgery. Common symptoms are pain, tenderness, erythema, and drainage at the site of injury or infection. Imaging studies usually show bone changes consistent with infection.	**Case 73-2 (Questions 1, 2), Table 73-1**
5 Secondary osteomyelitis is often polymicrobial. Surgical efforts should be instituted to reassess the site of bone injury and infection, with deep tissue or bone samples obtained for culture. Treatment is IV therapy for at least 4 weeks, and the antibiotics chosen should depend on the cultured organisms and their antibiotic susceptibilities.	**Case 73-2 (Questions 3, 4)**
6 Osteomyelitis associated with vascular insufficiency most often occurs in patients with diabetes mellitus. Neuropathy and impaired blood flow lead to the development of chronic lower extremity cellulitis and underlying osteomyelitis. Multiple gram-positive and gram-negative aerobic and anaerobic bacteria may be involved; thus, initial empiric treatment typically includes vancomycin and an antipseudomonal beta-lactam. Definitive therapy should be based on the results of deep surgical cultures. Duration of treatment should be 6 or more weeks, with chronic suppressive therapy considered thereafter.	**Case 73-3 (Questions 1, 2)**
7 Chronic osteomyelitis can present years later at a site of previous bone infection and is usually characterized by a draining sinus tract from bone to skin. Chronically infected dead bone is involved, and surgery is important in removing necrotic bone when possible. Chronic osteomyelitis is often polymicrobial, and the same organism (especially *S. aureus*) that was causative of a previous bone infection could still be involved in chronic infection. High-dose IV therapy directed at the results of bone cultures for at least 6 weeks is recommended to offer the best chances of preventing the extension of infection to adjacent uninfected bone.	**Case 73-4 (Questions 1–4)**

Continued

	CHAPTER CASES
8 Prosthetic joint infection with adjacent bone osteomyelitis usually requires surgical removal of the infected prosthesis for cure. Antibiotics should be directed at the cultured bacteria from a joint aspirate or from deep surgical specimens. The most common pathogens are *S. aureus* and coagulase-negative staphylococci. In a situation in which the prosthesis cannot be totally removed, lifelong, chronic suppressive oral therapy should be considered.	**Case 73-5 (Questions 1–3)**
SEPTIC ARTHRITIS	
1 Nongonococcal septic arthritis is characterized by fever, and the acute onset of joint pain and effusion in a single joint. Infection is typically acquired hematogenously from an originating site that may not always be easily identified. *S. aureus* is the most common pathogen. Duration of treatment should be 6 weeks, with oral therapy for the final 2 weeks.	**Case 73-6 (Questions 1, 2)**
2 *Neisseria gonorrhoeae* is the most common cause of polyarticular arthritis in a young, sexually active adult. Skin lesions may also be present in disseminated gonococcal infection (DGI). The diagnosis is frequently based on the clinical syndrome and sexual history, because joint fluid aspirate and blood cultures are frequently negative. Intravenous ceftriaxone is the treatment of choice and should be continued for 1 to 2 days after improvement begins. Treatment duration is 7–14 days.	**Case 73-7 (Questions 1–3)**

OSTEOMYELITIS

Osteomyelitis is an inflammation of the bone marrow and surrounding bone associated with infection. Any bone can be involved, and substantial morbidity is possible even with early diagnosis and treatment. Despite the continued refinement of diagnostic procedures (e.g., radionuclide imaging, computed tomography, magnetic resonance imaging), advances in antimicrobial therapy, and the use of prophylactic antibiotics before orthopedic procedures, osteomyelitis continues to be difficult to cure.

Osteomyelitis can affect all age groups. The most common causative microorganisms of acute osteomyelitis have historically been streptococci and staphylococci. *Staphylococcus aureus* remains the most causative organism, accounting for more than 50% of all cases, although the prevalence of infection caused by methicillin-resistant *S. aureus* (MRSA) is increasing across all age-groups. Additionally, osteomyelitis caused by gram-negative and anaerobic bacilli is becoming more common.[1]

Bone may be infected by three routes: hematogenous spread of bacteria from a distant infection site, direct infection of bone from an adjacent or contiguous source of infection, and infection of bone secondary to vascular insufficiency. Table 73-1 summarizes characteristics associated with osteomyelitis.[1–3] Patients with recurrent osteomyelitis are considered to have chronic osteomyelitis.

Bone Anatomy and Physiology

The bone is divided into three sections: the epiphysis, located at the end of the bone; the metaphysis (adjacent to the epiphysis and part of the epiphyseal growth plate); and the diaphysis (midsection of the bone). The rapidly growing area of the bone is supported by many blood vessels. Surrounding most of the bone is a fibrous, cellular envelope. The external portion of this envelope is the periosteum, and the internal portion is the endosteum.

Blood vessels that supply bone tissue are located predominantly in the epiphysis and metaphysis of the bone. Nutrient arteries enter the bone at the metaphyseal side of the epiphyseal growth plate and lead to capillaries that form sharp loops within the growth plate. These capillaries lead to large sinusoidal veins that eventually exit the metaphysis through a nutrient vein. Within the sinusoidal veins, blood flow is slowed considerably, and infection is possible with bacterial colonization.[4]

Differences in the vasculature of bone in different age groups lead to different forms of osteomyelitis. In neonates and adults, vascular communications are present between the metaphysis and epiphysis, which can allow infection to spread from bone to the adjacent joint. During childhood, however, this area often is protected from infection because the epiphyseal plate separates the vascular supply for these two regions.[4]

Hematogenous Osteomyelitis

Hematogenous osteomyelitis predominantly occurs in prepubertal children but may be seen in older adults, patients with indwelling central catheters, and intravenous drug users.[1] Osteomyelitis in children tends to be acute, hematogenous, and is often responsive to antibiotic therapy alone. In comparison, osteomyelitis in adults tends to be subacute or chronic, commonly results from trauma, infection of prosthetic devices, or other insult, and often requires surgical debridement in addition to antimicrobial therapy.[1–3]

Infection in children develops primarily in the metaphysis of the rapidly growing long bones of the body where the slowed blood flow allows bacteria to colonize and multiply. The acute infectious process (e.g., edema, inflammation, small vessel thrombosis) increases bone pressure, which compromises blood flow and eventually leads to necrosis. Released cytokines alter bone integrity by promoting osteoclast activity. Eventually, the elevated pressure and necrosis cause devitalized bone to fragment from healthy bone (sequestra). With continued spread of the infection into the outer layers of the bone and soft tissue, abscess and draining sinus tracts form.[1,3]

Hematogenous infection in children most commonly occurs in the long bones with a single focus in the femur and tibia.[1] Hematogenous osteomyelitis in neonates is an especially serious disease that often involves multiple bones, especially the long bones. Rapid infection spreading across the epiphyseal plate to the adjacent joint can lead to septic arthritis, necessitating immediate and aggressive treatment. Vertebrae involvement is seen more frequently in adults.[1–3]

The most common organism causing hematogenous osteomyelitis is *S. aureus*, responsible for up to 85% of pediatric cases.[4] The emergence of both hospital- and community-associated strains of MRSA has challenged the management of osteomyelitis. MRSA infections are associated with an increased risk of antibiotic treatment failures and complications, including abscess formation,

Table 73-1
Features of Osteomyelitis

Feature	Hematogenous	Adjacent/Contiguous Site of Infection	Vascular Insufficiency
Usual onset: pediatric or adult	Predominantly pediatric	Adult	Adult
Sites of infection	Tibia, femur (children); vertebrae (adults)	Femur, fibula, tibia, skull, mandible	Foot
Risk factors	Bacteremia	Surgery, trauma, cellulitis, joint prosthesis	Diabetes, peripheral vascular disease
Common bacteria	*S. aureus*, gram-negative bacilli; usually one organism	*S. aureus*, streptococci, gram-negative bacilli, anaerobic organisms; often polymicrobial	*S. aureus*, coagulase-negative staphylococci, streptococci, gram-negative bacilli, anaerobic organisms; often polymicrobial
Clinical findings	Fever, chills, local tenderness, swelling; limitation of motion	Fever, warmth, swelling; unstable joint	Pain, swelling, drainage, ulcer formation

deep vein thrombosis, and septic emboli.[5] Gram-negative bacilli (*Escherichia coli*, *Klebsiella*, *Proteus*, *Salmonella*, and *Pseudomonas*) are responsible for an increasing number of cases of osteomyelitis as well. *Pseudomonas aeruginosa* is more commonly seen in patients with indwelling central catheters and in intravenous (IV) drug users, whereas *S. aureus* and *Salmonella* species are common causes in patients with sickle cell anemia.[1]

Clinical features of hematogenous osteomyelitis vary, depending on the patient's age and the infection site. In children, infection usually is characterized by an abrupt onset of high fever and chills, localized pain, tenderness, and swelling. Systemic symptoms often are absent in neonates, potentially delaying the diagnosis. A diagnosis, therefore, must be made on the basis of localized symptoms such as edema and restricted limb movement. Systemic symptoms are also less common in adults, although patients with vertebral osteomyelitis can present with the insidious onset of localized back pain and tenderness.[1,3]

Acute Osteomyelitis

USUAL CLINICAL PRESENTATION

CASE 73-1

QUESTION 1: L.D., a 7-year-old girl, is unable to go to school today because of fever and worsening leg pain. Her upper left leg started to hurt 3 to 4 days ago, and last night she began limping. Her parents report no history of trauma to the area. Her past medical history is significant only for two episodes of otitis media at ages 2 and 5. In the pediatrician's office, maximal tenderness is localized over the left distal femur without knee joint effusion. No signs of swelling, warmth, or trauma are seen. Her white blood cell (WBC) count is 8,000/μL with a normal WBC differential. Plain radiographic studies of the left leg are normal, but the erythrocyte sedimentation rate (ESR) is 58 mm/hour (normal ≤30 mm/hour). Two blood samples are obtained for culture, and L.D. is sent home with directions for bed rest and use of acetaminophen as needed for fever. Two days later, she is admitted to the hospital with severe pain and tenderness in her left leg and a fever of 38.8°C. The blood cultures obtained 2 days ago are positive for *S. aureus* with susceptibilities still pending. C-reactive protein (CRP) is 14 mg/dL (normal, <2 mg/dL). Another plain radiographic study is normal, but a magnetic resonance imaging (MRI) scan reveals inflammation in her left distal femur. What findings in L.D. are consistent with hematogenous osteomyelitis?

L.D. displays the usual signs and symptoms of acute hematogenous osteomyelitis in children. She is a previously healthy child who experienced acute localized pain and tenderness of the left distal femur, abrupt onset of high fever, and an elevated ESR and CRP. Her plain radiographic studies were normal on two occasions; however, destructive changes to bone often do not appear on plain radiographs for at least 10 to 14 days after onset of infection.[1] Hence, a normal plain film does not rule out acute osteomyelitis if obtained within the first 2 weeks of infection. Diagnosis includes radionuclide imaging (bone scans), computed tomography (CT), or MRI.[1,4] MRI is more sensitive than CT for the assessment of soft tissue and detecting early bone marrow edema; however, it often requires sedation for children.[4] The sensitivity of bone scan detection of osteomyelitis has been lowest when the infection was caused by community-associated MRSA (CA-MRSA).[4] L.D.'s MRI scan on hospitalization detected inflammation in the left distal femur. Although L.D. did not have a bone biopsy sent for culture, her clinical picture, a positive MRI scan, and blood cultures positive for *S. aureus* establish the diagnosis of osteomyelitis. The specific event that caused bacteremia with dissemination to bone is unknown, as is often the case in children.[4]

Laboratory tests that should be routinely obtained in every child suspected of having osteomyelitis include a complete blood count (CBC), ESR, and serum CRP. Although these tests are not specific for the diagnosis of osteomyelitis, they help confirm the clinical diagnosis. An increased WBC count is consistent with osteomyelitis, but leukocytosis is absent in many children with osteomyelitis at the initial examination. Thus, L.D.'s WBC count of 8,000/μL is not unusual. In adults, leukocytosis is more common in an acute infection rather than with recurrent or chronic disease. Both ESR and CRP are nonspecific markers of systemic inflammation when elevated.

Predisposing factors for hematogenous osteomyelitis include any risk factors for bacteremia (e.g., indwelling catheters such as hemodialysis shunts and chronic central venous catheters). Other risk factors that can potentially lead to bacteremia and subsequently hematogenous osteomyelitis include IV drug use and a distant focus of infection in the gastrointestinal or urinary tract. None of these factors exist in L.D. In children such as L.D. who have no history of trauma, fractures, or penetrating injury, the most common cause of acute hematogenous osteomyelitis is *S. aureus* and the possibility of CA-MRSA must be considered.[1,5,6]

PATIENT WORKUP

CASE 73-1, QUESTION 2: What additional patient and diagnostic information should be obtained before L.D. receives her first dose of antibiotics?

Before L.D. receives antibiotic therapy, she should be assessed for drug allergies, especially penicillin allergy. Patient interviews, discussions with her parents, and a comprehensive review of her medical record are necessary, especially with a history of allergy. Details of an allergic reaction, including symptoms, onset of the reaction, probable causative agent, treatment, and exposure to related antimicrobials should be evaluated.

Cultures of blood and bone aspirate material optimally identify the pathogen and must be part of the initial workup prior to the start of antibiotics. Cultures taken after antibiotics have been initiated are often negative. Positive blood cultures are seen in 33%–50% of pediatric bone and joint infections.[6]

In L.D.'s case, the positive blood culture and MRI establish the diagnosis of osteomyelitis. If the blood cultures had been negative, however, a bone aspirate would be recommended to identify the pathogen.[1] Once material has been obtained for culture, empiric antibiotic therapy should start as soon as possible.

TREATMENT

Empiric Antibiotic Therapy

CASE 73-1, QUESTION 3: L.D. has no history of drug allergies. She took amoxicillin for the previous episodes of acute otitis media without incident. What empiric antibiotic(s) should be started? What is the relevance of bone concentrations or protein binding of antibiotics in the selection of therapy for osteomyelitis?

The chosen agent should be administered IV at high doses to optimize drug concentration in infected bone. Treatment should be initiated as soon as possible to improve the chances for complete eradication of infection and to avoid the need for surgery. Thus, empiric antibiotic therapy is often administered while bacterial cultures are pending or before antibiotic susceptibility results are known.

Although cultures are pending or with negative cultures, the age of the child can predict the likely pathogen and guide empiric antibiotic selection. For example, *S. aureus* and *Streptococcus* species are commonly responsible for osteomyelitis in the neonate.[1] *Kingella kingae*, a facultatively anaerobic, gram-negative hemolytic bacillus, is being detected with increasing frequency in children under 3 years of age, especially in the day care setting.[7,8] Table 73-2 summarizes the common causative organisms of acute hematogenous osteomyelitis in children and recommended drugs and doses for treatment.[2,4,9,10]

Considering the epidemiology of L.D.'s infection and the blood cultures, she should be treated for *S. aureus* osteomyelitis. In both children and adults, the number of acute osteomyelitis cases caused by MRSA continues to increase.[4,6] Empiric IV vancomycin should be administered pending susceptibility results. Alternative empiric therapy for L.D. with MRSA coverage includes daptomycin or linezolid.[9] Due to limited clinical experience, these two agents should be reserved for vancomycin-intolerant cases. Clindamycin is not an option for L.D., but may be used empirically for stable patients without bacteremia or intravascular infection.[9]

The importance of antibiotic bone concentration when treating osteomyelitis is unclear, and bone concentrations do not always predict outcome of therapy.[2,11] Theoretically, protein binding could influence clinical efficacy because free drug is thought to diffuse from plasma into bone tissue and protein-bound drug does not. However, cefazolin (for sensitive gram-positive cocci) and ceftriaxone (for sensitive gram-negative rods and streptococci), both highly protein-bound drugs, are well-established treatments for osteomyelitis when appropriate doses and duration are used. Therefore, antibiotic bone concentrations and protein binding of antibiotics (in appropriate doses) are not significant factors in the selection of appropriate therapy for osteomyelitis.[2,11]

Directed Antibiotic Therapy

CASE 73-1, QUESTION 4: The *S. aureus* grown from L.D.'s blood culture is methicillin sensitive. Considering these results, what is the optimal antibiotic regimen? Would other antibiotics given less frequently also be adequate?

L.D. is not allergic to penicillin. Although vancomycin is active against MSSA, it is inferior to β-lactams; thus, β-lactam-based therapy should be used for susceptible organisms.[1,6] De-escalating from vancomycin to oxacillin (or nafcillin) at 150 mg/kg/day every 6 hours is appropriate.[2] Nafcillin and oxacillin are therapeutically equivalent and are given in similar doses; therefore, selection typically depends on hospital formulary considerations. Her prior exposure to amoxicillin is irrelevant except to establish the absence of a penicillin allergy.

Continuing to treat L.D. with IV oxacillin (or nafcillin) every 6 hours follows treatment recommendations for MSSA osteomyelitis. Antistaphylococcal penicillins are effective therapy with appropriate doses and duration. Changing L.D. to cefazolin would allow slightly less frequent dosing (every 8 hours), a potential advantage for home treatment. Vancomycin use should be discouraged in L.D.'s case because cultures revealed a methicillin-sensitive organism, and vancomycin is more likely to be associated with treatment failure.[1,6] In the absence of susceptibility results or of methicillin resistance, IV vancomycin would be required for the duration of therapy. Although the logistics of outpatient therapy in L.D. are being investigated, she should remain on oxacillin while in the hospital.

Duration of Therapy

CASE 73-1, QUESTION 5: Both of L.D.'s parents are employed, and their work schedules prevent them from leaving their jobs to transport her to an outpatient antibiotic treatment center. Is L.D. a candidate for outpatient IV antibiotic therapy at home, or is oral antibiotic treatment an option? Must L.D. remain in the hospital to receive her oxacillin?

Initially, all patients should receive IV antibiotics because early, aggressive therapy offers the best chance to cure the infection. L.D., however, does not necessarily need to stay in the hospital for the duration of therapy. A peripherally inserted central catheter (PICC) can be placed, and antibiotics can be administered. The decision to use home IV antibiotic administration must be decided in concert with L.D.'s parents. If L.D.'s parents do not have the resources or are unwilling to oversee IV treatment at home, L.D. should remain hospitalized for a minimum of 1 week to assess the efficacy of IV treatment. Transition to oral therapy should be considered at discharge due to the frequency of PICC line complications and the cost and inconvenience of several weeks of IV therapy at home.[7,12]

As discussed below in Question 6, L.D. can complete most of her treatment with oral antibiotics, but oral therapy should not be given until the effectiveness of IV therapy can be assessed. Children with uncomplicated acute osteomyelitis are candidates for oral therapy when clinically improved, and the CRP has normalized, typically between 3 and 7 days.[13,14] Total duration of antibiotic therapy should be 3–4 weeks; however, current IDSA guidelines

Table 73-2
Empiric Intravenous Antibiotics for Acute Osteomyelitis in Children

Host	Likely Organisms	Antibiotics	Dose (mg/kg/day)	Dose (doses/day)
Neonate	*Staphylococcus aureus* Group B streptococci Gram-negative bacilli	Oxacillin (or nafcillin) *with*	25–50	2–4
		Cefotaxime	50	2–4
<3 years	*S. aureus*	Vancomycin *or*	40–60	4
		Linezolid *or*	30	3
		Daptomycin	6	1
	Haemophilus influenzae type b	Oxacillin (or nafcillin) *with*	150–200	4
		Cefotaxime	100–180	4–6
	Kingella kingae	Cefazolin *or*	50–100	3–4
		Cefuroxime	100–150	3–4
≥3 years	*S. aureus*	Vancomycin *or*	40–60	4
		Linezolid		
		≤12 years	30	3
		>12 years *or*	600 mg dose	2
		Daptomycin *or*	6	1
		Oxacillin (or nafcillin) *or*	150–200	4
		Cefazolin *or*	50–100	3–4
		Clindamycin	40	3–4
After puncture wound through shoe	*P. aeruginosa*	Ceftazidime	100–150	3
Child with sickle cell disease	*Salmonella* sp. *S. aureus*	Oxacillin (or nafcillin) *with*	150–200	4
		Cefotaxime *or*	100–180	4–6
		Vancomycin *with*	40–60	4
		Cefotaxime	100–180	4–6

recommend 4 to 6 weeks of therapy for children with MRSA osteomyelitis.[9,13,14] Neonatal cases warrant 4 weeks of IV antibiotics.[14]

Oral Antibiotics

CASE 73-1, QUESTION 6: After 1 week of IV nafcillin, L.D. is afebrile and reports that the pain and tenderness in her left leg are much improved. Her ESR is 40 mm/hour, and CRP is 6 mg/dL. The plan is to switch L.D. to oral antibiotics to complete a 4-week course of therapy at home. What would be an appropriate oral antibiotic regimen for L.D.? How often should she return to the clinic for evaluation?

Again, oral antibiotics are only appropriate if a clear clinical response has occurred within the first week of IV therapy, the patient's parents are aware of the vital importance of compliance, and the patient can swallow and tolerate oral therapy.

Assuming her parents agree to supervise treatment outside of the hospital, L.D. is a candidate for oral therapy. She has responded promptly to the IV therapy: her symptoms have improved, and the ESR and CRP are trending downward. Oral therapy will be effective only if L.D. consistently takes her medications; therefore, assurances must be in place to facilitate compliance. L.D.'s parents have made arrangements with her teacher to help her take her oral antibiotic during the day.

L.D. can complete her 4-week course of antibiotics with oral cephalexin capsules or suspension, which is more palatable (and is usually better tolerated) than dicloxacillin suspension. Cephalexin should begin at 37.5 mg/kg/dose every 6 hours. Weekly follow-up is necessary to monitor compliance and clinical response to therapy. Parenteral therapy should be reinitiated, and re-evaluation is warranted if L.D.'s compliance is not optimal, symptoms recur, or ESR or CRP increases.[4,14] Oral antibiotic doses for children with osteomyelitis are summarized in Table 73-3.[4,9]

Osteomyelitis Secondary to a Contiguous Source of Infection

CLINICAL PRESENTATION

CASE 73-2

QUESTION 1: M.K., a 30-year-old man, suffered an open left femur fracture 3 weeks ago in a motorcycle accident. His fracture was set by open reduction and internal fixation. M.K. had received prophylactic piperacillin/tazobactam for soft-tissue coverage of the

Table 73-3
Oral Antibiotic Doses for the Treatment of Osteomyelitis in Children

Drug	Dose (mg/kg/day)	Doses/day
Penicillin V	125	6
Dicloxacillin	100	4
Amoxicillin	100	4
Cephalexin	150	4
Clindamycin	40	3
Linezolid		
≤12 years	30	3
>12 years	600 mg dose	2

open fracture for 72 hours after hospitalization. His postoperative course was unremarkable until yesterday when he experienced left leg pain and spontaneous drainage from the surgical wound. On presentation, his left thigh is tender, warm, swollen, and erythematous, but he is afebrile. Laboratory data, including WBC count, serum creatinine, and blood urea nitrogen (BUN), are normal, but the ESR is 38 mm/hour and CRP is 8 mg/dL. Plain bone films and bone MRI show inflammation and nonhealing of the femur fracture. What findings in M.K. are characteristic of secondary osteomyelitis?

Few of the systemic signs and symptoms usually associated with acute osteomyelitis are seen in secondary osteomyelitis. The most common subjective complaint in acute contiguous osteomyelitis is pain in the area of infection, localized tenderness, swelling, erythema, and drainage. Considering several weeks might pass before the patient becomes symptomatic, radiographic studies at the time of diagnosis might reveal abnormalities consistent with bone deterioration.[1]

M.K.'s case is consistent with osteomyelitis secondary to a contiguous focus of infection. Infection likely is at the site of surgical repair of the left femur fracture. M.K.'s localized symptoms, along with the absence of fever and leukocytosis, are characteristic of secondary osteomyelitis. In these cases, bone becomes infected from an exogenous source or through spread of an infection from adjacent tissue to bone. Infection can result from any trauma with or without subsequent orthopedic procedure to fix a bone fracture. The bones most commonly involved are the tibia, fibula, femur, and hip.[1]

Unlike hematogenous osteomyelitis, which occurs mostly in children, acute contiguous infection occurs more often in adults. This finding is explained by the higher incidence of precipitating factors within this age-group, such as hip fractures, orthopedic procedures, oral cancers, sternotomy incisions for cardiac surgery, craniotomies, and trauma.[1] Other conditions potentially associated with secondary osteomyelitis include gunshot wounds, punctures, or soft-tissue infections.

Common Pathogens

Case 73-2, Question 2: What organisms are most likely causing infection in M.K.?

Whereas hematogenous osteomyelitis usually involves a single pathogen, polymicrobial infection is common in contiguous-spread osteomyelitis. Although *S. aureus* is the most common pathogen, it is often part of a mixed infection. Other common pathogens include *Pseudomonas*, *Proteus*, *Streptococcus*, and *Klebsiella* species, *E. coli*, and *S. epidermidis*. Most cases of osteomyelitis involving the mandible, pelvis, and small bones (e.g., those of the hands and feet) are caused by gram-negative organisms. *Pseudomonas* often is isolated from infections after puncture wounds of the foot.[1] Anaerobes also are associated with contiguous-spread osteomyelitis, and most commonly isolated are *Bacteroides* species and anaerobic cocci. Possible predisposing factors include previous fractures or injuries resulting from human bites. Adjacent soft-tissue infections can also lead to anaerobic bone infections, as in the case of sacral osteomyelitis secondary to severe decubitus ulcers. To identify the true pathogen(s), M.K. should have surgical re-evaluation and a biopsy of involved bone at the probable site of infection.[1] Bone films and the MRI scan will help localize the possible infectious process to direct the surgical biopsy.

Initial Treatment

Case 73-2, Question 3: M.K. returns to the operating room for surgical exploration, and bone tissue is obtained for culture. He has no drug allergies and weighs 90 kg. The initial postoperative antibiotic order is for vancomycin, 1 g IV every 12 hours. Is this adequate antibiotic treatment for M.K.?

M.K. has had surgery to obtain bone material for culture because cultures of adjacent wound or sinus tract material are not always predictive of the bacteria actually infecting the bone.[1] Broad empiric antibiotic coverage is necessary because *S. aureus* and polymicrobial gram-negative aerobic bacilli most likely are causing this infection.[1]

M.K. has been started on vancomycin for possible MRSA infection while awaiting results of bone tissue cultures. Many clinicians target goal trough concentrations between 15 and 20 mcg/mL for osteomyelitis.[9] Given his normal renal function and weight, M.K. will likely require at least 1.5 g IV every 12 hours of vancomycin (15 mg/kg/dose).

To cover possible pathogenic gram-negative aerobic bacilli, a third- or fourth-generation cephalosporin (cefotaxime, ceftriaxone, ceftazidime, or cefepime) or a quinolone (ciprofloxacin, levofloxacin) could be added. The choice of agent should, in part, be based on local susceptibility patterns. In locations in which quinolone gram-negative resistance approaches 30%, these agents have limited utility.

Anaerobic coverage should be initiated if an anaerobe is cultured from bone or anaerobes are suspected. Vancomycin has activity against gram-positive anaerobes, but not against the gram-negative anaerobe, *Bacteroides fragilis*. If *B. fragilis* is cultured from bone, additional therapy with metronidazole is indicated. Alternatively, combined, broad-spectrum aerobic (including *Pseudomonas*) and anaerobic gram-negative coverage could be provided by a β-lactam/β-lactamase inhibitor combination therapy with piperacillin/tazobactam or a carbapenem.

Although cultures are pending, M.K.'s antibiotic regimen is changed to vancomycin 1.5 g IV every 12 hours and cefepime 2 g IV every 8 hours.

DIRECTED THERAPY

Case 73-2, Question 4: The bone biopsy from M.K. grows MRSA that is sensitive to vancomycin, linezolid, and trimethoprim/sulfamethoxazole. His leg pain is no worse than it was 2 days ago, and he remains afebrile. How should M.K. now be treated? Is he a candidate for oral therapy?

Because no gram-negative organisms grew on culture, cefepime may be discontinued. Therapy should be directed against the MRSA. Thus, it is justified to continue treating M.K. with vancomycin (1.5 g IV every 12 hours) as long as he is monitored closely, following his symptoms, a vancomycin trough level between

 15 and 20 mg/L, weekly ESR or CRP concentrations, complete blood count, and metabolic panel. Vancomycin can be administered at home with the appropriate home health care. Studies have shown that oral antibiotics can achieve adequate concentrations in bone. Based on clinical improvement and provider preference, M.K. can be transitioned to oral linezolid (600 mg twice daily) or trimethoprim-sulfamethoxazole TMP-SMX (4 mg/kg/dose [TMP component] twice daily) in combination with rifampin (600 mg once daily) for a minimum of 8 total weeks of therapy.[9] He should be followed closely for at least 2 years to detect recurrent infection.

Osteomyelitis Associated with Vascular Insufficiency

CLINICAL PRESENTATION

CASE 73-3

QUESTION 1: M.S., a 55-year-old woman, presents to the diabetes clinic with an ulcer 2 cm wide × 1 cm deep on the left lateral aspect of her foot that she first noted a month ago. Her primary care physician had prescribed a 2-week course of ciprofloxacin and gave her instructions for regular wound care. A few days before her clinic visit, the callus surrounding the ulcer cracked open and a small piece of bone protruded from the wound. She reports mild swelling and redness but denies any pain, fever, or chills. Her past medical history includes type 2 diabetes mellitus, hypertension, peripheral neuropathy, and chronic kidney disease requiring hemodialysis 3 times a week. Laboratory findings include WBC 5,200/μL with normal differential, BUN 56 mg/dL, serum creatinine 5.6 mg/dL, fasting blood glucose 240 mg/dL, hemoglobin A_{1c} (Hb A_{1c}) 12.4%, and ESR 45 mm/hour. What findings in M.S. are consistent with osteomyelitis secondary to vascular insufficiency?

M.S. has chronic lower extremity vascular insufficiency as a result of type 2 diabetes. Patients with impaired blood flow may develop osteomyelitis in the toes or small bones of the feet. Infection often first presents as cellulitis, as in M.S.'s case, progressing to deep ulcers and finally to the underlying bone.

Similar to contiguous-spread osteomyelitis, systemic signs of infection (e.g., fever and leukocytosis) are often absent in patients who experience bone infection secondary to vascular insufficiency. Local symptoms such as pain, swelling, and erythema usually predominate, but there are no specific clinical findings.[15]

M.S. may have a bone infection under the chronic, cutaneous ulcer on the bottom of her left great toe. Because of peripheral neuropathy, the skin lesion may not be painful, and poor blood supply to the site likely contributed to the development of a chronic infection and possibly secondary osteomyelitis. The true depth of an ulcer is not always clinically apparent so careful physical examination and evaluation of patient risk factors are essential for diagnosis.[15] Infection is suggested by her elevated ESR, fasting glucose (consistent with infection), and Hb A_{1c} (indicating uncontrolled diabetes). In addition, diabetic foot ulcers with an area larger than 2 cm^2 or that penetrate to bone are often predictive for underlying osteomyelitis.[15]

ANTIBIOTIC SELECTION

CASE 73-3, QUESTION 2: M.S. is admitted into the hospital for diagnostic workup, wound care, and antibiotics. Plain films show destruction of the distal left fifth metatarsal with bony changes consistent with osteomyelitis. Her wound is debrided, and material obtained from a bone biopsy is sent to the microbiology laboratory for cultures. She has no drug allergies and is started on vancomycin (1 g IV every 12 hours) and oral ciprofloxacin (750 mg every 12 hours). Is this appropriate initial, empiric therapy?

In many cases of osteomyelitis associated with vascular insufficiency, multiple pathogens can be cultured from surgical specimens or the wound. The most commonly isolated pathogen is *S. aureus*; however, gram-negative and anaerobic bacteria are also often recovered. The bacteria isolated from a wound or soft-tissue culture may not correlate with bacteria found in a concomitant bone biopsy.[15,16] Therefore, empiric antibiotic therapy for osteomyelitis associated with vascular insufficiency should be active against both gram-positive and gram-negative aerobic bacteria and possibly anaerobes. No specific regimens have demonstrated superiority, so a broad-spectrum empiric regimen can be chosen based on local sensitivity patterns.[1] An antipseudomonal β-lactam (ceftazidime, cefepime) or quinolone (ciprofloxacin, levofloxacin) for gram-negative coverage is frequently used as an empiric regimen. If anaerobic bacteria are believed to be clinically involved (e.g., foul-smelling wound), metronidazole should be added to the regimen; alternatively an antipseudomonal β-lactam/β-lactamase inhibitor combination, such as piperacillin-tazobactam, can be used.

M.S. has risk factors for MRSA and resistant gram-negative bacilli because of her diabetes, hemodialysis, and recent course of antibiotics. The initial regimen of vancomycin and ciprofloxacin for M.S. is not optimal for several reasons. Because of her recent, prolonged ciprofloxacin exposure, a quinolone-resistant organism may be responsible for infection and a β-lactam-based antibiotic regimen would be more appropriate. Secondly, IV antibiotics should be used during initial treatment. Lastly, M.S. is dialysis-dependent, and the antibiotic regimen selected should be dose-adjusted according to her renal function. A more appropriate empiric regimen for M.S. would be vancomycin intermittently dosed based on serum drug concentrations and her dialysis regimen, and cefepime 1 g IV every 24 hours with the dose administered after dialysis on dialysis days.

Further antibiotic refinement should occur after the results of the deep wound swab culture are available. The optimal duration of IV therapy for diabetic foot osteomyelitis is patient-dependent, and some patients may require longer-term, oral suppressive therapy. The overall duration of antibiotic treatment can range from 6 weeks to many months depending on the degree of surgical debridement and the healing rate of the ulcer.[15] Oral linezolid (600 mg every 12 hours) has been used to treat MRSA osteomyelitis in diabetic patients, although long-term therapy can be associated with hematologic and neuropathic adverse effects.[17]

M.S. should be made aware that osteomyelitis associated with diabetic foot ulcers is difficult to treat. Despite adequate surgical debridement of the infection followed by appropriate treatment with long-term IV and oral antibiotic therapy, cure rates are low. Even minor amputations (one or two toes) are unsuccessful in eradicating infection. Radical surgical approaches, such as transmetatarsal, below-the-knee, or above-the-knee amputations, often are necessary to cure these infections.[1]

Chronic Osteomyelitis

CLINICAL PRESENTATION

CASE 73-4

QUESTION 1: J.F., a 52-year-old man, sustained a fracture of the right humerus in a farming accident 6 years ago. That fracture clinically healed without any immediate consequences; however, 1 year ago, a draining sinus tract developed at the site of the previous fracture without any antecedent events. He has taken various oral antibiotics during this last year, including amoxicillin and levofloxacin, which he stopped taking 2 months ago. Two weeks ago he noted increased sinus drainage, pain, swelling, and erythema of his left upper arm, and levofloxacin was restarted. A swab culture of the sinus drainage grew *S. epidermidis*, *E. coli*, *Peptostreptococcus micros*, and *Bacteroides* species. Surgical debridement of bone and tissue was performed because of increased drainage and poor appearance of the wound. Gentamicin-impregnated polymethylmethacrylate (PMMA) beads were placed in the tissue adjacent to the debrided bone during surgery. Bone cultures grew *Proteus mirabilis* and *B. fragilis*. The *Proteus* was resistant to ampicillin, cefazolin, levofloxacin, and tigecycline, but sensitive to cefotaxime, ceftriaxone, imipenem, gentamicin, and trimethoprim-sulfamethoxazole. Antibiotic susceptibilities for the *Bacteroides* were not tested. What aspects of J.F.'s case are characteristic of chronic osteomyelitis?

Inadequate treatment of an acute episode of osteomyelitis can lead to formation of necrotic, infected bone and recurrent symptoms consistent with chronic disease. Despite appropriate initial therapy, osteomyelitis can reactivate, even with organisms different from the initial episode. Some propose that previously infected bone might be a risk for reinfection. Persistent symptoms or signs lasting longer than 10 days are consistent with chronic osteomyelitis and the development of necrotic bone. Draining sinus tracts often develop from the bone to the skin with chronic osteomyelitis.[1,18]

J.F. probably experienced a chronic bone infection after the farming accident. The reappearance of sinus tract drainage in his left upper arm indicates an indolent infection of bone that was periodically suppressed, but not completely treated by oral antibiotics. Cultures of sinus drainage now reveal multiple organisms including normal skin flora. These sinus tract cultures usually do not correlate with the organisms actually causing bone infection. J.F.'s recurrent course of bone involvement with drainage and local symptoms, and lack of any remarkable systemic symptoms, suggests chronic osteomyelitis.[18]

SURGERY AND ORAL ANTIBIOTICS

CASE 73-4, QUESTION 2: Oral levofloxacin (500 mg daily) was restarted 2 weeks ago when J.F.'s left arm became more painful and drainage increased. Was his poor response to therapy unexpected? How should his case have been managed?

J.F.'s poor response should have been expected for at least two reasons: Antibiotic therapy was started before surgical debridement of avascular tissue, and he was given an antibiotic that was inactive against the cultured bone organisms.

Surgery plays an important role in the treatment of chronic osteomyelitis. Bone necrosis will continue to progress if decompression and drainage of the infected area is not carried out as soon as possible. Furthermore, without initial surgical removal of necrotic bone (sequestrum) and other poorly vascularized, infected material, even the most optimal IV antibiotics are likely to fail.

After surgery, antibiotic therapy directed against the pathogens isolated in the surgical specimens should be started. The regimen choice should not be based on the sinus tract culture results because these isolates may not correlate with the actual causative organisms. J.F. should be treated initially with IV antibiotics because of relatively poor blood flow at the infection site. Although the optimal duration of therapy for chronic osteomyelitis is not well established, the standard recommendation has been parenteral therapy for 6 weeks, followed by oral antibiotic therapy, depending on the healing rate.[19] However, based on more recent data with oral antibiotics in chronic osteomyelitis, the susceptibility of the antibiotic for the organism is more relevant than the route of administration.[19,20] J.F. should continue to be evaluated by an orthopedic surgeon because he may require further surgical treatment to eradicate chronically infected bone.

INTRAVENOUS ANTIBIOTICS

CASE 73-4, QUESTION 3: What would be reasonable antibiotic therapy for J.F.?

On the basis of the bone culture and sensitivity results, J.F. needs high-dose therapy directed at *P. mirabilis* and *B. fragilis*. For convenience and possible future home therapy, ceftriaxone (2 g IV every 24 hours) could be started for coverage of *Proteus* and metronidazole (500 mg IV every 8 hours) also should be started for coverage of *B. fragilis*. Because of excellent oral bioavailability, the metronidazole can be rapidly converted to oral therapy at the same dose before discharge. Ertapenem could be an alternative choice for home IV therapy assuming that the *Proteus* isolate is sensitive. This agent also provides excellent anaerobic activity, and its once-daily dosing (1 g IV every 24 hours) is convenient for home therapy.

After 6 to 8 weeks of home parenteral therapy, J.F. should be evaluated for response. If symptoms have abated, treatment with oral antibiotics (trimethoprim-sulfamethoxazole and metronidazole) may commence and should continue for an additional 6 to 8 weeks or longer depending on resolution of the sinus tract drainage, pain, and tenderness in J.F.'s arm. Under these circumstances, he should be monitored closely for possible long-term adverse drug effects (e.g., hepatitis, cytopenias, neuropathy). If the sinus tract does not heal or if J.F. remains symptomatic, surgical exploration and bone cultures must be repeated.

LOCAL ANTIBIOTICS

CASE 73-4, QUESTION 4: What is the rationale for and effectiveness of local antibiotic administration (the PMMA beads) inserted during J.F.'s orthopedic surgery?

To deliver high concentrations of antibiotics to poorly vascularized bone infection sites, various materials containing antibiotics can be placed at the infection site during surgery. Plaster pellets, fibrin, collagen, hydroxyapatite, and PMMA impregnated with antibiotic, usually an aminoglycoside or vancomycin, have been used. The dosage form is designed for the slow release of antibiotics from the material. The most commonly reported experience with local antibiotic delivery has been with antibiotic-impregnated PMMA cement or beads inserted during joint arthroplasty. Local delivery of antibiotics should not replace systemic antibiotics in the treatment of chronic osteomyelitis.[21]

Osteomyelitis Associated with Prosthetic Material

USUAL CLINICAL PRESENTATION

CASE 73-5

QUESTION 1: A.T., a 47-year-old woman, had a left knee replacement 1 year ago for osteoarthritis. She is seen today in the orthopedic clinic because of increasing left knee pain for the past 2 months. The knee is painful and warm. She is afebrile, and her peripheral WBC count is 9,800/μL. Aspiration of fluid from the knee reveals a total nucleated cell count of 78,000/μL with 90% neutrophils. A Gram stain of this fluid shows 4+ polymorphonuclear leukocytes (PMN) and 1+ gram-positive cocci. She is started on antibiotic therapy with vancomycin and ciprofloxacin pending culture results, and she is scheduled for operative evaluation and possible removal of her prosthetic joint. Does A.T. have a prosthetic joint infection?

Joint replacement surgery is commonly performed for patients with significant joint destruction as a result of arthritis and other disabling diseases. Prosthetic knee, shoulder, elbow, or hip devices made of metallic alloys are cemented to adjacent bone to re-establish joint function. Infection of these foreign bodies can occur because of exogenous inoculation of bacteria perioperatively, via hematogenous dissemination of bacteria, or by contiguous spread from a topical wound. Bacteria infect bone adjacent to the joint prosthesis, including the bone–cement interface, resulting in a loosened and less functional prosthesis.[22] *Staphylococcus* species including coagulase-negative species such as *S. epidermidis* are most commonly involved in prosthetic joint infections, followed by *Streptococcus* species, gram-negative bacilli, and anaerobes. Although coagulase-negative staphylococci are usually considered a contaminant in culture, this organism readily adheres to prosthetic material and should be considered pathogenic when cultured from prostheses. Coagulase-negative staphylococci are often methicillin-resistant but susceptible to vancomycin.

Chronic pain, swelling, erythema, and tenderness over a prosthetic joint are typical findings associated with prosthetic joint infection. Persistent wound drainage may also be present. A.T. has had a relatively lengthy duration of symptoms associated with her left knee, which could be caused by joint loosening, but the cell count and differential from the joint aspirate suggest joint infection. Consistent with infected prosthesis is also the predominance of neutrophils in her joint fluid and gram-positive cocci on a Gram stain. As is often the case, she has no obvious preceding source of infection from which bacteria may have originated. Occasionally, sources of infection with hematogenous dissemination to the prosthetic joint are identified, such as dental infections, cellulitis, or urinary tract infections. Given the Gram stain result, A.T. should receive coverage for *Staphylococcus* and *Streptococcus* species with vancomycin while awaiting the results of cultures and sensitivities. Because gram-negative bacteria also can infect these joints, gram-negative coverage is reasonable until the results of joint fluid cultures are available.

SURGERY

CASE 73-5, QUESTION 2: Does A.T. need surgery and antibiotics to cure her infection?

Surgical removal of A.T.'s knee prosthesis in conjunction with intravenous antibiotics for 6 weeks is the current recommendation for optimal eradication of prosthetic joint infection.[22,23] A two-stage orthopedic procedure is frequently used that involves removal of the infected prosthesis, placement of an antibiotic-filled spacer, joint immobilization, and antibiotics for 6 weeks. If the joint space remains culture negative after 2 weeks of antibiotics, a new joint prosthesis is then reinserted. Because avascular bone cement and prosthetic material can become seeded with bacteria, complete removal of this material is necessary to have the greatest chance of curing the infection. Six weeks of systemic antibiotic therapy in combination with orthopedic surgery results in restoration of joint function in 80% to 90% of cases. High rates of treatment failure occur if the joint prosthesis is not removed, if the antibiotic duration is too short, and if chronic suppressive antibiotics are not given.[22,23]

ANTIBIOTICS

CASE 73-5, QUESTION 3: The surgeon is unable to completely remove A.T.'s prosthetic joint. The removed lining material and three swabs of the left knee prosthesis grow MRSA. What antibiotic regimen could be used? How long should A.T. be treated?

Because A.T.'s prosthesis cannot be removed, she will need 2 to 6 weeks of vancomycin (15 mg/kg IV Q12 hours) plus oral rifampin (300–450 mg PO BID), followed by 6 months of oral antibiotics plus rifampin.[23] Daptomycin (6–10 mg/kg IV daily) or linezolid (600 mg PO/IV Q12 hours) may be considered alternatives to vancomycin, depending on pathogen susceptibility, drug allergies or intolerances, and potential drug–drug interactions.[23,24] However, these agents are not FDA-approved for prosthetic joint infections, and they require monitoring for adverse effects, such as creatine kinase elevations (daptomycin) and bone marrow suppression and neuropathy (linezolid).[22] Combination therapy with rifampin should be used for prosthetic joint infection caused by staphylococci, particularly if removal of the infected prosthesis is not possible, because rifampin penetrates bacterial membranes and biofilms to enhance the bactericidal activity of the antibiotic regimen. Monotherapy with rifampin should never be used because of rapid development of resistance.[25,26] Rifampin induces the metabolism of multiple other agents (e.g., warfarin, anticonvulsants, azole antifungals); therefore, a thorough review of A.T.'s medication profile is critical. A.T.'s baseline liver function should also be evaluated and rechecked at least monthly while she is taking rifampin.[27] Additionally, weekly assessment of A.T.'s complete blood count and renal function along with periodic vancomycin trough serum concentrations should be performed.[28]

SEPTIC ARTHRITIS

Septic arthritis or infectious arthritis is usually acquired hematogenously. The highly vascular synovium of the joint allows easy passage of bacteria from blood into the synovial space. Bacteremia, secondary to *Neisseria gonorrhoeae* or *S. aureus* in particular, often is associated with joint infections. Septic arthritis also can develop secondary to inoculation of pathogens due to trauma, including puncture (e.g., animal bites, nail) or surgery, as well as via contiguous spread from osteomyelitis.[29]

Several factors predispose patients to the development of infectious arthritis. Patients with abnormal joint structure, including rheumatoid arthritis (RA), prosthetic joints, or recent joint surgery, are more susceptible to the development of infection. Patients with age greater than 80 years, diabetes mellitus, and chronic illnesses such as malignancy and chronic renal failure are also at an increased risk. Gonococcal arthritis may occur in those who have been exposed to or are infected with *N. gonorrhoeae*.[29]

Clinical Presentation of Nongonococcal Arthritis

CASE 73-6

QUESTION 1: C.H., a 45-year-old man, is referred to the rheumatology clinic for left knee swelling. Two days ago, his left knee became painful and swollen, and he is unable to flex the joint. He also recorded temperatures at home of 100.7°F to 102°F for at least 4 days. In clinic, a joint effusion is noted, and fluid is aspirated for cell count, Gram stain, and culture. His medical history is unremarkable. C.H.'s WBC count is 16,000/μL, and his ESR is 42 mm/hour. The synovial fluid from his right knee contains 30,000 WBC/μL with 90% neutrophils, and the Gram stain shows gram-positive cocci in clusters. Culture results are pending. His temperature is 38.5°C. What findings in C.H. are consistent with septic arthritis?

C.H. has an acute onset of monoarticular joint pain and swelling, with reduced range of motion and fever. These findings are classic for septic, nongonococcal arthritis. The joint effusion shows a predominance of neutrophils, which confirms the diagnosis. C.H.'s knee has been infected hematogenously from a distant, unrecognized, source of infection. The knee is infected most frequently, and the most common causative pathogens are Gram-positive, including *Staphylococcus*, *Streptococcus*, and *Enterococcus* species.

A single joint is infected in 80% to 90% of nongonococcal arthritis cases. Other possible sites of infectious arthritis in adults besides the knee include the hip, shoulder, sternoclavicular, sacroiliac, and ankle joints.[29] Patients commonly present with fever, pain, swelling, redness, and decreased mobility of the involved joint.

As illustrated by C.H., most patients have joint effusion on physical examination. When evaluating a patient with possible septic arthritis, any purulent joint effusion should be considered septic until proven otherwise. Alternatively, noninfectious conditions may be present, such as single joint involvement with synovial effusions in acute RA, gout, or chondrocalcinosis.[29]

Aspirated joint fluid should be cultured because isolation of bacteria is the only definitive diagnostic test for bacterial arthritis. C.H.'s joint fluid picture is typical. The leukocyte count in the synovial fluid usually is elevated significantly, with counts above 50,000/μL with a predominance of neutrophils (>75%). Blood cultures are positive in 25% to 70% of patients.

Another laboratory finding in C.H. consistent with infectious arthritis is the elevated ESR and peripheral WBC count. CRP is frequently elevated as well, although both ESR and CRP are nonspecific markers of inflammation and can be elevated due to causes other than infectious arthritis.

The patient's age impacts the most common bacterial cause of infection. In adults older than 30 years of age such as C.H., and in children older than 2 years of age, *S. aureus* is the most common bacterial source. In sexually active young adults, *N. gonorrhoeae* is more likely to be the causative agent. Streptococci, such as group A β-hemolytic streptococci, can cause infection in children and adults. Other organisms, such as group B streptococci, anaerobic streptococci, and gram-negative bacteria, can also cause infection. Gram-negative bacilli are responsible for approximately 5% to 20% of cases and often infect multiple joints. Infections with gram-negative bacteria usually are associated with predisposing factors, such as RA, osteoarthritis, history of joint surgery, intra-articular injections, or intravenous drug use. An organism commonly isolated from patients with bacterial arthritis who have a history of IV drug use is *P. aeruginosa*.[29,30]

Initial Antimicrobial Therapy

Case 73-6, Question 2: How should C.H. be treated, and for how long? How should the efficacy of treatment be monitored?

Treatment of nongonococcal arthritis includes drainage of purulent joint fluid (by needle aspiration or surgery) and appropriate antibiotic therapy. Because of the increasing frequency of community-acquired MRSA causing infection, initial empiric therapy with vancomycin (15 mg/kg/dose IV every 12 hours, goal serum trough concentration 15–20 mg/L) should be initiated to provide coverage for this and streptococci in C.H. Daptomycin and linezolid are typically reserved for patients with vancomycin intermediate-susceptible or resistant gram-positive organisms or those patients with intolerance or allergy to vancomycin. Vancomycin can be changed on the basis of sensitivity testing to oxacillin, nafcillin, or cefazolin if the isolated organism is susceptible.[29,30]

DURATION OF THERAPY

No high-quality studies have been performed to determine the optimal duration of therapy for bacterial arthritis.[30] Previous recommendations based on early clinical trials recommended treating for 2 to 3 weeks.[31] However, current recommendations are to initiate therapy with at least 2 weeks of IV antibiotics, followed by oral antibiotics (if possible based on susceptibilities) for at least 4 more weeks.[29,30]

C.H. should be treated for at least 4 weeks.[29,30] His response to therapy should be monitored clinically (resolution of symptoms, fever, and falling ESR, CRP, or both) as well as by periodic evaluation of joint fluid. Frequent aspirations of joint fluid via closed-needle aspiration or following arthroscopic lavage, and debridement and insertion of drains will permit daily evaluation of cell count and fluid culture. Effective therapy should result in a decreasing WBC count in the joint fluid and negative cultures, usually within 3 to 4 days of treatment.[29]

Joint inflammation and other symptoms also should diminish during the first week of treatment. The duration of articular symptoms before antibiotic therapy begun correlates with the subsequent time required to sterilize the synovial fluid. Therefore, delay in initiating antibiotic treatment may necessitate a longer course of therapy.

Similar to hematogenous osteomyelitis, oral antibiotics have been used in septic arthritis to complete treatment if the initial response to IV therapy is adequate for some pathogens and in patients at lower risk for recurrent infection.[29,30] C.H. should be advised that parenteral treatment with vancomycin, which can be accomplished at home, would be the most effective mode of treatment if his cultures grow MRSA, because this pathogen typically requires 4 weeks of IV antibiotics. Finally, injections of antibiotics into the joint space are of no value. Most systemic antibiotics readily penetrate the joint space and enter the synovial fluid.

Gonococcal Arthritis

Polyarticular arthritis in a young, sexually active adult is caused most commonly by *N. gonorrhoeae*. Arthritis in multiple joints is a common feature of disseminated gonococcal infection (DGI). Unlike nongonococcal arthritis, which is almost exclusively monoarticular, gonococcal arthritis involves multiple joints in approximately 50% of cases. Women have a four-fold increased risk of developing gonococcal arthritis as compared with men, often due to delays in diagnosis of genital infection.[29,32] Clinically, patients present with a migratory polyarthralgia often with fever, dermatitis, and tenosynovitis. Skin lesions are an important clue to the diagnosis of DGI and often begin as tiny erythematous papules and develop into larger vesicles. As in hematogenously acquired nongonococcal arthritis, the synovial fluid leukocyte count usually is elevated, but often to a lesser degree. *N. gonorrhoeae* is recovered in approximately 50% of purulent joint effusions, but is detected using polymerase chain reaction (PCR) assays that have approximately 96% specificity and 80% sensitivity. These laboratory studies, coupled with the patient's clinical presentation, can be used to make a definitive diagnosis.[29,32]

CLINICAL PRESENTATION OF GONOCOCCAL ARTHRITIS

CASE 73-7

Question 1: E.D, a 21-year-old woman, presents to the walk-in clinic with right knee and right shoulder pain, nausea, and vomiting. On physical examination, her right knee is swollen and she has decreased range of motion of her right shoulder. Several erythematous, papular skin lesions are noted on both hands. She also has a vaginal discharge. Her temperature is 38.2°C, and her WBC count is 15,000/μL. She gives a history of having two recent sexual partners. Cultures of blood, joint fluid, and vaginal discharge are obtained; a joint fluid Gram stain shows 4+ PMNs, but no organisms are seen. Why is E.D. considered to have gonococcal arthritis?

E.D. has systemic signs of infection (fever, nausea, vomiting, leukocytosis), skin lesions, and multiple joint involvement, which are classic for DGI. Her history of recent sexual activity and the presence of a vaginal discharge are consistent with gonococcal infection, although evidence of mucosal infection with *N. gonorrhoeae* is not necessary for disseminated infection to occur.[29,32]

PATIENT WORKUP AND TREATMENT IN THE CLINIC

CASE 73-7, QUESTION 2: What additional workup should be done in E.D.? Can she be treated immediately in the clinic?

E.D. should be evaluated for other sexually transmitted diseases, specifically syphilis and HIV infection. Serologic testing for syphilis (rapid plasma reagent [RPR] or venereal disease research laboratory [VDRL] testing) and for antibody to HIV should be obtained. In addition, she should have a pregnancy test because some of the antibiotics that may be used are contraindicated during pregnancy, including doxycycline.

Because of possible penicillinase production by *N. gonorrhoeae*, recommended therapy is with ceftriaxone (1 g intramuscularly or IV every 24 hours) for at least 7 days. E.D. should receive her first dose of ceftriaxone in the clinic today. Conversion to oral antibiotics should be guided by antimicrobial susceptibility testing following 24 to 48 hours of clinical improvement by the patient.[33]

E.D.'s sexual partners should also be evaluated and treated for relevant sexually transmitted diseases. She should also be counseled on utilization of barrier methods (e.g., condoms) to prevent sexually transmitted infections.

FULL COURSE OF THERAPY

CASE 73-7, QUESTION 3: Results of RPR and pregnancy testing in E.D. are negative. How should she complete her course of therapy?

E.D.'s DGI should be treated for at least 7 days. E.D. also should begin treatment with azithromycin (1 g orally once) or doxycycline (100 mg orally twice daily for 7 days) for the possibility of concomitant chlamydial infection. Azithromycin is preferred because of increasing resistance with tetracyclines.[34] Treatment guidelines for DGI are also included in the gonorrhea section of Chapter 72, Sexually Transmitted Diseases.

KEY REFERENCES AND WEBSITES

A full list of references for this chapter can be found at http://thepoint.lww.com/AT11e. Below are the key references and website for this chapter, with the corresponding reference number in this chapter found in parentheses after the reference.

Key References

Berbari EF et al. Osteomyelitis. In: Mandell GL et al., eds. *Mandell, Douglas, and Bennett's Principles and Practice of Infectious Diseases*. 8th ed. Philadelphia, PA: Elsevier Churchill Livingstone; 2015:1318. (1)

Conterno LO, Turchi MD. Antibiotics for treating chronic osteomyelitis in adults (review). *Cochrane Database Syst Rev*. 2013;9:CD004439. (20)

Forrest GN, Tamura K. Rifampin combination therapy for nonmycobacterial infections. *Clin Microbiol Rev*. 2010;23(1):14. (25)

Keren R et al. Comparative effectiveness of intravenous vs oral antibiotics for postdischarge treatment of acute osteomyelitis in children. *JAMA Pediatr*. 2015;169(2):120–128. (12)

Lipsky BA et al. 2012 Infectious Diseases Society of America clinical practice guideline for the diagnosis and treatment of diabetic foot infections. *Clin Infect Dis*. 2012;54(12):e132–e173. (15)

Liu C et al. Clinical practice guidelines by the Infectious Diseases Society of America for the treatment of methicillin-resistant *Staphylococcus Aureus* infections in adults and children. *Clin Infect Dis*. 2011;52(3):e18–e55. (9)

Osmon DR et al. Diagnosis and management of prosthetic joint infection: clinical practice guidelines by the Infectious Diseases Society of America. *Clin Infect Dis*. 2013;56(1):e1. (23)

Spellberg B, Lipsky BA. Systemic antibiotic therapy for chronic osteomyelitis in adults. *Clin Infect Dis*. 2012;54(3):393–407. (19)

Zimmerli W, Sendi P. Orthopedic implant-associated infections. In: Bennett JE et al., eds. *Mandell, Douglas, and Bennett's Principles and Practice of Infectious Diseases*. 8th ed. Philadelphia, PA: Elsevier Churchill Livingstone; 2015:1328. (22)

Additional Reference

Berbari EF et al. 2015 Infectious Diseases Society of America (IDSA) clinical practice guidelines for the diagnosis and treatment of native vertebral osteomyelitis in adults. *Clin Infect Dis*. 2015;61(6):e26–e46.

Key Websites

Centers for Disease Control and Prevention, Sexually Transmitted Diseases Treatment Guidelines, 2015. http://www.cdc.gov/mmwr/preview/mmwrhtml/rr6403a1.htm. Accessed December 2, 2015.

74 Skin and Soft Tissue Infections

Cheryl R. Durand and Kristine C. Willett

CORE PRINCIPLES

	CHAPTER CASES
SKIN AND SOFT TISSUE INFECTIONS	
1 Cellulitis (an acute inflammation of the skin and subcutaneous fat) is characterized by local tenderness, pain, swelling, warmth, and erythema with or without a definite entry point.	**Case 74-1 (Question 1)**
2 Cellulitis is most often caused by group A β-hemolytic streptococci (*Streptococcus pyogenes*) and, less often, *Staphylococcus aureus*.	**Case 74-1 (Question 1), Table 74-1**
3 Community-acquired methicillin-resistant *S. aureus* (CA-MRSA) may be a causative pathogen, especially in high-risk patients (children, competitive athletes, prisoners, soldiers, selected ethnic populations, Native Americans/Alaska Natives, Pacific Islanders, intravenous drug users, men who have sex with men), and empiric treatment should have activity against CA-MRSA.	**Case 74-1 (Question 1)**
4 For most cases of cellulitis requiring antibiotics, the least expensive of dicloxacillin or cephalexin should be chosen. Cases of cellulitis as evidenced by signs of systemic infection require parenteral antibiotics. The duration of therapy should be at least 5 days.	**Case 74-1 (Questions 1, 4)** **Case 74-2 (Question 1)**
5 Conversion to oral antibiotic therapy should be considered when patients show signs of clinical improvement and are afebrile for at least 24 hours.	**Case 74-2 (Questions 3, 4)**
6 Abscesses, furuncles, and carbuncles are commonly caused by *S. aureus* and should be managed with incision and drainage. Antibiotic therapy is warranted when systemic inflammatory response syndrome is present.	**Case 74-3 (Questions 2, 3), Table 74-1**
ERYSIPELAS	
1 Oral or parenteral penicillins, with activity against group A streptococci, are the drugs of choice for treatment.	**Case 74-4 (Question 1), Table 74-1**
SKIN AND SOFT TISSUE INFECTIONS IN DIABETIC PATIENTS	
1 Skin and soft tissue infections are very common in diabetic patients with approximately 25% of patients reporting a history of skin and soft tissue infection.	**Case 74-5 (Question 1)**
2 Mild infections in diabetics can be treated similar to cellulitis (Gram-positive coverage), whereas moderate-to-severe infections require broad-spectrum coverage.	**Case 74-5 (Questions 1, 2) Table 74-1**
NECROTIZING SOFT TISSUE INFECTIONS	
1 Necrotizing soft tissue infections can progress rapidly to cause local (e.g., necrosis and loss of skin sensation) and severe systemic effects (e.g., hypotension, shock).	**Case 74-6 (Question 1)**
2 Initial treatment of necrotizing soft tissue infections involves extensive debridement to remove all necrotic tissue, fluid resuscitation, and broad-spectrum antibiotics.	**Case 74-6 (Question 1), Table 74-1**

Continued

	CHAPTER CASES
ANIMAL BITES	
1 The oral flora of animals (cats, dogs) necessitates irrigation to reduce risk of infection and may include aerobic or anaerobic organisms. Amoxicillin/clavulanate is the preferred first-line agent.	**Case 74-7 (Questions 1, 2) Table 74-1**
HUMAN BITES	
1 Treating a human bite is similar to any other laceration, including cleansing, irrigating, exploring, debriding, draining, excising, and suturing, as required. Human-bite infections can be caused by aerobic and anaerobic organisms and should be treated with amoxicillin/clavulanate or ampicillin/sulbactam, or ertapenem.	**Case 74-8 (Question 1), Table 74-1**

Skin and soft tissue infections may involve any or all layers of the skin (epidermis, dermis), subcutaneous fat, fascia, or muscle. Many terms or classifications are used to describe various skin and soft tissue infections, and these often are based on the site of infection and causative organism(s).[1] This chapter focuses on skin and soft tissue infections that are primarily the result of a break in the skin after an abrasion, skin puncture, ulceration, surgical wound, intentional or unintentional insertion of a foreign body, or blunt soft tissue contusion. Treatment of skin and soft tissue infections often is empiric and based on the severity and site of infection, presence of purulence, the patient's underlying immunocompetence, and the triggering event (e.g., abrasion, bite, insertion of a foreign object) because attempts to isolate the causative organism often are futile.

SKIN AND SOFT TISSUE INFECTIONS

Cellulitis (an acute inflammation of the skin and subcutaneous fat) is characterized by local tenderness, pain, swelling, warmth, and erythema with or without a definite entry point. Cellulitis is usually secondary to trauma or an underlying skin lesion that allows bacterial penetration into the skin and underlying tissues. Cellulitis is most often caused by group A β-hemolytic streptococci (*Streptococcus pyogenes*) and other streptococcus species (B, C, F, or G), and less often, *Staphylococcus aureus* (Table 74-1).[2] However, if the patient presents with abscess, purulence, or penetrating trauma, coverage of *S. aureus* is indicated.[2] Coverage for community-acquired methicillin-resistant *S. aureus* (CA-MRSA) may be warranted because the incidence has been increasing.[3] Gram-negative organisms (e.g., *Escherichia coli, Pseudomonas aeruginosa, Klebsiella pneumoniae*) also can cause cellulitis, but should be suspected only in immunocompromised patients or in patients who fail to respond to antibiotics that have activity limited to Gram-positive organisms. Wound cultures often are negative and fail to identify the causative organism.

Severity of infection is based upon presence of systemic signs of infection, failure of oral antibiotics, and immunocompetence. Cases of mild cellulitis without signs of systemic infection often require treatment with antibiotics active against streptococci. Patients with evidence of a systemic infection, suggesting a moderate-to-severe infection, will require intravenous [IV] antibiotics, in addition to local wound care. Severe infections occur in patients who have failed oral antibiotic therapy or those that are immunocompromised. Antibiotic selection is based on the suspected etiology as well as severity of infection.

In addition to cellulitis, skin and soft tissue infections include abscesses, furuncles, and carbuncles. A skin abscess is an infection and results in a collection of pus within the dermis and deep skin tissues.[2] Furuncles are abscesses that initiate in the hair follicle and penetrate into the surrounding subcutaneous tissue, whereas carbuncles are a coalescence of furuncles.

Table 74-1
Potential Organisms Causing Skin and Soft Tissue Infections

	Gram Positive		Gram Negative		Anaerobes			
	Staphylococcal	**Streptococcal**	***Escherichia coli, Klebsiella species, Proteus Species***	***Pasteurella multocida***	***Eikenella corrodens***	***Oral Anaerobes***	***Clostridium Species***	***Bacteroides fragilis***
Cellulitis	X	X						
Diabetic soft tissue	X	X	X					X
Necrotizing infections	X	X	X			X	X	X
Erysipelas		X						
Animal bites	X	X	X	X		X		
Human bites	X	X	X		X	X		

X, organisms that should be covered empirically with appropriate antibiotic therapy.

CASE 74-1

QUESTION 1: N.P., a 25-year-old woman, presents to her family doctor with a 2- to 3-day history of worsening pain, redness, and swelling on her left leg after an abrasion that occurred after falling while jogging in the park. The area is red, painful, nonpurulent, and warm to the touch. During the past 24 to 36 hours, the leg has become increasingly painful and "tight." N.P. denies having fever or chills. The presumptive diagnosis is a mild cellulitis, and dicloxacillin is prescribed. Why is dicloxacillin appropriate empiric treatment for N.P.?

Oral dicloxacillin is appropriate empiric therapy for cellulitis in an otherwise healthy individual with no signs or symptoms of systemic infection, regardless of presence of purulence. Dicloxacillin has predictable activity against streptococcus and methicillin-sensitive staphylococcus organisms and is better tolerated than erythromycin or clindamycin. Because the patient presents with nonpurulent cellulitis, penicillin VK is also an option; however, it lacks coverage against staphylococcus. If the cellulitis is well demarcated and nonpurulent, penicillin alone can be appropriate because the causative organism is likely to be *Streptococcus*. Many other available antibiotics that have activity against staphylococcus and streptococcus organisms have been evaluated for effectiveness in skin and soft tissue infections. A recent review concluded that the available evidence does not allow specific recommendations for the best antibiotic regimen for cellulitis.[3,4] Cephalexin is probably as effective and as well tolerated as dicloxacillin and is comparable in cost. However, the Gram-negative activity of cephalexin (not present with dicloxacillin) is not required for most cases of cellulitis in otherwise healthy patients. In this case, antibiotic treatment is required, and N.P. can receive dicloxacillin or cephalexin.

In geographic areas where the incidence of CA-MRSA has become clinically important (>10% of isolates), particularly with additional risk factors (children, competitive athletes, prisoners, soldiers, selected ethnic populations, Native Americans/Alaska Natives, Pacific Islanders, IV drug users, men who have sex with men), empiric treatment should include antibiotics with activity against CA-MRSA.[5] In cases in which there is an abscess without signs of systemic infection, drainage is often all that is needed because antibiotic therapy has been shown to be no better than placebo for uncomplicated skin abscesses in a population at risk for CA-MRSA infection.[6] At present, most CA-MRSA are still susceptible to trimethoprim-sulfamethoxazole, clindamycin, and doxycycline.[2] Although trimethoprim-sulfamethoxazole has good activity against *S. aureus,* its activity against *S. pyogenes,* that is group A streptococci, is weak, making this antibiotic undesirable alone as empiric therapy. If these agents are used, a reasonable suggestion would be to re-evaluate (by the patient if they are competent) within 24 to 48 hours to verify that an improvement is occurring. Some clinicians avoid the use of clindamycin because of concerns of inducible resistance. In areas with a clinically important incidence of CA-MRSA, laboratories should test for inducible clindamycin resistance. If N.P. is from an area of high CA-MRSA prevalence and has associated risk factors, the combination of trimethoprim-sulfamethoxazole or doxycycline with beta-lactam (penicillin, cephalexin, amoxicillin) would provide therapy for the anticipated pathogens. However, even in areas of high CA-MRSA prevalence, some investigations have found cephalexin to be as effective as therapy specifically targeted for CA-MRSA, although this has not been supported in all studies.[7–9] If CA-MRSA does not require antibacterial coverage, this practice may reduce antibacterial selection pressure and expense.[10]

CASE 74-1, QUESTION 2: What agents could be chosen if N.P. is allergic to penicillin?

Clindamycin could be chosen for patients with a documented history of penicillin or cephalosporin allergy.[2] In certain geographic areas, group A streptococci macrolide resistance approaches 15% to 20%, decreasing the potential value of this agent. Clindamycin is superior to macrolides with respect to group A streptococcal coverage; however, it causes diarrhea in 20% of patients and is one of the main agents responsible for antibiotic-associated colitis. Moxifloxacin and levofloxacin are potential alternatives that have the convenience of once-daily dosing.

CASE 74-1, QUESTION 3: What dose should be prescribed for N.P.?

The recommended dosage of dicloxacillin is 500 mg orally every 6 hours. The dosage for penicillin V is 250 to 500 mg orally every 6 hours; for oral clindamycin, the dosage is 300 to 450 mg every 6 hours. Because dicloxacillin is the drug chosen for N.P., a dosage of 500 mg orally every 6 hours is appropriate. The dose for doxycycline is 100 mg orally every 12 hours, and the dose for trimethoprim-sulfamethoxazole is one to two double-strength tablets orally every 12 hours. The recommended dose for moxifloxacin is 400 mg orally every 24 hours and 500 mg orally every 24 hours for levofloxacin.

CASE 74-1, QUESTION 4: What is the appropriate duration of therapy for N.P.?

Although the recommended duration of therapy for cellulitis is 5 days, treatment may be extended if clinical improvement is not seen.[2] A reasonable recommendation to the patient would be to continue oral antibiotics for 2 to 3 days after the patient has become afebrile and has clinically improved. N.P. should be counseled to expect a response within 1 to 2 days after therapy begins (although erythema may persist longer). In addition, she should be instructed to return for re-evaluation if the condition does not improve or worsens during the next few days.

CASE 74-1, QUESTION 5: What further diagnostic evaluation should be undertaken for N.P.?

In otherwise healthy individuals, identification of the causative organism in cases of mild cellulitis is unnecessary. Needle aspiration, fine-needle aspiration biopsy, and punch biopsy identify the causative organism in only 20% to 30% of patients.[2] Appropriate empiric treatment is effective in most patients, and an attempt to isolate the organism does not improve success of treatment and adds significantly to the cost of care. However, patients with moderate-to-severe purulent infection, patients who failed initial empiric therapy, immunocompromised patients, patients with potential joint or tendon damage, or patients with life-threatening infections requiring hospitalization may benefit from additional cultures. In these cases, a swab of the primary wound and a needle aspiration or punch biopsy of the leading edge of the cellulitis should be obtained for Gram stain and culture before initiating antimicrobial therapy. Blood and wound cultures should be drawn in these patients. Anaerobic cultures need to be drawn only when the wound contains necrotic tissue, the wound is foul smelling, or crepitus is present. Even if wound and blood cultures are obtained, many infections will be culture negative (74%). Blood culture results are positive in less than 5% of cellulitis cases. Culture information, in conjunction with clinical course, can be used to modify subsequent treatment. Because N.P. has only a mild cellulitis, cultures are not required and therapy should be given empirically. In addition to systemic therapy, N.P. should be instructed to keep the area clean with soap and water (if an open wound is present) and to protect the area. Treatment of cellulitis should also include rest, immobilization and elevation of the infected area, and surgical drainage or debridement, as required. The wound should be assessed daily for local tenderness, pain, erythema, swelling, ulceration, necrosis, and wound drainage.

CASE 74-1, QUESTION 6: Could topical antibiotics be used to treat N.P.'s cellulitis?

The value of topical antibiotics in treating skin infections is questionable.[11] Most topical antibiotics have not been evaluated in appropriately designed trials. Although mupirocin is superior to placebo in treating some types of wound infections, its value in more severe disease is uncertain. In patients with moderate-to-severe infections, mupirocin, or any topical antibiotics (neomycin, bacitracin, polymyxin B) should not be used to replace or augment systemic antibiotics. Topical antibiotics likely do little but add to the cost of therapy, and they occasionally cause a contact dermatitis. Therefore, N.P. should not be treated with topical antibiotics because her cellulitis should be managed adequately by her systemic antimicrobial therapy.

CASE 74-2

QUESTION 1: O.A., a 49-year-old man, presents to the ED with a 3- to 4-day history of increasing pain around his left hip, secondary to an injury he received falling on the sidewalk. In addition, he has a fever and feels weak, lethargic, and nauseated. Examination reveals a swollen, warm, and extremely tender hip. O.A. has a temperature of 39.8°C and appears quite ill. A diagnosis of moderate-to-severe cellulitis is made, and O.A. is hospitalized because of the severity of the infection. O.A. has no other underlying medical problems. What empiric antibiotic regimen would be reasonable for O.A.?

In moderate-to-severe ill patients, when hospitalization is required, antibiotics should be administered parenterally. The parenteral agent of choice is nafcillin or oxacillin.[2] Cefazolin (1–2 g IV every 8 hours) would be an appropriate alternative if it is less expensive than nafcillin. Second- and third-generation cephalosporins (cefuroxime, cefoxitin, ceftriaxone, cefotaxime) and some quinolones may be as effective as nafcillin, but provide no clinical advantages for most cellulitis. Patients with risk factors for MRSA (penetrating trauma, history of MRSA, nasal colonization, IV drug abuse, presence of systemic inflammatory response syndrome) should be treated with vancomycin or agents with activity against *Streptococci* and MRSA. One potential option is linezolid, but is limited by potential for drug interactions with serotonergic agents. Other agents include daptomycin, telavancin, dalbavancin, oritavancin, and ceftaroline. Although these agents are as effective in severe cellulitis, they are not used as commonly as vancomycin because of cost and formulary availability.

Therefore, O.A. should receive either nafcillin, oxacillin, or cefazolin, whichever is less expensive and more tolerable for the patient. Once O.A. has become afebrile and has evidence of clinical improvement, the parenteral antibiotic should be discontinued and appropriate oral therapy should be initiated to complete at least a 5-day course (or until clinical improvement).

CASE 74-2, QUESTION 2: Two days after starting therapy, O.A. develops a maculopapular skin rash. What alternative therapy should be chosen?

Regardless of when during the course of therapy a drug rash occurs (early or late), the precipitant drug should be discontinued because there is a chance, although small, that the reaction could worsen. In patients who have a penicillin allergy and who still require parenteral therapy, clindamycin, vancomycin, linezolid, moxifloxacin, or levofloxacin could be chosen. Because all of these agents are equally effective, the choice should be based on cost and dosing convenience and presence of risk factors for MRSA.

CASE 74-2, QUESTION 3: After 48 hours of therapy, culture and sensitivity results are available. What changes, if any, should be made in O.A.'s treatment?

If cultures show only streptococcus species in a patient who is not allergic to penicillin, therapy should be deescalated to penicillin because it is effective, well tolerated, and less expensive than nafcillin. If cultures grow staphylococcus species (*S. aureus*) that are sensitive to methicillin/oxacillin, the initial empiric therapy should be continued. If the organisms are resistant to methicillin/oxacillin, therapy should be switched to vancomycin 15 mg/kg IV every 12 hours or alternative agent as previously described. Because O.A. has a presumed penicillin allergy (due to maculopapular rash) and does not require therapy for MRSA, he should continue with clindamycin or vancomycin. Cefazolin may also be an option for penicillin-allergic patients who do not experience severe allergic reactions, such as urticaria and anaphylaxis.

CASE 74-2, QUESTION 4: After 72 hours of therapy, O.A. has improved considerably and has been afebrile for 24 hours. Can he be switched to oral therapy?

Once O.A. has been afebrile for at least 24 hours and is significantly improved, he can be switched to oral therapy, if tolerated. Clinicians should select the oral agent on the basis of culture results (if available), anticipated pathogens (if no culture results), convenience, and cost.

CASE 74-2, QUESTION 5: What is the role of anti-inflammatory agents as adjunctive treatment of cellulitis?

Anti-inflammatory agents, such as nonsteroidal anti-inflammatory agents and corticosteroids, have been shown to decrease time to resolution of cellulitis when given in conjunction with antibiotics to patients without diabetes.[2] Although supporting evidence is weak, a significantly quicker resolution of symptoms in patients on prednisolone 5 to 30 mg/day has been seen.[2,12,13]

CASE 74-3

QUESTION 1: M.C. is a 22-year-old college football player who presents to the ED with a 3- to 4-day history of pain in his left thigh. On examination, he has a swollen, erythematous, and purulent 2 × 3 cm abscess in the inner left thigh. The area is warm and tender to the touch. M.C. is afebrile with no signs of lymphangitis. What tests are needed to confirm the diagnosis?

In patients with abscesses, large furuncles (superficial skin abscess), and carbuncles (clusters of furuncles), Gram stain and culture of pus is recommended.[2] Though, typically cases may be adequately treated without further testing. M.C. has risk factors for CA-MRSA (competitive athlete); if CA-MRSA is identified, infection control measures should be implemented to prevent outbreak.[14] In febrile patients, blood cultures should be drawn before antibiotics are started to maximize the ability to isolate the pathogen.

CASE 74-3, QUESTION 2: Are the suspected organisms similar to those found in other patients with cellulitis?

Abscess, furuncles, and carbuncles are most commonly caused by staphylococci, predominately *S. aureus*.[2,6] Abscesses may also be polymicrobial. For patients who are IV drug abusers and present with abscess or cellulitis, the infecting bacteria are similar to those found in normal hosts. Intravenous drug use is also a risk factor for infection with CA-MRSA and should be particularly considered if the patient has had recurrent infections or has failed to respond to MSSA-directed antibiotic therapy.[14] Although *Staphylococcus epidermidis,* Gram-negative organisms, including *P. aeruginosa,* and anaerobes are rarely pathogens, they may be present and should be considered in patients who do not respond to initial therapy.

CASE 74-3, QUESTION 3: What is the appropriate empiric therapy?

Antibiotic therapy is often not required. Incision and drainage should be performed for all abscesses, large furuncles, and carbuncles.[2] Antibiotics may be considered as adjunct to incision and drainage when systemic inflammatory response syndrome is present, but has not been shown to improve cure rates in patients with cutaneous abscess. Antibiotic therapy should be directed toward CA-MRSA and based on severity of infection. Mild-to-moderate infection can be adequately treated with doxycycline or sulfamethoxazole/trimethoprim, whereas more severe disease should be empirically treated with vancomycin, daptomycin, linezolid, telavancin, or ceftaroline.[2,14] If treatment does not result in some resolution of inflammation within 48 hours, antimicrobial coverage should be expanded to cover Gram-negative organisms and resistant streptococci.

ERYSIPELAS

Erysipelas is a superficial skin infection caused by streptococci, predominantly group A, although groups C and G (and group B in children) also may cause the infection.[15,16] This skin infection affects approximately 1 in 1,000 persons/year and is associated with diabetes mellitus, chronic venous insufficiency, and cardiovascular disease.[16] Erysipelas is diagnosed based on characteristics of the skin lesion and concurrent systemic symptoms.[15] The lesion is a continuous, indurated, edematous area, with a clearly defined raised edge.[16] Early in the course, the lesion is bright red, but it may turn to brown as the lesion ages or grows. The lesion spreads peripherally with no islands of unaffected tissue. The initial lesion results from a small break in the skin that becomes infected, although signs of the initial wound often are not evident. Aspiration of the lesion or a superficial swab is not recommended because this has not been shown useful in detecting the pathogen.[15] Patients with erysipelas have associated systemic symptoms of high fever, chills, frequent history of rigors, and general malaise. This constellation of systemic symptoms differentiates erysipelas from other local skin disorders.

CASE 74-4

QUESTION 1: D.D., a 70-year-old man, presents to the ED with a red, swollen face. He describes the area as "a swollen red spot" that has appeared during the past 2 days. He also describes feeling unwell for the previous 3 days and having a fever. On examination, D.D. has a bright red, shiny, edematous lesion on his right cheek that is 0.4 cm wide. It is a continuous lesion with a clearly demarcated border. What antibiotic therapy should be initiated for D.D.?

Erysipelas will respond promptly to antibiotics with activity against group A streptococci.[17] Oral penicillin V 250 to 500 mg every 6 hours and for severe cases and parenteral penicillin G (2–4 million units IV every 6 hours) generally reduce the systemic symptoms (e.g., fever, malaise) within 24 to 48 hours[17]; however, it will take several more days for the skin lesion to resolve. If D.D.'s condition does not improve within 72 hours after initiation of antibiotics, he should be instructed to return for reassessment. If D.D. has an allergy to penicillins, then a macrolide, clindamycin, or an oral fluoroquinolone, such as moxifloxacin, is an alternative.[15,17] Ceftriaxone may also be an alternative in Penicillin allergic patients (without anaphylaxis) due to low (<1%) cross sensitivity risk. If the community has increased macrolide resistance to group A streptococci, these agents should not be part of empiric therapy. Antibiotic therapy should be continued for 10 days even if signs and symptoms resolve quickly to avoid a relapse, which could lead to chronic infection or scarring.

SKIN AND SOFT TISSUE INFECTIONS IN DIABETIC PATIENTS

Skin and soft tissue infections are common in patients with diabetes mellitus. Approximately 25% of diabetic patients report a history of skin and soft tissue infections, and 5% to 15% of diabetic patients may undergo limb amputation.[18] In addition to the cost associated with treating skin and soft tissue infections, functional disability may occur, which can significantly decrease the patient's quality of life. Diabetic patients are at particular risk for foot problems, primarily because of the neuropathies and peripheral vascular diseases associated with long-standing diabetes. The decreased pain sensation allows the patient to continue to bear weight in the presence of skin damage, thereby promoting the formation of an ulcer. In addition, minor trauma (e.g., cuts, foreign body insertion) can go unnoticed and, when left untreated, can become infected and extensive. Although these infections are common, preventive measures should reduce the frequency of amputations. Mild infections can be treated empirically with those agents used for soft tissue infections in nondiabetic patients because these are commonly caused by aerobic Gram-positive cocci. In moderate-to-severe infections, antibiotic coverage should be expanded because multiple organisms may be responsible for the infection. Although it is often difficult to determine colonizers from true pathogens, an average of two to six organisms are cultured from foot ulcers in patients with diabetes.[19,20] The following organisms (in no particular order) have been isolated in more than 20% of wounds in patients with diabetes: *S. aureus, S. epidermidis, Enterococcus faecalis,* other streptococci, *Proteus* species, *E. coli, Klebsiella* species, *Peptococcus* species, *Peptostreptococcus* species, and *Bacteroides* species.[20] These infections are often polymicrobic, but treatment can be effective even if not all cultured pathogens are covered.[19] To determine the pathogens most accurately, a specimen of infected deep tissue should be obtained after the wound has been cleaned. If this is not possible, cultures of purulent exudate or curettage should be obtained, versus superficial swab, to determine the true pathogens in the wound.[18] Although antibiotics have an important role, drainage and surgical debridement to remove necrotic tissue are essential and may be the mainstay of treatment.[19] Cultures of the affected areas may not be useful unless bone is infected. Although anaerobic organisms often are difficult to culture, they must be considered if an abscess or devitalized, necrotic, foul-smelling tissue is present or the wound is a result of abdominal surgery.

CASE 74-5

QUESTION 1: T.U. is a 67-year-old man with diabetes presenting to his general practitioner for a routine checkup and has no specific complaints. T.U. has a 15-year history of poorly controlled type 2 diabetes and a 3-year history of recurrent foot ulcers. On examination, the physician observes that an ulcer on the underside of the foot, which had previously healed over, is open and inflamed; purulent fluid can be expressed from the wound. T.U. reports no pain around the area and was unaware that the ulcer had worsened. He is currently febrile, and physical examination reveals mild lymphadenopathy and elevated white blood cell count. Does T.U. have an active infection, and is antibiotic therapy required?

All open wounds, in diabetic and nondiabetic patients, will become colonized with bacteria, but only infected wounds should be treated with antibiotic therapy.[19,20] Often it is difficult to determine whether an open wound is infected, but signs and symptoms (e.g., purulent drainage, erythema, pain, and swelling around the area) are suggestive of infection. Based on his symptoms, T.U. has an infection that requires treatment.

CASE 74-5, QUESTION 2: What treatment should T.U. receive?

Prior to initiating antibiotic therapy, the presence of a clinically infected wound must first be confirmed as often diabetic wounds may not be infected and thus do not require antimicrobial therapy. When determining appropriate antibiotic therapy for infected wounds, clinicians must consider the severity of infection (mild versus moderate to severe), whether the patient has risk factors for MRSA or *P. aeruginosa* or whether the patient has received any antibiotics within the past month. Mild diabetic foot infections should not be treated with topical antibiotic preparations because the evidence of efficacy is limited; the preparations do not allow sufficient penetration of antibiotic into the tissues; many preparations are detrimental to wound healing.[21] Mild infections can be treated empirically in a similar way to other soft tissue infections because these are commonly caused by aerobic Gram-positive cocci.[19] A penicillinase-resistant penicillin (e.g., dicloxacillin) or cephalexin will be effective in most cases. The choice between these agents should be based on tolerability and cost. Alternative agents include clindamycin, amoxicillin/clavulanate, or levofloxacin. If anaerobes are suspected (based on malodorous aroma, if the infection is severe or long-standing or has recently been treated with antibiotics), clindamycin or amoxicillin/clavulanate monotherapy can be used or metronidazole can be added to the regimen.[18] If metronidazole is selected, concurrent use of an antibiotic with good activity against aerobic pathogens is required, because metronidazole has no activity against aerobic bacteria. In patients with significant vascular compromise, crepitus, or gangrene, a radiograph should be taken to identify any bone involvement suggestive of osteomyelitis.

For treatment of moderate-to-severe infections, oral or parenteral antibiotics (IV recommended for severe) may be used depending on signs and symptoms and should be selected based on suspected organisms. For staphylococci, streptococci, and enterobacteriaceae, therapeutic options include levofloxacin, cefoxitin, ceftriaxone, ampicillin/sulbactam, moxifloxacin, ertapenem, and imipenem/cilastatin, or tigecycline.[20,21] Levofloxacin and ceftriaxone have no anaerobic coverage; thus, clindamycin or metronidazole should be added if anaerobes are suspected (ischemic or necrotic wounds).[22] It is important to consider that clindamycin may be more likely to cause *Clostridium difficile*-associated diarrhea.

Other considerations in antibiotic selection should include MRSA or *P. aeruginosa* when risk factors are present. Infections due to MRSA can be treated with vancomycin, daptomycin, or linezolid. Newer antibiotics, including dalbavancin, telavancin, oritavancin, and ceftaroline, have activity against MRSA skin and soft tissue infections, but there is a lack of efficacy data in diabetic foot infections.[23] Infections due to *P. aeruginosa* may be more common in patients in areas with high local prevalence, warmer climates, and frequent exposure of foot to water, and can be treated with piperacillin/tazobactam. Other antibiotics with activity against *P. aeruginosa* include, cefepime, ceftazidime, aztreonam, imipenem/cilastatin, meropenem, or doripenem. Aminoglycosides are associated with serious toxicity if used for an extended period and should probably be avoided in diabetic patients.

Because T.U. is an elderly diabetic patient with systemic signs and symptoms of infection (moderate to severe), empiric therapy with cefoxitin, ceftriaxone, ampicillin/sulbactam, levofloxacin, moxifloxacin, or ertapenem would be appropriate because he does not have risk factors for MRSA or *P. aeruginosa* infection.

CASE 74-5, QUESTION 3: Despite aggressive antibiotic therapy and debridement, T.U.'s infection spreads and an amputation is required. How long should antibiotics be prescribed for T.U. after surgery?

Antibiotics may be continued until signs and symptoms of infection have resolved. Typical treatment duration is 1 to 2 weeks; however, longer treatment duration (2–4 weeks) may be necessary in patients with moderate-to-severe infections or in patients with infections that are slow to resolve.[20] Oral therapy should be considered once the patient has clinically improved; treatment can be stopped even if the underlying ulcer has not completely healed.[18,20]

The best option for uncontrollable, life-threatening infections often is amputation to remove the infected area. Once the infected area has been removed, antibiotic therapy should be continued for 2 to 5 days.[20]

CASE 74-5, QUESTION 4: What measures could have been taken to prevent this complication in T.U.?

Many of the foot problems associated with diabetes can be prevented with proper foot care (Table 74-2), and these preventive measures must be emphasized. Diabetic patients with neuropathies or those who are elderly should carefully examine their feet every 1 to 2 days.

Necrotizing Soft Tissue Infections

Skin and soft tissue infections are described as *necrotizing* when the inflammation is rapidly progressing and necrosis of the skin or underlying tissue is present. The following clinical signs suggest necrotizing infections, as opposed to simple cellulitis: edema beyond the area of erythema, skin blisters or bullae, localized pallor or discoloration, gas in the subcutaneous tissues (crepitus), and the absence of lymphangitis and lymphadenitis. Common clinical features include high temperature, disorientation, lethargy, or the hard wood feel of the infected area.[2] Occasionally, a broad erythematous track along the route of infection may also be present. Necrotizing soft tissue infections can progress rapidly to cause additional local effects (e.g., necrosis and loss of skin sensation) and severe systemic effects (e.g., hypotension, shock).[24] Necrotizing soft tissue infections are rare, with approximately 1,000 cases/year in the United States, but they can be lethal.[25,26] Necrotizing infections can occur in healthy individuals, but are more commonly associated with IV or subcutaneous injections of illicit drugs.[27]

Table 74-2
Foot Care for the Diabetic Patient

Inspect feet daily for cuts, blisters, or scratches. Pay particular attention to the area between the toes and use a mirror to examine the bottom of the foot.
Wash feet daily in tepid water and dry thoroughly.
Apply lotion to feet to prevent calluses and cracking.
Ensure that shoes fit properly (not too tight or too loose) and inspect them daily.
Trim nails regularly, making sure to cut straight across the nail.
Do not use chemical agents to remove corns or calluses.

Necrotizing cellulitis involves the skin and subcutaneous tissues. Necrotizing fasciitis involves both superficial and deep fascia, and necrotizing infections involving the muscle are termed *myonecrosis*. Group A β-hemolytic streptococci, *S. aureus*, other staphylococci, *Pseudomonas* species, other Gram-negative organisms, *Clostridium perfringens*, *Peptostreptococcus*, *B. fragilis*, and *Vibrio* species can cause necrotizing infections.[24,28] Gas gangrene is myonecrosis caused by a *Clostridium* subspecies, most commonly *C. perfringens* (70%).[24] Gas in a wound is not necessarily indicative of gas gangrene caused by *C. perfringens*. Gram-negative organisms (e.g., *E. coli*, *Proteus* species, *Klebsiella* species) or anaerobic streptococci can produce gas in a wound. Air also could have been introduced at the time of the injury. Gas gangrene is characterized by acute onset of worsening pain that is usually out of proportion to the degree of injury. Clostridial myonecrosis (true gas gangrene), streptococcal gangrene (caused by group A β-hemolytic streptococci), and synergistic bacterial gangrene (caused by anaerobic and aerobic bacteria, usually Gram negative) are other terms used to describe necrotizing skin and soft tissue infections. Fournier gangrene (a type of synergistic bacterial gangrene of the scrotum), nonclostridial crepitant gangrene (nonclostridial gas gangrene), and necrotizing fasciitis (all necrotizing soft tissue infections other than clostridial myonecrosis, or sometimes just streptococcal gangrene) are other commonly used terms.[24] The primary treatment for necrotizing soft tissue infections involves extensive debridement of the area to remove all necrotic tissue and drainage. Early fluid resuscitation and broad-spectrum antibiotics are also imperative.[25]

CASE 74-6

QUESTION 1: M.T., a 45-year-old alcoholic homeless man, presents to the ED with a broken nose and facial lacerations, which he received after a fight outside one of the local taverns. On examination, in addition to the facial wounds, an area of severe inflammation, erythema, and necrosis is evident on his left calf. The area is very painful, crepitation is felt over the area, and a purulent discharge is present. M.T. states he believes the infection is because of a knife wound he experienced approximately 1 week ago. What antibacterial treatment should be provided?

In addition to setting the broken nose and suturing the facial lacerations, the clinician should evaluate the infection on M.T.'s calf. A Gram stain and culture of the purulent discharge should take place before initiating antimicrobial therapy. Because crepitus is present, the area should be incised, and a specimen of the infected tissue should be obtained for Gram stain and culture. Because the presence of crepitus may suggest a necrotizing infection, an immediate surgical consultation will be required for M.T. Pending the surgical evaluation, fluid resuscitation and IV antibiotics should be initiated. Gas in the tissues could be caused by many organisms, and empiric broad-spectrum antibiotic therapy with coverage against Gram-positive organisms, the enterobacteriaceae, and *B. fragilis* should be started. Initial therapy with piperacillin/tazobactam, ampicillin/sulbactam, or a carbapenem plus anti-MRSA antibiotic (vancomycin, daptomycin, or linezolid) should be used.[2] Clindamycin is often added for suspicion of group A streptococci, not for its antibacterial effects but because it inhibits protein synthesis, which may reduce toxin expression by the bacteria, and cytokine response by the host.[2,29] Alternative options include ceftriaxone plus metronidazole, or a fluoroquinolone plus metronidazole. If a Gram stain of the infected tissue clearly shows the predominance of Gram-positive cocci, consideration of narrowing the spectrum of antibiotic therapy is appropriate. Flesh-eating disease is usually a necrotizing fasciitis caused by virulent strains of group A streptococci. High-dose penicillin G (3 million units every 4 hours) plus clindamycin (900 mg IV every 8 hours) are the drugs of choice for this condition, as well as for gas clostridial myonecrosis.[2,29]

Potential adjunctive therapy for streptococcal necrotizing skin infections includes IV immunoglobulin G (IVIG) 2 g/kg as a single dose or 0.4 g/kg daily for 2 days. Alternative dosage regimens have included 1 g/kg on day 1 with 0.5 g/kg on days 2 and 3.[30] No clinical trials have proven the definitive benefit of IVIG, and the optimal dose, if used, is unknown. If it truly provides benefit, IVIG is thought to work by binding to the superantigens released by the streptococcal bacteria that are involved in the systemic effects of the infection.[30,31]

ANIMAL BITE WOUNDS

Any wound caused by an animal that results in the skin being cut or punctured should be examined to ensure no underlying tissue damage has occurred. This is especially true in patients with bites of the hand or around other joints. The wound should be washed thoroughly with clean water as soon as possible after the bite.[32] Irrigation of the wound, including puncture sites, should be extensive to reduce the risk of infection. Obtaining specimens for cultures is not required, and wound irrigation should begin as soon as possible.

Animal bites may develop bacterial infections due to aerobic or anaerobic organisms in up to 18% of cases.[33] Although purulent wounds or abscesses are likely to contain mixed aerobic and anaerobic organisms, nonpurulent wounds are more commonly caused by streptococci or staphylococci.[2] *Pasteurella multocida* is commonly isolated and is particularly significant in cat bites because it is present in up to 75% of the oral flora of cats.[2,33] Although antibiotic treatment is not required for some dog bites, reports of a greater than 75% incidence of infection after cat bites suggest that all patients with cat bites should receive antibiotics.[32]

CASE 74-7

QUESTION 1: P.J., a 18-year-old boy, presents to the ED 3 hours after being bitten on the leg by a neighbor's dog. He has a laceration, 14 cm long, on his medial calf. Four distinct puncture marks, suggestive of teeth marks, also are present on the calf. There is no suggestion of bone injury. P.J. was healthy before the attack and has no chronic illness. Should P.J. receive any treatment other than suturing of his laceration?

The standard of care for all bites involves wound irrigation and decontamination of the wound.[32] P.J.'s wound should be evaluated for deep tissue injury, devascularization of any tissue, and bone injury. Loose suturing or closure with adhesive strips is appropriate for lacerations after irrigation.[32] Although the safety of closure of bite wounds has been debated, a good therapeutic response has been obtained after the closure of wounds.

CASE 74-7, QUESTION 2: Because P.J. has several punctures that are difficult to irrigate, he is a candidate for antibiotic therapy. Which antibiotic(s) should he receive?

The need for antibiotics is controversial and guided by wound severity and patient immunocompetency.[2,34] The patient should receive a course of antibiotics if the wound involves the hand or is near joints, if it involves deep punctures or is difficult to irrigate, if the patient is immunocompromised (e.g., diabetes, splenectomy), or if the wound is not well perfused.

Antibiotics are not required for dog bites in which no deep tissue injury is present and the wound can be well irrigated, particularly if the wound is on the lower extremities in healthy adults or children.[32]

The selection of the appropriate antibiotic is based on the most likely pathogens from the specific animal bite. Although *P. multocida* often is considered the primary pathogen of dog bites, antibiotic coverage also must address the other common pathogens. Monotherapy with amoxicillin/clavulanate 875/125 mg orally every 12 hours is recommended.[2,32] Alternative options include second-generation cephalosporins (e.g., cefuroxime) plus an agent with anaerobic coverage (clindamycin or metronidazole). If the patient is allergic to penicillin, doxycycline, moxifloxacin, or a carbapenem provides adequate coverage.[2] In all cases, patients should be instructed to watch for improvement; if the wound does not heal or it worsens within 48 hours, the patient needs to be re-evaluated. Antibiotic treatment should not extend beyond 5 days unless signs of an infection remain. If the patient presents with an established infection, parenteral therapy is warranted if the infection is over a joint, has lymphatic spread, or involves the hand or head. Parenteral therapy should be continued until the infection has resolved, and therapy should then be continued with oral antibiotics for at least 7 days or until all clinical signs of the infection have resolved.

Prophylaxis for rabies is required only if the animal is from an area with endemic rabies or if the bite was the result of an unprovoked attack by a wild animal.[32] The local health board should be contacted to determine the recent rabies risk in the area. If P.J. has not received a tetanus toxoid booster within the past 5 years, a booster should be administered. If P.J. has never been immunized for tetanus, tetanus immune globulin should be administered in addition to the tetanus toxoid.

HUMAN BITE WOUNDS

CASE 74-8

QUESTION 1: C.K., a 40-year-old man, presents with a sore arm 24 hours after receiving a bite to his left forearm by his neighbor in a "discussion over property boundaries." C.K. was previously healthy and has no chronic diseases. A 6 × 8 cm area of his left forearm is swollen and erythematous, and includes several distinct puncture marks consistent with a human bite. No joint deformity or bone abnormality is detected on clinical examination. How should C.K. be treated?

Treating a human bite is similar to any other laceration, including cleansing, irrigating, exploring, debriding, draining, excising, and suturing, as required.[32] All human bites should be cleansed as soon as possible, and any lacerations or punctures irrigated copiously. Surgical exploration with debridement, drainage, or excision should be undertaken if deeper tissues may have been injured or if pus collection could have occurred. With evidence of pus accumulation in his wound, the area should be explored and drained. E.D. also should receive systemic antibiotic therapy to eradicate potential infecting organisms. If the wound is severe (i.e., involves subcutaneous tissues, a joint, or a large area) or if the patient is unlikely to be compliant with oral antibiotics, parenteral administration of antibiotics is required. The most common pathogens in human bites are β-hemolytic streptococci, *S. aureus, Eikenella corrodens, Fusobacterium, Peptostreptococcus, Prevotella*, and *Porphyromonas sp. Corynebacterium* subspecies.[2] Treatment with amoxicillin/clavulanate, ampicillin/sulbactam, or ertapenem is appropriate. For penicillin-allergic patients, alternatives include ciprofloxacin or levofloxacin plus metronidazole or moxifloxacin alone.

KEY REFERENCES AND WEBSITES

A full list of references for this chapter can be found at http://thepoint.lww.com/AT11e. Below are the key references and websites for this chapter, with the corresponding reference number in this chapter found in parentheses after the reference.

Key References

Bonnetblanc JM, Bedane C. Erysipelas: recognition and management. *Am J Clin Dermatol*. 2003;4:157. (15)

Kilburn SA et al. Interventions for cellulitis and erysipelas. *Cochrane Database Syst Rev*. 2010;(6):CD004299. (4)

Kosinski MA, Lipsky BA. Current medical management of diabetic foot infections. *Expert Rev Anti Infect Ther*. 2010;8(11):1293–1305. (23)

Lipsky BA. Medical treatment of diabetic foot infections. *Clin Infect Dis*. 2004;39(Suppl 2):S104. (22)

Lipsky BA et al. Clinical practice guidelines for the diagnosis and treatment of diabetic foot infections. *Clin Infect Dis*. 2012;54:e132–e173. (20)

Liu C et al. Clinical practice guidelines by the Infectious Diseases Society of America for the treatment of methicillin-resistant *Staphylococcus aureus* infections in adults and children. *Clin Infect Dis*. 2011;52:e18. (5)

Looke D, Dendle C. Bites (mammalian). *Clin Evid*. 2010;7:914. (33)

Matthews PC et al. Clinical management of diabetic foot infection: diagnostics, therapeutics and the future. *Expert Rev Anti Infect Ther*. 2007;5:117. (18)

Moran GJ et al. Antimicrobial prophylaxis for wounds and procedures in the emergency department. *Infect Dis Clin North Am*. 2008;22:117. (32)

Stevens DL et al. Practice guidelines for the diagnosis and management of skin and soft tissue infections: 2014 update by the Infectious Disease Society of America. *Clin Infect Dis*. 2014;59(2):e10–e52. (2)

75 Prevention and Treatment of Infections in Neutropenic Cancer Patients

Richard H. Drew

CORE PRINCIPLES

	CHAPTER CASES
DEFINITIONS	
1 As a consequence of select cancer chemotherapies, patients may experience neutropenia (defined as an absolute neutrophil count <500 cells/μL or anticipated to drop to <500 cells/μL within 48 hours) and fever (defined as a single oral temperature of ≥38.3°C [101°F] or a temperature of ≥38.0°C [100.4°F] for >1 hour).	**Case 75-1 (Question 4)**
2 Bacteria are the primary pathogens associated with infection in febrile neutropenic patients (especially those occurring early).	**Case 75-1 (Questions 1, 6)**
CLINICAL PRESENTATION	
1 Fever is usually the earliest (and often the only) sign of infection.	**Case 75-1 (Question 4)**
2 An accurate history and complete physical examination should be completed. Chest radiographs and oximetry should be completed if signs and symptoms point to the respiratory tract.	**Case 75-1 (Question 5)**
3 Before antibiotics are initiated, two sets of blood cultures (with each set consisting of two culture bottles) should be obtained. Additional site-specific cultures should also be obtained if such infections are suspected. A complete blood count, serum electrolytes, coagulation, C-reactive protein, urinalysis, and assessment of organ function (e.g., liver and kidney function) should be assessed.	**Case 75-1 (Question 5)**
KEY TREATMENT INFORMATION	
1 Risk stratification should be undertaken to identify patients most likely to experience significant infection-related complications. Patients at highest risk include those with prolonged (>7 days) and profound (<100 cells/μL) neutropenia or select comorbidities (hypotension, severe mucositis interfering with swallowing or causing diarrhea, pneumonia, new-onset abdominal pain, hepatic or renal insufficiency, or neurologic changes). Highest-risk patients should be considered for antibacterial and antifungal prophylaxis.	**Case 75-1 (Questions 2, 3, 7)**
2 In the absence of evidence of site- or pathogen-specific etiologies or clinical instability, initial empiric monotherapy is most commonly an antipseudomonal third-generation cephalosporin (e.g., ceftazidime), a fourth-generation cephalosporin (e.g., cefepime), or an antipseudomonal carbapenem (e.g., imipenem–cilastatin or meropenem). Prolonged infusion of β-lactam (3-4 hours) should be considered in order to optimize their pharmacodynamic properties. Additional agents may be added (such as vancomycin, an aminoglycoside, or fluoroquinolone) to initial therapy in patients who are hemodynamically unstable. Antiviral therapy is generally restricted to patients with serologic or clinical evidence of viral infection.	**Case 75-1 (Questions 7–9), Case 75-2 (Questions 1, 2, 4, 5), Case 75-4 (Question 4)**
MONITORING PARAMETERS	
1 The need for (and timing of) modification of the initial empiric therapy is dependent on the risk group (i.e., low vs. high risk), establishment of an infection site or causative pathogen, persistence or defervescence of fever, and clinical stability.	**Case 75-2 (Question 6)**

Continued

	CHAPTER CASES
2 High-risk patients unresponsive to initial empiric antibacterial therapy should be considered for the addition of antifungal therapy at days 4 through 7. In addition to coverage for *Candida* species, highest-risk patients with persistent or recurrent fever after 4 to 7 days of appropriate antibacterial therapy with prolonged (i.e., >10 days) neutropenia should be considered for antimold therapy. Low-risk patients who are clinically stable do not routinely need antifungal therapy.	**Case 75-3 (Questions 1, 2), Case 75-4 (Questions 1, 2)**
THERAPEUTIC CONTROVERSIES	
1 The role of vancomycin as part of the initial empiric regimen remains controversial. In general, routine use of vancomycin as part of initial empiric therapy for fever in neutropenic patients without other evidence of infection should be discouraged (except in clinically unstable patients).	**Case 75-2 (Question 3)**
2 The ideal initial empiric antifungal agent is debatable. However, patients receiving fluconazole prophylaxis requiring addition of empiric antifungals should be considered for antifungals with activity against azole-resistant *Candida* species and mold infections.	**Case 75-4 (Questions 3, 4)**
3 Although hematopoietic colony-stimulating factors prevent neutropenia in high-risk cancer patients, use of these agents as treatment of febrile neutropenia unresponsive to antibiotics remains controversial.	**Case 75-1 (Question 3), Case 75-4 (Question 5)**

Many patients with both solid tumor and hematologic malignancies have had their lives prolonged through therapeutic advances in chemotherapy, immunotherapy, and hematologic stem cell transplantation (HSCT). Despite such advances, infectious complications continue to be a major cause of morbidity and mortality in these patients. Risk assessment, prevention, rapid detection, and effective management of infections, while a major challenge, can lead to improved outcomes in such immunocompromised hosts.[1,2]

This chapter focuses on infectious complications in patients with immunosuppression as a consequence of cancer. The following topics are addressed: risks and epidemiology of infection, principles of prophylactic antimicrobials, empiric initial antibacterial selection, modification and duration of therapy, empiric antifungal and antiviral use, and the use of hematopoietic growth factors.

RISK FACTORS FOR INFECTION

Patients are rendered immunocompromised when there is a significant disruption or deficiency of one or more of the host defenses as a result of the underlying disease or chemotherapy. These risk factors include neutropenia and impairment in both humoral (antibody and complement) and cell-mediated immune defenses. Disruption of barriers to infection resulting from chemotherapy-related damage to skin and mucosal barriers further increases the risk of infection. As a result, bacteria, fungi, viruses, and (less commonly) protozoa may infect various sites (depending on the specific immunodeficiency).

Neutropenia

Granulocytes, or granular leukocytes, represent an important defense against bacterial and fungal infections. *Neutropenia* (a reduction in the number of circulating granulocytes or neutrophils) predisposes the host to infections. The terms *granulocytopenia* and *neutropenia* are often used interchangeably. The degree of neutropenia is expressed in terms of the absolute neutrophil count (ANC) or the total number of granulocytes (polymorphonuclear leukocytes and band forms) present in the circulating pool of white blood cells (WBCs).

For purposes of guideline development and clinical trials, neutropenia is most commonly defined as an ANC less than 500 cells/μL or less than 1,000 cells/μL with an anticipated to drop to less than 500 cells/μL within 48 hours.[2–4] The risk, severity, and type of infection in the neutropenic patient are proportional to the severity, rate of decline, and duration of neutropenia.[5] In general, the relative risk of infection is low when the ANC exceeds 1,000 cells/μL, with the frequency and severity of infection inversely proportional to the ANC.[3,5,6] Because the ANC drops to less than 500 cells/μL, the risk of infection rapidly increases. Conversely, recovery of the ANC is one of the most important factors determining the outcome of infectious complications in the neutropenic patient. Febrile patients with short durations of neutropenia (≤7 days) or in whom neutropenia is not severe (<100 cells/μL) less frequently experience serious, life-threatening infections.[2,3,7] In contrast, patients with severe neutropenia lasting more than 7 days are at significant risk of severe infection.[2,3,8]

Damage to Physical Barriers

The intact skin and mucosal surfaces of the body (GI, sinus, pulmonary, and genitourinary) constitute the host's primary physical defense against microbial invasion. The integrity of this physical barrier may be disrupted by tumor, treatment (e.g., surgery, radiation), or various medical procedures (e.g., insertion of intravenous [IV] or urinary catheters, venipuncture, measurement of rectal temperature). Device-related infections, including those associated with central venous catheters, are commonly caused by migration of skin flora (e.g., staphylococci) through the cutaneous insertion site. Infections secondary to damaged mucosal lining of the gastrointestinal (GI) tract such as mucositis (usually secondary to chemotherapy or graft-versus-host disease [GVHD]) are usually caused by enteric bacteria and fungi such as *Candida* species.

Malignancy-Related Alterations in the Immune System

Malignancies such as leukemia [acute and chronic], lymphoma (e.g., non-Hodgkin lymphoma) and myelodysplastic syndrome may invade bone marrow, resulting in leukopenia. This is most notable in patients with advanced or refractory malignancy, which may reflect either bone marrow invasion or as a consequence of multiple courses of immunosuppressive chemotherapy. In contrast, predisposition to infection in patients with solid tumors is often associated with anatomic abnormalities (such as obstruction or erosion). Such risks may be enhanced as a consequence of surgery, chemotherapy, and/or radiation to correct the underlying tumor.

Patients with immunoglobulin deficiencies (e.g., hypogammaglobulinemia, chronic lymphocytic leukemia, or splenectomy) are at increased risk for infections with encapsulated bacteria, which undergo antibody opsonization for efficient phagocytosis. Such bacteria include *Neisseria meningitidis, Haemophilus influenzae,* and *Streptococcus pneumoniae.* Hodgkin disease, organ transplantation, and human immunodeficiency virus (HIV) disease can disrupt the cellular immune system, increasing the risk for infections with obligate and facultative intracellular organisms such as mycobacteria, *Listeria, Toxoplasma,* viruses, and fungi. Certain hematologic malignancies and myelodysplastic syndromes may also be associated with immunodeficiencies secondary to replacement of leukocytes with malignant cells.

Medications Impacting Host Defenses

Some chemotherapeutic agents (such as fludarabine) have profound effects on both cellular and humoral defenses.[9,10] Corticosteroids exert their immunosuppressive effects on the cellular immune system, particularly at the T lymphocyte and macrophage level. Therefore, patients receiving corticosteroids (such as HSCT recipients with GVHD) have increased susceptibility to viral, bacterial, protozoal, and fungal infections.[11] Infectious complications secondary to glucocorticoids are dose-dependent. The risk of infection increases with daily doses greater than 10 mg or cumulative doses greater than 700 mg of prednisone or its equivalent.[11] Thus, patients receiving corticosteroids in either high doses (>20 mg prednisone or its equivalent daily) or for prolonged periods are at increased risk for infections caused by opportunistic pathogens. In addition, corticosteroids may blunt the usual signs of infection such as fever and inflammation. Severe cell-mediated immunodeficiency may also be caused by GVHD and its treatment.[2,3,9] More recently, chemotherapeutic monoclonal options (such as alemtuzumab, bortezomib, rituximab, and ofatumumab) significantly weaken the immune system, predisposing recipients to viral, bacterial, and fungal infections.[12,13]

Colonization or Prior Infection

Colonization is characterized as isolation of an organism from any particular site (e.g., stool, nasopharynx) without clinical signs of infection. Most infections in neutropenic patients are caused by either the host's endogenous microflora or hospital-acquired pathogens that have colonized the alimentary tract, upper respiratory tract, or skin. Therefore, microbial colonization can be a prerequisite to infection in neutropenic patients. This is perhaps best studied in patients colonized with methicillin-resistant *Staphylococcus aureus* (MRSA). Prior infection (especially in the pre-engraftment phase of HSCT recipients) is a risk factor for infection during immunosuppression, particularly for viral infections (such as cytomegalovirus [CMV], herpes simplex virus [HSV], and *Varicella zoster* virus [VZV]). Infections with these pathogens during immunosuppression are generally considered to be a consequence of latent infection rather than new infection.[2,3,9,14,15]

Hematopoietic Stem Cell Transplantation

Transplantation of bone marrow predisposes patients to the development of opportunistic infections secondary to both intensive immunosuppressive therapy and transmission.[9] These infections may be acquired or may represent reactivation of latent host infection. The introduction of new therapeutic approaches for treatment of the underlying malignancy (including nucleoside analogs and monoclonal antibodies to CD20 and CD52), along with use of unrelated stem cell donors, has increased the potential for infections in these patients.[9] When compared with autologous or syngeneic HSCT recipients, allogeneic HSCT patients have an increased risk of infection, particularly in those patients undergoing therapy for GVHD.[9] The pathogens causing infections vary with the time since transplantation. The use of immunosuppressives after transplantation (such as corticosteroids, antithymocyte globulin, and alemtuzumab) also significantly increases the risk for infection.[9]

Radiation Therapy

Side effects associated with the use of radiation therapy for the treatment of malignancy (e.g., mucositis, skin breakdown, or reduction in blood counts) also predispose a patient with neutropenia to infection.

Functional Asplenia

The spleen is responsible for production of opsonizing antibodies, assisting in protection against encapsulated bacteria (such as *S. pneumoniae, H. influenzae,* and *N. meningitidis*). Functional asplenia may occur secondary to irradiation or as a complication of GVHD.[3]

MOST COMMON PATHOGENS

CASE 75-1

QUESTION 1: B.C., a 41-year-old woman, was admitted to the cancer center for placement of a central IV catheter for administration of chemotherapy to treat acute nonlymphocytic leukemia in relapse. She was diagnosed 2 years ago and was treated with cytarabine plus daunorubicin, which resulted in a complete remission for 33 months. On this admission, she will be treated with high-dose cytarabine plus mitoxantrone for reinduction. What are the most likely pathogens to cause infection in patients like B.C. during periods of chemotherapy-induced neutropenia?

Bacteria are the primary pathogens associated with infection in febrile neutropenic patients, especially those occurring early.[16] Bacteremia (reported in approximately 25% of febrile neutropenic patients) is most often caused by aerobic gram-negative bacilli (including *Pseudomonas aeruginosa, Escherichia coli,* and *Klebsiella pneumoniae*) or aerobic gram-positive cocci (i.e., coagulase-negative staphylococci, *S. aureus,* enterococci, viridans streptococci).[17] Since the mid-1990s, the proportion of gram-negative infections has decreased with a proportional increase in gram-positive infections.[2,18] Gram-positive bacteria now account for approximately 60% to 70% of microbiologically documented infections in neutropenic cancer patients.[2,19] This is likely attributable (in part) to the frequent use of indwelling IV catheters, intensive chemotherapy, and widespread use of broad-spectrum antibiotics.

S. aureus (including MRSA) and coagulase-negative staphylococci, streptococci (including *S. pneumoniae* and viridans streptococci), and *Corynebacterium* species are increasingly important pathogens.[19] Moreover, enterococcal infections (including vancomycin-resistant enterococci [VRE]) are increasing in frequency. Meningitis caused by the intracellular organism *Listeria monocytogenes* can be observed in patients with defective cellular immunity caused by disease or prolonged corticosteroid use. In general, anaerobic bacteria are an infrequent cause of infection in granulocytopenic patients with hematologic malignancies.[20] However, they should be suspected in patients with GI malignancies or with significant disruption of the GI tract.[20] *Clostridium difficile* is another anaerobic pathogen that may cause infection in this population.

Pneumocystis jiroveci (formerly known as *Pneumocystis carinii* or PCP) is a pathogen responsible for lung infections primarily in patients with HIV infection. However, PCP can also be responsible for lung infections in some cancer patients.[21,22] Seen predominantly in patients with solid tumors or hematologic malignancies receiving long-term corticosteroids, PCP may present as subacute, febrile, hypoxemic, and diffuse pulmonary involvement.[21,22]

Invasive fungal infections (IFIs) are a major cause of morbidity and mortality among neutropenic cancer patients and patients undergoing HSCT.[23,24] The incidence of invasive fungal infections in febrile neutropenic patients varies widely because of differences in definitions, methods of detection, patient populations, and prior use of antifungal prophylaxis. In general, patients with hematologic malignancies have a higher incidence of fungal infections than those with solid tumors.[25] Similar to the risk of bacterial infections, the risk of invasive fungal infections is also related to the degree and duration of neutropenia. IFIs tend to occur later in the illness. Patients with prolonged neutropenia (>7 days) or with acute myelogenous leukemia (AML) undergoing intensive induction therapy, allogeneic HSCT recipients, and those undergoing therapy for GVHD are at increased risk of acquiring systemic fungal infections.[23,24] Up to 50% of patients who die during prolonged periods of neutropenia have evidence of deep-seated mycoses.[23] Before the use of fluconazole prophylaxis in selected populations, *Candida* species were responsible for most invasive fungal infections. Most fungal infections in neutropenic cancer patients are caused by *Candida* and *Aspergillus* species.[26–28] Other less common but important pathogenic fungi are those associated with zygomycosis (e.g., *Mucor* and *Rhizopus* species) and other emerging pathogens (non-albicans *Candida, Trichosporon beigelii, Malassezia* species, *Cryptococcus neoformans,* and *Fusarium* species).[26–28] Today, invasive infections attributable to *Aspergillus* species and other molds are a major cause of IFI-related death (particularly in those with prolonged neutropenia and GVHD).[23,29] Recent reports of improved survival from IFIs are likely related to newer prophylactic and treatment options and advances in cancer chemotherapy.[30]

As previously stated, most viral infections in neutropenic cancer patients are caused by a reactivation of latent infection rather than new infection.[2,3,9,14,15] These may include hepatitis B virus (HBV), herpes simplex virus (HSV), and *Varicella zoster* virus (VZV). Other viruses, such as CMV, can be either reactivation or newly acquired during HSCT. The risk of viral reactivation in these patients increases in patients who are seropositive prior to transplant. Respiratory viruses (e.g., respiratory syncytial virus [RSV], influenza, parainfluenza), GI viruses (such as rotavirus and norovirus), and other seasonal viruses may occasionally cause infection in this population.

STRATIFICATION FOR RISK OF INFECTION

Risk stratification to identify patients most likely to experience neutropenia has important implications for decisions about prevention, diagnostic strategies, empiric therapy (selection, route of administration, duration), and site of care.[2–4,9,14,15,31] In general, the underlying malignancy, status of disease (i.e., active vs. inactive), degree and duration of neutropenia, and chemotherapy type impact risk. Patients at highest risk of complications include those with prolonged (>7 days) and profound (<100 cells/μL) neutropenia or with select comorbidities (hypotension, severe mucositis interfering with swallowing or causing diarrhea, pneumonia, new-onset abdominal pain, hepatic or renal insufficiency, or neurologic changes).[3,4] In contrast, patients with shorter (≤7 days) anticipated durations of neutropenia without significant comorbidities are generally considered at low risk of complications of infection.[3,4,32] Patients without fever but exhibiting new signs of infection should also be treated as high risk. Presenting signs and symptoms, cancer type, chemotherapy regimen, medical comorbidities, and prior history of febrile neutropenia (especially if severe or prolonged) should also be considered. Patients with select solid tumors (breast, lung, colorectal, ovarian) and lymphoma most frequently experience neutropenic fever. Chemotherapeutic regimens associated with the highest (>20%) incidence of neutropenia are summarized in detail elsewhere[31] (see Section 17, Neoplastic Disorders).

The factors impacting risk have been utilized by the National Comprehensive Cancer Network in assigning infection risk in cancer patients as low, medium, and high.[3] Other risk assessment tools have been proposed,[3,14,15] including the Multinational Association for Supportive Care in Cancer (MASCC) index.[33] Age of at least 60 years, presence of hematologic malignancies with a history of prior fungal infections, severe symptoms (particularly hypotension), inpatient site of care, organ dysfunction (hepatic and renal), and presence of chronic obstructive pulmonary disease are important variables that result in a low MASCC score (i.e., <21), and (consequently) patients with any of these factors are considered at highest risk. Young patients (<20 years) with solid tumors and no or mild symptoms (including the absence of hypotension) or organ dysfunction are generally at low risk for complications.

PROPHYLAXIS AGAINST INFECTION

Infection Control

CASE 75-1, QUESTION 2: Should B.C. receive antimicrobial prophylaxis during the neutropenic period? If yes, which agents should be used?

Exogenous contamination can be prevented by strict protective isolation of patients in specially designed rooms that maintain a sterile environment. These laminar airflow rooms are ventilated with air that is passed through a high-efficiency particulate air filter, which removes greater than 99% of all particles larger than 3 μm. Total protective isolation is accomplished by strict isolation in conjunction with the administration of sterile food and water, local skin care, and intensive microbial surveillance. However, this regimen is burdensome, difficult to accomplish, and expensive, and is recommended only for high-risk patients (such as allogeneic HSCT recipients).[4] HSCT recipients and candidates undergoing conditioning therapy should avoid exposure to plants, flowers, and certain foods (such as uncooked fruits and vegetables), which increase the risk of exposure to fungi.[9,34] Close attention and adherence to adequate hand-washing procedures is essential. In addition, contact isolation is advocated in circumstances in which the patient may be colonized or infected with resistant organisms (such as MRSA, VRE, or multidrug-resistant gram-negative pathogens). Finally, isolating the patients from family or caregivers with potentially contagious respiratory viral illnesses is advocated.

Antimicrobial Prophylaxis

Early administration of antibiotics (i.e., antibacterials, antifungals, and antivirals) during the afebrile, neutropenic period in select high-risk patients may result in a reduction in the number of febrile episodes and subsequent risk of infection. The goals of such prophylactic regimens are intended to reduce pathogenic endogenous microflora or prevent the acquisition of new microorganisms. The potential benefits of such prophylaxis must outweigh the risks of antibiotic-related adverse effects including drug interactions, the development of resistance (most notable with antibacterials), and the potential for superinfection. Use of agents for prophylaxis (such as a fluoroquinolone for antibacterial prophylaxis) may also preclude the use of the class as empiric therapy for subsequent suspected or documented infections.

In general, lowest-risk cancer patients (such as those receiving standard chemotherapy for many solid tumors, and neutropenia anticipated to be <7 days) should not routinely receive antibacterial and antifungal prophylaxis.[3,4] Prophylactic administration of antivirals in such patients is generally restricted to those with a history of prior infection (such as HSV). In contrast, allogeneic HSCT recipients and those with acute leukemia, receipt of alemtuzumab therapy, GVHD requiring high-dose steroids, and prolonged (>10 days) neutropenia are at highest risk of infection and should receive antibacterial, antifungal, and (in select cases) antiviral prophylaxis.[3,4]

ANTIFUNGALS

CASE 75-1, QUESTION 3: Should antifungal prophylaxis be used in B.C.? What is the role of hematopoietic growth factors?

Routine antifungal prophylaxis is not indicated in patients with neutropenia at low risk of infection. However, select patients are at increased risk of developing systemic fungal infections.[23] Because of the frequency with which such infections are encountered, difficulties in establishing a diagnosis, poor response rates in patients with serious invasive infection who are immunocompromised, and effective prophylactic strategies are necessary in select intermediate and all high-risk patients. In patients for whom antifungal prophylaxis is indicated, the choice of the agent depends largely on the risk of invasive mold infections.

ANTIFUNGAL AGENTS

Nonabsorbable Antifungal Agents

Nonabsorbable antifungal agents, such as oral nystatin,[35,36] clotrimazole,[37] and oral amphotericin B,[38] have been studied. Although oral amphotericin B and clotrimazole reduce the frequency of oropharyngeal candidiasis, none of these antifungals has a role as primary prophylaxis of invasive fungal infections.[9] In attempts to enhance activity while minimizing side effects associated with IV administration, aerosolized delivery of amphotericin B deoxycholate has been investigated for the prevention of invasive fungal infections in this patient population,[39] and aerosolized liposomal amphotericin B has been used in leukemic and HSCT patients.[40] Although promising, the optimal dose, delivery device, and duration for aerosol administration of amphotericin B preparations have not yet been determined.

Amphotericin B

The use of systemic antifungals for prophylaxis has been summarized elsewhere.[41] Many of the earlier studies evaluated the prophylactic role of IV amphotericin B.[42–44] In general, use of amphotericin B deoxycholate is limited in this setting due to its toxicities (i.e., infusion-related reactions, nephrotoxicity, and electrolyte disturbances) relative to available options for prophylaxis. Consequently, amphotericin B is generally discouraged for primary prophylaxis in high-risk patients, unless the patient is unable to receive other mold-active prophylactic agents. If required, a lipid-based formulation would be preferred, especially in patients at increased risk of amphotericin B-induced nephrotoxicity.

Systemic Azole Antifungals

Systemic azole antifungals (e.g., itraconazole, fluconazole, voriconazole, posaconazole) may also be considered in select patients, but differ considerably in their spectrum of activity, adverse reaction profile, drug interactions, and need for serum concentration monitoring. The newest member of this class, isavuconazole, while representing potential advantages over comparator agents, has not yet been studied in such a setting.

Itraconazole has been well studied as an antifungal prophylaxis. In addition to in vitro activity against many *Candida* species (e.g., *Candida albicans*), itraconazole is active in vitro against *Aspergillus* species and reduces systemic *Candida* infections.[45–47] Although itraconazole oral solution demonstrates improved bioavailability over the capsule formulation, it is associated with significant GI intolerance.[48,49] Itraconazole is contraindicated in patients with reduced cardiac ejection fraction due to its negative inotropic effect. Use of newer azoles (such as posaconazole and voriconazole) has largely replaced the use of itraconazole for prophylaxis in patients at increased risk of mold infections (such as those patients undergoing immunosuppressive therapy for GVHD).

Fluconazole prophylaxis decreases the frequency of both superficial (e.g., oropharyngeal candidiasis) and systemic fungal infections in HSCT patients[50,51] but not in patients with leukemia.[7,52,53] Fluconazole is available as both oral and IV formulations, and its oral bioavailability is not significantly influenced by changes in gastric acidity. The IV formulation enables fluconazole to be administered to critically ill patients or patients who have difficulty swallowing. Although fluconazole is useful prophylactically, concern about its lack of reliable in vitro activity against molds limits its use in highest-risk patients. An increased frequency of isolation of non-albicans *Candida* (e.g., *Candida krusei, Candida glabrata, Candida parapsilosis*) has also been noted in some institutions.[54]

Posaconazole has demonstrated improved survival, a reduction in proven or probable IFI, and a reduction in invasive aspergillosis when compared with standard prophylaxis (either itraconazole or fluconazole) for the prevention of fungal infection in patients undergoing chemotherapy for AML or myelodysplastic syndrome.[55] Posaconazole was also effective prophylaxis in allogeneic HSCT recipients undergoing therapy for GVHD.[56] Posaconazole is currently available in both oral (solution and tablet) and parenteral (IV) formulations. The oral solution has been replaced largely by the tablet formulation due to its improved bioavailability and reduced dependency on the need for coadministration with high-fat meals for optimal absorption.[57,58] Absorption of oral posaconazole may be reduced in patients with mucositis and in patients receiving acid-suppressing therapy.[59] In addition, the use of IV posaconazole is not recommended in patients with significant renal impairment because of the potential toxicity of the vehicle.

Voriconazole's use as an antifungal prophylaxis in cancer patients at increased risk of mold infections is not well supported by clinical data despite its established use in the treatment of invasive aspergillosis.[60–62] Side effects (most notably hepatotoxicity, rash, phototoxicity) and the increased potential (relative to other azoles and the echinocandins) for drug interactions with voriconazole may limit its prophylactic use to patients at highest risk of mold infections. Similar to IV posaconazole, the use of IV voriconazole should be avoided in patients with significant renal impairment because of the potential toxicity of the vehicle. Oral voriconazole should be administered either 1 hour before or after a meal to optimize its absorption.

The echinocandins (e.g., caspofungin, micafungin, and anidulafungin) may be useful as a prophylactic strategy in high-risk patients. Micafungin has been compared with fluconazole in autologous and allogeneic HSCT recipients.[63] Based on a composite endpoint (which included absence of breakthrough fungal infection and absence of empiric modifications to the antifungal regimen owing to neutropenic fever), micafungin was found to be superior. Although breakthrough candidemia, survival, and adverse events were similar in both groups, a trend toward a reduction in invasive aspergillosis in the allogeneic HSCT population was noted in the micafungin group. Micafungin is currently US Food and Drug Administration (FDA)–approved for the prevention of *Candida* infections in HSCT patients.

SELECTION AND MONITORING OF PROPHYLACTIC ANTIFUNGALS

The use of primary antifungal prophylaxis in cancer patients with neutropenia should be reserved for patients at intermediate or high risk of invasive fungal infections (IFIs).[3,4] Patients with acute lymphocytic leukemia receiving remission or salvage induction chemotherapy are at intermediate risk and should be considered for prophylaxis. Although autologous HSCT recipients may not routinely benefit from fungal prophylaxis (most notably those without evidence of mucositis), those with prolonged neutropenia, mucosal damage, or receipt of purine analogs should receive primary prophylaxis.[9] Acceptable options for prophylaxis against *Candida* species include azoles (e.g., fluconazole, itraconazole, voriconazole, posaconazole) and the echinocandins (micafungin and caspofungin).[3,4] Of these options, fluconazole is the most commonly used agent. In the setting of colonization with fluconazole-resistant *Candida* species (such as *C. krusei, C. glabrata*), an echinocandin (such as micafungin) is preferred.[3,4,9,63] In contrast, patients with higher risk for mold infections (such as AML/MDS patients, or those with GVHD receiving intensive immunosuppressive therapy regardless of neutropenia) should be considered for prophylaxis with mold-active drugs (such as posaconazole, voriconazole, echinocandins, or amphotericin B) during periods of risk.[3,4,9] Mold-active agents are also recommended in the setting of anticipated periods of prolonged (at least 2 weeks) neutropenia, or prolonged neutropenia immediately before HSCT.[4]

Use of itraconazole, posaconazole, and voriconazole for prevention of fungal infections should be avoided in patients receiving vinca alkaloids (such as vincristine) due to their inhibition of the cytochrome P4503A4 (CYP3A4) isoenzyme and the resulting reduction in drug clearance of the vinca alkaloid. Fluconazole, while a CYP34A inhibitor, is less potent than these other azoles. Voriconazole also inhibits other cytochrome P450 isoenzymes to the greatest extent, expanding its potential for significant drug–drug interactions. The impact of isavuconazole on vinca alkaloids has not yet been report, but the potential for interactions does exist.

Prophylaxis is generally continued during the period of neutropenia. In those with acute leukemia, myelodysplastic syndrome (MDS), or autologous HSCT recipients, prophylaxis should continue until day 75 after transplant or through induction therapy for patients with leukemia.[64] Patients with a history of documented *Aspergillus* infection undergoing intensive chemotherapy should be considered for voriconazole.[9] Although the addition of a second prophylaxis (e.g., echinocandin) may be considered, the benefits of combination therapy for secondary prophylaxis are unknown.

Prophylactic use of antifungals may also be used in patients with a prior history of invasive disease due to *Candida* spp. or filamentous fungi. Such prevention (known as secondary prophylaxis) should be considered in such patients during subsequent chemotherapy or stem cell transplantation for the duration of immunosuppression.

In contrast to the predictable serum concentrations resulting from fluconazole administration, itraconazole, voriconazole, and posaconazole exhibit significant variability in drug concentration, most notably following oral administration. Therefore, serum concentration monitoring of these agents may help assure optimal drug exposure while reducing the potential for concentration-related toxicities. However, determination of definitive target concentrations for prophylactic use is hampered by the lack of controlled, prospective clinical trials. For itraconazole, steady-state trough concentrations of >0.5 mcg/mL or greater have been recommended. Voriconazole steady-state serum concentration of >0.5 to 4 mcg/mL has been recommended for use as prophylaxis. Studies regarding the optimal trough concentration of posaconazole for prophylaxis differ, but range between 0.5 and 0.7 mcg/mL.[65,66]

NONABSORBABLE ANTIBACTERIALS

Because the GI tract is an important reservoir of potential pathogens, gut decontamination has been investigated.[19] However, use of nonabsorbable antibacterial agents has been replaced by oral, absorbable antibiotics.[3,4]

ABSORBABLE (SYSTEMIC) ANTIBACTERIALS

Trimethoprim–Sulfamethoxazole

Although trimethoprim–sulfamethoxazole (TMP–SMX) decreases bacterial infections in neutropenic patients,[67,68] it may not reduce mortality in this patient population. The potential benefits of TMP–SMX prophylaxis must be carefully balanced against the potential for drug-induced bone marrow suppression, hypersensitivity reactions, hyperkalemia, nephrotoxicity, pancreatitis, the emergence of resistant organisms (e.g., *E. coli*), and the development of superinfections. In addition, leukemic patients receiving mucotoxic chemotherapy and TMP–SMX prophylaxis may be at increased risk for infections caused by viridans streptococci.[69,70] Therefore, TMP–SMX should not be routinely used for primary prophylaxis (except as noted below).

TMP–SMX prevents *P. jiroveci* (PCP) pneumonia in both ALL and HSCT patient populations. Patients with malignancy at highest risk for experiencing *P. jiroveci* (PCP) pneumonia (i.e., patients with acute lymphocytic leukemia receiving intensive chemotherapy, those with acquired immunodeficiency syndrome, allogeneic HSCT recipients, those receiving alemtuzumab, patients with GVHD, and those in whom neutropenia is anticipated to exceed 10 days) should receive TMP–SMX prophylaxis.[3,9] Recipients of T-cell-depleting agents (e.g., fludarabine or cladribine), cancer patients receiving prolonged or high-dose corticosteroids (>20 mg of prednisone or its equivalent daily), and autologous HSCT recipients should also be considered for prophylaxis with TMP–SMX.[9] In such settings, primary prevention should be continued for up to 6 months (in the case of HSCT recipients) or longer (in cases in which immunosuppression is continued). In the setting of alemtuzumab therapy, such prophylaxis would generally continue for at least 2 months and until the CD4 count exceeded 200 cells/μL.[3] In patients requiring PCP prophylaxis but unable to tolerate TMP–SMX, patients should receive alternate prophylaxis with either atovaquone, dapsone, or pentamidine (either IV or via aerosol).[3,9]

Fluoroquinolones

The fluoroquinolones ciprofloxacin and levofloxacin are used by some centers as prophylaxis for adult patients at high risk of infection.[71,72] Of concern, however, is the increasing frequency of gram-positive infections (including viridans streptococci) and resistant gram-negative bacilli (most notable in *P. aeruginosa* and *E. coli*)[73] in patients receiving fluoroquinolone prophylaxis.[69,70,74,75] Meta-analyses report reductions in mortality in high-risk patients receiving prophylaxis with these fluoroquinolones.[71,76] Because fluoroquinolone prophylaxis is offset by the emergence of resistant organisms, routine prophylactic use in low-risk patients should generally be avoided.[4] However, those at intermediate or high risk of bacterial infections (i.e., those patients with an ANC ≤100 neutrophils/μL for >7 days) should be considered for fluoroquinolone prophylaxis until either the onset of fever (at which time empiric antibacterials would be started) or resolution of severe neutropenia.[4,9] Levofloxacin has been recommended over ciprofloxacin in patients at increased risk of oral mucositis-related infection with invasive viridans streptococci.[4] Regardless of the fluoroquinolone chosen, local resistance patterns should be closely monitored before such prophylaxis is chosen.

Penicillin

Because of the increased risk of invasive pneumococcal infections, select patient populations (notably asplenic patients, allogeneic HSCT recipients [owing to functional asplenia and impaired B-cell immunity], and those undergoing immunosuppression for GVHD) should be considered for prophylaxis with penicillin. In patients with chronic GVHD, penicillin prophylaxis may be continued during the administration of immunosuppressives. In HSCT recipients, prophylaxis should begin 3 months after transplant and continue for 1 year after transplant. Alternative prophylaxis should be considered in areas where penicillin resistance in pneumococci is significant.

ANTIVIRALS

Most HSV disease in cancer patients is a consequence of reactivation from latent infection. High-risk patients (e.g., seropositive for HSV undergoing allogeneic HSCT or induction or re-induction therapy for acute leukemia) or patients previously requiring treatment for HSV reactivation should be given antiviral prophylaxis. Both oral or IV acyclovir and oral valacyclovir are appropriate initial choices in most patients. Published data for famciclovir for this indication are lacking. Those receiving foscarnet or ganciclovir (most commonly for prevention and treatment of CMV infection) do not require additional prophylaxis for HSV, given the activity of these against *H. simplex*. Prophylaxis should be administered during periods of neutropenia and for at least 1 month after HSCT.[3,4] The duration may be extended in those undergoing allogeneic HSCT with GVHD. Patients receiving alemtuzumab may also require extended prophylaxis of up to 2 months after completion of therapy or recovery of $CD4^+$ cells count >200 cells/μL, whichever is later.

Similar to HSV, VZV in cancer patients is most commonly reactivation. HSCT patients who are seropositive for VZV should also be given long-term prophylaxis (6–12 months for autologous HSCT and at least 1 year for allogeneic HSCT patients),[4] particularly with receipt of either bortezomib or alemtuzumab.[3] Extending prophylaxis in allogeneic HSCT patients should be considered in the setting of continued immunosuppressive therapy. Like for HSV, patients receiving alemtuzumab may also require extended prophylaxis of up to 2 months after completion of therapy or recovery of $CD4^+$ cells count >200 cells/μl, whichever is later. Agents active against HSV are also useful for VZV prevention. In one study, low-dose (i.e., 500 mg/day, 3 times weekly) valacyclovir prophylaxis after a 35-day course of IV acyclovir is safe and effective in allogeneic HSCT recipients.[77]

Patients at highest risk of either CMV reactivation or primary infection (e.g., allogeneic HSCT patients, those receiving alemtuzumab, and those with GVHD requiring high-dose steroids) should be considered for antiviral prophylaxis against this pathogen. One strategy is the administration of all patients at risk (universal prophylaxis). Given the toxicity of ganciclovir IV, valganciclovir PO, foscarnet IV, and cidofovir IV (the most potent agents for CMV), a second strategy, known as preemptive, involves administration of antivirals prior to symptoms by following serologic evidence (based on CMV pp65 antigen or two consecutive CMV PCR tests) of viral replication. Foscarnet and cidofovir IV are generally reserved as second-line agents for preemptive therapy (such as in the setting of neutropenia secondary to ganciclovir). The potential role of valganciclovir PO (an oral pro-drug of ganciclovir) as a preemptive strategy in this population has been evaluated and is now considered a viable option in the absence of GVHD involving the GI tract.[78–82] Finally, a third prevention strategy is to combine use of less effective yet safer agents (such as acyclovir or valacyclovir) together with active surveillance (up to 6 months in allogeneic HSCT patients) and, when serologic evidence of virus replication exists, initiate PO valganciclovir or ganciclovir IV therapy. Surveillance for CMV may be extended in patients with chronic GVHD receiving immunosuppressive therapy until recovery of $CD4^+$ count of 100 cells/μL or greater.

Patients with prior infections with hepatitis B virus (HBV) or hepatitis C virus (HCV) can experience reactivation of infection secondary to immunosuppressive therapy. Reactivation of infection can occur in patients infected with HBV undergoing immunosuppressive therapy (most notably in allogeneic HSCT recipients and those receiving anti-CD20 or anti-CD52 monoclonal antibodies). Therefore, serologic screening (utilizing testing for hepatitis B surface antigen [HBsAg] and hepatitis B core antibody [HBcAb]) is generally performed in patients at increased risk of infection. Prophylaxis should be considered in patients with positive tests. Patients with one or more of these screening tests positive often undergo further testing for active viral replication (utilizing a quantitative PCR test for HBV DNA). Preemptive therapy should be considered in patient with evidence of viral replication. Despite limited data in cancer patients, the nucleos(t)ide analogs adefovir and tenofovir have largely replaced lamivudine monotherapy in such settings due to the high incidence of viral resistance with this strategy. Other agents considered for HBV prophylaxis may include entecavir and telbivudine.

Respiratory tract infections caused by RSV, influenza, and parainfluenza are less commonly observed in patients with neutropenia. Although response to influenza virus vaccine may be attenuated, patients undergoing cancer treatment should receive annual vaccinations with inactivated influenza vaccine.[4] Whenever possible, the timing of such vaccinations may be best between cycles (>7 days after or >2 weeks before next treatment). In contrast, immunocompromised patients should not receive the intranasal live virus vaccine.[4]

Hematopoietic Growth Factors

Hematopoietic colony-stimulating factors (CSFs) such as granulocyte CSF (G-CSF; filgrastim), pegylated G-CSF (pegfilgrastim), or granulocyte-macrophage CSF (GM-CSF; sargramostim) are important adjuncts in cancer patients.[83,84] Studies in cancer patients receiving myelosuppressive or myeloablative chemotherapy have demonstrated that concurrent use of the CSFs can reduce the duration of neutropenia. The selection of one CSF agent over another is often based on practitioner preference rather than clinical data.

Hematopoietic growth factors (more specifically G-CSF [filgrastim] or pegylated G-CSF [pegfilgrastim]) reduce the risk of chemotherapy-induced febrile neutropenia.[10,31,85–87] Risk factors for neutropenia include age (i.e., >65 years), medical history (including prior history of febrile neutropenic episodes, nutritional status, unstable comorbidities, and presence of active infections), disease characteristics (especially those involving bone marrow resulting in cytopenias), and myelotoxicity of the regimen (including both chemotherapy and radiation) used to treat the underlying malignancy.[31,85–87] Routine use of CSFs for the prevention of febrile neutropenia should be discouraged in patients at low risk (<10%)

 of febrile neutropenia.[4,31,87] In contrast, guidelines advocate the use as primary prophylaxis in patients at high risk (>20%) of fever and neutropenia. Some guidelines also recommend administration of CSFs for primary prevention for patients >65 years with diffuse aggressive lymphoma treated with curative chemotherapy (especially in the setting of significant comorbidities and in those receiving select dose-dense chemotherapy regimens). Although benefits of CSFs are less clear in patients with intermediate risk (10%–20% risk of febrile neutropenia), they should be considered on a case-by-case basis.[84] CSFs are generally avoided as prophylaxis in patients undergoing radiation therapy concomitant with chemotherapy because of the potential for thrombocytopenia[88] or reductions in tumor response.[89] Administration is generally continued 3 to 4 days after chemotherapy administration and continued until a sufficient and stable postnadir ANC recovery is established.[10,84] Pegylated G-CSF may be preferred in some settings owing to the convenience of single administration.[31,90]

Consideration of the use of CSFs as secondary prophylaxis (i.e., prevention of febrile neutropenia in patients undergoing second or subsequent cycles of chemotherapy) should be based on repeated assessments of patient risk of febrile neutropenia.[84] Patients experiencing prior episodes of febrile neutropenia or neutropenia limiting the dose of chemotherapy without prior CSFs should be considered for secondary prophylaxis.[84]

Other Agents

Although beyond the scope of this chapter, select vaccinations have also been recommended for both autologous and allogeneic HSCT recipients (primarily caused by a decline in antibody titers to many vaccine-preventable diseases).[9] These include (but are not limited to) administration of pneumococcal, influenza virus and *H. influenzae* vaccines. Live vaccinations should be avoided in this population. However, because immune response may be altered immediately after transplant, delays of up to 3 months after cessation of immunosuppressive chemotherapy are recommended for many vaccines. In addition, serologic testing of antibody response is recommended in selected settings.[9]

Although data to support use are sparse, IV immunoglobulins have been recommended for HSCT recipients with severe hypogammaglobulinemia (i.e., serum immunoglobulin G level <400 mg/dL) and recurrent infections.[9] Intravenous immunoglobulins (IVIG) have been used as adjuncts in the prevention and treatment of CMV infections. In contrast, granulocyte transfusions have not been proven to be effective in either prevention or treatment of infection in the neutropenic cancer patient.[91]

INFECTIONS IN NEUTROPENIC CANCER PATIENTS

Clinical Signs and Symptoms

CASE 75-1, QUESTION 4: Seven days after completing chemotherapy, B.C. experienced a fever of 102°F (orally). Vital signs are blood pressure, 109/70 mm Hg; pulse, 102 beats/minute; and respirations, 25 breaths/minute. Physical examination demonstrates a clear oropharynx without exudates or plaques. Chest and cardiac examination are normal. The exit site for the Hickman catheter is clean and nontender without signs of erythema or induration. The perineum and rectum are nontender, and no masses are noted. Laboratory data are as follows:

Hematocrit, 20%
Hemoglobin, 7 g/dL
WBC count, 1,400 cells/μL, with 3% polymorphonuclear leukocytes (PMNs), 1% band forms, 70% lymphocytes, and 22% monocytes
Platelet count, 17,000 cells/L
Blood glucose, 160 mg/dL
Serum creatinine (SCr), 1.1 mg/dL
Blood urea nitrogen (BUN), 24 mg/dL

What are the signs and symptoms of infection in B.C.? What are the most common sites and sources of infection in patients such as B.C.?

B.C. has an ANC of 48 cells/μL (1,400 WBCs/μL × [0.03 PMNs + 0.01 bands]) and is therefore at high risk for infection.

Fever in neutropenic patients is defined as a single oral temperature of at least 38.3°C (101°F) or a temperature of at least 38.0°C (100.4°F) for more than 1 hour in the absence of an obvious cause.[3,4] It is the earliest (and often the only) sign of infection in neutropenic patients, because typical signs can be modified or absent in this patient population.[4] However, only 48% to 60% of patients with febrile neutropenia have occult or documented infections.[3] Noninfectious sources of fever in the neutropenic cancer patient include inflammation, tumor progression, tumor lysis, adverse drug reactions, and transfusion reactions.[3,14,15] Signs and symptoms consistent with a diagnosis of infection without fever should be considered to be infection in the neutropenic host until proven otherwise.[3]

In patients with documented infections, the most common sites are skin, mouth, throat, esophagus, sinuses, abdomen, rectum, liver, vascular access, lungs, and urinary tract.[3,92] Although the lung is the most common site of serious infection in neutropenic cancer patients, fever and dry cough are often the only presenting signs of pneumonia.[92] The impaired inflammatory response results in scant sputum production, and sputum Gram stains often contain few PMNs. Radiologic evidence of a pulmonary infection can be minimal or absent, and the chest examination is frequently not diagnostic.[93] Pneumonia is associated with high mortality in neutropenic patients, particularly in the setting of bacteremia. In the presence of shock, a mortality rate of approximately 80% has been observed in these patients.[94]

Invasive procedures such as venipuncture, central IV catheter placement (e.g., Hickman catheter), and skin biopsies are associated with cellulitis and systemic infections. However, the typical signs and symptoms of infection (e.g., pain, heat, erythema, swelling) are often absent in part owing to inadequate granulocytes.[92] Colonization of these lesions may result in local infection and the potential for systemic dissemination of bacteria and fungi. Bacteremia occurs primarily from entry of bacteria through the skin or through unrecognized ulcerations in the GI and perirectal areas.

Confirmation of Infection

CASE 75-1, QUESTION 5: How can an infection be confirmed in patients such as B.C.?

Because of the frequent lack of physical signs and symptoms of infection, the clinician must obtain an accurate history (including the cancer type and treatment regimen, new signs of infection, antimicrobial prophylaxis, prior infections, and comorbidities) and conduct a careful physical examination at the first sign of fever. A detailed search for subtle signs and symptoms of inflammation at the most common sites, such as the oropharynx, bone marrow aspiration sites, lung, periodontium, skin, vascular catheter access sites, nail beds, and perineum (including the anus) is necessary. Before antibiotics are initiated, two sets of blood cultures (with each set consisting of two culture bottles) should be obtained.[3,4,14] In patients with indwelling central venous catheters, one of the two sets of blood cultures should be obtained from the catheter to help rule out catheter-related infection.[4] Diarrheal stools may be tested for the presence of *C. difficile*. Additional Gram stain and cultures (e.g., stool, urine, skin, IV site, respiratory specimens) should be obtained depending on signs and symptoms.[4] The yield from such cultures, however, may be affected by the prior or concurrent administration of prophylaxis.[2] Chest radiographs and oximetry should be obtained in the presence of respiratory symptoms.[4] Respiratory virus testing should take place for patients with upper respiratory tract infection symptoms (i.e., coryza) or cough.[4] In settings in which pulmonary aspergillosis is suspected, further radiologic evaluations (such as computed tomography scans) should be considered.[29] A complete blood count, serum electrolytes, coagulation, C-reactive protein, urinalysis, and assessment of organ function (e.g., liver and kidney function) should be obtained to assist in drug dosing and monitoring for treatment-related toxicities.[4]

Recent advances have been made in nonculture-based diagnostic tests that help support (or in some cases eliminate) the diagnosis of infection in these patients.[95] Such studies include C-reactive protein[96–98] and procalcitonin.[98–100] However, these tests are not routinely ordered, and their role in the treatment of the neutropenic cancer patient has not yet been established.[4] Galactomannan (specific for aspergillosis)[101] and β-D-glucan testing may assist in the diagnosis of fungal infections.[102,103] Serial galactomannan testing has also been used preemptively to initiate antifungal therapy before overt signs and symptoms of invasive fungal infections occur.[104] In addition to other issues regarding sensitivity and specificity of these assays, both galactomannan and β-D-glucan are affected by prior or current receipt of antifungals.[29] At present, the use of these tests should be restricted to persistent fever despite other etiologic investigations.[4]

Significance of Colonization

CASE 75-1, QUESTION 6: Routine surveillance cultures of swabs taken from B.C.'s axillae, nasopharynx, and rectum grew *Corynebacterium jeikeium* (axillae), *S. aureus* (axillae and nasopharynx), and *Enterococcus faecium* (rectum). What is the significance of these culture results? Should routine, serial surveillance cultures be performed in patients such as B.C.?

Several factors influence the colonization and subsequent infection by microorganisms in cancer patients. Organisms isolated from infected patients can be found in endogenous flora or acquired during hospitalization.[105] Factors leading to colonization include staff-to-staff and patient-to-patient transmission (e.g., lack of frequent and adequate hand hygiene), direct transmission from the environment (e.g., inadequately disinfected bathtubs, sinks, toilet bowls), foods (e.g., raw fruits and vegetables), inhalation from contaminated fomites (e.g., respirators, ventilating systems), and IV access devices. In addition to immunosuppression, the underlying malignancy and associated chemotherapy diminish the cancer patient's resistance to colonization and infection.

The acquisition of and subsequent colonization by potentially pathogenic microbes may be detected by serial surveillance cultures of specimens obtained from various body sites such as the nasopharynx, axilla, urine, and rectum. Such surveillance cultures may be useful for infection control purposes. However, little clinically useful information is gained in the absence of infection. Therefore, surveillance cultures are generally restricted to select patients for infection control purposes. In such cases, culture of the anterior nares (for MRSA) or rectal samples (for VRE or multidrug-resistant gram-negative bacilli) may be performed.

In summary, B.C.'s surveillance culture results indicate that she is colonized with several potential pathogens associated with infection in the immunocompromised host, but these results are probably not useful in selecting empiric antibiotics for her fever.

EMPIRIC ANTIBIOTIC THERAPY

Rationale

CASE 75-1, QUESTION 7: Should B.C. be started on antibiotic therapy immediately? Is this rational in view of the fact that neither the source of her fever nor the pathogen has been established?

Neutropenic cancer patient with fever and/or other signs and symptoms of infection should undergo prompt risk assessment and initiation of antibiotic therapy. Once cultures are obtained, these patients should be emergently started on broad-spectrum antibacterials. Prompt institution should not be delayed if cultures cannot be obtained. Early studies confirmed high mortality in neutropenic patients with untreated gram-negative infections up to 24 to 48 hours after the onset of fever. Crude mortality rates secondary to *P. aeruginosa* bacteremia approached 91%.[6] Prompt use of empiric, broad-spectrum antibiotics has resulted in significant reductions in infectious mortality rates.

Initial Empiric Antibiotic Regimens

CASE 75-1, QUESTION 8: What pathogen- and patient-specific factors should be considered when initiating empiric therapy for B.C.?

Practice guidelines prepared by the National Comprehensive Cancer Network,[3] the Infectious Diseases Society of America,[4] and the European Society of Medical Oncology[14] identify antimicrobial options for the treatment of fever in the neutropenic cancer patient. The ideal antibiotic regimen for empiric management in this setting (i.e., those without evidence of site- or pathogen-specific infections) remains controversial. High-risk patients requiring IV therapy are often candidates for monotherapy regimens, including an antipseudomonal third-generation cephalosporin (e.g., ceftazidime), a fourth-generation cephalosporin (e.g., cefepime), or an antipseudomonal carbapenem (e.g., imipenem–cilastatin or meropenem).[3,4,14,15] Initial, empiric use of additional antibiotics (such as fluoroquinolones, aminoglycosides, and vancomycin) may be added to patients who are clinically unstable.[4] Alternative initial empiric parenteral regimens (excluding those containing vancomycin) have been investigated in this patient population.[3,4,14,15,34] However, because no significant differences exist among any of these empiric approaches, monotherapy is employed in most patients.

Optimal Antibacterial Spectrum

CASE 75-1, QUESTION 9: Given the lack of site-specific signs and symptoms of infection, what would be a reasonable initial empiric antibiotic regimen for B.C.?

Despite continued development in antibacterial drugs, the empiric management of febrile neutropenic patients is complicated by the changing spectrum of bacterial pathogens and their antimicrobial susceptibilities. Empiric antibiotic regimens should provide broad-spectrum coverage against the potential gram-negative bacilli most commonly isolated from neutropenic cancer patients (e.g., *E. coli, K. pneumoniae, P. aeruginosa*), staphylococci, and viridans streptococci.[3,13] Because mortality from untreated bacteremia caused by *P. aeruginosa* is so high,[65] empiric regimens have traditionally included antimicrobials with antipseudomonal activity.

Selecting an initial empiric regimen for a given patient should take into account the patient's risk of infection, likely pathogens, infection site-specific antibiotic efficacy, and institutional susceptibility patterns. This point is especially true in areas experiencing a growing frequency of multidrug-resistant organisms, such as MRSA, VRE, and extended-spectrum β-lactamase (ESBL)-producing organisms (such as *K. pneumoniae* and *E. coli*).[18] Patient-related considerations should include medical stability, allergies, prior and concomitant antimicrobials, and organ dysfunction (e.g., renal or hepatic). Attempts should be made to identify low-risk patients for whom oral antimicrobial therapy may be an option. Finally, dosing schedules, acquisition costs, and the potential for significant toxicities should be considered. In addition to broad-spectrum activity, antibacterial regimens should be bactericidal against the infecting pathogen. However, no adequately controlled comparative trials of bacteriostatic versus bactericidal antibiotics have been conducted in humans.

In summary, many organisms, including those recovered from surveillance cultures, may be pathogens in B.C. Those associated with a high mortality rate during the first 48 hours should be empirically treated pending culture and sensitivity results. Therefore, an empiric regimen with optimal activity against commonly isolated gram-negative bacilli (including *P. aeruginosa*) should be promptly administered to B.C.

ORAL ANTIBIOTICS

Carefully selected (i.e., low risk) adult febrile neutropenic patients may be candidates for oral antibiotic therapy, either as initial therapy or as follow-up to IV antibiotics (sequential therapy).[2,4,106–108] Patients must be able to tolerate oral medications. In general, patients considered for oral therapy must be without microbiologic or clinical evidence of infection (other than fever), clinically stable, and closely observed. Patients with severe (ANC < 100 cells/μL), or lasting anticipated ≥ 7 days, or those receiving prior fluoroquinolone prophylaxis would not be eligible. This would also exclude patients with any of the following: serious comorbidities, inpatient acquisition of infection, uncontrolled malignancy, pneumonia, recent HSCT, dehydration, hypotension, chronic lung disease, abnormal liver ($>3\times$ upper limits of normal) or renal function (serum creatinine >2 mg/dL), or signs and symptoms lasting longer than 7 days.[4] An international collaborative study established and validated a risk scoring system in adults that incorporated these principles to identify low-risk patients for whom oral therapy may be an option.[33]

Cefixime has been used effectively as an alternative regimen in low-risk pediatric patients initially receiving IV therapy,[109] but there is not adequate experience to recommend it at this time. It also lacks activity against *Pseudomonas* spp. Fluoroquinolone-containing regimens have been the mainstay of most oral regimens used in this setting. Patients already receiving fluoroquinolones as prophylaxis should be excluded from receiving this regimen. Oral ciprofloxacin in combination with amoxicillin–clavulanate (both administered every 8 hours) is useful in low-risk adult patients with febrile neutropenia[110,111] and is the most commonly used oral regimen. Oral levofloxacin may be used in place of ciprofloxacin, and oral clindamycin may be used in place of amoxicillin–clavulanate if the patient is allergic to β-lactam antibiotics. More recently, moxifloxacin has been evaluated in this patient population and demonstrates efficacy comparable to combination regimens containing ciprofloxacin.[112,113] However, although moxifloxacin permits simplification of the regimen, it lacks activity against *Pseudomonas* spp. Therefore, its use should be restricted to patients at low risk of pseudomonal infections.

Low-risk patients with adequate home support (e.g., access to emergency facilities, phone access) and the desire for home treatment may be treated as an outpatient (with either IV or oral therapy). Therapy is usually initiated in a clinic or hospital setting.[4] Monitoring in the outpatient setting should include either home nursing or office visits daily for 3 days to review progress and to screen for problems. Patients who are stable and responding after the initial observation period may continue to receive monitoring by phone contact.

Continued administration of antimicrobials in the outpatient setting initiated as an inpatient has been suggested in a subset of low-risk patients. The criteria used to define eligibility for outpatient therapy are generally similar to those established and previously discussed for oral therapy. Therefore, continued outpatient administration of parenteral antibiotics can be considered in a subset of low-risk patients with close medical follow-up.[4]

INTRAVENOUS MONOTHERAPY

In general, intravenous monotherapy with an antipseudomonal β-lactam (such as an antipseudomonal cephalosporin, carbapenem, or β-lactam and β-lactamase combination) is advocated as initial empiric therapy for most neutropenic cancer patients.[3,4] There are no convincing data to support one choice over the others as empiric monotherapy.

Antipseudomonal Cephalosporins

Ceftazidime monotherapy has been found to be as effective as combination therapy. However, in some of these trials, the efficacy of ceftazidime in patients with documented staphylococcal and streptococcal infections was suboptimal. Select clinical trials have empirically added antistaphylococcal coverage with a glycopeptide (e.g., vancomycin) and have shown improved outcomes in these patients. In addition, pathogens (particularly gram-negative pathogens) that produce either type 1 β-lactamase or ESBL (e.g., *K. pneumoniae*) are not likely to respond to ceftazidime monotherapy. These organisms are more likely with prolonged hospitalization or receipt of antimicrobial therapy. Therefore, local in vitro susceptibilities of common gram-negative pathogens should be examined before the routine use of ceftazidime as monotherapy.

Cefepime is a fourth-generation cephalosporin with an FDA-approved indication for monotherapy for empiric management of infection in patients with febrile neutropenia. The potential advantage of this agent compared with third-generation cephalosporins is its low affinity for major chromosomally mediated β-lactamases. Compared with ceftazidime, cefepime has more potent activity in vitro against select gram-positive bacteria (methicillin-susceptible *Staphylococcus* species, viridans streptococci, and *S. pneumoniae*). Similar to ceftazidime, numerous randomized, comparative studies have evaluated the role of cefepime as monotherapy in both adults and children with febrile neutropenia. The improved gram-positive activity (relative to ceftazidime) may decrease the empiric need for vancomycin in some patients. However, this advantage is less likely in institutions with a high rate of MRSA because cefepime and other cephalosporins (with the exception of ceftaroline) are inactive against this pathogen. Although a meta-analysis published in 2007 suggested increased all-cause mortality in neutropenic patients treated empirically with cefepime,[114,115] subsequent analysis by the FDA concluded no such differences existed when compared with control patients.

Carbapenems

The carbapenems are a unique class of antibiotics with broad-spectrum activity against numerous gram-positive and gram-negative bacteria, including anaerobes. In addition, carbapenems may be used in the setting in which the patient is at increased risk of ESBL-producing gram-negative pathogens (such as *K. pneumoniae* or *E. coli*). Imipenem (in combination with the dehydropeptidase inhibitor cilastatin) and meropenem are two currently available agents in this class that have been studied as monotherapy for febrile neutropenic patients.

Clinical outcomes with imipenem–cilastatin monotherapy have been comparable with those of the β-lactam plus aminoglycoside combinations. Although effective, imipenem–cilastatin has generally been associated with a higher incidence of nausea and vomiting compared with ceftazidime or meropenem.[116,117] The GI side effects are generally dose-related (3–4 g/day) and associated with the rate of IV administration. Therefore, dosages of 2 g/day (divided every 6 hours) are generally given to patients with normal renal function.

Meropenem monotherapy for febrile neutropenia has been evaluated in both adults and children, and the results have supported the value of meropenem as empiric monotherapy for use in febrile neutropenic patients. Meropenem may have advantages over imipenem–cilastatin in the treatment of central nervous system infections (owing to less associated seizure activity).

Although doripenem possesses comparable microbiologic activity, studies evaluating its administration in this population are lacking. Although ertapenem possesses microbiologic activity comparable to that of the other carbapenems, it lacks in vitro activity against *Acinetobacter* species and *Pseudomonas* spp., including *P. aeruginosa*. Considering this lack of activity, ertapenem would not be appropriate as empiric therapy for febrile neutropenic patients. Agents with increased anaerobic activity (including carbapenems) might be used as empiric therapy in cases in which an intra-abdominal infection is suspected.

Routine carbapenem use may be associated with increased drug acquisition cost (relative to cephalosporins) and increased potential for development of carbapenem resistance. Therefore, many institutions have elected to reserve the carbapenems for patients who have failed to respond to prior empiric therapy, have a history of infections with pathogens resistant to third- and fourth-generation cephalosporins, are clinically unstable, or have need for expanded anaerobic coverage.

β-Lactam/β-Lactamase Inhibitors

Randomized trials have compared piperacillin–tazobactam monotherapy to various antibiotics. Published trials have documented that piperacillin–tazobactam is not inferior to cefepime in this patient population.[118,119] Although experience with this agent as monotherapy is limited relative to that for the antipseudomonal carbapenems and antipseudomonal cephalosporins, it is considered to be an adequate choice for monotherapy.[4] Higher doses of piperacillin–tazobactam (i.e., 3.375 g IV every 4 hours or 4.5 g IV every 6 hours in adult patients with normal renal function) should be used because of the risk of pseudomonal infections.[3] Piperacillin–tazobactam may interfere with the galactomannan assay used in the diagnosis of select IFIs, including aspergillosis.

INITIAL ANTIMICROBIAL COMBINATIONS (EXCLUDING VANCOMYCIN)

CASE 75-2

QUESTION 1: B.L., a 13-year-old boy, presented with a 3-week history of "always being tired" and a persistent sore throat. Initial evaluation revealed anemia, thrombocytopenia, and a WBC count of 130,000 cells/L, with a predominance of immature lymphoblasts. Further evaluation demonstrated that B.L. had high-risk acute lymphocytic leukemia. Remission induction treatment was initiated with teniposide plus cytarabine followed by prednisone, vincristine, and L-asparaginase. Seven days after induction chemotherapy, B.L. experienced a fever (102°F) and chills. The ANC was 48 cells/μL. SCr and BUN were 1.0 and 15 mg/dL, respectively. The physician wants to empirically start B.L. on ceftazidime plus gentamicin combination regimen. What is the role of this combination in the empiric management of febrile neutropenia? Are there any differences in efficacy between these combinations?

Before the introduction of third- and fourth-generation cephalosporins and carbapenems, the empiric use of antibacterial combinations in febrile neutropenic cancer patients was favored because these regimens offered a broader spectrum of activity against bacteria commonly infecting cancer patients.[3,120] In addition, these combinations offered the potential for an additive or synergistic effect.[120,121] However, infections in neutropenic patients have shifted largely from gram-negative to gram-positive pathogens, for which these traditional combination regimens have limited efficacy. Despite this concern, some clinicians continue to favor antibiotic combinations as initial empiric therapy, especially in patients who are clinically unstable.[3] It is unknown whether combination therapy prevents the emergence of resistance.

Until the 1980s, most febrile neutropenic patients were treated with two-drug combination regimens that contained an aminoglycoside (gentamicin, tobramycin, or amikacin) plus a β-lactam antibiotic, such as antipseudomonal penicillin, or an antipseudomonal third-generation cephalosporin. This combination is one of the most established empiric treatment regimens for the management of febrile neutropenia.

Numerous studies have been conducted to evaluate the efficacy of combination therapy of an aminoglycoside with an antipseudomonal cephalosporin (ceftazidime and cefepime).[3] Antipseudomonal penicillins plus β-lactamase inhibitors (in combination with an aminoglycoside) would also be considered a comparable regimen. A better outcome was demonstrated with full-course amikacin plus ceftazidime than with a short course (3 days) of amikacin plus a full course of ceftazidime.[122] However, the longer course of the aminoglycoside is likely to be associated with more toxicity.

Because carbapenem antibiotics are more frequently evaluated as monotherapy in this patient population, there are limited studies examining the combination of an aminoglycoside with either imipenem–cilastatin or meropenem. However, in one such evaluation, the combination of imipenem–cilastatin plus amikacin was found to be superior to imipenem–cilastatin monotherapy.[123] Carbapenems (in combination with aminoglycosides and vancomycin) have been recommended as empiric initial therapy for patients who are clinically unstable.

Aminoglycosides have generally been considered the backbone of combination regimens because of their potential for bactericidal action against various bacteria. However, the addition of an aminoglycoside is associated with increased costs for therapeutic monitoring. The benefit of an aminoglycoside for empiric therapy has not been consistently demonstrated.[123,124] In addition, there is an increased potential for the development of nephrotoxicity and ototoxicity.[124] This concern is especially relevant in patients receiving concomitant nephrotoxins (such as cisplatin and cyclosporine).

CASE 75-2, QUESTION 2: Seven days into therapy, despite rehydration, B.L.'s SCr and BUN rose to 2.0 g/dL and 45 mg/dL, respectively. Because B.L. has nephrotoxicity (believed to be secondary to the aminoglycoside), what other combination regimens (excluding those containing aminoglycosides) could be used? Are these regimens as effective as aminoglycoside-containing regimens?

As previously stated, ciprofloxacin has been studied in combination with other antibacterials (either an aminoglycoside or a β-lactam, including an antipseudomonal penicillin) as initial empiric therapy for treatment of suspected infection in febrile neutropenic patients.[3,125–128] Ciprofloxacin in combination with clindamycin may also be useful in patients unable to receive β-lactam-containing combinations owing to the presence of immediate-type hypersensitivity reactions.[4] These studies, however, were associated with increased gram-positive infections in ciprofloxacin-treated patients. In addition, the in vitro activity of ciprofloxacin against *P. aeruginosa* has declined significantly (to <70% in many institutions). Therefore, if used as part of combination therapy, ciprofloxacin should be combined with an antimicrobial with favorable in vitro activity against this pathogen. Alternatively, the combination of aztreonam and vancomycin has been recognized as reasonable empiric combination therapy in patients with immediate-type hypersensitivity reactions to penicillin.[4]

Use of initial empiric therapy with combination antibiotic therapy is generally reserved for patients who are clinically unstable (hypotension, tachycardia, tachypnea, mental status changes, etc.). In such settings, intravenous therapy with an antipseudomonal *β*-lactam is generally combined with an aminoglycoside and vancomycin. Systemic antifungals (such as fluconazole or an echinocandin) may also be added in such settings, especially in patients not receiving antifungal prophylaxis.

EMPIRIC VANCOMYCIN

CASE 75-2, QUESTION 3: B.L. is begun on a two-drug regimen of ceftazidime and vancomycin. What is the rationale for adding vancomycin to the regimen?

As previously discussed, gram-positive bacteria are important pathogens in these patients. Because cephalosporins lack activity against methicillin-resistant staphylococci, vancomycin is often added to empiric regimens. A growing proportion of *S. aureus* infections are methicillin resistant (as many as 60% in some institutions). However, widespread use of vancomycin may be one factor associated with the rise in vancomycin resistance among enterococci. Furthermore, vancomycin intermediate-resistant *S. aureus* and rare case reports of *S. aureus* fully resistant to vancomycin have been reported. Vancomycin use has also been associated with a modest increase in the incidence of nephrotoxicity.

Primarily because of differences in the measured endpoints, the need for vancomycin as initial empiric therapy continues to be debated.[129] For example, febrile neutropenic patients with cancer had more rapid resolution of fever, fewer days of bacteremia, and a lower frequency of treatment failure when vancomycin was added to an initial regimen of antipseudomonal penicillin plus an aminoglycoside.[130,131] Similarly, the addition of vancomycin to ceftazidime showed improved results compared with ceftazidime alone or with a three-drug combination.[132] However, other studies have concluded that mortality was not increased when vancomycin therapy was delayed.[133–136] The mortality from staphylococcal (generally coagulase-negative staphylococci) infections is generally considered to be low (<4%) during the first 48 hours after the onset of fever. In contrast, the mortality associated with viridans streptococcal infections is higher among patients who are not initially treated with vancomycin.[137] Some strains of viridans streptococci are either resistant or tolerant to penicillin.[137,138] In general, vancomycin would represent a reasonable alternative treatment of such infections, or in patients allergic to penicillins.

There continues to be considerable debate about whether vancomycin should be included in the initial empiric regimen for febrile neutropenic patients.[129] In general, routine use of empiric vancomycin should be discouraged.[3,4] However, for institutions frequently isolating invasive gram-positive bacterial pathogens (e.g., those caused by viridans streptococci), vancomycin should be considered in the initial empiric regimen. In addition, patients at highest risk of serious, invasive infections with gram-positive organisms should be considered for initial vancomycin therapy. Such patients include suspected catheter-related infections, skin or soft-tissue infections, or pneumonia, those receiving intensive chemotherapy (e.g., high-dose cytarabine) resulting in substantial mucosal damage, patients receiving prior fluoroquinolone or TMP–SMX prophylaxis, those with prior history of colonization with *β*-lactam-resistant pneumococci or MRSA or with gram-positive bacteria in blood cultures (before identification and susceptibility testing), and those with sepsis without an identified pathogen should also be considered for vancomycin therapy.[4] The addition of vancomycin to an aminoglycoside-containing regimen should be done with caution because data support an increased risk of aminoglycoside-induced nephrotoxicity in patients receiving these agents concomitantly with vancomycin.[139] More recently, vancomycin has been shown to increase the risk of nephrotoxicity in patients receiving piperacillin–tazobactam.[8,140–142]

Alternatives to Vancomycin with Activity Against Gram-positive Pathogens

Options exist for the treatment of invasive gram-positive infections. Linezolid is an oxazolidinone that can be administered IV or orally. A randomized, double-blind trial comparing the use of linezolid with vancomycin for empiric therapy demonstrated comparable safety and efficacy.[143] It is associated with thrombocytopenia and secondary neutropenia, especially when given for prolonged periods (i.e., >14 days according to the product's package insert). Considering the reduced bone marrow reserve in cancer chemotherapy patients, these adverse events are of particular concern. In addition, it is currently not recommended for patients with catheter-related infections (including bacteremia). The emergence of linezolid-resistant enterococci is of concern in this patient population. Therefore, its primary role in this patient population would be as a treatment for resistant or refractory gram-positive infections (such as MRSA or VRE). Tedizolid, an oxazolidinone for IV and oral therapy, has more recently been approved in the US. Although advantages over linezolid include a potential reduction in hematologic adverse events and drug interactions, data are lacking to support tedizolid use in this population. In addition, tedizolid is not currently recommended in patients with neutropenia.

Quinupristin–dalfopristin is available for IV administration only, and concerns about potential drug interactions and patient tolerability (including myalgias and arthralgias) limit its use as empiric therapy in this setting. Daptomycin provides potent in vitro activity against many multidrug-resistant gram-positive pathogens (including VRE and MRSA). Compared to historical controls treated with vancomycin, daptomycin use in cancer patients with gram-positive catheter-related bacteremia was associated with earlier and overall improved response.[144,145] Daptomycin requires IV therapy and should not be used for the treatment of pneumonia. Tigecycline possesses activity in vitro against both MRSA and VRE (in addition to many gram-negative and anaerobic pathogens). However, it lacks activity against *P. aeruginosa* and therefore would not be considered a viable option for empiric monotherapy. Telavancin is a new lipoglycopeptide with potent activity in vitro against select gram-positive pathogens (including MRSA). However, experience to date in this population has not been published. Ceftaroline is a cephalosporin with activity against MRSA recently approved for the treatment of complicated skin and skin structure infections and community-acquired pneumonia. However, reports of the use of ceftaroline in this patient population are sparse. In addition, ceftaroline has infrequently been associated with neutropenia, most notably at higher doses and/or for prolonged courses of therapy.[146–148] Data are also lacking for the use of oritavancin and dalbavancin (also recently approved for IV therapy of MRSA infections) in these patients. Therefore, these alternative agents (daptomycin and linezolid) are generally reserved for situations in which vancomycin is inappropriate (because of resistance or intolerance).[3,4]

In the case of B.L., empiric use of vancomycin is not warranted based on the previous discussion, and it should be discontinued unless cultures indicate the need for this antibiotic.

ANTIBIOTIC DOSING, ADMINISTRATION, AND MONITORING CONSIDERATIONS

Intermittent versus Continuous versus Prolonged Infusion of Intravenous Antibiotics

CASE 75-2, QUESTION 4: Should B.L.'s antibiotics be given intermittently (i.e., divided doses) or as a continuous infusion?

β-Lactam antibiotics exhibit time-dependent (i.e., concentration-independent) pharmacodynamic activity, and in vitro models of infection suggest that prolonged exposure of bacteria to drug concentrations above the minimum inhibitory concentration is linked with improved bacterial killing and survival. On the basis of these observations and the poor prognosis of neutropenic cancer patients with bacteremia, noncomparative, open-label trials were conducted to evaluate the role of continuous infusions of β-lactams (i.e., ceftazidime) in the empiric treatment of suspected infection in cancer patients.[149–151] Additional studies in patients with febrile neutropenia have also been performed with meropenem suggesting a potential benefit of prolonged infusion over traditional administration.[152] However, this method of administration would require an IV line dedicated for continuous drug administration and limit B.L.'s ability to receive intermittent tobramycin infusions unless additional IV ports or lines are available for use. In contrast to continuous infusions, prolonged infusions (i.e., 3–4 hours) of select β-lactams (notably carbapenems, third- or fourth-generation cephalosporins, or piperacillin–tazobactam) have shown promise in a variety of pharmacodynamic models of infection (specifically with elevated minimum inhibitory concentrations) and tend to show better outcomes in observational studies. However, this has not been verified in prospective randomized, controlled trials. Prolonged infusions of β-lactams also have the potential to reduce the total dose and therefore result in drug acquisition cost savings. Although only limited clinical data exist to support such a strategy, such evaluations have not been tested specifically in the setting of infections in the neutropenic host.

Consolidated Interval (Extended-interval or "Once-daily") Aminoglycoside Dosing

CASE 75-2, QUESTION 5: What is the role of consolidated (once-daily) aminoglycoside dosing in febrile neutropenic patients such as B.L.?

Because of the concentration-dependent pharmacodynamic properties of aminoglycosides and the convenience of administration, studies have been conducted to describe both the pharmacokinetic properties and efficacy of consolidated dosing of aminoglycosides in animals and in neutropenic patients. Pharmacokinetic studies with amikacin[153,154] and gentamicin[155,156] have not revealed pharmacokinetic differences when compared with other populations. Several clinical studies have included consolidated aminoglycoside dosing for amikacin, gentamicin, and tobramycin.[157] However, most of the studies in this population were not designed to evaluate differences between consolidated aminoglycoside dosing compared with similar regimens using intermittent dosing. In general, the various studies suggest that consolidated dosing is as effective and possibly less nephrotoxic than traditional dosing. Therefore, consolidated dosing of aminoglycosides appears reasonable in empiric therapy of neutropenic patients.[157]

HOST FACTORS INFLUENCING RESPONSE TO THERAPY

CASE 75-2, QUESTION 6: What factors may have influenced B.L.'s clinical response to antimicrobial therapy?

The most important prognostic determinants of a favorable outcome in patients with neutropenia and infection are the recovery of the granulocyte count and (for the patient with infection) proper selection of antimicrobial therapy. Patients with profound, persistent neutropenia (<100 cells/μL that does not rise during therapy or an initial ANC of 100–500 cells/μL that declines during therapy) respond to antibiotics less favorably than patients whose bone marrow recovers. The initial granulocyte count appears to be less important than the trend toward granulocyte recovery. Although other evidence of bone marrow recovery (such as the absolute phagocyte count, absolute monocyte count, or reticulocyte fraction) may precede the ANC target of 500 cells/μL by several days, they are not as widely used clinically. The site of infection also influences outcome. Septic shock and pneumonia are associated with high mortality in bacteremic neutropenic patients.

MODIFYING INITIAL EMPIRIC ANTIBIOTIC THERAPY

CASE 75-3

QUESTION 1: M.H., a 24-year-old woman with a recent diagnosis of ovarian cancer, exhibited neutropenia (ANC <150 cells/μL) after chemotherapy. Five days after becoming neutropenic, she experienced a fever of 101°F and was begun on an empiric antibiotic regimen of ceftazidime 2 g IV every 8 hours. Although she remained febrile, her initial cultures remained negative at 48 hours. Should M.H. be continued on the same regimen, or should modifications be made? How do the culture results influence this decision? How long should empiric therapy be continued?

The need for modification of the initial empiric therapy is dependent on the risk group (i.e., low vs. high risk), establishment of an infection site or causative pathogen, response to initial therapy, and clinical stability. In the absence of worsening of clinical status or onset of new signs and symptoms of infection, 3 to 5 days of empiric treatment is generally required to determine initial efficacy after initiation of empiric antibiotics.[4] Defervescence in patients with hematologic malignancies, as well as HSCT recipients, may be delayed (up to 5 days). During this time, daily assessments should include history and physical examinations, review of laboratory results, assessment of response, and evaluation of any antibiotic-related toxicities. Adjustments to initial empiric antibiotic therapy should be made if a site-specific infection is identified, antimicrobial resistance is suspected or documented, or the patient's condition deteriorates.

Premature discontinuation of antibiotics may predispose these patients to recrudescence of bacterial infection and increase the risk of infection-related morbidity and mortality. Cancer patients with unexplained fever who became afebrile after empiric antibiotics were randomly assigned to continue or discontinue antibiotic therapy after 7 days.[158] The patients whose neutropenia resolved had no infectious sequelae regardless of whether antibiotics were continued or discontinued. However, for persistently neutropenic patients randomly assigned to continue or discontinue antibiotic therapy until their ANC was greater than 500 cells/μL, the percentages of patients remaining febrile without infections complications were 94% and 41%, respectively. Therefore, initial empiric therapy in responding patients without an identified source should be continued until the patient's ANC is >500 cells/μL and increasing, and the patient is well and afebrile for at least 24 hours. Patients who are afebrile and stable but whose neutropenia persists may be considered for continuation with oral antibiotics (such as ciprofloxacin plus amoxicillin/clavulanate). Patients whose initial empiric regimen appropriately included vancomycin should continue receiving such therapy. In contrast, those initiated inappropriately on vancomycin, or in whom cultures, diagnosis or condition does not support continued use should have vancomycin therapy discontinued.

Documented Infections

CASE 75-3, QUESTION 2: On day 3, M.H.'s temperature is normal (97.6°C). However, two sets of blood cultures drawn 3 days ago have grown *S. aureus* resistant to methicillin and susceptible to vancomycin. Her ANC is 170 cells/μL. How should therapy be modified in M.H.? For how long should antibiotics be continued?

As previously stated, modification of initial empiric therapy should be made based on culture results as well as site-specific signs and symptoms of infection (Table 75-1). For example, anaerobic coverage (often with a carbapenem or piperacillin–tazobactam

Table 75-1
Antibacterials and Antivirals in Patients with Neutropenia and Fever[a]

Condition	Therapy[b]
Initial Empiric Therapy (Site Unknown)	
Low Risk (Anticipated Neutropenia ≤7 Days, Clinically Stable, No Medical Comorbidities)	
Candidate for oral therapy	Adults: ciprofloxacin[a] + amoxicillin–clavulanate (alternate clindamycin if penicillin allergic), moxifloxacin Children: cefixime
Requires IV therapy	(see *High Risk* below)
High Risk (Anticipated Neutropenia >7 Days, Clinically Unstable, or Medical Comorbidities)	
	Piperacillin–tazobactam, antipseudomonal carbapenem,[c] ceftazidime, or cefepime Clinically unstable: consider addition of aminoglycoside, fluoroquinolone, or vancomycin to regimen above
Modifications of Initial Therapy	
Unexplained Fever	
Defervescence with negative cultures	Continue antibiotics Low-risk patients: if IV therapy initially, consider switch to oral therapy
Persistent fever (2–4 days) without clinical or microbiologic evidence of infection	Clinically stable: continue antibiotics Unstable: Hospitalize (if outpatient), IV therapy (if initially treated with oral), broaden antibacterial coverage to include anaerobes, resistant gram-negative rods, and resistant gram-positive organisms. Consider antifungal therapy for *Candida* species, or antimold therapy if previously receiving azole prophylaxis Consider empiric antifungal therapy on days 4–7, especially if neutropenia is expected to continue >7 days or the patient has other risk factors for fungal infections If initial regimen did not include vancomycin: re-evaluate risk factors for gram-positive infection, consider adding vancomycin
Documented Infection(s)	
Multidrug-resistant pathogen	MRSA: add vancomycin, linezolid or daptomycin[d] VRE: add linezolid or daptomycin ESBLs: switch to a carbapenem carbapenemase-producing Enterobacteriaceae: polymyxin-β-colistin or tigecycline
Head, Eyes, Ears, Nose, Throat	
Necrotizing ulceration	If initial regimen did not include anaerobic therapy (carbapenem or β-lactam/β-lactamase inhibitor; i.e., piperacillin–tazobactam), consider adding clindamycin or metronidazole or switch to antipseudomonal carbapenem (imipenem–cilastatin or meropenem) Consider adding antifungal or antiviral therapy for HSV
Oral vesicular lesions	Add antiviral therapy for HSV
Oral thrush	Add antifungal therapy (fluconazole) Consider extended-spectrum azoles (posaconazole, voriconazole) or an echinocandin if refractory to fluconazole

Table 75-1
Antibacterials in Patients with Neutropenia and Fever[a] (*continued*)

Condition	Therapy[b]
Esophagus	(See antifungal therapy for oral thrush) Consider acyclovir for HSV if laboratory or clinical suspicion of disease. Assess CMV risk and (if high) consider ganciclovir or foscarnet
Sinus tenderness, periorbital cellulitis, nasal ulceration	If suspicion of mold infection: add lipid-based formulation of amphotericin B. Reassess antistaphylococcal activity of empiric regimen; consider vancomycin Vancomycin for periorbital cellulitis
Gastrointestinal Tract	
Acute abdominal pain/perianal	If initial regimen did not include carbapenem or β-lactam/β-lactamase inhibitor (i.e., piperacillin–tazobactam), consider adding metronidazole, or switch to imipenem–cilastatin or meropenem. Assure pseudomonal coverage for perirectal infection For perirectal pain: consider enterococcal coverage for infection (not colonization) Consider antifungal
Diarrhea	Add metronidazole if *Clostridium difficile* documented or suspected. Oral vancomycin should be used for severe and/or complicated *C. difficile* infections. Contact isolation of rotavirus or norovirus documented
Respiratory Tract	
Pneumonia	Add fluoroquinolone or macrolide for atypical pathogens *(Mycoplasma, Legionella)*. Add vancomycin or linezolid. (Note: daptomycin is NOT indicated for pneumonia due to inactivation by lung surfactant) For patients with additional (pathogen-specific) risk factors or clinical/lab evidence of infection: Consider the addition of a mold-active antifungal (seasonal) Consider oseltamivir against influenza PCP: institute TMP–SMX or (for sulfa-allergic patients) CMV: add ganciclovir if high risk Consider growth factors (G-CSF, GM-CSF)
Vesicular lesions	HSV, VZV treatment: acyclovir, famciclovir, or valacyclovir
Cellulitis, wound infection	Consider adding vancomycin (or alternative MRSA) therapy
Vascular access device infection, tunnel tract infection	Remove catheter whenever possible. Add empiric vancomycin (or alternative MRSA therapy). Adjust based on culture and susceptibility results
Central nervous system	Antipseudomonal β-lactam (cefepime, ceftazidime, or meropenem) + vancomycin. Add ampicillin if meropenem not used
Encephalitis	High-dose acyclovir
Urinary tract	Change based on pathogen identification and susceptibility
Bloodstream infections	Gram negative: add aminoglycoside and switch to antipseudomonal carbapenem Gram positive: add vancomycin, linezolid or daptomycin

[a]Exclude option if patient received fluoroquinolone prophylaxis.
[b]All modifications should be based on clinical and microbiologic data.
[c]Antipseudomonal carbapenem is imipenem–cilastatin or meropenem. Doripenem provides comparable in vitro activity, but has not been investigated in this patient population.
[d]daptomycin excluded for pneumonia.
CMV, cytomegalovirus; ESBL, extended-spectrum β-lactamase; G-CSF, granulocyte colony-stimulating factor; GM-CSF, granulocyte-macrophage colony-stimulating factor; HSV, herpes simplex virus; IV, intravenous; KPCs, *Klebsiella* producing carbapenemases; MRSA, methicillin-resistant *Staphylococcus aureus*; PCP, *Pneumocystis jiroveci*; TMP–SMX, trimethoprim–sulfamethoxazole; VRE, vancomycin-resistant enterococcus; VZV, varicella-zoster virus.
Source: National Comprehensive Cancer Network. Myeloid growth factors (version 1.2015). **www.nccn.org**. Accessed September 4, 2015; Freifeld A et al. Clinical practice guideline for the use of antimicrobial agents in neutropenic patients with cancer: 2010 update by the Infectious Diseases Society of America. *Clin Infect Dis*. 2011;52:e56.

if not used for initial monotherapy) may be expanded in the setting of abdominal pain. Metronidazole or oral vancomycin should be initiated in the setting of diarrhea when *C. difficile* is suspected.[4] Vesicular lesions may be suggestive of viral infections (such as HSV or VZV) and may respond to the addition of acyclovir.[14] Suspected IV catheter infections should be managed with catheter removal (whenever possible), and this as well as skin and skin structure infections should be managed with treatment directed at MRSA.[4] For pneumonia, antibiotic coverage should be consistent with published guidelines for the treatment of health care-associated infections (see Chapter 67, Respiratory Tract Infections).[159] In the setting of severe or life-threatening pulmonary infections, antifungal therapy should also be included (see Table 75-1). Modifications of therapy may also be based on isolation of a resistant pathogen. For example, resistant gram-positive infections such as MRSA may be treated with vancomycin, linezolid, or daptomycin, whereas linezolid or daptomycin may be used for the treatment of VRE. For multidrug-resistant gram-negative pathogens, carbapenems are often used to treat ESBL-producing organisms, whereas carbapenemase-producing Enterobacteriaceae may require therapy with polymyxin, colistin, or tigecycline.

The duration of therapy is based on the infecting organism and site of infection (often up to 14 days), and should continue at least until the ANC is 500/μL or greater and rising.[4]

For patients with documented infections unresponsive to modification of therapy, new or worsening sites of infection should be suspected. Clinical, laboratory, and radiographic investigations should be undertaken or repeated. For hemodynamically unstable patients, antimicrobial therapy should be broadened and the patient should be considered for empiric antifungal therapy.[4]

No Etiology Identified

CASE 75-4

QUESTION 1: S.B. is a 55-year-old woman with chronic myelogenous leukemia. She was admitted to the hospital with a 4-day history of fevers and night sweats. On admission, her temperature was 102.3°F, and her WBC count was 100,000 cells/μL, with an ANC of 500 cells/μL. Blood and urine cultures were obtained, and cefepime was empirically started. For the next 3 days, S.B. remained persistently febrile and neutropenic. All cultures remained negative. How should she be treated?

Persistent fevers may be from noninfectious sources or from untreated infection. With the exception of consideration for antifungal therapy in some patients, those with persistent fever who are clinically stable do not routinely require a change in empiric therapy unless guided by clinical changes or culture results.[3,4] However, outpatients with persistent fever should be hospitalized and receive IV therapy. Empiric addition of vancomycin in patients with persistent fever does not decrease the time to fever resolution in this population[160] and should therefore be discouraged.[4] In contrast, persistently febrile patients who are hemodynamically unstable without a clear source of infection should have their initial therapy modified to broaden coverage against resistant gram-positive and gram-negative organisms, as well as anaerobes.[3,4] Patients with initial monotherapy with ceftazidime or cefepime can be switched to vancomycin with an antipseudomonal carbapenem (such as imipenem–cilastatin or meropenem) in combination with either an aminoglycoside, aztreonam, or ciprofloxacin.[3,4] Antifungal therapy targeting *Candida* species should also be considered (see Case 75-4, Question 3).

CASE 75-4, QUESTION 2: S.B., on day 4, continues to feel "lousy" and has started to complain of abdominal pains. What is the significance of this complaint? Should her antibiotic regimen be modified again?

Because S.B. has new abdominal pains suggestive of enterocolitis, her antibiotic regimen should be modified. Although cefepime provides excellent coverage against the common gram-negative pathogens, it has limited activity against select gram-positive pathogens (e.g., MRSA or VRE) and anaerobes. A change from cefepime to imipenem–cilastatin or another broad-spectrum regimen with both aerobic and anaerobic activity should be considered.

CASE 75-4, QUESTION 3: S.B.'s antibiotic regimen was changed to imipenem–cilastatin. Despite the change, she continues to have a low-grade fever and does not feel better. What is S.B.'s risk for having a systemic fungal infection? What is the significance of fungal infections in neutropenic cancer patients?

ANTIFUNGAL THERAPY

Early diagnosis and prompt treatment of systemic fungal diseases are critical to patient survival. However, significant challenges exist in making an accurate and timely diagnosis of invasive fungal infections. Therefore, patients who are neutropenic with protracted (4–7 days) fever despite the administration of broad-spectrum antibiotics should be considered for empiric antifungal therapy, especially patients whose neutropenia is anticipated to exceed 7 days.[4,161] Patients at highest risk of mold infections (i.e., those with prolonged neutropenia, allogeneic HSCT recipients, and/or those receiving high-dose corticosteroids) should be initiated on antifungals after 4 days of persistent fever unless they are currently receiving antimold prophylaxis. Considerations for earlier empiric antifungal therapy (i.e., days 2–4) should be made in patients with persistent fever and hemodynamic instability.[4]

Newer diagnostic tests (e.g., β-D-glucan tests or galactomannan assays), along with additional diagnostic support, may allow for early preemptive therapy (i.e., institution of therapy based on biomarker evidence of disease prior to the development of symptoms).[162] Such approaches may also be used to support decisions to withhold empiric antifungal therapy. As an example, persistently febrile patients on appropriate antibacterials who are clinically stable without clinical or radiographic signs of fungal infection have had negative serologic assays for invasive fungal infection and have had no recovery of fungi from any body site may have empiric antifungal agents withheld.[4,104]

Considerations about the choice of empiric antifungals should include prior or current antifungal prophylaxis, risk of mold infections, risks of antifungal-related toxicities, drug interactions, route of administration, clinical stability, and costs.[23] It is difficult to compare data among clinical trials evaluating empiric antifungal therapy in neutropenic cancer patients because of differences in trial design. Such differences may include inclusion of low-risk patients, lack of blinding, changes in concomitant antibacterials obscuring antifungal therapy end points, prior antifungal prophylaxis, use of composite end points of safety and efficacy, and different endpoint criteria.[25] Although select studies have also demonstrated that empiric antifungal therapy can decrease fungal-related deaths, overall mortality has not been affected.[23] This is the case particularly for patients with invasive disease and persistent neutropenia.

In patients requiring therapy, antifungal coverage should be directed at *Candida* species. Highest-risk patients with persistent or recurrent fever after 4 to 7 days of appropriate antibacterial therapy and anticipated to have prolonged (i.e., >10 days) neutropenia should be considered for antimold therapy.[4]

CASE 75-4, QUESTION 4: Should amphotericin B or acyclovir therapy be considered in S.B.?

Historically, amphotericin B deoxycholate (AmBD) was most commonly used in this setting because of its reliable activity in vitro against most *Candida* and *Aspergillus* species. Comparative trials have also evaluated the role of lipid-based formulations of amphotericin B in the treatment of suspected or documented infections in this population. Liposomal amphotericin B (LAmB),[163–166] amphotericin B lipid complex,[165] and amphotericin B colloidal dispersion[167] have demonstrated reductions in nephrotoxicity compared with AmBD. In addition, LAmB is least likely to be associated with infusion-related side effects.[164] Although there are limited data to suggest that the continuous infusion of AmBD may also reduce nephrotoxicity,[168] efficacy regarding this method of administration in patients with documented infections has not been established. Therefore, continuous infusion of AmBD cannot be routinely recommended at this time. Considering the availability of other agents, empiric amphotericin B products are generally reserved for patients at highest risk of mold infections unable to receive alternative antifungals. When initiated as empiric therapy, amphotericin B administration is often preceded by attempts to minimize nephrotoxicity (e.g., saline loading) and premedications to minimize infusion-related reactions. Close monitoring of tolerability, renal function, and electrolytes is required during administration.

In stable patients at low risk of mold infections or drug-resistant *Candida* species (e.g., *C. krusei* and some strains of *C. glabrata*), fluconazole may be preferable to amphotericin B.[4,169,170] Patients with suspected mold infections (e.g., aspergillosis), hemodynamic instability, or in whom an azole was used as prophylaxis should not receive fluconazole. Although itraconazole possesses enhanced activity in vitro against *Aspergillus* species and has reduced toxicity relative to amphotericin B, issues regarding tolerability with the oral solution, erratic bioavailability with the capsule formulation, potential for cross-resistance with other azoles, lack of a parenteral treatment option, and considerations of alternative treatment options generally limit its usefulness. Posaconazole possesses a broad spectrum of activity in vitro against a variety of yeasts and molds. It is currently available in both an oral and intravenous formulation. Voriconazole (an azole antifungal agent with increased activity against *Aspergillus* and non-albicans *Candida* relative to fluconazole) has been tested in this population. When compared with LAmB, voriconazole failed to meet the pre-established criteria for noninferiority.[166] However, some believe that voriconazole should be considered as an alternative to amphotericin B preparations for empiric therapy in patients requiring initial empiric antifungal therapy who are at increased risk of mold infections (owing to receipt of prior azole prophylaxis) or for those patients suspected of having invasive candidiasis.[161] Because of the increased potential (relative to fluconazole) for drug interactions (including immunosuppressives and chemotherapy) and adverse events (e.g., phototoxicity, hepatotoxicity), voriconazole therapy should be monitored closely. IV use of voriconazole is contraindicated in patients with severe renal dysfunction. In addition, serum drug concentration monitoring for posaconazole and voriconazole may be considered in patients with suspected malabsorption.[4,9] Most recently, isavuconazole (a broad-spectrum, triazole antifungal) has been approved for both oral and IV administration for the treatment of invasive aspergillosis and mucormycosis.[171] Potential advantages (relative to voriconazole) include improved oral bioavailability, predictable pharmacokinetics, and a reduction in the potential for drug interactions. For treatment of invasive aspergillosis, isavuconazole's efficacy was noninferior to that of voriconazole.

The echinocandins (e.g., caspofungin, micafungin, anidulafungin) possess in vitro activity against *Candida* species (including non-albicans *Candida*) and *Aspergillus* species. Caspofungin is at least as effective and better tolerated than LAmB as empiric therapy in this patient population.[172,173] Because of their safety profile and in vitro activity, echinocandins are often considered for patients requiring initial empiric antifungal therapy and who are at increased risk of mold infections (owing to receipt of prior azole prophylaxis). Caspofungin is currently FDA approved for such use. Published experience with other echinocandins (e.g., micafungin, anidulafungin) as empiric therapy in the febrile neutropenic patient is lacking at present.

In summary, empiric antifungal therapy is indicated for persistent (4–7 days) or recurrent fever on appropriate antibacterials if the duration of neutropenia exceeds 7 days.[4] Low-risk patients who are clinically stable do not routinely need antifungal therapy.[4] Persistently febrile patients who are clinically stable without computed tomography signs of infection and have no serologic or culture results suggestive of infection may have antifungal therapy withheld.[4] Patients receiving fluconazole prophylaxis requiring addition of empiric antifungals should be considered for antifungals with activity against azole-resistant *Candida* species and mold infections.[4] In the setting in which an antimold agent was used for prophylaxis, switching antifungal classes or conversion to IV therapy should be performed.[4]

ANTIVIRAL THERAPY

Empiric use of antiviral agents in the febrile neutropenic patient is not indicated without evidence of such disease.[4] In contrast, clinical evidence of HSV or VZV involving the skin or mucous membranes should be treated with antivirals (e.g., acyclovir, valacyclovir).[4] When oral therapy is used, valacyclovir is generally favored over acyclovir because of improved oral bioavailability and need for less frequent dosing. With the exception of patients undergoing bone marrow transplantation,[174] CMV is an uncommon source of infection in the febrile neutropenic patient. However, ganciclovir, valganciclovir, foscarnet, or less commonly cidofovir treatment should be initiated in patients with documented CMV infections (antigenemia, polymerase chain reaction for CMV DNA, or detection of CMV mRNA). Because both ganciclovir and valganciclovir can cause or worsen existing neutropenia, caution and close monitoring is warranted when these agents are prescribed in this setting. Treatment with neuraminidase inhibitors (such as oseltamivir or zanamivir) may be initiated empirically for influenza in the setting of exposure or outbreaks if the patient is presenting with an influenza-like illness.[4] Likewise, if RSV is identified, appropriate antiviral therapy should be initiated.[4]

ANTIMICROBIAL ADJUVANTS

CASE 75-4, QUESTION 5: S.B. became afebrile 2 days after micafungin was initiated, yet she remained neutropenic with an ANC of 480 cells/μL. An induction chemotherapy regimen consisting of idarubicin plus cytarabine was initiated for her chronic myelogenous leukemia. Because the chemotherapy will further reduce her ANC 7 to 10 days after treatment, is there any way to facilitate marrow recovery and reduce the duration of neutropenia in S.B.?

As previously discussed, the duration of neutropenia is the most important factor affecting outcome in neutropenic cancer patients. Because of this, there has been considerable interest in enhancing the immune system in these patients.

Granulocyte Transfusions

One of the earliest approaches used to boost the patient's defense against infections was the transfusion of WBCs. In the 1970s, granulocyte transfusions were used adjunctively in patients with persistent neutropenia and documented infections who, despite appropriate antibiotics, failed to respond after 24 to 48 hours. This approach had limited value because of the difficulties in obtaining adequate cells for transfusion, as well as the problems with alloimmunization and risk of infection transmission. In addition, the questionable efficacy of WBC transfusions has decreased the use of this strategy.[175] Therefore, granulocyte transfusions are not routinely indicated in this population. However, patients with progressive bacterial or fungal infections unresponsive to appropriate antimicrobial therapy may be considered as candidates.[3]

Hematopoietic Growth Factors

Because these agents have not demonstrated a consistent and significant effect on other infection-related parameters (e.g., duration of fever, use of antibiotics, costs of treatment), the use of CSFs as adjunctive therapy to antibiotics for febrile neutropenic patients is controversial.[4,31,83–85] Patients already receiving CSFs for primary or secondary prevention may be continued during treatment of febrile neutropenia.[84] Those patients administered pegfilgrastim for primary or secondary prevention should not require subsequent doses of CSFs due to persistence of high CSF concentrations for prolong periods.

Patients with high risks for infection-related complications not receiving CSFs for prophylaxis may be considered for therapy.[3,85] Such risks include expected prolonged (>7 days) and profound (<100 cells/μL) neutropenia in clinically unstable patients unresponsive to initial empiric therapy, age older than 65 years, uncontrolled malignancy, pneumonia, sepsis and multiorgan dysfunction (characteristic of sepsis syndrome), and invasive fungal infection.[84,85]

Immunoglobulins

Data regarding the use of immunoglobulins as adjunctive therapy for the treatment of select infections in the neutropenic cancer patient are primarily limited to case reports. Patients with pneumonia secondary to CMV may benefit from adjunctive immunoglobulin therapy (in combination with ganciclovir). In addition, IV immunoglobulin G should be considered in those patients with hypogammaglobulinemia.

G-CSF administration, although likely to reduce the duration of her chemotherapy-induced neutropenia, is not indicated in S.B., who is otherwise stable.

KEY REFERENCES AND WEBSITES

A full list of references for this chapter can be found at http://thepoint.lww.com/AT11e. Below are the key references and websites for this chapter, with the corresponding reference number in this chapter found in parentheses after the reference.

Key References

Averbuch D et al. European guidelines for empirical antibacterial therapy for febrile neutropenic patients in the era of growing resistance: summary of the 2011 4th European Conference on Infections in Leukemia. *Haematologica.* 2013;98:1826–1835. (176)

Flowers CR et al. Antimicrobial prophylaxis and outpatient management of fever and neutropenia in adults treated for malignancy: American Society of Clinical Oncology clinical practice guideline. *J Clin Oncol.* 2013;31:794–810. (32)

Lehrnbecher T et al. Guideline for the management of fever and neutropenia in children with cancer and/or undergoing hematopoietic stem-cell transplantation. *J Clin Oncol.* 2012;30:4427–4438. (177)

National Comprehensive Cancer Network. Myeloid growth factors (version 1.2015). www.nccn.org. Accessed September 4, 2015. (84)

Network Comprehensive Cancer Network. Prevention and treatment of cancer-related infections (v2.2015). www.nccn.org. Accessed September 3, 2015. (3)

Smith TJ et al. Recommendations for the use of white blood cell growth factors: American Society of Clinical Oncology Clinical Practice Guideline Update. *J Oncol Pract.* 2015. (83)

Key Websites

National Comprehensive Cancer Network. www.nccn.org.

American Society of Clinical Oncology. www.asco.org.

76 Pharmacotherapy of Human Immunodeficiency Virus Infection

Jessica L. Adams and Mackenzie L. Cottrell

CORE PRINCIPLES

	CHAPTER CASES
1 Acute retroviral syndrome is characterized by nonspecific symptoms, such as fever, lymphadenopathy, rash, fatigue, and night sweats that coincide with an initial burst of viremia. These symptoms, as well as the presence of an opportunistic infection, and high-risk sexual or drug-using behaviors, warrant human immunodeficiency virus (HIV) testing. With current antigen/antibody laboratory tests, HIV can be diagnosed as early as 2 weeks after infection. In patients in whom very early infection (<2 weeks) is suspected, nucleic acid tests for HIV RNA may be considered for diagnostic purposes.	**Case 76-1 (Question 1)**
2 HIV RNA viral load is measured to quantify the level of viral replication in the body and CD4 cell counts are followed to assess immune system function.	**Case 76-1 (Question 2)**
3 Antiretroviral therapy should be offered to all patients who are willing and able to commit to lifelong treatment after a discussion of the benefits and risks of highly active antiretroviral therapy (HAART) and the importance of adherence. Clinical situations which favor more urgent initiation of HAART include pregnancy; AIDS-defining condition such as an opportunistic infection; CD4 count of <200 cells/μL; HIV-associated nephropathy (HIVAN); hepatitis B and/or C infection; rapidly declining CD4 count (>100 cells/μL decrease per year); higher baseline viral load (>100,000 copies/mL); and acute/early HIV infection. US Department of Health and Human Services (DHHS) guidelines provide recommendations for optimal antiretroviral therapy.	**Case 76-1 (Question 3)**
4 Goals of antiretroviral therapy include suppression of viral load, preservation and strengthening of the immune system, limitation of drug adverse events, promotion of adherence, and prevention of HIV-related morbidity and mortality.	**Case 76-1 (Question 4)**
5 General rules of therapy involve selection of HAART-based regimen, optimization of the selected agents, and inclusion of quality of life in decisions.	**Case 76-1 (Questions 5, 6)**
6 After initiating a HAART regimen, short-term goals include resolution of symptoms, at least a threefold (0.5 log) decrease in HIV RNA at 1 month, a tenfold decrease (1.0 log) in HIV RNA at 2 months, and an increase in CD4 count at 3 to 4 months. Long-term assessments include the monitoring of HIV RNA and CD4 count every 3 to 6 months to identify treatment failures, assessment of medication adherence, and determination of tolerability and quality of life.	**Case 76-1 (Questions 7, 8)**
7 General rules for changing failing regimens include switching to at least two new active drugs (although all new drugs are preferable), as quickly as possible after treatment failure to avoid accumulation of resistance mutations. To avoid the development of further resistance, a single drug should never be added to a failing regimen. If one drug must be discontinued, the whole regimen should be stopped simultaneously. Finally, previously failed regimens should never be restarted because of the potential of archived resistance mutations.	**Case 76-1 (Questions 9, 10)**

Continued

		CHAPTER CASES
8	Considerations for treatment of antiretroviral-experienced patients include regimen tolerability, comorbid conditions, associated pharmacokinetic properties, antiretroviral histories, and resistance testing. Resistance testing should be performed when HIV RNA is greater than 1,000 copies/mL. Antiretroviral drug resistance is assessed through two methods: genotyping evaluates mutations in the virus genetic code and phenotyping involves growing virus in various concentrations of drug to determine viral susceptibilities. DHHS guidelines provide recommendations for treating antiretroviral-experienced patients.	**Case 76-2 (Question 1–3)**
9	Drug interactions between antiretrovirals and coadministered medications are common and should always be screened with the addition of any new medication.	**Case 76-3 (Question 1)**
10	Antiretrovirals are used in pregnancy for the health of the mother and to prevent transmission of HIV to the child. There are specific DHHS guidelines for antiretroviral use in pregnancy.	**Case 76-4 (Question 1)**
11	The use of antiretrovirals for pre-exposure prophylaxis in individuals who are HIV negative, but at high risk for acquiring HIV, has been shown to be safe and effective in clinical studies. The combination product of emtricitabine/tenofovir disoproxil fumarate is FDA approved for this use, and the Centers for Disease Control and Prevention has issued guidelines on the use and monitoring of the combination for this indication.	**Case 76-5 (Question 1)**
12	The use of antiretrovirals for occupational (e.g., needle sticks) and nonoccupational (e.g., high-risk behaviors) postexposure prophylaxis (PEP) may be warranted if initiated within 48 hours but no longer than 72 hours after exposure. There are Centers for Disease Control and Prevention guideline recommendations for the choice of antiretrovirals for PEP.	**Case 76-6 (Question 1)**

INTRODUCTION

Potent combinations of antiretroviral drugs (also called highly active antiretroviral therapy [HAART]) have dramatically altered the natural progression of human immunodeficiency virus (HIV) infection, and significantly improved patients' quality of life. As a result, the number of newly acquired immunodeficiency syndrome (AIDS)-related opportunistic infections and deaths has declined.[1,2] In most instances, the use of HAART has shifted HIV infection from a fatal disease to a manageable chronic disease. The most recent advances in HIV therapy include new and more potent antiretroviral agents in existing therapeutic drug classes, novel combinations of antiretrovirals, and new single tablet once daily regimens.

Despite the drastic improvements in HIV treatment over the last decade, successfully managing the HIV epidemic remains a challenge because of suboptimal patient compliance and the development of resistance, long-term adverse events, the price of antiretrovirals, and the rampant spread of HIV throughout resource-poor countries.

This chapter focuses on the antiretroviral treatment of HIV infection. Although many therapeutic options now exist, a thorough understanding of viral pathogenesis is essential for managing patients infected with HIV. By understanding the principles of therapy as they relate to viral pathogenesis, clinicians can rapidly assimilate new data as they become available. Consensus panel recommendations provide a framework for clinical decision making.[3–5] Given the complexity of therapy, this chapter focuses on treating adult HIV infections. A cursory introduction to the clinical concepts of perinatal transmission, pre-exposure prophylaxis (PrEP), and postexposure prophylaxis (PEP) for both occupational and nonoccupational HIV exposures are also provided. For more in-depth discussion of these concepts and the treatment of pediatric HIV, the reader is referred to the various consensus panel guidelines (http://www.aidsinfo.nih.gov/).

EPIDEMIOLOGY

Despite a dramatic decline in the number of AIDS-related opportunistic infections and deaths in industrialized countries,[2,6] HIV infection remains in the top 10 leading causes of death worldwide.[7] Access to newer, more potent antiretroviral regimens and monitoring are often limited by economics and politics. Infected patients residing in countries with a strong economic standing (North America, Western Europe, Australia, and New Zealand) have reasonable access to medications, whereas patients residing in countries with scarce resources (Africa, south and southeast Asia, the Pacific, and the Caribbean) do not. This is of significant concern given that most infected patients worldwide reside in these latter regions of the world.[6]

As of 2016, the worldwide estimate of persons living with HIV infection was 36.7 million: 34.5 million adults (52% of which are women) and 2.1 million children younger than 15 years of age.[6] The estimated incidence (1.8 million new HIV infections) decreased by 18% from 2010, and the estimated number of AIDS-related deaths (1.0 million) decreased by 33%. Approximately, two-thirds (70%) of all HIV-infected adults and children live in Africa, and approximately three-quarters (72%) of all AIDS-related deaths occurred there in 2016. Increasing access to HIV treatment in this region has led to a 52% reduction in the number of AIDS-related deaths since 2001. Universal access to HAART became a global priority in 2000 when the United Nations Millennium Declaration called for unprecedented action to halt and begin to reverse the AIDS epidemic. This call to action resulted in an increase of more than 13 million persons living with HIV in Africa (~54%) accessing HAART in 2016 (increased from <1% in 2000). With these global efforts, the percentage of all HIV infected persons worldwide on HAART is 53%.

In the United States, the availability of antiretroviral therapy resulted in a drastic decline (67%) in AIDS-related death rates between 1994 and 2007, and this percentage continues to drop albeit at a slower rate (20% decline from 2009 to 2012). Despite this success, 6,721 people in the United States still died from HIV attributable causes in 2014.[2] Racial and ethnic minorities continue to be disproportionately affected by HIV because of a complicated combination of poverty, disproportionate incarceration, and social and sexual network segregation.[8] In 2015 African Americans, who represented 12% of the US population, accounted for approximately 45% of all new HIV infections in adult and adolescents. Hispanics/Latinos, who constitute 18% of the U.S. population accounted for 24% of new infections in 2015. Compared with white men and women, the lifetime risk of HIV seroconversion is 6 times higher in African American men, 20 times higher in African American women, 3 times higher in Hispanic/Latino men, and 4 times higher in Hispanic/Latino women.[9] Transmission through sexual intercourse remains a predominant route of infection, with unprotected sex between men accounting for approximately 63% of cases, and heterosexual intercourse accounting for approximately 25% of cases in the United States.[9]

PATHOPHYSIOLOGY

Infection with HIV can be acquired through unprotected sexual intercourse (both anal and vaginal), injectable drug use, receipt of tainted blood products, and mother-to-infant transmission (both perinatal infection and postpartum through breast-feeding).[3] Infection can also be acquired from occupational exposures among health care workers after needle sticks or infected blood splashes from patients infected with HIV onto vulnerable mucosal membranes. Rarely, HIV infection has been documented following oral sex.[10,11]

Unprotected sexual intercourse accounts for approximately 80% of all documented HIV infections to date.[2,6] Transmission between sexual partners depends on a number of factors, including the HIV viral subtype, stage of infection in the index partner, genetic susceptibility to infection of the potential host, and the viral fitness (or pathogenicity) of the infecting strain. Perhaps one of the most important predictors of transmission is the amount of HIV RNA in the blood of the infected index patient (i.e., viral load). Recently, initiation of HAART treatment and subsequently suppressing infected patients' viral loads has been shown to decrease transmission rates by >95% among serodiscordant couples where one partner is HIV infected and the other is not.[12] Infectivity via receptive anal intercourse represents the greatest sexual risk factor followed by male-to-female vaginal transmission and then female-to-male penile transmission.[13]

During transmission, HIV binds to specific immune cells, including Langerhans cells, dendritic cells, T-cell lymphocytes (also known as $CD4^+$ T cells, helper T cells, or T cells), and macrophages.[13–16] However, recent reports indicate that the initial virus propagated during early infection (the HIV-1 transmitted founder virus) may not replicate efficiently in monocyte-derived macrophages raising questions regarding the importance of macrophages in initial transmission events.[17] HIV primarily enters target immune cells that express specific receptor proteins known as CD4 receptors to which HIV binds. However, evidence indicates that for some cells types like Langerhans cells compensatory mechanisms for viral entry exist.[18] Once bound to the CD4 receptor, co-receptor proteins (CCR5, CXCR-4) are required for fusion of the viral membrane to the immune cell membrane.[19,20] CCR5 co-receptors are found on both monocytes and T lymphocytes and are more abundant in patients newly infected with HIV.[21,22] CXCR-4 co-receptors are predominantly found on T lymphocytes and are more abundant in patients who have been on long-term antiretroviral therapy. The CD4–co-receptor complex causes conformational changes to key HIV proteins (gp41 and gp120) allowing for a more close association between the virus and the host cell.[22,23] HIV fuses with the cell and releases its contents into the host cell's cytoplasm: this includes the virus's RNA and specific enzymes necessary for replication (Fig. 76-1; see online animated images of HIV lifecycle and where the drugs act at http://biosingularity.wordpress.com/2007/03/04/3d-animation-of-hiv-replication/). The single-stranded viral RNA is transcribed via reverse transcriptase into a double-stranded proviral DNA that is subsequently incorporated into the host cell's genetic material via the integrase enzyme. HIV then uses the infected cell's machinery to translate, transcribe, and produce immature viral particles that bud and break from the infected cell. For these immature virions to become infectious, the HIV protease enzyme must cleave large precursor polypeptides into functional proteins.[24,25] Once complete, the mature virion is free to infect new host cells and subsequently produce more infectious virus.

Over time, HIV-infected host cells can be destroyed by a number of mechanisms: (a) a direct cytolytic effect of the virus (e.g., formation of syncytium induction, cellular dysfunction); (b) the identification and elimination of the infected cell by the host's immune response (e.g., via cytotoxic T-cell lymphocytes); or (c) the cell's natural life cycle coming to completion.[26] In addition, HIV infection can inhibit the production of new $CD4^+$ cells.[27]

Once a patient becomes infected, an initial burst of viremia occurs and causes latent infection in various tissues (e.g., lymph nodes) and cells (CD4, macrophages, and monocytes).[26,28] Most infectious HIV virions (~99%) reside inside lymph nodes and other immune-cell rich tissues found throughout the body.[14,26,29,30] The immune system reacts by producing antibodies against HIV; however, given the rapid production of new HIV particles and the development of many new and genetically diverse viral strains (a result of the error-prone HIV reverse transcriptase), the antibody response is inadequate.[31] After this burst of viremia, a transient depletion of $CD4^+$ cells occurs (Fig. 76-2). Initially, patients may complain of nonspecific symptoms, such as fever, lymphadenopathy, rash, fatigue, and night sweats.[3]

This phase of infection is known as the acute retroviral syndrome.

In most cases, patients are unaware that they are infected. Within 6 months, the host's immune response is able to control the infection to a point where the number of virus particles produced per day equals the number of particles destroyed per day. This steady-state is often referred to as the patient's viral "set point."

The higher a patient's viral set point, the greater the risk for disease progression. This is because there is a greater chance for more widespread viral infection and immune cell destruction with a larger replicating viral population. Why some patients establish higher or lower viral set points is currently under investigation, but this may be a consequence of differences in immune responses, cellular receptor populations, viral subtypes, viral fitness, or a combination of these factors. This understanding of viral pathogenesis has led to a new paradigm of therapy that prioritizes initiating HAART in the acute phase of infection[3] to lower viral set points and reduce the size of the viral reservoir (i.e., long-lived, latently infected memory T cells believed to be responsible for repopulating the virus in infected patients who stop HAART). A significant challenge is to identify these patients with acute infection who have nonspecific symptoms.[32]

Once the initial burst of viremia has been controlled and the viral set point established, infection with HIV results in a constant battle between viral replication and suppression of that replication by the immune system. Mathematical models have calculated the production of HIV at 10 billion particles per day.[14,33–35] To keep the infection controlled, the body must produce an equal immune response. Over time, HIV depletes the body of T cells, which places the host at an increased risk for opportunistic infections. Direct measurements of HIV RNA concentrations in plasma (also called "viral load") can predict disease progression (see subsequent discussion).[36–38] Higher viral load measurements represent an inability of the host to control viral replication, and a greater risk for immune cell destruction. Long-term "nonprogressors" (e.g., patients with asymptomatic HIV infection for >10 years; 5% of

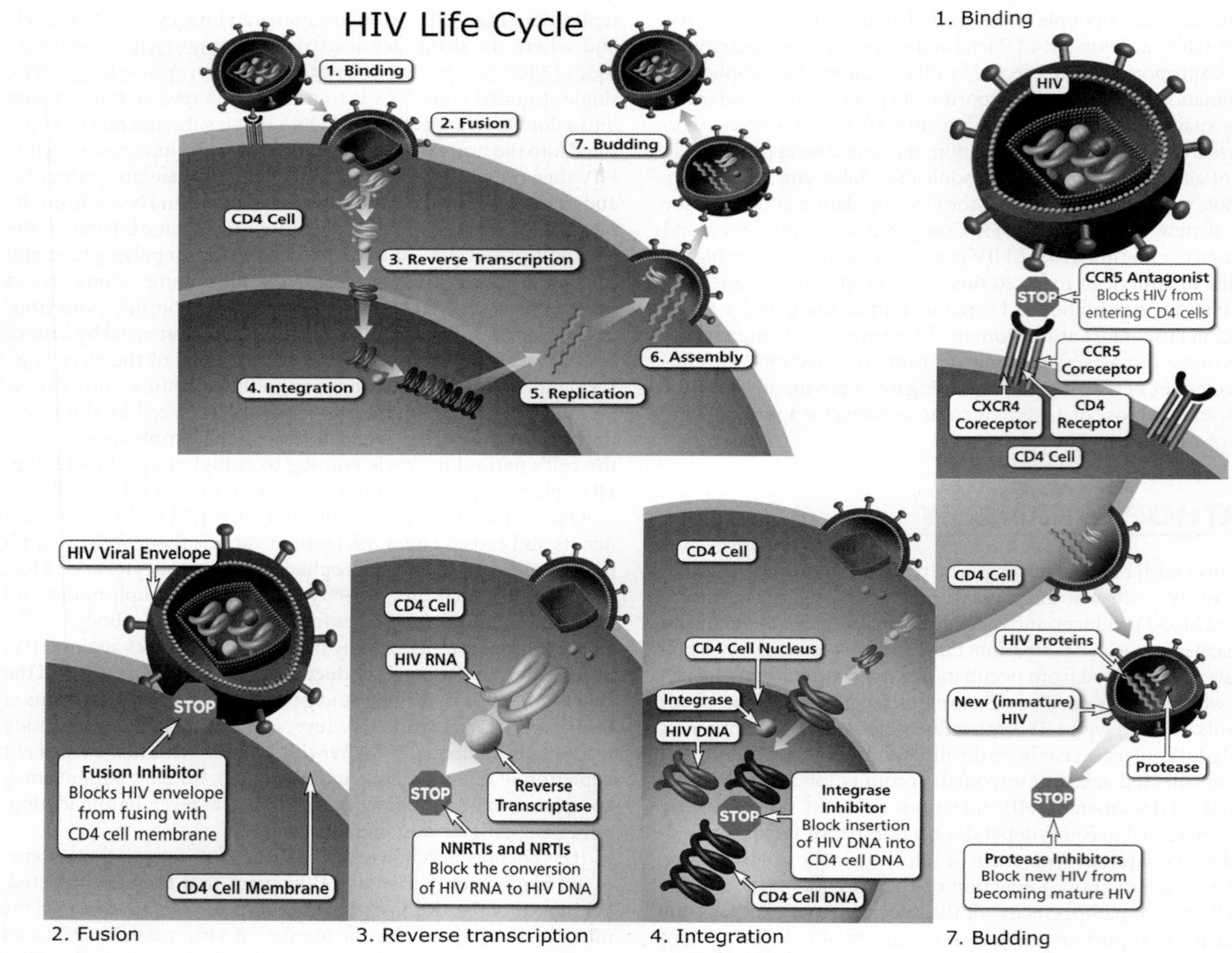

Figure 76-1 Schematic representation of the HIV-1 life cycle. Five classes of antiretroviral drugs are available at present. CCR5 antagonists and fusion inhibitors inhibit the entry of virions into a new target cell. The step of reverse transcription can be targeted, using nucleoside nucleotide analogs or non-nucleoside reverse-transcriptase inhibitors (NRTIs, NtRTI, and NNRTIs, respectively). The class of integrase inhibitors prevents integration of viral DNA into host cell DNA. The class of protease inhibitors interferes with the last state of the life cycle, the proteolytic processing of the viral proteins, which results in the production of noninfectious particles. (Adapted from education materials provided by the National Institutes of Health available on AIDSinfo.nih.gov.)

all HIV-infected patients) consistently have lower baseline viral loads than patients with rapidly progressive disease (e.g., AIDS within 5 years of infection; 20% of all HIV-infected patients).[39,40]

Without intervention, the natural progression of HIV infection results in depletion of 50 to 100 T cells/μL/year.[26] The severity of immune dysfunction, as evidenced by T-cell loss, is highly predictive of the potential for the development of specific types of opportunistic infections. For example, *Pneumocystis jirovecii* pneumonia rarely occurs when T-cell counts are greater than 200 cells/μL, whereas retinitis from cytomegalovirus infection rarely occurs in patients with CD4 counts greater than 75 cells/μL. The diagnosis of AIDS is made when a significant amount of immune deterioration has occurred, either by depletion of $CD4^+$ cells to less than 200 cells/μL or because of the development of new opportunistic infections (Tables 76-1 and 76-2). It is important to recognize that not every patient with HIV has a diagnosis of AIDS. On average, without appropriate drug therapy, death occurs within 10 to 15 years after infection.[26]

The interplay between viral load and CD4 T-cell counts is often compared with that of a train heading toward a particular destination. If the destination is immune system destruction (and eventually death), then the T-cell count is the distance of the train from this destination, and the viral load (concentration of HIV RNA in plasma) is the speed of the train. As both higher speeds and shorter distances reach destinations faster, so does a high viral load and low T-cell count result in quicker onset of immune destruction (and death). Potent antiretroviral regimens decrease viral replication and dramatically alter the natural course of infection by prolonging the time to opportunistic infection and death.[41]

PHARMACOTHERAPY

Pharmacotherapy of HIV has been directed at inhibiting key areas of the HIV life cycle (Fig. 76-1 and animations found at **http://biosingularity.wordpress.com/2007/03/04/3d-animation-of-hiv-replication/**; Table 76-3). Nucleoside RT inhibitors (NRTIs) include zidovudine, didanosine, lamivudine, abacavir, emtricitabine, and stavudine, while nucleotide RT inhibitors currently only include tenofovir. These agents inhibit this enzyme by incorporating false nucleic acids into the newly forming proviral DNA.[42] This results in an HIV DNA strand that cannot continue to elongate. Non-nucleoside reverse transcriptase inhibitors (NNRTIs; nevirapine, efavirenz, rilpivirine, and etravirine) inhibit reverse transcriptase by

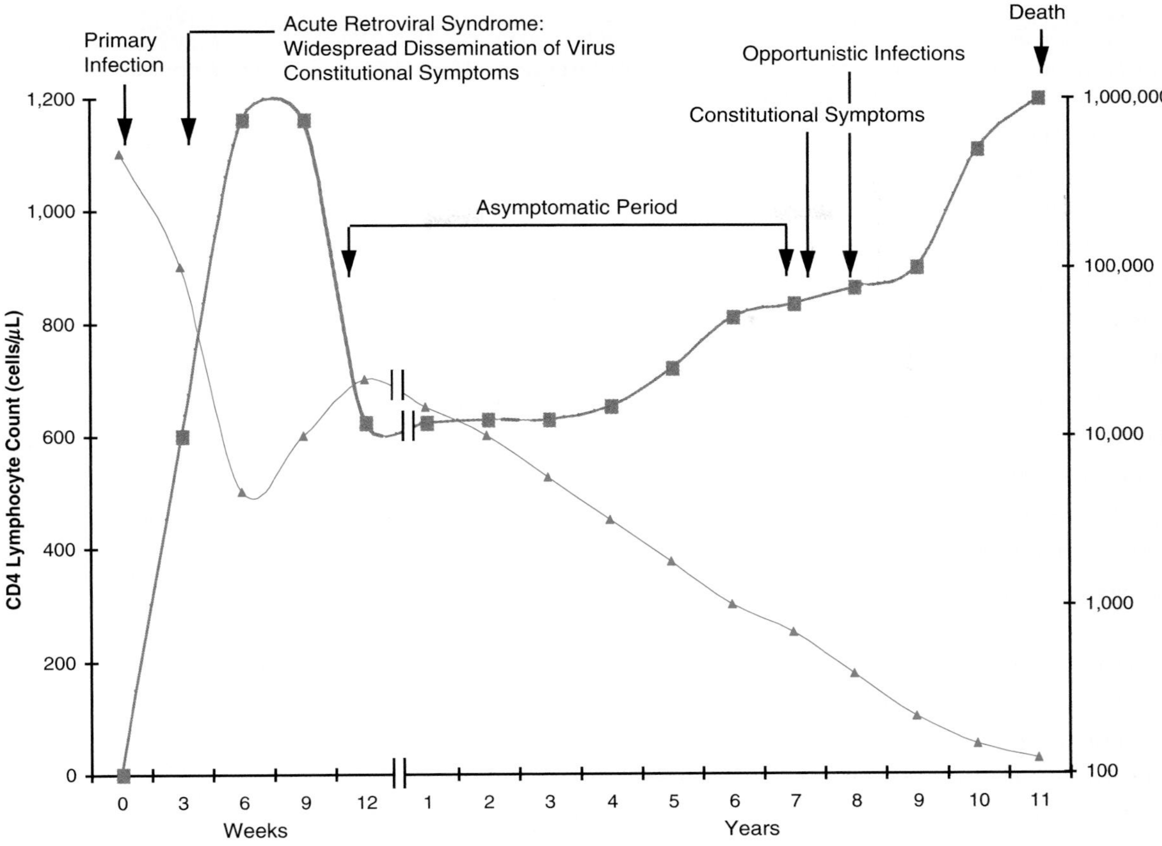

Figure 76-2 Sample disease course for an untreated HIV-infected individual showing the relationships among immunologic, virologic, and clinical outcomes over time. Constitutional symptoms include fever, night sweats, and weight loss. Viral load values; CD4 T lymphocytes. (Source: Fauci AS et al. Immunopathogenic mechanisms of HIV infection. *Ann Intern Med*. 1996;124:654; Perelson AS et al. HIV-1 dynamics in vivo: virion clearance rate, infected cell life-span, and viral generation time. *Science*. 1996;271:1582.)

Table 76-1
CDC MMWR Revised Surveillance Case Definition for HIV Infection—United States, 2014

HIV-infection stage[a] based on age-specific $CD4^+$ T-lymphocyte count or $CD4^+$ T-lymphocyte percentage of total lymphocytes

	Age on date of CD4+ T-lymphocyte test					
	<1 year		1–5 years		≥6 years	
Stage	**Cells/μL**	**%**	**Cells/μL**	**%**	**Cells/μL**	**%**
0[b]	Staging independent of CD4 count/% and age					
1	≥1,500	≥34	≥1,000	≥30	≥500	≥26
2	750–1,499	26–33	500–999	22–29	200–499	14–25
3	<750	<26	<500	<22	<200	<14

[a]Stage is based first on the $CD4^+$ T-lymphocyte count then on percentage if the count is unavailable. Three situations can dictate that staging is not based on count or percentage: (1) Stage 0 criteria are met meaning that the stage is 0 regardless of $CD4^+$ T-lymphocyte test results and the diagnosis of opportunistic infection; (2) if the criteria for stage 0 are not met and a stage-3 defining opportunistic illness has been diagnosed (see Table 76-2), meaning that the stage is 3 regardless of $CD4^+$ T-lymphocyte test results; or (3) if the criteria for stage 0 are not met and information on the above criteria for other stages is missing, then the stage is classified as unknown.

[b]Stage 0 can be established either:

1. Based on testing history (previous negative/indeterminate test results): a negative or indeterminate HIV test (antibody, combination antigen/antibody, or NAT) result within 180 days before the first confirmed positive HIV test result of any type. The first positive test result could be any time before the positive supplemental test result that confirms it or
2. Based on a testing algorithm: a sequence of tests performed as part of a laboratory testing algorithm that demonstrate the presence of HIV-specific viral markers such as p24 antigen or nucleic acid (RNA or DNA) 0 to 180 days before or after an antibody test that had a negative or indeterminate result.

Adapted from http://www.cdc.gov/mmwr/preview/mmwrhtml/rr6303a1.htm.

directly binding to the enzyme itself and prevent DNA transcription from RNA.[43] Protease inhibitors (PIs: saquinavir, fosamprenavir, nelfinavir, indinavir, lopinavir, atazanavir, ritonavir, tipranavir, and darunavir) directly bind to the catalytic site of HIV protease, inactivating the enzyme and preventing maturation of the HIV virion.[44,45] Unlike reverse transcription, which occurs early in the course of the HIV life cycle, protease enzyme activity occurs late in virion development. As a result, inactivation of the protease

Table 76-2

CDC MMWR Revised Surveillance Case Definition for HIV Infection—United States, 2014. Appendix Stage-3 Defining Opportunistic Illnesses in HIV Infection

Bacterial infections, multiple or recurrent[a]
Candidiasis of bronchi, trachea, or lungs
Candidiasis of esophagus
Cervical cancer, invasive[b]
Coccidioidomycosis, disseminated or extrapulmonary
Cryptococcosis, extrapulmonary
Cryptosporidiosis, chronic intestinal (>1 month's duration)
Cytomegalovirus disease (other than liver, spleen, or nodes), onset at age >1 month
Cytomegalovirus retinitis (with loss of vision)
Encephalopathy attributed to HIV[c]
Herpes simplex: chronic ulcers (>1 month's duration) or bronchitis, pneumonitis, or esophagitis (onset at age >1 month)
Histoplasmosis, disseminated or extrapulmonary
Isosporiasis, chronic intestinal (>1 month's duration)
Kaposi sarcoma
Lymphoma, Burkitt (or equivalent term)
Lymphoma, immunoblastic (or equivalent term)
Lymphoma, primary, of brain
Mycobacterium avium complex or Mycobacterium kansasii, disseminated or extrapulmonary
Mycobacterium tuberculosis of any site, pulmonary[b], disseminated or extrapulmonary
Mycobacterium, other species or unidentified species, disseminated or extrapulmonary
Pneumocystis jirovecii (previously known as *Pneumocystis carinii*) pneumonia
Pneumonia, recurrent[b]
Progressive multifocal leukoencephalopathy
Salmonella septicemia, recurrent
Toxoplasmosis of brain, onset at age >1 month
Wasting syndrome attributed to HIV[c]

[a]Only among children aged <6 years.
[b]Only among adults, adolescents, and children aged ≥6 years.
[c]Suggested diagnostic criteria for these illnesses, which might be particularly important for HIV encephalopathy and HIV wasting syndrome, are described in the following references: CDC. 1994 Revised classification system for human immunodeficiency virus infection in children less than 13 years of age. *MMWR*. 1994;43(RR-12):1–10; CDC. 1993 Revised classification system for HIV infection and expanded surveillance case definition for AIDS among adolescents and adults. *MMWR Recomm Rep*. 1992;41(RR-17)1–19.

Adapted from **http://www.cdc.gov/mmwr/preview/mmwrhtml/rr6303a1.htm.**

enzyme inhibits viral replication in any infected cell regardless of the current stage of HIV replication within that cell. In contrast, reverse transcriptase inhibitors can protect newly infected cells from becoming latently infected cells before the formation and insertion of proviral DNA into the host cell's genetic material. However, these agents provide no benefit for those infected cells that are actively producing new strains of virus.

Fusion inhibitors, such as enfuvirtide, prevent HIV and $CD4^+$ T cells from being pulled closer together after HIV binds to CD4 and CCR5 or CXCR-4 co-receptors. Enfuvirtide prevents fusion of the virus with the T-cell by binding to a double coil–coil complex at the gp41–gp120–CD4 receptor area.[46] The newest classes of antiretroviral agents are co-receptor blockers and integrase inhibitors. Maraviroc is a CCR5 co-receptor blocker which prevents HIV from fully binding to cells and causing infection.[47] Integrase strand transfer inhibitors (INSTIs: raltegravir, dolutegravir, and elvitegravir) prevent the integrase enzyme from integrating HIV DNA into the immune cell's genome.[48] The final class of agents used for HIV treatment, pharmacokinetic enhancers, are drugs that strongly inhibit CYP3A4, a liver enzyme responsible for metabolizing several PIs, NNRTIs, and INSTIs.[49] These agents are used with certain PIs and elvitegravir to impede metabolism and increase serum drug concentrations in order to decrease dosing requirements. Ritonavir, a PI itself, is now used primarily for its boosting effect rather than its anti-HIV activity. The newest pharmacokinetic enhancer, cobicistat, does not directly affect HIV replication.

With the development of newer, more potent antiretroviral regimens, researchers have speculated about the possibility of complete eradication of HIV from an infected patient. This outcome may require complete inhibition of viral replication in all cells and body stores where HIV resides.[13] However, a barrier to eradication is the varying half-lives of cell populations (e.g., 1–2 days for peripheral T cells vs. 14 days for macrophages).[50,51] In addition, extremely long-lived infected T cells with half-lives lasting more than 6 to 44 months have been identified.[52,53] Thus, it may

Table 76-3
Characteristics of Antiretroviral Agents for the Treatment of Adult Human Immunodeficiency Virus Infection[3,5]

Drug	Dose	Pharmacokinetic Parameters	Administration Considerations
Nucleoside Reverse Transcriptase Inhibitors			
Abacavir (ABC) **Ziagen** *Preparations* Tablets: 300 mg Oral solution: 20 mg/mL Epzicom: ABC 600 mg + 3TC 300 mg Trizivir: ABC 300 mg + ZDV 300 mg + 3TC 150 mg Triumeq: ABC 600 mg + 3TC 300 mg + DTG 50 mg	300 mg every 12 hours, or 600 mg daily Epzicom: one tablet daily Trizivir: one tablet BID Triumeq: one tablet daily	*Oral bioavailability*: 83% *Serum* $t_{1/2}$: 1.5 hours *Intracellular* $t_{1/2}$: 12–26 hours *Elimination*: alcohol dehydrogenase and glucuronyltransferase; 82% renal elimination of metabolites	Can be administered without regard to meals Alcohol raises abacavir exposure by 41% HLA testing required before administration
Lamivudine (3TC) **Epivir** *Preparations* Tablets: 150, 300 mg Solution: 10 mg/mL Combivir: 3TC 150 mg + ZDV 300 mg Epzicom: 3TC 300 mg + ABC 600 mg Trizivir: 3TC 150 mg + ZDV 300 mg + ABC 300 mg Triumeq: ABC 600 mg + 3TC 300 mg + DTG 50 mg	150 mg PO BID or 300 mg PO daily Combivir: one tablet BID Epzicom: one tablet BID Trizivir: one tablet BID Triumeq: one tablet daily	*Oral bioavailability*: 86% *Serum* $t_{1/2}$: 5–7 hours *Intracellular* $t_{1/2}$: 18–22 hours *Elimination*: 70% unchanged in urine	Can be administered without regard to meals
Emtricitabine (FTC) **Emtriva** *Preparations* Capsules: 200 mg Oral solution: 10 mg/mL Truvada: FTC 200 mg + TDF 300 mg Atripla: FTC 200 mg + TDF 300 mg + EFV 600 mg Complera: FTC 200 mg + RPV 25 mg + TDF 300 mg Stribild: FTC 200 mg + EVG/c 150/150 mg + TDF 300 mg Descovy: FTC 200 mg + TAF 300 mg Odefsey: FTC 200 mg + RPV 25 mg + TAF 25 mg Genvoya: FTC 200 mg + EVG/c 150/150 mg + TAF 10 mg	200 mg daily for patients with calculated CrCl >50 mL/minute Dose needs to be adjusted for renal dysfunction: CrCl 30–49 mL/minute: 200 mg every 48 hours CrCl 15–29 mL/minute: 200 mg every 72 hours CrCl <15 mL/minute: 200 mg every 96 hours Truvada: one tablet daily. Not for patients with CrCl <30 mL/minute Atripla: one tablet daily. Not for patients with CrCl <50 mL/minute Complera: one tablet daily Stribild: one tablet daily. Not for patients with CrCl <70 mL/minute Stribild: one tablet daily. Not for patients with CrCl <70 mL/minute	*Oral bioavailability*: 93% *Serum* $t_{1/2}$: 10 hours *Intracellular* $t_{1/2}$: >20 hours *Elimination*: 86% recovered in urine	Can be administered without regard to meals
Tenofovir Disoproxil Fumarate (TDF) **Viread** *Preparations* Tablets: 150, 200, 250, 300 mg Oral powder: 40 mg/g Truvada: TDF 300 mg + FTC 200 mg Atripla: TDF 300 mg + FTC 200 mg + EFV 600 mg Complera: FTC 200 mg + RPV 25 mg + TDF 300 mg Stribild: FTC 200 mg + EVG/c 150/150 mg + TDF 300 mg	300 mg daily for patients with CrCl >60 mL/minute Truvada: one tablet daily. Not for patients with CrCl <30 mL/minute Atripla: one tablet daily. Not for patients with CrCl <50 mL/minute Complera: one tablet daily Stribild: one tablet daily. Not for patients with CrCl <70 mL/minute	*Oral bioavailability*: 25% fasting; 39% with high-fat meal *Serum* $t_{1/2}$: 17 hours *Intracellular* $t_{1/2}$: >60 hours *Elimination:* primarily by glomerular filtration and active tubular secretion	Can be administered without regard to meals

(continued)

Table 76-3

Characteristics of Antiretroviral Agents for the Treatment of Adult Human Immunodeficiency Virus Infection[3,5] *(continued)*

Non-Preferred Nucleoside Reverse Transcriptase Inhibitors			
Tenofovir alafenamide (TAF) *Preparations* Descovy: TAF 25 mg + FTC 200 mg Odefsey: FTC 200 mg + RPV 25 mg + TAF 25 mg Genvoya: FTC 200 mg + EVG/c 150/150 mg + TAF 10 mg	25 mg for patients with CrCl >30 mL/min Descovy: one tablet daily Odefsey: one tablet daily Genvoya: one tablet daily	*Oral Bioavailability*: 40% *Serum* $t_{1/2}$: 0.51 hours Intracellular $t_{1/2}$: 150-180 hours Elimination: primarily by glomerular filtration and active tubular secretion	Can be administered without regard to meals
Zidovudine (ZDV) **Retrovir (R)** *Preparations* Oral Solution: 10 mg/mL Capsule: 100 mg Tablet: 300 mg IV Solution: 10 mg/mL Combivir: ZDV 300 mg + 3TC 150 mg Trizivir: ZDV 300 mg + 3TC 150 mg + ABC 300 mg	300 mg BID or 200 mg TID Combivir (R) or Trizivir (R): one tablet BID	*Oral bioavailability*: 60% *Serum* $t_{1/2}$: 1.1 hours *Intracellular* $t_{1/2}$: 3 hours *Elimination*: hepatic glucuronidation; renal excretion of glucuronide metabolite	Can be administered without regard to meals (manufacturer recommends administration 30 minutes before or 1 hour after a meal)
Didanosine (ddI) **Videx** *Preparations* Videx EC (R): 125, 200, 250, 400 mg capsule Pediatric powder for oral solution (when reconstituted as solution containing antacid): 10 mg/mL Generic ddI enteric-coated capsule also available	>60 kg: 400 mg daily (with TDF, use 250 mg daily) <60 kg: 250 mg daily (with TDF, use 200 mg daily)	*Oral bioavailability*: 30%–40% *Serum* $t_{1/2}$: 1.6 hours *Intracellular* $t_{1/2}$: 25–40 hours *Elimination*: renal excretion ~50%	Food decreases absorption (↓ 55%); administer ddI on empty stomach (1 hour before or 2 hours after meal) Separate ATV and TPV/r administration by at least 2 hours
Stavudine (d4T) **Zerit** *Preparations* Solution: 1 mg/mL Capsules: 15, 20, 30, 40 mg	>60 kg: 40 mg BID <60 kg: 30 mg BID Sustained release: >60 kg use 100 mg daily; <60 kg use 75 mg daily	*Oral bioavailability*: 86% *Serum* $t_{1/2}$: 1.0 hour *Intracellular* $t_{1/2}$: 3.5 hours *Elimination*: renal excretion ~50%	Can be administered without regard to meals
Non-Nucleoside Reverse Transcriptase Inhibitors[a]			
Rilpivirine (RPV) **Edurant** *Preparations* Tablets: 25 mg Complera: RPV 25 mg + TDF 300 mg + FTC 200 mg Odefsey: RPV 25 mg + TAF 25 mg + FTC 200 mg	25 mg daily Complera: one tablet daily	*Oral bioavailability*: not established *Serum* $t_{1/2}$: ~50 hours *Intracellular* $t_{1/2}$: unknown *Elimination*: hepatic metabolism primarily by CYP3A4 with 85% fecal excretion.	Take with moderate-to-high-calorie meal (increases absorption 40%)
Efavirenz (EFV) **Sustiva** *Preparations* Capsules: 50, 100, 200 mg Tablets: 600 mg Atripla: EFV 600 mg + TDF 300 mg + FTC 200 mg	600 mg at bedtime Atripla one tablet at bedtime. Not for patients with CrCl <50 mL/minute .	*Oral bioavailability*: ~60%–70% *Serum* $t_{1/2}$: 40–55 hours *Intracellular* $t_{1/2}$: unknown *Elimination*: hepatically metabolized by CYP2B6 and CYP3A4 (also CYP3A4 mixed inhibitor/inducer)	Avoid taking with high-fat meals, concentrations ↑ 50% (increased risk for CNS toxicity)
Etravirine (ETV) **Intelence** *Preparations* Tablets: 100, 200 mg	200 mg BID	*Oral bioavailability*: unknown *Serum* $t_{1/2}$: 40 ± 20 hours *Intracellular* $t_{1/2}$: unknown *Elimination*: hepatically metabolized by CYP3A4, CYP2C9, CYP2C19 (also 3A4 inducer, 2C9 and 2C19 inhibitors)	Take after a meal

Table 76-3
Characteristics of Antiretroviral Agents for the Treatment of Adult Human Immunodeficiency Virus Infection[3,5] (*continued*)

Non-Preferred Non-Nucleoside Reverse Transcriptase Inhibitors[a]			
Nevirapine (NVP) **Viramune** *Preparations* Suspension: 50 mg/5 mL Tablets: 200 mg	200 mg PO daily × 14 days, then 200 mg PO BID	*Oral bioavailability*: >90% *Serum* $t_{1/2}$: 25–30 hours *Intracellular* $t_{1/2}$: unknown *Elimination*: metabolized by CYP2B6 and CYP3A4 (also a CYP3A4 inducer) with 80% excreted in urine as the glucuronide metabolite	Can be administered without regard to meals
Protease Inhibitors			
Darunavir (DRV) **Prezista** *Preparations* Tablet: 75, 150, 600, 800 mg Suspension: 100 mg/ml Prezcobix: DRV 800 mg + COBI 150 mg	DRV 800 mg + RTV 100 mg daily In patients with ≥1 DRV resistance mutations: DRV 600 mg + RTV 100 mg BID Prezcobix: one tablet daily	*Oral bioavailability*: 37% alone, 82% with RTV *Serum* $t_{1/2}$: 15 hours *Intracellular* $t_{1/2}$: unknown *Elimination*: hepatic metabolism via CYP3A4 (inhibitor)	Food ↑ C_{max} and AUC by 30%: administer with food
Atazanavir (ATV) **Reyataz** *Preparations* Capsules: 100, 150, 200, 300 mg Evotaz: ATV 300 mg + COBI 150 mg	400 mg daily Atazanavir/RTV: 300/100 daily Evotaz: one tablet daily	*Oral bioavailability*: 60%–70% *Serum* $t_{1/2}$: 6–7 hours *Intracellular* $t_{1/2}$: unknown *Elimination*: hepatic metabolism via CYP3A4 (modest inhibitor)	Take with food, and avoid acid suppressing agents (which prevent ATV solubility and absorption)
Lopinavir (LPV)/ritonavir (RTV) **Kaletra** *Preparations* Tablet: LPV 200 mg + RTV 50 mg Solution: LPV 80 mg+ RTV 20 mg per mL	Two tablets or 5 mL BID or Four tablets or 10 mL daily (recommended for treatment-naïve patients only)	*Oral bioavailability*: not determined *Serum* $t_{1/2}$: 5–6 hours *Intracellular* $t_{1/2}$: unknown *Elimination*: hepatic metabolism via CYP3A4 (inhibitor)	Take with food (increases AUC by 48%). Tablet stable at room temperature
Non-Preferred Protease Inhibitors			
Indinavir (IDV) **Crixivan** *Preparations* Capsule: 200, 333, 400 mg	800 mg every 8 hours (BID dosing ineffective when sole protease inhibitor) IDV/RTV: IDV 800 mg + 100 mg or 200 mg RTV BID	*Oral bioavailability*: 65% *Serum* $t_{1/2}$: 1.5–2 hours *Intracellular* $t_{1/2}$: unknown *Elimination*: hepatically metabolized via CYP3A4 (also inhibitor of CYP3A4)	Must be taken on empty stomach (1 hour before or 2 hours after a meal); may be taken with skim milk or low-fat meal Adequate hydration necessary (at least 1.5 L/24 hours of liquid) to minimize risk of nephrolithiasis
Nelfinavir (NFV) **Viracept** *Preparations* Powder for oral suspension: 50 mg per one level scoop (200 mg per one level teaspoon) Tablets: 250 and 625 mg	750 mg TID or 1,250 mg BID	*Oral bioavailability*: 20%–80% *Serum* $t_{1/2}$: 3.5–5 hours *Intracellular* $t_{1/2}$: unknown *Elimination*: hepatic metabolism via CYP3A4	Administer with meal or light snack (exposure increased twofold to threefold)
Saquinavir (SQV) **Invirase** (hard gel capsules) *Preparations* Hard gel capsule: 200 mg Tablets: 500 mg	Unboosted saquinavir not recommended Saquinavir/ritonavir: 1,000/100 BID; 1,600/100 daily under investigation	*Oral bioavailability*: 4% (as the sole PI) *Serum* $t_{1/2}$: 1–2 hours *Intracellular* $t_{1/2}$: unknown *Elimination*: hepatic metabolism via CYP3A4 (inhibitor)	Take within 2 hours of a meal and take with RTV
Fosamprenavir (FPV) **Lexiva** Tablet: 700 mg	In ARV-naïve patients: FPV 1,400 mg BID or FPV 1,400 mg + RTV 200 mg daily or FPV 700 mg + RTV 100 mg BID In PI-experienced patients: FPV 700 mg + RTV 100 mg BID	*Oral bioavailability*: not determined *Serum* $t_{1/2}$: 7.1–10.6 hours (APV) *Intracellular* $t_{1/2}$: unknown *Elimination*: hepatic metabolism via CYP3A4 (inhibitor)	Can be taken without regard to meals but should not be taken with high-fat meals

(*continued*)

Table 76-3

Characteristics of Antiretroviral Agents for the Treatment of Adult Human Immunodeficiency Virus Infection[3,5] (*continued*)

Tipranavir (TPV) **Aptivus** Capsules: 250 mg	TPV 500 mg + RTV 200 mg BID DO NOT USE WITHOUT RTV	*Oral bioavailability*: not determined *Serum* $t_{1/2}$: 6 hours *Intracellular* $t_{1/2}$: unknown *Elimination*: hepatic metabolism via CYP3A4 (inhibitor and inducer)	Administer with food to increase bioavailability
Entry Inhibitors			
Enfuvirtide (T-20) Fuzeon	90 mg SC BID in upper arm, thigh, or abdomen	*Oral bioavailability*: 84.3% compared with IV *Serum* $t_{1/2}$: 3.8 hours *Intracellular* $t_{1/2}$: not applicable *Elimination*: non-renal, non-hepatic	Reconstitute with 1.1 mL sterile water for injection; gently tap vial for 10 seconds and then roll gently between hands to avoid foaming and ensure all drug is off vial walls After reconstitution, use immediately or refrigerate for 24 hours. Refrigerated T-20 should be brought to room temperature before injection
Chemokine Receptor Antagonists (CCR5)			
Maraviroc (MVC) **Selzentry** *Preparations* Tablet: 150, 300 mg	300 mg BID (with all NRTIs, NVP, TPV, ENF), 150 mg BID with CYP3A inhibitors (with or without a CYP3A inducer) including protease inhibitors (except tipranavir/ritonavir), delavirdine, ketoconazole, itraconazole, clarithromycin, and other strong CYP3A inhibitors (e.g., nefazodone, telithromycin) 600 mg BID with CYP3A inducers (without a strong CYP3A inhibitor) including Efavirenz, etravirine (TMC125), rifampin, carbamazepine, phenobarbital, and phenytoin	*Oral bioavailability*: ~33% *Serum* $t_{1/2}$: 14–18 hours *Elimination*: hepatic metabolism by CYP3A; 20% recovered in urine, 76% recovered in feces	Can be administered without regard to meals (high-fat meal decreases C_{max} and AUC by ~30%) Trofile assay must be performed before administration
Integrase Inhibitors			
Dolutegravir (DTG) **Tivicay** *Preparations* Tablet: 50 mg Triumeq: DTG 50 mg + ABC 600 mg + 3TC 300 mg	50 mg once daily 50 mg BID when coadministered with EFV, FPV/r, TPV/r, or Rifampin 50 mg BID when INSTI mutations present Triumeq: one tablet daily	*Oral bioavailability*: unknown *Serum* $t_{1/2}$: ~14 hours *Intracellular* $t_{1/2}$: unknown *Elimination*: hepatic metabolism by UGT1A1 (major) CYP3A4 (minor); 31% recovered in urine, 53% recovered in feces	Increased serum creatinine because of inhibition of tubular secretion not decreased renal glomerular filtration. Mean (range) increase from baseline = 0.15 (–0.32 to 0.65) mg/dL
Elvitegravir (EVG) **Vitekta** *Preparations* Tablet: 85, 150 mg Stribild: EVG 150 mg + COBI 150 mg + FTC 200 mg + TDF 300 mg Genvoya: EVG 150 mg + COBI 150 mg + FTC 200 mg + TAF 10 mg	85 mg once daily if coadministered with ATV/r or LPV/r 150 mg once daily if coadministered with DRV/r 600/100 mg BID, FPV/r 700/100 mg BID, or TPV/r 500/200 mg BID 50 mg BID when INSTI mutations present Stribild: one tablet daily	*Oral bioavailability*: not established *Serum* $t_{1/2}$: 9 hours when administered with RTV *Intracellular* $t_{1/2}$: unknown *Elimination*: hepatic metabolism by CYP3A, and UGT1A1/3; 6.7% recovered in urine, 94.8% recovered in feces	Vitekta must be administered with ritonavir unboosted EVG is not recommended Take with food

Table 76-3

Characteristics of Antiretroviral Agents for the Treatment of Adult Human Immunodeficiency Virus Infection[3,5] (continued)

Raltegravir (RAL) **Isentress** *Preparations* Tablet: 400 mg, 1,200 mg HD Chewable tablet: 25, 100 mg Single packet for oral suspension: 100 mg	400 mg BID or 1,200 mg (HD) daily	*Oral bioavailability*: not established *Serum* $t_{1/2}$: 9 hours *Intracellular* $t_{1/2}$: unknown *Elimination*: hepatic metabolism by UGT1A1 glucuronidation; 32% recovered in urine, 51% recovered in feces	Can be administered without regard to meals (high-fat meal decreases C_{max} by ~34% and increases AUC by ~19%)
Pharmacokinetic Enhancers			
Ritonavir (RTV) **Norvir** *Preparations* Oral solution: 80 mg/mL Capsules: 100 mg Tablets: 100 mg	RTV is a PI currently used as a pharmacokinetic enhancer for other PIs and EVG, using 100–400 mg/day in one to two divided doses	*Oral bioavailability*: Not determined *Serum* $t_{1/2}$: 3–5 hours *Intracellular* $t_{1/2}$: unknown *Elimination*: extensive hepatic metabolism via CYP3A4 (also potent CYP3A4 inhibitor and mixed inhibitor/inducer of other isozymes)	Take with food if possible to improve tolerability Dose should be titrated upward to minimize gastrointestinal adverse events Refrigerate capsules but not liquid or tablets Solution contains 43% alcohol
Tybost (COBI) **Cobicistat** *Preparations* Tablets: 150 mg Stribild: EVG 150 mg + COBI 150 mg + FTC 200 mg + TDF 300 mg Prezcobix: DRV 800 mg + COBI 150 mg Evotaz: ATV 300 mg + COBI 150 mg	150 mg daily when coadministered with ATV 300 mg daily 150 mg daily when coadministered with DRV 800 mg daily Stribild: one tablet daily. Not for patients with CrCl <70 mL/min Prezcobix: one tablet daily Evotaz: one tablet daily	*Oral bioavailability*: Not determined *Serum* $t_{1/2}$: 3–5 hours *Intracellular* $t_{1/2}$: unknown *Elimination*: extensive hepatic metabolism via CYP3A4 (also potent CYP3A4 inhibitor and mixed inhibitor/inducer of other isozymes) 8.2% recovered in urine, 86.2% recovered in feces	Not interchangeable with RTV Increased serum creatinine because of inhibition of tubular secretion not decreased renal glomerular filtration. Monitor for renal safety if increased from baseline >0.4 mg/dL

[a]In clinical trials, the NNRTIs were discontinued because of rash in 7% of patients taking nevirapine, 4.3% of patients taking delavirdine, and 1.7% of patients taking efavirenz. Rare cases of Stevens–Johnson syndrome have been reported with all three NNRTIs.

ABC, abacavir; ARV, antiretroviral; ATV, atazanavir; AUC, area under the curve; BID, twice daily; CNS, central nervous system; CrCl, creatinine clearance; COBI, cobicistat; ddI, didanosine; d4T, stavudine; DLV, delavirdine; DRV, darunavir; DTG, dolutegravir; EFV, efavirenz; ENF, enfuvirtide; ETV, etravirine; EVG, elvitegravir; FPV, fosamprenavir; FTC, emtricitabine; HLA, human leukocyte antigen; IDV, indinavir; IV, intravenous; LPV, lopinavir; MVC, maraviroc; NFV, nelfinavir; NNRTI, non-nucleoside reverse transcriptase inhibitor; NRTIs, nucleoside reverse transcriptase inhibitors; NVP, nevirapine; PI, protein inhibitor; PO, orally; QID, four times daily; RAL, raltegravir; RPV, rilpivirine; RTV, ritonavir; SC, subcutaneously; SQV, saquinavir; 3TC, lamivudine; TAF, tenofovir alafenamide; TDF, tenofovir disoproxil fumarate; TID, three times daily; TPV, tipranavir; TPV/r, tipranavir/ritonavir; T-20, enfuvirtide; ZDV, zidovudine.

require complete suppression of HIV replication for 60 years or more to eradicate HIV infection completely from the body.[52–54] Another complicating factor is the potential for HIV to reside in sites that achieve low antiretroviral concentrations, thereby serving as sanctuaries for HIV replication (e.g., central nervous system [CNS], testes). Once therapy is discontinued, these sites could theoretically release unaffected virions and repopulate the host. As a result, research has shifted toward immune-based therapies that can identify and destroy HIV-infected cells, in addition to preventing HIV acquisition.

DIAGNOSIS

CASE 76-1

Question 1: E.J. is a 27-year-old man who presents with new complaints of fevers, night sweats, weight loss, and white patches in his mouth. He states that these symptoms have been present for the past 4 to 6 weeks. E.J. admits to intravenous drug use in the past; however, he states that he has been "clean" for 3 years. E.J. is diagnosed with thrush caused by *Candida albicans*. HIV infection is suspected and consent for an HIV test is obtained. Why is HIV suspected and how is it confirmed?

In otherwise healthy, immunocompetent individuals, opportunistic infections, such as thrush, are rare because an intact cell-mediated immunity protects against infection. In immunosuppressed individuals, such as those infected with HIV, the immune system is significantly compromised and places patients at risk for opportunistic infections. Infections such as shingles (herpes zoster), tuberculosis, thrush, and recurrent candidal vaginal infections in an otherwise healthy person warrant further evaluation for the possibility of HIV infection. More advanced diseases, such as *P. jirovecii* pneumonia, *Mycobacterium avium* bacteremia, and cytomegalovirus retinitis infections, among others, generally occur in patients with severely depressed immune systems and strongly suggest HIV infection. This suggestion is especially true for those patients with risk factors for HIV infection. Despite E.J.'s discontinuation of intravenous drugs, his prior use places him at risk for HIV infection. Given his social history and current clinical presentation, an HIV test is warranted.

Laboratory methods used to diagnose HIV infection rely on detecting antigens produced by HIV viral replication or antibodies produced by the host's immune response to HIV infection. After HIV infection, there is an initial eclipse period where no antigen or antibody laboratory markers can be consistently detected.[55] The first laboratory marker that can be reliably detected in the plasma after infection is HIV RNA by nucleic acid tests (NAT) approximately 10 days after infection, then p24 (a protein produced during viral replication) approximately 4 to 10 days after HIV RNA can be detected. The immune response to HIV infection is characterized first by the production of anti-HIV immunoglobulin (Ig)M proteins (10–13 days after HIV RNA can be detected) then IgG (18–38 days after HIV RNA can be detected). The period between infection with HIV and the ability to detect these antibodies is known as the seroconversion window, and the duration of this window can vary based on assay sensitivity or antibody type. Established infection is characterized by a fully developed IgG response.

While early laboratory methods which utilized enzyme-linked immunosorbent assays (ELISA) and confirmatory Western blot to detect anti-HIV IgG antibodies were highly sensitive (>99%), the turnaround time for test results could be up to 1 to 2 weeks and the seroconversion window was 1 to 2 months long, making it difficult to diagnose early infections.[55] Third-generation HIV assays decreased the seroconversion window by including anti-HIV IgM.[55] Fourth-generation antigen/antibody combination assays further reduced this timeframe by testing for p24 antigen and anti-HIV-1 and -2 IgM/IgG. Current Center for Disease Control (CDC) guidelines recommend using of one of two US Food and Drug Administration (FDA)-approved fourth-generation antigen/antibody combination assays.[56,57] The sensitivity for these fourth-generation combination assays is >99.7%, and test results can be available within 3 hours which represents opportunity for more rapid engagement in clinical care upon a positive test result.[55] Unless there is reason to suspect very early infection, no further testing is required for a nonreactive antigen/antibody combination assay. Specimen with reactive antigen/antibody results should be further tested with an immunoassay to differentiate HIV-1 and HIV-2 antibodies. NATs for HIV RNA should be used to confirm an indeterminate antibody differentiation immunoassay or a negative antigen/antibody tests in patients where there is reason to suspect very early infection.[55]

SURROGATE MARKER DATA

While current guidelines recommend initiating therapeutic interventions for all HIV-infected persons ready to begin treatment,[3] the severity of immune damage and potential for disease progression should still be assessed to determine the clinical urgency for beginning treatment and if additional therapeutic interventions to prevent opportunistic infection are needed. As stated previously, HIV predominantly infects and destroys T cells. The larger the viral load, the greater the risk for T-cell destruction and opportunistic infections. Therefore, quantitative measurements of E.J.'s HIV viral load and T-cell counts will assist in "staging" the severity of infection, assessing the risk for disease progression, and providing a reference point (i.e., baseline) for future therapeutic decisions.

Identification and measurement of T-lymphocyte subsets (e.g., CD4, CD8) are based on flow cytometry readings of fluorescent-labeled monoclonal antibodies.[58] These values can vary widely on repeated laboratory evaluations, even in clinically stable patients. Patient samples can display up to 30% intralaboratory and interlaboratory variabilities.[3] Consequently, it is important to realize that assessment of T-cell measurements should always be interpreted as trends and not as individual values. Variability can also be minimized by using the same laboratory and by sampling patients at a consistent time of day.

The measurement of HIV viral load can be performed by one of three methods: reverse transcriptase–polymerase chain reaction (RT-PCR), branched-chain DNA assay, or nucleic acid sequence-based amplification.[59] Measurements using RT-PCR are obtained when viral RNA is amplified and counted. In contrast, branched-chain DNA amplifies and enumerates the signal from target probes attached to the viral RNA. Nucleic acid sequence-based amplification allows real-time, high throughput amplification of viral RNA. All methods report HIV RNA in plasma as the number of copies per milliliter but have differing lower limits of quantitation.[3] It should be recognized that plasma viral RNA values measure the amount of free virus in the periphery and not the lymph nodes. Because viral concentrations are substantially greater in the lymph node, plasma measurements of HIV indirectly reflect spillover from replication in that compartment.[60,61]

Similar to CD4 counts, viral load measurements (copies/milliliter) can vary by as much as threefold (0.5 log) in either direction.[3] When obtaining a patient's baseline value, a number of issues must be considered. On initial infection with HIV, a burst of viremia occurs until the host's immune responses are able to control the infection. Consequently, viral load measurements obtained during the first 6 months of infection may not accurately reflect a true baseline value.[3] In addition, factors that activate the immune system, such as the development of a new opportunistic infection or immunizations,[62] can result in transient elevations of viral load measurements. In these situations, concentrations obtained within 4 weeks of the event may not accurately reflect the baseline viral load measurement.[3]

Some clinicians would recommend that at least two separate viral load measurements, which are obtained within 1 to 4 weeks of each other, be performed before making decisions regarding therapeutic options.[3] As with T-cell values, viral load measurements should be evaluated as trends.

In addition to quantifying the viral load, baseline resistance testing should be performed, using either genotypic or phenotypic testing,[3] to guide the selection of the initial regimen. Resistance testing is recommended in most clinical situations before beginning treatment, because the rate of transmission of virus resistant to at least one drug (i.e., transmitted drug resistance) has been noted in up to 11% to 12% of HIV-infected patients who have never been on antiretroviral therapy in North America and Europe.[63] (see Resistance, Viral Genotyping, Phenotyping, and Viral Fitness section for further discussion).

CASE 76-1, QUESTION 2: E.J.'s HIV-1/2 antigen/antibody combination immunoassay is reactive and the antibody differentiation immunoassay detects HIV-1 antibodies. He is informed of his HIV status the next week at his follow-up examination. Before making any decisions regarding therapeutic options, what additional laboratory tests should be obtained?

E.J. should have a baseline T-cell count, viral load measurement, and viral genotype obtained. A complete blood count, electrolyte panel, renal, and liver function tests and hepatitis B and C serology should be performed. If specific therapies are being considered, such as abacavir and maraviroc, specific testing is available to guide the appropriate use of these agents. HLA-B5701 screening is performed before starting a patient on abacavir because of an increased risk for exhibiting a hypersensitivity reaction in patients positive for this allele. Co-receptor tropism assay is performed before initiating maraviroc to determine whether the patient has a virus that predominantly uses CCR5 receptors (vs. ones that use primarily CXCR-4 receptors or ones that can use both).[3] These laboratory results help in selecting therapeutic options (see subsequent discussion) and establish baseline values in the event that problems are encountered in the future.

ANTIRETROVIRAL THERAPY

CASE 76-1, QUESTION 3: E.J.'s T-cell count and viral load measurement return at 225 cells/μL and 145,000 copies/mL (by RT-PCR assay), respectively. Should antiretroviral therapy be initiated?

In deciding to initiate antiretroviral therapy, it is important to consider both the potential benefits of therapy and the potential risks of therapy, including both short-term and long-term side effects and potential for the development of drug resistance (and cross-resistance; see subsequent discussion). Antiretroviral therapy should be offered to all patients who are willing and able to commit to lifelong treatment after an in-depth discussion of the benefits and risks of HAART and the importance of adherence. Recently, the Department of Health and Human Services (DHHS) HIV Treatment Guideline Panel issued a statement modifying their 2015 guidelines. This modification was based on the results of two large randomized clinical trials (START; The Strategic Timing of AntiRetroviral Treatment and the TEMPRANO ARNS 12136 Study). These trials investigated the risks and benefits of initiating HAART at a CD4 count >500 cell/μL versus delaying until the CD4 count declined to <350 cell/μL. A significant increase in morbidity and mortality was observed when HAART was delayed prompting the Guideline Panel to upgrade the strength of their former recommendation to start HAART at any baseline CD4 count to the highest level of evidence (AI; strong recommendation supported by data from randomized controlled trials).[64] Previously, the strength of evidence in support of initiating HAART was prioritized across three categories of increasing baseline CD4 cell count (>500 cell/μL: lowest strength; 350–500 cell/μL: intermediate strength; <350 cell/μL: highest strength).[3] In further support of starting HAART regardless of baseline CD4 count, the 2015 guidelines recognize the benefits of initiating HAART for HIV prevention and support initiating HAART to prevent perinatal and heterosexual transmission (AI evidence rating) or other transmission risks (AIII evidence rating). Clinical situations which favor more urgent initiation of HAART include pregnancy; AIDS-defining condition such as an opportunistic infection; CD4 count of <200 cells/μL; HIV-associated nephropathy (HIVAN); hepatitis B and/or C coinfection; rapidly declining CD4 count (>100 cells/μL decrease per year); higher baseline viral load (>100,000 copies/mL); and acute/early HIV infection.[3] In patients who are asymptomatic, assessment of the patient's surrogate marker data (T-cell count, viral load measurements), concurrent medical conditions, medication adherence history (if any), and motivation to initiate therapy are necessary. The results of resistance testing should be considered before initiating therapy.

Knowledge of both the T-cell count and the baseline viral load values is important to "stage" the severity of infection (Table 76-1). In otherwise healthy, immunocompetent persons, T-cell measurements are greater than 1,200 cells/μL. In patients who have been chronically infected with HIV, significant T-cell destruction occurs. When T-cell counts fall to less than 500 cells/μL, patients are at increased risk for opportunistic infections. Data from both clinical trials and observational cohort studies have long shown a clear benefit for antiretroviral therapy when CD4 cell counts are ≤350 cells/μL, and many cohort analyses have shown benefit for starting therapy at CD4 counts ≤500 cells/μL.[3] Early, less definitive evidence also suggested initiating HAART in patients with CD4 counts of >500 cells/μL improves immune recovery, reduces HIV transmission risk, and potentially reduces the risk of non–AIDS-defining diseases. These suggestive data were recently confirmed by the two previously mentioned randomized trials, START and Temprano ANRS 12136 study, both of which found definitive benefit when initiating HAART at a CD4 Count >500 cells/μL versus delaying.[65,66] The risk of disease progression is closely tied to CD4 cell counts, with low CD4 counts (<200 cells/μL) predicting both short-term and long-term risk of disease progression.[67–69] High viral load (>100,000 copies/mL), increasing age, acquisition of infection through intravenous drug use, and a previous AIDS diagnosis also increase the risk of disease progression in observational cohorts.

The decision to initiate therapy should not be taken lightly. Antiretroviral regimens may improve the quality and duration of a patient's life, but they are not without risks. Once therapy is initiated, antiretroviral therapy is a lifetime commitment. For some patients, this may be a difficult realization, particularly if the patient is relatively healthy. In addition, the risk of adverse events/toxicities and the costs of HAART should be considered before beginning treatment. These guidelines, therefore, should be used to initiate discussions with the patient regarding the risks and benefits of therapy. It is critical for practitioners to talk openly with patients about their fears and concerns and make an assessment about their motivation to initiate therapy and ability to adhere to a lifelong regimen. The patient should always make the final decision after careful discussions with the practitioner.

E.J. has a number of significant risk factors for disease progression. He is clinically symptomatic with oral thrush and nonspecific constitutional symptoms (e.g., fevers, night sweats, and weight loss). His surrogate maker data place him at risk for greater disease progression (T-cell count <500 cells/μL and viral load >100,000 copies/mL). Based on these values, E.J. should be counseled on his risk of disease progression, potential adverse events associated with both starting and deferring treatment, and his willingness to adhere to a regimen.

Before developing a patient-specific regimen, it is important to recognize the benefits and limitations of therapy and identify obtainable and realistic goals.

CASE 76-1, QUESTION 4: After careful discussions, E.J. agrees to initiate therapy. What should be the goals of therapy? What other factors or information should be considered in selecting an appropriate regimen?

Goals of Therapy

GOAL 1: MAXIMALLY AND DURABLY SUPPRESS VIRAL LOAD

Maximal viral suppression often results in significant increases in T-cell counts and improved clinical outcomes. Based on our understanding of viral pathogenesis, this finding is not surprising. Lower amounts of replicating virus result in decreased risk for T-cell infection and destruction and, subsequently, a more intact immune response. Therefore, therapy should suppress viral replication to undetectable levels in the plasma (<50 copies/mL), for as long as possible.[3,5] The development of new antiretroviral agents with improved potency, higher genetic barrier to resistance, low adverse event profiles, and more convenient dosing regimens (including once daily single tablet regimens) makes viral suppression a reasonable goal in most patients, even those who previously have received multiple suboptimal regimens or failed therapy. In the treatment-experienced patient, however, special care must be given to designing a regimen that will suppress viral load, yet not contribute to the development of drug resistance that limits future treatment options. Consultation with an expert in antiretroviral resistance patterns is critical to designing a salvage regimen in such patients.

The development of drug resistance is also a consideration in the selection of regimens for patients who have not previously used antiretrovirals (antiretroviral naïve). In any given viral population, the potential exists for a spontaneous mutation to occur, which results in a resistant isolate. The larger the population, the greater the risk for mutations. HIV replication is a highly error-prone process, especially with the reverse transcriptase enzyme. Given the high rate of viral replication, the potential exists for the daily production of thousands of replication-competent viral mutations to each and every site on the HIV genome (~10,000 nucleotides in length).[4,35] Under selective pressures from inadequate antiretroviral therapies, spontaneously produced isolates with reduced susceptibility to the given regimen eventually flourish and repopulate the host. This fact is of particular concern given the potential for cross-resistance between antiretroviral agents (see the following discussion of resistance). Therefore, the use of a regimen that fully suppresses viral replication reduces the potential for mutations and the development of cross-resistance.

Although more than 20 FDA-approved antiretroviral agents are currently available to use in combination therapies, many of these agents display similar resistance profiles. Developing resistance to one or more agents in a given regimen may result in the loss of activity to other agents with similar resistance profiles (i.e., cross-resistance).[4] Whether or not drug resistance develops is determined by the genetic barrier associated with the individual antiretroviral drugs. Some drugs have low genetic barriers; that is, only one or two critical changes in the virus are necessary for resistance to occur. An example of a class of agents with a low genetic barrier is the NNRTIs. While a number of individual point mutations in the viral genome can confer the loss of activity for the first-generation NNRTIs (nevirapine and efavirenz), second-generation NNRTIs (rilpivirine and etravirine) exhibit improved barriers to resistance compared to these first-generation agents. In contrast, the PIs have a wide genetic barrier, which requires multiple changes to the viral genome to incur resistance.[4]

It should be recognized, however, that just because an agent has a low genetic barrier does not mean it is virologically inferior or less potent. Potent regimens containing NNRTIs are highly effective and provide durable treatment responses. The potency of the entire regimen[3] is critical to determining whether or not drug resistance develops. If viral replication is suppressed, the development of resistance will be minimal. When viral replication does occur, the greater the replication, the greater the risk for development of resistance. In those situations in which viral replication does occur, inclusion of a drug with a low genetic barrier in the antiretroviral regimen may be risky and could result in the loss of activity of the drug, the development of cross-resistance to other drugs, or both. As a result, an antiretroviral regimen should be selected that has a high likelihood of suppressing viral replication and to which the patient will strictly adhere.

GOAL 2: PRESERVE AND STRENGTHEN THE IMMUNE SYSTEM

Decreasing viral replication usually leads to increased CD4 cell counts, which strengthens and preserves the immune system. With increased cell counts, patients are at lower risk for exhibiting opportunistic infections and death. With newer and improved regimens, strengthening and preserving the immune system may be possible even in treatment-experienced patients, although drug regimens must be designed carefully to prevent developing further resistance. Full immune reconstitution may not be possible if the CD4 cell count is low for a long period of time; however, it is reasonable to try and restore immune function as fully as possible. Despite advances in drug therapy, it is important to remember that HIV remains an incurable condition.

GOAL 3: LIMIT DRUG ADVERSE EVENTS, PROMOTE ADHERENCE, AND IMPROVE QUALITY OF LIFE

Treatment with combination therapy has been shown to be highly effective in suppressing HIV replication and improving survival among patients who are HIV infected. Lifelong adherence to an antiretroviral regimen is required and can be a complex and difficult task, although advances in coformulation of drug products and the advent of ritonavir-boosted protease inhibitors have simplified HIV treatment considerably. Several once-daily regimens and single tablet regimens are recommended as first-line therapy (Tables 76-3 and 76-4). The patient's ability to adhere to therapy may, however, still be the difference between a regimen that fails and one that results in a clinical benefit. The first regimen generally provides the best chance for treatment success. Although newer antiretrovirals tend to exhibit better adverse event profiles compared to the early antiretrovirals, adverse events can still make tolerating these regimens difficult, and affect drug adherence and response to therapy. Changes in body composition (known as lipodystrophy), increases in lipids and triglycerides, bone and joint fractures, increased risks for cardiac disease, and the development of lactic acidosis are serious concerns.[3]

Limit Adverse Events

Although new antiretrovirals offer marked improvement over early generation agents' toxicity profiles, lifelong HAART is not without risk. Metabolic complications from antiretroviral therapy include abnormal distribution of body fat, lipid abnormalities (e.g., hypercholesterolemia, hypertriglyceridemia, increases in low-density lipoprotein [LDL] and decreases in high-density lipoprotein [HDL]), and new-onset diabetes.[70–72] Coronary artery disease, myocardial infarctions, and vascular complications among relatively young patients (30–40 years old) taking HAART-containing regimens have been reported.[73–78] Large observational studies suggest an increased risk for cardiovascular disease among patients taking HAART, particularly among those receiving protease inhibitors.[79–81] Additionally, nucleoside analogs can inhibit mitochondrial DNA polymerase and, as a result, have been implicated in lipoatrophy; however, this appears to be less of a concern for newer NRTIs.[82] Finally, metabolic abnormalities have also been reported in patients who are HIV infected before receiving HAART, and it may also be a consequence of HIV infection or preexisting metabolic disorders that are exacerbated by HAART.[71]

Up to 40% of patients on PI-based HAART are reported to experience impaired glucose tolerance because of significant insulin resistance.[83] Patients with type 2 diabetes mellitus are at increased risk, and PI-based regimens should be used with caution in these patients. Fasting glucose measures for all patients are recommended before and during therapy (e.g., every 3–6 months) with PI-based regimens.[3] Treatment of type 2 diabetes in HIV patients as a result of HAART therapy should be handled similarly to any other patient.

Elevations in serum levels of triglycerides, total cholesterol, and LDL, with mild decreases in HDL, are associated with HAART.[71,84,85] These abnormalities may be seen as early as 2 weeks after the initiation of therapy.[71] Although all PIs have been implicated, these laboratory abnormalities appear to occur more frequently in ritonavir-containing regimens, and less frequently in patients receiving atazanavir alone.[71] The NNRTIs can also cause lipid alterations, although their incidence is lower. Both efavirenz and nevirapine have been shown to increase HDL concentrations among patients receiving HAART. Nevirapine may have the least detrimental lipid profile (i.e., greater increases in HDL concentrations and less effect on LDL elevations).[86] Of the NRTIs, stavudine appears to affect

Table 76-4
Recommended Antiretroviral Agents for Initial Treatment of Established Human Immunodeficiency Virus Infection

	Preferred[a]	Alternatives
PIs (one or two PIs + two NRTIs)	Darunavir/ritonavir + emtricitabine/tenofovir disoproxil fumarate or emtricitabine/tenofovir alafenamide	Darunavir/ritonavir + abacavir/lamivudine[b]
		Darunavir/cobicistat[c] + abacavir/lamivudine[b] or emtricitabine/tenofovir disoproxil fumarate or emtricitabine/tenofovir alafenamide
		Atazanavir/ritonavir + emtricitabine/tenofovir disoproxil fumarate or emtricitabine/tenofovir alafenamide
		Atazanavir/cobicistat[c] + emtricitabine/tenofovir disoproxil fumarate or emtricitabine/tenofovir alafenamide
Integrase inhibitors	Raltegravir twice daily + emtricitabine/tenofovir disoproxil fumarate or emtricitabine/tenofovir alafenamide	
	Elvitegravir/cobicistat/emtricitabine/tenofovir disoproxil fumarate[c] *or* Elvitegravir/cobicistat/emtricitabine/tenofovir alafenamide	
	Dolutegravir + emtricitabine/tenofovir disoproxil fumarate or emtricitabine/tenofovir alafenamide	
	Dolutegravir/abacavir/lamivudine[b]	
NNRTIs (one NNRTI + two NRTIs)		Efavirenz/emtricitabine/tenofovir disoproxil fumarate
		Rilpivirine/emtricitabine/tenofovir disoproxil fumarate[d] or rilpivirine/emtricitabine/tenofovir alafenamide
Not recommended: Should not be offered	All monotherapies, dual-nucleoside regimens, triple-NRTI regimens	

[a]This table provides a guide to the use of available treatment regimens for individuals with no prior or limited experience on HIV therapy. In accordance with the established goals of HIV therapy, priority is given to regimens in which clinical trial data suggest the following: sustained suppression of HIV plasma RNA (particularly in patients with high baseline viral load), sustained increase in $CD4^+$ T-cell count (in most cases >48 weeks), and favorable clinical outcome (i.e., delayed progression to AIDS and death). Additional consideration is given to the regimen's pill burden, dosing frequency, food requirements, convenience, toxicity, and drug interaction profile compared with other regimens. It is important to note that all antiretroviral agents have potentially serious toxic and adverse events associated with their use.
[b]Only for patients who are HLA-B*5701 negative.
[c]Only for patients with pretreatment estimated CrCl >70 mL/minute.
[d]Only for patients with pretreatment HIV RNA <100,000 copies/mL and CD4 count >200 cells/μL.

AIDS, acquired immunodeficiency syndrome; HIV, human immunodeficiency virus; NRTI, nucleos(t)ide analog reverse transcriptase inhibitor; NNRTI, non-nucleos(t)ide analog reverse transcriptase inhibitor; PI, protease inhibitor.

lipid profiles to the greatest extent: two prospective clinical trials have shown greater increases in triglycerides and total cholesterol among patients receiving stavudine-based HAART compared with zidovudine- or tenofovir-based regimens.[88–93] The management of HAART-associated hyperlipidemias should be handled similarly to hyperlipidemia in other patients with close attention paid to preventing drug–drug interactions.

Up to 40% to 50% of patients have been reported to experience alterations in body composition (fat loss [arms, legs, face, buttocks] and fat accumulation [dorsocervical fatty deposits or "buffalo humps"], increased abdominal girth), although the exact rate is confounded by differences in definition and assessment.[71] Risk factors for this complication include higher baseline body mass index, increased duration of exposure to antiretroviral agents, lower CD4 nadir at time of initiation of HAART, increasing age, female sex, and prolonged duration of HIV infection. The nucleoside analogs are likely responsible for lipoatrophy, whereas the PIs are believed to be responsible for lipoaccumulation,[71] although it is difficult to precisely identify which class of agents is responsible for which adverse event because they are given in combination.

The causes of lipodystrophy are unknown. It appears that there is greater propensity for lipoatrophy by those nucleoside analogs which greatly inhibit mitochondrial DNA polymerase in vitro (e.g., stavudine). Although substituting stavudine with an alternate NRTI such as zidovudine, tenofovir, or abacavir is associated with significant increases in arm and leg fat, and decreases in trunk fat (using radiographic tests such as dual-energy x-ray absorptiometry, computed tomography scans), these improvements are so modest that they may not be clinically relevant.[72,89–93] The use of recombinant human growth hormone, an agent with lipolytic effects, decreases the size of buffalo humps and abdominal girth; however, the growth often returns once growth hormone therapy is stopped.[71] Tesamorelin, a growth hormone–releasing factor given as a 2-mg once daily subcutaneous injection, was approved in 2010. It is specifically indicated for the reduction of excess abdominal fat in HIV-infected patients with lipodystrophy.[94] Surgical excision or liposuction may be effective; however, recurrences, along with adverse events (intestinal perforation, intraperitoneal bleeding), have been reported.[95] For facial wasting, injection of fat or synthetic polymers into the recessed areas of the cheeks has shown good results, but it requires frequent costly administration and lacks long-term safety data.[96]

Other important long-term complications include nucleoside-associated lactic acidosis, osteonecrosis, and osteopenia.[71] Lactic acidosis has been predominantly associated with the use of older NRTIs (stavudine, zidovudine, and didanosine) which are no longer preferred antiretrovirals but has been reported with other nucleoside analogs. This complication is managed by discontinuing therapy until lactate levels return to normal and then reinitiating therapy with a non-stavudine or non-nucleoside analog-containing HAART regimen.[3] Tenofovir alafenamide (TAF), a novel formulation of tenofovir, is associated with improved long-term bone and renal outcomes compared to tenofovir disoproxil fumarate (TDF) in patients initiating therapy. [Ref 97: Wang H et al. The efficacy and safety of tenofovir alafenamide versus tenofovir disoproxil fumarate in antiretroviral regimens for HIV-1 therapy Meta-analysis. Medicine. 2016; 95:41(e5146).] With the availability of generic tenofovir disoproxil fumarate (FDA approved in June 2017), balancing lower cost vs improved safety will be an important consideration for clinicians in selecting a tenofovir based regimen.

Promote Adherence

While the exact degree of adherence required for clinical success is currently unknown and varies by antiretroviral class, taking 90% to 95% of prescribed doses is generally believed to be necessary to prevent the development of resistance. Data from studies evaluating adherence among HIV-infected patients indicates that approximately 62% of patients take ≥90% of the prescribed doses of antiretrovirals.[98] Although it is important to note that adherence patterns vary widely based on patient-specific factors. The four most common reasons for skipping antiretroviral doses are simple forgetfulness, a change in daily routine, being too busy with other things, and being away from home.[99] Factors associated with poor adherence include (a) the number of medications (the greater the number, the greater the likelihood of poor adherence); (b) the complexity of the regimen (special meal requirements, escalating or de-escalating doses, dose frequency); (c) special storage requirements; (d) interference of medication with lifestyle and daily activities; and (e) poor communication with primary care providers and other health care professionals. Comorbid psychiatric conditions, as well as substance abuse issues, are also significant barriers to adherence in the HIV-infected population. Incorporating these factors into the selection of a patient-specific regimen may improve adherence and, subsequently, the chance for an improved clinical outcome and quality of life.

To better address the complex, multidimensional, patient-specific structures that can influence adherence behavior and retention in care, the DHHS HIV Treatment Guidelines recommend that clinics adopt a multidisciplinary team approach which provides access to trustworthy case managers, pharmacists, social workers, nurses, psychiatric care providers, etc.[3] Additionally, before selecting an HIV treatment regimen clinicians should provide adherence-related education (including information regarding why adherence is important) and involve the patient in the antiretroviral selection process. Selecting a treatment plan that the patient can (1) understand and (2) commit to for the long term is critical for fostering lifelong adherence. Thus, considering the patient's daily schedule and their ability to comply with antiretroviral specific requirements (i.e., food requirements, drug interactions, etc.) is important. For example, rilpivirine should be consumed with a full meal (ideally ≥500 kcal) and therefore may not be the best option for a patient who frequently skips meals or does not have a consistent eating schedule. Efavirenz which may cause drowsiness and is generally taken before bed on an empty stomach to mitigate this CNS effect might not be the best option for a person who works night shifts where they are on for 7 days then off for 7 days. Involving patients in the selection of their antiretroviral regimen maximizes the possibility of selecting a regimen which is least burdensome to their daily routine and helps to reduce certain barriers which lead to poor adherence. After the antiretroviral regimen has been selected and treatment initiated, quickly identifying patients who are struggling with adherence (via patient self-report, pharmacy records, pill counts, etc.); identifying their specific barriers to adherence (i.e., pill fatigue, high co-pays, forgetfulness, etc.); and employing targeted interventions to improve adherence are essential. Examples of specific strategies to improve adherence can be found in Table 13 (https://aidsinfo.nih.gov/contentfiles/lvguidelines/AA_Tables.pdf) of the 2015 DHHS HIV treatment guidelines.[3]

GOAL 4: PREVENT HUMAN IMMUNODEFICIENCY VIRUS–RELATED MORBIDITY AND MORTALITY

By successfully treating HIV (suppressing viral load and restoring immune function), patients are at decreased risk for acquiring HIV-associated opportunistic infections. By achieving goals 1 through 3, goal 4 naturally follows, and truly this is the ultimate goal of the pharmacotherapy of HIV infection. With modern-day HAART therapy, patients infected with HIV are dying more frequently from non–HIV-related conditions common in the general population (i.e., cardiovascular disease, hepatic disease, non–HIV-associated malignancies).[100] Although this represents a significant achievement in care, it also provides increased complexity in caring for those who are both at risk for HIV-related illness and also receiving treatment for comorbid conditions. This increases the potential for drug–drug and drug–disease interactions.

The selection of a patient-specific regimen can be a complex decision. Many potential combinations can be used, but a number of general principles should be followed.[3,5]

General Rules of Therapy

Initiation of therapy should occur soon after diagnosis in most patients.[3,5] Many of the current regimens reduce viral replication to less than detectable levels, and result in durable treatment responses. Reasons for the current improved response rates include the simplification of the regimens (e.g., fewer pills per day, less frequent dosing per day, use of fixed-dose combination products), improvement in overall potency of the regimens, and minimization of short-term side effects. Consequently, if the correct patient-specific HAART regimen is selected as initial therapy, the patient should be able to adhere to therapy and gain both virologic and clinical benefits from the regimen.

CASE 76-1, QUESTION 5: On questioning, E.J. admits to having an occasional drink with dinner, but he is not currently using any illicit drugs and has not in 3 years. E.J. has no known drug allergies and is currently taking only omeprazole to help with stomach acid. He is employed as a construction worker and is extremely busy during the day, so he prefers to take medications only one time daily. His complete blood count, electrolyte, and liver and renal panel all return within normal limits. His baseline genotype does not indicate any transmitted drug resistance, and he is HLA-B*5701 negative. E.J. has no particular preference for a specific regimen and appears highly motivated to take control of his disease. What factors should be considered when selecting an appropriate antiretroviral regimen?

Select the type of antiretroviral regimen. In general, PI-based or INSTI-based combination HAART are preferred (Table 76-5). Currently, no evidence definitively recommends one regimen over another, and the selection is dependent on patient-specific factors, such as comorbid disease states, concomitant medications, and pill burden.

Avoid regimens that are not virologically additive or synergistic. Lamivudine and emtricitabine should not be used together because they have similar resistance profiles, and concomitant use will not confer any additional virologic benefit.

If PI-based HAART is desired, regimens combined with a pharmacoenhancer are preferred. Ritonavir, a potent inhibitor of cytochrome P-450 metabolism and P-glycoprotein (PGP) activity, interacts significantly with a number of agents, including other PIs. This inhibition can be exploited to decrease the metabolism or increase the absorption of the other PIs. In some cases, such as in the use of lopinavir, tipranavir, and darunavir, the use of coadministered ritonavir is required for virologically relevant concentrations. The result is a regimen with more potent viral suppression. In addition, boosting allows for less frequent dosing, often lowers the total daily pill burden, and removes the need for drug/food restrictions. The pharmacoenhancer, cobicistat, can also be combined with atazanavir or darunavir (as well as the INSTI, elvitegravir) to provide a similar boosting effect as ritonavir without providing any antiviral effect. Because ritonavir and cobicistat are potent inhibitors of CYP3A4, they interact with a number of medications. Concomitant medications may require dosage adjustments, depending on the severity of the interaction.[3,5]

Avoid regimens shown to be detrimental in specific patient populations. Examples include the use of efavirenz in women of childbearing potential who are not using reliable methods of birth control or who are in the first 8 weeks of pregnancy. Efavirenz is pregnancy category D because of an association with teratogenic effects in animals. Nevirapine has the potential for hepatotoxicity in patients with higher baseline CD4 cell counts (>250 cells/μL for women, >400 cells/μL for men).

Case 76-1, Question 6: What initial antiretroviral regimen should E.J. receive?

When selecting a patient-specific regimen, the following steps should be followed.

STEP 1: DETERMINE WHICH ANTIRETROVIRAL CLASS WILL BE USED

A careful review of the advantages and disadvantages of each regimen should occur (Table 76-5). For example, protease inhibitors may be less favored with a current medical condition consisting of coronary artery disease, hyperlipidemia, or diabetes mellitus because of their potential metabolic side effects.[3,71]

After discussions with E.J., it appears that he is highly motivated to take control of his disease and is willing to initiate therapy. Subsequently, the use of a combination regimen with either a PI-based or INSTI-based regimen is appropriate. Potential initial treatment options are listed in Table 76-4.

STEP 2: OPTIMIZE AGENTS IN THE REGIMEN

The next step requires the selection of agents for the regimen. In many situations, absolute contraindications and significant drug–drug interactions limit the agents available for use in the regimen. The nucleoside or nucleotide reverse transcriptase inhibitors, including lamivudine, tenofovir disoproxil fumarate or tenofovir alafenamide, emtricitabine, and abacavir, are all potential options for E.J. With respect to drug interactions, a PI or INSTI can be administered safely with omeprazole.

STEP 3: QUALITY-OF-LIFE CONSIDERATIONS

When selecting a regimen, assessment of quality-of-life issues, potential adverse drug events, and patient preference should receive as much consideration as drug–drug interactions and absolute contraindications. In some situations, these issues could mean the difference between a regimen that is effective and one that is not. Considering E.J.'s lifestyle and work requirements, it is best to select a regimen that will minimally interfere with his daily activities. The selection of a regimen with once-daily or twice-daily dosing is appropriate (Table 76-3), although once-daily dosing might be preferred. Potential regimens include the PI-based regimen, darunavir boosted with ritonavir plus emtricitabine/tenofovir disoproxil fumarate or emtricitabine/tenofovir alafenamide all once daily, or an INSTI-based regimen such as raltegravir twice daily with emtricitabine/tenofovir disoproxil fumarate or emtricitabine/tenofovir alafenamide once daily, elvitegravir/cobicistat/emtricitabine/tenofovir or elvitegravir/cobicistat/emtricitabine/tenofovir alafenamide as a combination tablet once daily, dolutegravir plus emtricitabine/tenofovir disoproxil fumarate or emtricitabine/

Table 76-5
Advantages and Disadvantages of Antiretroviral Components for Initial Antiretroviral Therapy

ARV[a] Class	Possible Advantages	Possible Disadvantages
Dual NRTI	■ Established backbone of combination antiretroviral therapy ■ Less fat maldistribution and dyslipidemia than PI-based regimens	■ Rare but serious cases of lactic acidosis with hepatic steatosis reported (d4T > ddI = ZDV > TDF or TAF = ABC = 3TC = FTC) ■ Low genetic barrier to resistance (single mutation confers resistance)
NNRTI	■ Long half-lives ■ Single tablet regimens available with EFV and RPV	■ Low genetic barrier to resistance ■ Cross resistance among first-generation NNRTIs ■ Skin rash ■ Potential for cytochrome P-450 drug interactions ■ Transmitted resistance to NNRTIs more common than with PIs and INSTIs
PI	■ Higher genetic barrier to resistance ■ PI resistance uncommon with failure (boosted PIs) ■ More forgiving to intermittent adherence	■ Metabolic complications (fat maldistribution, dyslipidemia, insulin resistance) ■ Cytochrome P-450 substrates, inhibitors, and inducers (potential for drug interactions)
INSTI	■ Well tolerated ■ Single tablet regimens available with EVG and DTG ■ Fewer drug–drug interactions with RAL and DTG than PI- or NNRTI-based regimens ■ Achieve rapid viral load suppression	■ Less long-term experience than with boosted PI-based regimens ■ Lower genetic barrier to resistance than boosted PI-based regimens

[a]Adapted from DHHS treatment guidelines July 2016. See full guidelines for discussion of the advantages and disadvantages of each individual ARV agent.

ABC, abacavir; ARV, antiretroviral; DHHS, Department of Health and Human Services; DTG, dolutegravir; EVG, elvitegravir; FTC, emtricitabine; NNRTI, non-nucleoside reverse transcriptase inhibitors; NRTI, nucleoside reverse transcriptase inhibitor; PI, protease inhibitor; INSTI, integrase strand transfer inhibitor; RAL, raltegravir; TAF, tenofovir alafenamide; TDF, tenofovir disoproxil fumarate; 3TC, lamivudine.

 tenofovir alafenamide all once daily, or dolutegravir/abacavir/lamivudine as a combination tablet once daily.

CASE 76-1, QUESTION 7: E.J. is starting emtricitabine, tenofovir, disoproxil fumarate, elvitegravir, and cobicistat (coformulated for once-daily dosing as Stribild). How should therapy be monitored? Are any additional laboratory tests necessary? What adherence support should be provided?

Short-Term Assessments

Three important criteria determine whether an antiretroviral regimen is effective: clinical assessment, surrogate marker responses, and regimen tolerability, including a patient's ability to adhere to the regimen.[3,5] In patients who are clinically symptomatic (e.g., constitutional symptoms such as fatigue, night sweats, and weight loss; new opportunistic infections), the initiation of an appropriate antiretroviral regimen often results in resolution of symptoms, increased strength and energy, and improvement in overall well-being. In some patients, however, the effect may not be as prominent. A careful assessment of clinical symptoms should therefore be regularly performed at all follow-up appointments.

In all patients, repeat viral load and T-cell measurements are necessary. This early value allows clinicians to assess the magnitude of response and ensures declining viral load measurements. Therapy with an effective regimen will result in at least a threefold (0.5 log) and tenfold decrease (1.0 log) in viral load counts by weeks 4 and 8, respectively.[3,5] The viral load should continue to decline during the next 12 to 16 weeks and, in most patients, it will become undetectable.[3,5] Long-term response to therapy correlates with the magnitude of viral suppression on initiation of a regimen. The greater the suppression, the greater the durability of response to that regimen.[101] The speed and magnitude of suppression, however, can be affected by a number of factors, including clinical status of the patient (e.g., more advanced disease–low T-cell counts, high viral load value), adherence to therapy, and overall potency of the regimen.[3,5]

In response to declining viral replication, T-cell destruction slows, and eventually cellular repopulation occurs. The magnitude of this T-cell increase can vary significantly, with some patients experiencing large increases (≥500 cells/μL) and others experiencing little or no change. Given that T-cell changes do not occur rapidly, once therapy is initiated, repeat T-cell counts should be obtained at 3-month to 4-month intervals.[3,5]

A seemingly worsening of symptoms may also occur after the initiation of potent antiretroviral therapies because of immune reconstitution.[102–104] In patients with advanced HIV disease (i.e., CD4 <100 cells/μL), significant immune dysfunction results in an inability to mount an appropriate response to subclinical infections. As a result, these infections replicate unimpeded and often undetected by the host (also known as quiescent disease). During the first 12 weeks of therapy, an increased immune response results from redistribution of memory cells,[105–107] and inflammation occurs at the site of infection. The immune reconstitution inflammatory syndrome can present in any organ system where quiescent disease exists (e.g., CNS, eyes, lymph nodes). Most cases occur within 1 to 4 weeks after the initiation of potent antiretroviral therapies.[3]

A patient's tolerability of the regimen, which includes involvement in the decision of what therapy to initiate, ease of administration, and avoidance of intolerable side effects, is vital to a patient's willingness and ability to adhere to an antiretroviral regimen. If the patient is not adherent, they are at risk for clinical failure and the development of resistance. Adherence should be evaluated at every clinic visit and the type and reason for identified non-adherence should be assessed. If adherence is not a present concern, then positive reinforcement and encouragement are recommended.[3]

CASE 76-1, QUESTION 8: After initiation of therapy, E.J.'s viral load values are 7,000 copies/mL at 4 weeks and less than 50 copies/mL (undetectable) at 14 weeks. His T-cell counts have increased from 225 to 525 cells/μL. In addition, E.J. states that his night sweats and fevers have disappeared, he "feels great," and that he has had no drug-related problems. Is the therapy effective? How should therapy be monitored?

E.J.'s response to elvitegravir/cobicistat/emtricitabine/tenofovir disoproxil fumarate does indicate efficacy. Clinically, his symptoms have subsided and his overall health is much improved. His viral load measurements have responded appropriately and are now less than the level of assay detection. T-cell counts have increased by 300 cells/μL. Finally, E.J. has experienced no drug-related adverse events. Given the response to date, no changes are required and the current regimen should be continued.

Long-Term Assessments

Once the prescribed regimen has been stabilized, the long-term goals are to maintain maximal viral suppression, sustain clinical and immunologic improvements, and maintain drug tolerability. Periodic assessments should be made of viral load and T-cell counts (every 3–6 months).[3,5] These surrogate marker data allow clinicians to monitor trends in viral activity and immunologic status and assist them in identifying early regimen failure. Clinical assessment of the patient questioning of tolerability and adherence to the prescribed regimen should occur at the 3- to 6-month follow-up visits.

Treatment Failure

CASE 76-1, QUESTION 9: E.J. has remained on elvitegravir/cobicistat/emtricitabine/tenofovir disoproxil fumarate for more than a year. To date, his T-cell counts have remained stable at 550 cells/μL, and his viral load measurements have remained less than the limit of assay detection. He presents with new complaints of fevers and malaise. E.J. reports that he has been compliant with therapy and has not started any new medications. Repeat laboratory tests now show E.J.'s viral load is 3,000 copies/mL and his T-cell count is 375 cells/μL (both repeated and validated). Should E.J.'s regimen be changed?

Assessment of regimen failure should be based on (a) clinical symptoms, (b) surrogate marker data, and (c) regimen tolerability and adherence.[3–5]

In some patients, the first sign of failure is a change in signs and symptoms. These changes can be subtle (e.g., increase in constitutional symptoms, new onset of oral thrush) or more severe (e.g., new opportunistic infections) and suggest a failing regimen and need to change therapy.

Assessment of efficacy should also involve evaluation of surrogate marker data (e.g., T cells and viral load). In many situations, changes to these markers occur before any noticeable clinical signs and symptoms. Therefore, careful evaluation of surrogate marker data may allow for intervention before any significant immune destruction occurs. Virologic failure, defined as new or continued viral replication despite appropriate antiretroviral therapy, suggests a failing regimen. For example, patients with repeated detection of virus in plasma after initial suppression to undetectable levels should be evaluated as potential treatment failures. In patients who do not achieve viral suppression to less than detectable levels, a significant increase in viral replication should also be viewed as a treatment failure.[3,4]

When assessing viral load, it is important to recognize that these values can increase from vaccinations or other concurrent

Table 76-6
Metabolism and Drug–Drug Interaction Potential of Antiretroviral Classes

Class	General Metabolism and Drug–Drug Interaction Considerations	Exceptions
NRTIs	Renally eliminated, few drug–drug interactions	ABC is metabolized by alcohol dehydrogenase and competes with alcohol for metabolism
NNRTIs	CYP3A4 substrates CYP3A4 inducers	RPV is a CYP3A4 substrate only ETR also a CYP2C9, CYP2C19 substrate/inhibitor
PIs	CYP3A4 & PGP substrates CYP3A4 inhibitors	RTV is also a CYP2D6 substrate/inhibitor ATV also inhibits UGT1A1 TPV is also a CYP2D6 inhibitor and PGP inducer
INSTI	UGT1A1	EVG is a CYP3A4 substrate, given with COBI a potent CYP3A4 inhibitor DTG is also a UGT1A3 and PGP substrate
CCR5	CYP3A4 substrate	

ABC, abacavir; CCR5, chemokine co-receptor 5; COBI, cobicistat; DTG, dolutegravir; EVG, elvitegravir; ETR, etravirine; INSTI, integrase strand transfer inhibitor; NRTI, nucleos(t)ide reverse transcriptase inhibitor; NNRTI, non-nucleoside reverse transcriptase inhibitor; PI, protease inhibitor; PGP, P-glycoprotein; RPV, rilpivirine; RTV, ritonavir; TPV, tipranavir.

infections (see Case 76-1, Question 2). Therefore, a thorough medical history should be taken to rule out other causes of increasing viral load. In addition, laboratory values should be interpreted as trends over time and not necessarily as individual measurements. A repeat viral load should be performed and evaluated within 4 weeks of the initial viral load increase. In some cases, transient viral "blips" occur (increases in viral load measurements just above the level of assay detection (e.g., 50–1,000 copies/mL), which become undetectable at the next visit.[107,108] The clinical significance of viral blips is unknown and, although they may not directly reflect treatment failure, they may represent near future viral breakthrough because of either patient non-adherence or insufficient antiretroviral potency.[109,110] Careful follow-up of these patients is required, because changes to the current HAART regimen may be necessary.

In response to increasing viral replication, T-cell destruction occurs. Persistently declining T-cell counts, with or without increasing viral load measurements, represent treatment failure and suggest a change in therapy is warranted.

Other potential causes for failure include non-adherence and drug–drug interactions. In the event of non-adherence, discussions regarding tolerability, number of doses missed, duration of non-adherence, and lifestyle changes should take place. The decision to reinitiate a prescribed regimen should take into account the future likelihood of adherence and the potential development of resistant strains. In those patients with a history of long-standing non-adherence, the success of reinitiating the prescribed regimen may be limited. Stopping all antiretrovirals at once poses less risk for the development of resistance than intermittent adherence to some or all of a regimen. The precise effect of the duration and extent of non-adherence on the development of resistance cannot be fully anticipated and is dependent on the barrier to resistance of the patient's ART. For the virus to mutate, sufficient drug pressure must be placed on the virus.

Significant drug interactions could also contribute to reduction in oral bioavailability or increased metabolism of the HIV medications leading to low serum concentrations, resulting in failure.[3] In addition, many medications require certain food requirements to allow maximal drug absorption. A careful review of all new medications and their potential for clinically significant drug interactions should be evaluated at all visits (Table 76-6).

Currently, E.J. has a number of signs and symptoms that suggest a failing regimen. E.J. is experiencing new symptoms of fevers and malaise not attributable to any other cause. E.J.'s viral load value has become detectable at 3,000 copies/mL without evidence of concurrent infections or vaccinations in the past 4 weeks. E.J.'s T-cell counts have declined from 550 to 375 cells/μL. Finally, it appears that E.J. has been adhering to his therapy and has not started any new medications that could affect the efficacy of his current regimen. Therefore, a change in therapy is necessary.

CASE 76-1, QUESTION 10: What potential antiretroviral regimen(s) can be considered for E.J.?

In addition to the general rules of therapy described in Case 76-1, Question 5, other issues should be considered when selecting an alternative regimen for a patient failing therapy.[3,4]

GENERAL RULES FOR CHANGING THERAPIES

1. If possible, the new regimen should contain at least two, preferably three fully active agents. The potential for cross-resistance between antiretroviral drugs should be considered when choosing new regimens, and therefore resistance testing should provide useful information (see Case 76-2, Question 2).
2. Given that antiretroviral drug resistance is more likely to occur with increased and prolonged viral replication in the presence of antiretroviral agents, changes to therapy should occur close to the time of treatment failure. Prolonged treatment with a failing regimen is likely to result in the accumulation of resistance mutations (particularly with protease inhibitors), which may limit future treatment options.
3. Resistance testing is recommended to guide the selection of future drug regimens. Optimally, testing via genotype, phenotype, or virtual phenotype should occur while the patient is taking the failing regimen, or within 4 weeks of discontinuation to increase the likelihood of detecting resistant isolates. These tests cannot reliably detect mutations at viral concentrations less than 1,000 copies/mL and may have limited usefulness in patients with persistent low-level viremia.
4. To prevent the development of resistance, one new drug should never be added to a failing regimen. An exception to this rule is if the initial response to a first regimen has been inadequate (e.g., undetectable viral load at 16–20 weeks). In this situation, some clinicians may intensify therapy with an additional agent provided that the viral load measurements were trending downward since initiation of therapy.
5. If possible, a regimen that has failed in the past should not be reinitiated, because an isolate resistant to the failed regimen could continue to reside within various compartments of the

body. If a regimen to which the patient had previously failed were restarted, unimpeded viral replication of the resistant strain would occur, repopulate the host, and eventually result in treatment failure. In some situations (e.g., patients with advanced disease, limited treatment options, and prior exposure to most antiretroviral agents), it may be necessary to reinitiate agents or regimens in combination with additional new agents with the goal of suppressing viral replication.

6. When treatment failure is a direct result of drug toxicity (rather than poor drug efficacy), the offending agent should be replaced with an alternative drug from a similar class, provided that the potential for cross-resistance is minimal.
7. If an agent in a given regimen must be stopped, it is recommended that all agents in the regimen be stopped and restarted simultaneously to prevent the development of resistance. An exception to this rule is when components of a regimen have differing half-lives, such as NNRTIs and NRTIs. In this situation, if all drugs are discontinued simultaneously, continued monotherapy exposure with the NNRTI is likely to result, because of the much longer NNRTI half-life. Consequently, some experts recommend continuing the NRTIs for 1 to 2 weeks past NNRTI discontinuation to provide combination therapy while the NNRTI is eliminated from the body (covering the "tail" of the pharmacokinetic profile).

It should be recognized that many alternative regimens are based on theoretical benefits or limited data. In addition, many potential options could be limited in some patients based on prior antiretroviral use, toxicity, or past intolerances. Therefore, the clinician should carefully discuss these issues with the patient before changing therapy.

Because E.J. is failing to respond to his current regimen, a new antiretroviral regimen must be chosen. In addition to selecting susceptible agents from resistance testing, the new regimen should take into consideration quality-of-life issues. In E.J.'s situation, it is reasonable to switch to a ritonavir-boosted PI regimen, with two or more nucleoside agents as dictated by the viral resistance profile.

Considerations in Antiretroviral-Experienced Patients

CASE 76-2

QUESTION 1: H.G. is a 56-year-old, HIV-positive man with an extensive history of treatment with a variety of antiretroviral agents. He took zidovudine monotherapy in the late 1980s and early 1990s. When lamivudine became available, he took the combination of zidovudine and lamivudine until he failed therapy about 20 years ago. At that time, he began experiencing zidovudine-induced myopathies. Since that time, H.G. has been "on and off" various regimens without sustained clinical benefit. He is currently taking emtricitabine/tenofovir disoproxil fumarate and atazanavir/ritonavir with a CD4 count and viral load measurement of 55 cells/μL and 48,000 copies/mL, respectively. These laboratory values have been stable for the last 9 months. How do patients with extensive antiretroviral histories differ from antiretroviral-naïve patients? Are there any special considerations when selecting therapeutic regimens for patients such as H.G.?

Patients who have been infected for 20 or more years may have been treated with many different regimens, both experimental and FDA approved. As a result, many potential regimens have already been exhausted; thus, there are fewer viable choices left. Agents with higher barriers to resistance that do not have cross resistance with older agents and agents with novel mechanisms of action are useful in these patients. Although, now a preferred agent in treatment naïve patients, darunavir was specifically marketed for highly treatment-experienced patients because of its high genetic barrier to resistance and limited cross resistance with other PIs.[3,4] The second-generation NNRTIs, etravirine and rilpivirine, have minimal cross resistance with the first-generation NNRTIs, efavirenz and nevirapine.[3,4] Maraviroc, the first CCR5 receptor antagonist approved by the FDA, is also an option for treatment-experienced patients infected with HIV-1 utilizing this co-receptor and failing current treatment. Maraviroc is not recommended for use in patients with dual-trophic viral populations (i.e., able to use CXCR-4 or CCR5 as co-receptors) or CXCR-4-trophic virus and, thus, patients with extensive treatment histories should undergo tropism testing before maraviroc is initiated. Additionally, INSTIs are newer agents with a novel mechanism of action that allow for use in patients with extensive reverse transcriptase or protease mutations. Some highly treatment-experienced individuals will have extensive resistance patterns that limit their therapeutic options. In such patients, full suppression of viral load and immune reconstitution may not be possible.[3,4]

Patients who have experienced several antiretroviral regimens present other unique challenges for clinicians and require consideration of the following factors.

1. *Regimen tolerability*: Patients with advanced HIV disease display decreased tolerability to many medications, including antiretroviral agents. Although this is not fully understood, it is probably a result of HIV-induced immune alterations and cytokine dysregulations. Subsequently, clinicians evaluating patients with advanced disease should be alert for possible drug-induced adverse events.
2. *Drug interactions*: Many patients with advanced disease take numerous medications for primary or secondary prophylaxis of various opportunistic infections, as well as other medications for comorbid disease states. Subsequently, the risk for a drug–drug interaction is increased. The addition of any new medication, either prescription or over-the-counter, should be carefully evaluated for potential interactions with the patient's current antiretroviral regimen (see Table 76-6). In addition, any change to the current antiretroviral regimen should also be checked against the patient's current medication list.
3. *Altered bioavailability*: Patients with advanced HIV infection may have unreliable absorption of many medications because of severe diarrhea, anorexia, weight loss, wasting, and gastric achlorhydria. As a result, the bioavailability of some agents, especially certain PIs that require specific dietary requirements, may be affected (Table 76-3). Any changes in dietary habits or bowel function should be carefully assessed in light of the potential impact on the antiretroviral regimen.
4. *Antiretroviral drug histories and resistance testing*: The most useful information to guide the choice of alternative regimens is a detailed drug history, in conjunction with appropriate resistance testing. Among patients with extensive prior antiretroviral use, it is critical to identify previously failed regimens and determine the precise cause of the failures. In an experienced patient who has taken many different regimens over a lifetime, the number of remaining viable agents and regimens may be limited. Therefore, it is important to determine whether prior regimens truly failed for virologic reasons or some other cause (e.g., regimen intolerability or an inadequate trial period). In addition, detailed knowledge of regimen intolerabilities and which agent(s) caused the adverse event will help in the selection of a new appropriate regimen. In some situations, the offending agent may be reinitiated if the adverse event was minimal or can be appropriately managed.

RESISTANCE, VIRAL GENOTYPING, PHENOTYPING, AND VIRAL FITNESS

CASE 76-2, QUESTION 2: Will viral genotyping and phenotyping assist in selecting an appropriate therapeutic regimen for H.G.? What are these tests? What are their limitations and when should they be used? What is viral fitness, and does it have a role in clinical decision making?

Viral genotyping and phenotyping reveal resistance patterns to antiretroviral agents. Genotyping evaluates mutations in the virus's genetic material, whereas phenotyping assesses the ability of the virus to grow in the presence of increasing concentrations of antiretroviral agents. The three potential causes for the development of resistance are as follows.

1. Initial infection with a resistant isolate[111–113]
2. Natural selection of a resistant isolate as a consequence of inefficient, error-susceptible viral replication[35]
3. Generation of resistant isolates via selective pressures from antiretroviral therapies that do not fully suppress viral replication[3,4]

Mutations are generated when naturally occurring amino acids in the HIV genome are replaced with alternative amino acids. For example, resistance to 3TC occurs when the amino acid methionine (M) is replaced by valine (V) at the 184th amino acid in the protein chain.[114,115] This mutation is subsequently referred to as an M184V mutation. These amino acid substitutions change the proteins that are produced and may alter the shape, size, or charge of the viral enzyme's substrate or primer.[115] Subsequently, antiretroviral drug binding to the active site is decreased, affinity for natural substrates is increased, or there is an increased removal of the antiretroviral agent from the enzyme by the virus (known as pyrophosphorylation).[113] Whether a mutation results in a clinically resistant, less viable, or indifferent isolate depends on which amino acid(s) is replaced. In addition, certain mutations or combination of mutations have been shown to produce viral isolates that display increased sensitivity to various antiretroviral agents (known as hypersusceptibility). Alterations to certain key amino acids can also result in cross-resistance between various antiretrovirals.[4,114]

Key enzymes have been extensively studied with regard to their potential for development of resistance: reverse transcriptase (RT), protease, and more recently, integrase. Replication by the RT enzyme is highly susceptible to errors. Given that the HIV genome is approximately 10,000 nucleotides in length and that mutations via the RT enzyme occur approximately once in every 10,000 nucleotides copied, it has been estimated that a mutation occurs with every viral replication cycle. With up to 10 billion particles of virus being produced per day, the potential exists for 1,000 to 10,000 mutations occurring at each site in the HIV genome every day.[35] Key mutations to the antiretroviral agents are updated periodically by expert panels of clinicians.[4]

Over time, countless viral subpopulations known as "quasi-species" develop. In any given host, at any given time, many different quasi-species can exist. In addition, within any compartment of the body (e.g., CNS, testes, lymph nodes), many different quasi-species can also exist. Because these mutant strains represent only a small number of isolates in the total viral population, they must have some replicative disadvantage when compared with the "wild-type" virus.[114] Under selective pressures from antiretroviral therapies, however, these mutant isolates can replicate. For example, if wild-type viral replication is inhibited by an antiretroviral regimen, and if any one viral strain of the quasi-species is more fit for growth in the presence of that regimen, then the viral mutant will have a competitive advantage.[114] It should be recognized that for resistance to develop, viral replication must occur. When viral replication is completely inhibited, the development of resistant isolates is unlikely.

Genotypic analysis involves sequencing the viral genetic material via PCR amplification. Mutations are identified by analysis of key sequences of the RT or protease enzymes. These tests can be rapidly processed; however, they detect mutations present only in more than 25% of all HIV isolates in the body and can only reliably detect resistance patterns in samples with HIV RNA greater than 1,000 copies/mL. Because pressures from antiretroviral therapies select resistant isolates, these tests may not provide information regarding rare, yet potentially clinically significant, isolates.[3,4]

Phenotypic analysis involves growing virus in the presence of various concentrations of drug and then determining viral susceptibilities (e.g., half-maximal inhibitory concentration [IC_{50}]). Phenotyping is limited because it evaluates only one viral isolate at a time and could fail to identify other clinically relevant isolates.[3]

One other measure available to clinicians is "viral fitness" or "replication capacity." The genetic changes that occur in a virus to become resistant to antiretroviral therapy often impair the virus' ability to replicate.[116,117] This measure is called "fitness" and is quantified as replication capacity during phenotypic evaluation. During amplification of the virus before the phenotype is measured, the replication capacity of the virus is evaluated and compared to a reference wild-type, drug-sensitive virus. A virus with normal fitness has a replication capacity between 70% and 120% of the reference viral strain; isolates with values less than 70% are considered to be less fit than wild-type virus. In general, the more mutations that occur to the virus, the more compromised the virus becomes, and the lower the fitness (although, in some situations, the interplay between mutations can result in a viral isolate that is relatively fit). Recent data have shown that, despite persistent viral replication, unfit viruses may not cause the same degree of immune destruction as fit viruses.[115] This finding is important for patients with limited treatment options because it may allow for continuation of a HAART regimen that is not completely suppressive, but that produces an unfit virus, with less T-cell depletion.

As with all clinical decisions made for those who are HIV infected, careful assessment of the results in combination with the treatment history are essential for proper clinical decision making. Consultation with an expert in antiretroviral drug resistance patterns is highly recommended.

Given H.G.'s extensive antiretroviral drug history and his current failure, a genotype or phenotype will likely provide some insights into potential therapeutic options.

SPECIAL CIRCUMSTANCES

Poor CD4 Cell Recovery

CASE 76-2, QUESTION 3: H.G. was started on a regimen of tenofovir alafenamide, emtricitabine, dolutegravir, and darunavir boosted with ritonavir. During the following 6 months, H.G.'s T-cell counts increased to 325 cells/μL and his viral load value declined to 5,000 copies/mL. At the last two clinic visits, H.G.'s viral load (copies/mL) and CD4 counts (cells/μL) were 2,000/275 and less than 20/225, respectively. H.G. reports no new clinical complaints or adverse drug events. In addition, H.G. states that he has been compliant with therapy. Are changes to therapy necessary?

In most cases, declines in viral load result in increases in CD4 cell counts; however, in some cases, CD4 cells fail to recover with viral load suppression.[5] In this situation, it may be wise to continue current treatment and monitor the patient closely. Adding an additional drug to intensify the regimen or changing to a different ART regimen does not consistently increase the CD4 cell count and is not recommended.[3]

Therapeutic Drug Monitoring

Pharmacokinetic evaluations of various antiretrovirals have shown interpatient variability in drug exposures among cohorts of patients taking the same dose of drug under the same conditions.[3,117–120] Many factors contribute to interpatient variability in drug exposure, such as pharmacogenetics, environment, different physiologic conditions, regimen adherence, and drug interactions. For most antiretrovirals, a drug exposure–response relationship exists (e.g., the higher the exposure, the faster and more prolonged the viral suppression). In addition, most antiretrovirals also have well-defined exposure–toxicity relationships.

Therapeutic drug monitoring (TDM) is currently recommended for selected clinical situations.[3,119] For patients with uncharacterized drug interactions and those with impairments in gastrointestinal, hepatic, or renal function, drug concentrations may help identify low or high exposure that can be corrected with a dosage adjustment. TDM may also be useful for assuring that a novel antiretroviral combination or dose does not have any unpredictable adverse drug interactions. In treatment-experienced patients, knowledge of drug exposure with viral susceptibility may assist in designing an optimal dosage regimen. Conversely, patients experiencing toxicities thought to be concentration-dependent (e.g., neuropsychiatric effects of efavirenz) may benefit from TDM. Monitoring adherence and evaluating pharmacokinetics in special populations, such as pregnant women or pediatric patients, are additional indications for TDM.

Pharmacology experts currently recommend obtaining trough concentrations immediately before the next antiretroviral dose. For efavirenz (which is usually taken in the evening), samples obtained 12 hours post-dose will closely reflect the concentration at 24 hours post-dose because of its long half-life. Many factors can affect the trough values of various antiretroviral agents. For proper interpretation of the concentrations, patients should provide a dosing history from the last several days, a list of concomitantly administered drugs to screen for interactions, and the exact time the last dose was taken. The exact time the TDM sample was collected should also be recorded. Another factor that can affect interpretation of drug concentrations over time is intrapatient variability. Outside of a clinical study, where patients take their medications under conditions that vary from day to day, the concentrations could be highly variable at clinic visits over time, and several samples might be required to determine trends in the drug exposure before making a dose adjustment. Finally, to minimize laboratory variability and error in measuring these concentrations, it is also recommended that a laboratory that routinely measures antiretrovirals and participates in both internal and external quality control programs be used. A list of such laboratories can be obtained from the Clinical Pharmacology Quality Assurance and Quality Control Program (**https://www.fstrf.org/apps/cfmx/apps/cpqa/cpqaDocs/public/index.html**).

Drug Interactions

CASE 76-3

QUESTION 1: J.F. is a 37-year-old HIV positive man who has been taking emtricitabine, tenofovir disoproxil fumarate, and darunavir boosted with ritonavir for the past 4 years. His most recent lipid panel showed markedly elevated triglycerides, LDL, and total cholesterol. What needs to be considered when starting a lipid lowering medication for J.F.?

Drug interactions are very common with antiretrovirals and need to be considered when changing HIV-related or non-related drug regimens. In this case, ritonavir will significantly increase the concentrations of HMG-CoA reductase inhibitors that are metabolized by CYP3A4 through inhibition of the CYP3A4 isoenzyme.[3] If increased concentrations of the HMG-CoA reductase inhibitor could put J.F. at risk for myalgia and rhabdomyolysis. J.F.'s lipids require treatment with an HMG-CoA reductase inhibitor, one that is only partially metabolized by CYP3A4 or metabolized by another pathway should be considered. Simvastatin and lovastatin are contraindicated in combination with ritonavir, but pravastatin, pitavastatin, rosuvastatin, and atorvastatin can be used at reduced doses.[3] The DHHS HIV adult treatment guidelines have extensive tables outlining specific drug interactions and recommendations for concomitant use of medications with the antiretrovirals.[3] Table 76-6 gives the general metabolism and transport effects of each of the classes of antiretrovirals and gives an idea of the drug interaction potential of each class.

Pregnancy and Breast-Feeding

CASE 76-4

QUESTION 1: T.D. is a 32-year-old woman infected with HIV, whose antiretroviral therapy includes the combination tablet dolutegravir/abacavir/lamivudine once daily. Her virus is fully suppressed and her CD4 cells count is 786/μL. She has had a positive home pregnancy test result. Is her current antiretroviral regimen appropriate for use during pregnancy and for prevention of mother-to-child transmission?

The current perinatal HIV guidelines[121] recommend that women receiving and tolerating a currently suppressive regimen when they become pregnant continue on that regimen. The guidelines state that "In general, the same regimens as recommended for treatment of non-pregnant adults should be used in pregnant women unless there are known adverse effects for women, fetuses, or infants that outweigh benefits." Efavirenz is the only antiretroviral that is currently pregnancy category D and is not recommended during the first 8 weeks of pregnancy. It has been shown to be teratogenic in animal studies, particularly in the first trimester of pregnancy, and retrospective case reports of neural tube defects in humans have been documented.[122–125] Perinatal transmission prevention guidelines recommend abacavir/lamivudine, emtricitabine/tenofovir disoproxil fumarate or lamivudine with tenofovir disoproxil fumarate as first-line NRTIs for HAART initiation in pregnancy. Atazanavir/ritonavir and daruanvir/ritonavir are the recommended PIs for initiation in pregnancy, and raltegravir is the first integrase inhibitor to be considered preferred for initiation in pregnancy. Alternative agents for initiation in pregnancy include zidovudine/lamivudine, lopinavir/ritonavir, efavirenz as long as it is initiated after 8 weeks of pregnancy, and rilpivirine.[120] Many of the pregnancy recommendations are based on those drugs which have the most safety and efficacy data available during pregnancy (both animal and human).[122]

In women who have a viral load persistently greater than 1,000 copies/mL, it is recommended that a planned 38-week cesarean section be performed to reduce the risk of mother-to-child transmission. In women with a viral load less than 1,000 copies/mL, there is little evidence to show that cesarean section decreases transmission rates compared to vaginal delivery. In this case, the decision is made at the discretion of the physician in consultation with the mother. Additionally, if the mother's viral load is >1,000 copies/mL or unknown at the time of delivery, it is recommended that intravenous zidovudine be administered to the mother at 2 mg/kg intravenously (IV) for 1 hour at the onset of labor, then given as a continuous infusion of 1 mg/kg/hour during the intrapartum period (during labor and postpartum). Once delivered, it is recommended that oral zidovudine at 2 mg/kg every 6 hours be started in all HIV-exposed infants immediately after birth and continued for 6 weeks. It is recommended that the infant undergo diagnostic virologic testing using either HIV DNA PCR or RNA virologic assays at a minimum at ages 14 to 21 days, 1 to 2 months, and 4 to 6 months. Antibody testing should not be performed on the infant because maternal HIV antibody crosses the placenta and will be detectable in all HIV-exposed infants up to 18 months of age.[122]

It is not recommended that HIV-positive women breast-feed their children in resource-rich settings where clean water and formula are reasonably available. The risk of transmission from breast-feeding is consistently higher than formula feeding even with the use of antiretroviral prophylaxis.[122,126]

Since J.F. is on a fully suppressive ARV regimen that she is tolerating, the guidelines recommend that she continue on her current regimen. If she continues to remain undetectable throughout her pregnancy, the decision whether to have a cesarean or a vaginal delivery will be at the discretion of J.F. and her physician.

Pre-Exposure Prophylaxis

CASE 76-5

QUESTION 1: F.C is a 22-year-old, HIV negative, healthy male with multiple male sex partners. He reports using condoms most of the time, but would like additional protection against the acquisition of HIV. What prevention methods can be offered to F.C.?

Pre-exposure prophylaxis (PrEP) is the use of antiretrovirals in HIV-uninfected individuals to prevent HIV infection. The fixed dose combination of emtricitabine 200 mg / tenofovir disoproxil fumarate 300 mg has been FDA approved for use as PrEP in HIV-uninfected individuals at high risk of HIV infection.[127] The Clinical Practice Guidelines for Preexposure Prophylaxis for HIV Prevention in the United States recommend PrEP as one prevention option for sexually active adult men who have sex with men, adult heterosexually active men and women, and adult injection drug users at substantial risk of HIV acquisition.[128] Additionally, the guidelines recommended that PrEP be discussed with HIV-uninfected heterosexual women and men whose partners are HIV infected as one of several options to protect the uninfected partner during conception and pregnancy. HIV testing should be done immediately before emtricitabine/tenofovir disoproxil fumarate is prescribed for PrEP and every 3 months while on emtricitabine/tenofovir disoproxil fumarate. If a patient is found to be HIV infected, emtricitabine/tenofovir disoproxil fumarate should immediately be stopped to avoid the development of resistance to emtricitabine and tenofovir. PrEP should always be provided in conjunction with behavioral risk reduction support and medication adherence counseling. In addition to regular HIV testing and risk reduction counseling, renal function testing should be performed at baseline, 3 months, and then every 6 months thereafter and sexually transmitted infections (STIs) should be screened for at baseline and every 6 months.[128]

Emtricitabine/tenofovir disoproxil fumarate one tablet daily can be considered for F.C. for the prevention of HIV. He will need to have baseline HIV, STI, and renal function testing as well as medication adherence and behavioral risk reduction counseling. He will need to follow up 3 months after emtricitabine/tenofovir disoproxil fumarate if prescribed for monitoring and repeat HIV testing.

Postexposure Prophylaxis

CASE 76-6

QUESTION 1: L.T. is a 47-year-old nurse at an HIV clinic. While drawing routine labs on a newly diagnosed HIV+ male patient, not yet started on HAART, she accidently stuck herself with a contaminated needle. Are interventions available to prevent L.T. from contracting HIV from the needlestick? What drugs should be utilized, and for how long?

Postexposure prophylaxis (PEP) is the use of ARVs to prevent HIV infection in individuals who have had an exposure to blood or body fluid either known to be infected with HIV or potentially infected with HIV. Occupational exposures require immediate evaluation with a first dose of ARVs offered within the first 2 hours following exposure.[129,130] PEP is more effective the earlier it can be initiated, and it should always be started within 72 hours of exposure. Percutaneous exposure poses more of a concern than mucous membrane exposure. A needle stick with a large hollow-bore needle is higher risk than a solid needle, a deep penetrating wound is considered a high-risk exposure compared to a superficial injury, and a exposure to a large volume of infectious fluid is more concerning than exposure to a low volume. Patient-specific factors must also be considered, such as whether the HIV-positive patient is on HAART therapy and has a suppressed viral load or whether the HIV-positive patient currently has a high viral load. Regardless of the type of exposure or risk factors, current guidelines recommend that PEP be offered to all health care workers with an exposure. If the source patient is known to be HIV positive or the HIV status is not known, PEP should be continued for a total of 4 weeks, or 28 days. If the source patient's status is unknown but is later determined to be HIV negative, then PEP can be discontinued prior to 28 days.[129,130]

Three-drug PEP is recommended for all health care workers exposed or possibly exposed to HIV. Recommended regimens include two NRTIs with either raltegravir or dolutegravir. Alternative regimens include two NRTIs with a boosted PI.[130]

In instances where the source patient is a known treatment experienced patient with HIV, the choice of agents to use for PEP is generally dependent on the patient's regimen and resistant profile.[129,130]

L.T. should start immediately a PEP regimen, preferably emtricitabine/tenofovir disoproxil fumarate once daily with raltegravir twice daily or dolutegravir once daily. This entire regimen should be continued for a total of 4 weeks. It would also be a good idea to look at the specific patient from which the exposure occurred. If he had a great deal of known antiretroviral drug resistance, then L.T. may need to be put on different antiretrovirals according to the patient's resistance profile. HIV antibody testing using ELISA should be performed on L.T. at baseline exposure, 6 weeks, 12 weeks, and 6 months after exposure. She should also have baseline and follow-up labs performed to assess antiretroviral toxicity. At a minimum, these should include a complete blood count, renal and hepatic function tests, and fasting glucose while on the protease inhibitor. Additional laboratory tests should be performed based on the individual drugs chosen.[129,130]

Additional guidelines exist for non-occupational HIV exposures and follow similar risk and stratification treatment paradigms. In those instances where a person seeks care within 72 hours of exposure to blood, genital secretions or other potentially infected body fluids of persons known to be HIV-infected and the exposure represents a substantial risk for HIV transmission then the person is started on PEP in a similar fashion as with an occupation exposure and continued for 4 weeks with similar monitoring and HIV testing.[131]

KEEPING CURRENT

The management of HIV infection continues to evolve. Additional important emerging data are in HIV prevention and cure.

Table 76-7
Human Immunodeficiency Virus Internet Resources

Government Sites
American Foundation for AIDS Research: http://www.amfar.org
Centers for Disease Control and Prevention: http://www.cdc.gov
Consensus Panel Guidelines Online: http://www.aidsinfo.nih.gov
Government HIV Mutation Charts: http://hiv-web.lanl.gov
National Institute of Allergy and Infectious Diseases: http://www.niaid.nih.gov
National Prevention Information Network: https://npin.cdc.gov/
United Nations AIDS Website: http://www.unaids.org/
University Sites
University of Stanford HIV Drug Resistance Database: http://hivdb.stanford.edu/
AIDS Treatment/Advocacy Groups
Project Inform: http://www.projectinform.org/
San Francisco AIDS Foundation: http://www.sfaf.org/index.html
Other Relevant Sites
The AIDS Map: http://www.aidsmap.com
Clinical Care Options: http://www.clinicalcareoptions.com
HIV Drug Interactions: http://www.hiv-druginteractions.org
HIV and Hepatitis: http://hivandhepatitis.com
HIV Treatment Information: http://i-base.info/
Medscape: http://www.medscape.com
Physician's Research Network: http://www.prn.org
The Body for Clinicians: http://www.thebodypro.com

The overwhelming data presented at scientific meetings and in journals have made staying informed about current issues and new developments a daunting task. As a result, many clinicians, even those actively caring for patients who are HIV infected, remain cautious and often confused regarding therapeutic options.

New technologies for the dissemination of medical information are constantly evolving. The Internet has allowed clinicians worldwide to exchange ideas, teach new concepts, and obtain access to limited resources. In addition, many research centers, patient advocacy groups, and academic institutions have posted sites on the Internet that have resulted in access to large amounts of high-quality medical information. This new technology has also allowed, however, for the dissemination of incomplete, misleading, or inaccurate information. Therefore, clinicians must remain cautious and carefully evaluate the information obtained from various websites.

When evaluating the quality of a website, clinicians should look for a few basic standards.

- *Author qualifications.* Is the author qualified to write the article or perform the research? Is his or her affiliation or relevant credentials provided?
- *Attribution.* Are references provided to confirm statements? Is all relevant copyrighted information noted?
- *Currency.* When was the content posted? Is the website updated regularly?
- *Disclosure.* Who owns the website? Is there a conflict of interest between what is being posted and any commercial interest?

Any Internet site that fails to meet these basic competencies should be viewed with caution. In general, the most accurate and informative websites for HIV-specific information come from academic institutions, government organizations, medical societies, and patient advocacy groups. Table 76-7 lists high-quality websites that provide timely and accurate information. A periodic evaluation of these sites often provides sufficient information to stay up-to-date on current issues and controversies.

CONCLUSION

Given the significant advances in antiretroviral therapy over the past 30 years, HIV-1 infection is now a manageable chronic disease for those who have access to antiretroviral therapies. The pharmacologic management of HIV continues to rapidly evolve, but a basic understanding of viral pathogenesis and drug interactions provides a framework that can be used to evaluate new information as it becomes available. Although a cure is still out of reach, methods for preventing infection via treatment as prevention, PrEP, PEP, and through the prevention of perinatal transmission, have become increasingly effective as alternative strategies for curbing the epidemic.

KEY REFERENCES AND WEBSITES

A full list of references for this chapter can be found at http://thepoint.lww.com/AT11e. Below are the key references and websites for this chapter, with the corresponding reference number in this chapter found in parentheses after the reference.

Key References

Cohen MS et al. Prevention of HIV-1 infection with early antiretroviral therapy. *N Engl J Med*. 2011;365:493. (12)

Gunthard HF et al. Antiretroviral Drugs for Treatment and Prevention of HIV Infection in Adults 2016 Recommendations of the International Antiviral Society–USA Panel. JAMA. 2016;316(2):191-210. (5)

INSIGHT START Study Group. Initiation of antiretroviral therapy in early asymptomatic HIV infection. *N Engl J Med*. 2015;373:795–807. (65)

Temprano ANRS 12136 Study Group. A trial of early antiretrovirals and isoniazid preventive therapy in Africa. *N Engl J Med*. 2015;373:808–822. (66)

Wensing AM et al. 2017 Update of the drug resistance mutations in HIV-1. *Top Antivir Med*. 2017;24(4):132-141. (4)

Key Websites

Centers for Disease Control and Prevention. HIV in the United States. 2015; https://www.cdc.gov/hiv/basics/index.html. Accessed June 15, 2015. (9)
Centers for Disease Control and Prevention.

Panel on Treatment of HIV-Infected Pregnant Women and Prevention of Perinatal Transmission. Recommendations for Use of Antiretroviral Drugs in Pregnant HIV-1-Infected Women for Maternal Health and Interventions to Reduce Perinatal HIV Transmission in the United States. https://aidsinfo.nih.gov/guidelines/html/3/perinatal-guidelines/0/#. Accessed August 7, 2017. (121)

Panel on Antiretroviral Guidelines for Adults and Adolescents. Guidelines for the use of antiretroviral agents in HIV-1-infected adults and adolescents. Department of Health and Human Services. https://aidsinfo.nih.gov/guidelines/html/1/adult-and-adolescent-treatment-guidelines/0/. Accessed August 7, 2017. (3)

US Public Health Service. Preexposure Prophylaxis for the Prevention of HIV Infection in the United States—2014 Clinical Practice Guideline. U.S. Department of Health and Human Services and Center for Disease Control. http://www.cdc.gov/hiv/pdf/PrEPguidelines2014.pdf. Accessed May 31, 2015. (128)

77 Opportunistic Infections in HIV-Infected Patients

Emily L. Heil and Amanda H. Corbett

CORE PRINCIPLES

	CORE PRINCIPLES	CHAPTER CASES
1	Acquired immunodeficiency syndrome (AIDS) is characterized by the gradual erosion of immune competence and the development of opportunistic infections (OIs) and malignancies. A decline in OIs and OI-related malignancies has been observed, which is associated with highly active antiretroviral therapy (HAART).	
2	*Pneumocystis jiroveci* pneumonia (PCP) should be treated with trimethoprim–sulfamethoxazole (TMP-SMX). The patients intolerant of sulfonamides should be treated with alternatives such as dapsone, atovaquone, or pentamidine. Steroids should be used to treat patients with moderate-to-severe diseases. Primary prophylaxis with these agents is recommended for patients with CD4 counts less than 200.	**Case 77-1 (Questions 1-5)**
3	Toxoplasmosis typically occurs in patients with CD4 counts less than 100, and primary prophylaxis is indicated in these patients who are also *Toxoplasma* immunoglobulin G (IgG)-positive. Alternatives for prophylaxis include TMP-SMX, dapsone + pyrimethamine + leucovorin, and atovaquone ± pyrimethamine + leucovorin. Treatment options include sulfadiazine + pyrimethamine + leucovorin, clindamycin + pyrimethamine + leucovorin, and TMP-SMX.	**Case 77-2 (Questions 1, 3, and 4)**
4	Cytomegalovirus (CMV) typically causes retinitis in human immunodeficiency virus (HIV)–infected patients with CD4 counts less than 50. Primary prophylaxis is usually not indicated, and treatment options include intravenous (IV) ganciclovir, valgancyclovir, IV foscarnet, IV cidofovir, and intraocular ganciclovir implants.	**Case 77-3 (Questions 1 and 2)**
5	Cryptococcal meningitis occurs typically in patients with CD4 counts less than 50, and primary prophylaxis is not typically recommended. First-line treatment includes amphotericin + flucytosine for induction therapy with subsequent addition of fluconazole for maintenance.	**Case 77-4 (Questions 1–5, 8)**
6	*Mycobacterium tuberculosis* infects HIV-infected patients at any CD4 count, sometimes with an atypical presentation. Isoniazid for 9 months is the preferred regimen for latent tuberculosis (TB) in HIV-infected patients. Initial treatment in drug-susceptible TB is with rifampin (or rifabutin) + isoniazid + pyrazinamide + ethambutol.	**Case 77-5 (Question 1), Case 77-6 (Question 1), and Case 77-7 (Question 1)**
7	*Mycobacterium avium* complex (MAC) can be localized to the lung or with disseminated infection in HIV-infected patients with CD4 counts less than 50. Primary prophylaxis is indicated with either azithromycin or clarithromycin. First-line treatment for acute infection consists of clarithromycin (or azithromycin) + ethambutol ± rifampin (or rifabutin).	**Case 77-8 (Questions 1, 5, and 7)**

INTRODUCTION

The AIDS is characterized by the gradual erosion of immune competence and the development of OIs. Since the advent of HAART, AIDS-related mortality has declined in the United States.[1,2] The overall 5-year survival probability after the first OI diagnosis has increased dramatically from 7% in the pre-HAART to 65% in the HAART era.[3] This decline in mortality has been associated with a decline in OIs and an increase in noninfectious AIDS-related mortality.[4] Patients with HIV infection are susceptible to an array of diseases, but most OIs are caused by a few common pathogens, including *P. jiroveci* (*carinii*), CMV, fungi, and mycobacteria.[5]

Chapter 77

The revised classification system for HIV infection and expanded surveillance case definition for AIDS included stratification for the CD4 lymphocyte count, as well as subgrouping by clinical categories (see Chapter 76, Pharmacotherapy of Human Immunodeficiency Virus Infection, Tables 76-1 and 76-2). These AIDS-defining OIs may also occur in asymptomatic HIV-infected patients.[5]

The Natural History of Opportunistic Infections

THE DECLINE OF THE CD4 LYMPHOCYTE

Within the immune system, the CD4 lymphocyte functions as a "helper cell" that modulates the actions of the other key cellular components of the immune system. The eventual loss of CD4 lymphocytes is the underlying pathophysiology that leads to AIDS. (See Chapter 76, Pharmacotherapy of Human Immunodeficiency Virus Infection, and comprehensive immunology texts for a more detailed explanation of immune function and inflammation associated with HIV infection.) The infected CD4 lymphocyte can function normally for a time but eventually becomes dysfunctional, as manifested by an abnormal response to soluble mitogens. It is this cellular functional deficit, compounded by the eventual decline in the absolute number of CD4 lymphocytes which leads to OIs and neurologic dysfunctions. The CD4 lymphocyte count declines gradually during several years in the untreated HIV-infected person. The average rate of decline in CD4 lymphocyte cells (CD4 slope) is approximately 40 to 80 cells/μL/year in the absence of antiretroviral therapy. An accelerated decline in the CD4 count occurs at 1.5 to 2 years, just before an AIDS-defining diagnosis.[6] Without therapy, the course of infection averages approximately 10 years from the time of initial infection to an AIDS-defining diagnosis.

The CD4 count dictates the need for OI prophylaxis, influences the differential diagnosis of the OI, and is an independent indicator of prognosis. For these reasons, the CD4 count has become a primary surrogate marker of immune suppression and antiretroviral activity. HIV-1 ribonucleic acid (RNA) is the other clinical surrogate marker, most predictive of survival and antiretroviral activity.

OIs range from relatively minor events (e.g., oral candidiasis or oral hairy leukoplakia) to sight-threatening episodes of CMV retinitis or life-threatening PCP. The risk for specific OIs varies with the degree of immunosuppression.[7] Asymptomatic patients with moderate immunosuppression (CD4 counts, 200–500) may become infected with herpes viruses and *Candida* species or develop pneumonia, enteric infection, and meningitis with more common pathogens. Massive destruction of the immune system occurs when the CD4 count drops below 200, which increases the risk of opportunistic pathogens (e.g., PCP), opportunistic tumors, wasting, and neurologic complications. With a CD4 count of 50 to 100, invasive candidiasis, cerebral toxoplasmosis, cryptococcosis, and various protozoal infections are observed. When the CD4 count falls below 50, the patient is in an advanced immunosuppressed state, which is associated with non-Hodgkin lymphoma, CMV, and disseminated MAC (Fig. 77-1). Without treatment, the median survival associated with a CD4 count less than 200 is 3.1 years, and the time to an AIDS-defining infection ranges from 18 to 24 months.[7] With the implementation of HAART, the 3-year probability of AIDS has dramatically declined; however, much of this decline may be associated with the use of OI prophylaxis.[8]

THE EFFECT OF OPPORTUNISTIC INFECTIONS ON VIRAL LOAD AND SURVIVAL

Acute OIs upregulate HIV replication, resulting in higher HIV-1 RNA concentrations in the plasma and lymphoid tissues of HIV-infected patients. This enhanced replication is presumably caused by antigen-mediated activation of HIV-1 replication in latently infected cells. To assess the impact of OIs on survival, data from a cohort of 2,081 HIV-infected patients followed up (in the pre–protease inhibitor era) for a mean of 30 months were analyzed.[9] CD4 counts and incidence of opportunistic disease were used as independent variables. These investigators found that PCP, CMV, MAC, esophageal candidiasis, Kaposi sarcoma (KS), non-Hodgkin lymphoma, progressive multifocal leukoencephalopathy (PML), dementia, wasting syndrome, toxoplasmosis, and cryptosporidiosis were independently associated with death.[9] Additionally, data from a prospective longitudinal study of HIV infection in homosexual men initiated in 1984 (Multicenter AIDS Cohort Study) demonstrated that plasma HIV-1 RNA concentrations strongly predict the rate of decline in the absolute CD4 count as well as clinical progression to AIDS and death.[10] More recent investigations in the era of HAART have demonstrated that CD4 count is the strongest prognostic factor in patients starting therapy.[8]

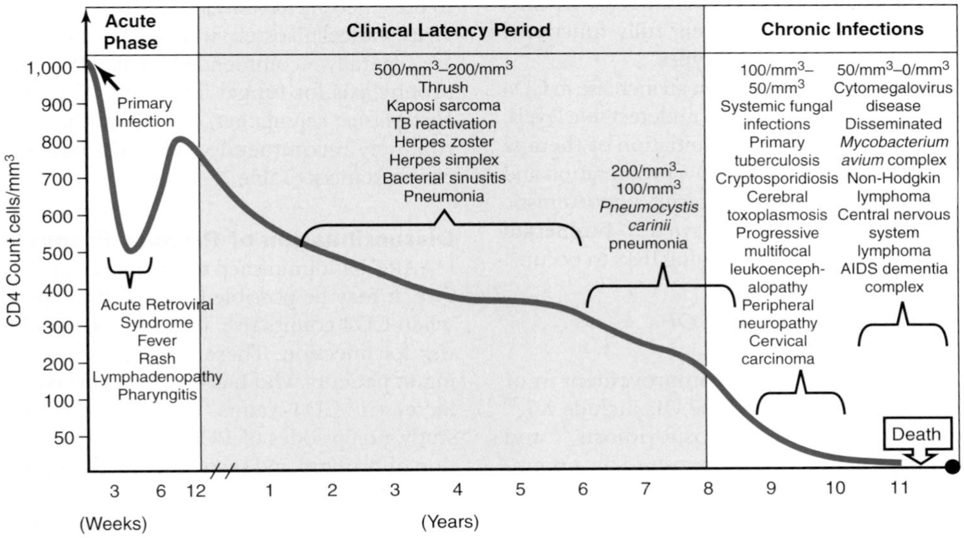

Figure 77-1 Natural history of CD4 cell count in the average HIV-infected patient without antiretroviral therapy, from the time of HIV transmissions to death. (Illustration by Mary Van, PharmD.)

IMPACT OF ANTIRETROVIRAL AGENTS ON THE NATURAL HISTORY OF OPPORTUNISTIC INFECTIONS

Reduction in the Incidence of Opportunistic Infections and Death

The introduction of protease inhibitors, combination therapy, prophylaxis therapy, and improved medical care has reduced the incidence of OIs and death resulting from AIDS in HIV-positive patients. HAART generally refers to an antiretroviral regimen that can be expected to reduce the viral load in antiretroviral-naïve patients to less than 50 copies/mL. A panel of experts convened by the US Department of Health and Human Services and the Henry J. Kaiser Family Foundation recommended HAART as the standard of care for all HIV-infected patients.[11] These potent antiretroviral agents and effective management of OIs have led to an improved quality of life and prolonged survival among HIV-infected US patients.[12] A significant decrease in the incidence of OIs and death was first reported in 1996, when preliminary data demonstrated that the addition of ritonavir to an existing reverse transcriptase regimen in severely immunocompromised patients decreased the incidence of OIs and death.[13] The steepest declines in the incidence of AIDS-defining OIs followed this introduction of HAART, but the declines have also continued into the late-HAART area.[14] A recent analysis demonstrated both a decline in opportunistic infections (89–13.3 per 1,000 person-years) and opportunistic malignancies (23.4–3.0 per 1,000 person-years) from 1994 to 2007.[2]

CHANGES IN THE NATURAL HISTORY OF OPPORTUNISTIC INFECTIONS

OIs result from long-standing immunosuppression from HIV infection.[7] For example, before HAART, approximately 40% of all AIDS patients exhibited CMV retinitis, with the most cases occurring at CD4 counts below 100. Since the implementation of HAART, a decrease in the incidence and progression of CMV retinitis have been noted.[15,16]

Ironically, HAART has also been associated with a worsening or an unmasking of occult OIs in patients with an advanced stage of AIDS. When antiretroviral therapy strengthens the immune system, inflammatory symptoms in response to infection are more clinically pronounced.[12] This syndrome has been referred to as immune reconstitution inflammatory syndrome (IRIS). IRIS incidence is estimated to be 10% to 40% in patients starting antiretroviral therapy, based primarily on retrospective observational data.[17–20] During IRIS, there is typically a rapid increase in CD4 lymphocytes; however, this does not represent fully functional cells, but rather an increase in memory subtypes.

The initiation of HAART typically results in an increase in CD4 lymphocytes and a decrease in HIV-1 RNA to undetectable levels. This initial increase in CD4 T cells after the initiation of therapy involves an increase in memory T cells with low proliferation and a decrease in functional or effector cells. As a result, opportunistic infections that are present in tissues are allowed to proliferate once the immune system is recovering, allowing IRIS to occur.[21]

IMPROVEMENT IN OR RESOLUTION OF OPPORTUNISTIC INFECTIONS

With the initiation of HAART, reports of improvement in or resolution of some OIs can occur.[22–26] These OIs include KS,[26] PML,[24] CMV,[15,16] microsporidiosis, cryptosporidiosis,[23] and molluscum contagiosum,[25] a viral infection caused by a member of the *Poxviridae* family. Furthermore, there are reports of restored immunity and clinical improvement in patients with chronic hepatitis B infection (not classified as a CDC-defined AIDS indicator condition) with the initiation of HAART.[22] However, these infections were not eradicated, and in some cases, improvement was only transient. Clinical resolution most likely results from immunologic improvement, and the protective immunity against OI is sustained only as long as HAART remains effective.

Pharmacotherapeutic Management of Opportunistic Infections

Successful pharmacotherapeutic management of OIs requires an understanding of the natural history of HIV-associated OIs, including the recognition that OIs occur with declining CD4 lymphocyte counts, the clinical presentation of each disease, diagnostic techniques, and effective treatment and preventive strategies. Management issues, complicated by multiple-drug therapy for OIs and HIV suppression, include adherence, toxicities, resistance, drug interactions, and cost. HIV-infected patients are usually less tolerant to drugs such as flucytosine, TMP-SMX, and pyrimethamine; however, alternative agents are available to overcome these barriers to treatment.

In 1995, the US Public Health Service (USPHS) and the Infectious Diseases Society of America (IDSA) issued guidelines for the prevention of OIs in HIV-infected patients; these were revised in 1997,[27] 1999,[28] and 2002.[29] Recommendations are included for preventing exposure to opportunistic pathogens, preventing first episodes of disease by chemoprophylaxis or vaccination (primary prophylaxis), and preventing disease recurrence (secondary prophylaxis). Additionally, in 2004, the CDC published the first edition of guidelines for the treatment of OIs.[30] In 2009, a combined set of guidelines for both prevention and treatment of more than 30 opportunistic infections was developed.[12] The most recent and any archived guidelines can be found at www.aidsinfo.nih.gov.

PRIMARY PROPHYLAXIS

Primary prophylaxis is defined as a therapy that is initiated before the appearance of an OI in high-risk asymptomatic persons to prevent the initial occurrence of an infection. Primary prevention of OIs is important, considering the inevitable immune depletion associated with chronic HIV infection.[31] PCP and MAC prophylaxis have significantly prolonged survival and delayed the onset of illness (see Prophylaxis sections for both PCP and MAC).[32,33]

The guidelines strongly recommend primary prophylaxis against PCP, toxoplasmosis, *M. tuberculosis*, and MAC. Vaccinations to prevent *Streptococcus pneumoniae*, hepatitis B virus, hepatitis A virus, varicella zoster virus (VZV), and influenza virus infection are generally recommended for all HIV-infected patients. Primary prophylaxis for fungal infections (*Cryptococcus neoformans* and *Histoplasma capsulatum*), CMV, and bacterial infections are not routinely recommended for most patients, except in unusual circumstances (Table 77-1).

Discontinuation of Primary Prophylaxis Therapy

HAART has diminished the incidence of several OIs.[16,23,26] Therefore, it may be possible to discontinue prophylactic OI therapy when CD4 counts rise above the threshold associated with the risk for infection. These data have been particularly encouraging in patients who had PCP prophylaxis discontinued with an increase in CD4 counts.[12] In one observational PCP prophylaxis study, no episodes of PCP were observed after the discontinuation of primary and secondary PCP prophylaxis.[34] These studies suggest that patients who respond to HAART with a sustained increase in CD4 count can have their primary prophylaxis safely discontinued. The OI prophylaxis guidelines suggest that primary PCP prophylaxis may be discontinued for patients on HAART

Table 77-1
Primary Prophylaxis of Opportunistic Infections in HIV-Infected Adults and Adolescents

		Preventive Regimens		
Pathogen	**Indication**	**First Choice**	**Alternatives**	**D/C Prophylaxis**
Strongly Recommended as Standard of Care				
Pneumocystis jiroveci (carinii)	CD4 count <200 or oropharyngeal candidiasis	TMP-SMX, 1 DS PO daily or TMP-SMX 1 SS PO daily	TMP-SMX 1 DS TIW Dapsone 50 mg BID or 100 mg/day; dapsone 50 mg daily + pyrimethamine 50 mg QW + leucovorin 25 mg PO QW; aerosolized pentamidine 300 mg QM via Respirgard II nebulizer, atovaquone 1,500 mg PO daily; atovaquone 1,500 mg PO + pyrimethamine 25 mg PO + leucovorin 25 mg PO daily	Patients on HAART with sustained CD4 >200 cells for ≥3 months may discontinue PCP prophylaxis. Reintroduce if CD4 <200.
Mycobacterium tuberculosis				
Isoniazid-sensitive	+ Diagnostic test for TB with no evidence of active TB, no prior treatment OR − Diagnostic test for TB, close contact with person with active TB and no personal active TB OR History of untreated or inadequately treated TB and no evidence of active TB	Isoniazid 300 mg PO daily OR isoniazid 900 mg PO BIW × 9 months both with pyridoxine 50 mg PO daily	Rifampin 600 mg PO daily × 4 months or rifabutin dose adjusted for antiretroviral therapy × 4 months	
Drug-resistant TB	Same; high probability of exposure to isoniazid-resistant tuberculosis	Choice of drugs requires consultation with public health authorities	None	
Toxoplasma gondii	IgG antibody to *Toxoplasma* and CD4 count <100	TMP-SMX, 1 DS PO daily	TMP-SMX, 1 SS PO daily; TMP-SMX 1 DS PO TIW; dapsone 50 mg PO daily + pyrimethamine 50 mg PO QW + leucovorin 25 mg PO QW; dapsone 200 mg PO QW + pyrimethamine 75 mg PO QW + leucovorin 25 mg PO QW; atovaquone 1,500 mg PO daily with or without pyrimethamine 25 mg PO daily + leucovorin 10 mg PO daily	Patients on HAART with sustained CD4 >200 for ≥3 months may discontinue toxoplasmosis prophylaxis. Restart if CD4 <100–200
MAC	CD4 count <50 after ruling out active infection	Azithromycin, 1,200 mg PO QW; clarithromycin 500 mg PO BID; azithromycin 600 mg PO BIW	Rifabutin, 300 mg PO daily	Patients on HAART with sustained CD4 >100 for ≥3 months may discontinue MAC prophylaxis. Restart if CD4 <50
VZV	Preexposure prevention: Patients with CD4 ≥200 who have not been vaccinated, have no history of varicella or herpes zoster or who are seronegative for VZV Postexposure prevention: Significant exposure to chicken pox or shingles for patients who are susceptible	Preexposure: Primary varicella vaccination, two doses administered 3 months apart Postexposure prevention: VZIG 125 international units per 10 kg (maximum of 635 international units) IM administered 96 hours after exposure		

(*continued*)

Table 77-1

Primary Prophylaxis of Opportunistic Infections in HIV-Infected Adults and Adolescents (*continued*)

Usually Recommended			
Streptococcus pneumoniae	Regardless of CD4 count followed by: If CD4 >200 If CD4 <200 For individuals who have previously received PPV23	PCV13 0.5 mL × 1 PPV23 0.5 mL IM at least 8 weeks after PCV13 PPV23 can be offered at least 8 weeks after receiving PCV13 or can wait until CD4 ≥200 One dose of PCV13 should be given at least 1 year after the last receipt of PPV23	None
HBV	All susceptible (anti-HBc-negative) patients	Hepatitis B vaccine three doses	None
HPV	Females aged 13–26 years Males aged 13–26 years	HPV quadrivalent vaccine 0.5 mL IM at Months 0, 1–2, and 6 OR HPV bivalent vaccine 0.5 mL IM at Months 0, 1–2, and 6 HPV quadrivalent vaccine 0.5 mL IM at Months 0, 1–2, and 6	
Influenza virus	All patients (annually before influenza season)	Inactivated influenza vaccine per recommendation for the season (note, live attenuated influenza vaccine is contraindicated in all HIV-infected patients)	
HAV	All susceptible (anti-HAV-negative) patients at an increased risk for HAV or patients with chronic liver disease (including HBV or HCV)	Hepatitis A vaccine; two doses	None
Not Recommended for Most Patients; Indicated for Use Only in Unusual Circumstances			
Bacteria	Neutropenia	G-CSF 510 mg/kg SC daily × 24 weeks or GM-CSF 250 mg/m² SC × 24 weeks	None
Cryptococcus neoformans	CD4 count <50	Fluconazole 100–200 mg PO daily	Itraconazole 200 mg PO daily
Histoplasma capsulatum	CD4 count <100, endemic geographic areas	Itraconazole 200 mg PO daily	None
CMV	CD4 count <50 and CMV antibody–positive	Valganciclovir 900 mg PO daily	None

BID, twice a day; BIW, twice weekly; CMV, cytomegalovirus; DS, double strength; G-CSF, granulocyte colony-stimulating factor; GM-CSF, granulocyte-macrophage colony-stimulating factor; HAART, highly active antiretroviral therapy; HAV, hepatitis A virus; HBc, hepatitis B core; HBV, hepatitis B virus; HPV, human papillomavirus; IM, intramuscularly; INH, isoniazid; MAC, *Mycobacterium avium* complex; PCV13, 13-valent pneumococcal conjugate vaccine; PO, orally; PPV23, 23-valent pneumococcal polysaccharides vaccine; QM, monthly; QW, weekly; RIF, rifampin; SC, subcutaneously; SS, single strength; TIW, three times a week; TMP-SMX, trimethoprim–sulfamethoxazole; TST, tuberculin skin test; VZIG, varicella zoster immune globulin; VZV, varicella zoster virus.

Source: Panel on Opportunistic Infections in HIV-infected Adults and Adolescents. Guidelines for prevention and treatment of opportunistic infections in HIV-infected adults and adolescents: recommendations from CDC, the National Institutes of Health, and the HIV Medicine Association of the Infectious Diseases Society of America. **https://aidsinfo.nih.gov/guidelines/html/4/adult-and-adolescent-oi-prevention-and-treatment-guidelines/**.

when the CD4 count is greater than 200 for at least 3 months. Primary prophylaxis for MAC may also be discontinued when the CD4 count increases to greater than 100.[12] In addition, the guidelines suggest discontinuing primary prophylaxis for toxoplasmosis when the CD4 count increases to greater than 200 for at least 3 months.[12]

ACUTE THERAPY

Prompt diagnosis and immediate initiation of therapy are essential for the management of acute infections. Most common OIs can be classified into one of two groups. The first group consists of infections that can be treated by conventional or investigational agents. These include PCP, TB, cryptococcosis, CMV, MAC, and histoplasmosis. Treatment may result in either effective or moderately effective resolution. These infections may recur if chronic suppressive or secondary prophylaxis is discontinued without an accompanying elevation in the CD4 count and viral load suppression. The second group includes pathogens for which no therapeutic regimen is currently effective. These include cryptosporidiosis, microsporidiosis, and PML.

SECONDARY PROPHYLAXIS OR CHRONIC SUPPRESSIVE THERAPY

Secondary prophylaxis is used to prevent recurrence of an OI once the patient has developed signs and symptoms of active infection. In some cases, secondary prophylaxis regimens can be discontinued after patients achieve a certain CD4 level. The USPHS and IDSA strongly recommend secondary prophylaxis for PCP, toxoplasmosis (reduced dosage), MAC, CMV, *Salmonella* species, and infections caused by endemic fungi and *C. neoformans.*[12]

Discontinuation of Secondary Prophylaxis or Chronic Suppressive Therapy

The USPHS/IDSA guidelines recommend discontinuing primary or secondary prophylaxis for certain pathogens with HAART-related increases in CD4 count to specified threshold levels.[12] Criteria for discontinuing chemoprophylaxis are based on specific clinical studies and vary by duration of CD4 count increase and duration of treatment of the initial episode of disease (in the case of secondary prophylaxis).

Secondary PCP prophylaxis may be discontinued among patients whose CD4 counts have increased to greater than 200 for more than 3 months while on HAART. Secondary prophylaxis for disseminated MAC may be discontinued among patients who have completed 12 months of MAC therapy, have no signs or symptoms of MAC, and have had a CD4 count of greater than 100 for more than or equal to 3 months in response to HAART. Similarly, secondary prophylaxis for toxoplasmosis may be discontinued in patients who have completed initial therapy, have no signs or symptoms of infection, and have had CD4 counts of greater than 200 for more than 3 months. Using the same criteria, patients with cryptococcosis can discontinue secondary prophylaxis if they have had CD4 counts of greater than or equal to 200 for more than 6 months. Maintenance therapy for CMV can be discontinued safely in patients who have maintained a CD4 count of greater than 100 for greater than 6 months on HAART.[12,16] The decision to stop CMV prophylaxis should be made in consultation with an ophthalmologist and is influenced by factors such as the magnitude and duration of CD4 increases and viral load suppression, anatomic location of retinal lesions, and vision in the contralateral eye.

Although there are considerable data concerning the discontinuation of primary and secondary prophylaxis, there are no data regarding restarting prophylaxis if the CD4 count decreases again to levels at which the patient is likely to again be at risk for OIs. For primary prophylaxis, the same CD4 count threshold for stopping or restarting therapy is recommended. For PCP prophylaxis, the current guidelines use a CD4 count of 200 as the threshold for restarting both primary and secondary prophylaxis. For toxoplasmosis, the CD4 threshold is 100 to 200, and for MAC, it is 50.[12]

PNEUMOCYSTIS *JIROVECI* PNEUMONIA

As an indication of the relative obscurity of this organism, no comprehensive text on PCP was available until 1983.[35] Since that time, this organism has been reclassified from a protozoan to a fungus on the basis of ribosomal RNA sequence comparisons. The morphologic resemblance of *P. carinii* to a protozoan has led to its life cycle being described as a cyst form, with up to eight sporozoites per cyst. The trophozoite or extracystic form has different staining characteristics (i.e., it does not stain with Toluidine Blue O or Grocott-Gomori stains) compared with the cyst or sporozoites. In addition, current literature refers to PCP as *P. jiroveci* as opposed to the original terminology of *Pneumocystis carinii*. The former species is the one responsible for infectivity in humans. *P. jiroveci* pneumonia is the second leading opportunistic infection affecting HIV-infected patients in the United States.[2] Hospitalizations and hospital mortality for AIDS-associated PCP have decreased significantly in the last 20 years; however, there has been a shift in the overall population at risk for PCP over time with a greater proportion of patients with PCP who are black, female, or from the southern region of the United States.[36]

Clinical Presentation

CASE 77-1

QUESTION 1: J.R. is a 38-year-old, HIV-seropositive man who was diagnosed 5 years ago when he had an outbreak of herpes zoster. He refused antiretroviral therapy and was determined to treat himself using natural teas and herbs. J.R. developed a mild, nonproductive cough that has persisted for the last 4 weeks. He has also had a low-grade fever but denies any chills or pleuritic chest pain. His chest radiograph demonstrates a diffuse, symmetric, interstitial infiltrate. Arterial oxygen partial pressure (Pa_{O_2}) is 80 mm Hg. His last CD4 count approximately 3 months ago was 180 cells/μL, and his viral load was 60,000 copies/mL. He refused primary PCP prophylaxis. After hypertonic saline nebulization for sputum induction and subsequent bronchoalveolar lavage, examination of the specimens with the modified Giemsa stain revealed both intracystic bodies and extracystic trophozoites. How is the clinical presentation of J.R. consistent with PCP?

The clinical features of PCP in AIDS patients differ from those of non-AIDS patients in that a more subtle onset, with mild fever, a cough, tachypnea, and dyspnea, is typically seen in HIV-infected patients.[12] J.R.'s low-grade fever and mild, nonproductive cough of 4 weeks' duration are consistent with this description of PCP. His history of HIV infection and the finding of trophozoites on Giemsa stain further support a diagnosis of PCP. The characteristic diffuse interstitial pulmonary infiltrates on J.R.'s chest radiograph are consistent with PCP. Limited data exist with regard to the latent state of *P. jiroveci* after host infection. Some investigators hypothesize that most persons are asymptomatic unless the host immune system becomes impaired. Others believe that the infection is caused by reinfection as opposed to reactivation.[37]

CASE 77-1, QUESTION 2: A diagnosis of PCP is made and J.R. agrees to be treated. What patient factors are important to consider when selecting an antimicrobial? What would be a reasonable drug for J.R., and how might his course of PCP be monitored?

The treatment of acute PCP is determined by the degree of clinical severity on presentation. The arterial oxygen status on presentation is an important indicator of overall outcome. Key factors to consider when initiating therapy for PCP include arterial blood gas findings, whether it is an initial or repeat episode of PCP, the need for parenteral therapy, and a prior history of adverse drug reactions or hypersensitivity. Concomitant therapy must also be considered.

Patients with PCP often can be classified as having mild, moderate, or severe disease, based on their oxygenation. Patients with mild PCP often have a room air alveolar-arterial (A-a) oxygen gradient of less than 35 or Pao_2 greater than 70 mm Hg, and patients with moderate or severe disease have an A-a greater than 35 mm Hg or Pao_2 greater than 70 mm Hg. With the advent of corticosteroid use for moderate-to-severe cases of PCP (discussed later), it is useful to calculate the A-a gradient or Pao_2. The A-a gradient (normal range, 5–15 mm Hg) can be calculated as $P_{IO_2} - (1.25 \times Paco_2) - Pao_2$, where P_{IO_2} is the partial pressure of inspired oxygen (150 mm Hg in room air), and $Paco_2$ and Pao_2 are arterial levels of CO_2 and O_2, respectively, expressed in mm Hg.

Several other clinical tests have been used to identify and monitor PCP. The lactate dehydrogenase concentration in serum or bronchoalveolar lavage fluid has been used to aid in diagnosis, monitor therapy, and to predict the outcome of PCP. However, it is a nonspecific value and should not be used alone. Chest radiographs also vary with PCP. The most common picture is one of bilateral diffuse interstitial pneumonitis, but atypical patterns, such as pleural effusion, cavities, pneumatoceles, and nodules, may also occur. A normal chest radiograph is associated with improved clinical outcome.

The natural course of PCP among untreated HIV-infected patients is progressive dyspnea and hypoxemia. Increasing patient age, subsequent episode of PCP, low hemoglobin, low partial pressure of oxygen breathing room air, the presence of medical comorbidity, and pulmonary KS are all early predictors of mortality from PCP at hospital admission.[38] The treatment of PCP in AIDS patients (compared with non–HIV-infected patients) indicates that a longer duration of therapy is needed.[35] Some patients may experience worsening hypoxemia during the first 3 to 5 days after the treatment is initiated. This period of clinical worsening is least tolerated by those patients with moderate-to-severe PCP (Pao_2 <70 mm Hg). In sicker patients, this period may lead to respiratory failure and the need for intubation. Although many would associate the need for intensive care unit admission as a poor prognostic factor, many patients do well despite the need for mechanical ventilation and IV antibiotics. In light of the role of corticosteroids, patients with PCP and respiratory failure may be viewed as manageable if treated aggressively (Table 77-2).

TRIMETHOPRIM–SULFAMETHOXAZOLE

The decision to hospitalize a patient is based on the severity of his or her illness. Patients who present with mild PCP with reasonable oxygenation and without evidence of clinical deterioration can be managed as outpatients. Patients with reasonably good gas exchange (i.e., Pao_2 >70 mm Hg) but with signs of clinical deterioration most often are admitted to the hospital and given oxygen by nasal cannula and are usually started on IV TMP-SMX (15–20 mg/kg/day TMP and 75–100 mg/kg/day SMX) for 21 days.[12,39] The dosing of IV TMP-SMX must be modified in patients with renal dysfunction. TMP reversibly inhibits dihydrofolate

Table 77-2
Treatment of *Pneumocystis jiroveci* Pneumonia

Regimen	Dose	Route	Adverse Effects/Comments
Approved			
TMP-SMX	15–20 mg/kg TMP (75–100 mg/kg SMX) daily administered IV or PO every 6–8 hours or two DS tablets TID	IV, PO	Hypersensitivity, hyperkalemia, rash, fever, neutropenia ↑LFTs, and nephrotoxicity (15 mg/kg/day preferred to 20 mg/kg/day because of reduced toxicity)
Pentamidine isethionate	4 mg/kg IV daily for 60–90 minutes × 21 days	IV	Pancreatitis, hypotension, hypoglycemia, hyperglycemia, and nephrotoxicity
Atovaquone[a]	750 mg BID with meals × 21 days (suspension)	PO	Headache, nausea, diarrhea, rash, fever, and ↑LFTs
TMP[a] + dapsone	15 mg/kg/day	PO	Pruritus, GI intolerance, and bone marrow suppression
	100 mg/day × 21 days	PO	Methemoglobinemia and hemolytic anemia (contraindicated in G6PD deficiency)
Clindamycin + primaquine	600 mg IV every 8 hours or 300–450 mg PO every 6 hours	PO or IV	Rash and diarrhea
	15–30 mg (base) daily × 21 days	PO	Methemoglobinemia and hemolytic anemia (contraindicated in G6PD deficiency)
Prednisone	Within 72 hours of anti-*Pneumocystis* therapy 40 mg every 12 hours × 5 days, then 40 mg daily × 5 days, then 20 mg/day × 11 days	PO	Initiation in patients with moderately severe or severe disease
			Pao_2 <70 mm Hg or A-a gradient >35 mm Hg

[a]Used only in mild to moderate *Pneumocystis jiroveci* pneumonia. A-a, alveolar-arterial gradient; BID, twice a day; CNS, central nervous system; DS, double strength; GI, gastrointestinal; G6PD, glucose-6 phosphate dehydrogenase; IV, intravenous; PO, oral; Pao_2, arterial partial pressure of oxygen; LFTs, liver function tests; TMP-SMX, trimethoprim–sulfamethoxazole.

reductase, and sulfamethoxazole competes with para-aminobenzoic acid in the production of dihydrofolate, synergistically blocking thymidine biosynthesis.

TMP-SMX is the drug of choice for PCP unless the patient has a history of life-threatening intolerance. In the treatment of PCP, TMP-SMX is either as effective as or superior to all alternative agents. A good response may be expected in more than 70% of patients receiving TMP-SMX. TMP-SMX is often prescribed orally (PO) because of its high bioavailability. The usual dose is 15 mg/kg (dosed by the TMP component) divided every 8 hours for 21 days. Because one double-strength tablet of TMP-SMX contains 160 mg TMP plus 800 mg SMX, a standard regimen is two double-strength tablets 3 times per day (or every 8 hours).

Although the TMP-SMX regimen is very efficacious, 25% to 50% of patients may be intolerant. Adverse effects include an erythematous, maculopapular, morbilliform rash, and, less commonly, severe urticaria, exfoliative dermatitis, and Stevens–Johnson syndrome. GI intolerance (nausea, vomiting, and abdominal pain) is common.[12] Hematologic side effects may include leukopenia, anemia, and thrombocytopenia. Neurologic toxicities, hyperkalemia, and hepatitis may also occur. Most patients who exhibit a mild hypersensitivity (skin rash) reaction can be managed with antipruritics or antihistamines without discontinuation of TMP-SMX. In some patients with mild hypersensitivity reactions, the agent can be restarted after the rash has resolved, using gradual dosage escalation or rapid oral desensitization to reduce adverse effects.[40] Patients with severe adverse reactions should be switched to another agent rather than being rechallenged with this drug (See also Chapter 32, Drug Hypersensitivity Reactions).

Because J.R. seems to have a mild-to-moderate case of PCP (Pao_2, 80 mm Hg), has not previously experienced an episode of PCP, and has no history of adverse effects to TMP-SMX, an outpatient course of TMP-SMX would be reasonable.

ALTERNATIVES TO TRIMETHOPRIM–SULFAMETHOXAZOLE

CASE 77-1, QUESTION 3: J.R. experienced exfoliative dermatitis on Day 7 of TMP-SMX treatment. What other drugs could be prescribed to treat his PCP?

Because J.R. presents with a serious adverse effect to TMP-SMX, it should be discontinued and he should not be rechallenged or desensitized. Instead, he should be treated with an alternative regimen (Table 77-2).

IV pentamidine isethionate can be used to treat acute PCP. The mechanism of action is unknown, but it may be related to interference with oxidative phosphorylation, inhibition of nucleic acid biosynthesis, or interference with dihydrofolate reductase. Pentamidine is generally more toxic than TMP-SMX.[41] In a 5-year review of 106 courses of IV pentamidine, 76 (72%) patients had adverse reactions (nephrotoxicity, dysglycemia, hepatotoxicity, hyperkalemia, and hyperamylasemia). Drug discontinuation occurred in 31 (18%) of the severe cases. Nephrotoxicity and hypoglycemia were the most common causes of drug discontinuation. Nephrotoxicity occurred in 25% to 50% of the patients with dehydration and concurrent nephrotoxic drugs among the risk factors. Hypoglycemia was noted in 5% to 10% of patients after 5 to 7 days of treatment or several days after discontinuation of treatment. Hyperglycemia is a consequence of decreased β-cells and results in diabetes mellitus in 2% to 9% of patients. Other less common adverse effects and toxicities include thrombocytopenia, orthostatic hypotension, ventricular tachycardia, leukopenia, nausea, vomiting, abdominal pain, and anorexia.[41]

Patients receiving IV pentamidine should be monitored closely, and serum concentrations of glucose, potassium, blood urea nitrogen (BUN), and creatinine should be obtained daily or every other day during treatment. Other tests for periodic monitoring include a complete blood count (CBC), liver function tests (LFTs), amylase, lipase, and calcium.[41] Renal toxicity often responds to a reduction in the dosage of pentamidine to 3 mg/kg/day or 4 mg/kg every 48 hours (creatinine clearance <10 mL/minute); however, the drug should be discontinued in patients who exhibit signs and symptoms of pancreatitis. Risk factors for pentamidine-induced pancreatitis include prior episodes of pancreatitis and concurrent therapy with other drugs known to cause pancreatitis. Nebulized pentamidine should not be considered as an alternative to IV pentamidine for the treatment of PCP.[42]

Atovaquone suspension, 750 mg twice a day (BID), is available for the treatment of mild-to-moderate PCP. Atovaquone interrupts protozoan pyrimidine synthesis and demonstrates activity against *P. jiroveci* and *Toxoplasma gondii* in animal models. Atovaquone is approved by the US Food and Drug Administration (FDA) for the treatment of mild-to-moderate PCP in patients intolerant of TMP-SMX. Atovaquone is also an alternative for primary and secondary prophylaxis for both PCP and toxoplasmosis.[12] Atovaquone is well tolerated compared with other PCP therapies. Adverse effects include rash, fever, elevated LFTs, and emesis. Atovaquone is safer, but less effective, than TMP-SMX in patients with mild-to-moderate PCP.[43] When compared with IV pentamidine in the treatment of mild-to-moderate PCP, atovaquone and pentamidine were equally efficacious; however, pentamidine was significantly more toxic.[44] Most atovaquone studies were performed using the moderately absorbed oral tablets; reformulation of this drug as a suspension has improved bioavailability by at least 30%. Concomitant administration of fatty foods with atovaquone doubles the absorption.

An oral regimen of dapsone plus TMP is another alternative to TMP-SMX. Dapsone–TMP can be used to treat mild-to-moderate PCP in patients intolerant of TMP-SMX. Dapsone is a sulfone antimicrobial that is used for leprosy. Although monotherapy (200 mg/day) with dapsone is ineffective for the treatment (not prophylaxis) of PCP, the addition of TMP (20 mg/kg/day) to dapsone (100 mg/day) is an effective alternative regimen.[45] In a small comparative trial of TMP–dapsone versus TMP-SMX, the response rates of 93% and 90% were observed, respectively.[46] When dapsone is coadministered with TMP, the resulting plasma concentrations for both drugs are higher than when either drug is taken alone. In combination with TMP, a pyrimidine, synergistic inhibition of folic acid synthesis occurs.[47] Dapsone–TMP should not be used in sulfonamide-allergic patients with a history of type I hypersensitivity reaction, toxic epidermal necrolysis, or Stevens–Johnson syndrome. Dapsone is associated with hematologic toxicities, including hemolytic anemia, methemoglobinemia, neutropenia, and thrombocytopenia. Patients with glucose-6-phosphate dehydrogenase (G6PD) deficiency cannot detoxify hydrogen peroxide and are at an increased risk for hematologic toxicity from dapsone.

Success rates of 70% to 100% have been reported with clindamycin (600 mg IV every 6 hours or 600 mg PO 3 times a day [TID]) given in conjunction with 30 mg/day of primaquine base. Although skin rashes are common with this combination, these often subside with continued therapy. Some patients experience toxicities (fever, rash, granulocytopenia, and methemoglobinemia) requiring discontinuation.[48–50] As with dapsone, before starting primaquine, patients should be screened for G6PD deficiency. Patients who test positive for G6PD deficiency are at a risk for developing hemolytic anemia.

A double-blind efficacy and toxicity study of 181 patients with mild-to-moderate PCP compared three oral drug regimens: TMP-SMX versus dapsone–TMP versus clindamycin–primaquine. The doses of TMP-SMX and dapsone–TMP were weight-based, and the dosage of clindamycin–primaquine was 600 mg clindamycin TID and primaquine 30 mg/day. All patients with moderately severe PCP (A-a oxygen gradient >45) were treated with prednisone (40 mg BID for 5 days, then once daily for 3 weeks). Rash was the most frequent dose-limiting toxicity (TMP-SMX, 19%; dapsone–TMP, 10%; clindamycin–primaquine, 21%). Hematologic toxicities were observed more frequently in the clindamycin–primaquine arm. Elevated LFTs (5 times above baseline) were more frequent in the TMP-SMX arm. The clindamycin–primaquine group demonstrated better quality of life scores at Day 7, but by Day 21, these differences became less significant.[45] TMP-SMX, dapsone–TMP, and clindamycin–primaquine demonstrated equal efficacy in patients with mild-to-moderate PCP.

J.R. should be hospitalized to better manage his severe adverse reaction and to complete his treatment of PCP. Because of his severe reaction to TMP-SMX, dapsone–TMP should not be administered because dapsone is a sulfone with a risk of cross-reactivity in patients with severe sulfonamide allergies. IV pentamidine is an option for J.R., but its toxicity suggests that it should be reserved for patients with more severe PCP presentation. Atovaquone is a reasonable option for patients with mild PCP who are intolerant of TMP-SMX and have no evidence of GI dysfunction, but it is not as effective as TMP-SMX or IV pentamidine. Clindamycin–primaquine is as efficacious as TMP-SMX for the treatment of mild-to-moderate PCP and can be administered PO. Consequently, it is the drug of choice in this patient.

The decision was made to start J.R. on oral clindamycin–primaquine for his mild-to-moderate PCP. J.R. tested negative for G6PD deficiency and was treated with clindamycin–primaquine for 14 days, completing a 21-day course of PCP therapy (Table 77-2).

Initiation of Corticosteroids

Case 77-1, Question 4: Should J.R. receive corticosteroid therapy with PCP treatment? If so, when should corticosteroids be initiated, and what would be a reasonable regimen for patients with PCP?

Corticosteroids have an important role in the management of patients with acute PCP who are clinically ill and have a low Po_2 (<70 mm Hg) or an A-a oxygen gradient greater than 35.[12] Many patients who are started on PCP therapy have an acute period of clinical deterioration, which may be associated with an acute inflammatory reaction to the rapid killing of *Pneumocystis*. Particularly among patients with moderate-to-severe PCP (A-a oxygen gradient >35 mm Hg or Pao_2 <70 mm Hg on room air), the use of prednisone during the first 72 hours of treatment may prevent fatal acute deterioration.[51] Corticosteroids may also have some benefits in patients exhibiting acute respiratory failure after 72 hours of conventional PCP therapy.[52] The recommended dose of prednisone is 40 mg given PO BID for 5 days, then 40 mg/day for 5 days, and then 20 mg/day for 11 days, for a total of 21 days.[53] Patients requiring IV corticosteroids may receive methylprednisolone at 75% of the prednisone dose. The major concern using glucocorticoids is the activation of latent infections (such as TB) or exacerbation of an active undiagnosed condition (especially fungal infections). However, the beneficial role of corticosteroids as adjunctive therapy outweighs the relative risk of short-term steroid use in this population.[54] More common side effects of short-term corticosteroids include ulcerative esophagitis, increased appetite, weight gain, sodium and fluid retention, headache, and elevated LFTs. Corticosteroids should be used with caution in the presence of uncontrolled diabetes, active GI bleeding, and uncontrolled hypertension.

Considering his mild hypoxemia (Pao_2, >70 mm Hg), J.R. is not a candidate for corticosteroid therapy.

Prophylaxis

Case 77-1, Question 5: J.R. was hospitalized and responded well to treatment. He now is a candidate for secondary prophylaxis. What secondary prophylaxis would be a good choice for J.R. when he is discharged from the hospital?

The early recognized efficacy of TMP-SMX prophylaxis[49] led to the eventual widespread application of prophylaxis and the development of guidelines for PCP prophylaxis (Table 77-2).[12] HIV-infected patients not receiving HAART or *Pneumocystis* prophylaxis were associated with a PCP prevalence of 8.4%, 18.4%, and 33.3% at 6, 12, and 36 months, respectively, in patients with a CD4 count of less than 200.[55] These data have formed the basis on which patients receive PCP prophylaxis. In addition to patients with CD4 counts of less than 200, other patients at a risk for PCP include those with a CD4 count of less than 14%, a history of an AIDS-defining illness, a history of oropharyngeal candidiasis, and possibly those with CD4 counts of 200 to 250.[12] J.R. refused primary prophylaxis and developed PCP. Secondary prophylaxis is necessary for J.R. to prevent recurrence and should be continued for life or until immune reconstitution occurs as a result of antiretroviral therapy.

The same agents and dosing schedules are recommended for primary (before an acute event) and secondary (after an acute event) prophylaxis of PCP.[12] TMP-SMX, one double-strength tablet daily, is the most efficacious prophylactic regimen; a single-strength tablet given daily is less toxic and nearly as efficacious. Patients with a history of non–life-threatening rash or fever caused by TMP-SMX may benefit from rechallenge with the original (or half) dose, or a dose escalation technique (desensitization regimen). Desensitization is preferred to switching to an alternative agent and is more successful than the direct rechallenge method.[56] Desensitization involves initiating very low doses of TMP-SMX and gradually increasing to the maximum dose over the course of days to weeks. In addition, patients who develop PCP while receiving prophylactic doses of TMP-SMX usually respond to full therapeutic doses for acute therapy. However, J.R. had a life-threatening reaction to TMP-SMX and should not be rechallenged or desensitized, and another agent should be chosen for prophylaxis.

The alternative agents used for prophylaxis include dapsone, dapsone plus pyrimethamine (with leucovorin), atovaquone suspension, and aerosolized pentamidine administered by the Respirgard II nebulizer (Table 77-2). TMP-SMX confers additional protection against toxoplasmosis and certain bacterial infections. Regimens containing dapsone plus pyrimethamine or atovaquone with or without pyrimethamine also protect against toxoplasmosis.[12] Although yet to be confirmed in clinical trials, other options include oral clindamycin–primaquine, intermittently administered IV pentamidine, oral pyrimethamine–sulfadiazine, and aerosolized pentamidine administered by other nebulizing devices.[12] TMP-SMX is more efficacious than dapsone or aerosolized pentamidine in the prevention of PCP.[57]

Extrapulmonary (e.g., lymph nodes, spleen, liver, bone marrow, adrenal gland, and GI tract) *P. carinii* has been noted in patients receiving inhaled pentamidine prophylaxis,[58] a finding rarely observed with IV administration. In addition, aerosolized pentamidine alters the usual chest radiograph findings associated with PCP, potentially complicating the diagnosis of this disease. Upper lobe infiltrates, cystic lesions, pneumothoraces, cavitary lesions with nodular infiltrates, and pleural effusions have been associated with aerosolized pentamidine prophylaxis.

The guidelines for primary prophylaxis suggest that prophylactic antimicrobial therapy can be discontinued when CD4 counts rise above the threshold associated with a risk for infection (i.e., <200 for PCP).[12] Many studies support the practice of discontinuing secondary PCP prophylaxis in patients whose CD4 counts have increased to greater than 200 for at least 3 months.[12] A European cohort study found that primary PCP rates were very low in patients with CD4 counts of 101 to 200 cells/μL and a viral load of less than 400 copies/mL regardless of prophylaxis, indicating that discontinuation of prophylaxis may be safe in patients with a CD4 count greater than 100 cells/μL who are on effective antiretrovirals.[59] The guidelines recommend that prophylaxis be reintroduced if the CD4 count decreases to less than 200 or if PCP recurs at a CD4 count of greater than 200.[12] J.R. responded well to his PCP treatment with clindamycin–primaquine in the hospital. However, because this regimen is unproven for secondary prophylaxis, it cannot be recommended. Considering his intolerance to TMP-SMX, the best selections would be dapsone (with or without pyrimethamine) or atovaquone suspension.

TOXOPLASMA GONDII ENCEPHALITIS

Clinical Presentation

CASE 77-2

QUESTION 1: W.O. is a 40-year-old man discovered to be HIV-positive during admission to a detoxification program for alcohol and heroin dependency. W.O. presented to the AIDS clinic with esophageal candidiasis, a CD4 count of 60 cells/μL (normal, approximately 1,000 cells/μL), a viral load of 150,000 copies/mL, and a *Toxoplasma* IgG titer of 1:256. W.O. was started on HAART. He remained well until 2 years later, when he presented to the emergency department reporting two seizures in the past 24 hours. His medications at that time included daily emtricitabine, tenofovir, darunavir/ritonavir, and inhaled pentamidine 300 mg monthly. His temperature was 100.1°F, and he was observed to have difficulty walking. His CD4 count is 90 cells/μL (previously 230 cells/μL), viral load is 70,000 copies/mL (previously 4,000), and white blood cell (WBC) count is 4,200 cells/L (normal, 3,800–9,800). A magnetic resonance image (MRI) of the head reveals several ring-shaped lesions in the brain stem. *Toxoplasma* encephalitis is presumptively diagnosed. Should W.O. be isolated from other patients and health-care workers to prevent the spread of this organism?

T. gondii is a parasitic protozoan that can infect people and is spread by environmental factors, such as the consumption of raw or undercooked meats and contact with cat feces. Immunocompetent persons infected with *T. gondii* may develop mild symptoms resembling infectious mononucleosis. However, these symptoms are generally transient and not associated with significant sequelae in immunocompetent patients (except in pregnant women). Recrudescent disease from *T. gondii* is problematic in patients with a suppressed cellular immune system, including those infected with HIV. Any HIV-positive patient infected with *T. gondii* is at a risk for developing clinical disease, particularly at CD4 counts less than 100, as illustrated by W.O.[12] W.O. presents with encephalitis (an inflammation of the brain or brainstem), the most frequent manifestation of *T. gondii* in HIV-positive patients.

All HIV-infected patients should be tested for IgG antibody to *T. gondii* after HIV diagnosis to detect latent infection. In the United States, as many as 70% of healthy adults are seropositive to *Toxoplasma*. The prevalence of *Toxoplasma* encephalitis among HIV-positive patients varies depending on the geographic region. In the United States, only 3% to 10% of AIDS patients actually develop encephalitis. In countries such as France, El Salvador, and Tahiti, where uncooked meat commonly is ingested, seropositivity is greater than 90% by the fourth decade of life. *Toxoplasma* encephalitis may develop in as many as 25% to 50% of AIDS patients in these countries.[60]

The two major routes of transmission of *Toxoplasma* to humans are oral and congenital. W.O. need not be isolated from other patients and health-care workers. HIV-infected patients should be advised not to eat raw and undercooked meat (internal temperature of meat should be at least 165°F–170°F), especially patients who are IgG-negative for *T. gondii*. Patients should wash their hands after touching uncooked meats and soil, and fruits and vegetables must be washed before eating. HIV-infected patients should avoid stray cats, keep their cats inside, and change the litter box daily. If no one else is available to change the litter box, patients should wash their hands thoroughly afterward.[12]

Diagnosis

CASE 77-2, QUESTION 2: Is there sufficient clinical evidence to establish a presumptive diagnosis of *Toxoplasma* encephalitis in W.O.?

The diagnosis of *Toxoplasma* encephalitis usually is presumptive because demonstration of cysts or trophozoites in brain tissue is required for a definitive diagnosis. The clinical signs and symptoms of *Toxoplasma* encephalitis can be either focal (indicating a specific region of the brain that is infected or inflamed) or generalized (indicating diffuse inflammation of the brain). *Toxoplasma* encephalitis usually occurs in patients with CD4 counts of less than 100. Serum titers of antibodies against *T. gondii* typically reflect past infection with the organism and unfortunately do not help delineate whether acute infection is present. In addition, cerebrospinal fluid (CSF) polymerase chain reaction for *Toxoplasma* is not always a reliable diagnostic tool. Most patients with encephalitis have single or multiple ring-enhancing lesions demonstrated on computed tomography scan or MRI of the head. Brain biopsy is reserved for patients with symptoms of encephalitis who are seronegative and for those who do not respond to presumptive antitoxoplasmosis therapy.[61] Because of the nonspecific diagnosis of *Toxoplasma* encephalitis, a high index of suspicion for other causes of encephalitis (e.g., central nervous system [CNS] lymphoma or TB) should be maintained throughout the treatment period for presumed *Toxoplasma* encephalitis. W.O. has overwhelming clinical evidence suggestive of *Toxoplasma* encephalitis. He is HIV-positive, has a CD4 count of less than 100, a positive *Toxoplasma* titer of 1:256 IgG, and a ring-shaped lesion in the brainstem on MRI. The development of this infection, in addition to the decline in CD4 T cells and the increase in plasma HIV RNA concentrations, may signal antiretroviral failure. W.O.'s current antiretroviral therapy should be reassessed, including his adherence to the regimen.

Prophylaxis

CASE 77-2, QUESTION 3: Should W.O. have been receiving prophylactic therapy for *T. gondii*?

Similar to many other OIs associated with HIV, therapy for toxoplasmosis can be categorized into primary prophylaxis, treatment of acute disease, and secondary prophylaxis. Primary prophylaxis is currently recommended for HIV-infected patients with CD4 counts of less than 100 who are also IgG-positive for *T. gondii* (Table 77-2). Many of the agents used to prevent PCP have activity against *T. gondii*: TMP-SMX, dapsone–pyrimethamine–leucovorin, and atovaquone with or without pyrimethamine/leucovorin are effective as primary prophylaxis for *T. gondii*.[12] The increased use of prophylaxis with these agents has significantly decreased the incidence of *Toxoplasma* encephalitis.[2,12] The double-strength TMP-SMX tablet once daily is recommended as the first-line prophylaxis. Data do not support the use of macrolides or aerosolized pentamidine for *Toxoplasma* prophylaxis. Similarly, data are conflicting regarding the efficacy of pyrimethamine as monotherapy for primary prophylaxis.[62,63]

Primary prophylaxis may be discontinued in patients who have responded to HAART with an increase in the CD4 counts to greater than 200 for more than 3 months. In addition, data support reinstituting primary prophylaxis when CD4 counts drop below 200.

W.O. is currently receiving inhaled pentamidine for PCP prophylaxis. Considering his CD4 count and IgG seropositivity, he should have received primary prophylaxis for *T. gondii*.

Treatment

ACUTE THERAPY

CASE 77-2, QUESTION 4: How should W.O.'s presumptive *Toxoplasma* encephalitis be treated?

The first-line treatment of acute *Toxoplasma* encephalitis consists of a combination of sulfadiazine 4 g/day in three or four daily divided doses and pyrimethamine as a single 200-mg loading dose, followed by 50 to 75 mg/day as a single daily dose plus leucovorin 10 to 25 mg PO every day.[12] Induction therapy should be continued for 6 weeks after resolution of symptoms (a treatment course of approximately 8 weeks) followed by maintenance therapy (secondary prophylaxis). Sulfadiazine toxicity may limit the completion of a full course of therapy in as many as 40% of patients.[64] However, successful desensitization has been documented.[65] W.O.'s clinical and radiologic response should be monitored closely, and other diagnoses should be considered if there is no improvement.

Alternative therapy includes pyrimethamine plus leucovorin with clindamycin 600 to 900 mg IV every 6 hours or 600 mg PO every 6 hours for at least 6 weeks. One controlled trial compared the efficacy and tolerability of pyrimethamine plus sulfadiazine versus pyrimethamine plus clindamycin. Although both regimens were effective, pyrimethamine–sulfadiazine was superior to pyrimethamine–clindamycin. The rate of adverse events was similar with both regimens; however, pyrimethamine–clindamycin led to fewer discontinuations than pyrimethamine–sulfadiazine (11% vs. 30%, respectively).[66] TMP-SMX may be considered a treatment option, particularly in patients who cannot take an oral regimen because the only widely available parenteral sulfonamide is the sulfamethoxazole component of TMP-SMX. However, there is less in vitro activity and less clinical data to support the use of TMP-SMX as monotherapy for toxoplasmosis.[67] Additionally, anticonvulsants should be given to patients with *Toxoplasma* encephalitis and a history of seizures, and corticosteroids may be warranted for focal lesions or edema but should be used cautiously.

CASE 77-2, QUESTION 5: W.O. is treated with sulfadiazine–pyrimethamine. What are the limitations to the use of the sulfadiazine component for the treatment of *Toxoplasma* encephalitis?

As with other sulfonamides in HIV-infected patients, rashes commonly occur with sulfadiazine therapy.[64] Similar to TMP-SMX, various desensitization regimens have been recommended[40,65]; however, it may be simpler to use alternative regimens.

Renal function should be monitored throughout therapy. Elevated serum creatinine (SCr) levels, hematuria, or decreased urine output may occur secondary to sulfadiazine-induced crystalluria. The water solubility of sulfadiazine is less than that of other sulfonamides; therefore, hydration (2–3 L/day) is needed to prevent crystalline nephropathy, and aggressive hydration and alkalinization can be used in cases of crystal formation.

CASE 77-2, QUESTION 6: What toxicities are associated with the pyrimethamine component?

Pyrimethamine can suppress bone marrow function; thus, concomitant therapy with other medications that suppress marrow function (e.g., zidovudine [AZT] or ganciclovir) may not be tolerated. Leucovorin (10–25 mg/day) is always given in conjunction with pyrimethamine to maintain bone marrow function, although it may not always be successful. Leucovorin doses can be increased to 50 to 100 mg/day in divided doses if needed to reverse bone marrow suppression.[12] Folic acid (not folinic acid) should be avoided because it can be used for growth by protozoal organisms, potentially antagonizing pyrimethamine–sulfadiazine activity.[68] Vitamin preparations containing large quantities of folic acid should be discontinued during therapy for *T. gondii*.

W.O. is not taking any medications that would make him particularly susceptible to the myelosuppressive effects of pyrimethamine, and he is not neutropenic. Consequently, he should be given sulfadiazine and pyrimethamine.

SUPPRESSIVE THERAPY (SECONDARY PROPHYLAXIS)

CASE 77-2, QUESTION 7: Once W.O. has completed acute therapy for his *Toxoplasma* encephalitis, should he receive suppressive therapy?

Most antiprotozoal agents do not eradicate the cyst form of *T. gondii*. Therefore, patients should be administered lifelong suppressive therapy unless immune reconstitution occurs as a consequence of HAART.[12] A commonly used regimen for patients who cannot tolerate sulfonamides is pyrimethamine plus clindamycin. However, only the combination of pyrimethamine plus sulfadiazine provides protection against PCP as well. Additionally, two small studies of patients receiving maintenance therapy for *Toxoplasma* encephalitis have suggested that sulfadiazine–pyrimethamine is more effective than clindamycin–pyrimethamine or pyrimethamine alone.[66] The use of atovaquone with or without pyrimethamine is also effective as prophylaxis for both *Toxoplasma* and PCP, but it is significantly more expensive and is only available as a less palatable liquid formulation.

Patients receiving secondary prophylaxis are at a low risk for recurrence of *Toxoplasma* encephalitis when they have completed their initial therapy, remain asymptomatic, and have a sustained increase in their CD4 count to greater than 200 after more than 6 months of HAART. Clinicians may obtain a brain MRI as part of the evaluation to determine the end point of therapy. Discontinuation of primary and secondary toxoplasmosis prophylaxis is safe if patients are receiving HAART and their CD4 count has increased to greater than 200 for at least 3 months. Secondary prophylaxis should be reintroduced if the CD4 count decreases to less than 200.[12]

W.O. will be continued on sulfadiazine–pyrimethamine for suppressive therapy for his *Toxoplasma* encephalitis because his CD4 count has decreased to less than 100. W.O. is currently receiving aerosolized pentamidine for PCP prophylaxis, but because sulfadiazine–pyrimethamine is also protective against PCP, the aerosolized pentamidine can be discontinued. Clindamycin–pyrimethamine is an inferior option because it does not protect against PCP.[12]

ALTERNATIVE THERAPIES

CASE 77-2, QUESTION 8: What treatment options exist for patients who cannot tolerate sulfadiazine and do not wish to undergo desensitization?

Clindamycin 1,200 mg IV or PO every 6 hours or 600 mg PO every 6 hours plus pyrimethamine and leucovorin at standard doses.[12] Combination therapy with pyrimethamine and leucovorin plus azithromycin (1.2–1.5 g/day), clarithromycin (1 g BID), or atovaquone (750 mg PO 4 times a day) has shown promise in a limited numbers of patients.[12]

CYTOMEGALOVIRUS DISEASE

Diagnosis

CASE 77-3

QUESTION 1: P.Z., a 39-year-old man with AIDS, complains of floating spots, light flashes, and difficulty reading road signs when he drives. His most recent laboratory results were as follows:

BUN, 17 mg/dL
SCr, 0.8 mg/dL
CD4 count, 40 cells/μL
Viral load, 80,000 copies/mL (3 months ago)
WBC count, 1,200 cells/L, with 63% polymorphonuclear neutrophil leukocytes

His current weight is 63 kg. P.Z.'s medications include tenofovir, emtricitabine, atazanavir, ritonavir, dapsone (PCP prophylaxis), and azithromycin (MAC prophylaxis). He has a history of hematologic intolerance to AZT and TMP-SMX. P.Z. is known to have a positive CMV IgG antibody titer. Funduscopic examination reveals alternating areas of hemorrhage and scar tissue (a "cottage cheese and ketchup" appearance) in the proximity of the retina in his left eye.

What is the likely cause of P.Z.'s visual problems?

P.Z. has an inflammation of the retina (retinitis), most likely because of CMV. Many HIV-infected patients have been previously infected with CMV, and reactivation typically occurs when CD4 counts are less than 50. Before HAART, the prevalence of CMV disease in patients with AIDS was 30%; however, the incidence of new cases of CMV end-organ disease has declined by 75% to 80% since the advent of HAART and is estimated to be less than 6 cases per 100 person-years.[12,69] Although CMV can cause colitis, pneumonitis, esophagitis, hepatitis, and neurologic disease, retinitis is the most common manifestation of active infection in AIDS patients, accounting for 75% to 85% of CMV end-organ disease. One investigation describing patients with CMV retinitis in the post-HAART era found a diverse demographic group with infection; most of them had received HAART, and as expected, they had very low CD4 counts.[70] In addition, the characteristics of the disease in this group were similar to those in the pre-HAART era. Diagnosis is usually presumptive because biopsy is difficult given the inaccessibility of the retina. Serology is indicative of previous CMV infection, but not an active disease. Cultures (serum, urine, and saliva) may be useful for monitoring therapy, considering that patients frequently have disseminated CMV disease. Patients with positive cultures for CMV while receiving therapy may be at a higher risk for relapse.[71] Typically, the diagnosis of CMV retinitis is based on observations made during a dilated retinal examination and indirect ophthalmoscopy, as was done for P.Z. Lesions appear as fluffy, white retinal patches with retinal hemorrhage.

Once CMV retinitis is diagnosed, the patient should be thoroughly examined for extraocular CMV disease. P.Z. will require regular ophthalmologic examinations, along with retinal photographs, for life. As with HIV therapy, CMV deoxyribonucleic acid (DNA) quantification in plasma or blood cells by polymerase chain reaction may have a role in evaluating treatment efficacy and predicting symptomatic development of CMV disease.[12]

Drug Therapy

CASE 77-3, QUESTION 2: What are the treatment options for CMV retinitis, and which one would be preferred for P.Z.?

Several treatment options exist for CMV retinitis: oral valganciclovir, IV ganciclovir, IV ganciclovir followed by oral valganciclovir, IV foscarnet, and IV cidofovir. Alternatives include combined IV ganciclovir plus foscarnet or intraocular injections of ganciclovir, foscarnet, or cidofovir.[12] The efficacy of combined parenteral ganciclovir and foscarnet is similar to that in monotherapy, but it is more toxic. This latter therapy should be reserved for patients with refractory disease (Table 77-3).[72]

Intraocular implants and intraocular injections of ganciclovir have similar efficacy in the treatment of CMV retinitis, but their benefit is localized to the infected eye and may lead to an increased risk of contralateral retinitis and extraocular CMV disease. Regimens consisting of systemic anti-CMV therapy have been associated with a 50% reduction in mortality compared with those using intraocular therapy alone.[73] Therefore, concomitant systemic anti-CMV therapy is recommended (e.g., oral valganciclovir or IV ganciclovir). The use of ganciclovir intraocular implants with oral valganciclovir has shown to be more effective at preventing relapse of retinitis than IV ganciclovir and likely oral valganciclovir.[12] Many providers prefer this as the first-line therapy in patients with immediate sight-threatening lesions, although others chose oral valganciclovir as the first-line treatment. The choice of agents typically depends on drug efficacy, toxicity, stage of disease, and quality-of-life issues.

GANCICLOVIR

Ganciclovir is an acyclic nucleoside with CMV activity superior to acyclovir. Similar to other nucleosides, ganciclovir must be taken into cells and phosphorylated before it can compete with endogenous nucleotides for binding to viral DNA polymerase. Ganciclovir is poorly absorbed PO (bioavailability, approximately 5%–9%), and the oral form is no longer marketed. The disposition of ganciclovir is biexponential after IV administration (terminal half-life, approximately 2.5 hours). The total body clearance is highly dependent on glomerular filtration and tubular secretion.

The dose-limiting toxicity is bone marrow suppression, with neutropenia occurring in approximately 50% of patients. Thrombocytopenia is also observed. Absolute neutrophil counts (ANCs) and platelets should be monitored weekly during ganciclovir therapy. If the ANC falls to less than 1,000 cells/μL or the platelet count falls to less than 50,000/μL, the monitoring frequency should be increased to twice weekly.[27,74] Ganciclovir is also available as an intraocular implant (Table 77-3). Dosage adjustments must be made in patients with renal dysfunction (Table 77-4).

Patients who develop ganciclovir-induced bone marrow suppression can be given granulocyte colony-stimulating factor (G-CSF). Both G-CSF (filgrastim) and granulocyte-macrophage colony-stimulating factor (GM-CSF [sargramostim])[75,76] have been used successfully in stimulating production of WBC. Although neither of these agents is FDA-approved for this indication, the use of the CSFs may allow for continuation of sight-saving or life-prolonging therapy. Because GM-CSF may stimulate HIV replication in macrophage cell lines,[77] patients should receive concomitant antiretroviral therapy.

VALGANCICLOVIR

Valganciclovir is an oral monovalyl ester prodrug that is rapidly hydrolyzed to ganciclovir. The absolute bioavailability of ganciclovir

Table 77-3
Treatment of Cytomegalovirus Retinitis

	IV Ganciclovir	Valganciclovir	IV Foscarnet	Combination IV Ganciclovir and IV Foscarnet Sodium	IV Cidofovir
Dosing regimens	*Induction:* 5 mg/kg every 12 hours for 14–21 days	*Induction:* 900 mg every 12 hours for 14–21 days	*Induction:* 90 mg/kg every 12 hours for 14–21 days	*Prior ganciclovir induction:* both IV foscarnet 90 mg/kg every 12 hours and IV ganciclovir 5 mg/kg daily for 14–21 days	*Induction:* 5 mg/kg every week for 2 weeks
	Maintenance: 5 mg/kg daily	*Maintenance:* 900 mg daily	*Maintenance:* 90–120 mg/kg daily; 750–1,000 mL of 0.9% saline or D_5W solution with each dose	*Maintenance:* both IV foscarnet 90–120 mg/kg and IV ganciclovir 5 mg/kg daily	
	Refractory disease induction: 7.5 mg/kg every 12 hours for 14–21 days	*Alternative regimen:* with ganciclovir intraocular implant 900 mg daily		*Prior foscarnet sodium induction:* both IV ganciclovir 5 mg/kg every 12 hours and IV foscarnet 90–120 mg/kg daily	
	Maintenance: 10 mg/kg daily (*Note:* dosage should be adjusted for creatinine clearance <70 mL/minute; see Table 77-4)			*Reinduction:* IV ganciclovir 5 mg/kg and IV foscarnet 90 mg/kg every 12 hours for 14–21 days	
Select adverse effects	Neutropenia, thrombocytopenia, and catheter sepsis	Same as ganciclovir	Nephrotoxicity, electrolyte abnormalities, anemia, catheter sepsis, nausea/irritability, and genital ulceration	Same as IV ganciclovir and IV foscarnet	Nephrotoxicity, neutropenia, probenecid adverse effects (rash, fever, nausea, and fatigue), uveitis, alopecia, and hypotonia
Important drug interactions	Neutropenia, with AZT, cancer chemotherapy didanosine levels	Same as ganciclovir	Nephrotoxicity with other nephrotoxic drugs (e.g., amphotericin B, aminoglycosides, and IV pentamidine)	Same as IV ganciclovir and IV foscarnet	Nephrotoxicity with other nephrotoxic drugs (e.g., amphotericin B, aminoglycosides, IV pentamidine, and NSAIDs) Probenecid: Level of most proximal tubular excreted drugs
Adjunctive therapy	G-CSF/GM-CSF effective for neutropenia	Same as ganciclovir	IV or oral hydration essential; potassium, calcium/magnesium supplements, and antiemetics may be required	Same as both IV ganciclovir and IV foscarnet	Probenecid and IV hydration essential; antiemetics, antihistamine, and acetaminophen premedication commonly used for probenecid toxicity
Advantages	Systemic therapy; anti-HSV activity	Increased bioavailability and decreased pill count compared with PO ganciclovir	Systemic therapy; anti-HSV (acyclovir-resistant) activity; anti-HIV activity	Increased efficacy compared with either IV ganciclovir or IV foscarnet alone; improved response for relapsed disease	Systemic therapy; no indwelling catheter required; infrequent dosing
Disadvantages	Hematologic toxicity; requires daily infusions; and indwelling catheter	Must have adequate GI absorption; less clinical data than with ganciclovir	Nephrotoxicity; requires daily infusions/indwelling catheter; supplemental hydration required; prolonged infusion time; and requires infusion pump or controlled rate infusion device	Same as IV ganciclovir and IV foscarnet; prolonged daily infusion time and impact on quality of life	Requires probenecid and IV hydration; probenecid toxicity; and nephrotoxicity (may be prolonged)

Table 77-3
Treatment of Cytomegalovirus Retinitis (*continued*)

Monitoring requirement	*Induction therapy:* (a) CBC with WBC differential, platelet count weekly; (b) SCr weekly	Same as ganciclovir	*Induction therapy:* (a) SCr twice weekly; (b) serum Ca^{2+}, albumin Mg^{2+}, phosphates, and K^+ twice weekly; and (c) Hgb and Hct weekly	Same as both IV ganciclovir and IV foscarnet	Within 48 hours before each induction and maintenance: (a) SCr quantitation proteinuria; and (b) WBC with differential cell count; monitor intraocular pressure and slit-lamp examination at least monthly
	Maintenance therapy: (a) CBC with WBC differential, platelet count weekly; and (b) SCr every 24 weeks		*Maintenance therapy:* (a) SCr weekly; (b) serum Ca^{2+}, albumin Mg^{2+}, phosphates, and K^+ weekly; and (c) Hgb and Hct every 24 weeks		
Precautions and contraindications	Moderate-to-severe thrombocytopenia (platelet counts $<25 \times 10^{10}$/L)	Same as ganciclovir	Concomitant use with other nephrotoxic drugs (e.g., amphotericin B, aminoglycosides, or IV pentamidine) or in patients with preexisting moderate-to-severe renal insufficiency (SCr >168 mmol/L or creatinine clearance <50 mL/minute)	Same as both IV ganciclovir and IV foscarnet	Same as IV foscarnet except parameters are baseline SCr level (>1.5 mg/dL) or creatinine clearance (<55 mL/minute), or 2+ proteinuria (after IV fluid); discontinue therapy for 3+ proteinuria, if SCr level increases by 0.5 mg/dL above baseline, or intraocular pressure decreases by 50% of baseline value

AZT, zidovudine; CBC, complete blood count; CMV, cytomegalovirus; G-CSF, granulocyte colony-stimulating factor; D_5W, 5% dextrose in water solution; GI, gastrointestinal; GM-CSF, granulocyte-macrophage colony-stimulating factor; Hct, hematocrit; Hgb, hemoglobin; HIV, human immunodeficiency virus; HSV, herpes simplex virus; IV, intravenously; NSAIDs, nonsteroidal anti-inflammatory drugs; PO, orally; SCr, serum creatinine; WBC, white blood cells.

Source: Whitley RJ et al. Guidelines for the treatment of cytomegalovirus diseases in patients with AIDS in the era of potent antiretroviral therapy: recommendations of an international panel. International AIDS Society-USA. *Arch Intern Med*. 1998;158:957; Panel on Opportunistic Infections in HIV-infected Adults and Adolescents. Guidelines for prevention and treatment of opportunistic infections in HIV-infected adults and adolescents: recommendations from CDC, the National Institutes of Health, and the HIV Medicine Association of the Infectious Diseases Society of America. **https://aidsinfo.nih.gov/guidelines/html/4/adult-and-adolescent-oi-prevention-and-treatment-guidelines/**; and product information.

from valganciclovir is 60%, and a dose of 900 mg results in ganciclovir blood concentrations similar to those obtained with a dose of 5 mg/kg of IV ganciclovir. Oral valganciclovir and IV ganciclovir are equally effective as induction therapy for newly diagnosed CMV retinitis in patients with AIDS.[78] The frequency and severity of adverse events were similar in the two groups. Based on these data, oral valganciclovir is as effective as and no more toxic than IV ganciclovir, and the convenience of the oral route suggests it be the drug of choice for the long-term management of CMV retinitis in patients with AIDS.

CIDOFOVIR

Cidofovir is a nucleotide analog that is phosphorylated intracellularly to an active diphosphate metabolite. It is the most potent of all the available anti-CMV compounds and is active against herpes simplex virus (HSV) and VZV, including acyclovir-resistant isolates. Cidofovir does not require viral activation. Because nucleotide analogs do not require virally encoded kinases for their activity, they remain a treatment option for patients who have failed to respond to ganciclovir. Cidofovir is poorly absorbed PO (bioavailability, <5%) and has an intracellular half-life of 17 to 65 hours, resulting in once-weekly induction and every-other-week maintenance therapy.

Eighty percent of this poorly soluble agent is excreted unchanged in the urine via filtration and tubular secretion. Cidofovir is nephrotoxic; however, the administration of probenecid (2 g administered 3 hours before the start of infusion and two 1-g doses administered at 2 and 8 hours after infusion) blocks tubular secretion and reduces nephrotoxicity. Prehydration with 1 L of normal saline is required 1 hour before each dose and, if tolerated, repeated concomitantly with or after the cidofovir infusion. Because nephrotoxicity is the most significant dose-limiting toxicity, other nephrotoxic agents should be discontinued (e.g., nonsteroidal anti-inflammatory drugs, and aminoglycosides), and renal function should be carefully monitored throughout therapy (BUN, SCr, and proteinuria; Table 77-4). Dosage adjustment must accompany any deterioration in renal function (Table 77-5).

The CBC should be checked at baseline because neutropenia has been reported in approximately 20% of patients in clinical trials. Hypotony (reduction in intraocular pressure) and uveitis (inflammation of the uveal tract of the eye) have also been reported. Thus, monthly ophthalmologic examinations of the retina are necessary.[12]

The role of cidofovir is limited. Although it offers the advantage of weekly and biweekly dosing, its toxicity greatly limits its utility. Cidofovir appears to be as efficacious as foscarnet and ganciclovir

Table 77-4
Dosage Adjustment for Cytomegalovirus Medications

Drug	Normal Dosage	CrCl (mL/minute/1.73 m^2)	Adjusted Dosage			
Cidofovir	*Induction dose:* 5 mg/kg IV QW × 2 doses	Increase in SCr of 0.3–0.4 above baseline	3 mg/kg per dose			
	Maintenance dose: 5 mg/kg IV QOW	Increase in SCr of 0.5 above baseline or 3+ proteinuria	Discontinue cidofovir			
		Cidofovir is contraindicated in patients with preexisting renal failure: 1. SCr concentrations >1.5 mg/dL 2. Calculated CrCl of <55 mL/minute 3. Urine protein 100 mg/dL (>2+ proteinuria)				
			Induction Dose		Maintenance Dose	
Foscarnet	*Induction dose:*	CrCl (mL/minute/kg)	Low Dose	High Dose	Low Dose	High Dose
	IV every 8 hours to 90 mg/kg	>1.4	60 mg/kg every 8 hours	90 mg/kg every 12 hours	90 mg/kg every 24 hours	120 mg/kg every 24 hours
	IV every 12 hours	1.0–1.4	45 mg/kg every 8 hours	70 mg/kg every 12 hours	70 mg/kg every 24 hours	90 mg/kg every 24 hours
	Maintenance dose: 90–120 mg/kg IV daily	0.8–1.0	50 mg/kg every 12 hours	50 mg/kg every 12 hours	50 mg/kg every 24 hours	65 mg/kg every 24 hours
		0.6–0.8	40 mg/kg every 12 hours	80 mg/kg every 24 hours	80 mg/kg every 48 hours	105 mg/kg every 48 hours
		0.5–0.6	60 mg/kg every 24 hours	60 mg/kg every 24 hours	60 mg/kg every 48 hours	80 mg/kg every 48 hours
		0.4–0.5	50 mg/kg every 24 hours	50 mg/kg every 24 hours	50 mg/kg every 48 hours	65 mg/kg every 48 hours
		<0.4	Not recommended		Not recommended	

Ganciclovir			Maintenance dose	
	IV			
	Induction dose: 5 mg/kg every 12 hours	CrCl (mL/minute)	Induction dose	Maintenance dose
		>70	5 mg/kg every 12 hours	5 mg/kg every 24 hours
	Maintenance dose: 5 mg/kg daily or 6 mg/kg daily × 5 day/week	50–69	2.5 mg/kg every 12 hours	2.5 mg/kg every 24 hours
		25–49	2.5 mg/kg every 24 hours	1.25 mg/kg every 24 hours
		10–24	1.25 mg/kg every 24 hours	0.625 mg/kg every 24 hours
		<10	1.25 mg/kg 3 × every week after hemodialysis	0.625 mg/kg 3 × every week after hemodialysis
Valganciclovir	*Induction dose:* 900 mg PO BID	CrCl (mL/minute)	Induction dose	Maintenance dose
	Maintenance dose: 900 mg PO daily	40–59	450 mg BID	450 mg daily
		25–39	450 mg daily	450 mg every other day
		10–25	450 mg every other day	450 mg BIW
		Hemodialysis	Not recommended	Not recommended

BID, twice a day; BIW, twice a week; CrCl, creatinine clearance; IV, intravenously; PO, orally; QOW, every other week; QW, weekly; SCr, serum creatinine; TID, three times a day; TIW, three times a week.

Source: Safrin S et al. Comparison of three regimens for treatment of mild to moderate *Pneumocystis carinii* pneumonia in patients with AIDS. A double-blind, randomized, trial of oral trimethoprim-sulfamethoxazole, dapsone-trimethoprim, and clindamycin-primaquine. ACTG 108 Study Group. *Ann Intern Med*. 1996;124:792; Lee BL et al. Dapsone, trimethoprim, and sulfamethoxazole plasma levels during treatment of *Pneumocystis* pneumonia in patients with the acquired immunodeficiency syndrome (AIDS). Evidence of drug interactions. *Ann Intern Med*. 1989;110:606; Panel on Opportunistic Infections in HIV-infected Adults and Adolescents. Guidelines for prevention and treatment of opportunistic infections in HIV-infected adults and adolescents: recommendations from CDC, the National Institutes of Health, and the HIV Medicine Association of the Infectious Diseases Society of America. **https://aidsinfo.nih.gov/guidelines/html/4/adult-and-adolescent-oi-prevention-and-treatment-guidelines/**; and product information.

Table 77-5
Tuberculosis Treatment Recommendations for Patients Coinfected with HIV and Tuberculosis

Induction	Maintenance	Comments
Rifampin-Based Therapy (no concurrent use of PIs, Nevirapine, Etravirine, Rilpivirine, or Elvitegravir)		
INH/RIF (OR RFB)/PZA/EMB (or SM) daily or 2–3 × per week × 2 months	INH/RIF (or RFB) daily or 2–3 × per week (duration dependent on location of TB)	RIF-containing regimens may have significant drug–drug interactions with antiretrovirals.

EMB, ethambutol; INH, isoniazid; NNRTI, non-nucleoside reverse transcriptase inhibitor; PI, protease inhibitor; PZA, pyrazinamide; RFB, rifabutin; RIF, rifampin; SM, streptomycin.

Source: Panel on Opportunistic Infections in HIV-infected Adults and Adolescents. Guidelines for prevention and treatment of opportunistic infections in HIV-infected adults and adolescents: recommendations from CDC, the National Institutes of Health, and the HIV Medicine Association of the Infectious Diseases Society of America. https://aidsinfo.nih.gov/guidelines/html/4/adult-and-adolescent-oi-prevention-and-treatment-guidelines/.

in the treatment of CMV retinitis, but limited comparative studies have been performed. Finally, the efficacy of cidofovir in the treatment of extraocular CMV (e.g., GI disease, pneumonitis, and encephalitis) remains to be established.

FOSCARNET

Foscarnet is a pyrophosphate analog that acts by selectively inhibiting viral DNA polymerases and reverse transcriptase. At doses currently recommended for induction therapy (60 mg/kg every 8 hours or 90 mg/kg IV every 12 hours), peak plasma foscarnet concentrations are higher than those that inhibit CMV in vitro (Table 77-4).[79] The dose-limiting toxicity of foscarnet is nephrotoxicity, probably because its poor solubility results in crystallization in nephrons.[74] In one trial, when compared with ganciclovir, patients treated with foscarnet survived approximately 4 months longer; however, foscarnet-treated patients with reduced creatinine clearance (<1.2 mL/minute/kg) had a poorer survival rate.[80]

Because P.Z. has a low ANC, the bone marrow–suppressive effects of ganciclovir and valganciclovir are of concern. Adjunctive therapy with G-CSF is an option. Because he has good renal function (SCr, 0.8 mg/dL), foscarnet or cidofovir would be an option.

Nephrotoxicity

CASE 77-3, QUESTION 3: P.Z. will receive foscarnet, 90 mg/kg IV for 2 hours every 12 hours. How can the risk of nephrotoxicity be minimized?

During foscarnet therapy, adequate hydration is important to prevent nephrotoxicity. To establish diuresis, 750 to 1,000 mL of normal saline or 5% dextrose should be administered before the first infusion of foscarnet. With subsequent infusions, 500 to 1,000 mL should be administered, depending on the foscarnet dose. Careful dosage titration based on P.Z.'s estimated creatinine clearance may also minimize nephrotoxicity (Table 77-5). The SCr clearance should be measured at least twice weekly and the dosage should be recalculated if the creatinine clearance changes. CMV infection itself may also cause an acute increase in the SCr owing to acute interstitial nephritis. Drugs with nephrotoxic potential, such as amphotericin B or aminoglycosides, should be avoided.

Adverse Effects

CASE 77-3, QUESTION 4: What toxicities other than nephrotoxicity have been associated with foscarnet therapy?

Hypocalcemia can occur because foscarnet, a pyrophosphate analog, can bind to unbound calcium. Electrolyte complications can be minimized by avoiding high foscarnet plasma concentrations with slow infusions over 1 to 2 hours.[81] Unbound serum calcium and phosphate levels should be monitored twice weekly during induction therapy and weekly during maintenance therapy, ideally when foscarnet is at its highest concentration. Fatal hypocalcemia has been reported in an AIDS patient receiving both foscarnet and parenteral pentamidine; thus, coadministration of these drugs should be avoided.[82]

Penile ulceration from foscarnet has been problematic, especially in uncircumcised men. Characterized as a fixed drug eruption, careful attention to genital hygiene may minimize the potential for penile ulceration. Other adverse events associated with foscarnet include seizures, hypomagnesemia, anemia, nausea, fever, and rash. Twice-weekly albumin, magnesium, and potassium levels are required during induction therapy and then weekly during maintenance therapy. In general, patients tolerate foscarnet less well than ganciclovir.[80]

Dosage Adjustments

CASE 77-3, QUESTION 5: After 12 days of foscarnet therapy, P.Z.'s SCr has increased from 0.8 to 1.2 mg/dL despite the coadministration of 2 L of normal saline daily. What dosage adjustments should be made for the remainder of the foscarnet treatment?

Valganciclovir, ganciclovir, foscarnet, and cidofovir are highly dependent on renal elimination, and dosages (or dosing intervals) should be adjusted for even a modest reduction in renal function (Table 77-5). Therefore, careful monitoring of renal function is important throughout CMV therapy. P.Z.'s estimated creatinine clearance is 1.2 mL/minute/kg; therefore, his foscarnet induction dosage should be adjusted to 70 mg/kg IV every 12 hours (Table 77-5).[12]

Suppression Therapy

CASE 77-3, QUESTION 6: P.Z. completes 21 days of foscarnet induction therapy. How can his CMV retinitis be suppressed in the future?

The currently available antiviral agents used to treat CMV disease are not curative. After induction therapy, chronic maintenance therapy is indicated for the remainder of P.Z.'s life, unless immune reconstitution occurs as a result of HAART. Effective suppressive regimens include parenteral or oral ganciclovir, parenteral foscarnet, combined parenteral ganciclovir and foscarnet, and parenteral cidofovir. The ganciclovir implant was also effective but is no longer manufactured (Table 77-4). Oral valganciclovir is approved for both acute induction and maintenance therapy, but the published clinical data are limited. In uncontrolled case series, repeated intravitreal injections of ganciclovir, foscarnet, and cidofovir have been shown to be effective for prophylaxis of CMV retinitis. However, because this therapy is effective only locally and does not protect the contralateral eye or other organ systems, it is usually combined with oral valganciclovir.

Guidelines suggest that discontinuation of prophylaxis may be considered in patients with CMV retinitis who are taking HAART with a sustained (>6 months) increase in the CD4 count to greater than 100 to 150 and have remained disease-free for more than 30 weeks. The decision to discontinue suppression should be based on the magnitude and duration of the CD4 increase and viral load suppression, the anatomic location of the retinal lesions, and the degree of vision loss.[12] All patients who have had anti-CMV maintenance therapy discontinued should continue to undergo regular ophthalmologic monitoring for early detection of CMV relapse as well as for immune reconstitution uveitis.

Relapse or Refractory Cytomegalovirus Retinitis

CASE 77-3, QUESTION 7: After 5 months of maintenance therapy with foscarnet, a routine funduscopic examination reveals retinal CMV disease progression. How should P.Z.'s retinitis be managed at this time?

Most patients with CMV not receiving HAART while undergoing maintenance treatment eventually relapse.[12] For the first relapse, repeat induction therapy followed by maintenance therapy with the same drug is beneficial in most patients. Because P.Z. has tolerated foscarnet therapy thus far, he should receive another course of induction therapy. After reinduction, P.Z. should receive a higher maintenance dosage (120 mg/kg/day).[12]

It is important to distinguish between relapse and refractory disease. Relapse, as in the case of P.Z., is defined as the recurrence of clinically apparent viral activity and is usually caused by a decline in immune function, insufficient delivery of drug into the eye, or resistant CMV strains. Relapse can effectively be managed by repeat induction therapy of the same drug. If the relapse is caused by a resistant virus, the patient may benefit from a change in therapy. Ganciclovir-resistant CMV strains occur by two mechanisms. DNA polymerase mutation at the *UL54* gene is observed in approximately 20% of ganciclovir-resistant strains. This mutation usually confers resistance to cidofovir and, to a lesser extent, foscarnet.[12] Most ganciclovir-resistant CMV strains have *UL97* mutations. *UL97* mutations are incapable of monophosphorylating ganciclovir. Cidofovir and foscarnet are appropriate alternatives to treat strains with *UL97* mutations. Patients who receive extensive ganciclovir treatment (>6–9 months) may present with highly ganciclovir-resistant strains containing *UL54* and *UL97* mutations.[83] Cidofovir may be considered in most patients who relapse while receiving ganciclovir or foscarnet. Although ganciclovir-resistant and foscarnet-resistant strains of CMV have been reported, their precise role in the clinical failure of these regimens is not known. Because of the different mechanisms of action of ganciclovir and foscarnet, strains resistant to one drug may retain sensitivity to the other.[84] Resistant or relapsing CMV retinitis may be treated by the administration of local ocular therapy via intravitreal injection of ganciclovir or foscarnet (see Local Treatment section).

Refractory CMV retinitis is defined by disease progression because of ineffective therapy. This phenomenon is observed in two clinical situations: when the disease persists with minimal or no response during induction therapy and when long-term control is inadequate with maintenance therapy. Refractory CMV disease has been defined in clinical trials as two relapses occurring within 10 weeks despite repeat induction and maintenance therapy. Treatment options for refractory CMV retinitis include reinduction with ganciclovir at higher dosages (7.5 mg/kg/dose every 12 hours, followed by maintenance doses of 10 mg/kg/day) or reinduction using combination therapy (IV ganciclovir plus foscarnet).[27] Refractory CMV retinitis can be treated with local ocular therapy via intravitreal injection of ganciclovir or foscarnet.[12]

Local Treatment

CASE 77-3, QUESTION 8: What is the role of intravitreal injections in CMV retinitis?

INTRAVITREAL INJECTIONS

Intravitreal administration of ganciclovir or foscarnet through a small-gauge needle is a method of selectively delivering the drug to the site of infection. Ganciclovir and foscarnet doses of 0.2 to 2 mg and 1.2 to 2 mg, respectively, are administered 2 or 3 times per week for active disease, followed by weekly maintenance injections.[27] Potential complications of intravitreal injections include bacterial endophthalmitis, vitreous hemorrhage, and retinal detachment. Intravitreal therapy is relatively uncommon because intraocular implants are available. Importantly, in contrast to systemic therapy, local instillation of a drug is associated with a higher risk of CMV disease developing in the contralateral eye as well as extraocular sites (Table 77-3).

Intraocular Ganciclovir Implants

CASE 77-3, QUESTION 9: Is P.Z. a candidate for ganciclovir intraocular implants?

The ganciclovir implant (no longer manufactured) was a surgically implanted reservoir of ganciclovir very effective in less severe vision loss, but ocular complications including cataract, vitreous hemorrhage, and retinal detachment were common.[85]

P.Z. should be reinduced with foscarnet therapy and maintained on a higher foscarnet dose. Neither alternating regimens nor intravitreal administration of antiviral agents is appropriate at present.

Valganciclovir

CASE 77-3, QUESTION 10: What is the role of valganciclovir for initial CMV prevention?

Valganciclovir has replaced oral ganciclovir, which is no longer marketed. This agent yields an area under the curve approximately equivalent to that associated with the IV administration of ganciclovir. The maintenance dosage is two 450-mg tablets of valganciclovir once daily.

Data from clinical trials conducted with oral ganciclovir have been extrapolated to valganciclovir, and all references in the OI treatment guidelines to oral ganciclovir have been substituted with valganciclovir. The role of oral ganciclovir for primary prophylaxis of CMV retinitis has been evaluated in two studies.[86,87] Oral ganciclovir decreased the 1-year incidence of disease by approximately 50% in one study[87] but was ineffective in another.[86] These two studies had important differences in study design that likely explains the disparate results. One cost-effectiveness study estimated that oral ganciclovir prophylaxis would cost more than $1.7 million per year of anticipated life expectancy.[88] Valganciclovir has not demonstrated a survival advantage in patients with CD4 count less than 50 using it for CMV primary prevention.[12] These issues, in addition to adverse effects such as neutropenia and anemia, the lack of proven survival benefit in HIV-infected patients, and the risk for inducing CMV resistance, are concerns that should be addressed when deciding whether to institute prophylaxis in individual patients. Prophylaxis with valganciclovir is not recommended as the standard of care (Table 77-2).[12]

CRYPTOCOCCOSIS

Clinical Presentation and Prognosis

CASE 77-4

QUESTION 1: A.S., aged 28, is infected with HIV. She weighs 48 kg. Her boyfriend was an IV drug user who died of AIDS 2 years ago. She presents with a fever (103°F) and a 2-week history of "splitting headaches." Laboratory test results include the following:

Hemoglobin, 11.2 g/dL
WBC count, 4,100 cells/μL
Platelets, 73,000/L
SCr, 0.9 mg/dL
Glucose, 94 mg/dL
CD4 count, 47 cells/μL

A.S. is highly nonadherent and has not been to the clinic in more than a year, at which time she was prescribed tenofovir, emtricitabine, atazanavir, and ritonavir. Physical examination reveals no nuchal rigidity. With the exception of moderate lethargy, her neurologic examination is unremarkable. Her chest radiograph and three sets of blood cultures for bacteria and fungi are negative. A computed tomography scan is nondiagnostic. Lumbar puncture reveals the following CSF findings:

Glucose, 45 mg/dL
Protein, 90 mg/dL
WBC count, 10 cells/μL
Cryptococcal antigen titer, 1:2,048 IU
Intracranial pressure (ICP), 24 cm H_2O (normal, 8–22 cm H_2O)

How is A.S.'s clinical presentation typical of a patient with AIDS and cryptococcal meningitis? What is her likely prognosis?

In the pre-HAART era, cryptococcosis developed in approximately 6% to 10% of AIDS patients in the United States, with meningitis being the most common clinical presentation.[89] In the era of HAART and azole prophylaxis, a significant decline in the incidence of cryptococcosis has been observed.[89] Based on a 2010 cohort study, cryptococcosis is the second most common CNS infection associated with AIDS.[2] The initial portal of entry is the lungs, where the organism is normally contained by an intact immune system. Cryptococcal disease typically develops in patients with profound defects in cell-mediated immunity (i.e., CD4 counts, <50). Unlike bacterial meningitis, cryptococcal CNS infection has a much more insidious onset; the most common symptoms are fever and headache. Less frequent signs and symptoms include nausea and vomiting, meningismus, photophobia, and altered mental status. Focal neurologic deficits and seizures are observed in less than 10% of patients. CSF glucose is decreased, whereas CSF proteins are usually elevated. CSF cryptococcal antigen titer and CSF culture are frequently positive. These findings, along with the clinical presentation, form the basis for the diagnosis. The overall outcome is poor, with a mean survival of 5 months in patients not receiving HAART. Relapse within 6 months occurs in 50% of patients who do not receive suppressive therapy. Altered mental status at baseline, CSF WBC count of less than 20 cells/μL, high CSF cryptococcal antigen titer (>1:1,000), and an elevated initial CSF opening pressure of greater than 20 cm H_2O have all been associated with a poor prognosis.[89]

A.S.'s CD4 count is 92. She has a temperature of 103°F and has experienced "splitting headaches" for about a week. Her clinical presentation is typical of an AIDS patient with cryptococcal meningitis. The CSF WBC count of 10 cells/μL, high cryptococcal antigen titer, and ICP greater than 20 cm H_2O suggest a poor prognosis.[90] If left untreated, cryptococcal meningitis is fatal.

Treatment

AMPHOTERICIN B

CASE 77-4, QUESTION 2: How should A.S.'s acute cryptococcal meningitis be managed?

The current treatment recommended for cryptococcal meningitis is amphotericin B, 0.7 mg/kg/day IV, plus flucytosine (100 mg/kg/day) given PO in four divided doses as induction therapy for 14 days. Once the patient is stable (e.g., afebrile, with the resolution of symptoms), then consolidation therapy with oral fluconazole 400 mg/day for 8 weeks or until CSF cultures are sterile can be initiated. After consolidation therapy, daily suppressive therapy with fluconazole 200 mg should be continued indefinitely unless immune reconstitution occurs with HAART.[90] Lipid-based formulations of amphotericin B (specifically liposomal amphotericin, dosed as 4–6 mg/kg/day) are also effective.[91,92]

Although the aforementioned regimen is highly effective, the ability to rapidly reduce A.S.'s ICP will also significantly improve her clinical course. Removal of 10 to 20 mL of spinal fluid by repeat lumbar puncture is recommended for patients with an ICP greater than 20 cm H_2O (A.S.'s ICP is 24 cm H_2O). An additional intervention to consider reducing A.S.'s elevated ICP is the insertion of an intraventricular shunt.[12]

CASE 77-4, QUESTION 3: What is the evidence for adding flucytosine to amphotericin B in the acute treatment of A.S.? What are the disadvantages of this combination?

Amphotericin B binds to sterols in the fungal cell membrane, resulting in leakage of cytoplasmic contents. Flucytosine is an antimetabolite type of antifungal drug that is activated by deamination within the fungal cells to 5-fluorouracil. It inhibits fungal protein synthesis by replacing uracil with 5-flurouracil in fungal RNA, and it also inhibits thymidylate synthase via 5-fluorodeoxy-uridine monophosphate, interfering with fungal DNA synthesis. Flucytosine, a purine analog, is approximately 10% converted to 5-fluorouracil, an antimetabolite, which is the mechanism for its potential bone marrow toxicity.

A classic prospective study conducted in HIV-negative patients favored the use of the combination.[93] The protocol randomly assigned patients to receive either amphotericin B monotherapy (0.4 mg/kg/day IV for 6 weeks followed by 0.8 mg/kg/day IV every other day for 4 weeks) or amphotericin B plus flucytosine (150 mg/kg/day PO divided every 6 hours) for 6 weeks. Fewer failures or relapses, more rapid CSF sterilization, and less nephrotoxicity occurred in the combination group, although overall mortality was not different. However, approximately one-fourth of the patients in the combination arm developed leukopenia, thrombocytopenia, or both.

If flucytosine is chosen as adjunctive therapy, renal function and CBCs should be monitored closely for these adverse effects. A.S. is at an increased risk of granulocytopenia because of her HIV infection and her concomitant myelotoxic AZT therapy.

The comparative trial forming the basis for the current recommendations for the treatment of acute cryptococcal meningitis in HIV-positive patients evaluated a higher dose of IV amphotericin B (0.7 mg/kg/day) with or without flucytosine given at a lower dose (25 mg/kg/dose PO every 6 hours) for 2 weeks.[90] The study evaluated 381 patients with an acute first episode of cryptococcal meningitis. The second part of this trial randomly reassigned stable or improved patients to either a fluconazole or an itraconazole treatment arm for an additional 8 weeks as consolidation therapy. Sixty percent and 51% of patients receiving amphotericin B plus flucytosine, and amphotericin B alone, respectively, had sterile CSF cultures at 2 weeks of therapy. No significant differences were noted between groups in the percentage of patients who were culture-negative at 2 weeks. Importantly, the addition of flucytosine to amphotericin B was not associated with a significant increase in drug toxicities at 2 weeks. Fluconazole and itraconazole were similar in efficacy. However, multivariate analysis revealed two factors that were independently associated with a higher rate of CSF sterilization: the addition of flucytosine and the randomization to fluconazole. A more recent trial randomized 299 patients to amphotericin B (1 mg/kg/day) for 4 weeks, amphotericin B (1 mg/kg/day) plus flucytosine (100 mg/kg/day divided) for 2 weeks, or amphotericin B (1 mg/kg/day) plus fluconazole (400 mg bid) for 2 weeks. Patients receiving amphotericin B and flucytosine had lower mortality rates and significantly increased rates of yeast clearance from CSF. Rates of adverse events were similar between groups with the exception of more frequent neutropenia in patients receiving a combination therapy. The addition of fluconazole provided no survival benefit.[94]

FLUCONAZOLE

CASE 77-4, QUESTION 4: Could A.S. be treated with fluconazole instead of amphotericin B for acute cryptococcal meningitis?

Fluconazole, one of the triazole antifungal agents, inhibits a fungal cytochrome P-450 enzyme necessary for the conversion of lanosterol to ergosterol. Without ergosterol, the fungal cell membrane becomes defective and loses its selective permeability properties. Unlike itraconazole, fluconazole is well absorbed PO even in the presence of an elevated gastric pH. Fluconazole has excellent CNS penetration and a good safety profile, but it is likely a secondary choice in the initial treatment of cryptococcal meningitis. In a prospective, randomized, multicenter trial, the National Institute of Allergy and Infectious Diseases Mycoses Study Group and the AIDS Clinical Trial Group compared amphotericin B with 200 mg/day of oral fluconazole (after a 400-mg loading dose) for 10 weeks in 194 patients.[95] The dose of amphotericin B (mean dose, 0.4–0.5 mg/kg/day) and the possible addition of flucytosine were left to the discretion of the individual investigators. Although the overall mortality was similar (14% for amphotericin B vs. 18% for fluconazole), more fluconazole-treated patients died during the first 2 weeks of treatment (15% vs. 8%; $p = 0.25$). Furthermore, the median time to the first negative CSF culture in the successfully treated patients was shorter in the amphotericin B group compared with fluconazole (16 vs. 30 days). In a small, prospective, randomized trial of 20 male patients with AIDS, oral fluconazole (400 mg/day) for 10 weeks was compared with IV amphotericin B (0.7 mg/kg/day for 1 week, followed by the same dose 3 times weekly for 9 weeks) combined with flucytosine (150 mg/kg/day).[96] There were four deaths in the fluconazole group and none in the amphotericin B group ($p = 0.27$). Eight of the 14 patients in the fluconazole group failed to respond to treatment, whereas none in the amphotericin B group failed to respond. The mean duration of positive CSF cultures was 41 days in the fluconazole group and 16 days in the amphotericin B group ($p = 0.02$). These results, taken together, have led most clinicians to choose amphotericin, with or without flucytosine, as initial treatment for severe cryptococcal meningitis. Although increased doses of fluconazole have been proposed, it is unknown whether these will result in improved outcomes. High doses of fluconazole are being investigated further for patients in the developing world where the use of IV amphotericin may not always be feasible. Considering the severity of her meningitis, A.S. should be treated acutely with amphotericin and not fluconazole.

DURATION OF THERAPY

CASE 77-4, QUESTION 5: How long should treatment continue for A.S.'s cryptococcal meningitis?

Once A.S. completes 2 weeks of acute induction therapy with amphotericin B and flucytosine, she should be switched, if stable, to oral fluconazole 400 mg/day for consolidation therapy. Consolidation should be continued for an additional 8 to 10 weeks, followed by lifelong suppressive therapy with fluconazole 200 mg/day[90] (see Maintenance Therapy section).

MAINTENANCE THERAPY

CASE 77-4, QUESTION 6: Should A.S. receive maintenance therapy after successful treatment?

After induction and consolidation treatment of cryptococcal meningitis, A.S. and all AIDS patients should receive maintenance therapy indefinitely, unless immune reconstitution occurs as a result of HAART.[12,89,90] A higher relapse rate and a shorter life expectancy have been observed in patients who did not receive chronic secondary prophylaxis.[97] Fluconazole (200 mg once daily) has emerged as the suppressive treatment of choice. In a randomized, placebo-controlled trial of 61 AIDS patients, four recurrent cases of meningitis developed in the placebo group and none in the fluconazole group.[98] A multicenter, comparative trial randomized patients to receive either weekly amphotericin B 1 mg/kg/day IV or 200 mg/day of fluconazole PO.[99] Of 189 patients enrolled, 18% of the patients in the amphotericin B group relapsed, compared with 2% in the fluconazole group. Serious toxicities were more frequent in the amphotericin B group.[90] The newer triazole antifungals, posaconazole and voriconazole, have limited experience as primary or maintenance therapy for patients with cryptococcosis and are associated with many drug interactions with antiretroviral therapy.[12]

According to the OI guidelines,[12] adult and adolescent patients are at a low risk for recurrence of cryptococcosis when they have completed a course of initial therapy, remain asymptomatic, and have a sustained increase (e.g., >6 months) in their CD4 counts to at least 200 after HAART. Thus, discontinuing chronic maintenance therapy among such patients is reasonable. Recurrences may occur, and some specialists recommend a repeat lumbar puncture to determine whether the CSF is culture-negative before stopping therapy. Maintenance therapy should be reinitiated if the CD4 count decreases to less than 200.

Primary Prophylaxis

CASE 77-4, QUESTION 7: What is the role of primary prophylaxis in cryptococcal meningitis?

Primary prophylaxis against cryptococcal disease in HIV-infected patients has been studied in a few clinical trials.[100,101] In an open-label study, fluconazole (100 mg/day) was administered to all patients (329 HIV-infected patients) with CD4 counts less than 68. These results were compared with 337 historical controls from the pre-HAART era.[100] Sixteen cases of cryptococcal meningitis occurred in the historical controls (4.8%) compared with only one case in the fluconazole group (0.3%). In a prospective, randomized AIDS Clinical Trial Group study, fluconazole 200 mg/day was compared with clotrimazole troches (10 mg 5 times a day) for the prevention of fungal infections in 428 patients with advanced HIV disease. After a median follow-up of 35 months, 32 cases of invasive fungal infection were confirmed. Of these, the majority (17 of 32) were cryptococcosis: 2 cases in the fluconazole group and 15 cases in the clotrimazole group. The greatest benefit derived from fluconazole was observed in patients with CD4 counts of less than 50.[101] However, no effect on survival was noted. A randomized, double-blind, placebo-controlled trial of fluconazole 200 mg 3 times weekly versus placebo in Ugandan adults with CD4 counts less than 200 found fluconazole prophylaxis to be effective prophylaxis against cryptococcal disease, with 18 patients in the placebo group developing cryptococcal disease versus one patient in the fluconazole group. There was no difference in all-cause mortality between the groups.[100]

Fluconazole resistance has been reported in HIV-infected patients receiving a long-term therapy.[102] In addition to the potential for resistance, other concerns include the lack of survival benefits associated with prophylaxis, the possibility of drug interactions, and cost. In light of these concerns, the guidelines currently do not recommend primary prophylaxis for this disease (Table 77-1).[12]

ADDITIONAL THERAPIES

CASE 77-4, QUESTION 8: What other acute therapies have been investigated for cryptococcal meningitis?

High-dose fluconazole alone (800–2,000 mg/day for up to 6 months) has been compared with high-dose fluconazole and flucytosine (100–150 mg/kg/day for 4 weeks) in multiple clinical trials.[103–105] These studies have shown that the combination of fluconazole and flucytosine is superior to fluconazole alone in terms of both survival and CSF culture clearance. The combination of fluconazole and flucytosine is useful because of their excellent oral bioavailability, cost-effectiveness, and safety, which are particularly important in developing countries. Additionally, higher doses of fluconazole in these settings (1,800–2,000 mg/day) may be the best option for patients owing to the limitations of obtaining and administering flucytosine.

MYCOBACTERIUM TUBERCULOSIS

Clinical Presentation

CASE 77-5

QUESTION 1: C.J., a 45-year-old male prison inmate with AIDS, presents with fever, cough, and occasional night sweats. A tuberculin purified protein derivative (PPD) skin test is negative. Two acid-fast bacilli (AFB) sputum smears are also negative. Chest radiograph reveals hilar adenopathy with a questionable right middle lobe localized infiltrate. No cavitary lesions are seen. Why is infection with *M. tuberculosis* a strong possibility in C.J.? His antiretroviral medications include abacavir, lamivudine, and dolutegravir. Three months ago, his CD4 count was 120 cells/μL, and his viral load was 5,200 copies/mL.

TB is the second leading cause of mortality caused by infection worldwide—second only to HIV—with 9 million infections in 2013 and 1.5 million deaths.[106] Low- to middle-income countries account for 95% of deaths from *M. tuberculosis*. Of the cases in 2013, 480,000 patients developed multidrug-resistant TB. In the United States, 9,582 cases of TB occurred in 2013, which was a 3.6% decline in the number of cases when compared with 2012.[107] The recognized link between HIV and TB, along with an increase in clinical and public health resources, has subsequently resulted in a decline in the incidence of TB in the United States.[107]

C.J. presents with fever, cough, night sweats, and a right middle lobe infiltrate with hilar adenopathy, consistent with TB. Furthermore, his HIV status in combination with his incarceration increases the probability of *M. tuberculosis* infection, including multidrug-resistant isolates. C.J. will be started with the standard four-drug regimen: isoniazid, rifampin (or rifabutin), pyrazinamide, and ethambutol.[12] (See Chapter 68, Tuberculosis, for a more comprehensive approach to TB treatment, and Table 77-5.)

CASE 77-5, QUESTION 2: Why are the negative tuberculin skin test, negative sputum smears for AFB, and lack of cavitary lesions in C.J. still consistent with *M. tuberculosis* infection?

HIV-infected patients with CD4 counts less than 200 commonly present with extrapulmonary TB, along with or in the absence of pulmonary disease. These extrapulmonary sites include lymph nodes, bone marrow, spleen, liver, CSF, and blood.[12] The chest radiograph in HIV-infected patients may reveal hilar or mediastinal adenopathy or localized infiltrates in the middle or lower lung fields.

In HIV-infected patients, it is unusual to see typical apical infiltrates or cavitations. Furthermore, concomitant PCP may confuse the interpretation of chest radiographs. Finally, anergy (a state of immune unresponsiveness) is common in HIV disease. Thus, definitive diagnosis of TB rests on positive cultures from sputum or other tissue and body fluid specimens.[12] Unlike many other AIDS-related opportunistic infections, CD4 count is not a reliable predictor of an increased risk for TB diseases, and patients can have relatively high CD4 counts at the time of TB development.

HIV-INFECTED PERSONS: DRUG-SUSCEPTIBLE TUBERCULOSIS

CASE 77-6

QUESTION 1: K.D., a 26-year-old HIV-infected man, comes in for a routine clinic visit. It is discovered that he is a household contact of a person known to have active, untreated, drug-susceptible TB. His CD4 count is 350 cells/μL. A tuberculin skin test (five tuberculin units of PPD) is administered, and he is instructed to return to the clinic in 48 hours. His PPD has been negative in the past, and he has demonstrated delayed hypersensitivity responsiveness. How should the results of K.D.'s skin tests be interpreted, and should he be treated for latent TB considering his known exposure to TB?

Current guidelines recommend 9 months of isoniazid prophylaxis (300 mg/day PO) plus pyridoxine (50 mg/day PO) for all HIV-infected persons who have at least a 5-mm induration reaction to PPD and no evidence of active TB (negative chest radiograph and no clinical symptoms), unless otherwise contraindicated and regardless of Bacillus Calmette–Guerin vaccination status.[12] The administration of Bacillus Calmette–Guerin vaccine to HIV-infected persons is contraindicated because of the potential to cause disseminated disease.[12] A greater than 5-mm reaction in HIV-infected persons is considered positive.[12] Few isoniazid prophylaxis failures have been reported, although this finding has not been systematically studied. Additional preferred regimens in instances of questionable compliance include isoniazid 900 mg twice weekly plus pyridoxine 50 mg twice weekly for 9 months, both administered under direct observed therapy. Persons who cannot take isoniazid or who have been exposed to a known isoniazid-resistant strain should use either rifampin or rifabutin alone for 4 months as alternatives, being mindful of potential drug interactions with antiretroviral therapy.[12,108] All HIV-infected persons, irrespective of age, PPD results, or prior course of chemoprophylaxis, should be given chemoprophylaxis if they are in close contact with persons who have active TB. Prophylaxis also

Table 77-6

Recommendations for Coadministering Rifampin and Rifabutin with Non-nucleoside Reverse Transcriptase Inhibitors, Protease Inhibitors, and Integrase Inhibitors

Antiretroviral	Use in Combination With Rifabutin	Use in Combination With Rifampin	Comments
All ritonavir- and cobicistat-boosted protease inhibitors	Dose as 150 mg every day or 300 mg 3 × per week. Therapeutic drug monitoring is recommended	Do not coadminister	
Fosamprenavir	Consider alternative ARV	Do not coadminister	
Atazanavir	Rifabutin 150 mg daily or 300 mg 3 × per week	Do not coadminister	
Nevirapine	Use caution at usual doses of rifabutin; however, there are no published clinical data	Do not coadminister	
Efavirenz	Rifabutin 450–600 mg daily or 600 mg 3 × per week unless coadministered with a protease inhibitor	Usual recommended dose of efavirenz is 600 mg daily. Some experts recommend increasing the efavirenz dose to 800 mg daily if efavirenz is used in combination with rifampin	
Etravirine	Rifabutin 300 mg daily unless coadministered with a boosted protease inhibitor, then do not coadminister	Do not coadminister	
Rilpivirine	Increase rilpivirine dose to 50 mg daily	Do not coadminister	
Maraviroc	Maraviroc 300 mg BID unless coadministered with a CYP3A4 inhibitor or inducer; rifabutin 300 mg daily	Coadministration not recommended; if used, then dose maraviroc 600 mg BID unless coadministered with a CYP3A4 inhibitor, then maraviroc 300 mg BID	
Raltegravir	No change in dosing	Raltegravir 800 mg BID and monitor closely for virologic response	
Dolutegravir	No change in dosing	Dolutegravir 50 mg BID unless INSTI resistance expected, then do not use with rifampin	
Elvitegravir/cobicistat/ tenofovir/emtricitabine	Do not coadminister	Do not coadminister	

BID, twice a day; CYP3A4, cytochrome P-450 3A4.

Source: Panel on Opportunistic Infections in HIV-infected Adults and Adolescents. Guidelines for prevention and treatment of opportunistic infections in HIV-infected adults and adolescents: recommendations from CDC, the National Institutes of Health, and the HIV Medicine Association of the Infectious Diseases Society of America. **https://aidsinfo.nih.gov/guidelines/html/4/adult-and-adolescent-oi-prevention-and-treatment-guidelines/**.

should be given for anergic, HIV-infected persons who have been in contact with patients known to have active TB.[108] Before the treatment of latent TB is begun, active TB needs to be ruled out. K.D. should undergo chest radiography and clinical evaluation to rule out active disease. The CDC no longer recommends routine anergy testing in these patients.[12]

HIV-INFECTED PERSONS: PROTEASE INHIBITORS, NONNUCLEOSIDE REVERSE TRANSCRIPTASE INHIBITORS, CCR5 ANTAGONISTS, AND INTEGRASE INHIBITORS

CASE 77-7

QUESTION 1: F.C., a 36-year-old HIV-infected woman, diagnosed 6 months ago, was found to have active TB (pulmonary infiltrates on chest radiographs, sputum AFB stain and culture positive, and culture pansensitive). She is taking tenofovir, emtricitabine, atazanavir, ritonavir, and fluconazole, and her CD4 count is 300 cells/μL. What factors must be considered when selecting TB therapy for F.C.?

The use of protease inhibitors in the treatment of HIV-infected patients coinfected with TB increases the potential for drug interactions with rifamycin derivatives (rifampin and rifabutin). Because the rifamycins are potent inducers of the hepatic cytochrome P-450 system (e.g., CYP3A4), they can induce metabolism of the protease inhibitors, resulting in subtherapeutic levels. Conversely, the protease inhibitors elevate rifamycin serum levels by inhibiting their metabolism and increasing toxicities, such as rifabutin-associated uveitis (inflammation of the uveal tract of the eye; see Chapter 68, Tuberculosis).

According to recent guidelines, rifampin should not be coadministered with any standard protease inhibitors (boosted or not with ritonavir or cobicistat), etravirine, nevirapine, rilpivirine, or elvitegravir.[11,108] Rifampin may be used with efavirenz at the standard 600-mg once-daily dose with close monitoring for virologic response to antiviral therapy. Some clinicians recommend an 800-mg dose of efavirenz for patients weighing greater than 60 kg.[11,108] When using rifampin with raltegravir, the recommended dose of raltegravir is 800 mg BID, and patients should be monitored closely for virologic response. Coadministration of rifampin and maraviroc is not recommended, but if necessary, maraviroc should be dosed 600 mg BID (or, if coadministered with a strong CYP3A inhibitor, maraviroc, 300 mg BID).[11] Dolutegravir should be dosed 50 mg twice daily if combined with rifampin.[11] Rifabutin should be given at 50% of the usual dose (i.e., reduced from 300 to 150 mg/day or 300 mg 3 times a week) with ritonavir- or cobicistat-boosted protease inhibitors.[11] Rifabutin should be given with efavirenz at dosages of 450 to 600 mg/day. Rifabutin can be used in full doses with nevirapine, etravirine, and rilpivirine; however, the rilpivirine dose should be increased to 50 mg daily.[108] If etravirine is coadministered with a ritonavir-boosted protease inhibitor, rifabutin should not be coadministered.[11] Tenofovir/emtricitabine/elvitegravir/cobicistat should not be coadministered with rifabutin; however, no dose adjustment is needed when combined with dolutegravir or raltegravir.[11] Sequential treatment of TB followed by HIV treatment is not recommended.[12] Three clinical trials have demonstrated a reduction in mortality and HIV-related diseases when antiretrovirals are given during TB treatment.[109–111]

Discontinuing the protease inhibitor for F.C. is not an option considering the rapid viral replication and the risk of developing resistant isolates, especially considering that she recently was started on protease inhibitor therapy and is clinically responsive. A reduced dose of rifabutin (150 mg daily or 300 mg 3 times per week) is recommended when coadministered with atazanavir + ritonavir. Considering that F.C. is receiving atazanavir + ritonavir, she will be treated with a rifabutin-based regimen. She will receive isoniazid, rifabutin, pyrazinamide, and ethambutol daily for 8 weeks followed by isoniazid and rifabutin daily or 3 times weekly for 6 months.

MYCOBACTERIUM AVIUM COMPLEX DISEASE

Clinical Presentation

CASE 77-8

QUESTION 1: M.E., an HIV-infected 38-year-old woman with a history of IV drug use, presents with fevers, drenching night sweats, a poor appetite, and a 20-pound weight loss (>15% of baseline) during the past 4 months. M.E. has refused all antiretroviral therapy for the past year because of drug intolerance. She has a past medical history of recurrent herpes zoster, PCP, and cryptococcal meningitis. Her current medications include one TMP-SMX double-strength tablet once daily and an occasional valacyclovir dose when she feels the herpes zoster "is beginning to start"; she refuses MAC prophylaxis therapy. Physical examination reveals a cachectic woman with mild hepatosplenomegaly. Pertinent laboratory test results include the following:

Hematocrit, 23%
WBC count, 3,500 cells/L, with 68% neutrophils, 2% bands, 22% lymphocytes, and 8% monocytes
Absolute CD4 count, 25 cells/μL
Viral load, 200,000 copies/mL
Aspartate transferase, 135 international units/L
Alanine aminotransferase, 95 international units/L
Alkaline phosphatase, 186 international units/L

Skin testing reveals anergy. The chest radiograph is unremarkable. Based on these findings, a presumptive diagnosis of MAC infection is made. Why is M.E.'s clinical presentation consistent with MAC infection?

Disseminated MAC infection is common in end-stage AIDS patients. On autopsy, MAC organisms are observed in the lungs and multiple other bodily tissues.[112] The predominant organism in HIV-positive patients is *M. avium* (>95% of typeable isolates).[12] The risk of developing disseminated MAC infection is highest in patients with a CD4 count less than 50.[12] Poor prognostic indicators include prior OI, high plasma HIV RNA levels, previous colonization of the respiratory or GI tract with MAC, and reduced in vitro lymphoproliferative immune responses to *M. avium* antigens.[12]

M. avium is a ubiquitous organism found in food, water, soil, and house dust. The most likely portal of entry is either the GI or respiratory tract. Common presenting symptoms associated with MAC infection include fever, night sweats, anorexia, malaise, profound weight loss (>10% body weight), anemia, lymphadenopathy, and diarrhea.[12] M.E.'s fevers, drenching night sweats, poor appetite, 20-pound weight loss, and mild hepatosplenomegaly are consistent with MAC infection. In particular, her CD4 count of 25 puts her at a risk for this OI.

Treatment

INITIATION

CASE 77-8, QUESTION 2: Why is it appropriate to initiate M.E.'s drug therapy before blood culture results have documented the presence of MAC?

Disseminated MAC is best diagnosed by peripheral blood cultures. However, initial testing often includes AFB on a blood smear.[12] Conventional culture methods using solid media may have a turnaround time of as long as 8 weeks; however, radiometric broth systems signaling the release of carbon 15-labeled CO_2 from mycobacteria may detect bacterial growth in 7 to 10 days.[113] Identification of the organism (*M. tuberculosis* vs. atypical mycobacteria) by conventional biochemical methods may take weeks to months. Techniques using DNA probes make diagnosis possible within several hours.[113] Quantitative blood cultures have been useful to monitor the effects of drug therapy but may not be practical on a routine clinical basis. Radiometric broth methods also may provide in vitro drug susceptibility in another 7 to 10 days. Even with the availability of all of these laboratory tests, results generally are not available for 2 to 3 weeks. In view of this lag time, empiric therapy should be initiated as quickly as possible. Although MAC is typically isolated from blood, the organism can also be demonstrated via acid-fast smears of lymph node, liver, or bone marrow biopsies. Because these organs are rich in monocytes (the target cells for MAC infection), the organism load may be high (up to 10^{11} colony-forming units/mL).

DRUG SUSCEPTIBILITY AS A BASIS FOR TREATMENT

CASE 77-8, QUESTION 3: Should M.E.'s therapy be based on in vitro drug susceptibility results?

Correlation between in vitro drug susceptibility results and clinical efficacy has not been clearly established for MAC.[113,114] In addition, drug susceptibility studies also may not correlate with clinical efficacy because in vitro results for individually tested drugs may show resistance, but combination therapy may be additive or synergistic. Finally, some antimycobacterial agents exhibit large differences between the minimum inhibitory concentration and maximum bactericidal concentration. This finding may reflect the difficulty in eradicating this organism, particularly in a severely immunocompromised host. Despite these limitations, in vitro drug susceptibility testing is only recommended for macrolide antibiotics because of the correlation with clinical outcomes.[115]

CASE 77-8, QUESTION 4: What drug regimens could be selected to treat M.E.?

The guidelines recommend a two-drug or more MAC regimen, because monotherapy can lead to breakthrough bacteremia and resistance; at least one of these drugs must be a macrolide. Clarithromycin (500 mg PO BID) is the preferred agent because there are more clinical data; however, if intolerable or significant drug interactions need to be avoided, azithromycin 500 to 600 mg PO QD is an alternative. Doses of clarithromycin greater than 1 g/ day in the treatment of MAC have been associated with increased mortality.[12] Ethambutol (15 mg/kg/day PO) is recommended as the second agent. Several drugs can be used as the third agent, including rifabutin (300 mg/day), amikacin (10–15 mg/kg/day), and fluoroquinolones. The choice of the third agent depends on the severity of the illness including high mycobacterial loads, CD4 count less than 50, drug interactions, hepatic and renal function, patient tolerability, patient compliance, and cost. Long-term therapy may be discontinued in patients who have completed a course of more than 12 months of treatment for MAC, remain asymptomatic, and have a sustained increase (e.g., >6 months) in their CD4 count to greater than 100 after HAART.[12]

Although four-drug regimens have been used, one study observed that a three-drug macrolide regimen (clarithromycin, ethambutol, and rifabutin) was more effective than a four-drug regimen (ciprofloxacin, clofazimine, ethambutol, and rifampin).[116] Benefits of the macrolide regimen included more rapid clearing of MAC bacteremia and a longer duration of survival. Rifabutin, at 600 mg/day, induced uveitis in approximately one-third of patients. Subsequently, the rifabutin dosage was lowered to 300 mg/day, and the incidence of uveitis decreased to 5.6%. Although clearance of bacteremia was superior at the higher rifabutin dose, no differences in survival were observed.

IRIS can also occur with MAC disease. IRIS-associated fever and lymphadenitis are difficult to differentiate from active MAC disease. IRIS most commonly occurs in patients with MAC and very low CD4 counts with the initiation of antiretroviral therapy. The disease is often self-limiting and requires no therapy; however, steroid therapy may be warranted in severe disease. For this reason, for patients not taking antiretroviral therapy, it may be warranted to administer MAC therapy for 2 weeks before the initiation of antiretroviral therapy to minimize the risk of IRIS.[12]

M.E. is placed on a regimen of clarithromycin 500 mg twice daily and ethambutol 15 mg/kg/day. The choice to use two drugs, rather than three, is based on M.E.'s poor adherence profile. Other considerations for the addition of a third-line agent include the severity of the illness, potential drug interactions, tolerability, hepatic and renal function, and cost. M.E. must be counseled regarding the slow response to treatment. If she improves, therapy should be continued and HAART should be reinstituted.

Monitoring Therapy

CASE 77-8, QUESTION 5: How should M.E. be monitored?

The primary goals of MAC therapy are to eradicate or reduce the number of *M. avium* organisms, decrease symptoms, enhance quality of life, and prolong survival. M.E. should be monitored for symptomatic relief (temperature spikes and frequency of night sweats), as well as a microbiologic response (colony-forming units/mL). Clinical response, as well as a decline in the quantity of mycobacteria, is expected in 2 to 4 weeks but may be delayed in patients with extensive disease. If no clinical response is seen in 4 to 8 weeks, repeat blood cultures for MAC should be obtained along with repeat susceptibility testing for clarithromycin and azithromycin. If resistance is observed or suspected, two new drugs should be added based on susceptibility testing with or without the macrolide. If the organism is found to be susceptible to macrolides, therapy should be continued and adherence, absorption, tolerance, and drug interactions should be considered.[12] If the problem is determined to be drug absorption, IV agents can be considered. M.E. should also be followed for the development of toxicities related to drug therapy. Furthermore, because many drugs used to treat MAC infections are associated with drug interactions, this issue must be considered each time a new drug is prescribed. In some cases, drug doses need to be modified or alternative drugs should be selected to prevent adverse events or therapeutic failures.[12,115]

CASE 77-8, QUESTION 6: What drug(s) should be used to provide primary prophylaxis against MAC infection?

Prophylaxis

The most recent official guidelines recommend oral therapy with clarithromycin (500 mg BID) or azithromycin 1,200 mg every week or 600 mg twice weekly for persons with a CD4 count less than 50. Although the combination of azithromycin and rifabutin is more effective than azithromycin alone, the increased cost, adverse events, potential for drug interactions with rifabutin, and the absence of a survival benefit preclude this regimen from being routinely recommended. If neither clarithromycin nor azithromycin is tolerated, rifabutin 300 mg/day may be used (Table 77-1).[12]

Six hundred eighty-two patients with AIDS, CD4 counts less than 100, and negative MAC blood cultures were randomly assigned to receive clarithromycin (500 mg PO BID) or placebo.[33] The clarithromycin arm had a 69% reduction in MAC bacteremia and fewer (16% vs. 6%) cases of MAC infection. Significantly more patients in the clarithromycin arm survived during the 10-month follow-up (68% vs. 59%), with an accompanying longer median duration of survival. This trial was the first prospective MAC prophylaxis study demonstrating a survival benefit and a reduced risk of disseminated MAC infection.[33]

Azithromycin 1,200 mg every week, rifabutin 300 mg/day, and a combination of both drugs in the same doses were compared in patients with AIDS and CD4 counts less than 100. The incidence of MAC bacteremia was 13.9% in the azithromycin monotherapy arm, 23.3% in the rifabutin monotherapy arm, and 8.3% in the azithromycin plus rifabutin combination arm. Time to death was not significantly different among the treatments; however, the combination arm had an increased incidence of adverse drug effects. Although combination therapy was superior to azithromycin alone, its use is considered second-line therapy because of the increased cost, toxicity, and lack of survival benefit.[117]

The decision to use clarithromycin or azithromycin (both first-line recommendations for primary prophylaxis) is based on patient compliance and the potential for drug interactions. Azithromycin (1,200 mg once weekly or 600 mg twice weekly) may be preferable for a patient who has difficulty with compliance. In contrast to clarithromycin, azithromycin does not affect the cytochrome P-450 enzyme system and is therefore less likely to interact with other drugs. M.E. would have benefited from MAC prophylaxis when her CD4 count decreased to less than 50.

Patients whose CD4 count increases from 100 for more than 3 months may discontinue primary prophylaxis (Table 77-2). However, prophylaxis should be reintroduced if the CD4 count decreases to less than 100.[12]

MUCOCUTANEOUS CANDIDIASIS

CASE 77-9

QUESTION 1: P.J. is a 45-year-old, HIV-positive man who was started on abacavir, lamivudine, and darunavir/cobicistat when he was diagnosed 1 year ago. P.J. is a heroin user and has not been seen in the clinic since his initial presentation. He appears today complaining of difficult, painful swallowing and diffuse pain. On examination, localized white plaques are observed in the oral cavity. His CD4 count is 280 cells/μL. What is the most likely cause of this patient's dysphagia and odynophagia?

Candida can cause both oropharyngitis and esophagitis in HIV-infected patients typically when CD4 counts are <200 cells/μL. Additionally, patients can present with CMV, HSV, or aphthous ulcers in the oropharynx. Symptoms include dysphagia, odynophagia, and thrush (with *Candida* infections). Oral ulcers are common with HSV, rare with *Candida*, and uncommon with CMV or aphthous ulcers. Pain is usually diffuse in *Candida* infections and more focused with HSV, CMV, and aphthous ulcers. Fever is primarily associated with CMV.[12]

Most infections are due to *Candida albicans*; however, because of the exposure of fluconazole, emergence of non-*albicans* species such as *Candida glabrata* has appeared and in some cases led to refractory candidiasis.[12] Patients with localized white plaques in the oral cavity likely have oral candidiasis (thrush) and should be started on antifungal therapy. Oral fluconazole (100 mg once daily) is considered the drug of choice for the treatment of oropharyngeal candidiasis because it is more convenient and better tolerated than topical therapies. Patients may also be treated with local antifungal therapy (e.g., "swish and swallow" nystatin suspension, 1 teaspoon 4 or 5 times daily, or clotrimazole troches 4 or 5 times daily). The preferred therapy for esophageal candidiasis is 14 to 21 days of fluconazole at higher doses (up to 400 mg PO or IV daily). Alternate therapies include itraconazole and posaconazole (for oropharyngeal disease) and voriconazole, anidulafungin, caspofungin, micafungin, and amphotericin B (for esophageal disease).[13] Primary prophylaxis is not recommended for candidiasis.[12]

A presumptive diagnosis of *Candida* esophagitis can be made for P.J. because he presents with oral pharyngeal candidiasis, dysphagia, and odynophagia. P.J. should be empirically treated with fluconazole 200 mg/day for 14 to 21 days. If he is unresponsive to fluconazole, endoscopy with biopsy and culture should be performed to confirm the diagnosis as well as *Candida* speciation. If candidiasis is confirmed, P.J. should be checked for medication adherence and potential drug interactions. If the patient is adherent and does not have malabsorption, posaconazole suspension or itraconazole solution should be considered. In addition, higher doses of fluconazole could be considered before the initiation of alternative IV therapy. Relapse is common in patients who do not receive secondary prophylaxis. Chronic suppressive therapy (fluconazole, 100–200 mg/day) could be considered in patients responsive to fluconazole therapy who have frequent or severe recurrent esophagitis; however, the risks of fluconazole resistance should be considered.[12]

ACKNOWLEDGMENTS

The authors acknowledge Angela D.M. Kashuba, Gene D. Morse, Alice M. O'Donnell, Marjorie Robinson, and Mark J. Shelton, for their contributions to this chapter in the previous editions.

KEY REFERENCES AND WEBSITES

A full list of references for this chapter can be found at http://thepoint.lww.com/AT11e. Below are the key references and website for this chapter, with the corresponding reference number in this chapter found in parentheses after the reference.

Key References

Buchacz K et al. AIDS-defining opportunistic illnesses in US patients, 1994–2007: a cohort study. *AIDS*. 2010;24:1549. (2)

Panel on Opportunistic Infections in HIV-infected Adults and Adolescents. Guidelines for prevention and treatment of opportunistic infections in HIV-infected adults and adolescents: recommendations from CDC, the National Institutes of Health, and the HIV Medicine Association of the Infectious Diseases Society of America. https://aidsinfo.nih.gov/guidelines/html/4/adult-and-adolescent-oi-prevention-and-treatment-guidelines/ 0 .

Selik RM et al. Revised surveillance case definition for HIV infection, United States, 2014. *MMWR Recomm Rep*. 2014;63(RR03);1–10. (5)

Key Websites

Centers for Disease Control and Prevention. HIV/AIDS. http://www.cdc.gov/hiv. Accessed June 5, 2015.

Centers for Disease Control. Managing Drug Interactions in the Treatment of HIV-Related Tuberculosis. 2013. http://www.cdc.gov/tb/publications/guidelines/tb_hiv_drugs/default.htm. Accessed June 5, 2015.

Panel on Antiretroviral Guidelines for Adults and Adolescents. Guidelines for the use of antiretroviral agents in HIV-1 infected adults and adolescents. Department of Health and Human Services. April 8, 2015. http://www.aidsinfo.nih.gov/contentfiles/adultandadolescentgl.pdf. Accessed June 5, 2015. (12)

US Department of Health and Human Services. AIDS Info. http://www.aidsinfo.nih.gov/. Accessed June 5, 2015.

78 Fungal Infections

John D. Cleary and Russell E. Lewis

CORE PRINCIPLES

		CHAPTER CASES
1	Owing to increased numbers of immunocompromised patients, the use of invasive devices, and an aging patient population, invasive fungal infections are the fourth most common nosocomial infection.	
2	Yeast infections are generally easier to treat than mold infections. However, mortality is still significant for both types of infection, even when treated appropriately.	**Table 78-2**
3	Most common risk factors for acquiring mycotic infections include immunocompromised host, the use of broad-spectrum antibacterials, and breakdown of physical barriers including invasive catheterization.	**Case 78-3 (Questions 1,3)**
4	Diagnostic tools (i.e., serum galactomannan or β-glucan) can be useful as monitoring parameters for therapeutic outcome assessment.	**Case 78-3 (Question 2)**
5	The Infectious Disease Society of America (IDSA) and the Mycoses Study Group are important sources for guidelines and evidence-based approaches to therapy.	**Case 78-5 (Question 1)**
6	Dermatophyte infection is most commonly associated with *Tinea* ringworm, and the most effective antifungal agents include itraconazole and terbinafine.	**Case 78-1 (Questions 1–3)**
7	Sporothrix is one of the most common fungal pathogens associated with subcutaneous infections. Amphotericin, terbinafine and itraconazole are useful treatments.	**Case 78-2 (Questions 1–3), Figure 78-1**
8	Candida represents the most common cause of systemic fungal infection in hospitalized patients. Candidemia must be treated promptly and appropriately. Delay in treatment or failure to adhere to IDSA guidelines results in a significant increase in mortality. Fluconazole and echinocandins are the most recommended prephylaxis and therapies for disseminated candidiasis.	**Case 78-3 (Questions 1–4 ,11), Table 78-4–78-6**
9	Fluconazole, although reliable against *Candida albicans*, is less reliable against certain non-albicans Candida species, including *Candida glabrata* and *Candida krusei*.	**Case 78-3 (Question 5)**
10	Conventional amphotericin is associated with significant infusion-related adverse events, nephrotoxicity, and electrolyte abnormalities. Consequently, other agents, including lipid-based amphotericin B, triazoles, and echinocandins, are drugs of choice for most deep-seated fungal infections.	**Case 78-3 (Questions 6–10), Table 78-3**
11	In patients with yeast identified in urine, the selection of drug therapy for a simple candiduria versus organ infection as a result of disseminated candidiasis is complicated by difficulties with diagnostics.	**Case 78-4 (Question 1)**
12	Blastomycosis, histoplasmosis, and coccidioides are associated with endemic infection from specific geographic areas. Long-term treatment with polyenes and/or azole antifungals is useful in the management of these diseases.	**Case 78-5 (Questions 1–3), Case 78-6 (Questions 1–3), Case 78-7 (Questions 1–3), Figures 78-2–78-4, Table 78-7**

Continued

		CHAPTER CASES
13	Aspergillus is the most significant fungal pathogen associated with severely immunocompromised patients. Aggressive, immediate treatment with voriconazole alone or in combination with other antifungals is the most effective therapy for disseminated disease.	Case 78-8 (Questions 1–3), Figure 78-5, Table 78-8
14	*Cryptococcus neoformans* is associated with opportunistic infection, particularly in acquired immunodeficiency syndrome (AIDS), and the central nervous system (CNS) is a common site of infection. Initial treatment of meningitis in AIDS should include amphotericin B plus flucytosine, followed by long-term fluconazole.	Case 78-9 (Questions 1–3)

Mycotic (fungal) infections are now the fourth most commonly encountered nosocomial infection. Attributable mortality associated with invasive yeast infections can approximate ~40%, whereas molds typically double that observed rate (i.e., invasive aspergillosis). This increase can be attributed, in part, to the growing numbers of immunocompromised hosts as a result of organ transplants, cancer-chemotherapy–associated neutropenia, and AIDS. This chapter reviews the mycology, diagnosis, and pharmacotherapeutics for common mycotic infections. For a more in-depth presentation of the basic biology of fungi, as well as the epidemiology, pathogenesis, immunology, diagnosis, and monitoring of mycotic infections, see *Clinical Mycology*.[1] You are referred to other chapters including Chapter 65, Central Nervous System Infections; Chapter 66, Endocarditis; Chapter 70, Intra-Abdominal Infections; Chapter 73, Osteomyelitis and Septic Arthritis; Chapter 75, Prevention and Treatment of Infections in Neutropenic Patients; Chapter 76, Pharmacotherapy of Human Immunodeficiency Virus Infection; and Chapter 77, Opportunistic Infections in HIV-Infected Patients for detailed pharmacotherapy in these human pathologies.

Table 78-1
Organism Classification

Hyphae (Molds)
Hyalohyphomycoses
Aspergillus species, *Pseudallescheria boydii*
Dermatophytes: *Epidermophyton floccosum*, *Trichophyton* species, *Microsporum* species
Phaeohyphomycoses
Alternaria species, *Anthopsis deltoidea*, *Bipolaris hawaiiensis*, *Cladosporium* species, *Curvularia geniculata*, *Exophiala* species, *Fonsecaea pedrosoi*, *Phialophora* species, *Fusarium* species
Zygomycetes
Rhizopus spp., *Mucor* spp., *Rhizomucor* spp. *Absidia corymbifera*
Dimorphic Fungi
Blastomyces species, *Coccidioides* species, *Paracoccidioides* species, *Histoplasma* species, *Sporothrix* species
Yeasts
Candida species, *Cryptococcus neoformans*

MYCOLOGY

Morphology

The pathogenic fungi that infect humans are nonmotile eukaryotes that are reproduced by sporulation, and they exist in two forms: filamentous molds and unicellular yeasts. These forms are not mutually exclusive, and depending on the growth conditions, a fungus may exist in one or even both of these forms (Table 78-1).

The dimorphic fungi (e.g., *Histoplasma capsulatum* and *Blastomyces dermatitidis*) grow as a mold in nature (27°C) but quickly convert to the pathogenic yeast form after infecting the host (37°C). This mycelium-to-yeast conversion is an important factor in the pathogenesis of disease caused by these organisms. Other pathogenic fungi, such as *Aspergillus* species, grow only in a mold form, whereas *C. neoformans* usually grows in a yeast form. *Candida* species grow with a modified form of budding whereby newly budded cells remain attached to the parent cells and form pseudohyphae. Fungi are aerobic and are easily grown on routine culture media similar to that used to grow bacteria. Most fungi grow best at 25°C to 35°C. Fungi that cause only cutaneous and subcutaneous disease grow poorly at temperatures greater than 37°C. This temperature-selective growth explains, at least in part, why these organisms rarely disseminate from a primary focus in the skin or subcutaneous tissues.

Classification

Fungal infections are best classified by the area of the body infected (Table 78-2). Superficial mycoses involve only the outermost keratinized layers of the skin (stratum corneum) and hair. The cutaneous mycoses extend deeper into the epidermis and may also infect the nails. The subcutaneous mycoses infect the dermis and subcutaneous tissues; entry into these sites is by the inoculation or implantation of dirt or vegetative matter. The systemic mycoses cause disease of the internal organs of the body. Standard definitions that are useful in daily patient care for invasive fungal infections have been developed for epidemiologic and clinical trials. The guidelines are referenced under each infection. The respiratory tract is the most common primary portal of entry, and lung infection may be symptomatic or asymptomatic. Systemic infection with *Candida* usually results from a primary focus on the gastrointestinal (GI) tract or skin. In each case, the organism may spread hematogenously from the primary focus throughout the body, resulting in disseminated disease. The opportunistic mycoses occur primarily in the immunocompromised host and require immediate and aggressive treatment. The list of fungi that cause opportunistic infection has expanded, especially with the AIDS epidemic; however, the now commonplace use of highly active antiretroviral therapy has resulted in some decrease in this incidence.[2] The nonopportunistic fungi (primary pathogens) usually cause disease in the immunologically normal host. Some primary pathogens, however, result in unique clinical syndromes when infection occurs in the immunocompromised host, such as histoplasmosis in AIDS.[1]

Pathogenesis of Infection

ENDOGENOUS

Fungal infection can be acquired from both exogenous and endogenous sources. The only pathogenic fungi identified as

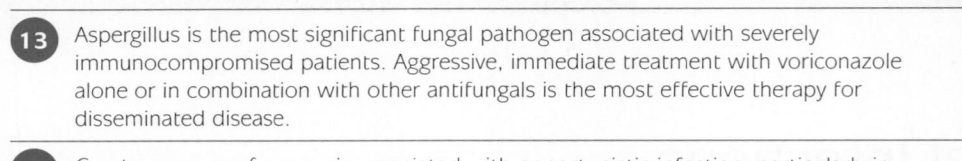

Table 78-2
Clinical Classification of Mycoses

Classification	Site Infected	Example	Potential Gene Deficiency
Superficial	Outermost skin and hair	Malasseziasis (tinea versicolor)	
Cutaneous	Deep epidermis and nails	Dermatophytosis	
Subcutaneous	Dermis and subcutaneous tissue	Sporotrichosis	
Systemic	Disease of more than one internal organ		
Opportunistic		Candidiasis	Mannose-binding Lectin-1 Toll-like Receptor 4
		Cryptococcosis	Dectin-1
		Aspergillosis	
		Mucormycosis	
Nonopportunistic		Histoplasmosis	
		Blastomycosis	
		Coccidioidomycosis	Interferon-γ receptor 1 Dectin-1 Mannose Binding Lectin-1

commensals within the human microbiome are *Pityrosporum orbiculare*, which causes the noninflammatory superficial condition of tinea versicolor, and *Candida* species. Infections with these yeasts primarily develop from the patient's own normal flora (endogenous infection). These endogenous fungal infections of the skin or mucous membranes generally occur when host resistance is lowered and the organism proliferates in high numbers. Excess heat and humidity, oral contraceptive use, pregnancy, diabetes, malnutrition, and immunosuppression facilitate endogenous local infection by both *Pityrosporum* and *Candida*. Systemic candidal infections occur in the immunocompromised or genetic deficient host (Table 78-2)[3,4] when the organism colonizing the patient's skin or GI tract disseminates hematogenously throughout the body.

EXOGENOUS

Exogenous infections occur when the fungus is acquired from an environmental source. In the case of dermatophytes (ringworm fungi), the organism can be acquired from dirt, animals, or another infected individual. The subcutaneous mycoses result from direct inoculation of infected material, often a thorn or other vegetable matter, through the skin. Infections of the skin and subcutaneous tissues by *Aspergillus* and zygomycetes (e.g., *Rhizopus*, *Absidia*, and *Mucor*) have resulted from contaminated wound dressings and cast materials.[1,5] Drug-induced disease has been observed secondary to *Saccharomyces cerevisiae* (nutraceutical) administration to healthy and immunocompromised patients or secondary to the administration of a contaminated sterile product (i.e., *Exserohilum rostratum*).

Exogenous fungi colonized or carried on the hands of health-care workers can infect patients; therefore, handwashing is emphasized for health-care workers, particularly in critically ill patients.[6] Other than candidal infections, the systemic mycoses are primarily the result of inhalation of dust contaminated by the infectious spores, with a primary focus of infection in the lungs.

If local or systemic host defenses do not control the primary infection, the organism can spread hematogenously to other organs. Some of the systemic mycoses have defined geographic (endemic) areas where the fungus is more commonly encountered. For example, histoplasmosis and blastomycosis occur most often in the regions of the Red, Mississippi, and Ohio River valleys, whereas coccidioidomycosis is endemic to the southwestern United States and the Central Valley of California.

Host Defenses

Host defenses against fungal infection involve both nonimmune (also known as nonspecific or natural resistance) and immune (also known as specific or acquired resistance) mechanisms. Nonimmune resistance plays a primary role in preventing colonization and invasion of a susceptible tissue. The normal bacterial flora of the skin and mucous membranes prevent colonization (colonization resistance) by more pathogenic bacteria and fungi. Patients treated with broad-spectrum antibiotics are at a greater risk for colonization and infection by fungi. The barrier function of the intact skin and mucous membranes is also an important defense. Skin defects (intravenous [IV] catheters, burns, surgery, or trauma) are risk factors for local invasion and fungemia, especially with *Candida* species. The translocation of yeast from the gut into the peritoneum during the trauma of a motor vehicle accident or post-GI surgery is also commonly associated with these infections. When these physical barriers are breached, the polymorphonuclear leukocyte (neutrophil) and monocytes along with defensive lectins (i.e., mannose-binding protein) provide early host defense. The antifungal activity of neutrophils involves phagocytosis and intracellular killing but also can include extracellular killing by secreted lysosomal enzymes. Neutropenia is the most common neutrophil defect predisposing to fungal infection, but functional defects of neutrophils, such as those occurring in patients with chronic granulomatous disease of childhood and myeloperoxidase deficiency, have also been associated with an increased frequency of fungal infections, especially with *Candida* and *Aspergillus*. Finally, endothermy/homeothermy and ultimately febrile responses are potent nonspecific immune defenses.

Antibody and complement have a potential role in the prevention of certain fungal infections, but they are not the primary effectors of acquired resistance. Cellular immunity, mediated by antigen-specific T lymphocytes, cytokines, and activated macrophages, is the primary acquired (immune) host defense against fungi. Patients with defective cellular immunity (e.g., immunosuppressed organ transplant recipients, patients with lymphoma and leukemia, patients with AIDS, and those treated with corticosteroids or cytotoxic agents) are at a greatest risk for fungal infection. Severe immunodeficiency often results in poor therapeutic outcome despite appropriate antifungal therapy. An additional factor associated with an increased risk for fungal infection is the use of total parenteral nutrition (TPN).[1] Interestingly, patients with specific T-cell dysfunction (i.e., HIV infection) appear to be at an isolated risk for mucosal *Candida* infection, but not systemic infections.

ANTIMYCOTICS

Mechanisms of Action

Table 78-3 lists the US Food and Drug Administration (FDA)-approved topical and systemic antimycotics for the treatment of fungal infections. Griseofulvin and potassium iodide have limited clinical utility and are not used to treat systemic fungal infections. Griseofulvin inhibits growth by inhibiting fungal cell mitosis caused by the polymerization of cell microtubules, thereby disrupting mitotic spindle formation. It has activity only against the dermatophyte fungi. The antifungal mechanism of potassium iodide is unclear. It is effective only in the treatment of lymphocutaneous sporotrichosis.

The 12 antifungal drugs used commonly for systemic disease fall into five structural classes that act by four mutually exclusive mechanisms. Amphotericin B (AmB) and nystatin (a polyene macrolide) act principally by binding to ergosterol in the fungal cell membrane, effectively creating pores in the cell membrane and leading to the depolarization of the membrane and cell leakage.[7] AmB binds with greater affinity to ergosterol than to cholesterol.[8] This phenomenon is believed to be mediated through both hydrophilic hydrogen bonding and hydrophobic, nonspecific van der Waals forces. Investigations using P^{32} nuclear magnetic resonance spectroscopy document that the presence of the double bond in the side chain of ergosterol (not present in cholesterol) accounts for the greater affinity of AmB for ergosterol.[7] AmB, however, also binds to sterols of mammalian cells (i.e., cholesterol), which may account for most of the toxic effects of AmB or reduced toxicity (i.e., circulating cholesterol). Alteration in the lipid content of the pathogens membrane may play a role in the development of resistance,[9] although other factors are also important.[10] The cidal antifungal effects of AmB are, however, not only owing to cell leakage resulting from ergosterol binding, but also owing to immune stimulation and oxygen-dependent killing.[8,11]

5-Flucytosine, a fluorinated cytosine analog, acts principally by inhibiting nucleic acid synthesis. It is actively transported into susceptible cells by the enzyme cytosine permease, where it is deaminated to the toxic metabolite 5-fluorouracil. Fluorouracil, when converted to 5-fluorouridine triphosphate, functions as an antimetabolite. It is incorporated into fungal RNA, where it is substituted for uracil and thereby disrupts protein synthesis. 5-Fluorouracil can also be converted to fluorodeoxyuridine monophosphate, which inhibits thymidylate synthase and thus disrupts DNA synthesis.[12]

The azole antifungals and the allylamines (naftifine and terbinafine) inhibit sterol biosynthesis by interference with either cytochrome (CYP) P450–dependent lanosterol C14-demethylase (azoles) or squalene epoxidase (allylamines), critical enzymes in the biosynthesis of ergosterol.[13,14] The superior affinity of the triazoles (fluconazole, itraconazole, isavuconazole, posaconazole, and voriconazole) for fungal versus mammalian

Table 78-3
Antifungal Agents Approved for Use

Agent (Brand Name)	Formulation
Systemic Agents	
Amphotericin B (Abelcet, AmBisome, Amphotec)	IV
Amphotericin B-deoxycholate (generic)	IV
Anidulafungin (Eraxis)	IV
Caspofungin (Cancidas)	IV
Fluconazole (Diflucan)	IV, tablet, oral suspension
Fluorocytosine [Flucytosine] (Ancobon)	Capsule
Griseofulvin (generic)	Tablet, oral suspension
Isavuconazole (Cresemba)	IV, oral capsule
Itraconazole (Sporanox)	IV, capsule, oral solution
Ketoconazole (Nizoral)	Tablet
Micafungin (Mycamine)	IV
Posaconazole (Noxafil)	IV, oral suspension, oral gastroresistant tablet
Potassium iodide	Solution
Terbinafine (Lamisil)	Tablet, oral granules
Voriconazole (Vfend)	IV, tablet, oral suspension
Topicals, Class I	
Amphotericin B	Cream, lotion, ointment, oral suspension[a]
Butenafine (Lotrimin Ultra)	Cream
Butoconazole (Gynazole)	Vaginal cream
Ciclopirox (Loprox)	Cream, gel, lotion, shampoo, solution, suspension
Clioquinol (Vioform)	Cream, ointment
Clotrimazole	Cream, lotion, lozenge, solution, tablet, vaginal cream
Econazole (Spectazole)	Cream
Ketoconazole (Nizoral)	Cream, foam, gel, shampoo
Miconazole	Aerosol liquid and powder, buccal tablet, cream, lotion, ointment, powder, suppository, vaginal tablet
Naftifine (Naftin)	Cream, gel
Nystatin	Cream, mouthwash, ointment, powder, suspension, tablet
Oxiconazole (Oxistat)	Cream, lotion
Povidone iodine	Aerosol, douche, gel, ointment, solution, suppository
Sodium thiosulfate (Exoderm)	Lotion
Sulconazole (Exelderm)	Cream, solution
Terbinafine (Lamisil)	Cream, spray
Terconazole (Terazol 7)	Cream, suppository
Tioconazole (Vagistat)	Ointment
Tolnaftate (generic)	Aerosol, cream, gel, powder, solution
Undecylenic acid	Powder

[a]No longer available in the United States.
IV, intravenous.

enzymes, as compared with the imidazoles (ketoconazole and miconazole), accounts for their reduced toxicity and improved efficacy.[13] The consequence of sterol biosynthesis inhibition is a faulty cell membrane with altered permeability. In general, the allylamines and older azoles are fungistatic. The newer triazoles (voriconazole and posaconazole) demonstrate fungicidal activity against some fungal species. The clinical relevance of in vitro fungicidal versus fungistatic action is the subject of considerable debate. Nevertheless, it seems logical that fungicidal action, if it can also be achieved in vivo, is preferred in immunosuppressed hosts.[15]

Lipopeptides, which are potent antifungal agents, include the structural class of echinocandins (anidulafungin, micafungin, and caspofungin). All share a common mechanism. They act by interfering with 1,3-β-D-glucan, preventing the synthesis of essential cell wall polysaccharides that protect the cell from osmotic and structural stresses. The result is inhibition of fungal cell wall biosynthesis. Targeting the cell wall (as opposed to the cell membrane, which is the target of polyene, azole, and allylamine antifungals) imparts greater selectivity for fungal versus mammalian cells; thus, echinocandins class of antifungals has fewer toxicities than other antifungal classes.[16]

Antifungal Spectrum and Susceptibility Testing

The Clinical and Laboratory Standards Institute (CLSI) recommends standardized broth dilution (M27-A3) and disk diffusion (M44-A2, M44-S3, and M51-A) methods for determining in vitro antifungal susceptibilities for yeasts.[17] These methods stipulate test medium, inoculum size and preparation, incubation time and temperature, end-point reading, and quality control limits for AmB, flucytosine, fluconazole, ketoconazole, and itraconazole. Minimum inhibitory concentration (MIC) values for use in clinical interpretation are specified for fluconazole, voriconazole, itraconazole, flucytosine, and the echinocandins against *Candida* species after 24 hours of incubation. For azole, a susceptible-dose-dependent (S-DD) break point was developed based on data supporting a trend toward better response with higher drug concentrations for isolates with higher MIC.[18] The fluconazole S-DD range is 4 to 8 mcg/mL for *C. albicans*, *Candida parapsilosis*, and *Candida tropicalis* and $\leq$32 mg/L for *C. glabrata*. Itraconazole and voriconazole S-DD ranges are 0.25 to 0.5 mg/L for *C. albicans*. Owing to the rapid development of resistance and limited data on correlation of MIC with outcome for flucytosine monotherapy, proposed interpretive break points for this agent are based on a combination of historic data and results from animal studies. *Candida* isolates with a flucytosine MIC $\leq$4 mcg/mL are considered susceptible, and isolates with MIC $>$16 mcg/mL are considered resistant. Limitations of the M27-A methodology have precluded the development of AmB interpretive break points nor have interpretive criteria been proposed for ketoconazole MIC. Candida are generally susceptible to MIC $<$0.25 mcg/mL and resistant to $>$1 mcg/mL, except for *C. parapsilosis* and *Candida guilliermondii* that have higher susceptibility ($<$2 mcg/mL) and resistant ($>$8 mcg/mL) values. Commercial kits are available for antifungal susceptibility testing ,which utilize broth microdilution, colorimetric, and agar-based techniques.[19–21] University of Texas Health Science Fungal Testing Laboratory has historically tested fungi susceptibilities and reports current break points and epidemiologic cutoff values.

An E-Test (AB Biodisk; Piscataway, NJ) is a commercially available antifungal gradient strip. Difficulties in end point determination using this method result from frequent, nonuniform growth of the fungus on the agar medium; yet, when properly performed, correlation between the E-Test and M27-A methods has been satisfactory for the azole antifungal agents against most *Candida*.[19] Other techniques under development for antifungal susceptibility testing for yeasts include flow cytometry and direct measurement of alterations in ergosterol synthesis.[20] Flow cytometry detects the activity of the test antifungal drug through identification of subtle dosage–response effects on specific cell parameters as cells within the prepared inoculum pass through a beam of light. Test results may be available in as few as 4 hours. Interlaboratory reproducibility or correlation between test results and clinical outcomes has not been well studied.[21]

The CLSI-recommended standardized broth dilution method for determining in vitro antifungal susceptibilities for certain spore-producing molds, namely *Aspergillus* species, *Fusarium* species, *Rhizopus* species, *Pseudallescheria boydii*, and *Sporothrix schenckii*, is the M38-A2 method.[15] An E-Test to evaluate mold susceptibilities is also commercially available (AB Biodisk) and correlates well with the CLSI M38-A method for AmB and itraconzole.[22] Colorimetric microdilution, flow cytometry, and agar-based testing methods are under development. Despite these recent advances, the determination of in vitro susceptibilities or resistance in clinical practice is of limited utility and not readily available for yeasts or molds in most institutions.

Susceptibility testing for clinical isolates is not routinely recommended because susceptibility is usually predictable. However, published data on the susceptibility of the identified species of yeasts or molds should guide the clinician's therapeutic choice. Clinical isolates from patients failing high-dose therapy (i.e., refractory oral pharyngeal candidiasis) or unusual pathogenic yeasts in patients with AIDS can be sent for testing.[20] Testing should be performed in a laboratory where the staff is trained in mycoses. Despite these limitations, certain patterns are common. First, AmB has broad in vitro activity and clinical efficacy against the yeasts and filamentous molds. The echinocandins have cidal activity in vitro versus *Candida* species and static activity for *Aspergillus* species; they are not active in vitro against *Cryptococcus* species and many endemic mycoses.[23] The azole antifungals are generally reliable against the yeasts and most dimorphic fungi. Additionally, itraconazole, voriconazole, and posaconazole have excellent in vitro activity against *Aspergillus* species, with associated clinical efficacy. Unlike other azoles, posaconazole and isavuconazole have some activity in vitro and reported clinical evidence of efficacy against zygomycetes, for which previously only AmB formulations were therapeutic options.[24,25]

Routine susceptibility testing of fluconazole, voriconazole, and an echinocandin against *C. glabrata* is increasing recommended, especially for isolates from blood normally sterile fluids, tissue, or abscess owing to recent reports of increasing echinocandin and multidrug resistance.[26–28] Additionally, any patient with invasive disease and clinical failure of initial therapy should be considered for susceptibility following consultation with an experience microbiologist.

New Frontiers for Antifungal Therapy

Various investigative efforts have been directed toward enhancing efficacy, reducing the toxicity, and improving the oral bioavailability of older antifungal drugs. Aerosol delivery of AmB products, itraconazole, voriconazole, and caspofungin in immunocompromised patients has been investigated for the prevention of invasive pulmonary aspergillosis. Reduction in invasive pulmonary aspergillosis was demonstrated in a randomized, placebo-controlled trial of aerosolized liposomal AmB.[29] Additional well-designed clinical trials are still needed to establish the role of aerosolized delivery of antifungal agents. Optimal antifungal dose and nebulized system required for

Table 78-4
Antimycotic Prophylaxis Regimens and Approximate Costs

Agent	Dose/Day	Formulation	Recommended Regimen	Cost ($)/day
Selective GI Decontamination				
Amphotericin B	400 mg	Oral suspension	Swish and swallow QID	9.75
Nystatin	4–12 million units	Oral suspension	Swish and swallow QID	38.50–115.25
Systemic				
Clotrimazole	30–80 mg	Troche	TID–QID	125–450
Ketoconazole	200–400 mg	Oral	Daily	0.75–1.50
Itraconazole	200–400 mg	Oral	Daily	18–36.25
Fluconazole	50–400 mg	Oral	Daily	4.50–35.25
Posaconazole	600–800 mg suspension 300 mg daily tablet 300 mg IV	Oral	Daily	175 636

GI, gastrointestinal; QID, four times daily; TID, three times daily.
Source: [No authors listed]. Red Book. Montvale, NJ: PDR Network, LLC; 2011.

effective prophylaxis have yet to be established compared with traditional GI regimens (Table 78-4).[29–31]

Identification of new antifungal compounds has been challenging. One significant barrier is that both mammalian cells and fungal cells are eukaryotes and share many similar biochemical processes, unlike bacterial cells, which are prokaryotes. Traditionally, the drug discovery process depended on the ability to detect compounds (either natural products or synthetic compounds) that selectively inhibit or destroy fungal cells. This process is accomplished by either or both of two approaches: (a) the evaluation of existing compounds (natural or synthetic) for potentially useful antifungal activity and (b) the design and synthesis of new compounds that selectively block fungal targets. Recent advances in genomic sequencing of *C. albicans*, *C. glabrata*, *Aspergillus fumigatus*, *Rhizopus* oryzae (delmar), and *C. neoformans* have facilitated the search for new targets. Other less conventional drug discovery approaches include targeting known traditional virulence factors (e.g., adhesions and secreted enzymes). This approach is based on the principle that killing of the microbe need not occur for an anti-infective agent to be efficacious. Promising lead compounds include nikkomycins, sordarins, lytic peptides, hydroxypyridones, and cathelicidins.[32–35]

SUPERFICIAL AND CUTANEOUS MYCOSES

Tinea Pedis: Treatment

CASE 78-1

QUESTION 1: C.W., a 28-year-old male construction worker, is evaluated for a chronic case of "athlete's foot." He wears boots all day at work and notes intense itching of both feet throughout the day. He has been using tolnaftate powder for 1 week with no real therapeutic benefit. On examination, the web spaces between all the toes are white, macerated, and cracked. A few vesicles are also present over the dorsum of the foot at the base of the toes. Scrapings of the lesions examined as a potassium hydroxide (KOH) preparation reveal branching, filamentous hyphae compatible with a dermatophyte infection. The diagnosis of athlete's foot is made. What therapeutic options are available for C.W.?

Selection of antifungal therapy should be based on the extent and type of infection.

Superficial or cutaneous infections should initially be approached topically. Any follicular, nail, or widespread (>20% of body surface area) infection should be treated systemically under medical supervision owing to poor penetration of topical applications. Topical antifungals have been reviewed as a class by the FDA advisory review panel on over-the-counter (OTC) antimicrobial drug products and on an individual basis as newer products have been released. To receive a class I recommendation, each agent (or combination) must have been tested in well-designed clinical trials that show that the drug is microbiologically and clinically effective against dermatophytosis or candidiasis with insignificant toxicity (irritation). Class I agents are listed in Table 78-3. Class II agents (camphor, candicidin, coal tar, menthol, phenolates, resorcinol, tannic acid, thymol, and tolindate) are considered to have higher risk–benefit ratios associated with their pharmacotherapy. Class III agents (benzoic acid, borates, caprylic acid, oxyquinolines, iodines, propionic acid, salicylates, triacetin, and gentian violet) lack adequate scientific data to determine efficacy. Topical therapy with any class I agent applied twice daily to the affected area for 2 to 6 weeks should be adequate. Therapy should be titrated to response.

C.W. could continue tolnaftate powder for 2 to 6 weeks or switch to an antifungal cream or lotion (e.g., miconazole and terbinafine), and these products should be applied to the web spaces between all the affected toes twice daily. C.W. should also be careful to use nonocclusive footwear (e.g., cotton rather than synthetic fiber socks and leather rather than vinyl boots). Application of an absorbent or antifungal powder to his footwear would also be helpful (see Chapter 39, Dermatotherapy and Drug-Induced Skin Disorders).

Tinea Unguium (Onychomycosis): Treatment

CASE 78-1, QUESTION 2: If C.W. also suffered from an infection of the toenail (onychomycosis), what additional therapy could be offered to him?

Onychomycosis is typically caused by a dermatophyte, a hyphal fungi, or *Candida*.

Nail scrapings and culture should be performed to help plan initial therapy. Once culture results are known, therapy can be initiated with either terbinafine 250 mg/day or itraconazole 200 mg/day for 6 (fingernail) to 12 (toenail) weeks. In some cases, however, successful therapy of tinea unguium can require 3 to 6 months for fingernails and 6 to 12 months for toenails. Therapy should be considered successful when several millimeters of healthy nail have emerged from the nailfold to the margin of infected nail or when a 25% reduction in the size of the infected site has been achieved.

For dermatophyte nail or paronychial infections, griseofulvin therapy could be used if an azole or allylamine is contraindicated. Griseofulvin (microsized or ultramicrosized) administered orally at 10 mg/kg/day and titrated to response should be effective.[25] Owing to the large doses given for prolonged periods, C.W. should be monitored closely at each prescription refill for signs and symptoms of adverse reactions. The most common adverse events associated with terbinafine or itraconazole are headache, rash, and GI distress. Griseofulvin is more toxic, often causing hypersensitivity (urticaria, angioedema, and type II hypersensitivity reactions), photosensitivity dermatitis, GI distress, and neurologic complications (headache, paresthesias, and altered sensorium).[25]

Antimycotic pulse therapy is a novel approach to the treatment of onychomycosis. An FDA-approved alternative to daily therapy can now include a course of itraconazole 200 mg twice daily for 1 week in two consecutive months for fingernail infections. Double-blind, placebo-controlled trials revealed that this regimen was associated with a 77% clinical response and 73% mycologic response.[36] Overall responses and toxicity to therapy were more desirable with pulse regimens than with traditional regimens. Comparative studies demonstrate promising results for itraconazole pulse therapy for toenail infections[37] and fluconazole pulse therapy administered as a 150- to 450-mg dose once weekly for up to 12 months for mild disease.[38,39] Relapse rates after pulse (intermittent) terbinafine for 4 months have been frequent, and longer courses of therapy are under study to enhance long-term efficacy.[40] Longer courses of therapy are being evaluated.

Removal of the nail as the sole therapy is not recommended because of the high relapse rate without concomitant systemic therapy. Likewise, IV antifungals are not indicated.

CASE 78-1, QUESTION 3: Describe the role of corticosteroids, antibacterials, or other additives to the antimycotic regimen in C.W.

Many patients with superficial, cutaneous, or nail fungal infections will have local inflammation and secondary bacterial infections. Inflammation is primarily a type IV hypersensitivity reaction. Topical corticosteroids in conjunction with antifungals can relieve itching and erythema secondary to inflammation. Bacterial (*Proteus* or *Pseudomonas* species) superinfection can also occur in these inflamed or macerated areas requiring concomitant topical antibacterial therapy. Pharmaceutical manufacturers of OTC preparations often combine a drying agent or astringent (e.g., alcohol, starch, talc, and camphor) to their preparations to increase desquamation of the stratum corneum. Hyperhidrosis also can be relieved by these pharmaceutical additions. Such combination treatments should not be used routinely, however, because they increase the risk of toxicity and do not increase efficacy. If required for symptomatic relief, they should be used only for the initial days of treatment.

The affected web spaces between C.W.'s toes are macerated and cracked, and vesicles are present at the base of his toes. A topical corticosteroid cream will probably facilitate the healing process and make him more comfortable during the first few days of antifungal therapy. The selection of topical corticosteroid formulations is presented in Chapter 39, Dermatotherapy and Drug-Induced Skin Disorders.

SUBCUTANEOUS MYCOSES

Sporotrichosis

TREATMENT OPTIONS

CASE 78-2

QUESTION 1: O.M., a 62-year-old man, has had a painless, slowly enlarging ulcer on his left hand for the past 4 months. He is an avid gardener but can identify no antecedent local trauma. The primary lesion began as a red papule that slowly enlarged and then ulcerated. At the same time that the ulcer developed, O.M. also noted painless, red nodules that spread proximally up his arm. He denies any chills, fever, weight loss, or cough. The ulcer has slowly enlarged despite the daily application of a povidone iodine ointment and 2 weeks of cephalexin treatment. On physical examination, O.M. is afebrile. A 1.5 cm^2 ulcer is present on the dorsum of the left hand. Extending proximally from the ulcer are a palpable cord and multiple nontender, erythematous nodules distributed linearly up the forearm, elbow, arm, and axilla. A culture of this ulcer obtained 4 weeks ago is now growing *S. schenckii*. What is the recommended therapy for O.M.?

S. schenckii is the dimorphic fungi found in the soil and on many plants. Infection is usually secondary to inoculation into the skin from a thorn or sharp plant matter. *S. schenckii* infection most commonly causes lymphocutaneous disease (Fig. 78-1) as illustrated by this case. Rarely, extracutaneous disease may occur and usually involves the lungs, bones, or joints.

HEAT TREATMENT

In the 1930s and 1940s, local heat was applied to very mild plaque or lymphocutaneous disease. Germination rates of this dimorphic fungus can actually be decreased by increased temperature, and heat therapy 1 hour/day for 3 months is effective in 90% of patients with plaques (very mild disease).[41] Heat treatment could be particularly useful in pregnant patients when pharmacotherapy may be contraindicated.

ITRACONAZOLE

Itraconazole is more active in vitro against *S. schenckii* than other imidazoles or saturated solution of potassium iodide. Saturated solution of potassium iodide is seldom used for therapy secondary to treatment-limiting toxicity. Cure rates for sporotrichosis cutaneous and lymphocutaneous disease are greater than 90% with itraconazole 100 to 200 mg/day for 3 to 6 months. For extracutaneous disease, higher dosages of itraconazole (200 mg twice a day

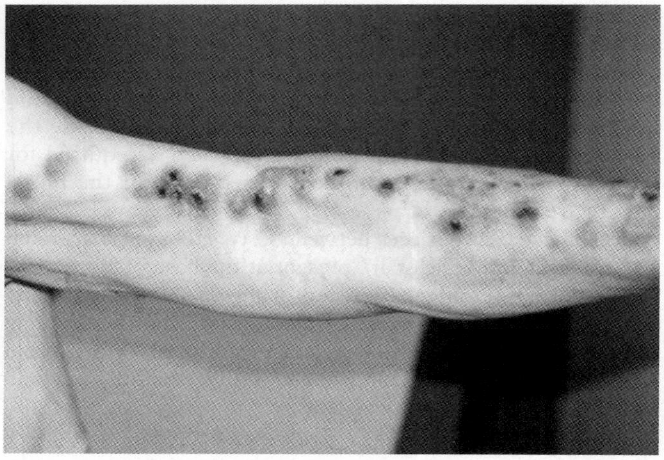

Figure 78-1 Lymphocutaneous sporotrichosis.

[BID]) for 1 to 2 years achieve response rates of 81%, but relapse frequently occurs (27%) after therapy is stopped.[41,42] Itraconazole is well tolerated in these patients. Patients with extracutaneous disease who are unable to tolerate the higher itraconazole dosages or whose disease continues to progress should be treated with AmB or a lipid-based amphotericin product. A total dose of 2.0 to 2.5 g is most often recommended if conventional AmB is used. Although voriconazole, posaconazole, and ravuconazole demonstrate in vitro activity against *S. schenckii* (albeit less than itraconazole), their role in the treatment of sporotrichosis has not been defined.[43] Neither ketoconazole nor fluconazole is effective in the treatment of sporotrichosis.

TERBINAFINE

Terbinafine has a good in vitro activity against *S. schenckii* and has been used clinically with some success.[44] An unpublished clinical trial comparing 250 or 500 mg BID for 3 months for lymphocutaneous disease appeared clinically equivalent to itraconazole. Adverse reactions include GI distress (dysgeusia, dyspepsia, and diarrhea), skin rash, and weight gain.

Therefore, in the case of lymphocutaneous disease, itraconazole 100 mg/day for a minimum of 3 months is the treatment of choice. If significant improvement is not observed in the first 6 weeks, the itraconazole dosage should be increased to 200 mg/day and continued for 6 months or until both the ulcer and lymphangitis have resolved. Most patients will respond to this dosage, but an occasional patient may require dosages of 300 or 400 mg/day.

Itraconazole Dosing

CASE 78-2, QUESTION 2: What instructions should O.M. receive for taking his antifungal agent?

The peak serum concentrations of itraconazole capsules are ninefold higher when the drug is taken with food (0.18 mcg/mL with food vs. 0.02 mcg/mL in fasting subjects).[45] The influence of food on absorption appears to be dependent on food type. High-carbohydrate meals decrease the absorption of itraconazole, and high-lipid-content meals increase itraconazole absorption.[46] Patients who have difficulty eating (e.g., patients with AIDS and those with cancer receiving antineoplastic therapy) or with hypochlorhydria may not absorb a sufficient amount from the capsule to achieve therapeutic plasma concentrations after a typical oral dose.[47] Although itraconazole manifests nonlinear serum pharmacokinetics (i.e., administering the total dose in two divided doses is associated with higher peak serum concentrations than a single larger dose), there is no clinical benefit in splitting the dose. Therefore, O.M. could be instructed to take his itraconazole capsule with his highest-fat-content meal of the day or itraconazole solution could be substituted to improve absorption.

Itraconazole oral solution is a cyclodextrin formulation that has 55% bioavailability in a fed patient; this increases in a fasting patient (Table 78-5). Furthermore, bioavailability of this formulation is not affected by level of gastric acidity. Average serum concentration in a cohort of patients with advanced HIV infection was 2.7 mcg/mL after a 28-day twice-daily dosing regimen.[48] O.M. should take his itraconazole solution on an empty stomach BID if this formulation is selected.

CASE 78-2, QUESTION 3: How would instructions for taking itraconazole capsules be modified if O.M. were achlorhydric as a result of medications or AIDS gastropathy? Should azole serum concentrations be monitored for an assessment of efficacy?

Itraconazole capsules, as with ketoconazole, require an acidic environment for dissolution and absorption. Thus, patients who are achlorhydric, as a result of medications, surgery, or underlying disease (e.g., AIDS gastropathy), may not absorb itraconazole capsules adequately.[47,49] The use of ketoconazole in achlorhydric patients has historically required concomitant administration of 4 mL, 0.2 N hydrochloric acid aqueous solution. Etching of tooth enamel by the acid can occur; thus, other alternatives have been explored. The administration of ketoconazole and itraconazole with a low pH liquid (e.g., 8–16 fluid ounces of a carbonated cola beverage or orange juice) improves absorption in 65.2% of healthy patients who are achlorhydric or taking H_2-blockers.[49] Refer to Azole–Drug Interactions section for more detailed information on problematic therapeutic combinations.

Voriconazole does not require an acidic environment for adequate oral absorption, but voriconazole should be administered 1 hour before or after meals because high-fat meals may reduce voriconazole serum concentrations.[50] In contrast, posaconazole plasma concentrations are fourfold higher after administration with food or a high-fat nutritional supplement. A newer formulation of posaconazole, which releases the drug in the pH-dependent manner in the duodenum, is not dependent on low gastric pH for dissolution and does not require administration with food to achieve therapeutic levels.[51–53] Isavuconazole is unique among triazole antifungals because it is administered IV or orally as a prodrug (isavuconazonium sulfate), which is rapidly cleaved by plasma esterases to the active antifungal, isavuconazole. Absorption of the prodrug is relatively complete (>90% bioavailability) and does not require low gastric pH or coadministration with food. IV isavuconazonium is water-soluble and, unlike voriconazole or posaconazole parenteral formulations, is not solubilized in hydroxypropyl-β-cyclodextrin.

Because serum ketoconazole, itraconazole, and voriconazole concentrations less than 0.25 to 1.0 mcg/mL have been associated with an increased risk of treatment failure and increased mortality in neutropenic patients, therapeutic drug monitoring is justified in patients in whom therapy is failing or suspected risk factors for low blood levels (i.e., poor gut function, drug interactions, and pediatric patients) or, in the case of voriconazole, suspected CNS toxicity, which is more frequent in patients with trough levels exceeding 5.5 mcg/mL.[54] Similarly, posaconazole serum concentrations less than 0.7 mcg/mL have been associated with an increased risk of breakthrough infection during prophylaxis, and trough or random levels approaching 1.5 mcg/mL have been associated with improved probability of treatment response in documented invasive aspergillosis.[54] Serum antimycotic concentrations may be more easily monitored in the future because assays, potentially

Table 78-5
Pharmacokinetic Properties of Systemically Active Non-polyene Antifungals

	Imidazoles		Triazoles					Echinocandins			Other	
Characteristic	MCZ	KCZ[a]	ITZ[a]	FCZ[a]	PCZ[a] Susp/ tablet	ICZ[a] (Cap)	VCZ[a]	AFG[a]	CFG[a]	MFG[a]	5FC[a]	TBF[a]
Absorption												
Relative bioavailability	<10	75[b]	99.8 (40)[b]	(85–92)[b]		>90	>90[d]	<10	<10	<10	75–90[b]	70
C_{max} (mcg/mL)	1.9	3.29	0.63	1.4	0.851/2.76	7.50	2.3–4.7[d]	7.5	12	7.1	70–80	1.34–1.7
T_{max} (hours)	1.0	2.6	4.0	1.0–4.0	3/4	3	<2	1	1	1	<2	1.5
AUC[c] (mcg/hour/mL)	ND	12.9 (13.6)	1.9(0.7)	42	8.619/51.62	121.4	9–11 (13)[d]	104.5	97.63–100.5	59.9	ND	4.74–10.48
Distribution												
Protein binding (%)	91–93	99	99.8	11	99	95	58	80	96.5	99.5	2–4	>99
CSF or serum concentration (%)	<10	<10	<10	60	ND	ND	~50	ND	ND	ND	60	<10
Excretion												
$\beta t_{1/2}$ (hours)	2.1	8.1[d]	17[d]	23–45	31	130	6	25.6	10	13	2.5–6.0	36
Active drug in urine (%)	1	2	<10	60–80	13	<1	<2	<1	2	1	0	80

[a]Given parameters are estimated from the administration of currently recommended doses. Miconazole (MCZ) 7.4–14.2 mg/kg/day (500–1,000 mg) parenterally; ketoconazole (KTZ) 2.8 mg/kg/day orally (200 mg); itraconazole (ITZ) 1.4–2.8 mg/kg/day orally (100–200 mg); fluconazole (FCZ) 0.7–1.4 mg/kg/day orally; voriconazole (VCZ) and posaconazole (PCZ) 400 mg twice daily orally; or 300 mg twice daily Day 1, then 300 mg daily; isavuconazole (ICZ) 200 mg (372 mg isavuconazonium sulfate) 3 times daily for 48 hours, then 300 mg daily anidulafungin (AFG) 200 mg parenterally; caspofungin (CFG) 70 (50) mg parenterally on Day 1 (2–14); micafungin (MFG) 70 mg parenterally; flucytosine (5FC) 150 mg/day parenterally; and terbinafine (TBF) 250 mg/day orally.
[b]With meals (fasting), absorption altered by gastric acidity.
[c]Dose-dependent and/or infusion-dependent.
[d]Absorption decreased when administered with high-fat meal; C_{max} and AUC reduced by 34% and 24%, respectively.

AUC, area under the concentration–time curve; C_{max}, maximum concentration; CSF, cerebrospinal fluid; ND, no data; T_{max}, time of maximum concentration; $t_{1/2}$, half-life.

performed at the point of care (patient bedside or clinic), become available, and correlations between concentration and efficacy or toxicity are more clearly established.[55]

SYSTEMIC MYCOSES

Candida Infection

CASE 78-3

QUESTION 1: L.K., a 21-year-old, 5-foot 8-inch, 170-pound, otherwise healthy man, was admitted to the hospital 16 days ago after a gunshot wound to the abdomen. He has undergone three exploratory laparotomies with repair and resection of damaged small intestine. He was placed on TPN to allow his bowel to rest and received stress doses of methylprednisolone Day 6 in hospital. Three days ago, he exhibited a fever of 39.1°C and chills; his blood pressure of 100/70 mm Hg had dropped more than 30 mm Hg (systolic). Vancomycin and meropenem were promptly begun after obtaining blood cultures. Despite 3 days of antibiotics, he remains febrile. His physical examination reveals a Hickman catheter in the right subclavian vein that is functioning normally; no inflammatory changes are evident at the exit site. A single erythematous nodule about 0.5 cm wide is noted near the left wrist. The funduscopic examination of both eyes is normal. A chest radiograph is also normal. The white blood cell (WBC) count is currently 10,950 cells/μL, and renal function is normal. What subjective and objective data in this case suggest a possible *Candida* infection?

EPIDEMIOLOGY

Although it is possible that L.K. might be infected with bacterial pathogens not susceptible to vancomycin and meropenem, the possibility of a candidal infection should be considered. *Candida* species are the most common nosocomial fungal pathogens. *Candida* species were responsible for 72.2% of mycoses in hospitalized cases, and *C. albicans* accounted for 55% of these cases in the Centers for Disease Control, National Nosocomial Infections Surveillance System. Attributable mortality associated with disseminated candidiasis from all species is 38% and it is ~12% for extremely low-birth-weight neonates.[56] These statistics may underestimate the true occurrence because systemic candidiasis is difficult to diagnose. To reinforce this point, the diagnosis of systemic candidal infection is made in 30% to 50% of neutropenic patients with hematologic malignancies at postmortem.[57] Therefore, the morbidity for systemic candidiasis may be even higher because of the limited ability to diagnose systemic disease.

CHARACTERISTICS

The diagnosis and monitoring of therapeutic outcomes for systemic candidal infection are difficult because the characteristics of systemic candidal infection are subtle. Salient clinical features include constitutional symptoms (e.g., fever, chills, and hypotension) and evidence of end-organ dissemination, such as nodular erythematous skin lesions, endophthalmitis, liver abscess, and spleen abscess. In addition, 50% of patients or fewer will have a single positive *Candida* blood culture. The Mycoses Study Group utilizes a single positive culture from a sterile body site and hypotension (systolic blood pressure [SBP] <100 mm Hg or a SBP decrease >30 mm Hg) or abnormal temperature (<35.5°C or >38.6°C on one occasion or >37.8°C on two separate occasions more than 4 hours apart), or inflammation at an infected site as diagnostic criteria.

RISK FACTORS

Risk factors for candidemia include central venous catheters, broad-spectrum antibiotic use, extensive surgical procedures, *Candida* colonization, TPN, pancreatitis, neutropenia or neutrophil dysfunction, and immunosuppression (e.g., premature infants, burn patients, patients with mannose-binding lectin deficiency, and patients with AIDS).[58]

L.K. has chills, a temperature of 39.1°C, and is hypotensive. He is probably immunosuppressed as a result of multiple surgical procedures and receipt of corticosteroids. His Hickman catheter is a possible portal of entry, and his broad-spectrum antibiotic therapy with vancomycin and meropenem should be adequate for most bacterial pathogens. Because L.K. still has manifestations of an infection despite 3 days of antibiotics, additional diagnostic studies are warranted.

DIAGNOSTIC TESTS

CASE 78-3, QUESTION 2: What diagnostic tests could be ordered for L.K. to evaluate a possible fungal infection?

The diagnosis of fungal infection may be made with varying levels of certainty. Sometimes, the diagnosis is absolutely certain, such as the isolation of a pathogenic fungus from a clinical specimen in an immunocompromised patient. Such a finding is referred to as a definitive or microbiologically confirmed diagnosis. At other times, only a high probability of infection can be determined, that is, a presumptive diagnosis. To illustrate this, a patient with a chest radiograph showing nodular lesions and a high complement fixation (CF) antibody against *H. capsulatum* would have a presumptive diagnosis of histoplasmosis. This finding may be as certain a diagnosis as is possible without performing a more invasive procedure to obtain lung tissue. In this event, a trial of drug therapy can be undertaken on the presumptive diagnosis alone. A diverse spectrum of tests is available for clinicians to diagnose and monitor therapeutic responses.

Direct Examination

Direct examination of the specimen is often useful in diagnosing fungal infection. Traditionally, the specimen is treated with 10% KOH to digest the cells and debris, resulting in clear visualization of the hyphae or yeast. Treatment of cerebrospinal fluid (CSF) specimens with KOH is not necessary because this fluid is naturally clear. India ink can be added to CSF to increase contrast and outline the organisms. Calcofluor white, a fluorescent fabric brightener that binds to fungi and fluoresces brilliantly when viewed under the ultraviolet microscope, can also be used to assist in the recognition of fungal elements.

Histologic examination of biopsy specimens is an important tool for diagnosing and monitoring fungal infection, but identifying the exact fungus may be difficult. This is because only the tissue phase can be observed, and the fungal organisms in the specimen may be few. Because recognizing a fungus in hematoxylin-stained or eosin-stained sections may be difficult, a number of special stains have been developed.[58] Periodic acid–Schiff staining binds linked sugar groups in the fungal cell wall. This intense magenta staining makes visualization of the fungal form easier. Likewise, several silver precipitation stains (e.g., Gomori methenamine silver) rely on the presence of a charged fungal surface to reduce oxidized silver to metallic silver. This process coats the fungus with a black layer, again outlining the form.[59] The mucicarmine stain imparts a deep red color to complex polysaccharides, such as mucin, which can stain the thick capsule of *C. neoformans*. Because no other yeast has a positive mucicarmine stain, the definitive diagnosis of cryptococcosis can be made.[60] The size of the organism, manner of budding, and the presence or absence of septae all assist in the diagnosis.

Monoclonal antibodies against many fungi are now available. Immunohistochemical procedures using these sera on biopsy specimens allow for the identification of a number of fungal pathogens.[60] Reagents for in situ oligonucleotide probe hybridization to detect fungi in tissue are being developed and will also be extremely helpful.[61]

Culture

The most definitive method for diagnosing or monitoring a fungal infection is using culture. Specimens should be inoculated onto several different types of fungal media, some of which contain antibiotics to inhibit bacterial overgrowth. Swab specimens have a very low yield, especially for hyphal fungi, and should be avoided in follow-up cultures. Yeast may grow rapidly and be isolated within 24 to 48 hours, but many fungi grow slowly, and 4 to 6 weeks of incubation may be necessary to isolate and identify the organism. After growth, yeasts are usually recognized by their patterns of metabolic activity on a variety of substrates, whereas mycelial organisms may produce characteristic spores and fruiting bodies that are used for identification. Occasionally, a mycelial organism will be slow in producing recognizable spores, and immunologic testing for a characteristic isoantigen may be used for identification. A peptide nucleic acid fluorescence in situ hybridization test more rapidly identifies *C. albicans* from blood-culture bottles.[62] It is unclear how cost-effective this test will be compared with traditional germ-tube testing.

Antigen Detection

Fungi synthesize polysaccharides that cannot be broken down by human enzymatic systems. These polysaccharides can accumulate within the body and can be excreted in the urine. These fungal antigens can be detected by using antibodies that specifically recognize a particular species of fungus, thereby providing a diagnosis. The most commonly used antigen detection test is a latex agglutination test for cryptococcal antigen. This assay can be performed on serum or CSF. Antigenemia is present in 80% to 100% of patients with culture-proved cryptococcal meningitis. This test can also be used to monitor patient response to therapy by determining the end point dilution for the positive reaction and following this end point over time when the patient is treated. If treatment is successful, the titer will decline.[63,64]

Tests (quantitative polymerase chain reaction, enzyme-linked immunosorbent assay [ELISA], and latex agglutination) for other fungal antigens are also not established. Latex particle agglutination tests to detect candidal antigens are available, but their utility has not been clearly demonstrated. Assays for detecting *H. capsulatum* antigen in serum and urine have been reported.[65] Antigen can be detected in the blood of 50% of patients and in the urine of 80% to 90% of patients with systemic histoplasmosis. Patients with blastomycosis and paracoccidioidomycosis, however, may also have positive cross-reactions. The ELISA for the detection of *Aspergillus* galactomannan antigen (Section 78-8) and *Candida* (1–3)-β-D-glucan has reported sensitivity (63%) and specificity (96%) of two consecutive (1–3)-β-D-glucan results greater than 7 pg/mL, which is clinically useful. Using these tests can result in a shorter time to diagnosis and leads to significantly shorter time of illness compared with other diagnostic tests. β-Glucan is most valuable for its negative predictive value.[66] Considering the presence of false-positives or false-negatives, it is unknown whether these assays will improve diagnostic capability for patients at a risk for these infections. False-positives may be caused by a myriad of products (IgG, albumen, cellulose filters, or gauze bandages) with variable outcomes associated with pipercillin/tazobactam manufactured antibiotics. Increasing or decreasing values can be used to monitor clinical response to antifungal therapy.[62]

Antibody Detection

The detection of antibody can be useful for some fungal diseases, but not for others. Serologic diagnosis of systemic candidiasis is complicated because most people have anti-*Candida* antibodies. A rising titer is not specific for infection and may indicate only colonization. Furthermore, dissemination of *Candida* is most likely in people who are immunocompromised and, therefore, may not respond by producing antibody.[67] On the other hand, seropositivity can be demonstrated in more than 90% of patients with symptomatic histoplasmosis.[68] The most important serologic tests use the CF, immunodiffusion, and enzyme immunoassay (EIA) techniques. The appropriate evolution of serologic results requires an understanding of the sensitivity, specificity, and predictive value of each methodology. In general, serologic tests allow only a presumptive diagnosis of mycotic infections.

Although any of the aforementioned tests could be ordered for L.K., a direct examination of his blood and urine specimens along with an assessment of signs and symptoms of disseminated candidiasis is a reasonable first step in his evaluation. A blood specimen from L.K. should also be cultured on different fungal media. Because a candidal infection is suspected, the culture could isolate *Candida* within 24 to 48 hours. Cultures and histopathologic examination of a biopsy specimen of skin lesions are often helpful not only in confirming a diagnosis of disseminated candidal infection, but also in monitoring response to therapy. The other fungal tests previously described need not be ordered immediately and should await the results from the direct examination and culture.

NECESSITY OF TREATMENT

CASE 78-3, QUESTION 3: The clinical laboratory reports that a single blood culture obtained 2 days ago is growing *Candida* species. Why is therapy necessary in L.K. with only a single positive blood culture?

Case–control studies of candidemia report an 85.6% mortality rate in untreated patients compared with a 41.8% mortality rate in patients who received early treatment. Isolation of *Candida* from a patient's bloodstream requires the initiation of immediate antifungal therapy. Delays in therapy are associated with a significant increase in mortality. In fact, delaying therapy 24 hours from the time a blood culture is positive or failure to follow IDSA treatment guidelines increases mortality nearly 50%.[69–71] Elimination of risk factors may improve the clinical outcome of candidemia, and the removal of central venous catheters reduces morbidity and mortality.[72,73] Although discontinuation of a centrally inserted catheter may complicate drug administration, it still should be removed. L.K.'s other risk factors (e.g., broad-spectrum antibacterials) are perhaps of even greater importance.

TREATMENT OPTIONS AND COMBINATION THERAPY

CASE 78-3, QUESTION 4: What therapeutic options are available to treat candidemia? Which option would be best for L.K.?

Therapeutic options are individualized and based on the competence of a patient's host defenses. In immunocompetent patients, AmB formulations, an echinocandin, or a triazole decreases morbidity and mortality associated with this disease.[74–78] Echinocandins have been demonstrated as effective as AmB formulations in neutropenic and non-neutropenic patients; however, AmB clears the bloodstream more rapidly.[79,80] In the largest, well-controlled comparative trial, 206 non-neutropenic patients were randomly assigned to AmB 0.5 to 0.6 mg/kg/day or fluconazole 400 mg/day for 14 days. Mortality was less than 9% in both the groups with no significant difference in successful outcomes (AmB, 80%; fluconazole, 72%). Less toxicity was noted in the fluconazole group, however.[75] Therefore, fluconazole 400 mg/day is as effective as AmB for non-neutropenic patients infected with susceptible *Candida*. Candidemic (or other mycotic infections discussed in this chapter) patients who are clinically stable and have no evidence of deep-seated infection should be initiated on a triazole or an echinocandin for at least 14 days. Patients who cannot be treated with an echinocandin or an azole can be treated with AmB 0.5 to 1.0 mg/kg/day or 3 to 5 mg/kg/day of a lipid formulation of AmB. Alternatively, a comparison of micafungin (100 or 150 mg) with caspofungin revealed no difference with micafungin 100 mg and caspofungin after 10 days of therapy. However, micafungin 150 mg trended toward poorer responses.[81]

High-dose fluconazole (12 mg/kg/day) alone or in combination with AmB for a minimum of 3 days, followed by step-down therapy to fluconazole, was evaluated. Outcomes were not different between treatment groups and consistent with the previously reported success rates. Notably, the fluconazole treatment group had higher Acute Physiology and Chronic Health Evaluation (APACHE II) scores, making evaluation of the comparison difficult.[79] In contrast, in another clinical trial, the combination of AmB and flucytosine was suggested to be more effective than single-agent therapy.[82,83] An AmB-containing regimen may be more effective in patients with APACHE II scores between 10 and 22.[79]

L.K. could be treated with an echinocandin, with the total duration based on clinical response and resolution of positive cultures (see Case 78-3, Question 6). Therapy typically should be continued for 14 days post–last positive blood culture. Some clinicians check cultures daily to assess this end point. Efficacy should be monitored using patient-specific signs and symptoms of candidemia. Combination therapy can be considered in those patients who are not responding clinically. More importantly, a complete examination for focal sites of infection (septic thrombi or intra-abdominal abscess) should take place.

CASE 78-3, QUESTION 5: This fungal species has now been identified as *C. non-albicans*. How does this affect the therapeutic options for L.K.?

Historically, the isolation of a non-albicans *Candida* from blood has resulted in a therapeutic dilemma caused by common in vitro resistance, which has been associated with poor clinical outcomes in animal models and uncontrolled case reports. Intrinsic resistance (i.e., *Candida lusitaniae* to AmB, *C. parapsilosis* to echinocandins, and *Candida krusei* to fluconazole) or acquired resistance (*C. tropicalis* or *glabrata* against fluconazole) has been reported.[76,82,83] Acquired in vitro fluconazole drug resistance is probably associated with altered fungal cell membrane permeability, antifungal efflux pumps, and changes in CYP450 enzymes. In observational studies, fluconazole resistance in vitro has been 9%.[76,82,83] A large, multicenter study of 232 non-neutropenic patients was unable, however, to demonstrate a relationship between yeast MIC and patient outcome.[76] An inability to demonstrate a relationship is probably a result of a limited understanding or inadequate management of risk factors for infection. For example, the removal of a colonized IV catheter is probably a more important predictor of outcome than the MIC of the isolated yeast. A disturbing increase in acquired *C. glabrata* resistance to the echinocandins via a *FKS* gene, first reported in 2008, should be suspected in echinocandin treatment failures.[27,84]

Therefore, the true rate of acquired clinical resistance to azoles and ultimate failure is unknown. Vigilant monitoring and aggressive therapy of infections caused by *Candida non-albicans* are recommended. In patients in whom susceptibilities are available, fluconazole should be avoided when the MIC is greater than 16 mcg/mL.

AMPHOTERICIN FORMULATIONS

Dosing

CASE 78-3, QUESTION 6: How should amphotericin B formulation be dosed and administered to L.K.?

The AmB formulation dose and duration of therapy should be individualized based on the severity of infection and immunocompetence of the patient. Once the patient is stable, therapy should be changed to one of the applicable regimens discussed previously. The dose of AmB formulations should be based on lean body mass. Owing to the difficulty in measuring lean body mass, many clinicians, however, use ideal body weight. Tissues that contain large numbers of macrophages sequester significant amounts of AmB (liver, 17.5%–40.3%; spleen, 0.7%–15.6%; kidney, 0.6%–4.1%; and lung, 0.4%–13%), but it does not distribute well into adipose tissue (<1.0%).[77,78] In fact, AmB formulations bound to cholesterol have been shown to bind to clathrin-coated pits (low-density lipoprotein receptors or receptors of endocytosis) on cells, facilitating intracellular incorporation and possibly reducing renal toxicity.[85] Because L.K. is 5-feet and 8-inches tall and not obese, his ideal body weight should be about 70 kg. Therefore, generic AmB 35 mg/day (0.5 mg/kg) should be initiated because L.K. is not clinically stable and may require increased doses. Half of the full dose should be given on the first day of therapy and the full dose given on subsequent days. In more seriously ill patients, the full dose of generic AmB can be initiated immediately. Although the optimal dosing regimen to initiate generic AmB is not well established, most clinicians gradually titrate the dose upward to minimize infusion-related reactions. Peak AmB serum concentrations achieved after parenteral administration are a function of dose, frequency of dosing, and the rate of infusion. When the AmB total dose is less than 50 mg, the serum concentration is directly proportional to the dose; doses greater than 50 mg are associated with a plateau in serum concentrations. After administration, AmB undergoes biphasic elimination: Peak serum concentrations drop rapidly (initial $t_{1/2}$, 24–48 hours), but low concentrations (0.5–1.0 mcg/mL) are detectable for up to 2 weeks (terminal $t_{1/2}$ 15 days).[86] The long terminal elimination half-life has been used as a justification for the common practice of less frequent AmB dosing, in which twice the daily dose is given every other day. Every-other-day regimens have not been carefully evaluated but are rationalized based on the potential for reduced nephrotoxicity. Administration of generic AmB 0.5 mg/kg/day or 1.0 mg/kg every other day results in trough AmB concentrations with sufficient postdose antifungal effects that inhibit the common pathogenic fungi.[87] Once L.K.'s clinical status has improved, the potential for renal toxicity could outweigh the concerns of potential reduced efficacy, and implementation of AmB every-other-day therapy should be considered.

Infusion Reactions

CASE 78-3, QUESTION 7: L.K. has no complaints except for fevers and shaking chills that occur during his 6- to 8-hour AmB infusion for the past 3 days. He has been receiving acetaminophen 650 mg 30 minutes before AmB infusion, but he has refused today's AmB dose. What measures can be taken to minimize these infusion-related reactions?

Adverse reactions, which are common with AmB formulation administration, are best classified as infusion-related, dose-related, or idiosyncratic reactions. Infusion-related reactions include an acute symptom complex of fever, chills, nausea, vomiting, headache, hypotension, and thrombophlebitis. Dose-related reactions also can be acute (e.g., cardiac arrhythmias) or chronic (e.g., renal dysfunction with secondary electrolyte imbalances and anemia). Premedication to prevent AmB formulation, infusion-related reactions, and a test dose of AmB formulations are not needed for L.K. Most practices of premedicating are performed out of ritual rather than predicated on a scientific study.[88] Test dosing with 1 mg before the first dose is not currently used because of the immeasurably low incidence of anaphylactoid reactions. Until clinical trials clarify the risk–benefit ratio of premedications, concomitant therapy should be restricted to acetaminophen for fever or headache and heparin to prevent thrombophlebitis when possible.

Many infusion-related reactions are mediated by AmB-induced cytokine (interleukin-1β, tumor necrosis factor, and prostaglandin E_2) expression by mononuclear cells.[89,90] Hydrocortisone is extremely effective in suppressing cytokine expression,[89] and it also blunts the fever and chills associated with AmB formulations.[91] Hydrocortisone, however, does not reduce the frequency of chronic dose-related toxicity such as renal insufficiency, and corticosteroid-induced immunosuppression could decrease AmB fungicidal activity.[92] Nonsteroidal anti-inflammatory drugs (NSAIDs) also prevent fever, most likely by the suppression of prostaglandin E_2 expression.[93] NSAIDs, however, cannot be recommended for routine use because of their potential for additive nephrotoxicity when used with AmB formulations.

The mild-to-moderate elevations in temperature and the other infusion-related symptoms usually subside when the infusion is completed, and tolerance to these effects develops over 3 to 5 days. L.K. initially should be counseled that these reactions will abate over the next few days without intervention. If assessment of the reactions suggests the need for more aggressive premedication, a short course of hydrocortisone 0.7 mg/kg prior to AmB or added to the infusion bag should be initiated.[91] Meperidine 25 to 50 mg by rapid IV infusion reduces AmB-induced rigors and can be repeated every 15 minutes as required while monitoring for signs and symptoms of opiate toxicity. Administration of an average meperidine dose of 45 mg has been found to resolve chills 3 times faster than placebo.[94]

Fast generic AmB infusion rates (< normal 4–6 hours) are associated with the earlier onset of infusion-related reactions, but not with more severe infusion reactions.[95,96] Many patients prefer rapid infusions (1–2 hours) because the infusion-related reactions abate quickly on the completion of the AmB infusion. Electrocardiographic evaluations of 1-hour infusions indicate that this rate of polyene infusion is safe at currently recommended doses in patients without renal or heart disease. Rapid infusions are not safe in all patients, however, because cardiac arrhythmias appear to be dose- and infusion rate–related. If infused too rapidly, high serum concentrations of AmB can precipitate severe cardiac adverse events. Arrhythmias have been reported most often in patients who are anuric or who have previous cardiac disease.[97] Continuous infusion is not recommended based on the pharmacodynamics of this agent and the concentration dependence of activity.

Nephrotoxicity

CASE 78-3, QUESTION 8: On Day 4 of therapy with AmB, L.K.'s serum creatinine (SCr) and blood urea nitrogen (BUN) are 2.3 mg/dL (SI units, 203.32 μmol/L) and 42 mg/dL (SI units, 14.99 mmol/L), respectively. How could AmB exacerbate L.K.'s renal dysfunction and how could it be prevented from worsening?

Renal dysfunction is the adverse event that most often limits treatment with AmB formulations. The renal toxicity results from AmB-mediated damage to renal tubules, which causes electrolyte wasting and disrupts the tubuloglomerular feedback mechanism. The clinical manifestations of AmB-induced renal damage include azotemia, renal tubular acidosis, hypokalemia, and hypomagnesemia.[88] The renal insult along with infusion-related reactions appears less severe in patients with higher serum cholesterol. This may be associated with the clathrin binding discussed earlier. Generally, AmB-related renal toxicity is reversible within 2 weeks after therapy has been discontinued. Administration of normal saline (250 mL) immediately before AmB administration reduces the risk for AmB-induced nephrotoxicity[98] and should be initiated before L.K.'s next dose. AmB formulations should not be admixed with normal saline, however, because sodium causes AmB to precipitate into an inactive particulate in IV admixture formulations.[99] Other nephrotoxins should be avoided (especially diuretics), and patients with already-compromised renal function should be closely monitored and alternate therapy should be considered.[99] Hypokalemia and hypomagnesemia should also be monitored closely. These measures to prevent further renal deterioration should be implemented, and the AmB therapy continued cautiously in this patient with systemic candidiasis. Anemia, associated with decreased renal production of erythropoietin, should resolve after AmB is discontinued and need not be treated.[100]

CASE 78-3, QUESTION 9: L.K. has exhibited significant renal dysfunction resulting from acute tubular necrosis. How should his dose of systemic antifungal drugs be altered?

Renal elimination of the antimycotics varies tremendously. For systemically administered AmB, only 5% to 10% of unchanged drug is eliminated in urine and bile during the first 24 hours,[88] and no evidence indicates that it is metabolized to a significant extent. Therefore, no substantial dosage adjustment is required for patients with chronic renal or hepatic failure. Although many clinicians will withhold AmB doses if acute renal dysfunction develops during therapy, concerns of drug-induced nephrotoxicity in L.K. must be balanced against the high likelihood of mortality in untreated patients with deep-seated infections.[55,56] Alternative systemic antifungal therapy (i.e., azoles or echinocandins) that is less nephrotoxic should also be considered. Dosing recommendations for echinocandins are unchanged in renal dysfunction or liver dysfunction, except for caspofungin. For patients with moderate hepatic insufficiency (Child–Turcotte–Pugh score 7–9), a change in the maintenance dose of caspofungin to 35 mg/day is recommended, even though the higher exposures expected with the standard dose are generally well tolerated. No data are available for caspofungin used in severe hepatic impairment, and a further dosage reduction should be considered.

Ketoconazole and itraconazole undergo first-pass metabolism and have a biphasic dose-dependent elimination.[45,46] These agents are extensively metabolized and excreted in the bile; small amounts of unchanged drug are excreted in the urine; therefore, no need exists to adjust dosages in patients with renal dysfunction or in patients undergoing dialysis.[101] Voriconazole is extensively metabolized by cytochrome P450 2C19 and to a lesser extend CYP3A4 to inactive metabolites excreted in the urine. However, the IV formulations of voriconazole and posaconazole are solubilized in sulfobutylether-β-cyclodextrin, which is eliminated via the kidneys. Accumulation of the cyclodextrin vehicle is associated with a theoretical potential for renal toxicity not reported to date in patients including those with renal impairment.[102,103] Therefore, oral therapy (or possibly isavuconazole) may be preferred in patients who require a broad-spectrum triazole but have impaired renal function. Fluconazole, unlike ketoconazole and itraconazole, is not extensively metabolized. More than 90% of a fluconazole dose is excreted in urine, of which about 80% is measured as unchanged drug and about 20% as metabolites.[104]

Because fluconazole is excreted primarily unchanged in the urine, dosages should be adjusted in patients with renal insufficiency (Table 78-5).[23,24,45–48,88,101–111] Fluconazole or voriconazole may be reasonable alternatives in L.K., but the dosage must be adjusted for renal function based on published nomograms.[105]

CASE 78-3, QUESTION 10: What is the role of an AmB formulated with a lipid?

Lipid formulations of AmB have been approved by the FDA for patients who are unable to tolerate generic AmB (Table 78-6). In addition, the admixture of AmB in 10% or 20% lipid emulsion has been used for treating systemic mycotic infections. The lipid carriers differ tremendously for each of the amphotericin formulations. The liposomal formulation is a spherical carrier that contains AmB on both the inside and outside of the vesicle. Imagine the lipid complex as a snowflake shape and the colloidal dispersion shaped like a Frisbee with AmB bound to the structure. The differences in structure appear to have no effect on therapeutic outcome but exhibit markedly different pharmacokinetics and rates of AMB release in vivo, which may account for difference in the rates of adverse effects observed with each formulation[112] AmB admixture with a lipid emulsion cannot be recommended until a stable formulation can be established.[113] Yet, similar in concept, some clinicians administer AmB formulations with breakfast (high-cholesterol meals) to simulate or enhance "lipid" coadministration, macrophage clathrin pit binding, and subsequent decreases in toxicity.

Limited data on AmB formulation comparisons are available to assist in the management of this case. A single large controlled trial has evaluated AmB lipid complex for the treatment of disseminated candidiasis. Generic AmB 0.6 to 1.0 mg/kg/day for 14 days was slightly, but not significantly, superior to the lipid complex formulation at 5 mg/kg/day for mycologic efficacy (68% vs. 63%) or survival.[114] Renal dysfunction defined as a doubling in SCr, however, was 47% with AmB and 28% with this lipid formulation. Because of the significant cost, some health-care facilities reserve lipid formulations for patients who have preexisting renal dysfunction or those who have severe adverse reactions to generic AmB. However, most centers use lipid formulations as their formulary polyene owing to patient acceptance and cost of AmB-associated renal dysfunction. Indications for the lipid formulations are further reviewed in the discussion of sections on aspergillosis, histoplasmosis, and cryptococcosis.

ANTIMYCOTIC PROPHYLAXIS

CASE 78-3, QUESTION 11: What measures could have been undertaken to prevent invasive fungal infections in L.K.?

In 2014, the National Institutes of Allergy and Infectious Diseases (NIAID)/Mycoses Study Group completed a randomized, double-blind, placebo-controlled trial of caspofungin prophylaxis followed by preemptive therapy for invasive candidiasis initiated on the basis of an antigen diagnostic test (β-D-glucan) among high-risk patients in the intensive care unit (ICU) setting.[115] The study utilized a validated risk-prediction score for invasive candidiasis that identified 18% of subjects admitted to the ICU with a predicted invasive candidiasis incidence rate of greater than 10%. Caspofungin prophylaxis was not associated with a reduction in the incidence of proven or probable invasive candidiasis or patient mortality. Therefore, prophylaxis among non-neutropenic patients at this time should be restricted to patient populations with proven benefit: post GI perforation, severe pancreatitis, liver/pancreas or small bowel transplant recipients, and extreme low-birth-weight neonates.[57]

Selective GI decontamination or systemic antimycotic pharmacotherapy can be used in high-risk, immunocompromised, or surgical patients to prevent the development of fungal infections and could have been used for L.K. In critically ill surgical patients, the risk of invasive infection, but not mortality, may be reduced by more than 50% with fluconazole prophylaxis.[116] Alternatively, a nonabsorbable antifungal such as AmB or nystatin is a possible option. Oral AmB decreases systemic candidal infections threefold to fivefold in high-risk patients.[117] Yet the problems of unreliable antifungal stool concentrations,[118] decreasing azole cost associated with the availability of generics, and poor compliance have led to preferential azole use. Azoles are also more effective in preventing oral pharyngeal candidiasis than placebo.[119,120] At the present time, no well-designed studies have compared azoles with polyene antifungals (e.g., AmB) for the prevention of oropharyngeal or systemic candidiasis.

Prophylaxis could be initiated and continued until L.K. is no longer immunocompromised. If L.K. is discharged from the hospital and treated as an outpatient, a systemic azole (imidazole or triazole) administered once daily is preferable to a polyene to improve adherence. To reemphasize, however, systemic therapy increases the risk of resistance, adverse effects, drug interactions, and potentially cost (Table 78-4). Therapeutic drug monitoring may be necessary in these patients.

Candiduria

TREATMENT

CASE 78-4

QUESTION 1: M.Y., a 24-year-old man, has been hospitalized in the surgical ICU with multiple traumatic injuries resulting from a motor vehicle accident. Shortly after admission, he underwent an exploratory laparotomy for a ruptured spleen and lacerated liver. He subsequently suffered from respiratory and renal failure. M.Y. is currently intubated and on mechanical ventilation. Since admission, he has been nutritionally supported with central hyperalimentation and has been receiving broad-spectrum antibiotics (gentamicin, ampicillin, and metronidazole). A Foley catheter is in place. Two recent urinalyses (UAs) show budding yeast, and cultures were positive for greater than 100,000 colony-forming units of *C. albicans*. M.Y. is currently afebrile, his funduscopic examination is normal, and no macronodular skin lesions are present. The WBC count is 8,900 cells/μL (SI units, WBC count, 8.9×10^9/L), and three sets of blood cultures drawn during the past 2 days are negative. How should M.Y.'s candiduria be treated?

It is difficult to differentiate among cystitis, urethritis, or systemic infection in the presence of funguria. Similarly, it is difficult to differentiate colonization from infection because candiduric patients are usually asymptomatic. Funguria cannot be used to determine the location or severity of invasion. Signs and symptoms of systemic disease should be monitored diligently until a diagnosis of colonization, cystitis, or urethritis is confirmed and the risk of dissemination is excluded.

Eradication of fungi in the urine (specifically *C. albicans*) should begin with the removal of the indwelling urinary catheter and alleviation of risk factors for fungal disease. If catheter removal does not clear the urine within 48 hours, pharmacotherapy should be considered. If M.Y. is scheduled for a genitourinary procedure, he should receive systemic therapy because the rate of candidemia after surgery is high (10.8%) in candiduric patients. In addition, any patient at a high risk for dissemination into the blood should be considered for treatment (e.g., patients with immunosuppression).[121]

Table 78-6

Amphotericin B Formulations

Category	Amphotericin B (Fungizone)	Amphotericin B Lipid Complex (Abelcet)	Amphotericin B Colloidal Dispersion (Amphotec)	Liposomal Amphotericin B (AmBisome)		Amphotericin B in Lipid Emulsion
FDA-approved indication	Life-threatening fungal infections Visceral leishmaniasis	Refractory or intolerant to AmB	Invasive Aspergillosis in patients refractory or intolerant to AmB	Empirical therapy in neutropenic FUO Refractory or intolerant to AmB Visceral leishmaniasis		NA
Formulation						
Sterol	None	None	Cholesterol sulfate	Cholesterol sulfate (5)[a]		Safflower and soybean oils
Phospholipid	None	DMPC and DMPG (7:3)[a]	None	EPC and DSPG (10:4)[a]		10–20 g/100 mL EPC > 2.21 g/100 mL Glycerin > 258 g/100 mL
Amphotericin B (Mole%)	34	33	50	10		Variable
Particle size (nm)	<10	1,600–11,000	122(±48)	80–120		333–500
Manufacturer	Generic	Enzon	Intermune	Fujisawa Pharmaceuticals		Not applicable
Stability	1 week at 2°C–8°C or 24 hours at 27°C	15 hours at 2°C–8°C or 6 hours at 27°C	24 hours at 2°C–8°C	24 hours at 2°C–8°C		Unstable
Dosage and rate	0.3–0.7 mg/kg/day during 1–6 hours[b]	5 mg/kg/day at 2.5 mg/kg/hour	3–4 mg/kg/day during 2 hours	3–5[c] mg/kg/day during 2 hours		Investigational: 1 mg/kg/day during 1–8 hours
Lethal dose 50%	3.3 mg/kg	10–25 mg/kg	68 mg/kg	175 mg/kg		Unknown
Pharmacokinetic Parameters						
Dose	0.5 mg/kg	5 mg/kg × 7 days	5 mg/kg × 7 days	2.5 mg/kg × 7 days	5 mg/kg × 7 days	0.8 mg/kg/day × 13 days
Serum Concentrations						
Peak	1.2 mcg/mL	1.7 mcg/mL	3.1 mcg/mL	31.4 mcg/mL	83.0 mcg/mL	2.13 mcg/mL
Trough	0.5 mcg/mL	0.7 mcg/mL		4.0 mcg/mL		0.42 mcg/mL
Half-life	91.1 hours	173.4 hours	28.5 hours	6.3 hours	6.8 hours	7.75 hours
Volume of distribution	5.0 L/kg	131.0 L/kg	4.3 L/kg	0.16 L/kg	0.10 L/kg	0.45 L/kg
Clearance	38.0 mL/hour/kg	436.0 mL/hour/kg	0.117 mL/hour/kg	22.0 mL/hour/kg	11.0 mL/hour/kg	37.0 m/hour/kg
AUC	14 mcg/mL·hour	17 mcg/mL·hour	43.0 mcg/mL·hour	197 mcg/mL·hour	555 mcg/mL·hour	26.37 mcg/mL·hour

[a]Molar ratio of each component, respectively.
[b]No benefit for longer infusions.
[c]Doses greater than 10 mg/kg have no benefit.

AmB, amphotericin B; AUC, area under the curve; DMPC, dimyristoylphosphatidycholine; DMPG, dimyristoylphosphatidyglycerol; DSPG, distearolyphosphatidyglycerol; EPC, egg phosphatidylcholine; FDA, US Food and Drug Administration; FUO, fever of unknown origin; NA, not applicable.

Bladder irrigation with AmB has been used in the past at concentrations of 150 mcg/mL, however has limited clinical utility, and is not recommended by the Infectious Diseases Society of America.[122] In two comparative studies, bladder irrigation for 5 days with AmB 50 mcg/mL was superior to fluconazole 100 mg/day as measured by microbiologic cure rates. Clinical cure rates at 2 to 4 weeks were equal—however, mortality rates were higher in the AmB-treated groups. It was suggested that AmB failures may have been associated with dissemination of yeast from the urinary tract.[123,124] Systemic antifungal therapy with flucytosine 100 to 150 mg/kg/day for 7 days[125] and azoles (fluconazole 0.6–1.4 mg/kg/day for 7 days)[126,127] also has been used in noncomparative or nonrandomized studies. Newer triazoles (voriconazole, posaconazole, and isavuconazole) or echinocandins are not recommended for the treatment of candiduria owing to their low concentrations in urine, even though some case series have suggested that clearance of positive cultures is possible on echinocandin therapy.[128]

Blastomycosis

ETIOLOGY

CASE 78-5

QUESTION 1: C.P., a 17-year-old girl from Arkansas, is admitted to the hospital with a chronic pneumonia that has not responded to antibiotics. Three months ago, she began to exhibit a chronic cough that eventually became productive of purulent sputum, which was occasionally streaked with blood. Two months ago, she began to exhibit "boils" on her lower extremities and back, which drained spontaneously. She was hospitalized at another hospital but failed to respond to amoxicillin and clarithromycin. C.P. denies fever, chills, or night sweats but has lost 11 pounds. Her temperature is 38.2°C. A 2 cm^2 subcutaneous, fluctuant, tender mass is seen over the right mandible and a second fluctuant mass about 4 cm wide on the lower back. In addition, several 0.5- to 1 cm^2 ulcers with heaped-up, hyperkeratotic margins are noted on the lower extremities (Fig. 78-2). Rales are heard at the right lung base. C.P.'s leukocyte count is slightly elevated at 13,500 cells/μL (SI units, WBC count, 13.5 × 10^9/L). A chest radiograph shows a mass-like infiltrate in the right mid-lung field (Fig. 78-3). A wet preparation of ulcer scrapings and material aspirated from a subcutaneous abscess reveal numerous broad-based, budding yeast forms with refractile cell walls and multiple nuclei typical of *B. dermatitidis*.

Cultures of sputum, skin scrapings, and abscess material eventually confirmed the diagnosis. What was the likely portal of entry for C.P.'s disseminated blastomycosis? Why should it be treated?

Typical of the other endemic mycoses, the primary portal of entry for *B. dermatitidis* is the lungs. A pulmonary origin for C.P.'s infection is supported by her history of cough with purulent, blood-streaked sputum, followed a month later with cutaneous lesions on her legs and back. An acute pulmonary infection is most often asymptomatic and, when symptomatic, usually requires only observation. Chronic pulmonary or extrapulmonary blastomycosis will develop in an unknown number of these patients. C.P.'s rales at the base of her right lung and persistent pneumonia unresponsive to antibacterials suggest a chronic pulmonary infection and a need for treatment. Chronic pulmonary disease often presents with radiographic studies often mistaken for tuberculosis or cancer; the mass-like infiltrate in her right lung on chest radiograph also is consistent with chronic pulmonary disease. Extrapulmonary infections can involve the skin (verrucous or ulcerative lesions), bone, genitourinary system (prostatitis and epididymo-orchitis), or CNS (meningitis or brain abscess). If untreated, these chronic pulmonary or extrapulmonary infections are fatal in at least 21% of patients.[129] Because C.P. presents with pulmonary and cutaneous evidence of blastomycosis, she should be treated.

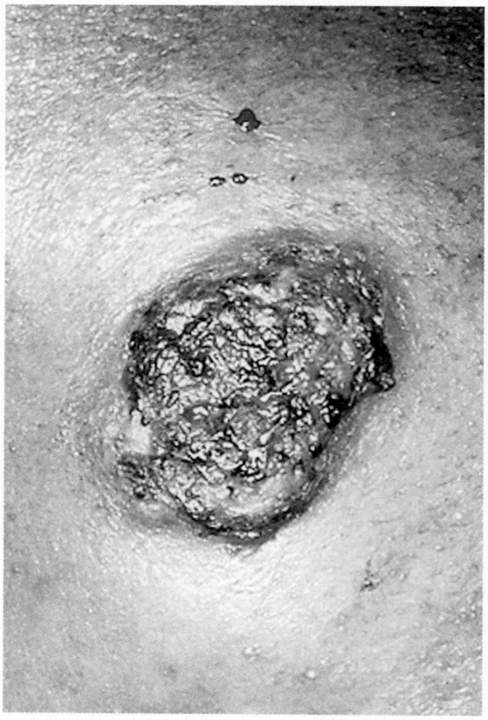

Figure 78-2 Disseminated *Blastomyces dermatitidis* skin ulcers.

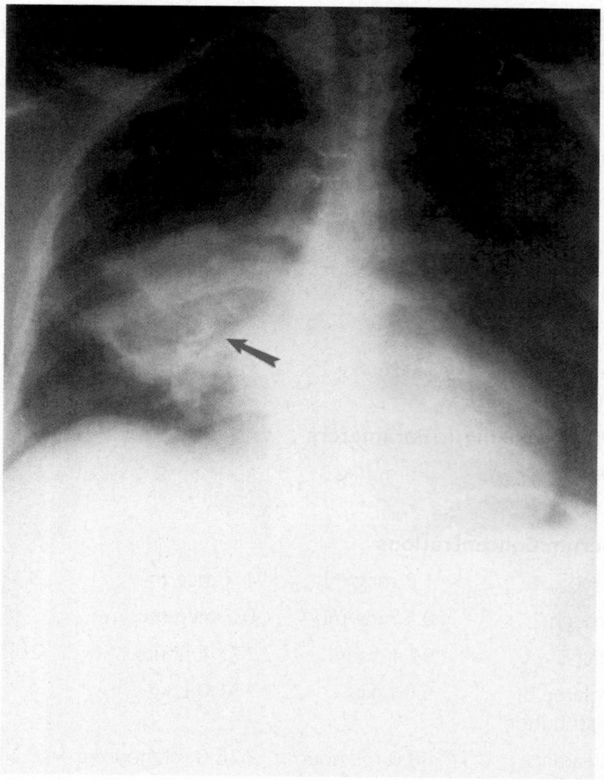

Figure 78-3 Chest radiograph of pulmonary *Blastomyces dermatitidis*. *Arrow* marks abnormality.

TREATMENT

CASE 78-5, QUESTION 2: What specific therapy should be initiated for C.P.?

Historically, AmB formulations were considered the treatment of choice for blastomycosis, and total doses of more than 2 g were associated with 97% cure rates, low relapse rates, but also, however, substantial associated toxicity.[129] Ketoconazole and itraconazole are safe, effective alternatives to AmB in patients with non–life-threatening, non-CNS infections. The NIAID–Mycoses Study Group[130] confirmed the effectiveness of azoles for the treatment of chronic pulmonary and extrapulmonary disease associated with blastomycosis and histoplasmosis. In uncontrolled evaluations of chronic pulmonary and extrapulmonary infections (excluding life-threatening or CNS), ketoconazole at dosages of 400 to 800 mg/day resulted in cure rates of about 89%, failure rates of about 6%, and relapse rates of about 5%.[130] In similar studies, itraconazole capsules 200 to 400 mg/day for a median of 6.2 months resulted in cure rates of 88% to 95%.[131] Fluconazole was ineffective at dosages less than 400 mg/day. Higher dosages (400–800 mg/day), however, are as effective as ketoconazole in non–life-threatening diseases.[132] Although these trials are neither comparative nor controlled, itraconazole is less toxic than ketoconazole and with the best benefit (efficacy) to risk (toxicity) ratio.

C.P. has mild-to-moderate disease and can be treated with an initial itraconazole dosage of 200 mg/day. If no clinical improvement is seen within 2 weeks or if the disease progresses, the dosage of itraconazole can be titrated upward in 100-mg increments to a maximal dosage of 400 mg/day. Treatment should be continued for at least 6 months. If C.P. experiences severe or meningeal disease, itraconazole should be discontinued and AmB or a lipid-based AmB product should be initiated. C.P. should be followed up for 12 months owing to the risk of relapse. Unlike histoplasmosis, skin test and serologic testing are not sufficiently sensitive to diagnose blastomycosis or evaluate the effectiveness of treatment.[130,133] Rather, patients should be evaluated closely for resolution of symptoms (constitutional and pulmonary), negative microbiologic samples, and improvement in radiographic studies.

ANTIFUNGALS IN PREGNANCY

Case 78-5, Question 3: C.P. reports she has not menstruated in 3 months, and a urine pregnancy test is positive. How does this information change the therapeutic options for her?

Data on the safety of antimycotics for treating patients who are pregnant or lactating are limited but are comprehensively reviewed according to FDA categories of the teratogenic risks of drugs (see Chapter 49, Obstetric Drug Therapy).[134,135] The systemic azoles are categorized with risk factor C. A recent Danish registration study did not find evidence of birth defects in women who took itraconazole during their first trimester.[136,137] However, the majority of women analyzed in this registry received low cumulative doses of triazoles for thrush. However, these agents should be avoided in pregnant or lactating women who are breastfeeding because of their potential teratogenicity and endocrine toxicity in the fetus or newborn. As with the azoles, griseofulvin and flucytosine have been classified with risk factor C. These agents should not be used in C.P. because the risk clearly outweighs the therapeutic benefit. Few or no data exist on the secretion of these agents in breast milk. Therefore, breastfeeding should be discouraged in women receiving these antifungal agents.

AmB and terbinafine are classified as risk factor B. Therapeutic agents in this category have no fetal risk based on animal studies, or when risk has been found in animals, controlled human studies have not confirmed the results. There are limited data regarding the use of terbinafine in pregnancy. Consequently, clinicians should avoid terbinafine use in pregnancy until published data support a B classification. Furthermore, considerable clinical experience with AmB formulations in pregnant women has documented successful treatment of systemic mycoses with no excess toxicity to either the mother or the fetus. Thus, AmB formulations have been the mainstay of antifungal therapy in pregnancy.

Histoplasmosis

TREATMENT

CASE 78-6

Question 1: J.N., a 47-year-old man with severe rheumatoid arthritis, has been maintained on daily prednisone for the past 6 years; his current dosage is 20 mg/day. For the past 4 weeks, he has experienced daily fevers to 38.4°C, drenching night sweats, anorexia, and an 8.2-kg weight loss. His prednisone dosage was increased to 40 mg/day with little clinical effect. On admission to the hospital, J.N. appears chronically ill and has many of the stigmata of chronic steroid therapy. His temperature is 37.8°C with an associated rapid heart rate of 105 beats/minute. A shallow mouth ulcer is present on the hard palate. The liver is enlarged to a total span of 18 cm, and the spleen is palpable 3 cm below the left costal margin. Stool is positive for occult blood. A chest radiograph shows bilateral interstitial infiltrates (Fig. 78-4A). He is pancytopenic, with the following laboratory results:

Hematocrit, 29% (normal, 39%–45% SI units, 0.29)
WBC count, 3,500 cells/μL (normal, 4,000–11,000 cells/μL) (SI units, 3.5 × 10^9/L)
Platelet count, 78,000 cells/μL (normal, 130 to 400,000 cells/μL)
UA, 8 to 10 WBC/high-power field
SCr, 1.9 mg/dL (SI units, 167.96 μmol/L)
BUN, 42 mg/dL (SI units, 14.99 mmol/L urea)

The bilirubin is normal, but the aminotransferases are elevated to about 1.5 times normal, and serum lactate dehydrogenase is 10 times greater than normal. A bone marrow aspirate and biopsy of the mouth ulcer reveal multiple, small intracellular yeast forms compatible with *H. capsulatum* in macrophages and polymorphonuclear leukocytes (Fig. 78-4B). Cultures of blood and urine, bone marrow aspirate, and mouth ulcer biopsy grew *H. capsulatum*. What is the optimal antifungal therapy in this case of systemic H. capsulatum? What clinical parameters should be monitored to assess the efficacy and toxicity of J.N.'s therapy?

The treatment benefits of antifungal therapy in systemic histoplasmosis have not been well investigated. Treatment options for histoplasmosis are outlined in Table 78-7.[138] Accordingly, J.N. should be treated with an IV amphotericin product or itraconazole 2.8 mg/kg/day, and his course of therapy should be monitored for both efficacy and toxicity. The decision was made to use conventional amphotericin for J.N.

Blood and urine cultures, WBC and platelet counts (histoplasma is associated with pancytopenia), constitutional symptoms, serum lactate dehydrogenase, and hepatosplenomegaly are useful measures for evaluating the outcome of antifungal therapy of J.N.'s histoplasmosis. Anemia and chest radiographs are poor measures of treatment response. Chest radiographs often reflect calcified granulomas in chronic disease with scarring, which rarely resolve even with extensive therapy. Therefore, evaluation of deterioration on radiograph, but not of improvement, is possible. In addition, AmB-induced renal disease with secondary anemia can confuse evaluation of disease resolution. Anemia must be excluded as a

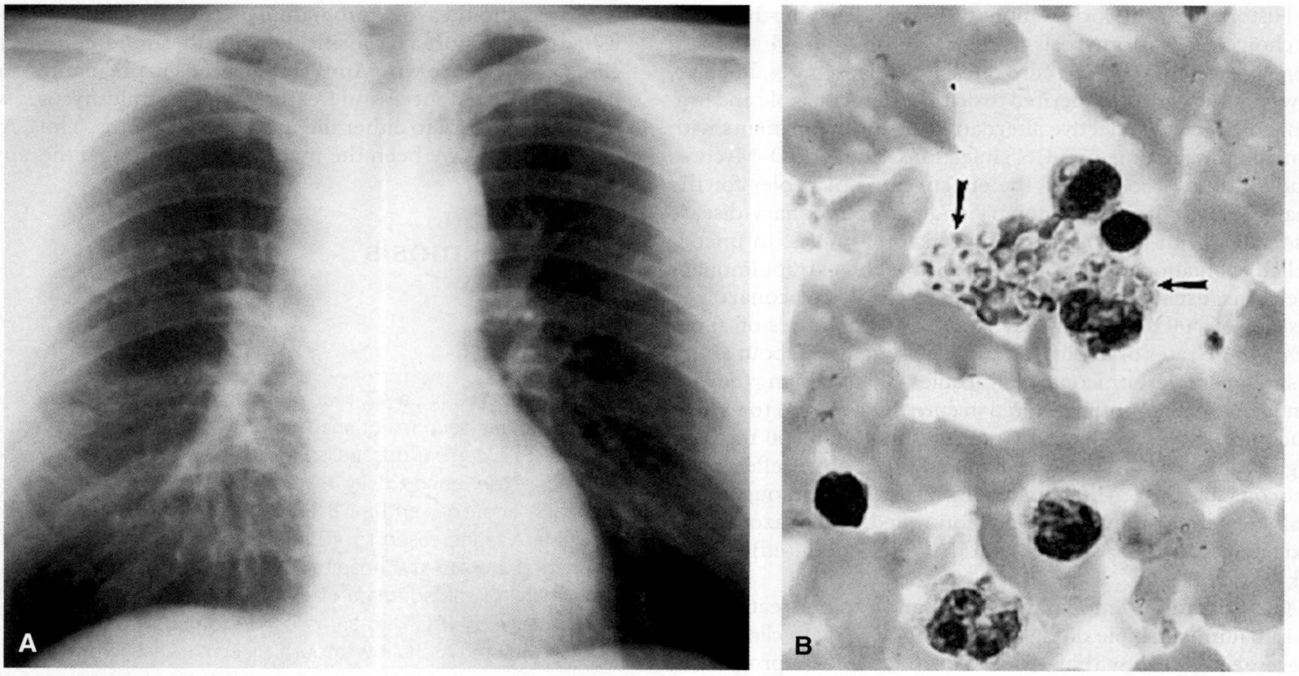

Figure 78-4 Histoplasmosis infection. **A:** Chest radiograph showing bilateral interstitial infiltrate. **B:** Gram stain of peripheral blood showing leukocytes with intracellular organisms.

Table 78-7
Treatment of Histoplasmosis

Disease	Primary	Secondary
Acute Pulmonary		
Prolonged symptomatology (>2 weeks)	Resolves spontaneously	N/A
Immunocompromised[a]	ITZ 50–100 mg/day (3–6 months)[b]	AmB 0.3–0.5 mg/kg/day[b]
Respiratory distress	AmB lipid formulation 3–5 mg/kg/day[a]	AmB 0.3–0.5 mg/kg/day
(Pao_2 <70 mm Hg)	AmB 0.5–1.0 mg/kg/day	ITZ 1.5–2.8 mg/kg/day (≥6 months)[b]
	(TD 250–500 mg) ± corticosteroids (methylprednisolone 0.5–1 mg/kg) × 1–2 weeks	ITZ (has not been investigated in life-threatening situations)
Chronic Pulmonary		
Active	ITZ (1.5–2.8 mg/kg/day 9 months)[b,c]	AmB 0.5 mg/kg/day[c]
Inactive		or KTZ 400 mg/day (≈6 mos)
Histoplasmoma	No treatment	N/A
Mediastinal fibrosis	Surgery[d]	N/A
Systemic Disease		
	AmB (TD recommended: 35 mg/kg) or lipid AmB then ITZ 2.8 mg/kg/day × up to 12 months[b]	Fluconazole 400–800 mg/day[e]

[a]Lipid formulations of amphotericin B are preferable to generic amphotericin B in HIV-infected patients.[148]
[b]Treatment should be continued until the patient is symptom-free and culture-negative for 3 months. The recommendations for duration of therapy or total doses should be used only as guides for initial therapy based upon the IDSA 2007 Guideline.[147]
[c]Indicated only for serious symptoms (i.e., hemoptysis).
[d]ITZ 200 mg daily or twice a day for 6–18 months for most patients.
[e]Fluconazole should only be used in patients who cannot take ITZ.

AmB, amphotericin B deoxycholate; ITZ, itraconazole; KTZ, ketoconazole; TD, total dose.

prognostic indicator in patients receiving AmB for durations of 3 weeks regardless of the dose.[100]

Diligent follow-up of patients is required because relapses occur in 5% to 15% of AmB-treated patients within 3 years. Relapses have occurred in patients who received less than 30 mg/kg total dose of generic AmB or had concomitant untreated Addison disease, immunosuppression, vascular infections (endocarditis, grafts, and aneurysms), or meningeal infections.[138] More than 90% of HIV-positive patients experience a relapse of histoplasmosis subsequent to adequate AmB therapy. A double-blind trial in immunocompromised patients (HIV) revealed that liposomal AmB was superior to AmB deoxycholate. It is not known how itraconazole is compared with liposomal AmB in those coinfected with HIV. If this patient was coinfected with HIV, a lipid-based amphotericin is preferred.[139] Even the initiation of subsequent immunosuppressive therapy is of particular concern because of the potential for reactivation (relapse) and dissemination of histoplasmosis from dormant foci, especially in patients with residual granulomas. The residual disease has been hypothesized to lead to chronic inflammatory responses and secondary strokes.[140]

Potential adverse effects to AmB should also be monitored in J.N. (e.g., infusion-related reactions, nephrotoxicity, anemia, hypokalemia, neurotoxicity, and thrombophlebitis). In addition, J.N.'s adrenal status should be monitored closely because of his long-term corticosteroid therapy and his histoplasmosis. Patients who are addisonian secondary to histoplasmosis infections appear to experience more episodes of AmB-induced acute hypotension.

AZOLE ADVERSE EFFECTS

CASE 78-6, QUESTION 2: After treatment with a total AmB dose of 750 mg, clinical improvement in J.N.'s histoplasmosis is subjectively and objectively documented. The clinician selected ketoconazole 400 mg/day as an oral substitute for his AmB regimen because of the patient's economic circumstances. Six weeks later, J.N. complains of impotence and wonders whether this could be caused by his medication. What is the likelihood that ketoconazole is the cause of J.N.'s impotence?

Ketoconazole has been associated with more adverse reactions and greater potential for drug interactions compared with itraconazole and fluconazole. The most common side effects of ketoconazole, however, are nausea and vomiting. GI distress is dose-related, with fewer GI effects with 400 mg/day compared with 800 mg/day.[138] Endocrine and hepatic toxicities are the most significant adverse effects of ketoconazole. Dose-splitting from daily to twice daily may decrease nausea and vomiting. Dose-related endocrinologic toxicities (hypoadrenalism, oligospermia, and diminished libido) have been observed during ketoconazole therapy secondary to the inhibition of mammalian sterol synthesis[13,141] and usually have been resolved with drug discontinuation. Therefore, J.N.'s complaints of impotence might well be attributed to his ketoconazole. Liver enzymes should also be monitored because an approximate 10% risk exists of elevation in transaminases and an occasional case of serious hepatitis and hepatic failure.[13,141]

The triazoles—itraconazole, fluconazole, and voriconazole—are much better tolerated and require less monitoring than ketoconazole therapy. This result has been attributed to the greater affinity of the triazoles for fungal cytochrome enzymes and less interference with mammalian enzymes.[142] Itraconazole, fluconazole (6 mg/kg/day), and voriconazole do not exhibit antiandrogenic effects, and nausea and vomiting are less common when compared with imidazoles. Abnormal elevations in liver function have been reported in 2.7% of patients receiving voriconazole during clinical trials. Abnormalities in liver function tests may be associated with higher azole dosages or serum concentrations but generally resolve either with continued therapy or dosage modification, including drug discontinuance. Liver function should be determined before and periodically throughout azole therapy because cases of serious hepatic reactions have been reported.[142] A unique adverse event associated with voriconazole is enhanced perception to light, which may be associated with higher plasma concentrations or doses. Generally, drug discontinuance is not required, although monitoring of visual acuity, visual field, and color perception is advised if therapy lasts longer than 28 days. Diarrhea, asthenia, flatulence, and eye pain have been reported with posaconazole therapy.[53] Based on these data, J.N. should be given a trial of itraconazole.

AZOLE–DRUG INTERACTIONS

CASE 78-6, QUESTION 3: J.N. chose to continue his ketoconazole therapy. He now returns with Cushingoid signs and symptoms. What potential drug or disease state interaction could be implicated as a cause of this serious problem in J.N.?

Drug interactions with systemic azoles and polyenes vary from mild inconveniences to life-threatening events. Historically, the interaction between azoles and nonsedating H_1-selective antihistamines has been serious, leading to QT prolongation and ventricular arrhythmias.[143] Although it is possible that concomitant use of corticosteroids could reduce antifungal efficacy, no clinical trial has addressed this important question. Corticosteroid serum concentrations can double with concomitant use of ketoconazole, leading to recommendations to decrease the steroid dose by 50% when ketoconazole is used. The interaction has been suggested between glucocorticoids and other azoles.[144] In addition, dexamethasone has been demonstrated to increase the clearance of caspofungin.

Other significant drug interactions with the azole antifungals involve their ability to inhibit the CYP450 enzyme system. All azoles inhibit CYP3A4, but with varying potency: Ketoconazole is the most potent inhibitor, followed by itraconazole and voriconazole, then posaconazole and fluconazole. Data on relative inhibition potency for isavuconazole are still pending. In addition to therapeutic interactions, numerous other agents are substrates to cytochrome CYP3A4 but have yet to be evaluated. Because azole antifungals could increase serum concentrations with associated potential toxicity, caution should be exercised during concomitant use. Adding complexity to voriconazole's interactions includes its propensity to inhibit CYP2C9 and CYP2C19, two isoenzymes exhibiting polymorphism, thus increasing concentrations of CYP2C9 or CYP2C19 substrates. Conversely, agents that either induce or inhibit the CYP450 system may decrease or increase, respectively, antifungal drug concentrations. Posaconazole is a substrate for *p*-glycoprotein efflux and is metabolized via uridine diphosphate glucuronidation; therefore, inhibitors or inducers of these clearance pathways may affect posaconazole concentrations.[51–53]

Although hundreds of drug interactions have been documented with antifungals (particularly azoles), the number of theoretical interactions probably exceeds 2000.[145] Therefore, patient medication profiles should be carefully screened before initiating and stopping antifungal therapy to assess the risk for serious drug interactions. Preferably, this screening should be performed with a frequently updated computerized interaction database, which are available commercially (Lexicomp) or free of cost (www.fungalpharmacology.org), including software for use on smartphones.

Coccidioidomycosis

SEROLOGIC TESTS

CASE 78-7

QUESTION 1: F.W., a 32-year-old Filipina woman and a lifelong resident of the Central Valley in California, is admitted to the hospital with a third recurrence of coccidioidal meningitis. Approximately 4 years ago, she was treated with a total AmB dose of 2.2 g, which resulted in a good clinical response. Nine months later, she relapsed and received a second course of AmB to a total of 1.6 g. She did well during the next 18 months and was able to return to work as a secretary. Over the past 4 months, however, F.W. has had chronic headaches, has been unable to concentrate at work, and is reported by family members to have a very labile personality. A computed tomography (CT) scan of the brain reveals mild hydrocephalus. An opening pressure of 19 mm Hg (normal, 10 mmHg) was documented at lumbar puncture. Analysis of the CSF showed:

110 WBC/μL (normal, 0 WBC/μL)
Glucose, 18 mg/dL (normal, 60% of serum glucose)
Protein, 190 mg/dL (normal, <50 mg/dL)

CF antibodies were positive in the CSF at a titer of 1:32. How should serologic tests for coccidioidomycosis be interpreted?

The most important serologic tests for fungal infections use CF, immunodiffusion, and EIA techniques. Tests for complement-fixing antibodies (i.e., CF) to the dimorphic fungi (Table 78-1) are well established, and various antigens have been used. Coccidioidin is the mycelial-phase antigen for *Coccidioides immitis*. Of patients with coccidioidomycosis, 61% will have coccidioidin CF titers of at least 1:32, and 41% will have titers of 1:64. Rising titers are a bad prognostic sign, and falling titers indicate clinical improvement. Therefore, F.W.'s CSF CF titer of 1:32 is consistent with active coccidioidomycosis. Immunodiffusion testing for coccidioidomycosis using coccidioidin reveals that seropositive results appear 1 to 3 weeks after the onset of primary infection in 75% of patients, and this positivity usually disappears within 4 months if the infection resolves.[146] IgG-specific and IgM-specific EIAs using a combination of antigens for *C. immitis* have been developed. These tests offer sensitivities of more than 92% and specificities of 98% for serum and CSF. EIA reactivity appears earlier than CF reactivity.[147,148]

ANTIFUNGAL CENTRAL NERVOUS SYSTEM PENETRATION

CASE 78-7, QUESTION 2: What is a pharmacokinetic explanation for the treatment failure of F.W.? How might this problem be overcome?

F.W. has received prolonged parenteral AmB administration, and the CSF still contains fungal organisms. Treatment failures in this case may partly be owing to the limited penetration of free AmB into the CSF.[88] Because generic AmB or lipid formulation–dissociated AmB is highly bound to lipid (90%–95%), CSF concentrations achieved are only 2% to 4% of the serum concentration[88,142]; peritoneal, synovial, and pleural fluid concentrations are less than 50% of the serum concentrations (Table 78-5). Flucytosine is not significantly bound to protein and penetrates the CSF, vitreous, and peritoneal fluids; its volume of distribution approximates that of total body water.[149] Flucytosine concentration in the CSF is 74% of the serum concentration, resulting in its extensive use in treatment of CNS mycoses, particularly cryptococcal meningitis. Flucytosine, however, has no activity in coccidioidomycosis and, therefore, cannot be used in F.W.

The volume of distribution of fluconazole approaches that of total body water,[150] and concentrations of fluconazole in CSF are approximately 60% of simultaneous serum concentrations. Ketoconazole penetrates CSF poorly, because it is highly bound to plasma proteins (>80%) and to erythrocytes (15%). Itraconazole is similar to ketoconazole in that it is greater than 99% protein-bound. Itraconazole concentrates intracellularly in host alveolar macrophages, which may account for its efficacy against some fungal CNS infections despite its inability to penetrate into the CSF.[151] Echinocandins also poorly (<5%) penetrate into the CSF. Reliable data on terbinafine, isavuconazole and posaconazole penetration are currently unavailable. Therefore, fluconazole might be an alternative to CNS instillation of AmB based upon pharmacokinetic considerations.[152,153]

Fluconazole, investigated at dosages of 400 mg/day, is useful in patients with coccidioidomycosis meningitis. Similar to amphotericin products, relapse rates are high once fluconazole therapy is stopped. Oral itraconazole 200 mg twice daily was not found to be superior to fluconazole in a controlled trial of nonmeningitis disease; however, a trend toward greater efficacy was observed, particularly in skeletal disease.[154]

INTRATHECAL AMPHOTERICIN

CASE 78-7, QUESTION 3: What adverse events might be observed with the intrathecal administration of an antifungal in F.W.?

Augmentation of systemic antifungal administration with intraventricular or intrathecal administration may improve the outcome for antifungals with poor penetration into the CSF. Intrathecal generic AmB doses in adults normally range from 0.25 to 0.5 mg diluted in 5 mL of 5% glucose.[155,156] A few studies suggest that doses larger than 0.7 mg improve the cure rate and decrease relapse. Cisternal or intraventricular administration is recommended as the routes of choice because of flow characteristics of CSF from the ventricles to the spinal cord. When lumbar administration has been necessary, agents are administered in a hypertonic solution of 10% glucose, and the patient is placed in a Trendelenburg position in an attempt to improve distribution of the drug to the basilar meninges and ventricles and reduce local toxicity. Voriconazole, caspofungin, and the lipid amphotericin formulations have been used, but not evaluated in controlled trials.

Cisternal antifungal administration has been associated with headaches, nausea, vomiting, cranial nerve paresis, and cisternal hemorrhage caused by needle trauma. An Ommaya reservoir often is used to facilitate intraventricular administration of AmB formulations. Common complications of these devices include shunt occlusion, bacterial colonization or bacterial meningitis, Parkinsonian symptoms, and seizures.[156–158] In the past, lumbar administration was used because it is simpler, but it often must be discontinued because of chemical arachnoiditis, headache, transient radiculitis, paresthesia, nerve pulses, difficulty voiding, impaired vision, vertigo, and tinnitus. Acute toxic delirium, demyelinating peripheral neuropathy, and spinal cord injury have also been reported.[159–162] Regardless of the substantial and serious adverse effects, intraventricular administration may be effective in treating patients with meningitis who have severe disease or who are pharmacologic nonresponders.

Aspergillosis

EMPIRIC THERAPY (NEUTROPENIC HOST)

CASE 78-8

QUESTION 1: M.Z., an otherwise healthy 29-year-old man, who received an allogeneic stem cell transplantation 12 days ago. He has had no serious complications associated with his chloroquine-induced aplastic anemia during his 7-month wait for transplant. On transplant Days 5 to 2, induction therapy was initiated with cyclophosphamide (50 mg/kg) and total body irradiation, and then bone marrow from his human leukocyte antigen–compatible brother was infused on Day 0. The onset of neutropenia was noted on Day 3, and the WBC count was 50 cells/μL. M.Z. has complained only of stomatitis and diarrhea before Day 5. On that morning, he was complaining of fever, chest pain, and headache. On physical examination, his temperature was 37°C. Empiric antibiotics were added, but by Day 8, he was not clinically improving. A CT scan of the chest and sinuses revealed a nodular pleural–based opacity with ground-glass attenuation (halo sign) in his right lung. What therapeutic options should be considered for this patient?

Empiric antifungal therapy in a neutropenic host should be initiated when a patient is febrile for more than 96 hours on appropriate antibiotics. Routine empiric therapy for a patient without evidence of deep-seated fungal infection was historically generic AmB 0.3 to 0.6 mg/kg/day or fluconazole 200 to 400 mg/day until the absolute neutrophil count is greater than 500 cells/μL.[163] Therapy results in resolution of signs and symptoms in up to 64% of patients.

CASE 78-8, QUESTION 2: What is the role of lipid formulations of AmB?

Because mold infections are of concern in this neutropenic patient who received an allogeneic stem cell transplant, mold-active antifungal therapy should be started immediately. A large, well-controlled, double-blind AmB 0.6 mg/kg/day was compared with liposomal AmB 3.0 mg/kg/day in febrile neutropenic patients. Patients who were febrile more than 96 hours and neutropenic (<500 cells/μL) experienced equal survival and clinical success of approximately 50% for both the agents.[164] Success rates have been similar with other agents, including liposomal AmB (34%), caspofungin (34%),[165] voriconazole, or itraconazole.[166,167] It is important to remember that fever is a late and insensitive measure of infection. Prevention of breakthrough invasive fungal infection may be the most important indicator of an agent's efficacy. Using this measure comparing the various trials, voriconazole appears to be the most effective agent, voriconazole versus liposomal AmB (1.9% vs. 5%) and AmB versus liposomal AmB (3.2% vs. 7.8%), although crude mortality rates were similar in the two patient groups (8% vs. 6%, respectively).[164,167] Selection of expensive, but less toxic, agents should be weighed against the morbidity and mortality associated with invasive fungal disease.

TREATMENT OF ASPERGILLOSIS

CASE 78-8, QUESTION 3: Fiberoptic bronchoscopy performed to evaluate the nodular lesion in chest CT revealed eroded bronchioles with necrotic tissue, and methenamine silver nitrate stain of a biopsy sample revealed fragmented, closely septated hyphal bodies branched at 45° angles. The samples were sent to microbiology for cultures. A galactomannan test from the bronchial wash was positive at an index of 1.1. All previous blood and sputum cultures have been negative. The diagnosis at this time is probable aspergillosis. What treatment steps should be taken?

Drug therapy should be approached by first determining whether the infection is likely to be invasive or noninvasive disease (Fig. 78-5). Most patients inhale *Aspergillus* species and never become symptomatic or exhibit only mild hypersensitivity pneumonitis. Pepper can be a common food source for *Aspergillus* exposure. Invasive infections are more likely to occur in immunocompromised patients, especially those with prolonged neutropenia or patients who receive high dose (i.e., more than 1 mg/kg/day prednisone equivalent) or corticosteroids or other T-cell immunosuppressive therapy (i.e., alemtuzumab and anti-thymocyte globulin) to treat acute graft versus host disease following stem cell transplantation or organ rejection after solid organ transplantation. Allogeneic hematopoietic stem cell transplantation (HSCT) has a much greater infection rate and mortality compared with autologous HSCT.[168] A classic observation reported by radiology is a "halo" sign or a "crescent" sign identified on CT, which is highly suggestive of invasive aspergillosis. However, the halo sign is not specific, because other bacterial viral, malignant, or autoimmune conditions can produce similar radiographic findings. The halo sign is also transient and is less common after 1-week of infection. Typically these nodular lesions will enlarge (even with effective antifungal therapy) and then cavitate when a patient's neutrophil count recovers, forming another distinguishing CT abnormality for invasive mold disease—the air crescent sign.[169]

A majority invasive aspergillosis cases are now diagnosed based on a compatible clinical and radiographic picture described above and the results of an ELISA antigen test for a cell wall polysaccharide in *Aspergillus* spp.-galactomannan. Serum galactomannan test is a fairly sensitive and specific test (80%–90%) in neutropenic patients with aspergillosis who rapidly progress to angioinvasive disease in the lung. The test is less sensitive in non-neutropenic patients who initially present with bronchial invasive patterns of pneumonia before angioinvasion or in patients receiving mold-active antifungal therapy.[170] In these populations, testing of bronchial alveolar lavage fluid for galactomannan antigen has better sensitivity than serum. False-positive test findings have been associated with *Bifidobacterium* sp. colonization in pediatric GI tracts, other eukaryotic infections (i.e., *Trichosporon*, *Fusarium*, *Saccharomyces*, *Hisplasma*, or *Acremonium*), and administration of piperacillin–tazobactam or calcium gluconate, which is of concern for clinicians using this test for screening in areas with low case rates. Galactomannan antigen is a useful prognostic indicator for therapeutic outcome in confirmed cases or as a screen in areas with high case rates. The subjective and objective data in this case clearly represent invasive symptomatic disease necessitating aggressive treatment.

Aspergillosis is a model for invasive mold infections that have a propensity to invade blood vessels and tissue. Antifungal therapy should be initiated rapidly and aggressively (Table 78-8) in conjunction with the removal or reversal of immunosuppression if possible. Definite or probable invasive aspergillosis should be treated with voriconazole, isavuconazole, or lipid amphotericin B formulation (i.e., liposomal AmB 3–5 mg/kg/day), or combination therapy.[171–173] In a recent European organization for research and treatment of cancer (EORTC)/Mycoses study group (MSG) trial performed in patients with probable or proven aspergillosis, a combination therapy with voriconazole plus anidulafungin for at least 2 weeks was associated with an 8% reduction in 6-week all-cause mortality versus voriconazole monotherapy alone, although this difference was not statistically different in the context of the design of the clinical trial.[174] Therefore, the optimal approach for using combination therapy in invasive aspergillosis remains unresolved. Despite early and intensive therapy, mortality from invasive aspergillosis can be greater than 50%.[175] In unresponsive patients, a lipid AmB formulation in combination therapy or possibly triazole should be considered.[171–177] Importantly, some less common molds intrinsically resistant to several antifungal classes (i.e., Mucorales, *Fusarium* spp. *Scedosporium* spp.) occasionally present as infections or breakthrough infections that may be indistinguishable from invasive aspergillosis.

Patients with mild-to-moderate *Aspergillus* should be treated with voriconazole or isavuconazole.[166] Clinical and microbiologic cure rates of 50% to 71% have been reported for voriconazole- or isavuconazole-treated invasive aspergillosis. In a comparative trial of voriconazole versus isavuconazole for patients with proven or probable aspergillosis, patients randomized to receive isavuconazole had similar clinical response and mortality rates as voriconazole-treated patients with lower rates of ocular, hepatic, and cutaneous adverse reactions.[178,179]

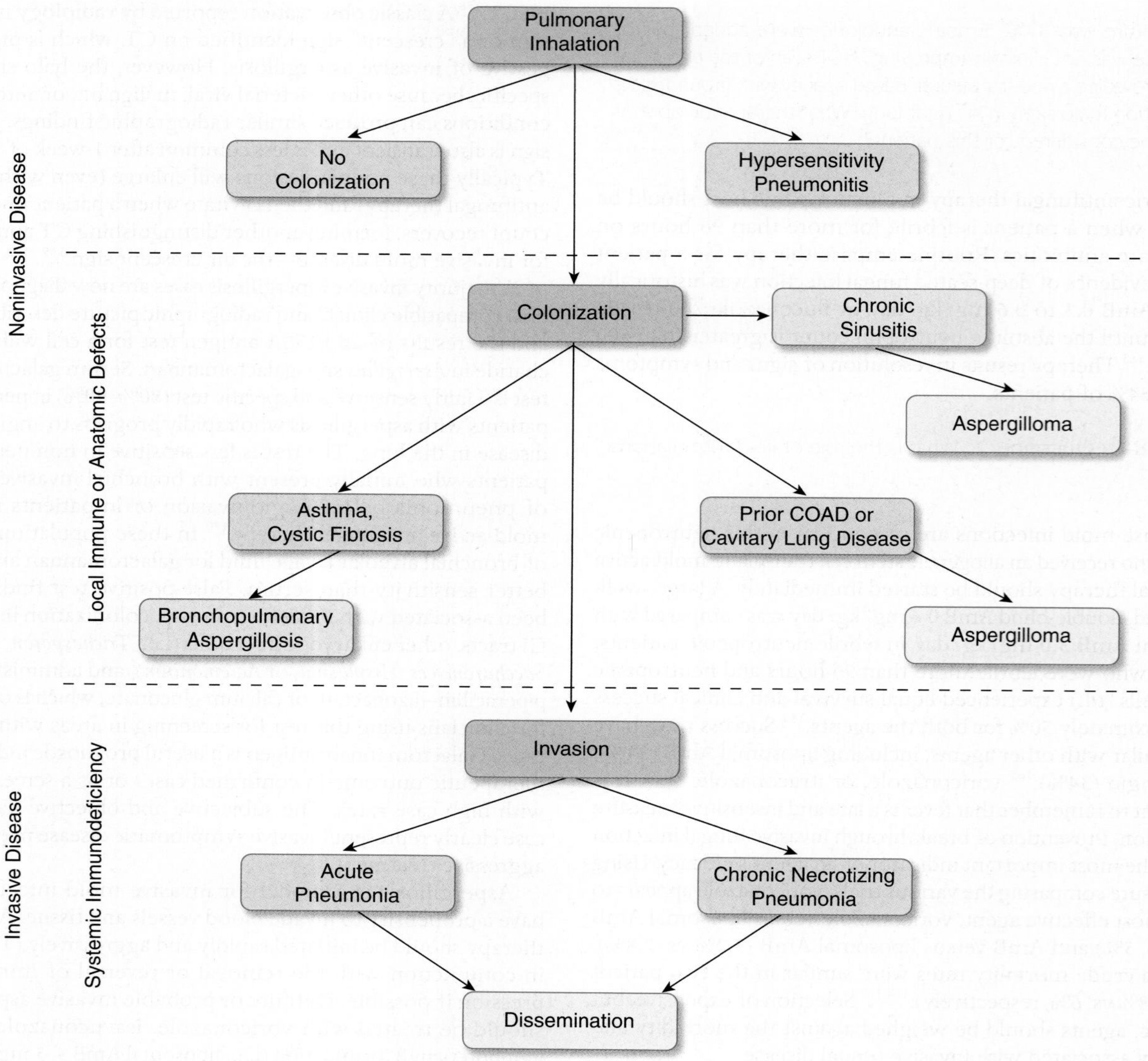

Figure 78-5 Classification of aspergillosis infections. COAD, chronic obstructive airway disease.

Table 78-8
Therapeutic Options for Treatment of Aspergillosis

Disease	Primary	Secondary
Hyalohyphomycetes		
Aspergillosis		
Allergic bronchopulmonary	Prednisone 1 mg/kg/day followed by 0.5 mg/kg/day or every other day × 3–6 months; no antifungal therapy	ITZ 200 mg BID × 4 months[a]
Aspergilloma	Observation	Surgery[b]
Systemic (invasive)	Isavuconazole 300 mg IV 3 times daily for 48 hours LD, then 300 mg daily	Amphotericin B lipid formulation[c], or Posaconazole 300 mg twice daily LD, then 300 mg daily or/and Combination therapy with an echinocandin[d]

[a]Treatment should be continued until the patient is symptom-free and culture-negative for 3 months. Noted durations or total doses should be used only as a compass to help guide therapy.
[b]Indicated only for serious symptoms (e.g., hemoptysis).
[c]Lipid formulations of amphotericin B should be utilized preferentially in these patients.
[d]anidulafungin (AFG) 200 mg parenterally; caspofungin (CFG) 70 (50) mg parenterally on Day 1 (2–14); micafungin (MFG) 70 mg parenterally; flucytosine (5FC) 150 mg/day parenterally.

AmB, amphotericin B; BID, twice daily; ITZ, itraconazole; LD, loading dose; TID, three times daily.

Cryptococcosis

CASE 78-9

QUESTION 1: D.W., a 48-year-old man, was hospitalized with fever and severe headache. His history was significant for Hodgkin lymphoma, which is in remission. Lumbar puncture revealed the following:

Opening pressure of 280 mm Hg (normal, 10 mm Hg)
WBC count, 50 leukocytes/μL (normal, 0 leukocytes/μL)
Positive India ink preparation
Cryptococcal antigen titer, 1:4,096

Serology for HIV infection was negative. Culture of the CSF eventually grew *C. neoformans*. The presumptive diagnosis is cryptococcal meningitis. What are the treatment options for D.W.?

Currently, only two therapeutic options exist for meningeal cryptococcal disease: an AmB formulation with or without flucytosine and fluconazole. Flucytosine cannot be used alone for therapy or prophylaxis because of the rapid development of resistance. This yeast is also resistant to echinocandins. Patients, whether infected with HIV or not, have improved treatment outcomes when the combination of AmB and flucytosine is used.[180,181] Furthermore, when flucytosine (100–150 mg/kg/day divided into four daily doses) is used in combination therapy, the dose of AmB may be reduced to 0.3 to 0.6 mg/kg/day, which decreases the frequency of dose-related AmB toxicity. In patients who cannot be treated with flucytosine, the dosage of AmB must be increased to more than 0.6 mg/kg/day. AmB 1 mg/kg/day is more rapidly fungicidal than 0.7 mg/kg/day when used with 5FC. Liposomal AmB 3 mg/kg/day can and probably should be used instead of the nonlipid formulations in this disease owing to presumed increase in safety.[182]

Fluconazole is an alternative to AmB in patients infected with HIV with cryptococcal meningitis. It is important to be mindful of the following caveats, however: Sterilization of the CSF occurs more rapidly, and mortality is lower during the first 2 weeks of therapy in patients treated with AmB as compared with fluconazole.[182] Early mortality was especially high in fluconazole-treated patients who presented with altered mental status.[183–185] Thus, initial therapy of cryptococcal meningitis in patients with mental status changes should be initiated with AmB for at least 2 weeks or until the patient has stabilized clinically.

A landmark study on patients with cryptococcal meningitis compared patients randomized to receive either amphotericin B 1 mg/kg/day for 4 weeks or a 2 week induction regimen of amphotericin B 1 mg/kg/day plus flucytosine (1 mg/kg/day) or fluconazole (400 mg twice daily).[185] At Day 70 after randomization, significantly fewer deaths were observed in patients receiving amphotericin B plus flucytosine versus patients receiving amphotericin B alone (hazard ratio: 0.61, 95% CI: 0.39–0.97, $P = 0.04$). Combination therapy with fluconazole did not significantly impact survival over amphotericin B monotherapy. Notably, the amphotericin B-flucytosine combination was associated with more rapid clearance of yeast from the CSF versus other regimens. Rates of adverse effects were similar in all groups even though neutropenia was slightly more common in patients receiving amphotericin B-flucytosine or amphotericin B-fluconazole combinations versus amphotericin B monotherapy (34% and 32% vs. 19%, $P = 0.04$).

Fluconazole 400 mg/day may be an acceptable option in patients with less severe disease in all other patients. Another alternative may include liposomal AmB 4 to 6 mg/kg/day for 21 days. Until larger clinical studies have been completed, however, this regimen cannot be recommended over generic AmB (see Chapter 77, Opportunistic Infections in HIV-Infected Patients).[181]

In D.W., initial treatment should focus on elimination of all factors leading to immunosuppression. Antifungal therapy should be initiated immediately with AmB 0.3 to 0.6 mg/kg/day plus flucytosine 100 to 150 mg/kg/for a minimum of 6 weeks to optimize the chance of a cure, especially in transplant recipients.[185] In addition, CSF hypertension, usually presenting as headache, should be resolved through therapeutic spinal tap. Acetazolamide should be avoided in these cases.[186] An unfortunate consequence of eliminating immune suppression is immune reconstitution syndrome (IRIS). This syndrome is most commonly observed in HIV-infected patients started on antiretrovirals who experience complications secondary to new onset inflammatory reactions from replenished leukocytes. IRIS may make it appear these patients are failing antifungal therapy.

CASE 78-9, QUESTION 2: What parameters should be monitored while D.W. is treated with flucytosine?

The most common side effect of flucytosine is GI distress (e.g., nausea, vomiting, and diarrhea). Although flucytosine is not metabolized per se by mammalian cells, gut flora may be responsible for metabolism of flucytosine to fluorouracil. This toxic metabolite has been speculated to account, in part, for the GI distress and bone marrow toxicity associated with flucytosine therapy.[187] Other flucytosine adverse effects include leukopenia, thrombocytopenia, and hepatotoxicity. Dose-dependent bone marrow suppression, which can be fatal, generally is seen in patients whose serum concentration of flucytosine is greater than 100 mcg/mL. Thus, it is important to monitor blood concentrations and maintain concentrations below this level.[181,183] If assays for flucytosine serum concentrations are unavailable, signs and symptoms of bone marrow suppression or worsening renal function should result in a dosage reduction or discontinuation of the drug. Flucytosine is eliminated by glomerular filtration, with 80% to 95% of the dose excreted unchanged in the urine. Renal excretion of flucytosine is directly related to creatinine clearance, and dosages should be adjusted based on creatinine clearance to prevent the accumulation to toxic concentrations in patients with renal impairment.[101] Patients with creatinine clearances of 10 to 40 mL/minute should have the dosage of flucytosine reduced by 50% (usual dose, 37.5 mg/kg every 12 hours). For patients with creatinine clearance less than 10 mL/minute, dosing should be initiated at 37.5 mg/kg/day, with frequent monitoring of flucytosine serum concentrations. Dosage adjustment and close monitoring also are required for patients receiving hemodialysis, and it is recommended that the dose be given postdialysis.

CASE 78-9, QUESTION 3: When is combination antifungal therapy indicated?

In vitro results of antifungal combinations against many common mycotic pathogens have been variable. These incomplete and inconsistent findings have been attributed to variable incubation times, variable concentrations of antifungal agents, and the sequence of antifungal addition. As a result, clinical decisions about combination therapy should be based on patient-specific in vivo evaluations. Because of the limited clinical data, combination antifungal therapy should be initiated cautiously. Except for the treatment of cryptococcal meningitis and disseminated aspergillosis, combination therapy should be reserved for cases of treatment failure (disseminated candidiasis) with no other established pharmacologic options for therapy or mold infections with high mortality rates.

KEY REFERENCES AND WEBSITES

A full list of references for this chapter can be found at http://thepoint.lww.com/AT11e. Below are the key references and website for this chapter, with the corresponding reference number in this chapter found in parentheses after the reference.

Key References

Herbrecht R et al. Voriconazole versus amphotericin B for primary therapy of invasive aspergillosis. *N Engl J Med*. 2002;347:408. (176)

Johnson PC et al. Safety and efficacy of liposomal amphotericin B compared with conventional amphotericin B for induction therapy of histoplasmosis in patients with AIDS. *Ann Intern Med*. 2002;137:105. (139)

Morrell M et al. Delaying the empiric treatment of candida bloodstream infection until positive blood culture results are obtained: a potential risk factor for hospital mortality. *Antimicrob Agents Chemother*. 2005;49:3640. (71)

Odom RB et al. A multicenter, placebo-controlled, double-blind study of intermittent therapy with itraconazole for the treatment of onychomycosis of the fingernail. *J Am Acad Dermatol*. 1997;36:231. (36)

Pappas PG et al. Clinical practice guidelines for the management of candidiasis: 2009 update by the Infectious Diseases Society of America. *Clin Infect Dis*. 2009;48(5):503. (57)

Patel M et al. Initial management of candidemia at an academic medical center: evaluation of the IDSA guidelines. *Diagn Microbiol Infect Dis*. 2005;52:26. (70)

Pelz RK et al. Double-blind placebo-controlled trial of fluconazole to prevent candidal infections in critically ill surgical patients. *Ann Surg*. 2001;233:542. (116)

Perfect JR et al. Clinical practice guidelines for the management of cryptococcal disease: 2010 update by the Infectious Diseases Society of America. *Clin Infect Dis*. 2010;50(3):291. (182)

Rex JH et al. Antifungal susceptibility testing: practical aspects and current challenges. *Clin Microbiol Rev*. 2001;14:643. (20)

Shepard JR et al. Multicenter evaluation of the *Candida albicans/Candida glabrata* peptide nucleic acid fluorescent in situ hybridization method for simultaneous dual-color identification of *C. albicans* and *C. glabrata* directly from blood culture bottles. *J Clin Microbiol*. 2008;46:50. (62)

Stevens DA et al. Practice guidelines for diseases caused by *Aspergillus*. Infectious Diseases Society of America. *Clin Infect Dis*. 2000;30:696.

79 Viral Infections

Milap C. Nahata, Neeta Bahal O'Mara, and Sandra Benavides

CORE PRINCIPLES

	CORE PRINCIPLES	CHAPTER CASES
1	Herpes simplex virus (HSV) encephalitis is associated with significant morbidity and mortality. Intravenous acyclovir for a 21-day period is the therapy of choice.	**Case 79-1 (Questions 2, 4)**
2	Neonatal herpes can present with mucocutaneous, ocular infection, as well as encephalitis and disseminated HSV infection. Transmission can be acquired during the first trimester of pregnancy or during vaginal delivery in an infected mother.	**Case 79-2 (Questions 1, 2)**
3	Herpes labialis is the most common oral-facial HSV infection and is usually self-limiting in an immunocompetent host. Patients who are immunocompromised must be treated with antiviral therapy, primarily oral or intravenous acyclovir or oral valacyclovir.	**Case 79-3 (Question 1), Case 79-4 (Question 1)**
4	Individuals with progressive varicella, those with extracutaneous complications, or those at high risk for developing complications to varicella infection benefit from antiviral therapy.	**Case 79-7 (Question 1), Case 79-8 (Question 1)**
5	The goal of pharmacotherapy of herpes zoster is to reduce pain and duration of rash and to prevent the development of postherpetic neuralgia (PHN). These outcomes can be accomplished with the use of oral acyclovir, famciclovir, or valacyclovir. For the treatment of PHN, topical capsaicin gels, creams and patches, topical lidocaine patches, and oral gabapentin and pregabalin are efficacious.	**Case 79-9 (Question 1)**
6	Neuraminidase inhibitors, such as zanamivir, oseltamivir, and peramivir, are indicated for the treatment of influenza if used within 48 hours after the onset of symptoms. Zanamivir is administered by oral inhalation with bronchospasm the most common adverse drug reaction. Oseltamivir is administered orally, with nausea, vomiting, and headache as common side effects. Peramivir is administered intravenously and has been associated with hypersensitivity reactions, such as Steven–Johnson syndrome.	**Case 79-11 (Question 2)**
7	Influenza vaccination is the most effective mechanism to prevent the flu. However, certain high-risk populations may require additional prophylaxis with oseltamivir or zanamivir.	**Case 79-10 (Question 2)**
8	Infants at high risk for severe disease caused by respiratory syncytial virus (RSV) should receive monthly intramuscular injections of palivizumab for a total of five doses during RSV season.	**Case 79-13 (Questions 1, 2)**
9	West Nile virus can cause disease ranging from a febrile infection to encephalitis. Treatment is supportive; however, ribavirin and interferon-α-2b have been tried in this patient population. Clinical trials evaluating the use of immunoglobulin, monoclonal antibodies, and vaccines are ongoing.	**Case 79-14 (Questions 1, 2)**
10	The common cold is the most prevalent viral infection. Numerous pathogens can cause this respiratory infection, including rhinovirus, coronavirus, parainfluenza, RSV, adenovirus, and enterovirus. There are currently no products that have been conclusively shown to prevent or treat the common cold.	**Case 79-15 (Question 1)**

Viral infections are common causes of human disease. An estimated 60% of illnesses in developed countries result from viruses, compared with only 15% from bacteria. These include the common cold, chickenpox, measles, mumps, influenza, bronchitis, gastroenteritis, hepatitis, poliomyelitis, rabies, and numerous diseases caused by the herpesvirus. Upper respiratory tract infections, such as the common cold or influenza, are among the most common reasons for visits to a health care professional.[1] Most of these patients have a self-limiting illness; however, certain viral infections, such as influenza, can cause significant mortality, particularly in the elderly. During the worldwide Spanish influenza epidemic of 1918 to 1920, 20 to 100 million people died.[2] Although influenza vaccines reduce the morbidity and mortality associated with this disease, for many other potentially severe viral infections, including herpes encephalitis and neonatal herpes, no vaccine is available.

Substantial progress has been made in antiviral chemotherapy as a result of advances in molecular virology and genetic engineering. Antiviral agents can be designed to inhibit functions specific to viruses, which maximizes their therapeutic benefits and minimizes adverse effects.

Current technology also permits rapid diagnosis of viral diseases. It is now possible to make a specific diagnosis of several viral illnesses within hours to a few days; previously, a specific diagnosis often took days to months. These improved diagnostics have facilitated rapid selection of an appropriate antiviral drug.

This chapter describes the etiology, pathogenesis, and treatment of common viral infections. Specific case presentations illustrate the optimal use of antiviral drugs in patients with viral infections.

HERPES SIMPLEX VIRUS INFECTIONS

Herpes viruses are responsible for a broad spectrum of diseases including acute life-threatening illness (herpes encephalitis and neonatal herpes), as well as more chronic, recurrent infection (genital herpes). Antivirals significantly decrease the morbidity and mortality in most of these infections.[3]

Herpes Encephalitis

Herpes simplex virus (HSV) encephalitis is the most common sporadic viral infection of the central nervous system (CNS). HSV encephalitis occurs in up to 500,000 people yearly, although this may be an underestimate owing to difficulties in diagnosis. It typically occurs in two populations, those 6 months to 20 years of age and those older than 50 years. It is characterized by the acute onset of fever, headache, decreased consciousness, and seizures. Any child with fever and altered behavior should be evaluated for HSV encephalitis. Without treatment, mortality approaches 70% and some morbidity is evident in 97% of survivors. Only 2.5% of patients recover sufficiently to lead normal lives.[3]

Herpes simplex virus type 1 (HSV-1) is the etiologic agent in most patients with herpes encephalitis, but herpes simplex virus type 2 (HSV-2) is more common in newborns. The infection may be localized to the brain or involve cutaneous and mucous membranes. Although any area of the brain can be involved, the orbital region of the frontal lobes and the temporal lobes are most often affected.[4]

Herpes encephalitis is often difficult to diagnose. A computed tomography (CT) scan is usually indicated to rule out other conditions, such as brain abscess or other space-occupying lesions. The CT or radionuclide scans may be unremarkable early in the course of the disease.

Cerebrospinal fluid (CSF) examination usually reveals pleocytosis (predominately lymphocytes) with 50 to 2,000 white blood cells (WBCs)/mcL. Polymorphonuclear leukocytosis and red blood cells (RBCs) may also be seen. Many patients have an elevated protein level in the CSF (median, 80 mg/dL; normal values differ per age, e.g., if ≥6 months, 15–45 mg/dL).

The electroencephalogram (EEG) is the most sensitive but least specific test. There are usually CT or brain scan abnormalities, but these may take a day or two longer to appear. The EEG, CT, and brain scan findings compatible with HSV encephalitis can be mimicked by other conditions, and a brain biopsy is required to clearly establish the diagnosis. Rapid diagnosis of herpes encephalitis by a polymerase chain reaction (PCR) assay of HSV DNA in the CSF is available at most medical centers. This is a highly sensitive, specific, and rapid method for diagnosing herpes encephalitis.[5]

CLINICAL PRESENTATION

CASE 79-1

QUESTION 1: R.F., a 7-year-old boy weighing 20 kg, was seen in the emergency department (ED) after a seizure. For the previous 3 days, R.F. had decreased appetite, headache, and fever (101°F–102°F), and was lethargic and disoriented. His leukocyte count was 13,000/mcL with a shift to the left. Ceftriaxone (50 mg/kg intravenously [IV] every 12 hours) and dexamethasone (0.15 mg/kg IV every 6 hours) were initiated for presumed bacterial meningitis. Phenobarbital (5 mg/kg IV every 24 hours) was given for seizure control. The CSF was normal, and no bacteria could be cultured. Acyclovir 20 mg/kg IV every 8 hours was started immediately. A PCR analysis of HSV-1 was positive. What findings in R.F. are consistent with the diagnosis of herpes encephalitis?

Fever, headache, lethargy, and disorientation are common features of herpes encephalitis. As illustrated by R.F., the CSF examination can be normal in some patients. A negative CSF culture suggests the absence of a bacterial infection.[6] However, the positive HSV-1 DNA by PCR analysis confirms the diagnosis of herpes encephalitis.

TREATMENT: ACYCLOVIR

CASE 79-1, QUESTION 2: What is the treatment of choice for R.F.'s herpes encephalitis?

Two studies comparing acyclovir and vidarabine (no longer marketed in the United States) have demonstrated that IV acyclovir (10 mg/kg every 8 hours for 10 days) is the treatment of choice in patients with herpes encephalitis.[7,8] The 12-month all-cause mortality was 25% in the acyclovir-treated group and 59% in the vidarabine-treated group. Notably, nearly one-third of the acyclovir-treated patients returned to normal life, compared with only 12% of those treated with vidarabine.[9]

Acyclovir is the treatment of choice for R.F. because it has been shown to decrease morbidity in patients with herpes encephalitis. Acyclovir should be started as soon as HSV encephalitis is suspected because early initiation of therapy is associated with improved outcome. Therapy should be continued for at least 21 days.[10] The role of corticosteroids in the treatment of herpes encephalitis is not well defined. One small, nonrandomized trial found that corticosteroid therapy, in combination with IV acyclovir, was associated with an improved outcome.[11] However, prospective, randomized trials are needed before routine use of corticosteroids can be recommended.[12] Acyclovir-resistant herpes is not an important consideration in the management of herpes encephalitis in most patients.

Adverse Effects

CASE 79-1, QUESTION 3: What adverse effects can occur with IV acyclovir therapy in R.F.? How should these be monitored, and how can they be minimized?

Acyclovir is a relatively safe drug, but renal toxicity associated with IV acyclovir is well described (Table 79-1). Blood urea nitrogen (BUN) and serum creatinine (SCr) levels can increase in 5% to 10% of patients; however, these changes are generally reversible. Acyclovir is relatively insoluble: maximal urine solubility at 37°C is 1.3 mg/mL. Consequently, the mechanism of acyclovir-associated renal disease is a transient crystal nephropathy, which may occur at high acyclovir concentrations.[9]

Other common adverse effects include gastrointestinal (GI) complaints, such as nausea and vomiting and, less commonly, neurologic disturbances, including lethargy, tremors, confusion, hallucinations, and seizures.[9,25] Neurotoxicity appears to be more common in patients with impaired renal function and is reversible. Finally, IV acyclovir can cause phlebitis and pain at the injection site.[9] This complication can be minimized by administering acyclovir at a concentration of 5 mg/mL (maximum, 7 mg/mL).[25]

Renal function tests, including BUN, SCr, and urine output, should be monitored in R.F. To minimize the risk of acyclovir nephrotoxicity, R.F. should be well hydrated, and each acyclovir dose should be infused for 1 hour. In addition, the IV infusion site should be inspected for inflammation and pain, and R.F. should be asked about pain at the infusion site.

Conversion to Oral Therapy

CASE 79-1, QUESTION 4: After 7 days of IV acyclovir, R.F. is alert, responsive, actively moving about, and eating a normal diet. The intern suggests switching him to oral acyclovir and discontinuing IV therapy. Is this appropriate?

Oral acyclovir therapy is inappropriate for R.F. On the basis of studies in adults, the absorption of acyclovir after oral administration is variable, slow, and incomplete. The relative bioavailability (F) of acyclovir is low ($F = 0.15–0.30$) and decreases with increasing doses.[26] The mean peak plasma concentration has ranged from only 0.83 to 1.61 mcg/mL after multiple acyclovir doses of 200 to 800 mg.[26] Thus, with only approximately 50% of acyclovir penetrating the blood–brain barrier, the concentrations of acyclovir in the CSF may be inadequate for R.F. There is only very limited information regarding the use of oral valacyclovir for therapy. A small pharmacokinetic trial of oral valacyclovir in patients with HSV encephalitis found that while therapeutic CSF

Table 79-1

Adverse Effects of US Food and Drug Administration (FDA)–Indicated Drugs for Various Viral Infections

Drug	Adverse Effects
Acyclovir[9]	Local irritation, phlebitis; increased SCr, BUN; nausea, vomiting; itching, rash; increased liver transaminases; CNS toxicity; hematologic abnormalities
Amantadine[13]	Nausea, dizziness (lightheadedness), insomnia (5%–10%); depression, anxiety, irritability, hallucination, confusion, dry mouth; constipation, ataxia, headache, peripheral edema, orthostatic hypotension (1%–5%); suicide ideation or attempt (<1%)
Cidofovir[14]	Nephrotoxicity; neutropenia; rash; headache; alopecia; anemia; abdominal pain; fever; infection; ocular hypotonia; nausea, vomiting; asthenia; diarrhea
Famciclovir[15]	Headache; nausea; diarrhea
Foscarnet[16]	Fever, nausea, vomiting; renal dysfunction; anemia; diarrhea; headache; electrolyte abnormalities; bone marrow suppression; seizure; anorexia; abdominal pain; mental status changes; paresthesia, peripheral neuropathy; cough, dyspnea; rash; first-degree AV block, ECG changes
Ganciclovir[17]	Increased SCr; anemia; neutropenia, pancytopenia, thrombocytopenia; abdominal pain, anorexia; diarrhea; nausea, vomiting; retinal detachment, vitreous hemorrhage, cataracts, corneal opacification; neuropathy; rash
Oseltamivir[18]	Nausea, vomiting; diarrhea; abdominal pain; dizziness, vertigo, insomnia; self-injury and psychosis
Ribavirin[19]	Worsening of respiratory status, bacterial pneumonia, pneumothorax, apnea, ventilator dependence; cardiac arrest, hypotension; rash; conjunctivitis
Rimantadine[20]	CNS (insomnia, dizziness, headache, nervousness, fatigue); GI (nausea, vomiting, anorexia, dry mouth, abdominal pain) (1%–3%)
Trifluridine[21]	Burning or stinging on instillation (4.6%); palpebral edema (2.8%); keratopathy; hypersensitivity reaction; stromal edema; hyperemia; increased intraocular pressure
Valacyclovir[22]	Headache (14%); nausea (15%); vomiting (6%); dizziness (3%); abdominal pain (3%)
Valganciclovir[23]	Neutropenia; thrombocytopenia; diarrhea; nausea, vomiting; abdominal pain; increased SCr; insomnia; peripheral neuropathy; paresthesias; CNS (ataxia, dizziness, seizures, psychosis, hallucinations, confusion, drowsiness); retinal detachment (during treatment of CMV retinitis); hypersensitivity
Zanamivir[24]	Bronchospasm; decline in respiratory function, especially if underlying respiratory disease; nasal or throat irritation or congestion; headache; cough; diarrhea; nausea, vomiting

AV, atrioventricular; BUN, blood urea nitrogen; CMV, cytomegalovirus; CNS, central nervous system; ECG, electrocardiogram; GI, gastrointestinal; SCr, serum creatinine.

 concentrations of valacyclovir were achieved, CSF concentrations dropped over time, likely because of resolution of inflammation of the blood–brain barrier. Consequently, switching to oral therapy cannot be recommended at this time and therapy with IV acyclovir should be continued to complete a 21-day course (Table 79-2).[27]

Neonatal Herpes

Most neonates acquire herpes from the infected genital secretions of the mother at delivery, and most cases are caused by HSV-2 virus.[28] The incidence ranges from 1 in 3,000 to 5,000 deliveries per year in the United States. The infection can present in one of three forms: localized to the skin, eye, and mouth (SEM) (45%); encephalitis (30%); or disseminated disease (25%). The effects of neonatal herpes can be devastating, and severe disabilities persist in many afflicted children.[28] With currently available antivirals, the mortality has ranged from 4% in those with CNS involvement to 29% in those with other disseminated disease.[28] Neonatal HSV-1 infections may also be acquired after birth through contact with family members with symptomatic or asymptomatic oral-labial HSV-1 infection or from nosocomial transmission. When the virus is transmitted from the mother, clinical evidence of infection in the neonate usually is present 5 to 17 days after birth. Although skin vesicles are the hallmark of infection, at least one-third to one-half of neonates never have skin lesions.[29] In 70% of patients, the disease may progress from isolated skin lesions to involve other organs, including the lungs, liver, spleen, CNS, and eyes.

Diagnosis can be made by direct fluorescent antibody examination of epithelial cells from the infant or the mother. Examination of the base of a vesicular lesion may show giant cells and intranuclear inclusions, which are characteristic of HSV infections. Serologic test results can support a diagnosis of neonatal herpes.

RISK FACTORS

CASE 79-2

QUESTION 1: S.P., an 18-year-old pregnant woman, was admitted to labor and delivery with premature rupture of the membranes. Four hours later, S.P. vaginally delivered a 2.5-kg baby boy, R.P., who had an estimated gestational age of 33 weeks. Twenty-four hours after delivery, S.P. reported the onset of vesicles in the genital area; she had a history of previous episodes of genital herpes. The last infection was during her first trimester of pregnancy. Is R.P. at risk of developing herpes infection?

R.P. is at risk of acquiring herpes infection because the mother had genital herpes during the first trimester and because he was delivered vaginally rather than by cesarean section.[30] The risk of a newborn acquiring the disease from an infected mother with primary disease is about 35%; that from a mother who has reactivation of disease is 3%.[30]

TREATMENT: ACYCLOVIR

CASE 79-2, QUESTION 2: Ten days after birth, R.P. exhibited poor feeding patterns, irritability, and respiratory distress. Three days later, skin lesions appeared. How should R.P. be treated?

R.P. is manifesting signs of HSV infection and should be treated with antiviral therapy (Table 79-2). The drug of choice for neonatal herpes simplex virus infections is IV acyclovir.[28,29] Vidarabine was the first antiviral agent used in the treatment of neonatal HSV. Because of the drastic reduction in morbidity, it became the standard of therapy to which other antiviral agents were compared. In clinical trials comparing vidarabine with acyclovir, acyclovir was shown to be as effective as vidarabine in infants with SEM involvement, encephalitis, and disseminated

Table 79-2
US Food and Drug Administration (FDA)–Indicated Drugs for Various Viral Infections

Disease	Drug	Dosage (Age Group)	Route	Duration
Herpes encephalitis	Acyclovir (Zovirax)[a]	>12 years: 10 mg/kg every 8 hours	IV	21 days
		3 months–12 years: 20 mg/kg every 8 hours	IV	21 days
Neonatal herpes	Acyclovir (Zovirax)	Birth–3 months: 10–20 mg/kg every 8 hours[a]	IV	14–21 days
Oral-facial herpes (for treatment of recurrent infection)	Acyclovir (Zovirax) Famciclovir (Famvir) Valacyclovir (Valtrex)	Adults: 400 mg 5 × per day Adults: 1,500 mg Adults: 2,000 mg BID	PO PO PO	5 days 1 dose 1 day
Oral-facial herpes[b] (immunocompromised patients)	Acyclovir (Zovirax)	>12 years: 5 mg/kg every 8 hours <12 years: 10 mg/kg every 8 hours	IV IV	7 days 7 days
	Famciclovir (Famvir)	Adults: 500 mg BID	PO	7 days
Herpes zoster[b] (immunocompetent patients)	Acyclovir (Zovirax) Famciclovir (Famvir) Valacyclovir (Valtrex)	Adults: 800 mg 5 × per day Adult: 500 mg every 8 hours Adult: 1,000 mg every 8 hours	PO PO PO	7–10 days 7 days 7 days
Herpes zoster[b] (immunocompromised patients)	Acyclovir (Zovirax)	>12 years: 10 mg/kg every 8 hours <12 years: 20 mg/kg every 8 hours	IV IV	7 days 7 days
Varicella (immunocompetent patient)	Acyclovir (Zovirax)	>40 kg: 800 mg QID >2 years and <40 kg: 20 mg/kg (max 800 mg) QID	PO PO	5 days 5–10 days

Table 79-2
US Food and Drug Administration (FDA)–Indicated Drugs for Various Viral Infections (*continued*)

Disease	Drug	Dosage (Age Group)	Route	Duration
Varicella (immunocompromised patients)		>12 years: 10 mg/kg every 8 hours <12 years: 500 mg/m² every 8 hours	IV IV	7–10 days 7–10 days
Cytomegalovirus retinitis (immunocompromised patients)	Ganciclovir (Cytovene)	5 mg/kg every 12 hours; then 5 mg/kg/day, 7days a week or 6 mg/kg/day, 5 days a week	IV	14–21 days for induction; maintenance
	Cidofovir (Vistide)	5 mg/kg every week for 2 weeks, then every 2 weeks	IV	Maintenance
	Foscarnet (Foscavir)	90 mg/kg every 12 hours; then 90 mg/kg every day	IV	Induction for 2 weeks; maintenance
	Valganciclovir (Valcyte)	900 mg BID; 900 mg every day	PO	Induction for 21 days; maintenance
Influenza A	Amantadine[c] (Symmetrel)	>9 years: 100 mg BID	PO	10 days (treatment), 14–28 days (protection with vaccine), 90 days (protection without vaccine)
		1–9 years: 4.4–8.8 mg/kg/day but <150 mg/day	PO	
	Rimantadine[c] (Flumadine)	>14 years: 100 mg BID	PO	7 days (treatment, not approved for treatment in children) up to 6 weeks for prophylaxis
		1–13 years: 100 mg BID	PO	Up to 6 weeks for prophylaxis
		1–9 years: 5 mg/kg div. every day BID (max 150 mg/day)	PO	
Influenza A and B	Oseltamivir (Tamiflu)	>13 years (or >40 kg): 75 mg BID	PO	5 days (treatment)
		>13 years (or >40 kg): 75 mg every day	PO	10 days (prophylaxis)
				Up to 6 weeks (community outbreaks)
		24–40 kg: 60 mg BID	PO	5 days (treatment)
		16–23 kg: 45 mg BID		
		>1 year–15 kg: 30 mg BID		
		24–40 kg: 60 mg every day	PO	10 days (prophylaxis)
		16–23 kg: 45 mg every day		
		>1 year–15 kg: 30 mg every day		
	Zanamivir (Relenza)	>7 years: 10 mg (2 inhalations) BID	Inhalation	5 days (treatment)
		Adolescent and adult: 10 mg (2 inhalations) every day	Inhalation	10 days (prophylaxis) 28 days (community outbreak)
		>5 years: 10 mg (2 inhalations) every day	Inhalation	10 days (prophylaxis)
Respiratory syncytial virus	Ribavirin (Virazole)	6 g in 300 mL for 12–18 hour/day	Inhalation	3–7 days

[a]FDA-approved dose is 10 mg/kg. Although doses of 15–20 mg/kg have been used, safety has not been established at these doses.
[b]Foscarnet 40 mg/kg IV every 8 hours is recommended for acyclovir-resistant herpes simplex virus or varicella-zoster virus.
[c]Amantadine and rimantadine are no longer recommended as drugs of choice for either prophylaxis or treatment of influenza A.
BID, 2 times day; IV, intravenously; PO, orally; QID, 4 times a day.

 HSV infection.[31] Although both agents were equally effective, acyclovir was safer and easier to administer, making it the standard of care for neonatal HSV.

Acylovir Administration

CASE 79-2, QUESTION 3: What dosage of acyclovir should R.P. receive?

Although an IV dosage of 30 mg/kg given in three divided doses has been shown to be effective in the treatment of neonatal herpes, the use of 60 mg/kg given in three divided doses is superior in decreasing morbidity and mortality. The higher dose of acyclovir is associated with a higher frequency of hematologic abnormalities, especially neutropenia.[9,32,33] The minimum duration of therapy should be 14 days for neonates with only SEM involvement, whereas longer courses (e.g., 21 days) are indicated in infants with CNS involvement or disseminated disease.[28]

The role of prolonged oral suppressive therapy in newborns with SEM involvement has been investigated.[34,35] Acyclovir, given orally (PO) at 300 mg/m^2 per dose 3 times a day (TID), resulted in a reduction in the recurrences of lesions. Half of these patients developed neutropenia. One patient had lesions resistant to acyclovir.[35] Because the long-term benefits cannot be fully attributed to the use of suppressive acyclovir, suppressive therapy for patients with SEM involvement is not recommended.[35]

Oral-Facial Herpes (Herpes Labialis)

Both primary and recurrent oral-facial HSV-1 infections can be asymptomatic. Gingivostomatitis and pharyngitis are the most common clinical manifestations of a first episode of HSV-1 infection, and recurrent herpes labialis is most commonly caused by reactivated HSV infection. Clinical features include fever, malaise, myalgia, inability to eat, and irritability. Immunocompromised patients with oral-facial herpes have severe pain, extensive lesions, and prolonged viral shedding; thus, they are candidates for antiviral therapy.

Herpes labialis (cold sores) is the most common oral-facial HSV infection. Clinical features include pain or paresthesia and erythematous or papular lesions followed by vesiculation and swelling. These lesions usually crust and heal in a few days. Viral cultures generally are positive within 2 to 3 days. Rapid diagnosis can be made by visualizing viral particles in vesicular fluid with electron microscopy or fluorescent antibody staining of cells from vesicles.

INDICATIONS FOR ANTIVIRAL TREATMENT

CASE 79-3

QUESTION 1: M.K., a 26-year-old man, experienced pain and erythematous skin lesions on his face and around his mouth during a 2-day period after contact with a person with active herpetic lesions. For the next 2 days, significant swelling was noted. He remembers similar episodes in the past. M.K. has no previous history of any other illness. Should he be treated with antiviral drugs?

Most patients with herpes labialis have a self-limiting benign course and the lesions heal within 10 days. Antiviral drugs (e.g., acyclovir, valacyclovir, famciclovir) are indicated only when the patient has a primary infection, an underlying illness, or a compromised immune system that may lead to prolonged illness or dissemination.

M.K. should not receive antiviral therapy. However, acetaminophen or nonsteroidal anti-inflammatory agents (NSAIDs) can be considered for symptomatic relief. Although ice, ether, lysine, silver nitrate, and smallpox vaccine have been used to treat cold sores, no data support their efficacy. Symptomatic treatment with ice or popsicles may also be beneficial.

CASE 79-4

QUESTION 1: P.L., a 16-year-old boy diagnosed with acute lymphocytic leukemia 8 months ago, is now admitted for a bone marrow transplant. Admission laboratory tests reveal that he has antibodies against HSV-1 and that 4 months ago, during a course of chemotherapy, he developed an oral-facial herpes infection. What is the significance of these findings for P.L., who is about to undergo a bone marrow transplant?

Immunosuppressed patients have more frequent and severe mucocutaneous HSV infections. Therefore, IV acyclovir should be considered to suppress the reactivation of oral-facial HSV infections.[36,37] Oral therapy with famciclovir is approved for use in HIV-infected patients,[38] but efficacy in other immunocompromised patients is not yet established.

Antiviral Treatment

CASE 79-4, QUESTION 2: P.L. did not receive antiviral therapy. Two weeks later, he developed malaise and painful oral-mucosal and skin lesions on his face. HSV was identified from the lesion by immunofluorescence. What is the treatment of choice for P.L.?

Acyclovir should be administered IV at 5 mg/kg every 8 hours for 7 days[9] or until the lesions are healed, followed by oral acyclovir 200 mg TID for about 6 months.[26] In patients with marrow transplants and culture-proven recurrent mucocutaneous herpes simplex, oral acyclovir (400 mg 5 times daily for 10 days) is significantly more effective than placebo in reducing pain, virus shedding, new lesion formation, and lesion healing time.[39] Valacyclovir and famciclovir have also been used in the transplant population.[40]

CASE 79-5

QUESTION 1: N.B., a 43-year-old woman, experiences 8 to 10 cold sores a year. These are typically preceded by "colds" or sun exposure. She requests a prescription for acyclovir to prevent cold sores when she feels one coming on. What is the role of antiviral medications in the acute treatment and prevention in immunocompetent patients with recurrent herpes labialis?

Topical agents approved by the US Food and Drug Administration (FDA) for the treatment of recurrent herpes labialis in immunocompetent patients include acyclovir 5% cream (Zovirax), acyclovir 5% and hydrocortisone 1% cream (Xerese), docosanol 10% cream (Abreva), and penciclovir 1% cream (Denavir). Clinical trials demonstrate that each agent modestly decreases healing time of herpes lesions when started at the first sign or symptom of a cold sore.[41–47] Although penciclovir cream may be more effective than acyclovir cream, the benefit is small.[44,45] An advantage of docosanol cream compared with the other agents is its availability without a prescription. The topical agents must be applied within 1 hour of the first sign or symptom of a cold sore and then every 2 hours for 4 days while awake.

Studies evaluating the use of oral antiviral agents have produced conflicting results. In some studies, oral antiviral medications have shown to decrease the duration of pain and healing time in immunocompetent patients. One study demonstrated that oral acyclovir 200 mg 5 times daily for 5 days had no benefit.[48] However, 400 mg 5 times daily for 5 days started within 1 hour of the development of a cold sore significantly decreased duration of pain and healing time in immunocompetent patients.[49] Valacyclovir

2 g at the first signs of a cold sore followed by 2 g 12 hours later, and famciclovir 1,500 mg as a single dose showed similar clinical efficacy.[50,51] No studies have directly compared the efficacy of the different oral antiviral medications.[52] Frequency of dosing and cost should be considered when choosing a particular agent.[9,15,22]

Daily suppressive therapy may be recommended in patients with six or more recurrences per year, in patients with frequent infection who do not experience a prodrome, or in patients with severe episodes. In immunocompetent patients with six or more episodes of herpes labialis, oral acyclovir 400 mg twice a day (BID) for 4 months was more effective than placebo in decreasing the number of recurrences.[53] Oral valacyclovir, 500 mg once daily or 1,000 mg once daily, is efficacious in decreasing the number of recurrences.[54] Controlled trials of famciclovir for chronic suppressive therapy of herpes labialis have not been performed.

N.B. should be treated with either a topical antiviral medication or an oral antiviral for the acute episode of herpes labialis. She should be instructed to start treatment as soon as the first sign or symptom of the cold sore appears. If suppressive therapy is desired, N.B. should be treated with oral acyclovir or valacyclovir.

RESISTANCE

The incidence of acyclovir-resistant herpes in patients with herpes labialis is greater in immunocompromised patients compared with immunocompetent patients. Current estimates of HSV resistance in the immunocompromised population are about 5%; some populations, such as bone marrow transplant patients, have a resistance rate approaching 30%.[55,56] IV foscarnet 40 mg/kg every 8 hours is more effective and less toxic than IV vidarabine 15 mg/kg/day in patients with AIDS and mucocutaneous herpetic lesions unresponsive to IV acyclovir.[57] More concerning, however, are the reports of foscarnet-resistant HSV, particularly in the bone marrow transplant population.[58,59] Cidofovir has been used with moderate success in such cases. In patients with recurrent acyclovir-resistant genital herpes, limited evidence suggests that topical imiquimod 5% cream may be effective.[60]

VARICELLA-ZOSTER INFECTIONS

Chickenpox

Chickenpox used to be a common childhood infection, but the incidence has decreased by up to 84% in states with moderate use of the varicella-zoster virus (VZV) vaccine since 1995.[61] This vaccine is now considered a routine childhood vaccine by the American Academy of Pediatrics. Unimmunized adolescents and adults who have not had chickenpox should also be vaccinated. Before the vaccine was available, approximately 4 million cases occurred per year in the United States: 90% of cases occurred in children and adolescents less than 15 years of age with the majority of cases occurring between 1 and 4 years of age.[62] In addition to a decline in cases of chickenpox, complications and mortality have also declined.[63] The population at risk for complications such as pneumonia and encephalitis, because of VZV, include immunocompromised individuals and pregnant women. Children with HIV are at an increased risk of mortality from VZV.[63]

Chickenpox is a contagious disease; the average incubation period is 14 to 16 days. Children are considered contagious from 1 to 2 days before the onset of rash until all vesicles have crusted (usually 4–6 days after the onset of rash).[63]

After household exposure, more than 90% of susceptible individuals become infected. Thus, a history of exposure is useful in making a diagnosis. A smear of cells scraped from the lesions will show multinucleated giant cells. Viruses also can be identified in vesicular lesions by electron microscopy, or antigen can be detected by countercurrent immunoelectrophoresis. Chickenpox is a primary varicella-zoster infection, whereas herpes zoster (shingles) is caused by reactivation of VZV.[63]

CLINICAL PRESENTATION

CASE 79-6

QUESTION 1: A.V., a 10-year-old boy, was admitted to the hospital for evaluation and treatment of possible recurrent chickenpox. According to his mother and his physician, he had a mild case of chickenpox at age 4 years and has not received the vaccine. At admission, A.V. had a 10-day history of progressive vesicular and pustular lesions that began on his neck and spread to his back, trunk, extremities, and face. Although he had been febrile (up to 40.5°C orally) for the past 3 days, his temperature on admission was 37°C. A.V. had episodes of vomiting during the 4 days before admission. On admission, he was alert, cooperative, and well oriented but had overt ataxia with abnormal cerebellar signs. Lesions consistent with VZV infection were extensive and confluent over the face, neck, chest, and back. Stages of lesions varied from tiny thin-walled vesicles with an erythematous base to umbilicated vesicles. Few crusted lesions were present. Blood analysis revealed the following results:

BUN, 9 mg/dL (normal, 5–18 mg/dL; 1.8–6.4 mmol/L)
SCr, 0.2 mg/dL (normal, 0.5–0.8 mg/dL; 44–71 μmol/L)
Serum aspartate aminotransferase, 65 international units/L (normal, 0–34 units/L)
Serum alanine aminotransferase 122 international units/L (normal, 0–34 units/L)

Because of the possibility of cerebellar involvement with VZV infection, therapy with acyclovir 550 mg IV every 8 hours (1,500 mg/m^2/day) was instituted. Oral diphenhydramine was also prescribed for itching, but A.V. required only two doses on the first hospital day.

New lesions were noted on the second day of acyclovir therapy, but by the third day no new lesions appeared and previous lesions were healing. The ataxia improved daily. He was discharged on day 7 with no further complaints of nausea and vomiting. Follow-up serologic evaluation demonstrated a fourfold rise in the optical density for the VZV enzyme-linked immunosorbent assay (ELISA) from day 20 to day 60 after the onset of infection. These results suggested primary VZV infection. Why is the use of acyclovir in A.V. appropriate?

ANTIVIRAL TREATMENT

Neonates, adults, immunocompromised hosts, patients with progressive varicella, and those with extracutaneous complications, benefit from acyclovir therapy. Acyclovir is effective in preventing dissemination of VZV infection, accelerating cutaneous healing, decreasing fever and pain, and reducing mortality.[64,65] A.V. had a prolonged progressive course of varicella and demonstrated an extracutaneous manifestation of varicella infection (e.g., ataxia with abnormal cerebellar signs). Because of the concern of possible cerebellar involvement, the use of IV acyclovir was appropriate in A.V.

CASE 79-7

QUESTION 1: C.J., an 8-year-old boy, developed a case of chickenpox and was kept home from school. Four days later, his 15-year-old brother, K.J., began to exhibit similar symptoms. What is the role of acyclovir in immunocompetent patients with chickenpox? Should C.J. or K.J. be treated with acyclovir?

Three studies in children (2–18 years of age) have shown that oral acyclovir 20 mg/kg (when initiated within 24 hours of disease onset) 4 times a day (QID) for 5 to 10 days accelerates healing and decreases the formation of new lesions, fever, and itching. However, the benefit is modest (usually healing 1 day sooner than placebo) and does not reduce the complications of varicella.[66] Thus, the American Academy of Pediatrics does not consider routine use of acyclovir in healthy children justified, and it is not indicated for C.J.[67]

Adolescents and adults are more likely to develop complications (e.g., pneumonia, encephalitis) than children. Others at higher risk for developing complications include those with chronic cutaneous or pulmonary disease, patients receiving chronic salicylate therapy, and patients receiving short, intermittent, or aerosolized corticosteroid therapy.[67] In these patients, acyclovir therapy may be warranted. Acyclovir 800 mg PO QID for 5 days in adolescents and adults (initiated within 24 hours of disease onset) decreases the number of lesions and reduces time for healing, fever, and itching. The effect of acyclovir on prevention of severe complications is unknown.[68–70] Thus, acyclovir therapy should be considered in those at increased risk of severe chickenpox, e.g., those like K.J. who are older than 14 years or those with chronic respiratory or skin disease.[71] There are no published clinical trials to support the use of famciclovir and valacyclovir in the treatment of chickenpox. However, valacyclovir or famciclovir may be preferred because of the need for less frequent administration for adolescents and adults at risk for moderate-to-severe complications.

SUPPORTIVE TREATMENT

CASE 79-7, QUESTION 2: What is the role of supportive treatment in C.J. and K.J.?

Cool baths and application of calamine or other topical antipruritic agents may decrease itching. Fingernails should be trimmed to avoid scratching and secondary bacterial infections. In severe cases, a systemic antipruritic and antihistamine preparation may be useful because some degree of sedation may be desired. In C.J. and K.J., aspirin should not be used because Reye syndrome has been associated with the use of salicylates in chickenpox or flulike illness (see Chapter 102, Pediatric Pharmacotherapy).

Shingles (Herpes Zoster)

Herpes zoster infections are caused by the reactivation of dormant VZV in the sensory neurons. Reactivation is believed to occur because of waning immunity. The incidence of herpes zoster is higher in immunocompromised patients (e.g., those with HIV or cancer or those receiving immunosuppressive medications), and the incidence of zoster increases with age. It tends to be more severe in the elderly.[72]

Acute herpes zoster infection is characterized by pain, which is described as a deep aching or burning pain. It may be accompanied by excessive sensitivity to touch. Many patients exhibit a rash that presents initially as erythematous patches and progresses to vesicles that crust in 7 to 10 days. By 1 month, the rash is usually gone, but scarring can occur.[72]

Postherpetic neuralgia (PHN) is the most common complication of acute herpes zoster characterized by pain that continues for more than 1 month after the onset of the rash. It is estimated that 10% to 70% of patients experience PHN, and its prevention is important because PHN pain is difficult to treat.[72]

The goal of pharmacotherapy in acute herpes zoster is to inhibit viral replication, to reduce pain and duration of rash. Ultimately, by inhibiting the virus, nerve damage can be prevented and the incidence and severity of PHN can be decreased. Unfortunately, no therapy can prevent all cases of PHN.

The herpes zoster vaccine (Zostavax) significantly reduces the incidence of herpes zoster and the associated resulting PHN (see Chapter 64, Vaccinations).

ANTIVIRAL THERAPY IN IMMUNOCOMPETENT PATIENTS

CASE 79-8

QUESTION 1: E.O. is a 72-year-old, previously healthy man who complains of a burning pain under his left arm for the last 2 days. The pain radiates across his chest. The pain is worse when the area is touched. This morning, he noticed a rash that starts under his arm and continues to his midline. Pertinent laboratory findings include BUN of 15 mg/dL (normal, 8–18) and SCr of 2.0 mg/dL (normal, 0.6–1.2). He has not received the herpes zoster vaccine. A diagnosis of herpes zoster is made. What therapy should be initiated?

Acyclovir is the standard antiviral agent against which new VZV therapies are compared. In immunocompetent patients, oral acyclovir 800 mg 5 times daily for 10 days is moderately beneficial in reducing acute pain during the first 28 days. Acyclovir therapy should be initiated within 72 hours of the onset of the rash. The benefit of acyclovir in reducing PHN and chronic pain is modest at best. Although a number of trials showed no benefit from acyclovir in reducing PHN, a meta-analysis of acyclovir treatment in herpes zoster concluded that acyclovir was effective, but that 6.3 patients would need to be treated to prevent one patient from having PHN 6 months after the outbreak of VZV.[73]

Famciclovir (Famvir) is approved for the treatment of acute herpes zoster infection. Famciclovir is a prodrug and is rapidly absorbed and converted to the active drug penciclovir in the intestine. The bioavailability of famciclovir is greater than acyclovir, resulting in higher concentrations of active drug in the infected cells. In addition, the intracellular half-life (10 hours) of penciclovir allows for less frequent administration.[74] Famciclovir 500 mg TID is as effective as acyclovir 800 mg 5 times a day in reducing the duration of acute pain and healing of the rash.[75] Although famciclovir does not decrease the incidence of PHN, it may reduce the duration of PHN.[76]

To overcome the poor oral bioavailability of acyclovir, valacyclovir (Valtrex), a prodrug of acyclovir, was developed. Valacyclovir is rapidly and extensively absorbed and converted to acyclovir after oral administration. Valacyclovir 1 g TID is as effective as acyclovir 800 mg 5 times a day in terms of reducing rash progression and time to rash healing, and valacyclovir is more effective than acyclovir in relieving zoster-associated pain.[77] Valacyclovir is comparable to famciclovir with respect to decreasing the duration of acute zoster-associated pain and PHN.[78]

E.O. should be started on either acyclovir, famciclovir, or valacyclovir. Famciclovir or valacyclovir may be preferred because adherence with a 3-times-daily regimen will likely be better than with acyclovir, which must be administered 5 times a day. Therapy should be initiated within 72 hours of the rash onset and continued for 10 days; the duration of therapy for famciclovir and valacyclovir is 7 days. Although therapy may not prevent PHN, it may decrease the duration of pain. Because these agents are renally eliminated, the dosage should be adjusted based on E.O.'s reduced creatinine clearance (Table 79-3).

For acute illness, E.O. may require pain control with medications such as nonsteroidal anti-inflammatory agents, opioids, or

Table 79-3

Clinical Pharmacokinetics of Antiviral Drugs

Drug	Type of Patient	Peak Serum Concentration (mcg/mL)	VD	Elimination			Comments
				% Recovered Unchanged in Urine	Total Clearance	Half-Life (hours)	
Acyclovir[9,25,26,79–82]	Adults	3.4–22.9 (based on a dose of 2.5–10 mg/kg IV) 0.83–1.61 (based on a dose of 200–800 mg PO)	59 L/1.73 m^2	69–91	327 mL/minute/1.73 m^2	2.5–3.3	Use 100% of recommended dose, but extend dosage interval to 12 and 24 hours if ClCr ranges from 25 to 50 and 10 to 25 mL/minute/1.73 m^2, respectively; use 50% of recommended dose every 24 hours if ClCr ranges from 0 to 10 mL/minute/1.73 m^2
	Neonates	N/A	24–30 L/1.73 m^2	N/A	98–122 mL/minute/1.73 m^2	3.2–4.1	
Amantadine[13]	Adults	0.2–0.5 (based on a dose of 100–200 mg PO)	3–8 L/kg	52–88	2.5–10.5 L/hour	20–41	Adjust doses in renal failure: 200 mg on day 1, then 100 mg/day if ClCr 30–50; 200 mg on day 1, then 100 mg every other day if ClCr 15–29; 200 mg every 7 days if ClCr <15 mL/minute/1.73 m^2
Famciclovir[15,83,84]	Adults	0.8–6.6 (based on a dose of 125–1,000 mg PO)	1.1 L/kg	73–94[a]	0.37–0.48 L/hour/kg	2.2–3.0	Use 100% of recommended dose, but extend dosage interval to 12 and 24 hours if ClCr ranges from 40 to 59 and 20 to 39 mL/minute, respectively; use 250 mg every 24 hours if ClCr <20 mL/minute
Oseltamivir[18,85–87]	Adults	0.6–3.5[b] (based on a dose of 75 mg PO)	23–26 L	99[b]	18.8 L/hour	6.0–10	Use 75 mg/day in patients if ClCr 10–30 mL/minute. The effect of hepatic impairment has not been determined
	Pediatrics (1–12 years)	0.06–0.8[b] (based on a dose of 2 mg/kg PO)	N/A	N/A	0.63 L/hour/kg	3.2–7.8	Dosage recommendations are based on body weight and age. Use 30 mg BID if patient is 15 kg and 1–3 years, 45 mg if patient is 15–23 kg and 4–7 years, 60 mg if patient is 23–40 kg and 8–12 years, and normal adult dose if >40 kg and older than 13 years
	Adolescents	N/A	N/A	N/A	0.32 L/hour/kg	8.1	
Rimantadine[20]	Adults	0.2–0.7 (based on a dose of 100–200 mg PO)	17–25 L/kg	20	20–48 L/hour	25–32	Because it undergoes extensive metabolism, dose may have to be adjusted in patients with severe liver disease. Dose adjustments may also be necessary in elderly and in those with severe renal failure (ClCr <10 mL/minute). Manufacturer recommends 50% reduction in such cases
Valacyclovir[22,88] (see Acyclovir [prodrug of acyclovir])	Adults	5.7–6.7[c] (based on a dose of 1,000 mg PO)	N/A	46–80[c]	N/A	2.5–3.3[c]	Use 100% of recommended dose, but extend dosage interval to 12 and 24 hours if ClCr ranges from 30 to 49 and 10 to 29 mL/minute, respectively; use 500 mg every 24 hours if ClCr <10 mL/minute
Zanamivir[24,89,90]	Adults	0.02–0.1 (based on a dose of 10 mg INH)	15.9 L	7–17	2.5–10.9 L/hour	2.5–5.1	4%–17% of inhaled dose systemically absorbed. Although only limited studies with renal or hepatic impairment, dosing adjustment likely unnecessary

[a]Pharmacokinetic properties of active metabolite penciclovir.
[b]Active metabolite oseltamivir carboxylate.
[c]Pharmacokinetic properties of active metabolite acyclovir.
BID, twice a day; ClCr, creatinine clearance; INH, inhalation; IV, intravenously; N/A, not available; PO, orally; VD, volume of distribution.

tramadol.[91,92] In addition, E.O. should be counseled to keep the area of the rash clean and dry and to avoid topical antibiotics. If the rash worsens or fever develops, he should contact his health care professional.

CASE 79-8, QUESTION 2: Should E.O. receive a corticosteroid to treat or prevent the pain associated with herpes zoster?

The decision to use corticosteroids, such as prednisone or prednisolone, remains controversial.[93] A number of studies have examined the effect of steroids on pain during acute neuralgia and on the development of PHN. Early studies revealed that steroids are effective for both acute pain and PHN, but these studies were small and uncontrolled, and used various corticosteroid regimens. Most studies suggest relief of the acute pain but no decrease in PHN.[94–97] Because of recent studies demonstrating a lack of benefit in preventing PHN, the theoretical concerns of herpes zoster dissemination, the development of secondary bacterial infections, and the beneficial effects of antiviral agents such as acyclovir, famciclovir, and valacyclovir for acute pain, corticosteroids should not be used in E.O.

CASE 79-8, QUESTION 3: Two months after the onset of the rash, E.O. continues to complain of pain. A diagnosis of PHN is made. What FDA-approved treatments for PHN should be prescribed for E.O.?

Although many different agents have been studied, the only FDA-approved treatments for PHN are topical capsaicin cream or gel, capsaicin patch 8% (Qutenza), topical lidocaine 5% patches (Lidoderm), and oral gabapentin (Neurontin) and pregabalin (Lyrica). Capsaicin depletes substance P, a mediator that transmits pain from the periphery to the CNS. The largest double-blind, placebo-controlled trial of capsaicin evaluated 143 patients with PHN for at least 6 months.[98] After 6 weeks of treatment with capsaicin 0.075% cream, pain scores were reduced in 21% and 6% of the capsaicin and placebo groups, respectively. After the double-blind phase of the study ended, a subset of patients continued to use capsaicin cream for up to 2 years, and most patients experienced prolonged pain relief.[98] Capsaicin should be applied 3 or 4 times per day. Qutenza is a capsaicin patch, which is applied by a health care professional. The patch is applied for 1 hour and cannot be repeated more frequently than every 3 months. Lidocaine 5% patches have only been compared with placebo and have been shown to relieve pain for 4 to 12 hours after administration. Either capsaicin cream or gel or lidocaine patches can be considered as a first-line option for E.O. A common adverse effect is a burning sensation after application of capsaicin, which is intolerable in up to one-third of patients. The burning sensation usually lessens with continued use.

If lidocaine patches are prescribed, E.O. should be instructed to apply up to three patches to the painful area. Patients should be instructed to wear the patches for a maximum of 12 hours a day, and proper disposal of used patches should be emphasized. Even a used patch contains a large amount of lidocaine, and small children or pets could suffer serious consequences from chewing or swallowing a used patch.[99]

Pregabalin is approved for the treatment of PHN, but it is associated with a greater risk of adverse effects. Pregabalin binds to a subunit of calcium channels, thereby decreasing calcium influx at nerve terminals and reducing the release of several neurotransmitters, including glutamate, norepinephrine, and substance P.[100] In clinical trials, dizziness was experienced by 29% of patients treated with pregabalin compared with 9% of placebo-treated patients; somnolence was noted in 22% of patients who received pregabalin compared with 8% of placebo-treated patients. Dizziness and somnolence usually occur soon after the pregabalin is started and is dose dependent.[100]

Other agents that have been used in the treatment of PHN include tricyclic antidepressants (e.g., amitriptyline, desipramine) and opioids.[101]

ANTIVIRAL THERAPY IN IMMUNOCOMPROMISED PATIENTS

CASE 79-9

QUESTION 1: R.F. is a 68-year-old woman with a chief complaint of vesicles on her face associated with severe pain. She has a history of polymyalgia rheumatica and possible temporal arteritis with headaches that are responsive to steroids. She had been having increasing headaches on the right side of her forehead 5 days before admission. Two days before admission, her family physician increased the dosage of prednisone from 30 to 60 mg/day. Vesicles developed on her face 1 day before admission. She was admitted for pain control and diagnosed with herpes zoster infection. Six hours after admission, R.F. began having visual hallucinations, hearing noises, and talking to herself. A lumbar puncture was performed with the following results:

WBCs, 3 (2 lymphocytes and 1 monocyte)
RBCs, 3
Protein, 84 mg/dL
Glucose, 86 mg/dL

VZV was isolated from the CSF and IV acyclovir was started at a dosage of 10 mg/kg every 8 hours. Why is antiviral therapy indicated in R.F.? Should her prednisone be continued or discontinued?

Antiviral therapy is indicated for R.F. Acyclovir may halt the progression of acute herpes zoster infection in immunocompromised hosts such as R.F., who has been taking large doses of corticosteroids.[102]

IV acyclovir 10 mg/kg every 8 hours is effective in severely immunocompromised patients. Alternatively, in less severely immunocompromised patients, oral therapy with acyclovir 800 mg 5 times a day, valacyclovir 1,000 mg TID, or famciclovir 500 mg TID, along with close monitoring, can be used.[103] Antiviral therapy is associated with more rapid clearance of the herpes zoster virus from vesicles. Acyclovir has little to no benefit in resolution of pain or prevention of PHN.[102] Initial data indicate that famciclovir or valacyclovir are effective in severe herpes zoster infection in an immunocompromised host.[104,105]

Systemic corticosteroids are of unproven usefulness and may slow the healing of lesions. Therefore, if possible, R.F.'s prednisone should be slowly tapered.

Acyclovir Toxicity

CASE 79-9, QUESTION 2: On the fourth day of acyclovir therapy, R.F. developed severe nausea and vomited 3 times. The laboratory data showed a BUN of 45 mg/dL and SCr of 3.2 mg/dL (baseline BUN, 10 mg/dL and SCr, 1.0 mg/dL). Why must R.F.'s acyclovir dosage be altered?

Nausea and vomiting have been reported with acyclovir therapy in patients with herpes zoster infections.[9] Similarly, elevations of SCr and BUN can occur in association with acyclovir therapy. This may be secondary to acyclovir crystallization in the renal tubules, particularly when fluid intake is inadequate (Table 79-1). Because R.F.'s creatinine clearance is between 10 and 25 mL/minute per 1.73 m^2, the acyclovir dosage interval should be extended to 24 hours. Every effort should be made to maintain adequate hydration for the duration of acyclovir therapy. (See Table 79-3 and Chapter 2, Interpretation of Clinical Laboratory Tests, for creatinine clearance calculation.)

INFLUENZA

Influenza is an acute infection caused by the virus of the Orthomyxoviridae family. Epidemics of influenza are usually caused by the type A virus; type B virus is generally associated with more sporadic infection. Infection is transmitted by the inhalation of virus-containing droplets ejected from the respiratory tract of a person with influenza. Influenza can be spread by direct contact, large droplets, or items recently contaminated by nasopharyngeal secretions. The incubation period is typically 2 days (range, 1–4 days).

Influenza A viruses are classified into subtypes of hemagglutinin (H) and neuraminidase (N) surface antigens. Three subtypes of hemagglutinin (H1, H2, H3) and two subtypes of neuraminidase (N1, N2) have caused influenza in humans. Infection with a virus of one subtype may confer little or no protection against viruses of other subtypes. In addition, significant antigenic variation (antigenic drift) within a subtype may occur with time. Thus, infection or vaccination with one strain may not protect against a distantly related strain of the same subtype. This is why major epidemics of influenza continue to occur, and influenza vaccines must be reformulated each year with the most likely viral strains to maximize vaccine benefit.[106]

The influenza vaccine is indicated for all individuals 6 months of age or older. However, there are a number of populations for which vaccination is vital. Persons at highest risk for influenza infection (Table 79-4) should receive the influenza vaccine each year. Two influenza virus vaccines are currently available, a trivalent vaccine which contains two type A strains and one type B strain, and a quadrivalent vaccine which contains two strains of type A and type B.[107] At this time, no recommendations exist regarding which vaccine is preferred in specific populations. Additionally, a high-dose influenza virus vaccine is available which is indicated for patients 65 years or older. The high-dose vaccine formulation contains 4 times the amount of antigen contained in other influenza vaccine products. The higher strength vaccine is intended to illicit a stronger immune response in the elderly, a population known to have a suboptimal response to the standard-dose influenza vaccine. Early trials with the higher strength vaccine found the high-dose vaccine was 24.2% more effective in preventing influenza in adults 65 years of age and older relative to a standard-dose vaccine.[108] Lastly, an intradermal influenza vaccine is injected subcutaneously rather than intramuscularly. The intradermal vaccine requires a smaller gauge needle for administration and less antigen to be as effective as the regular flu vaccine. It is indicated in adults 18 to 64 years of age.[109]

The efficacy of the influenza vaccine depends on the similarity of the components of the vaccine to the circulating viruses that year and the immunocompetence of the host. If there is a good match with the circulating viruses, the vaccine can prevent illness in approximately 70% to 90% of healthy adults and children. The vaccine is effective in preventing hospitalization and pneumonia in approximately 30% of elderly persons living in the community and in 40% of elderly persons residing in nursing homes.[110] Despite the lower efficacy, vaccination is still associated with less severe illness and fewer complications in vaccinated individuals.

Individuals at high risk for transmission to patients include physicians, nurses, and other personnel in both hospital and ambulatory settings; employees of nursing homes and chronic care facilities; providers of home care services; and household members, including children. It is vital that all the above individuals should be vaccinated annually. However, considering the morbidity and mortality associated with influenza, all individuals should receive an annual influenza vaccination.

The optimal time for vaccine administration is between mid-October and mid-November because influenza activity peaks between late December and early March in the United States. Vaccinating an individual too early in the season could result in waning antibody concentrations before the influenza season is over. However, influenza vaccine should be offered throughout the influenza season, even if outbreaks of influenza have already been documented in the community.[107]

Because the parenteral influenza vaccine is an inactivated vaccine and contains no infectious viruses, it cannot cause influenza. The most common adverse effect is soreness at the administration site lasting for up to 2 days.[111] Fever, malaise, myalgia, and other systemic reactions occur infrequently; these may develop within 6 to 12 hours after the vaccine is given and persist for 1 to 3 days.[110,111] Immediate hypersensitivity to egg protein (hives, angioedema, allergic asthma, or systemic anaphylaxis) rarely occurs. Persons with anaphylactic hypersensitivity and those with acute febrile illness should not be given the vaccine. However, minor illnesses with or without fever are not contraindications for the influenza vaccine, particularly in children with a mild upper respiratory tract infection or allergic rhinitis. When the vaccine is contraindicated, a neuraminidase inhibitor (oseltamivir or zanamivir) should be used for prophylaxis.[107] Amantadine and rimantadine are no longer recommended for prophylaxis of influenza because of widespread resistance in the United States.[107]

Clinically, it is impossible to differentiate between influenza A and B. Definitive diagnosis can be made by isolating the virus from throat washings or sputum and by a significant increase in antibody titers during the convalescent period.

Table 79-4
Persons Who Should Receive the Influenza Vaccine[97]

- All persons 6 months of age or older
- Nursing home or chronic care facility residents
- Children and adults with chronic pulmonary or cardiovascular disease
- Children and adults who have required medical follow-up because of chronic metabolic diseases (e.g., diabetes mellitus), renal dysfunction, hemoglobinopathies, or immunosuppression (as a result of medications or diseases such as HIV)
- Children and adults who are at risk for aspiration (e.g., cognitive dysfunction, spinal cord injuries, seizures)
- Children (6 months–18 years) receiving long-term aspirin therapy
- Women who will be pregnant during influenza season
- Health care workers
- Household members of persons in high-risk groups (including contacts of infants and children 0–59 months)

Clinical Presentation

CASE 79-10

QUESTION 1: K.B., a 40-year-old woman, comes into the pharmacy claiming she has "the flu." She recently started a new job and is afraid she will lose her job if she misses too many days from work. What questions would you ask her to differentiate the common cold from an influenza infection?

Although it can be difficult to differentiate the common cold from influenza, there are some clues that may suggest one viral infection from the other. Influenza infections typically occur from December through March in the United States. Patients with influenza generally experience more systemic symptoms, such as fever higher than 102°F, headache, myalgia, and cough. Rhinorrhea, nasal congestion, and sneezing are more pronounced in patients with the common cold. Sore throat can occur with both a cold and the flu. Bacterial sore throat (e.g., strep throat) is somewhat differentiated from a viral sore throat in that a viral sore throat usually has a slower onset and the throat pain is less severe. Lymph nodes are only slightly enlarged and not tender in a viral sore throat, whereas with a bacterial sore throat, lymph nodes are large and tender.[112]

K.B. should be questioned about her symptoms and exposure to ill contacts, and investigation into whether influenza has been documented in the community should be performed to help differentiate an influenza infection from the common cold.

Treatment

Case 79-10, Question 2: K.B. describes symptoms consistent with an influenza infection for the past 24 hours. What treatment options exist for the treatment of influenza? Why is she a candidate for a neuraminidase inhibitor agent such as zanamivir or oseltamivir?

Persons with suspected or confirmed influenza virus infection who are at high risk of developing complications (e.g., those with preexisting cardiac or pulmonary disease, unvaccinated infants and children, elderly, immunocompromised) may benefit from antiviral therapy if started within 48 hours after the onset of symptoms. Treatment is recommended regardless of influenza vaccination status and severity of illness in all patients who develop symptoms of influenza and who require hospitalization. Treatment should be considered in outpatients at high risk of complications with illness that is not improving or in patients who request antiviral therapy within 48 hours of onset of symptoms. Therapy will shorten the duration of illness and decrease the risk for transmission to others in close contact with persons at high risk of complications secondary to influenza infection. The benefits are less clear in patients who have had symptoms longer than 48 hours.[113]

The neuraminidase inhibitors, zanamivir (Relenza), oseltamivir (Tamiflu), and peramivir (Rapivab) are active against influenza A and B. These agents work by selectively inhibiting the enzyme neuraminidase, an enzyme necessary for viral replication and spread. Oral Oseltamivir is currently indicated for the prevention and treatment of influenza in patients 1 year of age and older; oral zanamivir is indicated for the prevention of influenza in patients 7 years of age and older and for the treatment of influenza in patients 5 years of age and older.[18,24] Peramivir, a parenteral formulation, is indicated in adults, greater than 18 years of age, and in patients who cannot tolerate or absorb orally administered oseltamivir or inhaled zanamivir.[114]

Zanamivir is available as an oral powder for inhalation. For the treatment of influenza infection in adults, 10 mg (two inhalations) BID for 5 days should be used. Patients should inhale two doses, separated by at least 2 hours, on the first day and then two doses, separated by 12 hours, on days 2 through 5.[24] Bronchospasm after use can occur, and if bronchodilators are also prescribed, the bronchodilator should be used before zanamivir.[24] Proper use of the delivery system (Rotadisk/Diskhaler) is important, and thus patients should be instructed by the pharmacist on proper delivery technique, with a demonstration device.

Oseltamivir is pharmacologically related to zanamivir but has significantly better oral bioavailability, allowing oral dosing. It is approved for children over 1 year of age and for adults. The dosage of oseltamivir for the treatment of influenza in adults is 75 mg BID for 5 days.[18] Oseltamivir is available as a suspension with pediatric dosing recommendations. As with zanamivir, treatment with oseltamivir must be started within 48 hours of the onset of symptoms. Common side effects include nausea, vomiting, and headache.[18] Of concern is that oseltamivir-resistant influenza has been reported.[115] In addition, there are reports, predominantly in children, of self-injury and delirium after the administration of oseltamivir.[116]

Peramivir is dosed at 600 mg once and is administered intramuscularly or intravenously as an infusion over 15 to 30 minutes. As the agent was primarily studied in patients with influenza A and moderate disease, efficacy is unknown for patients infected with influenza B or patients with severe infection requiring hospitalization. The most common side effect is diarrhea; however, severe dermatologic reactions and abnormal behaviors have been reported with its use.[114]

Resistance to amantadine and rimantadine has increased dramatically in recent years; consequently, these agents are no longer recommended for the routine prevention or treatment of influenza infections.[117]

When administered within 48 hours of onset of illness, zanamivir and oseltamivir reduce influenza symptoms by approximately 1 day.[118–120] Information regarding the effectiveness of the neuraminidase inhibitors in preventing serious complications of influenza, such as pneumonia or worsening of chronic diseases, is limited.[107] Considering the causative agent is unknown and symptoms have been present for only 24 hours, K.B. may benefit from a neuraminidase inhibitor. Oral oseltamivir is easier to administer than inhaled zanamivir, and the patient has no reason to not tolerate this drug. Although oseltamivir will not cure influenza, it may reduce the severity and duration of symptoms by about 1 day. She should be treated with a 5-day course of oseltamivir.

CASE 79-11

Question 1: J.T., a 74-year-old man, is brought to the ED from a nursing home with chief complaints of fever (103°F), shaking chills, cough, headache, malaise, anorexia, and photophobia. He has been ill for the past 48 hours but is much worse this evening. On physical examination, he appeared flushed, his skin was hot and moist, and he was having difficulty breathing. Vital signs included blood pressure, 150/90 mm Hg; pulse, 108 beats/minute; respiratory rate, 22 breaths/minute; and temperature, 103°F. Rales were audible on auscultation of both lungs. A chest roentgenogram showed bilateral infiltrates but no consolidation. Blood gas studies showed significant hypoxia, with a Pao_2 of 50 mm Hg and a $Paco_2$ of 50 mm Hg. J.T.'s medical history was significant for chronic bronchitis and a stroke 16 months ago. Blood, sputum, and urine cultures were obtained, and J.T. was started on antibiotics (ceftriaxone 1 g IV every 24 hours and azithromycin 500 mg IV every 24 hours). Gram stain of the sputum sample showed many WBCs but no bacteria. He was started on oxygen therapy at 4 L/minute via nasal cannula. Twenty-four hours later, his respiratory symptoms worsened, and his arterial blood gases deteriorated slightly (Pao_2, 40 mm Hg; $Paco_2$, 55 mm Hg). J.T. was intubated, and a sputum sample was obtained and sent to the virology laboratory. Three days later, influenza A virus was isolated from the sputum. Blood, urine, and sputum cultures were all negative for bacterial pathogens. Why is this presentation consistent with influenza infection? Is antiviral treatment appropriate in J.T.?

Although symptoms of influenza may vary depending on age, most patients with influenza A have an abrupt onset of fever, chills, cough, and headache. In elderly patients such as J.T. and those with underlying diseases, the course of influenza can worsen quickly, and patients are more likely to require hospitalization.

Antiviral therapy in J.T. is inappropriate. None of the antiviral agents has been studied in patients presenting with symptoms after 48 hours of onset. In addition, the antiviral agents have shown efficacy only in uncomplicated influenza.[107]

Prevention

INFLUENZA VACCINES

Case 79-11, Question 2: During the next 3 weeks, two other nursing home patients develop influenza A infections. What measures should be taken to prevent a further outbreak of influenza among other residents?

The nursing home residents and staff should receive influenza vaccine plus chemoprophylaxis with oseltamivir or zanamivir. The Centers for Disease Control and Prevention (CDC) recommends immunization of all individuals 6 months of age or older, and especially those in high-risk groups, primarily all individuals who are at high risk for influenza-related complications and their household contacts (Table 79-4).[107] Second in priority are otherwise healthy adults 50 years of age or older and children with chronic metabolic diseases severe enough to warrant regular follow-up during the preceding year. Any child younger than 9 years in whom the vaccine is indicated requires two doses of the vaccine for optimal effectiveness. The first dose should be administered as soon as the vaccine becomes available, if possible by October, and the second dose is given before influenza infection is present in the community. Vaccination should continue throughout the season, and can be given as late as February or March, depending on the duration of the influenza season. However, the efficacy of influenza vaccine is incomplete (70%).[120] Therefore, oseltamivir or zanamivir should be used in high-risk individuals who may not develop an adequate antibody response (e.g., patients with advanced HIV infection, residents of nursing homes) to supplement the protection by vaccine.[108,113]

A live, attenuated influenza vaccine (FluMist) is an option for healthy, nonpregnant individuals between the ages of 2 and 49 years. In clinical studies with matched influenza strains, live, attenuated influenza vaccine was approximately 87% effective in preventing influenza in children and provided 85% efficacy in adults.[121,122] Advantages of the intranasal route of administration include ease of administration and patient acceptability of an intranasal preparation compared with an intramuscular (IM) injection. However, because the vaccine is live, viral shedding can occur for 2 or more days after vaccination. Consequently, patients who are immunosuppressed and close contacts of patients who are severely immunocompromised (including health care workers who care for them) should not receive the live vaccine. Others who should not receive the live vaccine include patients with asthma or other chronic disorders of the pulmonary or cardiovascular systems, those with chronic metabolic diseases such as diabetes, renal dysfunction, or hemoglobinopathies, and children or adolescents who are receiving aspirin or other salicylates.[107]

OSELTAMIVIR AND ZANAMIVIR

Analysis of clinical trials of oseltamivir in the prevention of influenza showed a decreased incidence of laboratory-confirmed influenza: 4.8% in the placebo group and 1.2% in the treatment group.[123] The incidence of influenza in a skilled nursing facility was 4.4% in the placebo group and 0.4% in the oseltamivir group. In addition, oseltamivir lowered the rate of infection in patients exposed to influenza at home from 12% to 1%. Zanamivir has also been found to be effective in preventing infection.[124,125]

Comparative studies between neuraminidase inhibitors have not been published. Considering that oseltamivir is available in an oral formulation, it is easier to administer in nursing home patients compared with zanamivir, which requires proper use of the delivery device and a coordinated inspiratory effort.

RESPIRATORY SYNCYTIAL VIRUS INFECTIONS

Respiratory syncytial virus (RSV) causes bronchiolitis and bronchopneumonia in infants younger than 2 years. More than one-half of affected infants are infected in the first 2 years of life. Of these infants, approximately 1% to 2% will require hospitalization.[126] Children who are severely premature, immunocompromised, or with underlying congenital heart disease or lung disease may be at increased risk of mortality because of RSV.[127] Patients with RSV infection before 3 years of age are at increased risk of wheezing and asthma during childhood.[128]

RSV infections usually occur in the winter. The chest radiograph and blood gases are often abnormal, and the virus can be isolated in the nasopharyngeal secretions.

Clinical Presentation and Ribavirin Therapy

CASE 79-12

Question 1: J.R., a male 6-month-old infant who is lethargic, tachypneic, and cyanotic, is brought to the ED. J.R.'s medical history is significant for congenital HIV. He has a fever (102°F), his breathing is labored, and wheezing is audible on expiration. The chest roentgenograms reveal a flattened diaphragm and hyperinflated lung parenchyma. Because of hypoxemia and hypercarbia, J.R. is placed on ambient oxygen to maintain the alveolar oxygen pressure at greater than 60 mm Hg. RSV is present in the respiratory secretions. What therapy is indicated for J.R.?

The goal of RSV therapy is to increase oxygen saturation and decrease airway resistance in patients such as J.R.[129] Treatment of RSV is highly individualized, depending on the presenting signs and symptoms and associated comorbidities. Oxygen is first-line therapy. Although decreases in airway resistance are often achieved with the use of bronchodilators or corticosteroids in other conditions, such as asthma, they have not proven to be effective in the treatment of bronchiolitis.[130,131] Hypertonic saline, administered as a nebulized solution, is beneficial in increasing mucociliary clearance.[130] Infants and children admitted for bronchiolitis with an expected length of stay (LOS) of at least 3 days (moderate-to-severe presentation) may experience a shortened LOS by 1 day when prescribed 3% nebulized saline.[131] Adverse reactions include wheezing and excessive secretions.

Ribavirin (Virazole) is active against many DNA and RNA viruses, including RSV. However, its clinical benefit remains controversial. Early studies with ribavirin showed significant clinical improvement compared with placebo in both healthy children and those with underlying disease.[132] These studies reported benefit in terms of clinical recovery and improvement in arterial oxygenation. Subsequent studies found ribavirin to be ineffective in patients with a variety of risk factors.[133,134] Consequently, the routine use in previously healthy infants and children has not been clearly established. Whether ribavirin decreases the long-term sequelae and severity of illness in high-risk groups (including premature infants, patients with bronchopulmonary dysplasia, congenital heart disease, cystic fibrosis, and immunodeficiency) has not been determined.[135] Current recommendations include consideration for use of ribavirin in infants at risk for severe life-threatening infection.[135] Because J.R. has an underlying immunodeficiency, ribavirin may be considered if J.R.'s condition worsens.

ADMINISTRATION OF RIBAVIRIN

CASE 79-12, QUESTION 2: How is ribavirin administered, and what precautions should be taken during drug administration in J.R.?

Ribavirin is administered as an aerosol through a collision generator that generates particles small enough (1–2 μm wide) to reach the lower respiratory tract. The concentration of the ribavirin solution in the reservoir is 20 mg/mL (6 g in 300 mL of sterile water). The dose is administered over the course of 12 to 18 hours, although in nonventilated patients, 2 g during 2 hours TID (using a 60-mg/mL solution) has been successfully used.[132] Ribavirin therapy is continued for 3 to 7 days.[19]

Ribavirin is approved for use in patients requiring mechanical ventilation. However, ribavirin is hygroscopic, and aerosol particles can deposit in the tubing and around the expiratory valve of a ventilator. The precipitated drug can obstruct the expiratory valve and alter the peak end-expiratory pressure.[19] Ribavirin has been safely used in such patients,[136,137] but close monitoring of respiratory therapy is advised to prevent this problem. In addition to the inspection of tubing, modifications of standard ventilatory circuits have been suggested.[19]

ADVERSE EFFECTS

CASE 79-12, QUESTION 3: What are the important adverse effects of ribavirin?

The most common adverse effects of ribavirin are rash, initial mild bronchospasm, and reversible skin irritation.[138] Although long-term follow-up data are limited, a study evaluating the effects of ribavirin in patients 1 year after administration showed a reduction in the incidence and severity of reactive airway disease, as well as in hospitalizations related to respiratory illness.[139] Further long-term evaluation is still necessary.

Ribavirin is contraindicated in women who are or may become pregnant during exposure to the drug. Although there are no human data, ribavirin has been found to be teratogenic or lethal to embryos in nearly all animal species in which it has been tested. Teratogenesis was evident after a single oral dose of 2.5 mg/kg in hamsters and after daily oral doses of 10 mg/kg in rats. Malformation of the skull, palate, eye, jaw, skeleton, and GI tract have been documented in animals. Ribavirin has reduced the survival of fetuses and offspring of animals tested. It is lethal to rabbit embryos in daily oral doses as small as 1 mg/kg. There are no studies that address teratogenicity in humans, but hospital personnel who are pregnant or may become pregnant should avoid exposure to this drug.[19]

It is important to consider the environmental effects of ribavirin on the personnel involved with its administration. One study found no detectable plasma or urine concentrations of ribavirin in 19 nurses, whereas another reported its presence in the RBCs of a nurse caring for a patient who received ribavirin via oxygen tent.[140] The ribavirin concentration in the air was highest when it was administered via oxygen tent, followed by mist mask, and was lowest after administration via endotracheal tubes of mechanically ventilated patients. This has led to several recommendations: (a) ribavirin aerosol should be administered solely via endotracheal tube of mechanically ventilated patients in a closed filtered system[126]; (b) children receiving ribavirin should be placed in a containment chamber equipped with a high-efficiency particulate air filter exhaust in an isolation room with negative air pressure[19]; (c) disposable full-body coverings and either a powered air-purifying respirator or disposable particulate respirator should be made available to all health care personne[140]; and (d) men and women planning to have children should not care for patients receiving ribavirin via oxygen tents.[140] Valeant Pharmaceuticals markets an aerosol delivery system for oxygen and ribavirin that decreases the liberation of ribavirin into the environment.[19]

Prevention

CASE 79-13

QUESTION 1: S.N. is a 7-month-old boy born prematurely at 27 weeks' gestation. He has chronic lung disease of prematurity (CLD) and uses oxygen at home. RSV season will begin next month. What treatments to prevent RSV infection are available? Why is S.N. a candidate for such treatment?

Palivizumab (Synagis), a humanized monoclonal antibody made from recombinant DNA, is active against RSV and is indicated for children at risk of severe RSV respiratory tract infections (e.g., infants with CLD or a history of premature birth before 29 weeks' gestation). The efficacy of palivizumab has been demonstrated in children with a history of prematurity or CLD.[141] Children receiving monthly IM injections of palivizumab for 5 months during RSV season had a reduction in hospitalizations and intensive care admissions for RSV disease. Palivizumab has replaced the use of RSV-immunoglobulins in infants because it is easier to administer (IM vs. IV), does not interfere with the response of live vaccines such as measles–mumps–rubella or varicella vaccine, and is not likely to transmit blood-borne diseases because it is a synthetic product rather than one derived from human blood.[142]

Based on S.N.'s age and his CLD, he is a candidate for palivizumab therapy.[130]

PALIVIZUMAB DOSAGE AND ADMINISTRATION

CASE 79-13, QUESTION 2: How are the doses of palivizumab calculated, and how should it be administered?

The dose of palivizumab is 15 mg/kg given IM. The first dose is given before the start of the RSV season, and then monthly doses are given for a total of 5 months. In the Northern Hemisphere, the RSV season is typically November through April.

HANTAVIRUS

Infections

Rodents are the primary reservoir hosts of *Hantavirus*, and in the United States the deer mouse (*Peromyscus maniculatus*) is the main reservoir. These viruses apparently do not cause illness in the reservoir hosts, but infection in humans occurs when infected saliva, urine, and feces produced by the rodent are inhaled as aerosols. Most patients recall exposure to rodents or rodent feces within 6 weeks of the onset of illness.[143] Person-to-person transmission has not been documented.

The case definition includes clinical evidence of (a) febrile illness characterized by unexplained adult respiratory distress syndrome (ARDS) or acute bilateral pulmonary interstitial infiltrates, or (b) an autopsy finding of noncardiogenic pulmonary edema, resulting from an unexplained respiratory illness. In addition, laboratory evidence consists of (a) a positive serology (i.e., presence of hantavirus-specific immunoglobulin [Ig] M or rising titers of IgG), (b) positive immunohistochemistry for hantavirus antigen in a tissue specimen, or (c) positive PCR for hantavirus RNA in a tissue specimen.[144] Hantavirus infection can cause three different clinical diseases: hemorrhagic fever with renal syndrome, nephropathia epidemica, and hantavirus pulmonary syndrome (HPS). Hemorrhagic fever with renal syndrome and nephropathia epidemica occur in Asian and European countries. HPS occurs only in the Western Hemisphere, including North America.[145] From 1993 to 2013, 606 cases of HPS were reported in the United States, with 36% of the cases resulting in death.[146] Most have occurred in the southwestern United States during spring and summer.

Clinical Presentation

The clinical features of patients with HPS include fever, myalgia, headache, and cough. Abdominal pain, nausea, or vomiting may also be present. The physical examination has been unreliable. Laboratory abnormalities may include leukocytosis, thrombocytopenia, and hypoalbuminemia. The chest radiograph may initially be normal, but rapid disease progress may show bilateral infiltrates and ARDS. Other viral pneumonias do not typically progress to ARDS as rapidly as hantavirus infections. Because of the nonspecific signs and symptoms, some patients may be misdiagnosed as having influenza.[147]

Treatment

Supportive treatment is important. Oxygen therapy and mechanical ventilation may be necessary. Hypotension can be treated with vasopressor agents and judicious use of IV crystalloids (i.e., 0.9% NaCl) to prevent worsening of pulmonary edema. Universal precautions and respiratory isolation should be instituted.[145]

There is no FDA-approved drug to treat hantavirus infections. Based on one study in 242 patients, IV ribavirin was more effective than placebo in reducing morbidity (oliguria and hemorrhage) and mortality. IV ribavirin was given as a loading dose of 33 mg/kg, followed by 16 mg/kg every 6 hours for 4 days, and 8 mg/kg every 8 hours for the next 3 days.[148]

Two other clinical trials, however, did not show similar clinical efficacy in the treatment of HPS. One open-label trial conducted by the CDC showed a mortality rate of 47% in patients who received ribavirin compared with 50% to those who did not.[147] In addition, a small trial conducted at the National Institutes of Health could not demonstrate any benefit from ribavirin.[149]

WEST NILE VIRUS

West Nile virus (WNV) was first identified in the United States in 1999 in New York City. Since then, the virus has had rapid geographic expansion and has infected individuals in all states in the continental United States.[150] Although WNV normally occurs in tropical climates, the increase in international travel and changes in weather patterns have led to its spread.

WNV is a member of the Flaviviridae family. Culicine mosquitoes (including *Culex pipiens*, *Culex restuans*, and *Culex quinquefasciatus*) are the vectors, and they infect both birds and humans.[151] Infection with the virus involves direct inoculation by the infecting mosquito. Birds are reservoir hosts. WNV can infect a number of vertebrates, including horses. Transmission usually occurs from a mosquito bite; however, reports indicate that transmission of the infection has occurred through transfusions, organ transplantation, placental transfer, and via breast milk.[152] Because of the seasonal variations in the life cycle of the mosquito, cases are most commonly seen during the summer and early fall.

Diagnosis is usually made by high clinical suspicion and laboratory tests. WNV can cause a wide range of illness, from an asymptomatic disease to West Nile fever to encephalitis or meningitis. Mortality is low except in the neuroinvasive forms of the infection. Mortality rates in the elderly, particularly those older than 70 years, can be 9 times higher than in the general population.[153] The CDC laboratory criteria for diagnosis of WNV include (a) isolation of the WNV antigen or genomic sequence from a tissue, blood, CSF, or other body fluids; (b) WNV IgM antibody in a CSF sample; (c) a fourfold rise in the antibody titer to WNV; and (d) demonstration of an IgM or rising titers of IgG to WNV in a single serum sample.[154]

Clinical Presentation

CASE 79-14

QUESTION 1: A.G. is an 84-year-old woman. She is very active and runs the yearly flower festival in the community. She was brought to the ED by her granddaughter, who found her at home, confused and complaining of a headache, fatigue, and increasing muscle weakness. She has a temperature of 103°F, and her Mini-Mental Status Examination score is 21 of 30. She has decreasing muscle strength and an erythematous, macular, papular rash on her arms and legs. The complete blood count and electrolytes are normal, with the exception of slightly decreased sodium. The CSF reveals increased WBCs, increased protein, normal glucose, and positive IgM antibody to WNV. A CT scan shows no abnormalities. What signs and symptoms are indicative of WNV encephalitis?

Acute signs and symptoms of WNV include sudden onset of fever, anorexia, weakness, nausea, vomiting, eye pain, headache, altered mental status, and stiff neck. A rash may be present on the arms, legs, neck, and trunk. The rash is typically erythematous, macular, and papular with or without morbilliform eruption.[155] Laboratory parameters may show normal or elevated WBC counts. Low serum sodium concentrations may be seen in patients with encephalitis. CSF usually shows pleocytosis, mostly with an elevation of lymphocytes, elevated protein levels, and normal glucose levels.[155] Magnetic resonance imaging (MRI) shows some enhancement of the leptomeninges or the periventricular areas in approximately one-third of patients, but no other abnormalities or evidence of acute disease are present on either CT or MRI examination.[155]

With disease progression, further muscle weakness and hyporeflexia may be observed. Patients may progress to a diffuse, flaccid paralysis similar to Guillain–Barré syndrome. Ataxia, extrapyramidal symptoms, cranial nerve abnormalities, myelitis, optic neuritis, and seizures may be seen.

Treatment

CASE 79-14, QUESTION 2: What treatment options are available to A.G.?

Currently, treatment of WNV infection is supportive. Patients with febrile infection usually have a self-limiting course. In severe cases, patients with muscle weakness and signs of encephalitis will require admission to an intensive care unit, and many will need mechanical ventilation. The available antiviral medications do not have any activity against WNV in vivo, although ribavirin inhibits replication in vitro.[155] Combination therapy of high-dose ribavirin and interferon-α-2b has been used in patients with severe disease with limited success. Although optimal doses have not been established, the doses needed to inhibit the virus were 2 to

3 million units of interferon and 2,400 mg of ribavirin daily.[156–158] Current clinical trials investigate the efficacy and safety of intravenous immunoglobulin and humanized monoclonal antibodies for treatment and vaccines for the prevention of WNV.

SEVERE ACUTE RESPIRATORY DISTRESS SYNDROME

Severe acute respiratory distress syndrome (SARS), a highly infectious disease, was first identified in China in early 2003. Since then, the viral syndrome has been reported in several countries in East Asia, North America (particularly Canada), South America, and Europe. During the 2003 outbreak, approximately 8,000 cases were reported, with a case fatality rate of about 10%.[159,160] No cases of SARS have been reported worldwide since 2004. Many of the pre-2004 cases reported in Asia and Canada have been traced to a single index case, with outbreaks clustered in apartments, hotels, health care facilities, or biomedical facilities. There is some evidence to suggest that increased age (older than 60 years) may be associated with an increased mortality risk.[161]

The disease is easily spread by airborne microdroplets. Geography and a history of recent travel to affected areas are believed to be important to an individual's likelihood of contracting the disease. In a sample of 100 suspected patients in the United States, 94% traveled within the 10 days before illness onset to an area listed in SARS case definitions.[162] SARS is believed to be transmitted mostly by close contact with an infected person (e.g., sharing eating utensils, <3-foot conversations).

A novel coronavirus, SARS coronavirus (SARS-CoV), was isolated from patients and identified as the causative agent of SARS. Inoculations of a Vero E6 cell line with throat swab specimens from patients with the diagnosis of SARS showed cytopathologic features.[163] Although the natural reservoir of SARS-CoV has not been identified, the virus has been detected in the Himalayan masked palm civet, the Chinese ferret badger, and the raccoon dog.

Clinical Presentation

The case definition of SARS established by the CDC includes clinical, epidemiologic, laboratory, and exclusion criteria.[164] Symptoms of early disease include fever, chills, rigor, myalgia, headache, diarrhea, sore throat, or rhinorrhea. Mild-to-moderate illness includes temperature higher than 100.4°F and clinical findings of lower respiratory illness such as cough or shortness of breath. Severe illness is characterized by the previous criteria plus radiographic evidence of pneumonia or acute respiratory distress syndrome.

Probable or likely exposure to SARS-CoV is a critical component of the SARS case definition. Travel to a location with documented or suspected recent transmission of SARS-CoV and close contact with a person with mild-to-moderate or severe respiratory illness in the 10 days before the onset of symptoms are defined as possible exposures to SARS-CoV. Likely exposure is defined as close contact with a person with confirmed disease or symptoms of disease.[165]

For patients suspected of having SARS in the United States, laboratory diagnosis can be confirmed by an enzyme immunoassay detecting serum antibody to SARS-CoV, isolation of SARS-CoV from a clinical specimen, or detection of SARS-CoV RNA by a reverse transcriptase PCR. Both the enzyme immunoassay and the PCR are validated by the CDC.[163] Information regarding the most recent criteria for laboratory diagnosis can be found at the CDC website.

Although the majority of cases of infection are self-limited, initial symptoms may be followed by hypoxemia, which may progress to the need for intubation and mechanical ventilation. Typically, patients do not manifest neurologic or GI symptoms.

Treatment

Treatment for SARS during the 2002 through 2003 outbreak included broad-spectrum antibiotics, ribavirin, lopinavir/ritonavir, corticosteroids, interferon, and immunoglobulin.[165] Broad-spectrum antibiotics are recommended to cover other potential pathogens until infection attributable to SARS-CoV is confirmed. Ribavirin has been used in doses ranging from 400 mg IV every day to 2 g IV followed by 1 g IV every 6 hours with a duration of 4 to 14 days.[166] Interestingly, ribavirin does not inhibit SARS-CoV in vitro, and viral loads remained elevated after death despite therapy with ribavirin.[167,168] Furthermore, adverse drug reactions, including hemolytic anemia (61%), hypocalcemia (58%), and hypomagnesemia (46%), were common. Two of three in vitro studies of lopinavir and ritonavir showed activity against SARS-CoV. Lopinavir 400 mg PO BID with ritonavir 100 mg BID may be useful in the treatment of SARS, but data are limited.[165] Treatments with various corticosteroids, interferon, and immunoglobulin remain controversial. No treatment guidelines are available owing to the lack of prospective randomized controlled trials.

MIDDLE EAST RESPIRATORY SYNDROME

Middle East Respiratory Syndrome (MERS) was first reported in 2012 in Saudi Arabia. As of June 2015, a total of 1,130 cases have been reported, primarily in the Arabian Peninsula and most recently in the Republic of Korea.[169,170] To date, only two cases have been reported in the United States, both in health care workers who lived in Saudi Arabia and traveled to the United States. Both received supportive care at a hospital and were discharged.[171]

The causative organism of MERS is the Middle Eastern Respiratory Syndrome coronavirus (MERS-CoV). Symptoms of MERS include fever, cough, and shortness of breath. In some patients, gastrointestinal symptoms such as nausea, diarrhea, and vomiting have been reported. The infection progresses to complications including pneumonia and renal failure. Those at greatest risk for death have comorbid conditions, such as diabetes, cancer, heart disease, lung disease, or chronic kidney disease. Individuals with an underlying immunodeficiency may be at the greatest risk of death.[169]

MERS-CoV appears to be transmitted through close contact with an infected individual, likely through respiratory droplets. Most infections reported have occurred in hospitals or in individuals caring for or living with an infected individual.[169] Treatment of MERS is directed as supportive care for symptoms and complications.

ZIKA VIRUS

The Zika virus was first reported in 2007 in the Pacific Islands, with other rare outbreaks in Africa and Southeast Asia. In 2015, it was detected in Brazil and as of May 2016 reported areas of transmission include the Pacific Islands, the Caribbean, and South and Central America. Also as of May 2016, 503 cases related to travel have been reported in the United States.[172]

Zika is an RNA virus belonging to the *Flaviviridae* family. The most common symptoms of infection include fever, maculopapular rash, arthralgia, and conjunctivitis.[173] The infection is mild and self-limiting and generally resolves in 1 week. In some individuals, neurologic and autoimmune complications, such as Guillain–Barré syndrome, have been reported. Neonatal transmission in pregnant women infected with Zika virus has occurred resulting in microcephaly in the infant and loss of fetus in some instances.[173] Diagnosis is confirmed with RT-PCR, immunoglobulin M, and neutralizing antibody testing.

Zika is transmitted via a mosquito vector and can be transmitted sexually.[174] Women, particularly pregnant women, should use latex condoms or abstain from sexual activity with men who have traveled to an area with active Zika. The virus has been detected in the semen for up to 60 days after exposure.[175] Transmission from the female to the male has not been documented.[174] There is currently no vaccine or medication to prevent Zika virus infection. All travelers to or residents of areas with ongoing Zika virus transmission should follow steps to avoid mosquito bites because of the potential for exposure to Zika. Protective measures for prevention of infection with Zika include wearing long sleeve shirts and pants, remaining in air-conditioned areas with screens on windows, using insect repellent containing N,N-Diethyl-meta-toluamide (DEET), and sleeping in a mosquito net if traveling to an area with reported Zika.[176] Treatment of Zika virus is supportive.[177] Development of a vaccine against Zika virus is ongoing.

THE COMMON COLD

The most prevalent viral infection is the common cold. In the United States, approximately 62 million cases of the common cold occur annually.[178] An estimated 20 million and 22 million days of absence from work and school, respectively, occur. The frequency of the occurrence of a cold is greater in younger children and decreases with increasing age. Although the common cold is self-limiting, otitis media occurs in approximately 20% of children after infection.[179]

Many viruses have been isolated from patients with respiratory infections, but rhinovirus is the most common viral pathogen.[180] Rhinovirus accounts for approximately 34% of all respiratory illnesses. More than 100 different serotypes of rhinovirus exist, and the prevalence of each varies with time and geography. Other pathogens include coronavirus, parainfluenza, RSV, adenovirus, and enterovirus. Because of the number of pathogens known to cause the common cold, development of an effective vaccine remains difficult.

Treatment for the common cold is directed at pharmacologic treatment of symptoms. Nonsteroidal anti-inflammatory drugs, oral or intranasal decongestants, antihistamines, and antitussives may be used. However, these products provide minimal relief of symptoms and do not shorten the natural course of infection.[181–183] In pediatric patients younger than 4 years, the use of cough and cold medications is not recommended by the FDA because of the deaths associated with their use.[184–186] Currently, there are no specific antiviral treatments for the common cold.

Prevention

CASE 79-15

QUESTION 1: J.C. comes into the pharmacy asking for an herbal product that will help him prevent colds this upcoming cold season. He states that last year he had three colds and his neighbor had none. His neighbor had mentioned an herbal product he had been taking. J.C. cannot remember the name of the product but wonders whether there are any products that may be helpful.

ZINC

Zinc, a dietary supplement, has been studied in both the prevention and treatment of the common cold. The proposed mechanism of action is that the rhinovirus 3C protease is inhibited by zinc, and the inhibition of this enzyme prevents viral replication. In vitro, zinc has been shown to have antiviral activity. Several trials conducted in the past several decades have produced conflicting results on the benefits of zinc in decreasing symptom severity or duration. If started within 24 hours of symptom onset, zinc may shorten symptoms but not severity of the cold. Zinc lozenges, dosed at a minimum of 75 mg per day for the duration of cold symptoms, is recommended.[187] Patients who took zinc lozenges for the common cold complained of mouth irritation, unpleasant taste, feeling sick, and diarrhea. Daily administration of zinc is not currently recommended for prophylaxis of the common cold.

ECHINACEA

Echinacea is an herbal product extracted from the *Echinacea* plant, which belongs to the Compositae family. Echinacea is believed to stimulate the immune system, specifically phagocytosis. Some clinical trials using echinacea have shown positive results in decreasing the incidence of infection when compared with placebo, but the results remain inconclusive.[188] One study showed no benefit of echinacea versus placebo but did show an increased incidence of rash in the treatment group.[189] Because the current data are inconclusive and owing to the variability of echinacea concentrations in the available products, use of echinacea in the prevention and treatment of the common cold is not recommended.[190]

KEY REFERENCES AND WEBSITES

A full list of references for this chapter can be found at http://thepoint.lww.com/AT11e. Below are the key references and websites for this chapter, with the corresponding reference number in this chapter found in parentheses after the reference.

Key References

Chen N et al. Corticosteroids for preventing postherpetic neuralgia. *Cochrane Database Syst Rev*. 2010;(12):CD005582. (95)

Grohskopf LA et al. Prevention and control of influenza with vaccines: recommendations of the advisory committee on immunization practices, United States, 2015–16 influenza season. *MMWR Morb Mortal Wkly Rep*. 2015;64:818. (107)

Harpaz R et al. Prevention of herpes zoster. Recommendations of the Advisory Committee on Immunization Practices (ACIP). *MMWR Recomm Rep*. 2008;57(RR-5):1. (94)

James SH et al. Antiviral therapy for herpesvirus central nervous system infections: neonatal herpes simplex virus infection, herpes simplex encephalitis, and congenital cytomegalovirus infection. *Antiviral Res*. 2009;83:207. (10)

[No authors listed]. American Academy of Pediatrics Committee on Infectious Diseases: the use of acyclovir in otherwise healthy children with varicella. *Pediatrics*. 1993;91:674. (71)

Ralston SL et al. Clinical Practice Guideline: the diagnosis, management, and prevention of bronchiolitis. *Pediatrics*. 2014;134;e1474. (130)

Vassilev ZP et al. Safety and efficacy of over-the-counter cough and cold medicines for use in children. *Expert Opin Drug Saf*. 2010;9:233. (185)

Key Websites

Centers for Disease Control and Prevention. All About Hantaviruses. Hantavirus Pulmonary Syndrome (HPS). http://www.cdc.gov/hantavirus/. Accessed August 9, 2015.

Centers for Disease Control and Prevention. Severe Acute Respiratory Syndrome. http://www.cdc.gov/sars/index.html. Accessed August 9, 2015.

Centers for Disease Control and Prevention. West Nile Virus. http://www.cdc.gov/westnile/index.html. Accessed August 9, 2015.

80 Viral Hepatitis

Jerika T. Lam and Curtis D. Holt

CORE PRINCIPLES

	CORE PRINCIPLES	CHAPTER CASES
1	Hepatitis A virus (HAV) is a worldwide, acute self-limiting disease transmitted via the fecal–oral route. Hepatocyte injury is caused by a cytopathic and immunologic response, which can result in jaundice and increased liver function tests. Treatment measures are usually supportive and aimed toward prevention (pre-exposure and post-exposure) through vaccination.	**Case 80-1 (Questions 1–3), Case 80-2 (Question 1), Case 80-3 (Question 1)**
2	Hepatitis B virus (HBV) is a bloodborne pathogen that is transmitted through percutaneous or perinatal exposure, blood products, or sexual contact. HBV has an acute phase with resolution and a chronic phase. Over the course of decades, the chronic phase can lead to hepatic cirrhosis and death. Patients with chronic infection require treatment with peginterferon, nucleoside and nucleotide reverse transcriptase (RT) inhibitors. Several effective prophylactic strategies (immunizations and nucleoside or nucleotide RT inhibitors) are used to prevent HBV infection.	**Case 80-4 (Questions 1–4), Case 80-5 (Questions 1, 2), Case 80-6 (Questions 1–3), Case 80-7 (Question 1), Case 80-8 (Question 1), Case 80-9 (Question 1), Case 80-10 (Questions 1, 2), Case 80-11 (Question 1), Case 80-12 (Questions 1–14)**
3	Hepatitis C virus (HCV) is a bloodborne pathogen that is transmitted primarily through percutaneous exposure, blood products, or sexual contact. HCV has an acute and a chronic phase. The chronic phase can lead to cirrhosis, decompensated liver disease, hepatocellular carcinoma, and death. Acute clinical manifestations are similar to those for HAV and HBV. Treatment of chronic HCV infection (genotypes 1 to 6) is with direct-acting antivirals (DAAs).	**Case 80-13 (Question 1), Case 80-14 (Questions 1–3), Case 80-15 (Questions 1–3)**
4	Hepatitis D virus (HDV) is a small RNA virus that requires coinfection with HBV for replication. HDV transmission is most likely associated with percutaneous exposure. HDV, in combination with HBV, leads to a much higher risk of acute liver failure. Prevention strategies rely on successful immunization of HBV.	**No cases**
5	Hepatitis E virus is similar to HAV and is transmitted via the fecal–oral route, especially through contaminated water, which is found more common in developing countries. Recovery from acute illness usually occurs.	**No cases**

There are five distinctly separate hepatitis viruses that cause liver disease. A sixth virus also has been identified, but has yet to be implicated in liver disease. Four of these viruses are RNA viruses, and one is a DNA virus.[1] The individual virus types can be distinguished by serologic assays and, in some instances, by genotyping. Although progress in the area of disease prevention has improved, advances in treatment of certain viral infections have been limited because of the large amount of viruses produced and their rapid mutation. For instance, the hepatitis C virus (HCV) replicates approximately 1 trillion virus particles (virions) daily, compared with 100 billion HBV virions daily and 10 billion HIV virions daily.[1,2] This chapter reviews the virology, epidemiology, pathogenesis, natural history, diagnosis, clinical manifestations, prevention, and treatment strategies for viral hepatitis A through E.

CAUSATIVE AGENTS AND CHARACTERISTICS

Viral hepatitis is a major cause of morbidity and mortality in the United States.[1–3] At least five distinct pathogens are responsible for viral hepatitis. These hepatotrophic viruses are identified by the letters A through E as follows: (a) type A hepatitis caused by hepatitis A virus (HAV), (b) type B hepatitis caused by hepatitis B virus (HBV), (c) type C hepatitis caused by HCV, (d) type D or delta hepatitis caused by the HBV-associated hepatitis D virus (HDV), and (e) type E hepatitis caused by the hepatitis E virus (HEV). Hepatitis A through E viruses differ in their immunologic characteristics and epidemiologic patterns (Table 80-1).[4,5]

Table 80-1
Characteristics of Hepatitis Viruses[4,5]

Virus	Nucleic Acid	Routes of Transmission	Risk of Chronic Illness	Mortality
HAV	Nonenveloped SS RNA	Fecal–oral	None	Low
HBV	Enveloped DS DNA	Parenteral (sex, perinatal)	High	Moderate–High
HCV	Enveloped SS RNA	Parenteral (sex, perinatal)	High	Moderate–High
HDV	Enveloped SS RNA	Parenteral (sex, perinatal)	High	High
HEV	Nonenveloped SS RNA	Fecal–oral	None	Low–Moderate

HAV, hepatitis A virus; HBV, hepatitis B virus; HCV, hepatitis C virus; HDV, hepatitis D virus; HEV, hepatitis E virus; SS, single-stranded; RNA, ribonucleic acid; DNA, deoxyribonucleic acid.

Fecal–oral transmission is the primary mode of infection for HAV and HEV, whereas parenteral and sexual transmission is characteristic of HBV, HCV, and HDV infections.[1–3] Several other viruses primarily affect nonhepatic organ systems and may secondarily induce a hepatitis-like syndrome. These include the Epstein–Barr virus (infectious mononucleosis), cytomegalovirus, herpes simplex viruses, varicella-zoster virus, and rubella, rubeola, and mumps viruses.

Definitions of Acute and Chronic Hepatitis

Viral hepatitis can present as either an acute or chronic illness. Acute hepatitis is defined as an illness with a discrete date of onset with jaundice or increased serum aminotransferase concentrations greater than 10 times the upper limit of normal[1–3,5] and does not exceed 6 months. Chronic hepatitis is a prolonged inflammatory condition of the liver that involves ongoing hepatocellular necrosis for ≥6 months beyond the onset of acute illness.[4,5] The most common causes of chronic viral hepatitis are HBV and HCV.[3] Drug-induced and autoimmune chronic hepatitis occur less frequently; metabolic disorders and HDV chronic hepatitis are relatively rare.[6,7] HAV and HEV are self-limiting infections that rarely progress to chronic hepatitis.

Serologic Evaluation in Presumed Chronic Hepatitis

Serologies are useful in diagnosing viral hepatitis. Antibodies against hepatitis A virus (anti-HAV), hepatitis B surface antigen (HBsAg), and hepatitis C virus (anti-HCV) are useful diagnostic markers. A diagnosis of acute HAV infection includes the presence of immunoglobulin M (IgM) anti-HAV. If HBsAg is present, further testing for hepatitis B envelope antigen (HBeAg) and HBV DNA confirms the presence of active viral replication and viral load, respectively. Testing for hepatitis D antibody (anti-HDV) should also be performed in patients with HBV infection to evaluate the possibility of coinfection. If serology is negative, rare but treatable causes of chronic active hepatitis should be further ruled out. These include alcoholic liver disease, disease, alpha-1-antitrypsin deficiency, and drug-induced chronic active hepatitis. Drugs associated with reversible chronic active hepatitis syndrome include methyldopa,[8] nitrofurantoin,[9] isoniazid,[10] and, rarely, sulfonamides[11] and propylthiouracil.[12]

HEPATITIS A VIRUS

Virology and Epidemiology

Hepatitis A virus is an icosahedral, nonenveloped virus measuring 28 nm diameter. It is a single-stranded, positive-sense, linear RNA enterovirus of the Picornaviridae family (see Table 80-1).[2,4,5]

HAV has a worldwide distribution.[13,14] The prevalence of infection is related to the quality of the water supply, level of sanitation, and age.[14,15] Incidence data are unreliable because the disease is frequently mild and often unrecognized, resulting in under-reporting. The primary mode of transmission is from person to person via the fecal–oral route.[15,16] The virus is sturdy and resists degradation by drying, environmental conditions (temperatures as high as 56°C and as low as −20°C), gastric acid (pH 3.0), and digestive enzymes in the upper gastrointestinal (GI) tract. Therefore, HAV is easily spread within a population. Fecally contaminated water or food is a significant mode of transmission.[16,17] Children are considered a relatively common reservoir, but rarely exhibit clinical symptoms.[17,18]

In 2014, the overall incidence rate of HAV infection was 0.4 cases per 100,000 population in the United States.[19] HAV infection could occur from common-source outbreaks of fecally contaminated food or water, as well as uncooked HAV-contaminated foods. In developed countries with well-maintained sanitation and water supplies, waterborne outbreaks of HAV are uncommon.[19] Originally, HAV vaccination was recommended for persons at high risk of infection and children living in communities at high risk. However, due to the significant number of cases of HAV disease still occurring in the United States, HAV vaccination recommendations have expanded. In 2006, the Advisory Committee on Immunization Practices (ACIP) recommended routine vaccination for all children aged 12 to 23 months in the United States.[20]

Exceedingly rare causes of HAV include transfusion of blood or blood products collected from donors during the viremic phase of their infection and from contact with experimentally infected nonhuman primates.[16,21] Percutaneous transmission is rare because no asymptomatic carrier state for HAV exists and the incubation period is brief.[16] Occupations at risk for HAV infection include sewage workers, hospital cleaning personnel, day-care staff, and pediatric nurses.[18,19] HAV is the most common preventable (e.g., vaccination) infection in travelers visiting locations with poor hygienic conditions.[22]

Pathogenesis

Although the exact mechanism of injury is unknown,[17,23,24] viral replication occurs within the liver, or hepatocytes. Subsequent hepatocyte death results in viral elimination and eventual resolution of the clinical illness.[18]

Natural History

After exposure to HAV, usually via ingestion of HAV from material contaminated with feces, the virus resides and replicates in the hepatocytes within hours or days after infection. Following the translational and replication processes, HAV is released into the bile canaliculi and is transported to the intestine, where it is excreted in the feces at concentrations ranging up to 10^9 infectious virions per gram of feces.[17] This occurs during the subclinical stage (incubation period) or anicteric prodromal period (14–21 days) of the infection before alanine aminotransferase (ALT) levels become elevated and clinical symptoms or jaundice occurs.[18] The contagiousness of the infection is highest during this period and is significantly reduced following the onset of symptoms or jaundice. HAV infection could occur in two clinical courses varying from subclinical hepatitis (asymptomatic), usually observed in children, to anicteric hepatitis (symptoms without jaundice) or icteric hepatitis that occurs in adults and could result in fulminant hepatitis and death, especially among adults older than 50 years.[18] Chronic HAV infection usually does not manifest because of the robust humoral and cellular immune responses, particularly natural killer cells, $CD4^+$ and $CD8^+$ cytotoxic T cells.[18] Most important, humoral immunity plays a pivotal role in viral clearance leading to viremia declines after the presence of neutralizing antibodies.[25] Typically, the course of HAV includes an incubation phase, an acute hepatitis phase, and a convalescent phase. Complete clinical recovery is usually seen in all patients within 6 months after HAV infection.

Clinical Manifestations

CASE 80-1

QUESTION 1: E.T., a 34-year-old medical sales representative, presents to the emergency department (ED) with acute onset of jaundice and "dark urine." He was in good health until 2 weeks ago, when he noted feeling fatigued and weak, which he attributed to his demanding work schedule. He also recalled having a mild headache, loss of appetite, muscle pain, diarrhea, and low-grade fevers from 99°F to 101°F. He attributed these symptoms to the flu and took acetaminophen with plenty of fluids. His symptoms persisted until yesterday, when they seemed to resolve unexplainably. He then noted his urine was cola-colored. This morning, he noted jaundice of his eyes and skin and sought medical attention.

E.T.'s medical history includes a recent respiratory tract infection, treated successfully with levofloxacin. His social history is significant for frequenting the local oyster bar, where he regularly ingests raw oysters. He denies smoking and recent travel outside the United States, but admits to occasional alcohol consumption. E.T. has no history of sexual exposure, needle use, or transfusions. His current medications include oral (PO) diazepam 5 mg at bedtime (HS) as needed (PRN) for "muscle spasms," but he has not taken diazepam for "several months." He also has a seizure disorder sustained after a motorcycle accident 2 years before admission, for which he takes phenytoin 400 mg PO every HS.

Physical examination is significant for a well-developed, well-nourished man in no acute distress. He is alert and oriented, with a temperature of 99°F. His sclerae and skin are icteric, and his abdomen is positive for a tender, enlarged liver and right upper quadrant pain. Laboratory tests reveal the following values:

Hemoglobin (Hgb): 16 g/dL
Hematocrit (Hct): 44%
White blood cell (WBC) count: 5,500 cells/μL
Aspartate transaminase (AST): 120 units/L
Alanine aminotransferase (ALT): 240 units/L
Alkaline phosphatase: 86 units/L
Total bilirubin: 3.2 mg/dL
Direct bilirubin: 1.5 mg/dL
Phenytoin concentration: 12 mg/L (normal: 10–20 mg/L)

The albumin, prothrombin time (PT), blood glucose, and electrolytes all are within normal limits. E.T. is negative for anti-HCV, HBeAg, HBsAg, and hepatitis B core antibody (anti-HBc), but is positive for IgM anti-HAV. What clinical features and serologic markers are consistent with viral hepatitis in E.T.?

The incubation period for HAV is 15 to 50 days (average 28 days) after inoculation. The host is usually asymptomatic during this stage of the infection; thus, E.T. is beyond the inoculation phase of the disease. Because HAV titers are highest in the acute-phase fecal samples, the period of infectivity is 14 and 21 days, before the onset of jaundice, to 7 or 8 days after jaundice. Therefore, E.T. should be considered infectious at this time. In HAV infections, acute-phase serum and saliva are less infectious than fecal samples, whereas urine and semen samples are not infectious. Family members and persons recently in immediate contact with E.T. should be notified.[26]

The symptoms of acute viral hepatitis caused by HAV, HBV, HCV, HDV, and HEV are similar. The onset of symptoms in HAV infection, however, is less insidious than those seen with HBV and HCV infection.[5] Generally, symptoms of HAV infection present a week or more before the onset of jaundice. The likelihood of having symptoms is related to age. In children younger than 6 years of age, 70% of infections are asymptomatic, whereas older children and adults have symptomatic disease with jaundice occurring in more than 70% of cases.[18] E.T. has signs and symptoms of acute HAV infection, including the nonspecific prodromal symptoms of fatigue, weakness, anorexia, nausea, and vomiting. Abdominal pain and hepatomegaly are common. Less common symptoms include fever, headache, arthralgias, myalgias, and diarrhea. Within 1 to 2 weeks of the onset of prodromal symptoms, patients may enter an icteric phase with symptoms, including clay-colored stools, dark urine, scleral icterus, and jaundice. The dark urine is caused by bilirubin, generally occurring shortly before the onset of jaundice. E.T. should be questioned about the presence of pale stools (light gray or yellow), which usually is observed during the icteric phase. His scleral icterus is strongly suggestive of viral hepatitis. Icteric infections usually occur in adults and are 3.5 times more common than the nonicteric presentation that is seen in children.[16,26]

The results of E.T.'s liver function tests (e.g., elevations in AST, ALT, and total bilirubin) also are consistent with viral hepatitis. Serum transaminase concentrations increase during the prodromal phase (usually ALT > AST) of HAV infection, peaking before the onset of jaundice. These concentrations are often greater than 500 units/L and decline at an initial rate of 75%/week, followed by a slower rate of decline thereafter. Serum bilirubin peaks after aminotransferase activity and rarely exceeds 10 mg/dL. Total bilirubin levels decline more slowly than aminotransferases and generally normalize within 3 months. Right upper quadrant tenderness, mild liver enlargement, and splenomegaly may also be present in patients with acute HAV infection.[5,26]

Extrahepatic Manifestations

CASE 80-1, QUESTION 2: Are there any additional complications that E.T. could experience from his acute HAV infection?

With the appearance of jaundice, prodromal pruritus and extrahepatic manifestations can occur, usually in patients with a more protracted illness. E.T. should be monitored for additional manifestations of HAV infection, including immune complex-associated rash, leukocytoclastic vasculitis, glomerulonephritis, cryoglobulinemia (less likely than with HCV), and arthritis.[26]

Diagnosis and Serology

Diagnostic methods for detecting HAV antigen and anti-HAV are listed in Figure 80-1. Detection of IgM antibodies to HAV in a patient who presents with clinical characteristics of hepatitis, or in an asymptomatic patient with elevated transaminases, is consistent with acute HAV infection. HAV IgG appears after IgM and is indicative of previous exposure and immunity to HAV, whereas a rising IgG is consistent with recent exposure.[5,26] Anti-HAV IgM is commonly present throughout the disease course (16–40 weeks), usually peaking early and declining to undetectable levels 3 to 4 months after the initial infection.[26] One-quarter of patients infected with HAV have IgM present for up to 6 months and occasionally longer. HAV IgG appears early in the convalescent phase and is detectable for decades after the acute infection resolves, with a slowly declining titer.[16,26] Both enzyme-linked immunosorbent assay (ELISA) and radioimmunoassay methods of antibody detection are sensitive, specific, and reliable to diagnose acute HAV infection. E.T. has a positive IgM anti-HAV, consistent with acute HAV infection. He has a negative IgM anti-HBc test, ruling out acute HBV infection.[16,26]

Treatment

GENERAL MEASURES

HAV infection is usually a self-limiting disease and rarely leads to serious complications including fulminant liver failure and death.[27] Management involves supportive care and medical treatment of serious complications. Intravenous (IV) fluid and electrolyte replacement, nutritional support, and the use of antiemetics may be necessary for some patients. Antipyretics (acetaminophen) should not be used because the risk of fulminant hepatic failure (FHF) could increase. Considering that hemolysis or acute kidney injury is possible, a regular assessment of renal function with a complete blood count (CBC) should be performed. Patients should abstain from alcohol during the acute phase of the disease. After resolution of symptoms and serum biochemical abnormalities, moderate alcohol intake is no longer contraindicated. In general, prognosis after HAV infection is very good. Long-term immunity accompanies HAV infection, and recurrence or chronic hepatitis usually does not occur.

Adjustment of Medication Doses

CASE 80-1, QUESTION 3: Should E.T.'s medications be adjusted during the acute phase of HAV infection?

Dosage adjustments for hepatically eliminated drugs in the setting of liver disease are difficult to predict. This is because hepatic metabolism is complex, involving numerous oxidative and conjugative pathways that are variably affected in hepatic disease. In renal disease, creatinine serves as an endogenous marker to predict the clearance of renally eliminated drugs. In hepatic disease, however, no reliable endogenous markers exist to predict drug hepatic clearance. Laboratory tests that approximate the synthetic function of the liver (e.g., albumin, PT) and biliary clearance (bilirubin) are

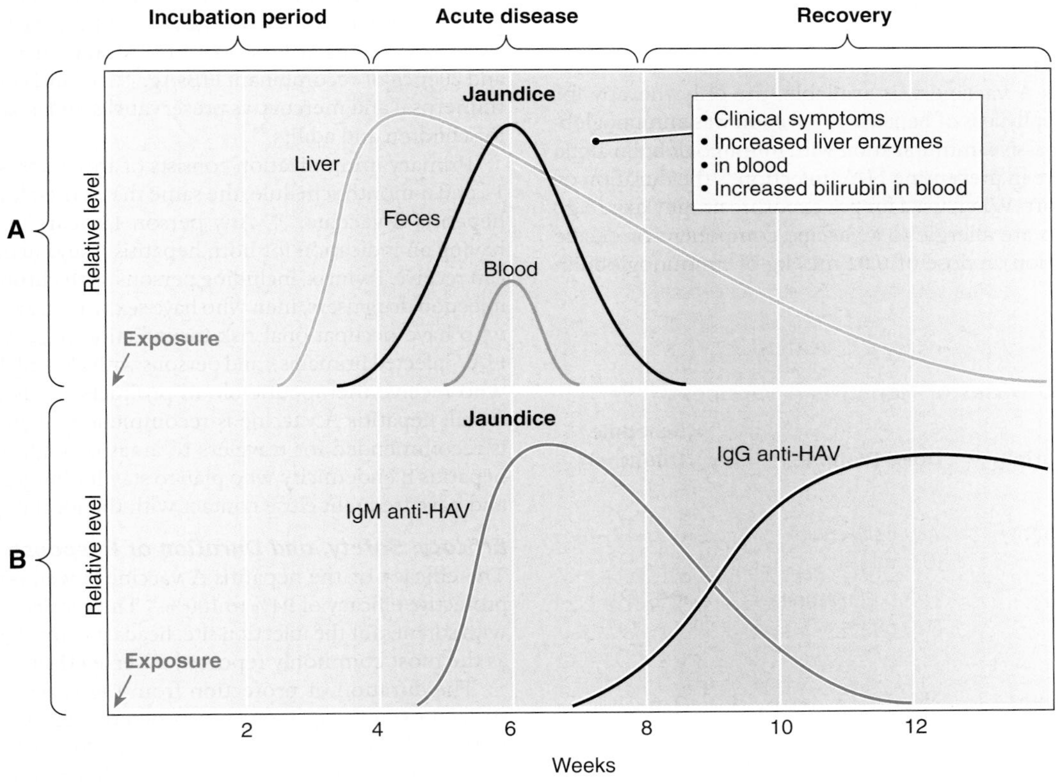

Figure 80-1 Typical course of hepatitis A. anti-HAV, antibody to HAV; HAV, hepatitis A virus. **A:** Presence of hepatitis A virus in liver, feces, and blood. **B:** Markers of hepatitis A virus in blood. (Adapted from McConnell TH, The *Nature of Disease Pathology for the Health Professions*. Philadelphia, PA: Lippincott Williams & Wilkins, 2007, with permission.)

used to estimate the degree of hepatic impairment, but these tests are not dependable in predicting alterations in pharmacokinetic parameters for hepatically metabolized drugs. Unnecessary and potentially hepatotoxic medications should be avoided during the acute phase of the illness. When drug therapy is indicated with agents that undergo hepatic elimination, it is prudent to use the lowest doses possible to achieve the desired therapeutic effect.

E.T. should be advised to discontinue diazepam because this medication undergoes extensive hepatic biotransformation and limited data suggest this agent accumulates in the setting of acute viral hepatitis.[28] If E.T. should require drug therapy for muscle spasms, he should either decrease the diazepam dose or consider using an alternative agent (e.g., lorazepam) that does not accumulate in acute viral hepatitis.[29] Patients with acute viral hepatitis do not require phenytoin dosage adjustments.[30] Because E.T.'s plasma phenytoin concentration is within the desired therapeutic range, no dosage adjustment is needed.

Prevention of Hepatitis A

Prevention of hepatitis A infection can be achieved through immunoprophylactic measures. Immunoprophylaxis may be passive, active, or a combination of both. In passive immunization, temporary protective antibody in the form of immunoglobulin is administered. In active immunization, a vaccine is administered to induce the formation of protective antibody.[20,31] Prophylaxis can be administered before (pre-exposure prophylaxis) or after exposure (post-exposure prophylaxis).

Pre-Exposure Prophylaxis

CASE 80-2

Question 1: M.D., a 22-year-old student, is preparing for a 2-week vacation to Thailand. He plans to travel 3 months from now and wonders whether he should receive prophylaxis for HAV.

Immunoglobulin

Before hepatitis A vaccine was available, the only therapy for pre-exposure prophylaxis of hepatitis A infection was immunoglobulin. Although passive immunization with immunoglobulin alone is highly effective in preventing HAV infection,[20] the duration of protection is short. When used for pre-exposure prophylaxis (e.g., in travelers who are allergic to a vaccine component or decide against vaccination), a dose of 0.02 mL/kg of immunoglobulin administered intramuscularly (IM) confers protection for less than 3 months, and an IM dose of 0.06 mL/kg confers protection for 5 months or longer.[19,20,26]

Table 80-2
Recommended Doses of Hepatitis A Vaccines[27,31,32]

Age at Vaccination	Dose (Volume)^a	Schedule (Months)^b
Havrix		
Children 12 months–18 years	720 ELISA units (0.5 mL)	0, 6–12
Adults >19 years	1,440 ELISA units (1.0 mL)	0, 6–12
Vaqta		
Children 12 months–18 years	25 units (0.5 mL)	0, 6–18
Adults >19 years	50 units (1.0 mL)	0, 6

^{a}Enzyme-linked immunosorbent assay (ELISA) units.
^{b}Zero months represent timing of the initial dose; subsequent numbers represent months after the initial dose.

Vaccine

Active immunization with hepatitis A vaccine has largely supplanted the use of immunoglobulin for pre-exposure prophylaxis of infection caused by HAV. Two types of the inactivated, monovalent hepatitis A vaccines are available in the United States and globally: Havrix and Vaqta. Both vaccines are formalin-inactivated preparations of attenuated HAV strains.[32] The manufacturers use differing units to express antigen content of their respective vaccines. Havrix dosages are expressed in ELISA units, and Vaqta dosages are expressed as units of hepatitis A antigen. These vaccines are developed to provide long-term immunity. They are free of thimerosal and mercury as preservatives and are safe and effective for children and adults.[33]

Dosing Regimen

Havrix is available in two formulations that differ according to age: for persons 12 months to 18 years of age, 720 ELISA units (0.5 mL)/dose in a two-dose schedule; and for persons 19 years and older, 1,440 ELISA units (1.0 mL)/dose in a two-dose schedule (Table 80-2).[27,31,32] Havrix is injected IM into the deltoid muscle with a booster dose administered 6 to 12 months later. The pediatric Havrix formulation (three-dose schedule) is no longer available. Vaqta is available in two formulations that differ according to the person's age: for persons 12 months to 18 years of age, 25 units (0.5 mL) in a two-dose schedule; and for persons 19 years and older, 50 units (1.0 mL) per dose in a two-dose schedule (Table 80-2).[27,31,32] Likewise, this vaccine is injected IM into the deltoid muscle with a booster dose administered 6 to 18 months later.[20,31,32]

Combination Vaccine

The US Food and Drug Administration (FDA) has also licensed a combined HAV and HBV vaccine (Twinrix) for use in persons aged 18 years and older. Twinrix is composed of the same antigenic components used in Havrix and Engerix-B. Each dose of Twinrix contains at least 720 ELISA units of inactivated HAV and 20 mcg of recombinant HBsAg.[34,35] Twinrix does not contain thimerosal and mercury as preservatives and is safe and effective for children and adults.[33]

Primary immunization consists of three doses, given on a 0-, 1-, and 6-month schedule, the same that is used for single-antigen hepatitis B vaccine.[34,35] Any person 18 years of age and older having an indication for both hepatitis A and hepatitis B vaccine can receive Twinrix, including persons with chronic liver disease, injection drug users, men who have sex with men (MSM), persons who have occupational risk for infection (e.g., who work with HAV-infected primates), and persons with clotting factor disorders who receive therapeutic blood products.[34,35] For international travel, hepatitis A vaccine is recommended; hepatitis B vaccine is recommended for travelers to areas of high or intermediate hepatitis B endemicity who plan to stay for longer than 6 months and have frequent close contact with the local population.[36]

Efficacy, Safety, and Duration of Response

The efficacy of the hepatitis A vaccine is well established, with protective efficacy of 94% to 100%.[34] The vaccine is well tolerated, with soreness at the injection site, headache, myalgias, and malaise as the most commonly reported adverse effects.

The duration of protection from the vaccines has not been studied extensively. However, protective levels of antibody to HAV could be present for at least 14 to 20 years in children and at least 25 years in adults.[32,34] The ACIP has no recommendations regarding the need for booster doses at this time. The safety of HAV vaccine during pregnancy has not been established. However, because the vaccine is produced from inactivated HAV, the theoretic risk to the developing fetus is low. The benefits versus risks associated with vaccination for HAV in women who might be at high risk for exposure to the infection should be discussed with her primary care physician and obstetrician.[19]

Indications

The ACIP recommends hepatitis A vaccination for several high-risk groups, including travelers to countries with high endemicity of infection (South and Central America, Africa, South and Southeast Asia, Caribbean, and the Middle East),[37–39] travelers to countries with intermediate endemicity of infection (Eastern and Southern Europe and the former Soviet Union), children living in communities with high rates of hepatitis A infection and periodic hepatitis A outbreaks (Alaskan Native villages, American Indian reservations), MSM, injection drug users, researchers or persons who have occupational risk for hepatitis A (healthcare workers), persons with clotting factor disorders, and persons with chronic liver disease who are at increased risk for fulminant hepatitis A.[20,27,31,32] Thus, M.D. should receive either Havrix 1,440 ELISA units or Vaqta 50 units. This initial injection will provide adequate protection from HAV infection during his travel, and he can receive the booster injection on his return, at least 6 months after the first injection. If M.D. decides to travel within the next 2 weeks, he should receive both vaccination and immunoglobulin before departure.[36]

POSTEXPOSURE PROPHYLAXIS

CASE 80-3

QUESTION 1: L.W., a 26-year-old man, recently was diagnosed with HAV infection. He attends college and works part-time as a retail clerk. He lives with his healthy, 25-year-old wife and 10-month-old infant daughter. Which of L.W.'s contacts require postexposure prophylaxis for HAV?

Although immune globulin has been recommended in the past for unvaccinated people recently exposed to HAV, hepatitis A vaccines (Havrix and Vaqta) are effective in preventing secondary HAV infection in healthy people. Twinrix is not recommended for postexposure prophylaxis.[19] A vaccine can be administered in healthy people age 12 months to 40 years within 2 weeks after exposure to HAV.[31,36] However, at this time, individuals outside of this age range or with significant comorbid conditions should receive immune globulin instead of the vaccine. Therefore, L.W.'s wife should receive prophylactic administration of HAV vaccine and his 10-month-old infected daughter should receive immune globulin at a dose of 0.02 mL/kg, administered IM as soon as possible but no later than 2 weeks after exposure. Contacts who have received a dose of hepatitis A vaccine at least 1 month before exposure do not need immune globulin, because protective antibody titers are achieved in greater than 95% of patients 1 month after vaccination.[20] Prophylaxis is not recommended for casual contacts at work or school.

Administration of immune globulin within 2 weeks after exposure to HAV is 80% to 90% effective in preventing acute HAV infection.[20,26] In most cases, when given early, immune globulin prevents both clinical and subclinical HAV illness. Protection after immune globulin administration is immediate and complete, but short-lived. Other situations in which immune globulin administration may be indicated include hepatitis A infection in day-care centers and in settings with infected persons who prepare and serve food. Immune globulin is recommended for all staff and children in day-care settings when a case of HAV infection is diagnosed among employees or attendees.[15,19,20] When a food handler is diagnosed with hepatitis A, immune globulin is recommended for other food handlers at the same location. Given the improbability of disease transmission to persons consuming food prepared or served by workers infected with hepatitis A, the routine administration of immune globulin in this setting is not recommended.[15,20]

When immune globulin is required for infants or pregnant women, preparations free of thimerosal should be used.[15] Although immune globulin does not impede the immune response to inactivated vaccines, oral poliovirus vaccine, or yellow fever vaccine, it may interfere with the response to live attenuated vaccines such as measles, mumps, rubella (MMR) vaccine and varicella vaccine. Therefore, MMR and varicella vaccines should be delayed for at least 3 months after administration of immune globulin for HAV prophylaxis. Immune globulin should not be given within 2 weeks after the administration of MMR or varicella vaccine. Finally, if immune globulin is administered within 2 weeks of MMR, the person requires revaccination, but not sooner than 3 months after the immune globulin administration for MMR.[15,19,20] Serologic tests for varicella vaccination should be performed 3 months after immune globulin administration to determine whether revaccination is required.

HEPATITIS B VIRUS

Virology

Hepatitis B virus is an icosahedral, enveloped, and encapsulated virus measuring 42 nm diameter and belongs to the Hepadnaviridae family of viruses.[40–43] The viral genome is a partially double-stranded, circular DNA linked to a DNA polymerase. Unlike HAV, HBV is antigenically complex and results in an acute illness with or without a chronic disease state. HBV infection can produce either asymptomatic or symptomatic infection. The average incubation period is 90 days (range: 60–150 days) from exposure to the onset of jaundice and 60 days (range: 40–90 days) from exposure to onset of abnormal serum ALT levels.[42–43]

The life cycle of HBV is described in Figure 80-2. Elucidation of the HBV life cycle has resulted in opportunities for drug development. Of special importance, the viral DNA polymerase functions as both a reverse transcriptase (RT) for synthesis of the negative DNA strand from genomic RNA and as an endogenous DNA polymerase. Because the HBV polymerase is remotely related to the RT enzymes of retroviruses (e.g., HIV), some inhibitors of HIV polymerase or RT also have activity against the HBV polymerase. Thus, several RT inhibitors have been evaluated for treating and preventing HBV; however, rapid emergence of resistance occurs with many of these agents.

Epidemiology

Globally, approximately 2 billion persons are infected with HBV, and between 350 and 400 million persons are living with chronic HBV infection.[44,45] HBV disease causes approximately 1 million deaths from cirrhosis, liver failure, and hepatocellular carcinoma (HCC).[46–48] In 2002, more than 600,000 persons died of HBV-associated acute and chronic liver disease.[44,45] In the United States, HBV infection affects an estimated 2.2 million persons and accounts for an estimated 5,500 deaths annually.[47,48]

Acute HBV infection is usually asymptomatic in infants and children aged less than 5 years compared to 30% to 50% of children older than 5 years and adults who could develop clinical signs and symptoms.[49] Clinical signs and symptoms can include anorexia, nausea, vomiting, abdominal pain, malaise and jaundice. Extrahepatic manifestations of HBV disease may include skin rashes, arthralgias, and arthritis.[50] Approximately 95% of primary infections in immunocompetent adults are self-limiting, with elimination of the virus from blood and subsequent lasting immunity to

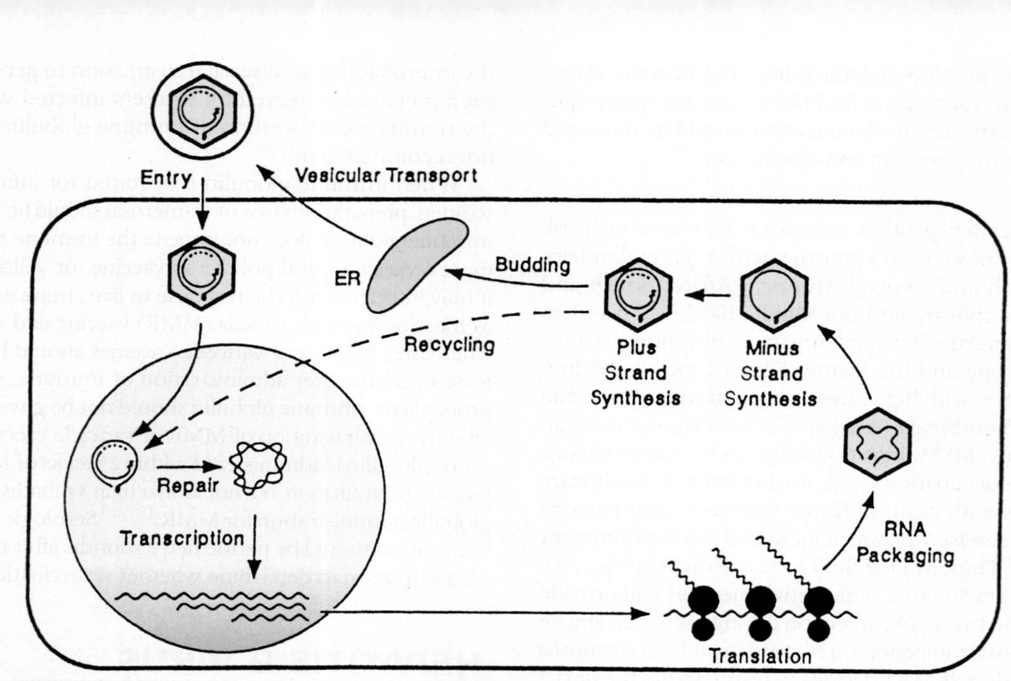

Figure 80-2 Life cycle of hepatitis B virus. ER, endoplasmic reticulum. (Reprinted from Ganem D. Hepadnaviridae: the viruses and their replication. In: Fields BN, ed. *Fundamental Virology*. 3rd ed. Philadelphia, PA: Lippincott-Raven; 1996:1199, with permission.)

reinfection. Progression from acute to chronic HBV infection is influenced by the person's age at acquisition of the virus. Chronic HBV infection occurs in approximately 30% of infected children younger than 5 years old, and less than 5% of infected persons older than 5 years.[49] Persons who are HBV infected and are at risk for developing chronic HBV disease include immunosuppressed persons (e.g., persons with diabetes, HIV, or on hemodialysis).[50]

With respect to HBV infection in certain parts of the world, HBV infection is acquired perinatally in Asia. The cellular immune responses to hepatocyte-membrane HBV proteins that are associated with acute hepatitis do not occur, and chronic, lifelong infection is established in more than 90% of persons infected in Asia.[51] On the other hand, most acute HBV infections that occur in the West are reported during adolescence and early adulthood because of behaviors and environments that favor the transmission of bloodborne infections, such as sexual activity, injection drug use, and occupational exposure. There are no specific treatment for acute HBV, and supportive care is the mainstay of therapy.[51,52]

Similar to HAV infection, chronic HBV infection is defined as persons positive for HBsAg for >6 months (Fig. 80-3). The incidence of acute HBV infection has declined in the United States by approximately 82% since 1991.[45,52–54] This reduction of infection occurs in all age, racial, ethnic, and high-risk groups, particularly among children and healthcare workers—the groups with the highest rate of vaccination. Less high-risk behaviors also have led to decreased transmission of infection. High-risk groups in the United States for acquiring HBV infection include certain ethnic groups (e.g., Alaskan Eskimos, Asian Pacific Islanders), first-generation immigrants from regions of high endemicity (e.g., India, Central and Southeast Asia), injection drug users, MSM, African-Americans, and males (more than females).[52–54] The most prominent risk factors associated with acute HBV infection include heterosexual contact (42%), MSM (15%), and injection drug use (21%).[52–54] HBV vaccination opportunities include clinics for sexually transmitted disease (STD), correctional facilities, and holding centers for incarceration.

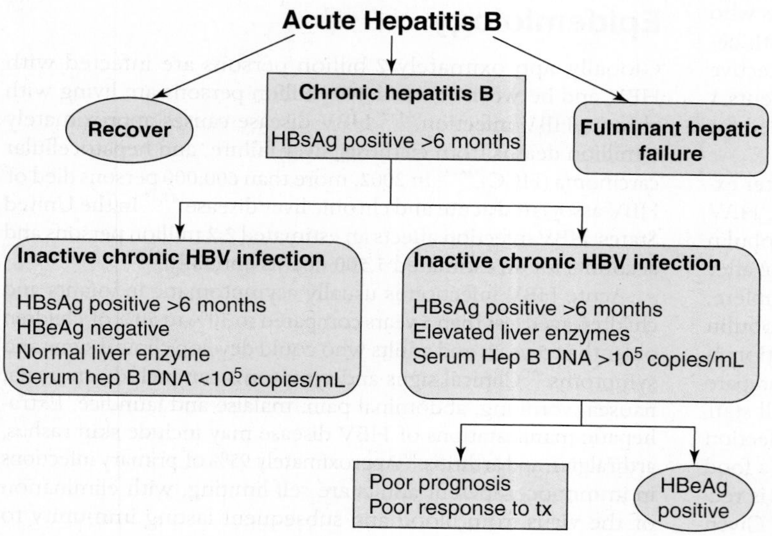

Figure 80-3 Acute hepatitis B virus infection. (Source: AASLD/IDSA Guidelines.)

Transmission

The transmission of HBV is from exposure to blood, semen, and other body fluids infected with HBV. Furthermore, HBV transmission could occur among unvaccinated adults with risky behaviors, including sexual contact, and percutaneous or perinatal exposure to infectious blood or body fluids. HBV is highly concentrated in serum with lower concentrations in semen and saliva.[49] The modes of HBV transmission include sexual, blood transfusion, perinatal transmission, and injection drug use are summarized in the following sections.

SEXUAL TRANSMISSION

Sexual activity, especially unprotected sex and having multiple sex partners, is the most significant mode of HBV transmission worldwide, including North America, where the prevalence of infection is low.[52–54] Heterosexual intercourse accounts for the majority of US infections (26%). In heterosexual persons, factors associated with an enhanced risk of HBV infection include duration of sexual activity, number of sexual partners, and history of STD. Sexual partners of injection drug users, sex workers, and clients of sex workers are at a very high risk for infection. Sexual partners of infected individuals are at high risk for infection, even in the absence of high-risk behavior. Because most patients with chronic HBV infection are unaware of their infection and are "silent carriers," sexual transmission is a significant mode of transmission. Many of the HBV infections could have been prevented through universal vaccination. The use of condoms appears to reduce the risk of sexual transmission.[52–54]

From 1980 to 1985, a very high rate of HBV infection was observed in MSM, accounting for 20% of all reported cases of infection.[52–54] Multiple sexual partners, anal-receptive intercourse, and duration of sexual activity were the most common factors associated with HBV acquisition in the MSM population. Current rates of HBV infection in this population have fallen and are estimated to be about 8%, possibly as a result of modifications of sexual behavior in response to HIV. Similar to heterosexuals, the use of condoms in this population has reduced the risk of sexual transmission.

BLOOD AND BLOOD PRODUCTS

Although the risk of transfusion-associated HBV infection has been greatly reduced with the screening of blood (tests for HBsAg and anti-HBc) and the exclusion of donors who engage in high-risk activities, it is estimated that 1 of 50,000 transfused units could transmit HBV infection.[52–54]

PERINATAL TRANSMISSION

Early-childhood exposure and perinatal exposure are additional modes of transmission of HBV infection. High serum concentrations of virus have been linked with increased risk of transmission by vertical routes (and needlestick exposure). Infants born to HBeAg-positive mothers with high viral replication (>80 pg/mL) have a 70% to 90% risk of perinatal HBV acquisition compared with a 10% to 40% risk in infants born to mothers infected with HBV who are HBeAg-negative.[52–54] Infection generally occurs via inoculation of the infant at the time of birth or soon thereafter, and even with active and passive immunization, 10% to 15% of babies acquire HBV infection at birth.

In developing countries with high prevalence rates and in regions of the United States with high endemicity, children born to HBsAg-positive mothers with HBV are at risk for acquiring HBV infection in the perinatal period, with infection rates reported to be between 7% and 13%.[48–50] In addition, children of HBsAg-positive mothers who are not infected at birth remain at very high risk of early-childhood infection, with 60% of those born to HBsAg-positive mothers becoming infected by the age of 5 years. The mechanism of the later infection, which is neither perinatal nor sexual, is not known however. Although HBsAg is detectable in breast milk, breast-feeding is not believed to be a primary mode of HBV transmission.

INJECTION DRUG USE

Recreational and illicit drug use in the United States and globally is a significant mode of HBV transmission, accounting for approximately 23% of all patients.[52–54] The risk increases with the duration of injection drug use; thus, serologic markers of ongoing or prior HBV infection are usually positive after 5 years of drug use.

OTHER MODES OF TRANSMISSION

Other risk factors for transmission of HBV include working in a healthcare setting, receiving blood transfusion (not properly screened) and dialysis, receiving acupuncture and tattoos from contaminated needles, traveling to regions of the world endemic for HBV infection, and living in correctional facilities or prisons.[52–54] Sporadic cases of HBV transmission have been attributed to nonpercutaneous transmission by way of small breaks in the skin, biting, or mucous membranes. Although HBsAg is found in bodily fluids (e.g., saliva, tears, sweat, semen, vaginal secretions, breast milk, cerebrospinal fluid, ascites, pleural fluid, synovial fluid, gastric juice, and urine), only semen, saliva, and serum actually contain infectious HBV.[55–58]

Pathogenesis

Similar to HAV infection, clinical observations suggest that host immune responses are more important than virologic factors in the pathogenesis of liver injury. Host cellular and humoral immune responses are linked to T lymphocytes, which enhance viral clearance from hepatocytes and cause liver injury.[55,56]

Diagnosis

The presence of HBsAg in serum is diagnostic for HBV infection. In 5% to 10% of acute cases in which the HBsAg levels fall below sensitivity thresholds of current assays, the presence of IgM anti-HBc in serum confirms a recent acute HBV infection. Another highly reliable marker of active HBV replication and diagnosis is the presence of HBV DNA in serum through qualitative or quantitative assays, detectable early during the course of acute HBV infection.[57–59] Persistent levels of HBV DNA indicate ongoing infection and a high degree of active viral replication and infectivity.

Serology

Antigens and antibodies associated with HBV infection include HBsAg and antibody to HBsAg (anti-HBs), hepatitis B core antigen (HBcAg), antibody to HBcAg (anti-HBc), hepatitis B e antigen (HBeAg), and antibody to HBeAg (anti-HBe). The serologic markers that differentiate between acute, resolving, and chronic infection are HBsAg, anti-HBc, and anti-HBs. HBeAg and anti-HBe screening are used for the management of patients with chronic infection.[49] Serologic patterns, general definitions, and diagnostic criteria of HBV infection are depicted in Table 80-3. Within the first several weeks after exposure (range: 2–10 weeks), HBsAg appears in the blood and is present for several weeks before serum concentrations of aminotransferases increase and symptoms (Fig. 80-4).[57–58] Clinical illness usually follows HBV exposure by 1 to 3 months. HBsAg can be detected in serum until the clinical illness resolves and usually becomes undetectable after 4 to 6 months. Persistence

TABLE 80-3
Hepatitis B Virus: Laboratory Markers and Interpretations[55,56]

Laboratory Marker	Interpretation
Hepatitis B surface antigen (HBsAg)	Marker of infection; presence indicates person is infectious
Hepatitis B surface antibody (anti-HBs)	Past infection, or person has been vaccinated
Hepatitis B core antibody (anti-HBc)	Marker of previous or ongoing infection
IgM antibody to Hepatitis B core antigen (IgM anti-HBc)	Indicates acute infection; first reaction of the body's immune response to HBV
Hepatitis B e antigen (HBeAg)	Marker of active replication of virus and infectiveness
Hepatitis B e antibody (HBeAb or anti-HBe)	Virus is no longer replicating; predictor of long-term clearance of HBV in patients undergoing antiviral therapy
Hepatitis B virus DNA (HBV-DNA)	Indicates active replication of virus; more accurate than HBeAg; used mainly for monitoring response to therapy

of HBsAg beyond 6 months implies progression to chronic HBV infection. The antibody to HBsAg (anti-HBs) often appears after a short "window" period during which neither HBsAg nor anti-HBs are detectable. In most patients, anti-HBs persists for years after HBV infection, conferring immunity to reinfection (see Fig. 80-4).

Interpretation of serologic markers is described in Table 80-4. A soluble viral protein, HBeAg, is detectable early during the acute phase of the disease and persists in chronic hepatitis B infection. HBeAg is a marker of active HBV replication, and its presence correlates with circulating HBV particles. The presence of both HBeAg and HBsAg indicates high levels of viral replication and infectivity and a need for antiviral therapy. Generally, seroconversion

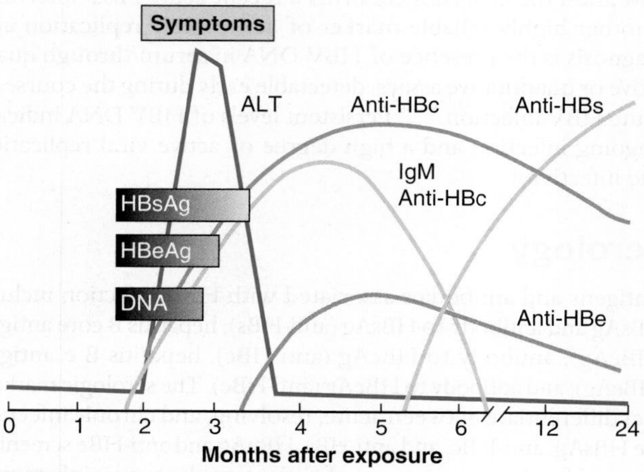

Figure 80-4 Sequence of events after acute hepatitis B virus infection with resolution. ALT, alanine aminotransferase; anti-HBc, hepatitis B core antibody; anti-HBe, hepatitis B envelope antibody; anti-HBs, hepatitis B surface antibody; HBeAg, hepatitis B envelope antigen; HBsAg, hepatitis B surface antigen; HBV DNA; hepatitis B virus DNA; IgM anti-HBc, immunoglobulin M antibody to hepatitis B core virus. (Adapted from Perrillo RP, Regenstein FG. Viral and immune hepatitis. In Kelley WN, ed. *Textbook of Internal Medicine*. 3rd ed. Philadelphia, PA: J.B. Lippincott; 1996, with permission.

TABLE 80-4
Hepatitis B Virus: Interpretation of Laboratory Results[45]

Laboratory Markers	Laboratory Results	Clinical Interpretation
HBsAg anti-HBc anti-HBs	Negative Negative Negative	Susceptible
HBsAg anti-HBc anti-HBs	Negative Positive Positive	Immune due to natural infection
HBsAg anti-HBc anti-HBs	Negative Negative Positive	Immune due to hepatitis B vaccination
HBsAg anti-HBc IgM anti-HBc anti-HBs	Positive Positive Positive Negative	Acute infection
HBsAg anti-HBc anti-HBs	Negative Positive Negative	Interpretation unclear; 4 possibilities: 1. Resolved infection (most common) 2. False-positive anti-HBc, thus susceptible 3. "Low-level" chronic infection 4. Resolving acute infection

from HBeAg to hepatitis B envelope antibody (anti-HBe) results in a reduction in HBV DNA and suggests resolution of HBV infection. Some patients may, however, continue to have active liver disease and detectable serum HBV DNA levels as a result of the presence of wild-type virus or the presence of precore or promoter mutations that impair HBeAg secretion (HBeAg-negative patients).

Hepatitis B core antigen does not circulate freely in the bloodstream and is not measured. Anti-HBc, the antibody directed against hepatitis B core antigen, is usually detected 1 to 2 weeks after the appearance of HBsAg and just before the onset of clinical symptoms, and it persists for life. The detection of IgM anti-HBc is the most sensitive diagnostic test for acute HBV infection. During the recovery phase of infection, the predominant form of anti-HBc is in the IgG class. The presence of this antibody suggests prior or ongoing infection with HBV. Furthermore, in areas where HBV is not endemic, isolated detection of anti-HBc in a patient's serum may correlate with low levels of HBV DNA. The presence of HBV DNA may enhance the risk of transmission of HBV and progression to cirrhosis and HCC. Patients immunized against HBV do not develop anti-HBc; therefore, the presence of this antibody differentiates successful vaccination from actual HBV infection.

Natural History

Of those patients with acute HBV infection, only 1% develop FHF with associated coagulopathy, encephalopathy, and cerebral edema.[60,61] The cause of fulminant infection is a heightened immune response to the virus, in the absence of HDV or HCV coinfections. Patients with ALF often have early clearance of HBsAg, which may complicate the diagnosis, but a positive IgM antibody to hepatitis B core antigen generally confirms the diagnosis.

Four phases of HBV infection are present: immune tolerance, immune clearance, low-level replication or nonreplication phase (inactive carrier), and reactivation phase. Up to 12% (average 5%) of immunocompetent patients acutely infected with HBV remain chronically infected (historically defined as detectable HBsAg in serum for 6 months or longer).[59,60] In these patients, HBsAg generally remains detectable indefinitely and anti-HBs fails to appear. The risk of chronicity after neonatally acquired infection is high (>90%), possibly because neonates have immature immune systems. Of infected neonates, 50% have evidence of active viral replication. Furthermore, patients who have a reduced ability to clear viral infections—including those receiving chronic hemodialysis, immunosuppression after transplantation, or chemotherapy, or patients with HIV infection—may have a greater risk for developing chronic HBV infection.[40,62] Ultimate outcomes are linked with the presence or absence of viral replication and by the severity of liver damage. Approximately 50% of all chronic carriers have ongoing viral replication, especially with elevated aminotransferases, and 15% to 20% of these develop cirrhosis within 5 years.[40–43,62] Spontaneous loss of HBeAg (7%–20%/year) has been reported, possibly as a result of the use of antiviral therapy, whereas loss of HBsAg occurs less frequently (1%–2%/year). In general, chronic carriers remain infected throughout their life.[40–43,62] Five-year survival rates decline depending on the severity of disease (55% survival with cirrhosis).[62] Asymptomatic HBV carriers tend to have mild disease manifestations with few complications, even with a long period of follow-up. Finally, the risk of HCC is increased up to 300 times in chronic carriers with active viral replication (HBeAg positive).[62,63]

Clinical Manifestations

CASE 80-4

QUESTION 1: W.H. is a 35-year-old man who developed nausea, vomiting, anorexia, scleral icterus, and jaundice within the past month. Within the past week he became increasingly lethargic, confused, and disoriented, and lapsed into a grade IV coma. He is admitted to the ED, intubated, and transferred to the intensive care unit.

W.H.'s social history is significant for IV drug use for the past 10 years and alcohol abuse (none for the previous 5 years). Physical findings include an older-than-age-appearing, hypertensive (blood pressure, 158/99 mm Hg), bradycardic (heart rate, 58 beats/minute) man in respiratory distress (respiratory rate, 26 breaths/minute) with severe jaundice, scleral icterus, and decreased hepatic dullness to percussion (reduced hepatic mass). He shows sluggish pupillary response and increasing muscle tone; neurologic examination reveals him to be stuporous and nonarousable.

The laboratory evaluation shows the following results:

Hct: 42%
Hgb: 14 g/dL
Platelets: 85,000/μL
PT: 25.8 seconds
International normalized ratio (INR): 3.8
AST: 555 units/L
ALT: 495 units/L
Alkaline phosphatase: 101 units/mL
Total bilirubin: 8.4 mg/dL
HBV DNA: 6,000,000 IU/mL

Hepatitis serologic tests are positive for HBsAg, HBeAg, IgM anti-HBc, and HBV DNA. IgM anti-HAV, IgM anti-HDV, and anti-HCV are negative. STAT blood gases reveal a metabolic acidosis with a compensatory respiratory alkalosis. W.H.'s serum creatinine is 1.8 mg/dL with a recent reduction in urine output.

What clinical findings does W.H. have that support the diagnosis of acute hepatitis and ALF?

The clinical features of acute HBV infection are similar to those described for HAV infection. W.H.'s initial symptoms included a recent history of nausea, vomiting, anorexia, scleral icterus, and jaundice. These are consistent with diagnosis of acute hepatitis B. His serologies, notably a positive IgM anti-HBc and HBV DNA, also support this diagnosis.

ACUTE LIVER FAILURE

The most significant complication of acute HBV infection is ALF, widely defined as a coagulation abnormality (INR >1.5) and any degree of mental alteration (encephalopathy) in a patient of less than 26 weeks' duration.[61,64] He has hepatic encephalopathy, lethargy, confusion, coma, coagulopathy, hemodynamic instability, declining liver function, and acidosis. Patients with ALF often have cerebral edema (80% mortality rate), a complication of a disrupted blood–brain barrier that allows protein-rich fluid to cross into the extracellular spaces of the brain tissue leading to edema and increased intracranial pressure (ICP) or intracranial hypertension (vasogenic model). Clinical symptoms (sluggish pupillary response and increasing muscle tone) develop when the ICP is greater than 30 mm Hg.[61,65–67] Cerebral edema in the confinement of the cranial vault raises the ICP, which may reduce intracerebral perfusion. The edema can result in cerebral ischemia if the cerebral perfusion pressure (systemic blood pressure minus ICP) is not maintained at greater than 40 mm Hg. Of note, intracranial hypertension in ALF is related to the severity of encephalopathy. Cerebral edema is rarely reported in patients with grade I or II encephalopathy but occurs in up to 75% of patients with grade IV coma.[68] Diagnostic head imaging tests (computerized tomography), elevation of the head of the bed, and intubation (and subsequent hyperventilation) may be necessary medical interventions in this setting.

W.H. has symptoms of cerebral edema and may benefit from 100 to 200 mL of a 20% solution of mannitol (0.5–1.0 g/kg) administered by rapid IV infusion to induce an osmotic diuresis with a subsequent decrease in ICP. The dose may be repeated at least once after several hours provided serum osmolality has not exceeded 320 mOsm/L.[67,68] Because W.H. also has a blood pressure of 158/99 mm Hg and a heart rate of 58 beats/minute, and is at risk for intracranial hemorrhage, an ICP monitoring device should be placed.[67,68] Although placement of this device is invasive and bleeding is a potential complication, ICP monitoring devices provide important prognostic information. Patients with a cerebral perfusion pressure of greater than 40 mm Hg that is refractory to mannitol therapy are not candidates for liver transplantation. W.H. also has a coagulopathy typical of ALF. Decreased levels of clotting factors II, V, VII, IX, and X normally synthesized by the liver account for his prolonged PT and elevated INR.[64–66] Recombinant activated factor VII has been used selectively in patients with ALF, but is usually reserved for administration before any invasive procedures. In addition, consumption of clotting factors by low-grade disseminated intravascular coagulation is common in ALF. W.H. is also thrombocytopenic and at risk for GI ulceration.[68,69] A platelet transfusion should be considered if his counts drop to less than 10,000/μL. Because he is not actively bleeding, fresh-frozen plasma is not indicated at this time.[68,69]

W.H. also should be monitored for cardiovascular and renal abnormalities as a result of his ALF.[64,67] Although W.H. is hypertensive, most patients with ALF are hypotensive and hypovolemic and present with interstitial edema owing to low levels of oncotic proteins. Functional renal failure, also known as hepatorenal syndrome or acute tubular necrosis, occurs in 43% to 55% of patients with ALF.[69,70] In hepatorenal syndrome, renal blood flow is reduced, renin and aldosterone levels are increased, and levels of atrial natriuretic factor are unchanged.[70]

As seen in W.H., patients may develop acid–base disturbances, including respiratory alkalosis as a result of central nervous system-mediated hyperventilation or a lactic acid-induced metabolic acidosis.[66,69] Hyponatremia, hypokalemia, hypocalcemia, hypomagnesemia, hypoglycemia, seizures, infections (bacterial or fungal), and pancreatitis are additional findings associated with ALF. Thus, sodium, potassium, calcium, magnesium, blood glucose, and amylase should be monitored closely in W.H.[66,69] Prophylactic antimicrobial therapy reduces the incidence of infections in selected groups of ALF patients, but no survival benefit has been demonstrated.[66,69] Therefore, if antibiotics are not initiated, surveillance for infection (via chest radiography and blood, urine, and sputum cultures) should be undertaken while having a low threshold for initiating appropriate antibacterial or antifungal therapy. Finally, pulmonary complications (hypoxemia, aspiration, adult respiratory distress syndrome, and pulmonary edema) may also occur in patients with ALF.[69,70]

PROGNOSIS

CASE 80-4, QUESTION 2: What is W.H.'s prognosis?

Although the incidence of ALF is less than 1%, the prognosis for these patients is poor once encephalopathy has developed.[70,71] Survival depends on the etiology and degree of hepatic destruction, the ability of the remaining liver cells to regenerate, and the management of complications that may develop during the course of illness. Survival rates often depend on the etiology of ALF. Non-A, non-B (NANB) hepatitis and halothane or drug hepatotoxicity have been associated with worse survivals compared with those with hepatitis A, hepatitis B, or acetaminophen overdose.[71] Age younger than 14 years, worsening grade of encephalopathy, reduced liver size, and significantly abnormal LFT values (e.g., serum bilirubin, aminotransferases, alkaline phosphatase, PT, and serum albumin) are also poor prognostic indicators in patients with ALF.[70,71] Because W.H. has evidence of encephalopathy, cerebral edema, and abnormal LFT values, he has a poor prognosis.

TREATMENT

CASE 80-4, QUESTION 3: Outline an appropriate treatment plan for W.H.'s ALF.

The primary therapy for ALF is supportive care for the comatose patient. Systemic therapies with heparin, prostaglandin, or insulin and glucagon have shown limited efficacy.[66] Blood or plasma exchange, hemodialysis, or other methods implemented to detoxify the blood or improve the coma grade do not result in long-term benefits if liver mass is not reconstituted as well. Thiopental may be useful in lowering ICP, but corticosteroids and prolonged hyperventilation are of no value.[66,69] W.H. could benefit from prophylactic histamine H_2-blockers because they have been shown to reduce the incidence of upper GI hemorrhage.[66] The role of proton-pump inhibitors has not been clearly defined, although limited data have also supported their role in this setting. Blood products (packed red blood cells, fresh-frozen plasma, or platelets) should be given as needed if W.H. develops active bleeding, and pulmonary artery monitoring should be implemented to guide management of intravascular volume and gas exchange. W.H. should be closely monitored for additional complications, especially cardiac abnormalities (arrhythmias), hemodynamic changes, renal failure, acidosis, pulmonary complications, and sepsis.

In cases in which prognostic information indicates less than 20% chance of survival without transplantation, liver transplantation is indicated. In patients with acetaminophen poisoning resulting in ALF, a pH less than 7.3, a PT longer than 100 seconds, and a serum creatinine greater than 3.4 mg/dL, with grade III or IV encephalopathy, usually require transplantation.[71] Other causes of ALF, a PT longer than 50 seconds, or any three of the following variables (irrespective of grade of encephalopathy)—age younger than 10 years or older than 40 years; liver failure caused by NANB hepatitis, halothane-induced hepatitis, or idiosyncratic drug reactions; duration of jaundice before encephalopathy more than 7 days; or serum bilirubin greater than 17.5 mg/dL—indicate a need for transplantation.[70,71] Although these criteria continue to be used worldwide, they are less reliable in patients with moderate illness; sensitivity is acceptable although specificity is poor. Therefore, other models and surrogate markers have emerged to predict survival, such as the model for end-stage liver disease, Acute Physiology and Chronic Health Evaluation II scoring system, and biomarkers such as Gc protein (also known as vitamin D_3-binding protein), α-fetoprotein, or troponin.[71] To date, none of these methods have been flawless in their ability to accurately predict outcome in ALF.

Coinfection with Human Immunodeficiency Virus (HIV)

CASE 80-4, QUESTION 4: What is the likelihood for HIV and HBV coinfection for W.H.?

Coinfection with other viruses has been reported in patients with HBV infection. For example, markers of prior or active HBV infection are present in more than 80% of patients with acquired immunodeficiency syndrome, with approximately 10% of these cases seropositive for HBsAg.[42,43] HIV has also been reported to coexist in up to 13% of patients with chronic HBV infection.[42,43] Compared with patients with HBV infection alone, patients coinfected with HBV and HIV have significantly higher levels of viral replication, lower ALT levels, and less severe histologic disease. HBV infection does not reduce survival in HIV-positive patients; however, because these patients live longer, hepatic decompensation and manifestations of HBV may occur.[50,52]

Prevention of Hepatitis B

Alterations in sexual behavior, screening of high-risk patients or settings (e.g., STD and HIV testing at treatment facilities, drug abuse treatment and prevention settings, healthcare settings targeting services to IV drug users, healthcare settings targeting services to MSM, and correctional facilities) and blood products, developing needle exchange programs, and cultural outreach and education may have an impact on HBV transmission. The goals of preventive therapy should be to identify all persons who require immunoprophylaxis for the prevention of infection and provide long-term protection through vaccination to decrease the risk of chronic HBV infection and its subsequent complications, as well as minimizing adverse effects and cost of therapy.

PRE-EXPOSURE PROPHYLAXIS

CASE 80-5

QUESTION 1: P.G., a 55-year-old nursing student, is going to start her clinical rotations. She has no history of hepatitis and has not yet been immunized. She is 5 feet 2 inches and weighs 80 kg. What prophylactic regimen should P.G. receive to prevent hepatitis secondary to HBV?

Manufactured using recombinant DNA technology, Recombivax HB (10 mg HBsAg/mL) and Engerix-B (20 mg HBsAg/mL) are yeast-derived HBV vaccines that induce an immunologic response.

Because P.G. will come in contact with potentially infectious bodily secretions during her rotations, she should be immunized against hepatitis B with either Recombivax HB or Engerix-B.[72,73]

Dosing Regimen

Relative potency comparisons are not clinically important because comparative trials using Recombivax HB and Engerix-B in the recommended dosages have demonstrated equivalent immunogenicity and tolerability. P.G. can be immunized with either product, provided she receives the manufacturer's recommended dosage with each injection. Hepatitis B vaccine is administered as an IM injection in the deltoid muscle of adults and children or in the anterolateral thigh muscle of neonates and infants. The immunogenicity of hepatitis B vaccine is significantly lower when injections are given in the buttocks, probably because the greater amount of fat tissue in the buttocks inhibits interfacing of vaccine and antigen-recognition leukocytes. The results of a small vaccination series suggest that healthy adults who do not respond to hepatitis B vaccine injection to the buttocks have a significantly higher response when vaccinated in the arm. P.G. should be immunized with either Recombivax HB (10 mcg) or Engerix-B (20 mcg) administered as a 1-mL IM injection in the deltoid muscle.[74–76]

Efficacy

Recombinant yeast-derived vaccines (e.g., Recombivax HB, Engerix-B) produce similar results.[71–73] A protective antibody response has been defined as anti-HBs levels of at least 10 IU/mL.[63,77] This threshold was derived from early HBV vaccine trials in homosexual men, in which vaccine recipients with serum antibody levels of at least 10 sample ratio units (SRUs) were protected from HBV infection.[74,75] A serum antibody level of 10 SRU is roughly equivalent to 10 milli-international units/mL when the international standard is used. For this reason, an anti-HBs level of at least 10 IU/mL is considered a protective antibody titer and is the standard used by the ACIP. Although HBV infections have occurred in vaccine recipients with a detectable immune response,. almost all infections have been asymptomatic, identified only through the presence of anti-HBc. These infections have been limited largely to patients with no response or a poor response to vaccination.[53]

Nonresponders

Case 80-5, Question 2: P.G. has completed her three-dose vaccination series with Engerix-B. Routine hepatitis serology testing, performed before volunteering for a drug study, reveals that P.G. is anti-HBs negative. Why did P.G. not respond to the hepatitis B vaccine, and how should she be managed?

Two important determinants of vaccine efficacy appear to be the age at vaccination and underlying immune function. In healthy recipients, the immune response to vaccination decreases with advancing age. In one study, 99% of patients aged 0 to 19 years, 93% of those aged 20 to 49 years, and 73% of those older than 50 years of age achieved protective anti-HBs levels (>10 SRU) after three doses of the hepatitis B vaccine.[53] Immunocompromised patients, including those receiving hemodialysis, those infected with HIV, or children receiving cytotoxic chemotherapy, respond poorly to the hepatitis B vaccine. Patients who smoke, or are obese, also have a reduced response.[74,75] P.G. has two risk factors for a poor response to the hepatitis B vaccine: She is older than 50 years of age, and she is moderately obese (ideal body weight for her height is 50 kg).

Vaccine recipients who respond poorly to hepatitis B vaccine have been classified either as hyporesponders who can probably be protected by additional doses of vaccine or as true nonresponders. Patients with inadequate initial response to the HBV vaccine series should be revaccinated. Of the hyporesponders (anti-HBs levels <10 IU/mL), 50% to 90% achieve a protective level after a single booster injection or after repeating the entire three-dose series.[76,77] Of patients not responding to a primary vaccination series with Engerix-B, 60% produced an immune response after a three-dose series with HBVax II (Recombivax), suggesting a repeat course with the alternative HBV vaccine may be a reasonable approach in some patients.[76,77] Revaccination of nonresponders (no detectable anti-HBs) is less successful, and protective levels, if achieved, are not sustained.[53] True nonresponders to HBV vaccination are rare in the immunocompetent population, and these persons may have a genetic predisposition toward nonresponsiveness.[76,78] P.G. should be revaccinated with a booster dose of hepatitis B vaccine. Her anti-HBs levels can be rechecked 1 month after the injection. If she still has not responded, it is reasonable to administer an additional two injections to complete a second vaccination series.

Interchangeability of Hepatitis B Virus Vaccines

CASE 80-6

Question 1: T.M., a 32-year-old hospital laboratory technician, received the first two doses of hepatitis B vaccine with Recombivax HB. He has relocated recently and is due for the third injection. The employee health service at his new job uses only Engerix-B for hepatitis B vaccination. Can hepatitis B vaccines produced by different manufacturers be used interchangeably?

Although it is recommended that patients receive the complete vaccination series with the same product, it is not absolutely necessary. To determine whether a hepatitis B vaccination series initiated with Recombivax HB could be completed with Engerix-B, healthy adults received 10 mcg of Recombivax HB at baseline and 1 month. At 6 months, the subjects were randomly assigned to receive either Engerix-B 20 mcg or Recombivax HB 10 mcg. One month after the third dose, 100% of those who had received Engerix-B and 92% of those who had received Recombivax HB had protective anti-HBs levels.[72,73]

Chan et al.[78] studied the booster response to either recombinant hepatitis B vaccine or plasma-derived vaccine in children who had been vaccinated originally with the plasma-derived product (Heptavax-B). Children were randomly assigned to receive either 5 mcg of the plasma-derived vaccine or 20 mcg of Engerix-B. One month after the booster injection, all vaccine recipients had significant elevations in their anti-HBs titers, suggesting recombinant hepatitis B vaccines elicit an adequate booster response in persons who originally received the plasma-derived vaccine. According to the ACIP, the immune response from one or two doses of a vaccine produced by one manufacturer, when followed by subsequent doses from a different manufacturer, is comparable with that resulting from a full course of vaccination with a single vaccine.[53]

T.M. may complete the hepatitis B vaccine series with Engerix-B provided he receives the recommended dosage of 20 mcg administered as a 1-mL IM injection to the deltoid region.

Duration of Response

Case 80-6, Question 2: Does T.M. require a booster injection for sustained protection from HBV infection?

The duration of vaccine-induced immunity has been evaluated in many long-term studies.[79–82] The duration of detectable anti-HBs appears proportional to the peak antibody response achieved after vaccination, and protective anti-HBs levels were sustained in 68% to 85% of patients receiving the plasma-derived HBV vaccine from 6 to 12 years.[79–82] Importantly, the protective efficacy of the HBV vaccine in these trials was high, even in patients with anti-HBs levels <10 IU/mL. HBsAg was only rarely detected, and most HBV events consisted of asymptomatic seroconversion to anti-HBc. These studies suggest that successful HBV vaccination is associated with long-lasting protection without the need for additional booster doses for up to 12 years.

The mechanism of sustained protection from HBV, despite low or undetectable anti-HBs levels, is thought to be related to the phenomenon of immunologic memory in previously sensitized B lymphocytes. This amnestic response, in combination with the long incubation period of HBV, may allow the synthesis of protective antibodies sufficiently quickly to block infection in patients rechallenged with HBV.[77]

In summary, no need exists for routine administration of HBV vaccine booster doses to immunocompetent persons after successful vaccination. Immunocompromised patients may require a persistent minimal level of protective antibody, and the ACIP does recommend annual antibody testing for patients receiving chronic hemodialysis with administration of a booster dose when antibody levels are less than 10 IU/mL.[53] Based on available evidence, T.M. does not require a scheduled booster dose of hepatitis B vaccine.

Indications

CASE 80-6, QUESTION 3: Why is it appropriate for T.M. to be vaccinated with hepatitis B vaccine, and who else should be vaccinated with this vaccine?

The ACIP has recommended pre-exposure hepatitis B vaccination for the following high-risk groups: Healthcare workers with exposure to blood, staff of institutions for the developmentally disabled, hemodialysis patients, recipients of blood products, household and sexual contacts of HBV carriers, international travelers to HBV-endemic areas, injecting drug users, sexually active homosexual men, bisexual men, and inmates of long-term correctional facilities.[53,83,84] Because T.M. is a hospital laboratory technician, he is at high risk for exposure to HBV and should be vaccinated.

Universal Hepatitis B Vaccination

In addition to the previously listed high-risk groups, all infants should receive hepatitis B vaccination. The practice of vaccinating only high-risk persons has resulted in little impact on the incidence of HBV disease. Populations at risk for HBV disease (injecting drug users, persons with multiple sexual partners) generally are not vaccinated before they begin engaging in high-risk behaviors. In addition, many persons who become infected have no identifiable risk factors for infection and thus would not be recognized as candidates for vaccination. A program designed to immunize children before they initiate high-risk behaviors is likely to have a greater impact in reducing the incidence of HBV infection. As a means to achieve this goal, the hepatitis B vaccine now is incorporated into the existing pediatric vaccination schedule. The first dose is administered during the newborn period (preferably before the infant is discharged from the hospital) but no later than 2 months of age.[52,53] The recommended vaccination schedule is shown in Table 80-5.

CASE 80-7

QUESTION 1: R.M. is a mother of two children aged 11 years and 2 months. Her infant daughter just received a second dose of hepatitis B vaccine as part of her routine well-baby care. R.M. wonders whether her son, who did not receive the hepatitis B vaccine during his normal childhood immunizations, should receive the vaccine now.

Table 80-5

Recommended Schedules of Hepatitis B Vaccination for Infants Born to HBsAg (−) Mothers[52,53]

Hepatitis B Vaccine	Age of Infant
Option 1	
Dose 1	Birth (before hospital discharge)
Dose 2	1–2 months[a]
Dose 3	6–18 months[a]
Option 2	
Dose 1	1–2 months[a]
Dose 2	4 months[a]
Dose 3	6–18 months[a]

[a]Hepatitis B vaccine can be administered simultaneously with diphtheria–tetanus–pertussis, *Haemophilus influenzae* type b conjugate, measles–mumps–rubella, and oral polio vaccines.

The Centers for Disease Control and Prevention (CDC) has addressed the issue of immunizing children and adolescents born before 1991 who are potentially at risk for hepatitis B infection. The current recommendations suggest that adolescents who have not received three doses of hepatitis B vaccine should initiate or complete the series at ages 11 to 15 years. A schedule of 0, 1 to 2, and 4 to 6 months is recommended.[52,53] It is anticipated that universal vaccination of all infants and previously unvaccinated adolescents aged 11 to 12 years, in addition to ongoing immunization of high-risk persons, will reduce the incidence of acute hepatitis B infection, hepatitis B-associated chronic liver disease, and HCC. R.M.'s son should receive either Recombivax HB 5 mcg or Engerix-B 10 mcg IM in the deltoid with repeat doses 1 to 2 months and 4 to 6 months from the initial injection.

Adverse Effects

HBV vaccination generally has been well tolerated. The most common side effect is pain at the injection site, observed in 3% to 29% of patients. Transient febrile reactions (defined as temperature >99.9°F) occur in less than 6% of recipients, and other reactions, including nausea, rash, headache, myalgias, and arthralgias, are observed in less than 1% of recipients. Ongoing monitoring of vaccine safety by the FDA and CDC is assessed through the Vaccine Safety Datalink project and Vaccine Adverse Events Reporting System.[52,53] On the basis of these reporting systems, additional "causal" adverse effects associated with vaccination include anaphylaxis (1 case/1.1 million vaccine doses), Guillain–Barré syndrome, and multiple sclerosis. Additional rare adverse events that have been reported but remain to be validated are chronic fatigue syndrome, neurologic disorders (leukoencephalitis, optic neuritis, and transverse myelitis), rheumatoid arthritis, type 1 diabetes, and autoimmune disease.

POSTEXPOSURE PROPHYLAXIS

Percutaneous Exposure

CASE 80-8

QUESTION 1: K.N., a 26-year-old medical student, presents to the ED after accidentally sticking herself with a contaminated needle while drawing blood from an HBsAg-positive patient. K.N. was not vaccinated previously and had no known prior episodes of hepatitis or liver disease. Her tetanus status is current. She weighs 56 kg. How should K.N. be treated for percutaneous exposure to hepatitis B?

After exposure to HBV, prophylactic treatment with hepatitis B vaccination and possibly passive immunization with hepatitis B immunoglobulin (HBIG) should be considered.[53] The ACIP recommends postexposure immunoprophylaxis after hepatitis B exposure. K.N.'s percutaneous exposure warrants active immunization with HBV and passive immunization with HBIG. The source of K.N.'s exposure is HBsAg positive, and K.N. had not been vaccinated previously with the hepatitis B vaccine. She should receive a single dose of HBIG 0.06 mL/kg (3.4 mL) as an IM injection in either the gluteal or deltoid region as soon as possible after exposure, preferably within 24 hours. HBIG is prepared from plasma of persons preselected for high-titer anti-HBs. The ratio of anti-HBs of HBIG in the United States is 1:100,000 as determined by radioimmunoassay. HBIG is superior to immunoglobulin in the prevention of hepatitis B infection after percutaneous exposure. K.N. also should receive active immunization with IM hepatitis B vaccine (at a separate site) simultaneously with HBIG. The second and third doses should be given 1 month and 6 months later. Passively acquired antibodies against HBV from HBIG or immunoglobulin will not interfere with active immunization via hepatitis B vaccine.[83]

If the HBsAg status of the donor source of a percutaneous exposure is unknown, recommendations for prophylaxis of HBV infection depend on whether the donor source is at high risk or at low risk for being HBsAg positive. High-risk donor sources include homosexual men, IV drug abusers, patients undergoing hemodialysis, residents of mental institutions, immigrants from endemic areas, and household contacts of HBV carriers.

Sexual Exposure

CASE 80-9

QUESTION 1: G.G. is a 20-year-old construction worker who had sexual contact with a partner who recently found out she was HBsAg positive. What are the current recommendations for a person who has had sexual contact with an HBsAg-positive person?

Sexual transmission of HBV is an important cause of HBV infection, accounting for approximately 30% to 60% of all new cases annually.[42,43,62] Passive immunization with a single 5-mL dose of HBIG was found highly effective in preventing HBV infection after sexual exposure when compared with a control globulin (with no anti-HBs activity).[63,83] The CDC recommends that susceptible persons exposed to HBV through sexual contact with a person who has acute or chronic HBV infection should receive postexposure prophylaxis with 0.06 mL/kg of HBIG as a single IM dose within 14 days of the last exposure.[19,83] Patients also should receive the standard three-dose immunization series with hepatitis B vaccine beginning at the time of HBIG administration.[53]

Perinatal Exposure

CASE 80-10

QUESTION 1: S.L., a 3.2-kg boy, was just born to an HBsAg-positive mother. Is S.L. at risk for acquiring HBV infection, and how should he be treated?

In many Asian and developing countries, perinatal (vertical) transmission accounts for most HBV infections. Infants born to HBV-infected mothers have a greater than 85% risk of acquiring HBV during the perinatal period. Of those who become infected, 80% to 90% become chronic HBsAg carriers.[62,84] Although fulminant cases have been reported, most hepatitis infections in neonates are asymptomatic. Despite the usually innocuous initial disease, significant adverse consequences are associated with chronic HBsAg carriage in neonates. Chronic hepatitis B infection is associated with chronic liver disease and has been clearly implicated as a major risk factor in the development of primary HCC.[62,63]

Mothers who are chronic carriers of HBV can transmit HBV to their infants. The risk is related to the presence of HBsAg and HBeAg (suggesting a high degree of viral replication and infectivity). The likelihood that S.L. will develop HBV infection is high. S.L. requires immediate therapy with HBIG to provide immediate high titers of circulating anti-HBs, and simultaneous vaccination with hepatitis B vaccine to induce long-lasting protective immunity. Screening pregnant women for the presence of HBeAg and administration of HBIG and hepatitis B vaccine is 85% to 98% effective in preventing HBV infection and the chronic carrier state.[63,77,83] This compares with a 71% efficacy rate for administration of HBIG alone. Simultaneous administration of HBIG and hepatitis B vaccine does not adversely affect the production of anti-HBs in neonates.[52,53,63,83]

Infants born to mothers who are HBsAg-positive should receive simultaneous IM injections of the appropriate doses of hepatitis B vaccine (Table 80-5) and HBIG (0.5 mL) within 12 hours of birth. The injections should be administered at separate sites. S.L. should receive HBIG (0.5 mL) as soon as possible after birth, administered as an IM injection. He also should receive 0.5 mL of either Recombivax HB (5 mcg) or Engerix-B (10 mcg) as an IM injection at a separate site.

CASE 80-10, QUESTION 2: What would the management plan be if the HBsAg status of S.L.'s mother was unknown?

The ACIP has developed recommendations for the prevention of perinatal HBV infection. This includes the routine testing of all pregnant women for HBsAg during an early prenatal visit. HBsAg testing should be repeated late in the pregnancy for women who are HBsAg negative, but who are at high risk of HBV infection or who have had clinically apparent hepatitis. Women admitted for delivery who have not had prenatal HBsAg testing should have blood drawn for testing. Although test results are pending, the infant should receive hepatitis B vaccine within 12 hours of birth. If the mother is found later to be HBsAg positive, her infant should receive HBIG as soon as possible within 7 days of birth. The second and third doses of vaccine should be administered at 1 and 6 months, respectively. If the mother is found to be HBsAg negative, her infant should continue to receive hepatitis B vaccine as part of the routine vaccination series.[63]

Evaluation and Management of Patients with Chronic Hepatitis B Virus Infection

CASE 80-11

QUESTION 1: E.A. is a 55-year-old woman who presents to the hepatology clinic with a recent history of mild jaundice. Her previous medical history is unremarkable except for a blood transfusion she received during childbirth in 1988. What initial and follow-up tests should be performed to assess the extent of HBV infection in E.A.?

Initially, a thorough history and physical examination should be performed with greater emphasis placed on risk factors for coinfection, alcohol use, and family history of HBV and liver cancer. Laboratory tests should include assessment of liver disease, markers of HBV replication, and screening tests for HCV, HDV, or HIV. Vaccinations for hepatitis A should also be administered as described above. The decision to perform a liver biopsy should be made based on knowledge of a patient's age, the ALT level, HBeAg status, HBV DNA levels, and additional clinical features

Overview of algorithm used to determine need for treatment of HBV

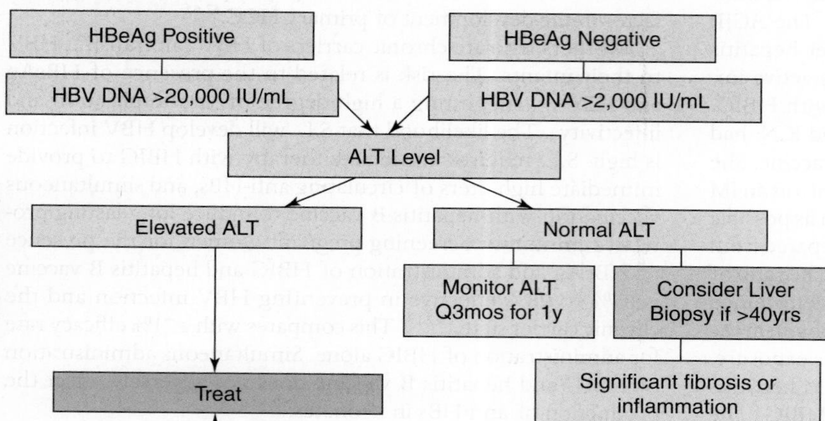

Figure 80-5 Overview of algorithm used to determine treatment of hepatitis B virus.

suggestive of chronic liver disease or portal hypertension. In patients who are not initially considered for treatment (inactive HBV carriers), a guideline for follow-up based on HBeAg status is described in Figure 80-5. Periodic screening for HCC should also be performed in high-risk populations such as Asian men older than 40 and Asian women older than 50 years of age, persons with cirrhosis, persons with a family history of HCC, blacks older than 20 years of age, and any carrier older than 40 years of age with persistent or intermittent ALT or HBV DNA elevations.

CASE 80-12

Question 1: C.R., a 48-year-old man, presents to the ED with jaundice, complaints of incapacitating fatigue, and vague intermittent abdominal pain for the past month. C.R. was diagnosed with HBV infection 12 years ago. His social history includes IV drug abuse (none in the past 2 years) and alcohol abuse (none in the past 2 years). Several weeks ago, C.R. noted darkening of his urine and yellowing of his eyes. Additionally, C.R. has a history of severe depression, managed with escitalopram.

Physical examination reveals a thin man in no apparent distress. He is afebrile, and his blood pressure, heart rate, and respiratory rate are within normal limits. Moderate scleral icterus is noted. The abdomen is soft and not distended. The liver is enlarged, nontender, and smooth with an edge palpable 5 cm below the costal margin and a span of 15 cm. The spleen is palpable. The cardiac, pulmonary, neurologic, and extremity examinations all are within normal limits.

C.R.'s laboratory evaluation is significant for the following:

Hct: 39%
Hgb: 11 g/dL
WBC count: 8.8 cells/μL
Platelets: 75,000/μL
PT: 15.4 seconds
INR: 2.1
AST: 326 units/L
ALT: 382 units/L
Alkaline phosphatase: 142 units/mL
Total bilirubin: 4.2 mg/dL
Albumin: 2.8 g/dL

Hepatitis serologic tests are positive for HBsAg, HBeAg, and anti-HBc, and negative for IgM anti-HBc, IgM anti-HAV, and anti-HCV. HBV DNA is reported as greater than 20,000 IU/mL. A liver biopsy reveals periportal inflammation as well as piecemeal and bridging necrosis. What clinical findings does C.R. have that support the diagnosis of chronic HBV infection?

The chronic occurrence of jaundice and hepatosplenomegaly with significantly elevated AST and ALT in a young patient such as C.R. is suggestive of chronic hepatitis. Although alcoholic hepatitis secondary to long-term alcohol use is consistent with these clinical features, his serologic tests are positive for HBV. Hepatitis serology with positive HBsAg and HBeAg suggests ongoing viral replication and a high degree of infectivity.

Serum concentrations of aminotransferases can range from slightly abnormal to greatly elevated, with ALT concentrations generally greater than AST. Serum bilirubin concentrations greater than 3.0 mg/dL are common, serum concentration of alkaline phosphatase usually is increased, and the PT may be prolonged. Patients such as C.R. with a prolonged PT, thrombocytopenia, and low serum albumin concentration generally have a more severe form of chronic hepatitis and can be considered to have decompensated liver disease.

Liver biopsy is important for the diagnosis, treatment, and prognosis of patients with chronic hepatitis. C.R.'s liver biopsy reveals the classic triad of periportal inflammation as well as piecemeal and bridging necrosis. The liver biopsy and hepatitis serologic test results are consistent with a diagnosis of chronic HBV infection. Treatment of chronic HBV infection requires knowledge of the natural history of the untreated disease and the potential benefits of intervention. Currently, six agents are approved by the FDA for treating chronic HBV infection.

Case 80-12, Question 2: Does C.R. require treatment for chronic hepatitis secondary to hepatitis B?

The decision to treat C.R. depends on the severity of symptoms, the serum biochemistries, and the liver biopsy results. C.R. has evidence of severe chronic HBV infection. He is symptomatic with jaundice, severe fatigue, and abdominal pain, and the results of his LFTs and HBV DNA levels suggest his disease is advanced (decreased albumin, elevated PT, low platelets). Therefore, he should be treated to reduce the replication of HBV, resolve the hepatocellular damage, and prevent long-term adverse hepatic sequelae.[62,84]

GOALS OF THERAPY

Case 80-12, Question 3: What are the goals of therapy for chronic hepatitis secondary to HBV?

Progression of chronic hepatitis to cirrhosis is likely because of continued replication of the HBV. Loss of active viral replication usually is associated with a decrease in infectivity, a reduction in inflammatory cells within the liver, and a fall of serum aminotransferase activities into the normal range. The disappearance of detectable HBeAg and HBV DNA is considered an indicator of loss of active viral replication.

The goals of therapy in chronic HBV infection are to achieve sustained suppression of HBV replication and remission of liver disease.[84,85] Ultimately, achieving these goals should lead to resolving ongoing hepatocellular damage and reducing the development of cirrhosis and HCC. Clinical trials for chronic HBV infection have used the following markers as end points for successful therapy: seroconversion from HBeAg positive to HBeAg negative (with appearance of anti-HBe), reductions in serum aminotransferase activity, elimination of circulating HBV DNA, and improvement in liver histology. The elimination of HBsAg (termination of HBV carrier state) has been difficult to achieve in clinical trials. Additionally, the responses to antiviral therapy of chronic HBV can be categorized as biochemical, virologic, or histologic, and as on therapy or sustained off therapy.

DRUG THERAPY

CASE 80-12, QUESTION 4: Would initiating therapy during the acute phase of the HBV infection have benefited C.R.?

Pharmacologic interventions in the management of acute hepatitis B have been disappointing. Early studies demonstrated a transient decrease in serum aminotransferase activity and bilirubin concentration associated with corticosteroids. More recent studies, however, have resulted in a higher incidence of relapse and mortality in patients receiving corticosteroids.[85–88] Other therapies, including HBIG and interferon alpha, have been ineffective in managing acute viral hepatitis secondary to HBV.[63,84] Nucleoside and nucleotide RT inhibitors reduce HBV DNA levels in patients with chronic disease,[88–92] but their use in acute HBV infection requires further investigation. Thus, administration of antivirals during the acute phase of HBV infection is not recommended in C.R.

Interferons

CASE 80-12, QUESTION 5: What drug therapy should C.R. receive to treat chronic HBV-associated infection?

Previously, the most effective agents for treating chronic hepatitis B have been interferons (IFNs),[89,90] which appear to activate their target cells by binding to specific cell surface receptors to induce synthesis of effector proteins.[89,91] These intracellular proteins induce the antiviral, antiproliferative, and immunomodulatory actions of the IFNs. Their antiviral activity possibly arises from their ability to abate viral entry into the host cells and modulate several steps of the viral replication cycle (e.g., viral uncoating, inhibition of messenger RNA, and protein synthesis). The only FDA-approved and commercially available IFN is pegylated IFN (PegIFN-α2a, Pegasys) for the treatment of chronic HBV infection. The formulation involves adding polyethylene glycol to IFN that leads to an increased serum half-life, resulting in a prolonged antiviral effect. As a result, the frequency in administration is extended from three times weekly to once a week.

Efficacy

Pegylated Interferon

Pegylated interferons (PegIFN-α2a) have the advantage of more convenient dosing and additional viral suppression for patients with HBV. Clinical data suggest that this agent has slightly enhanced efficacy than standard IFN formulations. PegIFN-α2a 180 mcg SQ weekly monotherapy was compared with PegIFN-α2a SQ weekly plus lamivudine 100 mg PO daily or lamivudine 100 mg PO daily alone.[90] At the end of the 24-week follow-up, significantly more patients who received PegIFN monotherapy or combination therapy than those who received lamivudine monotherapy had HBeAg conversion. PegIFN-α2a (alone or in combination) resulted in HBsAg conversion in 16 patients compared with none in the lamivudine monotherapy group ($p = 0.001$). Additionally, at the end of treatment, viral suppression was most pronounced in the group that received combination therapy. Similar results were reported in HBeAg-positive patients receiving PegIFN-α2b.[91] In the only published trial performed in HBeAg-negative patients, PegIFN-α2a 180 mcg weekly ($n = 177$) was compared with either PegIFN-α2a 180 mcg weekly plus 100 mg of lamivudine ($n = 179$) or 100 mg of lamivudine alone ($n = 181$). Viral suppression was greater in the combination group, but sustained response (HBV DNA and ALT levels at week 72) was comparable in the group that received PegIFN-α2a alone (or in combination), and superior to the lamivudine monotherapy group. Loss of HBsAg occurred in 12 patients in the PegIFN groups, as compared with none in the lamivudine group. Ultimately, the addition of lamivudine to PegIFN did not improve post-therapy response rates.[92]

Dosing Considerations

The recommended dose of PegIFN-α2a, the only pegylated IFN approved for the treatment of HBV infection in the United States, is 180 mcg SQ weekly for 48 weeks.[90–92] It is possible that more severe flu-like symptoms and headache occur with thrice-weekly dosing when compared with weekly administration. In contrast, severe bone marrow suppression tends to occur less often with thrice-weekly administration.[90,91]

Predictors of Response

CASE 80-12, QUESTION 6: Would C.R. be likely to respond to PegIFN-α2a therapy?

Certain patient variables can predict the response to therapy with PegIFN-α2a. The most reliable predictor of a positive response to PegIFN-α2a in HBeAg-positive patients is pretreatment ALT and HBV DNA levels.[90–92] Patients with high pretreatment ALT levels >2 times the upper limit of normal, and HBV DNA levels less than 20 IU/mL are more likely to respond to therapy.[90–93] HBeAg seroconversion with PegIFN treatment is associated with improved survival and reduced complications. Other predictors of a positive response include a short duration of disease, negative HIV status, and a high histologic activity index as demonstrated by liver biopsy or other diagnostic tools. No consistent predictor of sustained response in patients who are HBeAg negative exists. Thus, C.R. is not a reasonable candidate for PegIFN-α therapy. His liver biopsy is consistent with chronic disease, he has high pretreatment aminotransferase levels, his HBV DNA is greater than 20,000 IU/mL, and his duration of chronic hepatitis is long.

Adverse Effects

CASE 80-12, QUESTION 7: What are some additional reasons for avoiding PegIFN-α therapy in C.R.?

Adverse effects associated with PegIFN therapy can be categorized as early side effects that rarely limit the use of PegIFN, and late side effects that may necessitate dose reduction or discontinuation of therapy altogether.[90–92] The early side effects of PegIFN therapy generally appear hours after administration and resemble an influenza-like syndrome with fever, chills, anorexia, nausea, myalgias, fatigue, and headache. Virtually all patients receiving PegIFN experience these toxicities, and they tend to resolve after repeated exposure to the drug over time. Administration of PegIFN at bedtime may decrease the severity of early onset of the side effects. Acetaminophen can be used to treat early side effects of PegIFN therapy, but should be limited to 2 g/day to minimize the risk of hepatotoxicity. The late-onset side effects usually are observed after 2 to 4 weeks of therapy and are more serious. These toxicities, which limit the use of PegIFN, include worsening of the flu-like syndrome, alopecia, bone marrow suppression, bacterial infections, thyroid dysfunction (both hypothyroidism and hyperthyroidism), and psychiatric disturbances (emotional lability, irritability, depression, anxiety, delirium, and suicidal ideation). The use of PegIFN can also cause a flare (increase) in ALT levels in 30% to 40% of patients. These flares are considered to be a favorable prognostic indicator, but they have been reported to cause hepatic decompensation, especially in cirrhotic patients. C.R.'s history of severe depression should be considered a relative contraindication to treating him with PegIFN. Furthermore, the use of PegIFN in patients with decompensated liver disease may lead to FHF. Therefore, this agent, although approved for HBV, is not optimal for him.[90–92]

Nucleoside/Nucleotide Analogs

CASE 80-12, QUESTION 8: What other antiviral therapies are available to treat C.R.'s chronic HBV infection?

Although PegIFN-α2a have been important in the treatment of chronic HBV infection, patients included in most clinical trials represented a highly select group of chronic HBV carriers. Specifically, patients with decompensated liver disease were excluded because they often have leukopenia and thrombocytopenia as a result of hypersplenism, which limits the dose of PegIFN that can be administered. In addition to PegIFN-α2a, the FDA has approved several oral antiviral agents for treatment of chronic HBV infection (lamivudine, adefovir dipivoxil, entecavir, tenofovir disoproxil fumarate, and tenofovir alafenamide).

Lamivudine

Lamivudine (Epivir-HB) was the first oral nucleoside analog approved by the FDA for use in patients with compensated liver disease who had evidence of active viral replication and liver inflammation caused by chronic HBV infection. Nucleoside analogs represent an alternative approach to treatment in patients with decompensated liver disease.[85–87] Lamivudine, the (−) enantiomer of 3′-thiacytidine, is an oral 2′-,3′-dideoxynucleoside that inhibits DNA synthesis by terminating the nascent proviral DNA chain and interferes with the RT activity of HBV.[93–95] For chronic HBV treatment, Epivir-HB is administered as 100 mg orally daily. Lamivudine is well tolerated and reduces serum levels of HBV DNA.[85–87,93,95] Lamivudine is also used as an alternative nucleoside analog for HIV treatment and is administered at a higher dose of 600 mg orally once daily in combination with antiretrovirals.

Lamivudine Resistance

CASE 80-12, QUESTION 9: What is the risk of development of lamivudine resistance in C.R.?

Considering the high rate of viral turnover and the error-susceptible nature of the polymerase (particularly the RT), acquisition of resistance mutations is common. The most common mutation leading to lamivudine resistance is a specific point mutation in the highly conserved methionine motif of the HBV DNA polymerase.[96,97] In this mutation, the methionine residue is changed to a valine or isoleucine. These genotypic mutations in the YMDD locus associated with a reduced sensitivity to lamivudine occur after long-term therapy (e.g., 52 weeks). This motif is thought to be representative of the active site of the enzyme, similar to that associated with HIV RT, leading to lamivudine resistance.[96,97] Lamivudine-resistant HBV mutants generally are detectable after 6 months or more of continuous therapy. Integrated data from four studies show a 16% to 32% incidence at 1 year, increasing to 47% to 56% at 2 years of therapy and 69% to 75% at 3 years of therapy.[96,97] The presence of YMDD mutants results in a loss of the clinical response, a rise in ALT levels, and worsening of hepatic histology. Reports of continued improvement despite lamivudine resistance exist, but the long-term consequences of viral resistance (including hepatic decompensation and exacerbation of liver disease) are substantial. Thus, lamivudine has limited clinical utility in patients with chronic HBV and is currently considered a second-line agent.

CASE 80-12, QUESTION 10: What other nucleoside or nucleotide therapies are available for managing C.R.'s chronic HBV infection?

Adefovir

Adefovir dipivoxil (Hepsera) was approved for the oral treatment of chronic hepatitis B in adults with evidence of either active viral replication or persistent elevations in serum aminotransferases (ALT or AST) or histologically active disease.[98–100] Adefovir dipivoxil is the oral prodrug of an acyclic nucleotide monophosphate analog, 9-(2-phosphonylmethoxyethyl)-adenine. The active drug is a selective inhibitor of numerous species of viral nucleic acid polymerases and RTs. Previously, two trials reported the efficacy of adefovir 10 mg orally once daily for the treatment of patients who were HBeAg negative[99] and HBeAg positive.[100] Adverse effects from adefovir included abdominal pain, diarrhea, dyspepsia, headaches, nausea, and nephrotoxicity.

Resistance to adefovir occurs at a much slower rate compared with lamivudine. The cumulative probability of resistance in the HBeAg-negative patient trial was estimated to be 0%, 3%, 1%, 18%, and 29% at years 1, 2, 3, 4, and 5 years, respectively.[99] In the trial with HBeAg-positive patients, resistance was estimated to be 20% at 5 years.[100] Other reports have described adefovir resistance rates as high as 20% after 2 years of treatment.[98] Risk factors for adefovir resistance appear to be suboptimal viral suppression and sequential monotherapy. Thus, adefovir should also be considered a second-line therapy for C.R.

Entecavir

Entecavir (Baraclude) is an oral acyclic guanosine nucleoside derivative with potent activity against HBV.[101–103] The drug inhibits HBV replication at three different steps: (a) the priming of HBV DNA polymerase; (b) the RT of the negative-strand HBV DNA from the pregenomic RNA; and (c) the synthesis of positive-strand HBV DNA. In vitro studies have shown that the drug is more potent than lamivudine and adefovir and is highly effective against lamivudine-resistant HBV mutants.

In two published Phase III clinical trials, the efficacy of entecavir was reported in patients with HBeAg-positive[102] and HBeAg-negative[103] hepatitis B infection. Patients with compensated liver disease who had not previously received a nucleoside analog were assigned to receive entecavir 0.5 mg, or lamivudine 100 mg orally once daily for a minimum of 52 weeks. By week 48, HBeAg-positive patients receiving entecavir had higher rates of histologic (72% vs. 62%), virologic (HBV DNA undetectable by PCR; 67% vs. 36%), and biochemical (ALT normalization; 68% vs. 60%) responses when compared with lamivudine.[102] Of note, the seroconversion rates were similar among the two treatment groups (21% vs. 18%; entecavir vs. lamivudine, respectively). No viral resistance to entecavir was detected during the study period, but follow-up data suggest a low rate of resistance (3% by week 96 of therapy).[102] The authors concluded that entecavir was as safe and had significantly higher histologic, virologic, and biochemical response rates than HBeAg-positive patients treated with lamivudine. In patients who remained HBeAg positive with low levels of HBV DNA replication, a second year of entecavir and lamivudine therapy resulted in seroconversion in 11% and 13% of patients, respectively.[101,102]

In another trial of HBeAg-negative hepatitis B infection, patients received either entecavir 0.5 mg or 100 mg of lamivudine daily for a minimum of 52 weeks. At week 48, patients receiving entecavir had significantly higher rates of histologic (70% vs. 61%; $p < 0.01$), virologic (90% vs. 72%), and biochemical (78% vs. 71%) response rates.[103] No resistance was seen among patients receiving entecavir. Safety and adverse events were similar in the two groups. Thus, C.R. could receive entecavir 0.5 mg daily. As with all of the nucleoside agents, dosage adjustments should be implemented with changes in renal function. Furthermore, entecavir may be used for lamivudine-refractory or lamivudine-resistant patients. In these patients, lamivudine should be discontinued to reduce the risk of entecavir cross-resistance. The dose of entecavir used for lamivudine-resistant patients is 1 mg orally once daily. In these patients, entecavir resistance has been reported to be 51% after 5 years of therapy. Thus, alternatives may be warranted for these patients.[104–108] In regard to histologic liver improvement, entecavir was ranked superior over tenofovir disoproxil fumarate.[109]

Tenofovir disoproxil fumarate

Tenofovir disoproxil fumarate (Viread) is approved for the oral treatment of chronic HBV.[110–112] This agent is a potent nucleotide analog that is structurally similar, yet equipotent, but less nephrotoxic than adefovir. Clinical trials in HBeAg-positive and HBeAg-negative patients with chronic HBV infection have demonstrated the efficacy of tenofovir DF. In the first Phase III trial of HBeAg-positive patients with compensated liver disease, a significantly higher proportion of tenofovir-treated patients had undetectable HBV DNA (76% vs. 13%), ALT normalization (68% vs. 54%), and HBsAg loss (3% vs. 0%) at the end of therapy. Histologic response rates and HBeAg conversion were similar between the two groups. Of note, at the end of therapy, patients in the adefovir group were switched to tenofovir DF, and any patient who had detectable HBV DNA by week 72 had emtricitabine added to their regimen with subsequent additional serologic benefit.

In the second trial, HBeAg-negative patients with compensated liver disease were given a similar regimen (300 mg of tenofovir DF or 10 mg of adefovir daily for 48 weeks).[111] By week 48, a higher percentage of tenofovir-treated patients had undetectable serum HBV DNA than those treated with adefovir (93% vs. 63%). The proportions of patients having ALT normalization (76% vs. 77%) or histologic response (72% vs. 69%) were similar. No patients in the study became HBsAg negative. Again, at week 48, patients receiving adefovir were switched to tenofovir. Patients in both groups who still had detectable HBV DNA by 72 weeks were given emtricitabine. Similar to the HBeAg-positive group, the change to tenofovir DF led to additional viral suppression in the patients initially treated with adefovir. In the previous two trials, only 7 patients were observed to have virologic breakthrough during 96 weeks of therapy, but no tenofovir-resistant HBV mutations were detected. Current guidelines suggest and clinical data support tenofovir (300 mg PO every day) as a viable first-line agent for C.R.[112] Generally, tenofovir is well tolerated, but it has been reported to cause Fanconi syndrome, renal insufficiency, osteomalacia, and a decrease in bone density.[110] Similar to other agents in this class, the dose of tenofovir DF should be adjusted based on renal function.[110–112] Recommendations for treatment of chronic HBV can be found in Table 80-6.

TABLE 80-6
Treatments of HBV Infection[113,116]

Treatment	Preferred as First Choice	Comments
Entecavir	Yes (unless previous history of lamivudine resistance)	High potency, high genetic barrier to resistance
Tenofovir DF	Yes	High potency, high genetic barrier to resistance
TAF	Yes	High potency, high genetic barrier to resistance
PegIFN	Yes	Less safe in pts with cirrhosis
Adefovir	No	Low genetic barrier to resistance; nephrotoxic
Lamivudine	No	Low genetic barrier to resistance

Tenofovir DF, tenofovir disoproxil fumarate; TAF, tenofovir alafenamide; PegIFN, pegylated interferon alfa-2a.

Tenofovir alafenamide

Tenofovir alafenamide, or TAF (Vemlidy), is the latest oral antiviral approved for the treatment of chronic HBV infection. It is a nucleotide prodrug that is converted to tenofovir diphosphate in a two-step process, which inhibits replication of the HBV.[113] TAF has a similar antiviral profile as its sibling drug, tenofovir DF, but at a dose one-tenth less than 300 mg. Approved at 25 mg orally once daily, TAF exhibits greater plasma stability and more efficiently delivers tenofovir to hepatocytes and results in less tenofovir in the bloodstream, leading to improved renal (eGFR and renal tubular function) and bone safety parameters (smaller declines in spine and hip bone mineral density) compared to tenofovir DF.[113–115] Two pivotal international Phase III clinical studies (Studies 108 and 110) demonstrated TAF's efficacy among 1,298 treatment-naïve and treatment-experienced adults with chronic HBV infection over 48 weeks. Study 108 was a randomized, double-blind, active-controlled trial that showed TAF was noninferior to tenofovir DF in treatment-naïve and treatment-experienced patients with HBeAg-negative chronic HBV infection.[114] Study 110 randomized and treated 873 HBeAg-positive patients with either TAF or tenofovir DF. The study results were similar showing noninferiority to tenofovir DF based on the percentage of participants with a decline of HBV DNA below 29 IU/mL at 48 weeks and 96 weeks.[115] Upon further data analysis through 96 weeks, higher rates of ALT normalization occurred with participants in the TAF study arm compared to those in the tenofovir DF arm. No viral resistance developed with either TAF or tenofovir DF in the studies.[114,115]

TAF was generally well tolerated by the study participants, and discontinuations from adverse events were 1% compared to 1.2% of participants in the tenofovir DF arm. The most common adverse events (incidence ≥5%) reported for TAF included headache, fatigue, abdominal pain, cough, nausea, and back pain. Similar to tenofovir DF, TAF has a safety warning of risk of lactic acidosis/severe hepatomegaly with steatosis and post-treatment severe acute exacerbations of hepatitis B, especially upon discontinuation.[114,115] There have been no reported cases of Fanconi syndrome or proximal renal tubulopathy associated with TAF. Nevertheless, renal monitoring of the serum creatinine, phosphorus, creatinine clearance, urine glucose, and urine protein prior to initiating and during TAF treatment is clinically recommended. The antiviral has also been approved for HIV-1 treatment as part of a combination antiretroviral regimen with integrase strand transfer inhibitors. However, the safety and efficacy of TAF have not been established in patients with HBV and HIV coinfections. TAF is less nephrotoxic than tenofovir DF and, however, is not recommended for patients with CrCl <15 mL/minute. It is also not recommended for patients with decompensated (Child-Pugh B or C) hepatic impairment.[113–115]

Regarding the drug interaction profile of TAF, it is not recommended to be coadministered with anticonvulsants (i.e., oxcarbazepine, phenobarbital, and phenytoin), anti-tuberculosis medications (i.e., rifabutin, rifampin, and rifapentine), or Saint-John's-wort. Such coadministration will result in decreased serum levels of TAF, thus reducing its therapeutic effect. TAF is also a substrate of P-glycoprotein (P-gp) and breast cancer resistance protein (BCRP). Drugs that strongly affect P-gp and BCRP activity may lead to changes in TAF absorption.[113] Comparisons of PegIFN with the oral antivirals can be found in Table 80-7.

Combination Therapies

CASE 80-12, QUESTION 11: If C.R. fails therapy with entecavir or tenofovir DF, is combination therapy appropriate?

Combination therapy for HIV and HBV is more effective than monotherapy. The potential for additive or synergistic antiviral effects and reduced or delayed rates of viral resistance may also be possible in patients with HBV infection. Several combination therapies have been evaluated (PegIFN and lamivudine, lamivudine and adefovir, lamivudine and telbivudine), but none are superior to monotherapy.[116] Combination therapy is superior to lamivudine monotherapy in reducing the rate of resistance in patients. However, there is no such role for combination therapy for those agents (entecavir, tenofovir DF) associated with low resistance as monotherapy. Therefore, combination therapy is not appropriate for C.R. at this time.

LIVER TRANSPLANTATION

CASE 80-12, QUESTION 12: If C.R. fails therapy, continues to decompensate, and develops cirrhosis from his chronic HBV infection, what nonpharmacologic interventions are available?

TABLE 80-7
Comparison of HBV Treatments[85,86,96,97]

	PegIFN alfa-2a	Nucleos(t)ide Analogues
Advantages	Finite duration Lack or very little resistance Higher rates of HBeAg seroconversion within 12 months	Potent antiviral effect Well tolerated Oral ROA
Disadvantages	Moderate antiviral effect Inferior tolerability Bothersome adverse effects Subcutaneous injections	Indefinite duration Resistance risk Long-term safety unknown

PegIFN: pegylated interferon; ROA: route of administration.

One-year survival rates for patients with cholestatic or alcoholic liver disease who undergo liver transplantation are greater than 90% in most liver transplant centers.[117] Historical data for liver transplants in patients with chronic HBV infection indicated that the spontaneous risk for allograft reinfection was approximately 80%.[117–120] This reinfection rate was associated with the initial liver disease and the hepatitis B viral load at the time of transplantation, and with allograft failure, retransplantation, or death. However, with appropriate post-transplant HBV prophylactic management, overall survival rates of patients who received a liver transplant for HBV-related cirrhosis have exceeded 85% at 1 year and 75% at 5 years, making liver transplantation a viable alternative for C.R.

CASE 80-12, QUESTION 13: What are the current recommendations for prevention of recurrent HBV infection after liver transplantation?

The most efficacious approach to preventing HBV recurrence after transplantation historically was with high-dose IV HBIG given in the anhepatic and postoperative periods. Daily IV HBIG in the early postoperative period with maintenance of serum anti-HBs levels of 100 IU/L or more had an overall survival (84%) that approached that observed in other transplant recipients without HBV infection.[119,120] Furthermore, patients receiving long-term HBIG administration (>6 months) compared with patients receiving short-term HBIG (<6 months) had a lower risk for recurrent HBV infection (35% vs. 75%) and longer 3-year actuarial survival (78% vs. 48%).[119,120]

Hepatitis B Immunoglobulin Dosage, Administration, and Adverse Effects

Over the years, many liver transplant centers routinely administered immunoprophylaxis with IV HBIG 10,000 IU (10 vials, 50 mL in 250 mL of saline) given in the anhepatic (recipient liver excised) phase, then gave 10,000 IU (50 mL infused for 4–6 hours) for the next 6 days postoperatively. HBIG (10,000 IU) was generally administered on a monthly basis for life, or discontinued if HBsAg becomes positive, indicating treatment failure.[119,120] This regimen was able to achieve trough anti-HBs titers of approximately 500 IU/L and up to 2,000 IU/L, which provided protection from HBV recurrence in the majority of transplanted patients. Patients who received HBIG oftentimes experienced a serum sickness-like syndrome (fever, myalgias) and were managed by receiving premedication (i.e., acetaminophen, diphenhydramine), thus prolonging the HBIG infusion (up to 6 hours), or discontinuing HBIG therapy altogether.[119,120]

Long-term concerns associated with HBIG administration included the potential for treatment failure (HBV reinfection from extrahepatic sites despite adequate anti-HBs titers), emergence of mutant viruses, and the prohibitive high cost of therapy (>$60,000/year).[119,120] Some data suggested that pharmacokinetic modeling and use of maintenance therapy with IM administration of HBIG (e.g., 2.5–10 mL every 2–3 weeks) after a reduced induction dose (e.g., 10,000 IU anhepatically, then 2,000 IU intravenously for six doses) could achieve similar outcomes and reduce the cost associated with IV administration of the drug.[119,120]

CASE 80-12, QUESTION 14: What is the role of oral antiviral agents in liver transplant recipients with HBV?

The nucleoside and nucleotide analogs, such as lamivudine, adefovir, entecavir, tenofovir DF and, more recently, TAF, potentially prevent recurrence of HBV in patients who undergo transplants for chronic HBV infection.[120,121] Lamivudine monotherapy was proven successful in converting HBV DNA-positive patients to negative status before and after liver transplantation. Resistance in transplant and nontransplant recipients also has been observed.[120,121]

Nucleoside analogs are not FDA-approved for this prophylaxis in the United States. Several transplant centers, however, have implemented clinical protocols that administer adefovir, entecavir, or tenofovir DF before transplantation to achieve undetectable HBV DNA viral loads at the time of transplant, then combine one of these agents with HBIG in the postoperative setting.[120,121] Ultimately, these management strategies have emerged as a clinical standard in the preoperative and early postoperative period because they are effective and have low rates of resistance. Future considerations for preventing recurrent HBV infection after transplantation include combining oral nucleoside (adefovir, entecavir) with nucleotide (tenofovir DF) analogs, thus avoiding HBIG altogether.[121] At the moment, safety and efficacy data are very limited for TAF in liver transplant recipients.

HEPATITIS C VIRUS

Virology

HCV is recognized now as the most common cause of chronic NANB transfusion-associated hepatitis.[122,123] HCV is a positive-sense, single-stranded RNA virus in the *Flaviviridae* family that is 50 to 65 nm in diameter (see Table 80-1). It causes acute and chronic HCV infection in humans and chimpanzees. If untreated, chronic HCV can progress to cirrhosis and HCC in a subset of patients.[124] The infectious viral structure is comprised of envelope glycoproteins in a lipid bilayer that contain the viral core protein and RNA.[125] After entry into the hepatocyte, the viral RNA is translated through host machinery into a polyprotein, which is cleaved during and after translation by both host- and viral-encoded proteases into mature viral proteins and nonstructural (NS) proteins (Fig. 80-6).

Epidemiology

The worldwide prevalence estimated that up to 180 million people are infected with chronic hepatitis C. This estimate included high-risk populations, such as people who inject drugs, hemodialysis patients, cancer patients, and paid blood donors. Excluding the high-risk populations, the global prevalence of HCV infection, based on anti-HCV, was 1.6% (1.3%–2.1%) corresponding to 115 (92–149) million past viremic infections.[126–128] The estimated prevalence is conservative as it did not include high-risk populations (e.g., hemodialysis patients, cancer patients, paid blood donors, and injection drug users). The majority of these infections, 104 million, were among adults with an anti-HCV infection rate of 2.0%. There are six genotypes reported for HCV worldwide. Globally, the genotype 1 distribution is most common, accounting for 46% of all infections, followed by genotype 3 (22%), genotypes 2 and 4 (13% each). Subtype 1b accounted for 22% of all infections.[129] A further analysis of the genotype distribution across the global regions shows that genotype 1 is prevalent in Australia, Europe, Latin America, and North America (53%–71% of all cases), and genotype 3 accounting for 40% of all infections in Asia.[130–133] Genotype 4 is the most common (71%) in North America, Egypt, and the Middle East.[132]

HCV infection occurs among persons of all ages, but the highest incidence is among persons aged 20 to 39 years, with a male predominance. Blacks and whites have similar incidence rates of acute disease, whereas persons of Hispanic ethnicity have higher rates. In the general population, the highest prevalence rates of chronic HCV infection are found among persons aged 30 to 49 years and among males.[124,134,135] Unlike the racial or ethnic pattern of acute disease, blacks have a substantially higher prevalence of chronic HCV infection than do whites. In the United States, the predominant HCV genotype is type 1, with subtypes 1a and 1b accounting for 70% of cases.[134,136] Knowledge of the genotype or serotype (genotype-specific antibodies) of HCV is helpful in making recommendations and counseling regarding therapy. Once the genotype is identified, it need not to be tested again; genotypes do not change during the course of infection. Because HCV has a high mutation rate during replication, several so-called quasi-species, a heterogeneous population of HCV isolates that are closely related, may,

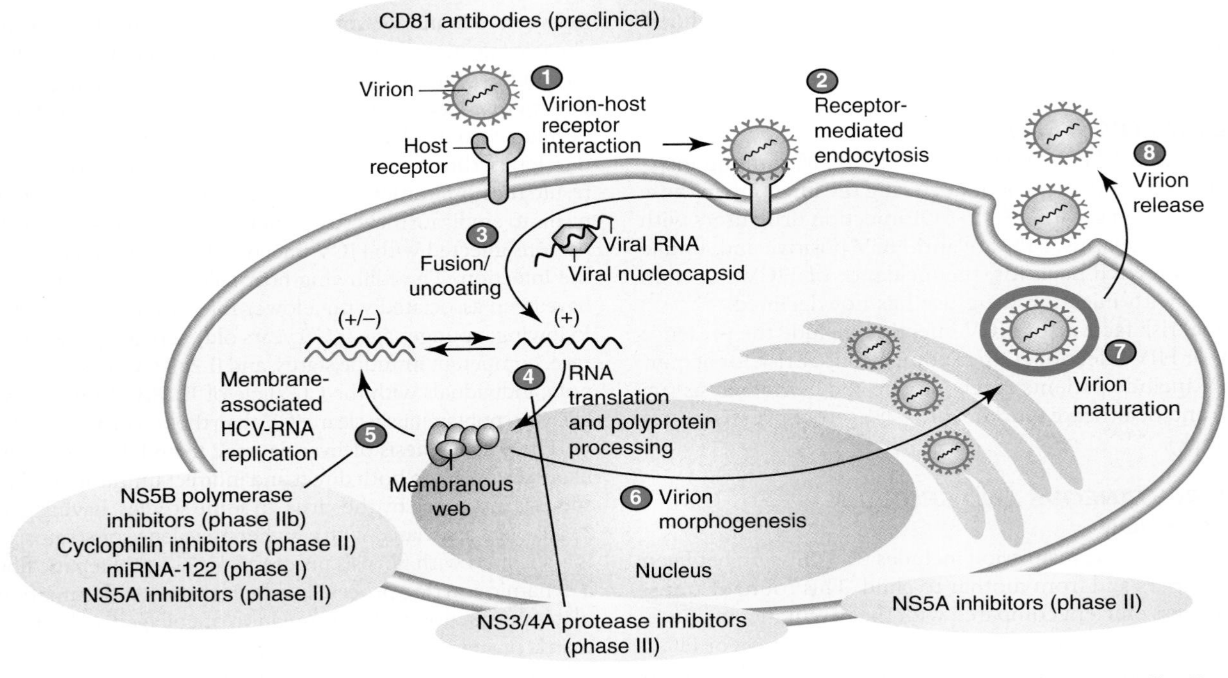

Figure 80-6 Hepatitis C virus life cycle. (Source: Ciesek S, Manns MP. Hepatitis in 2010: the dawn of a new era in HCV therapy. *Nat Rev Gastroenterol Hepatol*. 2011;8(2):69–71.)

however, exist in an infected individual.[134,136] The number of quasi-species increases during the course of infection, which allows HCV to escape the host's immune system, leading to persistent infection. In 2012, the CDC issued a new recommendation that all adults born from 1945 through 1965 (the "baby boomer" birth cohort) should undergo one-time hepatitis C testing without prior ascertainment of HCV risk status.[137] The specific cohort is selected based on data reporting HCV prevalence, disease burden, and cost-effectiveness analysis of routine screening.[138] The prevalence of anti-HCV found in this cohort is approximately 3.5%.[138,139] Furthermore, an estimated 70% of all hepatitis C-related deaths are attributed to this cohort. Birth cohort screening linked with effective hepatitis C treatment is presumed to significantly reduce future cases of decompensated cirrhosis, HCC, liver transplantation, and HCV-related deaths. The CDC screening recommendation for this cohort is also supported by the United States Preventive Services Task Force (USPSTF) and the American Association for the Study of Liver Disease, particularly for those with high-risk behaviors, risk exposure, and medical conditions associated with HCV acquisition.[140,141]

Similar to other hepatitis virus infections, acute HCV infection is defined as having an infection <6 months following acquisition of HCV. Acute HCV infection could occur whether or not the person develops clinical signs or symptoms of acute hepatitis. Six months is usually the time period to define an acute infection based on evidence that most individuals who clear HCV will do so by 6 months. Oftentimes, patients with acute HCV infection do not have a distinct symptomatic illness and most are not aware of their recent exposure to hepatitis C. If symptoms from acute infection develop, they usually develop within the first 4-12 weeks after infection and may persist between 2 and 12 weeks.[142,143] The clinical manifestations of acute HCV infection are similar to other types of viral hepatitis (e.g., jaundice, flu-like symptoms, dark urine and white stool, nausea, abdominal pain and malaise).[144] Approximately 15-20% of symptomatic acute liver disease in the United States is reported as resulting from acute HCV.[145] There are many potential sources of exposure to HCV, such as percutaneous transmission (e.g., blood transfusion, injection drug use, procedures involving potentially reused needles, tattooing, body-piercing and acupuncture) and nonpercutaneous transmission (e.g., sexual contact, high-risk sexual practices and exposure to nosocomial exposure to contaminated equipment).

PERCUTANEOUS TRANSMISSION

The incidence of HCV infection is 48% to 90% among injection drug users, and the risk of acquiring the infection in these persons is as high as 90%.[124,125,134] Of injection drug users with acute NANB hepatitis, 75% are anti-HCV positive and, unlike transfusion-related hepatitis, the incidence of HCV infection associated with injection drug use has not declined.[124,125,134] Additional risk factors for HCV infection include the presence of HBV or HIV infection. Other populations at risk for acquiring HCV include patients receiving chronic hemodialysis (up to 45%) and healthcare workers (0%–4% seroconversion after needlestick).[124,125,134]

NONPERCUTANEOUS AND SPORADIC TRANSMISSION

Nonpercutaneous transmission includes transmission between sexual partners and from mother to child. This route of transmission is less efficient compared with the percutaneous route, and is supported by data assessing sexual transmission of HCV. The risk of sexual transmission appears to be highest with male-to-male exposures, particularly with physically traumatic or rough sex.[142,143]

CASE 80-13

QUESTION 1: A 30-year-old woman presents to the clinic 3 months after having a diagnosis of chronic hepatitis C infection. Her past medical history shows that she was injecting crystal methamphetamine intermittently for 6 years, but denies using any drugs for 3 months. She is accompanied on the visit by her HCV-negative boyfriend and they ask you regarding her hepatitis C infection and her risk of transmitting hepatitis C to others. They have been together in a monogamous relationship for 2 years. What is her risk of transmitting hepatitis C to her boyfriend?

The couple do not need to alter their sexual practices. The CDC has issued recommendations regarding counseling recommendations for persons infected with hepatitis C. Patients should be counseled not to share needles or any of the injection materials, such as cookers, cottons, water, or the actual drug. The risk of HCV transmission among long-term, monogamous, discordant couples is very low. Therefore, the CDC recommends couples in that setting do not need to alter their sexual practices. The risk of HCV transmission among men who have sex with men is likely significant, especially with rough sexual activity. Household transmission of HCV can potentially occur via razors or toothbrushes, but it is not considered a risk to share food, water, or eating utensils.[141]

Compared with the high incidence of perinatal transmission of HBV from mothers to infants, perinatal transmission of HCV infection is relatively low. In general, it is considered safe for HCV-infected women to breastfeed their infants, with the exception that most experts recommend stopping breastfeeding if the mother's nipples (or surrounding area) are cracked and bleeding. The mother can temporarily pump her breast milk (and discard it) and then resume breastfeeding after the nipple region has healed.[141] Additional concerns and areas for investigation related to mother-to-infant transmission of HCV include the timing of transmission (in utero, time of birth) and the natural history of perinatally acquired infection.

Natural History and Pathogenesis

Between 75% and 85% of persons who acquire HCV will develop chronic infection.[146] The rate of viral production is high, between 10^{10} and 10^{12} virions daily, and the lack of proofreading by the viral polymerase leads to a broad genetic diversity. Among those who develop chronic HCV infection, approximately 20% to 25% will develop cirrhosis 20 to 30 years after HCV acquisition.[147–149] As a result, the host immune system has a major challenge in its mechanisms to eradicate the virus.[150] Nevertheless, a small percentage of persons infected with HCV infection have spontaneously cleared the infection. The following host factors or characteristics that have been associated with a lower rate of chronicity include the following: younger age (<20 years old), female gender, nonblack race, competent immune status, and IL28B CC genotype.[151,152] Of note, individuals with the CC allele of IL28B genotype are more likely to spontaneously clear HCV than those with CT or TT alleles.

The pathogenesis of liver damage from HCV infection most likely results from both direct and indirect immune-mediated responses instigated by the virus. In some studies, having genotype 3a has been associated with a higher prevalence of steatosis, which is associated with fibrosis progression.[147,153,154] Hepatic fibrosis is a dynamic scarring process in which chronic inflammation stimulates production and accumulation of collagen and extracellular matrix proteins. Over time, with chronic HCV infection, the total collagen content increases and fibrosis can develop, with potential progression to cirrhosis. Fibrosis is a precursor to cirrhosis.[153,154] For persons infected with HCV infection, factors that can influence an increased rate of progression of liver fibrosis include acquisition of HCV at an older age (>40 years old), male sex, heavy alcohol use, heavy marijuana use, coinfection with HIV or HBV, and metabolic factors (e.g., steatosis and insulin resistance).[155–160] For persons who develop hepatitis C-related cirrhosis, there is an estimated 1% to 4% risk per year of developing HCC.[149,161]

Diagnosis and Screening

Two classes of assays are used in the diagnosis and management of HCV. These include serologic assays that detect specific antibody to HCV (anti-HCV) and molecular assays that detect viral nucleic acid. These assays are not used to assess the severity of disease or predict prognosis in patients infected with HCV.

Screening for additional causes and contributors of liver disease and abnormal liver function tests should be part of the diagnosis process of liver disease. There are nonviral causes of hepatic inflammation, hereditary, and acquired conditions. Secondary causes of liver disease may include alcoholic liver disease, nonalcoholic fatty liver disease (NAFLD), α-1 antitrypsin (AAT) deficiency, hemochromatosis (excessive accumulation of iron in the liver), and autoimmune hepatitis.

LABORATORY STUDIES AND SEROLOGIC ASSAYS

The laboratory studies that are commonly used to evaluate HCV infection are HCV RNA, antibodies to HCV (anti-HCV), and ALT. Persons who become infected with HCV may develop abnormal laboratory findings in the following order: detectable HCV RNA, elevation in ALT, and anti-HCV.[162–163]

CASE 80-14

QUESTION 1: N.P. is a 27-year-old, law student who presents to clinic to his routine medical evaluation. He complains to his primary care physician of having recent flu-like symptoms and nausea. He also reports noticing dark urine color and was told by his friends that he is looking "yellow and pale." N.P. has a remote history of IV drug and alcohol use.

Recent laboratory tests reveal the following results:

ALT: 350 IU/L
Serum anti-HCV: positive
HCV RNA level: 1,100,000 IU/mL

What are the clinical and serologic features of acute HCV infection in N.P.?

N.P. clearly presents with a clinical picture consistent with acute HCV infection, including symptoms of fatigue, headache, and dark urine color. His laboratory tests show elevated ALT, positive anti-HCV, and detectable HCV RNA levels.

HCV RNA is usually detected in blood within 1 to 2 weeks after infection by a nucleic acid test (NAT). Qualitative, quantitative, and genotype test results are also performed for the HCV RNA. The period from infection until HCV RNA is detectable in plasma (by a commercially available assay) is referred to as the "eclipse phase," or "previremic phase." During this phase, the probability of establishment of HCV infection in susceptible hepatocytes is most likely. The eclipse phase is followed by an 8- to 10-day "ramp-up" phase in which HCV replication increases exponentially and readily becomes detectable in plasma. The "plateau phase" follows afterward with the HCV RNA viral load levels peaking 6 to 10 weeks after injection, and remains near these peak levels for approximately 40 to 60 days.[163,164] During an acute infection, detection of HCV RNA is not very reliable because RNA levels could fluctuate significantly. However, detectable HCV RNA levels are more uniform and present at the onset of symptoms.[142,165]

Between 4 and 12 weeks after infection, patients may have liver cell injury resulting in an elevation in serum ALT levels. Increases in ALT occur 1 to 2 weeks after detectable HCV RNA levels are present, and precede the development of anti-HCV. Usually, after an acute infection, the mean ALT could increase to 800 IU/L range. The CDC uses an ALT >200 IU/L during the period of acute illness as part of the diagnostic criteria.[162]

The last of the three abnormal laboratory findings associated with HCV infection is the presence of antibodies to HCV in the blood. Anti-HCV is usually detectable between 8 and 12 weeks after infection. Approximately after 12 weeks, >90% of patients will have positive anti-HCV. This is referred to as the "serologic window period," which describes the time period from initial infection until seroconversion.[143] Having detectable anti-HCV does not clearly differentiate acute from chronic HCV infection. Moreover, anti-HCV is not a reliable marker to diagnose acute HCV because only approximately 50% to 70% of patients have detectable anti-HCV at the onset of symptoms.[164,165]

CASE 80-14, QUESTION 2: After N.P. or any other person becomes infected with HCV, what is the typical sequence of laboratory findings?

Detectable HCV RNA, then increased aminotransferase levels, then anti-HCV positive.

The gold standard for the laboratory diagnosis of acute HCV infection is anti-HCV seroconversion (negative anti-HCV before suspected exposure and positive anti-HCV following exposure) combined with a positive HCV RNA viral load test.[145,164] However, because no many patients are unaware of their exposure or risk of infection, they may not present to their healthcare providers early enough to be evaluated and diagnosed. Oftentimes, acute HCV is diagnosed based on the first-time detection of HCV RNA and newly elevated ALT compared to negative laboratory results at baseline. Close follow-up of patients who have encountered high-risk exposures is recommended to establish the diagnosis and their treatment care. The laboratory testing for a known exposure to HCV is recommended as follows[162,166]:

- At initial presentation: anti-HCV, HCV RNA and ALT
- At 4 weeks from time of suspected exposure: anti-HCV, HCV RNA, and ALT
- At 12 weeks from time of suspected exposure: anti-HCV, HCV RNA, and ALT

CASE 80-14, QUESTION 3: According to the CDC 2016 case definition of acute hepatitis C, what level of increased ALT is required as part of the clinical description?

An ALT >200 IU/L. N.P.'s ALT result is 350 IU/L.

Acute HCV infection rarely causes a life-threatening illness. The CDC 2016 case definition for acute hepatitis C includes clinical and laboratory criteria, case classification as probable or confirmed, and criteria to distinguish a new case from an existing case.[162] Clinical criteria of acute hepatitis C is described as an illness with an onset of any sign or symptom consistent with acute viral hepatitis (e.g., fever, headache, abdominal pain, malaise, anorexia, nausea, vomiting, and diarrhea) combined with jaundice, or a peak-elevated serum ALT level >200 units/L during the acute illness phase.[162,165,166]

As part of the comprehensive patient work-up, a complete laboratory evaluation of the patient with chronic HCV infection includes the following[152,165,167]:

- General: CBC, platelet count, serum creatinine, and thyroid function tests (TSH). Because some studies have shown that persons with vitamin D deficiency have reduced response to hepatitis C treatment, some experts recommend obtaining baseline vitamin D levels (1,25-OH vitamin D).

- Hepatic inflammation and function: ALT or aspartate aminotransferase (AST), total and direct bilirubin, alkaline phosphatase, serum albumin, INR.
- Assays to detect coinfections: hepatitis A antibody, hepatitis B surface antigen, hepatitis B core antibody, hepatitis B surface antibody, HIV antibody.
- HCV RNA level (viral load): a quantitative HCV RNA viral load to confirm that the patient has chronic HCV infection, and to establish a pretreatment baseline level. In the absence of treatment, it is not necessary to repeatedly assess the HCV RNA levels because monitoring values over time does not provide useful prognostic information.
- HCV genotype: HCV exists as one of six distinct genotypes with significantly different clinical characteristics, mostly with respect to treatment response rates. In the United States, HCV genotype 1 is the most common, accounting for between 70% and 74% of prevalent cases. Knowing the HCV genotype is very important because response to antiviral therapy is very different among different genotypes and treatment protocols differ substantially.
- IL-28B testing: This is a single-nucleotide polymorphism (SNP) at the IL-28B locus that codes for interferon lambda and strongly correlates with HCV treatment response, especially with interferon-based therapies. Since the emergence and successful cure rates, or sustained virologic response (SVR) with the direct-acting antiviral (DAA) drugs, interferon-based therapies are no longer recommended for chronic HCV treatment. This test is now optional.

Serologic assays in terms of noninvasive, serum markers have clinical utility in predicting the presence or absence of significant fibrosis or cirrhosis and, however, are not useful in differentiating between intermediate stages of fibrosis. The indirect markers include the aspartate aminotransferase-to-platelet ratio index (APRI), FIB-4, FibroIndex, Forns Index, HepaScore (FibroScore), FibroSure, and FibroTest-ActiTest.

The APRI model is an easily calculated method to predict significant, severe fibrosis or cirrhosis. It is calculated using the patient's aspartate aminotransferase (AST) level and platelet count, and the upper limit of normal of AST level. A meta-analysis of 40 studies found that an APRI cut-off of greater than or equal to 0.7 had an estimated sensitivity (77%) and specificity (72%) for detection of significant hepatic fibrosis (greater than or equal to F2 by METAVIR). A cut-off score of a least 1.0 has an estimated sensitivity (61%–76%) and specificity (64%–72%) for detection of severe fibrosis/cirrhosis (F3–F4 by METAVIR). For detection of cirrhosis, a cut-off score of at least 2.0 was more specific (91%), but less sensitive (46%).[168–171] APRI has good diagnostic utility for predicting severe fibrosis or cirrhosis, but does not accurately differentiate intermediate fibrosis from mild or severe fibrosis. The liver guidelines recommend using APRI with other noninvasive markers of fibrosis.

The FIB-4 is a simple, quick, and inexpensive test that provides results immediately. The result is generated using age, AST, ALT, and platelet count. A cut-off value of less than 1.45 has a sensitivity (74%) and specificity (80%) in excluding significant fibrosis. A cut-off value >3.25 has a specificity (98%) in confirming cirrhosis. FIB-4 has valid utility in excluding or confirming cirrhosis; however, values between 1.45 and 3.25 do not clearly discriminate fibrosis.[172] Thus, additional methods to predict liver fibrosis are recommended.

The FibroIndex is a simple scoring method comprised of three biochemical markers: AST, platelet count, and gamma globulin. A cut-off value ≤ 1.25 has a sensitivity (40%) and specificity (94%) for mild fibrosis (F0 or F1 by METAVIR). In contrast, a cut-off value ≥ 2.25 has a sensitivity (36%) and specificity (97%) for significant fibrosis (F2 or F3 by METAVIR). Patients with F4 fibrosis were not included in the study.[173]

The Forns Index uses a complicated calculation method. It incorporates parameters, such as age, gamma glutamyltransferase (GGT), cholesterol, and platelet count. A cut-off value of <4.25 has a negative predictive value of 96% for excluding significant fibrosis (F2, F3, or F4). On the other hand, a cut-off of >6.9 has a positive predictive value of 66% for significant fibrosis (F2, F3, or F4). The Forns Index is useful and has good predictive value in selecting those with low risk of significant fibrosis, but does not reliably predict more advanced fibrosis or cirrhosis.[174] Patients with genotype 3 HCV infection may have varying cholesterol levels; thus, the Forns Index should not be used in these patients.

The HepaScore or FibroScore algorithm is more complex than other indirect markers. Additional fibrosis markers (i.e., age, sex, total bilirubin, GGT, α-2-macroglobulin, and hyaluronic acid levels) are included in the equation. Cut-off value ≤ 0.2 has a negative predictive value of 98% to exclude fibrosis. In contrast, cut-off value ≥ 0.8 has a positive predictive value of 62% for predicting cirrhosis.[175] The HepaScore has good utility at excluding significant fibrosis, but not as good at predicting cirrhosis.

The FibroSure and FibroTest-ActiTest are identical tests marketed in the United States and Europe. FibroSure is the test available in the United States. These tests are utilized to assess liver inflammation and fibrosis. The FibroSure provides estimates of grade and stage of fibrosis. It includes patient age and gender along with a composite of six biochemical markers associated with hepatic fibrosis: α-2-macroglobulin, haptoglobulin, GGT, apolipoprotein A1, total bilirubin, and ALT. The cut-off value <0.31 has a negative predictive value of 91% for the absence of clinical significant fibrosis. The positive predictive value for presence of significant fibrosis at a cut-off value >0.48 was 61% and cut-off of 0.72 was 76%.[176] There are contraindications to using the FibroSure test (e.g., Gilbert disease, acute hemolysis, extrahepatic cholestasis, post-transplantation, or renal insufficiency), which may result in inaccurate quantitative calculations and predictions.

Aside from the invasive, indirect markers for predicting liver fibrosis or cirrhosis, there are direct markers of fibrosis. Direct markers of fibrosis include procollagen type (II, III, IV), matrix metalloproteinases, cytokines, and chemokines. These markers exhibit variable effectiveness in predicting liver fibrosis. The FIBROSpect II is the only commercially available test that combines hyaluronic acid, tissue inhibitor of a metalloproteinase-1 (TIMP-1), and α-1-macroglobulin to predict fibrosis stages (F2–F4). An index score of >0.42 indicates the presence of stage F2 to F4 fibrosis. The cut-off values for sensitivity and specificity are 80.6% and 71.4%, respectively.[176,177] The FIBROSpect II test is a good tool to use to determine the presence of absence of cirrhosis in patients who have contraindications to liver biopsy, or those who refuse it. These markers may serve as reliable clinical alternatives in patients who are not candidates for liver biopsy. If noninvasive methods provide a clear assessment of hepatic fibrosis, then a liver biopsy may not be needed or warranted.

Radiologic imaging of the liver has been effective noninvasive, diagnostic techniques for identifying cirrhosis and stratifying the stages of liver fibrosis. Several techniques that are currently been used include hepatic ultrasound, transient ultrasound elastography, and magnetic resonance elastography.

BIOPSY

Liver biopsy with histologic analysis continues to be the gold standard for diagnosing other causes of liver disease and establishing severity of fibrosis. It provides information on both the grade (degree of inflammation associated with ongoing liver disease injury) and the stage (amount of currently established fibrosis). Some factors (e.g., alcohol consumption, increased hepatic iron concentration, and steatosis) are associated with accelerated fibrosis progression and may elicit concern for advanced fibrosis.[178–180] Some limitations of a liver biopsy include its invasive technique, associated risks of bleeding and complications, and the probability of incorrectly staging fibrosis in about 20% of patients.[178–180] Because of these limitations and the development of noninvasive tests that estimate hepatic fibrosis, liver biopsy is now used less frequently.

IMMUNOCOMPROMISED PATIENTS

Kidney transplant recipients also have a high incidence of HCV infection (6%–28%), which may be acquired through dialysis before transplant or from the allograft or blood products after transplantation.[181,182] After kidney transplantation, elevation in aminotransferases is more common in anti-HCV-positive compared with anti-HCV-negative patients (48% and 14%, respectively), and cirrhosis has been reported with the former.[181,182]

Clinical and Extrahepatic Manifestations

Most patients with acute HCV infection are asymptomatic.[126,134,135] In contrast, approximately 40% of patients with chronic HCV infection will develop at least one extrahepatic manifestation. Specific extrahepatic conditions may vary, and their prevalence is estimates derived from observational studies. Extrahepatic manifestations and conditions include cryoglobulinemic vasculitis, renal disorders with or without cryoglobulinemia, dermatologic manifestations including cutaneous leukocytoclastic vasculitis and porphyria cutanea tarda, diabetes mellitus and metabolic syndrome, and lymphomas.[183–190] Successful eradication of HCV may reduce the risk of some extrahepatic manifestations (i.e., lymphoma and diabetes) and conditions (i.e., cryoglobulinemic vasculitis and renal disease).

Prevention of Hepatitis C

PRE-EXPOSURE PROPHYLAXIS

No vaccines are effective against HCV, and current measures to prevent hepatitis C infection have largely focused on identifying high-risk uninfected persons and counseling them on risk-reducing strategies to prevent infection. The CDC and the National Institutes of Health have published recommendations that address these issues.[126,162] Suggested primary preventive measures are that in healthcare settings, adherence to universal (standard) precautions for the protection of medical personnel and patients be implemented and that HCV-positive individuals should refrain from donating blood, organs, tissues, or semen. In some situations, the use of organs and tissues from HCV-positive individuals may be considered. For example, in emergency situations, the use of a donor organ in which the HCV status is either positive or unknown may be considered in an HCV-negative recipient after full disclosure and informed consent. Strategies should be developed to identify prospective blood donors with any history of injection drug use. Such individuals must be deterred from donating blood.

Furthermore, safer sexual practices, including the use of latex condoms, should be strongly encouraged in persons with multiple sexual partners. In monogamous long-term relationships, transmission is rare.[126–128] Although HCV-positive individuals and their partners should be informed of the potential for transmission, insufficient data exist to recommend changes in current sexual practice in persons with a steady partner. It is recommended that sexual partners of infected patients should be tested for antibody to HCV.

In households with an HCV-positive member, sharing razors and toothbrushes should be avoided.[126–128] Covering open wounds is recommended. Injection needles should be carefully disposed of using universal precaution techniques. It is not necessary to avoid close contact with family members or to avoid sharing meals or utensils. No evidence justifies exclusion of HCV-positive children or adults from participation in social, educational, and employment activities.

Additionally, pregnancy is not contraindicated in HCV-infected individuals. Perinatal transmission from mother to baby occurs in less than 6% of instances.[126–128] No evidence indicates that breast-feeding transmits HCV from mother to baby; therefore, it is considered safe. Babies born to HCV-positive mothers should be tested for anti-HCV at 1 year.

Finally, needle exchange and other safer injection drug-use programs may be beneficial in reducing parenterally transmitted diseases.[126–128] Expansion of such programs should be considered in an effort to reduce the rate of transmission of hepatitis C. It is important that clear and evidence-based information be provided to both patients and physicians regarding the natural history, means of prevention, management, and therapy of hepatitis C.

GOALS OF THERAPY

CASE 80-15

QUESTION 1: K.C., a 20-year-old woman, presents to clinic for evaluation of liver enzyme elevation. She recently saw her gynecologist and labs revealed marked ALT/AST increase. She denies any recent symptoms or change in health other than flu-like illness a few months ago. She currently works as a waitress at Denny's. She denies prior medical problems and taking any prescribed medications and herbal/OTC medications. K.C. reports that she has been using IV heroin since she was 15 at the mall and that her best friend just died of an overdose. She went on a binge after he died and was not careful about needle sharing. She previously tested (about a year ago) for HCV and HIV by her physician. The laboratory results were both negative.

Upon physical examination, she has multiple tattoos and body piercings, as well as a few track marks on arms. Her physical examination is otherwise unremarkable. Liver is not enlarged, and there are no asterixis (no stigmata of liver disease), ascites, nor jaundice. Abdominal ultrasound is normal.

ALT: 45 units/L
AST: 64 units/L
Serum anti-HCV: positive
HCV RNA level: 6.1 million IU/mL
HCV genotype 1a
FibroSure: F1 (mild form of fibrosis; no cirrhosis)

K.C. and her parents decide they want her to be treated. They agree to continue support. K.C. agrees to go to Narcotics Anonymous and see psychological counseling. What is the goal of therapy for K.C. and the definition of a sustained virologic response 12 (SVR12)?

K.C. clearly has a clinical picture consistent with chronic HCV infection, including symptoms of flu-like symptoms, an elevated ALT, positive anti-HCV, and detectable HCV RNA levels. A SVR12 is defined as the HCV RNA level remaining undetectable for 12 weeks after completing therapy. The primary goal of HCV therapy is achieving virologic cure, or a SVR24 which is defined as the HCV RNA level remaining undetectable 24 weeks after completion of therapy. A negative HCV RNA level is <25 IU/mL, below the level of detection by sensitive test assays.

The primary goal of HCV therapy is to achieve SVR, which is an undetectable HCV RNA level using a sensitive assay (<25 IU/mL)

12 weeks after completion of therapy for hepatitis C.[126] This is referred to as a SVR12. Among persons who achieve a SVR12, more than 99% proceed to achieve SVR24.[191] A long-term follow-up of patients who achieve a SVR24 has demonstrated nearly 100% remain HCV RNA-negative years after therapy.[192–194] In clinical terms, achieving SVR24 is comparable to achieving virologic cure or total eradication of the HCV.

The impact of a SVR is remarkably positive because patients have an improvement in liver inflammation and fibrosis compared to those who do not achieve a SVR. Study data from pooled analysis of paired liver biopsies before and 1 month to 6 years after treatment with standard interferon monotherapy, PegIFN monotherapy, or PegIFN with ribavirin showed those patients who had a SVR were twice likely to have lower necroinflammatory scores after treatment versus patients who relapsed (67% vs. 32%).[195] Other studies have also confirmed the long-term histologic benefit.[192–194,196] In a study involving the general population, patients with advanced fibrosis who underwent antiviral therapy and achieved a SVR had reduction in overall mortality, liver-related death, liver failure, and HCC when compared with those who did not achieve a SVR.[197] Most of this survival benefit from successful treatment response was associated with improved clinical outcomes, primarily because of lower rates of liver failure. In a meta-analysis of 35 studies, investigators showed a clear benefit in the 5-year overall survival with HCV treatment, including patients with cirrhosis and with HIV coinfection.[198] With regard to the extrahepatic manifestations, successful treatment of HCV is associated with improvement or remission of insulin resistance and diabetes mellitus.[199,200] Overall, an SVR is associated with reversal of hepatic inflammation and fibrosis, and can reduce the chance of dying from hepatitis C by at least 60%.[201]

FACTORS THAT PREDICT RESPONSE TO THERAPY

CASE 80-15, QUESTION 2: K.C.'s parents have read about HCV infection and how treatment response may be affected by the person's genotype. They ask you if K.C.'s genotype could affect her successful response to HCV therapy?

In the DAA therapy era, K.C.'s genotype should not really affect her response to treatment. Treatment responses are high across all genotypes if a DAA-based combination appropriate for the genotype is used. There are viral and host factors that predict a person's response to therapy, such as the HCV genotype, HCV RNA level, IL28B genotype, race, age, gender, and degree of hepatic fibrosis. The HCV has six major genotypes, numbered 1 through 6. During the interferon era of treatment and prior to the emergence of the potent DAA drugs, the genotype was the predictor of obtaining an SVR.[202–204] In contrast, the role of HCV genotype in predicting treatment response has lessened in its influence as the DAAs are highly efficacious in their treatment of all genotypes.

The HCV RNA level had an influence in the successful treatment outcome in the interferon era. Patients with high RNA levels and genotype 1 infection had approximately 27% lower chance of achieving a SVR.[205] In the current DAA era, however, the baseline HCV RNA has little impact on achieving a SVR. Of note, in a post hoc analysis, a very high baseline RNA level of >6 million IU/mL is associated with reduced likelihood of SVR with shorter duration (8 weeks) of therapy with ledipasvir–sofosbuvir.[206]

The polymorphisms in the IL28B gene is associated with a difference in treatment response rates for persons receiving interferon-based therapies. The CT or TT alleles were associated with a 40% lower SVR rate compared to patients with the CC allele.[207] The majority of African-Americans have either the less favorable genotypes (CT or TT). On the other hand, Asians have the highest proportion of the CC genotype that may lead to better response to interferon-based therapy. In the DAA era, IL28B genotype does not seem to influence treatment response. Similarly, in the DAA era, a person's race, age, and gender do not appear to have a significant influence on treatment response for HCV infection.

The degree of hepatic fibrosis may still influence the SVR rates for persons receiving DAA therapies. Advanced fibrosis, defined as F3 (precirrhosis or bridging fibrosis), and F4 (cirrhosis) were associated with a much lower virologic cure rate across all genotypes (between 10% and 20% lower) during the interferon era.[202–204] This is similarly observed in patients receiving DAA therapies. Patients with decompensated cirrhosis (Child-Pugh class B or C) had lower SVR rates (86%–87%) with 12-week treatment of ledipasvir/sofosbuvir compared with SVR rates of >95% in similarly treated noncirrhotic patients.[208] Current strategies to improve the SVR rates for patients with cirrhosis include adding ribavirin to the DAA combination therapies and lengthening the duration of therapy.

CURRENT TREATMENT STRATEGIES OF CHRONIC HEPATITIS C

Historically, genotype 1 hepatitis C was considered the most difficult to treat hepatitis C genotype. From 1998 to 2013, therapy evolved from interferon monotherapy, to PegIFN monotherapy, to PegIFN plus ribavirin, to triple therapy with PegIFN plus ribavirin plus an NS3/4A protease inhibitor (boceprevir or telaprevir), the first-generation DAA serine protease inhibitors. Research methodologies for enhancing the effectiveness of HCV treatments and improving virologic cure rates, or SVR, primarily focused on genotype 1. The most promising of these explorations has been the development of the DAA agents. These oral compounds are developed to directly target the specific steps within the viral replication genome of hepatitis C. In late 2013 and most of 2014, the standard of care (SOC) for initial therapy of genotype 1 comprised of PegIFN plus ribavirin plus either sofosbuvir or simeprevir. Since 2015, the SOC for genotype 1 including the rest of the six genotypes consists of all-oral, interferon-free therapy with DAA combination regimens because of their significant high SVR rates and better tolerability profile. With the SOC changed from PegIFN to the DAAs, the treatment duration was also shortened from the traditional 48 weeks to 24 and then to 12 weeks. These oral compounds are developed to directly target the specific steps within the viral replication genome of hepatitis C. The four classes of DAAs are defined by their mechanism of action and therapeutic target, such as the NS proteins 3/4A (NS3/4A) serine protease inhibitors, NS5B nucleoside polymerase inhibitors, NS5B non-nucleoside polymerase inhibitors, and NS5A inhibitors.[209]

According to the AASLD/IDSA HCV guidance, treatment should be offered to all persons with chronic HCV infection because the DAAs are safer, better tolerated, and more effective in achieving virologic cure.[210] There are absolute contraindications for DAA treatment: persons with short life expectancies (<12 months); the use of ribavirin in pregnant women, women who may become pregnant, or men whose female partners are pregnant.[211,212] Persons with chronic HCV infection who are of reproductive age and are to receive treatment that includes ribavirin should be strongly advised to use two forms of contraception during treatment and for at least 6 months following the end of treatment. Similarly, there are relative contraindications to considerations for initiating HCV treatment. They include active severe substance abuse, psychiatric issues not controlled or stabilized, and social issues that may negatively affect a person's adherence to treatment, laboratory, and scheduled office visits.

Direct-Acting Antivirals

CASE 80-15, QUESTION 3: Genotyping of K.C.'s HCV infection shows that she has genotype 1a. What pharmacologic agents are effective treatments for patients with chronic HCV infection genotype 1a?

K.C. has a lot of treatment options with the DAA combination therapies. She has no signs of cirrhosis, or decompensated disease with splenomegaly, ascites, coagulopathy, and esophageal varices. Furthermore, she does not have HIV or HBV coinfections that could accelerate the progression of hepatitis C. The DAA combination therapies are highly potent and successful in achieving >90% SVR rates for persons with genotype 1 (1a and 1b) HCV infection (Table 80-8).

NS3/4A Protease Inhibitors

The NS3/4A protease inhibitors function through two mechanisms. They block the NS3/4A serine protease, an enzyme involved in post-translational processing and replication of HCV. They disrupt the virus replication process by blocking the NS3 catalytic site or the NS3/NS4A interaction.[213] The NS3/NS4A protease inhibitors also block the TRIF-mediated Toll-like receptor signaling and Cardif-mediated retinoic acid-inducible gene 1 (RIG-1) signaling, which result in impaired induction of interferons and blocking viral elimination (see Table 80-8).

Telaprevir and **boceprevir** were the first-generation NS3/4A protease inhibitors for HCV treatment. They were used in combination with PegIFN-α2a plus ribavirin for the treatment of genotype 1 infection. The clinical importance of telaprevir and boceprevir substantially diminished because of their cumbersome administration, substantial adverse effects, drug–drug interactions, and low barrier to resistance. As more-potent and better-tolerated protease inhibitors were developed and approved for HCV treatment without PegIFN-α2a and ribavirin, telaprevir and boceprevir eventually became clinically obsolete. The newer protease inhibitors have fewer drug–drug interactions, improved dosing schedules, and fewer severe adverse effects. In spite of their improved efficacy against genotype 1 infection, the newer protease inhibitors have limited efficacy against other genotypes and lower barrier to resistance.[214] The subsequent-generation protease inhibitors available in the United States include simeprevir, grazoprevir, and paritaprevir. Asunaprevir is available in Japan.

Simeprevir is the first second-generation, macrocyclic protease inhibitor. It is approved as 150-mg capsule for the use in combination with PegIFN-α2a plus ribavirin, or in combination with sofosbuvir with or without ribavirin for chronic HCV genotype 1 infection.[215] Simeprevir is administered orally once daily with food and should not be used as monotherapy. No dose adjustment is required in patients with renal impairment. Simeprevir cannot be used in patients with moderate (Child-Pugh class B) or severe (Child-Pugh class C) hepatic impairment because of two- to fivefold increases in drug exposure. Higher simeprevir exposure was reported in patients of East Asian ancestry; thus, simeprevir should be used with caution for this patient population.[216]

TABLE 80-8
Comparison of Direct-Acting Antiviral Agents for HCV Treatment[243]

	Protease Inhibitors	NS5B Polymerase Inhibitors	NNPI	NS5A Inhibitors
DAA agents	Grazoprevir Paritaprevir Simeprevir	Sofosbuvir	Dasabuvir	Daclatasvir Elbasvir Ledipasvir Ombitasvir Velpatasvir
MOA	Block the function of the NS3/NS4A serine protease	Block the function of the NS5B polymerase	Block the function of the NS5B polymerase	Block the replication complex and regulation
Activity against genotype	Grazoprevir: 1,4,6[a] Paritaprevir: 1 Simeprevir: 1	1–4	1	Daclatasvir: 1–3 Elbasvir: 1,4,6[a] Ledipasvir: 1,4,5,6 Ombitasvir: 1 Velpatasvir: 1–6
Potency	High (varies by GT)	Moderate-to-high (consistent across GTs)	Varies by GT	High (against multiple GTs)
Barrier to resistance	Low (GT 1a < GT 1b)	High (1a = 1b)	Very low (1a < 1b)	Low (1a < 1b)
Potential for drug interactions	High	Low	Variable	Low-to-moderate
Adverse effects	Rash, anemia, bilirubin increase	Mitochondrial toxicity; drug interactions with HIV drugs (NRTIs) and RBV	Variable	Variable
Dosing	Daily to 3 times daily	Daily to 2 times daily	Daily to 3 times daily	Daily
Comments	Future-generation PIs will have pangenotypic activity and will have higher barriers to resistance	Single target for binding at the active site of viral replication	Many targets for binding at allosteric sites	Multiple antiviral MOA

MOA, mechanism of action; NS5B, nonstructural protein 5B; NNPIs, non-nucleoside polymerase inhibitors; NS5A, nonstructural protein 5A; GT, genotype; HIV, human immunodeficiency virus; NRTIs, nucleos(t)ide RT inhibitors; RBV, ribavirin.
[a]Elbasvir/grazoprevir has activity against HCV genotype 6, but not FDA-approved for treating this genotype.

Simeprevir is overall well tolerated although pruritus and nausea have been reported. In clinical trials, treatment discontinuations from adverse effects were uncommon.[217,218] However, photosensitivity and rash have occurred that led to serious reactions requiring hospitalization for some patients in the trials. Patients taking simeprevir should be cautioned about the risk of photosensitivity and rash, and to use sun-protective measures and/or limit sun exposure while on treatment. If a severe rash or photosensitivity reaction occurs, simeprevir should be discontinued. Transient, mild elevations in bilirubin have been reported, which may result from decreased bilirubin elimination related to inhibition of the hepatic transporters OATP1B1 and MRP2. This does not suggest worsening of hepatic function.

With regard to drug interactions, simeprevir is oxidatively metabolized by CYP3A isoenzyme, primarily the hepatic and intestinal CYP3A4.[219] Coadministration with potent inducers and inhibitors of CYP3A4 will affect the serum levels of simeprevir. It is observed to inhibit the OATP1B1/3 transporter; therefore, serum levels of substrates of OATP1B1/3 (atorvastatin and rosuvastatin) could increase.[215]

The efficacy of simeprevir is affected by the presence of resistance mutations or polymorphisms of the NS3/4A protease. In particular, the presence of Q80K polymorphism was associated with a lower SVR rate (58% vs. 84% if the Q80K was not present).[216] However, data suggest that the Q80K mutation does not significantly affect SVR rates when simeprevir is coadministered with sofosbuvir, an NS5B polymerase inhibitor.[220] The emergence of other resistance mutations during unsuccessful treatment with either telaprevir or boceprevir, such as R155K and A156T/V, has been reported to affect the clinical response to simeprevir.[215]

Grazoprevir is a potent, second-generation protease inhibitor that is only available in combination with an NS5A inhibitor, elbasvir. Grazoprevir has activity against HCV genotypes 1, 4, and 6 and, however, is only FDA-approved for genotypes 1 and 4. (See elbasvir/grazoprevir section.)

Paritaprevir is the third, second-generation protease inhibitor FDA-approved for the treatment of HCV genotype 1 infection. It is coadministered with low-dose ritonavir, an HIV protease inhibitor, for pharmacokinetic enhancing effects via inhibition of CYP3A-mediated metabolism. Ritonavir does not have any anti-HCV activity. Paritaprevir and ritonavir are coformulated as a fixed-dose combination with ombitasvir, an NS5A inhibitor. (See paritaprevir/ritonavir/ombitasvir/dasabuvir section.)

NS5A Inhibitors

The NS5A inhibitors block the protein that has a role in viral replication and the assembly of the HCV (see Table 80-8).[221–222] The NS5A class is relatively potent and effective across all genotypes; however, it has a low barrier to resistance and variable toxicity profile. When coadministered with PegIFN and ribavirin, NS5A inhibitors can substantially reduce HCV RNA levels and improve SVR.[223] Available NS5A inhibitors in fixed-dose combinations with other DAAs comprise of ledipasvir, ombitasvir, and elbasvir. Daclatasvir is the only available, stand-alone NS5A inhibitor.

Daclatasvir (Daklinza) is a NS5A inhibitor mainly used in combination with sofosbuvir, a NS5B polymerase inhibitor. It has activity against HCV genotypes 1, 2, and 3. It is dosed as 60 mg orally once daily with or without food. It cannot be used as monotherapy and approved to be coadministered with sofosbuvir with or without ribavirin. If sofosbuvir is discontinued, daclatasvir should also be discontinued. Dose adjustments for patients with renal or hepatic impairment are not required. Daclatasvir is well tolerated with commonly reported adverse effects of headache, fatigue, and nausea from clinical trial data.[224,225]

Daclatasvir is metabolized via the CYP3A pathway and should not be coadministered with potent inducers, such as rifampin, phenytoin, carbamazepine, and Saint-John's-wort. The serum levels of daclatasvir will be significantly reduced to suboptimal efficacy. When coadministered with moderate CYP3A inducers (e.g., efavirenz, etravirine, dexamethasone, and nafcillin), the dose of daclatasvir should be increased to 90 mg once daily. On the other hand, when given with potent CYP3A inhibitors (e.g., HIV protease inhibitors, some azole agents, and clarithromycin), the dose of daclatasvir should be reduced to 30 mg once daily. Aside from the CYP450 system, daclatasvir also inhibits P-glycoprotein (P-gp), organic anion transporting polypeptide (OATP) 1B1 and 1B3, and the BCRP. Digoxin dose may need to be adjusted when coadministered with daclatasvir.

In vitro resistance mutations associated with daclatasvir include polymorphisms at M28, A30, L31, and Y93, which is the most clinically relevant. Based on the clinical trial data, the emergence of Y93H polymorphism was associated with lower SVR rates and responsible for several virologic failures.[225]

Elbasvir is a NS5A inhibitor only available as a fixed-dose combination with grazoprevir, a NS3/4A serine protease inhibitor. (See elbasvir/grazoprevir section.)

Ledipasvir is a NS5A inhibitor only available as a fixed-dose combination with sofosbuvir, a NS5B polymerase inhibitor. (See ledipasvir/sofosbuvir section.)

Ombitasvir is a NS5A inhibitor only available as a fixed-dose combination with the protease inhibitors paritaprevir and ritonavir, and administered in combination with dasabuvir, a NS5B non-nucleotide inhibitor. (See paritaprevir/ritonavir/ombitasvir with or without dasabuvir section.)

Velpatasvir is a NS5A inhibitor that has pangenotypic antiviral activity against genotypes 1 to 6. It is only available as a fixed-dose combination with sofosbuvir, a NS5B polymerase inhibitor. (See sofosbuvir/velpatasvir section.)

NS5B RNA-Dependent RNA Polymerase Inhibitors

NS5B is an RNA-dependent RNA polymerase involved in post-translational processing that is necessary for replication of HCV. The polymerase has a catalytic site for nucleoside binding and four other sites for non-nucleoside binding to cause an allosteric alteration. The enzyme structure is highly conserved across all six genotypes. Two classes of NS5B polymerase inhibitors include the nucleoside/nucleotide analogues (NPIs) and non-nucleoside analogues (NNPIs). The NPIs bind to the catalytic site of NS5B, whereas NNPIs function as allosteric inhibitors.[213,214]

Sofosbuvir (Sovaldi) is the first NS5B NPI available for HCV treatment. It should not be used as monotherapy and most effective when used in many combinations with other antivirals to treat different genotypes. Sofosbuvir is available as a 400-mg tablet and given orally once daily with or without food. It is primarily renally eliminated, however, pharmacokinetic studies suggest no dose adjustments are required for patients with mild or moderate renal impairment (eGFR >30 mL/minute/1.73 m^2).[226] Nevertheless, serum levels of sofosbuvir are increased in patients with severe renal impairment and receiving hemodialysis. There is insufficient data for dose-adjustment recommendations in these patients. Sofosbuvir can be given in patients with moderate (Child-Pugh class B) or severe (Child-Pugh class C) hepatic impairment and cirrhosis without dose adjustments.

Sofosbuvir is generally well tolerated. When given with PegIFN and ribavirin, the commonly reported adverse effects of sofosbuvir and ribavirin (with or without PegIFN) were fatigue, headache, nausea, insomnia, and anemia.[227,228] Concomitant use of sofosbuvir and sofosbuvir-containing regimens with amiodarone is contraindicated due to episodes of severe bradycardia and fatal cardiac arrest.[229,230]

As a substrate of the P-gp drug transporter, sofosbuvir has significant drug interactions with potent intestinal P-gp inducers that could decrease its serum levels. The coadministration of sofosbuvir with the anticonvulsants (e.g., carbamazepine, phenytoin, phenobarbital, oxcarbazepine), anti-tuberculosis drugs (e.g., rifampin, rifabutin, rifapentine), and Saint-John's-wort is contraindicated. Of note, the coadministration of sofosbuvir and amiodarone is also contraindicated.[229,230] In vitro resistance polymorphisms have been reported for sofosbuvir; however, their clinical significance is unclear.

Dasabuvir, unlike sofosbuvir, is a NS5B NNPI that is administered and packaged with paritaprevir/ritonavir/ombitasvir. (See paritaprevir/ritonavir/ombitasvir with or without dasabuvir section.) As a class, the NNPI class is less potent than the NPI class, is more specific for genotype 1, has a low-to-moderate barrier to resistance and a variable toxicity profile.[231]

CASE 80-15, QUESTION 4: According to the 2016 AASLD Guidelines, what fixed-dose DAA combination therapies could K.C. benefit from and for what duration length of treatment?

There are currently four FDA-approved fixed-dose combinations that are effective against HCV genotype 1 (and other genotypes). K.C. could benefit from either of the following:

- **a.** elbasvir 50 mg/grazoprevir 100 mg (Zepatier) 1 tablet orally once daily for 12 weeks;
- **b.** ledipasvir 90 mg/sofosbuvir 400 mg (Harvoni) 1 tablet orally once daily for 12 weeks;
- **c.** sofosbuvir 400 mg/velpatasvir 100 mg (Epclusa) 1 tablet orally once daily for 12 weeks; and
- **d.** paritaprevir 50 mg/ritonavir 33.33 mg/ombitasvir 8.33 mg plus dasabuvir 200 mg (PrOD; Viekira XR) 3 tablets orally once daily with food plus ribavirin (weight-based dosing) given in two divided doses for 12 weeks.

Fixed-Dose Combinations

Elbasvir/Grazoprevir

As a coformulated single tablet, elbasvir 50 mg plus grazoprevir 100 mg (Zepatier) is administered orally once daily for either 12 or 16 weeks.[232] This regimen is administered with or without weight-based ribavirin, depending on certain patient characteristics. Elbasvir/grazoprevir has been studied and approved for treatment of HCV and HIV coinfection. Patients should have documentation of baseline aminotransferases and be tested for current or previous HBV infection (HBsAg and anti-HBc) to ensure that there is no risk of HBV flares during HCV treatment. The regimen is the first of the newer DAA therapies that could be used in patients with renal impairment, including hemodialysis, without the need for dose adjustments. However, the regimen is contraindicated in patients with Child-Pugh class B or C cirrhosis. Prior to administering elbasvir/grazoprevir, patients with genotype 1a infection should be tested for the presence of NS5A resistance-associated substitutions (RASs) and NS3 protein polymorphisms. Preexisting NS5A polymorphisms that are associated with elbasvir resistance and lower SVR rates with the regimen in genotype 1a patients are found at positions M28, Q30, L31, and Y93.[233] Approximately 11% of genotype 1a viruses are estimated to harbor one of these polymorphisms prior to taking elbasvir/grazoprevir regimen. In the presence of one of the NS5A polymorphisms, ribavirin (weight-based) could be added to the regimen and the treatment course extended to improve the SVR rates. Of note, the polymorphisms do not affect the SVR rates in persons with genotype 1b virus infection. The polymorphisms in the NS3 protein, especially the Q80L polymorphism in genotype 1a virus, do not appear to affect treatment response and SVR rates. The other difference between the NS5A and NS3 polymorphisms appears to be the long persistence of the NS5A resistance mutations in the individuals after treatment.

Elbasvir/grazoprevir is overall well tolerated. From the large clinical trials, the most common adverse effects were headache, fatigue and nausea.[233,234] Approximately 1% of patients developed late aminotransferase elevations >5 times the upper limit of normal without associated bilirubin increases that resolved once the regimen was stopped. Aminotransferase monitoring at baseline and at week 8 of therapy (and at week 12, if the total duration is 16 weeks) is recommended.[232] The regimen should be discontinued if aminotransferase elevations are accompanied by other signs or symptoms of hepatic injury, such as jaundice, increased bilirubin, or INR. The regimen is primarily metabolized through CYP3A, and grazoprevir is a substrate of OATP1B1/3 transporters. The coadministration of elbasvir/grazoprevir is contraindicated with potent inducers (e.g., rifampin, phenytoin, carbamazepine, Saint-John's-wort, cyclosporine), efavirenz and HIV protease inhibitors. Furthermore, coadministration of the regimen is not recommended with ketoconazole, nafcillin, modafinil and antiretrovirals (etravirine or cobicistat).

Ledipasvir/Sofosbuvir

Sofosbuvir (400 mg) is combined with ledipasvir (90 mg), a NS5A inhibitor, as a fixed-dose combination (Harvoni) that is administered as a single tablet with or without food.[213] The regimen is given with or without weight-based ribavirin, depending on the patient population, and is active against HCV genotypes 1, 4, 5, and 6. The levels of sofosbuvir and its metabolite might accumulate in the setting of severe renal impairment (eGFR >30 mL/minute/1.73 m^2); thus, the combination should not be used until further data are available. Otherwise, no dose adjustment is needed for mild or moderate renal impairment, or in the setting of moderate (Child-Pugh class B) or severe (Child-Pugh class C) hepatic impairment.

Harvoni is well tolerated, and the common adverse effects include fatigue, headache, nausea, and insomnia. With regard to drug interactions, ledipasvir is also a substrate of the P-gp drug transporter. Similar to sofosbuvir, ledipasvir should not be coadministered with potent intestinal P-gp inducers because its serum levels will significantly decrease. Ledipasvir absorption is affected by gastric pH. The coadministration of ledipasvir with acid-suppressing agents could increase the gastric pH levels and decrease its absorption. If the regimen needs to be taken with proton pump inhibitors, the proton pump inhibitor dose should not exceed a dose comparable to omeprazole 20 mg daily. If the regimen is given with H_2 receptor antagonists, such as famotidine 40 mg or equivalent, both drugs should be administered twelve hours apart.[226]

The resistance profile of Harvoni has been associated with several NS5A mutations that reduce the susceptibility to ledipasvir, such as Q30R, Y93H/N and L31M in subtype 1a virus and Y93H in subtype 1b virus.[235] The presence of NS5A mutations does not require adjustment of duration or dosing of the combination regimen. Further data are warranted to make any clinical adjustments.

Sofosbuvir/Velpatasvir

Another fixed-dose combination regimen (Epclusa) comprises of sofosbuvir (400 mg) with velpatasvir (100 mg), a NS5A inhibitor. It is coformulated as a single tablet and administered once daily for 12 weeks with or without ribavirin. The regimen is active against all HCV genotypes. No dose adjustments are needed for mild-to-moderate renal impairment, or in the setting of moderate (Child-Pugh class B) or severe (Child-Pugh class C) hepatic impairment. The same renal precautions apply to this combination regimen because it contains sofosbuvir. The commonly reported adverse effects include headache, fatigue, nausea, nasopharyngitis, and insomnia.[236]

Similar to sofosbuvir, velpatasvir is a substrate of the P-gp drug transporter. Therefore, coadministration of the regimen with potent intestinal P-gp inducers can decrease both sofosbuvir and velpatasvir serum levels. The coadministration of Epclusa is contraindicated with anticonvulsants, anti-tuberculosis drugs, and Saint-John's-wort. Efavirenz can also significantly reduce the serum levels of velpatasvir and should not be coadministered. Velpatasvir is also an inhibitor of P-gp and thus may increase the absorption of P-gp substrates. Similar to ledipasvir, velpatasvir requires an acid gastric environment for optimal absorption. Proton pump inhibitors and H_2 receptor antagonists will increase the gastric pH levels, resulting in a decreased absorption of velpatasvir. If used with proton pump inhibitors, sofosbuvir/velpatasvir should be taken without food and 4 hours before omeprazole 20 mg or equivalent dose. The coadministration of amiodarone and sofosbuvir/velpatasvir is contraindicated because of severe bradycardia and cardiac arrest.[226] (See sofosbuvir section.)

Paritaprevir/Ritonavir/Ombitasvir plus Dasabuvir

The coformulated single tablet of paritaprevir/ritonavir/ombitasvir is given with dasabuvir, an NS5B non-nucleoside polymerase inhibitor. The regimen is called often referred to as PrOD (Viekira Pak, Viekira XR). PrOD can be taken with or without weight-based ribavirin, depending on the patient population, for the treatment of genotypes 1a and 1b without cirrhosis or with compensated cirrhosis. PrOD is also indicated in combination with ribavirin in liver transplant patients with any HCV genotype 1 subtype as long as hepatic function is normal and fibrosis is mild (Metavir score ≤2).[237] In contrast, the combination of paritaprevir/ritonavir/ombitasvir (Technivie) with ribavirin is approved for genotype 4 infections without cirrhosis. Technivie does not contain dasabuvir. Paritaprevir/ritonavir/ombitasvir, with or without dasabuvir, can be administered in HCV-infected patients with renal impairment. The administration of these regimens in patients with severe renal impairment (eGFR <30 mL/minute/1.73 m^2) has not been studied.[237] Dose adjustment for the regimens is not warranted for patients with mild (Child-Pugh class A) hepatic impairment. However, the regimens are contraindicated in patients with moderate-to-severe (Child-Pugh classes B and C) hepatic impairment. Hepatic decompensation was reported when the regimen is used, with or without dasabuvir, in patients with underlying cirrhosis.[238] Most of the reported cases occurred within 1 to 4 weeks of drug initiation, and some cases resulted in the need for liver transplantation or death.

PrOD is available in immediate-release and extended-release oral formulations. For the immediate-release formulation (Viekira Pak), two combination tablets (each containing 12.5 mg ombitasvir, 75 mg paritaprevir, and 50 mg ritonavir) are administered once daily. Dasabuvir is administered with the regimen as a single 250-mg tablet twice daily. For the extended-release formulation (Viekira XR), three tablets (each containing 8.33 mg ombitasvir, 50 mg paritaprevir, 33.33 mg ritonavir, and 200 mg dasabuvir) are administered once daily with ribavirin (weight-based dosing) in two divided doses with food. PrOD regimens should be taken with food and are generally well tolerated. The most commonly reported adverse effects in the trials that used the PrOD regimen with ribavirin included nausea, pruritus, insomnia, diarrhea, and asthenia.[239,240] Fatigue and headache were the most common side effects and may be attributable to the ribavirin component. Decreases in the hemoglobin level, by 2 to 2.5 g/dL, were also observed in patients taking regimens with ribavirin. The incidence of severe anemia (hemoglobin <8 g/dL) is uncommon.[239,240]

The components of PrOD are both substrates and inhibitors of CYP450 enzymes. The coadministration of paritaprevir/ritonavir/ombitasvir and dasabuvir is contraindicated with anticonvulsants, rifampin, Saint-John's-wort, oral contraceptives containing ethinyl estradiol and salmeterol.[237] Close monitoring and dose adjustments of certain drugs (e.g., HMG-CoAs, cyclosporine, tacrolimus, and antiarrhythmics) are recommended when given with the PrOD regimen.

The use of paritaprevir, ombitasvir, and dasabuvir can select for resistance mutations in NS3, NS5A, and NS5B, respectively, which will reduce the activity of a particular antiviral agent. In the clinical trials, the common resistance mutations that have emerged and/or caused treatment relapse among the genotype 1a infections were D168V in NS3, M28A/T/V and Q30E/K/R in NS5A, and S556G/R in NS5B.[239–242] In contrast, there were not many virologic failures in patients with HCV genotype 1b infection.

Future Treatment Options[243]

Several agents are currently under investigation for HCV genotype 1 infection, including voxilaprevir, ABT-493 plus ABT-530, and MK-3682 and MK-8408. Voxilaprevir is an investigational NS3/4A protease inhibitor currently studied in a coformulated combination with sofosbuvir-velpatasvir. This triple combination pill is intended to be used as short-duration treatment and as salvage therapy for DAA treatment failures.

The ABT-493 (NS3/4A protease inhibitor) plus ABT-530 (NS5A inhibitor) coformulated combination has pangenotypic activity currently under study as both an 8-week regimen for genotype 1 patients without cirrhosis and a 12-week salvage regimen for DAA-experienced patients.

The MK-3682 (NS5B inhibitor) plus MK-8408 (second generation NS5A inhibitor) are being studied in a variety of triple combinations with either grazoprevir or elbasvir as an 8-week regimen in genotype 1, 2, or 3 infection.

HEPATITIS D VIRUS

Virology and Epidemiology

HDV is a small, single-stranded circular RNA animal virus (36 nm) that is similar to defective RNA plant viruses (Table 80-1).[244–246] Between 15 and 20 million persons are infected with HDV globally, particularly in the Mediterranean basin, the Middle East, Central and Northern Asia, West and Central Africa, the Amazon basin, Colombia, Venezuela, Western Asia, and the South Pacific.[244–246] Vaccination for HBV significantly reduces the incidence of HDV. However, immigration from endemic areas, increased IV drug use, sexual practices, and body modification procedures have resulted in an increase in HDV prevalence in some regions. In the United States, an estimated 7,500 HDV cases occur annually.[247,248] The prevalence of HDV is greatest among persons with percutaneous exposure (e.g., injection drug users) and hemophiliacs (20%–53% and 48%–80%, respectively) and may be affected by additional factors such as duration of infection.[247,248] The modes of transmission of HDV are similar to those reported for HBV infection. Thus, HDV clearly represents a potential infectious hazard to patients susceptible to HBV and those who are chronic HBV carriers. Generally two major patterns of infection occur with HBV: coinfection and superinfection. Because infection by HDV requires the presence of active HBV, preventing HBV infection will prevent HDV infection in a susceptible patient.[248,249]

Pathogenesis

Limited data suggest that HDV antigen and HDV RNA are cytotoxic to hepatocytes; however, the immune response may also be important.[248,249] Furthermore, several autoantibodies associated with chronic HDV infection may play a role in propagating liver disease and could partially explain the differences in disease severity observed in patients with HDV plus HBV compared with those with HBV alone.

Diagnosis and Serology

Measuring HDV RNA (by RT-PCR) for HDV RNA confirms the presence of HDV and is currently the most accurate diagnostic tool available.[248,249] ELISA and radioimmunoassay tests for IgM anti-HDV are also commercially available. Measurement of anti-HDV is generally not useful for early diagnosis because detectable antibody levels are usually achieved late in the clinical course of the infection. Anti-HDV IgM is detectable before anti-HDV IgG in acute HDV coinfection and is diagnostic for acute HDV infection. Anti-HDV IgM levels are not sustained in self-limiting HDV infection but may persist in patients with chronic HDV infection. Also, anti-HDV IgM does not distinguish coinfection (HBV and HDV acquired simultaneously) from superinfection (HDV acquired in chronic HBV carrier).

Differentiation between coinfection and superinfection is made by the presence or absence of anti-HBc IgM. In acute coinfection, serum anti-HDV IgM and HDV RNA appear together with anti-HBc IgM, whereas in patients with superinfection, HDV markers are present in the absence of anti-HBc IgM. The presence and titer level of anti-HDV, in the case of persistent infection, also correlate with the severity of disease. Titers of anti-HDV IgG greater than 1:1,000 indicate ongoing viral replication.

HDV antigen is present in the serum in the late incubation period of acute infection and lasts into the symptomatic phase in up to 20% of patients. Because this antigen is transient, repeat testing may be required to detect its presence. HDV RNA is an early marker of infection in patients with both acute and chronic HDV infection.[248,249] HDV RNA is detectable in 90% of patients during the symptomatic phase of HDV infection. HDV RNA levels are not detectable after symptomatic resolution but remain elevated in chronic infection.

Natural History

Coinfection with HDV and HBV is correlated with a higher risk of severe or fulminant liver disease.[249,250] The rate of chronic disease after coinfection with HDV is similar to that of HBV infection alone, whereas superinfection with HDV is linked to a high rate of chronicity; however, the clinical course may be variable. Approximately 15% of patients superinfected with HDV develop rapidly progressive disease with hepatic decompensation (e.g., cirrhosis) within 12 months of the infection. Another 15% of patients have a benign course of illness. Most patients (70%) have a slow progression to cirrhosis, depending on age, IV drug use, and level of viral replication.[249] Finally, HBsAg-positive, HBeAg-positive patients who are superinfected with HDV are more likely to develop fulminant disease compared with those who are HBsAg-positive with anti-HBe and who are superinfected and develop chronic disease.[249,250]

Prevention

Hepatitis D virus replication is dependent on HBV replication; therefore, successful immunization with HBV vaccine also prevents HDV infection.[244–246] No immunoprophylactic therapies are available for patients with chronic HBV infection who are also at risk for superinfection with HDV. Prevention of HDV superinfection is based on behavioral modification, such as the use of condoms to prevent sexual transmission and needle exchange programs to minimize transmission by IV drug use.

Treatment

The goal of treatment is to eradicate HDV along with HBV. HDV is eradicated when both serum HDV RNA and HDV antigen in the liver become persistently undetectable. Notably, it is only when HBsAg clearance has taken place that complete clinical resolution occurs. Supportive care is the general strategy used to treat HDV infection. Because the development of FHF is more frequent with HDV infection, close monitoring for evidence of severe liver failure is warranted. Liver transplantation is the treatment of choice for patients with fulminant or end-stage liver disease after HDV infection. In patients with chronic HDV infection, antiviral therapy has been disappointing.[251–254]

In patients with decompensated cirrhosis caused by HDV, liver transplantation is the most appropriate intervention because IFN may precipitate hepatic decompensation.[251–254] The presence and amount of HBV DNA before transplantation is the most significant outcome marker, often predicting the post-transplant reinfection rate. Patients who receive a liver transplant for chronic HDV infection have a lower incidence of post-transplant HBV infection than do those with HBV infection alone (67% vs. 32%, respectively).[253,254] This is thought to be related to an inhibitory effect of HDV on HBV replication. Furthermore, 3-year survival is higher for patients with HDV cirrhosis than for patients undergoing transplantation for HBV cirrhosis alone (88% vs. 44%, respectively) and is similar to patients having liver transplantation for other indications.[117–119]

HEPATITIS E VIRUS

Virology, Epidemiology, Transmission, and Pathogenesis

HEV is an icosahedral, nonenveloped virus of the Hepeviridae family (Table 80-1). The HEV genome is a single-stranded polyadenylated RNA and, unlike HAV, has an RNA genome that encodes for NS proteins through overlapping open reading frames.[255,256] HEV sequences have been classified into four genotypes (1, 2, 3, and 4). Genotype 1 consists of epidemic strains in developing countries; genotype 2 has been found in Mexico; genotype 3 has been associated with acute cases of hepatitis and with domestic pigs in the United States, European countries, and Japan; and genotype 4 has been found in Asian countries.[257–260]

HEV occurs in endemic areas such as Africa, Southeast and Central Asia, Mexico, and Central and South America as both epidemic and sporadic infections.[258,259,261,262] Sporadic infections also occur in nonendemic areas and are usually associated with travel into areas of endemicity. The attack rate (the percentage of exposed patients who become infected) of HEV is low compared with HAV (1% vs. 10%, respectively). In endemic areas, outbreaks usually occur between 5 and 10 years apart and are often associated with times of heavy rainfall, after floods or monsoons, or after the recession of flood waters.[260–262] The overall case fatality rate for the general endemic population is 0.5% to 4%, whereas for reasons unknown, pregnant women have a much greater case fatality rate of 20%.[263] In particular, the fetal complication rate is increased, especially if the infection occurs in the third trimester of pregnancy. The frequency of death in utero and immediately after birth is also greater than that seen with acute hepatitis of other causes.[263]

Transmission of HEV is via the fecal–oral route, and the most common source of transmission is ingestion of fecally contaminated water.[261,262] Poor climactic conditions in conjunction with inadequate personal hygiene and sanitation have led to epidemics of HEV infection. Additional routes of transmission include consuming raw or undercooked meat of infected animals such as boar or deer and domestic animals such as pigs, vertical, and bloodborne transmission.[258,259]

Interference with the production of cellular macromolecules, alteration of cellular membranes, and alteration of lysosomal permeability are some of the proposed mechanisms of hepatic injury.[257,259] In addition, immune-mediated mechanisms are believed to be responsible for lysis of virally infected hepatocytes by direct lymphocyte cytotoxicity or antibody-mediated cytotoxicity.

Diagnosis

Initial assays for detection of anti-HEV used electron microscopy to detect HEV antigen on the surface of HEV particles in stool and serum and immunohistochemistry to detect the antigen in liver tissue.[257,259,260] Fluorescent antibody-blocking assay is currently used to detect anti-HEV reacting to HEV antigen in serum, but although highly specific, this assay lacks sensitivity (50%) in acute HEV infection.[257,259,260] Additional cloning and sequencing of HEV has led to the development of Western blot assays and ELISA that detect anti-HEV by using recombinant expressed proteins from the structural region of the virus. RT-PCR has also been used to confirm the diagnosis of HEV by detecting HEV RNA from serum, liver, or stool.[257,259,260] Clinically, HEV is a diagnosis of exclusion.

Clinical Manifestations and Natural History

Typical HEV clinical symptoms include jaundice, dark urine, tender and enlarged liver, elevated liver enzymes, abdominal pain, nausea, vomiting, and fever. Protracted coagulopathy and cholestasis have also been reported in more severe cases, possibly related to genotype 4.[257–259] Two phases of illness exist, including a prodromal and preicteric phase. Peak serum aminotransferase levels reflect the onset of the icteric phase and generally return to baseline by 6 weeks.[257–259] Stool is often positive for HEV RNA at the onset of the icteric phase and persists for an additional 10 days beyond this period. Viral shedding may occur for up to 52 days after the onset of icterus. Detection in the serum occurs during the preicteric phase, before detection of virus in the stool, and becomes undetectable after the peak in aminotransferase activity. Because HEV RNA is not detectable in the serum during symptoms, diagnostic tests using HEV RNA have limited utility, and a correlation between PCR detection and infectivity has not been observed. Serologically, HEV IgM becomes detectable before the peak rise in ALT, whereas antibody titers peak with peak ALT levels and subsequently decline. In most patients, HEV IgM is present for 5 to 6 months after the onset of illness. HEV IgG appears after HEV IgM and remains detectable for up to 14 years after acute infection; however, the duration of protective immunity has not been fully elucidated.[257–260]

In nonfatal cases, acute HEV hepatitis is followed by complete recovery without any chronic complications. There is protection from reinfection; however, the duration of protection is variable.

Prevention and Treatment

No immunoprophylactic measures exist for HEV disease, and effective prevention strategies are dependent on improved sanitation in endemic areas. Travelers going to endemic areas should be educated regarding the risks of drinking water, eating ice, or eating uncooked shellfish or uncooked and peeled fruits and vegetables. Drinking water should be boiled to inactivate HEV. No vaccines or postexposure prophylaxis treatments are currently available to prevent HEV infection.

SUMMARY

Viral hepatitis continues to be a significant worldwide infectious disease. To date, prevention strategies through universal vaccination are the most efficient methods for minimizing the incidence of HAV, HBV, and HDV coinfected with HBV. Patient education with respect to the common ways of spreading these infections may also result in behavioral modifications that reduce the overall incidence of infection. Once HBV and HCV progress to chronic infection, more efficacious and better-tolerated antiviral therapies are needed to treat these infections. Similarly, therapeutic modalities that reduce the progression of these diseases are necessary to prevent end-stage liver disease and the development of additional complications (encephalopathy, intractable ascites, coagulation disorders, and HCC). As a better understanding of viral replication is established, as well as appropriate models for study, new therapeutic agents are becoming available. Furthermore, viral kinetics and genomic-based approaches may optimize responses to drug therapies, especially in HCV-infected patients. The economic impact and quality of life of these patients remain to be fully elucidated.

KEY REFERENCES AND WEBSITES

A full list of references for this chapter can be found at http://thepoint.lww.com/AT11e. Below are the key references and website for this chapter, with the corresponding reference number in this chapter found in parentheses after the reference.

Key References

Advisory Committee on Immunization Practices (ACIP) Centers for Disease Control and Prevention (CDC). Update: prevention of hepatitis A after exposure to hepatitis A virus and in international travelers. Updated recommendations of the Advisory Committee on Immunization Practices (ACIP). *MMWR Morb Mortal Wkly Rep.* 2007;56:1080. (36)

Advisory Committee on Immunization Practices (ACIP) et al. Prevention of hepatitis A through active or passive immunization: recommendations of the Advisory Committee on Immunization Practices (ACIP). *MMWR Recomm Rep.* 2006;55:1–23. (20)

Aggarwal R. Hepatitis E: historical, contemporary and future perspectives. *J Gastroenterol Hepatol.* 2011;26(Suppl 1):72. (255)

Au JS, Pockros PJ. Novel therapeutic approaches for hepatitis C. *Clin Pharmacol Ther.* 2014;95:78–88. (231)

Chung RT. Acute hepatitis C virus infection. *Clin Infect Dis.* 2005;41(Suppl 1):S14–S17. (142)

Dienstag JL. Hepatitis B virus infection. *N Engl J Med.* 2008;359:1486–1500 (40)

Ghany MG, Strader DB, Thomas DL, et al. Diagnosis, management and treatment of hepatitis C: an update. *Hepatology.* 2009;49:1335–1374. (126)

Lok A, McMahon BJ. Chronic hepatitis B: update 2009. *Hepatology.* 2009;50:661. (42)

Rizzetto M. Hepatitis D: thirty years after. *J Hepatol.* 2009;50:1043 (245)

Scheel TK, Rice CM. Understanding the hepatitis C virus life cycle paves the way for highly effective therapies. *Nat Med.* 2013;19:837–849. (125)

Seeff LB. The history of the "natural history" of hepatitis C (1968–2009). *Liver Int.* 2009;29(Suppl 1):89. (127)

Terrault NAet al. AASLD guidelines for treatment of chronic hepatitis B. *Hepatology.* 2016;63:261–283. (23)

Zoulim F, Locarnini S. Hepatitis B virus resistance to nucleos(t)ide analogues. *Gastroenterology.* 2009;137:1593. (97)

Key Website

American Association for the Study of Liver Diseases (AASLD). http://www.aasld.org.

81 Parasitic Infections

Sheila Seed, Larry Goodyer, and Caroline S. Zeind

CORE PRINCIPLES

		CHAPTER CASES
MALARIA		
1	Malaria in humans is caused by protozoan parasites of the genus Plasmodium: *Plasmodium falciparum*, *P. vivax*, *P. ovale*, or *P. malariae*. Early symptoms of malaria are nonspecific with fever present in the majority of patients, and approximately two-thirds of infected persons may experience symptoms such as headache, muscle aches and pains, and malaise.	**Case 81-1 (Question 1)**
2	Travelers with symptoms of malaria should seek medical evaluation as soon as possible. Falciparum malaria is the most severe form of malaria and has the highest mortality. Mortality is higher in those with no immunity such as travelers from non-endemic areas, while adults living permanently in the country and exposed to malaria do develop semi-immunity. Suspected or confirmed malaria, especially *P. falciparum*, is a medical emergency necessitating early intervention. In instances when the traveler develops a febrile illness consistent with malaria and access to medical care is not readily available, a reliable supply of malaria treatment can be self-administered presumptively as a temporary measure.	**Case 81-1 (Questions 1, 2, 3, 5)**
3	Travelers to malaria-endemic areas need to understand the risk of malaria and know how to best prevent it with mosquito-avoidance measures and chemoprophylaxis (where appropriate). Pregnant women are at greater risk for malaria and its associated complications. Women who are pregnant or likely to become pregnant should be advised to avoid travel to endemic areas if possible. If travel cannot be deferred, use of an effective chemoprophylaxis regimen is essential.	**Case 81-1 (Question 4), Case 81-2 (Questions 1–3), Case 81-3 (Question 1), Tables 81-1 and 81-2**
4	Several factors must be considered when selecting a chemoprophylactic drug regimen, including drug resistance, patient-specific factors, adverse effects, precautions, and contraindications.	**Case 81-1 (Question 4), Case 81-2 (Questions 1–3), Case 81-3 (Question 1), Tables 81-1 and 81-2**
AMEBIASIS		
1	Amebiasis is caused by *Entamoeba histolytica* and implicated in amebic dysentery and hepatic abscesses. Diagnosis of amebic dysentery may include the following information: history of travel, stool and biopsy specimens, and ultrasound to exclude liver abscesses. Treatment for amebiasis calls for a combination of agents with both luminal-acting and extraintestinal effects. Amebic cyst passers and pregnant women must be treated to avoid invasive disease and transmission of the infection.	**Case 81-4 (Questions 1, 2), Case 81-5 (Questions 1, 2), Case 81-6 (Question 1), Case 81-7 (Question 1), Table 81-3**
GIARDIASIS		
1	The signs and symptoms of giardiasis could be insidious and vague, but patients usually present with diarrhea and bulky, foul-smelling stools along with laboratory confirmation of *Giardia lamblia*.	**Case 81-8 (Question 1)**
2	The major treatments for giardiasis are metronidazole and tinidazole or nitazoxanide.	**Case 81-8 (Question 2), Table 81-3**

Continued

	CHAPTER CASES
ENTEROBIASIS	
1 The signs and symptoms of the infection may be subtle, but the specific diagnostic test for *Enterobius vermicularis* is the cellophane tape swab. Therapy for enterobiasis includes the antihelminthic agents: albendazole, pyrantel pamoate, or mebendazole (not available in the United States). Household measures to eradicate the infection need to be addressed.	**Case 81-9 (Questions 1, 2), Table 81-3**
CESTODIASIS	
1 Primarily this includes *Taenia saginata* and *Taenia solium*, and symptoms of infections are nonspecific. It is critical to differentiate these two infections from other cestode infections. Praziquantel remains an effective agent for all species of Cestodes. Cysticercosis, a complication caused by the larval cysts of *T. solium* that may be associated with central nervous system infection (neurocysticercosis), is serious and requires separate diagnostic testing and controversial therapy. Praziquantel, which is indicated for most cestodiasis, is well tolerated.	**Case 81-10 (Questions 1, 2), Table 81-3**
PEDICULOSIS	
1 Head and body lice are associated with dermatologic reactions, which can be treated with a number of agents: permethrin, pyrethrin, malathion, and ivermectin. Special attention needs to be focused on correct application procedures, drug resistance, and lice decontamination measures.	**Case 81-11 (Questions 1, 2), Table 81-3 and 81-4**
SCABIES	
1 Scabies produces pruritic rash and excoriations of the interdigital area of the upper and lower limbs. Treatment includes lindane, permethrin, and crotamiton. Clothes and personal items of the infected person and family members need to laundered (>50°C) to avoid reinfection.	**Case 81-12 (Question 1), Table 81-3**

MALARIA

Epidemiology

According to World Health Organization (WHO) estimates, malaria was responsible for an estimated 214 million cases of malaria in 2015 with an estimated 438,000 deaths, which reflects an overall 60% reduction in malaria mortality rates since 2000.[1] The global malaria burden continues to be disproportionately high with approximately 89% of malaria cases and 91% of deaths in sub-Saharan Africa.[1] Within regions of high malaria transmission, children less than 5 years of age are particularly susceptible with more than two-thirds (70%) of all malaria deaths occurring in this age group.[1] Globally in children under the age of 5 years, the malaria death rate fell by 65% between 2000 and 2015. While malaria is no longer an endemic infectious disease in the industrialized countries of North America, Europe, Australia, New Zealand, and Japan, travel to malaria-endemic regions, as well as immigration and refugee migrations into non-endemic areas, have resulted in increases in the numbers of imported cases of malaria in industrialized countries.[2,3] Millions of US travelers visit malaria-endemic areas each year and approximately 1,500 cases of malaria are diagnosed in the United States annually, mostly in returned travelers.[4]

Distribution of Malaria Species

Malaria in humans is caused by protozoan parasites of the genus Plasmodium: *Plasmodium falciparum*, *P. vivax*, *P. ovale*, or *P. malariae*.[5] The distribution of the four *Plasmodium* species of malaria varies worldwide. However, the vast majority of imported cases are caused by *P. falciparum* or *P. vivax*[2]; the proportion of imported cases caused by *P. falciparum* or *P. vivax* within a country reflects both the destinations that travelers select and, to a larger degree, the nature of immigrant communities.[2] In most countries, only 5% or less of malaria cases are caused by *P. ovale* and *P. malariae*.[2] In addition, *P. knowlesi*, a species normally found in monkeys, has been documented as a cause of human infections and some deaths in forest fringe areas of Southeast Asia.[5]

Life Cycle of the Malaria Parasite and Transmission

The life cycle of the malaria parasites in the human host is complex. All species are transmitted by the bite of an infective female *Anopheles* mosquito that carries malaria-causing parasites and injects the asexual forms or sporozoites into the human bloodstream. Over a period of 5 to 16 days (depending on the species), the sporozoites grow, divide, and produce daughter cells, or merozoites, per liver cell. Infections caused by *P. vivax* and *P. ovale* may remain in a dormant stage for extended periods of time within the liver (hypnozoites) and cause relapses by invading the bloodstream for months or years later. The merozoites exit the liver cells and reenter the bloodstream and begin a cycle of invading red blood cells and asexual replication, thus producing and releasing newly formed merozoites from the red blood cells. Through this process symptoms can develop 1 week after being bitten by an infected mosquito, though in *falciparum* malaria this can occur up to 3 months or occasionally longer. The characteristic

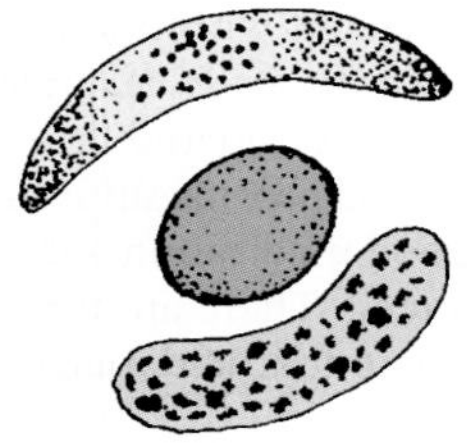

Figure 81-1 *Plasmodium falciparum* gametocytes.

malarial paroxysms of chills and fever usually coincide with the periodic release of merozoites and other pyrogens in the blood. In *P. falciparum* infections, this periodicity may not always be apparent. A subpopulation of merozoites differentiate into sexual forms of the parasite, resulting in male and female gametocytes that circulate in the bloodstream (Fig. 81-1). If the gametocytes in the host blood are ingested by a female *Anopheles* mosquito during a blood meal, fertilization and an asexual division in the mosquito midgut occurs where they develop into oocysts. Each oocyst grows and divides, producing thousands of active haploid forms, called sporozoites; once mature the oocyte bursts, releasing sporozoites, making their way to the mosquitos's salivary glands. Inoculation of the sporozoites into a new human host perpetuates the malaria life cycle.

While the majority of cases of malaria are transmitted by the bite of an infective female *Anopheles* mosquito, occasional transmission has occurred by blood transfusion, needle sharing, organ transplantation, or congenitally from mother to fetus.[2]

Drug Resistance

The development of drug resistance has emerged as one of greatest threats to malaria control.[1,2] Resistance to antimalarial drugs has been confirmed for two malaria species, *P. falciparum* and *P. vivax*, while the development of drug resistance is currently unknown for *P. malariae* or *P. ovale*. Of note, there have been two cases of chloroquine-resistant *P. malariae* reported from Indonesia, though the clinical significance remains undefined.[6]

Chloroquine-resistant *P. falciparum* (CRPf) has become widespread and is now found throughout most malaria-endemic areas, including all of sub-Saharan Africa, South America, the Indian subcontinent, Southeast Asia, and Oceania. Presently, CRPf, is not found in Mexico, the Caribbean, Central America, Argentina, and parts of the Middle East.[7] *P. falciparum* resistance has also developed to nearly all of the other currently available antimalarial agents, such as sulfadoxine/pyrimethamine, mefloquine, halofantrine, and quinine, along with the emergence of resistance to artemisinin derivatives in parts of Southeast Asia. In some parts of the world, the impact of multidrug-resistant malaria can be extensive.

Chloroquine-resistant *P. vivax* has also emerged as a global public health concern. First identified in 1989 among Australians living in or traveling to Papua New Guinea, chloroquine-resistant *P. vivax* has now been identified also in Southeast Asia, on the Indian subcontinent, and in South America. Since these areas are also co-endemic for CRPf, this has had minimal impact on chemoprophylactic recommendations because the antimalarial choice for these areas is not chloroquine.[3]

There are several online resources available to retrieve updated malaria information and country-specific risks from several sources, including the Centers for Disease Control and Prevention (CDC) and WHO.[1,3]

Acute Malaria

SIGNS AND SYMPTOMS

CASE 81-1

QUESTION 1: M.T., a 27-year-old male college student, presents to the emergency department (ED) with complaints of malaise, myalgia, headache, and fever of 5 days' duration. A native of Ghana, West Africa, he recently visited his parents who live in a remote area of Ghana, and he returned home to the United States 4 weeks ago. Two days prior to admission to the ED, he had an abrupt onset of coldness and chills, followed 1 hour later by a high fever, sweating, headache, nausea, and vomiting. The episode of chills and fever lasted about 24 hours, after which he became asymptomatic. On the afternoon of admission, he had another bout of chills that preceded a fever of 40°C.

When interviewed for his medical and travel history, he mentioned that he did not take malaria prophylaxis because he thought that he was protected since he was born and raised in Ghana and then as a teenager moved to the United States to live with relatives and to attend school. He also did not use mosquito-avoidance measures during his recent trip to Ghana.

Physical examination reveals a slender black man who is acutely ill and complaining of severe abdominal pain. Abdominal examination reveals a soft, tender spleen that is slightly enlarged. Blood pressure (BP) is 110/70 mm Hg; pulse, 120 beats/minute; respiration rate, 32 breaths/minute with crackles on pulmonary auscultation; and temperature, 40°C. Laboratory findings include the following:

Hemoglobin (Hgb), 11 g/dL
Hematocrit (Hct), 34%
White blood cell (WBC) count, 5,300 cells/μL with 76% neutrophils (normal, 45%–65%), 23% lymphocytes (normal, 15%–35%), and 1% monocytes. Platelets 26,000/microliter
Creatinine 1.5 mg/dL
CRP 228.9 mg/dL
Bilirubin, 1.0 mg/dL

Urinalysis reveals trace amounts of albumin and the presence of urobilinogen. Thick and thin films of M.T.'s blood are prepared and a parasitemia of 20% is reported. A Giemsa stain of the thin film demonstrates *P. falciparum* gametocytes.

Describe how M.T.'s presentation is consistent with *P. falciparum* malaria and explain his risk factors.

M.T. recently visited Ghana, West Africa, where *P. falciparum* is endemic. The incubation period ranges between 1 week and 3 months, though it may occur later in rare cases.[8,9] Early symptoms of malaria are nonspecific with fever presenting in most patients and is often accompanied by rigors, as in M.T.'s presentation. Approximately two-thirds of infected persons usually experience symptoms such as headache, muscle aches and pains, and malaise, while about one-third of patients experiencing dry cough in the absence of other respiratory symptoms, diarrhea, and other gastrointestinal (GI) symptoms.[6] M.T.'s presentation is consistent with the majority of malaria-infected travelers because approximately 90% of them do not become symptomatic until they return home.[10–12] Given the nonspecific symptomatology with malaria, it is important that a good travel history is obtained as part of the evaluation. M.T.'s history of travel to an endemic area, the cyclical paroxysmal episodes of chills and fever, the presence of thrombocytopenia, abdominal pain, splenomegaly, and the identification of *P. falciparum* gametocytes in M.T.'s blood confirm the diagnosis of malaria.

Because M.T. grew up in Ghana in his early years but has been living for over a decade in the United States (a non-endemic country), he is considered to be in a high-risk group known as "travelers visiting friends and relatives" or VFR travelers.[13] When he returned to Ghana, an endemic country, to visit his parents, his loss of immunity over a period of time, placed him in a high-risk group for malaria. Unfortunately, M.T. neglected to take malaria chemoprophylaxis because he thought his risk was low. Healthcare providers should raise awareness of the importance for malaria prophylaxis as well as other prevention strategies for VFR travelers.

TREATMENT

CASE 81-1, QUESTION 2: How should *P. falciparum* malaria in M.T. be treated?

Unfortunately, M.T. has acquired falciparum malaria, the most severe form of malaria with the highest mortality rate. Thus, M.T.'s treatment is a medical emergency, requiring immediate attention as mortality correlates with diagnostic and therapeutic delay.[8] M.T. would be classified as having a severe case of malaria with complications, which could result in organ damage, including cerebral malaria. This is a particular feature of *P. falciparum* which unlike the other forms causes red blood cell adhesion to blood vessel walls causing local damage and ischemia to end organs. His clinical symptoms along with the results of 20% parasitemia support a severe case of falciparum malaria.

Specific treatment guidelines for treatment of malaria in the United States are provided by the Centers for Disease Control and Prevention (CDC)[14] at **http://www.cdc.gov/malaria/diagnosis_treatment/treatment.html** and by the World Health Organization[15] available at **http://www.who.int/malaria/publications/atoz/9789241549127/en/.**

Because M.T.'s condition is critical, he should be admitted to an acute care unit and started on intravenous (IV) artesunate for at least 24 hours. According to WHO guidelines for severe malaria, intravenous or intramuscular artesunate is the drug of choice for treatment of severe malaria because it has demonstrated a greater reduction in mortality compared with parenteral quinine.[15] Many hospitals/institutions no longer stock intravenous quinidine gluconate for treatment of malaria and if used the drug requires careful cardiac monitoring. Parenteral artesunate can be obtained from the CDC (Malaria Hotline: 770-488-7788 or toll-free 855-856-4713 or after hours at 770-488-7100 for malaria clinician on call) as an investigational drug (IND). If parenteral artesunate is not available, an alternative agent would be the use of intramuscular artemether, which is preferred over the use of quinine for treatment of adults and children with malaria.

Once M.T. has received at least 24 hours of parenteral therapy and is able to tolerate oral therapy, he would complete 3 days of therapy with an artemisinin-based combination therapy (ACT), such as artemether–lumefantrine (Coartem). The artemisinin component is effective at rapidly clearing parasites from the blood. If an ACT is unavailable, other options can be used: artesunate + clindamycin, artesunate + doxycycline, quinine + clindamycin, or quinine + doxycycline, though tolerability and side effects of quinine are problematic. The risk of death is greatest within the first 24 hour, requiring careful monitoring for management of complications as well as supportive care.

Managing Other Plasmodium Species

CASE 81-1, QUESTION 3: How would M.T.'s treatment of malaria differ if it had been a different Plasmodium species?

If M.T. had been infected with one of the other species of *Plasmodium (P. vivax, P. ovale,* or *P. malariae)* treatment with an ACT for 3 days would be considered first-line treatment for all species.[15] This approach will provide sufficient efficacy for malaria treatment, promote good medication adherence, and minimize the risk of drug resistance. There are five ACTs recommended for the treatment of uncomplicated malaria:

- artemether + lumefantrine
- artesunate + amodiaquine
- artesunate + mefloquine
- artesunate + SP (sulfadoxine-pyrimethamine)
- dihyroartemisinin + piperaquine

It is important to check for chloroquine-resistant regions such as chloroquine-resistant *P. vivax*, which has been documented in Papua New Guinea and Indonesia, Brazil, Columbia, Ethiopia, Guatemala, Guyana, India, Myanmar, Peru, the Republic of Korea, Solomon Islands, Thailand, and Turkey.[8,16]

Patients with *P. ovale* and *P. vivax* should also be given primaquine to prevent relapses from the latent exoerythrocytic stages in the liver.[2] Before primaquine is used in any patient, glucose-6-phosphate dehydrogenase (G6PD) deficiency must be ruled out by laboratory testing because it can cause hemolysis that can be fatal in G6PD-deficient individuals.

PREVENTION OF MALARIA

CASE 81-1, QUESTION 4: What malaria chemoprophylaxis recommendation would have been options for M.T. prior to his travel to visit his parents in Ghana? Provide guidance to M.T. regarding antimalarial options, adverse effects, counseling parameters, and mosquito-avoidance measures.

Travelers to malaria-endemic areas, such as M.T., should receive malaria prophylaxis and should follow mosquito-avoidance measures.[7] The goal of malaria prevention is to prevent malaria caused not only by *P. falciparum* but also by all species. It is important to assess an individual's level of risk, which includes the destination country, the detailed itinerary, including specific activities (e.g., back-packing in the wilderness), types of accommodations, and style of travel. Pregnancy, lactation, and other conditions, HIV disease, other immunocompromised diseases, as well as drug resistance at the destination will impact the risk assessment.

Because M.T. is a first-generation immigrant living in a non-endemic country and was returning to Ghana, his country of origin, as a VFR traveler he was considered at high risk for contracting malaria. Recommendations for drugs used for malaria prophylaxis are provided by the CDC[17] at **https://wwwnc.cdc.gov/travel/yellowbook/2018/infectious-diseases-related-to-travel/malaria#3-10-chlor**

Given M.T.'s travel destination to Ghana with *P. falciparum* estimates at 90%, appropriate options for malaria prophylaxis are atovaquone–proguanil, doxycycline, or mefloquine. It is important that M.T. understands the differences in the agents, including proper administration, their adverse effect profile, and potential drug interactions. Table 81-1 provides a summary of the various agents for malaria prophylaxis and highlights adverse effects, contraindications, precautions, and potential drug interactions.[5,7,18] The importance of beginning chemoprophylaxis prior to travel should be emphasized. While medications for malaria prophylaxis may be available at the destination location, travelers are strongly discouraged from obtaining chemoprophylaxis medications while abroad because the quality of these products are not known. These products may be counterfeit or may have been manufactured using substandard manufacturing practices or may contain contaminants.[19,20]

Table 81-1
Antimalarial Drugs Used for Malaria Prophylaxis

Drug	Usage	Adverse Effects	Contraindications and Precautions	Drug Interactions
Atovaquone–proguanil (fixed drug combination)	Prophylaxis in all areas Begin 1–2 days before travel to malarious areas Take daily (same time each day) while in malarious area and for 7 days after leaving such areas Take with food or a milky drink In the United States and European Union, a pediatric formulation is available (quarter strength = 62.5 mg atovaquone and 25 mg proguanil). CDC sanctions atovaquone/proguanil for infants >5 kg. WHO allows use in infants weighing >11 kg Partial doses may need to be prepared by a pharmacist and dispensed in capsules	Nausea, vomiting, abdominal pain, increased transaminase, seizures, and rash	Contraindicated in severe renal impairment (creatinine clearance <30 mL/minute) Not recommended in pregnancy or breastfeeding (use only during pregnancy if potential benefits of therapy outweigh potential risk to infant)	Tetracycline, rifampin, and rifabutin significantly decrease atovaquone level (avoid concurrent use) May interact with antiretroviral protease inhibitors ritonavir, darunavir, atazanavir, indinavir, and lopinavir, in addition to the non-nucleoside reverse transcriptase inhibitors nevirapine, etravirine, and efavirenz; monitor when used Metoclopramide: may reduce bioavailability of atovaquone; avoid use of this agent as an antiemetic to treat vomiting that may occur with atovaquone at treatment doses Avoid use with cimetidine and fluvoxamine because of interference with proguanil's metabolism
Chloroquine phosphate	Prophylaxis only in areas with chloroquine-sensitive malaria Begin 1–2 weeks before travel to malarious areas. Take weekly (same day of the week) while in malarious area and for 4 weeks after leaving such areas Chloroquine sulfate (Nivaquine) is not available in the United States and Canada, but it is available in most malaria-endemic countries in both tablet and syrup forms	May exacerbate psoriasis; pruritus in black-skinned individuals, nausea, headache, skin eruptions, reversible corneal opacity, nail and mucous membrane discoloration, nerve deafness, photophobia, myopathy, retinopathy with daily use, blood dyscrasias, psychosis, seizures, and alopecia	Contraindications: Persons hypersensitive to 4-aminoquinoline compounds and in G6PD-deficient individuals (hemolysis is rare when given at prophylactic and therapeutic doses) Preexisting retinopathy, diseases of the central nervous system, myasthenia gravis, disorders of the blood-producing organs, a history of epilepsy or psychosis Dosage reduction may be required: hepatic function impairments	May increase risk of prolonged QTc interval when given with other QT-prolonging agents (e.g., sotalol, amiodarone, and lumefantrine); antiretroviral rilpivirine prolongs QTc; avoid combination of chloroquine with any of these agents Chloroquine inhibits CYP2D6 and when used concomitantly with substrates of this enzyme (e.g., metoprolol, propranolol, fluoxetine, paroxetine, and flecainide); increase monitoring for side effects Chloroquine absorption may be reduced by antacids or kaolin; space apart by ≥4 hours Avoid concomitant use of cimetidine and chloroquine as cimetidine can inhibit chloroquine's metabolism; avoid concurrent use of CYP3A4 inhibitors such as ritonavir, ketoconazole, and erythromycin as they may increase chloroquine levels Chloroquine may increase digoxin levels, requiring careful monitoring Use with caution with calcineurin inhibitors as their levels may be increased by chloroquine Chloroquine inhibits bioavailability of ampicillin; space apart doses by 2 hours. Chloroquine may decrease the bioavailability of ciprofloxacin and methotrexate

(continued)

Table 81-1

Antimalarial Drugs Used for Malaria Prophylaxis (*continued*)

Drug	Usage	Adverse Effects	Contraindications and Precautions	Drug Interactions
Doxycycline	Prophylaxis in all areas Begin 1–2 days before travel to malarious areas Take daily at the same time each day while in the malarious area and for 4 weeks after leaving such areas	GI upset (nausea, vomiting, abdominal pain, and diarrhea (less frequent than with other tetracycline agents); esophageal ulceration; vaginal candidiasis, photosensitivity, allergic reactions, blood dyscrasias, azotemia in renal diseases, and hepatitis	Contraindicated in children aged <8 years and in pregnant women Breastfeeding: excreted into breast milk; may cause permanent discoloration of teeth, damage to tooth enamel, impairment of skeletal growth, and photosensitivity in breastfed infants	Phenytoin, carbamazepine, and barbiturates may decrease doxycycline's half-life Anticoagulants: may require reduction in anticoagulant dose while taking doxycycline; close monitoring of prothrombin time Absorption may be impaired by concomitant ingestion of bismuth subsalicylate, preparations containing iron, calcium, magnesium, or aluminum; avoid taking these preparations within 3 hours of taking doxycycline Doxycycline may interfere with bactericidal activity of penicillin; avoid use of both drugs together
Hydroxy-chloroquine sulfate	An alternative to chloroquine for prophylaxis only in areas with chloroquine-sensitive malaria			
Mefloquine	Prophylaxis in areas with mefloquine-sensitive malaria Begin ≥2 weeks prior to travel to malarious areas Take weekly on the same day of the week while in the malarious area and for 4 weeks after leaving such areas Travelers should receive a copy of the FDA Medication Guide when receiving a prescription for mefloquine	Dizziness, diarrhea, nausea, vivid dreams, nightmares, irritability, mood alterations, headache, insomnia, anxiety, seizures, and psychosis	Contraindicated in persons allergic to mefloquine or related compounds (quinine, quinidine) and in persons with active depression, a recent history of depression, generalized anxiety disorder, psychosis, schizophrenia, other major psychiatric disorders, or seizures Caution: in persons with psychiatric disturbances or a previous history of depression Not recommended for persons with cardiac conduction abnormalities Use with caution or avoid in individuals taking antiarrhythmic or β-blocking agents, calcium channel blockers, antihistamines, H1-blocking agents, tricyclic antidepressants, or phenothiazines Use in second and third trimesters in pregnancy for women who cannot defer travel to high-risk areas is sanctioned by manufacturer, CDC, and WHO Breastfeeding: small amounts secreted in breast milk; effect on breastfed infants is unknown	May interact with antimalarial drugs that alter cardiac conduction; increased toxicities with lumefantrine (available in United States in fixed combination to treat uncomplicated *P. falciparum* malaria); avoid or use with caution because of potentially causing fatal prolongation of the QTc interval May lower plasma concentrations of anticonvulsant agents, such as valproic acid, carbamazepine, phenobarbital, and phenytoin; avoid concurrent use May increase levels of calcineurin inhibitors and mTOR inhibitors (tacrolimus, cyclosporine A, and sirolimus) Potent CYP3A4 inhibitors (e.g., clarithromycin, erythromycin, ketoconazole, voriconazole, and itraconazole, ritonavir, lopinavir, darunavir, atazanavir, and cobicistat) may increase the levels of mefloquine, increasing the risk of QT prolongation CYP3A4 inducers (e.g., efavirenz, nevirapine, etravirine, rifampin, and rifabutin) may reduce plasma concentrations of mefloquine and concurrent use should be avoided Avoid concurrent use with agents boceprevir and telaprevir (drugs used to treat hepatitis C)

Table 81-1
Antimalarial Drugs Used for Malaria Prophylaxis (*continued*)

Drug	Usage	Adverse Effects	Contraindications and Precautions	Drug Interactions
Primaquine	Prophylaxis for short-duration travel to areas with principally *P. vivax* Used for presumptive antirelapse therapy (terminal prophylaxis) to decrease the risk for relapses of *P. vivax* and *P. ovale* Start therapy 1–2 days before travel to malarious areas Take daily at the same time each day while in the malarious area and for 7 days after leaving such area A documented normal G6PD level should be obtained prior to starting primaquine therapy	GI upset; hemolysis in G6PD deficiency, methemo-globinemia	Contraindicated in individuals with G6PD deficiency (G6PD level should be obtained prior to starting primaquine therapy as G6PD deficiency must be ruled out by laboratory testing). Contraindicated during pregnancy and lactation (unless the infant being breastfed has a documented normal G6PD level)	

Sources: Arguin PM, Tan KR. Malaria. In: Centers for Disease Control and Prevention. CDC Health Information for International Travel 2016. New York, NY: Oxford University Press; 2016:242–255; Youngster I, Barnett ED. Interactions among travel vaccine & drugs. In: Centers for Disease Control and Prevention. CDC Health Information for International Travel 2016. New York, NY: Oxford University Press; 2016:54–57; Schlagenhauf P, Kain KC. Malaria prophylaxis. In: Keystone JS et al, eds. *Travel Medicine*. 3rd ed. Philadelphia, PA: Saunders Elsevier; 2013:146–147.

M.T. should be counseled regarding mosquito-avoidance measures, not only for malaria but also for protection against *Aedes* mosquitos (transitions of dengue, chikungunya, and the Zika viruses). Because malaria transmission occurs primarily between dusk and dawn, contact with mosquitos can be reduced by remaining in well-screened areas, using mosquito bed-nets (preferable insecticide-treated nets), using insecticide sprays, wearing clothes that cover most of the body, and treating clothing with permethrin. Table 81-2 summarizes strategies to optimize protection against mosquitos and items that travelers can include in a travel kit for malaria prevention.[21,22] In addition to mosquito-avoidance measures, it is important to emphasize to travelers, such as M.T., to inspect themselves and their clothing for ticks during outdoor activity and at the end of the day (see Chapter 82, Tick-Borne Diseases for further information).

STANDBY EMERGENCY TREATMENT

Given the risk of complications and deaths because of the delay initiating treatment of malaria, the concept of standby emergency treatment (SBET) was introduced in the late 1980s and then updated to provide travelers with a treatment dose of an appropriate antimalarial drug to be carried and taken in case of a febrile illness, when prompt medical attention is unavailable within 24 hours following the onset of symptoms.[23–25] The major issue with SBET is the difficulty for travelers to make a self-diagnosis of malaria based on clinical symptoms. For those situations in which the traveler does not have access to medical care and develops a febrile illness with symptoms consistent with malaria, a supply of medications could be administered presumptively until medical evaluation is available.

CASE 81-1, QUESTION 5: Would M.T. have been a candidate for SBET prior to his trip to Ghana?

In the United States, two malaria treatment regimens are available that could be prescribed for self-treatment: atovaquone–proguanil and artemether–lumefantrine. Because M.T. was traveling to a remote region in Ghana, discussing this option with a travel health provider would have been important in preparation for his trip. M.T. is a good candidate for SBET and could have taken a reasonable supply of a full-course of an approved malaria treatment regimen with him on his trip. It is important to note that the use of the same or related drugs that are taken for prophylaxis are not recommended to treat malaria. Thus, if M.T. was taking a reliable supply of atovaquone–proguanil as SBET, then atovaquone–proguanil would not be selected for malaria prophylaxis. Either mefloquine or doxycycline would be acceptable choices for malaria prophylaxis.

The introduction of rapid diagnostic tests (RDTs), which are based on the immunochromatographic detection of plasmodial proteins, has become an important component of the current global malaria control strategies, alongside ACTs for falciparium malaria across most areas of endemicity. The use of RDTs is being evaluated as a tool for self-use by travelers to determine if it will help them decide whether or not to use SBET.[23] Future directives will continue to evaluate the feasibility and utility of RDTs in providing guidance to travelers on whether to initiate SBET.

CASE 81-2

QUESTION 1: J.P., a 35-year-old male who owns a small business in the United States, is planning to visit his seriously ill grandmother who lives in eastern region of Indonesia. J.P. immigrated to the United States when he was 20 years old, and he has not previously had a chance to go back to Indonesia. Given his concern for his grandmother's health, his wife, R.T., who is 24 weeks pregnant, wants to join him and also bring their 6-year-old daughter. R.T. is also from Indonesia and moved to the United States 8 years ago. Assess the malaria risks of each member of the family.

Table 81-2
Mosquito Protection Measures

Protective Measures		Comments
Clothing	Wear a long-sleeved shirt, long pants, and socks Treat clothing with permethrin 24–48 hours prior to travel to allow them to dry or purchase pretreated clothing	Permethrin-treated clothing will retain repellant activity through multiple washes Repellants used on skin can also be applied to clothing and must be reapplied after laundering Clothing treated with other repellent products (e.g., DEET) provides protection from biting arthropods but will not last through washing and will require more frequent reapplications
Insecticides	Permethrin: highly effective insecticide–acaricide and repellent	
Repellents for use on skin and clothing	Apply lotion, liquid, or spray repellent to exposed skin Ensure adequate protection during times of the day when mosquitos are most active (malaria vector mosquitos bite mainly from dusk to dawn) Reapply repellants as protection wanes and mosquitos start to bite Purchase repellents before traveling	Repellents may be used with sunscreen. General recommendation: use separate products, applying sunscreen first and then applying the repellent. Combination sunscreen and repellent products are not recommended, because sunscreen may need to be reapplied more frequently and in larger amounts than repellents Travelers may need to reapply sunscreen more often as limited data show a one-third decrease in the sun protection factor of sunscreens when DEET-containing insect repellents are used after a sunscreen is applied
	DEET (chemical name: *N*,*N*-diethyl-m-toluamide or *N*,*N*-diethyl-3-methyl-benzamide) DEET formulations worldwide: concentrations range from 5% to 100%. For most activities, 10%–35% DEET will usually provide adequate protection	Gold standard of insect repellents for several decades In the United States registered for use by the general public since 1957 Can be applied to skin, clothing, mesh insect nets or shelters, window screens, tents, or sleeping bags
	Picaridin (KBR 3-23 [Bayrepel] and Picaridin outside of the United States; chemical name: 21-(2-hydroxyethylo)-1-piperidinecarboxylic acid 1-methylpropyl ester)	
	Oil of lemon eucalyptus (OLE) or PMD (chemical name: para-menthane-3,8-diol). The synthesized version of OLE.	Note that EPA-registered repellent products contain the active ingredient OLE (or PMD). "Pure" oil of lemon eucalyptus (essential oil is not formulated as a repellent) and not recommended because it has not undergone validated safety and efficacy testing and is not registered with the EPA as an insect repellent.
	IR3535 (chemical name: 3-[*N*-butyl-*N*-acetyl]-aminopropionic acid, ethyl ester).	

EPA, Environmental Protection Agency.
Source: Fradin MS. Insect protection. In: Keystone JS et al, eds. *Travel Medicine*. 3rd ed. Philadelphia, PA: Saunders Elsevier; 2013:51–61; Nasci RS et al. Protection against mosquitoes, ticks, & other arthropods. In: Centers for Disease Control and Prevention. CDC Health Information for International Travel 2016. New York, NY: Oxford University Press; 2016:94–99; Schlagenhauf P, Kain KC. Malaria prophylaxis. In: Keystone JS et al, eds. *Travel Medicine*. 3rd ed. Philadelphia, PA: Saunders Elsevier; 2013:143–144.

Malaria prevention strategies for both short-term and long-term travelers consist of a combination of mosquito-avoidance measures and chemoprophylaxis. It is important to assess the individual risk of each traveler, including a detailed itinerary of the specific cities, types of accommodations, and activities (e.g., backpackers, adventure travelers).

Similar to the previous case of M.T., (Case 81-1) VFR travelers, such as J.P. and R.T., are at high risk because they are first-generation immigrants living in non-endemic countries who are returning to their countries of origin. They may consider themselves to be at no risk because they were raised in a malarious country (Indonesia) and consider themselves immune. They should be advised that any acquired immunity is lost quickly and they are considered to have the same risk as nonimmune travelers. Because R.T. is pregnant, she should be advised that malaria infection in pregnant women can be more severe with increased risk for adverse pregnancy outcomes than in nonpregnant women. In particular, falciparum malaria acquired during pregnancy has been associated with an increased risk of miscarriage and still birth, intrauterine growth retardation, as well as other complications, and maternal mortality.[7] She should be advised to avoid travel to eastern Indonesia because it is an endemic region. Their 6-year-old daughter should also follow preventive measures because infants, children, and adolescents of any age can contract malaria and they are traveling to a malarious region.

Case 81-2, Question 2: J.P. and his wife R.T. have not finalized their decision if they will travel together to visit J.P.'s grandmother, and bring their daughter. They want to learn more about resources available to them and options for malaria prevention for this trip, so that they can weigh the risks and benefits of traveling to Indonesia.

In eastern Indonesia, including Papua New Guinea, chemoprophylaxis is recommended for J.P. and his family that will protect them against CRPf infections. The CDC *Health Information for International Travel*[26] (commonly referred to as the Yellow Book) serves as a useful resource for both travelers and clinicians regarding updated information on parasitic diseases and immunization requirements. In addition, travelers such as J.P. and his wife and clinicians can select the type of traveler on the program menu, which in their case they would select "traveling with children," "visiting friends or family," and also the "pregnant women" categories, which will provide them with additional relevant information for their special needs. In addition the CDC Malaria Hotline, mentioned previously provides malaria support. Other useful resources include the Morbidity and Mortality Weekly Reports and the WHO.

Non-Falciparum Prophylaxis

It is important to note that nearly all *P. falciparum* is chloroquine resistant and *P. vivax* and *P. falciparum* are the two most common encountered in travelers to eastern Indonesia (refer to section that follows for prophylaxis for P. falciparum). There have been reports confirming a high prevalence of chloroquine-resistant *P. vivax* in Papua New Guinea or Indonesia.[14] Therefore, antovaquone–proguanil, doxycycline, or mefloquine would be recommended as options for treatment, and mefloquine would be the appropriate choice during pregnancy. In addition, infections with *P. vivax* and *P. ovale* can relapse as a result of hypnozoites that remain dormant in the liver. Therefore, a 14-day course of primaquine therapy is recommended with appropriate screening for G6PD deficiency prior to treatment. Primaquine should be avoided during pregnancy.

Prophylaxis for Plasmodium falciparum

There are three broadly equally effective prophylactics for most regions where there is *P. falciparum*—atovaquone–proguanil, doxycycline, and mefloquine. Selection of an antimalarial agent depends on individual factors, patient preference regarding the regimen, the side effect profile, and contraindications (see Table 81-1).

Prophylaxis for *P. falciparum* can be achieved by taking the combination of atovaquone and proguanil administered once daily 1 to 2 days before entering malarious areas, continued for the duration of malaria exposure, and for 1 week after return. Mefloquine should be taken beginning at least 1 week prior to entering malarious areas, and continuing through 4 weeks after leaving the endemic area. A third option is doxycycline beginning 1 day before entering malarious areas, continued for the duration of the stay, and for 4 weeks after leaving the malarious area.

In pregnant patients, such as R.T., traveling to CRPf areas, mefloquine is the only medication recommended for malaria prophylaxis during pregnancy. Atovaquone–proguanil is not recommended for use during pregnancy because data are still lacking to fully evaluate its safety, and doxycycline is contraindicated. Given the prevalence of *P. falciparum* and *P. vivax* in eastern Indonesia, chloroquine would not be recommended and mefloquine would be an appropriate option for R.T. who is in her second trimester. As mentioned above, *P. vivax* resistance would also be a concern for travel to eastern Indonesia, and mefloquine would provide appropriate coverage.

Given the risks of acquiring malaria during pregnancy, J.P. and R.T. should reconsider their decision to travel together. With regard to their 6-year-old daughter, mefloquine and atovaquone–proguanil are options as doxycycline is contraindicated in children less than 8 years of age. Practical advice should be emphasized, including physical barriers (e.g., clothes, mosquito nets), insect repellent, and minimizing the stay in the endemic area also decrease the likelihood of transmission. Table 81-2 summarizes strategies to optimize protection against mosquitos and items that travelers can be advised to include in a traveler kit for malaria prevention. Considerations when selecting a drug for malaria prophylaxis are available by the CDC[17] at http://wwwnc.cdc.gov/travel/yellowbook/2018/infectious-diseases-related-to-travel/malaria.

MALARIA VACCINE

CASE 81-2, QUESTION 3: Could J.P. be vaccinated as an alternative to chemoprophylaxis?

Currently, no malaria vaccine is available because there have been numerous challenges in the development of a vaccine, including the technical complexity of developing a vaccine against a parasite and the lack of a traditional market.[27] As a result of successful in vitro *P. falciparum* cultivation and advances in genetic engineering and monoclonal antibody research, some progress has been made, but this vaccine is years from approval. The malaria parasite undergoes many transformations during its development, and each stage expresses a different plasmodial genome that generates a large number of antigens. The development of a malaria vaccine relies on the identification and characterization of these antigens and the subsequent production of monoclonal antibodies. Presently there are over a dozen vaccine candidates in clinical development that are being evaluated. A Malaria Vaccine Technology Roadmap has been designed by leading global health organizations that is focused on accelerating the development of a highly effective malaria vaccine.

CASE 81-3

QUESTION 1: C.S., a 29-year-old female, comes to the community pharmacy with a prescription for mefloquine that she obtained from a local travel medicine clinic. She explains that she will be traveling to sub-Saharan Africa for 6 weeks with a group of female friends, and she is concerned about experiencing adverse effects to mefloquine while she is on her 1-month safari trip. She also wants your advice regarding malaria prevention. She currently takes an oral contraceptive and also a multivitamin daily and has no known drug allergies. Provide guidance to C.S. regarding mefloquine and advice on approaches to malaria prevention.

It is important to consider patient-specific factors in C.S. and drug-related factors. Given her concerns, C.S. can be advised to start early with mefloquine prophylaxis (2.5–3 weeks before her trip), which will be taken weekly on the same day.[7] This will allow her to assess her tolerability to mefloquine as the majority of adverse effects occur within the first three doses. If there are any tolerability issues that occur, this will enable her to switch to another agent.

In terms of overall malaria prevention strategies, the importance of adherence to malaria prophylaxis should be emphasized, because C.S. will begin mefloquine prior to her trip and will continue therapy while she is in the malarious region, and for 4 weeks after leaving the area. Personal protection measures should be reviewed with C.S., including habitat avoidance, the use of insect repellants, protective clothing, and bed-nets (see Table 81-2).[21,22] For example, if C.S. selects a product containing DEET (*N,N*-diethyl-m-toluamide or *N,N*-diethyl-3-methylbenzamide), she should be counseled on using a sunscreen product separately (rather than a combination product). Sunscreen may need to be reapplied more often and in larger amounts than the insect repellent because limited data has shown a one-third decrease in the sun protection factor of sunscreens when DEET-containing insect repellents are used after a sunscreen is applied.[22]

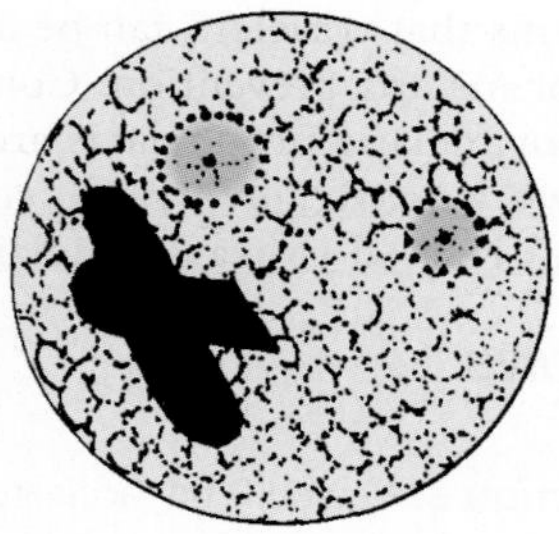

Figure 81-2 *Entamoeba histolytica*.

AMEBIASIS

Prevalence and Mortality

Amebiasis is an infection caused by the intestinal protozoan parasite *Entamoeba histolytica* (Fig. 81-2), resulting in diarrhea or amebic dysentery. Extraintestinal infections may occur when the parasite spreads to other organs, the most common being the liver, resulting in hepatic abscesses.[28,29] This parasitic infection is distributed globally, affecting more than 50 million people with over 100,000 deaths annually.[30] Those most affected are people living in, traveling to, or recent immigrants from endemic areas where there are suboptimal sanitary conditions, particularly in tropical or subtropical developing countries. Transmission occurs by the fecal–oral route via direct person-to-person contact or by consumption of contaminated food and water.[31] Risk factors include poor sanitary conditions, anal sexual exposure, and household contact with an infected person. Most individuals are infected with *E. dispar* (80%) or *E. moshkovskii*, which are antigenically different strains from the pathogenic *E. histolytica* (10%) and do not cause symptomatic invasive disease.[32,33] Amebiasis can be asymptomatic, or it may present as colitis or dysentery. Extraintestinal lesions include abscesses in the liver, lungs, skin, and, rarely, the brain.[28,29,31–33]

Life Cycle

Infection occurs by ingestion of mature cysts present in fecally contaminated water or food. Excystation occurs in the lumen of the small intestines where eight trophozoites are released from one cyst and migrate to the large intestine (Fig. 81-3). Trophozoites multiply by binary fission. In noninvasive infections, trophozoites remain in the intestinal lumen. In invasive infections, trophozoites invade the intestinal mucosa producing ulcerations, resulting in amebic dysentery.[34] Trophozoites may enter the bloodstream traveling to the liver, and in rare instances to the brain, lungs, and genitals forming abscesses. Both trophozoites and cysts are passed in the feces of an infected individual. Trophozoites do not survive outside the host body, if ingested they will be destroyed by gastric juices. The cyst form can survive days to weeks in the external environment, only killed by temperatures in excess of 55°C or hyperchlorinated water.[32,33,35]

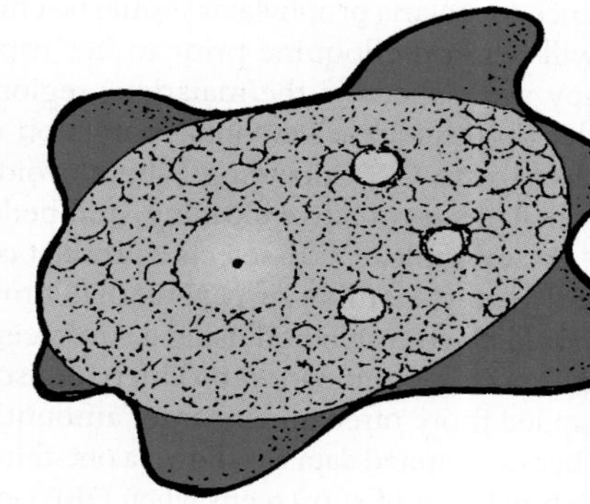

Figure 81-3 *Entamoeba histolytica* trophozoites.

Amebic Dysentery

DIAGNOSIS

CASE 81-4

QUESTION 1: B.W., a 39-year-old recent immigrant from rural India, presents to an urgent care clinic with a 14-day history of watery diarrhea with occasional blood, abdominal pain, and fever. On physical examination, he is a thin man complaining of abdominal discomfort and occasional nausea. His vital signs include blood pressure 150/90 mm Hg, heart rate 90 bpm, temperature 37.6°C. He has no signs of jaundice or lymphadenopathy. Examination is remarkable for slight abdominal distension and rebound tenderness in the right lower quadrant. Liver function tests are normal. Stool samples are collected and reveal stool positive for occult blood. Microscopic examination of stool for ova and parasites is ordered; light microscopy reveals trophozoites and cysts. Colonoscopy revealed flask-shaped intestinal mucosal ulcerations. A tissue biopsy of the ulceration showed trophozoites. Antigenic testing of stool samples confirmed presence of *E. histolytica*. What clinical findings does B.W. have that supports the diagnosis of amebic colitis?

Patients presenting with acute amebic colitis may present with bloody or watery diarrhea, abdominal pain, constipation, tenesmus, fever, rectal bleeding (especially in children), nausea, and anorexia.[36–39] On physical examination patients may present with elevated temperature, tachycardia, and hypertension in cases of severe colitis. Intestinal amebic dysentery may be suspected in patients from endemic areas with bloody or watery diarrhea, abdominal pain, and fever. Diarrhea lasting more than 10 days should be evaluated for intestinal parasites.[40] Almost all patients presenting with amebic colitis will have heme-positive stools. Microscopic examination of stool samples can only identify the presence of trophozoites or cysts but cannot differentiate between pathogenic or nonpathogenic strains of the *Entamoeba* species. Three stool samples from different days need to be collected, because cysts may be missed if only one sample is tested. Serology tests cannot determine between a current or past infection. There are various antigenic assay detection kits commercially available with varying specificity and sensitivity to differentiate the type of species found in the stool. B.W. is a recent immigrant from an endemic country and is presenting with symptoms consistent with amebic colitis. Antigenic examination of the stool confirmed B.W. has amebiasis, with the presence of *E. histolytica*.

CASE 81-4, QUESTION 2: What medications are available to treat B.W.'s symptomatic infection? What medication regimen is preferred?

Treatment is necessary if *E. histolytica* has been specifically identified. Treatment is not necessary with *E. dispar* infections.[36–38] Treatment involves the elimination of both trophozoites and cysts from the intestinal lumen. There are two classes of drugs to treat B.W.'s amebiasis: tissue amebicides and intraluminal amebicides. Those presenting with mild-to moderate intestinal symptoms or severe intestinal symptoms or extraintestinal disease should be treated with a tissue amebicide followed by a course of intraluminal amebicide therapy.[41] B.W.'s symptomatic amebic colitis needs to be treated with both a tissue amebicide and intraluminal agent. Tissue amebicides include nitroimidazoles, nitazoxanide

Table 81-3
Drug Therapy of Various Parasitic Infections[a]

Drug of Choice	Dosage	Adverse Effects	Warnings
Amebiasis			
Asymptomatic including cyst passers			
Luminal amebicides			
Paromomycin (drug of choice)	*Adults and children*: 25–35 mg/kg/day in three divided doses for 5–10 days	Nausea, vomiting, diarrhea, and cramps	Contraindicated in GI obstructions Use with caution in renal impairment
Iodoquinol	*Adults*: 650 mg PO TID × 20 days *Children*: 30–40 mg/kg/day PO TID × 20 days (max. 2 g/day)	Nausea, vomiting, and headache	Avoid use in elderly because of optic nerve damage
Diloxanide furoate (not available in the United States)	*Adults*: 500 mg PO TID × 10 days *Children*: 20 mg/kg/day in three divided doses × 10 days	Flatulence, nausea, and abdominal pain	
Symptomatic or invasive intestinal infections			
Tissue amebicides			
Metronidazole	*Adults*: 750 mg PO TID × 5–10 days *Children*: 35–50 mg/kg/day PO TID × 7–10 days	Nausea, headache, metallic taste, disulfiram reaction with alcohol, and abdominal discomfort	Avoid use in first trimester of pregnancy
Tinidazole	*Adults*: 2 g PO once daily × 3 days *Children*: 50 mg/kg (max. 2 g) × 3 days	Metallic or bitter taste, anorexia, nausea, vomiting, epigastric discomfort, and fatigue	Contraindicated in first trimester and those breast feeding
Followed by luminal amebicide: see above for dosing			
Amebic liver abscess			
Metronidazole	*Adults*: 750 mg PO/IV TID × 5–10 days *Children*: 35–50 mg/kg/day three divided doses × 5–10 days	Nausea, headache, metallic taste, disulfiram reaction with alcohol, and paresthesia	Avoid use in first trimester of pregnancy
Tinidazole	*Adults*: 2 g PO once daily × 3–5 days *Children*: 50 mg/kg (max. 2 g) × 5 days	Metallic or bitter taste, anorexia, nausea, vomiting, epigastric discomfort, and fatigue	Contraindicated in first trimester and those breast feeding
Followed by luminal amebicide agent to eliminate intestinal colonization—see above for dosing			
Ascariasis (Roundworm)			
Albendazole	*Adults and children*: 400 mg PO once	Nausea, vomiting, headache, and abnormal liver function tests	Avoid during pregnancy
Mebendazole (Withdrawn from market in the United States)	*Adults and children*: 100 mg BID PO × 3 days Or 500 mg PO single dose May repeat in 3 weeks if necessary	Headache, diarrhea, abdominal pain, and dizziness	Avoid during pregnancy Use with caution in hepatic disease and inflammatory bowel diseases
Enterobiasis (Pinworm)			
Mebendazole (withdrawn from market in the United States)	*Adults and children*: 100 mg PO once; repeat in 2 weeks	Diarrhea and abdominal pain	Avoid during pregnancy Use with caution in hepatic disease and inflammatory bowel diseases
Pyrantel pamoate	*Adults and children*: 11 mg/kg PO once (max. 1 g), repeat in 2 weeks	Nausea, vomiting, headache, dizziness, diarrhea, and abdominal cramps	Avoid in pregnancy Use with caution in hepatic disease
Albendazole	*Adults and children*: 400 mg PO once; repeat in 2 weeks	Nausea, vomiting, headache, and abnormal liver function tests	Avoid during pregnancy

(continued)

Table 81-3
Drug Therapy of Various Parasitic Infections (*continued*)

Drug of Choice	Dosage	Adverse Effects	Warnings
Filariasis			
Diethylcarbamazine	*Adults*: Day 1, 50 mg PO; day 2, 50 mg TID; day 3, 100 mg TID; days 4–14, 6 mg/kg/day in three doses *Children*: Day 1, 25–50 mg; day 2, 25–50 mg TID; day 3, 50–100 mg TID; days 4–14, 6 mg/kg/day in three doses	Severe allergic or febrile reactions, gastrointestinal disturbance, and rarely encephalopathy	
Albendazole	400 mg PO once daily for 10 days	Nausea, vomiting, headache, and abnormal liver function tests	Avoid during pregnancy
Flukes (Trematodes)[b]			
Praziquantel	*Adults and children*: 40 mg/kg PO 2 divided doses 4 hours apart (*S. haematobium*, *S. mansoni*, and *S. intercalatum*) 60 mg/kg PO in three divided doses 4 hours apart or two divided doses 6 hours apart (*S. japonicum* and *S. mekongi*)	Malaise, headache, dizziness, sedation, fever, and abdominal distress	Contraindicated with other strong CYP inducers (rifampin) Contraindicated in ocular cysticercosis
Giardiasis			
Metronidazole	*Adults*: 250 mg PO TID with meals × 5–7 days *Children*: 15 mg/kg/day PO TID × 5–7 days	Nausea, headache, metallic taste, and disulfiram reaction with alcohol	Avoid use in first trimester of pregnancy
Tinidazole	*Adults*: 2 g PO single dose *Children*: 50 mg/kg single dose	Metallic or bitter taste, anorexia, nausea, vomiting, epigastric discomfort, and fatigue	Contraindicated in first trimester and those breast feeding
Nitazoxanide	*Adults and children*: >12 years: 500 mg PO BID × 3 days *Children*: 7.5 mg/kg BID for 3 days in children <12 years old	Abdominal pain, diarrhea, vomiting, and headache	Use with caution in those with hepatic and renal impairment
Paromomycin (drug of choice in first trimester pregnancy)	*Adults*: 500 mg PO TID for 10 days *Children*: 25 mg/kg/day in three divided doses × 10 days	Nausea, vomiting, diarrhea, and cramps	Contraindicated in GI obstructions Use with caution in renal impairment
Albendazole	400 mg PO daily × 5 days	Nausea, vomiting, headache, and abnormal liver function tests	Avoid during pregnancy
Mebendazole	200 mg PO TID for 5 days	Headache, diarrhea, abdominal pain, dizziness	Avoid during pregnancy Use with caution in hepatic disease and inflammatory bowel diseases
Hookworm			
Mebendazole	*Adults and children*: 100 mg PO BID × 3 days OR 500 mg PO single dose	Headache, diarrhea, abdominal pain, and dizziness	Avoid during pregnancy Use with caution in hepatic disease and inflammatory bowel diseases
Albendazole	400 g PO single dose	Nausea, vomiting, headache, and abnormal liver function tests	Avoid during pregnancy
Lice			
1% Permethrin (Nix)	See Table 81-4 for instructions	Occasional allergic reaction, mild stinging, and erythema	Use with caution in those sensitive to chrysanthemums Not recommended for eyebrow or eyelashes infestations
Ivermectin	*Adults and children:* 200 mcg/kg × 3, day 1, 2, and 10	Fever, pruritus, sore lymph nodes, headache, joint pains, and rarely hypotension	Use with caution in those with severe asthma

Table 81-3
Drug Therapy of Various Parasitic Infections (*continued*)

Drug of Choice	Dosage	Adverse Effects	Warnings
Leishmaniasis			
Sodium stibogluconate	*Adults*: 20 mg /kg IV or IM × 20–28 days *Children*: Same as adults	Gastrointestinal, malaise, headache arthralgias, myalgias, anemia, neutropenia, and thrombocytopenia; ECG abnormalities (ST- and T-wave changes)	Use with caution in those with cardiac disease Use with caution on those with real or hepatic impairment
Liposomal Amphotericin B	Immunocompetent: 3 mg/kg/day on days 1–5, 14, and 21. Repeat if need Immunocompromised: 4 mg/kg/day on days 1 through 5, 10, 17, 24, 31, and 38. Seek advice if further therapy is needed	Hypotension, chills, headache, anemia, thrombocytopenia, fever, and elevated serum creatinine	
Scabies			
5% Permethrin (Elimite cream)	Apply topically to whole body. Remove cream by washing (shower or bath) after 8–14 hours.	Rash, edema, and erythema	Use with caution in those sensitive to chrysanthemums
Alternatives for scabies			
Ivermectin	*Adults*: 200 mcg/kg PO; repeat in 2 weeks	Nausea, diarrhea, dizziness, vertigo, and pruritus	Use with caution in those with severe asthma
Lindane (Kwell)	Apply topically once	Not recommended in pregnant women, infants, and patients with massively excoriated skin Second-line therapy when other alternatives have failed.	Not recommended by American Academy of Pediatrics Second-line only Black box warning because of neurologic toxicity Banned in California, United Kingdom, Australia
Crotamiton 10% (Eurax)	Apply topically to whole body especially folds and creases. May repeat in 24 hours. Cleansing bath 48 hours after last application	Local skin irritation	Do not apply to raw, weeping skin. Not to be swallowed
Tapeworm[c,d]			
Praziquantel	*Adults and children*: 5–10 mg/kg PO single dose	Malaise, headache, dizziness, sedation, eosinophilia, and fever	Contraindicated with other strong CYP inducers (e.g., rifampin) Contraindicated in ocular cysticercosis
Hydatid cysts[e]			
Albendazole	*Adults*: 400 mg BID × 8–30 days, repeat if necessary *Children*: 15 mg/kg/day × 28 days, repeat if necessary (surgical resection may precede drug therapy)	Diarrhea, abdominal pain, rarely hepatotoxicity, and leukopenia	Avoid use during pregnancy
Trichomoniasis			
Metronidazole	*Adults*: 2 g PO × 1 day or 250 mg PO TID × 7 days *Children*: 15 mg/kg/day PO TID × 7 days	Nausea, headache, metallic taste, disulfiram reaction with alcohol, and paresthesia	Avoid use in first trimester of pregnancy

[a]Does not include drugs used in the treatment and prophylaxis of malaria. (See Table 81-1 for the drugs used for malaria prophylaxis, as well as guidelines by the CDC and WHO for treatment and prophylaxis of malaria.)
[b]*Schistosoma haematobium*, *Schistosoma mansoni*, *Schistosoma japonicum*, *Clonorchis sinensis*, and *Paragonimus westermani*.
[c]Off-label use for tapeworms. Dose for *Hymenolepis nana* is 25 mg/kg single dose.
[d]*Diphyllobothrium latum* alternative treatment: adults, niclosamide 2 g orally once; children, 50 mg/kg (max. 2 g) orally once.
[e]*Echinococcus granulosus* and *Echinococcus multilocularis*.
BID, twice daily; IM, intramuscularly; IV, intravenously; PO, orally; TID, three times daily.
Source: Drug Facts and Comparisons. **https://fco-factsandcomparisons-com.ezproxymcp.flo.org/action/home?siteid=5&reauth**. St. Louis, MO: Wolters Kluwer Health, Inc. Accessed July 31, 2017.

(Alinia), and chloroquine. The drug of choice with a 90% cure rate are the 5-nitroimidazoles, metronidazole (Flagyl), and tinidazole (Tindamax).[29,39] Nitazoxanide shows promise, but the data are limited; chloroquine is ineffective in intestinal illnesses. Metronidazole will kill the trophozoites in the intestines and the tissues, but it does not eradicate the cysts from the intestine. To eradicate colonization, therapy should be followed with an intraluminal amebicide, such as paromomycin, diloxanide furoate (Furamide—not approved in the United States or Canada), or iodquinol (Yodoxin).

B.W.'s amebic colitis should be treated with metronidazole 750 mg orally or IV 3 times a day for 5 to 10 days.[34] Alternative treatment with tinidazole 2 g once daily for 3 days is often better tolerated because of its shorter duration of therapy. Common adverse effects of metronidazole are nausea, metallic taste, and abdominal discomfort. Patients should be warned of a possible disulfiram reaction with alcohol consumption during and up to 72 hours after the completion of therapy.[42] This should be followed by an intraluminal amebicide; the drug of choice is paromomycin 25 to 35 mg/kg/day orally in three divided doses for 5 to 10 days, second-line agents include diloxanide or iodoquinol[28] (see Table 81-3). The most common adverse effects of paromomycin are abdominal pain/cramping, nausea, and diarrhea. Paromomycin and metronidazole should not be taken simultaneously.

In those with a confirmed diagnosis of amebiasis, one study showed the addition of the probiotic *Saccharomyces boulardii* with metronidazole reduced the duration of bloody diarrhea and aided in the clearance of cysts when compared to metronidazole alone.[43]

B.W. must be monitored for the improvement of symptoms of diarrhea and abdominal pain. Follow-up should continue for 3 months after treatment. Three separate stool samples should be examined for cysts.[44]

Amebic Cyst Carrier

CASE 81-5

QUESTION 1: M.A., a 56-year-old man, presents to his PCP for a routine examination after multiple mission trips to Southeast Asia. M.A. is currently asymptotic, but his stool tested positive for *E. histolytica* cysts. Should M.A. be treated?

M.A. is an asymptomatic cyst passer. Cyst passers often do not develop invasive infections and sometimes can clear the infection spontaneously.[29] Detection of the nonpathogenic cyst *E. dispar* does not require treatment, but all asymptomatic patients with positive test results of *E. histolytica* must be treated to reduce the transmission to others.[28,29]

CASE 81-5, QUESTION 2: What medications should be used to treat M.A.?

Intraluminal amebicides are the drug of choice in the treatment of asymptomatic amebiasis. Paromomycin is the drug of choice, 25 to 35 mg/kg/day in three divided doses for 5 to 10 days with meals. Diloxanide furoate (not commercially available in the United States) or iodoquinol may also be recommended, but paromomycin has a higher efficacy rate when compared to diloxanide.[45] M.A.'s stools must be tested monthly for 3 months to assure eradication of the infection.[44]

Extraintestinal Infections

CASE 81-6

QUESTION 1: M.M. is a 26-year-old man presenting to the ED complaining of upper right quadrant abdominal pain, fever, and chills. Upon physical examination the patient shows signs of difficulty breathing during inspiration with pain radiating to the shoulder and back and abdominal tenderness. Rales at the right base could be heard on examination. Laboratory results are significant for leukocytosis with neutrophilia, mild anemia, elevated alkaline phosphate, and alanine aminotransferase. Blood serology shows high antibody titers for *Entamoeba*. Computed tomography (CT) confirmed presence of an abscess in the right lobe of the liver. How should M.M. be managed?

Extraintestinal infections occur in less than 1%, of which liver abscesses are the most common. The right hepatic lobe is the most frequently affected area because of the portal circulatory system of the colon.[38] M.M.'s clinical presentation and laboratory findings are consistent of a hepatic abscess. Only diarrhea is reported in approximately 50% of those infected.[38] The drug of choice for amebic liver abscess is metronidazole for 5 to 10 days followed with a luminal agent such as paromomycin.[37] Aspiration or drainage of the abscess is not recommended unless there is a failure to respond to therapy after 4 to 5 days, evidence of a secondary infection or impending rupture into the pericardium. After the completion of therapy, M.M. should be monitored for regression of the abscess with ultrasounds, and lesions may take up to 12 months to resolve. Complications of hepatic abscesses may include perforation of the abdominal cavity, septic shock, or superinfections. Infections outside of the intestines or liver are extremely rare (<0.1%), dissemination of the amebae to the brain or skin are almost always associated with amebic liver abscess. Because of the rarity of these infections, there are no definitive guidelines for treatment.[36,37]

Treatment During Pregnancy

CASE 81-7

QUESTION 1: S.W., a 26-year-old woman refugee from Sudan, presents to the clinic with an 8-day history of watery stools with blood streaks, abdominal cramping, and a fever. She is currently 12 weeks pregnant and has received no prenatal care prior to her arrival in the United States 4 weeks ago. Physical examination reveals a temperature of 38°C, HR 80 bpm, and blood pressure 140/85. An examination of fresh stools is positive for occult blood and trophozoites. Antigenic testing confirmed the presence of *E. histolytica*. Bacteria cultures are negative for *Campylobacter*, *salmonellosis*, and *shigellosis*. Ultrasound imaging and computed tomography (CT) are negative for the presence of liver abscesses. A diagnosis of intestinal amebiasis is made.

How would you manage S.W.'s infection? What are your concerns regarding her current condition?

S.W. needs to be treated for her intestinal amebiasis. The treatment of choice is metronidazole, but she is in her first trimester of pregnancy. Nitroimidazoles such as metronidazole and tinidazole should be avoided during the first trimester of pregnancy. Metronidazole readily crosses the placenta, and effects on the development of the fetus are unknown.[42] S.W. should be treated with paromomycin 25 to 35 mg/kg/day in three divided doses for 5 to 10 days. Paromomycin is an aminoglycoside that is poorly absorbed in the bowel with an excellent safety profile. The most common adverse effects are nausea, vomiting, and abdominal cramps. S.W.'s stools must be examined for 3 months to assure resolution of the infection.[36,37]

If S.W.'s infection does not resolve or progresses to fulminant colitis or amebic liver abscess, she will safely be beyond her first trimester and should be treated appropriately with a tissue amebicide such as metronidazole followed by a luminal agent such as paromomycin, or second-line agents such as iodoquinol or diloxamide furoate. If iodoquinol is chosen, the most common adverse effects are headache, nausea, and vomiting. Optic nerve damage is a concern with elderly patients and should be avoided. Reported cases of peripheral neuropathy have occurred in doses in excess of the recommended dose. Should diloxamide furoate be prescribed the most common adverse effect is flatulence, but it is not commercially available in the United States.[36]

GIARDIASIS

Prevalence and Transmission

Giardia is a globally endemic illness caused by the protozoa *Giardia lamblia*.[46] The highest number of cases are typically seen in developing countries with inadequate sanitary conditions, untreated water, or contaminated food. Although primarily seen in Asia, Africa, or South America, it is the most frequent parasitic intestinal disease in the United States.[34,47] Those at greatest risk live in rural areas with poor sanitation, low socioeconomic conditions, and have contact with infected individuals or travel internationally. *Giardia* is most prevalent in children and immunocompromised individuals. Presentation of illness varies between individuals from self-limiting diarrhea to more severe symptoms of chronic diarrhea, abdominal cramps, loose pale greasy stools that float, fatigue, weight loss and malabsorption of fat, lactose, vitamins A and B_{12}, but many present with no symptoms.[48] Severe *Giardia* infections may lead to mucosal damage in the small intestines.

Life Cycle

Infection occurs with the ingestion of cysts in contaminated water, food, or by the fecal–oral route. In the small intestine, excystation releases trophozoites (each cyst produces two trophozoites).[46] Trophozoites replicate in the lumen of the proximal small bowel where they can be free or attached to the mucosa by a ventral sucking disk. Encystation occurs as the parasites transit toward the colon and are excreted in the feces. The cysts are hardy, surviving in environmental elements such as cold water and chlorination for weeks (Fig. 81-4).[47,49]

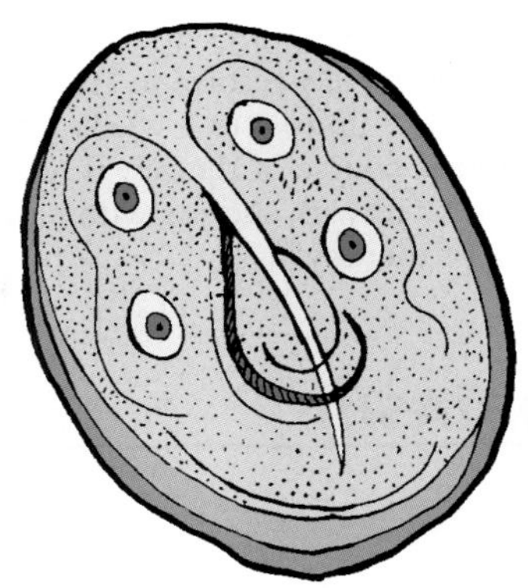

Figure 81-4 *Giardia lamblia* cyst.

Diagnosis

SIGNS AND SYMPTOMS

CASE 81-8

Question 1: P.C., a 23-year-old woman who returned 1 week ago from a mission trip from Zambia, presents to the clinic with complaints of diarrhea, pale-colored foul-smelling greasy stools, abdominal cramps, and fatigue. She states she has been having diarrhea with occasional constipation for about 2 months. She experienced other bouts of diarrhea while on her year-long mission, but it resolved itself quickly, and symptoms occurred typically after swimming in the lake. She has lost 17 pounds since the diarrhea started. She denies any blood or mucous in her stool and has no complaints of fever. Laboratory findings are the following: Fecal fat content >12 g (normal 7 g), complete blood counts (CBC) results are anemia with thrombocytopenia and low levels of vitamin B_{12}. Three separate stool sample were positive for *G. lamblia* cysts with antigenic tests confirming the presence of *G. lamblia*.

What clinical findings does P.C. have that support the diagnosis of Giardia?

Patients with *Giardia* may be asymptomatic, present with self-limiting diarrhea or with symptoms of chronic diarrhea with abdominal pain, yellowish greasy foul-smelling stools, abdominal distention, weight loss, or flatulence. Patients presenting with chronic diarrhea may suffer from dehydration and malabsorption of fat, lactose, and vitamins A and B_{12}.[47,50] The typical incubation period is 6 to 15 days after ingestion of the cysts. Infections may occur with as little as 10 cysts.[51] Confirmation of a giardiasis diagnosis is confirmed by signs and symptoms and the presence of cysts or trophozoites in stool samples. One stool sample may miss the presence of cysts, so it is recommended to test multiple stool samples (at least three). Antigenic testing of stool samples either ELISA or direct fluorescent antigen tests are more sensitive than traditional wet mount microscopy and should be performed if a patient presents with symptoms consistent with giardia but have multiple negative results for cysts. A differential diagnosis ruling out bacterial (*Salmonella*, *Shigella*, *Campylobacter*) and viral (rotavirus, norovirus) causes should be made because the presentation may be similar. *Giardia* differs from these infections by its length of illness (7–10 days before first presentation) and evidence of weight loss.[49]

P.C.'s history of missionary work in Zambia is considered high risk. She may have consumed contaminated food or water, particularly if she swallowed lake water. Her symptoms are consistent with chronic giardia: foul-smelling greasy stools, periods of diarrhea and constipation, fatigue, and abdominal cramps. Some patients will present with flatulence as well. Her laboratory results are consistent with malabsorption: fecal fat content is greater than 12 g (normal fecal fat content is <7 g)[50]; results greater than 7 is indicative of fat malabsorption resulting in steatorrhea.[52] Chronic infections may also present with anemia and low vitamin B_{12} levels. P.C. had *G. lamblia* cysts identified in the stool after three tests and confirmed with antigenic testing. A definitive diagnosis of *Giardia* can be made.

Case 81-8, Question 2: How should P.C. be treated?

Treatment of choice for P.C.'s giardiasis is a nitroimidazole. Metronidazole 250 mg orally 3 times a day for 5 to 7 days is the preferred option with efficacy rates from 52% to 100%.[53] Tinidazole 2 g as a single dose may be better tolerated because of the shorter duration of therapy with similar rate of efficacy. Alternative treatment options include nitazoxanide (Alinia) 500 mg orally twice a day for 3 days, paromomycin 500 mg 3 times daily for 10 days (drug of choice during the first trimester of pregnancy), albendazole (Albenza) 400 mg orally once daily for 5 days. Quinacrine[54] and furazolidone[55] are effective options but are not commercially available in the United States.

P.C. should be counseled to practice good hygiene, washing hands with soap and water for at least 20 seconds, to control transmission of disease.[56] Symptoms of diarrhea typically subside in 1 to 2 days and completely resolve in 10 days. Symptoms of malabsorption may take up to 4 to 8 weeks.[53,57–60] If treatment failure occurs, another course of therapy is necessary. Resistant strains have been treated with success with either higher doses or a longer course of therapy.[49]

ENTEROBIASIS

Prevalence

Human enterobiasis or pinworm infection is caused by the intestinal nematode, *Enterobius vermicularis.* It is the most common helminthic infection worldwide. The highest rate of infection occurs in school-aged children (5–10 years), institutionalized persons, and household members or caretakers of an infected individual. Unlike other helminth infections, all socioeconomic groups are affected. Transmission occurs via the fecal–oral route with finger sucking considered a source of infection for children. If one family member is infected, all members of the family must be treated.[61–63]

Life Cycle

Humans are the only host of *E. vermicularis*. The entire life cycle occurs in the gastrointestinal system for approximately 4 weeks. Infected eggs are ingested from contaminated hands that have scratched the perianal area, food, or water. Person-to-person transmission may occur from contaminated clothing or bed linens. Once eggs are ingested they hatch in the small intestine (duodenum), larvae migrates to the large intestine where they molt twice before becoming adult worms. Copulation occurs in the ileum, where the male typically dies and passes in the stool. The gravid female settles into the large intestine and caecum. The female body fills with approximately 11,000 eggs and makes nocturnal migrations to the rectum and anus where oxygen is needed for the maturation of eggs. Eggs are then deposited in the area around the anus causing severe pruritus.[64,65]

SIGNS AND SYMPTOMS

CASE 81-9

QUESTION 1: N.D. is a 5-year-old boy presenting to the pediatrician. N.D.'s mother states he has been scratching the perianal area for several days. The intense itching has been keeping him up at night and he is irritable during the day. N.D. is 3 feet 9 inches and weighs 19 kg. A cellophane tape swab is placed over the skin of the perianal area, evidence of *E. vermicularis* eggs are found under the microscope.

What signs and symptoms does N.D. exhibit to confirm a diagnosis of pinworm?

Many infected with pinworms are asymptomatic or present with mild symptoms; the most common symptom being nocturnal perianal pruritus and scratching because of the deposit of eggs to the perianal skin. The intense scratching may lead to secondary bacterial infections and sleep disturbances. Patients with major infestations may present with abdominal pain, anorexia, or insomnia. Enterobiasis infections rarely cause serious disease, but it may result in dysuria, appendicitis, or vaginal infections.[66,67]

N.D. is presenting with perianal itching, inability to sleep because of intense itching and a positive "tape test" showing *E. vermicularis* eggs indicative of a pinworm infestation.

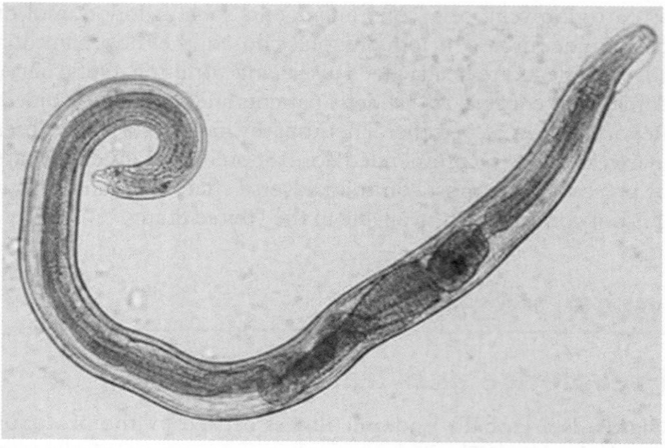

Figure 81-5 Adult male *Enterobius vermicularis image*. Centers for Disease Control and Prevention (CDC)-DpDx-Laboratory Identification of Parasitic Diseases of Public Concern. *Enterobiasis Image Gallery*. https://www.cdc.gov/dpdx/enterobiasis/index.html. Accessed July 31, 2017.

CASE 81-9, QUESTION 2: How should N.D.'s infection be managed? Should his parents be treated?

There are three options for the treatment of pinworm: albendazole (Albenza), pyrantel pamoate (PinX—available without a prescription), and mebendazole (not commercially available in the United States). Albendazole 400 mg as a single dose or pyrantael pamoate 11 mg/kg (maximum 1 g) are viable options for N.D.; a second dose must be repeated in 2 weeks. Mebendazole is currently not commercially available in the United States, but it is available internationally. Mebendazole is given as a single 100 mg dose and repeated in 2 weeks.

Albendazole and mebendazole are broad-spectrum antihelmites that selectively interferes with the microtubules in the intestinal cells of nematodes and glycogen depletion leading to their death.[68,69] Albendazole is considered the drug of choice in the treatment of enterobiasis with a 90% cure rate. Both albendazole and mebendazole are well tolerated with abdominal pain as the most common adverse effect reported. Pyrantel pamoate is a depolarizing neuromuscular agent that acts by paralyzing adult worms, resulting in their expulsion in the stool before eggs are laid.[69] The most common adverse effects are nausea and vomiting. The liquid formulation must be shaken well before use and may be mixed with fruit juice or milk.

All members of N.D.'s family needs to be treated simultaneously. Other preventative methods include proper hand hygiene, particularly after toilet use and before meals, trimming of fingernails, and frequent washing of bed linens and undergarments using hot water.[66]

CESTODIASIS

Description

Intestinal cestodes (tapeworms) are segmented worms; adults primarily live in the gastrointestinal tract, but larvae can live in any organ.[70] There are several species that affect humans: *Taenia saginata* (beef tapeworm), *Taenia solium* (pork tapeworm), *Diphyllobothrium latum* (broad or fish tapeworm), *Taenia asiatica* (Asian tapeworm), and *Hymenolepis nana* (dwarf tapeworm). Humans become infected by eating raw or undercooked meat (pork or beef) or fish (*Diphyllobothrium latum*).[71]

A tapeworm attaches to the mucosa of the intestines by a scolex, the anterior portion of the tapeworm "head of the tapeworm."[70–72] The crown of the scolex is referred to as the rostellum; it may be armed with hooklets or unarmed (no hooklets). Proglottids or segments form behind a short neck. As each proglottid matures, they form a chain called a strobili, giving the tapeworm its ribbon-like appearance. The length of the strobili varies by species (*T. saginata* may have over 2,000 proglottids). Mature proglottids contain eggs that are indistinguishable between species. A definitive diagnosis is made by examining the scolex, proglottids, and eggs.

Tapeworms obtain nutrients through their skin directly from the host, they do not invade the tissue mucosa or acquire blood; therefore, symptoms are often absent or mild in nature.[71] Typical symptoms involve the gastrointestinal tract, mild eosinophilia, and elevated IgE levels may be detected. *T. solium* infections may lead to cysticercosis; neurocysticercosis, the most serious form, involves the central nervous system. It is important, therefore, to seek treatment with any tapeworm infection.

Life Cycle

Humans are the only definitive host for *T. saginata* and *T. solium*. Cattle or pigs are infected by ingesting vegetation contaminated with eggs or gravid proglottids passed in feces. Eggs hatch and invade the intestinal wall and migrate to the muscles where they develop into cysticerci. Humans become infected by eating raw or undercooked meat. In humans, the cysticercus develop in the small intestines to an adult worm over a period of 2 months and can survive for years. Adult worms produce proglottids, which mature and become gravid, detach from the worm, and migrate to the anus or are passed in feces.[73]

Epidemiology

It is estimated that the prevalence of *Taenia* infections is approximately 170 to 200 million cases worldwide.[71] *T. solium* occurs worldwide where pigs are raised, but it is most prevalent in Latin America, sub-Saharan Africa, China, India, and Southeast Asia.[70–71] *T. saginata* can occur anywhere raw or undercooked beef is eaten. Most prevalent areas of occurrence are Eastern Europe, Russia, East Africa, Latin America, Indonesia, and China.[73] Rural and poor socioeconomic areas in developing countries with poor hygiene are at greatest risk.[74] Most cases of neurocysticercosis in industrial countries are primarily seen in refugees, immigrant populations, or travelers from endemic countries.

Cysticercosis

Cysticercosis is caused by the larval cysts of the *T. solium* tapeworm. The larvae migrate to muscle tissue, brain, subcutaneous tissue, or the eye. When the infection develops in the central nervous system it is called neurocysticercosis and is responsible for one-third of acquired epilepsy cases worldwide.[75] Signs and symptoms vary by location of the cyst. Clinical manifestations of cysts in the muscle may be absent other than a lump under the skin. Cysts that deposit in the eye may cause floaters in the eye or blurry vision.[76] Clinical manifestations of neurocysticercosis depends on how many cysts are found and the location; symptoms include seizures, focal neurologic deficits, cognitive decline, and increased intracranial pressure.[76,77]

Diagnosis of neurocysticercosis is made by clinical presentation and radiologic imaging such as magnetic resonance imaging (MRI) or CT scans.[74] Treatment should be customized for each patient, depending on the size, location, and stage of the cysticerci. Treatment includes use of antihelminthic agents, such as praziquantel and/or albendazole. Coadministration of corticosteroids and antiepileptic drugs are often used to manage seizures and the inflammatory response because of the cysticidal activity of praziquantel therapy. Severe cases may require surgery.[77–80]

Taenia Saginata and *Taenia Solium*

SIGNS AND SYMPTOMS

CASE 81-10

QUESTION 1: L.D. is a 28-year-old missionary who lived 12 months in Ethiopia. He has returned to the United States with complaints of perianal itching and diffuse abdominal discomfort (primarily cramping). He reports no fever, mild diarrhea, and states that he sees "moving pieces of rice-looking objects" in his stool. Laboratory tests show slightly elevated eosinophil count and IgE levels. Three stool samples, obtained on separate days, and a cellophane tape test of the perianal area revealed presence of *T. saginata*.

Are L.D.'s symptoms consistent with *Taenia* infection? How can infections be differentiated?

Patients presenting with tapeworm infections may present with a range of symptoms. Many present with no symptoms, but if symptoms are present then they are often mild. Symptoms include abdominal pain, cramps, flatulence, constipation, nausea, vomiting, headache, vitamin deficiency, or weight loss. More severe symptoms include appendicitis and pancreatitis. Patients may report the voiding of segments from the anus and in the feces. Some patients may present with moderate eosinophilia and elevated IgE because of the weak immunogenic activity of the adult worms.[72]

The eggs of *T. saginata* and *T. solium* are morphologically indistinguishable. A definitive diagnosis of species can be made by examining the scolex (in rare cases) or more likely mature gravid proglottids. Eggs and proglottids are only detected in the feces 2 to 3 months after the infection has been established. The CDC recommends three separate stool samples on different days to establish a diagnosis. *T. solium* scolex is characterized by a scolex with four large suckers and rostellum with two rows of hooks (see Fig. 81-6).[72,81,82] *T. saginata* has a scolex with four suckers but no rostellum or hooks (see Fig. 81-7).[81] Biomolecular assays are more accurate than microscopic stool examinations to distinguish between species but are only available in a research laboratory setting.[82]

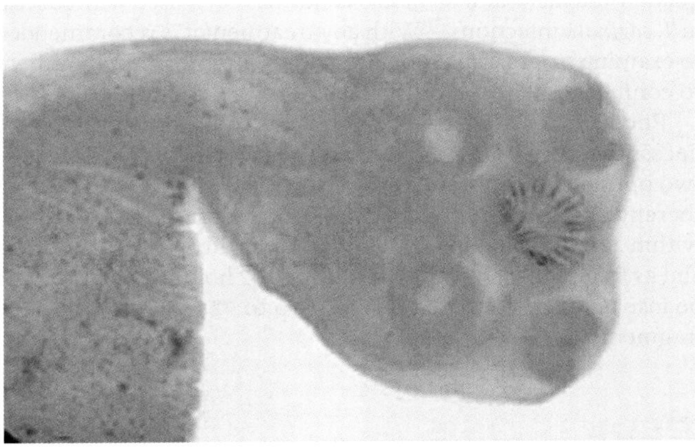

Figure 81-6 Scolex of T. *solium image*. (Source: Centers for Disease Control and Prevention (CDC)-DpDx-Laboratory Identification of Parasitic Diseases of Public Concern. *Taeniasis* Image Gallery. https://www.cdc.gov/dpdx/taeniasis/index.html. Accessed July 31, 2017.)

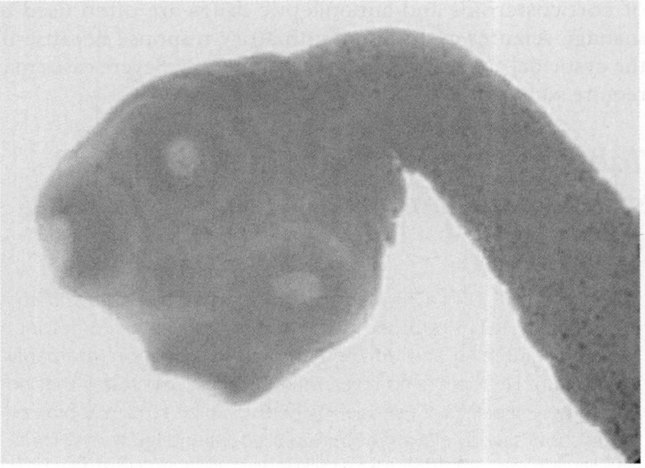

Figure 81-7 Scolex of *T. saginata* image. (Source: Centers for Disease Control and Prevention (CDC)-DpDx-Laboratory Identification of Parasitic Diseases of Public Concern. *Taeniasis* Image Gallery. **https://www.cdc.gov/dpdx/taeniasis/index.html**. Accessed July 31, 2017.)

CASE 81-10, QUESTION 2: How should L.D. be treated and how should it be evaluated?

The drug of choice for both *T. saginata* and *T. solium* infections is praziquantel (Biltricide) 5 to 10 mg/kg as a single dose.[83] Praziquantel works by killing the adult worm but does not destroy the eggs. Typical adverse effects include malaise, headache, dizziness, abdominal discomfort, and rarely urticaria. L.D. should be advised to swallow the tablet whole with water and a meal. The bitter taste of the tablet may cause L.D. to gag or vomit, so it is advisable to swallow the tablet promptly. Praziquantel cannot be chewed, but it may be halved or quartered. It is contraindicated to administer praziquantel with strong Cytochrome P450 (CYP450) inducers, such as rifampin, since adequate blood levels of praziquantel may not be achieved. L.D. should also be advised to not drive or operate heavy machinery on the day of treatment and the following day. Praziquantel has a high cure rate (up to 98%) in *T. saginata* and *T. solium* infections.[84]

An alternative regimen is niclosamide 2 g as a single oral dose for adults and 50 mg/kg in children. It is not available for human use in the United States. For those infections resistant to praziquantel and niclosamide, nitazoxanide has been used with success in *T. saginata* infections.[71] With any treatment it is recommended to examine stool samples for eggs 1 and 3 months after treatment to confirm eradication of the infection.

Recovery of the scolex for species identification may be necessary; purging of the bowel is recommended.[71] There are two options: administer electrolyte–polyethylene glycol prior to therapy or administer castor oil or magnesium sulfate solution within 2 hours of taking the anthelminthic drug. The tapeworm and its fragments should pass within 6 to 12 hours. Patients should be instructed to collect all feces for up to 72 hours to collect all fragments.

PEDICULOSIS

Prevalence

Pediculosis (lice infections) can be caused by *Pediculus humanus capitis* (head lice) (Fig. 81-8), *Pediculus humanus* (body lice), or *Pthirus pubis* (crab lice). Lice infections remain a major problem throughout the world, and infestations can be present in all socioeconomic groups.[85] It is estimated that treatment costs for head lice may exceed $1 billion in the Unites States.[86]

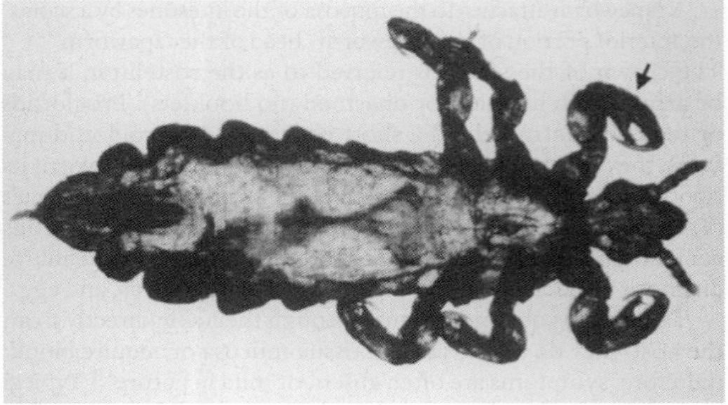

Figure 81-8 *Pediculus humanus capitis* (head lice).

Life Cycle

Head and body lice have similar life cycles, but their habitat preferences distinguish the two varieties. The life cycle of lice has three stages: egg, nymph, and adult. After fertilization, the female lays eggs (up to 10 a day), which attaches tightly to hair or seams of clothing. The eggs (nits) (see Fig. 81-9) hatch in 7 to 10 days and produce nymphs, which go through three molts to become adults. Louse feed by injecting a small amount of their saliva into the host and withdraw small amounts of blood; without these meals the louse will die. The lice penetrate the host skin via stylets within their head and attach themselves by a circlet of teeth on their proboscis. Crab lice are usually found in pubic hair, less frequently on facial hair, eyebrows, eyelashes, and axillary hairs.[85,87–89]

Epidemiology

The highest incidence of head lice is seen among schoolchildren aged 3 to 12 years and in household members. It is less common in African Americans because of different hair texture. The incidence of head lice infestation in the United States has been estimated to be as much as 12 million cases.[90] Body lice infest clothing by laying their eggs on the fabric. Head and crab lice infest hair by laying their eggs at the base of hair fibers. Hair and body lice are transferred between hosts by personal and clothing contact, whereas crab lice are transmitted by sexual contact.

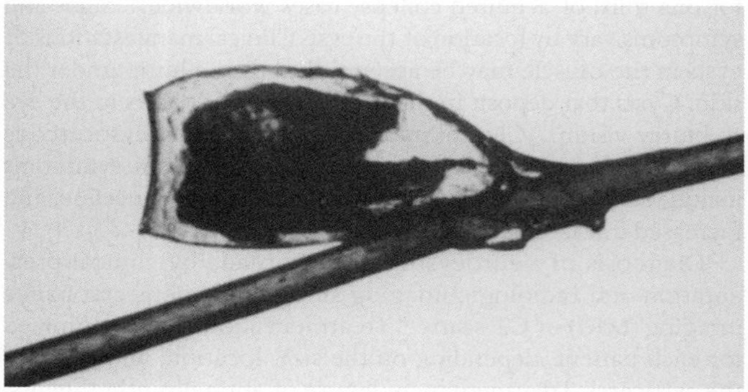

Figure 81-9 Nit or egg of lice on hair shaft.

SIGNS AND SYMPTOMS

CASE 81-11

QUESTION 1: W.L., a 30-year-old homeless man who primarily lives on the streets, presents to a free clinic complaining of intense itching all over his body. Upon examination it is noted that he has a number of pustular lesions all over his body. The skin is particularly thick and discolored around his midsection. The triage nurse says he has "lice all over his body."

Why are the symptoms in W.L. consistent with lice infection?

The most common complaint of patients with head and body lice is pruritus of the scalp, ears, neck, and other body parts. Chronic infestations may result in hyperpigmentation and thickening of the skin. These changes are often seen in the waist, groin, and upper thigh areas ("vagabond's disease"). In severe infestations, intractable itching and scratching can result in folliculitis, hemorrhagic macules or papules, or secondary bacterial infections.[85,91] In contrast, schoolchildren who are exposed frequently to head lice may have only minor pruritus affecting the scalp, ears, and neck.[92]

Treatment

CASE 81-11, QUESTION 2: How should W.L. be treated for lice infection of the head, body, and genital areas?

Concurrent treatment for the pustular bacterial lesions and lice infestation should be initiated in W.L. First-line treatment of head lice in both adults and children is permethrin 1% (Nix) rinse. Alternatives are 0.5% malathion (Ovide) lotion and pyrethrin 0.33% plus 4% piperonyl butoxide (Rid). Recent studies indicate that there may be differences in efficacy among the topical agents. Resistance of head lice to Ovide lotion (0.5% malathion) has been documented in the United Kingdom. The formula used in the United States contains terpineol, dipentene, and pine needle oil, possibly responsible for delaying resistance in the United States.[86,93] Lindane is FDA approved as a second-line therapy because of its neurologic toxicities, and it should be used only when other alternatives have failed (see Table 81-4).[86]

Body lice can be eliminated by bathing and laundering clothing in hot water. Because of W.L.'s severe infestation, he should also apply a topical pediculicide. Products for head lice may be used for body lice with treatment repeated in 7 to 10 days.[85,94] Oral medications such as ivermectin is not FDA approved but has shown to be more effective in some difficult-to-treat cases.[95] First-line treatment of pubic lice is permethrin 1% or pyrethrins plus piperonyl butoxide. Alternative regimes include malathion 0.5% lotion to be rinsed off after 8 to 12 hours or ivermectin 250 mcg/kg to be repeated in 14 days.[96] The pruritus in W.L. can be symptomatically treated with an antihistamine and a low-potency topical steroid.

Several "natural products" such as melaleuca plus lavender oil, coconut oil plus anise oil, tea tree oil, petrolatum shampoo, mayonnaise, and *Cetaphil* have been used in the management of lice.[97,98] None

Table 81-4
Application of Nonprescription and Prescription Options for Head Lice

	Nonprescription products[a,b]
Product	**Application directions**
Permethrin 1% (Nix)	Apply to damp hair that has been first shampooed with non-conditioning shampoo and towel dried. Leave on for 10 minutes and rinse off Repeat in 7–10 days if live lice are seen (re-treatment at 9 days is optimal) Alternative treatment schedule: 0, 7, and 13–15 days Conditioners and silicon-based products reduce residual effects of permethrin
Pyrethrins plus piperonyl butoxide (Rid) (available as mousse and shampoo)	Apply to dry hair and leave on for 10 minutes prior to rinsing off Retreatment schedules same as permethrin Significant resistance has been developed reducing its effectiveness
Prescription products	
Malathion 0.5% (Ovid) Lotion	Apply to dry hair, let air dry then wash off after 8–12 hours Repeat in 7–9 days if live lice are seen Highly flammable because of alcohol content. Instruct patients to let hair air dry uncovered—do not use hair driers, curling irons, or flat irons while hair is wet Resistance seen in the United Kingdom. Current US formulation differs from European formulation—less resistance seen in the United States
Benzyl Alcohol 5% (Ulesfia)	Apply a sufficient quantity to dry hair to saturate the scalp and the entire length of hair. Leave on for 10 minutes then rinse off Reapplication process is same as for permethrin
Spinosad 0.9% Suspension (Natroba)	Apply to dry hair to saturate the scalp and work out to end of hair (may require the entire contents of bottle). Leave on for 10 minutes and rinse off Retreat in 7 days if live lice are seen
Ivermectin 0.5% Lotion (Sklice)	Apply to dry hair and scalp, leave on for 10 minutes, and rinse off. Only one application is needed

[a]All topical products should be rinsed off over a sink with warm water—not in a shower or bath to limit exposure to the skin.
[b]Nits can be removed from the hair by using a sturdy fine-tooth comb.
There are various treatment options for head lice. Lack of adherence or failure to follow instructions may lead to resistance or failure to eradicate the louse.
Sources: Adapted from: Devore CD, Schutze GE. The Council on school health and committee on infectious diseases. Head lice. *Pediatrics*. 2015;135(5):e1355–e1365; Centers for Disease Control and Prevention (CDC) Head Lice Treatment. http://www.cdc.gov/parasites/lice/head/treatment.html. Accessed July 31, 2015.

are FDA approved and have not been proven to be more efficacious. Manual removal of nits by a fine-tooth comb can be a tedious task but necessary because none of the pediculicides are 100% ovicidal. Application of vinegar-based products 3 minutes prior to combing has been reported to make the process of "nit-picking" easier.[86]

Petrolatum

To remove lice from W.L.'s eyelids or eyelashes, ophthalmic grade petrolatum ointment can be used.[89] Petrolatum is applied to the eyelashes and lid margins with cotton swabs –2 to 4 times daily. This regimen will either suffocate the lice or physically remove them. Use of regular petrolatum may cause irritation to W.L.'s eyes.

Decontamination Measures

Treatment for pediculosis should include thorough decontamination to avoid reinfection. All personal articles of clothing, including bedding, should be washed and dried in temperatures >130°F or 54.4°C.[86] Items that cannot be washed can be dry-cleaned or placed in a plastic bag for 2 weeks. Furniture and carpeting should be vacuumed; pediculicide spray is not recommended. Hairbrushes, combs, and other plastic articles can be decontaminated by soaking in hot water.[99] In institutions and schools where lice infestations are a problem, outer clothing (coats, hats, scarves) of individuals should be isolated in separate plastic bags at the beginning of the day. This measure will reduce reinfection significantly.

SCABIES

Prevalence

Scabies is a contagious skin infestation caused by the female mite, *Sarcoptes scabiei var. hominis*. Infestations occur throughout the world and across all socioeconomic groups. The mite is transmitted by an infested individual through close skin contact.[96] Crusted scabies (Norwegian scabies), typically seen in immunocompromised individuals, is a more severe form that is highly infectious. Scabies outbreaks are often seen in institutional settings such as nursing homes and prisons.[100] Typical presentation is the presence of a pimple-like rash with intense itching. Those presenting with crusted scabies have thick crusts of skin containing a large number of mites and eggs.

Life Cycle

Adult females deposit eggs and feces (scybala) as they burrow under the skin. Once the eggs hatch, larvae are released which eventually mature to nymphs and adult mites. The female mite can live up to 6 weeks producing 2 to 4 eggs daily. The classic presentation of skin lesions are a result of the burrowing action of the mites and hypersensitivity reactions to their excrement. Most common sites of lesions are in the interdigital finger webs, wrists, elbows, buttock, and genitalia.[101–103]

Treatment

CASE 81-12

QUESTION 1: G.P., a 26-year-old nurse working at a nursing home, presents to her PCP with a pruritic rash with excoriations in the interdigital webs of her hands and wrists. Several patients and nurses in the same nursing home have similar symptoms as well as her 5-year-old son. Burrows were present in her finger webs with a definitive diagnosis made from a skin scraping test. Microscopic examination revealed eggs of *S. scabiei* and scybala.

How should G.P. and her family be treated? What special instructions and precautions should accompany therapy?

There are several treatment options available for scabies. The treatment of choice in patients 2 months or older is permethrin 5% cream.[102] A thin layer must be applied to the skin from the neck to toes for 8 to 14 hours and then washed off. Although not FDA approved, oral ivermectin 200 mg/kg as a single dose and repeated in 2 weeks is also considered first-line treatment. A repeat dose is needed because of its limited ovicidal activity.[104] Ivermectin is not recommended for children under the age of 5 years of age, <15 kg, pregnant, or lactating women.[102] Lindane should be considered only as a second-line therapy because of reported toxicities.[105] Lindane is useful if first-line therapies are not tolerated or if treatment fails.

Symptoms after exposure to scabies may take several weeks to appear for first-time infections. Sexual partners and any other person who have prolonged contact with an infested individual should be treated.[96] All members of the family should be treated at the same time to avoid reinfestation. Symptoms may persist for up to 2 weeks, if symptoms persist after 2 weeks evaluate for treatment failure.

G.P. must be educated on the non-pharmacologic measures to manage scabies. All bedding and clothing must be washed in hot water (140°F) and hot dried or dry-cleaned. Items that cannot be washed, such as stuffed toys, may be placed in a sealed plastic bag for 48 to 72 hours because mites cannot survive for more than 72 hours away from human skin.[96,106] Fumigation of living areas is not recommended.

ACKNOWLEDGMENT

The authors gratefully acknowledge Lin H. Chen, MD, Division of Infectious Diseases, Mount Auburn Hospital, for her expert review of this chapter.

KEY REFERENCES AND WEBSITES

A full list of references for this chapter can be found at http://thepoint.lww.com/AT11e. Below are the key references and websites for this chapter, with the corresponding reference number in this chapter found in parentheses after the reference.

Key References

Arguin PM, Tan KR. Malaria. In: Centers for Disease Control and Prevention. Health Information for international travel; 2016:236–255. (5)

Choudhuri G, Rangan M. Amebic infections in humans. *Indian J Gastroenterol*. 2012;31(4):153–162. (29)

Devore CD, Schutze GE. The Council on school health and committee on infectious diseases. Head lice. *Pediatrics*. 2015;135(5):e1355–e1365. (87)

Deye GA, Magill AJ. Malaria: epidemiology and risk to the traveler. In: Keystone JS et al, eds. Travel Medicine. 3rd ed. Philadelphia, PA: Saunders Elsevier; 2013:135–142. (2)

Escobeda AA et al. Giardiasis: the ever present threat of a neglected tropical disease. *Infect Disord Drug Targets*. 2010;10(5):329–348. (47)

Gardner TB, Hill DR. Treatment of giardia. *Clin Microbiol Rev*. 2001;14(1):114–128. (49)

Mendelson M. Approach to the patient with malaria. In: Keystone JS et al, eds. *Travel Medicine*. 3rd ed. Philadelphia, PA: Saunders Elsevier; 2013:173–177. (8)

Schlagenhauf P, Kain KC. Malaria chemoprophylaxis. In: Keystone JS et al, eds. *Travel Medicine*. 3rd ed. Philadelphia, PA: Saunders Elsevier; 2013:143–162. (7)

Stanley S. Amebiasis. *Lancet*. 2003;361(9362):1025–1034. (36)

White AC, Weller PF. Cestode infections. In: Kasper D et al, eds. *Harrison's Principles of Internal Medicine*. 19th ed. New York, NY: McGraw-Hill; 2014. http://accesspharmacy.mhmedical.com.ezproxymcp.flo.org/content.aspx?bookid=1130&sectionid=79741152. Accessed July 31, 2017. (70)

Key Websites

Centers for Disease Control and Prevention. Travelers' Health. http://www.cdc.gov/travel/.

Centers for Disease Control and Prevention. Parasites. http://www.cdc.gov/parasites/index.html.

Centers for Disease Control and Prevention. Sexually Transmitted Diseases 2015 Guidelines. http://www.cdc.gov/std/tg2015/default.htm.

World Health Organization. International travel and health. http://www.who.int/ith/en.

World Health Organization (WHO). Neglected Tropical Disease-Summary. http://www.who.int/neglected_diseases/diseases/summary/en/.

82 Tick-Borne Diseases

Caroline S. Zeind, Michelle L. Ceresia, and Lin H. Chen

CORE PRINCIPLES

		CHAPTER CASES
LYME DISEASE		
1	Lyme disease is a multisystem spirochetal disease caused by the bacterium *Borrelia burgdorferi* and is transmitted to humans through the bite of infected black-legged ticks. Geography, tick species, and duration of attachment are used to guide clinical decision-making.	**Case 82-1 (Question 1)**
2	Although clinical features of Lyme disease are diverse and vary with the stage and duration of infection, the presence of an erythema migrans (EM) skin rash is universally the most common feature.	**Case 82-2 (Questions 1, 2)**
3	Most cases of localized (early) Lyme disease can be treated effectively with a few weeks of antibiotics (range of 10–21 days); however, if left untreated, infection can spread to the joints, the heart, and the nervous system.	**Case 82-2 (Question 3, 4), Case 82-3 (Question 1), Case 82-4 (Question 1)**
RELAPSING FEVER		
1	Relapsing fever is a bacterial infection caused by certain species of Borrelia spirochetes. Of the two types of relapsing fever, tick-borne relapsing fever (TBRF) occurs in the western US and louse-borne relapsing fever (LBRF) is generally restricted to refugee settings in developing parts of the world.	**Case 82-6 (Question 1)**
BORRELIA MIYAMOTOI		
1	*Borrelia miyamotoi* is a recently identified tick-borne organism transmitted by Ixodes ticks and is endemic in the same areas as Lyme disease, anaplasmosis, and babesiosis.	**Case 82-6 (Question 2)**
SOUTHERN TICK-ASSOCIATED RASH ILLNESS		
1	Southern tick-associated rash illness (STARI) is a tick-borne disease transmitted by the lone star tick and whose etiology is unknown. Patients bitten may occasionally develop a rash similar to the rash of Lyme disease.	**Case 82-7 (Question 1)**
ANAPLASMOSIS		
1	Anaplasmosis, a tick-borne disease caused by the bacterium, *Anaplasma phagocytophilum*, was first recognized as a disease of humans in the United States in the mid-1990s. If not treated appropriately, illness can be severe and potentially fatal.	**Case 82-8 (Question 1)**
BABESIOSIS		
1	Babesiosis is an illness caused by parasites that infect red blood cells and are spread by certain ticks, with symptoms ranging from asymptomatic disease to potential fatality, especially in immunocompromised patients.	**Case 82-9 (Questions 1, 2)**
COLORADO TICK FEVER, TICK-BORNE ENCEPHALITIS, AND OTHER VIRALLY MEDIATED TICK-BORNE DISEASES		
1	Colorado tick fever (CTF) is a virally mediated tick-borne disease that can be more severe in children than in adults. Other virally medicated tick-borne diseases include those caused by Powassan, Bourbon, and Heartland viruses.	**Case 82-10 (Question 1)**

Continued

TICK PARALYSIS	
1 Tick paralysis occurs worldwide, affecting humans and livestock. It can be reversed by tick removal.	Case 82-11 (Question 1)
PREVENTION OF TICK-BORNE ILLNESSES	
1 Prevention of tick-borne diseases is always preferable to acquisition. Personal protective measures and other methodologies aid in prevention.	Case 82-5 (Question 1)

OVERVIEW

Currently, the majority of emerging infectious diseases are arthropod-borne and are caused by ticks and mosquitoes.[1] Unfortunately, with few exceptions, these emerging diseases cannot be prevented by vaccinations. Ticks belong to the class Arachnida, which includes scorpions, spiders, and mites.[2] Tick-borne diseases are a growing problem worldwide, transmitting pathogens that cause diseases in humans and animals.[3] As a vector of human illness worldwide, disease can be spread by ticks, either by transmission of microorganisms or by injection of tick toxin into a host. Bacterial, rickettsial, protozoal, and viral disease pathogens can be transmitted from ticks to humans (Table 82-1).[4,5]

Table 82-1
Tick-Borne Diseases

Disease	Causative Agent	Tick Vector	Host	Endemic Areas	Comments
Bacterial					
Anaplasmosis (Human granulocytic anaplasmosis (HGA))	*Anaplasma phagocytophilum*	*Ixodes scapularis, Ixodes pacificus*	Deer, elk, wild rodents	North America (upper Midwest and northeastern US)	Previously was known as human granulocytic ehrlichiosis (HGE) Reported in areas that correspond to the known geographic distribution of Lyme disease treatment: same as ehrlichiosis and RMSF
Ehrlichiosis	*Ehrlichia chaffeensis, Ehrlichia ewingii, Ehrlichia muris-like (EML)*	*Amblyomma americanum*	Deer, dogs	North America (southeastern and south-central US, from the eastern seaboard extending westward to Texas)	Similar clinical presentation as anaplasmosis but transmission by two different species of ticks and typically occur in different US regions New species EML was identified in 2009 in patients in the upper Midwest Treatment: same as anaplasmosis and RSMF
Lyme Disease	*Borrelia burgdorferi* *Borrelia mayonii*	*Ixodes scapularis, Ixodes pacificus*	Wild Rodents	North America: *Borrelia burgdorferi; Borrelia mayonii* (new species identified in Midwestern US; genetically distinct from *Borrelia burgdorferi, B. afzelii, and B. garinii*) Europe: more common in eastern and central Europe Asia: northern Asia *B. afzelii*, and *B. garinii*	Worldwide caused by three main species of bacteria: *Borrelia burgdorferi* (North America), and in Europe and Asia: *B. afzelii*, and *B. garinii*
Borrelia Miyamotoi Disease (BMD)	*Borrelia miyamotoi*	*Ixodes scapularis; Ixodes pacificus*			First BMD cases identified in North America in 2013

(continued)

Table 82-1
Tick-Borne Diseases (*continued*)

Disease	Causative Agent	Tick Vector	Host	Endemic Areas	Comments
Tick-borne Relapsing Fever (TBRF)	*Borrelia* species *Borrelia hermsii*, *B. parkerii*, or *B. Turicatae*	*O. hermsii* ticks; *O. parkerii*, and *O. turicata*	Rodents	North America (western states in the United States); Central America, South America, the Mediterranean, Central Asia, and much of Africa	Most cases occur in summer months in rodent-infested cabins but can occur in winter months when fires warming a cabin activate ticks resting in the walls/woodwork
Tick-borne Spotted Fever Rickettsial Infections, broadly grouped as "Spotted Fever group Rickettsia" (SFGR)[a]	*Rickettsia* species *Rickettsia parkeri* Worldwide: *Rickettsia* species including *R. conorii* and *R. africae*	various ticks depending on *Rickettesia* species		North America: United States: *R. parkeri* (Eastern and southern US); and *Rickettsia* species 364D (Northern California, Pacific coast) Worldwide: all continents except Antarctica; numerous Rickettsia species including *R. conorii* and *R. africae*	
Rocky Mountain Spotted Fever (RMSF)	*Rickettsia rickettsia*	*Dermacentor variabilis*, *Dermacentor andersoni*, *Rhipicephalus sanguineus*	Wild rodents, ticks	North America: United States >60% of cases occur in North Carolina, Oklahoma, Arkansas, Tennessee, and Missouri; reports increasing in certain parts of Arizona	United States: Reported throughout most of the contiguous states Treatment: same as anaplasmosis and ehrlichiosis.
Tularemia	*Francisella tularensis*	*Dermacentor variabilis*, *Dermacentor andersoni*, *Amblyomma americanum*	Rabbits, hares, and rodents; domestic cats	Most common in the south-central US, the Pacific Northwest, and parts of Massachusetts	United States: reported from all states except Hawaii Other transmission routes: inhalation and direct inoculation
Parasitic					
Babesiosis	*Babesia* species (most cases *Babesia microti*)	*Ixodes scapularis*	Mice, voles	North America (northeastern and upper Midwestern US where *Babesia microti* is endemic); also sporadic cases on West Coast	Transmission of *Babesia* parasites can occur by transfusion
Viral					
Colorado tick fever	*Coltivirus* species	*Dermacentor andersoni*	Wild rodents, mammals	North America: western US and southwestern Canada (at elevations of 4,000 to 10,000 feet)	Transmission can occur from person to person (rare)
Heartland virus	Phleboviruses	*Amblyomma americanum*		United States: Missouri and Tennessee	Worldwide

Table 82-1
Tick-Borne Diseases (*continued*)

Disease	Causative Agent	Tick Vector	Host	Endemic Areas	Comments
Tick-borne Encephalitis	Member of virus family *Flaviviridae*	*Ixodes ricinus, Ixodes persulcatus*	Rodents	Europe: temperate regions, forested areas Asia: northern Asia (temperate regions, forested areas)	May also be acquired by ingestion of unpasteurized dairy products from infected cows, goats, and sheep
Powassan virus	Member of virus family *Flaviviridae*	*Ixodes scapularis, Ixodes cookei*		North America: United States (northeastern states and Great Lakes region), Canada Europe: Russia	
Crimean–Congo Hemorrhagic Fever (CCHF) Virus	Nairo virus. Family *Bunyaviridae*	Ixodid ticks		Asia, Africa, and Europe	May also be inquired by contact with infected blood, saliva, or inhalation
Omsk Hemorrhagic Fever Virus (OHFV)	Member of virus family *Flaviviridae*	*Dermacentor reticulatus, Dermacentor marginatus, Ixodes persulcatus*		Europe: southwestern Russia	
Kyasanur Forest Disease Virus (KFDV)	Member of virus family *Flaviviridae*	*Hemaphysalis spinigera* (hard ticks)		Asia: southern India, Saudi Arabia (aka Alkhurma disease in Saudi Arabia)	Associated with exposure while harvesting agents
Other					
Southern Tick-Associated Rash Illness (STARI)		*Amblyomma americanum*		Eastern, southeastern, and south-central US	

[a]Refer to CDC for further information on Other Tick-borne SFGR transmitted internationally: http://www.cdc.gov/otherspottedfever/. Accessed January 17, 2017.
Source: Centers for Disease Control and Prevention. Tickborne diseases of the US: http://www.cdc.gov/ticks/diseases/. Accessed July 23, 2017.

Tick Genus

Only two of the three families of ticks are of medical significance to humans: the soft-bodied ticks, Argasidae, and the hard-bodied ticks, Ixodidae.[2] Four of the 13 genera of Ixodidae transmit disease in the United States: *Dermacentor, Ixodes, Amblyomma,* and *Rhipicephalus.* Among the five genera of Argasidae, only *Ornithodoros* are known to transmit pathogens to humans in the United States. Most hard ticks have a 2- to 3-year life cycle, comprising the larval, nymphal, and adult stages.[2] They require one blood meal during each stage before they can mature into the next stage, and they usually remain attached to a host for hours or days. In contrast, soft ticks may have multiple nymphal stages, and both nymphal and adult forms can feast on blood multiple times, usually for only 30 minutes. However, Argasidae can survive many years without blood sustenance and are long-lived.[2] Humans are the inadvertent hosts for the life cycle of almost all ticks and tick-borne diseases.

LYME DISEASE

Lyme disease, or more accurately Lyme borreliosis, is a multisystem spirochetal disease caused by several genospecies of the spirochete *Borrelia burgdorferi* sensu lato.[5,6] Lyme disease, which is transmitted by a tick bite, was first recognized in the United States in the mid-1970s, after a mysterious outbreak of arthritis near Lyme, Connecticut.[6] However, illness consistent with late manifestations of Lyme disease was described in Europe more than a century ago. In Europe and North America, Lyme disease is now recognized as the most commonly reported vector-borne disease.[6]

Etiologic Agent

Three genomic subgroups of *B. burgdorferi* worldwide account for most human infections: *B afzelii, B garinii,* and *B burgdorferi* sensu stricto (hereafter referred to as *B burgdorferi*).[6,7] Although all three groups have been found in Europe, most isolates are *Borrelia garinii* or *Borrelia afzelii,* the North American strains identified to date belong to the *B. burgdorferi* as the cause of Lyme disease.

Tick Vectors

There are four species of Ixodes ticks that commonly bite humans. In Europe and Asia, *I ricinus* and *I persulcatus* are principal vectors, respectively. In the United States, the black-legged or deer tick, *I scapularis,* is the principal vector in areas of the Northeastern, Mid-Atlantic, and North Central states, whereas *I. pacificus,* the western black-legged tick, is the principal human-biting vector in the western US.[6,7]

The tick acquires the *B. burgdorferi* spirochete from feeding on an infected reservoir host, such as mice, shrews, and other small mammals and various species of birds. The spirochete remains dormant in the tick's midgut until the tick feeds again. The spirochete then passes through the salivary ducts of the tick and is injected through the skin of the new host with the tick bite.[6,8,9]

Few spirochetes are transmitted from the tick to its host during the first 24 to 36 hours of attachment. An infected nymphal tick, however, invariably transfers spirochetes when attached to its host for more than 72 hours.

Most humans are infected through the bites of nymph ticks, which feed during the spring and summer months. Larval and nymph ticks are small, less than 3 mm, size of a freckle or poppy seed. Therefore, the tick often goes unnoticed, and fewer than half of patients with Lyme disease recall having been bitten by a tick. The tick feeds on small, medium, or large mammals, lizards, or birds during its larval and nymphal (immature) stages.[2] Larval ticks are not relevant vectors for Lyme disease, however, because they are rarely infected and become so only after feeding on an infected host.[3] Adult ticks parasitize only medium or large mammals.[2] Although adult ticks can also transmit Lyme disease bacteria, because they are much larger, individuals are more likely to discover and remove them prior to transmission of bacteria.

Humans are inadvertent hosts of any stage of the tick. Although the tick can feed on many different animals, each tick species has preferred hosts. The complex interplay of spirochete, host, and vector in a particular area influences the risk of Lyme disease after a tick bite. Lyme disease is not transmitted directly between people, and there has not been substantive evidence of human transmission through sexual contact, semen, urine, or breast milk.[6]

Clinical Features and Diagnosis

LOCALIZED (EARLY) STAGE

Although clinical features of Lyme disease are diverse and vary with the stage and duration of infection, the presence of an EM skin rash is universally the most common feature, occurring in 60% to 90% of cases in North America.[6] The development of an EM rash at the site of the tick bite is typically the first indication of transmission and early infection in most North American patients.[8] The EM rash, which reflects the innate immune response, occurs between 3 and 30 days (an average of 7 days). Fever, headache, fatigue, muscle and joint aches, and swollen lymph nodes, and the characteristic EM skin rash are the typical early signs and symptoms (3 to 30 days after the tick bite).[4]

Lyme disease is diagnosed based on patient symptoms, physical findings (e.g., EM rash), and the possibility of tick exposure.[4,8–10] Because it is a multisystem condition, if left untreated, infection can spread to the joints, the heart, and the nervous system. Although laboratory methods can be helpful if used correctly, serologic tests are insensitive during the first few weeks of infection. Though not necessary, in some cases, acute and convalescent titers may be helpful in some cases. During this stage, patient with an EM rash, systemic symptoms, and the possibility of tick exposure may be diagnosed clinically. Appropriate antibiotics should be initiated in early stages of Lyme disease.

DISSEMINATED STAGE

During the disseminated stage, serologic tests are usually positive and a standardized two-tier testing protocol is recommended.[4,8,11] The Lyme disease presentation and testing can be complex, and the reader is referred to the Centers for Disease Control and Prevention (CDC) and other resources for further information.[4] During this stage, a variety of manifestations may occur (Table 82-2).

Table 82-2
Lyme Disease Clinical Manifestations

Early Localized Stage
■ Erythema migrans (EM) skin rash: red ring-like or homogenous expanding rash
■ Flu-like symptoms—malaise, headache, fever, myalgia, arthralgia
■ Lymphadenopathy
Disseminated Stage
■ Flu-like symptoms
■ Lymphadenopathy
■ Multiple secondary annular rashes
Cardiac Manifestations
■ Myocarditis or pericarditis
■ Conduction defects, varying degrees of atrioventricular or bundle-branch block, but permanent pacing not indicated
Neurologic Manifestations
■ Bell's palsy or other cranial neuropathy
■ Meningitis
■ Radiculoneuritis, myelitis
■ Sensory or motor peripheral neuropathy
Rheumatologic Manifestations
■ Transient, migratory arthritis and effusion in one or multiple joints
■ Migratory pain in tendons, bursae, muscle, and bones
■ Baker cyst
■ Arthritis may recur in same or different joints (if untreated)
Additional Manifestations
■ Conjunctivitis, keratitis, uveitis
■ Mild hepatitis
■ Splenomegaly

Source: Centers for Disease Control and Prevention. *Tickborne Diseases of the United States. A Reference Manual for Health Care Providers*. 3rd ed. 2015.

Treatment

The clinical manifestations of Lyme disease should govern the treatment strategy.[4,11] Patients who receive appropriate treatment in the early stages of Lyme disease usually recover rapidly and completely. Oral treatment regimens commonly used in early-stage disease include doxycycline, amoxicillin, or cefuroxime axetil (Table 82-3).[5] Patients with disseminated (late) Lyme disease should be evaluated for severity and may require intravenous treatment.[4,11]

CASE 82-1

QUESTION 1: C.J., a 32-year-old male, visits his primary care physician (PCP) with symptoms of low-grade fever and muscle aches 2 days after camping in the western part of Massachusetts during the month of August. He explained that he was canoeing and hiking with his family in the woods, and on the last day of their trip, he noticed a small tick on his thigh and immediately destroyed it. A small, itchy spot that he felt at the site of the tick bite is no longer symptomatic. C.J. asks his PCP whether he needs any laboratory tests and/or preventive treatment. Given his presentation and tick bite history, what would be appropriate steps to management?

The routine use of antibiotic prophylaxis or serologic testing is not recommended for Lyme disease prevention following a recognized tick bite.[4,11] With regard to C.J.'s situation, the use of serologic testing is not recommended because the antibody

Table 82-3
Treatment Recommendations for Localized (Early) Lyme Disease

Adults: doxycycline 100 mg, 2 times/day orally × 14 days (14–21 days)
Or
Amoxicillin 500 mg, 3 times/day orally × 14 (14–21 days)
Or
Cefuroxime axetil 500 mg, 2 times/day orally × 14 (14–21 days)
Children: amoxicillin 50 mg/kg/day orally, divided into three doses (maximum, 500 mg/dose) × 14 days (14–21 days)
Children: cefuroxime 30 mg/kg/day, orally, divided into two doses (maximum, 500 mg/dose) × 14 days (14–21 days)
Children (>8 years): may use doxycycline 4 mg/kg/day orally, divided into two doses (maximum, 100 mg/dose) × 14 days (14–21 days)

Sources: Centers for Disease Control and Prevention. *Tickborne Diseases of the United States. A Reference Manual for Health Care Providers*. 3rd ed. 2015; Wormser GP et al. The clinical assessment, treatment, and prevention of Lyme Disease, Human Granulocytic Anaplasmosis, and Babesiosis: clinical practice guidelines by the Infectious Diseases Society of America. [published correction appears in *Clin Infect Dis*. 2007;45(7):941]. *Clin Infect Dis*. 2006;43:1089–1134.

response to *B. burgdorferi* is not detectable for the first few weeks after a tick bite. Therefore, the blood tests for antibodies to *B. burgdorferi* are unlikely to be positive, because C.J.'s tick bite occurred only 2 days ago.[8,10,11]

The risk of developing Lyme disease can be affected by the rate of transmission of the spirochete from infected ticks to humans, the length of time before the tick is removed during its bite, the degree of blood engorgement of the tick (scutal index), the prevalence of spirochete infestation of ticks in an area (which varies with the tick species), and the reservoir competency of host animals in the region.[3]

Although transmission rates of Lyme disease from an infected tick bite are estimated at approximately 10%, the risk is reduced dramatically if the tick is removed within 24 hours of attachment. The small, itchy spot experienced by C.J. may represent a hypersensitivity reaction to the bite. These erythematous, noninfectious skin lesions develop within 48 hours of tick detachment or may occur while the tick is still attached. They are usually less than 5 cm in diameter; they may have an urticarial appearance and usually disappear in 1 or 2 days.[4,6]

Prophylactic antibiotic preventive therapy with a single dose of 200 mg of oral doxycycline (children 8 years or older at 4 mg/kg to a maximum 200-mg dose) can be offered if all of the following criteria are met: (a) There are no contraindications to doxycycline use; (b) administration can start within 72 hours of tick removal; (c) the tick can be reliably identified as a nymphal or adult *I. scapularis* tick with certainty of the duration of attachment of 36 hours or more based on the degree of engorgement or time of exposure; and (d) the local rate of infection of ticks by *B. burgdorferi* in the area of exposure is 20% or greater based on current ecologic evidence.[3] Routine testing of ticks themselves for tick-borne infections is not recommended.[11]

Antibiotic prophylaxis after *I. pacificus* tick bites is generally not necessary because of relatively low prevalence of *B. burgdorferi* infestation of *I. pacificus* ticks.[11] However, C.J. had exposure in a region where *B. burgdorferi* is highly prevalent among *I. scapularis* ticks. If there is uncertainty regarding the duration of tick attachment, he may be offered a dose of doxycycline prophylaxis.

ERYTHEMA MIGRANS

Signs, Symptoms, and Disease Course

CASE 82-2

Question 1: M.K., a 37-year-old woman, presents with right knee pain and multiple, large, discrete skin rashes that she has had for the past 10 days. Three months ago, in July, she visited friends in Maine and spent much of her time engaged in outdoor activities. Two months ago, her husband noticed a circular area of intense redness, approximately 9 cm wide, in her left armpit. The rash grew considerably larger during the next 2 weeks and had a red outer border. M.K. attributed the expansion of the rash to having scratched the mildly itchy area. The rash gradually disappeared. In late August, M.K. experienced fatigue, nausea, and headache for a week and thought it was "summer flu." In early September, she experienced right knee pain; ibuprofen produced some relief.

On examination, she was afebrile and had mild soft tissue swelling of the right knee. Her white blood cell (WBC) count was normal. Serum samples contained antibody titers to *B. burgdorferi* demonstrated by a sensitive ELISA (enzyme immunoassay) followed by a Western blot for immunoglobulin M (IgM) and IgG. A Venereal Disease Research Laboratory (VDRL) test for syphilis and a pregnancy test were negative.

M.K. is started on a 4-week course of oral doxycycline 100 mg twice daily. What characteristics of M.K.'s skin rash are consistent with the EM of Lyme disease?

The EM of Lyme disease usually develops within 3 to 30 days (average 7 days) of a usually asymptomatic tick bite at the site of inoculation of the spirochete. The rash begins as an erythematous (red) macule or papule typically on the thigh, back, shoulder, calf, groin, popliteal fossa, flank, axilla, buttock, or upper arm.[4,6,11] In children, EM is often found on the head at the hairline, neck, arms, or legs. It expands outwardly at 2 to 3 cm/day to a diameter of 5 to 70 cm (mean, 16 cm), occasionally with some central clearing. Some cases of EM in the United States lack central clearing. The rash may be warm to the touch and is usually painless, but some patients have mild burning or itching. Up to 50% of patients with EM have multiple secondary lesions that most likely represent blood-borne spread of the spirochete to other skin sites rather than multiple tick bites.[5] If untreated, EM generally fades within several weeks; if treated, it usually resolves in several days.[4,6,11]

Low-grade fever and other nonspecific symptoms, such as malaise, headache, myalgias, or arthralgias, may accompany EM.[4,6,11] Some individuals may have no symptoms. Cough, rhinitis, sinusitis, and other respiratory symptoms do not usually occur in Lyme disease.[4] Pitfalls in the diagnosis of EM exist. Lesions are sometimes misdiagnosed. M.K.'s skin rash was large (>9 cm), red, and had a red outer border. It gradually faded over the course of a few weeks. These characteristics are consistent with a diagnosis of EM.

Serologic Testing

Case 82-2, Question 2: What might have been the rationale for the laboratory tests that were undertaken in M.K.?

Guidelines currently recommend a two-tier approach of ELISA and confirmatory Western blotting.[8,10,11] The sensitivity of such testing in Lyme arthritis cases is 97% to 100%.[9,11] However, routine use of serology testing for patients with early EM cannot be recommended presently. Syphilis and other known biologic causes (periodontal spirochetes) of false-positive serologic testing should be excluded. Rheumatoid factor or antinuclear antibody tests usually are negative in Lyme disease. These tests help differentiate rheumatoid arthritis or systemic lupus erythematosus from Lyme disease. The WBC count is normal or mildly elevated in Lyme disease. M.K. had a normal WBC. Pregnancy was ruled out before initiating a tetracycline. Most interesting in M.K. is the presence of secondary EM lesions representing disseminated infection.

The presence of EM as an early indicator of Lyme disease gives clinicians the best opportunity for early diagnosis and treatment.[4,11] In the United States, the expression of EM is the *only* manifestation of Lyme disease that is sufficiently distinctive to allow clinical diagnosis in the absence of confirmatory laboratory information.[4,11] Early treatment can prevent sequelae of disseminated disease.

LYME DISEASE TREATMENT

Antibiotics

CASE 82-2, QUESTION 3: Why was doxycycline selected to treat M.K.?

Borrelia burgdorferi is susceptible to amoxicillin, tetracyclines, and some second- and third-generation cephalosporins. It is only moderately sensitive to penicillin G and is resistant to first-generation cephalosporins, rifampin, cotrimoxazole, aminoglycosides, chloramphenicol, and the fluoroquinolones.[4,11]

Penicillin, tetracycline, and erythromycin historically were the drugs of choice for the treatment of Lyme disease because they can be administered orally; they are relatively inexpensive and appear to have good in vitro activity. However, this in vitro activity does not translate to in vivo efficacy. Doxycycline is an agent of choice for treatment of Lyme disease. Amoxicillin and cefuroxime axetil are also first-line options. In Europe, in contrast, penicillin still is used with continued success. A nondoxycycline regimen is preferred in pregnant or breast-feeding women and in children younger than 8 years of age.[4,11]

Compared with the third-generation cephalosporins, the oral second-generation drug cefuroxime axetil has good in vitro activity and efficacy. But it is more expensive than oral amoxicillin or doxycycline. Of the third-generation cephalosporins, ceftriaxone has the most potent in vitro activity and a long half-life for once-daily dosing in an outpatient program. Ceftriaxone is expensive, however, and has a higher incidence of diarrhea than other β-lactams, probably owing to extensive biliary excretion.

The macrolides clarithromycin and azithromycin are unpredictable in their in vitro activity.[4,11] Similar to erythromycin, they are less effective in the treatment of Lyme disease. The combination of a macrolide with lysosomotropic agents, especially hydroxychloroquine, anecdotally has been suggested to be associated with increased symptom relief probably related to combined anti-inflammatory activity rather than direct antimicrobial activity.[3] Doxycycline is well absorbed orally and is less expensive than parenteral ceftriaxone or cefotaxime. Doxycycline has a long serum half-life of 18 to 22 hours. In addition, doxycycline penetrates into the cerebrospinal fluid (CSF) at concentrations of at least 10% of serum levels, even in the absence of meningeal inflammation. Although not as significant as with tetracycline, doxycycline can complex with divalent or trivalent cations in the gut, with an associated decrease in oral absorption. On the other hand, administering doxycycline with food, to minimize nausea, is recommended.[3] Compared with other tetracyclines, doxycycline has the least affinity for divalent calcium cations, and oral absorption is reduced by only 20% if given with milk. The major side effect of doxycycline is phototoxicity, which is of concern because Lyme disease usually occurs during sunny times of the year. A less recognized side effect is the risk of doxycycline-induced esophageal ulceration. Patients should be instructed to never take doxycycline or other tetracyclines near bedtime and to take the medication while standing up with at least 240 mL of clear fluid, especially with the capsule formulation. Despite less in vitro activity compared with some β-lactam antibiotics, *B. burgdorferi* is sufficiently susceptible to doxycycline, and clinical experience with doxycycline has been very favorable. In conclusion, doxycycline was a suitable choice for M.K.

Chronic Lyme Arthritis

CASE 82-2, QUESTION 4: M.K. continues to have knee inflammation for 3 months after receiving a second course of antibiotic treatment and is now considered to have Lyme arthritis. Should antibiotic therapy be repeated for M.K.'s arthritis?

Acute Lyme arthritis occurs from the accumulation of neutrophils, cytokines, immune complexes, complement, and mononuclear cells induced by the spirochete.[12] Appropriate antimicrobial treatment of acute Lyme arthritis is usually successful, and doxycycline, amoxicillin, or cefuroxime axetil is recommended for adult patients, such as M.K., if there is no clinical evidence of neurologic disease.[11] Treatment for Lyme arthritis typically requires 28 days of therapy.[11] A minority subset of patients may have persistent Lyme arthritis.[12] It is very unlikely that this is attributable to the continued presence of *B. burgdorferi* in the joint, but rather to the patient's continued inflammatory response or autoimmunity.[12] Polymerase chain reaction (PCR) testing of synovial fluid can be considered, and if negative, symptomatic therapies may be offered rather than repeated antibiotic courses. Such patients often respond well to synovectomy, suggesting that the presence of synovitis may not be the result of persistence of the infection. Nonsteroidal anti-inflammatory agents, disease-modifying antirheumatic agents, intra-articular corticosteroid injections, or synovectomy may be offered.[3,11] However, it should be noted that before the antibiotic treatment era for Lyme disease, even the most prolonged cases of persistent Lyme arthritis eventually improved without treatment, although sometimes lasting for months to years.[12]

Neurologic Lyme Disease

CASE 82-3

QUESTION 1: E.T., a 57-year-old female, presents to her PCP with symptoms of early neurologic Lyme disease, including mild memory and cognitive deficits. Serum two-tier IgG seropositivity was confirmed. Should E.T. be treated with antibiotics? If so, how long should she be treated?

Although rare, late neurologic complications of Lyme disease may present as encephalopathy, peripheral neuropathy, or encephalomyelitis.[4,11] Although the Lyme *Borrelia* species found in Europe do not strictly overlap with those species found in the United States, there are no data to support a differential response to antibiotic.[10] Based on these studies, oral doxycycline can be considered as first-line therapy for neurologic Lyme disease in Europe and for ambulatory patients with early neurologic Lyme disease in the United States. An oral antibiotic treatment regimen may suffice in cases of early neurologic disease, but parenteral regimens are appropriate for severe cases.[13] In conclusion, E.T. can be treated with doxycycline administered orally and should be reassessed following treatment.

Post-Lyme Disease Syndromes

CASE 82-4

QUESTION 1: A friend who has been treated with a 4-week course of antibiotics for Lyme disease calls you to say that she has lingering symptoms and she thinks it's "chronic Lyme disease." She'd like more information about it. How should you respond?

Chronic Lyme disease is a confusing term, and most authorities agree that there may be "Post-Treatment Lyme Disease Syndrome," (PTLDS).[4] Although the exact cause is unknown, most medical experts believe that the lingering symptoms that can occur are the result of residual damage to tissues and the immune system. Clinical findings in patients may include fatigue, widespread musculoskeletal pain, cognitive difficulties, or subjective symptoms of such severity that a substantial reduction in quality of life has occurred. The subjective symptoms must include an onset within 6 months of the initial Lyme disease diagnosis and persistence for at least 6 months after completion of antimicrobial therapy. If adherence to a recommended Lyme treatment regimen is confirmed, the existence of symptomatic, chronic infection by *B. burgdorferi* is difficult to confirm. After appropriately targeted antibiotic therapy for early Lyme disease, treatment failure is exceedingly rare. The organism has not been shown to develop antibiotic resistance.[3] For these patients with chronic subjective symptoms for more than 6 months, repeated or prolonged antibiotic therapy is not useful or recommended.[4,11]

The friend should be encouraged to seek additional diagnostic workup for other diseases. Even in patients who have had verified Lyme disease, the aches and pains of daily living they experience appear to be more related to their post-treatment symptoms than to Lyme disease itself.[4]

Lyme Disease Prevention

CASE 82-5

QUESTION 1: A family living in a Lyme disease endemic area is concerned regarding their risk for contracting the disease. How would you advise them on Lyme disease prevention and overall protection from tick-borne disease?

Although some vector-borne diseases are prevented through vector control, this has proven difficult for tick-borne diseases because of a lack of efficacy or environmental concerns with the use of pesticides. Evaluated methods include habitat destruction by fire, chemical spraying agents such as acaricides to achieve tick eradication, culling or removal of host deer, or protection of mice from tick infestation.[13]

Currently, there are limited vaccines available for tick-borne and mosquito-borne illnesses.[14] A Lyme disease vaccine for humans is no longer available in the United States. Citing low demand, the U.S. manufacturer discontinued production in 2002. Clinical trials are currently underway for candidate *Lyme borreliosis* vaccines.[15]

The first step in prevention of Lyme disease is personal protection and tick avoidance.[16,17] Tick repellents may be applied to the skin or clothing. One basic chemical category of insect repellant is the synthetic agents, such as *N,N*-diethyl-*m*-toluamide (DEET), picaridin (also known as icaridin in Europe), and insect repellent (IR) 3535 (ethyl butylacetylaminopropionate). The second chemical category of repellant is the plant-derived oils and synthetics, such as oil of lemon eucalyptus or PMD (para-menthane-3,8-diol), which is an extract of the leaves of lemon eucalyptus, *Corymbia citriodora*, a synthesized version of oil of lemon eucalyptus.

The use of DEET skin repellent has evolved as the standard repellant for mosquito and tick-borne diseases. In combination with a permethrin clothing, DEET appears to offer adequate protection. DEET has been tested against *Ixodid* ticks for repellence and is more effective than dibutyl phthalate, dimethyl phthalate, pyrethrum, and two combination products.[16,17] DEET is generally safe; however, excessive DEET application has been associated with seizures in children.[17,18] These are rare events, however, and if the products are used according to their labeling, the adverse reaction risk is low, even for children older than 2 months of age.[3] Prolonged or excessive application is not recommended. It may be prudent to use the lowest effective concentration of DEET-containing repellents, such as those containing 20% to 30%. To minimize DEET toxicity, the product should be applied sparingly, inhalation or introduction into the eyes should be avoided, repellent-treated skin should be washed when coming inside, use on children's hands (that are likely to have contact with the eyes or mouth) should be avoided, and it should be applied only to intact skin or clothing.

Picaridin was developed in Europe in the 1990s and released in the United States about 10 years ago. A couple of advantages over DEET include the lack of a chemical odor and its nonsticky or greasy feel. It is also safe to use on plastics, whereas DEET may damage certain synthetics including eyeglass frames. IR3535, originally marketed in the United States as a skin emollient and moisturizer, was then adopted for use as an insect repellant. Plant-derived IRs, such as oil of lemon eucalyptus or PMD, have demonstrated efficacy against the tick vectors of Lyme disease (*Ixodes scapularis, Ixodes pacificus*) and Rocky Mountain spotted fever (*Dermacentor andersoni*).[1]

A literature review between 2000 and 2012 on the efficacy of repellants against various mosquito and tick species noted that there are only limited studies conducted on tick behavior and repellant efficacy against the tick species *Ixodes*.[18,19] The use of picaridin, IR 3535, and PMD were also reviewed as part of this study. Results of this study found that the use of IR 3535 provided the longest protection against *Ixodes scapularis*, whereas DEET and commercial products containing picaridin or PMD demonstrated a better response than IR 3535 against *Ixodes ricinus*.[18] In situations in which environmental exposure to disease-transmitting ticks, biting midges, sandflies, or blackflies is anticipated, topical repellants containing IR 3535, picaridin, or oil of eucalyptus (or PMD) would offer better protection than topical DEET alone.[1] (Refer to Chapter 81, Parasitic Infections, Table 81-2, Mosquito Protection Measures for additional information on insect repellants).

Physical barriers to ticks, such as wearing protective garments—long pants, and long-sleeved shirts—tucking shirts into pants and pants into boots, and wearing closed-toed shoes, prevent infection.[1] Ticks are easier to spot on light-colored clothing. Checking the body for ticks regularly is recommended; any that are found should be promptly removed. Avoiding tick habitats is the best protection against tick-borne diseases. Effective postexposure antibiotic prophylaxis can be administered in Lyme disease endemic areas after a tick bite.

RELAPSING FEVER

Relapsing fever, a bacterial infection caused by a variety of *Borrelia species,* causes episodes of fever, nausea, headache, and muscle and joint aches. Of the two types of relapsing fever, tick-borne relapsing fever (TBRF) occurs in the western US and louse-borne relapsing fever (LBRF) is generally restricted to refugee settings in developing parts of the world.[5]

Tick Vector

The predominant tick vector for relapsing fever is of the genus *Ornithodoros,* a soft-bodied tick. These ticks feed on wild rodents or domestic animals and, incidentally, on humans. In North America, three tick species carry the agents of endemic relapsing fever with apparent strict specificity. In fact, the names of the responsible *Borrelia* species have been adopted from the three tick species that transmit them: *Ornithodoros hermsii, Ornithodoros parkeri,* and *Ornithodoros turicata.*[20] Although the ticks themselves may serve as reservoir hosts, the *Borrelia* usually circulate among wild rodents, ticks, and possibly birds.[5] Similar to Lyme disease, greater worldwide variations of endemic cycles and vectors for TBRF may exist than in North America.

TICK GEOGRAPHY

In North America, relapsing fever is an uncommon disease largely confined to the geographic distribution of the tick species that harbor the *Borrelia.* In the United States, most cases of TBRF have occurred in 14 western states and are caused by *B. hermsii.*[5] These ticks are usually found in the remote natural settings of the mountains and semiarid plains of the far west and Mexico. TBRF can develop when people visit tick- or rodent-infested cabins or summer homes. While TBRF is spread by multiple tick species, *Ornithodoros hermsii* is the tick responsible for most cases in the United States usually at altitudes of 1,500 to 8,000 feet. The health significance of *O. parkeri* and *O. turicata* transmits its *Borrelia* at lower altitudes in the Southwest, where they inhabit caves and the borrows of ground squirrels, prairie dogs, and burrowing owls.

SPIROCHETAL BEHAVIOR

Ticks acquire spirochetes from blood feeding on small wild rodents. If high levels of *Borrelia* are present in the animal's blood, large numbers of spirochetes will be ingested by the tick and reside in the tick's midgut. During the next few days, the spirochetes invade the midgut wall, traverse the hemolymph system, and within a few weeks infect the salivary glands as well as other tick tissues and organs. Females may develop infected ovaries and transmit *Borrelia* to offspring in some *Ornithodoros* species, but this is rare in *O. hermsii.*[20] Having reached the tick's salivary glands, the spirochetes are poised to invade the tick's next host.

TICK BEHAVIOR

In contrast to the hard-bodied ticks, these soft ticks feed rapidly, often detaching after 30 to 90 minutes.[20,21] They feed at night while people are sleeping, and their bite is usually painless. Therefore, most people are unaware that they have been bitten.[18]

Disease Characterization

The hallmark of endemic relapsing fever is an abrupt onset of high fever (often >39°C) after an incubation period of 4 to 18 days.[20] The patient may experience shaking chills, severe headache, abdominal pain, myalgias, arthralgias, nausea, vomiting, and malaise. A few cases of acute respiratory distress syndrome have recently been recognized.[20] The fever usually breaks in 3 days (range, 12 hours to 17 days) in untreated patients.[20] After a variable afebrile period of 3 to 36 days (usually 7 days), cyclic periods of fever and constitutional symptoms reappear. Each febrile attack progressively diminishes in severity. Three to five relapses typically occur in untreated patients.

Routine laboratory testing is of little value. Moderate anemia and an increased erythrocyte sedimentation rate (ESR) are common. Leukocyte counts may be normal, yet moderate-to-severe thrombocytopenia is commonly observed but is considered nonspecific. The diagnosis of relapsing fever is made by direct observation of the spirochete on a peripheral blood smear while the patient is febrile.[20] Observation of the smear is enhanced with Wright or Giemsa staining. Few diagnostic laboratories perform antibody serology tests; however, these tests lack specificity.[20] Skin biopsy of a rash to identify the spirochete is unreliable. Direct culture of the spirochete from the blood into a special culture medium is the most specific diagnostic tool, but this is a slow technique confined to research laboratories.

TREATMENT

These Borrelia have not demonstrated antibiotic resistance. Successful treatment regimens usually include a 7- to 10-day course of antibiotics.[5,20] Tetracycline (500 mg every 6 hours for 10 days) is the preferred regimen. Erythromycin is an effective alternative at a dose of 500 mg (or 12.5 mg/kg) every 6 hours for 10 days. For individuals experiencing central nervous system (CNS) involvement, ceftriaxone (2 g/day for 10–14 days) is preferred. Hospitalization and administration of IV antibiotics may be required in severely ill patients.

CASE 82-6

QUESTION 1: T.J. is a 49-year-old man who visits his PCP with a sudden onset of high fever, severe headache, malaise, nausea, vomiting, and myalgias. He returned a week ago, at the end of August, from a stay in a rustic cabin on the north rim of the Grand Canyon. His PCP orders a manual complete blood count (CBC) and chemistry panel and asks the laboratory to observe a blood smear with Giemsa staining. T.J.'s recent visit and outdoor activities are consistent with areas with prior outbreaks where relapsing fever has been documented. After confirming the presence of *Borrelia* in the blood smear, the PCP prescribes a 10-day course of tetracycline. Two hours after the first dose, T.J.'s wife calls the physician's office with concerns that the disease is worsening. T.J. experiences an increased temperature, faintness, and chills, and has a rapid pulse and respiration rate. What do these symptoms represent? Is this an adverse drug reaction?

Up to 54% of patients with relapsing fever experience a reaction, a Jarisch–Herxheimer reaction, to the first dose of antibiotic (see Chapter 72 Sexually Transmitted Diseases).[21] It may occur in LBRF, TBRF, and in other spirochetal diseases such as syphilis or Lyme disease.[3] The dramatic reaction consists of a rise in temperature, chills, myalgias, tachycardia, hypotension, increased respiratory rate, and vasodilation.[20] Treatment of the reaction consists of supportive care. Severe reactions may require hospitalization for vital sign monitoring and management of hypovolemia. Although this is a reaction to the administration of an antibiotic drug, it is not an allergic response, and the antibiotic should be continued.

BORRELIA MIYAMOTOI

CASE 82-6, QUESTION 2: T.J. continues with antibiotic therapy and his symptom resolves. Given his clinical presentation and findings, his diagnosis and treatment were appropriate. How does *Borrelia miyamotoi* typically present and what treatment options are available?

Borrelia miyamotoi is a bacterial species that is closely related to the bacteria that cause TBRF and distantly related to *Borrelia burgdorferi* that causes Lyme disease. While first identified in 1995 in ticks from Japan, *B. miyamotoi* has been detected in two species of North American ticks, the black-legged or deer tick (*I. scapularis*) and the western black-legged tick (*I. pacificus*). The first human cases of infection were identified in Russia and described in 2011, followed by the first recognized cases in northeastern United States in 2013.[22] To date, there are less than 60 well-documented cases of *B. miyamotoi* in the United States. Because ticks are also known to transmit several diseases, including Lyme disease, anaplasmosis, and babesiosis, researchers and healthcare providers need to learn more about the transmission and signs and symptoms of this infection.

Patients with *B. miyamotoi* infection generally experience nonspecific symptoms such as fever, chills, headache, myalgia, and arthralgia.[22,23] Unlike Lyme diseases, rash was an uncommon finding, with only 4 out of 51 patients experiencing a rash. The blood tests that are used for Lyme disease are not helpful in the diagnosis of *B. miyamotoi* infections. Currently, the PCR tests that detect DNA from the organism or antibody-based tests are used for confirmatory diagnosis. Patients with *B. miyamotoi* have been successfully treated with a 2 to 4 week of doxycycline, and amoxicillin and ceftriaxone have also been used. *Borrelia miyamotoi* disease will continue to be evaluated, and it may be an emerging tick-borne infection in the northeastern region of the United States.

SOUTHERN TICK-ASSOCIATED RASH ILLNESS (STARI)

CASE 82-7

QUESTION 1: G.T., a 47-year-old man living in southern Missouri, recently experienced a rash resembling EM after a lone star tick bite. Because this tick is not a vector for Lyme disease, what could be the cause and how should he be managed?

Amblyomma americanum (the lone star tick) is found throughout the southeast and south-central US and along the Atlantic coast as far north as Maine, and its territory is expanding.[4] The lone star tick aggressively bites humans in the southern states, as opposed to *I. scapularis* ticks.[5,24] Spirochetes detected by microscopy and culture have been found in 1% to 5% of lone star ticks and are named *Borrelia lonestari*.[2,5,24] *B. lonestari* and *B. burgdorferi*, however, were ruled out as the cause of EM -like skin lesions known as STARI in one Missouri investigation.[5,24] Attempts to culture the agent of this Lyme-like illness, although exhaustive, have been unsuccessful.[24] The causative agent of STARI has not yet been confirmed. There are differences in the appearance and content of the rashes of STARI and the EM of Lyme disease. For example, Lyme EM rashes show an abundance of plasma cells contrasted with a predominantly lymphocytic infiltrate seen in STARI.[24]

G.T.'s diagnosis was based on symptoms, geographic location, and tick bite information. Because the cause of STARI is unknown, no diagnostic tests are available, nor is it known if antibiotic treatment is necessary or beneficial for patients. However, because STARI resembles Lyme disease, limited data support treating STARI with regimens similar to those used for Lyme disease.[24] For example, doxycycline may be given for 10 to 30 days, with longer durations reserved for evidence of dissemination beyond the rash, such as fever, severe headache, lymphadenopathy, or multiple rashes.[25]

OTHER BACTERIAL DISEASES: TULAREMIA

Tularemia

ETIOLOGY AND EPIDEMIOLOGY

In 1911, George W. McCoy and Charles W. Chapin from the US Public Health Service investigated a plague-like disease in wild ground squirrels harvested in Tulare County, California, and discovered the infectious etiology of tularemia.[25] The bacterium is a small, pleomorphic, catalase-positive, nonmotile, aerobic, nonencapsulated, gram-negative coccobacillus now named *Francisella tularensis* in honor of Edward Francis for his fieldwork and contributions to tularemia research. He proposed the terminology *tularemia* because the disease is associated with bacteremia.[25]

Although tularemia is found worldwide, it occurs primarily in the Northern Hemisphere.[22] The important reservoir hosts for *F. tularensis* are wild rabbits, ticks, and deer flies.[25] The North American tick vectors are *Dermacentor variabilis* (dog tick), *Amblyomma americanum* (lone star tick), and *Dermacentor andersoni* (wood tick). Tick-borne tularemia occurs most often in the spring and summer, matching the likelihood of exposure.[4] Before 1950, most human cases of the disease developed from direct contact with infected animals, usually hares or rabbits, and tularemia cases that occurred in the fall or winter were usually associated with hunting season exposure. Tick bite transmission, however, now accounts for more than half of tularemia cases west of the Mississippi River in the United States. In summer months, tick or fly bites appear to be the main mode of transmission of tularemia to humans. Other animals, such as domestic cats, are susceptible to tularemia and are known to have transmitted tularemia to humans.[4] Tularemia outbreaks have also occurred among hamsters purchased from pet shops. Individuals should be careful when handling any sick or dead animal. Other modes of transmission include ingestion of, or contact with, infected meat, water, or soil; inhalation of aerosolized bacteria; or bites from infected animals, mosquitoes, or deerflies.[25] Direct person-to-person transmission has not been reported.

CLINICAL PRESENTATION

The clinical manifestations of tularemia are related to the mode of transmission, patient characteristics, and bacterial subspecies causing infection.[25] Classically, six types of tularemia presentation have been identified: ulceroglandular, glandular, typhoidal, oculoglandular, oropharyngeal, and pneumonic. The last three forms were presumably not tick-borne, reflecting alternative avenues of transmission. Today, the clinical manifestations fall into two main groups: ulceroglandular and typhoidal.[25]

Ulceroglandular is the most common form of tularemia, accounting for approximately 75% of cases.[25] Sixty percent of ulceroglandular cases are characterized by an ulcer that forms at the site of entry, usually on the lower extremities, perineum, buttocks, or trunk from arthropods that tend to bite the lower extremities or on the upper extremities from mammalian bites.[22] The lesion starts as a firm, erythematous papule that ulcerates and heals over the course of several weeks. It is accompanied by regional, painful lymphadenopathy, usually inguinal or femoral. Typhoidal tularemia, occurring in approximately 25% of cases, is characterized by fever, chills, headache, debilitation, abdominal pain, and prostration. Fever and chills are common with all forms of tularemia.[25]

After exposure to the bacteria and an incubation period of 4 to 5 days, patients become ill with a sudden onset of fever, chills, headache, cough, arthralgias, myalgias, fatigue, and malaise. The severity of symptoms is quite variable, ranging from a mild, limited disease (probably type B tularemia) to rare cases of septic shock (probably type A tularemia). A hallmark manifestation is a high fever without an accompanying increase in pulse, or pulse–temperature disparity.[22] Common complications are mild hepatitis, secondary pneumonia, and pharyngitis. With antibiotic treatment of uncomplicated tularemia, mortality rates are only 1% to 3%. Increased morbidity and mortality are seen in the more rare typhoidal forms.[25] The most lethal form of tularemia is from pulmonary infection.[25] In the healthcare setting, standard precautions are all that is required when caring for tularemia-infected patients because they are not a source for secondary infection. However, any suspected outbreaks should be reported and investigated.[25]

DIAGNOSIS

Tularemia can be difficult to diagnose as routine laboratory testing is of little help in establishing a diagnosis and is limited to the demonstration of an antibody response to the bacteria. Because an antibody response to the illness requires 10 to 14 days for detection, treatment is usually empiric. The diagnosis is based on clinical suspicion from the epidemiologic history and the presence of compatible findings. The customary serologic test demonstrates *F. tularensis* antibody agglutination. Although a single-tube agglutination test with a titer of 1:160 or more (or 1:128 or more using a microagglutination study) in a suspected case is highly suggestive of a tularemia diagnosis, a fourfold or greater rise in titers between the acute and convalescent stages 2 weeks apart is diagnostic.[26] After a bout of tularemia, detectable antibodies may persist for many years.[25]

TREATMENT

Antibiotic treatment options for tularemia have included streptomycin, gentamicin, doxycycline, and ciprofloxacin. Streptomycin was historically the drug of choice for tularemia, but it is often unavailable commercially. Some clinicians believe that gentamicin is the best alternative aminoglycoside for the treatment of nonmeningitic tularemia. Its advantages compared with streptomycin include lower minimal inhibitory concentrations (MICs), less vestibular toxicity, and wider commercial availability. Although considered comparable in efficacy to streptomycin, gentamicin has been associated with increased treatment failure and relapse. Tobramycin is inferior to gentamicin or streptomycin and should not be used.

In many of the reported studies of antimicrobial therapy for tularemia, short courses of treatment were used. To prevent tularemia from worsening or relapsing, longer regimens (10–14 days) should be used, especially in more severe cases. Jarisch–Herxheimer reactions can occur with antibiotic treatment of tularemia. Antibiotic prophylaxis for people exposed to those with tularemia is not recommended, but prophylactic antibiotics might be used for suspected bioterrorism attacks of tularemia. Acute febrile illness with pneumonia and other signs of infection occur 3 to 5 days after exposure to airborne tularemia organisms from an intentionally set weapon. No tularemia vaccines are available in the United States. A partially protective one was developed in the former Soviet Union but was only used for at-risk personnel such as for certain laboratory workers.[23] Personal protective measures, as discussed for Lyme disease, should be used when spending time outdoors in endemic areas.[25]

THE RICKETTSIA: ROCKY MOUNTAIN SPOTTED FEVER, *RICKETTSIA PARKERI* INFECTION, EHRLICHIOSIS, AND ANAPLASMOSIS

Rocky Mountain Spotted Fever (RMSF)

Rocky Mountain spotted fever is the most prevalent and virulent rickettsial disease in the United States. As early as 1872, RMSF infected white settlers of the Northwest and it may have been prevalent in Native Americans of the region before that time. It was first described in residents of the Bitterroot, Snake, and Boise river valleys of Montana and Idaho in the late 1800s. Howard Ricketts discovered the causative agent, *Rickettsia rickettsii,* in 1908.[26] The rickettsia is a small (0.3 × 1 μm), pleomorphic, weakly gram-negative, obligate intracellular coccobacillus that can survive only briefly outside of a host.[26]

EPIDEMIOLOGY

RMSF is found throughout North America, including the United States, Canada, and Mexico, and in parts of Central and South America.[26] It has not been documented outside of the Western Hemisphere. The term "Rocky Mountain spotted fever" is actually a misnomer because the disease has shifted eastward from the Rocky Mountain states, and the greatest incidence of RMSF now occurs in North and South Carolina, Virginia, Oklahoma, Arkansas, and Tennessee.[26,27] Most RMSF infections arise from tick exposure in rural or suburban locations, although rare outbreaks in urban environments have occurred.

The prevalence of RMSF is highest in children with 5 to 9 years of age.[28] Another peak prevalence is seen in men older than 60 years. Risk factors include male sex, residence in wooded areas, and exposure to tick-infected dogs. RMSF, like other tick-borne diseases, is highly seasonal, with greatest incidence in late spring and early summer.[26]

TICK VECTORS AND HOSTS

In the east, south, and west coasts of the United States, the tick vector for RMSF has been identified as the dog tick, *Dermacentor variabilis.*[2] In the Rocky Mountain states, the wood tick, *D. andersoni,* is the vector.[24] In Mexico, the tick vectors are *Rhipicephalus sanguineus* and *Amblyomma cajennense,* with the latter also being responsible in Central and South America.[24] The brown dog tick, *R. sanguineus*, has been identified as a new tick vector for RMSF in a defined area of Arizona.[26–28]

Dermacentor ticks feed on humans only during their adult stage.[26] Larval *Dermacentor* ticks may be infected while feeding on small mammals that have sufficient rickettsemia for transmission, such as chipmunks, ground squirrels, cotton rats, snowshoe hares, and meadow voles. Dogs are not considered reservoirs for *R. rickettsii* but are susceptible to RMSF and may introduce infected ticks into households.[26,27] Adult ticks transmit the rickettsia transovarially to their progeny with high efficiency and establish newly infected tick lines. If the rickettsia burden is large in the adult tick, however, it may cause tick death, thereby reducing infected tick lines. Therefore, there must be nontick reservoirs, as mentioned previously, to develop newly infected tick generational lines; otherwise, RMSF would slowly disappear. In summary, ticks are both vectors and hosts for *R. rickettsii.*[26] Humans are dead-end accidental hosts of *R. rickettsii.*[26]

DISEASE COURSE, SYMPTOMS, AND FATALITIES

Rickettsia rickettsii is usually transmitted to humans from an infected tick bite.[26] The organism can also gain access to humans through broken skin if an infected tick is being crushed with bare fingers, and such crushing may generate infectious aerosols that might be inhaled. Conjunctival contact with infected tick tissues or feces provides another route for rickettsial entry. Contaminated blood transfusions and needle stick injuries have also transmitted *R. rickettsii.*[26]

After introduction of the organisms into the body, the rickettsia spread hematogenously with a predilection for the vascular endothelium, especially in capillaries and medium-sized blood vessels.[27] During an incubation period of 2 to 14 days, induced phagocytosis allows rickettsial entry into endothelial cells, where they replicate by binary fission in the cytoplasm and nuclei of infected cells. This induces a generalized vasculitis leading to activation of clotting factors, capillary leakage, and microinfarctions in various organs.[26] Exotoxins are not secreted by rickettsia; however, they do induce oxidative and peroxidative damage to host cell membranes, resulting in necrosis.[26] In severe infections, hypotension and intravascular coagulation may coexist and culminate in cell, tissue, or organ destruction.

Dehydration is an early sign of RMSF, followed by increased vascular permeability, edema, decreased plasma volume, hypoproteinemia, reduced serum oncotic pressure, and prerenal azotemia. RMSF is a multisystem disease, but a particular organ may be the major focus of the disease. If the brain or lungs are severely infected, death can ensue. An increased severity of illness is associated with edema, particularly in children, and hypoalbuminemia. Hypotension is present in 17% of patients and hyponatremia in 56%. Extensive infection of the pulmonary microvascular endothelium can cause noncardiogenic pulmonary edema.

A common finding in RMSF is myalgia (72%–83%) or muscular tenderness, which are manifestations of skeletal muscle necrosis. Striking creatinine kinase elevations have been described. Thrombocytopenia resulting from consumption of platelets during intravascular coagulation processes occurs in 35% to 52% of patients. True disseminated intravascular coagulation with attendant hypofibrinogenemia is exceptional, however, even in severe or fatal cases.[27] Blood loss or hemolysis in some may cause anemia, which is seen in 30% of patients and reflects blood vessel damage. Fatalities usually occur 8 to 15 days after illness onset if no treatment is given or is delayed. Long-term sequelae from severe forms of RMSF can include partial paralysis of the lower extremities, gangrene of extremities requiring amputation, deafness or hearing loss, incontinence, and movement or speech disorders, but these occur in a minority of patients who receive prompt antibiotic therapy.[26]

"Fulminant" RMSF is best defined as a disease with a rapidly fatal course with death occurring in approximately 5 days. This form of disease is characterized by an early onset of neurologic signs and late or absent skin rash; it is highly associated with glucose-6-phosphate dehydrogenase deficiency, advanced age, male sex, and possibly heavy alcohol use.[26,27] In the pre-antibiotic era, RMSF mortality rates were as high as 30%, but they have fallen to 5% in antibiotic-treated cases today.[2,27]

The classically defined triad of RMSF symptoms at initial presentation is fever, rash, and headache, but this is found in only up to 5% of cases during the first 3 days of illness and up to approximately 60% of cases 2 weeks after exposure.[26,28] The RMSF skin rash typically begins 2 to 4 days after fever onset as pink, 1- to 5-mm blanchable macules that later become papules.[27] It begins on the ankles, wrists, and forearms, and soon thereafter involves the palms or soles. It then spreads to the arms, thighs, and trunk, and typically evolves into a petechial exanthem. The utility of these findings in the differential diagnosis is limited because rash may be absent, transient, or late; it may never become petechial, or it may have an unusual distribution.

DIAGNOSIS

As for most tick-borne diseases, confirmatory serologic analysis is not particularly useful in early diagnosis of disease. The initial diagnosis is made based on clinical signs and symptoms and medical history. Because RMSF can be a severe or even fatal illness, antirickettsial treatment should begin immediately to prevent morbidity and mortality.[26,27] *R. rickettsii* is difficult to culture. Immunohistologic demonstration of *R. rickettsii* in biopsy specimens of rash lesions is the only approach that can yield diagnostic results in a timely manner, but this approach is applicable only to those presenting with a skin rash, and these tests are not readily available.[26]

The best serologic test for RMSF is the indirect immunofluorescence assay (IFA) test, but antibodies typically appear only after 10 to 14 days.[26] More striking laboratory abnormalities of RMSF disease include a normal leukocyte count with a shift to the left, hyponatremia, thrombocytopenia, elevated serum transaminases or creatinine kinase, and CSF pleocytosis. These findings are observed late in the disease course, however, and are not helpful in early disease recognition.

Clinical findings and history are essential to early diagnosis and successful treatment. Therapy must precede laboratory confirmation of RMSF.[26] In a febrile, tick-exposed person with a rash, RMSF should be considered. RMSF should be strongly considered in febrile children, adolescents, or men older than 60 years of age, especially if they reside in or have traveled to the southern Atlantic or south-central US from May through September. A delay in treatment for RMSF beyond 5 days of symptom onset increases the mortality rates from 5% to 22%.

TREATMENT

Doxycycline should be initiated immediately as first-line treatment for RMSF in both adults and children whenever RMSF is suspected. The recommended treatment is doxycycline 100 mg every 12 hours for children under 45 kg (100 lbs): 2.2 mg/kg body weight given twice a day. The standard duration of treatment is 7 to 14 days, including at least 3 days after the temperature has normalized.[4,5] The use of doxycycline to treat suspected RMSF in children is standard practice by the CDC and the American Academy of Pediatrics (AAP) Committee on Infectious Diseases as the use of alternative antibiotics increases the risk of death. Contraindications to doxycycline use include history of severe hypersensitivity reactions to tetracyclines, and in some pregnant patients in which the case of RMSF seems mild, chloramphenicol may be considered as an alternative antibiotic.[26] However, oral formulations of chloramphenicol are not available in the United States, and there are severe risks of adverse of effects with this agent, including gray baby syndrome and aplastic anemia.[26] The erythromycins, penicillins, sulfonamides, aminoglycosides, and cephalosporins are not effective for RMSF, and sulfa drugs may worsen infection.

A crucial component in the management of RMSF is appropriate supportive care.[4] Those with severe disease should be hospitalized and managed with hemodynamic, renal, pulmonary, and fluid support as needed.[4]

PREVENTION

In addition to the same guidelines for prevention of Lyme disease, keeping pets free of ticks can reduce exposure. Ticks must not be crushed in a way that might introduce rickettsia into cutaneous lesions, mucous membranes, or the conjunctiva. No RMSF vaccine is available.[26] Antirickettsial antibiotic prophylaxis after a tick bite is not warranted as there is no evidence that this approach is effective and it may delay the onset of the disease.

Spotted Fever Group *Rickettsia* (SFGR)

In addition to *Rickettsia rickettsii*, the agent of RMSF, many other rickettsial pathogens have been recognized and grouped broadly as "Spotted Fever group Rickettsia (SFGR)."[29] In the United States, these pathogens include *Rickettsia parkeri* and *Rickettsia* 364D, and internationally, there is a growing number of tick-borne SFGR that are pathogenic to humans.[4,30] Doxycycline treatment is effective and is the antibiotic of choice for tick-borne SFGR infections.[4]

Ehrlichiosis and Anaplasmosis

SPECIES IDENTIFICATION, TICK VECTORS, AND DISEASE HOSTS

Though ehrlichiosis and anaplasmosis are transmitted by two different species of ticks and generally occur in different regions of the United States, patients may have a similar clinical presentation.[4,5] The term "ehrlichiosis" may be more broadly applied to different infections, including *Ehrlichia chaffeensis* and *Ehrlichia ewingii*, which are transmitted by the lone star tick generally in the southeastern and south-central US, from the eastern seaboard extending westward to Texas. A third species, provisionally called Ehrlichia muris-like (EML), was identified among patients in the upper Midwest; however, the tick responsible for transmitting

EML is unknown and the clinical presentation is undifferentiated from other *Ehrlichia* species.

Anaplasmosis is a bacterial disease, caused by *Anaplasma phagocytophilum,* which was first recognized as a disease in humans in 1994.[4] Though previously known as human granulocytic ehrlichiosis (HGE), a taxonomic change in 2001 identified that this organism belongs to the genus Anaplasma and resulted in the name change to human granulocytic anaplasmosis (HGA). To date, the highest incidence of HGA in the United States is reported in the upper Midwest and northeastern states with transmission by the black-legged tick (*Ixodes scapularis*). Along the West Coast, it is transmitted by the western black-legged tick (*I. pacificus*).

CLINICAL AND LABORATORY FINDINGS

Human ehrlichiosis and anaplasmosis usually present as nonspecific, febrile, flu-like illnesses resembling RMSF. The symptoms caused by infection generally develop 1 to 2 weeks following the bite of an infected tick and are variable. Patients who are immunocompromised (e.g., receiving corticosteroids, cancer chemotherapy, long-term immunosuppressive therapy following organ transplant), or who have HIV infection or splenectomy may experience more severe disease and greater risk of mortality.

The following signs often are noted: hypertransaminemia, leukopenia (often with a shift to the left), and thrombocytopenia. A skin rash is an uncommon feature of ehrlichiosis and is rarely seen with anaplasmosis. However, up to 60% of children can experience a rash caused by *Ehrlichia chaffeensis.* The diagnosis of ehrlichiosis and anaplasmosis must be made based on clinical findings, as treatment should never be delayed pending the results of confirmatory laboratory testing or be withheld on the basis of an initial negative laboratory result. In patients presenting with known tick exposure, fever, thrombocytopenia, and increased liver function test, a peripheral smear should be performed. A peripheral blood smear showing neutrophilic morulae supports a provisional diagnosis, though this characteristic finding is not present in most cases. Confirmatory testing by serology or PCR or direct culture is still required to establish a diagnosis.[31] As with many other tick-borne diseases, serologic findings of antibody response to ehrlichiosis or anaplasmosis assist only by retrospectively confirming the diagnosis.

TREATMENT AND PREVENTION

CASE 82-8

QUESTION 1: G.C., a 68-year-old man living in northwest Wisconsin, presents with an influenza-like illness in late May. He has a two-day history of fever, shaking chills, headache, myalgias, nausea, and anorexia. On examination, his temperature is 39.4°C, but other physical findings are unremarkable. No skin rashes are found. G.C. states that he had multiple tick bites 1 week ago while he was fur trapping. The physician suspects anaplasmosis. Blood is drawn for serology, CBC with differential, chemistry profile, and a Wright stain microscopic examination. Immediately available abnormal results include neutrophilic morulae on microscopy, a WBC count of 2,500/μL, a platelet count of 80 × $10^3/\mu$L, C-reactive protein of 136 mg/L (normal, 4–8 mg/L), aspartate aminotransferase (AST) of 150 IU/L, and lactate dehydrogenase of 700 IU/L. Serology is still pending. What antibiotic treatment should be initiated?

G.C.'s history is significant for HGA. He was in the right place, the upper Midwestern US, and was outdoors during the right season; most patients are diagnosed with HGA in May through August, and his history fall within the usual 1- to 2-week incubation period from tick bite to onset of illness.

His symptoms are also important. Nearly 100% of patients with HGA have a fever of greater than 37.6°C. Other symptoms in G.C. consistent with HGA are rigors (shaking chills), headache, myalgias, nausea, and anorexia. Matching laboratory findings include neutrophilic morulae. The laboratory findings of leukopenia and thrombocytopenia strongly support the diagnosis of anaplasmosis. Evidence of mild-to-moderate hepatic injury, as seen by the elevated liver enzyme results, is helpful in HGA diagnosis.

Doxycycline is the first-line treatment for G.C. and should be used for both adults and children of all ages whenever anaplasmosis or ehrlichiosis is suspected.[4,5] In patients such as G.C. who are treated within the first 5 days of the disease, a good response to doxycycline occurs with fever resolution generally in 2 days.[32] Fever persisting for more than 2 days after doxycycline treatment suggests that the diagnosis is incorrect.

THE PROTOZOA: BABESIOSIS

Babesia, Ticks, and Hosts

There are more than 100 species of *Babesia* having a worldwide geographic range.[4] However, only relatively few species have caused documented cases of human infection, including *B. microti, B. divergens, B. duncani,* and currently an unnamed agent designated MO1.[4,32] The most common cause of human babesiosis is *B. microti,* which is transmitted by *Ixodes scapularis* ticks, primarily in the endemic regions in the Northeast and upper Midwest of the United States; however, sporadic cases of babesiosis have occurred in other regions, including the West Coast. In addition to the Ixodes ticks, *Babesia* species are also transmitted by *Dermacentor, Haemaphysalis,* and *Rhipicephalus* ticks. Because *B. microti* is typically transmitted by the nymphal stage of *I. scapularis* tick (about the size of a poppy seed), infected patients may not recall a tick bite.

SYMPTOMS AND DIAGNOSIS

CASE 82-9

QUESTION 1: H.W., age 68 years, lives in Martha's Vineyard in Massachusetts. During the month of July he enjoyed a day of boating, fishing and hiking at a nearby lake. About a week later, he felt fatigued and lost his appetite. He presents to his local PCP in the middle of August with complaints of fever, headache, drenching sweats, aches and pains, and occasional dark-colored urine. He does not recall a tick bite. On physical examination, he has splenomegaly and hepatomegaly. Laboratory tests show a severe normochromic, normocytic anemia, decreased hemoglobin, hemoglobinuria, thrombocytopenia, and increased liver enzymes. His temperature is 40°C. Examination of a Giemsa-stained thin blood smear reveals the presence of unpigmented ring-shaped intraerythrocytic parasites in more than 5% of his erythrocytes. The PCP institutes an atovaquone plus azithromycin regimen. What was the clue to the diagnosis of babesiosis?

The diagnosis of babesiosis was confirmed by the direct observation of the protozoan inside the red blood cells. Although the Giemsa-stain test is a commonly used tool, it is subject to false-negative results because the rate of parasitemia is typically low. Usually, multiple blood smears need to be examined because less than 1% of erythrocytes may be infected early in the course of the disease when most people seek medical help.[3,32] Because blood smear inspection is often not successful in diagnosing babesiosis or may only detect a few parasites, additional supportive laboratory results are advocated, such as serology using IFA for IgM and IgG antibabesial antibodies or PCR detection of babesial DNA in the blood.[3]

The clinical findings in patients with babesiosis are similar to those of malaria, ranging in severity from asymptomatic to severe complications and death.[11] Most patients with *B. microti* babesiosis are asymptomatic, though some people may develop nonspecific flu-like symptoms, such as fever, chills, sweats, headache, myalgias, and nausea. This form of babesiosis can be viewed as a distinct, occult, asymptomatic disease with few known sequelae.[32] A number of transfusion-acquired infections have been documented, reflecting the existence of an asymptomatic form of babesiosis in blood donors.

A second form of babesiosis has been termed a "mild-to-moderate viral-like illness."[33] It has a gradual onset of fatigue and malaise and later fever accompanied by one or more of these symptoms: chills, sweats, headache, arthralgias or myalgias, anorexia, or cough.[30] Rash is rare. It can last weeks to months, sometimes with a prolonged recovery time of up to a year or more.[33]

A third form of babesiosis is a potentially life-threatening hemolytic one that occurs in people predisposed to severe infection because of advanced age, immune suppression as a result of HIV disease or immunosuppressants, malignancy, or prior splenectomy.[32] Although babesial infection is as prevalent in children as it is in adults, it is more severe in adults older than 50 years of age. Complications seen in severe babesiosis include acute respiratory failure, disseminated intravascular coagulation, congestive heart failure, coma, and renal failure, with a 5% to 9% mortality rate.[3,32]

In the northeastern US, infections commonly occur in patients with spleens, as in H.W. Clinically apparent cases are most common in 50- to 60-year-old patients, many of whom do not recall a tick bite. Most symptoms of babesiosis are caused by hemolysis or the systemic inflammatory responses to parasitemia.[30] The usual incubation period is 1 to 6 weeks after a tick bite based on limited data.[34] Nonspecific, viral-like symptoms that are gradual in onset appear first, as in H.W.'s case, followed several days later by the other symptoms H.W. displayed. A hallmark of the disease is hemolytic anemia of varying severity. A high index of suspicion for babesiosis should be maintained in any patient with an unexplained febrile illness who lives in or has traveled to a region where the infection is endemic during June through August, as in H.W.'s case, particularly if there is a history of tick bite.

TREATMENT

CASE 82-9, QUESTION 2: Is atovaquone and azithromycin an appropriate treatment regimen for H.W.? What other drugs have been used?

The discovery of an original human babesiosis treatment regimen combining clindamycin and quinine was a fortuitous one. In 1982, an 8-week-old infant with presumed transfusion-acquired malaria was initially treated with chloroquine. Because of a lack of response, treatment was switched to quinine plus clindamycin, and the patient's fever decreased. A correct diagnosis of babesiosis was subsequently confirmed. Although this treatment combination is still used, frequent side effects (e.g., tinnitus, vertigo, and diarrhea) occur, often resulting in dose reduction or discontinuation.[3,32] Treatment failures with this regimen have occurred in splenectomized patients, patients with HIV infection, or those receiving concurrent corticosteroids.[3]

For mild-to-moderate babesiosis, atovaquone plus azithromycin is the regimen of choice, as H.W. received. This regimen has also achieved cures in pediatric cases, although a controlled trial study has not been performed.[32] On the other hand, persistent relapsing babesiosis and emergence of resistance have occurred in immunocompromised patients receiving this regimen.[33,35] It has been suggested that the usual 7- to 10-day course treatment regimen may not be adequate in these patients.[35] Combination therapy of azithromycin with atovaquone is better tolerated than clindamycin–quinine combinations. The dosing is atovaquone 750 mg orally every 12 hours and azithromycin 500 mg to 1,000 mg orally on day 1 and 250 mg to 1,000 mg on subsequent days for 7 to 10 days.[32] Increased azithromycin doses of 600 mg to 1,000 mg/day may be used in immunocompromised patients.[3,36] Children should receive atovaquone 20 mg/kg (maximum, 750 mg dose) every 12 hours *and* azithromycin 10 mg/kg (maximum, 500-mg dose) on day 1 and 5 mg/kg (maximum, 250-mg dose) orally thereafter for 7 to 10 days.[3,32]

For severe babesial illness, the intravenous clindamycin plus oral quinine should be given.[32] Dosing recommendations for adults are clindamycin 300 mg to 600 mg IV every 6 hours *plus* quinine 650 mg orally every 6 to 8 hours for 7 to 10 days; children should receive clindamycin 7 to 10 mg/kg (maximum, 600-mg dose) IV every 6 to 8 hours plus quinine 8 mg/kg (maximum, 650 mg dose) orally every 8 hours for 7 to 10 days.[3,32]

Antimicrobials should be used in all patients with symptomatic, active babesiosis once the diagnosis is confirmed by PCR or blood smear, owing to the risk of disease complications.[34] Antibody-seropositive, symptomatic patients without identifiable parasites on blood smear or PCR positivity should not be treated. Similarly, asymptomatic patients should not be treated regardless of serologic results, blood smear examinations, or PCR findings. A course of treatment should be considered in asymptomatic patients, however, if these tests are positive and repeat testing demonstrates persistent parasitemia for more than 3 months.[3,32]

Partial or complete red blood cell transfusions may be lifesaving in severe babesiosis for patients having high-grade parasitemia (10% or more infected erythrocytes), significant hemolysis, or pulmonary, renal, or hepatic compromise.[3] Rapidly increasing parasitemia leading to massive intravascular hemolysis and renal failure mandates immediate treatment for this form of the disease. Patients receiving antibiotic treatment, in particular those with severe or persistent symptoms, should be evaluated for coinfection with *B. burgdorferi* or *A. phagocytophilum* or both.

Babesiosis prevention is the same as for other tick-borne diseases. Asplenic patients should avoid areas where babesiosis is endemic. To date, no supportive data for the use of prophylactic antibiotics to prevent babesial infection after a tick bite are available.[32] Although developed for use in cattle, babesial vaccines are not available for humans.

THE VIRUSES: COLORADO TICK FEVER, TICK-BORNE ENCEPHALITIS, AND OTHER VIRALLY MEDIATED TICK-BORNE DISEASES

Colorado Tick Fever

VIRUS IDENTIFICATION, TICKS, AND HOST RESERVOIRS

"Mountain fever" has been described since the first immigrants arrived in the Rocky Mountains. It was later renamed Colorado tick fever (CTF), and the Colorado tick fever virus (CTFV) was identified as the cause.

CTF is caused by a double-stranded RNA *Coltivirus*. It is an intraerythrocytic virus. At least 22 strains of CTFV are known, but antigenic variation among human strains is low.[33] The virus is an arbovirus because it replicates inside ticks. The primary nidus of infection is thought to be CTFV invasion of hematopoietic progenitor erythroblasts, and it remains sheltered in mature erythrocytes.[37,38]

CTF is a viral illness transmitted by the bite of an infected tick.[37] Although at least eight tick species have been found to be infected with the virus, adult *D. andersoni* ticks are the primary tick vector that transmits CTF to humans.[37,38] *D. andersoni* feeds on numerous mammals, but ground squirrels, porcupines, and chipmunks are the primary reservoirs for CTFV as well as the ticks themselves.[37,38] Transstadial transmission of CTF virus within the tick ensures it is infected for life.[37]

PREVALENCE

CTF is contracted in forested mountain areas at higher elevations of the western Black Hills and Rocky Mountain regions of the United States and Canada, especially on the south-facing brush slopes and dry rocky surfaces of mountains east of the Continental Divide.[37,38] Although CTF can develop from March to October, May through July are peak incidence months.[4,5]

SYMPTOMS

CASE 82-10

QUESTION 1: T.P., a previously healthy 27-year-old native of Atlanta, Georgia, returns from a 1-week late-spring camping trip with her friends in the eastern Colorado Rocky Mountains. Four days later, she experiences fever, chills, headache, myalgias, conjunctivitis, and lethargy. She recalls no tick bites and has no skin rashes. Suspecting RMSF, her physician prescribes doxycycline. T.P.'s symptoms and fever initially resolve, but 2 days later her symptoms return. Physical examination at this time reveals a temperature of 39°C. Routine laboratory tests are normal, although leukopenia is observed with a WBC count of 2,400/μL. Explain how T.P.'s symptoms suggest a diagnosis of CTF?

Symptoms of CTF usually start 3 to 5 days after a tick bite, although more than half of patients do not remember being bitten.[37,38] The most common initial symptoms are fever of rapid onset, headache, chills without true rigors, and myalgias.[37] A rash, which may be petechial, maculopapular, or macular, can occur in 5% to 15% of patients.[38] About half of patients with fever experience a "biphasic" pattern of fever and other symptoms, which means they have several days of fever, then improve for several days, and then have a second period of fever and illness.[37,38] Sequelae are rare, although fatigue and malaise may last for months.[38] One- to three-week periods of convalescence are usual. Children, however, experience complications more frequently than adults. Patients with suspected CTF should defer from donating blood or bone marrow for at least 6 months after their illness because the virus may stay in red blood cells for several months and can be passed to others via blood transfusions.

LABORATORY FINDINGS

Moderate-to-significant leukopenia is the most important finding in CTF. Leukocyte counts are usually normal on the first day, but decrease to 2,000 to 4,000/μL by the fifth or sixth day of illness with a lymphocytic predominance.[38] In one-third of confirmed CTF cases, however, the leukocyte counts remained around 4,500/μL. Counts return to normal within a week of fever abatement in most cases. Thrombocytopenia may occur.[37,38] Although the CSF may show a lymphocytic pleocytosis, this does not distinguish CTF from other causes of meningoencephalitis.[38]

DIAGNOSIS AND TREATMENT

CTF diagnosis can be made serologically, either with IFA staining of erythrocytes, complement fixation, or ELISA.[37,38] The most sensitive isolation system is intracerebral injection of infected blood into suckling mice.[37,38] A reverse transcriptase PCR of specimens can be diagnostic within the first 5 days of illness, whereas serologic tests are more relevant for diagnosis 2 weeks after symptom onset.[38] There is no specific treatment available for patients with CTF infection, which is usually self-limiting. Supportive care should be provided. The best protection for CTF is tick prevention strategies.[38]

TICK-BORNE ENCEPHALITIS (TBE)

Tick-borne encephalitis, a life-threatening neurologic disease, is a growing public health concern in Europe and Asia as the incidence of TBE virus has significantly increased in the past decade.[4,34] TBE virus is divided into three subtypes: Central European (western subtype), Siberian, and Far Eastern (Russian spring–summer or eastern subtype), and is endemic to central and eastern Europe, Russia, and the Far East, with some overlap in geography.[4,34]

The etiologic agents are spherical, lipid-enveloped RNA viruses in the genus *Flavivirus*.[4,39] The western subtype is transmitted to humans by *I. ricinus*, and the Siberian and Far Eastern subtypes are transmitted by *I. persulcatus*, although *I. ovatus* is the vector in Japan.[40] A minority of TBE cases have followed the consumption of infected unpasteurized milk or cheese directly without a tick vector.[39] The main virus reservoirs are small rodents.[39] Ticks are vectors, and humans are accidental hosts of the virus. Ticks can become infected for life by the virus at larval, nymphal, or adult stages, can acquire it during mating, and can maintain the virus transovarially and transstadially.[39] TBE viruses are transmitted from the saliva of an infected tick very rapidly, within minutes of the bite, so early removal of the tick may not prevent subsequent encephalitis.

As the disease name implies, the ultimate outcome of the infectious process is manifested as CNS involvement, with symptoms of aseptic meningitis, meningoencephalitis, and meningoencephalomyelitis. TBE begins as a febrile headache with progression to CNS manifestations. There is no antiviral treatment available and treatment is supportive, including management of any complications. Two inactivated cell culture-derived preventive human TBE vaccines are available in Europe, in adult and pediatric formulations (FSME-IMMUN and Encepur).[4] The adult formulation of FSME-IMMUN is also licensed in Canada. Two other inactivated TBE vaccines are available in Russia (TBE-Moscow and EncVir). The reader is referred to the CDC for information regarding vaccination to TBE-endemic countries.[4]

POWASSAN DISEASE

Powassan virus infection is an RNA virus belonging to the genus *Flavivirus* that is related to West Nile, St. Louis encephalitis, and tick-borne encephalitis viruses.[4] Powassan disease is now recognized in the United States, Canada, and Russia. In the United States, approximately 60 cases have been reported in the past decade primarily from northeastern states and the Great Lakes region. The incubation period ranges from 1 week to 1 month. Many people who become infected are asymptomatic. Signs and symptoms of illness can include fever, headache, vomiting, and malaise. Because the Powassan virus can infect the CNS, progression of disease to meningoencephalitis with confusion, seizures, and memory loss may occur. There are currently no vaccines or treatment for Powassan disease. Supportive care should be provided to patients with suspected disease.

THE TOXINS: TICK PARALYSIS

Tick Paralysis

CASE 82-11

Question 1: C.M., a 7-year-old girl residing in Spokane, Washington, complains to her parents that she feels weakness in both legs. The next day, her mother notices that C.M. has worsened and immediately takes her to the pediatrician. The physician finds that C.M has begun experiencing flaccid paralysis in both legs and the lower trunk, although she is alert and oriented. The pediatrician finds that there is a tick attached to C.M.'s scalp under her hair and removes it. C.M. is back to full health in 2 days. What happened?

Tick paralysis (tick toxicosis) occurs worldwide in humans and many animals, and was first described by the explorer Hovell in Australia in 1824.[40] Although 60 tick species worldwide can produce tick paralysis in animals and humans, it is predominantly caused in humans by *D. andersoni* and *D. variabilis* in North America.[40] In Australia, *Ixodes holocyclus* is the culprit.[40]

Most human cases occur during the spring and summer in Australia and North America. In the United States, it is most common in the Pacific Northwest and adjacent areas of southwestern Canada and in the Rocky Mountain states.[40] In children, girls are more commonly affected; however, in adults, more men are affected.[40] Of epidemiologic significance, a young girl's long hair provides camouflage for feeding ticks.[40]

The cause of tick paralysis is the secretion of a neurotoxin present in the large salivary glands of female ticks. They must usually be attached to a host for 4 to 5 days before symptoms develop.[40] The toxin affects motor neurons, decreases acetylcholine release, and may have a mechanistic similarity to botulinum toxin.[40] Paresthesias and symmetric weakness in the lower extremities with motor difficulties progress to an ascending flaccid paralysis in several hours or days. Cerebral sensorium is usually spared, pain is absent, and the blood and CSF are normal.[40] If the tick is not removed, the toxicosis can progress to respiratory paralysis and death.[40] Initially reported mortality rates of 10% have fallen dramatically with our modern intensive care units and available respiratory care.[40] A Washington State case series of 33 patients conducted over the course of 50 years revealed a mortality rate of 6%, with the last two patients' deaths occurring in the 1940s.[40] Children are likely more vulnerable to tick paralysis than adults because the dose of neurotoxin present per kilogram of body weight is higher.[39] Diagnosis should include a complete body examination of the skin for the presence of an engorged tick.[39]

In North America, tick removal commonly results in complete recovery within hours to days. In Australia, the disease is more acute, and paralysis may continue to progress for 2 days after tick removal. Recovery from the disease in Australia may take several weeks. Treatment is supportive. Antitoxin derived from dogs is the treatment of choice for animals, but it also has been used occasionally in humans in Australia with severe tick paralysis.[40] Local experts must determine its use on a case-by-case basis because of the risk of serum sickness or acute allergic reactions.[39]

MIXED INFECTIONS

Because the tick vectors and mammalian hosts are the same for babesiosis, anaplasmosis, and Lyme disease in the northeastern US, all three diseases, theoretically, could be transmitted to a human from one tick bite. Human coinfection by the agents of Lyme disease, babesiosis, or anaplasmosis can occur, especially in endemic areas.[5] Coinfection may alter the natural course for each disease or increase clinical manifestations, especially flu-like symptoms, in concurrent Lyme disease with babesiosis or HGA. Because the same tick vector in Europe and Russia can carry Lyme disease and TBE, dual infection may result in more severe disease.[39]

Dual infection may affect the choice of initial antibiotic therapy. For example, although amoxicillin is sometimes used to treat early Lyme disease, it is not effective for HGA. Doxycycline, however, is useful in both of these diseases. Thus, some cases of Lyme disease that were believed to be treatment failures may actually have been confounded by coinfection. Patients with concurrent Lyme disease and babesiosis have more symptoms and a longer duration of illness compared with patients with single infections. When moderate-to-severe Lyme disease is diagnosed, the possibility of concomitant babesial or anaplasma infection should be considered in regions where both diseases are endemic. Neutropenia and thrombocytopenia are associated with anaplasmosis, anemia and thrombocytopenia are associated with babesiosis, and neither is routinely found in Lyme disease.[5] For patients with Lyme disease who experience a prolonged flu-like illness that fails to respond to appropriate antiborrelial therapy in an endemic area, clinicians should consider testing for babesiosis and anaplasmosis.[5]

SUMMARY

Most of the research into tick-borne human disease demonstrates a close historical relationship of endemic tick-deer-rodent cycles for various microorganisms. Tick-borne diseases have become increasingly challenging and a serious global problem. Scientists continue to search for improvements in diagnosing, treating and preventing tick-borne diseases, as well as controlling the tick populations that transmit microbes. We will continue to encounter increasing cases of tick-borne human disease of known or unknown causes. Because patients present frequently with nonspecific signs and symptoms, a high index of suspicion is crucial to include a tick-borne illness in the differential diagnosis of those presenting with symptoms compatible with a tick-borne illness. It is essential to obtain a careful history of possible tick exposure and consider the epidemiology of infected ticks when considering the possibility of tick-borne illnesses. It is important to increase awareness of personal protection strategies and tick avoidance.

ACKNOWLEDGMENT

The authors acknowledge Thomas E. Christian for his past contributions to this chapter of this text.

KEY REFERENCES AND WEBSITES

A full list of references for this chapter can be found at http://thepoint.lww.com/AT11e. Below are the key references and websites for this chapter, with the corresponding reference number in this chapter found in parentheses after the reference.

Key References

Alpern JD et al. Personal protection measures against mosquitoes, ticks, and other arthropods. *Med Clin N Am*. 2016(100):303–313. (16)

Centers for Disease Control and Prevention. Tickborne Diseases of the United States. A Reference Manual for Health Care Providers, 3rd ed. 2015. https://www.cdc.gov/lyme/resources/tickbornediseases.pdf. Accessed January 17, 2017. (5)

Diaz JH. Chemical and plant-based insect repellents: efficacy, safety, and toxicity. *Wilderness Environ Med.* 2016;27:153–163. (1)

Mead PS. Epidemiology of Lyme disease. *Infect Dis Clin N Am.* 2015(29):187–210. (6)

Sanchez E et al. Diagnosis, treatment, and prevention of Lyme disease, Human Granulocytic Anaplasmosis, and Babesiosis. A review. *JAMA.* 2016;315(16):1767–1777. (10)

Wormser GP et al. The clinical assessment, treatment, and prevention of Lyme Disease, Human Granulocytic Anaplasmosis, and Babesiosis: clinical practice guidelines by the Infectious Diseases Society of America. [published correction appears in *Clin Infect Dis*. 2007;45(7):941]. *Clin Infect Dis*. 2006;43:1089–1134. (11)

Key Websites

Centers for Disease Control and Prevention. Tickborne diseases of the U.S. http://www.cdc.gov/ticks/diseases/. (4)

SECTION 15 | Psychiatric Disorders and Substance Abuse

Section Editors: Michael C. Angelini and Michael G. Carvalho

83 Anxiety Disorders

Jolene R. Bostwick and Kristen N. Gardner

CORE PRINCIPLES

		CHAPTER CASES
CLINICAL ASSESSMENT AND DIFFERENTIAL DIAGNOSIS		
1	Anxiety disorders are characterized by anxiety that is out of proportion to any actual threat and is excessive for the situation or distressing to the point that it interferes with daily functioning. Both medical and medication-related factors can cause or exacerbate anxiety.	**Case 83-1 (Question 1), Table 83-2**
GENERALIZED ANXIETY DISORDER		
1	Generalized anxiety disorder (GAD) is defined in the *Diagnostic and Statistical Manual of Mental Disorders,* Fifth Edition, (*DSM-5*) as a chronic state of waxing and waning anxiety that is associated with an inability to control symptoms of anxiety and worry. The severity of anxiety and the degree of impairment in daily activities are the main determinants of whether medication should be used to treat GAD.	**Case 83-2 (Question 1), Table 83-3**
2	First-line therapies for the treatment of GAD may include medications such as venlafaxine, duloxetine, selective serotonin reuptake inhibitors (SSRIs), buspirone, or benzodiazepines, when a rapid onset is needed. Psychotherapy, such as cognitive behavioral therapy (CBT), can also be used alone or in combination with medications. Specific treatment for GAD should be chosen based on prior therapy, comorbid psychiatric disorders, pharmacokinetic drug properties, desired onset of effect, and patient preference.	**Case 83-2 (Questions 2, 3), Tables 83-4, 83-5, 83-6, 83-8**
3	When beginning treatment with benzodiazepines for GAD, patients should be educated about possible adverse effects, dependence liability, and drug–drug interactions. Possible effects on pregnancy, teratogenicity, and breast-feeding should also be discussed.	**Case 83-2 (Questions 4, 5), Case 83-3 (Question 1), Case 83-4 (Questions 1, 2), Case 83-5 (Question 1), Case 83-6 (Questions 1–3), Table 83-7**
4	Patients beginning treatment with SSRIs, venlafaxine, or duloxetine should be counseled regarding possible adverse effects that may occur early in treatment, as well as those that may occur later and display a more chronic time course. Additionally, all patients being treated with medications for GAD should be counseled regarding the duration of drug therapy.	**Case 83-2 (Question 6)**
PANIC DISORDER		
1	Panic disorder is characterized by short episodes of intense fear, associated with perceived physical symptoms such as increased heart rate or respiration, gastrointestinal disturbance, tremor, or feelings of disassociation with the physical body that are often not diagnosed or misdiagnosed because they are attributed by the patient to a medical illness.	**Case 83-7 (Question 1), Table 83-9**
2	Therapy for panic disorder includes CBT, medications (SSRIs, venlafaxine, TCAs, or benzodiazepines), or combination therapy. The expected short-term adverse effects such as jitteriness should prompt using a lower initial medication dose and be discussed with the patient.	**Case 83-7 (Questions 2–4), Table 83-5**

Continued

SOCIAL ANXIETY AND SPECIFIC PHOBIAS	CHAPTER CASES
1 Both social anxiety and specific phobias involve fears that are excessive and lead to avoidance behaviors to minimize fear. Social anxiety involves a generalized and intense anxiety involving social interactions, whereas specific phobias involve intense fear associated with specific objects or situations (e.g., spiders or elevators). SSRIs are first-line treatments for social anxiety, whereas psychotherapy is the primary treatment of specific phobias.	**Case 83-8 (Questions 1–3), Tables 83-5, 83-10**
POST-TRAUMATIC STRESS DISORDER AND ACUTE STRESS DISORDER	
1 Post-traumatic stress disorder (PTSD) and acute stress disorder occur in persons who have experienced a severely distressing traumatic event. Re-experiencing symptoms, avoidance, hyperarousal, and negative alterations in cognition and mood cause considerable psychological distress, as well as impairment in occupational functioning and personal relationships in PTSD.	**Case 83-9 (Question 1), Table 83-11**
2 Medications, primarily SSRIs, and CBT are used to treat PTSD. Adjunctive treatment for psychiatric comorbidities such as depression or sleep is often indicated. Treatment goals include reducing the core symptoms of PTSD and improving patient functioning.	**Case 83-9 (Questions 2, 3), Table 83-5**
OBSESSIVE–COMPULSIVE DISORDER	
1 Obsessive–compulsive disorder (OCD) is characterized by chronic obsessions and/or compulsions. Obsessions and compulsions can be extremely disabling and usually consume at least an hour a day. OCD can be treated with medications (SSRIs, clomipramine, or venlafaxine), psychotherapy (CBT with or without exposure therapy), or combined modalities for optimal therapy. Despite combination therapy, up to 40% of patients may continue to experience disabling symptoms.	**Case 83-10 (Questions 1–5), Table 83-5**
2 Owing to incomplete remission of symptoms with monotherapy in many patients suffering from OCD, augmentation strategies involving the combination of antidepressants or adjunctive antipsychotics may be considered with vigilant monitoring for increased adverse effects and drug–drug interactions.	**Case 83-11 (Questions 1–3)**

Anxiety can be described as an uncomfortable feeling of vague fear or apprehension accompanied by characteristic physical sensations. It is a normal reaction to a perceived threat to one's physical or psychological well-being. Anxiety is normally provoked by stress and involves activation of neurobiologic systems that, when activated, contribute to self-preservation. It involves two basic components: mental features (e.g., worry, fear, difficulty concentrating) and physical symptoms (e.g., racing heart, shortness of breath, trembling, pacing). Certain medical illnesses (e.g., pheochromocytoma or hyperthyroidism) and/or medications (e.g., sympathomimetics) can result in both the physical and psychological manifestations of anxiety. However, when the anxiety is attributable to an external cause such as a medical illness or a medication, the anxiety abates when the physiological cause is removed.[1]

If the anxiety is not the result of an external cause, is out of proportion to the actual threat, or persists beyond the presence of the threat, it may be classified as an anxiety disorder. Pathologic anxiety should be differentiated according to whether it occurs (a) as a primary anxiety disorder, (b) as a secondary anxiety disorder owing to medical causes or substances, (c) in response to acute stress (e.g., loss of a loved one, marital or financial problems), or (d) as a symptom associated with other psychiatric disorders to guide optimal treatment.[1]

Classification and Diagnosis of Anxiety Disorders

The *Diagnostic and Statistical Manual of Mental Disorders,* Fifth Edition (*DSM-5*) classifies primary anxiety disorders into seven types: generalized anxiety disorder (GAD), panic disorder, phobic disorders (including specific and social anxiety disorder), separation anxiety disorder, selective mutism, and agoraphobia.[1] Obsessive–compulsive disorder (OCD) and post-traumatic stress disorder (PTSD) are classified under new headings in *DSM-5*. Each disorder involves an unhealthy level of anxiety, but the characteristic type and severity of symptoms, course of illness, and efficacy of drug and nondrug treatments vary indicating underlying biologic differences. The *DSM-5* secondary anxiety disorders include "anxiety disorder due to a general medical condition" and "substance/medication-induced anxiety disorder."[1] Anxiety disorders often present in addition to other psychiatric disorders, such as mood disorders. Both are associated with dysregulations in the limbic system and, therefore, share similar symptoms, including fatigue, impaired concentration, restlessness, difficulties with sleep, and somatic symptoms, although mood disorders have a prominent mood factor.[2]

Neurobiology of Anxiety

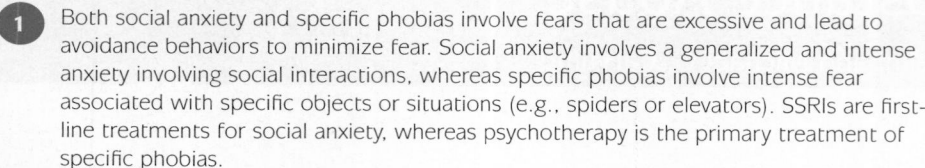

The limbic system, which is involved in emotion, learning, and memory, is composed of a set of structures integral to behavior, including the hippocampus and the amygdala. Hippocampal brain circuits are essential for conversion of short-term to long-term memory and for spatial memory, whereas the amygdala circuits are involved with emotion and its expression. A neurocircuit arising from the output pathways of the amygdala is believed to mediate fear and anxiety responses in humans.[3] Dysregulated or exaggerated output through various amygdala-related circuits may be a common element underlying the different anxiety disorders, but the specific type of dysfunction probably differs among the various disorders. If it is assumed a dysregulation of the stress response is the basis of anxiety disorders, then the genesis of anxiety is probably related primarily to interactions between neural pathways in and between the limbic system structures, the sympathetic nervous system, and the hypothalamic–pituitary–adrenocortical (HPA) axis.[2,4] Many neurotransmitter and neuroendocrine systems interact to modulate the actions of the limbic pathways, including the monoamine neurotransmitters, epinephrine and norepinephrine (NE); corticotrophin-releasing hormone (CRH); the indoleamine, serotonin (5-HT); the inhibitory amino acid, γ-aminobutyric acid (GABA); the excitatory amino acid, glutamate; and the neuropeptides, cholecystokinin (CCK), neuropeptide Y, and substance P.[3,5] As such, the genes from which these products are derived and regulated are an active area of research. Furthermore, epigenetic mechanisms are being investigated to explore the complex relationship between gene–environment interactions.[6]

Interaction of the Hypothalamic–Pituitary–Adrenocortical, Noradrenergic, and Serotonergic Systems

In the event of an acute threat, a fear stimulus is transmitted via the thalamus to the amygdala, which then projects to both the hypothalamus and the brainstem. This results in the peripheral reactions such as increased heart rate and heart stroke volume, and vasodilation of blood vessels carrying blood to the muscles. This is accompanied by a release of NE by the locus coeruleus (LC), the main nidus of NE cell bodies in the brain. Central release of NE results in vigilance, arousal, the ability to focus attention on the threat, and symptoms of anxiety (e.g., tachycardia, tremor, sweating). NE innervation of the hippocampus results in an increased state of memory formation, whereas innervation of the amygdala potentiates the formation of aversive memories.[4] Normally, this is important in allowing us to encode emotionally laden memories, but when overactive, it may result in a constant state of arousal and hypervigilance.

During a perceived threat, CRH is released in the hypothalamus, and it activates the anterior pituitary to release adrenocorticotropic hormone (ACTH). This stimulates the release of glucocorticoid steroids from the adrenal cortex. Although short-term elevation of glucocorticoids allows the body to adapt to a stressful situation by supporting HPA activation and mobilizing energy stores, prolonged elevation of the same glucocorticoids impairs neural plasticity and may even result in neuronal death. When CRH is infused into the LC in rodents, it causes anxiety-like behaviors.[2,4,7]

Although the inhibitory neurotransmitter 5-HT is involved in stress reactions, its role is not entirely clear. Serotonin has roles in sleep, appetite, memory, impulsivity, sexual behavior, mood, motor function, and seems to decrease aggressive behavior. The site of most 5-HT cell bodies in the brain is the raphe nuclei. There is considerable interconnectivity between the raphe nuclei and the LC, and they tend to mutually inhibit one another. Under normal circumstances, 5-HT connections from the hippocampus decrease activity in the amygdala, which would dampen fear and anxiety responses. However, under conditions of stress, the LC accelerates firing, inhibits the raphe nuclei firing, and increases CRH release—all of which sensitize the limbic system and cause arousal and sensitivity to memory of any stressful or aversive stimuli. This primes the system to a state of arousal to deal with the threat.[2]

Although the specific etiology of anxiety is only hypothesized, the current use of treatments activating the 5-HT system, or other inhibitory systems such as the GABA system, supports the hypothesis.

Epidemiology and Clinical Significance of Anxiety Disorders

As a group, anxiety disorders are the most common psychiatric illnesses. Epidemiologic surveys indicate 13% to 28% of Americans suffer from an anxiety disorder at some time in their lives, with similar prevalences in other parts of the world.[8,9] Anxiety disorders are more common in women than in men.[9]

Today, most anxiety disorders can be successfully treated with medications, cognitive or behavioral therapies, or combinations thereof. However, less than one-third of those affected seek help, and many who do are not properly diagnosed.[9] Most medical care for anxiety disorders is rendered in nonpsychiatric settings. Patients commonly present to primary-care providers complaining of physical symptoms that cannot be medically explained, leading to progression of the anxiety disorder. A significant portion of patients with anxiety does not believe in taking medication for emotional problems; others remain untreated because of an inappropriate diagnosis.[10]

Because anxiety is a feeling with which everyone is familiar, there is a tendency to trivialize the impact it can have on a sufferer's functioning and quality of life. An increased understanding about pathologic anxiety is needed in society and healthcare professionals, in particular, so that people seek and receive appropriate treatment. A list of consumer and professional resources for information about anxiety disorders and treatment can be found in Table 83-1.

Clinical Assessment and Differential Diagnosis of Anxiety

CASE 83-1

QUESTION 1: R.R., a 49-year-old woman, complains to her physician of having trouble sleeping, feeling tired and nervous, and worrying constantly. R.R. was divorced 2 years ago, and she retained custody of their 15-year-old daughter. Since her divorce, R.R. has returned to work as a nurse, but she worries constantly that she will not be able to earn enough money to support herself and her daughter. She has hypertension, asthma, and seasonal allergies for which she is prescribed hydrochlorothiazide 12.5 mg/day, losartan 50 mg/day, montelukast 10 mg/day, albuterol 1-2 puffs every 4-6 hours as needed (PRN) wheezing and shortness of breath, and pantoprazole 40 mg/day. She also takes over-the-counter (OTC) loratadine 10 mg/day and pseudoephedrine 60 mg every 4 to 6 hours PRN for allergies, naproxen 200 mg every 8 to 12 hours PRN for occasional back pain, and polyethylene glycol 17 g daily PRN for constipation. R.R. drinks three or four cups of coffee each morning and one or two glasses of wine four nights each week to help her calm down when she has had a stressful day. She denies any history of psychiatric illness but states she has always been a "worrier." What factors should be considered in the clinical assessment and differential diagnosis of R.R.'s symptoms of anxiety?

A diagnostic decision tree such as that in Figure 83-1 can be used to assist the clinician in differentiating among various causes of anxiety and different anxiety disorders. According to *DSM-5* criteria for primary anxiety disorders, the symptoms

Table 83-1
Resource Organizations for Anxiety Disorders

Anxiety Coach	Website: www.anxietycoach.com
Anxiety Disorders Association of America	Website: www.adaa.org
Freedom From Fear	Website: www.freedomfromfear.org
International OCD Foundation	Website: www.iocdf.org
Mental Health America	Website: www.nmha.org/
National Alliance on Mental Illness	Website: www.nami.org
PTSD Gateway	Website: www.ptsdinfo.org

should not be secondary to any medical (drug or disease) causes (Table 83-2).

SECONDARY CAUSES OF ANXIETY

A diagnosis of anxiety disorder attributable to a general medical condition is warranted when symptoms are believed to be the direct physiologic consequence of a medical condition.[1] A complete physical and laboratory workup, with a thorough medical and psychiatric history, is needed to exclude reversible causes before a primary anxiety disorder diagnosis is considered. Because new onset of anxiety disorders in elderly persons is rare, this can often be attributed to some medical or substance-related cause. The presence of anxiety may complicate the medical picture and have a negative impact on the course of illness. Also, it should be noted R.R. is 49 years old, and the median age for onset of menopause is 52 years. Although not a medical illness, menopausal symptoms also may include sleep disturbances and mood swings.

Medical illness is associated with higher rates of anxiety compared with the general population.[11] In some cases, the anxiety is physically induced by the medical condition, but reactional anxiety may also occur when faced with a medical illness. Successful management of the medical condition often relieves associated anxiety, but short-term anxiety treatment may be beneficial.

When evaluating for possible causes of anxiety, it is also important to consider all medications a person is taking, including OTC drugs such as cough and cold preparations.[12] A diagnosis of substance-induced anxiety disorder is warranted when anxiety symptoms occur in relation to substance intoxication or withdrawal or when medication use causes the symptoms. Among the medications R.R. is taking, pseudoephedrine might be contributing to her anxiety. Other medications that can cause anxiety are listed in Table 83-2. Psychoactive substance abuse, withdrawal from central nervous system (CNS) depressants (e.g., alcohol, barbiturates, benzodiazepines), excessive caffeine intake, and nicotine withdrawal may go unrecognized as underlying precipitants of anxiety. R.R.'s current pattern of alcohol use, although not excessive, may become problematic if she uses alcohol to self-medicate her anxiety symptoms.

Although anxiety symptoms are the hallmark characteristic of anxiety disorders, it is not unique to this diagnostic category. Virtually any psychiatric illness may present with these symptoms. If anxiety symptoms occur only in relation to another psychiatric disorder, then a separate anxiety disorder diagnosis is precluded. Anxiety in these cases may be alleviated with successful treatment of the primary psychiatric disorder. For example, R.R.'s difficulties with fatigue and sleeping may be target symptoms of either anxiety or depression, or possibly both. However, individuals with other psychiatric disorders can also have a primary anxiety disorder. In fact, comorbidity with anxiety disorders is the rule rather than the exception, particularly for depression.[7,13] Concurrent anxiety and depression are associated with greater disability, poorer treatment outcomes, and higher suicide rates than either depression or anxiety alone.

Anxiety in response to life stressors may be severe and functionally detrimental, but could be considered appropriate for the circumstances. Usually, this type of anxiety is self-limiting and brief, subsiding over days to weeks as the person adapts to the new situation. If the person has no history of an anxiety disorder and the symptoms last only a few months, a diagnosis of adjustment disorder with anxious mood may be appropriate. If the symptoms are severe and continue for a prolonged period, a primary anxiety disorder may be present. The initial onset of a chronic anxiety disorder often occurs during a stressful period. Short-term or intermittent therapy with anxiolytic medication or counseling can be extremely beneficial in helping persons cope during times of acute stress. In contrast, management of primary anxiety disorders usually requires more extended treatment.

In summary, the factors in R.R.'s case warranting further investigation before a primary anxiety disorder diagnosis can be made include her medical illness (asthma), possible onset of menopause, her use of pseudoephedrine and caffeine, and her adjustment to the recent life changes (divorce, returning to work, becoming a single mother). These factors need to be addressed and treated, if possible, before a diagnosis of an anxiety disorder can be applied and appropriately managed.

GENERALIZED ANXIETY DISORDER

Epidemiology and Clinical Course

Generalized anxiety disorder is one of the most common anxiety disorders, with a lifetime prevalence of about 9% and is twice as common in women than in men.[1,14] Onset is usually gradual and may be associated with increased life stressors. GAD usually begins between the mid-teens and mid-50s and the median age of onset is 30 years.[9,14] As such, GAD presents the latest of all anxiety disorders.[1] Whites are more likely to report anxiety symptoms than Asians, Hispanics, and African Americans.[15] The typical course of GAD is described as being chronic and recurrent, but much is unknown about the long-term course of illness. Without treatment, it appears that less than half of GAD cases undergo remission.

Most people with GAD have at least one other psychiatric disorder. Common comorbid disorders include panic or social anxiety disorder, simple phobia, OCD, and major depressive disorder.[8] Lastly, evidence suggests that GAD itself may be a risk factor for suicidal ideation, particularly among women, even when comorbid substance abuse and depression are considered.[16]

Diagnostic Criteria

GAD is characterized by excessive anxiety and worry about life issues for 6 months or longer.[1] The patient usually has great difficulty controlling the worry, which is accompanied by at least three of the associated symptoms listed in Table 83-3. Although some physical symptoms are similar between GAD and other anxiety disorders, if the anxiety is related solely to another anxiety

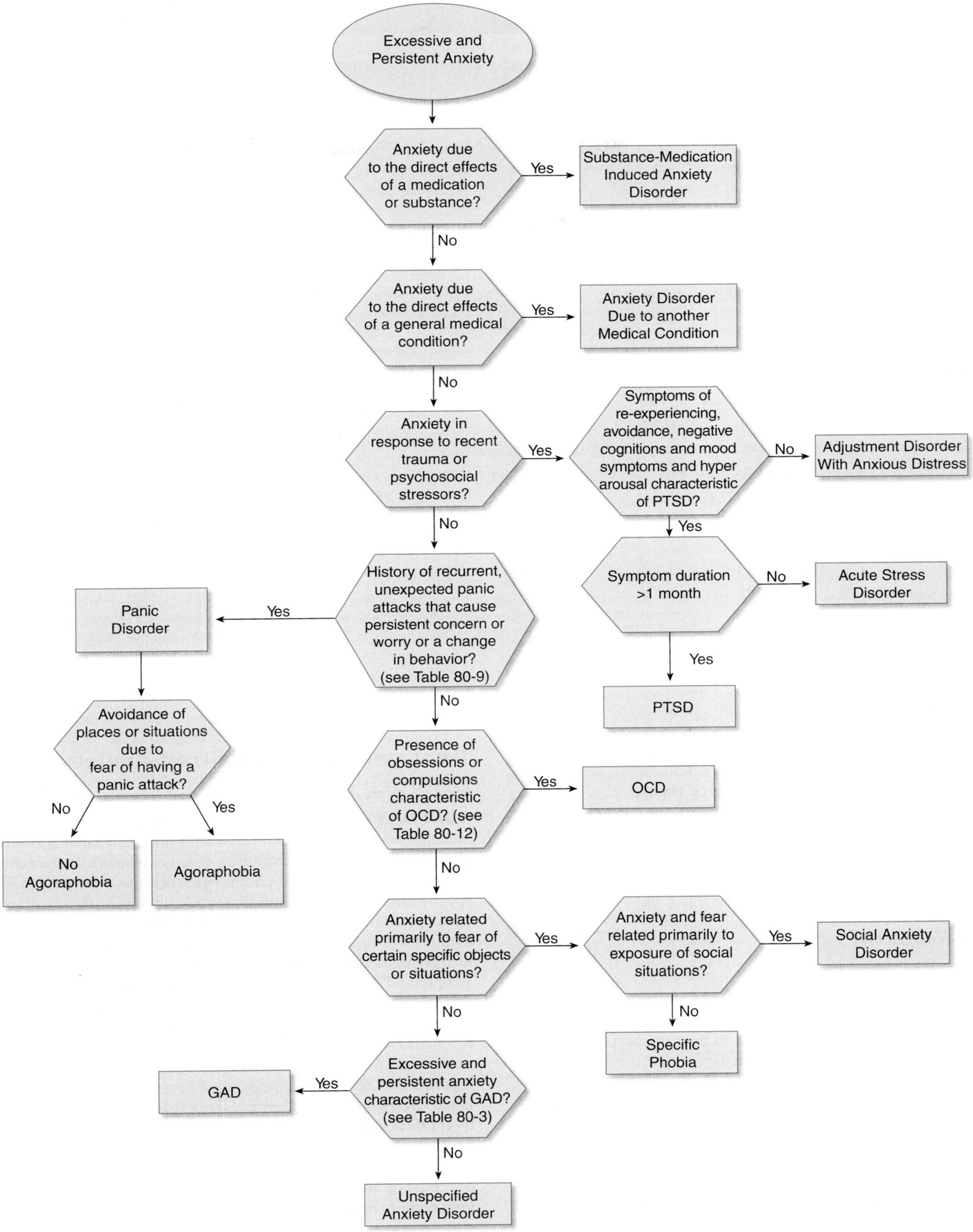

Figure 83-1 Diagnostic decision tree for anxiety disorders. GAD, generalized anxiety disorder; OCD, obsessive–compulsive disorder; PTSD, post-traumatic stress disorder.

Table 83-2
Secondary Causes of Anxiety

Medical Illnesses
Endocrine and metabolic disorders: hyperthyroidism, hypoglycemia, Addison disease, Cushing disease, pheochromocytoma, PMS, electrolyte abnormalities, acute intermittent porphyria, anemia
Neurologic: seizure disorders, multiple sclerosis, chronic pain syndromes, traumatic brain injury, CNS neoplasm, migraines, myasthenia gravis, Parkinson disease, vertigo, essential tremor
Cardiovascular: mitral valve prolapse, CHF, arrhythmias, post-MI, hyperdynamic β-adrenergic state, hypertension, angina pectoris, postcerebral infarction
GI: PUD, Crohn disease, ulcerative colitis, irritable bowel syndrome
Respiratory: COPD, asthma, pneumonia, pulmonary edema, respirator dependence, pulmonary embolus
Others: HIV infection, systemic lupus erythematosus
Psychiatric
Depression, mania, schizophrenia, adjustment disorder, personality disorders, delirium, dementia, eating disorders
Drugs
CNS stimulants: amphetamines, methylphenidate, caffeine, cocaine, diethylpropion, ephedrine, MDMA (Ecstasy), nicotine (and withdrawal), PCP, phenylephrine, pseudoephedrine
CNS depressant withdrawal: barbiturates, benzodiazepines, ethanol, opiates
Psychotropics: antipsychotics (akathisia), bupropion, buspirone, SNRIs, SSRIs, TCAs
Cardiovascular: captopril, enalapril, digoxin, disopyramide, hydralazine, procainamide, propafenone, reserpine
Others: albuterol, aminophylline, baclofen, bromocriptine, cycloserine, dapsone, dronabinol, efavirenz, fluoroquinolones, interferon-α, isoniazid, isoproterenol, levodopa, lidocaine, mefloquine, metoclopramide, monosodium glutamate, nicotinic acid, NSAIDs, pergolide, quinacrine, sibutramine, statins, steroids, theophylline, thyroid hormone, triptans, vinblastine, yohimbine

CHF, congestive heart failure; CNS, central nervous system; COPD, chronic obstructive pulmonary disease; GI, gastrointestinal; HIV, human immunodeficiency virus; MDMA, 3,4-methylenedioxymethamphetamine; MI, myocardial infarction; NSAIDs, nonsteroidal anti-inflammatory drugs; PCP, phencyclidine; PMS, premenstrual syndrome; PUD, peptic ulcer disease; SNRIs, serotonin and norepinephrine reuptake inhibitors; SSRIs, selective serotonin reuptake inhibitors; TCAs, tricyclic antidepressants.

Table 83-3
Symptoms of Generalized Anxiety Disorder[1]

Anxiety and worry are associated with at least three of the following symptoms (or one in children):

- Restlessness or feeling keyed up or on edge
- Easy fatigue
- Difficulty concentrating or mind going blank
- Irritability
- Muscle tension
- Sleep disturbances

disorder (e.g., obsession with germs, fear of social situations), a diagnosis of GAD is not warranted.

Etiology and Pathophysiology

Genetic factors play a significant role in the etiology of GAD. Genes involved in the hereditary development of GAD are believed to be the same as those for neuroticism and major depression, with environmental factors determining which disorder is expressed in an individual.[5,17,18] Biologic studies in GAD have found abnormalities in noradrenergic, serotonergic, and CCK and GABA-A receptor function.[5] Several studies report decreased α_2-adrenergic receptors in GAD patients, and this is believed to represent downregulation of receptors in response to high catecholamine levels.

Treatment of Generalized Anxiety Disorder

NONPHARMACOLOGIC TREATMENTS

Management of GAD can involve both nonpharmacologic and pharmacologic therapies. Nondrug treatments such as supportive psychotherapy, dynamic psychotherapy, cognitive behavioral therapy (including internet or computer based programs), relaxation training, and meditation are often helpful in relieving anxiety and improving coping skills.[19–21] Cognitive therapy is aimed at identifying negative thought patterns provoking or worsening anxiety and making them more positive. Cognitive behavioral therapy (CBT) has been associated with significant reductions in anxiety that are maintained for 6 to 12 months, as well as decreased psychiatric comorbidity in GAD.[19]

BENZODIAZEPINES

Benzodiazepines are widely prescribed anxiolytic agents, and their efficacy in treating GAD and other anxiety disorders, particularly in the short term, is well established.[22] Benzodiazepines offer rapid symptom relief, but are still associated with risks of dependence and withdrawal and are not recommended for the long-term management of GAD.

Mechanism of Action

Benzodiazepines have four distinct effects: anxiolytic, anticonvulsant, muscle relaxant, and sedative-hypnotic. Benzodiazepines potentiate GABA by binding to sites on the central GABA-A receptor which serve as the main inhibitory neurotransmitter in the

Table 83-4
Clinical Comparison of Benzodiazepine Agents

Drug (Trade Name, Generic)	FDA-Approved Indications	Usual Dosage Range Through 65 Years of Age	Maximal Recommended Dosage Through 65 Years of Age	Approximate Dosage Equivalencies
Alprazolam (Xanax, Xanax XR, Niravam orally disintegrating tablets, Intensol oral solution, generic)	Anxiety, anxiety associated with depression, panic disorder	0.5–6 mg/day (up to 10 mg/day for panic disorder)	2 mg/day	1
Chlordiazepoxide (Librium, Limbitrol,[a] Librax,[b] generic)	Anxiety, preoperative anxiety, acute alcohol withdrawal	15–100 mg/day	40 mg/day	50
Clonazepam (Klonopin, orally disintegrating tablets, generic)	Anticonvulsant, panic disorder	0.5–12 mg/day	3 mg/day	0.5
Clorazepate (Tranxene, Tranxene-SD, generic)	Anxiety, alcohol withdrawal, anticonvulsant	15–60 mg/day	30 mg/day	15
Diazepam (Valium, Intensol oral solution, Injection solution, generic)	Anxiety, muscle relaxant, acute alcohol withdrawal, preoperative anxiety, anticonvulsant	4–40 mg/day	20 mg/day	10
Estazolam (ProSom, generic)	Sedative-hypnotic	1–2 mg HS	1 mg HS	2
Flurazepam (Dalmane, generic)	Sedative-hypnotic	15–30 mg HS	15 mg HS	30
Lorazepam (Ativan, oral solution, injection solution, generic)	Anxiety, anxiety associated with depression, anticonvulsant, premedication for anesthetic procedure	2–6 mg/day	3 mg/day	1.5–2
Oxazepam (Serax, generic)	Anxiety, alcohol withdrawal	30–120 mg/day	60 mg/day	30
Quazepam (Doral)	Sedative-hypnotic	7.5–15 mg HS	7.5 mg HS	15
Temazepam (Restoril, generic)	Sedative-hypnotic	15–30 mg HS	15 mg HS	30
Triazolam (Halcion, generic)	Sedative-hypnotic	0.125–0.25 mg HS	0.125 mg HS	0.25

[a]Combination product containing amitriptyline.
[b]Combination product containing clidinium bromide (classified as a gastrointestinal antispasmodic agent).
FDA, US Food and Drug Administration; HS, at bedtime.

CNS.[23] These agents are used to treat a wide variety of medical and psychiatric conditions, including muscle spasms, seizures, anxiety disorders, acute agitation, and insomnia. Benzodiazepines with a rapid onset and short duration of action are commonly used to decrease anxiety and apprehension, as well as induce sedation before surgery and other medical procedures.

Clinical Comparison of Benzodiazepines

Of the 14 benzodiazepines commercially available in the United States, 7 are marketed as antianxiety agents, 6 as oral sedative-hypnotics., and 1 as an anticonvulsant. Indications reflect manufacturers' labeling decisions because anxiolytics can be effective sedatives and vice versa.

Table 83-4 compares the clinical profiles of marketed oral benzodiazepines. Midazolam and clobazam are not included in Table 83-4 as these agents are not used in the treatment of anxiety. Most benzodiazepines have unlabeled uses, including treatment of anxiety and agitation associated with medical or psychiatric illnesses; alcohol withdrawal; irritable bowel syndrome; premenstrual syndrome; chemotherapy-induced nausea and vomiting; catatonia; tetanus; involuntary movement disorders (restless legs syndrome, akathisia, tardive dyskinesia, essential tremor); and spasticity associated with various neurologic disorders (cerebral palsy, paraplegia).

ANTIDEPRESSANT AGENTS

Antidepressants are the recommended first-line treatment for most patients with GAD, though benzodiazepines are widely prescribed. One important distinction between these two medication classes is that the anxiolytic effects of benzodiazepines occur almost immediately, whereas the effects of antidepressants occur gradually over several weeks. Therefore, it is common for short-term benzodiazepine therapy to be prescribed in combination with an antidepressant during initial treatment of many anxiety disorders.[24]

As shown in Table 83-5, selective serotonin reuptake inhibitors (SSRIs) have since gained first-line status for treating all five primary anxiety disorders.[25] Use of these agents, in addition to serotonin and norepinephrine reuptake inhibitors (SNRIs), first line is increasingly common when compared to alternatives due to their tolerability profile as well as utility in treating the common comorbid presentation of depression.

Early controlled studies found trazodone, doxepin, imipramine, and amitriptyline comparably effective or superior to

Table 83-5

Summary of Comparative Medication Treatment Options for Anxiety Disorders

Disorder	FDA-Approved First-Line Treatments (Unless Otherwise Noted)	Second-Line Treatments	Possible Alternatives
Generalized anxiety disorder	Buspirone Benzodiazepines (short-term use only) Escitalopram Duloxetine Paroxetine Venlafaxine XR	Citalopram Pregabalin Sertraline	Atypical antipsychotics[c] Fluoxetine Mirtazapine Tricyclic antidepressants[b]
Panic disorder	Citalopram[a] Escitalopram[a] Fluoxetine Fluvoxamine[a] Paroxetine Sertraline Venlafaxine	Benzodiazepines (e.g., alprazolam, clonazepam, diazepam, lorazepam) Clomipramine Imipramine Mirtazapine	Anticonvulsants Atypical antipsychotics Phenelzine
Social anxiety disorder	Escitalopram[a] Fluvoxamine CR Paroxetine Venlafaxine XR Sertraline	Benzodiazepines (e.g., alprazolam, clonazepam) Citalopram Pregabalin	Atypical antipsychotics Duloxetine Fluoxetine Gabapentin Mirtazapine Phenelzine[b] Tranylcypromine[b]
Post-traumatic stress disorder	Paroxetine Venlafaxine XR[a] Sertraline	Citalopram Escitalopram Fluoxetine Fluvoxamine Mirtazapine	Amitriptyline[b] Anticonvulsants Atypical antipsychotics[c] Bupropion Duloxetine Imipramine[b] Nefazodone[b] Phenelzine[b] Prazosin
Obsessive–compulsive disorder	Escitalopram[a] Fluoxetine Fluvoxamine Fluvoxamine CR Paroxetine Sertraline	Citalopram Clomipramine[b] Venlafaxine	Anticonvulsants[c] Antipsychotic agents[c] Phenelzine

[a]Not US Food and Drug Administration (FDA) approved for the indication but evidence supports use
[b]Documented efficacy, but not recommended for first-line treatment because of undesirable clinical properties (side effects, potential toxicity, drug interactions).
[c]Adjunctive therapy only.

benzodiazepines in treating GAD.[22] Although benzodiazepines work quickly, and TCA treatment is often associated with initial increases in anxiety (especially with higher dosages), continued TCA therapy is usually effective if side effects are tolerated. However, TCAs are not widely used for treating anxiety disorders because attention has turned to other much safer and better tolerated antidepressants, including SSRIs and SNRIs.

Paroxetine and escitalopram are SSRIs approved for GAD by the US Food and Drug Administration (FDA). Sertraline and citalopram have also been studied for this indication and the former is the preferred first-line agent according to one guideline.[24] Overall, SSRIs and SNRIs are recommended for first-line use and specific agents should be selected based on patient-specific factors (e.g., risk for discontinuation syndrome, drug interactions, tolerability, and patient preference).[20,25]

Like TCAs, patients may experience an initial increase in anxiety during SSRI treatment, so lower-than-normal SSRI starting doses should be used in patients with GAD, particularly if fluoxetine is utilized, as it may be more likely than other SSRIs to cause anxiety as an initial side effect.[26]

SNRIs, venlafaxine and duloxetine, are FDA-approved for the treatment of GAD. Newer SNRIs including levomilnacipran, milnacipran, and venlafaxine's active metabolite, desvenlafaxine, have not been well studied in the management of anxiety. However, data suggest these agents may be useful for the treatment of anxiety symptoms associated with depression, although further randomized controlled trials are needed to confirm this finding.[27–29] The side effect profile of venlafaxine and other SNRIs is similar to that of the SSRIs, with dose-related nausea being the most common, and this usually subsides after 1 to 2 weeks of continued therapy. Similar to SSRIs, vigilance for worsening anxiety is required upon initiation of treatment and low doses should be utilized to mitigate this potential effect. Significant increases in blood pressure with venlafaxine are not usually seen within the dosage range used for GAD (75–225 mg/day), but can occur with higher doses. Long-term studies report remission of GAD during 6 months of continued treatment with venlafaxine XR.[30] Duloxetine's effectiveness has been demonstrated in short- and long-term trials, with the latter citing a decrease in relapse of GAD in patients treated with 60 to 120 mg/day.[31–35] In a noninferiority comparison of duloxetine 60 to 120 mg/day and venlafaxine XR 75 to 225 mg/day, these agents achieved criteria for noninferiority and demonstrated comparable tolerability.[36]

Mirtazapine is a non-SSRI antidepressant with limited controlled data in the treatment of GAD, though there is limited support in patients with comorbid major depression.[37,38] It is unlikely to cause anxiety as a side effect, owing to its 5-HT receptor type-2 blocking activity. (See Chapter 86, Depression for more information regarding the clinical use of various antidepressant agents.) Finally, vortioxetine has been studied in short- and long-term treatment of GAD with mixed results.[39–42] As mentioned previously, lower initial doses of antidepressants are recommended to avoid acute worsening of anxiety symptoms. Slow titration and patient education regarding adverse reactions associated with antidepressants, including the black-box warning for suicidality, are also recommended.[43] Although decreases in anxiety symptoms during antidepressant treatment may appear within the first 2 weeks, response is gradual and generally continues for 8 to 12 weeks or longer. Therefore, optimal trials of antidepressants in GAD should allow at least 8 weeks of adequate doses before a lack of response is determined. Continued improvements may occur for 4 to 6 months in some GAD patients treated with antidepressants.[44,45]

Overall, advantages of antidepressants compared with benzodiazepines in treating GAD include their superior efficacy for both cognitive symptoms, such as excessive worry, as well as for common comorbid disorders such as depression and other anxiety disorders. Antidepressants also lack potential for abuse and dependence, a safer withdrawal syndrome and no long-term cognitive impairments.

OTHER AGENTS USED TO TREAT GENERALIZED ANXIETY DISORDER

Buspirone was marketed in the United States as the first of a nonbenzodiazepine class of anxiolytics, the azapirones, and is FDA-approved for the treatment of GAD. Buspirone does not interact with GABA receptors and works as a partial agonist of the 5-HT type 1A receptor, reducing 5-HT neurotransmission.[46] In addition, buspirone enhances dopaminergic neurotransmission by blocking presynaptic dopamine receptor-2 autoreceptors and also facilitates noradrenergic activity.[47] Buspirone is effective in treating cognitive anxiety symptoms and is not associated with abuse or dependence; however, it has a delayed onset of anxiolytic effects and is not appropriate for as-needed use.

Pregabalin, a schedule V controlled substance, may be recommended as a second-line agent following use of SSRIs or SNRIs.[20,24] Pregabalin appears to be efficacious in managing somatic and psychic symptoms of GAD compared with active comparators, including benzodiazepines and venlafaxine.[43,48] Further, it has been studied as an adjunctive agent in combination with SSRIs or SNRIs.[49] Although there is a paucity of comparison studies with SSRIs or SNRIs, some guidelines support use of pregabalin as a first-line agent for GAD.[20,50] However, considerations need to made for the potential for weight gain associated with long-term use, as well as limitations with use in individuals with renal disease or those with a history of substance abuse.[25] Pregabalin exhibits a dose–response effect that appears to plateau at 300 mg/day, although one long-term continuation study of up to 24 weeks suggests pregabalin 450 mg/day may be effective in preventing relapse compared with placebo.[51] Further, an open-label study of doses up to 600 mg/day maintained response for up to 1 year.[52]

Finally, atypical antipsychotics are utilized off-label in patients with GAD, though current guidelines highlight that use of these agents should not be initiated in primary care and reserved after multiple antidepressant class failures.[24] Aripiprazole, olanzapine, quetiapine, risperidone, and ziprasidone have been studied for treatment-resistant GAD, with the bulk of evidence and current guidelines supporting use of quetiapine.[20,25,53] These agents may be useful in patients who fail to respond to first-line treatment options.[20,24,25]

Clinical Presentation and Assessment of Generalized Anxiety Disorder

CASE 83-2

QUESTION 1: L.V., a 32-year-old man, has been employed as a teacher for the past 10 years. He has had an excellent work record until 8 months ago, when excessive absences and a tendency to become easily upset at students and coworkers became noticeable. On clinical assessment, L.V. complains of being "on edge," irritable, and tense, with frequent stomach upset and diarrhea. He has no history of mental illness; however, he admits to being stressed and worrying too much about "insignificant things." He cannot seem to control these symptoms regardless of how hard he tries. L.V. denies any symptoms indicative of panic disorder or OCD.

L.V.'s physical examination is unremarkable, and his family history is only notable for his sister who is described as a "nervous person." L.V. denies past or present use of any illicit substances and drinks three to four beers at social events, which he has not enjoyed recently. His mental status examination reveals the following:

- *Appearance and behavior:* L.V. is neatly groomed and dressed and speaks coherently, but he constantly fidgets and taps his right foot.
- *Mood:* L.V. is anxious and worried about the clinician's evaluation and admits to occasionally feeling depressed and hopeless because of his anxiety. He often has difficulty falling asleep but generally remains asleep throughout the night.
- *Sensorium:* L.V. is oriented to person, place, and time.
- *Thoughts:* L.V. denies any auditory or visual hallucinations, or suicidal or homicidal ideation.

L.V. states, at times, that he is unable to relax, particularly in the classroom around his students. His work has been difficult for him lately, and the principal has told him that his job is in immediate jeopardy unless he improves his performance. L.V. states that he just wants to be able to perform his job like he used to and be able to "chill out" and get back to his old life. His insight and judgment are good, and he is motivated to obtain treatment. The physician's provisional diagnosis is GAD.

What clinical features of GAD are present in L.V., and how can his symptoms be assessed objectively?

L.V. exhibits the following target symptoms associated with GAD: excessive worry that is difficult to control, irritability, tension, and inability to relax. Other typical symptoms of anxiety present in L.V. include gastrointestinal (GI) problems (upset stomach and diarrhea), being startled easily, and fidgeting. These target symptoms are not necessarily diagnostic of any particular disorder, but other factors in association with these symptoms are consistent with GAD. The absence of physical or other psychiatric illnesses, as well as use of any illicit substances and lack of recent use of alcohol, excludes possible secondary causes of anxiety. The 8-month duration of symptoms is consistent with a diagnosis of GAD, and L.V.'s age is consistent with the usual onset of GAD. More importantly, the symptoms are causing significant occupational impairment for L.V. and interfering with his quality of life; therefore, a diagnosis of GAD is appropriate in L.V.

The Hamilton Anxiety Rating Scale (HAM-A) is a useful assessment tool to evaluate clinical anxiety, and it is the standard instrument used in GAD clinical trials. A HAM-A score of greater than 18 is generally correlated with significant anxiety, and a reduction of score to 7 to 10 is associated with no symptoms, defined as remission.[54] The HAM-A can be used to assess baseline anxiety symptoms in patients such as L.V. and to monitor response throughout treatment. The Sheehan Disability Scale is a patient-rated instrument, which is commonly used to assess functional impairment caused by GAD and other anxiety disorders. It measures 3 domains from 1 to 10. A score of 1 reflects mild disability whereas a score of 10 suggests severe impairment.[54]

Indications for and Selection of Treatment

CASE 83-2, QUESTION 2: Based on the information presented in L.V.'s case, how can it be determined whether treatment is indicated? What factors should be considered in choosing the most appropriate treatment for L.V.?

L.V. meets the diagnostic criteria for GAD and is suffering significant disability from his anxiety disorder. He also has insight into his illness and desires treatment that will enable him to improve his job performance and quality of life. Appropriate treatment of GAD can help achieve these goals and is therefore indicated for patients such as L.V.

Treatment options for GAD include both pharmacologic and nondrug therapies. Psychosocial treatments such as CBT can be effective in treating GAD, but use of these therapies alone is generally reserved for patients with mild-to-moderate symptoms. In L.V.'s case, prompt treatment is needed because his job is in immediate jeopardy owing to impairments associated with his anxiety. Therefore, pharmacotherapy in combination with psychological therapy, if available, is indicated in L.V.

Among potential drug therapies, short-term use of benzodiazepines, maintenance with SSRIs, SNRIs (duloxetine and venlafaxine), and buspirone are all considered first-line treatments for GAD.[20,24,25] A primary consideration when choosing among these options is whether any comorbid psychiatric conditions are present. Antidepressants are the recommended initial choice for patients with concurrent depression, which is common in GAD patients. Other medical or psychiatric disorders may also be present, which can guide selection toward a treatment that may be dually effective.

Another important consideration when selecting treatment for GAD is how quickly therapeutic effects are needed. Benzodiazepines reduce anxiety within a few hours, whereas antidepressants and buspirone have delayed onsets of anxiolytic effects. Medication cost is another potential factor, and generic benzodiazepines or SSRIs are inexpensive options.

In L.V.'s case, a benzodiazepine may be a good initial choice because of the need for quick symptom relief relating to his problems at work. L.V. is young and healthy with no past or present history of substance abuse or alcohol use that might make benzodiazepines unsuitable for him. Although L.V. drinks beer on occasion at social gatherings, he has not participated in these events recently, and he should continue to avoid alcohol if a benzodiazepine is initiated. GAD is often chronic, and antidepressants or buspirone are recommended over benzodiazepines for long-term treatment. Therefore, one of these agents would also be appropriate to use in this case.

Benzodiazepine Treatment

FACTORS INFLUENCING BENZODIAZEPINE SELECTION

CASE 83-2, QUESTION 3: The physician decides to treat L.V.'s GAD with paroxetine for maintenance and a benzodiazepine for quick control of his anxiety during the first several weeks until the onset of paroxetine's anxiolytic effects. What factors are important in the selection of a particular benzodiazepine agent for L.V.?

Of the available benzodiazepines, none have demonstrated clear superior efficacy in the treatment of GAD. However, certain agents have been used more extensively than others. Alprazolam, lorazepam, clonazepam, and diazepam have been successfully used in the treatment of GAD.

Because of similar overall anxiolytic efficacies of benzodiazepines, other factors must be considered when selecting one agent versus another. Benzodiazepines differ in their pharmacokinetic properties, and these are generally the main factors considered in drug selection (Table 83-6).

Benzodiazepines can be differentiated pharmacokinetically according to their elimination half-lives and their metabolism to active or inactive compounds (Table 83-6). Diazepam (Valium) and chlordiazepoxide (Librium) have half-lives between 10 and 40 hours, and are metabolized by hepatic oxidative pathways to the active metabolite desmethyldiazepam (DMDZ).[23] The metabolite DMDZ has a long half-life, and chronic dosing of benzodiazepines that get converted to DMDZ can result in drug accumulation and prolonged clinical effects.[55] This can be especially detrimental in the elderly, those with liver disease, persons taking other drugs interfering with benzodiazepine metabolism, or those who are poor metabolizers. Although long durations of action make once-daily dosing possible, small, divided daily doses are often used clinically to minimize side effects.

As highlighted in Table 83-6, the elimination half-life of clonazepam ranges from 20 to 50 hours, making once-daily dosing feasible. Alprazolam (Xanax, Niravam) and lorazepam (Ativan) have intermediate half-lives of 10 to 20 hours, and oxazepam (Serax) has a short to intermediate half-life of 5 to 14 hours. Alprazolam, lorazepam, and oxazepam usually need to be taken on a three times a day to four times a day dosing schedule for sustained clinical effects, but an extended-release (XR) preparation of alprazolam allows daily or twice-daily dosing. Alprazolam XR may be associated with fewer CNS side effects than the immediate-release form because peak alprazolam blood levels are lower.[56] Notably, lorazepam, temazepam, and oxazepam are free of active metabolites and are unlikely to accumulate with chronic administration; they are preferred over longer-acting agents in patients with liver disease and in the elderly. Unlike phase 1 oxidative metabolism, phase 2 glucuronidation processes, the pathway for these three agents, do not appear to decline with age.[57]

Benzodiazepines are readily absorbed after oral administration.[23] Lipid solubility varies among the agents, resulting in differences in rates of absorption and speed of onset, as well as duration of clinical effects (Table 83-6). Diazepam and clorazepate have the highest lipid solubilities and the quickest onset of action, which can be desirable when rapid anxiolysis is needed; however, both can produce a "drugged" or "high" feeling in some patients. Highly lipophilic benzodiazepines are also more quickly redistributed out of the brain, which decreases their duration of action acutely.

Diazepam, lorazepam, chlordiazepoxide, and midazolam are also available for parenteral (intravenous [IV] and intramuscular

Table 83-6
Pharmacokinetic Comparison of Benzodiazepine Agents

Drug	Elimination Half-Life (hours)[a]	Active Metabolites	Protein Binding (%)	Pathway of Metabolism	Rate of Onset After Oral Administration
Chlordiazepoxide	>100	Desmethyldiazepam	96	Oxidation	Intermediate
Diazepam	>100	Desmethyldiazepam	98	Oxidation (CYP3A4, CYP2C19)	Very fast
Oxazepam	5–14	None	87	Conjugation	Slow
Flurazepam	>100	Desalkylflurazepam, hydroxyethylflurazepam	97	Oxidation	Fast
Clorazepate	>100	Desmethyldiazepam	98	Oxidation	Fast
Lorazepam	10–20	None	85–90	Conjugation	Intermediate
Alprazolam	12–15	Insignificant	80	Oxidation (CYP3A4)	Fast
Temazepam	10–20	Insignificant	98	Conjugation	Intermediate
Triazolam	1.5–5	Insignificant	90	Oxidation (CYP3A4)	Intermediate
Quazepam	47–100	2-Oxoquazepam, *N*-desalkyl-2-oxoquazepam	>95	Oxidation	Fast
Estazolam	24	Insignificant	93	Oxidation	Intermediate
Clonazepam	20–50	Insignificant	85	Oxidation, reduction (CYP3A4)	Intermediate
Midazolam	1–4	None	97	Oxidation (CYP3A4)	NA

[a]Parent drug + active metabolite.
CYP, cytochrome P-450; NA, not applicable.

[IM]) administration[23] for treatment of severe agitation or seizures, or for induction of preoperative sedation and anxiolysis. IM injection of both chlordiazepoxide and diazepam can be very painful. Lorazepam is the preferred agent when IM dosing is needed for quick control of anxiety or agitation.

Cost is another important factor in benzodiazepine selection. Brand-name benzodiazepines can be relatively expensive, but all are available in less costly generic versions. Potential drug interactions should also be considered in the selection of an agent because they can alter pharmacokinetics and clinical effects (see Case 83-4, Question 1).

Because L.V. is young and healthy and is not taking any other medications, the clinician could choose any benzodiazepine. A shorter-acting high-potency agent, such as lorazepam or alprazolam, would be a reasonable option for L.V. Appropriate starting doses would be lorazepam 0.5 to 1 mg TID or alprazolam 0.25 to 0.5 mg TID. Dosages can be increased every 3 to 4 days, if needed, within the dosage ranges indicated in Table 83-4. L.V. should notice a decrease in his anxiety symptoms within the first few days of treatment. Prescription of a generic formulation is recommended to reduce treatment costs.

ADVERSE EFFECTS AND PATIENT COUNSELING

CASE 83-2, QUESTION 4: Alprazolam 0.25 mg TID is prescribed for L.V. in addition to paroxetine. What side effects may occur with benzodiazepine treatment, and how should L.V. be counseled regarding benzodiazepine therapy?

Overall, benzodiazepines are very safe and well tolerated. Sedation and feelings of tiredness are the most common side effects of benzodiazepines, but sedation can also be beneficial in alleviating insomnia that often accompanies anxiety. Tolerance usually develops to the sedative effects of benzodiazepines within 1 to 2 weeks of continued treatment; consequently, benzodiazepine sedative-hypnotics are recommended for only short-term use.[20,23,25] Tolerance does not appear to develop to the anxiolytic or muscle relaxant effects of benzodiazepines.

Benzodiazepines can cause cognitive impairment and anterograde amnesia (decreased memory for new information after taking the drug), which is dose-related and reversible on medication discontinuation. Tolerance often develops to the cognitive adverse effects, but they can also persist throughout therapy in some patients.[58] Newer studies have demonstrated a possible association with long-term benzodiazepine use and dementia.[59,60] Use of alcohol during benzodiazepine therapy greatly increases the risks for memory problems and sedation, as well as for other more dangerous effects, including respiratory depression. Elderly individuals are more sensitive to sedative, cognitive, and psychomotor effects of benzodiazepines, and tolerance to these effects may occur more slowly than in the nonelderly.[61]

Other psychomotor effects, such as problems with coordination and delayed reaction time, can also occur during benzodiazepine treatment.[23] These effects are also dose-related, but usually subside within a few weeks of continued treatment. Long-acting benzodiazepines taken the previous night may cause residual daytime effects, which can result in car accidents and hospitalization in older individuals receiving these medications.[62]

The link between benzodiazepine use and falls, especially in the elderly, is well documented.[63] Rapid dosage escalation and use of high doses have been identified as major risk factors, but even use of low doses of short-acting agents greatly increases the risk of falling in the elderly.[63–65]

Respiratory depression is another potential adverse effect of benzodiazepines, but it is usually clinically relevant only in patients with severe respiratory disease, in overdose situations (see Case 83-5, Question 1), or when combined with alcohol or substances that depress breathing, like opioids. It is recommended that benzodiazepines be avoided in patients with sleep apnea.

Respiratory complications are encountered most often with IV administration. Severe respiratory depression has also occurred with the concurrent use of benzodiazepines and olanzapine IM (Zyprexa), loxapine (Loxitane), or clozapine (Clozaril). Further, it should be noted benzodiazepines increase the risk of death in prescription drug overdoses, typically in combination with other medications or drugs of abuse.[66]

Paradoxical disinhibition, with increased anxiety, irritability, and agitation, can occur infrequently with benzodiazepines,[23] primarily in elderly or developmentally disabled individuals.[67] Other unusual behaviors, such as increased anger, hostility, depression, suicidal ideation, and rage, have been attributed to benzodiazepine use in a small number of cases.[23,68] Most of these reports were anecdotal and involved patients with preexisting psychiatric disorders such as bipolar disorder or schizophrenia. Overall, there is no convincing evidence that benzodiazepines actually cause violent or suicidal behaviors, but there is some evidence to the contrary.[23,67]

In summary, L.V. should be told he may experience sedation and difficulties in thinking, concentration, or memory during the first week or so of therapy, but these side effects should resolve once he experiences some tolerance to the drug. He should be extremely careful while driving or performing other tasks requiring psychomotor skills, especially during the first week, and he should avoid the use of alcohol while he is taking benzodiazepines.

BENZODIAZEPINE ABUSE AND DEPENDENCE

CASE 83-2, QUESTION 5: Two weeks later, L.V. contacts his clinician to discuss a medication concern. He reports the medication has been extremely effective in relieving his anxiety, and he is currently taking paroxetine 20 mg every morning and alprazolam, 0.25 mg TID, as directed by his physician. However, his friend has told him he will become addicted to alprazolam, and he wonders whether he should stop taking it because of this concern. What potential for abuse and dependence is associated with benzodiazepines? How should L.V. be counseled regarding "becoming addicted" to alprazolam?

Concerns related to abuse and dependence are one major drawback to the clinical use of benzodiazepines. These agents are classified as schedule IV controlled substances. Diazepam, alprazolam, and lorazepam are more likely to be abused than are oxazepam and chlordiazepoxide.[69] This difference is commonly attributed to the quicker onset of effect and high potency which may be associated with a subjective euphoric sensation. The XR alprazolam formulation is reported to have a lower abuse potential than immediate-release alprazolam because of its slower onset of effect smaller peak to trough ratio and lower maximal plasma concentrations.[56]

Patients without a history of substance abuse who take benzodiazepines for therapeutic purposes are unlikely to escalate doses or use them in ways characteristic of abuse.[69]

The potential problems with benzodiazepine abuse and dependence can be avoided or minimized in several ways. First is the identification of patients who have a history of alcohol or substance abuse and using nonbenzodiazepine treatments in such cases.[69] Second, patients should be counseled about the anticipated duration of benzodiazepine use, the possibility of withdrawal symptoms, and the importance of gradual drug tapering when therapy is discontinued. The distinction between "addiction" and appropriate therapeutic use, which may be accompanied by some degree of physical dependence, should be explained.

L.V. should be advised that as long as the medication is helping his anxiety and he is taking it according to his physician's instructions, his use of alprazolam does not constitute addiction. However, his body may develop some physiologic dependence to the drug, so if he stops taking alprazolam abruptly, he could experience increased anxiety and other withdrawal symptoms. When alprazolam is to be discontinued, the dose should be decreased gradually for a sufficient period to minimize withdrawal symptoms.

DURATION OF TREATMENT

CASE 83-2, QUESTION 6: Two weeks later at his clinic appointment, L.V. is still doing well and has shown further improvements in his GAD symptoms. He has been taking the prescribed alprazolam and paroxetine for 1 month, and his paroxetine has been increased to 40 mg/day during this time. How long should medication therapy continue?

GAD is a chronic disorder fluctuating in severity and often requires long-term treatment. Although long-term use of benzodiazepines can be safe and effective, it is desirable to limit treatment to the shortest duration necessary.[20,22,25] When benzodiazepines are used for acute anxiolytic effects during initiation of antidepressant treatment for GAD, they are commonly limited to short-term (2–6 weeks) therapy. L.V. has demonstrated good response after 1 month of combined alprazolam and paroxetine therapy. Because the anxiolytic effects of paroxetine usually occur between 2 and 4 weeks of therapy and he is taking a therapeutic paroxetine dose, it is appropriate to start discontinuing alprazolam at this time. While it is unlikely, L.V. may experience significant withdrawal symptoms even after only 1 month of treatment; thus, the dose should be gradually decreased for several weeks, according to tolerability of the taper.[70] In patients who are treated with short-acting benzodiazepines for longer durations, switching to an equivalent dose of a longer-acting benzodiazepine, like diazepam, may simplify the withdrawal schedule.[71]

There is no consensus about the optimal duration of drug therapy for GAD. However, recent recommendations suggest effective medication treatment be continued for at least 6 to 12 months after response.[22,72] Continuation treatment with antidepressants significantly reduces the risk of GAD relapse in 6 months.[73] Therefore, paroxetine therapy should be continued for another 5 to 11 months in L.V.'s case. After that time, gradual paroxetine discontinuation may be considered, and reinstitution of treatment is warranted if relapse occurs.

SYMPTOMS AND MANAGEMENT OF BENZODIAZEPINE WITHDRAWAL

CASE 83-3

QUESTION 1: T.B., a 48-year-old woman, has been taking diazepam 20 mg BID for 7 months for its muscle relaxant effects after sustaining back and other injuries from a collision with her road bike and an automobile. Five days ago, T.B. was unable to refill her prescription for financial reasons. A brief mental status examination reveals mild confusion and irritability. Physically, T.B. is trembling and complains of nausea and insomnia. Her medical history indicates no current medical problems or psychiatric illnesses, and T.B. denies the use of tobacco, alcohol, or other drugs of abuse. How should T.B. be treated?

Because T.B. has not taken her prescribed diazepam for five days, it is likely she is experiencing a withdrawal syndrome from long-term benzodiazepine use. Her mental and physical symptoms are consistent with benzodiazepine withdrawal. The benzodiazepine withdrawal syndrome implies some degree of physical dependence, and its onset, duration, and severity can vary according to dose, duration of treatment, speed of withdrawal,

Table 83-7
Symptoms of Benzodiazepine Withdrawal

Common	Less Common	Rare
Anxiety	Nausea	Confusion
Insomnia	Depression	Delirium
Irritability	Ataxia	Psychosis
Muscle aches or weakness	Hyperreflexia	Seizures
Tremor	Blurred vision	Catatonia
Loss of appetite	Fatigue	

and elimination half-life of the agent used.[69,70] Withdrawal symptoms that follow discontinuation of agents with short half-lives usually appear within 1 to 2 days and may be more intense and short-lived than after discontinuation of long-acting benzodiazepines. Withdrawal symptoms usually appear 4 to 7 days after discontinuation of long-acting agents and may last several weeks. Symptoms of benzodiazepine withdrawal, which are listed in Table 83-7, are generally mild when the drug is tapered gradually during discontinuation.[70] Rarely, serious symptoms such as seizures or psychosis may occur during benzodiazepine withdrawal. Risk factors for seizures include head injury, alcohol dependence, electroencephalogram abnormalities, and use of other drugs that lower the seizure threshold.

Diazepam 10 to 20 mg orally should be administered and repeated within 1 to 2 hours if needed. Resumption of her previous diazepam dosage of 40 mg/day should effectively treat her withdrawal symptoms. However, because her acute injury occurred 7 months ago, it may be desirable to begin tapering diazepam.

Various dosage reduction regimens have been proposed for benzodiazepine discontinuation. Even when managing withdrawal from low-dose benzodiazepine use, doses should be reduced slowly for 4 to 16 weeks.[70] The rate of the drug taper should be individualized to the patient, but a general recommendation is a 10% to 25% decrease in the dosage every 1 to 2 weeks. The first half of the benzodiazepine taper (down to 50% of the original dose) is generally easier and can proceed more quickly than the last half of the taper.[70] In T.B.'s case, the discontinuation period may take several months.

In general, the same benzodiazepine the patient has been taking should be used to manage withdrawal. However, because withdrawal symptoms are more severe during discontinuation of short-acting compared with long-acting benzodiazepines, a long-acting agent can be substituted at an equivalent dosage and then tapered.[70,71] In difficult cases, adjunctive medications, such as anticonvulsants, like carbamazepine or phenobarbital, or propranolol, have been used to ease tolerability of the gradual withdrawal, though the latter does not affect the associated anxiety or decrease the seizure risk.[70,74]

BENZODIAZEPINE DRUG INTERACTIONS

CASE 83-4

QUESTION 1: N.P., a 20-year-old female college student, has been taking alprazolam 1 mg TID PRN for treatment of GAD for the past 2 months. She states alprazolam has been very helpful for her GAD, but complains to her physician she is feeling especially stressed. She is having trouble balancing the increased workload of higher-level courses with her social life, which includes a new relationship. She has no medical illnesses, but states she has suffered from several episodes of heartburn recently, which may be stress-related. She is also interested in starting an oral contraceptive. N.P. smokes two packs of cigarettes per day and drinks up to three 12-ounce caffeinated sodas per day. An oral contraceptive (Yaz) is prescribed, and ranitidine is recommended for treatment of heartburn. What potential drug interactions with alprazolam are present in this case?

The most significant pharmacodynamic drug interactions involve other CNS depressants such as alcohol or barbiturates. These combinations can lead to additive CNS and respiratory depressant effects that can be deadly. Important pharmacokinetic drug interactions mainly involve agents that either inhibit or induce benzodiazepine metabolism.[75] One clinically significant drug interaction occurs with the use of azole antifungals in combination with benzodiazepines. Azole antifungals are potent CYP3A4 inhibitors that can cause a 170% increase in the area under the curve of alprazolam.[76] Therefore, the dosage of alprazolam should be reduced by about one-third in patients receiving this combination. Since benzodiazepines have a relatively wide margin of safety, elevated plasma levels or prolonged elimination half-lives are unlikely to cause serious toxicity. However, they can lead to increased sedative and psychomotor effects, which may be clinically significant in certain cases. Conversely, increased benzodiazepine metabolism by hepatic enzyme inducers may result in medication ineffectiveness. Most pharmacokinetic drug interactions with benzodiazepines involve CYP3A4- or CYP2C19-mediated mechanisms. Please refer to a drug interactions database, such as Facts & Comparisons (http://www.wolterskluwercdi.com/) for additional information.

In N.P.'s case, the most important drug interaction is between alprazolam and the newly prescribed oral contraceptive, Yaz. Estrogen-containing oral contraceptives can inhibit the CYP3A4 metabolism of benzodiazepines such as alprazolam, potentially resulting in increased side effects.[77,78] Thus, a reduction in the benzodiazepine dosage may be needed when oral contraceptives are added to ongoing benzodiazepine therapy, as in N.P.'s case. The clearance of benzodiazepines that undergo glucuronidation (lorazepam, oxazepam, and temazepam) can be accelerated by oral contraceptives, but this interaction is probably clinically insignificant.[57,77]

Cigarette smoking increases the clearance of some benzodiazepines (clorazepate, lorazepam, oxazepam), but has no effect on others (diazepam, midazolam, chlordiazepoxide).[79] Overall, the effect of smoking is unpredictable and is most likely to be important in patients who either stop or start smoking while taking a benzodiazepine. N.P. should be urged to quit smoking for the sake of her general health and to prevent substantial risks for serious cardiovascular events occurring in smokers taking oral contraceptives. If N.P. does quit, careful monitoring will be needed to determine whether any alprazolam dosage reduction is necessary.

N.P. should also be encouraged to decrease her soda consumption because caffeine can increase anxiety, thus decreasing the effectiveness of alprazolam. Caffeine has been shown to decrease diazepam concentrations by approximately 22%, but studies with other benzodiazepines are lacking.[75]

BENZODIAZEPINE USE IN PREGNANCY AND LACTATION

CASE 83-4, QUESTION 2: At her clinic visit 2 years later, N.P. is doing very well. She has graduated from college, is happily married, and states she and her husband have decided to start a family. N.P. has discontinued her oral contraceptive in hopes of becoming pregnant soon and has successfully quit smoking. N.P.

continues to take alprazolam 0.5 mg twice daily (BID) to TID as needed and wonders whether she should also stop taking this drug before she becomes pregnant. What is the teratogenic potential of alprazolam? What alternative treatments are available for the management of N.P.'s anxiety?

Early reports implicated diazepam in causing several birth deformities, including cleft lip or cleft palate and limb and digit malformations, but later studies failed to support this association.[80–84] Most benzodiazepine anxiolytics are classified as pregnancy category D (however, this language will be modified once the FDA labeling changes for pregnancy and lactation go into effect), indicating there is some evidence of fetal risk but the benefits of the medication may outweigh these risks in certain patients.[80,82] Available evidence suggests benzodiazepine use during the first trimester increases the risk for oral clefts by approximately 2.4-fold, but the absolute risk is increased only 0.01%. Benzodiazepines have not exhibited strong teratogenic effects, but it is always advisable to avoid drug use during pregnancy when possible, especially in the first trimester.[82,84] In patients such as N.P., the benzodiazepine should be tapered and discontinued before she becomes pregnant. Nondrug treatments for her GAD such as relaxation therapy, meditation, biofeedback, or cognitive therapy may be helpful. If necessary, single or repeated small doses of benzodiazepines during the second and third trimesters are unlikely to have important adverse effects on the fetus. In these instances, an agent with a short half-life, such as lorazepam, should be considered.[84] Chronic or large doses, especially of long-acting agents, should be avoided because they may accumulate in the fetus. Perinatal sequelae in newborns of mothers who took benzodiazepines during pregnancy include withdrawal symptoms, sedation, muscle weakness, hypotonia, apnea, poor feeding, low birth weight, and increased risk for preterm birth.[81,85]

The clinical situation of unexpected pregnancy in a woman maintained on benzodiazepines can also arise. The general course of action in such cases is often to discontinue all medications immediately. However, it is unwise to abruptly stop benzodiazepine treatment in someone who has been receiving chronic therapy because the resultant withdrawal syndromes can be detrimental to both mother and child. Benzodiazepine dosages should be tapered as quickly as possible to the lowest dosage necessary and discontinued if possible. The postpartum period is a time of heightened risk for recurrence of anxiety disorders, and new mothers should be monitored carefully for signs of relapse.[86] Benzodiazepines are excreted readily in breast milk, and they should be avoided by nursing mothers, when possible, but use is not absolutely contraindicated.[87] If benzodiazepines are used, short-acting agents with no active metabolites are recommended to avoid sedation, poor feeding, withdrawal, and other effects in the infant.[81,88]

BENZODIAZEPINE OVERDOSE AND USE OF FLUMAZENIL

CASE 83-5

QUESTION 1: S.P. is a 17-year-old young man who is brought to the hospital by his mother. S.P. is barely conscious, and his breathing is slow and shallow. His mother states he "took a whole bottle of diazepam" (5 mg, 30 pills) some time during the previous night. S.P.'s medical history is significant for a severe head injury sustained from a car accident 8 months ago. He currently takes carbamazepine (Tegretol) 200 mg TID for seizure prophylaxis. S.P.'s mother believes diazepam is the only drug he ingested because no other medications are missing. Toxicology is positive for benzodiazepines and negative for other substances. What signs and symptoms are consistent with benzodiazepine overdose? Why is it inappropriate to administer the benzodiazepine antagonist, flumazenil, in this case?

Benzodiazepine overdose is characterized by respiratory and CNS depression, both of which are evident in this case (S.P. is almost unconscious, with slow and shallow breathing). Overdose with benzodiazepines as the sole ingested agent is rarely life-threatening, and full recovery is the usual outcome.[89] Flumazenil is a benzodiazepine receptor antagonist effective in reversing sedation associated with benzodiazepine intoxication. Its effects on respiratory depression are inconsistent, but improved breathing may occur secondarily to increased consciousness.[89]

The primary use of flumazenil is in reversing benzodiazepine-induced conscious sedation (primarily with midazolam) in patients who have been sedated for minor surgical or diagnostic procedures. Flumazenil is also approved for treating benzodiazepine overdose, but this use is controversial because of potentially serious complications (e.g., supraventricular arrhythmia and seizure), and questions about its cost-effectiveness.[90,91] Flumazenil administration does not appear to decrease mortality or length of hospital stay in cases of benzodiazepine overdose; therefore, its use for this purpose has become limited.[90]

Flumazenil is contraindicated in overdoses of any agent that decreases the seizure threshold, such as TCAs. Toxicology screening and an electrocardiogram (ECG) should be performed before flumazenil is administered. Because of a risk of seizures, flumazenil should also be avoided in patients with increased intracranial pressure or a known history of seizures or head injury, in those who have been receiving chronic benzodiazepine therapy, and in patients with a history of recent illicit drug abuse (cocaine, heroin). Administration of flumazenil should occur only when acute seizure management measures are available.

Flumazenil reverses benzodiazepine-induced sedation or coma within 1 to 2 minutes after IV administration. The most common side effects include agitation, dizziness, nausea, general discomfort, tearfulness, anxiety, and a sensation of coldness.[89] Rapid or excessive infusion has been associated with tachycardia and hypertension. The elimination half-life of flumazenil is 41 to 79 minutes, and sedation may recur after 1 to 2 hours, especially when large doses of long-acting benzodiazepines are involved. Repeated flumazenil doses or an IV infusion may be indicated in these cases. Full recovery should be verified (3–4 hours of stable alertness) before patients are discharged after flumazenil administration, and they should be advised to avoid driving or performing other potentially hazardous activities for 24 hours. Flumazenil undergoes extensive hepatic metabolism to its glucuronide conjugate and de-ethylated free acid. Dosage reductions are recommended in patients with liver dysfunction.

Flumazenil is not appropriate in S.P.'s case because of his history of head injury and risk of post-traumatic seizures. Instead, management should involve general supportive measures and mechanical ventilation, if indicated. A psychiatric evaluation is also indicated in this case to identify and address the reasons for S.P.'s overdose.

PHYSIOLOGIC VARIABLES INFLUENCING BENZODIAZEPINES

CASE 83-6

QUESTION 1: B.G., a 68-year-old man, is brought to the emergency department (ED) by his wife after being involved as the driver in a minor car accident. He has no physical injuries except for several small abrasions caused by the car airbag deployment.

Table 83-8

Physiologic Factors Influencing Benzodiazepine Pharmacokinetics

Factor	Physiologic and Pharmacokinetic Effects	Clinical Significance or Comments
Aging	Increased elimination half-life as a result of increased Vd of all benzodiazepines[92]	Lower benzodiazepine dosages, and possibly less frequent dosing intervals, recommended in the elderly
	Decreased clearance of benzodiazepines that undergo oxidative hepatic metabolism (Table 83-6)[93]	Benzodiazepines that undergo glucuronidation (lorazepam, oxazepam) preferred in the elderly
	Decreased plasma proteins may lead to increased free fraction of highly protein-bound benzodiazepines (Table 83-6)	Possible increased clinical effects
	Decreased gastric acidity may lead to increased rate of benzodiazepine absorption	Possible faster onset of clinical effects
Sex	Age-related decrease in hepatic oxidative metabolism of benzodiazepines more pronounced in men	Elderly men may require especially low benzodiazepine dosages
	Increased CYP 3A4 and CYP 2C19 activity in premenopausal women may result in higher clearance of drugs that undergo oxidative metabolism[77]	Possible decreased plasma benzodiazepine concentrations and shorter duration of clinical effects of oxidatively metabolized agents in premenopausal women
	Decreased glucuronidation in women may result in slower clearance of benzodiazepines metabolized by conjugation[77]	Women may have longer elimination half-lives of lorazepam and temazepam and may require less-frequent dosing
	Increased Vd in women owing to lower lean body mass and increased adipose tissue[77]	Possible longer elimination half-lives in women, especially the elderly, and greater drug accumulation
	Lower plasma protein binding in women[77]	Clinical significance unknown
Obesity	Increased benzodiazepine elimination half-lives owing to increased Vd	Increased chance of drug accumulation in obese patients; dosage reductions may be indicated
Liver disease	Decreased clearance and increased elimination half-lives of long-acting benzodiazepines and alprazolam in cirrhosis and hepatitis; no changes with oxazepam or triazolam[57]	Avoid long-acting benzodiazepines, or use significantly lower doses to avoid drug accumulation
	Increased elimination half-life of lorazepam in cirrhosis but not acute hepatitis	Decreased lorazepam dose or increased dosing interval recommended in cirrhosis
Kidney disease	Decreased plasma protein binding may lead to increased free fraction of highly protein-bound benzodiazepines (Table 83-6)[94]	Dosage reductions may be necessary
Ethnicity	Decreased oxidative metabolism (via CYP 2C19) of diazepam and alprazolam in Asians[95]	Asians may require lower doses of diazepam, alprazolam, and possibly other benzodiazepines

CYP, cytochrome P-450; Vd, volume of distribution.

However, B.G. appears drowsy, is mildly confused, and has an unsteady gait. A toxicology screen reveals no alcohol or other substances, except for clonazepam, which his physician prescribed several months ago. B.G.'s wife states he has been taking 0.5 mg BID, and it has been remarkably effective in improving his mood and anxiety. B.G., who is 5 feet 8 inches tall and weighs 250 pounds, is a recovering alcoholic with moderate liver disease caused by years of heavy drinking. He has successfully maintained his sobriety for nearly 2 years. In addition to clonazepam, B.G. also occasionally takes OTC omeprazole and cimetidine for heartburn. It is determined B.G. is experiencing adverse effects of clonazepam, probably caused by drug accumulation. What factors could be influencing disposition of clonazepam in this patient?

Benzodiazepine pharmacokinetics can be affected by various physiologic factors, listed in Table 83-8.[57,77,92–95] Several of these factors are present in this case and may have contributed to the accumulation of clonazepam with resulting adverse consequences.

B.G.'s age may influence clonazepam disposition. Reductions in both CYP3A4 and CYP2C19 activity have been reported to occur with aging. The glucuronidation metabolic pathways are minimally affected with age, so no such effect is seen with lorazepam or oxazepam.[57] Other factors contributing to longer benzodiazepine half-lives in the elderly include decreased hepatic blood flow and increased volumes of distribution of lipid-soluble compounds (owing to decreased muscle mass and increased fat); the latter can increase a drug's half-life in the absence of any clearance changes. As described in Case 83-3, Question 4, older patients are more sensitive to the sedative and psychomotor and especially cognitive impairing effects of benzodiazepines. For these reasons, benzodiazepines should be avoided in the elderly but if necessary, then the recommended benzodiazepine dosages for patients older than 65 years are generally one-third to one-half of those used in healthy adults (Table 83-4).

Sex also may influence benzodiazepine clearance, but studies yield mixed results.[77,96,97] Women have been reported to have higher CYP3A4 and CYP2C19 activities than men, which may partially explain these findings. Increased CYP3A4 activity in women disappears after menopause, which may necessitate the use of lower benzodiazepine dosages during the postmenopausal period. Women have slower glucuronidation metabolic processes than men, resulting in lower clearance of agents such as temazepam and oxazepam.[57,77]

Obesity and liver impairment are other physiologic factors relevant to B.G.'s case. Obesity increases the volume of distribution of benzodiazepines and the extent of accumulation of long-acting agents. Significant changes in the elimination half-lives of lorazepam and oxazepam are not observed in obese patients. Liver dysfunction can reduce benzodiazepine elimination rates and prolong their half-lives, resulting in recommendations for decreased dosages. The pharmacokinetics of lorazepam, oxazepam, and temazepam are unaffected by liver disease.

Decreased protein binding of benzodiazepines can occur in patients with renal insufficiency, which may lead to increased free fractions of highly protein-bound agents. However, no significant changes in clearance or volume of distribution of free drug have been noted. Regarding ethnicity, up to 25% of Asians are CYP2C19 poor metabolizers. Decreased clearance of a variety of CYP2C19 substrates, including diazepam, has been reported in Asian subjects.[98]

In summary, the physiologic factors that can alter benzodiazepine disposition in B.G. are his age, obesity, male sex, and liver disease. Accumulation of clonazepam owing to these combined effects probably led to his mental status changes. In addition to these factors, cimetidine and omeprazole can both increase the exposure of clonazepam, resulting in decreased clearance and increased side effects.

If continued benzodiazepine therapy is deemed necessary for B.G., lorazepam or oxazepam would be preferred agents because they are least affected by aging, obesity, liver disease, or drug interactions. Benzodiazepine dosage equivalencies, which are based on relative potencies, can be used to determine an equivalent dose for the selected agent (Table 83-4). However, these equivalencies are inexact, and dosing conversions should take patient variables and usual dosage ranges into consideration. For example, B.G. had been taking 1 mg/day of clonazepam, so the calculated equivalent lorazepam dosage is 3 to 4 mg/day. Because of his age and recent reaction at this dose, a somewhat lower initial dose of 0.5 to 1 mg BID would be indicated, accompanied by careful monitoring for adverse effects or withdrawal symptoms. However, switching to a nonbenzodiazepine agent should be considered because this may be a better treatment option for B.G.

Buspirone Therapy

CASE 83-6, QUESTION 2: Several days after recovery from clonazepam intoxication, B.G. expresses a desire to discontinue benzodiazepine use. He is being criticized by his fellow Alcoholics Anonymous program members for taking a drug associated with dependency. The decision is made to switch B.G. from clonazepam to buspirone. How does the clinical profile of buspirone compare with benzodiazepines?

Buspirone lacks CNS depressant effects, sedation, cognitive or psychomotor impairment, respiratory depression, and muscle relaxant or anticonvulsant effects.[46] This makes buspirone useful in older patients who may have a variety of chronic medical conditions. Buspirone is generally well tolerated, and possible side effects include mild nausea, dizziness, headache, and initial nervousness.[99] Unlike many antidepressants, buspirone does not adversely affect sexual functioning and has actually improved sexual functioning in some patients with GAD.[47] Buspirone has minimal potential for abuse and is not classified as a controlled substance. It does not produce physical dependence or withdrawal syndromes on discontinuation, even after long-term therapy.[46,100] It also does not interact with alcohol or other CNS depressants and is relatively safe in overdose.[46]

Buspirone is a 5-HT1a receptor agonist/antagonist and is as effective as benzodiazepines such as alprazolam, oxazepam, lorazepam, diazepam, and clorazepate in the treatment of GAD.[99,100] Like antidepressants, buspirone is more effective than benzodiazepines in treating the cognitive symptoms of anxiety. However, the anxiolytic effects of buspirone have a more gradual onset than benzodiazepines. Initial effects are observed within the first 7 to 10 days, but 3 to 4 weeks may be needed for optimal results. Buspirone must be taken on an ongoing basis if it is effective, and the drug should not be taken "as needed."

SWITCHING FROM BENZODIAZEPINE TO BUSPIRONE THERAPY

CASE 83-6, QUESTION 3: How should B.G. be switched from benzodiazepine to buspirone therapy?

Because buspirone has no CNS depressant effects and is not cross-tolerant with the benzodiazepines, it is not effective in preventing or treating benzodiazepine withdrawal. Thus, when patients are converted from benzodiazepine to buspirone therapy, the benzodiazepine must be discontinued gradually. Because it takes several weeks for full therapeutic effects of buspirone to occur, it can be initiated before the benzodiazepine taper begins. This may indirectly ease benzodiazepine withdrawal by providing extra anxiolytic coverage during the benzodiazepine taper period.[101]

Administration with food may significantly increase bioavailability by decreasing the first-pass effect. Some of the side effects of buspirone, such as nervousness, are attributed to its active metabolite, 1-pyrimidinylpiperazine (1-PP).[46,102] The mean elimination half-life of buspirone is short, approximately 2 to 3 hours, but 1-PP is longer acting.

The clearance of buspirone is significantly reduced in patients with kidney or liver disease, but there is little change in side effects or tolerability.[46] Nevertheless, it is recommended that buspirone dosages be lowered in patients with compromised renal or hepatic function and that use of the drug be avoided in cases of severe impairment.

Buspirone is metabolized by CYP3A4, and coadministration of CYP3A4 inhibitors, including grapefruit juice, can result in significant increases in buspirone levels.[46] Because of buspirone's extremely wide margin of safety and tolerability, even very large increases in its plasma levels may be clinically insignificant. Buspirone should be avoided in patients taking MAOIs and used cautiously in combination with high-dose antidepressants because of the risk of serotonin syndrome.

Some studies suggest patients previously treated with benzodiazepines will not respond favorably to buspirone.[72,100] However, buspirone may provide benefit in this population as long as the benzodiazepine is tapered slowly enough to prevent withdrawal effects.[22] B.G. has been taking diazepam for several months and the drug needs to be withdrawn gradually during a period of at least several weeks. B.G. can be started on buspirone at this time. The usual recommended starting dosage of buspirone is 15 mg/day given in two to three divided doses, but a lower dosage (10 mg/day) is indicated in B.G. because of his liver disease. Twice-daily dosing is preferred to facilitate compliance and is comparable in efficacy and tolerability to three-times-daily dosing.[103] The daily dosage may be increased in 5-mg/day increments every 3 to 4 days. Optimal anxiolytic doses generally range from 20 to 30 mg/day, with 60 mg/day being the recommended maximum. There are no specific guidelines for adjusting dosages in patients with liver impairment; therefore, dosage titrations in B.G. should be made slowly, according to his response and side effects.

PANIC DISORDER

Diagnostic Criteria

The hallmark characteristic of panic disorder is the occurrence of sudden and distinct panic attacks, which are marked by an overwhelming wave of symptoms and feelings reaching their peak within 10 minutes. Symptoms are listed in Table 83-9. To meet diagnostic criteria, at least one of the attacks must be followed by symptoms lasting at least 1 month, including persistent worry or concern about the consequences of the attack or significant behavior change related to the attack.[1] Experiencing less than the four required symptoms to fulfill diagnostic criteria is termed a "limited symptom attack." Three types of panic attacks have been defined with regard to the context in which they occur: unexpected or uncued panic attacks (the attack is not associated with a situational trigger); situationally bound panic attacks (the attacks invariably occur on exposure to a situational trigger); and situationally predisposed panic attacks (the attacks are more likely to, but do not invariably, occur on exposure to a situational trigger).[1]

Although panic attacks are the hallmark symptom of panic disorder, their occurrence can also be associated with depressive and other anxiety disorders.[1] For example, situationally predisposed panic attacks may occur in either panic or phobic disorders. Nocturnal panic attacks, which awaken a person from sleep, are almost always indicative of panic disorder. Because panic attacks occur unpredictably, they often lead to generalized anxiety or constant fear of sudden attacks.

Epidemiology and Clinical Course

Although the estimated lifetime prevalence of panic disorder is 6.8%, approximately 10% of persons experience recurrent panic attacks that do not fulfill the diagnostic criteria for panic disorder and nearly 30% experience a single isolated panic attack at some point in their lives.[14] The onset of panic disorder often occurs during stressful periods, usually in the late teens to mid-30s, with rare first onset in the elderly population.[8,77] Women are affected two to three times more often than men.[77]

Panic disorder, like other anxiety disorders, is accompanied by marked degrees of psychiatric comorbidity. Common comorbidities include other anxiety disorders, affective disorders, personality disorders, and alcohol/substance use disorders with the majority of patients suffering a major depressive episode at some point.[1,14,104,105] Patients with psychiatric and medical comorbidities have more severe symptoms, respond more slowly to treatment, have a lower chance of reaching remission, and have a greater suicide risk (particularly when depression or substance abuse are present) than those with panic disorder alone.[106] Although most patients experience episodic periods of remission and relapse, nearly one in five suffer almost continuously.[107]

Table 83-9
Symptoms of Panic Disorder[1]

- Palpitations, pounding heart, or increased heart rate
- Sweating
- Trembling or shaking
- Sensations of shortness of breath or smothering
- Feeling of choking
- Chest pain or discomfort
- Nausea or abdominal distress
- Feeling dizzy, unsteady, lightheaded, or faint
- Derealization or depersonalization
- Fear of losing control or going crazy
- Fear of dying
- Paresthesias
- Chills or hot flushes

Panic disorder is associated with very high rates of healthcare service utilization.[106] The vast majority of patients with panic disorder do not complain of feeling anxious and report only physical symptoms, such as chest pain, GI problems, headache, dizziness, and shortness of breath, which contributes to misdiagnosis.[108] The poor recognition of panic disorder in primary-care settings further increases use of medical services. Panic disorder is the underlying cause of symptoms in an estimated 10% to 30% of patients referred to specialty vestibular, respiratory, or neurology clinics, and up to 60% of those referred for cardiology consultation.[1] It is not uncommon for patients to have been in the healthcare system for up to 10 years before they are correctly diagnosed.

Etiology and Pathophysiology

A neurobiologic model for panic disorder has been proposed in which the amygdala is the central hub of the fear circuit.[5,109] Various projections from the amygdala, including the hypothalamus and the locus coeruleus, trigger autonomic and neuroendocrine responses resulting in anxiety and panic attacks. Patients with panic disorder have a heightened anxiety sensitivity (fear of anxiety-related sensations), and a variety of substances and situations may activate the anxiety and panic response.[109] Acute panic attacks are believed to be caused by dysregulated firing in the LC as described previously (see Neurobiology of Anxiety section), and hyperresponsiveness of the NE system may be an underlying cause for panic disorder.[110]

Other neurobiologic research suggests patients with panic disorder have abnormal patterns of cerebral glucose metabolism in certain brain areas; abnormalities in GABA-A receptor, NE, 5-HT, and CCK functioning; decreased GABA-A benzodiazepine binding sites; abnormal regulation of neuroactive steroids that modulate GABA-A receptors; hyperactivation of the HPA axis; CCK-B receptor gene polymorphism; and are hypersensitive to carbon dioxide. These findings seem to predispose patients to panic attacks and require further study.[105,109–111]

Genetic and environmental influences both contribute to a familial pattern where people are 8 to 21 times more likely to develop panic disorder if they have a first-degree relative with the disorder.[1,17] The vulnerability is believed to involve heightened anxiety sensitivity whereby harmless normal physical sensations are misinterpreted as being dangerous and cause fear.[112] Several studies have shown distressing childhood events (e.g., separation from parents and abuse) and behavioral inhibition during childhood (e.g., excessive fear and avoidance of novel stimuli) are associated with markedly increased risks of developing panic disorder later in life.[109] No single biologic abnormality can explain panic disorder, and further research is needed to define the complex interplay of the various pathophysiological, genetic, and environmental findings in this illness.

Treatment of Panic Disorder

Approximately 70% to 90% of patients with panic disorder can experience substantial relief with currently available treatments, which include both pharmacologic therapies and CBT.[1,105] Medications and CBT both are beneficial for reducing panic attacks initially, and their effects on phobic avoidance generally occur later. First-line medication treatments for panic disorder are SSRIs and venlafaxine as TCAs are less tolerable and possess more safety and drug–drug interaction concerns.[20,25,112,113] Benzodiazepines also are effective but no longer recommended as first-line treatment given their abuse liability, cognitive and psychomotor impairments, and lack of efficacy at treating common comorbidities. The heightened anxiety sensitivity common in panic disorder makes patients especially vulnerable to initial SSRI and TCA side effects, such as anxiety and agitation. For this reason, lower-than-usual starting doses of antidepressants are recommended in patients with panic disorder.

SELECTIVE SEROTONIN REUPTAKE INHIBITORS

Paroxetine, sertraline, fluoxetine, and venlafaxine are FDA-approved for treating panic disorder although other SSRIs (fluvoxamine, citalopram, escitalopram) are also effective in reducing the frequency of panic attacks, anticipatory anxiety, and associated depression.[20,25,113] Although low starting dosages are recommended (10 mg/day for paroxetine and citalopram, 25 mg/day for sertraline, 5–10 mg/day for fluoxetine and escitalopram) to minimize side effects, higher doses relative to antidepressant doses are usually required for response. The recommended target dosage range is 20 to 40 mg/day for paroxetine, citalopram, and fluoxetine, 100 to 200 mg/day for sertraline and fluvoxamine, and 10 to 20 mg/day for escitalopram for panic disorder.[112] The initial dose of venlafaxine XR should be 37.5 mg/day with a recommended therapeutic dose of 150 to 225 mg/day.[112]

Response to SSRIs and other antidepressants in panic disorder occurs gradually, over the course of several weeks. Reduced frequency of panic attacks usually begins within 1 to 2 weeks. A trial period of at least 6 weeks should be allowed to fully assess response, and continued improvements may be seen during a treatment period of 6 months or longer.[112]

BENZODIAZEPINES

The benzodiazepines alprazolam and clonazepam are FDA-approved for treating panic disorder and are the most extensively studied agents of this class although lorazepam and diazepam, when used in equivalent doses, also appear effective.[108,112]

Optimal benzodiazepine dosing is an important issue in treating patients with panic disorder because these individuals may need higher doses for response than patients with other anxiety disorders.[114] This may be related to reduced sensitivity of benzodiazepine binding sites in panic disorder.[115] An alprazolam dosage range of 4 to 6 mg/day is effective for most panic disorder patients, but others may require up to 10 mg/day for optimal response. The total daily dose usually needs to be taken in three or four divided doses to minimize breakthrough anxiety or panic attacks before the next scheduled dose because of fluctuating serum levels given its relatively short duration of action. The extended-release alprazolam formulation (alprazolam XR) was developed to address this problem.[56] It may have a lower abuse liability than immediate-release alprazolam, but this remains unproven. Patients with panic disorder are especially sensitive to benzodiazepine withdrawal effects. For these reasons, using the longer-acting benzodiazepine clonazepam (1–2 mg/day dosed twice daily) may be preferred over alprazolam.[114]

TRICYCLIC ANTIDEPRESSANTS, MONOAMINE OXIDASE INHIBITORS, AND OTHER ANTIDEPRESSANTS

TCAs were the first medications widely used in the treatment of panic disorder. Imipramine (100–300 mg/day) and clomipramine (50–150 mg/day) are as effective as alprazolam, but are less well tolerated.[116] Evidence for most other TCAs is lacking.[20,25,112,113] Clomipramine appears to be more effective than other TCAs for panic disorder, perhaps because of its greater serotonergic effects.[117] Despite using lower initial doses to minimize anxiety-like side effect, many patients discontinue therapy because of poor tolerability.

Among the MAOIs, phenelzine is often heralded as being remarkably effective in the treatment of panic disorder, but this claim is based on studies conducted before the publication of the initial diagnostic criteria for panic disorder in 1980.[112] No recent MAOI studies are available to assess phenelzine's efficacy within the context of current diagnostic and treatment standards. It is generally an option of last resort for treatment-refractory cases because of the many clinical disadvantages of MAOIs relative to other antidepressants (see Chapter 86, Depression).

Preliminary reports suggest mirtazapine may also be beneficial in treating panic disorder.[20,112] This agent may be useful in patients who do not respond to SSRI therapy.[112]

MISCELLANEOUS AGENTS

Other medications that are reportedly effective in treating panic disorder include anticonvulsants (valproic acid and levetiracetam) and antipsychotics (primarily risperidone and olanzapine) as either monotherapy or adjunctive therapy used in combination with an SSRI.[20,112] More information is needed before any of these can be routinely recommended for treating panic disorder.

NONPHARMACOLOGIC TREATMENTS

CBT, including exposure treatment and relaxation training, is also established as being effective in panic disorder.[105,112] The cognitive theory of panic disorder is based on the observed heightened anxiety sensitivity in these patients and asserts that physical anxiety sensations are misinterpreted as being serious or life-threatening. These fears trigger a cycle of further worsening anxiety symptoms that finally progress to a panic attack. Reversing the cognitive component of this vicious cycle is an integral part of CBT and is important in producing lasting therapeutic effects of treatment.[112] Breathing retraining and exposure to fear cues are key components of behavioral therapy.

Some studies have found medications to be superior to CBT in the treatment of panic disorder, whereas others report opposite results.[112,118] Combining medication with CBT can be useful to increase response/remission rates in those with severe symptoms or a partial response as well as to improve relapse rates during pharmacotherapy discontinuation attempts.[20,114,119]

Clinical Presentation and Differential Diagnosis of Panic Disorder

CASE 83-7

QUESTION 1: S.K., a 24-year-old female graphic artist, presents to the ED complaining of chest pain, difficulty breathing, dizziness, and nausea. She describes feeling "as if my head is going off in space and I am outside my body." These attacks often escalate quickly peaking within 10 minutes and then start to subside within 30 minutes. She states she has been under extreme stress lately because of the poor economy and has conflicts with her landlord as a result of nonpayment of the rent on her art studio. S.K. fears she has had a heart attack or stroke brought on by her stressful life. S.K. recently visited her family physician for the same symptoms; however, a complete physical examination and laboratory workup yielded no abnormalities. She states her first "attack" occurred out of the blue about 5 months ago while she was shopping for oil paints at the art supply store, and she can never predict when they will occur. Since then, her symptoms have become more severe and frequent, and she has started isolating herself in her studio for fear they will return when she is in public. S.K. uses marijuana "to relax" and occasionally drinks alcohol (but only rarely). She has suffered from depression in the past and was hospitalized for one severe episode 2 years ago. An ECG is performed and found to be normal. The physician's diagnosis is panic disorder with agoraphobia. What clinical features of panic disorder does S.K. display, and what are the important factors in the differential diagnosis of panic disorder?

S.K. exhibits many typical characteristics of panic disorder. As illustrated in this case, the first panic attack typically occurs without warning while the person is involved in a normal everyday activity and lasts 10 to 30 minutes. Panic attacks are extremely terrifying and usually leave the sufferer feeling anxious and convinced something is medically wrong. As with S.K., it is not uncommon for persons to make ED visits after or during panic attacks, believing they have had a heart attack or other serious event. Unfortunately, panic disorder is often not recognized in primary-care settings, and no medical cause for the symptoms can be identified. Faced with findings that they are apparently healthy, persons may make repeated ED visits and consult different doctors and specialists in an attempt to uncover a physical explanation for their frightening symptoms.

S.K. exhibits the following target symptoms of panic disorder: chest pain, shortness of breath, dizziness, abdominal distress, and loss of control. Agoraphobia is present because she avoids leaving her studio because of her fear of having panic attacks. Other factors consistent with a diagnosis of panic disorder include her young age, female sex, and lack of abnormal physical findings. This case also illustrates the association between onset of panic disorder and stressful life events, its common association with depression, and the frequent lack of recognition of panic disorder in primary-care settings.

Because different substances or medical conditions can cause severe anxiety and panic, it is necessary to rule out these potential causes for panic attacks.[108] Notable triggers of panic attacks include caffeine, alcohol, nicotine, nonprescription cold preparations, cannabis, amphetamines, and cocaine (Table 83-2).[108] S.K. uses marijuana, which can be associated with panic symptoms. Although chronic moderate-to-severe use of marijuana may complicate the treatment of panic disorder, it appears infrequent marijuana use does not adversely affect treatment.[120,121] S.K. does not endorse chronic, severe marijuana abuse, but if she does not adequately respond to treatment, this might be further explored. Medical illnesses that can cause panic attacks include thyroid dysfunction, asthma, COPD, mitral valve prolapse, and seizure disorders.[122] Panic attacks can also occur with other anxiety disorders. However, in these cases, the panic attacks usually occur on exposure to a feared object or situation (in phobic disorders), an object of obsession (in OCD), or a stimulus associated with a traumatic stressor (in PTSD). S.K. reports her panic attacks occur unexpectedly, and situationally bound or predisposed attacks are not evident; therefore, the features are consistent with panic disorder.

Treatment Selection for Panic Disorder, Selective Serotonin Reuptake Inhibitor Dosing Issues, and Combination Selective Serotonin Reuptake Inhibitor–Benzodiazepine Therapy

CASE 83-7, QUESTION 2: S.K. is referred to a psychiatrist who decides to initiate treatment with paroxetine 20 mg every morning. Three days later, S.K. calls the doctor complaining that her anxiety and panic attacks have greatly increased since she started taking paroxetine. The psychiatrist prescribes alprazolam 0.5 mg (tablets) and instructs S.K. to take one tablet as needed for the anxiety. What factors should be considered in the selection of an initial medication treatment for panic disorder? Why is the prescribed treatment for S.K. inappropriate?

An SSRI is an appropriate first-line treatment for most panic disorder patients.[20] In patients such as S.K. who have a history of depression, SSRIs may also help prevent relapse of depression. Patients with severe or distressing symptoms may initially require concurrent benzodiazepine therapy, which provides quick relief from anxiety and panic attacks until the therapeutic effects of SSRIs are evident. At that time, usually after several weeks, the benzodiazepine can be gradually discontinued. An SSRI–benzodiazepine combination is still the most commonly prescribed initial treatment, even though guidelines recommend monotherapy unless initial anxiety is extremely high.[123] Although benzodiazepines are generally avoided in patients with a history of substance abuse, use of low doses for a limited time may be appropriate for some patients with disabling symptoms, as long as there is no current substance (especially alcohol) abuse.[20,69,112] Because of the levels of distress and impairment caused by S.K.'s panic disorder, combined SSRI–benzodiazepine therapy would have been the preferred initial treatment. Because panic attacks peak quickly and generally last less than 30 minutes, an as-needed benzodiazepine is not helpful to prevent panic attacks. As such, scheduled benzodiazepine dosing is preferred over as-needed dosing schedule during initial therapy.[112]

In choosing among SSRIs for the treatment of panic disorder, paroxetine or sertraline may be less anxiety provoking in some patients than a more activating SSRI such as fluoxetine.[26] When paroxetine is used, a very low initial dose of 10 mg/day should be used. In S.K.'s case, the prescribed 20-mg/day starting dose was too high. Also, scheduled versus as-needed benzodiazepine dosing would have been preferred. After 2 to 4 weeks, the benzodiazepine can be gradually discontinued while the SSRI therapy is continued and gradually titrated to the target effective dose. The potential for drug interactions must also be kept in mind when SSRI–benzodiazepine combinations are used because certain SSRIs can inhibit benzodiazepine metabolism, leading to increased benzodiazepine side effects (see Benzodiazepine Drug Interactions section).

Patient Counseling Information

Patients such as S.K. who are beginning SSRI therapy for the treatment of panic disorder should be counseled about possible increased anxiety during the first 1 or 2 weeks of treatment, as well as other common SSRI side effects, including nausea, headache, sexual dysfunction, and either insomnia or sedation. Because these are dose-related effects, patients should inform their clinician of any problems, and a dosage reduction may be indicated. These adverse effects (with the possible exception of sexual dysfunction) usually subside after 1 to 3 weeks of continued treatment. It is also important to inform patients it may take several weeks before beneficial effects of antidepressant treatment are seen, and 6 to 12 weeks or longer may be required for full response. Patients receiving benzodiazepines should be counseled about their use in providing anxiolytic coverage during the initial weeks of SSRI therapy, as well as their limited utility as long-term therapy. Other pertinent counseling information for benzodiazepine treatment should also be included (see Case 83-2, Question 4). The desired goals of therapy and likely duration of treatment should also be explained. Providing information about the nature of panic disorder, including reassurance that panic attacks are not life-threatening, is also important. Many clinicians recommend patients keep a "panic diary" in which they record frequency of panic attacks, along with symptoms experienced during attacks.

Clinical Assessment and Goals of Therapy

CASE 83-7, QUESTION 3: S.K. refuses to continue paroxetine, so escitalopram is prescribed instead. After 1 week of escitalopram therapy at the initial dosage of 5 mg/day, S.K. is tolerating the medication well. The plan is to gradually increase escitalopram to 10 mg, then to 20 mg/day during the next several weeks. S.K. is also taking alprazolam, 0.5 mg BID to TID. What are the desired goals of treatment in this case, and how can S.K.'s response to treatment be assessed?

Five domains in panic disorder have been identified in which treatment outcomes should be assessed: (a) frequency and severity of panic attacks, (b) anticipatory anxiety, (c) phobic avoidance behaviors, (d) overall well-being, and (e) illness-related disability in various areas (work, school, family).[112] The treatment goals in this case are first to stop S.K.'s panic attacks, then to reduce her anticipatory anxiety, followed by reversal of phobic avoidance.[54] These outcomes should allow her to more comfortably leave her studio when required and, secondarily, improve her overall functioning and quality of life.

Several different instruments have been used to assess outcomes of treatment in panic disorder.[54] In addition to the panic diary, others include the Fear Questionnaire, the Panic Appraisal Inventory, and the Panic Disorder Severity Scale. The latter is currently considered by many experts to be the most useful because it evaluates outcomes in all five identified target domains of panic disorder.[54,112]

Course and Duration of Therapy

Case 83-7, Question 4: After 3 months of escitalopram therapy, S.K. reports she has had no panic attacks in the past month and her functioning has improved dramatically. She is currently taking 20 mg/day of escitalopram and gradually stopped taking the alprazolam 3 to 4 weeks ago. S.K. reveals she is painting regularly, selling some of her paintings, paying her rent, and she has begun dating again. S.K. is experiencing no significant side effects from escitalopram except for some decrease in her sexual drive. She wonders how long she should continue taking it since she is doing so well. What is the recommended duration of treatment for panic disorder?

Long-term medication trials in panic disorder support the recommendation that treatment should continue for at least 6 to 12 months after acute response.[20,112] The benefits of maintenance pharmacotherapy in preventing relapse are well documented although the optimal duration of treatment is a subject of continued debate among panic researchers. Maintenance treatment gives patients time to resume normal lifestyles and to re-establish daily activities after acute cessation of panic attacks.

In this case, S.K.'s current escitalopram dosage of 20 mg/day is appropriate because this is within the effective dosage range for panic disorder. Escitalopram therapy should be continued at the current dosage for 3 to 6 more months. S.K.'s sexual dysfunction is not likely to decrease with continued treatment; therefore, specific remedies for SSRI-induced sexual dysfunction may be tried (see Chapter 86, Depression). After a successful period of full remission, a trial of medication discontinuation may be attempted to determine whether continued treatment is necessary. Medication should not be stopped in patients who are experiencing stressful life events or substantial residual problems in any of the five domains (frequency and severity of panic attacks, anticipatory anxiety, phobic avoidance behaviors, overall well-being, and illness-related disability in work, school, and family).[112] When a medication is discontinued, it should be withdrawn gradually over several months, regardless of the class. Because of the devastating impact panic disorder can have, reinstitution of drug treatment is indicated if relapse occurs. Long-term treatment with antidepressants, and benzodiazepines if necessary, is generally successful in maintaining treatment benefits without detrimental effects or dosage escalations.

SOCIAL ANXIETY DISORDER AND SPECIFIC PHOBIAS

Classification and Diagnosis of Phobic Disorders

The *DSM-5* includes two primary types of phobic disorders: specific phobia and social anxiety disorder (formerly social phobia) with symptoms presented in Table 83-10.[1] These disorders involve excessive or unreasonable fears and lead to avoidance behavior to minimize anxiety for a duration of at least 6 months. The main difference between specific phobias and social anxiety disorder is that the former involves fear and avoidance of specific stimuli and not a general fear of social situations.

SOCIAL ANXIETY DISORDER

Social anxiety disorder manifests as intense irrational fear, anxiety, or avoidance of scrutiny or evaluation by others in social situations because of concerns about humiliation or being made to appear ridiculous.[1] A defining feature is that the fears and anxiety are confined to social situations (e.g., speaking to people, attending social gatherings, eating or drinking in public, using public restrooms, public speaking), and patients are usually symptom-free when alone. If the fear is strictly confined to speaking or performing in public, a *performance-only* specifier is applied to the diagnosis. Common symptoms seen in social anxiety disorder include blushing, muscle twitching, and stuttering, in addition to other typical symptoms of anxiety. Panic attacks may also occur in either specific phobia or social anxiety disorder on exposure to the feared object or situation. However, social anxiety disorder is differentiated from panic disorder in that it involves the fear of scrutiny by others, rather than the fear of having a panic attack.

SPECIFIC PHOBIAS

Specific phobias are coded by one of five specifiers: animal (e.g., insects, dogs, spiders), natural environment (e.g., heights, water, storms), blood–injection–injury (e.g., blood, injury, medical procedures), situational (e.g., flying, bridges, elevators), or other.[1] Significant impairment of functioning or marked distress must be present for a diagnosis of specific phobia to be warranted. For example, fear of flying might constitute a diagnosis of specific phobia in a person whose job requires airplane travel, but it would not impair functioning in someone who never has occasion to fly.

First-line management of specific phobias involves avoidance of the stimuli or exposure-based psychotherapy, such as CBT or virtual reality exposure. Medications are not generally

Table 83-10

Symptoms of Social Anxiety Disorder (Social Phobia) (Items 1–5) and Specific Phobia (Items 2–5)[1]

1. Marked and constant fear of one or more social situations in which the person is exposed to unfamiliar people or possible scrutiny by others and the person fears humiliation or embarrassment
2. Experiencing the situation causes an immediate anxiety response
3. Feared situation is avoided or experienced with intense anxiety or distress
4. Feared situation exceeds the true risk associated with the social situation according to sociocultural norms
5. Fear or avoidance significantly interferes with the person's normal routine or activities or causes marked distress

considered beneficial, as pharmacotherapy for specific phobia is largely understudied and psychotherapy is extremely successful. Benzodiazepines effectively reduce anxiety associated with a phobic trigger, but they may also interfere with the efficacy of these exposure therapies.[20,25,113]

Social Anxiety Disorder

EPIDEMIOLOGY AND CLINICAL COURSE

In the United States, the lifetime and past-year prevalence of social anxiety disorder is approximately 13% and 7%, respectively.[14,124] The male-to-female prevalence ratio is approximately 2:3.[9] Social anxiety disorder usually begins early in life, with a mean onset between ages 14 and 16 years.[125] More than 50% of patients are affected before adolescence, and a history of shyness and behavioral inhibition throughout childhood is common.[125] Unless effectively treated, the clinical course is often chronic, unremitting, and lifelong, and only 20% to 40% of patients are reported to recover after 20 years of living with this condition.[124]

COMORBIDITY AND CLINICAL SIGNIFICANCE

Comorbidity in social anxiety disorder is high, with an estimated 70% to 90% of individuals having at least one other psychiatric disorder in their lifetime.[1,124,125] Common comorbid conditions include simple phobia, major depression, GAD, panic disorder, body dysmorphic disorder, and alcohol abuse. Because of its early onset, social anxiety disorder usually precedes the development of comorbid disorders. Alcohol is commonly used to decrease anxiety in social situations. The risk of suicide attempts is high, especially in those with both social anxiety disorder and another psychiatric illness, like depression.[9]

Because social anxiety disorder usually begins during the teenage years, it can seriously interfere with development of normal social skills, achievement of full academic and career potentials, and abilities to form interpersonal relationships.[126] This leads to functional disabilities that may persist for a lifetime. Social anxiety disorder is associated with unemployment, lower levels of education, and dependence on public financial support systems.[9] Persons with social anxiety disorder are less likely to marry, and more than half report moderate-to-severe impairments in their abilities to carry out ordinary daily activities.[126]

ETIOLOGY AND PATHOPHYSIOLOGY

Social anxiety disorder is a familial disease, but the relative contributions of genetic versus environmental influences have not been differentiated.[17] Early factors predisposing to its development include anxious behavior modeling in parents and parental overprotection.[1] Shyness in children, which is associated with later development of social anxiety disorder, has been linked to a specific genetic polymorphism of the serotonin transporter promoter region.[127]

Biologic studies suggest performance-only social anxiety disorder has a different underlying pathophysiology involving noradrenergic system dysfunction. Conversely, in nonperformance-only social anxiety disorder, there is substantial evidence for dopaminergic (decreased dopamine neurotransmission) and serotonergic dysfunction (5-HT type-2 receptor hypersensitivity).[128–130]

TREATMENT OF SOCIAL ANXIETY DISORDER

Early detection and treatment of social anxiety disorder are vital in reducing lifelong functional consequences and may prevent development of comorbid disorders. Because of the nature of the disorder, some sufferers are reluctant to seek treatment resulting in an average treatment delay of 16 years.[131] Those who seek help, even in psychiatric settings, are rarely diagnosed and treated appropriately.[125] Pharmacotherapy has become first line, but nonpharmacotherapy, particularly CBT, is also beneficial.[20] Data do not support the routine use of combined modalities in the management of social anxiety disorder; clinicians should determine whether combined therapy would be useful on a case-by-case basis.[132]

Selective Serotonin Reuptake Inhibitors and Serotonin and Norepinephrine Reuptake Inhibitors

As with other anxiety disorders, SSRIs, in addition to the SNRI venlafaxine, are considered the primary treatment option for most patients with social anxiety disorder[125] for which paroxetine, sertraline, fluvoxamine CR, and venlafaxine XR are FDA-approved.[132] Nonetheless, fluoxetine, citalopram, and escitalopram have also demonstrated efficacy in controlled clinical trials although fluoxetine has negative evidence as well.[20,132] Preliminary evidence with duloxetine suggests this agent may be useful.[133]

Unlike patients with GAD and panic disorder, those with social anxiety disorder often tolerate standard antidepressant starting doses. Target doses for social anxiety disorder are typically within the normal antidepressant dosage ranges. It is thought SSRIs exhibit a flat dose–response curve.[134] Fixed-dose studies of paroxetine (20, 40, and 60 mg/day) and duloxetine (≥60 mg/day) in social anxiety disorder found no overall difference in efficacy between doses.[133,135] Although some individuals may require higher dosages, adequate time (2–4 weeks) should be allowed before the dosage is increased. Response to SSRIs occurs gradually, and an adequate medication trial to assess response should last at least 8 to 10 weeks. Many who experience minimal response at week 8 may show a good response at week 12, and improvements have been found to continue throughout 16 weeks of treatment.[136]

Other Antidepressants

The MAOIs phenelzine (60–90 mg/day), tranylcypromine (30–60 mg/day), and selegiline (5 mg twice daily) have also demonstrated marked efficacy for social anxiety disorder but are reserved for SSRI nonresponders.[20,125,132]

Case reports and open studies suggest bupropion may be useful in treating social anxiety disorder, but controlled trials are needed to define its role.[125] Mirtazapine has conflicting evidence from small RCTs but may be considered in SSRI nonresponders.[20] Imipramine is ineffective for social anxiety disorder, and TCAs (except clomipramine) are not among the recommended treatment options.[20,125,132] Likewise, nefazodone is not recommended given the risk of hepatotoxicity and conflicting evidence, including one negative RCT.[20]

Benzodiazepines

Benzodiazepines are generally considered second-line therapy for social anxiety disorder, as they have limited efficacy in treating psychiatric comorbidities and abuse/dependence potential. In clinical practice, they are commonly used in combination with SSRI therapy on an as-needed basis before participation in stressful social situations.[132] However, the efficacy of adjunctive benzodiazepines to decrease time to response or increase response rate is unclear.[137] The high-potency benzodiazepines may be useful as monotherapy in select patients. Clonazepam (1–3 mg/day) was markedly efficacious in one controlled study, whereas alprazolam (1–6 mg/day) showed only modest efficacy compared with placebo.[132]

β-Blockers and Other Miscellaneous Agents

β-Adrenergic receptor blockers reduce peripheral autonomic symptoms of anxiety and, thus, are useful for performance-related social anxiety disorder.[125] Propranolol (10–80 mg) and atenolol (25–50 mg) are the two recommended agents and can be used on an as-needed basis (1–2 hours before the performance) to reduce performance anxiety symptoms such as tremors, palpitations, and blushing. A test dose should be tried before the actual occasion to assess tolerability.

Pregabalin is also considered to be an acceptable first-line agent, in the absence of comorbidities which would benefit from an SSRI, based on placebo-controlled trials for acute management and relapse prevention.[138] It appears a higher pregabalin dose (450–600 mg/day) may be necessary for effective treatment. Other anticonvulsants, antipsychotics, and miscellaneous agents have also been reported to be effective in the treatment of social anxiety disorder, but they are considered second- or third-line treatments.[20,43,132] These include gabapentin, tiagabine, topiramate, valproate derivatives, olanzapine monotherapy, adjunctive aripiprazole, adjunctive risperidone, and atomoxetine.

Nonpharmacologic Treatments

Several studies have demonstrated CBT to be comparable to medications in the treatment of social anxiety disorder.[139] Although medications may work faster, CBT is believed to result in longer-lasting treatment gains with effects persisting for 1 to 5 years. The cognitive therapy component changes maladaptive thought patterns, such as expectations of performing poorly and over concern about negative evaluation by others.[139] The behavioral therapy component, as in other anxiety disorders, involves repeated exposure and practice performing in those feared situations. Social skills training can also be beneficial in improving interpersonal communication skills.

CLINICAL PRESENTATION OF SOCIAL ANXIETY DISORDER

CASE 83-8

QUESTION 1: S.H., an 18-year-old man, is brought for psychiatric consultation by his mother who complains her son is extremely shy and she's concerned about his ability to "fit in" at college. S.H. was referred to the psychiatrist by his primary-care physician, who reports S.H. is physically healthy. S.H.'s mother states he is a very bright young man who made straight as in high school despite frequent absenteeism. He only has one close friend and has never been on a date. S.H.'s mother says during high school, S.H. rarely attended school social functions and spent much of his time in his room working on his computer. On graduation from high school, he received a full scholarship to a community college but is quite anxious about going and is debating whether he should turn down the scholarship. When questioned by the psychiatrist, S.H.'s face turns bright red, and his voice shakes when he speaks. S.H. admits his behavior is not normal but says he is afraid he might "do something stupid" when he is around people and becomes extremely embarrassed when he has to talk to anyone. He has wanted to ask a certain girl on a date for 3 years but experienced severe anxiety attacks on the few occasions he tried to approach her. S.H. is afraid of being turned down and believes no girl would ever want to date someone like him. The psychiatrist's diagnosis is social anxiety disorder. What clinical features of social anxiety disorder are present in S.H.?

S.H. exhibits many characteristic features of the generalized type of social anxiety disorder. S.H. admits he does not like being around people for fear of embarrassment, and he generally avoids social situations, which are classic traits of social anxiety disorder. Symptoms of blushing and shaking voice are also common in social anxiety disorder, as well as other typical anxiety symptoms such as palpitations, trembling, sweating, tense muscles, dry throat, hot/cold sensations, and a sinking feeling in the stomach. S.H. also displays hypersensitivity to rejection and low self-esteem, and he realizes his behavior and fears are unreasonable. These symptoms and S.H.'s young age are consistent with a diagnosis of social anxiety disorder.

S.H.'s case illustrates the substantial disability that can result from this illness. S.H.'s anxiety disorder has deprived him of normal social development, making friends, dating, participating in social functions regularly, and pursuit of higher education. Future impairments throughout S.H.'s life are likely to be significant unless his anxiety is treated successfully.

TREATMENT SELECTION FOR SOCIAL ANXIETY DISORDER

CASE 83-8, QUESTION 2: The physician decides to initiate sertraline 50 mg every morning for S.H. Is the prescribed pharmacotherapy appropriate in this case?

Because S.H.'s generalized social anxiety disorder is severely affecting his life, medication treatment is indicated. SSRIs are first-line therapy for treating social anxiety disorder, and sertraline is a good choice because it is FDA-approved for this indication and available as a generic. Although not applicable in this case, sertraline is also effective for many other psychiatric disorders commonly seen in patients with social anxiety disorder. The sertraline starting dose of 50 mg/day is appropriate for S.H., and 50-mg increment dosage increases can be made every 4 weeks according to response, up to a maximum of 200 mg/day. Signs of response may be seen within 2 to 4 weeks, but 8 to 12 weeks is usually required for optimal results. If available, CBT may also be combined with pharmacotherapy for S.H.

GOALS AND DURATION OF TREATMENT

CASE 83-8, QUESTION 3: What are the goals of treatment in this case, and how can S.H.'s response to treatment be objectively assessed? How long should effective therapy be continued?

Three principle domains of treatment outcomes have been defined for social anxiety disorder: symptoms, functionality, and overall well-being.[54] It is recommended that all three of these areas are assessed because even if all anxiety symptoms disappear, treatment is not clinically significant unless functioning also improves. The clinician-rated Liebowitz Social Anxiety Scale and the patient-rated Sheehan Disability Scale can be used for measuring improvements in symptom and functional ability domains, respectively.[54] In S.H.'s case, the desired outcomes of treatment include reducing fear and avoidance of social situations, enabling him to comfortably interact socially and attend college, and improving his quality of life.

Several studies have examined relapse rates after double-blind discontinuation of effective treatment in social anxiety disorder.[132,136,139] Long-term studies have shown sertraline, paroxetine, escitalopram, fluvoxamine CR, venlafaxine XR, pregabalin, and clonazepam prevent relapse of social anxiety disorder during continuation treatment.[20] Therefore, pharmacotherapy should be continued for at least 1 year after response.[125,132] After that time, a gradual medication discontinuation trial may be attempted with vigilant monitoring for signs of relapse.

POST-TRAUMATIC STRESS DISORDER AND ACUTE STRESS DISORDER

Diagnostic Criteria

PTSD and acute stress disorder occur in people who have experienced a severely distressing traumatic event. These disorders are characterized by symptoms of intrusive re-experiencing, avoidance features, autonomic hyperarousal, and negative cognitions and mood symptoms.[1] In addition to war veterans, PTSD also occurs in persons exposed to events such as natural disasters, serious accidents, criminal assault, rape, physical or sexual abuse, and political victimization (refugees, concentration camp survivors, hostages). The trauma does not have to involve physical injury to the PTSD victim. Witnessing someone else being injured or killed, being diagnosed with a life-threatening illness, and experiencing the unexpected death of a loved one are common types of trauma that may lead to PTSD.[1]

Symptoms of PTSD are presented in Table 83-11.[1] According to diagnostic criteria, the person must have exposure to actual or threatened death, serious injury, or sexual violence via directly experiencing the event, witnessing the event in person, learning the event occurred to a close family member or friend, or experiencing extreme exposure to aversive details of an event.[1] Specifiers indicate whether PTSD is delayed (after 6 months) onset in relation to the trauma and/or whether it is associated with dissociative symptoms.[1] Symptoms must persist for at least 1 month to meet the criteria for PTSD. *Acute stress disorder* is a separate diagnostic category in the *DSM-5* and refers to cases in which symptoms last less than 1 month (but at least 3 days).[1] It involves many of the same clinical features as PTSD, and like with PTSD, symptoms must be severe enough to interfere with functioning.

Epidemiology and Clinical Course

PTSD is associated with a lifetime prevalence in the general population of approximately 10% and up to 24% among deployed serviceman from Iraq and Afghanistan.[140] PTSD is twice as common in women, although overall, men are exposed to trauma more often.[141] Rates of PTSD are expected to rise as the frequency of traumatic events throughout the world continues to increase. An estimated 80% to 90% of individuals in the United States today will experience at least one event during their lifetime traumatic enough to lead to PTSD.[141]

Most people who are exposed to a traumatic event do not develop PTSD; approximately 90% of individuals experience a normal acute stress response to trauma and fully recover.[141] Risk factors for the development of PTSD include experiencing assaultive violence, more severe and chronic traumas, a history of depressive or anxiety disorders, lack of social support after the trauma, and experiencing dissociative or other intense symptoms during or soon after the trauma.[140–142] Previous exposure to trauma also increases the risk of developing PTSD after later traumas, and survivors of childhood sexual or physical abuse have been found to be especially vulnerable.[142,143]

Overall, 79% to 88% of PTSD patients also suffer from other disorders in their lifetime, including major depression, alcohol or other substance abuse, GAD, panic disorder, and phobic disorders.[140,141,143–145] The risk of suicidality in PTSD is high and likely influenced by comorbid major depression.[146] Recent studies have also found associations with PTSD and coronary heart disease, traumatic brain injury, and sexual dysfunction.[147–149] PTSD causes significant functional disability and has been associated with school failure, teenage pregnancy, unemployment, marital instability, legal problems, and impaired performance in the workplace.[150]

The course of PTSD is highly variable. Most patients who meet criteria for PTSD 1 month after trauma show spontaneous recovery within 6 to 9 months.[144] PTSD continues for years in a significant minority, estimated at 10% to 25%, and some sufferers experience a lifelong course of illness.

Etiology and Pathophysiology

Psychological trauma, especially that which occurs early in life or is chronic in duration, can cause persistent changes in various aspects of brain functioning and in neurobiologic responses to stress.[151] Evidence of altered NE, 5-HT, glutamatergic, GABA system, HPA axis, neuroendocrine, substance P, and opioid system functioning has been found in PTSD.[152–155] Stress-induced hyperactivity of central noradrenergic systems is believed to lead to the generalized anxiety and autonomic hyperarousal associated with PTSD.[153]

Neurobiologic consequences of stress and trauma result in both structural and functional changes in the brain, including reduced hippocampal volume and excessive activation of the amygdala.[156] Genetic factors may also play a role in influencing vulnerability to the damaging effects of stress.[157]

Table 83-11
Symptoms of Post-traumatic Stress Disorder for Individuals ≥6 Years of Age[1]

1. Intrusion (e.g., memories, dreams, dissociative reaction (like flashbacks), intense distress that is experienced on exposure to stimuli associated with the traumatic event, or physiologic reactions to internal or external cues that reflect the event)
2. Avoidance (e.g., avoidance of or efforts to avoid distressing memories, thoughts, or feelings or external reminders such as places, people, conversations about or related to the event)
3. Increased arousal including at least two of the following:
   - Sleep disturbances
   - Irritability or anger outbursts
   - Difficulty concentrating
   - Hypervigilance
   - Exaggerated startle response
   - Reckless of self-destructive behavior
4. Persistent negative alterations in cognition or mood associated with the event including at least two of the following:
   - Amnesia surrounding the event
   - Negative beliefs or expectations about oneself, others, or the world
   - Distorted cognitions about the cause or consequence of the event where the individual blames themselves or others
   - Negative emotional state
   - Diminished interest or participation in activities
   - Detachment or estrangement
   - Lack of ability to experience positive emotions

Treatment of Post-traumatic Stress Disorder

Both medications and CBT are useful in treating PTSD. Nonpharmacologic therapies alone may be appropriate for initial treatment of mild PTSD, but pharmacotherapy, either alone or in some instances in combination with psychological therapies, may be recommended for patients with moderate or severe illness.[25,142,143,150,158] When assessing various treatment options for PTSD, it is important to consider effects on all four core symptom clusters (re-experiencing or intrusive symptoms, avoidance, hyperarousal, or negative cognitions and mood symptoms). Not all PTSD treatments are effective for each domain.

The preferred first-line medications in PTSD are SSRIs or the SNRI, venlafaxine XR, but various other antidepressants may also be useful. Response to pharmacotherapy occurs very gradually, taking 8 to 12 weeks or longer. Partial response at 12 weeks of treatment may be followed by full remission after several more months of therapy; therefore, an adequate period should be allowed to fully determine response to a particular medication. Lack of improvement after 4 weeks of therapy indicates nonresponse, so alternative treatment strategies should be tried in these cases.[159] Although further research is needed, prevention of PTSD using various pharmacologic strategies has been evaluated in adults. A recent review highlights potential utility of hydrocortisone, but additional studies are needed.[160]

SELECTIVE SEROTONIN REUPTAKE INHIBITORS AND SEROTONIN AND NOREPINEPHRINE REUPTAKE INHIBITORS

Sertraline and paroxetine are currently the only FDA-approved SSRIs for PTSD. Large controlled studies have demonstrated that both agents, as well as venlafaxine, are effective and superior to placebo.[161] They also have beneficial effects on depression and general anxiety symptoms and have been associated with improvements in overall functioning and quality of life.[159,161] Use of fluoxetine also appears to be effective in treating PTSD in some patients, although study results have been mixed.[20,25] Citalopram, escitalopram, and fluvoxamine have shown efficacy in the treatment of PTSD in open trials, but randomized, double-blind, placebo-controlled studies have yielded negative results.[159,162] Finally, one small, naturalistic study in treatment-resistant men suggests duloxetine may be effective in managing comorbid depression and PTSD.[163] However, in another small, prospective study in military veterans suggests additional studies are warranted.[164]

OTHER ANTIDEPRESSANTS

Several open studies and case reports suggest nefazodone, mirtazapine, and bupropion are effective in treating core symptoms of PTSD.[155,165] Although supporting evidence for these antidepressants is not as strong, they may be considered appropriate alternatives to SSRIs or venlafaxine in certain patients. The TCAs amitriptyline and imipramine and the MAOI phenelzine have also been found to be effective for PTSD in controlled trials, but these agents are generally not recommended because of their poor tolerability and safety profiles.[143] Because of the relatively high risk of suicide in PTSD, TCAs can be especially dangerous in this population.

MISCELLANEOUS AGENTS

Various other medications have been used successfully in limited numbers of PTSD cases. Anticonvulsants carbamazepine, valproate, topiramate, tiagabine, gabapentin, oxcarbazepine, vigabatrin, pregabalin, levetiracetam, and lamotrigine have been studied with inconsistent results, mostly in case series and open-label trials.[20,25,161,165] These agents may be effective in certain patients and can be useful for reducing irritability, impulsivity, and anger or violent outbursts, particularly in patients with bipolar disorder.[166] Anticonvulsants may also be effective for intrusive, re-experiencing, and hyperarousal symptoms. Atypical antipsychotic agents (risperidone, quetiapine, olanzapine) have been used effectively to treat PTSD-related psychotic symptoms and sleep disturbances, though evidence is limited. One study failed to find benefit with adjunctive use of risperidone in treatment-resistant PTSD in military service personnel compared to placebo.[167] However, a recent meta-analysis suggests these agents may help target symptoms of intrusion.[168] The α_1-adrenergic antagonist, prazosin, may decrease nightmares, increase sleep time, and reduce other core symptoms in patients with PTSD.[155,169] Higher doses, up to 16 mg/day, may be needed to optimize efficacy.[170] Conflicting evidence exists for the use of the β-adrenergic antagonist, propranolol, which has been studied in blocking memory consolidation and therefore may prevent PTSD if administered within hours of the traumatic event.[171] Larger studies are needed to determine whether this is a useful preventive option. As previously mentioned, preliminary evidence supports the use of hydrocortisone for this indication, though additional studies are needed.[160] Benzodiazepines are generally ineffective in treating PTSD, and use of these agents is not recommended.[172]

NONPHARMACOLOGIC TREATMENTS

Various types of psychosocial therapies have been used in the treatment of PTSD, including anxiety management training to help patients cope with stress.[172] Trauma-focused CBT and eye movement desensitization and reprocessing treatment have both demonstrated effectiveness in PTSD, and either of these treatments are recommended for all patients with PTSD.[140,158] Cognitive therapies seem to be most effective for symptoms of demoralization, guilt, and shame, whereas exposure therapies are better for reducing intrusive thoughts, flashbacks, and avoidance behaviors. Studies are needed to further investigate the utility of virtual reality exposure therapy and transcranial magnetic stimulation in PTSD.[173,174] Trials of combined psychosocial therapies and medication are inconclusive and require further investigation to determine superior effectiveness compared with either treatment strategy alone.[175]

Clinical Presentation of Post-traumatic Stress Disorder

CASE 83-9

QUESTION 1: D.D. is a 42-year-old woman who was attacked and raped in the driveway of her home as she was getting out of her car 1 month ago. She did not seek medical treatment at the time and waited several days before reporting the incident to anyone, including her family. She presents to her physician complaining that she cannot sleep and she is irritable, anxious, and depressed. When asked about any recent stressors in her life, she finally tells her doctor about the rape. D.D. has no history of psychiatric illness, admits her symptoms have appeared since the attack, and says she has never had any psychiatric problems until now. She states she has nightly nightmares and becomes extremely anxious every time she comes home and gets out of her car at night (which she avoids doing when possible). She is startled when the phone rings or when someone approaches her unexpectedly, and she literally freezes if she sees a man who bears any physical resemblance to her attacker. D.D. also states that memories of the rape often flash through her mind for no reason, although she tries hard not to think about it. The assailant has not been caught, and D.D. feels extremely guilty for not promptly reporting the crime. Her symptoms are interfering significantly with her ability to work and have put a strain on her marriage. What clinical features of PTSD does D.D. display?

Individuals with PTSD often present with nonspecific complaints indicative of a generalized anxiety, depression, or substance use disorder. They may not realize or want to reveal an association between their symptoms and the trauma experienced. Careful evaluation by the clinician is required to elicit a pattern suggestive of PTSD. D.D. displays many target symptoms of PTSD, including re-experiencing/intrusive symptoms (nightmares, recurrent memories), avoidance of the activity reminding her of the trauma, symptoms of increased arousal (sleep difficulties, irritability, exaggerated startle response), and negative alterations in cognition (guilt). In addition, she is experiencing feelings of depression, distress, marital problems, and impairment in occupational functioning as a result of her symptoms. The lack of any previous psychiatric illness combined with the temporal relationship between the attack and her symptoms supports the presence of PTSD as opposed to another anxiety or depressive disorder. Since her trauma occurred 1 month ago, her condition would be classified as acute-onset PTSD.

Treatment Selection and Selective Serotonin Reuptake Inhibitor Dosing

CASE 83-9, QUESTION 2: What factors are important in the selection of an initial treatment for D.D.?

Because D.D. is exhibiting moderate-to-severe PTSD symptoms, pharmacotherapy is indicated. Medication treatment should be combined with CBT if it is available, but nonpharmacologic therapies alone are generally reserved for patients with mild symptoms. An SSRI is the preferred initial medication treatment for most patients.[161] Sertraline is an appropriate choice of treatment in this case and is FDA-approved for PTSD. Low initial SSRI doses are recommended in PTSD, so sertraline can be started at 25 mg/day and gradually increased to the target dosage range of 100 to 150 mg/day, according to response and tolerability.[165] Persistent sleep complaints during the first month after a traumatic experience may predispose the patient to chronic PTSD, so management of sleep disturbances is an important component of initial PTSD treatment.[175] If CBT for insomnia is available, this may be considered.[176]

Clinical Assessment and Goals of Therapy

CASE 83-9, QUESTION 3: What are the goals of treatment in this case, and how can D.D.'s symptoms be objectively assessed?

The first goal of treatment of PTSD is to reduce the core symptoms of re-experiencing/intrusion, avoidance, hyperarousal, and negative alterations in mood and cognitions. In D.D.'s case, these target symptoms include nightmares, intrusive memories, avoidance behaviors, irritability, hyperarousal, sleep difficulties, and guilt. Improvements should begin within the first 2 weeks and gradually continue over the course of 2 to 3 months. Secondary goals in this case include improving D.D.'s stress resilience, decreasing her work- and marriage-related disability, and improving her quality of life. Other general treatment goals in PTSD include decreasing detrimental behaviors (use of alcohol or substances, risky activities, violence) and treating comorbid psychiatric conditions.

Several different rating scales have been developed to assess response to treatments in PTSD.[54] The most commonly used clinician-rated scales are the Clinician Administered PTSD Scale and the Treatment Outcome PTSD Scale. The Clinician Administered PTSD Scale is most often used in clinical PTSD trials. The Sheehan Disability Scale is often used to assess functional impairment attributable to PTSD.

Course and Duration of Treatment

Good treatment response in PTSD is more likely to occur when treatment is started within 3 months of the trauma.[143,150] There is no well-established definition of response in PTSD, but a decrease in symptoms by 30% to 50%, along with substantial functional improvement, is commonly used in clinical trials. Full recovery during treatment of PTSD is fairly uncommon, and partial responders to either medication or psychosocial therapies may benefit from adding another treatment modality. When an initial SSRI trial is ineffective, the patient may be switched to another SSRI or another antidepressant shown to be effective in PTSD.[20] Partial responders may benefit from the addition of a second medication, depending on which core symptoms predominate (see Treatment of Post-traumatic Stress Disorder section).

For patients who respond, treatment should be continued for an additional 6 to 12 months for acute cases (when symptoms were present <3 months before treatment) and 12 to 24 months for chronic cases (when symptoms lasted >3 months before treatment).[143] Long-term SSRI treatment can prevent relapse of PTSD, especially in those who show good response during the first 3 months of therapy.[172] When pharmacotherapy is discontinued, it should be withdrawn gradually over the course of 1 to 3 months.

OBSESSIVE–COMPULSIVE DISORDER

Diagnostic Criteria

OCD is characterized by repetitive thoughts (obsessions) that cannot be ignored or suppressed voluntarily and/or repetitive behaviors (compulsions). The compulsions are designed to reduce anxiety associated with obsessions or to prevent some future event or situation; however, they are not actually connected to the obsessions in any realistic way or are excessive. Obsessions and compulsions result in marked distress, are time-consuming (greater than 1 hour/day), or significantly impair functional ability.[1] Both obsessions and compulsions are unpleasant and disturbing to the sufferer and are not associated with pleasure or gratification. This feature distinguishes OCD from certain other behaviors (e.g., excessive gambling or shopping) often described as "compulsive."

OCD is a clinically heterogeneous disorder involving a broad range of symptoms with four primary OCD symptom dimensions: symmetry obsessions and repeating, counting, and ordering compulsions; contamination obsessions and cleaning compulsions; hoarding obsessions and compulsions; aggressive, sexual, and religious and related compulsions. Although specific symptoms in an individual may change with time, they usually remain within the same dimension.[177]

Epidemiology and Clinical Course

OCD is one of the least common mood–anxiety disorders with a lifetime risk and 12-mo prevalence between 2% and 3%.[14] Although onset of illness ranges from very early childhood to adulthood, the mean onset of illness is 20 years, which is later than most anxiety disorders. Men tend to have an earlier onset of illness (childhood) than women (adulthood). Approximately one-fourth of patients experience symptoms by age 14, and onset after 30 years of age is rare.[1] Childhood onset OCD may be a distinct illness subtype.[177] There is usually a gradual onset of symptoms, although abrupt onset may occur during stressful periods and pregnancy.[1,178]

The course and severity of OCD are highly variable and unpredictable. The majority of patients with OCD will have a chronic course that waxes and wanes rather than an intermittent or episodic course. Less than 10% of patients will have a deteriorating course.[179] A 40-year naturalistic study found that although 83% of patients were improved at the end of the follow-up period, only 20% experienced full remission.[179]

OCD can have seriously detrimental effects on function such as abilities to socialize, study, work, make friends, and maintain good relationships with family and friends given the time spent obsessing and performing compulsions as well as avoiding situational triggers.[1,180] It is estimated that each person with OCD loses an average of 3 years' wages during his or her lifetime.[180] Quality-of-life ratings in OCD patients indicate marked impairments and are similar to those observed in patients with depression.

Although several effective treatments are currently available for OCD, there is an average delay of 7.5 years between onset and seeking medical evaluation for OCD.[180] This may be because most OCD patients realize their symptoms are senseless, so they attempt to hide their disorder because of embarrassment. People with OCD often carry out their rituals privately and may be very successful at concealing their symptoms from others. Initial treatment for OCD is commonly sought outside psychiatric settings, and the obsessive–compulsive symptoms are often missed. Clinicians across the health-care system can incorporate four simple OCD screening questions into their practice to improve detection: Do you have to wash your hands over and over? Do you have to check things repeatedly? Do you have recurrent distressing thoughts you cannot get rid of? Do you have to complete actions again and again or in a certain way?[181]

Psychiatric Comorbidity and Obsessive–Compulsive Spectrum Disorders

Identification of comorbid conditions with OCD is important because it can influence treatment decisions. As with other anxiety disorders, OCD is often accompanied by psychiatric comorbidity in 60% to 90% of patients with affective (e.g., depression, bipolar disorder), anxiety, and tic disorders being common.[1,20,25,179] Tics occur in 20% to 30% of OCD patients. These individuals believed to represent a distinct subtype of illness where patients are more likely to be male, have an earlier onset (before age 10 years), experience more severe symptoms, and have a poorer response to SSRIs than those with OCD alone.[182] Distinguishing from obsessive–compulsive personality disorder (OCPD), a personality pattern characterized by rigid and inflexible preoccupation with rules, lists, order, and perfectionism, can be difficult, and the two disorders co-occur in a small percentage of patients. OCPD, however, does not involve distressing obsessions and compulsions.

OCD is no longer classified as an anxiety disorder in the *DSM-5* but rather an illness within a new obsessive–compulsive and related disorders.[1] Other related disorders included are body dysmorphic disorder (preoccupation with an imagined or slight defect in appearance), trichotillomania (recurrent impulses to pull out one's hair), excoriation disorder (skin-picking), and hoarding disorder. Like OCD, many patients with these conditions have shown good response to treatment with serotonergic antidepressants such as clomipramine and SSRIs.[183]

Etiology and Pathophysiology

Since OCD displays such clinical heterogeneity, there may be several distinct etiologies for different subtypes of illness. Structural and functional brain imaging suggests that OCD is a neurologic disorder characterized by a hyperfunctioning circuit involving the frontal lobe and basal ganglia regions termed the frontostriatal circuit.[177] Abnormalities therein imply potential dysfunction in glutamatergic, dopaminergic, and serotonergic neurotransmission. In support of this hypothesis, these abnormalities normalize after successful treatment of OCD with SSRI monotherapy and antipsychotic augmentation. Preliminary evidence with glutamatergic agents suggests a role in treatment. Furthermore, neuromodulation therapies (e.g., deep brain stimulation, cycloserine-enhanced CBT) and neurosurgical techniques interrupting this circuit are often effective in the treatment of OCD. Aberrant activity in this system may lead to impaired executive function, decision-making, and memory as these cognitive domains are mediated by this system.

Besides biologic factors, twin and family studies support genetic influences, particularly in early-onset OCD cases.[17,184] Genetic studies have found associations between OCD and specific polymorphisms in the glutamatergic (high-affinity neuronal/epithelial excitatory amino acid transporters), dopaminergic (catechol-*O*-methyltransferase and dopamine D_4-receptor genes), and serotonergic (5-HT type 1Dβ and 5-HT type 2A receptor genes) pathways.[185–187] The heritability of OCD is estimated at 40% with the remaining variation purportedly mediated by environmental factors (e.g., perinatal events, trauma, stress, neuroinflammation).[177] An example of this is the autoimmune disease, called PANDAS (pediatric autoimmune neuropsychiatric disorders associated with streptococcal infection). Reports describe children who developed sudden and severe tics and obsessive–compulsive symptoms after strep throat infections.[188] These children may be better treated with other medications and modalities (e.g., antibiotics, corticosteroids, surgery). The possibility of a PANDAS correlation should be considered in any child who develops abrupt onset of obsessive–compulsive symptoms and has a history of pharyngitis within the past 6 months.

Treatment of Obsessive–Compulsive Disorder

Both medications and behavioral therapies are effective in the treatment of OCD. Behavioral therapy is vitally important for OCD, and the combination of drugs plus behavioral therapy provides optimal treatment. All medications consistently effective as monotherapy are potent inhibitors of serotonin reuptake. These include the SSRIs, clomipramine, and the SNRI venlafaxine.

SELECTIVE SEROTONIN REUPTAKE INHIBITORS AND SEROTONIN AND NOREPINEPHRINE REUPTAKE INHIBITORS

SSRIs are the only first-line medication treatments for OCD of which fluvoxamine, fluoxetine, paroxetine, and sertraline are FDA-approved based on double-blind, placebo-controlled studies.[189] Citalopram and escitalopram also are effective but with less evidence to support their use, particularly with the former. No single SSRI is considered to be more effective than the others in treating OCD, but some patients may respond to or tolerate one agent better than another.[189] Usual SSRI starting dosages can be used in OCD, but at least 4 weeks should be allowed before exceeding the targeted minimally effective dosages (fluvoxamine 200 mg/day, fluoxetine 40 mg/day, paroxetine 40 mg/day, and sertraline 100 mg/day).[189] SSRIs are generally considered to have a dose–response relationship such that higher SSRI doses may be required to effectively treat OCD.[25] Additionally, several controlled studies support the efficacy of venlafaxine in the treatment of OCD.[190] Although other SNRIs (duloxetine, desvenlafaxine, milnacipran, or levomilnacipran) may ultimately show efficacy in the treatment of OCD, no well-controlled studies have been conducted evaluating these medications in OCD.[191]

CLOMIPRAMINE

Clomipramine was the first drug FDA-approved for OCD treatment and was considered the standard treatment for several years until the SSRIs gained popularity. Many large well-controlled studies have documented that clomipramine is superior to placebo and significantly improves OCD symptoms in approximately 60% to 70% of patients.[179,190] Clomipramine is the only TCA recommended for OCD treatment as others have not proven efficacious[20,25,113,179,192] although there is some evidence to the contrary.[193] This is attributed to its more potent effects on 5-HT reuptake inhibition compared with other TCAs. Clomipramine is often referred to as a SRI (serotonin reuptake inhibitor), not a SSRI (*selective* serotonin reuptake inhibitor), because its major active metabolite, desmethylclomipramine, is a potent inhibitor of NE reuptake. Clomipramine also blocks adrenergic, histaminergic, and cholinergic receptors resulting in an adverse effect profile similar to other TCAs (see Chapter 86, Depression).

Although direct comparison studies have shown clomipramine to be similar in efficacy to various SSRIs in treating OCD, several meta-analyses have concluded clomipramine is superior to SSRIs overall.[190,194] Nonetheless, clomipramine is currently reserved as a second-line treatment option for patients who do not respond adequately to SSRI/venlafaxine therapy given its poorer tolerability (e.g., sedation, orthostatic hypotension, and anticholinergic side effects).[190] Details about the clinical use of clomipramine are discussed in Case 83-11, Question 1.

AUGMENTATION STRATEGIES

Other than venlafaxine, no other miscellaneous agents studied in OCD have demonstrated impressive efficacy as monotherapy. However, several agents appear to be useful as augmentation therapy to boost response to SSRIs or clomipramine in partial responders.[195] The combination of an SSRI plus clomipramine is one such option for patients who show partial response, although attention must be paid to potential drug interactions, which may lead to clomipramine toxicity (see Case 83-11, Questions 2 and 3).

Antipsychotic agents are the most studied pharmacologic augmentation strategy in OCD and may improve response in 30% of patients.[196] They may be particularly effective in four scenarios: treatment-refractory OCD, OCD with poor insight (often treatment refractory), comorbid tic disorders, and comorbid schizophrenia.[197] Several meta-analyses have been conducted on antipsychotic effectiveness.[196,198–200] Risperidone (0.5–4 mg/day) is generally considered to have the highest evidence base for antidepressant augmentation in OCD. Other reasonable agents include aripiprazole and haloperidol (of which haloperidol is less tolerated compared to second-generation antipsychotics). Conversely, quetiapine (up to 600 mg/day) and olanzapine (2.5–20 mg/day) use is controversial based on inconsistent evidence supporting their use in well-designed trials. Preliminary evidence suggests paliperidone may not be more effective than placebo, and ziprasidone may be less effective than quetiapine.[201,202] Recent evidence suggests antipsychotics are less effective than augmenting with CBT with exposure–response prevention (ERP) and, thus, may not be a preferred augmentation strategy.[203,204] Additionally, the use of antipsychotics must be weighed against tolerability and safety concerns such as metabolic dysfunction and extrapyramidal symptoms.

Anticonvulsants (e.g., topiramate, lamotrigine, pregabalin, gabapentin) may also be considered as augmentation agents although the evidence is limited to lower quality studies.[20,205] As such, this strategy should be one of last resort unless otherwise clinically indicated.

MISCELLANEOUS AGENTS

Benzodiazepines, although typically useful in other anxiety disorders, are generally not beneficial in treating OCD. There are several reports of clonazepam being effective as adjunctive therapy or monotherapy which may be explained by its serotonergic properties; however, double-blind placebo-controlled trials have been negative.[206] As such, clonazepam is not recommended by treatment guidelines.[179]

The MAOI phenelzine was one of the first medications studied for OCD. Early case reports of its use were favorable, but more recent findings suggest phenelzine is largely ineffective for OCD.[179]

NONPHARMACOLOGIC TREATMENTS

Cognitive Behavioral Therapies

CBT is an extremely important component of OCD treatment and should be incorporated into the treatment plan whenever possible. The combination of psychotherapy and medication is generally superior to pharmacotherapy alone but not to CBT alone.[20,179] CBT alone may be appropriate for mild OCD or in cases in which it is desirable to avoid medication (e.g., pregnancy, medical conditions). Treatment gains achieved with CBT often are maintained long after its discontinuation, which is an advantage versus pharmacotherapy, likely improving relapse prevention.[181]

The cognitive therapy component of CBT is aimed toward changing the detrimental thought patterns in OCD and is most helpful for obsessions such as scrupulosity, moral guilt, and pathologic doubt. The behavioral therapy aspect, ERP, involves exposure to feared objects or situations followed by prevention of the usual compulsive response. This type of therapy is most beneficial for patients with contamination fears, hoarding, and rituals involving symmetry, counting, or repeating. Because ERP is anxiety provoking and can be very distressing, patients may refuse to participate.[207]

Neurosurgery

Neurosurgical treatment of OCD has been practiced since the 1950s and is considered an option of last resort in treatment-refractory patients. Anterior cingulotomy and anterior capsulotomy are the most commonly used surgical procedures. Indications for neurosurgery include severe disability from symptoms and failed treatments (drugs and behavioral therapies) that have been tried systematically for at least 5 years.[208] Neurosurgery success rates range from 35% to 70%, complications (including potential infections, personality changes, cognitive impairment, and epilepsy) appear to be rare, and limited long-term follow-up studies indicate the benefit is maintained with mild-to-moderate impairments in neuropsychological performance.[208,209] Deep brain stimulation involving bilateral electrode implantation into the subthalamic nucleus and nucleus accumbens is gaining popularity for treatment-refractory OCD. Although this procedure is still experimental, overall preliminary results are positive.[210]

Defining Response to Therapy

Response to medication treatment in OCD is gradual and often delayed. Initial improvements usually begin to appear within the first month. Patients with unsatisfactory response by weeks 4 to 9 should have their SSRI dosages gradually increased to the manufacturer's recommended maximum. A trial of 8 to 12 weeks at maximal tolerated medication dosages is recommended before assessing therapeutic benefit and maximal response may take as long as 5 to 6 months..

Since complete elimination of symptoms is rare with current treatments, the primary goal of OCD treatment is to minimize functional impact of symptoms.[211] Most clinical trials in OCD define clinical response as a 25% to 35% reduction in Yale–Brown

Obsessive–Compulsive Symptom Checklist (Y-BOCS) scores. Therefore, even those classified as responders may be left with 65% to 75% of their original symptoms, and this may or may not result in significant improvements in functioning or quality of life. The Y-BOCS is an objective tool in the initial evaluation of those who present with symptoms of OCD. It is a 10-item scale with a maximal possible score of 40; a score of more than 15 is generally considered to represent clinically significant obsessive–compulsive symptoms.[212] This scale is a standard tool for evaluating drug efficacy in OCD clinical trials and is often used in clinical practice to assess response to treatments with a version designed for administration with children.

STRATEGIES FOR MANAGING NONRESPONSE AND PARTIAL RESPONSE

Approximately 40% to 60% of patients show clinically meaningful improvements during an initial (SSRI or clomipramine) medication trial, but only a small percentage exhibit marked response.[190] Predictors of poor response include poor insight; hoarding, sexual, religious, and symmetry dimension symptoms; prepubertal onset of illness; and presence of comorbid personality, mood, or eating disorders.[20] For nonresponsive patients, it is usually recommended to pursue a second SSRI trial, as approximately 20% of initial nonresponders will respond with a subsequent trial. Given this and tolerability concerns, clomipramine is typically reserved as a third-line treatment option, although its use second line would be reasonable given its efficacy in SSRI nonresponders.[181,190] Patients with partial response to an initial SSRI trial may be better served by adding an augmentation agent to preserve therapy benefits rather than switching to a new medication and risk losing any improvement already gained. Additionally, using SSRI doses beyond those FDA-approved may be beneficial for poor responders if tolerability is acceptable.[213–215]

Clinical Presentation and Assessment

CASE 83-10

QUESTION 1: R.G. is a 25-year-old woman whose husband complains she spends 1.5 hours a day cleaning the stove and takes four showers each day. The unusual behavior began about 1 year ago after the birth of their son but has continued to worsen, and R.G.'s husband states that he cannot deal with her "odd habits" any longer. R.G. recently lost her job as a secretary because of tardiness (it took her 3 hours to get ready for work) and spending too much time away from her desk in the ladies' room. R.G. admits that it is silly, but she has irresistible urges to make sure both she and her surroundings are completely free of germs so her child will not get sick. She also confines herself to one floor of their three-level house because she is afraid she will fall down the stairs while carrying her son. R.G. also states that she constantly has "what if" thoughts about horrible things happening to her family, which are very disturbing. The physician's diagnosis is OCD. What clinical features of OCD does R.G. display, and how can her symptoms be objectively evaluated?

R.G. displays many characteristic symptoms of OCD. The most commonly encountered clinical presentation of OCD involves excessive fear of contamination with dirt, germs, or toxins and repeated washing of hands or cleaning objects or surroundings. These persons also typically avoid touching possibly dirty objects (e.g., doorknobs, money) or shaking hands with people. Another common clinical presentation of OCD is the patient with pathologic doubt who constantly worries something bad will happen because of his or her negligence. Individuals can be afraid they have failed to lock the door, turn off the stove, shut the refrigerator door, or secure the medicine cabinet from children. As a result, they continuously check and recheck their actions.

R.G. displays obsessions of contamination and pathologic doubt, and compulsions of excessive cleaning and washing. These symptoms are time-consuming, cause significant distress, and have led to her unemployment and marital difficulties. As seen in this case, most persons present with a mixture of various obsessions and compulsions. R.G. also realizes her thoughts and behaviors are "silly," which most often is the case in OCD. This case also illustrates the onset of OCD during times of stressful or significant life events. Pregnancy, death of a relative, and marital discord have been identified as precipitating factors in the onset of OCD.[178,211,216]

Selective Serotonin Reuptake Inhibitor Treatment of Obsessive–Compulsive Disorder

CASE 83-10, QUESTION 2: On assessment, R.G.'s Y-BOCS score is found to be 33. Her physician prescribes fluvoxamine and instructs R.G. to take 100 mg every morning for 1 week and then 200 mg every morning thereafter. He also refers R.G. to a psychologist to receive CBT. Is this initial choice of therapy appropriate?

SELECTIVE SEROTONIN REUPTAKE INHIBITORS

Selection and Dosing

SSRIs such as fluvoxamine are considered the best choice of initial pharmacotherapy for OCD. The primary differences between SSRIs involve pharmacokinetic properties and potential for drug interactions (see Chapter 86, Depression). Because there are no overall differences in SSRI efficacy, fluvoxamine is a suitable selection for R.G. However, the prescribed dosing instructions for R.G. are not appropriate. The initial recommended dosage for fluvoxamine in adults is 50 mg/day (25 mg in children), and it is best taken in the evening because it tends to be sedating. Using higher-than-necessary dosages can increase both adverse effects and medication costs, and these factors can lead to early termination of therapy. The dosage can be increased by 50-mg increments every 3 to 4 days according to patient tolerability, up to the initial targeted dose of 200 mg/day and a maximum of 300 mg/day.[189] Daily doses exceeding 100 mg should be given in two divided doses if once-daily dosing is not well tolerated.

ADJUNCTIVE COGNITIVE BEHAVIORAL THERAPY

R.G.'s Y-BOCS score of 33 indicates a moderate-to-severe symptom severity, which supports using a combined treatment approach. The overall efficacy of these nonpharmacologic treatments is estimated to be 50% to 70% when used alone, and their use to complement pharmacotherapy is considered vital.[181] For R.G., ERP therapy might involve covering her hands with dirt and not allowing her to wash them for a certain time period. These behavioral techniques cause extreme anxiety and discomfort, which often lead to dropout from therapy or noncompliance with "homework assignments" (which involve continuation of the therapy principles outside the clinical setting), but are highly effective if the patient can adhere to treatment.

SELECTIVE SEROTONIN REUPTAKE INHIBITOR ADVERSE EFFECTS AND PATIENT COUNSELING

CASE 83-10, QUESTION 3: What patient counseling information should be provided to R.G. in conjunction with the prescribed treatments?

All OCD patients beginning treatment should be counseled that medication response occurs gradually and several weeks may elapse before beneficial effects become noticeable. It is important to emphasize that maximal response may take 3 months or longer and complete elimination of all symptoms is unlikely. Inform patients that a variety of other medications exist for those who do not respond adequately to an initial trial.

R.G. should be educated about possible fluvoxamine side effects, including nausea, sedation or insomnia, and headache. Medication should be taken with food to decrease these effects. Side effects are most common during the initial weeks of therapy, are usually dose-related, and often subside with continued treatment. Other aspects of SSRI therapy, including additional adverse effects and their management and drug–drug interactions, are discussed in Chapter 86, Depression. Patients should be encouraged to report any problems to their treatment provider. The importance of adhering to prescribed therapies, both pharmacologic and behavioral, should also be stressed.

CASE 83-10, QUESTION 4: After 4 weeks, R.G. is taking fluvoxamine 200 mg daily and tolerating the medication well. She complains she has not noticed much improvement, and her Y-BOCS score is slightly decreased at 30. R.G. has been to the cognitive behavioral therapist twice but is reluctant to return because the therapy was so stressful. R.G. requests to be switched to a more effective medication, and she also asks to be given some alprazolam to help calm her anxiety during behavioral therapy sessions. What is the best course of action for R.G. at this point?

Switching to another medication is not recommended at this point because not enough time has elapsed to assess fluvoxamine's efficacy. R.G. is tolerating fluvoxamine well and has shown a mild improvement, so this medication should be continued for at least another 4 weeks. Additional counseling information should be provided to R.G. to emphasize this fact. An increase in fluvoxamine dosage, up to 250 or 300 mg/day, may be considered after several more weeks because some patients may respond better to higher dosages. If R.G.'s symptoms continue to cause significant functional impairment after 10 to 12 weeks of higher-dose fluvoxamine therapy, a change in treatment (e.g., switching to another SSRI or augmentation therapy) will be indicated.

R.G. should be encouraged to continue CBT to optimize the chance for successful treatment. An anxiety response is integral to the therapeutic benefits of behavioral therapies; because benzodiazepines can blunt this response, they may reduce their efficacy. Therefore, alprazolam should be avoided, and a temporary reduction in the intensity of behavioral therapy may be indicated instead. Fluvoxamine can also inhibit the CYP3A4-mediated metabolism of alprazolam, resulting in more pronounced effects from a given dose.

Course and Duration of Therapy

CASE 83-10, QUESTION 5: After 5 months of treatment, R.G. is happy to report her OCD is much improved (Y-BOCS score of 11). She still has intermittent obsessions related to contamination and doubting, but they are less intense than before. She is usually able to resist urges to clean and wash excessively and is using the stairs in their home with only mild discomfort. Her previous employer has agreed to let her return to her secretarial position when she is ready, and she plans to do so soon. R.G.'s husband is extremely pleased with her progress. Their primary question at this visit is whether treatment can be discontinued now because R.G. is doing so well. What recommendations should be provided regarding the long-term course of therapy for R.G.?

This case illustrates a common outcome of OCD treatment, in which some symptoms persist (as evidenced by a Y-BOCS score of 11), but significant improvements in functioning occur. It is currently recommended that effective treatment for OCD be continued for at least 1 year after response to reduce the risk of relapse.[212,217] Therefore, continued drug treatment for at least 7 more months is indicated. Results from several studies suggest decreased medication doses (with SSRIs and clomipramine) during maintenance therapy are comparably as effective as full doses in preventing relapse.[212] If R.G. was experiencing any fluvoxamine-related problems, a decrease to the minimally effective dose (150 mg/day) during maintenance therapy might be recommended.

After a 1-year maintenance period, discontinuation of medication may be considered by carefully weighing the possible risks and benefits. When medication therapy for OCD is withdrawn, the dosage should be gradually decreased by approximately 25% every 1 to 2 months. Continuous monitoring for signs of relapse is required during this period. Gradual discontinuation also lessens the chance of the withdrawal syndrome often occurring after abrupt discontinuation of SSRI or TCA therapy (see Chapter 86, Depression). Long-term or even lifelong maintenance pharmacotherapy is usually recommended after two to four severe relapses or three to four less severe relapses.

Clomipramine Treatment

DOSING GUIDELINES

CASE 83-11

QUESTION 1: K.T. is an 18-year-old Asian man who was diagnosed with OCD 2 years ago and also suffers from moderate depression. His physician plans to start him on clomipramine therapy because he has failed previous trials with paroxetine and fluvoxamine. Is clomipramine an appropriate choice of therapy for this patient? What recommendations can be made regarding initiation of clomipramine treatment?

Current guidelines recommend clomipramine be reserved for OCD patients who fail at least two SSRI trials; therefore, its choice for this patient is appropriate.[179] One precaution relevant to this case is that clomipramine, like other TCAs, is highly dangerous in overdose situations. Because K.T. is depressed, he should be evaluated carefully for any suicidal thoughts before starting clomipramine. If suicidal ideation is detected, it would be preferable to try another SSRI. This case also illustrates the common comorbidity of depression with OCD. Fortunately, most effective treatments for OCD are antidepressants, and drug treatment can be beneficial for both conditions. Nevertheless, the responses of depression and OCD to treatment are independent of one another, so depression may respond completely to a certain medication while OCD symptoms persist.[212]

Clomipramine should be initiated at a low dosage of 25 to 50 mg/day administered with meals. Divided daily doses are sometimes used initially to minimize side effects, but the total daily dose can be given at bedtime after dose titration given its average elimination half-life of 24 hours.[189,218]

The clomipramine dosage should be increased to an initial target range of 150 to 200 mg/day during 2 to 4 weeks, guided by patient tolerability. The maximal recommended daily dosage of clomipramine is 250 mg/day because of the sharply increased risk of seizures (2.1%–3.4%) with higher dosages as compared with the risk with dosages less than 250 mg/day (0.24%–0.48%).[219] Longer duration of clomipramine therapy may also increase the risk of seizures. As such, use with caution in persons with a history of seizures, head injury, or other factors might lower the seizure threshold.

Side Effects and Monitoring Guidelines

CASE 83-11, QUESTION 2: What guidelines should be recommended for monitoring the outcomes (both therapeutic and adverse) of clomipramine therapy?

Clomipramine is less well tolerated than the SSRIs and can cause a number of significant adverse effects, especially during the first few weeks of therapy. The most common side effects, reported in more than half of those taking clomipramine, include sedation, dry mouth, dizziness, and tremor.[219] Constipation, nausea, blurred vision, insomnia, and headache also occur frequently. K.T. should be advised these usually subside with continued treatment.

Many patients receiving long-term clomipramine (and other TCA) therapy gain substantial amounts of weight. As with the SSRIs, sexual dysfunction can be a problem in both men and women. In men, clomipramine can cause ejaculation abnormalities, which can impair fertility. Patients taking clomipramine should also be counseled about the additive CNS depressant effects with alcohol and to be cautious about the possible sedative effects while driving or performing other potentially hazardous activities.

As with other TCAs, an ECG should be performed before starting clomipramine in individuals at risk for heart disease and in pediatric patients. Elevations in liver enzymes have been observed frequently during the first 3 months of clomipramine treatment, and baseline liver function tests should also be obtained before initiating treatment. The liver enzyme changes are reversible on discontinuation of clomipramine therapy.

No therapeutic range for plasma drug concentrations has been firmly established for clomipramine in OCD, but monitoring plasma levels may be clinically useful in certain patients to guide dosing and minimize drug toxicity. Clomipramine metabolism exhibits interpatient variability, and it is difficult to accurately predict the resulting clomipramine level from any given dose. The initial hepatic metabolism of tertiary TCAs such as clomipramine involves demethylation through various isozymes, including CYP1A2, CYP2C19, and CYP3A4.[218,220] Both the parent drug (clomipramine) and the primary active metabolite (*N*-desmethylclomipramine) then undergo CYP2D6-mediated hydroxylation. Therefore, the metabolism of clomipramine will be affected by combination with any agent inhibiting CYP1A2, CYP2C19, CYP3A4, or CYP2D6. Clinically significant drug interactions are possible with several of the SSRIs, including fluoxetine, paroxetine, fluvoxamine, and sertraline (see Chapter 86, Depression).

Although various studies have failed to find a correlation between clomipramine plasma level and clinical response, the ratio of clomipramine to *N*-desmethylclomipramine may be important.[221] Clomipramine is primarily serotonergic, whereas *N*-desmethylclomipramine is more noradrenergic; higher levels of *N*-desmethylclomipramine relative to clomipramine have been associated with poorer clinical response. Factors impairing the CYP2D6-mediated elimination of *N*-desmethylclomipramine (e.g., concurrent medications that are potent CYP2D6 inhibitors and CYP2D6 poor metabolizers) may possibly decrease the efficacy of clomipramine by shifting the metabolic ratio in an undesired direction.

Asian patients such as K.T. have been found to have significantly decreased clearance of clomipramine and higher clomipramine to *N*-desmethylclomipramine ratios compared with whites, which may necessitate use of lower doses.[222] This is probably caused by a genetic polymorphism of either CYP2C19 or CYP2D6, which results in decreased metabolic capacity via these metabolic pathways in the Asian population. Careful monitoring for possible signs of toxicity should accompany dose increases, and the clomipramine plasma level should be checked in those patients (Asian or otherwise) who show unexpected effects with usual doses. An opposite effect has been described in ultra-rapid CYP2D6 metabolizers, in which unusually high clomipramine dosages may be required for therapeutic efficacy.

Augmentation

CASE 83-11, QUESTION 3: After 10 weeks of taking clomipramine 100 mg at bedtime, K.T. has shown partial response. He continues to experience mild-to-moderate anticholinergic side effects and frequent daytime fatigue. His plasma clomipramine level is relatively high for the given dose at 453 ng/mL (clomipramine plus desmethylclomipramine; range 150–450 ng/mL).[223] The physician decides to add another drug to augment treatment. Considering K.T.'s current medication regimen and the evidence supporting the different augmentation strategies, which drug would be the best choice for K.T.?

When adding an SSRI to a TCA, the potential for drug interactions should always be considered. Clomipramine is metabolized by CYP1A2, CYP3A4, CYP2C19, and CYP2D6.[218,220,224,225] The CYP2D6 pathway is particularly important because it is the rate-limiting metabolic pathway for elimination of both clomipramine and desmethylclomipramine. Fluvoxamine, paroxetine, and fluoxetine are all strong inhibitors of clomipramine metabolism, whereas sertraline is a weak–moderate inhibitor. Alternatively, escitalopram and citalopram would not be likely to cause a significant drug interaction, but evidence for escitalopram as an augmenting agent in combination with clomipramine is lacking.[226] A combination less likely to be associated with a drug interaction is the combination of clomipramine and a second-generation antipsychotic; however, most trials combined antipsychotics with SSRIs rather than clomipramine. Nonetheless, antipsychotic augmentation with agents demonstrating more consistent efficacy in well-designed trials (e.g., risperidone and aripiprazole) is a reasonable strategy in patients requiring more improvement as previously discussed. Haloperidol would not be the optimal choice in K.T. because it inhibits clomipramine metabolism, and as a first-generation antipsychotic, it is associated with numerous side effects. Unfortunately, most of the well-designed studies are often small (15–45 patients).

KEY REFERENCES AND WEBSITES

A full list of references for this chapter can be found at http://thepoint.lww.com/AT11e. Below are the key references and websites for this chapter, with the corresponding reference number in this chapter found in parentheses after the reference.

Key References

ACOG Committee on Practice Bulletins—Obstetrics. ACOG Practice Bulletin: Clinical management guidelines for obstetrician-gynecologists number 92, April 2008 (replaces practice bulletin number 87, November 2007). Use of psychiatric medications during pregnancy and lactation. *Obstet Gynecol*. 2008;111:1001. (80)

American Psychiatric Association. *Diagnostic and Statistical Manual of Mental Disorders*. 5th ed. Washington, DC: American Psychiatric Association; 2013. (1)

American Psychiatric Association. *Practice Guideline for the Treatment of Patients with Obsessive-Compulsive Disorder*. Arlington, VA: American Psychiatric Association; 2007. (179)

Baldwin DS et al. Evidence-based pharmacological treatment of anxiety disorders, post-traumatic stress disorder and obsessive-compulsive disorder: a revision of the 2005 guidelines from the British Association for Psychopharmacology. *J Psychopharmacology.* 2014;1. (25)

Bellantuono C et al. Benzodiazepine exposure in pregnancy and risk of major malformations: a critical overview. *Gen Hosp Psychiatry.* 2013;35(1):3. (81)

Davidson JR et al. A psychopharmacological treatment algorithm for generalised anxiety disorder (GAD). *J Psychopharmacol.* 2010;24:3. (72)

Katzman MA et al. Canadian clinical practice guidelines for the management of anxiety, posttraumatic stress and obsessive-compulsive disorders. *BMC Psychiatry.* 2014;14(Suppl 1):S1. (20)

Kessler RC et al. Twelve-month and lifetime prevalence and lifetime morbid risk of anxiety and mood disorders in the US. Int J Methods Psychiatr Res 2012;21:169. (14)Muller JE et al. Anxiety and medical disorders. *Curr Psychiatry Rep.* 2005;7:245. (117)

National Institute for Health and Care Excellence (NICE). Generalised anxiety disorder and panic disorder (with or without agoraphobia) in adults: management in primary, secondary and community care. NICE clinical guideline 113. Available at http://www.nice.org.uk/CG113. Accessed July 6, 2015. (24)

Ravindran LN, Stein MB. The pharmacologic treatment of anxiety disorders: a review of progress. *J Clin Psychiatry.* 2010;71:839. (43)

Stein DJ et al. A 2010 evidence-based algorithm for the pharmacotherapy of social anxiety disorder. *Curr Psychiatry Rep.* 2010;12:471. (134)

Key Websites

National Institute for Health and Care Excellence (NICE). Generalised anxiety disorder and panic disorder (with or without agoraphobia) in adults: management in primary, secondary and community care. NICE clinical guideline 113. Available at http://www.nice.org.uk/CG113. Accessed July 6, 2015. (24)

National Institute for Health and Care Excellence (NICE). Obsessive-compulsive disorder: core interventions in the treatment of obsessive-compulsive disorder and body dysmorphic disorder. NICE clinical guideline 31. Available at http://www.nice.org.uk/cg31. Accessed August 11, 2015. (192)

National Institute for Health and Care Excellence. Antenatal and postnatal mental health: clinical management and service guidance. December 2014. http://www.nice.org.uk/guidance/cg192. (84)

Work Group on Panic Disorder et al. *Treatment of Patients with Panic Disorder.* 2nd ed. Available at http://psychiatryonline.org/pb/assets/raw/sitewide/practice_guidelines/guidelines/panicdisorder.pdf. Accessed August 12, 2015. (112)

84 Sleep Disorders

Devon A. Sherwood and Anna K. Morin

CORE PRINCIPLES

		CHAPTER CASES
INSOMNIA AND RESULTING DAYTIME SLEEPINESS		
1	Asking the right questions to investigate the type of insomnia (i.e., trouble falling asleep, staying asleep, or early morning awakening), possible causes (lifestyle issues, drugs), resulting impairment, and concomitant conditions are essential to determine proper management.	**Case 84-1 (Questions 1, 2) Table 84-1, 84-4, Figure 84-2**
2	Nonpharmacologic treatments such cognitive-behavioral interventions are recommended first-line therapy for managing insomnia in a variety of patients owing to high efficacy and avoidance of medication side effects.	**Case 84-1 (Questions 3, 4) Table 84-2**
3	Pharmacologic treatments for insomnia are selected based on their efficacy, tolerability, onset and duration of effect, potential for next-day hangover, and abuse potential.	**Case 84-1 (Questions 5–10) Table 84-3**
4	Insomnia concurrent with medical illness is frequently chronic (>1 month) and, if left untreated, may affect recovery from the medical condition. Treating both conditions at the same time is recommended.	**Case 84-2 (Questions 1–4) Table 84-5, Figure 84-2**
5	Insomnia concurrent with psychiatric illness requires optimization of psychiatric maintenance medications and the judicious use of hypnotic medications based on type of sleep complaint and substance abuse history.	**Case 84-3 (Questions 1–4) Figure 84-2**
6	Managing insomnia in an elderly individual involves consideration of age-related pharmacodynamic and pharmacokinetic changes and counseling regarding realistic treatment expectations. Medication doses lower than those used in younger individuals should be prescribed.	**Case 84-4 (Questions 1–5) Table 84-3**
7	If nonpharmacologic treatment is ineffective, diphenhydramine is considered safe for short-term use (<1 week) in pregnancy. Risks outweigh benefits for benzodiazepines and nonbenzodiazepine receptor agonists in pregnancy.	**Case 84-5 (Question 1)**
SLEEP APNEA		
1	Sleep apnea leads to excessive daytime sleepiness, fatigue, and increased risk of cardiovascular and cerebrovascular disease. Effective treatment with continuous positive airway pressure or surgical interventions can decrease cardiovascular disease and improve overall functioning and quality of life.	**Case 84-6 (Questions 1, 2)**
2	It is essential to avoid sedating medications in patients with sleep apnea because these agents interfere with mini-arousals that keep the patient alive.	**Case 84-6 (Question 3)**
NARCOLEPSY		
1	Narcolepsy is an incurable neurologic disease characterized by sleep attacks and cataplexy. Stimulants modafinil or armodafinil help decrease sleep attacks and promote daytime alertness but do not help with cataplexy or nocturnal insomnia.	**Case 84-7 (Questions 1, 2)**
2	Sodium oxybate is effective for cataplexy and improves nocturnal sleep, but it has high abuse potential and has been associated with psychiatric side effects.	**Case 84-7 (Questions 3, 4)**

OVERVIEW

Approximately one-third of the adult life is expended on sleep. The innate necessity of sleep is present in almost all mammals, though all the functions of sleep are not fully understood.[1,2] Naturally with human physiology devoted to sleep and the numerous factors that can disrupt this process, sleep disorders are remarkably common. Sleep deficiency, including insufficient sleep duration, irregular timing of sleep, poor sleep quality, and sleep or circadian rhythm disorders, is highly prevalent and threaten public safety.[3,4] Decades of scientific findings associate sleep deficiency with increased disease risk, including cardiovascular and metabolic disease, psychiatric illness, substance abuse, pregnancy complications, and impaired neurobehavioral and cognitive impairment.[4,5] At least 10% of the American population is reported to suffer from a sleep disorder that is clinically significant and of public health concern.[3] Major sleep disorders in the United States include insomnia ranging from 15% to 35%,[6,7] sleep apnea at 6% to 24%[8,9] periodic limb movements in sleep (PLMS, previously known as nocturnal myoclonus), and restless leg syndrome (RLS) ranging from 3% to 15%,[10,11] and narcolepsy at 0.025% to 0.05%.[12] Untreated sleep disorders, including chronic insomnia, sleep apnea, PLMS, and narcolepsy, are all associated with diminished mental and physical functioning and poor quality of life.[3,4,7]

Nightmares, nocturnal leg cramps, and snoring are more benign sleep disorders. Nightmares occur in 5% to 30% of children 3 to 6 years of age, and approximately 2% to 6% of adults have weekly nightmares.[13] Sleepwalking occurs in 1% to 2% of the population. Complex sleep behavior disorders, such as driving or eating while still half asleep, are uncommon to rare. These behaviors are more common in people taking hypnotics, and medication counseling should be provided for patients prescribed any sleep medication.[13,14]

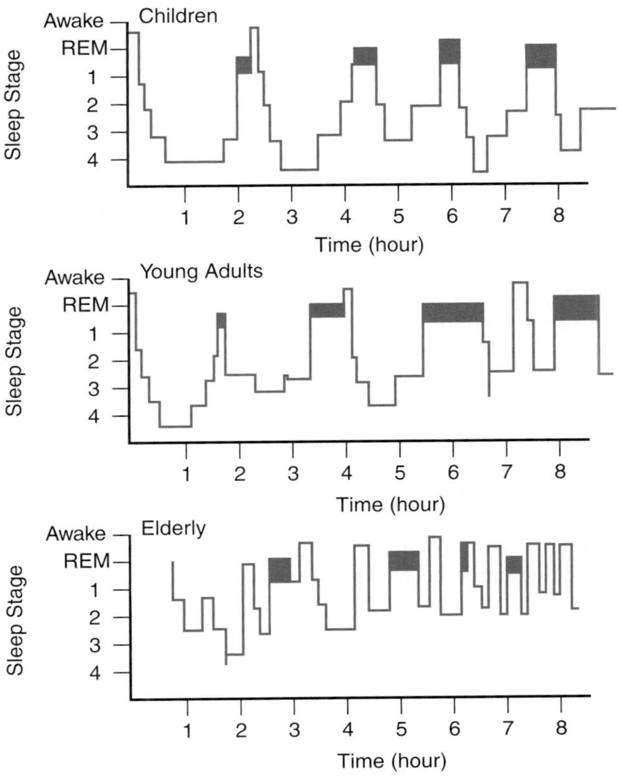

Figure 84-1 Normal sleep cycles.

CIRCADIAN RHYTHM AND SLEEP CYCLES

Sleep is a dynamic process with a cyclical recurrence and varying stages. The endogenous sleep–wake pattern of humans is based on the solar day–night cycle called the circadian rhythm. Circadian rhythm is controlled both by internal and external factors and sets the sleep–wake cycle at 24.2 hours. Sensory input (visual and acoustic) or other external factors modify the "internal clock" to a 24 hour day through working with the internal network and signaling brain centers to either wake or sleep. Thus, darkness is a visual cue that prepares the brain for sleep. Similarly, bright light serves to prepare the brain for wakefulness.[1,2]

Once sleep is initiated, it alternates between the two phases of rapid eye movement (REM) and nonrapid eye movement (NREM) sleep. These phases vary in length throughout the sleep cycles. During a normal night of sleep, a person generally has four to six cycles of sleep which last an average of 90 minutes (vary 70–120 minutes).[15] See Figure 84-1 for normal sleep cycles by age.

Polysomnography

Each sleep stage serves a physiologic function and can be monitored in sleep laboratories by polysomnography (PSG). PSG is the term used to describe three electrophysiologic measures: the electroencephalogram (EEG), the electromyogram, and the electrooculogram of each eye. It may also include an electrocardiogram, air thermistors, abdominal and thoracic strain belts, and oxygen saturation monitoring. The pattern of brain waves, muscle tone, and eye movements measured can be used to categorize the various sleep stages.[15,16]

Nonrapid Eye Movement Sleep

NREM sleep is divided into four stages, with different quantities of time and functions in each stage. Stage 1 is a transition between sleep and wakefulness known as *relaxed wakefulness*, which generally makes up approximately 2% to 5% of sleep. The function of stage 1 is to initiate sleep. Approximately 50% of total sleep time is spent in stage 2, which is rapid-wave (theta) or lighter sleep. Stage 2 provides rest for the muscles and brain through muscle atonia and low-voltage brain wave activity. Arousability from sleep is highest during stages 1 and 2. Stages 3 and 4 are slow-wave (delta) or deep sleep. Stage 3 occupies an average of 5% of sleep time, whereas stage 4 constitutes 10% to 15% of sleep time in young, healthy adults. In contrast to stages 1 and 2, it is difficult to awaken someone during stages 3 and 4, or delta sleep.[15] Delta sleep, also known as *restorative sleep*, is enhanced by serotonin, adenosine, cholecystokinin, and IL-1. The ability of IL-1 to promote slow-wave sleep supports a widely held theory linking deep sleep to the augmentation of immune function. Some hormones (e.g., somatostatin, growth hormone) are released mainly during slow-wave sleep. Deep sleep is most abundant in infants and children and tends to level off at approximately 4 hours a night during adolescence. At age 65, deep sleep accounts for only 10% of sleep, and at age 75, it is often nonexistent.[1,15–17]

Rapid Eye Movement Sleep

Whereas NREM sleep is necessary for rest and rejuvenation, the purpose of REM sleep remains a mystery. REM sleep is greatest in infants, accounting for about 50% of total sleep time. As aging occurs before 2 years and throughout adulthood, REM sleep is usually 20% to 25% of sleep. This percentage of total REM sleep is maintained into healthy old age, but can decline markedly in the presence of organic brain dysfunctions of the elderly. REM sleep is also called *paradoxical sleep* because it has aspects of both deep sleep and light sleep. Body and brainstem functions appear to be in a deep sleep state as muscle and sympathetic tone drop dramatically. In contrast, neurochemical processes and higher cortical brain function appear active. Dreaming is associated closely with REM sleep, and when a person is awakened from REM, alertness returns relatively quickly.[15]

Numerous physiologic functions are altered during REM sleep. Breathing is irregular, consisting of sudden changes in respiratory amplitude and frequency corresponding to bursts of REM. Temperature control is lost and the body temperature typically lowers. REM sleep brings on variability in heart rate, blood pressure (BP), cerebral blood flow, and metabolism. Cardiac output and urine volume decrease. Blood may become thicker as a result of autonomic instability and temperature changes.[1,15–17]

REM duration varies throughout the night but increases each cycle. In the last half of the night, REM becomes notably longer and more intense when body temperature is at its lowest, around 5 AM. The human body clearly needs REM sleep, although the reason it occurs is unknown. When deprived of REM sleep, whether through poor sleep, drugs, or disease states, the brain and body try to catch up. REM rebound occurs and may result in vivid dreams or an overall less restful sleep.[15–18]

NEUROCHEMISTRY OF SLEEP–WAKE CYCLE

Wakefulness- and Sleep-Promoting Neurochemicals

A basic understanding of brain neurochemistry is essential in understanding sleep disorders and the clinical use of hypnotics. Hypnotics exert their effects by modulating brain neurotransmitters and neuropeptides (e.g., serotonin, norepinephrine, acetylcholine, histamine, adenosine, and γaminobutyric acid [GABA]). The neuronal systems in which neurotransmitters and neuropeptides act to control the sleep–wake cycle lie in the brainstem, hypothalamus, and basal forebrain, with connections in the thalamus and cortex. Noradrenergic, histaminergic, and acetylcholine-containing neurons promote wakefulness as they modulate cortical and subcortical neurons.[18] Excitatory amino acids, such as glutamate and stimulating neuropeptides (e.g., substance P, thyrotropin-releasing factor, corticotropin-releasing factor) also promote wakefulness.[18] Hypocretin 1 and 2, also known as orexin A and B, are neuropeptides that modulate the sleep–wake cycle. Hypocretin 1 and 2 are deficient in people with narcolepsy and primary hypersomnia.[15,18–20]

Wakefulness and sleep are antagonistic states competing for control of brain activity. Sleep takes over as the wakefulness-maintaining neuronal systems weaken and sleep-promoting neurons become active. Serotonin-containing neurons of the brainstem raphe dampen sensory input and inhibit motor activity, promoting the emergence of slow-wave sleep.[15,16,18] Opiate peptides (e.g., enkephalin, endorphin) and GABA, an inhibitory neurotransmitter, also promote sleep.[15,21]

Drug-Induced Effects on Neurochemicals

The neurochemistry of sleep also can be understood by considering the effect of hypnotic drugs on specific neurotransmitters. GABA is facilitated when a benzodiazepine compound attaches to the GABA–chloride ionophore complex and causes chloride channels to open and inhibit overexcited areas of the brain.[22,23] GABA-facilitating hypnotics, such as benzodiazepines, induce sleep and decrease arousals between stages, providing more continuous stage 2 sleep.[18,22,24] Benzodiazepines, however, also may decrease stage 4 slow-wave sleep and suppress REM, leading to REM sleep rebound on abrupt discontinuation.[15,22,24] Antihistamines that promote sleep do so by blocking histamine-containing neurons involved in maintaining wakefulness. The excitatory effects of caffeine and other methylxanthines are attributed to their antagonism of adenosine receptors. Adenosine is a sleep-promoting neurotransmitter or neuromodulator.[18,20]

Neurotransmitter alteration may or may not affect REM sleep. Drug-induced noradrenergic and serotonergic modulation usually decreases REM sleep. An increase in dopaminergic neurotransmission can increase wakefulness but has no direct effect on REM sleep. In contrast, increased cholinergic neurotransmission triggers REM sleep.[18] It is useful to think of the brain centers, neurochemicals, and neuropeptides involved as an interactive network regulating our sleep–wake cycle. Hence, drugs or disease states that alter neurotransmission can have significant impact on the sleep–wake cycle.

Diagnosis

The International Classification of Sleep Disorders, Third Edition (ICSD-3)[25] and the Diagnostic and Statistical Manual of Mental Disorders, Fifth Edition (DSM-5)[26] are the latest editions of guides used for classification and diagnosis of sleep disorders. Both ICSD-3 and DSM-5 categorize sleep disorders largely based on pathophysiology and presumed etiology rather than numbers of hours of sleep. See Table 84-1 for DSM-5 classifications of sleep disorders.

INSOMNIA

During the course of a year, approximately one-third (30%–36%) of the population will experience insomnia, and 10% to 15% will consider the problem severe due to daytime consequences.[25] Sleep research also shows that chronic insomnia can predict untreated illness or may contribute to injury and illness.[2,27–29] Children, adolescents, and adults with persistent insomnia are twice as likely to develop anxiety and 4 times as likely to develop depression when compared to people without insomnia.[27] Chronic insomnia is also more common in individuals with high blood pressure, breathing difficulties, gastrointestinal (GI) disorders, cancer, and chronic pain, among other conditions.[27–29] Insomnia and excessive daytime sleepiness (EDS) in the elderly are leading predictors of institutionalization.[30]

To meet the criteria for insomnia disorder according to ICSD-3 and DSM 5, the sleep disturbance must cause significant distress or impairment in important areas of functioning (i.e., social, occupational, educational, academic, behavioral) and occur at least three nights per week over a 3-month period despite adequate opportunity for sleep.[25,26] The insomnia disorder can be further classified based on duration as follows: episodic (1–3 months), persistent (>3 months), and recurrent (two or more episodes in 1 year). Insomnia with duration less than 1 month, previously referred to as transient insomnia, would be classified as "other specified insomnia disorder."[25]

Patient Assessment

When first assessing a patient, it is important to determine whether the sleep problem is related to difficulty falling asleep, maintaining sleep, early morning awakening, nonrestorative–quality

Table 84-1
Classification of Sleep–Wake Disorders[26]

Insomnia disorder: too little or unrestful sleep; can have no identifiable underlying cause or be comorbid with a medical condition or another sleep or mental disorder
Hypersomnolence disorder: sleeping too much or experiencing drowsiness at times when individual should be alert
Narcolepsy/hypocretin deficiency: characterized by EDS, regardless of the time of day resulting in suddenly falling asleep; patients may also experience cataplexy, sleep paralysis, and hypnagogic hallucinations.
Breathing-related sleep disorders: most individuals with breathing problems that interfere with sleep experience fragmented sleep and complain of daytime drowsiness
Obstructive sleep apnea hypopnea
Central sleep apnea
Sleep-related hypoventilation
Circadian rhythm sleep–wake disorders
Sleep phase syndrome: falling asleep and waking earlier or later than desired
Irregular sleep–wake type: falling asleep and waking at irregular times
Non-24-hour sleep–wake type: falling asleep and waking progressively later than desired
Shift work type: sleep changes associated with work schedule
Non-REM sleep arousal disorders
Sleep terror type: individuals cry out in apparent fear during the first part of the sleep cycle but do not awaken; considered pathological only in adults
Sleep walking type: recurring sleepwalking, usually during the first part of the sleep cycle
Nightmare disorder: troubling dreams that awaken individuals or make them fearful of falling asleep
REM sleep behavior disorder: individuals may speak, thrash about, and/or awaken during REM sleep
Restless leg syndrome: individuals experience the need to move their legs during periods of inactivity, especially at night; can lead to fragmented sleep and daytime drowsiness
Substance/medication-induced sleep disorder: can result in insomnia or hypersomnolence
Other specified, or unspecified, sleep disorder: sleep–wake disorders that do not meet criteria for any of the above categories

EDS, Excessive daytime sleepiness; REM, Rapid eye movement.

sleep, excessive daytime sleepiness, or a combination of these problems. Answers to the questions, "How long does it take you to fall asleep, and how many hours do you sleep?" should be compared with the patient's normal sleep pattern to determine how it varies. Questions such as "How do you feel during the day: well rested, sleepy, or something else?" can help assess functional impairment. In addition, the patient's sleep schedule, including bed time, sleep onset latency, number and length of nighttime awakenings, time to sleep reinitiation, and total wake and sleep time should be reviewed.[31]

The next step involves investigating the possible causes of the sleep disorder and any concomitant conditions. All coexisting medical, psychiatric, drug, environmental, and social causes must be considered and treated along with the sleep disorder. Impact of the sleep disturbance on daytime functioning should be assessed to evaluate the severity of the disorder. A sleep diary in which the patient records bed and wake times, estimated time to fall asleep, number and duration or awakenings, time and type of medication / substance ingestion, time and duration of any naps, and sleep quality can help to elucidate the type of sleep disorder.[31]

Additionally to assessing patient symptoms and determining the cause of insomnia, it is important to discuss patient expectations. Not all patients need the same amount of sleep, and too much sleep can be as problematic as too little sleep.[26]

Table 84-2
Nonpharmacologic Treatments for Insomnia[32–34]

1. Cognitive-behavioral therapy: focus is on modifying behavioral and cognitive factors that lead to and foster sleep disturbances
   Cognitive: identify and stop thought patterns that interfere with sleep
   Behavioral: stimulus control, sleep restriction, relaxation, paradoxical intention.
   a. Stimulus control: train the brain to re-associate the bed and bedroom with sleep and re-establish a consistent sleep–wake schedule.
   b. Sleep restriction: create "sleep debt" by limiting amount of time in bed to only the total number of hours actually spent sleeping, then increasing time in bed as sleep efficiency improves.
   c. Relaxation therapy: target physiologic hyperarousal resulting from stress and tension (e.g., meditation, progressive tensing and relaxing of muscles, yoga, stretching).
   d. Paradoxical intention: encourage patient to engage in most feared behavior, "staying awake," to reduce performance anxiety associated with falling asleep.
2. Sleep hygiene: not considered effective on its own; useful adjunctive treatment.
   Avoid caffeine, stimulants, heavy meals, and alcohol at bedtime; exercise early in the day before dinner to relieve stress and prime brain for sleep; turn the face of the clock away from view; establish a before-bedtime ritual; use the bedroom only for sleep and intimacy; make sure bedroom is dark, quiet, comfortable; avoid daytime napping.

Nonpharmacologic Treatment

The first-line treatment for chronic insomnia should be psychological and behavioral therapies. Cognitive-behavioral therapies (CBTs) are effective, long-lasting interventions for insomnia and considered the standard of care.[32,33] They may be more effective than pharmacotherapy for sleep onset latency and sleep efficiency.[34,35] The sleep benefits of these interventions are not immediate and can take several weeks to successfully implement. Results vary depending on the individual and their severity and chronicity of insomnia.[34] Table 84-2 lists established cognitive and behavioral interventions with brief descriptions in addition to important sleep hygiene strategies to include in patient counseling.[32]

Pharmacologic Treatment

Pharmacotherapy is indicated for a variety of reasons, including when nondrug interventions fail or cannot be implemented, sleep disturbances produce significant distress or impairment and immediate symptom relief is required, patient preference is for drug therapy, or if insomnia is comorbid with another medical, sleep, or psychiatric disorder.[32] Patients often do not seek treatment for insomnia from their healthcare provider when pharmacologic treatment is warranted. Instead, alcohol or OTC sleep aids are used with unfavorable results that can worsen insomnia or next-day functioning.[35–37]

The ideal hypnotic has a rapid onset of effect (within 20 minutes, the natural time to fall asleep), helps the patient sleep throughout the night, does not cause daytime impairment, and carries no abuse potential. Currently, there are no ideal hypnotics. Hypnotics that are benzodiazepine receptor agonists come closest to the ideal.[35,38] Available agents vary in onset, duration, and potential for daytime impairment, mostly because of their individual pharmacokinetic profiles (Table 84-3).[39] The selection of an appropriate hypnotic should consider the type of insomnia to be treated and the physiologic characteristics of the patient. For example, if someone cannot fall asleep but has no trouble staying asleep and wants to prevent next-day carryover effects, a rapid-acting hypnotic with short half-life and no active metabolites is desirable.[35,38,39] Age, sex, socioeconomic status, and comorbidities also influence the hypnotic prescribed.[37–40]

INSOMNIA IN A NORMALLY HEALTHY PATIENT

CASE 84-1

QUESTION 1: P.B., a 36-year-old man, is requesting a medication for treatment of his sleep disorder. He returned to Boston, Massachusetts, from a month long business trip to California 2 days ago and is now having difficulty falling asleep. When he initially arrived in California 4 weeks ago, he went to sleep immediately at 7 PM and awoke at 3 AM. His sleep pattern adjusted during his 4-week visit in California, but upon returning to Boston, it now takes him 2 to 3 hours to fall asleep. He has difficulty awakening in the morning and, as a result, sleeps past 9 AM. He needs to be able to wake-up by 6 AM and be alert during the day in his job as an accountant.

What information provided by P.B. is important in the assessment of his sleep disorder? What additional information should be obtained from P.B. to assist in the assessment of his sleep disturbance?

P.B. describes a circadian rhythm sleep–wake disorder, specifically sleep phase syndrome related to a time-zone shift (previously referred to as "jet lag"). His major complaint is difficulty falling asleep and awakening later than desired, because he reports no trouble staying asleep or awakening too early. It is important for P.B. not to be sedated during the day so that he can fulfill his job obligations. Additional information needed from P.B. includes the duration of insomnia, methods already tried to relieve insomnia and their efficacy, concomitant medications, coexisting medical conditions or psychiatric disorders, alcohol use, caffeine use, and current life stressor. P.B. should be advised that assessing all of the aforementioned information is necessary in treating his sleep problem.

CASE 84-1, QUESTION 2: In response to your additional questions, you learn that P.B. has no medical problems and takes no prescription medications. He has been taking pseudoephedrine at night for nasal congestion since returning from California. He denies drinking alcoholic beverages and coffee but admits to recently increasing his cola intake from infrequent consumption of 1 to 2 cans between lunch and bedtime to try to stay awake. He denies a long history of sleep disorder, but adds, "I have not been able to sleep as well since traveling; I don't know why." What factors could be contributing to P.B.'s complaints?

Several factors are contributing to P.B.'s type of sleep disorder. His circadian rhythm has been disrupted because of travel, but he also takes a stimulating decongestant (i.e., pseudoephedrine) and drinks a caffeine-containing beverages (i.e., average can of cola has about 35 mg of caffeine; PB consumes 35–70 mg/day). In addition, he sleeps in new surroundings that may require time for adjustment. All these factors can contribute to difficulty in falling asleep. Circadian rhythm sleep disorder results from a mismatch between the sleep–wake schedule required by a person's environment and the circadian sleep–wake pattern.

NONPRESCRIPTION SLEEP AIDS

CASE 84-1, QUESTION 3: P.B. would like to purchase a nonprescription sleep medication. What would you recommend?

An individual risk-versus-benefit assessment is essential before recommending any medication, including OTC products. Although OTC products (i.e., antihistamines, melatonin, valerian, and other herbals) are commonly advertised as sleep aids, data supporting the use of these products are limited. Antihistamines can cause drowsiness and may help patients fall asleep. The ability to cause sedation does not necessarily lead to hypnotic efficacy. Some patients do not feel well rested the next day after taking an antihistamine, but instead feel slow, lethargic, and not mentally sharp. This "hangover effect" can be significant and may be related to the lipid solubility and central histaminic (H_1) and muscarinic blocking effects of the antihistamine.[35,41] Antihistamines with low lipid solubility (e.g., cetirizine, loratadine) do not cross the blood–brain barrier readily and do not cause sedation. Although diphenhydramine is the most common antihistamine found in nonprescription sleep medications, some preparations contain the antihistamines doxylamine or hydroxyzine.

CASE 84-1, QUESTION 4: What additional counseling is needed for P.B.?

Tolerance can develop to the sedative effects of antihistamines after 3 to 7 days of continued use.[35,37–38,41] Because of a high incidence of daytime sedation and risk of cognitive psychomotor impairment,[33] antihistamines are a poor choice for P.B., an accountant who must stay alert and functional throughout the day. Any attempt to manage P.B.'s sleep disorder should start with nonpharmacologic interventions before initiating any drug therapy.

TIME-ZONE SHIFT: NONPHARMACOLOGIC TREATMENT VERSUS TRIAZOLAM OR NONBENZODIAZEPINE RECEPTOR AGONISTS

CASE 84-1, QUESTION 5: P.B. asks whether he can try triazolam for the treatment of his sleep disturbances. What would you recommend?

P.B. should be informed about the likely causes of his sleep disturbances (i.e., time-zone shift, caffeine-containing beverages, pseudoephedrine, new surroundings). He also should understand that it may take 1 to 3 weeks for his system to readjust after traveling.[42] The importance of nonpharmacologic interventions, particularly those that pertain to reestablishing a desired sleep–wake cycle and sleep hygiene education, to improve sleep (Table 84-2) should be emphasized. In addition, an hour of bright light in the morning can serve as an environmental stimulus, normalizing the circadian rhythm.[42] If P.B.'s sleep disturbances persist despite adhering to cognitive-behavioral interventions, a prescription hypnotic may be necessary.

Table 84-3
Sedative-Hypnotic Agents FDA-Approved for Treatment of Insomnia[36–38,61]

Generic[a] (Brand Name)	Dose (mg)		Onset (minutes)	Half-Life (hours)	Duration of Action[b]	Insomnia Indication
	Healthy Adults	Elderly Hepatic Impairment				
Benzodiazepines						
Estazolam (generics)	1–2	0.5–1	60–120	10–24	Intermediate	Sleep onset and sleep maintenance[f]
Flurazepam (generics)	15–30	NR	60–120	>100[c]	Long	Sleep onset and sleep maintenance[f]
Quazepam (Doral, generics)	7.5–15	NR	30–60	47–100[c]	Long	Sleep onset and Sleep maintenance[f]
Temazepam (Restoril, generics)	7.5–30	7.5	60–120	3.5–18.4	Intermediate	Sleep onset and sleep maintenance[f]
Triazolam (Halcion, generics)	0.125–0.25	0.125	15–30	1.5–5.5	Short	Sleep onset[f]
Nonbenzodiazepine Receptor Agonists						
Zaleplon (Sonata)	10–20	5–10	30	1	Short	Sleep onset[f]
Zolpidem						
Oral tablet (Ambien)	5–10[d]	5	30	1.4–4.5	Short	Sleep onset[f]
ER oral tablet (Ambien CR)	6.25–12.5[d]	6.25	30	1.62–4.05	Intermediate	Sleep onset and sleep maintenance[g]
Sublingual tablet[e] (Intermezzo)	1.75–3.5[d]	1.75	20–38	1.4–3.6	Short	Middle-of-the-night-awakening[h]
Sublingual tablet[e] (Edluar)	5–10[d]	5	30	1.57–6.73	Intermediate	Sleep onset[f]
Mucous membrane spray (Zolpimist)[i]	5–10[d]	5	10	2.7–3	Short	Sleep onset[f]
Eszopiclone (Lunesta)	1–3 (start with 1 in all patients)	1–2	30	6	Intermediate	Sleep onset and sleep maintenance[g]
Melatonin Agonist						
Ramelteon (Rozerem)	8	8	30	1–5[c]	Short	Sleep onset[g,j]
Orexin Receptor Antagonists						
Suvorexant (Belsomra)	10–20 (5–10 with moderate CYP3A4 inhibitor)	Elderly—Not specified Severe hepatic dysfunction = NR	30	12	Intermediate	Sleep onset and maintenance[g]
Antidepressants						
Doxepin (Silenor)	6	3	30	15.3 (31[c])	Intermediate	Sleep maintenance[g,j]

[a]Dispense with a product-specific Medication Guide.
[b]Time the patient feels the effects after a single dose; usually approximates half-life with multiple doses; individual variability exists; and tolerance may develop with continued use, lessening the duration; short = 1 to 5 hours; intermediate = 5 to 12 hours; long = >12 hours.
[c]Half-life includes the parent compound and its active metabolites.
[d]In women start with the lower dose.
[e]To be dissolved under the tongue and not swallowed whole.
[f]FDA approved for short-term (7–10 consecutive days) treatment of insomnia.
[g]Not limited to short-term use.
[h]Take only if 4 hours remaining before planned wake time.
[i]To be sprayed over the tongue immediately before bedtime
[j]Not a controlled substance.

FDA, U.S. Food and Drug Administration; NR, Not recommended; ER, Extended-release.

Short-acting hypnotics (Table 84-3)[35,38,41,43] like triazolam are effective to induce and regulate sleep if the stay will be relatively short (<5 days) and if critical activities must be accomplished during the first 48 hours after arrival at the destination.[42] Triazolam, indicated for difficulties with sleep latency, has a rapid onset of sedative-hypnotic activity (within 15–30 minutes). Triazolam also has a short half-life of approximately 1.5 hours that does not contribute to next-day impairment at recommended doses (0.125–0.25 mg for healthy adults, 0.125 mg for elderly). Women may be more susceptible to the adverse effects of hypnotics than men, possibly due to greater oral bioavailability.[35,41] P.B. could ask his physician to prescribe triazolam 0.125 mg, as needed. Disadvantages of benzodiazepines, and triazolam in particular, include the impairment in new learning or anterograde amnesia and the potential for complex sleep behaviors (e.g., eating, sleeping, driving, or other activities while being asleep). These effects can interfere with daytime functioning and result in the inability to remember new information learned on the trip. P.B. should be cautioned regarding tolerance to the hypnosedative effects and physiologic dependence that can occur with long-term use of a benzodiazepine and the potential for rebound insomnia with abrupt discontinuation.[35,37,41] Of the benzodiazepine receptor–active hypnotics, triazolam is most commonly associated with rebound insomnia (i.e., daytime nervousness, jitteriness, and insomnia worse than before) if abruptly stopped after more than 7 to 10 days of continuous use and withdrawal problems, likely related to its high binding affinity at different gamma-aminobutyric acid $(GABA)_A$ receptor subtypes.[43–45] The pharmacologic properties of benzodiazepines, including sedation, anterograde amnesia, antianxiety and anticonvulsant activity, muscle relaxation, and ethanol potentiation, occur as a result of interaction with various $GABA_A$ receptor subunits. The sedative effects of benzodiazepines are primarily mediated via activity at the α_1-subunit of the $GABA_A$ receptor.[45] Nonbenzodiazepine hypnotics (NBRA; also known as Z-hypnotics) such as zaleplon, zolpidem, and eszopiclone have fewer reports of rebound insomnia and anterograde amnesia at recommended doses due to selectivity for the α_1-receptor subunit and also lack significant anxiolytic and muscle relaxant effects compared with triazolam.[43] Also, triazolam's short half-life and rapid decrease in blood levels create the potential for withdrawal symptoms including anxiety and insomnia. Triazolam is highly effective in inducing sleep when used on an as-needed basis. Long-acting hypnotics, such as flurazepam, may prevent the traveler from awakening in the morning and should be avoided.

MELATONIN

CASE 84-1, QUESTION 6: P.B. would like to try melatonin for improved sleep but wonders whether it is safe and effective. What information is available on the safety and efficacy of melatonin for circadian rhythm or other types of sleep disorders?

Melatonin is a naturally occurring hormone secreted by the pineal gland, located in the center of the brain. The pineal gland is connected to the retina via a nerve pathway that runs through the suprachiasmatic nucleus of the hypothalamus, the body's circadian clock. The pineal gland produces melatonin (a by-product of serotonin metabolism) only during the nocturnal phase of the circadian cycle and only in the presence of relative darkness.[41,46]

Studies in adults show that melatonin has at least mild sleep-promoting properties when administered before the period of natural increase in endogenous melatonin (~10 PM to midnight). It causes significantly more sleepiness when taken at 8 PM compared with 11:30 PM, theoretically because the brain's receptors are already saturated with melatonin late at night.[41,46] Doses between 0.5 and 5 mg taken close to the target bedtime in the new time zone can decrease sleep disturbances. A systematic review of 10 clinical trials showed melatonin was more effective for travel eastward crossing multiple time zones.[46] Melatonin 0.5 to 10 mg has been found effective for entraining the circadian rhythms in blind people, alleviating insomnia in developmentally disabled, handicapped, or autistic spectrum children and adults, and treating short-term, initial insomnia in children with attention deficit hyperactivity disorder (ADHD).[41,46,47] The safety and effectiveness of melatonin for long-term use or other sleep disorders has not been established. Consumers selecting melatonin products over the counter should be advised the purity of melatonin is not regulated by the FDA. Although doses of 0.5 to 5 mg melatonin are well tolerated, side effects include sleepiness, headache, and nausea.[41,46,47] Melatonin use has been associated with reports of depression, liver disease and vasoconstrictive, immunologic, and contraceptive effects.[41,46]

RAMELTEON

CASE 84-1, QUESTION 7: P.B.'s doctor gave him a prescription for ramelteon 8 mg at bedtime. How does ramelteon compare with melatonin?

Ramelteon is a highly selective melatonin agonist at melatonin 1 and 2 receptors (MT1, MT2). MT1 regulates sleepiness and MT2 adjusts circadian rhythms and regulates phase shifts from day to night.[48,49] Ramelteon is approved by the FDA for insomnia characterized by difficulty falling asleep. Clinical studies in primary insomnia show it decreases the time to fall asleep by 10 to 19 minutes, and it increases total sleep time by 8 to 22 minutes.[48–50] One controlled trial showed it was superior to placebo in decreasing time to fall asleep during a 6-month period, although ramelteon's onset was 15 minutes faster than placebo after week one but only 9 minutes faster at 6 months.[49] Its half-life ranges from 1 to 2.6 hours. The half-life of its active metabolite, M II, is 2 to 5 hours. Ramelteon undergoes hepatic metabolism by cytochrome P-450 isoenzyme CYP1A2. Increases in serum concentration occur even with mild liver disease, so caution is recommended for patients who have at least moderate liver disease. Fluvoxamine is a strong inhibitor of CYP1A2 and given with ramelteon dramatically increases its serum concentration. Coadministration with fluvoxamine or any potent CYP1A2 inhibitors should be avoided. The most common adverse events observed with ramelteon include headache (7%), dizziness (5%), somnolence (5%), fatigue (4%), and nausea (3%).[49,50]

In clinical trials, no evidence of cognitive impairment, rebound insomnia, withdrawal effects, or abuse potential was demonstrated even at doses up to 20 times the usual treatment dose.[51] These results were markedly different than the abuse potential and side effects of triazolam at treatment doses and doses up to 3 times higher than usual.[48,49,52] Of note, no study has directly compared ramelteon and another hypnotic for insomnia management.[52] Ramelteon is a reasonable option for patients with initial insomnia with no abuse potential and little to no risk of next-day impairment.

NONBENZODIAZEPINE RECEPTOR AGONISTS (ZOLPIDEM, ZALEPLON, AND ESZOPICLONE)

CASE 84-1, QUESTION 8: It has been a month since his return and P.B. continues to have difficulty falling asleep. What alternative medications (aside from triazolam and ramelteon) offer rapid onset, have low risk of daytime sedation, and can be administered safely for weeks to months if necessary?

Considering their rapid onset of action, NBRA medications (zaleplon, zolpidem, and eszopiclone) are all potential alternatives for P.B. They have varying degrees of selectivity for the α_1-subunit on the $GABA_A$ receptor. This selectivity imparts hypnotic efficacy with no significant anxiolytic, muscle relaxant, or anticonvulsant effects. Consequently, NBRAs have a lower risk of abuse, withdrawal, and tolerance compared with older nonselective benzodiazepines such as triazolam and temazepam. These attributes make NBRAs more desirable for the treatment of chronic insomnia. Both zolpidem controlled-release and eszopiclone are FDA-approved for chronic insomnia and are effective for up to 3 to 6 months of therapy.[38] Zolpidem has been studied up to 12 months and was not associated with rebound insomnia or withdrawal symptoms.[53]

Additionally, eszopiclone was studied for 12 months of nightly administration and found to be well tolerated with no tolerance observed.[54] Another potential advantage of NBRAs α_1-subunit selectivity is little to no change in sleep architecture or sleep stages. Temazepam and flurazepam increase the percentage of stage 2 sleep but can suppress REM and stage 3 and 4 deep restorative sleep. In contrast, NBRAs do not interfere with these sleep stages and have lower rates of uncomfortable REM rebound (vivid dreams, increased autonomic instability) on discontinuation.[38,44]

The NBRAs differ with respect to pharmacokinetics and adverse events. Zolpidem, the first NBRA, was marketed in the United States in 1991. It is absorbed rapidly, reaches peak serum levels in 1.5 hours, and is eliminated rapidly with an average half-life of approximately 2.5 hours.[42] For faster sleep onset, zolpidem should be taken on an empty stomach for faster absorption. A food-effect study demonstrated that administration of a zolpidem 10 mg tablet 20 minutes after a meal resulted in a decrease in AUC and C_{max} of 15% and 25%, respectively, and an increase in the T_{max} from 1.4 to 2.2 hours.[55] Zolpidem is metabolized by the oxidative cytochrome P-450 isoenzyme CYP3A4; therefore, drug interactions should be considered when zolpidem is coadministered with CYP3A4 inhibitors such as diltiazem or fluoxetine. Zolpidem has no active metabolites, and it has a low risk of residual daytime sedation in recommended doses.[38,43] Zolpidem controlled-release (CR) has no clear advantage over zolpidem, except that it may provide a slightly longer duration of sleep. Zolpidem CR is a bilayered tablet that has a first layer that dissolves quickly to induce sleep and a second layer that releases zolpidem more gradually to improve sleep maintenance. Serum concentrations peak in 2 hours compared with 1.5 hours for immediate-release zolpidem, with an associated longer latency to effect.[39] Of note, zolpidem has been approved as oral spray to help with sleep onset. Due to buccal absorption, it has a rapid-onset of action of 10 minutes.[56] In 2013, the FDA approved a new label change and dosing for zolpidem products to recommend avoiding driving the day after using zolpidem controlled-release. Also, gender metabolism differences exist where women metabolize zolpidem slower than men, resulting in blood levels nearly two-fold higher. As a result, in women or the elderly, the recommended starting dose is 5 mg zolpidem immediate-release or 6.25 mg zolpidem extended-release.[57] For P.B., though the usual adult dose in males for zolpidem immediate-release is 10 mg at bedtime, women, elderly, or patients such as P.B, who express concern that a medicine may be too strong, should begin with 5 mg at bedtime.

Zaleplon offers a shorter elimination half-life (approximately 1 hour) and duration of effect than zolpidem (see Table 84-3). It is least likely of all hypnotic agents to cause residual daytime sedation and has the least effect on memory and psychomotor performance. An assessment of psychomotor performance, arousal, memory, and cognitive functioning with zaleplon revealed no cognitive impairment.[38,43] The most common adverse effects with zaleplon include dizziness, headache, and somnolence.[58] In dose escalation studies using up to 60 mg, symptoms appear at approximately 30 minutes after dosing, peak at 1 to 2 hours, and are no longer evident after 4 hours. It can be taken in the middle of the night as long as the individual has 4 hours left in bed. Zaleplon is metabolized primarily via aldehyde oxidase, CYP3A4 is a secondary route of metabolism, and there are no active metabolites; it has less potential for drug or food interactions compared with zolpidem or eszopiclone.[41]

Eszopiclone maintains efficacy with no evidence of tolerance after 6 months of continuous use, resulting in FDA approval for long-term use.[59–62] Hypnotic efficacy has been demonstrated for up to 6 months in younger patients taking 2 to 3 mg nightly, and in elderly patients taking 1 to 2 mg nightly, although only the higher range of doses significantly improved sleep maintenance. As with zolpidem and zaleplon, eszopiclone has a rapid onset of effect, but differs in that it has a longer duration of effect (Table 84-3). Time to maximal concentration (T_{max}) is delayed up to 1 hour when eszopiclone is administered after a high-fat meal, potentially delaying the onset of sleep.[59,60]

Eszopiclone has less receptor selectivity than either zaleplon or zolpidem, potentially resulting in some anxiolytic, amnestic, and anticonvulsant activity.[61] Among the three Z-hypnotic drugs, eszopiclone has a dose-related unpleasant bitter taste noted by 16% to 34% of patients.[59,60] Headache and dizziness were reported more commonly with eszopiclone than placebo, and at higher doses, next-day confusion and memory impairment were reported in up to 3% of patients.[38,60] Eszopiclone is primarily metabolized by CYP3A4, so drugs that induce or inhibit this isoenzyme can have an impact on metabolism and a clinical effect.[60]

P.B. needs a medication that will hasten sleep onset, but does not need continued drug effect later in the night. Both zolpidem and zaleplon are useful alternatives for P.B. because of their efficacy for his sleep onset difficulty. However, zaleplon may be preferred due to quick onset and short half-life to mitigate the risk of next-day hangover. Among the NBRAs, eszopiclone has the longest half-life and the greatest risk for next-day impairment.

CASE 84-1, QUESTION 9: Zolpidem 5 mg is prescribed because of its rapid onset, low cost, and lower risk for next-day impairment. P.B. expresses concern about possible adverse effects owing to its labeling as a Schedule IV controlled substance and the FDA warning of complex sleep behaviors such as night eating and night driving. How should P.B.'s concerns be addressed?

Patient counseling is most effective when it is interactive with both patient and practitioner actively listening to each other while exchanging information. It is best to begin by emphasizing the benefits of zaleplon to improve his sleep and daytime functioning. Next, P.B. should be reassured that zaleplon is generally well tolerated and he will be prescribed the lowest dose to minimize the likelihood of adverse effects. Counseling should include a discussion of common and potentially serious adverse effects along with management strategies. Common possible adverse effects include headache (30%), abdominal pain (6%), asthenia (5%), somnolence (5%), and dizziness (7%).[38,58] Anaphylactoid reactions and nightmares have been reported in postmarketing studies. Additionally, P.B. should be encouraged to report both effectiveness and all adverse effects to his clinician. Alcohol should not be consumed together with zaleplon or any NBRA because it can cause excessive side effects and interfere with P.B.'s sleep.

To address P.B.'s concern regarding complex sleep behaviors, a reasonable response would be "rarely, individuals taking sleeping medication have been reported to be making phone calls, eating, having sex, or driving while half asleep. The risk for these potentially dangerous effects increases if consumers take a higher than the recommended dose, or drink alcohol or mix hypnotics with other sedating medications."[14] Another rare allergic reaction is facial swelling (angioedema). All manufacturers of hypnotic medication are required to include this information in their package inserts.[14]

Although the abuse potential of NBRAs is less than benzodiazepines, they are problematic in active substance abuse disorders. NBRAs are Schedule IV controlled substances with more potential for abuse than ramelteon or sedating antidepressants, like trazodone.[48] Tolerance and withdrawal associated with NBRAs is unlikely but reported with abrupt discontinuation and patients should be counseled of this possibility, particularly at high doses.

CASE 84-1, QUESTION 10: P.B. asks about a new sleep medication, suvorexant, and whether he could use this to help him sleep. What information can you provide P.B. regarding the safety and efficacy of suvorexant for insomnia?

Suvorexant is an orexin receptor antagonist FDA-approved in 2014 for treatment of insomnia characterized by difficulty falling asleep and/or maintaining sleep. The orexin signaling pathway promotes wakefulness and arousal; antagonism of orexin receptors can promote sleep. Studies show that suvorexant can decrease latency to onset of sleep and wake after sleep onset without disrupting the sleep architecture. The initial recommended daily dose is 10 mg within 30 minutes of bedtime and with at least 7 hours of sleep time available. Suvorexant should be taken on an empty stomach as time to sleep onset may be delayed by 1.5 hours if taken with or soon after a meal. If needed, the dose can be increased in 5 mg increments to the maximum recommended daily dose of 20 mg at bedtime. Suvorexant is a CYP3A substrate and a dose reduction of 5 mg daily is recommended when administered concurrently with a moderate CYP3A inhibitor; concurrent administration with a strong CYP3A inhibitor is not recommended.[63] No rebound insomnia or withdrawal symptoms have been observed following abrupt discontinuation.[64] When compared to zolpidem, suvorexant is associated with less abuse potential and like benzodiazepine receptor agonist hypnotics is a Schedule IV medication.[63] The most commonly reported adverse effect in clinical trials evaluating suvorexant was daytime somnolence. Complex sleep behaviors, a dose-dependent increase in suicidal ideation, sleep paralysis, hallucinations, and cataplexy-like symptoms have been reported with suvorexant. Suvorexant is contraindicated in patients with narcolepsy. Studies comparing suvorexant to other hypnotic agents, such as the Z-hypnotics, are lacking. The role of suvorexant in the treatment of sleep disorders has yet to be established.

INSOMNIA IN A MEDICALLY ILL PATIENT

Insomnia and Effect on Sleep Stages

CASE 84-2

QUESTION 1: A.T., a 42-year-old woman with a 5-year history of hypothyroidism and a 2-year history of hypertension and chronic lower back pain, was just transferred from the intensive care unit (ICU) into a medical unit. Her cardiac status is considered "stable" 2 days after a myocardial infarction (MI). She is 5 feet 9 inches tall and weighs 72 kg. She is receiving aspirin 81 mg (enteric-coated), levothyroxine 112 mcg, and felodipine 10 mg all taken by mouth 1 hour before breakfast every day. Her main complaint is insomnia, including difficulty falling asleep, difficulty maintaining sleep, and early morning awakenings. A.T. reports insomnia for 6 weeks before admission, which worsened during the hospitalization. What type of insomnia does A.T. have, and how might the insomnia affect her health?

A.T.'s insomnia is considered chronic because she experienced it for 6 weeks before hospital admission. It is severe because it involves difficulty falling asleep, maintaining sleep, and early morning awakening. Careful monitoring and effective treatment of A.T.'s sleep disturbance is crucial; studies show disrupted sleep can increase the risk of another adverse cardiac event owing to worsening autonomic instability and poor perfusion to the myocardium.[65]

Because normal sleep moves through all the stages of NREM and REM in a continuous cycle, a patient deprived of continuous sleep may not receive sufficient time in each sleep stage. When stage 2 is diminished, muscles have insufficient opportunity to rest and rejuvenate. If NREM stages 3 and 4 are eliminated, immune function and the healing process can be disrupted. If REM sleep is deprived or excessive, neurotransmitter function may be altered and physiologic homeostatic processes can be disrupted.[15,16,28]

Drug or Disease Etiologies

CASE 84-2, QUESTION 2: What individual drug or disease state factors should be assessed in A.T. before developing a treatment plan?

The Insomnia Treatment Algorithm in Figure 84-2 is useful in systematically addressing A.T.'s sleep complaint. It calls for thoroughly evaluating all concomitant conditions and the type of insomnia in each patient. Numerous medical disorders and primary sleep disorders are associated with difficulty falling asleep and maintaining sleep (Tables 84-4 and 84-5).[5,28,65] First, A.T. should be assessed for sleep apnea because untreated sleep apnea is a known etiology of cardiac disease and hypnotics can be dangerous in untreated sleep apnea (see Case 84-8, in the Sleep Apnea section). Second, A.T.'s pain management should be assessed for optimal efficacy. Acute post-MI pain adds to A.T.'s chronic lower back pain. Of patients with lower back pain, 50% experience chronic poor sleep patterns.[28,65] Third, A.T. was just transferred out of the ICU. Sleep deprivation in an ICU is common and is attributed to the continuous lighting, noise, and constant interventions. Sleep deprivation may prolong or worsen a disease process through diminished natural killer cell activity and decreased stages 3 and 4 of NREM sleep (when healing occurs).[41,66,67] Medications also may be contributing to A.T.'s insomnia (Table 84-4). Levothyroxine can overstimulate the CNS if given in excessive doses. A.T.'s thyroid status should be re-evaluated to ensure appropriateness of the thyroid dose, especially considering her post-MI status.[68] Calcium-channel blockers have been associated with occasional sleep disturbances; therefore, felodipine should be evaluated as a potential contributing factor.[68]

Another clue to a possible cause of A.T.'s sleep problem is her description of early morning awakening, which could be related to hospital activity during these hours or to the presence of a major depressive disorder. A.T. requires psychiatric evaluation to rule out depression, which occurs in about one-third of patients after an MI.[69] In general, patients with chronic illnesses are at increased risk of experiencing major depression, which typically presents with insomnia or hypersomnia. Interestingly, medical outcome studies of other chronic illnesses (cardiovascular, pulmonary, renal, neurologic disease) show a high prevalence of sleep disturbance even in those not suffering from depression.[28,65] Chronic insomnia related to multiple causes can be resistant to treatment; however, treatment of underlying causes increases the likelihood of insomnia resolution.

Comparing Available Hypnotics

CASE 84-2, QUESTION 3: A.T.'s pain is now under control, her levothyroxine dose is appropriate, and felodipine-induced sleep disturbance, sleep-disordered breathing, RLS, and PLMS have all been ruled out. A psychiatric evaluation finds that A.T. does not have major depression, but she is anxious about "life after a heart attack." She meets criteria for primary insomnia and adjustment disorder with anxiety. She continues to have trouble falling asleep and staying asleep. She will be discharged in 2 days. The psychiatric consultation suggests an adjunctive medication with anxiolytic properties that may also help with sleep. Which hypnotic is best for A.T., considering her individual clinical characteristics?

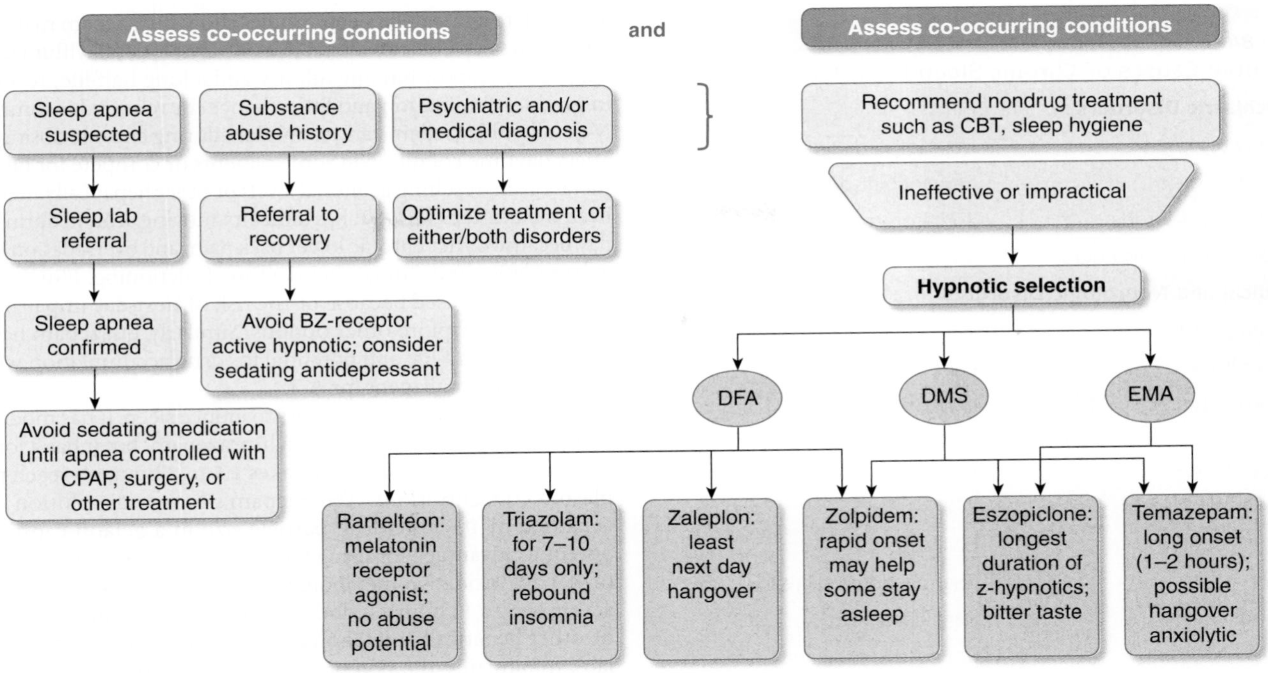

Figure 84-2 Algorithm for treatment of insomnia. DFA, difficulty falling asleep; DMS, difficulty maintaining sleep; EMA, early morning awakening.

Table 84-4
Potential Causes and Contributing Factors for Each Chronic Sleep Complaint[5,28,65]

Difficulty Falling Asleep (DFA)
Learned or conditioned activation (primary insomnia): restless legs syndrome (RLS)
Medications: methylphenidate, modafinil, fluoxetine, bupropion, steroid, β-blocker
Substances: caffeine, guarana, alcohol
Psychiatric disorders: schizophrenia, depression, anxiety disorder, bipolar disorder
Medical disorder: chronic pain, neuropathy, gastrointestinal disorder, cardiopulmonary disorders (particularly if in recumbent position)
Difficulty Maintaining Sleep (DMA)
Excessive time in bed
Psychiatric disorder: major depression, anxiety or bipolar disorder, substance abuse
Sleep-disordered breathing: sleep apnea, acute respiratory distress syndrome
Cardiac disease: atrial fibrillation, heart failure, angina
Neurologic disorder: dementia, Parkinson disease, multiple sclerosis
Early Morning Awakening (EMA)
Major depression
Advanced sleep phase syndrome: learned or conditioned activation (primary insomnia)
Forced to get up because of family or work obligations
Excessive Daytime Sleepiness
Medications: clonidine, antihistamines, antipsychotic, antidepressant, benzodiazepine, chloral hydrate, opioid, anticonvulsant, α_1-adrenergic blockers
Obstructive sleep apnea, central sleep apnea, narcolepsy
Chronic sleep deprivation

The ideal hypnotic for A.T. should act quickly and continue working throughout the night to provide her with uninterrupted sleep. A hypnotic that is not metabolized in the liver would have a lower potential for drug interactions and lessen the opportunity for systemic accumulation. If daytime drug concentrations are needed to calm anxiety, however, a hypnotic with slowly eliminated active metabolites may be desirable. The comparable doses of the hypnotic medications are listed in Table 84-3. When considering available hypnotic medications, differences in pharmacodynamic and pharmacokinetic properties should be considered (Table 84-3). Onset of effect is related to lipophilicity, receptor binding affinity, and T_{max}.[39,41]

Benzodiazepine Dependence and Tolerance

Case 84-2, Question 4: In further discussion with A.T., who prefers to try cognitive-behavioral interventions for anxiety reduction and sleep induction, temazepam 15 mg at bedtime is prescribed on an as-needed basis. A.T. will be monitored regularly as an outpatient for efficacy and tolerability. As A.T. is preparing to leave the hospital, her daughter expresses concerns about the potential for physical dependence on temazepam and the risk of A.T. becoming an addict. How would you respond to her concerns?

A benzodiazepine hypnotic that is nonselective is preferable in A.T. because of the need for anxiolytic properties in addition to hypnotic efficacy. NBRAs are not effective anxiolytic agents. The pharmacodynamic and pharmacokinetic properties of triazolam have already been presented. Its rapid onset is an advantage for A.T.; however, the duration of action would not be sufficient to help A.T. stay asleep. In addition, it should not be used for longer than 7 to 10 days because of the greater potential for adverse effects with prolonged use and the possibility of significant rebound insomnia on withdrawal.[41] A.T. may require a hypnotic for more than 7 to 10 days, which is the maximal duration for triazolam use.

Table 84-5
Potential Causes of Chronic Sleep Disorders[5,28,65,68]

Psychiatric Disorders	
Anxiety disorders	Depressive disorders
Bipolar disorder	Psychotic disorders
Personality disorders	Somatoform disorders
Organic mental disorders	Substance abuse
Medical and Neurologic Disorders	
Angina pectoris	Dementia
Bronchitis	Peptic ulcer disease
Chronic fatigue	Hyperthyroidism and hypothyroidism
Cystic fibrosis	Asthma
Huntington disease	COPD
Parkinson disease	Epilepsy
Hypertension	Gastroesophageal reflux
Arthritis	Renal insufficiency
Cardiac disease	Connective tissue disease
Chronic pain	
Cancer	
Sleep Disorders	
RLS	Sleep apnea (obstructive or central)
PLMS (nocturnal myoclonus)	Primary snoring
Circadian rhythm sleep disorder (jet lag, shift work, delayed sleep phase)	Narcolepsy
Drugs Associated With Sleep Disturbance	
Insomnia	Hypersomnia
Alcohol	Alcohol
Bupropion	Benzodiazepines
Fluoxetine	Antihypertensives
Sertraline	Clonidine
MAO inhibitors	α-Adrenergic blockers
TCA	ACE inhibitors
Thyroid supplements	β-Blockers
Calcium-channel blockers	Anticonvulsants
Decongestants	Analgesics
Appetite suppressants	Chloral hydrate
Theophylline	Antipsychotics
Corticosteroids	Antihistamines
Dopamine agonists	Opioids

ACE, angiotensin-converting enzyme; COPD, chronic obstructive pulmonary disease; MAO, monoamine oxidase; PLMS, periodic limb movements during sleep; RLS, restless legs syndrome; TCA, tricyclic antidepressants.

Flurazepam induces sleep within 15 to 45 minutes during chronic dosing. On the first night of use, however, flurazepam does not induce sleep as well as triazolam. It has intermediate fat solubility but depends on the plasma concentrations of its metabolite, *N*-desalkylflurazepam, for most of its activity.[41] *N*-desalkylflurazepam concentrations take approximately 24 hours to accumulate and induce sleep. Studies show flurazepam maintains efficacy in sleep induction for at least 30 days; *N*-desalkylflurazepam has weak receptor binding affinity and a long half-life, resulting in gradual elimination and little chance for rebound insomnia.[41] *N*-desalkylflurazepam can accumulate during chronic dosing and affect daytime cognition in some patients or compete for hepatic metabolism, resulting in altered levels of other hepatically metabolized medications.[41,68] A.T. has difficulty moving around during the day because of her chronic lower back pain, and oversedation from accumulation may impair her daytime functioning. Flurazepam is infrequently used because of the risk of next-day impairment; it is useful to explore other options. Similarly, quazepam having an extended half-life and potential for drug accumulation would not be an optimal agent for A.T.

Temazepam takes 1 to 2 hours to induce sleep. It has moderate fat solubility, similar to *N*-desalkylflurazepam, but it has a longer dissolution time. Temazepam takes 1.5 to 2 hours to reach peak plasma concentrations. Temazepam's longer dissolution time is caused by its large drug particle size in a gelatin capsule. A potential advantage for using temazepam in A.T.'s case is its lack of hepatic oxidative metabolism and intermediate duration of action of 8 to 12 hours. It does not interfere with the metabolism of other hepatically metabolized drugs and it does not accumulate, minimizing the potential for daytime impairment relative to flurazepam.[41,70] The long onset of action may be of concern, although A.T. could take the drug an hour before bedtime to optimize timing for sleep.

For A.T., the most appropriate choice is temazepam. Of the five approved benzodiazepine agents approved for insomnia (see Table 84-3), temazepam's advantages are intermediate duration of activity that would keep her asleep throughout the night, anxiolytic benefit, and low risk of daytime impairment owing to no known active metabolites.[41,70]

Fear of dependence and addiction to medications is a concern among the general public. Television station "medical experts" and popular magazine "health sections," while providing information, may increase the potential for confusion, erroneous impressions, and misinformation. For healthcare practitioners, it becomes even more crucial to provide sound drug information in common, easy-to-understand terms.

An example of the practitioner's response may be, "I'm glad you have expressed a concern; it gives us a chance to discuss temazepam therapy before your mother leaves the hospital." Temazepam has been prescribed for a medical reason, to improve your mother's sleep and to aid in her healing process. One therapeutic benefit of temazepam is an 8-hour duration of effect. Your mother will be able to sleep throughout the night so that she is well rested during the day. It also may decrease her anxiety over not sleeping, and that puts less stress on her heart.

"The possible side effects of temazepam include sedation, unsteadiness, and dizziness. She should let her doctor know if she experiences any adverse effects. Right now, it is unclear how long your mother will be taking temazepam. Duration of therapy needs to be assessed on an ongoing basis. If your mother takes temazepam every night for more than 4 weeks, two things could happen: (a) she may develop a tolerance and it may not help her sleep anymore, or (b) her system may develop a dependence in which she may have worse insomnia if she does not take it. The primary concern is not addiction but the possible dependence. This means your mother should not change her dose or stop on her own. Any changes in dose or stopping must be done slowly and with her doctor's involvement. These two scenarios do not always occur and are not likely because your mother will be taking it on an as-needed basis. If one or the other does happen, some other intervention may be tried to help with her sleep, or the temazepam dose can be gradually decreased to prevent withdrawal problems. It is important to advise your mother to avoid alcohol, and report any decrease in effectiveness or any adverse effects to her healthcare practitioner."

Patients taking benzodiazepines for longer than 1 year tend to be older, medically ill, and chronically dysphoric and have panic disorder or chronic insomnia. Most chronic use appears to be medically appropriate and does not lead to dose escalation or abuse. Among chronic dysphoric patients, the indications are less clear, and dose escalation is noted sometimes without notable therapeutic benefit. Benzodiazepine hypnotics rarely are taken alone for pleasure and generally are not likely to be abused. Among substance abusers, however, they frequently are taken as part of a polysubstance abuse pattern by alcoholics and narcotic, methadone, and cocaine users. In these groups, abuse is highly prevalent. Benzodiazepines are used to augment euphoria (narcotics and methadone users), to decrease anxiety and withdrawal symptoms (alcoholics), and to ease the "crash" from stimulant-induced euphoria (cocaine users).[71,72]

Physiologic dependence on benzodiazepines, resulting in a withdrawal and abstinence syndrome, develops usually after 2 to 4 months of daily use of the longer half-life benzodiazepines. Shorter half-life benzodiazepine use can result in physiologic dependence earlier (days to weeks) and may be associated with more withdrawal problems.[41,44] See Table 84-3 for a comparison of pharmacokinetic properties of hypnotics.

INSOMNIA AND PSYCHIATRIC DISORDERS

Stepwise Approach to Selecting a Hypnotic

CASE 84-3

QUESTION 1: M.B., a 33-year-old woman, is hospitalized after a suicide attempt in which she tried to overdose on sertraline, ibuprofen, and diphenhydramine. Before the suicide attempt, M. B. had been sober for 3 years. She is diagnosed with major depression and alcohol substance use disorder. After completing an interview with M.B., you learn she stopped taking fluoxetine 5 months ago due to insomnia. She reports doing well until 3 months ago where depression symptoms worsened during her divorce. Two weeks before admission, her outpatient primary-care doctor prescribed sertraline for depression and omeprazole for acid reflux. She went on a drinking binge 5 days ago that ended with the suicide attempt. Her target symptoms include early morning awakening, trouble falling asleep, 15-pound weight loss, apathy, social withdrawal, depressed mood, hopelessness, and anhedonia. Medications continued in the hospital include sertraline 100 mg daily and omeprazole 20 mg daily. M.B. currently reports feeling restless and sleeping only 3 to 4 hours a night. Use Tables 84-3 and Figure 84-2 to compare the clinically significant differences between available hypnotics and to demonstrate how such information can be used to develop a patient-specific treatment plan. What is the best approach to solving M.B.'s sleep problem?

The Insomnia Treatment Algorithm outlined in Figure 84-2 serves as a useful guide for the assessment and management of M.B.'s sleep complaint. Concomitant conditions and the type of insomnia (difficulty falling asleep, difficulty maintaining sleep, early morning awakening) are assessed simultaneously. Possible causes or contributing factors are identified and treated. The type of insomnia can aid in treatment selection. Cognitive-behavioral interventions can be implemented if M.B. is willing and able to participate.

Factors to consider in the drug selection process include substance abuse history, the need for rapid onset and duration of effect. For example, agents with long-acting metabolites (e.g., flurazepam) may accumulate or cause daytime hangover. If the hypnotic has no hepatic metabolism, it will not be subject to drug interactions with other agents that are hepatically metabolized. Also, if insomnia is chronic and resistant to hypnotic treatment, or if a low abuse potential agent is desired (e.g., for a person with an existing substance use disorder like M.B.), trazodone or another sedating antidepressant may be selected.

Sleep Disturbance of Depression

CASE 84-3, QUESTION 2: What type of insomnia does M.B. have, and how is it different from other types of insomnia?

M.B. has trouble falling asleep and early morning awakening, and sleep time has decreased to 3 or 4 hours a night. She is diagnosed with major depression, and sleep difficulty is part of the disorder. Generally, initial insomnia and early morning awakening are associated with depression, although difficulty maintaining sleep and next-day fatigue are common as well. M.B. is most bothered by trouble falling asleep, early morning awakening, and next-day fatigue. Up to 65% of outpatients with major depression report one or more symptoms of sleep disturbance, whereas 90% of inpatients with depression like M.B. report insomnia.[73]

The insomnia of depression is likely related to a dysregulation of neurotransmitters, such as serotonin, norepinephrine, and dopamine, in addition to dysregulation of the hypothalamic–pituitary axis. All are involved in regulating mood and the sleep–wake cycle.[16,66] Neurotransmitter activity is modified by the effects of antidepressants on REM sleep. Most pro-serotonergic antidepressants suppress REM, causing increased REM latency and decreased total REM time.[73,74] Indeed, REM sleep deprivation can elevate mood.[73,75] Depressed patients deliberately deprived of REM sleep have had a reduction in depressive symptoms. In addition to effects on REM, antidepressants redistribute slow-wave sleep to more physiologically natural patterns, with increased intensity in the first half of the night.[75] Sedating antidepressants with serotonin 2 (5-HT_2) antagonist properties, such as trazodone and mirtazapine, alleviate insomnia and improve sleep architecture.[73]

CASE 84-3, QUESTION 3: M.B. and the treatment team ask you what factors other than depression (i.e., medications, alcohol) may contribute to M.B.'s insomnia. How can her sleep problem be solved?

Treatment

The treatment for M.B.'s insomnia should begin with patient education. She should be informed that more than 90% of depressed patients have some sleep disturbance, either too little or too much, and her sleep should improve as depressive symptoms improve (in 2–8 weeks). Counseling on cognitive-behavioral interventions to improve sleep may be appropriate when M.B.'s depression begins to clear and she is more motivated to improve her sleep hygiene. In the meantime, the potential contribution of sertraline causing restlessness or insomnia should be assessed by confirming the drug is dosed in the early morning to minimize this effect.[70] A sedating antidepressant such as mirtazapine may be preferred unless M.B.'s history includes a positive response with sertraline that would justify ongoing treatment. M.B. also was using alcohol before admission. Alcohol disrupts sleep and can increase arousal when its sedative effects wear off, leading to more fragmented sleep.[37] All patients should be counseled to have their last alcoholic drink at least 3 hours before sleep. M.B. should avoid alcohol altogether given her history of abuse. Drug and alcohol withdrawal and the lingering "abstinence syndromes" often are associated with insomnia, although sometimes hypersomnia is the predominant symptom.[37,76]

HYPNOTICS

CASE 84-3, QUESTION 4: What is the evidence for trazodone's use in managing insomnia? What other antidepressants are used in the treatment of insomnia? Discuss the advantages and disadvantages of using sedating antidepressants for the treatment of insomnia in M.B.

Prescribing a hypnotic short-term or a sedating antidepressant is recommended for depressed patients with insomnia because a good night's sleep can improve treatment adherence and daytime functioning until antidepressant effects become apparent.[65,66] All antidepressants, including selective serotonin reuptake inhibitors (SSRIs), such as sertraline, can improve sleep as the depression lifts; however, most antidepressants like SSRIs, serotonin norepinephrine reuptake inhibitors (e.g., venlafaxine, desvenlafaxine, duloxetine), bupropion, and monoamine oxidase inhibitors can all cause insomnia as well.[68,73] Analysis of residual symptoms in partially treated depressed patients taking SSRIs shows continuing insomnia is present in 44%, requiring additional interventions such as trazodone or mirtazapine.

Hypnotics that act at benzodiazepine receptors are not recommended for M.B. due to her drug use history and recent alcohol abuse. Older nonselective benzodiazepines like temazepam can have a euphoric effect, are cross-tolerant with alcohol, and are likely to be abused by patients with alcohol and substance abuse problems.[41] Abuse, dependence, and withdrawal reactions have been reported with newer $GABA_A$ receptor α_1-subunit selective NBRAs (zolpidem, zaleplon, eszopiclone); therefore, neither class of drugs is appropriate for M.B.[38,58]

If the clinician determines that sertraline treatment is preferred, then trazodone may be added to alleviate insomnia.[77] The addition of trazodone to fluoxetine, bupropion, or monoamine oxidase inhibitors decreased time to sleep and increased duration of sleep but caused intolerable sedation in a few patients who received fluoxetine. Tolerance did not develop to the sedative effects of trazodone in short-term studies (<6 weeks) used adjunctively for depression; however, decreased benefit with time has been reported.[77] The 5-HT_2 antagonist properties of trazodone at low dosages, in addition to its antagonism at histamine-1 and α_1 adrenergic receptors, provide the rationale for its efficacy as a sedating agent.[78]

Trazodone is not thought to be a highly effective antidepressant medication because most people cannot tolerate an effective dose (300–600 mg/day). Because of its sedating properties, low-dose trazodone (50–200 mg/day at bedtime) has become a commonly prescribed adjunctive medication to induce sleep while awaiting the onset of another primary antidepressant's effect.[77] Trazodone has a half-life of approximately 6.4 hours in younger adults and 11.6 hours in the elderly. It undergoes hepatic metabolism via CYP2D6 and CYP3A4; thus, inhibitors of these isoenzymes can increase blood levels and worsen side effects. The most common side effects of trazodone include drowsiness (29.1%), dizziness (21.9%), and dry mouth (17.7%). Cardiac arrhythmias are possible at doses greater than 200 mg/day, as is priapism, a painful prolonged erection that occurs in 1 of 1,000 to 10,000 men. Although priapism is considered rare, it can lead to impotence if untreated; therefore, men should be counseled about priapism at any dose of trazodone.[77]

In the only placebo-controlled trial of trazodone conducted in primary insomnia, investigators compared the hypnotic efficacy of trazodone and zolpidem with placebo in 306 adults (21–65 years of age). Subjects were randomly assigned to receive trazodone 50 mg, zolpidem 10 mg, or placebo nightly for 2 weeks. Sleep parameters were assessed using a subjective sleep questionnaire, which patients completed each morning and at weekly office visits. Trazodone was found to be as effective as zolpidem for the first week of treatment, but during the second week, only zolpidem was more effective than placebo.[77] Tricyclic antidepressants (TCAs; e.g., amitriptyline, doxepin) were used to treat primary insomnia for years based on case reports describing efficacy in doses of 10 to 75 mg/night.[41,73] TCAs, however, increase the risk of cardiovascular problems and anticholinergic side effects in a dose-related manner (see Chapter 86 Depression).

Ultra-low-dose doxepin 3 and 6 mg tablets are now available (Silenor) for the treatment of insomnia characterized by difficulties with sleep maintenance. Doxepin is not a controlled substance, so it may be of value in patients with a history of substance abuse. Four clinical trials conducted in slightly more than 1,000 patients demonstrated ultra-low-dose doxepin's efficacy and safety in both younger adults and the elderly.[79] Doxepin demonstrated improved sleep efficiency during the final third of the night and in the seventh and eighth hours of sleep. Doxepin was well tolerated, with residual sedation and anticholinergic effects no different than placebo. There were no significant effects on next-day alertness, memory, or psychomotor function. Hypnotic efficacy with doxepin was demonstrated for up to 3 months. The primary disadvantage of this brand formulation is its cost. It remains to be seen whether these low-dose studies will prompt increased use of generic doxepin 10 mg, and whether any advantages can be demonstrated in using the branded formulation.

For M.B, a TCA raises additional safety concerns. M.B. has a history of substance abuse and prior suicide attempts. Both are risk factors for future suicide attempts. TCAs are more toxic in overdose when compared with trazodone, and there are multiple reports of TCA plasma levels increasing to toxic levels when administered in combination with CYP450 2D6 inhibitors (see Chapter 86, Depression).

Switching to mirtazapine as an antidepressant that offers more sedation is a reasonable consideration for M.B. If M.B. has a partial but significant response to sertraline at maximal tolerated doses and good tolerability except for insomnia at 4 weeks, mirtazapine can be added to facilitate remission. Mirtazapine has 5-HT_2 antagonist and antihistamine effects, which impart sedation, and it is safer than TCAs in overdose.[73] Mirtazapine is not associated with priapism, but it can cause weight gain.

INSOMNIA IN THE ELDERLY

CASE 84-4

QUESTION 1: S.D., a 77-year-old man, is seen for his initial geriatrics primary-care clinic visit. Vital signs include temperature, 98.8°F; heart rate, 58 beats/minute; respiratory rate, 18 breaths/minute; BP, 166/69 mm Hg; height, 5 feet 3 inches; and weight, 109 pounds. He was referred from an emergency department (ED) visit 4 days earlier with complaints of palpitations and anxiety. Before his ED visit, his medications included atenolol 50 mg daily, lorazepam 1 mg at bedtime, and saw palmetto 320 mg daily. At his ED visit, he stated he had taken lorazepam for sleep for more than 1 year, but did not take it the prior 2 nights and started feeling palpitations and anxiety. His electrocardiogram showed normal sinus rhythm at 67 beats/minute, and S.D.'s head computed tomography scan was negative for any hemorrhage. S.D. was told not to restart the lorazepam, but instead to take diphenhydramine 50 mg at bedtime. He took only one dose, felt "terrible" and fatigued for the next 2 days. On further questioning, he states that he falls asleep without difficulty, usually awakens 2 to 3 times each night to urinate, and often has difficulty falling back to sleep. In the past, lorazepam was helpful with his sleep difficulty. What considerations are important for the assessment and treatment of insomnia in an elderly patient such as S.D.?

Treatment of insomnia in the elderly represents a therapeutic dilemma. Evidence supports an increased need to treat insomnia in the elderly to reduce its potentially serious complications, yet many drug treatment options have potential for harm that may outweigh their benefit. In a large epidemiological study of sleep complaints in 9,282 individuals 65 years and older conducted by the National Institute on Aging, 57% of subjects indicated at least one sleep complaint occurring most of the time, 19% had difficulty falling asleep, 30% complained of awakening at night, and 19% complained of awakening too early.[80] Despite such high frequency of sleep complaints, these complaints are primarily thought to be more a marker of poor physical and mental health rather than caused by aging itself.[80,81]

Historically, it was accepted that age-related sleep changes begin in early adulthood and progress steadily across the adult lifespan.[82] However, in a meta-analysis of 65 studies of quantitative sleep parameters across the lifespan of individuals from ages 5 to 102 without sleep complaint, most changes in sleep were found to occur by age 60.[73] Changes in sleep latency are small and subtle, with an overall increase between 20 and 80 years of less than 10 minutes. Increases in percentages of stage 1 and 2 sleep, as well as decreases in total sleep time, percentage of slow-wave and REM sleep, and REM latency, were significant with aging up to age 60, but only minimal changes were seen after age 60. Only sleep efficiency was found to continue to significantly decrease after age 60. Therefore, identifying factors underlying sleep complaints in the elderly is critical and can lead to appropriate diagnosis and treatment. Elderly patients need not be resigned merely to getting the sleep that they do because they are "getting older."[82]

CASE 84-4, QUESTION 2: What are the more common underlying causes of sleep complaints in the elderly?

Common precipitants of acute insomnia in the elderly include acute medical illnesses, hospitalization, changes in the sleeping environment, medications, and acute or recurring psychological stressors. Chronic or long-term insomnia may be associated with a variety of underlying medical, behavioral, and environmental conditions, as well as a variety of medications.[83] Identification of treatable underlying causes should be the first step in management of insomnia, based on a medical and medication history, physical and mental status examination, and laboratory investigations including thyroid function, serum chemistry panel, and cardiopulmonary studies if indicated.[83,84] Special attention should be directed to chronic pain from any cause, pulmonary disease, chronic renal disease, neurologic disorders, and polyuria from urinary, prostate, or endocrine disorders. Medical conditions with a strong association with insomnia include heart disease, hypertension, diabetes, stomach ulcers, arthritis, migraine, asthma COPD neurological problems, menstrual problems, depression, and bipolar disorder.[85,86] Primary sleep disorders are RLS, sleep apnea, and circadian rhythm disorders.[65,81,86] The potential contribution of medications to the sleep complaint needs to be evaluated, and changes in medication or timing of administration should be considered. Many drugs with CNS effects can alter patterns of sleep and wakefulness, both during their use and their withdrawal.[36,80,86] Both prescribed and OTC medications must be evaluated. The more common drugs of concern include stimulants (caffeine, nicotine, and amphetamines), alcohol, activating antidepressants (e.g., SNRIs and bupropion), pseudoephedrine, bronchodilators, β-blockers, calcium-channel blockers, corticosteroids, and dopamine agonists. Evening administration of drugs like diuretics may also contribute to nighttime awakenings and sleep complaints.

Psychological Versus Drug Treatments for Insomnia

CASE 84-4, QUESTION 3: Which nondrug therapy treatment options might be appropriate for S.D.?

CBT is an effective and safe alternative to drug therapy for insomnia and has also been shown to be an effective augmenting treatment with drug therapy.[34,35] CBT limitations include that it is little known, not widely available, and more time-consuming than drug therapy. Both pharmacologic and nonpharmacologic approaches are effective for the short-term management of insomnia in late life, and current evidence suggests that sleep improvements are better sustained over time with behavioral treatment.[34] A comparative meta-analysis of 21 studies of pharmacotherapy and behavior therapy for persistent insomnia in adults found that both treatments similarly produced moderate to large improvements in number of awakenings, wake time after sleep onset, total sleep time, and sleep quality.[87] Behavior therapy, however, resulted in a greater reduction of sleep latency than pharmacotherapy. CBT was compared with pharmacotherapy (zolpidem) and its combination in 63 young and middle-aged adults with chronic sleep onset insomnia.[34] There was a significant difference in percent change in improved sleep onset latency (CBT 52%, combination therapies 52%, zolpidem 14%, placebo 17%). No significant differences were found among the groups in total sleep time. The authors concluded that CBT, alone or in combination with pharmacotherapy, was more effective than pharmacotherapy alone or placebo for the treatment of sleep onset insomnia. Avoidance of medications with their associated costs, adverse effects, and drug interactions is the primary advantage of CBT. Disadvantages of CBT include possible longer time to effective treatment, higher initial cost, and relative paucity of trained providers in many areas.[88]

CASE 84-4, QUESTION 4: What are the concerns about the use of lorazepam or another benzodiazepine in S.D.?

Specific concerns need to be addressed about the risks most associated with benzodiazepines in the elderly regarding dependence, risk of falls, cognitive dulling, and memory loss. Concern about dependence and the nontherapeutic use of benzodiazepines has been an important factor in limiting the long-term treatment of insomnia with hypnotic drugs.[89] In insomnia patients specifically, the risks of dependence and recreational use of benzodiazepines are relatively low. Dose escalation appears to occur only when treatment is ineffective, or when the patient has a history of substance abuse or anxiety. Although still controversial, the risk of dependence and abuse associated with the newer nonbenzodiazepine drugs may be lower than that associated with benzodiazepine hypnotic drugs. An even greater concern with benzodiazepine use in the elderly is the risk of falls and subsequent hip fractures. Using 42 months of Medicaid healthcare claims data in New Jersey for more than 125,000 individuals older than 65 years, the association of hip fractures and benzodiazepine use was evaluated.[90] Compared with not being exposed to a benzodiazepine, exposure to any benzodiazepine was associated with a 54% higher rate of hip fracture, and after adjusting for potential confounding variables, benzodiazepine use was associated with a 24% higher rate of hip fracture. Use of short half-life benzodiazepines was found to be no safer than use of long half-life benzodiazepines, and the risk of hip fracture was highest during the first 2 weeks after starting a benzodiazepine. These findings support the usual recommendation that the elderly should be given lower doses than their younger adult counterparts, but they challenge the suggestion that only long half-life drugs should be avoided in the elderly owing to clearance concerns. Elderly patients should also be monitored closely to prevent cognitive decline caused by benzodiazepines and avoid use when possible.[91]

CASE 84-4, QUESTION 5: What are the concerns about the use of diphenhydramine in S.D.?

Sedating antihistamines are not recommended for treating insomnia in the elderly, as there is no evidence of sustained benefit and they pose significant risk of anticholinergic effects, notably cognitive impairment, dry mouth, urinary retention, and constipation.[36,88,92] Duration of sedative effect efficacy from antihistamines is also problematic with tolerance to sedative effects developing quickly (3–7 days).[93,94]

S.D.'s primary sleep complaint is related to his nocturia. He is self-treating his urinary symptoms with saw palmetto, which he did not mention at his ED visit (perhaps because no one asked whether he used any OTC or herbal medications). His primary treatment, therefore, must be directed at assessing and more successfully treating his nocturia. S.D. also likely experienced lorazepam withdrawal symptoms. The many potential risks associated with benzodiazepines in the elderly led to a valid decision to discontinue lorazepam. The choice of diphenhydramine was poor, however, not only because of limited short-term efficacy but also because of its potential to worsen both urinary symptoms and memory impairment. Clinicians must ask patients about OTC and herbal medications they may be using to self-treat their symptoms. The best treatment of sleep complaints in elderly persons is to identify any underlying treatable cause, review and identify any sleep hygiene issues, and avoid using benzodiazepines or sedating antihistamines, whose risks often outweigh any benefit.

PEDIATRIC INSOMNIA

Typical sleep need in children varies from 12 to 14 hours in children 1 to 3 years of age to between 8.5 and 9.5 hours in adolescents.[95] All major sleep disorders can occur in youth, and therefore evaluation for insomnia, RLS, PLMS, sleep apnea, and narcolepsy are needed whenever symptoms warrant. Trouble initiating and maintaining sleep are more common in children with ADHD (25%–50%) and autism spectrum disorders (44%–83%). Of infants and toddlers, 10% to 30% have bedtime sleep resistance that can be managed behaviorally with parental education. Inconsistent bedtime, falling asleep away from bed, fears, and psychiatric and medical conditions can all contribute to poor sleep in children.[95]

At least 5% to 10% of high school students have delayed sleep phase syndrome, a physiologic condition in which they do not fall asleep until between 1 and 3 AM and they awaken between 9 AM and noon. School schedules dictate earlier awakening, resulting in chronic sleep deprivation. Poll data indicate that 28% of high school students fall asleep in school at least once a week, and 14% are late or miss school because of oversleeping.[95]

Behavioral interventions to promote good sleep habits (e.g., consistent bedtime and wake-time, before-bedtime ritual) should be initiated during childhood and continued throughout adolescence to promote a lifetime of healthy sleep. No hypnotics are FDA-approved for insomnia in children and adolescents, and significant data are lacking to guide clinicians on medications to improve sleep in youth. Diphenhydramine, clonidine and melatonin are commonly used in children and some adolescents; however, the use of Z-hypnotics is also increasing, although this class has not been well studied in this population.[96]

PREGNANCY AND LACTATION

CASE 84-5

QUESTION 1: J.J. is a 32-year-old woman who is 16-week pregnant. She is moving into a new home and has been experiencing difficulty falling asleep and staying asleep. She asks whether she can take zolpidem for insomnia like she did before she got pregnant. She also asks whether melatonin or other nonprescription medications are safer.

Pregnant women have insomnia symptoms more often than their nonpregnant counterparts, and many ingest hypnotic or sedating medications. Despite frequent usage of hypnotics, healthcare providers are often reluctant to prescribe medications to pregnant woman for fear of teratogenicity. Doxylamine is FDA pregnancy category A, though this indication derived from the treatment of hyperemesis gravidarum and not insomnia.[97] Diphenhydramine is in FDA pregnancy category B and is generally considered the safest sleeping medication in pregnancy.[94] Nevertheless, a pregnant woman should only use it on an as-needed basis. Sedating antihistamines are not compatible with breast-feeding as they have the potential to dry up milk supply due to anticholinergic effects.[99] Melatonin, ramelteon, and suvorexant should not be used because of unknown risks to the fetus.[98]

Regarding the most commonly prescribed hypnotic, zolpidem, The American Academy of Pediatrics considers zolpidem compatible with breast-feeding, but the risk versus benefit should be considered on an individual basis.[98,99] Other Z-hypnotics do not have sufficient data in pregnancy and lactation to make recommendations.

Benzodiazepine hypnotics are pregnancy category D or X. They should be avoided in pregnancy due to the risk of respiratory depression, neonatal flaccidity, and feeding difficulties if given in the second and third trimester and the controversial risk of cleft palate if benzodiazepines are given in the first trimester.[100] Benzodiazepines are not recommended in breast-feeding as the risks outweigh benefits in most cases.[99]

SLEEP APNEA

Clinical Presentation

CASE 84-6

QUESTION 1: E.S., a 52-year-old man, presents to an ambulatory-care clinic complaining of chronic fatigue, low energy, excessive snoring, and overall less restful sleep. When you ask what prompted E.S. to come to the clinic, he answers: "My wife and I have been sleeping in separate bedrooms for the last 6 months. She says my loud snoring and gasping to breathe keeps her awake. I'm tired all day and find myself nodding off a lot." His symptoms have worsened during the past year since early retirement. He has gained weight (6 feet, 220 pounds, body mass index 29.8 kg/m^2) and has developed hypertension. E.S.'s current BP reading is 145/92 mm Hg. Medications include lisinopril 10 mg and aspirin 81 mg both taken in the morning.

What are the possible causes of E.S.'s sleep disorder and why is it important for E.S. to have his problem evaluated in a sleep laboratory?

E.S. reports diminished sleep quality, excessive snoring, gasping for air, and weight gain. Although a number of causes could be responsible for E.S.'s symptoms, one of the most serious is sleep apnea. OSA is a neurologic disorder characterized by mini-episodes of breathing cessation lasting about 10 seconds. These mini-episodes generally occur multiple times in an hour. If there is a reduction in airflow but no cessation of breathing, it is termed *hypopnea*. The brain responds to episodes of apnea and hypopnea with mini-arousals, waking the individual to stimulate breathing.[101,102] These frequent mini-arousals prevent the individual from obtaining quality sleep by not allowing sufficient time in deep, slow-wave sleep, or REM. Obstructive sleep apnea (OSA), the most common type, may be induced when extra body weight (note E.S.'s weight gain) places pressure on the throat and uvula, narrowing the space into which air must travel; this results in the difficulty or cessation of breathing and excessive snoring. An estimated 3% to 7% of men and 2% to 5% of women meet the criteria for OSA.[102,103]

The apnea/hypopnea index (AHI), measured using polysomnography (i.e., EEG, electrooculogram, electromyogram), represents the number of episodes per hour. The AHI score accompanied by symptoms of excessive daytime sleepiness is used to diagnose OSA as follows: >5 to 14 (mild), 15 to 29 (moderate), and >30 (severe).[102]

Risk factor for OSA includes age 65 years and older, obesity (BMI >30), male gender, craniofacial anatomy that alters mechanical and neural properties of the upper airway, genetic predisposition, cigarette smoking, alcohol consumption before sleep, and comorbid conditions such as hypertension, diabetes mellitus, polycystic ovary syndrome, hypothyroidism, and pregnancy.[103] Hypertension and weight gain may be contributing to E.S.'s sleep difficulty. Untreated OSA is associated with an increased risk of hypertension, coronary artery disease, and cerebrovascular disease.[104–106] Although sleep apnea occurs in approximately 5% of women and 15% of men in the general population, it occurs in up to 40% of patients with hypertension.[104] Treatment of OSA can improve BP control and lead to more restful sleep. Of note, OSA also occurs in nonobese individuals and in all ages, including infants.[103,105] Sleep-disordered breathing, including snoring, is a significant risk factor for hypertension even in young individuals of normal weight.[104]

Overnight evaluation by polysomnography in a sleep laboratory would confirm or rule out sleep apnea and allow distinction between OSA and the less-common central sleep apnea.[102,105] Central sleep apnea results when breathing repeatedly starts and stops during sleep because the brain does not send proper signals to the muscles that control breathing (i.e., the diaphragm does not move in attempts to take in air).[105] Treatment of central sleep apnea requires continuous positive airway pressure (CPAP) as opposed to being alleviated through weight loss or anatomic manipulations. Central sleep apnea can occur along with OSA.

Drug Treatment Considerations

CASE 84-6, QUESTION 2: Results from the sleep laboratory study clearly document E.S.'s sleep problem as obstructive sleep apnea (OSA). He experiences an average of 65 apneic episodes per hour. E.S.'s weight gain and inactivity probably contribute to the problem. Both are serious, potentially life-threatening conditions. Why should E.S.'s sleeping difficulties not be treated with a hypnotic medication?

Hypnotics, alcohol, or any CNS depressant can be lethal for patients with sleep apnea and should not be prescribed for E.S. CNS depressants interfere with the mini-arousals required to stimulate breathing once it has stopped. In this case, the sleep laboratory study may have saved E.S. from a potential life-threatening breathing disorder that could have been exacerbated by a hypnotic with CNS depressant activity.

OSA can be treated by tracheostomy, nasal surgery, tonsillectomy, uvulopalatopharyngoplasty, and either nasally or orally administered continuous positive airway pressure CPAP.[98] Weight loss and CPAP therapy are the most effective treatments and must be maintained for continued therapeutic efficacy.[102,105] In CPAP, the patient wears a lightweight mask to bed each night, and a constant flow of air is provided mechanically to prevent breathing cessation and to allow for more restful sleep. Although CPAP is effective for both OSA and central sleep apnea, the results are short-lived, and apneic episodes typically reappear when CPAP therapy is stopped. Preliminary studies in individuals with nocturnal bradycardia and sleep apnea show that insertion of a permanent cardiac pacemaker significantly improved bradycardia and sleep apnea.[106] At this time, the best treatment for E.S.'s hypertension and sleep apnea is weight loss and CPAP.

CASE 84-6, QUESTION 3: If weight loss, surgery, and continuous positive airway pressure (CPAP) are all ineffective or impractical, what drug treatments are potentially effective for E.S.'s sleep apnea?

Modafinil and armodafinil agents approved for narcolepsy are also FDA-approved to treat EDS caused by OSA or shift work sleep disorder. For E.S., these agents are best used as an adjunct to nightly CPAP usage and morning administration of modafinil 200 to 400 mg or armodafinil 150 to 200 mg.[108,109] Protriptyline has dated evidence from the 1980's suggesting benefit by improving patients AHI, but it is not FDA-approved and has only been used in small numbers of patients with sleep apnea.[109]

NARCOLEPSY

Narcolepsy is an incurable neurologic disorder characterized by irrepressible sleep attacks typically occurring 3 to 5 times a day. These sleep attacks can intrude at any time during the individual's waking state. Narcolepsy may be present with or without cataplexy, although cataplexy is present in 60% to 90% of patients.[110] Cataplexy is the loss of muscle tone in the face or limb muscles and often is induced by emotions or laughter. Cataplexy can be subtle, with the patient limp and not moving, or dramatic, in which the patient collapses to the floor.[111] Hypnagogic hallucinations and sleep paralysis are other secondary symptoms not present in all persons with narcolepsy. Hypnagogic hallucinations are perceptual disturbances (i.e., auditory, visual, tactile) that occur while experiencing a sleep attack. The patient may see imaginary objects, hear sounds, or feel sensations. Sleep paralysis is a terrifying experience that can occur when falling asleep or when awakening and can last several minutes. Patients are unable to move their limbs, to speak, or even to breathe deeply. Narcoleptics learn, however, that sleep paralysis episodes are benign and brief (lasting <10 minutes). Between 10% and 20% of patients experience the tetrad of symptoms that include EDS, cataplexy, hypnagogic hallucinations, and sleep paralysis. Except for daytime sleepiness, these symptoms are thought to be expressions or partial expressions of REM sleep.[13,101,110]

Symptoms of narcolepsy often begin at puberty, but patients usually are not diagnosed until years later, in their late teens or early 20s. Early symptoms consist of excessive daytime sedation and poor sleep quality. The sleep cycle becomes progressively more erratic with frequent bursts of REM and decreased regularity of deep or slow-wave sleep. Polysomnography in a sleep laboratory is ideal to confirm narcolepsy. Sleep architecture is notably different. Instead of the 90-minute delay before REM, individuals with narcolepsy progress directly into REM sleep.[101,110] A cerebrospinal fluid hypocretin 1 level of less than 110 pg/mL is also diagnostic for narcolepsy. Postmortem brain studies of patients with narcolepsy show 85% to 95% decrease in hypocretin-containing neurons.[111]

An autoimmune response of unknown origin is thought to damage hypocretin/orexin-secreting cells in the hypothalamus. Without functional hypocretin/orexin cells, the sleep–wake cycle is disrupted. Hypocretin/orexin is also involved in control of body weight, water balance, and temperature.[101,110]

Comparing Treatments

Optimal treatment of narcolepsy involves treating both sleep attacks and cataplexy. Schedule II controlled substances, methylphenidate and dextroamphetamine, were the first drugs used to treat narcolepsy, with 65% to 85% of patients deriving significant improvements in wakefulness. Mixed amphetamine salts are also FDA-approved for narcolepsy.[101] The mechanism of action of methylphenidate and amphetamines is related to increasing neurotransmission of dopamine and norepinephrine. Modafinil, a Schedule C-IV controlled substance, is an effective treatment with less abuse potential. Its exact mode of action is not fully understood, but it is thought to increase wakefulness through noradrenergic, adrenergic, histaminergic, GABA-modulating, glutamatergic, and hypocretin/orexin-stimulating mechanisms.[101,110] Armodafinil is the dextroenantiomer of modafinil. Its therapeutic effect, side effect profile, half-life, and abuse potential are similar to those for modafinil.[110] In summary, these stimulating drugs decrease the number of sleep attacks, improve task performance, and increase the time to fall asleep, but they cannot eliminate sleep attacks altogether. Research is underway exploring the possible use of immunosuppression at the time of narcolepsy onset. One hypothesis suggests that immunosuppression therapy during a period of pathologic immune response could prevent or reduce damage to the hypocretin system that otherwise would lead to the development of narcolepsy.[101,110]

Cataplexy does not respond to psychostimulants or modafinil but may be lessened with low doses of antidepressants. TCAs (imipramine and clomipramine) were the first antidepressants used, but protriptyline, desipramine, and SSRIs (fluoxetine, sertraline, and paroxetine) are also used.[101] SSRIs and protriptyline offer the advantage of less daytime sedation, compared with tertiary TCAs. The effectiveness of antidepressants for the treatment of cataplexy is thought to be related to REM-suppressant effects. A Cochrane Database Review concluded that insufficient evidence exists to recommend antidepressants as effective treatments for cataplexy, given that most studies are small and uncontrolled.[114] It should be recognized, however, that large-scale studies on such a rare disorder are difficult to conduct.[101] Antidepressants are not considered effective in decreasing sleep attacks.[101,110,112]

Sodium oxybate (Xyrem), a salt form of the CNS depressant γ-hydroxybutyrate, is FDA-approved for treatment of cataplexy and EDS in narcolepsy. Its therapeutic effects are related to decreased REM, improved sleep consolidation, and increased stage 3 and 4 slow-wave sleep.[101,112] Sodium oxybate must be administered twice during the night while the patient is in bed to consolidate 6 to 8 hours of sleep. In two randomized, double-blind, placebo-controlled trials, sodium oxybate 9 g/night (i.e., 450 mg at bedtime, then 450 mg 2–4 hours later), but not 3 or 6 g/night, significantly reduced the median frequency of cataplexy attacks by 69% in patients with narcolepsy, whereas 4.5 to 9 g for 8 weeks significantly reduced the median frequency of cataplexy attacks by 57% to 85% in a dose-related manner. Both trials showed 6% to 30% reduction in EDS as measured on the Epworth Sleepiness Scale and 20% to 43% reduction in daytime sleep attacks.[107] Because of a significant abuse potential, sodium oxybate is a Schedule III controlled substance. It is only available through restricted distribution, the Xyrem Success Program, which uses only one central pharmacy in the United States for dispensing.[110,111]

Mixed Amphetamine Salts and Fluoxetine

CASE 84-7

QUESTION 1: G.B., a 23-year-old man with narcolepsy, has been taking mixed amphetamine salts extended-release 60 mg in the morning for sleep attacks associated with narcolepsy, and fluoxetine 20 mg daily will be started to treat cataplexy. What are the potential risks of using both mixed amphetamine salts and fluoxetine to treat G.B.?

Anorexia, gastrointestinal complaints (abdominal pain, nausea, vomiting, diarrhea), anxiety, irritability, insomnia, and headaches are common side effects of stimulant drugs.[101] Though rare, psychotic reactions can occur in narcoleptic patients taking stimulants at any dose; however, psychosis generally resolves when the stimulant is discontinued. Stimulants, even at high dosages (e.g., 80 mg methylphenidate), usually do not bring a patient to a normal level of alertness, and sometimes nocturnal sleep is disrupted. To prevent stimulant-induced insomnia, doses should be taken before 3 PM. Tolerance to the therapeutic effects of stimulants may, however, develop in some patients with narcolepsy.[101,110,113] Drug holidays may allow the patient to recapture therapeutic benefit; however, many patients opt for an increased stimulant dose instead. Exceeding maximal recommended doses of stimulant significantly increases the risk of psychosis, substance abuse, psychiatric hospitalization, tachyarrhythmia, and anorexia according to a case–control study in 116 patients with narcolepsy taking stimulants.[101,113] Seizures have also been reported.

Fluoxetine may improve cataplexy, but it can worsen nocturnal insomnia and contribute to restlessness, headache, nausea, and sexual side effects including anorgasmia.[73,112] In addition, fluoxetine is a potent CYP2D6 inhibitor resulting in higher levels of amphetamine.[114] G.B. should be monitored closely during the initiation of fluoxetine therapy, and the amphetamine dose should be lowered by 30% to 60% to minimize side effects and prevent toxicity. The optimal therapeutic dose of fluoxetine to manage cataplexy has not been established, but low doses may be effective and minimize the risk of side effects.

Modafinil and Sodium Oxybate

CASE 84-7, QUESTION 2: G.B. experiences intolerable nervousness, irritability, and nocturnal insomnia on mixed amphetamine salts and fluoxetine. There is no improvement in cataplexy with the addition of fluoxetine. He asks about switching to modafinil and sodium oxybate. Does the combination of modafinil and sodium oxybate offer any advantage for G.B.?

Modafinil's efficacy relative to other CNS stimulants has not been adequately assessed in controlled clinical trials; however, it has less potential for insomnia and adverse CNS reactions at recommended dosages between 200 and 400 mg/day administered in the morning.[115] It also has less abuse potential compared with stimulants and is a Schedule IV controlled substance. Headache was the only adverse experience rated significantly higher than placebo in 283 patients taking the recommended dose of either 200 or 400 mg/day of modafinil. Anorexia, nervousness, restlessness, and pulse and BP increases are dose-related side effects to discuss during counseling. The maximal tolerable single daily dose may be 600 mg/day, because 800 mg/day produced increased BP and pulse in one tolerability study.[116] Gradual dosage titration improves tolerability. Armodafinil, an active stereoisomer of modafinil, is effective at usual doses between 150 and 250 mg/day. It has a similar adverse effect profile as modafinil.[110,115]

Improved daytime wakefulness is an advantage of sodium oxybate compared with antidepressants. A controlled trial involving 278 patients showed an increase in slow-wave sleep (stages 3 and 4) and decreased nightly sleep disruption in patients taking sodium oxybate with modafinil compared with modafinil alone.[117] Sodium oxybate can be administered safely with stimulants and modafinil; however, coadministration with other CNS depressants, including hypnotic medication, is contraindicated because of the risk of respiratory depression.[111]

Case 84-7, Question 3: What counseling should G.B. receive as he switches to modafinil and sodium oxybate?

People taking modafinil should receive counseling regarding the potential for drug interactions. Modafinil induces CYP3A4 metabolism primarily in the gut and inhibits CYP2C19. Decreased levels of triazolam and ethinyl estradiol have been associated with modafinil coadministration.[118] Enzyme inhibition may also occur. Modafinil's inhibition of CYP2C19 is the proposed mechanism behind modafinil-associated clozapine toxicity.[119] Monitoring for drug interactions is crucial because modafinil and armodafinil are increasingly used for other indications, including daytime sleepiness associated with Parkinson disease, shift work, fibromyalgia, sleep apnea, fatigue associated with multiple sclerosis, and ADHD.[120–122]

Sodium oxybate should not be given to those with sleep-disordered breathing, sleep apnea, or an alcohol or substance abuse disorder.[112] Adverse effects include nausea, headache, dizziness, and enuresis. Safe coadministration of modafinil and sodium oxybate has been described in clinical trials[117]; however, cases of severe side effects including panic, psychosis, depression, and new-onset suicidal ideation have been described.[123] The risk of serious side effects versus benefits in managing cataplexy and nocturnal insomnia should be discussed with G.B. and his family. Close monitoring, particularly during the first weeks and months of treatment and when dosages are adjusted up or down, should be advised.[123] G.B. should be instructed how to properly administer sodium oxybate, drinking half the dose on an empty stomach immediately before bedtime and then setting his alarm for 4 hours later to take the midnocturnal dose.

Naps and Other Behavioral Interventions

Case 84-7, Question 4: The benefits, possible risks, and importance of regular physician assessment have been explained to G.B., and he agrees to report efficacy and adverse effects to his primary-care provider regularly. G.B. is reminded to take the medicine at regular intervals along with daytime naps. Why are naps helpful in the treatment of G.B., and what other behavioral interventions are useful in treating narcolepsy?

Strategically timed 15- to 20-minute naps taken at lunch and then again at 5:30 PM can be refreshing for patients with narcolepsy and increase their time between sleep attacks. Narcolepsy support groups are available and may help G.B. better cope with such a life-changing chronic illness. It also is important for G.B. to avoid alcohol and to regulate his bedtime and wake-up time in the attempt to normalize his sleep habits.[101,110]

ACKNOWLEDGMENT

The authors acknowledge Julie A Dopheide and Glen L. Stimmel for their contributions to this chapter in earlier editions.

KEY REFERENCES AND WEBSITES

A full list of references for this chapter can be found at http://thepoint.lww.com/AT11e. Below are the key references and websites for this chapter, with the corresponding reference number in this chapter found in parentheses after the reference.

Key References

Ahmed I, Thorpy M. Clinical features, diagnosis and treatment of narcolepsy. *Clin Chest Med*. 2010;31:371. (111)

Morgenthaler T et al. Practice parameter for the psychological and behavioral treatment of insomnia: an update. An American Academy of Sleep Medicine report. *Sleep*. 2006;29:1415. (32)

Morin CM et al. Chronic Insomnia. *Lancet*. 2012;379:1129. (37)

Moszczynski A et al. Neurobiological aspects of sleep physiology. *Neuro Clin*. 2012;30:963. (16)

Okun ML et al. A review of sleep-promoting medications used in pregnancy. *Am J Obstet Gynecol*. 2015;214:428. (98)

Key Websites

American Academy of Sleep Medicine. http://www.aasmnet.org/

American Sleep Apnea Association. http://www.sleepapnea.org/

National Sleep Foundation. http://www.sleepfoundation.org/

85 Schizophrenia

Richard J. Silvia, Robert L. Dufresne, and Justin C. Ellison

CORE PRINCIPLES

#	Core Principle	CHAPTER CASES
1	Schizophrenia is a persistent, heterogeneous syndrome, which includes both positive and negative symptoms. Together, these symptom clusters can have variable effects on patient quality of life, functional recovery, and prognosis. Prodromal symptoms preceding the first episode of psychosis may go unnoticed for many months. Onset of an initial psychotic episode can be an acute or insidious process that causes a significant impact on function and ability to perform activities of daily living.	**Case 85-1 (Questions 1, 2), Tables 85-1, 85-2, 85-3**
2	Treatment goals will vary based upon the stage of the patient. During an acute phase, stabilization and safety are primary. During a stable phase, maintaining stability and improving functional recovery are the main goals. Treatment modalities should include both pharmacologic and nonpharmacologic methods.	**Case 85-1 (Questions 3–5)**
3	Many factors need to be considered in selecting an appropriate medication regimen for a patient with schizophrenia. Patient factors such as comorbidities, target symptoms, adherence history, personal and family history of medication response, and others need to be assessed. Medication-related factors include efficacy, safety profile, pharmacokinetics and drug interactions, and economic considerations.	**Case 85-1 (Questions 6–7, 10–11, 14–15, 22, 26–27, 30, 33), Tables 85-5, 85-6, 85-7, 85-9**
4	Adverse effects of antipsychotics are varied. They may include acute and chronic extrapyramidal movement disorders, metabolic disturbances such as weight gain and alterations in serum glucose and lipids, and other adverse effects such as sedation and orthostasis. Monitoring and appropriate interventions for adverse effects should be ongoing throughout all stages of illness to ensure continued safety and avoid medication discontinuation.	**Case 85-1 (Questions 8–9, 15–25, 27–30), Tables 85-4, 85-5, 85-6, 85-7, 85-10, 85-11, 85-12, 85-13 Figure 85-1**
5	Patients who do not respond to an adequate antipsychotic trial should be assessed for adherence. Long-acting injectable antipsychotics may be an option to help maintain adherence. Clozapine is the treatment of choice in patients who are refractory to at least two adequate trials of antipsychotic medications. However, clozapine does require strict adherence to blood monitoring due to the risk of agranulocytosis and carries a significant adverse effect burden.	**Case 85-1 (Questions 12–14, 26, 30–32), Tables 85-8, 85-13**
6	Treatment of female patients of childbearing age may require special consideration. Untreated psychosis can result in poor self-care for the mother and inadequate prenatal care. There is also the concern for substance use, dangerous behaviors, and even suicide. Therefore, the risks and benefits of ongoing antipsychotic treatment should be carefully weighed by both the patient and the treatment team.	**Case 85-1 (Question 34)**
7	Early recognition of symptoms of first-episode psychosis (FEP) and referral to appropriate multidisciplinary, comprehensive treatment services are crucial to long-term functional recovery. This population is highly sensitive to adverse effects. Antipsychotics should be titrated to the minimum effective dose to decrease duration of untreated psychosis and improve long-term prognosis.	**Case 85-1 (Question 35), Figure 85-2**

Schizophrenia is a psychiatric illness that can lead to lifelong effects on a patient's functioning. Manifesting primarily as a thought disorder, patients often have problems with perception, maintaining contact with reality, thought processing, and behavior. These symptoms can lead to a variety of impairments across many domains, including social, occupational, and emotional. Due to these symptoms, patients may require hospitalizations to help maintain or restore functionality. Treatment of schizophrenia encompasses multiple modalities, all targeted on improving a patient's symptoms and functioning, decreasing hospitalizations, and preventing morbidity and mortality.

EPIDEMIOLOGY

Schizophrenia is a heterogeneous, genetically linked "spectrum" disorder that affects 0.7% of the population.[1] It is the ninth leading cause of disability in the world,[2] being found in all cultures and races. While often incorrectly assumed to be more common in men, there is no gender difference in the incidence of the illness. However, the onset of schizophrenia tends to occur between the ages of 18 to 25 in males and from 26 to 45 years old in females, and usually persists for a lifetime.[3] Overall, more severe symptoms are generally seen in males versus females.

ECONOMIC BURDEN

The economic burden of this devastating disease and its treatment is enormous.[4–7] In one estimate from 2002, US costs for schizophrenia totaled $62.7 billion. This included $30.3 billion in direct healthcare costs (of which medications accounted for $5.0 billion) and $32.4 billion in indirect costs, such as lost productivity and other costs incurred to the healthcare system.[3] Although progress has been made in treating the symptoms of schizophrenia and restoring moderate levels of functioning, there is as of yet no cure. As many patients present with an early age of onset, the lifetime burden of illness can be great. Many patients will need repeated hospitalizations and, when not hospitalized, will require significant outpatient services and treatment. Additionally, many patients require supportive living situations, either in facilities designed for these services or with family members, increasing the financial burden on their families as well.

ETIOLOGY

Multiple neurotransmitter and physiologic mechanisms have been hypothesized to explain the complex etiology of schizophrenia. Many theories on the role aberrant neurotransmitter systems play in schizophrenia are derived from the pharmacologic actions of the medications used to treat the illness in addition to direct analysis from biologic samples. Findings on neurologic scans and other measurements of neuroanatomy are also not consistent across patients to allow for these methods to be reliably employed in making a diagnosis of schizophrenia. Genetic markers have more recently been explored with advances in genetics, but these too are not all-encompassing. In this section, chemical, biologic, and environmental bases of schizophrenia will be presented.

Genetic and Environmental Risk Factors

A genetic component to schizophrenia has been hypothesized since the observation that family members of patients are more prone to develop schizophrenia than the general population. Rates of schizophrenia among family members vary (anywhere from 2% to 50%) based upon the relationship to the patient with schizophrenia.[1] Children born to parents who both have schizophrenia are affected in 40% to 60% of cases. Siblings of patients with schizophrenia, including dizygotic twins, are also affected in 10% to 15% of cases. However, monozygotic twins develop schizophrenia approximately 50% of the time if their twin also has the illness. Second- and third-degree relatives of patients more closely approximate the general population, but still develop the illness approximately 2% to 5% of the time. Many genes are thought to play a role in schizophrenia, but no gene has been found to be universal across patients. This finding suggests multiple genes may be involved in the etiology of schizophrenia. Although a genetic role appears to exist, it does not explain how all patients develop the illness. Approximately two-thirds of patients have no known familial history of the illness; therefore, other factors must play a role in these patients.[1] Certain environmental exposures in early development are associated with development of schizophrenia. Maternal infections, in particular influenza, stress, and malnutrition during the first and second trimesters, have shown a link to the child developing schizophrenia. Fetal or infant hypoxia during delivery or in the first few months of life has been shown to double the risk of schizophrenia. Childhood trauma and substance abuse have also been linked to the development of schizophrenia.

Pathophysiology

The actual nature of the pathophysiology of schizophrenia is both unknown and complex. It may be more appropriate to conceptualize it as a syndrome that may involve many different underlying disease mechanisms.[8] Although numerous deviations in brain structure and physiology have been noted, such as decreased gray matter volume, whole-brain volume, and enlarged ventricle size,[9] most treatments focus on antagonism of presupposed increased activity at dopamine-2 (D_2) receptors. The potency of typical antipsychotic medications has correlated with their antagonism of these receptors, although some atypical antipsychotics, such as clozapine, are extremely effective with a lesser degree of D_2 receptor blockade.[10] The initial *dopamine hypothesis* of schizophrenia theorized that positive symptoms of schizophrenia (e.g., conceptual disorganization and hallucinations) result from abnormally increased activity in the mesolimbic dopamine neurons and that negative and affective symptoms of schizophrenia result from subnormal mesocortical dopamine neuronal activity.[11] This remains a clinically useful, albeit simplistic, conceptual framework because many dopamine agonists tend to increase positive symptoms and oppose the effects of antipsychotics. The relation of negative symptoms to dopamine neurotransmission is even more complex. Some suggest that decreased dopamine in frontal areas is linked to negative symptoms and increased dopaminergic neurotransmission in striatal areas results in positive symptoms.[12] To explain the efficacy and lack of movement adverse effects, prolactin elevation, or secondary negative symptoms of antipsychotics such as clozapine and quetiapine, one theory proposes that they have a faster dissociation from the D_2 receptor than other antipsychotics.[13] It has also been suggested that 65% of D_2 receptor occupancy predicted response and 78% predicted extrapyramidal adverse effects.[14]

More recent thinking suggests involvement of glutamate and GABA, which are intertwined with the disturbances in dopaminergic neurotransmission.[15] While speculation that glutamate was involved in the pathophysiology of schizophrenia started in the 1980s, the demonstration that N-methyl-D-aspartate (NMDA) receptor antagonists best replicated all the major schizophrenic symptoms such as the positive, negative, and cognitive ones in healthy subjects lent credence to the "NMDA receptor hypofunction hypothesis." Because negative symptoms and cognitive deficits are not treated by D_2 receptor antagonists nor worsened by dopamine agonists, a theory that involves early disruption of glutamine transmission in schizophrenia is an appealing hypothesis. Also, unlike subcortical dopaminergic dysfunction, pathologic brain changes such as widespread dendritic and spine dysplasia along with cortical atrophy could possibly relate to NMDA receptor hypofunction.[16] Excitatory neurotransmission in the brain is predominantly glutamatergic, and glutamate dysfunction could possibly relate to dopamine dysfunction both in its prodrome and later on in the course of the illness.[17] In schizophrenia, it can be considered that dopaminergic changes are a final end mechanism where antipsychotics work in which increased mesocortical dopamine turnover and overactive mesolimbic dopaminergic over activity result from other preceding neurotransmitter changes.[10]

Gradual progressive NMDA receptor hypofunction would also be consistent with the altered neuroanatomy of schizophrenia.[18] Decreased brain volume in schizophrenia has been noted since the 1920s, and there are more recent findings to believe that there are changes in brain structure with reductions in the volume of certain areas of the brain as well as changes in connectivity.[8] Enlargement of cerebral ventricles is a typical finding in schizophrenia, and reduced dendritic spine density in cerebral cortical pyramidal neurons where NMDA subtypes of glutamate receptors are present has been noted.[19] Some of these neuroanatomic differences include impaired white matter integrity as well as reduced volume of gray matter in inferior parietal, prefrontal, superior, and medial temporal, thalamic, and striatal regions.[20] There are also a number of studies suggesting the importance of these white matter abnormalities in schizophrenia to dysconnectivity between functional tracts.[21]

CLINICAL PRESENTATION

Historical Concept of Schizophrenia

Schizophrenia was first characterized as "dementia praecox" by early psychiatrists Arnold Pick and Emil Kraepelin in the late 19th century,[22] and was described by Bleuler as a "disintegration of psychic functions."[23] Historically, schizophrenia has been a disease characterized by progressive deterioration of the brain. Although modern findings seem to corroborate this viewpoint, few patients with schizophrenia show the progressive incremental loss of function that is characteristic of neurodegenerative illnesses.[24] The demonstrated effectiveness of dopamine receptor antagonists in the treatment schizophrenia[25] resulted in the disorder being conceptualized as a heterogeneous syndrome characterized by D_2 receptor hyperfunction[26] predominately in mesolimbic regions of the brain.

Diagnosis and Differential Diagnosis

The diagnosis of schizophrenia in the recently introduced *DSM-5* requires that an individual has at least two persistent symptoms such as delusions, hallucinations, disorganized speech, or behavior over a 6-month period.[27] Also, in the *DSM-5,* subtypes of schizophrenia, such as paranoid or undifferentiated, have been removed. These distinctions were not clinically useful because patients often displayed characteristic symptoms from each subtype at various times in their illness, or even concurrently.[27] Patients presenting with either manic or depressive symptoms concomitantly with their typically schizophrenic ones are still diagnosed as having schizoaffective disorder (Table 85-1).

Table 85-1
***DSM-5* Criteria for Schizophrenia**

A. Characteristic Symptoms
Two (or more) of the following, each present for a significant portion of time during a 1-month period (or less if successfully treated). At least one of these must be 1, 2, or 3: 1. Delusions 2. Hallucinations 3. Disorganized speech (e.g., frequent derailment or incoherence) 4. Grossly disorganized or catatonic behavior 5. Negative symptoms (i.e., restricted affect or avolition)
B. Functional Disturbance
For a significant portion of the time since the onset of the disturbance, level of functioning in one or more major areas, such as work, interpersonal relations, or self-care, is markedly below the level achieved prior to the onset (or when the onset is in childhood or adolescence, there is failure to achieve expected level of interpersonal, academic, or occupational functioning).
C. Duration
Continuous signs of the disturbance persist for at least 6 months. This 6-month period must include at least 1 month of symptoms (or less if successfully treated) that meet Criterion A (i.e., active-phase symptoms) and may include periods of prodromal or residual symptoms. During these prodromal or residual periods, the signs of the disturbance may be manifested by only negative symptoms or by two or more symptoms listed in Criterion A present in an attenuated form (e.g., odd beliefs, unusual perceptual experiences).
D. Schizoaffective Disorder and Mood Disorder Exclusion
Schizoaffective disorder and depressive or bipolar disorder with psychotic features have been ruled out because either (1) no major depressive or manic episodes have occurred concurrently with the active-phase symptoms or (2) if mood episodes have occurred during active-phase symptoms, they have been present for a minority of the total duration of the active and residual periods of the illness.
E. Substance or General Medical Condition Exclusion
The disturbance is not attributable to the physiologic effects of a substance (e.g., a drug of abuse, a medication) or another medical condition.
F. Relationship to a Neurodevelopmental Disorder
If there is a history of autism spectrum disorder or a communication disorder of childhood onset, the additional diagnosis of schizophrenia is made only if prominent delusions or hallucinations, in addition to the other required symptoms of schizophrenia, also are present for at least 1 month (or less if successfully treated).

Reprinted from American Psychiatric Association. *Diagnostic and Statistical Manual of Mental Disorders*. 5th ed. Arlington, VA: American Psychiatric Publishing; 2013:87–122, with permission (Copyright 2013).

Numerous disorders are characterized by psychosis during exacerbation (Table 85-2). Schizophrenia differs in its presentation from bipolar disorder in that there are prominent signs of conceptual disorganization and hallucinations. Prominent "negative" symptoms such as apathy, avolition, poverty of speech, and emotional blunting may also be present. Schizoaffective disorder, bipolar type, may pertain to patients who present with both positive schizophrenic symptoms and either mania or depression. It is not uncommon for patients with schizophrenia to suffer from secondary depression at various times during the course of their illness as well.[28] Suicide in these patients is not uncommon.[29]

Table 85-2
Differential Diagnosis for Schizophrenia

Drug-induced Psychoses
Alcohol (or other sedative-hypnotics)
Amphetamine (or other stimulant)
Cocaine
Cannabis (marijuana)
Phencyclidine (PCP)
Lysergic acid diethylamide (LSD)
Anticholinergics (especially in overdose)
Anabolic and Corticosteroids
Other Psychiatric Disorders
Major depressive or bipolar disorder with psychotic features
Schizoaffective disorder
Schizophreniform disorder and brief psychotic disorder
Delusional disorder
Paranoid, Schizoid, or Schizotypal personality disorder
Obsessive-compulsive disorder and body dysmorphic disorder
Post-traumatic stress disorder
Autism spectrum disorder or communication disorders

Adapted from American Psychiatric Association. *Diagnostic and Statistical Manual of Mental Disorders*. 5th ed. Arlington, VA: American Psychiatric Publishing; 2013:87–122, with permission.

In new-onset psychosis, the treating clinician should be careful to rule out drug-induced (i.e., amphetamines, cocaine, "k2" synthetic cannabinoids, anticholinergics, LSD, phencyclidine) causes. Corticosteroids may induce a manic type of psychosis, whereas anabolic steroids may provoke a more aggressive type of psychotic presentation. Obtaining a toxicology screen may be prudent. A patient can have a brief psychotic disorder that comes on suddenly, last for up to one month, and remit with no recurrence of symptoms. A patient presenting with signs and symptoms of schizophrenia between one to 6 months is said to have a schizophreniform disorder. Furthermore, depression can present with mood congruent auditory hallucinations (often deprecatory) and delusions. Finally, patients with cluster A personality disorders can show some isolated symptoms such as paranoia or blunted affect, but do not meet full criteria of schizophrenia.[30]

Hallmark/Target Symptoms

The symptoms of schizophrenia are generally organized into two main domains: positive and negative (Table 85-3). Positive symptoms are usually what the public perceives when thinking about schizophrenia: hallucinations, delusions, and disorganization. Hallucinations can affect any of the five senses, but auditory are the most common. Delusions are fixed false beliefs that are persistent despite evidence to the contrary. Delusional subtypes include persecutory, erotomanic (e.g., delusion of love), delusions of grandeur (having special abilities), or somatic (i.e., delusion of being pregnant in context of negative pregnancy tests). Disorganization can manifest in the patient's speech, thought patterns, or behaviors. Some examples of disorganized speech can include made-up words (neologisms), rhyming words (clang speech), speaking words in a sentence in incorrect order (word salad), and repeating words said to them (echolalia). Examples of disorganized behaviors can include repeating the same activity needlessly (perseveration), repeating someone else's actions (echopraxia), dressing oddly for the setting or season of the year (wearing winter clothes in summer), or other odd behaviors based upon the setting the patient is in. Negative symptoms of schizophrenia include apathy, avolition, blunted affect, and poverty of speech.[31] A decreased ability to experience pleasure (known as anhedonia) and social withdrawal can lead to significant functional impairment, even when positive symptoms are relatively absent in a patient. During acute episodes, positive symptoms may predominate, whereas over the long term it may be negative symptoms that are more troubling and disabling to a patient. A third domain of cognitive symptoms can also present in schizophrenia. Symptoms include concrete thinking, inattention, problems with memory, learning and executive function, as well as conceptual disorganization.[32] When these cognitive symptoms are combined with negative symptoms over the patient's lifespan, significant impairment in function may result. Comorbid depression is also common in schizophrenia[33] and can be difficult to treat,[28,34,35] and symptoms can be predictive of relapse.[36,37] Depressive symptoms may be overlooked in the face of overwhelming positive symptoms, or confused with negative symptoms.

Table 85-3
Positive and Negative Symptoms of Schizophrenia

Positive	Negative
Hallucinations (auditory, visual, or other senses)	Diminished emotional expression (body language)
Delusions (persecutory, paranoid, grandiose, etc.)	Avolition/psychomotor retardation
Disorganized thinking/speech	Alogia (decreased speech)
Grossly disorganized or abnormal motor behavior (including catatonia)	Anhedonia (decreased ability to feel pleasure)
Unusual behavior	Asociality (lack of socialization)
Combativeness, agitation, and hostility	Affective flattening
Ideas of reference	

CASE 85-1

QUESTION 1: J.J., a 26-year-old, single female college student, was brought to the emergency department of the local hospital by her school's campus security at 3 am after she was found running naked through the campus screaming "They're after me and won't leave me alone! They keep telling me to run and hide!" J.J.'s roommate has accompanied her with the security officers.

History of Present Illness: J.J. is not a good historian, but her roommate is willing to provide information to help. When asked questions, J.J. provides indirect, tangential answers, repeating her concerns of "they are after me." When asked who is after her, she responds "the FBI of course! They think I'm a spy- but I am a spy for the CIA!" Various times during the interview, J.J. is found talking to someone not in the room. When asked about that, she says she hears the voice of her CIA supervisor through the "transmitter in my head" and needs to respond. She said the transmitter also allows her to read other people's minds, which is how she spies for the CIA. J.J.'s roommate states that JJ has been acting erratic for the past couple semesters, but she thought it was just from an online video game they had been playing. Once, she returned to their dorm room and J.J. had barricaded the door from the inside with furniture so no one would find her. She states J.J. is often up late at night on her computer, which she says is to "look for traces of the enemy spies."

Medical History: J.J. has no significant medical or psychiatric history. She has never been hospitalized or treated for any psychiatric condition in the past. Her roommate has known her since they started college together 3 years ago, and they have been roommates for the past 2 years. The roommate says J.J. was fairly normal—quiet and shy, getting good grades—until the unusual behavior started almost a year ago after they returned from summer break. She says J.J.'s behavior has gotten increasingly unusual and erratic since then.

Psychosocial History: A call to J.J.'s mother finds that her father has a history of alcoholism and domestic violence which led to their divorce when J.J. was 14. J.J.'s paternal uncle has been diagnosed with schizophrenia and has been hospitalized multiple times over his lifetime. J.J.'s mother says she has always been a very good student, but not very social when in high school, tending to isolate from her classmates. She screamed at them one day in school saying she would defend herself if they carried out their plans and the police were called. No charges were filed and J.J. was entered into the school's anger management program, to which she never showed up. J.J.'s roommate states she only drinks socially at occasional parties and denies any illicit substance abuse.

Physical Examination/Laboratory Tests: J.J.'s physical examination shows no significant or contributory findings other than some bruising on her knuckles from punching the walls. J.J. states this is from "fighting off the FBI agents" when they find her. Laboratory tests, including complete blood count (CBC), SMA-28 panel, and liver and thyroid function tests, all return normal. A urine drug screen returns all negative results. No other tests were ordered.

Mental Status Exam: *Appearance and Behavior:* J.J. is a tall, average build, neat but casually dressed young woman who appears her stated age. She shows signs of paranoia and agitation as she is constantly looking around the room and pacing. She constantly asks to be released "before they find me." *Mood:* J.J. is anxious and concerned that the "FBI will find me" and prevent her from completing her mission. Affect is animated due to his level of agitation. She does not report any depressive ideation. *Memory:* Long-term memory appears to be intact (confirmed by roommate) but patient will not cooperate with recall tests of immediate- and short-term memory as "this is a waste of time and I need to be released." *Orientation:* J.J. is oriented to person, place, time, and situation. *Thought Content:* J.J. is fixated on needing to leave in order to complete her mission. She is convinced the longer she stays the more likely the FBI will find her here and she will "need to fight my way out." She also states she is trying to use her implanted transmitter to read the thoughts of the people in the room. She denies any suicidal or homicidal ideation. She accuses you of keeping her there to help the FBI. *Thought Process:* J.J.'s speech is highly disorganized such that she can be difficult to comprehend. *Perception:* J.J. is clearly responding to internal stimuli and most likely auditory hallucinations. She also keeps asking the staff whether something is burning and where the smell is coming from. *Insight and Judgment:* J.J. has poor insight into her symptoms and mental state, and will most likely require inpatient hospitalization for psychosis.

Provisional diagnosis: psychotic episode, most likely due to schizophrenia.

What hallmark symptoms of schizophrenia is J.J. presenting with at this time? How might these symptoms be used in monitoring treatment?

J.J. currently presents with a number of hallmark symptoms of schizophrenia. She has olfactory as well as auditory hallucinations (hearing her CIA supervisor and others), delusions (she works for the CIA and the FBI is after her, having a transmitter in her head), and magical thinking (she can read people's thoughts). She shows conceptual disorganization in her speech. She is also agitated and uncooperative, and has acted out on her delusions by getting into arguments with people she feels are from the FBI. These symptoms should begin to decrease and subside with time as effective medication treatment is utilized, allowing us to determine whether J.J. is responding appropriately.

CASE 85-1, QUESTION 2: What information from J.J.'s history also contributes to a diagnosis of schizophrenia? What is the prognosis for J.J.?

Although J.J. has had no previous psychiatric treatment, she is in the age range for an initial psychotic episode of schizophrenia (late teens to mid-20s). J.J. has been showing increasingly unusual behavior for over 6 months, and possibly up to a year according to her roommate, with more drastic changes more recently. Prior to this, J.J. did show some prodromal symptoms, most notably some difficulty interacting with peers while in high school and isolating herself. There is also a family history of schizophrenia (paternal uncle) and alcoholism (father). J.J.'s prognosis is variable, because her young age of onset, family history of schizophrenia, and unstable home environment at a young age indicate a poor prognosis, but her relatively high baseline functioning and intelligence (she did very well in high school and is currently in college) would increase the chances for a better long-term outcome. As J.J. is early in her illness, it will take time to better determine her long-term prognosis more clearly.

Typical Course of the Illness and Prognosis

The course of schizophrenia can vary between individuals. However, a common pattern entails a premorbid phase with possible signs of cognitive, motor, and social deficits in childhood at 12 years old or under, a prodromal phase during adolescence and young adulthood (12–18 years old) including a functional decline with brief or attenuated positive symptoms, and then an active phase which includes florid positive symptoms as part of psychosis.[20,38] An improved prognosis is associated with female gender, a preponderance of positive and mood symptoms versus negative symptoms, rapid onset of symptoms, older age at symptom onset, and high premorbid functioning.[39,40]

Generally, the negative (or deficit) and cognitive symptoms of schizophrenia predominate earlier in the development of the disorder. Florid positive symptoms usually emerge between 18 to 25 years of age in men and 20 to 30 years of age in women.[22] During the prodromal phase, patients may show what resembles negative symptoms: blunted affect, decreased motivation and energy, social withdrawal, and others. Cognitive symptoms may also present, such as poor concentration and memory, which may manifest as declining school or work performance. Low-level positive symptoms may also be seen, mostly in the form of disorganized thinking. Other symptoms such as depression, anxiety, or irritability may also present. Often these symptoms will go unrecognized in adolescents and be mistaken for anything from puberty, relationship problems, or drug abuse. This phase may last from weeks to years and often is not attributed to schizophrenia until the first psychotic episode. In many instances, patients will convert to a full schizophrenia diagnosis with more significant positive symptoms and go months or more before receiving treatment. This delay may affect the long-term prognosis of the illness as early treatment can decrease later morbidity as response to treatment in first-episode schizophrenia in critical.[41]

After an active phase of schizophrenia, which can last a large part of adulthood, patients usually enter a residual phase of chronic disability. Later in this phase, symptoms may become somewhat similar to the prodromal phase. As the disease progresses, residual symptoms may increase between episodes and make normal day-to-day functioning difficult. As the patient ages, the medical complications of schizophrenia, treatment-emergent metabolic syndrome, and effects of tobacco use increasingly take hold.[38] Patients with schizophrenia have a life expectancy 9 to 10 years shorter (or more by some estimates) than the average population.[42] The disease often becomes characterized by a preponderance of negative symptoms and cognitive deficits in those living into the later years.[27] However, with early intervention and support, many patients can achieve symptom control and lead meaningful and fulfilling lives.

TREATMENT

Schizophrenia is generally considered a chronic, lifelong illness consisting of varying periods of illness severity, with resulting effects on patient functionality. Although pharmacotherapy can have positive effects on reducing symptoms of the illness and improving functionality, there are often symptoms that may not respond adequately to treatment. In addition, despite adequate treatment, patients may have relapses of their illness, leading to acute psychotic episodes needing more intensive treatment. Treatment is therefore usually lifelong and is often multidisciplinary in its approach, consisting of pharmacotherapy, psychosocial therapy, case management, and other methods.

Goals of Treatment

The overall goal for the treatment of schizophrenia is to reduce the symptoms of the illness in order to improve patient functionality and quality of life. Depending upon the patient's current level of acuity, the specific goals for the patient at that time may vary. Although similar pharmacotherapy and nonpharmacotherapy methods may be employed across the spectrum of severity of schizophrenia, they may be utilized differently. Patients are generally described as being in one of three treatment phases according to the American Psychiatric Association: acute, stabilization, and stable.[27] These phases are not static, and patients can move between these phases frequently over the course of their illness.

ACUTE PHASE

The primary goal of treatment in the acute phase of illness is to reduce the threat of harm to the patient or others. Patients experiencing acute psychosis will present with prominent positive symptoms and exhibit disorganized speech and/or behaviors. Negative symptoms and suicidal ideation may also be more pronounced and severe. This will often require a higher level of care than the outpatient setting can provide and necessitate inpatient psychiatric hospitalization where the patient is stabilized. Medications, including short-acting injectable antipsychotics and benzodiazepines, are usually required to target agitation in acute psychosis. However, psychosocial interventions and collaboration with family and caregivers for collateral information are also crucial in this phase of illness.[43] Antipsychotic should be initiated as soon as clinically possible to decrease duration of untreated psychosis and improve long-term prognosis.[44]

The reason for psychiatric decompensation should be ascertained through patient report and collateral information (e.g., caregiver insight, pharmacy fill records). Schizophrenia has a variable course. Exacerbations can occur even on a therapeutic regimen in the context of psychosocial stressors, illicit substance use, and other reasons. However, if the exacerbation was due to nonadherence, the reasons should be explored with the patient. If the patient was nonadherent due to intolerable adverse effects, a lower dose or alternative medication could be considered. If difficulty remembering to take medication was the issue, a long-acting injectable formulation could be considered. In either scenario, the decision to initiate or change the antipsychotic should be based on patient preference, prior history of response, tolerability, and relevant medical comorbidities.

STABILIZATION PHASE

The aim during the stabilization phase is to promote continued recovery, maintain symptom control, begin facilitating referrals for supportive outpatient services, and reduce adverse effects and likelihood of future relapse. The patient and involved caregivers should be educated on the timeline of symptom response, possible medication adverse effects and their management, importance of adherence, and recognizing early signs of symptom recurrence. Risk for relapse is highest within the first 6 months post initial psychotic episode. Therefore, medications should be maintained for at least 6 months at the dose found to be effective in reducing positive symptoms during the acute phase.[45] Patients and caregivers should be counseled that partial response, such as decreased volume, intensity, or frequency of auditory hallucinations, should not be considered a failure of treatment. Residual symptoms can persist beyond the acute and stabilization phases, but may remit with maintenance treatment.

STABLE PHASE

The main focus of the stable phase is quality of life and functional recovery. This is achieved through ensuring optimized treatment of symptoms, minimizing risk of adverse effects, and psychosocial interventions. The question of how long antipsychotics need to be continued is often raised by patients. Antipsychotics have been shown to significantly reduce rates of relapse at one year versus placebo.[46] Therefore, maintenance antipsychotic treatment should be continued for at least one year in all patients recovering from a psychotic episode. Caveats to this include intolerable adverse effects to the antipsychotic or uncertainty of the diagnosis of schizophrenia. Lifelong treatment is recommended in patients who have experienced multiple episodes of psychosis, at least two episodes within 5 years, or those who pose a significant risk to themselves or others when symptoms are left untreated. A slow, cautious taper off antipsychotics can be considered after one year in first-episode patients with close follow-up established.[45] Routine monitoring for adverse effects, especially EPS and metabolic syndrome, is recommended during the stable phase. Patients may not connect an adverse effect to their medications, particularly a somatic complaint when the main therapeutic target of their medication is in the CNS, so education and close follow-up are needed. The nonpharmacologic aspects of treatment are an important adjunct to pharmacologic management in functional recovery. Psychosocial interventions include assertive community treatment teams for high-risk patients, vocational training or supported employment, and cognitive behavioral therapy. Adjunctive treatments for comorbid conditions, such as depression and anxiety, should also be addressed during this phase.

Nonpharmacologic Interventions

In addition to medication-based treatments, there are a variety of nonpharmacologic treatments that have also been found to be useful in the treatment of schizophrenia. Most patients will benefit from a combination, multidisciplinary approach to treatment. Treatment guidelines for schizophrenia recommend a treatment plan that includes both pharmacologic and nonpharmacologic treatment.[45] Nonpharmacologic interventions may include individual or group psychological therapy as well as family therapy, cognitive skills training, vocational skills training, and others. When utilized, these interventions have increased patient understanding of their illness, decreased patient symptoms and relapse rates, and improved social and occupational functioning.

Selection of one of these interventions is based upon the patient's level of acuity and specific needs, but should be considered during all phases of the illness. For example, a patient having an acute episode of psychosis might not be appropriate for cognitive or vocational skills training, but might benefit from individual therapy to help develop insight into their illness and understand why they are being treated. During an acute phase, other, more simplistic interventions can also play a key role. For example, inpatient settings may utilize techniques to minimize stimulation or stress for patients, particularly those who are agitated or potentially aggressive. Group therapy sessions can assist patients with social interaction, something that might be difficult for many patients.

As the patient moves from an acute phase into a stabilization or stable phase, addition of skills training could be considered. Many patients will have lingering negative and cognitive symptoms that might not fully respond to pharmacotherapy. Cognitive skills training can assist with both of these areas, helping patients to overcome functional deficits arising from these symptoms. Vocational skills training can teach patients a variety of skills to prepare them to re-enter the workforce, even if only in a minor role.

Family therapy can be helpful for both patient and family. Many families are greatly affected when a family member is diagnosed with schizophrenia. Improving family understanding of the illness and how to interact appropriately with the patient can be of great impact to all involved. Additionally, the stress on the family can be mitigated through family therapy and assistance programs.

Pharmacists can also play a role in nonpharmacologic treatment by assisting with patient education (particularly in regard to medications) and patient adherence to medication. Assistance with adverse effects to medications is also an area in which pharmacists can play a role.

CASE 85-1, QUESTION 3: What are the management goals for J.J.?

First and foremost is to ensure J.J.'s safety. While not serious, she has already injured herself by punching her walls. She is also very argumentative due to her paranoia, which could inadvertently lead to an altercation. A reduction in J.J.'s symptoms is also desired, ideally leading to an improvement in her functionality and insight into her illness. In light of J.J.'s symptoms and lack of insight into her illness, she will most likely require hospitalization to both ensure her safety and effectively treat her symptoms.

CASE 85-1, QUESTION 4: What nonpharmacologic treatment would you recommend for J.J. at this time?

During the acute phase, especially while J.J. still displays prominent positive symptoms, nonpharmacologic treatment should center on stress reduction and education on her illness. By reducing her stress, the goal is that J.J.'s paranoia and agitation will decrease, allowing her to more meaningfully engage in treatment. Illness education can be accomplished through both individual and group therapy and education sessions. As J.J. moves from an acute phase into a stabilization phase, more specific interventions can be started, such as vocational skills training, depending upon her need and her level of functionality at that time.

J.J. would also benefit from medication education, such as from a pharmacist, once she is more stable in order to better understand her medications and any potential adverse effects.

CASE 85-1, QUESTION 5: How should J.J. be best communicated with by the staff treating her at this time? What recommendations would you provide her family and friends for communicating with her, both currently and once she is sent home?

The staff should attempt to use methods of communication that will not agitate J.J. or increase her paranoia. This includes both verbal and nonverbal (body language) communication. If J.J. does become paranoid or agitated, she should be approached with calmness in an attempt to deescalate the situation. Directly challenging her hallucinations and delusions will most likely only increase her paranoia, so this should be avoided. If possible, speak to J.J. during times when she is calm and having fewer symptoms and inquire about what methods she would prefer employed to calm her down when she does become agitated, such as being put in a room alone to relax, listening to music, conversing with a staff member, etc.

J.J.'s family and friends should be educated about her illness to help them understand how to avoid upsetting her and potentially increasing her symptoms, especially during the acute phase. Avoidance of topics that would make her upset would also be appropriate. Once J.J. is sent home, they should interact with her as they normally would, but being aware that her symptoms could return at any time and they should be vigilant for this. If they observe any significant change in her status, they should attempt to get J.J. to a medical provider to evaluate her situation.

Assessment

The issues and conducting a differential diagnosis of schizophrenia have been previously discussed above. Patients are assessed for the severity of their symptomatology after diagnosis using information from direct assessment via patient interview, discussions with family and friends of the patient as well as treatment staff, and review of the medical records. There are no laboratory tests to measure progress in schizophrenia at this time. It is important to obtain laboratory baseline monitoring tests that can be relevant for the differential diagnosis and for the monitoring of adverse effects of medications. First, it is important to obtain a complete psychiatric and medical history including all past medications. It is suggested that patients receive a physical examination and that clinical laboratory tests of thyroid, liver, and renal function be obtained. A complete cell blood count with differential as well as a urinalysis and urine toxicology screen (if drug abuse is suspected) should be obtained. A fasting blood glucose and serum hemoglobin A1c (HbA1c) level is useful considering the high rate of type 2 diabetes prevalent in patients with schizophrenia. Obtaining an electrocardiogram is also useful, especially if the patient is over 40 years of age or likely to receive a medication with significant QT_c prolongation effects.

The most prevalent way to record the results of a clinical assessment in the patient with schizophrenia would be via the mental status examination.[47] If a patient is to be treated in a clinical study, schizophrenic symptomatology may be assessed using the Positive and Negative Symptoms Scale (PANSS),[48] the Brief Psychiatric Rating Scale (BPRS)[49], and Clinical Global Impression (CGI) scale. Adverse effects to antipsychotic treatment can be assessed using instruments such as the Abnormal Involuntary Movements Scale (AIMS) or Dyskinesia Identification System Condensed User Scale (DISCUS) for tardive dyskinesia,[50] or the Simpson-Angus Rating Scale for drug-induced parkinsonism, and general adverse effects can be recorded via the Treatment

Emergent Symptoms Scale (TESS).[51] These are all scales suitable to measure the severity of these symptoms, but are not used as diagnostic instruments.

Pharmacotherapy Interventions

ANTIPSYCHOTICS

Classification and Nomenclature of the Antipsychotics

The first effective antipsychotic medication used in western medicine was chlorpromazine, a low-potency sedating "typical" antipsychotic first developed in 1951 to augment anesthesia, and was termed by its inventor Laborit to be a "vegetative stabilizer."[52] While its introduction resulted in a sharp decrease in the number of hospitalized patients with schizophrenia, it was imperfect in that it caused adverse effects such as drug-induced parkinsonism, acute dystonias, sedation, anticholinergic effects, and orthostasis. The knowledge that D_2 antagonism was a key in making effective agents for treating schizophrenia led to the development of a plethora of new agents, some of which were much more specific in selectively antagonizing these receptors. The medications with greater dopamine specificity tended to have fewer effects on other neurotransmitter systems (Fig. 85-1). Therefore, these "high-potency" first-generation antipsychotics (FGAs), such as haloperidol or fluphenazine, were less likely to cause related adverse effects such as sedation, increased appetite, dry mouth, constipation, and orthostasis than "low-potency" agents, such as chlorpromazine and thioridazine. However, high-potency FGAs have a greater propensity to cause acute dystonias and drug-induced parkinsonism than the low-potency agents. The middle-potency agents, such as loxapine, molindone, and perphenazine, have more moderate adverse effects. These medications have other unique properties that differentiate them. For example, molindone was found to induce modest weight loss,[53,54] and loxapine was thought to be somewhat atypical in its effects on serotonergic receptors. These recognized properties helped lead to the development of the second-generation antipsychotics (SGAs) or "atypical antipsychotics."[55]

The first SGA, clozapine, differed dramatically in its pharmacology from previous agents. It is a very potent antagonist of serotonin-2a (5-HT_{2a}) and serotonin-2c (5-HT_{2c}) receptors. It was later determined that the ability to antagonize serotonergic receptors was critical to creating other new "atypical" agents that could act in a manner similar to clozapine, but without its critically serious adverse effect profile. Clozapine was shown to have robust effectiveness in treating resistant schizophrenia[56], to cause agranulocytosis in about 1% to 2%[57] and to induce seizures in 6% of those taking it at higher dosages,[58] possesses nuisance side effects such as sialorrhea and constipation, and is even associated with myocarditis.[59–61] Because clozapine is restricted to only the

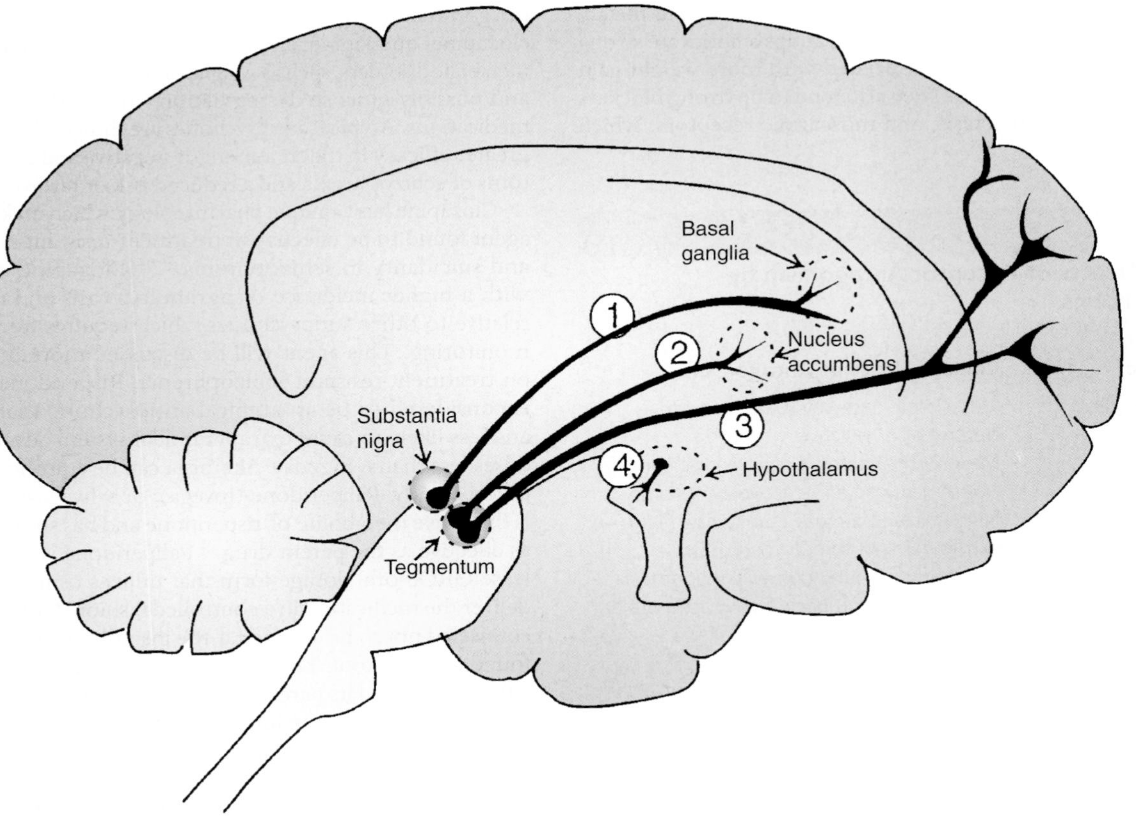

Figure 85-1 Four dopamine pathways in the brain. The neuroanatomy of dopamine neuronal pathways in the brain can explain both the therapeutic effects and the side effects of the known antipsychotic agents. (1) The nigrostriatal pathway projects from the substantia nigra to the basal ganglia and is thought to control movements. (2) The mesolimbic pathway projects from the midbrain ventral tegmental area to the nucleus accumbens, a part of the limbic system of the brain thought to be involved in many behaviors, such as pleasurable sensations and the powerful euphoria of drugs of abuse, as well as delusions and hallucinations of psychosis. (3) A pathway related to the mesolimbic pathway is the mesocortical pathway. It also projects from the midbrain ventral tegmental area, but sends its axons to the limbic cortex, where it may have a role in mediating positive and negative psychotic symptoms or cognitive side effects of neuroleptic antipsychotic medications. (4) The fourth dopamine pathway of interest is the one that controls prolactin secretion, called the tuberoinfundibular pathway. It projects from the hypothalamus to the anterior pituitary gland.

treatment-resistant or antipsychotic-intolerant patient, newer agents that were introduced, such as risperidone, olanzapine, quetiapine, and ziprasidone, were used with initial excitement. This excitement was tempered with caution when it was discovered that these agents could also be associated with obesity, hypertriglyceridemia, and even the onset of type 2 diabetes mellitus. Later, somewhat unique agents were introduced with possible advantages such as aripiprazole, lurasidone, paliperidone, iloperidone, asenapine, brexpiprazole, and cariprazine. The terms FGA and SGA will be utilized for clarity throughout the chapter.

General Differentiating Characteristics of Antipsychotics

It is sometimes useful to conceptualize the different antipsychotic medications in terms of their action at different receptor subtypes or by potency (Table 85-4). The second-generation antipsychotics (SGAs) are more potent at blocking 5-HT_{2a} serotonergic receptors than they are at blocking D_2 receptors. The SGAs are generally less likely to cause drug-induced parkinsonism and tardive dyskinesia than first-generation medications, but some of these agents may be more prone to cause metabolic issues than the FGAs.[52] Low-potency antipsychotics are often given in hundreds of milligrams per day and tend to have greater antihistaminic, anticholinergic, and α-1 antagonist effects than their high-potency (roughly 1–20 mg daily) counterparts.

Typical Antipsychotics or First-Generation Antipsychotics

Low-potency phenothiazine antipsychotics include the prototype antipsychotic chlorpromazine as well as thioridazine and its metabolite mesoridazine. Low-potency typical antipsychotics are strong histamine-1 blockers and are associated with more weight gain than the high-potency ones. They also tend to be strong blockers of α-1, inducing orthostasis, and muscarinic receptors, which results in dry mouth, blurred vision, and constipation. Thioridazine is distinctive in that it can cause a retinopathy in doses over 800 mg daily. Moreover, it has received a black box warning as it can cause prolonged QT_c intervals that can be clinically significant, especially if a 2D6 P450 isoenzyme antagonist (which increases its serum levels) is also being used.[63] Use of thioridazine is restricted to treatment-resistant patients due to these proarrhythmic effects, and use in clinical practice is uncommon.

Common middle-potency typical antipsychotics include molindone, loxapine, and perphenazine. Molindone is the only antipsychotic associated with weight loss.[53,54] Loxapine is regaining use due to its inhalation dose form, and perphenazine has had a resurgence in use of sorts due to it being the chosen typical antipsychotic in the CATIE-1 trial.[64] These agents tend to fall in between the high- and low-potency agents in terms of adverse effects.

The high-potency typical antipsychotics are very selective for D_2 receptor blockade, thus causing fewer adverse effects related to antihistaminic, anticholinergic, or α-1 receptor blocking effects. However, they are more likely to induce adverse extrapyramidal effects such as dystonia, drug-induced parkinsonism, and akathisia than the lower-potency typical agents. Their availability as long-lasting depot injections of haloperidol and fluphenazine and reduced rate of adverse metabolic effects encourage their continued use. Other, less often utilized high-potency agents include thiothixene and trifluoperazine (Table 85-5).

Table 85-4
Clinical Effects of Receptor Antagonism by Antipsychotics

Receptor (Subtype)	Clinical Effect of Antagonism
Dopamine (D_2)	Mesolimbic pathway (basal ganglia)—treatment of positive symptoms Mesocortical pathway (prefrontal cortex)—may worsen negative symptoms Nigrostriatal pathway (substantia nigra)—extrapyramidal symptoms (EPS) Tuberoinfundibular pathway (hypothalamus–anterior pituitary)—increased prolactin release
Serotonin (5-HT_{2a})	Treatment of negative symptoms; increased dopamine release in prefrontal cortex; may reduce mesolimbic dopamine release
Serotonin (5-HT_{2c})	Implicated in antipsychotic-associated weight gain
Muscarinic (M_1)	Anticholinergic side effects (dry mouth, constipation, urinary retention, blurred vision, hot/dry skin, memory impairment); sedation
Histamine (H_1)	Increased appetite, sedation
Alpha (α_1)	Orthostatic hypotension

Atypical or Second-Generation Antipsychotics

SGAs are agents that exert more effects on antagonism of 5-HT_{2a} subreceptors than on D_2 receptors and cause dramatically less drug-induced extrapyramidal symptoms. The SGAs such as clozapine, quetiapine, and olanzapine are more likely to induce metabolic disorders, such as weight gain,[65] hypertriglyceridemia,[66–70] and possibly glucose dysregulation[71] than other antipsychotic medications. Atypical antipsychotics are thought by many to have greater efficacy in the treatment of negative and cognitive symptoms of schizophrenia and a reduced risk of tardive dyskinesia.[62]

Clozapine has a unique pharmacology which makes it the only agent found to be effective in treatment-resistant schizophrenia and suicidality in schizophrenia.[56,62] Clozapine is associated with a higher incidence of agranulocytosis and neutropenia relative to other antipsychotics which requires frequent serum monitoring. This agent will be discussed more in the section on treatment-resistant schizophrenia. Risperidone (Risperdal) is considered to be an atypical antipsychotic that is effective and less likely to cause extrapyramidal system adverse effects at doses less than 6 mg/day. Akathisia can be a problem especially in the elderly. Paliperidone (Invega), or 9-hydroxyl risperidone, is the active metabolite of risperidone and has shown itself to be as effective as the parent drug.[72] Paliperidone is a controlled-release OROS oral dosage form that utilizes osmotic pressure to deliver the medication in a controlled fashion. Patients should be counseled not to be alarmed if the insoluble outer tablet shell is found in their stool. The long-acting injectable dosage forms of paliperidone and its parent compound risperidone are discussed in the section regarding long-acting agents.

Olanzapine (Zyprexa) is an atypical antipsychotic that is very effective, but it can cause significant weight gain with related glucose dysregulation as well as increased serum triglycerides.[68,73] Doses may need to be adjusted in smokers due to the induction of the cytochrome p450 1A2 isoenzyme system by the polycyclic aromatic hydrocarbons (PAHs) in cigarette smoke.[74] Quetiapine (Seroquel) is a low-potency D_2 antagonist.[64] Due to its minimal risk of drug-induced movement disorders, it is often utilized in patients with psychosis in Parkinson disease prior to use of clozapine.[75] It is recommended that patients be counseled regarding diet and exercise prior to and during the use of these agents and

Table 85-5
First-Generation Antipsychotics (FGAs)[279–287]

Medication Name (Generic/Brand); Potency—Chlorpromazine Equivalents; Class	Dosage Forms	Adult Dosing Schedules	Dose Adjustments
Haloperidol (Haldol) High—2 Butyrophenone	Tablet: 0.5, 1, 2, 5, 10, 20 mg Oral solution: 2 mg/mL Injectable (immediate-release): 5 mg/mL Injectable (long-acting): 50, 100 mg/mL	Initial: 0.5–5 mg BID or TID (depending on symptom severity) Usual range: 5–40 mg	Renal: No specific recommendations Hepatic: No specific recommendations
Fluphenazine (Prolixin) High—2 Phenothiazine	Tablet: 1, 2.5, 5, 10 Oral Elixir: 2.5 mg/mL Oral Solution: 5 mg/mL Injectable (immediate-release): 2.5 mg/mL Injectable (long-acting): 25 mg/mL	Initial: 2.5–10 mg q6–8 hours Usual range: 1–40 mg/day	Renal: Use with caution (nondialyzable) Hepatic: Use with caution
Thiothixene (Navane) High—4 Thioxanthene	Capsule: 1, 2, 5, 10 mg	Initial: 6–10 mg daily (divided doses) Usual range: 5–60 mg/day	Renal: Use with caution (nondialyzable) Hepatic: Consider dose reduction
Trifluoperazine (Stelazine) High—5 Phenothiazine	Tablet: 1, 2, 5, 10 mg	Initial: 2–5 mg BID Usual range: 15–20 mg/day	Renal: Use with caution (nondialyzable) Hepatic: Consider dose reduction
Perphenazine (Trilafon) Mid—8–10 Phenothiazine	Tablet: 2, 4, 8, 16 mg	Initial: 4–8 mg TID Usual range: 8–64 mg/day	Renal: No specific recommendations Hepatic: Consider dose reduction
Loxapine (Loxitane) Mid—10 Dibenzoxazepine	Capsule: 5, 10, 25, 50 mg Inhalation powder: 10 mg	Initial: 10 mg BID Usual range: 20–250 mg/day (PO)	Renal: No specific recommendations Hepatic: No specific recommendations
Chlorpromazine (Thorazine) Low—100 Phenothiazine	Tablet: 10, 25, 50, 100, 200 mg Injection (immediate-release): 25 mg/mL	Initial: 100–200 mg/day in divided doses; increase 20–50 mg/day q3–4 days as indicated	Renal: No specific recommendations Hepatic: Consider dose reduction
Thioridazine (Mellaril) Low—100 Phenothiazine	Tablet: 10, 25, 50, 100 mg	Initial: 50–100 mg TID with gradual dose increases Usual range: 50–800 mg/day	Renal: Use with caution (nondialyzable) Hepatic: Consider dose reduction

clozapine. Ziprasidone (Geodon) should be administered with at least 500 calories to ensure sufficient absorption.[76] It causes little weight gain or dyslipidemia and has minimal anticholinergic or extrapyramidal adverse effects. Although there were initial warnings about cardiac conduction delays (prolonged QT interval), there have been sparse reports linking the medication to death due to this concern.[77–79] An electrocardiogram prior to and during treatment is advised.[80]

Aripiprazole (Abilify) should be dosed in the morning as it may be activating in some patients due to its partial D_2 receptor agonism. Typical adverse effects include nausea, vomiting, and insomnia in the first weeks of treatment. It has a lower risk of weight gain, dyslipidemia, and QT delays, and can actually cause decreases in serum prolactin and triglycerides. In fact, it has been used as augmentation to remedy hyperprolactinemia induced by other antipsychotics.[81–83] It also seems to have a low risk of EPS. Although aripiprazole's unique differential effect on dopaminergic systems can be beneficial, dopamine-3 (D_3) partial agonism may induce an increase in risky, reward-based behaviors, such as gambling.[84,85] Brexpiprazole (Rexulti) is a recent addition to the antipsychotic armamentarium that showed superiority to placebo in both key clinical trials (at 4 mg daily) with pharmacologic and therapeutic similarities to aripiprazole.[86,87] It is a partial agonist at D_2 receptors and serotonin 5-HT_{1a} and antagonist at 5-HT_{2a} and noradrenergic α-1b and α-2c receptors.[88] It is metabolized by both 2D6 and 3A4 hepatic isoenzyme systems, and dose reductions are recommended if these systems are inhibited.[89] Cariprazine (Vraylar) is pharmacologically similar to aripiprazole and brexpiprazole in that it is an antagonist at the D_2 receptors and 5-HT_{2A} receptors and a "partial" agonist at 5-HT_{1A} receptors. However, it has about a 10-fold greater affinity for the D_3 receptor than the D_2 receptor.[90] It is unclear what differences will result from its stronger effects on D_3 receptors.[91–93]

Iloperidone (Fanapt) is less likely to cause drug-induced parkinsonism, akathisia, and hyperprolactinemia than the typical antipsychotics, but has a risk of moderate weight gain, orthostasis, and the potential to cause QT interval prolongation that can be of concern in some patients.[94,95] Asenapine (Saphris) needs to be administered sublingually for rapid and adequate absorption. It has an absolute bioavailability of 35% when taken sublingually and less than 2% when swallowed. The patient should be counseled not to eat or drink for 10 minutes after the sublingual administration. The most common adverse reactions (≥5% and at least twice the rate of placebo) are somnolence, dizziness, extrapyramidal symptoms other than akathisia, and weight gain.[96] Lurasidone (Latuda) is an effective agent with a low propensity to cause drug-induced parkinsonism, metabolic complications, or QT_c prolongation. It needs to be taken with food (about 350 calories or more) for adequate absorption. The most common adverse events associated with lurasidone treatment are nausea, vomiting, akathisia, dizziness, and sedation (Table 85-6).[97]

Mechanism of Drug Action

All antipsychotic medications have at least some D_2 antagonistic effects. These antipsychotic medications have been divided into two major classes depending on whether or not they substantially antagonize 5-HT_{2a} receptors as well as dopaminergic ones. Although activity in attenuating dopamine transmission in the mesolimbic pathway is seen as being beneficial in decreasing the severity of positive schizophrenic symptomatology, decreased activity of dopamine receptors in mesocortical pathways (sometimes due to antipsychotic medication) may relate to the severity of negative symptoms. Antagonism of 5-HT_2 receptors in the striatum by SGAs may balance decreased dopaminergic neurotransmission and decrease their relative propensity to cause tardive dyskinesia.[98]

Selection of an Antipsychotic

Antipsychotic choice is based upon a number of factors, many of which are patient specific. In making a selection, consider such patient factors as treatment history (if any), medical comorbidities and concurrent medications, patient preferences, and potential cost concerns. If the patient has a known history of being treated with antipsychotics, this can help guide current selection. Previous positive response to an antipsychotic is a good indicator of future response, just as previous lack of response would recommend against trying that agent in the future. History of adverse effects to particular agents is useful also. If a patient is known to have had an adverse event to a specific agent in the past that would preclude them from receiving this agent again (including a patient's stated preference for this reason), then this will help guide current medication selection. Additionally, if an adverse effect led to medication discontinuation or poor adherence in the past, an antipsychotic should be selected that has a minimal risk of causing that adverse effect in the future. If information about a patient is not available, particularly in newly diagnosed patients with no prior treatment, medication history for a first-degree relative with schizophrenia may be useful in selecting an agent for the patient in a similar manner.

One area of debate has been selecting between FGAs and SGAs. Studies comparing the two classes head-to-head have shown similar efficacy rates between them.[99,100] Where the older agents are more prone to cause movement disorders, such as extrapyramidal syndromes (EPSs), the newer agents are thought to be more prone to causing metabolic disturbances in patients. Although SGAs are widely considered first choice in clinical practice,[101] most treatment guidelines now consider either FGAs or SGAs (other than clozapine) as potential first-line choices for treatment, depending upon the patient factors described above.[102,103]

CASE 85-1, QUESTION 6: Which type of antipsychotic medication would you recommend for J.J. at this time? What factors would you use to select a treatment regimen for her?

As J.J. has never been treated with an antipsychotic before, most any type is potentially viable as a treatment. Atypical antipsychotics would most likely be preferable. Typical antipsychotics, while efficacious, might lead to significant extrapyramidal or other adverse effects that she might not tolerate well, possibly leading to nonadherence. Also, with chronic usage typical antipsychotics (FGAs) are more likely to cause tardive dyskinesia than SGAS. As she is young and fairly healthy, we would also want to select an atypical antipsychotic with minimal long-term risks of metabolic adverse effects, such as weight gain and glucose irregularities. Pharmacoeconomic considerations should also be taken into account, as some of the atypical antipsychotics are available generically and some are not.

CASE 85-1, QUESTION 7: What pharmacologic agents should be considered first to treat JJ considering her acute symptoms?

In light of J.J.'s acute psychotic symptoms and agitation, a combination of both antipsychotics and adjunctive agents should be considered at this time. Although antipsychotics are generally the mainstay of schizophrenia treatment, they may not reduce symptoms quickly enough. Benzodiazepines may also be useful, especially during periods of increased agitation. Use of adjunctive medications to treat any adverse effects, such as EPS, may also be needed. Depending upon J.J.'s compliance to oral medications or during any periods of increased agitation, intramuscular (IM) injections of medications, including antipsychotics, benzodiazepines, and side effect medications, may need to be utilized acutely.

EFFICACY

Although there are numerous studies demonstrating the efficacy of current antipsychotic medications in comparison with placebo and accepted treatment, more attention has been paid of late to effectiveness studies comparing currently available antipsychotics. These effectiveness trials are intended to show the comparative value of these agents in situations that are more comparable to routine clinical care by utilizing less stringent eligibility criteria, longer duration, prospective design, and large sample size.[104] Still, they are randomized double-blind trials using intent-to-treat analysis just as if they were efficacy studies. Interpreting these studies is a help in bridging the chasm between studies in ideal populations and routine clinical care.

One of the landmark effectiveness trials comparing antipsychotic agents is the National Institute of Mental Health (NIMH) funded Clinical Antipsychotic Trials of Intervention Effectiveness (CATIE) trial. The first phase of the CATIE trial compared the SGAs quetiapine ($n = 329$), ziprasidone ($n = 183$), risperidone ($n = 333$), and olanzapine ($n = 330$) with the middle-potency FGA perphenazine ($n = 257$). The main outcome variable was time to discontinuation of the antipsychotic for any cause. Overall, 74% of the patients discontinued treatment over the 18-month course of the study. This study showed significantly less medication discontinuation ($p < .001$) in olanzapine-treated patients (64%) than in those receiving quetiapine (82%) or risperidone (74%). After adjusting for multiple comparisons, the difference between olanzapine and ziprasidone or perphenazine did not reach significance. When analyzed separately, the discontinuation rates due to intolerability were substantially higher in the olanzapine-treated patients, but there was a significantly greater time to discontinuation with olanzapine compared to quetiapine, risperidone, and perphenazine. The lowered number of patients in the ziprasidone group reduced the power (and thus

Table 85-6
Second-Generation Antipsychotics (SGAs)[288–296]

Medication Name(Generic/Brand)	Dosage Forms	Adult Dosing Schedules	Dose Adjustments
Aripiprazole (Abilify)	Tablet: 2, 5, 10, 15, 20, 30 mg ODT: 10, 15 mg Injectable (short-acting): 9.75 mg/1.3 mL Injectable (long-acting): 300 mg/vial and 400 mg/vial Solution: 1 mg/mL	Initial: 10–15 mg/day, titrate at 2 week intervals Usual range: 15–40 mg Max: 30 mg/day	Renal/Hepatic: No dose adjustment necessary
Asenapine (Saphris)	Sublingual tablet: 5, 10 mg	Initial: 5 mg BID (no benefit demonstrated with higher doses)	Renal/Hepatic: No dose adjustments necessary; use not recommended in severe hepatic impairment
Brexpiprazole (Rexulti)	Tablet: 0.25, 0.5, 1, 2, 3, 4 mg	Initial: 1 mg days 1–4; 2 mg days 5–7; 4 mg day 8 Usual range: 4 mg daily	Renal: 3 mg max in CrCl < 60 mL/minute Hepatic: 3 mg max in Child-Pugh score ≥ 7
Cariprazine (Vraylar)	Capsule: 1.5, 3, 4.5, 6 mg	Initial: 1.5 mg day 1, inc. to 3 mg day 2, inc. in 1.5–3 mg increments as needed Usual range: 1.5–6 mg	Renal: Not recommended in CrCl <30 mL/minute Hepatic: Not recommended in severe impairment (Child-Pugh score 10–15)
Clozapine (Clozaril)	Tablet: 12.5, 25, 50, 100, 200 mg ODT: 12.5, 25, 100 mg	Initial: 12.5–25 mg/day, titrate by 25–50 mg/day to target of 300–450 mg/day Usual range: 350–600 mg Max: 900 mg/day	Renal/Hepatic: No specific recommendations
Iloperidone (Fanapt)	Tablet: 1, 2, 4, 6, 8, 10, 12 mg	Initial: 1 mg BID, increase by 2 mg/day to target dose of 12–24 mg/day Max: 24 mg/day	Renal: No adjustments necessary Hepatic: Use not recommended
Lurasidone (Latuda)	Tablet: 20, 40, 80, 120 mg	Initial: 40 mg daily taken with food Usual range: 40–160 mg/day Max: 160 mg/day	Renal: Initial dose of 20 mg/day and max of 80 mg/day in moderate–severe impairment Hepatic: Initial dose of 20 mg/day and max of 80 mg/day in moderate impairment and max of 40 mg in severe impairment
Olanzapine (Zyprexa)	Tablet: 2.5, 5, 7.5, 10, 15, 20 mg ODT: 5, 10, 15, 20 mg Injection (short-acting): 10mg/vial (5mg/ml after reconstitution) Injection (long-acting): 210, 300, 405 mg/vial	Initial: 2.5–10 mg/day Usual range: 20–40 mg/day Max: FDA recommended max is 20 mg/day	Renal: Initial dose of 5 mg/day should be considered Hepatic: Childs Pugh Class A and B, no adjustment necessary
Paliperidone (Invega)	Tablet (ER): 1.5, 3, 6, 9 mg Injectable (long-acting): 39, 78, 117, 156, 234 mg prefilled syringes	Initial: 6 mg/day; increases should not exceed 3 mg every 5 days Usual range: 9–12 mg Max: 12 mg/day	Renal: CrCl 50–79 mL/minute: initiate at 3 mg, max 6 mg/day CrCl 10–49 mL/minute: initiate at 1.5 mg, max 3 mg/day CrCl <10 ml/minute: use not recommended Hepatic: Child-Pugh Class A and B no adjustment required

(continued)

Table 85-6

Second-Generation Antipsychotics (SGAs)[288–296] (*continued*)

Medication Name(Generic/Brand)	Dosage Forms	Adult Dosing Schedules	Dose Adjustments
Quetiapine (Seroquel)	Tablet (IR): 25, 50, 100, 200, 300, 400 mg Tablet (ER): 50, 150, 200, 300, 400 mg	Initial (IR): 25 mg BID; titrate in 25–50 mg increments, given 2–3 times daily, to a target range of 300–400 mg/day by day 4; further adjustments at 25–50 mg increments with at least 2 days between adjustments; usual range 300–750 mg/day Initial (ER): 300 mg/day; target 400–800 mg/day Max: 800 mg/day	Renal: No specific recommendations Hepatic: Initiate IR tablets at 25 mg/day and increase by 25–50 mg/day increments/day; initiate ER tablets at 50 mg/day and increase by 50 mg/day increments
Risperidone (Risperdal)	Tablet: 0.25, 0.5, 1, 2, 3, 4 mg ODT: 0.5, 1, 2, 3, 4 Solution: 1 mg/mL Injectable (long-acting): 12.5, 25, 37.5, 50 mg	Initial: 1–2 mg/day; usual 4–6 mg/day Usual range: 4–8 mg/day Max: 16 mg/day	Renal/Hepatic: Recommend initial dose of 0.5 mg BID; may increase dose 0.5 mg BID; increases above 1.5 mg BID should be completed over 1 week intervals
Ziprasidone (Geodon)	Capsule: 20, 40, 60, 80 mg Injectable (short-acting): 20 mg/mL	Initial: 20 mg BID with food; dose adjustments at ≥48 hour intervals Max: 80 mg BID	Renal: No adj. necessary in mild-mod. Impairment use IM with caution Hepatic: No adj. necessary in mild-mod. impairment

chance to find difference) for comparisons with this agent and the others. The 18-month duration of the study could not yield information on the long-term effects of these agents in causing tardive dyskinesia or metabolic disorders.[64]

Patients who discontinued treatment were eligible for enrollment in phase two of the CATIE to receive a different antipsychotic if they dropped primarily for lack of tolerance or efficacy. Those primarily not responding in the earlier phase could instead enter in the phase two trial in which there was a clozapine treatment arm.[105] In the lack of tolerability arm, patients assigned to olanzapine ($n = 68$) or risperidone ($n = 70$) showed longer time to discontinuation rates than those receiving either quetiapine ($n = 63$) or ziprasidone ($n = 135$).[106] In the poor responder study arm, patients receiving clozapine (n = 45) showed a significantly lower ($p < .05$) time to discontinuation of treatment than those receiving either olanzapine ($n = 17$), quetiapine ($n = 14$), or risperidone ($n = 14$).[107] The third phase of the CATIE trial involved with the 270 patients who discontinued treatment in the earlier phases, who went on to receive either aripiprazole, clozapine, olanzapine, perphenazine, quetiapine, or risperidone. The lack of power made it difficult to show any differences in effectiveness between these agents, and in this open trial few patients received either perphenazine ($n = 4$) or fluphenazine decanoate ($n = 9$).[108] Of note, at each subsequent phase of CATIE, statistical power was reduced as compared to the original study due to subject attrition, thereby increasing type II error.

Another often cited study is the Cost Utility of the Latest Antipsychotic Drugs in Schizophrenia Study (CUtLASS 1) in which 227 patients were randomized to receive either FGAs ($n = 118$) or to be treated with a SGA ($n = 109$). This pragmatic, nonindustry-funded study was powered only to compare the overall differences between FGA and SGA groups and not the individual antipsychotics themselves. The hypothesis that second-generation medications would have an advantage on any quality of life measures over first-generation medications was disproven.[109] The CUtLASS 2 study was similarly designed and compared clozapine to other SGAs in patients who did not respond sufficiently to two prior treatments. Patients on clozapine showed significant improvements on PANSS scores ($p < .01$) and felt they did much better ($p < .05$), and there was a trend for improvement ($p = .08$) on their quality of life as measured on the QLS.[109,110]

SGAs have also shown better response and remission rates than haloperidol in first-episode patients.[111] Meta-analyses and related techniques have been utilized to attempt to overcome limitations of low power in comparative antipsychotic efficacy trials. One meta-analysis looked at 150 double-blind RCTs in over 20,000 patients and found only amisulpride (not available in USA.), clozapine, olanzapine, and risperidone to be more effective than the FGAs. The SGAs showed fewer EPS and, with the notable exception of aripiprazole and ziprasidone, caused more weight gain than haloperidol. However, there were no significant differences in weight gain between the low-potency typical antipsychotics such as chlorpromazine and the second-generation agents.[112]

One controversial topic not clearly covered by effectiveness trials or meta-analysis is the use of combinations of antipsychotic medications.[113] Although combination use is a relatively common practice,[114] it is not recommended due to the paucity of evidence for its safety and efficacy[115,116]; in fact, combination antipsychotic therapy is often targeted by quality improvement programs.[117] Although there are situations (i.e., adding aripiprazole to a patient stabilized on risperidone to attenuate hyperprolactinemia) in which this use can be logical and beneficial,[28,113,118,119] there are other times when treatment-resistant patients should receive alternative approved effective pharmacotherapy with clozapine.[120]

DOSAGE FORMS

Antipsychotics are commercially available in a variety of dosage forms to allow for different treatment situations and settings. The most common forms consist of orally administered products such as tablets/capsules (both short-acting and long-acting forms), orally disintegrating tablets (ODTs), and oral liquid solutions/suspensions. Many antipsychotics are also available as injectables, some as short-acting IM forms and some as long-acting IM forms. Selection of an appropriate dose form can depend upon factors such as the severity of the patient's illness and risk of imminent harm to themselves or others, willingness or ability to take medications, and treatment setting.

Alternate Oral Dose Forms

Although most every antipsychotic is available as a traditional tablet or capsule, many are available in other oral dosage forms. In an effort to help with adherence, several antipsychotics are available as either oral liquids or ODTs. The SGAs such as aripiprazole, risperidone, and ziprasidone are available as oral liquids, which may be useful in patients who have a hard time swallowing traditional tablets (or won't swallow them) or to achieve more specific dosing, such as might be needed for pediatric or geriatric patients. ODTs are formulated to dissolve rapidly when placed on the tongue, needing only for the patient to swallow their own saliva to obtain medication absorption in the gut. This formulation is particularly useful in the inpatient setting when "cheeking" or nonadherence is suspected. Aripiprazole, clozapine, olanzapine, and risperidone are available as ODTs, and asenapine is available only as a sublingually dissolving tablet.

Short-Acting Injectables

The short-acting injectable formulations of antipsychotics are frequently utilized in the acute phase of illness. Patients presenting to psychiatric emergency services are often in crisis and can be at risk of harm to themselves or others. If nonpharmacologic de-escalation techniques fail and the patient refuses PO medication, short-acting IM injections are effective in rapidly targeting agitation related to psychosis. IM formulations avoid first-pass metabolism and thus are approximately 2 to 4 times as potent as oral formulations and reach peak concentrations within 30 to 60 minutes.[121] The FGAs such as haloperidol, fluphenazine, and chlorpromazine, as well as the SGAs such as olanzapine, ziprasidone, and aripiprazole are currently available in short-acting IM formulations.

There are currently no head-to-head trials comparing the efficacy of the available short-acting IM SGAs. However, their efficacy and safety were evaluated in a review of nine double-blind, randomized controlled trials. Data were extracted to compare olanzapine, ziprasidone, and aripiprazole to either placebo or active comparator (haloperidol or lorazepam) in order to calculate number needed to treat (NNT) and number needed to harm (NNH).[122] All three of the agents demonstrated superior efficacy to placebo, and the NNT was lowest for olanzapine and ziprasidone. Olanzapine 10 mg demonstrated superiority compared to haloperidol 7.5 mg (NNT = 5). A low-dose of aripiprazole 1 mg IM was shown to be less effective compared to haloperidol 7.5 mg IM (NNT = −5).[122] The available RCTs for Ziprasidone IM did not have an active comparator such as haloperidol or lorazepam IM. The adverse effect profiles of the SGAs differed significantly in terms of NNH, though all three agents were associated with less EPS than haloperidol. Olanzapine was associated with a NNH of 50 for treatment-emergent hypotension.[122] This is in line with the manufacturer's recommendation to avoid concomitant administration with benzodiazepines. In one of the studies, aripiprazole demonstrated a NNH of 47 for akathisia when compared to placebo.[122] Data were not available to evaluate QT_c-prolonging effects of ziprasidone IM in terms of NNH. The manufacturer's guidance states ziprasidone IM is contraindicated in patients with a known history of QT prolongation, recent acute MI, or uncompensated heart failure. Caution should be taken when given with other medications known to increase the QT interval (i.e., Class Ia and III antiarrhythmics, thioridazine, chlorpromazine, moxifloxacin, etc.) and in patients with renal insufficiency due to the clearance of the cyclodextrin excipient through the kidney.[123]

Haloperidol short-acting IM is commonly the preferred agent on hospitals' acute agitation protocols because of its proven efficacy, low risk for orthostasis, and its ability to be administered with IM lorazepam, if necessary. The cost of haloperidol may also be advantageous versus the SGAs, but cost of IM anticholinergics (e.g., benztropine) must be taken into account with its higher risk of EPS. Overall, the short-acting IM dosage forms of the antipsychotic agents are a crucial piece of the treatment team's armamentarium and key to ensuring the safety of a patient with agitation related to acute psychosis (Table 85-7).

Table 85-7
Agents Used to Treat Acute Agitation[121,296–303]

Medication	Dosage Form	Dosing Schedule (As Needed)	Onset (minutes)	Max Dose/24 hours	Duration of Action (hours)
Lorazepam	PO (tablet), IM, IV	1–2 mg	60–90 (PO); 15 (IM)	10 mg	8–10
Typical Antipsychotics					
Haloperidol	PO (tablet), IM	5–10 mg every 0.5–2 hours	30–60 minutes	30 mg	Up to 24
Fluphenazine	PO (tablet), IM	1–2.5 mg every 6 hours (tablet); 1.25 mg every 6 hours (IM)	Not available	10 mg	6–8
Chlorpromazine	PO (tablet), IM	50 mg (IM); 100 mg (PO) every 1–4 hours	15–60	200 mg	Not available
Atypical Antipsychotics					
Olanzapine	PO (tablet), IM, ODT	5–10 mg every 2–4 hours	15–45	30 mg (IM), 20 mg (ODT)	24
Risperidone	PO (tablet, liquid), ODT	1–2 mg every 0.5–2 hours	60	4 mg	Not available
Ziprasidone	PO (tablet), IM	10–20 mg every 2–4 hours	30–60	40 mg	4
Aripiprazole	PO (tablet, liquid), IM, ODT	10–15 mg (tablet); 9.75 mg (IM) every 2 hours	1–3 hours	30 mg	Not available

IM, intramuscularly; IV, intravenously; ODT, oral disintegrating tablet; PO, orally.

Long-Acting Injectables

Long-acting injectable antipsychotics (LAIAs) are an option for patients with a history of medication nonadherence or in those patients that prefer LAIAs over once-daily oral antipsychotics. LAIAs allow the patient the option to decrease the frequency they need to make a decision to take medications. Oral antipsychotics require daily recommitment to be adherent versus biweekly, monthly, or quarterly with LAIAs. Lapses in adherence are also more apparent, and early interventions can be initiated if a patient fails to show for an injection appointment. Effectiveness and tolerability of the oral counterpart to an LAIA should be established prior conversion to the LAIA. Equivalent dosages of LAIAs do not pose greater risk for adverse effects than the oral antipsychotic with the exception of injection site pain.[124] LAIAs take months to reach steady state concentration; therefore, making dose adjustments to acutely target symptoms or manage adverse effects is inefficient.

A number of large-scale RCTs failed to demonstrate a significant benefit of LAIAs over oral antipsychotic medications in relapse prevention in schizophrenia.[125] A meta-analysis including a total of 5,176 patients enrolled in 21 RCTs of at least 6-month duration found LAIAs did not reduce relapse compared to oral antipsychotics.[126] This finding may be due in part to selection of a population of subjects with greater engagement in treatment, more insight, and high adherence to PO medications relative to the real-world patient population. Increased clinician contact, implicit or explicit efforts to monitor adherence, and free study medication also reduce the ability of RCTs to reflect relapse rates in more unstable patients who are often prescribed LAIAs. A 2-year, double-blind RCT, conducted by Rosenheck and colleagues, enrolled 369 patients with schizophrenia who were at risk of psychiatric hospitalization.[127] The patients were assigned to LAI risperidone or PO antipsychotic of clinician's choice. No significant differences in psychiatric hospitalization rates, symptoms of psychosis, or measures of social functioning were found between groups. Mirror-image studies, which compare periods of treatment with oral antipsychotics and LAIAs in the same patient, have been proposed as a better method to capture the real-world effectiveness of LAIAs. A systematic review and meta-analysis examined 25 mirror-image studies of 5,940 patients with schizophrenia greater than 12 months (greater than 6 months each of oral and LAIA treatment). LAIAs were superior to oral antipsychotics in preventing hospitalization (16 studies, RR = 0.43; 95% CI, 0.35–0.53; $p < .001$) as well as decreasing number of hospitalizations (15 studies, RR = 0.38; 95% CI, 0.28–0.51; $p < .001$). These results should be interpreted with caution because mirror-image studies can have intrinsic expectation bias and return to a stable status may reflect the natural course of illness.[125]

Patients with recent-onset schizophrenia have inherently less understanding of the importance of treatment and adherence and may benefit from treatment with LAIAs. One RCT of LAI risperidone versus oral risperidone in 86 patients with recent-onset schizophrenia demonstrated lower rates of relapse in the LAI risperidone group (5% vs. 33%).[128] Another prospective, open-label RCT randomized patients with first-episode schizophrenia, schizophreniform, or schizoaffective disorder in a 2:1 ratio to recommendation of switch to LAI risperidone ($n = 26$) or continuation of oral antipsychotic ($n = 11$). Patients were followed for up to 104 weeks, and an initial trend towards greater adherence was seen at 12 weeks ($p = 0.058$) for patients accepting LAI risperidone. However, no significant difference was seen in time to initial nonadherence during overall study duration.[129]

Two high-potency FGAs, fluphenazine and haloperidol, are available as decanoate ester long-acting injectable (LAI) formulations. Conversion to the LAI formulation of haloperidol can be achieved either by administering 10 times the oral dose the patient is stabilized on or by administering 20 times the oral dose for a loading dose regimen.[130] The loading dose regimen more rapidly achieves therapeutic serum levels of haloperidol and allows for earlier discontinuation of oral medication.[124,130] The standard conversion requires oral overlap with the current dose of oral haloperidol for at least one month prior to being gradually tapered.[124] Fluphenazine decanoate is released faster than the haloperidol decanoate and achieves Tmax in approximately 24 hours. It is recommended that the oral medication be decreased by 50% upon administration of the first injection and discontinued after the second injection.[124,131] There are not enough data to support a loading dose regimen for fluphenazine decanoate. The standard oral to LAI conversion is 1.25 times the oral dose administered every 2 to 4 weeks.[131] A double-blind study reported no difference in relapse, symptoms, or adverse effects between groups stabilized on every 2-week versus every 6-week injection intervals.[132] These results suggest dosing intervals longer than the usual 2 to 4 weeks may be an option to reduce antipsychotic exposure without risk of relapse. Both decanoate ester formulations require utilizing the "Z-track technique" for administration. This prevents loss of medication, abscess formation, or subcutaneous lumps. However, it is more painful than standard injections.

SGAs currently available in LAI formulations are aripiprazole (Abilify Maintena and Aristada), risperidone (Risperdal Consta), paliperidone (Invega Sustenna and Invega Trinza), and olanzapine (Zyprexa Relprevv). Aripiprazole monohydrate (Abilify Maintena) requires a 14-day oral overlap and is dosed monthly. Aripiprazole lauroxil (Aristada), a prodrug of aripiprazole, requires a 21-day oral overlap, but can be dosed every 4 weeks or every 6 weeks at the 882-mg dosage.[132] The normal starting dose of aripiprazole monohydrate for most patients will be 400 mg IM monthly. However, patients with renal impairment or concomitant administration with strong CYP3A4 and 2D6 inhibitors or inducers for greater than 14 days require dose adjustments which are detailed in Table 85-8. Dosing of aripiprazole lauroxil is converted from the oral dose requirement of each individual (i.e., 10-mg oral aripiprazole equates to 441-mg injection).

LAI risperidone is administered every 2 weeks and requires an oral overlap of 3 weeks due to delayed release of risperidone from suspension in copolymer microspheres. Less than 1% of the risperidone is released within the first 3 weeks postinjection. Paliperidone palmitate (Invega Sustenna) is dosed monthly and does not require oral overlap with the recommended loading regimen. In patients without renal impairment, the initial loading regimen consists of a 234-mg deltoid injection on day 1 followed by a 156-mg deltoid injection on day 8. Paliperidone palmitate should be avoided in severe renal impairment (CrCl <50 mL/minute). Paliperidone palmitate is also available in a formulation administered every three months (Invega Trinza) for patients stabilized on the monthly formulation for a minimum of 4 months. The dose of the 3-month formulation is 3.5-fold higher than the last dose of the monthly formulation. However, there is minimal difference in injection volume between the two formulations (1.5 mL for Invega Sustenna 234 mg vs. 2.625 mL for Invega Trinza 819 mg).

LAI olanzapine (Zyprexa Relprevv) has an associated risk evaluation and mitigation strategy (REMS) due to the risk of postinjection delirium/sedation syndrome (PDSS). PDSS results from supratherapeutic levels of olanzapine caused by accidental intravascular placement of the injection and rapid dissolution of olanzapine pamoate. Symptoms mimic olanzapine overdose and can include sedation, coma, and delirium. The administering facility must have available access to emergency response services and monitor the patient for at least 3 hours postinjection for signs and symptoms of PDSS. The risk of PDSS is 0.2% per injection, and history of prior tolerability does not translate to a lower

Table 85-8
Long-Acting Injectable Antipsychotics (LAIAs)[304–311]

	Available Dosages	PO to LAI conversion	Dosage	Interval	Loading Dose	PO overlap
Fluphenazine decanoate	25 mg/mL (5 mL multi-dose vial)	10 mg PO = 12.5 mg Q3weeks IM	Initial: 12.5–25 mg Target: 12.5–50 mg	Q2–4W	No	Decrease PO by 50% after 1st injection; d/c PO after 2nd injection
Haloperidol decanoate	50 mg/mL; 100 mg/mL (1 mL single-dose vial & 5 mL multi-dose vial)	10–20 × PO dose	10–15 × PO dose administered monthly; max 100 mg first injection if naive to haloperidol decanoate	Q4W	20x PO dose 1st injection then 10x PO dose maintenance	Continue PO × 2–3 injections if loading dose not used
Aripiprazole monohydrate (Abilify Maintena)	300 & 400 mg kits	400 mg IM Q month	Initial: 400 mg IM monthly; 300 mg IM monthly (poor CYP2D6 metabolizers, concomitant strong CYP2D6 or 3A4 inhibitors, or side effects at higher dose); 200 mg monthly (poor CYP2D6 metabolizers taking CYP3A4 inhibitors, concomitant strong CYP2D6 and 3A4 inhibitors)	Q month	No	Continue PO × 14 days
Aripiprazole lauroxil (Aristada)	441, 662, 882 mg	**PO Dose (mg)** / **IM Dose (mg)** 10 / 441 15 / 662 ≥20 / 882	Initial: 441, 662, or 882 mg monthly depending on PO dose 882 mg may be given Q6W	Q4–6W	No	21 days
Olanzapine pamoate (Zyprexa Relprevv)	210, 300, & 405 mg kits	PO dose / IM dose first 8 weeks / IM dose maintenance 10 mg/day / 210 mg Q2W or 405 mg Q4W / 150 mg Q2W or 300 mg Q4W 15 mg/day / 300 mg Q2W / 210 mg Q2W or 405 mg Q4W 20 mg/day / 300 mg Q2W / 300 mg Q2W	Initial: 150–300 mg IM Q2W or 405 mg Q4W Target: 300 mg Q2W or 405 mg Q4W	Q2W or Q4W	Yes	Not required

(continued)

Table 85-8

Long-Acting Injectable Antipsychotics (LAIAs)[304–311] *(continued)*

Paliperidone palmitate (Invega Sustenna)	39, 78, 117, 156, & 234 mg kits	Initiate with 234 mg IM on day 1 and 156 mg IM on day 8 (both deltoid) Mild renal impairment (CrCl ≥50 mL/minute and <80 mL/minute): Initiate with 156 mg IM on day 1 then 117 mg IM day 8	PO dose / IM dose: 3 mg/day — 39–78 mg 6 mg/day — 117 mg 12 mg/day — 234 mg Mild renal impairment — 78 mg	Q4W	Yes	Not required
Paliperidone palmitate (Invega Trinza)	273, 410, 546, 819 mg	Convert from Invega Sustenna dosage	Sustenna / Trinza: 78 — 273 117 — 410 156 — 546 234 — 819	Q3Months	No	Not required
Risperidone long-acting injection (Risperdal Consta)	12.5, 25, 37.5, 50 mg dose packs	PO dose / IM dose: 2–3 mg — 25 mg 4–5 mg — 37.5 mg 6 mg — 50 mg	Initial: 25 mg IM Q2W with PO overlap × 3W Target: 25–50 mg IM Q2W	Q2W	No	Continue PO × 3 weeks

risk of PDSS for future injections. LAI olanzapine distribution is restricted to the Zyprexa Relprevv Patient Care Program that requires the prescriber, facility, patient, and pharmacy be enrolled prior to releasing the injection. The high administrative burden placed on the facility and patient to coordinate the postinjection monitoring limits its use in clinical practice.

PHARMACOKINETICS AND DRUG INTERACTIONS

Pharmacokinetics and potential for drug–drug interactions are necessary considerations for the safe and effective dosing of antipsychotic medications. One key point to keep in mind is the difference between the time to therapeutic effect and time to steady state plasma concentration. Response of positive symptoms of schizophrenia can be seen within days of treatment initiation. However, it may take 4 to 7 days, or longer dependent on the half-life of the antipsychotic, to achieve steady state plasma concentrations. The half-life of an antipsychotic may also be misleading in determining dosing frequency. Most antipsychotics should be dosed once daily, with the exception of asenapine and ziprasidone due to issues with absorption. Ability to dose these agents once daily is in part due to higher concentration and longer receptor occupancy in the CNS as well as longer duration of pharmacologic effect than is reflected by the serum concentration.[134] During initial titration, split day dosing is appropriate when targeting acute agitation or as the patient develops tolerance to peak concentration-dependent adverse effects (i.e., sedation and orthostatic hypotension). Once the patient can safely tolerate the medication, the dose can be consolidated to bedtime to help reduce pill burden and increase patient adherence.[135]

Antipsychotic drug interactions can be mediated through direct pharmacokinetic (PK) interactions or by additive pharmacodynamic (PD) effects. PK interactions usually involve phase I oxidative metabolism through the cytochrome P450 (CYP) system; however, interactions can occasionally involve phase II metabolism (e.g., glucuronidation). Many antipsychotics undergo metabolism through CYP1A2, 2D6, and 3A4 hepatic isoenzymes (see Table 85-9). The inhibition or induction of these CYP enzymes can result in clinically relevant changes in antipsychotic serum levels. For example, inhibition of CYP1A2 by the antidepressant fluvoxamine can cause a significant elevation in clozapine serum level and place the patient at risk for serious adverse effects, such as seizures. The reverse would be true for CYP1A2 induction. To use the same example, if a patient were to begin taking a CYP1A2 inducer, such as carbamazepine or phenytoin, the clozapine serum level would drop and place the patient at risk for recurrence of psychotic symptoms. A common CYP1A2 inducer that deserves special mention is cigarette smoke and the polyaromatic hydrocarbons (PAHs) contained within that smoke. PAHs, not nicotine, are responsible for the induction; therefore, it is important to note when an inpatient is stabilized on an agent metabolized by CYP1A2 (e.g., clozapine, olanzapine, asenapine) the serum level can drop by up to 50% if they resume smoking upon discharge. Many antidepressants and mood stabilizers also have potent effects on CYP metabolism, so caution should be taken when adding them to an antipsychotic regimen.[136,137] PD interactions occur when an additional agent is added to a patient's regimen that enhances an effect of the antipsychotic activity at

Table 85-9
Pharmacokinetic Comparisons of Antipsychotics

Antipsychotic Agent	Mean Half-Life (hours)	Major Metabolic Pathway
First-Generation Antipsychotics (FGAs)		
Chlorpromazine	24	CYP 2D6
Fluphenazine	14–16	CYP 2D6
Haloperidol	18	CYP 2D6, CYP 3A4
Loxapine	6–8	None (minor—CYP 1A2, CYP 2D6, & CYP 3A4)
Perphenazine	9–12	CYP 2D6
Trifluoperazine	3–12	CYP 1A2
Thioridazine	5–27	CYP 2D6
Thiothixene	34	CYP 1A2
Second-Generation Antipsychotics (SGAs)		
Aripiprazole	75–94	CYP 2D6, CYP 3A4
Asenapine	24	UGT1A4, CYP 1A2
Brexpiprazole	86–91	CYP 2D6, CYP 3A4
Cariprazine	48–336	CYP 3A4
Clozapine	8–12	CYP 1A2, CYP 3A4
Iloperidone	18–33	CYP 2D6, CYP 3A4
Lurasidone	18	CYP 3A4
Olanzapine	21–54	CYP 1A2, CYP 2D6
Paliperidone	23	Limited CYP 2D6, CYP 3A4
Quetiapine	7	CYP 3A4
Risperidone	3–20	CYP 2D6
Ziprasidone	7	Aldehyde Oxidase, CYP 1A2, CYP 3A4

Adapted from Facts & Comparisons eAnswers. http://online.factsandcomparisons.com/MonoDisp.aspx?monoID=fandc-hcp10202. Accessed May 15, 2016, with permission.

the receptor site without directly affecting the serum level of the antipsychotic. For example, adding the potent anticholinergic agent benztropine to an SGA with anticholinergic properties, such as olanzapine or clozapine, will compound anticholinergic adverse effects such as constipation.

PHARMACOECONOMIC CONSIDERATIONS

When the SGAs were first introduced in the 1990s, there was great concern over their higher cost compared to the older antipsychotics. As the FGAs were all available in cheaper generic forms, the newly marketed SGAs were still under patent protection and therefore anywhere from 10 to 100 times higher the cost than their older counterparts.[138] From 1997 to 2007, the amount spent on outpatient antipsychotic prescriptions in the US (not including the Veterans Affairs system) increased from $1.7 billion/year to $7.4 billion/year.[139] This represents a large percentage of overall US mental health expenses over this time period. As the SGAs have slowly become available in generic forms, the concern about their higher costs has decreased slightly, but cost differences still remain.

Although actual medication cost is commonly scrutinized when examining schizophrenia treatment, it needs to be balanced against other costs associated with the illness. Factors such as hospitalizations rates, outpatient service utilizations, and patient functionality also need to be considered. One study examining the outcomes of formulary restrictions of SGAs in over 100,000 Medicaid patients with schizophrenia found that from 2001 to 2008 these restrictions increased hospitalization rates by 13%, inpatient costs by 23%, and total Medicaid expenditures by 16%, while only reducing medication expenses by 4%.[140] In selecting an antipsychotic, medication costs should be considered, especially in light of the costs to overall public health, along with other factors mentioned previously such as efficacy and adverse effect profile.

ADVERSE DRUG REACTIONS

One of the main factors in selecting an antipsychotic includes the adverse effect profile of the agents being considered. Although many of these adverse effects are common across most, if not all, antipsychotics, the incidence of these effects can vary greatly. The common, class-wide adverse effects seen with these agents include EPS, anticholinergic effects, cardiovascular effects, metabolic effects (including hyperprolactinemia), and others.

As in treating any illness, a careful balance must be maintained between efficacy and tolerability. When an adverse effect is discovered in a patient, evaluation of the benefit-to-risk ratio of the medication should take place. Medication factors such as the degree of benefit to the patient, the severity and frequency of the adverse effect, and level of discomfort or distress to the patient should all be considered. In any situation, the patient should be included in any decision regarding adverse effect management. Unresolved adverse effects that significantly bother a patient can lead to nonadherence and potential treatment failure.

If an adverse effect is determined to be fairly mild and cause minimal patient distress, then it may not require any intervention beyond close monitoring to ensure it does not worsen over time. Many adverse effects may be little more than a slight annoyance and can be approached like this. As an adverse effect becomes more severe or distressing to a patient, it may require more direct intervention. A reduction in antipsychotic dose may be needed or addition of a secondary medication to treat a particular adverse effect (described below) may be required. If truly warranted, the antipsychotic may need to be changed to another agent where the likelihood of the adverse effect might be lower. One potential factor to consider is the risk of decompensation when changing antipsychotics. Antipsychotics share similar pharmacologic effects and have similar efficacy rates, but not all antipsychotics may be effective for a given patient.

When determined that a change in antipsychotics is warranted, either due to adverse effects, poor efficacy, or both, there are several methods that can be employed for switching. In instances where the change needs to be abrupt, perhaps due to a serious or life-threatening adverse effect, an immediate discontinuation of the old agent and initiation of the new agent should be considered. When more time can be given to the change of agents, a cross-titration from one agent to the other can be performed. In these instances, either the new agent can be increased over time as the old agent is simultaneously reduced, or the new agent initiated at a therapeutic dose followed by a downward taper of the old agent over time. The rates of these medication increases and decreases are determined by the clinical presentation and concerns for patient safety (Table 85-10).

Extrapyramidal Adverse Effects and Tardive Syndromes

The blocking of D_2 receptors in the striatum by antipsychotics can also cause acute adverse reactions such as dystonias (involuntary contractions of skeletal muscles) and drug-induced parkinsonism (pseudoparkinsonism). Restoring the balance between acetylcholine and dopamine in the striatum can reduce EPS, which is why low-potency FGAs with appreciable anticholinergic activity (i.e., chlorpromazine and thioridazine) can be less problematic than high potency in this regard. This can also be done using anticholinergics such as benztropine or trihexyphenidyl, by using amantadine, by lowering the dose of the antipsychotic, or by using an SGA instead. However, some evidence suggests that changing patients to an SGA will not always lead to the improvement in these movement disorders to the degree expected.[141]

Dystonia

Acute dystonias are uncomfortable, sustained muscle contractions which can occur as torticollis (involving the neck), the trunk, the tongue, or as an oculogyric crisis (where the patient's eyes appear to roll up in the head). Oculogyric crisis and dystonias tend to present in the first few days of treatment. Symptoms are treated using anticholinergic medications via IM administration for rapid efficacy (i.e., benztropine 2 mg IM stat). Scheduled oral administration of the chosen anticholinergic agent is continued after acute symptom resolution. However, this rapid treatment often does not help the attitude of affected patients towards their caregivers when clinicians are trying to develop a therapeutic alliance with a patient who may already be prone to suspicion or paranoia.[142]

Parkinsonism

Drug-induced parkinsonism is the most common and reversible of adverse movement effects. It consists of rigidity, masked face, slowed gait, and tremor. These symptoms are short lived and easily treated. These occur most often in the first 3 months of treatment. Drug-induced parkinsonism is a separate entity from idiopathic Parkinson disease, which is a distinct illness on its own.

The high-potency FGAs are more likely to induce drug-induced parkinsonism than the low-potency agents. Increased dosages of FGAs in higher-risk patients (i.e., medication naïve, female, advanced age) increase this risk. SGAs are on the whole less likely to induce this syndrome. Clozapine and quetiapine are the least likely to induce drug-induced parkinsonism and often can be used without worsening the underlying movement disorder in patients with idiopathic Parkinson disease.[143–145] However, although clozapine has been robustly effective in these patients, reports with quetiapine are conflicting.[75]

Strategies for reducing or eliminating antipsychotic-induced parkinsonism include lowering the dose of antipsychotic, switching to an atypical antipsychotic (with the lowest risk choices being quetiapine or clozapine), or treating the patient with antiparkinsonian medication. The antiparkinsonian medications often

Table 85-10
Relative Incidence of Antipsychotic Adverse Effects

	Sedation	EPS	Anticholinergic	Orthostasis	Weight Gain
Typical—Low Potency					
Chlorpromazine	+++	++	++	+++	
Thioridazine	+++	+	+++	+++	
Typical—Mid-Potency					
Loxapine	+	++	+	+	
Perphenazine	++	++	+	+	
Typical—High Potency					
Fluphenazine	+	++++	+	+	
Haloperidol	+	++++	+	+	
Thiothixene	+	+++	+	+	
Trifluoperazine	+	+++	+	+	
Atypicals					
Aripiprazole	+	+	0 to +	+	+
Asenapine	++	+	0 to +	++	+
Clozapine	+++	0	+++	+++	++++
Iloperidone	++	+	+	++	+
Lurasidone	+	+++	0	+	++
Olanzapine	++	+	++	++	++++
Paliperidone	+	+	0 to +	+	+
Quetiapine	++	0	0 to +	++	+++
Risperidone	+	++	0 to +	++	+++
Ziprasidone	++	++	+	++	+

0, no effect; +, low; ++, moderate; +++, high; ++++, very high; EPS, extrapyramidal side effects.

Reprinted from Facts & Comparisons eAnswers. http://online.factsandcomparisons.com/MonoDisp.aspx?monoID=fandc-hcp10202. Accessed May 15, 2016, with permission.

used are anticholinergic agents such as benztropine (Cogentin; given from 0.5 mg BID to 2 mg TID), trihexyphenidyl (Artane), biperiden (Akineton), diphenhydramine, or the novel agent amantadine (Symmetrel; given from 100 to 400 mg daily in divided dosages). The anticholinergic agents add to adverse effect and pill burden, and continuation is often not necessary after 3 months. Amantadine causes less of these problems and works by an alternate mechanism of action; it is not as effective as the anticholinergics in many patients though.[142] Anticholinergic adverse effects are discussed in greater detail in the "Anticholinergic Adverse Effects" section.

Akathisia

Akathisia can present alone or in combination with drug-induced parkinsonism, or tardive dyskinesia.[146,147] It presents as an inability to remain still combined with an intense feeling of internal restlessness that can make the patient appear quite agitated.[148] In the unfortunate event akathisia is incorrectly interpreted as agitation, increased or "as needed" antipsychotic doses to target agitation will worsen the syndrome. Akathisia is best treated by a small reduction in antipsychotic dosage, addition of low dosage β-adrenergic blockers (i.e., propranolol 10 mg bid or tid), or addition of anticholinergic agents (especially if drug-induced parkinsonism is also present). Benzodiazepines can also be used in patients not responsive to the aforementioned strategies (Table 85-11).

CASE 85-1, QUESTION 8: J.J. is eventually stabilized on brexpiprazole 2 mg daily while hospitalized. During the admission, the staff notices that her psychotic symptoms have decreased but that her agitation has slowly increased over time. She is constantly pacing around on the unit, and when she does sit down she is always fidgety and unable to sit still. She says she feels uncomfortable most of the time. The unit staff have had to continue to give her lorazepam 1 mg several times a day for this agitation. What form of an EPS might J.J. be experiencing at this time? What information in her presentation supports this finding?

J.J. is most likely experiencing akathisia. As her symptoms did decrease when brexpiprazole was initiated, it is unlikely that it is agitation due to her schizophrenia that is causing the restlessness. Antipsychotics, even those that are D_2 partial agonists such as brexpiprazole, are known to cause akathisia as an adverse effect. Her symptoms also appear to be akathisia: constant pacing/movement, always fidgety, and feeling of inner restlessness. Although lorazepam would be expected to treat agitation, it is also a potential treatment for akathisia as well.

CASE 85-1, QUESTION 9: What would be the appropriate treatment for J.J.'s akathisia?

Table 85-11
Agents to Treat Antipsychotic-Induced Parkinsonism and Akathisia

Medication	Equivalent Dose (mg)	Dose/Day (mg/day)
Anticholinergic		
Benztropine (Cogentin)[a]	0.5	1–8
Biperiden (Akineton)[a]	0.5	2–8
Diphenhydramine (Benadryl)[a]	25	50–250
Procyclidine (Kemadrin)	1.5	10–20
Trihexyphenidyl (Artane)	1	2–15
Dopaminergic		
Amantadine	—	100–300
GABAminergic		
Diazepam (Valium)	10	5–40
Clonazepam (Klonopin)	2	1–3
Lorazepam (Ativan)[a]	2	1–3
Noradrenergic Blockers		
Propranolol (Inderal)	—	20–60 (max = 120)

[a]Oral dose or intramuscular (IM) injection can be used.

Adapted from Facts & Comparisons eAnswers. http://online.factsandcomparisons.com/MonoDisp.aspx?monoID=fandc-hcp10202. Accessed May 15, 2016, with permission.

First and foremost, it should be determined whether J.J. can be stabilized on a lower dose of her medication. Often a reduction in antipsychotic dose will resolve any EPS symptoms. If this is not possible and J.J. would destabilize as a result, then an additional medication will be needed to manage the problem. Although lorazepam would serve this purpose, the concerns about chronic daily administration of benzodiazepines must be considered. As J.J. may have akathisia with brexpiprazole as long as she is on the medication, she could require treatment for akathisia this entire time. Another option for treating this problem would be propranolol, the nonselective β-blocker. Propranolol has been found to be helpful in alleviating akathisia in low, subcardiac doses such as 10 to 20 mg twice daily. If this treatment is selected, then her blood pressure and heart rate should be monitored accordingly.

CASE 85-1, QUESTION 10: When arranging her discharge, the pharmacy that is called for her prescriptions informs you that her insurance plan will not pay for brexpiprazole. What medication would be appropriate to switch JJ to at this time?

Ideally, we would keep J.J. on the medication that stabilized her during her hospitalization. It might be possible to contact her insurance to obtain a prior authorization for this medication. If that cannot be done, then they should be asked whether aripiprazole is available for use with J.J. Aripiprazole is also a D_2 partial agonist, like brexpiprazole, so theoretically it should work in a similar manner as brexpiprazole. If her insurance will not pay for aripiprazole, then another atypical antipsychotic with a similar adverse effect profile should be considered. As brexpiprazole has lower rates of EPS and metabolic adverse effects, an agent such as ziprasidone might be considered as it has similar rates of EPS and metabolic effects but is available as a generic medication.

CASE 85-1, QUESTION 11: JJ has been stabilized on ziprasidone 40 mg twice daily with meals while in the hospital. When should her target symptoms start to respond to the medication? What else can be done to help improve JJ's prognosis once she is discharged?

Although J.J.'s symptoms should start to decrease within a few days of starting the medication, it may take a week or longer to see significant improvement. At this point she may be stable enough for discharge from the hospital, but still show some functional deficits. It may take several more weeks, possibly months, for her to return to her baseline prior to her symptoms starting, and she may never fully reach this point. The utilization of nonpharmacologic methods, including individual and group therapy modalities, could also help J.J.'s continued improvement and stabilization. Education for both her and her family could also be of benefit to her.

CASE 85-1, QUESTION 12: JJ returns home to her family, taking a leave from college for the remainder of the semester. She returns to school the following semester to resume classes, but notices she has a hard time focusing in class, which she attributes to the ziprasidone. As she has not had any psychotic symptoms since being released from the hospital approximately 5 months ago, she thinks she is cured and no longer needs to take the medication. She contacts her psychiatrist about stopping the medication. Should J.J. discontinue her medication at this time? What do practice guidelines state regarding J.J.'s treatment needs at this time?

J.J. should not stop her medication at this time. Although a medication adjustment might be needed, depending upon the nature and cause of her concentration, that is not a reason to stop the medication altogether. Most treatment guidelines recommend a minimum of 6 months, and preferably one year, of treatment after a psychotic episode. As she has only been symptom-free for 5 months, J.J.'s risk of relapse is very high without medication treatment.

CASE 85-1, QUESTION 13: Ultimately, J.J. decides to stop taking her ziprasidone and stops going to her psychiatrist appointments. In less than a month, she is brought to the ER by her parents as she has relapsed into another psychotic episode and admitted back into the hospital. Is J.J. a candidate for long-acting injectable antipsychotics (LAIAs) at this time?

J.J. is not a candidate for a LAIA currently as she has never tried an oral formulation of any of them to this point. Recommendations for use of a LAIA require at a minimum repeated dosages of the oral form of the medication to ensure a lack of an allergy to the med, or in some instances for the patient to be stable on an oral dose of the medication and the converted over to the LAIA form. However, she might benefit from the use of a LAIA if she truly intends to be nonadherent with oral forms of antipsychotics. As she has only shown nonadherence to one medication trial due to a potential misunderstanding of her illness and her treatment, she could benefit from education in these areas to improve her adherence. In addition, her family could be educated to help J.J. maintain her med adherence as well.

CASE 85-1, QUESTION 14: While on the inpatient unit for this most recent episode, JJ continues to remain nonadherent to oral medication. She eventually agrees to receive an LAIA, but after speaking with her insurance the only atypical antipsychotic LAIA they will pay for is risperidone LAIA. Is this an appropriate agent for JJ, and why or why not?

Assuming that J.J. has been administered oral risperidone in the past which ensures a lack of an allergy to the medication, it still would not be an appropriate option at this time. Due to the unique pharmacokinetic parameters of risperidone LAIA, it requires 3 weeks of overlap of oral medication (risperidone or otherwise) as the initial dose does not begin releasing medication until this time. Assuming J.J.'s nonadherence to oral medications will continue, this could lead to a poor outcome, especially if she is discharged from the hospital. J.J.'s insurance should be contacted to attempt to find an alternative atypical antipsychotic LAIA.

Tardive Dyskinesia

One of the more troubling potential adverse effects from chronic treatment with antipsychotics is the development of persistent choreoathetoid (sometimes described as snake-like) movements of the tongue, hands, feet, and in severe cases even the trunk of the patient.[149] Chronic blockade of striatal D_2 receptors by antipsychotics results in these receptors becoming supersensitive to available dopamine. Changes in interconnected neurotransmitter systems, such as GABAergic or muscarinic,[150] can result in dyskinesias that can often appear on withdrawal of antipsychotics, upon lowering of the dosage, or when a patient is changed to clozapine or quetiapine treatment from another antipsychotic. If these withdrawal dyskinesias persist, then the condition of persistent or tardive dyskinesia can result. Tardive dyskinesia can also present without any change in medication dose after many years of treatment. FGAs are considered to have a much greater risk (5% yearly incidence in long-term use in adults) of causing tardive dyskinesia than the SGAs, but reported incidences vary appreciably between studies.[151] Risk of developing tardive dyskinesia increases with cumulative lifetime dosage and duration of antipsychotic treatment, increased age, comorbid diabetes mellitus, traumatic brain injury, having an affective disorder, anticholinergic medication use, a history of drug-induced parkinsonism, and female gender.[152–155] Although the incidence rate for patients treated with typical antipsychotics is more substantial,[151] the atypical antipsychotics also carry this risk albeit at a lower but still not negligible rate.[156]

Although all dyskinetic movements seen on withdrawal of antipsychotic medication are not necessarily persistent or *tardive* dyskinesia, there are those cases of patients who do retain the potentially stigmatizing movements long after antipsychotic medications are tapered or changed. When this occurs, it is often very difficult to remediate these movements. Medication changes which decrease the effects of dopamine on striatal receptors tend to cause immediate improvement followed by long-term worsening of dyskinetic symptoms. Few double-blind studies show any benefit of augmenting with various agents, and agents which often have shown promise in early case reports and open studies (i.e., diazepam, donepezil, branched chain amino acids) often do not bear up to the scrutiny of a double-blind trial.[157–159] Even accepted strategies such as lowering antipsychotic dosages (or stopping them when possible) or changing to less offending second-generation agents such as clozapine or quetiapine do not always yield the desired outcome. Some limited evidence suggests that clonazepam and ginkgo biloba may prove helpful.[159] However, a better course of strategy appears to do what we can to prevent the occurrence of tardive dyskinesia by strategies such as keeping antipsychotic dosages as low as possible and using medications that are less likely to induce this syndrome,[150,151,160] and incorporating close monitoring for development of symptoms utilizing the Abnormal Involuntary Movement Scale (AIMS) examination. However, we do have the option to tailor our medication choice to the vulnerability of the patient. As the severity and prevalence of tardive dyskinesia is apparently on the decline,[150] there may be cause to be optimistic.

Anticholinergic

The low-potency FGAs and certain SGAs, particularly olanzapine and clozapine, are potent muscarinic receptor antagonists. The resultant anticholinergic effects can range from bothersome to potentially life-threatening. These effects include dry mouth, blurred vision, mydriasis, tachycardia, urinary retention, constipation, paralytic ileus, confusion, and delirium. Something that may appear merely bothersome, like dry mouth, can have more serious consequences if not addressed. Dry mouth can lead to dental caries or weight gain if thirst is quenched with sugary beverages. Additional sugar, in the form of gum or liquids, can also increase the risk of oral fungal infections. Patients can utilize sugar free hard candies or gum, or saliva substitute products if anticholinergic medication dosage cannot be reduced.[161] In general, patients with schizophrenia should be encouraged to connect with regular dental services. Another often overlooked anticholinergic adverse effect is constipation. Patients may not draw the connection between constipation and a medication that they are taking for their mental health. Consistent monitoring of patient's bowel habits and recommendation of a proper bowel regimen (e.g., diet, physical activity, bulk-forming laxatives, stool softeners) can be the difference between a week of unaddressed bowel discomfort progressing to paralytic ileus and patient expiration due to bowel rupture or aspiration of gastric contents.[162]

The patient's overall anticholinergic burden is often increased by the addition of anticholinergic medications, such as benztropine, for EPS prophylaxis or treatment. Indication for use of anticholinergic agents should be re-evaluated periodically during treatment and upon transitions in care. Failure to taper unnecessary anticholinergic medications can lead to decreased quality of life and preventable adverse effects.[163]

Cardiovascular Effects

Antipsychotic medications are thought to exert cardiovascular effects through direct antagonism of adrenergic and cholinergic receptors, as well as through indirect central autonomic effects and baroreceptor reflexes.[164] Three common antipsychotic-induced cardiovascular effects, orthostasis, tachycardia, and QT_c prolongation, are described below.

Orthostatic Hypotension

Orthostatic hypotension occurs in up to 40% of patients treated with antipsychotic medications.[164] It occurs frequently during the initial dose titration and disproportionately affects elderly patients. Orthostasis results from the blockade of vascular α_{1A}-adrenoceptors, which makes it difficult for patients to adapt to positional changes in blood pressure. Tolerance to orthostasis will usually develop within 2 to 3 weeks of antipsychotic initiation or dose increase. Antipsychotic agents with high affinity for α_{1A}-adrenoceptors relative to D_2 receptors (e.g., clozapine, risperidone) clinically display greater rates of orthostasis than agents with low α_{1A} affinity relative to D_2 affinity (i.e., haloperidol).[164] The risk for falls secondary to orthostasis can be mitigated by (1) slowing the rate of titration, (2) splitting the dose, and (3) counseling the patient to make slow transitions from prone and seated positions. Increasing fluid and salt intake and using support stockings are other nonpharmacologic interventions that may help alleviate orthostasis whereas the patient adapts to a change in dosage. More persistent orthostasis resulting from clozapine treatment can be managed with fludrocortisone or ephedrine if nonpharmacologic interventions are not clinically feasible.[165]

Tachycardia

Antipsychotic-associated tachycardia can occur as a direct effect of anticholinergic activity on vagal activity or as a compensatory mechanism related to orthostatic hypotension. Patients treated with clozapine tend to have a dose-related increase in heart rate of

20 to 25 beats/minute (bpm).[164] Dose reduction, slower titration, or addition of low-dose, preferably cardio-selective, β-blocker can be considered if tachycardia is bothersome to the patient or symptomatic.[165,166]

Electrocardiographic Changes

Prolongation of the QT interval, or QT_c interval when corrected for heart rate, is a variable risk associated with all antipsychotics. QT_c interval prolongation increases the risk for torsades de pointes (TdP), a malignant polymorphic ventricular tachycardia that is associated with syncope and sudden cardiac death.[164] The potential mechanism for this effect is believed to be mediated through blockade of the rapidly activating delayed rectifying current (I_{Kr}) which conducts potassium out of the cardiomyocytes to cause cardiac repolarization.[164,167] However, there are insufficient data to establish the direct causal relationship between antipsychotic-induced QT_c prolongation and sudden cardiac death.[164,167]

The Pfizer 054 study, developed in consultation with the FDA, demonstrated QT_c prolongation as a class effect for SGAs.[168] This prospective, randomized, parallel-group study conducted by Harrigan and associates examined the effect of steady state peak plasma concentrations of haloperidol 15 mg/day ($n = 27$), thioridazine 300 mg/day ($n = 30$), ziprasidone 160 mg/day ($n = 31$), quetiapine 750 mg/day ($n = 27$), olanzapine 20 mg/day ($n = 24$), or risperidone 6 to 8 mg/day increased to 16 mg/day ($n = 25/20$) on the QT_c interval in the presence or absence of metabolic inhibitors in patients with stable psychotic disorders. No patients were observed to have a QT_c interval greater than 500 ms, and mean QT_c changes from baseline were similar for monotherapy and with concomitant administration of a metabolic inhibitor. The antipsychotics associated with the greatest change in mean baseline QT_c were thioridazine (30.1 ms) and ziprasidone (15.9 ms). Haloperidol, quetiapine, risperidone 6 to 8 mg/day, risperidone 16 mg/day, and olanzapine were associated with mean QT_c changes of 7.5, 5.7, 3.9, 3.6, and 1.7 ms, respectively.[169] To add context, the mean diurnal variation in QT_c is approximately 75 to 100 ms and this may vary further based on sleep, diet, obesity, electrolyte disturbances, endocrine dysfunction, gender, and age.[164,167] No cases of torsades de pointes were observed in the 4,571 ziprasidone-treated patients included in the Pfizer 054 study and the ziprasidone database.[168] One of the newer SGAs, iloperidone, has also demonstrated a dose-dependent and drug interaction-dependent risk of QT_c prolongation similar to that of ziprasidone in both short- and long-term randomized trials.[170]

In clinical practice, concomitant administration of QT_c-prolonging agents should be avoided. If coadministration is necessary in a patient with no underlying cardiac abnormalities or risk factors for TdP, the patient should be monitored closely. The interacting medication should be discontinued if the QT_c interval extends beyond 500 ms. Use of antipsychotics with higher risk of QT_c prolongation, chlorpromazine or ziprasidone, should be avoided in patients with underlying cardiac issues, electrolyte abnormalities (hypokalemia or hypomagnesaemia), congenital long-QT syndrome, or those comedicated with agents affecting cardiac function (particularly antiarrhythmics of class Ia—disopyramide, procainamide, quinidine—and class III—amiodarone, dofetilide, sotalol).

CASE 85-1, QUESTION 15: After intensive education about her illness and need for treatment, as well as enlisting the help of her parents in ensuring she will take her medications, JJ eventually agrees to take oral medications and is restabilized on risperidone 2 mg twice daily again. After discharge, her outpatient psychiatrist notes that JJ is still responding to internal stimuli, and confirms she is still having some auditory hallucinations. JJ's parents confirm she is taking her doses, so the dose is increased to 3 mg twice daily. Within a few weeks at her next appointment, JJ's parents inform her psychiatrist that she can barely move, and she "walks like an old lady" at times. The psychiatrist examines JJ and notes she has some mild stiffness in her extremities, a mild tremor in her hands, and when she walks her gait is abnormally short and almost shuffling in appearance. Her hallucinations have subsided however. What is the probable cause of JJ's abnormal neurologic findings at this time? What information in her presentation supports this finding?

J.J. is most likely suffering from drug-induced parkinsonism, a type of EPS. All the abnormal findings noted in J.J. at this time, stiffness, tremor, and shuffling gate, are characteristic findings for drug-induced parkinsonism. Although risperidone, as an atypical antipsychotic, is less likely to cause this problem compared to the older, conventional antipsychotics, it can still cause it. One risk factor of parkinsonism with risperidone is increasing the dose, which occurred in J.J. recently. Although she was fine on the lower dose, the increase in dose to 6 mg/day caused enough D_2 receptor blockade in the nigrostriatal pathway to induce this EPS type.

CASE 85-1, QUESTION 16: How can J.J.'s drug-induced parkinsonism be treated?

Ideally the first choice would be to decrease the dose of the offending agent. As J.J.'s dose of risperidone was just increased to 6 mg/day due to lingering symptoms, this is most likely not an option as it is highly likely those symptoms would return. A change in antipsychotics could also be considered, but it appears that other than the EPS, J.J. is currently stable on this medication and dose. The only other option would be to add another medication to treat her parkinsonism. Some options include the use of anticholinergic medications, such as benztropine, or the use of amantadine.

CASE 85-1, QUESTION 17: J.J.'s drug-induced parkinsonism resolves with the addition of benztropine 0.5 mg twice daily. Will JJ need to stay on this medication indefinitely?

J.J. should be maintained on benztropine for at least 3 months once her parkinsonism resolves. If there are no other changes in her clinical status or her medication treatment for her schizophrenia, then the use of benztropine should be re-examined at that time. If the medication is then removed and her parkinsonism does not return, then she should not need the medication any longer. Should the EPS return, however, then she may need continued anticholinergic treatment.

CASE 85-1, QUESTION 18: What are some other adverse effects that should be monitored for in JJ, both specific to risperidone and for antipsychotics in general?

Any patient receiving an antipsychotic should be monitored for all types of EPS, including parkinsonism. Other EPS types, such as dystonia and akathisia, should be watched for as well as the development of any tardive dyskinesia. Although the risk of these concerns is lower with an atypical antipsychotic, such as risperidone, it is still possible. J.J.'s weight and serum glucose and lipids should also be monitored regularly both during the initiation of antipsychotic treatment and periodically throughout. Risperidone also can cause drug-induced orthostasis, so she should be monitored for dizziness, especially upon standing.

Metabolic Effects

Hyperprolactinemia

Prolactin is a polypeptide hormone secreted by lactotroph cells in the anterior pituitary. Dopamine acts as an inhibitor of prolactin release in the tuberoinfundibular dopamine tract which projects from the hypothalamus to the anterior pituitary. Blockade of D_2 receptors within this pathway leads to increased release of prolactin and potential effects on multiple organ systems and gene expression throughout the body. Agents that cause more potent D_2 blockade are associated with a greater risk of hyperprolactinemia.[171] A multiple-treatment meta-analysis by Leucht and associates stratified select antipsychotics based on their effect on the standardized mean difference in prolactin from baseline as follows: paliperidone (highest), risperidone, haloperidol, lurasidone, ziprasidone, iloperidone, chlorpromazine, olanzapine, asenapine, quetiapine, and aripiprazole (lowest/decreased prolactin).[172] Guidelines recommend baseline prolactin monitoring at the discretion of the clinician, screening for symptoms of excess prolactin at every visit for the first year of treatment and annually thereafter if symptoms are stable, and follow-up prolactin levels only if clinically indicated.[45,173,174] The upper limit of normal prolactin levels is 18 to 20 ng/mL in males and 24 ng/mL in females who are not pregnant or lactating.

Clinical sequelae from excess prolactin release include sexual dysfunction, gynecomastia, galactorrhea, amenorrhea, hypogonadism, and potential bone mineral density changes with long-term elevations. However, prolactin levels do not directly correlate with these adverse events and patients may remain asymptomatic. Considerations for treatment should only be addressed in actively symptomatic patients.[83,172] In symptomatic patients, dose reduction or switching to an agent with less potent D_2 blockade would be recommended first line. If these strategies fail to improve the symptoms or cannot be undertaken for clinical reasons, a dopamine agonist, such as bromocriptine, cabergoline, or amantadine, may be considered. However, the risk of potential exacerbation of psychosis must be weighed against potential benefit.[45,171,174,175] There is also growing evidence to support the use of adjunctive aripiprazole, a partial D_2 agonist, to improve hyperprolactinemia in patients who cannot be switched from a more potent agent.[81,83,176–178]

CASE 85-1, QUESTION 19: Over time J.J.'s dose of risperidone is increased to 4 mg twice a day due to lingering symptoms. At one of her follow-up appointments, JJ asks if it is safe to take the medication while she is pregnant. During the conversation, J.J. tells her psychiatrist that she is pregnant as she hasn't had her menstrual period in nearly 2 months, and her breasts have become larger and she has noticed she lactates periodically. The psychiatrist orders a pregnancy blood test which comes back negative, but her serum prolactin level is 115 ng/mL. What could explain why J.J. believes she is pregnant?

The negative pregnancy test proves J.J. is not pregnant (assuming no error by the laboratory). Her symptoms are indicative of hyperprolactinemia, another potential adverse effect of D_2 receptor antagonism from antipsychotic therapy. As her prolactin level increased, it caused J.J. to become amenorrheic and cause her to lactate. Although not a common adverse effect of most atypical antipsychotics, risperidone (and paliperidone) is similar to the typical antipsychotics in their propensity to increase serum prolactin.

CASE 85-1, QUESTION 20: How should J.J.'s hyperprolactinemia be treated?

Ideally the treatment of antipsychotic-induced hyperprolactinemia involves a dose reduction of the offending agent. As J.J. was increased to 4 mg twice daily due to an insufficient response to a lower dose, this may not be possible. If a dose reduction cannot be done safely, then a change in antipsychotic to one with a lower risk of hyperprolactinemia should be considered. If this too is not clinically appropriate for the patient, then addition of a dopaminergic agonist may be considered, such as amantadine. This should be done cautiously as a strong dopaminergic agonist, such as bromocriptine, may exacerbate her psychosis. There are also data available on using aripiprazole augmentation to treat hyperprolactinemia from antipsychotics, but this might be considered after other agents have been tried, unless J.J. appears to need a stronger antipsychotic regimen.

Weight Gain

Although the development of the SGAs was supposed to free us from the concern of the extrapyramidal adverse effects of the FGAs, many of the newer agents such as clozapine, olanzapine, quetiapine, and risperidone showed a tendency to, like the low-potency typical first-generation agents, cause substantial weight gain.[65] This substantial weight gain tended to occur to the greatest extent in the first few months of treatment, with a certain segment of those treated gaining more than 20 lb.[179] One study showed that 15.4% of those patients treated with olanzapine had weight gain greater than or equal to 7% of their body weight in the first 6 weeks of treatment.[180] It soon became apparent that clozapine and these newer SGAs had the potential to increase body weight and serum triglyceride levels,[65–68] and therefore potentially cause glucose dysregulation as well.[71,181,182] Patients suffering from schizophrenia are already prone to an earlier death than nonmentally ill patients due to their physical health and inherent sedentary lifestyle; therefore, weight gain may be an even more critical issue than the potentially stigmatizing occurrence of tardive dyskinesia.[156,183]

Numerous mechanisms have been theorized to explain the weight gain induced by the SGAs. These include histamine (H_1) receptor antagonism,[184,185] serotonin antagonism at 5-HT_{2c} with a possible genetic predisposition in some,[186,187] muscarinic antagonism which could possibly lead to increased consumption of sugary beverages or "thirsty" calories,[188] and impairments in plasma leptin secretion.[189–191] Concomitant medications, such as valproic acid, lithium, mirtazapine, some antihistamines, and tertiary tricyclic antidepressants, can also increase body weight by synergistic pharmacologic effects.[70,192]

Hyperglycemia and Diabetes Mellitus

It is unclear whether there are direct actions by SGAs involved in the development of diabetes mellitus. However, it is clear that weight gain, increased triglycerides, or decreased insulin sensitivity due to SGAs may cause an increased frequency or earlier onset of this endocrine disorder.[71,181,193–195] An early study showed a moderate correlation ($r = 0.60$, $p = .03$) between serum insulin and clozapine levels,[196] whereas Lund and associates showed an approximately 2.5 times greater risk of diabetes mellitus and hyperlipidemia in patients agents 20 to 34 years old treated with clozapine versus FGAs.[197] Other retrospective studies in veterans also suggested a slightly greater prevalence of diabetes in patients less than 40 years old on the SGAs clozapine, olanzapine, quetiapine, or risperidone (OR =1.09; CI=1.03–1.15) than those on FGAs[181] and an incidence of diabetes mellitus approximately 1.5 times greater in patients treated with olanzapine, risperidone, or quetiapine than with typical, mostly low-potency, antipsychotics.[71] Guidelines stress the need to monitor these patients routinely for glucose dysregulation, weight gain, and hyperlipidemia.[193,198]

Dyslipidemia

Treatment-emergent increases in both serum triglycerides and total serum cholesterol may occur with use of antipsychotics. The initial reports were of increased serum triglycerides with clozapine,[66,68,199] a notation of this phenomenon in the package insert for quetiapine, and reports of this occurring in patients taking olanzapine.[67] Risperidone does not raise serum triglycerides as severely as clozapine[199], and ziprasidone has negligible effects on serum triglycerides.[200,201] Aripiprazole resulted in lowered serum triglyceride levels compared to placebo in pooled double-blind trials.[202] Average serum triglycerides with clozapine, olanzapine, or quetiapine tended to increase by approximately 60 to 70 mg/dL between studies.[66–67,70] Extreme elevations in serum triglycerides (>1,000 mg/dL) have been noted in some patients and were often associated with acute pancreatitis (Table 85-12).[69]

CASE 85-1, QUESTION 21: What other metabolic effects need to be monitored in JJ while she is receiving antipsychotic treatment? What are the risks of these effects in patients receiving these medications?

J.J., as with all patients receiving antipsychotics, is at risk of developing potentially significant weight gain, glucose irregularities including diabetes mellitus type 2, and dyslipidemia, especially hypertriglyceridemia. The risk varies among the agents, with SGAs generally thought to be at a higher risk than with FGAs. Risperidone, which J.J. is currently receiving, is often considered to be at a mid-level risk of these effects compared to some of the other SGAs. Other possible risk factors include the patient's diet and exercise, family history of diabetes and cholesterol problems, and others.

CASE 85-1, QUESTION 22: The psychiatrist decides to change JJ from risperidone to an agent with a lower risk of hyperprolactinemia. He starts JJ on olanzapine, titrating up to 20 mg/day while removing the risperidone. What would be the appropriate monitoring for J.J. upon initiation of olanzapine?

As olanzapine has a high risk of causing metabolic adverse effects in patients, J.J. should be monitored closely for the development of these effects. Her weight should be checked very closely, especially at baseline and over the first few months of treatment. Monthly, if not more frequently, weights should be measured during this time. In addition, her serum glucose and/or HbA1c along with her serum lipid panel should be checked at baseline and then in 3 months for any changes, with an interim serum glucose measurement around 1 to 2 months. Her blood pressure should also be monitored for any changes, especially if her weight increases significantly. If any increases or abnormalities are noted in these parameters, they should be addressed appropriately before becoming a medical concern.

CASE 85-1, QUESTION 23: After 2 months on olanzapine, J.J. returns to the clinic complaining that she's always eating and doesn't fit into her clothes from last summer. Her weight today is 151 lb (BMI = 25.9 kg/m^2), an increase from her weight prior to olanzapine of 139 lb (BMI = 23.9 kg/m^2). J.J.'s parents are also concerned as they have never seen her eat this much in her life. She is currently doing well on the medication, with no psychotic symptoms noticed over this time. They ask whether this appetite and the weight gain are from the olanzapine, and whether there is anything that can be done about it.

Olanzapine could certainly be the cause of her recent weight gain, because it has one of the higher risks of causing weight gain among the SGAs. A 12-lb weight gain is certainly possible with this medication. As J.J., and her parents, has noticed an increase in her appetite since starting the medication, this makes it even more likely olanzapine is involved. Although there are no proven treatments for antipsychotic-induced weight gain, there are some interventions that could be implemented. J.J. should be given an appointment with a nutritionist to review her diet, and she should also be encouraged to increase her exercise on a regular basis, whether at a gym or even by adding 20- to 30-minute walks 4 to 5 days a week.

Table 85-12
Metabolic Monitoring Protocol for Antipsychotics

	Baseline	Week 4	Week 8	Week 12	Week 16	Week 20	Week 24	Quarterly	Annually
Personal or family history	X								X
Weight (BMI)[a]	X	X	X	X	X	X	X	X	
Waist circumference	X								X
Blood pressure	X			X					X
Fasting plasma glucose	X	X (once during this period)		X				X (for first year)	X
Fasting lipid profile	X			X			X		X

More frequent assessments may be warranted based on clinical status.

[a]Some references recommend weekly monitoring for first 6 weeks after initiation to determine patients at risk for more significant long-term weight gain, especially with agents with higher risk of causing weight gain.

Adapted from American Diabetes Association et al. Consensus development conference on antipsychotic drugs and obesity and diabetes. *Diabetes Care*. 2004;27(2):267–272; Hasnain M et al. Metabolic syndrome associated with schizophrenia and atypical antipsychotics. *Curr Diab Rep*. 2010;10(3):209–216. doi:10.1007/s11892-010-0112-8; Kinon BJ et al. Association between early and rapid weight gain and change in weight over one year of olanzapine therapy in patients with schizophrenia and related disorders. *J Clin Psychopharmacol*. 2005;25(3):255–258. doi:10.1097/01.jcp.0000161501.65890.22; and Marder SR et al. The Mount Sinai conference on the pharmacotherapy of schizophrenia. *Schizophr Bull*. 2002;28(1):5–16.

CASE 85-1, QUESTION 24: A month later, J.J. returns to the clinic. Blood work done a few days ago shows her fasting serum glucose to be 214 mg/dL, which is an increase from 132 mg/dL 4 months ago. Her HbA1c has also increased from 5.9% to 7.1% over this time. A serum lipid panel shows her total cholesterol is 256 mg/dL, her direct LDL cholesterol is 117 mg/dL, her HDL is 34 mg/dL, and her triglycerides are 997 mg/dL. Are these changes potentially related to J.J.'s antipsychotic treatment and if so, how should they be managed?

Increases in serum glucose and lipids, especially triglycerides, are possible with SGAs, and olanzapine in particular. As her glucose and A1c have increased since starting the medication, this makes it highly likely this is the cause. Although J.J.'s LDL and HDL cholesterol measurements are not ideal, they are not as concerning as her very elevated triglyceride level. At this high of a level of triglycerides, there is the concern of possible pancreatitis. J.J. should be asked about any upper abdominal pain or other possible symptoms.

Although we could treat her increased serum glucose and lipids with appropriate medications for each concern, another consideration would be to change J.J. from olanzapine to another SGA with a lower risk of metabolic problems. This would need to be done after considering the risk of J.J.'s possible psychiatric decompensation from changing her antipsychotic treatment.

Medical Comorbidity

Currently, metabolic syndrome is seen as a major concern when treating schizophrenia, and it is recommended that patients receiving SGAs must be routinely monitored for weight gain, changes in fasting serum lipids, or signs of glucose dysregulation.[193,198,203] Some estimates of the prevalence of metabolic syndrome in patients with schizophrenia range from 18.8% to approximately 40% of those tested.[204] As medication-naïve patients are already at a high risk for developing metabolic syndrome,[205] we should strive to minimize the chance or worsening their situation. Furthermore, since weight gain with antipsychotic medication and its secondary metabolic complications tends to occur rapidly, patients should receive more frequent assessments for this when they are first started or switched to a new antipsychotic medication. Medication use evaluations to make sure this necessary monitoring is performed may be helpful.[206]

Moreover, effective pharmacotherapy carries with it a potential for serious adverse metabolic effects such as obesity, hypertriglyceridemia, and resulting glucose dysregulation as well as movement disorders such as akathisia, drug-induced parkinsonism, and tardive dyskinesia. One study showed metabolic disorders occur more than 3 times (3.7; 95% CI = 1.5–9.0) as much in patients with schizophrenia as compared to nonpsychiatrically ill controls.[207] In fact, cardiovascular disorders are the main reason patients with schizophrenia tend to die at a younger age than their peers.[208]

Another concern is that, along with known genetic factors,[209] metabolic syndrome issues such as increased weight, serum leptin, lipids, and glucose are known risk factors for venous thromboembolism (VTE) which also may occur in association with antipsychotic pharmacotherapy.[210,211] The most established link is to the use of clozapine,[212] which is one of the most metabolically problematic agents. However, even more metabolically benign antipsychotics may eventually be linked to the increased occurrence of VTE.[213] Pulmonary embolism is a well-documented variant occurring with antipsychotics.[214,215] As VTE related to antipsychotics is likely rare, the benefit-to-risk ratio should be kept in perspective.[216]

Other cardiovascular effects can be problematic when utilizing antipsychotic pharmacotherapy. Of concern, olanzapine, risperidone, and quetiapine have been associated with a three-fold increased likelihood of cerebrovascular accidents (CVAs) and transient ischemic attacks during the first 6 months of treatment in elderly patients.[217,218] Other antipsychotics have also been implicated.[219] Such events could relate to the slightly higher risk of death in elderly patients receiving these medications.[220] As a result, all antipsychotics have a black box warning from the US FDA regarding an increased risk of CVAs in elderly patients taking these medications.

Neuroleptic Malignant Syndrome

Neuroleptic malignant syndrome (NMS) is a rare, but potentially fatal complication of antipsychotic therapy that can occur due to treatment with any antipsychotic or abrupt cessation of a dopamine agonist. Therefore, early recognition and management are crucial. There are numerous diagnostic scales to ensure accurate diagnosis of NMS for research purposes, but the most widely utilized in clinical practice is the *DSM-5* criteria. NMS is associated with high fever (103°F–104°F), muscular rigidity, altered consciousness, and highly elevated creatinine phosphokinase (CPK) often greater than 1,000 mcg/L. Other signs are drooling, difficulty swallowing, fast heart rate (greater than 100 bpm) profuse sweating, incontinence, and labile blood pressure. It is treated by immediate cessation of antipsychotic therapy, supportive care, and the administration of medications such as dantrolene sodium, biperiden, or bromocriptine. Combination antipsychotic therapy was found in 39% of all NMS cases.[221] Some believe that physical exhaustion and dehydration predispose a patient to develop NMS, so it is important that patients on antipsychotics be cautioned to take proper caution in hot weather. Also, the effects of antipsychotics on the hypothalamus (which regulates temperature and food intake among other activities) and the "body-secretion" drying activities of anticholinergic medications increase the danger of heat exhaustion in these patients.[222]

CASE 85-1, QUESTION 25: J.J.'s psychiatrist decides that in light of her weight gain and worsening glucose and lipid profiles, he is going to change her from olanzapine to lurasidone, titrating her up to 80 mg/day. She did well with the medication change. A few weeks after starting the lurasidone, her parents take JJ into the ER one evening concerned she has meningitis as she feels feverish, is sweating, seems confused, and has a stiff neck. The ER exam shows JJ has a fever of 103.1°F, blood pressure of 176/98 mm Hg, pulse of 136 bpm, respiratory rate of 36 bpm, a stiff neck that is not painful, and is sometimes incoherent when answering questions, but shows no outward signs of psychosis. She also is sweating profusely despite the air conditioning in the ER room. Laboratory work is ordered and returns a couple hours later. J.J.'s chemistries are normal except for a creatinine phosphokinase (CPK) of 5,960 mcg/L, a normal CBC, and a normal serum glucose. Repeat vital signs 2 hours after she comes to the ER show a fever of 103.2°F, blood pressure of 96/62 mmHg, pulse of 146 bpm, and a respiratory rate of 39 bpm. What is the most likely cause of J.J.'s presentation at this time and why? How should J.J. be managed?

J.J. is most likely suffering from neuroleptic malignant syndrome (NMS) from lurasidone. Although NMS can occur at any time during treatment with any antipsychotic, the timing of this episode shortly after beginning the medication makes it more likely. As she does not have pain in her neck or an elevated WBC, it is not likely meningitis as her parents feared (though this should be definitively ruled out). The high fever, labile blood pressure, tachycardia, sweating, confusion (without psychosis), and highly elevated CPK are indicative of NMS. J.J. will need to be admitted to the hospital as NMS can be life-threatening. As she will need to stop taking all antipsychotics for up to 2 weeks, she will most likely require hospitalization during this time as her psychosis is likely to return. During the acute treatment period, she will likely need treatment for the NMS with either dantrolene (for the fever) or bromocriptine (a dopamine agonist), as well as other measures as needed for her fever, elevated blood pressure, etc. During the longer period without antipsychotic treatment while waiting for the NMS to resolve, J.J. will likely need treatment with sedatives such as benzodiazepines as we cannot actively treat her schizophrenia.

CASE 85-1, QUESTION 26: During the subsequent admission for her episode of NMS, J.J. is eventually started on aripiprazole for her schizophrenia. A few days into titrating the medication to an effective dose, she develops some mild stiffness in her arms, most likely some mild parkinsonism. Fearful that this is the NMS returning, J.J. now refuses to take any antipsychotics. Her psychiatrist decides to start her on a LAIA form of aripiprazole, but notices there are two different versions of the medication available. Which of these two forms would be the better choice for J.J. at this time?

Ideally we would be able to stabilize J.J. on an oral form of aripiprazole prior to conversion to a LAIA form of the medication, but her nonadherence makes that unlikely. Both forms of aripiprazole LAIA require an overlap of oral medication during initiation: 14 days for the monohydrate salt and 21 days for the lauroxil salt. The main concern is the dosing of the LAIA, however. The monohydrate salt has a single dose for all patients, except in cases of renal impairment of P450 inhibitors or inducers. The lauroxil salt is dosed based upon a conversion from the dose of oral aripiprazole the patient is currently receiving. As J.J. was never stabilized on an oral dose of aripiprazole before she stopped taking the medication, it would be very difficult to convert her over to an equivalent dose of the lauroxil LAIA. Therefore, it would be easier to initiate the monohydrate salt version at its usual dose of 400 mg every month and then try to provide coverage for the initial 14-day window recommended for the product. Regardless of which form is used, J.J. should be monitored for the development of the parkinsonism she had when being titrated on the oral form of aripiprazole.

CASE 85-1, QUESTION 27: Over the next few months, J.J. is maintained on aripiprazole monohydrate LAIA 400 mg/month. As her symptoms improved but she was still showing some signs of daily auditory hallucinations, haloperidol 5 mg/day was added to her regimen. Her hallucinations subsided within a couple weeks after an increase to 10 mg/day of haloperidol, but now J.J. comes in with her parents to the ER attached to the clinic. J.J.'s neck is turned clockwise to her right shoulder, and she is unable to move her head back to her centerline and look forward. J.J. says her neck hurts a lot and she wants this feeling to go away. What is the most likely reason for J.J.'s current complaint and how should it be managed?

J.J. is most likely experiencing a dystonic reaction, or dystonia, from the recent addition and increase in her haloperidol dose. The specific type of dystonia she has is called torticollis, which is dystonia causing the muscles of the upper spine to contract and cause a twisting motion of the neck. This is another type of EPS, and as seen in J.J. here, can often be painful due to the strong muscle contraction. FGAs are more likely to cause this problem than SGAs, so the timing of the reaction to the addition of haloperidol makes sense.

Acutely, J.J.'s dystonia needs to be treated as quickly as possible as it is painful to her. Oral medications could take an hour or longer to work, so an injectable agent is preferred for more rapid action. As with drug-induced parkinsonism, the agent of choice is an anticholinergic medication to offset the EPS. Most ER's will have either benztropine or diphenhydramine (which has appreciable anticholinergic effects) readily available in an IM/IV form for a case like this. Atropine, while also likely available, is generally not used due to greater systemic and cardiac effects. Benzodiazepines can also be used in IM/IV forms if needed, as they too will help relax the contracted muscles and help J.J. calm down.

Additionally, J.J.'s medication regimen may need to be adjusted to prevent a future dystonic reaction. A reduction in her haloperidol dose may be needed, or adjunctive oral anticholinergics added to her regimen as prophylaxis.

CASE 85-1, QUESTION 28: J.J. has been continued on the combination of aripiprazole monohydrate LAIA and haloperidol over the next 8 years. Over time her symptoms have returned periodically, never requiring a hospitalization but necessitating gradual increases in her haloperidol to 15 mg/day. J.J. now presents to the clinic with "shakes in my hands" that are bothering her. During the physical examination, J.J. is noted to have facial grimacing, darting movements of her tongue, lip-smacking, and twisting movements in her hands. The movements in her hands seem to disappear when she grabs an object or performs other activities with her hands. What is the most likely cause of these movements in J.J.?

These movements are most likely an early form of tardive dyskinesia. Haloperidol, as a high-potency FGA, has a high risk of causing this movement disorder over time: approximately 3% to 5% per year of use, or 24% to 40% risk in J.J. The symptoms we are observing in J.J. are consistent with those movements seen in tardive dyskinesia which presents with arrhythmic choreoathetoid "snake-like" movements of the orofacial areas, limbs, and trunk. The fact that the irregular hand movements stop or decrease when J.J. performs a conscious task with her hands is also indicative of tardive dyskinesia.

CASE 85-1, QUESTION 29: What can be done to treat the tardive dyskinesia seen in J.J. at this time?

Although there are no definitive treatments for tardive dyskinesia, there are some strategies that might help to alleviate the problem. Slow decreases in her haloperidol dose over time may help these movements decrease; a rapid reduction in the dose may acutely worsen the problem, so this should be avoided. If the movements persist despite lowering the dosage or discontinuing the haloperidol, there are some data supporting the use of clozapine to treat the dyskinesia and schizophrenic symptoms. This should be considered cautiously in light of the other concerns related to clozapine treatment.

Inadequate Response

The patient with chronic schizophrenia must be evaluated in a systematic fashion to discern whether past medication trials were indeed medication failures. Medication nonadherence, intolerance, and inadequate dosing may often be documented as failed trials. Patients with schizophrenia have been shown to have a deficit in perspective habitual memory which may cause difficulty in remembering whether they took their medications.[223] This could result in either missed or doubled dosages. An in-depth assessment of medication adherence should be conducted in a nonpunitive and collaborative fashion with the patient. Outreach for collateral information should also be undertaken after acquiring appropriate releases of information. Clinical deterioration often occurs slowly and insidiously with incomplete medication adherence.[224] Poor therapeutic relationship and social supports may also lead to poor adherence in patients with schizophrenia.[225] Other important predictors include lack of insight, concomitant substance abuse, a short illness duration, issues with discharge planning and environment,[226] as well as higher levels of hostility.[227] Patients who have had difficulties with medication adherence in the past should be offered treatment with a long-acting injectable antipsychotic.

A trial of an antipsychotic should be continued for at least 4 to 6 weeks at a therapeutic dosage after initial partial response of symptoms. Switching and augmentation strategies should only be considered after symptoms fail to fully respond to an adequate trial. Patients may wind up in a stalled cross-titration, possibly due to a transition in care, and be continued on multiple antipsychotics. This highlights the need to carefully tease out the patient's medication experience and transition to effective monotherapy to avoid increased adverse effects, pill burden, and cost for the patient.

Between 20% and 30% of patients remain unresponsive despite multiple antipsychotic trials. The most commonly adopted and most stringent criteria for antipsychotic treatment refractoriness were proposed in the landmark trial conducted by Kane and colleagues that resulted in clozapine's approval in the U.S. market. Treatment refractoriness was defined as: (1) at least three periods of treatment in the preceding 5 years with antipsychotics from two chemical classes at dosages equivalent or greater to 1,000 mg/day of chlorpromazine for a period of 6 weeks, (2) no symptom-free period within 5 years, and (3) BPRS total score >45.[57,228]

Clozapine is the most efficacious medication in patients with treatment-resistant schizophrenia and should be considered in all patients who fail to respond to at least two adequate antipsychotic trials.[57,107,172,229] It is also the treatment of choice for those at high risk for suicide or violence, or in patients with TD.[102,230] Despite its superior efficacy, clozapine is often underutilized in the treatment of resistant schizophrenia due to its adverse effect burden. Close monitoring and follow-up are necessary to ensure safe and effective use of clozapine. Baseline monitoring should include a physical examination (weight, blood pressure, waist circumference), HbA1c or fasting blood glucose, a fasting lipid panel, liver function tests, serum creatinine, blood urea nitrogen levels and pregnancy test, if indicated. Clozapine has a unique adverse effect profile that ranges from common bothersome adverse effects to life-threatening adverse effects listed in its five black box warnings. The black box warnings caution for risk of agranulocytosis, seizures, myocarditis, other adverse cardiovascular and respiratory effects, and increased mortality in elderly patients with dementia-related psychosis.

Agranulocytosis is a rare, yet potentially life-threatening, hematologic reaction affecting approximately 1% of clozapine-treated patients. It is defined as a drop in neutrophil count below 500 cells/mm^3. Agranulocytosis is not dose-related and can occur at any point in treatment though the risk is higher within the first 6 months of therapy. Clozapine may also cause mild-to-severe neutropenia (ANC 500–2,000 cell/mm^3). Clozapine-induced neutropenia and agranulocytosis may be in part due to selective effect on precursors of polymorphonuclear leukocytes; however, the mechanism remains to be fully elucidated. Clozapine is only dispensed through the clozapine risk evaluation and monitoring strategy (REMS) to ensure ANC values are within range prior to dispensing clozapine. The pharmacy, patient, and provider must all be enrolled in the clozapine REMS program. Monitoring of the absolute neutrophil count (ANC) must occur 7 days prior to initiation of clozapine and weekly thereafter for the first 6 months. Monitoring frequency can be reduced to biweekly for the next 6 months if all ANC values are within range (>1,500/μL). Frequency of blood draws may be decreased to every 4 weeks if all values remain within range after 6 months of biweekly monitoring, and be maintained at every 4 weeks for the duration of clozapine treatment if no abnormalities are seen. Certain ethnic groups, including patients of African and Middle Eastern descent, may average a lower ANC value than normal ranges, called benign ethnic neutropenia (BEN). The clozapine REMS program allows for lower ANC values to compensate for patients diagnosed with BEN as they do not suffer from repeated or severe infections as a result of their low baseline ANC values. Severe neutropenia can be deadly due to the body's inability to fight off infection. This is a medical emergency that requires the abrupt discontinuation of clozapine. In other cases, clozapine should be discontinued gradually over a period of 2 weeks or longer, to prevent cholinergic rebound (sweating, headache, nausea, vomiting, diarrhea) or recurrence of psychotic symptoms. The patient should not be rechallenged on clozapine after agranulocytosis, but patients can be successfully rechallenged after neutropenia.[231] More information can be found at https://www.clozapinerems.com/ (Table 85-13).

Seizure risk associated with clozapine is a dose-related phenomenon. Risk of seizure is 4.4% at a dose of 600 mg and several case reports implicate serum levels greater than 500 to 1,300 ng/mL with higher risk of seizure.[232,233] Prophylactic use of antiepileptic drugs (AED) is generally not recommended.[234] However, patients that experience a seizure on clozapine can be safely continued on a lower dose of clozapine and initiated on an AED. Valproate and lamotrigine are preferred over carbamazepine due to its risk of agranulocytosis and extensive interaction profile.[233] Myocarditis is a potentially fatal hypersensitivity reaction that can occur approximately 3 weeks after initiation of clozapine. Diagnosis is confounded by the variable and nonspecific signs and symptoms of its presentation, but the incidence is estimated to fall between <0.1 and 3%.[235] The monitoring protocol proposed by Ronaldson and colleagues consists of obtaining baseline troponins, C-reactive protein (CRP), and an ECG, and then monitoring troponin and C-reactive protein on days 7, 14, 21, and 28 of treatment. In the case of mild elevation in troponins or CRP, persistent tachycardia, or signs or symptoms resembling infection, daily troponins and CRP should be drawn until symptom resolution. Clozapine should be discontinued if troponins reach twice the upper limit of normal or if CRP > 100 mg/L.[61] Successful rechallenge may be possible after symptoms resolve.[236,237]

The black box warning describing "other adverse cardiovascular and respiratory effects" references the risk of orthostatic hypotension associated with clozapine. Approximately 9% of patients will experience orthostatic hypotension, but tolerance develops over 4 to 6 weeks.[165] Risk is higher during initiation which necessitates the slow titration beginning at 12.5 mg twice daily and increasing at the rate of 25 to 50 mg/day or slower. Clozapine must also be retitrated after a gap in therapy of greater than 2 days to prevent significant orthostasis and risk of falls. Patients should be counseled to make slow transitions from prone or seated positions and maintain adequate fluid and salt intake. In patients with persistent dizziness and orthostasis after titration where dose reduction is not an option, treatment with the mineralocorticoid, fludrocortisone, may be an option.[165]

Clozapine is also associated with frequent, bothersome adverse effects that, if left unaddressed, can greatly impact quality of life. Constipation is a common, yet often overlooked adverse effect of clozapine that can result in serious complications including paralytic ileus, small-bowel perforation, or death secondary to aspiration of gastric contents. It affects between 14% and 60% of patients taking clozapine. Patients should be screened at every visit for bowel habits and providers should have a low threshold for initiating a bowel regimen. Bowel regimens consist of bulk-forming laxatives and increased fluid intake, stool softeners, or short-term use of stimulant laxatives or enemas. Anticholinergic adverse effects of clozapine can result in GI hypomotility, small-bowel obstruction, and ileus. These are serious concerns that may occur in up to 0.3% of clozapine-treated patients. Adjunctive anticholinergic agents and opioids should be limited and clozapine dose tentatively decreased, or held in cases of ileus. Sedation is usually more pronounced when first initiating clozapine and can be managed by slowing the rate

Table 85-13

Clozapine Monitoring Requirements

ANC Level	Treatment Recommendation	ANC Monitoring
Normal Range for a New Patient General Population ■ ANC ≥ 1,500/μL BEN Population ■ ANC ≥ 1,000/μL ■ Obtain at least two baseline ANC levels before initiating treatment	Initiate treatment ■ If treatment interrupted: ■ <30 days, continue monitoring as before ■ ≥30 days, monitor as if new patient	Weekly from initiation to 6 months ■ Every 2 weeks from 6 to 12 months ■ Monthly after 12 months
Mild neutropenia (1,000–1,499/μL)[a]	General Population ■ Continue treatment BEN Population ■ Mild neutropenia is normal range for BEN population, continue treatment ■ Obtain at least two baseline ANC levels before initiating treatment ■ If treatment interrupted ■ < 30 days, continue monitoring as before ■ ≥ 30 days, monitor as if new patient ■ Discontinuation for reasons other than neutropenia	General Population ■ Three times weekly until ANC ≥1,500/μL ■ Once ANC ≥1,500/μL return to patient's last "Normal Range" ANC monitoring interval[b] BEN Population ■ Weekly from initiation to 6 months ■ Every 2 weeks from 6 to 12 months ■ Monthly after 12 months
Moderate Neutropenia (500–999/μL)[a]	General Population ■ Recommend hematology consultation ■ Interrupt treatment for suspected clozapine-induced neutropenia ■ Resume treatment once ANC normalizes to ≥1,000/μL BEN Population ■ Recommend hematology consultation ■ Continue treatment	General Population ■ Daily until ANC ≥1,000/μL, then ■ Three times weekly until ANC ≥1,500/μL ■ Once ANC ≥1,500/μL check ANC weekly for 4 weeks, then return to patient's last "Normal Range" ANC monitoring interval[b] BEN Population ■ Three times weekly until ANC ≥1,000/μL or ≥patient's known baseline. ■ Once ANC ≥1,000/μL or patient's known baseline, check ANC weekly for 4 weeks, then return to patient's last "Normal BEN Range" ANC monitoring interval.[b]
Severe Neutropenia (<500/μL)[a]	General Population ■ Recommend hematology consultation ■ Interrupt treatment for suspected clozapine-induced neutropenia ■ Do not rechallenge unless prescriber determines benefits outweigh risks BEN Population ■ Recommend hematology consultation ■ Interrupt treatment for suspected clozapine-induced neutropenia ■ Do not rechallenge unless prescriber determines benefits outweigh risks	General Population ■ Daily until ANC ≥1,000/μL ■ Three times weekly until ANC ≥1,500/μL ■ If patient rechallenged, resume treatment as a new patient under "Normal Range" monitoring once ANC ≥1,500/μL BEN Population ■ Daily until ANC ≥500/μL ■ Three times weekly until ANC ≥ patients established baseline ■ If patient rechallenged, resume treatment as a new patient under "Normal Range" monitoring once ANC ≥1,000/μL or at patient's baseline

[a]Confirm all initial reports of ANC less than 1,500/μL (ANC <1,000/μL for BEN patients) with a repeat ANC measurement within 24 hours
[b]If clinically appropriate

BEN, Benign Ethnic Neutropenia

Clozaril (clozapine tablets) [package insert]. East Hanover, NJ: Novartis Pharmaceuticals Corporation; September 2015.

of titration and consolidating the dose to bedtime. As previously described, a benign tachycardia can also result from clozapine use, but patients also presenting with flu-like symptoms, dyspnea, fever, and chest pain should have further work-up for myocarditis. Sialorrhea is an embarrassing adverse effect that in the extreme can result in sleep disruption or aspiration pneumonia. Treatment options include tentative dose reduction or nonpharmacologic management, such as placing a towel on their pillow, as first line. Topical anticholinergic agents (ipratropium 0.03%–0.06% dosed 1–2 sprays sublingually or 1–2 atropine eye drops in 1 ounce of water swished and spit) are preferred over systemic anticholinergics (benztropine 0.5–2 mg HS or glycopyrrolate 1–2 mg) or the α-2 adrenergic agent, clonidine.[238] Serious cases may be treated with botulinum toxin injected into each parotid gland.[238] Nocturnal enuresis may also be underreported due to embarrassment. Management includes avoiding fluids in the evening, voiding prior to bed, and setting alarms to schedule nocturnal voiding. Desmopressin may also be effectively utilized, but the patient must be monitored for hyponatremia secondary to its use.[165]

CASE 85-1, QUESTION 30: J.J.'s psychiatrist decides to start J.J. on clozapine and remove all other antipsychotics in light of her tardive dyskinesia and past failures and adverse effects with other antipsychotics. What adverse effects of clozapine should be monitored for in J.J.?

Any patient started on clozapine should be monitored for agranulocytosis and metabolic adverse effects, among others. As J.J. has a history of metabolic adverse effects (weight gain, increased glucose, and increased triglycerides) with other antipsychotics, these are of particular concern with using clozapine with her as clozapine has the highest risk of these adverse effects. J.J. should also be counseled about orthostatic hypotension, sedation, anticholinergic effects (especially constipation), and sialorrhea.

CASE 85-1, QUESTION 31: Prior to initiating clozapine therapy, what laboratories and other tests should be performed on J.J.?

Clozapine therapy requires a baseline absolute neutrophil count (ANC) prior to starting the medication to ensure the patient has an adequate number of neutrophils prior to initiation. In addition, her weight, waist circumference, serum glucose/HbA1c, and lipid panel should be measured to monitor for the development of metabolic adverse effects. Baseline liver and kidney function tests should also be measured. A pregnancy test should also be performed, especially if there is any chance that J.J. could be pregnant.

CASE 85-1, QUESTION 32: Once J.J. is started on clozapine, how should she be monitored? What parameters should be checked and how frequently?

Clozapine treatment requires weekly ANC checks for at least the first 6 months of treatment. Assuming no problems with her ANC values (ANC $\geq$ 1,500/μL), she can then go to ANC checks every other week for 6 months, and then ANC checks once every 4 weeks thereafter. In addition, her weight should be monitored at least monthly (and perhaps weekly) for the first few months of treatment, along with at least quarterly serum glucose and lipid panel checks. She should also be asked about any problems with orthostasis (dizziness), constipation, sedation, and drooling during any office visits.

Serum Concentration Monitoring

Data supporting a strong correlation between antipsychotic serum concentrations and efficacy are lacking.[239] Therefore, routine therapeutic drug monitoring of antipsychotic serum concentration is not recommended in clinical practice. The exception is clozapine, which has sufficient data to support a higher rate of response at levels above 350 ng/mL.[173,240] Monitoring of serum levels is appropriate in the following clinical scenarios:

1. Psychiatric decompensation on a previously effective dose
2. Poor response to medication despite adequate dose and trial duration
3. Unexpected adverse effects while on a previously tolerated dose
4. Addition or withdrawal of an interacting medication
5. Patients with potentially altered PK (e.g., medically compromised, children, elderly)
6. Suspected medication nonadherence

Nonantipsychotic Agents

Antipsychotics are generally the treatment of choice for most patients with schizophrenia. However, in some situations, other medications may be needed and appropriate for use. Benzodiazepines may be appropriate in patients with acute agitation, as described previously. Other medications, such as mood stabilizers and antidepressants, may be useful for some patients based upon their clinical symptoms and presentation.

MOOD STABILIZERS

The mood stabilizers lithium, carbamazepine, valproic acid, and lamotrigine have been studied for use in schizophrenia. These medications are frequently used as an adjunct to antipsychotic treatment in schizophrenia in patients with affective symptomatology as well as core symptoms of schizophrenia. Evidence for these common practices is sometimes found to be equivocal or conflicting.

None of these mood stabilizers have shown efficacy as monotherapy for schizophrenia. Lamotrigine has been found to have modest effects in schizophrenic pathology as an adjunct to antipsychotic treatment but has little efficacy in treating the treatment-resistant patient.[241] Lithium was determined by a Cochrane review to have some benefit as an augmenting agent in lower quality studies, but replication in higher quality studies is needed.[242] A recent meta-analysis shows evidence that the practice of augmentation of antipsychotic medications with valproate yields significant improvements in patients treated for schizophrenia or schizoaffective disorder.[243] A recent Cochrane review does not recommend carbamazepine for augmentation of antipsychotics in the treatment of schizophrenia.[244] A need for further study of antipsychotic augmentation with mood stabilizers is warranted. Concomitant use should be carefully considered at this time given the potential for drug interactions, and additional adverse effect and pill burden.

ANTIDEPRESSANTS

Depression often presents in schizophrenia[37,245] and approximately 6% to 10% of patients with schizophrenia commit suicide in their lifetime.[29,246–248] Though controversial, there is evidence that antipsychotics may differ in their ability to treat depressive symptoms in schizophrenia[54,99,249,250] and many consider SGAs to be better for this syndrome than the FGAs.[250,251] Some of the advantages of SGAs in depression may be due in part to less antipsychotic-induced dysphoria or akinesia or effect on treating negative symptoms.[250,251] There is also substantial literature showing that adding an antidepressant may be a useful option in some depressed patients.[252] The divergent pattern of antidepressant response on numerous studies suggests that those patients whose positive symptoms are well controlled are more likely to respond favorably to antidepressant augmentation.[28] In one trial, the antidepressant bupropion did significantly worse than placebo in patients treated with thiothixene.[34]

Some also advocate for the possible effectiveness of antidepressant medication to decrease the severity of negative symptoms in schizophrenia.[253] One review found only 5 of 14 studies with SSRI antidepressants demonstrated efficacy in ameliorating negative symptoms; however, mirtazapine was promising in 4 of 6 trials.[252] Tricyclic antidepressants do not have robust evidence in treatment of negative symptoms.[254]

Case 85-1, Question 33: J.J. responds well to clozapine, taking a dose of 450 mg/day, with higher doses causing intolerable adverse effects in J.J. Over time, J.J. begins to become depressed as she realizes that her life has not gone the way she thought it would. Her psychiatrist assesses her as having depression secondary to her schizophrenia, and the decision is made to start her on paroxetine 20 mg daily. Is the addition of paroxetine appropriate for J.J.?

Although paroxetine is an appropriate treatment for depression, it is most likely not a good choice for J.J. There are data that show that paroxetine can cause anticholinergic adverse effects in patients, which could overlap any anticholinergic effects caused by clozapine. J.J. would need to be monitored for increased anticholinergic adverse effects, and possibly be treated for them (e.g., bowel regimen for constipation). Selection of an antidepressant with a lower risk of drug interactions, such as Escitalopram or Sertraline, would be more appropriate.

Treatment Guidelines for Schizophrenia

Clinical guidelines on the treatment of schizophrenia are published by a number of organizations. The most prolific and current guidelines at this time are the American Psychiatric Association (APA), Patient Outcomes Research Team on Schizophrenia (PORT), Texas Medication Algorithm Project (TMAP), and the National Institute for Health and Care Excellence (NICE) of the United Kingdom.[101–103,255] These guidelines are an excellent resource and starting point in ensuring evidence-based and safe care of patients with schizophrenia. However, it is important to keep in mind the level of evidence each organization requires to support a given treatment recommendation. The PORT guidelines have a threshold of at least two randomized controlled trials prior to publishing a treatment recommendation. The APA utilizes a less clearly defined process of systematically evaluating the literature, then rating clinical recommendations by the following coding system: (I) recommended with substantial clinical confidence, (II) recommended with moderate clinical confidence, and (III) may be recommended on the basis of individual circumstances. Other guidelines may also incorporate expert opinion[101,103] or consensus in areas which lack high level evidence, such as antipsychotic combination treatment or treatment after nonresponse to clozapine. The bottom-line is these guidelines provide a systematic framework for treatment, but should by no means be a substitute for clinical judgment and treating the unique clinical picture each individual presents. Any treatment decision should be aligned with the treatment team, caregivers, and most importantly—the patient. Even the most effective treatment is destined to fail unless the patient is invested and in agreement with their own treatment. Figure 85-2 is a consolidated view of the current guidelines on the use of antipsychotics in the treatment of schizophrenia.

CONSIDERATIONS IN SPECIFIC POPULATIONS

Pregnancy

The peak onset of schizophrenia in the female population coincides with peak childbearing age and unplanned pregnancies can be a

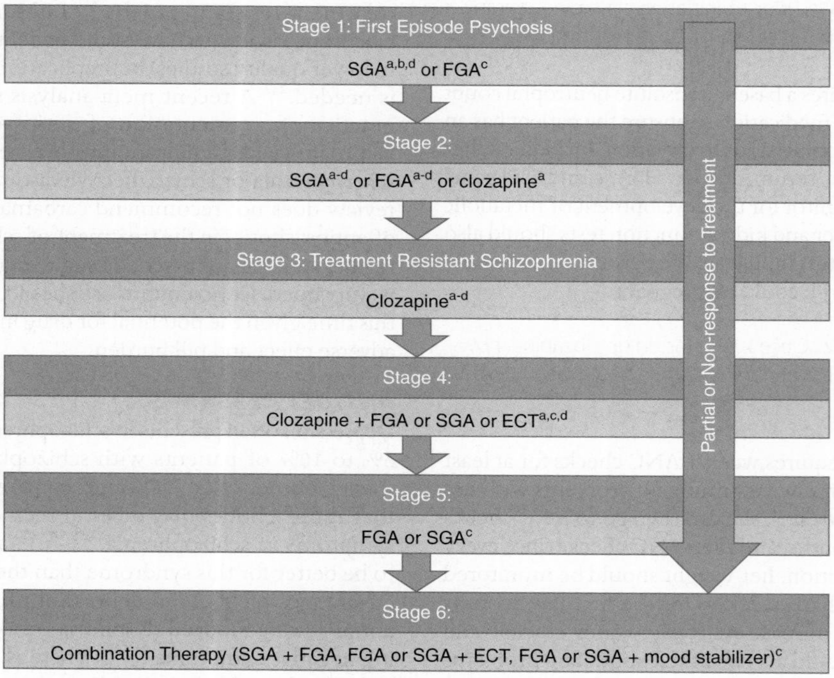

Figure 85-2 Summary of Current Treatment Guidelines on Schizophrenia. (Sources: [a]American Psychiatric Association [Lehman AF et al. Practice guideline for the treatment of patients with schizophrenia, second edition. *Am J Psychiatry*. 2004;161(2, Suppl):1–56. doi:10.1176/appi.books.9780890423363.45859.], [b]Patient Outcomes Research Team [Buchanan RW et al. The 2009 schizophrenia PORT psychopharmacologic treatment recommendations and summary statements. *Schizophr Bull*. 2010;36(1):71–93. doi:10.1093/schbul/sbp116.], [c]Texas Medication Algorithm Project [Moore T et al. The Texas medication algorithm project antipsychotic algorithm for schizophrenia: 2006 Update. *J Clin Psychiatry*. 2007;68(11):1751–1762. doi:10.4088/JCP.v65n0408.], [d]International Psychopharmacology Algorithm Project [IPAP Schizophrenia Algorithm. The International Psychopharmacology Algorithm Project website. **http://www.ipap.org/schiz/. Updated March 27, 2006.** Accessed February 1, 2016.])

concern.[256] Patients should be routinely educated on safe sexual practices, offered contraceptives if indicated, and receive pregnancy tests prior to prescription of antipsychotic medications. The general goals of treatment in pregnant patients are to thoroughly weigh the risks of teratogenicity with benefit of ongoing treatment and prevention of psychiatric decompensation. Untreated psychosis places both the patient and the fetus at significant risk. Effective treatment with an antipsychotic agent may enable the mother to carry out necessary self-care and prenatal care.[257] Ideally, treatment decisions should be made as part of a multidisciplinary team consisting of the patient, mental health provider, obstetrician, primary care provider, and pediatrician. General guidelines on treatment during pregnancy recommend[257]:

1. Utilizing antipsychotic monotherapy at an adequate dose versus combination therapy
2. Avoiding medication switching to minimize exposure to the fetus and risk of psychiatric relapse
3. Selecting appropriate treatment based on history of efficacy, prior exposure during pregnancy, and available evidence on safety
4. Choosing medications with fewer metabolites, fewer interactions, and higher protein binding are generally preferred

Data on the safety of antipsychotics during pregnancy are limited due to ethical barriers to conducting well-designed, prospective controlled trials. There is inconclusive evidence linking fetal exposure to antipsychotics and major congenital malformations, perinatal mortality, high birth weight (SGAs), and low birth weight (FGAs).[256] A large-scale prospective national pregnancy registry for atypicals antipsychotics reported three major fetal malformations in a cohort of 214 patients with first-trimester exposure to SGAs. The control group, which included 89 live births, had one major malformation. This translates to an OR of 1.25 (95% CI = 0.13–12.19) between exposed and unexposed infants. Although ongoing data collection is still underway, these results suggest SGA exposure would be unlikely to increase the risk of major malformations higher than 10-fold of that observed in control groups or the general population.[258] In 2011, the FDA implemented safety labeling changes concerning the use of antipsychotic agents during the third trimester of pregnancy. They reported a risk that newborns may experience withdrawal symptoms or EPS; however, many cases were confounded by comorbid substance use and concomitant psychotropic medications. Symptoms usually resolved within hours-days without intervention; however, some may require prolonged hospitalization.[259]

Case 85-1, Question 34: Several months later, the clinic receives word from J.J.'s primary care provider that J.J. is pregnant, as confirmed by blood test. J.J. is still receiving clozapine and is fairly stable psychiatrically on the medication, even working part-time in a supermarket. J.J. does not want to lose the baby, but is worried about the effect of being on medication despite knowing it is what is keeping her stable. Should J.J. be continued on clozapine, and what are the risks to her baby if she does or does not?

Treatment of schizophrenia with antipsychotics during pregnancy must be considered carefully. As J.J. is currently stable and functional while taking clozapine, there is a significant risk of relapse if she stops the medication. During this relapse, if she were to engage in high-risk behaviors, it could be quite dangerous to both her and her baby. Maintaining stability is of great importance, as if J.J. can take care of herself appropriately it is more likely she will also take care of her fetus simultaneously. However, antipsychotics do carry risks of teratogenicity, and J.J. should be counseled on these risks. Clozapine is rated as pregnancy category B by the US FDA, which is better than most antipsychotics but still with some risk involved. The decision to maintain J.J. on clozapine during her pregnancy should be made by her, her psychiatrist, obstetrician, and other care providers to determine whether continuation of clozapine, and presumptive stability of her illness, is appropriate.

First-Episode Psychosis and Early-Onset Schizophrenia

Child and adolescent patients presenting with early psychosis are exquisitely sensitive to EPS and metabolic adverse effects of antipsychotics.[260,261] In general, symptoms of first-episode psychosis (FEP) respond to lower antipsychotic dosages. Therefore, the minimum effective dose should be utilized to minimize adverse effect burden. The question of which interventions are appropriate to initiate and when is complicated. Multiple studies support the effectiveness of antipsychotics in the treatment of early psychosis.[262–265] However, the treatment of prodromal symptoms is an area of debate. Prompt recognition of prodromal symptoms and patients with psychosis risk syndrome is crucial. Features associated with greater rates of conversion to psychosis in patients at ultra-high risk of psychosis include: genetic risk for schizophrenia, high levels of unusual thought content, high levels of suspicion and paranoia, social impairment, and history of substance use.[266] There is emerging evidence to support early initiation of omega-3 fatty acids or antidepressants to reduce rates of conversion to psychosis in high-risk patients.[261,267,268] Early engagement with appropriate comprehensive, multidisciplinary clinics results in improved quality of life and psychopathology, greater involvement in educational and vocational pursuits, and increased treatment follow-up.[269,270] Reduction of the duration of untreated psychosis leads to improved long-term prognosis and greater likelihood of achieving symptom remission.[44,271,272] Neurocognitive impairment is also a key predictor of functional outcome in early schizophrenia. Unfortunately, available pharmacologic options have limited impact on neurocognition.[273] Cognitive enhancement therapy, in conjunction with antipsychotic medication, can lead to durable improvements in neurocognitive functioning, social adjustment, and employment for patients with early psychosis.[274,275]

After achieving initial remission, guidelines recommend continued maintenance treatment with an antipsychotic for at least 1 year.[44,102,255] Studies of medication discontinuation demonstrated 5 year relapse rates from 80%.[276] However, cautious dose reduction strategies as soon as 6 months after remission may improve long-term functional recovery. Wunderink and colleagues conducted a seven-year follow-up study of a two-year open RCT comparing maintenance therapy (MT) versus dose reduction/discontinuation (DR) after 6-month remission of FEP. In the initial RCT, 128 patients were randomized to MT or DR and followed for 18 months. The MT group showed benefit in short-term relapse rates over the DR group.[277] However, the DR group had approximately twice the recovery rate of patients in the MT group (40.4% vs. 17.6%, respectively) at the seven-year follow-up and there were no significant differences in long-term relapse rates.[278] A limitation to the generalizability of the study is the population who agreed to enrollment in the initial phase had a higher level of functioning, greater adherence, and was easier to engage. These findings demonstrate the potential impact of limiting total antipsychotic burden on functional recovery rates of patients with remitted FEP. The lower adverse effect burden from minimizing the antipsychotic dose allows for improved social engagement, improved therapeutic alliance, and lower risk of self-discontinuation due to tolerability issues. Functional recovery is the key treatment goal in the early course of schizophrenia. Getting patients engaged in treatment early on in the illness course, utilizing the lowest clinically effective dosages of antipsychotics, and providing psychoeducation can mean the difference in a patient recovering from a psychotic episode and completing college, returning to work, or engaging in meaningful social outlets.

CASE 85-1, QUESTION 35: J.J. gives birth to a son, R.J., who has a normal delivery. Over the course of time, R.J.'s pediatrician notes he is not socializing like other children, especially into adolescence. He is now age 15 and tends to isolate himself, does not have many peer friends, and recently has started performing poorly in school. His teachers have asked the pediatrician to evaluate R.J. for potential attention deficit hyperactivity disorder (ADHD) as he is often found not paying attention in class. J.J. also tells the pediatrician that she thinks R.J. still has "imaginary friends" as she often sees him alone in his room talking to people who are not there. What is potentially happening with R.J. and how should he be treated at this time?

R.J. is at higher risk for and potentially showing symptoms of early-onset schizophrenia. His lack of socialization and his isolation could be symptoms of the prodromal phase of schizophrenia. His "imaginary friends" could be R.J. responding to auditory and/or visual hallucinations; imaginary friends are not usually seen into adolescence. If these are hallucinations, this could also explain his lack of attention in school, which would not be ADHD. Considering his mother has schizophrenia, there is a definite genetic link to the illness in R.J. Once R.J. is evaluated for schizophrenia, it may be appropriate to initiate an antipsychotic at that time. If so, he should be started on an agent with minimal adverse effect burden at a minimal dose to control his symptoms. He should be evaluated regularly for possible medication discontinuation if warranted, but may require more long-term treatment depending upon his response and prognosis.

KEY REFERENCES AND WEBSITES

A full list of references for this chapter can be found at http://thepoint.lww.com/AT11e. Below are the key references and websites for this chapter, with the corresponding reference number in this chapter found in parentheses after the reference.

Key References

American Diabetes Association et al. Consensus development conference on antipsychotic drugs and obesity and diabetes. *Diabetes Care*. 2004;27:596. (193)

Buchanan RW et al. The 2009 schizophrenia PORT psychopharmacological treatment recommendations and summary statements. *Schizophr Bull*. 2010;36:71. (102)

Leucht S et al. Comparative efficacy and tolerability of 15 antipsychotic drugs in schizophrenia: a multiple-treatments meta-analysis. *Lancet*. 2013;382(9896):951–962. doi:10.1016/S0140-6736(13)60733-3. (172)

Lieberman JA et al. Effectiveness of antipsychotic drugs in patients with chronic schizophrenia. *N Engl J Med*. 2005;353(12):1209–1223. doi:10.1056/NEJMoa1404304. (64)

Marder SR et al. The Mount Sinai conference on the pharmacotherapy of schizophrenia. *Schizophr Bull*. 2002;28(1):5–16. (198)

Key Websites

American Psychiatric Association. Treatment of Patients With Schizophrenia, Second Edition. http://www.psychiatryonline.com/pracGuide/pracGuideTopic_6.aspx.

Clozapine REMS Program. https://www.clozapinerems.com/CpmgClozapineUI/home.u

National Institute for Health and Clinical Excellence. Schizophrenia (update). http://guidance.nice.org.uk/CG82.

National Institute of Mental Health. Schizophrenia. http://www.nimh.nih.gov/health/topics/schizophrenia/index.shtml

US Food and Drug Administration. FDA Drug Safety Communication: Antipsychotic drug labels updated on use during pregnancy and risk of abnormal muscle movements and withdrawal symptoms in newborns. http://www.fda.gov/Drugs/DrugSafety/ucm243903.htm. Accessed March 17, 2016.

86 Depressive Disorders

Michael C. Angelini

CORE PRINCIPLES

	Core Principle	CHAPTER CASES
1	Depression is a common and often chronic disorder that may manifest at any time in one's life. Diagnostic criteria for major depression include a minimum of five symptoms persisting for at least 2 weeks. One of these symptoms must be either depressed mood or anhedonia. Suicidal ideation should be assessed in all patients.	**Case 86-1 (Question 1), Table 86-4**
2	A variety of treatment modalities are available for the management of depression. These include prescription medications, psychotherapy, and somatic treatments. Prescription medications and/or psychotherapy are indicated for depressive symptoms that are moderate to severe in nature, whereas somatic treatments are for severe refractory cases.	**Case 86-1 (Question 2), Case 86-2 (Questions 1, 2), Case 86-3 (Question 2)**
3	All of the prescription medications that are currently available are equally effective and possess the same delayed onset of therapeutic effects. Selection of an antidepressant is based on many factors, including previous response to medication, age, reproduction status, and both medical and psychiatric comorbidities.	**Case 86-1 (Questions 2, 4), Case 86-2 (Question 2) Case 86-4 (Question 1), Table 86-6**
4	SSRIs are regarded as the initial treatment of choice for most depressed patients. They are inexpensive and effective for comorbid anxiety conditions, and possess a lower side effect burden than other antidepressants overall. Side effects are generally mild and transient.	**Case 86-1 (Question 2), Case 86-2 (Question 1)**
5	Educating the patient regarding side effects, how to monitor for efficacy, and the duration of treatment is important action for successful treatment.	**Case 86-1 (Question 3), Case 86-3 (Question 3), Table 86-10**
6	The goal of antidepressant treatment is remission of symptoms. Once remission is achieved, the general recommendation is to continue the effective antidepressant regimen for a minimum of 6 months.	**Case 86-1 (Question 3), Table 86-10**
7	Because only half of depressed patients will achieve remission with the first antidepressant selected, clinicians should have a comprehensive understanding of the role many antidepressants may have in optimizing outcomes. Clinicians should be familiar with switching antidepressants in patients with an incomplete response, and the merits of augmentation strategies.	**Case 86-2 (Questions 1–3)**
8	Untreated depression in children under 18 has a significant risk of suicide. Treatment consists of talking therapy and specific antidepressants, which is different than the broad options available to adults.	**Case 86-3 (Questions 1, 2)**
9	Depression and chronic pain are commonly comorbid, and pharmacologic treatment that addresses both is recommended. This makes the SNRI class of antidepressants preferred.	**Case 86-4 (Question 1)**

INTRODUCTION

In general, depressive disorders are enormous health concerns that are often misdiagnosed or undertreated. The physical and social dysfunction associated with depression is profound and is believed to outweigh many other chronic medical conditions, including hypertension, diabetes, and arthritis.[1] The Medical Outcomes Study determined that the degree of impairment in depressed individuals is comparable to that seen in patients with chronic heart disease.[2] The financial ramifications of depression are tremendous and place an overwhelming burden on our society. In 2000, the estimated cost of depression in the United States was $83.1 billion annually, with most of these costs ($51.5 billion) attributed to lost productivity and absenteeism in the workplace.[1,3]

Table 86-1

Classification of Depressive Disorders

1. Major depressive disorder
2. Persistent depressive disorder
3. Disruptive mood dysregulation disorder
4. Premenstrual dysphoric disorder
5. Substance/medication-induced depressive disorder
6. Depressive disorder due to another medical condition
7. Other specified depressive disorder
8. Unspecified depressive disorder

Adapted with permission from American Psychiatric Association. Diagnostic and Statistical Manual of Mental Disorders. 5th ed. Washington, DC: American Psychiatric Association; 2013.

Epidemiology

Since World War II, the lifetime incidence of depression has been rising steadily in studied populations. The annual incidence of all mood disorders is approximately 10% in the adult population, and 1 in 15 adults (6.7%) will suffer from an episode of major depression during any 12-month period.[4] Various studies from Europe and the United States have estimated the 1 year and lifetime prevalence to be 4.1% and 6.7%, respectively.[5] Although the incidence of depression is remarkably similar across various races and ethnic groups, the illness may be slightly more common in lower socioeconomic classes and women having double the incidence than men.[1,5]

The onset of depression occurs most commonly in the late 20s, but there is a wide range, and the first episode may actually present at any age. Genetic factors appear to play a major role in the cause of depression. The offspring of depressed individuals are 2.7 times more likely to have depression if one parent is afflicted, and 3.0 times more likely if both parents suffer from depression.[6] Concordance rates for monozygotic (identical) twins range from 54% to 65%, whereas the corresponding rates in dizygotic (fraternal) twins range from 14% to 24%.[7] Genetic factors may also predispose individuals to an earlier onset of depression (younger than 30 years of age).[8] Additionally, there is clear evidence that depression may occur as a result of stressful events (i.e., environmental factors) in one's life. These factors include a difficult childhood, physical or verbal abuse, pervasive low self-esteem, death of a loved one, loss of a job, and the end of a serious relationship. Acute depressive episodes are often attributed to a combination of environmental and genetic factors. For instance, individuals carrying a genetic predisposition to mood disorders may undergo a stressful experience that ultimately triggers the manifestation of depressive symptomatology. Depression may also occur spontaneously among people who appear to lack any obvious genetic or environmental predisposition.

Diagnosis and Classification

When assessing a person for depression, it is important to recognize the level of impairment due to the symptoms. Just as with all biologic systems, the body can function well within a particular range (e.g., serum potassium or BP). Mood is not different; as long as the depressive symptoms are not prolonged or impairing, there would be no reason to aggressively treat. Once the depression is severe enough to impact functioning or induce harm, it requires treatment.

Major depressive disorder (MDD) may manifest as a single episode, but it is more commonly a series of recurrent events. Thus, in most patients, depression is a chronic illness.[5] The frequency of recurrent episodes is highly variable, with some people experiencing discrete episodes separated by many years of relatively normal mood (euthymia), and others experiencing residual symptoms between episodes that may never completely remit. The risk of future episodes appears to increase disproportionately with the chronicity of the illness. For instance, after the first episode there is a 50% likelihood of a second episode. After the second, there is a 70% chance of a third, and with the third episode comes nearly a 90% incidence of a fourth.

The Diagnostic and Statistical Manual 5th edition (DSM-5) describes different types of depressed states. These include disruptive mood dysregulation disorder, MDD, persistent depressive disorder, premenstrual dysphoric disorder, substance/medication-induced depressive disorder, depressive disorder due to another medical condition, other specified depressive disorder, and unspecified depressive disorder (Table 86-1).[9] The different types of depressive disorders may then be subclassified using cross-sectional symptom features, or specifiers. For example, the phrase "with anxious distress" which infers that there are anxiety symptoms such as worry and feeling keyed up. The term "with mixed features" infers that there are manic or hypomanic symptoms. The term "with melancholic features" is used when patients possess primary neurovegetative symptoms, early morning awakening, marked psychomotor agitation or retardation, and significant anorexia or weight loss. Melancholia is often a more severe form of depression, and it often lacks apparent environmental triggers.[9,10] It may also be less likely than other forms of depression to remit spontaneously. The phrase "with atypical features" is used when depressive symptoms include weight gain, hypersomnia, leaden paralysis, or rejection sensitivity. When hallucinations or delusions occur in patients who are primarily depressed, the phrase "with mood congruent or mood incongruent psychotic features" is applicable to the mood disorder. Other diagnostic specifiers used in DSM-5 include "with catatonia," and "with peripartum onset," and "with seasonal pattern."

Persistent depressive disorder is a type of depressive illness characterized by fewer symptoms and less intensity than major depression, but the course is much more chronic with symptoms being present most of the time for at least 2 years. In practice, the detection of persistent depressive disorder may be difficult to make because patients often do not seek treatment because they are still functional (e.g., go to school, work, care for children) but they have significant morbidity. They will have less satisfaction with work and will get fewer promotions and poor raises. The treatment for persistent depressive disorder has traditionally focused on psychotherapy, but evidence suggests that antidepressant medications may actually be more effective.[11]

Differential Diagnosis

Symptoms of depression may be induced or exacerbated by numerous medical illnesses or medications (Tables 86-2 and

Table 86-2
Selected Medical Conditions That May Mimic Depression

Stroke
Parkinson disease
Dementia
Multiple sclerosis
Endocrine disorders
Metabolic conditions
Infectious diseases
Chronic pain

Source: Practice guideline for the treatment of patients with major depressive disorder. 3rd ed. Arlington, VA: American Psychiatric Association. 2010.

Table 86-3
Selected Medications That May Induce Depression

Benzodiazepines
Corticosteroids
Interferon
Interleukin-2
Gonadotropin-releasing hormone agonists
Mefloquine
Oral and implanted oral contraceptives
High-dose lipophilic β-blockers
Antiepileptics
Varenicline

Source: Patten SB, Barbui C. Drug-induced depression: a systematic review to inform clinical practice. *Psychother Psychosom*. 2004;73(4):207–215.

86-3).[1,5,10] Consequently, DSM-5 specifies that whenever an medical event is temporally related to the onset of depressive symptoms, the patient does not fit the criteria for major depression, even if all other criteria are met.[9] The rationale for this stipulation is that if the medical illness is successfully treated or the offending agent is discontinued, the depressive illness would spontaneously resolve, eliminating the need for psychiatric intervention. Although lists of medical illnesses or medications are helpful, the clinician should be aware that the actual evidence demonstrating an association between depression and specific organic causes is limited. If a medication or condition is suspected of causing depression, the chronologic association should be investigated rigorously before other action is taken. Additionally, a patient with a medical illness such as a hormonal abnormality may have depressive symptoms from the condition but can additionally have concomitant MDD. Treating the medical condition will likely lessen the severity but the MDD will still have to be treated as well.[1,5,10]

Clinical Presentation

For a diagnosis of MDD to be made, symptoms must be present for at least 2 weeks and must not be precipitated or influenced by a medical illness or medication (according to DSM-5 criteria). Individuals must possess at least five symptoms, one of which is either depressed mood or anhedonia (diminished interest or pleasure in activities). The other seven symptoms are as follows:

1. Change in appetite or significant weight loss or gain
2. insomnia or hypersomnia
3. Psychomotor agitation or retardation
4. Fatigue or loss of energy
5. Feelings of worthlessness or inappropriate guilt
6. Poor concentration (or difficulty making decisions)
7. Recurrent thoughts of death or suicidal

The diagnostic criteria also state that the mood disturbance must cause marked distress or result in clinically significant impairment of social or occupational functioning. Additionally, the symptoms cannot be due to a medical or organic illness (Table 86-4).

Pathophysiology

The monoamine hypothesis proposed that decreased synaptic concentrations of norepinephrine (NE) and/or serotonin (5-HT) caused depression. The NE depletion theory was originally based on the observation that reserpine, which depleted catecholamine stores in the central nervous system (CNS), was capable of causing depression.[12,13] This theory evolved into the permissive hypothesis, which emphasized a greater role for serotonin in promoting or "permitting" a decline in NE function. Specifically, this hypothesis suggests that low concentrations of serotonin or NE in the CNS precipitated depressive symptoms. Studies have shown that a 5-HT synthesis deficiency is correlated with depression. This has been shown in both persons genetically unable to produce 5-HT and those who have depleted precursors of 5-HT.[14,15] Selective serotonin reuptake inhibitor (SSRI) and serotonin and norepinephrine

Table 86-4
Diagnostic Criteria for Depressive Episode

- At least five of the following symptoms have been present during the same 2-week period and represent a change from previous functioning. One of the symptoms must be either depressed mood or loss of interest/pleasure.
  - Depressed mood most of the day, nearly every day
  - Loss of interest in pleasurable activities most of the day, nearly every day
  - Significant change in weight or appetite (increase or decrease) when not dieting
  - Insomnia or hypersomnia nearly every day
  - Fatigue or loss of energy nearly every day
  - Diminished ability to think or concentrate, or indecisiveness
  - Feelings of worthlessness or excessive or inappropriate guilt nearly every day
  - Psychomotor agitation or retardation nearly every day
  - Recurrent thoughts of death or suicidal ideation
- Symptoms cause clinically significant distress or impairment in social, occupational, or other important areas of functioning.
- Symptoms are not caused by an underlying medical condition or substance (e.g., medications or recreational drugs).
- For the diagnosis of major depressive disorder (MDD), this episode must not be part of schizophrenia, schizoaffective, delusional, or bipolar disorder.

Adapted with permission from American Psychiatric Association. Diagnostic and Statistical Manual of Mental Disorders. 5th ed. Washington, DC: American Psychiatric Association; 2013.

reuptake inhibitor (SNRI) antidepressants, which functionally include the tricyclic antidepressants (TCAs), are believed to relieve depression by inhibiting the reuptake of serotonin alone or serotonin and NE from the synapse up into the neuron, effectively increasing neurotransmitter concentrations in the synaptic cleft.[16,17] Mirtazapine and MAOIs work via different mechanisms, but also increase 5-HT and NE (and DA for the MAOIs).[16,17]

Depression has been associated with changes in presynaptic and postsynaptic receptor densities (or sensitivities) that have been described as being downregulated or desensitized.[18] Changes include a decrease in postsynaptic α-adrenergic receptor sensitivity, along with alterations in the sensitivities of the α-adrenergic, dopaminergic (D_2), and serotonin receptor subtypes (5-HT_{1A} and 5HT_{2A}). For example, SSRIs can increase the efficiency of serotonergic neurotransmission acutely (through reuptake blockade), but their therapeutic effects are linked temporally with increased release of serotonin through downregulation of presynaptic autoreceptors (5-HT_{1A}).[19] This downstream impact explains why there is a delay in maximal efficacy seen with all antidepressants.[14,15]

As our understanding of neurobiology increases, it has been found that other neurotransmitter systems can impact mood and this has resulted in research for non-5-HT direct-effect medications to supplement or replace the monoamine effecting antidepressants. Such mechanisms include blockade of substance P and antagonism of corticotropin-releasing factor or corticosteroid receptors.[20–23]

Neuroendocrine Findings

Along with dysregulated neurotransmitter systems, neuroendocrine abnormalities may contribute to the development of depression. Depressed patients often have abnormal thyroid function tests (including low triiodothyronine [T_3] and/or thyroxine [T_4] levels).[24] They also may exhibit an abnormal response to challenge with thyroid-releasing hormone, consisting of a blunted or exaggerated thyroid-stimulating hormone response.[25] Clinical hypothyroidism can also induce depressive symptoms, and thyroid supplementation can reverse this pathology, suggesting an indirect association between mood disorders and thyroid homeostasis.[26] The hypothalamic–pituitary–adrenal (HPA) axis may also influence the manifestation of depression, with a relative hyperactivity of this system commonly reported in depressed individuals.[27,28] Pituitary and adrenal glands are often enlarged in depressed patients, and concentrations of corticotropin-releasing factor are often elevated during depressive episodes and decline with the administration of antidepressant medications or electroconvulsive therapy (ECT).[22,29] Exogenous administration of corticotropin-releasing factor has elicited classic symptoms of depression in laboratory animals (including decreased appetite, anxiety, insomnia, and decreased libido).[23] In humans, medications that block postsynaptic corticosteroid receptors have also displayed antidepressant properties.[23,30,31] Interestingly, serotonin has been recognized as a strong influence on the HPA axis (and vice versa). Activation of the postsynaptic serotonin receptors (5-HT_2) along the hypothalamic paraventricular nucleus can stimulate corticotropin-releasing hormone–secreting neurons. Loss of hippocampal volume in major depression leads to increased levels of circulating glucocorticoids, which leads to neuronal apoptosis.[32] Hypercortisolemia due to chronic stimulation of the HPA axis has been implicated in potentially reducing gray matter loss in humans. It should be noted that the relationship between hippocampal volume and depression is not consistently observed and that various factors may affect these findings.[33] Corticosteroids can also modulate serotonin synthesis, metabolism, and reuptake.[22] However, the data in this area are inconsistent because different medications will have differing effects on cortisol despite being effective as well as depressive subtypes showing different effects on cortisol.[34,35] Increased inflammatory cytokines are seen in prospective and postmortem studies of depressed patients but, again, is not consistent.[27,36]

Genetic Studies

Over the last few years, significant scientific advances have been made in genetics and pharmacogenomics. Several genes have been implicated in predictive response or adverse effects to antidepressants. Pharmacodynamic targets have focused on serotonin transporters (5-HTTLPR), tryptophan hydroxylase enzymes 1 and 2 (TPH1 and TPH2), 5-HT_{1A} and 5-HT_{2A} receptors, brain-derived neurotrophic factor (BDNF), G-protein β-3 subunit (GNB3), and monoamine oxidase enzymes and p-glycoprotein; pharmacokinetic targets have been focused on polymorphic variations in CYP1A2, CYP2C19, CYP2D6, and CYP3A4 enzymes.[37–39] Variations in the serotonin transporter *SLC6A4* gene have been associated with remission and response rate in a meta-analysis of 1,435 patients.[38] Researchers found that patients with the *ss* genotype are less likely to reach remission during SSRI treatment and take longer to achieve 50% symptom improvement compared to those with the *ll* genotype. A recent review stated the genes *SLC6A4*, *HTR2A*, *BDNF*, *GNB3*, *FKBP5*, *ABCB1*, and cytochrome *P450* genes (*CYP2D6* and *CYP2C19*) as being the best correlated with depression.[40] A major challenge with pharmacogenomic studies lies in the difficulty of defining unambiguous drug response phenotypes in complex diseases, such as depression. Most likely there are multiple genes that are involved in disease phenotype, drug response, and toxicity. Gene–environment interactions undoubtedly also play a role in the determination of these phenotypes.

Imaging Studies

Imaging studies (including computed tomography, magnetic resonance imaging, positron emission tomography, and single-photon emission computed tomography) suggest that patients with depression have regional brain dysfunction, most often affecting the limbic structures and prefrontal cortex. Alterations in cerebral blood flow and/or metabolism in the frontal–temporal cortex and caudate nucleus are associated with common depressive symptoms such as dysphoria, anhedonia, hopelessness, and flat affect.[41] Increased firing of the amygdala in the left hemisphere has been linked in positron emission tomography studies with the future development of depression.[42] Because subtypes of depression have been linked to different regional dysfunctions, a network hypothesis began to emerge that may lead to improvements in depression diagnosis and targeted treatments.[43] There is also seemingly increased hippocampal loss that is consistent with severity and duration of illness.[44]

Patient Assessment Tools

Behavioral rating scales have been used for many years in drug efficacy studies and are widely advocated for routine use in the clinical arena today. Rating scales are helpful in assessing the severity of mental illness, quantifying changes in target symptoms, and determining treatment efficacy, but they are not diagnostic. Rating scales can vary in length, content, and format, and can be completed by providers, patients, researchers, family members, or conservators. Numerous depression scales have been developed, including the Hamilton Rating Scale for Depression (HAM-D_{17} or HAM-D_{21}), the Hospital Anxiety and Depression Scale (HADS), the Beck Depression Inventory (BDI), the Montgomery-Åsberg Depression Rating Scale (MADRS), the Center for Epidemiological Studies Depression (CES-D) Scale, the Patient Health Questionnaire (PHQ-9), and the Quick Inventory of Depressive Symptoms

Table 86-5
Comparison of Selected Depression Rating Scales

Instrument	Minimal	Mild	Moderate	Severe
Hamilton (HAM-D)—17 item (clinician rated)	<8	8–15	16–27	>27
Beck Depression Inventory (BDI)				
BDI (clinician rated)	<10	10–16	17–29	>29
BDI (patient rated)	<10	10–15	16–23	>23
Quick Inventory for Depressive Symptoms (QIDS)				
QIDS-C_{16} (clinician rated)	<6	6–10	11–15	>15
QIDS-SR_{16} (patient rated)	<6	6–10	11–15	>15
Patient Health Questionnaire (PHQ) (patient rated)	<10	11–14	15–19	>19
Montgomery-Åsberg Depression Rating Scale (MADRS) (clinician rated)	<7	7–19	20–34	>34

($QIDS_{16}$ or $QIDS_{30}$) (Table 86-5).[45–51] Because 30% to 50% of cases are not detected in primary care, enhancing education of the clinicians in this area has shown some benefit. Generally, a two-step process of screening with a simple questionnaire, such as the PHQ-9 or the HADS, and then a more thorough evaluation if the screening results in a positive score are the recommended methods of detecting depression severe enough to require treatment.[5,52]

Nondrug Therapies for Depression

PSYCHOTHERAPY

For the treatment of mild-to-moderate depression, psychotherapy has proved to be comparable to pharmacologic intervention and may be preferred by some patients. There are many types of psychotherapy, and experts suggest that cognitive behavioral therapy (CBT), behavioral activation (BA), and interpersonal psychotherapy (IPT) are effective with CBT being preferred for monotherapy.[5] For the acute treatment of severe depression, antidepressants appear to be more effective than psychotherapy alone and have a more rapid onset of therapeutic action.[5,26] The beneficial effects of psychotherapy, however, may persist longer than medication-related benefits after the interventions have been formally discontinued. In addition, psychotherapy may be particularly beneficial for preventing relapse among patients who previously demonstrated a therapeutic response to antidepressants.[53] Overall, the combination of treatments is superior to either intervention alone.[5,10]

SOMATIC INTERVENTIONS

ECT is a safe, rapid-acting, and highly effective therapeutic intervention. ECT was enormously popular during the 1940s and 1950s and was used without discretion to treat a wide variety of psychiatric conditions. This practice waned with the advent of effective psychotropic medications, and with the accumulation of case reports describing fractures and severe cognitive impairment in treated patients. Since the 1950s, the ECT procedure has undergone considerable transformation and refinement.[54] Adjunctive medications are now routinely administered to prevent adverse effects and reduce morbidity (e.g., a short-acting barbiturate for general anesthesia, an anticholinergic agent to prevent bradycardia and to dry excessive airway secretions, succinylcholine to prevent fractures from tonic–clonic contractions). The electric stimulus itself is no longer applied in one steady current but now consists of a series of brief pulses that have been shown to decrease the severity of postictal headaches and memory impairment.

Fundamentally, ECT features the induction of generalized seizures through an electric current delivered by bilateral or unilateral electrode placement. Medications that raise the seizure threshold or promote cognitive impairment (lithium) should be discontinued before the procedure although this is not always necessary. Adverse effects are generally minimal and consist mainly of transient anterograde amnesia (i.e., difficulty remembering events around the time of the procedure), retrograde amnesia, confusion, headaches, and muscle aches. Cardiovascular effects (e.g., ventricular arrhythmias, myocardial infarction [MI]) are the most ominous sequelae, but these events are extremely rare.[54]

ECT is recommended for patients with treatment-resistant depression, severe vegetative depression, psychotic depression, and severe depression in pregnancy. Overall response rates are impressive, ranging from 70% to 90%, and ECT has the distinct advantage of inducing a therapeutic response within the first week or two of treatments.[54–56] The recommended frequency of ECT treatments is variable. Most institutions have used three sessions weekly to induce a therapeutic response acutely, although evidence suggests that twice-weekly sessions are better tolerated and more cost-effective.[57] The frequency of treatments thereafter (i.e., maintenance therapy) is recommended that ECT be administered weekly for 1 month and less frequently thereafter may be as effective as aggressive pharmacotherapy in preventing relapse.[58]

Other somatic interventions have also been used successfully to treat depression. Repetitive transcranial magnetic stimulation (rTMS) is a noninvasive procedure involving the application of an electrical magnetic stimulus across the scalp, which ultimately generates an electrical field in the cerebral cortex.[59,60] Unlike ECT, rTMS does not generate an actual seizure, and it is very well tolerated, with common side effects consisting of transient scalp discomfort and headaches. Preliminary investigations successfully used repetitive high-frequency techniques in depressed subjects, and imaging studies have shown functional improvements consistent with antidepressant properties. However, not all studies have shown efficacy, and overall results show only a slight benefit for depression or treatment refractory depression.[56,61,62] In 2008, the US Food and Drug Administration (FDA) decided to allow the marketing of TMS for patients who failed a minimum of one prior antidepressant trial.

Vagus nerve stimulation involves the surgical implantation of an electrical device in the subcutaneous tissue below the clavicle, which sends an impulse along the left vagal nerve into the cerebral cortex. Setting adjustments are through a telemetric wand.[56,63] It is currently FDA-approved for the management of treatment-resistant depression although its effect takes time and cannot be considered an acute therapy. Implantation of the device is an invasive procedure with standard risks associated with this type of surgery. However, long-term safety has been shown in both epilepsy and depression studies. It may be useful when combined with medication treatment.[56]

Light therapy or phototherapy is particularly effective for relieving the irritability and malaise associated with seasonal affective disorder, a milder form of depression that has been attributed to decreases in natural sunlight found with seasonal variation.[10,64] Phototherapy is administered in the form of a light box delivering 1,500 to 10,000 lux for a period of 1 to 2 hours daily. It is extremely well tolerated.

LIFESTYLE ADJUSTMENTS

Any therapeutic approach to mood disorders should seek to reverse unhealthy or destructive lifestyle habits and promote other activities that may relieve stress and facilitate well-being. Alcohol and illicit drug use should be minimized (if not prohibited) in patients suffering from depressive disorders. Sleep habits should be evaluated and improved to ensure optimal rest. Dietary factors should be modified to promote diverse, balanced, and nutritional eating habits.

Increased physical activity and sustained cardiovascular exertion can impart a variety of health benefits, including improvement in depressive symptoms.[5] Although investigations examining the effectiveness of exercise for depression have met with mixed results, exercise can regulate appetite, improve sleep patterns, increase energy, enhance self-esteem, and promote a return to euthymic status.[65] Exercise has been shown to increase circulating concentrations of serotonin in the periphery and enhance neurogenesis in the hippocampus.[66] Other activities may also serve to relieve stress and help patients acquire insights into their emotional well-being. These pursuits can range from daily journal writing (journaling), meditation, yoga, and Tai chi. Classes in mindfulness-based meditation, in particular, are offered at many medical centers, and the health benefits of this approach have been demonstrated in a wide range of medical conditions including cancer, chronic pain syndromes, and human immunodeficiency virus (HIV) illness.[67]

MAJOR DEPRESSIVE DISORDER

CASE 86-1

QUESTION 1: A.R. is a 25-year-old female in graduate school who presents to the student health clinic for a routine physical examination. During her visit, A.R. states, "I've been feeling pretty down lately and just want to give up." Her physical examination is unremarkable, and all laboratory tests (complete blood count with differential, chemistry panel, and thyroid function tests) are within normal limits. A human chorionic gonadotropin test is negative. Her medical history is noncontributory, takes no medication, uses a daily multivitamin, and denies drinking alcohol, smoking cigarettes, or using illicit substances.

Diagnosis

When asked, A.R. states that she has had increasing periods of depressed mood during the past few months and often finds herself crying in the morning for no particular reason. She reports that she has no interest in her old hobbies (playing the piano, mountain biking, gardening). During the past 6 months, her appetite has decreased, and she has lost 15 pounds. She feels overwhelmed about all of her academic work and job and has difficulty sleeping, often waking in the middle of the night and being unable to fall back asleep. She has no energy during the day and finds it difficult to concentrate or make decisions. This is clearly impacting her ability to finish her graduate work as she is falling behind and has been getting extensions for her project due dates.

On examination, A.R. is an appropriately dressed woman who appears sad but who is alert, coherent, and logical. Her affect is constricted, apprehensive, and sad. Mood is depressed, and she admits having vague suicidal ideation but she has no specific plans. She is oriented to person, place, and time, but shows some recent memory deficits. Her intelligence is estimated to be above average. Concentration and abstractions (e.g., "don't cry over spilled milk," "a rolling stone gathers no moss") are satisfactory. She denies hearing voices or other hallucinations. She denies any symptoms of mania such as increased periods of energy, rapid speech, and racing thoughts (See Chapter 87, Bipolar Disorders). She has good insight and judgment into her illness. A.R. is asked to complete the PHQ-9 and has a total score of 15 with five different questions scoring 2 or more and as well as question one and two scoring 2 (i.e., moderate-to-severe symptoms). After reviewing the PHQ-9 results, a more in-depth interview is conducted and A.R. is diagnosed as having MDD. What nondrug options have shown efficacy?

From A.R.'s history, she appears to be exhibiting a dysphoric or depressed mood as well as anhedonia (lack of interest in hobbies or pleasurable activities). In addition, she demonstrates frequent episodes of crying, decreased appetite (with an unintentional 15-pound weight loss), poor concentration, low energy, suicidal ideation, worthlessness, and inappropriate guilt. Her mental status examination is consistent with these target symptoms, revealing a constricted, sad affect (physical manifestation of inner emotional states), and frequent crying episodes during the interview.

Based on the DSM-5 criteria (Table 86-4), A.R. has MDD. During the past 2 weeks, she has consistently exhibited at least five of the associated symptoms, one of which is depression or anhedonia. It does not appear that her symptoms are the result of any medical condition, medication, thought disorder, or uncomplicated bereavement. These are impacting functioning because she is not able to complete her school work assignments.

Psychotherapy has been shown to have beneficial effects on mild-to-moderate depression. Studies have also shown that combined with medication the beneficial effects are greater than either alone. ECT is an effective somatic treatment but typically reserved for more refractory cases. rTMS is currently being studied but has not been standardized yet. Lifestyle modifications such as exercise generally have benefit, but typically are not strong enough on their own to treat clinically significant depressed symptoms.

DRUG MANAGEMENT

Drug Selection: General Considerations

CASE 86-1, QUESTION 2: A.R. agrees to a therapeutic trial of an antidepressant. What are the drug options available for A.R.'s depressive symptoms? What considerations should be made when selecting antidepressant therapy?

In randomized, controlled trials (RCTs) of antidepressants, a therapeutic response is usually apparent in 60% to 70% of subjects receiving active medication (therapeutic response is defined as a ≥50% decline in depression rating scale score).[5,10]

Antidepressants can be divided into different categories:

1. Selective serotonin reuptake inhibitors (SSRIs)
2. Serotonin norepinephrine reuptake inhibitors (SNRIs)
3. Tricyclic antidepressants (TCAs)
4. Miscellaneous antidepressants (e.g., trazodone, nefazodone, mirtazapine, bupropion)
5. Monoamine oxidase inhibitors (MAOIs)
6. Serotonin reuptake inhibitor and receptor modulators (the newest group)

When comparing the impact of antidepressants on changes in depressive symptoms, all antidepressants are considered equal, regardless of class. It is possible that dual-acting antidepressants (SNRIs and TCAs) may be more effective in the severely depressed but this has not resulted in experts explicitly recommending them over other factors such as comorbid diseases, contraindications, or drug interactions (Tables 86-6 and 86-7)[5,10,26,68] Sertraline and escitalopram have the best efficacy to safety/tolerability ratio.[5,10,68,69] Thus, with no other factors influencing the selection of the medication, it may be easier to select either of these.

One of the first factors to consider is the patient's history of response to previous antidepressant drug therapy. If this history is unavailable (or the patient has never received an antidepressant before), the clinician should inquire about family history. If a first-degree relative had a successful course of antidepressant treatment with minimal adverse effects, that specific medication (or another from the same antidepressant class) would be a prudent choice for initial therapy. The potential impact of an antidepressant on concurrent medical conditions or disease states

Table 86-6
Factors to Consider in Selecting an Antidepressant

- History of prior response (personal or family member)
- Safety in overdose
- Adverse effect profiles
- Patient age
- Concurrent medical/psychiatric conditions
- Concurrent medications (e.g., potential for drug interactions)
- Convenience (e.g., minimal titration, once-daily dosing)
- Cost
- Patient preference

Table 86-7
Pharmacology of Antidepressant Medications

Medication	Serotonin	Norepinephrine	Dopamine	Bioavailability (Oral)	Protein Binding	Half-Life (hours) (Active Metabolite)
Selective Serotonin Reuptake Inhibitors						
Fluoxetine	++++	0/+	0	80%	95%	24–72 (146)
Sertraline	++++	0/+	+	>44%	95%	26 (66)
Paroxetine	++++	+	0	64%	99%	24
Citalopram	++++	0	0	80%	<80%	33
Escitalopram	++++	0	0	80%	56%	27–32
Serotonin Norepinephrine Reuptake Inhibitors						
Venlafaxine	++++	+++	0	92%	25%–29%	4 (10)
Desvenlafaxine	+++	+++	0	80%	30%	11 (0)
Duloxetine	++++	++++	0	50%	>90%	12 (8–17)
Levomilnacipran	+	++++	0	92%	22%	12
Dopamine/Norepinephrine Reuptake Inhibitors						
Bupropion	0/+	+	++	>90%	85%	10–21
Tricyclic Antidepressants						
Desipramine	+	++++	0/+	51%	90%	12–28
Nortriptyline	++	+++	0	46%–56%	92%	18–56
Amitriptyline	++++	++++	0	37%–49%	95%	9–46 (18–56)
Imipramine	+++	++	0/+	19%–35%	95%	6–28 (12–28)
Doxepin	+++	+	0	17%–37%	68%–85%	11–23
Others						
Mirtazapine	+++	++++	0	50%	85%	20–40
Nefazodone	+++	+	0	20%	99%	5
Vilazodone	++++	0	0	72%	98%	25
Vortioxetine	++++	0	0	75%	99%	60

0, negligible; +, very low; ++, low; +++, moderate; ++++, high.

Source: Practice guideline for the treatment of patients with major depressive disorder. 3rd ed. Arlington, VA: American Psychiatric Association; 2010; Deardorff WJ, Grossberg GT. A review of the clinical efficacy, safety and tolerability of the antidepressants vilazodone, levomilnacipran and vortioxetine. *Expert Opin Pharmacother*. 2014;15(17):2525–2542.

Table 86-8
Drug Interactions of the Cytochrome P-450 System

Relative Rank	CYP1A2	CYP2C9/19	CYP2D6	CYP3A4
Strong	Fluvoxamine	Fluvoxamine		
			Fluoxetine	
				Nefazodone
			Paroxetine	
Moderate			Duloxetine	
			Bupropion	
		Fluoxetine		Fluoxetine
				Fluvoxamine
Weak			Venlafaxine	
	Sertraline	Sertraline	Sertraline	Sertraline
			Escitalopram	
	Paroxetine	Paroxetine		Paroxetine
			Fluvoxamine	
			Citalopram	
	Fluoxetine			
			Nefazodone	

is often considered next. For example, certain antidepressants (e.g., TCA, paroxetine, mirtazapine) can cause significant weight gain and would not be desirable choices for obese patients, whereas bupropion should be avoided in patients with a history of seizures. Pharmacokinetic drug interactions will also help determine the preferred first-choice option. Among the SSRIs, fluoxetine and paroxetine have significant inhibitory effects on CYP450 2D6, whereas citalopram, escitalopram, sertraline, and fluvoxamine have minimally clinical inhibitory effects on 2D6. Fluvoxamine does have a strong impact on CYP1A1/2, and fluoxetine has a weak-to-moderate impact on 3A4 (Table 86-8).[70] Other important patient-specific factors to consider in the selection of an agent include safety in overdose, ease of administration (once-daily vs. divided doses), and necessity for dose titration, cost, and patient preference (Tables 86-6–86-9).[10]

Treatment Expectations

A similar delayed pattern of therapeutic response has been observed with all antidepressant medications. Patients often begin to show signs of clinical response during the first 1 or 2 weeks of active treatment and maximum improvement may not be evident until weeks 6-8.[5,26,71] The pattern of patient response can also be generalized, with neurovegetative symptoms often the first to subside (e.g., altered sleep or appetite, decreased energy, excessive worrying and irritability). Cognitive symptoms are slower to respond, and 3 to 4 weeks or more may elapse before improvements are evident. These symptoms include excessive guilt or pessimism, poor concentration, hopelessness or sadness, and decreased libido.

Selective Serotonin Reuptake Inhibitors

ADVERSE EFFECTS

There is a delay in onset of full efficacy, but side effects will occur soon after starting the medication. Common side effects of SSRIs are related to the fact that despite their neurotransmitter specificity to increasing the amount of serotonin in the synapse there are at least 14 different serotonin receptors having different effects.[15] Distinct side effect profiles have emerged, consisting of gastrointestinal (GI) complaints, CNS disturbances, and sexual dysfunction.

All of these medications may induce nausea, but this tends to be a transient effect that diminishes after the first week of treatment. Typically, SSRI-induced nausea occurs 1 to 2 hours after oral administration. Nausea with SSRIs can be a local effect but is also mediated centrally through the extra serotonin-stimulating serotonin receptors (5-HT_3) that activate the chemoreceptor trigger zone.[72] SSRIs may also cause transient and bothersome increases in GI motility. This diarrhea is generally limited to the first few weeks of treatment and is also related to the extra serotonin-stimulating 5-HT_3 receptors along the GI tract. As with nausea, this diminishes in the first few weeks of treatment unless the dose is increased. In contrast, paroxetine possesses a relatively mild anti-muscarinic effect that can manifest as constipation, dry mouth, or urinary hesitancy. Although this effect is mild, paroxetine use is often discouraged in patients with preexisting constipation or those where any anticholinergic effects are to be avoided such as the elderly.

SSRIs can have myriad effects on the CNS, with disturbances in sleep being a primary concern. SSRIs can have significant but highly variable effects on sleep architecture. In sleep studies, SSRIs have been shown to increase sleep latency and decrease sleep efficiency, often resulting in morning sleepiness or malaise. Many patients also notice that their dreams become more vivid and memorable, which may be an undesirable experience. REM stage sleep may be prolonged, resulting in less fitful sleep.[73] It should be emphasized, however, that sleep may eventually improve once the antidepressant properties of the medications are apparent and baseline depressive symptoms are relieved (e.g., midnocturnal insomnia).

The deleterious effects of SSRI on sexual function can often lead to medication nonadherence.[74] The reported incidence of sexual dysfunction ranges from 1.9% to 75%, reflecting the difficulty in appropriately measuring this adverse event.[75] The actual incidence of SSRI-induced sexual dysfunction is approximately

Table 86-9
Dosage Ranges of Commonly Prescribed Antidepressant Medications

Medication	Starting Dose (mg/day)	Usual Dosage (mg/day)
Selective Serotonin Reuptake Inhibitors		
Fluoxetine	20	20–60
Sertraline	50	50–200
Paroxetine	20	20–60
Paroxetine ER	12.5	25–75
Citalopram	20	20–60
Escitalopram	10	10–20
Serotonin Norepinephrine Reuptake Inhibitors		
Venlafaxine, IR	37.5	75–375
Venlafaxine, ER	37.5	75–375
Desvenlafaxine	50	50
Duloxetine	60	60–120
Levomilnacipran	20	40–120
Dopamine Reuptake Inhibitors		
Bupropion, IR	150	300–450
Bupropion, SR	150	300–400
Bupropion, ER	150	300–450
Tricyclic Antidepressants		
Imipramine	25–50	100–300
Desipramine	25–50	100–300
Amitriptyline	25–50	100–300
Nortriptyline	25	50–200
Others		
Mirtazapine	15	45
Nefazodone	50	150–300
Serotonin Reuptake Inhibitors and Receptor Modulators		
Vilazodone	10	20–40
Vortioxetine	10	20

Source: Practice guideline for the treatment of patients with major depressive disorder. 3rd ed. Arlington, VA: American Psychiatric Association; 2010; Deardorff WJ, Grossberg GT. A review of the clinical efficacy, safety and tolerability of the antidepressants vilazodone, levomilnacipran and vortioxetine. *Expert Opin Pharmacother*. 2014;15(17):2525–2542.

30% to 50%, and it appears to be slightly more common in men, but the severity may be worse in women.[75] Delayed orgasm is the most common sexual complaint attributed to SSRIs or SNRIs, and should be distinguished from decreases in desire or libido, which are considered to be an aspect of the psychopathology of depression itself. This iatrogenic effect on orgasms has actually been used to clinical advantage in treating men by delaying premature ejaculation, but most patients find it undesirable.[75] All SSRIs are at risk for causing sexual dysfunction, because it is due to the increased serotonin-stimulating 5-HT_{2c} receptors. Paroxetine has a higher rate than the others because it also inhibits nitric oxide synthase, reducing nitric oxide levels.[75] It also appears that this is a dose-dependent phenomenon, which may respond favorably to a decrease in daily dosage. Unlike the GI and CNS side effects reported with SSRIs, sexual dysfunction is not usually a transient adverse effect and must be addressed by clinicians if patients are to continue pharmacotherapy.

The detection and proper management of SSRI-induced sexual dysfunction can be one of the most important factors in ensuring medication adherence. Clinicians may be uncomfortable asking patients about their sexual activities and satisfaction, but the high incidence of this side effect (and low likelihood of patients volunteering this information) necessitates a thoughtful and direct approach. Some patients acknowledge sexual dysfunction but decide that improvements in mood and overall health outweigh limitations in sexual performance; however, others simply stop the medication if the side effect is never addressed.

It may be wise to advise patients that sexual function may change over time, depending on the type and etiology of sexual dysfunction experienced. Depression itself is associated with a decreased libido in 70% to 90% of untreated patients.[76] This symptom will most likely subside with a successful course of antidepressant treatment. Delayed ejaculation or anorgasmia, however, may be caused by SSRIs and SNRIs, often persisting and jeopardizing treatment.

Ordinarily, one of the first options in managing sexual dysfunction is to reduce the dosage, but this may induce a return in symptoms because increasing the dose initially was likely due to lack of full effect. It is also possible to introduce drug holidays. Small open-label studies with short-acting SSRIs (e.g., paroxetine) suggested that if patients skipped their doses on Friday and Saturday, sexual function would return to normal on the weekends.[77,78] Although this method was reported to be successful, it may also promote nonadherence with medication and lead to increased risk of relapse and withdrawal symptoms and is therefore not recommended.

If the patient has had a therapeutic response to the antidepressant, the next option in this setting is to consider antidotes to SSRI-induced sexual dysfunction. One option is to add the antidepressant bupropion. Clinical reports and controlled investigations suggest that the addition of bupropion can be helpful for restoring sexual desire and may relieve delayed orgasm or anorgasmia in approximately 50% of patients.[5,79–82] This therapeutic effect has been demonstrated in depressed and nondepressed patients alike. A common dosing technique is to start with 150 mg of bupropion daily. If unsuccessful, the dose can be increased to 150 mg of bupropion sustained release (SR) twice daily after several days (or 300 mg of the extended-release [XL] preparation). The mechanisms of SSRI-induced sexual dysfunction, and bupropion relief, are not well understood, but likely due to the pro-sexual effects of increasing DA.[83]

Other remedies have been prescribed for SSRI-induced sexual dysfunction. A large randomized, controlled trial examined the impact of sildenafil on male patients suffering from this side effect.[84] Overall, 54% of patients randomly assigned to sildenafil found it to be effective compared with a 4% response rate with placebo. Open-label trials of sildenafil in women experiencing SSRI-induced anorgasmia have also reported improvements. Tadalafil has also shown similar efficacy suggesting a class effect.[85]

Amantadine, buspirone, and yohimbine also have been used successfully to reverse delayed ejaculation or decreased libido, but the evidence for efficacy is limited.[86–88] One small double-blind study compared the effects of amantadine with buspirone or placebo among depressed patients experiencing sexual dysfunction on antidepressants.[89] All three study treatments improved sexual dysfunction to a comparable extent, and the only statistically significant finding was related to an increase in energy reported among patients receiving amantadine (vs. placebo). An open-label trial of Ginkgo biloba in men and women with sexual dysfunction reported very high success rates, but mixed results have been reported in clinical practice.[90] Mirtazapine is capable of blocking postsynaptic 5-HT_2 receptors and has been shown to have less sexual dysfunction than SSRIs.[91] The 5-HT and histamine receptor antagonist cyproheptadine has been shown to alleviate this adverse event. However, due to its broad effect on all 5-HT receptors, depression relapse and serotonin withdrawal can occur resulting in it not being recommended. Finally, stimulants such as methylphenidate or dextroamphetamine may increase libido in SSRI-treated patients, but the potential for dependence and abuse discourages their routine administration.[92]

All antidepressants have a black box warning regarding the possibility of an increase in suicidal thinking, specifically in persons 24 years old and younger. In regard to completed suicide, the rate is less in adult and pediatric patients treated with antidepressants than those who are not treated.[5,26,93,94] However, studies have shown a rate in suicidal thinking among children and young adults of 4% in the medication arms compared to 2% in placebo arms.[94] Therefore, in order to protect the patient, it is recommended that when an antidepressant is initiated in a child or adolescent, the patient should visit with the clinician every week in the first month, every 2 weeks in the second month, and then monthly for the next month. Adults should also be monitored frequently, and weekly visits initially have shown increased adherence rates. However, other factors may play a role in monitoring such as access to care and distance the patient needs to travel for the appointment. Therefore, it is recommended to at least speak with the adult patient (e.g., via telephone) at least every 1 to 2 weeks in the acute phase (initial 12 weeks) of treatment to assess suicidality but also to check for side effects and adherence.[5,10] SSRIs are dramatically safer in overdose compared to tricyclic antidepressants and are preferred for those with suicidal thinking or comorbidities that put them at risk for impulsive acts of self-harm such as substance misuse.

In addition to GI, CNS, and sexual side effects, a variety of other, less-common adverse sequelae have occurred with SSRIs. Headache can occur with SSRIs at a rate of approximately 10% to 15% with all agents similar and slightly greater than placebo, with discontinuations due to headache very low at 1% to 3%.[95] This may be due to the effects of serotonin on 5-HT_{1b} and $_{1d}$ receptors. It is important to note that SSRIs are actually recommended for migraine prophylaxis as a second-line agent.[96,97] Increased sweating has also been reported with SSRIs and can be particularly uncomfortable or embarrassing.[98] A dosage reduction may help relieve this adverse effect and should be tried first. Adjunctive treatment of α-blockers (e.g., terazosin, prazosin), cyproheptadine, and the anticholinergic benztropine has shown some success if a dose reduction is not possible.[99,100] Bruxism, or teeth grinding, can also be a consequence of SSRI treatment, leading to chipped or cracked teeth and generally poor dentition.[101] Often, patients may not be aware of this nocturnal effect and complain merely of a dull, persistent headache during the morning hours. This, too, may be a dose-dependent side effect of all SSRIs, and several antidotes have been prescribed (e.g., buspirone, benzodiazepines, gabapentin).[102,103] In small retrospective studies and several case reports, SSRIs have been linked to dilutional hyponatremia or syndrome of inappropriate antidiuretic hormone (SIADH).[104,105] All SSRIs and SNRIs have been associated with this phenomenon, and elderly patients appear to be uniquely at risk.

SSRIs have been rarely associated with extrapyramidal side (EPS) effects, consisting of akathisia, dystonias, and parkinsonian symptoms that are qualitatively identical to those seen with antipsychotics.[106–108] Although EPS reactions have been documented with all SSRIs, most case reports have correlated with aggressive dosing, often in a patient currently using a DA antagonistic medication, and during the first 1 to 4 weeks of initiation. The theory is that these EPS effects are mediated through the indirect influence of serotonergic neurons on dopaminergic activity.[107] In certain areas of the brain, serotonin and dopamine appear to have an inverse relationship, whereby central stimulation of serotonin receptors results in a net decline in dopaminergic transmission. Management of EPS effects induced by SSRI is identical to that of those precipitated by antipsychotics. Dystonias and parkinsonian side effects can be treated with anticholinergic agents and subsequent SSRI dosage reduction. Akathisia usually responds to a reduction in SSRI dosage and/or administration of low-dose β-blockers.[108]

The long-term effects of SSRIs on body weight are variable and difficult to predict. A problem with accurate measurement is because decreased appetite is one of the most common depressive symptoms and that a small weight gain after an antidepressant course may actually be viewed as a therapeutic effect of successful treatment. Conversely, early reports of weight loss with fluoxetine generated much optimism for the use of SSRIs in obesity, but longitudinal studies found this to be a brief, transient phenomenon.[109] All the SSRIs have been reported to cause significant weight gain in long-term use, but it is a rare phenomenon believed to be mediated by genetic markers that have not been conclusively identified. The exception is paroxetine, which has been implicated much more often than other SSRIs as a cause of weight gain. One long-term RCT compared the effects of fluoxetine, sertraline, and paroxetine on total body weight.[110] After 7 months of SSRI use, 25% of the patients receiving paroxetine gained a clinically significant amount of weight (defined as a >7% increase in total body weight) compared with 7% with fluoxetine and 4% with sertraline.[110] Long-term studies with citalopram and escitalopram suggest that 3% to 5% of patients will experience a significant weight gain. The risk of SSRI weight gain is minimal (except with paroxetine) and typically irrelevant, but because appetite changes are part of depression, it is best to monitor weight closely during long-term treatment for both disease- and drug-related reasons.

Epidemiologic studies have also linked SSRIs and SNRIs with an increased risk for upper GI hemorrhage, with a number needed to harm of 3,177.[111,112] Recent trials suggest that the risk is modest but can be increased significantly by concurrent ingestion of NSAIDs lowering the number needed to harm of 881.[112–114] Alcohol use can also increase the risk of bleeding.[113,114] The mechanism for SSRI-induced GI hemorrhage has been attributed to effects on decreasing platelet activation and aggregation. SSRIs and SNRIs should be avoided in patients with active GI bleeds, and the concurrent use of high-dose NSAID should be discouraged.

DOSAGE TITRATION

CASE 86-1, QUESTION 3: AR and the clinician agree to start escitalopram 10 mg QAM. What is considered the standard of care and expected outcomes for dosing and efficacy?

It is very important to establish realistic expectations for treatment with antidepressants from the beginning of therapy. Patients should be informed of the anticipated course of treatment and that the onset of side effects usually precedes that of therapeutic effects. Also, patients should be advised that, although antidepressants may relieve acute depressive symptoms and prevent relapse, they do not abolish environmental stressors such as an abusive relationship or an oppressive work setting.

After receiving the medication for 2 weeks, most improvement in A.R. is likely due to the support she is getting by being involved in treatment as placebo patients show a reduction in symptoms during this period. Medication will start to separate from placebo typically at the 2-week monitoring period and continue to enlarge that separation from placebo up until week 8. A.R. should be reminded that the optimal effects of antidepressants may not be evident for another 4 to 6 weeks. Therefore, a reasonable recommendation would be to continue with the current daily dose of 10 mg and to re-evaluate the medication's effects when she returns to clinic in 2 weeks. If there is no clear improvement at 4 weeks, then switching the medication is necessary. If there is a 25% or more improvement, then the clinician could continue for another 4 weeks (for 8 weeks of treatment) and decide whether the response is acceptable. If the improvement is small, such as just 25% to 30%, then one can increase the dose at this 4-week point and continue to monitor for another 8 weeks.[5,10,26]

DURATION OF TREATMENT

According to the guidelines issued by the Agency for Health Research and Quality, antidepressant treatment can be broken down into three stages (Table 86-10).[115] The first stage, acute treatment, lasts approximately 12 weeks; during this time, the clinician attempts to resolve the presenting symptoms and induce remission which is defined as no impairing symptoms of depression and a score of ≤7 on the $HAMD_{17}$ or ≤10 on the MADRS.[5,10] The second stage is commonly called continuation treatment because the patient continues to receive the same antidepressant regimen that induced the initial treatment response, and the clinician attempts to keep the acute symptoms in remission. The duration of continuation treatment is variable (4–9 months after initial treatment or response), but it is recommended that all patients suffering from major depression complete these first two stages. Therefore, the minimum duration of treatment is 7 months. Alternatively, others have advocated that the minimum duration of treatment should be for 6 months after the complete resolution of symptoms.[5]

Table 86-10
Duration of Antidepressant Treatment

Acute treatment phase	3 months
Continuation treatment phase	4–9 months
Maintenance treatment phase	Variable

- Acute and continuation treatment recommended for all patients with major depressive disorder (MDD) (i.e., minimal duration of treatment = 7 months)
- Decision to prescribe maintenance treatment is based on the following:
  - Number of previous episodes
  - Severity of previous episodes
  - Family history of depression
  - Patient age (worse prognosis if elderly)
  - Response to antidepressant
  - Persistence of environmental stressors
- Indefinite maintenance treatment is recommended if any one of the following criteria is met:
  - Three or more previous episodes (regardless of age)
  - Two or more previous episodes and age older than 50 years
  - One or more and age older than 60 years

The third stage of treatment, maintenance treatment or prophylaxis, is not indicated for all patients, and the necessity of continuing medication beyond the first 6 to 7 months depends on many patient-specific factors. One must consider the number of previous episodes, family history of depression, patient's age, severity of presenting symptoms, response to therapy, and persistence or anticipation of environmental stressors. There are specific populations for whom indefinite pharmacologic treatment is advocated: (a) individuals with three or more previous episodes of major depression, (b) individuals older than 50 years with two or more previous episodes, and (c) individuals older than 60 years with one or more previous episodes.[5,10] Continued antidepressant usage in the elderly is recommended to prevent relapse.[116]

Because A.R. is exhibiting a full therapeutic response to escitalopram, the recommendation would be for her to continue with the effective dosage (10 mg/day) for at least 7 consecutive months. At the end of this time frame, the clinician should review with the patient those considerations that enter into the decision to continue treatment. Ultimately, the decision to continue antidepressant medications is left to the patient's judgment, and he/she should be well informed of the potential consequences of stopping treatment.

In the future, if A.R. decides to discontinue her antidepressant she should fully disclose this to her prescriber so that an appropriate taper schedule and subsequent monitoring can occur. She should be advised of potential withdrawal symptoms (Table 86-11).[117] Abrupt discontinuation of chronic SSRI treatment (e.g., treatment >2 months) has been associated with dizziness, headache, anxiety, lethargy, dysphoria, and sleep problems.[5,117] The onset of these symptoms is generally within 36 to 72 hours of stopping treatment, and effects may persist for approximately a week. Withdrawal symptoms generally are mild and self-limiting but can be uncomfortable and alarming. Because of their relatively short half-life (and absence of long-acting metabolites), paroxetine, fluvoxamine, and venlafaxine have been associated with a more

Table 86-11
Discontinuation of Antidepressants

Withdrawal syndrome

- Worse with paroxetine, venlafaxine
- Symptoms: dizziness, nausea, paresthesias, anxiety/insomnia, flulike symptoms
- Onset: 36–72 hours
- Duration: 3–7 days

Note: Risk of depression relapse is greatest 1 to 6 months after discontinuation.

profound withdrawal presentation than other SSRIs and SNRIs. Due to its long half-life (and that of its active metabolite), fluoxetine has not been commonly associated with withdrawal symptoms. Nonetheless, it is advisable to taper slowly off all antidepressant medications after an extended treatment course to decrease the risk of withdrawal and subsequent relapse.[118] A defined time for taper has not been established. Switching therapies within classes can be done quickly (e.g., from sertraline to fluoxetine) without a cross-taper. When switching to another class or off antidepressant completely then a 6 to 8 week taper is standard as well as educating the patient to withdrawal symptoms and reassuring them that this is not a life-threatening event. Because withdrawal is not life-threatening, a much faster taper (3–7 days) can be completed with the patient's approval.[10,117]

Suicide Assessment

Patients with major depression should always be assessed for the presence of suicidal thoughts (e.g., "Do you ever feel like giving up?" "Are you thinking about hurting yourself?"). Reports have noted that completed suicide rates range from 2% to 15%. Up to 70% of suicides worldwide are persons with MDD.[5,119] Comments made by the patients alluding to suicide (e.g., "Life is not worth living anymore," "I am leaving and may never see you again") should be taken seriously. Several factors may place a person at greater risk for a suicide attempt. These include living alone, having a disabling illness, being unemployed, having a history of alcohol/drug abuse, chronic pain, anxiety, or having a family history of suicide.[10] Gender plays a role as well, with women much more likely to attempt suicide, although men are more likely to complete the act.[10]

For patients who are actively suicidal, hospitalization is often necessary and may be facilitated against the patients will in high-risk settings. Other life-saving interventions include establishing close contact with the patient's family and healthcare provider, convincing the patient to contract for his/her safety and ensuring that firearms and other lethal means are removed from the home. Antidepressants have different risks of lethality in overdose. Tricyclics are by far much more dangerous than SSRIs. Duloxetine, venlafaxine, and mirtazapine are a much lower risk than TCAs but higher than SSRIs. Among the SSRIs, citalopram has the greatest risk of cardiotoxicity in overdose but still less than venlafaxine.[5] For patients who are at risk for attempting suicide, TCAs and MAOIs are contraindicated.

A.R. is at some risk for suicide, although she does not have a detailed plan at present. She should be monitored closely during the first few weeks of therapy by friends or family members. If her suicidal ideation becomes severe, A.R. should be evaluated at a psychiatric emergency room for her own safety. Unfortunately, it is not always possible to predict whether A.R. (or any depressed patient) will attempt suicide. Even with the most conservative precautions, a small percentage of patients successfully complete their suicide attempts.

CASE 86-1, QUESTION 4: After A.R. has been treated for a year she is asking about coming off her escitalopram partly because she is getting married and considering becoming pregnant. What would be the most appropriate way to proceed with discontinuation and treatment of depression during pregnancy?

A.R.'s escitalopram should be tapered during several weeks (e.g., decrease to 5 mg daily for 2–4 weeks, then discontinue). The risk of relapse is relatively low during the first month off medication, but depressive symptoms often return during the second or third months. The risk of relapse is highest during the first 6 months after therapy is stopped.[120]

Antidepressants in Pregnancy and Lactation

The risk for depression is elevated during pregnancy and during the postpartum period.[121] A prospective investigation reported that women who discontinued their antidepressant on learning, when they were pregnant, were much more likely to relapse prior to delivery (68% relapse rate vs. 26% who continued treatment; hazard ratio, 5.0).[122]

Before deciding to treat with an antidepressant during pregnancy, one should make a careful inventory of the benefits and risks. The consequences of maternal depression on the mother and fetus must be compared with the potential risks of in utero medication exposure. From the mother's perspective, untreated depression carries with it a great deal of distress during an emotional time. Sleep and appetite may be compromised at a time when these functions are most important for the baby's development. Mothers may also be tempted to drink alcohol or abuse substances, and studies have also shown that depressed mothers are much less likely to attend prenatal clinic visits.[123] Depression during pregnancy is a very strong risk factor for postpartum depression.

Most of the SSRIs and newer antidepressants pose little risk for the development of serious fetal malformations, and they have been subsequently categorized as Class C by the FDA (suggesting that the risk to the fetus is not definitively known). Their relative safety has been corroborated by two large case–control studies in which very small increases in risks were reported.[124,125]

One notable exception is with paroxetine, which was reclassified as Class D by the FDA after the demonstration of an increased risk for congenital heart defects in newborns.[126] An additional concern with SSRIs and SNRIs in pregnancy is the risk for a neonatal serotonin withdrawal syndrome immediately after delivery. This has been reported with TCAs in the past as well. A small controlled investigation (n = 40) examined the effects of fluoxetine and citalopram on CNS effects in newborns and found a significant increase in restlessness, tremor, shivering, and hyper-reflexia during the first 4 days of life (vs. controls); these signs spontaneously remitted shortly thereafter.[127] Although some clinicians have interpreted these findings to suggest that antidepressants should be tapered and discontinued prior to delivery, others have argued that the delivery and the postpartum periods are major stressors for the new mother, and the risk of relapse during this time would be unacceptably high if the medication is withdrawn. Studies have also reported a small but significant decrease in birthweight among babies exposed in utero to SSRI although a prospective study found that neither depression or SSRI use effected infant growth.[128] Clinicians should be reminded, however, that both of these findings have been consistently reported with depression in the absence of antidepressant treatment, and attempts to distinguish the effects of the illness from medication effects in pregnant women have met with mixed results.[129] The safety of bupropion in pregnancy has not been extensively studied.

A recent review of animal studies uncovered an increased risk of congenital abnormalities, but retrospective reviews in humans have failed to identify an enhanced risk of fetal malformation or spontaneous abortions. Due to these findings in animal trials, the FDA recently changed bupropion to a Class C rating. Data are even more sparse with mirtazapine, venlafaxine, or duloxetine, but no obvious adverse effects have been identified among infants exposed to these antidepressants in utero. Similarly, fetal malformations have been rarely reported with TCAs and they are generally regarded as safe in pregnant women. MAOIs, however, should be avoided due to increased risks for hypertensive crises. Although screening for depression is not suggested in the general population, it is recommended specifically for those who are pregnant and postnatal.[130] If antidepressants need to be used, then monotherapy is best; avoid first-trimester exposure, do not stop the antidepressant abruptly, and do not discontinue prior to delivery due to the high risk of postpartum depression.[123]

For A.R., it is important to assess her risk for depression if she stops taking her antidepressant. This was her first episode of depression (which occurred under stressful circumstances), she is not currently symptomatic, and she does not have a strong genetic predisposition to mood disorders. If she is committed to starting a family, she should consider tapering off her escitalopram for several weeks before attempting to conceive. If she becomes pregnant and her depression returns, the risk to the fetus appears to be quite low with most SSRIs. Theoretically, this risk can be reduced further if the antidepressant is started after the first trimester (when most major fetal development occurs). An additional option for pregnant mothers suffering from mild-to-moderate symptoms would be to consider psychotherapy.[123,131]

Approximately 70% of new mothers report sadness or anxiety during the first few days after delivery (baby blues), but these feelings will usually resolve within 1 to 2 weeks and do not require treatment. Approximately 10% of mothers will experience unremitting symptoms postpartum that ultimately satisfy criteria for MDD. The onset of these symptoms can be quite variable, ranging from the immediate postpartum period to several months later. Although psychotherapy may be appealing and obviate the need for medication exposure via breast milk, it is often inconvenient and impractical for new mothers to leave the house on a weekly basis without their infants. Antidepressant medications, therefore, are frequently prescribed to manage postpartum mood disorders. Not treating depression postpartum results in symptom-related risks to the mother and newborn. Therefore, the priority is on reducing depression, and if an antidepressant is the most effective option for the mother then efforts should be placed on managing breast-feeding.[132]

Because breast-feeding is widely advocated, the passive transfer of medication from mother to infant must be considered. Studies with TCAs and SSRIs suggest that concentrations of some antidepressants in breast milk are measurable. However, subsequent concentrations in the infant's bloodstream are relatively low, and the sequelae from this exposure have been limited to scattered case reports of increased infant irritability. Among the available agents, fluoxetine and the tricyclic antidepressant doxepin have been associated with the highest concentrations in infants, and although the clinical or developmental consequences of this finding have not been elucidated, it has been recommended that these medications be avoided.[133] Recent studies with SSRIs suggest that the concentrations achieved in breast milk are lowest with sertraline, and that paroxetine, citalopram, escitalopram, bupropion, and venlafaxine are somewhere between the extremes of fluoxetine and sertraline.[132–134] If an antidepressant is to be continued in a mother who is breast-feeding, the lowest dosage should be prescribed. Concentrations of SSRIs in breast milk will generally peak approximately 4 to 8 hours after oral administration. If a new mother is particularly concerned about breast milk exposure, she can be advised to pump and save breast milk immediately prior to taking the antidepressant.

Drug Interactions

The SSRIs are inhibitors of the cytochrome P-450 isoenzymes, but important differences exist among the individual agents in their potency for specific metabolic pathways (Table 86-8). For instance, the cytochrome P-450 1A2 isoenzyme (or CYP1A2) is most sensitive to the inhibitory effects of fluvoxamine. Fluoxetine and paroxetine have the highest impact on CYP450 2D6 with fluoxetine resulting in approximately fourfold increase in TCAs and paroxetine a fivefold increase.[70,135] Fluoxetine's active metabolite has weak-to-moderate inhibitory effects on the CYP3A4 isoenzyme. In comparison, sertraline, citalopram, and escitalopram have a much lower potential for CYP450 2D6 drug interactions but still inhibit the metabolism of 2D6-dependent medications. The potency is typically between 30% and 50% increases in AUC and is often clinically irrelevant. Therefore, CYP450 2D6 drug interactions are less likely to cause harm with sertraline, escitalopram, citalopram, and fluvoxamine, but still require monitoring for a few weeks after the antidepressant is added to the patients' medication list.[70,135–138]

Although in vitro affinities of antidepressants for the respective isoenzymes can be very helpful for predicting potentially dangerous drug combinations, there is wide interpatient variability in the intensity of these interactions. Much of this variability can be attributed to genetic polymorphism. With CYP2D6, for example, approximately 5% to 10% of Caucasian patients and 1% to 2% of Asian patients are considered poor metabolizers via this isoenzyme.[139] CYP3A4 is the most abundant CYP enzyme found in the human body. Among the SSRIs, only fluoxetine and fluvoxamine have weak and moderate inhibitory effects on this isoenzyme, respectively. This has resulted in approximately 50% to 150% increase in AUC of the CYP450 3A4-dependent drug alprazolam.[70,137]

SEROTONIN SYNDROME

Serotonin syndrome is a rare but potentially fatal interaction due to excessive and prolonged serotonin within the synapse.[140] The syndrome includes a constellation of symptoms, including anxiety, shivering, diaphoresis, tremor, hyper-reflexia, and autonomic instability (increased/decreased blood pressure and pulse rate).[140] Fatalities have been attributed to malignant hyperthermia. It occurs due to excessive serotonin overstimulating 5-HT_{1a} receptors and possibly 5-HT_{2a} (hyperthermia, incoordination, and neuromuscular effects).[140] It can occur within hours of administration of medications that can cause the syndrome. With mild cases of serotonin syndrome, the symptoms ordinarily resolve 24 to 48 hours after the serotonergic agents have been discontinued. Supportive treatment may be necessary, and for more severe reactions, the serotonergic antagonist cyproheptadine is most commonly prescribed.[140] Dantrolene has been administered successfully to manage hyperthermia.[141]

Excessive serotonin can occur via four mechanisms: preventing its breakdown, preventing its reuptake into the neuron, increasing precursors or agonists, and increasing its release. Most case reports of serotonin syndrome (and most fatalities) have occurred with a combination of an MAOI and an SSRI, which is considered a contraindication. Other case reports involve the combination of an MAOI (or SSRI) with tryptophan, meperidine, SNRI, tricyclics, dextromethorphan, linezolid, and tramadol.[140] One case of serotonin syndrome was reportedly induced by the combination of clomipramine with S-adenosylmethionine (SAM-E).[142] Theoretically, the combination of an SSRI with Saint-John's-wort may also precipitate this pharmacodynamic interaction, but more recent evidence has suggested that the MAOI properties of the herbal preparation are minimal with therapeutic doses. Nonetheless, a case series of five older patients who exhibited symptoms reminiscent of serotonin syndrome has appeared in the literature, and, given the degree of uncertainty that persists, this combination of antidepressant agents is best avoided.[143] As noted by the previously described reports, the most concerning risk is combining agents that increase serotonin via differing mechanisms such as inhibiting the enzyme monoamine oxygenase and blocking the serotonin reuptake pump. Serotonin syndrome has also been reported with concurrent administration of multiple SSRIs; however, this would generally not be fatal. It is important to note that many medications have MAO inhibitory effects although they are not classified as an MAOI. This would include medications such as linezolid, dextromethorphan, and meperidine.

The combination of trazodone with an SSRI could possibly pose some concern because both classes of antidepressants augment serotonin activity in the CNS yet; because both are reuptake inhibitors, it is very unlikely. Trazodone has been associated with serotonin syndrome in two incidences, one involving the coadministration of buspirone and the other associated with a concomitant MAOI.[144] However, in practice, trazodone is recommended and is commonly prescribed to patients receiving an SSRI for the treatment of insomnia, with no confirmed cases of serotonin syndrome that have surfaced in the medical literature thus making it a possible risk only at very high doses.[145,146]

CASE 86-2

Question 1: M.G. is a 35 year old married female. She is diagnosed with MDD and has been tried on sertraline up to 100 mg QAM for 8 weeks which did not result in a response. She was then tried on fluoxetine 20 mg QAM for 8 weeks with only a partial response. What is the next step for M.G. who has not responded to two antidepressant trials at a therapeutic dose for a therapeutic duration?

Pooled results of clinical trials suggest that the majority of patients with major depression receiving an adequate trial of any antidepressant will have a therapeutic response, defined as at least a 50% reduction in depressive symptoms. However, for a patient who is severely depressed, a 50% reduction in symptoms still leaves him/her with significant psychopathology and associated disability. Consequently, full remission is the preferred therapeutic end point.[5] The STAR*D trials showed that after four stages of treatment (medication or psychotherapy), 33% of patients fail to reach remission.[147] In addition, with each course of antidepressants, people were less likely to achieve remission. One longitudinal investigation found that patients with residual symptoms were 3 times more likely to suffer relapse during the 12 months after treatment than those who had remitted.[148] Not surprisingly, patients with treatment-resistant depression have 40% higher direct medical costs than those without treatment-resistant depression, mainly due to medication and outpatient care costs.[149]

For M.G., the first step would be to confirm her diagnosis and rule out potential medical explanations for her symptoms, specifically bipolar disorder. Bipolar depression is diagnostically indistinguishable from MDD depressed episodes. Because antidepressants are minimally effective in bipolar depression, it would explain MGs lack of response if she were to have bipolar disorder. Iatrogenic causes should also be explored, such as any new medications or substance misuse. Assessing adherence to her previous medication trials is critical. A full therapeutic trial is considered to be a minimum of 4 weeks of treatment at a dosage shown to be clinically effective assuming the patient is compliant with therapy.

Drug Selection

SEROTONIN NOREPINEPHRINE REUPTAKE INHIBITORS

Because 30% to 40% of patients will effectively achieve remission and about 20% to 25% of patients will stop an antidepressant because of side effects, many patients started on a given antidepressant may eventually need a significant adjustment or change to their original regimen.[10]

In M.G.'s case, she has previously failed a therapeutic trial of sertraline and fluoxetine. Although she had failed a sertraline trial, large controlled investigations suggest that 50% to 70% of patients who are unresponsive or intolerant of one SSRI will experience a therapeutic response to a different SSRI.[150–152] For example, in the STAR*D trial, patients failing an initial course of citalopram were just as likely to respond whether they were randomly assigned to a subsequent trial of a different SSRI (sertraline) because they were to other antidepressant classes (venlafaxine and bupropion, specifically).[153] Because M.G. has now failed two SSRIs, it is recommended to try an antidepressant from a different class such as an SNRI, $\alpha 2$ antagonist, or DA reuptake inhibitor.[5,10] For M.G., it was recommended to use an SNRI and duloxetine was selected.

SNRIS

Venlafaxine, duloxetine, desvenlafaxine, and levomilnacipran are categorized as serotonin/norepinephrine reuptake inhibitors (SNRIs) (Table 86-7). At dosages less than 150 mg/day, venlafaxine's therapeutic effects are mediated exclusively from the blockade of serotonin reuptake. Therefore, associated adverse effects at these dosages are qualitatively and quantitatively very similar to those found with SSRIs: GI distress, sleep disturbances, and sexual dysfunction. At higher dosages, effects on NE occur, and this can lead to the emergence of different adverse effects (e.g., tachycardia and hypertension) and insomnia. NE effects occurring with duloxetine, desvenlafaxine, and levomilnacipran do not appear to be dose-dependent.[154] Levomilnacipran is an SNRI that has more potent effects on NE as compared to its 5-HT reuptake. However, its potency at NE reuptake is similar to duloxetine, and the ratio difference is due to its lower potency at 5-HT reuptake than the other SNRIs.[155,156] Venlafaxine, which is available as immediate- and extended-release formulations, has a relatively brief plasma half-life (5–8 hours) and is demethylated to an active metabolite (*O*-desmethyl-venlafaxine). This metabolite, desvenlafaxine, was approved by the FDA in 2008 for the treatment of depression. Desvenlafaxine is available as an extended-release tablet that has a similar mechanism of action as venlafaxine. It has no affinity for muscarinic, histaminic, cholinergic, or adrenergic receptors and has a terminal half-life of 11 hours.[157,158] Desvenlafaxine is not affected by CYP2D6 inhibitors; however, CYP3A4 inhibitors may reduce clearance of the drug.[138] Duloxetine also has a relatively short half-life (12 hours) and is metabolized via CYP450 1A1. Levomilnacipran is mainly metabolized by CYP3A4 with a terminal half-life of 12 hours and is available as an extended-release tablet.[159] Venlafaxine, desvenlafaxine, and levomilnacipran are not potent inhibitors of cytochrome P-450 isoenzymes. Duloxetine is a moderate inhibitor of the CYP2D6 isoenzyme.[138,159] As with SSRIs, SNRIs have been associated with serotonin syndrome. Additionally, increased BP will occur if combined with an MAOI.

As a class, all SNRIs have a risk of increasing blood pressure and heart rate thought to be due to the increase in NE. Venlafaxine averages an increase of 1 mm Hg and 3 bpm.[160] Duloxetine averages 1 mm Hg in BP and 3 bpm.[161] Desvenlafaxine averages an increase of 2 mm Hg and 4 bpm.[162,163] Levomilnacipran has the greatest risk and averages an increase of 4 mm Hg in BP and 8 bpm compared to placebo.[164] There will be some patients who have large changes in BP with any of the SNRIs; thus, monitoring of vital signs is necessary a few weeks after every dose increase.

Duloxetine has also been shown to increase LFTs 3 times the upper limit of normal by approximately 1.3% compared to 0.2% in placebo-treated patients.[165] Although these numbers are small and similar to other antidepressants, the FDA has given duloxetine a warning that it is not to be prescribed to patients with substantial alcohol use or evidence of chronic liver disease.[165] Levomilnacipran has also been shown to mildly increase LFTs at initiation of therapy.[159]

CASE 86-2, QUESTION 2: M.G. is given a prescription of duloxetine 30 mg QAM yet she has heard from television ads about a new antidepressant called Trintellix (vortioxetine) that is different than SSRIs. She asks if you can explain how this new antidepressant is different and if it is really better than the duloxetine she has just been prescribed.

SSRI and Serotonin Receptor Modulators

Vilazodone and vortioxetine are members of a new class of antidepressant. These medications have their primary effect on depression via inhibition of the serotonin reuptake pump, like the SSRIs (Table 86-10). These two agents also have potency at other serotonin receptors. Vilazodone is a partial agonist at the 5-HT_{1a} receptor.[166] Vortioxetine is a 5-HT_{1a} agonist, 5-HT_{1d}, 5-HT_3, 5-HT_7 antagonist, and 5-HT_{1b} partial agonist. Despite the potential for the added serotonin receptor effects, head-to-head trials with SSRIs and SNRIs have shown no greater efficacy advantage and similar side effect profiles.[164,166–168] In two separate studies, vortioxetine 20 mg showed a slightly less reduction in MADRS compared to duloxetine 60 mg QAM, –15.57 versus –16.9, respectively and –18.8 versus 21.2, respectively.[169,170]

Vilazodone should be taken with food as this increases absorption by about 50%. It is metabolized primarily by CYP450 3A4 and secondarily through 2C19. Inhibitors and inducers have a small effect on blood levels. Its half-life is approximately 25 hours.[171] Vilazodone seems to have no effect on CYP450 isoenzymes.[138] Vortioxetine is metabolized via multiple CYP 450 pathways with 2D6 being the primary one. It has a half-life of approximately 60 hours. It does not appear to effect the metabolism of other drugs using CYP450 (Tables 86-7 and 86-8).[172]

When speaking with M.G., it would be accurate to state that the new medication is not likely to be any better than her current prescription. Monitoring vital signs is more important with duloxetine than with vortioxetine although the change in vital signs with duloxetine is minimal and usually clinically irrelevant. Duloxetine has a potential for inhibiting CYP450 2D6 that is greater than vortioxetine. Duloxetine should be titrated to 60 mg QAM; thus, a dose increase is necessary to monitor for a therapeutic response (Table 86-9).

OTHER AGENTS: BUPROPION, MIRTAZAPINE, TRAZODONE, AND NEFAZODONE

Bupropion is an aminoketone with a mechanism of action that is clearly different from that of any other antidepressant because its therapeutic effect is due primarily to DA reuptake inhibition and has negligible effects on serotonin (Table 86-7).[173] This lack of serotonin provides a benefit in regard to both a lack of sexual dysfunction and sedation but has the negative effect in that it is definitively less anxiolytic as compared to the proserotonergic effect of the other antidepressants.[5] At therapeutic dosages, bupropion has a different adverse effect profile compared to SSRIs and SNRIs. Nausea, insomnia, agitation, and jitteriness are the most common, likely due to the stimulatory effect of DA. Seizures are a risk but are unlikely with therapeutic dosing of bupropion, provided that patients are not predisposed (e.g., history of epilepsy, bulimia, electrolyte abnormalities, or recent history of heavy drinking). Bupropion may decrease appetite. A randomized, placebo-controlled investigation of bupropion in depressed obese patients observing caloric restriction found that bupropion was much more likely to induce significant weight loss than placebo.[174] After 26 weeks of treatment, 40% of the bupropion-treated patients lost more than 5% of their total body weight versus 16% with placebo. This weight loss was positively correlated with an improvement in depressive symptoms. It has little-to-no negative effect on sexual function due to no stimulation of 5-HT receptors. For patients who develop sexual dysfunction from the SSRI or SNRI, bupropion has shown some benefit as an adjunctive treatment that reduces the side effect. It is also useful for poor responders as an adjunct to SSRI/SNRI due to its unique neurotransmitter effect.[5] Bupropion does not seem to affect cardiac rhythm or induce arrhythmias in susceptible patients.[175] Patients with hypertension should be monitored for increases in BP if bupropion is initiated.[176]

Bupropion is converted via the cytochrome CYP450 2B6 isoenzyme to an active metabolite (9 hydroxybupropion). Bupropion (and its metabolite) appears to have a moderate effect at inhibiting the CYP450 2D6 isoenzyme, and significant elevations of venlafaxine and metoprolol have been demonstrated to occur with concurrent administration (Table 86-8). Because of its short half-life (approximately 8 hours for the parent compound and 12 hours for the active metabolite), therapeutic doses of regular release bupropion must be administered in divided doses. The recommended starting dose is 100 mg twice a day (BID), increasing to 100 mg 3 times a day (TID) after at least 3 days. Individual doses must not exceed 150 mg and should be given at least 6 hours apart. For the SR formulation, initial daily doses are 150 mg every day, increased to 150 mg BID by the fourth day at the earliest. Individual doses of bupropion SR can be as large as 200 mg, and divided doses should be given at least 8 hours apart. The once-daily formulation is initiated at 150 mg daily and increasing to 300 mg daily as early as the fourth day. Maximum daily doses are 450 mg for regular and XL products, and 400 mg for SR products (Table 86-9). Maximum doses should be strictly followed due to the dose-dependent risk of seizures.[10]

Mirtazapine is a novel antidepressant capable of modulating serotonin and NE activity through a complex mechanism of action. In vitro studies reveal that mirtazapine is an antagonist at presynaptic α_2-autoreceptors and postsynaptic 5-HT_2 and 5-HT_3 receptors.[177] In addition, it appears to possess some mild inhibitory properties at serotonin reuptake transporters. Therefore, the net effect of mirtazapine is to enhance serotonin and NE in a manner that is clearly distinct from any other antidepressants (Table 86-8). In a comparative randomized trial with fluoxetine for moderate-to-severe depression, mirtazapine appeared to be much more effective than fluoxetine after 4 weeks of treatment (58% responders vs. 30% with fluoxetine; $P<0.05$), but the differences were no longer significant at 6 weeks (63% vs. 54%; $P = 0.67$).[178]

The most common adverse effects experienced with mirtazapine are sedation and weight gain. Because mirtazapine has potent antihistaminergic effects, it can be quite sedating and is often used as a hypnotic similar to trazodone. Unlike trazodone, antidepressant dosing is quite tolerable. Anecdotally, it has been reported that higher daily doses of mirtazapine (>30 mg) are less sedating than lower doses owing to a plateauing of antihistaminic effects at 15 mg but an increase in noradrenergic effects up to 60 mg. In addition to the substantial risk of increasing appetite and total body weight, mirtazapine has been associated with significant increases in total cholesterol and triglycerides. This is likely due to its combination of H_1 and 5-HT_{2c} antagonism, the pharmacology related to atypical antipsychotic metabolic effects.

This makes mirtazapine less preferred than SSRIs in the diabetic patient. Mirtazapine does not appear to affect cardiac rhythm or induce arrhythmias.[175] The recommended starting dosage is 15 mg at bedtime, and the therapeutic dosage ranges from 15 to 45 mg/day (Table 86-9).[179] Data from controlled trials have demonstrated safety and efficacy in doses up to 60 mg daily.[179–181] As with bupropion, mirtazapine is considered a top choice for antidepressant combination therapy in poorly responding patients on an SSRI/SNRI. Despite the fact that mirtazapine is increasing 5-HT and NE as do SNRIs, its unique method of doing this via $\alpha 2$ antagonism makes the combination with an SNRI or SSRI recommended.[5,10,182]

Nefazodone and trazodone have similar mechanisms of action. Both are serotonin reuptake inhibitors but nefazodone also has a mild NE reuptake inhibitory effect (Table 86-7). Both also block 5-HT_2 receptors.[17] This particular characteristic has resulted in very little sexual dysfunction, and switching studies have shown that patients who develop sexual side effects with SSRIs do not have this side effect with nefazodone.[183] Interestingly, trazodone does have the rare but well-documented side effect of priapism.[184] Trazodone, which comes as immediate-release and an extended-release caplet, is rarely used for depression due to its potency of H_1 antagonism centrally resulting in significant sedation and somnolence.[10,146,184] Antidepressive effects with trazodone occur above 150 mg a day with most patients requiring $>$300 mg a day, yet sedation occurs at low doses such as 25 mg.[184,185] This has caused clinicians to use trazodone as a hypnotic with other antidepressants instead of trying to titrate up and use it as monotherapy. It is also a potent $\alpha 1$ receptor antagonist and can cause orthostasis.[10,184] A reason that nefazodone has not been used more is due to its potential for hepatotoxicity.[5,10] This event is more common than any other antidepressant. With appropriate monitoring, such as LFTs q3 months for the first 18 to 24 months, this risk is nearly eliminated.[10] However, other drugs with hepatotoxic risks such as valproic acid increase this risk making nefazodone more difficult to use than most other antidepressants. Nefazodone is metabolized via CYP450 3A4 and is also a moderate-to-strong inhibitor of CYP450 3A4 (Table 86-8).[76,186]

TCAs

The SSRIs are recommended over TCAs in the treatment of mood disorders. The popularity of SSRIs can be attributed to numerous advantages over older compounds, including a lower side effect burden, safety in overdose, less dosage titration, and patient preference.[5,10,26] Results of a meta-analysis concluded that although the overall efficacy of the SSRI and TCA classes was comparable, primary care patients receiving an SSRI were much less likely to discontinue therapy prematurely due to side effects.[187] TCAs cause a variety of adverse effects, ranging from bothersome (dry mouth, sedation, constipation) to serious (cardiovascular effects), which often prevent patients from receiving therapeutic doses of medication.[188] Patient adherence with prescribed medication may also be compromised with TCAs.[189] Even though SSRIs and the newer SNRIs are preferred for treatment of depression, TCAs continue to be prescribed at low doses for other indications that are comorbid with depression (e.g., migraine prophylaxis, chronic neuropathic pain). This requires careful monitoring for drug interactions as TCAs as a class are primarily metabolized via CYP450 2D6 and, as noted previously, some SSRIs and SNRIs may inhibit this pathway substantially increasing the risk of TCA toxicity.

SIDE EFFECTS

Therapeutic effects of TCAs are primarily through their ability to inhibit the reuptake of serotonin and NE, functionally an SNRI (Table 86-7).[190] Additionally, TCAs have significant effects on acetylcholine, histamine, and α noradrenergic receptors all of which are considered potential for side effects. The intensity of these side effects has been shown to adversely affect adherence.[26] Although patients may develop tolerance to these effects, they may never disappear completely.

Due to the potent histamine 1 antagonism centrally, TCAs can be very sedating and are usually administered at bedtime to minimize functional impairments. Confusion or memory deficits may also occur with TCAs and can be particularly onerous in elderly patients. The secondary amines may be more tolerable in this regard, but all TCAs can impair concentration or alertness to some extent and are not recommended in geriatrics.[10] The sedating antihistaminic effect (along with orthostasis) increases the risk of falls. The risk of weight gain and constipation make TCAs undesirable in a patient with comorbid diabetes.

Orthostatic hypotension is the most common and troublesome cardiovascular effect of the TCAs (as well as MAOIs) because it can result in significant morbidity and mortality.[191,192] Major clinical consequences of orthostatic hypotension include falls leading to bone fractures, lacerations, and even MI. Patients with CHF and the elderly are at greatest risk for experiencing orthostatic hypotension. The tertiary amines (e.g., amitriptyline, imipramine) may cause more severe orthostatic hypotension than the secondary amines (e.g., nortriptyline, desipramine), and research supports the contention that nortriptyline has the lowest risk for causing orthostatic hypotension among TCAs.[193,194]

There are substantial differences among antidepressants (and antidepressant classes) in regard to overall cardiac safety and arrhythmogenic effects in particular. In general, the SSRIs appear to be relatively safe in patients with a history of arrhythmias or recent MI.[175] In a placebo-controlled investigation, hospitalized patients with unstable cardiac disease were randomly assigned to either sertraline or placebo.[195] Overall, both treatment arms were very well tolerated, and there was actually a lower risk of severe cardiac events reported in the sertraline group (vs. placebo). Retrospective data suggest that SSRIs may be somewhat cardioprotective in depressed patients with heart disease, a benefit that might be explained by their ability to decrease platelet activation.[196,197]

TCAs increase heart rate, probably via intrinsic anticholinergic properties that increase sinus node activity. Clinically, this effect is generally not significant, especially in medically healthy depressed patients.[10,198] However, it may be important in those with underlying conduction disease, coronary artery disease, or CHF. TCAs, even when used at therapeutic dosages for the treatment of depression, decrease premature atrial and ventricular contractions in both depressed and nondepressed patients.[199,200] Because TCAs have a Class 1A antiarrhythmic activity, they have arrhythmogenic activity and thus increase the chances of ventricular arrhythmias and even sudden death. This effect on rhythm and conduction is believed to be related to the inhibitory effects of TCAs on the fast sodium channels and a decrease in Purkinje fiber action potential amplitude, membrane responsiveness, and slowed conduction.[200] Even nortriptyline, which is believed to be one of the safer TCAs in patients with heart disease, was associated with a greater risk for adverse cardiac events than paroxetine.[201] In patients with preexisting conduction defects and in overdose, there is a greater risk for cardiac arrhythmias.[193] Therefore, patients should receive a baseline electrocardiogram (ECG) before therapy, and use in patients with preexisting cardiac conduction abnormalities should be avoided.[10]

Other risks associated with TCAs are a lowering of the seizure threshold. This seems to be worst with clomipramine and maprotiline compared to the others in the class.[10,202,203] This event is particularly risky in high doses, similar to bupropion. If patients are at risk of seizures or have a seizure disorder, SSRIs are much safer and are preferred over the TCAs.[10,202,203] TCAs have also been shown to produce photosensitivity; thus, excessive exposure to sunlight has resulted in severe sunburns. In patients who have had this reaction or whose lifestyle requires frequent contact with sunlight (e.g., lifeguard), switching to another class is recommended.[204]

MONOAMINE OXIDASE INHIBITORS

MAOIs are an alternative for patients who have failed multiple antidepressant trials. MAOIs are believed to relieve depressive symptoms by enhancing the activity of monoamines. This is done by blocking the enzyme monoamine oxidase which breaks down serotonin, dopamine, and NE. This is in contrast to SSRI/SNRI which increases 5-HT and/or NE by preventing its reuptake into the neuron. This may be desirable for refractory cases. Candidates for treatment should be chosen carefully, and MAOIs should be used only by specialist practitioners such as a psychiatrist.

Phenelzine, tranylcypromine, and isocarboxazid were commonly prescribed for the treatment of depression in the 1970s and 1980s, and their usefulness waned primarily because of the risks of serious drug–drug and drug–food interactions.[205] In standard treatment of depression, MAOIs are not recommended except for the treatment of atypical depression where this class appears to have a small efficacy advantage over other classes.[5,10] Data comparing TCAs with SSRIs for atypical depression suggest that the two classes are comparable in efficacy and both are superior to placebo and so SSRIs should still be tried first due to safety concerns.[10,206]

The "cheese reaction," which can manifest as a hypertensive crisis, is so named because it occurred in patients who were taking nonselective MAOIs and ingested foods high in tyramine, a by-product of tyrosine metabolism that is found in certain foods and beverages, such as aged cheese or Chianti wine (Table 86-12). When tyramine is ingested in the absence of an MAOI, it is rapidly metabolized by the MAO enzyme in the GI tract before systemic absorption. In the presence of an MAOI, more tyramine is absorbed and relatively high concentrations of tyramine may be achieved in circulation, resulting in the displacement of NE (and other catecholamines) from presynaptic storage granules. NE surges into the synapse, and as metabolic degradation is inhibited by the MAOI, a profound pressor response is triggered.[207] A slightly safer version of the MAOI class is the once-daily selegiline transdermal. By avoiding the GI tract, selegiline has less effect on the MAO that reduces tyramine from entering the bloodstream via food. Despite the improved safety of selegiline transdermal to oral MAOIs, there still remains a risk of food–drug interactions resulting in hypertensive reactions, particularly at higher doses, and so the FDA has recommended diet restrictions for doses over 6 mg/24 hours. Additionally, there are application site reactions that occur in approximately 35% of patients.[5,208,209] This agent is available in 6, 9, and 12 mg strengths. Selegiline transdermal as well as oral MAOIs are reserved for refractory cases and should be used only by skilled clinicians.[5,209]

Table 86-12
Foods Containing Tyramine

High Amounts of Tyramine[a]
Smoked, aged, or pickled meat or fish
Sauerkraut
Aged cheeses (e.g., Stilton, blue cheese)
Yeast extracts (e.g., marmite)
Fava beans
Moderate Amounts of Tyramine[b]
Beer (microbrewed > commercial)
Avocados
Meat extracts
Red wines such as Chianti
Low Amounts of Tyramine[c]
Caffeine-containing beverages
Distilled spirits
Chocolate
Soy sauce
Cottage and cream cheese
Yogurt and sour cream

[a]May not consume.
[b]May consume in moderation.
[c]May consume.

Adapted with permission from Shulman KI et al. Dietary restriction, tyramine, and the use of monoamine oxidase inhibitors. *J Clin Psychopharmacol*. 1989;9:397.

ADVERSE EFFECTS

Orthostatic hypotension, weight gain, edema, and sexual dysfunction are common during MAOI therapy.[191] As is the case with the TCAs, the nonselective MAOIs can cause clinically significant postural decreases in BP. However, with the MAOIs, the mechanism is believed to be a direct sympatholytic effect because both the lying and the standing systolic BP readings are decreased.[210,211] Phenelzine seems to cause orthostatic hypotension more commonly than does tranylcypromine.[212] Because the orthostatic hypotension appears to be dose-related, a reduction in dosage may be helpful.[213] Sexual dysfunction occurs in up to 20% of patients taking MAOIs but may diminish and disappear spontaneously over time.[214,215] A switch into mania has been reported in up to 10% of patients with a history of bipolar disorder. Therefore, MAOIs should be avoided in this population.[191] Although MAOIs are not known as antimuscarinic medications, some patients complain of anticholinergic-like side effects, including blurred near vision and urinary retention. Dosage reduction may be helpful, but these effects may also diminish over time. The nonselective MAOIs are not associated with proarrhythmic, antiarrhythmic, or contractility effects when used in therapeutic dosages. Like other MAOIs, selegiline can be quite activating, and insomnia is frequently reported.

Several potentially fatal drug–drug interactions occur with nonselective MAOI antidepressants. Like the reaction with tyramine, indirect sympathomimetics such as phenylpropanolamine and pseudoephedrine (common ingredients in over-the-counter cold preparations and diet pills) can cause a precipitous rise in BP that can result in stroke.

The potential for serotonin syndrome with the combined use of SSRIs and MAOI antidepressants or other medications with MAOI effect is well documented. A washout period of at least 14 days should separate the use of an SSRI and an MAOI. Because fluoxetine (and its primary active metabolite norfluoxetine) has a much longer half-life, the recommended washout period is at least 5 weeks after discontinuing this particular SSRI. Caution is advised when any other pro-serotonergic mediations are prescribed such as triptans and tramadol.[140]

CASE 86-2, QUESTION 3: M.G. still had some residual symptoms despite a therapeutic trial of duloxetine 60 mg QAM. An increase to 90 mg resulted in intolerable insomnia. She has had a partial response (approximately 40% reduction in symptoms) but is still impaired by her depression. What are possible next steps?

Antidepressant Augmentation with Non-Antidepressants

Treatment refractory depression (TRD) is considered to be a failure to reach remission with 2 or more antidepressant monotherapy trials that were given at a therapeutic dose and given for an appropriately therapeutic period. Generally, a therapeutic dose is for 4 to 8 weeks. This would not include the time it takes to titrate to a therapeutic dose.[216,217] A common strategy for TRD includes combining antidepressants such as an SSRI with bupropion or mirtazapine, as mentioned previously. Other strategies are augmenting an antidepressant with a medication from another class, or somatic treatments, particularly ECT.[5,10,26,216,217]

There are many options to augment an SSRI/SNRI if the patient has not achieved a full response. Some atypical antipsychotics, lithium and triiodothyronine, all have studies showing efficacy. Buspirone has less robust data but is still recommended.[5,216,217] The use of atypical antipsychotics for the management of treatment-resistant depression has become relatively common among mental health providers due to well-designed and replicated studies. Four atypical antipsychotics (olanzapine in combination with fluoxetine, aripiprazole, brexpiprazole, and quetiapine) have received FDA approval as adjunctive agents with SSRIs or SNRIs for depression that has poorly responded to monotherapy, and others have been reported to be effective as well.[5,216,217] Generally, lower doses of second-generation antipsychotics have been successfully used in trials for depression (vs. schizophrenia), and relatively rapid improvement was evident. Given the significant risk of metabolic side effects that have been reported, clinicians must carefully weigh the risks and benefits of recommending this augmentation strategy prior to maximizing antidepressant monotherapy trials and antidepressant combinatioms.[5,10] It is recommended that nonbehavioral health specialists use caution when using the atypical antipsychotics for poorly responding patients.[182]

One instance where the use of an atypical antipsychotic adjunct is given during the acute phase is with psychotic depression. Patients with psychosis during the depressed episode, as with multiple previous episodes and depression severity, are at greater risk of chronicity and suicidality.[10] Multiple studies have shown benefit of antipsychotic and antidepressant combination better than either monotherapy. Despite the fact that monotherapy may be appropriate for the maintenance phase, it is recommended to start an antipsychotic with the antidepressant during the acute phase and slowly taper off after the persons depression and psychosis remits.[5,10,218] The least preferred antidepressant is bupropion. Its prodopaminergic effect could worsen the psychosis.[10] ECT is also a recommended treatment.[5,10,218]

Lithium's antidepressant properties as an augmenting agent have primarily been conducted with TCAs.[217] Seven of nine antidepressant augmentation trials with lithium have reported positive therapeutic effects, usually within 1 week of achieving steady state dynamics (i.e., 3–7 days of daily dosing).[219] Effective lithium blood levels are generally within the range used to treat bipolar disorder (0.5–1.2 mEq/L). Lithium has a very narrow therapeutic index along with multiple significant drug interactions and should only be used by a clinician skilled in its use.[5]

Triiodothyronine (T_3) also has a long history of use in psychiatric circles for patients exhibiting partial or suboptimal responses to antidepressant monotherapy. Five of six RCTs support the use of T_3 supplementation for antidepressant augmentation, with an average effect size of 0.58 reported.[220] Triiodothyronine, at a dosage of 25 mg/day, can accelerate as well as augment antidepressant response, and superior effects have been reported in female patients, in particular. The response to the thyroid supplementation should be noticeable within 1 to 2 weeks, much like that found when lithium is used to augment therapy. Thyroxine (T_4) may also be effective with typical daily doses of 75 to 100 mcg daily often used. In the STAR*D trials, T_3 was compared to lithium for antidepressant augmentation with citalopram in patients with two previous treatment failures.[221] Remission rates were modest for both agents in this challenging population (24.7% with T_3 vs. 15.9% with lithium), and there was no significant difference between these two therapies.

In the STAR*D trial, augmentation with bupropion was compared to buspirone and both adjunctive treatments showed 30% remission rates.[221] Buspirone may be of benefit to patients with residual symptoms of anxiety, in particular, and titration up to daily doses of 30 to 60 mg daily is often required.[5,182] Stimulants and modafinil have generally shown no benefit on depressive symptoms overall.[182,222] However, they may provide temporary relief from excessive fatigue and somnolence while waiting for the full antidepressant effect of the primary treatments.[5,217]

Because M.G. had a failure to two monotherapies and some response to duloxetine, the option of adding a medication to the SNRI is the next step. Combinations of duloxetine with another antidepressant (mirtazapine or bupropion) or with an atypical antipsychotic are both recommended. Mirtazapine, quetiapine, and olanzapine would help if there is any insomnia and would protect against this side effect if duloxetine were to be increased in the future. Bupropion would possibly worsen the insomnia. Aripiprazole, brexpiprazole, mirtazapine, quetiapine, and olanzapine (least to most) all could cause weight gain worsen cholesterol. Discussing the risks of each option is critical and letting M.G. help decide which choice fits her lifestyle will ensure better adherence. M.G. decided to start aripiprazole 2 mg QAM and will increase her exercising to mitigate the possible weight gain and cholesterol increase.

Pediatric Depression

CASE 86-3

QUESTION 1: A.A. is a 15 year old male who has had a mood and behavior change over the last 6 months. A.A. is a sophomore in high school who averages B's in his classes. He was a member of the varsity lacrosse team, with many friends. Over the last 6 months he has been less involved with his friends to the point that he now doesn't want to go out. After lacrosse season was over he normally would participate in off season lacrosse camps. This year he didn't want to. His grades have dropped as he can't concentrate as well on his school work. He has missed some days of school lately because he doesn't want to get out of bed. Important rule outs are illicit drug use and recent trauma. Both have been ruled out. His medical history is unremarkable except for a 10 pound weight loss since last year, likely due to a poor appetite. His parents are very supportive. What are the recommendations for the treatment of pediatric depression?

Rates of pediatric depression are less than in adults. As a person ages, the risk of depression increases with rates of 0.5% in 3- to 5-year-olds increasing to 3.5% in 12- to 17-year-olds.[10,223] Diagnosing pediatric depression uses the same criteria from the DSM 5 as for adults; however, the interview questions may be slightly different. For example, poor concentration may be mislabeled as procrastination or anhedonia might be described as "being bored."[9] Treatment guidelines do differ compared to adults. One reason for this is that placebo rates are much higher in pediatric studies resulting in the medication not having as dramatic a difference when compared to the difference between placebo and drug in adult studies. Thus, there are many studies where SSRIs had strong response rates but placebo also did and the medication was not considered to be statistically different.[224–226] Due to this high response rate from placebo and the support given by being a subject in a research study, the expert guidelines recommend supportive care and formal talking therapy be the first option for mild-to-moderate depression.[227,228] Medications can be used if symptoms are moderate to severe. Pharmacotherapy options are limited, though, compared to adults. Fluoxetine is FDA-approved down to age 8, escitalopram to age 12. Clomipramine (10 and older), fluvoxamine (8 and older), and sertraline (6 and older) are FDA-approved for obsessive compulsive disorder but not depression. The SNRI duloxetine is approved for 7 years old and above for generalized anxiety disorder, and imipramine is approved for 6 and older for enuresis. To summarize, only two antidepressants are FDA-approved for depression in children although some other antidepressants do have nondepression indications in children.

CASE 86-3, QUESTION 2: The child psychiatrist's initial recommendation is to have A.A. meet with a psychologist. After 4 months of talking therapy A.A. is improved in general but is still having bouts of sadness that prevent him from going to school a couple days a month. It is decided to continue talk therapy but to add a medication. Which medication is the preferred agent?

Unlike adults where all antidepressants are similarly effective, pediatric depression guidelines have recommended that SSRIs particularly fluoxetine and escitalopram be the treatments of choice.[227,228] Fluoxetine's starting dose is 10 mg QAM with a target dose of 20 to 40 mg a day. Escitalopram's starting dose is 5 to 10 mg QAM with a target dose of 10 to 20 mg a day. Interestingly, the separation from placebo increases as the child ages for many of the SSRIs. For example, escitalopram did not statistically differ from placebo in the under 12 year old age group but did so in the adolescent age group.[224,229] Paroxetine is not recommended for depression due to overall lack of efficacy in any age group when studies are combined and a high dropout rate in the younger patient.[224,226] Bupropion, mirtazapine, venlafaxine and duloxetine have recommendations as treatment options but after failures to the SSRIs.[227] TCAs are not recommended primarily due to a high risk of harm being much greater than the small benefit on symptoms.[227,230]

CASE 86-3, QUESTION 3: A.A. is started on fluoxetine 10 mg QAM. What safety monitoring is required when starting a young adult or pediatric patient on an antidepressant?

Generally, the SSRIs are well tolerated in children. One black box warning is for suicidal thinking. As with adults, the clinician needs to monitor for suicidality, but in children there is a doubling of suicidal thoughts, not suicide attempts or completions, from 2% in the placebo arms to 4% in medication arms. It is important to note that actual suicides are much higher in untreated depressed youth compared to those taking antidepressants.[94,231–233] This risk diminishes as age groups increase. For patients over age 24, it is not required to be so vigilant regarding suicidal thinking although many guidelines recommend continuing to monitor throughout the age ranges due to the possibility of disease-related risk. In pediatrics and young adults, the experts recommend the use of antidepressants with the FDA-sanctioned monitoring for suicidal thinking of every week for the first week, every other week for the next 4 weeks, then monthly or as decided by the patient and clinician.[227,234] Talking therapy may have some protection against the side effect of increased suicidal thoughts.[235]

Geriatric Depression

Depression in late life is typically more difficult to recognize than depression in younger adults. Clinicians and patients may inappropriately attribute depressive symptoms to the "aging process" and minimize their significance. In addition, functional expectations are often lowered after retirement, making the degree of impairment difficult to evaluate. Because medical comorbidities are also more common in the elderly, depressive symptoms may be overlooked or misinterpreted in the workup as well.[116,236] In general, the elderly present with the same depressive target symptoms as younger adults, which is reflected in the fact that DSM-5 diagnosis for major depression in adults is not specific for age. However, qualitatively, the presentation of depression among the elderly may be quite different. For instance, older patients are more likely to present with psychomotor retardation and are less likely to acknowledge "depression" per se, preferring instead to dwell on somatic concerns (e.g., poor sleep, low energy, changes in bowel function, bodily aches and pains).[10] They are also much less likely to share or admit suicidal thoughts, and because elderly men have the highest suicide completion rate, an accurate assessment of depression and attendant risks is critical.[10,116,237] In assessing nonspecific behavioral and cognitive symptoms in the elderly, a careful differential diagnosis between medical and other psychiatric disorders is essential because numerous medical illnesses can mimic depressive symptoms. Anemia, malignancies, congestive heart failure (CHF), and endocrine abnormalities may all present in a manner similar to that in depressive illness.

Aging does result in decreased monoamine depletion as well as increased monoamine oxidase activity.[116] One of the more difficult differential diagnoses in this setting involves the distinction of depression from dementias.[238,239] Like depression, patients with dementia may present with apathy, poor memory or concentration, reduced facial expression, and lack of spontaneous interaction. The illnesses are often comorbid, as 30% to 70% of patients with dementia also suffer from major depression.[239] Some experts have suggested, in fact, that new-onset depression in elderly patients may actually be part of a prodrome toward the manifestation of Alzheimer dementia.[239,240] A longitudinal cohort study found that among elderly patients suffering from an acute episode of major depression, 57% were ultimately diagnosed with Alzheimer dementia within the next 3 years.[238] Diagnostically, there are three notable differences between dementia and depression: (a) the symptoms (slow and subtle changes with dementia, rapid with depression), (b) orientation (markedly impaired with dementia, intact with depression), and (c) principal CNS impairment (short-term memory with dementia, concentration with depression).

Drug Selection in the Elderly

A therapeutic trial of an antidepressant in a depressed individual with cognitive impairment may reverse the symptoms of the affective illness and restore functional capacity. Depression-related cognitive dysfunction will also improve to some degree. Moreover, because primary degenerative dementia is largely a diagnosis of exclusion, a successful trial of an antidepressant may help clarify the underlying pathologic condition and is strongly recommended in patients with a positive personal or family history of mood disorders.[241] The overall efficacy of antidepressants in elderly patients is believed to be comparable to that observed in younger subjects, although the response to treatment is somewhat slower (i.e., 6-week therapeutic trial usually warranted).[5] Psychotherapy may be somewhat more effective in the elderly particularly due to the emotional impact of medical comorbidities and neurodegeneration effects as long as there is no dementia hindering talking therapy's effect.[5] Similarly, the comparative therapeutic effects of individual antidepressants do not appear to differ qualitatively between elderly patients and the general population. The selection of antidepressants for geriatric depression is the same as the process for younger patients. The elderly are much more sensitive to side effects compared to the younger patient, and the presence of medical comorbidities and concurrent medications will have a greater influence on antidepressant selection. For example, the anticholinergic effects of TCAs preclude their use in elderly patients particularly if they are suffering from narrow angle glaucoma, chronic constipation, or urinary hesitancy. Anticholinergic impact on memory and the cardiac-related effects such as arrhythmias, orthostasis, and tachycardia are other critical reasons not to use the TCAs in the elderly. As noted previously, the risk of falls from TCAs due to antihistaminic, anticholinergic, and α receptor antagonistic properties is another reason not to use them in the elderly population.

SSRIs are recommended as first line but among this list paroxetine is considered the worst option due to its anticholinergic effects (albeit mild) compared to no effect from the others. SNRIs also have data showing efficacy.[5,10,26] There does seem to be more dropouts with venlafaxine compared to the SSRIs.[5] Although sedating antidepressants such as mirtazapine may serve to promote sleep in depressed patients suffering from insomnia, other geriatric clients may be candidates for more activating medications that can increase energy or enhance alertness (e.g., bupropion).

All antidepressants have a risk of causing the syndrome of antidiuretic hormone secretion (SIADH) with SSRIs being the group with the highest reported cases. Elderly patients, compared to younger patients, are at a much greater risk of this event with some reviews reporting hyponatremia up to 32%.[10,242] As with other medications used in the elderly, the antidepressants should be started at lower initial doses compared to adults.[5,10,116] Titration to a known therapeutic target dose has the best evidence even if the geriatric seems to be responding to a subtherapeutic dose.[5]

Therapeutic Blood Level Monitoring

Attempts to demonstrate an association between plasma concentrations and therapeutic response for SSRIs and SNRIs have been largely unsuccessful. In contrast, the serum concentration of some TCAs correlates well with clinical response. Nortriptyline exhibits a curvilinear effect, whereas imipramine demonstrates a sigmoidal relationship between serum levels and clinical response.[243,244] Maximum benefit of imipramine is usually associated with serum levels of imipramine plus its demethylated metabolite, desipramine, in excess of 250 ng/mL. The relationship between plasma concentration of desipramine and clinical response is less clear, but a linear relationship is likely.[245] The most controversy surrounds amitriptyline; studies have shown a linear relationship, a curvilinear relationship, and no relationship between serum concentration and outcome.[246–248] The APA Task Force on the Use of Laboratory Tests in Psychiatry recommends plasma concentration monitoring of TCAs when patients are elderly, not responding to therapy, nonadherent, experiencing adverse effects, or on multiple medications that may result in a possible drug interaction.[249] Plasma concentrations of imipramine, nortriptyline, and desipramine should be obtained after at least 1 week of a constant dosage when steady state has been achieved. Samples should be drawn 12 hours after the last dose has been administered. Routine therapeutic blood monitoring of other antidepressants is not recommended because information concerning their usefulness is limited; however, serum levels may be useful for evaluating adherence in some patients or ruling out serious toxicities.[250]

Antidepressants and Chronic Pain

CASE 86-4

QUESTION 1: D.C. is a 42-year-old woman with a history of chronic lower back and left leg pain who has noted increased crying spells and a decreased interest in social activities during the course of the last 4 months. She attributes this downturn to the stress she is experiencing as she cares for her disabled mother who recently moved in with her. When asked, she also notes significant decreases in energy and concentration, and difficulties in falling and staying asleep.

In the past, D.C. recalls one previous episode of depression 8 years ago, when she was treated initially with venlafaxine (discontinued due to nausea) and ultimately responded to a course of psychotherapy. Her past medical history is significant for chronic pain from a car accident 7 years ago which continues to bother her on a daily basis (she rates pain at 5 of 10 currently), hypertension and hyperlipidemia. Her current medications include lisinopril 10 mg QAM and atorvastatin 10 mg QHS. In addition, she started amitriptyline 50 mg at bedtime 2 months ago for her insomnia but noticed a 12-pound weight gain and recently discontinued. In the meantime, she has continued to see her therapist on a weekly basis during this time frame.

What considerations may influence treatment selection in this patient with chronic pain? What treatment should be recommended?

There is a strong and complex association between chronic pain syndromes and mood disorders. Epidemiologic investigations report that 50% of patients with chronic pain will satisfy the criteria for a depressive disorder.[251] Anxiety disorders are also commonly reported in this population as well. On the other hand, 65% of individuals with major depression will experience some symptoms of somatic pain, often presenting with pain as their chief complaint. Researchers have theorized that this comorbid phenomenon can be explained by deficiencies in the neurotransmitters serotonin and NE, which influence mood disorders in the prefrontal cortex and limbic system, as well as module pain sensitivity via descending projections down the spinal column. Other theories implicate elevations in cytokine activity, which commonly occur during the course of mood disorders, as well as mediating inflammatory activity occurring within the context of chronic pain.[251,252]

Treatment plans for depressed patients with chronic pain should target both of these conditions in order to achieve optimal outcomes. In regard to the selection of antidepressants, preference is often given to medications that can address both sets of symptoms associated with these comorbid conditions. For instance, antidepressant agents with pain-relieving properties and agents that promote sleep and relieve anxiety are often preferred. Antidepressants that enhance 5-HT and NE (TCAs and SNRIs) have proven to be quite effective for the management of neuropathic pain conditions, in addition to their benefits on anxiety and depression.[5,251,252] SSRIs are much less effective primarily due to the lack of NE enhancement which is critical for analgesia.[5]

Drug interactions are often a major consideration in the selection of antidepressants. For example, the combination of SNRI antidepressants with the analgesic tramadol has been linked to a few case reports of serotonin syndrome, and concomitant use of these agents should be discouraged. Certain opioid analgesics are prodrugs and require metabolic transformation to generate the active species. These analgesics include codeine (metabolized to morphine), hydrocodone (active metabolite: hydromorphone), and oxycodone (oxymorphone), as well as tramadol (*o*-desmethyl tramadol). Patients who require these medications would benefit from antidepressants that do not effect CYP 450 (Table 86-8).

D.C. meets the criteria for an acute episode of major depression, and medication is clearly indicated. Among the alternatives, SSRIs have not proven to be effective for neuropathic pain. SNRIs and TCAs are effective for neuropathic pain conditions, as well as depression and anxiety. However, there are substantial tolerability and toxicity risks with TCAs not shown with the SNRI class. Additionally, she has experienced significant weight gain with a low-dose TCA (50 mg amitriptyline). An SNRI would be a good choice for the treatment of her depression and chronic pain. Given

D.C.'s history of nausea from venlafaxine, an alternate SNRI, such as levomilnacipran or duloxetine, should be initiated. Duloxetine inhibits CYP450 2D6, and this should be taken into consideration if other medication changes are considered in the future.

Summary

Depressive episodes have a significant morbidity impact and can result in mortality, usually via suicide. Treatment has been shown to reduce acute impact and prevent future episodes. All antidepressants are considered generally equal in regard to efficacy. Comorbid drug–disease and drug–drug interactions help identify best first-choice options. Overall, SSRIs are considered the best first choice due to good tolerability, safety in overdose, and low cost. Of these, sertraline and escitalopram may have a slight advantage. Previous treatment successes or failures and family history of medication response are important determining factors when disease and drug issues are not present. Minimal treatment duration should be 6 months after remission has been achieved though many patients will require lifelong pharmacotherapy. Patient education and safety monitoring are critical aspects once the patient enters into treatment. Outcomes for treatment are predictably beneficial with improvements in quality of life and reduction of suicidal events.

KEY REFERENCES AND WEBSITES

A full list of references for this chapter can be found at http://thepoint.lww.com/AT11e. Below are the key references and websites for this chapter, with the corresponding reference number in this chapter found in parentheses after the reference.

Key References

Cleare A et al. Evidenced based guidelines for treating depressive disorders with antidepressants: a revision of the 2008 British Association for Psychopharmacology guidelines. *J Psychopharmacol*. 2015;29(5):459–525. (5)

Practice Guideline for the Treatment of Patients with Major Depressive Disorder. 3rd ed. Arlington, VA: American Psychiatric Association. 2010. (10)

Spina E et al. Clinically significant drug interactions with newer antidepressants. *CNS Drugs*. 2012;26(1):39–67. (138)

Key Websites

American Psychiatric Association. http://www.psychiatryonline.org.
National Alliance on Mental Illness. http://www.nami.org.
National Institute of Mental Health. http://www.nimh.nih.gov.

87 Bipolar Disorders

Megan J. Ehret and Charles F. Caley

CORE PRINCIPLES

		CHAPTER CASES
1	Bipolar disorder is a chronic progressive illness that occurs in approximately 4% of the population. It is characterized by recurrent mood episodes of mania and depression. Life stressors, substance use, treatment non-adherence, and medications are common precipitants of these mood episodes.	**Case 87-1 (Questions 1–3)**
2	Manic episodes are characterized by elevated mood, irritability, increased goal-directed activity, inflated self-esteem, poor judgment, and excessive motor activity.	**Case 87-1 (Question 1), Case 87-2 (Question 1)**
3	Depressive episodes of bipolar share the same diagnostic criteria as major depressive disorder, including depressed mood, decreased interest, feelings of worthlessness, diminished ability to concentrate, and recurrent thoughts of death.	**Case 87-7 (Question 1)**
4	Valproate, lithium, or atypical antipsychotics are appropriate first-line treatments for acute mania. Depending on the severity of symptoms, these agents may be used alone or in combination.	**Case 87-1 (Questions 4, 5), Case 87-2 (Question 1), Case 87-5 (Question 2), Case 87-6 (Question 1)**
5	Lithium, lamotrigine, quetiapine, lurasidone, or the combination of these agents is appropriate treatments for bipolar depression.	**Case 87-7 (Question 1)**
6	Maintenance treatment of bipolar disorder is imperative to prevent disease progression. The standard of practive is to continue the acute-phase treatment with gradual simplification toward monotherapy, if possible, with lithium, lamotrigine, valproate, or atypical antipsychotics.	**Case 87-5 (Question 1), Case 87-8 (Questions 1, 2)**
7	Medications used to treat bipolar disorder have a wide range of adverse effects that may impact adherence. The history of response, patient preference, and long-term tolerability profile are important considerations when selecting an agent. Therapeutic blood level monitoring, as well as laboratory monitoring for adverse effects, is commonly required for certain medications.	**Case 87-1 (Questions 6–8), Case 87-2 (Questions 1–8), Case 87-3 (Questions 1, 2), Case 87-4 (Questions 1, 2)**
8	Non-pharmacologic treatments including electroconvulsive therapy (ECT) and herbal supplements are important considerations for the treatment of bipolar disorder.	**Case 87-8 (Questions 3, 4)**

INTRODUCTION

Bipolar disorder (BD), once known as manic depression, is a severe life-threatening psychiatric condition that is commonly misdiagnosed and too often insufficiently treated.[1,2] BD is associated with high rates of healthcare utilization, suicidal behavior, and use of public assistance.[3] The global burden of BD is immense, exceeding many chronic diseases including human immunodeficiency virus, diabetes mellitus, and asthma.[4]

Epidemiology

Using DSM-IV-TR criteria, the 12-month prevalence of bipolar I disorder is estimated to be 0.6%; bipolar II disorder is marginally more common at 0.8%.[5] The prevalence rate for the bipolar spectrum of illnesses, which include bipolar I, bipolar II, and subthreshold BD (i.e., Bipolar Disorder Not Otherwise Specified [NOS]), is 4.4%.[6] Bipolar I and II are more common in women than in men, whereas subthreshold illness predominates in men.[6] The familial nature of BD has been well established with an

11-fold increased risk in first-degree relatives.[7] Twin studies add further support to the genetic linkage. Goodwin and Jamison reported a 63% concordance rate (rate of illness in co-twin of affected proband) for monozygotic twins compared with 13% for dizygotic twins.[7]

The estimated total U.S. economic burden of BD between 1991 and 2009 was reported to be $151 billion.[8] Direct costs, such as hospitalization, outpatient visits, and medications, accounted for 20% of the total. The remaining 80% was attributable to indirect costs such as lost productivity by patients and caregivers.

The mean age of onset of symptoms for the bipolar spectrum of illnesses is 21 years.[6] Bipolar I is the earliest in onset at age 18, compared with bipolar II at age 20 and subthreshold BD occurring at age 22.[6] Approximately 20% to 30% of new cases occur in children between 10 and 15 years old.[9,10] Late-life onset of BD is rare. After age 60, there is a sharp reduction in the new onset of BD; therefore, a presentation of mania at this age should alert the clinician to an underlying medical problem as the possible cause.[11]

Patients may present initially with any affective episode, but it is important to note that 75% of patients report having had multiple episodes of depression before the development of a manic episode.[9] Not surprisingly, misdiagnosis (primarily as major depressive disorder) is common, occurring in roughly 70% of patients.[9] By some accounts, one in four patients visit as many as five physicians before an accurate diagnosis is made. A significant contribution to misdiagnosis is the underreporting of manic symptoms, which are not considered to be particularly problematic by patients.[9]

BD is a recurrent illness; single episodes of mania, unrelated to BD, occur in fewer than 10%.[12] Most patients with BD suffer multiple episodes of mania, hypomania, or depression separated by periods of euthymia (stable mood) throughout the course of their lives. In the majority, mania occurs just before or immediately after a depressive episode.[12] There may be a 5- to 10-year period from the onset of illness until the first hospitalization or diagnosis of BD.[11]

The course of illness is characterized by the type of episode(s), duration of euthymic intervals, frequency of relapse, severity of episodes, and predominant syndrome (mania, hypomania, or depression). These factors do not remain fixed throughout an individual's illness. For instance, individuals may experience episodes of dysphoria and depression before ever experiencing hypomania or mania. Often, the euthymic interval and cycle length decrease with additional episodes. With time, a course of alternating recurrent depression interspersed with manic or hypomanic episodes and no intervening euthymic periods can develop.

A specifier of BD, termed rapid cycling, occurs in both bipolar I and bipolar II disorder and is defined as a patient experiencing four or more mood episodes per year. Rapid cycling is common, occurring in 20% of cases; women are more often affected than men.[13] The rapid cycling type of BD is often refractory to conventional treatment and carries significant morbidity and mortality because of rapid changes in mood states.

The prognosis, even for treated BD, is concerning, with 73% experiencing a recurrent mood episode within 5 years. Furthermore, nearly half of patients continue to have significant mood symptoms between episodes, whereas less than 20% are euthymic or have minimal symptoms.[14]

Pathophysiology

BD is a complex disease involving developmental, genetic, neurobiologic, and psychological factors.[15] Neuroimaging studies have demonstrated neurochemical, anatomic, and functional abnormalities in those with a diagnosis of BD.[16] Recent studies have demonstrated that altered synaptic and circuit functioning accounts for mood and cognitive changes rather than the previous theory of dysfunction of individual neurotransmitters.[17] Environmental, or psychosocial, stressors, immunologic factors, and sleep dysfunction have been associated with BD and can negatively influence the course of illness.[18–22]

Clinical Presentation

Risk factors for BD include family history of mood disorders, perinatal stress, head trauma, environmental factors (including circadian rhythm disorders), and psychosocial and physical stressors. A recent systematic review of 16 published reports with varying study designs suggested that early phases and suspected precursor states for those who develop BD include: early-onset panic attacks and disorder, separation anxiety, generalized anxiety disorders, attention deficient hyperactivity disorder, and conduct symptoms and disorder.[23]

A manic episode usually begins with a change in sleep patterns along with mood elevation. Presenting symptoms include talkativeness, lack of sleep, and bursts of energy during which projects are begun but rarely completed. Mania often is characterized by thought disturbances exhibited by "flight of ideas" (rapid speech that switches among multiple ideas or topics) and grandiose delusions (false beliefs of wealth, special powers, knowledge, abilities, importance, or identity). The behavior of manic patients is characterized as being intrusive, loud, intense, irritable, at times suspicious, and even challenging. Patients often exercise poor judgment, which may include spending large sums of money in business deals that ultimately fail, becoming sexually promiscuous, using substances of abuse, or failing to obey laws.

The symptoms of mania usually develop gradually over the course of several days to more than a week and are defined in three stages.[24] Stage I is characterized by euphoria, irritability, labile affect, grandiosity, overconfidence, racing thoughts, increased psychomotor activity, and an increase in the rate and amount of speech. This stage corresponds to an episode of hypomania. Stage II features increased dysphoria (a feeling of extreme discomfort and unrest), hostility, anger, delusions, and cognitive disorganization. This stage corresponds to acute mania. Many patients progress no further than this stage. Others may proceed to stage III, in which the manic episode progresses to an undifferentiated psychotic state. Individuals in stage III experience terror and panic, their behavior is bizarre, and psychomotor activity is frenzied. They may experience hallucinations. What were once simply disorganized thoughts become incoherent; disorientation to time and place occurs. Just as the manic episode gradually builds, it often declines in a gradual manner. Psychotic symptoms usually resolve first, whereas irritability, paranoia, and excessive behavior persist. Remaining symptoms such as talkativeness, seductiveness, and dysphoria slowly decrease with time.

Depressive episodes of BD share the diagnostic criteria with unipolar depression; however, the presentation of bipolar depression has some distinguishing features. In particular, bipolar depression (type I specifically) is more likely to be associated with mood lability, psychotic features, psychomotor retardation, and comorbid substance use.[25] This contrasts with unipolar depression, which is more likely to be associated with anxiety, agitation, insomnia, somatic complaints, and weight loss.[25]

Mixed states appear to be common and could represent a more severe phase of bipolar illness. These episodes have been associated with a younger age of onset, more frequent occurrence of psychotic symptoms, major risk for suicide, higher rate of comorbidities, and longer time to achieve remission.[26–28]

A review by Salvatore et al.[29] identified three important presentations of mixed states: manic stupor, agitated depression, and unproductive mania. Manic stupor, "the most important of the mixed states," is characterized by mood elevation with a deficit in psychomotor activity (stupor) and slowed thoughts.[29] Agitated depression occurs when depressed mood is experienced with psychomotor activation and flight of ideas. Unproductive mania consists of mood elevation, psychomotor activation, and thought retardation. Mixed states can occur abruptly or serve as a transitional phase to a depressed or manic episode. The duration may be short-lived, lasting only days, or may take on a chronic course of weeks to months.

Patients with BD have higher rates of mortality from both natural and unnatural causes. Higher rates of natural deaths largely result from cardiovascular disease.[30] Mortality due to cardiovascular disease in BD has been estimated to be twice as frequent as the general population.[31–33] Rates of cerebrovascular disease, coronary heart disease / acute myocardial infarction, and cardiac arrest / ventricular fibrillation are all estimated to be increased in BD patients.[33] Suicide (more likely during depressive and mixed states) and excessive risk-taking behaviors (more likely to occur during manic or hypomanic episodes) also contribute to the high mortality rate. Suicidal behavior is a complex issue that likely depends on both environmental circumstances and risk factors inherent to BD, and current evidence regarding suicide risk is likely confounded by multiple risk factors.[34] Lifetime risk for an attempted suicide is reported to occur in as many as 25% to 50% of patients with BD, while the lifetime risk of a completed suicide may be as high as 17% to 19%.[35] The most rigorously determined estimate for completed suicide in BD reports rates of 7.8% in men and 4.8% in women.[36] Previous suicide attempts and the presence of hopelessness are primary risk factors for completed suicide.[37] Non-lethal suicidal behavior also has risk factors that are multifactorial and include a family history of suicide, younger age at onset, greater severity of mood episodes, the presence of mixed episode, rapid cycling, comorbid psychiatric conditions, and substance use.[37] Fortunately, overall mortality as well as deaths owing to suicide or cardiovascular disease are significantly reduced when BD is adequately treated.[14]

Approximately 42% of patients with BD have comorbid substance use disorders.[6] The estimated lifetime prevalence of a comorbid substance use disorder in BD patients is 40% for bipolar I and 20% for bipolar II.[38] Comorbid alcohol use in BD is estimated at 50%, while comorbid cannabis use is estimated at 30%.[39,40] Those with rapid cycling and dysphoric mania have the highest rates of substance use.[41] BD becomes difficult to treat in the face of active substance use. Constant intoxication and withdrawal not only impact the course of BD but masquerade as mood episodes. Symptoms are highly recurrent, and treatment resistance is common, as is violence and suicidal behavior.[42] The best outcome is achieved with aggressive simultaneous management of both BD and the concurrent substance use disorder.

Individuals with BD are likely to experience stress and upheaval in many areas of their lives, including relationships, employment, and finances. Of patients with BD, 88% have been hospitalized once and 66% at least 2 times.[43] Divorce rates in those with BD are two- to threefold higher than those found in non-affected populations. Patients often report having poor relationships with family members, and nearly 75% report that their family members have a limited understanding of BD.[9] Employment problems may result from bizarre, inappropriate, or unreliable behavior. In one study, 60% of patients reported being unemployed, 88% felt the disease affected how well they performed at work, and 63% felt that they were treated differently from their peers.[9] Financial and legal problems are tied to excessive spending, involvement in schemes, substance abuse, and risk-taking behavior.

Diagnosis

Mood disorders like BD are diagnosed using the criteria established in the Diagnostic and Statistical Manual of Mental Disorders, Fifth Edition (DSM-5).[12] Discrete periods of mood disturbance associated with BD are defined as manic episodes, hypomanic episodes, or major depressive episodes with various specifiers including mixed features and rapid cycling.

Manic or hypomanic episodes (Table 87-1) are periods of abnormally and persistently elevated, expansive, or irritable mood and persistently increased goal-directed activity or energy.[12] Hypomanic episodes are less intense than manic episodes, but are severe enough to impair functioning (self-care, occupational, social), complicate a medical condition, result in psychotic features, or require hospitalization.[12] Although manic and hypomanic episodes are characteristic symptoms of BD, it is depressive episodes that predominate and are ordinarily the initial presenting symptom.[44,45] Major depressive episodes share the same criteria with major depressive disorder (see Chapter 86, Depression).[12]

A person who has experienced one or more manic episodes with or without a depressive episode is diagnosed as having bipolar I disorder. An individual who has experienced one or more episodes of both hypomania and depression (without a history of manic episodes) is diagnosed as having bipolar II disorder.[12]

Table 87-1

DSM-5 Criteria for a Manic Episode

1. A distinct period of abnormally and persistently elevated, expansive, or irritable mood, and persistently increased goal-directed activity or energy lasting ≥1 week (or of any duration if hospitalization is necessary).[a]
2. During the period of mood disturbance and increased energy or activity, at least three of the following symptoms have persisted (four if the mood is only irritable) and have been present to a significant degree:
   - Inflated self-esteem or grandiosity
   - Decreased need for sleep (e.g., feels rested after only 3 hours of sleep)
   - More talkative than usual or pressure to keep talking
   - Flight of ideas or subjective experience that thoughts are racing
   - Distractibility (i.e., attention too easily drawn to unimportant or irrelevant external stimuli)
   - Increase in goal-directed activity (either social, at work, at school, or sexually) or psychomotor agitation
   - Excessive involvement in pleasurable activities that have a high potential for painful consequences (e.g., the person engages in unrestrained buying sprees, sexual indiscretions, or foolish business investing)
3. The mood disturbance is sufficiently severe to cause marked impairment in occupational functioning or in usual social activities or relationships with others, or to necessitate hospitalization to prevent harm to self or others, or there are psychotic features.
4. The symptoms are not caused by the direct physiologic effects of a substance (e.g., a drug of abuse, a medication, or other treatment) or a general medical condition (e.g., hyperthyroidism).

[a]Criteria for a hypomanic episode are identical to a manic episode; however, the symptoms need only be present for 4 days and are not severe enough to cause marked impairment in social or occupational functioning, necessitate hospitalization, or for psychotic features to be present.

Manic-like or hypomanic-like episodes that are clearly caused by somatic antidepressant treatment (e.g., medication, electroconvulsive therapy, light therapy) should not count toward a diagnosis of bipolar disorder.

Source: American Psychiatric Association. Mood disorders. In: American Psychiatric Association, ed. *Diagnostic and Statistical Manual of Mental Disorders*. 5th ed. Text Revision. Washington, DC: American Psychiatric Association; 2013;123:124.

The diagnosis of a cyclothymic disorder is for a person who has experienced at least 2 years of both hypomanic and dysthymic periods without ever fulfilling the criteria for an episode of mania, hypomania, or major depression.

The DSM-5 also uses a series of descriptors called specifiers to further characterize the course of illness and the most recent type of episode experienced by the individual. Recent episodes are first classified as hypomanic, manic, or depressed. A mixed specifier is diagnosed when a patient meets criteria for either manic or hypomanic episode with at least 3 depressive symptoms being present during the current or most recent episode of mania or hypomania or when a patient meets criteria for depressive episode with at least 3 manic or hypomanic symptoms being present during the current or most recent episode of depression.[12] They may be described further in terms of severity (mild, moderate, severe), the presence of psychotic features (in partial or full remission), with or without catatonic features, or with peripartum onset. Other specifiers convey information regarding the pattern of illness. For example, some individuals experience major depressive episodes at a characteristic time of the year (usually the winter) or switch from depression to mania during a particular season, "with seasonal pattern". The rapid cycling specifier applies to those who experience at least four mood episodes in the previous 12 months that meet criteria for manic, hypomanic, or major depressive episode.[12]

Overview of Treatment

During the previous 15 to 20 years, several treatment guidelines have been published. Recent treatment guidelines have been published by the Department of Veterans Affairs (2010), the British Association for Psychopharmacology (2016), Canadian Network for Mood and Anxiety Treatments (CANMAT), World Federation of Societies of Biological Psychiatry (WFSBP), and the Harvard South Shore Program (2010/14).[35,46–50] The reader is advised that published efficacy research is categorized by bipolar type (I vs. II), mood episode (manic vs. mixed vs. depressed), and treatment phase (acute vs. maintenance). As such, treatment guidelines may reflect these specifiers, depending upon their date of publication. Additionally, there is often an uneven amount of published evidence supporting treatment recommendations in these clinical categories.

The reader is advised that when considering the published efficacy research and guidelines for bipolar disorder, it is necessary to first consider acute versus chronic treatment, and then manic versus depressed episode.

The goals of treatment across the phases of illness are numerous, including the control of acute symptoms, achieving symptomatic remission, returning to a normal level of functioning, prevention of relapses, and prevention of suicide.[11] Both the acute treatment of manic and depressive episodes and the maintenance treatment for prevention of future episodes require individualization of therapy. Treatment decisions should take into account presenting symptoms, medication history, patient preference, and comorbid medical or substance use conditions.

Initial treatment for acute hypomanic or manic episodes should be with one of the well-established antimanic agents such as lithium, valproate (VPA), or one of several atypical antipsychotics (AAP). During episodes of mania, short-term adjunctive use of benzodiazepines is often useful to reduce agitation and promote sleep.[11] In the case of severe manic symptoms or in those only partially responsive to an adequate trial of monotherapy (generally 1–2 weeks), a two-drug combination of lithium, valproate, or an AAP is recommended.[46] Carbamazepine (CBZ) and a typical antipsychotic, alone or in combination with a preferred antimanic drug, are potential alternatives. For treatment-resistant cases, electroconvulsive therapy (ECT), clozapine, and a three-drug combination of lithium plus an anticonvulsant (CBZ or VPA) plus an AAP are recommended. When drug combinations are used, the individual agents should be from different medication classes. Lamotrigine is not recommended for the treatment of acute mania.

In the case of acute mixed states, VPA or an AAP is preferred over lithium because of its poor efficacy. If monotherapy with VPA or an AAP is ineffective or undesirable, then a combination of the two is advised.

Medications for the treatment of bipolar depression ideally produce an acute antidepressant response and prevent future depressive episodes, all while not inducing mania or mood cycling. Long-term tolerability is critical because of the chronic recurrent nature of depressive episodes in BD. First-line treatment options vary based on the chosen guideline, but it includes choices of lithium, lamotrigine, lurasidone, olanzapine or quetiapine monotherapy or lithium or valproic acid or olanzapine with a selective serotonin reuptake inhibitor (SSRI), lithium plus valproic acid, or lithium or valproic acid plus bupropion.[47–52] Subsequent treatment trials again vary on guideline, but include different combinations of the above choices. Additional options include adjunctive modafinil or other antidepressants. Third-line treatment includes carbamazepine, ECT, or lithium plus pramipexole or a monoamine oxidase inhibitor (MAOI) or a tricyclic antidepressant (TCA). Readers are referred to individual guidelines for complete details.

Maintenance treatment of BD should include continuing the acute-phase treatment while periodically simplifying and moving toward monotherapy with lithium, VPA, or lamotrigine if possible. Many AAPs are effective in maintenance treatment of BD; however, they must be used cautiously because of the long-term risk of metabolic and neurologic complications.[48] Olanzapine, quetiapine, aripiprazole, and long-acting injectable risperidone are effective. Regardless of the regimen selected, medication adherence is critical to long-term recovery. Patients and caregivers must be actively engaged in discussing causes of non-adherence, including ambivalence, adverse effects, lack of insight, and a strong desire to achieve the euphoria and energy of manic episodes.[11] Patients should also be advised to maintain regular patterns of daily activities, a consistent sleep–wake cycle, meals, exercise routines, and other schedules to promote stability.

CLINICAL ASSESSMENT

Clinical Presentation and Diagnosis

CASE 87-1

QUESTION 1: T.R. is a 25-year-old man, accompanied to the clinic by his wife, A.R. She called the clinic before bringing him in and reported much of the following information. T.R. states that he was doing well until about 3 weeks ago, when he returned home from a crab fishing trip where he works for the winter months. Given the stress of the job, he borrowed some "nerve pills" from his fellow co-worker. Since then, T.R. has been acting increasingly "wild." He has been staying up later at night and often bursts into the bedroom at 2 or 3 AM and loudly awakens A.R. Sometimes, he presents her with expensive gifts, which they cannot afford. He often jumps on the bed and starts singing her love songs in a loud voice. A.R. notes that T.R. then almost always demands sex, after which he sleeps for 2 to 3 hours and then loudly gets up and leaves the house.

During the last several weeks, he was noted to be driving his car recklessly and well beyond the speed limit. The police have pulled him over several times and given him multiple tickets for not only speeding, but for running red lights and passing on the double yellow lines. Last week, when his boss called to express concern about his behavior, T.R. said he was quitting his job. He wrote an rambling, disorganized resignation note, which was at least 10 pages long, called an overnight air delivery service to send the note to his employer (who is located only 3 miles from his home), and then left the house before the driver arrived to pick it up. T.R. returned several hours later with a brand new car and wearing an expensive new suit, red cowboy boots, and a bright green hat with a large feather. He told A.R. that he had a new job, which was going to make him a millionaire. Last night, she found a large sum of money in his pants pocket when emptying the clothes hamper. He did not come home at all, but he called her at 4 AM to tell her to pack for Dallas, where he was going to become the new head coach of the professional football team.

On arriving at the clinic, T.R. insists, "I don't need no doc. I am supercalifragilistic!" He then bursts into song. He is dressed flamboyantly but needs a shave and shower. He gives the examiner (a stranger) a bear hug and has trouble sitting still, listening, or allowing others to talk. His speech is pressured and loud; he often fails to complete sentences or communicate entire ideas, and he is rhyming and punning. His mood obviously is elevated, but he becomes increasingly irritable throughout the examination. He is oriented to person and place, but thinks it is tomorrow. Intelligence seems average. When asked to interpret a proverb, T.R. becomes angry and throws a chair across the room. How is T.R.'s presentation consistent with the diagnosis of a manic episode?

The hallmark of a manic episode is changes in mood, behavior, cognition, and perception (Table 87-1).[24] T.R. demonstrates an elevated mood. He is exuberant and notes how great he feels. Nevertheless, manic patients often demonstrate lability in their mood, and they may become irritable and easily frustrated, especially when challenged. In this case, T.R. becomes irritable and resentful when questioned by the examiner. His quick displays of anger further demonstrate the volatility of his mood.

T.R. displays behavior and speech typical of acute mania. He has a reduced need for sleep, behaves recklessly, and is overactive. His speech is pressured, loud, and full of rhymes and puns, and he sings to express his emotions and skips from topic to topic reflecting a flight of ideas. Behavior often is characterized as being excessive. T.R. dresses flamboyantly, hugs his examiner, writes an unnecessarily lengthy letter of resignation, seeks an overnight courier service for local delivery, and presents his wife with lavish gifts.

Delusions are often present in acute mania and are grandiose or religious in nature and deal with inflated abilities, self-importance, wealth, or special missions in life. T.R. makes unrealistic comments about his money-making schemes, his singing ability, and his position as the coach of a professional football team.

Patients with acute mania are often disorganized and do not complete tasks. They tend to skip from idea to idea and scheme to scheme. In this case, T.R. neglects his hygiene and neglects sending out his resignation letter.

Precipitating Factors

Case 87-1, Question 2: What factors make T.R. vulnerable to the occurrence of a manic episode at this time?

T.R. is at the age at which his disorder would likely first manifest itself. In addition, manic episodes are often precipitated by psychosocial and recurring life stressors.[7] Working long hours with reduced sleep may have served as a predisposing factor for the development of a manic episode.

Table 87-2
Selected Drugs Reported to Induce Mania[53–74]

Anticonvulsants	Gabapentin, lamotrigine, topiramate
Antidepressants	Monoamine oxidase inhibitors, TCAs, SSRIs, SNRIs, bupropion, nefazodone, trazodone, mirtazapine, vortioxetine
Antimicrobials	Clarithromycin, ofloxacin, cotrimoxazole, erythromycin, isoniazid, metronidazole, zidovudine, efavirenz
Antiparkinsonian drugs	Levodopa, amantadine, bromocriptine
Anxiolytics/hypnotics	Buspirone, alprazolam, triazolam
Atypical antipsychotics	Aripiprazole, olanzapine, quetiapine, risperidone, ziprasidone
CNS stimulants	Caffeine, cocaine, methylphenidate, amphetamine
Drugs of abuse	Marijuana, PCP, LSD
Endocrine	Corticosteroids, thyroid supplements, androgens
Herbals	Saint-John's-wort, SAMe, ma-huang, omega-3 fatty acids, tryptophan
Sympathomimetics	Ephedrine, phenylpropanolamine, pseudoephedrine, phenylephrine
Miscellaneous	Cimetidine, tramadol, sibutramine

CNS, central nervous system; LSD, lysergic acid diethylamide; PCP, phencyclidine; SAMe, *S*-adenosyl-L-methionine; SNRI, serotonin and norepinephrine reuptake inhibitor; SSRI, selective serotonin reuptake inhibitor; TCA, tricyclic antidepressant.

A variety of medications and clinical states can induce or precipitate manic episodes (Table 87-2).[53–74] The drugs that most commonly precipitate mania affect monoamine neurotransmitters, such as antidepressants and stimulants.[53] Corticosteroids, anabolic steroids, isoniazid, levodopa, caffeine, and over-the-counter stimulants can induce or aggravate mania.

Case 87-1, Question 3: If the "nerve pills" borrowed by T.R. were antidepressants, could they have contributed to the development of his manic episode?

Antidepressants are commonly prescribed for patients with bipolar depression (35%–40%).[47] Their use is controversial though with criticisms that they lack efficacy or that they destabilize mood and can cause a switch to mania. All of the major classes of antidepressants including monoamine oxidase inhibitors, tricyclic antidepressants (TCAs), SSRIs, and SNRIs have been associated with precipitating mania in patients with BD.[54] Despite this risk, up to 50% of patients with BD are treated with antidepressants of which only half are receiving a concurrent mood stabilizer.[75] There are numerous case reports of mania or hypomania with antidepressant treatment, but few controlled studies, making it difficult to make comparisons across antidepressant classes.[76] See Case 87-7 for complete details of the use of antidepressants in bipolar depression.

A comparison of the monoamine oxidase inhibitor, tranylcypromine, and the TCA, imipramine, found a similar rate of treatment emergent mania (21% and 25%, respectively).[77] A meta-analysis found a higher "switch" to mania rate for TCAs (11%) than for SSRIs (4%).[78] A controlled trial with bupropion, sertraline, and venlafaxine (all in combination with a mood stabilizer) found an overall switch rate of 19% during acute treatment and 37% during the continuation phase of the study with no difference among agents.[79] Antidepressants may also cause cycle acceleration, which effectively decreases the time between mood episodes. The risk for cycle acceleration may be heightened for patients who experience manic or hypomanic symptoms on antidepressants despite receiving antimanic treatment concurrently.[80] Other recent literature has suggested that adjunctive antidepressants to mood stabilizers versus placebo are not associated with an increased efficacy or with increased risks of treatment emergent affective switches.[81] In the case of T.R., an antidepressant may have precipitated the manic episode or shortened his cycle, moving him into an episode of mania from a preexisting state of depression or euthymia.[82] Any patient presenting with an acute manic episode should have a review of medications completed to determine the risk of continuing antidepressant medications.[35]

Current guidelines state that the dual-action monoamine reuptake inhibitors carry a greater risk of precipitating a switch to mania than single action drugs. Additionally, they state that antidepressant medications medications appear unlikely to induce mania when used in combination with a drug for mania.[47]

TREATMENT OF ACUTE MANIA

CASE 87-1, QUESTION 4: Why does T.R. require treatment?

Manic episodes have a number of severe complications. Left untreated, severe mania can result in confusion, fever, exhaustion, and even death. The impairment in judgment, the excesses, and the risk-taking that occur during manic episodes may be devastating. Detriments to relationships, careers, and finances and physical harm or loss of life may occur. Manic individuals may engage in illegal activities or behave in a manner that result in a violation of the law. T.R. drives recklessly; may have lost his job; spends excessive amounts of money on gifts, clothing, and automobiles; and plans to participate in a variety of money-making schemes. He has acquired a great deal of cash suddenly, perhaps from withdrawing all of his family's savings or from some type of illegal enterprise. Manic patients may engage in risky sexual encounters, leading to infection with sexually transmitted diseases including human immunodeficiency virus. Alcohol and substance abuse are common and may exacerbate or even precipitate mood episodes. Irritability, such as that demonstrated by T.R., can lead to episodes of violence, resulting in potential harm to the patient or to others. The goals of treatment are to reduce the severity and duration of the current mood episode as well as to prevent recurrence of future episodes.

Valproate (Divalproex Sodium, Valproic Acid)

CASE 87-1, QUESTION 5: What is the appropriate treatment for T.R.'s acute manic episode?

Depending on the type and severity of mania, first-line treatment involves selecting from lithium, VPA, AAPs, or a combination of these agents.[46–50] If psychosis is present, an AAP would be an appropriate choice either as monotherapy or in combination with a mood stabilizer. VPA is an ideal choice for T.R. considering the rapid onset, tolerability, and the established efficacy of this agent for preventing future mood episodes.[83–85]

DOSING AND MONITORING

CASE 87-1, QUESTION 6: VPA was chosen for the management of T.R.'s mania. How should VPA be initiated, and what baseline tests are necessary? How will T.R.'s response to therapy be monitored?

The initial dose of VPA for T.R. should be 250 mg 3 times per day.[11] The dosage should then be increased by 250 to 500 mg every 2 to 3 days to obtain steady-state serum VPA levels between 50 and 125 mcg/mL or a maximum dosage of 60 mg/kg/day.[86] An alternative strategy is to use an oral loading dose regimen of 20 to 30 mg/kg/day given on a 3 times a day schedule during an acute episode of mania. This approach has been used during inpatient management and may result in a more rapid onset of effect.[87] VPA levels of 50 mcg/mL are the minimum threshold with higher concentrations offering greater benefit. In fact, those exceeding a serum concentration of 84 mcg/mL by the third day of treatment may have greater early symptom improvement.[88] A pooled analysis demonstrated a linear relationship between serum concentration and efficacy with the greatest improvement found in patients with VPA levels in excess of 94 mcg/mL.[89] VPA levels greater than 125 mcg/mL are more often associated with side effects and should be avoided.[83]

Before VPA is initiated, baseline laboratory tests, including a complete blood count (CBC) with differential and platelets, and liver function tests should be measured. T.R.'s baseline weight and neurologic status should be recorded. In premenopausal women who have not undergone surgical sterilization, a baseline pregnancy test is warranted since VPA is a known teratogen. Attention should be given to any medications that might be administered concurrently. Interactions with aspirin, lorazepam, phenytoin, phenobarbital, lamotrigine, rifampin, warfarin, felbamate, and CBZ are cited frequently (also see Chapter 60, Seizure Disorders).

VPA should decrease the severity and duration of T.R.'s current manic episode, decrease the frequency of subsequent episodes, and increase his time spent in a euthymic state. Once treatment has started, T.R. should be monitored for response of his initial target symptoms, including grandiosity, decreased need for sleep, pressured speech, distractibility, and impulsivity. Initial symptom improvement with VPA can be expected in approximately 5 days.[89]

Side Effects

CASE 87-1, QUESTION 7: What are the potential side effects of VPA therapy? How should T.R. be monitored for these possible effects?

T.R. should be monitored for potential dose-related adverse reactions of VPA including various gastrointestinal complaints (nausea, diarrhea, dyspepsia, anorexia), sedation, ataxia, tremor, transaminase elevations, and thrombocytopenia. Reducing the dosage, changing to an extended-release preparation,[90] or administering an antacid or histamine H2-antagonist may mitigate gastrointestinal complaints. Central nervous system effects such as ataxia and sedation may respond to dosage reduction, although sedation may resolve with continued treatment. If a tremor is bothersome or interferes with the patient's functioning, a dosage reduction or change to the extended-release preparation may provide relief.[86] Small elevations in transaminases are considered benign; however, VPA should be discontinued if elevations are more than 2 to 3 times the upper limit of normal.[91]

Weight gain occurs in up to 20% of patients receiving VPA.[83] The increase in body weight is particularly distressing to some patients and may contribute to medication non-adherence. Weight gain has been associated with VPA at different concentrations, so a dosage reduction may not be helpful.[83,92] In women, VPA has been associated with the development of polycystic ovary syndrome.[93] Core features of polycystic ovary syndrome include oligomenorrhea and hyperandrogenism, which develop in about 10% of women with BD taking VPA. Alopecia occurs in 0.5% to 12% of patients and may improve with dose reduction.[94]

There are several reports of VPA-induced hyperammonemic encephalopathy in psychiatric patients.[95,96] Patients presenting with coma or mental status changes should have serum ammonia and liver functions tests ordered. If VPA-induced hyperammonemic encephalopathy is suspected, then VPA should be discontinued. Other serious adverse events with VPA include fulminant hepatic failure, agranulocytosis, and pancreatitis. All of these adverse events require immediate discontinuation of therapy.

In January 2008, the U.S. Food and Drug Administration (FDA) issued a warning to healthcare professionals about the potential for an increased risk of suicidality associated with antiepileptic drugs (AEDs), including VPA. For its analysis, FDA used data from 199 randomized clinical trials of 11 AEDs involving 43,892 study participants with either psychiatric or neurologic disorders. In the "Warnings and Precautions" section of AED product labels, it is stated that the risk of suicidality for those treated with AEDs during clinical trials was approximately twice that of placebo treatment (0.43% vs. 0.24%; adjusted relative risk = 1.8, 95% CI = 1.2, 2.7; number needed to harm = 530). In these clinical trials, there were a total of four suicides in AED-treated patients, and zero suicides in placebo-treated patients. As a result, practitioners are advised to inform patients and caregivers to be vigilant about the emergence or worsening of signs and symptoms of depression or mood/behavior changes, especially if they involve thoughts or behaviors centered on self-harm when patients receive AED treatment.[97]

Once VPA therapy is initiated, liver function tests, VPA serum levels, and CBCs with differential and platelets should be monitored at least monthly for the first 3 months and every 3 to 6 months thereafter.[11] Body weight should also be determined at baseline and monitored monthly during therapy.

CASE 87-1, QUESTION 8: T.R. was titrated to a total daily VPA dosage of 2,500 mg/day and determined to have a steady-state plasma concentration of 95 mcg/mL after 1 month of treatment. A routine CBC with differential and platelet count was ordered at this time, and the following data were reported:

Red blood cells, 5.2 × 106/μL
Hemoglobin, 14.5 g/dL
Hematocrit, 43%
White blood cell count, 8.5 × 103/μL
Neutrophils, 59%
Lymphocytes, 27%
Monocytes, 6%
Eosinophils, 2%
Basophils, 0.5%
Platelets, 75 × 10^3/μL

How should T.R.'s VPA-induced thrombocytopenia be managed?

VPA-induced thrombocytopenia occurs in 18% of patients and is associated with female gender and higher VPA levels (>100 mcg/mL in women and >130 mcg/mL in men).[98] Clinicians should educate patients to look for signs such as easy bruising or bleeding. In most patients, thrombocytopenia is asymptomatic and responds to a lowering of the VPA dosage; complete discontinuation of the drug is usually unnecessary.[99] T.R.'s dosage should be reduced, and his platelet count should be monitored closely. In addition, he should be observed for reemerging symptoms of mania.

LITHIUM

Prelithium Workup

CASE 87-2

QUESTION 1: C.N., a 21-year-old woman, was diagnosed with her first episode of mania 3 weeks ago. At that time, she was hospitalized and treated with olanzapine 15 mg daily. C.N.'s was stabilized, and after 10 days, she was discharged from the hospital. She was scheduled to see an outpatient psychiatrist for follow-up 1 week later, but she failed to keep the appointment. Today, C.N. arrives at the emergency department at the request of her mother. C.N. is grabbing her mother's hair and kicking wildly as she is pulled from the car. She can be heard screaming "The FBI is after me, Mom! You want them to find me, don't you? I would have made it out of the country if you hadn't gotten in the way! I was going to marry Prince Charles and become the new queen of England." On evaluation, C.N.'s mood is irritable, and she is pacing around the interviewer. She is dressed in a short skirt and high heels and is wearing an excessive amount of makeup and costume jewelry. During the interview, she interrupts the examiner, smiles, and says in a loud, provocative voice, "Let's you and me get out of here!" Her mother states that after C.N. was discharged from the hospital, she stopped taking her olanzapine due to gaining some weight and, within several days, stopped attending her classes at the local community college. She began staying out late, playing her radio loudly, and driving recklessly, finally hitting the side of the garage while parking early this morning. The clinician would like to admit C.N. to the inpatient unit and initiate lithium treatment. What laboratory tests are required before initiating lithium therapy for C.N.?

Because lithium can affect many organ systems, baseline laboratory values must be evaluated before therapy is initiated. Baseline laboratory tests are useful in determining contraindications to the use of lithium or conditions that may require an adjustment in dosage. As a young, healthy female, C.N.'s prescreening laboratory battery should include electrolytes, blood urea nitrogen, creatinine, urine specific gravity, thyroid-stimulating hormone (TSH), thyroxine (T_4), and a CBC (Table 87-3). Also, a pregnancy test should be obtained before starting therapy since lithium is a known teratogen.

Table 87-3
Routine Monitoring During Lithium Therapy

	Baseline	Every 1–3 Months	Yearly
CBC	X		
Electrolytes	X		X
Renal function[a]	X		X
ECG[b]	X		X
Urine	X		
Thyroid function	X		X
Lithium level[c]		X	
Weight or BMI	X		X
Pregnancy[d]	X		

[a]Monitor more often in patients with history of kidney disease.
[b]Patients ≥45 years or those with history of cardiac disease.
[c]Weekly monitoring during the first month of treatment is often recommended.
[d]Women of childbearing potential.

BMI, body mass index; CBC, complete blood count; ECG, electrocardiogram.

Dosing

Case 87-2, Question 2: C.N.'s baseline laboratory parameters were normal, and her pregnancy test was negative. How should lithium treatment for C.N. be initiated?

Although there are many strategies for calculating lithium dosage requirements, it is simplest to begin C.N. at a dosage of 300 mg twice daily. This is a common starting dose for a healthy adult patient.

Patients experiencing an acute manic episode require higher lithium levels compared with maintenance therapy. The goal for the acute management of C.N. is a serum level between 0.8 and 1.2 mEq/L.[11] Because lithium is not immediately effective, C.N.'s lithium dosage can be adjusted based on the results of lithium serum levels checked weekly until the manic episode resolves. As she recovers and enters the maintenance phase of treatment, both C.N.'s lithium dosage and her lithium levels will require re-evaluation (see Case 87-8, Question 1).

Case 87-2, Question 3: How long will it take for C.N. to get the full effect of lithium?

The half-life of lithium in a young patient with normal renal function is approximately 24 hours; therefore, steady-state concentrations are typically achieved in approximately 5 days. The onset of action is slow, taking as long as 1 to 2 weeks to fully exert its therapeutic effects.[11] Because of the delay in onset, it is appropriate to use an adjunctive medication to help reduce C.N.'s acute symptoms. Both benzodiazepines and antipsychotics have been used in this manner.[11] AAPs are preferred over typical antipsychotics (see also Chapter 85, Schizophrenia) and have been demonstrated to enhance efficacy and accelerate time to response when used in combination with lithium in acute mania.[48] Benzodiazepines work rapidly to reduce agitation, anxiety, and decreased need for sleep.[100]

Adverse Effects

Case 87-2, Question 4: After 3 weeks of lithium therapy, C.N. is demonstrating significant improvement in her sleep, impulsivity, delusions, and activity level. She has achieved a lithium carbonate dose of 1,200 mg/day, and her lithium level is 0.8 mEq/L. Today she is complaining to the clinical staff that she has developed a hand tremor. Soon after her clinician arrives to evaluate her, C.N. asks to be excused so that she can go to the bathroom. How might C.N.'s presentation be related to her medication?

When considering adverse effect management early in lithium therapy, it becomes important to monitor lithium levels closely. When patients start to recover from acute mania, the rate of lithium clearance may decrease and patients may demonstrate an increase in lithium levels and worsening side effects (Table 87-4). This does not seem to be the case with C.N. because her lithium level is within the accepted range for the management of acute mania.

C.N. is complaining of a hand tremor. She should be interviewed and examined to determine its origin. Lithium-induced tremor occurs in 10% to 65% of treated patients and is characteristically rapid, regular, and fine in amplitude.[100,101] Often, this tremor occurs early in therapy and improves with time. Caffeine, personal or family history of tremor, alcoholism, anxiety, antidepressants, antipsychotics, and possibly older age enhance the risk of lithium-induced tremor.[101] The tremor is more common in patients with higher serum concentrations and may be worse at times of peak lithium levels.[11] If C.N. is not bothered by the tremor and suffers no impairment, treatment is not necessary.

Table 87-4
Lithium Adverse Effects

Adverse Effect	Considerations
ECG changes	T-wave suppression, delayed or irregular rhythm, increase in PVCs; SSNS; myocarditis
Edema	Primarily ankles and feet; transient or intermittent; secondary to effects on sodium and carbohydrate metabolism; caution about diuretics and sodium restriction to avoid lithium toxicity
Acne	Worsens
Psoriasis	Treatment-refractory worsening
Rashes	Maculopapular and follicular
Hypothyroidism	About 5% goiter; about 30% clinically significant hypothyroidism; may diminish sex drive
Hyperparathyroidism	Clinically not significant
Teratogenicity	Ebstein anomaly (tricuspid valve malformation, atrial septal defect); educate female patients, encourage advanced planning regarding pregnancy.
Anorexia, nausea (10%–30%)	Usually early in treatment and usually transient; may be early sign of toxicity
Diarrhea (5%–20%)	Slow-release preparations may help
Leukocytosis	May be useful in disorders such as Felty syndrome, iatrogenic neutropenia
Tremor (10%–65%)	Dose-related; men > women; worse with antidepressants and antipsychotics; reduce dose or use β-blocker
Cognitive disruption (10%)	Worsens compliance; perceived as "mental dulling"
Fatigue or weakness	May be early toxicity; may mimic depression
Polyuria-polydipsia (nephrogenic diabetes insipidus)	May be an indication of morphological changes; requires adequate hydration

CBZ, carbamazepine; ECG, electrocardiogram; PVC, premature ventricular contraction; SSNS, sick sinus node syndrome.

If the tremor becomes problematic, her lithium dosage may be reduced or a β-adrenergic blocking agent can be added. Propranolol is the most commonly used. Additionally, switching to a sustained-release lithium preparation may reduce peak serum levels and ameliorate tremors if associated with peak concentrations.[11] Because it is early in treatment and C.N. has only a moderate lithium level, it is reasonable to add propranolol 10 mg 3 times a day rather than to reduce the lithium dosage (if an intervention is required). Propranolol usually is effective at dosages less than 160 mg/day.[101] C.N. should be educated about her tremor, the adverse effects of propranolol (see Chapter 9, Essential Hypertension) and instructed to minimize her caffeine consumption.

In addition, C.N. should be asked about her trip to the bathroom during this clinic visit because lithium may cause both diarrhea and polyuria. Polyuria and polydipsia are common, occurring in up to 60% of patients.[102] Nephrogenic diabetes insipidus is less common, affecting about 10% of patients on long-term treatment.[103] Nephrogenic diabetes insipidus (see Chapter 53, Diabetes Mellitus) is dose dependent, so C.N. can be told that a lower lithium dose may minimize the symptoms. Although the advantages of once-daily administration of lithium are not universally accepted, switching a stabilized patient to this schedule with its lower trough levels may help to reduce urine volume.[11] If C.N. were to fail to respond to either of these interventions, amiloride could be administered, which minimizes lithium's effect on free water clearance.[11,104]

If C.N.'s trip to the bathroom was because of diarrhea, lithium should be evaluated as a possible cause; up to 20% of patients started on lithium experience diarrhea, epigastric bloating, and sometimes stomach pain early in therapy.[105] Diarrhea from lithium is associated with high serum levels, once-daily dosing, and rapidly absorbed preparations; therefore, divided doses may help to alleviate the problem. Use of lower doses and switching to sustained-release preparations are alternative strategies that could be used if C.N. is experiencing diarrhea or polyuria. Her fluid status and lithium level also should be monitored closely. Dehydration leads to increased lithium reabsorption in the proximal tubule and could result in accumulation and lithium toxicity.

CASE 87-2, QUESTION 5: What should C.N. be told regarding potential renal damage from lithium?

C.N. should be informed that lithium could adversely affect her kidneys. Long-term treatment has been associated with reduced kidney function and, rarely, end-stage renal disease.[106] Routine monitoring of renal function (Table 87-3) allows for the identification of patients with precipitous declines in glomerular filtration. In such patients, lithium should be discontinued to prevent progression to end-stage renal disease. Risk factors for renal insufficiency include episodes of lithium intoxication, medical conditions that impair glomerular filtration (e.g., hypertension, diabetes mellitus), and concurrent medications that are damaging to the kidney.[107] Communication with her physician about situations that increase the risk of lithium toxicity (see Case 87-2, Question 7) and cooperation with regular lithium and renal function monitoring can vastly reduce the risk of renal disease. Finally, C.N. must be informed that polyuria is not related to any of the more serious renal side effects.

Patient Education

CASE 87-2, QUESTION 6: What lithium education should C.N. receive prior to discharge from the hospital?

As with all medications, C.N. should be instructed to disclose all medications she is taking to each of her healthcare providers. She should be informed that dehydration, fever, vomiting, or sodium-restricted diets could lead to increases in her lithium level. Therefore, she needs to drink plenty of fluids and should avoid restricting sodium.

C.N. should be instructed to contact her physician if she starts to experience any symptoms of lithium toxicity, including worsening tremor, slurred speech, muscle weakness or twitches, or difficulty walking. C.N. should be told to use caution in selecting over-the-counter medications. Specifically, she should be warned to avoid the use of preparations containing nonsteroidal anti-inflammatory drugs, which can increase lithium levels.[108] C.N. should know that caffeine can sometimes be troublesome in patients taking lithium, worsening tremor on a short-term basis and lowering lithium levels during the long term.[108] With regard to serum lithium level monitoring, C.N. needs to know that lithium levels usually are drawn approximately 12 hours after a dose of lithium. If she is taking lithium in the evening and the morning, she should take her evening dose and then report for a blood sample to be drawn in the morning before taking her morning dose.

Toxicity

CASE 87-2, QUESTION 7: About 6 months after discharge, C.N.'s mother calls, concerned that C.N. has been complaining of nausea, vomiting, and diarrhea for several days. During the past few hours, C.N. has become confused and has developed a coarse tremor and slurred speech. It has been 4 months since C.N.'s lithium level has been checked. The only change is that C.N. recently started taking naproxen for headaches. What action should be taken?

There is a strong possibility that C.N. is suffering from lithium toxicity, which can occur acutely from an overdose or insidiously from reduced lithium clearance. Mild toxicity at levels less than 1.5 mEq/L causes feelings of apathy, lethargy, and muscle weakness accompanied by nausea and irritability. Moderate toxicity occurs between 1.5 and 2.5 mEq/L with symptoms progressing to coarse tremor, slurred speech, unsteady gait, drowsiness, confusion, muscle twitches, and blurred vision. Severe toxicity at levels greater than 2.5 mEq/L can result in seizures, stupor, coma, renal failure, and cardiovascular collapse. C.N. seems to be experiencing moderate lithium toxicity. She should stop any medications that can decrease lithium clearance and the lithium itself until instructed to resume it. She should be taken to the emergency department immediately, where stat laboratory tests, including a lithium level, electrolytes, and renal function tests, should be ordered. There is no antidote for lithium intoxication. Intravenous solutions should be started to ensure that C.N. is hydrated adequately, and electrolyte abnormalities should be corrected promptly. Depending on the results of physical examination and laboratory tests, cardiac monitoring should be instituted and hemodialysis should be considered. Hemodialysis is used to shorten the exposure of different tissues of the body to the elevated lithium concentration and to lower the lithium level to 1.0 mEq/L. Mohandas and Ramjmohan suggest that candidates for hemodialysis include those with: compromised renal function, severe (irreversible) neurological symptoms, acute lithium ingestions where symptoms are clear and serum levels are greater than 4.0 mEq/L, or a chronic toxicity where lithium levels exceed the therapeutic values with a clearly manifested clinical picture.[109]

Hypothyroidism

CASE 87-2, QUESTION 8: After receiving lithium 1,200 mg/day for 1 year, C.N. returns complaining that the lithium is slowing her down. She is tired and has gained weight in recent weeks and thinks that she is becoming depressed. In the examining room, C.N. complains that the temperature is too cold. What is the most likely cause of C.N.'s complaints? What treatment should be instituted?

C.N.'s symptoms are consistent with those of hypothyroidism.

Lithium affects the incorporation of iodine into thyroid hormone, interferes with secretion of thyroid hormones, and may interfere with the peripheral conversion of T_4 to T_3 (triiodothyronine).[110] According to laboratory indices, the incidence of hypothyroidism in lithium-treated patients with BD ranges from 28% to 32% compared with 6% to 11% in patients not taking lithium.[111] Risk factors for lithium-induced hypothyroidism include female gender, family history of hypothyroidism or thyroid illness in first-degree relatives, weight gain, elevated baseline TSH, preexisting autoantibodies, an iodine-deficient diet, rapid cycling, and elevated lithium levels.[112] For women, the first 2 years of treatment is a period of heightened risk as well as for any middle-aged patient starting lithium.[112]

Thyroid function tests should be ordered to evaluate C.N.'s current symptoms. If she is found to be hypothyroid, discontinuation of lithium is not necessary. She should receive levothyroxine in doses that normalize her thyroid function tests. Even if she has an elevated TSH with normal levels of T_3 and T_4, low-dose thyroid supplementation may help to resolve her symptoms, and prevent breakthrough depression.[110]

Drug and Dietary Interactions

CASE 87-3

QUESTION 1: T.J., a 35-year-old man, is hospitalized and treated with lithium for a severe manic episode. He had a stable lithium level of 0.84 mEq/L for several weeks, but his last two levels were 0.65 and 0.61 mEq/L without any change in his drug therapy. T.J. insists that he is taking the medication as prescribed. The nursing staff believes that he is adherent with his medication but notes that he is spending more time off the unit and in the cafeteria. What factors could contribute to a decrease in T.J.'s lithium levels?

Drug interactions are a common cause of changes in lithium levels, but there have been no changes in T.J.'s regimen (Table 87-5 provides a list of clinically significant drug interactions). Changes in formulation or brand may sometimes have an impact on lithium levels. Nevertheless, lithium is relatively well absorbed and has a long elimination half-life, so this usually does not result in large changes in the 12-hour postdose lithium level. Occasionally, patients switched from lithium citrate to solid dosage forms experience small changes in lithium levels.

T.J. should be questioned about his visits to the cafeteria because diet can have a major influence on lithium excretion. If T.J. is consuming large amounts of caffeinated beverages or salty snacks, a reduction in lithium levels could occur. Increases in dietary sodium intake and the ingestion of methylxanthines (e.g., caffeine, theophylline) can increase lithium clearance.[108]

Finally, acute mania can increase lithium clearance.[7] If T.J. was showing signs of a relapse, his decrease in lithium levels might be attributable to his return to a manic state.

Lithium in Pregnancy

CASE 87-4

QUESTION 1: A.J., a 36-year-old woman, has been maintained successfully on lithium therapy for 5 years for BD. She asks whether she should stay on lithium because she plans to become pregnant in the near future.

While there is considerable disagreement about the importance of lithium as a teratogen, it has been associated with a variety of congenital malformations, including the rare cardiac malformation, Ebstein anomaly.[113] Lithium was originally thought to increase the risk of Ebstein anomaly 400 times; however, the risk is more likely 20 to 40 times higher than in the general population.[114] The current estimated overall risk for congenital malformations related to lithium treatment is approximately 4% to 12% (compared with 2%–4% in controls).[115] Because malformations are most likely to occur in the first trimester of pregnancy, it is advisable for patients to avoid lithium, when possible, during this high-risk period.

In addition to cardiac malformations, infants exposed to lithium have been reported to have hypotonia, nephrogenic diabetes insipidus, and thyroid abnormalities.[113] Lithium administration during pregnancy increases the risk of premature delivery by a factor of two to three.[116] Unfortunately, the relative safety of other

Table 87-5
Lithium Drug Interactions of Clinical Significance

Drugs That Increase Lithium Levels
NSAIDs
Many NSAIDs have been reported to increase lithium levels as much as 50%–60%. This probably is owing to an enhanced reabsorption of sodium and lithium secondary to inhibition of prostaglandin synthesis.
Diuretics
All diuretics can contribute to sodium depletion. Sodium depletion can result in an increased proximal tubular reabsorption of sodium and lithium. Thiazide-like diuretics cause the greatest increase in lithium levels, whereas loop diuretics and potassium-sparing diuretics seem to be somewhat safer.
Angiotensin-Converting Enzyme (ACE) inhibitors
ACE inhibitors and lithium both result in volume depletion and a reduction in glomerular filtration rate. This results in reduced lithium excretion.
Angiotensin II Receptor Blockers (ARBs)
ARBs decrease in sodium and reabsorption via AT_1 blockade results in reduced lithium excretion.
Drugs That Decrease Lithium Levels
Theophylline, caffeine
Theophylline and caffeine may increase renal clearance of lithium and result in a decrease in levels in the range of 20%.
Acetazolamide
Acetazolamide may impair proximal tubular reabsorption of lithium ions.
Sodium
High dietary sodium intake promotes the renal clearance of lithium.
Drugs That Increase Lithium Toxicity
Methyldopa
Cases of sedation, dysphoria, and confusion owing to the combined use of lithium and methyldopa have been reported.
Carbamazepine
Cases of neurotoxicity involving the combined use of lithium and carbamazepine have been reported in patients with normal lithium levels.
Calcium-channel antagonists
Cases of neurotoxicity involving the combined use of lithium and the calcium-channel blockers verapamil and diltiazem have been reported. Lithium interferes with calcium transport across cells.
Antipsychotics
Cases of neurotoxicity (encephalopathic syndrome, extrapyramidal effects, cerebellar effect, EEG abnormalities) have been reported owing to the combined use of lithium and various antipsychotics. The interaction may be related to increase in phenothiazine levels, changes in tissue uptake of lithium, or dopamine-blocking effects of lithium. Studies attempting to demonstrate this effect have yielded differing results.
Serotonin-selective reuptake inhibitors
Fluvoxamine and fluoxetine have been reported to result in toxicity when added to lithium. Sertraline has been reported to cause nausea and tremor in lithium recipients.

ACE, angiotensin-converting enzyme; EEG, electroencephalogram; NSAIDs, nonsteroidal anti-inflammatory drugs.

psychotropic agents commonly used in BD is either not ideal or unknown. VPA and CBZ are categorized as US Food and Drug Administration (FDA) category D during pregnancy; the general consensus is that these medications are genuine teratogens and should be avoided.[117] Among 1,558 exposures, lamotrigine, FDA category C, had 35 major congenital malformations among first trimester monotherapy exposures (2.2%, 95% CI = 1.6%–3.1%).[118]

Typical and most atypical antipsychotics are classified as pregnancy category C, suggesting that adverse morphologic outcomes are less common with these treatments than with mood stabilizers. Clozapine and lurasidone are pregnancy category B. In a comparison of AAPs of placental passage, olanzapine was associated with the highest exposure (72% ratio of umbilical cord-to-maternal plasma concentrations), followed by haloperidol (65%), risperidone (49%), and quetiapine (24%).[119] Olanzapine was also associated with the highest rates of low birth weight and neonatal intensive care unit admissions.

A.J. and her physician should discuss her individual risks related to lithium treatment. In addition to the risks of teratogenicity, they must consider the harm that could result from the possible recurrence of episodes of mania or depression and the risks inherent in discontinuing lithium or switching to another antimanic agent. Also, A.J. should be actively involved in the decision-making process.

If A.J. and her physician decide that she is to remain on lithium, her serum levels must be monitored closely during pregnancy and her dosage adjusted accordingly. Lithium clearance increases during the third trimester by 30% to 50%, resulting in a reduction in lithium levels and a need for dosage adjustment.[114] Approximately 16 to 18 weeks after conception, screening tests, high-resolution ultrasound, and fetal echocardiography can be used to determine whether cardiac defects have developed.[114] If possible, A.J.'s physician should consider decreasing the lithium dose before delivery to minimize lithium levels in the newborn and to offset the reduction in lithium excretion that occurs after delivery.[114]

If A.J. and her physician decide that she is to discontinue lithium, they must be prepared to deal with the risks of lithium discontinuation. Several cases of presumed rebound mania have occurred after abrupt cessation of lithium therapy. If lithium is to be discontinued in A.J., it should be gradually reduced over at least 4 weeks.

CASE 87-4, QUESTION 2: A.J. did not use lithium throughout her pregnancy. After delivery, A.J. and her physician decide to restart lithium. How soon can lithium be reinitiated in A.J.?

Lithium can be restarted as soon as A.J.'s urine output is established and she is fully hydrated. However, this decision also may be affected by whether or not A.J. chooses to breastfeed her child because lithium passes into breast milk and is present in concentrations up to 72% of that found in the maternal blood.[114] Risks to the newborn include hypothyroidism, cyanosis, hypotonia, lethargy, and cardiac dysrhythmias. Hydration status must be closely monitored because lithium toxicity may develop during infantile illnesses. Thus, A.J. and her physician must discuss the advantages of breastfeeding versus the risks of exposing the newborn to lithium or withholding lithium during the postpartum period. A.J. should be informed that approximately 40% to 70% of women with BD experience affective episodes after delivery.[114–119]

If A.J. chooses to breastfeed while taking lithium, she should consider using infant formula when the child becomes ill because febrile illness, vomiting, and diarrhea can increase the risk of lithium toxicity. She also should be instructed to contact her pediatrician if the infant experiences diarrhea, vomiting, hypotonia, poor sucking, muscle twitches, restlessness, or other unexplained changes in behavior.

Atypical Antipsychotics

CASE 87-5

QUESTION 1: D.W., a 34-year-old female singer and musician, recently experienced her fourth hospital admission for a manic episode. Her past medical history includes psoriasis and asthma. A trial of lithium led to worsening of her psoriasis and an unacceptable tremor, which interfered with her guitar playing. Use of propranolol was not considered because of her asthma. She was subsequently switched to VPA monotherapy; however, tremor has again become problematic. Furthermore, she is concerned about her appearance because she has begun to experience weight gain and hair loss from the VPA. What other drugs are available for the treatment of acute mania?

AAPs can be selected as first-line choices for the treatment of acute mania.

Three recent systematic reviews and meta-analyses support the efficacy of AAPs as a class.[120–122] Perlis et al.[120] reviewed data from 12 randomized, placebo-controlled, monotherapy studies and six adjunctive studies and found a collective response rate of 53% for AAPs compared with 30% for placebo. There was no difference in response between the individual AAPs. In adjunctive studies, the mean odds ratio was 2.4 for a 50% improvement with the addition of an AAP to a mood stabilizer (primarily lithium or VPA). Scherk et al.[121] conducted a meta-analysis of 24 randomized controlled trials and found superiority of AAPs for acute mania in comparison with placebo and equal efficacy to lithium, VPA, and haloperidol. In this analysis, the addition of an AAP to lithium, VPA, or CBZ was found to be more effective in reducing manic symptoms and yield less treatment discontinuation than lithium or the anticonvulsant alone. The results of a different meta-analysis specifically designed to evaluate combination treatment of AAPs with lithium or an anticonvulsant also found greater efficacy for the combined regimen.[122] In most combination therapy studies, AAPs were limited to patients having no response or only a partial response to lithium or an anticonvulsant. Thus, the utility of drug combinations as initial therapy cannot be directly assessed.

In a more recent systematic review of 68 randomized controlled trials [eliminate "to"] comparing the efficacy and acceptability of antimanic drugs either against placebo or against one another in the treatment of acute mania was completed via a multiple-treatment meta-analysis. Fourteen treatment options were analyzed including: aripiprazole, asenapine, carbamazepine, valproic acid, gabapentin, haloperidol, lamotrigine, lithium, olanzapine, paliperidone, quetiapine, risperidone, topiramate, ziprasidone, and placebo. All of the antipsychotic drugs were found to be significantly more effective than mood stabilizers in the treatment of acute mania, with risperidone and olanzapine being ranked as superior for efficacy and tolerability. Lamotrigine, topiramate, and gabapentin were not significantly better than placebo in terms of efficacy and should not have a place in the treatment of acute mania.[123]

Additionally, a comparative analysis of 32 placebo-controlled trials demonstrated that YMRS scores improved significantly more with second-generation antipyschotics than mood stabilizers but the efficacy needs to be balanced against anticipated common adverse effects.[124] A significant concern about the use of AAPs is the risk of metabolic complications, including weight gain, glucose dysregulation, and dyslipidemia (see also Chapter 85, Schizophrenia). Clozapine and olanzapine have the highest risk for metabolic complications, quetiapine, iloperidone, paliperidone, and risperidone are associated with an intermediate risk, and ziprasidone, brexpiprazole, cariprazine, asenapine, lurasidone, and aripiprazole appear to have the lowest risk.[48,125] Clozapine is also associated with significant safety concerns, including agranulocytosis, seizures, sialorrhea, anticholinergic side effects, and orthostasis. Efficacy data with clozapine are limited compared with the other AAPs, but clozapine appears to be effective in treatment-resistant mania and in long-term mood stabilization.[126–128]

Sedation is common with clozapine, olanzapine, asenapine, and quetiapine, and this effect may be beneficial in the treatment of acute mania; however, sedation can also lead to non-adherence with long-term use.[129] Aripiprazole and ziprasidone are less sedating; thus, the adjunctive use of a benzodiazepine is often necessary in the acute management of mania with these AAPs. Adjunctive benzodiazepines may also benefit treatment of emergent akathisia, which occurs in 11% to 18% of patients treated with aripiprazole.[130,131] Cariprazine has also been associated with treatment emergent akathisia and extrapyramidal disorders (>10%).[132] Asenapine can cause dysgeusia or oral hypoesthesia, although a black-cherry formulation can help with the unpleasant taste.[133] Ziprasidone may cause activation; however, this effect is attenuated at doses of 120 mg/day or more.[134] Risperidone may overall be the best tolerated of the AAPs, but this drug carries a higher risk for serum prolactin elevation and extrapyramidal symptoms.[135]

D.W.'s concern about her weight gain makes aripiprazole, cariprazine, asenapine, or ziprasidone rational choices for her manic episode. In addition to symptom response, D.W. should be monitored for characteristic antipsychotic side effects, such as movement disorders, and metabolic complications. If D.W. fails to respond to the initially selected AAP, a switch to a different AAP may prove beneficial given the variability in individual response.[47] Table 87-6 provides dosing information for AAPs approved for the treatment of acute mania.

CASE 87-5, QUESTION 2: What alternative agents are available for acute mania if lithium, VPA, or an AAP fail?

Anticonvulsants

CBZ represents an alternative treatment for the management of acute mania when lithium, VPA, and AAPs fail.[11,46,47] In 2005, the FDA-approved extended-release CBZ for the treatment of acute manic and mixed episodes based on the results of two double-blind, randomized, placebo-controlled trials.[136] A meta-analysis of four randomized, controlled trials (n = 464 patients) found that maintenance treatment with carbamazepine has similar efficacy as, and fewer discontinuations due to adverse effects than, lithium.[137] Despite demonstrated efficacy, CBZ remains a less than popular choice in BD due to significant tolerability and drug–drug interaction risks. If elected for treatment, CBZ should be started at 100 to 200 mg twice daily. The dose should be increased by 200 mg every 3 to 4 days until adequate serum levels have been reached.[11] Although no correlation between CBZ serum levels and response in BD has been established, serum levels greater than 12 mcg/mL are associated with sedation and ataxia. The recommended target serum level for seizure prophylaxis is 4 to 12 mcg/mL.[11] Average daily doses for maintenance therapy range from 200 to 1,600 mg/day (see Chapter 60, Seizure Disorders).

Oxcarbazepine, a structural analog of CBZ, offers some advantages over CBZ, including improved tolerability and fewer drug interactions; however, there is a paucity of well-designed clinical trials in BD.[138] Cochrane reviews suggest that there are insufficient trials of adequate methodological quality to recommend use for either acute or maintenance treatment for bipolar disorder.[139,140]

Other anticonvulsants studied in mania include lamotrigine, gabapentin, topiramate, tiagabine, zonisamide, and levetiracetam. Initial open-label studies of lamotrigine in mania were promising, but two unpublished trials were negative.[141] Currently, experts doubt that lamotrigine has any significant effect in acute mania. Open trials and case reports suggested adjunctive treatment with gabapentin was effective in manic, hypomanic, and depressive states of BD.[142–144] A more recent controlled trial found no benefit of gabapentin.[145] In this double-blind, placebo-controlled trial, gabapentin was administered as an adjunctive treatment in patients with bipolar I disorder whose current episode was manic, hypomanic, or mixed. At 12 weeks, gabapentin failed to show any significant benefit compared with placebo. In fact, the placebo group did significantly better than the gabapentin-treated patients.

In four double-blind, placebo-controlled trials, topiramate did not separate from placebo and was less effective than lithium in the treatment of acute mania.[146,147] Tiagabine, levetiracetam, and zonisamide have been studied in BD but lack adequate safety or efficacy data to receive any formal evaluation.

Table 87-6
Atypical Antipsychotic Dosing in Acute Mania

Atypical Antipsychotic	Initial Dose	Titration	Effective Dose Range
Aripiprazole	15 mg/day	Not required	15–30 mg/day
Asenapine	10 mg twice daily	5 mg twice daily	5–10 mg twice daily
Cariprazine	1.5 mg/day	Increase to 3 mg on day 2, then increase as needed in 1.5 or 3 mg increments	3–6 mg/day
Olanzapine	10–15 mg/day	5 mg/day	5–20 mg/day
Quetiapine	50 mg twice daily	50 mg twice daily	200–400 mg twice daily
Quetiapine XR	300 mg/day	300 mg/day	400–800 mg/day
Risperidone	2–3 mg/day	1 mg/day	1–6 mg/day
Ziprasidone	40 mg twice daily	20–40 mg twice daily	40–80 mg twice daily

Source: Abilify (aripiprazole) [package insert]. Tokyo, Japan: Otsuka Pharmaceutical; February 2012; Saphris (asenapine) [package insert]. Whitehouse Station, NJ: Merck & Company; Vraylar (cariprazine) [package insert]. Parsippany, NJ: Allergan; April 2015; March 2015; Zyprexa (olanzapine) [package insert]. Indianapolis, IN: Eli Lilly and Company; December 2014; Seroquel (quetiapine) [package insert]. Wilmington, DE: Astra Zeneca Pharmaceuticals; October 2013; Seroquel Extended Release (quetiapine fumarate) [package insert]. Wilmington, DE: Astra Zeneca Pharmaceuticals; October 2013; Risperdal (risperidone) [package insert]. Titusville, NJ: Janssen, LP; April 2014; Geodon (ziprasidone) [package insert]. New York, NY: Pfizer; December 2014.

COMBINATION TREATMENT

Despite the array of treatments available for the management of acute mania, large numbers of patients fail to respond to monotherapy, and combination therapy is becoming a first-line treatment option.[148] Potentially useful combinations include lithium plus AAPs, VPA plus AAPs, and lithium plus VPA.[35,46] A combination to be avoided is CBZ and clozapine owing to the increased risk of hematologic adverse effects. Also combinations of CBZ with either olanzapine or with risperidone result in more side effects and decreased efficacy; therefore, these combinations are not recommended.[47]

BENZODIAZEPINES AND ANTIPSYCHOTICS FOR ACUTE AGITATION

CASE 87-6

QUESTION 1: M.B. is a 39-year-old man hospitalized for an acute manic episode, but is refusing all medications, reporting "I will be robbed of my superpowers." He is found pacing around the inpatient unit shouting orders for his release. When asked to return to his room by the clinical staff, he becomes agitated, picks up a chair, and begins swinging it wildly at anyone who approaches him. In the past, M.B. experienced a documented acute dystonic reaction to haloperidol. M.B. has a medical history of diabetes mellitus and hypertension. What is an appropriate pharmacologic intervention for M.B.?

Benzodiazepines and antipsychotics are useful in treating agitation, irritability, and hyperactivity associated with acute manic episodes. Oral formulations are preferred and are favored by patients in psychiatric emergencies.[149] Oral dose delivery can be facilitated with liquid concentrates and orally disintegrating tablets. Patients refusing oral medications may require intramuscular (IM) injections.[150] Traditionally, the combination of IM haloperidol and IM lorazepam has been used. Currently, ziprasidone, aripiprazole, and olanzapine are available in rapid-acting IM dosage forms. IM ziprasidone at doses of 10 and 20 mg is effective in psychotic agitation.[151,152] IM aripiprazole at doses of 9.75 or 15 mg and IM olanzapine 10 mg are effective for manic or mixed-state agitation.[153,154] Repeat doses of IM ziprasidone, aripiprazole, and olanzapine can be administered 2 to 4 hours after the first dose, if needed. The concurrent use of a benzodiazepine with an antipsychotic is generally safe and potentially more effective than either agent alone. In the case of IM olanzapine, concurrent benzodiazepines should not be used because the combination may cause excessive sedation and cardiorespiratory depression.[155,156]

Lorazepam is the preferred benzodiazepine for acute manic agitation. Advantages of lorazepam include availability as both an IM and oral formulation (tablet and concentrate), lack of active metabolites, and safety in hepatic and renal impairment. The Expert Consensus Guideline recommends dosing lorazepam at 1 to 3 mg orally or 0.5 to 3 mg IM, with repeat doses at least 60 minutes apart. The maximal dose should not exceed 10 to 12 mg in the first 24 hours.[157] The primary concern regarding the use of benzodiazepines for agitated mania is sedation. The risk of abuse and addiction is minimal with short-term inpatient use.

M.B. is uncooperative and an immediate danger to others, thus warranting IM therapy. Because of M.B.'s history of acute dystonia to haloperidol, an IM AAP (such as olanzapine, ziprasidone, or aripiprazole) should be used. The combination of ziprasidone 10 mg IM and lorazepam 2 mg IM is an appropriate intervention. IM administration of aripiprazole and lorazepam may also be used. As M.B. becomes calmer and more receptive to treatment, he can be transitioned to oral therapy.

TREATMENT OF ACUTE BIPOLAR DEPRESSION

CASE 87-7

QUESTION 1: H.C., a 31-year-old woman, was hospitalized for treatment of an acute manic episode 3 months ago. She was discharged on VPA 1,750 mg/day with a favorable response. Starting about 2 weeks ago, her parents become concerned because H.C. started spending most of the day in bed. When out of bed, H.C. sits on the couch without moving for hours. She only nibbles at the food her parents offer her. She has no other signs or symptoms of physical illness and has not taken any additional medications, alcohol, or drugs of abuse to her parents' knowledge. They report that H.C. was diagnosed with diabetes mellitus type 2 last year. Her serum glucose has been controlled by diet. On further questioning, H.C.'s parents report that she has been intermittently tearful and expressed remorse for her behavior when she was manic. They also recall her as saying "I am as low as I can go, and I just want to die." Hence, they suspect she is suicidal. H.C.'s parents report that she is taking VPA as prescribed and that the last time she experienced this level of depression, the addition of lithium to VPA did not seem to help. Her VPA level on discharge was 84 mcg/mL. What change in H.C.'s treatment should be instituted at this time?

Bipolar depression is both recurrent and chronic, accounting for three-quarters of the time spent ill in BD.[158] Depression is often difficult to treat and puts patients at significant risk for suicide, which occurs at a rate 15 times greater than that of the general population.[159]

In bipolar depression, complete remission of symptoms is the primary goal of treatment. The ideal regimen should target acute depressive symptoms, decrease suicide risk, and prevent future mood episodes (both manic and depressive). These goals should be achieved without precipitating mania (switching) or mood cycling. Because simply addressing the acute depressive symptoms is often shortsighted in an illness with recurrent depressive episodes, the ability to prevent future depressive episodes and the long-term tolerability are important considerations.[160]

A logical first step in the management of bipolar depression is to verify adherence and optimize the dose of the current mood stabilizer.[35] For H.C., she is already on a therapeutic level of VPA; thus, no change in dose is needed.

Lithium

Lithium remains a first-line treatment for bipolar depression.[47,48] The CANMAT guidelines recommend a level of 0.8 mEq/L or more for optimal response.[49] The benefit of lithium was demonstrated in seven of eight placebo-controlled crossover studies with a mean response rate of 76%.[161] Lithium may also be effective for preventing depressive episodes. A 6-year follow-up study of patients maintained on lithium found a reduction in the annual rate of depressive episodes by 46% and the time spent ill by 53%.[162] A meta-analysis of 1- or 2-year-long studies found a 22% relative risk reduction for a depressive relapse compared with placebo (risk ratio, 0.78; 95% CI = 0.60–1.01).[163] The difference from placebo was not statistically significant.[156] Beyond antidepressant effects in BD, lithium also has the vital benefit of reducing the risk of suicide, deliberate self-harm, and all-cause mortality.[164,165]

Lamotrigine

Lamotrigine is recommended as a first-line treatment for bipolar depression by both the World Federation of Societies of Biological

Psychiatry (WFSBP) and CANMAT guidelines; however, more recent data from five double-blind, placebo-controlled trials have brought this recommendation into question.[47,49] These studies did not detect any benefit from lamotrigine on the primary end points (change in Hamilton Depression Rating Scale [HAM-D], or Montgomery–Åsberg Depression Rating Scale [MADRS]) relative to placebo. An independent meta-analysis of the same five studies found significant (but only modest) benefits for lamotrigine with a relative risk of response of 1.27 for the HAM-D and 1.22 for the MADRS.[166] The ability of lamotrigine to reduce the risk of relapse to depression is less controversial. A pooled analysis of two long-term studies (up to 18 months) with lamotrigine found a 36% reduction in the risk of relapse to depression.[167] Lamotrigine was well tolerated with no difference from placebo in any side effect. Because lamotrigine has limited antimanic properties, patients with a history of severe, recent, or recurrent mania should only take lamotrigine in combination with an antimanic drug, such as lithium.[46]

The combination of lamotrigine and lithium may confer additional benefits on reducing depressive symptoms and should be considered for bipolar depression. Patients stabilized on lithium (predefined range of 0.6–1.2 mEq/L, mostly >3 months' duration) were randomly assigned to receive lamotrigine (200 mg/day) or placebo. The lithium–lamotrigine group had a response rate of 52% (based on MADRS scores) compared with 32% for the lithium–placebo group.[168] From the results of this study, clinical experience, and the need for long-term tolerability, the combination of lamotrigine and lithium is an appropriate treatment when monotherapy with these drugs has failed.

Due to valproate's inhibition of UGT2B7, it can increase lamotrigine's AUC by 2.6-fold. Clinicians should pay particular attention to the dosing with initiating or discontinuing either medication in the presence of the other medication.[91]

Atypical Antipsychotics

AAPs offer another option for the treatment of bipolar depression. Quetiapine has demonstrated efficacy in a total of four 8-week double-blind, placebo-controlled studies (300 or 600 mg/day).[169–172] Response rates ranged from 58% to 69% for the 300-mg dose, and 58% to 70% for the 600-mg dose. Both doses were commonly associated with sedation, somnolence, dry mouth, and dizziness. Clinically significant weight gain (≥7% of baseline weight) was detected in roughly 5% to 10% of subjects receiving quetiapine.

The combination of olanzapine with fluoxetine is effective for patients with bipolar depression.[173] In a 7-week acute-phase treatment, OFC was superior to lamotrigine in symptom improvement but not significantly different in response rate (69% with OFC vs. 60% with lamotrigine).[174] The rate of relapse to depression during the 6-month study was low and similar between OFC and lamotrigine (14% vs. 18%). In an extension of this study (for a total of 6 months), OFC caused significant elevations in all metabolic parameters (weight, glucose, prolactin, cholesterol).[175] Most alarming was a 34% incidence of clinically significant weight gain in the OFC group (vs. 2% with lamotrigine). Therefore, the risk of metabolic complications should be taken into consideration when selecting this treatment.

Lurasidone has demonstrated efficacy in two 6-week, randomized, double-blind controlled clinical trials as monotherapy at either 20 to 60 mg/day and 80 to 120 mg/day. Response rates were 53% for the low dose, 51% for the high dose, and 30% for placebo. An additional study with a similar design failed to separate from placebo. An adjunct to lithium or VPA trial demonstrated response rates of 57% of lurasidone with either lithium or VPA compared to 42% of placebo with either lithium or VPA.[176–178] Table 87-7 provides dosing information for AAPs approved for the treatment of bipolar depression.

Despite its efficacy in treatment-resistant unipolar depression, aripiprazole does not appear to be effective for bipolar depression on the basis of two randomized, controlled trials.[172, 179] Considering these findings, the CANMAT guidelines have listed aripiprazole as not recommended for acute bipolar depression.[49] Other AAPs have not been systematically studied in bipolar depression.

Antidepressants

The use of antidepressants in BD has been hotly debated. Some guidelines recommend restrictive use of antidepressants because of concerns about mood switching and cycle acceleration.[48] Other guidelines recommend early treatment with antidepressants, particularly SSRIs, to address the recurrent depressive episodes.[47] In either case, there is agreement that antidepressants should only be used in combination with antimanic agents such as VPA, lithium, or an AAP.[47,48] The largest controlled trial of antidepressant augmentation in bipolar depression was conducted as part of the Systematic Treatment Enhancement Program for Bipolar Disorder (STEP-BD) study. This study was a naturalistic 26-week, double-blind, placebo-controlled trial comparing antidepressants (bupropion or paroxetine) with placebo as adjunctive treatment to an antimanic agent.[81] The primary end point of durable recovery (euthymia for 8 weeks) was achieved in 24% of antidepressant-treated subjects compared with 27% receiving placebo. There was no significant difference between groups in treatment emergent mood switch. A recent meta-analysis of 15 studies, primarily with bupropion or SSRIs, found that antidepressants were no more effective than placebo for acute (<16 weeks) bipolar depression.[180] This study also did not find an increased risk of mood switch. Therefore, although it appeared to be safe to add the antidepressant in regard to switching into mania, there is question about whether there is a large benefit on depressive symptoms.

Table 87-7

Atypical Antipsychotic Dosing in Bipolar Depression

Atypical Antipsychotic	Initial Dose	Titration	Effective Dose Range
Lurasidone	20 mg/day	20 mg every 2 days	20–120 mg/day
Olanzapine/Fluoxetine	6/25 mg/day	As indicated	12/50 mg/day
Quetiapine (IR and XR)	50 mg/day	100 mg Day 2 200 mg Day 3 300 mg Day 4	300 mg/day

Source: Latuda (lurasidone) [package insert]. Marlborough, MA: Sunovion Pharmaceuticals; July 2013; Symbyax (olanzapine/fluoxetine) [package insert]. Indianapolis, IN: Lilly USA, LLC.; January 2015; Seroquel XR (quetiapine XR) [package insert]. Wilmington, DE: AstraZeneca; July 2009.

Because H.C. did not respond to lithium in combination with VPA during her past depressive episode, an alternative first-line agent such as lamotrigine is a reasonable choice. OFC or quetiapine may compromise her type 2 diabetes control and thus are not appropriate options. Lurasidone would also be an alternate choice, although no current data exist in comparing it to lamotrigine, quetiapine, or OFC for the treatment in bipolar depression. Dosing of lamotrigine needs to account for H.C.'s concurrent use of VPA, which is known to inhibit the metabolism of lamotrigine. Therefore, the initial dose for H.C. is 25 mg every other day for weeks 1 and 2 followed by an increase to 25 mg/day for weeks 3 and 4. The dose can be increased to 50 mg/day for week 5 and then to a maximum of 100 mg/day beginning at week 6. In the absence of VPA, the recommended target dose of lamotrigine is 200 mg/day. In patients taking enzyme inducers (e.g., CBZ), the target dose is 200 mg twice daily.[181] The appropriate titration schedule must be followed for lamotrigine (see also Chapter 60, Seizure Disorders) because of the risk of skin rash, which may progress to the life-threatening Stevens–Johnson syndrome. The combination of lamotrigine and VPA is a risk factor for the development of this dangerous cutaneous reaction; therefore, H.C. should be instructed to contact her physician immediately if a skin rash develops.

MAINTENANCE THERAPY OF BIPOLAR DISORDER

CASE 87-8

QUESTION 1: R.L., a 33-year-old man, has been treated for an episode of acute mania with lithium 600 mg twice a day for 3 weeks. He is no longer overtly manic. Because of R.L.'s past episodes of depression and mania, his physician decides to institute prophylactic (maintenance) lithium therapy. What are the goals of maintenance lithium therapy for R.L.? How should he be monitored during this maintenance phase? How long should R.L. be maintained on lithium?

Recurrent episodes are associated with decreased quality of life, poorer response to treatment, longer hospitalizations, and cognitive impairment.[35] Thus, early maintenance (prophylactic) treatment is indicated to prevent disease progression. Appropriate goals for maintenance therapy include an increase in the interval between episodes, a decrease in the frequency of episodes, and a reduction in the duration and severity of mood episodes. In most cases, patients will have been started on an acute treatment for a manic or depressive episode. These agents should generally be continued because abrupt switches in medications may predict poorer treatment outcomes.[35]

Lithium

The aforementioned meta-analysis (Case 87-7, Question 1) of long-term lithium therapy for relapse prevention in BD included five randomized, placebo-controlled studies.[163] Although lithium did not effectively reduce the risk of relapse to depression, it did reduce the risk of relapse to any mood episode (risk ratio, 0.66) and to manic episodes specifically (risk ratio, 0.62). The average risk of relapse to any mood episode on lithium was 40% versus 60% for placebo. The average risk of relapse to a manic episode was 14% for lithium versus 24% for placebo.

In the case of R.L., he should be continued on lithium. The target levels for maintenance therapy with lithium should be in the range of 0.5 to 0.8 mEq/L.[11] Higher levels ranging from 0.8 to 1.0 mEq/L are associated with a reduced number of relapses (compared with levels between 0.4 and 0.6 mEq/L) but also have an elevated risk of side effects.[182]

In addition to determining an appropriate maintenance lithium level for R.L., it is important to consider whether once-daily administration of lithium can improve adherence or adverse effects. During periods of dosage readjustment, R.L. will require monitoring of his lithium serum level more frequently. Once stabilized, the monitoring frequency can be reduced to quarterly. See Table 87-3 for recommended lithium monitoring guidelines.

CASE 87-8, QUESTION 2: What other maintenance treatments for BD are available should R.L. fail to respond to lithium?

Anticonvulsants

VPA and lamotrigine are reasonable alternatives to lithium that have shown efficacy in BD maintenance therapy. In the first controlled trial of VPA for the maintenance treatment of BD, patients were randomly assigned to receive VPA, lithium, or placebo and followed for 52 weeks.[183] The three groups did not differ with regard to the primary outcome of time to any mood episode. However, a lower percentage of patients discontinued treatment for any reason in the VPA group (62%) than lithium (76%) or placebo (75%); patients on VPA remained in the study longer (198 days) than patients on lithium (152 days) but not placebo (165 days). The mean VPA serum concentration was 85 mcg/mL. Lamotrigine has been studied rigorously in the maintenance treatment of BD. A pooled analysis of two placebo-controlled studies found that lamotrigine and lithium more than doubled the time to intervention (e.g., addition of pharmacotherapy or ECT) for any mood episode compared with placebo (see Case 87-7, Question 1).[167] The time to intervention was 197 days for lamotrigine, 187 days for lithium, and 86 days for placebo. Lithium preferentially prevented manic relapses, whereas lamotrigine preferentially prevented depressive episodes.

Atypical Antipsychotics

AAPs have become increasingly popular alternatives and adjunctive treatments for maintenance therapy of BD. To date, aripiprazole, olanzapine, quetiapine (adjunctive), risperidone long-acting injection, and ziprasidone (adjunctive) have received FDA approval for the maintenance treatment of BD (Table 87-8). A meta-analysis evaluated 20 trials ($n = 5364$) in the efficacy of maintenance treatments for BD. No monotherapy options were associated with significantly reduced risk for both manic/mixed and depressive poles compared to each other, while the only combination, quetiapine plus lithium or VPA demonstrated significant reduction in risk versus the comparator of placebo in reduced risk for both poles.[184] The long-term risk of side effects, including metabolic complications and EPS, should be the primary consideration for selecting one AAP over another (see Case 87-5, Question 1).

CASE 87-8, QUESTION 3: What is the role of psychotherapy in BD?

Psychotherapy can have a profound effect on the prevention of acute illness, as well as a sustained effect on maintenance treatments. Excessive stress, for example, is often implicated in the onset of affective episodes, particularly early in the lifetime course of BD.[7] If individuals and their families can learn to avoid these triggers or to develop coping skills, the acute impact can be minimized and future episodes averted.

Therapy may also help the family to cope with the extreme emotions and disruption that are the hallmark of acute manic and depressive episodes. Violent outbursts, infidelity, financial debts, substance abuse, suicidal thinking, and loss of self-esteem may all be a byproduct of mood recurrence, and family members must

Table 87-8
FDA-Approved Medications for Bipolar Disorder

Drug	Mania	Mixed	Depression	Maintenance
Carbamazepine (extended-release capsule)	X	X		
Lamotrigine				X
Lithium	X			X
Valproate (divalproex sodium)	X	X		
Asenapine	X	X		
Aripiprazole	X	X		X
Lurasidone			X[a]	
Olanzapine	X	X		X
Olanzapine–fluoxetine			X	
Quetiapine	X		X	X[a]
Quetiapine XR	X	X	X	X[a]
Risperidone long-acting injection				X
Risperidone	X	X		
Ziprasidone	X	X		X[a]

[a]Monotherapy or adjunct to lithium or valproate.

FDA, Food and Drug Administration.

come to terms with such calamities, as well as fears surrounding future episodes. Regular sleep–wake cycles seem vital to the maintenance of euthymic states; thus, improvements in sleep hygiene may be encouraged in these sessions. Last, sustained medication adherence must also be emphasized; individuals with BD will often stop their medications in an effort to resume the "highs" of mania or because of the cumulative side effect burden of complex psychotropic regimens.

The specific psychotherapeutic approach to BD is generally quite similar to interventions offered to individuals with schizophrenia. Family-focused therapy seems to be quite effective, as are cognitive-behavioral and interpersonal and social rhythm therapy. Collaborative care models have been extensively studied for unipolar depression in primary-care settings, but the effectiveness of collaborative care models for bipolar illness is less clear. In fact, in the STEP-BD trials, collaborative care was the least effective intervention.[185] Reported response rates were 77% with family-focused therapy, 64% with interpersonal and social rhythm therapy, 60% with cognitive-behavioral therapy, and 54% with collaborative care. Experts contend that the collaborative care intervention was comparatively less intensive than the other three treatment modalities in this report.

Although most experts advocate for regular physical activity to prevent bipolar mood swings, the body of literature supporting such an approach is very limited. Lifestyle surveys have demonstrated that people afflicted with BD are less likely to exercise and more likely to exhibit poor dietary habits than those without a serious mental illness.[186] Theoretically, exercise may improve dietary habits, regulate sleep, increase energy, and promote euthymic moods. As a result, increased physical activity would be expected to improve the prognosis of bipolar illness and should be encouraged at the very least for the physical health benefits.

CASE 87-8, QUESTION 4: Are there other treatment options for BD?

Alternative Medicines

A wide variety of herbal preparations and dietary supplements have been studied for the treatment of BD. A meta-analysis of double-blind, placebo-controlled trials of combined bipolar and unipolar depression found significant benefit of omega-3 fatty acid supplementation compared with placebo in patients with depressive episodes.[187] In most cases, omega-3 fatty acid supplementation, including eicosapentaenoic acid alone or in combination with docosahexaenoic acid, was used as adjunctive treatment. The doses studied ranged from 1 g/day of eicosapentaenoic acid to 9.6 g/day of combined eicosapentaenoic acid and docosahexaenoic acid.

Inositol was recently compared with lamotrigine and risperidone in an augmentation trial for bipolar depression.[188] The three treatments were equivalent with regard to recovery from depression; however, the study was open label and the sample size was small (n = 66). Saint-John's-wort and *S*-adenosyl-L-methionine may be effective for depressive episodes; however, these agents, like traditional antidepressants, should generally be avoided in BD owing to the risk of mood destabilization.[55,56]

Electroconvulsive Therapy

ECT is effective in all phases of BD and continues to play a vital role in the contemporary treatment of mood disorders. The efficacy of ECT in bipolar depression is equivalent to unipolar depression with approximately 80% of patients achieving a response and 60% meeting criteria for remission.[189] The benefits of ECT in acute mania are similarly impressive. In a review spanning 50 years of research, "remission or marked clinical improvement" was achieved in 80% of patients.[190,191]

BD medication regimens need to be carefully evaluated before ECT treatment. Anticonvulsants and benzodiazepines raise the seizure threshold and interfere with the effectiveness of ECT. A retrospective analysis found that patients taking anticonvulsants achieved the same overall clinical response but required more ECT treatments and a longer hospital stay.[192] An exception is the concurrent use of lamotrigine, which appears to have no significant effect on electrical stimulus dose or seizure duration.[193] Lithium use with ECT has been discouraged on the basis of early reports of organic brain syndrome; however, a more recent prospective study found the combination to be safe in a younger population without risk factors for ECT complications.[194,195] Small case series and clinical experience suggest that AAPs are safe to use during ECT.[196–198]

ECT remains an effective and important tool for the treatment of BD, particularly bipolar depression, which is highly recurrent and has limited safe and effective treatment options. All patients failing to respond to standard BD pharmacotherapy, presenting with severe mood symptoms, or not otherwise appropriate for medication treatment should be considered for ECT.

KEY REFERENCES AND WEBSITES

A full list of references for this chapter can be found at http://thepoint.lww.com/AT11e. Below are the key references and websites for this chapter, with the corresponding reference number in this chapter found in parentheses after the reference.

Key References

American Diabetes Association et al. Consensus development conference on antipsychotic drugs and obesity and diabetes. *Diabetes Care.* 2004;27:596. (125)

American Psychiatric Association. Mood disorders. In: American Psychiatric Association, ed. *Diagnostic and Statistical Manual of Mental Disorders.* 5th ed. Text Revision. Washington, DC: American Psychiatric Association; 2013:123. (5)

Cipriani A et al. Comparative efficacy and acceptability of antimanic drugs in acute mania: a multiple-treatments meta-analysis. *Lancet.* 2011;378:1306–1315. (123)

Cipriani A et al. Lithium in the prevention of suicidal behavior and all-cause mortality in patients with mood disorders: a systematic review of randomized trials. *Am J Psychiatry.* 2005;162:1805. (164)

Crismon ML et al. *Texas Medication Algorithm Project Procedural Manual: Bipolar Disorder Algorithms.* Austin, TX: The Texas Department of State Health Services; 2007.

Goodwin FK, Jamison KR. Medical treatment of hypomania, mania, and mixed states. In: Jamison FK, Jamison KP, eds. *Manic-Depressive Illness: Bipolar Illness and Recurrent Depression.* New York, NY: Oxford University Press; 2007:721. (7)

Goodwin GM et al. Evidence-based guidelines for treating bipolar disorder: revised third edition recommendations from the British Association for Psychopharmacology. *J Psychopharmacol.* 2016;30:495–553. (47)

Grunze H et al. The world federation of societies of biological psychiatry (WFSBP) guidelines for the biological treatment of bipolar disorder. *World J Biol Psychiatry.* 2013;14:154–219. (50)

Mohammad O, Osser DN. The psychopharmacology algorithm project at the Harvard South Shore Program: an algorithm for acute mania. *Harv Rev Psychiatry.* 2014;22(5):274–294. (46)

Sidor MM, Macqueen GM. Antidepressants for the acute treatment of bipolar depression: a systematic review and meta-analysis. *J Clin Psychiatry.* 2011;72:156. (174)

Suppes T et al. The Texas implementation of medication algorithms: update to the algorithms for treatment of bipolar I disorder. *J Clin Psychiatry.* 2005;66:870.

Yatham LN et al. Canadian Network for Mood and Anxiety Treatments (CANMAT) and International Society for Bipolar Disorders (ISBD) collaborative update of CANMAT guidelines for the management of patients with bipolar disorder: update 2009. *Bipolar Disord.* 2013;15:1–44. (49)

Key Websites

Depression and Bipolar Support Alliance. http://www.dbsalliance.org.
National Alliance on Mental Illness. http://www.nami.org.
National Institute of Mental Health. http://www.nimh.nih.gov.

88 Developmental Disorders

Lee A. Robinson and Kimberly Lenz

CORE PRINCIPLES

	CHAPTER CASES
1 Developmental disorders are a group of conditions in which early brain development is impaired. This very large group of disorders includes diagnoses such as intellectual disability (ID) and autism spectrum disorder (ASD). The core diagnostic features of ASD include impairment in reciprocal social communication and social interaction, and restricted, repetitive patterns of behavior, interests, or activities. These symptoms must be present from early childhood and impair everyday functioning. ASD is diagnosed clinically, though standardized behavioral diagnostic instruments can assist this process. ASD is more common in boys than girls, and the core diagnostic features can be addressed through multiple different types of nonpharmacologic interventions, including specialized education, physical therapy, occupational therapy, speech and language therapy, and behavioral therapy, such as applied behavior analysis (ABA).	**Case 88-1 (Question 1), Table 88-1**
2 Individuals with ID/ASD have high rates of comorbid ADHD. Treatment of ADHD, especially hyperactivity, in individuals with ID/ASD is similar to the treatment of ADHD in neurotypical individuals, and includes stimulants, α_2 agonists, and atomoxetine. Compared to their neurotypical peers though, individuals with ID/ASD and comorbid ADHD experience lower effect sizes with ADHD treatment, lower tolerated doses of ADHD medication, and more risk of adverse effects, including increased rates of decreased appetite, insomnia, depressive symptoms, irritability, and social withdrawal.	**Case 88-1 (Question 2)**
3 Some individuals with developmental disorders demonstrate symptoms of irritability and aggression, which can sometimes be helped with a pharmacologic intervention if nonpharmacologic interventions are ineffective. The strongest evidence for the pharmacologic treatment of irritability/aggression in individuals with developmental disorders exists for the use of risperidone and aripiprazole to treat irritability in children with ASD. Doses for this purpose are likely lower than those used to treat schizophrenia or bipolar disorder, and adverse events are relatively common and may include sedation, weight gain, and extrapyramidal symptoms.	**Case 88-2 (Question 1)**
4 Individuals with developmental disorders are at high risk of having comorbid anxiety and depression. Although no large prospective, randomized, controlled trials (RCTs) exist to support the use of selective serotonin reuptake inhibitors (SSRI) for this purpose, case studies and open-label studies have shown possible benefits. RCTs of SSRIs for the treatment of repetitive behavior in children with developmental disorders have shown mixed results, although they have demonstrated that individuals with developmental disorders may be at increased risk of emotional and behavioral adverse events from SSRIs, and therefore, target dosing should be lower than in individuals with typical development.	**Case 88-3 (Questions 1, 2)**
5 Individuals with developmental disorders have high rates of comorbid medical and psychiatric disorders, and therefore may often be prescribed multiple different concurrent medications. Precaution should be taken to avoid any pharmacodynamic or pharmacokinetic drug–drug interactions, and such interactions should always be considered to describe any adverse events.	**Case 88-3 (Questions 1, 2)**
6 Sleep disturbances are common in individuals with developmental disorders. Melatonin has the strongest body of evidence for being a safe and effective treatment of sleep disturbances in this population.	**Case 88-4 (Question 1)**

Developmental disorders are a group of conditions characterized by impaired early brain development, resulting in deficits of cognitive, communicative, behavioral, sensory, or motor functioning. This broad group of disorders includes diagnoses such as intellectual disability, and autism spectrum disorder (ASD), which will be the focus of this chapter, attention-deficit/hyperactivity disorder (ADHD) and tic disorder, which are covered in another chapter, and communication disorders, learning disorders, cerebral palsy, congenital hearing loss, and congenital blindness. Intellectual disability (ID), previously labeled mental retardation, is a disorder with deficits in intellectual and adaptive functioning. Although ID is typically reserved for older children, for whom intellectual testing is more valid and reliable, global developmental delay (GDD) is the diagnosis given to younger children in which delays exist in two or more developmental domains. ASD, which includes prior diagnoses of autistic disorder, Asperger disorder, and pervasive developmental disorder (PDD) not otherwise specified, is a condition involving deficits in social communication, as well as the presence of restricted and repetitive patterns of behavior, interests, or activities.[1]

EPIDEMIOLOGY, NATURAL COURSE OF THE DISEASE, AND PROGNOSIS

Developmental disorders are common in the community, affecting as many as 15% of children in the U.S., based on parent report.[2] Collectively, developmental disorders are nearly twice as likely in boys and children insured by Medicaid, relative to girls and those insured by private insurance, respectively.[2] Additionally, a higher prevalence of developmental disorders is reported by families with incomes below the federal poverty level and with lower maternal education (any educational attainment less than a college degree).[2]

For ID and GDD, the overall prevalence is estimated to be between 1% and 3% of the population, though with considerable variability depending on how the diagnosis is defined and reported in the literature.[3,4] Intellectual disability is more prevalent in males versus females, and in low- and middle-income countries relative to high-income countries.[3]

ASD is increasing in prevalence, with the Centers for Disease Control and Prevention reporting about 1 in 68 children (1.47%) being identified with the disorder.[5] Although around one-third of children with ASD may also qualify for intellectual disability, the proportion of children with average or above average intelligence being diagnosed with ASD has been steadily increasing over the years and may explain some of the increase in overall ASD prevalence.[5] The proportion of children with ASD who are boys has consistently been 4 to 5 times that of girls.[5] In the United States, around 30% of children with ASD have some level of ID.[5]

The course and prognosis of both ID and ASD vary considerably depending on the severity of the deficits, the impact of comorbid medical and psychiatric conditions, and the access to services and treatments. Many individuals will go on to live rich and fulfilling lives, with minimal required assistance in daily life functioning, though some will require constant supervision in supportive group housing, and assistance for basic tasks of daily living.

PATHOPHYSIOLOGY: DISEASE ETIOLOGY, ANATOMY, AND PHYSIOLOGY

Many different known and unknown genetic and environmental factors can lead to the impairment in early brain development associated with developmental disorders.

For both ID and ASD, risk factors include preterm birth, low birth weight, small for gestational age, and low Apgar scores, though all of these are associated more strongly with ID.[6] For ID specifically, risk factors may differ depending on the severity of ID. Studies have shown risk factors for mild ID to include mothers under the age of 20 years or older than 30 years, paternal age greater than 40 years, increasing birth order, increasing social disadvantage, maternal education less than high school, being part of a multiple birth, and being second or later in the birth order.[7,8] The risk of severe ID was consistently increased with increasing maternal age and decreasing level of maternal education.[7] For ASD without ID, additional risk factors include mothers aged 35 years or older, first-born infants, male infants, and increasing socioeconomic advantage.[8]

In only about half of all cases of ID can a specific etiology be identified and may include genetic anomalies, intrapartum asphyxia, cerebral dysgenesis, and environmental causes.[9] In only about 30% of children with ASD can an identifiable genetic etiology be determined.[10] Although inherited genetic forms of ID likely represent a minority of identified cases, ASD on the other hand is widely considered to be one of the most heritable neuropsychiatric conditions with heritability estimates of 60% to 90%.[11] For parents with one child with ASD, the recurrence rate in future siblings is thought to be 5% to 20%, with higher rates if the original child with ASD is female.[12] This recurrence rate increases to about 33% if a family already has two children with ASD.[12]

For inherited genetic anomalies, X-linked gene defects account for 10% to 12% of all ID cases in males, with fragile X syndrome being the most common.[13] Fragile X syndrome, marked by a CGG triplet repeat expansion in the *FMR1* gene on the X chromosome, is also the most common single-gene cause of ID, accounting for about 0.5% to 3% of individuals with ID,[14] and ASD, accounting for around 1% to 3% of cases.[10,15] Single-gene disorders, some heritable like fragile X syndrome, account for about 5% to 7% of ASD cases and include *PTEN* macrocephaly syndrome (~1%), tuberous sclerosis complex (~1%), and Rett syndrome (~1%).[10,15] Other inherited causes of ID and ASD include inherited metabolic disorders, such as phenylketonuria, adenylosuccinate lyase deficiency, and Smith–Lemli–Opitz syndrome.[15] Although inherited metabolic disorders are relatively rare, accounting for only 1% to 5% of cases of ID, the potential for positive prognosis with treatment is high.[4]

Other genetic anomalies that can lead to ID and ASD include noninherited, or de novo, single-gene mutations, chromosomal aberrations, and imprinting/epigenetic disorders.[14] Chromosomal aberrations may account for up to 25% of individuals with ID, about 8% or 9% of which is due to trisomy 21, or Down syndrome, the most common known cause of ID.[14,16] Prader–Willi and Angelman syndromes, both associated with developmental delays, are two examples of disorders involving imprinted genes.

Environmental causes of ID range in the literature from 2% to 13% and include antenatal toxin exposure (e.g., fetal alcohol spectrum disorders), antenatal infection (e.g., TORCH infections), and early severe psychosocial deprivation.[17,18] Environmental causes of ASD include first trimester intrauterine exposure to valproic acid, thalidomide, misoprostol, the organophosphate insecticide chlorpyrifos, and phthalates, in addition to first trimester rubella infection.[19] While receiving much scrutiny, multiple studies have shown no support linking vaccines to autism.[20]

CLINICAL PRESENTATION

Developmental disorders are typically recognized clinically once it becomes clear that a child is delayed in meeting one or more developmental milestones. Primary care providers have been tasked by the American Academy of Pediatrics (AAP) to assess development at every routine preventative visit throughout childhood.[21] Additionally, the AAP encourages pediatricians to use standardized developmental screening tools (e.g., Ages and Stages Questionnaires—ASQ and Parents' Evaluation of Developmental Status—PEDS) at the 9-, 18-, and 24- or 30-month visit, and an autism-specific screening tool at the 18- and 24-month visits (e.g., Modified Checklist for Autism in Toddlers—MCHAT).[21,22] Once concerns are raised by routine surveillance or screening measures, children should be referred to early intervention and early childhood programs, as well as to developmental specialists, when indicated.[21]

Early recognition of developmental disorders depends on children having access to preventative medical care, and almost 25% of children with special health care needs might not have that access.[23] The nature and severity of the developmental deficits also contribute to the age at recognition. The sensitivity of developmental and autism screening measures rarely reaches 0.9,[21] and so relatively mild developmental deficits may go undetected. For children with ASD, the mean age of diagnosis has been around 53 months,[5] though children with intellectual disability and those diagnosed with autistic disorder are typically diagnosed earlier; children with higher IQ scores and those eventually diagnosed with Asperger disorder, whose limitations do not include communication delays, are typically diagnosed later.[5] Some individuals with particularly subtle deficits may not be diagnosed until adulthood. Individual symptoms that may lead to an earlier diagnosis of ASD may include severe language deficits, hand flapping, toe walking, and sustained odd play.[24]

DIAGNOSIS

ID is defined by both the American Psychiatric Association and the American Association on Intellectual and Developmental Disability (AAIDD) as a disorder with deficits in intellectual and adaptive functioning in conceptual, social, and practical domains.[1,25] The Diagnostic and Statistical Manual of Mental Disorders, Fifth Edition (DSM-V) requires that the disability has onset "during the developmental period," whereas the AAIDD requires the disability to start before age 18 years. Intellectual functioning is assessed clinically and by standardized tests of intelligence, like IQ testing (e.g., Wechsler Intelligence Scale for Children and the Stanford–Binet Intelligence Scale), with a cutoff being two standard deviations below the mean for the general population, or a score of around 65 to 75, for disability.[1] Older references focused diagnosis primarily around IQ scores, and subcategories of intellectual disability (then called mental retardation) were set to specific IQ scores.[1] Current methods of diagnosis focus more on measures of adaptive functioning, because this is more relevant to planning treatment and supports. Adaptive functioning is also assessed clinically or with standardized tests of adaptive functioning (e.g., Vineland Adaptive Behavior Scales). Subcategories for intellectual disability in the DSM-V are now based on levels of adaptive functioning, mild, moderate, severe, and profound. As standardized testing for intellectual and adaptive functioning is typically valid for children above the age of 5 years, for children younger than 5 years, the diagnosis of GDD is used and describes significant delays in two or more developmental domains, including gross/fine motor, speech/language, cognition, social/personal, and activities of daily living.[26]

ASD is defined by the DSM-V as the presence of persistent impairment in reciprocal social communication and social interaction, and restricted, repetitive patterns of behavior, interests, or activities, present from early childhood, and impairing everyday functioning (Table 88-1).[1] The diagnosis is made clinically, though standardized behavioral diagnostic instruments, including caregiver interviews, questionnaires, and clinician observation measures

Table 88-1
***DSM-V* Criteria for ASD[1]**

A. Persistent deficits in social communication and social interaction across multiple contexts, as manifested by all of the following, currently or by history (examples below):
  1. Deficits in social–emotional reciprocity, ranging, for example, from abnormal social approach and failure of normal back-and-forth conversation; to reduced sharing of interests, emotions, or affect; to failure to initiate or respond to social interactions.
  2. Deficits in nonverbal communicative behaviors used for social interaction, ranging, for example, from poorly integrated verbal and nonverbal communication; to abnormalities in eye contact and body language or deficits in understanding and use of gestures; to a total lack of facial expressions and nonverbal communication.
  3. Deficits in developing, maintaining, and understanding relationships, ranging, for example, from difficulties adjusting behavior to suit various social contexts; to difficulties in sharing imaginative play or in making friends; to absence of interest in peers.

B. Restricted, repetitive patterns of behavior, interests, or activities, as manifested by at least two of the following, currently or by history (examples below):
  1. Stereotyped or repetitive motor movements, use of objects, or speech (e.g., simple motor stereotypies, lining up toys or flipping objects, echolalia, idiosyncratic phrases).
  2. Insistence on sameness, inflexible adherence to routines, or ritualized patterns or verbal nonverbal behavior (e.g., extreme distress at small changes, difficulties with transitions, rigid thinking patterns, greeting rituals, need to take same route or eat food every day).
  3. Highly restricted, fixated interests that are abnormal in intensity or focus (e.g., strong attachment to or preoccupation with unusual objects, excessively circumscribed or perseverative interest).
  4. Hyper- or hyporeactivity to sensory input or unusual interests in sensory aspects of the environment (e.g., apparent indifference to pain/temperature, adverse response to specific sounds or textures, excessive smelling or touching of objects, visual fascination with lights or movement).

  Severity is based on social communication impairments and restricted, repetitive patterns of behavior [Level 1 (requiring support), Level 2 (requiring substantial support), Level 3 (requiring very substantial support)]

C. Symptoms must be present in the early developmental period (but may not become fully manifest until social demands exceed limited capacities, or may be masked by learned strategies in later life).

D. Symptoms cause clinically significant impairment in social, occupational, or other important areas of current functioning.

E. These disturbances are not better explained by intellectual disability (intellectual developmental disorder) or global developmental delay. Intellectual disability and autism spectrum disorder frequently co-occur; to make comorbid diagnoses of autism spectrum disorder and intellectual disability, social communication should be below that expected for general developmental level.

(e.g., Autism Diagnostic Interview and Autism Diagnostic Observation Schedule), are available to potentially assist in diagnosis.

After a child is identified to have a developmental disorder, further diagnostic workup is warranted to identify an etiologic cause, because some causes may be treatable (e.g., metabolic disorder), some may inform of other potential comorbid medical problems (e.g., cardiac conditions in Down syndrome and fragile X syndrome), and some may help inform parents of risks for future children. This further etiologic workup should include a thorough medical history (including prenatal and birth history), a family history going back three or more generations, and a physical and neurologic examination focused on findings consistent with recognizable syndromes.[4]

If children with ID or GDD still do not have a known etiologic cause after this workup, they should be referred for chromosomal microarray and possibly screening for inborn errors of metabolism given the treatable nature of some metabolic disorders.[4] The American College of Medical Genetics and Genomics proposes that in the event of a diagnosis of ASD without a known cause despite the above workup, all children should undergo chromosomal microarray, those children with clinical indicators should undergo metabolic or mitochondrial testing, fragile X testing should be performed for all boys, MECP2 (Rett syndrome) testing should be performed in all girls, PTEN testing in children with macrocephaly, and neuroimaging only if specific clinical indicators (e.g., seizures, regression, history of stupor/coma, microcephaly).[27]

CASE 88-1

Question 1: L.B. is a 3-year-old boy who is brought to his pediatrician for a well-child visit. During the behavioral health screening, his mother notes that L.B. speaks very few words, does not express many different emotions on his face, does not seem to share enjoyment in activities, and remains fairly unmotivated to interact with other children in daycare. He has more recently been making repetitive loud "woop"-ing sounds that are nonprompted and occur multiple times per day. He also becomes quite aggressive during any transitions. During the visit, the pediatrician completes the Childhood Autism Rating Scale, Second Edition (CARS-2). The result is a score of 32, suggesting a diagnosis of autism spectrum disorder (ASD). The pediatrician refers L.B. and his mother to a developmental pediatrician, who specializes in ASD, for further evaluation. After a thorough evaluation, and review of the differential diagnosis, L.B. is given a diagnosis of ASD and is referred for applied behavior analysis (ABA) services.

What signs and symptoms of autism spectrum disorder does L.B. demonstrate?

Based on the DSM-5 criteria for ASD, L.B. is showing persistent deficits in social communication and social interaction in multiple settings, as demonstrated by his deficits in nonverbal communication (poor facial expressions), lack of relationship building with children, and poor social–emotional reciprocity (lack of shared enjoyment). L.B. also demonstrates restricted, repetitive patterns of behavior with his stereotyped "woop"-ing noises and his inflexible insistence on sameness, with aggression associated with transitions.

OVERVIEW OF TREATMENT

Therapy and Psychosocial Interventions

Individuals with ID or ASD can benefit from many different services to help with issues of communication, social skills, sensory integration, behavior modification, gross and fine motor, executive functioning, and adaptive functioning. Most of these services are provided to children through the public education system, at no cost to the families, as ensured by the Individuals with Disabilities Education Act (IDEA). The IDEA provides all states with grants to provide early intervention services for children with developmental delays under the age of 3. Services vary between states, though each child and family are evaluated and given an Individualized Family Service Plan (IFSP), which spells out the services to be provided, which may include, but are not limited to, physical therapy, occupational therapy, speech and language therapy, and behavioral therapy. For children reaching the age of 3 years, and still eligible for specialized education, an Individualized Education Plan (IEP) is drafted, which outlines the services to be provided in the school setting, starting in preschool. IEP services could include all of the same types of services as above, as well academic support, social skills groups, social pragmatics counseling, vocational training, and emotional counseling. IEPs are required to be reevaluated every 3 years, with updated testing and evaluation. Families must consent to both IFSPs and IEPs, and if they disagree with the supports proposed, there is a process by which they can appeal to have changes made.

Despite the services assured by the IDEA, children and families with developmental disabilities also often receive psychosocial services in their communities. In fact, in the 2011 Survey of Pathways to Diagnosis and Services, almost two-thirds of children with ASD and/or ID were receiving a community-based service.[28] The odds of using any school- or community-based service were almost 8 times more likely for children with ASD, and over 9 times more likely for children with ID, compared to children without those respective diagnoses.[28]

To address the core symptoms of ASD, which include social communication deficits and repetitive, restricted behaviors and interest, the most prevalent treatment modality has been applied behavior analysis (ABA). ABA is a behavioral therapy rooted in the concepts of operant conditioning, in which an antecedent leads to a behavior, which results in a consequence. In ABA, preferred behavior, such as an appropriate social response, is reinforced with an incentive. Classic ABA employs the use of discrete trial training (DTT), in which specific skills are broken down into discrete components and systematically taught in highly structured settings, often using incentives like food and stickers. Critics of this form of ABA worry that children with ASD are unlikely to apply the learned skills outside of the trial setting. As a result, multiple different therapy approaches have been created, such as Pivotal Response Therapy and the Early Start Denver Model, both derivations of ABA, and the Developmental, Individual-differences, Relationship-based (DIR) Floortime approach, which all operate in more naturalistic settings, focus more on building child initiation and motivation, and employ natural incentives like positive affect and affection. The research evidence to support such interventions for children and young adults with ASD varies widely, as is explored in Wong et al.'s[29] comprehensive recent review. Operant conditioning though, and the principles of manipulating antecedents, behavior, and reinforcements, remains the mainstay for the treatment of aggressive behaviors in individuals with developmental disabilities.[30]

Individuals with ID often require the same types of interventions as individuals with ASD, though perhaps with a stronger emphasis on adaptive functioning training, and building skills of independent living. Likewise, for individuals with ID, the evidence base for psychological interventions is varied. One recent review and meta-analysis of psychological therapies for individuals with ID showed that in the literature, individual therapy seems to be superior to group interventions, and moderate to large effect sizes exist for therapy for depression and anger, though there is no evidence that therapy has an effect on interpersonal functioning.[31]

Pharmacologic Interventions

The evidence supporting psychopharmacologic interventions in individuals with ID/ASD is relatively limited. There are only a few large double-blind, randomized, placebo-controlled trials (RCTs), many of which were funded by, or affiliated with, the manufacturers of the particular study medications. Most of the existing RCTs are for individuals with ASD and are of children and adolescents, likely, in part, because of the complications involved in consenting adults with ID/ASD to participate in research. Additionally, the targets for medication intervention with the strongest research evidence are behaviors, which relay little about any possible underlying emotional etiology for the individual.

Despite the limitations of the evidence, clinicians working with individuals with ID/ASD know that medications can often serve a very important role as part of a comprehensive treatment plan. Although much of the literature is of studies of children with ASD, it should be noted that a large percentage of these studies contained many individuals with comorbid ID (76%,[32] 71%,[33] 53%,[34] mean IQ, 63[35,36]). However, the literature confirms that individuals with ID/ASD are more sensitive to adverse events from medications compared to their neurotypical peers, and therefore, pharmacologic interventions should be performed with caution.

At the time of this writing, there are no medications approved by the U.S. Food and Drug Administration (FDA) to treat any of the core diagnostic elements of ID/ASD. The target symptom behaviors with the most research evidence include hyperactivity, irritability, repetitive behaviors, and self-injurious behavior. As anxiety disorders are the most common comorbid psychiatric conditions in individuals with ID/ASD, anxiety/depression is another frequent target for psychopharmacologic intervention, though with considerably less research support. Sleep disturbances are also remarkably common in individuals with developmental disabilities and often are a target for medication intervention.

Hyperactivity

Individuals with ID/ASD have high rates of comorbid ADHD, with literature in children with ASD showing prevalence rates of about 30% for children derived from community, nonclinical, populations (28%[37] and 31%[38]), and 41% to 78% for children evaluated in the clinical setting.[39] The mainstay of treatment for symptoms of ADHD in individuals with ID/ASD, like their neurotypical peers, includes stimulants, α_2 agonists, and atomoxetine.

Stimulants

Stimulants are a group of medications derived either from methylphenidate or amphetamine that act by increasing the amount of dopamine and norepinephrine in the neuronal synaptic cleft. This increase in dopamine and norepinephrine is the result of blocking the reuptake of dopamine and norepinephrine (methylphenidate and amphetamine) and increasing the release of dopamine and norepinephrine (amphetamine).

Reichow et al.,[40] in their recent meta-analysis of pharmacologic treatments of symptoms of ADHD in children with PDD, found four RCTs of stimulant medications. All four RCTs studied methylphenidate and found it to be superior to placebo for the treatment of global ADHD symptomatology and specifically hyperactivity. In the largest of the four RCTs ($n = 66$),[41] effect sizes for hyperactivity and impulsivity symptoms were greater than for inattention symptoms (0.77 vs. 0.60 for parent rating; 0.48 vs. 0.35 for teacher rating).[35]

The effect size for the treatment of ADHD symptoms in children with PDD (0.67 for methylphenidate),[40] however, was lower than estimates in a meta-analysis of stimulant treatment of typically developing children with ADHD (0.77 for methylphenidate and 1.03 for amphetamine).[42] In the study conducted by the Research Unit on Pediatric Psychopharmacology (RUPP) group,[41] 49% of children experienced a therapeutic response, compared to 69% in the Multimodal Treatment Study of Children with ADHD (MTA), which studied mostly neurotypical children (ID was an exclusion criteria, and ASD was not mentioned as a comorbid diagnosis in any participants).[43]

Adverse events were more common in children with PDD treated with methylphenidate versus placebo, with increased rates of decreased appetite, insomnia, depressive symptoms, irritability, and social withdrawal.[40] Rates of adverse events with methylphenidate were also larger in children with PDD compared to typically developing children, as evidenced by 18% of RUPP study participants[41] discontinuing the medication due to adverse events (primarily irritability), compared to 1.4% in the MTA study.[43]

Mean dosage in the four RCTs ranged from 0.29 to 0.45 mg/kg/dose.[40] Secondary analysis of the RUPP study data showed that methylphenidate doses of 0.25 and 0.5 mg/kg/dose were more consistently effective for treating ADHD symptoms than the lower 0.125 mg/kg/dose.[35] The highest dose used in the RUPP study was 0.625 mg/kg/dose, compared to the MTA study, in which the highest dose used was 0.8 mg/kg/dose.[41]

Daily methylphenidate doses may be titrated weekly, until an optimal dose is obtained. Improvement in symptoms should be noted within the first week.[44]

Overall, the research literature shows that methylphenidate can be used to improve ADHD symptoms, especially hyperactivity, in children with PDD, though with lower effect sizes, lower tolerated doses, and more risk of adverse effects than children without developmental disabilities.

Although no RCTs have been conducted studying the effects of amphetamine-derived stimulants for the treatment of ADHD in children with ASD, consensus guidelines suggest that amphetamine salts can be an option for children demonstrating insufficient benefit or dose-limiting adverse events from methylphenidate.[45]

α_2 Agonists

Although the exact mechanism in ADHD is unknown, α_2 agonists are thought to work by stimulating the α_2 adrenoceptors on norepinephrine-containing neuron cell bodies in the locus coeruleus which modulates the tonic and phasic firing to the prefrontal cortex. This allows the person to have increased attention on the desired task.[46]

α_2 Agonists include clonidine, a nonselective α_2 adrenergic receptor agonist, and guanfacine, a selective α_2A adrenergic receptor agonist. α_2 Agonists were initially marketed for the treatment of hypertension, though have been shown to also improve symptoms of ADHD.

For clonidine, one small study ($n = 8$)[47] was identified by Reichow et al.[40] looking at clonidine versus placebo for the treatment of ADHD in children with PDD. Although the original study found no statistically significant results, the effect size calculated by Reichow et al.[40] for improvement in ADHD symptoms and irritability was in the medium range ($g = 0.51$ and 0.64, respectively) and smaller for improvements in hyperactivity ($g = 0.30$) and stereotypic behavior (0.24). The authors of the original study[47] report increased rates of hypotension and drowsiness in some children who took clonidine. Mean dosage ranged from 0.15 to 0.20 mg/day.

One small pilot RCT ($n = 11$) looking at guanfacine treatment in children with developmental disabilities showed statistically significant reductions in hyperactivity subscales and global rating of improvement, with 5 of the 11 participants deemed to be responders.[48] In this study, adverse events included drowsiness, irritability, and enuresis, as well as diarrhea, constipation, and social withdrawal; additional adverse events from an open-label study of guanfacine in children with PDD include sleep disturbance (insomnia or midsleep awakening).[49] Doses in both studies ranged from 1 to 3 mg/day.

Overall, a small collection of literature suggests that clonidine and guanfacine may be beneficial for the treatment of ADHD symptoms in children with ASD/ID, with similar adverse events as reported in neurotypical children, though more evidence is needed to draw any more extensive conclusions about the use of these medications in the ID/ASD population.

Atomoxetine

Atomoxetine is a medication for ADHD that acts by inhibiting the reuptake of norepinephrine, therefore increasing the amount of norepinephrine in the synaptic cleft. Dosing is generally once daily, with adjustments after a minimum of 3 days to a target daily dose. Clinical benefit has been noted within the first 1 to 2 weeks.[50]

Reichow et al.'s[40] meta-analysis found two RCTs comparing atomoxetine to placebo in children with PDD, though only the larger of the two ($n = 97$)[51] showed statistically significant benefits for the treatment of global ADHD symptoms and hyperactivity (effect sizes calculated by Reichow et al.[40] of $g = 0.83$ and g 0.80, respectively). In this study by Harfterkamp et al.,[51] changes in the subscales of inattention and oppositional behavior did not reach statistical significance for children on atomoxetine compared to placebo.

Children with PDD in the Harfterkamp et al.[51] study demonstrated increased rates of nausea, decreased appetite, and early morning awakening compared to study participants taking placebo. Mean dosage in the two studies was 1.2 mg/kg/day[51] and 44.2 mg/day.[52] This dosing is perhaps only slightly lower than other large studies of atomoxetine in children with ADHD without developmental disorders (mean final atomoxetine dose was 1.45 mg/kg/day, 53.0 mg/day[53]), though documentation from the drug manufacturer's studies, of presumably mostly neurotypical children with ADHD, indicates no additional benefits for doses above 1.2 mg/kg/day.[50]

Similar to the α_2 agonists, it seems that atomoxetine shows benefits in the literature for addressing ADHD symptoms in children with PDD, particularly for hyperactive symptoms, with similar dosing and adverse events to children with ADHD without developmental disorders.

Other Medications

Tricyclic antidepressants (TCA), which primarily act as serotonin–norepinephrine reuptake inhibitors (SNRIs), had been a part of older treatment algorithms for the treatment of ADHD in typically developing children[54] and, as a result, have also been studied in children with ASD. In Gordon et al.'s crossover RCT of clomipramine and desipramine versus placebo[55] (5 weeks each intervention), both drugs were significantly superior to placebo for reducing the hyperactivity domain of the Children's Psychiatric Rating Scale (CPRS) Autism Relevant Subscale, though no different from each other. TCAs are known for adverse effects, primarily antimuscarinic in nature, which includes dry mouth, blurred vision, decreased gastrointestinal motility, and urinary retention. TCAs can also cause irregular heart rhythms, tachycardia and hypotension, and should be used in caution in patients with preexisting cardiac conditions and can be fatal with just small excesses in dose. TCAs are also highly metabolized by the cytochrome P450 hepatic enzymes, including 3A4 and 2D6. Therefore, inhibitors of these enzymes can lead to increased concentrations and higher risk of side effects including cardiac abnormalities.

Although antipsychotic medications are not typically part of the treatment algorithm for ADHD in children with typical development,[54,56] studies of risperidone and aripiprazole for the treatment of children with ASD and irritability/aggression symptoms did show statistically significant improvement in hyperactivity subscales (Risperidone[32–34]; Aripiprazole[57,58]). As a result, atypical antipsychotics are part of a treatment algorithm developed by the Autism Speaks Autism Treatment Network Psychopharmacology Committee Medication Choice Subcommittee for symptoms of ADHD in individuals with ASD, if they have not shown adequate improvement from stimulants, atomoxetine, and α_2 agonists.[45]

Other medications, which have not yet been included in standard practice, though have shown some promising evidence for improvement in hyperactivity symptoms in RCTs of children with ASD, include omega-3 fatty acids,[59] tianeptine,[60] and adjunctive pentoxifylline[61] and topiramate,[62] when each added to risperidone.

CASE 88-1, QUESTION 2: L.B., now 5 years of age, has been receiving ABA services for nearly 2 years and has been progressing well. At home though, L.B. has become increasingly disobedient and hyperactive. In school, his teachers note that he is inattentive, wandering around the classroom and staring out the windows. In addition, during story time and craft time, he is disruptive and hyperactive, running around the room. In response, L.B.'s pediatrician facilitates an increase in the number of hours of in-home ABA services, whose providers also work with L.B.'s parents' teaching behavioral management techniques. The pediatrician also recommends certain classroom modifications to help with attention. This, however, does not reduce the outbursts or inattentive and hyperactive behavior, both at home and school. The pediatrician believes that a trial of pharmacotherapy may be helpful. The pediatrician consults you, the clinical pharmacist, to discuss an appropriate treatment plan.

What pharmacotherapy and formulation would be most appropriate for L.B.'s target symptoms?

Clinical trials have shown that stimulants can be a very effective treatment option for children with attention-deficit/hyperactivity disorder (ADHD). The American Academy of Child and Adolescent Psychiatry (AACAP) and the American Academy of Pediatrics (AAP) recommend the use of methylphenidate, over that of amphetamines or nonstimulant medication, in preschool children where behavioral modification therapy has not been adequate. The metabolism of methylphenidate in preschool children is slower than that of older children, and therefore the starting dose is lower, and the optimal dose is likely lower than in older children.

Based on this information, you recommend starting L.B. on methylphenidate IR solution 1.25 mg twice daily, with an increase to 2.5 mg twice daily on day 3, with subsequent dose increases every 3 days to reduce target symptoms, up to a maximum of 7.5 mg 3 times daily. You recommend that the parents keep a journal of the responses and possible experienced adverse effects during this period with a report back to the pediatrician at the end of the week.

Irritability/Aggression

Irritability/aggression is the pharmacologic target behavior with the most robust RCT evidence in children with ASD. Most of this evidence comes from four large RCTs of either risperidone or aripiprazole.[32,33,57,58] In this context, risperidone and aripiprazole are the only two medications with FDA approval for the use in individuals with developmental disabilities. Specifically, each has an FDA-approved indication for the treatment of autistic disorder-associated irritability in children and adolescents (risperidone—age 5–17 years; aripiprazole—age 6–17 years).

Risperidone

Both McCracken et al.'s[32] and Shea et al.'s[33] studies of risperidone were 8 weeks in duration, in a population of children and adolescents with either solely autistic disorder,[32] or mostly autistic disorder[33] (70% of study population had autistic disorder; rest were diagnosed with either PDD NOS, Asperger disorder, or childhood disintegrative disorder), and with mostly comorbid ID (64% of study population[33]; 81% of study population[32]). Both showed risperidone to have statistically significant improvements, compared to placebo, in the Irritability subscale of the Aberrant Behavior Checklist (ABC-I) (ABC-I is a 15-item subscale that includes items such as "injures self," "physical violence to self," "aggressive to other children and adults," "irritable," "temper outbursts," "depressed mood," "mood changes," and "yells" or "screams" inappropriately; individual items are rated on a scale ranging from 0—not at all a problem, to 3—severe),[58] as well as the ABC subscales for hyperactivity and stereotypy. The subscales for social withdrawal and inappropriate speech only showed statistically significant improvements for risperidone compared to placebo in Shea et al.'s study.[33] The definition of "response" was different in each study. In McCracken et al.,[32] positive response was defined as at least a 25% decrease in the ABC-I score and a rating of much improved or very much improved on the Clinical Global Impression rating scale (CGI), improvement subscale (CGI-I). With this definition, 69% were responders in the risperidone group and 12% in the placebo group. In Shea et al.,[33] a responder was defined as having a 50% or greater decrease from baseline in at least two of the five ABC subscales with none of the other subscales presenting a 10% or larger increase. With this definition, 69% of subjects in the risperidone group were responders, compared to 40% in the placebo group.

In McCracken et al.,[32] study participants in the risperidone group, compared to placebo, experienced significantly higher rates of increased appetite, fatigue, drowsiness, dizziness, and drooling, with trends of increased rates of tremor, tachycardia, and constipation ($P = 0.06$). In a 16-week open-label extension of McCracken et al.'s[32] study, the most common adverse events were excessive appetite, enuresis, tired during day, dry mouth, excess saliva, rhinitis, coughing, and anxiety.[63] Risperidone-treated participants in Shea et al.'s study[33] experienced significantly greater increases in weight, pulse rate, and systolic blood pressure and had a significantly higher rate of reported somnolence (73% risperidone vs. 8% placebo). Extrapyramidal symptoms (EPS) were endorsed by 28% of the risperidone-treated participants in Shea et al.,[33] compared to 13% in the placebo group. Mean weight gain in both 8-week studies for those taking risperidone was 2.7 kg. Mean final daily risperidone dose was 1.8[32] and 1.48 mg,[33] which is in contrast to the mean final daily risperidone dose of 2.8 mg in a large RCT of the antipsychotic treatment of early-onset schizophrenia and schizoaffective disorder in children and adolescents (ID was an exclusion criteria).[64]

Although prolactin was not mentioned in either 8-week study of risperidone, a long-term follow-up of the McCracken et al.[32] study confirmed that risperidone treatment was associated with a 2- to 4-fold increase in serum prolactin levels.[65]

McDougle et al.'s[66] study of risperidone in adults with ASD showed similarly beneficial findings for the reduction in aggressive behavior, compared to placebo, and common adverse events also included sedation and weight gain. The mean final daily dose of risperidone was 2.9 mg, which is in contrast to the mean daily dose of risperidone of 3.9 mg in a large RCT of adults with schizophrenia.[67]

Aripiprazole

Both Marcus et al.'s[58] and Owen et al.'s[57] studies of aripiprazole versus placebo in children and adolescents with autistic disorder were 8 weeks in duration. Prevalence of comorbid ID was not mentioned in either study. Both studies showed statistically significant improvement in children treated with aripiprazole, compared to placebo, for ABC-I, CGI-I, as well as ABC subscales of hyperactivity and stereotypy. Although Owen et al.'s[57] flexible dosing schedule showed statistically significant improvements in the ABC subscale for inappropriate speech with aripiprazole versus placebo, in Marcus et al.'s[58] fixed-dose study, only the 15 mg/day dose of aripiprazole showed statistically significant improvement in inappropriate speech. Neither study showed statistically significant improvement for aripiprazole, versus placebo for the ABC lethargy/social withdrawal subscale. Both studies defined response as at least a 25% reduction from baseline to endpoint in the ABC-I subscale and a CGI-I score of 1 (very much improved) or 2 (much improved) at endpoint. With this definition, response rate was 52.2% for aripiprazole in Owen et al.'s study[57] (14.3% for placebo) and although response rates for each dose of aripiprazole (5 mg—55.8%*, 10 mg—49.2%, 15 mg—52.8%) were higher than placebo (34.7%) in Marcus et al.'s study,[58] only the response rate at 5 mg/day separated from placebo with statistical significance.

In Marcus et al.'s study,[58] the three most common adverse events leading to discontinuation of aripiprazole were sedation, drooling, and tremor, none of which were reported in the placebo group. The most common adverse events reported in the aripiprazole group of Owen et al.'s study[57] were fatigue, somnolence, vomiting, increased appetite, and sedation. In Owen et al.,[57] 14.9% of aripiprazole-treated subjects (vs. 8% for placebo) endorsed EPS symptoms, with the most common being tremor (8.5%). In Marcus et al.,[58] EPS symptoms were reported at roughly twice the rate in all aripiprazole doses (5 mg/day—23.1%, 10 mg/day—22.0%, and 15 mg/day—22.2%) compared to placebo (11.8%), the most common of which were tremor and extrapyramidal disorder. Aripiprazole was associated with statistically significant gains in weight compared to placebo after 8 weeks, with the mean weight gain on aripiprazole in Owen et al.[57] being 2.0 kg, and for Marcus et al.,[58] 1.3 kg (5 mg/day), 1.3 kg (10 mg/day), and 1.5 kg (15 mg/day). Interestingly, both studies showed aripiprazole to have statistically significant reductions in prolactin levels compared to placebo. Mean final daily dosing for aripiprazole in Owen et al.[57] was 8.9 mg/day. In a 52-week open-label follow-up study of participants from both Owen et al.[57] and Marcus et al.,[58] as well as newly enrolled subjects, mean final daily dosing of aripiprazole was 10.6 mg/day.[68] In a 2-month RCT of aripiprazole versus risperidone in children with ASD, the mean final daily dose of aripiprazole was 5.5 mg.[69] Manufacturer recommended daily dosing of aripiprazole in pediatric patients with schizophrenia or bipolar disorder is 10 mg/day.[70]

Overall, the literature shows that risperidone and aripiprazole, in doses likely lower than that used in children with schizophrenia or bipolar disorder, can be used effectively to reduce symptoms of irritability and aggressive behavior in children and adolescents with ASD, though treatment should be monitored closely for relatively common adverse events of sedation, weight gain, and EPS. Of note, although risperidone has been shown to consistently increase prolactin levels, aripiprazole was shown to consistently lower prolactin levels.

Although risperidone and aripiprazole are the two antipsychotic medications with FDA approval for the treatment of irritability in children with ASD, other typical and atypical antipsychotics have also demonstrated benefits for treating symptoms of irritability in children with ASD. Haloperidol, dosed in the range of 0.5 to 4.0 mg/day, has shown benefits in four RCTs and two long-term follow-up studies, though with significant rates of dyskinesia (34%).[71] One RCT supports the benefits of pimozide, one RCT supports the use of olanzapine, and either open-label studies or case reports exist to support the benefits of olanzapine, clozapine, quetiapine, ziprasidone, and paliperidone.[72] A head-to-head comparison RCT of risperidone and haloperidol in children with autistic disorder showed risperidone to be significantly more effective than haloperidol at reducing aberrant behavior and symptoms of PDD.[73] An RCT though comparing risperidone, haloperidol, and placebo for the treatment of aggression in adults with ID showed all three treatment arms to decrease aggression, though no significant difference between any of the three treatments.[74]

Other Medications

VALPROATE

Two RCTs of similar size ($n = 30$[75] and $n = 27$[36]) looked at valproate versus placebo in children and adolescents with ASD and irritability/aggression with somewhat conflicting results. Hellings et al.[75] found no significant difference in improvement of irritability or aggression (including ABC-I and CGI-I) between valproate and placebo after 8 weeks, whereas Hollander et al.,[36] after 12 weeks, showed valproate to be significantly superior to placebo at improving CGI-I and the rate of improvement of ABC-I. While in Hollander et al.,[36] no significant differences existed in adverse events between valproate and placebo, in Hellings et al.,[75] there was a significantly increased rate of endorsed appetite increase in the valproate group, and two individuals in the valproate group developed elevated ammonia levels, one with clinically associated symptoms. Both studies had target blood valproate levels (at least 50 mcg/mL,[36] 70–100 mcg/mL[75]).

Additional medications with either limited RCT data, open-label studies, or case reports to support its use for irritability in individuals with ASD include buspirone, clomipramine, clonidine, levetiracetam, memantine, mirtazapine, pioglitazone, topiramate (when added to risperidone), riluzole, sertraline, and trazodone,[72] as well as fluvoxamine[76] and lithium.[77] In Reichow et al. recent meta-analysis of medications for the treatment of ADHD symptoms in children with PDD, methylphenidate had moderate, though not statistically significant, benefits in treating irritability.[40]

CASE 88-2

QUESTION 1: C.Y., a 9-year-old girl with ASD has been well maintained on risperidone for the last 3 years. At the most recent checkup, the prescriber notes that she has gained ~25 lbs over the last 2 years (note that average weight gain for a 9-year-old child is approximately 5 lbs/year). The majority of weight gained seems to be in the abdominal area. Blood tests note an elevated hemoglobin A1C of 8.4%. The provider discusses diet and exercise, but C.Y.'s mother notes no change over the last few years. She believes her weight gain started with the addition of risperidone, which is now at 4 mg/day.

The prescriber asks you for a recommendation based on your knowledge of the metabolic profiles of atypical antipsychotics. You make the following recommendation.

Although risperidone and aripiprazole are not necessarily interchangeable, both are indicated for the treatment of irritability in children with ASD, and aripiprazole may convey less of a risk for weight gain than risperidone. This potential benefit may outweigh the potential risk of aripiprazole being less clinically efficacious than risperidone in some patients. In this context, you may recommend for the prescriber to decrease risperidone by 1 mg every other week, while starting aripiprazole 2 mg/day for 7 days followed by an increase to 5 mg daily. Additional 5 mg dose increases can be made weekly up to a maximum of 15 mg/day. C.Y. should be monitored for tolerability during both the cross-taper/titration period and beyond.

REPETITIVE BEHAVIORS

Numerous different types of medications have been studied for the treatment of repetitive behaviors in individuals with ASD. Selective serotonin reuptake inhibitors (SSRIs) and TCAs have been studied likely due to perceived similarities between the repetitive behaviors and compulsions exhibited in children with obsessive–compulsive disorder, as well as the clinical observation that repetitive behaviors may increase in children with PDD due to underlying anxiety. However, the literature is mixed to support the use of SSRIs or TCAs for this indication.

Selective Serotonin Reuptake Inhibitors

Two RCTs looking at SSRIs for children with ASD and repetitive behavior demonstrate conflicting results. Hollander et al.'s[78] crossover trial ($n = 39$, mean age, 8.2 years) showed that low-dose liquid fluoxetine was superior to placebo for treating repetitive behaviors, as measured by the Children's Yale-Brown Obsessive Compulsive Scale (CY-BOCS) compulsion subscale, with a medium to large effect size (0.76), though did not separate from placebo for improvements in other aspects of global autism severity. In King et al.'s[79] large study of citalopram ($n = 73$) versus placebo ($n = 76$) to target repetitive behaviors in children with ASD, there were no statistically significant differences between citalopram and placebo in improvements in overall symptomatology (CGI-I) or repetitive behaviors on the modified CY-BOCS-PDD rating scale. An RCT of fluvoxamine versus placebo in adults with ASD ($n = 15$ each group), however, did show fluvoxamine to be significantly superior to placebo for improving repetitive thoughts and behavior.[76] [See below in anxiety/depression for more details on SSRI prescribing in children with ASD].

TCAs

Clomipramine was studied in Gordon et al.'s[55] RCT, in which it was shown to be significantly superior to both placebo and desipramine for the treatment of repetitive behavior in children with ASD as shown by the Modified CPRS OCD subscale, the modified National Institute of Mental Health (NIMH) OCD Scale, and the modified NIMH Global OCD and Anxiety scales. The mean final week daily dose of clomipramine was 152 mg; the mean final week clomipramine blood level was 235 ng/mL and desmethyl clomipramine level was 422 ng/mL. Overall adverse events were relatively minor, though in those taking clomipramine, one person had a seizure, and two had cardiac adverse events, one with a prolonged corrected QT interval (0.45 seconds) and the other with severe tachycardia (160–170 beats/minute), both of which resolved with reduction in dose. In Remington et al.'s[80] crossover RCT (7 weeks each intervention) comparing clomipramine to haloperidol in children with autistic disorder, the most striking finding was that only 37.5% of participants taking clomipramine finished the study (compared to 69.7% haloperidol and 65.6% for placebo), with adverse events contributing to discontinuation including behavioral problems, fatigue or lethargy, tremors, tachycardia, insomnia, diaphoresis, nausea or vomiting, and decreased appetite. The mean daily dose of clomipramine was 128.4 mg, range 100 to 150 mg.

Overall, for the reduction of repetitive behaviors, SSRIs, specifically fluoxetine, and TCAs, specifically clomipramine, may be helpful in children with ASD, though adverse events may be particularly limiting for clomipramine. For adults with ASD, SSRIs, specifically fluvoxamine, may be helpful in reducing repetitive behaviors.

Antipsychotics

Antipsychotics have shown the most robust evidence in reducing repetitive behaviors in children with ASD. Nearly all of the data to support antipsychotics for this purpose come from the same studies that targeted irritability. Both aripiprazole[57,58] and risperidone[32,33] were superior to placebo for reducing the score on the ABC Stereotypy subscale. In McDougle et al.'s[81] secondary analysis of the 8-week RUPP Risperidone trial,[32] risperidone resulted in significantly greater reductions, compared to placebo, in the scores on the modified compulsion subscale of the CY-BOCS (effect size, 0.55), and the sensory motor behaviors subscale of the Ritvo–Freeman Real Life Rating Scale (effect size, 0.45). Similar findings for risperidone's benefit for reducing repetitive behaviors have been found in adults with ASD, including McDougle et al.'s RCT,[66] which found statistically significant reductions in the modified version of the Y-BOCS (focusing only on repetitive behavior, not thoughts).

Stimulants

In Reichow et al. recent meta-analysis of medications for the treatment of ADHD symptoms in children with PDD, methylphenidate had moderate, though not statistically significant, benefits in treating stereotypies.[40]

Other Medications

Despite valproate demonstrating efficacy for the treatment of irritability in Hollander et al.'s study of children with ASD, it showed no significant improvement in repetitive behavior, compared to placebo.[36] One small RCT of 1.5 g/day of omega-3 fatty acids (fish oil $n = 7$, placebo $n = 5$) showed no significant difference compared to placebo in reduction of ABC Stereotypy, though effect size was 0.72.[59]

SELF-INJURIOUS BEHAVIOR

Depending on the rating scale or etiologic theory, self-injurious behavior is commonly thought of as either an act of aggression toward the self, or as a repetitive, stereotyped behavior. Consequently, pharmacologic approaches to the treatment of self-injury have been rooted in the approaches for the treatment of aggression or repetitive behavior. Self-injurious behavior has its own literature base though, with similar and dissimilar findings.

Typical and Atypical Antipsychotics

RCTs of typical antipsychotics for the reduction of self-injurious behavior in individuals with developmental disabilities have had mixed findings. There has been relatively unconvincing data for the benefit of haloperidol, fluphenazine, chlorpromazine, or thioridazine in reducing self-injurious behavior.[82] Risperidone is the atypical antipsychotic with the most robust RCT data for improving self-injurious behavior, with two relatively large RCTs in children with ID showing improvement in the self-injury/stereotypic subscale of the Nisonger Child Behavior Rating Form,[83,84] one of which was statistically significant,[84] and statistically significant reductions in self-injurious behavior in adults with ASD, as measured by the Self-injurious Behavior Questionnaire.[66] Similar to studies in children with ASD, weight gain and somnolence were markedly higher in children taking risperidone than placebo.

Antidepressants

Clomipramine has been shown to be effective in reducing self-injurious behavior, but again with significant adverse effects.[82] Fluoxetine has been shown to be effective at reducing compulsive skin picking in two RCTs,[85,86] and fluvoxamine has been effective for reducing repetitive behavior and aggression in adults with ASD.[76] Case reports and open-label studies have shown possible benefit for buspirone and paroxetine as well.[82]

Naltrexone

A recent systemic review of naltrexone used in adults with intellectual disability showed 8 out of 10 RCTs demonstrating a reduction in the frequency of self-injurious behavior.[87] More specifically, 50% of participants had improvement in self-injury, with improvement being more pronounced in individuals with severe and profound ID. Nine percent experienced minor adverse events, which included weight loss, loss of appetite, thirst, yawning, mild liver function test abnormalities, nausea, and tiredness. Dosing ranged from 0.5 to 2 mg/kg, and doses from 25 to 100 mg.

Overall, despite very limited evidence, it seems the literature supports the use of risperidone, naltrexone, and clomipramine for the reduction of self-injurious behavior in individuals with developmental disabilities. Additionally, fluoxetine and fluvoxamine may have benefits as well, though less well evidenced.

ANXIETY/DEPRESSION

Selective Serotonin Reuptake Inhibitors

Studies have found that individuals with PDDs are at high risk of comorbid anxiety and mood disorders.[37,38] Due to the demonstrated benefits and relative safety of SSRIs in typically developing children, SSRIs are very commonly prescribed for anxiety and depression in children with developmental disorders. No large double-blind, placebo-controlled trials have been conducted looking at the use of SSRIs for depression or anxiety in children with developmental disorders, though the literature has numerous case reports and open-label studies demonstrating SSRI-induced improvements in anxiety in individuals with ASD.[88,89]

Overall, the literature indicates that children with DD may respond differently to SSRIs compared to children with typical development. Three areas in which response to SSRIs may differ include risk of adverse events, dosing requirements, and target symptoms.

Adverse Events

Compared to children with typical development, children with DD are more likely to experience adverse events to SSRIs and specifically are more likely to endorse emotional/behavioral adverse events. The only two RCTs looking at SSRIs in children with DD evaluated fluoxetine[78] and citalopram[79] for the treatment of repetitive behaviors. In the crossover study (8 weeks each phase) of low-dose fluoxetine by Hollander et al.[78] ($n = 39$, mean age, 8.2 years), although there was no statistically significant difference in treatment-emergent adverse events between fluoxetine and placebo, the most common adverse events emerging during fluoxetine treatment were agitation (46%), insomnia (36%), and anxiety/nervousness (16%). Additionally, 16% of subjects required a dose reduction due to agitation while on fluoxetine, compared to 5% on placebo.

In contrast, both Geller et al.[90] and Liebowitz et al.[91] conducted RCTs of fluoxetine for the treatment of OCD in typically developing children (Geller: 13 weeks; $n = 71$ fluoxetine, 32 placebo; mean age 11.4 years/Liebowitz: 8-week acute phase; $n = 21$ fluoxetine, 22 placebo; mean age, 12–13). In Geller et al.,[90] there was no statistically significant difference in reported adverse events, and the most common adverse events reported in the fluoxetine group were headache (28%), rhinitis (27%), and abdominal pain (16%), with no reports of agitation. In Liebowitz et al.,[91] six adverse events occurred significantly more frequently in the fluoxetine group: palpitations, weight loss, drowsiness, tremors, nightmares, and muscle aches, and the most common adverse events reported by those taking fluoxetine were headache (52%), abdominal pain (43%), decreased appetite (38%), difficulty staying asleep (38%), and drowsiness (38%).

For citalopram, in the 12-week study by King et al.[79] ($n = 73$ citalopram, 76 placebo; mean age ~9 years), 97.3% of subjects with ASD treated with citalopram experienced at least one treatment emergent adverse event. They were significantly more likely to experience adverse events compared to those treated with placebo, specifically: increased energy level (38%), impulsiveness (19%), decreased concentration (12%), hyperactivity (12%), stereotypy (11%), diarrhea (26%), insomnia (23.3%), and dry skin or pruritus (12%).

In contrast, in RCTs of citalopram for the treatment of depression in children and adolescents with typical development, the most commonly reported adverse events were headache, gastrointestinal issues, and insomnia.[92] Specifically in the 8-week RCT by Wagner et al.[93] of citalopram for typically developing children with depression ($n = 89$ citalopram, 85 placebo; mean age, 12 years), rhinitis (14%), nausea (14%), and abdominal pain (11%) were the only adverse events reported in >10% of subjects taking citalopram, and in the 12-week RCT by von Knorring et al.[94] of citalopram for typically developing adolescents with depression ($n = 124$ citalopram, 120 placebo; mean age, 16 years), headache (26% and 25%), nausea (19% and 15%), and insomnia (13% and 11%) were the most common in both groups (citalopram and placebo, respectively), with only fatigue being the adverse event reported significantly more often in the citalopram group (6%) than the placebo group (1%).

Dosing

Children with PDD typically require smaller doses of SSRIs compared to children with typical development and may experience adverse emotional/behavioral events at higher doses. For fluoxetine, the mean final daily dose of fluoxetine in Hollander et al.'s study[78] of children with PDD was 9.9 mg, or 0.36 mg/kg. This is compared to Geller et al.[90] and Liebowitz et al.'s[91] studies of typically developing children with OCD, in which mean final daily fluoxetine dose was 24.6 and 64.8 mg (after the acute phase), respectively. Additionally, in RCTs of typically developing children with depression and other forms of anxiety, fluoxetine was well tolerated at mean daily doses of 20 mg,[95–97] 28.4 mg and 33.3 mg,[98] and 40 mg.[99]

For citalopram, the mean daily dose in the King et al. study[79] of children with ASD and repetitive behavior was 16.5 mg. In studies of citalopram use in typically developing children and adolescents with depression, citalopram was tolerated at mean daily doses of 24[93] and 26 mg.[94]

The issue of individuals with PDD requiring lower dosages of SSRI might diminish in adulthood, because RCTs of SSRIs in adults with ASD demonstrate mean daily doses close to that expected for typically developing adults: fluoxetine—36.7[101] and 64.8 mg[101]; fluvoxamine 276.7 mg.[76]

CASE 88-3

QUESTION 1: N.W. is a 6-year-old girl with a history of supraventricular tachycardia (SVT) at birth, well controlled on propranolol since infancy. N.W. also has a diagnosis of ASD. Over the past year, she has been trialed on varying stimulant formulations and doses for the treatment of ADHD symptoms. However, N.W.'s mom reports only small improvement, but significant worsening of repetitive behavior and aggression. N.W. has been pushing, hitting, and throwing things at school and home. Additionally, N.W. has had a decrease in appetite and lost ~4 lb. At home, N.W. has recently developed a lot of anxiety, refusing to go to school and participate in outdoor activities. Her mother notes that N.W. appears to be isolating herself more and not enjoying activities that used to make her happy. The prescriber discontinues methylphenidate and starts N.W. on risperidone 1 mg/day for aggression and repetitive behaviors. She also starts her on fluoxetine 10 mg/day for depression and anxiety.

You get a call from N.W.'s mother 3 days after N.W. starts the new medication regimen. N.W.'s mother reports that N.W. is extremely lethargic, and seems confused. She fell the last few times she tried to get out of bed. You have the mother use a blood pressure cuff she has at home to measure N.W.'s vital signs. Based on the results, N.W. is bradycardic and hypotensive. What is your recommendation?

The dose of risperidone that N.W. was started on is high. Additionally, you know that fluoxetine is a strong 2D6 inhibitor, although risperidone and propranolol are 2D6 substrates. Therefore, fluoxetine may be decreasing the clearance of both the risperidone and propranolol. You decide to call the provider and discuss the interaction and adverse effects that N.W. is experiencing.

CASE 88-3, QUESTION 2: The prescriber is thankful for the call and asks for your advice on altering the current regimen. What changes would you recommend?

You recommend discontinuation of the fluoxetine and initiation of sertraline 12.5 mg/day, because sertraline is a weaker inhibitor of 2D6. You would recommend the continuation of risperidone at a reduced dose of 0.5 mg/day.

Target Symptoms

Most studies looking at symptoms of anxiety and depression in children with ASD have used rating scales validated in typically developing children. For anxiety, predictors that children with ASD will manifest a high level of parent-reported anxiety include the following: IQ > 70,[102–104] higher levels of parent-rated social impairment,[102,103] and increased age[103]; additionally, it seems that children with IQ < 70 might experience higher levels of parent-reported anxiety if they demonstrate more adaptive social behaviors.[102,103] For depression, higher IQ and age seem correlated with higher depression ratings[105] and both seem to predict lower self-perceived social competence in children with ASD.[106] Lower self-perceived social competence, in turn, seems to predict high levels of depression symptomatology.[106] Additionally, it seems that adults with ASD with less social impairment (higher social functioning) were more likely to be categorized as depressed.[107] All of this seems to indicate that the more individuals with ASD are aware of social impairments, or exposed to social interactions, the more likely they are to demonstrate classically recognizable symptoms of anxiety or depression.

However, this body of literature, due to the scales that are used, only addresses anxiety and depressive mood symptoms that are also seen in typically developing individuals. Clinicians who work with individuals with PDD are well aware that anxiety and depression might manifest in alternative ways in this population. Individuals with ASD often have impaired abilities to communicate their emotional experiences to others and can have significant trouble managing their emotions. This routinely leads to alternative manifestations of emotions like anxiety and depression, in the forms of rigidity, tantrums, oppositionality, social avoidance, hyperactivity, repetitive behaviors, irritability, aggression, and self-injury. As mentioned above, studies of SSRIs to target some of these behaviors, have been mixed.

Overall though, it seems that case studies and open-label trials have shown possible benefits for the use of SSRIs in children with PDD for the treatment of classically recognized symptoms of anxiety and depression. To avoid significant emotional and behavioral adverse events though, target dosing should be lower than in children with typical development.

SLEEP

Melatonin

The medication with the strongest research backing for the treatment of sleep disturbance in individuals with developmental disabilities is melatonin. Hollway and Aman's excellent review[108] found thirteen RCTs of individuals with sleep disturbance, many of which also with developmental disabilities. All thirteen RCTs had positive findings, particularly for sleep initiation and sleep maintenance, with the longest trial being 10 weeks in duration. The effect sizes for sleep onset latency ranged from .25 to 1.63, and for total sleep time from .25 to 1.0. Adverse effects were generally mild and similar to placebo. Doses ranged from 2.5 to 10 mg.

Ramelteon

The MT_1/MT_2 melatonin receptor agonist has limited evidence in children with developmental disabilities, though considerable positive findings in adults with typical development, specifically in primary insomnia and sleep maintenance.[108] Adverse effects were mild and similar to placebo, and doses ranged from 4 to 64 mg.

Clonidine

Although no RCTs have been conducted in children with developmental disabilities and sleep disturbance, retrospective reviews have shown benefits in helping with sleep disturbance, with doses ranging from 0.05 to 0.1 mg.[108]

Trazodone

Although no RCTs have been conducted in children with sleep disorders, four open-label studies in children and two in adults showed benefits for improving sleep, including sleep architecture.[108] Doses ranged from 25 to 150 mg.

Mirtazapine

One open-label study in children and one RCT in adults showed benefits for the treatment of sleep problems, with mild adverse effects, which included increased appetite, irritability, and sedation.[108] Doses ranged from 7.5 to 45 mg.

Diphenhydramine

Despite its abundant use in pediatric patients for sleep disturbance, only three RCTs were identified by Hollway and Aman for its use in pediatric subjects.[108] Two of the studies were negative, one showed benefit, and none of them were specifically in children with developmental disabilities.

Zolpidem

Studies are limited, and none seem to have studied individuals with developmental disabilities, though benefits seem greater in adolescents and adults, and less effective in children.[108]

Benzodiazepines

In partially or uncontrolled studies in children, and controlled studies in adults, it seems that benzodiazepines may be most effective at helping sleep disturbances associated with parasomnias (e.g., periodic limb movement disorder, tongue biting, REM sleep behavior disorder) though with considerable risks of adverse effects, including tolerance, dependence, rebound insomnia, daytime sedation, and cognitive impairment.[108]

Overall, it seems that melatonin is the most well-studied, effective, and safe medication option for treating sleep disturbance in individuals with developmental disabilities. Although promising evidence for ramelteon, trazodone, mirtazapine, and clonidine exists, further research is needed in individuals with developmental disabilities. Research evidence does not seem to support the wide use of diphenhydramine for sleep disorders in children, and although zolpidem and benzodiazepines may be of benefit for sleep in some, they should be used with caution, and primarily in adults for zolpidem, and those with parasomnias for benzodiazepines.

CASE 88-4

QUESTION 1: T.T. is a 10-year-old boy with ASD and significant sleep disturbances. His father has tried diphenhydramine for the last few weeks but has not seen any meaningful improvement in T.T.'s total sleep time. Last year, T.T. had a trial of melatonin 2.5 mg daily with only a small recognized improvement. T.T.'s clinician is thinking about starting a low-dose benzodiazepine, however, is weighing the concerns for adverse effects. T.T.'s clinician asks for your opinion.

You note that the dose of melatonin last year may have been on the lower range and you would recommend another trial of melatonin before considering a controlled substance. The dose you would recommend is 5 mg taken approximately 1 hour to T.T.'s bedtime. You note that this dose can be increased to 10 mg if an adequate response is not seen.

Table 88-2
Summary of Target Symptoms and Pharmacologic Treatment

Target Symptom	Treatment Medications/Classes to Consider
Hyperactivity	Stimulants, atomoxetine, α_2 agonists
Irritability/aggression	Risperidone, aripiprazole
Repetitive behaviors	Risperidone, aripiprazole, fluoxetine, clomipramine, fluvoxamine,
Self-injurious behavior	Risperidone, clomipramine, naltrexone
Anxiety/depression	SSRIs
Sleep	Melatonin, ramelteon, clonidine, trazodone, mirtazapine, zolpidem, benzodiazepines

SSRI, selective serotonin reuptake inhibitors.

KEY REFERENCES AND WEBSITES

A full list of references for this chapter can be found at http://thepoint.lww.com/AT11e. Below are the key references and websites for this chapter, with the corresponding reference number in this chapter found in parentheses after the reference.

Key References

Doyle CA, McDougle CJ. Pharmacotherapy to control behavioral symptoms in children with autism. *Expert Opin Pharmacother.* 2012;13(11):1615–1629. (72)

Hollway JA, Aman MG. Pharmacological treatment of sleep disturbance in developmental disabilities: a review of the literature. *Res Dev Disabil.* 2011;32:939–962. (108)

Mahajan R et al. Clinical practice pathways for evaluation and medication choice for attention-deficit/hyperactivity disorder symptoms in autism spectrum disorders. *Pediatrics*. 2012;130:s125–s138. (45)

Minshawi NF et al. Multidisciplinary assessment and treatment of self-injurious behavior in autism spectrum disorder and intellectual disability: integration of psychological and biological theory and approach. *J Autism Dev Disord*. 2015;45:1541–1568. (82)

Volkmar F et al. Practice parameter for the assessment and treatment of children and adolescents with autism spectrum disorder. *J Am Acad Child Adolesc Psychiatry*. 2014;53(2):237–257.

Wong C et al. Evidence-based practices for children, youth, and young adults with autism spectrum disorder: a comprehensive review. *J Autism Dev Disord*. 2015;45:1951–1966. (29)

89 Attention Deficit Hyperactivity Disorder in Children, Adolescents, and Adults

Michael C. Angelini and Joel Goldstein

CORE PRINCIPLES

		CHAPTER CASES
1	Attention deficit hyperactivity disorder (ADHD) is a heterogeneous psychiatric disorder that consists of multiple subtypes, including inattention, hyperactivity/impulsivity, and a combination of these two types. For diagnostic criteria to be met, there must be evidence that these symptoms are present in multiple settings and that the individual exhibited this psychopathology before the age of 12 years. These symptoms cannot be because of other illnesses.	**Case 89-1 (Question 1), Table 89-1**
2	Behavioral therapy is an important component of any effective treatment plan and typically includes educational interventions, creation of a structured environment for the child, and introducing contingency training.	**Case 89-1 (Questions 1-3)**
3	Stimulant medications are highly effective for the rapid relief of ADHD symptoms and substantially improve a child's prognosis. Individuals who fail to respond adequately to one type of stimulant will often do well with another, suggesting that subtle differences exist in the pharmacologic mode of action. Although the duration of pharmacologic action is relatively brief for stimulants, a variety of preparations have been approved that can prolong the relief of ADHD symptoms and permit once-daily dosing.	**Case 89-1 (Questions 3-5), Table 89-2**
4	There are a number of non-stimulant medications that have proven to be effective for ADHD over the years, including atomoxetine a NE reuptake inhibitor, and α-agonists. These medications may be viable options for the management of treatment-resistant illness as well as in patients with a history of substance abuse. They also possess a different side effect profile than stimulants and have a delay until therapeutic effects are evident.	**Case 89-1 (Question 6), Table 89-2**
5	Many people are reluctant to consider stimulant medications for ADHD treatment because of unfounded fears about drug tolerability and abuse. As a result, there have been a wide variety of alternative treatments considered for use, including changes in dietary habits, ingestion of herbs and supplements, and other somatic interventions. At the present time, the evidence supporting these options is sparse, although the rigor of investigations has steadily improved in recent years, and there is hope that some of these options may prove to be beneficial.	**Case 89-2 (Question 1)**
6	ADHD is commonly associated with several psychiatric and medical comorbidities, and these concurrent conditions often influence treatment plans. Tic disorders such as Tourette syndrome are frequently found in children with ADHD, but research evidence suggests that stimulants are not only safe but also effective in this particular population.	**Case 89-1 (Question 1)**
7	Some children with ADHD will continue to have symptoms of their illness well into their adult years, usually of the inattention subtype. There is a growing awareness that adults with ADHD have significant social and occupational impairments. Fortunately, medications used to treat ADHD in children appear to be equally effective in adults. Stimulants are the most effective agents but have the unique side effect risk of abuse and diversion. Monitoring for this is essential. If abuse or diversion occurs then a reevaluation of the diagnosis is necessary as well as a change to a medication with less risk of misuse.	**Case 89-2 (Question 2)**

Although the diagnosis and treatment of attention deficit and hyperactivity disorder (ADHD) have been associated with considerable controversy, ADHD is a serious psychiatric condition that has been well described in the medical literature for more than two centuries.[1] There are highly effective pharmacologic treatments that ameliorate the core symptoms of the illness. These agents are generally safe and have been shown to improve long-term prognosis.[2]

By definition, ADHD symptoms manifest in childhood and will often persist into adulthood in many cases. If left untreated, ADHD can produce significant impairments in academic performance and social functioning; adults with ADHD are often hindered in occupational settings as well.[3] Psychiatric comorbidities are commonly encountered among individuals suffering from ADHD, including developmental disorders, mood disorders, and substance abuse.

Although hyperactivity had been recognized as a troublesome childhood behavior for many years, ADHD was not formally described in the *Diagnostic and Statistical Manual of Mental Disorders* until the third edition was released in 1980. The recently released *DSM-5* describes three different subtypes of ADHD including "Predominantly inattentive presentation," "Predominantly hyperactive/impulsive presentation," and "Combined presentation."[4] The *DSM-5* also requires the diagnosis by age 12, in contrast to *DSM IV* that required the onset of impairment before age 7. Qualitatively the core symptoms of ADHD will differ according to gender, with boys more likely to exhibit the hyperactive/impulsive subtype (vs. girls).[5] These symptoms often change with time as hyperactive and impulsive behaviors recede during adolescence, and inattention predominates among adolescents and adults with ADHD.[6]

Although the effectiveness of pharmacologic treatments for ADHD has been widely replicated, many children and adolescents with ADHD will receive suboptimal treatment for a variety of reasons, including parental reluctance to consider psychotropic medications, the perceived stigma of mental illness, and well-described deficiencies in the delivery of health care to persons with psychiatric conditions.[7] It is important to note that ADHD poses a huge economic burden to Western society. A meta-analysis by Doshi et al. reports overall national incremental costs of $143 to $266 billion in the United States.[8] The economic impact related to adults with the disorder from productivity and income loss is greatest, although there are also significant costs associated with youth with the disorder from educational and health expenses. Further, the study documents significant "spillover costs" for family members of individuals with ADHD.[8]

Stimulants such as methylphenidate and amphetamine have been the mainstay of ADHD treatment in children for more than 30 years, and recent studies have demonstrated acute and long-term benefits in adolescents as well as adults.[1,9-11] Unfortunately, stimulants have not been consistently shown to decrease delinquency rates. They have also been implicated with rare but serious side effects, and they carry an elevated risk of diversion and abuse.[11-13] Pharmacologic alternatives to stimulants have been identified in recent years and have proven to be useful, albeit often as second-line agents among individuals who have significant side effects and those with medical or psychiatric comorbidities.[11] The benefits of cognitive behavioral psychotherapy have also been emphasized in recent years, and most experts now contend that the combination of pharmacotherapy with family-based cognitive behavioral interventions will generate the best long-term prognosis for individuals with this disorder.[2]

Recent landmark studies have helped clarify important aspects of diagnosis and treatment with regard to ADHD. The Multimodal Treatment of Attention Deficit Hyperactivity Disorder Study (MTA) is considered a groundbreaking study of ADHD treatments and outcomes. The main findings were released in 1999, but additional findings have been subsequently released. MTA was a multisite study that differed from earlier studies of ADHD in that the duration of the study was significantly longer (up to 14 months) and that the study compared the use of both medication and cognitive behavior therapy, both alone and in combination with routine community-based treatment. The central findings of MTA included the following: (1) Medication alone and in combination with CBT was more effective than intensive behavioral treatment alone or routine community-based care, (2) youth receiving combined treatment required lower doses of medication, and (3) youth with associated mental health issues, in addition to ADHD, had better outcomes with combined treatment than with medication alone.[14,15]

The question of medication treatment for preschool children presenting with ADHD symptoms is a controversial issue. The "Preschool ADHD Treatment Study" (PATS) is considered a landmark study in this arena. The majority of the findings were released in 2006. The central findings include (1) preschool children tend to respond better and with fewer adverse effects with lower doses of medication and (2) preschool children are more sensitive to the adverse effects of psychostimulants and require closer monitoring. In particular, younger children tend to have more emotional adverse effects such as irritability and a tendency toward crying.[16,17]

EPIDEMIOLOGY

ADHD is a chronic neurobehavioral disorder, with an overall estimated prevalence of 6% to 12% in school-aged children worldwide.[18] The Centers for Disease Control and Prevention analyzed data from the 2006 National Survey of Children's Health and reported that the incidence of ADHD diagnoses has risen annually by an average of 3% between 1997 and 2006.[19] In 2006, 7.4% of US children aged 4 to 17 years were diagnosed with ADHD. The *DSM-5* reports that "ADHD occurs in most cultures in about 5% of children and about 2.5% of adults." The diagnosis is more common in males with a ratio of 2:1 in children and 1.6:1 in adults.[4] It is hypothesized, however, that this gender predominance may be exaggerated because the more overt hyperactive subtype is more common in boys and the less overt inattentive subtype is more common in girls. As ADHD transitions into adulthood, the prevalence falls to 4.4% (standard error 0.6), with a higher risk found in previously married men who are unemployed and non-Hispanic white.[19]

PATHOPHYSIOLOGY

Various abnormal genetic and neurochemical abnormalities are associated with ADHD. Estimates of heritability of ADHD range in the area of 0.7, indicating that ADHD is one of the most heritable conditions in psychiatry.[20] Family studies have demonstrated that the relative risk of ADHD is 6 to 8 times higher among first-degree relatives of persons with ADHD compared with the general ADHD population.[21] Several candidate genes associated with ADHD have been identified, such as the dopamine receptor, dopamine-transporter receptor, and serotonin transporter gene.[22,23] Despite a small causal effect, no single gene is responsible for the symptoms seen with ADHD, but rather these symptoms are likely the result of interactions among several genes, which influence multiple neurotransmitters, including serotonin, dopamine, and norepinephrine.[22]

Multiple neuroimaging studies have documented consistent abnormalities in brain structure and development with youth and adults with ADHD. Subjects with ADHD have been shown to have reductions in global brain volume.[24] Specifically, the reduction in volume is most prominent in the prefrontal cortex, basal ganglia, cerebellum, and parieto-temporal regions.[24] Functional magnetic resonance imaging studies have also shown hypoperfusion with memory tests in the anterior cingulate areas in ADHD patients.[25] This area of the brain is responsible for behavioral and functional abilities that may manifest in patients with ADHD as difficulties in organization, mood, motivation, self-regulation, and ability to retain specific information while performing a particular task, which are abilities referred to as executive functioning. These findings are research population–based findings. These studies are not yet useful in clinical practice for accurate diagnosis.

Etiology

ADHD is a heterogeneous behavioral disorder with a variety of theorized etiologies. Clearly, the research suggests a strong genetic component. However, to this point, no specific genetic risk factor has been identified.[20] As a result, other environmental and congenital etiologies have been considered and studied. Examples of studied etiologies for ADHD include maternal smoking, dietary factors, prematurity/low birth weight, and family environment/parenting behavior. Of these proposed factors, low birth rate is the factor with the most confirming research evidence.[20,26] The potential impact of parenting behavior, in particular, is a complex question as youth with ADHD often present more significant challenges to parents. Further, as ADHD is highly heritable, many parents of youth with ADHD may have ADHD themselves.

DIAGNOSIS, SIGNS, AND SYMPTOMS

The diagnosis of ADHD is a clinical diagnosis that may be supported by various types of screening tools and neuropsychologic assessment. The diagnosis of ADHD in a child is based upon the *DSM-5* criteria (Table 89-1). The evaluation should include clinical interviews with the patient and/or parent, physical examination (including neurologic status), obtaining history regarding functional pattern in school or daycare setting, evaluation for comorbid psychiatric disorders, and review of the patient's medical, social and family histories.[2] Other sources of valuable information include performance reports (e.g., report cards or job reviews) and ADHD rating scales scored in two different settings.[4] There are a number of validated rating scales available both proprietarily and in the public domain. Some of the rating scales have different versions for parents and teachers. Rating scales are helpful both for diagnosis and for monitoring treatment outcome.

The recent publication of *DSM-5* included a number of revisions to the diagnostic criteria for ADHD. To meet criteria for ADHD, the child must have six or more symptoms present in two different settings (e.g., home, school, etc.) for a minimum of 6 months. Furthermore, there must be evidence that these symptoms were present before the age of 12 years. Based on these criteria, three types of ADHD are identified: predominantly inattentive, predominately hyperactive/impulsive, and combined. The diagnostic criteria require that the symptoms interfere with or impact functioning in daily life so that care providers will look for symptoms that have a negative impact on the child's education, relationships, or social life (see Table 89-1). On occasion, however, parents or teachers may "pressure" clinicians into writing psychostimulant prescriptions for a "let's see if it helps" trial. If the medication is helpful, they may assume incorrectly that the diagnosis of ADHD is validated. Additionally, *DSM-5* eliminated the exclusion criteria for Autism Spectrum Disorder. However, the *DSM-5* mandates that the symptoms of ADHD "do not occur exclusively during the course" of another psychiatric disorder.[4]

Establishing a diagnosis of ADHD in an adult who has never been treated for the disorder during childhood is difficult. In adults, ADHD is a clinical diagnosis that relies on their recollection of ADHD symptoms as a child to which *DSM-5* criteria validated for children are applied. Unlike teachers who are ordinarily familiar with the symptoms associated with ADHD in children, spouses, coworkers, and employers are often unfamiliar with ADHD as a disorder that can also affect adults. They may attribute the individual's difficulties to being lazy or to underachievement.

Table 89-1
Diagnostic Criteria for Attention Deficit Hyperactivity Disorder

Inattention Factor
(Six or more of the following nine behaviors need to be present for ≥6 months in two or more settings, such as home, school, or physician's office.)
1. Careless mistakes or inattention to detail
2. Reduced attention span
3. Poor listener
4. Cannot follow instructions and does not complete tasks
5. Difficulty organizing tasks and activities
6. Avoids and/or dislikes chores or homework
7. Loses things needed for tasks and activities
8. Easily distracted by extraneous stimuli
9. Forgetful in daily activities
Hyperactivity/Impulsivity Factor
(Six or more of the following nine behaviors need to be present for ≥6 months in two or more settings, such as home, school, or physician's office.)
Hyperactivity
1. Fidgets with hands/feet or squirms in chair
2. Cannot remain seated in the classroom
3. Uncontrollable/inappropriate restlessness
4. Difficulty in engaging in play or leisure activities quietly
5. Often on the go and appearing driven by a motor
6. Excessive talking
Impulsivity
7. Blurts out answer prior to completion of question
8. Difficulty waiting turn
9. Interrupts or intrudes on others

Reprinted with permission from American Psychiatric Association. *Diagnostic and Statistical Manual of Mental Disorders*. 4th ed. Text Revision (*DSM-5*). Arlington, VA: American Psychiatric Association Press; 2015.

COMORBIDITY AND PROGNOSIS

Between the ages of 10 and 25 years, the signs and symptoms of ADHD decrease in frequency and severity by about 50% every 5 years but will generally persist into adulthood.[6] In the differential diagnosis of ADHD, it is critically important to distinguish ADHD from various behavioral, developmental, or medical conditions. Psychiatric comorbidity is more common with ADHD as up to 87% of children will be diagnosed with at least one additional psychiatric disorder and 67% have at least two or more disorders.[27]

Other psychiatric conditions that frequently coexist or imitate symptoms of ADHD include conduct disorder, oppositional defiant disorder, Tourette syndrome, depression, anxiety disorders, and obsessive–compulsive disorder. Of these conditions, anxiety disorders and mood disorders are most commonly misdiagnosed as ADHD. The comorbidity of ADHD and learning disabilities is both complex and often leads to significant academic challenges. Studies suggest that 25% to 35% of youth with ADHD will also have language-based or other learning disabilities.[27] Clinical wisdom suggests that ADHD often presents early in the child's academic career (e.g., kindergarten or first grade), whereas learning disabilities may present later in the elementary years, when children are "reading to learn" rather than "learning to read." Medication is a central treatment component for ADHD, whereas learning support and specialized teaching strategies are the interventions of choice for youth with learning disabilities. Medications are not helpful for the treatment of learning disabilities.

It has been known for decades that family histories from first-degree relatives of probands with ADHD reveal increased rates of ADHD (25% concordance rate), polysubstance dependence, antisocial personality disorder, depression, and anxiety disorders.[28] Children with ADHD are at an increased risk of having antisocial behavior, depression, and substance abuse problems as adults. ADHD symptoms persist into adulthood in the majority of these comorbid patients.[11] Adults with ADHD are usually self-sufficient, but they have poorer academic performance, poorer job performance, and lower socioeconomic status than do their siblings. They also have more frequent divorces, job changes, and car accidents. Most adults with ADHD report a high level of subjective distress (79%) and interpersonal problems (75%).[29]

Medical conditions often complicate the diagnosis of ADHD and should be excluded before initiating treatment. These medical conditions include head injuries, seizure disorders, metabolic disorders, cerebral infection, toxic exposures (e.g., chronic lead exposure), sleep problems, substance abuse, and hyperthyroidism.

CASE 89-1

QUESTION 1: M.T. is a 12-year-old girl who recently started middle school. M.T.'s mother calls the pediatrician looking for advice. M.T. was adopted at 2 months of age from Guatemala and little is known about prenatal care or her life before the adoption. M.T. is having a good deal of difficulty with the transition to middle school. She seems overwhelmed with the amount of work and has become withdrawn and angry. The guidance counselor has called the parents because M.T. has missed most of her homework assignments. M.T.'s mother feels at a loss because M.T. now has many more teachers and they don't seem to know her or to support her in the same way as the teachers in the elementary school. M.T. has begun counseling with a social worker in the community but does not want to go. Her mother is interested to know if medication may be of help. How do you think about the differential diagnosis?

Depression is the most prominent diagnosis that comes to mind. However, it is important to remember that comorbidity is quite common in youth with psychiatric disorders. It is important to consider if there are underlying, less obvious disorders or circumstances that may be contributing.

CASE 89-1, QUESTION 2: What are the next steps in the evaluation?

The pediatrician refers M.T. to a child/adolescent psychiatrist for evaluation. The professionals help the parents request an educational assessment through the school. The latter includes both an academic and psychologic assessments. The assessments suggest underlying poor self-esteem. However, there is also evidence of slow processing speed and other evidence of ADHD and executive functioning deficits. The Vanderbilt rating scales confirm the diagnosis of ADHD.

There are a number of validated instruments to assist with the diagnosis and clinical management of ADHD. Often, these instruments have a parent and teacher version. Commonly used instruments include the Conners Global Index, the SNAP IV, DuPaul Rating Scale for ADHD, and the Vanderbilt Rating Scale. Some rating scales are proprietary and others such as the Vanderbilt is in the public domain.[30]

CASE 89-1, QUESTION 3: What are the first-line interventions?

The psychiatrist provides psychoeducation to M.T. and her parents about ADHD. They discuss that ADHD may be missed more commonly in girls, and that youth with ADHD often develop concurrent depression, anxiety, conduct disorders, and substance-use disorders because their experience in school and activities often leads to feelings of inadequacy. Additionally, an Individualized Educational Plan (IEP) is developed for M.T. to provide more supports in the school setting. Special accommodations such as added time for exams, a seat in the front of the class, and the availability of fidget toys are specified in the IEP.

M.T. continues in counseling with the social worker, in which they focus on cognitive and behavioral strategies to manage both her ADHD symptoms and her depression and poor self-esteem. All agree that it is prudent to hold off on any medication for depression to see if the other interventions are effective in alleviating the symptoms of depression.

The ADHD symptoms are tracked with Vanderbilt rating scales completed by parents and teachers. Medication treatments for ADHD are discussed. With informed consent, a trial of a psychostimulant is begun.

TREATMENT

Optimal strategies to manage ADHD symptoms that are moderate to severe in nature should focus on the combined use of behavioral and pharmacotherapy interventions. It is important to recognize that ADHD is a chronic disorder with symptoms that frequently continue into adolescence and adulthood. Before developing a treatment plan, defined and realistic treatment goals should be established collaboratively with the child, parent, and school.

Several ADHD consensus statements, practice parameters, and guidelines have been developed, based on both evidence-based literature evaluation and expert opinions, to assist clinicians in evaluating, diagnosing, and managing patients with ADHD in a consistent manner.[2,31–34]

Behavioral Therapy

During the years, numerous psychosocial or educational programs have been studied for their potential benefit in controlling ADHD symptoms and maximizing function.[2] Behavioral interventions have been among the most popular nonpharmacologic approaches, with programs emphasizing the creation of a structured environment containing minimal distractions both at home and in school. Contingency training is another common component of behavioral therapy for ADHD, with children receiving tokens for specific tasks or achievements, as well as punishments (e.g., revoking privileges) for maladaptive behaviors. Although most treatment guidelines continue to advocate trying some type of structured behavioral modification, the empiric evidence that such programs improve functioning or prognosis is certainly not as strong as it is for pharmacotherapy.[33]

The previously mentioned Multimodal Treatment Study of Children with ADHD was a landmark study in reviewing the relative impact of medication and nonpharmacologic treatment.[14] The MTA Cooperative Group study, as it is commonly known, was designed to compare long-term medication and behavioral treatments with respect to efficacy and acceptability. A group of 579 children between 7 and 10 years of age with the combined type of ADHD were recruited and randomly assigned to four different treatment groups: medication management, behavioral treatment, medication plus behavioral treatment, or typical community treatment. Behavioral interventions were delivered in a group-based recreational setting and included an 8-week, 5-days/week, 9-hours/day, intensive program administered by a counselor or aide. Once school started, the subjects in this arm of the study received 60 school days of a part-time, behaviorally trained, paraprofessional aide who worked directly with the child. In addition, the child's teacher received 10 to 16 sessions of biweekly consultation that focused on classroom behavior management strategies. Daily behavior report cards were sent home to parents. At the same time, families were involved in 27 group therapy meetings plus 8 individual family meetings. Of the children receiving medication, 75% received methylphenidate, 10% received dextroamphetamine, and 15% received pemoline, imipramine, clonidine, guanfacine, or bupropion. After the 14-month study, it was concluded that drug treatment was more effective than behavioral treatment according to parents' and teachers' ratings of inattention, and teachers' ratings of hyperactivity/impulsivity. Combined treatment (drug treatment plus behavioral modification) was preferred by parents, but the therapeutic advantage versus medication did not achieve statistical significance. Combined treatment was significantly more effective than behavioral treatment and community care for reducing ADHD symptoms, according to both parent and teacher reports, but a subgroup analysis of children with comorbid conditions (e.g., conduct, oppositional defiant, anxiety, or affective disorders) found behavior management to be as effective as monotherapy. A 3-year follow-up study revealed that all four interventions were equally effective in improving academic performance and social functioning with time, but given the costly and labor-intensive nature of the behavioral modification, in particular pharmacotherapy, it continues to be regarded as the first-line treatment for children with at least moderate ADHD symptoms.[15] There have been a variety of school-based, clinic-based, and home-based interventions to address ADHD symptoms, mainly with positive results. Additionally, specialized summer treatment programs have been established to provide more intensive intervention when school is not in session.[35]

Pharmacotherapy

STIMULANTS

Stimulants are considered the most effective option to treat ADHD, with more than 60 years of clinical experience accrued. Currently there are two basic types of stimulants marketed in the United States, methylphenidate based and amphetamine based, and they have all been reported to improve academic performance and behavior in children with ADHD (Table 89-2).[32]

Table 89-2
Overview of Common Drugs to Treat Attention Deficit Hyperactivity Disorder

Drug		Duration of Action	Pediatric Dose	Adult Dose	
Stimulants					
Methylphenidate C-II	Aptenso XR	Long	20–60 mg a day	20–60 mg a day	Adult doses may need to be higher and can be titrated up based on tolerability
	Concerta (generic)	Long	18–72 mg a day	18–72 mg a day	
	Metadate CD	Long	20–60 mg a day	20–60 mg a day	
	Metadate ER	Intermediate	20–60 mg a day	20–60 mg a day	
	Methylin ER	Intermediate	20–60 mg a day	20–60 mg a day	
	Quillichew ER	Long	20–60 mg a day	20–60 mg a day	
	Quillivant XR	Long	20–60 mg a day	20–60 mg a day	
	Ritalin IR	Short	20–60 mg a day	20–60 mg a day	
	Ritalin SR	Intermediate	20–60 mg a day	20–60 mg a day	
	Ritalin LA	Long	20–60 mg a day	20–60 mg a day	
	Daytrana Transdermal Patch	Long	10–30 mg per 9 hour patch	10–30 mg per 9 hour patch	
Dexmethylphenidate C-II	Focalin	Short	5–20 mg a day	20 mg a day	
	Focalin XR	Long	5–20 mg a day	20 mg a day	
Amphetamine C-II	Adzenys XR ODT	Long	6.3–18.8 mg a day	No approved max. dose	Adult doses likely to be similar to pediatric doses and titrated as tolerated
	Dynanavel XR	Long	20 mg a day	No approved max dose	
	Evekeo	Long	2.5–40 mg a day	No approved max. dose	
Amphetamine/Dextroamphetamine C-II	Adderall	Short	10–40 mg a day	10–40 mg a day	Doses may be increased as tolerated
	Adderall XR	Long	10–30 mg a day	10–20 mg	
Dextroamphetamine C-II	Dexedrine	Short	5–40 mg a day	5–40 mg a day	
	Dexedrine XR	Long	5–40 mg a day	5–40 mg a day	
	ProCentra	Short	5–40 mg a day	5–40 mg a day	
	Zenzedi	Short	5–40 mg a day	5–40 mg a day	

(continued)

Table 89-2

Overview of Common Drugs to Treat Attention Deficit Hyperactivity Disorder (*continued*)

Drug		Duration of Action	Pediatric Dose	Adult Dose	
Lisdexamfetamine C-II	Vyvanse	Long	30–70 mg a day	30–70 mg a day	
Methamphetamine	Desoxyn	Long	5–25 mg a day	No approved dose	Strongly recommended not to use this product
Non-stimulants					
Noradrenergic Reuptake Inhibitor					
Atomoxetine	Strattera	Long	40–100 mg a day	40–100 mg a day	
α-2 Receptor Agonist					
Clonidine	Clonidine	Short	0.1–0.3 mg a day	0.1–0.3 mg a day	Use in adults not well studied. Higher doses have been used for control of BP. Monitoring for hypotension is recommended
Guanfacine	Kapvay	Long	0.1–0.4 mg a day	0.1–0.4 mg a day	
	Guanfacine	Short	1–4 mg a day	1–4 mg a day	
	Intuniv	Long	1–4 mg a day	1–4 mg a day	

BP, blood pressure; IR, immediate release; SR, sustained release; ER and XR, extended release; ODT, orally disintegrating tablet; CD, controlled delivery.

A review of short-term clinical trials that evaluated the safety and efficacy of stimulants in nearly 6,000 children and adults with ADHD showed a 75% to 80% improvement in patients treated with stimulants compared with 5% to 30% treated with placebo.[36] Although stimulant drugs are grouped as a class based on their pharmacologic effect of increasing dopamine and norepinephrine levels in the synapse, the mechanisms by which stimulant drugs exert this effect varies slightly. These subtle differences in the mechanism of action support the possibility that patients who respond partially to one stimulant may respond completely to another. In fact, approximately 20% to 25% of those who respond poorly to one medication will respond positively to another and up to 90% of children will respond if both are tried.[37] Stimulants also are rapid acting and have predictable effects, with response typically within 2 hours.[38]

Methylphenidate and dexmethylphenidate block the reuptake of dopamine from the synaptic cleft into the presynaptic neuron via the dopamine transporter protein. Methylphenidate is metabolized into ritalinic acid via carboxylesterase CES1A1, a non CYP450 enzymatic pathway.[39,40]

The most common side effects of methylphenidate include appetite suppression, insomnia, headache, nausea and vomiting, and abdominal pain.[40]

A long-acting methylphenidate transdermal formulation is available. As with any transdermal system, drug delivery can vary greatly because of heat and site-related skin porosity differences. AUC and Cmax can increase 300% if the patch is applied to an inflamed area and 250% if the patch area is exposed to heat such as going outside and exercising in the sun.[2,41–43] The patch is applied to the hip area for 9 hours, and methylphenidate is steadily released and absorbed into the circulation for about 11.5 hours. When compared to the oral long-acting Oros release system, methylphenidate's side effects were similar between the two products but numerically higher in the transdermal arm compared to the oral arm. One side effect exclusive to the patch is skin irritation which can occur from 3% to 40%.[41]

Amphetamines, including mixed amphetamine salts, dextroamphetamine, and lisdexamfetamine, enhance the release of both dopamine and norepinephrine from storage vesicles in the presynaptic neuron and block their storage in addition to blocking their reuptake from the synaptic cleft. They also have a weak MAOI effect.[44,45]

Dextroamphetamine is metabolized via CYP2D6. A strong inhibitor of 2D6 could increase levels twofold. The long-acting prodrug lisdexamfetamine requires enzymatic hydrolysis in the blood to cleave off the L-lysine portion of the molecule. This leaves just dexamphetamine available for activity.[46,47] Lisdexamfetamine is rapidly absorbed, but the step of hydrolysis results in a delayed release of dextroamphetamine in the circulation allowing for once a day dosing.

Since approximately two-thirds of children and adolescents with ADHD respond equally to methylphenidate or amphetamine products, the preferred agent should be based on duration of action, formulation preferences, and cost.[33] As shown in Table 89-2, stimulant preparations are classified based on duration (i.e., immediate [2–5 hours], intermediate [6–8 hours], and long-acting [10–12 hours]) and available delivery systems. Long-acting formulations are preferable to intermediate and short acting, because it provides uninterrupted benefit allowing the child to avoid going to the school nurse for doses or lack of effect between doses.[48] Many long-acting options are biphasic, which provides an immediate-release (IR) dose then a second long-acting dose a few hours later. For example, Ritalin LA, Metadate CD, Focalin XR, and Adderall XR all contain both immediate and enteric-coated, delayed-release beads that mimic the blood concentrations seen with immediate-release stimulant preparations given twice daily. Although a prescription methamphetamine product does have FDA approval for treatment of ADHD, no expert guidelines recommend it because of high-abuse liability and neurotoxicity.

Adverse Effects

Both types of stimulants are similar in their side effect profiles. Adverse drug reactions such as insomnia and appetite loss are mild, and tolerance often develops within a few days. These reactions can be easily managed by adjustment in dose and timing if necessary (Table 89-3). In a double-blind, crossover study comparing side effects of methylphenidate and dextroamphetamine, surveyed parents reported worsening appetite (vs. baseline) with methylphenidate; severe insomnia and appetite suppression were reported with

Table 89-3
Managing Adverse Effects of Stimulants Used in Children with Attention Deficit Hyperactivity Disorder

Adverse Effect	Management
Decreased appetite, nausea, or growth impairment	■ Schedule evening meals after medication has worn off ■ Take drug after meals ■ Encourage foods with high caloric density or nutritional supplements ■ Encourage evening/bedtime snack ■ Switch from long-acting to short-acting preparation ■ Consider a drug holiday when appropriate
Sleep disturbance	■ Administer doses earlier in the day ■ If using a sustained-release product, consider changing to a short-acting preparation ■ Discontinue afternoon/evening dose
Behavioral rebound	■ If using short-acting preparation, consider changing to a long-acting preparation ■ Overlap stimulant dosing

Irritability	■ Assess time of symptoms:
	  ■ Related to peak: reduce dose or try long-acting preparation
	  ■ Related to withdrawal: change to long-acting preparation
	■ Evaluate for comorbid diagnosis

Dysphoria, moodiness, agitation, dazed, or withdrawn behavior	■ Decrease dose or change to long-acting preparation ■ Consider comorbid diagnosis
Dizziness	■ Monitor blood pressure ■ Encourage fluid intake ■ Lower dose or change to long-acting preparation to reduce peak effects
Development or increase in tic disorder	■ Stop stimulant ■ Consider trial of clonidine or guanfacine ■ Consider referral to physician

dextroamphetamine.[49] Side effects that were significantly more severe with methylphenidate (vs. dextroamphetamine) included insomnia, appetite suppression, irritability, proneness to crying, anxiety, dysphoria, and nightmares.[49] Only 3.2% of patients treated with either drug discontinued the medication because of side effects. Another head-to-head trial showed similar types and rates of adverse effects for IR methylphenidate and IR dextro/levo amphetamine.[50]

There is an association between stimulant use and growth retardation. The relative impact of this seems minimal and can be reduced or eliminated with drug holidays.[51–53] There seems to be no loss of efficacy if the child does have a drug holiday and stops the medication over weekends holidays or summer months.[54] The risk of drug holidays is a worsening of symptoms and this may have impact on social maturation.

There was concern that the stimulants may have a cardiotoxicity risk. Population studies suggest, however, that the overall risk of sudden death associated with stimulant use has been shown to be the same, if not lower, than that of the general population.[55] Slight increases in BP and HR are seen with methylphenidate and amphetamines, although ECG changes are very rare.[56–58] Clinicians should follow current recommendations suggested by the American Academy of Pediatrics and the American Heart Association, which advocate screening for a personal or family history of cardiovascular disease in all children with ADHD. Continual monitoring for these risks along with routine blood pressure and heart rate assessments should be performed.[59] Pretreatment ECGs are not required but recommended by the AHA as general practice for all children. Stimulants should not be used in those with known structural cardiac abnormalities.[60]

NON-STIMULANTS

For patients with ADHD only, it is recommended to initiate treatment with either a methylphenidate or an amphetamine.[2,32–34] For patients who fail both types of stimulants or when stimulants are not preferred, a trial of a non-stimulant is warranted (Table 89-2). Non-stimulants are less effective than stimulants and usually require at least 4 weeks until a full response is evident. A meta-analysis of 29 double-blind, placebo-controlled trials evaluated the efficacy of stimulant and non-stimulant agents using 17 outcome measures in 4,465 children and adolescents with ADHD.[61] It found that the effect size of amphetamine and methylphenidate was significantly greater than that for atomoxetine, bupropion, and modafinil ($p = 0.02$).[61] If atomoxetine fails or is not indicated, the α_2-adrenergic agonists clonidine and guanfacine should be considered.[31–33]

Atomoxetine

Atomoxetine inhibits the presynaptic norepinephrine transporter and is classified as norepinephrine reuptake inhibitor (NRI). Clinical trials have shown that atomoxetine is superior to placebo in reducing the symptoms of ADHD in children, adolescents, and adults.[62,63] However, trials comparing atomoxetine with stimulants have found atomoxetine to be less effective.[2,64–67]

Atomoxetine is likely to have some immediate benefit after initiation but unlike the stimulants a longer trial of 6 to 8 weeks is recommended as efficacy continues to grow. Atomoxetine requires a 10- to 14-day titration to achieve a therapeutic dose of 1 to 1.5 mg/kg/day to avoid nausea (12%), vomiting (15%), and asthenia (11%).[68] As with stimulants, atomoxetine can also raise blood pressure and heart rate, with reports of high systolic and diastolic blood pressures occurring in 8.6% and 5.2% of pediatric subjects, respectively. Increases in heart rate of more than 110 beats/minute and more than 25 beats/minute above baseline were observed in 3.6% of patients.[68] Atomoxetine is metabolized via CYP 450 2D6, with the major metabolite being 4-hydroxyatomoxetine which is also a potent inhibitor of NE reuptake but at low concentration levels. It has a half-life of 4 to 5 hours but can be extended by about 3 hours with a high fat meal.[69]

There have been postmarketing cases of reversible hepatic injury in association with atomoxetine, but this is quite rare.[70] Baseline liver enzyme testing should be performed, and evidence of jaundice or liver injury should warrant immediate discontinuation. Atomoxetine also contains the warning regarding increased risk of suicidal thoughts that are part of all antidepressant class labeling. However, a meta-analysis of 14 trials found that no subject committed suicide. Suicidal ideation in the atomoxetine group was 5/1,357 (0.37%) and placebo group was 0/851 (0%).[71] So, despite the low risk, monitoring frequently for the first 3 months of treatment is required by the FDA.

α_2-Agonists

Clonidine and guanfacine are α_2-agonists that have been used for years off-label to control hyperactive/impulsive or aggressive symptoms and insomnia.[72] They are believed to directly stimulate the postsynaptic norepinephrine receptors in the prefrontal cortex and locus coeruleus. Guanfacine is most specific for the α-2a receptor, while clonidine is less specific and agonizes α-2a, b, and c. The FDA has approved extended-release formulations for clonidine and guanfacine both as monotherapy and as adjuncts to stimulants. Clonidine and guanfacine are also approved as adjuncts to stimulants for ADHD. Although they are a monotherapy option, they are not considered as first line as they are less effective than stimulants. They are particularly useful for behavioral comorbidities, such as aggression and tics.[31–34,73–75]

Guanfacine is primarily metabolized via CYP 3A4, and potent inhibitors can increase blood levels by 200%. Guanfacine extended release provides approximately 60% of the serum levels of the immediate-release version. Clonidine is partially metabolized via CYP 2D6, although inhibitors of this pathway have only minor changes in serum levels.[76] The extended-release version has an AUC approximately 89% of the immediate release.

The side effect profile of α-2 agonists is quite different than the stimulants and atomoxetine. Sedation and related side effects can occur in nearly 40% for both. Reductions in BP and HR can occur and need to be monitored. Bradycardia (HR $<$ 60 bpm) can occur in up to 20% of children with clonidine and is a side effect of guanfacine also but to a lesser degree. This is likely because of guanfacine's specificity to α2a. Rebound hypertension can occur if either of these medications are stopped abruptly.[73]

Despite positive studies with immediate-release formulations, the short duration of action makes them less desirable than the QD dosing of guanfacine ER and the BID dosing clonidine extended-release formulation.[32]

CASE 89-1, QUESTION 4: It is agreed upon by the parents and the pediatrician that M.T., the 12-year-old female, will begin using a medication for her ADHD symptoms. What would be the first-line option for M.T.?

Either stimulant groups are considered first line and in this case methylphenidate 10 mg qam is tried. After steadily increasing the dose to 30 mg qam the parents feel that there is minimal change in attention, but that there are significant side effects of nausea and loss of appetite.

CASE 89-1, QUESTION 5: What would be the next trial of medication for M.T.?

Expert guidelines state that if medication is decided upon then the greatest efficacy is from the stimulants. Neither stimulant is considered superior to the other and initial choice should be based on the comfort level of the clinician and patient/parent acceptance. If the initial choice of stimulant is ineffective, it is recommended to trial the other stimulant class. By doing this 90% of children will display efficacy. Therefore, the next trial for M.T. should be the initiation of dextroamphetamine 5 mg qam and titrate as tolerated to a maximum of 40 mg a day.

CASE 89-1, QUESTION 6: M.T. is showing some improvement on 10 mg qam of immediate-release dextroamphetamine, but it is clearly wearing off about 4 hours after dosing. Dosing of 10 mg BID was tried during a school vacation and found to be somewhat effective; thus, the pediatrician decided to switch to long-acting dextroamphetamine spansules 20 mg qam. This clearly has shown to last throughout M.T.'s school day, but efficacy is not maximized and some residual symptoms of poor attention and hyperactivity exists. What is the next step of pharmacotherapy for M.T.?

Increasing the dose to 30 mg qam is possible. Although a switch from a stimulant to atomoxetine could be tried, data have shown that atomoxetine is less effective than stimulants. Experts recommend that combination therapy of a stimulant and an α-2 agonist is appropriate, and studies have shown an increase in efficacy from monotherapy to combination therapy.

Comorbidities

TOURETTE'S SYNDROME AND TIC DISORDER

Tourette's syndrome is neuropsychiatric condition which has tics as a hallmark symptom. Children with ADHD have a higher risk of comorbid tic disorder than the general population; however, stimulants are relatively safe in this population. As an example, the Tourette's Syndrome Study Group contrasted the effect of methylphenidate, clonidine, and the combination of the two to placebo in the treatment of 136 children (7–14 years old) diagnosed with ADHD and Tourette syndrome.[77] The group concluded that prior recommendations to avoid methylphenidate in these children because of concerns of worsening tics were unsupported. As such, expert recommendations are that a child with ADHD should start on methylphenidate, and if tics emerge or worsen then a switch to atomoxetine or clonidine is warranted. A meta-analysis of studies with subjects who have ADHD and Tourette's syndrome concluded that methylphenidate shows the greatest improvement in ADHD symptoms without worsening tics in most kids. α-2 Agonists offer less efficacy in ADHD symptoms but greater control over tics compared to methylphenidate. Atomoxetine offers benefit on both groups of symptoms and is an option.[32,74,75] Amphetamines should be avoided because although they do treat ADHD symptoms, they have a higher chance of worsening tics compared to methylphenidate.[74,75]

A review regarding treatment of tic disorders without comorbid ADHD states that the α-2 agonists guanfacine and clonidine are recommended as first-line options. Guanfacine may be preferred because of less sedation than clonidine.[78]

ANXIETY DISORDER

Anxiety disorders are more frequently comorbid in the ADHD child (approximately ninefold) and adult (approximately fourfold) compared to the frequency seen in the general population. Despite the fact that the anxiety disorder may be a separate illness, anxiety symptoms in the child can be directly related to poor performance because of ADHD symptoms. Treatment with a stimulant that subsequently improves performance will reduce the anxiety. However, some children after a trial with a stimulant will not have an anxiety reduction or it may even worsen. At this point a trial with atomoxetine is recommended over treating the anxiety with an SSRI and continuing the stimulant.[2,79]

SUBSTANCE ABUSE

Despite the fact that stimulants are medications with an abuse risk, multiple studies have shown a protective effect against developing a substance-use disorder with children who derive a benefit to their ADHD symptoms from the medication. A meta-analysis of epidemiologic literature led to the conclusion that stimulant-treated patients with a diagnosis of ADHD were less likely to be diagnosed with substance-use disorder than those not treated with stimulants.[80] Using a stimulant for ADHD in a current substance abuser has contradictory results. Stimulants do treat the ADHD symptoms but not as robustly as those without a concurrent substance-use disorder. They do not seem to reduce the substance use but clearly do not worsen it.[81] Expert opinion suggests that those with current substance-use disorders should be tried on non-stimulant options first, but stimulants are not fully contraindicated and can be used with close monitoring. There is growing data to support that there is a high rate of diversion of stimulants in the college population. One report correlated an increased incidence of diversion with increased difficulty of the academic program.[32,82,83]

If misuse and diversion are of concern, methylphenidate comes as a transdermal patch formulation, and dextroamphetamine is available as a hard to abuse prodrug lisdexamfetamine.[32,34,43,44,46]

Despite the potential for being less effective than a stimulant, atomoxetine has preferred benefits in specific patient subtypes. Because it is not a stimulant, its risk of abuse and diversion are low and is preferred in patients with an addictions disorder history or living in a household where someone other than the patient (e.g., parent or sibling) has an addiction disorder and may take the patients medications.

PSYCHOSIS

Stimulants may cause psychosis. This is because of the enhancement of DA centrally. If the child is acknowledging hallucinations or exhibiting bizarre behavior then cessation of the stimulant is required. A rechallenge can occur but at a lower dose. If a child stabilized on the medication starts to exhibit psychotic symptoms then one should assess for drug interactions. The methylphenidate transdermal patch formulation can have greater unexpected fluctuations in blood levels because of a greater range of absorption compared to the oral formulations.[42,43] The absorption of the transdermal patch is influenced by placement site and temperature of the skin. Treating this side effect with an antipsychotic is not recommended.[32]

Other Non-FDA Pharmacotherapy

BUPROPION

Bupropion has been shown to be effective compared to placebo, but it is less effective than stimulants in treatment of ADHD.[67] Randomized, controlled trials have established the effectiveness of bupropion as an alternative to the psychostimulants in the treatment of ADHD in children, adolescents, and adults.[84–86] The two most common adverse effects encountered with bupropion in ADHD studies were dermatologic reactions and seizures. Dermatologic reactions occurred twice as often with bupropion compared with placebo. Severe bupropion-induced urticaria required discontinuation in 5.5% (4 of 72) of the patients in one study.[87] In adults, the risk of seizures increases by about fourfold if extended-release doses of greater than 450 mg/day or greater than 400 mg/day sustained-release doses of bupropion doses are exceeded.[88] Although there are no case reports of seizures in children receiving therapeutic doses of bupropion, it is recommended to limit doses to less than 6 mg/kg/day in the treatment of ADHD and to avoid using bupropion in patients with a history of seizure disorders.

MODAFINIL

Modafinil has been found to be effective in the treatment of prepubescent, adolescent, and adult patients with ADHD.[89,90] The 2006 Pediatric FDA advisory committee reviewed the efficacy and safety of modafinil for ADHD and determined the drug was effective but rejected its approval for ADHD based on concerns about safety. Twelve of 933 patients developed a skin rash, with one case thought to be Stevens–Johnson syndrome.[91]

TRICYCLIC ANTIDEPRESSANTS (TCAS) AND SEROTONIN AND NOREPINEPHRINE REUPTAKE INHIBITORS (SNRIs)

As recently as 2007 guidelines reported, TCAs could be an option for ADHD. However, their poor tolerability and dangerous effect on cardiac conduction has resulted in more recently published guidelines in 2011 and 2014 to not recommend them.[2,32–34]

The SNRI venlafaxine has shown efficacy in both adolescents and adults with ADHD. This is a legitimate choice for comorbid anxious or depressed older patients, but because of antidepressants having a risk of increasing suicidal thinking in children, other options should be tried first. Adults often have this comorbidity and venlafaxine in that population is more likely to be used.[32]

Alternative Therapy

There have been a number of studies that have tried to discern if certain diets may result in ADHD. One of the most famous regimens is the Feingold Diet. Recent reviews on the topic have found the evidence to be of low quality and of small benefit. Most studies have not been blinded and when efficacy is noted it is of lower rates than the FDA-approved pharmacotherapies. Additionally, there is a practical limitation to the implementation of these diets as it eliminates many of the foods that are regular parts of American meals. At this time it does seem reasonable to assume that some children's ADHD-like behavior may be related to intolerance to certain dyes, artificial sweeteners, and flavors. One should not discourage a parent to promote healthier food selection for their child, but the effectiveness of lowering their symptoms is marginal. Additionally, if a child has a delay in administration of pharmacotherapy because of trials of different types of diets then this could result in persistency of symptoms longer than is necessary.[92]

Many companies have created dietary supplements that have been touted as effective remedies for treating and preventing ADHD, but convincing results derived from rigorous trials are currently lacking and are likely to benefit a very few children with food allergies or intolerances.[92–94] For instance, the use of very high doses of vitamins or minerals has been promoted as a possible intervention, but all randomized, controlled trials conducted to evaluate the effectiveness of megavitamin therapy have been negative to date.[95] Omega-3 fatty acids have been considered as possible treatments for ADHD, based largely on population studies demonstrating an association between high dietary intake and a reduced risk of various neuropsychiatric disorders. Omega-3 supplementation, specifically EPA content, may have a small benefit as monotherapy. Studies of omega-3 as an adjunct to stimulants have shown little added benefit.[96,97] Similarly, there have been reports of zinc, iron, magnesium, *Hypericum* (St. John's wort), and gingko all relieving ADHD symptoms, but the evidence to support these interventions is very limited at the present time.[98]

There have been other somatic treatments aimed at relieving ADHD symptoms that may prove to be beneficial in the years ahead.[98] Several small randomized studies have reported benefits with neurofeedback, in which children are trained to modify certain brain activities demonstrated on electroencephalographic tracings (e.g., increased slow wave or α activity). Preliminary evidence also supports the exploration of meditation as an effective intervention for ADHD, particularly mindfulness-based methods that have proven to be particularly helpful for depression and chronic pain conditions.[99] Clinic-based interventions have included cognitive-behavioral therapy, social skills training programs and computer-based cognitive training programs. Early studies of some of these intervention strategies have been promising and there is need for further research to establish efficacy.[35] Regarding acupuncture a recent systematic review failed to find any studies of sufficient rigor to include in their analysis.[100]

ADULTS WITH ATTENTION DEFICIT HYPERACTIVITY DISORDER

CASE 89-2

Question 1: K.C. is a 27-year-old female who is an adjunct professor in a pharmacy program and comes to a retail pharmacy wanting to fill a prescription for dextroamphetamine IR 10 mg tid #90. What are the treatment recommendations for an adult with ADHD?

It is estimated that two-thirds of children with ADHD will continue to have significant symptomatology as adults.[11] Often the hyperactivity/impulsivity aspect of the illness becomes less pronounced once the child hits adolescence, but the symptoms of inattention persist into adulthood.[6] Even though many of the children with ADHD may no longer satisfy strict diagnostic criteria for ADHD as adults, the severity and persistence of inattentive symptoms can continue to cause considerable social and functional disability. One investigation followed 128 children with ADHD for several years and reported that hyperactivity and impulsivity symptoms were seen to decline at a higher rate than inattention symptoms.[6] Other researchers have followed children with ADHD to adulthood by comparing the academic records of control subjects and ADHD adults. The latter had significantly higher rates of repeated grades, tutoring, placement in special classes, and reading disability.[101,102] Children with ADHD will have greater morbidity in psychosocial and educational areas in adulthood compared to adults who did not have ADHD as children.[103] Adults with ADHD have been found to achieve lower socioeconomic status and experience more work difficulties and more frequent job changes.[104] Adults with ADHD reported more psychologic maladjustment, more speeding violations, and more frequent changes in employment.[105] More adults with ADHD had their driver's licenses suspended, had performed more poorly at work, and had quit or been fired from their job. Adults with ADHD were also more likely to have had multiple marriages.[11]

The diagnostic criteria for ADHD in adults are the same as for children and adolescents (*DSM-5*).[4] However, only five of either hyperactivity/impulsivity or inattention must be present for a minimum of 6 months, impairing function in two or more settings. A diagnosis of ADHD in adults also requires evidence that symptoms were present before the age of 12. One study compared the functional outcomes of adults with ADHD before age 7 with adults, who had the requisite symptoms but lacked conclusive evidence of childhood onset. The investigators found no difference between the two groups in primary outcomes such as learning disabilities, arrests, motor vehicle accidents, and divorce.[106]

Current treatment recommendations for ADHD in adults continue to support pharmacotherapy as the first-line option for moderate-to-severe symptoms.[32] Although benefits have been noted for psychotherapeutic approaches such as cognitive behavioral therapy and dialectic behavioral therapy, these interventions are recommended only for adults exhibiting suboptimal response to approved medications.[107,108]

A variety of medications have been reported to be beneficial for ADHD in adults, including methylphenidate, dexmethylphenidate, mixed amphetamine salts, lisdexamfetamine, desipramine, bupropion, atomoxetine α-2 agonists, venlafaxine, and modafinil.[85,90,109–116] The stimulants and atomoxetine are FDA approved in adults.[32] In general, the effect sizes for these ADHD medications in adults have been very similar to what has traditionally been reported in children. A meta-analysis of medications for ADHD in adults found that long-acting stimulants were significantly more effective than non-stimulant drugs, but that the effectiveness of shorter-acting stimulants was comparable to the latter.[9] The authors also noted that lower doses appeared to be more effective for inattention than hyperactivity. For example, doses for immediate-release methylphenidate were more conservative (0.3 mg/kg per dose in adults) when inattention was the predominate feature. In contrast, doses of up to 0.6 mg/kg immediate-release methylphenidate were often necessary to optimally control the behavioral feature of the disorder in children.[117] These methylphenidate doses are consistent with 0.5 to 1.0 mg/kg/day doses found to be effective in children.[110] Mixed amphetamine salts were effective in doses of 20 to 60 mg/day.[111] The effective dose of desipramine was approximately 150 mg/day.[114] Bupropion was generally dosed at 3 mg/kg/day.[85] The two large studies of atomoxetine used doses that ranged from 60 to 120 mg/day.[114,115] The mean effective dose for modafinil was 207 mg/day.[90]

Treatment with stimulants or atomoxetine have shown improvements in reduced criminality and driving accidents.[118–121]

Case 89-2, Question 2: Before filling the prescription for K.C. the pharmacist reviews it and finds that it is written within 30 days. He also checks the prescription drug monitoring program in his state and finds that she has filled a prescription for the same drug and directions 25, 28, 54, and 56 days ago at other retail pharmacies. These double fills are also written by two different physicians.

What would be an appropriate response by the pharmacist to K.C.'s request?

As noted above, ADHD symptoms can persist into adulthood for many children. A positive history of either an ADHD diagnosis or untreated symptoms in childhood is required for an adult to be diagnosed with ADHD. However, many other diseases can lead to a false positive. Complete blood counts, urine toxicology, and head injury must all be evaluated along with psychiatric conditions such as bipolar disorder, anxiety disorders, and major depressive disorder.[122] Also, one cannot rule out the possibility of substance-use disorder. As with other drugs that have an abuse liability, stimulants can either be abused by the patient or diverted and sold to those who want to use them for their euphoria-inducing effect instead of helping treat ADHD. There is an increasing amount of data reporting the intermittent use of stimulants by college students for study enhancement and abuse, particularly when mixed with a sedating drug of abuse. Therefore, the pharmacist should consult with the clinician who wrote the prescription alerting him to the recent fill at another pharmacy. It is quite possible that this new prescription is legitimate, but it is also possible that K.C. is misusing the dextroamphetamine herself or diverting them to others. A reevaluation of her diagnosis is necessary. If it is confirmed that the patient does have ADHD then options would be to switch to a less abusable stimulant such as lisdexamfetamine or methylphenidate transdermal patch. Switching to the non-abusable atomoxetine is recommended because even though these stimulant formulations are less abusable they are not devoid of abuse risk. Atomoxetine or the non-FDA adult approved agents such as α-2 agonists or bupropion, venlafaxine, and modafinil will likely be less effective than the stimulant for ADHD but provide a safer abuse-risk possibility.

KEY REFERENCES AND WEBSITES

A full list of references for this chapter can be found at http://thepoint.lww.com/AT11e. Below are the key references and websites for this chapter, with the corresponding reference number in this chapter found in parentheses after the reference.

Key References

Bolea-Alamanac B et al. Evidence-based guidelines for the pharmacologic management of attention deficit hyperactivity disorder: update on recommendations from the British Association for Psychopharmacology. *J Psychopharmacol*. 2014;1–25. (32)

Canadian Attention Deficit Hyperactivity Disorder Resource Alliance (CADDRA). *Canadian ADHD Practice Guidelines*. 3rd ed. Toronto, ON: CADDRA; 2011. (34)

Clinical Practice Guideline ADHD. Clinical practice guideline for the diagnosis evaluation, and treatment of attention-deficit/hyperactivity disorder in children and adolescents. *Pediatrics*. 2011;128(5):1–16. (33)

Key Websites

American Academy of Child and Adolescent Psychiatry. http://www.aacap.org.

National Alliance on Mental Illness. http://www.nami.org.

National Institute of Mental Health. http://www.nimh.nih.gov.

NIMH website. http://www.nimh.nih.gov/funding/clinical-research/practical/mta/the-multimodal-treatment-of-attention-deficit-hyperactivity-disorder-study-mta-questions-and-answers.shtml.

90 Substance Use Disorders

Michael C. Angelini

CORE PRINCIPLES		CHAPTER CASES
1	Substance use disorder is a chronic disease with progressive deterioration of psychological and physiologic activity secondary to the habitual use of a drug. This complex disease disrupts many if not all aspects of an individual's life; therefore, multimodal treatment is necessary.	**Case 90-1 (Question 1), Case 90-11 (Question 1), Table 90-1**
2	Opioid misuse includes illicit drugs, such as heroin, and the nonmedical use of prescription pain relievers. Opioid withdrawal is characterized as a flu-like syndrome, involving nausea, vomiting, sweats, diarrhea, pain, and elevations in pulse and blood pressure. The full agonist methadone, partial agonist buprenorphine, and antagonist naltrexone all can be used as maintenance therapy to reduce relapses. Treatment considerations during pregnancy consist of fetal risks if the mother goes into opiate withdrawal or if the mother relapses into addictive behavior. Neonatal abstinence syndrome occurs in the newborn if the mother has been maintained on methadone or buprenorphine.	**Case 90-2 (Question 1), Case 90-3 (Question 1), Case 90-4 (Question 1), Case 90-5 (Question 1), Table 90-2**
3	Sedative-hypnotic drugs of abuse include benzodiazepines, barbiturates, some skeletal muscle relaxants, such as carisoprodol, and γ-hydroxybutyric acid (GHB). Withdrawal symptoms, similar to those of alcohol withdrawal, may include tremors, insomnia, anxiety, elevations in pulse and blood pressure, seizures, and hallucinations, and may be potentially life-threatening. In clinical practice, three general medication strategies are used for withdrawing patients from sedative-hypnotics: gradual tapering of the drug of abuse, substituting and gradually tapering phenobarbital, and substituting and gradually tapering a long-acting benzodiazepine.	**Case 90-6 (Question 1), Table 90-3**
4	Major central nervous system (CNS) stimulants of abuse include cocaine and amphetamines. These drugs are associated with serious acute and chronic adverse effects, such as hyperthermia, paranoia, psychosis, hypertension, arrhythmias, myocardial infarction, seizures, and strokes. Withdrawal from stimulants is not associated with severe symptoms. Primarily, withdrawal consists of fatigue and hypersomnolence. There is currently no US Food and Drug Administration (FDA)-approved treatment for withdrawal or maintenance treatment of stimulant use disorder.	**Case 90-7 (Questions 1, 2)**
5	The use of hallucinogens, including LSD, psilocybin, mescaline, and MDMA, may result in psychological, but not physical, dependency. Adverse reactions during intoxication, such as anxiety, paranoia, and fear, may necessitate benzodiazepine or antipsychotic therapy, but are best managed using a "talk-down" method.	**Case 90-8 (Questions 1–3)**
6	Marijuana is a widely used substance. The withdrawal syndrome is generally mild, characterized by anxiety, depression, irritability, and insomnia, and does not require treatment. Chronic use has been shown to result in increased risks of car accidents, pulmonary complications, psychosis, and anxiety.	**Case 90-9 (Questions 1–3)**

Continued

	CHAPTER CASES
7 Alcohol use disorder is defined by acute and chronic alcohol use. It can result in toxicity, withdrawal, and addiction. Alcohol toxicity is an acute, life-threatening condition that requires aggressive medical attention. Symptoms include a strong smell of alcohol, risk of aspiration, depressed and shallow respiration, and cardiac arrest. Management generally consists of respiratory support and a thorough diagnostic evaluation to rule out coingestion of other drugs or other underlying medical conditions that may also need attention.	**Case 90-10 (Question 1), Tables 90-4, 90-5**
8 Alcohol withdrawal is the neurobiological syndrome associated with increased tolerance or physical dependence resulting from chronic alcohol consumption. This syndrome results in a continuum of signs or symptoms including paresthesias, headache, nausea, anxiety, shaking, increased heart rate and blood pressure, and seizures. Symptom-triggered assessment and treatment of alcohol withdrawal is extremely important since untreated withdrawal can result in death. Treatment may be complicated not only by the physical or cognitive deterioration that can occur but also by the lack of attention to other serious medical or psychological conditions that could be contributing to, or resulting from, chronic alcohol use. Adjunctive treatments including fluid (e.g., normal saline solution), nutritional (e.g., thiamine, folic acid, multivitamins), and electrolyte (e.g., magnesium, potassium) replacement should also be initiated to address the physiological consequences of chronic alcohol use.	**Case 90-10 (Questions 2–4), Table 90-6**
9 Chronic alcohol use disorder (alcohol dependence) is a life-long relapsing disorder that consists of signs of alcohol abuse (continued drinking despite alcohol-related physical, social, psychological, or occupational problems, or drinking in dangerous situations, such as while driving) to the extent that the person also experiences at least three of the following seven symptoms: neglect of other activities, excessive use of alcohol, impaired control of alcohol consumption, persistence of alcohol use, large amounts of time spent in alcohol-related activities, withdrawal symptoms, and tolerance of alcohol. Approved pharmacotherapies include disulfiram, naltrexone (tablets and injection), and acamprosate. Which option is best is determined by many factors such as home support, medical comorbidities, and concomitant medications.	**Case 90-11 (Question 1), Tables 90-4, 90-6**

SUBSTANCE USE DISORDER

Physical dependence occurs when repeated administration of a drug causes an altered physiologic state (neuroadaptation). After neuroadaptation, a characteristic set of withdrawal symptoms occurs when the drug is abruptly discontinued. Psychological addiction or psychological dependence refers to a "maladaptive pattern of substance use leading to clinically significant impairment or distress."[1] Habituation is a state of either chronic or periodic drug use characterized by a desire (but not a compulsion) to continue using the drug, no tendency to increase the dose, and an absence of physical symptoms despite some degree of psychological dependence. A different clinical syndrome is associated with each drug, but all involve a chronic process with progressive deterioration of psychological and physiologic activity secondary to the habitual use of a drug. Addiction is not a diagnosis but is defined by the American Society of Addiction Medicine as a chronic disease of brain reward, motivation, memory, and related circuitry. Dysfunction in these circuits has biological, psychological, social, and spiritual effects. There is a pathologic pursuit of the substance with an inability to abstain, loss of control, craving, and diminished recognition of the intensity of the problem. It is cyclical with periods of relapse and remission. Without treatment, it is significantly disabling and will result in premature death. Addiction is frequently used as a descriptor of the most disabling and intense form of a substance use disorder.[2] Although the neurochemistry of the addictive process is possibly the same for all drugs, the psychosocial and pharmacokinetic aspects vary from drug to drug. Evidence, consistent with models established for alcoholism, indicates that genetically inherited traits may result in expression of addictive disease when the person is exposed to certain drugs and other habituating psychic stimuli.[3]

CASE 90-1

QUESTION 1: R.L., age 26, was recently arrested for possession and driving under the influence (DUI) oxycodone. This is his second DUI offense in the last year. R.L. does not use oxycodone daily, but admits to weekly use. Does R.L. meet the criteria for a diagnosis of a substance use disorder?

The *Diagnostic and Statistical Manual of Mental Disorders,* fifth edition (*DSM-5*) cites criteria for substance-related disorders and divides them into two groups: the substance use disorders Table 90-1) and the substance-induced disorders (intoxication, withdrawal, and others).[1] In 2014, an estimated 27 million persons age 12 or older were classified as current illicit drug users.[4]

Pharmacologic treatment is only one aspect of the management of substance use disorders. Treatment of withdrawal (when needed depending on the chemical of abuse) is the first step in management and should be followed by individualized, psychosocial treatment that is effective in the least restrictive and most cost-effective manner. A strong therapeutic alliance between care provider and patient based on a supportive, empathic, nonjudgmental, clinically appropriate relationship is predictive of successful therapy outcomes. Substance use disorder is a complex disease that disrupts many if not all aspects of an individual's life. Therefore, multimodal treatment is necessary. Psychosocial therapies that may or may not include pharmacologic agents consist of individual as well as group counseling, cognitive-behavioral therapies (learning triggers for use, new coping mechanisms, and relapse prevention), motivational enhancement therapies, family counseling, and voucher-based reinforcement therapy among others. These therapies are often augmented with involvement in support groups, such as 12-step programs.[3]

Table 90-1
American Psychiatric Association, *Diagnostic and Statistical Manual of Mental Disorders*, Criteria for Substance Use Disorders

The patient must display 2 of the following in the last 12 months
Consuming larger amounts of the substance[a] or over a longer period of time than was intended
Persistent desire to reduce substance use or unsuccessful efforts to cut down or control use
A great deal of time is spent in activities necessary to obtain, use, or recover from the effects of the substance
Craving or a strong urge to use the substance
Recurrent use results in failures to fulfill obligations at work, school, or home
Continued substance use despite having persistent social and interpersonal problems created or made worse by the use of the substance
Important social, occupational, or recreational activities are given up or reduced because of the substance use
Recurrent substance use in situations that are physically hazardous
Substance use is continued despite knowledge of having persistent or recurrent physical or psychological problems caused or worsened by the substance
Tolerance defined by either of the following:
A need for increased amounts of the substance to achieve intoxication or desired effects
A markedly diminished effect with continued use of the same amount of the substance
Withdrawal as defined by either of the following:
The characteristic withdrawal syndrome for the substance
The withdrawal syndrome is alleviated by taken a closely related substance (e.g., using a benzodiazepine for alcohol withdrawal)

[a]Substance is defined as any drug, including alcohol.
Source: American Psychiatric Association. *Diagnostic and Statistical Manual of Mental Disorders, (DSM-5)*. 5th ed. Washington, DC: American Psychiatric Publishing; 2013.

R.L. has a pattern of oxycodone use in situations in which it is physically hazardous, as well as two arrests in the last year for DUI. R.L. meets the *DSM-5* criteria for substance use disorder.

OPIOIDS

Abuse of opioids includes illicit drugs, such as heroin, and the nonmedical use of prescription pain relievers. According to the Drug Enforcement Administration (DEA), prescription pain relievers appear to be increasingly diverted from legitimate and illegitimate sources of supply via the internet.[5] The 2014 National Survey on Drug Use and Health reports, among persons age 12 years or older, that there are 4.3 million nonmedical use of pain relievers.[4] The non–FDA-approved opiate heroin is produced in four major source areas, South America, Mexico, Southeast Asia, and Southwest Asia. Mexico has been the predominant supplier to the west coast of the United States and is expanding distribution in eastern US markets as South American production has decreased.[6] Mexican heroin black tar is potent, 40% to 80% pure, but contains more plant impurities than the white powder refined heroin from Asia or South America.[7] The purity of available heroin enables a new, younger user population, who can smoke or snort this high purity heroin and avoid the stigma and hazards associated with needle use. As the substance use disorder intensifies and the user's "habit" (amount used daily) increases, the user will often begin injecting the drug. The Centers for Disease and Prevention (CDC) estimates there are roughly 900,000 persons who have used heroin in the last year in the United States. The 2014 National Survey on Drug Use and Health found that usage of heroin has increased since the early 2000s mostly driven by the 18- to 25-year age group.[4] Some prescription opioid abusers will eventually switch to using heroin, because it is less expensive.

Opioid Use Disorder

Physical dependence occurs in any patient after a few days of continuous administration of an opioid. In the management of acute pain, opioid dependence is generally not clinically significant because the patient is tapered off opioid analgesics naturally because the pain condition resolves. If the opioid is abruptly stopped, the patient may experience withdrawal symptoms; however, the intensity of those symptoms varies depending on the individual's physiology, as well as the dose and duration of use of the opioid. Although the exact dose and duration of opioid administration required to produce clinically significant physical dependence is not known, higher doses and longer times of administration correlate with more severe symptoms of withdrawal on cessation of opioid use.

Physical dependence is defined as a neurobiological adaptation that occurs with chronic exposure and occurs with many drug classes regardless if they have an abuse potential (e.g., β-blockers, steroids, SSRIs). Physical dependence and tolerance (the need for increasing doses to achieve the initial effects of the drug) can occur in the setting of substance use disorder, but are also expected, nonpathological sequelae of chronic opioid therapy.

Most studies evaluating the occurrence of opioid use disorder resulting from the therapeutic treatment of pain have concluded the risk is low.[8] Historically, a much greater problem has been the undertreatment of pain. Yet, people at risk environmentally or predisposed genetically for substance use disorder may have their first exposure through a legitimate, therapeutically dosed prescription of an opiate for an acute pain syndrome. This then progresses to an inappropriate use of the opiate and resultant substance use disorder. Thus, pain management with opiates needs careful monitoring (see Pain Management Chapter 55).

Certain pharmacologic properties, such as high potency, rapid onset and shorter duration of action, and water solubility, may increase the likelihood of abuse of that medication. Although all opioids have some abuse liability, some are intrinsically more abusable than others. For example, the controlled-release formulations have been promoted as less likely to cause substance use disorder than immediate-release products, because some of the reinforcing properties, like multiple peaks and troughs, of the opioid are reduced. When tablets, such as OxyContin, are crushed, however, the drug's controlled-release properties are compromised, and the result is much higher dosages than what is available in the immediate-release formulation tablets. Despite the manufacturer's attempts at altering the formulation of OxyContin to make it harder to tamper with, this product can still be abused. Mixed agonist–antagonist opioids (pentazocine, nalbuphine, butorphanol, buprenorphine) have less potential for misuse than the pure mu agonists (e.g., morphine, hydromorphone, oxycodone); however, misuse to all has been observed.[8] Other options to reduce diversion and misuse are formulary management strategies that help the clinician limit opiate prescriptions.[9,10] In total, the best method of reducing this problem is a combination of psychosocial therapy, pharmacotherapy, and policy.

The term "pseudoaddiction" has been coined to describe the inaccurate interpretation of certain "drug-seeking behaviors" in patients who are inadequately treated for pain.[8] Their preoccupation actually reflects a need for pain relief, but is erroneously interpreted as a severe substance use disorder (addiction).

Medical Complications

The common practice of sharing needles and syringes between friends has resulted in transmission of various infectious diseases. Chief among those is viral hepatitis, specifically the hepatitis C virus (HCV). According to the CDC, in the United States, human immunodeficiency virus (HIV) infection caused by injection drug use had an overall prevalence of 6% in 2015.[11] Other infectious diseases such as syphilis, tetanus, botulism, and malaria can be transmitted in a similar manner and should be considered when evaluating these patients. When heroin is prepared for self-administration, cotton is used as a filter to trap adulterants; thus, some of the drug remains trapped in the cotton. These crude filters are saved, and when money or drug availability is poor, water or other solvents are added to the "old cottons" to extract any remaining drug for intravenous (IV) use. "Cotton fever" is an acute febrile reaction. The onset is within 30 minutes of injection, with shaking chills, diaphoresis, postural hypotension, tachycardia, and low-grade fever. These symptoms are initially suggestive of sepsis, but most of the symptoms resolve without treatment in 2 to 4 hours, with complete recovery in 1 day. The causal agent is probably *Pantoea* (formerly *Enterobacter*) *agglomerans*, via a heat-stable endotoxin.[12] Cotton and cotton plants are heavily colonized with *P. agglomerans*.[13] IV drug users will often use the term *cotton fever* to describe any short-term illness characterized by fever, chills, aches, and pains.[14]

Opioid Toxicity/Overdose

CASE 90-2

QUESTION 1: T.F., a 21-year-old man, was found unconscious after an alleged "OD" (overdose) on heroin. He had a decreased respiratory rate of 4 breaths/minute, cyanosis, symmetrically "pinned" (maximally miotic or pinpoint) pupils, and a slightly decreased blood pressure, 117/72 mm Hg. He has one needle puncture wound and several old needle marks and healed scars in the antecubital fossa area. What is the immediate treatment of choice for this patient?

Immediate treatment includes airway management, cardiorespiratory support, and opioid reversal with naloxone. Naloxone is a full opioid competitive antagonist that rapidly reverses the respiratory depression and hypotension associated with overdose. The preferred route of administration is IV; if access cannot be gained, it may be given intramuscularly (IM), subcutaneously (SC), intranasally, or by endotracheal tube. Intranasal use by first responders and friends or family members of those who have overdosed has shown to have saved lives.[15–17]

Initial IV administration of 0.2 to 0.4 mg naloxone should be slow and should be discontinued if T.F. responds. It is not necessary to precipitate opioid withdrawal symptoms; the end point of naloxone therapy is a relative stabilization of the patient's vital signs. A naloxone-precipitated, sudden-onset withdrawal syndrome is more severe than the symptoms produced by abstinence alone. Repetitive doses should be given if the patient remains unresponsive, up to a maximal dose of 10 mg of naloxone.[15] If the patient still has not responded, the diagnosis of opioid overdose should be reconsidered.[15]

The duration of action of naloxone ranges from 20 to 60 minutes, depending on the dose and route of administration. Treatment of the methadone-overdosed patient will require serial dosing of naloxone every 20 to 60 minutes because the toxic effects of this long-acting opiate recur.[15] The patient must be carefully observed after the termination of naloxone therapy to detect any reappearance of opioid intoxication. An IV infusion of naloxone may be appropriate if high doses are needed or if the patient has recurrent respiratory depression.

Treatment of Opioid Withdrawal Syndrome

OPIOID WITHDRAWAL

CASE 90-3

QUESTION 1: D.J. arrives at the detoxification clinic 10 hours after his last dose of heroin. He is sweating and shaking and keeps yawning. His pulse is 92 and his blood pressure is 130/86 mm Hg. He is a 28-year-old who has been injecting two "quarter bags" ($25 worth) of heroin daily for about a month. He explains he began smoking the heroin but has now progressed to injecting it. D.J. developed a "big habit" (tolerance developed, and his daily requirement of drug to maintain euphoria had increased). He could not afford his daily use. When he tried stopping, his use abruptly became "dope sick" (typical heroin withdrawal symptoms). Describe D.J.'s withdrawal symptoms and what treatment options there are available for detoxification.

Abstinence precipitated a withdrawal syndrome in D.J.; therefore, he is physically dependent on heroin. The powerful ability of the drug to rapidly alleviate withdrawal symptoms results in reinforcement to continue using the drug. D.J.'s ongoing desire to continue using heroin despite his inability to afford it and his all-day hustling constitutes a psychological dependence on heroin. Noticeable opioid physical dependence is highly variable, but it is assumed that the potential for an abstinence syndrome exists after repeated administration for only a few days.[2,18]

Six to twelve hours after the last dose of morphine or heroin (diacetylmorphine), patients physically dependent will experience symptoms of anxiety, hyperactivity, restlessness, and insomnia with yawning, sialorrhea, rhinorrhea, and lacrimation. There may also be profuse diaphoresis with concurrent shaking chills and pilomotor activity resulting in waves of gooseflesh of the skin (thus, the term *cold turkey*). Anorexia, nausea, vomiting, abdominal cramps, and diarrhea may occur. Severe back pain may accompany muscle spasms that cause kicking movements ("kicking the habit"). These symptoms are most severe 48 to 72 hours after the last opioid dose. D.J. is exhibiting typical heroin withdrawal symptoms, and supportive therapy would be appropriate.

During withdrawal, the heart rate and blood pressure may be elevated. Inadequate nutrition and hydration, combined with vomiting, sweating, and diarrhea, can result in marked weight loss, dehydration, ketosis, and acid–base imbalance. Rarely, cardiovascular collapse has occurred during the peak phase of opiate withdrawal. The more dramatic symptoms of heroin withdrawal subside after 7 to 14 days of abstinence even without treatment; however, a return to complete physiologic equilibrium may require months or longer.[2,3]

The character, severity, and time course of withdrawal symptoms that appear when an opioid drug is discontinued depend on many factors, including the particular opioid, total daily dose, interval between doses, duration of use, and the health and personality of the user. Unlike the withdrawal symptoms from sedative-hypnotic drugs, opioid withdrawal symptoms are seldom life-threatening.

Physiologic withdrawal symptoms from all opioid drugs are qualitatively similar but quantitatively different in onset, duration, and severity. Opioids with shorter durations of action tend to produce brief, intense abstinence syndromes, whereas those eliminated from the body at much slower rates produce prolonged but milder withdrawal syndromes.

Treatment options for detoxification usually involve either an abrupt cessation of the opioid with supportive nonopioid pharmacotherapeutic options or opioid substitution. Currently, methadone and buprenorphine are FDA-approved for the opiate substitution indications. The nonopiate approach involves symptomatic treatment of withdrawal. The mainstay of this approach is the α_2-agonist clonidine. A third approach uses rapid detoxification precipitated by an opioid antagonist under general anesthesia.[2,18]

METHADONE DETOXIFICATION

Methadone is a synthetic oral opiate agonist with a prolonged duration of action of 12 to 24 hours. Pharmacologically, it is qualitatively identical to morphine and other opioid analgesics. Methadone detoxification involves stabilizing the patient on a daily methadone dose that is determined by the patient's response based on objective symptoms of withdrawal. This may involve the use of standard rating scales for withdrawal, such as the Clinical Opiate Withdrawal Scale.[19] Initially, methadone may be given in 5-mg increments up to a total of 10 to 20 mg during the first 24 hours.[19] Larger methadone doses (i.e., a 20-mg starting dose) may be required for patients with larger habits. If initial withdrawal symptoms persist 2 to 4 hours after initial dose administration, the dose can be supplemented with an additional 5 to 10 mg. Federal regulations allow a maximum of 40 mg as an initial dose unless a program physician documents that 40 mg was insufficient to suppress opioid withdrawal symptoms.[20] Once a stabilizing dose has been reached (usually, 40–60 mg/day, but may be as high as 120 mg/day), methadone is tapered by 20% a day for inpatients or 5% a day for outpatients.[15,19,20] Studies have suggested that slow tapers are associated with better outcomes. The duration of the taper varies, but a period of 3 to 4 weeks is generally used. The gradual taper may last as long as 6 months. The most common side effects of methadone are constipation, sweating, and sexual dysfunction.[15,19] A Cochrane review of studies comparing methadone tapers with other detoxification methods (adrenergic agonists and other opioid agonists) found that programs vary widely in design, duration, and treatment objectives, but overall the effectiveness of the treatments was similar.[21] A reasonable starting dose of methadone would be 20 mg orally. An additional 5 to 10 mg could be administered after 2 to 4 hours for persistent withdrawal symptoms. The daily dose should be titrated upward every third day by 10 mg until stabilized on a methadone dose of 60 mg/day.

BUPRENORPHINE DETOXIFICATION

Buprenorphine, a synthetic partial opioid agonist, was approved by the FDA in October 2002 for the treatment of opioid dependence. It is a partial agonist at mu receptors, and in opioid-dependent patients, it prevents withdrawal symptoms. Because of its partial effects, it produces maximal "ceiling" analgesia with sublingual doses of 24 to 32 mg, a dosage equivalent to approximately 60 to 70 mg of oral methadone. Buprenorphine is associated with a milder withdrawal syndrome compared with full opioid agonists.[22]

Because buprenorphine is a schedule III medication, it can be prescribed in an office-based setting under the Drug Addiction Treatment Act of 2000. The film and tablets contain buprenorphine hydrochloride alone or in combination with naloxone. The naloxone is poorly absorbed orally, and its presence in the combination tablets is to discourage the IV abuse of buprenorphine. Both forms can be used in an inpatient setting, but the combination product is preferred in the outpatient setting to decrease the risk of diversion. When initiating buprenorphine, the first dose should not be given until more than 4 hours after the last dose of a short-acting opioid, such as heroin, or 24 hours after a long-acting opioid, such as methadone. As previously discussed, evaluation of objective opioid withdrawal signs may involve use of standard rating scales. Induction dosing should begin with 2 or 4 mg on the first day, which can be repeated every 2 to 4 hours if withdrawal symptoms subside and then reappear, up to a maximum of 8 mg. The dose can then be titrated the second day in 2- to 4-mg increments to a dose of 12 to 16 mg.[22] Higher doses during induction may precipitate withdrawal symptoms. In the inpatient setting, the patient may be stabilized on a relatively low daily dose (e.g., 8 mg/day) and then tapered in increments of 2 mg/day over the course of several days.[15] In the outpatient setting, the patient should be initially stabilized on a daily dose (probably 8–32 mg/day) of buprenorphine that suppresses withdrawal. The dose should then be gradually tapered during a period of 10 to 14 days. Buprenorphine is not associated with any significant adverse effects when used to manage opioid withdrawal. Buprenorphine (and methadone) detoxification should be accompanied by psychosocial treatments and support groups as mentioned.[3]

A Cochrane review found that relative to clonidine, buprenorphine is more effective in alleviating opioid withdrawal symptoms; patients treated with buprenorphine stay in treatment longer, and are more likely to complete treatment.[23] The severity of withdrawal appears to be similar for withdrawal managed with buprenorphine or methadone, but withdrawal symptoms may resolve more quickly with buprenorphine. The authors of the meta-analysis concluded that although there is limited evidence comparing buprenorphine with methadone, both agents have similar effectiveness in the management of opioid withdrawal.

Nonopiate Symptomatic Therapy of Opioid Withdrawal

Although opiate replacement has shown to provide a safe withdrawal, treatment with opiates is not always necessary. The ability of the α_2-adrenergic agonist, clonidine, to ameliorate some of the opioid withdrawal symptoms, has led to its widespread use as a nonopioid alternative. Other α_2-adrenergic agonists (lofexidine, guanfacine, guanabenz acetate) have also been investigated.[2,3,24] Noradrenergic outflow from the locus coeruleus is increased during opioid withdrawal and is blocked by administration of mu agonist opioids. Symptoms of opioid withdrawal, therefore, are partly caused by excessive sympathetic activity in the locus coeruleus. Central α_2-adrenergic agonists inhibit locus coeruleus noradrenergic outflow opioid withdrawal, thereby significantly reducing some of the symptoms.

Clonidine is therefore best used in a multidrug regimen. Contraindications to clonidine use include diastolic blood pressure less than 70 mm Hg, concurrent dependence on sedative-hypnotics, and clonidine hypersensitivity or previous intolerance. The most common adverse effects are sedation and hypotension. A Cochrane review examined studies comparing clonidine with methadone taper and found no significant difference in efficacy between the two for the treatment of heroin or methadone withdrawal.[24] A separate Cochrane review did find buprenorphine to be more effective than clonidine in alleviating opioid withdrawal symptoms.[23]

A sublingual or oral test dose of 0.1 mg (0.2 mg for patients >91 kg) of clonidine is given: if diastolic blood pressure remains more than 70 mm Hg, additional doses may be instituted. Oral clonidine can be used at a dose of 0.1 to 0.2 mg/dose 2 to 4 times daily to a maximum of approximately 1 mg/day for 2 to 4 days after cessation of opioids, then tapered and discontinued by 7 to 10 days.[24] Because opiate withdrawal consists of other effects such as musculoskeletal aches and pains, anxiety, insomnia, and gastrointestinal disorders, it is common to use medications such as dicyclomine, loperamide, and ibuprofen as adjuncts. This is particularly true when the detox protocol does not contain opiates.[2,18] (Table 90-2)

Table 90-2
Symptomatic Therapy of Opiate Withdrawal

Symptom	Medication
Bone, muscle, joint or other pain	Ibuprofen, naproxen, other NSAID
Insomnia, anxiety	Benzodiazepine
Gastrointestinal hyperactivity	Loperamide, dicyclomine
Nausea	Prochlorperazine, ondansetron

Sources: Schuckit MA. Treatment of opioid-use disorders. *N Engl J Med*. 2016;375:357–368 and ASAM Public Policy Statement on Treatment for Alcohol and Other Drug Addiction, Adopted May 1, 1980, Revised: January 1, 2010. http://www.asam.org/quality-practice/definition-of-addiction.

D.J.'s blood pressure and drug history should be evaluated for clonidine therapy. Provided his diastolic blood pressure is greater than 70 mm Hg after the clonidine test dose, he can receive oral clonidine 0.1 mg with additional medications to treat his withdrawal symptoms, along with psychosocial counseling.

Ultrarapid Opiate Detoxification

Ultrarapid opiate detoxification (UROD) is a method to shorten the opioid detoxification period by precipitating withdrawal with an opioid antagonist. The opioid antagonist causes rapid stripping of agonist from opioid receptors. UROD is performed under heavy sedation or general anesthesia so the patient does not consciously experience the acute withdrawal symptoms. The protocols for UROD vary in terms of the setting of the procedure (inpatient or outpatient), opioid antagonist (naloxone, nalmefene, or naltrexone), anesthetic agent, adjunctive medications, and duration of anesthesia.[25]

The UROD procedure includes risks, such as vomiting with aspiration; cardiovascular complications, including cardiac arrest; pulmonary edema; and death.[25] Some patients have reported residual withdrawal symptoms for several days. Little information exists regarding referral to ongoing treatment or relapse rates after UROD.[26] A review of five randomized, controlled trials found no benefit of UROD compared with safer, less expensive treatments.[26] UROD has been criticized for being simply a "quick fix" that fails to address the underlying behavior changes necessary for recovery. Additionally, it subjects patients to possible morbidity and mortality when safer, established procedures are available. The high cost of UROD limits its accessibility. The American Society of Addiction Medicine recommends against this method of treating opiate withdrawal due to cardiac complications and anesthesia related events.[2]

Pharmacotherapies for maintenance treatment of Opioid Use Disorder

MAINTENANCE THERAPY

The ultimate goal of outpatient substance use disorder programs is to assist the addicted patient into a drug-free healthy lifestyle. This results in reductions in medical conditions for the patient and reduced crime and health care cost for societal members. Methadone for maintenance treatment of opioid substance use disorder is federally regulated and is only available through specially licensed opioid treatment programs. The Drug Addiction Treatment Act of 2000 allows qualified physicians to prescribe Schedule III, IV, and V medications approved for the treatment of opioid dependence in an office-based setting.[27] Currently, only buprenorphine, a Schedule III medication, is approved for this indication.

CASE 90-4

QUESTION 1: A.X., a 27-year-old man, has a severe opiate use disorder (addiction) to heroin for the last 3 years but is tired of the street scene and wants to "get clean" (complete abstinence). He can no longer afford his growing daily habit but is not sure he can stop using opioids. He seems willing and determined to receive treatment for his heroin dependence. What therapeutic options are available to him?

The goal of eliminating illicit opiate use is the gold standard; however, a more realistic expectation is reduced use and subsequent harm reduction. Even temporary reductions in heroin use are a benefit due to reduced risk of developing major health (HIV, hepatitis C) and social (crime) issues.[2] Medical management of opioid dependence should be accompanied by psychosocial treatments, such as cognitive-behavioral therapies, behavioral therapies, and self-help groups, such as Narcotics Anonymous (NA).

Methadone maintenance is the most common form of pharmacologic treatment for opioid dependence. During methadone maintenance, heroin-dependent patients are stabilized on a dose of methadone that will be sufficient to suppress cravings for 12 to 24 hours without producing euphoria. Studies have shown that patients maintained on methadone doses of 60 mg or more had better outcomes than those maintained on lower doses.[28] Most patients do well on a dose range of 60 to 120 mg/ day, although some patients require more and some require less.[20] Because methadone is metabolized via CYP450 3A4 drugs that induce, this pathway can precipitate withdrawal in patients maintained on methadone. Drugs that inhibit this pathway extend the duration of methadone's effects. The half-life of methadone is typically 25 hours (15–60) but can extend up to 120 hours with frequent dosing.[29] The drug is administered daily at the clinic in a single liquid oral dose. With the aid of daily counseling and rehabilitation, the goal is to eventually taper the patient from methadone as well. Patients who relapse repeatedly despite supportive treatment will require long-term maintenance therapy. This may take years, and it is shown that longer duration in treatment correlates with better outcomes. Methadone's efficacy comes from the fact that it reduces cravings without producing euphoria itself, primarily due to its slow time to peak. This produces a high degree of cross-tolerance to other opioids so that it is extremely difficult to obtain euphoria with IV injection of other opioids. But, patients have been able to reach euphoric states through the concomitant IV administration of other opioids. The higher purity heroin available today has required even higher doses of methadone to achieve cross-tolerance.[28] It is often cut (mixed) with fentanyl to increase the opiate effect.

Buprenorphine has the advantage of office-based availability, thus removing the stigma associated with attending a methadone clinic and providing more places for patients to receive treatment because methadone clinics are limited as to how many patients can enroll and may be hundreds of miles away from the patient's home. Buprenorphine, and high-dose methadone (60–100 mg) therapies were compared with low-dose methadone (20 mg), all three therapies were effective in treating opioid dependence and were superior to low-dose methadone.[30] Trials comparing 12 to 16 mg/ day of buprenorphine with moderate doses of methadone (50–60 mg/ day) have generally shown comparable outcomes, although higher doses of methadone (>80 mg) appear to be superior to buprenorphine.[30] Low-dose buprenorphine seems to have worse outcomes compared to low-dose methadone.[31] Buprenorphine patients are more likely to be employed, have less medical comorbidity, and a shorter duration of drug use compared to methadone clinic patients.[32,33] There are multiple formulations of buccal and sublingual buprenorphine and absorption rates are different between some of them. All are compared to the original buprenorphine sublingual tablet (Subutex and Suboxone) regarding pharmacokinetics, blood levels and efficacy. There is also a buprenorphine implant available which was found similarly effective to lower doses of buprenorphine sublingual.[34] For maintenance treatment buprenorphine combined with naloxone is the standard of care with pregnancy or allergy to naloxone the only two reasons not to use the combination.[2]

Buprenorphine has a long half-life of around 35 hours (24–60 hours) and it produces a relatively mild withdrawal when discontinued.[35] It is believed to be a safer alternative to methadone because life-threatening respiratory depression is much less likely to occur than with a pure mu agonist, unless another CNS depressant is taken concurrently. Most deaths involving buprenorphine have been caused by a combination of the drug with benzodiazepines and through injection of the monotherapy formulation.[22,36] Naloxone bolus doses often are ineffective in reversing respiratory depression caused by buprenorphine because of its prolonged occupancy on mu receptors. Continuous infusion of naloxone is necessary to overcome buprenorphine-induced respiratory depression.[37] Another safety advantage compared to methadone is the lower risk of prolonging QTc.[29] Similar to methadone, buprenorphine is also metabolized by CYP450 3A4.

The narcotic antagonist naltrexone can block the euphoriant effects of heroin and other opiates, prevent the development of physical dependence, and afford protection from opioid overdose deaths. Although naloxone is similar to naltrexone, it is impractical because of its short duration of action and its extremely poor absorption when taken orally. Naltrexone is orally active and provides a dose-related duration of opioid blockade. An oral dose of 100 mg of naltrexone will block opiate effects for 2 days, and 150 mg for 3 days. Thus, dosing on Monday, Wednesday, and Friday is possible; however, it is recommended to use 50 mg QAM because it is easier to remember for the patient and will result in better adherence. Naltrexone is also available in an injectable extended-release formulation for once-monthly use.[38] Patients selected for naltrexone therapy must be opioid free to avoid precipitation of withdrawal. For heroin- or morphine-dependent patients, a 4- to 7-day wait is recommended, whereas longer half-life opiates can require a 10- to 14-day wait. Patients who are highly motivated to abstain have been most successfully treated with this drug.

Because A.X. has had a short duration of opiate misuse, he is a good candidate for outpatient buprenorphine/naloxone or naltrexone. Methadone is equally effective but does require enrollment into a clinic, which may or may not be practical for him. Methadone clinics are considered more effective than the other choices because the addiction becomes more severe.

Research suggests that physicians consume more opioids, sedatives, and alcohol than the general public, but less tobacco.[39] The risk is largely based on access to drugs of abuse, and drug dependence is described as an occupational hazard for healthcare providers. Fentanyl (injectable as well as transdermal formulations) and meperidine are primarily, but not exclusively, drugs of abuse among health care providers. Hospice workers and veterinarians also have access to high-potency opioids. Studies have noted that substance use was highest in psychiatrists and emergency medicine physicians and lowest in surgeons and pediatricians.[39] Fentanyl is associated with rapid development of dependence, intense tolerance, and drug-seeking behavior in addicted physicians for a period of months rather than years.

A comprehensive assessment of addicted health care providers is necessary to determine whether professional impairment is present, and whether issues involving public health and safety or violations of ethical standards, such as professional boundary violations or improprieties, require that the heath care provider be reported to his or her respective medical board. A physician's registration with the federal DEA may need to be suspended. It generally is accepted that health care providers require longer durations of treatment because they are held to a higher standard of recovery owing to concerns of public safety, and they may be clever at concealing their illness.[39]

Health care providers are often good candidates for naltrexone therapy (particularly the long action injection) because of the need to remain drug-free despite continued access to opioids at work.

Opiate Use Disorder Treatment in Pregnancy

CASE 90-5

QUESTION 1: J.R., a 28-year-old woman, has been maintained on 100 mg of methadone daily for the past year. J.R.'s last menstrual period was 8 weeks ago, and she took a home pregnancy test yesterday, which was positive. What is the recommend treatment for pregnant patients?

Methadone has been accepted since the late 1970s to treat opioid use disorder during pregnancy.[20] Methadone maintenance was determined to be the standard of care for pregnant women with opioid use disorder by a 1998 National Institutes of Health (NIH) consensus panel.[40] Currently, methadone is the only opioid medication approved by the FDA for medication-assisted treatment of opioid use disorder in pregnant patients. Women maintained on methadone frequently have regular menstrual periods, ovulate, conceive, and have normal pregnancies. Heroin-addicted mothers, however, generally experience more complicated pregnancies because their lifestyles often predispose them to a poor general state of health and precludes adequate prenatal medical care.[22] Infants born to heroin-addicted mothers may also be exposed to other substances (e.g., alcohol, cocaine, tobacco). These infants tend to be smaller, to weigh less at birth, and to be born prematurely compared with the children of women not using opiates.[22]

WITHDRAWAL DURING PREGNANCY

J.R. should continue methadone maintenance to avoid precipitating a withdrawal syndrome or a relapse to opiate addiction. Both relapse and withdrawal syndrome could lead to a spontaneous abortion.[20] A structured methadone maintenance program provides access to counseling and perinatal medical care which are additional benefits. The dose of methadone should be titrated individually throughout the pregnancy and may even need to be increased and switched from QD to BID dosing due to changes in kinetics that occur during pregnancy.[2] The neonate can be managed for either opioid-induced CNS depression or methadone withdrawal after delivery, as needed.

Methadone continues to be the standard of care for the management of opioid dependence in pregnancy; however, a growing body of evidence suggests buprenorphine may be a reasonably safe alternative.[15] Also most evidence suggests that infants born to buprenorphine-maintained women have a lower incidence of neonatal abstinence syndrome and shorter hospital stays.[41–43]

NEONATAL ABSTINENCE SYNDROME (NAS)

CASE 90-5, QUESTION 2: Because methadone crosses the placental barrier, will J.R.'s infant exhibit opioid withdrawal symptoms after birth, and if so, how should they be managed?

Methadone crosses the placental barrier and can cause CNS and respiratory depression as well as opioid withdrawal in the newborn. In general, the most common opioid NAS symptoms include restlessness, tremors, a high-pitched cry, hypertonicity, increased reflexes, regurgitation, tachypnea, diarrhea, and sneezing. Seizures are associated with, but not necessarily caused directly by, opioid withdrawal in the neonate.[44]

Management of the neonate's opioid withdrawal syndrome entails careful attention to hydration with demand feeding and symptomatic care. Treatment of opioid NAS should begin when symptoms occur; prophylactic therapy is not recommended. Mild withdrawal symptoms generally do not need therapy, but moderate to severe symptoms may require 14 or more days of treatment.[44]

Symptoms of physiologic withdrawal are usually apparent within 48 hours of birth. At this time, treatment can be initiated. Currently, NAS is treated with morphine.[41,44–46] Morphine can be started at a dose of 50 mcg/kg given orally four times daily and titrated to control symptoms. Once the NAS symptoms have stabilized, the dose can be decreased daily by 20% until discontinuation of the drug. Phenobarbital is preferred for the treatment of NAS in cases of combined dependence or benzodiazepine dependence or if maximum doses of opiate have been used.[41] If used, phenobarbital is instituted in doses of 5 to 10 mg/kg/day in the first 24 hours, then tapered symptomatically, usually about 20%/day.

If J.R.'s infant displays opioid withdrawal symptoms (e.g., feeds poorly, becomes tremulous or agitated), morphine at a dosage of 50 mcg/kg orally given four times daily would be an appropriate intervention. This dosage is given until symptoms stabilize and then gradually tapered (e.g., 20% each day) during the next week. Buprenorphine has also shown positive data supporting its use and is a potential option if morphine is unacceptable.[44]

BREAST-FEEDING

Methadone is excreted into the breast milk of methadone-maintained mothers. The amount of methadone in the breast milk is unlikely, however, to have adverse effects on the infant.[47] Furthermore, studies have found minimal transfer of methadone into breast milk.[20] There are little data regarding the safety of buprenorphine in breast-feeding. One study found low levels of buprenorphine and its active metabolite, nalbuphine, in infants' urine.[48] Breast milk offers advantages clearly beneficial to infants, and J.R. should be encouraged to breast-feed her infant.

SEDATIVE-HYPNOTICS (NON-ETOH)

The sedative-hypnotics are a diverse group of compounds with broad clinical uses, including anesthesia, treatment of anxiety, and treatment of insomnia. Ethanol, also a sedative-hypnotic agent, continues to be the most widely abused substance in the United States and will be discussed later. Benzodiazepines have become the prototypical sedative-hypnotic drugs of abuse. Other abused sedative-hypnotic drugs include carisoprodol and γ-hydroxybutyric acid (GHB). Carisoprodol, a nonscheduled skeletal muscle relaxant, has an active metabolite meprobamate, a sedative-hypnotic agent with known abuse potential.[49] GHB is a putative neurotransmitter abused for its euphoric and sedative-hypnotic effects. Although sedative-hypnotics can be abused as monotherapy, they are more commonly used as adjuncts to other chemicals such as opiates and EtOH.

Abstinence Syndromes Associated with Sedative-Hypnotic Dependence

CASE 90-6

QUESTION 1: During a year of therapy for anxiety, B.J. increased his dose of alprazolam to two 1-mg tablets 5 times a day. He has admitted to "doctor shopping" and buying alprazolam on the street. He states he uses the benzodiazepine to get high but he also becomes extremely anxious if he doesn't use any alprazolam for more than an afternoon. Will he experience withdrawal symptoms if he suddenly discontinues alprazolam?

Patients who have been on long-term courses of therapeutic doses of sedative-hypnotics often experience withdrawal symptoms on abrupt discontinuation of therapy. Withdrawal syndromes seen with sedative-hypnotics are similar to those seen with alcohol withdrawal and can include insomnia, anxiety, tremors, headaches, restlessness, nausea, vomiting, hypertension, tachycardia, hypersensitivity to light, sound, and touch, and perceptual distortions.[50] Generalized tonic–clonic seizures can occur as isolated seizures or as status epilepticus. The psychoses that develop resemble the delirium tremens produced by alcohol withdrawal and are usually characterized by disorientation, agitation, delusions, and hallucinations. During the delirium, hyperthermia and agitation can lead to exhaustion, rhabdomyolysis, cardiovascular collapse, and death. Abstinence from short-acting barbiturates and meprobamate produces symptoms that peak within 1 to 5 days. Discontinuation of short-acting benzodiazepines (e.g., lorazepam, oxazepam, alprazolam, temazepam) results in the abrupt onset of withdrawal symptoms, usually within 12 to 24 hours after the last dose. Long-acting agents, and those with active metabolites, have a gradual onset of milder withdrawal symptoms compared with the short-acting agents. Withdrawal symptoms after chronic use of long-acting benzodiazepines typically occur within 5 days of cessation and peak at 1 to 9 days after the last dose.[50]

B.J. has been abusing alprazolam, taking more than the recommended maximal dose. Likely, he will experience withdrawal, possibly including seizures, if he were to abruptly discontinue the alprazolam. His withdrawal from this medication should be medically managed.

Treatment of Sedative Withdrawal

Three general medication strategies are used for withdrawing patients from sedative-hypnotics: tapering; substituting (and gradual taper) of phenobarbital for the drug of dependence; and the substituting (and gradual taper) of a long-acting benzodiazepine for the drug of dependence.[51] Gradual tapering of the drug of dependence is appropriate for patients with therapeutic dose dependence or those taking long-acting sedative-hypnotics, who are not currently abusing alcohol or other substances. A recent meta-analysis suggests that management of benzodiazepine mono-dependence by gradual taper is preferable to abrupt discontinuation.[52] The patient who is abusing sedative-hypnotics already has a strong association between the drug of choice and certain desired effects. Therefore, to minimize exacerbating addictive disease, substitution and taper with a long-acting therapeutic agent is preferred.

The phenobarbital method is used in some drug treatment programs. The pharmacologic rationale for phenobarbital substitution is that it is long acting, producing little changes in serum levels between doses, thereby preventing breakthrough withdrawal symptoms. Lethal doses are many times higher than toxic doses, and dysphoria occurs with elevated dose, rendering it less desirable for abusers.

The standard method involves calculating a phenobarbital replacement dose for the total daily dose of the sedative-hypnotic being abused. The calculation is based on phenobarbital equivalents (Table 90-3). If multiple sedative-hypnotics are being used, the totals for each drug and alcohol (amount of pure ethanol) are summated. The total phenobarbital substitution dose should be given in divided doses, 3 or 4 times daily (to avoid dysphoria). Because the calculated dosage is an estimate based on patient history, which may be inaccurate, it is advisable to administer a test dose if the calculated replacement dose is more than 180 mg/day. The test dose, generally one-third the total dose, is given to the patient, who is then observed for 1 to 2 hours. The patient is observed for mitigation of withdrawal symptoms as well as signs of

Table 90-3
Hypnotic Dose Equivalent to 30-mg Phenobarbital

Pure ethanol 30–60 mL	Clonazepam 1–2 mg	Pentobarbital 100 mg
Alprazolam 0.5–1 mg	Diazepam 10 mg	Secobarbital 100 mg
Butalbital 100 mg	Flunitrazepam 1–2 mg[a]	Temazepam 15 mg
Carisoprodol 700 mg	Lorazepam 2 mg	Triazolam 0.25–0.5 mg
Chlordiazepoxide 25 mg	Oxazepam 10–15 mg	Zolpidem 5 mg

[a]Not approved for use in the United States.
Source: Dickinson WE, Eickelberg SJ. Management of sedative-hypnotic intoxication and withdrawal. In: Ries RK et al. eds. Principles of Addiction Medicine, 4th ed. Philadelphia, PA: Lippincott Williams & Wilkins; 2009:573.

overmedication, such as somnolence or incoordination. Once an appropriate dose is determined, the patient is usually stabilized on that dose for 1 to 2 weeks. After stabilization, a gradual taper of phenobarbital is instituted, with dosages reduced by 15 mg weekly or every other week, or 10% of the current (starting) dose per week. For the last 25% to 35% of the taper, the rate is slowed to keep the patient stabilized. The taper should be held for a few days if withdrawal symptoms occur.[50]

B.J. has a substance use disorder to alprazolam. Tapering of alprazolam or conversion to phenobarbital will both result in a safe withdrawal. His total dose of alprazolam is 10 mg/day, so if phenobarbital is used he should receive 300 mg divided 3 or 4 times a day. The total daily phenobarbital dose or alprazolam dose should be tapered by 10% of the dose per week as tolerated.

γ-Hydroxybutyric Acid

γ-Hydroxybutyric acid (GHB), commonly referred to as "liquid ecstasy," is a potent "club drug." Once available as an over-the-counter nutritional supplement, primarily used by bodybuilders for its muscle building effect, the FDA removed it from the retail market in 1990 because of widespread reports of poisoning. In 2000, it was classified as a schedule I drug; however, a GHB-containing product, sodium oxybate, is available as a schedule III prescription drug for the treatment of cataplexy associated with narcolepsy. GHB is found in mammalian brain tissue, where it is derived from conversion of its parent neurotransmitter, γ-aminobutyric acid (GABA).[53] It is believed to be a neurotransmitter. Experimental evidence suggests that the mechanism of action of exogenously administered GHB involves agonist activity at the $GABA_B$ receptor.[53]

γ-Hydroxybutyric acid has CNS depressant effects and is abused for its euphorigenic properties, disinhibition, and enhanced sensuality. Its psychic effects are similar to those of alcohol, and include increased libido, short-term anterograde amnesia, and a dreamy, altered sensorium. It has a steep dose-response curve, and common adverse effects include dizziness, nausea, weakness, agitation, hallucinations, seizures, respiratory depression, and coma. Its effects are synergistic with alcohol. GHB overdose may be fatal, and there is no antidote. Treatment for GHB overdose is primarily supportive.

Highly addictive, tolerance and physical dependence can occur with regular use of GHB, and a withdrawal syndrome has been seen in people who have taken high doses of it (~18 g/day or more, although doses are variable in solution form) with frequent dosing (every 1–3 hours).[53] Withdrawal symptoms can include muscle cramps, nausea, vomiting, tremor, anxiety, insomnia, tachycardia, restlessness, and delirium or frank psychosis. Death caused by pulmonary edema has been reported. Treatment of withdrawal involves supportive care, including use of benzodiazepines (e.g., lorazepam or diazepam) for sedation. Withdrawal can last up to 2 weeks.[53]

Misrepresented sometimes as a natural and safe hypnotic, the low therapeutic index and the unknown purity of illicit supplies, particularly when sold in solution, make GHB a potentially dangerous drug. Physical dependency is a possibility as well. GHB, along with the benzodiazepine flunitrazepam, are considered "date rape" drugs because they cause profound hypnosis and amnesia. This is intensified when mixed with alcohol which is often how the sexual predator gives it to his victim.

CENTRAL NERVOUS SYSTEM STIMULANTS

Cocaine

Cocaine is a naturally occurring alkaloid derived from the *Erythroxylon coca* plant, found mainly in the Andes Mountains of South America. Cocaine was first isolated in the 1800s and was a common ingredient in tonics and elixirs of the 1900s. The Harrison Narcotic Act of 1914 prohibited nonmedical use, and in 1970 it became a schedule II controlled substance. According to the 2014 National Survey on Drug Use and Health, nearly 1 million people in the continental United States have a diagnosed cocaine use disorder within the last year which is similar to the rate in 2009.[4] Cocaine is a CNS stimulant and has vasoconstrictive and local anesthetic properties. Cocaine's stimulant effects are primarily caused by blockade of the reuptake of dopamine, norepinephrine, with a small effect on serotonin. It also facilitates the release of dopamine and norepinephrine. This results in an overall increase in availability of neurotransmitters. Cocaine also has other indirect effects on neurophysiology, including effects on the endogenous opioid systems.[54,55] Cocaine is associated with compulsive use. The powerful reinforcing effects of cocaine have been identified as occurring in brain regions rich in dopaminergic nerve terminals.

DOSAGE FORMS AND ROUTES OF ADMINISTRATION

In the manufacture of cocaine, organic solvents are used to solubilize the alkaloidal bases from the leaves, which are then precipitated to form a sticky material, called "pasta" or "cocaine paste." The benzoylmethylecgonine (cocaine) in this "pasta" is separated from most of the other plant alkaloids, converted to the hydrochloride or other salts, precipitated, and dried. This product is the white cocaine hydrochloride powder usually seen in the illicit market. The final product is usually "stepped on" or "cut" (diluted) with various adulterants to increase profits for the dealers. According to the DEA, in 2009 the average purity of cocaine was down from 68.1% in 2006 to 46.2%.[56] Powdered cocaine is generally snorted. Usually 10 to 25 mg of powdered cocaine is placed on a mirror or flat surface, formed into a line, and then insufflated through a straw or rolled dollar bill. A typical low to moderate user may consume 1 to 3 g/week. Cocaine powder can also be used for IV injection. The highly water-soluble powder is usually mixed with water and injected. When cocaine is injected simultaneously with heroin, this is known as a "speedball."

Cocaine hydrochloride melts at a high temperature, destroying much of its psychoactivity in the process. Therefore, it is inefficient to smoke cocaine hydrochloride in this form. The use of "freebase" cocaine became popular during the late 1970s, because this form of cocaine has a lower melting point and can therefore be smoked, producing an intense rush. For freebase, the cocaine hydrochloride is dissolved into ethyl ether. The synthesis of freebase is dangerous, and the resultant product may contain residual organic solvents, thus making it highly volatile and putting the user at risk of burns.

In the mid-1980s a safer, easier method for extracting the cocaine base supplanted the traditional freebase process. In the manufacture of "crack," cocaine hydrochloride is dissolved in water. When alkali (bleach or sodium bicarbonate) is added to this aqueous solution, the free alkaloidal base ("crack") precipitates out whereas the salts and some adulterants stay in aqueous solution. The precipitate is commonly referred to as a "rock." The size of the rock varies but generally ranges from one-tenth of a gram to a half a gram.

PHARMACOKINETICS AND EFFECTS

Cocaine generally produces a euphoriant action with a rapid onset and short duration. Snorting cocaine generally produces euphoria and stimulation within 2 minutes; smoking produces these effects within 6 to 8 seconds. Cocaine has a short elimination half-life of approximately 30 minutes owing to its rapid metabolism by esterases in the plasma, liver, brain, and other tissues.[54] When alcohol and cocaine are consumed together, a metabolite, cocaethylene, is formed. Cocaethylene intensifies the euphoric as well as the toxic effects of cocaine. The risk of death from cocaethylene is 18 to 25 times greater than with cocaine alone.[56]

An initial relaxed, euphoric, gregarious, talkative, hyperactive state characterizes the "high" of cocaine. Additionally, the person may report increased interest in sexual matters, diminished short-term memory, periods of intense concentration on one limited subject, diminished hunger, hypervigilance, and a peculiar, slightly out-of-body sense of one's actions. Without additional doses of cocaine, these feelings usually resolve into a state of mild depression, fatigue, hunger, and sleepiness by 1 to 3 hours. Physiologic manifestations include mydriasis, sinus tachycardia, vasoconstriction with hypertension, bruxism, repetitive behavior, hyperthermia, and talkativeness. After a few hours, continuous self-administration of cocaine will begin to progress from euphoria to dysphoria and hallucinosis and then to psychosis. Some users engage in nonstop binges of self-administration until psychological toxicity develops.[57]

ADVERSE EFFECTS

In 2007, 553,530 cocaine-related visits to an emergency department were reported in the United States.[58] The potential adverse effects associated with both acute and chronic use of cocaine are numerous and involve most organ systems in the body.

The cardiac complications associated with cocaine use include hypertension, arrhythmias, myocardial ischemia and infarction, dilated and hypertrophic cardiomyopathy, myocarditis, aortic dissection, and acceleration of atherosclerosis. These cardiac effects have occurred in individuals with and without underlying heart disease who have taken large or small doses by all routes of administration and may be associated with acute or chronic use. The cardiac events can occur before, during, or after other toxicities, such as seizures, and can be fatal. The mechanism of cocaine-induced myocardial infarction is most likely multifactorial, involving one or more of the following processes: coronary artery vasoconstriction, increased myocardial oxygen demand related to increased blood pressure and increased heart rate, increased platelet aggregation and thrombus formation, coronary vasospasm, and arrhythmia. The risk is greatest within the first hour after use.[59] Studies have shown 6% of patients presenting to emergency departments with chest pain after cocaine use have myocardial infarctions.[56,57,59]

The medical management of acute coronary syndromes differs when cocaine is the cause. Specifically, nonselective β-blocker therapy (i.e., propranolol) is contraindicated due to unopposed alpha affects, thrombolysis should be used with caution, and nitroglycerine and benzodiazepines are part of first-line therapy.[56,57,59] In patients with cocaine-associated chest pain, a 12-hour observation period to rule out myocardial infarction or ischemia is probably sufficient before discharge from a medical facility.[57]

Cocaine has also been associated with cerebrovascular catastrophes. Stroke can occur as a result of increased blood pressure, vasoconstriction, or thrombosis. Seizures are another CNS complication. Seizures can occur with first use and are most often single, generalized tonic–clonic seizures. Most occur within 90 minutes of drug use, when drug plasma concentrations are highest.[54]

The route of cocaine administration also affects the nature of the adverse effects. For example, pulmonary complications, including pneumomediastinum, pneumothorax, pneumopericardium, acute exacerbation of asthma, diffuse alveolar hemorrhage, pulmonary edema, and "crack lung," are associated with smoking crack cocaine. Crack lung is a syndrome of acute pulmonary infiltrates associated with a spectrum of clinical and histologic findings.[56] Snorting cocaine can lead to perforation of the nasal septum because of the drug's local anesthetic and vasoconstrictive effects. IV use of cocaine has been associated with renal infarction, wound botulism, viral hepatitis, HIV infection, bacterial endocarditis, sepsis, and other infectious complications.

COCAINE USE DISORDER

A person who uses cocaine despite adverse consequences (emergency department visit), uses it compulsively, suffers withdrawal symptoms, and alleviates symptoms with further use is diagnosed with cocaine use disorder per the *DSM-5*. Prolonged or heavy use of cocaine has been associated with the development of tolerance to some of its central effects. Tolerance is caused by adaptive changes in the brain.[54] A withdrawal syndrome may follow long-term or binge use. The initial, acute symptoms, referred to as the "crash," consist of depression, fatigue, craving, hypersomnolence, and anxiety. Anhedonia and hyperphagia soon follow. Although most symptoms are mild and resolve within 1 to 2 weeks, the dysphoria and anhedonia can persist for weeks. These symptoms do not produce profound physiologic changes and are generally not life-threatening.[57]

TREATMENT OF COCAINE USE DISORDER

Most cases of simple cocaine withdrawal do not require medical treatment. However, multiple pharmacologic therapies to facilitate abstinence from cocaine have been, and continue to be, under investigation. Most studies have yielded variable results, and to date no drug exists that is proven effective in treating cocaine dependence.[15] Studies of dopamine agonists (amantadine, selegiline, levodopa / carbidopa, pergolide), antidepressants (desipramine, fluoxetine, bupropion), and carbamazepine have yielded inconsistent findings. Methylphenidate has been investigated as "maintenance treatment" to satisfy the cocaine addict's desire for further enhancement of mood; however, methylphenidate also can stimulate a powerful craving for the more intense euphoria of cocaine and has significant abuse potential. Recent research shows promise for topiramate, baclofen, tiagabine, and modafinil, but these findings require replication.[15] A cocaine vaccine is currently under investigation. Psychosocial treatments focusing on abstinence have been effective in the treatment of cocaine dependence.[15] Cognitive-behavioral therapies and behavioral therapies, such as contingency management, along with 12-step–oriented individual counseling can be useful, although the efficacy of these therapies varies. Participation in a 12-step self-help group (AA, NA), as an adjunct to treatment, seems to predict less cocaine use.[3,15]

Amphetamines

Central nervous system stimulants have been used both with and without social acceptance for thousands of years. The Chinese prepared ephedrine-containing products from a plant called Ma-Huang (*Ephedra vulgaris*).[7] People in East Africa and the Arabian Peninsula chew the leaves of the khat bush (*Catha edulis*) for the stimulating effects of the alkaloid cathinone.[54] Caffeine is consumed worldwide in a usually socially acceptable manner in the form of coffee and energy drinks. Amphetamine was synthesized in 1887, and methamphetamine in 1919. The legal sanctions against widespread prescribing of amphetamines in the 1970s restricted their supply and fostered a black market thriving on the illicit production of methamphetamine powder ("speed," "meth," "crank," "crystal meth"). During the 1990s, California and the West Coast experienced a dramatic resurgence of methamphetamine-related hospital admissions, poison center calls, and law enforcement actions. Methamphetamine misuse has since become a nationwide problem, prompting government restrictions on retail sales of ephedrine and pseudoephedrine (precursor chemicals used in the manufacture of methamphetamine). A new marketing tool developed by savvy drug dealers aimed at younger, new users involves bright coloring and flavoring (strawberry, cola, cherry, orange) added to crystal methamphetamine to help mask the bitter taste. According to the National Survey on Drug Use and Health for 2014, there were 569,000 current users of methamphetamine in America.[4]

PHYSICAL AND PSYCHOLOGICAL EFFECTS

CASE 90-7

QUESTION 1: D.C., a college student, used amphetamine this past weekend when partying with his friends. He has a midterm examination in 2 days and is too tired to study, so one of his friends suggests snorting some more amphetamine and then hitting the books. D.C. finds amphetamine very much to his liking and begins to use it daily. He goes many days at a time without sleeping or showering and starts losing weight because he seldom has an appetite. He believes his friends are working with the DEA and tapping his phone. Are these symptoms of a stimulant use disorder?

Methamphetamine produces CNS stimulation by enhancing the effects of norepinephrine, serotonin, and dopamine. This is accomplished by both blocking the reuptake and stimulating release of these neurotransmitters. These effects are greater for dopamine and norepinephrine than for serotonin.[47]

The powerful stimulating effects of amphetamine and methamphetamine have made their use popular among a wide variety of groups, including students, athletes, the military, dieters, and long-distance truck drivers. Initially, the user may experience alertness, euphoria, increased energy, the illusion of increased productivity, sociability, and decreased appetite. Continuous dosing, however, produces stereotypical grooming and other repetitive motions. Physiologic effects include bruxism, tremor, muscle twitching, mydriasis, hypertension, diaphoresis, elevated body temperature, nausea, dry mouth, weight loss, and malnutrition. Continued use for several days decreases productivity and is associated with disordered thoughts, paranoia, and psychosis. Tolerance develops very rapidly after continued use.[54]

Illicit methamphetamine is commonly insufflated or injected and, less commonly, taken orally. In a pattern similar to that seen with smoking cocaine, users freebase methamphetamine and smoke it. Heating the crystals and smoking the vapor of "crystal meth," as with crack, is a common route of administration; however, snorting and IV administration are also used. Absorption is rapid after smoking, and the effects can last as long as 24 hours. Methamphetamine-induced psychosis may occur more frequently with smoking.

D.C. will probably be able to stay awake to study if he uses more methamphetamine; however, if he is up for too many days without sleep, his performance on the examination will suffer.

ADVERSE EFFECTS AND TOXICITIES

D.C. is exhibiting classic signs of chronic methamphetamine abuse, which will likely progress if he continues using. A "speed freak" or "tweaker" (chronic methamphetamine user) is generally regarded even by other drug users as mentally unstable, aggressive, and emotionally labile, with unpredictable periods of violent, even homicidal, behavior. Chronic users characteristically develop complex paranoid delusional systems with hallucinations during extended periods of intoxication that may involve several sleepless days and nights of continuous methamphetamine administration. This "speed psychosis" may include tactile hallucinations, such as formication (the sensation of something crawling under the skin). The initial treatment approach for stimulant-induced adverse psychologic effects is nonpharmacologic. The distressed patient may be calmed by reducing environmental stimuli and using the "ART" approach developed by the Haight-Ashbury Free Clinic in San Francisco: **A**cceptance of the patient's immediate needs; calm **R**eassurance that the condition is caused by the drug and will resolve eventually; and **T**alk-down, which involves reassuring, reality-oriented communication.[57] An extremely agitated, anxious, psychotic user, however, will often require administration of a benzodiazepine, such as diazepam (10 to 30 mg orally or 2 to 10 mg intramuscularly or intravenously) or lorazepam (2 to 4 mg orally, intramuscularly, or intravenously). If psychosis persists, a high-potency neuroleptic, such as haloperidol (5 to 10 mg orally, intramuscularly, or intravenously) or risperidone (2 to 4 mg orally), is preferred owing to its minimal anticholinergic activity. Low-potency neuroleptics, such as chlorpromazine, with higher anticholinergic activity, may worsen symptoms of delirium and hyperthermia.[57]

The physiologic toxicity of stimulant drugs includes hypertension, stroke, seizures, hyperthermia, sexual dysfunction, dental caries, rhabdomyolysis, renal failure, cardiac arrhythmias and cardiomyopathies, myocardial infarction, and malnutrition.

The development of neurotoxicities involving dopaminergic and serotonergic neurons (possibly through interference with monoamine transport and increased production of reactive oxygen species) has been demonstrated in animals. It also appears to cause permanent neuronal toxicity with prolonged use.[60]

WITHDRAWAL AND TREATMENT

CASE 90-7, QUESTION 2: D.C. is arrested for assault after a bar fight. He is held in the county jail and is unable to post bail. What withdrawal symptoms might he experience during incarceration?

D.C. will probably suffer intense cravings for methamphetamine and initial agitation, followed by fatigue and hypersomnolence. A withdrawal state after acute cessation of chronic stimulant use is generally the same as that previously described for cocaine. As with cocaine, the crash is notable for marked fatigue, depression, and anhedonia. Most symptoms are mild and will resolve within 1 to 2 weeks, although anhedonia and depression may persist.

Clinical studies investigating treatments for methamphetamine dependence is similar to cocaine treatments. Currently, no pharmacologic treatments have been proved effective for methamphetamine dependence. The most effective treatment so far appears to be psychosocial therapies, such as cognitive-behavioral therapy and contingency management.[57]

DISSOCIATIVE DRUGS: PHENCYCLIDINE, KETAMINE, AND DEXTROMETHORPHAN

Phencyclidine (phenylcyclohexylpiperidine) and ketamine are arylcycloalkylamine, dissociative, anesthetic agents. Phencyclidine (PCP) at one time was marketed as an IV anesthetic agent under the trade name of Sernyl.[61] Subsequent reports of postanesthetic dysphoric reactions caused the drug to be withdrawn in 1965. It was reintroduced in 1967 as Sernylan and marketed as a veterinary anesthetic until 1978, when the manufacture and sale of the drug became illegal. Ketamine is currently used clinically as an anesthetic in both animals and humans. There is some data supporting its use in treatment refractory depression but common side effect of dissociation has confounded the blinding of studies and is a significant side effect. More research is necessary but it is possible that it could be used for very short-term treatment during the efficacy lag of established antidepressants.[62] Ketamine is shorter acting and somewhat less potent than PCP.

Abuse of arylcycloalkylamines occurs primarily in large metropolitan areas. PCP is relatively easy to synthesize and is inexpensive; therefore, it is often misrepresented as other street drugs, such as lysergic acid diethylamide (LSD), amphetamine, mescaline, or Δ-9-tetrahydrocannabinol (THC). Ketamine ("K," "Special K," "Super K," "cat valium") is commonly used as a "club drug" and is sometimes misrepresented as 3,4-methylenedioxymethamphetamine (MDMA; ecstasy). Ketamine is often diverted from veterinarian supplies. PCP ("angel dust," "dust") in powdered form is often applied to parsley, marijuana ("dusted joint," "superweed"), or tobacco cigarettes and smoked. Oral, intranasal and parenteral routes of administration are used by some. The combination of cocaine and PCP in a freebase smoking mixture is called "SpaceBase." Although ketamine is manufactured as an injectable liquid, it is frequently evaporated to a powder. The powder can be snorted or compressed into tablets.

Dextromethorphan is an antitussive agent found in some over-the-counter cough remedies. Its appeal as a drug of abuse may be because it is inexpensive, licit, lacks social disapproval associated with other drugs, and available over-the-counter, and abusers believe it to be safe because it is produced by a pharmaceutical company. Street names include "Skittles," "DXM," "Dex," "Robo," "C-C-C," and "Red Devils." Use is referred to as "dexing," "robotripping," and "robodosing." Dextromethorphan is the D-isomer of the codeine analog of levorphanol. The metabolic byproduct of dextromethorphan, dextrorphan, has weak *N*-methyl-D-aspartate (NMDA) antagonist properties.[61] When dextromethorphan is ingested in large doses, it produces effects similar to PCP or ketamine. When abused, doses range from 300 to 1,800 mg. The most commonly abused form is Coricidin HBP Cough and Cold (called "C-C-C" on the street) because it contains the highest concentration of dextromethorphan per dosage unit on the market (30 mg). Dextromethorphan is also available for sale on the internet in powdered form, which can be ingested orally or snorted. The dextromethorphan "high" can last 3 to 6 hours and can consist of euphoria, dissociation, hallucinosis, increased perceptual awareness, altered time perception, hyperexcitability, pressure of thought, and disorientation; increased blood pressure, heart rate, and body temperature; and blurry vision.[61] Other ingredients found in the over-the-counter preparations, such as acetaminophen, chlorpheniramine, guaifenesin, and alcohol, may be problematic when ingested in large doses. PCP is considered the typical dissociative drug, and review of its effects largely applies to ketamine and dextromethorphan as well.

Phencyclidine

PHENCYCLIDINE INTOXICATION

Persons who use PCP may appear agitated, diaphoretic, and disoriented. There is an increase in blood pressure, pulse, and temperature, and the person may experience vertical and horizontal nystagmus. These symptoms are consistent with PCP intoxication. PCP and ketamine are noncompetitive antagonists of the NMDA receptor subtype of the major excitatory neurotransmitter, glutamate. The dose, route of administration, and serum concentration of phencyclidine all influence the pharmacologic effects of this drug and, thus, the symptoms of intoxication.[61] PCP in low doses causes inebriation, ataxia, changes in body image, numbness, and a mind–body dissociative feeling. Horizontal or vertical nystagmus or both are often present, and the anesthetic effect of the drug raises the pain threshold. Amnesia can occur after intoxication.

As the dose of PCP increases, the patient may manifest agitation, combativeness, catatonia (ketamine users refer to this as a "k-hole"), and psychosis. The action of PCP on the autonomic nervous system becomes more prominent and is characterized by a confusing combination of adrenergic, cholinergic, and dopaminergic effects. A hypertensive response is typically encountered. Tachycardia, tachypnea, and hyperthermia may also be noted in the moderately intoxicated patient. The agitated, combative patient often has feelings of great strength. This, combined with the anesthetic effect of PCP, can result in serious injury because there is no pain sensation to stop the physical activity.

With large doses of PCP, marked CNS depression occurs, and nystagmus may no longer be present. In addition to the physiologic effects noted earlier, respiratory depression, seizures, acidosis, and rhabdomyolysis may further compromise the patient's condition. Rhabdomyolysis, particularly in the presence of acidemia, can result in acute renal failure.[57] Opisthotonic posturing and muscular rigidity occur frequently in the severely intoxicated patient.

MEDICAL MANAGEMENT OF INTOXICATION

Diagnosis of PCP intoxication should be confirmed through a blood or urine specimen. Currently, no clinically useful antidote to PCP exists, and treatment should be supportive. Environmental stimuli should be minimized. Even attempts to talk down the patient may trigger a combative response, and chemical restraints may be indicated. Physical restraints may increase risk of rhabdomyolysis and should be reserved for patients who pose threat of great danger to themselves or others. Benzodiazepines are useful in the management of the anxious, agitated patient with mild to moderate PCP intoxication. If benzodiazepines are insufficient, haloperidol (5 mg IM) is effective.[57] Low-potency neuroleptics should be avoided because a greater possibility of precipitating a hypotensive response or a seizure exists.

Hypertension may be managed with β-blockers or calcium-channel blockers. Diazepam (5 to 10 mg intravenously to 30 mg total) is a useful anticonvulsant for the management of PCP-induced seizures.[57] Because extreme agitation, seizures, and hyperthermia can initiate rhabdomyolysis and secondarily cause myocardial, renal, or hepatic dysfunction, anxiolytics, neuroleptics, anticonvulsants, and cooling measures should be used as needed.

The urinary excretion of PCP (a basic compound) is enhanced when the urine is acidic; however, this approach is not recommended because it may exacerbate myoglobinuric renal failure.[51] Activated charcoal in a dose of 50 to 150 g initially, then 30 to 40 g every 6 to 8 hours, can prevent the intestinal reabsorption of this drug and promote its elimination.[57]

PSYCHOLOGICAL AND PROLONGED EFFECTS

Chronic PCP use can result in prolonged residual psychological symptoms, including anxiety, depression, and psychosis.[57]

Pharmacotherapy for these symptoms may be necessary. Prolonged psychiatric sequelae are almost always associated with premorbid psychopathology. Perceptual disorders, including auditory and visual hallucinations, such as after images seen following moving objects ("trails"), may also occur. Flashbacks (discussed in detail in the subsequent section on LSD) have been reported after PCP use.

The *DSM-5* does not recognize PCP withdrawal; however, about one-fourth of heavy PCP users report symptoms after discontinuation of use.[57] These symptoms include depression, anxiety, irritability, hypersomnolence, diaphoresis, and tremor. Animal studies have described a withdrawal syndrome, but it is unclear whether a true withdrawal syndrome occurs in humans.[57] Currently, no pharmacologic treatments for PCP use disorder exist. Some animal data indicate neurotoxicity; however, the long-term consequences and significance for humans are unknown and require further study. Chronic users often complain of feeling "spaced"; they may be irritable and antisocial and feel depersonalized and isolated from people. Memory lapses, speech and visual disturbances, and confusion have been described in long-term users as well.

HALLUCINOGENS

Hallucinogens can be categorized as indole alkylamines (e.g., LSD, psilocybin, and dimethyltryptamine) or phenethylamines (e.g., mescaline; MDMA). LSD is considered the prototype hallucinogen. Although MDMA is classified as a phenethylamine, it has structural similarities to amphetamine and mescaline. It has been labeled an entactogen or empathogen because of its strong empathy-producing effects and mild hallucinogenic effects. The term *entactogen* can be translated as "a touching within." Hallucinogens are commonly referred to as *psychedelics*.

In 2014, 1.2 million Americans were current hallucinogen users. The popularity of MDMA (ecstasy, X) has risen dramatically in recent years, partly because of its use as a "club drug." In 2014, 609,000 Americans reported using MDMA sometime in the past month.[4] The usual pattern of use for hallucinogens is occasional self-administration for enhancement of recreational activities, such as dancing, or for "mind expansion." Certain individuals may develop psychological dependence and use hallucinogens in a more chronic and compulsive manner.

LSD

EFFECTS

Perhaps the most famous of all hallucinogens, LSD-25 was first synthesized by Albert Hofmann of Sandoz Laboratories in 1938. It was developed as an analeptic agent but produced significant uterine stimulation and caused experimental animals to become excited or cataleptic. Five years later, while resynthesizing LSD-25 for further pharmacologic testing, Dr. Hofmann experienced a restlessness that forced him to go home. This was followed by 2 hours of intense visual hallucinations of kaleidoscopic images and colors. Later, he identified LSD-25 as a potent hallucinogen. Clinical experimentation produced hundreds of papers describing LSD as a drug that could facilitate psychotherapy, particularly in the management of addictive behavior. Widespread public self-experimentation with LSD for recreation and self-exploration, coupled with growing attention to adverse psychological consequences, led Sandoz to discontinue production of LSD-25 (as well as psilocybin, psilocin, and related congeners) in August 1965. The United States made LSD a schedule I controlled substance in 1970 after the proliferation of illicit suppliers to meet the huge public demand for this drug.

Although the mechanism of action of classic hallucinogens is not fully understood, they appear to predominately act as agonists or partial agonists at serotonin (5-HT) receptors, specifically the 5-HT_2 receptor.[63] LSD, one of the most potent hallucinogens known, is active at doses of 25 to 250 mcg. Most users take about 100 to 150 mcg of LSD for a significant effect. This dose produces mild to moderate sympathomimetic effects, profound visual hallucinosis, and the sensation of disordered integration of sensory input. For example, sounds and music are perceived as visual imagery, odors are felt, and inanimate objects assume lifelike qualities. In addition to these sensory-perceptual effects, psychic effects occur, such as depersonalization, dreamlike feelings, and rapid alterations of affect. These are accompanied by somatic effects, including dizziness, nausea, weakness, tremor, and tingling skin.[63] These combined effects begin within an hour of ingestion of LSD and usually peak in intensity during the first 2 to 4 hours. After taking LSD, most people feel they have returned to a normal psychological state by 10 to 12 hours.[64] Within an hour after ingestion, a person will begin to experience altered sensations of his/her surroundings, in addition to some psychic and somatic effects.

ADVERSE EFFECTS

The most frequently encountered adverse reaction associated with the hallucinogenic drugs is a mental state of acute anxiety and fear, typically referred to as a "bad trip." The hallucinogen experience is influenced by set (the user's mental state and expectations of drug effects) and setting (the environment in which drug use takes place, including the social conditions). Users may be able to calm themselves without outside intervention. The initial therapy of people undergoing a bad trip is frequently called "reality therapy" and consists of talking down the fear and panic. This consists of getting the person to a quiet, relaxed setting and helping him or her focus on explanations for the uncertainties that are causing the panic. This process also tends to reassure the person that he or she is in a safe physical environment and that the drug effects will diminish in a few hours. Most of these bad trips are resolved during the state of intoxication (generally, 6–12 hours), but some last as long as 24 to 48 hours.[57]

If the talk-down approach is not successful in resolving the panic, drug therapy can be considered. Sedation with an oral benzodiazepine (i.e., diazepam 10–30 mg) or a parenteral benzodiazepine (i.e., lorazepam 2 mg IM) will frequently alleviate the panic.[57] Supportive talking down should be continued because the benzodiazepine will not stop the trip; it will simply sedate the patient. Haloperidol 2 mg IM may also be used if benzodiazepines are insufficient. Phenothiazines should not be used for initial management of bad trips because they have been associated with poor outcomes.[57]

Regarding adverse physical effects, classic hallucinogens have a high margin of safety, although patients should be monitored for seizures or elevations in body temperature, which may indicate a potential hyperthermic crisis. Anticonvulsant therapy may not be effective until body temperature has been lowered.[57]

FLASHBACKS AND LONG-TERM EFFECTS

Use of hallucinogens can trigger a transient psychosis or unmask an underlying psychiatric disorder; however, a true psychotic episode is rare. Psychiatric conditions after hallucinogen use that persist more than a month are likely caused by preexisting psychopathology.[57] Hallucinogen use does not seem to be associated with any cognitive impairment.[64]

Hallucinogen persisting perceptual disorder (HPPD), commonly referred to as *flashbacks*, is characterized by recurrences of part or all of the hallucinogenic drug experiences after a period of normal consciousness in a person who used the drug previously. The flashbacks may last from minutes to days or months (usually a few hours). The estimated prevalence of flashbacks varies widely in studies, and the etiology is still unclear.[65] Flashbacks can occur spontaneously or be triggered by exercise, stress, or another drug (e.g., marijuana).[64] Treatment remains anecdotal; no randomized, controlled trials have evaluated the efficacy of pharmacotherapy for HPPD.

LSD and other classic hallucinogens have low potential for chronic use disorder. There does not appear to be a clinically important withdrawal syndrome associated with their use. The rapid development of tolerance that occurs with these drugs may explain the intermittent use patterns commonly seen.

MDMA

CASE 90-8

QUESTION 1: R.X. and her friend P.B. go to "raves" (all-night dance parties) every weekend and usually take ecstasy (MDMA). R.X. says it makes her feel like "I love everyone around me," and P.B. likes to be able to "dance all night without getting tired." Are these effects common with MDMA?

Merck Pharmaceuticals patented MDMA in 1914, but it was not until the 1950s that its use was examined in animal studies, when the US Army Intelligence investigated it as a "brainwashing" agent. By the late 1970s, a few therapists and psychiatrists began using the drug with reported success in patients with a wide range of conditions.[66] MDMA produces a very manageable and comfortable entactogenic effect, during which the person has a clear sensorium. The experience can be recalled in detail, and the insights gained during the session can be incorporated into normal life. The public gave several names to this drug, such as ecstasy, XTC, Adam, and M&Ms. The media became aware of the anecdotal reports from both psychiatrists and people self-experimenting with MDMA. In 1985, the DEA made MDMA a schedule I drug. Subsequently, supplies of the drug proliferated in the public illicit marketplace, and its popularity soared. In 2001, after successful lobbying by researchers interested in reinstituting MDMA in clinical practice, the FDA granted approval for a pilot study investigating the therapeutic use of MDMA in the treatment of posttraumatic stress disorder (PTSD). Results of this placebo-controlled study indicate that MDMA is very effective (83% vs. 25%) in treating PTSD.[67] The effects of MDMA are mainly exerted by three neurochemical mechanisms: blockade of serotonin reuptake, stimulation of serotonin release, and stimulation of dopamine release.[68] The common psychological effects of MDMA intoxication include an overall heightened sense of empathy, interpersonal closeness, increased acceptance of others, and a powerful sense of well-being.[69] The experience is influenced by set and setting. The amphetamine-like side effects include mydriasis, tachycardia, sweating, increased energy and alertness, bruxism, nausea, and anorexia.[70] Users generally ingest MDMA in tablet form, and the onset of action is usually after 30 to 60 minutes. Some users take a "booster" dose after 2 hours. The usual duration of action of MDMA is 4 to 6 hours, and the half-life is approximately 8 hours. MDMA users in the rave scene often "stack" multiple doses, and polydrug use is common. The combined use of ecstasy and LSD is referred to as "candy flipping."[68]

R.X.'s feelings of love for everyone are consistent with the empathogenic effects of MDMA, whereas P.B. is enjoying the amphetamine-like effects of increased energy to dance all night.

ADVERSE EFFECTS

CASE 90-8, QUESTION 2: Several hours after taking MDMA, P.B. is still dancing. She begins to feel hot and realizes she is profusely sweating. On her way to the bar for a drink, she begins to feel confused and collapses to the floor. Her friends witness her having a seizure and call 9-1-1. What is happening to P.B.?

The rave scene, with its crowded conditions and often-high ambient temperatures, has contributed to many adverse effects associated with MDMA ingestion. Because of their increased physical activity, the ravers may become dehydrated. Additionally, supplies of MDMA have been notoriously unreliable. Many other drugs have been misrepresented as MDMA, including other phenethylamines such as 3,4-methylenedioxy-amphetamine (MDA) and paramethoxyamphetamine (PMA); amphetamine; cocaine; opiates; ketamine; and dextromethorphan. The common polydrug use practiced at raves compounds the problem. Dextromethorphan taken at high doses for its dissociative properties competes with MDMA for hepatic metabolism, and its anticholinergic effects block perspiration, potentially leading to overheating.[66]

The most dangerous adverse physical effect of MDMA is hyperthermia. MDMA has a slight affinity for the 5-HT_2 receptor, and the increased body temperature may be the result of this activation.[68] The hyperthermia has led to rhabdomyolysis, and acute renal and hepatic failure, disseminated intravascular coagulation (DIC), and death.[71] DIC has been the most common cause of death. Treatment of hyperthermia involves cooling measures and IV fluids. Benzodiazepines (e.g., lorazepam 2 mg IM or IV) and dantrolene (1 mg/kg IV) may be helpful. Other adverse physical effects can include hypertension, cardiac arrhythmias, convulsions, cerebrovascular accident, hepatitis, and hyponatremia (from over ingestion of water as a harm reduction measure to avoid hyperthermia).[70,71] In 2011, there were 22,498, emergency department visits associated with MDMA use.[72] Adverse psychological effects are also possible, including anxiety, depression, panic attacks, agitation, paranoia, and rarely psychosis. The treatment of these psychological adverse effects is the same as for those associated with the classic hallucinogens, including talk-down therapy and benzodiazepine administration. P.B. may be suffering from MDMA-induced hyperthermia and needs urgent medical evaluation.

LONG-TERM EFFECTS

CASE 90-8, QUESTION 3: R.X. has read in the newspaper that MDMA is associated with "brain damage" and is worried that she has caused permanent damage to her brain. What are the long-term effects of MDMA?

Animal studies have consistently demonstrated long-term MDMA-induced serotonin depletion. This has been evidenced by lower levels of serotonin, decreased metabolite levels, lowered levels of tryptophan hydroxylase, and loss of serotonin reuptake transporters.[66] This may explain the induction of panic attacks for chronic users. MDMA damages serotonin axonal projections; axonal resprouting and regeneration do occur, but it is unclear whether these new projections are damaged.[66,73] Both hepatotoxicity and neuronal toxicity occur with MDMA use and is suspected to be due to oxidative stress, mitochondrial dysfunction, and excitotoxicity.[60]

Several retrospective studies in humans have claimed lowered cognitive performance in MDMA users compared with nonusers. These studies have confounding variables, such as other drug use and adulterant exposure and lifestyle factors.[66,73]

Use of MDMA does not appear to produce physical dependence, but some users may become psychologically dependent. Tolerance to the empathogenic effects develops rapidly and may last 24 to 36 hours. This may explain in part the more common practice of sporadic dosing of the drug.[57,69] No distinctive withdrawal syndrome has been described that would require pharmacologic treatment.

MARIJUANA

Marijuana is the most widely used illicit substance in the United States. In 2014, 35.1 million Americans reported using marijuana in the past year.[4] The main psychoactive ingredient in the *Cannabis sativa* plant is Δ-9-tetrahydrocannabinol (THC), although the plant is known to contain more than 70 cannabinoids.[74] In the United States, the dried, chopped leaves and flowers of the *Cannabis* plant (grass, pot, weed, green bud, chronic, mary jane) are rolled into a cigarette paper (marijuana cigarette, known as a joint or blunt; a "roach" is the butt of the marijuana cigarette) or smoked in a pipe or water pipe ("bong"). Each joint usually weighs 0.5 to 1 g, for a THC content of about 5 mg (very weak), 30 mg (average), or 150 mg (highest-quality sinsemilla). The sinsemilla (Spanish for "without seeds") growing technique involves separating the female plants from the males before pollination occurs. This results in female plants with higher amounts of THC, up to 14%.[75]

The raw resin of the *Cannabis* plant can be pressed into cakes, balls, or sticks, called hashish ("hash," "temple balls"), which is smoked or eaten. Hashish can contain up to 8% THC. The oils can be extracted from the plant with organic solvents to produce "hash oil," perhaps the most potent *Cannabis* derivative, with THC concentrations of up to 50%.[75]

Researchers in cannabinoid neurobiology have discovered two cannabinoid receptors in the CNS: CB_1 and CB_2; however, additional receptors have been proposed. Research has demonstrated that the main pharmacologic and addictive effects are almost completely mediated by the CB_1 receptor.[75] In addition, five endogenous cannabinoids (endocannabinoids) that act at the cannabinoid receptors have been discovered.[76] The best known are arachidonic acid ethanolamide (anandamide) and 2-arachidonoylglycerol (2-AG).[76] Considerable evidence exists supporting the role of THC–opioid interactions with enhanced antinociception. Cannabinoids have been shown to release endogenous opioids, and cannabinoid receptors colocalize with substance P (the neurotransmitter responsible for transmitting pain information) receptors in the striatum. Subsequently, investigation of THC as an adjunct to opioid treatment of pain, prevention of opioid tolerance, and dependence is underway.[75]

Marijuana's therapeutic potential has been the center of much public controversy. Research on the effects of cannabinoids has led to several potential therapeutic uses, including relief of nausea and vomiting, appetite stimulation, and treatment of pain, epilepsy, glaucoma, and movement disorders (Parkinson disease, Huntington disease, Tourette syndrome, multiple sclerosis).[75,77] In 1999, the State of California passed the law SB847, which commissioned the University of California to establish the Center for Medicinal Cannabis Research (CMCR) to expand scientific knowledge on purported therapeutic usages of marijuana. The center's 2010 report to the California legislature and governor presented clinical trial findings demonstrating that cannabis has analgesic effects in pain conditions secondary to injury or disease and that cannabis reduces MS spasticity.[78] A synthetic form of THC, dronabinol, is available as prescription tablets, and a synthetic cannabinoid, nabilone (Cesamet), is available as capsules, but advocates of medicinal marijuana use argue that inhalation allows for faster onset and easier titration of the dose. In addition, nauseated patients want to avoid the oral route of administration. Future research focuses on developing a safer delivery system that will be reliable, rapid, and safe. An oromucosal spray, Sativex, derived from botanical material, is under investigation in the United States. The principal active components are THC and cannabidiol. This cannabis extract spray has been approved in Canada, and is also being used in the United Kingdom. A capsule formulation containing a mixed ratio of THC and cannabidiol produced by Cannador in Germany is also available.[75] Other alternative delivery methods may include vaporization, patches, and suppositories.

Effects

CASE 90-9

QUESTION 1: P.H. is a 16-year-old male who is offered a marijuana cigarette (joint) by one of his friends. He smokes it and begins to feel light-headed and euphoric. He begins laughing at everything around him. Thirty minutes later he and his friend become very hungry ("the munchies") and eat several candy bars. Which of P.H.'s symptoms are consistent with marijuana use?

The pharmacologic effects sought by most users of cannabis products are sedation, mental relaxation, euphoria, and mild hallucinogenic effects, and these effects depend on set and setting. Other common effects that are usually perceived as pleasurable include silliness, subjective slowing of time, gregariousness, hunger, and mild perceptual changes of all the senses that engender an absorbing fascination with music, eating, and other sensual and sensory activities. The state of mind generated is referred to as "stoned," "high," "loaded," "wasted," and many other colloquial terms. Smoking marijuana typically causes numbness and tingling of the extremities, light-headedness, loss of concentration, and a floating sensation in the first 3 or 4 minutes. Some of these effects are probably caused by the hyperventilation associated with deep inhalation of the smoke (referred to as a "hit" or "toke") and breath holding to allow maximal absorption from the lungs. During the first 10 to 30 minutes, the user may experience tachycardia (possibly palpitations), mild diaphoresis, conjunctival injection ("red eye"), drying of the mouth, weakness, postural hypotension, periods of tremulousness, incoordination, and ataxia along with euphoria and the mental effects described above. These effects usually resolve by 1 to 3 hours and are followed by a 30- to 60-minute period of sleepiness before complete clearing and return to normal consciousness. Oral ingestion of cannabis products may delay the onset of effects by 45 to 60 minutes and prolong the duration.[75] P.H. is experiencing euphoria, giddiness, and increased appetite, consistent with marijuana intoxication.

Adverse Effects

CASE 90-9, QUESTION 2: P.H. smokes more marijuana with his friend. He liked it so much the first time, he decides to take several "hits" this time. He begins to think his friend is laughing at him and notices his heart is beating rapidly. He starts to panic. Is P.H.'s reaction caused by the marijuana?

Consistent with its widespread use, marijuana was the second most frequently mentioned illicit substance in emergency department episodes in the United States in 2007. A total of 308,547 marijuana-related emergency department (ED) visits were reported in 2007.[58] These visits include marijuana in combination with other drugs. As the percentage of THC has increased in marijuana, so have the ED visits. The majority of ED visits are from unexpected reactions, such as anxiety, paranoia, and panic attacks. Despite these numbers, there are no documented cases of fatality in humans from marijuana overdose, and adverse effects tend to be self-limiting and often do not require medical treatment.

A syndrome consisting of anxiety, paranoia, depersonalization, disorientation, and confusion that can lead to panic states and incapacitating fear is perhaps the most frequently reported adverse effect of marijuana. Comforting reassurance (talk-down) and reducing stressful stimuli can alleviate this condition. The dysphoria and anxiety usually resolve in a few hours or less with such an approach. More severe incidents that evolve into panic reactions that are not resolved by sympathetic counseling may be relieved with oral benzodiazepine therapy in a dose equivalent to 5 to 10 mg of diazepam.[57] These adverse psychological reactions to cannabis products commonly occur with inexperienced users, high doses, concomitant use of other psychoactive drugs, and overtly stressful situations. Severe reactions requiring pharmacologic therapy are rare. A review of the literature found that cannabis use increases the risk of developing psychotic disorders among vulnerable or predisposed individuals and negatively affects the course of preexisting chronic psychosis.[79]

Other adverse effects can include slowed psychomotor responses and short-term memory loss. Slowed psychomotor responses have been shown in certain groups of acutely intoxicated subjects and chronic users. Even medical marijuana users have shown a steep increase in automobile accidents. Short-term memory loss is a frequently documented acute, reversible effect of marijuana intoxication as well.

The paranoid ideation and panic reaction of P.H. could certainly be caused by the high dose and his inexperience with marijuana.

Long-Term Effects

CASE 90-9, QUESTION 3: P.H. continues to smoke marijuana daily. What are possible long-term effects of marijuana use?

Chronic use of cannabis has been alleged to produce an "amotivational syndrome" characterized by apathy, lack of long-term goal achievement, inability to manage stress, and generalized laziness.[75,80,81] Cognitive impairment can occur after heavy marijuana use, but appears to be reversible with abstinence.[82] However, the adolescent brain has shown a drop in IQ related to marijuana use that does not reverse even after 1 year of abstinence.[83] The impairment is more pronounced the longer the drug is used.[67] Other concurrent drug use may also contribute to cognitive impairment associated with marijuana use. As noted above, there is a dose-dependent risk of chronic use resulting in an increased risk of developing a psychotic illness later in life.[79,84] Chronic users will have worse periodontal health.[85] The pulmonary complications of chronic heavy marijuana use are potentially significant. Chronic cough, sputum, wheezing, bronchitis, and cellular changes typical of chronic tobacco smokers are reported in chronic cannabis smokers.[75,86] THC has been shown to be a potent bronchodilator. Both oral and smoked THCs were shown to produce significant bronchodilation when given to healthy subjects. The bronchodilatory response in asthmatics given THC has been shown to be less vigorous.[87] Tolerance to these effects can develop after some weeks, and chronic marijuana smoking results in increased airway resistance and decreased pulmonary function.[75] Many of the same carcinogens in nicotine cigarettes are also found in marijuana smoke and risk of some cancers is increased compared to nonusers.[75,81] *Aspergillus*-contaminated marijuana has been reported to cause pulmonary fungal infections in immunocompromised patients, who may be using the drug for its medicinal value.[88]

Tolerance to the psychoactive effects of marijuana does develop. Chronic users may not experience the full range of effects as new users unless they abstain for several days or weeks to regain initial sensitivity to the cannabis, and chronic users can tolerate large doses that generally are toxic to novices. Tolerance develops rapidly to both physiologic and psychological effects of cannabis. Dependence characterized by a physical withdrawal syndrome occurs after chronic high-dose use of cannabis. The withdrawal syndrome can involve anxiety, depression, irritability, restlessness, anorexia, insomnia and vivid or disturbing dreams, sweating, tremor, nausea, vomiting, and diarrhea.[57,75,83] Dysphoria and malaise similar to that experienced with influenza can also occur. The cumulative dose of cannabis and duration of use necessary to produce dependence is unknown. The withdrawal syndrome is generally mild and self-limiting, and pharmacologic treatments usually are not required.

Marijuana has been labeled as a "gateway drug," meaning that it will lead to the use of "harder" drugs, such as cocaine or heroin. Marijuana is the most widely used illicit drug, but use of drugs such as alcohol and tobacco often predates marijuana use. No studies have conclusively demonstrated a causal link between marijuana use and subsequent other drug use.[75]

There are clear acute and chronic risks involved with marijuana use. As more states legalize it for recreational and "medical" purposes, researchers will be able to define and predict the fullness of these problems.

INHALANTS

The introduction of anesthetics (nitrous oxide, chloroform, and ether) to medicine in the early 1800s also promoted the widespread and popular recreational use of these inhalants for mind-altering recreational purposes. Today, abused inhalants include a wide variety of chemicals that are found readily in homes or workplaces, or purchased at retail establishments. Inhalants are commonly subdivided into three main categories: the volatile solvents (mostly hydrocarbons); volatile nitrites (amyl, butyl, isobutyl, cyclohexyl); and nitrous oxide (laughing gas). The fumes or vapors of these liquids, or paste in the case of glue, are directly inhaled out of their containers ("sniffing"); poured onto a rag that is held to the nose ("huffing"); poured into a plastic bag ("bagging"); or merely cupped in the hands and inhaled. Aerosols and gaseous substances such as nitrous oxide are also used to inflate a balloon and then inhaled out of the balloon by the user. These products can also be ingested orally or sprayed directly into the mouth. Volatile solvents include gasoline, toluene, kerosene, alcohols, airplane glue, lacquer thinner, acetone (nail polish remover), benzene (nail polish remover, model cement), naphtha (lighter fluid), plastic cement, liquid paper (i.e., White Out, usually containing 1,1,1-trichloroethane, also trichloroethylene and perchloroethylene), and many others. The volatile nitrites, once widely available, are prohibited by the Consumer Product Safety Commission but can still be found, sold in small bottles, labeled as "video head cleaner" or "room odorizer." Amyl nitrite is used medically as a vasodilator for treatment of angina and requires a prescription. The volatile nitrites are commonly referred to as "poppers," because of the sound made when an ampule of amyl nitrite is broken open. The most commonly used inhalants are glue, shoe polish, toluene, and gasoline.[89] The use of multiple products is common. Silver and gold paints are popular because they contain more toluene than paints of other colors.[90]

Inhalant use is most common among younger individuals (consistently highest annual prevalence among 8th graders) and tends to decline as youth grow older. The decline likely reflects that other drugs become available and are substituted. Abuse of inhalants is believed to be popular among children and adolescents because of their low cost, easy availability, rapid onset, and low threat of legal intervention. Additionally, they are easily concealed.

The 2009 Monitoring the Future (MTF) study found that 12.5% of 8th, 10th, and 12th graders have abused inhalants.[91] The MTF and other national surveys of adolescents have found that after marijuana, inhalants are the second most widely used class of illicit drugs for 8th graders. Most inhalant users, however, have used alcohol or cigarettes previously.[92] These surveys, most of which are administered in schools, likely underestimate the true prevalence, as a small but high-risk group (incarcerated, homeless, and transient adolescents) are not included in the surveys.

Effects of Inhalants

Inhalant abuse includes a broad range of chemicals, and they likely have different pharmacologic effects. In fact, the mechanisms of action of the volatile inhalants are poorly understood. Nearly all have CNS depressant effects. Evidence from animal studies suggests the effects and mechanism of action of volatile solvents are similar to those of alcohol and sedative-hypnotics.[93]

Gases and vapors are rapidly absorbed when inhaled and, because of their high lipophilicity, tend to distribute preferentially to lipid-rich organs such as the brain and liver.[93] Expired air is the major route of elimination, and most are metabolized to some extent. Inhalation of these products produces a temporary stimulation and reduced inhibitions before the depressive CNS effects occur. Acute intoxication is associated with euphoria, giddiness, dizziness, slurred speech, unsteady gait, and drowsiness.[90] As the CNS becomes more deeply affected, illusions, hallucinations, and delusions develop. The user experiences a euphoric, dreamy high that culminates in a short period of sleep. The intoxicated state lasts a few minutes, but users may continue to inhale repeatedly for several hours. Nitrous oxide is an antagonist of the NMDA subtype of the glutamate receptor.[61] Its pharmacologic effects are poorly understood. It produces euphoria and symptoms of intoxication similar to those described for the volatile solvents.

The major effect of the volatile nitrites is the relaxation of all smooth muscles in the body, including the blood vessels. This usually allows a greater volume of blood to flow to the brain. The onset of effects takes 7 or 8 seconds and the effects last about 30 seconds. A certain "rush" occurs, which may be followed by a severe headache, dizziness, and giddiness. The volatile nitrites are frequently used in the context of sexual activity, because of the effect of increased tumescence and relaxation of smooth muscle.[93]

Acute and Chronic Toxicities Associated with Inhalants

The wide variety of chemicals inhaled causes a tremendous range of toxicities. Toxicity depends on the chemical, and on the magnitude and duration of exposure. Complications can result from the effects of the solvents or other toxic ingredients, such as lead in gasoline. The lipophilicity of the volatiles enhances their toxicity. Injuries to the brain, liver, kidney, bone marrow, and particularly the lungs can occur, and they may result from the effect of heavy exposure or hypersensitivity. Inhalant abusers may develop irritation of the eyes, nose, and mouth, including rhinitis, conjunctivitis, and rash.[93] Methemoglobinemia has been associated with volatile nitrite use.

Deaths from inhalant use are well documented and may occur from overdose or trauma (falls, drowning, hanging). Death from overdose is often caused by respiratory problems or suffocation after CNS depression.[93] Deaths caused by asphyxiation, convulsions, coma, and aspiration of gastric contents have occurred.[90] Acute cardiotoxicity resulting in cardiac arrest may cause sudden death. Referred to as "sudden sniffing death," it is likely caused by sensitization of the myocardium to catecholamines, exacerbated by physical exercise, resulting in fatal ventricular arrhythmias.

Many of the inhalants produce neurotoxicity, which can range from mild impairment to severe dementia. Neurologic deficits include cognitive impairment, ataxia, optic neuropathy, deafness, and disorders of equilibrium. Loss of white matter, brain atrophy, and damage to specific neural pathways can result from chronic exposure to some inhalants. Some damage to the nervous system and other organs may be at least partially reversible when inhalant use is discontinued.[90]

Inhalant Abuse and Dependence

Compulsive use has been documented with inhalants, although inhalant abuse and dependence is a neglected area of research. Animal studies have shown some of the abused inhalants to have reinforcing properties.[93,94] It is unclear whether a true withdrawal syndrome occurs with chronic use of inhalants. Inhalant use is typically episodic in nature, and thus users may not be exposed to levels with sufficient frequency necessary to develop physical dependence or tolerance.

ALCOHOL USE DISORDERS

Alcohol Content and Definitions

Beverages containing alcohol (ethanol) have a wide range of ethanol content. Alcoholic proof is a measure of how much ethanol is in an alcoholic beverage, and is twice the percentage of alcohol by volume (ABV), the unit that is commonly used as percent. This system dates to the 18th century, and perhaps earlier, when spirits were graded along with gunpowder. A solution of water and alcohol "proved" itself when it could be poured on a pinch of gunpowder and the wet powder could still be ignited. If the gunpowder did not ignite, the solution had too much water in it and the proof was considered insufficient. A "proven" solution was defined as 100 degrees proof (100).[95,96] In the United States, the proof is twice the percentage of alcohol content measured by volume at a temperature of 60°F. Therefore "80 proof" is 40% ABV, and pure alcohol (100%) is "200 proof." One hundred percent ethanol does not stay 100% because it is hygroscopic and absorbs water from the atmosphere.

Legally, in the United States, beers containing up to 0.5% ABV can be called nonalcoholic. Light beers range from 2% to about 4% ABV; beers range from 4% to 6% ABV; ales, stouts, and specialty brews can be as high as 10% ABV. Wines are produced at about 14% to 16% (28–32 proof), because that is the point in the fermentation process at which the alcohol concentration denatures the yeast. Stronger liquors are distilled after fermentation is complete to separate the alcoholic liquid from the remains of the source of sugar (e.g., grain, fruit). Distilled liquor cannot be stronger than 95% (190 proof). A standard drink in the United States is considered to be 0.5 ounces or contain 15 g (0.5 fl oz of absolute alcohol) of alcohol. This is equal to 12 ounces (355 mL) of 5% beer, 5 ounces (148 mL) of 12% wine, or 1.5 ounces (44 mL) of 40% spirits.[95,96]

Epidemiology

Slightly more than half (52.7%) of Americans age 12 or older reported being current drinkers (at least one drink in the past 30 days) of alcohol in the 2014 National Survey on Drug Use and Health survey.[4] This translates to an estimated 137 million people, which is similar to the 2005 estimate of 126 million people (51.8%). In 2014, heavy drinking (five or more drinks on the same occasion on each of 5 or more days in the past 30 days) was reported by 6.2% of the population age 12 or older.[4]

Approximately 10% of Americans will be affected by alcohol use disorder sometime during their lives.[97,98] Treatment of alcohol dependence consists mainly of psychological, social, and pharmacotherapy interventions aimed at reducing alcohol-related problems.[99] Treatment usually consists of two phases: detoxification and maintenance.

The rationale for pharmacotherapy is based on several considerations. Advances in neurobiology have identified neurotransmitter systems that initiate and sustain alcohol drinking; pharmacologic modification of these neurotransmitters or their receptors may alter dependence.[100] Promising genetic research confirms that alcoholics are a heterogeneous population and that several gene variations can predispose some to increased alcohol use whereas other gene variations can confer protection.[100] Animal models have identified pharmacologic agents that reduce alcohol consumption in animals, suggesting similar agents could reduce alcohol consumption in humans.

Risks and Benefits of Alcohol Consumption

The role of alcohol in the development of medical problems such as cardiovascular disease, hepatic cirrhosis, and fetal abnormalities is well documented. Alcohol use and abuse contribute to thousands of injuries, auto collisions, and violence.[101] Alcohol can dramatically affect worker productivity and absenteeism, family interactions, and school performance.[102] Some studies suggest, however, that individuals who abstain from using alcohol may also be at greater risk for a variety of conditions, particularly coronary heart disease (CHD), than people who consume small to moderate amounts of alcohol.[103]

A number of studies have documented an association between moderate alcohol consumption and lower risk for CHD and myocardial infarction (MI).[104,105] Binge drinking after an MI, however, increases the risk of mortality.[106] US guidelines define moderate drinking as one drink or less daily for women or people age 65 and older, and two drinks or less per day for men.[107] An association between moderate drinking and lower risk of CHD does not mean that alcohol is the cause of the lower risk. A review of population studies indicates that the higher mortality risk among abstainers may be attributable to socioeconomic and employment status, mental health, and overall health, rather than abstinence from alcohol use.[108] Benefits of moderate drinking on CHD mortality are offset at higher drinking levels by increased risk of death because of other types of heart disease, cancer, cirrhosis, and trauma. The risk of a disease outcome from low to moderate drinking is less than the risk from either no drinking at all or heavier drinking. This produces a U-shaped curve when examining the association of alcohol consumption with rates of deaths from all causes.[103]

The exact mechanism by which alcohol use may be protective against morbidity in those with CHD is not clear. Some evidence indicates that different types of alcoholic beverages, such as red wines, which are high in tannins, may lower blood lipids and fats by increasing antioxidants.[106] Specifically, the mechanisms by which alcohol may reduce the risk of CHD include increasing levels of high-density lipoprotein cholesterol, decreasing levels of low-density lipoprotein cholesterol, prevention of clot formation, reduction in platelet aggregation, and lowering of plasma apolipoprotein(a) concentration, resulting in the attenuation of the formation of atheroma and decreasing the rate of blood coagulation.[109,110] It is also possible, however, that how a person drinks alcoholic beverages matters as well. For example, wines are ingested more slowly as they are typically consumed in moderate amounts with food. Binge drinking of any type of beverage, however, increases the risk of mortality from CHD in particular.[106]

Pharmacokinetics and Pharmacology

When consumed in amounts typical of normal social drinking, the absorption of ethanol from the stomach, small intestine, and colon is complete; however, the rate is variable. Peak blood ethanol concentrations after oral doses in fasting subjects generally are reached in 30 to 75 minutes, but several factors can influence the rate and extent of absorption.[111] The most rapidly absorbed formulations are carbonated beverages containing 10% to 30% ethanol. In contrast, high concentrations of alcohol can produce vasoconstriction in the gastrointestinal (GI) mucosa, which results in slowed or even incomplete absorption of ethanol. Absorption of ethanol from the small intestine appears to be more rapid than any other part of the GI tract and does not depend on the presence or absence of food. Factors that control the rate of gastric emptying significantly control the rate of absorption by controlling the rate at which ethanol is delivered to the small intestine.[112,113] For example, food in the stomach slows the absorption of ethanol, probably by slowing gastric emptying. The level of intoxication achieved is not solely related to the plasma concentration. For any particular plasma concentration, greater cognitive impairment is seen during times when the plasma level is rising compared with when ethanol is primarily being eliminated. The degree of intoxication also appears to be directly related to the rate at which pharmacologically active plasma concentrations are attained. Alcohol negatively affects cognitive performance and has a differential effect on the descending versus ascending limb of the blood alcohol concentration (BAC) curve. The latter finding may have important ramifications relating to the detrimental consequences of alcohol intoxication.[114]

The blood alcohol level (BAL) or BAC is calculated using the weight of ethanol in milligrams and the volume of blood in deciliters. This yields a BAC expressed as a proportion (i.e., 100 mg/dL or 1.0 g/L) or as a percentage (i.e., 0.10% alcohol). Ethanol concentrations are usually converted to equivalent BACs for standardization purposes when measured in other body fluids.

The alcohol dehydrogenase (ADH) pathway is the major enzyme system responsible for alcohol metabolism in humans. The main alcohol metabolism occurs with ADH isoenzymes, in the stomach (ADH6 and ADH7) and in the liver (ADH1, ADH2, and ADH3). The pathway involves conversion of ethanol to acetaldehyde by these ADH isoenzymes, resulting in the reduction of nicotinamide adenine dinucleotide (NAD) to NADH. In the second step, acetaldehyde is converted to acetate via the enzyme aldehyde dehydrogenase, which also reduces NAD to NADH. These are the rate-limiting steps in ethanol metabolism, and this route becomes saturated when large amounts of ethanol deplete NAD.[115] Acetate ultimately is converted to carbon dioxide and water. An additional pathway that is more involved in alcohol-dependent individuals than those who are not involves the catalase pathway of peroxisomes and the microsomal ethanol oxidizing system (MEOS), in the smooth endoplasmic reticulum. The main functional component of the MEOS is the cytochrome-P450 (CYP) 2E1.

Of a dose of ethanol, 90% to 98% is oxidized in the liver, with the remaining drug excreted unchanged in the alveolar air and urine. Ethanol metabolism formerly was described by zero-order kinetics; however, Michaelis–Menten and other nonlinear, concentration-dependent models are more accurate.[116,117] In some situations, a portion of the absorbed dose of ethanol does not appear to enter the systemic circulation, suggesting first-pass metabolism. The relative contribution of hepatic versus gastric ADH to this response continues to be debated, however.[118,119] Using a two-compartment, Michaelis–Menten pharmacokinetic model as well as experimental data, it appears that gastric metabolism contributes negligibly to first-pass metabolism.[120–122] They believe that gastric metabolism accounts for sex and ethnic differences in first-pass metabolism. Estimates of total gastric ADH suggest that the enzyme can metabolize 0.9 to 1.8 g/hour of ethanol, depending on the concentration of ethanol consumed.[123] The extent of first-pass extraction tends to decrease as the dose of alcohol increases. This is likely because of saturation of ADH, regardless of the source. When plasma ethanol levels are greater than 0.2 g/mL, the ADH system becomes saturated. As hepatic ADH becomes saturated, there is increased unchanged excretion of alcohol. This results in a more intense odor of alcohol on the breath as the plasma ethanol concentration increases. The metabolism of alcohol also then tends to become nonlinear because of stimulation of CYP2E1, which produces metabolic tolerance to ethanol in chronic users.

Lower first-pass metabolism has been found in alcohol-dependent individuals, women, the elderly, and Japanese subjects.[120,122] Gastric ADH may also play a role in the effect of food in reducing ethanol bioavailability. Food, by delaying gastric emptying, allows for more extensive gastric metabolism.[123]

The accepted average rate of ethanol oxidation is 0.15 g/mL/hour for men and 0.18 g/mL/hour for women.[124] Although this rate still is widely used for both legal and medical purposes, other data suggest wide variability in ethanol metabolism. For example, wide differences in ADH activity have been demonstrated and attributed to heredity and other causes.[125,126] Chronic heavy drinkers frequently oxidize ethanol at twice the normal rates, with their metabolic rates returning to baseline after a period of abstinence.[127] The rate of oxidation in chronic heavy drinkers may also increase with elevated blood ethanol levels.[127] In contrast, patients with end-stage liver disease may progress to the point at which they have almost no metabolic capacity.

Chronic alcohol use is associated with characteristic changes in the liver. Hyperlipidemia and fat deposition in the liver occur because of shunting of the excess hydrogen into fatty acid synthesis and direct oxidation of ethanol for energy instead of body fat stores being used for energy. Fatty liver is the first step in a sequence of events that ultimately leads to alcoholic cirrhosis. Accumulated acetaldehyde, which interferes with mitochondrial function by shortening and thickening microtubules, has been implicated as playing a role in the hepatotoxic process. The damaged microtubules then inhibit the secretory functions of the hepatocytes, which results in an increase in size and weight of the liver.[128] Nutritional deficits and impaired hepatic protein metabolism may contribute as mechanisms of hepatotoxicity in chronic ethanol consumers.[129,130]

Acetaldehyde is believed to play a role in most actions of alcohol.[131] Elevated acetaldehyde concentrations during ethanol intoxication cause the commonly seen sensitivity reactions, including vasodilatation and facial flushing, increased skin temperature, increased heart and respiration rates, and lowered blood pressure. Acetaldehyde also contributes to the sensations of dry mouth and throat associated with bronchoconstriction and allergic-type reactions, as well as nausea and headache. These adverse effects mediated by acetaldehyde have the potential to protect drinkers against the excessive ingestion of alcohol, but acetaldehyde also has the potential to produce euphoric effects that may reinforce alcohol consumption. Acetaldehyde also contributes to the increased incidence of GI and upper airway cancers that are seen with increased incidence in heavy consumers of alcohol and which may also play a role in the pathogenesis of liver cirrhosis.[132]

Ethanol ingestion can depress the CNS through all the different stages of anesthesia. Tolerance to this effect occurs after chronic use such that a blood ethanol level of 0.150 g/mL will not produce apparent behavioral or neurologic dysfunction in persons who drink a pint or more of 80-proof liquor (or its equivalent) daily for several years.

Neurobiological Basis of Alcohol Dependence

Proteins that are particularly sensitive to alcohol include ion channels, neurotransmitter receptors, and enzymes involved in signal transduction.[133] Notable neurotransmitters, hormones, and neuropeptides include adenosine, cannabinoid receptors, corticotropin-releasing factor (CRF), dopamine (DA), γ-aminobutyric acid (GABA), ghrelin, glutamate, neurokinin-1 (NK1), neuropeptide Y (NPY), norepinephrine, opioid peptides, and serotonin (5-HT). The key inhibitory neurotransmitter in the CNS is GABA, which is associated with a chloride-ion channel that is affected by low concentrations of alcohol. Normally, when GABA binds to the $GABA_A$ receptor, the chloride channel opens, allowing negatively charged chloride ions to enter the cell and inhibiting neuronal cell activity. In the presence of alcohol, GABA release accentuates the anxiolytic effect of both combined.[134] Receptor compensation for continual inhibition by alcohol is to reduce $GABA_A$ receptor subunits.[135] Other sedative medications, such as benzodiazepines, also bind to the chloride channel at slightly different sites and facilitate GABA inhibition. The existence of a common receptor mechanism for the actions of alcohol and sedative-hypnotics accounts for the cross-tolerance between these substances.

Glutamate is the major excitatory neurotransmitter in the CNS. Low doses of alcohol strongly inhibit NMDA receptors and inhibit neuronal activity.[136] After continual exposure to high doses of alcohol, NMDA receptors upregulate in an attempt to balance alcohol's inhibitory action. Thus, the combined effect of alcohol on $GABA_A$ and glutamate is to inhibit excitation and facilitate sedation.

Alcohol also affects several other ion channels and receptors. The $5\text{-}HT_3$ receptor subtype is particularly sensitive to the action of low doses of alcohol, and may result in activation of 5-HT and DA. Alcohol also modifies the activity of β-adrenergic and adenosine neurotransmitter receptors linked to adenylate cyclase through membrane-bound G-proteins. Low doses of alcohol can facilitate the activity of norepinephrine, 5-HT, DA, endocannabinoid signaling system, and other neurotransmitter receptors linked to G-proteins.[137–139]

On a neurobiological behavioral level, the mesolimbic dopaminergic pathway from the ventral tegmental area to the nucleus accumbens is activated by most dependence-producing drugs, including alcohol, cocaine, opiates, and nicotine.[140,141] Putatively, activation of this pathway mediates drug reward and is responsible for the dependence-producing properties of all drugs of abuse.[142] Repeated alcohol use sensitizes the system, so that behavioral stimuli associated with alcohol also begin to release dopamine and to facilitate additional alcohol use.[143] Dopamine released by drugs of abuse are 2- to 10-fold that of natural rewards.[144] This sensitization may account for the craving and preoccupation with drugs of abuse.

Cessation of chronic alcohol use results in a withdrawal state of nervous system excitation that is dysphoric and negatively reinforcing. It has been suggested that abstinence contributes to alcohol craving and the preoccupation with alcohol use, in that dependent individuals will continue alcohol use to avoid this state.[145] As noted, chronic alcohol use causes $GABA_A$ downregulation and NMDA upregulation, leading to CNS hyperactivity. The locus coeruleus, a nucleus of norepinephrine-containing cells in the pons, becomes hyperactive during withdrawal, and is proposed as mediating some of the negative effects of withdrawal. Chronic alcohol and drug use alters gene expression and increases levels of adenylyl cyclase, upregulates cyclic adenosine monophosphate (cAMP)-dependent protein kinases, and activates cAMP-response element binding protein (CREB) and several phosphoproteins in this brain region mediating tolerance and dependence.[146]

ALCOHOL TOXICITY

Toxicology

In the medulla, ethanol can depress respirations by inhibiting the passive neuronal flux of sodium via a mechanism similar to that of general anesthetic agents.[147] The enzyme Na^+/K^+-adenosine triphosphatase (ATPase) is inhibited, cAMP concentrations are reduced, and GABA synthesis is impaired. Ethanol is a CNS depressant, and even the uninhibited behavior associated with its use is caused by preferential suppression of inhibitory neurons. More global neuronal inhibition is seen at high ethanol concentrations.

Treatment of alcohol intoxication is essentially supportive. In highly intoxicated patients, however, the prolonged slowing of the respiratory rate can lead to arrhythmias, cardiac arrest, and death, often accompanied by aspiration of vomitus. Respiratory depression is responsible for the respiratory acidosis acid–base abnormality. Even when blood ethanol levels are below those associated with medullary paralysis, a blunted respiratory response to hypercapnia and hypoxia is seen.[148,149] This makes the assessment of respiratory status a primary concern in severely intoxicated patients.

Highly intoxicated patients with depressed respiration require immediate supportive care that may include endotracheal intubation for respiratory support. This should be sufficient to restore acid–base balance to within normal limits. When metabolic acidosis is a significant component of the acid–base disturbance, it may be necessary to administer sodium bicarbonate. This should be done only in conjunction with appropriate respiratory support to prevent the development of hypercapnia.

Serum Ethanol Concentration

Chronic use of alcohol can produce significant tolerance; therefore, the BAL cannot be used as a sole determinant of physiologic status. By contrast, for the alcohol naïve, a BAC in the 0.30 mg% range can be fatal, although chronic drinkers can be awake and alert at even higher levels. The blood ethanol concentration generally correlates with the clinical presentation of the patient (Table 90-4), but tolerance varies among individuals. Impairment in motor function may become observable at levels of 0.05 mg%. Moderate motor impairment usually is seen at 0.08 mg%, which is the legal definition of intoxication in all states when driving. Respiratory depression may occur with ethanol concentrations 0.45 mg%.[150] The accepted median lethal dose (LD_{50}) for ethanol in humans is a blood concentration of 0.50 mg%, although fatalities have been reported with ethanol concentrations ranging from 0.295 to 0.699 mg%.[151,152]

Factors that may be associated with fatalities at lower ethanol concentrations include lack of tolerance to alcohol, ingestion of other drugs, heart disease, and pulmonary aspiration. For example, patients who died of combined ethanol and barbiturate ingestions had a mean ethanol concentration of only 0.359 mg%, a mechanism that is applicable to other more commonly used drugs that also depress respiration such as anxiolytics and opioids.[152,153] Therefore, the clinician should order a toxicologic urine screen to rule out possible concurrent drug ingestion.

Table 90-4
Relationship of Blood Alcohol Concentration to Clinical Status

Blood Ethanol Concentration	Clinical Presentation[a]
50 mg/dL (0.05 mg%)	Motor function impairment observable
80 mg/dL (0.08 mg%)	Moderate impairment; legal definition of intoxication in all states when driving
450 mg/dL (0.45 mg%)	Respiratory depression
500 mg/dL (0.50 mg%)	LD_{50} for ethanol

[a]Tolerance to alcohol varies among individuals.
LD_{50}, median lethal dose.

Acute Management

In the alert intoxicated patient, general management is supportive and protective. Volume depletion resulting in hypotension often occurs in ethanol-intoxicated patients. Hypothermia also is a complication of severe intoxication and can contribute to hypotension. Hypoglycemia most often occurs in conjunction with reduced carbohydrate intake. This situation is common in malnourished alcoholics but also might be particularly pronounced if a patient was dieting. If intravenous (IV) fluids are given, thiamine administration should precede that of glucose to prevent Wernicke's encephalopathy. Administration of a short-acting benzodiazepine, such as lorazepam, should be considered.

Gastric lavage may be useful if ingestion of other drugs is expected, or when the large consumption of alcohol is very recent. Activated charcoal absorbs ethanol poorly but should be administered when coingestion of other drugs is suspected. Hemodialysis rapidly removes ethanol from the body.[154] In uncomplicated cases, it has been suggested that dialysis be initiated immediately when the blood ethanol concentration is greater than 0.6 mg%.[151] Ventilatory assistance and good supportive care usually are most important because respiratory depression is the primary cause of death in ethanol intoxication. With good supportive care, dialysis is generally unnecessary. Dialysis may be considered if the patient cannot be stabilized or has other complicating factors, such as coexisting disease states (e.g., renal dysfunction) or ingestion of other drugs (Table 90-5).

ALCOHOL WITHDRAWAL

CASE 90-10

QUESTION 1: J.M. is a chef at a nursing home where his wife is the administrator. He drinks at work and was found unconscious and brought to the hospital. His wife states that J.M. regularly drinks half a gallon of vodka daily and has suffered an alcohol withdrawal seizure in the past. J.M.'s wife states that she does not believe that he ever abused street or prescription drugs. His blood alcohol concentration (BAC) on admission was 0.52 mg%. J.M. has a history of hepatic insufficiency secondary to cirrhosis. The following laboratory results are reported:

Sodium, 143 mEq/L	Albumin, 4.7 g/dL
Potassium, 4.2 mEq/L	Cholesterol, 423 mg/dL
CO_2, 25.2 mEq/L	CK, 1,344 units/L
Chloride, 107 mEq/L	Total bilirubin, 2.3 mg/dL
BUN, 18 mg/dL	Direct bilirubin, 0.3 mg/dL
Creatinine, 0.8 mg/dL	ALP, 74 units/L
Glucose, 101 mg/dL	AST, 288 units/L
Calcium, 9.9 mg/dL	ALT, 148 units/L
Magnesium, 0.9 mg/dL	GGT, 992 units/L
Uric acid, 6.3 mg/dL	

What signs and symptoms evident in a clinical diagnosis of alcohol withdrawal need to be monitored in J.M.?

Table 90-5
Acute Alcohol Intoxication: Symptoms and Treatment

Symptom	Course	Treatment
Respiratory acidosis	Alcohol-induced respiratory depression; blunted response to hypercapnia and hypoxia	Endotracheal intubation for respiratory support
Coma	Alcohol-induced CNS depression; ingestion of other drugs	Gastric lavage, naloxone (Narcan) 1 mg, repeat every 2–3 minutes up to 10 doses, depending on response and suspicion of ingestion. Dialysis possible
Hypotension	Hypovolemia	IV fluid replacement
Hypoglycemia	Most often occurs in malnourished patients. Pyruvate is converted to lactate, rather than glucose, through gluconeogenesis	50% glucose (50 mL) by IV push

CNS, central nervous system; IV, intravenous.

For many alcohol-dependent individuals with significant physical dependence, a cluster of withdrawal symptoms known as "alcohol withdrawal syndrome" (AWS) may occur on cessation or reduction of alcohol consumption. Depending directly on the degree of physical dependence, AWS can range from creating significant discomfort to mild tremor to alcohol withdrawal-related delirium, hallucinosis, seizures, and potentially death.[155,156] A gamma-glutamyl transferase (GGT) of 992 units/L in combination with the patient's medical history suggests that J.M. is a heavy drinker. Although J.M.'s AST, ALT, and total bilirubin are elevated, his direct (unconjugated) bilirubin is within normal limits, suggesting a problem with bilirubin excretion as would be consistent with viral hepatitis or cirrhosis.

Patients may present with AWS in a variety of settings, because alcohol-dependent patients may be unrecognized and experience withdrawal after inpatient hospital admission for unrelated medical reasons. For example, a sample from a primary care practice indicated that 15% of patients presented with at-risk drinking patterns or identified alcohol-related problems.[157] Surgical patients should be screened preoperatively for possible alcohol dependence, to prevent and adequately treat AWS-related complications during and after surgery.[158]

Diagnosis requires cessation or reduction in alcohol use that has been heavy and prolonged, and two or more of the following symptoms developing within several hours to a few days after the cessation: autonomic hyperactivity, hand tremor, insomnia, nausea or vomiting, transient hallucinations or illusions (tactile, visual, or auditory), psychomotor agitation, anxiety, and generalized tonic–clonic seizures.[1] These symptoms must cause significant distress or impairment of important areas of functioning, and not be caused by a general medical condition or another mental disorder. Withdrawal-related seizure is considered a more severe manifestation of withdrawal, as is alcohol withdrawal delirium (AWD), or delirium tremens as it is traditionally called. AWD is estimated to have a mortality rate of approximately 5% of patients who go into alcohol withdrawal.[159] Recognized predictors for AWS complications include the duration of alcohol consumption, total number of prior detoxifications from alcohol, and previous withdrawal-related seizures and episodes of AWD.[160]

CASE 90-10, QUESTION 2: How could the severity of J.M.'s withdrawal symptoms be quantitatively assessed?

Of currently used instruments available for measuring the degree of withdrawal in an alcohol-dependent patient, the most commonly used is the revised Clinical Institute Withdrawal Assessment (CIWA-Ar).[161] Additionally the Sedation-Agitation Scale (SAS) could be used to assess agitation.[162] The CIWA-Ar is a validated ten-item scale used for grading severity of AWS that is often used as an inpatient assessment of withdrawal. The CIWA-Ar provides a final score with a maximum of 67 points assessing the extent of headache, nausea, tremors, agitation, paresthesia, sweats, audio and visual disturbances, and lack of awareness of time or location. Treatment of AWS can be initiated based on a patient's CIWA-Ar score. A CIWA-Ar rating of 8 points or less represents mild withdrawal and needs little pharmacologic support. A rating of 9 to 15 is associated with moderate withdrawal and may require some pharmacotherapy. A rating more than 15 corresponds to severe withdrawal, with an increased risk of seizures and AWD. Providers should also consider concomitant illnesses and medications when interpreting CIWA-Ar scores because individual items in the scale are not specific to AWS, and likewise some manifestations of withdrawal may be blunted. The SAS can be used in combination with the CIWA-Ar to evaluate the level of agitation and consciousness of a patient, and be linked to administer benzodiazepines on a symptom-triggered regimen when a patient becomes agitated (for scores >4 on a 7-point scale).

Management of withdrawal

CASE 90-10, QUESTION 3: What drugs are demonstrated to be the most clinically effective for alcohol withdrawal, particularly in a patient such as J.M. with evidence of cirrhosis?

Benzodiazepines

Benzodiazepines modulate anxiolysis by stimulating $GABA_A$ receptors and, in doing so, substitute pharmacologically for alcohol.[163] They are considered the drugs of choice for alcohol withdrawal,[158,163,164] long-acting benzodiazepines (e.g., chlordiazepoxide and diazepam) and short-acting agents (e.g., lorazepam and oxazepam) represent the most efficacious pharmacotherapies for the treatment of acute alcohol withdrawal.[157] They are effective in preventing both first seizures and subsequent seizures during alcohol withdrawal.[165] Longer-acting benzodiazepines may provide for easier weaning because they gradually self-taper on metabolism and excretion; this allows for less fluctuation in plasma drug levels.[166] Longer-acting benzodiazepines also cause fewer rebound effects and withdrawal seizures on discontinuation. Shorter-acting agents (e.g., lorazepam or oxazepam), which undergo phase II hepatic metabolism to inactive metabolites, require more frequent dosing but may be more appropriate for alcoholics with liver disease and the elderly.[164,167] When used appropriately, all benzodiazepines appear equally effective in ameliorating the signs and symptoms of alcohol withdrawal; however, the choice of a benzodiazepine is dependent on factors such as pharmacokinetic properties, dosage formulation, presence of liver impairment, and ease of dosage titration.[168] (Table 90-6)

Table 90-6

Suggested Treatment Strategies for Alcohol Withdrawal Syndrome

Protocol	Clinical Rationale	Drug	Dosing Regimen (Example)	Considerations
Fixed-Schedule Regimen	The patient receives a fixed dose of medication for 2–3 days regardless of the severity of symptoms. This approach is generally used in severe alcohol withdrawal.	Chlordiazepoxide	25 to 100 mg orally every 2–6 hours or 25 mg IV every 2–4 hours	Protocol fixed dose and time parameters are decided beforehand. Additional medication is provided as needed when symptoms are not controlled (e.g., the CIWA-Ar score remains at least 8–10).
		Diazepam	10 mg orally every 1–2 hours (maximum 60 mg) or 5–10 mg IV 20–120 minutes (maximum 100 mg/hour or 250 mg/8 hour)	
		Lorazepam	On days 1 and 2 give 2–4 mg PO 4 times a day. On days 3 and 4 give 1–2 mg PO 4 times a day. On day 5 give 1 mg PO twice a day. May use IV or IM (maximum 20 mg/hour or 50 mg/8 hour).	
Symptom-Triggered Regimen	The patient is assessed every hour using the CIWA-Ar to determine the need for medication. The primary advantage of this approach is that less medication is used to achieve the same control and less sedation.	Chlordiazepoxide	50–100 mg	Less abuse potential for outpatients, low cost; long acting 24–48 hours.
		Diazepam	10–20 mg	Long duration of action (20–50 hours), which provides a smooth treatment course with less break-through symptoms.
		Lorazepam	2–4 mg	Shorter duration of action may be more appropriate for patients at risk for prolonged sedation (e.g., elderly, hepatic impairment).
Alternative Therapies	In patients with benzodiazepine allergy or when use of a benzodiazepine is deemed medically inappropriate.	Carbamazepine	Taper from 600–800 mg on day 1 down to 200 mg over 5 days. 400 mg PO TID for 3 days, then 400 mg PO BID for 1 day, then 400 mg PO for 1 day	Both carbamazepine and baclofen are nonaddicting. Few drug interactions. Cause relatively little cognitive impairment.
	May be equally efficacious as benzodiazepines.	Baclofen	5 mg PO TID for 3 days and then increase to 10 mg TID	Known to lower the seizure threshold; more information is needed before its routine use in alcohol withdrawal.
Adjunctive Therapies	Adrenergic hyperactivity	Clonidine	0.1 mg PO BID as needed	For mild to moderate hyperactivity.
	Adrenergic hyperactivity	β-Blockers: Atenolol Metoprolol	50 mg PO daily 2.5–5 mg IV	May improve vital signs faster than oxazepam alone. Up to 3 doses about 2 minutes apart; use parameters for HR and blood pressure.
	Agitation, hallucinations, delirium	Neuroleptics: Haloperidol Olanzapine	0.5–5 mg PO/IM/IV every hour; maximal dose 100 mg/day 10 mg IM	Rapid onset but note QTc prolongation (e.g., >450 ms); recommend baseline ECG before using IV. Maximal dosing, three 10-mg doses given 2–4 hours apart; monitor for orthostatic hypotension before the administration of repeated doses.

BID, 2 times daily; CIWA-Ar, Clinical Institute Withdrawal Assessment; ECG, electrocardiogram; HR, heart rate; IM, intramuscular; IV, intravenous; PO, oral; TID, 3 times daily.

Source: Guirguis AB, Kenna GA. Treatment considerations for alcohol withdrawal syndrome. *US Pharm*. 2005;30:71; Mayo-Smith MF, et al. Management of alcohol withdrawal delirium. An evidence-based guideline [published correction appears in *Arch Intern Med*. 2004;164:2068. Dosage error in article text]. *Arch Intern Med*. 2004;164:1405.

Two strategies for dosing benzodiazepines in AWS include fixed-schedule and symptom-triggered regimens. Fixed-schedule regimens involve a set dose and interval for the agent chosen, which is to be tapered off at specific times, usually starting on the second day of treatment. Symptom-triggered regimens depend on the use of a rating scale of withdrawal severity, such as the CIWA-Ar previously noted, which is repeated at set intervals. Medication is only administered if the scoring from the scale is above a predetermined threshold value for treatment. In this way, the risk of undermedicating or overmedicating patients may be minimized, because the degree of withdrawal symptoms guides dosing. Several studies confirm that symptom-triggered regimens compared with fixed-dose regimens appear to result in a shorter duration of necessary therapy and less medication administered in total without any loss of efficacy.[168]

The treatment challenge associated with individuals who are in alcohol withdrawal with a comorbid medical illness is illustrated by the case of a patient with AWS who has coronary artery disease. Such a patient may be more aggressively treated for withdrawal-related hypertension and thus treated with a β-blocker or clonidine. The result of such adjuvant treatment may be a reduced sensitivity of the CIWA-Ar owing to a masking of the patient's autonomic manifestations of withdrawal. This could then lead to a higher likelihood of undermedicating the patient for withdrawal and may put the patient at higher risk for severe sequelae from withdrawal. Because of these exclusion criteria, the symptom-triggered approach has not been tested in such populations or those with histories of severe withdrawal including seizures or delirium. Therefore, traditional fixed-dose regimens are recommended in these populations.[168] An effective approach is most likely to consider combining these two dosing strategies. For example, a low-risk patient (no history of AWS or AWD, the patient consumes low weekly amounts of alcohol and has no signs or symptoms of early AWS) receives a symptom-triggered regimen (e.g., lorazepam 1 mg every hour as needed). Alternatively, a high-risk patient (history of AWS, AWD, or withdrawal seizures, consumes large daily amounts of alcohol, has signs or symptoms of early AWS) receives fixed-dose lorazepam or diazepam with a tapering dose schedule and as needed benzodiazepine administration for uncontrolled alcohol withdrawal signs or symptoms. Importantly, phenobarbital, dexmedetomidine and propofol are useful adjuncts to benzodiazepines if an inpatient has severe symptoms.[168]

CONTRAINDICATIONS, WARNINGS, AND INTERACTIONS

Elderly patients, those with hepatic or renal insufficiency, and those with medical (e.g., diabetes, cirrhosis) or other psychiatric illnesses (e.g., dementia) require close observation to prevent overmedication. As noted above, patients receiving calcium-channel blockers, β-blockers, and α_2-adrenergic agonists, some signs of withdrawal such as hypertension, tachycardia, and tremor may not be apparent.

Patients with a history of severe withdrawal symptoms, withdrawal seizures, or delirium tremens; multiple previous detoxifications; concomitant psychiatric or medical illness; recent high levels of alcohol consumption; pregnancy; and lack of a reliable support network should be considered for inpatient treatment regardless of the severity of their symptoms.[168]

Lorazepam is the only benzodiazepine with predictable intramuscular absorption (if intramuscular administration is necessary). Rarely, it is necessary to use extremely high dosages of benzodiazepines to control the symptoms of alcohol withdrawal. Controlled studies comparing the advantages and disadvantages of the various benzodiazepines in alcohol detoxification have not been performed, and no evidence exists to definitively support the use of lorazepam as the first-line agent in the treatment of AWS.[168,169]

In most patients with mild to moderate withdrawal symptoms, outpatient detoxification is safe and effective, and costs less than inpatient treatment. If outpatient treatment is chosen, the patient and support person(s) should be instructed on how to take the prescribed medication, its side effects, the expected withdrawal symptoms, and what to do if symptoms worsen. Small quantities of the withdrawal medication, especially benzodiazepines, should be prescribed at each visit. Because close monitoring is not available in outpatient treatment, a fixed-schedule regimen should be used.

Given J.M.'s elevated liver enzymes, a reasonable approach would be to start with lorazepam. Shorter-acting agents, such as lorazepam, which do not undergo extensive hepatic metabolism, are more appropriate for patients with evidence of hepatic insufficiency.

ADJUNCTIVE TREATMENTS

CASE 90-10, QUESTION 4: What adjunctive therapeutic support might be considered for J.M.?

The hydration, electrolyte (especially potassium and magnesium), and nutritional status of patients should be assessed at presentation. Support with IV fluids may be necessary in those patients with excessive losses through vomiting, sweating, and hyperthermia.[170] Thiamine and multivitamins as well as folate 1mg should be routinely administered to patients in alcohol withdrawal. If IV fluids are given, to prevent precipitation of Wernicke encephalopathy thiamine administration should precede that of glucose.[160] Alcohol-dependent patients are deficient of thiamine and have a higher risk for developing Wernicke encephalopathy.[171] The condition is a triad of acute mental confusion, ataxia, and ophthalmoplegia. Korsakoff amnestic syndrome is a late neuropsychiatric manifestation of Wernicke encephalopathy with memory loss and confabulation; hence, the condition is referred to as Wernicke–Korsakoff syndrome. It is most often seen in chronic alcohol use disorder patients, but it can also be seen in disorders associated with malnutrition, e.g., long-term hemodialysis or patients with acquired immunodeficiency syndrome (AIDS).[172]

Thiamine deficiency results in a decrease in cerebral glucose utilization. The body usually stores about 3 weeks of thiamine with daily requirements of about 1.5 mg. Rapid correction of brain thiamine deficiency can occur with high plasma concentrations of thiamine, achieved by parenteral supplementation only because absorption of the oral thiamine by the GI tract is minimal (<5%), even with massive oral daily dosing.[171] Patients should receive at least 200-500mg TID IV for 3 days to prevent the neuropsychiatric effects of thiamine deficiency.[172]

Several adjunctive medications, aside from the sedative-hypnotics, may serve ancillary roles in the therapy of AWS. Their selection should be based on treating specific symptoms associated with the syndrome. For instance, β-blockers (propranolol,[173] atenolol[174]) or α_2-adrenergic agonists (e.g., clonidine[175] or dexmedetomidine if in an ICU) can be used for moderate to severe hypertension or other autonomic manifestations. α_2-adrenergic agonists are preferred because it reduces NE outflow from the nerve and addresses all hyperadrenergic effects instead of just effecting the β receptors with a β-blocker, and delirium seems to be more common with the β-blocker use.[168,169] Antipsychotics (e.g., haloperidol, quetiapine) can be used for managing hallucinations and severe agitation, but care must be used because these drugs can reduce the seizure threshold.[163,168,176]

PHARMACOTHERAPY OF ALCOHOL DEPENDENCE

CASE 90-11

QUESTION 1: R.M. is a 55-year-old man, weighing 140 lb, who used to drink about 60 drinks a week before going through alcohol detoxification. R.M. is married and has a good job, and he is now committed to remain alcohol abstinent. R.M. heard about a drug called disulfiram from a friend and is interested in using this medication to help him abstain from drinking. Laboratory values obtained today include the following:

Sodium, 132 mEq/L	AST, 30 units/L
Potassium, 3.3 mEq/L	ALT, 35 units/L
CO_2, 22.6 mEq/mL	Uric acid, 9.1 mg/dL
Chloride, 109 mEq/L	Calcium, 8.7 mg/dL
BUN, 14 mg/dL	Magnesium, 1.7 mg/dL
Creatinine, 1.0 mg/dL	Albumin, 4.0 g/dL
Glucose, 123 mg/dL	Cholesterol, 255 mg/dL
Total bilirubin, 0.3 mg/dL	CK, 78 units/L
Direct bilirubin, 0.1 mg/dL	GGT, 30 units/L
ALP, 53 units/L	

Is disulfiram an appropriate agent to consider for R.M.?

In order to assess alcohol use disorder treatments an accurate medical history, including laboratory test results. In addition, several instruments are available to screen and delineate the extent of a patient's alcohol use. Ultimately, time and purpose for use are always major factors when deciding which instrument to use. The simplest screen to assess risk of alcohol abuse is to ask the patient, during the past year on how many occasions have you had five or more drinks (for a man) or four or more drinks (for a woman) at one time?[177] An affirmative answer would suggest that further follow-up of the patient's alcohol use history is needed. A second tool called the **C-A-G-E** consists of four questions: (1) Have you ever felt you should **c**ut down on your drinking?; (2) Have people **a**nnoyed you by criticizing your drinking?; (3) Have you ever felt bad or **g**uilty about your drinking?; and (4) Have you ever felt you needed a drink first thing in the morning to steady your nerves or get rid of a hangover (**e**ye opener)? Positive responses to two questions suggest an alcohol problem (Table 90-7).[178] The Alcohol Use Disorders Identification Test (AUDIT), which was developed by the World Health Organization, has also been shown to be effective in screening individuals and distinguishing problem drinkers from others.[179]

Pharmacotherapy

The pharmacologic treatments of alcohol dependence focus on relapse prevention once detoxification is complete and the patient has achieved a few days of abstinence. Treatment is intended to be an adjunct to psychosocial treatments and not used alone.[180] To date, disulfiram, acamprosate, and naltrexone tablet and injection have been FDA-approved for the treatment of alcohol dependence. In addition, several other drugs have shown varying degrees of success such as quetiapine, ondansetron, and others. [180–202] Yet much is still unknown about the long-term rates of abstinence, how long these drugs should be used once patients are in treatment, the optimal doses, and whether the drugs are more effective in men or women or for which specific subpopulations.[203]

Table 90-7
Useful Screens for Assessing Alcohol Problems

The C-A-G-E Screening Questions (CAGE)
Have you ever felt you should *c*ut down on your drinking?
Have other people *a*nnoyed you by criticizing your drinking?
Have you ever felt *g*uilty about drinking?
Have you ever taken a drink in the morning to calm your nerves or get rid of a hangover (*e*ye opener)?
Methods for Determining Recent Alcohol Consumption
Acute consumption ■ Blood alcohol concentration ■ Urine (ethyl glucuronide) ■ Saliva ■ Breath alcohol concentration
Recent heavy consumption ■ Gamma-glutamyl transferase (GGT) ■ Carbohydrate-deficient transferrin (CDT) ■ Mean corpuscular volume (MCV)

DISULFIRAM

Disulfiram is an irreversible acetaldehyde dehydrogenase inhibitor that blocks alcohol metabolism, leading to an accumulation of acetaldehyde. Disulfiram reinforces an individual's desire to stop drinking by providing a disincentive associated with increased acetaldehyde levels, resulting in headache, palpitations, hypotension, flushing, nausea, and vomiting when patients consume alcohol. The primary predictor of success with disulfiram is the patient's commitment to total abstinence from alcohol. Although anecdotal reports of success are common, clinical evidence suggests disulfiram appears to be most effective for alcoholics who are involved in special high-risk situations (e.g., weddings, graduations) and is particularly effective when administration is supervised.[3,180]

Controlled clinical trials of disulfiram have clearly shown efficacy, yet this has not been a consistent finding.[180] Double-blind, placebo-controlled studies using disulfiram are difficult because the psychological deterrent to use alcohol is experienced by both treatment groups and those who relapse will be unblinded when they experience the pharmacologic interaction.

In the most rigorous clinical trial conducted in a population of veterans, no significant difference in abstinence rates was demonstrated between patients taking placebo or 1 mg or 250 mg of disulfiram.[181] Patients randomly assigned to receive 250 mg of disulfiram daily drank less frequently (significantly fewer drinking days per year), however. Patients who were middle-aged and had social stability were more likely to benefit from disulfiram. In another trial in which administration was supervised, patients receiving disulfiram drank less alcohol and less frequently; however, on randomization, patients were unblinded to their drug.[204]

The efficacy of disulfiram compared with acamprosate and naltrexone shows definitive efficacy advantage for disulfiram when the patients are assigned to supportive care that verifies adherence.[205,206] Although no advantage was seen for combining disulfiram with naltrexone in dually diagnosed alcohol-dependent patients.[207] In one study, disulfiram combined with acamprosate resulted in increased days of cumulative abstinence.[208]

Dosing

The recommended starting dose of disulfiram is 250 mg once daily, with a range of 125 to 500 mg/day.[207] If a patient drinks and does not experience a disulfiram–ethanol reaction, the dose can be increased to 500 mg, because a significant proportion of patients may not experience a disulfiram–alcohol reaction at the usual 250-mg daily dose.[209,210] Side effects are increased, however, at doses exceeding 250 mg. Dosing starts at least 12 to 24 hours after abstinence initiation (when the blood or breath alcohol concentration is zero). Treatment continues, depending on the particular needs of the individual, but is generally at least 90 days, and maintenance therapy may be required for years.

Contraindications, Warnings, and Interactions

Because of the intense cardiovascular and physical changes that occur in the disulfiram–ethanol interaction, disulfiram is contraindicated in patients with cardiac disease, coronary occlusion, cerebrovascular disease, and renal or hepatic failure. At somewhat higher doses, psychotic reactions have occurred. It is not definitive that disulfiram causes fetal abnormalities when administered during pregnancy but some data are found regarding limb reduction anomalies in infants born to disulfiram-treated mothers taking disulfiram during the first trimester of pregnancy.[211,212] Thus, disulfiram should only be used during pregnancy if the expected benefit to the mother and fetus is greater than the possible risk to the fetus; however, it should be avoided in the first trimester (category C). No information is available about the safety of this medicine during breast-feeding.

Disulfiram can also be hepatotoxic and should be used cautiously in patients with liver disease. Liver function should be established at baseline and after 14 days of treatment, and a complete blood count (CBC) and liver function tests (LFTs) should be obtained every 6 months.[213]

R.M. has normal hepatic function; however, LFTs should be monitored at baseline and periodically during treatment. Although not all clinicians agree, most would recommend—at minimum—baseline LFTs: ALT, AST, and GGT and withholding disulfiram when LFTs are more than three times upper limits of normal.[213] If elevated, repeat LFTs every 1 to 2 weeks until normal, and then every 3 to 6 months if no elevations, with an awareness that increased LFT results may signal a return to drinking rather than disulfiram toxicity.[214,215] Persistently elevated LFTs may also indicate viral hepatitis (B or C), for which alcoholics have a higher risk, and thus the need to order a hepatitis profile. Currently, guidelines point out that a reduction in alcohol use will lead to more normalized LFTs. Psychiatric adverse effects include disorientation, agitation, depression, and behavioral changes such as paranoia, withdrawal and bizarre behaviors, and worsening of schizophrenia, especially at doses greater than 250 mg daily.[216,217] Disulfiram should be avoided or used very cautiously in persons with these conditions although it can be used safely at a dose of 250 mg daily in alcohol-dependent patients with concomitant psychiatric disorders, including schizophrenia.[207,218,219] Common side effects of disulfiram include drowsiness, particularly in the first few weeks of treatment, a metallic or garlic taste, and sexual dysfunction. The dose can be taken at bedtime if drowsiness or tiredness occurs.

Disulfiram is a potent inhibitor of the CYP2E1 oxidase and can interact with anticoagulants (warfarin), antiepileptics (phenytoin, carbamazepine), some benzodiazepines (e.g., diazepam), and tricyclic antidepressants (amitriptyline, desipramine), potentially increasing the toxicity of these medications. Delirium can result in combination with monoamine oxidase inhibitors. Adverse effects with disulfiram that mimic the alcohol–disulfiram interaction can also occur with metronidazole and omeprazole.[220]

To receive optimal results with disulfiram, patients must receive regular counseling and be closely monitored for any changes in hepatic function. Having someone participate in helping to validate the administration process is known to lead to better outcomes. Discontinuation of disulfiram should occur only after consultation with the prescriber and counselor involved. Patients must stop the medication for at least 3 days (up to 14 days in some) before being exposed to products containing alcohol. It is important to educate patients taking disulfiram about the dangers of consuming even small amounts of alcohol in foods, over-the-counter medications, mouthwashes, and topical lotions. The patient should report any respiratory difficulty, nausea, vomiting, decreased appetite, dark colored urine, or a change in pigmentation in the skin or eyes (primarily yellowing).

Summary

Generally, given the special circumstances needed for success, disulfiram is not the drug of choice for treating alcoholism. The social, medical, and psychiatric status of a candidate is an important consideration in the use of disulfiram. R.M. would appear to be a reasonable candidate for disulfiram given he has agreed to have his medication administration supervised (in this case by his wife), his steady employment, and his motivation to sustain abstinence. R.M. should also receive counseling and support services on a regular basis.

ACAMPROSATE

Acamprosate (Campral) has multiple actions, but is principally a glutamate and GABA modulator. The key mechanism of action is considered to be as a weak functional antagonist of the glutamate NMDA receptor, possibly mediated through indirect modulation of the receptor site via antagonism at the mGluR5 receptor.[221] A series of meta-analyses and systematic reviews demonstrated that when used as an adjunct to psychosocial interventions, acamprosate improves drinking outcomes such as the length and rate of abstinence.[180,222–224] This effect is less likely if acamprosate is not initiated quickly after a detoxification.[225,226] Evidence indicates that the effect of acamprosate on abstinence lasts after the treatment is stopped.[227] Acamprosate appears to be especially useful in a therapeutic regimen targeted at promoting abstinence and can be used in primary care settings as well as specialized addiction treatment programs.[228] Few contraindications to treatment exist. Little consistent information is found about patient characteristics that predict improvement while taking acamprosate. In a meta-analysis of all US and European studies, predictors of abstinence were motivation, readiness to change, baseline abstinence, initial first week compliance, and living with a partner or child.[229] A pooled analysis of seven European trials, however, found no significant predictors of the abstinence outcome measures.[230] Candidates for acamprosate should be committed to abstinence and begin the medication after being abstinent from alcohol.[231,232]

In a systematic review of the efficacy data related to acamprosate, proof for efficacy of acamprosate was strong.[231] Moreover, several acamprosate studies have reported positive results. For example, in a study of 272 severely dependent alcoholics, patients receiving acamprosate showed a significantly higher continuous abstinence rate within the first 2 months of treatment compared with patients receiving placebo.[184] Of acamprosate-treated patients, 40% were continuously abstinent for a 48-week period compared with 17% of those who received placebo.

Acamprosate has also been studied for periods of up to a year. In a long-term follow-up (12 months) after trial completion, acamprosate still maintained an effect on abstinence rates, but not on nondrinking days. Some studies have found limited to no efficacy,[191,233–236] although two of the studies may have been underpowered.[191,233–236] One of these studies also had a short treatment period, and the other had a long delay in initiating treatment.[234,235] In summary, most studies suggest that acamprosate is a safe and well-tolerated drug for the promotion of alcohol abstinence.[237]

Dose

Acamprosate is dispensed in 333-mg tablets and the usual dose is 666 mg/day 3 times daily.[238] Patients can be started on the full dose without titration. Acamprosate is not well absorbed from the GI tract and with a terminal half-life of around 30 hours it takes several days to achieve desired blood levels of the medication.[238] The medication appears to be safe and effective in alcoholics, with minimal side effects. It does not appear to produce sedation and does not cause drug dependence. Main adverse effects of acamprosate appear to be GI, including nausea, diarrhea, and bloating. Nausea or diarrhea can be easily managed, but if symptoms are severe or persistent, the dose should be reduced by one-third to one-half. The duration of therapy ultimately depends on treatment success and the willingness of the patient to continue therapy indefinitely.

Contraindications, Warnings, and Interactions

Acamprosate is excreted unchanged in the urine and should not be used in patients with impaired kidney function (creatinine clearance [CrCl] <30 mL/minute) or in patients who previously exhibited hypersensitivity to acamprosate.[238] The dose should be 333 mg 3 times daily in patients with moderate renal impairment (CrCl 30–50 mL/minute). Acamprosate should only be used during pregnancy when the benefit clearly outweighs the risk as the drug has been shown to be teratogenic (category C) in rats.[238] Tetracyclines may be inactivated by the calcium component in acamprosate during concurrent administration.[238] Naltrexone increases plasma levels of acamprosate, although the clinical significance of this interaction is unknown and the two can be safely used together.[238,239] Suicidal ideation and attempted and completed suicides have occurred in patients taking acamprosate.

Acamprosate must be used in combination with a psychosocial program such as cognitive-behavioral therapy (CBT) or regular Alcoholics Anonymous (AA) meetings. Acamprosate may be taken without regard to meals. The tablets should not be crushed and should be taken whole. Although no interaction with alcohol occurs, abstinence in combination with counseling and social support is required to attain optimal treatment. Patients should report persistent diarrhea, sudden or excessive weight gain, swelling of the extremities, respiratory difficulties, fainting, or thoughts of suicide.

A retrospective long-term study in 353 alcohol-dependent patients, supervised disulfiram was found to be superior to acamprosate, particularly in patients with a long history of alcohol dependence.[206]

NALTREXONE

Naltrexone blocks the action of endorphins when alcohol is consumed, and this results in an attenuation of the dopamine release at the nucleus accumbens thought to be crucially important to positive reinforcement, reward, and craving.[145] Although naltrexone therapy has been recommended for all alcohol-dependent patients who do not have a medical contraindication to its use, a survey of 1,388 US physicians specializing in addiction reported that they prescribed naltrexone to an average of only 13% of their patients.[240] The main self-reported reasons why physicians did not prescribe naltrexone to more patients were that patients refused to take the medication or comply with prescribing regimens (23%), and that patients could not afford the medication (21%).

Evidence seems to support the use of naltrexone as an adjunct to psychosocial interventions, with higher abstinence rates in short-term treatment, and as a deterrent to progressing from a lapse to a full-blown relapse.[180,209,241,242] Naltrexone is as efficacious as disulfiram and probably more efficacious than acamprosate.[191,242–244]

Several studies indicate that naltrexone is most effective in patients with strong craving,[182,245] poor cognitive status at study entry,[246] and high compliance.[247,248] This observation is consistent with the demonstrated effect of naltrexone in reducing craving. Evidence also indicates that persons with a family history for alcoholism, early age at onset of drinking, and comorbid use of other drugs are more likely to benefit from naltrexone.[249]

Comprehensive reviews of pharmacotherapies for alcoholism concluded that oral naltrexone produced a consistent decrease in the relapse rate to heavy drinking and in drinking frequency, although it did not enhance absolute abstinence rates.[232,250,251] More specifically, several studies using naltrexone report the opioid antagonist to be more effective than placebo in reducing relapse rates, in increasing the percent of nondrinking days,[182,183,247] and in reducing craving in heavy drinkers.[252] Yet other studies fail to demonstrate a significant difference with placebo.[253,254] Several factors may explain the discrepancies in results of the different clinical trials with naltrexone. Many of the studies included small sample sizes and may lack the statistical power to demonstrate treatment effects.[235] Several large sufficiently powered studies also reported negative results.[253–255]

The COMBINE trial[191] clearly supports the effectiveness of naltrexone in that each of the groups of patients receiving naltrexone in conjunction with medical management had a higher percentage of days abstinent than those receiving placebo plus medical management without naltrexone or combined behavioral intervention (CBI). Naltrexone also reduced the risk of heavy drinking. Extended-release naltrexone injection 380 mg is safe and well tolerated in alcohol-dependent individuals.[256] In two double-blind, randomized, placebo-controlled trials, the efficacy of once-monthly extended-release injectable or depot forms of naltrexone was demonstrated.[198,257,258] which suggests the advantage of increased compliance. Garbutt et al.[198] reported that men receiving naltrexone injection had significantly better treatment outcomes than women, and women who received naltrexone demonstrated no difference from those who received placebo. Additionally, because a robust effect was seen for naltrexone injection compared with placebo for people coming into the study abstinent, the FDA required the manufacturer to place a requirement for abstinence when starting the medication on its product information. In the primary care setting, naltrexone injection given for 3 months and offered with physician-delivered medical management was found to be effective in the treatment of alcohol dependence.[259]

Dose

Naltrexone has been approved for use in the first 90 days of abstinence when the risk of relapse is highest. It has also been shown to be safe and well tolerated by patients for periods of up to a year. Treatment with naltrexone should continue based on the response to the medication. Discontinuation should only be considered in consultation with the health care provider. The usual dose of naltrexone is 50 mg daily, although doses of 25 mg to 100 mg daily have been reported to be effective, particularly in those with lower blood concentrations of the drug.[259] Side effects, such as nausea or headache, are more common in the initial few days of therapy. Starting with a 25-mg dose (half a tablet) for the first two to four daily doses may reduce the incidence of side effects. Because of its long half-life (4 hours, or 13 hours for 6-β-naltrexol, naltrexone's active metabolite), naltrexone has been studied as three times weekly doses of 100 mg on Mondays, 100 mg on Wednesdays, and 150 mg on Fridays (or the equivalent of 50 mg daily).[202] This method may facilitate supervised or observed administration of naltrexone, because only three (versus seven) observations are required per week. However, this schedule is not recommended for most cases.

The extended-release injection (380 mg) should be administered by deep IM injection every 4 weeks deep into a gluteal muscle, alternating buttocks each injection. No dose adjustment is required for mild or moderate renal or hepatic impairment, but naltrexone has not been studied in severe renal or hepatic impairment.[198]

Contraindications, Warnings, and Interactions

Naltrexone is contraindicated in patients with a history of sensitivity to naltrexone with acute hepatitis or liver failure; in those who are physically dependent on opioids, receiving opioid analgesics, or in acute opioid withdrawal. The benefit of using naltrexone during pregnancy should clearly outweigh the risk. The concurrent administration of naltrexone and opioid analgesics is contraindicated. To avoid triggering an acute abstinence syndrome, patients must be opioid free for a minimum of 7 to 14 days before initiating treatment with naltrexone, as substantiated with a urine drug test. Although rarely performed, a naloxone challenge test can be used before treatment with naltrexone to rule out concurrent use of opioids. Naltrexone is in the FDA pregnancy category C, and it is unknown whether naltrexone passes into breast milk.

A possible clinical concern with naltrexone tablets or long-acting injectable naltrexone is pain management. Any attempt to overcome the opioid blockade produced by naltrexone using exogenous opioids may result in fatal overdose. Should a patient be in pain after receiving an injection, the first drug of choice should be a nonopioid, such as a nonsteroidal anti-inflammatory drug (NSAID). If the patient is still in pain, an opiate can be used, but it will most likely have to be administered in a higher dose and more frequently. When reversal of naltrexone blockade is required for pain management, patients should be monitored in a setting equipped and staffed for cardiopulmonary resuscitation and monitored for signs of respiratory depression.

In a yearlong safety study, the most common side effects were nausea, dizziness, sedation, headache, anxiety, and blurred vision.[260] Should such side effects occur, reducing the dosage by one-half often reduces the side effects. Large doses (e.g., 200 mg) of naltrexone can cause liver failure. Patients should report excessive tiredness, unusual bleeding or bruising, loss of appetite, pain in the upper right part of the stomach, any discoloration of the skin or eyes, a change in stool color or urine, thoughts of suicide, or signs of pneumonia. Patients receiving extended-release naltrexone injection must also monitor the injection site for any type of reaction, e.g., swelling, tenderness, bruising, or redness-69% for naltrexone v 50% for placebo). Reactions that do not resolve in 2 weeks may result in induration, cellulitis, abscess, sterile abscess, or necrosis. Some patients may need to be evaluated for surgical intervention.[260]

COMBINATION PHARMACOTHERAPY

The rationale for combining medications is that acamprosate reduces negative reinforcement and naltrexone attenuates positive reinforcement.[141] To test this hypothesis, a randomized, controlled study of 160 patients performed in Europe demonstrated that although combining naltrexone and acamprosate was more effective than either placebo or acamprosate alone, adding acamprosate was not significantly more effective than naltrexone alone.[244] In the much larger study, the COMBINE trial randomized more than 1,300 individuals in a double-blind fashion to receive placebo, naltrexone, or acamprosate alone or in combination with medical management or CBI.[191] Results from this study suggest that acamprosate has no significant effect on drinking versus placebo, either by itself or with any combination of the other treatments in the study. Furthermore, patients receiving placebo and medical management (MM) from a health care professional had better outcomes than patients receiving CBI (a CBT-like therapy that includes 12-step facilitation) alone. From the available evidence, it is acceptable to combine acamprosate with naltrexone with the expectation that in some patients it may not be any more effective than naltrexone alone.

Topiramate

Topiramate has multiple mechanisms of action, including enhanced $GABA_A$ inhibition that results in decreased dopamine facilitation in the midbrain, thought to be of potential benefit in the treatment of alcohol use disorder, maintenance treatment.[261] Additionally, it causes antagonism of kainate to activate the kainate/AMPA glutamate receptor subtypes and inhibition of type II and IV carbonic anhydrase isoenzymes.[262] Topiramate is not FDA-approved for the treatment of alcohol use disorder.

A randomized, double-blind, placebo-controlled trial used an escalating dose from 25 to 300 mg/day of topiramate or matching placebo in 150 alcohol-dependent men and women during the first 8 weeks of a 12-week period.[190] Patients stayed at the same dose for the last 4 weeks of the study. All patients in the study received brief behavioral compliance enhancement therapy (BBCET) that was a 10- to 15-minute meeting with a health care professional that focused on resolving side effect issues and facilitated adherence. Participants receiving topiramate reported significantly fewer drinks per day and drinks per drinking day, significantly fewer drinking days, significantly more days of abstinence, and significantly less craving than those on placebo. The evidence suggests that although abstinence was not a goal at the start of the topiramate study, the medication may be more beneficial during the abstinence initiation phase of treatment.[263] In a phase II clinical trial, the use of topiramate for alcohol dependence treatment was confirmed by outcomes demonstrating that topiramate recipients showed a significantly greater lowering of percentage of heavy drinking days and drinks per drinking day, and a higher percentage of days abstinent.

In the treatment of alcohol dependence, topiramate is titrated from 25 mg/day up to 300 mg/day over a 6-week period (100 mg in the morning; 200 mg in the afternoon) or to the patient's maximal tolerable dose. Abrupt discontinuation of topiramate has been associated with seizures in patients without a history of seizures, and for this reason, gradual withdrawal of the drug (e.g., a 25% decrease in the dosage every 4 days for 16 days) is recommended.

In addition to paresthesias (tingling in the extremities), other prominent side effects include mental confusion, slowness in thinking, depression, and somnolence, which may be attenuated by titration when initiating therapy, and the development of renal calculi in about 1.5% of patients.[264] Adequate hydration is encouraged, particularly in patients who may be at risk for developing calculi. Topiramate can cause drowsiness, dizziness, changes in memory, a change in taste (particularly with carbonated beverages), vision changes (particularly associated with increased intraocular pressure), pressure to the touch, loss of appetite or weight loss, and sudden changes in mood.

CONTRAINDICATIONS, WARNINGS, AND INTERACTIONS

Topiramate is contraindicated in those hypersensitive to the drug. Topiramate should be used with caution in those who have a history of urolithiasis, paresthesias, secondary angle closure glaucoma, renal or hepatic impairment, and conditions or therapies that predispose to acidosis (e.g., renal disease, severe respiratory disorders, status epilepticus, diarrhea, surgery, ketogenic diet, or drugs). Monitoring for hyperchloremic non–ionic-gap metabolic acidosis is essential, and therefore baseline chemistry (e.g., HCO_3^- and pH) should be assessed and monitored regularly thereafter. Metabolic acidosis can cause symptoms such as tiredness and loss of appetite, or more serious conditions including arrhythmia or coma. Topiramate has been found to be teratogenic in animal studies and is a pregnancy category C medication.[264]

Concomitant use of oral contraceptives, phenytoin, carbamazepine, and valproic acid has been found to interact with topiramate.[220] Coadministration of another carbonic anhydrase inhibitor, such as acetazolamide, may increase the possibility of renal stone formation and should be avoided.

COMORBIDITIES IN ALCOHOL USE DISORDER

It is quite common for patients who are involved in harmful drinking to have comorbid medical issues. Alcohol has significant drug interactions with many medications (Table 90-8). Clinicians must also consider the potential for comorbid psychiatric disorders,

Table 90-8
Ethanol–Drug Interactions

Acetaminophen	Chronic excessive alcohol consumption increases susceptibility to acetaminophen-induced hepatotoxicity. Acute intoxication theoretically protects against acetaminophen toxicity because less hepatotoxic metabolite is generated.
Anticoagulants (oral)	Chronic ethanol consumption induces hepatic metabolism of warfarin, decreasing hypoprothrombinemic effect. Very large acute ethanol doses (>3 drinks/day) may impair the metabolism of warfarin and increase hypothrombinemic effect. Vitamin K-dependent clotting factors may be reduced in alcoholics with liver disease, also affecting coagulation.
Antidepressants	Enhanced sedative effects of alcohol and psychomotor impairment are possible. Acute ethanol impairs metabolism. Fluoxetine, paroxetine, fluvoxamine, and probably other serotonin reuptake inhibitors (SSRIs) do not interfere with psychomotor or subjective effects of ethanol.
Ascorbic acid	Ascorbic acid increases ethanol clearance and serum triglyceride levels and improves motor coordination and color discrimination after ethanol consumption.
Barbiturates	Phenobarbital decreases blood ethanol concentration; acute intoxication inhibits pentobarbital metabolism; chronic intoxication enhances hepatic pentobarbital metabolism.
Benzodiazepines	Psychomotor impairment increases with the combination.
Bromocriptine	Ethanol increases gastrointestinal side effects of bromocriptine.
Caffeine	Caffeine has no effect on ethanol-induced psychomotor impairment.
Calcium-channel blockers	Verapamil inhibits ethanol metabolism and increases intoxication.
Cephalosporin antibiotics	Ethanol produces flushing, nausea, headaches, tachycardia, and hypotension. Cephalosporin antibiotics that have an ethyl tetrazole thiol side chain produce this disulfiram-like reaction (e.g., cefoperazone, cefamandole, cefotetan).
Chloral hydrate	Elevation of plasma trichloroethanol (a chloral hydrate metabolite) and blood ethanol may occur. Combined central nervous system (CNS) depression. Vasodilation, tachycardia, headache.
Chloroform	Ethanol increases chloroform hepatotoxicity.
Doxycycline	Chronic consumption of ethanol induces hepatic metabolism of doxycycline and may lower serum concentration of the antibiotic.
Erythromycin	Ethanol may interfere with absorption of the ethylsuccinate salt. Effects on other formulations are unknown.
Furazolidone	When ethanol is ingested, nausea, flushing, light-headedness, and dyspnea may occur (i.e., a disulfiram-like reaction).
H_2 antagonists	Cimetidine potentiates ethanol effects. Increases peak plasma ethanol concentrations and area under the plasma ethanol concentration–time curve. CNS toxicity from increased cimetidine serum concentration. Nizatidine and ranitidine may also increase blood alcohol levels (BALs) slightly by inhibiting gastric alcohol dehydrogenase. Famotidine does not affect BALs.
Isoniazid	Consumption of ethanol with isoniazid increases risk of hepatotoxicity. Tyramine-containing alcoholic beverages may cause hypertensive reaction.
Ketoconazole and metronidazole	When ethanol is ingested, nausea, flushing, light-headedness, and dyspnea may occur (i.e., a disulfiram-like reaction may occur with metronidazole). A sunburn-like rash has been reported with ethanol consumption and ketoconazole. A similar reaction may occur with itraconazole, although no reports exist.
Meprobamate	Synergistic CNS depression may occur.

(continued)

Table 90-8
Ethanol–Drug Interactions (*continued*)

Metoclopramide	Enhances sedative effects of ethanol.
Monoamine oxidase inhibitors	Tyramine-containing alcoholic beverages (e.g., wines, beer) may cause a hypertensive crisis. Pargyline may inhibit aldehyde dehydrogenase and cause a disulfiram-like interaction with ethanol.
Narcotic analgesics	Volume of distribution of intravenous meperidine increases with increasing ethanol consumption. Clinical significance unknown. Potential for enhanced CNS depression.
Oral hypoglycemic agents	Chlorpropamide, tolbutamide, and tolazamide may cause flushing, light-headedness, nausea, and dyspnea if alcohol is ingested (i.e., a disulfiram-like reaction).
Paraldehyde	Possible metabolic acidosis may occur.
Phenothiazines	Potentiates psychomotor effects of ethanol.
Quinacrine	Possibly inhibits acetaldehyde oxidation.
Salicylates	Increases gastric bleeding associated with aspirin; may increase chance of gastrointestinal hemorrhage.
Tetrachloroethylene	Combined CNS depression may occur.
Trichloroethylene	Flushing, lacrimation, blurred vision, and tachypnea may occur when patients exposed to trichloroethylene drink alcohol.

Adapted from Ciraulo D, Shader RI, Greenblatt DJ, Creelman WL. *Drug Interactions in Psychiatry*. 3rd ed. Philadelphia, PA: Lippincott Williams & Wilkins; 2006, with permission.

(also known as dual diagnosis, e.g., depression, bipolar disorder, or schizophrenia) combined with a substance use disorders. Tobacco and caffeine dependence are common.[265] Increased comorbid conditions lead to a poorer treatment prognosis for both medical and psychiatric conditions.

Principles for the optimal treatment of patients with a dual diagnosis include the following: (a) flexibility (e.g., although the goal of treatment may be abstinence, for some patents, movement in the right direction is just as important to keep the person engaged in treatment); (b) repetition (e.g., a constant refocusing of attention for avoiding alcohol and for confronting their psychiatric symptoms is a priority); and (c) counseling (e.g., matching patients to the appropriate intervention). These factors are all fundamental to long-lasting treatment success. Medications, when appropriate (e.g., early and vigorous drug intervention with nonaddictive medications), may also help the patient stay in treatment; however, every effort must be made to use medications that do not induce euphoria or cause dependence, and are effective and safe even during relapse.[2,3]

Patients with both drug use and psychiatric disorders constitute a substantial and challenging subpopulation. Treating the alcohol use disorder alone predicts a poorer outcome for other disorders including early relapse. Early and aggressive treatment for each condition should be implemented. Furthermore, care must be taken to ensure that the medications prescribed are safe if combined with alcohol.[3]

ACKNOWLEDGMENT

The author acknowledges the authors for their contributions to the following chapters in previous versions of the textbook: Wendy O. Zizzo and Paolo V. Zizzo for their chapter on Drug Abuse and George A. Kenna for his chapter on Alcohol Use Disorders.

KEY REFERENCES AND WEBSITES

A full list of references for this chapter can be found at http://thepoint.lww.com/AT11e. Below are the key references and website for this chapter, with the corresponding reference number in this chapter found in parentheses after the reference.

Key References

American Psychiatric Association. *Diagnostic and Statistical Manual of Mental Disorders (DSM-5)*. 5th ed. Washington, DC: American Psychiatric Publishing; 2013. (1)

Perry EC. Inpatient management of acute alcohol withdrawal syndrome. *CNS Drugs*. 2014;28:401–410. (168)

Lingford-Hughes AR, et al. BAP updated guidelines: evidenced guideline for the pharmacologic management of substance abuse, harmful use, addiction and comorbidity: recommendations from BAP. *J Psychopharmacol*. 2012;26(7):899–952 (3)

Key Websites

Center for Behavioral Health Statistics and Quality. (2015). *Behavioral health trends in the United States: Results from the 2014 National Survey on Drug Use and Health* (HHS Publication No. SMA 15-4927, NSDUH Series H-50). Retrieved from http://www.samhsa.gov/data/. (4)

Alcoholic Anonymous. http://www.aa.org.

The National Institute on Alcohol Abuse and Alcoholism. http://www.niaaa.nih.gov.

Research Society on Alcoholism. http://www.rsoa.org.

ASAM Public Policy Statement on Treatment for Alcohol and Other Drug Addiction, Adopted: May 1, 1980, Revised: January 1, 2010. http://www.asam.org/quality-practice/definition-of-addiction. (2)

91 Tobacco Use and Dependence

Andrea S. Franks and Sarah E. McBane

CORE PRINCIPLES

		CHAPTER CASES
1	Cigarette smoking is the single most preventable cause of premature death in the United States. Smoking harms nearly every organ of the body, causing many diseases (including, but not limited to, cardiovascular disease, pulmonary disease, and cancers) and reducing the health of smokers in general. Quitting smoking has immediate as well as long-term benefits, reducing risks for diseases caused by smoking and improving health in general.	**Case 91-2 (Questions 1, 4), Case 91-3 (Question 1), Case 91-5 (Question 1), Case 91-6 (Question 1)**
2	Tobacco products are effective delivery systems for the drug nicotine. Nicotine is a highly addictive drug that activates the dopamine reward pathway in the brain that reinforces continued tobacco use. Nicotine withdrawal symptoms (e.g., irritability, anxiety, difficulty concentrating, restlessness, depressed mood, insomnia, impaired performance, increased appetite or weight gain, cravings) generally occur when nicotine is discontinued.	**Case 91-1 (Questions 2, 4), Case 91-3 (Question 1), Case 91-6 (Questions 1, 2)**
3	Constituents in tobacco smoke are associated with a number of clinically significant drug interactions.	**Case 91-4 (Questions 1, 3), Case 91-6 (Question 3)**
4	Tobacco dependence, a chronic disease that often requires repeated intervention and multiple attempts to quit, is characterized by physiologic dependence (addiction to nicotine) and behavioral habit of using tobacco.	**Case 91-1 (Question 5), Case 91-2 (Question 3), Case 91-3 (Question 1)**
5	Numerous effective medications, as delineated in the Clinical Practice Guideline, are available for treating tobacco use and dependence. Most patients should be encouraged to use one or more first-line agents, which include the nicotine patch, nicotine gum, nicotine lozenge, nicotine nasal spray, nicotine oral inhaler, sustained-release bupropion, and varenicline. All first-line agents approximately double quit rates, and therefore, the choice of therapy is based largely on contraindications, precautions, patient preference, and tolerability. In some cases, medications can be combined or used for extended durations. Although alternative therapies are available, these are not recommended because of insufficient evidence of efficacy.	**Case 91-1 (Questions 1–3), Case 91-2 (Questions 3, 4), Case 91-3 (Question 1), Case 91-4 (Question 2), Case 91-6 (Questions 1, 4)**
6	Comprehensive counseling, as defined by the Clinical Practice Guideline, includes asking about tobacco use, advising patients to quit, assessing readiness to quit, assisting patients with quitting, and arranging follow-up. This approach is referred to as "The 5 A's." Counseling and support can be provided a variety of ways, such as through individual counseling, group programs, telephone, or the Internet. Two components of counseling are especially effective and should be applied when assisting patients with quitting: practical counseling (problem solving or skills training) and social support delivered as part of treatment. Relapse is common, and clinicians should work with patients throughout the quit attempt to increase the chances for long-term abstinence.	**Case 91-1 (Questions 2, 5), Case 91-3 (Question 1), Case 91-5 (Question 1), Case 91-6 (Questions 1, 2, 4)**
7	Brief tobacco dependence treatment (<3 minutes) is effective. In the absence of time or expertise, ask about tobacco use, advise patients to quit, and refer patients to other resources (e.g., telephone quitlines, web-based support, local programs) for additional assistance. This approach is referred to as "Ask-Advise-Refer."	**Case 91-5 (Question 1)**

Continued

	CHAPTER CASES
8 Patients with psychiatric disorders exhibit a higher prevalence of tobacco use and a disproportionately high level of tobacco-related morbidity and mortality.	**Case 91-6 (Question 1)**
9 Cigarettes are the most common form of tobacco used in the United States; however, other forms of tobacco exist (spit tobacco, pipes, cigars, bidis, hookah). All forms of tobacco are harmful.	**Case 91-2 (Question 2), Narrated PowerPoint slides on Forms of Tobacco**

Tobacco is a detrimental substance, and its use dramatically increases a person's odds of dependence, disease, disability, and death. Cigarettes are the only marketed consumable product that when used as intended will contribute to the death of half or more of its users.[1] Tobacco products are carefully engineered formulations that optimize the delivery of nicotine, a chemical that meets the criteria for an addictive substance: (a) nicotine induces psychoactive effects, (b) it is used in a highly controlled or compulsive manner, and (c) behavioral patterns of tobacco use are reinforced by the pharmacologic effects of nicotine.[2] As a major risk factor for a wide range of diseases, including cardiovascular conditions, cancers, and pulmonary disorders, tobacco is the primary known preventable cause of premature death and disease in our society.[3] Since the Surgeon General's first report on smoking in 1964, over 20 million American deaths have been attributed to smoking or secondhand smoke exposure.[3] Globally, almost 7 million people die annually from smoking (6 million) or being exposed to secondhand smoke (890,000).[4]

In the United States, smoking is responsible for more than 480,000 premature deaths each year.[3] In addition to the harm imposed on users of tobacco, exposure to secondhand smoke results in an estimated 50,000 deaths annually.[5,6] According to the Office of the US Surgeon General, there is no risk-free level of exposure to tobacco smoke.[2] Because of the health and societal burdens that it imposes, tobacco use and dependence should be addressed during each clinical encounter with all tobacco users.[7]

EPIDEMIOLOGY OF TOBACCO USE AND DEPENDENCE

In the United States, cigarettes are the most common form of tobacco that is consumed, but other forms are also prevalent: smokeless tobacco (chewing tobacco, oral snuff), pipes, cigars, clove cigarettes, bidis, and hookah. Electronic cigarettes (e-cigarettes) are growing in popularity. Electronic cigarettes, electronic nicotine delivery systems (ENDS), contain a liquid consisting of nicotine and other substances that is heated by an atomizer and inhaled as a vapor. Among adults, smoking prevalence varies by sociodemographic factors, including sex, race or ethnicity, education level, age, and poverty level. The Centers for Disease Control and Prevention (CDC) reported that in 2014, 21.3% of adults in the United States used a tobacco product every day or some days, with 17% reporting cigarette use.[8] Smoking prevalence is increased among persons with mental illness, with over one-third smoking cigarettes.[9]

Factors Contributing to Tobacco Use

Tobacco addiction is maintained by nicotine dependence.[10,11] Nicotine induces a variety of pharmacologic effects that lead to dependence.[12] However, tobacco dependence is not simply a matter of nicotine pharmacology—it is a result of the interplay of complex processes, including the desire for the direct pharmacologic actions of nicotine, the relief of withdrawal, learned associations, and environmental cues (e.g., advertising, the smell of a cigarette, or observing others who are smoking).[11] Physiologic factors, such as preexisting medical conditions (e.g., psychiatric comorbidities[9,11] and one's genetic profile), also can predispose individuals to tobacco use.[12,13]

Nicotine, the addictive component of tobacco, is rapidly absorbed and passes through the blood–brain barrier, contributing to its addictive nature. After inhalation, nicotine reaches the brain within seconds.[10] As such, smokers experience nearly immediate onset of the positive effects of nicotine, including pleasure, relief of anxiety, improved task performance, improved memory, mood modulation, and skeletal muscle relaxation.[10] These effects, mediated by alterations in neurotransmitter levels, reinforce continued use of nicotine-containing products.[10,11]

Nicotine Pharmacology

Nicotine (*Nicotiana tabacum*) is one of the few natural alkaloids that exist in the liquid state. Nicotine is a clear, weak base with a pK_a of 8.0.[14] In acidic media, nicotine is ionized and poorly absorbed; conversely, in alkaline media, nicotine is nonionized and well absorbed. Under physiologic conditions (pH = 7.4), a large proportion of nicotine is nonionized and readily crosses cell membranes.[14] Given the relation between pH and absorption, the tobacco industry and pharmaceutical companies are able to titrate the pH of their tobacco products and nicotine replacement therapy (NRT) products to maximize the absorption potential of nicotine.[14–16]

Once absorbed, nicotine induces a variety of central nervous system, cardiovascular, and metabolic effects. Nicotine stimulates the release of several neurotransmitters, inducing a range of pharmacologic effects such as pleasure (dopamine), arousal (acetylcholine, norepinephrine), cognitive enhancement (acetylcholine), appetite suppression (dopamine, norepinephrine, serotonin), learning (glutamate), memory enhancement (glutamate), mood modulation (serotonin), and reduction of anxiety and tension (β-endorphin and γ-aminobutyric acid [GABA]).[17] The dopamine reward pathway, a network that elicits feelings of pleasure in response to certain stimuli, is central to drug-induced reward. The neurons of the ventral tegmental area contain the neurotransmitter dopamine, which is released in the nucleus accumbens and in the prefrontal cortex. Immediately after inhalation, a bolus of nicotine enters the brain, stimulating the release of dopamine, which induces nearly immediate feelings of pleasure, along with relief of the symptoms of nicotine withdrawal. This rapid dose response reinforces repeated administration of the drug and perpetuates the smoking behavior.[11,17]

Chronic administration of nicotine has been shown to increase the number of nicotine receptors in specific regions of the brain.[18] This may represent upregulation in response to nicotine-mediated desensitization of the receptors and could play a role in nicotine tolerance and dependence.[17,18] Chronic nicotine administration also leads to tolerance of its behavioral and cardiovascular effects during the course of the day; however, tobacco users regain sensitivity to the effects of nicotine after overnight abstinence from nicotine,[10,11] as shown in Figure 91-1.[19] After smoking the first cigarette of the day, the smoker experiences marked pharmacologic effects, particularly arousal. No other cigarette throughout the day produces the same degree of pleasure or

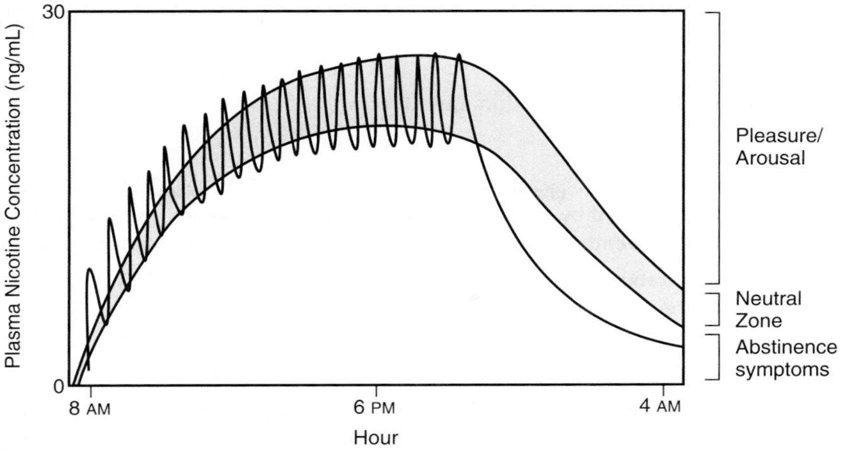

Figure 91-1 Nicotine addiction cycle throughout the day. The *sawtooth line* represents venous plasma concentrations of nicotine because a cigarette is smoked every 40 minutes between 8 AM and 9 PM. The *upper solid line* indicates the threshold concentration for nicotine to produce pleasure or arousal. The *lower solid line* indicates the concentrations at which symptoms of abstinence (i.e., withdrawal symptoms) from nicotine occur. The *shaded area* represents the zone of nicotine concentrations (neutral zone) in which the smoker is comfortable without experiencing either pleasure and arousal or abstinence symptoms. (Reprinted with permission from Benowitz NL. Cigarette smoking and nicotine addiction. *Med Clin North Am*. 1992;76(2):415.)

arousal. For this reason, many smokers describe the first cigarette as the most important one of the day. Shortly after the initial cigarette, tolerance begins to develop. Accordingly, the threshold levels for both pleasure or arousal and abstinence rise progressively throughout the day because the smoker becomes tolerant to the effects of nicotine. With continued smoking, nicotine accumulates, leading to an even greater degree of tolerance. Later in the day, each individual cigarette produces only limited pleasure or arousal; instead, smoking primarily alleviates nicotine withdrawal symptoms. Lack of exposure to nicotine overnight results in resensitization of drug responses (i.e., loss of tolerance). Most dependent smokers tend to smoke a certain number of cigarettes / day and tend to consume sufficient nicotine / day to achieve the desired effects of cigarette smoking and minimize the symptoms of nicotine withdrawal.[11,19] Withdrawal symptoms, which include anger, anxiety, depression, difficulty concentrating, impatience, insomnia, and restlessness, typically manifest within a few days after quitting, peak within a week, and subside within 2 to 4 weeks.[20] Tobacco users become adept at titrating their nicotine levels throughout the day to avoid withdrawal symptoms, maintain pleasure and arousal, and modulate mood.

Nicotine is extensively metabolized in the liver and, to a lesser extent, in the kidney and lung. Approximately 70% to 80% of nicotine is metabolized to cotinine, an inactive metabolite.[14] The rapid metabolism of nicotine (half-life [$t_{1/2}$] = 2 hours) to inactive compounds underlies tobacco users' needs for frequent, repeated administration. The half-life of cotinine, however, is much longer ($t_{1/2}$ = 18–20 hours), and for this reason, cotinine is commonly used as a marker of tobacco use as well as a marker for exposure to secondhand smoke.[14] Measurement of cotinine cannot, however, differentiate between the nicotine from tobacco products and the nicotine from NRT products. Nicotine and other metabolites are excreted in the urine. Urinary excretion is pH dependent; the excretion rate is increased in acidic urine.[14] Nicotine crosses the placenta and accumulates in breast milk.[14]

Drug Interactions with Smoking

It is widely recognized that polycyclic aromatic hydrocarbons (PAHs) in tobacco smoke are responsible for most drug interactions with smoking.[21,22] PAHs, which result from incomplete combustion of tobacco, are potent inducers of several hepatic cytochrome-P450 microsomal enzymes (CYP1A1, CYP1A2, and possibly CYP2E1). Although other substances in tobacco smoke, including acetone, pyridines, benzene, nicotine, carbon monoxide, and heavy metals (e.g., cadmium), might also interact with hepatic enzymes, their effects appear to be less significant. Most drug interactions with tobacco smoke are pharmacokinetic, resulting from the induction of drug-metabolizing enzymes (especially CYP1A2) by compounds in tobacco smoke. Table 91-1 summarizes key interactions with smoking.[21,22,23] Patients who begin smoking, quit smoking, or dramatically alter their level of smoking might require dosage adjustments for some medications.

Health Consequences of Tobacco Use

All forms of tobacco are harmful, and there is no safe level of exposure to tobacco products. Smoking has a causal or contributory role in the development of a variety of medical conditions, affecting almost every organ in the body.[2,3]

SECONDHAND SMOKE EXPOSURE

Exposure to secondhand smoke, which includes the smoke from burning tobacco and that exhaled by the smoker, affects an estimated 88 million nonsmokers older than the age of 3 in the United States.[24] Secondhand smoke exposure causes disease and premature death in children and adults who do not smoke resulting in an estimated 50,000 deaths annually.[6] Millions of American children and adults are still exposed to secondhand smoke in their homes and workplaces despite substantial progress in tobacco control. Evidence indicates that there is no risk-free level of exposure to secondhand smoke. Only completely eliminating smoking in indoor spaces fully protects nonsmokers from exposure to secondhand smoke. Separating smokers from nonsmokers, cleaning the air, and ventilating buildings cannot eliminate exposure of nonsmokers to secondhand smoke.

Benefits of Quitting

Benefits of smoking cessation incurred soon after quitting (e.g., within 2 weeks–3 months) include improvements in pulmonary function, circulation, and ambulation. Smoking cessation results in measurable improvements in lung function (see Chapter 19, Chronic Obstructive Pulmonary Disease). One year after cessation,

Table 91-1
Drug Interactions with Tobacco Smoke

Drug/Class	Mechanism of Interaction and Effects
Pharmacokinetic Interactions	
Alprazolam (Xanax)	■ Conflicting data on significance, but possible ↓ plasma concentrations (up to 50%); ↓ half-life (35%).
Bendamustine (Treanda)	■ **Metabolized by CYP1A2. Manufacturer recommends using with caution in smokers due to likely ↓ bendamustine concentrations, with ↑ concentrations of its two active metabolites.**
Caffeine	■ **↑ Metabolism (induction of CYP1A2); ↑ clearance (56%).** ■ **Caffeine levels likely increase after cessation.**
Chlorpromazine (Thorazine)	■ ↓ AUC (36%) and serum concentrations (24%). ■ ↓ Sedation and hypotension possible in smokers; smokers may require ↑ dosages.
Clopidogrel (Plavix)	■ **↑ Metabolism (induction of CYP1A2) of clopidogrel to its active metabolite.** ■ **Clopidogrel's effects are enhanced in smokers (≥10 cigarettes/day): significant ↑ platelet inhibition, ↓ platelet aggregation; although improved clinical outcomes have been shown, may also ↑ risk of bleeding.**
Clozapine (Clozaril)	■ **↑ Metabolism (induction of CYP1A2); ↓ plasma concentrations (18%).** ■ **↑ Levels on cessation may occur; closely monitor drug levels and reduce dose as required to avoid toxicity.**
Erlotinib (Tarceva)	■ **↑ Clearance (24%); ↓ trough serum concentrations (2-fold).**
Flecainide (Tambocor)	■ ↑ Clearance (61%); ↓ trough serum concentrations (25%). ■ Smokers may need ↑ dosages.
Fluvoxamine (Luvox)	■ **↑ Metabolism (induction of CYP1A2); ↑ clearance (24%); ↓ AUC (31%); ↓ Cmax (32%) and Css (by 39%).** ■ **Dosage modifications not routinely recommended but smokers may need ↑ dosages.**
Haloperidol (Haldol)	■ **↑ Clearance (44%); ↓ serum concentrations (70%); data are inconsistent therefore clinical significance is unclear.**
Heparin	■ Mechanism unknown but ↑ clearance and ↓ half-life are observed. Smoking has prothrombotic effects. ■ Smokers may need ↑ dosages because of PK and PD interactions.
Insulin, subcutaneous	■ Possible ↓ insulin absorption secondary to peripheral vasoconstriction; smoking may cause release of endogenous substances that cause insulin resistance. ■ PK and PD interactions likely not clinically significant but smokers may need ↑ dosages.
Irinotecan (Camptosar)	■ **↑ Clearance (18%); ↓ serum concentrations of active metabolite SN-38 (~40%; via induction of glucuronidation); ↓ systemic exposure resulting in lower hematologic toxicity and may reduce efficacy.** ■ **Smokers may need ↑ dosages.**
Methadone	■ Possible increase ↑ metabolism (induction of CYP1A2, a minor pathway for methadone.)- Carefully monitor response upon cessation.
Mexiletine (Mexitil)	■ ↑ Clearance (25%; via oxidation and glucuronidation); ↓ half-life (36%).
Olanzapine (Zyprexa)	■ **↑ Metabolism (induction of CYP1A2); ↑ clearance (98%); ↓ serum concentrations (12%).** ■ **Dosage modifications not routinely recommended but smokers may need ↑ dosages.**
Propranolol (Inderal)	■ ↑ Clearance (77%; via side-chain oxidation and glucuronidation).
Riociguat (Adempas)	■ **↓ Plasma concentrations (by 50%–60%)** ■ **Smokers may require dosages higher than 2.5 mg 3 times daily; consider dose reduction upon cessation.**
Ropinirole (Requip)	■ **↓ C_{max} (30%) and AUC (38%) in study with patients with restless legs syndrome.** ■ **Smokers may need ↑ dosages.**
Tacrine (Cognex)	■ Increase ↑ metabolism (induction of CYP1A2); decrease ↓ half-life (50%); serum concentrations 3-fold lower. -Smokers may need increased ↑ dosages.
Tasimelteon (Hetlioz)	■ Increased ↑ Metabolism (induction of CYP1A2); drug exposure decreased ↓ by 40%. -Smokers may need increased ↑ dosages.
Theophylline (Theo-Dur, etc.)	■ **↑ Metabolism (induction of CYP1A2); ↑ clearance (58%–100%); ↓ half-life (63%).** ■ **Levels should be monitored if smoking is initiated, discontinued, or changed.** ■ **↑ Clearance with secondhand smoke exposure.** ■ **Maintenance doses are considerably higher in smokers; ↑ Clearance also with secondhand smoke exposure.**
Tizanidine (Zanaflex)	■ ↓ AUC (30%–40%) and ↓ half-life (10%) observed in male smokers.

Table 91-1
Drug Interactions with Tobacco Smoke (*continued*)

Drug/Class	Mechanism of Interaction and Effects
Tricyclic antidepressants (e.g., imipramine, nortriptyline)	■ Possible interaction with tricyclic antidepressants in the direction of ↓ blood levels, but the clinical significance is not established.
Warfarin	■ ↑ Metabolism (induction of CYP1A2) of *R*-enantiomer; however, *S*-enantiomer is more potent and effect on INR is inconclusive. Consider monitoring INR on smoking cessation.
Pharmacodynamic Interactions	
Benzodiazepines (diazepam, chlordiazepoxide)	■ ↓ Sedation and drowsiness, possibly caused by nicotine stimulation of central nervous system.
β-Blockers	■ Less effective antihypertensive and heart rate control effects; possibly caused by nicotine-mediated sympathetic activation. ■ Smokers may need ↑ dosages.
Corticosteroids, inhaled	■ **Smokers with asthma may have less of a response to inhaled corticosteroids.**
Hormonal contraceptives (combined)	■ **↑ Risk of cardiovascular adverse effects (e.g., stroke, myocardial infarction, thromboembolism) in women who smoke and use combined hormonal contraceptives.** ■ **↑ Risk with age and with heavy smoking (15 or more cigarettes/day) and is quite marked in women aged 35 and older.**
Serotonin 5-HT1 receptor agonists (triptans)	■ This class of drugs may cause coronary vasospasm; caution for use in smokers due to possible unrecognized CAD.

Bold rows indicate the most clinically significant interactions.
AUC, area under the curve; C_{max}, maximal concentration; Css, steady state concentration; INR, international normalized ratio; PD, pharmacodynamics; PK, pharmacokinetics.
Adapted with permission from *Rx for Change: Clinician-Assisted Tobacco Cessation*.

the excess risk of coronary heart disease is reduced to half that of continuing smokers. After 5 to 15 years, the risk of stroke is reduced to a rate similar to that of people who are lifetime nonsmokers, and 10 years after quitting, the chance of dying of lung cancer is approximately half that of continuing smokers. In addition, the risk of developing mouth, throat, esophagus, bladder, kidney, or pancreatic cancer is decreased. Finally, 15 years after quitting, the risk of coronary heart disease is reduced to a rate that is similar to that of people who have never smoked.[25] Similarly, more recent data suggest that smokers who quit for good over a sustained period have an overall mortality rate and death rate associated with cardiovascular disease, ischemic heart disease, and stroke that is similar to individuals who have never smoked. In contrast, individuals who had successfully quit, but later resumed smoking, had mortality risks that were significantly higher than lifetime nonsmokers.[26]

Quitting at ages 30, 40, 50, and 60 results in 10, 9, 6, and 3 years of life gained, respectively.[1] On average, cigarette smokers die approximately 10 years younger than do nonsmokers, and of those who continue smoking, at least half will eventually die as a result of a tobacco-related disease. Persons who quit before age 35 add 10 years of life and have a life expectancy similar to men who had never smoked.[1] A reduction in smoking does not equate to a reduction in harm,[27] and even low levels of smoking (e.g., 1–4 cigarettes/day) have documented risks.[28,29] Therefore, decreasing the number of cigarettes smoked/day should be viewed as a positive step toward quitting, but should not be recommended as a targeted end point. For any patient who uses tobacco, the goal is complete, long-term abstinence from all nicotine-containing products.

Tobacco Use and Dependence: Treatment Approaches

Most tobacco users attempt to quit without assistance, despite the fact that persons who receive assistance are more likely to be successful in quitting.[7,30] Given the complexity of the tobacco dependence syndrome and the constellation of factors that contribute to tobacco use, treatment requires a multifaceted approach. To assist clinicians and other specialists in providing cessation treatment to patients who use tobacco, the US Public Health Service published the Clinical Practice Guideline for Treating Tobacco Use and Dependence. This document, which represents a distillation of more than 8,700 published articles,[7] specifies that clinicians can have an important impact on their patients' ability to quit. A meta-analysis of 29 studies[7] estimated that compared with patients who do not receive an intervention from a clinician, patients who receive a tobacco-cessation intervention from a physician clinician or a nonphysician clinician are 2.2 and 1.7 times, respectively, more likely to quit (at 5 or more months after cessation). Although even brief advice from a clinician has been shown to lead to increased odds of quitting,[7] more intensive counseling yields more dramatic increases in quit rates.[7] Other effective methods for delivery of counseling include group programs[7,31] and telephone counseling.[32] Internet-based interventions have become more prevalent in recent years, but a meta-analysis of 28 trials revealed inconsistent results.[33]

Numerous effective medications are available for tobacco dependence, and clinicians should encourage their use by all patients attempting to quit smoking—except when medically contraindicated or with specific populations for which there is insufficient evidence of effectiveness (i.e., pregnant women, smokeless tobacco users, light smokers, adolescents).[7] Although both pharmacotherapy and behavioral counseling are effective independently, patients' odds of quitting are substantially increased when the two approaches are used simultaneously.[34] Clinicians can have a significant impact on a patient's likelihood of success by recommending pharmacotherapy agents and by supplementing medication use with behavioral counseling as described later in this chapter.

Assisting Patients with Quitting

BEHAVIORAL COUNSELING STRATEGIES

According to the Clinical Practice Guideline,[7] five key components constitute comprehensive counseling for tobacco cessation: (a) asking patients whether they use tobacco, (b) advising tobacco users to quit, (c) assessing patients' readiness to quit, (d) assisting patients with quitting, and (e) arranging follow-up care. These steps are referred to as the "5 A's" and are described, in brief, as follows. Figure 91-2 can be used as a guide for structuring counseling interactions.

- **Ask:** Screening for tobacco use is essential and should be a routine component of clinical care. The following question can be used to identify tobacco users: *"Do you ever smoke or use any type of tobacco?"* At a minimum, tobacco use status (current, former, never user) and level of use (e.g., number of cigarettes smoked/day) should be assessed and documented in the medical record. Also, patients should be asked about exposure to secondhand smoke.
- **Advise:** Tobacco users should be advised to consider quitting; the advice should be clear and compelling, yet delivered with sensitivity and a tone of voice that communicates concern and a willingness to assist with quitting. When possible, messages should be personalized by relating advice to factors such as a patient's health status, medication regimen, personal reasons for wanting to quit, or the impact of tobacco use on others. For example, *"I'm concerned because you are on two different inhalers for your emphysema. Quitting smoking is the single most important treatment to improve your breathing. I strongly encourage you to quit. Would you be interested in having me help you with this?"*
- **Assess:** Key to the provision of appropriate counseling interventions is the assessment of a patient's readiness to quit. Patients should be categorized as being (a) not ready to quit in the next month; (b) ready to quit in the next month; (c) a recent quitter, having quit in the past 6 months; or (d) a former user, having quit more than 6 months ago.[7,35] This classification defines the clinician's next step, which is to provide counseling that is tailored to the patient's level of readiness to quit. As an example for a current smoker: *"Mr. Malkin, what are your thoughts about quitting, and would you consider quitting sometime in the next month?"* The counseling interventions for patients who are ready to quit will be different from those for patients who are not considering quitting.
- **Assist:** When counseling tobacco users, it is important that clinicians and patients view quitting as a process that might take months or even years to achieve. The goal is to promote forward progress in the process of change, with the target end point being sustained abstinence from all nicotine-containing products.

When counseling patients who are not ready to quit, an important first step is to foster motivation. Some patients are not convinced that quitting is important, but most recognize the need to quit and are simply not ready to make the commitment to do so. Often, patients have tried to quit multiple times and failed, and thus are too discouraged to try again. The "5 R's" can be applied to enhance motivation to quit[7] (Table 91-2) by clinicians offering to work closely with the patient in designing a treatment plan. Although it might be useful to educate patients about the pharmacotherapy options, it is inappropriate to prescribe a treatment regimen for patients who are not ready to quit. For patients

STEP One: ASK about Tobacco Use

➲ Suggested Dialogue

- "Do you ever smoke or use any type of tobacco, such as e-cigarettes?"
- "I take time to talk with all of my patients about tobacco use—because it's important."
- "Medication X often is used for conditions linked with or caused by smoking. Do you, or does someone in your household smoke?"
- "Condition X often is caused or worsened by exposure to tobacco smoke. Do you, or does someone in your household smoke?"

STEP Two: Strongly ADVISE to Quit

➲ Suggested Dialogue

- Quitting is the most important thing you can do to protect your health now and in the future. I have training to help my patients quit, and when you are ready I would be more than happy to work with you to design a treatment plan.
- What are your thoughts about quitting?
- Might you consider quitting sometime in the next month?
- Prior to imparting advice, consider asking the patient for permission to do so – e.g., "May I tell you why this concerns me?" {then elaborate on patient-specific concerns}.

STEP Three: ASSESS Readiness to Quit

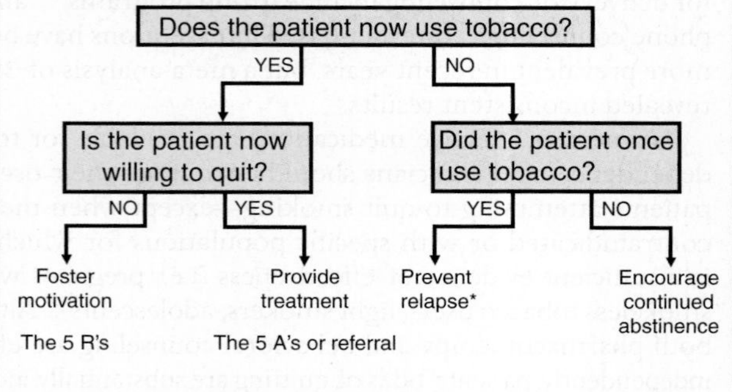

* Relapse prevention interventions not necessary in the case of the adult who has not used tobacco for many years and is not at risk for re-initiation.

Fiore MC, Jaen CR, Baker TB, et al. Treating Tobacco Use and Dependence: 2008 Update. Clinical Practice Guideline. Rockville, MD: U.S. Department of Health and Human Services, Public Health Service. May 2008.

STEP Four: ASSIST with Quitting

✓ **Assess Tobacco Use History**
- Current use: type(s) of tobacco used, brand, amount
- Past use:
  - Duration of tobacco use
  - Changes in levels of use recently
- Past quit attempts:
  - Number of attempts, date of most recent attempt, duration
  - Methods used previously—What did or didn't work? Why or why not?
  - Prior medication administration, dose, compliance, duration of treatment
  - Reasons for relapse

✓ **Discuss Key Issues** (for the upcoming or current quit attempt)
- Reasons/motivation for wanting to quit(or avoid relapse)
- Confidence in ability to quit (or avoid relapse)
- Triggers for tobacco use
- Routines and situations associated with tobacco use
- Stress-related tobacco use
- Social support for quitting
- Concerns about weight gain
- Concerns about withdrawal symptoms

✓ **Facilitate Quitting Process**
- Discuss methods for quitting: pros and cons of the different methods
- Set a quit date: ideally, less than 2 weeks away
- Recommend completion ofa Tobacco Use Log
- Discuss coping strategies (cognitive, behavioral) for key issues
- Discuss withdrawal symptoms
- Discuss concept of "slip" versus relapse
- Provide medication counseling: compliance, properuse, with demonstration
- Offer to assist throughout the quit attempt

✓ **Evaluate the Quit Attempt** (at follow-up)
- Status of attempt
- Inquire about "slips" and relapse
- Medication compliance and plans for discontinuation

STEP Five: ARRANGE Follow-up Counseling

✓ Monitor patients' progress throughout the quit attempt. Follow-up contact should occur during the first week after quitting. A second follow-up contact is recommended in the first month. Additional contacts should be scheduled as needed. Counseling contacts can occur face-to-face, by telephone, or by e-mail. Keep patient progress notes.

✓ Address temptations and triggers; discuss strategies to prevent relapse.

✓ Congratulate patients for continued success.

Figure 91-2 Tobacco-cessation counseling guide sheet. (Reprinted with permission from *Rx for Change: Clinician-Assisted Tobacco Cessation.* Copyright © 1999–2017. The Regents of the University of California. All rights reserved.)

Table 91-2
Enhancing Motivation to Quit: The "5 R's" for Tobacco-Cessation Counseling

- **Relevance**—Encourage patients to think about the reasons why quitting is important. Counseling should be framed such that it relates to the patient's risk for disease or exacerbation of disease, family or social situations (e.g., having children with asthma), health concerns, age, or other patient factors, such as prior experience with quitting.
- **Risks**—Ask patients to identify potential negative health consequences of smoking, such as acute risks (shortness of breath, asthma exacerbations, harm to pregnancy, infertility), long-term risks (cancer, cardiac, and pulmonary disease), and environmental risks (promoting smoking among children by being a negative role model; effects of secondhand smoke on others, including children and pets).
- **Rewards**—Ask patients to identify potential benefits that they anticipate from quitting, such as improved health, enhanced physical performance, enhanced taste and smell, reduced expenditures for tobacco, less time wasted or work missed, reduced health risks to others (fetus, children, housemates), and reduced aging of the skin.
- **Roadblocks**—Help patients identify barriers to quitting and assist in developing coping strategies (Table 91-4) for addressing each barrier. Common barriers include nicotine withdrawal symptoms, fear of failure, a need for social support while quitting, depression, weight gain, and a sense of deprivation or loss.
- **Repetition**—Continue to work with patients who are successful in their quit attempt. Discuss circumstances in which smoking occurred to identify the trigger(s) for relapse; this is part of the learning process and will be useful information for the next quit attempt. Repeat interventions when possible.

Reprinted from Fiore MC et al. *Treating Tobacco Use and Dependence: 2008 Update*. Clinical Practice Guideline. Rockville, MD: Public Health Service, U.S. Department of Health and Human Services; 2008.

who are not ready to quit in the next 30 days, encourage them to seriously consider quitting and ask the following questions:

1. *Do you ever plan to quit?*
   If the patient responds "no," the clinician should ask, "*What would have to change for you to decide to quit?*" If the patient responds "nothing," then offer to assist, if or when the patient changes his or her mind. If the patient responds "yes," the clinician should continue with question 2.
2. *What might be some benefits of quitting now, instead of later?*
   The longer a patient smokes, quitting generally becomes more difficult. Most patients will agree that there is never an ideal time to quit, and procrastinating a quit date has more negative effects than positive.
3. *What would have to change for you to decide to quit sooner?*
   This question probes patients' perceptions of quitting, which reveals some of the barriers to quitting that can then be discussed.

For patients who are ready to quit (i.e., in the next month), the goal is to work with the patient in designing an individualized treatment plan, addressing the key issues listed under the "Assist" component of Figure 91-2.[23] The first steps are to discuss the patient's tobacco use history, inquiring about levels of smoking, number of years smoked, methods used previously for quitting (what worked, what did not work and why), and reason(s) for previous failed quit attempts. Clinicians should elicit patients' opinions about the different medications for quitting and should work with patients in selecting the quitting methods (e.g., medications, behavioral counseling programs). Although it is important to recognize that pharmaceutical agents might not be appropriate, desirable, or affordable for all patients, clinicians should educate patients that medications, when taken correctly, can substantially increase the likelihood of success.

Patients should select a quit date, ideally within the next 2 weeks. This allows sufficient time to prepare for the quit attempt, including mental preparation, preparation of the environment, removing all tobacco products and ashtrays from the home, car, and workspace, and soliciting support their family, friends, and coworkers. Additional strategies for coping with quitting are shown in Table 91-3. Patients should be counseled about withdrawal symptoms, medication use, and the importance of receiving behavioral counseling throughout the quit attempt. Finally, patients should be commended for taking important steps toward improving their health.

- **Arrange:** Because patients' ability to quit increases when multiple counseling interactions are provided, arranging follow-up counseling is an important element of treatment for tobacco dependence. Follow-up contact should occur soon after the quit date, preferably during the first week. A second follow-up contact is recommended within the first month after quitting.[7] Additional follow-up contacts should occur to monitor patient progress, assess compliance with pharmacotherapy regimens, and provide additional support.

Relapse prevention counseling should be part of every follow-up contact with patients who have recently quit smoking. When counseling recent quitters, it is important to address challenges in countering withdrawal symptoms and cravings or temptations to use tobacco. A list of strategies for key triggers or temptations for tobacco use is provided in Table 91-3.[23] Importantly, because tobacco use is a habitual behavior, patients should be advised to alter their daily routines; this helps disassociate specific behaviors from the use of tobacco. Patients who slip and smoke a cigarette (or use any form of tobacco) or experience a full relapse back to habitual tobacco use should be encouraged to think through the scenario in which tobacco use first occurred and identify the trigger(s) for relapse. This process provides valuable information for future quit attempts.

PHARMACOTHERAPY OPTIONS

All smokers who are trying to quit should be encouraged to use one or more US Food and Drug Administration (FDA)-approved pharmacologic aids for cessation. Potential exceptions that require special consideration include medical contraindications or use in specific populations for which there is insufficient evidence of effectiveness (i.e., pregnant women, smokeless tobacco users, light smokers, adolescents).[7] Pharmacotherapy should always be combined with behavioral support and counseling. Currently, the FDA-approved first-line agents that have been shown to be effective in promoting smoking cessation include five NRT dosage forms, sustained-release bupropion, and varenicline.[7] The choice of therapy is dictated by considerations such as patient preference for a given agent, previous experience with cessation medications, current medical conditions, previous levels of smoking, medication adherence issues, and the patient's out-of-pocket costs. Dosing information, precautions, and adverse effects for the first-line agents are shown in Table 91-4.

Table 91-3

Cognitive and Behavioral Strategies for Tobacco Cessation

Cognitive Strategies	
Focus on *retraining the way a patient thinks*. Often, patients will deliberate on the fact that they are thinking about a cigarette, and this leads to relapse. Patients must recognize that thinking about a cigarette does not mean they need to have one.	
Review commitment to quit	Each morning, say, "I am proud that I made it through another day without tobacco!" Remind oneself that cravings and temptations are temporary and will pass. Announce, either silently or aloud, "I am a nonsmoker, and the temptation will pass."
Distractive thinking	Deliberate, immediate refocusing of thinking toward other thoughts when cued by thoughts about tobacco use.
Positive self-talks, "pep talks"	Say "I can do this" and remind oneself of previous difficult situations in which tobacco use was avoided.
Relaxation through imagery	Center mind toward positive, relaxing thoughts.
Mental rehearsal, visualization	Preparing for situations that might arise by envisioning how best to handle them. For example, envision what would happen if offered a cigarette by a friend—mentally craft and rehearse a response, and perhaps even practice it by saying it aloud.
Behavioral Strategies	
Involve *specific actions to reduce risk for relapse*. These strategies should be considered prior to quitting, after determining patient-specific triggers and routines or situations associated with tobacco use. Below are strategies for several of the common cues or causes for relapse.	
Stress	Anticipate upcoming challenges at work, at school, or in personal life. Develop a substitute plan for tobacco use during times of stress (e.g., use deep breathing, take a break or leave the situation, call a supportive friend or family member, or use nicotine replacement therapy to manage situational cravings).
Alcohol	Drinking alcohol can lead to relapse. Consider limiting or abstaining from alcohol during the early stages of quitting.
Other tobacco users	Quitting is more difficult when around other tobacco users. This is especially difficult if there is another tobacco user in the household. During the early stages of quitting, limit prolonged contact with individuals who are using tobacco. Ask coworkers, friends, and housemates not to smoke or use tobacco in your presence.
Oral gratification needs	Have nontobacco oral substitutes (e.g., gum, sugarless candy, straws, toothpicks, lip balm, toothbrush, nicotine replacement therapy, bottled water) readily available.
Automatic smoking routines	Anticipate routines that are associated with tobacco use and develop an alternative plan.
	Examples:
	Morning coffee: change morning routine, drink tea instead of coffee, take shower before drinking coffee, take a brisk walk shortly after awakening.
	While driving: remove all tobacco from car, have car interior detailed, listen to an audio book or talk radio, use oral substitutes.
	While on the phone: stand while talking, limit call duration, change phone location, keep hands occupied by doodling or sketching.
	After meals: get up and immediately do dishes or take a brisk walk after eating, call supportive friend.
Postcessation weight gain	Do not attempt to modify multiple behaviors at one time. If weight gain is a barrier to quitting, engage in regular physical activity and adhere to a healthful diet (as opposed to strict dieting). Carefully plan and prepare meals, increase fruit and water intake to create a feeling of fullness, and chew sugarless gum or eat sugarless candies. Consider use of pharmacotherapy shown to delay weight gain (e.g., nicotine gum, lozenge, or sustained-release bupropion).
Cravings for tobacco	Cravings for tobacco are temporary and usually pass within 5–10 minutes. Handle cravings through distractive thinking, take a break, do something else, take deep breaths.

Reprinted with permission from *Rx for Change: Clinician-Assisted Tobacco Cessation*.

FIRST-LINE AGENTS

Nicotine Replacement Therapy

NRT improves cessation rates by reducing the physical withdrawal symptoms associated with tobacco cessation whereas the patient focuses on behavior modification and coping with the psychological aspects of quitting. In addition, because the onset of action for NRT is not as rapid as that of nicotine obtained through smoking, patients become less accustomed to the nearly immediate, reinforcing effects of inhaled nicotine. A meta-analysis found that all NRT formulations result in statistically significant improvements in abstinence rates when compared with placebo. Patients using NRT are 1.6 times as likely to quit

Table 91-4
Pharmacologic Product Guide: FDA-Approved Medications for Smoking Cessation

NRT Formulations					Bupropion SR	Varenicline
Gum	**Lozenge**	**Transdermal Patch**	**Nasal Spray**	**Oral Inhaler**		
Product						
Nicorette,[a] ZONNIC[b] generic	Nicorette Lozenge[a]; Nicorette Mini Lozenge[a], (standard and mini),[a] generic	NicoDerm CQ,[a] generic	Nicotrol NS[c]	Nicotrol inhaler[c]	Zyban,[a] generic	Chantix[c]
OTC	OTC	OTC (NicoDerm CQ, generic)	Rx	Rx	Rx	Rx
2 and 4 mg	2 and 4 mg	Rx (generic)	Metered spray	10-mg cartridge	150-mg sustained-release tablet	0.5- and 1-mg tablet
Original, cinnamon, fruit, mint	Cherry, mint	7, 14, and 21 mg (24-hour release)	10 mg/mL aqueous solution	Delivers 4 mg of inhaled nicotine vapor		
Precautions, Warnings, and Contraindications						
■ Recent (≤2 weeks) myocardial infarction ■ Serious underlying arrhythmias ■ Serious or worsening angina pectoris ■ Temporomandibular joint disease ■ Pregnancy[d] and breast-feeding ■ Adolescents (<18 years)	■ Recent (≤2 weeks) myocardial infarction ■ Serious underlying arrhythmias ■ Serious or worsening angina pectoris ■ Pregnancy[d] and breast-feeding ■ Adolescents (<18 years)	■ Recent (≤2 weeks) myocardial infarction ■ Serious underlying arrhythmias ■ Serious or worsening angina pectoris ■ Pregnancy[d] (Rx formulations, category D) and breast-feeding ■ Adolescents (<18 years)	■ Recent (≤2 weeks) myocardial infarction ■ Serious underlying arrhythmias ■ Serious or worsening angina pectoris ■ Underlying chronic nasal disorders (rhinitis, nasal polyps, sinusitis) ■ Severe reactive airway disease ■ Pregnancy[d] (category D) and breast-feeding ■ Adolescents (<18 years)	■ Recent (≤2 weeks) myocardial infarction ■ Serious underlying arrhythmias ■ Serious of worsening angina pectoris ■ Bronchospastic disease ■ Pregnancy[d] (category D) and breast-feeding ■ Adolescents (<18 years)	■ Concomitant therapy with medications or medical conditions known to lower seizure threshold ■ Hepatic impairment ■ Pregnancy[d] (category C) and breast-feeding ■ Adolescents (<18 years) ■ Treatment-emergent neuropsychiatric symptoms[e] ■ **Contraindications:** ■ Seizure disorder ■ Concomitant bupropion (e.g., Wellbutrin) therapy ■ Current or prior diagnosis of bulimia or anorexia nervosa ■ Simultaneous abrupt discontinuation of alcohol or sedatives (including benzodiazepines) ■ Monoamine oxidase inhibitor therapy in previous 14 days	■ Severe renal impairment (dosage adjustment is necessary) ■ Pregnancy[d] (category C) and breast-feeding ■ Adolescents (<18 years) ■ Treatment-emergent neuropsychiatric symptoms[e]

(continued)

Table 91-4
Pharmacologic Product Guide: FDA-Approved Medications for Smoking Cessation (*continued*)

NRT Formulations					Bupropion SR	Varenicline
Gum	**Lozenge**	**Transdermal Patch**	**Nasal Spray**	**Oral Inhaler**		
Dosing[f]						
First cigarette ≤30 minutes after waking: 4 mg *First cigarette >30 minutes after waking:* 2 mg Weeks 1–6: 1 piece every 1–2 hours Weeks 7–9: 1 piece every 2–4 hours Weeks 10–12: 1 piece every 4–8 hours ■ Maximum, 24 pieces/day ■ Chew each piece slowly ■ Park between cheek and gum when peppery or tingling sensation appears (~15–30 chews) ■ Resume chewing when tingle fades ■ Repeat chew and park steps until most of nicotine is gone (tingle does not return; generally 30 minutes) ■ Park in different areas of mouth ■ No food or beverages 15 minutes before or during use ■ Duration: up to 12 weeks	*First cigarette ≤30 minutes after waking:* 4 mg *First cigarette >30 minutes after waking:* 2 mg Weeks 1–6: 1 lozenge every 1–2 hours Weeks 7–9: 1 lozenge every 2–4 hours Weeks 10–12: 1 lozenge every 4–8 hours ■ Maximum, 20 lozenges/day ■ Allow to dissolve slowly (20–30 minutes for standard; 10 minutes for mini) ■ Nicotine release may cause a warm, tingling sensation ■ Do not chew or swallow ■ Occasionally rotate to different areas of the mouth ■ No food or beverages 15 minutes before or during use ■ Duration: up to 12 weeks	*>10 cigarettes/day:* 21 mg/day × 4 weeks (generic) × 6 weeks (NicoDerm CQ) 14 mg/day × 2 weeks 7 mg/day × 2 weeks *≤10 cigarettes/day:* 14 mg/day × 6 weeks 7 mg/day × 2 weeks ■ Rotate patch application site daily; do not apply a new patch tot he same skin site for at least one week. ■ May wear patch for 16 hours if patient experiences sleep disturbances (remove at bedtime) ■ Duration: 8–10 weeks	1–2 doses/hour (8–40 doses/day) One dose = 2 sprays (one in *each* nostril); each spray delivers 0.5 mg of nicotine to the nasal mucosa ■ Maximum ■ –5 doses/hour or ■ –40 doses/day ■ For best results, initially use at least 8 doses/day ■ Do not sniff, swallow, or inhale through the nose as the spray is being administered ■ Duration: 3–6 months	6–16 cartridges/day Individualize dosing; initially use 1 cartridge every 1–2 hours ■ Best effects with continuous puffing for 20 minutes ■ Initially use at least 6 cartridges/day ■ Nicotine in cartridge is depleted after 20 minutes of active puffing ■ Inhale into back of throat or puff in short breaths ■ Do NOT inhale into the lungs (like a cigarette) but "puff" as if lighting a pipe ■ Open cartridge retains potency for 24 hours ■ No food or beverages 15 minutes before or during use ■ Duration: 3–6 months	150 mg PO every morning × 3 days, then increase to 150 mg PO BID Do not exceed 300 mg/day ■ Begin therapy 1–2 weeks *before* quit date ■ Allow at least 8 hours between doses ■ Avoid bedtime dosing to minimize insomnia ■ Dose tapering is not necessary ■ Duration: 7–12 weeks, with maintenance up to 6 months in selected patients	Days 1–3: 0.5 mg PO every morning Days 4–7: 0.5 mg PO BID Weeks 2–12: 1 mg PO BID ■ Begin therapy 1 week *before* quit date. ■ Take dose after eating and with a full glass of water ■ Dose tapering is not necessary ■ Dosing adjustment is recommended for patients with severe renal impairment ■ Duration: 12 weeks; an additional 12-week course may be used in selected patients ■ May initiate up to 35 days before target quit date OR may reduce smoking over a 12-week period of treatment prior to quitting and continue treatment for an additional 12 weeks.

Adverse Effects						
■ Mouth or jaw soreness ■ Hiccups ■ Dyspepsia ■ Hypersalivation ■ Effects associated with incorrect chewing technique: ■ Lightheadedness ■ Nausea or vomiting ■ Throat and mouth irritation	■ Nausea ■ Hiccups ■ Mouth Irritation ■ Heartburn ■ Headache ■ Sore throat ■ dizziness	■ Local skin reactions (erythema, pruritus, burning) ■ Headache ■ Sleep disturbances (insomnia, abnormal or vivid dreams); associated with nocturnal nicotine absorption	■ Nasal or throat irritation (hot, peppery, or burning sensation) ■ Rhinitis ■ Tearing ■ Sneezing ■ Cough ■ Headache	■ Mouth or throat irritation ■ Cough ■ Headache ■ Rhinitis ■ Dyspepsia ■ Hiccups	■ Insomnia ■ Dry mouth ■ Nervousness or difficulty concentrating ■ Rash ■ Constipation ■ Seizures (risk is ~0.1%) ■ Neuropsychiatric symptoms (rare; see PRECAUTIONS)	■ Nausea ■ Sleep disturbances (insomnia, abnormal or vivid dreams) ■ Constipation ■ Flatulence ■ Vomiting ■ Neuropsychiatric symptoms (rare; see PRECAUTIONS)

[a]Marketed by GlaxoSmithKline.
[b]*Marketed by Niconovum USA (a subsidiary of Reynolds American, Inc.).*
[c]Marketed by Pfizer.
[d]The US Clinical Practice Guideline states that pregnant smokers should be encouraged to quit without medication based on insufficient evidence of effectiveness and theoretic concerns with safety. Pregnant smokers should be offered behavioral counseling interventions that exceed minimal advice to quit.
[e]In July 2009, the FDA mandated that the prescribing information for all bupropion- and varenicline-containing products includes a black-boxed warning highlighting the risk of serious neuropsychiatric symptoms, including changes in behavior, hostility, agitation, depressed mood, suicidal thoughts and behavior, and attempted suicide. Clinicians should advise patients to stop taking varenicline or bupropion SR and contact a healthcare provider immediately if they experience agitation, depressed mood, and any changes in behavior that are not typical of nicotine withdrawal, or if they experience suicidal thoughts or behavior. If treatment is stopped because of neuropsychiatric symptoms, patients should be monitored until the symptoms resolve.Based on results of a mandated clinical trial, the FDA removed this boxed warning in December 2016.
[f]For complete prescribing information, refer to the manufacturers' package inserts.
NRT, nicotine replacement therapy; OTC, over-the-counter (nonprescription); Rx, prescription; SR, sustained-release.
Adapted with permission from *Rx for Change: Clinician-Assisted Tobacco Cessation*.

smoking than are those receiving placebo.[36] Figure 91-3 depicts the concentration–time curves for the various NRT formulations, compared with a cigarette and snuff, a smokeless form of tobacco.[37–39] Nicotine nasal spray reaches its peak concentration most rapidly. The nicotine gum, lozenge, and oral inhaler have similar concentration curves, and the nicotine transdermal patch has the slowest onset, but offers more consistent blood levels of nicotine for a sustained period. Although ideally tobacco use stops when NRT is initiated, some patients may continue to occasionally use tobacco products after beginning NRT. This allows patients more flexibility with continuing to use NRT if they slip and use tobacco products, or with initiating NRT in an effort to decrease the number of cigarettes smoked prior to complete cessation.(the "reduce to quit" method)[34,40,41] Initiating nicotine patch prior to a quit attempt may be more effective than applying the patch on the quit date. However, data are conflicting, and the evidence does not support using other forms of NRT prior to the quit date.[41]

Sustained-release Bupropion

Sustained-release bupropion is an atypical antidepressant medication hypothesized to promote smoking cessation by blocking the reuptake of dopamine and norepinephrine in the central nervous system[7] and possibly by acting as a nicotine receptor antagonist.[42] These neurochemical effects are believed to modulate the dopamine reward pathway and reduce cravings for nicotine and symptoms of withdrawal.[7] Use of sustained-release bupropion approximately doubles the long-term abstinence rate when compared with placebo.[7,43]

Varenicline

Varenicline is a partial agonist that binds with high affinity and selectivity at $\alpha_4\beta_2$ neuronal nicotinic acetylcholine receptors.[44] The efficacy of varenicline in smoking cessation is believed to be the result of sustained, low-level agonist activity at the receptor site combined with competitive inhibition of nicotine binding. The partial agonist activity induces modest receptor stimulation, leading to increased dopamine levels, which attenuates the symptoms of nicotine withdrawal. In addition, by blocking the ability of nicotine to activate $\alpha_4\beta_2$ nicotinic acetylcholine receptors, varenicline inhibits the surges of dopamine release that are believed to be responsible for the reinforcement and reward associated with smoking.[44,45] Use of varenicline more than doubles the chances of quitting when compared to placebo.[7,46] Patients should be monitored for neuropsychiatric symptoms, including changes in behavior, mood, or suicidal thoughts and behavior.[47]

SECOND-LINE AGENTS

Although not FDA-approved specifically for smoking cessation, the prescription medications clonidine and nortriptyline are recommended as second-line agents.[7] Lack of an FDA-approved indication for smoking cessation and less desirable side-effect profiles currently prohibit these agents from achieving first-line classification.[7]

PHARMACOTHERAPY FOR TREATING TOBACCO USE AND DEPENDENCE

Transdermal Nicotine Patch

CASE 91-1

QUESTION 1: T.B. is a 32-year-old woman who is enrolled in a worksite smoking-cessation program. During the previous group session, the cessation counselor discussed the various medications for cessation. T.B. has set her quit date for 1 week from today, and she is interested in starting the nicotine transdermal patch. She is currently smoking 1.5 packs/day (PPD), which is a reduction from the 2 PPD she had been smoking for the past 10 years. T.B. reports she smokes several cigarettes in succession immediately after waking in the morning. She takes no medications and has no medical problems. Which nicotine transdermal product should T.B. select, and how should it be used?

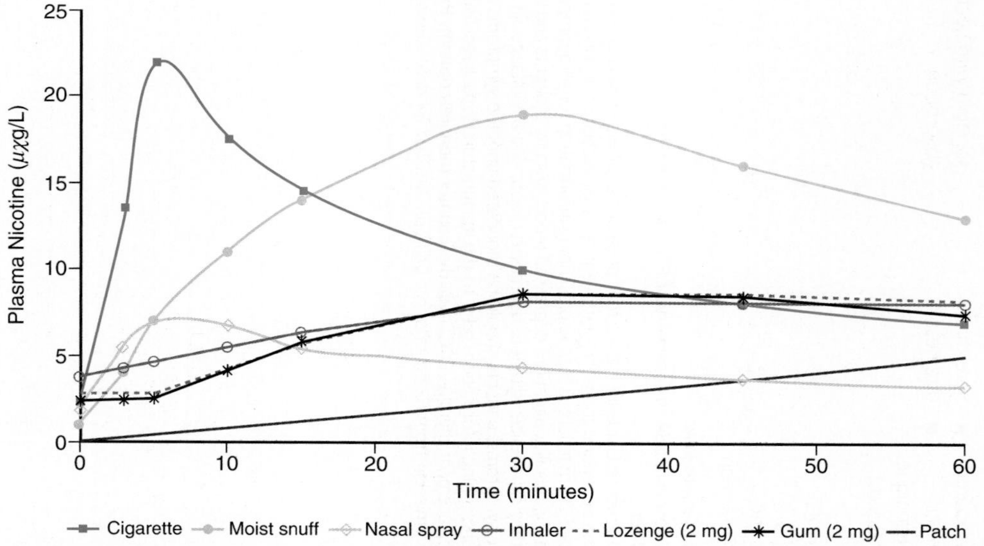

Figure 91-3 Plasma nicotine concentrations for various nicotine-containing products. (Reprinted with permission from *Rx for Change: Clinician-Assisted Tobacco Cessation*. Copyright © 1999–2017. The Regents of the University of California. All rights reserved. Plasma nicotine concentration curves derived from Choi JH et al. Pharmacokinetics of a nicotine polacrilex lozenge. *Nicotine Tob Res*. 2003;5(5):635; Schneider NG et al. The nicotine inhaler: clinical pharmacokinetics and comparison with other nicotine treatments. *Clin Pharmacokinet*. 2001;40(9):661; and Fant RV et al. Pharmacokinetics and pharmacodynamics of moist snuff in humans. *Tob Control*. 1999;8(4):387.)

Transdermal nicotine delivery systems consist of an impermeable surface layer, a nicotine reservoir, an adhesive layer, and a removable protective liner. Although the transdermal delivery technology varies by manufacturer, nicotine is well absorbed, with 68% to 82% of the dose released from 24-hour patch formulations systemically bioavailable across the skin. Plasma nicotine concentrations from the patch rise slowly during 1 to 4 hours and peak within 3 to 12 hours after application.[14] Levels of nicotine achieved with the transdermal patch are lower and fluctuate less than do those achieved with tobacco products or other NRT formulations (Fig. 91-3).

The transdermal nicotine patch exhibits significantly improved abstinence rates relative to placebo.[7,35] A meta-analysis of 25 randomized, controlled trials found treatment with the nicotine patch (6–14 weeks) approximately doubled the likelihood of long-term abstinence compared with placebo.[7]

DOSING

The manufacturers' recommended dosages are listed in Table 91-4. In general, higher levels of smoking necessitate the use of higher-strength formulations and a longer duration of therapy. Ultimately, the starting dose, rate of tapering, and total duration of therapy must be individualized to the patient's baseline smoking levels, development of side effects (e.g., nausea, dyspepsia, nervousness, dizziness, sweating), and the presence or absence of withdrawal symptoms. T.B. currently smokes 30 cigarettes/day, and thus she should initiate the regimen using the 21-mg/day patch.

PATIENT EDUCATION

T.B. should be instructed to apply the patch to a clean, dry, hairless area of skin on the upper body or the upper outer part of her arm at approximately the same time each day. To minimize the potential for local skin reactions, the patch application site should be rotated daily, and the same area should not be used again for at least 1 week. After patch application, T.B. should ensure that the patch adheres well to the skin, especially around the edges. The clinician should reassure T.B. that water will not reduce the effectiveness of the nicotine patch if it is applied correctly, and she may bathe, shower, swim, or exercise while wearing the patch. Finally, T.B. should be advised to discontinue use of the nicotine patch and contact a healthcare provider if skin redness caused by the patch does not resolve after 4 days; if the skin swells or a rash develops; if irregular heartbeat or palpitations occur; or if she experiences symptoms of nicotine overdose such as nausea, vomiting, dizziness, diarrhea, sweating, weakness, or rapid heartbeat.

ADVERSE REACTIONS

CASE 91-1, QUESTION 2: Ten days later, T.B. calls to complain of an itchy rash that she believes is caused by the nicotine patch. She noticed the rash yesterday when she removed the first patch from her left upper arm. This morning, after removing the second patch from her right upper arm, she noticed a similar rash. T.B. describes the skin on her right arm as slightly red but not swollen; the rash on her left arm has only a faint trace of pink discoloration. Her last cigarette was 2 days ago. How should T.B. be managed at this time?

The most common side effects associated with the nicotine patch are local reactions (erythema, burning, and pruritus) at the skin application site. These reactions are generally caused by skin occlusion or sensitivity to the patch adhesives. Rotating the patch application sites on a daily basis minimizes skin irritation; nonetheless, skin reactions to the patch adhesives occur in up to 50% of patch users. Fewer than 5% of patients discontinue therapy because of a skin reaction.[7]

T.B. appears to be experiencing a mild skin reaction and should be reassured that it is common for the skin to appear erythematous for up to 24 to 48 hours after the patch is removed. T.B. can apply topical hydrocortisone cream (0.5% or 1%) or triamcinolone cream (0.5%), or she can take an oral antihistamine for symptomatic treatment.[7] Another option would be to try a different brand of patch as the adhesive may vary. Because the rash on her left arm has nearly resolved, it is reasonable for T.B. to continue using the nicotine transdermal patch provided that the erythema is not too bothersome.

Other less common side effects associated with the transdermal nicotine patch include vivid or abnormal dreams, insomnia, and headache. Sleep disturbances likely result from nocturnal nicotine absorption. Patients experiencing troublesome sleep disturbances should be instructed to remove the patch before bedtime and apply a new patch as soon as possible after waking the following morning.[7]

The clinician should also provide behavioral counseling support by asking T.B. about the current quit attempt. Appropriate issues to address include her confidence in remaining tobacco free, situations in which she has been tempted to smoke and potential triggers for relapse, nicotine withdrawal symptoms, her social support system for quitting, and any other questions or concerns she might have. It is reasonable to review potential coping strategies (behavioral and cognitive; Table 91-4) and schedule a future follow-up call. The clinician should commend T.B. for her decision to quit, congratulate her for remaining free of cigarettes for 48 hours, and reassure her that skin irritation is a common, yet generally manageable, complication with the nicotine patch.

PRODUCT SELECTION CONSIDERATIONS

The primary advantage of the transdermal nicotine patch compared with other NRT formulations is that the patch is easy to use, releases a continuous dose of nicotine throughout the day, and requires administration only once daily. Disadvantages of the patch include a high incidence of skin irritation associated with the patch adhesives and the inability to acutely adjust the dose of nicotine to alleviate symptoms of withdrawal. Finally, patients with underlying dermatologic conditions (e.g., psoriasis, eczema, atopic dermatitis) should not use the patch because they are more likely to experience skin irritation.[7]

CASE 91-1, QUESTION 3: T.B. would like to discontinue the nicotine transdermal patch. She would like to purchase a nonprescription smoking-cessation medication and wants to know whether the gum or lozenge is an effective alternative. What options would you recommend? What factors should be considered?

Nicotine Gum

Nicotine polacrilex gum is a resin complex of nicotine and polacrilin in a chewing gum base that provides slow release and absorption of nicotine across the oral mucosa. The product is available in 2- and 4-mg strengths, and in multiple flavors. The gum has a distinct, tobacco-like, slightly peppery, minty, or fruity taste and contains buffering agents to increase the salivary pH, which enhances the buccal absorption of nicotine. The amount of nicotine absorbed from each piece is variable, but when used properly, approximately 1.6 and 2.2 mg of nicotine is absorbed from each 2- and 4-mg piece of gum, respectively.[14] Peak plasma concentrations of nicotine are achieved approximately 30 minutes after chewing a single piece of gum and then slowly decline thereafter (Fig. 91-3). Patients using nicotine gum are significantly more likely to remain abstinent compared with those receiving placebo.[7,35]

DOSING

Table 91-4 outlines the manufacturers' recommended dosing schedule for the nicotine gum. The recommended dosage of the nicotine gum is based on the "time to first cigarette" (TTFC) of the day. Having a strong desire or need to smoke soon after waking is viewed as a key indicator of nicotine dependence.[48] Therefore, patients who smoke their first cigarette of the day within 30 minutes of waking are likely to be more highly dependent on nicotine and require higher dosages than those who delay smoking for more than 30 minutes after waking (Table 91-4). The "chew and park" method (Table 91-4) allows for the slow, consistent release of nicotine. Patients can use additional pieces of gum (to the daily maximum of 24 pieces/day) if cravings occur between scheduled doses. In general, patients who smoke a greater number of cigarettes/day will require more nicotine gum to alleviate their cravings than will patients who smoke fewer cigarettes/day. It is preferable to use the gum on a fixed schedule of administration, tapering during 1 to 3 months rather than using it only as needed to control cravings.[7]

PATIENT EDUCATION

Proper chewing technique is crucial when using the nicotine gum, using the "chew and park" method (Table 91-4). The chew and park steps should be repeated until most of the nicotine is extracted; this generally occurs after 30 minutes and becomes obvious when chewing no longer elicits the characteristic taste or tingling sensation.

Patients should be warned that the absorption and therefore the effectiveness of nicotine gum might be reduced by acidic beverages (e.g., coffee, juices, wine, soft drinks),[49] which transiently reduce the salivary pH. To prevent this interaction, patients should be advised not to eat or drink (except water) for 15 minutes before or while using the nicotine gum.

ADVERSE REACTIONS

Most of the common side effects (Table 91-4) can be minimized or prevented by using proper chewing technique.[7] Patients should be warned that chewing the gum too rapidly may result in excessive release of nicotine, leading to lightheadedness, nausea, vomiting, irritation of the throat and mouth, hiccups, and indigestion.

PRODUCT SELECTION CONSIDERATIONS

Advantages of nicotine gum include the fact that this formulation may be used to satisfy oral cravings and the 4-mg strength might delay weight gain.[7] For these reasons, the gum may be particularly beneficial for patients who have weight-gain concerns or for patients who report boredom as a trigger for smoking. The gum might also be advantageous for patients who desire flexibility in dosing and prefer the ability to self-regulate nicotine levels to manage withdrawal symptoms. Some patients may find that the viscous consistency of the gum makes it difficult to use because it sticks to dental work. Others may find it difficult or socially unacceptable to chew the gum so frequently. Nicotine gum should not be used by patients with temporomandibular joint (TMJ) conditions.

Nicotine Lozenge

The nicotine polacrilex lozenge is a resin complex of nicotine and polacrilin in a sugar-free, flavored lozenge. The product is available in 2- and 4-mg strengths, which are meant to be consumed like hard candy or other medicinal lozenges (e.g., sucked and moved from side to side in the mouth until fully dissolved). A mini-lozenge is also available. Because the nicotine lozenge dissolves completely, it delivers approximately 25% more nicotine than does an equivalent dose of nicotine gum.[35] Like the nicotine gum, the lozenge also contains buffering agents (sodium carbonate and potassium bicarbonate) to increase salivary pH, thereby enhancing buccal absorption of the nicotine. Peak nicotine concentrations of nicotine with the lozenge are achieved after 30 to 60 minutes of use and then slowly decline thereafter (Fig. 91-3). The nicotine lozenge approximately doubles 6-month abstinence rates compared with placebo.[35]

DOSING

Table 91-4 outlines the manufacturers' recommended dosing schedule for the nicotine lozenge. Like the nicotine gum, the lozenge is dosed based on the TTFC. Patients are more likely to succeed if they use the lozenge on a fixed schedule rather than as needed. Patients can use additional lozenges (up to 5 lozenges in 6 hours or a maximum of 20 lozenges/day) if cravings occur between scheduled doses.

PATIENT EDUCATION

Similar to the gum, the nicotine lozenge is a specially formulated nicotine delivery system that must be used properly for optimal results. The lozenge should be allowed to dissolve slowly in the mouth; when nicotine is released, a warm, tingling sensation may be experienced. The patient should occasionally rotate the lozenge to different areas of the mouth to reduce the potential for mucosal irritation. When used correctly, the lozenge should completely dissolve within 30 minutes. Patients should be counseled not to chew or swallow the lozenge because this increases the incidence of gastrointestinal-related side effects.

As with the gum, patients should be cautioned that the effectiveness of the nicotine lozenge may be reduced by acidic beverages such as coffee, juices, wine, or soft drinks.[49] Patients should be advised not to eat or drink (except water) for 15 minutes before or while using the nicotine lozenge.

ADVERSE REACTIONS

In general, the nicotine lozenge is well tolerated. The most common side effects include nausea, hiccups, cough, dyspepsia, headache, and flatulence. Patients who use more than one lozenge at a time, continuously use one lozenge after another, or chew or swallow the lozenge are more likely to experience dyspepsia or hiccups.

PRODUCT SELECTION CONSIDERATIONS

The nicotine lozenge is similar to the nicotine gum formulation in that it may be used to satisfy oral cravings, the 4-mg strength might delay weight gain,[7,49] and patients can self-titrate therapy to acutely manage withdrawal symptoms. Because the lozenge does not require chewing, many patients find this to be a more discreet nicotine delivery system. The disadvantages of the lozenge are the fact that it requires frequent dosing, and the gastrointestinal side effects (nausea, hiccups, and heartburn) may be bothersome.

T.B. has expressed interest in either the nicotine gum or lozenge formulation for her quit attempt. Both agents are effective, and the choice of therapy is dependent on the patient's perceptions and expectations regarding treatment, including the ability to comply with the regimen, previous experience with cessation medications, and other concerns (e.g., adverse effects, weight gain, cost of medications). T.B. would be a candidate for either agent provided she is able to comply with the frequent dosing schedule (one lozenge or piece of gum every 1–2 hours while she is awake). T.B. smokes her first cigarette of the day immediately after waking in the morning and she smokes approximately 30 cigarettes/day; this smoking pattern suggests a higher degree of nicotine dependence, and therefore T.B. would benefit from a higher dose of NRT. T.B. should initiate treatment with the 4-mg strength of either the nicotine lozenge or nicotine gum dosed every 1 to 2 hours while she is awake and tapered according to the schedule outlined in Table 91-4.

Postcessation Weight Gain

Case 91-1, Question 4: T.B. is very concerned about gaining weight after she quits smoking. Is weight gain common after quitting, and if so, how can this be prevented?

Most tobacco users gain weight after quitting, and clinicians should neither deny the likelihood of weight gain nor minimize its significance.[7] For nearly all patients, the health risks associated with postcessation weight gain are negligible compared with the risks of continued smoking.

Most quitters gain fewer than 10 lb, but there is a broad range of weight gain reported, with up to 10% of quitters gaining as much as 30 lb.[7] In general, women tend to gain more weight than men. In a study of nearly 6,000 smokers who were followed for 5 years after quitting, the average weight gain during the follow-up period was 19.2 and 16.7 lb among women and men, respectively.[50]

The weight-suppressing effects of tobacco are well known. However, the mechanisms to explain why most successful quitters gain weight are not completely understood. Smokers have been found to have an approximately 10% higher metabolic rate compared with nonsmokers.[51] Increased postcessation caloric intake might result from an increase in appetite, improved sense of taste, or a change in the hand-to-mouth ritual through the substitution of tobacco with food.

In general, a patient is less likely to be successful if he or she attempts to change multiple behaviors at once. For most patients, strict dieting to prevent weight gain, especially during the early stages of quitting, is generally not recommended.[7] T.B. should be counseled that the average weight gain of fewer than 10 lb is less detrimental to her overall health than is continued smoking. Although exercise interventions have not been shown to reduce weight gain among quitters,[52] it should not be ruled out as a recommendation for T.B. because she expresses significant concern about weight gain, and this might be a barrier to her quitting. Modest increases in activity can help with weight gain and exercise can serve as a behavioral substitution for tobacco use. Furthermore, T.B. should be advised to plan her meals in advance to avoid binge eating, increase her water intake to create a feeling of fullness, chew sugarless gum, and limit alcohol consumption. T.B. may consider pharmacotherapy options that have been shown to delay weight gain including NRT, varenicline, or sustained-release bupropion.[7,52] It is important to note, however, that none of the medications have been shown to prevent weight gain in the long term.[7,52]

Relapse Back to Smoking

Case 91-1, Question 5: During a follow-up contact, the clinician learns that T.B. smoked half a pack of cigarettes at a party over the weekend and has relapsed to her previous smoking levels after not having smoked for more than a month. How should the clinician respond?

The clinician should thank T.B. for being honest about her smoking and ask whether she is comfortable discussing the circumstances during which the smoking occurred. At the time of her smoking, where was she, who was she with, how did she get access to cigarettes, and how was she feeling at the time? What, specifically, were the triggers for her relapse (e.g., alcohol, depression, friends who were smoking around her)? It is important that the clinician help the patient to use this information as part of the learning process, but it also is important to focus on the "positive," such as T.B.'s ability to have remained tobacco free for more than 1 month. Four weeks after quitting, most physical effects of nicotine withdrawal have completely resolved, and thus, the relapse trigger for T.B. likely was psychological or situational and could be abated through application of effective coping techniques. After an informative discussion about the situation in which the smoking occurred, it is important that the clinician works with the patient in identifying strategies for avoiding relapse in the future (Table 91-3).

Smoking and Cardiovascular Disease

CASE 91-2

Question 1: P.J. is a 62-year-old man admitted for an elective coronary artery bypass graft (CABG) procedure. His medical history is significant for angina, hypertension, dyslipidemia, peripheral vascular disease (PVD), and allergic rhinitis. He underwent a bilateral carotid endarterectomy procedure 2 years ago and had iliac artery angioplasty with stent placement 5 years ago for PVD. P.J.'s social history is significant for tobacco use (2 PPD) and alcohol (3–4 drinks/day). He is approximately 10 lb overweight. His preoperative laboratory results are significant for a total cholesterol of 270 mg/dL (desirable, <200), low-density lipoprotein cholesterol (LDL-C) of 163 mg/dL (optimal, <70), high-density lipoprotein cholesterol (HDL-C) of 35 mg/dL (low, <40), and triglycerides of 350 mg/dL (normal, <150). His medications before admission include atenolol 50 mg daily, aspirin 81 mg daily, isosorbide dinitrate 20 mg TID, atorvastatin 20 mg daily, fluticasone nasal spray (50 mcg/spray) 1 spray/nostril daily, and nitroglycerin 0.4 mg sublingually as needed. Which of P.J.'s chronic medical conditions may be caused or exacerbated by his tobacco use?

A wealth of evidence suggests that cigarette smoking is a major cause of cardiovascular disease and is responsible for approximately 128,000 premature cardiovascular-related deaths each year.[3,5,53]

There are numerous plausible pathophysiologic mechanisms by which tobacco smoking contributes to the development of cardiovascular disease.[7] Oxidant gases and other compounds in tobacco smoke are believed to induce a hypercoagulable state characterized by increased platelet aggregation and thrombosis, which substantially increases the risk of myocardial infarction (MI) and sudden death.[53,54] The carbon monoxide in smoke reduces the amount of oxygen available to tissues and organs, including myocardial tissue, and may reduce the ventricular fibrillation threshold.[53] Smoking may accelerate atherosclerosis through effects on serum lipids; smokers tend to have higher levels of total cholesterol, LDL-C, and triglycerides and lower HDL-C than nonsmokers.[3] Smoking increases the levels of inflammatory mediators (C-reactive protein, leukocytes, and fibrinogen), which might contribute to the development and progression of atherosclerosis.[55] Finally, smoking stimulates the release of neurotransmitters (e.g., epinephrine, norepinephrine) that increase myocardial workload and induce coronary vasoconstriction, leading to ischemia, arrhythmias, and sudden death.[3,53]

P.J.'s hospital admission for a CABG procedure for coronary heart disease and angina, and previous procedures for peripheral vascular disease (angioplasty with stent placement) and cerebrovascular disease (bilateral carotid endarterectomy) are all conditions associated with chronic tobacco use. His elevated total cholesterol, LDL-C, and triglycerides, and reduced HDL-C levels are consistent with smoking-induced dyslipidemia. Cigarette smoking in combination with P.J.'s other established cardiovascular risk factors (hypertension, dyslipidemia) has synergistically increased his risk for serious cardiovascular disease.[3,53] Fortunately, the effects of smoking on lipids, coagulation, myocardial workload, and coronary blood flow appear to be reversible, and P.J.'s risk of developing further cardiovascular-related complications will markedly decrease if he is able to quit smoking.[25,56]

Smoking cessation is associated with a 36% reduction in the risk of death among patients with established coronary heart disease. The reduced mortality risk associated with quitting smoking is comparable to that observed with other established secondary preventative approaches such as therapies for hyperlipidemia and hypertension.[57] The clinician should approach this hospitalization as an opportunity to assist P.J. with quitting smoking.[7] Furthermore, published data suggest that initiation of intensive cessation counseling interventions for hospitalized patients is effective in achieving long-term abstinence.[58]

Noncigarette Forms of Tobacco

CASE 91-2, QUESTION 2: The cardiothoracic surgeon has strongly advised P.J. to quit smoking. P.J. would like to know whether cutting down to one to two cigars a day is an acceptable alternative to his current one to two packs of cigarettes/day.

The adverse health effects of cigar smoking have been well described and include an increased risk of cancer of the lung, oral cavity, larynx, esophagus, and pancreas. In addition, cigar smokers who inhale deeply are at increased risk for developing cardiovascular disease and chronic obstructive pulmonary disease (COPD).[59,60] Cigarette smokers who switch to smoking only cigars decrease their risk of developing lung cancer, but their risk is markedly higher than if they were to quit smoking altogether.[60]

Cigar weight and nicotine content vary widely from brand to brand and from cigar to cigar. Most cigars range in weight from about 1 to 22 g, and a typical cigarette weighs less than 1 g. The nicotine content of 10 commercially available cigars studied in 1996 ranged from 10 to 444 mg. In comparison, US cigarettes have a relatively narrow total nicotine content range (mean, 13.5 ± 0.1 mg)/cigarette.[61] It is possible for one large cigar to contain as much tobacco as an entire pack of cigarettes and deliver enough nicotine to establish and maintain dependence.[62]

The amount of nicotine delivered by one to two cigars/day is capable of sustaining his dependence on nicotine. Furthermore, former cigarette smokers are more likely to inhale deeply, which further increases the risk of cancer and cardiovascular and pulmonary disease. The clinician should strongly advise P.J. to quit smoking cigarettes and that switching to cigars is not a safe alternative.

CASE 91-2, QUESTION 3: P.J. is willing to quit completely, but he is worried because he has tried to quit smoking "hundreds of times" and has never been able to quit for longer than 1 week. He expresses a desire for a medication to assist him during this quit attempt. He has tried the nicotine gum and transdermal patch during three previous quit attempts. He did not like the gum because it made his jaw sore. He had temporary success with the nicotine patch but found it to be less flexible than the gum. For example, when he needed extra nicotine during stressful situations, he could not apply a second patch. What treatment alternatives are reasonable for P.J.?

P.J. has inadequately responded to treatment with the transdermal patch and experienced intolerable jaw soreness with the nicotine gum. Newer formulations of the nicotine gum are less viscous, and therefore easier to chew, than earlier formulations of the gum; however, other options are available. First-line treatment options that he has not tried include the nicotine lozenge (see Case 91-1, Question 3), nicotine nasal spray, nicotine inhaler, sustained-release bupropion, varenicline, or an effective combination of first-line agents (see Case 91-3, Question 1).

Nicotine Nasal Spray

The nicotine nasal spray is an aqueous solution of nicotine available in a metered-spray pump for administration to the nasal mucosa. Each actuation delivers a metered 50-μL spray containing 0.5 mg of nicotine. Nicotine in the nasal spray is more rapidly absorbed than other NRT formulations (Fig. 91-3), with peak venous nicotine concentrations achieved within 11 to 18 minutes after administration.[14] Use of the nicotine nasal spray more than doubles long-term abstinence rates when compared with placebo).[7,35]

DOSING

Table 91-4 outlines the manufacturers' recommended dosing schedule for the nicotine nasal spray. A dose of nicotine (1 mg) is administered as two sprays, one (0.5-mg spray) in *each* nostril. For best results, patients should be encouraged to use at least eight doses/day during the initial 6 to 8 weeks of therapy because less frequent administration may be less effective. The initial regimen may be increased, as needed, to a maximum recommended dosage of five doses/hour or 40 mg/day. After 6 to 8 weeks, the dose should be gradually decreased during an additional 4 to 6 weeks.

PATIENT EDUCATION

Before using the nasal spray for the first time, the nicotine nasal spray pump must be primed. This is done by actuating the device into a tissue until a fine spray is visible (about 6–8 times). When administering a dose, the patient should tilt the head back slightly and insert the tip of the bottle into the nostril as far as is comfortable. After actuation of the pump, the patient should not sniff, swallow, or inhale through the nose because this increases the irritant effects of the spray. The spray increases the likelihood of tearing, coughing, and sneezing, so patients should wait 5 minutes before driving or operating heavy machinery.

ADVERSE REACTIONS

In clinical trials, 94% of patients report moderate–severe nasal irritation during the first 2 days of therapy; 81% of patients still reported mild to moderate nasal irritation after 3 weeks of therapy. Nasal congestion and transient changes in taste and smell have also been reported.[7] Despite the high incidence of local adverse effects (Table 91-4), most patients become tolerant to the irritant effects of the spray during the first week.[63]

PRODUCT SELECTION CONSIDERATIONS

The primary advantage in using the nicotine nasal spray is the ability to rapidly titrate therapy to manage withdrawal symptoms. However, because nicotine from the spray more rapidly penetrates the central nervous system, there may be a higher likelihood of developing dependence during treatment. The nicotine nasal spray has a dependence potential intermediate between tobacco products and other NRT products. Individuals with chronic nasal disorders (e.g., rhinitis, polyps, sinusitis) or severe reactive airway disease should not use the nicotine nasal spray because of its irritant effects. Exacerbation of asthma has been reported after use of the nicotine nasal spray.[64]

Nicotine Inhaler

The nicotine oral inhaler consists of a plastic mouthpiece and a disposable cartridge containing a porous plug containing 10 mg of nicotine and 1 mg of menthol. Menthol is added to reduce the irritant effect of nicotine.

Given that the usual pack-a-day smoker repeats the hand-to-mouth motion up to 200 times per, it is not surprising that many smokers find they miss the physical manipulation of the cigarette and associated behaviors that accompany smoking. The nicotine inhaler was designed to provide nicotine replacement in a manner similar to smoking while addressing the sensory and ritualistic factors that are important to many patients who smoke.[36]

As a patient inhales through the mouthpiece, nicotine vapor is released from the cartridge and is distributed throughout the oral cavity. When the inhaler is used correctly, approximately 4 mg of nicotine vapor is released from the cartridge and 2 mg is absorbed across the buccal mucosa.[65] Peak plasma nicotine concentrations with the inhaler are achieved after approximate 30 minutes of use[14] and then slowly decline thereafter (Fig. 91-3). Use of the nicotine inhaler approximately doubles long-term abstinence rates when compared with placebo (Table 91-4).[7,35]

DOSING

Table 91-4 outlines the manufacturers' recommended dosing schedule for the nicotine inhaler. During the initial 3 to 6 weeks of treatment, the patient should use 1 cartridge every 1 to 2 hours while awake. This should be increased, as needed, to a maximum of 16 cartridges/day. The manufacturer recommends that each cartridge be depleted of nicotine by frequent continuous puffing for 20 minutes. The recommended duration of treatment is 3 months, after which patients may be weaned from the inhaler by gradual reduction of the daily dose during the following 6 to 12 weeks.

PATIENT EDUCATION

To minimize the likelihood of throat irritation, patients should be instructed to inhale shallowly (as if puffing a pipe). When used correctly, 100 shallow puffs from the inhaler mouthpiece during 20 minutes approximate 10 puffs from one cigarette during 5 minutes.[36] The release of nicotine from the inhaler is temperature dependent and significantly reduced at temperatures less than 40°F.[7,36] In cold conditions, patients should store the inhaler and cartridges in a warm place (e.g., inside pocket).[7] Conversely, under warmer conditions, more nicotine is released/puff. However, nicotine plasma concentrations achieved using the inhaler in hot climates at maximal doses will not exceed levels normally achieved with smoking.[36]

As with all forms of NRT that are absorbed across the buccal mucosa, the effectiveness of the nicotine inhaler is reduced by acidic foods and beverages, such as coffee, juices, wine, or soft drinks. Therefore, patients should be instructed not to eat or drink anything (except water) for 15 minutes before or while using the inhaler.

ADVERSE REACTIONS

The most common side effects associated with the nicotine inhaler include mouth or throat irritation (40%) and cough (32%).[7] Most patients rated cough and mouth and throat irritation symptoms as mild, decreasing with continued use. Other less common side effects are rhinitis, dyspepsia, hiccups, and headache. Adverse reactions necessitating discontinuation of treatment occurred in less than 5% of patients using the inhaler.

PRODUCT SELECTION CONSIDERATIONS

Patients who express a preference for therapy that can be easily titrated to manage withdrawal symptoms or one that mimics the hand-to-mouth ritual of smoking may find the nicotine inhaler to be an appealing option. Patients with underlying bronchospastic conditions should use the nicotine inhaler with caution, because the nicotine vapor can be irritating and might induce bronchospasm.

Sustained-release Bupropion

Sustained-release bupropion increases long-term abstinence rates relative to placebo. (RR 1.62; Table 91-4).[7,43]

DOSING

Because approximately 1 week of treatment is necessary to achieve steady state blood levels, sustained-release bupropion should be initiated while the patient is still smoking (Table 91-4). Patients should set a target quit date that falls within the first 2 weeks of treatment, generally in the second week. The starting dose of sustained-release bupropion is one 150-mg tablet each morning for the first 3 days. If the initial dose is tolerated, the dosage should be increased on the fourth day to the recommended maximal dosage of 300 mg/day (150 mg BID). Therapy should be continued for 7 to 12 weeks after the quit date.

PATIENT EDUCATION

Patients experiencing insomnia should avoid taking the second dose close to bedtime. Patients should be informed that bupropion might cause dizziness or drowsiness, and should exercise caution when driving or operating machinery. Patients should avoid or drink alcohol only in moderation while taking bupropion as alcohol use can increase the risk of seizures. Abrupt cessation of alcohol use while taking bupropion might increase the risk of seizure. Patients should also be advised not to take Zyban[66] and Wellbutrin or generic bupropion formulations concomitantly to avoid dose-related adverse effects, including seizures.

ADVERSE REACTIONS

The most common adverse effects associated with bupropion therapy include insomnia (35%–40%) and dry mouth (10%)[8]; these usually lessen with continued use. Taking the second daily dose in the early evening, but no sooner than 8 hours after the first dose, might reduce insomnia. Less common side effects include headache, nausea, tremors, and rash. Seizures are a dose-related toxicity associated with bupropion therapy. For this reason, bupropion is contraindicated in patients with underlying seizure disorders and those receiving concurrent therapy with other forms of bupropion (Wellbutrin, Wellbutrin SR, and Wellbutrin XL). Bupropion also is contraindicated in patients with anorexia or bulimia nervosa, patients undergoing abrupt discontinuation of alcohol or sedatives (including benzodiazepines), and patients currently taking monoamine oxidase inhibitors owing to the increased potential for seizures in these populations.[67] In clinical trials for smoking cessation, seizure frequency with sustained-release bupropion was less than 0.1% (seven seizures among 8,000 bupropion-treated patients), which is comparable to the reported incidence of seizures (0.1%) with the sustained-release formulation when used for the treatment of depression.[68] For this reason, bupropion should be used with extreme caution in patients with a history of seizures or cranial trauma, in individuals taking medications that may lower the seizure threshold, and in patients with underlying severe hepatic cirrhosis. The manufacturer recommends that patients space the doses at least 8 hours apart and limit the total daily dose to no more than 300 mg. Although a boxed warning has been removed, clinicians should monitor patients for serious psychiatric symptoms while taking bupropion.

PRODUCT SELECTION CONSIDERATIONS

Sustained-release bupropion may be the drug of choice for patients who prefer to take oral medications (an alternative oral option is varenicline, described below). Because sustained-release bupropion tablets require twice daily administration, this agent may be preferable for patients with adherence concerns (e.g., those unable to consistently use short-acting NRT formulations that require multiple daily doses). Sustained-release bupropion might be beneficial for use in patients with coexisting depression or in individuals with a history of depressive symptoms during a previous quit attempt. Finally, sustained-release bupropion has been found to reduce postcessation weight gain during treatment,[7,52] and this might be of short-term benefit in selected patients with concerns about weight gain after quitting. Disadvantages of sustained-release bupropion include a high prevalence of insomnia and several contraindications and precautions mentioned above.

Varenicline

Data from meta-analyses indicate that varenicline significantly increases long-term abstinence rates relative to placebo,[7,46] NRT,[46] and sustained-release bupropion.[7,46] The pooled risk ratio for long-term abstinence (≥6 months) for varenicline compared with placebo was 2.24 (95% CI, 2.06-2.43). The pooled risk ratio for varenicline versus sustained-release bupropion at 1-year follow-up was 1.39 (95% CI, 1.25 -1.54). At 24 weeks, the pooled risk ratio for varenicline compared to NRT was 1.25 (95% CI, 1.14 -1.37).[46] Lower doses and longer durations of varenicline have been shown to be safe and effective in clinical trials.[46]

PHARMACOKINETICS

Varenicline absorption is virtually complete after oral administration, and oral bioavailability is unaffected by food. Once absorbed, varenicline undergoes minimal metabolism, with 92% excreted unchanged in the urine. Renal elimination is primarily through glomerular filtration, along with active tubular secretion.[69] The half-life is approximately 24 hours, and following administration of multiple oral doses, steady state conditions are reached within 4 days.[69]

DOSING

Treatment with varenicline (Table 91-4) should be initiated 1 week before the patient stops smoking. This dosing regimen allows for gradual titration of the dose to minimize treatment-related nausea and insomnia. The recommended dosage titration for varenicline is as follows: 0.5 mg daily days 1 to 3, 0.5 mg twice daily days 4 to 7, and 1 mg twice daily weeks 2 to 12. For patients who have successfully quit smoking at the end of 12 weeks, an additional course of 12 weeks may be considered to increase the likelihood of long-term abstinence. An alternative approach is to set a quit date 8 to 35 days after starting varenicline. Patients should be advised to decrease their smoking over the first 12 weeks and then continue varenicline for 12 additional weeks.[69] Varenicline should be used with caution in patients with impaired renal function. For patients with severe renal dysfunction (estimated creatinine clearance <30 mL/minute), the recommended maximal dose of varenicline is 0.5 mg twice daily. In patients with end-stage renal disease undergoing hemodialysis, a maximal dose of 0.5 mg daily is recommended.[69]

PATIENT EDUCATION

The tablets are to be taken after eating and with 8 ounces of water. Nausea and insomnia are side effects that are usually temporary. Patients should be advised to discontinue varenicline and contact their healthcare provider immediately if they experience agitation, hostility, depressed mood, or changes in behavior or thinking that are not typical for them (see adverse reactions below).

ADVERSE REACTIONS

Varenicline is generally well tolerated. Common side effects (≥5% and twice the rate observed in placebo-treated patients) include nausea (30%), sleep disturbance (insomnia 18%; abnormal dreams 13%), constipation (8%), flatulence (6%), and vomiting (5%). Nausea is dose dependent and generally described as mild or moderate and often transient; however, for some patients, it persists for several months. Initial dose titration was beneficial in reducing the occurrence of nausea. Approximately 3% of subjects receiving varenicline 1 mg BID discontinued treatment prematurely because of nausea. For patients with intolerable nausea, dose reduction should be considered.[69]

The FDA recommends that (a) patients tell their healthcare providers about any history of psychiatric illness before starting varenicline, and (b) clinicians and patients monitor for changes in mood and behavior during treatment with varenicline.[69] A large, randomized, controlled trial that included a cohort of smokers with current or past psychiatric disorders evaluated the neuropsychiatric safety of varenicline, bupropion, nicotine patch, and placebo. No difference in neuropsychiatric adverse events was reported between groups.[70] Additionally, a review of published cases and clinical trials using varenicline in patients with schizophrenia and schizoaffective disorder concluded that psychiatric symptoms were not worsened significantly in stable, carefully monitored patients with these conditions.[71] The prescribing information for varenicline was revised to include warning for a possible increased risk of cardiovascular events (MI, ischemic and hemorrhagic stroke) in patients with stable cardiovascular disease.[69] However, a published meta-analyses examining the risk concluded that there is no significant increase in the risk of serious cardiovascular events with varenicline in tobacco cessation.[72] Seizures have been reported in patients treated with varenicline, most often within the first month of therapy. These events occurred in individuals who had no seizure history, as well as in those with a remote history or well-controlled seizure disorder.[69]

PRODUCT SELECTION CONSIDERATIONS

Varenicline is a first-line agent for the treatment of tobacco use and dependence.[7,23] It offers a convenient oral dosing regimen and a new mechanism of action that might be particularly appealing for patients who have failed quit attempts with other first-line agents (e.g., NRT or sustained-release bupropion). Given its potential for inducing negative neuropsychiatric effects, varenicline should be used with extreme caution in patients with a current or past history of psychiatric illness.

P.J. has tried the nicotine gum and transdermal patch during previous quit attempts. Because he was intolerant to the nicotine gum (sore jaw), this form of NRT is not appropriate. P.J.'s experience with the transdermal patch suggests he may benefit from a short-acting NRT formulation that enables active administration and titration of drug as needed to alleviate symptoms of withdrawal and situational cravings. Other first-line therapies include the nicotine nasal spray, inhaler, and lozenge; sustained-release bupropion; or varenicline. P.J. should not use the nicotine nasal spray because he has allergic rhinitis and may be more susceptible to the irritant effects of the spray. In addition, some data suggest that the bioavailability of nicotine is reduced in patients with rhinitis.[63] Furthermore, the safety and efficacy of the nasal spray in patients with chronic nasal disorders have not been adequately studied. Reasonable choices for P.J. therefore include sustained-release bupropion, nicotine lozenge, nicotine inhaler, or varenicline. Any of these options are reasonable, and the choice of therapy should be dictated by P.J.'s individual preference. If varenicline is chosen, given P.J. has underlying cardiovascular disease, he should be instructed to notify a healthcare provider for new or worsening cardiovascular symptoms and to seek immediate medical attention if he experiences signs and symptoms of myocardial infarction. Finally, it is reasonable to consider combination therapy (see Case 91-3, Question 1).

Safety of Nicotine Replacement Therapy Among Patients with Cardiovascular Disease

CASE 91-2, QUESTION 4: P.J. would like to try the nicotine inhaler. Is NRT safe for use in patients with cardiovascular disease?

Nicotine activates the sympathetic nervous system, leading to an increase in heart rate, blood pressure, and myocardial contractility. Nicotine also may cause coronary artery vasoconstriction.[74] These known hemodynamic effects of nicotine have led to doubts about the safety of using NRT in patients with established cardiovascular disease, particularly those with serious arrhythmias, unstable angina, or recent MI.

Soon after the nicotine patch was approved, anecdotal case reports in the lay press linked NRT (patch and gum) with adverse cardiovascular events (i.e., arrhythmias, MI, stroke). Since then, several randomized, controlled trials have evaluated the safety of NRT in patients with cardiovascular disease.[75–77] The results of these trials suggest no significant increase in the incidence of cardiovascular events or mortality among patients receiving the nicotine patch when compared with placebo. However, because these trials specifically excluded patients with unstable angina, serious arrhythmias, and recent MI, the manufacturers of NRT products recommend that these agents be used with caution among patients in the immediate (within 2 weeks) post-MI period, those with serious arrhythmias, and those with unstable angina.[7]

Although two small, retrospective studies have raised questions regarding the safety of NRT use in intensive care settings,[77,78] NRT use in patients with cardiovascular disease has been the subject of numerous reviews, and it is widely believed by experts in the field that the risks of NRT in this patient population are small in relation to the risks of continued tobacco use.[2,53,72,74,75] The 2008 Clinical Practice Guideline concludes that there is no evidence of increased cardiovascular risk with these medications.[7] Although the use of NRT may pose some theoretic risk in a patient like P.J., cigarette smoking is far more hazardous to his health. Cigarettes, unlike NRT, deliver numerous toxins that induce a hypercoagulable state, reduce the oxygen-carrying capacity of hemoglobin, and adversely affect serum lipids. The amount of nicotine that P.J. would receive using the recommended dose of any NRT product will not exceed the amount he previously obtained from his 2 PPD smoking habit. The clinician should strongly encourage pharmacotherapy during P.J.'s current quit attempt. P.J. is 10 lb overweight; the additional risk imposed by a modest weight gain after smoking cessation likely will not be of clinical significance compared with that of continued smoking.

Combination Therapy for Tobacco Dependence

CASE 91-3

QUESTION 1: J.B. is a 60-year-old man referred to the pulmonary clinic for further evaluation and management of his chronic obstructive pulmonary disease (COPD). He complains of decreased exercise tolerance and has noted increasing shortness of breath (SOB) with minimal exertion (e.g., while golfing or climbing stairs). He currently uses an albuterol inhaler (90 mcg/puff), 2 puffs every 4 hours regularly for SOB. His medical history is otherwise unremarkable except for osteoarthritis controlled with acetaminophen 1 g TID. He has smoked approximately 1.5 to 2 PPD for more than 40 years. J.B. indicates he has made several quit attempts during the past year. On the first attempt (quitting "cold turkey"), J.B. relapsed within 2 days. J.B. successfully quit for nearly 2 weeks on his second attempt (using the 4-mg nicotine lozenge), but he found it difficult to adhere to the frequent dosing schedule and relapsed shortly after discontinuing the lozenge. His most recent quit attempt was 6 months ago using varenicline. After 1 month of abstinence, J.B. self-terminated varenicline (I thought I didn't need it anymore) and relapsed within 1 week. On further questioning, J.B. states that he did not enroll in a behavioral counseling program or seek additional assistance (other than pharmacotherapy) during any of his quit attempts. He expresses an interest in smoking cessation but is discouraged by his prior lack of success. On physical examination, coarse breath sounds that clear after coughing are noted. A chest radiograph obtained in the office shows no infiltrates. J.B. is concerned about his worsening pulmonary function and is committed to making another effort to quit. What treatment options are appropriate for J.B.?

Tobacco smoking is the single most important risk factor for the development of COPD,[3] and nearly all patients diagnosed with COPD are current or former smokers.[79] Given his escalating pulmonary symptoms, it is imperative that he stop smoking as soon as possible. J.B. should be advised that medications for COPD offer only limited symptomatic relief, and the most important component of his treatment is smoking cessation.[79,80] The clinician should commend J.B. for his interest in quitting and help him devise a patient-specific treatment plan.

Plasma levels of nicotine achieved with standard doses of NRT are generally much lower than those attained with regular smoking.[63,81] As such, conventionally dosed NRT may deliver subtherapeutic nicotine levels for some individuals, and in particular, for moderate-to-heavy smokers.

Combination NRT regimens, which typically consist of a long-acting agent (nicotine patch) in combination with a short-acting formulation (i.e., gum, lozenge, inhaler, or nasal spray), are often used as initial therapy. The long-acting formulation, which delivers nicotine at a relatively constant level, is used to prevent the onset of severe withdrawal symptoms, and the short-acting formulation, which delivers nicotine at a more rapid rate, is used as needed to control withdrawal symptoms that may occur during potential relapse situations (e.g., after meals, during times of stress, when around other smokers).

Controlled trials suggest that the nicotine patch in combination with short-acting NRT formulations (i.e., gum, lozenge, nasal spray, or inhaler) significantly increase quit rates relative to placebo. Similar results have been observed in trials using combination therapy with sustained-release bupropion and the nicotine patch. Aggressive combination regimens including triple-agent NRT (e.g., patch, inhaler, and nasal spray) with or without sustained-release bupropion, triple-combination therapy (e.g., patch, inhaler, and sustained-release bupropion)[82] may be a safe and effective treatment approach. Some data suggest that adding varenicline alone[83] or sustained-release bupropion and varenicline to nicotine patch,[84,85] therapy may improve cessation rates; however, addition of bupropion sustained-release to varenicline had little effect on long-term abstinence and increased rates of depression and anxiety.[85]

Clinicians should be aware that although the combination of the nicotine patch and sustained-release bupropion has been approved by the FDA, the concurrent use of multiple NRT products is not FDA-approved for tobacco cessation. Furthermore, the optimal agents, dosages, and durations of therapy for NRT combination therapy are currently unknown.

Given the severity of J.B.'s condition and his willingness to quit now, the clinician should initiate treatment as soon as possible. His treatment should consist of pharmacotherapy in conjunction with behavioral counseling and appropriate follow-up.

The clinician should work with J.B. to select the most appropriate pharmacotherapy. As noted previously, appropriate options would include the various NRT formulations, sustained-release bupropion, varenicline, or an effective combination of first-line agents. For patients reporting a positive experience with a given medication, retreatment with the same agent or a combination of agents might be appropriate, with consideration given to increasing the dose, frequency, or duration of therapy. For patients reporting a negative experience with pharmacotherapy (e.g., poor adherence, side effects, palatability issues, cost), an alternative agent should be considered. Given J.B.'s previous adherence issues with the nicotine lozenge as monotherapy, it might be preferable to use a long-acting cessation medication such as the nicotine patch, sustained-release bupropion, or varenicline. Combination therapy might also be appropriate.

BEHAVIORAL COUNSELING

Although medications are effective alone in helping patients quit smoking, the combination with pharmacotherapy maximizes patients' chances for a long-term, successful quit attempt. J.B.'s previous 1-month-long quit attempt highlights the success of varenicline in this patient; however, J.B.'s relapse likely is attributable to a shortened course of therapy and the absence of a behavioral change program. J.B. should be advised that the medications are designed to make patients more comfortable while quitting and that behavioral counseling is needed to address the "habit" of smoking by helping him cope with difficult situations and triggers for relapse. J.B. should be advised to JB should be advised to pursue behavioral therapy options in addition to pharmacotherapy. J.B. should be reminded that adherence with the medication regimen—daily adherence, as well as duration of therapy—will increase his chances of quitting for good. Clinician-delivered counseling might also include a personalized message to further enhance his motivation to quit. For example, the clinician could perform pulmonary function testing and translate J.B.'s spirometry results into an effective "lung age" (e.g., the age of the average healthy individual with similar spirometry values). This educational approach has been found to significantly increase long-term (12-month) quit rates in a recent controlled trial.[86]

Drug Interactions with Smoking

CASE 91-4

Question 1: M.K. is a new patient requesting Ortho Cyclen (norgestimate/ethinyl estradiol). The new patient history form completed by M.K. reveals that she is 32 years old, weighs 65 kg, and is 70 inches tall. She takes no prescription medications but occasionally uses loratadine 10 mg as needed for allergies, and ibuprofen 400 mg as needed for dysmenorrhea. She has no significant medical history. Her father has hypertension and suffered an MI last year. Her mother has type 2 diabetes and dyslipidemia. Her social history is significant for tobacco use (1 PPD for 15 years), alcohol (1 glass of wine/night), and caffeine (3–4 cups of coffee daily). Are there any potential drug interactions with M.K.'s new prescription?

SMOKING AND COMBINED HORMONAL CONTRACEPTIVES

One of the most important precautions to consider with oral contraceptive use is the potential interaction between tobacco smoke and estrogens in combination hormonal contraceptives (see Chapter 47, Contraception). Estrogens are known to promote coagulation by altering clotting factor levels and increasing platelet aggregation. As described in Case 91-2, Question 1, substances present in tobacco smoke induce a hypercoagulable state, increasing the risk of acute cardiovascular events. Exposure to both factors (smoking and high levels of estrogen) greatly increases the risk of thromboembolic and thrombotic disorders. Considerable epidemiologic evidence indicates that cigarette smoking substantially increases the risk of adverse cardiovascular events, including stroke, MI, and thromboembolism in women who use oral combination hormonal contraceptive agents.[87,88] This risk is age-related, in that the absolute risk of death as a result of cardiovascular disease in oral contraceptive users who smoke is 3.3/100,000 women ages 15 to 34 years compared with 29.4/100,000 women ages 35 to 44 years. To put this in perspective, the corresponding risk of death as a result of cardiovascular disease in *nonsmoking* women who use oral contraceptives is much lower, with a death rate of 0.65/100,000 women ages 15 to 34 years and 6.21/100,000 women ages 35 to 44 years.[89] Because of the increased risk of adverse cardiovascular events, current guidelines[89] state that combination estrogen–progestin contraceptives should not be used in women who are older than 35 years of age and smoke, and progestin-only or nonhormonal contraceptives are recommended for use in this population. M.K. is 32 years of age, and despite smoking 20 cigarettes/day, oral contraceptive use is not contraindicated at this time. However, the clinician should strongly advise M.K. to quit smoking and assess her readiness to do so. M.K. should be informed that if she continues to smoke while using oral combined hormonal contraceptives, her risk of developing a blood clot, stroke, or heart attack will continue to increase with time.

ALTERNATIVE THERAPIES

Case 91-4, Question 2: M.K. asks whether e-cigarettes or vapes are effective for smoking cessation.

Some patients or clinicians may ask about the efficacy of electronic nicotine delivery systems (ENDS) in tobacco cessation. These devices seem to offer an attractive solution in that they may eliminate exposure to the toxic substances inhaled when tobacco is burned in cigarettes. Little data are available to support use of ENDS as a tobacco-cessation therapy. A systematic review concluded that ENDS may help smokers successfully stop smoking, although more robust data on the safety and efficacy of ENDS are needed.[90] Preliminary data suggest that adding ENDS use to cigarettes does not increase cessation.[91] Data are unclear on the safety of ENDS as a cessation method, although to date few adverse events have been reported.[90,91] M.K. should be advised that the efficacy of ENDS as cessation therapies is not well established, and use of these agents cannot be recommended at this time.

Although many herbal and homeopathic products are available to help people quit smoking, data that support their safety and efficacy are lacking. Furthermore, patients should be cautioned that herbal cigarettes are not safe alternatives because they result in the inhalation of other toxins present in smoke.

Case 91-4, Question 3: M.K. is not considering quitting smoking in the next 30 days. She cannot discontinue her oral contraceptives because she is sexually active and needs a reliable form of birth control. She wonders whether the new low-dose birth control pills or other formulations (e.g., patch, vaginal ring) are safer for smokers.

Combined oral contraceptives available in the United States contain estrogen in doses ranging from 20 to 50 mcg of ethinyl estradiol. Higher doses of ethinyl estradiol appear to have greater procoagulant effects.[92–94]

In 2001, the US Surgeon General stated that lower-dose oral contraceptives may be associated with a reduced risk for coronary heart disease (CHD) compared with higher-dose formulations. Despite this conclusion, the report cautioned that heavy smokers who use oral contraceptives still have a greatly elevated risk for CHD.[94]

Serum estrogen levels obtained with the vaginal ring are significantly lower than those achieved with either transdermal or oral combined contraceptive formulations, and data have not shown the patch or the ring to be safer options for women who smoke. Current guidelines apply the same precautions to all contraceptives containing estrogen.[89]

M.K.'s prescribed oral contraceptive agent (Ortho Tri-Cyclen) contains 35 mcg of ethinyl estradiol in combination with 0.25 mg norgestimate. Although some clinicians recommend the use of low-dose (20 mcg) estrogen preparations in smokers, the available evidence suggests that the prescribed regimen poses no additional risk in M.K. The clinician should inform M.K. that there are currently no studies demonstrating a reduced risk of adverse cardiovascular events in smokers using oral contraceptives containing low doses (e.g., 20 mcg) of estrogen or the newer transdermal and vaginal ring formulations.[95] In the absence of published data, only smoking cessation can be advocated to definitively reduce the risk of stroke, MI, and thromboembolism in women who use combined hormonal contraceptives.

BEHAVIORAL COUNSELING

Although M.K. is not considering quitting at this time, it is appropriate for the clinician to apply the 5 R's (Table 91-2) to promote motivation to quit. This counseling should be *relevant* to M.K.'s situation and should highlight the *risks* of continued tobacco use, such as her elevated risk for thromboembolic and thrombotic disorders (associated with continued use of oral contraceptives). M.K. should be asked to think about the *rewards* of quitting and any potential *roadblocks* to quitting. At subsequent encounters, the clinician should sensitively assess M.K.'s tobacco use status and motivation to quit, and offer assistance with quitting when M.K. is ready. If M.K. decides to quit, it would be important to reassess her caffeine intake because caffeine, which is metabolized via CYP450 1A, levels have been reported to increase by 56% in patients who quit smoking.[21]

Brief Interventions to Promote Tobacco Cessation

CASE 91-5

QUESTION 1: J.C. is a 52-year-old man with a history of asthma requesting a refill of his albuterol inhaler prescription. This is the third request for an albuterol inhaler (200 doses/inhaler) during the past 2 months. Before this period, his last refill was more than a year ago. J.C. reports that he has been using albuterol on most days of the week for coughing and SOB. He has no other medical conditions and takes no other medications. His social history is significant for tobacco use (smokes 1.5 PPD; he recently started smoking again after starting a new job where "everyone smokes"). J.C. previously quit smoking 20 years ago using the "cold turkey" approach (e.g., no medications or counseling), and although he was successful, he was miserable for weeks and he expresses reluctance to "go through this again" during a stressful job transition.

The clinician is running behind schedule and does not have the time to provide comprehensive smoking-cessation counseling during this patient encounter. What brief smoking-cessation interventions can the clinician provide to J.C. to assist him with quitting?

TELEPHONE QUITLINES

Clinicians should become aware of local, community-based resources for tobacco cessation, including telephone quitlines. When time or expertise does not afford provision of comprehensive tobacco-cessation counseling during a patient visit, clinicians are encouraged to apply a truncated 5 A's model, whereby they *ask* about tobacco use, *advise* tobacco users to quit, and *refer* patients who are ready to quit to a telephone quitline. Effective brief interventions can generally be accomplished in fewer than 3 minutes. Telephone services provide low-cost interventions that can reach patients who might otherwise have limited access to medical treatment because of geographic location or lack of insurance or financial resources. Data support the efficacy of quitline counseling in promoting abstinence.[30,32] The addition of medication to quitline counseling significantly improves abstinence rates compared with medication alone.[7] In addition, preliminary evidence suggests that quitlines are also effective for smokeless tobacco cessation.[96] The telephone number for the toll-free tobacco quitline is 1-800-QUIT NOW.

J.C.'s asthma is not well controlled (e.g., increased use of short-acting bronchodilator). The change in J.C.'s asthma control is temporally related to his recent job change and relapse to daily smoking. Exposure to tobacco smoke is a potent trigger for asthma exacerbations and an important cause of poor asthma control. Given that the clinician is unable to provide comprehensive smoking-cessation counseling at this time, a brief intervention is appropriate. The clinician should strongly advise J.C. to quit as a key component of his asthma management plan and refer him to a telephone quitline or to other resources that are available within the community (e.g., local individual or group counseling programs). The clinician should briefly explain that pharmacologic treatment combined with support should increase the likelihood of a successful quit attempt compared to his previous, "cold turkey" experience. clinician could address J.C.'s previous negative experience with quitting by educating on the benefits of medications in reducing nicotine withdrawal symptoms.

Smoking Among Individuals with Mental Illness

CASE 91-6

QUESTION 1: J.D. is a 42-year-old woman presenting to clinic for follow-up of her depression management. Nine months ago, she was started on venlafaxine XR 75 mg daily. At her 3-month follow-up visit, she was stable on venlafaxine XR 150 mg daily, and her depressive symptoms had improved. She also reported that she was sleeping much better. J.D. has no other significant past medical history, and she takes no other medications. Her social history is positive for current tobacco use (1 PPD for 25 years) and caffeine use (1–2 Diet Cokes a day). She does not drink alcohol. During the appointment, J.D. indicates that she would like to quit smoking because her depression is better, and she knows that her overall health will improve if she quits. She also states that the last time she attempted to quit (several years ago, using the nicotine gum), she felt "down and had difficulty concentrating and couldn't sleep." She is now fearful that her depression will return if she quits. Is smoking cessation appropriate for J.D. at this time, and what are her treatment options?

Although persons with mental illness constitute 20% of the US population, nearly 36% smoke cigarettes.[9] In the past, the mental health community has not addressed smoking cessation with their patients, but increasing evidence suggests that quitting is possible and should be promoted. For patients with mental illness to achieve wellness, smoking-cessation intervention is an essential component of the overall care plan.[97]

Given that J.D. is currently willing to quit, and her depression has been stabilized for more than 4 months, it is appropriate for the clinician to discuss a quitting plan with J.D. and initiate therapy. The therapeutic approach should include counseling and pharmacotherapy, with ongoing monitoring of progress toward quitting and depressive symptoms.

TREATMENT SELECTION

Pharmacotherapy

Because no contraindications are present, any of the FDA-approved medications for cessation are appropriate. Although data are mixed on efficacy of varenicline in patients with psychiatric illness,[98] varenicline seems to be safe. In a pooled analysis of patients without psychiatric disorders, only sleep disorders and disturbances exhibited a higher incidence in patients treated with varenicline.[98]

Regardless of whether sustained-release bupropion, varenicline, or NRT product(s) are selected, the clinician should monitor J.D. closely to assess incidence of depressive symptomatology. If sustained-release bupropion or varenicline is selected, J.D. should be advised to stop taking the medication and contact the clinician immediately if she experiences agitation, depressed mood, and any changes in behavior that are not typical of nicotine withdrawal, or if she experiences suicidal thoughts or behavior.

BEHAVIORAL COUNSELING

Because J.D. has indicated that she is ready to quit, the clinician should commend her for making the important decision that will positively impact her overall health. J.D. should be advised that quitting is a process, and it will be important for them to work closely together to address the physiologic as well as psychological aspects of quitting during the upcoming months.

CASE 91-6, QUESTION 2: After discussing the various treatment options with the clinician, J.D. decides that she would like to add sustained-release bupropion to her regimen because the nicotine gum by itself did not help her much last time. She also thinks that the combination of venlafaxine with bupropion might help to "keep her depression more stable" whereas she is quitting. She confides in the clinician that her biggest fear is the ability to avoid smoking when she is stressed because of her job. She is a survey researcher and must meet client-induced deadlines. How can J.D. cope with stressful situations?

A variety of coping mechanisms can be applied to alleviate the need to smoke during stressful situations or when exposed to other triggers for smoking (Table 91-3). The clinician should encourage J.D. to think about strategies that would be effective for her in these situations, such as deep breathing or calling a supportive friend. Additionally, the clinician should consider suggesting use of a short-acting NRT product (e.g., nicotine gum, lozenge, inhaler, or nasal spray) as needed to alleviate situational cravings to smoke. Appropriate dosing of sustained-release bupropion should be reviewed (Table 91-4). A follow-up appointment should be scheduled for approximately 3 months after the quit date, and the patient should be advised to contact the clinician if she encounters any difficulties before then.

CASE 91-6, QUESTION 3: Four weeks later, J.D. calls and reports that she has a dry mouth, is having difficulty sleeping, and feels jittery and anxious. She also is currently using nicotine gum (2 mg), approximately four pieces daily. How should J.D. be managed?

As noted above, insomnia and dry mouth are commonly associated with sustained-release bupropion therapy and usually lessen with continued use.[67] The nicotine gum dose is low and not likely contributing to this condition. To address insomnia, J.D. can be advised to take the second dose of the day earlier, but not less than 8 hours after the first dose of the day. Alternatively, the clinician could consider reducing the daily dose to 150 mg in the morning and omitting the evening dose. Although the manufacturer recommends 300 mg/day, the 150-mg dose has been shown to have comparable outcomes with those of the 300-mg dose and is better tolerated.[99, 100] The clinician also should assess J.D.'s caffeine consumption patterns and, if appropriate, suggest that she reduce her caffeine intake by 50% and not drink caffeinated beverages after 12 noon so her system is clear of its stimulatory properties before sleep.[22]

Extended-Use Medications for Cessation

CASE 91-6, QUESTION 4: J.D. returns to the clinician's office 3 months later and indicates that she is doing well but had a few "slips" and smoked four times. She has not felt depressed and has been handling her stress at work through deep-breathing exercises. She uses the nicotine gum a few times a week and does not feel ready to discontinue the sustained-release bupropion. She wonders whether it is possible to continue the therapy for a bit longer, until she feels more stable as a nonsmoker.

Extended-duration medication therapy appears to be safe and effective. Long-term follow-up data indicate that approximately 15% of long-term quitters continued nicotine gum therapy with no serious side effects.[101] The 2008 Clinical Practice Guideline states that extended use of medications might be beneficial in individuals who report persistent withdrawal symptoms during treatment, those who have relapsed shortly after medication discontinuation, or those who are interested in long-term therapy.[7]

Clinicians should be aware that although many of the medications (sustained-release bupropion, varenicline, nicotine nasal spray, and inhaler) are approved by the FDA for long-term (6-month) use, the effectiveness of additional weeks on therapy is not well established. A meta-analysis of eight trials found that extended treatment with varenicline might prevent relapse, extended treatment with bupropion is unlikely to have a clinically important effect, and studies of extended treatment with nicotine replacement are needed.[102] Given J.D.'s current depression and because she is interested in continuing therapy, it is reasonable for the clinician to recommend continuation of therapy for an additional 12 weeks and reassess progress at that time. If JD does decide to discontinue her bupropion, then it should be with close monitoring by her mental health professional to assess for any rebound depressive symptoms.

KEY REFERENCES AND WEBSITES

A full list of references for this chapter can be found at http://thepoint.lww.com/AT11e. Below are the key references and websites for this chapter, with the corresponding reference number in this chapter found in parentheses after the reference.

Key References

Benowitz NL. Nicotine addiction. *N Engl J Med.* 2010;362(24):2295. (19)

Benowitz NL et al. Nicotine chemistry, metabolism, kinetics and biomarkers. *Handb Exp Pharmacol.* 2009;(192):29. (22)

Cahill K, Lindson-Hawley N, Thomas KH, Fanshawe TR, Lancaster T. Nicotine receptor partial agonists for smoking cessation. *Cochrane Database of Sys Rev*. 2016(5):CD006103. (46)

Fiore MC et al. *Treating Tobacco Use and Dependence: 2008 Update. Clinical Practice Guideline*. Rockville, MD: Public Health Service, U.S. Department of Health and Human Services; 2008. (7)

Hughes JR et al. Antidepressants for smoking cessation. *Cochrane Database Syst Rev*. 2014;(1):CD000031. doi:10.1002/14651858.CD000031.pub4. (43)

Kroon LA. Drug interactions with smoking. *Am J Health Syst Pharm*. 2007;64(18):1917. (22)

Hartmann-Boyce J, McRobbie H, Bullen C, Begh R, Stead LF, Hajek P. Electronic cigarettes for smoking cessation. *Cochrane Database of Sys Rev*. 2016(9):CD010216. (90).

National Center for Chronic Disease Prevention and Health Promotion, Office on Smoking and Health. *The Health Consequences of Involuntary Exposure to Tobacco Smoke: A Report of the Surgeon General*. Atlanta, GA: Office on Smoking and Health, National Center for Chronic Disease Prevention and Health Promotion, Centers for Disease Control and Prevention, U.S. Department of Health and Human Services; 2006. (6)

National Center for Chronic Disease Prevention and Health Promotion, Office on Smoking and Health. *The Health Consequences of Smoking—50 Years of Progress: A Report of the Surgeon General*. Atlanta, GA: Office on Smoking and Health, National Center for Chronic Disease Prevention and Health Promotion, Centers for Disease Control and Prevention, U.S. Department of Health and Human Services; 2014.(3)

Stead LF et al. Nicotine replacement therapy for smoking cessation. *Cochrane Database Syst Rev*. 2012;(11):CD000146. doi:10.1002/14651858.CD000146.pub4. (35)

Key Websites

Rx for Change: Clinician-Assisted Tobacco Cessation. San Francisco, CA: The Regents of the University of California; 1999–2017. http://rxforchange.ucsf.edu/. (23)

92 Anemias

Cindy L. O'Bryant, Ashley E. Glode, and Lisa A. Thompson

CORE PRINCIPLES

		CHAPTER CASES
1	Anemias arise from multiple etiologies. A full laboratory evaluation is necessary to appropriately diagnose and determine the cause of anemia.	**Case 92-1 (Questions 1, 2), Case 92-2 (Question 1), Case 92-5 (Question 2), Figure 92-1, Table 92-2 and 92-3**
2	Iron deficiency is the most common nutritional deficiency worldwide and is associated with symptoms of pallor, cardiovascular, respiratory, cognitive complications, and decreased quality of life.	**Case 92-1 (Question 2)**
3	Oral or parenteral iron is used to treat iron deficiency anemia. The goal of therapy is an increased hemoglobin of 1 to 2 g/dL within 2 to 4 weeks of the initiation of therapy.	**Case 92-1 (Questions 1, 3-5, 7–9), Table 92-6 and 92-8**
4	Distinguishing between vitamin B_{12}-deficient and folic acid-deficient megaloblastic anemia is important to minimize potentially permanent effects of these deficiencies.	**Case 92-2 (Questions 1, 2), Case 92-3 (Question 1), Case 92-5 (Questions 1, 2)**
5	Patients with sickle cell disease should receive appropriate preventive care, including infection prophylaxis with penicillin and routine immunizations.	**Case 92-6 (Questions 1, 2)**
6	Acute sickle cell crises are an urgent situation and should be managed with pain control, transfusions, oxygen, or antibiotic therapy as appropriate.	**Case 92-7 (Questions 1–3)**
7	Anemia of inflammation is associated with the upregulation of inflammatory cytokines that results in shortened red blood cell survival and decreased production. Treatment focuses on the underlying disease and the use of erythropoietin (EPO).	**Case 92-8 (Question 1)**
8	Response to EPO depends on the dose and underlying cause of anemia. Lack of response to treatment with erythropoiesis-stimulating agents (ESAs) is commonly associated with functional or absolute iron deficiency. Safety concerns with the use of ESAs have resulted in a Risk Evaluation and Mitigation Strategy (REMS) program for the use of these agents.	**Case 92-8 (Question 1)**

ANEMIAS

Definition

Anemia is a reduction in red blood cell (RBC) mass. It is often described as a decrease in the number of RBCs per microliter (μL) or as a decrease in the hemoglobin (Hgb) concentration in blood to a level below the normal physiologic requirement for adequate tissue oxygenation. The term *anemia* is not a diagnosis, but rather an objective sign of a disease. Diagnostic terminology for anemia requires the inclusion of the pathogenesis (e.g., megaloblastic anemia secondary to folate deficiency, microcytic anemia secondary to iron deficiency) in order to implement the appropriate specific therapy to correct the anemia.

Pathophysiology

Anemia is a symptom of many pathologic conditions. It is associated with nutritional deficiencies, acute and chronic diseases, and may be drug-induced. Anemia is also caused by decreased RBC production, increased RBC destruction, or increased RBC loss. When anemia is caused by decreased RBC production, it may be the result of disturbances in stem cell proliferation or

Table 92-1
Classifications of Anemia

Pathophysiologic (Classifies Anemias Based on Pathophysiologic Presentation)
Blood Loss
Acute: trauma, ulcer, hemorrhoids
Chronic: ulcer, vaginal bleeding, aspirin ingestion
Inadequate Red Blood Cell Production
Nutritional deficiency: vitamin B_{12}, folic acid, iron
Erythroblast deficiency: bone marrow failure (aplastic anemia, irradiation, chemotherapy, folic acid antagonists) or bone marrow infiltration (leukemia, lymphoma, myeloma, metastatic solid tumors, myelofibrosis)
Endocrine deficiency: pituitary, adrenal, thyroid, testicular
Chronic disease: renal, liver, infection, granulomatous, collagen vascular
Excessive Red Blood Cell Destruction
Intrinsic factors: hereditary (G6PD), abnormal hemoglobin synthesis
Extrinsic factors: autoimmune reactions, drug reactions, infection (endotoxin)
Morphologic (Classifies Anemias by Red Blood Cell Size [Microcytic, Normocytic, Macrocytic] and Hemoglobin Content [Hypochromic, Normochromic, Hyperchromic])
Macrocytic
Defective maturation with decreased production
Megaloblastic: pernicious (vitamin B_{12} deficiency), folic acid deficiency
Normochromic, Normocytic
Recent blood loss
Hemolysis
Chronic disease
Renal failure
Autoimmune
Endocrine
Microcytic, Hyperchromic
Iron deficiency
Genetic abnormalities: sickle cell, thalassemia

G6PD, glucose-6-phosphate dehydrogenase.

differentiation. Anemias caused by increased RBC destruction can be secondary to hemolysis, whereas increased RBC loss may be caused by acute or chronic bleeding. Anemias associated with acute blood loss, those that are iron-related, and those caused by inflammation constitute most anemias.[1] Classifications of anemias according to pathophysiologic and morphologic characteristics are shown in Table 92-1.

Normally, RBC mass is maintained by feedback mechanisms that regulate levels of erythropoietin (EPO), a hormone that stimulates proliferation and differentiation of erythroid precursors in the bone marrow. Two types of erythroid precursors reside in the bone marrow: the burst forming unit–erythrocyte cell (BFUe) and colony forming unit–erythrocyte cell (CFUe). The BFUe is the earliest progenitor, which eventually develops into a CFUe. The BFUe is moderately sensitive to EPO and is under the influence of other cytokines (e.g., interleukin [IL] 3, granulocyte-macrophage colony-stimulating factor [GM-CSF]). In contrast, the CFUe is highly sensitive to EPO and differentiates into erythroblasts and reticulocytes. The kidneys produce 90% of EPO; liver synthesis accounts for the remainder. Reduced oxygen-carrying capacity is sensed by renal peritubular cells, which stimulates release of EPO into the bloodstream. Patients with chronic anemia may have a blunted and inadequate EPO response for the degree of anemia present.

Detection

SIGNS AND SYMPTOMS

Signs and symptoms of anemia vary with the degree of RBC reduction as well as with the time to development. The decreased oxygen-carrying capacity of the reduced RBC mass results in tissue hypoxia followed by decreased perfusion to nonvital tissues (e.g., skin, mucous membranes, extremities) in order to sustain tissue perfusion of vital organs (e.g., brain, heart, kidneys). Slowly developing anemias can be asymptomatic initially or include symptoms such as slight exertional dyspnea, increased angina, fatigue, or malaise.[1,2]

In severe anemia (Hgb <8 g/dL), heart rate and stroke volume often increase in an attempt to improve oxygen delivery to tissues. These changes in heart rate and stroke volume can result in systolic murmurs, angina pectoris, high-output heart failure, pulmonary congestion, ascites, and edema. Thus, anemia is generally not well tolerated in patients with cardiac disease. Skin and mucous membrane pallor, jaundice, smooth or beefy tongue, cheilosis, and spoon-shaped nails (koilonychia) also may be associated with severe anemia of different etiologies.

HISTORY

A thorough history, including a time line of onset of symptoms and current clinical status, and physical examination are essential because of the complexity of the pathologic conditions associated with anemia. When evaluating a patient for the diagnosis of anemia, histories should include: (a) past and current Hgb or hematocrit (Hct) values; (b) transfusion history; (c) family history, because longstanding anemias can indicate hereditary disorders; (d) occupational, environmental, and social histories; and (e) medication history, to eliminate drug reactions or interactions as the cause of the anemia.

PHYSICAL EXAMINATION

Pallor is most easily observed in the conjunctiva, mucous membranes, nail beds, and palmar creases of the hand. In addition, postural hypotension and tachycardia can be seen when hypovolemia (acute blood loss) is the primary cause of anemia. Patients with vitamin B_{12} deficiency may exhibit neurologic findings consistent with nerve fiber demyelination, which may include changes in deep tendon reflexes, ataxia, and loss of vibration and position sense. Patients with anemia from hemolysis may be slightly jaundiced from bilirubin release. Manifestations of hemorrhage can include petechiae, ecchymoses, hematomas, epistaxis, bleeding gums, and blood in the urine or the stool.

LABORATORY EVALUATION

Although anemia may be suspected from the history and physical examination, a full laboratory evaluation is necessary to confirm the diagnosis, establish severity, and determine the cause. A list of the routine laboratory evaluations used in the workup for anemia is found in Table 92-2. The cornerstone of this evaluation is the complete blood count (CBC). Other evaluations assessing nutritional deficiencies, including iron studies, vitamin B_{12}, and folate as well as EPO levels may also provide insight into the cause of

Table 92-2
Routine Laboratory Evaluation for Anemia Workup

Complete blood count (CBC): Hgb, Hct, RBC count, RBC indices (MCV, MCH, MCHC), WBC count (and differential)
Platelet count
RBC morphology
Reticulocyte count
Bilirubin and LDH
Serum iron, TIBC, serum ferritin, transferrin saturation
Peripheral blood smear examination
Stool examination for occult blood
Bone marrow aspiration and biopsy[a]

[a]Performed in patients with abnormal peripheral blood smears.
Hgb, hemoglobin; Hct, hematocrit; RBC, red blood cell; MCV, mean corpuscular volume; MCH, mean corpuscular hemoglobin; MCHC, mean corpuscular hemoglobin concentration; WBC, white blood cell; RBC, red blood cell; LDH, lactate dehydrogenase; TIBC, total iron-binding capacity.

Table 92-3
Supplemental Hematology Values

	Pediatric	Adult	
Laboratory Test	1–15 years	Male	Female
Erythropoietin (milliunits/mL)	4–26	4–26	4–26
Reticulocyte count (%)	0.5–1.5	0.5–1.5	0.5–1.5
TIBC (mg/dL)	250–400	250–400	250–400
Fe (mg/dL)	50–120	50–160	40–150
Fe/TIBC (%)	20–30	20–40	16–38
Ferritin (ng/mL)	7–140	15–200	12–150
Folate (ng/mL)	7–25	7–25	7–25
RBC folate (ng/mL)	—	140–960	140–960
Vitamin B_{12} (pg/mL)	>200	>200	>200

Fe, iron; RBC, red blood cell; TIBC, total iron-binding capacity.

anemia as shown in Table 92-3. Males have higher normal Hgb and Hct values than do females. The Hgb and Hct are increased in individuals living at altitudes greater than 4,000 feet in response to the diminished oxygen content of the atmosphere and blood.

The morphologic appearance of the RBC found in RBC indices included as part of the CBC, including mean corpuscular volume (MCV), mean cell Hgb (MCH), and mean cell Hgb concentration (MCHC), provide useful information about the nature of the anemia. Note: corpuscular and cell may be used interchangeably when referring to MCV, MCH, etc. Microscopic evaluation of the peripheral blood smear can detect the presence of macrocytic (large) RBCs, which are associated with vitamin B_{12} or folic acid deficiency, or microcytic (small) RBCs, typically associated with iron deficiency anemia. Acute blood loss generally is associated with normocytic cells.

The history and physical examination and laboratory evaluation typically provide sufficient information to distinguish among the most common forms of anemia (Fig. 92-1). If not identified after

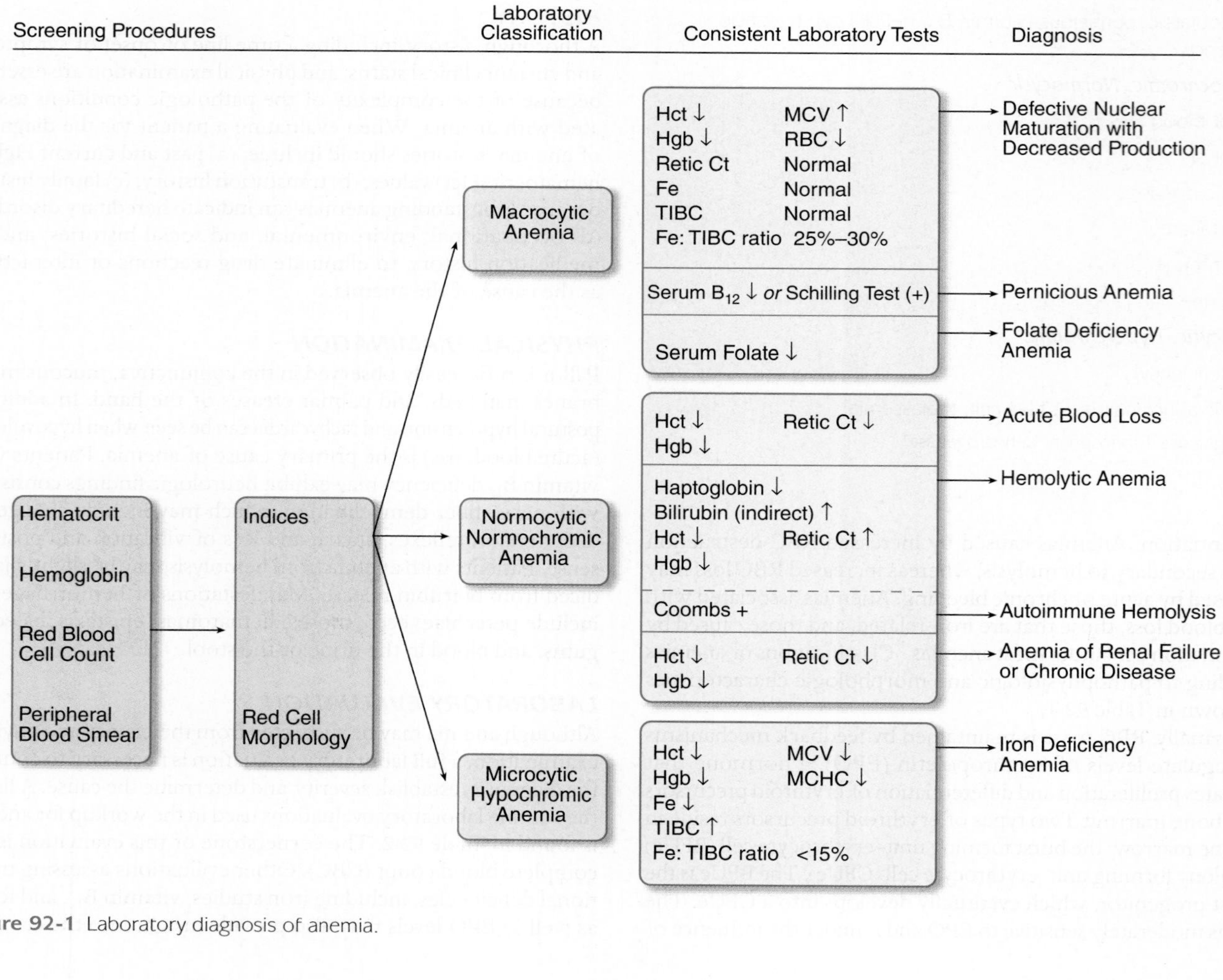

Figure 92-1 Laboratory diagnosis of anemia.

routine evaluation, problems such as autoimmune disease, collagen vascular disease, chronic infection, or endocrine disorders may be causing the anemia. When uncertainty exists or an abnormal peripheral blood smear is noted, a bone marrow aspiration with biopsy is indicated.

There are many causes of anemia. This chapter is limited to the most common anemias and their medication management. Hemolytic anemias will not be discussed. Before proceeding, the reader should review the basic hematologic laboratory tests used to evaluate and monitor anemia (see Chapter 2, Interpretation of Clinical Laboratory Tests).

IRON DEFICIENCY ANEMIA

Iron deficiency is a state of negative iron balance in which the daily iron intake and stores are unable to meet the RBC and other body tissue needs.[3] This is not the same as iron-deficient erythropoiesis, which is a decreased supply of plasma iron to the marrow for RBC synthesis, which can occur with normal or elevated amounts of stored iron. The body contains approximately 3 to 4 g of iron, of which 2.5 g is found in RBCs.[4,5] Only a small fraction of iron is found in plasma and most is bound to transferrin, the transport protein.[4]

Despite the continuing turnover of RBCs, iron stores are well preserved because the iron is recovered and reused in new erythrocytes. Only about 1 to 2 mg/ day of iron is lost from minor bleeding, urine, sweat, and the sloughing of intestinal mucosal cells that contain ferritin in men and in nonmenstruating women.[4] Menstruating women lose approximately an additional 1 mg of iron per day.[6] Pregnancy and lactation are other common sources of iron loss (see Chapter 49, Obstetric Drug Therapy).

Individuals with normal iron stores absorb roughly 10% of ingested dietary iron. The average American diet contains 5 to 15 mg of elemental iron and 1 to 5 mg of heme iron, resulting in 1 to 2 mg of absorbed iron from the intestines. For menstruating, pregnant, or lactating women, however, the daily iron intake requirement may be as high as 20 to 30 mg.[7]

Iron is absorbed from the duodenum and upper jejunum by an active transport mechanism. Dietary iron exists primarily in the ferric state and is converted to the more readily absorbed ferrous form in the acidic environment of the stomach. The ferrous form binds to transferrin for transport to the bone marrow, where it is incorporated into the Hgb of mature erythrocytes.

Gastrointestinal (GI) absorption of iron is increased as much as three- to fivefold in iron deficiency states or when erythropoiesis occurs at a more rapid rate.[6] Animal sources of iron (heme iron) are better absorbed than plant sources (nonheme iron). A number of issues, including gastrointestinal diseases, surgical bypass, a hypochloric state, infections, or drug–food complexes, can alter the absorption of iron.[7] Anemia caused by iron deficiency is the most common nutritional deficiency worldwide.[6] Although iron deficiency anemia has many causes (Table 92-4), blood loss is considered one of the more common. Common causes of chronic blood loss include peptic ulcer disease, hemorrhoids, ingestion of GI irritants, menstruation, multiple pregnancies, and multiple blood donations.[8]

Dietary reference intakes (DRI) for iron are listed in Table 92-5.[9,10] The increased amounts of iron required by pregnant or lactating women are difficult to obtain through diet alone; thus, oral iron supplementation generally is necessary. Although maternal iron usually provides term infants with sufficient stored iron for the first 6 months, infants 6 months to 3 years of age experience rapid growth and a threefold increase in blood volume, which can increase the risk of iron deficiency. Premature infants have reduced iron stores and thus require replacement therapy.

Table 92-4
Iron Deficiency Anemia Causes[8]

Blood Loss
Menstruation, gastrointestinal (e.g., peptic ulcer), trauma, blood donation
Decreased Absorption
Medications, gastrectomy, bariatric surgery, celiac, regional enteritis
Increased Requirement
Infancy, pregnant/lactating women, adolescence
Impaired Utilization
Hereditary, iron use
Environmental
Insufficient intake, diet (e.g., vegetarian)

Table 92-5
Dietary Reference Intake for Iron[9,10]

	mg/day
Healthy, nonmenstruating adults	8
Menstruating women	18
Pregnant women	27
Lactating women	9
Vegetarians	16[a]
Preterm Infants	2–4
Term Infants (Birth to 6 months)	0.27
Term Infants (7–12 months)	11
Toddlers (1–3 years)	7

[a]Twofold higher than those not consuming a vegetarian diet.

Predisposing Factors

CASE 92-1

QUESTION 1: H.P. is a 31-year-old woman seen in the clinic. Her chief complaints include weakness, dizziness, and epigastric pain. She has a 5-year history of peptic ulcer disease, a 10-year history of heavy menstrual bleeding, and a 15-year history of chronic headaches. She has two children who are 1 and 3 years of age. H.P. is currently taking minocycline 100 mg twice daily (BID) for acne, ibuprofen 400 mg as needed for headaches, and esomeprazole 40 mg daily. Her review of systems is positive for decreased exercise tolerance. Physical examination reveals a pale, lethargic, white woman appearing older than her stated age. Her vital signs are within normal limits; her heart rate is regular at 100 beats/minute. Her examination is notable for pale nail beds and splenomegaly.

Significant laboratory results include the following:

Hgb, 8 g/dL
Hct, 26%
Platelet count, 500,000/μL
Reticulocyte count, 0.2%
MCV, 75 femtoliters (fL)
MCH, 23 pg/cell
MCHC, 300 g/L
Serum iron, 40 mcg/dL
Serum ferritin, 9 ng/mL

Total iron-binding capacity (TIBC), 450 g/dL
4+ stool guaiac (normal, negative)

Iron deficiency is determined to be the cause of H.P.'s anemia. An upper GI series with a small bowel follow-through are planned to evaluate her persistent epigastric pain.

What factors predispose H.P. to iron deficiency anemia?

Several factors predispose H.P. to iron deficiency anemia. Her history of heavy menstrual bleeding and the 4+ stool guaiac indicate menstrual and GI sources of blood loss. The GI blood loss may be secondary to H.P.'s chronic use of nonsteroidal anti-inflammatory drugs, recurrent peptic ulcer disease, or both.

Many women of childbearing age have a borderline iron deficiency that becomes more evident during pregnancy because of the increased iron requirements.[3] H.P. has given birth to two children. Therefore, her iron stores have been repeatedly taxed in recent years. In addition, absorption of dietary iron may be compromised by her use of proton pump inhibitors and minocycline (see Case 92-1, Question 6).

Signs, Symptoms, and Laboratory Tests

CASE 92-1, QUESTION 2: What subjective or objective signs, symptoms, and laboratory tests are typical of iron deficiency in H.P.?

H.P.'s constitutional symptoms of weakness and dizziness could be a result of her severe anemia. Generally, until the anemia is severe, such symptoms occur with equal frequency in the nonanemic population. The most important signs and symptoms of iron deficiency anemia are related to the cardiovascular system and are a reflection of the imbalance between the ongoing demands for oxygen against a diminishing oxygen supply.

H.P.'s increased heart rate, decreased exercise tolerance, and pale appearance are consistent with tissue anoxia and the cardiovascular response that may be seen in iron deficiency anemia. H.P.'s iron deficiency has advanced to symptomatic anemia. In patients who are not yet symptomatic, however, depletion of iron stores can be detected by measuring ferritin, the iron storage compound. Although ferritin is primarily an intracellular protein, serum concentrations of ferritin correlate closely with iron stores with only a few exceptions.[7] Ferritin, an acute-phase reactant, is generally found in higher levels in patients with inflammatory disorders, infection, malignancy, liver disease, and chronic renal failure.[3,7] H.P. has a serum ferritin level of 9 ng/mL; less than 12 ng/mL is consistent with iron deficiency. An increased TIBC also can reflect depletion of storage iron, but it is less sensitive than serum ferritin. Thus, in iron deficiency, the serum ferritin concentration is low, whereas the TIBC is usually high; both of these parameters can be detected before the clinical manifestations of anemia are apparent. These abnormalities persist and worsen because anemia develops as illustrated by H.P.'s laboratory values. If the TIBC is low or normal, rather than high, in association with a low serum ferritin, other causes of anemia should be considered and evaluated with additional labs and bone marrow examination.

H.P.'s low serum iron, low serum ferritin, and elevated TIBC are typical of the laboratory findings associated with iron deficiency anemia. Serum transferrin receptor levels, which reflect the amount of RBC precursors available for active proliferation, are increased in iron deficiency. After stored iron is depleted, heme and Hgb synthesis is decreased. In severe iron deficiency, the RBCs become hypochromic (low MCHC) and microcytic (low MCV).[5]

Usually, the RBC indices do not become abnormal until the Hgb concentration falls to less than 10 g/dL. H.P.'s corpuscular indices indicate that her anemia is hypochromic and microcytic.

The reticulocyte count provides an estimate of effective RBC production and is usually normal or low in iron deficiency anemia. H.P. has a reticulocyte count of 0.2%, which also is compatible with iron deficiency anemia.

In the workup of a microcytic, hypochromic anemia, the stool should be examined for occult blood. H.P. has a 4+ stool guaiac, which suggests blood loss via the GI tract. Further diagnostic evaluations (e.g., endoscopy, abdominal X-rays) are necessary to determine the underlying problem. In summary, H.P.'s signs, symptoms, and laboratory findings all support the diagnosis of an iron deficiency anemia.

Iron Therapy

ORAL IRON DOSING

CASE 92-1, QUESTION 3: How should H.P.'s iron deficiency be managed? What dose of iron should be given to treat H.P.'s iron deficiency anemia?

The primary treatment for H.P. should be directed toward control of the underlying causes of anemia; GI blood loss, multiple childbirths, heavy menstrual flow, decreased dietary iron absorption, and perhaps, an inadequate diet. The cause of her GI blood loss should be corrected, her dietary intake should be analyzed and modified and supplemental iron should be prescribed to replenish her stores and correct the anemia.

The usual adult dose of ferrous sulfate is 325 mg (one tablet) administered 3 times daily between meals. However, because of limited absorption of iron in the intestines, repletion with lower doses of iron has been shown to be effective, potentially minimizing side effects and improving compliance.[7] If no iron is being lost through bleeding, the required daily dose of elemental iron can be calculated using a formula that assumes that 0.25 g/dL/day is the maximal rate of Hgb regeneration.

$$\text{Elemental iron (mg/day)} = 0.25\text{g Hgb}/100\text{ mL blood/day}\ (5{,}000\text{ mL blood})(3.4,\text{ mg Fe}/1\text{ g Hgb}) \quad \text{(Eq. 92-1)}$$

$$= 40\text{ mg Fe/day}/20\%\text{ absorption (approximate absorption rate in iron-deficient states)}$$
$$= 200\text{ mg Fe/day}$$
$$= 1{,}000\text{ mg ferrous sulfate/day (ferrous sulfate contains 20\% elemental iron)}$$
$$= 325\text{ mg 3 times daily (TID) ferrous sulfate} \quad \text{(Eq. 92-2)}$$

PRODUCT SELECTION

CASE 92-1, QUESTION 4: What are the differences between iron products? Which is the product of choice?

The ferrous form of iron is absorbed 3 times more readily than the ferric form. Although ferrous sulfate, ferrous gluconate, and ferrous fumarate are absorbed almost equally, each contains a different amount of elemental iron that is available for absorption.[11] Carbonyl iron, another iron product, is available but its use may be limited owing to the fact that iron in this form must be solubilized by gastric acid to be absorbed. Table 92-6 compares the iron content of several oral iron preparations to assist in making appropriate treatment choices for patients.

Product Formulation

Product formulation is of considerable importance in product selection. Sustained release (SR) and enteric coated preparations

Table 92-6
Comparisons of Oral Iron Preparations[11]

Preparation	Dose (mg)	Fe^{2+} Content (mg)	Fe (%)
Ferrous sulfate	325	65	20
Ferrous fumarate	324	106	33
Ferrous gluconate	240	29	12
Carbonyl iron	—	45	—
Ferrous sulfate (time-released)	160	50	32

Note: This is a representative list of example oral iron preparations that may be utilized.

may increase GI tolerance or decrease side effects, increase bioavailability, and also may have additives claimed to enhance absorption. Because these products can be given once daily, increased adherence is an additional claim.

Anecdotal claims that SR iron preparations cause fewer GI side effects have not been substantiated by controlled studies. These products transport iron past the duodenum and proximal jejunum, thereby reducing the absorption of iron.[5,7] Because poor absorption and poor hematologic responses might occur with SR formulations, caution should be used if chosen for initial treatment.

Adjuvants are incorporated into iron preparations in an attempt to enhance absorption or mitigate side effects. An acidic environment is needed for absorption in the duodenum and upper jejunum. Ascorbic acid (vitamin C), given in doses up to 1 gram, is able to increase iron absorption by approximately 7%; however, smaller doses of vitamin C (e.g., 25 mg) do not significantly alter iron absorption.[12] To decrease the side effect of constipation, stool softeners are also sometimes added to iron preparations.[5] The stool softener dose may not be appropriate and additional doses may need to be taken. In summary, H.P. should take the least expensive iron preparation containing ferrous sulfate, gluconate, or fumarate.

GOALS OF THERAPY

CASE 92-1, QUESTION 5: What are the goals of iron therapy? How long should H.P. be treated? How should H.P. be monitored?

The goals of iron therapy are to normalize the Hgb and Hct concentrations and to replete iron stores. Initially, if the doses of iron are adequate, the reticulocyte count will begin to increase by the 3rd to 4th day and peak by the seventh to 10th day of therapy. By the end of the second week of iron therapy, the reticulocyte count will fall back to normal. The Hgb response is a convenient index to monitor in outpatients. Hematologic response is usually seen in 2 to 3 weeks with a 1 to 2 g/dL increase in Hgb and a 6% increase in the hematocrit. H.P.'s anemia can be expected to resolve in 1 to 2 months; however, iron therapy should be continued for 3 to 6 months after the Hgb is normalized to replete iron stores.[7] Therapy duration is related to the absorption pattern of iron with more iron being absorbed during the first month of therapy; because iron stores are repleted, less is absorbed.

PATIENT INFORMATION

CASE 92-1, QUESTION 6: What information should be provided to H.P. when dispensing oral iron? What can be done if she experiences intolerable GI symptoms (e.g., nausea, epigastric pain)?

Iron should be dispensed in a childproof container and H.P. should be counseled to store it in a safe place, inaccessible to her young children. Accidental ingestion of oral iron can cause serious consequences in small children[13] (see Chapter 5, Managing Drug Overdoses and Poisoning). H.P. should be told that oral iron therapy produces dark stools. She should try to take her iron on an empty stomach because food, especially dairy products, decreases the absorption by up to 50%.[11]

Gastric side effects, which occur in 5% to 20% of patients, include nausea, epigastric pain, constipation, abdominal cramps, and diarrhea. Constipation does not appear to be dose-related but side effects (e.g., nausea and epigastric pain) occur more frequently because the quantity of soluble elemental iron in contact with the stomach and duodenum increases.[5] To minimize gastric intolerance, oral iron therapy can be initiated with a single tablet of ferrous sulfate 325 mg/day and increased by increments of one tablet per day every 2 to 3 days until the full therapeutic dose of 325 mg 3 times daily can be administered.

H.P. also should be educated about potential drug interactions that can occur with iron therapy. Currently, she is taking a proton pump inhibitor, which is thought to inhibit serum iron absorption by increasing the pH of the stomach and decreasing the solubility of ferrous salts. In addition, antacids can increase stomach pH, and certain anions (carbonate and hydroxide) also are thought to form insoluble complexes when combined with iron. Table 92-7 provides additional drug interactions to be considered.

H.P. is also taking minocycline for the treatment of acne. Because the absorptions of both iron and minocycline are decreased when administered concomitantly, the minocycline should be taken at least 2 hours apart.[11]

PARENTERAL IRON THERAPY

Indications

CASE 92-1, QUESTION 7: When would parenteral iron therapy be indicated for H.P.?

Several indications exist for parenteral iron administration. Causes of oral therapy failure can include nonadherence, misdiagnosis, inflammatory conditions, malabsorption (e.g., atrophic gastritis, radiation enteritis, gastric bypass, celiac disease), the need for rapid iron repletion, and continuing blood loss equal to or greater than the rate of RBC production.[3,4] Besides failure to respond to oral therapy, other indications for parenteral iron administration include intolerance to oral therapy, required antacid therapy, or significant blood loss in patients refusing transfusion. In H.P.'s case, intolerance, continued blood loss, long-term antacid therapy, and malabsorption may be potential indications for use and, if documented, she would be a candidate for injectable iron.

Preferred Route

CASE 92-1, QUESTION 8: What is the preferred formulation of parenteral iron administration?

Iron can be given parenterally in the form of ferric gluconate, iron dextran, iron sucrose, ferric carboxymaltose, and ferumoxytol (Table 92-8).[14] Comparison between agents reveals similar efficacy with differences in cost analysis from diverse administration schedules. Iron dextran and ferric carboxymaltose are US Food and Drug Administration (FDA)-approved for the treatment of iron deficiency when oral supplementation is impossible or ineffective. All parenteral iron products can be administered undiluted slowly as an intravenous (IV) push, or diluted and administered by infusion; although not included in the FDA-approved labeling, iron dextran injection is commonly diluted in 500 mL of 0.9%

Table 92-7
Drug Interactions with Iron Salts

Iron Salts Drug Interactions			
Precipitant drug	**Object drug**[a]		**Description**
Acetohydroxamic acid (AHA)	Iron salts	↓	AHA chelates heavy metals, notably iron. The absorption of iron may be decreased. When iron is indicated, administer intramuscularly (IM).
Antacids	Iron salts	↓	GI absorption of iron may be reduced.
Ascorbic acid	Iron salts	↑	Ascorbic acid at doses ≥200 mg have been shown to enhance the absorption of iron ≥30%.
Calcium salts	Iron salts	↓	GI absorption of iron may be reduced. When possible, separate administration times.
Chloramphenicol	Iron salts	↑	Serum iron levels may be increased.
Digestive enzymes	Iron salts	↓	The serum iron response to oral iron may be decreased by concomitant pancreatic extracts.
H_2 antagonists	Iron salts	↓	GI absorption of iron may be reduced.
Proton pump inhibitors	Iron salts	↓	GI absorption of iron may be reduced.
Trientine	Iron salts	↓	The 2 agents inhibit the absorption of each other. If iron is needed, administer the agents at least 2 hours apart.
Iron salts	Trientine		
Iron salts	Captopril	↓	Concomitant use within 2 hours may promote formation of inactive captopril disulfide dimer.
Iron salts	Cephalosporins (e.g., cefdinir)	↓	Iron supplements and foods fortified with iron may reduce the absorption of cefdinir 80% and 30%, respectively. If iron supplements are needed during cefdinir therapy, cefdinir should be taken 2 hours before or after the supplement. Iron-fortified infant formula (elemental iron 2.2 mg per 6 oz) has no effect on cefdinir absorption.
Iron salts	Fluoroquinolones (e.g., ciprofloxacin)	↓	GI absorption of fluoroquinolones may be decreased because of formation of iron–quinolone complex. Avoid coadministration of these drugs. (See individual fluoroquinolone monographs for administration recommendations.)
Iron salts	Levodopa	↓	Levodopa appears to form chelates with iron salts, decreasing levodopa absorption and serum levels.
Iron salts	Levothyroxine	↓	The efficacy of levothyroxine may be decreased, resulting in hypothyroidism. Avoid coadministration.
Iron salts	Methyldopa	↓	Extent of methyldopa absorption may be decreased, possibly resulting in decreased efficacy.
Iron salts	Mycophenolate mofetil	↓	Absorption of mycophenolate mofetil may be decreased. Avoid simultaneous administration.
Iron salts	Penicillamine	↓	Marked reduction in GI absorption of penicillamine may occur, possibly because of chelation.
Iron salts	Tetracyclines	↓	Concomitant use within 2 hours may decrease absorption and serum levels of tetracyclines. Absorption of iron salts also may be decreased.
Tetracyclines	Iron salts		
Iron salts	Thyroid hormones	↓	Absorption of thyroid hormones may be decreased. Avoid coadministration.

[a]↑ = object drug increased; ↓ = object drug decreased.
Source: Facts & Comparisons eAnswers. **http://online.factsandcomparisons.com/MonoDisp.aspx?monoID=fandc-hcp11143#IronSaltsDrugInteractions**. Accessed June 12, 2015.

NaCl and administered by IV infusion.[3] Iron dextran is also the only product that may be given intramuscularly (IM). This route may be preferred in a few instances, such as in patients with limited IV access. Although the data are limited, infusion of the total dose (total estimated iron deficit) of iron dextran is given in clinical practice and has proved to be effective and convenient.[15] The total dose method of administration can be associated with a higher prevalence of fever, malaise, flushing, and myalgias. Because of the potential for anaphylaxis with iron dextran, an IM or IV test dose should be given. The test dose for adults is 25 mg of iron dextran. Although anaphylactic reactions usually are evident within a few minutes if they occur, it is recommended that a period of 1 hour or longer elapse before the remaining portion of the initial dose be given. Subsequent use of test doses should be considered during iron dextran therapy but is not required.

Ferric gluconate, iron sucrose, and ferumoxytol are parenteral iron formulations that are FDA-approved for the treatment of iron deficiency anemia in patients with chronic kidney disease undergoing chronic hemodialysis. Ferric carboxymaltose is indicated for treatment of iron deficiency anemia in nondialysis-dependent

Table 92-8
Comparison of Parenteral Iron Preparations

Preparation	Dosage Form	Usual Dose	Maximum Dose
Ferric carboxymaltose	Solution for injection: 50 mg/mL (elemental iron)	Weight ≥50 kg: 750 mg per dose Weight <50 kg: 15 mg/kg per dose Repeat dose ≥7 days	1,500 mg (cumulative per treatment course)
Ferumoxytol	Solution for injection: 30 mg/mL (elemental iron)	510 mg per dose; repeat once 3–8 days later	N/A
Iron dextran	Solution for injection: 50 mg/mL (elemental iron)	Test dose: 25 mg; followed by up to 75 mg (dose based on patient weight)	100 mg per day
Iron sucrose	Solution for injection: 20 mg/mL (elemental iron)	**HD:** 100 mg during consecutive HD sessions for 10 doses **CKD, nondialysis:** 200 mg on 5 different occasions over 14 days; 500 mg once on days 1 and 14 **CKD, PD:** 300 mg IV days 1 and 14, then 400 mg on day 28	N/A
Sodium ferric gluconate complex	Solution for injection: 12.5 mg/mL (elemental iron)	125 mg per dose (usually repeated to cumulative dose of 1,000 mg)	N/A

CKD: chronic kidney disease; HD: hemodialysis; PD: peritoneal dialysis.
Source: Facts & Comparisons eAnswers. http://online.factsandcomparisons.com/MonoDisp.aspx?monoid=fandc-hcp15283&book=DFC&search=83228%7c24&isStemmed=True&fromtop=true&section=table-list#IRONPARENTERALProductTable. Accessed June 6, 2015.

chronic kidney disease. A test dose is not required for these agents due to the lower incidence of serious anaphylactoid reactions. Iron requirements in these patients typically exceed 1 to 2 g and, therefore, multiple doses of ferric gluconate and iron sucrose are needed to achieve the total dose of iron.

In general, rates of adverse effects are similar among agents. Patients should be monitored for hypersensitivity reactions for at least 30 minutes after administration of any parenteral iron compound.

Dosage Calculation

Case 92-1, Question 9: What is the total dose of iron dextran for IV infusion that would be needed to achieve a normal Hgb value for H.P. and to replenish her iron stores? How quickly should she respond?

The total dose of iron dextran to be administered can be determined using the following equation.

$$\text{Iron (mg)} = \text{Weight (pounds)} \times 0.3\ \{100 - [100(\text{Hgb})/14.8]\} \quad \text{(Eq. 92-3)}$$

where Hgb is the patient's measured Hgb (g/dL).

The equation uses the person's weight (in pounds) and assumes that an Hgb of 14.8 g/dL is 100% of normal. Children weighing less than 30 pounds should be given 80% of the calculated dose because the normal mean Hgb in this population is lower.

For patients with anemia resulting from blood loss (e.g., hemorrhagic diathesis) or patients receiving chronic dialysis, the iron requirement is based on the estimate of iron contained in the blood lost. In this case, the following equation should be used:

$$\text{Iron (mg)} = \text{Blood loss (mL)} \times \text{Hct (the patient's measured Hct expressed as a decimal fraction)} \quad \text{(Eq. 92-4)}$$

This formula assumes that 1 mL of normochromic blood contains 1 mg of iron.

After parenteral administration, iron dextran is cleared by the reticuloendothelial cells and processed. The iron is then released back into the plasma and bone marrow. Because the rate of iron incorporation into Hgb does not exceed that achieved by oral iron therapy, the response time is similar to that of oral iron therapy, and the Hgb can be expected to increase at a rate of 1 to 2 g/dL/week during the first 2 weeks and by 0.7 to 1 g/dL/week thereafter until normal values are attained.

Side Effects

Case 92-1, Question 10: What side effects can be expected from parenteral iron therapy?

Overall adverse reactions reported with parenteral iron administration are rare.[16] Anaphylactoid reactions occur in less than 1% of patients treated with parenteral iron therapy and are more commonly associated with iron dextran and ferumoxytol than with ferric gluconate and iron sucrose.[16,17] In a small study comparing iron dextran to ferric carboxymaltose, patients experienced significantly fewer immune-related adverse reactions.[18] Other side effects seen with parenteral iron agents include chest pain, headache, hypotension, nausea and vomiting, cramps, and diarrhea.

MEGALOBLASTIC ANEMIAS

Megaloblastic anemia is a common disorder that can have several causes, including anemias associated with vitamin B_{12} or folic acid deficiency or metabolic or inherited defects associated with a decreased ability to use vitamin B_{12} or folic acid.[19,20]

Megaloblastosis results from impaired DNA synthesis in replicating cells, which is signaled by a large immature nucleus.[19] RNA and protein synthesis remain unaffected, and the cytoplasm matures normally. Megaloblastic changes can be observed microscopically in RBC and in proliferating cells (e.g., in the cervix, skin, GI tract). The extent of RBC macrocytosis is reported as MCV, calculated as shown below.

$$\text{MCV (fL)} = [\text{Hct (percent)} \times 10]/[\text{RBC count } (10^6/\mu L)] \quad \text{(Eq. 93-5)}$$

Although the clinical effects of vitamin B_{12} and folic acid deficiencies can differ in various organ systems, they are similar in their effects on the hematopoietic system. Typically, macrocytic anemia develops slowly and can be identified by large, oval, well-hemoglobinized RBCs; anisocytosis; and nuclear remnants. The reticulocyte count is low and the bilirubin level is elevated. If biopsied, the bone marrow is markedly hypercellular. Nuclear immaturity is present, but the megaloblasts have normal maturation of the cytoplasm. Iron stores in the marrow are increased as a result of the intramedullary hemolysis. Symptoms include fatigue; exaggeration of preexisting cardiovascular or pulmonary problems; a sore, pale, smooth tongue; diarrhea or constipation; and anorexia.[21,22]

Vitamin B_{12} Deficiency Anemia

VITAMIN B_{12} METABOLISM

Deficiency and poor utilization of vitamin B_{12} are two mechanisms for the development of megaloblastic anemia.[22] Vitamin B_{12} (cobalamin) is naturally synthesized by microorganisms, but humans are incapable of doing so and must obtain vitamin B_{12} in their diet. Animal protein and fortified foods provide the majority of dietary vitamin B_{12}.[23] The typical Western diet contains 3.5 to 5 mcg/day of vitamin B_{12}, an amount sufficient to replace the up to 1 mcg lost daily through urine, sweat, and other body secretions.

In the stomach, vitamin B_{12} is released from protein complexes and bound to intrinsic factor, which protects it from degradation by GI microorganisms. Intrinsic factor is essential for the absorption of vitamin B_{12}. Specific mucosal receptors in the distal small ileum allow for attachment of the intrinsic factor–vitamin B_{12} complex. Vitamin B_{12} is then transferred to the ileal cell and finally to portal vein blood.

After vitamin B_{12} is absorbed, it is bound to specific β-globulin transport proteins, transcobalamins I, II, and III. Transcobalamin II is responsible for transporting absorbed vitamin B_{12} through cell membranes and delivering it to the liver and other organs. In the liver, vitamin B_{12} is converted to coenzyme B_{12}, which is essential for hematopoiesis, maintenance of myelin throughout the entire nervous system and production of epithelial cells.

Total body stores of vitamin B_{12} range from 2,000 to 3,000 mcg, approximately 50% of which is stored in the liver. Because body stores are extensive, 5 to 10 years are required before symptoms of vitamin B_{12} deficiency develop.[21]

PATHOGENESIS AND EVALUATION OF VITAMIN B_{12} DEFICIENCY

Vitamin B_{12} deficiency can result from decreased supply (reduced intake, absorption, transport, or utilization) or increased requirement (greater metabolic consumption, destruction, and excretion). Other causes of vitamin B_{12} deficiency include inadequate proteolytic degradation of vitamin B_{12} from protein, or congenital intrinsic factor deficiency. In addition, the gastric mucosa may be unable to produce intrinsic factor under conditions such as partial gastrectomy, autoimmune destruction (e.g., Addisonian or juvenile pernicious anemia), or destruction of the gastric mucosa from caustic agents.

Pernicious anemia can result in vitamin B_{12} deficiency.[24,25] It can be caused by chronic atrophic gastritis accompanied by reduced intrinsic factor and hydrochloric acid secretion or acquired as a result of gastrectomy, pancreatic disease, or malnutrition. Pernicious anemia occurs commonly in patients with thyrotoxicosis, autoimmune thyroiditis, vitiligo, rheumatoid arthritis, or gastric cancer. Intrinsic factor and parietal cell autoantibodies may be observed in the serum of patients with pernicious anemia.

The onset of the pernicious anemia is insidious. Patients generally do not feel well for months and often complain of at least two of the following symptoms: weakness, sore tongue, and symmetric numbness or tingling in the extremities. The neurologic symptoms of vitamin B_{12} deficiency are associated with a defect in myelin synthesis and often are described as peripheral neuropathy or nonspecific complaints (e.g., tinnitus, neuritis, vertigo, headaches).

LABORATORY EVALUATION

In general, the serum vitamin B_{12} level reliably reflects vitamin B_{12} tissue stores. Falsely low vitamin B_{12} concentrations may be observed in patients with folic acid deficiency, transcobalamin I deficiency, multiple myeloma, or pregnancy.[21] Falsely normal levels may be observed in patients with myeloproliferative, liver, or renal disease. Measuring serum methylmalonic acid and homocysteine levels may also differentiate between folate and vitamin B_{12} deficiency. Once vitamin B_{12} therapy has been instituted, serum levels of these chemicals decrease if true vitamin B_{12} deficiency is present.

The cause of vitamin B_{12} deficiency may be determined by the use of antibody testing (antiparietal cells and anti-intrinsic factor antibodies).[25,26] Patients with pernicious anemia are not able to absorb vitamin B_{12} because intrinsic factor is not available for binding. Some patients produce intrinsic factor but are still unable to absorb dietary vitamin B_{12}. Malabsorption, which occurs more commonly in the elderly, can be caused by intestinal bacteria that usurp vitamin B_{12}, achlorhydria, chronic acid suppression therapy, pancreatic insufficiency, alcohol abuse, inadequate disassociation of vitamin B_{12} from proteins, or lack of intrinsic factor receptors secondary to ileal loops, bypass, or surgical resection.[27]

PERNICIOUS ANEMIA

Signs, Symptoms, and Laboratory Findings

CASE 92-2

QUESTION 1: C.L. is a 63-year-old Scandinavian man that is seen by a private physician. C.L. has a 1-year history of weakness and emotional instability. He also complains of a painful tongue, alternating constipation and diarrhea, and a tingling sensation in both feet. Pertinent findings on physical examination include pallor, red tongue, vibratory sensory loss in the lower extremities, disorientation, muscle weakness, and ataxia.

Significant laboratory findings include the following:

Hgb, 8.7 g/dL
Hct, 27%
MCV, 115 fL
MCH, 38 pg/cell
MCHC, 340 g/L
Reticulocytes, 0.4%
Poikilocytosis and anisocytosis on the blood smear
White blood cell (WBC) count, 4,000/μL
Platelets, 100,000/μL
Serum iron, 90 mcg/dL
TIBC, 350 g/dL
Ferritin, 140 ng/mL
RBC folate, 300 ng/mL
Serum vitamin B_{12}, 90 pg/mL
Intrinsic factor antibody positive

What signs, symptoms, and laboratory findings in C.L. are typical of pernicious anemia?

C.L.'s signs and symptoms are classic for pernicious anemia. This disease occurs equally in both sexes (primarily in individuals of northern European descent), with an average onset of 60 years.[28] Pernicious anemia develops from a lack of gastric intrinsic factor production which causes vitamin B_{12} malabsorption and, ultimately, vitamin B_{12} deficiency. C.L.'s signs and symptoms of vitamin B_{12} deficiency include painful red tongue, loss of lower extremity vibratory sense, vertigo, and emotional instability. The elevated MCV suggests megaloblastic anemia.

Folate and iron are two other factors that can affect the MCV and should be evaluated during the workup of a patient for anemia. In this case, C.L.'s folate and iron levels are normal, but his serum vitamin B_{12} level is low. The presence of poikilocytosis and anisocytosis observed in the blood smear represents ineffective erythropoiesis. Other cell lineages also may be affected in the bone marrow. Erythroid hypercellularity, along with a decrease in the myeloid cells (leukocytes and platelets), increases the erythroid to myeloid ratio in C.L. The patient's low Hgb, elevated MCV, low serum vitamin B_{12} levels, and presence of intrinsic factor antibodies are compatible with the diagnosis of pernicious anemia, which is often associated with atrophic body gastritis. The Schilling test, which confirms intestinal malabsorption of vitamin B_{12}, is no longer available in the United States.[21]

Treatment

CASE 92-2, QUESTION 2: How should C.L.'s pernicious anemia be treated? How soon can a response be expected?

C.L. should receive parenteral vitamin B_{12} in a dose sufficient to provide the daily requirement of approximately 2 mcg and the amount needed to replenish tissue stores (about 2,000–5,000 mcg; average, 4,000 mcg). To replete vitamin B_{12} stores, cyanocobalamin can be given IM in accordance with various regimens as shown in Table 92-9.[29] Intramuscular or deep subcutaneous administration provides SR of vitamin B_{12} with better utilization compared with rapid IV infusion. An oral tablet or intranasal cyanocobalamin solution is also available for maintenance therapy, after the patient has normalized blood counts.

Treatment with vitamin B_{12} should completely reverse the hematologic complications of pernicious anemia.[22,23] The reticulocyte count increases within the first week of treatment and the megaloblastic anemia resolves within 6 to 8 weeks. Neurologic symptoms may worsen at first and then resolve over weeks to months. Some symptoms may never resolve completely. Because the rapid production of RBCs can increase potassium demand, serum potassium should be monitored and potassium supplementation provided as necessary. Peripheral blood counts should be obtained every 3 to 6 months to evaluate the adequacy of therapy. If maintenance therapy is discontinued, pernicious anemia will recur within years, making patient adherence vital to long-term success.

Oral Vitamin B_{12}

CASE 92-2, QUESTION 3: What factors affect the oral absorption of vitamin B_{12}? When might oral vitamin B_{12} therapy an effective alternative to parenteral therapy for C.L.?

The amount of vitamin B_{12} that can be absorbed orally from a single dose or meal ranges from 1 to 5 mcg; approximately 5 mcg of vitamin B_{12} is absorbed daily from the average American diet.[23] The percentage of vitamin B_{12} absorbed decreases with increasing doses: 50% of a 1 mcg dose and 5% of a 20 mcg dose. Overall, oral vitamin B_{12} therapy is considered safe and effective,[30] although because of lack of long-term efficacy data, oral supplementation is not routinely used in the acute treatment of vitamin B_{12} deficiency.[27] Oral therapy for pernicious anemia using high dosages of oral cyanocobalamin may be indicated in certain patients, especially those who refuse or cannot receive parenteral therapy.[27,31] Issues of nonadherence or lack of response with oral therapy places the patient at substantial risk for significant neurologic damage. Patients receiving oral vitamin B_{12} therapy should be monitored more frequently to ensure adherence to therapy.

Anemias After Gastrectomy

CASE 92-3

QUESTION 1: F.M. has just undergone a total gastrectomy for recurrent nonhealing ulcers. What form(s) of anemia would be expected to develop in a patient after gastrectomy? Should F.M. receive prophylactic vitamin B_{12}?

Partial or total gastrectomy often results in anemia, particularly pernicious anemia, because the loss of intrinsic factor impairs oral vitamin B_{12} absorption. The hematologic and neurologic abnormalities associated with vitamin B_{12} deficiency do not develop until existing vitamin B_{12} stores are depleted (about 2–3 years). Nevertheless, prophylactic vitamin B_{12} should be administered in this patient after total gastrectomy.[32] Because the vitamin B_{12} stores are not currently depleted, maintenance therapy, as discussed in Case 92-2, Question 2, should be adequate for F.M.

Table 92-9
Cyanocobalamin (Vitamin B_{12}) Supplementation Regimens for Macrocytic Anemia[29]

	Initial Supplementation			Chronic Supplementation (lifelong)		
Patient Population	**Dose**	**Frequency**	**Route**	**Dose**	**Frequency**	**Route**
Adults	100 mcg	Daily for 7 days, then on alternate days for 14 days, then q 3–4 days for 2–3 weeks	IM or SC	100–200 mcg	Monthly	IM or SQ
Severe Deficiency	100–1,000 mcg	Daily or every other day for 1–2 weeks	IM or SC	100–1,000 mcg	every 1–3 months	IM or SQ
				500 mcg	Weekly	Intranasal
	1,000–2,000 mcg	Daily for 1–2 weeks	Oral	1,000 mcg[a]	Daily	Oral

[a]In patients with normal gastrointestinal absorption, doses of 1–25 mcg daily are considered sufficient as a dietary supplement.
IM, intramuscular; SC, subcutaneous.

CASE 92-4

QUESTION 1: P.G. is a 48-year-old female scheduled to have laparoscopic Roux-en-Y gastric bypass (RYGB) surgery for morbid obesity with a body mass index (BMI) >40.

What forms of anemia would be expected to develop in P.G.?

When a RYGB procedure is performed, the stomach is decreased in size, and the small intestine is manipulated creating a gastrojejunostomy and jejunojejunostomy.[33] This results in bypassing the duodenum and proximal jejunum where iron is absorbed, resulting in iron deficiency anemia. The gastric pouch is no longer an acidic environment which impairs iron bioavailability and functioning of iron transport mechanisms. Patients are also recommended to avoid red meat which is a common dietary source of iron. An acidic environment is also needed for the bioavailability of vitamin B_{12} leading to decreased absorption. The diagnosis of vitamin B_{12} deficiency following bariatric surgery is rare due to the large amount stored in the body. Folate deficiency may occur from reduced dietary folate intake. The majority of folate is absorbed from the upper third of the small intestine, but may occur at any location. Iron deficiency anemia is the most common cause for anemia in bariatric surgery patients; however, other micronutrient deficiencies may also contribute.

CASE 92-4, QUESTION 2: What prophylactic strategies might P.G. employ to prevent anemia?

Following bariatric surgery, patients will need to take lifelong multivitamin and micronutrient supplementation.[34] Patients should take a high potency multivitamin with 100% of the recommended daily value for at least 75% of the nutrients. It should have a minimum of 18 mg iron, 400 mcg folic acid, selenium, and zinc.[35] Patients should be instructed to take an additional 1 to 2 tablets per day of an iron salt, ferrous sulfate, or ferrous fumarate to prevent iron deficiency anemia. In addition to a high potency multivitamin, patients should take 350 to 500 mcg/day of oral cyanocobalamin or receive 1,000 mcg injections monthly.

Folic Acid Deficiency Anemia

FOLIC ACID METABOLISM

Folate is abundant in virtually all food sources, especially fresh green vegetables, fruits, yeast, and animal protein. As a result of food fortification, the average American diet provides 50 to 2,000 mcg of folate per day; however, excessive or prolonged cooking (>15 minutes) in large quantities of water may reduce the folate contained in food.[36] Human requirements for folate vary with age and depend on the rate of metabolism and cell turnover but are generally 3 mcg/kg/day.[36] The minimal daily adult requirement of folate is 50 mcg but, because absorption from food is incomplete, a daily intake of 200 mcg is recommended. Folate requirements are increased in conditions in which the metabolic rate and rate of cellular division are increased (e.g., pregnancy, infancy, infection, malignancies, hemolytic anemia). The following are estimates of daily folate requirements based on age and growth demands: children, 80 to 400 mcg; infants, 65 mcg; pregnant or lactating women, 600 mcg.[37]

Dietary folic acid is in the polyglutamate form and must be enzymatically deconjugated in the GI tract to the monoglutamate form before it is absorbed. Once absorbed, the inactive dihydrofolate must be converted to active tetrahydrofolate (folinic acid) by dihydrofolate reductase.

In contrast to the large stores of vitamin B_{12}, the body's folate stores are relatively small (about 5–10 mg). Therefore, deficiency and subsequent megaloblastic anemia can occur within 3 to 4 months of decreased folate intake.

PREDISPOSING FACTORS

Folate deficiency is most commonly associated with alcoholism, rapid cell turnover, and dietary deficiency. In alcoholics, the daily intake of the folate contained in food may be restricted or absent. In addition, enterohepatic recirculation of folate can become impaired by the toxic effect of alcohol on hepatocytes. Folate deficiency may also develop during the third trimester of pregnancy as a result of a marginal diet and rapid fetal metabolism. Folate coenzymes are required for most metabolic pathways (Fig. 92-2). Therefore, folate deficiency will develop in any condition of rapid cellular turnover (e.g., hemolytic anemias, hemoglobinopathies, sideroblastic anemia, leukemias, lymphomas, multiple myeloma) or a diet lacking in folate (e.g., food faddism or a weight-loss diet). Folate deficiency also can occur with chronic hemodialysis, diseases that impair absorption from the small intestine (e.g., sprue, regional enteritis), extensive jejunal resections, and drugs that alter folate metabolism (e.g., trimethoprim, pyrimethamine, methotrexate, sulfasalazine, oral contraceptives, anticonvulsants).[38,39] Few patients have inborn errors of folate metabolism.[40]

The evaluation of megaloblastic anemia must be thorough because indiscriminate use of nondirected therapy can be dangerous. Large doses of folate can partially reverse hematologic abnormalities caused by vitamin B_{12} deficiency; however, folate cannot correct neurologic damage caused by vitamin B_{12} deficiency. Therefore, folate deficiency must be differentiated from vitamin B_{12} deficiency *before* folate therapy is initiated. Otherwise, progression of the neurologic sequelae of vitamin B_{12} deficiency can occur.

CASE 92-5

QUESTION 1: D.H. is a malnourished-appearing woman in her second trimester of pregnancy who presents to the local health clinic for her regular checkup. She is a multiparous, 26-year-old woman with a 7-year history of excessive alcohol intake and has been using cocaine frequently for 3 years. She lives with her boyfriend and her 19-month-old daughter. During both pregnancies, D.H. lost 8 to 10 pounds during the first trimester secondary to nausea, vomiting, and anorexia. Her only complaints are dyspnea on exertion, palpitations, and diarrhea.

Pertinent laboratory values include the following:

Hct, 25.5%
MCV, 112 fL
MCH, 34 pg/cell
RBC, $1.1 \times 10^6/\mu L$
Iron, 179 mcg/dL
Folate, 40 ng/mL
Serum vitamin B_{12}, 350 pg/mL (normal, 200–1,000)
Reticulocytes, 1%
Platelets, 70,000/μL
WBC count, 2,000/μL with hypersegmented polymorphonuclear neutrophils (PMN)
LDH, 425 units/L
Bilirubin, 1.2 mg/dL

D.H. is not taking any prescription medications. What factors make D.H. at risk for folate deficiency?

As with most patients who are folate deficient, D.H. has more than one risk factor. Cocaine and alcohol, together with multiparity complicated by anorexia, nausea, and vomiting, could lead to poor nutrition. Alcohol has toxic effects on the intestinal mucosa and

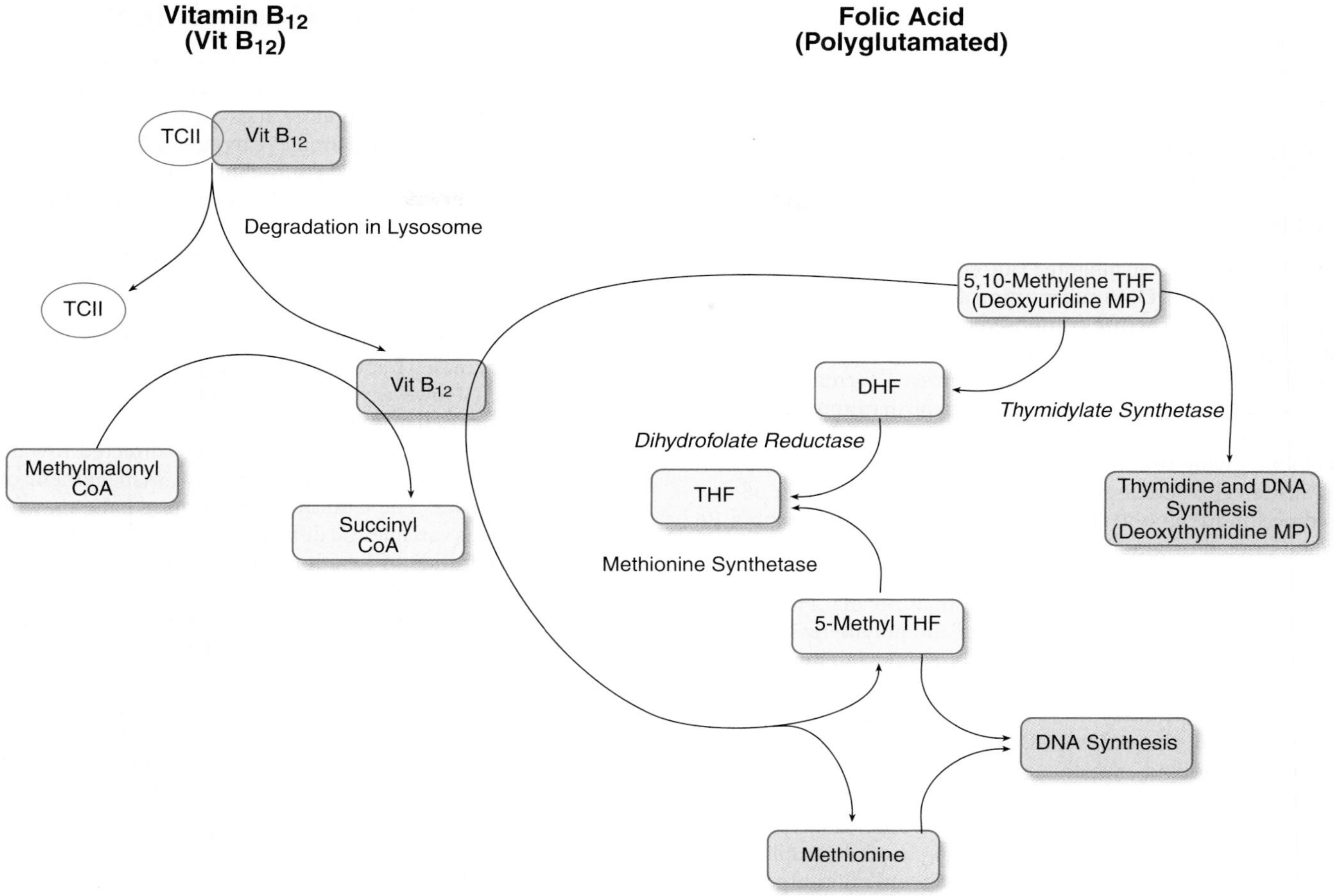

Figure 92-2 Intracellular metabolic pathways. Vitamin B_{12} and folic acid are both necessary for nucleic acid precursors used for DNA synthesis. DHF, dihydrofolate; MP, monophosphate; TCII, transcobalamin II; THF, tetrahydrofolate.

interferes with folate utilization by the bone marrow. D.H. should be asked specifically about her dietary habits and recent weight history. She may have a folate-poor diet for financial reasons or because she is overcooking her food. Alternatively, cocaine may be causing anorexia. The nutritional intake of people who abuse alcohol and drugs is often poor. The diagnosis of folate deficiency is plausible, considering folate deficiency can develop in a matter of weeks to months.

DIAGNOSIS AND MANAGEMENT

Case 92-5, Question 2: Which laboratory values support the diagnosis of folate deficiency? How should D.H. be treated and monitored?

D.H.'s laboratory values reflect macrocytic anemia (Hct, 25.5%; MCV, 112 fL) with pancytopenia (reduced number of RBCs, WBCs, and platelets). Serum vitamin B_{12} concentrations reflect normal vitamin B_{12} stores, but folate stores are inadequate as exemplified by the low RBC folate concentration, pancytopenia, and macrocytic anemia.

Serum folate concentrations generally reflect folate balance during the past 3 weeks although one balanced meal can raise serum levels and falsely elevate body stores. Tissue folate stores are more accurately reflected by the RBC polyglutamated folate content, which is approximately 10 to 30 times the corresponding serum folate concentrations.[41] Hemolysis or vitamin B_{12} deficiency causes leakage of monoglutamated folates from cells, thereby falsely elevating serum folate levels.[42]

D.H. should be counseled regarding her nutritional and social habits. Because the estimated total body folate store is only about 5 to 10 mg, 1 mg of folic acid given daily for 2 to 3 weeks should be more than adequate to replace her storage pool of folate. Higher dosages (up to 5 mg) may be needed, however, if absorption is compromised by alcohol or other factors.[38] Once stores are replenished, D.H. should continue folate supplements throughout her pregnancy and lactation period. She should be reassessed after the course of therapy to determine response to therapy and whether the cause of the folate deficiency has been corrected. Supplementation with folic acid 1 mg/day may be required as long as risk factors are present. D.H.'s fetus is unlikely to develop folate deficiency because maternal folate is preferentially delivered to the fetus; however, sustained folate deficiency during pregnancy can cause birth defects in the newborns (see Chapter 49, Obstetric Drug Therapy).

D.H.'s response to therapy can be monitored by several different parameters. Although bone marrow aspirates are not obtained routinely, the RBC morphology should begin to revert back to normal within 24 to 48 hours after therapy is initiated, and hypersegmented neutrophils should disappear in the periphery in about 1 week. Serum chemistry and hemogram studies should begin to normalize within 10 days. The reticulocyte count should increase by day 2 to 3 and peak by day 10. Bilirubin and LDH values should normalize in 1 to 3 weeks. Finally, the anemia should be corrected in 1 to 2 months. Once anemia is corrected, 100 mcg daily of folate as a nutritional supplement should be adequate for maintenance treatment (independent of the patient's pregnancy/lactation status).

SICKLE CELL ANEMIA

Pathogenesis

Sickle cell anemia is an inherited, autosomal recessive Hgb disorder characterized by a DNA substitution at the β-globin gene.[43] Hgb is a quaternary structure composed of two α-globin chains and two β-globin chains ($\alpha 2\beta 2$) in adults. During fetal development, the γ-globin is the primary β-globin expressed, forming fetal Hgb (HbF or $\alpha 2\gamma 2$). Normally, the period from birth to approximately 3 to 6 months of age is marked by the replacement of γ-globin with β-globin, giving rise to the adult form of Hgb (HbA, $\alpha 2\beta 2$).[44,45]

Sickle cell anemia results from a DNA substitution of thymidine for adenine in the glutamic acid codon, forming a B6 valine instead of glutamic acid.[45] βS represents the inheritance of the sickle β-globin gene.[46] The Hgb produced from this substitution has a more negative charge than normal HbA and in the deoxygenated state will aggregate and polymerize, forming sickled RBCs.[44,45] Sickled RBCs are more rigid and may become "lodged" when passing through the microvasculature, resulting in vascular occlusions.

In addition, the sickled RBC surface contains rearranged aminophospholipids, which augment the ability of the RBC to initiate coagulation, adhere to vascular endothelium, and activate complement. Abnormal interactions with other cell types cause hemolysis and vaso-occlusion, producing several complications such as anemia, pain, increased infections, and multi-organ damage.[44] For these reasons, much effort has been focused on neonatal diagnosis to reduce morbidity and mortality in children younger than 3 years of age.[47]

More than one inheritance pattern results in abnormal Hgb polymerization. Patients with sickle cell anemia are homozygous, inheriting a sickle gene from each parent ($\alpha 2\beta S2$), whereas patients with sickle cell trait are heterozygous and have inherited the sickle cell gene from one parent and the HbA gene from the other parent ($\alpha 2\beta A\beta S$). Other inheritance patterns include patients with a sickle cell gene and a hemoglobin C (HbC) gene (in which glutamic acid is substituted for lysine B6 [$\alpha 2\beta S\beta C$]). Patients may also inherit the sickle cell gene and the β-thalassemic gene ($\alpha 2\beta S\beta S$thal), in which case the clinical course is less severe than with patients diagnosed with sickle cell anemia.[48] Hematologic abnormalities are more commonly observed in patients with sickle cell anemia and less often in those with sickle cell HbC disease or sickle cell β_0-thalassemia.[44,45]

Laboratory Evaluation

In patients with sickle cell disease, the WBC and platelet counts often are elevated, but the WBC differential is normal.[44] The reticulocyte count can range from 5% to 15%, and the MCV may be elevated. If MCV values are within the normal range, iron deficiency or β_0-thalassemia must be considered. Sickled cells may be visually observed in poorly oxygenated blood of a patient with sickle cell anemia. In contrast, a patient with the sickle cell trait should have normal RBC morphology and WBC, reticulocyte, and platelet counts. Sickled cells are rarely observed. In patients with sickle cell β_0-thalassemia, hematologic abnormalities vary depending on the amount of HbA present. This form may be difficult to distinguish from sickle cell anemia; RBC microcytosis may be the only differentiating parameter.[44]

Clinical Course and Management

Part of efforts to improve outcomes in this population include routine screening for sickle cell anemia or sickle cell trait in newborns in the United States. Therefore, most patients are diagnosed during their first year of life. Families carrying sickle cell trait or disease are referred for genetic counseling. Patients with sickle cell disease are referred to a hematologist and multidisciplinary team for medical management.

Patients carrying the sickle cell trait experience milder symptoms than those with sickle cell anemia. The kidney is commonly affected by microinfarction, which occurs in the renal medulla and impairs the kidney's ability to concentrate urine. During pregnancy, an increased frequency of urinary tract infections and hematuria is seen. However, vaso-occlusive events are uncommon and are usually caused by hypoxic conditions.

Treatment of sickle cell anemia is largely directed toward prophylaxis against infections and supportive management of vaso-occlusive crises. The clinical course among patients with sickle cell disease is variable and difficult to predict. Some patients experience a multitude of health problems. Organs such as the kidneys, retina, spleen, and bones are frequent sites of vaso-occlusive events because these sites have a relatively low pH and oxygen tension. Cardiac, pulmonary, neurologic, hepatobiliary, obstetric/gynecologic, ocular, dermatologic, or orthopedic complications can also occur. The management of these complications is organ specific and primarily aimed at supportive interventions.

Sickle cell HbC disease is usually associated with few clinical complications. These patients may have normal physical examination findings with only splenomegaly. Patients are at risk for bacterial infections and, because of elevated Hgb levels, they may experience ocular, orthopedic, and pulmonary vaso-occlusive events.[44,48]

INFECTIONS

CASE 92-6

QUESTION 1: B.C. is a 4-month-old girl who has recently been diagnosed with sickle cell anemia (both parents positive for sickle cell trait). Her older sibling is positive for sickle cell trait but is asymptomatic.

How does B.C.'s diagnosis affect her risk of infections?

B.C. is at an increased risk for infections because sickle cell anemia causes defects in splenic function, complement activation, granulocyte function, and B-cell immunity, as well as micronutrient deficiencies.[49] Impaired splenic function increases B.C.'s risk for infection from polysaccharide-encapsulated bacteria such as *Streptococcus pneumoniae*, *Haemophilus influenzae*, *Neisseria meningitidis*, and *Salmonella typhimurium*. These infections occur most frequently in early childhood, although B.C. will have a lifelong increased risk of infection. Pneumonia caused by *S. pneumoniae*, mycoplasma, or viruses can worsen hypoxia, causing progression to vaso-occlusion and acute chest syndrome (discussed in more depth below). Pulmonary complications from pneumonia or vascular occlusion can also lead to right-sided heart failure. Other infectious conditions such as osteomyelitis from *Staphylococcus aureus* or *S. typhimurium* or urinary tract infections caused by *Escherichia coli* are common complications in patients with sickle cell anemia.[44,46]

CASE 92-6, QUESTION 2: What preventive measures should be taken to prevent infections in B.C.?

Patients with sickle cell anemia should use general preventive measures, such as frequent hand-washing, avoiding sick contacts, and thoroughly cooking foods that may carry *Salmonella* (e.g., chicken or eggs).[49] Children should be closely monitored for symptoms and antibiotic therapy should be instituted at the earliest sign of infection. Prophylactic administration of penicillin has significantly reduced morbidity and mortality from pneumonia in children younger than 3 years of age[50] and is recommended to be continued through age 5.[46] Patients such as B.C. should receive 62.5 mg twice daily during the first year of life, increased to 125 mg twice daily for ages 1 through 3, then 250 mg twice daily until the age of 5. The US guidelines recommend discontinuing penicillin prophylaxis at age 5 unless the child has undergone splenectomy or has had an invasive pneumococcal infection.[51]

Vaccines that are recommended for patients with homozygous sickle cell include all standard pediatric and adult vaccines. B.C. also should receive the pneumococcal 23-valent polysaccharide vaccine at 2 and 5 years of age with a booster every 10 years throughout her life.[47] Because patients with sickle cell typically respond poorly, only 50% of patients will be protected by vaccination. Therefore, there is a continued need for penicillin prophylaxis in young children.[52]

CASE 92-6, QUESTION 3: B.C. is now 3 years old and presents with pallor and significantly decreased activity. Her mother notes that some of B.C.'s daycare classmates have been experiencing a mild viral illness and rash. Her pediatrician obtains a CBC with the following results:

Hgb, 6.2 g/dL
Hct, 18.1%
Platelets, 97,000/μL
Reticulocyte count, 0.5%
WBC count, 6,000/μL

What is a potential cause of B.C.'s symptoms and how should they be managed?

Human parvovirus (HPV) B19 is a common cause of transient RBC aplasia, with up to 67% of infections resulting in a hematologic change typical of aplasia.[53] It is a common, highly contagious childhood infection with more than 70% of adults testing seropositive.[49] Nearly 70% of all homozygous sickle cell patients are HPV B19 seropositive by 20 years of age.[54] In normal individuals, the infection is asymptomatic or presents as mild flu-like symptoms with or without a generalized maculopapular rash. The virus also infects RBC progenitor cells in the bone marrow, causing a temporary 7- to 10-day cessation of erythropoiesis in 65% to 80% of infected individuals. In normal individuals, RBC lifespan is 120 days and this does not typically produce symptoms. Patients with sickle cell anemia have an RBC lifespan of 5 to 15 days, so the temporary break in erythropoiesis leads to a severe anemia. Thrombocytopenia has been noted in approximately one-fourth of those infected with less than 20% of patients experiencing neutropenia. Although most children recover within 2 weeks, the majority will require blood transfusions to manage anemia.

Vaso-occlusive Complications

CASE 92-7

QUESTION 1: J.T. is an 18-year-old man with sickle cell anemia who presented to the emergency department with rapid onset of abdominal pain and shortness of breath.

During early childhood, he experienced several episodes of acute pain, swelling of the hands and feet, and jaundice. Three years before this admission, J.T. required a left hip replacement due to osteonecrosis caused by sickle cell anemia. Recently, frequent blood transfusions have reduced the frequency of sickling crises.

Physical examination reveals J.T. as a thin black man in acute distress and with scleral icterus. He has a pulse of 118 beats/minute, a respiratory rate of 17 breaths/minute, and a temperature of 98.8°F. His lungs are clear. Splenomegaly is noted, and a chest radiograph reveals only cardiomegaly.

A CBC is obtained. Notable results include the following:

Hgb, 5.9 g/dL
Hct, 27%
WBC count, 5,000/μL
Platelets, 335,000/μL
Reticulocyte count, 1%
Bilirubin, 5.8 mg/dL
Serum creatinine, 3.1 mg/dL
Blood urea nitrogen, 54 mg/dL

The peripheral blood smear shows target cells with an occasional sickled cell. What signs and symptoms are consistent with sickle cell anemia? What is J.T.'s current complication?

Vaso-occlusive crisis, or "sickle cell crisis," is caused by severe pain and organ damage. These may be precipitated by many factors including hypoxia, dehydration, infection, and pregnancy.[55] Based on the presence of splenomegaly and anemia with target and sickled cells, J.T. currently is presenting with an acute splenic sequestration crisis. Acute splenic sequestration is caused by the trapping of RBCs within the spleen. This causes splenomegaly and progressive anemia. The low reticulocyte count is consistent with acute sequestration because a reticulocyte response would be expected if the anemia had developed in recent days. J.T.'s inadequate reticulocyte response may reflect rapid progression of the anemia, HPV B19 infection, or a blunted EPO response secondary to compromised renal dysfunction.

CASE 92-7, QUESTION 2: How should J.T. be treated?

J.T.'s signs and symptoms are sufficiently serious to justify transfusion therapy.[51] In addition, J.T. should be adequately hydrated, considering his elevated serum creatinine and blood urea nitrogen. Because patients with sickle cell anemia often lose the ability to concentrate urine, they may become dehydrated, which further contributes to cell sickling. The pain associated with a crisis typically lasts at least 2 to 6 days and should be managed with analgesics including parenteral opioids for severe pain. Pain control should be aggressively instituted for J.T.'s comfort and should be continued for a few days after hospital discharge (also see Chapter 55, Pain Management). It is important not to withhold opioids because of a fear of addiction.[55]

Splenectomy may be indicated in instances of severe splenomegaly, repeated infarction, or pain in adults and it is indicated when crises occur in children. Those patients with sickle cell anemia who are bedridden should be placed on chronic heparin therapy to prevent vascular occlusions and deep vein thrombosis.

CASE 92-7, QUESTION 3: J.T. presents to the emergency department 3 months later with complaints of fever, cough, and severe throbbing pain in his chest and abdomen beginning 2 days prior. This is his third admission within the last year. Notable laboratory results include the following:

Hgb, 6.6 g/dL
Hct, 18.9%

Platelets, 218,000/μL
WBC, 19,700/μL
Bilirubin, 4.7 mg/dL
Serum creatinine, 1.1 mg/dL

His chest radiograph shows diffuse interstitial infiltrates in both lung fields. His vital signs are as follows: blood pressure, 98/53 mm Hg; heart rate, 102 beats/minute; respiratory rate, 23 breaths/minute; temperature, 101.4°F; and oxygen saturation, 93%. What complication of sickle cell disease is J.T. experiencing and how should he be treated for this condition?

J.T. is experiencing acute chest syndrome, a leading cause of morbidity and mortality in patients with sickle cell disease. The diagnosis of acute chest syndrome is determined by new pulmonary infiltrates on chest radiograph with one or more of the following: fever, cough, worsening anemia, and pleuritic or nonpleuritic chest pain. Patients may also experience shortness of breath, rales, hypoxia, and wheezing (more commonly in children).[51] Causes of acute chest syndrome include pulmonary fat embolism, pulmonary infarction, and infection.[3] Commonly implicated organisms include *Chlamydia pneumoniae*, *Mycoplasma pneumoniae*, *S. pneumoniae*, *Haemophilus influenzae*, and various viruses.

The primary goal of treatment is to prevent progression to acute respiratory failure; therefore, treatment should involve pain management, hydration, oxygen supplementation, incentive spirometry, antibiotics, and, potentially, transfusion.[51] Optimal pain control and incentive spirometry are important to prevent hypoventilation and atelectasis, as well as to increase patient comfort. Oxygen should be administered nasally to patients who are moderately hypoxemic (O_2 saturation, 92%–95%; Pao_2, 70–80 mm Hg), as J.T. is. Patients who are febrile or severely ill should receive IV broad-spectrum antibiotics as it is difficult to exclude bacterial causes of acute chest syndrome. Empiric antibiotic therapy should take into account the commonly implicated organisms described above.

Transfusions are used to increase the oxygen affinity of blood and are indicated in patients with hypoxemia or whose clinical status is deteriorating and with a hemoglobin >1.0 g/dL less than baseline. J.T. should be monitored closely for deteriorating respiratory function and should receive transfusions if his clinical status does not improve.

TREATMENT FOR FREQUENT VASO-OCCLUSIVE CRISES

CASE 92-7, QUESTION 4: What preventive therapies exist for J.T. that will reduce occurrences of vaso-occlusive crises?

Hemoglobin F has a protective effect against Hgb polymerization. Investigators have observed that patients with HbF levels greater than 20% experience a relatively mild or benign course with fewer vaso-occlusive crises.[55] Hydroxyurea has been found to increase HbF synthesis which may decrease RBC sickling and the occurrence of disease-related complications.[56–58] Hydroxyurea is used prophylactically in patients with recurrent moderate-to-severe vaso-occlusive crises but not in acute treatment. The use of hydroxyurea in the sickle cell population should be carefully weighed for risk versus benefit, because it is a cytotoxic agent associated with bone marrow suppression. The US guidelines recommend hydroxyurea for adult patients who have three or more sickle cell-associated moderate-to-severe pain crises in a 12-month period.[51] Patients taking hydroxyurea should have bone marrow studies performed before therapy and periodically during therapy. Other adverse effects of hydroxyurea include GI effects (nausea, vomiting, diarrhea), dermatologic effects (maculopapular rash, pruritus), and potential risk of developing a secondary neoplasm (leukemia) with prolonged use. The treatment dose of hydroxyurea for sickle cell anemia is 15 to 35 mg/kg/day. Goals of therapy include improvement in pain and well-being, increase in HbF, increased Hgb (if severely anemic), and maintenance of acceptable platelet and granulocyte counts. After initiation of therapy, blood counts should be monitored closely and the dose adjusted based on efficacy and tolerability. Several clinical trials evaluating hydroxyurea show improvement in the clinical course of patients with sickle cell anemia.[57,59] Other areas of potential promise for the treatment of sickle cell anemia include bone marrow transplantation and gene therapy.[60,61]

IRON CHELATION THERAPY

CASE 92-7, QUESTION 5: Despite optimal treatment with hydroxyurea, J.T. continues to experience exacerbations of his sickle cell disease requiring blood transfusions. J.T. estimates he has required six such transfusions in the last 2 years and at least 25 units of blood in his lifetime. During a visit with his hematologist, J.T.'s serum ferritin is noted to be 1,050 mcg/L. What potential adverse effect of treatment is the hematologist's concern? What other tests may be performed to detect this?

Patients requiring chronic transfusions of PRBCs are at an increased risk for iron toxicity due to iron overload.[62] Normally, plasma iron binds with transferrin; however, if transferrin becomes saturated, patients will have higher levels of toxic nontransferrin-bound iron. As nontransferrin-bound iron increases, it deposits in other organs, most frequently the liver. Therefore, nontransferrin-bound iron produces free radicals, causing tissue damage and fibrosis.

Patients with sickle cell disease should be monitored for iron overload.[51] Obtaining a serum ferritin level is the most commonly used method of screening for iron overload, although the accuracy of this test is affected by inflammatory processes. Thus, serial serum ferritin values should be obtained when patients are not experiencing an acute crisis (i.e., steady-state values). More specific tests such as magnetic resonance imaging measure iron levels in organs such as the heart, liver, pancreas, and spleen although may not be routinely used because of cost.[62] The gold standard for assessing iron overload is liver iron concentration by biopsy, although this is an invasive procedure that should be performed by specialists.

CASE 92-7, QUESTION 6: J.T. returns for continued assessment of iron overload. His repeat serum ferritin levels are 1,357 mcg/L and 1,500 mcg/L (3 months apart). Liver iron concentration is 7.8 mg/g dry weight. Does J.T. meet the criteria to receive iron chelation therapy? What options are available?

J.T. meets criteria for iron chelation therapy because of his steady-state serum ferritin levels being consistently more than 1,000 mcg/L and his liver iron concentration being greater than 7 mg/g dry weight.[51] Other considerations for a patient to receive iron chelation therapy include transfusion of approximately 100 mL/kg of PRBCs, or 20 units for a 40-kg or more patient.

There are three iron chelators currently approved for use in patients with sickle cell disease; their dosing and adverse effects are summarized in Table 92-10. These agents work by binding free iron present in circulation and tissues. The iron is then excreted in the urine and bile.

Deferoxamine (DFO) is the oldest agent and has the most clinical experience. Deferoxamine and deferasirox have been studied in patients with sickle cell disease who are as young as 2 years

Table 92-10
FDA-Approved Iron Chelation Therapies

Medication	Dose	Frequency	Route	Common/Serious Adverse Effects	Notes
Deferoxamine (DFO)	25–50 mg/kg/day, titrate to effect (Maximal dose 40 mg/kg for children)	Daily, Monday–Friday	SC for 8–12 hours	*Common:* headache, upper respiratory tract infection, abdominal pain, nausea, vomiting, pyrexia, pain, arthralgia, cough, nasopharyngitis, constipation, chest pain, injection site reactions, muscle spasms, viral infection *Serious:* audiotoxicity, hepatotoxicity, nephrotoxicity, ocular toxicity, hypotension, anaphylaxis, respiratory distress syndrome, growth retardation	Requires a syringe pump or balloon infuser; Rotate sites to prevent scarring
Deferasirox	Exjade: 20 mg/kg, titrate to effect Jadenu: 14 mg/kg, titrate to effect	Once daily	Exjade: oral drink Jadenu: oral tablet	*Common:* headache, abdominal pain, nausea, pyrexia, vomiting, diarrhea, back pain, upper respiratory tract infection, arthralgia, pain, cough, nasopharyngitis, rash, constipation, chest pain *Serious:* nephrotoxicity, cytopenias, hepatic failure, GI hemorrhage, anaphylaxis, ocular disturbances	Exjade should be dissolved in juice for administration
Deferiprone	75 mg/kg/day (divided into 3 doses of 25 mg/kg), titrate to effect (max dose 99 mg/kg/day)	3 times daily	Oral tablet	*Common:* chromaturia, nausea, vomiting, abdominal pain, ALT increased, arthralgia, neutropenia *Serious:* agranulocytosis/neutropenia, hepatotoxicity, zinc deficiency	Urine may be discolored red-brown. Pregnancy category D

FDA, Food and Drug Administration; GI, gastrointestinal; SC, subcutaneously.

old; deferiprone is not approved for use in children. Because of its short half-life, DFO must be administered daily via continuous IV or subcutaneous infusion for 5 days. Deferasirox has a longer half-life, allowing for once-daily oral administration and enhanced patient convenience and adherence. A study of 195 patients with sickle cell disease observed similar reductions in iron levels between patients receiving DFO and patients receiving deferasirox at comparable doses.[63] Additionally, more patients in the deferasirox group reported their treatment was convenient.[62] Deferiprone has predominantly been studied in patients with transfusional iron overload with inadequate response to other iron chelating therapies although it has been shown to be similar to deferasirox in patients with sickle cell anemia.[64] Deferoxamine is associated with more dose-dependent oculotoxicity and audiotoxicity, although both agents may cause this.[65,66] Deferasirox has been associated with more nephrotoxicity, hepatotoxicity, and cytopenias. Either DFO or deferasirox is appropriate for J.T. at this time.

J.T. should also receive appropriate monitoring consisting of serial serum ferritin levels and annual audiology and ophthalmology assessments. Some centers obtain a liver biopsy every 2 years during treatment to assess efficacy.[51] Patients receiving deferasirox should have serum creatinine monitored weekly for the first month after initiation or a dose alteration and monthly thereafter.[51] Monthly monitoring for proteinuria and assessment of liver function tests should also be initiated for patients receiving deferasirox.

Other Complications of Sickle Cell Disease

NEUROLOGIC COMPLICATIONS

Neurologic complications are age dependent. Stroke most commonly occurs in the first decade of life, whereas intracerebral hemorrhage is a complication associated with adulthood. Primary prevention of stroke with RBC transfusions targeted to maintain HbS level less than 30% reduces the incidence of stroke in high-risk patients by 92%.[67] If a stroke occurs, approximately 50% of patients experience recurrent strokes within 3 years unless they are treated by chronic RBC transfusion therapy.[45] A concern with RBC transfusion therapy is iron overload. Conflicting evidence exists regarding the benefit of chronic hydroxyurea plus phlebotomy (removal of blood to reduce iron burden) as an alternative option to prevent secondary stroke.[68,69]

RENAL AND GENITAL COMPLICATIONS

Renal and genital complications are common in sickle cell disease because the environment (hypoxic, acidotic, and hypertonic) predisposes the renal medulla or corpus cavernosum to infarction. As a result, patients might experience reduced potassium excretion, hyperuricemia, hematuria, hyposthenuria, and renal failure. Patients with renal disease generally have inappropriately low levels of EPO as well. Men experiencing occlusion of the corpus cavernosum can experience acute or chronic priapism. Conservative management includes IV fluid administration and pain control. Refractory cases may require surgery.[44,46]

MICROINFARCTIONS

Microinfarctions often produce ophthalmic, hepatic, orthopedic, and obstetric/gynecologic complications as well. Patients with sickle cell anemia may require screening to detect these complications.[51]

ANEMIA OF INFLAMMATION

Anemia of inflammation (AI), also known as anemia of chronic disease, refers to a mild-to-moderate anemia that results from decreased RBC survival and production and generally occurs over months to years.[70] It has been associated with a number of disorders (e.g., autoimmune disorders, acute and chronic infections, chronic kidney disease, and malignancy).[71] Because of the common occurrence of such conditions, AI is encountered frequently and has been estimated to be the second most common anemia after iron deficiency. Most often, AI is a normochromic, normocytic anemia, although RBCs may be hypochromic and microcytic in less than a quarter of patients.[72] A prominent feature of AI is the altered availability of iron which is not reliably reflected in iron indices due to an increase of hepcidin, a hormone that regulates iron metabolism.[73] Additionally, the EPO response may be inappropriate for the degree of anemia.[74]

The pathogenesis of AI is not well understood. It appears the production of inflammatory cytokines such as interferon-γ, tumor necrosis factor-α, IL-6, and IL-1 leads to either activation of macrophages that consume and destroy erythrocytes or the suppression of erythropoiesis by inhibition of RBC precursors, such as BFUe.[75] In response to inflammation, elevated levels of IL-6 upregulate hepcidin production through the JAK-STAT pathway, inhibiting the release of iron stores to the plasma. This high concentration leads to hypoferremia (functional iron deficiency) and blunted erythrocyte production.[73] Hepcidin can further alter iron hemostasis by decreasing duodenal iron absorption.[72] A review of iron studies is important to distinguish AI from iron deficiency anemia. In AI, serum iron, transferrin saturation, and TIBC are low with an increased serum ferritin. Conversely, in iron deficiency anemia, serum iron, transferrin saturation, and serum ferritin are low with an increased TIBC. However, it is important to recognize that both forms of anemia may be seen concurrently in patients with AI.

Management of mild-to-moderate AI usually focuses on the underlying disease process. Anemia of inflammation is not usually progressive or life threatening, although it generally affects a patient's quality of life. Patients may require blood transfusions for symptomatic anemia which are associated with risks such as hepatitis, viral infections, iron overload, treatment-related acute lung injury, and immunogenic reactions. Unless a concurrent deficiency of vitamin B_{12} or folate exists, administration of vitamin supplements for AI is not of value. Iron supplementation may be warranted in patients with a functional or absolute iron deficiency anemia. Erythropoiesis-stimulating agents (ESAs) have been used successfully to treat AI in patients with rheumatoid arthritis, acquired immunodeficiency syndrome (AIDS), malignancy, and chronic kidney disease; however, medication costs and increased safety risks can be significant and risk versus benefits should be assessed when determining treatment.[72,74]

Erythropoietic Therapy

Erythropoietic therapy is indicated for use in anemia associated with chronic kidney disease, drug-induced anemia (myelosuppressive chemotherapy and zidovudine therapy), and autologous blood transfusions for elective noncardiac, nonvascular surgery.[76–78] Response to ESAs is dependent on both dose and the underlying cause of anemia and may take days to weeks to be seen. Currently, there are two ESAs, epoetin alfa (Procrit, Epogen) and darbepoetin alfa (Aranesp), approved for use in the United States. Darbepoetin differs from epoetin alfa by the addition of two carbohydrate chains. The significance of the additional carbohydrate chains is an increased sialic acid content resulting in decreased clearance and a serum half-life 3 times longer than that of epoetin alfa. These kinetic differences allow darbepoetin alfa to be administered less frequently. Table 92-11 illustrates current therapeutic uses of epoetin alfa and darbepoetin alfa. Lack of response to erythropoietic therapy (ESA hyporesponsiveness) in all patient populations is most commonly associated with iron deficiency.

Although some studies assessing the use of ESAs in the treatment of chronic kidney disease and chemotherapy-induced anemia (CIA) have shown benefit (i.e., decreased RBC transfusions), there is also evidence that use increases the risk for cardiovascular events, stroke, thrombosis, shortened overall survival, and/or increased the risk of tumor progression or recurrence in the respective patient populations.[79,80] In 2011, the FDA mandated a Risk Evaluation and Mitigation Strategy (REMS) program based on studies that identified safety concerns with the use of epoetin alpha and darbepoetin alpha. Recently the FDA performed an evaluation of the ESA REMS requirements and found that the requirements had minimal impact on ESA utilization beyond that of CMS coverage determinations and other FDA regulatory

Table 92-11
Therapeutic Uses and Regimens for Recombinant Human Erythropoietin (rhEPO)[a]

	Epoetin Alfa		Darbepoetin Alfa	
Anemia Pathogenesis	**Dose (units/kg)**	**Frequency**	**Dose (mcg/kg)**	**Frequency**
Zidovudine-induced	100	3 ×/week	—	—
Chemotherapy-induced	150 or 40,000 units (total dose)	3 ×/week or once a week, respectively	2.25 or 500 mcg (total dose)	Once a week or once every 3 weeks, respectively
Chronic kidney disease	50–100	3 ×/week	On dialysis 0.45 or 0.75 Not on dialysis 0.45	Once a week or once every 2 weeks, respectively Once every 4 weeks

[a]Adult dosing.

actions. As a result, in 2017, the FDA determined that it is no longer necessary to require the ESA REMS requirements and the risk and benefits of the medications can be communicated by the current product prescribing information. Healthcare providers are encouraged to discuss the risks and benefits of using ESAs with each patient prior to initiating use.

Renal Insufficiency-Related Anemia

The cause of renal insufficiency-related anemia is complex but involves reduced EPO production and a shortened RBC life span. Repeated transfusions are a possible treatment but can lead to complications and should be avoided unless rapid Hgb correction is needed. Because EPO is secreted in the kidney in response to anoxia and is responsible for normal differentiation of RBCs from other stem cells, erythropoietic therapy is used to treat anemia in patients with renal failure who are undergoing hemodialysis.[79,81] A dose-dependent rise in Hct is observed in patients with end-stage renal disease at approved doses of epoetin alfa or darbepoetin alfa (See Table 92-11). Targeting higher concentrations of Hgb (>13 g/dL) is associated with increased mortality and adverse effects. A FDA mandated black-box warning for these drugs states to individualize treatment to maintain use of the lowest dose of an ESA necessary to decrease the need for transfusion.[76–78] This target Hgb differs from the current kidney disease guidelines.[79,82] Refer to Chapter 28, Chronic Kidney Disease, for further information on treatment target goals as well as the appropriate use of ESAs and IV iron in patients with renal insufficiency-related anemia.

Malignancy-Related Anemia

CASE 92-8

QUESTION 1: P.M is a 62-year-old woman diagnosed with Stage IV ovarian cancer. She is being seen for her fourth cycle of chemotherapy with carboplatin and paclitaxel. She reports shortness of breath and fatigue when she walks up stairs but otherwise has a good performance status. Her CBC indicates the following:

Hgb, 9.7 g/dL
Hct, 29%
MCV, 90 mcm^3
Reticulocytes, 100 × 10^3/mcL

The peripheral smear shows normochromic and normocytic RBCs and iron studies are within normal limits. What is the most likely cause of P.M.'s anemia? What is the appropriate treatment?

P.M. appears to have malignancy-related anemia, which can be characterized as AI or CIA. Anemia is common in cancer occurring in up to 30% to 90% of patients.[83] The etiology of anemia in cancer patients is frequently complex and a conglomeration of various attributing factors such as comorbidities, malignancy, blood loss, nutritional deficiencies, and treatment with radiation and/or chemotherapy.[84] Chemotherapy-induced anemia is the result of hematopoietic impairment affecting RBC production and nephrotoxic effects of chemotherapy agents, such a platinum-containing agents, decreasing erythropoietin production.[80] It is generally normocytic and normochromic and develops over the course of treatment.[85] As with P.M., the CIA is often classified as mild to moderate and patients present as asymptomatic or mildly symptomatic (weakness, decreased exercise tolerance).[86] Factors that can influence the incidence of malignancy-related anemia in patients with cancer are the type of malignancy and the stage and duration of disease; the type, schedule, and intensity of treatment; and history of prior myelosuppressive chemotherapy or radiation. Cancer patients receiving chemotherapy should be routinely screened for CIA with a CBC. As per the NCCN Clinical Practice Guidelines in Oncology (NCCN Guidelines), evaluation for CIA should begin at an Hgb ≤11 g/dL. Additional tests including a peripheral blood smear and reticulocyte count as well as other potential causes of anemia should be performed.

The recommended treatment for CIA is comprised of transfusion or use of ESAs with or without iron supplementation.[80] Therapy should be directed to the underlying disease, if possible. When considering treatment options, transfusion with packed red blood cells (PRBC) should be used when rapid correction of Hgb is warranted with an expected 1 g/dL increase in Hgb and 3% increase in Hct with a single unit of PRBC. The use of transfusion for chronic management is associated with known risks, notably an increased risk of thromboembolic events in patients with cancer.[87] Conflicting data exist regarding the effect of transfusion on mortality.[80] ESAs with or without iron supplementation should be considered for long-term management of anemia in a patient with cancer because it has been shown to reduce transfusion requirements. Large, randomized, multicenter trials have failed to show a clinical benefit to using ESAs in anemia that is not chemotherapy-induced. The reported increased risk of mortality and tumor progression in clinical trials of anemic patients with head and neck, breast, nonsmall cell lung, lymphoid, and cervical cancers receiving ESAs resulted in a black-box warning being added to all ESA product information to advise about these and other increases in serious adverse events.[88] ESAs are recommended for anemic patients with cancer who are receiving myelosuppressive chemotherapy and the intent of treatment is not curative, with the possible exception of small cell lung cancer as there are no clinical trials reporting a deleterious impact on survival. As recommended by the FDA, treatment with an ESA should not be initiated until the Hgb is less than 10 g/dL and there is an additional 2 months of chemotherapy planned. The lowest dose needed to avoid RBC transfusion should be given, and use should be discontinued at the end of chemotherapy treatment.[76–78] Although response rates to ESAs have been reported upwards of 70% to 80% in clinical trials, not all patients will respond to treatment.[89] The most common cause of nonresponse to erythropoietic therapy is absolute or functional iron deficiency. Iron studies should be evaluated before and during therapy with supplementation given if needed. Oral or intravenous iron may be used for supplementation but data from clinical trials show intravenous iron is superior when given with an ESA.[80]

In P.M.'s case, the clinician may choose from a number of anemia management options. For example, the current course of chemotherapy can be delayed to allow for hematologic recovery and resolution of anemia symptoms. Alternatively, an RBC transfusion can be given to relieve her symptoms and allow her to better tolerate chemotherapy. Erythropoietic therapy with epoetin alfa or darbepoetin alfa also should be considered because the patient has metastatic disease (not curative) and will continue on chemotherapy until disease progression. Treatment with epoetin alfa or darbepoetin alfa increases Hgb and decreases the need for blood transfusions. If treatment with epoetin alfa is desired for P.M., therapy can be administered at an initial dose of 150 units/kg subcutaneously 3 times a week or 40,000 units once a weekly.[77,78] Alternative dosing regimens, 80,000 units every 2 weeks or 120,000 units every 3 weeks, have proved to be safe and effective in terms of hematopoietic and transfusion effects.[80,90] Darbepoetin alfa is also a treatment option for P.M. Initial dosing of darbepoetin alfa is 2.25 mcg/kg subcutaneously once a week or 500 mcg every 3 weeks.[76,91] Alternative dosing regimens of darbepoetin alfa 100 mcg once weekly, 200 mcg every 2 weeks and 300 mcg every 3 weeks have reported similar beneficial effects seen with epoetin alfa.[93–94] Response of ESAs is monitored by measuring Hgb weekly until stabilization. During this time, the dose should be titrated to the lowest dose needed to avoid transfusion. A minimum of 2 weeks is required before an increase in RBCs is seen. A reduction in dose (25% for epoetin alfa and 40% for darbepoetin alfa) is required if there is a greater than 1 g/dL rise in the Hgb in any 2 week period or the Hgb reaches a level to avoid transfusion. If no response (less than 1 g/dL rise in Hgb and Hgb remains below 10 g/dL) is seen in 4 weeks with epoetin alfa or 6 weeks with darbepoetin alfa, a dose increase should be considered. Common dose escalation schedules for epoetin alfa include escalating to 300 units/kg 3 times a week if initially treated with 150 units/kg 3 times a week or 60,000 units once a week if initially on 40,000 units once a week. Dose escalation for darbepoetin would consist of an increase to 4.5 mcg/kg once weekly if prior treatment was 2.25 mcg/kg weekly. The need for iron supplementation should also be considered at this time. Response should again be assessed at week 8 or 9 and appropriate dose reductions made based on Hgb level or transfusion avoidance. If no Hgb response is noted after 8 or 9 weeks of treatment or transfusions are still required, the drug should be discontinued.[76–78]

Human Immunodeficiency Virus (HIV)-Related Anemia

Anemia is a common finding in patients with HIV and correlates with the severity of disease as well as clinical outcomes.[95] In this patient population, anemia that has been identified is an independent prognostic factor for increased morbidity and mortality.[96] It has also been shown to be a marker of treatment failure in patients who do not achieve viral suppression and thus should be monitored as part of treatment.[97] Several factors may lead to the development of anemia in HIV patients including infections, malignancies, the presence of genetic disorders of hemoglobin, nutritional deficiencies, and the use of combination antiretroviral therapy (cART). Examples of infections includes bacteria (*Mycobacterium avium* complex disease), fungus (Histoplasmosis), and viruses (CMV, herpes simplex viruses type 1 and 2, and HPV B19). The use of myelosuppressive cART drugs such as zidovudine, zalcitabine, didanosine, lamivudine, and other medications often used to treat AIDS-associated illnesses (e.g., bone marrow suppressive chemotherapy, ganciclovir, trimethoprim–sulfamethoxazole, dapsone) also contributes. Additionally conditions like malignancies, Kaposi's sarcoma, and lymphoma, all of which impair normal bone marrow function, predispose these patients to anemia.[98] Vitamin B_{12} deficiency is a contributing cause to anemia in up to a third of patients[97] and is correlated with progression to AIDS.[99] Vitamin B_{12} malabsorption can result from HIV-infected mononuclear cells within the ileum and altered gastric mucosal functioning caused by infection.[100] Alterations in the utilization of vitamin B_{12} and folate[101] can place a patient at risk for hematologic toxicity from drugs such as zidovudine and trimethoprim. More recently, evidence suggests the actual virus may play a role in the pathophysiology resulting in decreased erythropoiesis and erythropoietic response.[95] Common features of HIV-related anemia are comprised of a decreased reticulocyte count, morphologically normochromic and normocytic RBCs, adequate iron stores, and impaired response to erythropoietin.[95]

Treatment for HIV-related anemia consists of erythropoietic therapy or removal of the offending drug, if possible. Erythropoietic therapy has demonstrated increases in Hgb and quality of life in HIV-infected adult patients, regardless of drug therapy, $CD4^+$ count, or viral load.[100] While no longer first-line treatment for HIV in the United States, zidovudine is still used in pregnant women and children as well as in developing countries. Its use is associated with the development of cytopenias, primarily anemia, that occur within 3 to 6 months of beginning treatment.[102] Clinical studies show patients taking zidovudine who have baseline erythropoietin levels less than 500 units/L experience a significant reduction in transfusion requirements.[103] Epoetin alfa therapy may be initiated in patients with zidovudine-induced anemia at 100 units/kg 3 times weekly. RBC indices should be closely monitored. If the Hgb exceeds 12 g/dL, then the dose should be held until it declines to less than 11 g/dL. At that time a dose reduction of 25% or to the lowest dose necessary to prevent RBC transfusion is recommended. If a patient has no response after 8 weeks of therapy, the dose should be increased by 50 to 100 units/kg 3 times weekly at 4- to 8-week intervals or increased to 300 units/kg 3 times weekly. If no response is seen at a dose of 300 units/kg for 8 weeks, it is unlikely that the patient will benefit from further therapy and the drug should be discontinued.[76–78] Alternative once-weekly dosing with epoetin alfa has been evaluated at starting doses of 40,000 units.[104] The use of darbepoetin alfa has been assessed in HIV patients receiving hemodialysis and is as safe and effective as epoetin alfa for treating anemia.[105]

KEY REFERENCES AND WEBSITES

A full list of references for this chapter can be found at http://thepoint.lww.com/AT11e. Below are the key references and websites for this chapter, with the corresponding reference number in this chapter found in parentheses after the reference.

Key References

Booth C et al. Infection in sickle cell disease: a review. *Int J Infect Dis*. 2010;14:e2. (49)

Camaschella C. Iron-deficiency anemia. *New Engl J Med*. 2015;1832:1843. (8)

Gangat N, Wolanskyj AP. Anemia of chronic disease. *Semin Hematol*. 2013;50:232. (72)

KDOQI. KDOQI Clinical Practice Guideline and Clinical Practice Recommendations for anemia in chronic kidney disease: 2007 update of hemoglobin target. *Am J Kidney Dis*. 2007;50:471. (83)

National Comprehensive Cancer Network. NCCN guidelines for cancer- and chemotherapy-induced anemia v1.2018. http://www.nccn.org. Accessed August 3, 2017. (80)

Redding-Lallinger R, Knoll C. Sickle cell disease—pathophysiology and treatment. *Curr Probl Pediatr Adolesc Health Care*. 2006;36:346. (46)

Redig AJ et al. Pathogenesis and clinical implications of HIV-related anemia in 2013. *Hematology Am Soc Hematol Educ Program*. 2013;2013:377. (96)

Snow CF. Laboratory diagnosis of vitamin B_{12} and folate deficiency: a guide for the primary care physician. *Arch Intern Med*. 1999;159:1289. (42)

Stabler SP. Vitamin B_{12} deficiency. *New Eng J Med*. 2013;149–160. (22)

Waldvogel-Abramowski S et al. Physiology of iron metabolism. *Transf Med Hemother*. 2014;41:000. (4)

Key Websites

Kidney Disease Improving Global Outcomes. KIDGO Clinical Practice Guidelines for Anemia in Chronic Kidney Disease. http://www.kdigo.org/clinical_practice_guidelines/pdf/KDIGO-Anemia%20GL.pdf. Accessed June 16, 2015. (79)

National Institutes of Health. National Heart, Lung, and Blood Institute Division of Blood Diseases and Resources. *Evidence-based management of sickle cell disease: Expert Panel Report, 2014*. https://www.nhlbi.nih.gov/sites/www.nhlbi.nih.gov/files/sickle-cell-disease-report.pdf. Accessed June 15, 2015. (51)

93 Neoplastic Disorders and Their Treatment: General Principles

Jaime E. Anderson, Andrea S. Dickens, and Katherine Tipton Patel

CORE PRINCIPLES

	CORE PRINCIPLES	CHAPTER CASES
1	Cancer is a group of diseases characterized by uncontrolled growth and spread of abnormal cells. Tumor metastases to distant sites generally have a greater effect than the primary tumor on the frequency of complications and the patient's quality of life and mortality.	**Case 93-1 (Question 1)**
2	Avoiding known risk factors may prevent cancer. Cancer may also be prevented by appropriate use of vaccines and chemoprevention in selected groups of high-risk patients.	**Case 93-2 (Question 1)**
3	The histologic diagnosis of a tumor is the most important determinant of how a malignancy will be treated. The stage of cancer and the diagnosis influence the treatment and prognosis. As part of staging, diagnostic imaging facilitates identification of disease metastases.	**Case 93-3 (Question 1)**
4	The initial signs and symptoms of malignant disease are variable and depend on histology, location, and tumor size. This may influence treatment options if they affect performance status, which is a measure of a patient's functional capacity.	**Case 93-4 (Question 1)**
5	Cancer is predominately treated with three modalities: surgery, radiation, and systemic therapy. The goal of therapy should always be to cure the patient when possible.	**Case 93-5 (Question 1)**
6	Biochemical resistance to chemotherapy is the major impediment to successful treatment with most cancers. Resistance can occur de novo in cancer cells or develop during cell division as a result of mutation.	**Case 93-6 (Question 1)**
7	There are different types of systemic therapy: chemotherapy, targeted agents, endocrine therapy, and biologic response modifiers. Systemic therapy may be used in varying combinations and different settings. Use depends on histology, cancer stage, and the patient's predicted tolerance of the treatment.	**Case 93-7 (Question 1), Case 93-8 (Question 1), Case 93-9 (Question 1)**
8	Response to treatment is assessed by evaluating therapy's antitumor and toxic effects, including impact on the patient's overall quality of life. Evaluation should occur at scheduled intervals and include physical examination, laboratory tests, and repeat diagnostic imaging.	**Case 93-10 (Question 1)**
9	Systemic therapies used to treat cancer are potentially carcinogenic, teratogenic, or mutagenic. Handling and administering these agents poses a risk to healthcare workers. Appropriate policies and procedures must be in place to maximize safety and minimize risk while following national guidelines and standards.	**Case 93-11 (Questions 1–4)**

INTRODUCTION TO NEOPLASTIC DISORDERS

Cancer (neoplasm, tumor, or malignancy) is not a single disease. It is a group of diseases characterized by uncontrolled growth and spread of abnormal cells. Cancer cells do not respond to the normal processes that regulate cell growth, proliferation, and survival, and they cannot carry out the physiologic functions of their normal counterparts. Other characteristics of cancer cells include their ability to invade adjacent normal tissues and break away from the primary tumor (metastasize) and travel through the blood or lymph to establish new tumors (metastases) at a distant site. Their ability to stimulate the formation of new blood vessels (angiogenesis) and their endless replication potential further contribute to their continued growth and survival.[1] Cancers can arise in any tissue in the body. If cancer cells are allowed to grow uncontrollably, they can eventually result in the death of the patient.

Cancer Statistics

Each year, the American Cancer Society publishes an estimate for the number of new cases and number of cancer-related deaths. The National Cancer Institute publishes cancer statistics that include cancer risk, prevalence, and survival information.[2] The American Cancer Society estimates that 1 of 2 American men and 1 of 3 American women will eventually develop cancer and that approximately 1,658,370 new cases of cancer will be diagnosed in 2015.[3] The most common cancers and causes of cancer-related deaths in adult Americans are listed in Table 93-1. The incidence of cancer and cancer-related deaths can be affected by both age and ethnic background, with the incidence greater in the elderly and African-American populations.[3] Other factors that are associated with an individual's increased risk for cancer include environmental and lifestyle factors, genetic predisposition, immunosuppression, and exposure to one or more potential carcinogens.[4]

Etiology

Cancers arise from the transformation of a single normal cell. Damage or mutation to the cell's DNA is caused by an initial "event." These events may include lifestyle, environmental, or occupational factors, as well as some medical therapies (e.g., cytotoxic chemotherapy, immunosuppressive or radiation therapy) and hereditary factors. Cigarette smoking is probably the single largest factor that contributes to cancer development, responsible for approximately 30% of cancer deaths per year. Other preventable causes, including physical inactivity, obesity, and nutrition, are estimated to cause an additional 30% of cancer deaths per year.[5] An estimated two million skin cancers diagnosed yearly are also potentially preventable with adequate skin protection.[6]

Cancer is a genetic disease. Two gene classes, oncogenes and tumor suppressor genes, are important in the pathogenesis of cancer. Damage to cellular DNA can result in mutations that lead to the development of oncogenes and loss or inactivation of tumor suppressor genes. Oncogenes are genes whose overactivity or presence in certain forms can lead to the development of cancer. Oncogenes arise from normal genes called proto-oncogenes through genetic alterations such as chromosomal translocations, deletions, insertions, and point mutations.

Table 93-1

Estimated Sites of New Cancer Cases and Deaths in the United States, 2015[3]

Estimated New Cases

Males		Females	
Prostate	220,800 (26%)	Breast	231,840 (29%)
Lung and bronchus	115,610 (14%)	Lung and bronchus	105,590 (13%)
Colon and rectum	69,090 (8%)	Colon and rectum	63,610 (8%)
Urinary bladder	56,320 (7%)	Uterine corpus	54,870 (7%)
Melanoma of the skin	42,670 (5%)	Thyroid	47,230 (6%)
Non-Hodgkin lymphoma	39,850 (5%)	Non-Hodgkin lymphoma	32,000 (4%)
Kidney and renal pelvis	38,270 (5%)	Melanoma of the skin	31,200 (4%)
Oral cavity and pharynx	32,670 (4%)	Pancreas	24,120 (3%)
Leukemia	30,900 (4%)	Leukemia	23,370 (3%)
Liver and intrahepatic bile duct	25,510 (3%)	Kidney and renal pelvis	23,290 (3%)
All sites	**848,200(100%)**	**All sites**	**810,170 (100%)**

Estimated Deaths

Males		Females	
Lung and bronchus	86,380 (28%)	Lung and bronchus	71,660 (26%)
Prostate	27,540 (9%)	Breast	40,290 (15%)
Colon and rectum	26,100 (8%)	Colon and rectum	23,600 (9%)
Pancreas	20,710 (7%)	Pancreas	19,850 (7%)
Liver and intrahepatic bile duct	17,030 (5%)	Ovary	14,180 (5%)
Leukemia	14,210 (5%)	Leukemia	10,240 (4%)
Esophagus	12,600 (4%)	Uterine corpus	10,170 (4%)
Urinary bladder	11,510 (4%)	Non-Hodgkin lymphoma	8,310 (3%)
Non-Hodgkin lymphoma	11,480 (4%)	Liver and intrahepatic bile duct	7,520 (3%)
Kidney and renal pelvis	9,070 (3%)	Brain and other nervous system	6,380 (2%)
All sites	**312,150 (100%)**	**All sites**	**277,280 (100%)**

Source: Siegel RL et al. Cancer statistics, 2015. *CA Cancer J Clin*. 2015:65(1):5–29.

Section 16 Hematology and Oncology

Growth and proliferation of normal cells are influenced by proteins, known as growth factors. When growth factors bind to receptors on the cell surface, they activate a series of enzymes within the cell that stimulate cell signaling pathways and gene transcription. These genes encode for proteins that regulate cell growth and proliferation. The coordination and integration of cellular signaling processes are referred to as signal transduction. Proto-oncogenes are responsible for encoding several components of signal transduction pathways, including growth factors, growth factor receptors, signaling enzymes, and DNA transcription factors. Abnormal forms or excessive quantities of these stimulatory proteins disrupt normal cell growth signaling pathways, leading to excessive growth and proliferation and, ultimately, a malignant transformation.

Tumor suppressor genes are normal genes that encode for proteins that suppress inappropriate cell division or growth. Gene deletions or mutations can cause these proteins to become inactivated, eliminating the normal inhibition of cell division. Alterations in a third class of genes, DNA repair genes, are also implicated in cancer. DNA repair genes encode for proteins that correct errors that may arise during DNA duplication. Mutations in these genes further contribute to the accumulation of genetic changes that promote cancer progression.

Cancer development is a multistep process. Therefore, multiple genetic mutations, including activation of oncogenes and loss or inactivation of tumor suppressor genes within a cell, are necessary for malignant transformation.[7] Additional genetic changes are required for tumor invasion of normal tissues and metastases.

Tumor Growth

CELL CYCLE

Cancer cells, like normal cells, proceed through a specific and orderly set of events during cellular replication referred to as the cell cycle (Fig. 93-1). The cell cycle contains four phases (M, G_1, S, and G_2), each responsible for a different task necessary for cell division. During the first activity phase, the M phase, the cell undergoes mitosis, the process of cell division. After mitosis, the cell enters the first gap or resting phase (G_1). During the G_1 resting (or gap) phase, the cell makes the enzymes necessary for DNA synthesis. The synthesis of DNA occurs during the S phase. After S phase, the cell enters a second resting phase (G_2). RNA and other proteins are synthesized to prepare for cell division during M phase. Cells that complete mitosis may either continue to proceed through the cell cycle to divide again, differentiate or mature into specialized cells and eventually die, or enter a third resting phase called G_0.[8]

Proliferation of normal cells is carefully controlled to balance the loss of mature functional cells with the production of new cells. As mentioned, proto-oncogenes and tumor suppressor genes provide the stimulatory and inhibitory signals, respectively, that regulate the cell cycle. The transition of cells through the cell cycle is an ordered, tightly regulated process, which involves a series of checkpoints that assess these signals and the number and integrity of the cells.[8] Cyclins, a group of interacting proteins found in the nucleus, and cyclin-dependent kinases (CDKs) make up the molecular machinery that regulates passage of cells through various phases of the cell cycle. The cyclins combine with CDKs to form complexes that act as molecular switches. One of these molecular switches regulates whether a cell moves through a critical restriction point that occurs late in G_1 phase to S phase. If insufficient amounts of cyclins or CDK are present during G_1 phase, the cell will not enter S phase to start cell division. Cells that pass through this restriction point are irreversibly committed to the next phase of the cell cycle.[8] A decline in the level of the CDK complex signals the end of the phase. The balance of regulation of cyclins and CDKs is influenced by several factors, including cyclin gene transcription, cyclin degradation, CDK inhibitors,

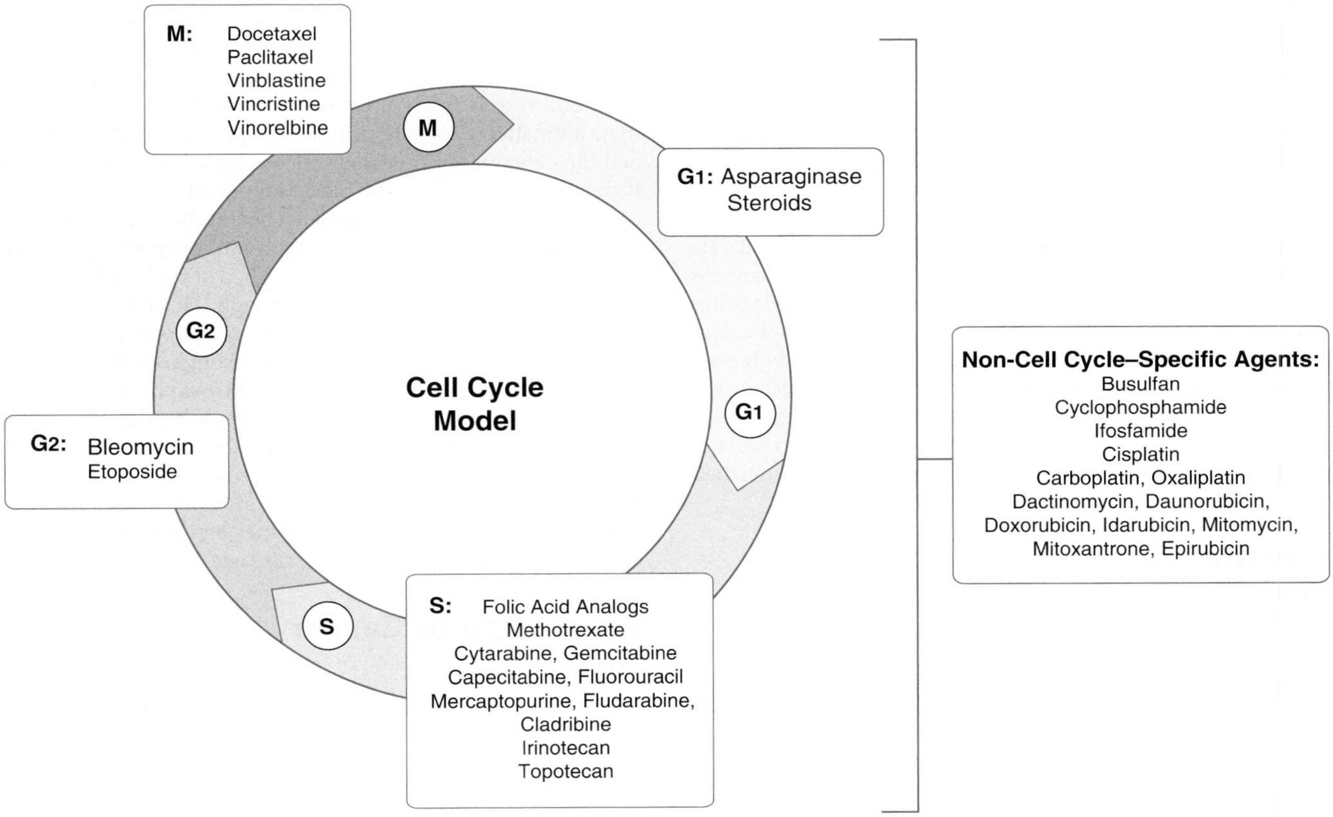

Figure 93-1 Cell cycle and effects of representative cytotoxic drugs on phases of the cell cycle.

and the transfer of phosphate groups to various proteins and enzymes. Activating signals from the cell's external environment are transmitted to the nucleus via growth factor receptor signaling pathways, which influence formation of cyclins and cyclin–CDK complexes. The complexes generate phosphate groups from molecules of adenosine triphosphate (ATP) and transfer them to a protein called a retinoblastoma protein (pRb). If pRb acquires enough phosphate groups, it will release the transcription factors the cell needs to make proteins essential for a cell division. In other words, phosphorylated pRb promotes cell cycle progression from G_1 to S and, subsequently, cell division. Other signaling pathways inhibit cell proliferation through endogenous CDK inhibitors, which result in dephosphorylated pRb.

In cancer cells, the regulation and function of cyclins, CDK, and inhibitory proteins may be disrupted by malignant transformation, or these proteins can undergo changes that cause malignant transformation. Examples of defects in these processes include deletion of the *Rb* gene, a tumor suppressor gene that encodes for pRb, and dysregulation of the CDK through overactivation or loss of CDK inhibitors.[9] As mentioned above, pRb regulates cell cycle transition from the G_1 to the S phase and, if this molecule becomes inactive, excessive cell proliferation can occur. In normal cells, the *p53* gene is responsible for temporarily arresting cell growth in response to biochemical or molecular damage until the DNA damage can be repaired.[10] If the damage cannot be repaired, apoptosis (programmed cell death) occurs to prevent genetically damaged cells from growing uncontrollably. Loss or mutation of a second tumor suppressor gene, *p53*, is also common in human cancers and is associated with the resistance of cancer cells to undergo cell cycle arrest or apoptosis.

Carcinogenesis

Carcinogenesis is the process by which normal cells are transformed into cancer cells. If the balance of stimulatory and inhibitory growth signals becomes dysregulated, carcinogenesis may occur. In carcinogenesis, normal mechanisms such as apoptosis and senescence (aging) do not function properly and cannot control excessive cell division. Because abnormalities in the proto-oncogenes and tumor suppressor genes regulating these processes are present in cancer cells, the balance between cell renewal and loss of mature (senescent) cells is disrupted. Cancer cells are also less dependent on receiving stimulatory signals from external growth factors.[10] Furthermore, cancer cells possess unlimited replication potential, owing to their ability to activate telomerase.[1,11] Telomerase is an enzyme that synthesizes sequences of telomeres, thereby enabling cells to proliferate endlessly. The expression of telomerase in most normal human cells is suppressed, but is reactivated in most cancer cells.[10,11] Telomeres are repeats of DNA and DNA-binding proteins that form the ends of eukaryotic chromosomes.[11] Telomere loss occurs with each successive cell replication, and after a critical length is reached, the cell undergoes irreversible growth arrest (replicative senescence).[11] Unlike normal cells, in which a finite telomere sequence regulates their life span, cancer cells are capable of immortality through their ability to maintain their telomeres indefinitely.

Metastasis

CASE 93-1

QUESTION 1: S.T., a 16-year-old boy, presented to the emergency department with a painful, swollen right leg. X-ray examination confirmed a fracture that appeared to be caused by a tumor mass in the bone. Biopsy of the bone mass confirmed osteogenic sarcoma. A chest x-ray study showed three nodules that were also believed to be malignant tumors. Does S.T. also have lung cancer or are the tumors in S.T.'s lungs metastases from the sarcoma in his leg?

S.T. does not have lung cancer. Tumor nodules in his lung are most likely metastases from the sarcoma in his leg. The ability of cancer cells to disseminate and form metastases represents their most malignant characteristic. Tumor metastases to distant sites generally have a greater effect than the primary tumor on frequency of complications and patient's quality of life. Metastases also have a greater impact than the primary tumor on mortality, with metastases associated with most cancer-related deaths. Consequently, individuals diagnosed with metastases face a worse prognosis.

Cancer cells must develop new blood vessels to obtain nutrients and spread to distant sites (metastasize). In response to low oxygen supply (hypoxia) and other factors, cancer cells and surrounding tissues secrete growth factors that stimulate growth of new blood vessels (angiogenesis) from existing blood vessels in surrounding normal host tissue. Vascular endothelial growth factor (VEGF), platelet-derived growth factor (PDGF), and basic fibroblast growth factor (bFGF) are growth factors needed for sustained endothelial cell growth. Once released by tumor cells, these growth factors bind to tyrosine kinase receptors on the surface of endothelial cells of existing blood vessels and activate a series of intracellular relay proteins that transmit signals to genes in the nucleus to produce factors required for new endothelial cell growth.[12] Once older endothelial cells become activated by growth factors, they begin making matrix metalloproteinase (MMP) enzymes. These enzymes destroy the extracellular matrix of surrounding cells, allowing older endothelial cells to invade the extracellular matrix and begin cell division.[12] This process of invasion and proliferation is repeated several times until new blood vessels are formed.

Tumor cells can use these newly formed blood vessels to facilitate their spread to distant locations. Cells must break away from the primary tumor and travel to other sites in the body to form metastases. Normally, cells adhere to one another and the extracellular matrix. The cell-to-cell adhesion molecules are called *cadherins*, and the cell-to-extracellular matrix molecules are called *integrins*. In cancer cells, these molecules are often absent, allowing tumor cells to easily move away from the primary tumor mass.

Once a tumor cell leaves the primary mass, it travels through the blood vessels and lymphatic system within the body to form metastatic site(s). Usually, tumor cells spread to the first capillary bed they encounter after their release from the primary tumor. If the primary site drains its blood supply into the vena cava, the cancer cells will reach the capillary bed in the lung. Similarly, if the primary site drains its blood supply into the portal circulation, the cancer cells will reach the capillary bed in the liver. In addition, cancer cells can potentially pass through the first capillary bed they encounter and enter the arterial circulation where they can distribute to other organs and tissues throughout the body.

Growth conditions (e.g., growth factors, physiologic conditions) within a tissue or organ also can determine the location of a metastatic site. After a cancer cell establishes a metastatic site, it must again undergo angiogenesis to ensure continued growth. Together, angiogenesis and hematogenous or lymphatic spread help cancer cells invade healthy tissues and increase morbidity and mortality associated with the disease.

Prevention of Cancer

TOBACCO

Cigarette smoking is probably the single largest factor that contributes to cancer development, increasing risk for multiple cancer types including lung, head and neck, gastrointestinal, bladder, and cervical cancers.[5] Therefore, tobacco cessation and abstinence play an important role in prevention of cancer. For more information, visit the following page on the American

Cancer Society's website: https://www.cancer.org/cancer/cancer-causes/tobacco-and-cancer.html. For review of tobacco dependence and methods for cessation see Chapter 88, Tobacco Use and Dependence.

CHEMOPREVENTION

Chemoprevention is the use of a drug or substance to reverse, inhibit, or prevent the development of cancer. Use of chemoprevention is helpful in selected groups of high-risk patients with breast, colorectal, and prostate cancers.[13] For discussion of chemoprevention for these cancers, see Chapter 97, Breast Cancer, Chapter 99, Colorectal Cancer, and Chapter 100, Prostate Cancer.

HUMAN PAPILLOMA VIRUS (HPV) VACCINES

CASE 93-2

QUESTION 1: M.M., a 44-year-old woman, asks you about vaccines to prevent cervical cancer. Should M.M. consider vaccination for her daughter or her son? Would this substitute for Pap smear screening for her daughter?

The human papilloma virus is primarily transmitted through sexual contact; serotypes 16 and 18 (HPV-16, -18) cause approximately 70% of cervical cancers.[14] There are three different HPV vaccines available, each requiring three intramuscular injections over the course of 6 months. The HPV bivalent vaccine (Cervarix) includes HPV types 16 and 18 whereas the HPV quadrivalent vaccine (Gardasil) includes HPV types 6, 11, 16, and 18. Both vaccines demonstrated efficacy in reducing the incidence of cervical intraepithelial neoplasia (CIN), a premalignant lesion that can lead to cervical cancer.[15–17] Because the progression of HPV infection to invasive cervical cancer requires several years to possibly decades, CIN is utilized as a surrogate efficacy endpoint in HPV vaccine clinical trials. It is anticipated that the use of HPV vaccines will ultimately lead to a reduction in the incidence of cervical cancer.

The HPV 9-valent vaccine (Gardasil 9) includes the same HPV types as the bivalent and quadrivalent vaccines (6, 11, 16, 18) but with five additional HPV types (31, 33, 45, 52, 58), increasing prevention to approximately 90% of cervical cancers.[18] The HPV quadrivalent and 9-valent vaccines are also approved for the prevention of vulvar intraepithelial neoplasia (VIN) and vaginal intraepithelial neoplasia (VAIN) in females as well as prevention of HPV-related genital warts and anal cancer in males. However, there are no data to support the use of these vaccines to prevent other cancers associated with HPV, such as penile cancer or head and neck cancers.

Routine Pap smear and HPV screening should continue for vaccinated women because the vaccines do not prevent all oncogenic types of HPV. The duration of vaccine-induced anti-HPV immunity is also unknown.

M.M. should consider HPV vaccination for her daughter. All three vaccines are indicated in females of 9 to 26 years of age, but the vaccines are most effective if initiated before sexual activity. Whether or not M.M.'s daughter is vaccinated, she should still receive routine Pap smear screening according to current guidelines.[19] The HPV quadrivalent and 9-valent vaccines are approved in males of 9 to 26 years of age; therefore, M.M. should also consider vaccination for her son. The Centers for Disease Control recommends HPV vaccination for all females and males at the age of 11 to 12 years.[20]

DIET

Diet has been linked to the development of colon, prostate, and breast cancers. The American Cancer Society advocates a healthy diet that consists of vegetables, fruit, whole grains, and fi ber and is low in fat and red meat.[21] For more information, visit the following page on the American Cancer Society's website: http://www.cancer.org/Cancer/CancerCauses/DietandPhysicalActivity/index.

Migrant studies suggest that diet, environmental, or social factors play a role in the development of prostate cancer and that the incidence of colon cancer in a population increases as individuals migrate from a low-incidence region to a high-incidence region.[22,23] In women, the risk of breast cancer is increased with obesity and physical inactivity, but an association with a high-fat diet is less clear.[24] Moderate alcohol consumption has also been associated with an increased risk of breast cancer.[25] For more information, visit the following page on the American Cancer Society's website: http://www.cancer.org/Healthy/EatHealthyGetActive/index.

SUN AND ULTRAVIOLET RADIATION EXPOSURE

Most risk factors associated with skin cancer are uncontrollable, with the exception of sun exposure and other forms of ultraviolet (UV) radiation. The interaction between UV radiation and skin cancers is complex, because nonmelanomas (e.g., basal cell and squamous cell carcinomas) are associated with cumulative UV radiation exposure and certain cutaneous melanomas are associated with excessive, intermittent UV radiation exposure.[26] The risk of melanoma is further increased in people who have a history of five or more severe sunburns in their lifetime, particularly during adolescence, or history of tanning bed use.[26,27] Depletion of the ozone layer in the stratosphere may also contribute to the increased incidence of melanoma.[26]

Prevention of skin cancer is based on limiting sun and UV radiation exposure. The American Cancer Society guidelines recommend avoiding or limiting sun exposure from 10 AM to 4 PM when the UV rays are the strongest, and avoiding tanning bed or sun lamp use. Protective clothing (hat, sunglasses, long-sleeved shirt, pants) and sunscreens are also advised to minimize exposure.[27] However, the protective effects of sunscreens alone against melanoma, particularly for intentional sun exposure, are controversial and should not be used to prolong time in the sun.[27,28]

Screening and Early Detection of Cancer

Standardized screening tests help identify disease in asymptomatic individuals (screening) or diagnose disease in symptomatic individuals (early detection). The cancer screening tests recommended by the American Cancer Society meet four basic requirements: (a) There must be good evidence that the test is effective in reducing morbidity or mortality; (b) benefits of the test should outweigh its risks; (c) costs of the test should be in balance with its presumed benefits; and (d) the test should be practical and feasible within the existing healthcare setting. For more information, visit the following page on the American Cancer Society's website: http://www.cancer.org/Healthy/FindCancerEarly/CancerScreeningGuidelines/american-cancer-society-guidelines-for-the-early-detection-of-cancer.

Screening guidelines are updated frequently, and newest guidelines should be consulted when counseling patients. Professional organizations including the American Cancer Society (http://www.cancer.org) and National Comprehensive Cancer Network (NCCN) (http://www.nccn.org) regularly publish recommendations for screening of breast, cervical, colon, lung, and prostate cancers.[29]

Diagnosis and Staging of Cancer

The histologic diagnosis of a tumor is the most important determinant of treatment selection. This is because its histologic classification influences its natural history, pattern of progression, and responsiveness to treatment. A biopsy followed by a microscopic and biochemical evaluation by a pathologist can provide the most accurate histologic diagnosis. Thereafter, staging can begin.

CASE 93-3

QUESTION 1: J.S. is diagnosed with breast cancer after a biopsy of a large breast mass. Chemotherapy, radiation, and surgery are commonly used to treat patients diagnosed with breast cancer. What information is needed to select a treatment plan for J.S.?

The stage of the cancer, as well as the histologic diagnosis, influences both the treatment selection and prognosis. Staging is the process that determines the extent or spread of the disease.

Determining the stage of the cancer typically requires tests that can physically or radiographically measure the size of the primary tumor and assess for evidence of tumor spread (e.g., radiographs, computed tomography [CT] scans, magnetic resonance imaging [MRI] scans, or positron emission tomography [PET] scans) and pathologically examine regional lymph nodes.[30] Clinicians also evaluate symptoms (e.g., pain) or signs (e.g., swelling, abnormal laboratory findings) that may indicate tumor involvement at a distant site. Common sites of tumor metastases are shown in Table 93-2.

Staging schemas have been developed for all major types of cancers. For solid tumors, the most widely used and accepted staging classification is the TNM system, which incorporates the size of the primary tumor (T), the extent of regional lymph node spread (N), and the presence or absence of metastatic spread to distant organs (M). Within each TNM category, the extent of cancer involvement is related to prognosis. Most solid tumor staging systems also incorporate the TNM classification into broader groups, called stages, to facilitate treatment decisions and comparison among patient populations. Classification of stages differs among solid tumors types. Please refer to malignancy-specific chapters for TNM staging of breast, lung, prostate, and colorectal cancers.

Whereas the TNM system enables staging of solid tumors, it does not enable staging for hematologic malignancies, including leukemias, lymphomas, and multiple myeloma. Because hematologic malignancies occur in the blood cells and lymphatic tissues that are widely distributed throughout the body, the TNM staging system cannot sufficiently describe these diseases. To define the extent of disease, guide treatment, and provide prognostic information, specific staging systems have been developed for various hematologic malignancies. Staging systems for hematologic malignancies are discussed in further detail in Chapter 96, Adult Hematologic Malignancies.

Table 93-2
Common Sites of Metastases for Selected Tumors

Cancer Type	Common Sites of Metastases
Breast	Bone (osteolytic lesions), lung, liver, brain. ER-positive tumors preferentially spread to bone; ER-negative tumors may metastasize to visceral organs
Lung	Liver, brain, adrenals, pancreas, contralateral lung, and bone
Prostate	Bone (osteoblastic lesions)
Colon	The portal circulation pattern favors dissemination to the liver and peritoneal cavity, but metastasis also occurs in the lungs
Ovarian	Local spread in the peritoneal cavity
Myeloma	Bone (osteolytic lesions), sometimes spreading to other organs

ER, estrogen receptor.

Staging systems for some tumors also include other characteristics to further determine the stage and prognosis of the disease, such as clinical signs and symptoms, biochemical characteristics of the tumor, or other laboratory tests. For example, the staging system used for Hodgkin lymphoma includes constitutional symptoms (i.e., fever, night sweats, and weight loss). These symptoms confer a poorer prognosis and could indicate the need for more intensive therapy.

Tumor staging is done at the time of initial diagnosis and periodically during treatment to assess the patient's response to therapy. Staging should also be repeated (a) when evidence shows that the cancer has progressed during treatment or recurred after therapy to establish the most appropriate next-line therapy, and (b) to enable measurement of response to that therapy.

J.S. needs to undergo the appropriate imaging scans, laboratory studies, and clinical evaluation so that her breast cancer can be staged. These tests may include blood tests (e.g., complete blood cell and platelet count, liver function tests), mammograms or breast ultrasounds, determination of tumor ER/PR and HER2 status, breast MRI, bone scan, abdominal scans, and chest imaging. Once staging is completed, treatment recommendations and options can then be determined. Treatment options for breast cancer based on stage are further discussed in Chapter 97, Breast Cancer.

CLINICAL PRESENTATION AND COMPLICATIONS OF MALIGNANCY

The initial signs and symptoms of malignant disease are variable and predominantly depend on histologic diagnosis, location (including metastases), and size of the tumor. Pain secondary to compression, obstruction, and destruction of adjacent tissues and organs is the most common presenting symptom. Other common initial symptoms reported by patients with cancer include anorexia, weight loss, and fatigue. Certain symptoms, however, may be obscured by a concomitant illness, such as chronic lung disease in patients with lung cancer. Some tumors cause signs and symptoms early in the course of the disease, whereas others may not cause symptoms until late in the course of the disease and after significant tumor growth. In either of these circumstances, early diagnosis may be difficult. Individuals at a higher-than-average risk for certain malignancies should be screened regularly to help detect early disease. Tumor involvement of the liver, kidneys, or lungs can complicate therapy by causing significant organ dysfunction and metabolic disturbances. In addition, compression or obstruction could produce a "mass effect" by impairing normal organ or tissue function and causing pain or other uncomfortable physical effects. Life-threatening complications that require immediate intervention include obstruction of the superior vena cava, spinal cord compression, and brain metastases.

CASE 93-4

QUESTION 1: P.N., a 59 year-old woman, presents with shortness of breath, fatigue, anorexia, weight loss, and abdominal pain and distension that have worsened significantly during the previous 3 weeks. A CT scan of her abdomen shows a large mass surrounding the head of her pancreas with biopsy results that confirm pancreatic adenocarcinoma. The staging workup confirms the presence of distant metastases. Her husband states that she was previously an active person, but that she most recently has been unable to dress herself or participate in normal daily activities. He states that she spends most of the day in bed. Will her activity level influence the type of treatment that she can receive?

Cancer can have a profound effect on a patient's quality of life and his/her ability to tolerate appropriate therapy. Patients with malnutrition secondary to anorexia, mechanical obstruction, or pain may not tolerate some therapies because of significant physical debility. Performance status is a measure of functional capacity and reflects a patient's ability to ambulate, care for himself/herself, and carry out normal activities. For several cancers, poor pretreatment performance status is associated with decreased ability to tolerate treatment, decreased tumor response to treatment, and worsened clinical outcome. In these cases, especially if the cancer is not known to respond well to treatment, a less aggressive treatment regimen may be recommended. For this reason, performance status is important to assess at the time of staging evaluation and periodically during treatment. Different scales (i.e., Karnofsky score, Eastern Cooperative Oncology Group [ECOG]) can be used to determine performance status. The Karnofsky and ECOG performance scales are depicted in Table 93-3.[31] Because P.N. has a poor performance status (ECOG grade 3) and may not tolerate chemotherapy well, her oncologist may recommend a less toxic treatment plan. Because other conditions, such as depression, could contribute to her symptoms, P.N. should undergo comprehensive evaluation.

TREATMENT

CASE 93-5

QUESTION 1: T.J., a 40-year-old man with no significant medical history, presents to his physician with complaints of abdominal pain, nausea and vomiting, weakness, and weight loss. On physical examination, he is noted to be slightly jaundiced. A CT scan of his abdomen reveals a mass present in the peripancreatic area that is suggestive of malignancy. Once diagnosed and staged, T.J. asks the surgeon how will this malignancy be treated? And what is the goal of therapy?

The choice of specific therapy and its goals depends not only on the histology and stage of the cancer but also on the patient's predicted tolerance of the side effects of the various treatment options. The goal of therapy should always be to cure the patient when possible. The likelihood of cure is greater when the tumor burden is low (i.e., lower stage). When using therapy with curative intent is not possible, therapy becomes palliative in nature, with disease control and symptom management the priority. Goals of therapy should be balanced so that quantity and quality of life are both adequately considered.

Cancer is predominately treated with three modalities: surgery, radiation, and systemic therapy (including chemotherapy, targeted therapy, biologic response modifiers, etc.). Systemic therapy is the primary treatment modality for hematologic malignancies. In most solid tumor malignancies, early-stage and localized disease is treated with either surgery or radiation therapy. Sometimes, combinations of modalities may be used to maximize the potential for cure or disease control (e.g., radiation given in combination with chemotherapy). For advanced disease (presence of metastases or recurrence after initial therapy), solid tumor malignancies are usually treated with systemic therapy as the primary treatment modality. T.J.'s treatment will be dependent on tumor histology, stage, and expected prognosis. If T.J. has potentially curable disease, he should be treated with curative intent therapy, whereas if T.J. has advanced disease that denotes a poor prognosis, he should be treated with palliative therapy.

Surgery

Surgery is an important treatment option for patients diagnosed with certain solid tumors. With the recent advances in surgical techniques (e.g., minimally invasive procedures) and improved

Table 93-3
Performance Status Scales[31]

Eastern Cooperative Group (ECOG)		Karnofsky	
Grade	**Description**	**Grade**	**Description**
0	Fully active, able to carry on all predisease performance without restriction	100	Normal, no complaints; no evidence of disease
		90	Able to carry on normal activity; minor signs or symptoms of disease
1	Restricted in physically strenuous activity but ambulatory and able to carry out work of a light or sedentary nature	80	Normal activity with effort, some signs of symptoms of disease
		70	Cares for self but unable to carry on normal activity or do active work
2	Ambulatory and capable of all self-care but unable to carry out any work activities. Up and about more than 50% of waking hours	60	Requires occasional assistance but is able to care for most of personal needs
		50	Requires considerable assistance and frequent medical care
3	Capable of only limited self-care, confined to bed or chair more than 50% of waking hours	40	Disabled; requires special care and assistance
		30	Severely disabled; hospitalization is indicated although death not imminent
4	Completely disabled. Cannot carry on any self-care. Totally confined to bed or chair.	20	Very ill; hospitalization and active supportive care necessary
		10	Moribund
5	Dead	0	Dead

(continued)

understanding of patterns of tumor growth and spread, successful resections are possible for an increasing number of patients. Surgery may be used as preventive therapy (e.g., removal of colonic polyps or cervical dysplasia) or diagnostic treatment, or staging of some cancers.

Surgery can be used to manage both localized and advanced tumors. When surgery provides curative therapy for a localized tumor, the surgeon removes the tumor plus a margin of normal tissue surrounding the tumor. For extensive, localized tumors that cannot be completely removed, selected patients may undergo cytoreductive surgery to resect the tumor partially in an attempt to improve the likelihood that subsequent chemotherapy or radiation therapy may successfully kill the tumor.

Patients with metastatic disease may have palliative surgery to relieve pain or improve functional abnormalities caused by the advanced tumor (e.g., gastrointestinal obstruction). Palliative surgery may improve quality of life without prolonging survival.

Radiation

Radiation may be administered as either curative or palliative therapy for solid tumors. Radiation is administered in varying doses depending on the type of tissue (e.g., bone, lung, breast, liver, brain) being treated and the intent of therapy (palliative or curative). A limit exists to the total amount of radiation that can be delivered to the area being treated dependent on the type of tissue. Damaging effects of radiation on the normal tissues that surround the tumor can be dramatic, and may be exacerbated if given concomitantly with chemotherapy. Chemotherapy that follows completion of radiation therapy can produce "radiation recall" of local toxicity that manifests as skin redness, swelling, and peeling at the radiation site.

Not all cancers are sensitive to radiation, so this modality has limited application in these cases. For radiation-sensitive tumors (Table 93-4), potential advantages exist over surgery. For instance, radiation therapy may encompass a wider area around the tumor and treat tumors in regions of the body where surgery cannot safely be performed. Radiation therapy also can be used when surgery could result in considerable disability or disfigurement. Patients may receive radiation therapy to multiple sites simultaneously.

Multiple methods are used to administer radiation to tumors. External-beam radiotherapy and brachytherapy are two types that are commonly used. Newer radiation therapy techniques, including intraoperative radiation, hyperfractionated radiation, stereotactic radiosurgery, intensity-modulated radiation therapy, charged-particle (proton) radiation therapy, and computerized three-dimensional conformal treatment planning, may reduce associated toxicities, enhance tumor responsiveness, and improve the clinical usefulness of radiation.[32,33]

Table 93-4
Cancers Frequently Treated with Radiation Therapy

Acute lymphocytic leukemia (central nervous system radiation)
Brain and central nervous system
Breast
Head and neck cancers, squamous cell
Lung
Lymphomas
Neuroblastoma
Prostate
Rectal
Testicular, seminoma

Systemic Therapy

Not all cancers can be treated by surgery or radiation therapy. Patients may present with widespread metastatic disease at diagnosis or recur following primary treatment with surgery or radiation. Patients may also have residual tumor following initial surgery or radiation, requiring additional treatment. In these circumstances, systemic treatments including chemotherapy, targeted therapy, endocrine therapy, and biologic response modifiers generally offer the only hope of controlling disease.

CHEMOTHERAPY

The National Cancer Institute defines chemotherapy as drugs that treat cancer cells.[34] For the purposes of this chapter, chemotherapy will be defined as cytotoxic therapy that is directed toward rapidly dividing cells. Chemotherapy kills cancer cells by damaging DNA, interfering with DNA synthesis, or inhibiting cell division. Chemotherapy agents are classified by their effect on the cell cycle or mechanism of action. Agents that affect a specific phase of the cell cycle are referred to as phase-specific agents or schedule-dependent agents. In contrast, agents that affect any phase of the cell cycle are referred to as phase-nonspecific agents or dose-dependent agents (Fig. 93-1). The specific mechanisms of action for several chemotherapy agents are described in Table 93-5.[35]

Factors that Influence Response to Chemotherapy

Cell Kill

Studies using rodent animal models during the 1960s demonstrated that the number of tumor cells killed by chemotherapy is proportional to the dose when the growth fraction is 100% (i.e., all cells are dividing) and the tumor cells are sensitive to the agent.[36,37] For example, if a dose of chemotherapy reduces the tumor burden from 10^{10} to 10^8 cells, the same dose administered when only 10^7 cells are present should reduce the tumor burden to 10^5 cells. This theory has become known as the cell-kill or log-kill hypothesis (Fig. 93-2).

In the clinical setting, tumor cells do not always decrease predictably with each successive course of chemotherapy. This is because the growth fraction of human tumors is not 100% and the cell population is heterogeneous, with some cells that are resistant to chemotherapy.

Dose Intensity

Dose intensity is defined as the chemotherapy dose per unit time during which treatment is given (e.g., mg/m^2/week). Drug resistance might be overcome by increasing the dose of chemotherapy. Evidence suggests that reducing a dose can cause treatment failure in patients with chemotherapy-sensitive tumors who are having their first chemotherapy treatment.[38] A direct relationship between dose intensity and response rate also has been reported in several human tumors including breast cancer, lymphomas, ovarian cancer, and small-cell lung cancer.[39,40] However, dose-intensive therapy has not consistently improved the overall cure rate of most solid tumors.

The dose intensity for most chemotherapy regimens is limited by the major dose-related toxicity, bone marrow suppression. To minimize this toxicity and administer higher doses, patients may receive hematopoietic growth factors, autologous stem cell transplantation, or altered schedules of drug delivery.[41,42]

Schedule Dependency

Chemotherapy is administered in cycles (e.g., every 2, 3, or 4 weeks) with recovery periods between cycles. A typical course of chemotherapy usually consists of several cycles. The interval of time between cycles depends on the type of cancer and the drugs being used.

Table 93-5
Chemotherapy Agents

Subclass	Agent (Trade Name)	Mechanism of Action	Route of Administration	Notable Toxicities
Alkylating Agents				
Nitrogen mustards (and related agents)		Cross-links DNA strands leading to cell death		Myelosuppression; nausea, vomiting; fatigue
	Bendamustine (Treanda)	Nitrogen mustard analog	IV	Also: hepatic dysfunction; fever; headache
	Chlorambucil (Leukeran)		PO	Also: rash; hepatic dysfunction; pulmonary fibrosis; myoclonus, hallucinations
	Cyclophosphamide (Cytoxan)		IV, PO	Also: immunosuppression; hemorrhagic cystitis; alopecia; cardiomyopathy
	Ifosfamide (Ifex)		IV	Also: hemorrhagic cystitis (coadministered with mesna); encephalopathy; alopecia
	Melphalan (Alkeran)		IV, PO	Also: stomatitis
	Thiotepa (Thioplex)	Ethylenimine-type related to nitrogen mustard	IV, IT, intracavitary	Also: anaphylaxis, rash, blurred vision; dizziness; alopecia
Nitrosoureas		Interferes with normal cellular function via cross-linking of DNA and RNA strands		Myelosuppression; nausea, vomiting; pulmonary toxicity; hepatic and renal dysfunction
	Carmustine (BiCNU)		IV, brain implant	
	Lomustine (CeeNU)		PO	Also: ocular changes
Platinum analogs		Reacts with nucleophilic sites on DNA forming cross-links		Myelosuppression, nausea, vomiting; peripheral neuropathy; delayed hypersensitivity reactions; secondary malignancy
	Carboplatin (Paraplatin)		IV	Also: electrolyte abnormalities
	Cisplatin (Platinol)		IV, IP	Also: renal dysfunction; ototoxicity; electrolyte abnormalities; vesicant
	Oxaliplatin (Eloxatin)		IV	Also: sensitivity to cold, jaw spasm, dysphagia; diarrhea; pulmonary fibrosis
Triazenes		Alkylates DNA leading to double-strand breaks and cell death		Myelosuppression; nausea, vomiting, anorexia; fatigue; headache; alopecia
	Dacarbazine (DTIC-Dome)	Prodrug (activated by CYP)	IV	Also: flu-like syndrome
	Temozolomide (Temodar)	Prodrug of dacarbazine (spontaneously hydrolyzed)	IV, PO	Also: constipation
Other				
	Busulfan (Myleran, Busulfex)	Cross-links DNA strands, interfering with normal function	IV, PO	Myelosuppression; pulmonary fibrosis; hyperpigmentation; hepatic dysfunction; seizures and veno-occlusive disease (high dose)
	Procarbazine (Matulane)	Inhibits DNA and RNA synthesis through transmethylation of methionine	PO	Myelosuppression; nausea, vomiting; neurologic toxicity; hepatic dysfunction; secondary malignancy

(continued)

Table 93-5
Chemotherapy Agents (*continued*)

Subclass	Agent (Trade Name)	Mechanism of Action	Route of Administration	Notable Toxicities
Antimetabolites				
DNA demethylation agents		Incorporates into RNA and DNA and inhibits methylation		Myelosuppression; nausea, vomiting, diarrhea; bruising, petechiae; fatigue, fever
	Azacitidine (Vidaza)		IV or SC	Also: injection-site reaction
	Decitabine (Dacogen)		IV	Also: electrolyte abnormalities; edema; psychiatric changes
	Nelarabine (Arranon)		IV	Also: somnolence, dizziness, seizure, peripheral neuropathy; edema
Folic acid antagonists		Inhibits dihydrofolate reductase; interferes with DNA synthesis, repair, and cellular replication		Myelosuppression; stomatitis; nausea; fatigue; hepatic dysfunction
	Methotrexate (Trexall)		IV, PO	Also: renal dysfunction; photosensitivity; pulmonary toxicity; neurotoxicity
	Pemetrexed (Alimta)	Also: inhibits additional enzymes involved in folate metabolism	IV	Also: rash
	Pralatrexate (Folotyn)	Also: selectively enters cells expressing reduced folate carrier-1	IV	Also: fever; edema; diarrhea; cough, rash
Purine analogs		Inhibits DNA synthesis and repair by incorporating into DNA		Myelosuppression; nausea, vomiting, anorexia; fatigue
	Cladribine (Leustatin)	Prodrug (intracellular phosphorylation)	IV	Also: fever; fatigue; headache; rash; injection-site reaction
	Clofarabine (Clolar)	Also: inhibits ribonucleotide reductase	IV	Also: headache; rash, pruritus; anxiety; fever; tachycardia, hypotension; diarrhea; hepatic and renal dysfunction
	Fludarabine (Fludara)	Also: inhibition of DNA polymerase and ribonucleotide reductase	IV	Also: fever, chills; edema; cough; rash
	Mercaptopurine (Purinethol)	Also: S phase specific; converted to a ribonucleotide	PO	Also: rash; drug fever; hepatic dysfunction
	Thioguanine (Tabloid)	Also: complete cross-resistance with mercaptopurine	PO	Also: hepatotoxicity, veno-occlusive disease; stomatitis; hyperuricemia; fluid retention
Other				
	Hydroxyurea (Hydrea, Droxia)	Holds cells in the G_1 phase of cell cycle	PO	Myelosuppression; dermatologic toxicity; nausea, vomiting, diarrhea
Pyrimidine analogs		Incorporates into RNA and DNA; interferes with RNA function		Myelosuppression; nausea, vomiting, stomatitis, diarrhea
	Capecitabine (Xeloda)	Also: prodrug metabolized to fluorouracil; inhibits thymidylate synthase	PO	Also: hand-foot syndrome; anorexia
	Cytarabine (Cytosar-U, Ara-C)	Also: inhibits DNA polymerase	IV, IT (liposomal)	Also: cytarabine syndrome (fever, myalgia, bone pain, rash, conjunctivitis); hepatic dysfunction
	Fluorouracil (Adrucil)	Also: inhibits thymidylate synthase	IV	Also: alopecia; hand-foot syndrome

Table 93-5
Chemotherapy Agents (*continued*)

Subclass	Agent (Trade Name)	Mechanism of Action	Route of Administration	Notable Toxicities
	Gemcitabine (Gemzar)	Also: inhibits DNA polymerase and ribonucleotide reductase	IV	Also: flu-like syndrome; rash, edema
Antimitotic Agents				
Epothilones		Binds directly to β-tubulin; promotes stabilization of microtubules		Alopecia; myelosuppression; peripheral neuropathy; arthralgia, myalgia; stomatitis, nausea, vomiting, diarrhea
	Ixabepilone (Ixempra)		IV	
Taxanes (and related agents)		Binds to β-tubulin; promotes stabilization and suppresses disassembly of microtubules		Myelosuppression; alopecia; nausea, vomiting, diarrhea; peripheral neuropathy; myalgia, arthralgia; fatigue
	Cabazitaxel (Jevtana)		IV	
	Docetaxel (Taxotere)		IV	Also: hand-foot syndrome; edema; hypersensitivity reaction
	Paclitaxel (Taxol)		IV, IP	Also: hypersensitivity reaction
	Paclitaxel, albumin-bound (Abraxane)		IV	
Vinca alkaloids		Binds to tubulin interfering with microtubule assembly and mitotic spindle formation		Myelosuppression; constipation; bone pain; neurotoxicity, neuropathies; vesicant
	Vinblastine (Velban)		IV	
	Vincristine (Vincasar, Oncovin)		IV	Also: autonomic neuropathies (high dose); fever; nausea; constipation; SIADH
	Vinorelbine (Navelbine)		IV	Also: fatigue; liver dysfunction
Halichondrin B analog		Disrupts microtubule polymerization		Myelosuppression; alopecia; nausea, constipation; peripheral neuropathy; fatigue
	Eribulin (Halaven)		IV	
Other				
	Estramustine (Emcyt)	Stabilizes microtubule formation	PO	Gynecomastia; hepatic dysfunction; edema; nausea, diarrhea
Antitumor Antibiotics				
Anthracyclines		Stabilizes the cleavable complex between topoisomerase II and DNA, causing single- and double-strand DNA breaks		Myelosuppression; mucositis; alopecia; nausea, vomiting; cumulative cardiac toxicity; secondary malignancy
	Daunorubicin (Cerubidine)		IV	Also: vesicant
	Daunorubicin, liposomal (DaunoXome)		IV	Also: diarrhea; fatigue, rigors, neuropathy; dyspnea
	Doxorubicin (Adriamycin, Rubex)		IV	Also: acute cardiac toxicity; vesicant
	Doxorubicin, liposomal (Doxil)		IV	Also: fatigue; stomatitis; rash, hand-foot syndrome
	Epirubicin (Ellence)		IV	Also: mucositis, alopecia; vesicant

(continued)

Table 93-5
Chemotherapy Agents (*continued*)

Subclass	Agent (Trade Name)	Mechanism of Action	Route of Administration	Notable Toxicities
	Idarubicin (Idamycin)		IV	Also: diarrhea; alopecia; vesicant
	Valrubicin (Valstar)		Intravesical	Urinary urgency; urinary frequency, dysuria, hematuria
Other				
	Bleomycin (Blenoxane)	Binds to DNA, producing single- and double-strand DNA breaks	IV	Erythema, hyperpigmentation; pulmonary toxicity; fever, chills
	Dactinomycin (Cosmegen)	Intercalates DNA, inhibiting DNA synthesis and DNA-dependent RNA synthesis	IV	Myelosuppression; nausea, vomiting; hepatic dysfunction; vesicant; radiation recall
Miscellaneous				
Cephalotaxine		Inhibits ribosome function, impairing protein synthesis		Myelosuppression; diarrhea, nausea; infusion-related reaction, injection-site reaction; hyperuricemia; infection, fever, fatigue
	Omacetaxine (Synribo)		SC	
Differentiation Agents		Promotes myeloid differentiation and maturation		Nausea, vomiting, diarrhea; dermatologic toxicity; headache, fatigue, edema; bone pain
	Arsenic trioxide (Trisenox)	Also: causes morphologic changes and DNA fragmentation	IV	Also: RA-APL syndrome, myelosuppression, leukocytosis; cardiac effects; psychiatric changes; electrolyte abnormalities
	Tretinoin (Vesanoid)		PO	Also: RA-APL syndrome, leukocytosis; cardiac effects; psychiatric; lipid abnormalities
	Bexarotene (Targretin)		PO	Also: lipid abnormalities; hypothyroidism; myelosuppression
DNA Topoisomerase Inhibitors		Inhibits topoisomerases, leading to DNA strand breaks		Myelosuppression, fatigue; alopecia
	Etoposide (VePesid)	Inhibits topoisomerase II	IV, PO	Also: nausea, vomiting; hypersensitivity reaction; secondary malignancy
	Irinotecan (Camptosar)	Inhibits topoisomerase I	IV	Also: diarrhea, cholinergic syndrome; hepatic dysfunction
	Topotecan (Hycamtin)	Inhibits topoisomerase I	IV, PO	Also: nausea, vomiting, diarrhea
Other				
	Asparaginase (Elspar, Erwinase)	Depletes asparagine, leading to inhibition of protein synthesis	IV	Hypersensitivity reaction; nausea, vomiting; decreased clotting factors; renal dysfunction

CYP, cytochrome; DNA, deoxyribonucleic acid; IP, intraperitoneal; IT, intrathecal; IV, intravenous; PO, oral; RA-APL, retinoic acid–acute promyelocytic leukemia; RNA, ribonucleic acid; SC, subcutaneous; SIADH, syndrome of inappropriate antidiuretic hormone.

The optimal schedule is also influenced by the pharmacokinetics of the agent. For example, phase-specific agents exert their cytotoxic effects only when the cell is in a particular phase of the cell cycle. If a phase-specific agent with a short half-life is administered by intravenous bolus, a significant number of tumor cells will not be in the vulnerable phase of the cell cycle during exposure to the agent. Comparatively, the same agent administered by frequent intravenous bolus or continuous infusion could expose more cells to the agent during the vulnerable phase.[43]

Drug Resistance

CASE 93-6

QUESTION 1: B.C. is a 39-year-old male with aggressive non-Hodgkin lymphoma (NHL). At the time of diagnosis, B.C. had enlarged cervical lymph nodes, dyspnea, and a large mediastinal mass noted on chest x-ray examination. Chemotherapy was initiated with rituximab, cyclophosphamide, doxorubicin, vincristine, and prednisone (RCHOP).

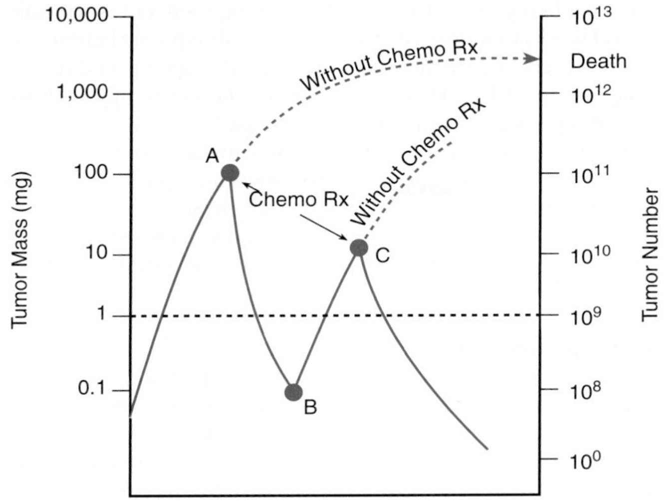

Figure 93-2 Log-kill hypothesis. The growth rate of a tumor is initially very rapid and eventually slows as it approaches 10^{11} cells. Two trillion (2×10^{12}) cells or 2 kg of tumor is lethal to humans. An effective chemotherapy treatment (Chemo Rx) given at point A will decrease the tumor number to point B. Regrowth of the tumor will occur during the recovery period until further chemotherapy is given at point C.

After the first cycle of chemotherapy, B.C.'s lymphadenopathy was greatly reduced. Chest x-ray examination repeated after the second cycle of therapy showed marked improvement. When he returned for his fifth cycle of chemotherapy, recurrent lymphadenopathy was noted and the chest radiograph confirmed enlargement of the mediastinal mass. Why is B.C.'s cancer growing despite continued chemotherapy and how should his treatment be altered?

Most likely, B.C.'s cancer is now growing because the tumor has become resistant to the chemotherapy. Therefore, it would be wise to discontinue the current regimen. Biochemical resistance to chemotherapy is the major impediment to successful treatment with most cancers.[38] Resistance can occur de novo in cancer cells or develop during cell division as a result of mutation.[38] In 1979, a proposed mathematical model known as the Goldie–Coldman hypothesis predicted that tumor cells mutate at a rate related to the genetic instability of the tumor.[44] Thus, the probability that a tumor mass will contain resistant clones is related to both the rate of mutation and the size of the tumor. Many mechanisms have been identified by which cancer cells resist the activity of cytotoxic agents.

Some cell lines that become resistant to a single chemotherapy agent may also be resistant to structurally unrelated cytotoxic compounds. This phenomenon is called pleiotropic drug resistance or multidrug resistance (MDR).[45] Cell lines that display this type of resistance are generally resistant to natural product cytotoxic agents such as the vinca alkaloids, antitumor antibiotics, epipodophyllotoxins, camptothecins, and taxanes. The primary mechanism believed to be responsible for MDR is an increase in efflux transporters such as P-glycoprotein in the cell membrane. These proteins mediate efflux of the chemotherapy agent, causing decreased accumulation of drug within the cell and decreased cytotoxicity.[45] Other transport proteins (e.g., breast cancer resistance protein) have been implicated in resistance to chemotherapy as well.[46]

Another type of MDR is resistance caused by changes or mutations of drug targets, for example, the altered binding of topoisomerase II, an enzyme that promotes DNA strand breaks in the presence of anthracyclines and epipodophyllotoxins.[47] Because of the likelihood of MDR, B.C. should receive a chemotherapy regimen that does not include agents transported from tumor cells by the MDR mechanism. An alternative regimen such as gemcitabine or oxaliplatin, with or without rituximab, may be a reasonable option because this regimen is active against NHL and these drugs are not known substrates for various efflux transporters.

Tumor Site

The cytotoxic effects of chemotherapy agents are related to the time the tumor is exposed to an effective concentration of the agent (i.e., concentration × time [C × T]). The drug dose, infusion rate, route of administration, lipophilicity, and protein binding can influence the concentration–time product. Other factors, such as tumor size and location, can also critically affect an agent's cytotoxicity. As tumors grow larger, their degree of vascularity lessens, making it more difficult for agents to penetrate the entire tumor mass. Tumors located in sites of the body with poor drug penetration (e.g., the brain) may not receive a sufficient concentration to provide effective kill.

Pharmacogenetics

Antitumor activity and adverse effects of chemotherapy agents are associated with the presence of genetic polymorphisms that can affect the metabolism and disposition of drug. See Chapter 97, Breast Cancer, and Chapter 99, Colorectal Cancer, for a more detailed discussion of genetic polymorphisms associated with UGT1A1, CY2D6, and HER2/neu receptor positivity.

Combination Chemotherapy

CASE 93-7

Question 1: K.K. has newly diagnosed stage II, bulky Hodgkin lymphoma. She initially presented with asymptomatic lymphadenopathy, night sweats, and a 15% weight loss in the previous 2 months. K.K. is to begin chemotherapy today with doxorubicin, bleomycin, vinblastine, and dacarbazine. All of these chemotherapy agents have activity in Hodgkin lymphoma. Why is it recommended that K.K. receive all four drugs, rather than just one drug?

Although single-agent chemotherapy can cause significant early regression of Hodgkin lymphoma, acute lymphocytic leukemia, and adult NHL, some tumors show only a partial, very short response to single-agent therapy. In Hodgkin lymphoma, the use of combination chemotherapy results in long-term, disease-free survival for more than 60% of patients. If K.K. were to receive single-agent therapy, her disease would not be cured. Combination chemotherapy is recommended to provide her with the best chance for long-term, disease-free survival.

Combination chemotherapy provides broader coverage against resistant cell lines within the heterogeneous tumor mass. Several principles provide the basis for selecting the agents to be included in a chemotherapy regimen:

- Agents with demonstrable single-agent activity against the specific type of tumor should be used in combination therapy.
- Agents in the regimen should have different mechanisms of action.
- Agents should not have overlapping toxicities so that the severity and duration of acute and chronic toxicities are minimized.
- Agents in the regimen should be used in their optimal dose and schedule.

Subsequent chapters will provide examples of commonly used systemic regimens in the treatment of hematologic and solid tumor malignancies.

Primary treatment is the first-line therapy, and in certain tumor types may be referred to as induction therapy. Choice of primary treatment is governed by observations made from clinical trials that demonstrate that a given regimen has the highest known activity against the tumor. These regimens may include chemotherapy, targeted agents, endocrine agents, or biologic response modifiers. Second-line treatment is administered after the tumor has become refractory to primary therapy or if the patient is unable to tolerate first-line therapy. Systemic therapy is frequently used in different ways during the course of an individual's malignancy. Primary treatment can be either curative or palliative, depending on the specific type of tumor (Table 93-6).[48] After primary therapy, patients may receive additional treatment in an attempt to further eradicate residual disease and improve their chances for long-term survival. This treatment may be termed consolidation, intensification, or maintenance therapy. See subsequent chapters for specific discussion of the use of primary, consolidation, or maintenance therapy in the treatment of hematologic and solid tumor malignancies.

Adjuvant Therapy

CASE 93-8

QUESTION 1: F.R., a 58-year-old woman with no other medical problems, recently underwent surgical resection for stage III ovarian cancer. She has been told that she currently has no evidence of cancer; however, she also is told that she should now receive 6 months of chemotherapy. Why would chemotherapy be recommended now when she has no detectable disease?

Micrometastases or residual disease may still be present in some patients after primary treatment. These patients have a high probability of disease recurrence, even though the primary treatment may have successfully removed all visual evidence of the primary tumor. To eradicate any undetectable tumor in these patients, systemic therapy after initial curative surgery (or radiation therapy) may be recommended. Systemic treatment administered after primary therapy (in the case of F.R., primary therapy was surgery) is referred to as adjuvant therapy. Because the tumor burden is relatively low at this time, adjuvant therapy should immediately follow primary therapy. For adjuvant therapy to provide benefit, the risk of tumor recurrence must be high, and effective agents must be available to eradicate the tumor. Adjuvant therapy is considered standard of care for some stages of breast, lung, and colorectal cancer, but it also has benefited selected patients with ovarian cancer, Ewing sarcoma, Wilms tumor, and other malignancies (Table 93-7).[48] The duration of administration of adjuvant therapy varies depending on the type of cancer being treated and the drugs being used, but is typically several weeks to months in duration. See subsequent chapters for specific discussion of the use of adjuvant therapy in solid tumor malignancies. F.R. will receive adjuvant chemotherapy with six to eight cycles of carboplatin and paclitaxel.

Because it is difficult to detect micrometastases or residual disease, it is a challenge to determine which patients should receive adjuvant therapy. To help with these decisions, clinicians frequently consider histologic and cytogenetic characteristics of the primary tumor that are associated with high risk of relapse.

Table 93-7
Neoplasms for Which Adjuvant Systemic Therapy is Indicated After Primary Treatment

Anaplastic astrocytoma
Breast cancer
Colorectal cancer
Gastric cancer
Melanoma
Non-small-cell lung cancer
Osteogenic sarcoma
Ovarian cancer

Reprinted from DeVita VT Jr, Chu E. Principles of medical oncology: basic principles. In: DeVita VT Jr et al, eds. *DeVita, Hellman, and Rosenberg's Cancer: Principles & Practice of Oncology*. 8th ed. Philadelphia, PA: Lippincott Williams & Wilkins; 2008:339, with permission.

Neoadjuvant Therapy

Neoadjuvant therapy is given before the primary treatment (typically surgery or radiation) in patients who present with locally advanced tumors (e.g., large tumors or those that are impinging on surrounding vital structures) that are unlikely to be cured with primary therapy alone. The objective of neoadjuvant therapy is to reduce the tumor mass, thereby increasing the likelihood of eradication by subsequent surgery or radiation. Neoadjuvant therapy also can lessen the amount of radical surgery the patient needs, which can preserve cosmetic appearance and function of the surrounding normal tissues. The tumor can be resistant to neoadjuvant therapy and continue to grow, however, making surgery or radiation even more difficult. Patients may also experience toxicities with neoadjuvant therapy that may delay surgery or impair postsurgical healing. Locally advanced tumors in which neoadjuvant therapy has been shown to improve survival rates include non-small-cell lung cancer, breast cancer, sarcomas, esophageal cancers, laryngeal cancer, bladder cancer, and osteogenic sarcoma (Table 93-8).[48] See subsequent chapters for specific discussion of the use of neoadjuvant therapy in solid tumors.

CASE 93-9

QUESTION 1: H.P. is a 57-year-old man who is currently undergoing a staging workup for a presumed diagnosis of metastatic adenocarcinoma of the lung. He has heard that cytotoxic "chemotherapy is the only thing available to treat metastatic cancer." What other agents are being used to treat cancer besides those that are considered cytotoxic?

TARGETED THERAPY

By understanding the mechanisms by which cancer cells exhibit unregulated growth and immortality and possess the ability to invade tissues and metastasize, it has been possible to design drugs that inhibit these processes.

Monoclonal Antibodies

Directed at specific receptors associated with cancer, monoclonal antibodies block ligands from binding to their targets. Unlike traditional chemotherapy, monoclonal antibodies selectively target receptors or their ligands known to potentiate cancer pathways, and as a result, minimize toxicity to noncancer cells. Table 93-9 provides a list of monoclonal antibodies currently approved by the US Food and Drug Administration to treat malignancy.[35]

Tyrosine Kinase Inhibitors

Tyrosine kinase inhibitors (TKIs) are small molecules that directly inhibit tyrosine kinase activation by competing with ATP for binding to the intracellular tyrosine kinase domain. Advantages of these inhibitors include inhibiting cells that may not overexpress the receptor on their surface or have mutated forms of the receptor that result in its activation and direct inhibition of cell signaling. Even though most TKIs are designed to inhibit a single target, they

Table 93-8

Neoplasms for Which Neoadjuvant Systemic Therapy is Indicated for Locally Advanced Disease

Anal cancer
Bladder cancer
Breast cancer
Cervical cancer
Gastroesophageal cancer
Lung cancer
Head and neck cancer
Ovarian cancer
Osteogenic sarcoma
Pancreatic cancer

Reprinted with permission from DeVita VT, Jr, Chu E. Principles of medical oncology: basic principles. In: DeVita VT, Jr et al, eds. *DeVita, Hellman, and Rosenberg's Cancer: Principles & Practice of Oncology*. 8th ed. Philadelphia, PA: Lippincott Williams & Wilkins; 2008:338.

often have inhibitory properties for additional molecules, which could affect an internal cascade of biologic activity resulting in antitumor activity and toxicity.

This class of drug is taken orally. Due to varying pharmacokinetics, specific instructions on self-administration should be provided to patients (i.e., take on an empty stomach, take with a full meal). Additionally, many TKIs are substrates, inhibitors, and inducers of CYP P450 enzymes. Attention to potential drug interaction is crucial to safe medication use.

Table 93-10 provides the TKIs currently approved by the US Food and Drug Administration to treat malignancies.[35]

Other Targeted Therapy

Because more information is learned regarding signal transduction pathways and cellular growth and proliferation, more drugs are being developed that target these key molecules. Histone deacetylase (HDAC) inhibitors, mammalian target of rapamycin (mTOR) inhibitors, and proteasome inhibitors are examples of drugs that have novel mechanism(s) of action. Table 93-11 lists these and other targeted agents currently approved by the US Food and Drug Administration to treat malignancies.[35]

Combination Therapy with Targeted Agents

The optimal activity of adding targeted agents to cytotoxic chemotherapy is difficult to predict. Knowledge about how to combine targeted agents with chemotherapy is limited, although clinical investigations are ongoing. See subsequent chapters for specific discussion of the use of targeted therapy with chemotherapy in solid tumor and hematologic malignancies.

ENDOCRINE THERAPY

Endocrine therapy can be used to treat several common cancers, including breast, prostate, and endometrial cancers, which arise from hormone-sensitive tissues (Table 93-12). These tumors grow in response to endogenous hormones that trigger growth signals. Current endocrine therapies inhibit tumor growth by blocking hormone receptors or by eliminating endogenous hormone feeding the tumor. Not all tumors arising from hormone-sensitive tissues respond to endocrine manipulation. Lack of response may be associated with hormone-resistant tumor cells or inadequate suppression of the endogenous feeding hormones.[49]

IMMUNOTHERAPY

Immune therapy is comprised of substances that stimulate the body's immune system to identify circulating tumor cells. Some agents target certain cells of the immune system; other agents are more nonspecific.[34] An individual's immune system plays a crucial role in developing or eradicating cancer. Normally, an intact immune system can protect the host against malignant cells and infectious pathogens, but current evidence shows that individuals with "weakened" immune systems are at an increased risk of developing cancer. Immunotherapy can include vaccines, cytokines, and checkpoint inhibitors.

Table 93-9

Monoclonal Antibodies

Class[a]	Agent (Trade Name)	Mechanism of Action	Notable Toxicities
Anti-CD19, Anti-CD3	Blinatumomab (Blincyto)	Binds to CD19 on B cells and CD3 on T cells; causes formation of cytolytic synapses between B and T cells	Neurotoxicity; infection; tremor; fever; edema, rash; nausea, diarrhea, constipation; cytokine release syndrome
Anti-CD20	Obinutuzumab (Gazyva)	Binds to CD20 on B cells; induces cell death via ADCC, CDC, and antibody-dependent cellular phagocytosis	Myelosuppression; hepatic and renal dysfunction; electrolyte abnormalities; infection; infusion reaction
	Ofatumumab (Arzerra)	Binds to CD20 on B cells at different binding sites than rituximab; induces cell death via ADCC and CDC	Cough; diarrhea, nausea; fatigue; myelosuppression; hypersensitivity reaction, pyrexia; rash; infection
	Rituximab (Rituxan)	Binds to CD20 on B cells; induces cell death via ADCC and CDC	Hypersensitivity reaction; myelosuppression; infection; tumor lysis syndrome
Anti-CD20 Radiation	Ibritumomab tiuxetan (Zevalin)	Yttrium-90 (Y-90) linked to rituximab; binds to CD20 on B cells and releases radiation (β particles); induces cell damage via free radicals	Infusion-related reaction; chills, nausea; fatigue; myelosuppression; see notable toxicities for rituximab
	Tositumomab (Bexxar)	Iodine-131 linked to rituximab; binds to CD20 on B cells and releases radiation; induces cell death via ADCC and CDC	Infusion-related reaction; nausea; myelosuppression, infection; hypothyroidism; see notable toxicities for rituximab

(continued)

Table 93-9
Monoclonal Antibodies (*continued*)

Class[a]	Agent (Trade Name)	Mechanism of Action	Notable Toxicities
Anti-CD30	Brentuximab vedotin (Adcetris)	Three-component antibody drug conjugate; binds to cells expressing CD30 and is internalized; monomethyl auristatin E is then released which disrupts the microtubule network	Myelosuppression; peripheral neuropathy; fatigue; nausea, vomiting, diarrhea; fever; rash; upper respiratory infection
Anti-CD52	Alemtuzumab (Campath)	Binds to CD52, leading to lysis of CD52-positive leukemic cells	Hypersensitivity reaction; myelosuppression, opportunistic infection, fever; nausea, rash
Anti-EGFR	Cetuximab (Erbitux)	Binds to EGFR, preventing activation and inhibiting cell proliferation	Papulopustular rash; hypersensitivity reaction; fatigue; nausea, vomiting, stomatitis; hypomagnesemia
	Panitumumab (Vectibix)	Binds to EGFR with higher affinity than cetuximab, preventing activation and inhibiting cell proliferation	Papulopustular rash, pruritus; fatigue; hypersensitivity reactions; abdominal pain, nausea, diarrhea; hypomagnesemia; paronychia
Anti-HER2	Ado-Trastuzumab emtansine (Kadcyla)	HER2-antibody drug conjugate of trastuzumab and microtubule inhibitor DM1; binds to HER2 inducing cell cycle arrest and cell death	Myelosuppression, nausea, constipation, diarrhea; fatigue, peripheral neuropathy; hypokalemia, fever
	Pertuzumab (Perjeta)	Binds to HER2, inhibiting HER2 dimerization and downstream signaling, halting cell growth	Myelosuppression; cardiomyopathy; fatigue, alopecia; nausea, vomiting, diarrhea
	Trastuzumab (Herceptin)	Binds to HER2; induces cell death via ADCC	Cardiomyopathy; nausea, vomiting, diarrhea; infusion-related reaction
Anti-VEGF	Bevacizumab (Avastin)	Binds to and inhibits VEGF ligand interaction with receptors, blocking angiogenesis	Hypertension; bleeding, thrombosis; gastrointestinal perforation; impaired wound healing; proteinuria
	Ramucirumab (Cyramza)	Binds to and inhibits VEGF2 ligand interaction with receptors (VEGF-A, VEGF-C, VEGF-D), blocking angiogenesis	Hypertension; proteinuria; infusion-related reaction; bleeding; thrombosis; gastrointestinal perforation
Immune Checkpoint Inhibitors	Ipilimumab (Yervoy)	Enhances T-cell activation and proliferation by inhibiting CTLA-4; restoring antitumor immune response	Fatigue; nausea, anorexia, diarrhea, colitis; pruritus, rash; hepatic dysfunction; hypophysitis
	Nivolumab (Opdivo)	Enhances T-cell activation and proliferation by inhibiting PD-1 activity, which is a negative regulator of T-cell pathways; restores antitumor immune response	Rash, pruritus; nausea, constipation, diarrhea; fatigue; electrolyte abnormalities; hepatic dysfunction; musculoskeletal pain; cough, pneumonitis
	Pembrolizumab (Keytruda)		Fatigue; pruritus, rash; electrolyte abnormalities; hepatic dysfunction; nausea, constipation, diarrhea; arthralgia; cough, pneumonitis
Other	Dinutuximab (Unituxin)	Cell lysis of GD-2-expressing neuroblastoma cells via ADCC and CDC	Myelosuppression; urticaria; diarrhea, nausea, vomiting; hepatotoxicity; fever; capillary leak syndrome; infusion-related reaction; peripheral neuropathy

[a]All monoclonal antibodies are administered intravenously, IV.
ADCC, antibody-dependent cellular toxicity; CDC, complement-dependent cytotoxicity; CTLA-4, cytotoxic T-lymphocyte-associated antigen-4; EGFR, epidermal growth factor receptor; HER, human epidermal growth factor receptor; PD-1, programmed cell death-1; VEGF, vascular endothelial growth factor.

Sipuleucel-T (Provenge) is a cancer vaccine approved for patients with metastatic prostate cancer that is resistant to prior endocrine therapy.[50] The immune system is stimulated to recognize the patient's own cancer cells. The cytokines, interferon-α and interleukin 2, were the first immune-modulating therapies available. They nonspecifically stimulate B- and T-cell proliferation and differentiation along with activity on other immune functions.[51–56] Immune checkpoint inhibitors release the brakes on the immune system, allowing it to identify and kill cancer cells better.[34]

If H.P. is in fact diagnosed with stage IV adenocarcinoma of the lung, he may receive other agents besides chemotherapy during

Table 93-10
Tyrosine Kinase Inhibitors

Class[a]	Agent (Trade Name)	Mechanism of Action	Notable Toxicities
ALK inhibitor		Inhibits ALK thereby reducing tumor cell proliferation in cells expressing ALK fusion protein; also inhibits ROS1 kinase	Myelosuppression, visual disturbances; liver enzyme elevations; diarrhea, nausea, vomiting; fatigue
	Ceritinib (Zykadia)	Also inhibits IGF-1R, insulin receptor kinases	Also: increased creatinine; hyperglycemia
	Crizotinib (Xalkori)		Also: dysgeusia; edema; bradycardia
BCR-ABL inhibitor		Inhibits BCR-ABL kinase, c-KIT, and PDGFR kinases	Myelosuppression; nausea, vomiting, diarrhea; fatigue; dermatologic toxicity
	Bosutinib (Bosulif)	Includes activity against most imatinib-resistant BCR-ABL mutations and SRC kinases	Also: electrolyte disturbances; liver enzyme elevations; fever; cough, dyspnea
	Dasatinib (Sprycel)	Inhibits most imatinib-resistant BCR-ABL mutation kinases and SRC kinases	Also: headache; fluid retention, pleural effusion
	Imatinib mesylate (Gleevec)		Also: fluid retention; headache; hepatic toxicity; musculoskeletal pain
	Nilotinib (Tasigna)	Inhibits most imatinib-resistant BCR-ABL mutation kinases	Also: musculoskeletal pain; hepatic toxicity; hyperglycemia; QT prolongation
	Ponatinib (Iclusig)	Inhibits most imatinib-resistant BCR-ABL mutation kinases and VEGFR, SRC RET, and FLT3 kinases	Also: hypertension; edema, arterial ischemia; headache; arthralgias; constipation; hepatic dysfunction; dyspnea, pleural effusion
BTK inhibitor		Irreversibly inhibits the BTK of the B-cell receptor signaling pathway	Myelosuppression; nausea, diarrhea; fatigue, edema, fever; dermatologic toxicity; musculoskeletal pain; tumor lysis syndrome
	Ibrutinib (Imbruvica)		
EGFR inhibitor		Inhibits EGFR TK; resulting tumor growth inhibition	Rash, dry skin, pruritis; paronychia; diarrhea
	Afatinib (Gilotrif)	Irreversible inhibitor of EGFR as well as HER2 and HER4	Also: stomatitis, decreased appetite
	Erlotinib (Tarceva)	Reversible inhibitor of EGFR	
HER2 inhibitor		Reversibly inhibits HER2 and EGFR TK	Nausea, diarrhea; dermatologic toxicity; myelosuppression; hepatic toxicity; cardiomyopathy, QT prolongation; pulmonary toxicity
	Lapatinib (Tykerb)		
MEK inhibitor		Decreased cell proliferation and increased apoptosis by inhibiting MEK activation, which is a downstream effector of BRAF (mutant)	Cardiomyopathy; acneiform rash; diarrhea; hepatic dysfunction; edema; QT prolongation; hypoalbuminemia
	Trametinib (Mekinist)		
PI3K inhibitor		Inhibits PI3K expressed on B cells	Myelosuppression; nausea, diarrhea, colitis, gastrointestinal perforation; fatigue; hepatic toxicity; pulmonary toxicity
	Idelalisib (Zydelig)		
VEGF inhibitor		Inhibits VEGF receptor tyrosine kinases thereby blocking angiogenesis and tumor growth	Hypertension; diarrhea, nausea, vomiting
	Axitinib (Inlyta)		Also: electrolyte disturbances; creatinine increased; fatigue; myelosuppression; proteinuria
	Cabozantinib (Cometriq)	Also inhibits FLT-3, KIT, MET, RET kinases	Also: liver enzyme elevation; stomatitis, weight loss, anorexia; fatigue; electrolyte disturbances; hand-foot syndrome, hair color changes
	Lenvatinib (Lenvima)	Also inhibits PDGFR, KIT, and RET kinases	Also: palmar-plantar erythrodysesthesia; proteinuria; thrombosis, bleeding; hepatic toxicity; gastrointestinal perforation

(continued)

Table 93-10
Tyrosine Kinase Inhibitors (*continued*)

Class[a]	Agent (Trade Name)	Mechanism of Action	Notable Toxicities
	Pazopanib (Votrient)	Also inhibits c-KIT, PDGFR, FGFR kinases	Also: depigmentation of hair and skin; dysgeusia, visual disturbances; muscle spasms; alopecia, rash
	Regorafenib (Stivarga)	Also inhibits PDGFR-α and -β, RET, RAF-1 kinases	Also: mucositis; fatigue; proteinuria; palmar-plantar erythrodysesthesia: rash; dysphonia; fever; myelosuppression; infection
	Sorafenib (Nexavar)	Also inhibits RAF kinases, PDGFR-β, FLT-3, c-KIT, RET kinases	Also: rash, palmar-plantar erythrodysesthesia; myelosuppression
	Sunitinib (Sutent)	Also inhibits PDGFR-α and -FLT-3 kinases	Also: Myelosuppression; prolonged QT interval; palmar-plantar erythrodysesthesia, skin discoloration
	Vandetanib (Caprelsa)	Also inhibits EGFR, RET, SRC kinases	Also: QT prolongation; headache; colitis; hepatic dysfunction; leukopenia; rash, photosensitivity

[a] All tyrosine kinase inhibitors are administered orally, PO.
ALK, anaplastic lymphoma kinase; ROS1, c-ros oncogene 1; IGF-1R, insulin-like growth factor 1 receptor; BCR-ABL, breakpoint cluster region-ABL1 gene fusion gene; KIT, tyrosine-protein kinase kit; PDGFR, platelet-derived growth factor; SRC, steroid receptor coactivator; VEGFR, vascular endothelial growth factor receptor; RET, c-RET oncogene; FLT-3, Fms-like tyrosine kinase 3; BTK, Bruton tyrosine kinase; EGFR, epidermal growth factor receptor; TK, tyrosine kinase; HER2, human epidermal growth factor receptor 2; HER4, human epidermal growth factor receptor 4; MEK, mitogen-activated protein kinase (MAPK)/ extracellular signal-regulated kinase (ERK) kinase; BRAF, proto-oncogene b-Raf; PI3K, phosphatidylinositol 3-kinase; MET, proto-oncogene c-Met; FGFR, fibroblast growth factor receptor; RAF, MAPK 3 kinase

the course of treatment for his disease. For specific discussion of which noncytotoxic agents H.P may receive, refer to Chapter 98, Lung Cancer.

Administration

Systemic

Systemic chemotherapy is most commonly administered by the intravenous route, either as a bolus injection (generally <15 minutes), short infusion (15 minutes to several hours), or as a continuous infusion (lasting 24 hours to several weeks). Some chemotherapy can also be administered orally, intramuscularly, or subcutaneously.

Targeted agents are most commonly administered intravenously or orally. Monoclonal antibodies are primarily administered intravenously, whereas small-molecule TKIs are primarily administered by mouth. Endocrine agents are primarily administered orally or subcutaneously.

Although chemotherapy was initially developed for systemic use, techniques have been developed to administer agents directly to specific sites of the body affected by the tumor (Table 93-13). Regionally or locally administered chemotherapy allows for high concentrations of drug at the tumor site while reducing systemic exposure and subsequent toxicity. However, a potential disadvantage is that distant micrometastases may not be exposed to chemotherapy, allowing continued growth of tumor cells.

Assessing Response to Therapy

CASE 93-10

QUESTION 1: G.K. is a 67-year-old woman who was recently diagnosed with metastatic breast cancer. Her symptoms include widespread pain, anorexia, and fatigue. She has received two cycles of treatment with a combination chemotherapy regimen. A recent CT scan of her abdomen showed marked shrinkage at several tumor sites and her pain has decreased. How long should she continue to receive this chemotherapy?

An important step in the treatment process is assessing response to treatment. This assessment should include evaluation of efficacy as well as toxicity, including impact on the patient's overall quality of life. Re-evaluation should occur at regularly scheduled intervals and include physical examination, laboratory tests, and repeat diagnostic imaging.

Response Evaluation Criteria in Solid Tumors (RECIST) was introduced in 2000 to unify response assessment criteria, define how to choose evaluable tumors, and enable the use of new imaging technologies (spiral CT and MRI). The World Health Organization, National Cancer Institute, and European Organization for Research and Treatment of Cancer have adopted RECIST criteria as the standard for evaluating tumor response (Table 93-14).[57]

Several standardized toxicity grading scales are available to assess toxicity associated with chemotherapy. However, the National Cancer Institute Common Toxicity Criteria for Adverse Events is the most commonly used.[31,58] Toxic effects of systemic therapy will be further discussed in Chapter 94, Adverse Effects of Chemotherapy and Targeted Agents.

Because toxicities associated with systemic therapy are potentially severe, it is important to evaluate the risks and benefits. The benefits of a treatment regimen should outweigh the negative effects it has on the physical, mental, and social well-being of the patient. To monitor a patient's quality of life, several comprehensive assessment tools have been developed.[59] In addition, other clinical benefits (e.g., reduced pain, decreased use of analgesics, weight gain, improved performance status) have been recognized by the US Food and Drug Administration as acceptable criteria for measuring quality of life. These criteria are also considered when evaluating new agents for approval.

G.K. should continue to receive the same therapy as long as her tumor is responding and she does not experience intolerable or life-threatening treatment-related toxicities. For some cancers, continued therapy after a certain number of cycles is not associated with further benefit because toxicity becomes an overriding issue.

Tumor Markers

Tumor markers are substances found in tumor tissue or released from tumor into the blood or other body fluids (e.g., urine).[34]

Table 93-11
Other Targeted and Miscellaneous Agents

Class	Agent (Trade Name)	Mechanism of Action	Route of Administration	Notable Toxicities
HDAC inhibitors		Inhibits HDAC resulting in accumulation of acetyl groups, cell cycle arrest, and apoptosis		Nausea, vomiting; fatigue; myelosuppression; fever; peripheral edema; EKG changes
	Belinostat (Beleodaq)		IV	
	Panobinostat (Farydak)		PO	Also: diarrhea; electrolyte abnormalities; increased creatinine; fever
	Romidepsin (Istodax)		IV	Also: anorexia, dysgeusia; pruritis, dermatitis; infection
	Vorinostat (Zolinza)		PO	Also: diarrhea, anorexia, weight loss, dysgeusia; proteinuria; pruritis, alopecia
Proteasome inhibitor		Inhibits proteasomes, enzymes that regulate protein homeostasis within cells		Nausea, diarrhea, constipation; peripheral neuropathy; headache, fatigue, fever; myelosuppression; herpes zoster reactivation
	Bortezomib (Velcade)		IV and SC	
	Carfilzomib (Kyprolis)		IV	Also: edema, dyspnea; cardiac toxicity; hypersensitivity reactions
mTOR inhibitors		Inhibits mTOR kinase, VEGFR		Fatigue, nausea, anorexia; dermatologic toxicity; hyperlipidemia, hyperglycemia, electrolyte abnormalities; stomatitis; myelosuppression, infection; pneumonitis
	Everolimus (Afinitor)		PO	
	Temsirolimus (Torisel)		IV	Also: gastrointestinal perforation
Immunomodulating Agents		Immunomodulatory and angiogenic effects		Fatigue; teratogenic potential; thromboembolism; arthralgias
	Lenalidomide (Revlimid)	Inhibits secretion of proinflammatory cytokines; induces cell cycle arrest and apoptosis in myeloma cells	PO	Also: thrombocytopenia, neutropenia, pruritus; rash; diarrhea, pyrexia; dizziness
	Pomalidomide (Pomalyst)	Induces cell cycle arrest and apoptosis in myeloma cells; enhances T-cell- and NK-cell-mediated cytotoxicity	PO	Also: rash; peripheral edema; constipation, nausea, diarrhea; myelosuppression; muscle spasms; dyspnea, renal dysfunction
	Thalidomide (Thalomid)		PO	Also: bradycardia; dizziness; somnolence; neutropenia, peripheral neuropathy
BRAF inhibitor		Blocks cellular proliferation of mutated BRAF		Dermatologic toxicity; nausea, diarrhea; edema; headache; hepatic dysfunction; fever, chills; secondary skin cancer
	Dabrafenib (Tafinlar)		PO	Also: electrolyte abnormalities, hyperglycemia; myelosuppression
	Vemurafenib (Zelboraf)		PO	Also: fatigue; arthralgias; anorexia
Other				
CDK inhibitor	Palbociclib (Ibrance)	Reversibly inhibits CDK	PO	Myelosuppression, infection, fatigue; nausea, vomiting, diarrhea; stomatitis, alopecia; thrombosis
Hedgehog inhibitor	Vismodegib (Erivedge)	Selectively binds and inhibits the transmembrane protein in Hedgehog signal transduction pathway; inhibits unrestricted proliferation of skin basal cells	PO	Fatigue; alopecia; anorexia, nausea, diarrhea, constipation; muscle spasms; arthralgias

(continued)

Table 93-11
Other Targeted and Miscellaneous Agents (*continued*)

Class	Agent (Trade Name)	Mechanism of Action	Route of Administration	Notable Toxicities
IL-2 receptor inhibitor	Denileukin diftitox (Ontak)	Fusion protein containing diphtheria toxin and IL-2 segments; directs cytocidal action of diphtheria toxin to IL-2 receptor-expressing cells leading to inhibition of protein synthesis, cell death	IV	Hypersensitivity reaction; nausea, vomiting, diarrhea; fatigue; rash; fever, rigors, capillary leak syndrome; peripheral edema
PARP inhibitor	Olaparib (Lynparza)	Inhibits the PARP enzyme, inducing synthetic lethiality in BRCA deficient cells	PO	Nausea, vomiting, fatigue; myelosuppression; musculoskeletal pain; thrombosis; upper respiratory infection; interstitial lung disease; secondary malignancy
VEGF inhibitor	Ziv-Aflibercept (Zaltrap)	Fusion protein comprised of VEGF receptor binding domains, acting as a decoy receptor for VEGF, inhibiting angiogenesis	IV	Fatigue, diarrhea, stomatitis; myelosuppression; hypertension, proteinuria; bleeding, impaired wound healing; thrombosis; gastrointestinal perforation

IV, intravenous; PO, oral; SC, subcutaneous; HDAC, histone deacetylase; mTOR, mammalian target of rapamycin; VEGF, vascular endothelial growth factor; NK, natural killer; BRAF, proto-oncogene b-Raf; CDK, cyclin-dependent kinase; IL-2, interleukin 2; PARP, poly ADP-ribose polymerase.

Table 93-12
Endocrine Therapies

Class	Agent	Mechanism of Action	Route of Administration	Notable Toxicities
Androgens		Synthetic derivative of testosterone; suppresses GnRH, LH, FSH by a negative feedback system		Deepening voice, alopecia, hirsutism, facial or truncal acne, fluid retention, menstrual irregularities, cholestatic jaundice
	Fluoxymesterone (Androxy)		PO	
Antiandrogens				Hot flashes; breast tenderness; hepatic dysfunction, diarrhea; fatigue; edema; hypertension; arthralgia
	Abiraterone (Zytiga)	Inhibits formation of testosterone precursors (DHEA, androstenedione); selectively inhibits CYP17	PO	Also: hypertriglyceridemia; electrolyte abnormalities
	Bicalutamide (Casodex)	Nonsteroidal androgen receptor inhibitor	PO	Also: gynecomastia; back pain; constipation; infection
	Enzalutamide (Xtandi)	Inhibits androgen receptor translocation, leading to cellular apoptosis	PO	Also: constipation; neutropenia
	Flutamide (Eulexin)	Inhibits androgen uptake and binding in tissue; nonsteroidal	PO	Also: galactorrhea; decreased libido; impotence; rectal hemorrhage
	Nilutamide (Nilandron)	Nonsteroidal androgen receptor inhibitor	PO	Also: insomnia; headache; constipation; flu-like syndrome; decreased libido
Antiestrogens		Competitive binding of estrogen receptors produces downregulation of estrogen receptors		Liver enzyme elevation; hot flashes; myalgia, arthralgia; nausea, vomiting; thromboembolism
	Fulvestrant (Faslodex)		IM	
	Tamoxifen (Nolvadex, Soltamox)		PO	Also: nausea, vomiting; edema, endometrial cancer

Table 93-12
Endocrine Therapies (*continued*)

Class	Agent	Mechanism of Action	Route of Administration	Notable Toxicities
Aromatase inhibitors		Inhibits aromatase preventing androgen conversion to estrogen		Hot flashes; nausea; fatigue, insomnia; increased risk of bone fractures, arthralgia
	Anastrozole (Arimidex)		PO	
	Exemestane (Aromasin)		PO	
	Letrozole (Femara)		PO	Also: hypercholesterolemia
Estrogens		Suppresses androgen synthesis, as well as secretions of gonadotropins, FSH and LH via negative feedback system		Nausea, vomiting, fluid retention, hot flashes, anorexia, thromboembolism, hepatic dysfunction
	Ethinyl estradiol (Estradiol)		PO	
	Conjugated estrogens (Premarin)		PO	Also: headache
GnRH analogs (LHRH agonists)		Downregulates GnRH receptor on the pituitary gland, decreasing secretion of FSH and LH		Amenorrhea, hot flashes, sexual dysfunction; nausea, edema; tumor flare; injection-site reaction; osteoporosis
	Goserelin (Zoladex)		SC	Also: headache, emotional lability, cystitis, vaginitis
	Histrelin (Vantas)		SC	
	Leuprolide (Lupron, Eligard)		IM, SC	Also: vaginitis
	Triptorelin (Trelstar)		IM	
GnRH antagonists		Binds to GHRH receptors on the pituitary gland, blocking secretion of FSH and LH		Hot flashes; hepatic toxicity; injection-site reaction
	Degarelix (Firmagon)		SC	
Progestins		Promotes differentiation and maintenance of endometrial tissue		Weight gain, edema; hot flashes, vaginal bleeding; thrombosis
	Medroxyprogesterone (Provera)		PO	Also: emotional lability
	Megestrol acetate (Megace)	Also: may suppress LH and enhance estrogen metabolism	PO	

CYP, cytochrome; DHEA, dehydroepianderosterone; FSH, follicle-stimulating hormone; GnRH, gonadotropin-releasing hormone; IM, intramuscular; LH, luteinizing hormone; LHRH, luteinizing hormone-releasing hormone; PO, oral; SC, subcutaneous.

Table 93-13
Regional or Local Routes of Chemotherapy Administration

Route of Administration	Cancer Managed With Alternative Route
Intrathecal or intraventricular	Leukemia, lymphoma
Intravesicular	Bladder
Intraperitoneal	Ovarian
Intrapleural	Malignant pleural effusions
Intra-arterial	Melanoma, sarcoma
Hepatic artery	Liver metastases
Chemoembolization (intra-arterial or intravenous)	Colon, rectal, carcinoid, liver metastases

However, not all cancers have relevant tumor markers. The ideal tumor marker should be produced and released primarily by cancer cells (or by other tissues in response to tumor) at levels proportional to the tumor mass. Surgical removal of the tumor, radiation therapy, or therapeutic response to systemic therapy should result in a reduction in the level of the marker. In addition, the ideal tumor marker should be measurable at very low levels, allowing for detection of tumor at lower volumes than conventional diagnostic imaging permits.[60] Tumor markers may therefore be used to monitor patients in remission and to detect recurrent disease. Unfortunately, few tumor markers fulfill these criteria sufficiently to be clinically useful as the sole screening or diagnostic test. Most tumor markers lack specificity for tumor and may be elevated due to other causes. Table 93-15 lists some of the common tumor markers used in practice.

Table 93-14
Response Criteria for Evaluating Effects of Chemotherapy of Target Lesion (RECIST version 1.1)

Complete Response
Disappearance of all target lesions. Any pathologic lymph nodes (whether target or nontarget) must have reduction in short axis to <10 mm

Partial Response
At least a 30% decrease in the sum of diameters of target lesions, taking as reference the baseline sum diameters

Progressive Disease
At least a 20% increase in the sum of diameters of target lesions, taking as reference the smallest sum on study (this includes the baseline sum if that is the smallest on study). In addition to the relative increase of 20%, the sum must also demonstrate an absolute increase of at least 5 mm. The appearance of one or more new lesions is also considered progression

Stable Disease
Neither sufficient shrinkage to qualify for partial response nor sufficient increase to qualify for progressive disease, taking as reference the smallest sum diameters while on study

Table 93-15
Clinically Useful Tumor Markers

Tumor Markers	Cancers Commonly Associated With Increased Markers
CA-19-9	Pancreatic
CA-15-3, CA-27-29	Breast
α-Fetoprotein (AFP)	Liver, testicular, ovarian
CA-125	Ovarian
Carcinoembryonic antigen (CEA)	Colon, lung
Human chorionic gonadotropin (hCG)	Trophoblastic, testicular
β_2-Microglobulin	Multiple myeloma
Prostate-specific antigen (PSA)	Prostate

HANDLING OF CYTOTOXIC DRUGS

Impact on the Pharmacy

CASE 93-11

QUESTION 1: The administrator of an outpatient care clinic recently announced that two medical oncologists will be joining the staff. Previously, patients were referred to outside oncologists and no cytotoxic drugs were prepared or administered at this clinic. What implications will the addition of these physicians have on the pharmacy department?

Addition of cancer treatment to institutional services will affect three areas of the pharmacy department: budget, policies and procedures for safe drug handling and disposal, and the staff education program. The pharmacy department will need to increase its budget to accommodate additional personnel and purchase new equipment, supplies, supportive care medicines, and chemotherapy agents. To estimate the projected budget increase, pharmacy leadership should meet with the oncologists to discuss anticipated volume of chemotherapy orders including systemic therapy and supportive care medicines (e.g., antiemetic therapy, analgesics, growth factors) likely to be prescribed. All new systemic therapy agents and supportive care medicines should be added to the institutional formulary. In addition, projected use of investigational agents, clinical pharmacy services needed, and any plans to develop an ambulatory infusion program should be determined. Institutional policies and procedures to ensure safe handling of chemotherapy agents must be created. These should be conveyed to all personnel affected through a staff education program because safe handling of chemotherapy agents is critical in decreasing the risk of medication errors and injuries.

Medication Errors

Several chemotherapy-related medication errors resulting in death or permanent disability have been highly publicized. These devastating events have brought significant attention to the entire drug use process in oncology and have identified several factors that appear to contribute to the risk. Use of abbreviations, verbal orders, multiple-day regimens, incorrect references and protocols, and illegible medication orders has contributed to medication errors. Increasing use of computerized prescriber order entry and standardized preprinted orders have helped eliminate many errors. Several groups have responded to the problem by issuing policy recommendations to minimize such errors.[61–66]

Risks

CASE 93-11, QUESTION 2: What are the potential risks of handling cytotoxic drugs? What resources are available to assist the pharmacy director and the pharmacy staff in the development of policies and procedures?

Many of these agents are carcinogenic, teratogenic, or mutagenic in animal models and in humans at therapeutic doses.[66] Danger to healthcare personnel handling such agents results from inherent toxicities of the agents and the extent (i.e., amount and length of time) to which the workers are exposed during drug handling.[66] Various studies have attempted to assess the effect of occupational exposure to hazardous drugs on healthcare workers. These studies measured urine mutagenicity, chromosomal damage, blood concentrations, and the level of contamination that occurs in the work areas used for drug preparation and administration.[66–68] These studies indicate urine mutagenicity and chromosomal damage in workers may be a direct result of cytotoxic exposure. Other reports have correlated reproductive risks (e.g., infertility or increased risk of miscarriage) and birth defects in pregnant workers handling cytotoxic drugs.[67,69] Findings from these reports together with the toxicities observed in patients receiving therapeutic doses led the American Society of Health-System Pharmacists to conclude that healthcare workers exposed to hazardous drugs may be absorbing or inhaling these drugs and may be at risk for adverse outcomes.[66]

In response to concerns regarding occupational exposure to hazardous drugs, several groups have published guidelines for the safe handling of these agents in the workplace (i.e., storage, preparation, administration, and disposal).[66,68] These guidelines will be helpful to the pharmacy department when developing policies and procedures.

Policies and Procedures

CASE 93-11, QUESTION 3: What specific policies and procedures are necessary? What other departments should be consulted during the development and implementation of the handling guidelines?

Policies must be developed that address the entire scope of potential occupational exposures within the workplace. These policies should include (a) a worker's "right to know" regarding potential hazards; (b) education and training for workers involved with hazardous drug handling; (c) quality assurance to monitor adherence to safe handling procedures; and (d) guidelines for workers who are attempting to conceive a child, become pregnant, or are nursing.

Specific procedures that outline appropriate handling of hazardous agents during all aspects of institutional storage, use, and disposal should be developed. These procedures should address appropriate (a) storage in the receiving and storeroom areas, (b) preparation and administration of parenteral formulations, (c) manipulation and dispensing of oral and topical formulations, (d) cleanup of spills, (e) management of acute exposures, and (f) disposal of hazardous agents and supplies used to prepare and dispense chemotherapy. If the oncology program includes ambulatory infusion or home-care components, procedures should also be developed for appropriate handling and disposal of these products in the home. Handling of oral chemotherapy and biotherapy must also be specifically addressed. Policies should include processes for cleaning of tools and nondisposable items used to dispense oral cytotoxic agents to minimize contamination with other drugs.[70]

Other departments may be affected by these guidelines including medical staff, nursing, environmental services staff (in the cleanup of spills and equipment), maintenance (upkeep of equipment), and the receiving area (where cytotoxic drugs may be received from suppliers). The institutional safety office and legal staff also should be consulted to help devise the policies and procedures.

Necessary Equipment and Supplies

Case 93-11, Question 4: What equipment and supplies are necessary for handling hazardous drugs?

Proper equipment and supplies can minimize occupational exposure in the healthcare workplace by protecting both the worker and the environment. All handling guidelines recommend that manipulations (e.g., reconstitution, admixing) of hazardous drugs be done in a class II biologic safety cabinet (BSC) to provide maximal protection for the worker and the work environment. Workers also should wear gloves (one or two pairs), protective boot covers, hair cover, mask, and a disposable gown of lint-free, low-permeability fabric with long sleeves, knit cuffs, and back closure. In addition, only syringes and intravenous sets with threaded Luer lock connections should be used. Final products (e.g., syringes, intravenous bags or bottles) should be placed in sealable containers such as zipper-closure plastic bags to prevent accidental spillage and clearly labeled as a hazardous drug. The United States Pharmacopeia dictates guidelines for compounding sterile products including appropriate facilities for preparation.[71]

Disposal of hazardous waste requires specific receptacles, which should be placed in all areas where workers handle these drugs. Disposal of these agents should follow institutional, state, and local regulations. Materials for the cleanup of spills (e.g., absorbent material, plastic bags or containers, protective garments) also must be available in all areas where hazardous drugs are stored, prepared, or administered.

KEY REFERENCES AND WEBSITES

A full list of references for this chapter can be found at http://thepoint.lww.com/AT11e. Below are the key references and websites for this chapter, with the corresponding reference number in this chapter found in parentheses after the reference.

Key References

DeVita VT, Jr et al, eds. *DeVita, Hellman, and Rosenberg's Cancer: Principles & Practice of Oncology*. 9th ed. Philadelphia, PA: Lippincott Williams & Wilkins; 2011.

Siegel RL et al. Cancer statistics, 2015. *CA Cancer J Clin*. 2015:65(1):5–29.

Key Websites

American Cancer Society. http://www.cancer.org.

American Society of Health-Systems Pharmacists. *The ASHP Discussion Guide on USP Chapter for Compounding Sterile Preparations. Summary of Revisions to USP Chapter.* https://www.ashp.org/-/media/assets/policy-guidelines/docs/guidelines-compounding-sterile-preparations.ashx. (78)

American Society of Health-Systems Pharmacist. ASHP Guidelines on Handling Hazardous Drugs. https://www.ashp.org/-/media/assets/policy-guidelines/docs/guidelines-handling-hazardous-drugs.ashx.

National Cancer Institute. http://www.cancer.gov.

National Cancer Institute. Surveillance, Epidemiology and End Results. http://seer.cancer.gov.

94 Adverse Effects of Chemotherapy and Targeted Agents

Amy Hatfield Seung and Emily Mackler

CORE PRINCIPLES

		CHAPTER CASES
1	Myelosuppression is one of the most common toxicities of cytotoxic anticancer therapy. Cytotoxic therapy may affect any one or all of the bone marrow cell lines including erythrocytes, neutrophils, and platelets. Complications from anemia, neutropenia, and thrombocytopenia can cause significant morbidity and mortality, including complications from bleeding and infections. Prophylactic administration of growth factors may protect against the myelosuppressive effects of chemotherapy.	**Case 94-1 (Questions 1–4)**
2	The upper and lower gastrointestinal (GI) tract is highly susceptible to cytotoxic chemotherapy, and toxicities can include nausea and vomiting, mucositis, xerostomia, constipation, and diarrhea. Efficacy of preventive strategies is limited; thus, supportive treatment is a foundation for managing adverse effects in patients.	**Case 94-2 (Questions 1–3), Case 94-3 (Question 1)**
3	Dermatologic toxicities from anticancer therapies include alopecia, nail changes, hyperpigmentation, radiation sensitivities, hand-foot syndrome, dry skin, and papular–pustular (acneiform) rash. Most of the toxicities are cosmetic and resolve upon discontinuation of the agent. Onset and duration of dermatologic toxicities depend on the causative agent. Treatment is supportive.	**Case 94-4 (Questions 1–4), Tables 94-1 and 94-2**
4	Extravasation is the unintended infiltration of an agent into the tissue area surrounding the vein during an infusion. Several anticancer agents demonstrate vesicant properties that can cause tissue necrosis and permanent damage to the extravasated area. Cases of extravasation require emergency treatment that is agent-specific, including elevation of the extremity, extraction of the agent, hot or cold treatment, and potential antidotes.	**Case 94-4 (Questions 5–7), Tables 94-3–94-5**
5	Many anticancer therapies are associated with immunoglobulin-E-mediated hypersensitivity reactions. Monoclonal antibodies including rituximab, trastuzumab, cetuximab, and ofatumumab are among some of the agents most commonly associated with reactions. Reactions commonly occur with the first dose, and they may be minimized with premedications such as acetaminophen, diphenhydramine, and corticosteroids.	**Case 94-5 (Question 1), Tables 94-6 and 94-7**
6	Multiple types of central nervous system (CNS) toxicity, including encephalopathy, cerebellar toxicity, and peripheral neuropathy, are associated with anticancer agents and differ in presentation between various agents. Most of the symptoms of neurotoxicity are reversible over time, but modifications to regimens including discontinuation of agents or reduction of doses may be necessary.	**Case 94-6 (Questions 1–4), Table 94-8**
7	Cardiomyopathy, arrhythmias, and hypertension are common types of cardiotoxicity observed in patients receiving infusion and oral anticancer therapies. Anthracycline-induced cardiomyopathy is closely linked to a patient's cumulative dose and may be treated with current heart failure medications.	**Case 94-7 (Questions 1–4)**

Continued

		CHAPTER CASES
8	Several anticancer agents carry severe risks of nephrotoxicity and bladder toxicity for which preventive measures are necessary. Cisplatin is one of the most nephrotoxic agents. Preventive strategies for cisplatin nephrotoxicity include normal saline hydration, mannitol, and amifostine, and methotrexate-induced nephrotoxicity may be prevented with alkalinization of the urine and leucovorin rescue. Ifosfamide-induced hemorrhagic cystitis may be prevented with concomitant use of mesna.	**Case 94-8 (Questions 1, 2), Case 94-9 (Questions 1–3), Table 94-9**
9	Many anticancer medications demonstrate organ-specific toxicities, such as pulmonary fibrosis caused by bleomycin and transaminitis caused by cytarabine. Specific treatments for resolution of these toxicities do not exist; rather, supportive care for symptoms is necessary. If adverse effects do not resolve, discontinuation of therapy or dose modifications may be warranted.	**Case 94-10 (Questions 1–4), Case 94-11 (Question 1), Tables 94-10–94-13**
10	Many anticancer agents cause long-term complications after therapy, including treatment-related acute myeloid leukemia, lymphomas, bladder cancer, and bone sarcoma. The risks of secondary malignancies should be considered in assessing the adverse effect profile within the risks and benefits of specific types of therapy.	**Case 94-12 (Questions 1, 2)**
11	Cytotoxic chemotherapy is potentially gonadotoxic with use of specific agents. Sex, age, agent, and cumulative dose are factors in determining the risk of infertility. Methods of preserving fertility should be discussed with patients before initiating therapy.	**Case 94-13 (Question 1), Case 94-14 (Questions 1–3)**

Cytotoxic, targeted anticancer and immunotherapy agents are toxic to cancer cells and also to various host tissues and organs. The adverse effects of anticancer therapies are considered for both infusional and oral therapies and can be classified as common and acute toxicities, specific organ toxicities, and long-term complications. Common and acute toxicities generally occur as a result of inhibition of host-cell division. Host tissues most susceptible to cytotoxic agents include tissues with renewal cell populations, such as lymphoid tissues, bone marrow, and epithelium of the GI tract and skin. Some other common and acute toxicities (e.g., nausea and vomiting, hypersensitivity reactions) frequently occur in patients shortly after therapy. Specific organ toxicities often are attributed to a unique uptake or a selective toxicity of the anticancer agent to the organ. Long-term complications are toxicities that occur months to years after anticancer therapy. These long-term toxicities occur secondary to continued immunodeficiencies or from permanent damage to the organ cells from the specific therapy. Regardless of the type of toxicities observed, most are classified for severity by the National Cancer Institute (NCI) Common Terminology Criteria for Adverse Events. This classification creates a common method for classification of events in clinical trials and for management of toxicities that occur for patients receiving standard of care regimens.[1] These criteria may be accessed at the NCI website (**http://ctep.cancer.gov/protocolDevelopment/electronic_applications/ctc.htm**).

The toxicities associated with anticancer therapies are the most important factors limiting the use of potentially curative doses. Therefore, all discussions regarding the benefits of anticancer agents must include a discussion of toxicities associated with their use. Concerns regarding the toxicities of therapy include the incidence, predictability, severity, and reversibility of the adverse effects. In addition, the specific agent, dose intensity, and treatment duration can influence the incidence of several adverse effects. Although the incidence and predictability may be well defined in specific patient populations, the incidence often varies depending on individual susceptibility. The specific adverse effects that an individual patient will experience may be difficult to predict. Because several toxicities have well-defined characteristics, clinicians should be aware of the most common adverse effects.

Clinicians should also be aware of patient-specific factors, such as the stage of disease, concomitant illnesses, and concurrent medications, which could cause signs or symptoms that mimic the adverse effects associated with anticancer therapy. Many patients have disease involvement which may impair organ function. In addition, most patients with cancer receive many other medications, including antibiotics and analgesics, which may cause additional adverse effects or interact with anticancer agents. When a patient reports a new symptom, it may be difficult to determine whether it is secondary to anticancer therapy, concurrent medications, or disease progression.

COMMON AND ACUTE TOXICITIES

Hematologic Toxicities

The bone marrow contains a population of pluripotent stem cells capable of self-renewal and differentiation into any mature blood cell. Their progeny commits to either the myeloid or the lymphoid cell line. The myeloid stem cell further commits to developing into an erythrocyte (red blood cell (RBC)), megakaryocyte (platelet), or granulocyte (white blood cell (WBC)). Multiple types of granulocytes exist including neutrophils, basophils, and eosinophils, although neutrophils are the most common type.

After committing to a particular cell line, bone marrow precursor cells undergo a series of divisions (mitosis) to increase the number of cells. The cells then undergo several developmental stages to mature and differentiate into their final forms (postmitotic) and leave the bone marrow. The total time required for a cell to pass through the mitotic and postmitotic pool under normal resting conditions is approximately 10 to 14 days. This process is regulated by several cytokines; although many cytokines have been identified, only a few growth factors are now produced through recombinant DNA technology. These growth factors can expand the mitotic pool and accelerate maturation and differentiation. Ultimately, these growth factors decrease the total time spent in these stages to approximately 5 to 7 days.

The development and circulating life span of hematopoietic cell lines determine the severity of the depression of that cell line (nadir, lowest point) and the time course of peripheral cytopenias. Because RBCs survive approximately 120 days in the peripheral blood, clinically significant anemia is unlikely if production is impaired for a short period of time. Instead, anemia usually develops slowly after several courses of cytotoxic therapy. In contrast, platelets survive approximately 10 days, and granulocytes survive only 6 to 8 hours. Hence, neutropenia generally occurs before thrombocytopenia, but both may be observed after the first or subsequent courses of cytotoxic chemotherapy. The clinician may have to adjust the subsequent chemotherapy dosage based on nadir depth and slow recovery. Life-threatening neutropenia or thrombocytopenia often necessitates some action to minimize the risk of adverse effects with additional courses of cytotoxic chemotherapy. To diminish these effects, one can reduce the dose, delay therapy until recovery, or administer colony-stimulating factors (CSFs). The availability of CSFs provides an alternative approach to preventing severe neutropenia.

MYELOSUPPRESSION

CASE 94-1

QUESTION 1: J.T., a 68-year-old, 59-kg man with no significant past medical history, presents to the university hospital with complaints of cough and shortness of breath (SOB). Chest radiograph reveals a lesion in the right upper lobe; surgical resection and cytologic examination are positive for non-small-cell lung cancer (NSCLC). A workup for metastases is negative. J.T. is diagnosed with early-stage (stage II) NSCLC. His physicians plan to initiate adjuvant chemotherapy of carboplatin targeted to an area under the concentration–time curve (AUC) of 6 mg/mL × minute and paclitaxel 135 mg/m^2 on day 1. Discuss the toxicities that might be expected to occur with this regimen. What effects on the bone marrow can be anticipated and how might they clinically appear in J.T.? What factors can influence the incidence and severity of these adverse effects? When can J.T. expect these effects to occur?

Although several toxicities are commonly associated with carboplatin and paclitaxel, the most predictable and severe toxicity associated with this regimen is myelosuppression. This chemotherapy regimen can significantly affect any cell line, including RBCs, neutrophils, and platelets, and the cytopenias can cause significant morbidity or mortality. Decreased RBCs can cause anemia, and patients usually present with fatigue and decreased exercise tolerance. Having low neutrophil counts significantly increases a patient's risk for bacterial infections. Moreover, reduced platelets can cause thrombocytopenia, which can cause bleeding from the GI and genitourinary tracts.

Both patient-related and agent-related factors can significantly influence the degree of cytopenia a patient faces after cytotoxic therapy. Agent-related factors include the specific agent, dose intensity, and dose density. Because most anticancer treatments are not given as a single agent, the effects of concurrent cytotoxic therapies may intensify the myelosuppressive effect of an individual agent. Host factors that specifically may affect the cellularity of the bone marrow compartment also influence the degree of cytopenia. They include the following:

1. Patient age. Younger patients are generally better able to tolerate cytotoxic chemotherapy than elderly patients because they have a more cellular marrow with a decreased percentage of marrow fat.
2. Bone marrow reserve. Certain diseases might present with tumor cells in the bone marrow, such as leukemias and some lymphomas, in which case the bone marrow does not have a healthy reserve of normal hematopoietic cells to help in the recovery process.
3. The degree of myelosuppression from previous cytotoxic chemotherapy, radiation therapy, or both. Prior cytotoxic chemotherapy and radiation therapy to fields involving marrow-producing bone (pelvic bone and sternum) reduce bone marrow reserves.
4. The ability of the liver or kidney to metabolize and excrete the compounds administered. If agents are administered to patients with specific organ insufficiencies (i.e., renal or hepatic), slower clearance, resulting in increased systemic exposure, can occur. This can cause greater toxicities, including longer cytopenias.

These factors, along with the kinetics of the stem cells, can help clinicians predict the severity and duration of cytopenia observed after therapy.

With most myelosuppressive agents, the patient's WBC and platelet counts begin to fall within 5 to 7 days of cytotoxic therapy administration, reach a nadir within 7 to 10 days, and recover within 14 to 26 days. Phase-specific cytotoxic chemotherapy agents, such as the vinca alkaloids and antimetabolites, cause a fairly rapid onset of cytopenia that recovers faster than those occurring after treatment with phase-nonspecific agents, such as alkylating agents and anthracyclines. For poorly understood reasons, nitrosoureas typically produce severe, delayed neutropenia and thrombocytopenia 4 to 6 weeks after therapy. Other agents that exhibit this pattern include mitomycin and mechlorethamine. All of these anticancer agents exert their cytotoxic effects during the resting phase of the cell cycle. The nitrosoureas, as well as mitomycin and mechlorethamine, can cause two neutropenic nadirs; the first nadir occurs at the conventional time expected for phase-nonspecific agents and the second nadir occurs approximately 4 to 6 weeks after therapy. Many combination regimens with these agents are therefore given for 6-week cycles to avoid treatment before the second nadir. However, most other myelosuppressive regimens can be safely given every 3 to 4 weeks. The majority of the targeted therapies do not suppress bone marrow production, because they are designed to inhibit a specific molecular pathway rather than proliferating cells in general. Because of their minimal myelosuppressive effects, they may be desirable agents to add to regimens that are known to cause cytopenias.

Each of the agents included in J.T.'s regimen has marked myelosuppressive activity. His elderly age may place him at higher risk for exhibiting myelosuppression. J.T. should be carefully counseled to contact his physician or report to the emergency department if he experiences signs or symptoms of an infection (including fever) or bleeding. Typically, these symptoms occur 10 to 14 days after the first day of chemotherapy.

Prevention of Neutropenia

CASE 94-1, QUESTION 2: About 9 days after the first course of cytotoxic chemotherapy, J.T. experienced a severe sore throat and fever. He was admitted to the hospital and treated with intravenous (IV) antibiotics. At the time, his WBC count was 300 cells/μL; absolute neutrophil count (ANC), 50 cells/μL; platelets, 102,000 cells/μL; and hemoglobin (Hgb), 11 g/dL. His fever resolved after 3 days, and all cultures were negative for bacterial growth. It is now 3 weeks after chemotherapy, and he is scheduled to receive a second course. Should he receive the same doses he was given initially?

One option would be to reduce (usually by 25%) the dose of each agent for all subsequent cycles. Although a dose reduction can clearly cause less neutropenia, it can also compromise the response and survival of patients with chemotherapy-sensitive tumors. Because J.T.'s cancer (i.e., early-stage NSCLC) is both chemosensitive and potentially curable, a dosage reduction is undesirable. To minimize the risk of neutropenia with future therapy, CSFs can be administered to J.T. to prevent potential complications associated with neutropenia.

Prophylactic administration of CSFs can be used to reduce the myelosuppressive effects of cytotoxic chemotherapy. Several CSFs—granulocyte colony-stimulating factors (G-CSFs [filgrastim, tbo-filgrastim, and filgrastim-sndz]), granulocyte-macrophage colony-stimulating factor (GM-CSF [sargramostim]), and a pegylated long-acting form of filgrastim, pegfilgrastim—are available in the United States. Pegfilgrastim was developed with the aim of providing the same pharmacologic benefit as filgrastim while offering the advantage and convenience of fewer injections. The FDA approved filgrastim-sndz as the first biosimilar in the United States in March 2015. Although tbo-filgrastim was FDA-approved in 2012, it is not considered a biosimilar because it was filed as a Biologics License Application, prior to the establishment of the FDA biologics approval pathway. Clinical safety, particularly related to immunogenicity, is a concern with new approval of biosimilars, and assessment of tolerability and safety should occur in clinical practice.[2] The evidence-based clinical practice guidelines for the use of CSFs have been developed by the American Society of Clinical Oncology (ASCO).[3] These guidelines recommend primary prophylaxis for all patients receiving chemotherapy regimens that have been previously reported to cause a febrile neutropenia incidence of approximately 20%. A CSF used in these patients can reduce both the incidence of febrile neutropenia and need for hospitalizations and broad-spectrum antibiotics. However, CSF usage has not been shown to lead to better tumor response or higher overall survival. Two randomized Phase III clinical trials have shown that the risk of neutropenic fever is reduced when primary prophylaxis is used in regimens with a known neutropenia incidence of approximately 20%. In one trial, 928 patients with breast cancer receiving docetaxel 100 mg/m^2 every 21 days were randomly assigned to receive placebo or pegfilgrastim 6 mg subcutaneously (SC) 24 hours after chemotherapy. Patients who received pegfilgrastim had a lower incidence of febrile neutropenia (1% vs. 17%, respectively) and hospitalizations (1% vs. 14%, respectively).[4] A trial in patients ($n = 171$) with small-cell lung cancer (SCLC) receiving a dose-intense regimen containing cyclophosphamide 1,000 mg/m^2 on day 1, doxorubicin 45 mg/m^2 on day 1, and etoposide 100 mg/m^2 on days 1 to 3 every 21 days was conducted. Patients were randomly assigned to receive prophylactic antibiotics with or without filgrastim. The rate of febrile neutropenia over all five cycles was 32% with prophylactic antibiotics without filgrastim versus 18% with antibiotics and filgrastim.[5] A meta-analysis of 17 randomized trials including 3,493 adult patients with solid tumors and lymphomas showed that the use of filgrastim as primary prophylaxis reduced the risk of febrile neutropenia and improved the rate of full-dose cytotoxic chemotherapy given on schedule. Additionally, the investigators in the meta-analysis observed a significant reduction in the risk of infection-related mortality.[6] The use of CSFs for secondary prophylaxis is recommended by ASCO for those patients who experience a neutropenic complication from the prior cycle, where primary CSF was not used, when a reduced dose or treatment delay may negatively impact the survival/treatment outcome.[3] Because the regimen J.T. received does not typically produce a 20% incidence of febrile neutropenia, a CSF was not recommended for him after his first course of cytotoxic chemotherapy. Now that J.T. has experienced febrile neutropenia and he has a potentially curable malignancy, a CSF is indicated with subsequent courses of chemotherapy to prevent additional febrile episodes.

Dosing of Colony-Stimulating Factors

Case 94-1, Question 3: How should a CSF be dosed in J.T. to reduce the severity of chemotherapy-induced neutropenia?

The recommended initial dose of filgrastim, tbo-filgrastim or filgrastim-sndz, is 5 mcg/kg/day as a single daily subcutaneous (SC) injection, and of sargramostim, 250 mcg/m^2/day SC beginning 24 to 72 hours following the administration of myelotoxic chemotherapy. The ASCO guidelines state that rounding the dose of either weight-based filgrastim or sargramostim to the nearest vial size may enhance patient convenience and reduce cost without clinical detriment. Because commercially available vials or syringes contain either 300 or 480 mcg of filgrastim, adult patients weighing less than 75 kg should receive 300 mcg daily and adult patients weighing more than 75 kg should receive 480 mcg daily.[3] Because of differences in commercially available vial sizes, the weight break point for sargramostim is slightly different; patients who weigh more than 60 kg should receive 500 mcg daily and patients who weigh less than 60 kg should receive 250 mcg daily. Pegfilgrastim is given once per cycle, 24 to 72 hours following administration of myelotoxic chemotherapy and not less than 14 days prior to the next treatment, as 6 mg SC in adult patients regardless of patient weight. A new formulation of pegfilgrastim was recently approved that is a timed automated-inject device that delivers the medication 27 hours after it is activated.[7]

The ASCO guidelines also recommend a shorter duration of treatment than the manufacturers. The manufacturers recommend that therapy with filgrastim or sargramostim continues until the patient's neutrophil count is greater than 10,000 cells/μL after the expected chemotherapy nadir. This is based on the observation that the neutrophil count falls roughly 50% after discontinuing a CSF. The risk of bacterial infection is highest, however, in patients with neutrophil counts of less than 500 to 1,000 cells/μL; patients with neutrophil counts greater than that are not thought to be at high risk for experiencing bacterial infections. Thus, many clinicians elect to discontinue the CSF when the neutrophil count reaches 2,000 to 4,000 cells/μL after the chemotherapy nadir. This reduces the number of treatment days and the cost associated with therapy while concurrently reducing the excessive risk for bacterial infections. The ASCO guidelines support this recommendation to discontinue CSF earlier.

In summary, J.T. should be given either filgrastim, tbo-filgrastim or filgrastim-sndz 300 mcg/day, or sargramostim 250 mcg/day SC beginning the day after his last dose of chemotherapy. Treatment should continue until the ANC is greater than 2,000 to 4,000 cells/μL. Filgrastim is used much more widely than sargramostim. Alternatively, J.T. could receive a single 6-mg injection of pegfilgrastim the day after chemotherapy administration. This more convenient administration is due to pegfilgrastim's favorable pharmacokinetics. Self-regulation of pegfilgrastim serum levels, related to its pegylation, is almost entirely dependent on neutrophil receptor-mediated clearance. Serum levels of pegfilgrastim will remain elevated during neutropenia induced by chemotherapy, and decline on recovery of neutrophil counts.[8] Aside from high cost and inconvenience, the only negative effect of filgrastim or sargramostim therapy is mild transient bone pain. Bone pain is most commonly experienced when patients begin to recover peripheral blood cells after their nadir. The proposed mechanism suggests the stimulatory effect of CSF on granulopoiesis causes the pain. Most patients commonly report pain in bone marrow-rich areas, such as the sternum and pelvic regions. They should be advised that the bone pain experienced during marrow recovery is normal and usually is relieved with analgesic agents.

Treatment of Fever and Neutropenia with a Colony-Stimulating Factor

Case 94-1, Question 4: If J.T. was not given filgrastim and presented with febrile neutropenia, would CSF therapy be helpful?

Febrile neutropenia leads to increased hospital admissions and lengths of stay as well as greater morbidity and mortality, so the optimal indication for CSFs is as prophylaxis; however, CSFs have been studied as part of the treatment of neutropenic fever. Because the duration of neutropenia is the most significant prognostic factor in patients with established febrile neutropenia, the major benefit of CSFs is their ability to reduce the duration of neutropenia. CSFs accelerate hematopoiesis by expanding the mitotic pool of committed progenitor cells and shortening the time spent in the postmitotic pool from 6 days to 1 day. If CSFs reduce the duration of neutropenia in patients who present with febrile neutropenia, then morbidity, mortality, and cost should be significantly reduced.

The ability of CSFs to reduce the duration of neutropenia in patients with established febrile neutropenia has been addressed in numerous randomized, double-blind, placebo-controlled trials[9] and two meta-analyses.[3,10,11] The combined data for filgrastim and sargramostim reveal minimal-to-moderate benefit in reducing hospital stays and no differences in mortality. Furthermore, questions have been raised as to whether all patients with febrile neutropenia require hospitalization. Several studies have shown equal efficacy and safety with increased cost effectiveness of outpatient treatment of febrile neutropenia.[12–14] Although CSFs do appear to hasten neutrophil recovery, the true cost–benefit ratio associated with the use of these products in established febrile neutropenia remains to be determined. The ASCO guidelines currently do not support routine use of CSFs in patients with febrile neutropenia, although they do recognize that certain patients with febrile neutropenia and high-risk features predictive of clinical deterioration (e.g., age >65 years, pneumonia, fungal infection, hypotension, sepsis syndrome, uncontrolled primary disease) may benefit from use of CSFs.[3]

Thrombocytopenia

The reduction in platelets is another common myelosuppressive toxicity seen with chemotherapy. Most commonly, thrombocytopenia is managed via the use of platelet transfusions and modifications to the chemotherapy dosing scheme. Although oprelvekin, a thrombopoietic growth factor, is indicated to prevent severe thrombocytopenia and reduce the need for platelet transfusions after myelosuppressive chemotherapy in patients with nonmyeloid malignancies at high risk for developing severe thrombocytopenia, it is rarely utilized in clinical practice due to limited efficacy and potential adverse effects.[15,16] The majority of clinicians do not incorporate the use of oprelvekin into care for patients with chemotherapy-induced thrombocytopenia, and use is not considered part of the standard of care. The use of thrombopoietin receptor agonists, romiplostim and eltrombopag, is being investigated. These agents are both approved for the treatment of idiopathic thrombocytopenia purpura (ITP), but only case reports and Phase I trials have looked at the use of these agents for chemotherapy-induced thrombocytopenia[17] and are not to be utilized in this setting.

Anemia

Anemia usually is not a dose-limiting toxicity commonly associated with cytotoxic chemotherapy, because RBCs survive approximately 120 days. Chemotherapy predominantly affects RBCs by causing anisocytosis and macrocytosis. These effects are related to inhibition of DNA synthesis, and they predominantly occur after treatment with antimetabolites, including folic acid analogs, hydroxyurea, purine antagonists, and pyrimidine antagonists. Anemia commonly does not accompany these changes in RBC size. In addition, chemotherapy-induced effects on RBCs are rarely the sole factor contributing to the low Hgb levels that necessitate an RBC transfusion. See Chapter 92, Anemias, for additional information on anemias and their treatment.

COAGULOPATHIES

Patients with cancer can exhibit bleeding secondary to chemotherapy-induced thrombocytopenia or thrombosis after chemotherapy. Bleeding can occur after treatment with asparaginase or the pegylated formulation, pegaspargase, due to inhibition of the synthesis of fibrinogen and other specific coagulation factors produced by the liver under the influence of vitamin K.[18–20] Asparaginase has a widespread effect on protein synthesis, and many plasma protein factors are depressed shortly after treatment. A patient receiving asparaginase can often exhibit a prolonged prothrombin time (PT) and partial thromboplastin time (PTT). Bleeding or thrombosis occurring as a direct result of changes in coagulation factors has not been frequently reported or conclusively documented. Coagulation factors may return to normal levels with continued administration of the agent, which suggests that the impairment of protein synthesis created by asparaginase is partially overcome by the liver. Specific treatment of prolonged PT and PTT with coagulation factors, fibrinogen, or vitamin K is not indicated.[21]

Thrombotic Events

The risk of venous thrombotic events is markedly elevated in patients with cancer. Possible pathophysiologic mechanisms include hypercoagulability marked by abnormalities in clotting factors and the coagulation cascade, vessel wall damage, and vessel wall compression by tumor masses. Many risk factors for thromboembolic events include the type of cancer, stage of cancer, comorbidities, mobility, and type of systemic anticancer therapy received, among others. Pancreatic, stomach, kidney, lung, brain, and uterine cancers are associated with the highest risk.[22] Use of systemic anticancer therapy has been associated with a 2.2-fold increased risk compared with patients not using these treatment modalities.[23]

Trousseau[24] first reported an increased incidence of venous thrombosis in patients with cancer, and many investigators have since confirmed the relationship of multiple or migratory venous thrombosis in patients with cancer. Up to one-third of apparently healthy adults who exhibit otherwise unexplained deep vein thrombosis eventually are proved to have a malignancy.[25,26]

Initiating treatment for acute promyelocytic leukemia (APL) commonly is associated with disseminated intravascular coagulation (DIC).[27,28] DIC is a systemic process that results from a large activation of the clotting cascade and presents as overlapping bleeding and thrombotic events. These events can result in end-organ damage. The lysed tumor cells in patients with APL appear to release procoagulant materials after anticancer therapy causing both hemorrhagic and thrombotic events. The foundation of treatment for DIC is to treat the underlying disease. Use of heparin and antifibrinolytics to minimize risk of coagulation is controversial. Other treatment is primarily supportive with blood products including platelets and cryoprecipitate.[28]

Several anticancer agents have been associated with an increased thrombosis risk, including cytotoxic chemotherapy (cisplatin, fluorouracil), hormonal targets (tamoxifen, aromatase inhibitors), antiangiogenic therapies (bevacizumab), and the immunomodulatory agents, thalidomide and lenalidomide.[29] Thalidomide and lenalidomide, in combination with other agents including dexamethasone and doxorubicin, have been associated with venous thromboembolic events when used in the treatment of multiple myeloma and other diseases.[30–32] Prophylaxis is warranted when these combinations are used. There are several guidelines and reviews discussing both prophylaxis, including the use of low-molecular-weight heparin or warfarin, and treatment in this patient population.[30] The use of direct-acting oral anticoagulants such as rivaroxaban or apixaban is not well studied nor currently recommended for prophylaxis in this population. Bevacizumab is associated with both arterial thrombosis and bleeding events. A retrospective analysis of five trials of patients receiving chemotherapy for colorectal, breast, or NSCLC showed a 3.8% incidence of arterial thrombosis in patients receiving chemotherapy and bevacizumab versus 1.7% in chemotherapy alone.[33] Most bleeding events associated with bevacizumab are minor. However, severe major bleeding events have been reported in patients with metastatic colorectal and lung cancer.[34] Different types of thrombotic events have been identified in patients receiving bevacizumab for other types of cancers.[35]

Other factors can cause patients to experience thrombosis. Many patients receiving cancer chemotherapy often have other illnesses that may predispose them to exhibiting thrombosis. In addition, surgical procedures and bed rest can increase the risk of thrombosis. Clinicians should maintain a high index of suspicion when a patient with cancer presents with signs or symptoms of thrombosis. Several reviews summarize risk factors and recommendations and provide further insight for specific clinical scenarios.[30,36,37]

Gastrointestinal Tract Toxicities

The GI tract may be second only to bone marrow in its susceptibility to toxic effects produced by cytotoxic chemotherapy. GI toxicities include nausea and vomiting, oral complications, esophagitis, and lower bowel disturbances.

NAUSEA AND VOMITING

Nausea and vomiting are common and serious toxicities associated with many cytotoxic and targeted anticancer agents. Anticancer agents or their metabolites may stimulate dopamine or serotonin receptors in the GI tract, the chemoreceptor trigger zone, or the CNS, which ultimately act on the vomiting center. Emesis most commonly occurs on the first day of chemotherapy and often persists for several days thereafter.[38] Most patients who receive traditional cytotoxic chemotherapy agents require antiemetics before and after chemotherapy for several days to control these symptoms. The most appropriate antiemetic regimen is based on patient-specific and agent-specific factors. Some of the targeted therapy agents carry some risk of emetogenicity, although it is generally milder. Guidelines are beginning to incorporate these targeted agents into their emetogenic classification schema based on incidence of nausea and vomiting in clinical trials (see Chapter 22, Nausea and Vomiting, for antiemetic algorithms and emetogenic potential of the cancer agents).

COMPLICATIONS OF THE ORAL CAVITY

Complications of the oral cavity include mucositis (or stomatitis), xerostomia (dry mouth), infection, and bleeding. The incidence of severe oral mucositis varies with the anticancer therapies given. Doxorubicin and continuous-infusion fluorouracil are among the agents at highest risk for causing severe mucositis. Virtually, all patients who receive myeloablative hematopoietic cell transplantation (HCT) or have radiation therapy to the head and neck experience oral complications.[39] These toxicities occur because of the nonspecific effects of chemotherapy on cells undergoing rapid division, including the cells of the mouth that undergo rapid renewal with a turnover time equal to 7 to 14 days. Cytotoxic therapy reduces the renewal rate of the basal epithelium and can cause mucosal atrophy, as well as glandular and collagen degeneration.[39,10] Radiation therapy to the head and neck also causes mucosal atrophy by decreasing cell renewal. Radiation can also cause fibrosis of the salivary glands, muscles, ligaments, and blood vessels, and damage to the taste buds.[40] The combined effects of chemotherapy and radiation therapy on the oral mucosa can also cause infection and bleeding in the oral cavity. Infection and bleeding occurs when treatment causes bone marrow suppression, including thrombocytopenia and neutropenia. Because the oral mucosa is highly vascular and frequently traumatized, bleeding occurs commonly with thrombocytopenia. In addition, cytotoxic chemotherapy and neutropenia can alter the extensive microbial flora harbored in the oral cavity, thus leading to oral infections. Oral complications often compound one another. For example, xerostomia can accelerate the development of mucositis as well as the formation of dental caries and local infection. Mucositis can clearly predispose the oral cavity to local bleeding and infection, as well as systemic infections leading to sepsis. These oral complications can also cause varying degrees of discomfort and adversely affect the patient's ability to eat, which potentially may lead to a compromised nutritional status. Topical treatments of oral complications are reviewed extensively in guidelines.[41]

Xerostomia

CASE 94-2

QUESTION 1: J.B. is a 55-year-old man with newly diagnosed, locally advanced head and neck cancer. His planned therapy includes cisplatin and fluorouracil given with concurrent radiation for a total of 6 weeks after surgical resection. A review of systems suggests that J.B. has poor oral hygiene, and a decision is made to consult the dental department of the university hospital before initiating radiation and chemotherapy. Is J.B. at risk for experiencing oral complications of chemotherapy? Is there anything that should be completed at this point to decrease his risk?

J.B. is at high risk for several of the oral complications previously described. Xerostomia, one of the most frequent side effects of radiation therapy to the head and neck, occurs secondary to radiation-induced changes to the salivary glands.[42] Evidence supports a direct relationship between the dose of radiation to the salivary glands and the extent of glandular changes.[43] In most patients treated with less than 6,000 rad (radiation absorbed dose), radiation-induced changes to the salivary glands are reversible within 6 to 12 months after the end of therapy. J.B. will also be receiving chemotherapy agents (i.e., cisplatin) that can cause xerostomia and enhance the toxicity to the salivary glands. Clinically, xerostomia has been caused by as little as two to three radiation doses of 200 rad.[43]

Damage to the salivary glands causes various effects, including a loss of salivary buffering capacity, lower salivary pH, no mechanical flushing, decreased salivary immunoglobulin A, and reduction of saliva production. In addition, xerostomia can alter the sense of taste, causing some patients to lose their ability to differentiate between sweet and salty foods and others to report a bitter taste. Xerostomia also commonly causes caries. Caries and decalcification may become sufficiently severe to compromise tooth integrity and cause fracture. Because saliva is no longer available to help clear bacteria from the mouth, xerostomia also predisposes patients to infection secondary to the increases in oral bacteria.

Treatments and Prevention

Amifostine, an organic thiophosphate chemoprotectant agent, is approved to reduce the incidence of moderate-to-severe xerostomia in patients having postoperative radiation treatment for head and neck cancer. Guidelines published by ASCO support the use of amifostine to reduce the incidence of acute and late xerostomia in patients receiving fractionated radiation therapy without concurrent chemotherapy for head and neck cancer.[44] However, amifostine is not widely used due to its cost and adverse effect profile. If xerostomia occurs, treatment strategies can include stimulation of existing salivary flow and replacement of lost secretions. Relatively low doses of systemically administered pilocarpine (5–10 mg orally 3 times daily) may stimulate salivary flow and produce clinically significant benefits in patients with postradiation xerostomia.[45] Results demonstrating pilocarpine's benefit are inconsistent. Dose-related adverse effects include cholinergic effects, such as sweating, rhinitis, headache, nausea, and abdominal cramps. A review on the oral complications of cancer therapy suggests that cevimeline (30 mg orally 3 times daily) and bethanechol (25 mg orally 3 times daily) may have fewer side effects than those seen with pilocarpine.[42] Sucrose-free hard candy and sugar-free chewing gum can also stimulate salivation, but these treatments are typically considered oral comfort agents. Saliva substitutes can also provide oral comfort to patients with xerostomia. Commercially available saliva substitutes generally are recommended for use before meals and at bedtime. They are available in several formulations, including sprays, rinses, and chewing gums. Patients who find one product or formulation unacceptable or unsuccessful may benefit from experimenting with other formulations or product lines. Studies have shown that salivary substitutes containing carboxymethyl cellulose or hydroxyethyl cellulose are more effective in relieving dryness than water-based or glycerin-based solutions.[46,47]

Prevention of radiation-induced cavities is best accomplished by aggressively using fluorides.[48] Generally, acidulated fluorides are the most effective, although neutral fluorides may be more acceptable to patients with mucositis. Patients are instructed to rinse daily for 1 minute with 5 to 10 mL of a fluoride rinse. Stannous fluoride gels 0.4% or sodium fluoride gel 1.1% tooth brushing agents may also be used by patients to minimize their risk of caries. Meticulous attention to oral hygiene with regular dental checkups and avoidance of sucrose is essential to minimize the development of caries.

In general, a dentist should see patients who will be receiving radiation therapy to the head and neck or chemotherapy agents with a high risk of oral complications before starting therapy. This includes patients with hematologic malignancies who will most likely experience severe myelosuppression for prolonged periods. Oral evaluation before therapy, intervention to eliminate potential sources of infection or irritation before therapy, and preventive measures taken during therapy can dramatically decrease the frequency of oral complications.[48,49] Given J.B.'s risk factors, including the dose of radiation he will receive and concomitant therapy with cisplatin, a dental examination is indicated before initiating therapy.

Mucositis and Stomatitis

CASE 94-2, QUESTION 2: J.B. successfully completed his first 2 weeks of combined chemotherapy and radiation therapy; however, 3 days into his third week, he complains of generalized burning, discomfort, and pain on the ventral surface of his tongue. On clinical observation, both the ventral surface of his tongue and the floor of his mouth appear erythematous, and several discrete lesions are present in both areas. What is the most likely explanation for J.B.'s new onset of symptoms? What treatment is indicated at this time?

Mucositis occurs as a nonspecific effect of chemotherapy and radiation therapy on the basal epithelium of the mouth. Nonkeratinized mucosa is affected most often. Thus, the buccal, labial, and soft palate mucosa, the ventral surface of the tongue, and the floor of the mouth are the most common sites of involvement. Although lesions are usually discrete initially, they often progress to produce large areas of ulceration. The lesions typically do not progress outside the mouth, but they may extend to the esophagus and involve the entire GI tract. The terms of stomatitis and oral mucositis may be used interchangeably. Mucositis may occur anywhere along the full GI tract. Signs and symptoms generally occur about 5 to 7 days after chemotherapy or at almost any point during radiation therapy. The antimetabolites (e.g., methotrexate, fluorouracil, capecitabine, and cytarabine) and the antitumor antibiotics are the chemotherapy agents that most commonly produce direct effects on the epithelial cells of the GI tract. Lesions generally regress and resolve completely in approximately 1 to 3 weeks, depending on their severity. Unlike oral toxicity seen with conventional chemotherapy, aphthous-like mucositis or stomatitis is a prevalent toxicity distinctly seen with mTOR (mammalian target of rapamycin) inhibitor therapy. Lesions typically appear during the first cycle of therapy, within the first week. Management often consists of supportive care measures and dose reductions.[50]

In severe cases, mucositis may require parenteral opioid analgesics for relief. Other signs or symptoms include decreased ability to eat and speak. Mucositis may be confused with an oral infection (particularly thrush), or mucositis and oral infections may occur concurrently. Local and systemic bacterial, fungal, or viral infections can occur and can cause a characteristic lesion; however, the lesion's appearance usually does not always correlate with the infectious agent. This particularly occurs in patients with neutropenia who cannot mount a full inflammatory response. In these individuals, the clinical appearance of an infected lesion may be muted relative to the presence or number of pathogens. Under normal conditions, the mucosa provides a natural barrier to the entry of normal oral flora, but the ulcerated mucosa allows pathogens access to the bloodstream. The patient could experience life-threatening infection or sepsis in addition to a local infection.

Treatments and Prevention

Treatment of mucositis is palliative. Topical anesthetics, including viscous lidocaine or dyclonine hydrochloride 0.5% or 1%, are often recommended. Equal portions of lidocaine, diphenhydramine, and magnesium-containing or aluminum-containing antacids can be used for their anesthetic and astringent properties. Many institutions compound mouthwash products containing these ingredients as well as antibiotics, nystatin, or corticosteroids. Corticosteroids provide anti-inflammatory properties, and the antibiotics and antifungals provide antibacterial or antifungal properties. Another topical agent, sucralfate, may provide some benefit by coating the lesion and reducing discomfort. All of these topical products provide symptom control only, and data supporting superior efficacy of one product over another in relieving pain are lacking. Furthermore, these topical products are only effective in oral and throat lesions because lesions lower in the GI tract are not reached with these local products.

All the topical anesthetic-containing preparations are recommended for use as "swish-and-spit" preparations. Generally, 5 to 10 mL is used three to 6 times a day. The longer the patient can hold the solution in the mouth, the longer the contact, and, theoretically, the better the symptom relief. Therefore, patients should be advised to hold and swish the solution around the mouth for as long as possible before spitting it out. The risk of systemic effects from topical anesthetic preparations is slim if patients were to swallow them; however, large quantities swallowed could induce sedation and possible arrhythmias. Other palliative treatment options include topical benzocaine and ice chips. For small localized lesions, ointments such as benzocaine may be applied after the affected area has been dried with a sponge. Patients may also find ice chips soothing by allowing them to melt in their mouth. Most patients, however, require systemic analgesics to alleviate the pain. Table 94-1 provides guidelines to manage mucositis.[41]

Gelclair is a bioadherent oral gel containing polyvinylpyrrolidone, hyaluronic acid, and glycyrrhetinic acid (but no alcohol or anesthetic agent). It provides an adherent barrier over the mucosal surfaces, thereby shielding oral lesions from the effect of food, liquids, and saliva.[51] Controlled clinical data are lacking. In a study of 20 patients with head and neck cancer undergoing radiation therapy presenting with mucositis, Gelclair was compared with standard of care, including sucralfate and lidocaine. No significant difference was found between the Gelclair and standard of care in relieving general pain.[52]

J.B. appears to have a mild case of stomatitis or mucositis at this time. J.B. should be encouraged to maintain good mouth care by keeping his mouth clean. Additionally, topical anesthetics are indicated for J.B. Topical lidocaine or a mixture of topical lidocaine with diphenhydramine and an antacid, 5 to 10 mL swish and spit 3 to 6 times/day, should be recommended. If the lesions progress during the next several days, systemic opioids may be necessary. J.B. should also be carefully assessed for local infections within his mouth.

CASE 94-2, QUESTION 3: Could J.B.'s mucositis have been prevented?

Historically, treatment of chemotherapy-induced and radiation-induced mucositis has been aimed at reducing symptoms once they occur and avoiding further trauma to the oral mucosa. Cryotherapy has been marginally effective in reducing the severity of chemotherapy-induced mucositis.[53] Ice chips are placed in the mouth 5 minutes before chemotherapy begins and retained for 30 minutes. Theoretically, this will reduce blood flow to the mouth, thereby protecting the dividing cell population from toxins. Chlorhexidine gluconate 0.12% also may reduce the frequency and severity of mucositis infection,[54,55] although not all studies have shown a benefit. This solution should be used twice daily as a rinse. Side effects include occasional burning (thought to be caused by the product's alcohol content, which can be reduced by diluting it with water) and superficial brown tooth staining, which polishes off easily. Chlorhexidine may reduce the frequency and severity of mucositis by eliminating microorganisms in the oral cavity.

Despite these prophylactic measures, none of these aforementioned methods have a definitive benefit. To date, the only medication with proven efficacy is palifermin, a keratinocyte growth factor, approved for patients with hematologic malignancies undergoing HCT to reduce the incidence and duration of severe oral mucositis. For further discussion, see Chapter 101, Hematopoietic Cell Transplantation.

Other methods for decreasing the incidence and severity of mucositis symptoms include reducing the dose of radiation or cytotoxic therapy, but doing so comes at the risk of compromising treatment outcomes. Mucositis remains the dose-limiting toxicity for several anticancer regimens. Unfortunately, there are no prevention strategies that would reduce the chance of J.B. experiencing mucositis from his chemotherapy and radiation, and thus, treatment for J.B. is targeted toward relief of symptoms.

Table 94-1
Guidelines for the Management of Mucositis[43]

An oral care protocol which may include the following:

1. Remove dentures to prevent further irritation and tissue damage
   Maintain gentle brushing of teeth with a soft toothbrush
   Avoid mouthwashes or rinses that contain alcohol because they may be painful and cause drying of the mucosa. Consider normal saline or sodium bicarbonate oral swishes
2. Apply local anesthetics for localized pain control, especially before meals (may add an antacid or an antihistamine).
   Systemic opioid analgesics, including transdermal fentanyl, may be required to control pain associated with severe mucositis. Acetaminophen is often avoided because it may mask fevers in neutropenic patients, and ibuprofen is often avoided because it may cause more bleeding in patients with thrombocytopenia
3. Ensure that adequate hydration and nutrition are maintained:
   Eat a bland diet, avoiding spiced, acidic, and salted foods
   Avoid rough food; process in a blender if necessary
   Use sugar-free gum or sugar-free hard candy to stimulate salivation and facilitate mastication
   If necessary, provide intravenous (IV) nutritional support
   Avoid extremely hot or cold foods
   Use shakes with nutritional supplements or ice cream

ESOPHAGITIS

Cytotoxic chemotherapy and radiation therapy can also damage the mucosal lining of the esophagus. Although dysphagia is a common symptom reported by patients with esophagitis, other causes of dysphagia should be excluded. Because patients receiving myelosuppressive cytotoxic therapy may exhibit infectious esophagitis, bacterial, viral, and fungal cultures should be completed to search for infectious causes before starting treatment for esophagitis. Symptomatic management of esophagitis is similar to the management of mucositis. Other treatment modalities, including behavioral modifications (e.g., elimination of acidic and irritating foods) and other medications (e.g., histamine-2 [H_2] receptor antagonist, antacids, and proton pump inhibitors), may help reduce esophageal irritation and improve comfort. Patients with severe esophagitis should be carefully monitored to ensure adequate oral hydration and nutritional intake, and instructed to avoid acidic or irritating foods. Symptoms should resolve in 1 to 2 weeks as myelosuppression resolves.

LOWER GASTROINTESTINAL TRACT COMPLICATIONS

Lower GI tract complications associated with anticancer therapy include malabsorption, diarrhea, and constipation. These complications may be related to structural changes that occur to the GI tract after cytotoxic or radiation therapy. Several investigators noted villus atrophy and cessation of mitosis within GI crypts in patients and animals treated with combination cytotoxic therapy.[56–58] Other investigators noted swelling and dilation of mitochondria and endoplasmic reticulum and shortening of the microvilli. These or other changes to the small and large bowel can cause decreased absorption of medications that are primarily absorbed in the upper portion of the small intestine.

Cytotoxic-induced intestinal changes also may be responsible for diarrhea, which frequently occurs with regimens containing irinotecan, high-dose cytarabine, or fluorouracil. Unlike diarrhea, constipation is rare. The vinca alkaloids, which produce colicky abdominal pain, constipation, and adynamic ileus caused by autonomic nerve dysfunction (see Neurotoxicity section), can cause chemotherapy-induced constipation. Additionally, constipation is a problematic side effect of therapy with thalidomide. Constipation should be treated prophylactically with stool softeners and mild stimulants. The true incidence of diarrhea and constipation associated with chemotherapy is difficult to discern, because many medications (e.g., opioid analgesics, antiemetics, antacids) and clinical conditions (e.g., immobility, spinal cord compression) commonly associated with cancer and anticancer therapies can cause these symptoms as well.

Diarrhea

CASE 94-3

QUESTION 1: B.G., a 60-year-old woman with recurrent colorectal cancer refractory to FOLFOX (fluorouracil, leucovorin, and oxaliplatin), is beginning her first course of cetuximab and irinotecan. What instructions should she receive regarding the management of diarrhea if she experiences this complication?

Diarrhea is a common toxicity seen during cancer treatment. It is most prevalent in patients treated with fluoropyrimidines and irinotecan. In addition, it is one of the most common side effects seen with new targeted therapies. A recent review provides an excellent summary of targeted therapy-induced diarrhea.[59] Diarrhea is a toxicity in which patient education is paramount. Patients who do not recognize potentially serious symptoms, understand the role of self-management, or understand when to contact their provider are at risk of life-threatening consequences. The mechanism of diarrhea is not completely understood, is likely multifactorial, and varies depending on the therapy. Diarrhea may result from direct effects on the GI mucosa, secretory factors, dysmotility, and immunotherapy-related (ipilimumab) and parasympathetic (irinotecan) effects. Irinotecan can cause severe diarrhea, both early and late, in the course of therapy. The early-onset diarrhea and late-onset diarrhea appear to be mediated by different mechanisms. Unique to irinotecan, the early-onset diarrhea (within 24 hours after treatment) may be mediated by parasympathetic stimulation. Patients often report other cholinergic symptoms, such as rhinitis, increased salivation, miosis, lacrimation, diaphoresis, flushing, and abdominal cramping as well. These symptoms can be prevented or managed with atropine IV or SC 0.25 to 1 mg. Late-onset diarrhea (generally occurring >24 hours after treatment) can be prolonged leading to dehydration, electrolyte imbalances, and significant morbidity. In irinotecan-induced diarrhea, patients should promptly receive loperamide 4 mg with the first episode of diarrhea and repeat doses of 2 mg every 2 hours until 12 hours have passed without a bowel movement.[60] The maximum dose of loperamide (16 mg in 24 hours) does not apply for irinotecan-induced diarrhea. Fluid and electrolyte replacement should also be administered, if necessary. With the potential severe complications associated with chemotherapy-associated diarrhea, prompt treatment cannot be overemphasized.

If a patient fails to respond to adequate doses of loperamide, the somatostatin analog, octreotide, can be used to manage the diarrhea. Randomized trials comparing loperamide with octreotide in patients with acute leukemia or those undergoing HCT found loperamide to be more effective.[61,62] Nevertheless, some evidence shows that octreotide may be used to successfully manage diarrhea associated with fluorouracil and other high-dose chemotherapy regimens.[63,64] These findings have been inconsistent. Several trials in patients with colorectal cancer receiving chemoradiation or chemotherapy failed to show benefit of decreasing diarrhea with long-acting octreotide.[64,65] Octreotide produces antisecretory activity in the gut and promotes the absorption of sodium, chloride, and water from luminal content. Patients should receive doses ranging from 100 to 2,000 mcg SC 3 times daily or 20 to 40 mg of long-acting octreotide.[64,65] Although responses seem to correlate with octreotide dose, more studies are needed to determine the optimal dose. Based on current evidence, octreotide should be limited to second-line therapy for cytotoxic therapy-associated diarrhea. Other treatment options, including antibiotics, opioids, and corticosteroids, have been evaluated and are summarized in review articles.[59,66]

B.G. should be counseled on the diarrhea that is often seen with irinotecan. She should be instructed to call her clinic if she starts experiencing any diarrhea within 24 hours after administration of irinotecan so she can receive prompt atropine therapy. Additionally, she should be given a prescription and instructions for loperamide administration and oral hydration recommendations for diarrhea occurring beyond the initial 24 hours after chemotherapy.

Dermatologic Toxicities

Dermatologic toxicities associated with anticancer therapies include alopecia, hyperpigmentation, radiation recall, photosensitivity, nail changes, hand-foot syndrome, acneiform rashes, hypersensitivity reactions, and extravasations. Several reviews serve as excellent references and provide detail related to dermatologic toxicities of targeted agents.[67–70]

ALOPECIA

CASE 94-4

QUESTION 1: C.W. is a 45-year-old woman with recently diagnosed breast cancer, who underwent lymph node dissection and lumpectomy. She will receive 20 fractions, or courses, of radiation therapy to the affected breast. She will also receive chemotherapy to minimize her risk of recurrence. She is in the clinic today to receive the first of four cycles of doxorubicin and cyclophosphamide (AC). Although C.W. had minimal problems with surgery, she particularly fears receiving combination chemotherapy. You counsel C.W. about the most common toxicities by reviewing the likelihood and management of myelosuppression, nausea, and vomiting. C.W. is appropriately attentive as you discuss these issues with her; however, her overriding concern is whether or not she will lose her hair. Is C.W.'s concern typical of most cancer patients? How would you respond?

C.W.'s concern regarding hair loss is typical of cancer patients starting chemotherapy. In fact, several investigators have reported that hair loss ranks second only to nausea and vomiting as a patient's greatest fear. Because hair bulb cells replicate every 12 to 24 hours, the cells are susceptible to various cytotoxic chemotherapy agents. Normally, hair follicles independently move cyclically through phases of growth (anagen), involution or transition (catagen), and rest (telogen). Although most persons normally lose about 100 scalp hairs a day, patients with cancer can lose substantially more. Because approximately 85% to 90% of hair follicles are in the anagen phase, chemotherapy agents may partially or completely inhibit mitosis or impair metabolic processes in the hair matrix. These effects can cause a thinned or weakened hair shaft or failure to form hair. Even mild trauma, such as normal hair grooming or rubbing the head on a pillow, can fracture the thinned hair shaft and cause hair loss. Hair loss usually begins 7 to 10 days after one treatment, with prominent hair loss noted within 1 or 2 months.

Other terminal hairs, such as beards, eyebrows, eyelashes, and axillary and pubic hair, can be affected; however, these effects are somewhat variable, depending on the rate of mitosis and the percentage of hairs in the anagen phase.[71,72]

C.W. should be informed about the expected onset of hair loss, and she should be reassured that alopecia caused by cytotoxic chemotherapy is reversible. She can expect her hair to begin regenerating 1 to 2 months after therapy is completed. The color and texture of her hair may be altered; the new hair may be lighter, darker, or curlier as it regrows.

Several interventions have been proposed to prevent scalp hair loss during chemotherapy. These procedures attempt to prevent chemotherapy agents from circulating to the hair follicles with either an occlusive scalp tourniquet or an ice cap that produces a localized hypothermia and vasoconstriction. Recognizing that such devices create a refuge for tumor cells, these procedures are contraindicated in patients with hematologic malignancies and in others at risk for scalp metastases. Concerns regarding the efficacy and safety of these devices have prevented them from availability in the US market.[72,73] Topical minoxidil has been studied with unimpressive results to date.[74]

C.W.'s concern is a legitimate one expressed by many patients with cancer, not just patients with breast cancer. C.W. is likely to experience near or complete hair loss, depending on the thickness of her hair and its growth rate. She should be told how to minimize the effect of alopecia on her appearance through the use of hair pieces or stylish head scarves, turbans, or hats. She also should be referred to volunteer groups and organizations that can help her through this difficult time. Hair pieces are tax deductible as a medical expense and are covered by some health insurance policies. If C.W. thinks she will use a hair piece, she should be advised to select a wig before hair loss begins.

CASE 94-4, QUESTION 2: Besides alopecia, what other skin or nail changes should C.W. anticipate?

NAIL AND SKIN CHANGES

Several skin and nail changes have been associated with cytotoxic and targeted anticancer agents, which C.W. may find disturbing.

The major consequences of these toxicities are cosmetic, however, and they usually resolve within 6 to 12 months after discontinuing or completing therapy.

Nail Changes

The growth of fingernails and toenails is arrested in a manner similar to hair growth. A reduction or a cessation of mitotic activity in the nail matrix causes a horizontal depression of the nail plate. Within weeks, these pale horizontal lines (Beau lines) begin to appear in the nail beds. They are most commonly seen in patients receiving chemotherapy for more than 6 months. These growth arrest lines move distally as the nail grows and normally disappears from the fingernails in approximately 6 months. Nail changes including hemorrhagic onycholysis, discoloration, and acute exudative paronychia are seen in approximately 40% of patients receiving paclitaxel and docetaxel.[67,75] Some other nail pigmentation changes that can occur after therapy with cyclophosphamide, fluorouracil, daunorubicin, doxorubicin, and bleomycin are less well understood.[76,77] Brown or blue lines deposit as horizontal or vertical bands in the nails. These lines are seen more commonly in dark-skinned patients. As with Beau lines, these pigmentation lines generally grow out with the nail. Standardized treatment recommendations for nail-related adverse events do not exist. Oral antibiotics and corticosteroids may be considered.

Dermatologic Pigment Changes

Dermatologic pigment changes are among the most common and least well-understood side effects of chemotherapy. Hypopigmentation has been reported occasionally in patients receiving cytotoxic therapy, but hyperpigmentation is more frequently reported. Usually, hyperpigmentation is not associated with an identifiable cause or systemic toxicity. It usually occurs after treatment with a wide variety of cytotoxic agents, including anthracyclines, alkylating agents, and antimetabolites. Most agents cause a diffuse, generalized hyperpigmentation, but the pigmentation changes can also be localized, involving only the mucous membrane, hair, or nails. Busulfan, cyclophosphamide, fluorouracil, dactinomycin, and hydroxyurea are examples of specific agents that can cause widespread cutaneous hyperpigmentation.[67]

Various chemotherapy agents can cause diverse patterns of hyperpigmentation. A peculiar serpiginous hyperpigmentation can occur over veins used to administer fluorouracil and bleomycin.[78,79] Some investigators have attributed this phenomenon to a subclinical phlebitis. Hyperpigmentation has also been noted over pressure points after the use of bleomycin. Thiotepa has been reported to cause hyperpigmentation in areas of skin occluded by bandages, which may be caused by secretion of thiotepa in sweat.[80] Interestingly, skin contact with thiotepa and mechlorethamine has been reported to cause hypopigmentation.[81,82] Although hyperpigmentation reactions commonly affect the skin, some rare reactions are noted in hair. Methotrexate can cause hyperpigmented banding of light-colored hair. This phenomenon has been described in a patient receiving intermittent high-dose methotrexate and has been referred to by some investigators as the "flag sign" of chemotherapy.[83] Alternatively, depigmentation of hair has been seen with several tyrosine kinase inhibitors including sunitinib, imatinib, and pazopanib. This adverse effect is attributed to c-KIT signal inhibition leading to decreased melanin synthesis.[84] To minimize a patient's concern regarding these pigment changes, they should receive counseling before treatment.

As previously stated, pigment changes that occur in patients receiving cytotoxic chemotherapy are basically a cosmetic concern. It is important to anticipate these distressing side effects and educate patients in appropriate cases. At this time, C.W. should receive counseling, explaining that these side effects may occur because she will be receiving several agents that have been implicated in producing diffuse, as well as localized, cutaneous nail hyperpigmentation. She should be reassured that pigment changes usually resolve with time.

Hand-Foot Syndrome

Some patients receiving chemotherapy may exhibit tender, erythematous skin on the palms of their hands and sometimes on the soles of their feet. Patients may also complain of tingling, burning, or shooting sensations in their hands or feet usually not described as painful. These signs and symptoms may resolve after several days, or they may progress to bullous lesions that can desquamate. This reaction is referred to as chemotherapy-associated acral erythema or the palmar-plantar erythrodysesthesia syndrome. Agents most commonly reported to cause this reaction include cytarabine, fluorouracil, doxorubicin, liposomal doxorubicin, docetaxel, capecitabine, sorafenib, sunitinib, pazopanib, regorafenib, axitinib, and vemurafenib.[85,86] There is evidence that the application of urea-based cream may be effective in prevention of hand-foot syndrome based on study results in patients receiving capecitabine and sorafenib. Both study populations utilized 10% urea-based cream 3 times daily for 6 to 12 weeks and saw a decrease in the incidence of hand-foot syndrome.[87,88] Treatment is primarily focused on symptom control, and discontinuation of the medication or treatment interruption will help to resolve the reaction. After resolution, the medication may be initiated at a lower dose.

Acneiform–Erythematous Rash

The most common toxicities reported with the epidermal growth factor receptor (EGFR) inhibitors and EGFR monoclonal antibodies are skin related and are probably due to inhibition of the tyrosine kinase pathways in EGFR-dependent tissues, including keratinocytes in the skin. Erlotinib, gefitinib, afatinib, and lapatinib are small-molecule tyrosine kinase inhibitors that target the intracellular domain of the EGFR, and cetuximab and panitumumab are monoclonal antibodies that target the extracellular domain of EGFR. These agents are associated with skin toxicities. Skin effects occur in greater than 50% of patients who receive these treatments and are dose-dependent. A pustular or maculopapular eruption typically appears on the upper body, face, and scalp in the first 1 to 2 weeks of treatment.

The rashes are predominantly grade 1 or 2 in severity, may be associated with dry skin and itching, and completely resolve without sequelae when the drug is discontinued.[69,89] Evidence suggests that the severity of the skin rash is associated with increased efficacy of this class of agents. In a retrospective analysis of a Phase III trial in patients with NSCLC receiving erlotinib, those who experienced a rash had a significantly longer survival time than those who did not. Survival was reported to be 1.5 months in patients with no development of skin rash versus 8.5 months in those with grade 1 rash, and 19.6 months in patients exhibiting a grade 2 or 3 rash.[90] Evidence of a correlation between skin rashes and higher response rates has also been observed in patients receiving cetuximab for colorectal cancer.[91] Multiple therapies have been studied in hopes of reducing or preventing this bothersome side effect. Patients should be advised to minimize sun exposure and to keep the rash moist with lotions and creams, avoiding drying agents.[92–95] The Multinational Association of Supportive Care in Cancer (MASCC) has developed an EGFR Inhibitor Skin Toxicity Tool to assist clinicians in monitoring and reporting EGFR-induced dermatologic toxicities. In addition, MASCC has published both patient information and clinical practice guidelines for the prevention and treatment of EGFR inhibitor-associated dermatologic toxicities. Because of the prevalence and significant discomfort associated with the rash, prevention is recommended in the majority of patients in the first 6 to 8 weeks of therapy and consists of hydrocortisone 1% cream with moisturizer, sunscreen, and either minocycline or doxycycline therapy.[95]

Dry Skin

Many cytotoxic anticancer agents (especially bleomycin, hydroxyurea, and fluorouracil) and several targeted therapies (EGFR inhibitors) can cause dry skin with fine scaling on the surface. Normally, sebaceous and sweat glands provide lipids, lactates, and other products that contribute to the pliability and moisture retention of the stratum corneum. In patients receiving cytotoxic therapy, the dry skin may be caused by the cytostatic effect of agents on sebaceous and sweat glands. Topical application of emollient creams may provide some symptomatic relief of this dryness.

INTERACTIONS WITH RADIATION THERAPY

Case 94-4, Question 3: C.W. recently completed her course of total breast radiation therapy. She plans to leave for a 1-week vacation in Florida 3 days after this clinic visit. Are there any interactions between radiation therapy and sunlight exposure with cytotoxic anticancer agents? Are there any specific precautions C.W. should take, or signs and symptoms of toxicity that she should know about?

The interactions between cytotoxic therapy and radiation therapy or ultraviolet (UV) light (from both external beam and natural sources) can be divided into radiation sensitization, radiation recall, photosensitivity reactions, and sunburn reactivation (Table 94-2).

Table 94-2

Chemotherapy-Associated and Radiation-Associated Reactions

Radiation Sensitivity Reactions		
Bleomycin	Doxorubicin	Hydroxyurea
Dactinomycin	Fluorouracil	Methotrexate
Etoposide	Gemcitabine	
Radiation-Recall Reactions		
All of the above plus		
Vinblastine	Epirubicin	Capecitabine
Etoposide	Paclitaxel	Oxaliplatin
	Docetaxel	
Reactions with Ultraviolet Light		
Phototoxic Sensitivity		
Dacarbazine	Thioguanine	Methotrexate
Fluorouracil	Vinblastine	Mitomycin
Sunburn Reactivation		
Methotrexate		

Source: Payne AS et al. Dermatologic toxicity of chemotherapeutic agents. *Semin Oncol*. 2006;33:86; Yeo W, Johnson PJ. Radiation-recall skin disorders associated with the use of antineoplastic drugs: pathogenesis, prevalence, and management. *Am J Clin Dermatol*. 2000;1:113; Alley E et al. Cutaneous toxicities of cancer therapy. *Curr Opin Oncol*. 2002;14:212.

Several excellent reviews are available that describe each of these interactions in detail. A discussion of the important principles of the interaction between radiation therapy and cytotoxic therapy follows.[96–98] A synergistic interaction between a small number of cytotoxic agents and radiation therapy results in an enhanced radiation effect. This may be caused by an agent's ability to interfere with radiation repair. Radiation therapy can alter the molecular structure of DNA, but excision repair allows cells to remove small, damaged portions of one strand of DNA and insert new bases using the other strand as a template. This repair mechanism requires several enzymes, including DNA polymerase. Cytotoxic therapy agents can interfere with some of the enzymes and synthetic mechanisms needed to repair damaged cells. Although the synergistic effects of radiation therapy and cytotoxic therapy are often exploited therapeutically for the treatment of solid tumors, these reactions can inadvertently cause undesirable reactions in nontumor tissues, such as the skin, esophagus, lung, and GI tract. The skin is the most common target of radiation reactions.

These reactions can produce severe tissue necrosis, which can compromise organ function and delay or mandate discontinuation of future treatment courses. These reactions may be further classified as either radiation sensitivity or radiation-recall reactions. The primary distinction between radiation sensitivity reactions and radiation-recall reactions lies in the temporal relationship between radiation therapy and chemotherapy. Generally, sensitivity reactions occur when chemotherapy is given concurrently or within 1 week of radiation therapy. In comparison, recall reactions occur several weeks to years after radiation therapy, when the administration of chemotherapy induces an inflammatory reaction in tissues previously treated with radiation. Radiation recall is independent of previous, clinically apparent radiation damage. Not surprisingly, the chemotherapy agents that have been associated with radiation-recall reactions are the same as those that cause radiation sensitivity reactions. Management of reactions is supportive and consists primarily of topical agents including corticosteroids.[96,98–101]

Because UV light has sufficient energy to cause photochemical changes in biologic molecules, cytotoxic agents can interact with it. The subsequent reactions are usually less severe than reactions that occur with radiation therapy, and they may be caused by a different mechanism. Photosensitivity reactions, defined as enhanced erythema responses to UV light, have been reported with specific agents (Table 94-2). Methotrexate can also reactivate sunburns, causing a similar, but less severe reaction compared with the radiation-recall reactions described previously. The reaction can be more severe than the initial sunburn, resulting in severe blisters, and it usually occurs only in patients who receive large doses of methotrexate. Although the precise incidences of photosensitivity reactions caused by chemotherapy agents are unknown, they may be more common than generally believed. For example, photosensitivity may account for many of the erythematous periodic rashes attributed to allergy.[67,102]

C.W. received doxorubicin which can interact with radiation therapy. Although not commonly reported, doxorubicin also can cause some increased erythema in the specific area of skin treated with radiation. Because C.W. may have an increased risk for a photosensitivity reaction, she should be advised to avoid direct exposure to the sunlight for several days to a week after chemotherapy. Although no data exist regarding the efficacy of sunscreens in this patient population, C.W. should be advised to use a protective sunscreen with a high sun protective factor when she cannot avoid sun exposure. Protective clothing and a hat can provide additional protection for C.W. Furthermore, she should periodically assess her skin's reaction to the sun with intermittent periods of rest and observation throughout the day.

CASE 94-4, QUESTION 4: How will C.W. know whether she has a radiation reaction? How should she be treated if such a reaction occurs?

If C.W. has a radiation reaction, she will experience "easy burning" and erythema or redness, followed by dry desquamation. With a more severe reaction, small blisters (vesicles) and oozing can develop. Necrosis with persistent painful ulceration can also occur in severe cases. Postinflammatory hyperpigmentation or depigmentation may follow. Treatment options vary, depending on reaction severity. Milder cases can be treated with topical steroids in an emollient cream base and cool wet compresses. Necrosis and ulcers are notoriously difficult to treat, however, because radiated skin does not heal well. Ulcers are often treated with surgical debridement to keep the ulcer clean. Even when the ulcers are clean, exudation and bacterial contamination can be persistent. Radiation reactions that occur in tissues other than the skin (e.g., the lungs, esophagus, GI tract) often are treated with oral corticosteroids, although data regarding the efficacy of these agents in ameliorating the symptoms or reducing the extent of damage are lacking. If C.W. experiences any of these signs or symptoms, she should immediately seek medical attention.

IRRITANT AND VESICANT REACTIONS

CASE 94-4, QUESTION 5: C.W. complained of pain and burning at the injection site immediately after the administration of her third course of IV chemotherapy with doxorubicin and cyclophosphamide. She described the sensation as being distinctly different from the mild discomfort she had experienced with previous courses. Physical examination of the injection site revealed mild erythema and slight induration. What types of local reactions can occur after the administration of chemotherapy?

Several distinct types of local reactions (ranging from transient local irritation to severe tissue necrosis of the skin, surrounding vasculature, and supporting structures) have been reported after cytotoxic chemotherapy[68,103,104] (Table 94-3). Some reactions are characterized by immediate local burning, itching, and erythema. Some patients may also experience a "flare" reaction along the length of the vein used for treatment. More severe reactions, including irritation of the vein (or phlebitis) caused by the irritant properties of an agent or a diluent, and possibly extravasation, can occur after cytotoxic chemotherapy.[68,103] Extravasation, a potentially serious local reaction, is seen in approximately 1% of chemotherapy administration and occurs when IV medications are accidentally administered into the surrounding tissue, either by leakage or by a needle puncturing the vein, causing direct exposure and damage to surrounding tissues.

Reactions resulting from the extravasation of agents with vesicant or irritant properties are more severe. All agents with vesicant properties potentially can produce devastating reactions. Agents known to bind to DNA (i.e., the anthracyclines) have the propensity to produce the most severe damage. Treatment with a cytotoxic agent with these properties can produce phlebitis and pain; however, extravasations can cause severe local irritation or soft tissue ulcers, depending on the agent and the amount and concentration of the extravasated drug. In addition, no clear agreement exists regarding the vesicant potential of many cytotoxic chemotherapy agents, and various references may categorize agents differently based on their vesicant or irritant properties. Initially, it may be impossible to distinguish a local irritant reaction from a vesicant extravasation; therefore, if an agent with vesicant or irritant properties has been administered, the reaction should be treated as a potential extravasation.

Patients who experience an extravasation can show a range of different signs or symptoms. Infiltration of a vesicant into tissue often produces a severe burning sensation that may persist for hours. In some cases, no immediate symptoms or signs are evident. However, in the days to weeks that follow, the skin overlying the extravasation site may become reddened and firm. The redness may gradually diminish or progress to ulceration and necrosis.[103]

Table 94-3
Chemotherapeutic Drugs Reported to Produce Local Toxicities

Potential Vesicants	
Dactinomycin	Epirubicin
Daunorubicin	Streptozocin
Doxorubicin	Vinblastine
Idarubicin	Vincristine
Mechlorethamine	Paclitaxel
Mitomycin	Oxaliplatin
Potential Irritants	
Carmustine	Etoposide
Cisplatin	Mitoxantrone
Dacarbazine	Melphalan
Vinorelbine	Vindesine
Cyclophosphamide	Teniposide

Source: Doellman D et al. Infiltration and extravasation: update on prevention and management. *J Infus Nurs*. 2009;32:203; Boulanger J et al. Management of the extravasation of antineoplastic agents. *Support Care Cancer*. 2015;23(5):1459.

Case 94-4, Question 6: What factors in C.W. increase her risk of extravasation, and what administration techniques and precautions can minimize these risks?

Several factors have been associated with an increased risk of extravasation and subsequent tissue damage after administration of cytotoxic chemotherapy. Risk factors include generalized vascular disease commonly found in elderly and debilitated patients or in patients who have undergone frequent venipuncture and treatment with irritating chemotherapy (the latter causes venous fragility and instability or decreased local blood flow); elevated venous pressure, which typically occurs in patients with an obstructed superior vena cava or venous drainage after axillary dissection; prior radiation therapy to the injection site; recent venipuncture in the same vein; use of injection sites over joints, which increases the risk of needle dislodgement; and others.[68,103]

Tissue damage may be more severe if extravasation occurs in areas with only a small amount of subcutaneous tissue (e.g., the back of the hand or wrist) because wound healing is more difficult and exposure of deeper structures, such as the tendons, is increased.[103] These risks have led to the increased use of central catheters in patients receiving vesicant chemotherapy.

C.W. has several risks for extravasation. She had an axillary lymph node dissection for her breast cancer, which places her at higher risk for obstructed venous drainage. Additionally, she has had multiple venous punctures, and she is a thin woman with relatively small amounts of subcutaneous tissue.

Extravasations of agents with vesicant properties can produce devastating tissue damage that can potentially cause loss of an extremity or death. To prevent significant morbidity or mortality, major emphasis must be placed on prevention. All caretakers who administer agents with vesicant or irritant properties should be skilled in IV drug administration and receive special instruction before administering these agents. The patient also must be told how agent administration should feel and to report immediately any change in sensation, including pain, burning, or itching.

Case 94-4, Question 7: C.W.'s oncology nurse believes that the doxorubicin may have extravasated during administration. How should this be managed? Do management strategies differ for other vesicant agents?

Immediate management of a potential vesicant extravasation should include stopping the injection if the entire agent has not been administered. Various other recommended measures may minimize vesicant exposure and subsequent tissue damage (Table 94-4). These include application of cold compresses to the extravasation site and elevation of the extremity. Cold compresses have been shown to cause vasoconstriction, which can help to localize the extravasation and allow time for local vessels to displace the extravasated agent, whereas warm compresses are thought to induce vasodilation, increase drug distribution and absorption, therefore decreasing the concentration of the offending agent around the immediate site. Warm compresses are recommended for vinca alkaloids and epipodophyllotoxins.[103,104] With the exception of these two classes of agents, cooling has been shown to be more effective than warm compresses. Specific antidotes thought to inactivate the extravasated chemotherapy have been suggested; however, many of these antidotes are based on observations in a few patients or animal models, and their effectiveness, in many cases, is unsubstantiated. Antidotes recommended in some guidelines may actually worsen tissue damage (e.g., sodium bicarbonate for doxorubicin). Recommended treatments for suspected extravasation of vesicant agents are outlined in Table 94-5.[103,104]

Table 94-4

Suggested Procedures for Management of Suspected Extravasation of Vesicant Drugs

1. Stop the infusion immediately, but do not remove the needle. Any drug remaining in the tubing or needle, as well as the infiltrated area, should be aspirated
2. Contact a physician as soon as possible
3. If deemed appropriate, instill an antidote in the infiltrated areas (via the extravasated intravenous (IV) needle if possible)
4. Remove the needle
5. Apply ice to the site and elevate the extremity for the first 24–48 hours (if vinca or epipodophyllotoxin, use warm compresses)
6. Document the drug, suspected volume extravasated, and the treatment in the patient's medical record
7. Check the site frequently for 5–7 days
8. Consult a surgeon familiar with extravasations early so that the surgeon can periodically review the site, and, if ulceration begins, the surgeon can rapidly assess if surgical debridement or excision is necessary

Source: Doellman D et al. Infiltration and extravasation: update on prevention and management. *J Infus Nurs*. 2009;32:203; Boulanger J et al. Management of the extravasation of antineoplastic agents. *Support Care Cancer*. 2015;23(5):1459.

Dexrazoxane has been established as a reliable antidote for anthracycline extravasations. Dexrazoxane, an iron chelator, was studied based on evidence that it protects cardiac tissue from anthracycline-induced toxicities. Two prospective, multicenter, single-arm trials were conducted in a total of 54 evaluable patients with anthracycline extravasations. In 98.2% of patients, surgical intervention was avoided and 71% of patients were able to continue treatment regimen without any delays. Hospitalization of 41% of patients was necessary secondary to their extravasation. Toxicities included myelosuppression, increased liver function tests, nausea, and pain at the dexrazoxane infusion site.[105] Based on these results, dexrazoxane is approved for the treatment of anthracycline extravasations. Dexrazoxane is given once daily for 3 days at a dose of 1,000 mg/m^2 IV on days 1 and 2, and 500 mg/m^2 IV on day 3. Administration should start within 6 hours of extravasation.[106]

HYPERSENSITIVITY REACTIONS

Almost all anticancer agents have produced at least an isolated instance of a hypersensitivity reaction. All types of hypersensitivity reactions can occur with anticancer agents, although type I is the most common reaction documented. Type I hypersensitivity reactions are immediate reactions that are most often immunologically mediated, although there are other possible mechanisms for type I hypersensitivities. Anaphylactic or immunoglobulin E (IgE)-mediated reactions occur when an antigen interacts with IgE bound to a mast cell membrane, causing degranulation of mast cells. Major signs and symptoms of type I reactions include urticaria, angioedema, rash, bronchospasm, abdominal cramping, and hypotension. Although many reactions associated with anticancer agents probably are immunologically mediated, other mechanisms may cause type I reactions. Those include the degranulation of mast cells and basophils through a direct effect on the cell surface that releases histamine and other vasoactive substances. Activation of the alternative complement pathway can also release vasoactive substances from mast cells. When

Table 94-5
Recommended Extravasation Antidotes

Class/Specific Agents	Local/Systemic Antidote Recommended	Specific Procedure
Alkylating Agents Cisplatin[a] Oxaliplatin Mechlorethamine	1/6-M solution sodium thiosulfate	Mix 4 mL 10% sodium thiosulfate USP with 6 mL of sterile water for injection, USP for a 1/6-M solution. Into site, inject 2 mL for each mg of mechlorethamine or 100 mg of cisplatin extravasated
Mitomycin-C	Dimethyl sulfoxide 99% (w/v)	Apply 1–2 mL to the site every 6 hours for 14 days. Allow to air dry; do not cover
Anthracyclines	Cold compresses	Apply immediately for 30–60 minutes on first day
Doxorubicin Daunorubicin	Dexrazoxane	Once daily for 3 days. First dose should be given within the first 6 hours. Day 1: 1,000 mg/m^2 IV Day 2: 1,000 mg/m^2 IV Day 3: 500 mg/m^2 IV
Vinca alkaloids Vinblastine Vincristine	Warm compresses Hyaluronidase	Apply immediately for 30–60 minutes, then alternate off/on every 15 minutes for 1 day Inject 150 units into site
Epipodophyllotoxins[a]	Warm compresses	Apply immediately for 30–60 minutes, then alternate off/on every 15 minutes for 1 day
Etoposide	Hyaluronidase	Inject 150 units into site
Taxanes	Cold compresses	Apply immediately for 30–60 minutes every 6 hours for 1 day
Docetaxel	Hyaluronidase	Inject 150 units into site
Paclitaxel		

[a]Treatment indicated only for large extravasations (e.g., doses one-half or more of the planned total dose for the course of therapy).
IV, intravenous; w/v, weight per volume.
Source: Goolsby TV, Lombardo FA. Extravasation of chemotherapeutic agents: prevention and treatment. *Semin Oncol*. 2006;33:139; Doellman D et al. Infiltration and extravasation: update on prevention and management. *J Infus Nurs*. 2009;32:203; Totect (dexrazoxane injection) [package insert]. Rockaway NTTU, Inc.; 2011.

non-IgE-mediated mechanisms account for the symptoms of a type I reaction, it is called an anaphylactoid reaction (see Chapter 32, Drug Hypersensitivity Reactions).

Many of the type I hypersensitivity reactions produced by anticancer medications appear to be mediated by non-IgE mechanisms. Although little research has been conducted on the mechanism of these reactions, two features suggest that they are not mediated by IgE. First, many reactions occur during or immediately after administration of the first dose. This is in contrast to immunologic reactions that require prior exposure (i.e., one must be sensitized before becoming hypersensitized). In addition, certain symptoms or symptom complexes are more diagnostic of immunologically mediated disorders. These symptoms include urticaria, angioedema, bronchospasm, laryngeal spasm, cytopenias, arthritis, mucositis, vasculitic syndromes, and vesicular dermatitis. Although the spectrum of symptoms and their severity vary widely in the case reports, most hypersensitivity reactions that occur with anticancer agents are classified as grade 1 (transient rash, mild) or grade 2 (mild bronchospasm, moderate) by the NCI Common Terminology Criteria for Adverse Events.[1] Furthermore, a patient who has had a reaction to an agent that is not immunologically mediated can safely receive future courses of anticancer therapy if he or she receives appropriate premedication. For example, appropriate premedication allows many (>60%) patients who have previously experienced a hypersensitivity reaction secondary to paclitaxel to continue therapy; this also reduces the incidence of hypersensitivity reactions associated with short-duration infusions (i.e., 3 hours). Some agents can commonly cause hypersensitivity reactions after the first and subsequent doses of therapy.

The other types of hypersensitivity reactions are less commonly documented with cytotoxic and targeted therapy administration. Type II is hemolytic anemia. Type III results from deposition of antigen–antibody complexes that form intravascularly and in tissues that can result in tissue injury. Sensitized T lymphocytes that react with antigens causing a release of lymphokines are responsible for type IV reactions.[107] Anticancer agents most frequently reported to produce hypersensitivity reactions and their characteristic reactions are listed in Table 94-6.[108–134] Most valuable information stems from patient series and case reports. However, they often provide conflicting and contradictory information, particularly with respect to incidence, severity, characteristic symptoms, time course, and the success of rechallenge. If a patient experiences a hypersensitivity reaction and the clinician decides to continue therapy with this regimen, a full review of all of the relevant literature as well as manufacturer's data is advised. Several reviews are available to assist in this effort.[107,135,136]

Monoclonal Antibodies

CASE 94-5

Question 1: S.R., a 58-year-old man with metastatic colorectal cancer, previously progressed after four cycles of FOLFOX (oxaliplatin 85 mg/m^2 IV on day 1, leucovorin 100 mg/m^2 IV on days 1 and 2, and fluorouracil 400 mg/m^2 IV bolus, followed by 600 mg/m^2 IV for 22 hours on days 1 and 2) plus bevacizumab 5 mg/kg. He also recently progressed after two cycles of second-line FOLFIRI (irinotecan 180 mg/m^2 on day 1, leucovorin 100 mg/m^2 IV on days 1 and 2, and fluorouracil 400 mg/m^2 IV bolus, followed by 600 mg/m^2 IV for 22 hours on days 1 and 2). S.R. now presents to the clinic for his first weekly dose of cetuximab (400 mg/m^2 IV load, followed by 250 mg/m^2 IV weekly). Discuss the toxicities that S.R. may expect and when they might appear. How should these side effects be managed? S.R. asks how these side effects can be prevented.

Table 94-6
Cancer Chemotherapeutic Agents Commonly Causing Hypersensitivity

Drug	Frequency	Risk Factors	Manifestations	Mechanism	Comments
Asparaginase[107]	10%–20%	Increasing doses; interval (weeks to months) between doses; IV administration; history of atopy or allergy; use without prednisone, mercaptopurine and/or vincristine	Pruritus, dyspnea, agitation, urticaria, angioedema, laryngeal spasm	Type I	Substitute pegaspargase, but up to 32% may demonstrate mild hypersensitivity
Paclitaxel[107,108]	Up to 10% first or second dose	None known	Rashes, dyspnea, bronchospasm, hypotension	Nonspecific release of mediators; Cremophor EL	Premedicate with diphenhydramine corticosteroids, and H_2 receptor antagonists Paclitaxel protein-bound particles (Abraxane) may be substituted and better tolerated in some patients
Cisplatin[109–113]	Up to 20% intravesicular, 5%–10% systemic; case reports of hemolytic anemia	Increasing number of doses (typically > dose 6) Anemia: none known	Rash, urticaria, bronchospasm Anemia: hemolytic anemia	Type I Anemia: type III	Carboplatin may be substituted in some cases but cross-reactivity has been reported
Procarbazine[116–118]	Up to 15%, case reports	None known	Urticaria pneumonitis	Type I Type III	All patients rechallenged have prompt return of symptoms
Anthracyclines[119–123,125]	1%–15% depending on anthracycline	None known	Dyspnea, bronchospasm, angioedema	Unknown; nonspecific release	Cross-reactivity documented, but incidence and likelihood unknown
Bleomycin[126–128]	Common	Lymphoma	Fever (up to 42°C), tachypnea	Endogenous pyrogen release	Not technically classified as HSR; premedicate with acetaminophen and diphenhydramine
Rituximab[129]	First treatment 80%; subsequent treatments 40%	Female sex, pulmonary infiltrates, CLL or mantle cell lymphoma	Fevers, chills, occasional nausea, urticaria, fatigue, HA, pain, pruritus, bronchospasm, SOB, angioedema, rhinitis, vomiting, ↓ BP, flushing	Unknown; related to manufacturing process	Stop or ↓ infusion rate by 50%; provide supportive care with IV fluids, acetaminophen, diphenhydramine, vasopressors PRN
Trastuzumab[130]	First treatment 40%; subsequent treatments rare	None known	Chills, fever, occasional nausea or vomiting; pain, rigors, HAs, dizziness, SOB, ↓ BP, rash, asthenia	Unknown, related to manufacturing process	Manage with acetaminophen, diphenhydramine, meperidine

Cetuximab[131]	First treatment, 15%–20%; grades 3–4, 3%; subsequent treatments uncommon	None known	Airway obstruction (bronchospasm, stridor, hoarseness), urticaria, hypotension, or cardiac arrest		Premedicate with diphenhydramine; stop or decrease infusion rate; provide supportive care with epinephrine, corticosteroids, IV antihistamines, bronchodilators, and oxygen PRN
Alemtuzumab[132]	~90% with IV administration in first week	None known	Hypotension, rigors, fever, SOB, bronchospasm, chills, rash	Unknown	Dose titration during several days; substitute with SC administration rather than IV; premedicate with acetaminophen, diphenhydramine, meperidine
Docetaxel[133]	0.9% with premedication	None known	↓ BP, bronchospasm, rash, flushing, pruritus, SOB, pain, fever, chills	Unknown	Premedicate with acetaminophen, dexamethasone, and diphenhydramine
Doxorubicin[134] liposomal	6.8%	None known	Flushing, SOB, angioedema, HA, chills, ↓ BP	Unknown, related liposomal components	Stop infusion; restart at a lower rate

Type I: Antigen interaction with IgE bound to mast cell membrane causes degranulation. Drug binding to mast cell surface causes degranulation. Activation of classic or alternative complement pathways produces anaphylatoxins. Neurogenic release of vasoactive substances. Type III: Antigen–antibody complexes form intravascularly and deposit in or on tissues.

BP, blood pressure; CLL, chronic lymphocytic leukemia; HA, headache; HSR, hypersensitivity reaction; IV, intravenous; PRN, as needed; SC, subcutaneous; SOB, shortness of breath.

The most common toxicities observed in patients receiving cetuximab include rash, diarrhea, hypomagnesemia, headache, nausea, and hypersensitivity reactions. Infusion-related reactions occur in 15% to 20% of patients receiving their first infusion. However, severe hypersensitivity reactions (including allergic and anaphylactic reactions) occur in 1% to 3% of patients. The reactions are related to the infusion of cetuximab and generally occur during or within 1 hour of completing the first dose. Patients should be premedicated with diphenhydramine before the infusion. The infusion can be stopped or the rate decreased if S.R. begins experiencing these effects. The skin rash and dry skin occurring after cetuximab administration are related to the inhibition of EGFR and were the most common side effect seen in clinical trials. The rash occurred in approximately 80% of patients and appeared in the first 1 to 3 weeks of therapy. Grade 3 or 4 skin rashes occurred in 5% to 10% of patients.[137]

Several of the monoclonal antibodies (e.g., rituximab, trastuzumab, cetuximab, ofatumumab) are associated with a higher incidence of hypersensitivity reactions than traditional cytotoxic agents. These agents are genetically engineered humanized monoclonal antibodies containing foreign proteins that can trigger the reaction. During the first infusion with trastuzumab, approximately 40% of patients experience a symptom complex, mild to moderate in severity, which consists of chills, fever, or both. These symptoms usually do not recur with subsequent injections.[135] In comparison, approximately 80% of patients receiving rituximab may experience an infusion-related reaction ranging from fever, chills, and rigors to severe reactions (7%) characterized by hypoxia, pulmonary infiltrates, adult respiratory distress syndrome, myocardial infarction, ventricular fibrillation, or cardiogenic shock with the first dose. Approximately 40% of patients receiving rituximab experience infusion-related reactions with subsequent infusions (5%–10% severe).[135] Treatment of these reactions follows the recommendations for treatment of hypersensitivity reactions that occur with more traditional agents.

Table 94-7
Prophylaxis and Treatment of Hypersensitivity Reactions from Anticancer Drugs

Prophylaxis
IV access must be established
BP monitoring must be available
Premedication
Dexamethasone 20 mg PO and diphenhydramine 50 mg PO 12 and 6 hours before treatment, then the same dose IV immediately before treatment
Consider addition of H_2 antagonist with schedule similar to dexamethasone
Have epinephrine and diphenhydramine readily available for use in case of a reaction
Observe the patient up to 2 hours after discontinuing treatment
Treatment
Discontinue the drug (immediately if being administered IV)
Administer epinephrine 0.3 mg IM or SC minutes until reaction subsides
Administer diphenhydramine 50 mg IV
If hypotension is present that does not respond to epinephrine, administer IV fluids
If wheezing is present that does not respond to epinephrine, administer nebulized albuterol solution
Although corticosteroids have no effect on the initial reaction, they can block late allergic symptoms. Thus, administer methylprednisolone 125 mg (or its equivalent) IV to prevent recurrent allergic manifestations

BP, blood pressure; IV, intravenous; PO, orally.

Treatment

Recommended treatment of hypersensitivity reactions is reviewed in Table 94-7. If a patient experiences a severe type I hypersensitivity reaction to any anticancer agent, the treatment should be stopped. If a structural analog or another agent in the same chemical class is an effective treatment for the same cancer, subsequent therapy should use the analog or other agent to minimize the risk of future reactions. If the reaction is mild or moderate, the patient may continue with the same therapy if treatment is preceded by methods to prevent or minimize hypersensitivity reactions. General recommendations for preventing hypersensitivity reactions are found in Table 94-7. Pretreatment with corticosteroids and diphenhydramine significantly decreases the frequency and severity of hypersensitivity reactions; however, the effect of H_2 receptor antagonists and epinephrine remains controversial. Because the success of these preventive measures depends on the cause of the reaction (immunologic or anaphylactoid), the aforementioned characteristics of type I reactions should be used to assess the underlying pathogenesis. In addition, other chemicals present in the formulation or other agents administered concomitantly with the chemotherapy can cause the hypersensitivity reaction. Potential allergens included in the diluent or formulation of chemotherapy agents include Cremophor EL (present in paclitaxel), polysorbate 80 (present in docetaxel and etoposide), benzyl alcohol (present in the parenteral form of methotrexate, cytarabine, and etoposide), and methoxypolyethylene glycol (present in liposomal doxorubicin). Recognizing potential allergens can significantly affect treatment of the current reaction and minimize the risk of future reactions.

To reduce the hypersensitivity reactions observed with paclitaxel, paclitaxel protein-bound particles (Abraxane), an albumin-bound formulation of paclitaxel, has been created. Because paclitaxel protein-bound particles formulation is Cremophor EL-free and less likely to cause hypersensitivity than traditional paclitaxel, it is not necessary to premedicate patients with steroids and antihistamines. Doses between the two agents are not comparable. Although fewer hypersensitivity reactions are associated with this formulation, myelosuppression remains a dose-limiting toxicity.[108,138]

Specific Organ Toxicities

NEUROTOXICITY

Specific Agents

CASE 94-6

Question 1: A.L., a 39-year-old woman with acute lymphocytic leukemia, has been admitted to the hospital for induction chemotherapy. Methotrexate 3 g/m^2 IV once on day 1, cytarabine 2 g/m^2 IV every 12 hours on days 2 and 3 for four doses, vincristine 2 mg IV on days 1 and 8 for two doses, and dexamethasone 20 mg orally daily for on days 1 through 5 are ordered. Laboratory data obtained on admission include a WBC count of 120,000 cells/μL with 9% neutrophils, 11% lymphocytes, and 80% blasts. On day 3, A.L. is confused and she has difficulty performing a finger-to-nose neurologic examination. On day 10, she complains of numbness in her hands and feet. In addition, the clinician notes an eyelid lag and ataxia. A.L. also complains of severe constipation. What signs and symptoms of neurotoxicity is A.L. experiencing? Should the leukemia regimen be modified for future courses?

Methotrexate, Cytarabine, and Vincristine

Methotrexate causes little or no neurotoxicity when administered orally or intravenously in doses less than 1 g/m^2; however, high-dose IV methotrexate (usually >1 g/m^2) can occasionally cause acute encephalopathy. The encephalopathy that occurs after therapy with methotrexate is usually transient and reversible. Some patients may experience a progressive leukoencephalopathy after high-dose IV methotrexate. The risk of leukoencephalopathy increases with higher cumulative doses of methotrexate and concomitant cranial radiation therapy.[139,140] Posterior reversible encephalopathy syndrome has also been associated with high-dose methotrexate and intrathecal methotrexate. Chemical meningitis can occur with intrathecal administration of methotrexate and, less frequently, myelopathy or paraplegia may be observed[141] (see Chapter 95, Pediatric Malignancies). Patients receiving intrathecal therapy or high-dose methotrexate should be carefully monitored for signs and symptoms associated with neurotoxicity.

High doses of cytarabine (>1 g/m^2 in multiple doses) are associated with CNS toxicity in 8% to 37% of patients.[142,143] These neurotoxicities are dose-related and schedule-related. Doses greater than 18 g/m^2 per course increase the frequency of neurotoxicity. Older patients are more susceptible than younger patients, and the prevalence seems higher in subsequent versus initial courses of therapy. As illustrated by A.L., neurotoxicity may become evident within a few days after treatment with cytarabine and, most commonly, the neurotoxicity is manifested by a generalized encephalopathy with symptoms such as confusion, obtundation, seizures, and coma. Cerebellar dysfunction, presenting as ataxia, gait and coordination difficulties, and dysmetria (inability to arrest muscular movement when desired and lack of harmonious action between muscles when executing voluntary movement), is also commonly observed in patients receiving high-dose cytarabine therapy. These neurologic symptoms may partially resolve over days to weeks after discontinuation of therapy. Other neurologic toxicities reported with cytarabine include progressive leukoencephalopathy and chemical meningitis. Intrathecal administration of cytarabine, including the liposomal formulation, may also cause a chemical meningitis or arachnoiditis.[141,144] Leukoencephalopathy typically presents with progressive personality and intellectual decline, dementia, hemiparesis, and, sometimes, seizures. These neurotoxicities also can occur after treatment with other chemotherapy agents.

Asparaginase and pegaspargase can cause encephalopathy, which presents most commonly as lethargy and confusion. These agents are used in acute lymphocytic leukemia regimens. Severe cerebral dysfunction occurs occasionally, and patients may present with stupor, coma, excessive somnolence, disorientation, hallucination, or severe depression. Symptoms can occur early (within days of administration of asparaginase) or late, depending on the treatment schedule.[145,146] The suspected mechanism is the direct neurocytotoxic effect of aspartic acid, glutamic acid, and ammonia. The neurotoxicity is usually reversible with the acute syndrome clearing rapidly and a delayed syndrome lasting several weeks.

A.L.'s symptoms most likely are the result of CNS toxicity caused by both high-dose methotrexate and cytarabine. A decision regarding further treatment with these agents is complicated because omitting a dose or decreasing the dose of either of these agents could compromise the likelihood of a complete remission. High-dose cytarabine cerebellar toxicity may be irreversible. Therefore, the clinician may decide to discontinue cytarabine in A.L.'s future regimens. Additionally, modifications of methotrexate including dose reductions may be necessary in future therapy for A.L.

Multiple other anticancer agents including fluorouracil, fludarabine, nelarabine, procarbazine, and ifosfamide produce an encephalopathic toxicity (Table 94-8). Recognition of neurotoxicity resulting from cytotoxic chemotherapy is often difficult because of comorbid conditions such as metastatic disease and other paraneoplastic syndromes, but it is important in assessing the need for potential dose modifications or even discontinuation of the agent. Several reviews provide detailed explanations

Table 94-8
Neurotoxicity of Selected Chemotherapeutic Agents

Acute Encephalopathy	Chronic Encephalopathic Syndrome	Cerebellar Neuropathy	Peripheral Neuropathy	Cranial Neuropathy	Arachnoiditis (Intrathecal Therapy)	Autonomic Neuropathy	SIADH
Asparaginase	Cytarabine	Cytarabine	Bortezomib	Fluorouracil	Cytarabine	Vinblastine	Cyclophosphamide
Cisplatin	Methotrexate	Cisplatin	Brentuximab	Ifosfamide	Methotrexate	Vincristine	Vinblastine
Cytarabine	Nelarabine	Fludarabine	Cisplatin		Thiotepa	Vinorelbine	Vincristine
Fludarabine	Thiotepa	Fluorouracil	Docetaxel				Vinorelbine
Ifosfamide		Ifosfamide	Fluorouracil				
Methotrexate			Ifosfamide				
Nelarabine			Lenalidomide				
Procarbazine			Nelarabine				
			Paclitaxel				
			Thalidomide				
			Vinblastine				
			Vincristine				
			Vinorelbine				

SIADH, syndrome of inappropriate secretion of antidiuretic hormone.
Sources: Newton HB. Neurological complications of chemotherapy to the central nervous system. *Handbook of Clinical Neurology.* 2012;105:903–916; Magge RS, DeAngelis LM. The double-edged sword: Neurotoxicity of chemotherapy. *Blood Rev.* 2015;29(2):93–100.

of signs and symptoms, mechanisms, and potential treatments for chemotherapy-induced neurotoxicities.[145,147] When a patient presents with any signs or symptoms of neurotoxicity, the patient should receive a neurologic examination followed by a dose reduction or discontinuation of therapy.

Fluorouracil

Fluorouracil can cause acute cerebellar dysfunction characterized by the rapid onset of gait ataxia, limb incoordination, dysarthria, and nystagmus. Cerebellar dysfunction occurs in approximately 5% to 10% of patients receiving fluorouracil at all treatment schedules in common use and can present weeks to months after beginning therapy. A more diffuse encephalopathy presenting as headache, confusion, disorientation, lethargy, and seizures can also occur. These symptoms can be reversed if fluorouracil is discontinued or the dose is reduced. Reports of cerebellar ataxia have also been reported with capecitabine, an oral prodrug of fluorouracil.[148,150]

Fludarabine and Nelarabine

Fludarabine can cause severe neurotoxicity when used at doses greater than 90 mg/m^2 for 5 to 7 days.[145,151,152] Symptoms include altered mental status, photophobia, amaurosis (blindness that usually is temporary without change in the eye itself), generalized seizures, spastic or flaccid paralysis, quadriparesis, and coma. Patients may progress to death even when therapy is discontinued. This neurotoxicity, however, is not common with the current recommended dosage of 20-30 mg/m^2/day for 5 days. Mild neurologic symptoms are typically reported, but severe neurotoxicity,[145,151] and optic demyelination occurs only occasionally.[153] Patients with signs or symptoms suggestive of significant neurotoxicity should receive a neurologic examination and, if warranted, therapy should be discontinued without rechallenging with a dose reduction. Nelarabine, another purine analog has dose-limiting neurotoxicity, and 18% to 37% of patients in Phase II trials showed severe grade 3 or 4 neurotoxicies.[154,155] The clinical presentation includes severe somnolence, convulsions, and peripheral neuropathy ranging from paresthesias to motor weakness. Several cases of ascending peripheral neuropathies and demyelination have been reported.[156] Therapy should be stopped if grade 2 toxicity is present because some cases have been irreversible.[157]

Ifosfamide

Ifosfamide is associated with an encephalopathy thought to result from one of its metabolites, chloroacetaldehyde. The incidence ranges from 10% to 20%; it presents hours to days after initiation of treatment with confusion and disorientation and is generally self-limiting. Methylene blue, albumin, and thiamine have been used for both prevention and treatment. Conclusive evidence to promote routine prophylaxis is not available.[158] Reported risk factors for this complication include a history of ifosfamide-induced encephalopathy, prior cisplatin exposure, concomitant opioids, concomitant CYP2B6 inhibitors, renal dysfunction, low serum albumin, increased hemoglobin, and abdominal disease.[159,160]

CASE 94-6, QUESTION 2: What is the most likely medication causing A.L.'s numbness?

Peripheral Neuropathy

Paresthesia (numbness and tingling) involving the feet and/or hands is an early subjective symptom of vincristine neurotoxicity, which often appears within the first days to weeks of therapy. Because A.L. received vincristine on days 1 and 8, it is reasonable to assume that her presentation of numbness in her extremities is secondary to her vincristine. This peripheral nerve toxicity commonly is bilateral and symmetric and is often referred to as a "stocking-glove" neuropathy. Symptoms initially consist of paresthesias, loss of ankle jerks, and depression of deep tendon reflexes. Areflexia (absent reflexes) typically occurs in about 50% to 70% of patients treated with a cumulative dose greater than 6 to 8 mg. Although older patients appear to be more susceptible to paresthesias than younger ones, almost all complain of paresthesias after combination chemotherapy that incorporates vincristine or vinblastine. Pain and temperature sensory loss are usually more pronounced than vibration and proprioception sensory loss. Patients also may display motor weakness with a foot drop or muscle atrophy. Motor weakness, which can become the most disabling symptom associated with vincristine neurotoxicity, can occasionally cause muscle wasting. Although some patients exhibit muscle atrophy, true muscle weakness seldom occurs after treatment with vincristine. Stumbling and falling that can occur with this peripheral neuropathy is not usually caused by muscle weakness; instead, it occurs in the dark when patients lose proprioception because they lack visual orientation. These complications are either partially or completely reversible, but recovery often takes several months.[161]

Other agents that often share the peripheral nerve toxicity of vincristine include vinblastine, vinorelbine, cisplatin, etoposide, oxaliplatin, paclitaxel, docetaxel, cabazitaxel, ixabepilone, bortezomib, thalidomide, and lenalidomide among others.[147] Unlike the vinca alkaloids, most of these agents cause numbness only and not a loss of reflexes, or weakness. Patients may report sensory loss and pain, however. The incidence may be related to cumulative doses as well as individual risk factors such as history of diabetic neuropathy.[162–164] Many preventive strategies have been evaluated including amifostine, glutamine, glutathione, vitamin E, and others, but many of the studies are limited by small sample sizes and are lacking placebo-controlled randomized designs.[165] The serotonin–norepinephrine reuptake inhibitor (SNRI), venlafaxine, was evaluated for the prevention of neuropathy in a randomized, double-blind, placebo-controlled Phase III trial of 48 patients receiving an oxaliplatin-based regimen. The primary endpoint was the percentage of patients with no acute neurotoxicity, which was significantly higher in the venlafaxine-treated group compared with patients receiving placebo (31.3% vs. 5.3%, respectively; $p = 0.03$). Due to the small study population and ongoing concerns about compromise of chemotherapy efficacy, this preventive strategy is not routine practice. Treatment strategies are only palliative and include adjuvant pain medications such as tricyclic antidepressants, anticonvulsants (pregabalin and gabapentin), and topical agents. Peripheral neuropathy is usually reversible, although resolution may take months. Several reviews provide detailed references for this information.[165–167]

Oxaliplatin causes peripheral neuropathies that differ from other anticancer agents. Oxaliplatin-induced neurotoxicity manifests as an acute neurosensory complex as well as a cumulative sensory neuropathy. Hyperexcitability of peripheral nerves causes an 85% to 95% incidence of paresthesia and dysesthesias of the hands, feet, and the perioral region. Laryngeal dysesthesias have been described as well. These effects are precipitated by exposure to cold. The cumulative dose-limiting chronic neuropathy is described as a sensory neuropathy that is reversible several months after completion of therapy. Dose modifications for patients with persistent neurotoxicities have been developed and typically involves delaying therapy until their condition improves.[168,169] Prevention of these toxicities with infusions of magnesium and calcium has been evaluated in a prospective, randomized double-blind study of patients ($n = 102$) with colon cancer receiving adjuvant therapy with oxaliplatin, fluorouracil, and leucovorin. Patients received either calcium gluconate 1 g IV and magnesium sulfate 1 g IV 15 minutes before and immediately after completion of the oxaliplatin administration or placebo infusions. Calcium and magnesium infusions reduced the incidence of grade 2 of greater sensory neurotoxicity significantly over placebo (22% vs. 41%, respectively).[170] An additional Phase III randomized trial of 353 patients randomly assigned to receive calcium and magnesium pre-and postoxaliplatin showed no statistically significant differences in the incidence of peripheral neuropathy compared to placebo.[171] Decreased efficacy of this anticancer regimen has been reported with use of the calcium and magnesium infusions.[172] Therefore, the use of calcium and magnesium infusions remains controversial.

CASE 94-6, QUESTION 3: What is the significance of A.L.'s lid lag?

Cranial Nerve Toxicity

Cranial nerve toxicity occurs in 1% to 10% of patients receiving vinca alkaloids, and most patients present with ptosis or ophthalmoplegia,[173,174] probably related to damage to the third cranial nerve. Toxicity to other cranial nerves can cause trigeminal neuralgia, facial palsy, depressed corneal reflexes, and vocal cord paralysis—and may occur in the first few days to weeks after administration.[175] Other nerve toxicities associated with the vinca alkaloids include jaw pain, which can occur as early as after the first or second injection[176]; the pain usually resolves spontaneously and does not recur with subsequent doses. Several of the cranial nerve toxicities, especially with vincristine, may be dose-limiting because evidence shows an increased prevalence with increasing doses. A.L.'s eyelid lag probably is caused by vincristine.

Ifosfamide, vinblastine, and cisplatin have been reported to cause cranial neuropathies. Intra-arterial administration of chemotherapy agents such as carmustine may increase the risk of encephalopathy and cranial neuropathies.

Ototoxicity, characterized by a progressive, high-frequency, sensorineural hearing loss, commonly occurs with cisplatin,[177,178] most likely as a result of a direct toxic effect on the cochlea. Ototoxicity occurs more frequently at higher dosages, worsens with concurrent cranial radiation therapy, and appears to be more pronounced in children. The reversibility of cisplatin ototoxicity is questionable. At some centers, routine audiometric tests are performed in patients receiving cisplatin; as a result, these centers have a greater percentage of patients with documented decreases in audio acuity than others. Early cessation of cisplatin may result in greater hearing improvement. Although ototoxicity appears to be a major toxicity associated with cisplatin, it has been reported in patients receiving carboplatin.[178] If ototoxicity is suspected, a hearing test should be performed and therapy discontinued if alternate treatments are available.

Autonomic Neuropathy

CASE 94-6, QUESTION 4: What is the cause of A.L.'s constipation, and how might this problem have been prevented?

Vincristine, as well as vinblastine, commonly causes an autonomic neuropathy. The earliest symptoms (colicky abdominal pain with or without constipation) are reported by one-third to one-half of patients receiving these agents.[147,173] Because severe constipation can progress to or include adynamic ileus, prophylactic laxatives are recommended on a regular basis for patients receiving vincristine and vinblastine. Stimulant laxatives such as the senna derivatives or bisacodyl are believed to be the most effective agents, and stool softeners also may be used concurrently. No compelling evidence suggests, however, that laxatives prevent constipation. Other less frequent manifestations of autonomic dysfunction associated with vinca alkaloids include bladder atony with urinary retention, impotence, and orthostatic hypotension.[179,180] Patients should be monitored carefully for these signs or symptoms and receive appropriate management after diagnosis.

CARDIOTOXICITY

Cardiomyopathy

Doxorubicin

CASE 94-7

QUESTION 1: D.A., a 35-year-old man with stage IV Hodgkin lymphoma, is receiving ABVD (doxorubicin 25 mg/m^2 IV days 1, 15, bleomycin 10 units/m^2 IV on days 1, 15, vinblastine 6 mg/m^2 IV on days 1, 15, and dacarbazine 375 mg/m^2 IV on days 1 and 15) and concurrent radiation therapy to a large mediastinal mass. He comes to the clinic to receive his fifth cycle of ABVD and complains of tachycardia, SOB, and a nonproductive cough. Physical examination reveals neck vein distension, pulmonary rales, and ankle edema. Past medical history is significant for controlled hypertension. What is the most likely cause of D.A.'s current symptoms?

D.A. is experiencing symptoms of congestive heart failure (CHF) most likely caused by doxorubicin therapy. Doxorubicin, an anthracycline, can cause a dose-dependent cardiomyopathy that generally occurs with repeated administration. Doxorubicin causes myocyte damage by a mechanism that differs from its cytotoxic effect on tumor cells. Because myocytes stop dividing in infancy, they presumably would not be affected by an agent whose cytotoxicity relies on actively cycling cells. Many mechanisms have been proposed to explain the cardiac toxicity associated with anthracyclines including the formation of reactive oxygen species.[181–184] The association of anthracycline-induced cardiotoxicity with other agents administered concomitantly, monitoring techniques, and therapies to prevent and treat this condition have been reviewed.[181,185,186]

D.A.'s presentation is fairly typical of doxorubicin-induced cardiomyopathy, although he has no significant risk factors usually associated with CHF. The total cumulative dose of doxorubicin is the most clearly established risk factor for CHF.[187] Patients, such as D.A., who are receiving bolus doses of doxorubicin at the standard 3-week interval face little risk of CHF until a total dose of 450 to 550 mg/m^2 has been reached. After a patient has received a total dose greater than 550 mg/m^2, the risk of CHF rises rapidly. Patients receiving less than 550 mg/m^2 of doxorubicin face a 0.1% to 1.2% risk of experiencing CHF. Comparatively, patients receiving greater than 550 mg/m^2 face a risk that rises more or less linearly; the probability of CHF in patients receiving a total dose of 1,000/m^2 may be nearly 50%.[187]

Other factors that could increase D.A.'s risk of experiencing doxorubicin cardiomyopathy include mediastinal radiation therapy, preexisting cardiac disease, and hypertension. Young children, as well as older patients, are likely to experience CHF at a lower cumulative dose. Concurrent chemotherapy agents (e.g., cyclophosphamide, etoposide, mitomycin, melphalan, trastuzumab, paclitaxel, vincristine, bleomycin) may also potentiate doxorubicin cardiac toxicity.[181,185] When patients receive paclitaxel and doxorubicin, the risk of cardiac toxicity appears to be related to the sequence and proximity of the infusions. In a pharmacokinetic study, paclitaxel increased the AUC of doxorubicin and its active metabolite, doxorubicinol, when paclitaxel administration immediately preceded doxorubicin. Therefore, doxorubicin should be given at least 30 minutes before paclitaxel. The relationship between risk factors and the total cumulative dose of doxorubicin is sufficiently strong to warrant guidelines restricting the total cumulative dose of doxorubicin to 450 mg/m^2 in patients with one or more identified risk factors including mediastinal radiation, elderly age, and preexisting cardiovascular disease (high-risk patients) and to 550 mg/m^2 in patients without any of these aforementioned risk factors (low-risk patients).

It is unusual that D.A., a 35-year-old man who has received a cumulative dose of only 200 mg/m^2 of doxorubicin, would be presenting with symptoms of CHF. Mediastinal radiation therapy, or an undiagnosed cardiac disease may, however, have contributed to this event. In addition, Hodgkin lymphoma involving the myocardium may be responsible for this presentation.

Cardiac Monitoring

CASE 94-7, QUESTION 2: Should D.A. receive routine cardiac monitoring while he is receiving doxorubicin?

Doxorubicin

Prevention of cardiomyopathy is achieved primarily by limiting the total cumulative dose. Limiting the total dose, however, cannot entirely prevent the cardiomyopathy for two reasons. First, individual tolerance to doxorubicin varies such that cardiotoxicity may occur before the arbitrary dose limit; second, some clinical situations warrant exceeding the dose limit to achieve positive chemotherapeutic outcomes.

Early efforts to prevent cardiomyopathy focused on monitoring systolic time intervals, QRS voltage loss, or ST-T segment changes on an electrocardiogram. These changes were too nonspecific or occurred too late to be useful; however, serial echocardiography (ECHO) has been useful. Current monitoring for anthracycline cardiomyopathy includes assessment of a patient's left ventricular ejection fraction (LVEF), which is a measure of the heart's systolic function by ECHO, radionuclide cardiac angiography (multiple gated acquisition [MUGA]), or endomyocardial biopsy. The use of MUGA for early detection of doxorubicin-induced cardiac dysfunction has been investigated extensively.[188] A MUGA can accurately detect functional cardiac status, but it is not particularly sensitive in detecting patients who have early myocyte damage. Augmenting the MUGA with exercise appears to give a more accurate picture of functional cardiac reserve. Because myocyte damage usually occurs days to weeks after treatment with doxorubicin, the MUGA should be obtained just before, rather than just after, a course of the agent. Although guidelines vary, most suggest regular cardiac function assessment by evaluation of LVEF by either ECHO or MUGA.[185]

D.A. should have received a baseline assessment of his LVEF either by ECHO or MUGA before his first cycle of ABVD. During courses of therapy, LVEF monitoring for D.A. would not have been routinely recommended unless he was approaching his lifetime cumulative dose or there were clinical signs or symptoms of CHF. Because D.A. presented before his fifth cycle of ABVD with symptoms of CHF, another ECHO should be performed, and his doxorubicin should be discontinued.

Additional assessments should be obtained when a patient shows signs or symptoms of CHF or when low-risk patients receive cumulative doxorubicin doses greater than 450 mg/m^2 or high-risk patients receive greater than 350 mg/m^2, if additional doses are planned. Most guidelines recommend stopping doxorubicin or obtaining an endomyocardial biopsy when there is an absolute decrease in the LVEF of greater than 10% to 20%, the LVEF is less than 40%, or the LVEF fails to increase greater than 5% with exercise. Endomyocardial biopsies, along with a quantitative assessment of morphologic changes, provide the most specific evaluation of myocardial damage induced by anthracyclines. Progressive myocardial pathology is graded on a scale (the Billingham score) of 0 (no change from normal) to 3 (diffuse cell damage in >35% of total number of cells with marked change in cardiac ultrastructure).[189] Abnormal MUGA findings and the appearance of signs and symptoms of CHF correlate with biopsy scores. Usually, a significant change in cardiac function is not seen with scores less than 2 to 2.5. Several investigators have evaluated the predictive value of this technique. With a score of 2, a patient has less than a 10% chance of experiencing heart failure if 100 mg more of doxorubicin is given.[190] The most significant risk associated with endomyocardial biopsy is perforation of the right ventricle with associated tamponade; this occurs rarely and depends largely on the experience of the individual performing the biopsy.

Other Anthracyclines

Daunorubicin differs structurally from doxorubicin only by hydroxylation of the fourteenth carbon. Cardiac toxicities are similar for both drugs, although somewhat higher cumulative doses of daunorubicin are typically tolerated.[191] Although idarubicin appears less cardiotoxic than doxorubicin in animal models and daunorubicin in some early clinical trials, other studies show equivalent myelosuppressive doses can cause cardiotoxicity comparable to that of doxorubicin and daunorubicin.[192–194] Epirubicin also has an incidence of demonstrated CHF.[195] For all of the agents in the anthracycline class, risk factors for CHF appear to be the same, and similar assessments should be undertaken to monitor for cardiotoxicity. Mitoxantrone is an anthracenedione that is structurally similar to the anthracyclines. Guidelines for monitoring doxorubicin-induced cardiotoxicity should also be followed with mitoxantrone therapy to minimize the risk for CHF.[185]

Prevention

CASE 94-7, QUESTION 3: Could D.A.'s CHF be prevented by the use of a different dose or dosing schedule or by an agent that protects the myocardium?

Altering the dose schedule of doxorubicin to more frequent, smaller doses while maintaining dose intensity has consistently resulted in reduction of cardiotoxicity without obvious compromise of antitumor effects.[196–200] Several reports suggest that peak plasma levels, as well as cumulative dose, have an important relationship to doxorubicin cardiotoxicity. Low doses of doxorubicin administered weekly or prolonged continuous IV infusions (48–96 hours) can be relatively cardiac sparing, allowing higher cumulative doses to be administered. In a retrospective, uncontrolled study of 1,000 patients receiving weekly doxorubicin, a total dose of 900 to 1,200 mg/m^2 of doxorubicin given in weekly fractions had the equivalent cardiotoxicity of 550 mg/m^2 given in every-3-week fractions.[197] Although well-designed studies comparing cardiac toxicity after bolus doses with fractionated therapy or continuous infusion are lacking, treatment that incorporates these alternative schedules should be considered in patients with preexisting risk factors who will be receiving doses greater than 450 mg/m^2 or in patients without risk factors who will be receiving doses greater than 550 mg/m^2. In patients with preexisting CHF or those who have exhibited CHF, a continuous-infusion schedule of anthracyclines rather than bolus doses may be considered. The concurrent use of drugs that might minimize the risk of cardiotoxicity without compromising efficacy can be considered as well.

Dexrazoxane is a chemoprotectant that reduces the incidence and severity of cardiomyopathy. It is indicated in women with metastatic breast cancer who have received a cumulative doxorubicin dose of 300 mg/m^2. The recommended dosing ratio of dexrazoxane to doxorubicin is 10:1 slow IV push 30 minutes before starting doxorubicin. Currently, the ASCO guidelines do not support the routine use of dexrazoxane in patients unless a plan exists to continue doxorubicin beyond a total cumulative dose greater than 300 mg/m^2.[44] Clinical trials have evaluated the benefits of dexrazoxane in children and patients receiving other anthracyclines. A meta-analysis including 10 trials with a total of 1,619 patients evaluated the use of dexrazoxane in anthracycline therapy and observed a decreased risk of clinical HF (relative risk 0.18, CI 0.1–0.32, $p < 0.001$), but there was no effect on overall survival.[201] Despite data suggesting cardioprotection with the use of dexrazoxane, it is not used routinely. Concerns exist about a possible decrease in efficacy of anthracyclines with its use as well as the potential for an increase in secondary leukemias. In the meta-analysis, there was no difference in tumor response rate reported and toxicities attributed to dexrazoxane only included an increased frequency of risk of neutropenia that resolved with count recovery.[201]

To reduce cardiotoxicity, doxorubicin that is encapsulated in liposomes can be given instead. A Phase III trial of women ($n = 509$) with metastatic breast cancer showed that efficacy with liposomal pegylated doxorubicin may be similar to conventional doxorubicin with decreased cardiotoxicity.[202] A review and meta-analysis of 55 randomized control trials in patients receiving anthracyclines showed that the risk of cardiotoxicity was significantly decreased with liposomal doxorubicin versus conventional doxorubicin (odds ratio, 0.18; 95% confidence interval, 0.08–0.38).[203] The majority of patients were women with advanced breast cancer. Despite reduced cardiotoxicity, liposomal doxorubicin has not replaced standard doxorubicin in current treatment regimens secondary to high cost and lack of evidence showing equivalency. An established equivalent dose of liposomal preparations to conventional doxorubicin is not confirmed and is variable depending on the disease state and regimen.

D.A.'s CHF may have been prevented with continuous-infusion doxorubicin or the use of dexrazoxane; however, because he had not approached a cumulative dose that warranted alternative strategies, this would not have been part of the standard management plan for a patient receiving their first several cycles of ABVD.

Management

CASE 94-7, QUESTION 4: How should D.A.'s doxorubicin-induced CHF be managed clinically?

Anthracycline-induced CHF presents similarly to other forms of biventricular CHF and occurs between 0 and 231 days after the last dose of doxorubicin (mean, 33 days). Anthracycline-induced CHF should be treated with a similar approach to cardiomyopathy induced by other means. Often these measures are ineffective. The clinical course varies, with some patients showing stable disease and others showing improvement. Before cardiotoxicity was a widely recognized toxicity, the course of anthracycline-induced CHF was characterized by a rapid progression that generally led to death in a few weeks. The clinical outcome is better now, likely because anthracycline therapy is promptly discontinued after initial presentation and there are better treatments for CHF. These include the use of spironolactone, β-blockers, angiotensin-converting enzyme (ACE) inhibitors, angiotensin II receptor blockers, and diuretics, which have decreased morbidity and mortality in non-anthracycline-induced CHF. Enalapril was evaluated to determine whether it would prevent cardiac function decline in a randomized, double-blind, placebo-controlled study of pediatric cancer patients who were at least 2 years out from treatment with anthracyclines and had evidence of CHF. Patients received enalapril at 0.05 mg/kg/day and this dose was progressively escalated to 0.10 mg/kg/day, and finally 0.15 mg/kg/day if there were no side effects. Although enalapril did not increase exercise intolerance, it did increase left ventricular end-systolic wall stress in the first year of treatment. Side effects included dizziness, hypotension, and fatigue.[204,205] An additional trial evaluated 201 patients with anthracycline-induced cardiomyopathy. Enalapril and carvedilol were initiated as tolerated as soon as LVEF impairment was observed. Complete resolution of CHF was observed in 85 (42%) of patients, and an additional 26 (13%) demonstrated a partial response. Patients who had heart failure therapy initiated closer to the time of observation of their LVEF impairment had better response. No responses were observed in patients who had heart failure therapy initiated greater than 6 months from the end of their anthracycline regimen.[206] D.A.'s cardiomyopathy should be managed conservatively with an ACE inhibitor such as enalapril and fluid restriction with the addition of diuretics as necessary.[183]

Trastuzumab

In addition to anthracyclines, trastuzumab has also been associated with increased cardiotoxicity, likely through a different mechanism. Signs and symptoms of CHF (e.g., dyspnea, increased cough, peripheral edema, S_3 gallop, and reduced ejection fraction) have been reported in 3% to 7% of patients receiving trastuzumab single-agent therapy. Of these patients, 5% had New York Heart Association (NYHA) class III or IV heart failure. The use of trastuzumab in combination with chemotherapy in patients ($n = 469$) with metastatic breast cancer was associated with a 27% incidence of cardiotoxicity compared with an overall 8% incidence in the anthracycline-alone arm. In these same patients, the incidence of NYHA class III or IV heart failure was 16% in the trastuzumab and chemotherapy arm versus 3% in patients receiving anthracyclines alone. Additionally, heart failure occurred in the combination paclitaxel and trastuzumab arm with an overall incidence of 13% and 2% (classes III and IV, respectively) versus a 1% incidence in the paclitaxel-alone arm.[207] A meta-analysis of five randomized trials of adjuvant trastuzumab also showed a 2.5 higher risk of cardiotoxicity following trastuzumab administration.[208] The toxicity seems to be direct and not dependent on cumulative dose or treatment duration. Trastuzumab-associated cardiac toxicity usually responds to standard medical treatment or discontinuation of the drug.[181] Before, and periodically during treatment with trastuzumab, patients should undergo cardiac evaluation to assess left ventricular ejection fraction. Therapy should be discontinued if patients exhibit a clinically significant decrease in left ventricular function.

Multitargeted Tyrosine Kinase Inhibitors

The multitargeted tyrosine kinase inhibitors exhibit a range of cardiovascular toxicities. Because these agents are dosed chronically, toxicities may develop relatively late in the course of therapy. Imatinib has been associated with the development of CHF. A single-institution series reviewed all patients ($n = 1,276$) who had received imatinib within their institution. Twenty-two patients (1.2%) exhibited CHF. Eleven patients continued imatinib with the addition of diuretics, β-blockers, and ACE inhibitors. Five of those who continued therapy with imatinib had dose reductions. The remaining eleven discontinued imatinib (3 secondary to disease progression, 6 secondary to CHF, and 2 were deaths).[209] Patients receiving imatinib should be monitored for symptoms and signs of heart failure.[210] Dasatinib has also been associated with heart failure and ventricular dysfunction.[211] Sorafenib and sunitinib have been associated with a decline in cardiac ejection fraction in 5% and 14%, respectively, in 86 patients treated for metastatic renal cell cancer.[212] A decline in cardiac function has also been reported in a pooled analysis of 3,689 patients with breast cancer receiving lapatinib. The incidence was 1.6% (60 patients). Twelve of the patients had prior anthracyclines and fourteen had received prior trastuzumab.[213] There have been additional oral oncolytic agents associated with CHF including pazopanib and vemurafenib.[185] Patients experiencing cardiomyopathy on targeted agents are treated similarly to those patients with anthracycline-induced cardiomyopathy. Discontinuation of the offending agent or reduction of dose with concurrent pharmacologic management of CHF is warranted. Two reviews of proposed mechanisms and reported incidence of targeted therapy-induced cardiomyopathy therapies provide a summary of current evidence.[181,214]

Arrhythmias

Electrocardiographic (ECG) changes have been observed during or after treatment with doxorubicin, other anthracyclines, cisplatin, etoposide, paclitaxel, cyclophosphamide, mechlorethamine, and arsenic. ST-T segment changes, decreases in voltage, T-wave flattening, and atrial and ventricular ectopy are most common. Arrhythmias may occur in 6% to 40% of patients receiving bolus doxorubicin.[215] Paclitaxel also caused significant arrhythmias and conduction defects in Phase I and II trials[216]; most patients experienced sinus bradycardia. Doxorubicin and paclitaxel are used in many outpatient regimens, so this toxicity is seen frequently. Arsenic, used in the treatment of APL, can cause QT interval prolongation and complete atrioventricular block. Dasatinib, nilotinib, lapatinib, pazopanib, and sunitinib have also demonstrated QT prolongation.[185] The underlying mechanisms for these prolongations are not yet understood. Nilotinib, with a reported incidence of 1% to 10%, carries a black box warning regarding prolongation of the QT interval. The package insert gives specific recommendations for monitoring of ECGs; baseline, 7 days after initiation, after any change of dose, and routinely thereafter.[217] QT prolongation can lead to a torsade de pointes-type ventricular arrhythmia. Before initiating therapy, an ECG should be performed, and serum electrolytes, including potassium and magnesium, should be assessed and corrected. Additionally, all medications, both anticancer and other supportive care medications that are known to prolong the QT interval, should be discontinued.[185] Many other anticancer agents not mentioned previously occasionally cause a rhythm disturbance, but these are limited to a few scattered reports and should not be considered clinically significant. Therapy should not be discontinued unless the patient experiences a serious cardiac arrhythmia.

Hypertension

An increased incidence of hypertension has been observed in patients receiving VEGF-targeted therapy including bevacizumab, sunitinib, sorafenib, axitinib, regorafenib, and pazopanib among others. Bevacizumab-related hypertension may be dose-related; it can occur at any time during therapy and is reported to have a 22% to 32% incidence. Hypertension is usually grade 3 or less and can be controlled with antihypertensive medications.[218] An increased risk of myocardial ischemia and infarction has been observed with the use of sorafenib in patients with metastatic renal cell cancer in a Phase III study.[219] Patients receiving these agents should be routinely monitored for hypertension and antihypertensives promptly initiated. In patients with uncontrolled hypertension, anticancer therapy medication may need to be dose-reduced or discontinued. Several consensus statements and guidelines have been published to assist in the hypertension management of patients in VEGF inhibitors.[220,221]

Angina and Myocardial Infarction

Fluorouracil and capecitabine have been associated with angina pectoris and myocardial infarction. In a systematic review including 30 studies, symptomatic cardiotoxicity occurred in 0% to 20% of the patients treated with fluorouracil and in 3% to 35% with capecitabine. The most common symptom was chest pain (0%–18.6%) followed by palpitations (0%–23.1%), dyspnea (0%–7.6%), and hypotension (0%–6%). It appears to occur more frequently in patients receiving multiple-day continuous infusions.[222] Direct myocyte damage is observed from animal studies; however, human studies suggest that coronary artery spasm is the most likely cause of angina. Because the chest pain associated with fluorouracil responds to nitrates, this problem, theoretically, could be managed prophylactically or therapeutically with long-acting nitrates or calcium-channel blockers.[221] Other agents have been associated with myocardial ischemia (including, but not limited to temsirolimus, docetaxel, paclitaxel, and imatinib) based on case reports in the literature.[185]

NEPHROTOXICITY

Cisplatin

CASE 94-8

QUESTION 1: T.J., a 58-year-old man with nonresectable head and neck cancer, is being treated with cisplatin 100 mg/m^2 IV on day 1 and fluorouracil 1 g/m^2/day IV on days 1 to 4. He received 1 L of normal saline (NS) before and 1 L of NS after his cisplatin on day 1. He presents today for the third cycle of this regimen. T.J.'s labs reveal an estimated creatinine clearance (CrCl) of 75 mL/minute, decreased from 110 mL/minute at baseline. Other abnormalities include serum magnesium of 1.2 mEq/L; all other electrolyte values are within normal range. Is cisplatin responsible for T.J.'s decreased glomerular filtration rate (GFR) and serum magnesium levels?

Cisplatin, a platinum heavy metal complex, is active against many solid tumors and remains as part of first-line therapy for lung, head and neck, and testicular cancers. The major dose-limiting toxicity of cisplatin is nephrotoxicity, and various renal and electrolyte disorders, both acute and chronic, have been associated with cisplatin. In the early 1970s, before the need for vigorous hydration was recognized, cisplatin often caused acute renal failure. Today, with the use of vigorous hydration, acute renal failure is uncommon; however, tubular dysfunction and decreased GFR remain problematic.

Morphologic damage is greatest in the straight segment of the proximal renal tubules where the highest concentration of platinum occurs. Acute and cumulative renal tubular damage has been demonstrated by increased urinary excretion of proximal tubular enzymes, such as β_2-microglobulin, alanine aminopeptidase, and *N*-acetyl glucosamine. Acute renal failure occurs from acute proximal tubular damage and presents as polyuria in the first 24 to 48 hours when urine osmolality declines, but GFR is normal. Polyuria will decline, and then 72 to 96 hours later polyuria increases again, urine osmolality declines, and the GFR declines as well and is persistent. Increases in proximal tubular enzymes correlate well with urinary excretion of protein and magnesium as well as decreased reabsorption of salt and water in the proximal tubules. T.J. has hypomagnesemia, which is the most common electrolyte abnormality caused by cisplatin. Hypomagnesemia appears to be dose-related and may occur after a single treatment. Despite replacement with oral magnesium, renal losses of magnesium and decreased serum magnesium levels can persist for months or even years after completion of cisplatin therapy. Hypocalcemia, hyponatremia, and hypokalemia occur less frequently. The cause of these electrolyte abnormalities is thought to be similar to that of hypomagnesemia in that a proximal tubular defect occurs that interferes with reabsorption of these electrolytes.[223,224]

Chronic renal toxicity associated with cisplatin presents as a decrease in the GFR. Published reports suggest that the GFR decreases by 12% to 25% in most patients receiving multiple courses.[224] The decrease appears to be persistent and only partially reversible. An increase in serum creatinine or a decrease in CrCl does not necessarily reflect the decline in GFR. T.J. is at risk for chronic renal toxicity because he has previously received two other cycles. The renal function of patients receiving cisplatin therapy should be evaluated, because dosage reductions of cisplatin may be necessary if the CrCl decreases. T.J.'s decreased GFR and low serum magnesium likely are caused by repeated cycles of cisplatin therapy. Although a dose reduction of cisplatin generally is not recommended for creatinine clearances that are greater than 60 mL/minute, the clinician should provide T.J. with adequate and aggressive hydration to prevent cisplatin nephrotoxicity. Despite preventive methods, many patients will still experience declines in GFR as seen in T.J. In addition, T.J. should receive an oral magnesium supplement. When large doses of magnesium are necessary, diarrhea often limits the use of oral supplementation. IV administration should be used if higher magnesium doses are required. Patients should undergo frequent measurements of their electrolytes, including magnesium, to minimize potential complications.

Prevention

CASE 94-8, QUESTION 2: What measures should be taken to prevent further cisplatin nephrotoxicity in T.J.?

Several measures are used to minimize or prevent cisplatin-induced nephrotoxicity, including hydration with saline and prophylactic magnesium. Incorporation of hydration with saline and magnesium is the standard of care for all patients receiving cisplatin. The patient should be vigorously hydrated with 2 to 3 L of normal saline over 8 to 12 hours to maintain a urine output of 100 to 200 mL/hour for at least 6 hours after treatment with cisplatin.[223–225] A loop diuretic (e.g., furosemide) may be required in elderly patients to eliminate excess sodium or in patients with compromised cardiac reserve, but these diuretics should not be used routinely to prevent nephrotoxicity. Additionally, mannitol (25–50 g) may be administered just before chemotherapy to prevent cisplatin-induced renal artery vasoconstriction, which can increase the concentration of platinum in the renal tubules. The use of mannitol is controversial and is not given in all practice settings. Most patients may also benefit from prophylactic magnesium supplementation. Patients who received prophylactic magnesium 16 mEq IV daily during a 5-day course of cisplatin followed by 60 mEq orally (20 mEq 3 times daily) between courses experienced less nephrotoxicity compared with those who received no supplements in a prospective trial of 16 patients with testicular carcinoma.[226] T.J. should be encouraged to increase his oral hydration to 2 to 3 L/day for several days after this cycle of chemotherapy. Additionally, he should take oral magnesium supplementation between courses. For cycle 4 of his chemotherapy, he should receive 3 to 4 L of saline the day of cisplatin administration. He may also receive 25 to 50 g of IV mannitol before cisplatin to reduce his risk of further nephrotoxicity.

Patients who experience renal dysfunction commonly have the dose of cisplatin reduced. Guidelines to modify the dosage of cisplatin in patients with decreased renal function are available. Most suggest a 50% dosage reduction when the GFR decreases to 30 to 60 mL/minute and discontinuation when the GFR falls to less than 10 to 30 mL/minute. Percentage dose reductions are relative to the recommended dose for a specific cancer in a given combination chemotherapy regimen.[227] Because the cisplatin dose ranges from 50 to 120 mg/m^2, the precise dose for a patient with a GFR of less than 60 mL/minute must be individualized to the situation. T.J. should have another SCr drawn to estimate CrCl before his next cycle. As long as his CrCl is maintained above 60 mL/minute, then no dose reductions of his cisplatin are necessary. If a tumor type is known to be responsive to carboplatin and efficacy will not likely be compromised, substitution of carboplatin should be considered because it does not cause nephrotoxicity. Carboplatin is excreted primarily by the kidneys and the dose is calculated by the Calvert equation,[228] which accounts for decreased GFR (discussed further in Chapter 98, Lung Cancer). Therefore, patients who have decreased renal function receive lower doses than those with normal function. Other agents requiring dose adjustments or omission for renal dysfunction are shared in Table 94-9.

Other Nephrotoxic Agents

Proximal Tubule Dysfunction

Other agents reported to cause renal tubular defects include lomustine, carmustine, ifosfamide, pemetrexed, and azacytidine.[223,225] Nephrotoxicity appears to be related to the total cumulative dose for carmustine and lomustine, but not necessarily for ifosfamide. Renal abnormalities associated with high doses of bolus ifosfamide have led to the use of fractionated doses and a reduced incidence of toxicity.[223] Most patients show signs and symptoms consistent with proximal tubular dysfunction.

The primary renal lesion associated with each of these agents occurs in the proximal renal tubule and patients experience several electrolyte imbalances, such as loss of protein, glucose, bicarbonate, and potassium. Serum creatinine, bicarbonate, potassium, urinary pH, protein, and glucose should be monitored closely in patients receiving these agents. Because the reversibility of the lesions is reported to be highly variable and a significant number of patients who exhibit severe renal toxicity with these agents require dialysis,[223] patients should discontinue treatment with these agents if they show any changes in serum creatinine or electrolytes.

Proteinuria

Bevacizumab, an anti-VEGF monoclonal antibody, is associated with proteinuria and the reported incidence ranges from 21% to 46% of patients.[229] While bevacizumab is the anti-VEGF agent most noted with this toxicity, oral tyrosine kinase inhibitors that affect the VEGF receptor such as axitinib have also been associated

Table 94-9

Anticancer Agents Requiring Dosage Modifications or Dosage Omissions in Renal Insufficiency

Bleomycin	Lenalidomide
Capecitabine	Lomustine
Carboplatin	Melphalan
Carmustine	Methotrexate
Cisplatin	Mitomycin
Cytarabine	Pemetrexed
Dacarbazine	Pentostatin
Fludarabine	Topotecan
Ifosfamide	

Sources: Kintzel PE, Dorr RT. Anticancer drug renal toxicity and elimination: dosing guidelines for altered renal function. *Cancer Treat Rev*. 1995;21:33; Launay-Vacher V et al. Prevalence of renal insufficiency in cancer patients and implications for anticancer drug management: the renal insufficiency and anticancer medications (IRMA) study. *Cancer*. 2007;110:1376; Li YF et al. Systemic anticancer therapy in gynecologic cancer patients with renal dysfunction. *Int J Gynecol Cancer*. 2007;17:739.

with proteinuria.[230] Mechanisms for this toxicity include microcirculatory angiogenesis and inhibition of nitric oxide synthesis. This may lead to an increase in peripheral resistance and endothelial dysfunction. Glomerular injury from VEGF inhibition may also lead to renal thrombotic microangiopathy and glomerulonephritis. Severe nephrotic syndrome has been observed in 1% to 2% of patients.[221,229,231] Patients receiving bevacizumab should be monitored routinely for proteinuria by dipstick urinalysis. The manufacturer recommends that patients with a 2+ or greater urine dipstick reading undergo further assessment with a 24-hour urine collection. Additionally, it is recommended to delay further administration of bevacizumab when greater than 2 g of proteinuria in 24 hours is observed. Therapy may be reinitiated when the proteinuria observed is less than 2 g in 24 hours. Proteinuria is most often mild in patients and is usually reversible upon discontinuation of the agent. The highest incidence of severe proteinuria requiring permanent discontinuation has been seen in patients with metastatic renal cell carcinoma.[232]

CASE 94-9

QUESTION 1: J.R., a 15-year-old boy with osteogenic sarcoma of the right knee, is to be treated with chemotherapy consisting of high-dose methotrexate with leucovorin rescue, doxorubicin, and cisplatin. The dose of methotrexate is 12 g/m^2 IV administered over 4 hours. What precautions are necessary to prevent the renal and other toxicities associated with high-dose methotrexate therapy in J.R.?

Methotrexate normally is not nephrotoxic, although 90% of the agent is excreted unchanged in the urine; however, acute tubular obstruction can occur with high-dose methotrexate if appropriate precautions are not taken. Acute tubular obstruction is caused by tubular precipitation of methotrexate, which is poorly soluble at a pH less than 7.0. To prevent this, J.R. should receive hydration and brisk diuresis to produce urine output of 100 to 200 mL/hour for at least 24 hours after administration. A urine pH greater than 7.0 usually can be ensured by administration of 25 to 150 mEq/L sodium bicarbonate within the hydration fluid. J.R.'s urine output and pH must be monitored closely to prevent acute tubular obstruction during this period.[233] In addition, intrapatient and interpatient variability in methotrexate clearance is considerable, particularly with high doses of methotrexate therapy. Renal excretion of methotrexate is a complex process involving glomerular filtration, tubular reabsorption, and secretion. Acute tubular obstruction associated with high-dose methotrexate therapy can be prevented only by appropriate attention to optimal urinary output before, and for at least 24 hours after, high-dose methotrexate administration and urinary alkalization.[233]

If J.R. has existing renal insufficiency, methotrexate excretion will be decreased, leading to higher systemic exposure. As a result, myelosuppression and mucositis can become more problematic. Leucovorin (folinic acid) is a reduced form of folic acid given after methotrexate administration to selectively rescue normal cells from adverse effects such as myelosuppression and mucositis. Because leucovorin is already in reduced form, it can bypass the action of dihydrofolate reductase and not interfere with methotrexate's inhibition of this enzyme. Therefore, it is important that leucovorin rescue is initiated 24 hours after the high-dose methotrexate infusion. Blood concentrations of methotrexate obtained within 24 hours after the infusion often are not predictive of concentrations at 48 hours. Therefore, methotrexate concentrations between 24 and 48 hours after infusion must be monitored in J.R. and in all patients receiving high-dose therapy. Methotrexate levels are necessary to guide leucovorin dosing. Leucovorin rescue does not affect the renal clearance of methotrexate. A rescue agent, glucarpidase, is indicated for the treatment of toxic methotrexate concentrations in patients with delayed methotrexate clearance due to impaired renal function. Glucarpidase is a recombinant bacterial carboxypeptidase enzyme that converts methotrexate to its inactive metabolites, and provides an alternative route for methotrexate elimination in patients with renal dysfunction and signs or symptoms of methotrexate toxicity.[234]

HEMORRHAGIC CYSTITIS

Ifosfamide

CASE 94-9, QUESTION 2: After J.R.'s surgery, it is decided to add ifosfamide to his treatment. What bladder toxicity occurs with ifosfamide that requires attention before its administration?

Pathogenesis

Ifosfamide is a structural analog of cyclophosphamide belonging to the oxazaphosphorine class of antitumor alkylating agents, which must be hydroxylated and activated by the cytochrome P-450 3A4/3A5 and 2B6 enzymes in the liver. The 4-hydroxy metabolite spontaneously liberates acrolein, which is excreted in high concentrations in the urine. Acrolein is responsible for urotoxicity causing a direct irritation of the bladder mucosa. Both ifosfamide and cyclophosphamide can produce cystitis, which ranges from mild-to-severe bladder damage and hemorrhage. Cystitis is characterized by tissue edema and ulceration followed by sloughing of mucosal epithelial cells, necrosis of smooth muscle fibers and arteries, and culminating in focal hemorrhage.

Clinical Presentation

Patients with acrolein-induced hemorrhagic cystitis initially go through an asymptomatic stage characterized by complaints of brief episodes of painful urination, frequency, and hematuria. The symptoms may subside over a period of several days or weeks after discontinuing the agent. The course of acrolein-induced hemorrhagic cystitis usually is relatively benign, although death from massive refractory hemorrhage has occurred.[235] The primary factors that may predispose J.R. to hemorrhagic cystitis include the dose of ifosfamide he is receiving.

Prevention

Historically, forced hydration was the primary method used to prevent hemorrhagic cystitis in patients treated with cyclophosphamide therapy. Theoretically, hydration flushes the toxic acrolein metabolite out of the bladder so that insufficient contact time is available to set up the tissue reaction. The more urotoxic agent, ifosfamide, was introduced to the market with a uroprotective agent, mesna. This agent contains a free thiol group, which can neutralize acrolein in the bladder. When administered in an appropriate dosing schedule, mesna can prevent the bladder toxicity completely, and thus use of mesna is the current standard of care.[225,235]

The ASCO guidelines recommend a parenteral mesna dose of 20% of the ifosfamide dose given at zero, 4, and 8 hours after ifosfamide (for a total mesna dose of 60% of the ifosfamide dose).[44] The goal is to maintain prolonged mesna concentrations within the urinary tract that are uroprotective. Repeated administration is required because mesna has a much shorter elimination half-life (<1 hour) than ifosfamide. If patients receive a continuous infusion of ifosfamide, a different dosing strategy for mesna is required. To prolong mesna's protective effects, ASCO guidelines recommend an IV bolus mesna dose that is 20% of the ifosfamide dose, followed by a mesna continuous infusion that is an additional equivalent of 40% given during and for 12 to 24 hours after the end of the ifosfamide infusion.[46] This regimen ensures that mesna remains in the bladder for an extended amount of time after the end of the ifosfamide infusion.

Various other mesna dosing schedules are clinically used, but no trials have compared the different regimens. Many clinicians use a 1:1 mg dose of mesna to ifosfamide when administered by continuous infusion. The dosing guidelines become less well defined, however, when patients receive higher dosages of ifosfamide ($>2.5\ g/m^2$). The lack of data and the unique pharmacokinetic properties of ifosfamide have caused some concerns about the current dosing guidelines. The pharmacokinetics of ifosfamide are nonlinear. For example, the elimination half-life associated with doses of $2.5\ g/m^2$ is 6 to 8 hours, whereas with doses of 3.5 to $5\ g/m^2$, it is 14 to 16 hours. The current recommendations for mesna administration enable protection for approximately 12 hours after an IV bolus; thus, with higher dosages of ifosfamide, mesna should be infused beyond the recommended 8 hours after ifosfamide to maintain bladder protection.[235] Also, concern exists that the 4-hour dosing interval used with lower doses may be inadequate to maintain sufficient mesna concentrations within the bladder. To ensure maximal protection against urotoxicity, ASCO currently recommends more frequent or prolonged mesna dosage regimens to account for its short half-life.[44] Ifosfamide and mesna are compatible in solution; therefore, they can be infused together, offering greater patient convenience.

Because mesna works in the bladder, frequent urination may diminish its efficacy. Patients may be reminded to try to empty their bladder every few hours. Although forced hydration has been the mainstay for prevention of cyclophosphamide-induced hemorrhagic cystitis, it is unnecessary and potentially disadvantageous when mesna is used. This is because forced hydration can increase urination and thus the evacuation of mesna from the bladder.

Mesna is usually given IV but an oral formulation is available. The oral bioavailability of mesna is approximately 50%; therefore, patients should receive twice the standard IV dose (e.g., oral mesna 40% of the IV ifosfamide dose) 2 hours before and 4 and 8 hours after ifosfamide.[236] Others have recommended that an oral dose also be given with the ifosfamide dose. Many centers administer the first dose of mesna IV followed by oral doses at 4 and 8 hours, particularly in the outpatient clinic setting.[44] All patients receiving cyclophosphamide should receive saline diuresis or forced saline diuresis to protect urothelial tissue. When patients receive cyclophosphamide for an HCT, it is at high dose; therefore, they receive mesna and hydration. Other practices to prevent this complication include hyperhydration and the use of continuous bladder irrigation. Data comparing these methods are controversial and report varying rates of hematuria and severe hemorrhagic cystitis. These recommendations are currently supported by the ASCO consensus guideline[44] (see Chapter 101, Hematopoietic Cell Transplantation). J.R. will receive mesna at a dose of 20% of the ifosfamide dose given immediately before ifosfamide, and at 4 and 8 hours after ifosfamide (for a total mesna dose of 60% of the ifosfamide dose).

Treatment

CASE 94-9, QUESTION 3: If J.R. exhibits hemorrhagic cystitis, how should it be treated?

Once hemorrhagic cystitis develops, the agent causing the disorder must be discontinued and vigorous hydration started. If gross hematuria occurs, a large-bore urinary catheter should be inserted to avoid obstruction of the urethra by clots. Some clinicians also use continuous silver nitrate irrigation, local instillation of formalin or alum, or electrocauterization of bladder blood vessels to control bleeding. There is no consensus as to which of these methods is superior. If these measures fail, surgical intervention may be necessary to divert urine flow away from the bladder.[235,237]

PULMONARY TOXICITIES

Bleomycin and Other Agents

CASE 94-10

QUESTION 1: J.A., a 54-year-old man with stage III Hodgkin lymphoma, has received ABVD (doxorubicin 25 mg/m² IV days 1 and 15, bleomycin 10 units/m² IV on days 1 and 15, vinblastine 6 mg/m² IV on days 1 and 15, and dacarbazine 375 mg/m² IV on days 1 and 15) for six cycles. He presents to the clinic 6 months after his last cycle with dyspnea, a nonproductive cough, and fever. Chest radiograph showed diffuse bilateral infiltrates; his respiratory rate was 36 breaths/minute; and his arterial blood gases (ABG) were as follows:

pH, 7.50
Po_2, 62 mm Hg
Pco_2, 28 mm Hg
O_2 saturation, 92%

What are the possible causes of his new pulmonary findings?

J.A. is at risk for several processes that could produce diffuse pulmonary infiltrates and dyspnea. He is immunosuppressed secondary to his lymphoma and the therapy; therefore, J.A. has an increased risk for infection and may have pneumonia. In addition, the infiltrates may represent a relapse of his disease. Pulmonary infiltrates also may represent toxicity from one or more of the cytotoxic agents he received. Further diagnostic workup is necessary to establish the cause.

CASE 94-10, QUESTION 2: A bronchoscopy with bronchoalveolar lavage and a biopsy with pathologic and microbiologic evaluations were performed. Bacterial, fungal, and viral cultures were negative, and the biopsy revealed inflammation and fibrosis with no evidence of lymphoma. These results are highly suggestive of chemotherapy-induced pulmonary damage. Which of the agents that J.A. received is associated with pulmonary toxicity?

J.A. has received bleomycin and that places him at risk for pulmonary toxicity. As part of initial workup before initiating chemotherapy with ABVD, J.A. had pulmonary function tests, which were normal. Many chemotherapy agents have been associated with pulmonary toxicity and the varying types of mechanisms and clinical presentations have been reviewed (Table 94-10).[238–250] Several reviews discuss the different types of pulmonary toxicities associated with anticancer agents.[238–240,250]

Among all chemotherapy agents, bleomycin is associated with the highest incidence of pulmonary toxicity. Although several types have been reported, the most frequent is interstitial pneumonitis followed by pulmonary fibrosis.[238,243,251] Patients generally present with a nonproductive cough and dyspnea. Clinicians may detect only fine crackling bibasilar rales that often progress to coarse rales. The chest radiograph may be normal in the early stages, but patients can exhibit bilateral alveolar and interstitial infiltrates. Arterial blood gases show hypoxia and pulmonary function tests generally reveal a progressive fall in the diffusing capacity without a significant decrease in the forced vital capacity.[243,251] The most significant factor associated with the development of pulmonary toxicity is the cumulative dose of bleomycin. At total doses less than 400 units, fewer than 10% of patients may experience pulmonary toxicity. When the cumulative dose reaches 450 to 500 units, the incidence is higher. A rarer, hypersensitivity reaction produces fever, eosinophilia, and diffuse infiltrates, and this pulmonary toxicity is not dose-related. The mortality associated with bleomycin pulmonary toxicity is about 50%.[238,251] If bleomycin is discontinued while symptoms are minimal and before pulmonary function has decompensated significantly, the damage may not

Table 94-10
Chemotherapy-Induced Pulmonary Toxicity

Drug	Histopathology	Clinical Features	Treatment/Outcome
Aldesleukin[241]	Capillary leak, pulmonary edema	*Clinical presentation:* ↓ BP, fever, SOB, anorexia, rash, mucositis	Stop infusion; provide supportive care to cause a quick resolution of symptoms
Bleomycin[243,251]	Interstitial edema and hyaline membrane formation, mononuclear cell infiltration pneumonitis with progression to fibrosis, eosinophilic infiltrations seen in patients with suspected hypersensitivity-type reactions	Cumulative dose-related toxicity with risk increasing substantially with total dose >450 mg or 200 units/m^2; may occur during or after treatment *Clinical presentation:* cough, fever, dyspnea, tachypnea, rales, hypoxemia, bilateral infiltrates, dose-related ↓ in diffusing capacity	Recovery if bleomycin is discontinued while symptoms and radiologic changes still minimal; progressive and usually fatal if symptoms severe. Avoid cumulative doses >200 mg/m^2; monitor serial pulmonary function tests. Discontinue therapy if diffusing capacity ≤40% of baseline, FVC <25% of baseline, or if any signs or symptoms suggestive of pulmonary toxicity occur. Steroids may be helpful if toxicity is result of hypersensitivity
Busulfan[238]	Pneumocyte dysplasia; mononuclear cell infiltrations, fibrosis	Does not appear to be dose-related, but no cases reported with total doses <500 mg *Clinical presentation:* insidious onset of dyspnea, dry cough, fever, tachypnea, rales, hypoxemia, diffuse linear infiltrate, ↓ in diffusing capacity	Fatal in most patients; progressive despite discontinuation of busulfan. High-dose steroids (50–100 mg prednisone daily) have been helpful in a few cases
Carmustine[242]		Dose-related; usually occurs with doses >1,400 mg/m^2 *Clinical presentation:* dyspnea, tachypnea, dry hacking cough, bibasilar rales, hypoxemia, interstitial infiltrates; spontaneous pneumothorax has been reported	May continue to progress after carmustine discontinued. No evidence that steroids improve or alter incidence. High mortality rate if symptoms severe. Serial pulmonary function studies recommended. Total cumulative dose should not exceed 1,400 mg/m^2
Chlorambucil[240]	Pneumocyte dysplasia, fibrosis	Usually occurs after at least 6 months of treatment with total cumulative doses of >2 g *Clinical presentation:* dyspnea, dry cough, anorexia, fatigue, fever, hypoxemia, bibasilar rales, localized infiltrates progressing to diffusing involvement of both lung fields	Fatal in most cases despite discontinuation of chlorambucil and treatment with high-dose steroids
Cyclophosphamide[239]	Endothelial swelling, pneumocyte dysplasia, lymphocyte infiltration, fibrosis	Does not appear to be schedule-related or dose-related and may occur after discontinuation *Clinical presentation:* progressive dyspnea, fever, dry cough, tachypnea, fine rales, ↓ diffusing capacity and restrictive ventilatory defect, bilateral interstitial infiltrates	Clinical recovery reported in about 50% of patients within 1–8 weeks if therapy stopped. Some of these patients received steroid therapy; however, others have died despite steroid therapy. Occasionally, therapy has been restarted without recurrence
Cytarabine[244]	Pulmonary edema, capillary leak	*Clinical presentation:* tachypnea, hypoxemia, interstitial or alveolar infiltrates	Not always fatal
Gemcitabine[245]	Pulmonary edema, rare interstitial pneumonitis	Dyspnea was reported in 23% of patients; severe dyspnea in 3%; dyspnea occasionally accompanied by bronchospasm (<2% of patients); rare reports of parenchymal lung toxicity consistent with drug-induced pneumonitis	Treatment is supportive care measures. Symptoms resolve and are usually not seen with rechallenge

Table 94-10
Chemotherapy-Induced Pulmonary Toxicity (*continued*)

Drug	Histopathology	Clinical Features	Treatment/Outcome
Fludarabine[240]	Interstitial infiltrates, alveolitis, centrilobular emphysema	*Clinical presentation:* fever, dyspnea, cough, hypoxia; onset 3–28 days after third or fourth course; bilateral infiltrates and effusions	Resolves spontaneously during several weeks with or without corticosteroids
Melphalan[238]	Pneumocyte dysplasia	Not dose-related *Clinical presentation:* dyspnea, dry cough, fever, tachypnea, rales, pleuritic chest pain, hypoxemia	Most patients die because of progressive pulmonary disease. Most reported cases occurred while patients were receiving concomitant prednisone therapy Usually progresses rapidly
Methotrexate[247] Delayed	Nonspecific changes, occasional fibrosis	No evidence that it is dose-related; daily or weekly schedules more likely to cause toxicity than monthly dosing *Clinical presentation:* headache, malaise prodrome, dyspnea, dry cough, fever, hypoxemia, tachypnea, rales, eosinophilia, cyanosis in up to 50% of patients, interstitial infiltrates, ↓ diffusing capacity, restrictive ventilatory defect	Most patients recover within 1–6 weeks (some may have persistent infiltrates or ↓ pulmonary function parameters). Steroids may produce more rapid resolution. May resolve despite continuation of methotrexate, but discontinuation may speed resolution. Rarely fatal
Noncardiac pulmonary edema	Acute pulmonary edema	Occurs very rarely 6–12 hours after PO or IT methotrexate	May be fatal
Pleuritic chest pain		Not related to other methotrexate toxicities or serum levels; may not occur with each course of therapy *Clinical presentation:* right-sided chest pain, occasional pleural effusion or collapse of lung, thickened pleural densities	Usually resolves within 3–5 days
Mitomycin[273]	Similar to bleomycin	*Clinical presentation:* dyspnea, dry cough, basilar rales, hypoxemia, bilateral interstitial or finely nodular infiltrates, ↓ diffusing capacity	Fatal in ~50% of cases. Complete resolution reported in some patients, including some who received steroid therapy

BP, blood pressure; FVC, forced vital capacity; IT, intrathecal; PO, oral; SOB, shortness of breath.

progress. In contrast, patients with prominent physical and radiographic findings generally die because of pulmonary complications. Other anticancer agents can potentially exacerbate the pulmonary toxicity associated with bleomycin. J.A.'s pulmonary findings are most likely suggestive of bleomycin toxicity. Unfortunately, there are no methods for reversing the pulmonary toxicity seen with bleomycin and treatment consists of supportive measures such as oxygen and steroids.

CASE 94-10, QUESTION 3: Why are routine pulmonary evaluations indicated in patients such as J.A. who receive bleomycin or other pulmonary toxic agents?

Dose-related decreases in diffusing capacity can occur before the onset of clinical symptoms; therefore, routine baseline and serial pulmonary function studies are recommended.[243] Bleomycin therapy should be withheld if the diffusing capacity falls to less than 40% of the baseline value, if the forced vital capacity falls to less than 75% of the baseline value, or if patients exhibit any signs or symptoms of pulmonary damage.[238,251] Some practitioners also recommend limiting the total cumulative lifetime dose to less than or equal to 450 units. Specific screening is not routinely recommended for patients receiving other pulmonary toxic agents; however, if patients exhibit any symptoms or clinical findings, therapy should be withheld until the cause can be determined. J.A. received pulmonary function tests before his first cycle of ABVD. Further tests are usually not completed, unless the patient shows signs or symptoms of SOB or difficulty breathing. J.A. did not receive any further studies during his chemotherapy courses because he had no pulmonary symptoms until 6 months after his six cycles of ABVD.

Management

CASE 94-10, QUESTION 4: How should J.A.'s agent-induced pulmonary toxicity be managed?

If pulmonary toxicity becomes evident, all suspected agents should be discontinued and the patient should receive symptomatic support based on their physical condition. As illustrated by J.A., other treatable causes of pulmonary infiltrates (e.g., infection) also should be eliminated. Often, pulmonary toxicity is irreversible and progressive, and effective treatments are unavailable. Corticosteroids are administered but probably are effective only in cases of hypersensitivity-associated pulmonary damage. Nevertheless, because other effective treatments are lacking, a trial of steroids generally is indicated for all patients; if steroids are discontinued, they must be tapered carefully to avoid clinical deterioration.

HEPATOTOXICITY

CASE 94-11

QUESTION 1: J.D., a 56-year-old man, has received two courses of therapy with cytarabine for acute myeloid leukemia. Before his therapy was started, his liver function tests (LFT) and coagulation studies were within normal limits. His current laboratory values on day 10 of his second cycle of high-dose cytarabine include the following:

Aspartate aminotransferase, 204 units/L
Alanine aminotransferase, 197 units/L
Lactate dehydrogenase, 795 units/L
Alkaline phosphatase, 285 units/L
Bilirubin, 1.2 mg/dL

Why could J.D.'s cytarabine be responsible for these laboratory abnormalities?

Elevated LFTs occur frequently in cancer patients and their causes are listed in Table 94-11. Other signs and symptoms of hepatotoxicity include jaundice, nausea, vomiting, abdominal pain, and, rarely, encephalopathy. Patients should receive an extensive workup to determine whether they require immediate attention for tumor involvement of the liver or possible infection. In addition, patients should discontinue any nonessential medications that can potentially cause hepatotoxicity. The clinician may also discontinue chemotherapy if this is the suspected cause.

Several anticancer agents, including cytarabine, have been associated with hepatocellular damage (Table 94-12).[252–263] Some agents commonly associated with hepatotoxicity include asparaginase, carmustine, cytarabine, mercaptopurine, methotrexate, irinotecan, oxaliplatin, clofarabine, and imatinib. A review of 537 cancer patients with tyrosine kinase-associated liver enzyme elevations observe that clinically significant abnormalities were unusual and transient.[264] Multiple agents have black box warnings regarding potential hepatotoxicity. The onset of hepatotoxicity with these drugs is usually within 2 months of treatment initiation and is reversible in the majority of cases. Although death from hepatotoxicity in these cases is uncommon, there have been reports of cirrhosis.[264] All of these drugs come in contact with the liver by entering the liver's blood supply; the liver uniquely receives a dual blood supply from the portal and superior mesenteric veins. The liver detoxifies or inactivates noxious substances and metabolizes many anticancer agents. The exact mechanisms by which cytotoxic and targeted agents cause hepatotoxicity are unknown, but most agents probably cause it by (a) interfering with the mitochondrial function of the hepatocyte, (b) depleting hepatic glutathione stores, (c) eliciting hypersensitivity reactions, (d) decreasing bile flow, or (e) causing phlebitis of the central hepatic vein to produce sinusoidal obstructive syndrome (also known as veno-occlusive disease). Several articles serve as excellent resources for anticancer therapy-induced hepatotoxicity.[252,253]

Several laboratory tests can serve as indicators of liver structure and function. Serum transaminases, alkaline phosphatase, and bilirubin levels should be monitored routinely in patients receiving hepatotoxic chemotherapy. Although these laboratory indices are sensitive, they are nonspecific for the type of liver disease and do not necessarily correlate with hepatic function. Serum levels of proteins produced by the liver (e.g., ferritin, albumin, pre-albumin, or retinol-binding protein) also may be helpful in assessing liver function. The decision to continue or discontinue chemotherapy in patients with apparent hepatic dysfunction can be difficult. If the chemotherapy is the suspected cause, therapy should be withheld until LFTs are within normal ranges. The clinician should also consider alternative (nonhepatotoxic) chemotherapy for future treatment. In addition, agents that are cleared predominantly via the liver may require dosage adjustments and should be administered cautiously (Table 94-13). J.A.'s cytarabine is likely responsible for his elevated liver enzymes. Therefore, costly workup should be deferred to allow recovery of liver function.

Table 94-11
Common Causes of Elevated Liver Function Tests in Patients with Cancer

Primary or metastatic tumor involvement of the liver
Hepatotoxic drugs (e.g., cytotoxics, hormones [estrogens, androgens], antimicrobials [trimethoprim–sulfamethoxazole, voriconazole])
Infections (e.g., hepatic candidiasis, viral hepatitis)
Parenteral nutrition
Portal vein thrombosis
Paraneoplastic syndrome
History of liver disease (including hepatitis B and hepatitis C)

Table 94-12
Hepatotoxicity From Select Antineoplastic Drugs

Drug	Type
Asparaginase[254]	Hepatocellular fatty metamorphosis
Busulfan[255]	Veno-occlusive disease
Carmustine[252]	Hepatocellular
Clofarabine[257]	Hepatocellular
Cytarabine[258]	Cholestatic
Etoposide[259]	Hepatocellular
Imatinib[253]	Hepatocellular
Mercaptopurine[261]	Cholestatic and hepatocellular
Methotrexate[262]	Hepatocellular
Streptozocin[263]	Hepatocellular

Table 94-13
Select Anticancer Agents[a] Requiring Dose Modification in Hepatic Dysfunction

Fluorouracil	Methotrexate
Daunorubicin	Paclitaxel
Docetaxel	Vinblastine
Epirubicin	Vincristine
Etoposide	

[a]The agents listed in this table are examples and are not meant to be an exhaustive list of agents that may need dose adjustments. Additionally, specific dose reductions may depend on multiple factors including treatment goals (curative versus palliative), performance status, and specific protocols.

Sources: Thatishetty AV et al. Chemotherapy-induced hepatotoxicity. *Clin Liver Dis*. 2013;17(4):671–686, ix–x.; Bahirwani R, Reddy KR. Drug-induced liver injury due to cancer chemotherapeutic agents. *Semin Liver Dis*. 2014;34(2):162–171.

Recovery should occur within 2 weeks of chemotherapy. If full recovery does not occur, further therapy (agents, doses, or both) may require modifications.

LONG-TERM COMPLICATIONS OF ANTICANCER THERAPY

Secondary Malignancies After Anticancer Therapy

CASE 94-12

QUESTION 1: T.D., a 55-year-old woman, was diagnosed with an early-stage breast cancer and successfully treated with radical mastectomy followed by four cycles of adjuvant AC (doxorubicin 60 mg/m^2 IV on day 1, cyclophosphamide 600 mg/m^2 IV on day 1). Eighteen months after her breast cancer therapy was completed, T.D. presents to her primary care physician with complaints of fatigue, SOB, easy bruising, and sinusitis. A peripheral blood smear shows a WBC count of 120,000 cells/μL with a differential of greater than 90% leukemic blasts and a bone marrow biopsy confirms acute myeloid leukemia (AML). Subsequent cytogenetic analysis revealed abnormalities involving chromosome 11q23. What factors support the diagnosis of anticancer therapy-associated acute leukemia in T.D.?

Acute leukemia has been associated with cytotoxic therapies used to treat hematologic malignancies, solid tumors, and nonmalignant diseases.[265] It has been reported after combination chemotherapy that involves topoisomerase inhibitors, including etoposide and anthracyclines. These leukemias usually occur 1 to 3 years after the completion of chemotherapy, and myelodysplasia does not usually occur before the leukemia. Other characteristics include chromosomal abnormalities involving chromosome 11q23.[265] This challenge is an important area for research given the widespread use of these agents for many curable diseases such as Hodgkin lymphoma, breast cancer, and testicular cancer.

Acute myeloid leukemia has also been reported in patients who have had previous exposure to alkylating agents. It usually occurs 5 to 7 years after the patient finishes chemotherapy. Myelodysplastic syndrome (preleukemia changes) commonly occurs in 50% of patients before overt acute leukemia. Although all alkylating agents can cause acute leukemia, melphalan appears to be the most potent leukemogenic agent in this class; other classes of chemotherapy agents do not appear to carry as significant a risk. Large doses, continuous daily dosing, prolonged treatment periods, age older than 40 years, and concomitant radiation therapy may increase the risk of exhibiting acute leukemia. Several additional factors may increase a patient's risk of exhibiting acute leukemia.[265]

Evidence that cytotoxic agents can cause secondary lymphoid malignancies, particularly non-Hodgkin lymphoma, is also strong. Immunosuppression from the disease and its treatment rather than the particular agent may be the primary cause of non-Hodgkin lymphoma. Other secondary malignancies can occur after anticancer treatment as well. Solid tumors have been associated with superficial bladder cancer in patients treated with daily oral cyclophosphamide, and bone sarcoma has occurred after treatment with alkylating agents.[266,267] The secondary solid tumors in patients treated with other cytotoxic agents are considered coincidental.

T.D.'s AML probably occurred secondary to her previous doxorubicin. The chemotherapy agent, as well as the time course for her acute leukemia, is consistent with topoisomerase-II agent-induced malignancies. The use of adjuvant AC has been associated with an acute leukemia incidence of 0.2%. In addition, cytogenetic abnormalities occur in more than 90% of those patients who have received chemotherapy or radiation therapy and have subsequently experienced therapy-related myelodysplastic syndrome or AML.[265] Abnormalities in chromosome 11q23 are involved in many of the cases with cytogenetic abnormalities from topoisomerase inhibitors.[265] The chromosomal abnormalities of 11q23 in T.D. strongly support the diagnosis of chemotherapy-associated acute leukemia rather than de novo leukemia.

CASE 94-12, QUESTION 2: Are the therapy and prognosis of T.D. with treatment-associated AML similar to those of patients with de novo AML?

Therapy for patients with treatment-associated AML is much less effective than that of patients with de novo leukemia. Complete remissions with standard cytarabine and daunorubicin regimens are obtained in less than half of patients with treatment-associated AML compared with a complete remission rate of 70% to 80% in patients with de novo leukemia[265] (see Chapter 96, Adult Hematologic Malignancies).

The best "treatment" of therapy-associated AML is prevention. In patients such as T.D. receiving adjuvant chemotherapy for a curable malignancy, avoiding the use of agents that cause treatment-related AML should be discussed in conjunction with the benefits of therapy. Use of alternative regimens is increasing as more is learned about secondary leukemias.

Fertility and Teratogenicity

EFFECTS ON OOGENESIS

CASE 94-13

QUESTION 1: C.L., a 32-year-old woman with recently diagnosed stage II breast cancer, underwent a lumpectomy and external beam radiation therapy and is scheduled to begin adjuvant chemotherapy with doxorubicin and cyclophosphamide followed by paclitaxel (AC-T). C.L. was married 12 months before her diagnosis and wishes to have children. What are C.L.'s prospects for fertility after adjuvant chemotherapy?

Cytotoxic chemotherapy is potentially gonadotoxic in humans. Ovarian biopsies taken from women treated for cancer demonstrate loss of ova and follicular elements. This injury is evident even in prepubertal female patients treated for cancer. Ova die or become nonfunctional by direct injury to the ova or by indirect injury resulting from loss of supporting follicular cells. If the damage to the follicular elements is extensive and irreversible, fertility is impaired even if the ova are spared.

Agent-induced injury to ova and follicular elements reduces ovarian estrogen and progesterone secretion in menstruating women. This causes the hypothalamus and pituitary to secrete more follicle-stimulating hormone (FSH) and luteinizing hormone (LH), which in turn increase follicular recruitment and the number of follicles vulnerable to cytotoxic chemotherapy agents. If the gonadal toxicity is severe or prolonged, permanent ovarian failure can occur secondary to depletion of ova and follicles. Recovery of some of the affected follicles often occurs, however, and this may be manifested by irregular menses or delayed recovery of menses. If the ova are spared and follicular cells recover sufficiently, ovulation and pregnancy might occur, but premature ovarian failure is inevitable in most women treated with large doses of gonadotoxic agents given for long periods.[268]

Prepubertal girls have a greater reserve of primary follicles. Because their ovaries are not producing estrogen and progesterone, increases in FSH and LH with resultant recruitment of follicular elements do not occur. For this reason, prepubertal girls can tolerate large doses without apparent effects even if the pathology previously described occurs. The gonadal effects of cytotoxic chemotherapy in women and girls have been described in several reviews.[268–270]

C.L. is going to receive one of the alkylating agents, which are the most potent gonadotoxic agents. Cyclophosphamide is well known for producing infertility in men and women and gonadal failure even in children. The effect is influenced strongly by the total dose of cyclophosphamide and the patient's age at the onset of chemotherapy. Nearly 100% of women older than 20 years of age experience amenorrhea when the mean total dose is 20 to 50 g. The same consequence can be expected in women older than 35 years of age who receive greater than 6 to 10 g and in women 40 years of age and older who receive more than 5 g.[271] Depending on the exact dose of cyclophosphamide in the AC-T regimen planned, C.L. may or may not fall into a dose range that would be expected to produce permanent amenorrhea.

The clinician also must consider that a synergistic gonadotoxic effect has been reported when doxorubicin is combined with cyclophosphamide. Aside from the alkylating agents, the only agents with strong evidence of gonadal toxicity include vinblastine, etoposide, and cisplatin. Several resources discuss the doses of chemotherapy agents, used both alone and in combination, and specific incidences of associated gonadotoxicity, as well as the prevalence of temporary and permanent amenorrhea.[269,271,272]

C.L. most likely will experience amenorrhea along with the signs and symptoms of menopause as both estrogen and progesterone production diminishes during cytotoxic chemotherapy. C.L. may recover from chemotherapy-induced amenorrhea months to years after completion of her therapy. Recovery may be manifested as amenorrhea interspersed with normal menstrual periods.

Pregnancy is possible during periods of normal menstruation because ovulation does occur in most instances. Premature menopause is inevitable, however. Because the greatest risk of pregnancy exists early in the course of therapy, C.L. should be counseled to practice birth control while receiving cytotoxic chemotherapy. Because oral contraceptives are contraindicated in patients with breast cancer, barrier methods (i.e., diaphragm, condoms, spermicide) should be advised.

EFFECTS ON SPERMATOGENESIS

CASE 94-14

QUESTION 1: J.K., a 25-year-old man with recently diagnosed testicular cancer, will receive systemic chemotherapy with bleomycin, etoposide, and cisplatin. What effect does systemic chemotherapy have on male gonadal function?

The primary gonadal toxic effect of cytotoxic chemotherapy agents in male patients is a progressive dose-related depletion of the germinal epithelium lining the seminiferous tubule. The clinical manifestations of germinal depletion include a marked reduction in testicular volume and azoospermia. The Leydig cells responsible for testosterone production remain morphologically intact, although mild functional impairment occurs rarely. The major toxicity of chemotherapy in men is loss of reproductive capacity. During treatment, libido and sexual activity may decline, but most men report a return to pretreatment sexual function after chemotherapy.[273]

Of the cytotoxic chemotherapy agents, alkylating agents are associated most commonly with azoospermia. Progressive dose-related oligospermia occurs in men receiving chlorambucil,[274,275] cyclophosphamide,[276,277] melphalan, busulfan, procarbazine, and nitrosoureas; procarbazine appears to be the most gonadotoxic alkylating agent in men. Doxorubicin, vinblastine, cytarabine, and cisplatin also have been associated with azoospermia,[278] and doxorubicin appears to have a synergistic toxic effect in men when given with cyclophosphamide similar to that previously described in women. Phase-specific agents, such as antimetabolites and vinca alkaloids, seem unlikely to produce azoospermia when used alone, but may play a minor role in combination chemotherapy regimens.[279]

In contrast to oogenesis, in which women are born with a full complement of ova, spermatogenesis occurs in a continuous cycle of regeneration, differentiation, and maturation beginning in the second month of embryogenesis and continuing through old age. Although different cytotoxic chemotherapy agents appear to exert more damage to germ cells in specific phases of spermatogenesis in animal models, in humans, gonadotoxic agents generally are used in sufficiently large doses to affect varying proportions of maturing sperm cells in any stage of development. This has two realistic implications. The first is that because spermatogenesis must start at the beginning after agent-induced azoospermia occurs, the length of recovery is prolonged, usually lasting at least 2 to 3 years. The second is that the relationship of age to the development of azoospermia is far less clear than the relationship of age to ovarian suppression. Although conventional wisdom holds that prepubertal boys are less likely to be affected by chemotherapy agents than adult men, the reserve of primitive sperm cells in male children is far less than it is in adults. Therefore, the spermatogenesis potential in prepubertal testes may make them more vulnerable to cytotoxic damage than those of adults. A review of the literature regarding the effects of cytotoxic chemotherapy administered to male children concluded that agents and regimens known to be toxic in men should be considered toxic in young boys.[272,273] Short of a testicular biopsy, the damage cannot be detected until puberty.

The two diseases most likely to affect young men who are concerned with their fertility are Hodgkin lymphoma and testicular cancer. The standard treatment for advanced Hodgkin disease is ABVD. Azoospermia has been observed in 35% of patients receiving ABVD and spermatogenesis nearly always recovered in these patients.[278] A similar scenario exists in patients about to start on chemotherapy for testicular cancer. Evidence to date suggests that therapy-induced azoospermia that follows treatment with vinblastine, bleomycin, and cisplatin for nonseminomatous testicular carcinoma is reversible within 2 to 3 years in approximately 50% of patients treated and that those who recover spermatogenesis are capable of impregnating their partners.[280,281] In this particular patient population, it is important to recognize that retroperitoneal lymph node dissection, which results in retrograde ejaculation, as well as cryptorchidism, which predisposes to infertility, may contribute to the lack of full recovery of fertility potential.

CASE 94-14, QUESTION 2: Aside from the use of anticancer therapy agents with less gonadal toxicity, are there means of circumventing infertility in young patients such as J.K. receiving therapy?

Sperm or gamete cryopreservation should be considered in males. A major limitation of this approach has been the finding of diminished sperm counts, sperm volume, and sperm motility in young men affected with Hodgkin lymphoma and testicular cancer even before combination chemotherapy is initiated. Although published studies suggest that the quantity and motility of sperm are important determinants of successful artificial insemination, pregnancies have been reported. Thus, sperm banking should be considered even in oligospermic men.[273,279] Oocyte cryopreservation and embryo cryopreservation now are feasible options for young women about to undergo cytotoxic chemotherapy. Even in the face of cytotoxic chemotherapy-induced ovarian failure, in vitro fertilization of an ovum and implantation into the endometrium with proper hormonal support can successfully accommodate a term pregnancy. This may be an option for females.[270,282]

In both sexes, it has been hypothesized that gonadal toxicity from cytotoxic chemotherapy could be decreased by inhibiting spermatogenesis or follicular development during therapy. Methods used to suppress gonadal function have included administration of testosterone in men, oral contraceptives in women, and gonadotropin-releasing hormone analogs in both men and women. Several reviews describe these approaches in detail,[269,270,273] and ASCO provides recommendations on preserving fertility in cancer patients.[282]

TERATOGENICITY

CASE 94-14, QUESTION 3: If J.K. regains fertility after his planned combination chemotherapy regimens, is he at risk for producing offspring with congenital abnormalities or an excess risk of cancer?

Most of the agents used to treat cancer are designed specifically to interfere with DNA synthesis, cellular metabolism, and cell division. Thus, reason exists to suspect that they may cause mutation of ova or spermatocytes exposed to these effects. The actual outcomes of pregnancies in survivors of cancer are published as case reports, small series, and retrospective case series. Nearly 1,600 children have been born to 1,078 patients previously treated for malignancy in childhood or as adults. A review of the published information suggests no evidence that spontaneous abortion, genetic disease, or congenital anomalies occur more frequently in the progeny of cancer survivors. Similarly, there does not appear to be an increased risk of malignancy in the offspring of patients treated for cancer.[272] The likely explanation for this is that ova and sperm cells affected by cytotoxic chemotherapy usually are killed. The risk of producing an abnormal offspring thus would be highest at the time of chemotherapy. Men and women should be explicitly discouraged from conception during chemotherapy. In general, adults surviving cancer should be advised to wait at least 2 years after completion of therapy before attempting to parent a child; this theoretically allows time for elimination of damaged germ cells. This also provides time to assess the likelihood of the necessity for further treatment that would have grave consequences on the fetus, particularly in the case of female patients.

KEY REFERENCES AND WEBSITES

A full list of references for this chapter can be found at http://thepoint.lww.com/AT11e. Below are the key references and websites for this chapter, with the corresponding reference number in this chapter found in parentheses after the reference.

Key References

Bahirwani R, Reddy KR. Drug-induced liver injury due to cancer chemotherapeutic agents. *Semin Liv Dis.* 2014;34(2):162–171. (253)

Boulanger J et al. Management of the extravasation of anti-neoplastic agents. *Support Care Cancer.* 2015;23(5):1459 (106)

Churpek JE, Larson RA. The evolving challenge of therapy-related myeloid neoplasms. *Best Pract Res Clin Haematol.* 2013;26(4):309–317. (265)

Heidary N et al. Chemotherapeutic agents and the skin: an update. J Am Acad Dermatol. 2008;58:545. (70)

Hensley ML et al. American Society of Clinical Oncology 2008 clinical practice guideline update: use of chemotherapy and radiation therapy protectants. *J Clin Oncol.* 2009;27:127. (44)

Kwong YL et al. Intrathecal chemotherapy for hematologic malignancies: drugs and toxicities. *Ann Hematol.* 2009;88:193. (141)

Lacouture ME, Anadkat MJ, Bensadoun RJ, et al. Clinical practice guidelines for the prevention and treatment of EGFR inhibitor-associated dermatologic toxicities. *Support Care Cancer.* 2011;19(8):1079–1095. (95)

Lalla RV et al. MASCC/ISOO clinical practice guidelines for the management of mucositis secondary to cancer therapy. *Cancer.* 2014;120(10):1453–1461. (41)

Loren AW et al. Fertility preservation for patients with cancer: American Society of Clinical Oncology clinical practice guideline update. *J Clin Oncol.* 2013;31(19):2500–2510. (282)

Lyman GH et al. Venous thromboembolism prophylaxis and treatment in patients with cancer: American society of clinical oncology clinical practice guideline update 2014. *J Clin Oncol.* 2015;33(6):654–656.(37)

Magge RS, DeAngelis LM. The double-edged sword: neurotoxicity of chemotherapy. *Blood Rev.* 2015;29(2):93–100. (147)

Perazella MA. Onco-nephrology: renal toxicities of chemotherapeutic agents. *Clin J Am Soc Nephrol.* 2012;7(10):1713–1721. (225)

Piccolo J, Kolesar JM. Prevention and treatment of chemotherapy-induced peripheral neuropathy. *Am J Health-Syst Pharm.* 2014;71(1):19–25. (165)

Sadowska AM et al. Antineoplastic therapy-induced pulmonary toxicity. *Exp Rev Anticancer Ther.* 2013;13(8):997–1006. (238)

Smith TJ et al. Recommendations for the use of WBC growth factors: American Society of Clinical Oncology Clinical Practice Guideline Update. *J Clin Oncol.* 2015. (3)

Truong J, Yan AT, Cramarossa G, Chan KK. Chemotherapy-induced cardiotoxicity: detection, prevention, and management. *Can J Cardiol.* 2014;30(8):869–878. (185)

Key Websites

American Society of Clinical Oncology (ASCO). http://www.asco.org.

American Society of Hematology (ASH). http://www.hematology.org.

Cancer Therapy Evaluation Program, National Cancer Institute. Common Terminology Criteria for Adverse Events (CTCAE). http://ctep.cancer.gov/protocolDevelopment/electronic_applications/ctc.htm.

Oncology Nursing Society (ONS). http://www.ons.org.

95 Pediatric Malignancies

David W. Henry and Nicole A. Kaiser

CORE PRINCIPLES

		CHAPTER CASES
1	Micrometastases are present in most solid tumors at the time of diagnosis. Neoadjuvant therapy was designed to treat micrometastatic disease before surgery, in hopes of increasing survival. Although it is not clear whether neoadjuvant therapy increases survival, residual viable tumor serves as a marker of response to chemotherapy, and neoadjuvant therapy may reduce tumor size to allow more surgical options in the patient.	**Case 95-3 (Question 1)**
2	When monitoring therapy in children, one has to remember the age-related differences in measured parameters and large differences in size. Blood pressures are lower and heart rates and respirations are higher in younger children. Intake and output need to be considered in relationship to the patient's size.	**Case 95-1 (Question 3)**
3	It is important to adjust creatinine clearance measurements or estimates to adult size (i.e., per 1.73 m^2) to correctly adjust drug doses for renal function in children.	**Case 95-1 (Question 4)**
4	Infants have larger body surface area–weight ratios than older children. Further, organ function changes rapidly during the first year of life. Therefore, chemotherapy dosing guidelines in protocols generally specify how to calculate doses for smaller children and infants (i.e., converting to mg/kg dosing from mg/m^2, or halving doses).	**Case 95-2 (Question 2)**
5	Leucovorin, when used with methotrexate, reduces methotrexate-related toxicities to rapidly proliferating cells. In treating children with high-dose methotrexate and leucovorin rescue, serum methotrexate concentrations are measured so that leucovorin will be discontinued at the correct time. Renal dysfunction, fluid accumulation in the patient, or drug interactions can slow methotrexate excretion and require prolonged leucovorin rescue.	**Case 95-3 (Questions 3, 4)**
6	Rhabdomyosarcoma is a soft tissue tumor of skeletal muscle origin, and it is the most common soft tissue sarcoma of childhood, occurring in 3% of all children with cancer. The two most common histologic types in children are embryonal and alveolar. Using the combination of vincristine, dactinomycin, and cyclophosphamide with local control of surgery or radiation, it is associated with an approximate 75% failure-free survival for patients with non-metastatic disease.	**Case 95-4 (Question 1)**
7	Acute lymphoblastic leukemia (ALL) involves replacement of normal bone marrow elements because of abnormalities in cellular proliferation. Signs and symptoms relate to the deficiency in normal bone marrow elements.	**Case 95-5 (Question 1)**
8	Important prognostic variables in ALL are based on clinical and laboratory findings, including age and white blood cells at diagnosis, sex, race, immunologic classification, cytogenetics, and early treatment response/minimal residual disease.	**Case 95-5 (Question 1)**
9	The treatment of ALL is divided into phases, including remission induction therapy, central nervous system (CNS) preventive therapy, consolidation/intensification phases, and maintenance therapy. All phases are different, each using multiple agents, schedules, and toxicity.	**Case 95-5 (Questions 3, 5, 6, 10–12)**

Continued

10 Induction treatment is a combination of systemic and intrathecal chemotherapy that is administered to induce a complete remission. Given disease-induced morbidity and treatment-related complications, this early phase of therapy can be associated with considerable complications.	Case 95-5 (Questions 2, 3)
11 Central nervous system preventive therapy is a key component of ALL treatment. Contemporary treatment/preventive regimens are composed of intrathecal administration of antimetabolite chemotherapy. Central nervous system radiation is reserved for special situations.	Case 95-5 (Questions 4, 5, 7, 8)
12 The post-induction phase consists of intensified chemotherapy treatments that are tailored to the specific type of leukemia and the patient's response to prior induction therapy.	Case 95-5 (Question 9), Case 95-6 (Question 4)
13 Maintenance therapy is the longest phase of ALL treatment and consists mainly of oral antimetabolite therapy that is less myelosuppressive than therapies given during the consolidation/intensification phase. Because of its prolonged length and low disease-related morbidity, this phase is associated with the highest rates of noncompliance.	Case 95-5 (Questions 10–12)
14 Patients with relapsed ALL will often achieve a second remission of their disease but have a high likelihood of further relapses. Various approaches including intensified chemotherapy or stem cell transplantation have been used in the treatment of relapse.	Case 95-6 (Questions 1–3)
15 Non-Hodgkin lymphoma accounts for 10% of childhood cancers. It has a cure rate of more than 80%. It often presents as a mass in the mediastinum or as pleural effusions. Masses may be large; therefore, adjunctive therapies to prevent tumor lysis syndrome and nephropathy are necessary.	Case 95-7 (Question 1)

PEDIATRIC MALIGNANCIES

In the United States, cancer is the leading cause of disease-related death for children between 1 and 14 years of age.[1] However, 5-year survival rates for children diagnosed with many common cancers have improved to greater than 80% because of the advent of chemotherapy. Approximately 10,270 new malignancies are expected to occur in children in the year 2017. Acute leukemias are the most common malignancies of childhood (Table 95-1), and the solid tumors discussed in this chapter represent 2.5% to 7.0% of all childhood malignancies.[1] Many common pediatric solid tumors are uncommon in adults. Likewise, many tumors common in adults occur infrequently in children. In general, sarcomas and embryonal tumors are common in children, whereas carcinomas predominate in adults.

Small Round Cell Malignancies

Several pediatric malignancies present similarly to one another as small round cells, making morphologic diagnosis by traditional light microscopy difficult. The less typical forms of these diseases, such as peripheral primitive neuroectodermal tumors, extraosseous Ewing sarcoma, extranodal lymphoma, rhabdomyosarcoma, metastatic neuroblastoma, and some bone sarcomas, are even more challenging.[2] Therefore, newer techniques aimed at detecting tumor-specific antigens or chromosomal aberrations have been developed. This information may prove useful in identifying prognostic subgroups and tumor types in children and adults with cancer. For example, identification of the t(11;22) chromosomal translocation in both peripheral primitive neuroectodermal tumors and Ewing sarcomas has resulted in the classification of both into the Ewing sarcoma family of tumors.

Table 95-1
Relative Incidence of Malignancies in Children 0 to 14 Years of Age[1]

Malignancy	Relative Incidence (%)
Acute lymphoblastic leukemia	26
Central nervous system	21
Neuroblastoma	7
Non-Hodgkin lymphoma	6
Wilms tumor	5
Acute myeloid leukemia	5
Hodgkin lymphoma	4
Rhabdomyosarcoma	3
Retinoblastoma	3
Osteosarcoma	2.5
Ewing sarcoma	1.5
Other histologic types	20

Genetics

Similar to adult cancers, the association of many pediatric cancers with chromosomal aberrations or genetic defects is well confirmed. Examples include the association of Wilms tumor with congenital malformations, acute leukemias with Down syndrome, and the association of some pediatric cancers with loss of the p53 or retinoblastoma tumor suppressor genes.[2–4]

Carcinogens

The role of carcinogens in pediatric cancer is probably less prominent than in adults because of the long latency periods required. Carcinogens, however, are implicated in the etiology of some childhood cancers.[5] Postnatal exposure to ionizing radiation is associated with increased risks for acute leukemias, chronic myelogenous leukemia, and solid tumors such as brain, thyroid, bone, and other sarcomas. Treatment of pediatric malignancies with alkylators or topoisomerase II inhibitors such as etoposide or doxorubicin is associated with an increased risk of acute leukemias. Treatment of childhood acute lymphoblastic leukemia (ALL), especially in those younger than 5 years of age who received radiation, results in an increased risk of central nervous system (CNS) neoplasms, leukemia, lymphoma, and other neoplasms later in life. The only well-documented prenatal carcinogen is diethylstilbestrol, which is associated with an increased risk of vaginal or cervical cancer in offspring.[6]

Patient Age

Patient age can be a factor in pediatric cancer prognoses and their treatments. Neuroblastoma is the most common malignancy in infants; however, an infant's prognosis is typically better than a child's, which is attributed to the biology of the disease in this age group.[7] In contrast, infants with ALL tend to have a worse prognosis than children. The biology and location of rhabdomyosarcomas are often different in younger versus older children, with younger children having better overall survival.[8]

Age may also be associated with treatment-related toxicity. Children may have higher susceptibility to radiation-related toxicity than adults. Normal organ development may be disrupted; the skeletal system and, in children younger than 4 years of age, the brain are particularly susceptible.[7] Prepubertal girls may have a decreased risk of fertility problems from chemotherapy and, conversely, children appear to have a greater risk for anthracycline cardiovascular toxicity than adults.[9,10]

Treatment of adolescents and young adults has become an interesting issue in recent years.[11] Because of various referral practices, several of the malignancies that are most common in this age group (acute leukemias, lymphomas, sarcomas) are treated by both adult and pediatric oncologists. Historically, this has divided the available patient data for this population; thus, minimal new treatment-related information is published. Outcomes for adolescent and young adult patients have not improved as much in the last 30 years as for either younger or older patients. This age group has generally had better results when treated on pediatric protocols; the reasons are not clear, although suggestions have been made that pediatric protocols are more aggressive, pediatric oncologists are less likely to reduce doses for toxicity, biology is at higher risk, and fewer data are available on how to determine appropriate dosages in adolescents and young adults. This dilemma has led to the Children's Oncology Group (COG) (described in the next paragraph) and adult cooperative groups joining together on investigational protocols to pool data collected from this population so that more meaningful conclusions might be drawn.

Multi-Institutional Research Groups

With the exception of a few pediatric oncology centers, most treatment centers do not have sufficient numbers of patients with specific diagnoses to scientifically establish the efficacy of therapeutic regimens within a reasonable time frame. Thus, most pediatric centers join the COG, the largest pediatric multi-institutional research group in the United States, Canada, Australia, and New Zealand. Through this mechanism, clinical trials often can be finished in 3 to 4 years, allowing for more rapid progress in the treatment of pediatric cancers. The majority of pediatric hematology and oncology patients in the United States are either treated on a COG protocol or treated based on the standard treatment arm of a current protocol. There are also trials available through smaller consortia that specialize in early phase clinical trials or pilot studies. Unlike the more common adult cancers, few alternative chemotherapy regimens are available for pediatric malignancies. With the number of childhood cancer survivors increasing, research is focusing on reducing the long-term risks and complications of treatment modalities. It is important to determine which patients are at greatest risk from their cancer and to stratify treatments according to prognoses. Ideally, the minimal treatment needed to produce cure would be given when the prognoses are good. On the other extreme, maximal treatment would be given when the prognoses are poor, and potential benefits outweigh the treatment-associated risks. Progress is already being made in this direction, and the future holds promise, especially with rapid gains in our understanding of the biology of cancers.

Late Effects

Late effects can be described as toxicities or complications that either persist or occur after therapy is finished. Most of the early data on late effects are from adult Hodgkin lymphoma patients or from children with cancer. Both groups receive aggressive therapy and often live for years or decades after treatment. Examples of late effects include joint or bone problems, heart failure, second malignancies, strokes, and cognitive dysfunction.[12] A group of pediatric institutions have been collecting data on thousands of pediatric cancer survivors and a sample of their siblings, comparing the health problems of the two groups. This study is known as the Childhood Cancer Survivor Study. In 2006, Oeffinger reported data from the study showing that more than 60% of the survivors had at least one chronic medical problem, and 27% had a severe or life-threatening health problem.[12] The overall relative risk of a health problem compared to siblings was 3.3-fold, with specific risks as high as 54-fold for joint replacements and 15-fold for heart failure. This type of knowledge has reemphasized the need for clinicians to limit therapies for low-risk patients and thus reduce late effects and enhance quality of life for survivors. A website hosted by St. Jude Children's Research Hospital contains a listing of all published studies from the Childhood Cancer Survivor Study (www.stjude.org/ccss). A CureSearch and Children's Oncology Group–sponsored website (www.survivorshipguidelines.org) contains an extensive set of guidelines for the screening and management of childhood cancer survivors. An important recommendation relating to care of cancer survivors is to ensure that they have a record of their treatments that they can keep and provide to their health care providers for the remainder of their lives.[13] This will enable the health care providers to use publications and guidelines that might help the survivor's care.

PEDIATRIC SOLID TUMORS

Neuroblastoma

DESCRIPTION, INCIDENCE, AND EPIDEMIOLOGY

Neuroblastoma is a tumor which develops from immature cells originating from the sympathetic nervous system.[14] It is the most common extracranial tumor during childhood, representing 7% of all childhood cancers. The median age at diagnosis is 19 months; 36% occur in children younger than 1 year of age and 89% before 5 years of age.[14] Of neuroblastomas, 65% are abdominal (half of these adrenal) and 20% are thoracic.[14] The majority of children older than 1 year of age at diagnosis have metastatic disease at diagnosis. Lower-risk patients, which mostly includes infants with stage 1, 2, or 4S, may have spontaneous remissions or at least a 75% to greater than 90% 5-year event-free survival.[15] Intermediate-risk patients have a 50% to 75% event-free survival, and high-risk patients a 19% to 42% 5-year event-free survival.[16] With evolving therapies for high-risk patients (see below), survival may be improved over these numbers.

PATHOPHYSIOLOGY

Neural tumors related to neuroblastoma can be ganglioneuroma (benign) or ganglioneuroblastoma (mixed benign and malignant) or pure neuroblastoma. At biopsy, multiple specimens may be required to fully assess the malignant potential of the tumor. As with other cancers, neuroblastoma results from the loss of cell-growth control because of oncogene activation, tumor suppressor gene inactivation, and related malignant processes. The association of MYCN oncogene amplification with aggressive, poor-prognosis disease was the first key genetic alteration to be identified. Recently, reports suggest that patients whose tumor is characterized by hyperdiploidy with increases in whole chromosome copy number to approximately triploidy generally have excellent outcomes, whereas segmental alterations of chromosomes resulting in diploidy or tetraploidy are associated with poor prognosis.[17,18] The latter includes loss of 1p or loss of heterozygosity at 11q, both of which are being studied in current COG protocols as risk factors that may require more aggressive treatments for patients otherwise categorized as intermediate-risk. The explanations for these correlations are not clear, but this new biology may lead to better understanding of this disease and its treatment.

CLINICAL PRESENTATION, DIAGNOSIS, STAGING, AND OTHER PROGNOSTIC FACTORS

Patients with neuroblastoma often present with a fixed, hard, abdominal mass noted on physical examination by the family or physician, and possibly other signs or symptoms, depending on the location of the primary tumor and metastases.

For example, gastrointestinal (GI) fullness, discomfort, or dysfunction can occur. Other less common but characteristic signs include proptosis with periorbital ecchymoses, increased renin hypertension, secretory diarrhea with increased vasoactive intestinal peptide, respiratory distress, nerve root compression, opsomyoclonus, and unilateral ptosis.[14] The most common sites of metastases are the bone marrow, bone, liver, and skin.[14] Because bone marrow can be involved (distant metastases), it is necessary to do a bone marrow aspirate to rule out bone marrow involvement.

A ^{123}I metaiodobenzylguanidine (MIBG) test is an important diagnostic tool for neuroblastoma because of its high uptake into the tumor tissue (including metastatic sites). The catecholamine metabolites vanillylmandelic acid (VMA) and homovanillic acid (HVA) are elevated in the urine of 90% of patients with neuroblastoma and are also useful in diagnosis.[14] Because infants have a better prognosis than older children with neuroblastoma, efforts have been made to screen infants using urinary concentrations of VMA and HVA.[19] To date, these efforts have resulted in the diagnosis of more infants with good-risk disease but have not reduced the number of older children diagnosed with poor-risk disease. This is thought to reflect two distinct types of biology: a relatively benign biology in infants and a relatively malignant biology in patients older than 12 to 18 months old.

Table 95-2
International Neuroblastoma Staging System (Abbreviated)

Stage 1	Local tumor with complete gross excision
Stage 2A	Unilateral localized tumor with incomplete gross excision
Stage 2B	Unilateral localized tumor, complete or incomplete excision, with ipsilateral non-adherent lymph node spread
Stage 3	Involves both sides of the midline
Stage 4	Distant lymph node or organ involvement
Stage 4S	Infants younger than 1 year of age with localized primary tumor (stage 1 or 2) with dissemination limited to liver, skin, or less than 10% of bone marrow

Source: National Cancer Institute PDQ® Neuroblastoma Treatment. Bethesda, Maryland: National Cancer Institute. Date last modified 12/15/2014. http://cancer.gov/cancertopics/pdq/treatment/neuroblastoma/HealthProfessional. Accessed May 14, 2015.

A simplified description of the international staging system is shown in Table 95-2. Twenty percent (20%) of infants (<1 year) and 59% of children have stage 4 disease at the time of diagnosis. A newer staging system has been designed by the International Neuroblastoma Risk Group task force, but it is only used in the most recent COG protocols. The new system has the designations L1, L2, M, and MS. M and MS are the same as International Neuroblastoma Risk Group stages 4 and 4S. L1 and L2 are more localized disease and are differentiated by a list of "image-defined risk factors."[20]

A large number of prognostic factors have been identified and are discussed elsewhere.[14,19] Patients are currently stratified for treatment based on age, stage, MYCN amplification, histology, and diploidy, or by the new staging system with good or bad genomics and histology. COG guidelines divide low-risk and intermediate-risk patients into four groups for the purpose of assigning treatments (Table 95-3).[19] Infants have better outcomes than older children for the same stage of disease and low-stage infants have a significant incidence of spontaneous regression or regression with minimal treatment.[14,19]

OVERVIEW OF TREATMENT

In current US clinical trials, patients with low-risk disease are typically treated with observation or surgery (groups 1 and 2, Table 95-3). Progression or recurrence may be treated with surgery, unless disease is unresectable, in which case chemotherapy is used. Two to four courses of chemotherapy may be used with initial surgery if organ-threatening symptoms are present. Intermediate-risk disease is treated with surgery and four to eight courses of chemotherapy (groups 3 and 4, Table 95-3, and chemotherapy in Table 95-4) for favorable or unfavorable histology and ploidy.[19,21] Chemotherapy for patients with low-risk or intermediate-risk disease avoids cisplatin to reduce nephrotoxicity and ototoxicity, limits the total doxorubicin dose to avoid cardiac toxicity, limits the total etoposide dose to reduce the risk of secondary acute myelogenous leukemia, and avoids ifosfamide to eliminate Fanconi renal syndrome. Radiation therapy is used only for poor responders.

Table 95-3

Example of Children's Oncology Group Neuroblastoma Risk Groups and Treatment for Low-Risk, Intermediate-Risk, and High-Risk Patients

Low-Risk; Surgery and Observation
All stage 1 patients
Patients with stages 2A or 2B, >50% resected and MYCN not amplified[a]
Infants with 4S with MYCN not amplified, favorable histology, and hyperdiploidy
Low-Risk, Group 2; Receive 2 Cycles of Chemotherapy with Surgery
Stage 2A/2B, <50% resected, or biopsy only and MYCN not amplified
Infants with Stage 3 or symptomatic 4S, MYCN not amplified, favorable histology, and hyperdiploid; increase one group if loss of heterozygosity at 1p or 11q
Stage 3, >1 year old, MYCN not amplified, favorable histology
Intermediate-Risk, Group 3; 4 Cycles of Chemotherapy with Surgerya
Infants with stage 3, MYCN not amplified, and diploidy or unfavorable histology
Stage 4, up to 18 months old, MYCN not amplified (good genomics)
Infants with stages 4S and MYCN not amplified, and either diploidy or unfavorable histology
Intermediate-Risk, Group 4; 8 Cycles of Chemotherapy with Surgery
Infants with stage 4S, unknown biology
Infants with stage 4, MYCN not amplified, with diploidy or unfavorable histology
Stage 3, up to 18 months old, MYCN not amplified and unfavorable histology
High-Risk
Biopsy, 5–6 cycles of chemotherapy, followed by definitive surgery, high-dose chemotherapy with autologous progenitor cell rescue, radiation to the primary site, and maintenance therapy. Induction chemotherapy: Vincristine, doxorubicin, and cyclophosphamide for cycles 1, 2, 4, and 6; cisplatin and etoposide for cycles 3 and 5. Consolidation: high-dose chemotherapy (carboplatin, etoposide, and melphalan) followed by autologous progenitor cell rescue. Maintenance therapy: 6 cycles of isotretinoin (2 weeks on; 2 weeks off for each cycle) concurrent with 5 cycles of dinutuximab with GM-CSF on cycles 1, 3, 5 or interleukin-2 on cycles 2 and 4.[b]
MYCN amplified and not included in previous groups.

Consult current protocols as classifications and treatment recommendations are changing rapidly. Typical correlations with the newer staging terminology: L1 and MS patients with good genomics would be in the low-risk group; L2 patients with good genomics would be in the intermediate-risk group but bad genomics in the high-risk group; MS patients with good genomics would be lower risk or with bad genomics would be high risk; M patients would be in the high risk unless they are less than 18 months old with good genomics. See Table 95-4 for details of chemotherapy regimens in low-risk and intermediate-risk patients.

[a]MYCN is an oncogene that is associated with more aggressive higher-risk neuroblastomas.

[b]GM-CSF is granulocyte-macrophage colony stimulating factor.

Sources: Brodeur GM et al. Neuroblastoma. In: Pizzo PA, Poplack DG, eds. *Principles and Practice of Pediatric Oncology*. 6th ed. Philadelphia, PA: Lippincott Williams & Wilkins; 2010:886; National Cancer Institute PDQ® Neuroblastoma Treatment. Bethesda, MD: National Cancer Institute. Date last modified 12/15/2014. **http://cancer.gov/cancertopics/pdq/treatment/neuroblastoma/Health Professional. Accessed May 14, 2015.**

Therapy for high-risk disease generally involves a first surgery for biopsy, aggressive chemotherapy, second-look surgery for residual tumor resection, either additional aggressive chemotherapy or high-dose chemotherapy with autologous progenitor cell rescue, radiation to the tumor bed, and maintenance therapy (Table 95-3.)[16,19] High-dose chemotherapy with autologous progenitor cell rescue raised 5-year, disease progression–free survival to 49% from historic values of 10% to 20%; however, relapses can occur later with 7-year disease progression–free survival of only 26%.[22,23] Survival can be improved (46% vs. 29% 5-year post-chemotherapy disease-free survival) for patients with higher-risk disease if standard-dose or high-dose chemotherapy is followed by maintenance with six cycles of isotretinoin 80 mg/m^2 given orally twice daily for 14 days of each 28-day cycle.[22] Addition of the anti-GD2 monoclonal antibody, dinutuximab (ch14.18), along with interleukin-2 and granulocyte-macrophage colony stimulating factor (GM-CSF), to the maintenance regimen has been shown to further increase survival.[24] Typical conditioning regimens preceding autologous progenitor cell rescue include carboplatin and etoposide with either cyclophosphamide or melphalan, or thiotepa and cyclophosphamide.

CLINICAL PRESENTATION AND DIAGNOSIS

CASE 95-1

QUESTION 1: H.K. is a 2-year-old girl with a 3-month history of constipation and progressive abdominal distension. She has a decreased appetite, 1-week history of vomiting, and she is pale and tired. She has a large retroperitoneal mass and multiple bilateral enlarged inguinal lymph nodes. Her WBC count, differential and platelets are within normal limits. Serum sodium, potassium, chloride, creatinine, and glucose are within normal limits. Her laboratory test results also include the following:

Hemoglobin (Hgb), 5.1 g/dL (normal, 11–14 g/dL)
Lactate dehydrogenase (LDH), 424 units/L
Albumin, 2.3 g/dL
Urine HVA, 570 mg/g creatinine (normal, <26 mg/g)
Urine VMA, 31 mg/g creatinine (normal, <11 mg/g)

Biopsies of the abdominal mass and bone marrow are positive for neuroblastoma cells that are MYCN amplified. The lymph nodes are negative for neuroblastoma. Scans are negative for other sites of disease. Which of these signs, symptoms, and laboratory results are consistent with a diagnosis of neuroblastoma?

Table 95-4
Typical Cycles of Chemotherapy Used in Children's Oncology Group Low-Risk and Intermediate-Risk Neuroblastoma

Cycle[a]	Drugs
1	Carboplatin, etoposide
2	Carboplatin, cyclophosphamide, doxorubicin
3	Cyclophosphamide, etoposide
4	Carboplatin, doxorubicin, etoposide
5	Cyclophosphamide, etoposide
6	Carboplatin, cyclophosphamide, doxorubicin
7	Carboplatin, etoposide
8	Cyclophosphamide, doxorubicin

[a]Each row represents a single 21-day cycle of therapy. Generally, the first four cycles are used in patients at intermediate risk with favorable histology disease, and all eight for patients with unfavorable histology. Patients at low risk whose disease is potentially organ-threatening may receive the first two to four cycles plus surgery. See Table 95-3 for common chemotherapy guidelines for neuroblastoma patients.

Source: Brodeur GM et al. Neuroblastoma. In: Pizzo PA, Poplack DG, eds. *Principles and Practice of Pediatric Oncology*. 6th ed. Philadelphia, PA: Lippincott Williams & Wilkins; 2010:886; National Cancer Institute PDQ® Neuroblastoma Treatment. Bethesda, MD: National Cancer Institute. Date last modified 12/15/2014. http://cancer.gov/cancertopics/pdq/treatment/neuroblastoma/Health Professional. Accessed May 14, 2015.

Virtually all of H.K.'s findings are consistent with neuroblastoma. The low hemoglobin and albumin and high LDH, however, are not specific for this cancer. In addition to the biopsy, the elevated urine VMA and HVA are most helpful in confirming the diagnosis of neuroblastoma. In H.K., biopsies of the bone marrow, lymph nodes, and primary tumor were necessary to demonstrate the presence or absence of neuroblastoma at more than one site for staging purposes.

TREATMENT

CASE 95-1, QUESTION 2: What stage of disease does H.K. have? What treatment will she receive?

H.K.'s abdominal disease with distant bone marrow involvement indicates stage 4 (or M) disease. Considering her age and disease stage, H.K. has a high risk of dying from her disease. Her MYCN also was amplified. Therefore, she is started on chemotherapy consisting of vincristine, doxorubicin, and cyclophosphamide for cycles 1, 2, 4, and 6, and cisplatin and etoposide for cycles 3 and 5.

CASE 95-1, QUESTION 3: H.K. is 81.5 cm tall, weighs 11.65 kg, and has a body surface area of 0.5 m^2. For her third chemotherapy cycle, consisting of cisplatin 50 mg/m^2/day on days 1 through 4 and etoposide 200 mg/m^2/day on days 1 through 3, she is given hydration fluids of 5% dextrose with 0.45% sodium chloride at 62.5 mL/hour. Urine output is 4 mL/kg/hour. How does monitoring of H.K.'s chemotherapy differ from that of an adult?

Monitoring Vital Signs for Etoposide

Although prevention and monitoring of toxicities from chemotherapy agents in children follow the same basic rules as in adults, there are some differences. When monitoring vital signs for hypotensive reactions to etoposide, normal blood pressure will be lower (hypotension is defined as a systolic blood pressure under 74 mm Hg for a 2-year-old girl) and the pulse higher (mean, 119 beats/minute for a 2-year-old) than in adults.[25] It is important to have baseline vital signs so that hypotension or tachycardia will be recognized.

Monitoring Hydration for Cisplatin

In adults receiving cisplatin, hydration is often standardized with 1 to 2 L of intravenous (IV) fluids given before the drug, 1 to 2 L with the drug, and then continuous hydration for at least 24 hours after the dose.[26] In children, hydration volumes should be calculated based on the child's size. To decrease the risk of cisplatin nephrotoxicity, most pediatric protocols recommend IV fluids at twice maintenance rates to maintain urine outputs of at least 2 to 3 mL/kg/hour. The COG calculates maintenance fluids as 1,500 mL/m^2/24 hours, so H.K. should receive 3,000 mL/0.5 m^2 = 1,500 mL during 24 hours (62.5 mL/hour). H.K.'s measured urine output is 4 mL/kg/hour, which should be adequate to prevent nephrotoxicity. Weight should also be monitored throughout cisplatin administration to assure fluid balance. Acute weight gain may require diuretics to prevent overhydration, and weight loss may indicate dehydration with impending reduction of urine output that could lead to acute nephrotoxicity. Increased IV fluids would help prevent the latter.

Adjustment of Creatinine Clearance to Adult Size

CASE 95-1, QUESTION 4: H.K.'s measured creatinine clearance (CrCl) is 39 mL/minute. Should her cisplatin be withheld or the dose adjusted because of low creatinine clearance?

Cisplatin is either not administered or administered at a reduced dosage when the creatinine clearance is less than 50 to 60 mL/minute/1.73 m^2.[27] Although H.K.'s creatinine clearance of 39 mL/minute appears to be low, it is relative to the patient's size (i.e., 39 mL/minute/0.5 m^2). Guidelines for dosing drugs cleared by glomerular filtration are based on creatinine clearance for normal adult body size, 1.73 m^2. Therefore, it is important to correct H.K.'s creatinine clearance to adult body size.[28] Multiplying by 1.73/0.5, her creatinine clearance is 135 mL/minute/1.73 m^2, so this is not a reason to withhold cisplatin. One precaution is that the accuracy of serum creatinine and creatinine clearance in assessing renal function during cisplatin therapy in children has been questioned.[29]

Partial Response and Hematopoietic Progenitor Cell Rescue

CASE 95-1, QUESTION 5: H.K. obtains a partial response to the aforementioned initial chemotherapy regimen with reduction of urine VMA and HVA concentrations and a 50% decrease in the size of the primary tumor in the abdomen. Second-look surgery is performed to debulk the tumor, and pathology results indicate that the residual tumor contains 95% mature (benign) ganglioneuroma cells, but neuroblastoma cells are still present. What further treatment has the most potential benefit for H.K.?

The best chance for prolonged disease-free survival for H.K. is dose-intensive chemotherapy combined with autologous peripheral blood progenitor cell rescue. The regimen she is receiving was designed to be followed by high-dose chemotherapy and stem cell rescue. The 2- to 3-year disease-free survival is better with high-dose chemotherapy followed by autologous progenitor cell rescue.[14,16,19,22,23] The plan for H.K. is to proceed to high-dose chemotherapy (carboplatin, etoposide, and melphalan) with an autologous progenitor cell rescue. If a complete response is achieved, she would then receive radiation to the bed of the primary tumor, followed by 6 monthly cycles of isotretinoin (cis-retinoic acid) and 5 cycles of dinutuximab with granulocyte-macrophage colony stimulating factor (GM-CSF cycles 1, 3, 5) and interleukin-2 (cycles 2, 4). All three of these treatments, dose-intensive chemotherapy with progenitor cell rescue, isotretinoin, and the dinutuximab regimen, have been shown to independently increase survival.

Further Treatments Based on Disease Biology

With rapid advances in neuroblastoma biology being made, future alternatives may include more biologic treatments. One agent in clinical trials is ^{131}I-MIBG, a compound that delivers radiation directly to catecholamine-secreting cells such as neuroblastoma. Studies have used ^{131}I-MIBG as part of the conditioning regimen before progenitor cell rescue in patients with neuroblastoma.[30] Crizotinib, an anaplastic lymphoma kinase receptor tyrosine kinase inhibitor, has entered phase I–II clinical trials in pediatric patients and shows some promise for a small percentage of patients with neuroblastoma.[31]

Wilms Tumor

DESCRIPTION, EPIDEMIOLOGY, AND PATHOPHYSIOLOGY

Wilms tumor, also known as nephroblastoma, is a kidney tumor composed of various kidney cell types at different stages of maturation.[32] Approximately 5% of all childhood cancers are Wilms tumor, making it the most common intra-abdominal tumor of childhood.[1] The peak incidence occurs at 3 to 4 years of age.[32] Overall, Wilms tumor has an excellent prognosis. Four-year relapse free survival is greater than 50% for all categories of Wilms tumor except stage IV with diffuse anaplasia. For low-stage patients, 4-year relapse-free survival is generally greater than 86%.[32] Histology is the most important indicator of likely outcomes with diffuse anaplasia being distinctly worse than either focal anaplasia or favorable histology.

The relationship of genetic factors to Wilms tumor is demonstrated by the approximately 1.5% of patients with Wilms tumor who have family members with the disease and the approximately 10% who have aniridia, hemihypertrophy, or genitourinary anomalies.[32,33] Chromosomal aberrations at 11p13 and 11p15, known respectively as WT1 and WT2, and WTX on the X chromosome, are associated with nonfamilial Wilms tumor. Genes at these sites are involved with normal development of the urinary tract and other tissues involved in the anomalies. It is thought that the relationship between congenital anomalies and Wilms tumor may relate to methylation and inactivation of a set of neighboring genes involved with the two medical conditions.[32] The familial syndrome is related to FWT1 (17q12-21) and FWT2 (19q13.4), which have been identified more recently and about which less is known.[33] Loss of heterozygosity (LOH) at 1p and 16q correlates with increased risk of recurrence in stage III or IV disease with favorable histology. Treatment guidelines suggest increased chemotherapy for patients with these findings (Table 95-5).

CLINICAL PRESENTATION

Patients with Wilms tumor frequently present with an asymptomatic abdominal mass, although malaise and pain may be reported.[32] Hematuria and high renin hypertension each occur in approximately 25% of patients. Metastases, when present at diagnosis, most commonly involve the lungs (80%) or liver (15%).

DIAGNOSIS, STAGING, AND OVERVIEW OF TREATMENT

Diagnosis of Wilms tumor is based on biopsy and computed tomography (CT) of chest and abdomen to rule out metastatic disease. Treatment in the United States is based mostly on disease stage after surgical resection or debulking and favorable histology versus focal or diffuse anaplasia. Surgical resection is the primary treatment, followed by adjuvant chemotherapy (Table 95-5). A simplified description of the staging is as follows: stage I is limited to the kidney and can be completely removed surgically; stage II is extended beyond the kidney but can be completely excised; stage III is characterized by residual tumor confined to the abdomen; stage IV is distant metastases; and stage V is bilateral disease.[33] Metastases are present in only 15% of patients at diagnosis, and even these patients have relatively good prognoses. Notably, in Europe the majority of treatments use neoadjuvant chemotherapy before surgery. The benefits and risks of each method have been discussed elsewhere.[34] COG studies suggest surgery followed by adjuvant chemotherapy except in stage V (bilateral disease), where neoadjuvant chemotherapy is used in an attempt to preserve kidney function. Current protocols use newer regimens and also examine the possibility of surgery without chemotherapy for some very-low-risk patients.[33]

Table 95-5
Wilms Tumor Treatment Regimens by Stage and Histology

Stage I, Any Histology, and Stage II, Favorable Histology
Surgery followed by 18 weeks of vincristine and dactinomycin. Add abdominal radiation for either focal or diffuse anaplasia.[a]
Stage III or IV, Favorable Histology; Stages II, III, or IV Focal Anaplasia
Surgery followed by 24 weeks of vincristine, dactinomycin, and doxorubicin, with abdominal radiation.[b] Add pulmonary radiation if chest CT (computed tomography) shows metastases, unless there is complete resolution after chemotherapy.
Stages II through IV, Diffuse Anaplasia
Surgery followed by 24 weeks of vincristine, doxorubicin, etoposide, and cyclophosphamide with mesna, plus or minus dactinomycin and carboplatin, abdominal radiation. Stage IV: Add pulmonary radiation if chest CT (computed tomography) shows metastases, unless there is complete resolution after chemotherapy.
Stage V
Biopsy followed by neoadjuvant vincristine, dactinomycin, and doxorubicin, then complete resection or debulking followed by more chemotherapy and, if a poor response, radiation therapy; more aggressive treatment if unfavorable histology.

[a]Stage I with tumor <550 g in a patient <24 months of age: surgery alone has been used investigationally with some success.
[b]Stage III or IV with favorable histology but loss of heterozygosity at 1p and 16q: higher risk, use vincristine, dactinomycin, doxorubicin, plus outpatient cyclophosphamide and etoposide.
Source: National Cancer Institute: PDQ® Wilms tumor and other childhood kidney tumors treatment. Bethesda, MD: National Cancer Institute. Date last modified August 15, 2014. http://cancer.gov/cancertopics/pdq/treatment/wilms/HealthProfessional. Accessed May 14, 2015

CLINICAL PRESENTATION AND TREATMENT

CASE 95-2

QUESTION 1: B.N. is a 34-month-old boy who is pale and irritable. He has had abdominal complaints with decreased bowel movements and reduced oral intake for 2 weeks. He has played less than normal for the last 4 weeks. B.N.'s blood pressure has intermittently been as high as 146/87 mm Hg (normal, 90th percentile, 106/69). His laboratory results include the following:

Hgb, 7.9 g/dL (normal, 11.5–13.5)
Erythrocyte sedimentation rate, 139 mm/hour (normal, <10)

B.N. has a history of hypospadias and left hydronephrosis. Scans show a right kidney mass extending through the capsule plus two distant metastases in the peritoneum. Chest radiography shows one nodule in the lung as well. Pathology from a biopsy sample shows favorable histology Wilms tumor. What treatment should B.N. receive?

B.N. has stage IV disease with favorable histology and the cells are negative for loss of heterozygosity at 1p and 16q. The expected treatment for him is 24 weeks of vincristine, dactinomycin, and doxorubicin, assuming findings at surgery are consistent with pretreatment scans. He will receive abdominal radiation; he would also receive pulmonary radiation unless the lung metastases completely disappear with chemotherapy. The series of five National Wilms Tumor studies have sought to progressively minimize toxicities from radiation and chemotherapy while maintaining the excellent cure rate. The fourth National Wilms Tumor Study Group (NWTS-4) study demonstrated that intermittent, higher doses of dactinomycin allowed higher dose intensity with less myelosuppression than lower doses given daily for 5 days. Using greater dose intensity and dose density, 6 months of therapy was shown to be as effective as 15 months of therapy given the traditional way.[35] Also, fewer clinic visits were made and estimated costs were reduced by 50%.[35,36] The NWTS-5 evaluated surgery followed by 18 to 24 weeks of chemotherapy. Chemotherapy was determined by the stage and histology findings (Table 95-5). Abdominal radiation therapy was added to chemotherapy for stage II disease with unfavorable histology (focal or diffuse anaplasia) or stages III or IV with any histology; pulmonary radiation was added for stage IV disease if the chest radiograph was positive for metastases. The latter part of the guideline has now changed to depend on whether or not the pulmonary nodules clear with chemotherapy or not. For patients with stage V, or those with inoperable tumors, surgery could be delayed until neoadjuvant chemotherapy reduces the tumor size.

Dosing Chemotherapy in Infants and Young Children

CASE 95-2, QUESTION 2: Are there any special precautions for dosing chemotherapy in B.N.?

The NWTS-2 study noted an excessive number of toxic deaths in infants with good prognosis, and this resulted in a dosing change.[37] After chemotherapy doses were decreased by 50%, severe hematologic toxicity, toxic deaths, and pulmonary and hepatic complications were reduced.[38] Importantly, no decrease in therapeutic effect was noted. Reduction of chemotherapy doses in infants is a consideration for other pediatric cancers as well.[39–41] Reasons for increased toxicity in infants may include altered pharmacokinetics or organ sensitivity as well as the larger body surface area/kilogram relative to older children and adults.[37] In NWTS-5, dosages of chemotherapy agents for Wilms tumor patients who are less than 30 kg were converted from mg/m^2 to mg/kg. By assuming the average 1-m^2 child weighs 30 kg, the dose/m^2 can be divided by 30 to arrive at a dose/kilogram, which can be used in dosing calculations. This adjustment lowers the dose by 20% to 50% in children who weigh less than 15 kg. In NWTS-5, infants younger than 12 months of age received doses that were further reduced by halving the milligram/kilogram dose.

Interaction of Chemotherapy with Radiation

CASE 95-2, QUESTION 3: Are there any dosing precautions required because of potential interactions between B.N.'s treatments?

Another medication-related problem that may arise in B.N. is the interaction of dactinomycin and doxorubicin with radiation therapy.[42–46] Two effects have been reported. One is acute enhancement of radiation effects, and the other is recurrence (recall) of radiation effects up to several weeks later, especially to skin and mucous membranes. Because B.N. is to receive abdominal and lung irradiation during his chemotherapy treatment, concurrent doses of dactinomycin and doxorubicin will need to be reduced by 50%, and held if wet desquamation of the skin at the radiation site occurs. In many of the Ewing sarcoma and rhabdomyosarcoma protocols, dactinomycin or doxorubicin is stopped during concurrent radiation treatments.

Doxorubicin Cardiotoxicity in Pediatrics

CASE 95-2, QUESTION 4: When B.N. receives lung radiation for his metastases, how will it affect the doxorubicin he is scheduled to receive?

Although it is well known that mediastinal radiation can increase the risk of anthracycline-induced cardiac toxicity,[47] the only adjustment for B.N. would be a temporary reduction of doxorubicin doses (same reductions as described in Case 95-2, Question 3). The total doxorubicin dose should be limited to no more than 5 mg/kg (150 mg/m^2 in larger children). In earlier Wilms tumor studies, the risk of congestive heart failure was 4.4% at 20 years, or up to 17.4% in patients who relapsed and received more doxorubicin.[48] Thus, cardiovascular toxicity can develop as long as 20 years after therapy is completed, with an apparent decrease in left ventricular wall thickness and increased ventricular afterload, probably related to inadequate numbers of myocytes.[49] These reports emphasize the need to minimize chemotherapy in patients with good prognosis, as the Wilms tumor studies are doing. New recommendations include better standardization of cardiac monitoring and continuation of monitoring throughout life in survivors of childhood cancer who receive cardiotoxic agents.

Dactinomycin Hepatotoxicity

CASE 95-2, QUESTION 5: B.N. is to receive vincristine 0.05 mg/kg weekly for 10 weeks; doxorubicin 1.5 mg/kg at weeks 3 and 9; 1 mg/kg at weeks 15 and 21; and dactinomycin 0.045 mg/kg at weeks 0, 6, 12, 18, and 24. During the third week of treatment, his alanine aminotransferase (ALT) is elevated to 78 units/dL. Is this related to his drug therapy?

Early in the NWTS-4, an increased incidence (14.3%) of severe hepatotoxicity (elevation of alanine aminotransferase or ALT 10 times normal with or without ascites) was reported with the pulse-intensive dactinomycin doses (0.060 mg/kg/single dose) in patients receiving no abdominal radiation.[50] Subsequently, dactinomycin doses were reduced. Still, the incidence of hepatotoxicity in patients receiving the newer 0.045-mg/kg pulse doses (3.7%), as well as those receiving the standard 0.015 mg/kg/day for 5 days (2.8%), remained elevated relative to the NWTS-3 results (0.4%), which used the same 0.015 mg/kg/day for 5 days.[51] The reasons for the increased hepatotoxicity are not known. Liver function usually returns to baseline within 1 to 2 weeks after discontinuation of chemotherapy, although more severe problems with sinusoidal obstructive syndrome (hepatopathy, veno-occlusive disease) have also been reported.[33] Chemotherapy was restarted in some patients, although frequently at lower doses or without dactinomycin. B.N. should be monitored closely in case his liver enzymes continue to rise, especially because he will receive abdominal radiation treatments that may increase the risk of hepatic toxicity. If his ALT rises to 2 to 5 times normal, or his total bilirubin is 3 to 5 mg/dL, doses of all three of his drugs should be reduced by 50%. If his ALT or bilirubin rises above 2 to 5 times normal, the drugs should be withheld until laboratory values return to lower than the aforementioned ranges.

Osteosarcoma

DEFINITION, EPIDEMIOLOGY, PATHOPHYSIOLOGY, AND COURSE OF THE DISEASE

Osteosarcoma is a malignant osteoid-producing bone tumor that occurs most commonly in adolescents or young adults in the second or third decade of life.[52–54] A second peak incidence occurs in patients older than 50 to 60 years old. The most common manifestation at diagnosis is pain at the site, which can sometimes be present for several weeks to months. It occurs most frequently in the metaphyseal ends of the distal femur, proximal tibia, or proximal humerus, but it can occur in the flat bones as well.

The age range and bones involved suggest a malignant response associated with normal childhood growth spurts. Osteosarcoma has been associated with Paget disease in the elderly, another condition with rapid bone turnover.[53] Radiation from treatments or nuclear disasters has also been linked to osteosarcoma. Mutation of the retinoblastoma gene increases the risk of osteosarcoma, and retinoblastoma survivors and carriers need to be monitored for osteosarcoma. There are a number of other uncommon inherited conditions that are associated with an increased risk of osteosarcoma.

Typical staging systems are not used for osteosarcoma; however, presence of clinically detectable metastatic disease at diagnosis, resectability of the tumor, and tumor grade (high vs. low) are important to outcomes. Low-grade tumors are not likely to metastasize and are not treated with chemotherapy in contrast to high-grade tumors. Clinically detectable metastases are present in 15% to 20% of patients, usually in the lungs but occasionally in the same or other bones. If surgery alone is used for treatment, 80% of patients will die within 5 years of recurrent metastatic disease, indicating the presence of subclinical micrometastases at the time of diagnosis.[52–54] The degree of tumor necrosis at surgical resection is an indicator of chemosensitivity of the tumor and risk of relapse. Greater than 90% necrosis at the time of surgery after six cycles of neoadjuvant chemotherapy is associated with a 70% to 80% chance of long-term survival for non-metastatic disease, with survival dropping to around 50% for non-metastatic disease with less than 90% necrosis.

CLINICAL PRESENTATION AND DIAGNOSIS

Because osteosarcoma usually presents close to a joint in long bones, it most commonly presents with pain or a limp. It is often thought to be an athletic injury at first. In some patients, a broken arm or leg will occur, bringing attention to the mass on radiographs. Diagnosis is based on pathology from a biopsy, which should be obtained by the surgeon performing the definitive surgery; therefore, the biopsy tract can be resected with the tumor.

TREATMENT OVERVIEW

Although surgery is the main treatment of the primary tumor, chemotherapy is used to prevent development of metastases in patients with high-grade osteosarcoma. Drugs frequently used for osteosarcoma include high-dose methotrexate, cisplatin, doxorubicin, and ifosfamide. Regimens have changed minimally in the last 25 years, with the current standard treatment in COG being cisplatin and doxorubicin alternating with two cycles of high-dose methotrexate. Neoadjuvant chemotherapy is commonly given for 6 cycles and continued after surgery for 12 more cycles (for a total of 29 weeks). The tumor is relatively resistant to radiation therapy, which is usually reserved for cases in which local control cannot be achieved surgically.[54] Surgical procedures usually fit into two categories: limb preservation or salvages, or amputation with prosthetics. There are a number of versions of each type of surgery.[52,53] When chemotherapy is used with surgery in non-metastatic patients, long-term (2–5 years) disease-free survival is 50% to 85%.[52–54]

ROLE OF CHEMOTHERAPY IN TREATMENT

CASE 95-3

QUESTION 1: G.C. is an 18-year-old man with a 2- to 3-month history of left shoulder pain. A tumor is found on radiograph, and biopsy confirms a high-grade conventional osteosarcoma of the left proximal humerus. No apparent metastases are found with CT and bone scans. Renal function, left ventricular ejection fraction, and hearing tests are all within normal limits. G.C. begins neoadjuvant chemotherapy consisting of high-dose methotrexate alternating with cisplatin and doxorubicin. Six cycles of this chemotherapy (cisplatin/doxorubicin twice and high-dose methotrexate 4 times) will be given before his surgery, after which he will receive two more cycles of cisplatin/doxorubicin, each followed by two cycles of methotrexate, then two more cycles of doxorubicin, each followed by two cycles of methotrexate. What is the goal of chemotherapy? What is the role of presurgical (neoadjuvant) chemotherapy in G.C.?

Because G.C.'s osteosarcoma is in his proximal humerus, the surgeon can remove the primary tumor using one of the various operations described in the literature.[52,53] Limb salvages typically work well in the upper extremities, with fewer complications than when they are used for lower extremities. Because patients with osteosarcoma usually die from metastases, the goal of the chemotherapy is to eradicate micrometastases, which are present more than 80% of the time, as discussed in the previous section. Neoadjuvant chemotherapy of osteosarcoma was developed to treat micrometastases while waiting for limb salvage surgeries to be arranged, performed, and healed. Neoadjuvant therapy may improve limb-sparing surgery by shrinking the tumor; it also allows histologic grading of the response to initial chemotherapy at surgery, a prognostic factor for risk of relapse (see Case 95-3, Question 2). However, no convincing evidence to date indicates that disease-free survival is better for patients who receive neoadjuvant chemotherapy relative to those who receive their chemotherapy as adjuvant therapy.[54] In G.C., a titanium bone implant was placed where the diseased humerus was removed. The ease of doing this surgery may have been enhanced by neoadjuvant chemotherapy–induced shrinkage of the tumor.

PROGNOSTIC FACTORS

CASE 95-3, QUESTION 2: At surgery, G.C.'s tumor shows excellent histologic response, shown by 99% necrosis of the tumor sample. At diagnosis, his LDH was 220 units/L. How do these prognostic factors affect the choice of therapy in osteosarcoma?

Conventional staging systems do not correlate well with prognosis for most bone cancers. Clinically apparent metastases or a location that does not allow complete surgical removal of the primary tumor are associated with a poor prognosis.[52–54] Newer surgical techniques and treatments have improved the prognosis with 20% to 30% of metastatic patients cured using neoadjuvant chemotherapy and surgery. Other potential prognostic factors have been identified; however, few of these factors have been used to stratify patients to different treatment regimens. G.C. has a minimally elevated LDH consistent with a relatively small tumor mass, although this is not used to stratify for treatment. The percentage necrosis of the tumor at surgery correlates with risk of recurrence. In current studies, patients with greater than 90% tumor necrosis after six cycles of neoadjuvant chemotherapy are considered good risk and are treated with standard chemotherapy such as G.C. is receiving. Patients whose tumors have less necrosis at surgery are considered to be standard risk, and they have a higher risk of treatment failure. No treatment modifications to date have demonstrated better outcomes for these patients than the good risk protocol described above.

DELAYED CLEARANCE AFTER HIGH-DOSE METHOTREXATE

CASE 95-3, QUESTION 3: After reconstructive surgery using a titanium implant, G.C. restarts his chemotherapy. During his fourth cycle of chemotherapy, after high-dose methotrexate is given, G.C.'s peak methotrexate concentration is 1,300 micromolar (μM) and the 72-hour concentration is 0.22 μM (normal, <0.1 μM at 72 hours). Recorded urine-specific gravities are less than 1.010, urine pH is between 7 and 8, and urine output is greater than 2 to 3 mL/kg/hour, which, according to guidelines, suggest a reduced risk of methotrexate-induced nephrotoxicity. His creatinine has increased from 0.9 to 1.1 mg/dL (creatinine clearance of 106 mL/minute/1.73 m^2); however, he does not have any signs or symptoms of methotrexate toxicity in spite of his delayed clearance. Leucovorin rescue (15 mg IV every 6 hours beginning at hour 24) is continued. What potential problems could be causing his retention of methotrexate?

Accumulations of protein-containing fluids (called third-spaces), such as pleural effusion and ascites, or GI obstruction, may retain methotrexate and slow the terminal excretion.[55–58] Slow excretion of methotrexate allows more proliferating cells to be exposed to methotrexate during the S phase of the cell cycle, increasing the cytotoxicity and resulting in more mucositis and myelosuppression. Many drugs interact with methotrexate, which can also slow its excretion. Cisplatin reportedly reduces the excretion of methotrexate because of nephrotoxicity, especially at cumulative cisplatin doses greater than 300 mg/m^2.[59] G.C. has received four doses of 120 mg/m^2 (480 mg/m^2 total dose) of cisplatin, which may have contributed to the reduced methotrexate excretion. He has not received concomitant nephrotoxins, such as aminoglycosides or amphotericin B. Weak organic acids, such as salicylates, nonsteroidal anti-inflammatory drugs (NSAIDs), penicillins, or trimethoprim–sulfamethoxazole (TMP–SMX), can compete with methotrexate for renal tubular secretion via the organic anion transport system.[59,60] Proton pump inhibitors are thought to more directly inhibit transporter proteins and have been reported to delay methotrexate excretion.[59,61]

Although G.C.'s serum creatinine appears to be the same that it was at diagnosis (1.1 mg/dL), serum creatinine is not always a good indicator of renal function, so it is possible that G.C. has had some renal damage that is not apparent from his serum creatinine concentrations.[29] A measured creatinine clearance was 176 mL/minute/1.73 m^2 at diagnosis, and a repeat at this point is 106 mL/minute/1.73 m^2. Even measured creatinine clearance may not always be accurate when compared with Cr-ethylenediaminetetraacetic acid measurement of glomerular filtration rate.[29] Although the reduced renal clearance may be contributing, it is not clear why G.C. is retaining methotrexate; future courses of methotrexate need close monitoring.

LEUCOVORIN RESCUE

CASE 95-3, QUESTION 4: How long should leucovorin be administered to G.C.?

Leucovorin is a tetrahydrofolate that bypasses methotrexate's block of dihydrofolate reductase and reduces the toxicities of high-dose methotrexate. It, therefore, can be used as a form of methotrexate rescue. Cytotoxic effects of methotrexate depend on concentration and duration of exposure.[62] Many high-dose methotrexate protocols continue leucovorin rescue until serum methotrexate concentrations are 0.1 μM, which would be expected to occur approximately 72 hours after a 12 g/m^2 dose infused over 4 hours. Because G.C. has delayed methotrexate clearance with persistence of methotrexate levels still above 0.1 μM at 72 hours, prevention of GI and bone marrow cytotoxicity may require continuation of leucovorin rescue until methotrexate concentrations are less than 0.05 μM.[62] For G.C., methotrexate concentrations did not fall below 0.1 μM until 108 hours after his dose; thus, leucovorin was continued 24 hours past that time to ensure presence until methotrexate fell below 0.05 μM. Other considerations may also be important in patients receiving leucovorin rescue. Because of the competitive nature of leucovorin rescue, higher leucovorin doses may be needed for patients with excessively high methotrexate concentrations.

Petros and Evans[56] describe in Figure 95-1 that the methotrexate concentrations (those above the blue-shaded area) place patients at

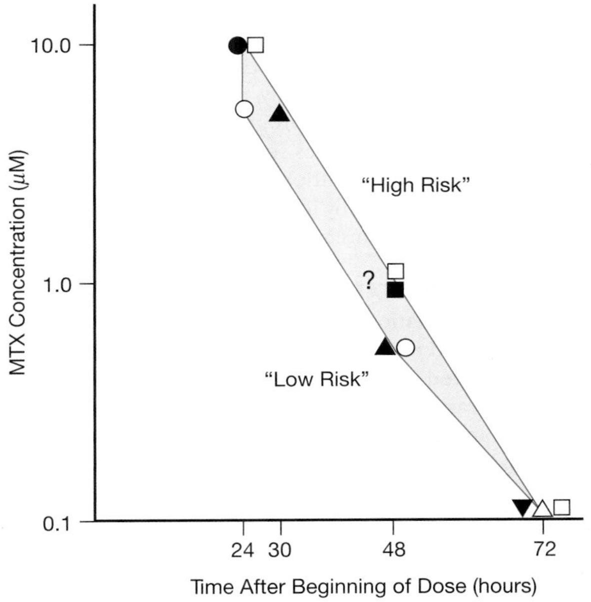

Figure 95-1 Composite semi-logarithmic plot of serum methotrexate (MTX) concentrations versus time. Several research groups have proposed threshold MTX concentrations over time that enable clinicians to identify patients at "high risk" for experiencing toxicity after high-dose MTX plus conventional low-dose leucovorin administration. Data for the figure were obtained from reports of (▲) Evans,[63] (△) Tattersal,[64] (●) Isacoff,[65] (○) Isacoff,[66] (□) Nirenberg,[67] (■) Stoller,[68] and (▼) Rechnitzer.[69] (Source: Petros WP, Evans WE. Anticancer agents. In: Burton ME et al, eds. *Applied Pharmacokinetics & Pharmacodynamics*. 4th ed. Philadelphia, PA: Lippincott Williams & Wilkins; 2006:617.)

high risk for methotrexate toxicity if given the usual low-rescue doses of leucovorin.[56,63–69] Methotrexate doses (12 g/m^2) infused over 4 hours are designed to produce peak methotrexate concentrations in the blood of 1,000 μM, followed by less than 10 μM at 24 hours, 1 μM at 48 hours, and 0.1 μM at 72 hours. Higher concentrations may result in greater toxicity and additional leucovorin doses may be necessary. If G.C.'s methotrexate concentrations had remained more than 1 μM 48 hours after the beginning of the infusion, current COG recommendations are to increase the leucovorin dose to 15 mg/m^2 every 3 hours until methotrexate concentrations fall below 0.5 μM. If concentrations exceed 5 μM 48 hours or more after the methotrexate dose, higher doses of leucovorin are recommended (150 mg/m^2 every 3 hours). Oral leucovorin administration should not be used when the patient has emesis or requires large oral doses (>50 mg), which are often poorly absorbed.[56] If a patient on high-dose methotrexate experiences renal failure and has elevated concentrations of methotrexate, glucarpidase (carboxypeptidase G2) may be used in addition to the leucovorin. Glucarpidase hydrolyzes methotrexate into inactive compounds and is very effective at quickly lowering methotrexate concentrations; however, it generally needs to be administered within the first 96 hours after the methotrexate dose. In spite of rapid reduction of methotrexate concentrations, it is not clear the extent to which it lowers morbidity or mortality from the high levels and delayed clearance.[70]

Rhabdomyosarcoma

DESCRIPTION, EPIDEMIOLOGY, AND PATHOPHYSIOLOGY

Rhabdomyosarcoma is a soft tissue tumor of skeletal muscle. It is the most common soft tissue sarcoma of childhood, occurring in 3% of all children with cancer.[1] The two most common histologic types in children are embryonal and alveolar.[71]

Embryonal rhabdomyosarcoma cells resemble striated muscle and occur most frequently in young children with involvement in the head and neck or genitourinary tract. Alveolar rhabdomyosarcoma cells resemble lung parenchymal cells and occur more frequently in older children or adolescents with involvement of the trunk or extremities. Generally, patients with alveolar rhabdomyosarcoma have a poorer prognosis than patients with the embryonal type. Recent studies suggest that alveolar-appearing rhabdomyosarcoma cells without the *PAX/FOXO1* fusion gene are molecularly and clinically identical to embryonal and may be treated as such, although this is not current practice in protocols.[72,73]

CLINICAL PRESENTATION AND DIAGNOSIS

The clinical presentation of rhabdomyosarcoma varies with its location (head and neck, genitourinary, parameningeal, extremity, orbit, as noted above). Diagnosis involves a biopsy of the tumor, which can be examined for appearance under an electron microscope, and a number of tests are run to identify molecular markers to differentiate it from other small round cell tumors.[71]

TREATMENT OVERVIEW

Treatment combines surgery, radiation, and chemotherapy. Complete surgical removal is often difficult, given the locations and infiltrative characteristics of rhabdomyosarcoma. Because good local control improves the prognosis,[71] radiation is generally administered after the surgery. Combination chemotherapy is necessary because the 5-year survival with local control alone is only 10% to 30%. Vincristine, dactinomycin, and cyclophosphamide (VAC regimen) have been used extensively to treat rhabdomyosarcoma.[71] Other agents producing responses include combinations of vincristine, doxorubicin, and cyclophosphamide; ifosfamide and etoposide; and vincristine and irinotecan.[71] Using the combination of vincristine, dactinomycin, and cyclophosphamide with local control of surgery or radiation in the fourth Intergroup Rhabdomyosarcoma Study (IRS) resulted in a 76% failure-free survival for patients with non-metastatic disease.[74]

CLINICAL PRESENTATION, PROGNOSTIC FACTORS, AND TREATMENT

CASE 95-4

QUESTION 1: F.J. is a 2-year-old girl with a rapidly enlarging mass on the lateral head of the gastrocnemius muscle in the right calf. F.J. has no other complaints. Bone marrow and scans are negative for metastatic disease. The diagnosis is embryonal rhabdomyosarcoma, stage III (unfavorable site and >5 cm mass). Initial expectations were that gross residual tumor would remain after the surgery, consistent with clinical group III. Chemotherapy consists of 3-week cycles of vincristine 0.05 mg/kg (days 1, 8, and 15 of some cycles but day 1 only of some cycles); dactinomycin 0.045 mg/kg on day 1 of each cycle; and cyclophosphamide 73 mg/kg on day 1 of each cycle with mesna to reduce the risk of hemorrhagic cystitis. Because of reports of hepatotoxicity during a prior study, especially in patients younger than 3 years of age, the protocol recommends all three drugs be dosed in milligram/kilogram for children younger than 3 years of age. Prophylactic TMP–SMX is begun at 150 mg/m^2/day (TMP) divided twice daily for three consecutive days/week. After each course of chemotherapy, F.J. is to receive filgrastim 5 mcg/kg/day subcutaneously for 14 days or until the absolute neutrophil count (ANC) is greater than 750 cells/μL. What factors in F.J. are associated with a good prognosis? What chemotherapy treatment would be most appropriate for F.J.?

The embryonal histopathologic classification has a better prognosis than the alveolar one, although evidence indicates that the location of the primary tumor is more important than the histology.[71] The primary site affects resectability, route of spread, and how early the diagnosis is made. Additionally, age between 1 and 9 years is associated with a better prognosis. The IRS have used a clinical grouping system (groups I–IV), which is based on spread of the disease and extent of resection. This system has been useful because of its correlation with prognosis where complete surgical removal and lack of metastases both correlate with good prognosis.[71] The fourth and fifth IRS studies compared the clinical grouping system with a TNM (tumor, lymph node, metastasis) staging system similar to that used in adult cancers. Although the two systems may result in different disease stages for a specific patient, both are considered valuable and current protocols use both systems.

In rhabdomyosarcoma, the tumor site is one important part of the T rating in the staging system. F.J.'s tumor involves an unfavorable site (the calf) and is greater than 5 cm, making it stage III. Although her tumor was expected to be clinical group III, after a good response to neoadjuvant chemotherapy, a complete resection was performed, making it clinical group I. This suggests that she has an 80% to 90% chance of 3-year survival based on the IRS-II, IRS-III, and IRS-IV results.[71,74–76] The IRS-V classified patients as having low-risk, intermediate-risk, or high-risk disease. Patients at low-risk include those with embryonal rhabdomyosarcoma at favorable sites, or at unfavorable sites with no more than microscopic residual tumor.[71] Patients at intermediate risk have the embryonal subtype with gross residual tumor or the alveolar subtype without metastatic disease. Patients at high risk include those with metastatic alveolar or embryonal disease.

Chemotherapy for many patients at low risk is limited to vincristine and dactinomycin.[71] Most at intermediate risk are treated with vincristine, dactinomycin, and cyclophosphamide.

Patients at high risk have not responded well in the past and are candidates for trials with newer drugs added to the vincristine, dactinomycin, and cyclophosphamide. A recent study added courses of vincristine and irinotecan, ifosfamide and etoposide and vincristine, doxorubicin, and cyclophosphamide (COG ARST0431), and 3-year event free survival appears good compared to historical data for patients with 0 to 1 higher-risk features.[77] F.J. would be in the low-risk group; however, her large initial tumor justifies adding cyclophosphamide to the vincristine and dactinomycin as in the intermediate-risk regimen. Because radiation to her leg would stop bone growth and her surgical margins were tumor free, no radiation is being administered.

TRIMETHOPRIM-SULFAMETHOXAZOLE PROPHYLAXIS AND FILGRASTIM FOR MYELOSUPPRESSION

CASE 95-4, QUESTION 2: What are the reasons for treating F.J. with TMP–SMX and filgrastim?

F.J.'s VAC regimen was associated with a high incidence of neutropenic fevers even during the pilot studies. Because of the frequency of severe myelosuppression, TMP–SMX is used until 6 months after chemotherapy for prophylaxis against *Pneumocystis jirovecii*, an opportunistic pathogen. Filgrastim is used to minimize neutropenia so that the chemotherapy dose intensity can be maintained.

RENAL FANCONI SYNDROME WITH IFOSFAMIDE

CASE 95-4, QUESTION 3: F.J.'s mother read on the Internet about a patient with rhabdomyosarcoma who had received vincristine, ifosfamide, and etoposide and was cured. She wants to know why that regimen is not being used for her daughter. Explain the rationale for F.J.'s regimen.

The IRS-IV results for local or regional disease (intermediate risk) demonstrated no advantages of vincristine, ifosfamide, and etoposide or vincristine, dactinomycin, and ifosfamide over the standard vincristine, dactinomycin, and cyclophosphamide treatment.[74] Additionally, the ifosfamide-containing regimens caused more toxicity. Ifosfamide has been associated with renal Fanconi syndrome, a proximal tubular defect that is characterized by wasting of electrolytes, glucose, and amino acids, as well as renal tubular acidosis and, in a minority of cases, an increased serum creatinine. Data suggest that the risk of Fanconi syndrome is increased in children that are younger than 3 years of age; have received total ifosfamide doses greater than 72 to 100 g/m^2; have hydronephrosis, a single kidney, or an elevated serum creatinine; or have received previous platinum therapy.[78–81] During each course of her chemotherapy, F.J. exhibits ketonuria; however, this is not a toxicity of her chemotherapy. Ketonuria is caused by her mesna therapy, which has been reported to routinely cause false-positive ketone tests.[82]

ACUTE LYMPHOBLASTIC LEUKEMIA OF CHILDHOOD

Acute leukemia is a malignancy of blood-forming cells involving the lymphoid and myeloid cell lines. The two most common types of childhood leukemia are ALL and acute myelogenous leukemia (AML), with the former accounting for 75% of cases and the latter for approximately 15%. Acute lymphoblastic leukemia is the most common childhood cancer, accounting for approximately 26% of all malignancies in children.[83] Approximately 2,600 new cases of childhood ALL occur each year in the United States in children younger than 19 years of age.[83]

A distinct peak incidence occurs at ages 2 to 3 years for ALL (>80 cases/million) and then decreases substantially for 8- to 10-year-olds (20 cases/million). A higher incidence of ALL is seen in white children than in African American children. This racial difference is most apparent in the 2- to 3-year-old age group, with a nearly threefold greater incidence rate for white children.[84]

Before the early 1970s, ALL was a fatal illness with most children succumbing to their disease within 2 to 3 months after diagnosis. Today, more than 80% of children achieve prolonged survival with antileukemic therapy.[83,84] New innovations in therapy for ALL continue to improve survival while decreasing the long-term morbidity associated with current treatment regimens.[85]

Epidemiology and Etiology

The etiology of ALL is unknown; however, several interesting associations have been discovered. A high incidence of leukemia was found among survivors of the atom bomb explosion in Japan during World War II, and those closest to the epicenter of the blast were at greatest risk.[86,87] Leukemia also occurs in children exposed to radiation in utero.[88] Other unproven factors that have been suggested to cause ALL include exposure to electromagnetic fields, pesticides, maternal use of alcohol, contraceptives, and cigarette smoking.[89–92] Viruses have not been proven to cause childhood ALL.[93] In particular, the incidence of childhood ALL has not increased markedly over the past 40 years during a time when electricity use has seen a large increase.[94]

Pathophysiology

The pathophysiology of ALL involves the replacement of normal bone marrow elements with a clone of immature lymphoid cells. The essential lesion in ALL is a stabilization of a malignant cell in the lymphocyte differentiation process. Many factors are involved in the control of normal cellular proliferation. Leukemia may represent a disruption in one or more of the normal relationships within the cell proliferation pathway, such as an abnormal response to lymphoid cell growth factors.[95]

With the availability of classification systems of lymphoblasts based on morphology, immunology, and cytogenetics, it has become clear that ALL is a heterogeneous disease. This is especially true with regard to cytogenetic abnormalities. The immunologic heterogeneity results from leukemic transformation at various stages of lymphocyte differentiation. In addition, an emerging classification involving gene expression profiling may allow for further classification of ALL cytogenetic subtypes, potentially allowing for prediction of response and adverse events.[96] As discussed later in this section, these classifications have important prognostic value.

Clinical Presentation

The signs and symptoms of ALL are nonspecific and many are shared with other childhood diseases such as juvenile rheumatoid arthritis (JRA). This occasionally leads to a child with ALL being mistakenly treated with corticosteroids for JRA. As a general rule, children should not be treated with corticosteroids without first performing a complete blood count (CBC) or a bone marrow aspirate. These signs and symptoms reflect the uncontrolled growth and differentiation of the leukemic clone and the resulting deficiency in normal bone marrow elements, namely neutrophils, red blood cells (RBCs), and platelets. Frequent clinical findings include fever (61%), bleeding (48%), and bone pain (23%).[97] Bone pain is believed to be the result of hypercellular bone marrow and infiltration of leukemic lymphoblasts into pain-sensitive structures such as the periosteum. Although bone pain may be severe, it quickly resolves once chemotherapy is initiated. On physical examination, many patients have lymphadenopathy (50%), splenomegaly (63%), or hepatosplenomegaly (68%).[97]

At diagnosis, at least 59% of patients have a normal or low white blood cell (WBC) count; the remainder have elevated counts.[97] The WBC differential typically shows a low percentage of neutrophils and bands with a marked lymphocytosis. Lymphoblasts may be present in the peripheral blood even with a low WBC count (e.g., 2,000–4,000 cells/μL), but they are more likely when the WBC count is elevated.[98] A normochromic, normocytic anemia, along with thrombocytopenia, is present in most patients.[97]

Diagnosis

A bone marrow aspirate and biopsy are usually necessary to confirm the diagnosis of ALL. In patients with elevated WBC counts, the diagnosis can be confirmed by studies of lymphoblasts in the peripheral blood. The diagnosis of ALL is made when at least 25% of lymphoid cells in the bone marrow are blasts.[99] Most ALL patients have far greater than 25% blasts and many have complete replacement of bone marrow with lymphoblasts. Once a child is diagnosed with ALL, it is important to determine the disease characteristics that influence treatment decisions and prognosis.

Prognostic Variables

CLINICAL VARIABLES

Certain clinical and laboratory findings present at diagnosis are important predictors of prognosis and are used to determine risk stratification. Children with ALL are classified by their risk of relapse into one of the following categories: standard, high, or very high risk. Debate continues over which variables most strongly influences patient outcome. Upon initial presentation, the most important risk-defining features of childhood ALL are age and initial WBC count.[98] Ongoing investigations are likely to further refine what constitutes different ALL risk populations.

White Blood Cell Count

The initial WBC count is considered to be among the most important predictors of outcome in childhood ALL. Its importance as a prognostic feature is often retained after the adjustment for other important prognostic criteria.[99] Children with the highest WBC counts at presentation have the shortest duration of complete remissions.[100–102] There appears to be a linear relationship between the duration of remission and the WBC count at presentation. Although exactly where the demarcation line is for predicting a good or a poor prognosis is unknown, an initial WBC count greater than 50,000 cells/μL is generally associated with a poor prognosis.[98]

Age

Patients younger than 1 year or older than 9.99 years of age at diagnosis tend to have worse prognoses.[98] At least one trial has demonstrated that more intensive therapy may overcome the adverse prognostic factor of adolescent age.[103] These investigators reported that young adults (16–21 years of age) with ALL have an event-free survival of approximately 60% at 6 years, which is similar to that of patients 10 to 15 years of age and superior to that achieved in most trials of older adults.[103] For adolescents 15 to 20 years of age, treatment on intensive pediatric leukemia protocols has demonstrated superiority over that achieved on adult treatment protocols, with one study showing an estimated event-free survival of 67% with the pediatric protocol versus 41% for the adult protocol.[104]

Age is the strongest predictor of prognosis with regard to infants, a group in which survival is exceedingly poor compared with other age groups.[105–107] For infants, even with intensified chemotherapy regimens, long-term, disease-free survival is usually less than 50%, especially when associated with cytogenetic aberrations involving the mixed lineage leukemia (MLL) locus.[108]

Race

Although African Americans have a lower incidence of ALL, several studies have shown that these children appear to have a higher relapse rate than Caucasian children.[84,109–113] Data from the National Cancer Institute's Surveillance, Epidemiology, and End Results (SEER) Program demonstrate a 5-year survival rate of 64% versus 78% for African American and Caucasian children, respectively. The differences in outcome for African Americans appear to be the result of a more severe form of ALL in this patient population.[113] However, intensified therapy showed that 10-year survival rates are equal between African American and Caucasian children.[113] It has also been demonstrated in a SEER update that the incidence rate for Hispanics was greater than for non-Hispanics and was the highest of all racial subgroups.[112] An analysis of racial and ethnic differences in outcome with contemporary therapy also demonstrated a difference in survival among groups, with the greatest survival for Asian children and lowest for African Americans and Hispanics.[113]

IMMUNOLOGIC VARIABLES

Acute lymphoblastic leukemia is classified into different immunologic subsets based on cell surface markers or antigens present on the leukemic lymphoblasts at diagnosis. These can be categorized as cells of B-cell and T-cell origin. The B-cell lineage is further classified into various subtypes through the use of monoclonal antibodies. These subtypes reflect the various stages of differentiation at which leukemia may develop. Approximately 15% to 20% of children with ALL have leukemia with a T-cell lineage,[114,115] and 1% to 2% of patients have leukemia with a mature B-cell origin.[116,117] Using more sophisticated diagnostic techniques, the majority of patients who were previously classified as non–T-cell ALL or non–B-cell ALL (null cell ALL) are now known to have leukemia of a more immature B-cell lineage.[118–120] Most patients with B-cell lineage ALL (80%) have cells that are positive for the common ALL antigen (CALLA, designated CD10) on their surface,[121] this is referred to as common ALL. Additional markers, including CD19 and cytoplasmic immunoglobulin, have been used to further determine the level of differentiation of leukemic cells of the B-cell lineage. Intermediate cells of the B-cell lineage (pre–B cells) possess these markers but more immature cells (early pre–B cells) do not.[121,122] More than 60% of children with ALL have a leukemia of the early pre–B subtype and approximately 20% have a leukemia of pre–B cells.

Mature B-cell ALL (or Burkitt ALL) has traditionally been associated with a poor prognosis, but prognosis has improved greatly with the advent of short-term, very intensive chemotherapy.[117,123,124] Although differences in outcome have been noted among the B-cell subtypes,[123] when other prognostic factors are considered and when effective therapy is used, these differences may no longer be evident.[125] At present, immunologic features that differentiate B-cell precursor, T-cell, and mature B-cell ALL are believed to be clinically important because different types of chemotherapeutic strategies are used for these three immunophenotypes.[85,126]

Patients with T-cell ALL have several distinguishing features, including a greater likelihood of being older males with high initial WBC counts and the presence of a mediastinal mass or initial leukemic involvement of the CNS.[127,128] Patients with T-cell ALL historically have had a decreased survival, although more intensive treatment is improving their outcomes.[125] Studies with more intensified therapy also demonstrate no difference in relapse between T-cell and B-cell lineage ALL, although T-cell ALL patients tend to relapse much earlier.[127,128] T-cell lymphoblasts are less efficient at polyglutamation of methotrexate because these cells have lower concentrations of the methotrexate polyglutamate synthesizing enzyme, folylpolyglutamate synthetase.[129] This has been proposed as a possible explanation for the relative chemotherapy resistance and the need for increased methotrexate dose intensity in patients with T-cell ALL.[85]

CYTOGENETIC VARIABLES

Advances in chromosomal analysis have improved the understanding of ALL biology. Abnormalities in either chromosome number (ploidy) or structure of the leukemic clone have been found in 60% to 75% of ALL cases.[85] Many of these abnormalities appear to have prognostic importance.[85] Ploidy is represented by the DNA index. A value of 1.0 indicates a normal number of chromosomes, and a value greater than 1.0 indicates an increased number of chromosomes by a multiplication factor of the normal chromosome number. Children with leukemia blasts containing more than 52 chromosomes (DNA index >1.16, hyperdiploid) appear to have an increased probability of continuous complete remission versus patients with leukemia blasts containing a diploid chromosome complement or with a DNA index less than 1.16.[130] An in-vitro study of hyperdiploid versus non-hyperdiploid ALL revealed that those cells with a higher DNA index were more sensitive to antimetabolites (e.g., mercaptopurine) and asparaginase.[130,131] Also, B-precursor hyperdiploid ALL cells contain more reduced folate carriers than diploid B-precursor blasts. Hyperdiploid cells have elevated levels of gene expression for these carriers, which may account for the higher levels of methotrexate polyglutamates noted in these cells as compared to patients with B-precursor diploid ALL.[131–134] In contrast, patients with hypodiploidy (<45 chromosomes and, in particular, those with 24–28 chromosomes) have a significantly worse outcome than non-hypodiploid patients.[135]

Translocations are the most common structural abnormalities occurring in leukemic cells[136] and occur in approximately 75% of childhood ALL cases.[137] Certain translocations are associated with treatment failure and relapse.[85] The translocations most commonly associated with treatment failure are the *MLL* rearrangements [t(4;11), t(11;19), and t(1;11)] and the *BCR-ABL* fusion transcript [t(9;22), Philadelphia chromosome]. Historically, children with the Philadelphia chromosome rearrangement were considered to represent a population at very high risk of relapse and allogeneic stem cell transplantation was often part of their initial therapy. This translocation occurs in approximately 2% to 5% of childhood ALL cases. A published study added imatinib, a tyrosine kinase inhibitor directed against the Philadelphia chromosome fusion product, to aggressive leukemia therapy. They treated 28 patients with chemotherapy and imatinib and compared them to children receiving a matched sibling transplant (21 patients) or a transplant from an unrelated donor (13 patients). The 5-year event-free survival was similar (70%, 65%, 59%) respectively, and the authors concluded that allogeneic stem cell transplant now provides no role in the upfront treatment of children with Philadelphia chromosome positive ALL.[136–139]

Once a patient achieves complete remission, abnormalities of both ploidy and structure are not evident in the patient's recovered bone marrow by morphologic assessment, although a leukemic cell burden as large as 10^9 may remain. However, newer techniques based on polymerase chain reaction (PCR) assays can detect minimal residual disease (MRD) in many patients. If relapse does occur, the leukemic cell cytogenetic characteristics are usually identical to those observed at diagnosis.[140,141]

EARLY RESPONSE

An additional factor of prognostic importance in childhood ALL is that of early response to therapy. Several investigations have noted that early response, as measured by either clearance of blasts from the peripheral blood or morphologic bone marrow remission (e.g., $<5\%$ bone marrow blasts) on day 7 or 14 of therapy, is predictive of long-term disease-free survival. In a review of 15 trials, early response was an independent prognostic factor in each study.[141] Response was most commonly measured based on morphologic evaluation of day 14 bone marrow results, and it appeared that assessment of early response was more sensitive with bone marrow studies. Children who were slow early responders were 2.7 times more likely to have a relapse than those with more rapid clearance of blasts. Interestingly, the rapidity of response maintained its prognostic significance adjusting for the initial WBC count, providing further evidence that this variable is an important independent marker of prognosis. The rapidity of response is an intuitive marker of treatment sensitivity. However, the use of morphologic criteria to assign responder status still includes patients with a significant disease burden. It is important to note that such tests of bone marrow burden may represent a dilute sample or a decrease in marrow cellularity and may not reflect the total leukemia burden in the body. It is estimated that these measures of early response may detect up to 25% of children at risk for early relapse.[145] Rapid early response has been defined as clearance of bone marrow blasts by day 15 of induction, whereas slow early response refers to the converse. Whether patients are rapid or slow early responders is now being used to determine the type and intensity of further chemotherapy because slow early responders benefit from more intensive post-induction chemotherapy.[133] Other groups have examined response to initial treatment with a 7-day course of prednisone (initiated before the start of systemic induction chemotherapy) in children with high-risk ALL. Prednisone-poor response, defined as patients with greater than 1,000 blast cells/μL in peripheral blood after 7 days, was a predictor of poor outcome and was used to intensify induction therapy with a consequent improvement in event-free survival.[142]

MINIMAL RESIDUAL DISEASE

Several investigators have examined the prognostic value of detecting MRD in bone marrow samples through the use of sophisticated PCR and flow-cytometry. A variety of lymphoblast characteristics, including gene fusion transcripts, immunophenotype, and antigen receptor gene rearrangements, may be relied on for MRD detection in children with ALL. Although specific fusion transcripts can be relied on as PCR targets in only one-third of childhood ALL cases, clonal antigen receptor gene rearrangements occur in virtually all cases.[140] Using various techniques, approximately 50% of children with ALL are MRD positive at the completion of induction therapy, and roughly 45% of these patients will experience a relapse. The association of a negative test for MRD at the completion of induction therapy appears stronger because it has a negative predictive value of 92.5% and a positive predictive value of 44.5%. In patients positive for MRD, there is a continuous decrease in MRD during the months of chemotherapy treatment. Persistence of MRD beyond 4 to 6 months or reemergence of MRD is almost always predictive of future relapse. It is now established that the presence of MRD is an important prognostic factor, regardless of the patient's initial WBC count or age at presentation.[140] A large study of the prognostic value of MRD for day 7 blood samples and for bone marrow samples at both the end of the induction and consolidation phases demonstrated that MRD at the end of the induction phase was the most important predictor of prognosis when compared to other laboratory and clinical factors. Day 7 MRD findings had additional prognostic value. Data from this study for end of induction MRD demonstrated major differences in event-free survival as follows:

88% for MRD negative, 59% for MRD of 0.01% to 0.1%, 49% for MRD of 0.1% to 1%, and 30% for MRD greater than 1%. MRD predicted relapse that occurred early in treatment and late relapses as well. Monitoring of MRD is now established in the management of childhood ALL and is being used to risk-stratify treatment in current front-line leukemia studies.[143,144]

Overview of Treatment

The treatment for pediatric ALL is organized into different phases of chemotherapy. Treatment begins with induction therapy, which typically includes three or four systemic agents in addition to CNS preventive therapy. The intensity of induction therapy is based on the biology of the ALL, and today the main variables used for determining this phase of therapy are the child's age and WBC count at diagnosis. Induction therapy is designed to induce a complete remission and typically lasts 28 days. After induction therapy, the next phase of therapy can be defined as post-induction therapy and consists of a number of different cycles of chemotherapy referred to by such terms as consolidation, delayed intensification, and interim maintenance therapies. This phase of intensive chemotherapy usually uses combination approaches that are somewhat different than induction therapy and that are designed to kill leukemia cells in the cell cycle that were not destroyed by induction therapy. This phase of therapy is continuing to undergo substantial revision as studies determine which therapy components are optimal for various patients. The duration and intensity of the post-induction phase of therapy is tailored based on certain prognostic features of the leukemia as outlined above. The third phase of therapy is termed the maintenance phase, and it represents the longest phase of chemotherapy for these patients, often taking approximately 2 years to complete. Maintenance therapy is typically less intensive than the previous phases and consists mostly of continuous oral chemotherapy with infrequent intravenous and CNS therapy. In general, treatment intensity diminishes from the induction/consolidation phase to the maintenance phase.

REMISSION INDUCTION THERAPY

Goal of Induction

CASE 95-5

QUESTION 1: J.B. is a 4-year-old Hispanic boy presenting with a 2-week history of an upper respiratory tract infection and a 1-week history of otitis media. His symptoms have worsened, and he now presents with a nosebleed and fatigue. Physical examination reveals appreciable pallor and hepatosplenomegaly. A CBC with differential reveals a normochromic, normocytic anemia with the following:

Hematocrit (Hct), 15.7%
Hgb, 5.7 g/dL
WBC count, 4,300 cells/μL
Platelet count, 13,000 cells/μL

A differential on the WBC count reveals 82% lymphocytes (normal, 30%–40%), 7% neutrophils (normal, 50%–60%), and 11% lymphoblasts (normal, 0%). Based on these findings, a bone marrow biopsy is performed which reveals 95% lymphoblasts. A diagnosis of ALL is made. The immunologic class is early pre–B cell based on CD10 and CD19 positivity. Radiography of the chest does not reveal a mediastinal mass and a lumbar puncture shows that there are no leukemic lymphoblasts in the cerebrospinal fluid. J.B. is hydrated, alkalinized, and treated with oral allopurinol 200 mg/m^2/day, with a plan to institute induction therapy the next day. Within a few days, J.B. will be treated with several drugs for his leukemia.

What is the goal of the induction therapy that J.B. will receive?

The goal of induction therapy is complete remission (i.e., the inability to detect leukemic cells in the peripheral blood or the bone marrow by morphologic microscopic evaluation). J.B.'s peripheral blood values must be within the normal range and the bone marrow must reveal less than 5% lymphoblasts. This definition also assumes the absence of lymphoblasts in the cerebrospinal fluid (CSF). In addition, based on what is now known regarding MRD, achievement of an MRD measurement of less than 0.01% by the end of induction therapy (i.e., day 29) would now be an additional goal of this first phase of therapy. Although these findings indicate an adequate response to chemotherapy, they do not indicate a cure. Most patients have a total of 10^{12} cells at diagnosis and successful induction regimens reduce this cell load by 99% to 10^9.[145,146] Therefore, continuation of therapy will be required for J.B. to further reduce the leukemic cell population and to increase his chances of long-term survival. Without continuation of therapy, the majority of patients with ALL will relapse within a few months.[147]

Induction Combination Chemotherapy

CASE 95-5, QUESTION 2: Which agents should be used to achieve complete remission?

The agents most commonly used in remission induction therapy are vincristine, prednisone, dexamethasone, asparaginase, pegaspargase, and daunorubicin (Table 95-6). The prednisone or dexamethasone dose is not routinely tapered at the end of induction treatment.[148–151] Dexamethasone has supplanted prednisone as the corticosteroid used during induction therapy or throughout therapy. This is based on earlier work showing that dexamethasone has greater CSF penetration.[152] In patients with standard-risk ALL, a randomized comparison of dexamethasone to prednisone for induction therapy showed a lower CNS relapse rate in the dexamethasone group.[150] However, the use of a 28-day course of dexamethasone during induction for patients with high-risk ALL was also associated with an increased risk of infectious complications and avascular necrosis of the joints in adolescent patients.[153] This has led to removal or alteration of dexamethasone use during induction therapy in high-risk patients.

Table 95-6
Systemic Induction Regimens for Childhood Acute Lymphocytic Leukemia

Agent	Route	Dose/Schedule
Three-Drug Induction Regimen		
Prednisone	PO	60 mg/m^2/day × 28 days
Or		
Dexamethasone	PO	6 mg/m^2/day × 14 days
With		
Vincristine	IV	1.5 mg/m^2/week (max 2 mg) × 4 doses
And		
Pegaspargase	IM	2,500 units/m^2 × 1 dose
If Four-Drug Induction		
Daunorubicin	IV	25 mg/m^2/week × 4 doses

IM, intramuscularly; IV, intravenously; PO, orally.
Sources: Pui CH et al. Treatment of acute lymphoblastic leukemia. *N Engl J Med*. 2006;166–178; Bassen R et al. Modern therapy of acute lymphoblastic leukemia. *J Clin Oncol*. 2011;29:532.

It is plausible that the addition of dexamethasone to a more intensive chemotherapy backbone that is used for induction therapy of high-risk ALL may significantly increase the risk of infection in this more myelosuppressive regimen.

No chemotherapy drug meets the criteria of an ideal agent (i.e., toxic to leukemic cells only and active in all phases of the cell cycle). Corticosteroids, vincristine, and various asparaginase products come closest to this ideal in terms of activity, primarily against lymphoblastic leukemia, because these agents are selectively toxic to the leukemia cells while sparing normal bone marrow elements. To improve the success in attaining complete remission, additional agents have been added to vincristine, prednisone, and asparaginase (Table 95-6). The most frequently used additional agent is an anthracycline, such as daunorubicin or doxorubicin. Use of at least a three-drug induction regimen is the current standard of care for children at low or intermediate risk of relapse and results in improvements in both remission rate and duration versus less intensive therapy.[154–156] Currently, a four-drug regimen, or an even more intensive induction regimen consisting of more than four drugs, and often for a duration of more than 4 weeks, is used for children at high risk of relapse and adult ALL patients.[148,157–159]

If complete remission is not achieved with three agents by the end of induction, patients are treated with additional agents (e.g., an additional 2–4 weeks of daunorubicin and prednisone; initiation of cytarabine with additional asparaginase; vincristine and prednisone for 1–2 weeks). Because this occurs rarely, there is no consensus about the most effective agents or schedules to use in this situation. Most of these patients have a decreased survival and a higher relapse rate.

Intensive induction treatment has benefits for the majority of children with ALL. This treatment strategy supports the hypothesis of Goldie and Coldman[160] that intensification of early treatment may decrease the chance that drug resistance will develop. This may therefore increase the proportion of long-term relapse-free survivors. Induction therapy is determined based on clinical findings, such as age at diagnosis and initial WBC count. Based on these prognostic variables, J.B. is a patient with a low risk of relapse. A three-drug induction regimen consisting of vincristine, dexamethasone, and pegaspargase is recommended to optimize his chances for long-term disease-free survival.[149,150,161] Additional laboratory testing (e.g., bone marrow analysis for remission and MRD) will be relied on to design his post-induction therapy.

Vincristine Toxicity

CASE 95-5, QUESTION 3: J.B. is discharged from the hospital during the second week of induction chemotherapy. Results of his CBC and differential indicate that he is responding well to his chemotherapy (i.e., WBC count 2,600 cells/μL, neutrophils 69%, lymphocytes 22%, platelets 229,000 cells/μL, Hct 28.6%, and blastocytes 0). However, during the third week of induction chemotherapy, J.B. exhibits severe abdominal pain. It is discovered that he has not had a bowel movement in 6 days. J.B. has also been exhibiting "acting out" behaviors in recent days. How might these symptoms be explained?

The use of vincristine is associated with an autonomic neuropathy, which may substantially reduce GI motility;[162] in severe cases, paralytic ileus may result. Constipation is often accompanied by colicky abdominal pain, which may be quite distressing.[163] These symptoms usually become apparent 3 to 10 days after drug administration and resolve over several days. Prophylactic use of a stool softener (docusate) or laxative (polyethylene glycol) may lessen the severity of J.B.'s constipation and facilitate regular stooling. This regimen should have been instituted soon after the first dose of vincristine.

J.B.'s emotional changes are likely the result of the dexamethasone he is receiving. Emotional lability, sleep disturbances, depressed mood, and listlessness have occurred during corticosteroid therapy in children with ALL.[164] These behavioral changes can be quite disruptive, and parents should be prepared for them in advance. Behavioral disturbances typically resolve within 2 weeks after corticosteroid discontinuation.[164]

INTRATHECAL CHEMOTHERAPY PROPHYLAXIS

CASE 95-5, QUESTION 4: In addition to the aforementioned drugs, J.B. also receives intrathecal (IT) chemotherapy for CNS prophylaxis with methotrexate at the beginning (week 1) and end (week 4) of induction therapy. What is the purpose of IT chemotherapy?

IT or CNS preventive therapy decreases the chance of relapse within the CNS and increases J.B.'s chance of long-term survival. Before CNS preventive therapy was routine, the CNS was the most common site of leukemic relapse and thus predicted bone marrow relapse.[165,166] Patients at greatest risk for CNS relapse include those with very high initial WBC counts, T-cell ALL, and infants.[167,168] However, because all patients with ALL are at risk for CNS relapse, one of the largest incremental improvements in disease-free survival has been the routine use of CNS preventive therapy.[85] Because many antileukemic agents do not distribute well into the CSF, this area becomes a sanctuary site for leukemic lymphoblasts. The aim is to eradicate any CNS leukemic lymphoblasts present at diagnosis and to prevent the emergence of a relapse within the CNS.

Central Nervous System Preventive Therapy Options

CASE 95-5, QUESTION 5: What are the various treatments available for CNS preventive therapy? What factors determine which treatment is selected for J.B.?

All treatment protocols for childhood ALL use some form of CNS preventive therapy, although different regimens are used. The first successful CNS prophylaxis treatments were 2,400 cGy of craniospinal radiation with or without IT methotrexate, which markedly reduced the CNS relapse rate.[169] However, the adverse effects of cranial irradiation were problematic. These included decreased intellectual function, dysfunctions of the neuroendocrine system, and poorer psychosocial functioning.[170–175] As a result, clinicians sought alternative, potentially safer forms of CNS preventive therapy. For example, lower doses (1,800 cGy) of cranial irradiation were combined with IT methotrexate to reduce the CNS effects, which proved to be equivalent to 2,400 cGy in preventing CNS relapse.[168,173] Nevertheless, because concerns regarding the long-term toxicity of cranial radiation remain, especially for younger children, it is currently reserved for patients with detectable CNS disease on presentation, some patients with T-cell ALL, and patients with CNS relapse. Currently, CNS preventive therapy includes IT methotrexate alone, triple IT chemotherapy (methotrexate, cytarabine, and hydrocortisone), or IT methotrexate combined with systemic-dose–intensified methotrexate.[174–176]

Because patients differ in their risk for developing CNS leukemia, CNS preventive therapy should be tailored accordingly. Children with standard ALL have equivalent CNS protection rates with either cranial radiation or IT chemotherapy, as long as adequate intensive systemic therapy is provided.[177–179] These patients are treated with triple IT chemotherapy or IT methotrexate, depending on the institutional protocol.[180]

Intrathecal Chemotherapy: Chronic Adverse Effects

CASE 95-5, QUESTION 6: What are the chronic adverse effects of IT chemotherapy?

The chronic toxicities of IT chemotherapy are now being determined. When examined for effects on growth, triple IT chemotherapy demonstrated no effect on the final height achieved by children in contrast to a reduced final height in patients receiving cranial irradiation.[181] Limited evidence suggests that IT chemotherapy may be associated with some neuropsychologic deficits. At least one study of patients receiving IT chemotherapy without cranial irradiation has demonstrated deficits in higher-order cognitive function tasks and learning disabilities in mathematics.[182] Another study has demonstrated that children who were treated with IT chemotherapy before age 5 years had deficits in the cerebellar-frontal brain subsystem and in neuropsychologic performance.[183] It is unclear whether these deficits translate into significant long-term consequences.

CASE 95-5, QUESTION 7: J.B. is at a low risk for CNS relapse, and the decision is made to treat him with IT methotrexate. What dose of IT methotrexate should J.B. receive?

Intrathecal Methotrexate Dose

High chemotherapy concentrations can be attained within the CSF with relatively low doses because the CSF volume of distribution is small in contrast to the peripheral plasma volume (140 vs. 3,500 mL).[184,185] Drug exposure is also maximized by the longer half-life of most drugs in the CSF.[186] The approach used for IT dosing differs from systemic administration, the latter of which is based on body weight or body surface area. CSF methotrexate concentrations appear to correlate better with patient age than size.[187] The CSF volume in children approaches that of an adult by the age of 3 years. Because CSF volume does not correlate with body surface area, IT doses based on body size result in subtherapeutic concentrations in young children and potentially toxic concentrations in older children and adults. The age-based dosing regimens shown in Table 95-7 are less neurotoxic and are associated with a lower rate of CNS relapse than doses based on size.[187] Using this dosing regimen, J.B.'s dose of IT methotrexate should be 12 mg. If triple IT therapy were used, the doses of IT cytarabine and hydrocortisone would be 24 and 12 mg, respectively. These latter doses are also based on age, but no literature exists to support how they were derived. Nevertheless, empiric evidence supports their efficacy.

Dangers of Intrathecal Vincristine

CASE 95-5, QUESTION 8: J.B.'s IT methotrexate is to be administered on the same day as his vincristine dose. Are there any special precautions that should be taken when these medications are administered in close proximity?

Table 95-7
Dosage Regimen for Intrathecal Chemotherapy Based on Patient Age

Patient Age (years)	Methotrexate (mg)	Hydrocortisone (mg)	Cytarabine (mg)
<1	6	6	12
1	8	8	16
2	10	10	20
3	12	12	24
≥9	15	15	30

Inadvertent administration of vincristine into the IT space is almost uniformly fatal,[188–192] although there is at least one report of a patient in whom death but not serious sequelae was prevented. Despite widespread educational efforts in hospitals and clinics, and numerous precautionary measures, deaths from the inadvertent IT administration of vincristine still occur. The clinical course in patients mistakenly given IT vincristine has typically progressed from backache and headache on day 1, muscle weakness (generalized) on day 2, apnea on day 5, loss of evidence of electroencephalographic activity by days 7 to 9, and death on day 12.[190] To avoid the tragedy of IT vincristine administration, vincristine should be admixed separately or at a different time from IT medications, specially labeled and mixed as a small volume parenteral (i.e., minibag) rather than in a syringe, and preferably delivered to the patient area for IV infusion after the administration of IT medications.

TAILORING OF POST-INDUCTION THERAPY

CASE 95-5, QUESTION 9: An analysis of the chromosomes from J.B.'s bone marrow reveals the TEL-AML1 translocation and a DNA index of 1.0. His MRD findings reveal the following: blood on day 8 is less than 1% of cells and bone marrow on day 29 shows 0.15% of cells. Based on his day 29 (end of induction) bone marrow positive MRD finding, J.B. is scheduled to receive a more aggressive post-induction chemotherapy regimen. This treatment is chosen because MRD findings are more predictive of the chance for relapse than are his cytogenetics. Although J.B. had bone marrow MRD performed at day 8 and at the completion of induction treatment on day 29 that both indicated a complete morphologic remission, his MRD findings at the end of induction take precedence in defining his further therapy. After completion of the induction phase, J.B. was scheduled to receive an intensified phase of post-induction chemotherapy known as augmented interim maintenance. What is the purpose of post-induction treatment and what are some examples of effective regimens for this phase of treatment?

Post-induction chemotherapy consists of a variety of combinations of different agents typically given on a 2 to 6 week treatment cycle. These different phases of post-induction therapy are known as consolidation, interim maintenance, and delayed intensification.

Post-induction treatment has proven to be an important strategy for the prevention of relapse in children with ALL and has helped produce event-free survival of greater than 80% in low-risk childhood ALL.[85,193] To date, the optimum post-induction regimens have yet to be determined. However, a few interesting findings from investigations of consolidation therapy are briefly mentioned. A comparison between high-dose methotrexate 5 g/m^2 IV every 2 weeks for four doses and escalating "Capizzi" dose methotrexate (every 10 days, increase by 50 mg/m^2 until toxicity is seen) showed improved 5-year event-free survival (EFS) (82 $\pm$3.5% vs. 75.4 $\pm$3.6% $p = 0.006$) and no increased toxicity. In fact, there was a lower incidence of febrile neutropenia in the high-dose methotrexate group compared to the escalating-dose group; 5.2% versus 8.2% respectively ($p = 0.005$). This advantage was shown in high-risk patients and is currently being studied in standard-risk patients to evaluate if there is a survival advantage in that group as well.[194] Another trial comparing either longer duration or more intensive post-induction regimens for children with high-risk ALL found that a higher intensity treatment regimen improved outcome, whereas the longer duration regimen did not. In this study, the higher intensity post-induction treatment was made up of greater use of pegaspargase, vincristine, and escalating-dose methotrexate (Table 95-8).

Table 95-8
Acute Lymphoblastic Leukemia Post-Induction Regimen Components

Schedule
Vincristine 1.5 mg/m^2 IV on days 0, 10, 20, 30, and 40
Methotrexate 5000 mg/m^2 IV over 24 hours, followed by leucovorin rescue. Given every 14 days × 4 doses
Pegaspargase 2,500 units/m^2 IM on days 1 and 21
Methotrexate IT on days 0 and 30
Cyclophosphamide 1 g/m^2 IV on days 0 and 28
Cytarabine 75 mg/m^2 SC or IV on days 1–4, 8–11, 29–32, and 36–39
Mercaptopurine 60 mg/m^2 PO daily on days 0–13, and 28–41
Methotrexate IT on days 1, 8, 15, and 22
Pegaspargase 2,500 units/m^2 IM on days 14 and 42
Vincristine 1.5 mg/m^2 IV on days 14, 21, 42, and 49
Vincristine 1.5 mg/m^2 IV on weeks 8, 9, 17, and 18
Prednisone 40 mg/m^2 PO daily × 7 days on weeks 8 and 17
Dexamethasone 10 mg/m^2 PO daily on days 0–7, 14–20
Vincristine 1.5 mg/m^2 IV on days 0, 7, and 14
Pegaspargase 2,500 units/m^2 IM on day 3
Doxorubicin 25 mg/m^2 IV on days 0, 7, and 14

IV, intravenously; IM, intramuscularly; PO, orally; SC, subcutaneously; IT, intrathecally.
Source: Borowitz MJ et al. Prognostic significance of minimal residual disease in high rick B-ALL: a report from the Children's Oncology Group Study AALL0232. *Blood*. 2015;126(8):964–971.

MAINTENANCE CHEMOTHERAPY REGIMENS

CASE 95-5, QUESTION 10: After completion of his induction and post-induction treatments, J.B. is scheduled to receive maintenance (continuation) treatment for a total therapy duration of 2.5 years from the start of his induction therapy. His parents question why treatment will be of such a long duration and ask whether this is necessary because J.B. is already in remission. What is the purpose of J.B.'s maintenance or continuation treatment for ALL? Which agents should be used in J.B. for this phase of therapy?

Maintenance or continuation treatment sustains the complete remission achieved from induction chemotherapy. Early trials have shown that without maintenance treatment, the majority of ALL patients will relapse. Patients who have successfully responded to induction and post-induction therapy may still have a high leukemic cell burden (although undetectable), which must be eradicated by additional treatment. This is supported by the results of bone marrow biopsies from patients who have experienced relapse after several months to years of treatment. The cytogenetic characteristics of the leukemic cells in relapsed patients are identical to those at the time of diagnosis.[195,196] Maintenance therapy is also supported by the results of MRD studies, which demonstrate that some amount of measurable leukemic cells are still present months after the completion of induction therapy.[140–144]

Drugs that are effective during induction therapy cannot, by themselves, sustain remission during maintenance therapy.[9] However, other agents are effective in sustaining a complete remission. Two of the most effective drugs are mercaptopurine and methotrexate. Methotrexate is most effective and least toxic when administered intermittently, usually on a weekly basis in oral doses of 20 mg/m^2/week. Mercaptopurine is effective and well tolerated orally when dosed daily, usually at a dose of 50 to 75 mg/m^2/day.[197–199]

Other agents have been added to standard maintenance therapy with mercaptopurine and methotrexate to improve remission duration and to increase a patient's chances for long-term survival. There is evidence that monthly pulses of vincristine and prednisone offer advantages (lower bone marrow and testicular relapse rates) in standard-risk patients as well. At present, most contemporary treatment regimens for childhood ALL have intensified induction and post-induction phases during approximately the first 6 months. These early intensive treatments typically are followed by a less intensive maintenance therapy consisting of methotrexate and mercaptopurine in combination with periodic IT chemotherapy treatments, either with or without intermittent vincristine/prednisone pulses.[200–206]

The available evidence suggests that a patient like J.B. with standard-risk ALL will benefit from use of daily mercaptopurine 50 to 75 mg/m^2 orally (PO) and weekly methotrexate 20 mg/m^2 PO or IV, along with periodic pulse therapy with vincristine 1.5 mg/m^2 for 1 day and either prednisone 40 mg/m^2 or dexamethasone 6 mg/m^2 PO for 7 days every 4 weeks. In addition, IT methotrexate should be repeated every 8 to 12 weeks.

Dosing of Methotrexate and Mercaptopurine Maintenance

CASE 95-5, QUESTION 11: After 8 weeks of maintenance therapy with the aforementioned regimen, J.B. has had an ANC that has ranged between 2,000 and 3,500 cells/μL for more than 6 weeks. Other hematologic and chemistry findings are also within normal limits. Should any changes in his maintenance therapy be considered at this time? Are there any potential problems with mercaptopurine and methotrexate that could explain his ANC values? Could normal ANCs increase his risk of treatment failure?

Diurnal variation of methotrexate concentration and marked interpatient variability in absorption and metabolism of mercaptopurine have been described, which may explain the varied response among patients to standard doses.[201–207] Most patients are able to tolerate full doses of mercaptopurine, which is inactivated by the enzyme thiopurine-*S*-methyltransferase (TPMT). It is known that approximately 89% to 94% of patients have high TPMT activity, 6% to 11% have intermediate activity, and 0.3% have deficient activity. Patients with deficient TPMT activity experience severe and even fatal toxicity with standard mercaptopurine doses and require very low doses (approximately 10 mg/m^2 3 times/week) for avoidance of profound myelosuppression.[201,208–210]

Patients receiving half doses of these agents have shorter remission durations;[210] however, even those who tolerate maximal protocol dosages may also be at greater risk of relapse. Patients who are able to tolerate maximal doses without significant myelosuppression may require doses that are higher than protocol initiation doses. Some protocols allow for dosage increases of methotrexate or mercaptopurine every 4 to 6 weeks to maintain a target ANC in the range of 300 to 2,000 cells/μL. This is usually accomplished by alternately increasing the doses of mercaptopurine and methotrexate by 25%. In this situation, dose increases of one of these agents are performed every 4 to 6 weeks.[211]

J.B. has a normal ANC and is tolerating therapy; therefore, it is reasonable to attempt to intensify his chemotherapy dosing. For J.B., this means an increase in mercaptopurine from 50 mg/m^2/day, or an increased methotrexate dose from 20 to 25 mg/m^2/week. Although parenteral administration of methotrexate provides more predictable levels and improved compliance, it does not consistently improve the results of therapy.[212] To assess whether J.B. is receiving an adequate dose, weekly WBC counts are essential. This allows his treatment team to accurately appraise the adequacy of his dose and to follow his disease status to ensure that remission is continuing. If an inadequate degree of myelosuppression is demonstrated, J.B.'s compliance should be investigated because decreased compliance is a frequent problem in the therapy of childhood ALL. At least one investigation has found improved compliance with evening administration of mercaptopurine.[213–215]

Duration of Therapy

Case 95-5, Question 12: How long should J.B.'s maintenance therapy be continued?

Most centers treat children with ALL until a total therapy duration of approximately 2.5 years for females and 3.5 years for males. Most patients who experience relapse do so during therapy or within the first year of completing therapy. After the second year of therapy and for every year thereafter, relapses become much less common but are occasionally observed. Some centers are exploring whether more intensive treatment protocols could decrease the duration of maintenance treatment because the current duration is based on data from less aggressive protocols. Until there is more conclusive evidence regarding the duration of ALL maintenance therapy, patients with J.B.'s characteristics should receive chemotherapy for approximately 2.5 years.

Asparaginase Preparations

Asparaginase is available from two natural sources, *Escherichia coli* and *Erwinia chrysanthemi*. These two preparations are not 100% cross-reactive, so the *Erwinia* product may be substituted for the *E. coli* product when hypersensitivity reactions occur. However, one should be aware that cross-reactions occur in 17% to 26% of patients.[216,217] Because of the shorter half-life of the *Erwinia* product, a dosage increase of *Erwinia* asparaginase is necessary to equal the activity of the *E. coli* product. Of note, patients receiving equivalent doses of *Erwinia* asparaginase have a poorer remission rate and survival than those patients receiving the *E. coli* asparaginase. In contemporary protocols, the dose of *Erwinia* asparaginase is typically about 2.5 times greater than the *E. coli* asparaginase dose. The incidences of rash and silent immune clearance appear to be equivalent for these two preparations.

E. coli–derived asparaginase is available in a long-acting form known as pegaspargase. This agent is formed by covalently linking monomethoxy PEG to *E. coli* asparaginase. Pegaspargase has a prolonged half-life of 5.8 days compared with 1.2 days for *E. coli* asparaginase and appears to be safe and effective, even in patients with prior reactions to *E. coli* and *Erwinia* asparaginase. The prolonged half-life allows for less frequent (i.e., every 2 weeks) dosing of pegaspargase than for the natural source asparaginase products (i.e., 3 times a week). Asparaginase compounds derived from different *E. coli* strains may differ in both enzyme activity and half-life. At least one study has reported an unexpected mortality rate in childhood ALL associated with an assumption of equivalence among different *E. coli* asparaginase preparations.[218–222]

Relapsed Acute Lymphoblastic Leukemia

PROGNOSIS

CASE 95-6

Question 1: N.B. is a 12-year-old boy with T-cell acute lymphoblastic leukemia. Initially he responded to therapy and achieved a complete remission. However, about 17 months after his initial diagnosis, N.B. undergoes a routine lumbar puncture as part of his planned maintenance therapy. Analysis of the CSF indicates the presence of numerous lymphoblasts. A CBC reveals the following:

Hct, 29.5%
Platelet count, 120,000 cells/μL
WBC, 5,300 cells/μL, with 45% lymphocytes, 50% neutrophils, and 5% bands

A bone marrow biopsy confirms relapsed ALL with 53% lymphoblasts. What are N.B.'s chances of achieving a second remission and long-term survival? Are there specific features about N.B.'s relapse which confer a worse prognosis?

N.B. is asymptomatic at the time of relapse, as are most patients experiencing a relapse of ALL. Most of these patients are diagnosed by routine CBCs or lumbar punctures. Although ALL patients typically have excellent responses to treatment after relapse, 20% to 25% of patients will relapse again, and most will not be long-time survivors. Routine bone marrow biopsies may identify bone marrow relapses before they become evident on a CBC, but it has not been demonstrated that earlier identification of bone marrow relapse by morphologic criteria impacts long-term survival.[223–225]

At least 80% of relapsed ALL patients will achieve a second remission with salvage chemotherapy. Unfortunately, bone marrow relapse in childhood ALL is associated with poor long-term survival and most patients will not be cured of their disease. Rates of 5-year disease-free survival vary from 6% to 60% for patients with bone marrow relapse and are dependent on multiple variables. N.B.'s situation has several features which confer a worse prognosis on relapse including male sex, both marrow and CNS relapse, T-cell disease, and relapse less than 18 months from initial diagnosis.[225–229]

TREATMENT OF RELAPSED ACUTE LYMPHOBLASTIC LEUKEMIA

Case 95-6, Question 2: Which treatments could be used in an attempt to attain a complete remission and improve N.B.'s chances of long-term survival?

Agents used in salvage regimens are similar to those used in high-risk ALL regimens. In general, treatment usually consists of an intensive four-agent induction regimen of vincristine, prednisone, daunorubicin, and asparaginase. This is accompanied by radiation therapy to sites of local relapse (e.g., testis, CNS) and IT chemotherapy.[229–231] After this regimen has been completed, the patient may continue with courses of intensification therapy, continuation therapy, and IT therapy. Relapsed regimens will include more intensive chemotherapy, including high-dose methotrexate and high-dose cytarabine (HiDAC), as well as etoposide and cyclophosphamide. High-dose methotrexate has excellent penetration into the central nervous system and can be used to treat and prevent CNS leukemia relapses. HiDAC (3 g/m^2 every 12 hours for four doses) in conjunction with standard-dose asparaginase may be used to induce a remission in patients who fail re-induction therapy. This approach has been successful in approximately 40% of patients, although the median duration of second remission was only 3 months.[232,233] The selection of a salvage regimen will depend on how intensive the patient's initial therapy was, whether or not the relapse occurred while on therapy and sites of relapse. In N.B.'s case, his regimen should include intensive therapy, preferably with chemotherapy drugs and regimens to which he has not been previously exposed, because his relapse occurred while he was on therapy. Additionally, he will have CNS radiation and IT chemotherapy aimed at treating his specific sites of relapse.

CASE 95-6, QUESTION 3: N.B.'s family is quite concerned about the poor prognosis associated with his relapse and inquire about the role of hematopoietic cell transplantation (HCT) in his relapse treatment. Should he be considered for HCT at this point? Knowing the potential morbidity and mortality associated with allogeneic transplantation, would autologous transplant be a more appropriate option for N.B?

Allogeneic HCT is emerging as a superior treatment option for children with relapsed ALL who have high-risk and intermediate-risk features. In patients who receive a matched sibling HCT during their second complete remission for relapsed ALL, event-free survival rates of 52% at 5 years have been reported versus chemotherapy alone producing 5% event-free survival at 5 years.[234–237] Autologous HCT does not appear to be superior to standard chemotherapy for children with ALL in second remission and should not be offered.[236] N.B.'s family should be offered the option of allogeneic HCT, and his family should be tested for an appropriate sibling match as this offers lower morbidity than an unrelated donor. Because his outcome in transplant improves if performed during a second complete remission, he should begin re-induction chemotherapy, while HCT is being arranged. If HCT does not prove to be a feasible option for N.B., novel therapies may be considered. Nelarabine is a purine analog approved for the treatment of relapsed T-cell leukemias and lymphomas, and it has shown response rates (complete and partial remission) as high as 55% in pediatric populations.[237,238]

PEDIATRIC NON-HODGKIN LYMPHOMA

Lymphomas are a collection of diseases originating in cells and organs of the immune system. Lymphomas account for approximately 10% to 15% of all childhood malignancies, but they are less common in children than in adults. Children younger than 16 years account for only 3% of all lymphoma cases. The malignancy can occur in any lymphoid cell at any level of differentiation and appears to be a consequence of a genetic alteration. Non-Hodgkin lymphoma (NHL) is the most common form of lymphoma in children younger than 10 years of age, whereas Hodgkin lymphoma is most common in children 15 to 19 years of age. This section will focus on NHL. Considerable progress has been made in the treatment of children with NHL and currently approximately 80% are cured.[239]

Classification

Numerous classification systems for NHL exist, and there is considerable variation in terminology among these systems.[239] Pediatric NHLs are best classified using histopathology, which divides them into three different categories: B-cell lymphomas, lymphoblastic lymphomas, and anaplastic large-cell lymphomas.[240–243] This is a narrower range of histologic types than in adults.

Lymphoblastic lymphomas account for approximately 30% of childhood NHLs, B-cell lymphomas for about 50%, and large-cell lymphomas for the remainder[1] The lymphoblastic lymphomas are usually immature T-cells that are histologically identical to the cells of ALL. The distinction between lymphoblastic lymphoma and ALL is made on the basis of bone marrow involvement, with ALL being diagnosed if there is greater than 25% bone marrow infiltration. B-cell lymphomas may be further divided into Burkitt, Burkitt-like, and large B-cell lymphomas. Anaplastic large-cell lymphomas may be T-cell or null cell in origin.[240–243]

Clinical Presentation

Pediatric patients with NHL may present with a number of different symptoms, many of which are related to the type of NHL. In general, these symptoms differ from those in adults because of the propensity of pediatric NHLs to be extranodal in origin in contrast to the common nodal presentation of adult NHL. Patients with lymphoblastic lymphoma commonly present with a mediastinal mass or pleural effusions. They also may have pain, dyspnea, or swelling of the face and upper arms if superior vena cava obstruction is present. Lymphoblastic lymphoma also has a predilection for the bone marrow and the CNS.[244,245] Lymphadenopathy in patients with lymphoblastic lymphoma tends to be supradiaphragmatic. Patients with B-cell NHL typically present with an abdominal tumor, abdominal pain, an alteration in bowel function, and possibly nausea and vomiting. In addition, many patients with B-cell NHL present with bone marrow involvement. Lymphadenopathy in these patients typically occurs below the diaphragm in the inguinal or iliac area. Anaplastic large-cell lymphomas may involve the gut or unusual sites such as the lung, skin, face, or CNS.[246,247]

Staging

Several staging systems for pediatric NHLs are used. A commonly used staging system for pediatric NHL is the St. Jude staging system.[244] This staging system includes four stages, with stage I being a single tumor or a single nodal area, and higher stages including cases with regional involvement or more than one anatomical site involved. The highest stage (stage IV) refers to patients with bone marrow or CNS involvement. The main predictor of outcome in pediatric patients with NHL has historically been determined by tumor burden at presentation.[247] However, with modern chemotherapy regimens that are tailored to the extent of disease, patients with higher-stage disease may achieve a similar event-free survival to that achieved in patients with lower-stage disease. A higher LDH is correlated with greater tumor burden, and it has been demonstrated that serum LDH greater than or equal to 500 to 1,000 units/L is a significant predictor of poorer outcome.[247]

Overview of Treatment

LYMPHOBLASTIC (T-CELL) LYMPHOMAS

The primary treatment for all stages and histologic types of pediatric NHL is combination chemotherapy because it is a generalized disease at the time of diagnosis.[248,249] A wide variety of chemotherapy agents have activity in childhood NHL. At present, the best results to date are reported by the Berlin–Frankfurt–Muenster (BFM) group, with an estimated 5-year event-free survival of approximately 92% (Table 95-9). This regimen uses an intensive scheme of multi-agent chemotherapy administered over 24 months. Patients with lymphoblastic lymphoma require longer treatment duration than patients with B-cell or anaplastic large-cell lymphoma. This chemotherapy plan is similar to that used in the treatment of ALL, and it is designed to deliver continuous or weekly therapy. All patients with lymphoblastic lymphoma are given CNS preventive therapy, regardless of stage. Few patients with lymphoblastic lymphoma present with limited disease (stages I and II), thus making it difficult

Table 95-9
Berlin–Frankfurt–Muenster (BFM) Group Treatment Protocols for T-Cell Lymphoblastic Lymphoma

Drug	Dose	Days of Administration
Induction Protocol I (All Stages)		
Prednisone (PO)	60 mg/m^2	1–28, then taper
Vincristine (IV)	1.5 mg/m^2 (max 2 mg)	8, 15, 22, 29
Daunorubicin (IV over 1 hour)	30 mg/m^2	8, 15, 22, 29
L-asparaginase (IV[a] over 1 hour)	10,000 IU/m^2	12, 15, 18, 21, 24, 27, 30, 33
Cyclophosphamide[b] (IV over 1 hour)	1,000 mg/m^2	36, 64
Cytarabine (IV)	75 mg/m^2	38–41, 45–48, 52–55, 59–62
6-Mercaptopurine (PO)	60 mg/m^2	36–63
Methotrexate (IT)[c]	12 mg	1, 15, 29, 45, 59
Protocol M (Typically Stages I and II)		
Mercaptopurine (PO)	25 mg/m^2	1–56
Methotrexate (IV)	5 g/m^2	8, 22, 36, 50
Methotrexate (IT)	12 mg	8, 22, 36, 50
Re-induction Protocol II (Stages III and IV Only)		
Dexamethasone (PO)	10 mg/m^2	1–21, then taper
Vincristine (IV)	1.5 mg/m^2 (max 2 mg)	8, 15, 22, 29
Doxorubicin (IV over 1 hour)	30 mg/m^2	8, 15, 22, 29
L-asparaginase (IV[a] over 1 hour)	10,000 IU/m^2	8, 11, 15, 18
Cyclophosphamide[b] (IV over 1 hour)	1,000 mg/m^2	36
Cytarabine (IV)	75 mg/m^2	38–41, 45–48
Thioguanine (PO)	60 mg/m^2	36–49
Methotrexate (IT)	12 mg	38, 45
Maintenance (All Stages)		
Mercaptopurine (PO)	50 mg/m^2	Daily until month 24 of therapy
Methotrexate (PO)	20 mg/m^2	Weekly until month 24 of therapy

Note: IT methotrexate doses were adjusted for children younger than 3 years. Ten percent (of the 5 g/m^2 methotrexate dose in Protocol M was given for 30 minutes, and 90% was given as a 23.5-hour continuous IV infusion. Leucovorin rescue: 30 mg/m^2 IV at hour 42; 15 mg/m^2 IV at hours 48 and 54.
[a]This agent is typically administered intramuscularly in most treatment protocols in the United States.
[b]With mesna.
[c]Additional intrathecal chemotherapy doses are given on days 8 and 22 for CNS-positive patients.
CNS, central nervous system; IT, intrathecally; IV, intravenously; PO, orally.
Source: Watanabe A et al. Undifferentiated lymphoma, non-Burkitt's type: meningeal and bone marrow involvement in children. *Am J Dis Child.* 1973;125:57.

to conduct adequate studies in this patient population. Attempts to shorten the duration of therapy for patients with limited-stage disease have been unsuccessful, although less-intensive therapy is administered to patients with early-stage disease on some protocols.

B-CELL LYMPHOMAS

The main differences between the treatment of lymphoblastic and B-cell lymphoma are the use of more agents and longer treatment duration in the former. The trend in the treatment of B-cell lymphomas has been toward short-duration, intensive therapy with alkylating agents in conjunction with high-dose antimetabolite therapy (e.g., methotrexate, cytarabine). Chemotherapy is administered in rapid succession with limited recovery from neutropenia (i.e., ANC 500 cells/μL) between cycles. Patients with localized B-cell lymphomas respond as adequately to a four-drug regimen (consisting of cyclophosphamide, vincristine, methotrexate, and prednisone) as they do to more aggressive regimens.[249,250]

Evidence suggests that a 6-month course is as efficacious as an 18-month course for patients with localized B-cell lymphomas. Studies indicate that even 6 months of chemotherapy may be unnecessary for patients with limited-stage disease because it has been demonstrated that maintenance treatment offered no additional benefit after 9 weeks of combination chemotherapy. Contemporary chemotherapy regimens include varying degrees of treatment intensity from three to seven cycles, depending on whether the tumor is completely resected, on bone marrow and CNS involvement, and the serum LDH.[250]

With the addition of high-dose methotrexate, ifosfamide, etoposide, and HiDAC to the standard regimen, patients with stage III disease are now achieving survival rates comparable to those of patients with limited-stage disease. Patients with bone marrow disease also benefit from these intensive therapeutic strategies and have achieved impressive survival rates of approximately 80%.[1] Currently, patients with advanced-stage disease are treated with a total of six to eight cycles of chemotherapy, and these treatment protocols achieve superior results to those of a much longer duration (e.g., 1–2 years) used previously. Although rituximab is now a standard therapy component for B-cell lymphomas in adults, it has yet to be routinely used in front-line treatment in the pediatric arena. Case reports demonstrate the utility of this agent when added to a standard chemotherapy backbone for children with relapsed disease.[250–252]

LARGE-CELL LYMPHOMAS

Large-cell lymphomas have responded well to both types of regimens.[253,254] Thus, the use of shorter, less complicated, B-cell protocols is appropriate. Patients who fail to respond may be treated with additional courses of their prescribed protocol in hopes of eventually inducing a response. Patients who relapse may be re-induced with intensive chemotherapy, but their prognosis for long-term survival is unfavorable.

Lymphoblastic Lymphoma

ACUTE TREATMENT

CASE 95-7

QUESTION 1: D.B., a 16-year-old girl, presents with a history of shortness of breath and chest pain for 3 weeks before admission. A mediastinal mass is found, and a biopsy confirms a lymphoblastic (T-cell) lymphoma. Radiography of the chest reveals a right pleural effusion. Laboratory values show the following results:

Erythrocyte sedimentation rate, 35
WBC count, 22,000 cells/μL
Uric acid, 7 mg/dL
LDH, 1,259 units/L

The bone marrow, CNS, and abdomen are negative for lymphoma. How should D.B. be managed acutely? Besides chemotherapy, what types of adjunctive therapies should be initiated to minimize the acute effects of treatment?

Given D.B.'s shortness of breath and chest pain, it is likely that her mediastinal mass may be obstructing the superior vena cava. To alleviate this obstruction, the most appropriate course of action is to decrease the tumor mass by initiating chemotherapy as soon as possible. Radiation therapy offers no additional benefit in patients such as D.B. with a tumor such as NHL, which is highly responsive to chemotherapy.[255] Because of the high cell kill that will result from the initial chemotherapy treatment, tumor lysis syndrome and uric acid nephropathy are possible. However, the risk of this complication is probably greater in patients with B-cell NHL in whom the fraction of cells in S phase is higher.[256,257]

Alkaline diuresis and allopurinol should be instituted before chemotherapy to prevent tumor lysis syndrome. Because D.B. has a pleural effusion, fluids may collect in this third space, resulting in weight gain and decreased urine output. Thus, in addition to placement of a chest tube with suction, D.B. should be given diuretics to maintain an adequate urine output. To minimize intravascular volume depletion and maintain electrolyte balances, fluid input and output, body weight, and electrolyte panels should be monitored daily. These values should be used to make appropriate adjustments in D.B.'s electrolyte and fluid balance. See Chapter 96, Hematologic Malignancies, for a complete discussion of tumor lysis syndrome.

Adverse Effects

CASE 95-7, QUESTION 2: D.B. is treated with the BFM combination chemotherapy regimen. Because of her intrathoracic mass, her disease is characterized as stage III. She is to receive induction therapy (Induction Protocol I) for 8 weeks, as outlined in Table 95-9. Which acute adverse effects is D.B. likely to experience with these agents? How can they be monitored, minimized, and treated?

Several toxicities are expected with these chemotherapy agents. For vincristine, both constipation and neuropathy are likely to appear during or after the 4 weeks of therapy.[163] Constipation can be prevented or minimized by use of stool softeners with or without a laxative. Neuropathy may be painful (especially when jaw pain occurs) but can be managed with mild analgesic regimens consisting of NSAIDs or acetaminophen with codeine. Both toxicities are self-limiting and are not reasons to discontinue or decrease the dosage of vincristine unless neuromuscular toxicity, as evidenced by motor weakness, develops. The incidence of jaw pain and foot drop is higher in pediatric populations as compared to adults. Asparaginase can cause several types of toxicities (e.g., hypersensitivity reaction, coagulation disorders, pancreatitis), most of which are not thought to be preventable.

Prednisone is likely to increase D.B.'s appetite and may cause gastritis, although divided doses will help decrease stomach upset. In addition, prednisone-induced behavioral disturbances, such as hyperactivity, are common in children.[164] Unlike prednisone and vincristine, daunorubicin, cyclophosphamide, cytarabine, and mercaptopurine produce significant myelosuppression. Leukopenia is common with the nadir occurring in approximately 8 to 14 days, and recovery occurring by approximately day 21 after administration. Because the goal of induction therapy is achievement of remission, doses of daunorubicin will not be held for uncomplicated myelosuppression during the first 4 weeks of induction therapy, although during the latter 4 weeks, the combination of cyclophosphamide, cytarabine, and mercaptopurine are typically held until hematologic recovery occurs.

Hemorrhagic cystitis may occur with cyclophosphamide, but it is usually associated with high-dose therapy or with prolonged administration, which D.B. is not receiving. Vigorous IV hydration to maintain urine output of approximately 50 to 100 mL/m^2/hour should reduce the risk of this toxicity at this dose. In addition, this chemotherapy protocol also includes mesna, which will bind to urotoxic metabolites of cyclophosphamide and also reduce the risk of hemorrhagic cystitis. Because most of the induction regimen will be administered on an outpatient basis, patients or parents should be instructed to report signs or symptoms of infection (e.g., febrile episodes) immediately so that proper treatment may be instituted as soon as possible. To decrease the risk of hemorrhagic cystitis, parents should be instructed to report whether patients are urinating regularly after cyclophosphamide. See Chapter 94, Adverse Effects and their Treatment, for further discussion of these adverse effects.

Nausea and vomiting are likely to be induced by both daunorubicin and cyclophosphamide/cytarabine. D.B.'s chemotherapy regimen includes a corticosteroid (prednisone), which may provide some antiemetic activity during the initial 4 weeks.[258] However, to maximize tolerance to her chemotherapy, D.B. should receive a 5-HT_3 serotonin antagonist. D.B. is unlikely to require additional corticosteroids during the first 4 weeks of induction therapy. However, during the second portion of induction, D.B. will benefit from a few doses of dexamethasone at the time of cyclophosphamide administration.[259] See Chapter 22, Nausea and Vomiting, for further discussion of chemotherapy-induced nausea and vomiting.

Central Nervous System Prophylaxis

CASE 95-7, QUESTION 3: What is the importance of CNS prophylaxis for D.B. and what type of treatment regimen is typically used?

All pediatric patients with lymphoblastic lymphoma should receive some form of CNS prophylaxis. Although lymphoblastic lymphoma rarely presents with CNS involvement, as illustrated by D.B., it was a common site of relapse before CNS prophylaxis was included as a routine part of the chemotherapy regimen.[250,251] Recurrence of NHL within the CNS is rare when IT methotrexate or cytarabine is given.[245] D.B. will be treated with IT methotrexate periodically, as outlined in Table 95-9.

Myelosuppression and Hematopoietic Recovery

CASE 95-7, QUESTION 4: After completion of induction therapy, the chemotherapy plan for D.B. consists of protocol M and re-induction protocol II, as outlined in Table 95-9. How should D.B.'s hematopoietic recovery be managed, and what guidelines may be used to determine when it is appropriate for her to receive the next sequence of the treatment cycle? Would D.B. benefit from a colony-stimulating factor to aid with hematopoietic recovery?

Protocol M will likely not produce significant myelosuppression because leucovorin rescue will reduce the myelosuppression from the high-dose methotrexate. The most challenging problems with this phase of treatment will be to confirm that the methotrexate has been properly eliminated and to continue aggressive hydration, alkalinization, and leucovorin dosing until the methotrexate level is nontoxic. Owing to D.B.'s pleural effusion at the time of diagnosis, it should be confirmed that this has resolved before administration of high-dose methotrexate to avoid significantly delayed clearance because the pleural effusion could allow for third spacing of high doses of methotrexate. Pleural effusions are a relative contraindication to high-dose methotrexate. Methotrexate elimination has high interpatient and intrapatient variability, and necessitates close monitoring of methotrexate concentrations and renal function after each dose. Refer to the discussion of high-dose methotrexate earlier in this chapter.

Protocol II will result in significant myelosuppression. However, as with protocol I, dosing of doxorubicin will not be held for uncomplicated myelosuppression. Similarly, during the second phase of this protocol, dosing of cytarabine and thioguanine will also not be held for uncomplicated myelosuppression. However, before initiating the second phase on day 36, clinicians will assure adequate hematologic recovery, typically defined as an ANC greater than 750 cells/μL and platelets greater than 100,000 cells/μL. It is unlikely that D.B. will benefit from a colony-stimulating factor during these phases of therapy. When myelosuppressive chemotherapy is given fairly continuously, as is the case with protocol II, there is little room for inserting doses of colony-stimulating factors on days where myelosuppressive chemotherapy is not being administered.

KEY REFERENCES AND WEBSITES

A full list of references for this chapter can be found at http://thepoint.lww.com/AT11e. Below are the key references and websites for this chapter, with the corresponding reference number in this chapter found in parentheses after the reference..

Key References

Bassen R et al. Modern therapy of acute lymphoblastic leukemia. *J Clin Oncol*. 2011;29:532.

Boissel N et al. Should adolescents with acute lymphoblastic leukemia be treated as old children or young adults? Comparison of the French FRALLE-93 and LALA-94 trials. *J Clin Oncol*. 2003;21:774. (104)

Borowitz MJ et al. Clinical significance of minimal residual disease in childhood acute lymphoblastic leukemia and its relationship to other prognostic factors: a Children's Oncology Group study. *Blood*. 2008;111:5477. (144)

Fernandez CV et al. Intrathecal vincristine: an analysis of reasons for recurrent fatal chemotherapeutic error with recommendations for prevention. *J Pediatr Hematol Oncol*. 1998;20:587. (192)

Holdsworth MT et al. Acute and delayed nausea and emesis control in pediatric oncology patients. *Cancer*. 2006;106:931. (258)

Hurwitz CA et al. Substituting dexamethasone for prednisone complicates remission induction in children with acute lymphoblastic leukemia. *Cancer*. 2000;88:1964. (153)

Lipshultz SE et al. Chronic progressive cardiac dysfunction years after doxorubicin therapy for childhood acute lymphoblastic leukemia. *J Clin Oncol*. 2005;23:2629. (49)

Mahoney DH et al. Intermediate-dose intravenous methotrexate with intravenous mercaptopurine is superior to repetitive low-dose oral methotrexate with intravenous mercaptopurine for children with lower-risk B-lineage acute lymphoblastic leukemia: a Pediatric Oncology Group phase III trial. *J Clin Oncol*. 1998;16:246. (193)

Maris JM. Recent advances in neuroblastoma. *N Engl J Med*. 2010;362:2202.

McNeil DE et al. SEER update of incidence and trends in pediatric malignancies: acute lymphoblastic leukemia. *Med Pediatr Oncol*. 2002;39:554. (112)

Nguyen K et al. Factors influencing survival after relapse from acute lyphoblastic leukemia: a Children's Oncology Group Study. *Leukemia*. 2008;22:2142. (226)

Oeffinger KC et al. Chronic health conditions in adult survivors of childhood cancer. *N Engl J Med*. 2006;355:1572. (12)

Pizzo PA, Poplack DG, eds. *Principles and Practice of Pediatric Oncology*. 6th ed. Philadelphia, PA: Lippincott Williams & Wilkins; 2010. (239)

Pollock BH. Where adolescents and young adults with cancer receive their care: does it matter? *J Clin Oncol*. 2007;25:4522. (11)

Pui C et al. Biology, risk stratification, and therapy of pediatric acute leukemias: an update. *J Clin Oncol*. 2011;29:551.

Rosoff PM. The two-edged sword of curing childhood cancer. *N Engl J Med*. 2006;355:1522. (13)

Schmiegelow K et al. The degree of myelosuppression during maintenance therapy of adolescents with B-lineage intermediate risk acute lymphoblastic leukemia predicts risk of relapse. *Leukemia*. 2010;24:715. (197)

Seibel NL et al. Early postinduction intensification therapy improves survival for children and adolescents with high-risk acute lymphoblastic leukemia: a report from the Children's Oncology Group. *Blood*. 2008;111:2548.

Key Websites

Childhood Cancer Survivor Study. www.stjude.org/ccss.

Children's Oncology Group Cure Search. Screening and management guidelines for survivors. www.survivorshipguidelines.org.

96 Adult Hematologic Malignancies

Lynn Weber, Jacob K. Kettle, Andy Kurtzweil, Casey B. Williams, Rachel Elsey, and Katie A. Won

CORE PRINCIPLES

	CHAPTER CASES
ACUTE MYELOID LEUKEMIA	
1 Acute myeloid leukemia (AML) generally appears suddenly and progresses rapidly. Death as a result of infection or bleeding occurs within weeks to months if the patient is not effectively treated.	**Case 96-1 (Questions 1, 2)**
2 Although more than 60% of patients treated for AML achieve complete remission after induction therapy, the median duration of the remission is only about 12 to 18 months, and only 20%–40% of patients have a disease-free survival (DFS) exceeding 5 years. Short remissions have been attributed to proliferation of clinically undetectable leukemic cells. Thus, the rationale for administering chemotherapy after remission is to eradicate these residual cells.	**Case 96-1 (Questions 6, 7)**
3 The incidence of AML increases with advancing age. At age 40 years, there is only 1 case of AML per 100,000, but the annual incidence increases to 15% at age greater than 75 years. The prognosis of patients with AML is directly related to age.	**Case 96-1 (Question 8)**
4 Elderly patients do not tolerate intensive induction and postremission chemotherapy as well as younger patients. Older patients often have comorbid medical conditions and a poor performance status, which are associated with worse outcomes with conventional therapy.	**Case 96-1 (Question 8)**
5 In younger patients, failure to achieve remission or disease relapse remains the major cause of treatment failure. This reflects both the failure of current salvage regimens and the absence of effective strategies to secure long-term DFS in those patients who achieve a second hematologic remission. A wide range of salvage options have been studied, but with less than 50% of patients achieving a second remission and median survival ranging from 3 to 12 months, there remains considerable room for improvement.	**Case 96-2 (Question 1)**
CHRONIC MYELOGENOUS LEUKEMIA	
1 Many patients are asymptomatic at presentation but are evaluated because of an abnormally high leukocyte count. The cytogenetic hallmark of chronic myelogenous leukemia (CML) is the Philadelphia chromosome. The chromosomal translocation generates a fusion gene called BCR-ABL that becomes inappropriately expressed, leading to CML. Identifying the Philadelphia chromosome is important in confirming the diagnosis of CML.	**Case 96-3 (Question 1)**
2 Hematopoietic stem cell transplantation is the only curative therapy for CML, but it is seldom recommended as first-line therapy for patients in chronic-phase CML. Imatinib, nilotinib, and dasatinib are all small-molecule tyrosine kinase (TK) inhibitors of the BCR-ABL protein and are all approved as initial first-line treatment.	**Case 96-3 (Question 3)**

Continued

CHRONIC LYMPHOCYTIC LEUKEMIA	CHAPTER CASES
1 Common treatment regimens for chronic lymphocytic leukemia (CLL) in patients without significant comorbidities include combinations of rituximab with fludarabine, cyclophosphamide, or bendamustine. Patients unable to tolerate a purine analog are treated with a monoclonal antibody in combination with chlorambucil.	**Case 96-4 (Question 3)**
2 Infectious complications are common in patients with CLL. For recurrent infections, immune globulin treatment may be indicated. Vaccinations to prevent influenza and pneumococcus are indicated. Live vaccines, including varicella zoster virus, must be avoided.	**Case 96-4 (Question 5)**
MULTIPLE MYELOMA	
1 Multiple myeloma (MM) generally begins as a benign condition known as monoclonal gammopathy of undetermined significance (MGUS). This condition may precede MM by years before transforming into a malignant disorder with clinical manifestations.	**Case 96-5 (Question 1)**
2 Induction therapy followed by hematopoietic cell transplantation (HCT) in eligible patients is the standard of care and has increased overall survival (OS) in those with MM.	**Case 96-5 (Question 2)**
3 Supportive care of patients with MM includes the prevention and treatment of skeletal disease and should be considered in conjunction with induction therapy.	**Case 96-5 (Question 3)**
4 Multiple myeloma is not generally curable, even with maintenance therapy. Therefore, relapse usually occurs, and salvage therapies are commonly used.	**Case 96-5 (Questions 4, 5)**
LYMPHOMA	
1 The lymphomas are a diverse collection of hematologic malignancies originating from lymphoid tissues. Lymphomas are classified as either Hodgkin lymphoma (HL) or non-Hodgkin lymphoma (NHL). The NHLs can be further divided into aggressive or indolent subgroups. Symptoms include painless lymphadenopathy along with nonspecific findings of generalized malaise and fatigue. Advanced complications arise from the infiltration of the disease into extramedullary tissues including the lungs, central nervous system (CNS), and bone marrow.	**Case 96-6 (Questions 1)**
2 Hodgkin lymphoma (HL) is B-cell neoplasm and is highly responsive to chemotherapy and often curable with modern treatments. A combination of doxorubicin, bleomycin, vinblastine, and dacarbazine (ABVD) is the most frequently used chemotherapy regimen. Delayed consequences of therapy have a heightened importance in management of this disease due to the expected long-term survival for most patients.	**Case 96-7 (Questions 1, 2)**
3 Aggressive NHLs such as diffuse large B-cell lymphoma (DLBCL) progress rapidly and are treated with intensive combination chemotherapy regimens administered with a curative intent. Chemoimmunotherapy with rituximab, cyclophosphamide, doxorubicin, vincristine, and prednisone (R-CHOP) is conventional therapy for DLBCL.	**Case 96-8 (Questions 1, 2)**
4 Although indolent NHLs including follicular lymphoma (FL) are generally incurable, these diseases develop slowly and are initially responsive to numerous therapies. Treatment is aimed at reducing disease burden and prolonging survival and is often reserved until the patient is symptomatic. A combination of bendamustine and rituximab (BR) is commonly used in the management of these neoplasms.	**Case 96-9 (Questions 1, 2)**

ACUTE MYELOID LEUKEMIA

Epidemiology

Acute myeloid leukemia (AML) consists of a group of relatively well-defined hematopoietic neoplasms involving precursor cells committed to the myeloid line of cellular development.

In the United States and Europe, the incidence has been stable at 3 to 5 cases per 100,000. AML is the most common acute leukemia in adults and accounts for approximately 80% of cases in this group of neoplasms. In contrast, AML accounts for less than 10% of acute leukemias in children younger than 10 years of age. In adults, the median age at diagnosis is approximately 67 years. The incidence increases with age with approximately 1.3 and 12.2 cases per 100,000 for those younger than or older than 65 years, respectively. The male-to-female ratio is approximately 5:3.[1,2]

Pathophysiology

AML is characterized by a clonal proliferation of myeloid precursors with a reduced capacity to differentiate into mature

Table 96-1

Pretreatment Molecular Entities Shown to Predict Disease Outcome in Adults with Acute Myeloid Leukemia and a Normal Karyotype

Gene	Mutation Frequency (%)	Prognosis
NPM1	45–63	Favorable
FLT3	23–33	Poor
C/EBPα	8–19	Favorable
MLL	5–30	Poor

Source: Baldus CD et al. Clinical outcome of de novo acute myeloid leukemia patients with normal cytogenetics is affected by molecular genetic alterations: a concise review. *Br J Haematol.* 2007;137:387.

myeloid cells. As a result, there is an accumulation of leukemic blasts in the bone marrow, peripheral blood, and occasionally in other tissues, with a variable reduction in the production of normal red blood cells, platelets, and mature granulocytes. The proliferation of malignant cells, along with a reduction in normal hematopoietic cells, results in a variety of systemic consequences including anemia, bleeding, and an increased risk of infection.

Based on karyotype status (characterization of the chromosome such as shape, type, or number), two major groups of AML can be identified: (a) those with an abnormal karyotype, which accounts for approximately 50% to 60% of patients, and (b) those that demonstrate a normal karyotype by conventional cytogenetic testing, which accounts for the remainder of AML patients.[3,4]

The outcomes of patients with an abnormal karyotype are generally poor regardless of the molecular findings. However, the prognosis of patients with normal karyotype in the presence of each of these mutations is different as shown in Table 96-1.

Clinical Presentation and Diagnosis

Patients with AML generally present with symptoms related to complications of pancytopenia (e.g., anemia, neutropenia, and thrombocytopenia), including weakness and easy fatigability, infections of variable severity, and hemorrhagic findings such as gingival bleeding, ecchymosis, epistaxis, or menorrhagia. Combinations of these symptoms are common. It is often difficult to date the onset of AML precisely, at least in part because individuals have different symptomatic thresholds for seeking medical attention. It is likely that most patients have had more subtle evidence of bone marrow involvement for weeks, or perhaps months, before diagnosis. Although a presumptive diagnosis of AML can be made by examination of the peripheral blood smear when there are circulating leukemic blasts, a definitive diagnosis usually requires a bone marrow aspiration and biopsy. Morphologic, immunophenotypic, cytogenetic, and molecular studies must be performed in every case. The information derived from these studies is critical for making the correct diagnosis as well as determining prognosis.

Overview of Treatment

Once the diagnosis of AML is established, induction chemotherapy is given with the goal of rapidly restoring normal bone marrow function. Treatment regimens and outcomes differ between younger and older adults. Although there is no clear dividing line between younger and older adults when dealing with AML, in most studies "older adults" are defined as older than 60 years of age.

The objective of induction therapy is to reduce the total body leukemia cell population from approximately 10^{12} to less than the cytologically detectable level of about 10^9 cells. It is generally assumed, however, that a substantial burden of leukemia cells persists undetected (i.e., presence of "minimal residual disease"), leading to relapse within a few weeks or months if no further therapy was administered. The traditional goal of treatment of AML is to produce and maintain a complete remission. Criteria for this are platelet count higher than 100,000 cells/μL, neutrophil count higher than 1,000 cells/μL, and bone marrow specimen with less than 5% blasts.[5]

The most commonly used induction regimens for AML are the "7+3" regimens, which combine a 7-day continuous intravenous (IV) infusion of cytarabine (100 or 200 mg/m^2/day) with a short infusion or bolus of an anthracycline given on days 1 through 3. The most commonly used anthracycline in this regimen is daunorubicin, but idarubicin may be used instead.

Sixty to 80% of adult patients with newly diagnosed AML will attain a complete remission with intensive induction chemotherapy. However, without additional cytotoxic therapy, virtually all of these patients will relapse within a median of 4 to 8 months. In contrast, patients who receive postremission therapy may expect 4-year survival rates as high as 40% in young and middle-aged adults with good-risk disease.[6] High-dose cytarabine (HiDAC) has been the consolidation chemotherapy of choice for more than a decade for younger patients with good- or intermediate-risk disease. Attempts to improve on survival rates attained with HiDAC by substituting other agents with different mechanisms of action have not been successful.[7] For patients with an abnormal karyotype or with adverse molecular mutations, consolidation with HiDAC followed by an allogeneic hematopoietic cell transplantation (HCT) with a suitably matched donor is the treatment of choice whenever possible. For patients older than 75 years of age, there is no specific standard of care except to enroll in a clinical trial when available. For the large number of patients who are 60 to 75 years of age, most clinicians will base induction and consolidation therapy recommendations on a patient's performance status, patient's wishes, and prognostic factors such as cytogenetics and mutation analysis.[8]

Twenty to 30% of young adult patients and 50% of older adult patients with newly diagnosed AML will fail to attain a complete response (CR) with intensive induction chemotherapy as a result of drug resistance or death. In addition, a large percentage of patients who initially attain a CR will relapse. The therapy that provides the best chance to cure a patient with relapsed or refractory AML is an allogeneic HCT. The best outcomes appear to be with a myeloablative preparative regimen administered after attaining a CR. However, some patients may be cured with myeloablative HCT even without attaining a CR although their chance of long-term survival is reduced. Nonmyeloablative preparative regimens are considered for patients who are not candidates for myeloablative HCT but have attained a CR.[9] See Chapter 101, Hematopoietic Cell Transplantation, for a complete discussion of HCT for leukemia. Please refer to the following online reference for more details about the treatment and prognosis of AML: http://www.cancer.gov/cancertopics/pdq/treatment/adultAML/healthprofessional/page4.

Signs and Symptoms

CASE 96-1

QUESTION 1: J.V., a 57-year-old man, presented to the emergency department with increasing fatigue and fever and an inability to eat. This past week, a peripheral blood smear (complete blood count [CBC]) revealed a white blood cell (WBC) count of 180,000 cells/μL with a differential of more than 90% leukemic blasts (normal, 0%), a hemoglobin (Hgb) of 7.8 g/dL, and a platelet count of 46,000 cells/μL. A bone marrow aspirate and biopsy confirmed the diagnosis of AML (FAB-M2, myeloid with maturation; 60% blasts, myeloperoxidase positive; CD13 and CD33 positive). All serum chemistry values were within normal limits, with the exception of potassium (K), 3.2 mEq/L; phosphorus, 5.5 mg/dL; and lactate dehydrogenase (LDH), 3,500 units/mL. Physical examination was remarkable for oral leukoplakia from oral candidiasis and poor dentition. Which signs and symptoms exhibited by J.V. are consistent with AML?

J.V.'s symptoms of increasing fatigue and fever of 1 week's duration are consistent with a rapid reduction in red blood cells leading to anemia (Hgb, 7.8 g/dL) and a low neutrophil count leading to infection (oral candidiasis). Although his WBC count is high, the differential reveals that more than 90% are blasts, which are immature, nonfunctional cells of myeloid or lymphoid origin. Circulating blast cells are typically not present in early chronic leukemias or mild-to-moderate infections. However, blasts may be observed on the peripheral blood smear in patients with anemia associated with primary bone marrow dysfunction (myelodysplastic syndromes). Blasts are also present in patients with severe infection, stress, or trauma, and in those with chronic myelogenous leukemia (CML) in transformation to acute leukemia. J.V.'s platelet count is also low, which may lead to bleeding or bruising. Collectively, these are presenting signs and symptoms of acute leukemia.

J.V.'s symptoms are consistent with either AML or acute lymphocytic leukemia (ALL). However, patients with ALL also commonly present with lymphadenopathy and hepatosplenomegaly, which J.V. does not have. It is important to distinguish between these two disorders because treatment regimens differ greatly. AML is more common in adults than in children. For additional information on ALL, see Acute Lymphoblastic Leukemia of Childhood section in Chapter 95, Pediatric Malignancies.

Classification and Diagnosis

For a definitive diagnosis of AML, the bone marrow aspirate must contain more than 20% leukemic blast cells. A normal bone marrow aspirate would typically contain less than 5% blasts. Eight major variants of AML are defined by the French–American–British (FAB) classification system based on morphologic characteristics. More recently, the World Health Organization (WHO) has developed a classification system that expands the number of AML subtypes and better incorporates genotypic information, which is important in determining prognosis.[10]

Cells of myeloid origin commonly contain myeloperoxidase enzymes and express surface markers CD13, CD33, CD14, and CD15. Specific clonal chromosomal abnormalities are associated with several AML subtypes. These aberrations include gains or losses of whole chromosomes on the long (q) or short (p) arms, as well as a variety of structural rearrangements (e.g., translocations, inversions, insertions). A number of cytogenetic abnormalities in AML are associated with molecular-clinical syndromes, which are now under investigation at the genetic level. The translocation t(15;17) is the cytogenetic hallmark of acute promyelocytic leukemia (APL or AML-M3). This translocation splits the retinoic acid receptor gene on chromosome 17 and blocks expression of retinoic acid-controlled genes required for cell differentiation. Treating patients who have APL with all-*trans* retinoic acid (ATRA, tretinoin) has resulted in complete morphologic responses. This example shows how defining cytogenetic or chromosomal abnormalities in acute leukemia can be critical to understanding its pathophysiology and identifying optimal treatments. Currently, three chromosomal abnormalities are recognized as being associated with a better prognosis: t(8;21), t(15;17), and inversion (inv) 16.[11,12] In contrast, several chromosomal abnormalities have been associated with a relatively poor prognosis, including inv 3, deletion (del) 5, del(5q), del(7), and del(7q); trisomy 8; and complex (three or more unrelated cytogenetic abnormalities) cytogenetics. Additionally, molecular abnormalities such as *FLT3*, which is generally unfavorable, and *NPM1* and *C/EBPa,* which are generally favorable, are central in the evaluation of AML patients.[13] These findings are increasingly being used to guide treatment decisions. For example, patients with cytogenetic and molecular findings associated with a poor prognosis may be considered for more aggressive postremission therapy such as high-dose chemotherapy with HCT. Other poor prognostic signs in AML include age older than 60 years at the time of diagnosis, a preexisting hematologic disorder (e.g., myelodysplastic syndrome), prior exposure to a chemotherapy agent (e.g., a secondary leukemia), and poor baseline performance status.[14]

J.V. has FAB-M2 (myelomonocytic) AML. Approximately 10% to 20% of patients with FAB-M2 acute leukemia have a translocation of t(8;21)(q22;q22).[11] This translocation is usually seen in young patients such as J.V. and is associated with a better response to therapy. J.V.'s bone marrow has been sent for cytogenetic and molecular analysis; however, results will not be available for approximately a week. Although neither the cytogenetic nor the molecular analysis will alter the planned induction therapy for J.V., these findings in combination with other prognostic features, as discussed previously, will influence postremission therapy recommendations.

Treatment

GOAL OF THERAPY

CASE 96-1, QUESTION 2: What is the goal of treatment and what type of therapy is indicated for J.V. at this time?

The leukemic cells populating J.V.'s blood are abnormal and incapable of fighting infection. Their rapid proliferation is suppressing red blood cell and megakaryocyte production in the bone marrow. J.V. is at substantial risk for life-threatening infections and bleeding complications. The goal of the initial chemotherapy is to clear the bone marrow and peripheral blood of all blast cells in the hope that normal blood cell components can regenerate.

INDUCTION THERAPY

Standard induction chemotherapy for AML includes an anthracycline (either daunorubicin or idarubicin) and cytarabine, an antimetabolite. One commonly used regimen includes idarubicin 12 mg/m^2/day on days 1 to 3 as an IV bolus injection, plus cytarabine 100 mg/m^2/day as a continuous IV infusion on days 1 to 7.[15–17] This combination (7 + 3) is one of the most effective chemotherapy regimens used to treat adult AML, with CR rates of 60% to 80%.[11] Continuous infusions of cytarabine are preferred because these regimens produce higher response rates than bolus injections during induction therapy.[18,19]

If a patient presents with a very high WBC count, he or she may experience complications associated with hyperviscosity of the blood (e.g., ringing ears, stroke, blindness, or headache as a result of impaired oxygen delivery to the central nervous system

[CNS], pulmonary infarction). Because it may take several days for cytarabine and idarubicin to substantially decrease the WBC count, the patient may receive hydroxyurea 2 to 4 grams orally or undergo leukapheresis to rapidly reduce the WBC count. Leukapheresis is not routinely done unless the patient is experiencing symptoms of hyperviscosity or has a WBC 100,000 cells/μL or greater on diagnosis.

Because J.V.'s initial WBC was 180,000 cells/μL, leukapheresis was initiated together with concomitant hydroxyurea 2 grams twice daily. Approximately 12 hours after initiating leukapheresis, J.V.'s WBC had decreased to 85,000 cells/μL and he was stable enough to proceed to induction therapy with idarubicin and cytarabine. The leukapheresis and hydroxyurea were subsequently discontinued.

Tretinoin and Arsenic Trioxide for Acute Promyelocytic Leukemia

CASE 96-1, QUESTION 3: Would induction therapy for other subtypes of AML differ from that described previously?

Induction therapy with 7 + 3 is standard for all types of AML, with one exception: APL (also called AML-M3). APL is uniquely characterized by the t(15;17) translocation that fuses the *PML* gene on chromosome 15 to the retinoic acid receptor-alpha (*RAR-α*) gene on chromosome 17. In clinical trials, tretinoin has induced complete remission in approximately 90% of patients with APL.[20] Serial bone marrow aspirations after initiation of tretinoin therapy demonstrate progressive differentiation without hypoplasia.[20,21] Unfortunately, tretinoin typically induces brief remissions. A number of trials have investigated combination treatment with chemotherapy and tretinoin.[22,23] Current evidence supports the use of concurrent tretinoin with arsenic trioxide[24–26] or an anthracycline with or without cytarabine for induction in the treatment of low-risk APL. For high-risk APL, conventional chemotherapy remains the standard of care.[24] In addition, postremission therapy should include at least two cycles of an anthracycline-based regimen. Maintenance therapy with intermittent tretinoin has been shown to decrease the relapse rate.[22,27]

Tretinoin therapy, although avoiding life-threatening myelosuppression, can produce significant toxicities, including the differentiation syndrome (formerly called retinoic acid syndrome), which manifests as fever, weight gain, respiratory distress, lung infiltrates, pleural or pericardial effusion, hypotension, and acute renal failure.[28,29] If this syndrome develops, corticosteroid therapy (dexamethasone 10 mg twice a day for 3 to 5 days with a taper over 2 weeks) should be initiated.[24,30] Tretinoin also causes dryness of the lining of the mouth, rectum, and skin; hair loss; skin rash; blepharoconjunctivitis; corneal erosions; muscle weakness; nail changes; depression; elevated liver enzymes; and high cholesterol. Despite the risk of serious complications and death during induction therapy, the long-term disease-free survival (DFS) rate of patients with APL is superior compared with other AML subtypes. Approximately 75% of patients who receive tretinoin-based induction and maintenance therapy are alive 3 to 5 years after diagnosis.[27]

Complications of Induction Therapy

Tumor Lysis Syndrome

CASE 96-1, QUESTION 4: Twenty-four hours after J.V.'s induction chemotherapy was initiated, the following laboratory values were obtained:

WBC count, 78,000 cells/μL
K, 5.3 mEq/L
Phosphorus, 6.0 mg/dL
Uric acid, 9.8 mg/dL
Calcium, 6.0 mg/dL
Creatinine, 1.6 mg/dL

Why have these laboratory values changed so suddenly? Could this have been minimized or prevented? How should these metabolic disturbances be managed?

J.V. presented with a very high number of peripheral blood blasts. On administration of chemotherapy, patients with a hypercellular bone marrow and high number of blast cells can have a rapid lysis of the blast cells and the release of cellular contents. This can result in tumor lysis syndrome (TLS), which is associated with metabolic abnormalities such as hyperuricemia, hyperphosphatemia, hypocalcemia, and uremia. These disturbances may lead to arrhythmias and acute renal failure. In most cases, TLS occurs 12 to 24 hours after chemotherapy is initiated. TLS may occur after therapy for other malignancies, particularly in those with a high tumor burden, such as high-grade lymphomas and ALL; it rarely occurs after therapy for solid tumors.

Patients should receive IV hydration (3–4 L/day) beginning 24 to 48 hours before chemotherapy to maintain renal perfusion, optimize the solubility of tumor lysis products, and compensate for fluid losses caused by fever or vomiting. Alkalinization of the urine with the addition of sodium bicarbonate to the IV fluids may also reduce or prevent uric acid from precipitating in the renal tubules and collection ducts by maintaining the urate in its ionized state, but is not currently recommended for all patients. This is because the increased pH may increase the risk of precipitating calcium phosphate in both soft tissue and kidney tubules, and it may aggravate hypocalcemia.[31,32]

Allopurinol, a xanthine oxidase inhibitor that blocks the production of uric acid, should be started before chemotherapy to prevent or minimize the complications of TLS. The recommended adult dosage is 300 to 600 mg/day. J.V.'s serum uric acid and electrolytes should be monitored at least 2 to 3 times a day for 24 to 48 hours after initiating chemotherapy. If severe abnormalities occur, more aggressive measures should be initiated. Allopurinol may be discontinued if the serum uric acid is within normal limits, the LDH has normalized, and the WBC count is low. Rasburicase, a recombinant urate oxidase product, can also be used as prophylaxis in patients who are at high risk of developing TLS or for the treatment of patients who present with or develop TLS. Rasburicase acts as a catalyst in the enzymatic oxidation of uric acid to allantoin, which is 5 to 10 times more soluble than uric acid and undergoes rapid renal excretion. The recommended dose of rasburicase for both prevention and treatment of TLS is 0.2 mg/kg/dose IV. Rasburicase results in a rapid reduction in serum uric acid (within 4 hours of administration) and is generally well tolerated.[33] In many adult centers, doses of 3 or 6 mg are commonly used.[34–38] Although rasburicase has demonstrated excellent efficacy and tolerability, its optimal role in the prevention and management of hyperuricemia in adults remains to be defined because of its high cost and lack of a randomized trial comparing its effect with other interventions.

Although J.V.'s serum potassium was low on admission, it has increased significantly as a result of TLS. For this reason, replacement potassium therapy by any method is not recommended before chemotherapy in patients in whom TLS is highly likely. In extreme circumstances, dialysis may be required to correct severe metabolic and electrolyte disturbances associated with TLS. J.V.'s kidneys continued to function throughout. Even though J.V.'s creatinine was above the normal range, his urine output did not decline substantially and he was able to proceed without further intervention.

CASE 96-1, QUESTION 5: J.V. received allopurinol therapy and aggressive hydration throughout his induction chemotherapy. The metabolic abnormalities gradually resolved as his WBC count declined and tumor lysis diminished. What other complications may occur during induction therapy and can they be treated?

Patients receiving cytarabine and idarubicin induction therapy develop profound anemia, granulocytopenia (e.g., WBC count <100 cells/μL), and thrombocytopenia (<20,000 platelets/μL) shortly after therapy is initiated, which usually persist for approximately 21 to 28 days. Additionally, all infectious complications must be considered life-threatening in severely immunocompromised patients such as J.V.

Filgrastim (granulocyte colony-stimulating factor [G-CSF]) and sargramostim (granulocyte-macrophage colony-stimulating factor [GM-CSF]) stimulate leukemic cells as well as normal granulocyte precursors in vitro; however, several studies have demonstrated that these agents, when used as an adjunct to AML chemotherapy, are safe and do not adversely affect disease outcome.[39,40] Most studies have demonstrated that colony-stimulating factors (CSFs) can modestly decrease the length of profound neutropenia and sometimes reduce the incidence of infection-related morbidity, the duration of systemic antibiotic and antifungal therapy, and the number of hospitalization days. Despite the reduction in short-term neutropenia-related complications, administration of CSFs after induction chemotherapy does not appear to have an impact on the rate of CR or the long-term outcomes of the disease. Refer to Chapter 94, Adverse Effects of Chemotherapy and Targeted Agents, for additional information about CSFs.

Severe thrombocytopenia may result in bleeding episodes that range in severity from oozing gums to massive hemorrhage. Serious bleeding complications can usually be avoided if patients receive platelet transfusions when their platelet counts decrease to less than 10,000 cells/μL or when patients experience bleeding.

Other common drug-induced complications that may occur during induction therapy include nausea and vomiting, mucositis, fever, and skin rash (see Chapter 22, Nausea and Vomiting, Chapter 55, Pain and Its Management, and Chapter 94, Adverse Effects of Chemotherapy and Targeted Therapy, for additional information and their management).

Postremission Therapy

CASE 96-1, QUESTION 6: After completion of his induction chemotherapy, J.V.'s WBC count fell to less than 100 cells/μL and his platelet count fell to 5,000 cells/μL. He received platelet transfusions approximately every 2 to 3 days to prevent bleeding complications. On day 9, he developed a fever of 38.8°C. He was started immediately on empiric, broad-spectrum antibiotic therapy for fever and neutropenia, and it subsequently resolved. On day 29, his WBC count was 5,600 cells/μL with a normal differential, and his platelet count was 168,000 cells/μL. He received packed red blood cell transfusions on two separate occasions when his Hgb fell to less than 7 mg/dL. A repeat bone marrow aspirate showed no evidence of persistent leukemia, and J.V. was told that his leukemia was in remission. Nevertheless, his hematologist recommended additional chemotherapy, and J.V. questions why this is necessary. Is postremission therapy necessary, and if so, what therapeutic options are available to J.V.?

RATIONALE

Although greater than 60% of patients treated for AML achieve CR after induction therapy, the median duration of the remission is only about 12 to 18 months, and only 20% to 40% of patients have a DFS exceeding 5 years.[41] Short remissions have been attributed to proliferation of clinically undetectable leukemic cells. Thus, the rationale for administering chemotherapy after remission is to eradicate these residual cells.

In adult AML, postremission therapy (also referred to as consolidation therapy) includes three to four cycles of chemotherapy. Clinical trials have shown that high-dose postremission therapy results in a higher percentage (30%–40%) of long-term (>2–5 years) disease-free survivors than either no or low-dose postremission chemotherapy in patients generally younger than 60 years of age.[42,43] Postremission therapy regimens usually include HiDAC alone or in combination with one or more agents such as an anthracycline or etoposide. Patients 60 years of age and older or those with comorbid disease may not be able to tolerate this intensive postremission therapy. In these circumstances, the risk of life-threatening toxicity may outweigh the potential benefits of postremission chemotherapy. Allogeneic HCT has also been studied in the postremission treatment of AML and is addressed in Chapter 101, Hematopoietic Cell Transplantation.

In conclusion, J.V. should receive consolidation therapy after HiDAC induction because this has been shown to give him the best chance of long-term survival. Additionally, because J.V. was fortunate enough to be diagnosed with good-risk disease, he will not require an allogeneic HCT. He will be followed closely with at least bimonthly CBCs and a bone marrow biopsy at least every year for 5 years after consolidation. This close follow-up is vital for catching relapse as early as possible with the intent of going immediately to an allogeneic HCT and minimizing additional reinduction therapy if relapse occurs.

HIGH-DOSE CYTARABINE

CASE 96-1, QUESTION 7: Because J.V. does not require an allogeneic HCT at this time, his hematologist recommends three courses of HiDAC as postremission therapy. One week after he was declared to be in remission, J.V. is readmitted to the hospital to receive HiDAC 3 grams/m² every 12 hours, over 3 hours, on days 1, 3, and 5. What are the potential acute and delayed toxicities associated with HiDAC, and how can these effects be prevented?

At conventional dosages of 100 to 200 mg/m²/day, adverse effects associated with cytarabine include myelosuppression, fever, and skin rashes. Occasionally, liver enzymes rise transiently. The side effect profile for HiDAC (>1 g/m²/day) by contrast is very different and can produce major cerebellar, ocular, and skin toxicities that present as rash or palmar-plantar erythrodysesthesia (PPE).[44,45]

Cerebellar and Ocular Toxicity

Cerebellar toxicity is a significant problem in patients receiving HiDAC therapy. See Chapter 94, Adverse Effects of Chemotherapy and Targeted Agents, for details regarding cerebellar toxicity. Ocular toxicity results from damage to the corneal epithelium, occurring when cytarabine penetrates the epithelium through the anterior chamber of the eye or tears. Symptoms include conjunctivitis, excessive lacrimation, "burning" ocular pain, photophobia, and blurred vision. Artificial tears (two drops every 4–6 hours) administered concurrently with HiDAC generally prevent these symptoms. Corticosteroid eye drops can be used as an alternative to artificial tears or if symptoms of conjunctivitis occur.[46]

ACUTE MYELOID LEUKEMIA IN THE ELDERLY

CASE 96-1, QUESTION 8: Would recommendations for induction and postremission therapy differ if J.V. were elderly (60 years of age or older)?

As mentioned earlier, the incidence of AML increases with advancing age. At age 40 years, there is only 1 case of AML per 100,000, but the annual incidence increases to 15% at ages older than 75 years. The prognosis of patients with AML is also directly related to age. Older patients are generally less able to tolerate intensive induction and postremission chemotherapy. Older patients often have comorbid medical conditions and a poor performance status, which are directly associated with worse outcomes with conventional AML therapy.[47,48]

Many single-institution and cooperative group studies exclude elderly patients with AML or treat them on a separate, less-intensive protocol. Elderly patients are often judged to be poor-risk candidates for intensive chemotherapy without objective review of available criteria. Because the median age of patients with AML and myelodysplastic syndrome is 67 years, the results of regimens studied in younger patients may not be applicable to the elderly. Some hematologists believe that it is most appropriate to offer older patients supportive care only, low-intensity therapy, or investigational treatment. Others believe that moderately intensive chemotherapy is beneficial in some candidates. However, most physicians feel uncomfortable offering intensive chemotherapy to elderly patients because of the high risk of induction mortality. Several studies have addressed the outcome of elderly patients.[49–56]

The selection of postremission therapy is difficult in elderly patients because they have a higher risk of morbidity and mortality, and more important, no clinical trials have demonstrated the benefit of postremission therapy specifically in the elderly. The intensity of the regimens must often be attenuated because there is risk of serious toxicities. This is particularly true with HiDAC therapy because of the increased risk of cerebellar toxicity in the elderly. Studies have shown that postremission therapy with low-dose cytarabine (100 mg/m^2 by continuous infusion for 5 days) is as effective as HiDAC and better tolerated in elderly patients.[42]

Refractory or Resistant Acute Myeloid Leukemia

CASE 96-2

QUESTION 1: A.W., a 55-year-old man, is approximately 40 days after induction therapy with 7 + 3. Initially, his counts recovered on day 25, and a bone marrow biopsy on day 28 revealed less than 5% blasts; therefore, he was in remission. Thereafter, a recent CBC showed a significant drop in his platelet count from 150,000 cells/μL on day 30 to 90,000 cells/μL 10 days later. A subsequent bone marrow biopsy reveals 60% blasts, confirming the diagnosis of relapsed AML. What are treatment options for A.W. at this time?

In younger patients, failure to achieve remission or disease relapse remains the major cause of treatment failure. This reflects both the failure of current salvage regimens and the absence of effective strategies to secure long-term DFS in those patients who achieve a second hematologic remission. A wide range of salvage options have been studied, but with less than 50% of patients achieving a second remission and median survival figures ranging from 3 to 12 months, there remains considerable room for improvement.[57]

The treatment of relapse in a patient younger than 75 years of age with a good performance status generally comprises one of several salvage options, including clofarabine, intermediate-dose cytarabine to HiDAC, or combination regimens such as fludarabine, cytarabine, and filgrastim (FLAG), or cladribine, cytarabine, and filgrastim (CLAG), followed by allogeneic HCT.

Future Chemotherapy in Acute Myeloid Leukemia: Targeted Therapies?

CASE 96-2, QUESTION 2: The results of A.W.'s cytogenetic and molecular analysis show that his leukemia is *FLT3* positive. What would be the next step for A.W.?

Whereas some clinical factors have an impact on response to treatment, it is the cytogenetic and molecular heterogeneity of AML that is the major determinant of treatment success or failure. For A.W., the finding that his AML has a mutation in the *FLT3* gene portends a poor likelihood of long-term survival without new therapies. The estimated 5-year survival is approximately 10% to 15% among patients with a *FLT3* internal tandem duplication mutation.[58] Therefore, it is an attractive molecular target for the development of new therapeutics. Although several molecules have been reported to have inhibitory activity against *FLT3*,[59,60] only a few have clinical trials to assess their efficacy in AML patients: lestaurtinib,[60–62] midostaurin,[63–65] quizartinib,[60] sorafenib,[66–68] and sunitinib.[69]

To date, *FLT3* inhibitors have shown only modest efficacy as monotherapy in patients with relapsed or refractory disease. However, in vitro studies suggest synergism between *FLT3* inhibitors and conventional chemotherapy. As a result, clinical trials are being conducted to investigate the combination of *FLT3* inhibitors in combination with conventional chemotherapy like daunorubicin and cytarabine along with hypomethylating agents such as decitabine and azacitidine with the hope of improving the outcomes of patients with *FLT3* mutations in both the initial and relapse setting.[70] Some trials have been shown that there may be an increased risk for toxicity and infectious complications with combination therapy and further research will be necessary to find improved combinations that can maximize efficacy and minimize adverse effects of treatment.[67,68]

For A.W., the best option would be to enroll in an investigational trial that incorporates one of the available *FLT3* inhibitors with chemotherapy. If a trial is not available, then HiDAC or a combination regimen containing clofarabine or fludarabine followed by an allogeneic HCT would be his best option.

CHRONIC MYELOGENOUS LEUKEMIA

Epidemiology and Pathophysiology

Chronic myeloid leukemia is a myeloproliferative disorder characterized by unregulated stem cell proliferation in the bone marrow and an increase in mature granulocytes in the peripheral blood. The disease is relatively rare, representing only 0.4% of all cancer cases and 12% of new leukemia cases.[71,72] The median age of diagnosis is 64 years and the current estimated 10-year survival rate is 80% to 90%.[71,73]

Clinical Presentation and Diagnosis

Approximately 30% to 50% of patients are asymptomatic at presentation with the most common physical finding of splenomegaly occurring in 50% to 60% of patients.[73] Additional symptoms may include fatigue, abdominal fullness, fever, anorexia, and weight loss. For many patients, the suspicion for CML is based solely on an abnormal CBC with a confirmatory bone marrow biopsy revealing the hallmark of CML, the Philadelphia (Ph) chromosome. Cytogenetic analysis reveals the presence of the Ph chromosome which is a translocation of chromosomes 9 and 22 t(9;22)(q34;q11).[74] This translocation creates a new protein (BCR-ABL) that has unregulated tyrosine kinase (TK) activity. The three major mechanisms that have been implicated in the malignant transformation by unregulated TK include abnormal cell cycling, inhibition of apoptosis, and increased proliferation of cells.[74] The natural history of CML can be divided into three distinct phases: chronic phase, accelerated phase, and blast phase. The greatest number of patients is diagnosed in chronic phase, which is the earliest phase of the disease.

Treatment

Hematopoietic stem cell transplant (HCT) remains the only curative therapy for CML. However, due to its substantial risks of morbidity and mortality, TK inhibitors have become first-line therapy in most patients. Patients in accelerated or blast phase at presentation or those progressing during TK inhibitor therapy are generally referred for HCT.[75] Though the exact timing of HCT remains controversial, patient outcomes are dependent on disease stage with patients having better 3-year survival rates if transplanted in chronic phase (91%) as compared to accelerated (59%) or blast phase.[76] Use of HCT for CML has declined since 2001 when the FDA approved the first TK inhibitor but the indication has remained for patients who fail these therapies or for those who obtain suboptimal response. Additional information regarding HCT for CML can be found in Chapter 101, Hematopoietic Cell Transplantation.

The primary goals of the TK inhibitors are to prevent progression from chronic phase to accelerated or blast phase while achieving a complete cytogenetic response (CCyR) within 12 to 18 months of therapy initiation.[74] Assessment of response to TK inhibitors is based on hematologic, cytogenetic, and molecular responses. Hematologic response (Table 96-2) is defined by normalization of peripheral blood, platelet count, and splenomegaly whereas cytogenetic response (Table 96-3) is determined by the amount of Ph chromosomes within the bone marrow. Complete molecular response is defined quantitatively by polymerase chain reaction assay with no detectable BCR-ABL mRNA identified to 4.5 logs below the standard baseline.[74]

Table 96-2
Definition of Hematologic Response in Chronic Myelogenous Leukemia

	Partial Response	Complete Response (CR)
Peripheral leukocyte count	$<10 \times 10^9$/L	$<10 \times 10^9$/L
Platelet count	<50% pretreatment count (but >450 $\times 10^9$/L)	$<450 \times 10^9$/L
Immature cells	Present	Absent
Splenomegaly	Present (but <50% pretreatment extent)	Absent

Adapted with permission from NCCN Clinical Practice Guidelines in Oncology (NCCN Guidelines). Chronic myelogenous leukemia. 2015;V1.2015. Available at: http://www.nccn.org/professionals/physician_gls/f_guidelines.asp. Accessed May 17, 2015.

Table 96-3
Definition of Cytogenetic Response in Chronic Myelogenous Leukemia

Cytogenetic Response	Philadelphia (Ph) Chromosome-Positive Metaphase Cells (%)
Complete	0
Partial	1–35
Major (includes complete and partial responses)	0–35
Minor	>35

Adapted with permission from NCCN Clinical Practice Guidelines in Oncology (NCCN Guidelines). Chronic myelogenous leukemia. 2015; V1.2015. Available at: http://www.nccn.org/professionals/physician_gls/f_guidelines.asp. Accessed May 17, 2015.

Cytogenetic monitoring is an evaluation of the reduction in Ph-positive (Ph+) metaphases within the bone marrow and is the most widely used technique for monitoring patient response to TK inhibitor therapy.[74] Quantitative polymerase chain reaction (QPCR) assay is widely used at three-month intervals to monitor BCR-ABL transcript levels for failure of treatment or recurrence of CML disease.[73,74] BCR-ABL transcript levels >10% signify medication failure and more than one measurement is needed to support a change to an alternative therapy.[77,78]

Signs and Symptoms

CASE 96-3

Question 1: S.E., a 66-year-old white woman, recently had a routine CBC drawn during her annual checkup. Her CBC showed a WBC count of 152,000 cells/μL with 15% basophils, a hematocrit of 32%, and a platelet count of 300,000 cells/μL. The only pertinent physical finding was splenomegaly. On further workup, a bone marrow aspirate revealed a hypercellular marrow with less than 10% blasts. Cytogenetic analysis confirmed a diagnosis of Ph+ CML in chronic phase. S.E. was asymptomatic at diagnosis even though her WBC count was very high. What are the possible clinical consequences of this abnormally high value?

S.E.'s labs indicate hyperleukocytosis, which would be a white blood count (WBC) greater than 100,000 cells/μL. A major consequence of hyperleukocytosis can be leukostasis which may manifest as dizziness, dyspnea, priapism, headaches, tinnitus, and cerebrovascular accidents.[79] Interestingly, S.E. is asymptomatic except for splenomegaly, which occurs in 50% to 60% of newly diagnosed CML patients. The presence of Ph chromosomes within S.E.'s bone marrow established her diagnosis as CML and the percentage of blasts and basophils confirm her stage. Less than 10% of blasts in the bone marrow and less than 20% of basophils in the peripheral blood space place S.E. in chronic phase using the WHO Criteria for CML Staging.[74] Please see Table 96-4 for these criteria.

Clinical Course and Prognosis

Case 96-3, Question 2: What is the prognosis for S.E. and others with newly diagnosed CML?

S.E. has been diagnosed with chronic-phase CML, which may range in duration from a few months to many years. Because symptoms can be nonspecific and relatively minor, CML may remain undiagnosed until patients progress into more advanced

Table 96-4

World Health Organization Criteria for CML staging

Chronic phase	■ None of the criteria for blast or accelerated phase
Accelerated phase	■ Blasts 10%–19% of peripheral white blood cells or nucleated bone marrow cells ■ Peripheral blood basophils >20% ■ Persistent thrombocytopenia (<100 × 10^9/L) not related to therapy or persistent thrombocytosis (>1,000 × 10^9/L) unresponsive to therapy ■ Increasing spleen size and increasing WBC count, unresponsive to therapy ■ Cytogenetic evidence of clonal evolution
Blast phase	■ Blasts >20% of peripheral white blood cells or nucleated bone marrow cells. ■ Extramedullary blast proliferation ■ Large foci or clusters of blasts in the bone marrow biopsy

Adapted from Vardiman JW et al. The World Health Organization (WHO) classification of myeloid neoplasms. *Blood*. 2002;100:2292.; Cortes J, Kantarjian H. How I treat newly diagnosed chronic-phase CML. *Blood*. 2012;120:1390.

stages. S.E.'s prognosis is good and her projected 10-year overall survival (OS) is 80% to 90% if treated with a TK inhibitor.[73]

If S.E.'s leukocytosis progresses despite therapy, an increased number of immature leukocytes (blasts) would appear in the peripheral blood signaling the second phase of the disease, the accelerated phase. The accelerated phase can progress quickly to blast phase if left untreated. The estimated 4-year OS is 40% to 55% for those patient with accelerated phase CML who are started on a TK inhibitor.[73] The final phase of the disease (blast phase or blast crisis) is defined as 20% or more blasts in the peripheral blood or bone marrow by the WHO or 30% or more blasts in the blood or bone marrow by the European Leukemia Net.[79] During this phase, CML is indistinguishable from AML with the exception of cytogenetics and is often refractory to conventional induction chemotherapy regimens for AML when treated. The median survival for patients in this phase is approximately 9 to 12 months with allogeneic HCT considered a good first-line treatment option.[73]

Treatment

CASE 96-3, QUESTION 3: What therapy is appropriate for S.E.'s chronic-phase disease?

With the approval of the TK inhibitors, treatment of CML has shifted towards disease management. Because S.E. was asymptomatic upon presentation, she will receive one of the TK inhibitors approved for first-line management of chronic-phase CML.

TYROSINE KINASE INHIBITORS

Imatinib, a first-generation TK inhibitor, inhibits BCR-ABL kinase, which prevents phosphorylation of substrates that are involved in regulating the cell cycle.[73] Approval was based on the pivotal International Randomized Study of Interferon and STI571 (IRIS) trial, which compared imatinib with the combination of interferon (IFN)-α plus low-dose cytarabine in patients with newly diagnosed CML in the chronic phase. A total of 1,106 patients were randomized to either imatinib (400 mg orally daily) or IFN/cytarabine.[80] All primary and secondary end points of the trial demonstrated superiority of imatinib versus IFN/cytarabine. Based on the results of this trial, TK inhibitors became standard of care as first-line therapy for patients with newly diagnosed CML in chronic phase. At the 8-year follow-up of the IRIS trial, 55% of the patients were still taking imatinib, and the estimated OS was 85%.[81] The most common toxicities reported with imatinib are superficial edema, nausea, muscle cramps, and rashes.

Dasatinib is a second-generation TK inhibitor that binds the BCR-ABL protein in the active confirmation, making it 325 times more potent than imatinib.[82] Approval was based on the international DASISION (Dasatinib versus imatinib study in treatment-naïve CML patients) trial, which compared dasatinib with imatinib in 519 patients with chronic-phase CML.[83] The primary objective of CCyR at 12 months and the secondary objective of a major molecular response by 12 months were statistically superior for dasatinib versus imatinib. Dasatinib demonstrates a similar safety profile compared with imatinib but with a higher incidence of pleural effusion, pulmonary hypertension, and thrombocytopenia as well as a lower incidence of rash and diarrhea.[82,84]

Nilotinib is a second-generation TK inhibitor which is structurally similar to imatinib but 30 times more potent as a result of an improved structural fit in the receptor pocket.[82] Approval was based on the international ENESTnd (Evaluating Nilotinib Efficacy And Safety In Clinical Trials—Newly Diagnosed Patients) trial, which randomly assigned 846 patients with chronic-phase CML to either imatinib or two strengths of nilotinib. At 12 months, both doses of nilotinib were statistically superior for molecular response and CCyR compared with imatinib.[85] Upon follow-up, molecular remission rates between the nilotinib arms and the imatinib arm increased from 6% to 10% at 1 year to approximately 21% to 23% by 5 years.[86] Nilotinib demonstrates a similar safety profile compared with the other TK inhibitors, with a higher incidence of rash, headache, pruritus, and alopecia and a lower incidence of nausea, diarrhea, vomiting, edema, and muscle spasm.[85]

Clinicians and patients must carefully evaluate the potential risks and benefits of each treatment modality to make the best therapeutic decision for each individual situation. The following online video discusses the current treatment strategies for CML: https://www.youtube.com/watch?v=Lvz-C6QRNQc. Because S.E. presented in chronic-phase CML, initiation of either imatinib, nilotinib, or dasatinib is an appropriate choice but S.E.'s physician chose to start her on imatinib 400 mg once daily.

Relapsed and Refractory Disease

CASE 96-3, QUESTION 4: On routine follow-up at 3 months, S.E. is found to have an 11% BCR-ABL transcript level. Her side effects and compliance were evaluated, where she was found to be 90% compliant due to nausea. She was counseled on medication adherence as well as what she can take for nausea and then re-evaluated at 6 months. The BCR-ABL level was measured at 15% and her bone marrow revealed 36% Ph+ metaphases. Because S.E.'s compliance had improved, the disease appeared to be resistant to imatinib. Imatinib was discontinued and dasatinib was initiated at 100 mg once a day. S.E. maintained low BCR-ABL assay levels until 12 months when her level was measured at 12%. Cytogenetic analysis revealed that S.E. had become resistant to dasatinib. What treatment options are available for S.E. at this time?

Primary cytogenetic resistance is defined as failure of the patient to achieve any level of cytogenetic response at 6 months, major cytogenetic response at 12 months, or CCyR at 18 months.[74] Just like 15% to 25% of all patients who start on imatinib therapy, S.E. appeared to have primary cytogenetic resistance at 6 months which prompted therapy discontinuation.[74] Medication adherence can affect resistance rates as well as outcomes.[87] In the ADAGIO study, one-third of patients were noted to be nonadherent to imatinib therapy with suboptimal response occurring in those with higher rates of nonadherence.[88] In S.E.'s case, adherence improved but nausea was problematic, so a dose escalation of imatinib from 400 mg daily to 400 mg twice daily did not seem prudent, given her symptoms and cytogenetics.

Although S.E. has relapsed, she has multiple options for treatment: dasatinib, nilotinib, bosutinib, ponatinib, and omacetaxine. Both nilotinib and bosutinib can be used for second-line treatment while ponatinib and omacetaxineare generally reserved for patients with resistance or intolerance to at least two TK inhibitor therapies. Bosutinib is a TK inhibitor that has shown effectiveness in patients with resistant CML. Of the 118 patients pretreated with imatinib, dasatinib, and/or nilotinib, 24% achieved CCyR with bosutinib, thus estimating the 2-year OS to be 83%.[89] Ponatinib is a TK inhibitor which can be used in patients who have exhausted other TK inhibitor options or in patients with a particular gene mutation (T315I).[74] In the PACE study, which evaluated heavily pretreated patients, major cytogenetic response was achieved and maintained for 2 years in 89% of patients and OS was 86% at 2 years.[90] Omacetaxine is a protein synthesis inhibitor which can be used in patients who have failed at least two TK inhibitors.[74] An average cytogenetic response of 20.5% was found in one study of TK inhibitor-resistant patients who were given omacetaxine.[91] S.E.'s next treatment would likely be based on her tolerability of the first two therapies, her genetic mutations, her concomitant medications, and her comorbidities.

CHRONIC LYMPHOCYTIC LEUKEMIA

Epidemiology and Pathophysiology

Chronic lymphocytic leukemia (CLL) is a disorder of mature but functionally incompetent lymphocytes. Lymphomas are also disorders of lymphocytes; therefore, some molecular abnormalities are shared between the diseases. CLL is the most common type of leukemia in adults, with approximately 15,000 new cases annually and 4,700 deaths.[92] It is a disease of the older population, and the median age at diagnosis is 65 years, with 90% of patients older than age 50 at diagnosis.[93,94] This disease is characterized by overproduction of functionally incompetent B-cell lymphocytes derived from a single stem cell clone in the bone marrow. These lymphocytes accumulate in the blood, bone marrow, lymph nodes, and spleen.

Presentation, Diagnosis, and Overview of Treatment

Chronic leukemias follow a relatively insidious onset and course compared with acute leukemias. Approximately 40% of patients are asymptomatic at presentation and are diagnosed by routine CBC (lymphocytosis, anemia, or thrombocytopenia).[95] Symptomatic patients commonly experience night sweats, fatigue, weight loss, fever, and painful lymphadenopathy. Patients often seek medical attention for infection caused by immune suppression or bleeding caused by thrombocytopenia.

Predicting the clinical course of CLL remains a challenge because some patients experience an indolent course and maintain a good quality of life, whereas others experience more aggressive disease and debilitation. Therefore, survival is variable and depends on the stage of disease at diagnosis. CLL is staged based on peripheral lymphocyte counts; enlargement of lymph nodes, liver, and spleen; and the presence of anemia or thrombocytopenia. The two most commonly used staging systems in clinical practice are the Rai classification and the Binet system. The Rai classification is used in national treatment guidelines and is shown in Table 96-5. The Rai classification is the most clinically useful because it contains prognostic information. Low-risk patients (Rai Stage 0) have survival similar to that of age-matched control subjects. Intermediate-risk patients (Stages I and II) have shorter survival, and high-risk patients (Stages III and IV) have poor prognosis.

Selection of therapy is in part determined by the presence or absence of cytogenetic abnormalities such as del(11q) or del(17p) which are unfavorable, comorbidities, and age. Common first-line therapies include targeted monoclonal antibodies in combination with chlorambucil, bendamustine, fludarabine, or cyclophosphamide. Relapsed disease is often treated with combinations of the same drugs used for initial treatment. Although patients with CLL may survive for years with suppressive therapies, these disorders are curable in only a fraction of patients who are candidates for immune-based approaches using chemotherapy and HCT.

Signs and Symptoms

CASE 96-4

QUESTION 1: G.R., a 66-year-old man, presents to his physician with a persistent semiproductive cough and increased fatigue. A routine CBC revealed an Hgb of 13.0 g/dL, a WBC count of 34,000 cells/μL (80% lymphocytes), and a platelet count of 175,000 cells/μL.

Table 96-5
Modified Rai Classification

Risk	Stage	Lymphocytosis[a]	Anemia[b]	Thrombocytopenia[c]	Lymphadenopathy	Hepatomegaly or Splenomegaly	Median Survival (Years)
Low	0	+	–	–	–	–	10
Intermediate	I	+	–	–	+	–	7
	II	+	–	–	±	+	
High	III	+	+	–	±	±	1.5–4
	IV	+	±	+	±	±	

[a]Lymphocytes >5,000/μL in peripheral blood and >30% of total cells in the bone marrow.
[b]Hemoglobin <11 g/dL excluding immune-mediated etiology.
[c]Platelets <100,000/μL.
Source: Rai KR et al. Clinical staging of chronic lymphocytic leukemia. *Blood*. 1975;46:219.

Blood pressure was 120/70 mm Hg, heart rate 64 beats/minute, and respiratory rate 23 breaths/minute. He was afebrile. Physical examination was unremarkable. He was prescribed azithromycin for possible community-acquired pneumonia and scheduled for a return visit in 3 weeks. At that time, his CBC results were Hgb 13.2 g/dL, WBC count 32,000 cells/μL (82% lymphocytes), and platelets 168,000 cells/μL. Physical examination was unchanged, the chest radiograph was clear, and his cough had resolved. G.R. was referred to a hematologist for evaluation of his persistent lymphocytosis. What is the most likely cause of persistent lymphocytosis in G.R.?

CLL is usually included in the differential diagnosis of any adult with persistent lymphocytosis (>5,000 lymphocytes/μL in peripheral blood). Additional causes of lymphocytosis include transient reactions to acute infections such as influenza or mononucleosis, as well as other hematologic malignancies.

To differentiate between benign and malignant lymphocytosis, examination of the peripheral blood or bone marrow morphology may be required. Patients with CLL commonly have lymphocytosis in both the peripheral blood and bone marrow, whereas patients with other disorders have a high percentage of atypical lymphocytes in the peripheral blood alone. The absence of fever or additional signs of infection without significant diagnostic or physical examination findings, together with the presence of mature peripheral blood lymphocytes, make CLL the most likely diagnosis for G.R. Immunophenotyping and cytogenetics of involved cells are required to establish the diagnosis, to provide prognostic information, and to determine therapy. Bone marrow biopsy with aspirate may be useful to determine the definitive diagnosis.[95]

Staging and Prognosis

CASE 96-4, QUESTION 2: G.R.'s bone marrow examination reveals normal cellularity with greater than 40% of nucleated cells lymphocytes. The immunophenotype indicates that peripheral blood lymphocytes are predominately B cells and are positive for CD5, CD19, and CD20. A diagnosis of CLL is confirmed. Is G.R.'s presentation consistent with CLL? What is the prognosis for G.R.'s disease? What treatment is indicated at this time? G.R.'s cells were sent for routine cytogenetic analysis, which revealed a chromosome abnormality (deletion 11q). How does this affect his management?

G.R. has fatigue, infection, and lymphocytosis without lymphadenopathy, and these are consistent with low-risk CLL based on his modified Rai stage. Given his stage, G.R. has an expected survival of at least 10 years.[93,96]

An accepted treatment modality for early-stage disease includes a conservative, watchful waiting approach. No clear advantage has been demonstrated in treating asymptomatic patients in early-stage disease with alkylator-based chemotherapy as compared with deferred treatment.[97] The survival of patients with smoldering CLL is similar to an age- and sex-matched normal population.[98,99]

There is significant heterogeneity in the clinical course of CLL that is in part attributable to the biologic differences between tumors. Scientific advances have led to the discovery of chromosomal abnormalities (deletions 11q or 17p), gene mutations (unmutated immunoglobulin variable region and p53), and serum or cell surface markers (increased β_2 microglobulin, zeta-associated protein-70, and CD38 expression) that may confer poor prognosis.[100–102] The deletion 13q is the most common cytogenetic abnormality, occurring in 55% of patients, and it has a favorable prognosis (survival >10 years). The deletion 11q and deletion 17p occur in 18% and 7%, respectively, with shorter survival times of approximately 7 and 3 years, respectively. Current national guidelines take into account some of these factors in their treatment recommendations.

Despite his early stage by the modified Rai classification, G.R. had an 11q deletion, conferring a worse prognosis; he would be encouraged to start treatment. However, as a result of having minimal symptoms, G.R. chooses to delay treatment until he becomes symptomatic.

Treatment

CASE 96-4, QUESTION 3: G.R. returns to the hematologist every 3 months and has no new symptoms or infectious complications for about 2 years. At that time, physical examination reveals enlargement of cervical, inguinal, and axillary lymph nodes; hepatomegaly; and splenomegaly. His WBC has increased from 34,000 cells/μL 6 months ago to 68,000 cells/μL today (85% lymphocytes). His Hgb is 11.7 g/dL, and his platelet count is 140,000 cells/μL. What treatment is now indicated?

Indications for treatment initiation in CLL include significant anemia or thrombocytopenia, progressive disease demonstrated by lymphadenopathy, hepatomegaly, splenomegaly, a lymphocyte doubling time of less than 6 months, persistent B symptoms (fever, night sweats, and weight loss), threatened end-organ function, and recurrent infection. Patient performance status, comorbid conditions, pharmacoeconomic variables, and social support should all be taken into consideration when selecting treatment. Cytogenetic results will also be considered. Because G.R. has experienced significant lymphadenopathy and hepatosplenomegaly, he should initiate treatment at this time to prevent further deterioration of his hematologic and immune function.

INITIAL THERAPY

Chlorambucil

Therapy for CLL has historically included use of an alkylating agent, most often oral chlorambucil or cyclophosphamide, with or without prednisone. A variety of daily and intermittent dosing schedules have been reported. The overall response (OR) rate to chlorambucil was approximately 40% to 60%, but only 3% to 5% achieved a CR.[94] Chlorambucil use has diminished, and the use of purine analogs, such as fludarabine, is more common in clinical practice; however, chlorambucil is recommended for patients older than or equal to 70 years, or in younger patients if they have significant comorbidities.[101] Chlorambucil is often used in combination with monoclonal antibodies.[101]

Fludarabine

Fludarabine is an active agent in the treatment of CLL. Fludarabine monotherapy at a dose range of 25 to 30 mg/m^2/dose IV × 5 days has shown a 70% to 80% OR rate, and CR rates of 20% to 30% with increased progression-free survival (PFS).[103–107] Fludarabine may have improved OS compared with chlorambucil, but results are inconsistent across studies.[107,108] Toxicities associated with fludarabine are typically mild and include fever and immunosuppression. Increased incidence of infection and autoimmune hemolytic anemia are also associated with fludarabine therapy. Infection prophylaxis should be considered in elderly patients and patients with advanced disease or renal dysfunction.

Fludarabine has been combined with other chemotherapy and monoclonal antibodies, including cyclophosphamide and rituximab, in an effort to prevent multidrug resistance and increase response. Although combination regimens including fludarabine have demonstrated higher response rates and PFS, no difference in OS has been consistently demonstrated.[109–110] Additional toxicities of the combination regimens include higher rates of leukopenia, thrombocytopenia, nausea, vomiting, and alopecia.

Bendamustine

Bendamustine, a nitrogen mustard/alkylating agent, was approved in 2008 for the treatment of CLL. In clinical studies, it has been shown to be superior to chlorambucil with OR and CR rates of 68% and 31%, respectively.[111] A typical dose and schedule is 100 mg/m^2 IV on days 1 and 2. Toxicities include infusion reactions and myelosuppression. It is often used in combination with rituximab and primarily in patients older than or equal to 70 years or those with comorbidities.[101]

Rituximab

Rituximab is a chimeric human–murine anti-CD20 monoclonal antibody. The CD20 surface antigen is expressed on a high percentage of CLL cells. Rituximab monotherapy as initial therapy for untreated patients at a dose of 375 mg/m^2 weekly for four doses yielded OR rates of 58% and CR rates of 9%; these are lower than those seen with cytotoxic therapy, with a disappointing duration of response.[112] Therefore, rituximab monotherapy is reserved for patients with significant comorbidity. Generally, it is used in combination therapy with cytotoxic agents.

Combination Regimens

A regimen for initial treatment is the combination of FCR. In a study of first-line treatment of CLL, patients were treated with fludarabine 25 mg/m^2 IV on days 1 to 3, cyclophosphamide 250 mg/m^2 IV on days 1 to 3, and rituximab 375 mg/m^2 IV on day 1 of cycle 1, escalated to 500 mg/m^2 in subsequent cycles. OR rate was 96%. Toxicity of this regimen included infusion-related reactions, nausea, vomiting, and myelosuppression. Grade 3 or 4 neutropenia was frequently noted with an infection rate of 20%.[113] The FCR regimen is recommended in patients younger than 70 years without significant comorbidities or older patients without comorbidities, and in any patient with the unfavorable del(17p) cytogenetic abnormality.[93]

Results for a bendamustine plus rituximab (BR) combination regimen have recently been reported. In a study of 117 patients with previously untreated CLL, patients were given bendamustine 90 mg/m^2 IV on days 1 and 2, and rituximab 375 mg/m^2 IV on day 1 of cycle 1, escalated to 500 mg/m^2 in subsequent cycles for up to 6 cycles. OR was 90% and CR 33%.[114] Trials are ongoing to compare this combination with FCR as first-line therapy for CLL patients who are able to tolerate combination chemotherapy. A published interim analysis showed an ORR that was identical in both groups at 98%. However, the adverse effect profile favored BR with a higher rate of toxicity in the FCR group (91% for FCR vs. 79% for BR).[115] The BR regimen, like chlorambucil with or without prednisone, is commonly used in patients older than or equal to 70 years or in younger patients with comorbidities.[101]

In summary, first-line therapy for patients older than or equal to 70 years old or with significant comorbidities generally includes BR or chlorambucil. For younger patients without comorbidities, three-drug combinations such as FCR may be offered. G.R. is now 68 years old with no significant comorbidities and is likely to tolerate treatment with FCR.

RELAPSED OR REFRACTORY THERAPY

CASE 96-4, QUESTION 4: G.R. receives FCR as initial CLL therapy. After the third cycle, he has complete regression of his lymphadenopathy and hepatosplenomegaly, and his WBC count decreases to 9,000 cells/μL. He finishes six cycles in total. G.R. comes to clinic 1.5 years after completion of therapy. A CBC is obtained that reveals a WBC count of 55,000 cells/μL (70% lymphocytes), Hgb of 10 g/dL, and platelet count of 90,000 cells/μL. On physical examination, G.R. is found to have cervical, inguinal, and axillary lymphadenopathy with no palpable splenomegaly. He complains of excessive fatigue and fever. Therefore, G.R. has recurrent disease. What therapies may be helpful to him at this point?

Second-line therapy should be selected based on criteria similar to those used for initial management. Relapsed patients are classified as treatment-sensitive if the disease relapses more than 3 years after FCR treatment.[101] G.R.'s relapse occurred less than 2 years from completion of FCR therapy. He is classified as refractory to his first-line regimen. He is still younger than 70 years old with minimal comorbidities and is a candidate for aggressive second-line treatment.

TREATMENT SENSITIVE

Treatment-sensitive patients are retreated with the same regimen given for first-line therapy as long as they are expected to tolerate treatment. For patients who are older than 70 years or those who have comorbidities, the regimen may be changed to one with less toxicity. These less toxic regimens include dose-reduced FCR, obinituzumab, chlorambucil, ibrutinib, BR, single-agent rituximab, or cyclophosphamide–prednisone–rituximab.[101]

TREATMENT REFRACTORY

Treatment-refractory patients will be offered a regimen containing at least one anticancer agent not previously given. For patients older than 70 years with comorbidities, options include chemo-immunotherapy combinations: dose-reduced FCR, dose-reduced pentostatin–cyclophosphamide–rituximab, rituximab–chlorambucil, BR, and high-dose methylprednisolone–rituximab. Other options are ofatumumab, obinutuzumab, and ibrutinib. Patients younger than 70 years old without significant comorbidities have several options, including combination chemotherapy, chemoimmuno-therapy, ibrutinib, and monoclonal antibodies and consideration of allogeneic HCT.[101]

In conclusion, G.R.'s disease relapsed within 18 months of completing initial therapy and is treatment refractory; therefore, he should receive a second-line regimen, which includes an agent to which he has not been previously exposed. G.R. received FCR as his initial treatment; therefore, the BR regimen is a good choice for him now. In addition, he is younger than 70, in relatively good health, and should tolerate combination therapy.

Infectious Complications

CASE 96-4, QUESTION 5: Six weeks after the initiation of BR, G.R. complains of progressive shortness of breath and fever. On questioning, he reveals that he quit taking his trimethoprim–sulfamethoxazole and valacyclovir because "I felt fine." Radiography of the chest reveals bilateral infiltrates. G.R. is admitted to the hospital for further evaluation and treatment. A CBC reveals a WBC count of 22,000 cells/μL (80% lymphocytes) and an absolute neutrophil count of 800 cells/μL, Hgb of 11 g/dL, and platelet count of 70,000 cells/μL. Quantification of serum immunoglobulins reveals profound hypogammaglobulinemia. What are the possible causes of G.R.'s pneumonia, and what treatment is indicated?

Infections contribute significantly to morbidity and mortality in patients with CLL. The immune compromise of CLL is attributable to immunoglobulin deficiency, abnormal T-cell function, neutropenia, and chemotherapy, which contribute to the increased rate of both common and opportunistic infections.[116] Up to 80% of patients will develop an infectious complication; therefore, the use of IV immune globulin, antibacterials (trimethoprim–sulfamethoxazole), and antivirals (acyclovir for herpes simplex virus), and vaccinations (influenza, pneumococcal) are common. Opportunistic infections are particularly common in patients receiving a purine analog. The use of supplemental IV immune globulin for prophylaxis of future infection is often used in patients with low immunoglobulin levels (IgG $<$500 mg/dL) and recurrent infections requiring hospitalization.[117]

Hospitalization is warranted for G.R. so he can receive broad-spectrum antimicrobials for neutropenic fever and a thorough workup for opportunistic etiologies. Because G.R. has a significant pulmonary infection requiring hospitalization with a documented hypogammaglobulinemia, prophylactic IV immune globulin therapy should be considered to prevent future infections.

MULTIPLE MYELOMA

Incidence and Epidemiology

Multiple myeloma (MM) is defined as a malignancy of "plasma cells," terminally differentiated B lymphocytes responsible for the production of antibodies and for the rapid immune response to antigen exposure.[118,119] In the United States, an estimated 26,850 new cases of MM will be diagnosed in 2015, accounting for 1% of all cancers.[120] MM occurs nearly twice as often in African-Americans compared to whites, is slightly more common in males than in females, and is diagnosed at a median age of 65 years.[118,121]

Pathophysiology

Although MM may present as a de novo diagnosis, most cases are believed to arise from a benign precursor condition known as monoclonal gammopathy of undetermined significance (MGUS). It is characterized by the accumulation of abnormal clonal plasma cells and may be differentiated from MM by the serum concentration of M-protein (<3 g/dL) and the lack of clinical manifestations typically associated with MM (osteolytic bone lesions, hypercalcemia, renal dysfunction, etc.).[122,123] By way of a complex multistep process involving a variety of genetic events and changes in the plasma cell's microenvironment, a transformation from MGUS to smoldering MM or symptomatic MM occurs at a rate of approximately 1% of patients/year.[124,125] Cellular events promoting the growth of malignant plasma cells, i.e., induction of angiogenesis, suppression of immunity, and the production of osteoclast-activating factors (e.g., IL-6, tumor necrosis factor, parathyroid hormone-related peptide), occur during the conversion of benign plasma cells to their malignant counterparts.[126,127]

Smoldering myeloma represents an indolent form of the disease in which patients produce M-protein ≥3 g/dL and/or have 10% to 60% plasma cells in the bone marrow, but remain asymptomatic.[122,126] Smoldering myeloma progresses to MM at a rate of 10%/year for the first 5 years after diagnosis, 3%/year for the next 5 years, and 1%/year for the next 10 years.[126]

Clinical Presentation

Patients presenting initially with symptomatic MM frequently complain of bone pain, fatigue, and recurrent infections. Patients may also have end-organ damage, including hyper<u>c</u>alcemia, <u>r</u>enal dysfunction, <u>a</u>nemia, and <u>b</u>one lesions (which may be remembered using the mnemonic *CRAB*). Because MM is not generally considered to be a curable malignancy, the goal of treatment is to achieve and maintain a clinical response through the combination of induction therapy, hematopoietic stem cell transplant (HCT), and maintenance therapy. See the following video for more general information on MM: http://www.youtube.com/watch?v=uxdgFn1ZMRk.

CASE 96-5

QUESTION 1: B.B. is a 62-year-old, otherwise healthy man who presents with acute back pain after performing light maintenance work. He was initially prescribed nonsteroidal anti-inflammatory drugs (NSAIDs) but has achieved little relief. Computed tomography (CT) scan of the spine reveals osteolytic bone lesions from T6 to T11. Further workup reveals an Hgb of 7 g/dL, serum calcium of 11.8 mg/dL, and serum creatinine of 1.9 mg/dL. Serum and urine protein electrophoresis reveals M-protein typed as IgG-kappa of 5.3 g/dL. A serum β_2 microglobulin was 4.4 mg/L. Bone marrow biopsy reveals 90% plasma cells, and cytogenetics reveal that he has a t(4;14) translocation. Skeletal survey shows additional lesions in the ribs. A diagnosis of MM Stage II is made. Is this presentation consistent with the diagnosis of MM?

B.B. presents with a number of the classic features of MM. Bone pain and skeletal disease are common and occur when plasma cells infiltrate the bone marrow and secrete osteoclast-activating factors. Plain radiographic films will reveal osteopenia or multiple osteolytic bone lesions. Patients with smoldering MM should have more extensive imaging scans done with magnetic resonance imaging (MRI), positron emission tomography (PET), and/or CT, to help determine the presence of MM bone lesions.[122] Hypercalcemia and pathologic fractures often accompany the osteolytic lesions. When plasma cells infiltrate the bone marrow, they can also lead to a normocytic normochromic anemia in up to 70% of patients, although neutropenia and thrombocytopenia are relatively rare. Renal dysfunction is generally attributable to deposition of kappa or lambda light chains of immunoglobulin in the distal tubule, and up to 40% of patients have or will develop renal insufficiency with the disease.[128] Renal dysfunction can be further complicated by dehydration secondary to hypercalcemia, the use of NSAIDs, and the use of contrast dyes in radiographic evaluation. B.B. should receive hydration to restore euvolemia and reduce his calcium; he should avoid NSAIDs and other nephrotoxic therapies. Excessive immunoglobulin production may also cause hyperviscosity syndrome, which may lead to CNS, renal, cardiac, or pulmonary symptoms. Plasmapheresis may be used to alleviate life-threatening cases. Patients may experience recurrent infections as a result of depressed production of other immunoglobulin classes, leading to an inability to opsonize bacteria.

Diagnosis, Staging, and Risk Stratification

Diagnostic criteria for plasma cell disorders are shown in Table 96-6. B.B. clearly meets the criteria for MM. Two staging systems have been used for patients with MM: the older Durie–Salmon system, developed in 1975, and the newer international staging system (ISS).[122,129] The ISS was validated in a large international study demonstrating that prognosis can be predicted reliably from serum β_2 microglobulin (a light chain protein expressed on all nucleated cells) and albumin (Table 96-7). Based on the ISS, B.B. has Stage II MM. Further classifying patients as having standard or high-risk disease based on cytogenetic markers can also help determine a patient's prognosis and help guide treatment decisions.[130]

Treatment

INITIAL THERAPY

Patients with MM are candidates for systemic chemotherapy (Table 96-8). The most effective treatment is induction followed by autologous HCT; therefore, eligibility for HCT helps determine the most appropriate treatment option.[131] Determination of HCT eligibility includes consideration of patient age (typically 65 years of age or younger) and comorbidities. In the case of B.B., his age (62 years) and relative good health make him a candidate for further consideration of HCT as a component of his MM management. Those who are eligible for HCT should not be

Table 96-6
Diagnostic Criteria for Plasma Cell Disorders

Multiple Myeloma
Biopsy-proven plasmacytoma or bone marrow clonal plasmacytosis ≥10%, plus 1 or more of the following:
1. End-organ damage (CRAB features) related to plasma cell proliferation, including the following:
Elevated calcium (1 mg/dL above the upper limit of the normal range, or >11 mg/dL)
Renal insufficiency (creatinine >2 mg/dL or creatinine clearance <40 mL/minute)
Anemia (2 g/dL below the lower limit of normal range, or <10 g/dL)
Bone lesions (lytic lesions or osteoporosis with compression fractures)
2. Presence of any one of the following biomarkers:
Bone marrow clonal plasmacytosis ≥60%
Serum free light chain ratio ≥100 (involved: uninvolved)
MRI studies with >1 lesion of ≥5 mm in size
Asymptomatic (Smoldering) Multiple Myeloma
1. Serum monoclonal immunoglobulin ≥3 g/dL or urine monoclonal protein ≥500 mg/24 hours and/or clonal bone marrow plasmacytosis 10%–60%
2. No end-organ damage related to plasma cell proliferation
Monoclonal Gammopathy of Undetermined Significance (MGUS)
1. Serum monoclonal immunoglobulin <3 g/dL
2. Bone marrow plasma cells <10%
3. No end-organ damage related to plasma cell proliferation

Source: Rajkumar SV, et al. International Myeloma Working Group updated criteria for the diagnosis of multiple myeloma. *Lancet Oncol*. 2014;15:e538.[122]

Table 96-7
International Staging System for Multiple Myeloma

Stage I—β_2 microglobulin <3.5 mg/L and serum albumin ≥3.5 g/dL
Stage II—neither Stage I nor Stage III
Stage III—β_2 microglobulin ≥5.5 mg/L

Source: Greipp PR et al. International staging system for multiple myeloma. *J Clin Oncol*. 2005;23:3412.[129]

treated with agents such as melphalan, which may compromise the ability to collect a sufficient number of hematopoietic stem cells necessary to perform the autologous HCT. More aggressive 3 drug combination regimens may be advantageous in high-risk patients to help increase the chance of developing a CR.[130]

CASE 96-5, QUESTION 2: The decision is made to begin B.B. on treatment with a regimen including bortezomib, lenalidomide, and dexamethasone. What advantages and disadvantages does this regimen have compared with others?

The proteasome inhibitor bortezomib acts by inhibiting the 26S proteasome, a multienzyme complex responsible for regulation of proteins that promote cell survival, stimulate growth, and reduce susceptibility to programmed cell death.[146] Bortezomib is commonly used in combination with thalidomide, lenalidomide, cyclophosphamide, and/or dexamethasone. Patients should be monitored for common adverse events, including fatigue, diarrhea, mild nausea, thrombocytopenia, and peripheral neuropathy (the most common cause of discontinuation of bortezomib in clinical trials).[133] Subcutaneous administration significantly reduces the incidence of neuropathy and may be a preferred route for many patients.[147,148] Reactivation of herpes zoster has been observed in greater than 10% of patients treated with bortezomib; therefore, concomitant antiviral prophylaxis should be utilized.[149,150] An additional benefit of bortezomib is the ability to induce responses in patients with del(13) and t(4;14).[151,152] B.B. has the t(4;14) and would benefit from the use of bortezomib.

Thalidomide and lenalidomide are immunomodulatory drugs (IMiDs) commonly used in the initial treatment of MM. They possess complex antiangiogenic, anti-inflammatory, and immunomodulatory properties that make them active in MM.[153] Common adverse effects of lenalidomide include hematologic toxicities, muscle weakness, fatigue, and rash.[154] Several studies have also revealed a small but concerning risk of secondary malignancies, which may be associated with combined oral melphalan use.[155] Although this concern should not prohibit the use of lenalidomide, patients should be made aware of this risk. In comparison with lenalidomide, thalidomide is less potent and has a less favorable toxicity profile with sedation and peripheral neuropathy being common in addition to constipation. Both thalidomide and lenalidomide have a risk of thromboembolism, and venous thrombotic embolism prophylaxis is recommended.[156] Thalidomide and lenalidomide are only available via a restricted access prescription programs due to the risk of teratogenicity.

Dexamethasone is an active treatment option for MM, mostly used in combination regimens. It does have significant adverse effects, including hyperglycemia, insomnia, and increased infection risk. Although response rates are increased with higher doses, lower doses are often more beneficial. When combined with lenalidomide, low-dose dexamethasone (120 mg/cycle) improved 1-year OS compared to high-dose dexamethasone (480 mg/cycle) (96% vs. 87%, $p = 0.0002$).[131]

Several 2 or 3 drug combination regimens are effective and appropriate for the initial treatment of MM. The combination of lenalidomide, bortezomib, and dexamethasone (RVD) has demonstrated response rates up to 100% in patients with newly diagnosed MM and is well tolerated with sensory neuropathy, fatigue, and hematologic toxicities being the most commonly reported.[134] The most current National Comprehensive Cancer Network (NCCN) Clinical Practice Guidelines In Oncology (NCCN Guidelines) recommend RVD as a preferred initial induction therapy option along with several other regimens, some of which are outlined in Table 96-8.[157] Independent of the choice of induction regimen, patients commonly receive 3 to 6 cycles of treatment before HCT.[158]

In patients ineligible for autologous HCT, melphalan-based regimens are appropriate for induction therapy. Melphalan and prednisone (MP), combined with either bortezomib (MPB), thalidomide (MPT), or lenalidomide (MPR), have all been proven to be more effective than MP alone.[137–139] The MPT regimen may have limited utility due to the increased risk of toxicities compared to MP, including thromboembolism, neuropathy, constipation, and infection. In addition to melphalan-based regimens, lenalidomide plus low-dose dexamethasone or bortezomib plus dexamethasone are also considered preferred initial induction therapy options for transplant ineligible MM.[157]

HEMATOPOIETIC CELL TRANSPLANTATION

Efforts to improve the outcome of MM treatment have led to the investigation of high-dose chemotherapy (e.g., melphalan 200 mg/m^2) with autologous HCT. Randomized comparisons of autologous HCT and conventional chemotherapy in previously untreated patients demonstrated higher response rates and improved survival

Table 96-8
Multiple Myeloma Treatment Regimens

Regimen[a]	Agents
Induction Therapy	
Eligible for High-Dose Chemotherapy with Autologous HCT	
Rd[b,c,132]	Lenalidomide 25mg PO daily, days 1–21 Dexamethasone 40mg PO daily, days 1, 8, 15, and 22 Repeat cycle every 28 days
BD[d,130,133]	Bortezomib 1.3 mg/m² IV days 1, 4, 8, and 11 Dexamethasone 20 mg PO daily, days 1–2, 4–5, 8–9, 11–12 Repeat cycle every 21 days
RVD[b,c,d,134]	Lenalidomide 25 mg PO daily, days 1–14 Bortezomib 1.3 mg/m² IV days 1, 4, 8 and 11 Dexamethasone 20 mg PO daily, days 1–2, 4–5, 8–9, 11–12 Repeat cycle every 21 days
VTD[b,d,135]	Bortezomib 1.3 mg/m² IV days 1, 4, 8, and 11 Thalidomide 200 mg PO daily, days 1–21 Dexamethasone 40 mg PO daily, days 1–4 and 9–12 Repeat cycle every 21 days
CyBorD[d,130,136]	Cyclophosphamide 300 mg/m² PO daily, days 1, 8, 15, and 22 Bortezomib 1.3 mg/m² IV days 1, 8, 15, and 22 Dexamethasone 40 mg PO daily, days 1, 8, 15, and 22 Repeat cycle every 28 days
Ineligible for High-Dose Chemotherapy with Autologous HCT	
MPB[d,137]	Melphalan 9 mg/m² PO daily, days 1–4 Prednisone 60 mg/m² PO daily, days 1–4 Bortezomib 1.3 mg/m² IV days 1, 4, 8, 11, 22, 25, 29, 32 for the first 4 cycles, then days 1, 8, 22, 29 in subsequent cycles Repeat cycle every 42 days
MPR[b,c,138]	Melphalan 0.18 mg/m² PO daily, days 1–4 Prednisone 2 mg/kg PO daily, days 1–4 Lenalidomide 10 mg PO daily, days 1–21 Repeat cycle every 28 days
MPT[b,139]	Melphalan 4 mg/m² PO daily, days 1–7 Prednisone 40 mg/m² PO daily, days 1–7 Thalidomide 100 mg PO daily, days 1–28 Repeat cycle every 28 days
Rd[b,c] and BD[d] are also appropriate treatment options for patients ineligible for HCT	
Salvage Therapy	
Carfilzomib + dexamethasone ± lenalidomide[b,d,140,141]	Carfilzomib 20 mg/m² (days 1 and 2 of cycle 1) or 27 mg/m² (doses thereafter) IV days 1, 2, 8, 9, 15, and 16 Dexamethasone 40mg PO daily, days 1, 8, 15, and 22 Lenalidomide 25 mg PO daily, days 1–21 Repeat cycle every 28 days
Pomalidomide + dexamethasone[b,142,143]	Pomalidomide 4 mg PO daily, days 1–21 Dexamethasone 40 mg PO daily, days 1, 8, 15, and 22 Repeat cycle every 28 days
Panobinostat + bortezomib + dexamethasone[d,144]	Panobinostat 20 mg PO daily, days 1, 3, 5, 8, 10, and 12 Bortezomib 1.3 mg/m² IV days 1, 4, 8, and 11 Dexamethasone 20 mg PO daily, days 1, 2, 4, 5, 8, 9, 11, and 12 Repeat cycle every 21 days
Bortezomib + liposomal doxorubicin[d,145]	Bortezomib 1.3 mg/m² IV days 1, 4, 8, and 11 Liposomal doxorubicin 30 mg/m² IV once on day 4 Repeat cycle every 21 days
Additional single or combination regimens, including several utilized as induction treatments, can also be appropriate salvage therapy options	

[a]List of regimens is not all inclusive. Additional combination regimens exist that may be appropriate for the treatment of MM.
[b]Antithrombotic prophylaxis is recommended when on lenalidomide, pomalidomide, or thalidomide, especially when combined with glucocorticosteroids.
[c]Lenalidomide dose adjustments are recommended if creatinine clearance is <50 mL/minute.
[d]Antiviral prophylaxis against herpes virus is recommended while on bortezomib or carfilzomib.

HCT, hematopoietic cell transplantation; IV, intravenously; PO, orally.

in patients assigned to receive autologous HCT.[159–162] Younger age, chemosensitive disease, and fewer pretransplant therapies have emerged as important predictive factors for response to autologous HCT.[131] Currently, autologous HCT is considered an integral component of the overall treatment of MM and should be performed in conjunction with induction therapy in eligible patients.[163] The use of allogeneic HCT in MM is a potentially curative option, although it has shown mixed results and is often associated with excessive morbidity and mortality (see Chapter 101, Hematopoietic Cell Transplantation).[164–166] B.B. will receive three cycles of RVD and will be evaluated for HCT.

BISPHOSPHONATES

CASE 96-5, QUESTION 3: Zoledronic acid 4 mg IV over 15 minutes every 28 days is ordered for B.B. What is the rationale for bisphosphonate therapy in the presence of normal serum calcium? What benefits and toxicities are associated with bisphosphonate therapy?

Osteolytic bone lesions or osteopenia occurs in nearly 80% of all patients with MM and represents one of the most significant challenges to quality of life in this patient population.[124] Although the bone manifestations of MM may occur throughout the body, they are most commonly identified in the vertebral column, where they may lead to clinically significant issues, including fracture.[118]

The efficacy of pamidronate and zoledronic acid for the prevention of skeletal-related events and improvement in OS has been established in MM patients, irrespective of the presence of osteolytic bone lesions.[167,168] Equivalent efficacy with monthly infusions has been shown with pamidronate and zoledronic acid. Because bisphosphonates can negatively affect kidney function, serum creatinine should be monitored monthly and treatment should be held if creatinine increases by more than 0.5 mg/dL above baseline. Higher doses and shorter infusion times have been associated with renal damage. Patients with creatinine clearances between 30 and 60 mL/minute should receive reduced doses of zoledronic acid and pamidronate over 4 to 6 hours is recommended if the creatinine is more than 3 mg/dL. Osteonecrosis of the jaw (ONJ) is a rare but serious complication of bisphosphonate therapy. Zoledronic acid is associated with a 9.5-fold increased risk of ONJ compared with pamidronate.[169] Baseline dental examinations and avoidance of invasive dental procedures during therapy are recommended. All patients with responsive or stable disease should be strongly considered for bisphosphonate discontinuation after 2 years of treatment.

Denosumab is a monoclonal antibody that binds to RANK ligand, which results in decreased osteoclast function and a reduction in bone resorption and bone destruction. Although the efficacy and side effect profile of denosumab are appealing, it cannot be recommended at this time to replace bisphosphonates in the management of MM patients because of an increased risk of mortality observed in a planned subgroup analysis.[170]

B.B. is a candidate for bisphosphonate therapy because he has symptomatic MM and osteolytic disease in the spine and ribs.

MAINTENANCE THERAPY

CASE 96-5, QUESTION 4: B.B. receives three cycles of RVD, followed by autologous HCT. He returns to clinic today 8 weeks after HCT. Should he receive any additional treatment at this time?

Given the near certainty that MM will progress after autologous HCT, maintenance therapies are utilized to extend the duration of response. Two Phase III studies have evaluated the benefit of lenalidomide in this setting. In the CALGB 100104 and IFM 2005-02 studies, lenalidomide 10 to 15 mg/day significantly improved PFS with the CALGB study also demonstrating an OS advantage.[171,172] Although thalidomide has also demonstrated some efficacy as maintenance therapy, its side effect profile limits its use long term. Therefore, lenalidomide may be preferred as a result of its improved toxicity profile although the risk of secondary malignancies should be discussed with patients. Bortezomib has also shown efficacy in the maintenance setting. Compared with thalidomide, bortezomib, at a dose of 1.3 mg/m^2 every 2 weeks, significantly improved PFS and OS.[173] Although neuropathy is a long-term toxicity that may limit its use in some patients, bortezomib may be considered a treatment option in the maintenance setting as well.

The decision was made that B.B. would receive maintenance therapy with lenalidomide 10 mg daily until disease progression was documented.

Relapsed and Refractory Disease

CASE 96-5, QUESTION 5: Four years after autologous HCT, B.B. is found to have relapsed disease. What other therapies may offer benefit for his myeloma?

The number of treatment options for relapsed or refractory MM is continuing to grow. When deciding on treatment, many factors need to be taken into consideration such as chromosomal abnormalities, prior regimen exposure and toxicities, response to prior regimens, and comorbidities.[174] For patients presenting with relapsed MM more than 6 months after initial induction therapy, it is reasonable to re-treat using the same regimen. For those patients with early relapse or refractory MM, bortezomib- or lenalidomide-containing regimens are acceptable options. When either of these agents was studied in combination with dexamethasone, they demonstrated significantly improved time to progression and OS compared to dexamethasone alone.[175,176] Bortezomib may also be combined with pegylated liposomal doxorubicin as an effective salvage regimen with cytopenias, diarrhea, and fatigue being common toxicities.[145]

Carfilzomib and pomalidomide are 2 newer agents, both approved in the relapsed or refractory setting with ongoing studies as initial therapy options. Carfilzomib is a proteasome inhibitor that binds irreversibly and more selectively than bortezomib, leading to decreased neuropathy and activity in some bortezomib-resistant patients. Common adverse effects include fatigue, anemia, nausea, and thrombocytopenia. Peripheral neuropathy occurs in 12.4% of patient with only 1.1% being grade 3 or higher.[140] Carfilzomib also has significant efficacy when combined with lenalidomide and dexamethasone, as demonstrated in the Phase III ASPIRE trial.[141] Dexamethasone premedication is recommended with each dose during cycle 1 and with any dose increase due to the risk of infusion reactions. Hydration is also recommended with each dose during cycle 1 to decrease the risk of TLS. Pomalidomide is the new IMiD structurally similar to thalidomide and lenalidomide.[153] Phase II and III trials have demonstrated significant activity and a manageable toxicity profile when used with or without dexamethasone in the relapsed/refractory setting.[142,143] Pomalidomide is dosed at 4 mg daily for 21 days of each 28 day cycle, although lower doses may be effective. Myelosuppression is the most common toxicity.

The histone deacetylase inhibitor, panobinostat, has also been approved for use in the relapsed and refractory setting in combination with bortezomib and dexamethasone based on the favorable result of the Phase III PANORAMA-1 trial.[144] Side effects, including cytopenias, diarrhea, and peripheral neuropathy, may limit the use of panobinostat. The NCCN considers a variety of combinations as preferred regimens for the management of patients with relapsed or refractory MM, some of which are listed in Table 96-8.[157]

LYMPHOMA

The lymphomas represent a dramatically diverse collection of hematologic malignancies originating from lymphoid tissues. The heterogeneity among these lymphoproliferative disorders is manifest by variations in pathophysiologic features, disease course, and therapeutic approach. Disease may present within the lymph nodes or in extranodal sites such as gastrointestinal tract, skin, bone marrow, sinus or CNS. Lymphomas are classified as either Hodgkin lymphoma (HL) or non-Hodgkin lymphoma (NHL). The NHLs are further divided into more than 20 subtypes according to factors such as cell of origin, histology, and natural history. A review of lymphoma classifications is presented in Table 96-9. Refer to Chapter 95, Pediatric Malignancies, for further discussion of pediatric lymphomas.

Epidemiology, Pathophysiology, and Etiology

The lymphomas impact pediatric through elderly populations with prevalence differing not only according to disease type but also additional factors such as geographic region, ethnicity, and socioeconomic status.[72,177] Causality is often not established; however, certain viral infections including Epstein–Barr virus and human immunodeficiency virus as well as immunosuppression, autoimmune disease, and family history contribute to an increased risk.[178–182]

Table 96-9
Simplified Classification of Lymphomas

	Cell of Origin
Hodgkin Lymphomas	
Classical Hodgkin lymphoma	B cell
Nodular lymphocyte predominant	B cell
Aggressive Non-Hodgkin Lymphomas	
Diffuse large B-cell lymphoma	B cell
Burkitt lymphoma	B cell
Mantle cell lymphoma	B cell
AIDS-related B-cell lymphoma	B cell
Primary central nervous systemlymphoma	B cell
Precursor lymphoblastic leukemia/lymphoma	B or T cell
Peripheral T-cell lymphomas	T cell
Anaplastic large-cell lymphoma	T cell
Adult T-cell leukemia/lymphoma	T cell
Extranodal NK/T-cell lymphoma	NK/T cell
Indolent Non-Hodgkin Lymphoma	
Follicular lymphoma	B cell
Cutaneous T-cell lymphomas	T cell
Marginal zone lymphoma	B cell

Adapted from Harris NL et al. World Health Organization classification of neoplastic diseases of the hematopoietic and lymphoid tissues: Report of the Clinical Advisory Committee meeting-Airlie House, Virginia, November 1997. *J Clin Oncol*. 1999;17:3835.

Clinical Presentation and Diagnosis

CASE 96-6

QUESTION 1: E.A. is a 35-year-old female with a two-week history of fevers, lymphadenopathy, malaise, and shortness of breath that was initially treated with antibiotics for suspected pneumonia. Progressive symptoms resulted in a hospital admission where radiologic evaluation revealed diffuse lymph node enlargement. Are E.A.'s symptoms consistent with aggressive or indolent lymphoma?

E.A.'s presenting symptoms of fevers, lymphadenopathy, and malaise are all generalized signs of lymphoma with the respiratory symptoms being consistent with pulmonary infiltration of malignant cells. The rapid onset and extensive disease involvement at presentation is suggestive of aggressive lymphoma. A biopsy of an involved node is essential to establish a definitive diagnosis and determine the subtype of lymphoma.

CASE 96-6, QUESTION 2: What diagnostic evaluation is necessary to establish the diagnosis of lymphoma for E.A.?

Suspicion of lymphoma requires a confirmatory biopsy of the lymph node or involved tissues. Morphology, immunophenotyping, flow cytometry, and cytogenetic techniques are utilized to refine the diagnosis. Additional patient assessment should include a complete history and physical examination with a focus on lymph node bearing areas along with laboratory analysis including CBC, comprehensive metabolic panel, and human immunodeficiency virus serology. Radiologic evaluation includes computerized tomography or PET to evaluate the extent of disease. Staging is based on the Ann Arbor system for HL or the Lugano modifications for NHL.[183] A simplified version of these schema is shown in Table 96-10. A bone marrow biopsy or lumbar puncture may be advisable under certain clinical circumstances. Assessment of baseline cardiac and pulmonary function is necessary for all patients expected to be treated with anthracyclines or bleomycin, respectively.

Treatment

Chemotherapy, immunotherapy, radiation, and bone marrow transplant are used in various combinations and sequences in lymphoma therapy. Selection of treatment is guided according to each specific classification of disease. Aggressive lymphomas, such as diffuse large B-cell lymphoma (DLBCL) and Hodgkin lymphoma, are treated with intensive combination chemotherapy regimens administered with a curative intent. In contrast, indolent lymphomas such as follicular lymphoma (FL) are essentially incurable and are regularly managed with an approach aimed at reducing disease burden and prolonging survival. Individual patient characteristics, including comorbid conditions and performance status, must be carefully considered in order to optimize outcomes. An overview of chemotherapy regimens is presented in Tables 96-11 and 96-12.

A biopsy of a supraclavicular lymph node confirms the diagnosis of aggressive NHL for E.A.

CASE 96-6, QUESTION 3: What are some important supportive care considerations with lymphoma therapy?

Beyond selecting the optimal chemotherapy regimen, care for E.A. will require proper supportive care focused on addressing both treatment- and disease-related complications. Prophylaxis and treatment of TLS is vital upon therapy initiation particularly for cases like this involving aggressive and bulky disease. Adequate

Table 96-10

Simplified Staging of Lymphoma

Stage		Description
Early	I	Disease limited to a single lymph node region
	II	Multiple lymph node regions involved on the same side of the diaphragm
Advanced	III	Lymph node regions involved on both sides of the diaphragm
	IV	Diffuse disease involving one or more extranodal organs
A: absence of any of the B symptoms; B: unexplained fever, drenching night sweats, or unexplained weight loss >10% of body weight during the previous 6 months		

Adapted from Cheson BD et al. Recommendations for initial evaluation, staging, and response assessment of Hodgkin and non-Hodgkin lymphoma: the Lugano classification. *J Clin Oncol*. 2014;32:3059.

antiemetics must accompany all chemotherapy. While common to virtually all lymphoma therapies, regimens designed for aggressive lymphoma are associated with significant hematologic toxicity and risk for infectious complications. As such, appropriate support with granulocyte colony-stimulating factors, antibiotics, and blood product transfusions is imperative. Although the urgent need for treatment may preclude opportunities, fertility counseling for a patient of childbearing age like E.A. should be offered. Delayed effects of both chemotherapy and radiation may develop more than a decade after conclusion of therapy and include secondary malignancy, cardiovascular disease, and pulmonary dysfunction. Subsequently, survivorship programs designed to monitor for delayed complications of treatment are increasingly valuable when treating theoretically curative diseases.

Table 96-12

Summary of Select Alternative Initial or Relapsed/Refractory Regimens for Lymphoma Therapy

Regimen	Chemotherapy
Stanford V	Mechlorethamine, doxorubicin, vinblastine, prednisone, Vincristine, bleomycin, and etoposide
BEACOPP	Bleomycin, etoposide, doxorubicin, cyclophosphamide, Vincristine, procarbazine, and prednisone
ESHAP ± R	Etoposide, methylprednisolone, cytarabine, cisplatin
DHAP ± R	Dexamethasone, cytarabine, cisplatin
ICE ± R	Ifosfamide, carboplatin, etoposide
CVP ± R	Cyclophosphamide, vincristine, prednisone
Hyper-CVAD ± R	Cyclophosphamide, vincristine, doxorubicin, and dexamethasone (Part A) alternating with methotrexate and cytarabine (Part B)
McGrath Protocol ± R	Cyclophosphamide, vincristine, doxorubicin, methotrexate (CODOX-M) alternating with ifosfamide, etoposide, cytarabine (IVAC)

R, rituximab

Table 96-11

Summary of Essential Initial Chemotherapy Regimens for Lymphoma Therapy

Regimen	Medication	Dose	Days	Cycle Length (days)
ABVD	Doxorubicin	25 mg/m^2 IV	1, 15	28
	Bleomycin	10 units/m^2 IV	1, 15	
	Vinblastine	6 mg/m^2 IV	1, 15	
	Dacarbazine	375 mg/m^2 IV	1, 15	
R-CHOP	Rituximab	375 mg/m^2 IV	1	21
	Cyclophosphamide	750 mg/m^2 IV	1	
	Doxorubicin	50 mg/m^2 IV	1	
	Vincristine[a]	1.4 mg/m^2 IV	1	
	Prednisone	100 mg PO	1–5	
EPOCH-R	Etoposide[b]	50 mg/m^2 IV	1–4	21
	Prednisone	60 mg/m^2 PO	1–5	
	Vincristine[b]	0.4 mg/m^2 IV	1–4	
	Cyclophosphamide	750 mg/m^2 IV	5	
	Doxorubicin[b]	10 mg/m^2 IV	1–4	
	Rituximab	375 mg/m^2 IV	1	
BR	Bendamustine	90 mg/m^2 IV	1, 2	28
	Rituximab	375 mg/m^2 IV	1	

[a]Maximum dose is 2 mg

[b]Etoposide, vincristine, and doxorubicin are infused over 24 hours

Hodgkin Lymphoma

CASE 96-7

QUESTION 1: L.G. is a 26-year-old woman with a month-long history of painless swelling around her collarbone and drenching night sweats. She reports increased fatigue and "feeling unwell" over the past 6 months. Radiography revealed a cervical, mediastinal, and inguinal lymph node enlargement. Excisional biopsy of the cervical lymph node revealed nodular sclerosing HL. Because of anemia and thrombocytopenia on presentation, a bone marrow biopsy was performed and found to be positive for lymphoma cells. All other laboratory values are normal and she is otherwise in very good health. What is the goal of therapy for L.G.?

Hodgkin lymphoma, formerly referred to as Hodgkin disease, is a B-cell neoplasm consisting of characteristic Reed–Sternberg cells within an inflammatory background. HL represents approximately 10% of lymphomas and will account for an estimated 9,050 new diagnoses in 2015 in the United States.[71,72] Occurrence of HL displays a bimodal age distribution primarily occurring in young adults with a second peak at approximately age 65.[184] Although once a uniformly fatal disease, improvements in treatment over the last 50 years represent a remarkable success story as now three out of every four new cases can be cured.[185] Given that long-term survival is expected for most patients, delayed consequences of therapy have a heightened importance in management of this disease.[186,187]

Hodgkin lymphoma is categorized as either classical HL or nodular lymphocyte predominant according to the appearance of tumor cells and the composition of the tumor microenvironment.[188] Classical HL is further subdivided, in order of prevalence, as nodular sclerosing, mixed cellularity, lymphocyte rich, and lymphocyte depleted.[189] Nodular lymphocyte-predominant HL accounts for only 5% of all HL and has a unique immunophenotypic profile and therapeutic approach. The remainder of this section will focus on classical HL.

Prognosis is multifactorial and incorporates systemic symptoms, stage of disease, and the size of the mass. The International Prognostic Score (IPS) for HL describes hypoalbuminemia (albumin $<$ 4 g/dL), anemia (Hgb $<$ 10.5 g/dL), male gender, age $>$ 45, Stage IV disease, leukocytosis (WBC $>$ 15,000/mm^3), and lymphocytosis (lymphocyte count $<$8%) as adverse indicators.[190] According to the IPS for HL, L.G. has two adverse indicators—anemia and Stage IV disease. This suggests that, while she presented with advanced disease, she maintains favorable long-term prognosis.

INITIAL THERAPY

CASE 96-7, QUESTION 2: What is appropriate initial therapy for L.G.?

The objective of initial therapy in HL is to maximize the potential for disease eradication while simultaneously limiting the risk of late effects. This requires stratifying patients according to prognostic factors. European Organization for the Research and Treatment of Cancer (EORTC) criterion is commonly employed to divide patients into one of three groups—early-stage favorable, early-stage unfavorable, and advanced disease. Early-stage favorable patients have Stage I or II disease and have no large mediastinal adenopathy, an erythrocyte sedimentation rate $<$50 mm/hour, $\leq$ 3 involved nodes, and are age $\leq$50. Patients with Stage I or II disease not meeting this criterion are classified as early-stage unfavorable; patients with Stage III or IV HL are considered to have advanced disease.

Radiation alone was the standard of care for decades in early-stage disease. Although effective, the utility of this approach is limited by substantial long-term toxicity.[191,192] The incorporation of combination chemotherapy into HL protocols has both improved long-term disease control and enhanced tolerability. Consequently, radiation therapy alone is no longer an acceptable approach. The regimen ABVD (doxorubicin, bleomycin, vinblastine, and dacarbazine) is the most commonly used regimen in modern practice and supplanted the previous standard, MOPP (mechlorethamine, vincristine, procarbazine, and prednisone), by demonstrating superior efficacy with reduced incidence both of acute toxicities and long-term complications such as secondary leukemia and sterility.[193,194] In early-stage favorable HL, chemotherapy with ABVD can either be given for four to six cycles alone or for two to four cycles followed by sequential radiation therapy.[195–197] Neither approach is considered superior because OS appears to be equivalent. Comparative studies suggest that chemotherapy alone portends a reduced risk of latent adverse events whereas dual therapy provides a lower rate of disease recurrence.[198–200] Patients with early unfavorable disease require a longer duration of therapy (four to six cycles), and incorporation of radiation therapy becomes essential.[201] For patients with advanced disease, chemotherapy becomes the mainstay of treatment and the duration of ABVD is increased to six to eight cycles.[202–204] Radiation is conventionally reserved to augment therapy for poor responders or patients requiring rapid debulking.[205] A distinctive feature of ABVD is the general avoidance of dose reductions or delays secondary to leukopenia due to the heightened importance of maintaining dose intensity in this disease.[206,207]

The Stanford V regimen incorporates a shorter duration of chemotherapy with an increased reliance on radiation.[208] While less commonly utilized, it represents a suitable alternative to ABVD and can be utilized in both early and advanced HL.[203,209,210] Advantages to the regimen include reduced cumulative doses of doxorubicin and bleomycin and thereby a reduced incidence of late effects of these antineoplastics.[211,212]

Select patients may benefit from escalating therapy to the BEACOPP regimen. This intensive chemotherapy regimen appears to improve tumor control, although a definitive survival advantage has yet to be elucidated.[204,213,214] Individuals with four or more adverse IPS factors and the physical capacity to tolerate the markedly increased toxicity of the combination are likely to derive the greatest potential advantage from this approach.

Given the multiple nodal sites on both sides of the diaphragm and the involvement of the bone marrow, L.G. has Stage IV HL and should be treated with six to eight cycles of ABVD. Although she has advanced disease, she has a favorable prognosis and long-term remission would be anticipated.

RELAPSED AND REFRACTORY DISEASE

CASE 96-7, QUESTION 3: On routine follow-up 9 months after completion of therapy, L.G. is found to have an extensive recurrence of nodal enlargement which is confirmed to be relapsed disease. What are appropriate treatment options for L.G.?

Unlike numerous malignant diseases, patients with HL maintain a reasonable likelihood of attaining cure in the setting of relapsed or refractory disease. Relapses consisting of minimal disease occurring more than 12 months after documented remission suggest a better prognosis. Salvage chemotherapy alone or with radiation is often sufficient therapy.[215,216] Patients with an early or extensive relapse or primary refractory disease generally require second-line chemotherapy followed by autologous bone marrow transplant. Selection of therapy is dependent on individual patient characteristics and provider preference because there is currently no standard of care. Effective regimens in this setting mimic those used in relapsed NHL, and include DHAP,

ESHAP, and ICE.[217] Repetition of initial therapy or use of an alternative first-line regimen may be reasonable in a minority of patients.[218,219] Brentuximab vedotin is a CD30-targeted monoclonal antibody linked to an antitubulin antineoplastic agent that has demonstrated activity in heavily pretreated patients failing bone marrow transplant and/or two prior lines of chemotherapy.[220]

L.G. should likely receive a salvage regimen such as ESHAP followed by autologous stem cell transplant given her early and extensive relapse. The aim of her therapy should remain curative.

Non-Hodgkin Lymphoma

Non-Hodgkin lymphoma (NHL) is a spectrum of lymphoid malignancies distinguished by variations in clinical features and responsiveness to treatment. These diseases combined will account for an estimated 71,850 new cases and 19,790 deaths in the United States in 2015.[71] Although various histopathologic classification schemes for NHL have been developed and modified as the cellular understanding of NHL has improved, NHLs can essentially be classified as either aggressive or indolent. Approximately 90% of all lymphomas arise from B lymphocytes with the remaining cases developing from T-lymphocytes or, rarely, natural killer (NK) cells. DLBCL and FL are the two most frequently occurring subtypes of NHL and, as such, will be the focus of this section.

AGGRESSIVE LYMPHOMA

Aggressive lymphomas include DLBCL and Burkitt lymphoma. Although these diseases are rapidly fatal if untreated and require intensive treatments, the prospect of attaining cure is reasonable for many patients receiving modern therapy.

CASE 96-8

QUESTION 1: P.A., a 64-year-old male, presents with complaints of swollen lymph nodes and occasional fevers and night sweats during the past month. Physical examination reveals marked cervical, supraclavicular, and inguinal lymphadenopathy. Laboratory values are normal with the exception of a mild anemia and an elevated LDH. Excisional biopsy of a supraclavicular lymph node confirms a diagnosis of DLBCL. Flow cytometry is positive for CD10, CD19, and CD20 surface markers. He does not have any identifiable extranodal disease. Is P.A.'s disease considered curable?

DLBCL represents about 25% to 30% of all cases of NHL and is the most common type of lymphoma.[10,189,221] Incidence of DLBCL increases with age with the median age at diagnosis occurring in the sixth decade of life.[222] Anticipated 5-year survival rates range from 21% to 76% depending on various prognostic indicators. Adverse indicators include age >60, elevated LDH, multiple extranodal sites, advanced clinical stage, and poor performance status.[223,224] Although the potential for relapse is relatively high given his numerous adverse indicators, the goal of therapy for P.A. is, nonetheless, curative.

Initial Therapy

CASE 96-8, QUESTION 2: Given this information, what is generally considered the standard of care for P.A.?

A combination of chemotherapy and immunotherapy with or without radiation is the foundation of therapy for DLBCL. The cyclophosphamide, doxorubicin, vincristine, and prednisone (CHOP) protocol has been the prevailing chemotherapy backbone in DLBCL for decades owing to its activity, tolerability, and simplicity in comparison with previously utilized regimens.[225] The inclusion of rituximab, a CD20-targeted monoclonal antibody, with CHOP therapy (R-CHOP) increases survival by approximately 10 to 15% with only a nominal increase in adverse effects.[226–228] Likewise, immunotherapy with rituximab is integrated into virtually all therapy for DLBCL. For patients with Stage I or II disease, a treatment course consists of three cycles of R-CHOP followed by involved field radiation.[229,230] If relative contraindications or aversions to radiotherapy are present, adequate results can typically be obtained by omitting radiation and extending chemotherapy duration. The large size and/or extent of disease limit the utility of radiation in patients with advanced disease (Stage III/IV or bulky tumors). As such, administration of R-CHOP for a total of six to eight cycles is the predominant practice in this setting.

Chemotherapy with CHOP plus rituximab (because his lymphoma is CD20 positive) for six to eight cycles would be ideal for P.A. The addition of radiation treatment is not beneficial in this setting because P.A. has Stage III disease.

Unique Circumstances

CASE 96-8, QUESTION 3: During completion of pretreatment assessment, P.A. is found to have a past medical history significant for cardiac disease. His ejection fraction is revealed to be 45% following an echocardiogram. Final cytogenetic analysis reveals his lymphoma is positive for c-Myc and BCL-2. Do any of these findings change the therapeutic approach for P.A? If so, how?

Notwithstanding its proven reliability, therapy with R-CHOP is not applicable to all patients with DLBCL. Anthracyclines, such as doxorubicin, are a cornerstone of numerous lymphoma regimens. This presents a significant clinical challenge for patients with underlying cardiovascular disease. Replacing the doxorubicin in CHOP with either liposomal doxorubicin or mitoxantrone may be reasonable options to limit cardiovascular toxicity although efficacy is compromised.[231,232] The EPOCH regimen has substantial efficacy in DLBCL and employs infusional doxorubicin which is thought to minimize cardiac effects.[233] If the anthracyclines and related compounds must be avoided entirely, the CEPP regimen (cyclophosphamide, etoposide, prednisone, procarbazine) is feasible.[234] Alternatively, etoposide or gemcitabine serves as acceptable replacements for doxorubicin in the CHOP regimen.[235,236] Treatment of very frail or elderly patients with DLBCL represents a similar challenge to those with cardiac disease. Maintaining dose intensity is ideal given the curative intent of therapy; however, this is not attainable for all patients and use of reduced intensity therapy may be required.[237,238]

The presence of c-Myc and BCL-2 typically appears in NHL with features intermediate between DLBCL and Burkitt lymphoma. These findings, often referred to as "double-hit" lymphomas, are indicative of a poorer prognosis and reduced responsiveness to conventional therapy.[239,240] Escalation from CHOP to EPOCH, a protocol with known activity in Burkitt lymphoma, appears to increase response rates with acceptable tolerability in this subset of DLBCL patients.[241,242]

A change from R-CHOP to EPOCH plus rituximab might be advantageous for P.A. because this treatment is potentially superior given his cytogenetic abnormalities and may be associated with reduced cardiac complications.

Relapsed and Refractory Disease

CASE 96-8, QUESTION 4: Four years after completing therapy, P.A. experiences a relapse of disease. In addition to his lymphoma recurrence, his physical condition has significantly deteriorated since his first therapy due to worsening of comorbid disease unrelated to his cancer.

What is the goal of additional therapy for P.A. now that his disease has recurred?

Eligibility for bone marrow transplant is a critical component in decision-making for the management of relapsed or refractory disease. The aim of therapy for appropriate candidates is administration of aggressive chemotherapy to induce maximal response followed promptly by autologous transplant.[243,244] Comparatively, the approach to patients that are not transplant appropriate, fail to respond to therapy, or relapse following transplant is largely palliative. Numerous intensive regimens have been successfully used to induce remission prior to autologous transplant (Table 96-11).[245–247] No option has proven superior to another, and all are associated with significant hematologic and nonhematologic toxicity. Although efficacy data are limited, rituximab is frequently included into these salvage regimens. Treatment with less-intensive therapy such as gemcitabine plus oxaliplatin (GemOx) or BR is ideal for patients not pursuing stem cell transplant.[248,249] Low doses of single-agent chemotherapy may be a useful approach to palliate symptoms caused by large masses.

Now at age 68 and in suboptimal physical condition, P.A. is not likely a candidate for aggressive salvage therapy followed by bone marrow transplant. A reduced intensity treatment such as BR may be beneficial at controlling disease, though the aim of therapy in this setting would be palliative.

Other Aggressive NHL Subtypes

Burkitt lymphoma is a quintessential aggressive malignancy that demonstrates an exceptionally rapid proliferation rate. Urgent therapy is crucial and must be more vigorous than conventional DLBCL protocols.[250] Active regimens include the McGrath protocol, Hyper-CVAD, or various Cancer and Leukemia Group B (CALGB) protocols.[251–254] Although many of these regimens were developed in the pre-rituximab era, the monoclonal antibody is generally included given the limited impact on toxicity and evidence suggesting improved responses. The EPOCH regimen is a viable therapeutic option with improved tolerability and comparative efficacy to other commonly used regimens.[255] Given the predilection of the disease to involve the CNS, prophylaxis with either intrathecal chemotherapy or high-dose methotrexate and cytarabine is an imperative component to Burkitt lymphoma treatment.[256] While treatment-related complications can be severe, durable remission is attained in 60% to 90% of pediatric and young adult cases.[257] This favorable prognosis dissipates when the disease occurs in older populations.[258]

Mantle cell lymphoma harbors the incurable nature of indolent lymphoma while displaying the capability for rapid proliferation of aggressive disease.[259] Therapy for the disease reflects this dual nature because therapy ranges from low-intensity indolent regimens to high-intensity aggressive regimens. While there is no current standard of care, conventional practice is to administer intensive regimens such as Hyper-CVAD with rituximab to young and medically fit patients based on the perceived advantage in disease response.[260] Protocols such as BR or R-CHOP are ideal for elderly patients or those with significant comorbid disease.[261–263] Various combinations of antineoplastics or single-agent therapy with ibrutinib, a Bruton TK inhibitor, have shown efficacy in the relapsed/refractory setting.[264–266] Autologous or allogeneic bone marrow transplant may be considered for carefully selected individuals.[267]

INDOLENT LYMPHOMA

In contrast to the aggressive lymphomas, indolent varieties are subject to slow growth and typically do not require treatment until the patient is symptomatic.[268] Although numerous effective treatments are available, indolent lymphomas are frequently incurable and prone to recurrent relapses. Treatment is aimed at prolonging survival and palliating symptoms by reducing disease burden until the malignancy either becomes resistant to therapy and/or transforms to a more aggressive lymphoma.[269]

CASE 96-9

QUESTION 1: T.M. is a 61-year-old male in generally good health who is presenting with a three month history of painless axillary lymphadenopathy that seems to "come and go." He is otherwise asymptomatic. An excisional biopsy and pathologic examination revealed follicular B-cell lymphoma, a type of indolent lymphoma. A CT scans showed axillary, mediastinal, and iliac lymphadenopathy. Laboratory values are normal. What is the goal of therapy for T.M.?

FL is the second most common form of NHL and comprises approximately 70% of all indolent lymphomas.[270] The condition predominantly appears in patients over 50 years of age though pediatric variants have been described. A reasonable percentage of patients will survive a decade or longer with disease. The Follicular Lymphoma International Prognostic Index (FLIPI) identifies age >60, elevated LDH, Stage III or IV disease, Hgb <12, and more than four involved nodes as adverse indicators.[271]

Initial Therapy

Myriad treatment options are available for FL though no absolute standard of care has been established. For a small subset of patients presenting with early disease, treatment may consist of radiation therapy alone which is potentially curative in rare instances.[272–275] Under most circumstances, however, initial treatment of FL involves chemoimmunotherapy. Similar to B-cell-related aggressive NHL, the availability of rituximab has dramatically shaped therapy for FL in the modern era.[276,277] Preferred initial treatment regimens are BR, R-CHOP, or R-CVP (rituximab, cyclophosphamide, vincristine, prednisone). Bendamustine, an alkylating agent with additional properties similar to purine analogs, in combination with rituximab is perhaps the most commonly applied regimen for FL today. In comparison with alternatives such as R-CHOP, BR provides improved PFS and has a lower incidence of myelosuppression, infections, and alopecia.[263,278] Although BR is currently favored by many practitioners, R-CHOP is supported by extensive experience and remains a reasonable therapy particularly for patients with advanced presentations.[279] For patients unable to tolerate anthracyclines, R-CVP has favorable tolerability compared to R-CHOP but compromised efficacy secondary to the removal of doxorubicin.[276] Single-agent rituximab elicits significant response rates with minimal toxicity and is an ideal treatment for patients unable to tolerate the rigors of cytotoxic therapy.[280,281] Administration of maintenance rituximab in various schedules following completion of initial therapy shows an increase in PFS.[282,283]

CASE 96-9, QUESTION 2: When should treatment be initiated for T.M.?

Distinct from aggressive lymphoma therapy, active treatment of FL can be withheld until the development of disease-related symptoms without compromising outcomes.[268,284] Advantages to the "watchful waiting" approach include cost avoidance, minimizing treatment complications, and theoretically limiting future drug resistance. Localized symptoms due to nodal disease, compromised organ function secondary to lymphoma infiltration, B symptoms, cytopenias from bone marrow involvement, or an aggressive tempo are generally considered indications to initiate therapy.

Because his disease is presently asymptomatic, a "watchful waiting" approach is reasonable for T.M. Once criteria for treatment are met, therapy can be initiated with the goal being to reduce disease-related symptoms and to prolong survival.

CASE 96-9, QUESTION 3: T.M. eventually requires treatment for his FL and maintains a durable remission after therapy with the BR regimen. Three years later, he has a rapid onset of recurrent disease in multiple nodal regions accompanied by unintentional weight loss and night sweats. Laboratory evaluation reveals thrombocytopenia and neutropenia. Given the characteristics of his relapse, what additional diagnostic tests must be considered prior to providing therapy for T.M?

Nearly one in three FLs will transform into an aggressive lymphoma at the time of relapse.[285] In the event of aggressive presentation, a repeat biopsy is required to determine conversion to alternate histology.[286] If transformation is documented, treatment must be intensified to a protocol consistent with aggressive lymphoma therapy.

CASE 96-9, QUESTION 4: What treatment options are available for T.M.?

For simple relapses of FL, rituximab maintains a pivotal role in relapsed disease and is effective both as a single agent or in combination with chemotherapy.[287,288] Re-challenge with a previously administered regimen is reasonable for patients attaining a durable remission with minimal symptoms. Alternative first-line regimens may also be effectively used in the relapsed setting. Treatment regimens containing bortezomib, mitoxantrone, and fludarabine have additionally demonstrated activity in patients with prior chemotherapy.[289–292] Hematopoietic stem cell transplant is an important treatment option for young and medically fit patients.

The rapid nature of disease relapse in T.M. is an important finding and concerning for transformation to a more aggressive lymphoma. A repeat lymph node biopsy is indicated in this case. If disease has not transformed, a regimen such as R-CHOP may be ideal considering his more advanced presentation.

KEY REFERENCES AND WEBSITES

A full list of references for this chapter can be found at http://thepoint.lww.com/AT11e. Below are the key references and websites for this chapter, with the corresponding reference number in this chapter found in parentheses after the reference.

Key References

Baccarani M et al. European LeukemiaNet recommendations for the management of chronic myeloid leukemia: 2013. *Blood*. 2013:872–884. (77)

Bonfante V et al. ABVD in the treatment of Hodgkin's disease. *Semin Oncol*. 1992;19:38. (202)

Burnett A et al. Therapeutic advances in acute myeloid leukemia [published correction appears in *J Clin Oncol*. 2011;29:2293]. *J Clin Oncol*. 2011;29:487. (15)

Cheson BD et al. Recommendations for initial evaluation, staging, and response assessment of Hodgkin and non-Hodgkin lymphoma: the Lugano classification. *J Clin Oncol*. 2014;32:3059. (183)

Flinn IW et al. Randomized trial of bendamustine-rituximab or R-CHOP/R-CVP in first-line treatment of indolent NHL or MCL: the BRIGHT study. *Blood*. 2014;123:2944. (278)

Hallek M. Chronic lymphocytic leukemia for the clinician. *Ann Oncol*. 2011;22(Suppl 4):iv54. (116)

Harris NL et al. World Health Organization classification of neoplastic diseases of the hematopoietic and lymphoid tissues: report of the Clinical Advisory Committee meeting-Airlie House, Virginia, November 1997. *J Clin Oncol*. 1999;17:3835. (10)

Jabbour E, Kantarjian H. Chronic myeloid leukemia: 2014 update on diagnosis, monitoring, and management. *Am J Hematol*. 2014;89:548–556. (73)

Kindler T et al. *FLT3* as a therapeutic target in AML: still challenging after all these years. *Blood*. 2010;116:5089. (70)

Marcucci G et al. Molecular genetics of adult acute myeloid leukemia: prognostic and therapeutic implications [published correction appears in *J Clin Oncol*. 2011;29:1798]. *J Clin Oncol*. 2011;29:475. (14)

Munshi NC, Anderson KC. Plasma cell neoplasms. In: DeVita VT et al, eds. *Cancer: Principles and Practice of Oncology*. 9th ed. Philadelphia, PA: Lippincott Williams & Wilkins; 2011:1998. (118)

Pollyea DA et al. Acute myeloid leukaemia in the elderly: a review. *Br J Haematol*. 2011;152:524. (48)

Rajkukmar SV et al. Lenalidomide plus high-dose dexamethasone versus lenalidomide plus low-dose dexamethasone as initial therapy for newly diagnosed multiple myeloma: an open-label randomized controlled trial. *Lancet Oncol*. 2010;11:29. (132)

Rajkumar SV. Multiple Myeloma: 2014 update on diagnosis, risk-stratification, and management. *Am J Hematol*. 2014;89:999. (130)

Sehn LH et al. Introduction of combined CHOP plus rituximab therapy dramatically improved outcome of diffuse large B-cell lymphoma in British Columbia. *J Clin Oncol*. 2005;23:5027. (226)

Key Websites

American Society of Hematology. *Hematology. Education Program Book*. 2010. http://www.asheducationbook.org.

The National Comprehensive Cancer Network® (NCCN®). NCCN Clinical Practice Guidelines in Oncology (NCCN Guidelines®). http://www.nccn.org.

97 Breast Cancer

Kellie Jones Weddle

CORE PRINCIPLES

	CORE PRINCIPLES	CHAPTER CASES
1	Mammography and clinical breast examinations are common screening modalities used in patients with an average risk of developing breast cancer.	**Case 97-1 (Question 1)**
2	Prevention can include both surgery (prophylactic mastectomy ± bilateral oophorectomy) and chemoprevention. Tamoxifen and raloxifene are two agents approved for breast cancer prevention.	**Case 97-1 (Question 2)**
3	Breast cancer is the most common cancer diagnosed in American women. Many risk factors have been associated with the development of breast cancer; however, the two most common risk factors are gender and age.	**Case 97-2 (Question 1), Case 97-3 (Question 1)**
4	A painless mass is a common presenting symptom for patients. To diagnose the disease and determine the histology, a mammogram and a biopsy are performed. Staging is also performed to determine the extent of disease.	**Case 97-3 (Questions 2–4)**
5	Tumor-specific characteristics help guide treatment selection and contribute to prognosis. The most significant factors are hormonal status (estrogen and progesterone receptor status) and human epidermal growth factor receptor 2 (HER2) status.	**Case 97-3 (Question 5)**
6	Local and systemic treatment can include surgery, radiation, hormonal therapy, chemotherapy, and/or biologic therapy.	**Case 97-3 (Questions 6–9)**
7	Early-stage disease is highly curable. In the adjuvant setting (after surgery), patients can receive hormonal therapy or biologic therapy, depending on tumor-specific factors and may receive chemotherapy, depending on the size of the disease and the presence of positive axillary lymph nodes.	**Case 97-3 (Questions 7–9)**
8	Adjuvant chemotherapy can include regimens containing anthracyclines, cyclophosphamide, and taxanes. Biologic therapy such as trastuzumab can be incorporated if the patient has HER2-positive disease.	**Case 97-3 (Questions 6–8)**
9	Metastatic disease is considered incurable. Decisions regarding therapy will depend on the hormonal status of the tumor, toxicities from previous treatment, or other preexisting comorbidities. Therapies could include systemic therapy (hormonal therapy, chemotherapy, or biologic therapy) or local treatment (radiation therapy or surgery).	**Case 97-4 (Questions 1–5)**

BREAST CANCER

Incidence, Prevalence, and Epidemiology

Breast cancer is the most common malignancy in American women and is second to lung cancer in mortality rates. It arises from the tissues of the breast, usually the ducts (tubes that carry milk to the nipple) and lobules (glands that make milk). In 2017, it is estimated that 255,180 individuals will be diagnosed with breast cancer, and approximately 41,070 are expected to die from their disease. Approximately 2,470 cases are estimated to be diagnosed in men, indicating this is not a disease solely of women.[1]

The incidence of breast cancer has continued to decline from 1999 through 2004 due to the decreased use of hormone-replacement therapy. This decline follows the results of the Women's Health Initiative study, which demonstrated increased risk of breast cancer in those receiving hormone-replacement therapy.[2] One in eight women are expected to develop the disease over the course of their lifetime. However, this frequently quoted statistic may overestimate the risk of breast cancer because it is derived from women who live to 110 years of age.[3]

If breast cancer is diagnosed early, it is curable. The likelihood of diagnosing breast cancer is increased by the use of standardized screening methods. Currently, many different guidelines are available for breast cancer screening including recommendations from the American Cancer Society (ACS), National Comprehensive Cancer Network (NCCN), and the US Preventive Services Task Force (USPSTF).

Pathophysiology

The breast itself is composed of many different structures including fat, muscle, ducts, and lobules (Fig. 97-1). Lobules arise from glandular tissue that forms into a spoke-like formation to constitute a lobule of two layers of epithelial cells. The ducts connect the milk-secreting lobules to the nipple.[4] A breast cancer is defined by where the tumor cells originate. The two most common histologic types of breast cancer are ductal and lobular carcinoma. Ductal tumors may be classified as either invasive ductal carcinoma (IDC) if it has invaded through the basement membrane of the duct, or ductal carcinoma in situ (DCIS) if it has not. Likewise, lobular tumors may be classified similarly (i.e., invasive lobular carcinoma [ILC] or lobular carcinoma in situ [LCIS]). Other types of breast cancers include inflammatory (which will be discussed later in the chapter) and rare histologies such as tubular or medullary carcinomas or sarcomas.

Clinical Presentation and Diagnosis

Most patients will present with early-stage disease, where the 5-year survival rate is approximately 98%.[5] Many present with a painless lump found upon breast examination (either by themselves or by a clinician) or with a small mass found only on routine mammogram. Patients who present with metastatic

Figure 97-1 Anatomy of the breast. (Asset provided by Anatomical Chart Co.)

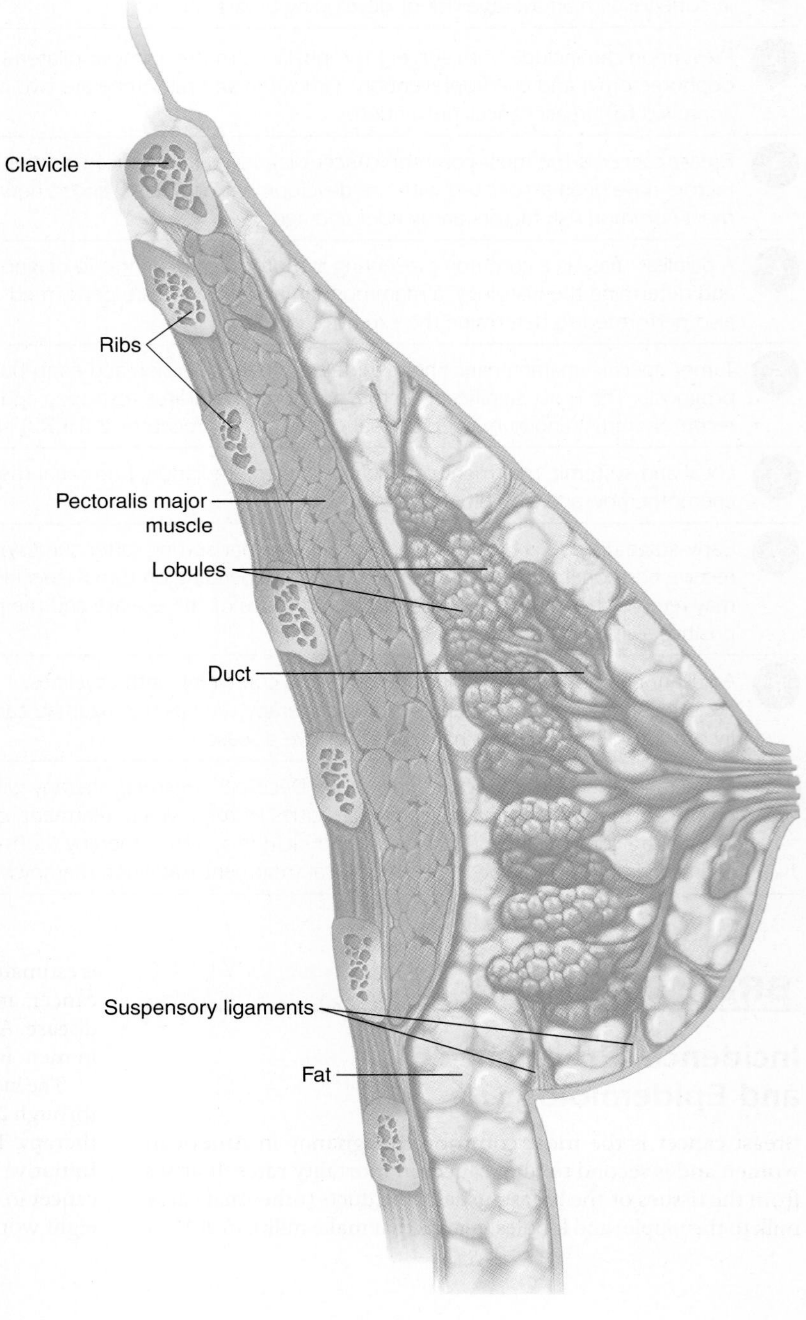

disease typically present with symptoms of their disease based on the metastatic site (such as bone pain with bone metastases or shortness of breath with lung metastases).

Treatment will be determined based on the stage of disease. Staging is completed by evaluating the size of the tumor (either radiographically or from the surgical specimen), the extent of positive lymph nodes (on physical examination and surgical removal through an axillary lymph node dissection or sentinel lymph node dissection), and the extent of disease (through radiologic examinations including computed tomography [CT] scan of the chest, abdomen, and pelvis and a bone scan to identify any metastatic disease).

Overview of Treatment

The treatment of breast cancer includes multiple modalities. Surgery, radiation therapy, hormonal therapy, chemotherapy, and biologic therapy can all be used in many different combinations based on a patient's specific disease. If therapy is given before surgery, it is called neoadjuvant therapy, and if treatment is administered after surgery it is termed adjuvant therapy. Early-stage disease may be treated with surgery; other factors will determine whether additional therapy is needed. The staging of a patient's tumor may require radiation and/or chemotherapy, and tumor-specific characteristics decide whether hormonal or biologic therapy will be added. In patients with metastatic disease, the goal is palliation of symptoms and improvement in quality of life.

SCREENING

CASE 97-1

QUESTION 1: M.P. is a 42-year-old woman with no personal history of breast cancer. She has a cousin who was diagnosed with breast cancer at the age of 65 years. M.P. is in her doctor's office today to discuss routine breast cancer screening. Based on M.P.'s personal and family history, would M.P. be considered an average-risk or high-risk patient and what modalities of screening are recommended for average-risk and high-risk patients?

The guidelines for cancer screening for breast cancer were recently updated in 2015 and led to major changes in the recommended screening modalities and intervals of obtainment for women of average risk of developing breast cancer.6 For the average risk patient, screening involves a mammogram and a breast self-examination (if the woman chooses to do so). Although the risk of breast cancer is low in one's 20s, breast self-examination allows a woman to become more familiar with her body and better able to discern changes as she ages. Clinical breast examinations have long been part of the screening guidelines, but with the new changes in recommendations, this component of screening has been removed due to a lack of benefit of detecting breast cancer in a woman with average risk.

Screening mammography has been the gold standard for breast cancer for many decades. With the newer recommendations, a change has occurred as to when to start mammograms and the intervals in which they should be obtained. In the older recommendations, mammography was recommended annually starting at the age of 40. In the newer guidelines, women of average risk should have the opportunity to begin annual mammograms between the ages of 40 to 44 and then annual mammograms should commence at the age of 45 through 54. Once a woman turns 55, she should transition to biennial screening or have the opportunity to continue annual screening. The guidelines also recommend for women to continue screening mammograms as long as their overall health is good and their life expectancy is 10 or more years.

For many years, there has been controversy regarding the utility of mammography and when screening should begin (40 or 50 years of age). This controversy has stemmed from recommendations by the USPSTF.7 Their newest recommendations state that the decision to start screening mammograms before the age of 50, should be an individual decision. Women may choose to begin biennial screening between the ages of 40-49, but that this may lead to more false positive results and unnecessary biopsies. The guidelines state that the largest benefit for screening mammograms occur in women ages 50 to 74 and there are insufficient data to support the utility of annual mammograms in women greater than or equal to the age of 75. While these screening recommendations can be confusing, the controversy that has stemmed from the changes has heightened the awareness to the general public of the importance of breast cancer screening.

M.P. has no first-degree relatives with breast cancer or other family members affected by early breast cancer. M.P. is an average-risk patient, and she should start standard screening modalities and intervals of testing with annual mammograms and clinical breast examinations. She may also decide to do breast self-examinations.

Individuals considered high risk include those that (a) have a known *BRCA* gene mutation, (b) are untested for the *BRCA* gene mutation but have a first-degree relative with a *BRCA* mutation, (c) have a lifetime risk of experiencing breast cancer of approximately 20% to 25% or more based on risk estimation models, or (d) have a strong family history of breast cancer.[6] Screening with breast magnetic resonance imaging (MRI) is recommended in high-risk individuals. Annual mammography and breast MRIs should be initiated starting at the age of 30 years in this population. An MRI allows a radiologist to see a contrasted view of the breast and is more sensitive to detecting breast cancer. In addition, breast tissue in younger patients can be denser due to higher levels of estrogen, making mammography less sensitive.[8]

PREVENTION

CASE 97-1, QUESTION 2: M.P. works at her local hospital as a nurse and is volunteering this year at their breast cancer awareness seminar that is offered by her hospital. She was asked to prepare a talk for the event about breast cancer awareness. She wants to discuss breast cancer prevention. What are the common modalities of breast cancer prevention that M.P. should address and what chemopreventive agents should she include?

Prevention is key with any cancer. Women who are considered high risk for breast cancer may decide to undergo prophylactic mastectomy with reconstruction as an alternative to living with the prospect that they may develop breast cancer in their life. This modality of prevention is very successful, but does not completely eliminate the risk for developing breast cancer.[9] In addition, prophylactic oophorectomy may also be completed to remove the largest source of estrogen in a premenopausal patient. This does not however eliminate the risk completely from developing breast cancer.[10]

Chemoprevention is also another option. Two agents approved for prevention are tamoxifen and raloxifene, both are selective estrogen receptor modulators (SERMs). The Breast Cancer Prevention Trial (or P1 trial) was conducted in more than 13,000 high-risk women, who were randomly assigned into three groups: those older than 60 years, 35 to 59 years of age with an increased risk of breast cancer based on a score of at least 1.66 as determined by the Gail risk model, or older than 35 years with a history of LCIS (a risk factor for developing invasive breast cancer).[11] Women received tamoxifen 20 mg daily or placebo for 5 years of therapy. Tamoxifen significantly decreased the risk of developing breast cancer ($p < 0.00001$). In addition, this study illustrated toxicities associated with tamoxifen therapy, especially in women older than 50 years of age. In those patients, a higher risk of deep vein thrombosis, stroke, pulmonary embolism, and endometrial cancers was identified.[11]

Raloxifene was also approved for chemoprevention in breast cancer. This originated from observations made in osteoporosis studies with raloxifene where patients who had received raloxifene therapy had a decreased risk of breast cancer. With this information, a large randomized chemoprevention trial of more than 19,000 postmenopausal women was conducted evaluating the use of raloxifene 60 mg daily compared to tamoxifen 20 mg daily for 5 years.[12,13] There was no difference in the number of invasive breast cancers diagnosed in the two treatment arms (relative risk, 1.02; 95% confidence interval, 0.82–1.28). Interestingly, more noninvasive breast cancers were identified in the raloxifene group (80 cases) compared with tamoxifen (57 cases); however, the clinical significance of this difference is unknown. The tamoxifen arm reported more hot flashes and endometrial cancer, and the raloxifene arm demonstrated fewer thromboembolic events and cataracts but more musculoskeletal problems and weight gain. Based on the results of this trial, raloxifene received an indication for chemoprevention in high-risk women. The aromatase inhibitors, exemestane and anastrozole, have been studied in the chemopreventive setting in postmenopausal patients (NCIC CTG MAP III trial and IBIS II trial, respectively). Although both trials demonstrated reductions in breast cancer incidences, neither agent has been compared with tamoxifen or raloxifene and so they are not approved for use as a preventive therapy at this time.[14,15]

M.P. should include information on prophylactic mastectomy and both tamoxifen (for pre- and postmenopausal patients) and raloxifene (in only postmenopausal patients) in her talk for women with a high risk of breast cancer but not exemestane or anastrozole.

RISK FACTORS

CASE 97-2

Question 1: B.W., a 55-year-old woman, is found to have a 2.2 cm mass in the upper, outer quadrant of her left breast during a routine screening mammogram. The rest of her physical examination is unremarkable, and she has no complaints. All laboratory values, including the complete blood count and liver function tests, are within normal limits. A chest X-ray is negative. B.W. reports that she had her first menstrual cycle at the age of 10 years and has had regular periods since that time. She is married but has never been pregnant. What are B.W.'s risk factors for developing breast cancer?

Many different risk factors have been identified to be associated with the development of breast cancer. However, in greater than 50% of patients, there are no identifiable risk factors beyond increased age and female gender[16] (Table 97-1). One's risk increases with each decade of life, and the median age of diagnosis is between 60 and 65 years of age. If the patient has had a previous history of breast cancer or atypical hyperplasia from previous breast biopsies, this increases her risk of developing breast cancer.

Breast cancer is a hormonally mediated disease, and many factors are associated with hormonal influences. Early menarche (generally defined as younger than 12 years of age) and late menopause (generally defined as older than 55 years of age) expose a woman to more estrogen throughout her lifetime, increasing her risk (Relative risk [RR] = 1.5 for age <12 years and RR = 2 for ages >55 for late menopause).[17] Based on the results of the Women's Health Initiative, the use of hormone-replacement therapy was shown to increase one's risk of breast cancer.[18] Nulliparity, or having children after the age of 30 years, has been associated with an increased risk (RR increased up to 3.5).[17] Oral contraceptives have long been thought to increase the risk of breast cancer. Earlier forms of oral contraceptives contained much higher doses of estrogen compared with products today. The dose of estrogens in those products was thought to increase a woman's risk of developing breast cancer. However, a meta-analysis demonstrated no difference in risk no matter the dose of estrogen in the oral contraceptives.[19] Hereditary breast cancers (one or more first-degree relatives with the disease) only account for approximately 10% of breast cancer cases; however, these individuals have the highest risk of developing breast cancer.[20]

Table 97-1
Risk Factors for Developing Breast Cancer

Known Risk Factors
Gender: female > male
Personal history of breast cancer
Family history of breast cancer (first-degree relatives)
Benign breast "cancer" (i.e., atypical hyperplasia)
Early menarche (<12 years of age), late menopause (>55 years of age)
Late first pregnancy (≥30 years) or no pregnancy
Advancing age
Long-term use of hormone-replacement therapy (estrogen)
Previous chest wall irradiation
Possible Risk Factors
Alcohol
Obesity
High-fat diet

Sources: Carlson RW, Allred DC, Anderson BO, et al. Invasive breast cancer. *J Natl Compr Canc Netw*. 2011; 9:136; Chlebowski RT, Hendrix SL, Langer RD, et al. Influence of estrogen plus progestin on breast cancer and mammography in healthy postmenopausal women: the Women's Health Initiative randomized trial. *JAMA*. 2003; 289:3243.

B.W. has risk factors that increase her risk of developing breast cancer. B.W. started menses early at the age of 10 years and therefore has been exposed longer to estrogen, and she does not have any children. She is also 55 years of age, and the risk of breast cancer increases with each decade of life. Therefore, all of these are considered risk factors for B.W.

INHERITED BREAST CANCER MUTATIONS

CASE 97-3

Question 1: C.D., a 37-year-old woman, is found to have a 2.2 cm mass in the outer quadrant of her right breast during a mammogram. All of her laboratory values were normal, and her chest X-ray was negative. Her family history is significant in that her mother died of breast cancer at the age of 42 years and her 44-year-old sister had a breast tumor removed 5 years ago. With C.D.'s family history, what genetic testing could be performed for her or for anyone else in her family? If C.D. did not have a family history of breast cancer, what other tests could be conducted to estimate her risk of developing breast cancer?

C.D. has two first-degree relatives with early-age breast cancer. This would indicate a possible inherited genetic mutation. Genetic testing for the presence of *BRCA1* and *BRCA2* mutations should be discussed with C.D. By the age of 70, a person with a BRCA1 mutation has a ~60% risk of developing breast cancer and a 40% risk of developing ovarian cancer.

BRCA2 mutation carriers have a slightly lower risk of breast cancer (~40%) and a lower risk of developing ovarian cancer

(~20%).[20,21] One population with a high incidence of *BRCA* mutations is those of Ashkenazi Jewish descent, where 1 in 50 individuals are *BRCA* carriers.[22] C.D. should meet with a genetic counselor to discuss risks and benefits of genetic testing for her and her family members. The results would then play a role in future screening and preventive strategies.

Patients can assess their risk of developing breast cancer by using validated risk tools. One such instrument for average-risk patients is the Gail model, which takes into account numerous factors such as age at menarche, age of first live birth, presence of atypical hyperplasia, and number of previous breast biopsies. This model is available online (www.cancer.gov/bcrisktool/). Other models that have been validated include BRCAPRO and the Breast Cancer Risk Assessment Tool (for average-risk patients).[23,24] BRCAPRO is a statistical program that uses information from both affected and unaffected relatives to predict the likelihood if a person would have an inherited mutation in *BRCA1* or *BRCA2*.[21] This tool would be used in an individual with a high risk of developing breast cancer. There are numerous resources for patients and family members to help understand their risk of developing breast cancer. Concerned individuals should have a conversation with their physician regarding their risk of breast cancer and the utility of these risk assessment tools based on their personal and family history.

Clinical Presentation

CASE 97-3, QUESTION 2: What are the typical signs and symptoms of breast cancer and does C.D. have any?

Typical presentation involves the identification of a painless lump on clinical examination by a healthcare professional, by the patient, or by visualization of a painless lump on mammography. Other symptoms are nipple discharge or retraction, or skin changes of the breast.[25,26] Less than 10% of patients will present with metastatic disease. Symptoms upon presentation can reflect their metastatic disease (i.e., back pain: bone metastases; headaches/nausea/vomiting: brain metastases; dyspnea: lung metastases; or abdominal pain: liver metastases).[25,26] C.D. had a painless lump identified on mammogram as her presenting sign.

Diagnosis

CASE 97-3, QUESTION 3: After the identification of C.D.'s breast mass on mammogram, what diagnostic procedures should be done to determine C.D.'s type and stage of breast cancer?

Workup for breast cancer includes radiographic examinations, patient history, and a physical examination. If a mass is palpated, a mammogram is completed to identify the abnormality. A breast ultrasound can also be added after the mammogram to differentiate fluid-filled cysts (which are usually benign) versus discreet masses. Once identified, a biopsy would then be performed to diagnose the disease. This is achieved with a core biopsy—the standard method used to obtain a tissue sample. This procedure uses a large bore needle for tissue collection and allows for distinguishing invasive versus noninvasive disease. Other methods are available for tissue diagnosis such as fine-needle aspiration and excisional biopsy, but the core biopsy is considered the standard approach.[25,26]

Full radiologic testing should also be completed including a CT scan of the chest, abdomen, and pelvis, and bone scan to assess for metastatic disease. The most common places for breast cancer to metastasize are the bone, lung, liver, lymph nodes, and the brain.[27] Evaluation for brain metastases will usually be performed if the patient is experiencing signs and symptoms such as blurry or double vision, uncontrolled nausea/vomiting, headaches, and unsteady gait. These tests are used to determine the extent and stage of the disease and ultimately help determine the prognosis and treatment of the patient. C.D. will need to undergo a biopsy and full staging with a CT scan of the chest, abdomen, and pelvis, and a bone scan.

Types of Breast Cancer and Staging

CASE 97-3, QUESTION 4: C.D. had a core biopsy performed which revealed IDC. Other staging tests included a CT scan of the chest, abdomen, and pelvis and a bone scan. All tests were negative. Physical examination revealed ipsilateral lymph node involvement. Mammogram revealed a 2.2 cm mass in the right breast. What are the common types of breast cancer and what stage is C.D.'s breast cancer?

The histology of breast cancer is typically divided into two categories: invasive and noninvasive (in situ) disease. IDC is the most common type found (~75% of cases) and ILC is second (~5%–10%). The noninvasive tumors are less common (DCIS and LCIS; ductal carcinoma in situ and lobular carcinoma in situ, respectively).[25,26] Other less common histologies include medullary, mucinous, tubular, and papillary. One of the most aggressive forms of breast cancer is inflammatory breast cancer, which is distinctly different from the other types of breast cancer mentioned. Breast cancer can take years to develop into a mass that is identifiable on physical examination or mammogram. In contrast, the onset of inflammatory breast cancer is sudden and can develop in weeks. Presentation includes a breast that looks "inflamed," red, and has the look of an orange peel (peau d'orange). The diagnosis may be delayed because the skin has the appearance of cellulitis with antibiotics prescribed first; however, the symptoms do not improve with treatment.

Staging is conducted to evaluate the extent of disease. This is completed to understand a patient's prognosis and to help to determine the best treatment course. Staging of breast cancer is determined using the TNM (T, tumor size; N, nodal status; M, any site of metastatic disease) classification. This information is determined by both clinical and pathologic examination. In 2010, the breast cancer staging system was updated by the American Joint Commission on Cancer.[28] Stage I disease involves small tumors (< 2 cm) with no lymph node involvement and is highly curable (~98% 5-year survival). Stage II includes small tumors with lymph node involvement or larger tumors (>2 cm and ≤ 5 cm) with no lymph node involvement. Stage III tumors are larger (>5 cm) with lymph node involvement with a 5-year survival of approximately 80%. Stage IV disease has metastasized to other distant organs and has the poorest prognosis with a 5-year survival of approximately 26% (Table 97-2).[25,26,29] Most patients will present with stage I or II disease due to routine screening. Based on C.D.'s clinical staging, she is considered to have stage II disease based on the size of her disease and the involvement of ipsilateral lymph nodes.

Prognostic Factors

CASE 97-3, QUESTION 5: Further pathologic analysis of C.D.'s breast tumor reveals estrogen receptor (ER)-positive and progesterone receptor (PR)-positive disease. Human epidermal growth factor receptor (HER2) testing of the tumor was negative. What routine prognostic factors are evaluated in all breast cancer patients?

Table 97-2
American Joint Committee on Cancer Staging for Breast Cancer

Stage	T	N	M
0	Tis	N0	M0
IA–B	T1–T1a	N0-N1mi	M0
IIA–B	T0–T3	N0–N1b	M0
IIIA	T0–T3	N1–N2	M0
IIIB	T4	N0–N2	M0
IIIC	Any T	N3	M0
IV	Any T	Any N	M1

T, tumor size and/or invasion; N, presence of lymph nodes; M, metastatic disease; N0, no lymph node involvement; N1, movable ipsilateral lymph nodes; mi, micrometastasis; N2, ipsilateral axillary lymph nodes (fixed or matted), or clinical ipsilateral internal mammary nodes with no axillary lymph node involvement; N3, ipsilateral infraclavicular lymph nodes, clinical ipsilateral internal mammary lymph nodes, clinical axillary lymph nodes, or ipsilateral supraclavicular lymph nodes with or without axillary or internal mammary lymph node involvement; Tis, carcinoma in situ; T1, ≤2 cm; T2, >2 to 5 cm; T3, >5 cm; T4, any size with skin invasion or direct invasion to the chest wall; T0 and T1 tumors with nodal micrometastasis only are excluded from stage IIA and are classified as stage IB.
Source: American Joint Committee on Cancer. Breast Cancer. In: Edge S, et al, eds. *AJCC Cancer Staging Manual*. 7th ed. New York, NY: Springer-Verlag; 2010:347.

In addition to staging, other prognostic factors should be evaluated to help determine a patient's treatment course. Prognostic factors such as size of the tumor and lymph node status are important. A larger tumor size denotes a poorer prognosis than a smaller tumor size, and the presence of disease in the lymph nodes leads to a poorer prognosis than lymph node-negative disease. Further, presence of a high number of positive lymph nodes is directly related to a poorer prognosis. Pathologic testing of the breast tumor gives important prognostic factors such as ER and PR and HER2 status.[30] Tumors that are ER- or PR-positive tend to denote a slower-growing, indolent disease and have a more favorable prognosis than ER- and/or PR-negative disease. Approximately two-thirds of breast cancer patients diagnosed have ER- and/or PR-positive disease. If a patient has ER- and/or PR-positive disease, hormonal therapy is a treatment option. Tumors that are HER2-positive generally denote more aggressive disease. Approximately 25% of breast cancers test positive for HER2 gene amplification. Although this is indicative of a more aggressive disease, it is a positive predictor for response to trastuzumab.

HER2 positivity is determined by two different methods, immunohistochemistry or fluorescence in situ hybridization (FISH). Either method could be used to determine HER2 status. Immunohistochemistry determines the overexpression of the HER2 protein, and results are reported as 1+, 2+, and 3+. Patients with 3+ overexpression are considered positive for HER2 and will respond to trastuzumab therapy or other HER2-targeted therapies. If a patient is determined to have 2+ overexpression (an equivocal test), then further testing would be conducted with FISH. FISH testing evaluates the HER2 gene amplification by denoting a ratio of the number of gene copies of HER2 compared to the control, and only those patients with positive FISH testing will respond to HER2-targeted therapies.[30]

Other pathologic tests are completed such as nuclear grade (which determines the degree of differentiation of the tumor cells) as well as tests to evaluate the growth fraction of the disease (such as S-phase fraction, Ki-67, and mitotic index). Clinicians use all of these factors (positive and negative) to determine a patient's prognosis and treatment course.

Other tools allow clinicians to take a more individualized approach (i.e., hormonal therapy alone, chemotherapy alone, or a combination of chemotherapy and hormonal therapy) to treatment. One such tool is Adjuvant!Online (www.Adjuvantonline.com), which can be used in early-stage breast cancer patients after surgery to evaluate their individual risk factors and determine treatment benefit versus risk of recurrence. This tool uses clinical factors to estimate an individual's percent risk reduction in recurrence after adjuvant treatment (the benefit with hormonal therapy alone versus the benefit of hormonal therapy and chemotherapy). In addition, genetic profiling has led to the creation of gene arrays to evaluate a patient's risk of recurrence based on their treatment course. Many patients today present with early-stage disease, which is highly curable. Clinicians can use these tests to determine which patients should receive more or less therapy based on their recurrence score. One such test is the Oncotype DX assay for patients with ER- and/or PR-positive and lymph node-negative disease and assigns a patient a recurrence score.[31] Based on the score, clinicians and patients can decide the best treatment course such as hormonal therapy alone versus the combination of hormonal therapy and chemotherapy.

Treatment

CASE 97-3, QUESTION 6: C.D. was diagnosed with a stage II, ER-positive and PR-positive, HER 2-negative IDC of the right breast. Her staging workup was negative as indicated previously with a negative CT scan of the chest, abdomen, and pelvis, and a negative bone scan. Based on this information what would be C.D.'s likely treatment course?

LOCAL TREATMENT (SURGERY AND RADIATION THERAPY)

Surgery is the definitive treatment in early-stage breast cancer. Many years ago, a more radical approach to the surgical removal of breast cancer was used. This approach, called a radical mastectomy, involved the removal of the entire breast, both the major and minor pectoralis muscle, and a full axillary lymph node dissection on the side of the breast cancer. Increased morbidity was associated with this approach such as shoulder dysfunction and a poor cosmetic appearance. Today, a modified radical mastectomy is used that removes the entire breast along with an axillary lymph node dissection while leaving the pectoralis muscles intact. This approach leads to equivalent survival compared with the radical surgery.[32–34] Radiation may be offered in addition to a modified radical mastectomy if the tumor is greater than 5 cm in size, if the patient has greater than four positive lymph nodes, or if positive tissue margins were present after surgery.[35,36] This further improves the local control of the disease. These guidelines are widely debated and the subject of numerous studies evaluating patient populations who would benefit from adjuvant radiation therapy.

Conservative approaches to surgery, such as lumpectomy, segmental mastectomy, or quadrantectomy, are also available. If a patient has a small tumor and wishes to preserve the breast, this surgical approach could be used; however, not all patients are candidates for this procedure. Those who are not candidates can include those with multicentric disease (numerous tumors throughout the breast), large tumors in relation to the size of the breast, and inflammatory breast cancer.[25,26] If the decision is to proceed with breast-conserving surgery, the patient must also undergo adjuvant radiation therapy. Because the surgery only removes the primary tumor, the rest of the breast should be treated with radiation therapy to prevent recurrence of disease. Similar survival rates are observed with modified radical mastectomy versus breast-conserving surgery plus radiation therapy.[33,37]

Larger tumors do not preclude a patient from undergoing breast-conservative surgery. However, to be eligible for this surgery, patients would receive neoadjuvant chemotherapy to help shrink the tumor to a size conducive to breast-conserving techniques. Neoadjuvant chemotherapy also allows the oncologist to assess response to treatment whereas the tumor is still in place and allows the opportunity to discontinue a particular chemotherapy regimen if the patient is not responding. Most patients will respond to chemotherapy; however, for those who do not, further chemotherapy (with a different regimen) or radiation therapy may be offered.[37]

The presence and extent of nodal disease is assessed through an axillary lymph node dissection. This involves the removal of at least 10 lymph nodes on the same side of the primary tumor to assess for the presence of breast cancer. Lymph node dissection may result in lymphedema, thromboembolism, and infection.[38–40] Sentinel lymph node biopsy is one way to avoid the comorbidities associated with the axillary lymph node dissection. In this procedure, a blue dye (labeled with a radiocolloid) is injected around the breast tumor. Time is given for the dye to drain from the tumor to the lymph nodes. The surgeon is able to identify the sentinel nodes because of the presence of radiocolloid and the blue color. The breast (and presumably the cancer) drains first into the sentinel lymph nodes. Only one or two of the sentinel lymph nodes will be removed, reducing the risk of lymphedema, thromboembolism, and infection.

Many consider this procedure the standard of care for assessment of the axillary lymph nodes.[38,41–43]

C.D. could either undergo breast-conserving surgery plus radiation therapy or a modified radical mastectomy, but with C.D.'s family history she may also choose to undergo bilateral mastectomies to prevent the development of contralateral breast cancer.

SYSTEMIC THERAPY (CHEMOTHERAPY, HORMONAL THERAPY, AND BIOLOGIC THERAPY)

Surgery and radiation therapy eradicates most tumor cells; however, microscopic disease is difficult to detect and treat locally. Microscopic cancer deposits can migrate throughout the body and serve as sites for disease recurrence. To diminish the chance of recurrence, systemic adjuvant chemotherapy, hormonal therapy, and/or biologic therapy is given. The determination of which single modality or combination of therapies is based on the patient's prognostic factors: ER/PR status and HER2 positivity. As mentioned earlier, tools such as the Oncotype DX genetic assay can estimate risk recurrence based on these tumor-specific characteristics and assist in determination of therapy.

The size of the tumor and other prognostic factors are also evaluated to determine the course of therapy; see Table 97-3. The NCCN provides treatment guidelines to help with treatment planning.[37] Patients with small tumors (0.6–1 cm) and negative lymph nodes can be further divided into two groups based on favorable and unfavorable prognostic features. Favorable prognostic features would include hormone-positive disease. These patients can be offered hormonal therapy without chemotherapy. Those individuals with poor prognostic features (tumors with lymphatic invasion, high nuclear grade, hormone receptor-negative, or HER2-positive disease) would be offered chemotherapy with or without trastuzumab therapy.[25,26]

Tumors greater than 1 cm in size are generally offered treatment with systemic chemotherapy. If the patient is ER- and/or PR-positive, they are additionally treated with hormonal therapy after chemotherapy. Biologic therapy with trastuzumab is added to chemotherapy if the patient has HER2-positive disease and assuming there are no contraindications such as cardiac disease. Patients should be fully informed of the absolute benefit of chemotherapy, because in those with early-stage disease the benefit from chemotherapy could be as low as 2% to 3%. The Early Breast Cancer Trialists' Collaborative Group conducts an overview analysis every 5 years on the effects of chemotherapy and hormonal therapy in breast cancer randomized trials. In 2005, the 15-year survival updates were published.[44] Although no standard regimen has been identified, combination regimens are superior to single-agent therapy (recurrence rates and mortality for combination chemotherapy, respectively: hazard ratio (HR), 0.77; $p < 0.00001$ and HR, 0.83; $p < 0.0001$, respectively; single-agent therapy recurrence rates and mortality: HR, 0.86; $p = 0.001$ and HR, 0.96; $p = 0.4$, respectively).[44,45] Updated meta-analyses have also included the use of taxanes to fixed anthracycline-based regimens. In the previous EBCTCG trial, taxanes were not included in the data analysis. With the incorporation of taxane therapy, breast cancer mortality was reduced: RR (event rate ratio: newer treatment versus control) = 0.86, SE (standard error) = 0.04, $p = 0.0005$.[46] This demonstrated the benefit of adding taxane therapy to standard adjuvant therapy for specific patients.

Table 97-3
Overview of the Selection of Adjuvant Treatment

	Adjuvant Hormonal Therapy		Adjuvant Chemotherapy[b]
Lymph Node-Negative Disease	**ER/PR (+)**	**ER/PR (−)**	
<0.5 cm	Yes	No	No
0.6–1 cm[a]	Yes	No	Consider
>1 cm	Yes	No	Yes
Lymph Node-Positive Disease	**ER/PR (+)**	**ER/PR (−)**	
	Yes	No	Yes

[a]Consider Oncotype DX testing: low recurrence score (<18) = adjuvant hormonal therapy; intermediate recurrence score (18–30) = adjuvant hormonal therapy ± chemotherapy; high recurrence score (≥31) = adjuvant hormonal therapy + chemotherapy.
[b]Give trastuzumab therapy if the patient is HER2 (+) and no contraindications.
Source: NCCN Guidelines. Breast Cancer. V2 http://www.nccn.org/professionals/physicians_gls/pdf/breast.pdf. Accessed August 2,2017

Looking back at C.D.'s tumor characteristics, she has stage II (2.2 cm with lymph node involvement), ER-positive, PR-positive, and HER2-negative breast cancer. Based on this information, C.D. would be a candidate for surgery and chemotherapy (based on the tumor size and lymph node-positive disease), followed by hormonal therapy due to her ER/PR-positive disease.

ADJUVANT CHEMOTHERAPY

CASE 97-3, QUESTION 7: C.D. underwent a right modified radical mastectomy and axillary lymph node dissection. She had 2 of 15 lymph nodes positive for disease. Her adjuvant treatment will consist of chemotherapy (due to the larger size of the tumor and positive lymph nodes). What are typical adjuvant chemotherapy regimens for the treatment of early-stage breast cancer, and what should C.D. receive?

Many different combination chemotherapy regimens are used in the adjuvant setting (Table 97-4). Anthracycline-containing regimens are commonly used. Doxorubicin or epirubicin in combination with an alkylating agent (cyclophosphamide) plus or minus fluorouracil is a typical regimen. In the most recent Early Breast Cancer Trialist' Cancer Group analysis, anthracycline-based regimens had significantly lower recurrence rates and death compared to traditional cyclophosphamide, methotrexate, and fluorouracil (recurrence rate ratio, 0.89; $p = 0.001$; and cancer death rate ratio, 0.84; $p < 0.00001$, respectively).[44] A large pooled analysis demonstrated improved disease-free ($p < 0.00001$) and overall survival ($p < 0.0001$) with the addition of a taxane.[46] Updated meta-analyses have also included the use of taxanes to fixed anthracycline-based regimens. As discussed earlier, the optimal taxane regimen has yet to be identified, and the full benefit of the utility of taxane therapy in lymph node-negative disease is yet to be determined; however, the benefit is apparent in lymph node-positive disease and taxanes should be incorporated into the treatment regimen of those with lymph node-positive disease.

Congestive heart failure is a well-known toxicity associated with anthracycline chemotherapy. If a patient has heart failure or other preexisting cardiac disease, anthracyclines must be used cautiously. To avoid potential toxicity, taxane regimens such as docetaxel and cyclophosphamide have been compared to a standard anthracycline-containing regimens, doxorubicin and cyclophosphamide. After 7 years of follow-up, both disease-free and overall survival were significantly better in the taxane arm compared with the anthracycline arm (81% vs. 75%; $p = 0.033$ and 87% vs. 82%; $p = 0.032$, respectively).[47] Although the results are encouraging, these data do not have the track record of the anthracycline-containing regimens that are still considered the mainstay of therapy for adjuvant chemotherapy in early-stage breast cancer. Studies are currently underway to identify specific populations that may not respond to anthracycline therapy, thereby avoiding the risk of cardiac toxicity in these individuals.[48] If these specific cases are identified, more nonanthracycline-based chemotherapy regimens will be incorporated into clinical practice. Based on C.D.'s lymph node–positive breast cancer, a typical adjuvant chemotherapy regimen would consist of doxorubicin and cyclophosphamide (AC) or fluorouracil and doxorubicin and cyclophosphamide (FAC) given every 3 weeks for four cycles followed by a taxane such as paclitaxel weekly for 12 weeks (see Table 97-4 for commonly used adjuvant chemotherapy regimens).

Trastuzumab therapy can be incorporated into a patient's adjuvant chemotherapy regimen if the tumor is HER2-positive. Trastuzumab was first studied in the metastatic setting and demonstrated improved overall survival when added concurrently with chemotherapy.[49] Because of its robust activity in the metastatic setting, it was then studied in early breast cancer to see whether the same benefit could be achieved. Two large trials were conducted concurrently addressing different questions regarding the use of concurrent, sequential, and maintenance trastuzumab.[50,51] Patients received the classic AC regimen for four cycles followed by paclitaxel weekly given either sequentially or concurrently. Trastuzumab therapy was started after the completion of the AC regimen to reduce potential cardiac toxicities associated with doxorubicin and trastuzumab.[50,51] The results of these trials were combined and published in full. Disease-free and overall survival were significantly improved with the addition of trastuzumab (52% decrease in recurrence rates, $p < 0.0001$; and 33% reduction in mortality, $p = 0.015$, respectively).[50,51] Four-year follow-up data continued to demonstrate significant improvements with trastuzumab compared to chemotherapy alone. Based on these data, trastuzumab was approved for use in early-stage, HER2-positive disease after the completion of AC therapy followed by sequential paclitaxel therapy for 1 year.[52] The use of maintenance trastuzumab was further studied in the HERA Trial (Herceptin Adjuvant Trial).[53] In that trial, patients were randomly assigned to complete 1 or 2 years of maintenance trastuzumab therapy. One year of trastuzumab therapy is the current standard of practice for maintenance therapy in the adjuvant setting. Because C.D. does not have HER2-positive disease, trastuzumab therapy should not be used.

Table 97-4
Common Neoadjuvant and Adjuvant Chemotherapy Regimens

Regimen
HER2-Negative Disease
Dose dense[a] AC → paclitaxel every 2 weeks
Dose dense[a] AC → paclitaxel weekly
TC
CMF, classic (oral) or intravenous
CAF (oral/intravenous)
CEF
TAC
AC
AC → paclitaxel weekly
AC → docetaxel every 3 weeks
FEC/CEF followed by paclitaxel or docetaxel
FAC followed by paclitaxel or docetaxel
HER2-Positive Disease
AC → paclitaxel + trastuzumab ± pertuzumab
TCH ± pertuzumab
AC → docetaxel + trastuzumab ± pertuzumab
Docetaxel + cyclophosphamide + trastuzumab
FEC → paclitaxel or docetaxel + pertuzumab
Paclitaxel + trastuzumab
Pertuzumab + trastuzumab + docetaxel or paclitaxel → FEC

[a]Dose dense, given every 2 weeks instead of every 3 weeks. See source document for specific dosing; TCH, docetaxel, carboplatin, trastuzumab.
A, adriamycin; C, cyclophosphamide; E, epirubicin; F, fluorouracil; M, methotrexate; P, paclitaxel; T, docetaxel; →, followed by.
Source: NCCN Guidelines Breast Cancer. V2. http://www.nccn.org/professionals/physicians_gls/pdf/breast.pdf. Accessed August 2, 2017.

CHEMOTHERAPY TOXICITY

CASE 97-3, QUESTION 8: C.D. is to undergo four cycles of AC chemotherapy followed by weekly paclitaxel for 12 weeks. What are the common toxicities associated with this treatment course? If the tumor was HER2-positive and C.D. received trastuzumab, what toxicities would be associated with its use?

Doxorubicin is an anthracycline chemotherapy agent. It works through multiple mechanisms, but inhibition of topoisomerase II may be most important.[54] By inhibiting this enzyme, double-strand DNA breaks occur. Common toxicities include myelosuppression, nausea/vomiting, and alopecia. A well-known toxicity of anthracyclines is the risk of cardiomyopathy due to the formation of oxygen free radicals and doxorubicin metal complexes. These toxicities can be acute (with symptoms similar to an arrhythmia or myocardial infarction) or chronic (with a patient demonstrating symptoms of congestive heart failure).[55] The risk of cardiotoxicity increases with larger anthracycline cumulative doses.[56,57] With the typical doses of anthracyclines used in the adjuvant setting, a patient will not reach the cumulative doses known to increase the risk of cardiotoxicity. If a patient has underlying cardiac dysfunction, baseline evaluation of ejection fraction through either an echocardiogram or a multigated acquisition scan should be completed.[56,58,59] Other known risk factors for the development of anthracycline-induced cardiotoxicity include age older than 70 years, hypertension, preexisting coronary artery disease, and previous cardiac irradiation or anthracycline exposure, which may warrant cardiac evaluation.[60,61]

Cyclophosphamide is an alkylating agent that works by forming cross-links in DNA, thus inhibiting DNA synthesis.[54] Common toxicities are nausea/vomiting, myelosuppression, and alopecia. The alkylating agents, although rare, are also associated with a risk of secondary leukemias.[54]

Paclitaxel, a taxane chemotherapy derived from the Pacific yew tree, works by binding to the β-tubulin subunit of microtubules, preventing disassembly and ultimately causing inhibition of mitosis. Common toxicities associated with paclitaxel include nausea/vomiting, myelosuppression, neuropathy, and hypersensitivity reactions due to the modified polyoxyethylated castor oil (Cremophor EL) solvent in paclitaxel. All patients should be premedicated with dexamethasone and H_1 and H_2 blockers to prevent hypersensitivity.[62]

Trastuzumab is a monoclonal antibody targeted against the extracellular HER2 protein. The classic toxicity associated with trastuzumab is cardiac toxicity, but is different from that with anthracyclines. Trastuzumab cardiotoxicity is considered reversible and believed to be a result of HER2 blockade (HER2 signaling is responsible for cardiomyocyte growth, repair, and survival).[60,61] In those patients who will receive long-term trastuzumab therapy, baseline cardiac function should be evaluated similar to doxorubicin and then periodically with echocardiogram or a multigated acquisition scan during therapy. C.D. does not have a history of cardiac disease, so a baseline cardiac evaluation before AC therapy may not occur. C.D. should be counseled on the common toxicities associated with her chemotherapy, such as myelosuppression, nausea/vomiting, alopecia, neuropathy, cardiomyopathy, and hypersensitivity reactions.

HORMONAL THERAPY

CASE 97-3, QUESTION 9: After the completion of her adjuvant chemotherapy, C.D. will receive hormonal therapy because her disease is ER/PR-positive. What are the common adjuvant hormonal regimens used? What regimen would be appropriate for C.D.?

Breast cancer is a hormonally mediated disease, and therapies that alter hormonal levels are an integral component to the treatment plan. This therapy is offered to patients with ER- and/or PR-positive disease. Therapeutic options include SERMs, luteinizing hormone-releasing hormone (LH-RH) agonists, and AIs. Menopausal status of the patient is used to help guide selection of therapy.

Traditionally, tamoxifen has been the gold standard for adjuvant hormonal therapy. Tamoxifen is a SERM, which works by blocking estrogen from binding to the ER. It does not alter estrogen production. Tamoxifen has antiestrogenic activity in the breast, although it has estrogenic effects in other areas such as bone.[63,64] Tamoxifen can be used in both premenopausal and postmenopausal women and is given 20 mg orally daily for 5 years based on the data from the National Surgical Adjuvant Breast and Bowel Project B-14 trial.[65] Tamoxifen should be initiated after chemotherapy because it can antagonize the antitumor activity of chemotherapy if given concurrently.[66] Common toxicities associated with therapy are hot flashes and vaginal discharge. More thrombosis, pulmonary embolisms, and strokes can occur in patients (older than 50 years of age) receiving tamoxifen compared to placebo (risk ratio, 1.60, 3.19, 1.59, respectively).[11]

Ovarian suppression is an alternative therapy for premenopausal patients because the ovaries are the largest source of estrogen. This is typically achieved through the use of LH-RH agonists. Surgery or radiation can also induce ovarian ablation; however, surgery is irreversible and offers an immediate effect whereas radiation may offer an incomplete response and slower onset.[67] If a woman would like to maintain fertility throughout chemotherapy, a thorough discussion with her physician should occur. Studies with the use of LH-RH agents have been tested as a means to preserve fertility but have shown mixed results.[68] Combination data with an LH-RH agonist with tamoxifen have not shown significantly better outcomes than each modality alone.[68,69]

Postmenopausal patients also have the option of AI therapy. Aromatase inhibitors inhibit the production of estrogen by preventing the conversion of androstenedione and testosterone to estrone and estradiol. There are two classes of agents: nonsteroidal AIs (anastrozole and letrozole) and the steroidal AI, exemestane. These agents are highly selective for the aromatase enzyme and have less toxicity than tamoxifen and other hormonal agents. Aromatase inhibitors should only be used in postmenopausal women. If used in the premenopausal setting, initial surges of estrogen occur due to the body's compensation mechanisms (i.e., hypothalamic–pituitary axis) and negative feedback loop. Table 97-5 provides a list of adjuvant hormonal therapies that can be used. If used as single therapy, AIs are given for 5 years.

The optimal hormonal therapy regimen for the adjuvant setting has not been identified. In premenopausal women, the options are 5 years of tamoxifen therapy plus or minus ovarian suppression with an LH-RH agonist. If the patient continues to be premenopausal at the end of 5 years of adjuvant tamoxifen therapy, the patient may consider five additional years of therapy. There are conflicting data to support this recommendation. Based on newer data, the American Society of Clinical Oncology published an updated practice guideline for adjuvant hormonal therapy.[70–72]

If, after 2 to 3 years, the patient becomes postmenopausal, then 2 to 3 years of an AI may be given to complete a total of 5 years of therapy. If the patient is postmenopausal at the beginning of adjuvant hormonal therapy, an option would be to take an AI for 5 years. There have been no prospective comparisons of the AIs with each other; therefore, any can be used as first-line treatment.[73,74] Another clinical option is 5 years of tamoxifen, and, if the patient is postmenopausal after the end of 5 years, an additional 5 years of an AI can be given. This was found to be beneficial in an extended study of hormonal therapy (the BIG 1–98 trial). At

Table 97-5
Adjuvant Hormonal Therapies

Type	Dose	Toxicities
Nonsteroidal		
Anastrozole Letrozole	1 mg daily PO 2.5 mg daily PO	Common toxicities: myalgias/arthralgias, hot flashes, osteoporosis
Steroidal		
Exemestane	25 mg daily PO	Common toxicities: myalgias/arthralgias, hot flashes, osteoporosis
SERMs		
Tamoxifen	20 mg daily PO	Common toxicities: hot flashes, vaginal discharge Rare but serious side effects: deep vein thrombosis, pulmonary embolism, abnormal uterine bleeding

Source: Jones KL, Buzdar AU. A review of adjuvant hormonal therapy in breast cancer. *Endocr Relat Cancer*. 2004;11:391; Buzdar AU, Howell A. Advances in aromatase inhibitors: clinical efficacy and tolerability in the treatment of breast cancer. *Clin Cancer Res*. 2001;7:2620.

the 2.4-year follow-up, additional letrozole therapy was associated with a superior 4-year disease-free survival (93% with extended letrozole vs. 87% in the tamoxifen arm; $p < 0.001$).[75] However, in the 8.1-year follow-up data, the additional letrozole therapy did not improve outcomes compared with letrozole monotherapy in terms of disease-free and overall survival.[76] Each individual's length of therapy should be determined based on the patient's risk of recurrence and their ability to tolerate therapy. Table 97-6 lists adjuvant hormonal therapy options.

C.D. is premenopausal, so she would start with tamoxifen therapy. If after 2 to 3 years of therapy, C.D. becomes postmenopausal, she could continue the tamoxifen for a total of 5 years or convert to an AI to complete a total of 5 years of therapy then continuing the AI for an additional 5 years. Because of her age, she will likely continue to be premenopausal after chemotherapy and be maintained on tamoxifen for 5 years. If she remains premenopausal, she should have a discussion with her physician on the merits of continuing tamoxifen for a total of 10 years. If she completes 5 years of tamoxifen therapy and is postmenopausal at that time, then extended use of an AI for an additional 5 years would be recommended. At this time, ovarian suppression with an LH-RH agonist could also be added because she is premenopausal to chemically suppress her ovarian function.

METASTATIC BREAST CANCER

Treatment—Endocrine Therapy

CASE 97-4

Question 1: T.R. is a 65-year-old, postmenopausal woman diagnosed with breast cancer at the age of 48 years. At the time of diagnosis she was premenopausal. She underwent surgery with a modified radical mastectomy and was found to have a 1.5-cm IDC of the right breast. She had 2 of 10 lymph nodes positive. Her breast cancer was ER-positive, PR-positive and HER2-negative. T.R. went on to complete adjuvant chemotherapy with AC therapy for four cycles followed by weekly paclitaxel for 12 weeks. After completion of her chemotherapy, she received 5 years of tamoxifen therapy. Ten years after completing her therapy, she experiences pain in her right arm and rib cage. A bone scan revealed metastatic breast cancer. What would be an appropriate treatment regimen for T.R. at this time?

Early-stage breast cancer is curable. However, if a patient develops metastatic disease, the goal of treatment shifts from cure to palliation and stabilization of disease. Treatment is offered to improve quality of life and alleviate symptoms from treatment or disease. The mean survival time after diagnosis of metastatic disease is approximately 2 to 4 years; however, this can range from months to many years depending on the site of the metastases.[77] The choice of therapy is based on the site of disease and

Table 97-6
Overview of Adjuvant Hormonal Therapy

Option 1	Option 2	Option 3
Premenopausal at time of therapy initiation (Patients can complete one of 3 different options)		
Tamoxifen × 5 years ± LH-RH agonist or ovarian ablation	If still premenopausal after 2–3 years of tamoxifen therapy, complete a total of 5 years of tamoxifen	If still premenopausal after 5 years of tamoxifen, consider an additional 5 years of tamoxifen
	If postmenopausal after 2–3 years: **A.** Complete 5 years of tamoxifen followed by 5 additional years of an AI OR **B.** Convert to an AI × 2–3 years for a total of 5 years of hormonal therapy	If postmenopausal after 5 years of therapy, give AI × 5 additional years
Postmenopausal at time of therapy initiation (Preferred to start with an AI if the patient is postmenopausal at the onset of therapy)		
Any AI × 5 years	Tamoxifen × 2–3 years then an AI to complete a total of 5 years	Tamoxifen × 4–6 years then an AI for 5 additional years

AI, aromatase inhibitor; LH-RH, luteinizing hormone-releasing hormone.
Source: NCCN Guidelines. Breast Cancer. V2. http://www.nccn.org/professionals/physicians_gls/pdf/breast.pdf. Accessed August 2, 2017.

other factors that help guide therapy such as ER and PR status. Endocrine therapy is more likely to be effective in patients with bone-only disease whereas chemotherapy may be used when there is visceral disease (i.e., liver or lung). Patients with organ involvement tend to have more rapidly growing disease that generally requires therapy with a quicker onset of action such as chemotherapy.[25] In addition to systemic therapy (chemotherapy and/or hormonal and/or biologic therapy), the clinician needs to determine whether or not local therapy (such as radiation or surgery) would be appropriate for a patient. Radiation therapy can be used to target painful bone metastases, to prevent further tumor growth, and to relieve pain. Surgery may be performed on bones with impending fractures, spinal cord compression, or brain metastases for palliation. These modalities of treatment only affect the local site of disease, so a combination of local and systemic therapy would need to be administered to fully treat the patient. If a patient is experiencing worsening symptoms such as shortness of breath due to lung metastases or increased abdominal pain due to liver metastases, the use of chemotherapy may be preferred over hormonal therapy because of its quicker onset of action.[78] Disease recurrence greater than 5 years after diagnosis illustrates a more indolent-growing disease and is a favorable prognostic factor. Tumors with ER- and/or PR-positive characteristics would also be considered a good prognostic factor. Once therapy is initiated, response to therapy should be monitored periodically. Tumor markers such as CA.27.29 and CA.15.3 are commonly monitored in metastatic breast cancer. A clinical examination in combination with radiologic tests and tumor markers is assessed to determine response to therapy. Based on T.R.'s metastatic bone disease and ER/PR-positive tumor characteristics, the use of hormonal therapy would be the most appropriate agent to initiate. T.R. received tamoxifen therapy in the adjuvant setting. Because she progressed after taking tamoxifen therapy, this would not be reinitiated. An AI would be started because she is postmenopausal and should be continued until there is evidence of progression of disease via radiologic findings or increases in tumor markers.

CASE 97-4, QUESTION 2: T.R. is started on anastrozole 1 mg orally daily. What are other hormonal agents that can be used in the treatment of metastatic breast cancer?

Hormonal therapy in the metastatic setting can provide long progression-free survival in patients. If the patient responds for an extended period of time, the likelihood of response to another hormonal agent is high.[74] A patient may take multiple hormonal therapies before ever having to receive chemotherapy. As before, the decision regarding which hormonal agent to use is based on one's menopausal status. If the patient is premenopausal, the options include tamoxifen and LH-RH agonists; however, if the patient has received a SERM in the adjuvant setting, this would not be used again in the metastatic setting. Aromatase inhibitors are indicated for use in first-line therapy in the metastatic setting for postmenopausal women. If an AI is chosen as the first-line agent in the metastatic setting, use of another AI after progression would include one from another category (i.e., nonsteroidal vs. steroidal AI). For example, if anastrozole was used as first-line therapy for metastatic disease, then when the patient progresses, exemestane can be used.

Many other hormonal agents are available for use. The pure antiestrogen, fulvestrant, is the only drug in a unique category of agents. It exerts its mechanism via binding and blocking of the ER and downregulates the number of ER s. Fulvestrant is administered as an intramuscular injection and is dosed initially as 500 mg on days 1, 14, and 28, then 500 mg monthly.[79,80] It is approved for use after failure of tamoxifen therapy in the metastatic setting.[79] This is an alternative for patients with compliance issues due to its once-monthly intramuscular dosing. Other hormonal agents used in metastatic disease are megestrol acetate, progestins, and high-dose estrogens (higher doses have been found to inhibit cancer cell growth). These agents were used routinely before the approval of AIs. Now they are reserved for use after multiple hormonal therapy failures due to the toxicities associated with these therapies such as weight gain, vaginal bleeding, and thromboembolic events.[25]

Newer data have evaluated a class a drugs called the mTOR (mammalian target of rapamycin) inhibitors.[81] These agents have demonstrated the ability to block resistance pathways of endocrine therapy. In the BOLERO-2 trial, patients who had failed previous AI therapy were randomized to everolimus 10 mg orally daily plus exemestane 25 mg orally daily versus exemestane plus placebo.[82] Progression-free survival was statistically significantly better in the combination arm, but follow-up overall survival results did not demonstrate the same results.[82] FDA approval was granted to this combination therapy in the metastatic setting after patients have failed a nonsteroidal AI.

Another new class of agents just recently approved in the first-line metastatic setting for HER2-negative, ER-positive patients is the cyclin-dependent kinase (CDK) inhibitors. Palbociclib, in combination with letrozole, was found to increase PFS in the phase II, Paloma-1 trial.[83] Overall survival has yet to be determined, and a large phase III trial is currently underway. This agent targets the inhibition of CDK 4 and 6 and inhibits cell growth and division. Serious side effects identified included neutropenia, pulmonary embolism (3 patients), back pain (2 patients), and diarrhea (2 patients).[83] T.R. was started on anastrozole therapy. She could have been initiated on any of the AIs. If her disease progresses, options include sequential exemestane, exemestane plus everolimus, fulvestrant, and then other agents such as megestrol acetate, high-dose estrogens, or androgens. The goal is to continue T.R. on multiple lines of hormonal therapy (as long as she is responding) before administering chemotherapy.

Prevention of Skeletal Events

CASE 97-4, QUESTION 3: In addition to anastrozole therapy, what other supportive care medicines should be added to T.R.'s regimen?

Patients with bone metastases are commonly treated with bisphosphonate therapy to decrease the risk of skeletal-related events (i.e., pathologic fractures, spinal cord compression, need for surgery, or radiation to the bone). Bisphosphonates act by inhibiting bone resorption. This ultimately will halt osteoclastic activity leading to stabilization of bony involvement, prevention of fractures, and reduction in calcium levels.[84,85] Bisphosphonates used are pamidronate 90 mg intravenously (IV) for 2 hours or zoledronic acid 4 mg IV for 15 minutes. Either of these agents can be administered once a month. Bisphosphonates are typically well tolerated although they may cause nausea, increased bone pain, and fever. Reduced doses should be used in patients with underlying renal dysfunction. A more well-known but uncommon side effect is osteonecrosis of the jaw.[86] The mechanism by which this occurs is not fully understood, but prevention is critical. If dental extractions or surgery is needed, patients should not be initiated on bisphosphonate therapy until these procedures are completed. If these procedures are required after initiation of therapy, an oral maxillofacial surgeon should be consulted.

A more recently approved agent for use in the prevention of skeletal-related events in solid tumors is the humanized monoclonal antibody, denosumab. This therapy offers a unique mechanism of action, targeting the RANK ligand, which is a mediator in osteoclast activity. Inhibition of osteoclastic activity by denosumab reduces bone pathology in osseous metastases. Denosumab has been compared prospectively with zoledronic acid in metastatic breast cancer patients and demonstrated significant delays in and prevention of skeletal-related events.[87] Denosumab is administered as a subcutaneous injection and is given once a month. It has similar toxicities to zoledronic acid, but the dose does not require adjustments for declining renal function. Denosumab has been added to the American Society of Clinical Oncology guidelines for the prevention of skeletal events in metastatic breast cancer and other solid tumors.[88] T.R. can start on bisphosphonate therapy with zoledronic acid 4 mg IV or denosumab 120 mcg SC once a month to help prevent skeletal-related events.

Progression of Disease

CASE 97-4, QUESTION 4: T.R. has a long progression-free survival on hormonal therapy. Over the course of 4 years, she progresses on sequential anastrozole, then fulvestrant, then exemestane plus everolimus, and eventually, megestrol acetate. Each time she has progressed, the progression-free interval has shortened. Follow-up staging tests now reveal new liver lesions measuring 1 cm × 1 cm and 2 cm × 1 cm. A CT scan of the chest was negative. She is not currently experiencing any symptoms of her disease. What should the treatment course include now that T.R. has progressed after numerous lines of endocrine therapy?

Because T.R. has progressed through multiple lines of hormonal therapy and the progression-free interval has shortened with each treatment course, chemotherapy would now likely be the best option. Patients with a good performance status, little previous treatment, prolonged progression-free intervals, and limited metastatic disease are more likely to respond to further treatment with chemotherapy.[78] Chemotherapy is continued as long as the person is receiving benefit and is tolerating toxicities associated with treatment. If the disease progresses or the toxicities become intolerable, therapy should be changed or stopped. Patients experiencing toxicities may be placed on a chemotherapy holiday until toxicities are resolved or until therapy is tolerable.

In the metastatic setting, stabilization of disease and palliation of symptoms are considered when deciding what chemotherapy regimen to use. Sequential (single agent) versus combination chemotherapy should be discussed. Combination chemotherapy is generally associated with more toxicities than sequential treatment; however, it provides improved response rates.[25,89–91] Patients with substantial symptoms from their disease may initially be given combination therapy to rapidly shrink the tumor. Combination therapies that have demonstrated improvements in survival are docetaxel and capecitabine, paclitaxel and gemcitabine, and doxorubicin and paclitaxel. Based on T.R.'s lack of symptoms, sequential therapy would be the best option for her at this time. This would offer her less toxicity and reserve other chemotherapeutic agents for the future.

Chemotherapy decisions can be very complex. There is no one standard regimen, and decisions should be made on an individual basis based on the patient's prior treatment, concurrent comorbidities, and time from adjuvant therapy to metastatic disease.

Most individuals today will have received anthracycline and taxane chemotherapy in the adjuvant setting. If the patient's disease recurs quickly after adjuvant therapy (i.e., less than one year), the disease is considered resistant to that treatment and different agents should be selected. If a patient receives adjuvant paclitaxel and progresses on therapy, there are data to support the use of docetaxel in the treatment of metastatic disease because of the lack of cross-resistance between taxanes.[92,93] Other chemotherapeutic agents with mechanisms similar to taxanes, such as eribulin or ixabepilone, have been approved for use in previous taxane failures. These agents offer additional options to patients who had responded to previous therapies.[25]

Previous toxicity is also considered when selecting therapy. In patients with preexisting neuropathies either from diabetes or previous chemotherapy, taxanes may not be an appropriate choice because these agents can also cause neuropathy. Additionally, capecitabine may be chosen over intravenous chemotherapy because this agent is administered orally. Table 97-7 provides a list of commonly used agents/regimens in the metastatic setting. Clinical trials are always an option for patients if they have a good performance status. Many clinical trials are available and should be discussed with the patient if clinical trials are a possibility. Because T.R. has received an anthracycline and taxane agent in the adjuvant setting, an agent such as capecitabine would be an appropriate choice. This is an oral agent and also has the indication for first-line treatment of metastatic disease after failure of anthracycline and taxane chemotherapy.

Table 97-7
Commonly Used Chemotherapy Agents in the Metastatic Setting

HER2-Negative	
Sequential or single agent	Doxorubicin, epirubicin, liposomal doxorubicin, paclitaxel, docetaxel, capecitabine, vinorelbine, gemcitabine, albumin-bound paclitaxel, eribulin, ixabepilone
Combination chemotherapy	FAC, CAF, FEC AC, EC, CMF, GT docetaxel/capecitabine, gemcitabine/carboplatin
HER2-Positive	
Chemotherapy + trastuzumab	Pertuzumab/trastuzumab/docetaxel, pertuzumab/trastuzumab/paclitaxel, paclitaxel/carboplatin, docetaxel, vinorelbine, capecitabine
If previously received trastuzumab	Lapatinib/capecitabine, trastuzumab + other first-line agents, trastuzumab/capecitabine, trastuzumab/lapatinib, ado-trastuzumab emtansine
Single-agent therapy used after failing standard options listed here	Cyclophosphamide, mitoxantrone, cisplatin, etoposide (oral), vinblastine, fluorouracil (continuous infusion), ixabepilone

A, doxorubicin; C, cyclophosphamide; E, epirubicin; F, fluorouracil; G, gemcitabine; H, trastuzumab; M, methotrexate; T, paclitaxel.
Source: NCCN Guidelines. Breast Cancer. V2. **http://www.nccn.org/professionals/physicians_gls/pdf/breast.pdf**. Accessed August 2, 2017.

CASE 97-4, QUESTION 5: Would T.R. be a candidate for any biologic therapy for the treatment of her metastatic breast cancer if she was HER2-positive?

Trastuzumab revolutionized the treatment of HER2-positive breast cancer. Newer biologic therapies are also available for use in the metastatic setting. Trastuzumab is a fully humanized monoclonal antibody that binds to the extracellular HER2 receptor and works via antigen-dependent cellular cytotoxicity. When chemotherapy alone was compared with chemotherapy plus trastuzumab in HER2-positive metastatic breast cancer, the addition of trastuzumab therapy significantly increased survival.[49] This was the first study of its kind using biologic therapy and demonstrating survival benefit in metastatic breast cancer. Current practice is to continue the trastuzumab in patients who progress on a chemotherapy regimen but switch to an alternative chemotherapy agent.

As with all chemotherapeutic agents, breast cancer can become resistant to therapy. Trastuzumab provided significant improvement in overall survival for patients with HER2-positive disease; however, trastuzumab resistance occurs. Newer pathways and resistance patterns have been identified to help clinicians understand the complexity of this disease. Two therapies are now approved for use in HER2-positive patients.[94] Pertuzumab offers a novel mechanism of action for HER2-positive patients. This agent is a monoclonal antibody similar to trastuzumab but blocks the extracellular domain on the HER2 receptor and blocks ligand-dependent heterodimerization with HER1, HER3, and HER4. The binding is different from trastuzumab in that trastuzumab binds to domain IV while pertuzumab binds to domain II of the HER2 receptor. The CLEOPATRA trial evaluated pertuzumab in combination with docetaxel and trastuzumab versus docetaxel and trastuzumab and placebo for the first-line treatment of metastatic breast cancer.[95] At a median follow-up of 50 months, the pertuzumab arm demonstrated improved OS of 56.5 months versus 40.8 months in the docetaxel + trastuzumab arm (HR, 0.68; 95% CI, 0.56 to 0.84; $p < 0.001$).[95] Those treated with pertuzumab experienced more diarrhea, rash, mucosal inflammation, and febrile neutropenia. Pertuzumab is approved for use in the first-line metastatic setting and the neoadjuvant setting in combination with docetaxel and trastuzumab.

Because pertuzumab does target the HER2 receptor, there is a concern regarding cardiac toxicity associated with its use. In the cardiac assessment of the CLEOPATRA trial, the incidence of cardiac adverse events (all grades) was similar between arms: 16.4% versus 14.5% in the placebo arm and the pertuzumab arm, respectively. Most patients experienced asymptomatic decreases in left-ventricular ejection fraction which resolved upon removal of the drug.[95,96]

Ado-trastuzumab emtansine (also known as TDM-1) is a unique formulation of an antibody–drug conjugate: Trastuzumab linked to DM1, a maytansine derivative. Maytansine is a potent microtubular inhibitor. Once the drug binds to the HER2 receptor, it is internalized and then undergoes degradation, releasing the cytotoxic agent to induce apoptosis. This agent was approved based on the results from the EMILIA trial comparing ado-trastuzumab to capecitabine and lapatinib in patients who had failed previous taxanes and trastuzumab.[97] Ado-trastuzumab improved both PFS and OS. Common toxicities for this agent include peripheral neuropathy, fatigue, anemia, increased liver enzymes, and myelosuppression. As with other HER2-targeted therapies, the concern for cardiac toxicity was evaluated. Less cardiotoxicity was identified in the ado-trastuzumab group compared to the combination arm (1.8% vs. 3.3%, respectively). This drug's name is very similar to traditional trastuzumab and hence the FDA recommendation for the addition of the prefix ado- to the name.[98] The approved indication of this agent includes use in patients with HER2-positive metastatic breast cancer who have previously received trastuzumab and a taxane, separately or in combination.

Lapatinib was the second HER2 target agent approved after trastuzumab. It is an oral tyrosine kinase inhibitor (small molecule) that inhibits both the activity of HER2 and the epidermal growth factor receptor. Lapatinib received approval based on a study in which capecitabine was compared with capecitabine plus lapatinib.[99] This trial included patients whose disease had progressed during or after an anthracycline, taxane, and trastuzumab therapy. Time to progression was statistically significantly better with the combination therapy compared to capecitabine alone (HR, 0.46; 95% confidence interval, 0.34–0.71; $p < 0.001$).[99]

Toxicities commonly associated with lapatinib are diarrhea and rash. Concerns of cardiotoxicity associated with lapatinib have been closely monitored in these trials. Because one of the mechanisms of lapatinib is blockade of HER2 (like trastuzumab), there is concern regarding its cardiotoxicity potential. Currently, data do not demonstrate an increased risk of cardiac dysfunction with lapatinib; however, long-term data are needed.[100] Lapatinib's approved indications include use in combination with capecitabine or combined with letrozole therapy or in those who have failed prior anthracyclines, taxanes, and trastuzumab for metastatic breast cancer.

One concern with lapatinib is its inhibition of the cytochrome P-450 (CYP) 3A4 and 2C8 isoenzymes. Because of this, when a patient is initiated on therapy, a full review of medications should occur to ensure no drug–drug interactions. Recommendations are included in the package insert for use and dosing of lapatinib with CYP3A4 inhibitors and inducers.[101]

If TR had HER2-positive disease, a common first-line regimen to use in the metastatic setting would be pertuzumab, trastuzumab, in combination with docetaxel based from the data of the CLEOPATRA trial. Second-line therapy in those that are exposed to previous trastuzumab therapy could include ado-trastuzumab emtansine or lapatinib in combination with capecitabine therapy.

Other unique targeted therapies are being evaluated in metastatic breast cancer. Poly-ADP-ribose polymerase (PARP) inhibitors potentially offer unique activity for patients with triple-negative breast cancers (ER/PR/HER2-negative disease). These tumors are typically refractory to chemotherapy and difficult to treat. PARP is an enzyme that repairs DNA breaks and is overexpressed in triple-negative breast cancers. Hence, this class of investigational inhibitors is expected to enhance the activity for cytotoxic therapies such as DNA-damaging agents. Initial studies have been promising, and currently phase III trials are underway to evaluate the antitumor activity of PARP inhibitors in the metastatic setting.[102] Other agents in the pipeline are mTOR (mammalian target of rapamycin) inhibitors, HSP90 (heat shock protein 90) inhibitors, multitargeted inhibitors of vascular endothelial growth factor receptor, and platelet-derived growth factor as well as other monoclonal antibodies.[102]

KEY REFERENCES AND WEBSITES

A full list of references for this chapter can be found at http://thepoint.lww.com/AT11e. Below are the key references and websites for this chapter, with the corresponding reference number in this chapter found in parentheses after the reference.

Key References

Briest S, Stearns V. Chemotherapeutic strategies for advanced breast cancer. *Oncology* (Williston Park). 2007;21:1325. (78)

Burnstein HJ et al. Adjuvant endocrine therapy for women with hormone receptor-positive breast cancer: American Society of Clinical Oncology clinical practice guideline focused update. *J Clin Oncol*. 2014;32(21):2259–2269. (72)

Carlson RW et al. Invasive breast cancer. *J Natl Compr Canc Netw*. 2011;9:136. (16)

Early Breast Cancer Trialists' Collaborative Group (EBCTCG). Effects of chemotherapy and hormonal therapy for early breast cancer on recurrence and 15-year survival: an overview of the randomised trials. *Lancet*. 2005;365:1687. (43)

Fisher B et al. Tamoxifen for prevention of breast cancer: report of the National Surgical Adjuvant Breast and Bowel Project P-1 study. *J Natl Cancer Inst*. 1998;90:1371. (11)

Lyman GH et al. Sentinel lymph node biopsy for patients with early stage breast cancer: American Society of Clinical Oncology clinical practice guideline update. *J Clin Oncol*. 2014;32:1365–1383. (42)

Romond EH et al. Trastuzumab plus adjuvant chemotherapy for operable HER2-positive breast cancer. *N Engl J Med*. 2005;353:1673. (50)

Slamon DJ et al. Use of chemotherapy plus a monoclonal antibody against HER2 for metastatic breast cancer that overexpresses HER2. *N Engl J Med*. 2001;344:783. (49)

Van Poznak CH et al. American Society of Clinical Oncology executive summary of the clinical practice guideline update on the role of bone-modifying agents in metastatic breast cancer. *J Clin Oncol*. 2011;29:1221. (88)

Yang SH et al. Breast conservation therapy for stage I or stage II breast cancer: A meta-analysis of randomized controlled trials. *Ann Oncol*. 2008;19:1039–1044. (36)

Key Websites

NCCN Guidelines. Breast Cancer. V2. http://www.nccn.org/professionals/physicians_gls/pdf/breast.pdf. Accessed August 2, 2017. (36)

98 Lung Cancer

Sara K. Butler

CORE PRINCIPLES

	CHAPTER CASES
1 Non-small-cell lung cancer (NSCLC) and small-cell lung cancer (SCLC) together account for more cancer-related deaths than any other malignancy for both men and women. Smoking is the biggest risk factor, and is proportional to the number of pack years. For former smokers, the risk for developing the disease decreases over time after smoking cessation.	**Case 98-1 (Question 1)**
2 Chances for survival are increased for those whose disease is detected early. The U.S. Preventive Services Task Force recommends annual screening with low-dose computed tomography in patients 55–80 years old with at least a 30-pack-year smoking history in current smokers or those who have quit within 15 years as this did increase detection and improve survival.	**Case 98-1 (Question 1), Table 98-3**
3 The initial signs and symptoms vary according to location and stage of the disease. Many patients are asymptomatic upon initial diagnosis, or signs and symptoms may be masked by other concurrent conditions such as chronic obstructive pulmonary disease.	**Case 98-1 (Question 2), Case 98-2 (Question 1), Table 98-1**
4 Surgery, radiotherapy, and chemotherapy are all modalities used in the treatment of NSCLC. Treatment decisions are individualized according to disease stage, tumor histology (e.g., adenocarcinoma, squamous), presence or absence of molecular marker mutations (e.g., epidermal growth factor receptor (EGFR), anaplastic lymphoma kinase (ALK)), performance status, comorbidities, and patient preference.	**Case 98-1 (Questions 2, 3), Case 98-2 (Questions 1–7), Tables 98-4–98-6**
5 Small-cell lung cancer tumors generally have a higher proliferation rate than NSCLC tumors. Hence, chemotherapy and radiotherapy are the primary treatments. These tumors tend to grow more centrally and rapidly than NSCLC tumors; therefore, surgical resection is usually not performed.	**Case 98-3 (Questions 1–4)**
6 Most NSCLC cytotoxic chemotherapy regimens are cisplatin-based or carboplatin-based doublets, which are given for 4–6 cycles. Maintenance therapy has been shown to be beneficial for patients receiving pemetrexed, bevacizumab, and erlotinib therapies. Targeted therapies are currently limited to the treatment of some late stage inoperable NSCLCs, but their use is under investigation for patients diagnosed with earlier stages of the disease.	**Case 98-1 (Question 4), Case 98-2 (Questions 1–3), Tables 98-4–98-6**
7 Most SCLC cytotoxic chemotherapy regimens are cisplatin-based or carboplatin-based doublets in combination with etoposide or sometimes irinotecan if extensive-stage disease. Investigations have not shown the utility for targeted agents in treating this disease.	**Case 98-3 (Questions 3–6)**

Lung cancers may be referred to as non-small-cell lung cancer (NSCLC) or small-cell lung cancer (SCLC) and, although there are many similarities between these two, treatments will often differ. Approximately 85% of lung cancers are classified as NSCLC and the remaining are classified as SCLC.[1] This chapter will initially focus on the presentation, diagnosis, and treatment of NSCLC, followed by a shorter section that describes SCLC.

Non-Small-Cell Lung Cancer

EPIDEMIOLOGY

Incidence for NSCLC in the United States is second to prostate cancer in men and breast cancer for women. Lung cancer is the leading cause of death relative to all of the other cancers. As with most solid tumors, survival is better for patients diagnosed with early-stage disease than it is for those with more advanced disease.[2] However, for many patients, the disease often goes undetected either due to the lack of noticeable symptoms or because they may be masked by concurrent diseases with similar symptoms such as chronic obstructive pulmonary disease (COPD).

PATHOPHYSIOLOGY

Non-small-cell lung cancer tumorigenesis is a multistep process in which neoplastic tissue arises from bronchial epithelium. These cells, which form the inner lining of bronchial tissue, develop genetic lesions to proto-oncogenes and tumor suppressor genes, resulting in the dysregulation of key molecular signaling pathways. As a result, cellular proliferation occurs and responsiveness to apoptotic signaling is often diminished. Eventually, accumulation of additional genetic abnormalities can influence the cell's ability to metastasize, resulting in the spread of tumorous tissue locally or to more distant sites in the lymph nodes and organs.

Non-small-cell lung tumors are classified further according to tumor tissue histology. The three major histologic types include squamous cell carcinoma, adenocarcinoma, and large cell carcinomas. Although these different variants were identified several decades ago, recently it has been demonstrated that the histology impacts chemotherapeutic agent selection. These three may be subcategorized further and other variants of NSCLC also exist; however, discussion in this chapter will be limited to these three. The adenocarcinomas and large cell carcinomas are commonly grouped together as nonsquamous carcinomas. These tumors commonly arise in the periphery of the lung and the smaller airways. After various periods of growth in the lung parenchyma or bronchial wall, these primary tumors invade the vascular and lymphatic system, enabling metastases to regional lymph nodes and more distant sites.[1]

RISK FACTORS AND CLINICAL PRESENTATION

There are several risk factors for developing lung cancer, but the biggest factor is cigarette smoking, which is estimated to increase the risk by up to 30-fold. The prevalence of smoking peaked in the early 1960s and has steadily decreased in the United States due to increased awareness of the harm of smoking. Death rates from lung cancer in both men and women have also followed this downward trend. For men, deaths due to lung cancer peaked in the 1980s and has since steadily decreased. For women, deaths due to lung cancer began to decline in the mid-2000s. Other risk factors include secondhand smoke, cigar and pipe smoking, occupational and environmental exposures, radon, asbestos, certain metals such as chromium and cadmium, various organic chemicals, radiation, air pollution, history of tuberculosis, and genetic factors. The latter appears to be related to those who exhibit the disease early in life. The probability of developing invasive lung cancer increases with age and peaks during the seventh decade of life.[2–4]

Table 98-1
Common Selected Signs and Symptoms for Lung Cancer

Cough
Hemoptysis
Wheeze
Dyspnea
Pain (e.g., chest wall)
Obstruction of vital structures (e.g., esophagus, superior vena cava)

Symptoms are highly dependent on tumor size, location within the chest cavity, and presence of metastases.

The disease is detected either when a person presents with signs and symptoms commonly associated with lung cancer or by chance, when the patient is under evaluation for other disorders or procedures. Selected signs and symptoms are listed in Table 98-1, but vary widely between patients according to tumor size, stage, and location.

DIAGNOSIS

If a malignancy comes under consideration, a computed tomography (CT) or positron emission tomography (PET)-CT scan of the abdomen and thoracic region is usually performed to identify any possible primary lesions and to look for possible metastases to lymph nodes and other organs or contralateral lung. If located, a pathologic evaluation is performed to confirm the diagnosis. Magnetic resonance imaging (MRI) of the head may be ordered if brain metastases are suspected. Preoperatively, specimens may be obtained through methods such as bronchial brushings, bronchial washings, fine needle aspiration biopsy, core needle biopsy, endobronchial biopsy, and transbronchial biopsy. Mediastinal lymph nodes are also sampled via mediastinoscopy to determine staging. If surgery is performed, specimens are evaluated during the procedure to determine the resection margin status, diagnose incidental nodules discovered during surgery, and sampling of regional lymph nodes. Postoperative evaluation provides pathology characteristics necessary for classifying tumor type and staging.[1]

Staging is performed to determine prognosis and to guide treatment decision-making. In general, the prognosis declines with increasing disease stage at initial diagnosis. Five-year overall survival rates are 54% for patients with disease that is locally limited and 4% for metastatic disease. For all stages, 5-year overall survival has only marginally improved over the last 30 years to 18%. Unfortunately, the disease has already metastasized in greater than 50% of patients upon initial presentation. However, earlier detection with spiral CT is promising and has resulted in a decrease in disease-related death in patients with at least a 30-pack-year smoking history.[2,4] Staging classification is reliant on anatomic characteristics and was updated by the International Association for the Study of Lung Cancer (IASLC) and adopted by the American Joint Committee on Cancer staging in 2010. Even though clinicians are placing more importance on molecular markers such as epidermal growth factor receptor (EGFR) mutations and tumor histology, the revised system still relies strictly on the TNM system of staging and places an emphasis on tumor size.[5,6] Table 98-2[5–7] illustrates how the TNM classification is used to determine the clinical stage.

OVERVIEW OF TREATMENT

Surgery, radiation, and systemic therapy (i.e., cytotoxic chemotherapy and targeted therapy) are all treatment modalities used in the

Table 98-2

Clinical Staging for Non-Small-Cell Lung Cancer[5–7]

Clinical Stage	Tumor Characteristics
Stage I	Tumor ≤5 cm in greatest diameter with no nodal involvement
Stage II	Tumor >5 cm, but ≤7 cm in greatest diameter with no nodal involvement Tumor ≤7 cm with adjacent lymph nodes involved Tumor >7 cm or invading local structure (i.e., chest wall) with no nodal involvement
Stage III	Any tumor size with adjacent lymph nodes involved or ipsilateral mediastinal and/or subcarinal lymph nodes Tumor invading mediastinum, heart, great vessels, esophagus, or another tumor nodule in different ipsilateral lobe
Stage IV	Any tumor size, any nodal involvement and metastasis to the contralateral lobe, malignant pleural effusions or distant metastasis

treatment of NSCLC. If caught in the early stages of the disease, surgery offers the best chance of cure. Chemotherapy is associated with enhanced survival depending on the stage of disease. The remaining discussion of NSCLC in this chapter will outline the key aspects in the treatment of early and late stages of the disease.

Early Stage Non-Small-Cell Lung Cancer

CASE 98-1

QUESTION 1: A 69-year-old male patient, J.W., was found to have a 3-cm nodule on a chest X-ray done prior to an elective cataract surgery. The patient was a lifelong cigarette smoker, having started smoking in his early 20s, approximately one pack of cigarettes per day. He quit smoking 9 years ago. What screening methods might be available to detect the disease in asymptomatic patients? What risk factors does J.W. have for lung cancer?

The National Lung Screening Trial (NLST) was a randomized study comparing low-dose CT scans with chest radiography in over 50,000 patients with a heavy smoking history, examining lung cancer mortality.[8,9] The NLST did result in a higher incidence of confirmed diagnoses of lung cancer with low-dose CT, resulting in a 20% relative reduction in the rate of death from lung cancer. However, low-dose CT scans did result in a higher rate of false positives than chest radiography.[10] The NLST did result in the U.S. Preventive Service Task Force making a recommendation of annual screening for lung cancer with low-dose CT scans in adults 55 to 80 years old with a 30-pack-year smoking history and currently smoke or have quit within the last 15 years.[11]

The probability for developing the disease increases with age, and J.W.'s age is close to the median age of peak incidence. Men also have a slightly higher risk than women as discussed previously. Smoking is the largest risk factor for lung cancer development; however, what if a person stops smoking? Does the risk decrease with time? These questions are important for healthcare providers to address whether they are encouraging smoking cessation for their patients. In J.W.'s case, he stopped 9 years ago, so what impact would this smoking history have on development of the disease? In general, people who stop smoking, even well into middle age, avoid almost 90% of the risk attributable to tobacco. Shown in Table 98-3 are data demonstrating the relation between the age at which a person stops smoking and the cumulative percent risk (at age 75) for developing lung cancer.[12] J.W. stopped when he was approximately 60 years old; therefore, based on this table, the cumulative risk would approach 10% if he were 75 years old. Because he is 69 years old, his risk would be decreased but not to the extent that it would if a longer period of time had elapsed. If he were still smoking the risk would be expected to be closer to 16%. Hence, smoking cessation is an effective means for lowering the risk over time. He smoked for approximately 35 to 40 pack-years, so the total number of cigarettes would also increase his risk. According to data from the same studies, risk of disease for a one pack per day smoker would be approximately twice that of someone who smoked less than a half pack per day. Survival from the disease is also better for nonsmokers than for smokers.[12,13]

Table 98-3

Cumulative Risk (%) of Death from Lung Cancer at Age 75 Years

Smoking Status	Risk at Age 75
Lifelong nonsmoker	<1
Stopped at age 30	<2
Stopped at age 40	3
Stopped at age 50	6
Stopped at age 60	10
Continuing smoker	16

Frequently, patients will experience remorsefulness for having smoked, but it is never possible to attribute one's disease to a single factor such as smoking. In fact, 90% of smokers never exhibit the disease. Furthermore, 15% of men and 53% of all women with lung cancer worldwide are never smokers.[14] This suggests that other factors such as genetics are associated with the development of the disease. Research has been directed at identifying genomic associated factors that have the potential to lead to the development of lung cancer in both smokers and nonsmokers. It has been shown that there can be some genetic associations, but the true impact of these genetic polymorphisms has not been fully elucidated.[3,15–18]

A more thorough history from J.W. would be helpful but recall for exposure to pollution, chemicals, and secondhand smoke exposure is difficult to quantify. Hence, the view held by much of society that lung cancer is a self-inflicted disease is not entirely true. In summary, there is limited history on J.W.'s exposure to environmental hazards such as radon and secondhand smoke. His age is close to that of peak incidence. Although he stopped smoking almost a decade ago, there is still some residual risk associated with past smoking history, and this would be expected to be higher for those with many pack-years history. Due to his heavy smoking history, J.W. may have benefited from low-dose CT scan screening to potentially provide earlier detection of lung cancer.

CASE 98-1, QUESTION 2: A CT scan was ordered for further evaluation and it showed an isolated spiculated nodule in the right upper lobe with no mediastinal or hilar adenopathy. The nodule showed no calcification. A CT-guided needle biopsy was performed which showed a well-differentiated adenocarcinoma consistent with a primary NSCLC. Further staging was carried out with PET scanning that demonstrated no additional areas of disease except for the nodule. What would be the best treatment plan for J.W., given the current information? Would surgery or neoadjuvant therapy be indicated?

The goals of therapy for this patient are to achieve a cure, especially since the disease appears to be in the early stage. Surgery is the best treatment modality for patients with stages I and II disease because these tumors are limited to one hemithorax and can be readily removed by excision. In most instances, lobectomy with node dissection is sufficient for local control. During surgery, the nodes would be sampled for presence of the disease and to confirm staging. J.W. appears to have limited disease, and so lobectomy would be recommended for him. For patients whose primary tumor or lymph node involvement extends to the proximal bronchus or proximal pulmonary artery, or crosses the major fissure, then a more extensive pneumonectomy is performed. Therefore, surgery is the treatment of choice, and final staging during surgery will guide further adjunct treatments. The tumors can often spread to mediastinal lymph nodes and for those patients (stage IIIA), then neoadjuvant chemotherapy can be recommended to reduce the tumor burden prior to surgery. If neoadjuvant therapy is chosen, the regimen is usually similar to those used in the adjuvant setting (Table 98-4).[19–24] Therefore, surgery is the primary treatment modality for patients with stages I, II, and early stage III disease. J.W.'s disease appears to be localized; therefore, surgical removal of the tumor would be indicated, and neoadjuvant chemotherapy would not be indicated because there does not appear to be disease in the mediastinum.[7]

CASE 98-1, QUESTION 3: J.W. was referred to a thoracic surgeon for resection. A right upper lobe lobectomy was performed with lymph node dissection. The pathology report revealed a 3.2 × 4 cm adenocarcinoma with three associated peribronchial lymph nodes containing cancer cells. Lymph nodes sampled from the mediastinum demonstrated no cancer. The patient's tumor was staged as a T2N1M0 (stage IIA) NSCLC. Now that the tumor is removed and staging of the disease is finalized, what additional therapy, if any, is recommended?

Although NSCLC tumors are minimally responsive to chemotherapy, evidence from several studies (Table 98-4) demonstrates that adjuvant treatment enhances patient survival, and therefore should be considered as part of the treatment plan for the patient. Though adjuvant treatment is often recommended, results from two other studies indicate that adjuvant treatment is not always effective.[25] This suggests that there is a need to identify subsets of patients who would likely benefit from treatment, and one group that does not seem to gain benefit are those with stage I disease. In the CALGB 9633 study, patients were randomly assigned to receive carboplatin and paclitaxel or placebo and a survival benefit was observed for those receiving chemotherapy. However, this survival was not uniform across the entire cohort. Subgroup analysis showed that adjuvant chemotherapy should not be considered standard of care for patients with stage IB disease unless the tumor size is greater than 4 cm. Collectively, these studies show that patients with stages II and IIIA disease gain the most benefit from adjuvant chemotherapy.[23] As summarized in Table 98-4, this chemotherapy usually includes cisplatin or, if the patient is unable to tolerate it, then carboplatin. A second agent, usually selected from one of those listed in Table 98-4, is added as doublet therapy, and the goal is for patients to receive four cycles. Toxicity often becomes worse beyond four cycles and benefits are diminished thereafter. Therefore, cytotoxic chemotherapy is beneficial but has its limitations.

Radiation therapy is frequently used in the treatment of malignancies including later stages of NSCLC; however, it has no proven benefit for the treatment of early-stage disease. The PORT Group conducted a meta-analysis from nine randomized trials to evaluate the possible role of postoperative radiotherapy in patients with completely resected NSCLC. There were 707 deaths among 1,056 patients assigned postoperative radiotherapy and 661 among 1,072 assigned surgery alone (hazard ratio, 1.21 [95% confidence interval, 1.08–1.34]). This 21% relative increase in the risk of death with radiotherapy is equivalent to a reduction in overall survival from 55% to 48%. Subgroup analysis showed that the increased risk of death was greatest for patients with stage I/II, N0 or N1, but no clear evidence for those with stage III, N2 disease.[26] Separately, another postoperative radiotherapy study was conducted, using data from 7,465 patients in the Surveillance, Epidemiology, and End Results (SEER) database. The investigators for this study also found no benefit for radiotherapy, especially for patients with N1 and N0 nodal disease. However, an increase in survival was associated with radiotherapy for patients who had N2 nodal disease.[27] Consequently, radiation therapy is reserved for patients with more advanced NSCLC. In summary, adjuvant cytotoxic chemotherapy is recommended for all patients found to have stage II or III NSCLC at surgery, as well as for larger (>4 cm) tumors. Multiple prospective phase 3 studies have shown that platinum-based chemotherapy after surgery will increase the survival rate of patients after surgery by about 10%. Because J.W. has stage IIA disease, four cycles of a platinum-based doublet regimen would be indicated after surgery; however, he should not receive radiotherapy at this time.

Table 98-4
Adjuvant Chemotherapy Regimens for Non-Small-Cell Lung Cancer

Regimen	Schedule
Cisplatin, days 1 and 8 Vinorelbine, days 1, 8, 15, 22	Every 28 days for 4 cycles[20]
Cisplatin, day 1 Vinorelbine, days 1, 8, 15, 22	Every 28 days for 4 cycles[21,22]
Cisplatin, day 1 Vinorelbine, days 1, 8	Every 21 days for 4 cycles[20]
Cisplatin, day 1 Etoposide, days 1–3	Every 28 days for 4 cycles[22]
Cisplatin, days 1, 22, 43, 64 Vinblastine, days 1, 8, 15, 22, then every 2 weeks after day 43	Every 21 days for 4 cycles[22]
Paclitaxel, day 1 Carboplatin, day 1	Every 21 days[23]
Other Acceptable Regimens	
Cisplatin, day 1 Gemcitabine, days 1, 8	Every 21 days[7]
Cisplatin, day 1 Docetaxel, day 1	Every 21 days[24]
Pemetrexed, day 1 Cisplatin, day 1 *nonsquamous etiology	Every 21 days for 4 cycles[7]

NSCLC, non-small-cell lung cancer.

Late Stage Non-Small-Cell Lung Cancer

CASE 98-2

QUESTION 1: L.L., an 85-year-old woman, presented with a mild cough, productive with nonbloody sputum, shortness of breath, and fever. She was initially seen by primary care physicians who treated her with antibiotics for possible pneumonia; however, the radiogram of the chest showed a persisting infiltrate in the left upper lung. This was later confirmed on a CT scan with the presence of a 6 × 3 × 3.6 cm mass in the left upper lobe. Mediastinal adenopathy and multiple pulmonary nodules were seen in the right upper lobe with associated scarring, the largest of them measuring 14 × 9 mm in the right upper lobe anteriorly. Transbronchial biopsy led to a diagnosis of adenocarcinoma. Because of the spread of disease to the contralateral lung, disease was staged as IV. Pertinent patient history included hypertension and hyperlipidemia. The patient also had a hemangioma of the brain resected in 1950 and a history of cervical cancer treated with an abdominal hysterectomy in 1952. She has never smoked. Upon evaluation, she was found to have a hemoglobin that was slightly low at 11.3 g/dL with a white blood cell count of 5,200 cells/μL and a platelet count of 245,000/μL. The electrolytes showed normal sodium of 143 mEq/L, normal potassium of 4.4 mEq/L, and creatinine of 1.08 mg/dL, with estimated creatinine clearance of 48 mL/minute. Her performance status was 0–1. What are the treatment options for patients such as L.L. with advanced (stages IIIB and IV) disease?

SURGERY

In general, tumors in patients with stages IIIB and IV disease are inoperable. These tumors often invade the carina, great vessels, vertebral bodies, more distant lymph nodes, metastases, and are frequently associated with malignant pleural effusions. Hence, combined-modality treatments such as cytotoxic chemotherapy and radiation are the preferred treatments for patients with advanced-stage disease.[28,29] Surgery to remove solitary metastatic sites may also be considered in selected patients, especially in patients with a solitary brain metastasis.[30]

RADIATION

Radiotherapy is the primary local treatment (i.e., definitive radiotherapy) for inoperable nonmetastatic NSCLC and is also used as a palliative modality for patients with incurable disease with symptoms such as pain or shortness of breath. For tumors classified as stage III, radiotherapy is often given concurrently with chemotherapy, as this has been shown to be superior to both radiation alone and also sequential radiation followed by chemotherapy.[7] The radiation dose, in combination with chemotherapy, usually ranges between 60 and 65 Gray (Gy), given in 2-Gy fractions. The recommended chemotherapy regimen for stage III disease with radiation is either cisplatin and etoposide or carboplatin and paclitaxel. If the patient has adenocarcinoma, then pemetrexed may be substituted for the etoposide or paclitaxel.[31–36] See Table 98-5 for specific chemoradiation regimens. Metastases may also be treated locally with radiotherapy. For example, brain metastases, spinal cord compression, and impending fractures of weight-bearing bones can be treated with radiation or surgery before systemic therapy commences. In contrast to patients with stage III disease, those with stage IV disease usually receive local treatment with radiotherapy, either before or after chemotherapy, because therapy given concurrently is often not well tolerated by patients with this stage of disease.

CHEMOTHERAPY

Patients with advanced disease and good performance status usually benefit from chemotherapy. Similar to early-stage disease, these tumors often respond to treatment with platinum-based doublet cytotoxic combination therapy, which refers to treatment with either cisplatin or carboplatin plus a second cytotoxic agent.[37–46]

Non-small-cell lung cancer was treated as a single disease despite recognition of its histologic and molecular heterogeneity,

Table 98-5

Representative Chemoradiation Regimens for Inoperable Stage III Non-Small-Cell Lung Cancer

Regimen	Schedule
Cisplatin, days 1, 8, 29 and 36 Etoposide days 1–5, 29–33	Concurrent radiation of 45 Gy administered in 25 daily 1.8 Gy fractions over 5 weeks[31,32]
Cisplatin days 1 and 29 Vinblastine weekly × 5 doses	Concurrent radiation of 45 Gy administered in 25 daily 1.8 Gy fractions over 5 weeks[33]
Carboplatin AUC 5 on day 1 Pemetrexed on day 1 *nonsquamous etiology	Every 21 days for 4 cycles[34] Concurrent radiation of 70 Gy administered in 35 daily 2 Gy fractions over 7 weeks
Cisplatin on day 1 Pemetrexed on day 1 *nonsquamous etiology	Every 21 days for 3 cycles[35] Concurrent radiation of 66 Gy in 33 daily 2 Gy fractions over 6.5 weeks
Paclitaxel weekly for 7 weeks Carboplatin AUC 2 weekly for 7 weeks followed by Paclitaxel day 1 and carboplatin day 1	Concurrent radiation of 63 Gy in 34 daily 1.8 Gy fractions over 7 weeks Followed by consolidative chemotherapy every 21 days for 2 cycles[36]

but recent clinical trials demonstrate that histology is an important factor for individualizing treatment based on either safety or efficacy outcomes. Hence, once the biopsy is obtained, it is crucial to differentiate the histologic subtype (i.e., squamous vs. nonsquamous). The role of histology in the management of advanced NSCLC is reviewed more extensively elsewhere.[37] In developed countries, an increasing incidence of adenocarcinoma and a decline in squamous cell carcinomas have been observed in recent years. This appears to be correlated to declines in smoking rates. Many agents are effective against all histologic types such as cisplatin, carboplatin, gemcitabine, and paclitaxel. However, other agents such as bevacizumab and pemetrexed are only indicated for use in patients who have the nonsquamous histology (see Table 98-6). Squamous cell histology is associated with increased risk for severe pulmonary hemorrhage compared with adenocarcinoma.[45] For pemetrexed, significant association between improved efficacy and the nonsquamous subtype has been reported.[47,48]

Characterization of advanced NSCLC tumors at the molecular level has also become part of clinical practice. It is recommended that tumor tissues from patients with nonsquamous histology tumors should be analyzed for the presence of EGFR and ALK mutation status.[7] Tumors that are positive for EGFR somatic mutations are often more responsive to erlotinib therapy and have become the standard front-line treatment over cytotoxic chemotherapy.[49] This analysis is limited to patients with stages IIIB or IV disease, because erlotinib has not been proven to be beneficial in patients with earlier stage disease and EGFR mutations.[50] For the advanced disease setting, therefore, treatment decisions are becoming more individualized on the basis of tumor histology and somatic mutations. As more targeted therapies, designed to inhibit other targets, are approved, it is likely that their use will be based upon at least some of these same principles.

Patients who respond to treatment or achieve stable disease after four to six cycles may be given maintenance therapy. The intention of such additional treatment would be to prolong the response and survival made possible by first-line treatment, while

Table 98-6
Representative Initial Regimens for Advanced or Metastatic Non-Small-Cell Lung Cancer

Regimen	Schedule
Paclitaxel, day 1 Carboplatin, day 1	Every 21 days[38]
Cisplatin, day 1 Paclitaxel, day 1	Every 21 days[38]
Cisplatin, day 1 Gemcitabine, days 1, 8, 15 *squamous etiology	Every 28 days[38,39]
Cisplatin, day 1 Docetaxel, day 1	Every 21 days[38]
Pemetrexed, day 1 Cisplatin, day 1 *nonsquamous etiology	Every 21 days[39]
Pemetrexed, day 1 Carboplatin, day 1	Every 21 days[40]
Nab-paclitaxel days 1, 8, 15 Carboplatin, day 1	Every 21 days[41]
Cisplatin, day 1 Vinorelbine, days 1, 8 Cetuximab weekly *nonsquamous etiology	Every 21 days[42]
Cisplatin, day 1 Gemcitabine, days 1, 8 Bevacizumab, day 1 *nonsquamous etiology	Every 21 days[43]
Paclitaxel, day 1 Carboplatin, day 1 Bevacizumab, day 1 *nonsquamous etiology	Every 21 days[43,45]
Pemetrexed, day 1 Cisplatin, day 1 Bevacizumab, day 1 *nonsquamous etiology	Every 21 days[46]

minimizing the chances for toxicity associated with platinum-based doublet regimens. Maintenance therapy differs from second-line therapy in that second-line treatment is only used when the patient has progressed during or after first-line treatment or is unable to tolerate it. Maintenance may be given as continuation maintenance, which refers to the use of one of the agents given in first line. Often, biologic agents that were given as part of the first-line regimen (e.g., bevacizumab or cetuximab) are continued due to their better tolerability relative to the cytotoxic agents.[44,51] For adenocarcinoma, pemetrexed should be given as continuation maintenance treatment due to an improved overall survival compared to placebo.[52] Alternatively, the agent may be different from those used in first-line treatment and is referred to as switch maintenance. Pemetrexed, erlotinib, and docetaxel are three agents for which there is supportive clinical trial data in the switch maintenance setting.[7,47,53] The first two agents are associated with an improvement in overall survival and have an indication for use in this setting.[54]

PALLIATION

Patients with metastatic NSCLC receive benefit from palliative care early after diagnosis, rather than waiting until end-of-life care. This palliative care includes helping the patient cope with the psychosocial aspects of their disease through methods such as counseling (e.g., expectation of treatment outcomes and affordability of treatment). In a study of patients with metastatic disease, subjects were randomly assigned to receive either early palliative care integrated with standard oncologic care vs. standard oncologic care alone. Patients assigned to early palliative care experienced a better quality of life and survival (11.6 vs. 8.9 months) than patients assigned to standard care alone. They also experienced fewer depressive symptoms (16% vs. 38%). The results show that palliative care is appropriate and potentially beneficial when it is introduced at the time of diagnosis at the same time as other beneficial therapies.[55]

In conclusion, L.L. would not likely receive benefit from surgical removal of the primary tumor or metastatic site. Instead, chemotherapy is the treatment of choice with a pemetrexed-based regimen along with maintenance pemetrexed for controlling disease that has already spread. Consideration for palliative care would also be beneficial.

CASE 98-2, QUESTION 2: The tumor tissue was sent out for analysis of the presence of an EGFR mutation. What characteristics in L.L. would prompt a decision to send a tumor specimen for analysis of an EGFR mutation?

The importance of this analysis is underscored by the fact that patients with EGFR mutation-positive advanced-stage tumors respond better to treatment with erlotinib than they do with conventional chemotherapy.[49] Furthermore, erlotinib is better tolerated than doublet platinum-based therapies; therefore, patients with EGFR mutation-positive tumors would be expected to experience better outcomes related to both tumor response and tolerability.[56] Soon after erlotinib was approved by the US Food and Drug Administration (FDA), investigators noticed that patients who were women, Asian, and nonsmokers tended to respond to erlotinib therapy more frequently than other populations. However, it was subsequently realized that presence of mutations in EGFR was a better predictor of response to erlotinib therapy than demographic factors and smoking status. The prevalence of EGFR mutations is between 10% and 15% for the overall population, but is 35% in white nonsmokers, and 65% for Asian nonsmokers.[57] Hence, the probability that L.L., a nonsmoking white woman, has a tumor with this somatic mutation is higher than for other categories of patients such as smokers or men. Further, the observed incidence of these mutations is less than 3% for patients with squamous cell histology; therefore, it is not recommended to test patients with this histology.[7] L.L. was diagnosed with adenocarcinoma, which is a nonsquamous subtype, and mutation testing is thus warranted on that basis alone.

The question arises that patients who fall into the category with multiple clinical predictors of response could be started empirically on erlotinib therapy without the need to test for EGFR mutations. In L.L.'s case, she would be classified as having three of these clinical predictors: female, nonsmoker, and adenocarcinoma. However, studies with populations of patients from developed countries with NSCLC showed that those who had three or more of these characteristics experienced a 49% response rate, whereas those with sensitizing EGFR mutations experienced a much higher 67% response rate.[58] This indicates that EGFR mutation is a better predictor of response to erlotinib therapy than presence of multiple clinical predictors.

Additionally, a second EGFR inhibitor, afatinib, is now available for patients with activating mutations of EGFR. Afatinib is an irreversible inhibitor of EGFR (whereas erlotinib is reversible) that has been shown to be superior to treatment with conventional chemotherapy as well as a second-line option for patients who have progressed on front-line erlotinib therapy.[59–62]

Application of this EGFR testing is useful for small molecule tyrosine kinase inhibitors (e.g., erlotinib, afatinib), but not for antibody molecules (e.g., cetuximab) that also block EGFR. The antibody molecules function to block the receptor external to the cell surface, and they also stimulate immune responses (e.g., antibody-dependent cell-mediated cytotoxicity, complement) against the tumor. It is likely that even without presence of the mutation(s), the antibody molecule still binds and can function through several mechanisms to promote an antitumor effect.[43] Small molecule inhibitors, however, also bind the receptor internal to the cell surface and can inhibit the active ATP binding region, which is constitutively activated in tumors with EGFR mutations.

CASE 98-2, QUESTION 3: L.L. was started on erlotinib therapy based on a positive EGFR mutation and, within 8 weeks of therapy, had obtained a partial response. What benefit from erlotinib therapy can L.L. expect in terms of prolonged survival?

Although there is short-term benefit for patients with EGFR mutation-positive tumors to receive erlotinib, it is not yet clear if there is a longer-term benefit. The response rate for erlotinib treatment is approximately 67%, time to disease progression is 11.8 months, and overall survival is approximately 24 months. As of yet, there are no data to support that treatment with small molecule inhibitors prolongs overall survival relative to doublet platinum-based therapy.[49] It is much easier to demonstrate an effect on tumor response and time to progression (such as with erlotinib) than it is for overall survival in most cancer studies. Showing improvement in overall survival is difficult because study subjects who are randomly assigned to one arm of a study can exhibit progressive disease and could hypothetically cross over to receive the competing treatment once they are classified as off study. The competing treatment could prolong overall survival and confound interpretation of the overall survival benefit for the test treatment (e.g., erlotinib). Further study is required to establish the benefit of erlotinib or afatinib treatment on overall survival. There is also no evidence to show that addition of erlotinib to chemotherapy is superior to either treatment alone. Hence, at this time, treatment for L.L. (single-agent erlotinib) would be expected to prolong her progression-free survival, but it is not yet known whether erlotinib prolongs overall survival.

CASE 98-2, QUESTION 4: If L.L.'s tumor was classified as having wild-type EGFR instead, what treatment should L.L. receive?

If the biopsy results had shown that the tumor EGFR was wild type (i.e., no mutation), then L.L. would be considered for a platinum-based doublet such as one shown in Table 98-6. Because her disease is nonsquamous, the adjunct agent selected would most likely be pemetrexed. Scagliotti et al. randomly assigned patients with advanced stage NSCLC to receive either cisplatin plus gemcitabine versus cisplatin plus pemetrexed. Although the median survival time was similar between the two arms, there were differences depending on tumor histology. Patients who received pemetrexed and had adenocarcinoma experienced a median overall survival of 12.6 months, whereas those who received gemcitabine had shorter survival. In contrast, those with squamous carcinoma who received pemetrexed experienced a 9.4-month median overall survival, whereas those who received gemcitabine had longer survival.[39] Therefore, if L.L.'s tumor had been wild type for EGFR, she could receive cisplatin and pemetrexed as first-line treatment because her disease is adenocarcinoma. Consideration could also be given for using cisplatin and paclitaxel together with bevacizumab. As mentioned previously, the latter agent is approved for use only in patients with nonsquamous cell NSCLC.[44] Those who respond to treatment with four to six cycles of cytotoxic therapy should receive maintenance therapy with pemetrexed and bevacizumab afterward based on the AVAPERL trial.[46]

CASE 98-2, QUESTION 5: As discussed in Chapter 94, Adverse Effects of Chemotherapy and Targeted Agents, the adverse effect profiles for cisplatin and carboplatin differ from each other. If a platinum-based regimen had been selected instead of erlotinib for L.L., what characteristics about L.L. could be used to guide the selection of carboplatin versus cisplatin?

Cisplatin is predominantly associated with ototoxicity, nephrotoxicity, and neurotoxicity, whereas carboplatin is predominantly associated with myelosuppression. This would be her first cycle of chemotherapy; therefore, she is not expected to have depleted reserves of myeloid progenitor cells. Her estimated creatinine clearance is 48 mL/minute and, based upon this, would be considered to have moderate renal impairment. In this case, carboplatin may be preferred over cisplatin because it is associated with less renal toxicity and it is dosed according to the Calvert formula, which accounts for renal function:

$$\text{Total carboplatin dose (mg)} = \text{AUC}\,(\text{GFR} + 25) \quad \text{(Eq. 98-1)}$$

where AUC is the area under the concentration–time curve and GFR is glomerular filtration rate.[63] A typical dose of carboplatin in this setting would be determined based on an AUC to account for renal function instead of the typical weight (or m^2)-based dosing. The AUC targets are commonly 4 to 6 mg/mL × minute for most doublet regimens. If a patient with moderate renal function were to receive a fixed dose that is similar to that given to a patient with normal renal function, then systemic exposure would be higher. This higher exposure could result in greater toxicity, notably greater myelosuppression. By dosing the drug according to the patient's renal function, the risk for overdosing a patient with decreased renal function is minimized. For example, if L.L.'s carboplatin dose is ordered as AUC 5 mg/mL × min, then her dose would be calculated as dose = 5 mg/mL × minute (48 mL/min + 25), which is 365 mg. In contrast, if her renal function were within normal range for estimated creatinine clearance (e.g., 100 mL/minute), her carboplatin dose would be 625 mg (~70% higher). Several different methods may be used to estimate renal function, such as the Cockroft and Gault equation, and the dose calculations will differ according to the method chosen. The American Society of Clinical Oncology (ASCO) has developed recommendations for the dosing of carboplatin. It is recommended to cap the GFR or CrCl at 125 mL/minute within the Calvert equation.[64] Usually, the choice of method is institution specific, because there is no evidence to show that one estimation method is superior to the other. By consistently using the same formula, providers reduce variability in systemic exposure and thus increase the predictability of tolerance to the drug. If the patient's GFR is estimated based upon serum creatinine measurements by the isotope dilution mass spectrometry method, then the GFR should be capped to a maximum of 125 mL/minute, because serum creatinine values can be underestimated when they fall below 0.7 mg/mL, as can happen in some patients. The FDA issued this safety alert to avoid administration of high doses to patients with normal renal function and thus likely avoiding drug-related toxicity.[64]

In conclusion, L.L. should receive erlotinib as first-line therapy. If her tumor had contained wild-type EGFR (instead of mutant), then a platinum-based doublet (i.e., cisplatin or carboplatin) could be considered with pemetrexed therapy. She has moderate renal impairment; therefore, an agent such as cisplatin would not be favored because it is associated with a high incidence of renal toxicity. Carboplatin would be a safer choice because the dose would be selected based upon her renal function, and is associated with a lower incidence of renal toxicity than cisplatin.

CASE 98-2, QUESTION 6: L.L. experienced minor grade diarrhea and skin rash and otherwise tolerated erlotinib treatment very well without any impact on her daily activities and quality of life. L.L. continued erlotinib therapy, and at 9 months, there is no evidence of disease progression. The plan is to continue this therapy until the disease relapses. What types of side effects should L.L. be monitored while receiving erlotinib therapy?

In general, therapy with erlotinib is well tolerated, especially relative to cytotoxic chemotherapy. Diarrhea and rash are the two most common adverse effects of EGFR TKI therapy.[65] The diarrhea can be treated with loperamide in most cases. Rash requires intervention in approximately one-third of cases, and it is desirable to treat it with agents such as 2% topical clindamycin, minocycline, or doxycycline, and topical 1% hydrocortisone (discussed in Chapter 94, Adverse Effects of Chemotherapy and Targeted Agents). Erlotinib dose reduction (in 50-mg decrements) could also be considered, although this would likely shorten the anticancer benefit experienced with this agent.[65]

As mentioned earlier, NSCLC is primarily a disease in those older than 60 years. L.L. is 85 years old, and there is concern that patients, particularly more than 80 years old, may not tolerate cytotoxic chemotherapy as well as younger patients. Hence, elderly patients are often undertreated. However, recent studies suggest that survival benefits are greater in elderly patients who receive doublet therapy versus single agent.[66] More studies of various regimens are needed that would focus on treatment of elderly patients, particularly effects on survival, quality of life, and tolerability. Such studies would investigate the best clinical parameters that enable prediction of response and tolerability to therapies, and also the doses associated with the best outcomes. Because the majority of patients have wild-type EGFR, cytotoxic chemotherapy is first line. Therefore, considerations must be given to patient preferences, comorbidities, and performance status. It is not uncommon for those with advanced age to live alone. Caretakers who could help the patient monitor for and treat adverse effects of chemotherapy (dehydration from diarrhea or vomiting, febrile neutropenia, etc.) would be an essential consideration, particularly in this population. Even though L.L. is able to continue treatment beyond 9 months, most patients eventually exhibit progressive disease within 1 to 2 years. These patients can often be re-biopsied. Approximately 40% of these cases develop secondary mutations in EGFR that render the tumor resistant to erlotinib treatment.[67] At such time, consideration can be given for second-line treatment with afatinib.

CASE 98-2, QUESTION 7: In addition to EGFR mutation testing, L.L.'s pathology was analyzed for ALK fusion rearrangement. If this returned positive, how would that impact the initial choice of treatment for L.L.?

Anaplastic lymphoma kinase (ALK) rearrangement consisting of a fusion of EML4 and ALK is a predictive marker that is present in 2% to 7% of NSCLCs and has been validated to identify patients who may benefit from ALK inhibitors such as oral crizotinib or ceritinib. Patients are more likely to be ALK-positive if they are never smokers or have adenocarcinoma histology. Therefore, it is standard of care to determine whether ALK rearrangement is present in all patients with adenocarcinoma histology.[68,69] Initial therapy with crizotinib resulted in an improvement in progression-free survival of 10.9 months versus 7.0 months for patients receiving platinum-pemetrexed doublet chemotherapy.[70] Additionally, crizotinib has been shown to improve progression-free survival over chemotherapy in patients who have already received chemotherapy in the first-line setting.[71] Recently, a new oral ALK inhibitor that is 20 times more potent than crizotinib, ceritinib, was approved for treatment of patients after progression on therapy with crizotinib.[72]

The ALK inhibitors are generally well tolerated with the main adverse events being visual disorders, nausea, vomiting, diarrhea, and fatigue. The visual disorders usually present within the first 2 weeks of therapy and most commonly present as flashing or trailing lights and the presence of floaters.[73]

In conclusion, initial therapy for NSCLC is predominately focused on initial staging, role of therapy, and then histology present. After progression of disease, there are many chemotherapeutic options that may result in some progression-free survival although overall survival is still dismal. Recently, a new targeted approach to the treatment of progressive NSCLC was introduced with the approval of nivolumab. Nivolumab is a programmed cell death 1 (PD-1) receptor inhibitor that gained FDA approval for advanced, previously treated squamous cell NSCLC based on the CheckMate 017 trial. This trial demonstrated an improved overall survival in patients receiving nivolumab over docetaxel (1-year OS 42% with nivolumab vs. 24% with docetaxel, HR for death, 0.59, $p < 0.001$).[74] It is expected that the use of PD-1 inhibitors will expand beyond squamous histology as well as exploring a role in first-line therapy.

Small-Cell Lung Cancer

EPIDEMIOLOGY

Small-cell lung cancer (SCLC) accounts for approximately 13% of all lung cancer histology and affects both sexes in equal distribution. The disease is much more highly attributable to smoking than NSCLC. As the numbers of people who smoke have decreased in the United States since its peak in the 1960s, the incidence of SCLC has also declined, resulting in ~2.4% decrease per year.[75] Relative to NSCLC, these tumors generally have a more rapid doubling time, a higher growth fraction, and early development of widespread metastases. As a consequence, SCLC is highly sensitive to chemotherapy and radiotherapy; however, most patients eventually die from recurrent disease.[76,77]

PATHOPHYSIOLOGY

Small-cell lung cancer is a malignancy thought to be derived from neuroendocrine cells in the bronchus and is readily diagnosed on small specimens such as bronchoscopic biopsies, fine needle aspirates, core biopsies, and cytology. As the name suggests, these tumors consist of small cells that may be round, oval, or spindle-shaped, with limited volume of cytoplasm, poorly defined cell borders, and finely granular chromatin.[78]

CLINICAL PRESENTATION

Most SCLCs usually arise centrally and present as a large hilar mass with bulky mediastinal lymphadenopathy that can cause cough and dyspnea. Very rarely do patients diagnosed with SCLC present with the primary tumor located in the lung periphery, as can be the case with adenocarcinoma NSCLC. Due to smoking, patients with lung cancer may have had previously existing symptoms such as cough and dyspnea that are related to the presence of other smoking-related diseases such as COPD. Therefore, these symptoms may not prompt patients to seek medical attention quickly.[79]

DIAGNOSIS AND OVERVIEW OF TREATMENT

In general, diagnostic procedures are similar to those used to diagnose NSCLC. Staging of SCLC is used to determine prognosis and treatment. The median overall survival for patients with limited-stage disease ranges from 17 to 26 months and, for extensive stage, 3 to 12 months.[79] (These data were collected from an analysis of 14 studies of SCLC, and thus wide ranges for survival are reported.) Surgery (e.g., thoracotomy) is appropriate for less than 5% of patients with early stage disease, mainly due to the tendency for these tumors to be bulky and to metastasize quickly. The limited role for surgery, therefore, enables the use of a simple two-stage system instead of the TNM system used for other solid tumors. In the Veterans Administration Lung Study Group staging system, limited-stage disease is defined as disease confined to the ipsilateral hemithorax and encompassed in a tolerable radiation field, and extensive disease is defined as disease beyond the ipsilateral hemithorax including malignant pleural effusions or hematogenous metastases.[80–82] As discussed subsequently, patients with limited-stage disease are treated with a combined-modality approach (i.e., chemotherapy and radiation), and extensive stage is treated with chemotherapy. Only approximately 30% of patients present with limited stage and the rest with extensive-stage disease.[75]

CLINICAL PRESENTATION AND PATHOPHYSIOLOGY OF SMALL-CELL LUNG CANCER

CASE 98-3

QUESTION 1: M.W. is a 63-year-old woman who presented to her primary doctor with a complaint of heartburn and pain in the right side of her upper abdomen; she also had a feeling of gas in the stomach. In addition, she noticed a 20-lb weight loss within 3 months, although she attributed this to changes in her diet. She was not complaining of any coughing. There was no shortness of breath. The evaluation with chest radiograph demonstrated the presence of a large mass in the right perihilar region with extension to the mediastinum and significant mediastinal adenopathy with narrowing of the trachea and its displacement to the left by the mass. The follow-up PET-CT scan confirmed presence of that large mass and no other areas of abnormality within the abdomen or pelvis. The patient also had a brain MRI that showed no evidence of metastatic disease. After that, the patient had a bronchoscopic evaluation and a biopsy of the mediastinal mass. Pathology came back positive for small-cell lung carcinoma histology. Having disease only limited to the chest and mediastinum, the patient was diagnosed with limited-stage SCLC. Peripheral blood chemistry, LDH, and counts were normal. What features of M.W.'s disease are suggestive for SCLC?

M.W.'s chief complaints were heartburn and pain in the upper right side of her abdomen, not necessarily common symptoms of SCLC. Location of the tumor is a determining factor in specific symptoms that a patient can experience, and can serve as an indicator of the invasiveness of the disease. Although M.W. did not complain of cough, her presentation is representative of patients diagnosed with this disease in that the tumor was centrally located with spread to the mediastinum. She also experienced weight loss and, although she attributed this to her diet, it is a symptom experienced by patients with rapidly growing disease and associated with appetite suppression.

M.W. did not experience all of the symptoms that are frequently found in patients. Fatigue, especially together with decreased physical activity, is a common complaint as well as hemoptysis.[83] Owing to the central location of most of these tumors, approximately 10% of patients can experience superior vena cava syndrome (SVCS). This is a very serious complication and requires immediate medical attention as a result of the growing tumor impinging upon the superior vena cava. This can restrict blood return to the heart, resulting in head and facial swelling.[84,85]

CASE 98-3, QUESTION 2: What potential complications might patients such as M.W. experience during the course of their disease?

Patients with SCLC frequently experience paraneoplastic syndromes as a result of their disease, and these often differ from patients who have NSCLC. For example, patients with NSCLC have a higher tendency to develop hypertrophic pulmonary osteoarthropathy and hypercalcemia. On the other hand, patients with SCLC have higher incidence rates for hyponatremia, Cushing syndrome, and neurologic paraneoplastic syndrome. The serum concentrations of antidiuretic hormone are often elevated in SCLC, but few of these cases fulfill the criteria for SIADH and are mostly asymptomatic. In some cases, ectopic production of atrial natriuretic factor contributes to the disorder in sodium homeostasis. Because SCLC is usually responsive to cytotoxic agents, the treatment of choice for hyponatremia is chemotherapy. If further management is needed (i.e., if the cancer is nonresponsive to chemotherapy or symptomatic), fluid restriction, intravenous hypertonic saline, and treatment with demeclocycline are options, depending on severity.[1] The serum concentrations of adrenocorticotropic hormone are elevated in approximately half of patients with lung cancer but Cushing syndrome develops in only 5% of those with SCLC. Low serum sodium and Cushing syndrome are both poor prognostic indicators for the disease.[86]

Unlike M.W., most patients already have metastatic disease at diagnosis, and the most common sites include bone, liver, adrenal glands, and brain. Patients with hepatic and adrenal lesions do not usually experience symptoms, even if they have elevations of bilirubin, alkaline phosphatase, or hepatic transaminases.[87] In contrast, brain metastases are symptomatic in more than 90% of cases, and patients can often present with central nervous system complications (e.g., seizures) as the first sign of the disease.[1]

CASE 98-3, QUESTION 3: M.W. reads about various treatments for her disease online. What is the utility for each of the three treatment modalities (i.e., surgery, radiation, and chemotherapy) for the treatment of her disease?

TREATMENT MODALITIES FOR SMALL-CELL LUNG CANCER

Surgery

As mentioned earlier, surgery has a very limited role as part of the treatment for patients with SCLC. In general, patients with tumors larger than 3 to 7 cm and presence of any disease in the lymph nodes or distant metastases do not benefit from surgery.[88] The percentage of patients who fit this category is less than 5%. If surgery is chosen, the procedure usually includes lobectomy with mediastinal nodal dissection and sampling. Thereafter, patients would receive adjuvant radiation and chemotherapy and then prophylactic cranial irradiation as described in the subsequent sections.

Radiation

Small-cell lung cancer is responsive to radiation therapy; therefore, it is useful in treating patients with limited-stage disease. These treatments are usually given as fractionated doses over the course of 3 to 7 weeks, and total dosage targets range between 45 and 70 Gray (Gy). The optimal dose and frequency of administration of radiation is still under investigation. Three-dimensional conformal radiation (intensity modulated radiation therapy) is the preferred method and the radiation is delivered from an external source concurrently with multidimensional imaging to assure tumor movement of less than 1 cm is achievable (movement as a result of breathing during the procedure).[89–92] In addition to their cytotoxic effects, many chemotherapeutic agents also sensitize tumors to radiation. Hence, radiotherapy should start concurrently with chemotherapy, usually at the first or second cycle. Due to the high incidence of metastases to the brain (i.e., greater than 50% of patients with SCLC), prophylactic cranial irradiation consisting of 25 to 30 Gy given for 10 to 15 fractions is the standard of treatment for patients with limited-stage and extensive-stage disease after completion of initial chemotherapy or chemoradiation and minimal residual systemic disease.[93,94]

Chemotherapy

The proliferative indices for SCLC cells are high and early metastatic spread is common. Therefore, systemic chemotherapy is the treatment of choice for its utility in treating metastases and because it is effective for tumor cells progressing through the cell cycle. In general, most of the regimens are platinum-based combinations with etoposide or, less commonly, irinotecan (the latter proven to be efficacious in Japanese patients) as outlined in Table 98-7.[95] If a tumor response is observed, the benefit is usually seen early in the treatment course. Prolongation of treatment beyond six cycles is usually not recommended for this disease because the maximum effect of the treatment is achieved in this time frame. Further, toxicity after treatment with these agents accumulates and diminishes the overall benefit to the patient beyond six courses.[99,100] Hence, treatment is usually stopped after four to six cycles and the patient is closely monitored for recurrence of the disease.

As mentioned previously, SCLC has a very high rate of recurrence; therefore, second-line therapy is usually implemented. Several choices of agents are available as shown in Table 98-7, and the selection is dependent on the overall condition of the patient (e.g., performance status, toxicity from previous regimen) and the length of time after the first-line regimen was completed. Many of these agents are given as single-agent therapy except for the CAV regimen. In general, a recurrence that occurs within 6 months of treatment with first-line therapy is considered resistant and other agents are selected. If recurrence occurs after 6 months, then the same agents used for the first-line regimen may be used again. To date, no targeted agents are approved for use in treating SCLC.

In conclusion, M.W.'s disease would not be a good candidate for surgical removal because there is lack of proven benefit. Small-cell lung tumor cells proliferate rapidly; therefore, they are usually responsive to chemotherapy and radiation treatment. This systemic therapy would also be favored because the tumor tends to metastasize quickly and it provides a way to eradicate disease that may have spread.

Table 98-7
Representative Chemotherapy Regimens for Small-Cell Lung Cancer

Limited-Stage SCLC (maximum 4–6 cycles)
Cisplatin, day 1 Etoposide, days 1–3, then every 21 days[91]
Carboplatin, day 1 Etoposide, days 1–3, then every 21 days[69]
Extensive-Stage SCLC (maximum 4–6 cycles)
Cisplatin, day 1 Etoposide days 1–3, then every 21 days[71]
Carboplatin, day 1 Etoposide, days 1, 2, 3, then every 21 days[96]
Cisplatin, day 1 Irinotecan days 1, 8, 15, then every 28 days[97]
Cisplatin, day 1 Irinotecan days 1, 8, then every 21 days[98]
Chemotherapy for Relapsed Disease[78]
Clinical trial preferred
If relapse occurs <2–3 months after first line and PS 0–2: paclitaxel, docetaxel, gemcitabine, irinotecan, or topotecan (oral or IV), ifosfamide
If relapse occurs >2–3 months up to 6 months: topotecan (oral or IV), irinotecan, paclitaxel, docetaxel, oral etoposide, vinorelbine, gemcitabine, or cyclophosphamide/doxorubicin/vincristine (CAV)
If relapse occurs >6 months: original regimen

PS, performance status; SCLC, small-cell lung cancer.

Case 98-3, Question 4: M.W. begins therapy with intravenous cisplatin on day 1 combined with etoposide on days 1 to 3 given in a 21-day cycle. Four to six cycles are planned, and she will also receive concurrent radiation.[92,101] For M.W., what is the goal of therapy? What objective baseline data should be acquired prior to starting treatment? What monitoring parameters should be utilized?

TREATMENT WITH CHEMOTHERAPY AND RADIATION

The goal of therapy for a patient with limited-stage disease such as M.W. would be to increase overall survival and achieve a potential cure. In patients with limited-stage disease, response rates of 70% to 90% are expected after a regimen such as the one M.W. is receiving, whereas response rates of 60% to 70% are expected for patients with extensive-stage disease.[78] If M.W. had been diagnosed with extensive-stage disease, then the goals would have been to increase overall survival and for palliation of symptoms. Given the complications that can arise as a result of SCLC, treatment could be used to minimize these adverse events. For example, radiotherapy is often used in treating patients with SVCS because it would reduce tumor size and enable resumption of more normal blood flow. Therefore, if a patient has acceptable performance status (e.g., 0–2) and minimal to no comorbidities, then treatment such as the one that M.W. is receiving is the best course of action.

A treatment regimen such as cisplatin and etoposide plus radiation is tolerated by most patients, especially because the number of cycles is usually limited to six. However, administration of these cytotoxic agents is associated with several adverse effects, some of which can be life-threatening. Hence, the clinician is expected to anticipate these events and plan treatment accordingly to minimize complications. The patient is receiving cisplatin, which causes several different adverse effects such as renal insufficiency, sensory neuropathy, ototoxicity, and is considered highly emetogenic (refer to Chapter 94, Adverse Effects of Chemotherapy and Targeted Agents). Hydration and diuresis are required with cisplatin doses greater than 40 mg/m^2 to maintain a urine output of 100 to 150 mL/hour before administration of the drug. The intravenous fluids are often supplemented with potassium and magnesium to counteract electrolyte wasting from cisplatin. Monitoring of serum creatinine, electrolytes including magnesium and calcium, is performed usually before each infusion of chemotherapeutics. An appropriate antiemetic regimen must be implemented to prevent both acute and delayed nausea and vomiting. For etoposide, neutropenia is usually the dose-limiting toxicity. Therefore, monitoring of absolute neutrophil count (ANC) is important and, if the counts do not recover before the next dose is due, then delays in treatment or dosage reductions occur. In phase III clinical trials for this regimen, grade 4 leukopenia occurred in approximately 35% to 40% of patients, and any grade fever and infection in greater than 20%.[90,91] Therefore, consideration must be given toward the use of colony-stimulating factors to manage this latter event, usually after radiation is completed (refer to Chapter 94, Adverse Effects of Chemotherapy and Targeted Agents).

In conclusion, the goal of M.W.'s therapy is a potential cure. Hydration with fluids supplemented with potassium and magnesium must be initiated prior to cisplatin therapy to prevent cisplatin-induced renal toxicity. During therapy, clinicians must observe for decreased ANC due to etoposide and may need to implement delays in therapy or use of a colony-stimulating factor (e.g., granulocyte colony-stimulating factor, filgrastim). Supportive care such as anti-emetics during therapy to prevent or manage cisplatin-associated acute- and delayed-phase nausea and vomiting will also be essential.

CASE 98-3, QUESTION 5: M.W. tolerated therapy very well with mild esophagitis and cough during treatment. She did not experience any vomiting due to aggressive antiemetic use, nor did she exhibit any neuropathy or hearing loss. What adverse conditions that M.W. experienced are associated with her treatment?

Both esophagitis and cough are likely attributable to radiation effects. If esophagitis worsens to grade 3 or more, patients can lose the ability to swallow and may require a feeding tube. During therapy, cough can develop and patients may become concerned that it is a sign of worsening disease. Radiation-induced pneumonitis, acute (in first 3 months) and chronic (4–12 months), can be a frequent cause of the new onset of cough, which can be ameliorated with corticosteroid treatment.

CASE 98-3, QUESTION 6: After two cycles of chemotherapy with concurrent radiotherapy, a CT scan indicates a partial response. Therefore, an additional four cycles of cisplatin and etoposide were planned. How is the course of M.W.'s disease likely to proceed?

The chances for long-term survival greater than 5 years are very low, even for the patient with no other comorbidities and limited-stage disease such as M.W. At the completion of chemotherapy, M.W. should be offered therapy with prophylactic cranial irradiation because brain metastases occur in greater than 50% of patients with SCLC. Prophylactic cranial irradiation not only reduces the incidence of metastatic disease but also increases overall survival.[93] Within a year of completing therapy, most patients experience progressive or relapsed disease. The duration of the remission is the single largest predictor of outcome and patients are classified as having either sensitive or refractory disease, depending on length of this duration. Approximately half of those tumors that are deemed sensitive in this setting will respond to second-line therapy.[100] Therefore, most SCLC tumors become resistant to therapy either during first-line or salvage therapy. Patients can also exhibit second primary tumors, especially NSCLC, during the course of the disease.

ACKNOWLEDGMENT

The author acknowledges Mark N. Kirstein, Robert A. Kratzke, and Arkadiusz Z. Dudek for their contributions to the version of this chapter found in previous editions.

KEY REFERENCES AND WEBSITES

A full list of references for this chapter can be found at http://thepoint.lww.com/AT11e. Below are the key references and websites for this chapter, with the corresponding reference number in this chapter found in parentheses after the reference.

Key References

Brahmer J, Reckamp KL, Baas P et al. Nivolumab versus docetaxel in advanced squamous-cell non-small cell-lung cancer. *N Engl J Med.* 2015;373:123–135. (74)

DeVita VT et al, eds. *DeVita, Hellman, and Rosenberg's Cancer: Principles and Practice of Oncology*. 10th ed. Philadelphia, PA: Lippincott Williams & Wilkins; 2014. (1)

Doll R et al. Mortality in relation to smoking: 50 years' observations on male British doctors. *BMJ*. 2004;328:1519. (13)

Gandhi L, Johnson BE. Paraneoplastic syndromes associated with small cell lung cancer. *J Natl Compr Canc Net*. 2006;4:631–638. (86)

Langer CJ et al. The evolving role of histology in the management of advanced non-small-cell lung cancer. *J Clin Oncol*. 2010;28:5311. (37)

Pirker R. Adjuvant chemotherapy in patients with completely resected non-small cell lung cancer. *Transl Lung Cancer Res*. 2014;3:305. (19)

Solomon BJ, Mok T, Kim DW et al. First-line crizotinib versus chemotherapy in ALK-positive lung cancer. *N Engl J Med*. 2014;371:2167. (70)

Socinski MA, Bogart JA. Limited-stage small-cell lung cancer: the current status of combined-modality therapy. *J Clin Oncol*. 2007;25:4137. (101)

Subramanian J, Govindan R. Lung cancer in never smokers: a review. *J Clin Oncol*. 2007;25:561. (14)

Key Websites

NCCN Clinical Practice Guidelines in Oncology (NCCN Guidelines®). Small cell lung cancer. http://www.nccn.org/professionals/physician_gls/f_guidelines.asp. Accessed June 10, 2015. (78)

NCCN Clinical Practice Guidelines in Oncology (NCCN Guidelines®). Non–small cell lung cancer. http://www.nccn.org/professionals/physician_gls/f_guidelines.asp. Accessed June 10, 2015. (7)

99 Colorectal Cancer

Marlo Blazer

CORE PRINCIPLES

		CHAPTER CASES
1	Family history, patient-specific factors, and environmental factors are identified as risk factors for colorectal cancer. Environmental factors could be modified to reduce the risk of colorectal cancer.	Case 99-1 (Question 1)
2	Early detection of colorectal cancer through screening reduces cancer-related mortality. Most patients at low risk of colorectal cancer are recommended to begin screening at the age of 50 years.	Case 99-1 (Question 2)
3	Patients may be asymptomatic at diagnosis or have nonspecific symptoms. Carcinoembryonic antigen may be elevated in patients with colorectal cancer, but it cannot be used alone for diagnosis.	Case 99-2 (Question 1)
4	Adjuvant combination chemotherapy with fluorouracil and oxaliplatin is currently considered the standard of care for patients with stage III colorectal cancer after surgery with curative intent.	Case 99-2 (Questions 2, 3)
5	All patients diagnosed with localized colorectal cancer should undergo routine surveillance visits with their oncologist for a period of 5 years after completion of their definitive therapy.	Case 99-2 (Question 5)
6	During the last decade, newer chemotherapy agents (oxaliplatin, irinotecan) and targeted therapies (bevacizumab, ramucirumab, ziv-aflibercept, cetuximab, panitumumab, regorafenib) have increased the overall survival of patients with metastatic colorectal cancer. Fluoropyrimidines (fluorouracil or capecitabine) remain the backbone of therapy in the first- and second-line treatment of advanced cancer. The right combination and sequencing of these agents is vital to improving the care of patients with colorectal cancer.	Case 99-3 (Question 1)
7	Utilization of specific predictive markers helps maximize the desired outcome in colorectal cancer. Patients with *RAS* mutant tumors do not derive any benefit from anti–epidermal growth factor receptor (EGFR) monoclonal antibody therapy.	Case 99-3 (Question 4)
8	Myelosuppression, diarrhea, and peripheral neuropathy are potential dose-limiting toxicities associated with chemotherapy agents used in the treatment of colon and rectal cancers. Prevention strategies, diligent monitoring, and adequate supportive-care measures are vital to effective toxicity management and should be used to maintain patient safety and enhance quality of life.	Case 99-2 (Questions 3, 4), Case 99-3 (Question 3)
9	Severe, life-threatening adverse effects are uncommon, but potential hazards are associated with targeted colorectal cancer therapies and avoiding their use is warranted in patients at increased risk of experiencing these complications. Prevention and treatment strategies are available for common adverse effects such as hypertension associated with vascular endothelial growth factor therapy or EGFR inhibitor–induced dermatologic toxicity.	Case 99-3 (Questions 3, 5, 6)
10	Certain genetic variants of key enzymes involved in the catabolism of fluorouracil and irinotecan are associated with increased toxicity from these agents. The clinical utility of identifying these variants in an effort to avoid or manage these toxicities continues to be elucidated.	Case 99-3 (Question 2)

COLORECTAL CANCER

Epidemiology, Etiology, and Pathophysiology

Colorectal cancer is the malignant growth of tumor that begins from the inner wall of the colon or rectum. It is the third most commonly diagnosed cancer in the United States and the second leading cause of cancer-related deaths. In 2015, it is estimated that there will be 132,700 new cases of colon and rectum cancer with the median age at diagnosis of 68 years, and 49,700 people will die from this disease. During the last decade, new agents and better predictive markers have enabled improvement in the detection, safety, and survival of patients with colorectal cancer. The age-adjusted 5-year relative survival rate in 1975 (based on 1975–2007 data) was 48.6% and is estimated to be 64.9% in 2015 (2005–2011 data).[1]

The formation of colorectal cancer is a multistep process. It begins with an abnormal growth of tissue known as a polyp (adenoma) originating from the innermost wall of the colon. The process of transformation from a polyp to malignant disease can take up to 10 to 15 years.[1] Once this transformation occurs, the cancer begins to spread through the wall of the colon or rectum, where it can eventually invade the blood, lymph nodes, or other organs directly. The vast majority of colon and rectal cancers are classified as adenocarcinomas, meaning that they arise from the glandular tissue responsible for producing the secretions of the gastrointestinal tract. Approximately two-thirds of these cancers will arise from the colon, and the remainder will form in the rectum. Colorectal cancer is among the few cancers that can be prevented by removal of precancerous tissue; therefore, early detection is crucial.

The etiology of colorectal cancer is complex, involving patient-specific, environmental, and genetic factors. Of these, age is considered the most important risk because greater than 90% of patients diagnosed are older than 50 years of age.[2] Other patient-specific risk factors are family history of colon cancer, history of previous colonic polyps, and inflammatory bowel disease (ulcerative colitis or Crohn's disease). Environmental factors like a diet consisting primarily of red meat, high fat, and low fiber can also increase the risk of colorectal cancer, as can a sedentary lifestyle, obesity, excessive alcohol consumption, and long-term smoking.[2,3] Smoking, particularly early in life, has been shown to increase the risk of developing colorectal cancer. Patients who smoked more than 12 pack-years of cigarettes before the age of 30 are at increased risk of recurrence after a diagnosis of stage III colon cancer.[3]

Hereditary syndromes account for 5% to 6% of all colorectal cancers.[4] Specific inherited syndromes include hereditary nonpolyposis colon cancer, also known as Lynch syndrome, and familial adenomatous polyposis (FAP). Although accounting for <1% of all colorectal cancer cases, FAP is associated with a lifetime risk of colorectal cancer of greater than 90% because of an autosomal dominant germline mutation causing the development of 10s to 1,000s of polyps distributed in the colon and rectum, usually beginning in adolescents.[5] Lynch syndrome accounts for 2% to 3% of colorectal cancers.[5] It is an autosomal dominant disorder that also has an early age of onset (age 20–25 years) and is associated with an increased risk of other cancers, such as endometrial cancer, cancers of the urinary tract, small intestine, ovary, stomach, pancreas, biliary tract, brain, and skin. Screening for both of these inherited syndromes begins at an early age (age 10–12 years for FAP and age 20–25 for Lynch syndrome).[5]

Celecoxib, a cyclo-oxygenase-2 inhibitor, is US Food and Drug Administration (FDA) approved for the treatment of patients with known FAP. However, the routine use of NSAIDs for the prevention of colorectal cancer in the general population is not recommended because of concerns of toxicity.

Clinical Presentation and Diagnosis

Symptoms associated with the development of colon and rectal cancers are often subtle and can mimic "generalized" symptoms associated with numerous other benign conditions, such as abdominal pain, constipation, diarrhea, bloating, rectal bleeding, and other sudden changes in bowel habits or caliber. Unintentional weight loss, anemia, and weakness may also be present, particularly in advanced stages of the disease. A diagnosis is made once a colonoscopy or sigmoidoscopy is performed and a biopsy is obtained to confirm the presence of cancer. Additional diagnostic procedures would be performed before initiating treatment, including a computed tomography (CT) scan of the chest, abdomen, and pelvis as well as laboratory collection of blood to obtain a baseline carcinoembryonic antigen (CEA) level. These determine the extent of disease and provide a means to monitor for recurrence or progression after or on treatment. For cancers of the rectum, an endoscopic ultrasound may also be performed to aid in the preoperative or clinical staging of the tumor. Definitive or pathologic staging for all tumors of the colon and rectum takes place during surgical resection.

Treatment Overview

The therapeutic modalities available to the patient with colorectal cancer are similar to those used in other solid tumors. Surgery, radiation, and chemotherapy all have roles in both localized and advanced disease, but how each of these strategies is used, and sequencing, depends on the location and extent of disease and on the goal of therapy. In general, surgery is utilized as the primary initial modality for patients with stages I, II, and III disease. It may also be employed in selected patients with metastatic stage IV disease at some point during their treatment course. Radiation is usually reserved for patients with rectal cancer. This chapter will primarily focus on the use of systemic therapy (i.e., chemotherapy and targeted therapy) for patients diagnosed with colon and rectal cancer.

Stage of disease at diagnosis determines the initial treatment. Colorectal cancer, like other solid tumors, utilizes the TNM staging system, but it is unique in that it is the depth of invasion of the primary tumor and not its size that determines the "T" in the TNM staging. Like other solid tumors, the remaining components of this classification system are lymph node involvement (N) and metastatic spread (M). Colon and rectal cancers are staged in the exact same manner; however, rectal tumors lie in closer proximity to the anal sphincter, therefore the risk of localized treatment failure and of recurrence at the initial site of disease is increased. An area of controversy in the management of colon cancer is whether or not all patients with stage II disease should receive adjuvant therapy. Although the routine use of adjuvant chemotherapy in this setting is not recommended, it should be considered for stage II patients with the following high-risk features: T4 lesions, bowel obstruction or local perforation at presentation, poorly differentiated histology, lymphovascular invasion, inadequate lymph node sampling, and positive margins after surgery.[5]

Etiology

CASE 99-1

QUESTION 1: O.B., a 35-year-old woman, recently learned that her 58-year-old father was diagnosed with colon cancer. O.B. is obese and smokes a half-pack of cigarettes per day. She loves eating out and spends most of her evening watching TV at home. O.B. would like to know the risk factors for colorectal cancer. She would also like to know whether there is anything she can do to reduce her risk of developing colorectal cancer in the future.

O.B. is at an increased risk of developing colorectal cancer given her family history of colon cancer. In addition, she is obese, lives a sedentary lifestyle, and smokes. She eats out, but no information is given about her diet. There are modifiable risk factors, which she could address to lower her risk of developing colorectal cancer. O.B. can lose weight through exercise and adopt a high-fiber, low-fat diet. In addition, she can stop smoking, which can help reduce the risk of colorectal as well as other cancers.

Screening

Case 99-1, Question 2: O.B. would like to know whether there is a way to screen for colorectal cancer. If there is, does this method detect cancer early? Her father had a colon cancer diagnosis; therefore, O.B. wonders when she should get screened for colorectal cancer.

Colon and rectal cancers are among the few cancers that can be prevented by removal of precancerous tissue; therefore, early detection is crucial. As described above, formation of colorectal cancers is a multistep process, and the early precancerous tissue is identifiable and can be removed. Colorectal cancer is not always asymptomatic, but early detection of colorectal cancer through screening has been proven to reduce mortality. A variety of screening methods exist, including fecal screening tests, digital rectal examination, barium enemas, endoscopy, and CT colonography. Fecal screening tests are designed to detect occult blood in the stool and are relatively inexpensive and noninvasive. There are two main types: the fecal occult blood test (FOBT) and the fecal immunochemical test (FIT). The FOBT been shown to reduce mortality from colorectal cancer by 33%, but the test does require diet restrictions prior to sampling.[6] The FIT uses antibodies to detect hemoglobin or other blood components and, compared with FOBT, has no drug or food interactions. Screening guidelines acknowledge that FIT may be more sensitive than FOBT[7]; however, neither is preferred over the other, possibly because of a lack of mortality data with FIT along with potential cost/out-of-pocket difference between the two tests. Endoscopic screening for colorectal cancer includes either flexible sigmoidoscopy or colonoscopy, and both offer the ability to remove polyps and obtain biopsy samples during the procedure. The advantages of sigmoidoscopy are that no sedation is required, a simple preparation (two Fleet enemas) is used, and it can be performed in various settings. Patients may choose flexible sigmoidoscopy over colonoscopy if they do not want to go under sedation or undergo an extensive bowel preparation. Sigmoidoscopy has been shown to reduce incidence of colorectal cancer by 33% and mortality because of colorectal cancer by 43%.[8] However, flexible sigmoidoscopy allows for examination only of the sigmoid colon and rectum, while colonoscopy examines the entire colon. As such, colonoscopy is the most widely accepted screening tool; it has been shown to reduce the incidence of colorectal cancer by 77% and is associated with significant risk reduction in both right- and left-sided colon cancer incidences.[7,9] A relatively new method known as CT colonography provides two- and three-dimensional images of the colon. As with endoscopic procedures, it requires complete bowel preparation to remove feces from the intestine. This screening technique has demonstrated an approximate 80% sensitivity to detect polyps >6 mm in size and 90% sensitivity for polyps >1 cm.[10] However, any cancerous lesion detected will ultimately necessitate an examination by colonoscopy.

CEA is a tumor marker that is detected in the blood and has been evaluated as a screening tool, but its primary utility is in monitoring response to treatment and not screening. Healthy smokers are likely to have twice the CEA level compared with nonsmokers. Further, administration of therapies given for metastatic colon cancer can cause false elevation of CEA without disease progression, so even in monitoring response to treatment, it is only used in conjunction with other modalities.

The American Cancer Society, the US Multi-Society Task Force on Colorectal Cancer, and the American College of Radiology have jointly published screening recommendations for the early detection of colorectal cancer.[11] According to their recommendations, any man or woman at average risk of developing colorectal cancer should begin screening at age of 50 years (Table 99-1). Patients at average risk of developing colorectal cancer will not have genetic predisposition or history of a family member with colorectal cancer. In addition, patients in this category will have no history of polyps, previous history of colorectal cancer, inflammatory bowel disease, chronic ulcerative colitis, or Crohn's colitis.

O.B. is a 35-year-old woman with a first-degree relative with a diagnosis of colon cancer at the age of 58. It is less likely she would develop colorectal cancer through a hereditary syndrome because her father was diagnosed after the age of 50. She does, however, have nearly double the life time risk of developing colorectal cancer because a first-degree relative had colorectal cancer.[12] Because O.B.'s father had colorectal cancer diagnosed before the age of 60, she is at increased risk for developing the disease and should consider initiating a colorectal screening program at the age of 48 or 10 years earlier than her father was diagnosed (at age 58).[10]

Table 99-1
American Cancer Society Screening Recommendation for Colorectal Cancer by Age and Risk

Average Risk	Begin screening at age of 50 years Annual DRE and FOBT or FIT (stool DNA test, interval uncertain) and one of the following: ■ Sigmoidoscopy every 5 years[a] ■ CT colonography every 5 years[a] ■ Colonoscopy every 10 years[a] ■ Barium enema every 5 years[a]
Family History	Begin screening at age of 40 years or 10 years younger from first-degree relative colorectal cancer diagnosis
Hereditary nonpolyposis colon cancer	Begin screening at age of 20–25 years or 10 years younger from first-degree relative colorectal cancer diagnosis
Familial adenomatous polyposis	Begin screening at age of 10–12 years
Inflammatory bowel disease, Chronic ulcerative colitis, or Crohn's colitis	Begin screening at 8–15 years after diagnosis

[a]Interval of surveillance is shown for negative findings. If polyps are found at screening, interval of surveillance may change based on biopsy results.[8]

CT, computed tomography; DRE, digital rectal examination; FIT, fecal immunochemical test; FOBT, fecal occult blood test.

Clinical Presentation

CASE 99-2

QUESTION 1: B.R. is a 66-year-old white man who was in his usual state of health until recently, when he decided to visit his general practitioner owing to progressively worsening gastrointestinal symptoms, including abdominal cramping and changing bowel habits. He admits to also having some blood in his stool at times, which he attributes to his hemorrhoids. His family history is notable for a paternal uncle with gastric cancer. He occasionally drinks alcohol and has never smoked nor used illicit or recreational drugs. On physical examination he is a well-nourished, well-developed man who is afebrile, alert and oriented, and in no apparent distress. He has no palpable masses and no hepatomegaly, and his abdomen is soft and nontender with normal active bowel sounds. The rest of his review of systems is unremarkable. His performance status is excellent. He does have a history of type II diabetes mellitus and hypercholesterolemia, which are both controlled on his current medication regimen. Vital signs and laboratory values obtained are as follows:

Blood pressure, 108/71 mm Hg
Heart rate, 95 beats/minute
Respiratory rate, 18 breaths/minute
White blood cell (WBC) count, 4.8×10^3 cells/μL
Hemoglobin, 11.6 g/dL
Hematocrit, 35.1%
Platelet count, 208×10^3 cells/μL
Total bilirubin, 0.3 mg/dL
Serum creatinine, 0.8 mg/dL
Blood urea nitrogen, 15 mg/dL
Alkaline phosphatase, 61 IU/L
Lactate dehydrogenase, 366 IU/L
Albumin, 4.2 g/dL
Hemoglobin A1C, 6.2%

Are any of the symptoms that B.R. is exhibiting associated with colorectal cancer?

Although the symptoms B.R. is describing are nonspecific in nature, the changes in bowel habits in addition to the blood in his stools are symptoms associated with the development of colorectal cancer. Given his age, symptoms, and lack of prior cancer screening, additional workup is warranted with one of the screening modalities mentioned earlier in this chapter, preferably colonoscopy.

Chemotherapy for Localized Colorectal Cancer

ADJUVANT THERAPY

CASE 99-2, QUESTION 2: After a colonoscopy, B.R. is found to have a moderately differentiated adenocarcinoma of the colon lying 18 cm from the anal verge invading through the muscularis propria with lymphovascular invasion and involvement of 8 of 25 regional lymph nodes. A CT scan of his chest, abdomen, and pelvis shows no evidence of metastatic disease. A baseline CEA level of 8.0 ng/mL (normal range, 0–3.0 ng/mL for nonsmokers and 0–6.0 ng/mL for smokers) is reported. After surgical resection, would B.R. benefit from adjuvant chemotherapy? Which chemotherapy agents or regimen gives B.R. the best chance to avoid a future recurrence?

Historically, fluorouracil (also known as 5-fluorouracil and often abbreviated as 5-FU), a fluoropyrimidine, combined with leucovorin was considered the standard chemotherapy for adjuvant treatment of stage III colon cancer based on studies that showed both an improvement in disease-free survival (DFS) and overall survival (OS) over no chemotherapy after surgery.[13] For patients with Stage II disease, only those with certain high risk features (tumors that were adherent to or invaded other organs, were obstructive, or in patients that experienced bowel perforation) appeared to gain any benefit from fluorouracil/leucovorin given after surgery.[13] Leucovorin stabilizes the binding of an active metabolite of fluorouracil known as fluorodeoxyuridine monophosphate to its intracellular target thymidylate synthase, ultimately enhancing the cytotoxicity of fluorouracil. Fluorouracil is administered primarily in two different ways—as a bolus injection over 3 to 5 minutes, and this is followed by a continuous infusion over 24 to 46 hours (depending on the regimen). Single-agent capecitabine, an oral prodrug of fluorouracil, offers convenient administration and is as effective as intravenous (fluorouracil modulated with leucovorin).[14] At present, the combination of fluorouracil and leucovorin or capecitabine monotherapy are the preferred adjuvant regimes for stage III colon cancer for patients that are over the age of 70, because this population does not seem to benefit from the addition of other cytotoxic agents to this fluoropyrimidine backbone.[15,16]

For patients younger than 70 years of age, the addition of oxaliplatin, a platinum agent, to the fluoropyrimidine backbone (either capecitabine alone or fluorouracil with leucovorin) is considered the current standard of care in the adjuvant setting for patients with stage III disease, because several landmark trials have shown the addition of oxaliplatin in this population can improve both DFS and OS over fluorouracil and leucovorin alone.[17,18] The increase in DFS and in OS with the addition of oxaliplatin was less pronounced for those patients with Stage II (node negative) disease, and so the use of oxaliplatin in this population is controversial.[15] There were several fluorouracil and oxaliplatin regimens historically used in clinical practice. However, more current practices recommend that when combining fluorouracil with additional cytotoxic agents, the infusional modality be primarily utilized rather than bolus (IV push) regimens to maximize efficacy while minimizing toxicity, although the infusional regimens do still contain a small portion of the entire fluorouracil dose given as an initial bolus injection.[19]

As stated, oxaliplatin may also be combined with capecitabine as the fluoropyrimidine backbone. This is considered equally effective to the combination with fluorouracil modulated with leucovorin, with the main difference seen in toxicity patterns. Capecitabine is given orally typically as a twice daily dose for 14 days of each 21-day cycle. Often the decision of which fluoropyrimidine to choose is multifactorial owing to the nuances of clinical practice. Potential factors that play a role in the agent chosen can include, but are not limited to, toxicity differences, institutional resources (ambulatory pump availability, etc.), insurance coverage, and patient preference. Additional factors that could influence the selection of a capecitabine-based regimen include the presence of renal impairment and relevant drug–drug interactions, particularly concomitant warfarin use. Regimens that are commonly used in the adjuvant treatment of colon cancer are noted in Table 99-2.

Irinotecan in combination with fluorouracil and leucovorin has been evaluated in the adjuvant setting for stage III colon cancer. The use of irinotecan did not produce any benefit in terms of DFS; however, toxicities were increased with the combination of irinotecan and fluorouracil versus fluorouracil alone.[20] Therefore, irinotecan is not an agent used at present time in the adjuvant setting for colorectal cancer. In addition, some of the biologics available for the treatment of metastatic colon cancer, such as bevacizumab and cetuximab, have been studied in the adjuvant setting as well. To date, none of the biologics approved for metastatic colon cancer (bevacizumab, ramucirumab, ziv-aflibercept, cetuximab, panitumumab, or regorafenib) are approved or recommended in the adjuvant setting.[17]

Table 99-2

Selected Regimens Used in Metastatic or Advanced Colorectal Cancer

Selected Colorectal Cancer Treatment Regimens—Metastatic Disease	
Regimen	**Dosing**
Oxaliplatin-Based Regimens	
mFOLFOX6[a]	■ Oxaliplatin 85 mg/m^2 IV over 2 hours, day 1 ■ Leucovorin 400 mg/m^2 IV over 2 hours, day 1 ■ Fluorouracil 400 mg/m^2 IV bolus on day 1, then 1,200 mg/m^2/day × 2 days (total 2,400 mg/m^2 over 46–48 hours) IV continuous infusion Repeat every 2 weeks
mFOLFOX6 + Bevacizumab	■ Oxaliplatin 85 mg/m^2 IV over 2 hours, day 1 ■ Leucovorin 400 mg/m^2 IV over 2 hours, day 1 ■ Fluorouracil 400 mg/m^2 IV bolus on day 1, then 1,200 mg/m^2/day × 2 days (total 2,400 mg/m^2 over 46–48 hours) IV continuous infusion ■ Bevacizumab 5 mg/kg IV, day 1 Repeat every 2 weeks
mFOLFOX6 + Panitumumab	■ Oxaliplatin 85 mg/m^2 IV over 2 hours, day 1 ■ Leucovorin 400 mg/m^2 IV over 2 hours, day 1 ■ Fluorouracil 400 mg/m^2 IV bolus on day 1, then 1,200 mg/m^2/day × 2 days (total 2,400 mg/m^2 over 46–48 hours) IV continuous infusion ■ Panitumumab 6 mg/kg IV over 60 minutes, day 1 Repeat every 2 weeks
CapeOX[a,b]	■ Oxaliplatin 130 mg/m^2 IV over 2 hours, day 1 ■ Capecitabine 850–1,000 mg/m^2 twice daily PO for 14 days Repeat every 3 weeks
CapeOX[b] + Bevacizumab	■ Oxaliplatin 130 mg/m^2 IV over 2 hours, day 1 ■ Capecitabine 850–1,000 mg/m^2 PO twice daily for 14 days ■ Bevacizumab 7.5 mg/kg IV, day 1 Repeat every 3 weeks
Irinotecan-Based Treatment Regimens	
FOLFIRI	■ Irinotecan 180 mg/m^2 IV over 30–90 minutes, day 1 ■ Leucovorin 400 mg/m^2 IV infusion to match duration of irinotecan infusion, day 1 ■ Fluorouracil 400 mg/m^2 IV bolus day 1, then 1,200 mg/m^2/day × 2 days (total 2,400 mg/m^2 over 46–48 hours) continuous infusion Repeat every 2 weeks
FOLFIRI + Bevacizumab	■ Irinotecan 180 mg/m^2 IV over 30–90 minutes, day 1 ■ Leucovorin 400 mg/m^2 IV infusion to match duration of irinotecan infusion, day 1 ■ Fluorouracil 400 mg/m^2 IV bolus day 1, then 1,200 mg/m^2/day × 2 days (total 2,400 mg/m^2 over 46–48 hours) IV continuous infusion ■ Bevacizumab 5 mg/kg IV, day 1 Repeat every 2 weeks
FOLFIRI + Cetuximab	■ Irinotecan 180 mg/m^2 IV over 30–90 minutes, day 1 ■ Leucovorin 400 mg/m^2 IV infusion to match duration of irinotecan infusion, day 1 ■ Fluorouracil 400 mg/m^2 IV bolus day 1, then 1,200 mg/m^2/day × 2 days (total 2,400 mg/m^2 over 46–48 hours) IV continuous infusion ■ Repeat every 2 weeks ■ Cetuximab 400 mg/m^2 IV over 2 hours first infusion, then 250 mg/m^2 IV over 60 minutes weekly ■ OR ■ Cetuximab 500 mg/m^2 IV over 2 hours, day 1, every 2 weeks
FOLFIRI + Panitumumab	■ Irinotecan 180 mg/m^2 IV over 30–90 minutes, day 1 ■ Leucovorin 400 mg/m^2 IV infusion to match duration of irinotecan infusion, day 1 ■ Fluorouracil 400 mg/m^2 IV bolus day 1, then 1,200 mg/m^2/day × 2 days (total 2,400 mg/m^2 over 46–48 hours) IV continuous infusion ■ Panitumumab 6 mg/kg IV over 60 minutes, day 1 Repeat every 2 weeks

(continued)

Table 99-2

Selected Regimens Used in Metastatic or Advanced Colorectal Cancer (*continued*)

Selected Colorectal Cancer Treatment Regimens—Metastatic Disease	
Regimen	**Dosing**
FOLFIRI + ziv-aflibercept Currently approved only in the second-line setting	■ Irinotecan 180 mg/m² IV over 30–90 minutes, day 1 ■ Leucovorin 400 mg/m² IV infusion to match duration of irinotecan infusion, day 1 ■ Fluorouracil 400 mg/m² IV bolus day 1, then 1,200 mg/m²/day × 2 days (total 2,400 mg/m² over 46–48 hours) continuous infusion ■ Ziv-aflibercept 4 mg/kg IV over 60 minutes Repeat every 2 weeks
FOLFIRI + Ramucirumab Currently approved only in the 2nd line setting	■ Irinotecan 180 mg/m² IV over 30–90 minutes, day 1 ■ Leucovorin 400 mg/m² IV infusion to match duration of irinotecan infusion, day 1 ■ Fluorouracil 400 mg/m² IV bolus day 1, then 1,200 mg/m²/day × 2 days (total 2,400 mg/m² over 46–48 hours) continuous infusion ■ Ramucirumab 8 mg/kg IV over 60 minutes ■ Repeat every 2 weeks
Fluoropyrimidine Treatment Regimens[b]	
Capecitabine[d] ± Bevacizumab	■ Capecitabine 850–1,250 mg/m² PO twice daily, days 1–14 ■ ± Bevacizumab 7.5 mg/kg IV, day 1 Repeat every 3 weeks
Bolus or infusional 5-FU/leucovorin (Roswell Park regimen)	■ Leucovorin 500 mg/m² IV over 2 hours, days 1, 8, 15, 22, 29, and 36 ■ Fluorouracil 500 mg/m² IV bolus 1 hour after start of leucovorin, days 1, 8, 15, 22, 29, and 36 Repeat every 8 weeks
Simplified biweekly infusional 5-FU/leucovorin[d] ± Bevacizumab	■ Leucovorin 400 mg/m² IV over 2 hours on day 1 ■ Fluorouracil bolus 400 mg/m² IV and then 1,200 mg/m²/day × 2 days (total 2,400 mg/m² over 46–48 hours) continuous infusion ± Bevacizumab 5 mg/kg IV on day 1
Miscellaneous Combination Regimens	
IROX Shown to be inferior in the first line to FOLFOX-based therapy	■ Oxaliplatin 85 mg/m² IV over 2 hours ■ Irinotecan 200 mg/m² over 30 or 90 minutes every 3 weeks
FOLFOXIRI ± Bevacizumab Increased PFS vs. FOLFIRI alone; however, no data regarding superiority vs. sequencing patients from FOLFOX to FOLFIRI or vice versa (± Bevacizumab)	■ Irinotecan 165 mg/m² IV day 1 ■ Oxaliplatin 85 mg/m² day 1 ■ Leucovorin 400 mg/m² day 1 ■ Fluorouracil 1,200 mg/m²/day × 2 days (total 2,400 mg/m² over 48 hours) continuous infusion starting on day 1 Repeat every 2 weeks ■ ± Bevacizumab 5 mg/kg IV, day 1
Salvage Therapy	
Regorafenib Used post progression on irinotecan, oxaliplatin, fluorouracil, and an EGFR-inhibitor (if *RAS* wild-type)	160 mg PO daily in the morning with a low-fat breakfast on days 1–21. Repeat every 28 days
Trifluridine/Tipiracil Used post-progression on irinotecan, oxaliplatin, fluorouracil, and an EGFR-inhibitor (if *RAS* wild-type)	35 mg/m² orally twice daily, after morning and evening meals, on days 1–5 and days 8–12 of each 28-day cycle Dose is based on trifluridine content of combination tablets BSA was capped at 2.3 m² in registrational trial

[a]Oxaliplatin combined with either fluorouracil or capecitabine (as in mFOLFOX6 or CapeOX) for 6 months of therapy is also used in the adjuvant setting (post-surgery) for Stage III colon cancer.
[b]Phase II data exists for bi-weekly regimens with oxaliplatin given at 85 mg/m² every two weeks and capecitabine given on day 1 to 7 and days 15 to 21.
[c]Fluorouracil or capecitabine ± bevacizumab is an appropriate therapy in a poor performance status patient where concerns of the added toxicity of oxaliplatin or irinotecan outweigh benefit.
[d]Capecitabine alone or fluorouracil with leucovorin alone for 6 months of therapy are also appropriate as adjuvant therapy for high-risk stage II colon cancer patient or as adjuvant therapy for patients older than 70 years old with stage III colon cancer post-surgery.

B.R. has extensive lymph node involvement, and this means he has stage IIIC disease (refer to key websites #3 and #4 for more information on staging guidelines), which places him at a high risk of recurrence; therefore, he should receive adjuvant chemotherapy after surgery. The goal of adjuvant therapy is to eradicate any residual, undetectable disease left behind after surgery and to reduce his risk of recurrence. The initial cycle of B.R.'s adjuvant chemotherapy should begin approximately 4 to 6 weeks after his surgery and continue for a total of 6 months.

ADVERSE EFFECTS OF FLUOROURACIL AND OXALIPLATIN

CASE 99-2, QUESTION 3: B.R. is scheduled to receive a modified FOLFOX6 (mFOLFOX6) regimen in the adjuvant setting. What potential adverse effects should B.R. be made aware of before receiving this regimen? Are any dose-limiting side effects associated with this therapy? Are there any preventive measures that can be taken to limit the severity of these adverse effects?

The goal of therapy in this setting is a cure; therefore, clinicians typically try to remain aggressive and limit chemotherapy dose reductions or delays while trying to maintain an acceptable toxicity profile. There are a number of chemotherapy-related toxicities that may occur during adjuvant therapy or after its completion.

Toxicities related to fluoropyrimidines include hand-foot syndrome (HFS, also called palmar-plantar erythrodysesthesia), mucositis, diarrhea, hematologic toxicities (neutropenia), photosensitivity, and rarely, cardiac toxicity (vasospastic angina). HFS is managed primarily with supportive-care measures, such as the application of topical moisturizers in addition to temporary withdrawal of fluorouracil-based therapy to allow time to heal. (See Chapter 94, Adverse Effects of Chemotherapy and Targeted Therapy for further discussion of HFS.) Once healed or decreased in its severity, fluorouracil-based therapy is often resumed at a reduced dose. The frequency and severity of HFS is increased with capecitabine versus fluorouracil.[21] Severe neutropenia is typically managed with chemotherapy dose reductions or delays, and in some cases clinicians may use the administration of granulocyte colony-stimulating factors, such as filgrastim or pegfilgrastim, to prevent febrile neutropenia while maintaining dose intensity. The incidence of neutropenia is higher with bolus fluorouracil than with infusional fluorouracil or with capecitabine.[22,23] Severe mucositis is uncommon and is mainly associated with bolus fluorouracil.[20,21] Moderate-to-mild symptoms can also occur, however, with capecitabine or infusional fluorouracil, and these can be managed with supportive-care measures, such as mild narcotic pain medications or mouthwashes that contain a local anesthetic such as lidocaine. Strategies for preventing this complication are also important and include stressing the importance of good oral hygiene and avoidance of harsh substances, which may irritate the oral mucosa or inhibit saliva production, such as alcohol, alcohol-based mouthwashes or rinses, spicy foods, and anticholinergic medications. As is the case with many fluorinated pharmaceutical agents, fluorouracil and capecitabine cause photosensitivity, which may result in mild-to-severe sunburns after sun exposure. Therefore, during fluoropyrimidine therapy, prolonged exposure to direct sunlight should be avoided and use of a sun block of SPF-15 or higher during outdoor activities is recommended.

Oxaliplatin is the newest member of the platinum family of antineoplastics, and it offers a different antitumor profile and resistance pattern than cisplatin or carboplatin. Of the three agents, oxaliplatin is highly active against colorectal tumors. Myelosuppression, primarily neutropenia and thrombocytopenia, and neurotoxicity are dose-limiting toxicities associated with its use. Oxaliplatin causes an acute, reversible neuropathy consisting of either paresthesias or dysesthesias and in some instances muscle spasms. One particular phenomenon that is distressing for patients is an involuntary laryngopharyngeal dysesthesia that can create the sensation of an inability to swallow or breathe. The acute phenomenon is reported to occur in greater than 90% of patients receiving oxaliplatin.[24,25] Although our understanding of the event is limited, it is known to be triggered by direct contact with anything cold. This sensitivity to cold as well as the aforementioned reactions generally occur within minutes of receiving the infusion and can persist up to 7 days. Avoidance of cold objects, including the eating or drinking of cold foods and beverages, should be emphasized to patients after each dose of oxaliplatin. The use of gloves, socks, and scarves can also be recommended, especially in cold weather. Delayed, cumulative neurotoxicity may also occur, and it is potentially irreversible and occurs in a dose-dependent manner. It initially develops in the distal extremities and slowly progresses in a glove and stocking distribution pattern. It is typically characterized by a persistent sensation of numbness, tingling, or burning in the extremities.

Hypersensitivity reactions have also been observed with oxaliplatin use with a reported incidence of 10% to 25%, and although the appearance of the reaction is arbitrary in that it can manifest with any dose, the median number of doses reported in those that have reacted is 7 to 9.[26] Typically, the symptoms of hypersensitivity occur during the infusion, but delayed reactions are also possible. The severity of these allergic reactions can range from mild itching or flushing to anaphylaxis. After a reaction, mild cases are often managed through premedication with antihistamines or corticosteroids (e.g., diphenhydramine 50 mg IV or orally and either dexamethasone 20 mg or another corticosteroid 15 minutes before oxaliplatin IV) in addition to prolonging the infusion of oxaliplatin. More severe reactions generally warrant discontinuation of the drug; however, there are reports in which desensitization protocols have been used successfully, allowing for continued administration.[27,28] Regardless of what is chosen, this strategy accompanies all subsequent doses of oxaliplatin.

Liver toxicity has also been reported with oxaliplatin and is mainly characterized by sinusoidal injury. This can occur in as high as 51% of patients, although blatant liver failure with oxaliplatin is rare. Splenomegaly has been reported to correlate with sinusoidal liver injury and this manifestation may also contribute to thrombocytopenia that may last long after oxaliplatin is discontinued.[29]

The primary role of chemotherapy in this setting is to reduce the risk of relapse and prolong DFS by eradicating residual, undetectable disease. A total of 6 months of adjuvant therapy is considered the current standard of care after surgery with curative intent (12 cycles of an every 2-week regimen like FOLFOX, or 8 cycles of an every 3-week strategy of capecitabine with or without oxaliplatin). A large ongoing trial is currently evaluating the necessity of 6 months versus 3 months of therapy, but the results are pending.[30] Because B.R. will receive a combination of fluorouracil and oxaliplatin in the adjuvant setting, the toxicities of these agents should be discussed before initiation of therapy. The toxicity of fluorouracil will vary depending on its dose, route, and schedule of administration. At doses used in the treatment of colorectal cancer, bolus administration is associated with more severe neutropenia and mucositis, whereas continuous infusion administration is associated with more severe HFS. Fluorouracil is also associated with photosensitivity, so B.R. should be counseled on the use of SPF-15 or greater sunscreen when outdoors because of the increased risk of sunburn. The main toxicities of oxaliplatin are thrombocytopenia, neuropathy, liver toxicity, and hypersensitivity reactions. To minimize the acute neuropathy after each dose, B.R. should be counseled on the avoidance of cold objects, including the eating or drinking of cold foods and beverages. The use of gloves, socks, and scarves can also be recommended, especially in cold weather. B.R. will also have labs drawn at regular intervals prior to administration of chemotherapy to ensure that his neutrophils and platelets are at a sufficient level to give chemotherapy and to monitor for changes in liver function that can occur with oxaliplatin.

PERIPHERAL SENSORY NEUROPATHY

CASE 99-2, QUESTION 4: After eight treatments of adjuvant therapy, B.R. begins complaining of a constant numbness and tingling in his toes bilaterally. It is not interfering with his daily activities but is described as more of a nuisance. Which drug is most likely responsible for this and what course of action should be taken?

As explained earlier, the severity of peripheral sensory neuropathy (PSN) can worsen with continued doses of oxaliplatin and is not readily reversible; therefore, it is imperative that clinicians and patients work together to minimize its negative impact on various activities of daily living such as being able to button a shirt, walking up or down stairs, or realizing whether one's foot is actually touching the brake pedal as the car approaches a red light. In the hallmark clinical trial in the adjuvant setting, during the 6 months of therapy with oxaliplatin, fluorouracil, and leucovorin, 12.5% of patients reported grade 3 PSN; however, this increased to 24.1% in the 18 months after treatment assessment, indicating that PSN will continue to worsen even after cessation of oxaliplatin.[17] It does appear that over time PSN can improve off oxaliplatin as at 4 years post-adjuvant treatment grade 1, 2, and 3 PSN was observed in 11.9%, 2.8%, and 0.7%, respectively.[24] In the metastatic setting a "stop-and-go" approach to limit exposure to oxaliplatin while retaining its antitumor effects and has been shown to be beneficial in delaying the development of PSN without adversely affecting the outcomes of PFS and OS.[31,32] In this approach, oxaliplatin is withdrawn from therapy in patients with metastatic disease and is reinitiated when disease progression is noted. However, in the adjuvant setting where the goal is cure, the benefits of stopping therapy to decrease the risk of permanent PSN must be weighed against the risk of recurrent disease. Newer trials in the adjuvant setting recommend holding oxaliplatin for a period of 4 weeks in the setting of persistent grade >2 neuropathy (defined as persisting between treatments) and resuming at a dose reduction once PSN resolves to grade <1.[23] Further, permanent discontinuation of oxaliplatin is recommended for grade >2 neuropathy that does not resolve within 4 weeks.[23]

Several small trials have been conducted to evaluate the effectiveness of certain pharmaceutical agents in the management of chemotherapy-induced peripheral neuropathy. These trials have focused on either the prevention or treatment of chemotherapy-induced peripheral neuropathy and as a whole have yielded disappointing results. To date, no agent is recommended as a chemoprotectant for the prevention of oxaliplatin-induced PSN. Duloxetine, an antidepressant, has been studied in a randomized clinical trial and has shown to decrease specifically the pain component experienced by some patients with PSN including oxaliplatin-induced PSN.[33] In addition, tricyclic antidepressants such as nortriptyline and amitriptyline or an anticonvulsant such as gabapentin and pregabalin could be considered as these agents have proven beneficial and are recommended as initial therapy in other neuropathic pain settings.[34,35] It is important to note that when using adjunctive agents such as these to manage neuropathic pain, doses typically require upward titration after initiation. This strategy enables the clinician to find the dose that provides the greatest benefit. It is important to explain to the patient that these agents may take several weeks before a response is seen, and that the indication is for the *pain* associated with PSN—these agents have not been shown to improve numbness or tingling. Symptom relief generally requires continued daily use of these agents on a scheduled basis; however, it is important to consider weaning them with time if neuropathic symptoms either improve or show no improvement despite optimal dosing.

The timing of the symptoms that B.R. is experiencing is indicative of the cumulative toxicity oxaliplatin exerts on peripheral sensory nerves. Because B.R. has completed 8 of a planned 12 cycles of his adjuvant therapy and because his symptoms just started, the reaction would be graded as relatively mild in its severity at this point. He will likely benefit most from continued administration of oxaliplatin at a reduced dosage with diligent monitoring of his neuropathy.

Microsatellite Instability and BRAF

The ultimate goal of treatment is to individualize therapy based on patient and tumor characteristics. Prognostic markers provide information on disease outcome regardless of treatment provided. Predictive markers provide information on disease outcome based on treatment provided. As stated previously, in stage II disease, adjuvant therapy is only offered in those patients with high-risk disease. The definition of "high risk" stage II disease varies among different national guidelines but in general includes T4 tumors, less than 12 lymph nodes examined at surgery, poorly differentiated histology, perforation, and obstruction.[36] There has been increased interest in looking at microsatellite instability and mutations in *BRAF* to determine what stage II patients would benefit from adjuvant therapy.

Microsatellites are short repeating nucleotide sequences that are under surveillance by the mismatch repair (MMR) system. The MMR system is responsible for repair of errors that occur during DNA synthesis. Tumors are found to have microsatellite instability (MSI) if they have a defect in their MMR system. This defect results in the accumulation of mutations of microsatellites. In a pooled analysis of 5 trials of stage II and III patients where no adjuvant therapy was given, patients with MSI had a longer DFS than those that were microsatellite stable.[31] In addition, in the Stage II patients that were MSI, those treated with fluorouracil actually did worse in terms of DFS than those that were only treated with surgery.[37] At this time, it appears that MSI is prognostic in that it appears to convey a DFS benefit in stage II disease. It further appears that fluorouracil/leucovorin alone does not convey any benefit in stage II MSI disease. The benefit of adding oxaliplatin to a high-risk stage II MSI patient is unknown, and currently cannot be recommended based on MSI status alone.

The *BRAF* oncogene is downstream from the EGFR receptor. Mutations in *BRAF* have been associated with a poor prognosis, but to date, they lack any predictive value in both early stage and in advanced disease.[38,39]

Clinical Surveillance for Recurrence

CASE 99-2, QUESTION 5: After completing his treatment, how often and for how long should B.R. be monitored for recurrence of his disease?

Because the majority of recurrences occur within the first 2 to 3 years after completion of adjuvant therapy, both the American Society of Clinical Oncology and the National Comprehensive

Cancer Network (NCCN) have published guidelines that address the importance of patient follow-up and surveillance after definitive therapy for localized disease.[17,40] Both organizations agree that patients treated definitively for localized disease should be monitored regularly for at least 5 years. Because most recurrences occur relatively soon, surveillance screening should be more frequent for the first 2 years and include a history and physical examination, and CEA level performed every 3 to 6 months for these first 2 years, then semiannually thereafter for up to 5 years. In addition, future recommended imaging includes CT scan of the chest, abdomen, and pelvis performed at least annually for up to 5 years and colonoscopy within a year of surgical resection (or approximately 1 year from the original colonoscopy) and then repeated again in 3 years if no high grade adenomas are identified. During the surveillance period, development of a concerning symptom on physical examination, an abnormality on a CT scan, or a rise in CEA level above the upper limit of normal (3 ng/mL for nonsmokers or 6 ng/mL for smokers) would necessitate further evaluation for disease recurrence. After the 5-year surveillance period, an increased risk for recurrent disease remains; therefore, screening for colorectal cancer every 5 years in these patients will continue rather than the every 10-year screening recommended for the average-risk population.

B.R. should be monitored regularly for at least 5 years. Should B.R. remain disease-free throughout this 5-year surveillance period, he will be considered cured of his cancer. Because most recurrences occur relatively soon, his surveillance visits will be more frequent for the first 2 years with a history and physical examination and CEA level performed every 3 to 6 months, then semiannually thereafter. He should also have a CT scan of his chest, abdomen, and pelvis performed at least annually for 3 years. Another colonoscopy should be performed within a year of his surgical resection or approximately 1 year from his original colonoscopy, and then repeated again in 3 years.

Chemotherapy for Metastatic Colorectal Cancer

CASE 99-3

QUESTION 1: K.T. is a 64-year-old man treated approximately 2 years ago with adjuvant chemotherapy for colon cancer, which he tolerated well. On a routine surveillance visit, his CT scan shows a colon mass, two discrete liver nodules, and a nodule in the left lung that are consistent with metastatic disease. The biopsy of the liver was positive for adenocarcinoma of the colon. K.T. is feeling well and has been asymptomatic. No cytogenetics on the tumor was performed at this time. K.T.'s CBC and chemistry values were as follows:

WBC count, 7.8×10^3 cells/μL
Hemoglobin, 13.2 g/dL
Platelet count, 252×10^3 cells/μL
Serum creatinine, 1.1 mg/dL
Blood urea nitrogen, 15 mg/dL
Aspartate aminotransferase, 28 units/L
Alanine aminotransferase, 35 units/L
Alkaline phosphatase, 135 units/L
Total bilirubin, 0.8 mg/dL

K.T.'s CEA concentration was 22 ng/mL. What is the role of chemotherapy now that K.T. has a metastatic recurrence?

Metastatic colorectal cancer affects a substantial number of patients. Approximately 20% of patients have metastatic disease at initial presentation, and ~50% of patients diagnosed at any stage will eventually develop metastatic disease.[1,2]

Significant treatment advances have been made over the last decade for cases of advanced colorectal cancer such that the median OS is currently over 2 years in treated patients.[41–43] Treatments tend to include combination therapy (a fluoropyrimidine plus either irinotecan or oxaliplatin) for good performance status (PS) patients and mono-cytotoxic therapy (fluorouracil or capecitabine or irinotecan) for poor PS patients.[17] Further, agents directed against the vascular endothelial growth factor (VEGF) (e.g., the monoclonal antibodies, bevacizumab and ramucirumab, and the soluble decoy receptor, ziv-aflibercept) or against the epidermal growth factor receptor (EGFR) (cetuximab and panitumumab, both monoclonal antibodies) can be added to the chemotherapy backbone in qualifying patients. Given the number of agents currently available and that we tend to talk in terms of regimens (i.e., combining agents together) in the treatment of metastatic colorectal cancer, it is imperative to consider which agents have greater synergy and less toxicity when combined and how best to sequence these agents, because patients will most likely remain on some type of therapy throughout their disease course.

Irinotecan has been studied combined with a bolus regimen of fluorouracil and leucovorin (IFL) and an infusional regimen (FOLFIRI) as well as with capecitabine (XELIRI or CAPIRI). In general, both IFL and CAPIRI/XELIRI have fallen out of favor because of exorbitant toxicities and less efficacy than FOLFIRI.[17]

Oxaliplatin, as in the early stages of colon cancer, has been studied with both infusional fluorouracil, and leucovorin (FOLFOX) or with capecitabine (XELOX or CAPOX) in the metastatic setting. Both strategies of combining oxaliplatin with a fluoropyrimidine in the metastatic setting are equally efficacious, with again, the main differences being the toxicity profile of capecitabine versus fluorouracil /leucovorin.[19,44]

The decision to start with an oxaliplatin-based regimen (FOLFOX or XELOX) or an irinotecan-based regimen (FOLFIRI) tends to reflect differences in clinical practice rather than clinical outcomes, because sequencing studies and the results of multiple individual studies seem to indicate that both regimens are equally efficacious in the first line.[17,31–45] With the optimal sequencing of these regimens remaining unclear, the decision regarding the choice of combination therapy for first- or second-line therapy is based on prior therapy, quality of life, preexisting toxicities, comorbid conditions, and clinical practice where the patient is first seen. Surgery is typically not an option in extensive metastatic disease.

In the past decade, biologic therapies targeting VEGF (bevacizumab, ziv-aflibercept, and ramucirumab) and EGFR (cetuximab and panitumumab) have been incorporated into the treatment of many cases of metastatic colorectal cancer. In addition, regorafenib, a multi-targeted, orally administered tyrosine kinase inhibitor (TKI) and trifluridine/tipiracil (TAS-102), an orally administered cytotoxic agent, have both been shown to modestly improve OS over placebo as monotherapy in the salvage setting.

TARGETING VASCULAR ENDOTHELIAL GROWTH FACTOR

Bevacizumab is a humanized monoclonal antibody that binds to the ligand of the VEGF-2 receptor, VEGF-A. The addition to bevacizumab in the first line to oxaliplatin-based regimens FOLFOX or XELOX or irinotecan-based FOLFIRI has been shown to increase progression-free survival (PFS) versus chemotherapy alone, and OS was also improved although this seems more pronounced with FOLFIRI than with oxaliplatin-based regimens.[17,33] Bevacizumab, when continued beyond progression in the second-line setting, with either FOLFOX or FOLFIRI has shown a modest survival benefit of the addition of 1.4 months versus placebo.[46]

Two newer anti-VEGF agents, ziv-aflibercept and ramucirumab, have also been shown to provide a survival benefit to the chemotherapy backbones with which they were studied. However, the differences in how they were studied is important to note in order to apply them in clinical practice. Ramucirumab, a fully human monoclonal antibody that binds to the extracellular domain of the VEGF-2 receptor, has been shown to increase survival versus placebo by 1.6 months when combined with FOLFIRI in patients that progressed on bevacizumab plus FOLFOX.[47] Ziv-aflibercept, a soluble decoy receptor that targets the ligands VEGF-A, VEGF-B, and placental growth factor (PIGF), has also been shown to increase survival versus placebo when combined with FOLFIRI in the second-line setting after progression on oxaliplatin-based therapy; however, in the patients that had previously received bevacizumab, this benefit was less pronounced (around 0.8 months).[48]

TARGETING THE EPIDERMAL GROWTH FACTOR RECEPTOR

The EGFR receptor is overexpressed in the majority of colorectal cancers, making it an attractive target for therapy. However, 56% to 63% of these tumors will possess a downstream mutation in the *RAS* oncogene, a predictive biomarker for a lack of response to EGFR targeted therapy.[32,40,41] Therefore, prior to consideration of EGFR therapy in any metastatic colorectal patient, analysis must be undertaken to determine *RAS* status, with EGFR therapy only being offered to those that are *RAS* wild-type.

Cetuximab is a chimeric monoclonal antibody against the extracellular domain of EGFR. It has been studied in the first line with both FOLFIRI and with oxaliplatin-based therapy and is currently approved in combination with FOLFIRI only in the first line for patients that are *RAS* wild-type.[32,49] It is also active as a single agent or in combination with irinotecan even in patients with irinotecan-refractory malignancies.[50] Panitumumab, a fully human monoclonal antibody also targeting the extracellular domain of EGFR, has been shown in *RAS* wild-type patients to improve OS in the first-line setting when combined with FOLFOX and in the second-line setting combined with FOLFIRI in patients that had progressed on an oxaliplatin and bevacizumab containing regimen.[51,52] It may also be used as monotherapy in patients that have progressed on oxaliplatin- and irinotecan-based therapy. The trials of combining cetuximab or panitumumab with bevacizumab and chemotherapy have resulted in a decrease in PFS and increased toxicity, so this combination should not be utilized.[53,54] The choice of whether cetuximab or panitumumab is chosen as the anti-EGFR agent is more a matter of local practice and differences in prescribing habits than being data driven. They have been compared to each other in the salvage setting as monotherapy and are considered equally efficacious with the main difference being a slightly higher rate of infusion reactions with cetuximab versus panitumumab (13% vs. 3%).[55] In addition, there is currently no data to support the use of one of these agents after proven progression on the other agent.

K.T. has stage IV colon cancer with metastasis to the liver and lung. The goal of therapy for K.T. is prolongation of survival. At this point, K.T.'s cancer is not curable. Because tumor cytogenetics was not performed, K.T.'s *RAS* status is unknown. Therefore, EGFR monoclonal antibody at this point is not considered a first-line treatment option. K.T. should receive combination chemotherapy. Standard first-line chemotherapy involves a fluoropyrimidine in combination with oxaliplatin or irinotecan. Addition of bevacizumab to this regimen will further improve response rate and survival of K.T. In this case, K.T. is scheduled to receive the FOLFIRI plus bevacizumab regimen, which is given every 2 weeks. He will receive this chemotherapy regimen until disease progression. The FOLFIRI plus bevacizumab is given as bevacizumab 5 mg/kg IV for 10 to 30 minutes, leucovorin 200 mg/m^2 IV for 2 hours, irinotecan 180 mg/m^2 IV for 90 minutes, and fluorouracil 400 mg/m^2 given as a bolus, which is then followed by 2,400 mg/m^2 infused for 46 hours.

IMMUNOTHERAPY FOR MSI-H TUMORS

Immunotherapies have broadly made their way into different areas of oncology; however, until recently, colorectal cancer patients, did not seem to benefit from these agents.[56] Two new drugs have been approved in metastatic colorectal cancer, specifically for patients with mismatch repair deficient tumors. Pembrolizumab, given as a single agent, was granted accelerated approval from the FDA on May 23, 2017 for treatment of metastatic colorectal cancer that is deficient in MMR and has progressed following treatment with a fluorpyrimidine, oxaliplation, and irinotecan; nivolumab, given as a single agent, was granted accelerated approval for this group of patients on July 31, 2017.[57,58] Approval for both was based on tumor response rate, and as a condition of accelerated approval, further studies are required to confirm the clinical benefit of these two agents for this indication.[57,58] However, while promising, patients with mismatch repair deficient colorectal cancer represent only a small subset of patients with metastatic disease (~3% of the population vs ~22% of those with stage II colon cancer and ~12% of those with stage III colon cancer).[56]

HEPATIC METASTASES

Colorectal-related metastases most commonly arise in the liver, and 20% of patients are diagnosed with synchronous liver metastases.[2] Surgical resection, if possible, offers the potential for long-term survival in colorectal patients with isolated liver metastases.[59,60] Further, because liver metastases derive most of their blood supply from the hepatic artery, direct administration of anticancer drugs into the artery can provide high drug concentrations to the area of tumor involvement and, as such, has been an area of therapeutic interest. Hepatic intra-arterial administration of floxuridine (FUDR), a fluoropyrimidine with a high first-pass metabolism, offers the ability to deliver chemotherapy to the liver metastases with virtually no systemic exposure or side effects.[61] However, the hepatobiliary toxic effects of hepatic arterial FUDR include elevations in AST, alkaline phosphatase, and bilirubin levels, and in severe cases can evoke changes similar to sclerosing cholangitis.[62] To prevent this, FUDR is infused with dexamethasone for its anti-inflammatory effect.[63] Hepatic intra-arterial therapy is usually restricted to treatment centers that have expertise for this modality. The major limitation for such treatment is that undetected metastases located elsewhere would not be exposed to the agents as they would after systemic administration. Further, there is a paucity of data related to giving FUDR via the hepatic artery in combination with systemic chemotherapy but, from the limited data available, it does seem that coadministration with systemic bevacizumab may increase the risk of biliary toxicity.[64]

Pharmacogenomics of Irinotecan and Fluorouracil

Case 99-3, Question 2: Fourteen days after receiving FOLFIRI plus bevacizumab, K.T. presented to the emergency room complaining of fever (101.2°F). On further evaluation, K.T. was identified as having febrile neutropenia with a WBC count of 1.2 × 10^3 cells/μL and an absolute neutrophil count of 650 cells/μL. He was admitted to the hospital for treatment. Is there an accurate method for predicting this outcome in K.T.? Can K.T. continue to receive this therapy?

Recent discoveries in the field of pharmacogenomics have identified several important genetic variations (polymorphisms) that partly account for inter-patient variability regarding the tolerability and efficacy of some drug therapies. Dihydropyrimidine dehydrogenase (DPD) is the rate-limiting enzyme responsible for the breakdown of fluorouracil to dihydrouracil and eventually to fluorinated ß-alanine. The cytotoxic effects of both fluorouracil and capecitabine can only occur after conversion to active metabolites, and the amount of fluorouracil available for this conversion is determined by the extent of its breakdown.[65] DPD is subject to genetic polymorphism, which can lead to a deficiency in its activity.[66] Approximately 3% to 5% of the population will have a partial DPD deficiency, with 0.2% of the population estimated to have complete loss.[60,67] While several tests are currently available that attempt to identify this deficiency, no single test has the specificity and positive/negative predictive values to accurately predict a true lack of enzyme activity.[68] Further, most studies to date that evaluated testing for DPD deficiency prior to administration of fluorouracil-based therapy only addressed reduced toxicity but not whether dose reduction was actually necessary.[62,69,70]

Uridine diphosphate glucuronosyltransferase (UGT) enzymes are responsible for the glucuronidation of bilirubin and other endogenous substrates as well as drugs and other toxins.[71] The enzyme UGT1A1 is responsible for the glucuronidation of SN-38, the active metabolite of irinotecan. Reductions in glucuronidation and accumulation of SN-38 are associated with greater toxicity. Of the known genetic polymorphisms of UGT1A1, one polymorphism in particular (UGT1A1*28) has been associated with decreased glucuronidation and therefore prolonged exposure to SN-38.[72,73] Studies have shown that those homozygous for the UGT1A1*28 allele are at an increased risk of neutropenia.[72] Although not consistently observed among trials, severe diarrhea has also been observed with genetic polymorphisms of UGT1A1.[72] However, while the ability to test for this polymorphism is available, the low sensitivity (i.e., the ability of this test to correctly identify all patients at risk of severe neutropenia) and the lack of consensus guidelines that outline how to use the results limit its widespread use in clinical practice.[72] However, practitioners should still exercise caution when treating patients with either a known or suspected deficiency in dihydropyrimidine dehydrogenase or a known polymorphism in UGT1A1.

K.T. should receive empiric antibiotic therapy and his chemotherapy should be held until both his fever and neutropenia resolve. Because he did not experience febrile neutropenia with his previous adjuvant therapy, it is unlikely he would harbor a DPD deficiency. A dose reduction of fluorouracil could be considered. More importantly, a reduction of his irinotecan dose is warranted before resuming his chemotherapy to reduce the risk of fever and neutropenia with consecutive cycles. The FDA-approved Invader UGT1A1 molecular assay is commercially available to detect the UGT1A1*28 polymorphism. If it is known that a patient has this polymorphism, an empiric reduction in the dose of irinotecan is recommended; however, its use is not generally recommended for determining reductions of subsequent doses of irinotecan after a toxic event.

Adverse Effects of Fluorouracil, Irinotecan, and the Vascular Endothelial Growth Factor Inhibitors

CASE 99-3, QUESTION 3: K.T. was discharged from the hospital after 4 days without identification of any infection. K.T. presents to clinic to receive a second cycle of FOLFIRI plus bevacizumab. He is now more cognizant of chemotherapy's adverse effects. He states that after his first cycle of chemotherapy, he also experienced abdominal cramping followed by profuse watery bowel movements for 3 days. He reported periods of nose bleeds lasting up to 2 weeks as well, which he never had in the past. The following laboratory values were also noted:

WBC count, 4.5 × 10^3 cells/μL
Hemoglobin, 12.5 g/dL
Platelet count, 210,000 cells/μL
Serum creatinine, 1.3 mg/dL

What can be done to alleviate or avoid these symptoms? K.T. would like to know more information about the side effects of chemotherapy agents he is receiving.

The incidence of irinotecan-induced diarrhea varies depending on the dosing schedule used and its combination with other chemotherapeutic agents. Trials in metastatic colorectal cancer have reported rates of grade 3 or 4 diarrhea of 20% to 30% depending on which irinotecan-based regimen is used.[28,74] The active metabolite of irinotecan, SN-38, is capable of producing acute abdominal cramping and diarrhea, which is a cholinergic-mediated process. Administration of subcutaneous or IV atropine at doses typically lower than those used in the cardiac setting is recommended for the treatment of acute diarrhea caused by irinotecan. The occurrence of diarrhea can also be delayed; thus, the use of an oral antidiarrheal is recommended if this occurs. A regimen of oral loperamide 4 mg with the first loose bowel movement, followed by 2 mg every 2 hours during the day or 4 mg every 4 hours in the evening, is recommended until the patient is diarrhea-free for a period of 12 hours.[75] If severe diarrhea symptoms persist for more than 48 hours in spite of these measures, patients should be instructed to seek emergency medical attention. Insufficient hydration resulting from diarrhea may lead to electrolyte losses and life-threatening consequences.

The key adverse effects of fluorouracil, oxaliplatin, and irinotecan are discussed under Case 99-2, Questions 3 and 4, and Case 99-3, Question 2. Although the VEGF inhibitors (bevacizumab, ziv-aflibercept, and ramucirumab) may share some overlapping toxicities with traditional chemotherapy, the majority of their effects are unique. Although cytotoxic agents are associated with myelosuppression, antiangiogenesis agents (i.e., VEGF inhibitors) do not target proliferating cells. Hence, they do not cause this type of toxicity. All VEGF inhibitors carry the risk of grade 3 or 4 bleeding events and gastrointestinal perforation which, while severe and require immediate medical attention, are also relatively rare (<3% and <2% with bevacizumab, respectively).[76] Other adverse events deemed as VEGF inhibitor-related are arterial thrombosis, hypertension, proteinuria, and wound-healing complications.[77] Monitoring of blood pressure and the pharmacologic management of diagnosed hypertension while on VEGF-inhibitor therapy is essential. In addition, because of the wound-healing complications, the use of VEGF-inhibitors should be stopped at least 6 to 8 weeks prior to planned surgery and should not be resumed until the patient has fully healed (at least 4–6 weeks).[78,79] Finally, a rare but serious side effect of posterior reversible encephalopathy syndrome (PRES) has been reported with agents that target VEGF including bevacizumab, requiring immediate medical attention and discontinuation of therapy.[80,81]

The epistaxis K.T. is experiencing with this cycle of chemotherapy may be attributed directly or indirectly to his current regimen. Although fluorouracil and irinotecan may also cause bleeding, this is usually related to their myelosuppressive effects on platelet progenitors. Because K.T. has a platelet count of 210,000 cells/μL on his recent laboratory work, this bleeding is more likely associated with bevacizumab use.

CASE 99-3, QUESTION 4: About 10 months into his treatment, K.T. had a CT scan that suggested progression of the liver and lung masses. Cytogenetic analysis of tissue from his old tumor biopsy was requested. The cytogenetic results suggested wild-type *RAS* and no mutation of *BRAF*. What should be the best second-line treatment option for K.T.'s metastatic disease?

K.T. has not received anti-EGFR monoclonal antibody–based chemotherapy. A tumor tissue analysis now reveals that it contains wild-type *RAS* and negative *BRAF* cytogenetics. Therefore, K.T. may receive benefit from anti-EGFR monoclonal antibodies. In addition, irinotecan in combination with EGFR antibodies have synergistic activity; therefore, a regimen of irinotecan and anti-EGFR (cetuximab or panitumumab) combination would be a good choice. In many cases the fluoropyrimidine is continued as well.

Adverse Effects of Epidermal Growth Factor Receptor Inhibitors

DERMATOLOGIC REACTIONS

CASE 99-3, QUESTION 5: K.T. will receive the following combination chemotherapy regimen: FOLFIRI (dosed as before with the dose reductions for irinotecan as previously noted because of his episode of febrile neutropenia) and cetuximab at 500 mg/m^2. Each cycle is to be repeated every 2 weeks. What is the most common adverse effect KT is likely to experience with his new anti-EGFR therapy? How can this toxicity be minimized?

In addition to diarrhea, dermatologic toxicity related to EGFR therapy occurs in more than 90% of metastatic colorectal cancer patients treated with these agents. Epidermal growth factor receptor skin reactions typically occur within 7 to 10 days of therapy, and most often present as a maculopapular rash on the face or upper torso of patients.[82] The rash may cause discomfort and reduce quality of life. Both cetuximab and panitumumab have recommendations for dose reductions or the withholding of therapy based on rash severity. Collaborative efforts have been made across clinical disciplines to develop treatment strategies for EGFR-induced dermatologic toxicities based on their severity. Strategies for preventing or limiting the severity of EGFR dermatologic toxicities have also been explored, including the use of a daily regimen of skin moisturizer, sunscreen, topical 1% hydrocortisone cream, and doxycycline.[83] In addition to their antimicrobial properties, the tetracycline class of antibiotics possesses anti-inflammatory properties and anti-proliferative effects on lymphocytes, which makes it a reasonable class of agents to consider given the proposed mechanisms involved in EGFR rash development. Two studies have revealed that the use of either minocycline or doxycycline as preemptive treatment (i.e., given prior to the first dose of either cetuximab or panitumumab and continued throughout therapy) can significantly reduce the severity of the rash but not the overall incidence of occurrence.[84,85]

K.T. would most likely develop an EGFR-inhibitor rash. A strategy focused on skin moisturization and protection combined with a daily application of hydrocortisone cream and the administration of doxycycline 100 mg twice daily or another tetracycline derivative could also be considered.

INFUSION-RELATED REACTIONS

CASE 99-3, QUESTION 6: K.T. comes in for his first dose of cetuximab with FOLFIRI. Within minutes of receiving the initial cetuximab infusion, K.T. becomes hypotensive and begins having difficulty breathing. What measures should be taken as quickly as possible?

The incidence of grade 3 or 4 infusion-related reactions reported in clinical trials is less than 3.5% with cetuximab and even less for panitumumab.[50,51,86,87] Because cetuximab is a chimeric monoclonal antibody, the higher incidence of reactions is not surprising. Therefore, cetuximab administration requires premedication with diphenhydramine, whereas panitumumab does not. Although the incidence estimate for hypersensitivity is less than 5%, these reactions may be underestimated, especially in the middle southern region of the United States where a higher incidence has been observed.[88] It is not currently known why there is a greater propensity for severe hypersensitivity reactions in patients in this region of the country.

Because of the severe nature of the reaction experienced by K.T., rechallenging with cetuximab at this point would be contraindicated.

Salvage Therapy in Metastatic Colorectal Cancer

Regorafenib, a multi-kinase inhibitor targeting VEGF, as well as multiple other protein kinases (KIT, RET, BRAF, PDGFR, and FGFR) was approved in the United States for use in metastatic colon cancer. It is currently utilized as salvage therapy (i.e., in patients who have been previously treated with fluoropyrimidine-, oxaliplatin-, and irinotecan-based chemotherapy, with an anti-VEGF therapy, and, if *RAS* wild-type, with an anti-EGFR therapy). Regorafenib has been shown versus placebo to provide a modest survival advantage of 1.4 months in this patient population. However, toxicity and its management are very important with the most common grade 3 or higher adverse events being HFS, fatigue, diarrhea, hypertension, and rash.[89] Regorafenib has a half-life of 26 to 28 hours with two active metabolites (M2 and M5) with M5 having a half-life of 48 hours which, owing to its anti-VEGF properties, is important to consider as the same precautions apply for bleeding risk and wound healing issues as for the traditional VEGF inhibitors.

Trifluridine, a thymidine-based nucleic acid analog, combined with tipiracil hydrochloride, a thymidine phosphorylase inhibitor, is another oral agent approved in the salvage setting for metastatic colon cancer. Trifluridine is the active cytotoxic agent, and tipiracil prevents the rapid degradation of trifluridine once administered, and the combination is abbreviated as TAS-102.[90,91] It is administered at a dose of 35 mg/m^2 orally once daily on days 1 to 5 and days 8 to 12 of each 28-day cycle. Compared with placebo in the salvage setting, it has also been shown to convey a modest survival benefit of 1.8 months; however, unlike targeted therapy, TAS-102 is cytotoxic, and as such has more of the traditional chemotherapy side effects.[92] The main grade 3 or higher toxicities associated with TAS-102 were hematologic (i.e., neutropenia, anemia, and thrombocytopenia).[93]

CHEMOTHERAPY AND RADIATION FOR EARLY-STAGE RECTAL CANCER

Approximately one-third of newly diagnosed colorectal cancers originate from the rectum.[3] The differentiation between cancers of the colon and rectum lies in their location and their propensity for recurrence at or near the site of origin after treatment. If the location of B.R.'s tumor had been within 12 to 15 cm from the anal verge, he would have been diagnosed with rectal cancer (Case 99-2). The main difference between rectal cancer and colon cancer treatment lies primarily in patients with stage II or stage III disease. Unless contraindicated, radiation therapy is incorporated into the treatment plan of patients with stage II or stage III disease of the rectum. In addition, slightly different surgical techniques are used and a short course of fluorouracil or capecitabine chemotherapy is administered in combination with the radiation until it is complete. When combined with chemotherapy, radiation can significantly reduce local recurrence rates.[93–95] An area of debate is the timing of chemoradiotherapy and whether it should be started before (neoadjuvant) or after surgery (adjuvant). Both strategies appear to be equally effective, so other issues are considered when choosing one modality over the other. Adjuvant chemoradiotherapy may avoid overtreatment of disease, whereas a neoadjuvant approach of chemoradiotherapy before surgery has the advantage of potentially shrinking the tumor and giving the surgeon a greater chance of obtaining negative margins, perhaps allowing for a less radical procedure and preservation of the anal sphincter. Another difference between tumors of the rectum and colon is the vascular drainage by the venous system. The colon is drained by the mesenteric veins of the hepatic portal system, whereas more distal portions of the rectum are drained by veins that empty into the inferior vena cava. This plays a role in the initial site of metastatic development for each disease. Although the liver is the most common overall site of colorectal cancer metastasis, when compared with the colon, cancers of the distal rectum are more likely to metastasize to the lungs because of the differences in their respective vasculature.

ACKNOWLEDGMENT

The author acknowledges Sachin R. Shah and Julian Hoyt Slade, III for their contributions to the version of this chapter found in previous editions.

KEY REFERENCES AND WEBSITES

A full list of references for this chapter can be found at http://thepoint.lww.com/AT11e. Below are the key references and websites for this chapter, with the corresponding reference number in this chapter found in parentheses after the reference.

Key References

André T et al. Improved overall survival with oxaliplatin, fluorouracil, and leucovorin as adjuvant treatment in stage II or III colon cancer in the MOSAIC trial. *J Clin Oncol*. 2009;27(19):3109–3116. (17)

Bennouna J et al. Continuation of bevacizumab after first progression in metastatic colorectal cancer (ML18147): a randomised phase 3 trial. *Lancet Oncol*. 2013;14:29–37. (46)

Benson AB 3rd et al. Recommended guidelines for the treatment of cancer treatment-induced diarrhea. *J Clin Oncol*. 2004;22:2918–2926. (72)

Gammon D et al. Hypersensitivity reactions to oxaliplatin and the application of a desensitization protocol. *Oncologist*. 2004;9:546–549. (27)

Grothey A. Oxaliplatin-safety profile: neurotoxicity. *Semin Oncol*. 2003;30(4, Suppl 15):5–13. (24)

Grothey A et al. Regorafenib monotherapy for previously treated metastatic colorectal cancer (CORRECT): an international, multicentre, randomised, placebo-controlled, phase 3 trial. *Lancet*. 2013;381(9863):303–312. (89)

Levin B et al. Screening and surveillance for the early detection of colorectal cancer and adenomatous polyps, 2008: a joint guideline from the American Cancer Society, the US Multi-Society Task Force on Colorectal Cancer, and the American College of Radiology. *CA Cancer J Clin*. 2008;58:130–160. (11)

Mayer RJ et al. Randomized trial of TAS-102 for refractory metastatic colorectal cancer. *N Engl J Med*. 2015;372:1909–1919. (92)

Meyerhardt JA et al. Follow-up care, surveillance protocol, and secondary prevention measures for survivors of colorectal cancer: American Society of Clinical Oncology clinical practice guideline endorsement. *J Clin Oncol*.2013;31:1–8. (40)

Price TJ et al. Panitumumab versus cetuximab in patients with chemotherapy-refractory wild-type KRAS exon 2 metastatic colorectal cancer (ASPECCT): a randomised, multicentre, open-label, non-inferiority phase 3 study. *Lancet Oncol*. 2014; 15: 569–579. (55)

Tabernero J et al. Ramucirumab versus placebo in combination with second line FOLFIRI in patients with metastatic colorectal carcinoma that progressed during or after first-line therapy with bevacizumab, oxaliplatin, and a fluoropyrimidine (RAISE): a randomised, double-blind, multicentre, phase 3 study. *Lancet Oncol*. 2015;16:499–508. (47)

Tabernero J et al. Aflibercept versus placebo in combination with fluorouracil, leucovorin and irinotecan in the treatment of previously treated metastatic colorectal cancer: prespecified subgroup analyses from the VELOUR trial. *Eur J Cancer*. 2014;50:320–331. (48)

Tournigand C et al. Adjuvant therapy with fluorouracil and oxaliplatin in stage II and elderly patients (between ages 70 and 75 years) with colon cancer: subgroup analyses of the Multicenter International Study of Oxaliplatin, Fluorouracil, and Leucovorin in the Adjuvant Treatment of Colon Cancer trial. *J Clin Oncol*. 2012:30:3353–3360. (15)

Tournigand C et al. FOLFIRI Followed by FOLFOX6 or the Reverse Sequence in Advanced Colorectal Cancer: A Randomized GERCOR Study. *J Clin Oncol*. 2004;22:229–237. (45)

Key Websites

American Cancer Society. Cancer Facts & Figures 2015. Available at the website: http://www.cancer.org/research/cancerfactsstatistics/cancerfactsfigures2015/

American Society of Clinical Oncology Practice Guidelines on Gastrointestinal Cancers available at: http://www.instituteforquality.org/practice-guidelines

http://cancerstaging.org/references-tools/quickreferences/documents/colonmedium.pdf

NCCN Clinical Practice Guidelines in Oncology (NCCN Guidelines®) By Site available at: http://www.nccn.org/professionals/physician_gls/f_guidelines.asp#site

100 Prostate Cancer

Marina D. Kaymakcalan and Christy S. Harris

CORE PRINCIPLES

		CHAPTER CASES
1	Risk factors for the development of prostate cancer include age, family history, ethnicity, and diet.	Case 100-1 (Questions 1, 2), Figure 100-1, Figure 100-2
2	Screening through the use of prostate specific antigen (PSA) testing and digital rectal exams allows for early identification of prostate cancer. There is now concern that prostate cancer is being overdiagnosed.	Case 100-1 (Question 3), Case 100-2 (Question 1), Table 100-1
3	The PSA, Gleason score, and tumor stage can determine how aggressive the prostate cancer is and are considered prognostic factors for the risk of recurrence.	Case 100-2 (Questions 2,3), Table 100-2, Figure 100-3
4	Most prostate cancers are slow growing and some men may not ever develop symptoms of disease. Therefore, observation and active surveillance are options for certain men with early stage disease and shorter life expectancies.	Case 100-2 (Question 4), Table 100-3
5	Treatment of localized disease includes surgery, radiation, and/or androgen deprivation therapy. Androgen deprivation therapy is first line treatment for advanced prostate cancers. It lowers testosterone in the body to a castration level of ≤ 50 ng/ml. This can be accomplished through surgical (orchiectomy) or chemical (gonadotropin-releasing hormone analogs) means.	Case100-2 (Question 5), Case 100-3 (Questions 1,2), Table 100-4, Figure 100-4
6	Castration-resistant prostate cancer occurs when the cancer has acquired a mechanism of resistance in the presence of hormonal therapy and is no longer responding to hormonal therapy manipulation alone.	Case 100-3 (Questions 3)
7	Cytotoxic chemotherapy or immunotherapy may be used in metastatic disease. Metastases often occur in the bone, requiring therapy to decrease skeletal-related events.	Case 100-4 (Questions 1,2), Table 100-5
8	Adverse effects of prostate cancer include urinary and sexual issues but are often not a problem until the disease is advanced. Complications of therapy include cardiovascular and metabolic issues.	Case 100-5 (Question 1), Case 100-6 (Question 1), Table 100-6
9	Prevention of prostate cancer with finasteride or dutasteride has been studied and may be an option for select men with high risk.	Case 100-7 (Question 1)

INCIDENCE, PREVALENCE, AND EPIDEMIOLOGY

Prostate adenocarcinoma is the most common malignancy in American men and is the second leading cause of cancer death in men in the United States. It is a disease occurring mainly in older men with the average age of diagnosis being 66 years.[1] The incidence of prostate cancer is estimated to be 220,800 cases with 27,540 deaths in 2015,[2] which correlates to 1 chance in 7 of eventually being diagnosed with prostate cancer and about 1 chance in 38 of eventually dying of it.[1] Progress in treatment and increased public awareness has improved the 5-year overall survival to 98.9% with rates of new diagnoses falling an average of 4.3% each year over the last 10 years.[1] Because of the widespread use of screening, prostate cancer is being found in earlier stages, which allows for the possibility of earlier treatment that is less invasive with fewer adverse effects. However, the screening guidelines are changing because of what is perceived as an overdiagnosis of the cancer with a risk of overtreatment.

PATHOPHYSIOLOGY

The prostate is a walnut-shaped gland that sits directly below the bladder and is anterior to the rectum with the urethra running through the center. This location gives rise to many of the urinary, rectal, and sexual symptoms that men may experience in advanced cancer. The prostate consists of lobular glands that produce the fluid that protects and nourishes the sperm cells within the semen. This fluid is also rich in prostate-specific antigen (PSA), a glycoprotein that enhances sperm motility.[3] Cells within the prostate convert testosterone into the more potent dihydrotestosterone (DHT) by the enzyme 5-α-reductase, which stimulates growth of the cells within the prostate. Cancer can often be found confined within the capsule of the prostate if discovered early or may extend out of the capsule into the surrounding seminal vesicles and bladder neck. Eventually, systemic spread can occur via the lymphatics to involve the bone, lung, or liver.[4]

CLINICAL PRESENTATION AND DIAGNOSIS

Because of the ability to screen for prostate cancer for early identification, symptoms are rarely present at the time of diagnosis. Symptoms usually manifest after the cancer has spread beyond the prostate. At that point, the most common sign in men older than 50 years of age is bladder outlet obstruction, including hesitancy, nocturia, incomplete emptying, and diminished urinary stream. In metastatic disease, bone pain, anemia, or pancytopenia may be present.[4]

The use of routine PSA testing in men at risk for prostate cancer allows for early detection and diagnosis of prostate cancer, although rises in the serum PSA do not automatically indicate cancer. Although PSA is highly specific to the prostate, it is not specific to cancer with an overall sensitivity of ~50% to 70%.[5] Normal PSA levels in the blood are generally considered to be <4 ng/mL but begin to rise in men as they age, often in the setting of benign prostatic hypertrophy (BPH). Median PSA levels are 0.7 ng/mL in ages 40 to 49 and 0.9 ng/mL in ages 50 to 59.[6] Factors that can falsely elevate PSA levels are inflammation of the prostate, urinary retention, prostatic infection, ejaculation, or trauma.

Certain medications and supplements can affect PSA levels, which warrant careful review of a patient's medication history. The 5-α-reductase inhibitors can cause a decrease in the serum PSA by up to 50% within 6 to 12 months after initiation. Some herbal supplements, such as saw palmetto, may also falsely lower the PSA.[5] Men with PSA levels of 4 to 10 ng/mL have a 30% to 35% chance of having prostate cancer. If the level increases above 10 ng/mL, there is over a 67% risk of a prostate cancer diagnosis.[6] However, the use of PSA alone may not be adequate for screening and diagnosis as PSA elevations are not observed in up to 15% of men with prostate cancer.[1] A digital rectal exam (DRE) may be performed in conjunction with the PSA level. The placement of the prostate directly in front of the rectum allows the practitioner to feel the outside of the prostate, which should be smooth with any nodules, indurations, or asymmetry felt being suspicious for cancer.

To definitively diagnose prostate cancer, trans-rectal ultrasound (TRUS)-guided needle biopsies are used. It is important to obtain 10 or more core biopsies in a single setting as differences in pathology can be seen within different cores. Treatment will be decided by the extent and aggressiveness of the disease along with the overall health and life expectancy of the patient. Staging of prostate cancer determines the extent of the disease using the TNM (T, tumor size, N, node status, and M, sites of metastases) classification from the American Joint Committee on Cancer, although clinically it is usually referred to as local, locally advanced, and metastatic. Aggressiveness is determined by the grade and rate of growth of the cancer cells.[4,6]

OVERVIEW OF TREATMENT

Treatment modalities of prostate cancer can include surgical removal of the prostate, radiation therapy, hormonal therapy, and chemotherapy. Because prostate cancer is fueled primarily by DHT, hormonal therapy will comprise the mainstay of treatment. Only in the metastatic setting, after the failure of hormonal therapy will cytotoxic chemotherapy be utilized. As well, the option to simply observe the patient is an alternative in certain situations. Prostate cancer can be a very slow-growing disease and, if the right men are chosen, may be monitored with no treatment.

For patients diagnosed with cancer confined to the prostate, removal of the prostate, prostatectomy, or radiation to the prostate are the primary treatment options for definitive local therapy. Radiation therapies most commonly used in practice include external beam and brachytherapy. Brachytherapy consists of small pellets of radioactive material that can be placed into the prostate in small volume disease. These treatments can provide an opportunity for cure in patients with locally confined prostate cancer. Eighty percent of patients will be diagnosed in this stage and have a 5-year survival of 100%. With more advanced cancer, in which there is an increased risk of recurrence, the addition of gonadotropin-releasing hormone (GnRH) therapy to radiation may be necessary. Locally advanced cancer is diagnosed in 12% of patients and also has a 100% 5-year survival rate. Only after failure of hormonal therapy will chemotherapy be used. A number of cytotoxic agents as well as immunologic therapy are available for the treatment of castration-resistant metastatic disease. Although only 4% of patients are initially diagnosed with metastatic disease, their 5-year survival is only 28%.[7] Therapy in the different stages of prostate cancer will be discussed in more detail in the following.

RISK FACTORS

CASE 100-1

QUESTION 1: S.J. is a 50-year-old African-American male who has never been screened for prostate cancer. He has no comorbidities, does not smoke, exercises regularly, and has a diet consisting mainly of red meat 4 to 5 times a week with few vegetables and fruit. What are S.J.'s risk factors for prostate cancer?

Age

Risk factors are important in identifying those men who are most likely to develop prostate cancer and also helps identify those who will most benefit from screening. Age is the most important factor with over half of all cases occurring after the age of 65 and rarely occurs before 40 years of age. Median age at time of death is 80.[1]

Ethnicity

The risk for development of prostate cancer begins to increase after the age of 50 in white men and after age 40 in black men. In the United States, the highest risk is in African Americans with lower survival rates (Fig. 100-1). Prostate cancer also has one of the largest disparities in death rates between black and white men, which is about 2.5× higher in black men.[2] This ratio was seen

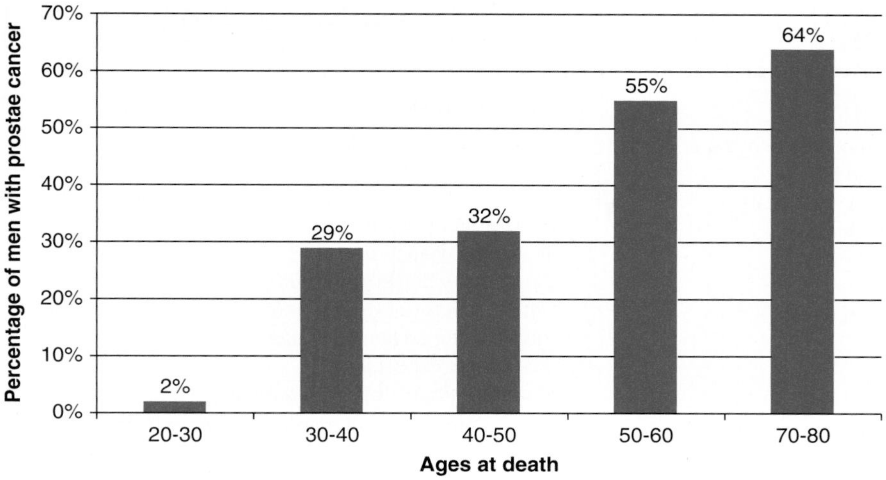

Figure 100-1 Percentage of men found to have prostate cancers at autopsy after dying of unrelated causes in the era prior to standardized PSA testing.[16]

in previous decades before the era of PSA testing as well. Black men tend to be diagnosed at a younger age with more advanced tumors having a 1.5-fold higher incidence of metastatic disease at presentation.[6] It is suggested that sub-Saharan ancestry may be more relevant than geographic location in a study of African and Caribbean men. Japanese men have the lowest risk and are also known to have a lower level of 5-α-reductase activity. However, it is unknown whether these differences in incidence among ethnicities are really because of genetic or environmental causes.[4]

Family History

Family history confers up to a 2.5-fold increased risk if a man's brother or father has been diagnosed by age 60.[6] If two or more first-degree relatives develop prostate cancer, then the risk is increased sevenfold to eightfold compared to the general population. Younger age at diagnosis in a family member is a higher risk than a family member who is diagnosed later in life.[1,4]

Diet and Lifestyle

Diet and lifestyle are also associated with a risk of prostate cancer. Those men having a diet with any of the following have a higher risk of developing prostate cancer: diet high in saturated fats and red meat and low intake of fruits, vegetables, tomato products, fish, or soy.[1,4] Vitamin D, calcium, lycopene, zinc, omega-3 fatty acids, a-linoleic fatty acids, selenium, vitamin E, statins, and nonsteroidal anti-inflammatory medications have been correlated with decreased risk in observational studies, but it is not sure in what way they affect the disease.[4] Several of these agents have been investigated as dietary supplements in prospective trials, but the studies did not show a benefit.

Genetic Syndromes

Germline BRCA2 mutations are associated with a twofold to sixfold increase in the risk of prostate cancer. It is not known exactly how much the BRCA1 mutation affects prostate cancer, although the two are often considered together. Cancers in men with these mutations are more aggressive, occur earlier, and are associated with a significantly reduced survival time.

Men with Lynch syndrome (germline mutations in MLH1, MSH2, MSH6, PMS2, or EPCAM) have a twofold to fivefold increase in the risk of prostate cancer. However, these cancers act similarly to those cancers without the mutation, so they are not more aggressive or occur at any earlier age.[1]

S.J. has the following risk factors for the development of prostate cancer: race and diet. Modifiable risk factors include maintaining his exercise regimen and making some changes to his diet, with less red meat and incorporating fish into his regular diet, as well as more fruits and vegetables.

CASE 100-1, QUESTION 2: S.J. has learned that his 47-year-old brother was just diagnosed with advanced prostate cancer. How has S.J.'s risk changed?

Because S.J. now has a first-degree relative who has been diagnosed with prostate cancer, especially before the age of 60, his risk has increased substantially (2.5-fold).

SCREENING

CASE 100-1, QUESTION 3: After S.J.'s brother's diagnosis, he becomes concerned and makes an appointment with his primary care office to discuss screening. Should S.J. begin routine screening for prostate cancer?

In the past 25 years, 5-year survival rates increased from 68.3% to 99.9%, attributed in part to early detection, with a 10-year survival rate of 97.8% and a 15-year rate of 91.4%.[8] There are several guidelines for the screening of prostate cancer, including those of the American Cancer Society,[9] National Comprehensive Cancer Network (NCCN),[5] and the American Urological Association[10] (Table 100-1). Historically, men over the age of 50 were encouraged to have a PSA screening yearly. There was a steep rise in the diagnosis of prostate cancer once PSA screening was put into effect in the early 1990s; from <100 cases per age-adjusted 100,000 in 1975 and peaking at 240 cases per 100,000 in 1992, at the time of writing it is fairly constant rate of 158 cases per 100,000.[4] However, there is now some controversy among different entities regarding the appropriate recommendations for PSA screening. Prostate cancer is a relatively slow-growing cancer that may not be life threatening to some patients and potentially would not need treatment. Because it occurs primarily in older men, a number of males might not ever have symptoms of the disease that would cause them to be tested if not for routine screening.

The Prostate, Lung, Colorectal, and Ovarian (PLCO) Screening Trial randomized over 76,000 US men to strict annual PSA and DRE screening or to standard practice. It was found that prostate cancer was identified more often in the annual screening group, but that it did not change the rate of fatal disease.[11] However, a European study that randomized over 182,000 men to yearly screening or to no screening found that in the screening group, the relative reduction in risk of death was 21% at a median follow up of 11 years. To

Table 100-1
Prostate Cancer Screening Guidelines for Average and Elevated Risk Patients

	Average Risk	Elevated Risk
ACS,[9] 2010	≥10 year life expectancy: Informed and shared decision-making beginning at age 50 If PSA <2.5 ng/mL, repeat every 2 years If PSA ≥2.5 ng/mL, repeat annually If PSA ≥4 ng/mL, consider biopsy <10 year life expectancy: If asymptomatic, offer no screening	Higher risk (African American, family history of diagnosis <65 years of age), ≥10 year life expectancy: Informed and shared decision-making beginning at age 45 <10 yr life expectancy: If asymptomatic, offer no screening Appreciably higher risk (multiple family members diagnosed before age 65), Informed and shared decision-making beginning at age 40 <10 yr life expectancy: If asymptomatic, offer no screening
NCCN 1.2017[5]	Begin testing at age 45 in men expected to live >10 years From age 45-75: If PSA ≥ 1.0 ng/mL, repeat every 1-2 year intervals If PSA <1.0, ng/mL, repeat every 2-4 year intervals If PSA >3 ng/mL or very suspicious DRE, consider biopsy Individualize after age 75 in select patients who are very healthy with no comorbidities: If PSA <4 ng/mL, repeat every 1-4 years If PSA ≥4 ng/mL or very suspicious DRE, consider biopsy	African American and men with a family history Screening is not different than average risk but discussion with providers should occur several years earlier; consider screening every year instead of every other year BRCA2 (and BRCA1); begin discussion of screening at age 40
AUA,[10] 2013	Age 55–69—shared decision-making; every 2+ years No screening ≥70 if life expectancy less than 10–15 years	High risk (African American or family history)—≤55 individualized decision
USPSTF,[14] 2012	Do not recommend routine screening with PSA	

prevent one death from prostate cancer, 1,055 men would need to be screened and 37 cancers would need to be detected.[12] Therefore, it is being recognized that prostate cancer may be overdiagnosed (over-detection), especially at older ages. Overdiagnosis is typically defined as detecting a disease when it would not otherwise have shortened lifespan or resulted in adverse effects.[13] The United States Preventive Services Task Force analyzed data from several trials and concluded that for every 1,000 men between the ages of 55 and 69 who were screened, 0 to 1 death from prostate cancer would be avoided, and that 110 men would be diagnosed with prostate cancer. However, 100 to 120 men would have a false positive that would result in an unnecessary biopsy.[14] There are risks associated with any potential diagnosis, including risks during biopsy such as infection, bleeding, and dysuria, along with risks associated with unnecessary treatment, which need to be taken into account in the risk-to-benefit ratio of screening. These studies highlight the need for selective screening to avoid overdiagnosis and overtreatment while not compromising long-term survival.

Guidelines are consistent in their recommendation that men over the age or 70 to 75 do not need to be screened as they have not been diagnosed with cancer at this time and are more likely to die of unrelated causes before ever having any symptoms in this slow-growing cancer. Guidelines emphasize considering the life expectancy of the patient and not screening those whose expectancy is less than 10 to 15 years. For those at an elevated risk of developing prostate cancer (e.g., family, ethnicity, or other risk factors), screening may begin earlier. However, many of the guidelines are advocating that men should have a discussion with their doctor regarding any risk factors that they have and together decide whether they should undergo screening and at what age to start, depending on their risk factors, comorbidities, and personal preferences.[5,9,10] For S.J., because of his elevated risk due to his brother's diagnosis and his ethnicity, as well as his modifiable risk factors, it may be considered prudent to begin screening. However, this should be discussed with his doctor to ensure that he recognizes all of the benefits and risks of screening.

PROGNOSTIC FACTORS

CASE 100-2

QUESTION 1: C.W. is a 67-year-old man who began routine screening for prostate cancer with his primary care physician 15 years ago. His PSA history is listed below. His PSA drawn on August 5, 2012 is 6.68 ng/mL. DRE is negative. He has an excellent performance status being fully active and able to carry out all pre-disease activities without restriction. On physical exam he is well appearing with no apparent signs of distress. He has no known family history of prostate cancer. When asked about his social history, he said that he drinks socially with an average of 1 to 2 drinks every month and has never smoked or used illicit drugs. His past medical history is significant for hypercholesterolemia, hypertension, and depression.

Medications: atorvastatin, lisinopril, and sertraline; no known allergies.

PSA History:

Date	PSA Level (ng/mL)
08/05/2012	6.68
09/22/2011	3.11
09/25/2010	2.52
08/29/2009	2.43
08/27/2008	2.27
09/03/2007	2.02
08/19/2006	1.98
08/15/2005	1.82
09/01/2004	1.52
08/28/2003	1.38
09/09/2002	1.25
08/20/2001	1.17

From the assessment above, what would have prompted C.W.'s primary care physician to refer the patient to an urologist?

Using prognostic factors to stratify the risk of the cancer recurring is essential to better characterize the cancer and to determine the optimal treatment. This is particularly important with a heterogeneous disease like prostate cancer. Patients with a high risk of recurrence will need more aggressive treatment, whereas those with low risk can benefit from a more conservative approach. Stage of the tumor, PSA, and Gleason score are prognostic factors that can be used by the provider to calculate the probability of a patient recurring in the next 5 to 10 years. Utilizing these factors and incorporating the patient's life expectancy will help the physician to determine the best therapies for their patient while maximizing quality of life.

LIFE EXPECTANCY

There are a number of men who will die with, not of, their prostate cancer. Autopsy data has shown that as many as 7 out of every 10 men who died of various causes had prostate cancer at time of death that was undiagnosed[15,16] (Fig. 100-2). Estimation of a patient's life expectancy can help determine the extent of benefit of potential life gained from treatment. Men with short life expectancies are at low risk of developing any symptoms of disease, or morbidity, before their demise from another unrelated event, and therefore will likely not benefit from definitive treatment. Conversely, younger men otherwise in good health are likely to need treatment as they have a longer lifetime in which to develop a recurrence of cancer that can be a cause of morbidity and mortality. Although insurance life expectancy charts (Minnesota Metropolitan or the Social Security Administration Life Insurance Tables) can be used to determine potential life expectancy, it often is a comprehensive clinical determination by the patient's healthcare team, weighing a number of factors, including their overall health, quality of life, comorbid conditions, and family history when determining a treatment plan.[4] The Social Security Administration Life Insurance Tables can be found at www.ssa.gov/OACT/STATS/table4c6.html.

Prostate Specific Antigen

As previously discussed, serum PSA level is used in screening for prostate cancer detection. It is also a prognostic factor used as an aid to determine treatment because a higher PSA level is associated with an increased risk of more advanced and potential progression of disease. The more prostate cancer cells there are, the more PSA is being made. Being able to determine how fast the level is rising is another way to assess the cancer's ability to potentially recur and progress. However, it is also known that not all prostate cancers will produce elevated PSA levels. It is another tool that may help the practitioner to assess the risk of recurrence in a specific patient. As mentioned previously, men with PSA levels of 4 to 10 ng/mL have a 30% to 35% chance of having prostate cancer; that risk doubles if the level increases above 10 ng/mL.[6] A number of other screening modalities have been developed in order to better define a patient's risk for prostate cancer.

Observing the time over which the PSA level rises, or PSA velocity, is a way of potentially identifying those men with prostate cancer versus those with an elevated PSA because of other causes. Determining the PSA velocity may help further ascertain those men who should have a biopsy performed. Upon diagnosis, a rapid PSA velocity can also suggest more rapid progression and can serve as a guide for treatment decisions. However, it is important to know the normal PSA ranges by age and that fluctuations in levels can exist because of the laboratory controls.[4]

Because of the fact that C.W. had a PSA level of 3.21 in 2011 and 6.68 in 2012, there is concern that he may have developed prostate cancer. The Prostate Cancer Prevention Trial (PCPT) found that 15% of men with PSA $\leq$4.0 ng/mL and a normal DRE were diagnosed with prostate cancer. This percentage doubles with PSA levels between 4 to 10 ng/mL.[5] C.W.'s change in PSA from 2010 to 2011 and 2011 to 2012 indicated an increased PSA velocity, which can also suggest that further evaluation is necessary. The Baltimore Longitudinal Study of Aging (PLSA) trial of 980 men demonstrated an increased relative risk of prostate cancer death in men with a PSA velocity $>$0.35 ng/mL/year compared to those with a PSA velocity $\leq$0.35 ng/mL/year (p = .02).[5]

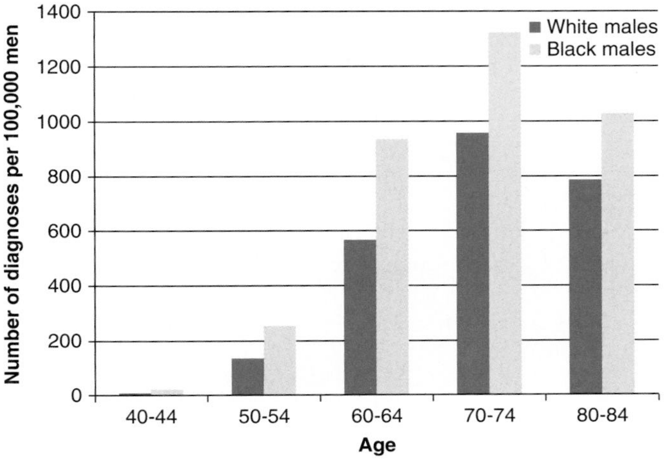

Figure 100-2 The Incidence of New Cases of Prostate Cancer by Race and Age.[4]

CASE 100-2, QUESTION 2: C.W. is referred to the urologist for further evaluation. What additional diagnostic procedures can be done to definitively diagnose prostate cancer? What assessments can be done from the procedure for better prognostication of the disease?

Tumor Staging

The American Joint Committee on Cancer (AJCC) developed a staging system for newly diagnosed prostate cancer. This AJCC TNM staging system classifies the extent of the tumor according to the size of the tumor (T), the extent of lymph node involvement (N), and the absence or presence of distant metastases (M). In general, if the cancer remains within the prostatic capsule, it is considered localized disease. If it has spread outside of the capsule or has invaded the adjacent structures, it is locally advanced and the cancer is considered metastatic if it has spread to other parts of the body.

Gleason Score

A Gleason score is the histologic grading of the tumor biopsy. It is calculated by adding the most common to the second most common growth patterns found in the core biopsies. This score is one of the most important factors when determining treatment and prognosis as it corresponds to how aggressive the tumor is behaving. An aggressive tumor is one that will grow faster and have a higher risk of metastasizing, increasing the likelihood of recurrence after localized treatment. There are five distinct patterns of growth from well (1) to poorly (5) differentiated with progressive loss of glandular formation (Fig. 100-3).[18] Well-differentiated cancer cells are those that are most similar to the normal prostate cells and tend to grow and spread at a slower rate than poorly differentiated tumor cells that are more aggressive. Up to 50% of prostate tumors demonstrate more than one histologic pattern.[19] By assessing several of the biopsy samples to find the most common growth patterns, the aggressive behavior of the tumor can

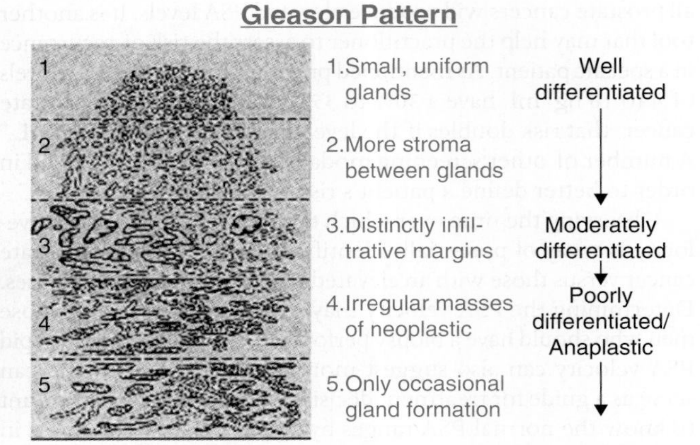

Figure 100-3 Gleason histologic grading of prostate cancer demonstrating progressive loss of glandular formation with increasing score. (Adapted with permission from Scher HI et al. Cancer of the Prostate. In: DeVita VT et al, eds. *Cancer: Principles and Practice of Oncology*. 10th ed. Philadelphia, PA: Lippincott Williams & Wilkins; 2015.)

be more accurately estimated. The added value of the first and second most common patterns can theoretically range from 2 to 10 with the majority of tumors ranging from 5 to 10. Cancer with a Gleason score of 6 or less, which is relatively well-differentiated and less aggressive, is considered low-grade. A Gleason score of 7 is considered intermediate grade cancer, and a Gleason score greater than 7 is considered poorly differentiated, high grade. For someone with a Gleason score of 2 to 4, there is a 4% to 7% chance of dying of their disease within 15 years. A man with a Gleason score of 8 to 10 has a 87% risk of dying within 15 years if untreated.[4]

Risk stratification tools that incorporate stage, PSA level, and Gleason score have been developed and validated as they identify those men who are associated with an increased risk of recurrence and worse outcomes after localized treatment. These systems group patients who are yet to receive treatment as very low, low, intermediate, high, or very high risk to be used as a basis for providers, along with life expectancy and overall health of the patient, in the selection of initial treatment (Table 100-2).[6,20]

A trans-rectal ultrasound guided needle biopsy can be done to definitively diagnose prostate cancer. The biopsy specimen can be used in conjunction with DRE results to determine the prognostic factors of clinical stage and the Gleason score.

CASE 100-2, QUESTION 3: C.W.'s biopsy revealed a Gleason 3 + 3 = 6, stage T1c (no suspected nodal or distant metastases) prostate cancer in 3 of 10 cores. Based on C.W.'s prognostic factors, what is C.W.'s risk group?

C.W. has stage T1cN0M0 prostate cancer with a Gleason score ≤6 and a PSA <10 ng/mL. With these prognostic factors and with 3 of 10 positive cores, he is considered to have low-risk prostate cancer.

TREATMENT

Observation versus Active Surveillance

CASE 100-2, QUESTION 4: C.W. consulted with a medical oncologist about his treatment options for low-risk prostate cancer. The oncologist explained that C.W. is an overall healthy patient with a long life expectancy and that his prostate cancer is relatively slow growing. What is C.W.'s conservative option for the management of his prostate cancer?

Studies have aimed to identify those select men who will have a good outcome with a very conservative approach of observation with no immediate, definitive intervention for their cancer. This is because we are now seeing what some call an overtreatment of prostate cancer. Over-screening, as discussed earlier, plays a role with some models estimating between 23% and 42% of all US screen-detected cancers are being overtreated.[6] This approach of not treating the cancer immediately has subtle distinctions according to differences in patient status.

Table 100-2
Prostate Cancer Risk Groups[6]

Risk	Stage	PSA (ng/mL)	Gleason	Other
Clinically Localized				
Very Low	T1c	<10	≤6	Fewer than three prostate biopsy cores positive, ≤ 50% cancer in each core; PSA density: <0.15 ng/mL/g
Low	T1–T2a	<10	≤6	
Intermediate	T2b–T2c	10–20	7	
High	T3a	>20	8–10	
Locally Advanced				
Very high	T3b–T4		5 > 4 cores with a score of 8–10	
Metastatic				
Metastatic	Any T, N1 or Any T, Any N, M1			

Patients are assigned a risk group according to their most severe prognostic factor. Patients with multiple adverse factors may be shifted into the next highest risk group.

Observation involves no cancer intervention, such as additional biopsies, scans, surgery or treatment but simply monitors the patient with the plan to only deliver palliative therapy if the patient becomes symptomatic. This is an option for men with low or intermediate risk prostate cancers with a life expectancy of less than 10 years due to concurrent comorbid conditions or diseases that will most likely outcompete their prostate cancer, providing no benefit from treatment.[6]

Active surveillance is different from observation as these men are actively monitored with routine PSA levels and, potentially, DREs with the expectation of intervention if it looks like the cancer is progressing with a goal of deferring side effects from treatment without missing the opportunity for cure. For this reason, it is preferred in patients with a life expectancy of less than 20 years and very low risk prostate cancer or in patients with a life expectancy greater than 10 years and low-risk prostate cancer.[6] A study of almost 1,000 men with favorable or intermediate risk prostate cancer on active surveillance were followed for a median 6.4 years (range, 0.2 to 19.8 years). They were offered treatment if their PSA doubled in less than 3 years, if their Gleason score was higher based on another biopsy or if they had clinical progression. Of those 993 study participants, 15% had died but only 15 patients (1.5%) died from prostate cancer. There were an additional 13 patients (1.3%) who developed metastases but only 4 had died at the time of analysis. At 5, 10, and 15 years, 75.7%, 63.5%, and 55% of patients, respectively, were untreated and continued surveillance.[21] In another study of over 5,500 men with low-risk and favorable intermediate-risk prostate cancer treated with brachytherapy and then active surveillance, 605 men had died, but only 5.6% of those deaths were because of prostate cancer.[22] These studies illustrate the potential to delay therapy in some men without compromising survival. The decision of observation or active surveillance should be made after a full discussion between the patient and the physician of the advantages and disadvantages of this approach (Table 100-3).

Because C.W. has low-risk prostate cancer and an excellent performance status without precluding comorbidities, giving him a long life expectancy (≥10 years), he would be eligible for active surveillance. He would not be a candidate for observation given his age and long life expectancy.

Table 100-3
Advantages and Disadvantages of Observation and Active Surveillance[6]

Advantages	Disadvantages
Avoidance of potential side effects	Chance of missed opportunity for cure
Quality of life	Risk of progression and/or metastases
Unnecessary treatment possibly avoided	Future therapy, if necessary, will be more complex with more side effects
	Nerve sparing surgery will be more difficult
	Increased anxiety
	Frequent medical exams and biopsies

Adapted with permission from Zelefsky MJ, Eastham JA, Sartor AO. Cancer of the Prostate. In: DeVita VT et al, eds. Cancer: *Principles and Practice of Oncology*. 10th ed. Philadelphia, PA: Lippincott Williams & Wilkins, 2014. Accessed November 15, 2015

Definitive Local Therapy

Treatments for early stage disease can include radiation, mainly in the form of either brachytherapy or external beam radiation therapy (EBRT) and radical prostatectomy. These localized treatments are used because the cancer is thought to still be confined to the prostate. Choice of therapy is dependent upon risk stratification, which takes into account extent of disease, pathologic stage and PSA, along with life expectancy, patient preference, and potential comorbidities that may cause complications and impact treatment outcomes. If treatment is successful and if the correct patients are selected, these local therapies can potentially provide a cure from the disease.

Surgery

Radical prostatectomy is the surgical removal of the prostate gland and possibly some surrounding tissue. It is generally recommended only for patients with clinically confined prostate cancer who have a life expectancy of 10 years or more and no comorbidities precluding their ability to undergo an operation.[6] A study using the SEER Medicare database looked at outcomes after surgery among hospitals and surgeons. In a study of 11,522 men between 1992 and 1996, it was found that postoperative complications correlated with the volume of procedures performed by the surgeon and the volume done at the institution. Postoperative morbidity was lower in very high-volume hospitals compared to low-volume hospitals (27% vs. 32%; $p = .03$) and was also lower when performed by high-volume surgeons as compared to low-volume surgeons (26% vs. 32%; $p < .001$). There was no link between surgeon/institution and death.[23] Another study found that surgeon experience was linked to a lower risk of recurrence ($p < .001$) when adjusted for tumor characteristics and year of surgery in patients who received no other therapy. Five-year probability of recurrence was 17.8% in early phase of career (10 prior operations) compared to 10.9% later on (>250 operations).[24] These findings confirm that experience is a critical factor in the success of radical prostatectomy. Surgery can be done as either an open or laparoscopic radical prostatectomy and can also include the removal of surrounding lymph nodes if there is suspicion of nodal metastases. Laparoscopic removal of the prostate is less invasive and usually a shorter hospital stay and a quicker recovery. With experienced surgeons, the outcomes of either are thought to be comparable, but long-term results are still needed.[1]

Additional information from the surgery can provide more accurate prognostic information on the grade or any extension into the surrounding tissue or lymph nodes. This information is used to determine if further treatment is necessary. In addition to providing more accurate prognostic information, radical prostatectomy also has the benefit of being a short treatment with a hospital admission typically being 1 day. It does, however, have the risks of erectile dysfunction, urinary incontinence, and morbidities associated with any major surgery. Because of these risks, radical prostatectomy is indicated for very low risk patients with >20-year life expectancy, in low- and intermediate-risk patients with >10-year life expectancy, and in higher-risk patients without evidence of fixation of disease to adjacent tissue outside of the prostate.[6]

RADIATION THERAPY

Radiation therapy uses high-energy beams in the case of external beam (EBRT), or radioactive particles in the case of brachytherapy, to kill cancer cells. With brachytherapy, the radiation sources are placed directly into the prostate for a direct action with minimal effect to surrounding tissue. This form of radiation is given as either low dose or high dose and is indicated as monotherapy for low- risk cancers or can be given as an adjunct to EBRT in intermediate and particularly in higher-risk cancers.[6] In low-risk cancers, brachytherapy demonstrated comparable control rates to radical prostatectomy.[25] Brachytherapy has the advantage of a short 1-day course of therapy and minimal risk of incontinence and erectile dysfunction, but it can cause acute urinary retention.

Current EBRT techniques use three-dimensional conformal radiation therapy (3D-CRT) to deliver radiation under the guidance of computer-generated images of a patient's anatomy. Intensity-modulated radiation therapy (IMRT) is the second iteration of 3D-CRT that uses various intensities of radiation according to the needs of the treatment area. Image-guided radiation therapy (IGRT) is a 3D-CRT that more accurately localizes the treatment area. Both IMRT and IGRT techniques are the standard of care for EBRT treatment that allows for higher doses of radiation to be delivered more precisely to lower the risk of adverse effects. Because of the proximity of the prostate to the bladder and rectum, treatment with EBRT can cause rectal urgency and increased bowel frequency, urinary frequency and incontinence, and erectile dysfunction. Although these symptoms are most often experienced short-term and the risk is lessened with newer techniques, they can persist for the long-term in a low percentage of patients. Unlike radical prostatectomy, EBRT avoids surgery and anesthesia complications, such as bleeding, myocardial infarction, or pulmonary embolism. External beam radiation therapy is an option for low-risk, intermediate-risk, and in higher-risk cancers. It is typically combined with a short course of ADT for intermediate risk and a longer course with ADT in higher risk cancers (see next section on androgen deprivation therapy).

Other modalities of radiation therapy, such as proton beam and stereotactic body radiation, have been used in the treatment of localized prostate cancer. However, their benefits over the current standards have not been established in the first-line setting of definitive localized treatment.[26]

There are no prospective, randomized trials to directly compare treatment outcomes of radiation versus prostatectomy in localized prostate cancer. A retrospective study of patients compared outcomes of 766 patients treated with EBRT to 888 patients treated with surgery and found no statistically significant difference in disease-free survival across all disease groups.[27] Several other retrospective studies have not found a difference between EBRT and prostatectomy.[28,29] Until prospective, randomized trials can definitively compare efficacy between these treatment options, physicians must compare the advantages and disadvantages of each treatment along with patient-specific factors to determine the most appropriate therapy.

ANDROGEN DEPRIVATION THERAPY

Androgen deprivation therapy (ADT) is the suppression of androgen production. It can be used in combination with radiation therapy for intermediate-risk patients and is used as a standard in combination with radiation in higher-risk patients. Androgen deprivation therapy can be done either through orchiectomy, because ~90% of androgens will come from the testes and called surgical castration, or by adding a GnRH analog, called medical castration. Both should decrease the body's testosterone production to castration levels, usually less than 50 ng/mL. As both methods are equally effective, most men will start GnRH therapy; however, orchiectomy can be useful for immediate decreases in testosterone when patients present with highly symptomatic disease or when adherence, cost, or availability is prohibitive. Table 100-4 includes the GnRH agonists, which include leuprolide, goserelin, histrelin, buserelin, and triptorelin as well as one GnRH antagonist, degarelix.

GnRH agonists work by binding to GnRH receptors to suppress luteinizing hormone (LH) and follicle stimulating hormone (FSH) production in the pituitary, decrease testicular testosterone and, subsequently, dihydrotestosterone. They bind to the GnRH receptors and initially cause a rise in LH and FSH and a surge in testosterone for up to a week until the continuous pituitary overstimulation eventually downregulates GnRH receptors and decreases hormone levels[30] (Fig. 100-4). This initial, transient surge in testosterone, called a tumor flare, can negatively impact patients presenting with symptoms, including bone pain and bladder obstruction. The flare can be prevented with the addition of antiandrogen therapy for a short course of at least 7 days.

Antiandrogens used in this setting are androgen receptor blockers that work by binding to androgen receptors to competitively inhibit their interaction with testosterone and dihydrotestosterone. These oral medications include flutamide, nilutamide, and bicalutamide. The combination of castration with a GnRH agonist or orchiectomy and an antiandrogen is called a combined androgen blockade (CAB). In addition to its initial use to prevent tumor flare in definitive local treatment, combined androgen blockade can also be used later in the treatment of recurrent disease.

Because GnRH antagonists directly block the receptors, there is an immediate decrease in LH and FSH production and subsequent testosterone suppression, avoiding a tumor flare and the need for antiandrogens, which may be most useful in symptomatic patients who would have experienced an increase in symptoms during this period.

Adding ADT to radiation improved overall survival in several clinical trials of men with intermediate-risk prostate cancer and is an option for some patients, particularly those thought to have characteristics of higher-risk prostate cancer.[6] These trials support the use of a short-term course of ADT of 4 to 6 months when added to radiation in intermediate-risk patients.[31–33] In high-risk or very high-risk patients, combining ADT with radiation therapy improved survival with studies favoring long-term ADT (2–3 years) over short-term (4–6 months). The addition of ADT to radiation is thought to have an additive synergistic cytotoxic effect on cancer cells that can possibly reduce the size of the prostate and the amount of radiation needed.[34] For this reason, ADT is often initiated up to 2 months prior to radiation. Androgen deprivation monotherapy, without concomitant radiation, has not been shown to be beneficial in patients with localized prostate cancer. Neoadjuvant or adjuvant ADT does not give added benefit with radical prostatectomy.

Traditionally, studies in the treatment of localized prostate cancer with radiation therapy plus ADT were done using combined androgen blockade for the entire ADT portion of treatment. Whether the addition of an antiandrogen is necessary is still unknown. Meta-analyses suggest that bicalutamide may provide an incremental relative improvement in overall survival by 5% to 20% over GnRH agonist monotherapy, but more clinical trials are needed to definitively confirm its utility in the localized treatment setting.[35,36] Antiandrogen monotherapy is less effective than medical/surgical castration and is not recommended for use in the treatment of localized prostate cancer.

Using ADT to disrupt the production of testosterone and dihydrotestosterone can cause a range of symptoms that can impact quality of life, particularly in patients using ADT for prolonged periods. These side effects include hot flashes, decreased libido, erectile dysfunction, gynecomastia, behavioral changes, and burning at injection site. Androgen deprivation therapy decreases bone mineral density after 6 months of use that can cause osteoporosis.[37] It can also cause cardiovascular and metabolic abnormalities, such as increased body fat, decreased muscle strength, and decreased insulin sensitivity leading to hyperlipidemia and hyperglycemia. The incidence of diabetes is increased up to 44% with the use of ADT.[38]

Table 100-4
Androgen Deprivation Agents

Agent	Route	Dose
GnRH Agonists		
Leuprolide (Eligard)	Subcutaneous	7.5 mg every month 22.5 mg every 3 months 30 mg every 4 months 45 mg every 6 months
Leuprolide (Lupron Depot)	Intramuscular	7.5 mg every month 22.5 mg every 3 months 30 mg every 4 months 45 mg every 6 months 3.75 mg
Triptorelin (Trelstar or Trelstar Mixject)	Intramuscular; suspension (reconstituted)	3.75 mg every 4 weeks 11.25 mg every 12 weeks 22.5 mg every 24 weeks
Goserelin (Zoladex)	Subcutaneous implant	3.6 mg every 28 days, 10.8 mg every 12 weeks
Histrelin (Vantas)	Subcutaneous implant	50 mg every 12 months
Buserelin (Suprefact)	Subcutaneous	500 mcg every 8 hours for 7 days. Maintenance 200 mcg once daily
Buserelin (Suprefac Depot)	Subcutaneous implant	6.3 mg every 2 months 9.45 mg every 3 months
GnRH Antagonist		
Degarelix (Firmagon)	Subcutaneous	Loading dose: 240 mg administered as two 120 mg injections Maintenance dose: 80 mg every 28 days (beginning 28 days after initial loading dose)
Antiandrogens		
Bicalutamide (Casodex)	Oral	50 mg once daily (with GnRH analog) 150 mg once daily (monotherapy)
Nilutamide (Nilandron)	Oral	300 mg once daily × 30 days, followed by 150 mg once daily
Flutamide (Eulexin)	Oral	250 mg three times daily

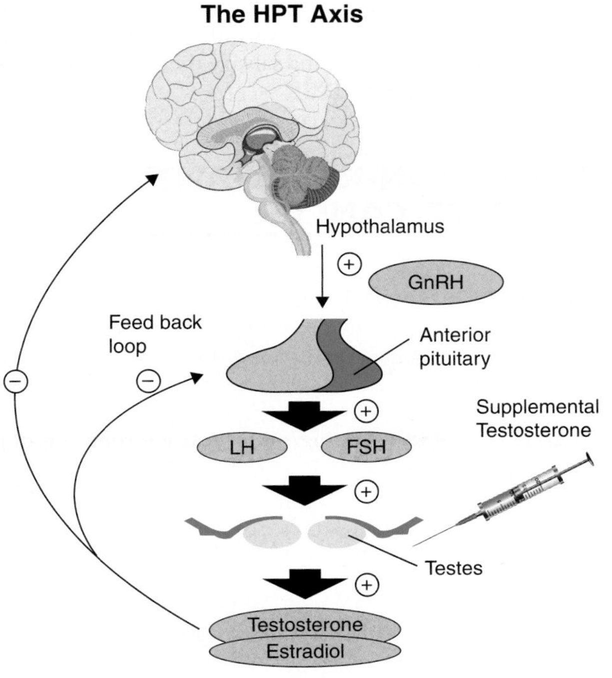

Figure 100-4 The hypothalamic-pituitary-thyroid axis is continuously stimulated by GnRH agonists to suppress testosterone through negative feedback.

CASE 100-2, QUESTION 5: C.W. is elected to proceed with active surveillance. His medical oncologist had scheduled appointments and PSA checks every 3 months and DREs every 6 months. His results are as follows:

Date	PSA Level (ng/mL)	DRE
01/13/2013	7.16	Negative
04/27/2013	7.45	
7/12/2013	7.74	Negative
11/03/2013	8.08	
04/10/2014	8.75	Negative
10/29/2014	9.05	
01/30/2015	10.70	Negative
03/20/2015	11.19	
07/02/2015	11.70	Negative

C.W.'s PSA continued to rise; however, his overall health remained excellent and he did not have any symptoms from his disease. C.W. began to get anxious and the medical oncologist decided to do a repeat biopsy to reassess the tumor and treatment plan. The results revealed a Gleason 4 + 3 = 7 in 4 of 12 cores. What are the possible treatment options for C.W.?

C.W. now has T1cN0M0, Gleason 7, PSA 11.7 prostate cancer placing him into the intermediate-risk group. His options for definitive local treatment are radical prostatectomy or EBRT plus ADT with the possibility of adding brachytherapy. Because of the results of several trials investigating the use of ADT with radiation in intermediate- risk patient,[31–33] EBRT would be given with a short course of 4 to 6 months of ADT.

Locally Advanced Disease

CASE 100-3

QUESTION 1: Patient H.L. is a 63-year-old male with a clinical stage T1cN0M0, PSA 9.2, Gleason 4 + 3 = 7 prostate cancer. His past medical history is unremarkable and he has an excellent performance status. He has no known allergies and is not on any medications. His labs are not clinically significant other than his PSA level. When presented with his options, H.L. decided to undergo a radical prostatectomy for definitive local treatment, which revealed a pathologic stage T2cN0M0. He was monitored after surgery and after 6 months had no symptoms from the procedure or the disease. His PSA was monitored and his nadir after surgery was 0.32 ng/mL. The medical oncologist believes that the cancer is still present but does not think there is any indication of disseminated disease. H.L. has what type of cancer progression?

Recurrence and Progression

For patients who have definitive local treatment with either radiation or surgery, about 25% to 33% of patients will experience a recurrence of their cancer. After the completion of local therapy, patients are monitored by periodically checking PSA for the detection of biochemical recurrence, which is recurrence of disease as indicated by rising PSA with no other signs or symptoms. The threshold for PSA recurrence is dependent upon the initial treatment given. Because a radical prostatectomy involves the removal of all prostate tissue, serum PSA after the procedure should become undetectable. A PSA level of ≥0.2 ng/mL following a radical prostatectomy is considered a biochemical recurrence. Risk factors for the development of a recurrence after radical prostatectomy are the Gleason score, positive surgical margins, and elevated postoperative PSA levels.[39] A biochemical recurrence after EBRT is defined as a rise in PSA level by ≥2 ng/mL above the nadir, or lowest achieved PSA, or three consecutive PSA rises above the nadir according to the American Society of Radiation Oncology (ASTRO) criteria. Risk factors for recurrence after EBRT include large volume of disease, short time to PSA recurrence, invasion of extraprostatic organs, and high Gleason score.[40] As H.L. is not symptomatic and his only evidence of disease is his PSA rise that never became undetectable post prostatectomy. He has biochemically recurrent prostate cancer.

CASE 100-3, QUESTION 2: What is the most appropriate treatment for which H.L. may be eligible?

A biochemical recurrence can indicate that a patient has either a local or metastatic recurrence. A patient thought to have local recurrence may be eligible to again receive local therapy, called local salvage therapy, providing a chance for a cure or a delay in progression. A patient with a biochemical recurrence after a radical prostatectomy with no indication of distant metastases may be a candidate for salvage radiation therapy with or without ADT. Conversely, a patient initially treated with radiation therapy may be a candidate for salvage prostatectomy. In addition to salvage prostatectomy, cryotherapy, which is a procedure that freezes cancer cells, and brachytherapy, if EBRT was first used, are also salvage therapy options post radiation therapy. Careful consideration of the characteristics of both the disease and the patient must be assessed in order to determine the appropriateness for salvage therapy.[6]

In patients with clinical features suggesting that the disease is no longer confined to the prostate, called disseminated prostate cancer, systemic therapy is indicated. As prostate cancer is hormonally driven, ADT is the initial standard treatment in recurrent prostate cancer. At this point in the disease, patients are considered castrate-sensitive as their cancer is still being suppressed by the lowering of testosterone to castrate levels with ADT. Androgen deprivation therapy is palliative, but it can control or delay symptoms and complications, improving patient quality of life.[6]

Because the benefit of ADT for biochemical recurrence is still not fully known, when to initiate ADT is still not clear. Observation until evidence of progression is an option; however, patients with rapidly progressing disease, as indicated by the presence of symptoms, an elevated PSA, or a rapid PSA velocity with a long life expectancy, should initiate ADT earlier. With long-term use of ADT, cost and the extensive side effect profile may be limiting and will impact the quality of life for some patients. Intermittent ADT, once there is response to treatment, rather than continuous administration, is an approach that can minimize side effects and improve quality of life. With this approach, patients continue ADT until maximal PSA response and then temporarily stop ADT until a set PSA threshold is reached at which point ADT is reinitiated.[41] The full benefit of intermittent ADT is still not known. A trial done by Crook and colleagues assigned 1,386 men with rising PSA after radiation therapy to either intermittent ADT or continuous ADT. The intermittent ADT approach was non-inferior in terms of overall survival (8.8 vs. 9.1 years; HR 1.02, 95% CI 0.86–1.21), but more patients in this group died from prostate cancer (120/690 vs. 94/696). The trial demonstrated an improvement in quality of life with intermittent ADT; however, more research must be done to determine the true impact on survival. This approach may be considered for well-informed patients without metastatic disease.[42] The duration of response from ADT varies, but eventually the cancer becomes resistant to ADT and most patients progress.

At this point in the disease, H.L. has recurrent prostate cancer without evidence of disseminated disease. Because it is thought that the disease is a local recurrence, he may still have an opportunity for a cure with local salvage therapy. He was initially treated with a prostatectomy, and salvage therapy should consist of EBRT with or without ADT.

CASTRATION-RESISTANT PROSTATE CANCER

CASE 100-3, QUESTIONS 3: H.L. undergoes local salvage therapy with EBRT and ADT with leuprolide. After EBRT is completed, he is monitored while continuing ADT therapy. His pertinent laboratory results are as follows:

Date	PSA Level (ng/mL)	Testosterone (ng/dL)
04/27/2014	1.56	
07/09/2014	0.36	
10/17/2014	0.31	<50
01/23/2015	0.57	
04/19/2015	1.08	<50
07/10//2015	0.74	
10/02/2015	2.45	<50

H.L. continues to be in good health other than experiencing mild depression and 3 to 4 hot flashes a day. Bone density scan results on 04/19/2015 shows osteopenia with a T-score of −1.5. Bicalutamide was added to his ADT treatment plan on 04/19/2015. How has H.L's cancer progressed? What should H.L.'s medical oncologist do next?

Castration-resistant prostate cancer (CRPC) occurs when the cancer no longer responds to ADT alone, and the cancer is progressing despite castrate levels of testosterone. This is indicated by a rising PSA or by new or progression of existing metastases. At that time, there are a number of different therapies that can be used, including chemotherapy and immunotherapy. CRPC has acquired mechanisms of resistance that upregulate androgens and/or androgen receptors, enabling the cancer to grow in the presence of ADT. This continued dependence on the androgen pathway allows for CRPC to be sensitive to additional agents that affect androgens and the inhibition of androgen receptors, despite its name suggesting tumor resistance to further androgen manipulation. A GnRH agonist or antagonist should be continued indefinitely while undergoing any other therapies to continue its inhibitory effect on testosterone and dihydrotestosterone.

If a patient has a rising PSA level while on ADT, a testosterone level should be rechecked to make sure it is below castration levels. If it is not, then ADT is not adequately blocking the production of androgens, and a change in medication or an orchiectomy is usually recommended. If the testosterone level is below 50 ng/mL, the patient is confirmed to be castrate resistant and additional systemic treatment will be necessary (Table 100-5).[6]

SECONDARY HORMONAL THERAPIES

Despite the fact that the cancer is now labeled castration resistant, many cells are still very dependent on the androgen receptor and can continue to be targeted throughout the disease. For a patient who has adequate castration levels (<50 ng/dL) while on a GnRH analog and has a significant rise in PSA level or clinical recurrence, they will typically be responsive to secondary hormonal manipulations, such as antiandrogens, antiandrogen withdrawal, ketoconazole, glucocorticoids, and estrogens. These agents can delay disease progression and postpone the need for therapies with increased toxicities; however, they have not shown a survival benefit. It is possible to use these agents sequentially prior to initiating a different approach.[6]

The addition of an antiandrogen for combined androgen blockade is a common initial treatment for CRPC patients. As mentioned earlier, there are three approved antiandrogens that are used in this setting: bicalutamide, nilutamide, and flutamide. Because of the multiple daily dosing of flutamide and the additional side effect of delayed dark vision adaptation of nilutamide, bicalutamide is typically the preferred agent. Although these agents are generally well tolerated, adverse effects can include hepatic toxicities with elevations in liver enzymes. Monitoring of liver function tests are recommended with the use of these agents. Gastrointestinal toxicities can occur with these agents, particularly flutamide. Nilutamide has the highest rate of pulmonary-associated side effects although it is rare with any of the antiandrogens.[4]

Discontinuation of an antiandrogen after progression on combined androgen blockade can result in a decline in PSA level, called "antiandrogen withdrawal syndrome." This response can be seen in approximately 20% of patients and should be attempted prior to initiation of another treatment.[43]

Ketoconazole is an antifungal agent that is an inhibitor of adrenal androgen synthesis. The testes produce nearly 90% of testosterone in males with the remaining 10% derived from the androgens produced in the adrenal glands. The androgens are subsequently converted to testosterone and dihydrotestosterone. In the setting of prostate cancer, ketoconazole is administered orally as 400 mg three times daily under low gastric pH conditions to allow for maximal absorption along with a low-dose glucocorticoid. The

Table 100-5

Survival and Quality of Life Advantages with Therapies for Metastatic Castration-Resistant Prostate Cancer

Therapy	Overall Survival Advantage	Quality of Life Advantage
Abiraterone 1000 mg PO once daily Days 1–28 and Prednisone 5 mg PO twice daily Days 1–28 Repeat every 28 days	X	X
Enzalutamide 160 mg once daily Days 1–28 Repeat every 28 days	X	X
Radium-223 50 kBq/kg (1.35 microcurie/kg) Repeat every 4 weeks for 6 doses	X	X
Docetaxel 75 mg/m² IV Day 1 and Prednisone 5 mg twice daily Days 1–21 Repeat every 21 days	X	X
Sipuleucel-T doses about every 2 weeks Total of 3 doses	X	
Cabazitaxel 25 mg/m² IV Day 1 and Prednisone 10 mg daily Days 1–21 Repeat every 21 days	X	
Mitoxantrone 12 mg/m² IV Day 1 and Prednisone 5 mg PO twice daily Repeat every 21 days		X

PO, daily; kBq, kiloBecquerel; IV, intravenous.

PSA can be reduced by 50% or more in up to 71% of patients.[4] This drug has an increased potential for drug interactions as it is a potent inhibitor of CYP3A4. Toxicities include nausea, vomiting, rash, and fatigue and are often limiting for patients.

Several different glucocorticoids and estrogens have historically been utilized in the treatment of prostate cancer. It is still unknown exactly how these agents act in CRPC. It is thought that estrogen can cause suppression of LH release from the pituitary to then reduce testosterone production in the testes. They may also have a direct cytotoxic effect on cancer cells. Conjugated estrogens and estramustine have also shown response rates of 24% to 42%. Glucocorticoids, such as hydrocortisone, dexamethasone, and prednisone may suppress adrenal androgen synthesis by reducing the production of adrenocorticotropic hormone (ACTH) in the pituitary. These agents have somewhat fallen out of favor given their toxicities and the increased number of options that are now available.[4]

H.L. now has castrate-resistant prostate cancer confirmed by the rise in PSA despite testosterone below castrate level. The medical oncologist had added an antiandrogen to H.L's treatment plan, which he initially responded to as indicated by his PSA, but at his next evaluation his PSA rose because of an acquired mechanism of resistance. The next step for H.L. would be to discontinue his antiandrogen for a withdrawal response.

Metastatic Disease

When metastatic disease occurs, performance status and extent of disease should be evaluated and a discussion started regarding the goals of treatment as the patient is no longer considered curable. Metastatic disease is most likely to be seen in the bones, lung, and liver. Symptoms are more common in metastatic disease and are often related to the sites of metastases. For a patient who is first diagnosed with metastatic prostate cancer, treatment begins with ADT, just as it does in earlier stages with secondary hormonal therapy used at progression or recurrence. Androgen deprivation therapy will be continued concomitantly, while other agents are used through the progression of the disease.

Once a patient is castrate resistant, men who are in good health and have asymptomatic disease may be treated with sipuleucel-T, an immunotherapy. For castrate-resistant disease that is symptomatic, cytotoxic chemotherapy would generally be considered first line. Newer antiandrogens are approved in metastatic CPRC and can be given before or after chemotherapy. Appropriate sequencing of these agents is still not known; however, patients with poor performance status, advanced age, rapidly progressing disease, or a need to delay cytotoxic chemotherapy can benefit from receiving the relatively tolerable antiandrogens sooner rather than later. A discussion regarding the benefits of each therapy, along with potential adverse effects is important in deciding if and when these therapies should be implemented.[44]

CYTOTOXIC CHEMOTHERAPY

CASE 100-4

QUESTION 1: E.S. is a 70-year-old male who has been receiving leuprolide every 3 months since December 2005 for a biochemical recurrence after radical prostatectomy in 2004. He was started on bicalutamide in March 2013 for a rising PSA of 0.47 from 0.12, which he initially responded to. However, the PSA subsequently rose to 2.16 in July 2013, at which point the bicalutamide was discontinued. His pertinent laboratory results are as follows:

Date	PSA Level (ng/mL)
07/27/2013	2.16
10/20/2013	3.01
01/10/2014	3.32
04/12/2014	3.67
07/14/2014	3.93
10/26/2014	4.42
01/14/2015	4.77
04/17/2015	5.06
07/23/2015	5.51
10/02/2015	10.79

He continued leuprolide and clinical monitoring every 3 months (pertinent laboratory findings below). He comes to the medical oncologist's office for a routine follow-up appointment and complains of increased fatigue as well as a new pain in his hip. Besides this new pain, he is otherwise in good health and exercises by walking 3 miles a day. He has no known drug allergies and is only taking lisinopril 10 mg daily for high blood pressure. The medical oncologist orders a CT scan of the chest, abdomen, and pelvis, which reveals a new pelvis mass. What would be the best treatment recommendation for E.S.?

Taxanes

Taxanes are the only class of chemotherapy that have shown an overall survival benefit in the treatment of CRPC. These agents are microtubule inhibitors, which promote assembly of microtubules and inhibit disassembly, thereby stabilizing microtubules and arresting the cell cycle. Prior to their development, chemotherapy was generally not effective, with mitoxantrone only providing a relief of symptoms.

Docetaxel

Docetaxel in combination with prednisone is considered to be first-line therapy for symptomatic, metastatic CRPC when cytotoxic chemotherapy is indicated. Docetaxel-based regimens were found to improve overall survival in two randomized phase III studies. Docetaxel plus prednisone was compared to the previous standard of care, mitoxantrone plus prednisone, which had not conferred any survival benefit but had improved quality of life. When docetaxel-based regimens were given every 3 weeks with prednisone versus mitoxantrone plus prednisone in over 1,000 men, there was an increase in overall survival of about 2 months (TAX327: 18.9 vs. 16.5 months, $p = .009$ and SWOG9916: 17.5 vs. 15.6 months, $p = .02$). Quality of life was similar in both arms of each study.[45–47] Tolerability was improved when docetaxel was switched to a lower dose every 2 weeks with less febrile neutropenia and other toxicities.[48] This every 2-week regimen may be considered in patients unable to tolerate docetaxel on an every 3-week schedule.

There is recent data to support the early use of docetaxel in men with advanced or metastatic, hormone-sensitive prostate cancer. The CHAARTED trial illustrated that in men with a high metastatic burden indicated by the presence of visceral disease or high bone burden of disease, early initiation of docetaxel plus prednisone for six cycles in addition to ADT improved survival. The median overall survival was 13.6 months longer with a combination of ADT and docetaxel over ADT alone (57.6 vs. 44 months, $p < 0.001$). The time to progression was 20.2 months compared with 11.7 months ($p < 0.001$). A subgroup analysis of men with high-volume disease had a median overall survival of 49.2 versus

32.2 months ($p = 0.0006$); this benefit was not seen as much in men with less disease volume. Adverse effects seen in the combination group included febrile neutropenia and neuropathy.[49]

The STAMPEDE trial demonstrated an average overall survival of 10 months longer (77 vs. 67 months) with the addition of six cycles of docetaxel than those who only received standard therapy in men with newly diagnosed advanced prostate cancer. In men with metastatic disease, the overall survival was an additional 22 months (43 vs. 65 months).[50] These studies provide evidence of a survival advantage with the early use of docetaxel that suggest a new treatment strategy of chemotherapy in the setting. Experience with its use in this setting will confirm its role in metastatic, hormone-sensitive prostate cancer.

Cabazitaxel

Cabazitaxel in combination with prednisone can be utilized after progression on docetaxel-based regimens. In a randomized phase III study of cabazitaxel plus prednisone versus mitoxantrone plus prednisone in metastatic CRPC patients who were docetaxel refractory, there was a 2.4 month improvement in overall survival ($p = .0001$), but more severe adverse effects were seen. Death occurred in 4.9% of patients (vs. 1.9% in the mitoxantrone-containing regimen), mostly because of sepsis and renal failure. Other adverse effects included febrile neutropenia, severe diarrhea, anemia, nausea, vomiting, and fatigue.[51] With the increased frequency and severity of toxicities associated with cabazitaxel, the risks versus the benefits for an individual patient should be assessed prior to use.

Mitoxantrone

Prior to the introduction of docetaxel as first-line cytotoxic chemotherapy, mitoxantrone plus prednisone was considered the only chemotherapy regimen that provided benefit in metastatic CRPC. It did not improve overall survival, but it did increase quality of life, as measured by a 29% pain response rate versus 12% with prednisone alone.[52] Because of its lack of benefit in overall and progression free survival, it has been relegated to last line therapy in which there are no other viable therapies for symptomatic relief of advanced metastatic CRPC.

IMMUNOTHERAPY

Sipuleucel-T

Sipuleucel-T is the first cancer vaccine to be approved by the FDA. Unlike vaccines that prevent infection by allowing the immune system to recognize the virus or bacteria, a cancer vaccine treats the cancer. This cancer vaccine stimulates a patient's own immune system against the prostatic acid phosphatase (PAP) antigen that is expressed in most prostate cancer tissues. Collection of a white blood cell fraction containing antigen-presenting cells are taken from the patient and then exposed to PAP-granulocyte macrophage colony-stimulating factor (PAP–GM–CSF recombinant fusion protein). The activated cells are then reinfused into the patient 3 days after collection. The infusion is repeated every 2 weeks for a total of three treatments. The randomized, double-blind, placebo-controlled phase III study was conducted in over 500 men with minimally symptomatic or asymptomatic metastatic CRPC. Median overall survival was 25.8 versus 21.7 months in the placebo group ($p = .03$). Treatment was well-tolerated with common adverse effects of mild-to-moderate chills (54.1%), pyrexia (29.3%), and headache (16%).) Unlike other treatments for metastatic CRPC, sipuleucel-T does not elicit a change in PSA level that can be used as an objective measure of response.[53]

NEXT GENERATION ANTIANDROGEN THERAPY

An increased understanding of the role of androgens in prostate cancer has clarified the concept that the androgen pathway is still active in CRPC. This has led to the development of new agents with proven efficacy in metastatic CRPC that work to inhibit androgen receptors or the enzymes needed for androgen synthesis. Phase III trials have confirmed their utility in metastatic CRPC both before and after docetaxel. Because of their tolerable toxicity profile and ease of oral administration, they can be used prior to docetaxel in patients who are ineligible to receive or unable to tolerate chemotherapy.

Abiraterone

Abiraterone is an androgen synthesis inhibitor that irreversibly inhibits CYP17 (17 alpha-hydroxylase/C17,20-lyase), an enzyme that is required for androgen biosynthesis and is expressed in prostatic, testicular, and adrenal tissue. It inhibits testosterone precursors, dehydroepiandrosterone and androstenedione. When given in combination with prednisone in men with metastatic CRPC who had progressed on docetaxel, a phase III, randomized, placebo-controlled trial found that median overall survival could be prolonged over 4 months compared to prednisone alone (15.8 vs. 11.2 months, $p < .001$).[54,55] There was also a statistically significant improvement in palliation of pain because of bone metastases, PSA response rate, and time to PSA progression.[56]

Abiraterone was studied prior to docetaxel therapy in another randomized phase III trial. Patients with asymptomatic or minimally symptomatic metastatic CRPC had a progression-free survival that was doubled compared to prednisone alone (16.5 vs. 8.3 months, $p < .001$). Progression of pain intensity was delayed from 18.4 months to 26.7 months.[57] This is a reasonable option in a patient who cannot tolerate, wishes to delay use, or chooses not to receive docetaxel.

Because of the inhibition of abiraterone on CYP17, increased mineralocorticoid production by the adrenals can occur, causing side effects such as hypertension, hypokalemia, and fluid retention and should be monitored. Concomitant use of prednisone can reduce the incidence and intensity of these side effects. The most common adverse effects associated with abiraterone include fatigue (39%) back/joint discomfort (28%–32%), and peripheral edema (28%). Diarrhea, nausea, constipation, hot flashes, and hypertension all occurred in around 22% of patients and were severe in only 4% of patients. Atrial fibrillation also occurred rarely (4%) and the most common reasons for discontinuation were liver enzyme elevations or cardiac disorders. When a patient is started on abiraterone, liver function, electrolytes (potassium and phosphorus), and blood pressure should be monitored at least monthly.[54–57]

Enzalutamide

Enzalutamide is an androgen-receptor inhibitor that inhibits androgen receptor translocation and binding to nuclear DNA to inhibit prostate cancer cell proliferation. Initial studies were done in men with metastatic CRPC who had received prior docetaxel therapy as the standard of care.

In the AFFIRM trial, men were randomized in a 2 to 1 fashion to either enzalutamide or placebo. The study was stopped early and patients on placebo were allowed to begin treatment with enzalutamide because of the results seen at the interim analysis. Median overall survival was 18.4 months versus 13.6 months in the placebo arm ($p < .001$). Quality of life was improved and there was a greater than 50% decrease in PSA level in 54% of patients ($p < .001$).[58] Adverse effects in the treatment arm versus placebo included fatigue (34% vs. 29%), diarrhea (21% vs. 18%), hot flushes (20% vs. 10%), and headache (12% vs. 6%). Seizures occurred very rarely (<1%) with enzalutamide and the incidence of cardiovascular disorders was not different.[58,59] Enzalutamide is currently the only agent that is not given in conjunction with prednisone in the metastatic CRPC setting.

When given in the first-line setting prior to any docetaxel treatment, the phase III PREVAIL trial was also halted early because of the better progression-free survival seen in the treatment arm (65% vs. 14%, $p < .001$). Overall survival was also increased (32.4 months vs. 30.2 months ($p < .001$).[60]

RADIUM-223

In patients with CRPC and symptomatic bone metastases and no known visceral metastases, radium-223 dichloride has been shown to increase median overall survival (14.9 months with radium-223 vs. 11.3 months with placebo) and to reduce pain when given every 4 weeks for six cycles. It also delayed time to first skeletal event (15.6 vs. 9.8 months, $p <.001$). It emits high-energy alpha particles that target bone metastases by binding to areas of increased bone turnover. The short-range radiation creates a localized toxic effect of double-stranded DNA breaks in these targeted areas. Adverse effects were consistently similar between the active and placebo arms, although there was a slightly higher rate of myelosuppression with radium-223. More participants in the placebo arm discontinued the study drug because of adverse events.[61]

E.S. has castrate-resistant, metastatic prostate cancer. He is symptomatic and his PSA is rapidly rising since last visit. Docetaxel is the standard of care for symptomatic, metastatic prostate cancer, and this would be the most appropriate choice for E.S. without any comorbidities or conditions that would prohibit its use.

BONE METASTASES

CASE 100-4, QUESTION 2: Now that E.S. has symptomatic bone metastases, what recommendations can be made to decrease the risk of skeletal related events?

Bone metastases occur in around 90% of men who develop metastatic prostate cancer and are a common complication in advanced disease. They may be asymptomatic but can frequently cause pain, decreased mobility, and diminished quality of life. These metastases can also cause skeletal-related events, which include pathologic fractures, need for radiation or surgery to the bone, and spinal cord compression. Prostate cancer bone metastases are primarily osteoblastic lesions, in which there is increased bone formation around tumor deposits. Additionally, there is increased osteoblastic bone resorption, or osteolysis.[4] There are several therapies proven to have benefit in bone metastases by improving symptoms, preventing complications, or improving survival.

Bisphosphonates

The only bisphosphonate shown to be of benefit in patients with CRPC and bone metastases is zoledronic acid. In a phase III study, zoledronic acid was shown to demonstrate a delay in skeletal related events, including radiation to the bone, time to pathologic fracture, and bone pain. However, the study did not show an improvement in quality of life or a decrease in the development of new metastases. It is dosed at 4 mg intravenously every 3 to 4 weeks but must be dose-reduced in renal dysfunction, and it is not recommended to use if renal clearance is <30 mL/minute. Patients should take calcium and vitamin D as necessary to prevent hypocalcemia. An uncommon but serious adverse effect of osteonecrosis of the jaw can occur with zoledronic acid use.[4]

RANKL Inhibitors

Denosumab is a monoclonal antibody for the receptor activator of nuclear factor-kB ligand (RANKL), which is involved in osteoclast-mediated bone resorption and remodeling. When compared to zoledronic acid in CRPC with bone metastases, denosumab was more effective at preventing the skeletal-related events of pathologic fractures, need for radiation or surgery to bone metastases, or spinal cord compression. Denosumab also restored bone density.[4] The serious adverse effect of concern associated with denosumab is the same as that with bisphosphonates, osteonecrosis of the jaw, and it also has a higher rate of hypocalcemia. Renal adjustment is not necessary for denosumab dosing; however, renal function should be monitored because of the increased risk of hypocalcemia in patients with renal clearance <30 mL/minute. For bone metastases occurring in patients with CRPC, denosumab is given as 120 mg subcutaneously every 4 weeks. Patients should take calcium and vitamin D as necessary to prevent hypocalcemia.[62]

Systemic Radiotherapy

Systemic radiotherapy may be used, with radium-223 delaying time to first skeletal event in symptomatic bone metastases as discussed previously. It is the only bone targeting agent with a survival benefit and can be a good choice for patients with extensive bone disease with otherwise minimal disease. Two beta-emitting radiotherapy agents that have been utilized are strontium-89 or samarium-153 in patients with painful bone metastases that is not responsive to palliative chemotherapy and pain medications. However, they have no survival benefit, and myelosuppression is a major concern that must be factored into the future plan if additional chemotherapy is to be used.

External beam radiation therapy, although not systemic radiotherapy, is an option for one or a few symptomatic sites of bone metastases. It is most often used to provide symptomatic relief.[6]

Hormonal Agents

Abiraterone was shown, in the phase III trial discussed earlier, to improve bone-related pain and delay the time to first skeletal-related event (13.3 months vs. 16.7 months).[56,58] The PREVAIL study of enzalutamide prior to docetaxel therapy also showed an increase in time to first skeletal-related event.[60]

E.S. should start taking calcium and vitamin D supplementation and can add weight bearing exercises to his daily walking. In addition, his medical oncologist can recommend either zoledronic acid every 3 to 4 weeks or denosumab every 4 weeks.

Adverse Effects of Prostate Cancer Therapy

Because of the large number of men who are diagnosed with prostate cancer, as well as the continuously increasing numbers of those who live a considerable amount of time after therapy, the adverse effects of cancer therapy should remain a consideration for the remainder of the patient's life. It should be recognized that these effects include both short- and long-term issues. Patients should be aware of these potential adverse effects and their management strategies in a discussion with their physician. Guidelines from the American Cancer Society are now available for the primary care physician regarding long-term survivorship of patients with a prior diagnosis of prostate cancer.[8]

Androgen Deprivation Therapy

The loss of the majority of testosterone with the use of ADT in a male can instigate symptoms much as loss of estrogen does in the postmenopausal female. The large number of men living after a diagnosis of cancer should be aware of the long-term adverse effects of this therapy. The American Society of Clinical Oncologists (ASCO) survivorship guidelines recognize these problems and give recommendations for their monitoring. These include health promotion, screening for secondary cancers, rectal and urinary symptoms, cardiovascular and metabolic effects, anemia, bone health, sexual dysfunction, and vasomotor symptoms.[63]

CASE 100-5

QUESTION 1: P.L. is a 63-year-old male who has been on ADT therapy for just over a year and is experiencing hot flashes and mild depression. He also had a bone mineral density scan, indicating ADT-induced osteopenia. What can P.L.'s medical oncologist offer him to alleviate some of the side effects and complications he is experiencing from ADT treatment?

VASOMOTOR SYMPTOMS

Vasomotor symptoms will bother most men for the duration of their treatment with ADT. Hot flashes are characterized by an intense heat sensation, flushing and diaphoresis, involving the face and trunk and may also include anxiety and palpitations. These effects can vary in frequency, intensity, and duration. The mechanism may be because of a withdrawal of androgens, disrupting the equilibrium of the norepinephrine and serotonin neurotransmitters. Data has been taken from women as well as men in the efficacy of these agents because most therapies have seen similar efficacy in both men and women. These agents include, among others, estrogens, gabapentin, pregabalin, and venlafaxine.[63]

Gabapentin has been one of the most studied drugs for the treatment of hot flashes in men. Gabapentin at doses of up to 900 mg/day in men on ADT showed a significant reduction in hot flashes. Titration recommendations are to start at 300 mg daily and increase at increments of 300 mg to achieve the final dose. Pregabalin has shown some benefit in women at doses of 150 to 300 mg/day and has not been studied in men but may be a reasonable option starting at doses of 75 mg twice daily.

Serotonin and serotonin–norepinephrine reuptake inhibitors have also shown benefit in men on ADT, although no placebo-controlled, randomized trials have been done to date. Venlafaxine at doses of 75 mg/day has been the most extensively studied from this drug class. Paroxetine has also been studied in men on ADT. The use of other agents in these classes have also been reported.

Estrogens have also been used to treat hot flashes. Diethylstilbestrol and transdermal estrogen have resulted in good responses. Thrombotic events were not seen but gynecomastia occurred in a number of men. Megestrol and medroxyprogesterone have also been studied and one trial revealed a better response with medroxyprogesterone than with venlafaxine. However, there is concern that it might stimulate prostate cancer growth, similar to what is seen with an androgen receptor antagonist and the agent should be stopped if cancer growth does occur.

Alternative therapies have also been used to treat hot flashes. Acupuncture has shown some promise in small studies. Soy and herbal products have also been used; however, randomized controlled studies must be done to determine the true benefit of these therapies.[64]

CARDIOVASCULAR AND METABOLIC ADVERSE EFFECTS

There is concern of an association between ADT and risk of mortality from cardiovascular disease. However, this has not been consistently seen in clinical trials. Congestive heart failure and myocardial infarction have been identified as a risk highest in those who already have a risk of cardiovascular disease. A meta-analysis of studies with non-metastatic and non-CRPC did not find a significant difference in cardiovascular death in those men treated with ADT versus those who were not. The American Heart Association advisory panel concluded that links remain controversial and do not recommend periodic cardiac testing, but screening for cardiovascular risk factors should occur and monitoring of blood pressure, lipid profiles, and serum glucose should be routine, especially in those men who receive more than 6 months of ADT.[65]

Androgen deprivation has been shown to increase the risk of obesity, decrease lean muscle mass, decrease insulin sensitivity, increase high-density lipoprotein levels, and increase subcutaneous fat accumulation. Screening for diabetes and hypercholesterolemia is necessary, particularly with long-term use of ADT.[8,66–71]

SEXUAL ADVERSE EFFECTS

Loss of libido and erectile dysfunction are expected adverse effects of ADT, occurring in up to 85% of men treated with ADT. The impact of ADT therapy may be delayed with full effect occurring up to 2 years later.[72] Recovery from erectile dysfunction will usually occur after cessation of therapy. However, for patients on long-term therapy, there should be open dialog between the healthcare team and the patient regarding options available to help in mitigating these effects.[8] Other factors that may be contributing to erectile dysfunction should also be considered, including a history of diabetes or cardiovascular disease as well as whether the patient has had a previous prostatectomy. There is no consensus regarding the best therapy for this adverse effect. Phosphodiesterase inhibitors can be tried as 44% of patients reported a benefit in one study.[72]

PSYCHOLOGIC/COGNITIVE ADVERSE EFFECTS

Psychosocial adverse effects such as distress, depression, and cognitive impairment may occur. It has been estimated that up to 30% experience distress, 25% have increased anxiety, and almost 10% have a major depressive disorder. Low testosterone levels can affect mood in some men, causing depression and short temper. Routine assessment is crucial to identifying those patients experiencing these effects that can have a major impact on survivorship and quality of life with referral for behavioral intervention considered, as necessary.[8,73,74]

BONE HEALTH ADVERSE EFFECTS

Patients treated with ADT are more susceptible to decreased bone mineral density and bone fractures. In a study looking retrospectively at men diagnosed with prostate cancer from 1992 to 1997, those men who received ADT therapy were compared to those who did not and were found to have a higher incidence of fractures (19.4% vs. 12.6%, $p < .001$). Androgen deprivation therapy increases bone turnover and decreases bone mineral density with a 21% to 54% relative increase in fracture risk. Rapid loss of bone mineral density is seen within the first 6 to 12 months.[75]

The Prostate Cancer Survival Guidelines of the American Society of Clinical Oncologists (ASCO) suggest that all men who have received ADT should be assessed for the risk of fracture, using a baseline dual energy x-ray absorptiometry (DEXA) scan and calculation of a FRAX (fracture risk assessment) score.[8] For those men who are determined to be high risk, there are a number of options. Alendronate 70 mg weekly, zoledronic acid 5 mg annually, or denosumab 60 mg every 6 months are available for use in this setting.[6]

Osteonecrosis of the jaw is considered to be the most serious adverse effect of the agents used to improve bone health. Patients are recommended to undergo a baseline dental evaluation prior to the start of a bisphosphonate or denosumab with any invasive dental surgery done and completely healed before these agents are started. Good oral hygiene should also be stressed.

P.L.'s medical oncologist can offer P.L. an antidepressant. Gabapentin, venlafaxine, estrogens, and acupuncture have been shown to have some benefit for vasomotor symptoms, such as hot flashes. If P.L. is interested in being treated for both his depression and hot flashes, venlafaxine may be a good option as it can treat both side effects at the appropriate dose. As for P.L's osteopenia, weight-bearing exercises, supplementation of vitamin D and calcium, and the addition of yearly zoledronic acid or biyearly denosumab can be given to prevent complications that can arise from bone loss.

Radiation Effects

CASE 100-6

Question 1: K.A. has been recently diagnosed with prostate cancer after a biopsy. The results revealed a Gleason 4 + 3 = 7 in 5 of 12 cores. He discusses his options for definitive local treatment with the medical oncologist, radiation oncologist, and urologist. He decides to undergo radiation, and the radiation oncologist plans to treat him with EBRT in conjunction with 6 months of ADT. What side effects from treatment can C.W. expect? What concerns will the medical oncologist have regarding side effects and his history (PMH, FH, and SH)?

SEXUAL SIDE EFFECTS

Erectile dysfunction is the most commonly seen sexual adverse effect of radiation but can include decreased volume of ejaculate, absence of ejaculate, decreased intensity of orgasm, and decreased libido. Erectile dysfunction 3 or more years after EBRT occurs in 36% to 68% of patients and 50% to 60% of men have some extent of erectile dysfunction with brachytherapy. With radical prostatectomy, erectile dysfunction is seen soon after surgery but may improve over time. This is the opposite of what is seen with radiation, where it is more of a slow decline.

In one study, 80% of patients receiving radiation therapy responded well to sildenafil. It was seen that 74% of patients in another study continued to respond after 4 years. Additional factors that may contribute to erectile dysfunction should be considered, such as coronary artery disease and diabetes as well as patient age. Some patients will not respond and should be referred to an urologist or sexual health expert to evaluate other options for treatment.[4,72]

EXTERNAL BEAM RADIATION THERAPY

Radiation treatment for definitive local treatment is typically 4 to 6 weeks long with acute symptoms usually occurring around the third week and resolving within days to weeks after completion of treatment. Symptoms such as diarrhea can be treated with standard agents (e.g., loperamide, diphenoxylate/atropine). Internal or external hemorrhoids can become inflamed and sitz baths and hydrocortisone suppositories can help alleviate symptoms. Also, acute urinary symptoms may occur with agents such as phenazopyridine and alpha-blockers such as tamsulosin providing benefit.

Late rectal toxicities from radiation therapy can occur 12 to 18 months after completion of EBRT and persist for several years, although developing adverse effects after 5 years is rare. These adverse effects can include rectal bleeding, mucous discharge, and mild incontinence of stool. Rectal bleeding can be controlled with increased fiber in the diet, steroid suppositories, and sitz baths with rectal ulcers and fistulas occurring in less than 1% of patients.

Late urinary toxicities consist of chronic urethritis in 10% to 15% of patients and urethral strictures in 2% to 3%.[4]

BRACHYTHERAPY

Brachytherapy allows for the radiation of small areas of the prostate, which decreases some of the adverse effects of EBRT. In low-dose brachytherapy, acute urinary retention is known to occur in 6% to 15%, although better identification of risk factors for its development have decreased the incidence to ~6% in recent years. Transient urinary effects that occur include radiation-induced urethritis or prostatitis, urinary frequency, urgency, and dysuria. Symptoms will peak about 1 to 3 months after brachytherapy is placed and gradually resolve over the subsequent couple of months. Alpha-blockers such as tamsulosin help relieve some of these symptoms.[4]

C.W. may experience some of the common symptoms from EBRT, which include diarrhea and hemorrhoids. Other urinary and rectal symptoms include rectal urgency, increased urinary and bowel frequency, and erectile dysfunction may also occur. Androgen deprivation therapy can cause many side effects as listed in Table 100-6. The most common adverse effects include loss of libido, erectile dysfunction, hot flashes, weight gain, and muscle loss. Because C.W. already has hypercholesterolemia and suffers from depression, which can be impacted by the use of ADT, C.W.'s medical oncologist must closely monitor for changes in these comorbidities and be proactive about treating them if needed.

PREVENTION

CASE 100-7

Question 1: A.G. is a 42-year-old, African-American male who has come to his doctor's office to discuss potential ways to decrease his risk of prostate cancer. His father was diagnosed with prostate cancer at the age of 49, and his brother has just been diagnosed at the age of 45. Beyond lifestyle and diet modifications, what should A.G.'s physician discuss with him about the use of 5-α-reductase inhibitors?

Because of the large number of men who develop prostate cancer, interest has turned to the possibility of prevention. There are modifiable risk factors that can be addressed, but there is also interest in the potential of drugs or supplements that can at least lower the risk or possibly prevent the occurrence of prostate cancer.

The largest trials to date have involved the 5-α-reductase inhibitors, finasteride and dutasteride. Finasteride is a competitive inhibitor of type II 5-α-reductase that blocks the conversion of testosterone to DHT in prostatic cells. In the Prostate Cancer Prevention Trial (PCPT), over 18,000 men aged 55 or older were included if they had a baseline PSA of $\leq$3 and a normal DRE. They were randomized to finasteride 5 mg daily or placebo and had annual DREs and PSA measurements. At 7-years follow-up, a 24.8% reduction in the prevalence of prostate cancer was seen for those men on finasteride. In the finasteride cohort, there were 803 cancers of the 4,368 men; the placebo cohort had 1,147 cancers in 4,692 men. There were more reports of sexual side effects but were less likely to have lower urinary tract symptoms, which can be attributed to finasteride's mechanism of action and it use for BPH. However, for those men on finasteride, there was a higher proportion of cancers considered to be high grade (Gleason score of 7 or more) with 280 high grade tumors diagnosed in the finasteride group and 237 on placebo.[76] There was concern that these cancers would be more aggressive. The risk was considered too high and few considered its use for prevention. At 18 years from the start of the trial, a post hoc analysis of survival was assessed again to see whether there was an increased risk of death in the finasteride group because of the higher grade cancers diagnosed. The 10-year survival rates in men with low-grade cancers was 83% with finasteride and 80.9% in placebo group ($p = 0.46$), and in high-grade cancers survival was 73% in the finasteride group versus 73.6% in placebo group. Updated data at 15 years found that prostate cancer had been diagnosed in 10.5% versus 14.9% of finasteride and placebo patients, respectively ($p < 0.001$). In the finasteride cohort, 3.5% were found to be high grade and 3% were high grade in the placebo arm ($p = 0.05$). At 15 years, the survival was 78% in the finasteride arm and 78.2% in the placebo

Table 100-6

Adverse Effects of Androgen Deprivation, Approximate Frequency, and Potential Therapeutic Options for Amelioration

Effect	Approximate Frequency	Potential Corrective Actions
Libido loss	Universal	None known
Erectile dysfunction	Universal	None known
Hot flashes	50%–80%	Venlafaxine, estrogens, progestins
Muscle loss	Common, duration-dependent	Exercise
Weight gain	Common	Exercise/diet
Facial/body hair loss	Very common	None known
Fatigue	Not defined	Exercise
Emotional liability	Not defined	None known
Depression	0%–30%	Various antidepressants
Cognitive dysfunction	Not defined	None known
Gynecomastia	Up to 20%	Preemptive radiation
Breast tenderness	Not defined	Aromatase inhibitors
Osteoporosis	Common, duration-dependent	Exercise/bisphosphonates
Anemia	5%–13%	Erythropoietin not recommended
Hyperlipidemia	10%	Diet, statins
Diabetes	0.8%/year increase	Exercise, oral agents
Myocardial infarction	0.25%/year increase	Treatment of risk factors
Coronary heart disease	1%/year increase	Treatment of risk factors

A number of events are poorly defined in frequency as a consequence of a lack of controlled studies, quantitative assessments, and/or agreed on definitions. Adapted from Scher HI et al. Cancer of the Prostate. In: DeVita VT et al, eds. *Cancer: Principles and Practice of Oncology*. 10th ed. Philadelphia, PA: Lippincott Williams & Wilkins; 2015, with permission.

arm. The hazard ratio for death in the finasteride arm was 1.02 ($p = 0.46$). The difference in the risk of death was not significant between the two groups. Overall, finasteride reduced the risk of prostate cancer by about one-third.[77]

Dutasteride, a type I and II 5-α-reductase inhibitor, was studied in a 4-year randomized, double-blind, placebo-controlled trial in which men were given either dutasteride 0.5 mg daily or placebo. These men were between the ages of 50 and 75 with a PSA between 2.5 and 10 ng/mL and one negative prostate biopsy within 6 months. There were 6,729 men who participated and cancer was found in 659 of 3,305 men in the dutasteride arm and 858 of 3,424 men diagnosed in the placebo arm. This was a relative risk reduction of 22.8% over the 4-year period ($p < 0.001$). The difference between those with a high-grade tumor was not significant between the two groups. Erectile dysfunction was seen in 9% and 5.7% of men in the dutasteride and placebo arms, respectively ($p < 0.001$). Decreased libido was also seen (3.3% vs. 1.6%), although the symptoms of BPH were less in the dutasteride group. Less than 5% of men discontinued the study drug because of drug-related adverse events.[78]

The SELECT trial assessed the use of selenium and vitamin E in the prevention of prostate cancer. Research has indicated that reactive oxygen species may be associated with the onset and progression of various malignancies, including prostate cancer. This was a phase III, randomized, double-blind, placebo-controlled trial to assess the efficacy of selenium 200 mcg daily and vitamin E 400 IU daily, either alone or in combination. Over 35,000 men were included in this study who had a normal DRE and a PSA level <4 ng/mL. At a median of 5.46 years, no difference was seen among the groups.[79]

S.J.'s physician should explain that the 5-α-reductase inhibitors did show a significant decrease in the incidence of prostate cancer, but that it is still not clear what impact they have on prostate cancer survival and may have a negative impact on the incidence of high-grade cancers. In addition, there are side effects that patients may experience with these medications, such as erectile dysfunction and decreased libido.

SURVIVORSHIP

Because of the large numbers of prostate cancer diagnoses as well as the generally slow growth of the tumor, there are a large number of men who are living with or after a diagnosis of prostate cancer. They account for about 20% of all cancer survivors. It is recognized that physical and psychosocial effects can occur long after treatment is complete. The American Cancer Society created guidelines, last updated in 2014 and endorsed by ASCO in 2015, for the primary care physician to monitor the health of prostate cancer survivors.[8,64]

Quality of life should be assessed at baseline and monitored at least annually using one of the validated surveys for this purpose, 5-item Sexual Health Inventory for Men or International Index of Erectile Function.[8] These are beneficial for identifying side effect burden or other adverse effects that are of concern to the patient.

Healthy Lifestyle

Guidelines include an emphasis on reminding patients of the benefit of achieving and maintaining a healthy weight, getting enough physical exercise, and eating a diet that is high in fruits, vegetables, and whole grains. For those patients with residual bowel problems that impact absorption, they should be referred to a registered dietitian. Guidelines also include cautions on avoiding alcohol or limiting it to no more than 2 drinks a day as well as tobacco use and offering cessation counseling if necessary. Smoking increases the chance of recurrence as well as second cancers.

Obesity is associated with increased prostate cancer–specific mortality and biochemical recurrence. Body mass index and healthy food choices along with physical activity should be addressed and encouraged by the primary care physician.

Physical activity has been shown to improve cancer-specific and overall survival, help speed up recovery from short-term effects of therapy, and prevent some long-term effects. Exercise can improve fatigue, anxiety, depressive symptoms, self-esteem, happiness, and quality of life. Patients should be encouraged to engage in at least 150 minutes of physical activity per week.[8]

Surveillance

Once treatment is complete, the PSA should be monitored every 6 to 12 months for the first 5 years and then monitored annually. An annual DRE is also appropriate, especially as some patients will not have a PSA elevation in the setting of cancer. As well, those patients who have received pelvic radiation are at an increased risk of bladder and colorectal cancers. They should have routine screening and any signs of hematuria and rectal bleeding or pain should be referred back to their treating radiation oncologist for evaluation.[4]

KEY REFERENCES AND WEBSITES

A full list of references for this chapter can be found at http://thepoint.lww.com/AT11e. Below are the key references and websites for this chapter, with the corresponding reference number in this chapter found in parentheses after the reference.

Key References

Basch E et al. Systemic therapy in men with metastatic castration-resistant prostate cancer: American Society of Clinical Oncology and Cancer Care Ontario Clinical Practice Guideline. *J Oncol Pract*. 2014;10(6):e418–e420.(52)

Skolaris TA et al. American Cancer Society Prostate Cancer Survivorship Care guidelines. *CA Cancer J Clin*. 2014;64:225–249. (8)

Valencia LB et al. Sequencing current therapies in the treatment of metastatic prostate cancer. *Cancer Treat Rev*. 2015;41:332–340. (44)

Scher HI et al. Cancer of the Prostate. In: DeVita VT et al, eds. *Cancer: Principles and Practice of Oncology*. 10th ed. Philadelphia, PA: Lippincott Williams & Wilkins; 2015. (4)

Key Websites

American Cancer Society. www.cancer.org (1)

NCCN Clinical Practice Guidelines in Oncology (NCCN Guidelines)for prostate cancer early detection v2.2015, www.nccn.org. Accessed December 21, 2015 (5)

NCCN Clinical Practice Guidelines in Oncology (NCCN Guidelines) for prostate cancer v1.2015, www.nccn.org. Accessed December 21, 2015 (6)

101 Hematopoietic Cell Transplantation

Valerie Relias

CORE PRINCIPLES

	CORE PRINCIPLES	CHAPTER CASES
1	Hematopoietic cell transplantation (HCT) is a life-saving medical procedure involving the infusion of hematopoietic stem cells into a patient, the HCT recipient, to treat malignant and nonmalignant diseases and/or restore normal hematopoiesis and lymphopoiesis.	**Case 101-1 (Question 1), Case 101-2 (Question 1)**
2	In autologous HCT, the donor and recipient are the same individual, eliminating the need for pretransplantation and posttransplantation immunosuppression. Autologous hematopoietic cells must be obtained (i.e., harvested) before the myeloablative preparative regimen is administered and subsequently stored for administration after the preparative regimen.	**Case 101-1 (Questions 2, 3)**
3	Post-transplantation pharmacotherapy for autologous HCT includes hematopoietic growth factors to stimulate the proliferation of committed progenitor cells and to accelerate hematopoietic recovery.	**Case 101-1 (Question 6), Case 101-2 (Question 8)**
4	Common complications after autologous HCT are infections and organ failure, which occur in less than 5% of patients. The most common cause of death after autologous HCT is recurrence of the primary disease.	**Case 101-1 (Question 5)**
5	Allogeneic HCT involves the transplantation of hematopoietic stem cells obtained from a donor's bone marrow, peripheral blood progenitor cells (PBPCs), or umbilical cord blood to a patient. The donor for an allogeneic HCT may be an unrelated or related individual. Histocompatibility determination between donors and recipients must be performed through human leukocyte antigen (HLA) typing. The preparative regimen is, in part, determined by the degree of mismatch between the donor and the recipient.	**Case 101-2 (Questions 2, 3)**
6	The function of the preparative regimens for autologous HCT is to eradicate residual malignancy. The function of the preparative regimen in allogeneic HCT is to eradicate the residual malignancy, but also to provide immunosuppression, allowing the transplanted stem cells to grow and create a graft-vs.-tumor effect.	**Case 101-1 (Question 4)**
7	Choice of preparative regimens for HCT depends on factors such as underlying disease, degree of HLA matching, stem cell source, patient age, and comorbid conditions. Preparative regimens differ in intensity and are distinguished as myeloablative or nonmyeloablative.	**Case 101-2 (Questions 5, 6)**
8	Post-transplantation immunosuppressive therapy is necessary for allogeneic HCT to prevent both graft rejection and acute and/or chronic graft-vs.-host disease (aGVHD/cGVHD). Some immunosuppressants require therapeutic drug monitoring to ensure effectiveness while minimizing toxicity.	**Case 101-2 (Question 7), Case 101-4 (Question 1), Case 101-5 (Questions 1–9)**
9	Post-transplantation complications of myeloablative preparation regimens such as hemorrhagic cystitis, mucositis, and Sinusoidal obstructive syndrome (SOS)/veno-occlusive disease (VOD) require pharmaceutical management.	**Case 101-2 (Questions 8, 9), Case 101-3 (Questions 1–9)**
10	Opportunistic infections are a major cause of morbidity and mortality after myeloablative and nonmyeloablative HCT. The primary pathogens vary based on the time post-transplant and include bacterial, fungal, and viral species.	**Case 101-6 (Questions 1–3), Case 101-7 (Questions 1–5)**
11	Long-term complications of HCT include cGVHD, endocrine dysfunction, and secondary cancers.	**Case 101-5 (Questions 7–9), Case 101-8 (Question 1)**

OVERVIEW

Worldwide, more than 32,000 autologous and 25,000 allogeneic hematopoietic cell transplantations (HCTs) are performed annually.[1] The rationale behind the use of HCT is based on the steep dose response of chemotherapy; however, with increasing doses of chemotherapy, bone marrow suppression becomes a dose-limiting side effect. The administration of HCT provides recovery of the bone marrow.

Hematopoietic stem cell transplant is a procedure that involves the infusion of hematopoietic stems cells into patients who have received high doses of chemotherapy and/or radiation. Variations of this procedure depend on the donor of these stem cells, self-versus nonself, and the source of the stem cells. Autologous stem cell transplants are ones in which the patient serves as the donor of hematopoietic stem cells whereas, in allogeneic transplants, the donor is another related individual such as a sibling, or an unrelated donor. The source of the hematopoietic stem cells may be from peripheral blood progenitor cells (PBPCs), bone marrow (BM), or umbilical cord blood.

The type of HCT performed depends on a number of factors, including type and status of the disease, patient age, performance status, and organ function and, if allogeneic transplant is needed, the availability of a compatible donor. Characteristics of autologous and allogeneic transplantation, with either myeloablative or nonmyeloablative preparative regimens, are compared in Table 101-1.[2] Many diseases are treated with autologous or allogeneic HCT and are listed in Table 101-2.[2] Modifications to the basic schema for HCT are necessary based on the immunologic source (i.e., allogeneic or autologous) and the anatomic source (i.e., bone marrow, PBPCs, or umbilical cord blood) of the hematopoietic stem cells infused.

Hematopoietic cell transplantation (HCT) may be the only treatment available to many patients; however, it is associated with considerable morbidity and mortality, with approximately 40% of advanced cancer patients who undergo HCT dying of its complications.[2] The basic schema for HCT is illustrated in Figure 101-1. A combination of chemotherapy and/or radiation administered before infusion of the hematopoietic stem cells is referred to as the preparative or conditioning regimen.[2] The days leading up to the infusion of the hematopoietic stem cells are counted in the negative (i.e., −3, −2, −1), the day of HCT infusion is termed day 0, and the days following the transplant are counted in the positive (+1, +2, etc.). Although the preparative regimen may use the same agents that are used in conventional chemotherapy regimens, the doses are higher. The purpose of the preparative regimen is to eradicate the residual malignancy and, in the setting of an allogeneic HCT, to suppress the recipient's immune system.[2] Only myeloablative preparative regimens are used for autologous HCT; however, myeloablative, reduced-intensity or nonmyeloablative preparative regimens may be used with allogeneic HCT. Myeloablative preparative regimens involve administration of near-lethal doses of chemotherapy and/or radiation, which ablate the bone marrow; this may be followed by a 1- to 2-day rest. After completion of the preparative regimen, the HCT takes place. Myeloablative preparative regimens have significant regimen-related toxicity and morbidity and thus are usually limited to healthy, younger (i.e., usually younger than 60 years) patients.[3] Alternatively, reduced-intensity or nonmyeloablative transplants are performed with the hope of curing more cancer patients without the complication of preparative-related toxicity. Nonmyeloablative regimens make use of the graft-versus-tumor (GVT) effect allowing for donor lymphocyte-induced tumor eradication (see graft-vs.-tumor section). For most chemotherapy-based preparative regimens, a rest period is necessary to allow for elimination of toxic metabolites from the chemotherapy that could damage infused cells. After chemotherapy and/or radiation, a period of pancytopenia lasts until the infused hematopoietic stem cells re-establish functional hematopoiesis. Engraftment, when functional hematopoiesis is established, is commonly defined as the point at which a patient can maintain a sustained absolute neutrophil count (ANC) of more than 500 cells/μL and a sustained platelet count of at least 20,000/μL lasting three consecutive days without transfusions.[4] Graft rejection occurs when the patient cannot maintain functional hematopoiesis and may occur after autologous or allogeneic HCT.

AUTOLOGOUS HEMATOPOIETIC STEM CELL TRANSPLANTATION

The defining characteristic of autologous HCT is that the donor and the recipient are the same individual, making post-transplantation immunosuppression unnecessary. Autologous hematopoietic stem cells must be obtained (i.e., harvested) before the myeloablative preparative regimen is administered and subsequently stored for administration after the preparative regimen. Essentially, these hematopoietic stem cells are administered as a rescue intervention

Table 101-1
Comparison of Types of Hematopoietic Cell Transplants

	Myeloablative		Nonmyeloablative
Risk[a]	Autologous	Allogeneic	Allogeneic
Relapse after HCT	+++	+	+
Rejection	–	+	++
Delayed engraftment	++	+	+
GVHD	–	+	++
Infection	+	++ to +++[b]	++ to +++[b]
Transplant-related morbidity	+	+++	++
Transplant-related mortality	+	++	+
Cost of procedure	++	+++	++ to +++

[a]Risk varies depending on underlying disease, patient characteristics, and previous medical history.
[b]Risk of infection increases with intensity and duration of immunosuppression and/or chronic GVHD.
GVHD, graft-versus-host disease; HCT, hematopoietic cell transplants.

Section 16 Hematology and Oncology

Table 101-2
Diseases Commonly Treated with Hematopoietic Cell Transplantation (HCT)

Allogeneic
Nonmalignant
Aplastic anemia
Thalassemia major
Severe combined immunodeficiency disease
Wiskott–Aldrich syndrome
Fanconi anemia
Inborn errors of metabolism
Malignant
AML
Acute lymphoblastic leukemia
Chronic myeloid leukemia
Myelodysplastic syndrome
Myeloproliferative disorders
NHL
Hodgkin disease
Chronic lymphocytic leukemia
Multiple myeloma
Juvenile myelomonocytic leukemia
Autologous
Malignant
NHL
Multiple myeloma
AML
Hodgkin disease
Neuroblastoma
Germ-cell tumors
Other diseases
Autoimmune disorders
Amyloidosis

Timing of HCT relative to diagnosis varies with disease.
AML, acute myelogenous leukemia; NHL, non-Hodgkin lymphoma.
Source: Copelan EA. Hematopoietic stem-cell transplantation. *N Engl J Med*. 2006;354:1813; Vaughan W et al. The principles and overview of autologous hematopoietic stem cell transplantation. *Cancer Treat Res*. 2009;144:23.

to re-establish bone marrow function and avoid long-lasting, life-threatening marrow aplasia that results from the myeloablative preparative regimen.[5] Incomplete tumor eradication by the high-intensity treatment prior to transplant remains the main cause of relapse after transplant.[6]

Indications for Autologous Hematopoietic Cell Transplantation

CASE 101-1

QUESTION 1: P.J., a 46-year-old man, has diffuse large B-cell non-Hodgkin lymphoma (NHL) in first relapse after a complete remission of 1 year. An 80% reduction in measurable disease is noted after two cycles of dexamethasone, high-dose cytarabine, and cisplatin (DHAP) salvage chemotherapy. P.J.'s bone marrow biopsy and lumbar puncture are negative for malignant cells. Is a myeloablative preparative regimen with autologous HCT indicated for P.J.?

Autologous HCT is used to treat a variety of malignancies (Table 101-2). NHL and multiple myeloma are the most common indications for this procedure and represent more than two-thirds of all autologous HCT.[2] Nearly all patients who undergo autologous HCT have failed standard chemotherapy regimens; therefore, their hematopoietic stem cells have been exposed to prior chemotherapy leading to less abundant and viable stem cells.

The primary use of autologous HCT is in diseases that have aggressive features but are still chemotherapy-sensitive.[7] In a randomized, controlled trial,[8] autologous bone marrow transplant (BMT), compared with conventional chemotherapy with DHAP, resulted in a 5-year event-free survival of 46% versus 12%, respectively ($p = 0.001$). Overall 5-year survival was 53% in the BMT group and 32% in the conventional chemotherapy patients ($p = 0.038$).[8]

Whereas HCT is delayed until relapse after primary treatment in NHL, in some malignancies, autologous HCT is indicated as primary therapy to improve overall survival and progression-free survival.[7,9–10]

Prospective studies comparing preparative regimens, stem cell mobilization techniques, and stem cell source (i.e., BMT vs. PBPCT) are not available; however, autologous PBPCT has become the preferred source of stem cells, most likely owing to the improved outcomes with PBPCT in other disease settings.[11] PBPCs, defined as cells that express the CD34 antigen (e.g., CD34$^+$), are continuously circulating in the blood; however, their numbers are too low to easily collect the amount needed in transplant. Mobilization refers to the techniques used to move the stem cells out of the bone marrow compartment, increasing their numbers in circulation. Mobilization can be accomplished using growth factors or chemotherapy (see Mobilization and Collection of Autologous Peripheral Blood Progenitor Cells section).

P.J. has minimal residual disease that has demonstrated chemotherapy sensitivity (i.e., he had an 80% response to chemotherapy). His long-term prognosis will be improved with autologous PBPCT rather than with further conventional chemotherapy, as described previously. Thus, autologous PBPCT is indicated, owing to the greater likelihood that higher-dose chemotherapy may eradicate his tumor.

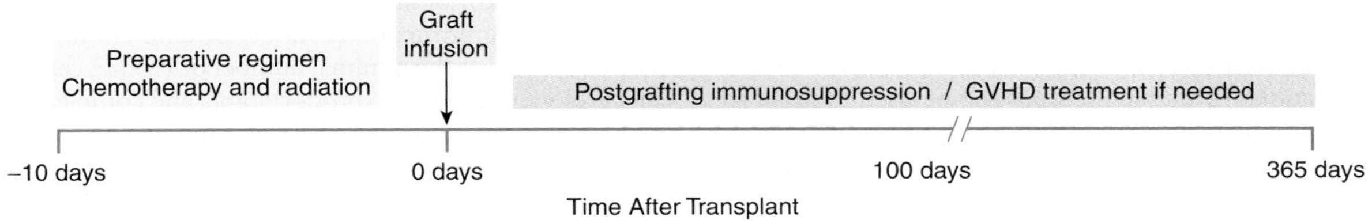

Figure 101-1 Basic schema for hematopoietic stem cell transplantation. Day 0 = bone marrow, peripheral blood progenitor cell (PBPC), or umbilical cord blood infusion. Postgraft immunosuppression or graft-versus-host disease (GVHD) prophylaxis for allogeneic grafts only.

Harvesting Autologous Hematopoietic Stem Cells

CASE 101-1, QUESTION 2: What is the best way to harvest and preserve harvested hematopoietic stem cells for P.J.?

PBPCs have essentially replaced bone marrow as the source of stem cells at many HCT centers, accounting for 98% of autologous transplants in adults from 2004 to 2008.[1] PBPCs result in more rapid engraftment than bone marrow and fewer days of neutropenia.[12] Collection of PBPCs occurs before administering the preparative regimen; thus, autologous hematopoietic stem cells must be cryopreserved.[2] Hematopoietic stem cells are frozen below −120°C and used within a few weeks; although, when frozen, they are viable for years.[2] Dimethyl sulfoxide (DMSO) is the cryopreservative commonly used to protect hematopoietic stem cells from damage during freezing and thawing. Infusion of hematopoietic stem cells stored in DMSO can be associated with toxicities due to the DMSO itself. During infusion, DMSO is associated with skin flushing, nausea, diarrhea, dyspnea, hypotension, arrhythmias and, rarely, anaphylactic reactions.[13] The presence of undetectable tumor cells in the transplanted cells contributes to relapse of hematologic cancers; unfortunately, purging the grafts of tumor cells does not improve survival.[2]

Relative to bone marrow harvest, collection of PBPCs requires less invasive collection methods and contains up to 5 times more hematopoietic stem cells. This results in a PBPC HCT having more rapid neutrophil and platelet recovery (i.e., a shorter duration of neutropenia or thrombocytopenia), fewer platelet transfusions, fewer days of intravenous antibiotics, and a shorter duration of hospitalization compared to a bone marrow HCT. Thus, the shift to the use of PBPCs instead of bone marrow for autologous HCT is primarily because of the more rapid engraftment and less invasive collection methods.[11] Therefore, it would be best for P.J. to undergo pheresis for PBPC collection. These cells would be bathed in DMSO and frozen at −120°C.

Mobilization and Collection of Autologous Peripheral Blood Progenitor Cells

CASE 101-1, QUESTION 3: For PBPC mobilization, P.J. received one dose of cyclophosphamide 4 g/m^2 IV on day 1, followed by filgrastim 10 mcg/kg/day subcutaneously (SC) beginning on day 2 and continuing through completion of pheresis. Twelve days after receiving cyclophosphamide, P.J.'s white blood cell count recovered to 3,000 cells/μL and pheresis was begun. An adequate number of PBPCs is collected after two pheresis sessions. P.J.'s cells are processed and stored. What was the rationale for administering filgrastim and cyclophosphamide? What determines the duration of pheresis?

Normally, low numbers of PBPCs are found in the peripheral circulation; therefore, it is necessary to "mobilize" PBPC from the marrow compartment into the systemic circulation. Mobilization leads to a collection of sufficient numbers of autologous PBPCs in most patients, although a minority of patients may still have poor mobilization.[11] Multiple methods can be used to mobilize PBPCs. Hematopoietic growth factors alone or in combination with myelosuppressive chemotherapy are used to mobilize PBPCs.[11] After administration of the mobilizing agent(s), the patient undergoes pheresis, an outpatient procedure similar to dialysis in order to collect PBPCs.[12]

Granulocyte–macrophage colony-stimulating factor (GM-CSF, sargramostim) and granulocyte colony-stimulating factor (G-CSF, filgrastim) are both hematopoietic growth factors and are used as mobilizing agents for PBPC collection.[11,14] Both reliably mobilize PBPCs, with filgrastim providing a higher PBPC yield.[11] The most frequently used filgrastim doses for autologous PBPC mobilization are in the range of 10 to 24 mcg/kg/day subcutaneously.[11,14] PBPC yield is higher when pheresis is started at day 5 (vs. day 6), with the optimal yield being around 10 hours after filgrastim administration.[11]

Myelosuppressive chemotherapy stimulates stem cell and progenitor cell proliferation. The combination of chemotherapy with filgrastim enhances PBPC mobilization relative to filgrastim alone. A benefit of using chemotherapy is that it also treats the underlying malignancy.[11] Examples of PBPC mobilization chemotherapy regimens include single-agent cyclophosphamide or melphalan. No mobilization chemotherapy regimen is clearly superior, which has led to incorporating PBPC mobilization into a cycle of disease-specific chemotherapy, such as using a single cycle of R-ICE (rituximab, ifosfamide, carboplatin, etoposide) therapy as the mobilization regimen for a NHL patient whose disease is responsive to R-ICE treatment.[11] By administering chemotherapy to the patient, the body's repair mechanism accelerates the cell division of stem cells and releases them into the circulation. This is a delicate balance, because the more the chemotherapy that is given to mobilize the stem cells the greater the potential for damage to the stem cells and a decreased yield at collection. Stem cell toxic agents, such as carmustine, should be avoided because they lower the quantity and quality of PBPCs. The hematopoietic growth factor is initiated 24 to 72 hours after completion of chemotherapy. Pheresis begins when the peripheral WBC count recovers to greater than 1 to 3 × 10^3 cells/μL.[11]

Certain patients fail to mobilize sufficient PBPC due to extensive prior therapy or therapy with marrow toxic agents. In these patients, plerixafor, an inhibitor of the CXCR4 chemokine receptor, can be used. Plerixafor was approved by the US Food and Drug Administration (FDA) in 2008 for use in stem cell mobilization in conjunction with filgrastim. It is known that CD34 is an adhesion molecule involved in promoting adherence of hematopoietic stem cells to the bone marrow microenvironment. Stromal cell-derived factor-1 (SDF-1) is a chemo-attractant agent for hematopoietic stem cells; its presence in circulation causes rapid migration of these stem cells to the peripheral blood.[11] Inhibition of the CXCR4 by plerixafor blocks the ligand SDF-1 from binding to the CXCR4 receptor, thus releasing CD34$^+$ cells from the bone marrow. In two randomized studies, 59% of NHL patients and 72% of multiple myeloma patients had sufficient CD34$^+$ cell collection for autologous transplant using plerixafor and filgrastim in four or fewer pheresis sessions, compared to 24% and 34%, respectively, in those using filgrastim alone.[15] Plerixafor is administered to the patient approximately 10 to 18 hours prior to each pheresis beginning four days after initiation of daily filgrastim 10 mcg/kg. Pheresis is continued daily until the target number of PBPCs per kilogram of the recipients' weight is obtained.[11] Typically, 1 to 2 large volume pheresis sessions are needed to collect adequate numbers of CD34$^+$ cells.[16] For adult recipients, the number of cells infused that are CD34$^+$ is the most reliable indicator of an adequate PBPC collection and predictor of durable engraftment.[11] A variety of different thresholds have been identified as the minimal number of CD34$^+$ cells needed for an autologous PBPCT to produce rapid and complete (i.e., white blood cells, red blood cell, platelet) engraftment in adults. The minimum threshold range has varied from 1 to 3 × 10^6 CD34$^+$ cells/kg of recipient weight, with more rapid platelet and neutrophil engraftment occurring with greater than or equal to 5 to 8 × 10^6 CD34$^+$ cells/kg of recipient weight.[11]

There are a number of factors that can affect the yield of CD34+ cells, including the timing and amount of myelosuppressive treatments received prior to mobilization; both chemotherapy and radiation negatively impact mobilization. The type of chemotherapy, number of different regimens, and overall duration of chemotherapy treatment affect the ability to collect stem cells. Additionally, hypocellular marrow and refractory disease can lead to a poor PBPC harvest.[11] There is a paucity of information regarding the parameters associated with engraftment in children undergoing an autologous PBPCT.[17] After pheresis, the cells are cryopreserved, stored, thawed, and infused into the patient as described in the Harvesting Autologous Hematopoietic Stem Cells section. Because P.J. has been in remission for a year after initial treatment for his disease, he received no radiation treatment, and his salvage therapy did not contain alkylating agents, his cell collection can be expected to be good and of short duration.

Myeloablative Preparative Regimens

CASE 101-1, QUESTION 4: What are the goals and characteristics of agents used for myeloablative preparative regimens in patients like P.J.?

The primary goal of P.J.'s high-dose, myeloablative preparative regimen followed by autologous transplant is to eradicate residual malignancy that is not treatable with standard chemotherapy. With autologous HCT, there is no need for immunosuppression because the donor and recipient are genetically identical.[2] Combination chemotherapy with multiple alkylating agents constitutes the most common high-dose regimens before autologous HCT. Alkylating agents are used because they exhibit a steep dose–response curve for various malignancies to overcome resistance to treatment, and are characterized by dose-limiting bone marrow suppression.[18] Ideally, combinations of antineoplastics should have nonhematologic toxicities that do not overlap and that are not life-threatening. Examples of common myeloablative regimens are illustrated in Table 101-3.[19–23] The early and late toxicities to myeloablative regimens are listed in Table 101-4.[2–4]

Table 101-4
Common Toxicities Associated with Myeloablative Allogeneic Hematopoietic Stem Cell Transplantation

Early Post-transplant (<100 days)	Late Post-transplant (>100 days)
Febrile neutropenia	Increased susceptibility to infections
Nausea, vomiting, diarrhea Mucositis Veno-occlusive disease (VOD) Renal dysfunction Cardiotoxicity	Endocrine disorders (hypothyroidism, hemorrhagic cystitis, infertility, growth retardation) Neurocognitive changes
Pneumonitis	Secondary malignant neoplasms
Graft rejection	Chronic GVHD
Acute GVHD	Cataracts

GVHD, graft-versus-host disease.

Complications of Autologous Hematopoietic Cell Transplantation

CASE 101-1, QUESTION 5: What complications must be anticipated as a consequence of autologous HCT? How can these be minimized? How can treatment be provided in an outpatient setting?

The most common cause of death after autologous HCT is relapse of the primary disease. The most common toxicities seen during autologous HCT are the result of the pancytopenia induced by high-dose chemotherapy. Because autologous HCT is not complicated by profound immunosuppression or GVHD, supportive-care strategies differ from allogeneic HCT. Isolation and use of laminar air flow rooms are unnecessary. The use of autologous PBSCT is associated with shorter periods of neutropenia and less need for clinical resources; thus, some HCT centers have developed programs that incorporate outpatient care into

Table 101-3
Representative Myeloablative Preparative Regimens Used in Hematopoietic Stem Cell Transplantation

Type of HCT	Disease State	Regimen	Dose/Schedule
Allogeneic[75]	Hematologic malignancies[a]	CY/TBI	CY 60 mg/kg/day IV on 2 consecutive days before TBI 1,000–1,575 rads fractionated for 1–7 days
Autologous[92,93]	Acute and chronic leukemias	BU/CY	BU adult 1 mg/kg/dose PO or 0.8 mg/kg/dose IV every 6 hours for 16 doses
			BU children <12 kg 1.1 mg/kg/dose IV every 6 hours for 16 doses
			CY 50 mg/kg/day IV daily for 4 days or 60 mg/kg/day IV daily for 2 days after BU
Autologous[23]	Non-Hodgkin lymphoma, Hodgkin disease	BEAM (carmustine/etoposide/cytarabine/melphalan)	Carmustine 300 mg/m²/day IV, 1 dose
			etoposide 200 mg/m²/day BID IV for 3 days
			Cytarabine 200 mg/m²/day IV BID for 4 days
			Melphalan 140 mg/m² 1 dose

[a]Includes acute myelogenous leukemia (AML), acute lymphocytic leukemia, chronic myelogenous leukemia, non-Hodgkin lymphoma, and Hodgkin disease.
BID, twice a day; BU, busulfan; CY, cyclophosphamide; IV, intravenously; PO, orally; TBI, total body irradiation.

the initial recovery. These outpatient programs also offer cost savings to the payer for health services.[24,25] Successful outpatient care during autologous HCT requires careful development and implementation of the necessary supportive-care strategies to prevent or minimize infection, chemotherapy-induced nausea and vomiting, infection, pain, and transfusion requirements. It is also necessary to develop admission criteria for patients with more severe complications.

Use of prophylactic oral antibiotics and once-daily IV antibiotics to prevent or treat febrile neutropenia has facilitated outpatient care and prevented many patients from being hospitalized.[26]

In addition, outpatient care during autologous HCT demands that HCT centers have appropriate resources, facilities, and staff to provide 24-hour patient care coverage. Patients undergoing outpatient care must meet eligibility criteria, including the availability of caregivers 24 hours a day and housing within close proximity to the HCT center.

Hematopoietic Growth Factors After Autologous Peripheral Blood Progenitor Cell Infusion

CASE 101-1, QUESTION 6: Ten days after the collection of PBSC, P.J. is admitted for his autologous HCT. He receives a myeloablative preparative regimen with cyclophosphamide, carmustine, and etoposide with an autologous PBPC graft. An order is written to begin filgrastim 5 mcg/kg/day subcutaneously, beginning on day 0 and continuing until the ANC has recovered to 500 cells/μL for two consecutive days. What is the rationale for filgrastim in P.J. after the transplant procedure?

Autologous HCTs, regardless of the stem cell source, are associated with profound aplasia due to the myeloablative preparative regimen (Table 101-3). Aplasia typically lasts 14 to 21 days after an autologous BMT and 10 to 14 days after an autologous PBPCT.[21] During this period of pancytopenia, patients are at high risk for complications such as bleeding and infection. In order to lessen the complications of pancytopenia, hematopoietic growth factors, such as filgrastim and sargramostim, may be used. These drugs exert their effects by stimulating the proliferation of committed progenitor cells. The benefits of the hematopoietic growth factor have been shown in several large multicenter, randomized, double-blind, placebo-controlled trials.[27–29] The majority of the trials suggest hematopoietic growth factor administration is associated with a shorter time to neutrophil engraftment (by 4–7 days), less infectious complications, shorter hospitalization after autologous BMT, and therefore decreased resource utilization.[27,28,30] However, the use of these agents does not affect overall survival.[27,29]

Although studies in the autologous PBPCT setting note more rapid neutrophil recovery after hematopoietic growth factor use, others report no difference in infection rates and minimal decreases in associated resource use such as the duration of hospitalization.[28,30–32] Although clinical practice guidelines for hematopoietic growth factors support their use after autologous transplant, pharmacoeconomic analyses are needed to further evaluate the true benefit of hematopoietic growth factors after autologous PBPCT.

Filgrastim is preferred for accelerating neutrophil engraftment in clinical practice. The reason most commonly cited is the desire to avoid febrile reactions associated with sargramostim, which complicates interpretation of febrile neutropenia. Although sargramostim or filgrastim theoretically may stimulate proliferation of leukemia myeloblasts, no evidence to date suggests that the incidence of leukemia relapse is higher in patients who receive these hematopoietic growth factors after autologous or allogeneic HCT.[33,34]

Although both filgrastim and sargramostim successfully hasten neutrophil recovery, neither agent stimulates platelet production or augments platelet recovery.[27,28] At this time, there is no established role for erythropoietin stimulating agents or platelet growth factors in the care of these patients. In summary, P.J. is undergoing autologous PBPCT for the treatment of a lymphoid malignancy. Thus, either sargramostim or filgrastim is an acceptable option for accelerating engraftment. Whether the addition of either agent will reduce infection and improve other clinically relevant outcomes is debatable.[14] A complete blood cell (CBC) count with differential should be obtained daily. Filgrastim should be continued until neutrophil recovery is achieved.

ALLOGENEIC HEMATOPOIETIC STEM CELL TRANSPLANTATION

Allogeneic HCT involves the transplantation of hematopoietic stem cells obtained from a donor's bone marrow, PBPCs, or umbilical cord blood to a patient. Fifty-one percent (51%) of all transplants performed in North America in 2008 used unrelated donors.[1] Thus, to understand the application of and complications after allogeneic HCT, a working knowledge of immunology and the major histocompatibility complex (MHC) and human leukocyte antigen (HLA) in humans is necessary.

Indications for Allogeneic Hematopoietic Stem Cell Transplantation

CASE 101-2

QUESTION 1: B.S., a 22-year-old man, has acute myelogenous leukemia (AML) in first remission after induction chemotherapy with standard doses of cytarabine and daunorubicin and consolidation with high-dose cytarabine. B.S. has poor risk cytogenetics, with abnormalities of 11q23 and inversion 3. Thus, he will receive an allogeneic HCT as part of postremission therapy. Typing performed on family members has identified a fully HLA-matched sibling donor. B.S. returns to the clinic today for a pretransplantation workup. At this time, his physical examination is noncontributory. All laboratory values are within normal limits. A bone marrow biopsy reveals less than 5% blasts. B.S. has a normal electrocardiogram and cardiac wall motion study. His renal, hepatic, and pulmonary function tests are normal. Is an allogeneic HCT indicated for B.S.?

The primary indications for allogeneic HCT include treatment of otherwise fatal diseases of the bone marrow or immune system (Table 101-2). The optimal role and timing of allogeneic HCT, in contrast to other therapies, remains controversial,[35] especially because treatment options for AML have increased. The National Comprehensive Cancer Network treatment guidelines for AML include the use of allogeneic HCT. A matched sibling or alternative donor (e.g., matched unrelated donor [MUD]) HCT is recommended as part of postremission therapy in patients with preceding hematologic disease (e.g., myelodysplasia, secondary AML) or poor risk cytogenetics, as in the case of B.S.[36] Current research efforts focus on the use of reduced-intensity preparative regimens and the utility of HCT relative to novel targeted agents in the hope of improving the outcome of allogeneic HCT.[36] B.S. is eligible for allogeneic HCT by virtue of his cytogenetics and the availability of a histocompatible donor. In addition, he meets age and organ function eligibility requirements and is in complete remission with minimal residual disease.

Histocompatibility

CASE 101-2, QUESTION 2: Why is histocompatibility important in selection of the donor in patients like B.S. who undergo an allogeneic HCT?

Because the tissue transplanted in allogeneic HCT is immunologically active, there is potential for bidirectional graft rejection.[2] In the first scenario, cytotoxic T cells and natural killer (NK) cells belonging to the host (recipient) recognize MHC antigens of the graft (donor hematopoietic stem cells) and elicit a graft rejection response. This results in ineffective hematopoiesis (i.e., inadequate ANC and/or platelet counts) post-transplant. In the second scenario, immunologically active cells in the graft recognize host MHC antigens and elicit an immune response, referred to as GVHD. Therefore, an essential first step for patients eligible for HCT is finding an HLA-compatible graft with an acceptable risk of rejection and GVHD.

Determination of histocompatibility between potential donors and the patient is completed before allogeneic HCT.[37] Initially, HLA typing is performed using tissue (buccal swab) and blood samples. Compatibility at class I MHC antigens (HLA-A, HLA-B, and HLA-C) is determined through serologic and DNA-based testing methods.[38,39] Currently, most clinical and research laboratories are also performing molecular DNA typing.[38–47] A donor–recipient pair with different HLA antigens (i.e., "antigen mismatched") always has different alleles, whereas pairs with the same allele always have the same antigen and are termed "matched." However, some pairs have the same HLA antigen but different alleles and are thus "allele mismatched." (See Chapter 34, Kidney and Liver Transplantation, for additional discussion of histocompatibility.)

Graft rejection is least likely to occur with a syngeneic donor, meaning that the recipient and host are identical (monozygotic) twins. Identical twins occur spontaneously in nature in approximately 1 in 100 births; thus, it is unlikely that a patient would have a syngeneic donor. In those patients without a syngeneic donor, initial HLA typing is conducted on family members because the likelihood of a complete histocompatibility match between unrelated individuals is remote. Siblings are the most likely to be histocompatible within a family; however, only 25% of potential HCT recipients will have an HLA-identical sibling.[38]

Lack of an HLA-matched sibling donor can be a barrier to allogeneic HCT. Alternative sources of allogeneic hematopoietic stem cells, such as related donors mismatched at one or more HLA loci, or MUDs, are used.[40] Establishment of the National Marrow Donor Program has helped increase the pool of potential donors for allogeneic HCT.[40] Through this program, an HLA-matched unrelated volunteer donor might be identified. Recipients of an unrelated graft are more likely to experience graft failure and acute GVHD relative to recipients of a matched sibling donor.[41] Thus, work is ongoing to identify factors that predict graft failure or GVHD to improve the availability and safety of unrelated donor transplants (see Graft Rejection section).[42]

The preparative regimen and/or GVHD prophylaxis may be altered based on the mismatch between the donor and the recipient. The risk of graft failure decreases with better matches, and although mismatching in a single HLA allele does not appear to impact overall survival, mismatching in more than one allele significantly impairs overall survival. The most important alleles to match are the HLA class I antigens (HLA-A, HLA-B, HLA-C) and the HLA class II antigens (HLA-DRB1, HLA-DPB1, HLA-DQB1).[43–45] This field is continually evolving with current data suggesting that mismatches at HLA-DPB1confer an increased risk of mortality.[46]

Eligibility criteria for allogeneic HCT vary between institutions. Having a matched sibling donor is no longer a requirement for allogeneic HCT, because improved immunosuppressive regimens and the National Marrow Donor Program have allowed an increase in the use of unrelated or related matched or mismatched HCT.[41] Potential donors also include haploidentical donors, who are a parent, sibling, or child of a parent with only one identical HLA haplotype. Hematopoietic cell transplant with a haploidentical donor was initially associated with high rates of graft failure and GVHD, but recent technologic advances have improved outcomes. Haploidentical HCT involves another alloreactive mechanism involving NK cells, which may be associated with reduced relapse rates in AML patients.[2]

Normal renal, hepatic, pulmonary, and cardiac functions are necessary for eligibility at most centers. Historically, patients older than 55 years were excluded from allogeneic HCT because they were more likely to succumb to transplantation-related complications. However, many centers are now considering patients up to 65 years old and basing their selection criteria on physiologic rather than biologic age.

Harvesting, Preparing, and Transplanting Allogeneic Hematopoietic Stem Cells

CASE 101-2, QUESTION 3: What methods can be used to harvest hematopoietic stem cells from B.S.'s histocompatible sibling and prepare them for transplant? Are there any advantages to the use of bone marrow, PBPCs, or umbilical cord blood as a source for hematopoietic stem cells?

The method of harvesting allogeneic hematopoietic stem cells varies according to the site of harvest (i.e., bone marrow, peripheral blood, or umbilical cord blood). ABO incompatibility increases the complexity of HCT, but is not an obstacle to HCT. The hematopoietic stem cells may need additional processing to reduce the RBCs infused with the HCT product if the donor and recipient are ABO-incompatible, which occurs in 30% to 40% of sibling donor HCTs and is higher in unrelated donor HCT.[47] Various strategies post-transplant used to manage blood support for ABO-incompatible HCT recipients include the infusion of donor-type fresh frozen plasma to provide a noncellular source of A or B antigens, as well as transfusing-type volume reduced RBCs and platelets or O RBCs to minimize the risk of immune-mediated hemolytic anemia and thrombotic microangiopathic syndromes.[47]

BONE MARROW

Harvesting bone marrow entails a surgical procedure in which marrow is obtained from the iliac crests. Allogeneic bone marrow is obtained from the donor under local or general anesthesia on day 0 of BMT.[2] The number of nucleated marrow cells harvested varies depending on disease being treated, conditioning regimen, and preinfusion manipulation, and is usually 1 to 3×10^8 infused cells/kg of recipient weight.[17] These cells are obtained through multiple aspirations of marrow from the posterior iliac crests. The marrow is then processed to remove fat or marrow emboli and is usually immediately infused intravenously into the patient. If immediate transplant is not possible, the bone marrow is frozen until it can be infused. Once infused into circulation, through the mechanism of the chemokine SDF-1/CXCR4 receptor, the stem cells migrate to the bone marrow compartment where they will eventually reside.

PERIPHERAL BLOOD PROGENITOR CELLS

As mentioned earlier, hematopoietic stem cells continuously detach, enter the circulation, and return to the marrow; thus, the peripheral blood is a convenient source of hematopoietic stem cells. The number of PBPCs is estimated by using the cell surface molecule CD34 as a surrogate marker. The number of circulating $CD34^+$ cells in blood is increased by mobilizing them from the marrow. The most commonly used regimen to mobilize allogeneic (healthy) donors is a 4- to 5-day course of filgrastim 10 to 16 mcg/kg/day subcutaneously, followed by pheresis on the fourth or fifth day when peripheral blood levels of $CD34^+$ cells peak.[9] An adequate number of hematopoietic stem cells is usually obtained with one to two pheresis collections. The optimal number of $CD34^+$ required is 4 to 10 $\times$ 10^6 cells/kg of recipient body weight for a HLA-identical sibling donor transplant with haploidentical transplants requiring greater numbers.[10,48,49] Higher cell doses have been associated with not only more rapid engraftment but also fewer fungal infections and improved overall survival.[50] Hematopoietic stem cells obtained from the peripheral blood are processed like bone marrow-derived stem cells and may be infused immediately into the recipient or frozen for future use. Compared to bone marrow, PBPC infusions are associated with quicker neutrophil and platelet engraftment.[2] In patients with a hematologic malignancy and a matched sibling donor, PBPCT is also associated with lower relapse rates and increased disease-free survival rates.[51] However, PBPC grafts contain more T cells than do bone marrow grafts.[2] Therefore, PBPCT has a similar incidence of acute GVHD, but an approximately 20% higher incidence of extensive stage and overall chronic GVHD.[51]

UMBILICAL CORD BLOOD

Blood from the umbilical cord and the placenta is rich in hematopoietic stem cells but limited in volume.[52] Thus, umbilical cord blood offers an alternative stem cell source to those patients who do not have a suitable related donor. After consent is obtained, the cord blood cells are obtained in the delivery room after birth, typically after the delivery of the placenta.[53]

The cord blood is then processed, and, if it matches certain pre-established criteria (e.g., minimum nucleated cell content, sterility), a sample is sent for HLA typing and cryopreserved for future use. An estimated 20,000 HCTs with cord blood donors have been performed with more than 300,000 cord blood units banked worldwide. It is unknown how long cryopreserved cord blood is viable.[54]

HCT with an unrelated cord blood donor has several potential advantages over unrelated marrow or PBPC donors.[52] Specifically, (a) cord blood is readily available, which leads to a more rapid time to HCT; (b) lack of stem cell exposure to the thymus allows for greater degrees of HLA disparity as compared to bone marrow or PBPC[53]; and (c) despite the less-stringent HLA matching, mismatched cord blood cells are less likely to cause GVHD while still maintaining GVT activity. The less-stringent HLA requirements increase the likelihood of identifying a suitable allogeneic donor, which is particularly beneficial for minority populations who are underrepresented in adult registries and often lack matched stem cell sources. Outcomes in umbilical cord blood recipients are improved with fewer HLA mismatches and greater numbers of $CD34^+$ cells.[55] However, the limited number of hematopoietic stem cells in cord blood is a disadvantage in particular when considering adult patients.[56] In order to overcome the cell dose limitation and improve engraftment, researchers have been studying infusing two cord blood units,[57] coinfusing a cord blood unit with highly purified $CD34^+$ cells from haploidentical donors,[58] and ex vivo expansion of cord blood progenitors,[59] delivery of the cord blood unit directly into the bone marrow space,[60–62] and priming of cord blood with agents that may facilitate homing to the bone marrow.[63]

As an adequate cell dose is critical for engraftment after cord blood transplantation and the cell dose of a single cord blood unit is limited, progress in the field of cord blood transplantation for the treatment of adults has been slower.[56] However, recent data showed that when a single cord blood unit with an adequate cell dose is available, the outcomes of adults with leukemia are similar to those receiving unrelated bone marrow or peripheral blood grafts.[64]

Moreover, for those adults with leukemia who do not have a single cord blood unit with a suitable cell dose, the use of two partially matched cord blood units to compose the graft also provides outcomes similar to that of related and unrelated donors.[65] These data associated with the promising outcomes when using umbilical cord blood in the context of reduced-intensity conditioning have significantly increased the utilization of cord blood as a source of hematopoietic progenitors for the treatment of adult patients.[66,67]

In summary, the utilization of cord blood as a source of hematopoietic stem cells for transplantation has substantially expanded in the last decade. Novel methodologies to improve engraftment, promote immune reconstitution, and improve outcomes after cord blood transplantation are under investigation and are likely to further extend its availability to patients who require a potentially curative allogeneic transplant but lack a suitable related donor.

Therefore, it is most reasonable to harvest PBPCs from B.S.'s sibling to use for his myeloablative HCT because his sibling is fully HLA-matched. A PBPC transplant is preferred to BMT due to the expectations of increased speed of neutrophil and platelet engraftment and disease-free survival rate and lower relapse rate.

Graft-versus-Tumor Effect

CASE 101-2, QUESTION 4: B.S. will receive an allogeneic HCT from his histocompatible sibling with the hope of inducing GVT effect to help in treating his malignancy. What is the GVT effect? Which tumors are most responsive to this effect?

Graft-vs.-tumor refers to the phenomenon where the donor's cytotoxic T lymphocytes suppress or eliminate the recipient's malignancy. Initial clinical evidence of a GVT effect came from the observation that patients with GVHD had lower relapse rates compared with those who did not.[68,69] This suggested a GVT effect due to the donor lymphocytes. Lymphocyte involvement in GVT was further supported by the effectiveness of donor lymphocyte infusions in treating patients who experienced relapse of their malignancies after allogeneic HCT.[70,71] Eradication of the recurrent malignancy is due to either specific targeting of the tumor antigens or to GVHD, which may affect cancer cells preferentially. Different illnesses vary in their responsiveness to donor lymphocyte infusions, with chronic myelogenous leukemia (CML) and acute leukemias being the most and least responsive, respectively.[72] Patients with certain solid tumors (e.g., renal cell carcinoma) also appear to benefit from a GVT effect.[73] These data are the platform on which the use of reduced-intensity and nonmyeloablative preparative regimens are based.

Preparative Regimens for Allogeneic Hematopoietic Stem Cell Transplantation

MYELOABLATIVE PREPARATIVE REGIMENS

CASE 101-2, QUESTION 5: What is the rationale for using myeloablative preparative regimens for patients like B.S. who are to receive an allogeneic HCT? What types of regimens are used, and what is recommended for B.S.?

The combination of chemotherapy and/or radiation used in allogeneic HCT is referred to as the preparative or conditioning regimen. The rationale for high-dose myeloablative preparative regimens is similar to that discussed in the Autologous Hematopoietic Stem Cell Transplantation section. Infusion of hematopoietic stem cells restores hematopoiesis induced by dose-limiting myelosuppression of chemotherapy, maximizing the potential value of the steep dose–response curve to alkylating agents and radiation[18], and suppressing the host immune system. The preparative regimen is also designed to eradicate immunologically active host tissues (lymphoid tissue and macrophages) and to prevent or minimize the development of host-versus-graft reactions (i.e., graft rejection). Conversely, patients undergoing syngeneic transplantation do not require immunosuppressive preparative regimens before HCT because the donor and the patient are genetically identical; thus, there is no potential for host-versus-graft reactions. Therefore, preparative regimens are tailored to the primary disease and to HLA compatibility between the recipient–donor pair.

Examples of common preparative regimens for allogeneic HCT are shown in Table 101-3.[8,20,74] Table 101-4 lists the common toxicities associated with myeloablative allogeneic HCT. Most allogeneic preparative regimens for the treatment of hematologic malignancies contain cyclophosphamide, radiation, or both. The combination of cyclophosphamide and total body irradiation (TBI) was one of the first preparative regimens used, and it is still used widely today. This regimen is immunosuppressive and has inherent activity against hematologic malignancies (e.g., leukemias, lymphomas). TBI is myeloablative and immunosuppressive, does not have cross-resistance to chemotherapy, and reaches sites not affected by chemotherapy (e.g., the central nervous system).[2] The toxicity of TBI and the scarcity of facilities for its delivery have led to the development of radiation-free preparative regimens. Modifications of the cyclophosphamide–TBI (CY/TBI) preparative regimen include replacing TBI with other agents such as busulfan and adding other chemotherapeutic or monoclonal agents such as alemtuzumab to the existing regimen. These measures are designed to minimize the long-term toxicities associated with TBI (e.g., growth retardation in children, cataracts) or to provide additional antitumor activity. The long-term outcomes of busulfan/cyclophosphamide (BU/CY) and CY/TBI in patients with AML and CML have been compared in a meta-analysis of four clinical trials.[75] Equivalent rates of long-term complications were present between the two preparative regimens, except for a greater risk of cataracts with CY/TBI and alopecia with BU/CY. Overall and disease-free survival rates were similar in patients with CML although there was a trend for improved disease-free survival with CY/TBI in AML patients. In the case of a mismatched allogeneic HCT with an increased chance of graft rejection, antithymocyte globulin (ATG) may also be added to the preparative regimen to further immunosuppress the recipient.

Based on these data, the CY/TBI preparative regimen is preferred for B.S. because he has AML with poor cytogenetics and has a matched sibling available. Because of the high relapse rates seen in AML, myeloablative allogeneic transplant is indicated in first remission for patients less than 60 years old with good performance status due to the decrease in likelihood of achieving a complete response to reinduction chemotherapy and the expected reduced duration of a second remission.

REDUCED-INTENSITY OR NONMYELOABLATIVE PREPARATIVE REGIMENS

CASE 101-2, QUESTION 6: Describe the rationale for nonmyeloablative preparative regimens. Is B.S. a candidate for such a regimen?

The regimen-related toxicity of a myeloablative preparative regimen (Table 101-4) limits the use of allogeneic HCT to younger patients who have minimal comorbidities. Because many patients with hematologic malignancies are older and have comorbidities, myeloablative HCT cannot be offered to a substantial portion of them.[76] The observation that patients with GVHD have less relapses and an improved understanding of the GVT effect led to the development of strongly immunosuppressive but not myeloablative (i.e., a reduced-intensity or nonmyeloablative) preparative regimens.[2] Currently, reduced-intensity preparative regimens account for 30% of allogeneic transplants.[77] More than 60% of patients receiving reduced-intensity preparative regimens are older than 50 years.[1,77]

There is a wide spectrum of reduced-intensity preparative regimens, with the nonmyeloablative regimens causing the least amount of myelosuppression. In general, more intensive preparative regimens are required for engraftment in the setting of unrelated donor or HLA-mismatched related HCT.[78] Reduced-intensity regimens do not completely eliminate the host's normal hematologic and malignant cells and therefore depend on the GVT effect to eradicate remaining cancer. The newly transplanted donor cells slowly replace host hematopoiesis, and elicit GVT effects.[73] After engraftment, mixed chimerism is generally present. Chimerism can be defined as the ability to detect both donor-derived and recipient-derived hematopoietic cells; both donor and patient cells coexist together for a period of time in the patient. If the graft is rejected, typically only recipient cells are present. After a reduced-intensity preparative regimen, mixed chimerism (defined as 5%–95% donor T cells present in the peripheral blood) between the host and recipient develops, allowing for a GVT effect as the primary form of therapy. Chimerism is evaluated to monitor disease response and engraftment post-transplant. Chimerism is assessed within T cells and granulocytes in the peripheral blood and bone marrow using conventional (e.g., using sex chromosomes for opposite sex donors) and molecular (e.g., variable number of tandem repeats for same sex donors) methods. The methods used to characterize chimerism after HCT are reviewed elsewhere.[79–81] A few months after HCT, donor lymphocytes can be infused (called a "donor lymphocyte infusion") to augment the GVT activity.[2] The use of donor lymphocyte infusions is dependent on the availability of the donor and is highly center specific. The challenge is to maximize the GVT effect while minimizing the risk of GVHD. Therefore, GVHD prophylaxis, although different from that used with myeloablative regimens, is still necessary. Although reduced-intensity preparative regimens have led to lower treatment-related mortality rates, they may be offset by higher relapse rates.[2,82] The safety and efficacy of these regimens have led to their wider application to nonmalignant conditions.[2] Because most of the data for reduced-intensity preparative regimens are derived from older patients or those with comorbid conditions, they cannot be compared with data for myeloablative preparative regimens.[82] It is unclear if reduced-intensity preparative regimens improve long-term survival of patients with malignant or nonmalignant diseases who are younger or without comorbid conditions. Prospective controlled trials are needed with stratification based on comorbidities, disease characteristics, pretransplant therapy, and hematopoietic stem cell source.[82]

There is a paucity of data regarding the optimal source of hematopoietic stem cells after reduced-intensity preparative regimens. Most case series have combined data from PBPC and marrow grafts. But some data suggest that, compared to bone marrow grafts, PBPC is associated with quicker engraftment, earlier T-cell chimerism, longer progression-free survival, and a lower risk of graft rejection.[83,84]

B.S. is young and healthy enough to receive a myeloablative allogeneic HCT. Presently, reduced-intensity HCT is only indicated as first-line therapy for patients ineligible for myleoablative regimens due to age, extensive prior treatments, or other contraindications. It is not an option for B.S.

Post-transplantation Immunosuppressive Therapy

CASE 101-2, QUESTION 7: What is the rationale for immunosuppressive therapy after an allogeneic HCT? What is recommended for B.S.?

After infusion of hematopoietic stem cells, immunosuppressive therapy is administered to prevent or minimize GVHD. Patients receiving syngeneic transplants or a T-cell-depleted histocompatible allogeneic transplant generally do not receive post-transplantation immunosuppressive therapy. In syngeneic transplantation, the donor and the patient are genetically identical, and GVHD should not be elicited. In T-cell-depleted transplantation, the volume of donor T cells infused into the patient is usually insufficient to elicit significant GVHD.[70,85] Numerous immunosuppressive agents given alone or in combination have been evaluated for the prevention of GVHD. Commonly used regimens after myeloablative HCT include cyclosporine or tacrolimus administered with a short course of low-dose methotrexate.[86] Graft-versus-host disease (GVHD) prophylaxis varies in reduced-intensity protocols and can be found in Table 101-5.[87] Corticosteroids may also be used to prevent GVHD, but they are more commonly used to treat GVHD. In allogeneic HCT recipients without GVHD, immunosuppressive therapy is slowly tapered and discontinued over the course of 6 months to 1 year. Over time, the immunologically active tissue between host and recipient become tolerant of one another and cease recognizing the other as foreign, negating the need for immunosuppression. In contrast, solid organ transplant recipients usually continue immunosuppressive therapy for the duration of the recipient's life.

In patients without a matched related or unrelated donor who undergo HCT with a haploidentical donor, the use of cyclophosphamide posthematopoietic stem cell infusion may be used. The cyclophosphamide is typically given approximately 4 days after HCT. It has been shown that the cyclophosphamide does not affect the hematopoietic stem cells but does exert its effect on alloreactive T cells, thereby reducing the risk of GVHD development.[88] Current trials are ongoing to assess the usefulness of this approach.

B.S. is receiving a myeloablative preparative regimen with allogeneic transplant and will receive cyclosporine administered for 6 months, followed by a taper, with a short course of methotrexate 15 mg/m^2 on day +1 and 10 mg/m^2 on day +3, +6, and +11 for post-transplant immunosuppression. This combination regimen will lower the risk of GVHD. Assuming B.S. does not experience any serious complications, he will likely be immunosuppressant free by 9 months post-transplant. The cyclosporine will require therapeutic drug monitoring.

Table 101-5
Common Reduced-Intensity Preparative or Nonmyeloablative Regimens and Post-grafting Immunosuppresion[102]

Preparative Regimens	Postgraft Immunosuppression
Fludarabine 30 mg/m^2/day IV on 3 consecutive days (−4, −3, −2), TBI 2 Gy as single fraction on day 0	Cyclosporine 6.25 mg/kg PO BID, days −3 to day +100 with taper from day +100 to +180
Fludarabine 25 mg/m^2/day IV for 5 days and melphalan 90 mg/m^2/d IV for 2 days	Mycophenolate mofetil 15 mg/kg PO BID or TID, day +0 to +40 with taper from day +40 to +90
Fludarabine 25–30 mg/m^2/day IV for 3–5 days, busulfan ≤9 mg/kg/total dose	Tacrolimus to maintain trough blood concentration of 5–10 ng/mL with methotrexate 5 mg/m^2/day IV days +1, +3, +6, +11

BID, 2 times a day; IV, intravenous; PO, orally; TBI, total body irradiation; TID, 3 times a day.

Comparison of Supportive-Care Strategies Between Autologous and Allogeneic Myeloablative Hematopoietic Stem Cell Transplantation

CASE 101-2, QUESTION 8: How do supportive-care strategies used for myeloablative preparative regimens with an autologous graft differ from an allogeneic graft? What supportive care will B.S. likely require?

Supportive-care strategies common to patients receiving a myeloablative preparative regimen, regardless of whether they have received an autologous or allogeneic HCT, include use of indwelling central venous catheters; blood product support; and pharmacologic management of chemotherapy-induced nausea and vomiting, mucositis, and pain. These similarities are a function of the side effects of a myeloablative preparative regimen.

Because of the different needs for immunosuppression with an autologous and allogeneic HCT, the supportive care differs. Allogeneic HCT patients experience an initial period of pancytopenia followed by a more prolonged period of immunosuppression, which substantially increases the risk of bacterial infections, but more importantly, fungal, viral, and other opportunistic infections.[4] The risk of infection increases as additional immunosuppressive therapy is incorporated to prevent or treat GVHD. Supportive strategies designed to minimize infection during immunosuppression are essential after allogeneic HCT (see Infectious Complications section).

B.S. received a myeloablative allogeneic transplant; therefore, he will have a central venous catheter inserted at admission. He will most likely require multiple RBC and platelet transfusions until engraftment occurs. He is at increased risk of infection because he will be immunosuppressed for months after the transplant. Also, if he were to develop GVHD, additional supportive care would be required. GVHD prophylaxis with cyclosporine and methotrexate will place him at risk for additional drug-related toxicities that will require monitoring. Had he received an autologous transplant the duration of neutropenia would be less, no immunosuppressive medications would be required, and the risk of developing complications from GVHD would have been avoided.

Comparison of Supportive-Care Strategies Between Allogeneic Myeloablative and Nonmyeloablative Hematopoietic Cell Transplantation

CASE 101-2, QUESTION 9: How do supportive-care strategies used for myeloablative and nonmyeloablative preparative regimens with an allogeneic graft differ?

A direct comparison of the toxicities between a myeloablative and nonmyeloablative preparative regimen is difficult because the latter is offered only to patients who are not candidates for myeloablative allogeneic HCT. The preparative regimens differ substantially in terms of the chemotherapy agents used (Tables 101-3 and 101-5) and the degree of myelosuppression. Nonmyeloablative HCT may have a different time pattern for infectious complications but there is a similar incidence and severity of acute GVHD. This makes comparisons between the preparative regimens challenging because of the differences in the pre-HCT health of the recipients.[78] Clinical research is focusing on designing optimal preparative regimens with acceptable efficacy and toxicity. Thus, as compared to myeloablative HCT, the preparative regimens and immunosuppression used after hematopoietic stem cell infusion are more variable for reduced-intensity and nonmyeloablative HCT.

COMPLICATIONS ASSOCIATED WITH HEMATOPOIETIC CELL TRANSPLANTATION

CASE 101-3

QUESTION 1: K.M. is a 36-year-old woman with CML in accelerated phase. After her initial diagnosis, a successful search for an unrelated 6/6 HLA-matched allogeneic donor was conducted. K.M. is being admitted for myeloablative allogeneic PBPCT. Orders for K.M.'s preparative regimen are written as follows: busulfan, 16 mg/kg total dose to be administered over 4 days (1 mg/kg/dose orally [PO] every 6 hours for 16 doses, days −7, −6, −5, and −4). Cyclophosphamide 60 mg/kg/day IV to be administered on days −3 and −2. Day −1 is a "rest" day, followed by infusion of PBPC on day 0. What toxicities associated with myeloablative preparative regimen should be anticipated in K.M.? Are they similar to those anticipated after standard-dose chemotherapy?

Myelosuppression is a frequent dose-limiting toxicity for chemotherapy when administered in conventional doses used to treat cancer. However, because myelosuppression is circumvented with hematopoietic rescue in the case of patients receiving HCT, the dose-limiting toxicities of these myeloablative preparative regimens are nonhematologic (i.e., extramedullary) in nature. The toxicities vary with the preparative regimen used. Most patients undergoing HCT experience toxicities commonly associated with chemotherapy, such as alopecia, mucositis, chemotherapy-induced nausea and vomiting, infertility, and pulmonary toxicity (see Chapter 94, Adverse Effects of Chemotherapy and Targeted Agents). However, these drug-related toxicities are magnified in the HCT population.

Table 101-4 depicts a range of toxicities that can occur after myeloablative preparative regimen for HCT, and Figure 101-2 depicts the time course for complications after HCT. Selected toxicities are discussed in the following sections.

Busulfan Seizures

CASE 101-3, QUESTION 2: In addition to her preparative regimen, the following supportive-care agents and monitoring parameters are prescribed for K.M.: on the day of admission (day −8), administer levetiracetam 500 mg PO twice daily from days −8 to −3. Busulfan pharmacokinetic blood sampling is to occur after dose 1 to a target busulfan concentration at steady state (C_{SS}) greater than 900 ng/mL. Begin normal saline hydration 3,000 mL/m^2/day 4 hours before cyclophosphamide and continue for 24 hours after the last cyclophosphamide dose. Mesna is to be given concurrently with cyclophosphamide as 10% of the cyclophosphamide dose administered intravenously 30 minutes before starting the cyclophosphamide dose, then as 100% of cyclophosphamide dose administered as a continuous IV infusion for 24 hours after

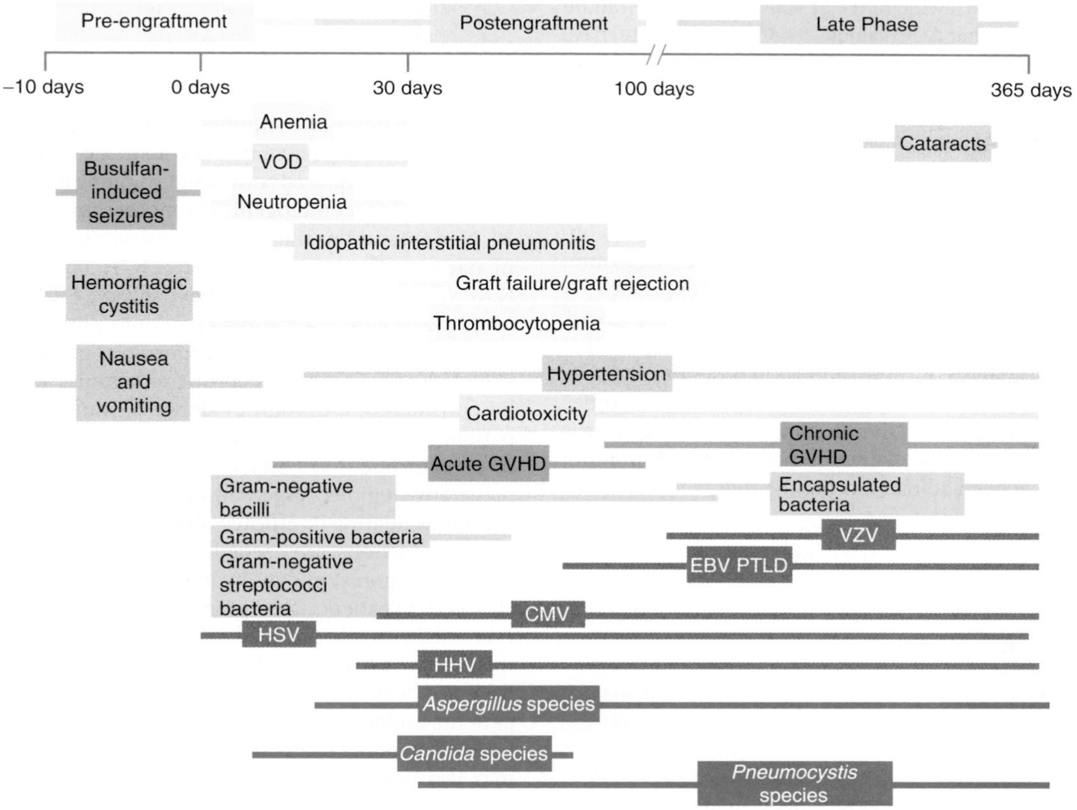

Figure 101-2 Complications after hematopoietic stem cell transplantation (HCT) by time for patients undergoing myeloablative allogeneic HCT only. CMV, cytomegalovirus; EBV, Epstein-Barr virus; GVHD, graft-versus-host disease; HHV, human herpes virus; HSV, herpes simplex virus; PTLD, post-transplantation lymphoproliferative disease; VOD, veno-occlusive disease; VZV, varicella-zoster virus.

each dose of cyclophosphamide. Beginning on day −5, weigh patient twice daily, check fluid input and urinary output every 4 hours, and monitor urine for RBCs daily until 24 hours after the last cyclophosphamide dose. If urine output drops below 300 mL for 2 hours, administer an IV bolus of 250 mL normal saline and give furosemide 10 mg/m^2, not to exceed 20 mg IV. What is the rationale for these supportive-care therapies and monitoring parameters prescribed for K.M. as they relate to busulfan therapy?

Seizures occur in approximately 10% of patients receiving high-dose busulfan in HCT preparative regimens. Busulfan is highly lipophilic and readily crosses the blood–brain barrier with an average cerebrospinal fluid:plasma ratio of 1 or higher. Seizures are probably a direct neurotoxic effect[89]; therefore, seizure prophylaxis is used. Many HCT centers have moved from phenytoin to levetiracetam for seizure prophylaxis, although benzodiazepines (e.g., lorazepam or clonazepam) also have been used.[90] Seizure prophylaxis is started at least 12 hours before the first busulfan dose and is usually discontinued 24 to 48 hours after administering the last busulfan dose. Seizures can occur despite the use of seizure prophylaxis, but they usually do not result in permanent neurologic deficits.

Adaptive Dosing of Busulfan

CASE 101-3, QUESTION 3: What dosing strategies can be used to minimize busulfan toxicities?

Intravenous busulfan is commonly used in combination with cyclophosphamide as a preparative regimen before allogeneic HCT for CML. The FDA-approved dose is 0.8 mg/kg IV every 6 hours for 16 doses, which is similar to the oral busulfan dose of 1 mg/kg, assuming a fraction absorbed of 90%.[91] Intravenous busulfan, at 0.8 mg/kg of actual body weight, produces an average AUC of 1,200 μM/minute, within a wide range of 900 to 1,500 μM/minute in 80% of patients.[92] Higher AUC values (>1,500 μM/minute) have been associated with an increased risk of developing veno-occlusive disease (VOD) of the liver; therefore, monitoring of busulfan AUC is warranted. Target AUCs are commonly between 900 and 1,350 μM/minute after the first dose. This minimizes the risk of VOD and graft failure and minimizes the risk of disease recurrence.[93] (See Case 101-3, Questions 7–9 for information on VOD.)

To minimize adverse events from IV busulfan, an AUC is obtained with the first dose of busulfan to analyze K.M.'s exposure. Samples are drawn at the end of the 2-hour infusion, then 1, 2, and 4 hours after the first sample. Many centers are not capable of analyzing IV busulfan levels; therefore, prior arrangements must be made for timely analysis of these samples in order to adjust the dose after the second or third dose, if needed. K.M.'s AUC comes back 12 hours later at 1,225 μM/minute and, therefore, her dose is not changed. Had the AUC been greater than 1,350 μM/minute; her dose could have been adjusted using the following formula:

$$\text{Adjusted dose (mg)} = \text{Actual Dose (mg)} \times \text{Target AUC } (\mu M/\text{min}) / \text{Actual AUC } (\mu M/\text{min}) \quad \text{(Eq. 101-1)}$$

Hemorrhagic Cystitis

CASE 101-3, QUESTION 4: What is the rationale for these supportive-care therapies and monitoring parameters prescribed for K.M. as they relate to cyclophosphamide therapy?

In HCT patients receiving cyclophosphamide, moderate-to-severe hemorrhagic cystitis occurs in 4% to 20% of patients receiving hydration alone.[94] Development of hemorrhagic cystitis is thought to be due to the bladder toxin acrolein, a metabolite of cyclophosphamide.[95] The chemoprotectant mesna donates free thiol groups which bind acrolein and reduce its toxicity. The American Society of Clinical Oncology (ASCO) Guidelines for the Use of Chemotherapy and Radiotherapy Protectants recommends the use of mesna plus saline diuresis or forced saline diuresis to lower the incidence of urothelial toxicity with high-dose cyclophosphamide in the setting of HCT.[96] It is important to note that hematuria or hemorrhagic cystitis can occur despite the use of any of these methods.

The optimal mesna dose with high-dose cyclophosphamide in preparation for myeloablative HCT is unknown. A variety of different regimens have been used, including intermittent bolus dosing (mesna dose 20%–40% of cyclophosphamide dose, administered for up to five doses) or continuous infusion regimens (mesna dose 80%–160% of cyclophosphamide dose).[94,97,98] Mesna should be continued for 24 to 48 hours after the last cyclophosphamide dose, such that mesna is present within the bladder at the same time as the urotoxic metabolite acrolein. After IV administration of mesna, most of it (i.e., 60%–100%) is excreted within the urine over the course of 4 hours.[99] Cyclophosphamide has an average half-life of 7 hours after administration of 60 mg/kg,[100] and acrolein may be present within the urine for 24 to 48 hours after cyclophosphamide administration.[101]

Thus, K.M. is receiving hydration with normal saline and mesna, administered as a continuous infusion, to minimize her risk of hemorrhagic cystitis due to cyclophosphamide. K.M. should be monitored for any RBCs present in the urine, along with her urinary output, to allow for rapid intervention if hemorrhagic cystitis occurs.

Chemotherapy-Induced Gastrointestinal Effects

CASE 101-3, QUESTION 5: What other end-organ toxicities must be watched for? Should any medications be ordered for K.M. to prevent and treat the gastrointestinal (GI) effects associated with myeloablative therapy?

The high doses of chemotherapy in preparative regimens cause most patients to be nauseated and anorexic until day +10 to +15. Chemotherapy-induced nausea and vomiting in HCT recipients can be due to highly emetogenic chemotherapy agents (see Chapter 22, Nausea and Vomiting), TBI administration, and poor control of nausea and vomiting prior to HCT. Thus, patients such as K.M. who are undergoing a myeloablative HCT should be given prophylaxis with a serotonin antagonist plus a corticosteroid.[102]

American Society of Clinical Oncology guidelines state that the use of the neurokinin receptor-1 antagonist, aprepitant, should be considered, although evidence to support its use in HCT patients is lacking.[102] Because aprepitant is a moderate inhibitor of cytochrome P-450 3A4, it may theoretically interact with the preparative regimen, especially cyclophosphamide. Well-controlled studies evaluating its efficacy, along with its potential for causing drug interactions, are needed.[102] Some data suggest that the serotonin antagonist ondansetron may increase cyclophosphamide clearance in patients undergoing a myeloablative HCT.[103,104] However, further work is needed to identify the clinical implications of this finding because, to date, cyclophosphamide concentrations have not been consistently associated with clinical outcomes in patients undergoing a myeloablative HCT.[19,91]

Most patients receiving a myeloablative preparative regimen may also experience mucositis due to its effects on rapidly dividing cells of the oral epithelium. The use of methotrexate as GVHD prophylaxis also contributes to mucositis.[105] Oral mucositis may also contribute to the development of nausea and anorexia.

In severe cases, parenteral opioid analgesics for pain relief[106] and total parenteral nutrition (TPN) may be needed. Because mucositis can be worsened by superinfection, good oral hygiene should be practiced. Soft toothbrushes should be used and replaced often.[107] Oral mucositis can be decreased with the use of recombinant human keratinocyte growth factor palifermin. The Multinational Association of Supportive Care in Cancer and International Society for Oral Oncology Guidelines recommend palifermin to prevent mucositis for patients with hematologic malignancies receiving myeloablative chemotherapy and TBI with autologous HCT. Palifermin 60 mcg/kg/day is given for 3 days immediately prior to administering the preparative regimen and for 3 days after infusion of the hematopoietic stem cell graft (i.e., days 0, +1, +2).[108] In these patients, palifermin lowered the incidence and average duration of clinically meaningful oral mucositis. The incidence of blood-borne infections and the use of parenteral opioids were also diminished in patients using palifermin.[108]

Myelosuppression and Growth Factor Use

CASE 101-3, QUESTION 6: An order is written to begin filgrastim on day +5 and to continue administration until the ANC has recovered to 500/μL for 2 consecutive days. Is this therapy appropriate for K.M.?

The use of hematopoietic growth factors after infusion of allogeneic PBPC is controversial and is not recommended by ASCO Guidelines.[14] Administration of hematopoietic growth factors after allogeneic graft infusion decreases the duration of neutropenia, but has not been demonstrated to decrease cost, length of hospitalization, or antibiotic use. Hematopoietic growth factor administration may increase the incidence of severe GVHD and lower survival.[109] K.M. is receiving an allogeneic PBPC graft and thus should not receive filgrastim.

Sinusoidal Obstructive Syndrome (SOS)/Veno-Occlusive Disease of the Liver

CASE 101-3, QUESTION 7: K.M.'s pretransplantation admission laboratory values are within normal limits. Her weight on admission is 80 kg. During the first 5 days after marrow infusion, K.M.'s weight begins to increase by approximately 0.5 kg/day, her inputs exceed her outputs by about 500 to 1,000 mL/day, and she is mildly febrile with an axillary temperature of 38°C. Blood and urine cultures are all negative. On day +6, her weight is 85 kg. Laboratory values on day +7 are significant for the following:

Total bilirubin, 1.5 mg/dL
Aspartate aminotransferase (AST), 40 units/L
Alkaline phosphatase, 120 units/L

By day +10, K.M. is complaining of mid-epigastric, right upper quadrant pain, and a liver that is tender to palpation. During the next few days, K.M. begins to look icteric. Her liver function tests continue to rise slowly, until day +18 when they reach the following peak values:

Total bilirubin, 5 mg/dL
AST, 150 units/L
Alkaline phosphatase, 180 units/L

On day +18, K.M.'s weight is 90 kg. "Rule out SOS of the liver" is included on her problem list in the medical record. What is SOS?

Sinusoidal obstructive syndrome (SOS), formerly known as VOD, is a syndrome consisting of fluid retention, right upper quadrant pain, and hyperbilirubinemia. In severe cases, it results in renal failure, encephalopathy, multiorgan failure, and ultimately may result in death. The incidence of SOS/VOD varies depending on the definition used to diagnose the syndrome; however, it is most commonly associated with high-dose chemotherapy with HCT. It has been reported to occur in 5% to 55% of patients undergoing myeloablative HCT.[110,111] The major risk factor for the development of SOS/VOD is high-dose chemotherapy associated with myeloablative transplants. Preparative regimens including busulfan, cyclophosphamide, and/or TBI greater than 13.2 Gy have been associated with higher SOS/VOD rates.[19,112] Patient-specific factors such as older age, impaired performance status, and advanced disease have also been reported to increase SOS/VOD risk.

Although the exact pathophysiology underlying the development of SOS/VOD is not fully understood, it is known that damage to the sinusoidal endothelial cells in the liver is the initial insult which initiates the process. Damage continues and leads to sloughing of the endothelial lining of the sinusoids ultimately resulting in embolism and obstruction of sinusoidal flow.[113] This obstruction of flow within the liver contributes to postsinusoidal portal hypertension and worsening liver dysfunction, usually manifested by increased bilirubin and ascites.

CLINICAL PRESENTATION AND DIAGNOSIS

CASE 101-3, QUESTION 8: What signs and symptoms in K.M. are consistent with a diagnosis of SOS/VOD?

The initial signs and symptoms of SOS/VOD can occur anytime within the first 15 to 30 days post-transplant. Insidious weight gain exceeding 5% of baseline may be one of the first manifestations of impending SOS/VOD, occurring in more than 90% of patients within 3 to 6 days after marrow infusion.[111] Weight gain is caused by sodium and water retention, as evidenced by decreased renal sodium excretion. New onset of transfusion refractory thrombocytopenia may also be an early sign of impending SOS/VOD. Hyperbilirubinemia, which also occurs in virtually all patients, follows the onset of weight gain and usually appears within 10 days after hematopoietic stem cell infusion. Other liver function test abnormalities usually occur after hyperbilirubinemia and include elevations in AST and alkaline phosphatase. Ascites, right upper quadrant pain, and encephalopathy lag behind changes in liver function tests and develop within 10 to 15 days after infusion of hematopoietic stem cells.[111]

Although liver biopsy is the gold standard for diagnosis of SOS/VOD, its use is limited due to the risk of bleeding during the procedure. Other noninvasive criteria have been developed to help diagnosis SOS/VOD after HCT. Two sets of clinical criteria call for an evaluation of hyperbilirubinemia, ascites/weight gain, and right upper quadrant pain not attributable to other causes such as medications, acute GVHD, or infection.[111,114] Along with these criteria, ultrasound may be useful in determining whether there is reversed hepatic venous flow and to confirm ascites and/or hepatomegaly.

CASE 101-3, QUESTION 9: What is the likelihood that K.M. will recover from her SOS/VOD? How should she be treated?

There is no standard treatment for SOS/VOD although many patients with SOS/VOD (70%–85%) spontaneously recover. Preventive measures look to control patient risk factors, and pharmacologic prevention strategies have also been used. Patient-specific risk factors are often not reversible; however, selection of appropriate preparative regimens such as nonmyeloablative regimens, avoidance of concomitant hepatotoxic drugs, use of fractionated TBI, and the use of adaptive busulfan dosing may reduce risk. Preventive medications have also been investigated. The use of prophylactic heparin has shown varied results in clinical trials; therefore, its use is still controversial.[115] The data for the use of ursodeoxycholic acid are also inconclusive. However, some trials have shown a benefit in reducing the incidence of SOS/VOD with its use. According to one trial, patients who received ursodeoxycholic acid were shown to have decreased hepatotoxicity, less acute GVHD, and better survival.[116]

Other treatments consist of supportive-care measures such as management of sodium and water balance, and paracentesis, in severe cases, for ascites that is associated with pain and pulmonary compromise.[105] Volume expanders such as albumin and colloids may be used to maintain intravascular volume, spironolactone may be used to minimize extravascular fluid accumulation, and protein restriction and lactulose may be used if encephalopathy develops. Unfortunately, improved outcomes with these measures have not been confirmed. In patients with severe SOS/VOD and multiorgan failure, available treatment options are limited. Thrombolytic therapy with recombinant human tissue plasminogen activator and heparin have had mixed results in terms of efficacy and can cause fatal intracerebral or pulmonary bleeding.[105] Defibrotide, an investigational drug, has shown promising results in the treatment of SOS/VOD.[117–119] Defibrotide, a ribonucleotide, has antithrombotic, anti-ischemic, and thrombolytic activity without producing significant systemic anticoagulation. In a compassionate use trial of 88 patients with severe SOS/VOD and associated organ dysfunction, 36% of patients had complete resolution of SOS/VOD and 35% survived past day 100 after HCT.[119]

Although the use of defibrotide in treating SOS/VOD appears to be effective, little is known about whether prophylactic defibrotide could be beneficial in high-risk patients. Corbacioglu et al. explored this question in children with malignant infantile osteopetrosis undergoing stem cell transplantation. Previously 7/11 or 63.6% ($n = 20$) of the children in their center between 1996 and 2001 experienced SOS/VOD. Defibrotide prophylaxis was initiated in nine consecutive patients between 2001 and 2005 and in this group 1/9 (11.1%) was diagnosed with moderate SOS/VOD, suggesting a significant benefit from prophylactic defibrotide. To further explore this question, a US National Institutes of Health-sponsored prospective randomized trial has been undertaken to answer the question as to whether prophylactic defibrotide is superior to therapeutic defibrotide in children at high risk for experiencing SOS/VOD during stem cell transplantation.[120]

Because K.M. does not meet the criteria for severe SOS/VOD, she should be managed conservatively with fluid restriction and spironolactone for fluid diuresis. Her signs and symptoms should resolve during the next 2 weeks. Because she has mild SOS/VOD, she is likely to recover completely without sequelae.

Graft Rejection

CASE 101-4

QUESTION 1: E.R. is a 65-year-old woman diagnosed with myelodysplastic syndrome. Past medical history is significant for type I diabetes and renal dysfunction. After her initial diagnosis, a search for a completely HLA-matched unrelated donor was conducted. A donor was found in the National Marrow Donor Registry and E.R. will receive a nonmyeloablative allogeneic HCT using bone marrow from an unrelated male donor. E.R.'s preparative regimen is as follows: fludarabine 30 mg/m^2/day on days −4, −3 and −2 and 2 Gy TBI on the day of marrow infusion with post-transplant cyclosporine and mycophenolate mofetil. It is now day +28 and E.R.'s CBC shows the following:

WBC count, 500 cells/μL
Differential, no granulocytes or monocytes detected
Platelets, 100,000/μL
Hematocrit (Hct), 30%
Donor T-cell chimerism is <5%. What is E.R. experiencing and how should she be treated?

Reduced-intensity regimens typically consist of fludarabine in combination with an alkylating agent or low-dose TBI (Fig. 101-3). With the nonmyeloablative fludarabine/TBI regimen, there is minimal neutropenia, thrombocytopenia, and other nonhematologic toxicities.[2] Engraftment is usually evident within the first 30 days in patients receiving a nonmyeloablative preparative regimen; however, rejection can occur after initial engraftment.[121] Mixed chimerism, a state where both host and donor cells coexist, generally develops after nonmyeloablative HCT. E.R. has low donor T-cell chimerism on day +28, placing her at high risk of graft rejection.

Graft rejection occurs particularly after nonmyeloablative allogeneic HCT. A delicate balance exists between host and donor effector cells. This is established with myelosuppressive chemotherapy and immunosuppressants to decrease the risk of excessive host-versus-graft effects that could lead to graft rejection. The incidence of graft rejection is higher in patients with aplastic anemia and in patients undergoing HCT with histoincompatible marrow or T-cell-depleted marrow. There are limited therapeutic options for the treatment of graft rejection. A second HCT is the most definitive therapy, assuming donor cells are available, although the toxicities are formidable.[122] In patients receiving myeloablative allogeneic HCT, graft rejection is best managed with immunosuppressants such as ATG. In patients receiving a reduced-intensity regimen, graft rejection may require a second HCT.

E.R. received nonmyeloablative conditioning, and thus, she should have mixed chimerism post-transplant; however, she has fewer than 5% donor T cells. Current research is focusing on quantitative chimerism monitoring, specifically evaluating the percent donor chimerism, which may be used as a tool with which to base clinical interventions.[80] Donor chimerism is evaluated in different cell types (e.g., T cells, NK cells, granulocytes) although the cell type most predictive of outcome is not known. The changes in the percent donor chimerism over time post-transplant, termed "engraftment kinetics," are influenced by several factors such as type of HCT conditioning, stem cell source, and intensity of postgrafting immunosuppression.[80,123] A balance between the recipient's and donor's cells is needed to maximize the GVT effect, which lowers the risk of relapse while minimizing the risk of GVHD.[80,123] Based on E.R.'s state of chimerism, she will not benefit from the GVT effect due to the lack of the donor's cytotoxic T lymphocytes that suppress the recipient's malignancy.

E.R. is at high risk of graft rejection and therefore may not benefit from the transplant. A trial of discontinuing cyclosporine and mycophenolate mofetil, in an attempt to shift the balance toward donor graft growth and away from recipient T-cell growth, is an option. E.R.'s T-cell chimerism should be monitored periodically and hematopoietic function should be monitored with daily CBC and a bone marrow biopsy as clinically indicated.

GRAFT-VERSUS-HOST DISEASE

Graft-versus-host disease is caused by activation of donor lymphocytes, leading to immune-mediated damage to the recipient. Histocompatibility differences between donor and recipient

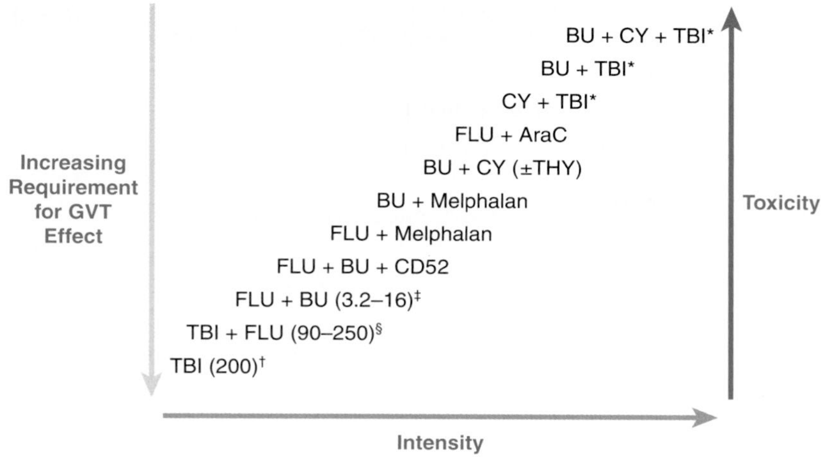

Figure 101-3 Partial spectrum of preparative regimens of various intensities, their impact on toxicity, and their dependence on graft-versus-tumor (GVT) effects for success of hematopoietic stem cell transplantation. AraC, cytarabine; BU, busulfan; CD52, anti-CD52 antibody (alemtuzumab); CY, cyclophosphamide; FLU, fludarabine; TBI, total body irradiation; THY, thymoglobulin. *TBI >1,200 cGy; †200 cGy; ‡3.2 to 16 mg/kg; §90 to 250 mg/m². (Adapted from Deeg HJ et al. Optimization of allogeneic transplant conditioning: not the time for dogma. *Leukemia*. 2006;20:1701, with permission.)

necessitate post-transplantation immunosuppression after allogeneic HCT because considerable morbidity and mortality are associated with graft rejection and GVHD. Therefore, immunosuppression or GVHD prophylaxis is used after allogeneic HCT. However, because allogeneic transplantation offers the potential for a GVT effect in which immune effector cells from the donor recognize and eliminate residual tumor in the recipient, research is focusing on immune suppression manipulations that allow sufficient GVT effects while not increasing the risk of graft rejection and GVHD.[124]

Graft-versus-host disease is the most important complication of allogeneic HCT and limits the use of this lifesaving treatment in patients without histocompatible donors.[2,125] GVHD can occur after allogeneic HCT, regardless of the preparative regimen used. The pathophysiology of GVHD is not completely understood, but the current view of its development is described by a three-step process, including (a) the preparative regimen causing tissue damage and release of inflammatory cytokines into the circulation; (b) recipient and donor antigen presenting cells and inflammatory cytokines triggering activation of donor-derived T cells; and (c) activated donor T cells mediating cytotoxicity through a variety of mechanisms, which leads to tissue damage characteristic of acute GVHD (aGVHD).[126]

Graft-versus-host disease has traditionally been divided into two forms (i.e., acute or chronic) based on time points and clinical manifestations. Acute GVHD, defined as occurring during the first 100 days post-transplant, damages the skin, GI tract, and liver.[2] In contrast, chronic GVHD (cGVHD) may affect almost any organ system, closely resembles several autoimmune diseases, and occurs after day 100. With the introduction of nonmyeloablative HCT, the time course of GVHD has shifted and a late-onset aGVHD occurring after day 100 is possible; however, in these individuals, acute and chronic GVHD symptoms may both be present. As such, consensus criteria developed by The National Institutes of Health have classified GVHD based on clinical manifestations and not time after HCT.[127]

The majority of the data regarding the prevention and treatment of GVHD have been obtained after myeloablative preparative regimens. Therefore, the subsequent section refers only to trials conducted in recipients of a myeloablative allogeneic HCT.

Acute Graft-versus-Host Disease

RISK FACTORS

CASE 101-5

QUESTION 1: M.P., a 22-year-old, 70-kg man, undergoes a one-antigen mismatched allogeneic HCT from his sister for the diagnosis of Philadelphia chromosome-positive (Ph⁺) AML. After a myeloablative preparative regimen of CY/TBI, the following immunosuppressive regimen is ordered: cyclosporine 2.5 mg/kg every 12 hours from day −3 until tolerating oral medications, then switch to cyclosporine 4 mg/kg PO every 12 hours until day +50. Methotrexate 15 mg/m² IV on day +1, then 10 mg/m² on days +3, +6, and +11. What factors are associated with an increased risk of acute GVHD?

The single most important factor associated with the development of GVHD is the degree of histocompatibility between donor and recipient.[2] Clinically relevant grade II–IV acute GVHD occurs in 20% to 50% of HLA-matched sibling grafts and 50% to 80% of HLA-mismatched sibling or HLA-identical unrelated donors.[128] The onset of aGVHD is earlier and severity is increased in mismatched grafts relative to matched grafts, and also in MUDs relative to matched sibling donors.[41,129] Other factors that increase the risk of experiencing aGVHD include increasing recipient (and possibly donor) age, greater intensity of the preparative regimen, use of PBPC rather than bone marrow, and donor/recipient sex mismatch.[126] Umbilical cord transplants have a lower risk of aGVHD.[130–132]

M.P. is receiving allogeneic bone marrow from a female sibling donor that is mismatched at one HLA antigen. These two factors increase his risk of exhibiting aGVHD. Therefore good immunosuppressive therapy is critical in preventing its development.

CLINICAL PRESENTATION

CASE 101-5, QUESTION 2: On day +14, the time at which engraftment has occurred, M.P. is noted to have a diffuse maculopapular rash on his arms, hands, and front trunk. He does not have diarrhea, and his liver function tests are within normal limits. At the onset of his rash, M.P.'s empiric antibiotics are changed from cefepime to meropenem. Despite the change in antibiotics, M.P.'s rash persists. How is M.P.'s presentation consistent with acute GVHD?

The primary targets of immune-mediated destruction of host tissue by donor lymphocytes in aGVHD are the skin followed by the GI tract (diarrhea) and the liver.[128,133] Acute GVHD of the skin, the most common site of aGVHD, usually manifests as a diffuse maculopapular, pruritic rash that starts on the palms of the hands, soles of the feet, or the face. In more severe cases, skin aGVHD can progress to a generalized total body erythroderma, bullous formation, and skin desquamation.

The earliest symptoms of aGVHD of the GI tract are usually loss of appetite followed by nausea and vomiting.[105] Abdominal

Table 101-6
Modified Glucksberg Grading of Acute Graft-versus-Host Disease

Organ Stage	Skin[a]	Liver	Intestinal Tract[b]
1	Maculopapular rash <25% of body surface	Bilirubin 2–2.9 mg/dL	500–1,000 mL/day diarrhea or biopsy-proven upper GI involvement
2	Maculopapular rash 25%–50% body surface	Bilirubin 3–6 mg/dL	1,000–1,500 mL/day diarrhea
3	Maculopapular rash >50% body surface	Bilirubin 6.1–15 mg/dL	1,500–2,000 mL/day diarrhea
4	Generalized erythroderma with bullae	Bilirubin >15 mg/dL	>2,000 mL/day diarrhea or severe abdominal pain with or without ileus

[a]Extent of rash determined by "rule of nines."
[b]Diarrhea volume applies to adults.
Source: Cutler C, Antin JH. Manifestations and treatment of acute graft-versus-host disease. In: Blume KG et al, eds. *Thomas' Hematopoietic Cell Transplantation*. 4th ed. Malden, MA: Blackwell; 2009:1291.

pain and watery or bloody diarrhea also occur, which can result in electrolyte abnormalities, dehydration, or ileus in severe cases. Liver GVHD usually follows skin and/or GI GVHD. Clinical symptoms of liver GVHD include a gradual rise in total bilirubin, alkaline phosphatase, and hepatic transaminases.[105] Acute GVHD is usually not evident until the time of engraftment, when donor lymphoid elements begin to proliferate. The skin is usually the first organ to be involved. The onset of liver or GI GVHD usually lags behind the onset of skin GVHD by approximately 1 week and infrequently occurs without skin GVHD.

Acute GVHD must be distinguished accurately from other causes of skin, liver, or GI toxicity in the HCT patient. For example, a maculopapular rash, which may occur as a manifestation of an allergic reaction to antibiotics, usually begins on the trunk or upper extremities and is rarely present on the palms of the hands or soles of the feet. Diarrhea can be caused by chemotherapy, radiation, infection, or antibiotic therapy.[105] However, diarrhea caused by the preparative regimen is rarely bloody and usually resolves within 3 to 7 days after discontinuation of drugs and radiation. Diarrhea caused by infectious agents such as *Clostridium difficile* or cytomegalovirus (CMV) should be distinguished from GVHD. Liver GVHD must be distinguished primarily from SOS/VOD and, to a lesser extent, hepatitis induced by drugs, blood products, or parenteral nutrition. Although liver function test abnormalities between these syndromes are similar, liver GVHD is rarely associated with insidious weight gain or right upper quadrant pain.[105] A tissue biopsy of the affected organ in conjunction with clinical evidence is the only way to definitively diagnose aGVHD, though biopsy of the gut or liver is rarely done due to the increased risks associated with thrombocytopenia early in the post-transplant phase. Acute GVHD is associated with characteristic histologic changes to affected organs. A staging system based on clinical criteria is used to grade aGVHD. The severity of organ involvement is determined first (Table 101-6), and then an overall grade is established based on number and extent of involved organs (Table 101-7).

M.P. developed a rash at the time of engraftment that could have been consistent with either an antibiotic-induced rash or aGVHD. Although it was appropriate to change antibiotics, the fact that M.P.'s rash did not improve is suggestive of aGVHD. M.P.'s rash is present on 36% of his body, but because there are no signs of GI or liver involvement at this time, M.P. is likely to have grade I aGVHD (Tables 101-6 and Table 101-7).

Table 101-7
Modified Glucksberg versus International Bone Marrow Transplant Registry Overall Grading of Acute Graft-versus-Host Disease Severity

Organ Stage	Skin	Liver	Gut
Glucksberg Grading			
I—Mild	Stage 1–2	None	None
II—Moderate	Stage 3 or	Stage 1 or	Stage 1
III—Severe		Stage 2–3 or	Stage 2–4
IV—Life-threatening	Stage 4 or	Stage 4	—
IBMTR Grading			
A—Mild	Stage 1	None	None
B—Moderate	Stage 2	Stage 1 or 2	Stage 1 or 2
C—Severe	Stage 3	Stage 3	Stage 3
D—Life-threatening	Stage 4	Stage 4	Stage 4

Source: Cutler C, Antin JH. Manifestations and treatment of acute graft-versus-host disease. In: Blume KG et al, eds. *Thomas' Hematopoietic Cell Transplantation*. 4th ed. Malden, MA: Blackwell; 2009:1291.
IBMTR, International Blood and Marrow Transplant Registry.

IMMUNOSUPPRESSIVE PROPHYLAXIS

Case 101-5, Question 3: Why did M.P. receive prophylactic immunosuppressive therapy with cyclosporine and methotrexate?

Graft-versus-host disease is a leading cause of morbidity and mortality after allogeneic HCT. Without immunosuppression, serious aGVHD would occur in almost every allogeneic HCT recipient.[2] The most common method used to minimize GVHD risk is to administer prophylactic immunosuppressive therapies and most patients receive multi-drug GVHD prophylaxis.

Historically, aGVHD was prevented with single-drug therapy using ATG, cyclophosphamide, methotrexate, or cyclosporine.[134–136] ATG binds nonspecifically to mononuclear cells and depletes hematopoietic progenitor cells in addition to lymphocytes. Consequently, ATG is generally avoided as a prophylactic agent due to the risk of graft failure.[134] The risk of GVHD is greatly reduced by two-drug combination immunosuppression (Table 101-8). Although the most widely published regimen is short-course methotrexate plus cyclosporine,[136] there is no consensus with regard to the most effective regimen. Several randomized clinical trials have compared tacrolimus and short-course methotrexate with cyclosporine plus short-course methotrexate in patients undergoing allogeneic

Table 101-8

Combination Immunosuppression Regimens for Prophylaxis of Acute Graft-versus-Host Disease in Myeloablative Transplant[137]

Drug	Dosing Examples
Cyclosporine/short-term methotrexate	1.5 mg/kg IV or 4 mg/kg (Neoral) PO every 12 hours, days −1 to +50, then taper 5% per week and discontinue by day +180
	Methotrexate 10 mg/m^2 IV, days +3, +6, +11
Tacrolimus/short term	Tacrolimus 0.03 mg/kg/d continuous IV infusion or 0.12 mg/kg/d PO BID
Methotrexate[136]	Methotrexate 15 mg/m^2 IV day +1; 10 mg/m^2 IV, days +3, +6, +11
Cyclosporine/methotrexate/prednisone	Cyclosporine 5 mg/kg/d IV continuous infusion, days –2 to +3, then 3–3.75 mg/kg IV until day +35; then 7 mg/kg/d (Neoral) PO, dose adjusted to cyclosporine concentrations (via radioimmunoassay) of 200–400 ng/mL. Taper by 20% every 2 weeks; then discontinue by day +180
	Methotrexate 15 mg/m^2 IV day +1; 10 mg/m^2 IV days +3, +6
	Methylprednisolone 0.5 mg/kg/day IV day +7 until day +14; then 1 mg/kg/d IV until day +28; then prednisone 0.8 mg/kg/day PO until day +42; then taper slowly and discontinue by day +180

BID, twice a day; IV, intravenous; PO, orally.

HCT using HLA-matched siblings[137,138] and unrelated donors.[86] Recipients of matched sibling grafts treated with tacrolimus had a lower incidence of grade II to IV aGVHD but a similar incidence of cGVHD.[137] Overall survival was lower in the tacrolimus group as a result of more toxic deaths in patients with advanced stage disease; however, a higher number of advanced stage disease patients in the tacrolimus/methotrexate group make the results of this trial somewhat difficult to interpret.[137]

Subsequently, the International Blood and Marrow Transplant Registry conducted a matched control study, which suggested that the survival difference between the two arms of tacrolimus plus short-course methotrexate and cyclosporine plus short-course methotrexate was in fact due to the imbalance in the underlying risk factors.[138] In patients receiving HLA-matched or slightly mismatched unrelated grafts, those given tacrolimus had a lower incidence of grade II to IV aGVHD, a similar incidence of cGVHD, and similar disease-free and overall survival rates.[86] Both regimens are currently used in allogeneic HCT after myeloablative preparative regimens.

More recently, the use of mycophenolate mofetil has been studied in allogeneic transplants with myeloablative conditioning used in combination with cyclosporine. It appears to have a similar incidence of aGVHD and 100-day survival as methotrexate/cyclosporine, yet significantly less severe mucositis and more rapid neutrophil engraftment than the methotrexate/cyclosporine arm.[139,140] Mycophenolate mofetil is now commonly used in clinical practice in combination with cyclosporine or tacrolimus.

M.P. received acute GVHD prophylaxis with a two-drug regimen of short-course methotrexate and cyclosporine, the most common regimen for myeloablative allogeneic conditioning regimens. Using two drugs with different mechanisms of immunosuppression, one blocking the activation of T cells (cyclosporine) and the other (methotrexate) blocking the division and clonal expansion of activated T cells, is more effective in decreasing the likelihood of GVHD than one of these agents alone.

CASE 101-5, QUESTION 4: What principles are used in dosing medications used for acute GVHD prophylaxis?

Although the various combination immunosuppressive regimens vary slightly by drug, dose, and combination, several guidelines are consistent throughout all regimens. First, methotrexate used for prophylaxis of aGVHD is withheld or given in reduced doses if mucositis is severe or the patient experiences excessive fluid retention.[136,141] Fluid retention sites act as a depot for methotrexate accumulation, increasing duration of exposure. Methotrexate for GVHD prophylaxis can delay engraftment, increase the incidence and severity of mucositis, and cause liver function test elevations. The methotrexate dose is reduced in the setting of renal or liver impairment.[136,142]

The calcineurin inhibitors (i.e., cyclosporine, tacrolimus) should be initiated before or immediately after donor cell infusion (day −3 to 0) when used for GVHD prophylaxis. This schedule is recommended because of the known mechanism of action of these agents, which entails blocking the proliferation of cytotoxic T cells by inhibiting production of helper T-cell-derived interleukin-2 (IL-2). Administering cyclosporine before the donor cell infusion allows inhibition of IL-2 secretion to occur before a rejection response has been initiated.

Cyclosporine is usually administered intravenously until the GI toxicity from a myeloablative preparative regimen has resolved (e.g., for 7–21 days).[136] This is because GI effects of the preparative regimen (e.g., chemotherapy-induced nausea and vomiting, diarrhea) and GVHD affect the oral absorption of microemulsion cyclosporine and may result in inconsistent blood concentrations.[143] Most centers use the microemulsion oral formulation (Neoral) or other new generic microemulsion formulations that have improved bioavailability. With the microemulsion oral formulation, an IV to PO dosing ratio of 1:2 or 1:3 is appropriate. The most common ratio used when converting tacrolimus from IV to oral is 1:4. Empiric dose adjustments may be required when patients are receiving concomitant medications (e.g., voriconazole) that affect cytochrome CYP3A4 or P-glycoprotein, which are involved in the metabolism and transport of the calcineurin inhibitors. Thus, careful monitoring for drug interactions with the calcineurin inhibitors is warranted.[144]

The dose of cyclosporine or tacrolimus is adjusted based on serum drug levels and the serum creatinine (SCr) concentration. Although the calcineurin inhibitors do not contribute to myelosuppression, common adverse effects to these agents include electrolyte abnormalities, neurotoxicity, hypertension, and/or nephrotoxicity.[89]

Tapering schedules for GVHD prophylaxis vary widely among institutions. The general goal is to keep calcineurin inhibitor doses stable until day +50 and then slowly taper with the intent of discontinuing all immunosuppressive agents by 6 months after HCT. By this time, immunologic tolerance has developed, and patients no longer require immunosuppressive therapy. This can only be accomplished if the patient is not experiencing GVHD.

ADAPTIVE DOSING OF CALCINEURIN INHIBITORS

CASE 101-5, QUESTION 5: On day +18, a cyclosporine concentration is measured right before the morning dose (trough) and is reported as 392 ng/mL. Why are cyclosporine concentrations being obtained for M.P.?

The role of pharmacokinetic monitoring of the calcineurin inhibitors in HCT patients is not well defined but is commonly performed because of the established pharmacodynamic associations within solid organ transplant recipients. It is standard practice for HCT centers to adjust cyclosporine or tacrolimus doses based on trough blood concentrations.[145] An association between cyclosporine concentrations and aGVHD was not found in early studies; however, other studies have suggested that cyclosporine trough concentrations for 12-hour dosing of 200 to 400 ng/mL in adult patients minimize the risk of aGVHD and the risk of cyclosporine-induced nephrotoxicity.[146–148] For continuously infused cyclosporine, higher target blood concentrations of 300 to 500 ng/mL have been required to prevent GVHD in order to provide an equivalent AUC of exposure to intermittent dosing.[149,150] It is important to note that cyclosporine-induced nephrotoxicity may occur despite low or normal concentrations of cyclosporine and may be a consequence of other drug- or disease-related factors known to influence the development of nephrotoxicity. Additionally, recent studies suggest that trough concentrations do not correlate well with exposure to cyclosporine and that a peak level is better correlated to the $AUC_{(0-12)}$. A peak concentration of greater than 800 ng/mL may be required to prevent GVHD. Despite this, the data are limited and the routine use of peaks for therapeutic drug monitoring is not recommended.[151] Desired tacrolimus trough concentrations are 5 to 15 ng/mL. Tacrolimus concentrations greater than 20 ng/mL have been associated with increased risk of toxicity, primarily nephrotoxicity.[145,152] Adjustments in tacrolimus dosing for increased SCr should be made in a manner similar to that described for cyclosporine.

It is reasonable to adjust M.P.'s doses to maintain cyclosporine trough concentrations between 200 and 400 ng/mL, as in all patients undergoing allogeneic HCT with a myeloablative preparative regimen. Recommendations for dose adjustments should be based on cyclosporine concentrations and SCr level. No standard dosage adjustment schedule exists, but most centers adopt their own standardized approach. M.P. has a normal SCr, and his cyclosporine trough is 392 ng/mL. Therefore, his cyclosporine dose should be maintained and the trough repeated in a few days. It may be repeated sooner if an interacting drug is added or discontinued, or if there are toxicity concerns.

TREATMENT OF ESTABLISHED ACUTE GRAFT-VERSUS-HOST DISEASE

CASE 101-5, QUESTION 6: In the third week post-transplant, M.P. experiences a pruritic rash on his shoulders and neck which spreads to the palms of his hands and looks like a sunburn. On day +19, the suspicion of acute skin GVHD is confirmed by biopsy. On the same day, M.P. develops diarrhea (1,000 mL over 24 hours) and is noted to have a bilirubin of 2.8 mg/dL. He is started on methylprednisolone 1 mg/kg IV every 12 hours. What is the rationale for methylprednisolone therapy in M.P.?

Preventing the development of aGVHD is the most effective way to treat this HCT complication. In patients who develop aGVHD, first-line treatment is a corticosteroid added to their current immune suppression regimen.[126] For this reason, aGVHD and its treatment cause profound immunodeficiency.[2,153] The combination of aGVHD and infectious complications is the leading cause of mortality for allogeneic HCT patients.

The route of corticosteroid administration is determined by the severity of the aGVHD. Those patients with only skin involvement of less than 50% of their body surface area may be treated with topical steroid creams, whereas involvement of other organs, or stage 3 or 4 skin disease, requires systemic corticosteroids. A complete response occurs in up to 25% to 40% of patients, with a lower likelihood of response in more severe cases of aGVHD.[126,153] Patients with mild-to-moderate (grades I–III) aGVHD who respond to initial therapy have a significantly better survival advantage than patients with severe aGVHD who do not respond to initial therapy. Patients who do not respond to corticosteroid therapy or have ongoing severe GVHD usually die from a combination of GVHD and infectious complications.[154]

Corticosteroids used in the treatment of aGVHD are generally tapered based on response. There is no consensus on the optimal method for tapering the corticosteroids,[153] and the tapering rate depends on the patient. Patients who experience aGVHD or who experience flares of existing GVHD during a tapering trial will have their dosages increased or tapered more slowly as tolerated.

Because M.P. had objective evidence of established aGVHD, he was given systemic IV corticosteroids. This was appropriate because single-agent corticosteroids are considered the therapy of choice for established aGVHD.[153] Corticosteroids indirectly halt the progression of immune-mediated destruction of host tissues by blocking macrophage-derived interleukin-1 secretion. Interleukin-1 is a primary stimulus for helper T-cell-induced secretion of IL-2, which in turn is responsible for stimulating proliferation of cytotoxic T lymphocytes. The recommended dosage of methylprednisolone for the treatment of established aGVHD is 1 to 2 mg/kg/day, given intravenously or orally in divided doses, followed by a tapering schedule that is determined by response.[154,155] Trials that compared higher doses of corticosteroids (i.e., 10 mg/kg/day) to 2 mg/kg/day as initial treatment of aGVHD showed no advantage.[156] Monitoring for rash, diarrhea, and bilirubin levels to asses aGVHD response should occur daily.[126] M.P. was receiving cyclosporine for GVHD prophylaxis at the time the aGVHD developed. Although the cyclosporine was not effective in preventing the aGVHD, it is typical for patients to remain on their prophylactic immune suppressants.

A significant portion of patients do not respond to corticosteroids, and they are said to have steroid-refractory GVHD.[126] If aGVHD symptoms worsen during 3 days of treatment and if the skin does not improve by 5 days, it is unlikely that a response will be achieved in a timely manner, and secondary therapy should be considered.[126] Patients with steroid-refractory aGVHD have a poorer prognosis. A variety of medications are being studied for "salvage" or secondary therapy. The salvage therapy depends on the organs affected. For example, phototherapy is used as salvage therapy for skin GVHD, and nonabsorbable corticosteroids are used for GI GVHD. Other options for salvage therapy include ATG, denileukin diftitox, and TNF-α blockers (e.g., infliximab, etanercept).[126,157] The most effective dose, timing, or combination of these salvage therapies is still unknown.

M.P. should be evaluated for response to methylprednisolone after 4 to 7 days. If his aGVHD has improved or stabilized, he should be continued on therapy at this dose for a total of 14 days. If M.P. responds to therapy, his methylprednisolone dose should be tapered slowly over a minimum of 1 month, and he should be monitored for any evidence of recurrent GVHD. If the GVHD flares during his steroid taper as evidenced by worsening skin reactions, increased bilirubin, or increased diarrhea volume, the dose should be increased again until his disease is stable; the subsequent taper should be initiated at a slower rate. If M.P. fails to respond to first-line therapy with methylprednisolone, he should receive salvage therapy.

Chronic Graft-versus-Host Disease

CLINICAL PRESENTATION

CASE 101-5, QUESTION 7: M.P. was successfully treated for his aGVHD, is no longer taking corticosteroids, and is currently tapering off his cyclosporine. On day +200, M.P. comes to clinic for follow-up after a 2-week vacation in Florida. On examination, M.P. is found to have a mild skin rash on his arms and legs, hyperpigmentation of the tissue surrounding the eyes, and white plaque-like lesions in his mouth. He is also complaining of dry eyes. Laboratory tests reveal an increased alkaline phosphatase and total bilirubin concentration. What is the most likely cause of M.P.'s findings?

Chronic GVHD (cGVHD), the most common late complication of allogeneic HCT, occurs in 20% to 70% of patients surviving more than 100 days.[158] Chronic GVHD is a major cause of nonrelapse morbidity and mortality.[2] Risk factors for cGVHD include recipient, donor, and transplant factors. Nonmodifiable recipient risk factors include older age, certain diagnoses (e.g., CML), and lack of an HLA-matched donor. Modifiable factors that may lower the risk of cGVHD include selecting a younger donor, avoiding a multiparous female donor, using umbilical cord blood or a bone marrow graft rather than PBPC, and limiting the $CD34^+$ and T-cell dose infused.[158] Development of aGVHD is a major predictor of cGVHD; 70% to 80% of those with grade II to IV aGVHD go on to develop cGVHD.[158]

Chronic GVHD is not a continuation of aGVHD. Traditionally, the boundary between the two was based on time, but now they are classified based on different clinical symptoms.[158] Signs and symptoms of cGVHD in various organ systems are listed in Table 101-9.

A consensus guideline for the diagnosis and scoring of cGVHD has been published.[127] The diagnosis of cGVHD requires (a) being

Table 101-9
Selected Signs and Symptoms of Chronic Graft-versus-Host Disease

Affected Organ	Diagnostic	Distinctive	Other Features[a]	Seen With Both Acute and Chronic GVHD
Eyes		New-onset dry, gritty, or painful eyes[b]	Photophobia	
		Cicatricial conjunctivitis Keratoconjunctivitis sicca[b]	Periorbital hyperpigmentation	
		Confluent areas of punctuate keratopathy, tear formation, dry eyes, burning, photophobia	Erythema of the eyelids with edema	
Gastrointestinal tract	Esophageal web		Pancreatic insufficiency	Anorexia
	Stricture or stenosis in the upper- to mid-third of the esophagus[c]			Nausea Vomiting Diarrhea Weight loss
				Failure to thrive (infants and children)
Liver				Total bilirubin, alkaline phosphatase >2 × upper limit of normal[c]
Lung	Bronchiolitis obliterans diagnosed with lung biopsy	Bronchiolitis obliterans diagnosed with pulmonary function tests and radiology[b]		Bronchiolitis obliterans organizing pneumonia
Skin	Poikiloderma	Depigmentation	Seat impairment ichthyosis	Erythema
	Lichen planus-like features		Keratosis pilaris	Maculopapular rash Pruritus
	Sclerotic features		Hypopigmentation	
	Morphea-like features		Hyperpigmentation	
	Lichen sclerosus-like features			

Signs and symptoms for hematopoietic and immune differences, as well as for nails; scalp and body hair; mouth; genitalia; muscles, fascia, and joints; and other organs, are also described by Filipovich et al.[152]
[a]Part of chronic GVHD symptomatology if the diagnosis is confirmed.
[b]Diagnosis of chronic GVHD requires biopsy or radiology confirmation (or Schirmer test for eyes).
[c]Infection, drug effects, malignancy, or other causes must be excluded.
GVHD, graft-versus-host disease.

distinct from aGVHD, (b) having at least one diagnostic clinical sign of cGVHD or at least one distinctive manifestation confirmed by pertinent biopsy or other relevant tests, and (c) exclusion of other possible diagnoses. The clinical scoring system uses a numerical value of 0 to 3, with more severe symptoms having a higher number. A global score is calculated by including the number of organs involved and the severity within each affected organ. The global score reflects the expected effect of cGVHD on the patient's performance status and can be used to evaluate whether treatment with systemic immunosuppression is required. The grading and prognosis of cGVHD can define and predict high-risk patient groups.[159]

The signs and symptoms of cGVHD in M.P. include a rash in sun-exposed areas of the skin, hyperpigmentation of tissues surrounding his eyes, white plaque-like lesions in the mouth, dry mucous membranes, and increased alkaline phosphatase and total bilirubin levels. These symptoms appeared after a period of complete resolution of aGVHD and during a taper of the cyclosporine. Thus, M.P. has moderate-involvement, quiescent cGVHD.[127]

PHARMACOLOGIC MANAGEMENT

CASE 101-5, QUESTION 8: M.P. is started on prednisone 1 mg/kg PO daily for the treatment of his chronic GVHD. His cyclosporine taper is stopped, and the dosage is raised to therapeutic concentrations. Is this therapy rational? What other agents are available to treat cGVHD?

There is no specific prophylactic therapy for cGVHD, and the optimal treatment remains controversial. The mainstay of therapy for cGVHD is long-term immunosuppressive therapy. Survival for patients with cGVHD is improved by extended corticosteroid therapy, although there are multiple long-term adverse effects associated with the corticosteroids.[158,160] A typical regimen is prednisone 1 mg/kg/day, administered orally in divided doses for 14 days and then converted slowly to alternate-day therapy by increasing the "on-day" and decreasing the "off-day" dose until a total of 1 mg/kg/day on alternate days is administered.[160] Alternate-day therapy is preferred to minimize adrenocortical suppression. Once therapy is initiated, 1 to 2 months may pass before an improvement in clinical symptoms is noted. Therapy is usually continued for 9 to 12 months and then slowly tapered after signs and symptoms of cGVHD have resolved. The median duration of treatment has been reported to be 23 months.[161] If cGVHD worsens during the tapering or after discontinuation of prednisone, immunosuppressive therapy is restarted. Other potential approaches for patients with refractory cGVHD include mycophenolate mofetil, daclizumab, sirolimus, pentostatin, and extracorporeal photophoresis.[160]

When immunosuppressive therapy is administered for long periods, the patient must be monitored closely for chronic toxicity. Cushingoid effects, aseptic necrosis of the joints, and diabetes can develop with long-term corticosteroid use. Other severe complications include a high incidence of infection with encapsulated organisms and atypical pathogens such as *Pneumocystis jiroveci (P. jiroveci)* pneumonia, CMV, and herpes zoster.

It is reasonable to start M.P. on single-agent prednisone for cGVHD treatment at 1 mg/kg daily for 2 weeks and then convert to every other day as described.

ADJUVANT THERAPIES

CASE 101-5, QUESTION 9: Suggest some adjuvant therapies that should be instituted in a patient like M.P. with chronic GVHD.

Patients who are being treated for cGVHD should receive trimethoprim–sulfamethoxazole for prophylaxis of *P. jiroveci* and encapsulated organisms, such as *Streptococcus pneumoniae* and *Haemophilus influenzae*. Ensuring optimal prophylactic antibiotics in cGVHD patients is critical because infection is the primary cause of death during treatment.[161] Artificial tears and saliva may improve lubrication and decrease the occurrence of cracking and fissures in mucous membranes. Newer therapies such as cyclosporine ophthalmic emulsion and autologous serum tears have provided relief for chronic ocular GVHD.[162] If nutritional intake is poor, consultation with a clinical nutritionist and use of oral nutritional supplementation may be advisable. Patients should be instructed to apply sunscreens to exposed areas whenever prolonged sun exposure is anticipated. Liver function abnormalities have been improved by up to 30% with the use of ursodiol as bile acid displacement therapy.[163–165] Calcium supplements, estrogen replacement, or other anti-osteoporosis agents should be considered in women or other patients at risk for fracture or bone loss while receiving prolonged regimens with immunosuppressant therapy.[166] Patient education regarding the gradual resolution of symptoms such as skin sclerosis, fatigue and muscle weakness, anticipated duration of therapy, and importance of compliance with oral immunosuppressive therapy is essential.

INFECTIOUS COMPLICATIONS

Opportunistic infections are a major cause of morbidity and mortality after myeloablative and nonmyeloablative HCT. There are three general periods of infectious risk (Fig. 101-2). During the early period pre-engraftment, particularly for patients undergoing myeloablative HCT, the primary pathogens are aerobic bacteria, *Candida* spp., and herpes simplex virus (HSV). Chemotherapy-induced mucosal damage creates a portal of entry into the bloodstream for many organisms, such as viridans group *Streptococcus*, *Candida*, and aerobic gram-negative bacteria. Catheter-associated infections have become the leading cause of bacteremia, most notably in the early post-transplant period.[159,161] The routine use of antiviral prophylaxis has decreased the incidence of HSV. Respiratory viruses such as respiratory syncytial virus (RSV), influenza, adenovirus, and parainfluenza are increasingly recognized as pathogens causing pneumonia, particularly during community outbreaks of infection.[167] To reduce potential exposure of HCT recipients to these pathogens, visitors and staff members with signs and symptoms of a viral respiratory illness may not be allowed direct contact with patients.

A potential advantage of reduced-intensity or nonmyeloablative preparative regimens is reduced toxicity of the preparative regimen compared to myeloablative HCT. Reduced-intensity or nonmyeloablative preparative regimens frequently do not result in true neutropenia,[5] and the incidence of mucositis during the early period is reduced.[168] In a matched controlled study, the incidence of bacteremia during the first 30 days post-HCT in the nonmyeloablative recipients was significantly reduced compared to myeloablative recipients.[168] Moreover, nonmyeloablative HCT recipients experienced significantly fewer infections attributable to mucositis during the early period.

The second or middle (Fig. 101-2) period of infectious risk includes the time from engraftment to post-transplant day +100. Pathogens such as CMV, adenovirus, and *Aspergillus* are common. Adenovirus, CMV, *Aspergillus*, and *P. jiroveci* frequently cause interstitial pneumonitis. Patients undergoing reduced-intensity or nonmyeloablative preparative regimens that experience acute GVHD and are treated with corticosteroids have a similar risk of infection during this time period as those undergoing myeloablative HCT.[168]

During the late period (after day +100), the predominant pathogens are the encapsulated bacteria (e.g., *S. pneumoniae*, *H. influenzae*, *Neisseria meningitidis*), fungi/mold, and varicella-zoster virus (VZV). The encapsulated bacteria commonly cause sinopulmonary infections. The risk of infection during this late period is increased in patients with cGVHD as a result of prolonged immunosuppression.

Because of the morbidity associated with opportunistic infection in HCT recipients, optimal pharmacotherapy for prevention and treatment is critical. In 2009, the US Centers for Disease Control and Prevention (CDC) published guidelines for prevention of opportunistic infection in HCT recipients.[4,169] These guidelines were constructed from available data by an expert panel from the CDC, the Infectious Disease Society of America, and the American Society for Blood and Marrow Transplantation. The following discussion incorporates recommendations from the CDC guidelines and also provides information on the pharmacotherapy of opportunistic infections in all types of HCT.

Prevention and Treatment of Bacterial and Fungal Infections

CASE 101-6

QUESTION 1: S.D. is a 26-year-old woman with Ph^+ acute lymphocytic leukemia in first complete remission who is admitted for allogeneic myeloablative HCT. The following orders are written: Admit to a room with a positive-pressure HEPA filter. Flush double-lumen Hickman catheter per protocol. Immunosuppressed patient diet as tolerated. Begin fluconazole 400 mg PO every 24 hours and levofloxacin 500 mg PO every 24 hours on admission. Begin ceftazidime 2 g IV every 8 hours with first fever when ANC is less than 500 cells/μL. Transfuse 2 units of packed RBCs for hematocrit less than 25% and 1 unit of single-donor platelets for platelet count less than 20,000/μL. What is the rationale for these supportive measures?

As a result of disease-related immunosuppression, intensive preparative regimens, and post-transplant immunosuppressive therapy, patients undergoing allogeneic HCT require careful monitoring for regimen-related toxicities and intensive supportive care directed at maintaining adequate blood counts, preventing or treating infection, and providing optimum nutrition.

Placement of a double-lumen or triple-lumen central venous catheter is mandatory in all patients. The need for administration of chemotherapy, blood products, antibiotics, parenteral nutrition, and adjunctive medications over a prolonged period of time precludes the use of peripheral access sites. The use of a central venous catheter allows delivery of maximum concentrations of all medications into a high-flow blood vessel. Administration time is reduced and daily fluid infusion is minimized.

After administration of the preparative regimen and before successful engraftment, allogeneic myeloablative HCT patients undergo a period of pancytopenia lasting from 2 to 6 weeks. During this time, patients may require multiple RBC and platelet transfusions. Packed RBCs and platelets are usually given for a hematocrit less than 25% and a platelet count less than 10,000/μL or 20,000/μL. Transfusions with multiple blood products put patients at risk for blood product-derived infection (e.g., CMV, hepatitis). In addition, sensitization to foreign leukocyte HLA antigens (alloimmunization) may cause immune-mediated thrombocytopenia. Thus, blood product support in the myeloablative allogeneic HCT patient must incorporate strategies that reduce the risk of viral infection and alloimmunization. Effective methods include minimizing the number of pretransplant infusions, using single-donor rather than pooled-donor blood products, irradiating blood products, and filtering blood products with leukocyte reduction filters.

Patients receiving reduced-intensity or nonmyeloablative preparative regimens may or may not experience neutropenia and generally have reduced requirements for blood products. In fact, many centers perform reduced-intensity or nonmyeloablative HCT in the outpatient setting and admit patients to the hospital only for complications requiring more aggressive management.

Several measures are recommended to minimize the risk of infection in autologous and allogeneic myeloablative HCT patients. Private reverse isolation rooms equipped with positive-pressure HEPA filters and adherence to strict handwashing techniques reduce the incidence of bacterial and fungal infections.[4] To reduce exposure to exogenous sources of bacteria in immunosuppressed patients, low microbial diets (Table 101-10) may be instituted on hospital admission, and visitors are prohibited from bringing

Table 101-10
Foods Posing Infection Risk in Neutropenic Patients

High-Risk Foods to Avoid When Neutropenic	Infection Risk
Salad	Gram-negative bacillus including *Pseudomonas aeruginosa* and *Campylobacter*
Tomatoes, radishes, celery, and carrots	*Pseudomonas aeruginosa*
Raw eggs	*Campylobacter jejuni, Salmonella*
Unpasteurized cheeses	*Listeria monocytogenes* Enterococci
Cold, loose meats	*Listeria, Clostridium perfringens, Campylobacter jejuni*
Undercooked meat	*Salmonella, Listeria, Escherichia coli*
Uncooked nuts	*Aspergillus niger, Aspergillus flavus*
Black pepper/uncooked herbs and spices	*Aspergillus* spp.
Raw shellfish/sushi	*Vibrio vulnificus*, Norwalk virus
Bottled water	*Pseudomonas, Cytophaga, Campylobacter*
Prepared foods that are cooked and then eaten chilled	*Listeria*
Ice machines	*P. aeruginosa, Stenotrophomonas maltophilia*

plants or flowers into the patient's room. Patients are encouraged to maintain good oral hygiene because the mouth can be a source of bacterial or fungal infection. Frequent (4–6 times daily) mouth rinses with sterile water, normal saline, or sodium bicarbonate are effective.[4] Brushing or flossing teeth is avoided during periods of thrombocytopenia and neutropenia.

Aggressive use of antibacterial, antifungal, and antiviral therapy, both prophylactically and for documented infection, is an important aspect of patient management. Antibiotics with a broad gram-negative spectrum may be instituted prophylactically once the patient becomes neutropenic (ANC $<$1,000 cells/μL), or empirically after the patient is neutropenic and experiences fever (oral temperature $>$38°C). Some transplant centers administer a prophylactic fluoroquinolone such as levofloxacin on admission especially if the neutropenic period is expected to extend beyond 7 days.[170–174]

Fluoroquinolone prophylaxis during periods of neutropenia significantly reduces the incidence of gram-negative bacteremia but generally does not affect mortality.[4] Concerns regarding prophylactic fluoroquinolone use include the emergence of resistant organisms and an increased risk of streptococcal infection.[4,175] In fact, the incidence of *Viridians* group of streptococci has been increasing.[4,176] Prophylactic antibiotics (e.g., penicillin, vancomycin) are not recommended due to their lack of proven efficacy in preventing streptococcal infections and the concern about antibiotic-resistant bacteria.[4] Regardless of prophylactic strategies, patients who become febrile during neutropenia should immediately receive broad-spectrum IV antibiotic(s) (e.g., ceftazidime, cefepime, imipenem, or meropenem) and prophylaxis should be discontinued.[4,177]

Antifungal prophylactic agents are commonly used in HCT recipients. S.D. is prescribed fluconazole 400 mg/day on admission because prophylactic use until day +75 post-transplant decreases the incidence of systemic fungal infection and fungal death in patients undergoing HCT.[178,179] The use of prophylactic fluconazole has been linked to reports of breakthrough infections with resistant fungi such as *C. glabrata* and *Aspergillus*.[180,181]

When broader yeast and mold prophylaxis is required, either posaconazole or voriconazole may be used; however, data are limited in the transplant setting. If S.D. were to require mold prophylaxis, voriconazole 200 mg twice daily would be a reasonable choice. Voriconazole 200 mg twice daily was compared to fluconazole 400 mg once daily in a randomized double-blind trial for prevention of invasive fungal infections in standard risk HCT. No significant differences were seen in fungus-free survival, relapse-free status, and overall survival at 6 months. Toxicities were similar, and there was a trend toward reduced aspergillus infections and less empiric antifungal therapy in the voriconazole arm.[182] Posaconazole has also been used for mold prophylaxis in HCT based on its efficacy as prophylaxis in neutropenic patients.[183] However, data in HCT are very limited. Both azoles affect the CYP3A4 isoenzyme, and their use with calcineurin inhibitors requires judicious monitoring. The use of broader spectrum azoles has also resulted in the development of breakthrough zygomycosis infections, particularly with the use of voriconazole.[184]

The echinocandins have also been used for broader yeast and mold prophylaxis in HCT. Micafungin (50 mg IV every 24 hours) and fluconazole (400 mg IV every 24 hours) were compared in a randomized, double-blind study of patients undergoing HCT. Overall success was defined as the absence of suspected, proven, or probable systemic fungal infection through the end of therapy and as the absence of proven or probable systemic fungal infection through the end of the 4-week post-treatment period. The overall efficacy was greater in the patients who received micafungin (80.0% vs. 73.5% $p = 0.03$). Fewer episodes of aspergillosis occurred in patients treated with micafungin.[185]

Prevention of Herpes Simplex Virus and Varicella-Zoster Virus

CASE 101-6, QUESTION 2: On routine screening before transplantation, S.D. is found to be HSV-seropositive (≥1.11 index value) and VZV-seropositive (≥1 index value). How will this affect her management?

Up to 70% of HSV-seropositive patients undergoing myeloablative allogeneic HCT will experience reactivation of HSV.[186] Prophylactic acyclovir is commonly used in HSV-seropositive patients undergoing allogeneic or autologous HCT to prevent viral reactivation.[4,187] Dosing regimens for prophylactic acyclovir vary widely; the dose of IV acyclovir is typically 250 mg/m^2 IV every 8 hours, whereas oral doses of acyclovir range from 600 to 1,600 mg/day.[4] The recommended duration of acyclovir prophylaxis for HSV varies from day +30 to day +365 post-transplant or longer, depending on the specific type of HCT and other risk factors. Valacyclovir, a prodrug of acyclovir with improved bioavailability, provides sufficient blood concentrations to prevent HSV in patients with mucositis or GI aGVHD.[188] Prophylactic valacyclovir is commonly used at a dose of 500 mg PO every 12 hours.[189,190]

Varicella-zoster virus (VZV)-seropositive patients are at risk for developing herpes zoster, particularly after day +100 post-transplant.[191] Prophylactic acyclovir reduces the risk of VZV reactivation.[192] As with prophylaxis for HSV reactivation, the optimum duration of VZV prophylaxis is controversial, often extending to day +365 post-transplant or longer.

Patients who are HSV-seronegative or VZV-seronegative rarely exhibit primary HSV or VZV infection and are therefore not administered prophylactic acyclovir. If HSV does occur, lesions usually appear on the oral mucosa, nasolabial mucous membranes, or genital mucocutaneous area and can be managed with acyclovir at standard treatment doses.

Because S.D. is HSV- and VZV-seropositive, she is at risk for viral reactivation and should receive prophylactic acyclovir 400 mg PO twice daily, beginning 4 days prior to transplant and continuing until her ANC is greater than 2,500 cells/μL for at least 2 days.

Prevention of Cytomegalovirus Disease

CASE 101-6, QUESTION 3: S.D. is also CMV-seropositive. What is the significance of this finding and what measures can be taken to prevent reactivation of CMV?

Cytomegalovirus has the ability to establish lifelong latent infection after primary exposure. In immunocompromised patients, the virus may reactivate, resulting in asymptomatic shedding or the development of CMV disease. The incidence of CMV infection (defined as isolation of the virus or detection of viral proteins or nucleic acid in any body fluid without clinical symptoms) and CMV disease (signs and symptoms consistent with CMV invasion into a tissue) in HCT recipients is 15% to 60% and 20% to 35%, respectively. The most common manifestations of CMV disease after allogeneic HCT are pneumonitis, fever, and GI infection.[193]

In the CMV-seronegative HCT recipient, primary CMV infection or disease can be prevented by selecting a CMV-seronegative donor and using only blood products from CMV-seronegative donors. No anti-CMV prophylaxis is required in these recipients. In patients who are CMV-seropositive or who have received a CMV-seropositive graft, antiviral drugs are essential to minimize morbidity associated with CMV reactivation or secondary infection. Two general strategies are possible. Universal prophylaxis involves the administration of ganciclovir from the time of engraftment until approximately day +100 post-transplant. This strategy significantly decreases the incidence of CMV infection and disease compared with placebo.[194] However, prophylactic ganciclovir therapy is associated with neutropenia in 30% of patients, which contributes to an increased risk of invasive bacterial and fungal infections.[194,195] Neutropenia secondary to ganciclovir may lead to interruptions in antiviral therapy or necessitate administration of filgrastim daily or several times per week to maintain adequate neutrophil counts. The other strategy involves preemptive therapy, or risk-adjusted therapy.[188,196] Using this strategy, patients begin therapy only if they have early reactivation of CMV detected through the assay of blood for CMV antigens (e.g., pp65), or viral nucleic acid using polymerase chain reaction (PCR) testing. Using preemptive therapy selectively administers ganciclovir to only those HCT patients at greatest risk for development of CMV disease.[197–199] Antigenemia-based preemptive therapy is as effective as universal ganciclovir prophylaxis for prevention of CMV disease and is associated with reduced CMV mortality.[195,200–203] The induction dose of ganciclovir is typically 5 mg/kg IV every 12 hours for 7 to 14 days, followed by a maintenance dose of 5 mg/kg IV daily until 2 to 3 weeks after the last occurrence of antigenemia or until day +100 post-transplantation.[4] Preemptive therapy limits patient exposure to the potential toxicity of ganciclovir and thus reduces overall cost.[191] Recent data suggest that oral valganciclovir is a safe and effective alternative to ganciclovir for preemptive therapy.[204,205] Foscarnet may also be administered in lieu of ganciclovir, but its use is complicated by nephrotoxicity and electrolyte wasting.[203,206] Monitoring and correction of electrolyte and fluid imbalances are essential when foscarnet is initiated.

Cidofovir is used to treat CMV in HCT patients but is reserved for use when ganciclovir or foscarnet has failed.[207] Dose-related renal dysfunction, which can be seen after even 1 or 2 doses, limits the number of patients able to receive cidofovir.[207] An advantage of cidofovir is its infrequent dosing making it conducive to clinic administration. Monitoring renal function, electrolytes, WBC, and intraocular pressure are essential monitoring parameters.

Autologous HCT recipients who are CMV-seropositive pretransplant should receive antiviral treatment preemptively as described previously.[4,208] Nonmyeloablative or reduced-intensity HCT recipients should also receive preemptive antiviral treatment. Because host T cells may persist in the peripheral blood for up to 6 months after reduced-intensity or nonmyeloablative preparative regimens, their presence may provide some protection against early CMV disease. A matched controlled study comparing the incidence and outcome of CMV infection in myeloablative and nonmyeloablative HCT demonstrated that although the time to onset of CMV antigenemia was similar in the two groups, fewer nonmyeloablative HCT recipients experienced CMV disease in the early period.[209] The overall 1-year incidence of CMV disease was also similar, suggesting that nonmyeloablative HCT recipients are at increased risk for exhibiting late CMV disease (>100 days after transplantation) compared to their myeloablative counterparts.[209] It is therefore recommended that nonmyeloablative HCT patients receive preemptive antiviral therapy and be monitored for development of CMV antigenemia for 1 year after HCT.[209,210]

S.D.'s ANC recovers to greater than 1,000 cells/μL on day +20, and on day +32, her weekly surveillance blood sample is positive for CMV by PCR. Preemptive ganciclovir induction is initiated at 5 mg/kg IV every 12 hours for 2 weeks followed by maintenance dosing of 5 mg/kg daily. After 3 weeks of therapy, S.D.'s surveillance samples are negative and ganciclovir is discontinued. Weekly surveillance sampling continues until day +100. If surveillance samples again become positive for CMV, ganciclovir therapy should be reinstituted.

Diagnosis and Treatment of *Aspergillus* Infection

RISK FACTORS

CASE 101-7

QUESTION 1: A.W., a 60-kg, 165-cm, 15-year-old boy, is day +79 after a matched, unrelated, nonmyeloablative PBPC transplant for acute lymphocytic leukemia in third complete remission. He presents to the clinic for evaluation of a temperature of 102.3°F and a 3-day history of nonproductive cough. Significant medical history includes skin and GI GVHD (stable on his current regimen of cyclosporine, mycophenolate mofetil, and prednisone) and congestive heart failure believed to be secondary to anthracycline exposure. A.W. has chronic low-grade nausea and hypomagnesemia necessitating daily IV hydration with magnesium supplementation. Relevant laboratory values are as follows:

Na, 138 mEq/L
K, 4.2 mEq/L
Cl, 100 mEq/L
CO_2, 23 mEq/L
Blood urea nitrogen, 18 mg/dL
SCr, 0.8 mg/dL
Total bilirubin, 0.6 mg/dL
Mg, 1.5 mg/dL
WBC count, 3,500 cells/μL
Platelets, 78,000/μL
ANC, 1,810 cells/μL
Hemoglobin, 10.8 g/dL

He was CMV-seropositive and HSV-seropositive before HCT. Oral medications include cyclosporine 275 mg every 12 hours, mycophenolate mofetil 900 mg every 12 hours, prednisone 60 mg every morning and 12.5 mg every evening (tapering), trimethoprim–sulfamethoxazole (TMP/SMX) 160 mg/800 mg twice daily on Monday and Tuesday, fluconazole 400 mg every morning, valacyclovir 500 mg BID, digoxin 0.125 mg every 12 hours, enalapril 10 mg every 12 hours, and a multivitamin every morning.

On physical examination, A.W. is a chronically ill-appearing child with "moon" face, dry skin with thickened areas, a pleural friction rub, and thinning hair. Blood cultures, urinalysis, and chest X-ray are obtained. Chest X-ray reveals several small cavitary lesions worrisome for fungal disease. A.W. is admitted for further workup and management of presumed *Aspergillus* infection. What risk factors does A.W. have for developing an infection with *Aspergillus*?

Invasive molds (most commonly *Aspergillus* spp., but also *Fusarium* spp., *Scedosporium*, and *Zygomycetes*) are an increasing cause of morbidity and mortality after allogeneic and autologous HCT. Factors contributing to this trend include (a) more effective prevention of bacterial and viral infection which promote mold overgrowth, as described previously; and (b) the use of fluconazole prophylaxis, which has reduced the incidence of candidemia and Candida-related mortality.[178–180,211,212] *Aspergillus* infection is reported in up to 26% of HCT recipients, and the mortality rate of invasive aspergillosis (IA) is 74% to 92%.[185]

Several risk factors for development of invasive fungal infection have been identified.[211,212] Given that neutrophils are critical for host defense, prolonged neutropenia is considered the single most important predictor of infection at any point after HCT.[181,211] GVHD (acute and chronic) and treatment with corticosteroids are also important risk factors, particularly for aspergillosis, presumably as a result of neutrophil dysfunction.[185,211–213] In addition, the widespread use of fluconazole prophylaxis (400 mg/day) for prevention of invasive candidiasis in transplant patients since the early 1990s has led to a substantial increase in the incidence of invasive aspergillosis and also fluconazole-resistant *Candida* species such as *Candida krusei* and *Candida glabrata*.[211,213,214]

A.W. is receiving corticosteroid treatment for GVHD and fluconazole prophylaxis. These therapies increase his risk for exhibiting invasive aspergillosis.

TREATMENT

CASE 101-7, QUESTION 2: A.W. undergoes bronchoalveolar lavage to identify the organism responsible for his pulmonary infection. Pathologic examination of the fluid obtained reveals septate, branching hyphae, and culture results confirm the diagnosis of *Aspergillus fumigatus* infection. Imaging scans are negative for extrapulmonary involvement. How is aspergillosis usually diagnosed, and what are the acceptable alternatives for treating this infection?

Early diagnosis and treatment of invasive aspergillosis, which rely on tissue or fluid obtained from the infected site followed by aggressive antifungal therapy, may improve patient survival.[215] Although the lower respiratory tract is frequently the primary focus of infection, *Aspergillus* may invade blood vessels and spread hematogenously to other organs, including the brain, liver, kidneys, spleen, and skin.[191] Head, chest, abdomen, and pelvic computed tomography scans assist in assessing the extent of disease, treatment options, and overall prognosis. Cultures of respiratory tract secretions lack sensitivity for detecting *Aspergillus,* and the medical condition of the patient may preclude invasive diagnostic procedures altogether. Many clinicians have adopted the European Organization for Research and Treatment of Cancer criteria for diagnosis of proven, probable, and possible invasive aspergillosis.[216]

Newer diagnostic tests based on the detection of fungal antigens or metabolites, such as galactomannan, 1,3-β-D-glucan, and fungal DNA detection by PCR, are being developed. Galactomannan is a polysaccharide component of the *Aspergillus* cell wall that is released during fungal cell growth. Galactomannan detection by enzyme-linked immunoassay (GM-EIA) has proved to be a sensitive and specific tool for early detection of *Aspergillus* infection. The test is useful not only for serum samples but also for bronchoalveolar lavage and cerebrospinal fluid. Concomitant antifungal therapy may cause false-negative results, whereas antibiotics of fungal origin (e.g., piperacillin/tazobactam) have been associated with false positives.[185,217]

ANTIFUNGALS

Outcomes for patients with invasive aspergillosis after HCT are often poor, with approximately 20% of patients alive after 1 year.[211] Treatment success depends not only on the use of intensive antifungal agents but also on recovery of the host immune system and/or reduction of immunosuppression.[215,218] Conventional amphotericin B had traditionally been the gold standard antifungal therapy for invasive aspergillosis with response rates in the range of 28% to 51%, depending on the severity of the underlying immunosuppression; however, 65% of responders eventually died of their infection.[215] Fortunately, broad-spectrum triazoles and echinocandins are available as alternatives. The treatment of invasive aspergillosis has moved away from the use of amphotericin to the use of broad-spectrum azoles for its treatment.

Three broad-spectrum triazole agents (itraconazole, voriconazole, posaconazole) are available for patients. In an early compassionate use trial of invasive aspergillosis unresponsive to amphotericin B, 27% of patients had a complete response to itraconazole, and another 35% experienced improvement in their infection.[219] Patients who had undergone HCT had response rates similar to patients who were less immunocompromised. Unfortunately, oral itraconazole capsules exhibit erratic absorption and the IV form is complicated by the risk of drug precipitation in the IV line.[218] In addition, itraconazole is a potent inhibitor of common CYP isoforms and also has negative inotropic properties.[220,221]

Voriconazole is one of the newer broad-spectrum azoles whose advantage is its excellent (96%) oral bioavailability. Voriconazole has been compared to conventional amphotericin B in a randomized, unblinded trial as primary therapy for established invasive aspergillosis in an immunocompromised host.[222] The primary objective was to demonstrate the noninferiority of voriconazole compared with conventional amphotericin B after 12 weeks of therapy in patients with definite or probable invasive aspergillosis. Patients received voriconazole 6 mg/kg IV every 12 hours for two doses followed by 4 mg/kg IV every 12 hours for at least 7 days, followed by oral voriconazole 200 mg every 12 hours or amphotericin B at a dose of 1 to 1.5 mg/kg/day. Patients refractory to or intolerant of initial therapy could receive other antifungal drugs. Of 144 evaluable patients who received voriconazole, 76 (52.8%) had a partial or complete response compared to 42 of 133 (31.6%) patients treated with amphotericin B. The median duration of therapy for patients treated with voriconazole was 77 days, and 52 of 144 patients switched to an alternative agent. In contrast, the median duration of therapy for patients receiving amphotericin B was 10 days, and 107 of 133 patients switched to another agent (most commonly, a lipid formulation of amphotericin B). The survival rate at 12 weeks in the voriconazole group was 70.8% compared to 57.9% ($p = 0.02$). These results of initial therapy with voriconazole indicate superior response and improved survival in immunocompromised patients, such as allogeneic HCT recipients, with invasive aspergillosis. Voriconazole-treated patients also experienced fewer drug-related adverse effects; however, drug interactions due to P450 3A4 inhibition should be closely monitored.

Posaconazole, a newer broad-spectrum triazole, is available as an oral suspension, oral tablets and an intravenous formulation. The oral suspension has a more variable absorption as compared to the tablet formulation. In general, posaconazole has the lowest minimum inhibitory concentration of any available triazole against *Aspergillus* spp., including *Aspergillus terreus*. It is the only triazole with activity against the *Zygomycetes*. Published clinical experience with posaconazole is limited; however, in an open-label externally controlled trial in patients with invasive aspergillosis refractory to or intolerant of other therapies, the overall success rate was 42% in posaconazole-treated patients compared to 26% for controls ($p = 0.006$).[223]

Echinocandin antifungal agents (caspofungin, micafungin) inhibit the synthesis of β-(1,3)-glucan, an important component of the fungal cell wall. No prospective randomized trials have documented the efficacy of any echinocandin for primary therapy of invasive aspergillosis, and only caspofungin is approved for salvage therapy. An open-label, noncomparative trial evaluated the efficacy of caspofungin in 69 patients who had failed or were intolerant of at least 7 days of standard antifungal therapy.[224] Patients received 70 mg IV of caspofungin on day 1 followed by 50 mg IV daily. Of the 63 evaluable patients, 26 (43%) responded favorably to treatment. Twenty-six of 52 patients (50%) who had received at least 7 days of therapy had a favorable response. In another open-label, noncomparative trial, Denning et al. evaluated the safety and efficacy of micafungin (alone or in combination) in patients with proven or probable aspergillosis. Eighty of 225 patients (35.6%) had a favorable response. Most patients received combination therapy; the 34 patients treated with monotherapy had a similar response rate.[225] Amphotericin B is no longer first-line therapy for the treatment of invasive aspergillosis. It is typically reserved for patients who develop mold infections, such as cryptococcus, that are resistant to the azoles.

In summary, the number of agents available to manage invasive aspergillosis has expanded greatly in the past decade. Although some experts believe that voriconazole is the drug of first choice, considerable controversy still exists regarding acquiring resistance, selecting out other species of molds, and side effect tolerance due to the lack of definitive studies. Therapy should be tailored to the individual patient based on response, tolerability, and cost.

ANTIFUNGAL TOXICITIES AND LENGTH OF ANTIFUNGAL THERAPY AND COMBINATION ANTIFUNGAL THERAPY

CASE 101-7, QUESTION 3: A.W. is started on voriconazole 6 mg/kg IV every 12 hours for two doses, followed by 4 mg/kg IV every 12 hours, plus caspofungin 70 mg IV on day 1 and 50 mg IV daily thereafter. What toxicities can be expected with azole treatment? What is the rationale for combination therapy and how should the patient be monitored? How long should A.W. receive antifungal therapy?

Common toxicities reported with voriconazole include reversible visual disturbances (blurred vision, altered color perception, photophobia, visual hallucinations), skin reactions (rash, pruritus, photosensitivity), elevations in hepatic transaminase enzymes and alkaline phosphatase, nausea, and headache.[222,226,227] Caspofungin has fewer adverse effects. Vein irritation and headache are most common; dermatologic reactions related to histamine release (flushing, erythema, wheals) have also been reported. Increased hepatic transaminase enzymes occur in approximately 6% of patients treated with caspofungin.[224] A.W. should be monitored for changes in liver function and counseled regarding the potential visual side effects of voriconazole. The azoles are also known inhibitors of the CYP3A4 isoenzyme; therefore, drug interaction monitoring is imperative. The major interaction seen in patients undergoing allogeneic HCT is an increase in calcineurin inhibitor levels. Careful monitoring is warranted.

Data supporting improved outcomes with two-drug combinations of triazoles, echinocandins, and polyenes in patients with aspergillosis are sparse. However, *in vitro* and animal data suggest that an echinocandin plus voriconazole or a polyene may be synergistic.[228–231] Given the overall poor prognosis of invasive aspergillosis in severely immunocompromised patients, many practitioners choose to treat patients with two-drug combination therapy. Voriconazole in combination with caspofungin is thus a reasonable alternative for A.W.

The optimum duration of antifungal therapy for treatment of invasive aspergillosis has not been established.[218] Important considerations include the status of the patient's immune system and the extent of response to treatment. Many clinicians continue aggressive antifungal therapy until the infection has stabilized radiographically and then proceed with less aggressive "maintenance" therapy (e.g., single-agent oral voriconazole) until restoration of the immune system has taken place. It is not uncommon for a patient to require several months of antifungal therapy for effective management of invasive aspergillosis.

Prevention of *Pneumocystis jiroveci* Pneumonia

CASE 101-7, QUESTION 5: A.W. is receiving TMP/SMX, one double-strength tablet PO BID on Monday and Thursday. What is the rationale for its use?

Pneumocystis jiroveci is a common pathogen that causes *Pneumocystis* pneumonia (PCP) in patients who have undergone allogeneic HCT. PCP is a potentially lethal infection, and prophylaxis is routinely administered. The optimum prophylactic regimen has not been established, but most centers administer TMP/SMX for PCP prophylaxis.[4] Dapsone and aerosolized pentamidine are alternatives for patients who are allergic to sulfonamides or do not tolerate TMP/SMX for other reasons such as hematologic toxicities. PCP prophylaxis is usually begun after neutrophil recovery because (a) PCP most commonly occurs after engraftment and (b) TMP/SMX is potentially myelosuppressive. Patients should be closely monitored for unexplained neutropenia or thrombocytopenia.

ISSUES OF SURVIVORSHIP AFTER HEMATOPOIETIC CELL TRANSPLANTATION

CASE 101-8

QUESTION 1: H.O. is a 32-year-old woman who received a BU/CY preparative regimen and an HLA-matched sibling HCT for treatment of chronic phase CML at age 21 years. H.O. received her HCT more than 10 years ago, is disease-free, and has not had chronic GVHD for 9 years. Her only medication is one multivitamin tablet daily. What issues of cancer survivorship are of concern to H.O.?

A greater proportion of HCT recipients are surviving their cancer diagnosis without evidence of their primary malignancy, but they are at risk for long-term physical and emotional sequelae of their cancer treatments.[2] Many long-term HCT survivors are no longer under the care of an HCT center and their healthcare providers may be unfamiliar with the complications of HCT. To facilitate the clinical care of long-term HCT recipients, recommendations for screening and preventive practices have been created for adult and pediatric HCT survivors.[232,233] These guidelines should facilitate the provision of health care to HCT recipients. The following paragraphs describe various concerns associated with the morbidity of long-term HCT survivors.[232–234] Long-term HCT survivors should be regularly screened for the development of secondary malignancies, complications of GVHD that affect the oral mucosa, liver, respiratory, endocrine, ocular, skeletal, nervous system, kidney, and vascular systems. The psychosocial health of HCT survivors should also be evaluated.

Immune function can take more than 2 years to recover, even after discontinuation of immunosuppressants.[235] Treatment of GVHD exacerbates immune system defects, necessitating prophylaxis and vigilant monitoring for infectious complications. Fevers should be rapidly assessed and treated to prevent fatal infections. Recipients of HCT also lose protective antibodies to vaccine-preventable diseases; therefore, HCT survivors need to be revaccinated for selected infectious diseases with due consideration for the risk of vaccination.

Hematopoietic cell transplant survivors have a greater risk of secondary malignant neoplasms.[2] An increased incidence of cancer of the skin, oral mucosa, brain, thyroid, and bone is observed after allogeneic HCT, and an increased incidence of myelodysplasia and acute leukemia can occur after autologous HCT for NHL.[2] Survivors should avoid carcinogens (e.g., tobacco) and be screened for secondary malignant neoplasms indefinitely.[2] Long-term impairment of end-organ function may be due to the preparative regimen, infectious complications (either autologous or allogeneic grafts), and post-transplant immunosuppression (allogeneic grafts only).[232,234] Endocrine dysfunction, specifically of the thyroid, gonads, and growth velocity, is common.[232,233] Adrenal insufficiency can result from long-term corticosteroid therapy used to treat GVHD. Infertility is commonly observed after myeloablative HCT secondary to the high doses of alkylating agents and radiation administered. Frequently, men become azoospermic, and chemically induced menopause develops in women.[2] However, pregnancies have occurred after HCT.[2] Up to 60% of HCT recipients have osteopenia, most likely resulting from gonadal dysfunction and corticosteroid administration; avascular necrosis due to corticosteroids can also occur.[236] A significant portion (15%–40%) of HCT survivors exhibit pulmonary dysfunction with variable symptoms (e.g., restrictive, chronic obstructive lung disease) from multiple causes.[236] Hepatic infections can occur in HCT recipients through blood transfusions or, more commonly, because recipients or donors have a latent hepatitis viral infection. The prevalence of chronic hepatitis C ranges from 5% to 70% in long-term HCT survivors.[237] Because of this, cirrhosis and its complications may become an important late complication of HCT.[237] Hepatic dysfunction can also result from iron overload, which may occur secondary to multiple red blood cell transfusions administered during aplasia after myeloablative preparative regimens and before HCT. Alopecia is a common late effect with BU/CY, as are cataracts with CY/TBI.[75]

H.O. should be routinely monitored for signs of relapse and chronic GVHD. To lower the risk of infectious complications, she should be counseled to obtain prompt medical care for fevers or signs of an infection, and she should be revaccinated if she has not done so since receiving her myeloablative HCT. Thorough evaluation of end-organ function, including renal, hepatic, thyroid, and ovarian function, should be assessed at regular intervals. In addition, her bone mineral density should be determined, and H.O. should be counseled on preventive measures for osteopenia (e.g., calcium supplementation). In addition to standard cancer screening tests, H.O. should be closely monitored for secondary malignant neoplasms.[2]

KEY REFERENCES AND WEBSITES

A full list of references for this chapter can be found at http://thepoint.lww.com/AT11e. Below are the key references and websites for this chapter, with the corresponding reference number in this chapter found in parentheses after the reference.

Key References

Appelbaum FR et al. Haematopoietic cell transplantation as immunotherapy. *Nature*. 2001;411:385. (4)

Copelan EA et al. Hematopoietic stem-cell transplantation. *N Engl J Med*. 2006;354:1813. (2)

Pasquini MC, Wang Z. Current use and outcome of hematopoietic stem cell transplantation: CIBMTR Summary Slides. Center for International Blood and Marrow Transplant Research. http://www.cibmtr.org/ReferenceCenter/SlidesReports/SummarySlides/pages/index.aspx. Accessed August 8, 2015. (1)

Blume KG et al, eds. *Thomas' Hematopoietic Cell Transplantation*. 4th ed. Malden, MA: Blackwell; 2009. (11, 13, 38, 47, 49, 53, 79, 89, 105)

Key Websites

Health Resources and Services Administration (HRSA). http://www.hrsa.gov/. Accessed July 7, 2015.

Center for International Blood and Marrow Transplant Research (CIBMTR) https://www.cibmtr.org/. Accessed July 7, 2015.

National Marrow Donor Program. https://bethematch.org. Accessed August 4, 2015.

American Society for Blood and Marrow Transplantation (ASBMT). http://www.asbmt.org/. Accessed July 7, 2015.

Section Editor: Marcia L. Buck

102 Pediatric Pharmacotherapy

Marcia L. Buck

CORE PRINCIPLES

		CHAPTER CASES
GROWTH AND DEVELOPMENT		
1	Children undergo considerable physiologic changes between birth and adulthood. Although most follow the same general pattern of growth, the timing of maturation varies from child to child.	**Case 102-1 (Question 1), Table 102-1**
PHARMACOKINETIC DIFFERENCES		
1	All aspects of pharmacokinetics are affected by growth and development. Drug absorption is altered by a variety of mechanisms, with the most significant differences noted during the first months of life.	**Case 102-2 (Question 1), Case 102-3 (Questions 1–4)**
2	Drug distribution is affected by changes in relative organ size, body water content, fat stores, plasma protein concentrations, acid–base balance, cardiac output, and tissue perfusion. The greatest degree of change occurs during the first year of life.	**Case 102-3 (Questions 5, 6), Table 102-2**
3	Metabolic function is highly dependent on patient age. This has been demonstrated in a number of recent studies, which have identified significant differences in half-life during infancy, childhood, and adolescence.	**Case 102-4 (Questions 1–4)**
4	Elimination is reduced during infancy, resulting in slower rates of clearance for many commonly used drugs. Glomerular filtration rate increases throughout childhood. Use of creatinine clearance as an estimate of glomerular filtration rate requires different equations than those used in adults.	**Case 102-5 (Questions 1, 2), Case 102-6 (Question 1)**
5	Adolescence is not simply a link between childhood and adulthood; it is a distinct period of significant physiologic change. The effects of puberty can alter the efficacy or toxicity of many drugs administered during this period.	**Case 102-7 (Question 1)**
PHARMACODYNAMIC DIFFERENCES		
1	Although less well understood than pharmacokinetic differences between children and adults, there are significant age-related effects on pharmacodynamics as well. Children may exhibit differences in both therapeutic response and adverse effect profiles.	**Case 102-8 (Question 1), Case 102-9 (Questions 1, 2)**
MEDICATION DOSING IN CHILDREN		
1	The differences in pharmacokinetics and pharmacodynamics observed in children influence the choice of drug dose and dosing interval. For most dose calculations, weight is used to account for growth and development.	**Case 102-10 (Question 1)**
2	All pediatric prescriptions and medication orders must be checked for the appropriateness of the dose, route, and frequency with a pediatric dosing reference.	**Case 102-10 (Question 1)**

Continued

	CHAPTER CASES
PREVENTING MEDICATION ERRORS IN CHILDREN	
1 Children are at a greater risk for medication errors than adults, as a result of the need to calculate drug doses and alter dosage formulations.	**Case 102-10 (Question 2)**
2 Electronic prescribing, standardization of drug doses and concentrations, and the introduction of smart-pump technology have been shown to reduce errors in many children's hospitals. One of the most effective methods to avoid errors is the inclusion of pediatric pharmacists in the medication ordering and review process.	**Case 102-10 (Question 3), Table 102-3**
INCREASING PEDIATRIC MEDICATION INFORMATION	
1 A number of governmental programs are increasing the availability of pediatric medication information and improving the ability of pediatric healthcare professionals to provide safe and effective drug therapy for children.	**Case 102-10 (Question 4)**

Providing care for children can be one of the most challenging, but rewarding, aspects of pharmacy practice. Although a relatively small number of healthcare providers pursue specialty training in pediatrics and work exclusively with children, most clinicians will provide care for children every day in the community or hospital setting. According to recent population estimates, approximately one-quarter of the US population is younger than 20 years of age, with 6% younger than 5 years of age.[1] Although most children are healthy, this segment of the population still uses a significant amount of healthcare resources. In a recent telephone survey, one in five parents reported giving their child one or more prescription medications within the previous week.[2] A survey conducted in pediatricians' offices found that 53% of children left their visit with a prescription.[3]

Pediatrics, as a specialty, encompasses a very diverse patient population. Patients range in age from premature neonates to adolescents and can vary in weight by 100-fold, from a 0.5-kg premature neonate to a 50-kg 16-year-old. Further complicating the care of children is the relative lack of information on drug dosing and monitoring. Because of the small numbers of children requiring medical treatment and the difficulty in conducting research in these patients, fewer than half of the drugs currently available in the United States are approved by the Food and Drug Administration (FDA) for pediatric use.[4,5] As a result, as many as 60% of all prescriptions written by pediatricians are for "off-label" uses.[6] Dosing and monitoring information for off-label uses is often based on case series and clinical trials published in the medical literature and may not be readily available in general drug references.

Healthcare providers caring for children must be capable of assessing the appropriateness of drug doses for this diverse population and providing recommendations for dosage adjustments and patient monitoring with limited resources. This requires knowledge of the pharmacokinetic and pharmacodynamic differences between children and adults and how these differences impact both therapeutic and adverse drug effects.

Table 102-1
Commonly Used Age Definitions

Premature neonate	**Born at <36 weeks' gestational age**
Term neonate	Born at ≥36 weeks' gestational age
Neonate	Birth–1 month of age
Infant	>1 month–1 year of age
Child	>1–11 years of age
Adolescent	12–16 years of age

GROWTH AND DEVELOPMENT DURING CHILDHOOD

CASE 102-1

QUESTION 1: C.J. is a 4-month-old, 6.5 kg baby boy who has recently started teething. His parents ask for advice on a medication to alleviate C.J.'s pain. What factors will influence your decision about the choice of medication and dosing regimen for C.J.? What medication and dose will you recommend to his parents?

Children undergo considerable physiologic changes between birth and adulthood. Although many changes are easily observed, such as the ability to walk or the development of language, others are less evident. C.J.'s analgesic dose will be based on his age and weight, as estimates of the numerous pharmacokinetic and pharmacodynamic differences between children and adults. To discuss the changes that occur with growth and development, pediatric patients are typically grouped by age (Table 102-1). These definitions are helpful to provide a consistent framework for dosing recommendations, but it should be kept in mind that they are arbitrary and can oversimplify the differences among individual patients. Although children tend to grow and develop in a relatively similar manner, the timing of maturation varies from child to child. Children do not grow in a predictable, linear fashion, but rather in periodic bursts, with additional variation caused by differences in genetic predisposition, nutritional intake, and environment.[7,8] Research on the impact of growth and development on pharmacokinetics and pharmacodynamics, often referred to as developmental pharmacology, has grown considerably during the past several decades, improving our ability to optimize the efficacy of drug therapy in children while minimizing adverse effects.

The most appropriate analgesic for C.J. would be acetaminophen. Aspirin is no longer used as an analgesic in children because of its association with Reye syndrome, a rare condition causing mitochondrial damage and resulting in hepatic failure. Nonsteroidal anti-inflammatory drugs, such as ibuprofen, are not recommended for use in infants younger than 6 months of age because of an increased risk for renal impairment. C.J. should receive an acetaminophen dose of 10 to 15 mg/kg given every 4 to 6 hours as needed, with no more than five doses or 75 mg/kg given in a 24-hour period. Based on his age and weight, an appropriate recommendation for C.J. would be to give 65 mg (2 mL) of the acetaminophen 160 mg/5 mL oral suspension by mouth every 6 hours as needed. If C.J. continues to need medication for more than 24 hours, his parents should contact C.J.'s primary healthcare provider.

PEDIATRIC PHARMACOKINETIC DIFFERENCES

All aspects of pharmacokinetics are affected by growth and physical maturation, beginning during gestation (pregnancy) and ending in adulthood. These changes are complex, and their timing can vary widely from patient to patient.

Drug Absorption

ORAL DRUG ABSORPTION

CASE 102-2

QUESTION 1: A.H., a 1.5-kg, 4-week-old infant girl born at 29 weeks' gestational age, is being treated with phenobarbital for seizures associated with a period of asphyxia at birth. She is currently receiving a maintenance dose of 7.5 mg (5 mg/kg) given intravenously (IV) once daily. The team wishes to transition her to oral therapy now that she is receiving full enteral feeds. A trough serum phenobarbital concentration obtained during IV therapy was 17.5 mcg/mL, within the desired range of 15 to 40 mcg/mL. Switching the patient to phenobarbital elixir 7.5 mg given orally once daily results in a serum concentration of only 8.9 mcg/mL after 1 week of therapy. What factors might explain the lower concentration, and how should A.H. be managed?

Enteral absorption of drugs is altered at birth and does not approximate adult patterns for several months.[7,8] Gastric fluid volume is greatly reduced at birth. Gastric acid production is decreased, giving the neonate a higher, nearly neutral pH in the stomach. This results in a greater absorption of acid-labile drugs such as penicillin G and erythromycin, but reduced absorption of weakly acidic drugs such as phenobarbital and phenytoin. Gastric acid output increases during the first 1 to 2 weeks of life, but only reaches adult values at 2 to 3 years of age. Transport of bile acids into the gastrointestinal lumen and pancreatic enzyme production are also reduced, further altering the absorption of pH-sensitive drugs and reducing enterohepatic recirculation. Amylase activity is minimal at birth and remains low until the third month of life.[9] Pancreatic lipase activity is detectable by 32 weeks' gestational age, but remains low at birth and throughout the next 2 to 3 months. In contrast, gastric lipase is present at birth and accounts for a greater percentage of fat absorption during early life. In addition to these differences, neonates are also born with relatively sterile gastrointestinal tracts. Normal bacterial colonization typically occurs within days for term infants, but may be delayed in premature infants who reside in the more sterile environment of an intensive care unit. The effectiveness of drugs that rely on gastrointestinal flora for activation or degradation may be significantly altered during this period.

Gastric emptying time is delayed and intestinal transit time is prolonged at birth, but both quickly increase within the first few days of life because contractions in the stomach become more coordinated and intestinal contractions become more frequent, stronger, and sustained. Premature infants have delayed development of normal gastric emptying and intestinal transit, as shown in a study of acetaminophen dosing in which premature infants at 28 weeks' gestational age had a 2-hour delay in absorption compared with older infants.[10] Adult values for gastric emptying and intestinal transit time are generally reached by 4 to 8 months of age.

Chapter 102

For drugs absorbed through passive diffusion, reduced splanchnic blood flow during the first weeks of life can reduce the rate and extent of absorption by altering concentration gradients across the intestinal villi.[7] Reduction in blood flow may also place neonates at risk for damage to the gut lining from hyperosmolar drug formulations. As a result, many institutions delay use of the enteral route for drug administration until the patient is receiving at least one-quarter to half of their nutritional needs through enteral feedings. This allows dilution of drug doses and may reduce the risk for mucosal damage. Lower levels of metabolic enzyme activity in the intestine may reduce first-pass metabolism of drugs given enterally.[11,12] Boucher et al.[12] found that the bioavailability of zidovudine decreased from 89% in neonates during the first 2 weeks of life to 61% in older infants, reflecting increased first-pass metabolism in the older patients. Intestinal enzymatic activity does not approach adult values until 2 to 3 years of age.

The lower phenobarbital serum concentration after A.H. was placed on enteral therapy is most likely the result of reduced drug absorption in the gastrointestinal tract, resulting from the higher gastric pH and reduced splanchnic blood flow. The maintenance phenobarbital dose for A.H. should be increased to achieve a trough serum concentration within the desired range. An increase of the oral dose to 10 mg would be appropriate, with a plan to obtain a trough concentration within 3 to 5 days. Although this value will not yet reflect the steady state concentration, due to the long half-life of the drug, it will be useful to guide additional dosing changes.

INTRAMUSCULAR DRUG ABSORPTION

CASE 102-3

QUESTION 1: C.B. is a 3.6-kg newborn boy, born at 39 weeks' gestational age, who was transferred to the newborn nursery after delivery. Routine care for neonates during the first hours of life generally includes administration of erythromycin eye ointment for prevention of neonatal ophthalmia and 1 mg of phytonadione (vitamin K_1) given intramuscularly (IM) to prevent vitamin K-deficiency bleeding of the newborn. C.B.'s parents question the need to give their baby a shot so soon after birth. How would you explain the rationale for giving phytonadione IM rather than orally?

In the United States, phytonadione is typically given by IM injection after birth. Drug administration by IM injection typically results in a delay in time to reach peak serum concentrations in neonates. This delay is related to reduced muscle size, weaker muscle contractions, and an immature vasculature resulting in more erratic blood flow to and from the muscle.[7,8] Although considered a disadvantage when rapid absorption is needed, such as with antibiotic administration, the delay in systemic absorption after IM injection is used as an advantage for the administration of phytonadione after birth. The delayed absorption from muscle results in a depot-like effect, providing a slow release of the drug into the systemic circulation until the infant's dietary intake is adequate to maintain necessary vitamin K serum concentrations.[13] A similar delay in drug absorption may occur with subcutaneous injection because of the lower percentage of body fat in neonates. The delay in absorption seen with IM and subcutaneous administration becomes negligible after the first months of life. When counseling C.B.'s parents, it will be important to stress the benefit of the slower absorption of vitamin K with IM administration compared with the rapid absorption and clearance of a single oral dose. A single IM injection of vitamin K will protect their son from bleeding until he is approximately a month old, when he should be taking in enough breast milk or infant formula to maintain adequate vitamin K concentrations.

TRANSDERMAL DRUG ABSORPTION

CASE 102-3, QUESTION 2: C.B. is scheduled for a circumcision before discharge. The surgical site will be prepped with a 10% povidone–iodine solution. What factors influence the absorption of medications via this route in the neonatal patient? Based on these factors, how should the povidone–iodine be applied to minimize toxicity?

In contrast to enteral, IM, and subcutaneous administration, transdermal or percutaneous administration results in greater drug absorption in neonates than it does in older children and adults. Enhanced absorption results from a greater skin to body surface area ratio, approximately 3 times that of adults, as well as a thinner stratum corneum, better epidermis hydration, and greater perfusion.[7,8] The greater degree of percutaneous absorption in infants has resulted in significant toxicity. Hexachlorophene, when used routinely to bathe infants, has resulted in seizures and is now considered contraindicated in this age range. Application of povidone–iodine as a topical disinfectant before surgery has been linked to neonatal thyroid dysfunction and, as a result, is now used only in limited quantities for brief periods to limit percutaneous iodine absorption. In spite of the knowledge of this adverse effect, cases continue to be reported in the medical literature.[14] Even relatively common topical products can produce systemic toxicity. Frequent use of diaper rash products containing hydrocortisone can produce suppression of the hypothalamus–pituitary–adrenal axis in as little as 2 weeks.

Cleaning and disinfecting the skin before surgery in a neonate requires special attention to the selection of agent, surface area affected, and the length of skin contact. For C.B., a 10% povidone–iodine solution should be gently applied to the penis and surrounding skin immediately before surgery and removed as soon as the 5- to 10-minute circumcision has been completed to minimize the risk for systemic toxicity resulting from enhanced percutaneous iodine absorption.

CASE 102-3, QUESTION 3: Are transdermal anesthetics an appropriate option for use before C.B.'s procedure?

Both 4% lidocaine and eutectic mixture of local anesthetics (EMLA) cream, which contain lidocaine and prilocaine, are widely used as topical anesthetics for infants and children before venipuncture, IV catheter placement, or circumcision. Both have been shown in clinical trials to be safe and effective.[15] The low concentration of the active ingredients and the limited duration of contact, 30 to 60 minutes, prevent excessive systemic absorption when applied to intact skin. Either analgesic cream would be appropriate for C.B. EMLA should be applied an hour before the start of the circumcision, whereas 4% lidocaine cream should be applied 30 minutes before the procedure. A thin layer of cream should be applied, without an occlusive dressing, and the baby diapered until the start of the procedure. The cream should be completely removed before the application of the 10% povidone–iodine solution.

Other transdermal medications should be avoided or used with caution for only limited periods in infants. After the first year of life, transdermal application becomes a more useful route of administration for several medications. Methylphenidate and clonidine patches are used in the treatment of attention deficit hyperactivity disorder (ADHD) in school-aged children, and both lidocaine and fentanyl patches are used for the treatment of older children and adolescents with severe pain.

RECTAL DRUG ABSORPTION

CASE 102-3, QUESTION 4: A week after C.B.'s discharge from the hospital, he is brought into the emergency department after becoming lethargic and febrile at home. His parents have tried giving him oral acetaminophen, but he is vomiting and unable to take liquids. Is rectal administration of acetaminophen an acceptable option for C.B. in the hospital after he has been stabilized?

Rectal administration is a useful route of drug delivery for many pediatric patients. Most drugs are well absorbed by this route, but the strong rectal contractions in infants can result in an inability to retain suppositories for the length of time needed to achieve optimal absorption.[7,8] Gels and liquid dosage preparations that do not require an extended time for dissolution are better options. Rectal diazepam gel is often used by parents of children with seizure disorders to provide rapid control of worsening seizures while awaiting emergency medical personnel. In an observational trial of 358 children, the median time from administration of rectal diazepam by a parent to cessation of seizures was 4.3 minutes.[16]

Rectal acetaminophen would be a viable option for C.B. It is rapidly absorbed through this route. Many drug dosing references recommend a slightly higher rectal acetaminophen dose (10–20 mg/kg) to account for a potentially lower bioavailability.

Drug Distribution

Growth and development also affect drug distribution. Organ size, body water content, fat stores, plasma protein concentrations, acid–base balance, cardiac output, and tissue perfusion all change throughout childhood, altering the pattern of distribution and extent of drug penetration.[7] The greatest degree of change occurs during the first year of life.

CASE 102-3, QUESTION 5: In the emergency department, C.B. is refusing to breast-feed and is having difficulty breathing. Neonatal sepsis with possible meningitis is suspected. Laboratory values and vital signs include the following:

Temperature, 39.4°C
Heart rate, 202 beats/minute (normal 107–182 beats/minute)
Blood pressure, 85/62 mm Hg (normal systolic 70–75 mm Hg, diastolic 50–55 mm Hg)

He currently weighs 3.4 kg and appears slightly dehydrated. His parents report that C.B. has had fewer wet diapers than usual during the last 24 hours. What physiologic differences in the neonatal period would affect your choice of empiric antibiotics for the treatment of neonatal central nervous system infections? What drugs would you select and what doses would you recommend?

Empiric antibiotic therapy for sepsis and meningitis for C.B. typically consists of ampicillin and aminoglycoside. Although not commonly used in adults because of the relatively low degree of penetration across the blood–brain barrier, this combination is very effective in the neonatal period when drug distribution into the central nervous system is higher. Constituting only 2% of total body weight in an adult, the brain makes up 10% to 12% of the weight of an infant. As a result, the brain serves as a much larger potential compartment for drug distribution. In addition, the percentage of systemic blood flow that reaches the cerebral vasculature is greater. These factors, along with a potential for greater passive diffusion of drugs across the functionally immature blood–brain barrier, can result in higher drug concentrations within the central nervous system of infants compared with older children and adults.[7,8] This can produce both benefit and risk to the infant. Drugs given to treat meningitis or seizures are more likely to achieve therapeutic concentrations within the central nervous system, but there is also a greater potential risk for drug-induced neurotoxicity.

BODY WATER

One of the most significant differences in drug distribution during childhood is the decrease in total body water content with increasing age. Approximately 85% of a premature newborn's weight and 70% to 80% of a term newborn's weight are body water, compared with only 60% to 65% in a 1-year-old.[7,8] After a year of age, the percentage declines from 50% to 60% and remains relatively constant. Extracellular water decreases in a similar manner, from 40%–45% in the newborn to 20%–25% by the end of the first year of life. Intracellular water content, however, remains relatively stable. These changes result in a much greater distribution of highly water-soluble drugs, such as the aminoglycosides or linezolid, and a reduced accumulation of highly lipid-soluble drugs, such as amphotericin, amiodarone, benzodiazepines, or digoxin.

The pharmacokinetic profile of gentamicin has been well described in infants and children as a result of its role in empiric antibiotic therapy for neonatal sepsis and meningitis. The volume of distribution of gentamicin in premature neonates ranges from 0.5 to 0.7 L/kg, reflecting the higher extracellular water content at this age. This value falls to 0.4 L/kg by the end of the first year of life and further declines from 0.2 to 0.3 L/kg by adulthood.[17] As a result of their higher volume of distribution, the weight-based dose for an infant is often much higher than a comparable dose in an adult. Based on C.B.'s age and weight, the *Pediatric Dosage Handbook*,[17] one of the most widely used pediatric drug references, recommends an ampicillin dose of 170 mg (50 mg/kg) given IV every 6 hours and a gentamicin dose of 8.5 mg (2.5 mg/kg) given IV every 8 hours, or if using extended-interval dosing, 13.6 mg (4 mg/kg) every 24 hours. Using these same weight-based doses in a 70-kg adult would result in doses much higher than the typical recommended adult dose.

BODY FAT

Whereas the effects of growth and development on changes in body water content are well defined and typically require adjustments in drug dosing only during infancy, the effects of changes in body fat are not yet well understood. Body fat increases throughout gestation and infancy. A premature neonate may have as little as 1% to 2% body fat, whereas a term infant will have closer to 10%–15% body fat. A 1-year-old will have a body fat of 20% to 25%, similar to that of an adult. Children following normal growth patterns have relatively little change in their body fat percentage between the second year of life and the onset of puberty. However, the increasing rate of childhood obesity has generated concern about the efficacy and safety of current weight-based dosing strategies.[18] In a 2010 retrospective study of 699 children between 5 and 12 years of age admitted to a children's hospital during a 6-month period, overweight children (defined as having a body mass index greater than the 85th percentile for age) accounted for 33% of the admissions.[19] Evaluation of their medication orders revealed that 8.5% of the doses ordered were for less than the recommended dose, whereas 2.8% were for an excessive dose. The need to make dosage adjustments in these children remains controversial; only limited research is available documenting the effects of childhood obesity on the pharmacokinetics and pharmacodynamics of commonly used pediatric medications.

PROTEIN BINDING

CASE 102-3, QUESTION 6: On the third day of admission, the microbiology laboratory reports the culture and sensitivity results for C.B. Although the cerebrospinal fluid and urine cultures were negative, the peripheral blood culture grew *Escherichia coli*. The organism appears to be sensitive to a wide range of antibiotics, including penicillins, cephalosporins, gentamicin, and sulfamethoxazole-trimethoprim. What would your recommendation be for C.B.'s continuing treatment?

Many of the drugs that would treat C.B.'s infection are highly protein bound. Plasma protein binding is reduced in neonates as a result of decreased circulating levels of both albumin and α_1-acid glycoprotein, as well as decreased binding affinity.[7,8,11] With the known susceptibilities and their long history of efficacy and safety, continuing C.B.'s current ampicillin and gentamicin regimen for 7 to 10 days would be an appropriate choice. Although ampicillin is known to be present in higher unbound concentrations in infants compared with adults (Table 102-2), use of standard dosing recommendations for C.B. based on age should be adequate to prevent toxicity. Sulfamethoxazole-trimethoprim would not be appropriate. Administration of drugs with a high binding affinity for albumin, such as the sulfonamides, during the neonatal period can result in competition with bilirubin for binding sites. The resulting increase in unbound bilirubin can lead to kernicterus, neurologic damage caused by deposition of bilirubin in the brain, primarily in the basal ganglia.[20] For this reason, sulfonamides are not recommended for neonates and are not approved by the FDA for use in infants younger than 2 months of age. Ceftriaxone, another possible option for C.B., also is known to be highly protein bound. Although approved for use in neonates, it is contraindicated in those with hyperbilirubinemia. As a precaution, many hospitals restrict its use in the neonatal population to only those patients who have infections resistant to other antibiotics.

The clinical impact of changes in protein binding can be difficult to predict. Separation and measurement of the unbound (free) fraction can be used to guide therapy for drugs such as valproic acid or phenytoin, but this process is more labor-intensive and expensive and, as a result, may not be available at all hospitals. Larger blood sample volumes may also be required, which can lead to excessive blood loss in premature infants. An estimation of the unbound concentration can be made from total serum drug concentrations, but may not be accurate in infants. Methods to estimate unbound serum valproic acid concentrations from total concentrations that were developed for adults have been found to be ineffective in predicting free levels in neonates and infants.[21]

Table 102-2
Examples of Drugs Present in Greater Unbound Concentrations in Neonates than in Adults

Alfentanil	Penicillin G
Ampicillin	Phenobarbital
Ceftriaxone	Phenytoin
Cefuroxime	Propranolol
Diazepam	Salicylates
Digoxin	Sulfonamides
Lidocaine	Theophylline
Ketamine	Valproic acid
Morphine	
Nafcillin	

Metabolism

Much of the research currently being conducted in developmental pharmacology is focused on changes in metabolic function.[7,8,11,22–49] Our understanding of the ontogeny of metabolic enzymes is improving rapidly, because in vitro data gathered from studies quantifying hepatic microsomal proteins and determining levels of enzymatic activity are combined with information obtained through pharmacokinetic and pharmacogenomic research. It is clear that the onset of function varies among enzymes; whereas some exhibit metabolic activity in utero, others demonstrate activity only after several months of life. The development of metabolic enzyme function continues during the first years of life and does not appear to be complete until after puberty. There appears to be considerable interpatient variability. Enzyme development can be affected by the underlying health of the child, nutritional status, and exposure to substrate. Metabolic activity also reflects genetic polymorphisms, just as in adults.

PHASE I DRUG METABOLISM

CASE 102-4

QUESTION 1: N.M. is a 1.38-kg, 3-week-old girl who was born at 28 weeks' gestational age. She has recently been started on nasogastric feedings, but has had repeated episodes of emesis and is not producing regular stools. Erythromycin is recommended to increase her gastric motility. What can you tell your team about the ability of N.M. to metabolize this drug? What dose of erythromycin would you recommend for N.M.?

Phase I reactions, which include oxidation, reduction, hydroxylation, and hydrolysis, develop at varying rates during childhood, resulting in the wide range of half-lives reported for many drugs. The cytochrome P-450 (CYP) 3A enzymes, which play a major role in drug metabolism, including that of erythromycin, develop early in life.[7,8,11,22–27] The earliest isozyme in this group to show activity is CYP3A7, the primary metabolic enzyme present in utero. It has been found on the endoplasmic reticulum of fetal hepatocytes by the end of the first trimester and serves a role in the transformation of fetal dehydroepiandrosterone and the detoxification of retinoic acid derivatives transferred from maternal serum across the placenta.[22,23,25–27] Enzymatic activity of CYP3A7 declines rapidly after birth, with a 50% reduction during the first month of life. Levels continue to decline at a slower rate through the next 6 months and are typically undetectable after 1 year of age. As levels of CYP3A7 decline, CYP3A4 and CYP3A5 levels rise. Although present during fetal development, the level of CYP3A4 activity is nearly 100-fold less than that of CYP3A7 until after birth.[22,27] Increases in CYP3A4 occur over the first months of life, often reaching levels of enzymatic activity higher than that seen in adults during early childhood. Development of CYP3A5 function is highly variable among infants and children and does not appear to be related to patient age.

It can be anticipated that N.M. will have a slower rate of erythromycin metabolism as a result of lower levels of CYP3A4 activity, so a more conservative approach to dosing is often used. An oral erythromycin dose of 7 mg (5 mg/kg) given every 8 hours would be an appropriate starting dose for N.M. In addition to increasing the risk for adverse effects, higher serum erythromycin concentrations can lead to greater inhibition of CYP3A4. This may place N.M. at risk for toxicity from accumulation of other drugs metabolized via CYP3A4, such as fentanyl and midazolam.

Upregulation of CYP2D6 appears to begin in the last stage of gestation as a part of the complex transition of the baby to extrauterine life.[22–24,28] In fetal liver tissue samples obtained early in gestation, CYP2D6 activity has been reported to be only 1% to 5% of adult values.[22] Earlier studies suggested that levels of enzymatic activity remained low during infancy, but more recent research has demonstrated that CYP2D6 activity increases rapidly during the third trimester, and by the second week of life, values are similar to values in adults.[23] CYP2D6 levels remain relatively constant throughout childhood. The impact of genetic polymorphisms of CYP2D6 on elimination half-life in children is comparable to that demonstrated in adults and appears to play a greater role in determining metabolic function than ontogeny.[23,24,28] A study of atomoxetine response in children and adolescents with ADHD found that CYP2D6 poor metabolizers had greater increases in heart rate and blood pressure and impaired weight gain compared with extensive metabolizers taking comparable doses, reflecting higher serum concentrations with the poor metabolizer phenotype.[29]

The enzymatic activity of CYP2C9 and CYP2C19 develops throughout childhood.[22,23,30] Studies of fetal hepatocytes demonstrated CYP2C9 activity at only 1% of adult values from 8 to 24 weeks' gestation, with an increase from 10% to 20% between 25 and 40 weeks. Enzyme activity continues to increase after birth, reaching 25% of adult values by approximately 5 months of age. Unlike other enzymes, CYP2C9 activity remains at only 50% of adult values until after puberty. The development of CYP2C9 activity is illustrated by the change in the rate of metabolism of phenytoin with advancing age. The apparent (calculated Michaelis–Menten) half-life of phenytoin in premature infants is approximately 75 hours, compared with 20 hours in a term neonate and 8 hours in a 2-week-old.[31]

Development of CYP2C19 function also occurs in utero, with enzyme activity 10% to 20% that of adults at birth.[23] Enzymatic activity increases gradually during the first 3 months of life to near full adult values. As with CYP2D6, genetic polymorphisms for CYP2C9 and CYP2C19 play an important role in determining individual patient response. Population modeling of pantoprazole pharmacokinetics in term neonates and premature infants revealed a longer elimination half-life than that reported in adults, supporting the lower levels of CYP2C19 activity in this age group.[32] The study also demonstrated significantly greater drug concentrations in the patients who had the poor metabolizer genotype.

The ontogeny of CYP2E1 has been studied in conjunction with the ability of infants to metabolize acetaminophen. Fetal hepatic CYP2E1 concentrations are typically undetectable during the first trimester, but begin to increase during the second trimester.[33] Levels are approximately 10% to 20% of adult values at birth. Enzyme concentrations continue to increase at a more gradual pace, until by 3 months of age, CYP2E1 expression becomes similar to that in adults. The increase in CYP2E1 metabolic capacity, along with maturation of glucuronidation, is responsible for the changing patterns of acetaminophen metabolite formation during infancy.

CASE 102-4, QUESTION 2: N.M. is now tolerating her enteral feedings and was recently extubated. However, she has had increasing episodes of apnea, a pause in breathing of 20 seconds or greater frequently present in premature newborns, during the past 2 days. Based on current dosing guidelines, you have recommended a caffeine citrate loading dose of 20 mg/kg given IV to be followed by a maintenance dose of 5 mg/kg given once daily to treat her apnea.[34] While reviewing the dosing information, you note that the elimination half-life for caffeine in neonates is approximately 70 to 100 hours, whereas the half-life for older infants, children, and adults is only 5 hours. What would explain that dramatic difference in half-life?

The changing elimination half-life of caffeine reflects the onset and maturation of CYP1A2 activity. The metabolism of caffeine during infancy has been extensively studied because many neonates are exposed in utero as a result of maternal intake and premature infants often receive caffeine for the treatment for apnea.[22–23,34,35] Studies have shown that CYP1A2 activity is negligible in fetal liver tissue and in newborns who were not exposed to it in utero.[35] The lower levels of enzymatic activity result in a longer caffeine half-life and allow once-daily dosing.[36] In contrast, newborns exposed to caffeine during gestation have higher levels of CYP1A2 activity at birth. Enzymatic activity rises progressively during the first months of life. By 6 months of age, it may exceed adult values, giving the infant a caffeine half-life of only 4 to 5 hours and necessitating more frequent dosing.

Case 102-4, Question 3: While N.M. was receiving mechanical ventilation during her first weeks of life, she was sedated with an infusion of midazolam. Many IV products, including some brands of midazolam, contain benzyl alcohol as a preservative and are labeled "Not for Use in Infants." What is the rationale for restricting the use of benzyl alcohol in the neonatal population?

Alcohol dehydrogenase, another Phase I enzyme, is present in utero, but in concentrations less than 5% of adult values.[23] Enzymatic activity does not approach functional maturity until approximately 5 years of age. The lack of alcohol dehydrogenase activity has a profound impact on the ability of newborns to metabolize benzyl alcohol, a common preservative in injectable drug products. In 1982, five neonates died after developing gasping respirations that progressed to respiratory failure, severe metabolic acidosis, renal and hepatic failure, thrombocytopenia, and cardiovascular collapse.[37] All of the infants had been repeatedly exposed to benzyl alcohol as a preservative in IV flush solutions. This toxicity, termed *gasping syndrome*, resulted from accumulation of the parent compound, as well as the benzoic acid metabolite. Another series of ten patient deaths was reported from a second institution.[38] From these case series, the threshold for toxicity was estimated to be a total daily exposure of 99 mg/kg/day. Within months of these reports, the FDA issued a safety alert calling attention to this reaction and recommending use of preservative-free products or preparations with alternative preservatives in newborns.[39] This change in practice led to the virtual elimination of gasping syndrome and brought to light the significance of differences in neonatal metabolism on drug toxicity. Pediatric clinicians continue to be vigilant for benzyl alcohol exposure, because several drugs routinely used in premature and critically ill neonates are not available in preservative-free preparations.[40]

PHASE II DRUG METABOLISM

Phase II reactions, including glucuronidation, sulfation, and acetylation, also undergo change throughout childhood. Present in low levels in fetal hepatic and renal tissues, the uridine 5'-diphosphate glucuronosyltransferase (UGT) enzymes responsible for the glucuronidation of both drugs and endogenous substances have minimal metabolic activity. A gradual increase in UGT expression occurs in the first 6 months of life, but still remains lower than that of adults for the first 2 to 3 years of life. Genetic polymorphisms produce additional variation in UGT expression.[11,22,23,41–44] The reduced ability of infants to perform glucuronidation has been known for many years as a result of the chloramphenicol "gray baby syndrome." Chloramphenicol was a widely used antibiotic during the 1950s. Within several years of its introduction, case reports began to appear in the medical literature describing emesis, abdominal distension, and cyanosis followed by cardiovascular collapse in infants given the drug.[46] The mechanism for this toxic effect was later found to be reduced activity of UGT2B7, the primary enzyme responsible for chloramphenicol metabolism, that allowed accumulation of the parent compound.[23,41]

Case 102-4, Question 4: N.M. also received morphine as an infusion during mechanical ventilation. Careful attention is needed when administering opioids to neonates to avoid drug accumulation. What differences in metabolism might affect the dosing requirements of morphine in the premature neonate such as N.M.?

Glucuronidation of morphine to morphine-6-glucuronide and morphine-3-glucuronide via UGT2B7 can be demonstrated in premature neonates born as early as 24 weeks' gestational age, but at a much slower rate than that of term neonates.[23,43,47,48] Studies of fetal liver microsomes have confirmed the presence of UGT2B7, with a rate of enzymatic activity only 10% to 20% of adult values.[22] Morphine metabolism increases rapidly during the last trimester of intrauterine life and the first weeks after birth. Clearance has been estimated to increase fourfold between 24 and 40 weeks' postconceptional age, but remains substantially slower than that of adults until approximately 3 years of age.[47,48]

Sulfation is a more important pathway in the metabolism of morphine during early infancy than later in life. Unlike UGT enzymes, sulfotransferases (SULTs) develop extensively in utero, reaching levels of enzyme activity similar to that of adults at birth.[22,23,49] Intrauterine expression of SULT1A1, which is responsible for fetal metabolism of thyroid hormones, SULT2A1, the enzyme that metabolizes steroid hormones, and SULT1A3, which metabolizes catecholamines, occurs early in gestation and remains relatively constant thereafter. Not all SULT enzyme development takes place in the liver. Expression of SULT2A1 occurs primarily in the fetal adrenal gland.

The reliance on sulfation during infancy is found with several drugs besides morphine, including catecholamines, thyroid hormones, theophylline, and acetaminophen. Glucuronidation of acetaminophen via UGT1A6 and UGT1A9 is decreased in infants, and as a result, the primary route of acetaminophen metabolism is formation of sulfate conjugates for the first year of life.[23,45] Glucuronide pathways begin to predominate later in infancy and eventually surpass sulfation as the predominate route for acetaminophen metabolism.

Because of the slower rate of morphine clearance in neonates, particularly those born prematurely, morphine should be initiated at lower doses than those recommended for older infants and children. An appropriate starting dose for N.M.'s morphine infusion would be 0.005 to 0.01 mg/kg/hour. N.M. should be closely monitored for adverse effects, including hypotension, respiratory depression after extubation, and constipation.

Elimination

CASE 102-5

Question 1: E.C. is a 1.85-kg infant girl born at 30 weeks' gestation. As with the other neonates described earlier, she is started on empiric antibiotic therapy with ampicillin and gentamicin shortly after birth. E.C. is given ampicillin 92.5 mg (50 mg/kg) IV every 12 hours and gentamicin 4.6 mg (2.5 mg/kg) IV every 24 hours. In the next bed, N.M., now 2 months old and 2.6 kg, is on the same regimen for a fever and elevated white blood cell count during the past 24 hours. N.M. is given ampicillin 130 mg (50 mg/kg) IV every 6 hours and gentamicin 6.5 mg (2.5 mg/kg) IV every 8 hours. What is the rationale for the differences in these patients' dosing intervals?

GLOMERULAR FILTRATION

Like the liver, the kidneys are not fully developed at birth. The ability to filter, excrete, and reabsorb substances is not maximized until 1 year of age.[7,8,50,51] At birth, full-term neonates have an average glomerular filtration rate (GFR) of only 2 to 4 mL/minute/1.73 m^2; in premature infants, the value may be even lower (0.6–0.8 mL/minute/1.73 m^2). There is a rapid rise in GFR during the first 2 weeks of life, with values increasing from 20 to 40 mL/minute/1.73 m^2 as a result of increased renal blood flow, increased function of the existing nephrons, and the appearance of additional nephrons, all of which may be timed to coincide with birth.[51] GFR increases from 80 to 110 mL/minute/1.73 m^2 by 6 months of age and continues to increase in a linear manner until it approaches adult values of 100 to 120 mL/minute/1.73 m^2 by 1 year of age. The impact of this increase in GFR can be seen in the neonatal dosing recommendations for many renally eliminated drugs, including the aminoglycosides and vancomycin. To account for reduced renal function, most pediatric references use a combination of patient weight and age (postnatal, postconceptional, or postmenstrual) to determine gentamicin dosing in neonates.[17] As a premature newborn, E.C. is likely to have significantly reduced glomerular filtration. E.C.'s gentamicin regimen will consist of the standard neonatal dose (2.5 mg/kg) given at a less frequent interval than that of 2-month-old N.M. to compensate for her renal insufficiency.

TUBULAR SECRETION

The elimination of ampicillin is also affected by changes in the rate of tubular secretion.[7,8,50] Like GFR, tubular secretion is reduced immediately after birth, but gradually increases during the first year of life. In addition to the penicillins, a reduction in tubular secretion also results in a prolonged elimination half-life for cephalosporins, furosemide, and digoxin. Digoxin has been used for many years in the management of supraventricular tachycardia in neonates. The half-life of digoxin decreases from approximately 30–40 hours in a term neonate to 20–25 hours in a 1-year-old as renal function matures. Selection of a digoxin dose must take into account the difference in elimination. The recommended oral digoxin maintenance dose for a neonate is 5 mcg/kg/day, whereas a 2-year-old would need to receive twice that amount to achieve target serum digoxin concentrations.[52] Ampicillin doses are typically adjusted by lengthening the dosing interval to compensate for reduced tubular secretion. E.C. (a newborn delivered at 30 weeks' gestation) would be dosed every 12 hours, whereas an older child such as N.M. would be expected to clear ampicillin more rapidly and would be dosed every 6 hours.

CASE 102-5, QUESTION 2: How should renal function be assessed in E.C. and N.M.?

As with adults, renal function should be closely monitored in children and drug doses adjusted accordingly. Unlike adults, blood urea nitrogen and serum creatinine values are not always useful as indicators of renal function. In the first days after birth, serum creatinine values reflect maternal creatinine transferred through the placenta and may appear falsely elevated. After the first week, serum creatinine values are typically low as a result of less muscle mass, especially in premature neonates, and may not accurately represent renal function.[8] Urine output is often used as an additional measure of renal function in this population. Diaper weights can be used to estimate output in E.C. and N.M., with values greater than 1 mL/kg/hour considered adequate renal function. At the time of initiation of therapy, if both babies are maintaining urine output values greater than 1 mL/kg/hour, the dosing regimens recommended in the *Pediatric Dosage Handbook*[17] can be used without further alteration. If urine output falls, the dosing intervals of both antibiotics may require adjustment. A trough serum gentamicin concentration should be obtained to further guide dosing.

CASE 102-6

QUESTION 1: H.G. is a 10-year-old boy admitted with osteomyelitis in his left ankle. The team plans to treat H.G. with vancomycin for 6 weeks. He is 140 cm (55 inches) tall and weighs 32 kg (70 pounds). His serum creatinine is 0.5 mg/dL (normal for age 0.5–1.5 mg/dL). Determine H.G.'s creatinine clearance.

After infancy, serum creatinine may be used to estimate clearance. The equations used in adults, such as Cockroft–Gault, Jellife, or the Modification of Diet in Renal Disease (MDRD), are not appropriate for patients younger than 18 years of age.[8,53,54] There are several equations designed for pediatric use; the National Kidney Disease Education Program (NKDEP) and the National Kidney Foundation recommend the bedside isotope dilution mass spectroscopy (IDMS) Schwartz equation[53,54]:

$$CL_{Cr} = (0.14 \times Ht)/S_{Cr} \qquad \text{(Eq. 102-1)}$$

where CL_{Cr} is creatinine clearance (mL/minute/1.73 m^2), Ht is height (cm), and S_{Cr} is serum creatinine (mg/dL).

Using this method, H.G. has a calculated creatinine clearance of 116 mL/minute/1.73 m^2, indicating normal renal function. As with patients of any age, this equation should be used only as an estimate of renal function. It should be interpreted with caution in patients with little muscle mass or those who are dehydrated.

Pharmacokinetic Changes During Puberty

CASE 102-7

QUESTION 1: A.M. is a 16-year-old, 67-kg boy with osteosarcoma. He has received morphine for pain throughout his numerous hospitalizations for surgery and chemotherapy during the past 2 years, requiring an infusion rate as high as 0.5 mg/kg/hour. During this period, he has also progressed through puberty and is now a mature adult male. During his last admission, it was noted that his pain was well controlled on an adult morphine infusion rate of 10 mg/hour, equivalent to 0.15 mg/kg/hour. It was noted by the medical team that A.M.'s morphine infusion requirements were actually lower than in earlier admissions, although his pain scores have been unchanged. What might explain the change in A.M.'s response to morphine?

Although developmental pharmacology has traditionally focused on the differences in neonatal pharmacokinetics, there is growing interest in the influence of puberty on drug disposition.[55–57] Adolescence is not simply a link between childhood and adulthood, but is a distinct period of significant physiologic change. Hormonal fluctuations and sexual maturation can alter the efficacy or toxicity of many drugs administered during this period. Drug distribution can be altered as a result of an increase in body fat. Rapid increases in serum protein concentrations that occur during puberty alter drug binding characteristics.[56] Renal function, as measured by GFR, may exceed average adult values, resulting in rapid clearance of renally eliminated drugs such as aminoglycosides and vancomycin. Metabolic activity changes as well.[57] A study conducted in adolescents receiving morphine during a sickle cell crisis revealed a reduction in drug clearance with advancing sexual maturation.[58] Postpubertal adolescents, such as A.M., had weight-normalized clearance values 30% lower than younger patients during early puberty, suggesting a possible reduction in UGT2B7 activity. The titration of A.M.'s morphine must encompass not only the changes in drug clearance resulting from growth and development but also the progression of his disease and his need for pain control. Assessment of pain, using frequent self-report or a standardized pain scale, as well as heart rate, blood pressure, and respiratory rate, is essential for appropriate adjustment of A.M.'s morphine infusion.

A second example comes from a recent study of lopinavir pharmacokinetics in children who exhibited identified age- and sex-related differences in drug clearance.[59] When normalized for weight, there was no significant difference in clearance between prepubertal boys and girls. After the age of 12, boys had a mean rate of lopinavir clearance 39% greater than girls. The area under the concentration–time curve in boys was only half that of the girls. The authors suggest that this difference may reflect a reduction in CYP3A4 in girls that becomes apparent only with sexual maturation. Similar sex-related results have been reported in lopinavir studies conducted in adults. Caffeine metabolism via CYP1A2 has also been found to differ by sex in adolescents.[60] The rate of *N*-demethylation slows in both sexes after puberty, but appears to decrease earlier in puberty for girls than for boys. Other investigators have identified pharmacokinetic changes during adolescence with acetaminophen, alprazolam, carbamazepine, digoxin, isoniazid, lamotrigine, lorazepam, and theophylline.[56]

PEDIATRIC PHARMACODYNAMIC DIFFERENCES

Although not as well studied as pharmacokinetics, developmental changes in pharmacodynamics during growth may have equally significant effects on response to drug therapy in children.

CASE 102-8

QUESTION 1: S.L. is a 0.725-kg infant boy with an estimated gestational age of 24 weeks. He was brought to the neonatal intensive care unit immediately after birth with severe hypotension. A dopamine infusion was started at a rate of 10 mcg/kg/minute and quickly titrated to 20 mcg/kg/minute without significant benefit. What might explain S.L.'s lack of response, and how should his hypotension be managed?

Maturational changes in receptor conformation, density, and affinity, as well as signal transduction, can result in clinically significant differences in response to common therapies.[61] Although a dopamine infusion of 20 mcg/kg/minute will produce an adequate increase in myocardial contractility and elevate systemic vascular resistance in most children and adults, infants may not have a significant change in cardiovascular response. Infants have long been suspected to be relatively resistant to the effects of β-adrenergic agonists, including dopamine, dobutamine, and epinephrine. Recent research suggests the lack of response is related to a relative reduction in adrenergic receptor density or a downregulation of receptors within the myocardium of premature and critically ill neonates.[62] A higher dopamine infusion rate, up to 40 mcg/kg/minute, may be necessary to achieve an adequate blood pressure for S.L. If the dopamine is increased, S.L.'s extremities must be closely monitored for any signs of excessive peripheral vasoconstriction. Supplemental therapy with hydrocortisone, at a dose of 0.7 mg (1 mg/kg) IV every 8 hours, may also be used to manage his hypotension.

CASE 102-9

QUESTION 1: You will be counseling the parents of E.S., a 7-year-old girl with refractory seizures as a result of Lennox-Gastaut syndrome, on the use of lamotrigine. While preparing for your discussion, you notice in the manufacturer's prescribing information a black box warning regarding the risk for serious skin rashes. The incidence is listed as 0.8% in children 2 to 16 years of age, but only 0.3% in adults.[63] What might explain the difference in the incidence of an adverse effect by age?

Differences in pharmacodynamics resulting from growth and development can alter more than just therapeutic response. A drug's adverse effect profile may be distinctly different during childhood. A classic example of this phenomenon is the higher incidence of serious dermatologic reactions, including toxic epidermal necrolysis, in children taking lamotrigine compared with that of adults.[64–66] This was first suspected during initial pediatric clinical trials and appeared to be associated with rapid dose titration during the first several months of treatment, which had been based on previous studies in adults.[65] The slower dose escalation, now recommended for pediatric patients, is starting E.S.'s lamotrigine dose at 0.15 mg/kg/day and increasing by 0.15- to 0.3-mg/kg/day increments every 2 weeks, and may reduce the likelihood for these reactions.

CASE 102-9, QUESTION 2: What is the possible mechanism(s) for the increased risk for toxicity with lamotrigine in children such as E.S.?

Research has led to several theories for the greater incidence of serious dermatologic reactions in children. Some investigators have suggested that this is a dose-related toxicity more evident in children who have a limited capacity to metabolize lamotrigine through glucuronidation to its inactive metabolites.[65] This theory, however, does not explain why other patient groups known to have higher serum lamotrigine concentrations during treatment, such as the elderly, are not at increased risk. Others have speculated that this represents an immune-mediated hypersensitivity response, because many of the affected patients reported have had previous reactions with other antiepileptic drugs.[66] Children with refractory seizures, such as those with Lennox-Gastaut syndrome, who are often treated with multiple agents beginning in the first years of life may be more likely to develop hypersensitivity. Although the mechanism underlying the age-related difference in the incidence of lamotrigine-associated rashes is not yet well understood, the importance of patient counseling is clear. The caregivers of all children receiving lamotrigine should be made aware of the risk and the need to seek medical care as soon as any signs of rash or erythema are noted.

MEDICATION DOSING IN CHILDREN

CASE 102-10

QUESTION 1: A.K. is a 7-year-old, 20-kg boy recently diagnosed with ADHD. After developing insomnia when treated with methylphenidate, he was switched to clonidine by his pediatrician. The recommended starting dose for clonidine in children is 5 mcg/kg/day divided and given in two to four doses.[67] His prescription is for clonidine 0.05 mg by mouth twice daily. Because A.K. does not yet swallow tablets easily, he will need a solution made from the tablets. It will be prepared from a published extemporaneous formulation with a final concentration of 0.1 mg/mL. What steps are necessary to ensure the accuracy of this prescription?

The differences in pharmacokinetics and pharmacodynamics observed in children influence the choice of dose and dosing interval.[68] Because incorporating all of these variables would result in dosing calculations too difficult for practical use, weight has traditionally been chosen as the single best estimate of growth. Pediatric drug references provide most doses in units per weight, such as mg/kg/day or mcg/kg/dose. Among the exceptions to this are chemotherapeutic agents, which are dosed by body surface area, incorporating height as an additional variable. Because of the difficulty in accurately determining height (or length) in young children, it is not commonly used for other drugs.

Age can be an important variable, especially for premature infants, in whom it can be used to account for differences in volume of distribution and elimination half-life. For example, neonatal gentamicin dosing is often based on a rubric of gestational or postconceptional age, postnatal age, and weight.[17] A recent study of clonidine clearance in the early postnatal period suggests that both age and weight should be used to optimize clonidine doses in newborns being treated for neonatal abstinence syndrome.[69] In the future, pediatric dosing recommendations for many drugs may be based on more than just weight to incorporate new pharmacokinetic data.[70]

Medication orders or prescriptions with doses outside of the dosing range listed in a pediatric drug reference should always be questioned for appropriateness. Older children and adolescents should transition to adult dosing whenever the calculated weight-based dose exceeds the usual adult dose. When evaluating a pediatric prescription or medication order, determining whether the dose is appropriate for the patient's weight is not the only step undertaken by the pharmacist. As with all patients, allergies, underlying diseases, and concomitant therapy must be taken into account as well.

A.K.'s clonidine dose of 0.05 mg twice daily is equivalent to 5 mcg/kg/day, the appropriate starting dose for a child. Using a 0.1-mg/mL extemporaneous solution, his dose will be 0.5 mL twice daily. The label on A.K.'s clonidine bottle should include the concentration of the formulation, as well as the dose in both mg and mL. Before the start of treatment, A.K.'s parents should be counseled about the drug, the dose, and potential adverse effects. They should be given or have access to an oral dosing syringe or spoon to accurately measure the dose.

PREVENTING MEDICATION ERRORS IN CHILDREN

CASE 102-10, QUESTION 2: After 2 days of therapy, A.K. returns to his pediatrician's office with his parents. He is lethargic and feels dizzy when getting out of bed. His blood pressure is 90/54 mm Hg (normal for age and weight is 99/59 mm Hg), suggesting a possible clonidine overdose. As you begin to investigate the potential cause of A.K.'s symptoms, what factors may have led to an error in A.K.'s case?

Medication errors pose a significant risk for infants and children.[71–75] Whereas the rate of medication errors reported in studies of adults is approximately 5%, rates in many pediatric studies have ranged from 10% to 15%.[71–73] The need to calculate weight-based doses can lead to mathematic errors. In A.K.'s case, the dose must be multiplied by the patient's weight, divided into individual doses, and converted from micrograms to milligrams. Unit conversions and decimal point errors are particularly dangerous in pediatrics, because a 10-fold overdose of a drug with a narrow dosing range such as clonidine, digoxin, morphine, or fentanyl can be fatal.[76] In addition to prescribing errors, dosage formulation manipulation, such as the preparation of an extemporaneous liquid in this case, increases the risk for drug preparation errors. Oral liquid medications also present a risk for administration errors. Healthcare providers and caregivers in the home must be aware of the potential for errors and the need for precise dose measurement. A.K.'s medical history must include information on how the clonidine had been prepared by the pharmacy as well as how his parents were preparing and administering his doses.

CASE 102-10, QUESTION 3: What steps could have been taken to prevent the medication error that occurred with A.K.?

There are a number of methods to reduce the potential for medication errors, including recommendations from the Joint Commission, the American Academy of Pediatrics, and a recent Cochrane review (Table 102-3).[74,75,77–82] Use of standard

Table 102-3
Methods for Reducing Pediatric Medication Errors

Improve Ordering and Preparation
Perform careful medication histories, including assessment of oral liquid concentrations
Provide access to current pediatric medication information
Include patient weight (in kg) on all medication orders and prescriptions
Include dosage calculations on orders and prescriptions
Limit the number of concentrations available for high-risk medications
Use accurate measuring devices, in both the hospital and home settings
Implement Appropriate Technology
Adopt weight-based electronic prescribing or dose-checking software
Employ barcode technology to reduce patient identification and medication administration errors
Use smart-pump technology (programmable IV pumps with weight-based dosing limits)
Use Staff Expertise
Provide pediatric-specific continuing education for all staff on a routine basis
Develop pediatric-specific medication orders and protocols to guide care
Assign staff with pediatric expertise to all committees involved in medication management
Involve Families and Other Caregivers
Encourage all caregivers to ask questions about their child's medications
Recommend that all caregivers know the names and doses of their children's medications or carry information about their medications
Remind caregivers to include nutritional supplements, herbal or complementary therapies, and over-the-counter medications when giving a medication history
Ensure that caregivers can accurately prepare the medication dose

IV, intravenous.

concentrations for IV products and oral liquids, smart-pump technology, bar coding, and electronic prescribing with clinical decision support tools have been found to significantly reduce errors in pediatric hospitals. In the outpatient setting, medication errors can be reduced by the inclusion of patient-specific information on prescriptions, including diagnosis and patient weight.[83] The product label, whether it is a prescription or over-the-counter medication, should include all the information needed to correctly prepare and administer the dose. Caregivers should have access to the appropriate tools for measuring liquid medications, such as oral dosing spoons or syringes, and the opportunity to practice preparing a dose under the supervision of a healthcare provider to ensure that they are able to prepare the dose correctly.[84]

One of the most effective methods to prevent medication errors has been to include pharmacists in the medication ordering and review process.[83,85] The value of pharmacists in reducing pediatric medication errors was demonstrated by Folli et al.[85] In this landmark study, clinical pharmacists performed prospective evaluations of medication orders at two children's hospitals for a 6-month period. The overall rate of medication errors detected by the pharmacists averaged 4.7 per 1,000 medication orders. Of these, 5.6% were considered potentially lethal. The majority of the errors (64.3%) occurred in children younger than 2 years of age. The most common type of error identified by the pharmacists was incorrect dosage. The authors concluded that pharmacy intervention had a significant effect on medication error prevention, a finding that resulted in the expansion of pediatric clinical pharmacy services in many institutions. Pharmacists in the community provide the same benefit when reviewing pediatric prescriptions and play a significant role in caregiver medication education.

INCREASING AVAILABILITY OF PEDIATRIC MEDICATION INFORMATION

Case 102-10, Question 4: Although the dose of clonidine for the treatment of ADHD is available in most pediatric dosing references, it is not found in the manufacturer's prescribing information (package insert) for the drug because the treatment of ADHD is not currently an FDA-approved indication. What is being done to increase the availability of pediatric drug information?

Although the availability of pediatric drug information has been limited in the past, several recent initiatives from the FDA are increasing the number of clinical trials being conducted in infants and children. The Pediatric Exclusivity Program, part of the FDA Modernization Act of 1997, was developed to address the lack of pediatric study data, including medication prescribing information.[8,86–88] The Exclusivity Program provides pharmaceutical manufacturers with incentives to study their products in children, including a 6-month extension at the end of a drug's patent life if a pediatric study is conducted. The 1998 Pediatric Rule and the Research Equity Act of 2003 authorized the FDA to require that manufacturers conduct clinical trials of drugs that would be used in a significant number of patients. The Best Pharmaceuticals for Children Act supplements the previous incentives by the creation of a mechanism for funding studies of older, off-patent medications that are often used in children.

These programs have been successful in adding pediatric dosing and adverse effect information to the prescribing information of many drugs routinely used in children. As of June 2017, the FDA had issued 430 written requests for pediatric studies, and 241 drugs had been granted a patent extension under the Exclusivity Program.[86] An assessment of the first 7 years of the program found that 50% of the studies conducted resulted in the new information supporting the use of the drug in children.[87] In spite of this success, much work remains to be done. Modifications in clinical trial design to incorporate pharmacogenomic studies and the use of combined pharmacokinetic–pharmacodynamic analyses have been recommended to further refine our knowledge of drug disposition in children.[87,88] The emphasis on the needs of pediatric patients has not been limited to just the United States; similar programs are in place in the European Union and throughout Asia. With the growing interest in developmental pharmacology and pharmacogenomics, as well as the increased funding and support for pediatric clinical trials worldwide, our understanding of the unique differences in how children respond to drug therapy continues to improve.

KEY REFERENCES AND WEBSITES

A full list of references for this chapter can be found at http://thepoint.lww.com/AT11e. Below are the key references and websites for this chapter, with the corresponding reference number in this chapter found in parentheses after the reference.

Key References

Kearns GL et al. Developmental pharmacology—drug disposition, action, and therapy in infants and children. *N Engl J Med*. 2003;349:1157. (7)

Leeder JS et al. Understanding the relative roles of pharmacogenetics and ontogeny in pediatric drug development and regulatory science. *J Clin Pharmacol*. 2010;50:1377. (24)

Maaskant JM et al. Interventions for reducing medication errors in children in hospital. *Cochrane Database Syst Rev*. 2015;3:CD006208.

MacLeod S. Therapeutic drug monitoring in pediatrics: how do children differ? *Ther Drug Monit*. 2010;32:253. (88)

Schwartz GJ et al. New equations to estimate GFT in children with CKD. *J Am Soc Nephrol*. 2009;20:629. (54)

Taketomo CK et al. *Pediatric Dosage Handbook*. 21st ed. Hudson, OH: Lexi-Comp; 2014. (17)

Key Websites

American Academy of Pediatrics. Ages and Stages. http://www.healthychildren.org.

The Joint Commission. Sentinel event alert: preventing pediatric medication errors. http://www.jointcommission.org/assets/1/18/SEA_39.PDF. (74)

U.S. Department of Health and Human Services, Food and Drug Administration. Pediatric Drug Development. http://www.fda.gov/Drugs/DevelopmentApprovalProcess/DevelopmentResources/ucm049867.htm. (86)

103 Pediatric Fluid, Electrolytes, and Nutrition

Michael F. Chicella and Jennifer W. Chow

CORE PRINCIPLES

	CORE PRINCIPLES	CHAPTER CASES
1	Fluid requirements and calories normalized to body weight are much greater in very small children than in older children and adults. It is important to understand how to calculate the normal fluid and caloric needs of children, and how fluid and caloric needs change with changes in clinical status.	**Case 103-1 (Question 1), Case 103-2 (Questions 1–3), Case 103-3 (Questions 1–3), Tables 103-1–103-6**
2	Human milk is the ideal food for a human infant. In addition to meeting the infant's nutritional requirements, human milk provides the infant with protection against a wide variety of infectious diseases and noninfectious disorders. Solid foods are generally introduced at 4 to 6 months of age, and pure cow's milk is generally introduced after 1 year.	**Case 103-4 (Questions 1, 2, 4, 5)**
3	Infant formula is available in three different formulations: cow's milk based, soy based, and protein hydrolysate (elemental). Cow's milk-based formulas are the standard for most infants. Soy-based and protein hydrolysate formulas are primarily intended for infants who are intolerant of cow's milk-based formulas. Other therapeutic formulas are available or can be made for infants with disease states that preclude the use of one of these three main types of formula.	**Case 103-4 (Question 3), Case 103-5 (Question 1), Case 103-6 (Questions 2, 3), Table 103-5**
4	Growth assessment is an important focus of pediatric health care, especially during the first year of life. With the exception of the intrauterine period, the most rapid growth occurs during the first year.	**Case 103-6 (Question 1)**
5	Parenteral nutrition in infants and children is usually initiated below estimated caloric needs and advanced as tolerated over the course of 3 or more days until goal caloric needs are met.	**Case 103-6 (Question 4)**
6	Parenteral nutrition can be used to supply sufficient nutrients to promote healing and a normal rate of growth in sick infants and children. However, parenteral nutrition is associated with clinically significant risks and complications.	**Case 103-7 (Questions 1–5, 7–9), Table 103-6**
7	Specialized pediatric amino acid solutions are available for infants younger than 1 year of age. These products were designed to produce plasma amino acid patterns closely matching those of human milk-fed infants.	**Case 103-7 (Question 6)**
8	Irreversible liver damage can occur with long-term parenteral nutrition. Parenteral nutrition-associated liver disease usually presents as an elevated direct (conjugated) hyperbilirubinemia and can occur as early as 2 weeks after beginning parenteral nutrition.	**Case 103-7 (Questions 10, 11)**
9	A number of modifications can be made to the patient's parenteral nutrition regimen to alleviate or slow the progression of cholestasis. The initiation of enteral feeding, even if limited to low-volume trophic feeding, appears to be the most effective method for preventing cholestasis.	**Case 103-7 (Question 11)**

Adequate nutrition is an essential component of the health maintenance of children and, in part, has been responsible for the dramatic reduction of infant mortality seen in the United States during the 20th century. Clinical experience has confirmed the value of optimal nutrition in resisting the effects of disease and trauma and in improving the response to medical and surgical therapy. The metabolic demands of rapid growth and maturation, in addition to the low nutritional reserves present during infancy, make the potential benefit of good nutrition to critically ill pediatric patients even greater.

Breast-feeding is the ideal method of feeding an infant and should be continued for at least the first year of life whenever possible. When this is not feasible, various infant formulas are available that provide appropriate nutrients for infants using the oral route. A pediatric patient who has a functioning intestinal tract, but is unable to achieve adequate oral intake, can be fed enterally using a tube inserted into the stomach or small intestine. Indications for providing specialized enteral nutrition include malnutrition, malabsorption, hypermetabolism, failure to thrive, prematurity, and disorders of absorption, digestion, excretion, or utilization of nutrients.

Despite the many formulas and feeding techniques available, several medical and gastrointestinal (GI) dilemmas that limit the use of the GI tract for nutritional support can occur in infants and children. Premature infants with severe respiratory disease, congenital abnormalities of the GI tract, or necrotizing enterocolitis are typical candidates for support with parenteral nutrition (PN). Older children with short bowel syndrome, severe malnutrition, intractable diarrhea, or inflammatory bowel disease have been treated successfully with PN therapy. Pediatric patients receiving chemotherapy for the treatment of malignancies or bone marrow transplant and children with severe cardiac failure also have been successfully rehabilitated with PN.

Many disorders that adversely affect nutrient intake or absorption also have an adverse impact on fluid and electrolyte status. Consequently, fluid, electrolyte, and nutrient management should be approached in an integrated manner. This chapter reviews selected aspects of fluid and electrolyte management and nutrition therapy for the pediatric population.

FLUID AND ELECTROLYTE MAINTENANCE

Management of fluid and electrolyte disturbances involves providing normal daily maintenance requirements and replacing deficits and ongoing losses. To design rational fluid therapy, it is necessary to know the normal composition of body water and to understand the routes through which water and solutes are lost from the body and the effects of disease and medications on water and electrolytes. Sodium-containing fluids are often referred to as fractions of normal saline (NS) (0.9% NaCl). Normal saline contains 154 mEq/L of sodium chloride.

Calculation of Maintenance Fluid and Electrolyte Requirements

CASE 103-1

QUESTION 1: P.J., a 2-day-old, 3.5-kg term female infant has developed abdominal distension, and her oral feedings have been stopped. Calculate a maintenance fluid and electrolyte prescription for her. Her serum electrolytes include the following:

Sodium, 137 mEq/L
Potassium, 4.2 mEq/L
Chloride, 105 mEq/L
CO_2, 23 mEq/L

While P.J. receives nothing by mouth (NPO), her fluid and electrolyte needs must be met intravenously. Estimate her requirements.

General recommendations for calculating maintenance fluid have not changed significantly since first outlined by Holliday and Segar in 1957.[1] Similarly, electrolyte and nutrient replacement is still based on guidelines published in 1988 by Greene et al.[2] Fluid, electrolyte, and nutrient requirements on the basis of weight are provided in Table 103-1. Although a commercially available intravenous (IV) solution will be used, each component of the solution can be calculated separately. Using the guidelines in Table 103-1, P.J.'s maintenance requirements can be estimated as follows:

Fluid $100\ mL/kg/day \times 3.5\ kg = 350\ mL/day$ or 15 mL/hour (Eq. 103-1)

Sodium $2\text{–}4\ mEq/kg/day \times 3.5\ kg = 7\text{–}14\ mEq/day$ (Eq. 103-2)

Potassium $2\text{–}3\ mEq/kg/day \times 3.5\ kg = 7\text{–}10.5\ mEq/day$ (Eq. 103-3)

Fluid and electrolyte requirements can be met by infusing a solution of 5% dextrose with one-quarter NS (38 mEq/L) and 20 mEq/L of KCl at 15 mL/hour. This provides 12 mEq (3.4 mEq/kg/day) of NaCl and 7 mEq (2 mEq/kg/day) of KCl in 360 mL (103 mL/kg/day) of fluid per day.

Additionally, fluid and electrolyte requirements can also be altered when fluid and electrolyte losses are increase or when excretion is impaired. When abnormal fluid losses are present, they must be given back to the patient daily. Replacement fluid is generally 1 mL for every 1 mL lost, but can be more or less based on the patient's clinical status. In general, NS can be initially used for most replacement fluids.

The requirements for fluid and calories normalized to body weight are much greater in very small children than in older children and adults as can be seen in Table 103-1. This is because infants have a much larger body surface area relative to weight, lose more fluid through evaporation, and dissipate more heat per kilogram than their older counterparts. Furthermore, very low-birth-weight (VLBW) infants cannot concentrate urine and are at increased risk for dehydration if inadequate fluids are provided.

Dehydration

CASE 103-2

QUESTION 1: H.S. is a 2-year-old lethargic girl with a 2-day history of vomiting and minimal oral intake. Yesterday, she required only three diaper changes instead of her usual eight and has needed only one change today. Her vital signs are as follows:

Temperature, 39°C
Pulse, 140 beats/minute (normal, 80–130 beats/minute)
Respiratory rate, 30 breaths/minute (normal, 30–35 breaths/minute)
Blood pressure (BP), 80/45 mm Hg (normal, 80–115 mm Hg systolic and 50–80 mm Hg diastolic)

On physical examination, her eyes appear sunken, her mucous membranes are dry, and her skin is dry and cool to touch. Although she is crying, there are no tears, and the skin over her sternum tents when pinched. Her weight today is 11.4 kg; 3 weeks ago, it was 12.9 kg. What do these findings represent? What immediate treatment should be provided?

Table 103-1
Daily Parenteral Nutrient Requirements in Children

Nutrient	Weight/Age	Requirement
Fluid	<1.5 kg	150 mL/kg
	1.5–2.5 kg	120 mL/kg
	2.5–10 kg	100 mL/kg
	10–20 kg	1,000 mL + 50 mL/kg for each kg >10 kg
	>20 kg	1,500 mL + 20 mL/kg for each kg >20 kg
Calories	Up to 10 kg	100 kcal/kg
	20 kg	1,000 kcal + 50 kcal/kg for each kg >10 kg
	>20 kg	1,500 kcal + 20 kcal/kg for each kg >20 kg
Protein[a]	Infants	2–3 g/kg
	Older children	1.5–2.0 g/kg
	Adolescents and older	1.0–1.5 g/kg
Fat[b]	Infants and children	Initially 0.5–1 g/kg and then increase by 0.5–1 g/kg (maximum of 3 g/kg in preterm neonates, 4 g/kg older infants and children) (≥4% of calories as linoleic acid)
	>50 kg	One 500-mL bottle (100 g fat)
Electrolytes and Minerals[c]		
Sodium	Infants and children	2–4 mEq/kg
Potassium	Infants and children	2–3 mEq/kg
Chloride	Infants and children	2–4 mEq/kg
Magnesium	Preterm and term infants	0.25–0.5 mEq/kg
	Children >1 year (or >12 kg)	4–12 mEq
Calcium	Preterm and term infants	2–3 mEq/kg
	Children >1 year (or >12 kg)	10–20 mEq
Phosphorus	Preterm and term infants	1.0–1.5 mmol/kg
	Children >1 year (or >12 kg)	10–20 mmol
Trace Elements		
Zinc	Preterm infants	400 mcg/kg
	Term infants	
	<3 mos	250 mcg/kg
	>3 mos	100 mcg/kg
	Children	50 mcg/kg (up to 5 mg)
Copper	Infants and children	20 mcg/kg (up to 300 mcg)
Manganese	Infants and children	1 mcg/kg (up to 50 mcg)
Chromium	Infants and children	0.2 mcg/kg (up to 5 mcg)
Selenium	Infants and children	2 mcg/kg (up to 80 mcg)

[a]"Infant" amino acids contain histidine, taurine, tyrosine, and cysteine, which are essential in infants but not older patients.
[b]Because linoleic acid represents 54% of the fatty acid in soy bean oil and 77% in safflower oil, 7% to 10% of calories must be provided as fat emulsion. This can be given daily over the course of 24 hours (preferred in patients predisposed to sepsis and preterm infants) or 2 to 3 times weekly.
[c]These doses are guidelines and all patients should be evaluated individually for appropriateness of dosing. For example, patients with short bowel syndrome may require large doses of magnesium, and patients with renal insufficiency may require none to low amounts of potassium, calcium, phosphorous, and magnesium.
Source: Holliday MA, Segar WE. The maintenance need for water in parenteral fluid therapy. *Pediatrics*. 1957;19(5):823–832; Greene HL, Hambidge KM, Schanler R, Tsang RC. Guidelines for the use of vitamins, trace elements, calcium, magnesium, and phosphorus in infants and children receiving total parenteral nutrition: report of the Subcommittee on Pediatric Parenteral Nutrient Requirements from the Committee on Clinical Practice Issues of the American Society for Clinical Nutrition [published corrections appear in *Am J Clin Nutr.* 1989;49(6):1332; *Am J Clin Nutr.* 1989;50(3):560]. *Am J Clin Nutr*. 1988;48(5):1324–1342.

H.S.'s lethargy, decreased urine output, tearless crying, dry mucous membranes, dry skin with fever, sunken eyes, mild tachycardia with low normal blood pressure, and poor skin turgor are all signs of dehydration. This is consistent with her 2-day history of vomiting and poor intake. Her weight loss of 1.5 kg gives a further clue to the extent of dehydration. Dehydration or fluid loss is determined most accurately by weight loss. Because 1 g of body weight is approximately equal to 1 mL, her fluid deficit

Table 103-2
Clinical Signs of Dehydration

Severity	Dehydration (%)	Psyche	Thirst	Mucous Membranes	Tears	Anterior Fontanel	Skin	Urine Specific Gravity
Mild	<5	Normal	Slight	Normal to dry	Present	Flat	Normal	Slight change
Moderate	6–10	Irritable	Moderate	Dry	±	±	±	Increased
Severe	10–15	Hyperirritable to lethargic	Intense	Parched	Absent	Sunken	Tenting	Greatly increased

is estimated to be 1,500 mL. The percentage dehydration is estimated using the following formula:

$$\% \text{ Dehydration} = \text{Normal body weight} - \text{Actual body weight} / \text{Normal body weight} \times 100 \quad \text{(Eq. 103-4)}$$

If recent weights are unavailable, the extent of dehydration can be approximated from physical findings as described in Table 103-2. Tachycardia and marginal blood pressure dictate the need for immediate IV rehydration. Normal serum sodium concentration ranges from 135 to 145 mEq/L of sodium; thus, normal saline approximates the sodium concentration of plasma and is often used as a volume expander. In this patient, 10 to 20 mL/kg of normal saline (12.9 kg × 10–20 mL/kg = 129–258 mL) should be infused as rapidly as possible to establish normal blood pressure. For symptomatic patients, including those with seizures, the serum sodium concentration should be increased acutely only to the degree necessary to abate symptoms.

CASE 103-2, QUESTION 2: Calculate H.S.'s fluid and electrolyte needs and provide recommendations for her fluid orders to the team. Her serum electrolyte results were as follows:

Sodium, 128 mEq/L (normal, 135–145 mEq/L)
Potassium, 3.1 mEq/L (normal, 3.5–5 mEq/L)
Chloride, 88 mEq/L (normal, 102–109 mEq/L)
HCO_3^-, 30 mEq/L (normal, 22–29 mEq/L)

In addition to normal maintenance fluids, H.S. must be provided with fluids and electrolytes to replace her deficit secondary to dehydration and compensate for increased insensible water loss because of fever. Each component of the fluid can be calculated separately, using Equations 103-5 to 103-7.

$$\text{Fluid deficit} = \text{Weight loss (kg)} \times 1{,}000 \text{ mL/kg} \quad \text{(Eq. 103-5)}$$

$$\text{Fever adjustment} = 10\% \times \text{Maintenance for each } ^\circ\text{C} \geq 37^\circ\text{C} \quad \text{(Eq. 103-6)}$$

$$(\text{CD} - \text{CO}) \times F_d \times \text{Weight} = \text{mEq required} \quad \text{(Eq. 103-7)}$$

where CD is the concentration of sodium desired (mEq/L), CO is the concentration observed (mEq/L), F_d is the apparent distribution factor as a fraction of body weight (Table 103-3), and weight is the baseline weight before illness (kg). In consideration of both maintenance needs and current deficits, fluid and electrolyte requirements for H.S. would be estimated as follows.

FLUID

Maintenance	1,000 mL + (50 × 2.9) = 1,145 mL
Fever	2°C × 0.1 (1,145) = 229 mL
Deficit	1.5 kg × 1,000 mL/kg = 1,500 mL
	Total fluid = 2,874 mL

(Eq. 103-8)

Table 103-3
Electrolytes and Apparent Distribution

Electrolyte	F_d (L/kg)
Sodium	0.6–0.7
Bicarbonate	0.4–0.5
Chloride	0.2–0.3

F_d, apparent distribution factor as a fraction of body weight.

SODIUM

Maintenance 3 mEq/kg × 12.9 kg = 38.7

Deficit (135 – 128 mEq/L) × 0.6 L/kg × 12.9 kg = 54.2

Total sodium ~ 93 mEq (Eq. 103-9)

CHLORIDE

H.S. has a mild metabolic alkalosis as evidenced by her serum chloride of 88 mEq/L and her serum bicarbonate of 30 mEq/L. This is most likely because of the loss of hydrogen and chloride in her vomitus. Thus, both the sodium and potassium replacements should be administered as chloride salts.

POTASSIUM

Potassium is primarily an intracellular ion. It moves in and out of cells in exchange for hydrogen ions to maintain a normal blood pH. Therefore, in metabolic alkalosis, the intracellular shift of potassium will decrease the serum potassium concentration. When the pH normalizes, as will occur with rehydration, the hydrogen ions will move intracellularly and the potassium will move extracellularly, thus causing the serum potassium concentration to increase. Additionally, potassium is also excreted by the kidney in exchange for hydrogen ion conservation. These factors make the serum potassium concentration difficult to interpret. Intravascular volume depletion causes hypoperfusion of the kidney and can result in acute renal failure; therefore, the prudent approach is to give no potassium until urine output is clearly established. Then, only maintenance doses of potassium should be administered until a normal acid–base and fluid status are established and the serum potassium can be assessed more accurately. Hence, H.S. should receive approximately 26 to 39 mEq of potassium (2–3 mEq/kg × 12.9 kg) once urine flow is established.

Administration of Fluid Requirements

CASE 103-2, QUESTION 3: J.H.'s nurse asks for details of how the fluid therapy should be administered. How should these calculated needs be given?

Requirements for the first 24 hours of parenteral fluid therapy should provide approximately 2,875 mL of fluid to account for maintenance fluid needs, fever replacement, and deficit replacement. In addition to fluid, at least 93 mEq of sodium (maintenance needs plus deficit replacement) should be provided in the first 24 hours. It is important to provide sufficient amounts of sodium and water.

Rehydration fluids are usually dispensed in volumes less than the 24-hour requirement. This is to prevent wasting IV fluids caused by changes in electrolyte needs during replacement therapy. Because this patient requires approximately 3 L of fluid, only 1 L would be prepared initially, and this would likely consist of dextrose 5% and 0.2% NS (or greater). Approximately 15 mEq/L of potassium would be added to the next liter of IV solution if the patient had a reasonable urine output.

The infusion rate should be calculated to provide one-third of the daily maintenance fluid plus one-half of the deficit replacement during the first 8 hours. The remainder of the maintenance fluid (adjusted for fever) and deficit replacement should be administered during the next 16 hours. Usually, serum electrolytes are monitored every 6 to 8 hours during rehydration therapy to ensure that appropriate electrolytes are being provided. Usually, the concentration of serum electrolytes is monitored frequently during fluid replacement therapy of deficits. In general, the serum sodium concentration should not be increased by more than 10 to 12 mEq/L/day. After the initial fluid deficits are replaced, the infusion rate of the IV fluid would be decreased to 48 mL/hour (1,152 mL or approximately maintenance fluid rate).

Dehydration Associated with Diarrhea

CASE 103-3

QUESTION 1: S.B. is a 4-month-old, 5.9-kg boy presenting with a 4-day history of diarrhea (five to eight large, liquid stools each day). On a well-child visit 4 weeks ago, his weight was 6 kg. Since the onset of diarrhea, he has only been receiving oral rehydration fluids. Physical examination reveals the following:

Temperature, 38.8°C
Pulse, 110 beats/minute (normal, 80–160 beats/minute)
Respirations, 45 breaths/minute (normal, 20–40 breaths/minute)
BP, 100/58 mm Hg (normal, 75–105 mm Hg systolic and 40–65 mm Hg diastolic)
His skin is pale, warm, and dry. He is very irritable, and his mucous membranes are dry. S.B.'s laboratory values are as follows:
Sodium, 159 mEq/L
Potassium, 3.3 mEq/L
Chloride, 114 mEq/L
CO_2, 12 mEq/L
Blood urea nitrogen (BUN), 22 mg/dL
Creatinine, 0.9 mg/dL
Correlate S.B.'s history and physical findings with the reported laboratory values.

Diarrheal fluid losses commonly contain high concentrations of bicarbonate, accounting for S.B.'s metabolic acidosis. This, in turn, has resulted in a rapid respiratory rate as the body attempts to compensate for the acidosis by eliminating carbon dioxide. The increased insensible water losses of fever and tachypnea have resulted in the loss of water in excess of sodium, producing hypernatremia.

CASE 103-3, QUESTION 2: How should S.B.'s dehydration be managed?

S.B. has relatively normal vital signs and will not require rapid fluid replacement to correct hypotension. Hypernatremia in S.B. indicates fluid losses in excess of sodium and this should be corrected. With hypernatremia, the central nervous system (CNS) increases intracellular osmolarity load to prevent intracellular dehydration of cells in the CNS. Rapid correction of hypernatremia can cause excessive movement of water into the cells of the CNS and has been associated with seizures. Therefore, S.B.'s fluid and electrolyte deficits should be corrected over the course of 2 to 3 days at a consistent rate, rather than rapidly. In general, serum sodium should not be decreased more than 2 mEq/hour (maximum, 15 mEq/L/day).

S.B.'s requirements are estimated using the same methods described previously. First, the approximate extent of dehydration must be estimated. S.B.'s weight of 6 kg at the time of his well-child visit at 3 months of age was at the 50th percentile. If his growth has continued at this rate, his current pre-illness weight should be approximately 6.5 kg.[3] This weight should be used to calculate his maintenance requirements. Thus, his water deficit is approximately 0.6 L, or 9%. Using this approximation, his fluid and electrolyte requirements can be estimated as follows.

FLUID

Maintenance	6.5 × 100 mL/kg = 650 mL/24 hours
Fever	1.8°C × 0.1 (650 mL) = 117 mL/24 hours
	600 mL/3 days = 200 mL/24 hours
Deficit	Total daily needs = 967 mL or 40 mL/hour

(Eq. 103-10)

SODIUM

Maintenance	3 mEq/kg × 6.5 kg = 19.5 mEq/24 hours
Deficit	This is calculated as total body deficit (normal–actual)
Normal	145 mEq/L × 0.6 L/kg × 6.5 kg = 566 mEq
Actual	159 mEq/L × 0.6 L/kg × 5.9 kg = 563 mEq
Deficit	= 3 mEq or 1 mEq/day

(Eq. 103-11)

POTASSIUM

As discussed in Case 103-2, Question 2, the serum potassium value of 3.3 mEq/L may not be indicative of S.B.'s total body potassium status. A metabolic acidosis in S.B. should have facilitated the movement of hydrogen ions into the cells and the movement of potassium from the intracellular to the extracellular space. Thus, the serum potassium of 3.3 mEq/L probably indicates a total body deficit. Therefore, a maintenance potassium dosage of 13 to 20 mEq/day (approximately 2 to 3 mEq/kg) of potassium should be added to the intravenous fluid. Serum electrolytes should be measured every 8 to 12 hours, and the intake of all electrolytes should be readjusted based on the results.

BICARBONATE

With metabolic acidosis, bicarbonate should be administered as well. No maintenance amount is customarily given, but deficit replacement is calculated in a manner similar to that used for sodium (Table 103-3). The volume of distribution of bicarbonate is 0.5 L/kg. For S.B., the bicarbonate deficit is as follows:

$$\text{Calculated Deficit Requirement} = (\text{Normal} - \text{Actual}) \times V_d \times W_t$$
$$= (23\text{–}12)\ \text{mEq/L} \times 0.5\ \text{L/kg} \times 6.5\ \text{kg}$$
$$= 36\ \text{mEq} \qquad \text{(Eq. 103-12)}$$

Initially, about half this amount should be added to the intravenous fluid and replaced during the first 8 to 12 hours. His serum electrolytes then should be reassessed, and the dosages adjusted accordingly. The entire bicarbonate deficit need not be replaced at once because other compensatory mechanisms will contribute to endogenous bicarbonate sparing.

CASE 103-3, QUESTION 3: Recommend an appropriate replacement fluid for S.B.'s therapy.

S.B.'s fluid and electrolyte maintenance requirements and deficits should be corrected with dextrose 5% and approximately 0.2% NS with half as the chloride salt and half as $NaHCO_3$. An infusion of this solution at 43 mL/hour should correct approximately one-half the calculated fluid and bicarbonate deficits within 24 hours in addition to his normal daily doses. After he urinates, 15 mEq/L KCl can be added to the next liter of solution to provide approximately 2.6 mEq/kg/day to this patient. The concentration of serum electrolytes should be measured often, and the concentration of electrolytes in the replacement fluid should be adjusted every 8 to 12 hours based on laboratory results. The amount of fluid replacement should be modified based on whether this patient's diarrhea has resolved and fever has subsided.

Rehydration of the dehydrated patient may be achieved by either the oral or intravenous route. In some patients, vomiting may preclude effective oral rehydration. If the losses are diarrheal and no problem with vomiting exists, the oral route may be a cost-effective alternative to the parenteral route. Various solutions have been used to rehydrate children orally. In an asymptomatic dehydrated child, the sodium concentration of an oral rehydration fluid should contain at least 70 mEq/L of sodium.[4]

The composition of several products is shown in Table 103-4. A glucose concentration of 2% optimizes water and electrolyte absorption from the GI tract[4]; more concentrated glucose solutions can worsen rather than ameliorate diarrhea. Use of the oral route and the more concentrated sodium solutions may allow safe rehydration of hypernatremic dehydration in a shorter time frame than the 2 to 3 days previously noted.[4]

INFANT ENTERAL NUTRITION

Caloric requirements of infants can be estimated using the formula provided in Table 103-1. The American Heart Association has suggested that infant feeding be divided into three stages.[5] In the nursing period, only liquids are provided. During the transitional period, solid foods are introduced, but human milk, or commercially prepared infant formula, still provides the major source of the infant's caloric and nutrient supply. In the modified adult period, most nutrition is derived from the solid foods consumed by other household members.

At birth, the human GI tract is adapted for the consumption of a human milk-based diet. Intestinal lactase is present from 36 weeks' gestation and exhibits its maximal activity during infancy. Pancreatic amylase secretion is low, and the bile salt pool is decreased relative to that of older persons, resulting in decreased fat absorption.[6] Human milk provides nutrients in their most usable form for the developing GI tract.

Human Milk Feeding

CASE 103-4

QUESTION 1: M.E. is a 1-day-old full-term infant. M.E.'s mother will breast-feed her infant. What are the nutritional implications of this decision for M.E.?

Human milk is the ideal food for a human infant and should be encouraged to be continued for the first year of life as long as mutually desired by both mother and child.[7] There are three phases to human milk production. During the first 5 days of lactation, a viscous, yellow liquid known as *colostrum* is produced. Colostrum is rich in protein, minerals, and other substances (e.g., immunoglobulins). During the next 5 days, transitional milk is produced; in the last phase, mature human milk is produced. The exact nutritional content of human milk varies from mother to mother; however, mature human milk provides sufficient protein, minerals, and calories regardless of the mother's nutritional status. Mature human milk generally provides 70 kcal/100 mL, and fat accounts for more than 50% of the caloric content.[8] The fat in human milk is highly digestible and absorbable.[8] An additional 40% of calories is provided as carbohydrates, primarily in the form of lactose, and the remaining 10% is provided as protein. Whey and casein are the two primary proteins in mature human milk, with whey being the major protein component (whey-to-casein ratio of 60:40).[9] Human milk is of such biologic quality and bioavailability that adequate growth can be attained with a lower overall intake of protein than is provided by commercially prepared infant formulas, which contain lower whey-to-casein ratios.[9]

The iron content of human milk is inadequate for term infants; however, supplementation generally is unnecessary in the breast-fed infant.[10] Regardless of maternal status, the vitamin D content of human milk is inadequate. Thus, M.E. will require 400 international units of vitamin D while she is exclusively breast-fed.[11]

Additionally, human milk provides the infant with protection against a wide variety of infectious diseases, including otitis media, diarrhea, pneumonia, and bronchiolitis. Evidence further suggests that human milk provides protection against noninfectious disorders, such as allergies, inflammatory bowel disease, insulin-dependent diabetes mellitus, and sudden infant death syndrome.[7,8] Human milk contains immunologically active cellular components and antibodies. These include secretory IgA, both T and B lymphocytes, macrophages, and neutrophils.[7,8] The

Table 103-4
Composition of Oral Rehydration Products[4]

Product	Na^+ (mEq/L)	K^+ (mEq/L)	Cl^- (mEq/L)	Bicarbonate Source (mEq/L)	Carbohydrate (%)
Enfalyte	50	25	45	34 citrate	3
Rehydralyte	75	20	65	30 citrate	2.5
Pedialyte	45	20	35	30 citrate	2.5
Gatorade	23.5	<1	17	—	4.6
WHO salts	75	20	65	10 bicarbonate	2

WHO, World Health Organization.

lipases and amylase present in human milk may facilitate digestion of fat and carbohydrates in the still developing GI tract. Proteins present in human milk serve as carriers for trace minerals and facilitate their absorption.[9] Oligosaccharides and glycopeptides may promote the colonization of the GI tract by *Lactobacilli* and decrease colonization by *Bacteroides*, *Clostridia*, enterococci, and gram-negative rods, all of which may be pathogenic.[8]

CASE 103-4, QUESTION 2: What potential complications are associated with breast-feeding? What instructions should be given to M.E.'s mother?

Complications associated with breast-feeding are few; however, there are some potential problems. "Breast milk jaundice" associated with an indirect (unconjugated) hyperbilirubinemia can occur in the breast-fed infant during the first week of life and generally resolves by the fourth week of life. Although the infant's skin, sclera, and palate become yellow, this is generally not a dangerous condition. Nevertheless, if the bilirubin level becomes too high, the infant could develop an encephalopathy known as kernicterus. However, it is generally not necessary for the mother to stop breast-feeding while the infant has jaundice. The American Academy of Pediatrics (AAP) recommends that infants nurse at least 8 to 12 times daily while jaundiced.[12] Some maternal infections have the potential to be transmitted to the infant during breast-feeding. Human immunodeficiency virus (HIV) and human T-lymphotropic virus 1 (HTLV-1) can be transmitted via breast milk, and therefore, maternal infections with these viruses are contraindications to breast-feeding.[7,8] Other viruses, such as herpes simplex virus, can be transmitted if contact with active lesions occurs during breast-feeding. Similarly, some medications taken by the mother are detectable in her breast milk. Only a few agents (e.g., antineoplastics, radiopharmaceuticals, ergot alkaloids, iodides, atropine, lithium, cyclosporine, chloramphenicol, bromocriptine), however, are absolute contraindications to breast-feeding.[7,8]

CASE 103-4, QUESTION 3: M.E.'s mother suffers from migraine headaches, which have increased in frequency since M.E.'s birth. M.E.'s mother takes an ergot alkaloid for the acute management of her headaches and therefore has decided not to breast-feed M.E. She will be using infant formula instead. How are these products prepared and how do they differ from human milk?

Because of the excretion of ergot alkaloids into breast milk and the risk for toxicity to the infant, it is advisable to either select an alternative medication or discontinue breast-feeding and use an infant formula. Examples of infant formulas are provided in Table 103-5. According to AAP guidelines for commercially prepared infant formula composition, formula should provide 20 kcal/ounce, osmolality should be between 300 and 400 mOsm/L, protein quantity should be a minimum of 1.8 g/100 kcal and should not exceed 4.5 g/100 kcal, and fat quantity should be between 3.3 and 6 g/100 kcal, supplying between 30% and 54% of calories. Infant formulas generally begin with a cow's milk base; however, intolerance to pure cow's milk has resulted in several modifications. The predominant protein in cow's milk is casein, which is more difficult for infants to digest than the human milk protein, whey. Consequently, infant formulas generally have less casein than cow's milk, although not to the level of human milk. The casein present in cow's milk formulas also may be heat-denatured to improve its digestibility. In addition, the fat source in cow's milk is replaced by one of several vegetable oils, allowing for easier digestion. Last, the carbohydrate source in cow's milk-based formula is supplemented with lactose or sucrose because the lactose content of cow's milk is only 50% to 70% of that in human milk. Soy-based and protein hydrolysate formulas are available for infants who are intolerant of cow's milk-based formulas.

Soy-based formulas use soybean as the protein source.[13] The soy is heat-treated to enhance protein digestibility and improve the bioavailability of some nutrients. Although nutrients, such as methionine, zinc, and carnitine, are still present, their concentrations are relatively low. Therefore, the manufacturer routinely adds methionine to all soy-based formulas. Zinc and carnitine may not be added, and exogenous supplementation may be necessary. Soy-based formulas substitute sucrose, corn syrup, or a combination of the two for lactose as the carbohydrate source. Additionally, soy protein formulas are more expensive than cow's milk-based formulas. The AAP recommends that the use of soy-based formula be limited to patients with primary lactase deficiency (galactosemia), patients with secondary lactose intolerance from enteric infections or other causes, vegetarian families in which animal protein formulas are not desired, and infants who are potentially cow's milk protein allergic, but who have not demonstrated clinical manifestations of allergy. Long-term use of soy-based formulas in premature and low-birth-weight infants should not be recommended. Soy-based formulas have aluminum contamination and have been associated with the development of rickets. Soy-based formulas are also not recommended for infants with documented allergic reactions to cow's milk protein because of the potential for cross-antigenicity between the two proteins. Additionally, soy protein formulas are not recommended for the routine management of colic.

Elemental formulas, made with hydrolysate formulas, are another option for infants who are intolerant of cow's milk-based formulas. The milk proteins (i.e., casein and whey) are heat-treated and enzymatically hydrolyzed to enhance

Table 103-5
Infant Formulas

Cow's Milk-Based Formulas	Soy-Based, Lactose-free Formulas	Protein Hydrolysate, Elemental, Premature Infant Formulas
Enfamil with iron	Isomil	Alimentum
Similac with iron	Nursoy	Nutramigen
Gerber Good Start	ProSobee	Pregestimil
	Alsoy	NeoCate
	Gerber Soy Plus	Neosure Advance
	Similac Sensitive	Enfamil Premature
		Similac Special Care

digestibility of protein hydrolysate formulas, which are fortified with additional amino acids that are lost during processing. As with soy protein formulas, protein hydrolysates substitute sucrose, tapioca, or corn syrup for lactose as the carbohydrate source. Protein hydrolysate formulas often include significant amounts of medium-chain triglycerides because they are easily absorbed. Because the proteins are extensively hydrolyzed, these formulas probably are the least allergenic of the infant formulas and, therefore, may be appropriate for infants with true allergy to cow's milk protein. Nevertheless, prospective studies on the safety of such a substitution in human infants have not been undertaken because it would be unethical to intentionally expose infants with documented allergies to a potential allergen. Protein hydrolysate formulas are the least palatable of the available pediatric formulas and are more costly than other formulas.[14]

Infant formula is available from the manufacturers in three forms: ready-to-feed formula, powder for reconstitution, and concentrated liquid. The ready-to-feed form is the most convenient but also the most expensive. The powder and the concentrated liquid are less expensive; however, both require that predetermined amounts of boiled water be added before use. To save money, some parents will dilute infant formula to a greater extent than is recommended to make the formula last longer. This practice should be discouraged because excessive free water intake by infants younger than 1 year of age may result in hyponatremia and, ultimately, seizures. Similarly, supplementing an infant's diet with free water, for whatever reason, may also result in hyponatremia and seizures and should be discouraged. Periodically, manufacturing problems can occur, resulting in the recall of a product from the market.[15] Therefore, it is important for the patient's healthcare providers to stay abreast of manufacturers' recalls.

Introduction of Pure Cow's Milk

Case 103-4, Question 4: At 2 months of age, M.E. is found to have a hematocrit (Hct) of 33% (normal, 35%–45%). After questioning her mother, you learn that M.E. was taken off infant formula 1 month ago and changed to whole cow's milk to decrease food costs. How are these two findings related, and how should M.E. be managed?

Pure cow's milk, straight from the dairy counter in the grocery store, is not recommended for infants younger than 1 year of age. Unlike human milk, the iron in cow's milk is present in inadequate concentrations and absorbed poorly from the human GI tract. For this reason, most infant formulas are fortified with iron. Cow's milk has been associated with GI blood loss in infants younger than 140 days of age.[16] When the milk is heated to a higher temperature than the usual pasteurization temperature, as it is in formula preparation, the association of cow's milk with GI bleeding is no longer present; therefore, the component responsible for the blood loss appears to be a heat-labile protein. Furthermore, cow's milk contains excessive amounts of solute that cannot be eliminated by the immature kidney. Also, cow's milk does not contain taurine, an amino acid that is important in retinal development.

To treat M.E.'s anemia, iron should be added to her diet. This can be done by changing back to an iron-fortified infant formula, feeding her an iron-fortified cereal, or giving a therapeutic ferrous sulfate liquid medication. The appropriate iron replacement dose for severe anemia is 4 to 6 mg/kg/day of elemental iron in divided doses with follow-up of the infant's hemoglobin and hematocrit.

Introduction of Solid Foods

Case 103-4, Question 5: At 4 months of age, M.E.'s mother asks about the introduction of "baby foods" into M.E.'s diet. How should the clinician respond?

Human milk or commercially prepared infant formula provides adequate nutrition for an infant for the first 12 months of life. Introduction of solid foods before the age of 4 months, although common in the past, is discouraged because the younger infant is unprepared to swallow foods other than liquids. Solids (first cereals, then fruits, and vegetables) should be introduced when the child has good control of the head and neck movements (i.e., usually at the age of 4–6 months).[5] Preferably, one new food should be introduced at a time, at 1-week intervals, to allow assessment of food allergy.

Therapeutic Formulas

CASE 103-5

Question 1: L.B. is a 2-week-old infant whose newborn screen is positive for phenylketonuria (PKU). Discuss the concepts behind the production of therapeutic formulas and the dietary management of patients with inborn errors of metabolism. How should L.B.'s diet be modified?

Inborn errors of metabolism are disorders in which an enzyme or its cofactor is absent or insufficient to meet metabolic demands.[17] As a result, one or more precursor compounds in a metabolic pathway can accumulate before the defective step. Correspondingly, one or more metabolic products that normally would have been generated after the defective step in the metabolic pathway are not sufficiently available.

The dietary management of metabolic errors is based on the following strategies:

- Reduce the intake of a precursor compound that cannot be metabolized.
- Supplement the deficient compounds that would have been produced if the normal metabolic pathway had not been blocked.
- Add a substrate that provides an alternative pathway for elimination of an accumulated toxin.

Therapeutic formulas are designed to reduce the intake of precursor compounds or to provide the deficient metabolic end product.

When hydroxylation of phenylalanine to tyrosine does not take place, phenylalanine accumulates in the blood and results in mental retardation. Because PKU has been diagnosed in L.B., his diet should be modified using a formula containing little or no phenylalanine. The tyrosine deficiency of PKU also can be managed by the addition of tyrosine to the phenylalanine-free therapeutic formulas that are available for patients with PKU. When L.B. progresses to solid foods, it will be important to limit or avoid foods that contain high levels of protein such as eggs and soybeans.

Other metabolic errors present in infancy include galactosemia (galactose cannot be metabolized to glucose), homocystinuria (methionine is not converted to cysteine), urea cycle disorders (ammonia detoxification is impaired), and maple syrup urine disease (metabolism of the branched-chain amino acids leucine, isoleucine, and valine is blocked).

These metabolic errors are managed by manipulating the diet.[17] In galactosemia, the carbohydrate source should not contain galactose or lactose. In homocystinuria, methionine should be present only in quantities sufficient to meet basic requirements, and cysteine should be supplemented. In the urea cycle disorders, protein often is provided only as essential amino acids, and a high-energy diet is provided to maximize the formation of nonessential amino acids from nitrogen and to minimize ammonia production. In maple syrup urine disease, natural protein is fed in small quantities to provide the minimal requirement of branched-chain amino acids, and a branched-chain amino acid-free supplement is added to provide adequate protein intake.

Route of Administration

Nutritional support using the GI tract is the preferred approach when possible. Enteral nutrition provides several advantages. First, interposition of the GI mucosa between the nutrient supply and the circulation allows absorptive function to provide a homeostatic control. Second, the flow of nutrients from the GI tract to the liver via the portal circulation before reaching the systemic circulation also assists homeostatic control. Third, the lack of enteral nutrition allows normal GI tract flora to overgrow and translocate into the blood, ultimately resulting in bacteremia. Finally, the intestinal mucosa depends on intraluminal absorption for much of its energy supply. Hence, provision of at least a small amount of enteral feeding, referred to as trophic feeds, helps to ensure a healthy GI tract and may facilitate advancement to full enteral feedings at the appropriate time.[18]

Normal oral feeding is the most basic method for patients who are willing and able to eat or drink. Patients whose GI motility, structure, and function are normal but whose oral feeding is prevented by an altered state of consciousness, uncoordinated sucking and swallowing, or other conditions that prevent adequate oral ingestion can be fed by a GI tube in intermittent boluses or by continuous infusion.

Bolus tube feedings more closely mimic the normal state. They periodically distend the stomach, which aids in gastric secretion and emptying. When bolus tube feeding is undertaken, the volume of formula or expressed breast milk required to provide sufficient calories for a 24-hour period is administered through the tube in equal aliquots every 2, 3, 4, or 6 hours. The frequency of administration depends on the patient's age, gastric capacity, and the infant's ability to maintain a normal serum glucose concentration between feedings. In general, younger and more premature infants require more frequent feedings. Intolerance to bolus tube feedings can be manifested as diarrhea, gastroesophageal reflux with emesis, or poor motility. Poor motility usually is apparent when large volumes of feeding, referred to as residuals, remain in the stomach when the next feeding is due.

Continuous tube feedings can be given at a constant rate of infusion by pump into the stomach or duodenum when bolus feedings have failed. This approach may be better tolerated by premature infants and children with diarrhea.

Patients with intrinsic GI disease (Table 103-6) or malabsorption may require total or supplemental PN. Concurrent administration of low-volume, trophic enteral feedings may provide important nutrients to the gut mucosa even when the parenteral route supplies all of the necessary systemic nutrients.[18] Administration of PN into a peripheral vein is limited to those patients expected to require parenteral feeding only for a short time (i.e., 2 weeks) because the amount of nutrients that can be safely infused peripherally is limited. In patients who require long-term PN, the IV solution is more concentrated and must be administered into a central vein.

Nutritional Assessment

CASE 103-6

QUESTION 1: T.C. is a 4-month-old, lethargic boy. On examination, he has a moderately distended abdomen and dry mucous membranes. No other remarkable abnormalities are noted. His weight is 6.5 kg (50th–75th percentile for age). Previously, when he was 2 months old, T.C. weighed 5.6 kg (75th percentile for age), and his length was 57 cm (50th percentile for age). His mother reports that for the past 5 to 7 days, he has had five to eight large, liquid stools per day. His infant formula has not changed. He is to be hospitalized for evaluation of his diarrhea and weight loss and for fluid and nutritional management.

After correction of his initial fluid and electrolyte deficits, an assessment of his nutritional status shows the following:

Weight, 6.5 kg (50th–75th percentile)
Length, 62 cm (50th percentile)
Albumin, 3.8 g/dL (normal, 4–5.3 g/dL)
Prealbumin, 7 mg/dL (normal, 20–50 mg/dL)
How would you assess T.C.'s nutritional status?

Growth assessment is an important focus of pediatric health care, especially during the first year of life. With the exception of the intrauterine period, the most rapid growth occurs during the first year. On average, a normally growing infant gains approximately 30 g/day. Typically, healthy infants weigh approximately 3 times their birth weight by their first birthday.

The patient's nutritional status should be assessed before beginning a nutritional support regimen and reassessed at regular intervals during the course of treatment. If the patient previously was well nourished, the goal is to maintain that status until a normal diet can be resumed. In a child who was previously malnourished, an effort should be made to promote "catch-up" growth and to normalize the biochemical nutritional measures. One in five children admitted to the hospital experience acute or chronic malnutrition.[19] Malnutrition in children is a risk factor for decreased social skills and impaired intellectual development.[20]

Factors used to determine nutritional status in children include dietary history, weight, height, and visceral protein measurements (e.g., albumin, prealbumin). Other measurements used in adults, such as 24-hour creatinine excretion, 24-hour nitrogen excretion, and nitrogen balance, are reserved for older children because complete collections of urine are difficult to obtain and because the percentage of non-urea nitrogen present in urine is variable in infants.

Anthropometric measurements can also be used to assess T.C.'s nutritional status. Height, weight, and head circumference are used to determine nutritional status in infants and children. Standards for these measurements have been derived from pediatric patients in the United States and compiled into graphs referred to as growth curves (http://www.cdc.gov/growthcharts).[3] An individual patient's measurements are compared with the graph of normal values for that specific age group. As prematurely born infants age, a standard growth curve adjusted for prematurity can be used. Using these measurements, comparisons with standards are possible: weight for age, height for age, and weight for height.[3] A weight that is below the fifth percentile for the patient's height is considered an indication of acute malnutrition. Similarly, a height and weight that are below the fifth percentile for the patient's age indicate chronic malnutrition. It is important to consider the height and weight of the child's parents because genetics are important determinants of the height and weight that a child may ultimately achieve. Additionally, the revised growth charts

Table 103-6

Common Indications for Parenteral Nutrition Support[a]

Extreme prematurity
Respiratory distress
Congenital GI anomalies
Duodenal atresia
Jejunal atresia
Esophageal atresia
Tracheoesophageal fistula
Pyloric stenosis
Congenital webs
Hirschsprung disease
Malrotation
Volvulus
Abdominal wall defects
Omphalocele (herniation of viscera into the umbilical cord base)
Gastroschisis (defect of abdominal wall, any location except umbilical cord)
Congenital diaphragmatic hernia
Necrotizing enterocolitis
Chronic diarrhea
Inflammatory bowel disease
Chylothorax
Pseudoobstruction
Megacystis microcolon
Abdominal trauma involving viscera
Adverse effects of treating neoplastic disease
Radiation enteritis
Nausea and vomiting
Stomatitis, glossitis, and esophagitis
Anorexia nervosa
Cystic fibrosis
Chronic renal failure
Hepatic failure
Metabolic errors

[a]Other indications for parenteral nutrition may exist.
GI, gastrointestinal.

include the body mass index (BMI) for age for children older than 2 years. The BMI helps identify children at risk for obesity and type 2 diabetes, two problems that have recently become concerns in children.[3]

Numerous biochemical indices are also used in the assessment of nutritional status. Of these, the most readily available and widely used is the serum albumin concentration. Although a low serum albumin can be a specific indicator of protein-calorie malnutrition, its long half-life (20 days)[19] makes it an insensitive indicator for developing and resolving malnutrition.

Prealbumin can also function as a biochemical marker of nutritional status.[19] Because of its shorter half-life, prealbumin has the advantage of being more sensitive than albumin to acute nutritional changes, and it is still useful when exogenous albumin infusions are given.[19]

CASE 103-6, QUESTION 2: After initial IV rehydration and receiving nothing by mouth (NPO) for 48 hours, T.C.'s stool output has decreased dramatically. Is this characteristic of infants with chronic diarrhea? How should T.C.'s enteral diet be initiated?

A prompt decrease in stool output when enteral intake is stopped is typical of infants with chronic diarrhea. Nonetheless, evaluation of bowel function and adaptation has shown that enteral nutrition is superior to PN with regard to histologic recovery, improvement of D-xylose absorption, protein absorption, and disaccharidase activity.[21] In fact, improvement in histology or absorptive function might not occur until enteral nutrients are given.[18] Thus, for T.C., every effort should be made to provide some nutrition enterally.

The enteral regimen should be initiated with a lactose-free formula, such as an elemental formula or a soy-based formula. Although any soy-based formula would be appropriate, Isomil DF is a soy-based formula with added fiber that is indicated for infants with diarrhea. Infants with chronic diarrhea can have small bowel mucosal damage and decreased disaccharidase activity.[4] Carbohydrate absorption depends on digestion of disaccharides and polysaccharides to monosaccharides through disaccharidase activity in the intestinal lumen. Substitution of free glucose orally may overcome the problem of carbohydrate digestion and absorption. Administration of large amounts of oral glucose should be limited, however, because of its osmotic effect and potential to worsen diarrhea. Furthermore, incompletely absorbed carbohydrate is available to colonic bacteria for fermentation, the end products of which can produce diarrhea through colonic irritation.

Unlike carbohydrate, protein rarely causes diarrhea, but the mucosal damage present in patients with chronic diarrhea, such as T.C., can reduce the absorptive surface area so that protein malabsorption may occur. This can be minimized through the administration of a formula containing protein in the form of dipeptides and tripeptides, which are absorbed more efficiently than free amino acids.

Dilution of hypertonic formulas to half strength may improve formula tolerance. The concentration is increased in a stepwise fashion to full strength if there is no carbohydrate malabsorption and if stool output is not excessive. Tolerance may be improved by continuous infusion of the enteral product. If enteral refeeding results in the return of diarrhea, fluid and electrolytes must be replaced with an equal volume of an IV solution of similar electrolyte composition to the stool loss.

CASE 103-6, QUESTION 3: How can T.C.'s tolerance to the formula and his recovery of intestinal function be assessed?

Malabsorption or formula intolerance can be assessed by stool studies, which would include assessing for the presence of reducing substances and stool pH. Lactose is a reducing sugar and its presence in stool is an assessment of carbohydrate absorption. The bacterial fermentation products of malabsorbed carbohydrates can result in a decreased stool pH, which suggests malabsorption. To further evaluate carbohydrate absorption, D-xylose may be given orally; a blood sample is drawn 4 to 5 hours later to determine the amount absorbed. This test may be of initial prognostic value in predicting which patients will require prolonged courses of treatment.[21] More than 5% of ingested fat in a stool collection (typically obtained for 3 days) is indicative of fat malabsorption. All these tests can be evaluated during outpatient visits to guide the refeeding process.

Once the diarrhea has resolved, standard infant formula feedings should be established using an enteral elemental or soy-based formula. Regardless of the time chosen, a gradual stepwise conversion is suggested. A small volume of standard formula is substituted for an equal volume of elemental or soy-based formula, and the substitution volume is increased daily until the elemental or soy-based formula is eliminated completely from the regimen. If a specific nutrient intolerance has been identified, a standard formula that does not contain that nutrient must be selected. For example, a patient with cow's milk protein intolerance may require a soy protein formula or an elemental formula.

Pediatric Parenteral Nutrition

The basic requirements for a parenteral nutrient regimen are listed in Table 103-1. These guidelines for the initiation of a nutrient regimen should be individualized to specific patient needs. The correct regimen for any specific patient is that which supplies sufficient nutrients to promote a normal rate of growth without toxicity. In particular, patients with ongoing, abnormal nutrient losses may require much larger doses of certain nutrients. Individualization of the nutrient prescription cannot be overemphasized. Many of the requirements listed in Table 103-1 apply to nutrients administered by the enteral route as well. In some instances, the absorption of a particular nutrient from the GI mucosa is incomplete, and enteral requirements are substantially higher. This is particularly true of the major minerals (calcium, magnesium, and iron) and trace elements.

Indications

Parenteral nutrition is indicated for any infant or child unable to take in sufficient nourishment to maintain normal growth. Some specific indications are listed in Table 103-6.

VERY LOW-BIRTH-WEIGHT INFANTS

Extremely premature or VLBW infants require specialized nutritional support for two distinct reasons. First, the third trimester in utero is a time of rapid growth and accumulation of protein, glycogen, fat, and minerals.[22] The infant born in the very early stages of the third trimester does not accumulate these stores and, therefore, must receive nutrients earlier than a more mature infant. Second, extreme prematurity is associated with poor coordination of the suck and swallow reflex, poor GI motility, and incomplete absorption. Therefore, enteral nutrients may need to be administered via an orogastric or nasogastric tube, and PN supplementation probably will be needed. PN, especially of amino acids, should be initiated soon after birth to duplicate intrauterine growth and prevent a catabolic state in the first few days of life. The fetus has a continuous supply of amino acids that is immediately stopped after preterm birth.[23] A standardized solution containing amino acids and dextrose can be used for infants weighing less than 1 kg in the first 24 hours of life. There has been some reluctance to administer amino acids this soon after birth because of increased risk of hyperammonemia, uremia, and metabolic acidosis. Several studies, however, have shown early introduction of amino acids is safe, provides a positive nitrogen balance, and promotes better health outcomes.[24,25]

RESPIRATORY DISTRESS

Respiratory distress may preclude the ability to consume sufficient nutrients enterally because high respiratory rates prevent coordinated breathing and swallowing. In infants who are hypoxic, or at high risk for hypoxia, aggressive enteral feedings during the acute phase of their illness can increase the likelihood of bowel ischemia. Often, these situations are resolved in 3 to 5 days, but this can rarely be predicted at the outset. Trophic feedings (1–5 mL/hour) are often implemented to maintain GI tract integrity. Nutritional support in such cases is initiated by giving parenteral fluids, which provide dextrose as a caloric source. This allows the infant to conserve endogenous energy substrates, an important consideration for the VLBW infant whose entire body composition may contain as little as a 3- to 4-day energy supply.[22] PN should be initiated as soon as it becomes clear the enteral feeding will not be possible for at least 3 to 5 days, or when several days have elapsed and no clear time frame can be determined for the establishment of enteral feeding. Although a short course (5 days or less) of PN may be used, the quantity of nutrients supplied during the process of initiation and gradual increase to full requirements is so low that extremely short courses may be difficult to justify. Peripheral PN using fat emulsion as a significant source of calories, however, can provide up to 70 kcal/kg and, with appropriate types and amounts of protein, result in modest weight gain and nitrogen equilibrium.

GASTROINTESTINAL ANOMALIES

Infants with GI anomalies often require PN because the implementation of enteral feedings may be delayed. For example, GI tract atresia or stenosis can obstruct, or partially obstruct, the lumen of the GI tract. This prevents or slows the passage of fluids and nutrients and can result in vomiting, depending on the location of the obstruction. Similarly, infants with necrotizing enterocolitis have zones of ischemic bowel and are at risk for bowel perforation if fed enterally.[26] Infants with these disorders need PN until the viability of the entire GI tract can be assured.

CHRONIC RENAL FAILURE AND HEPATIC DISEASE

Chronic renal or hepatic disease requires modification of a normal diet to account for the impaired elimination of nitrogenous waste or impaired protein metabolism. Careful caloric supplementation with a reduced amount of protein may permit normal growth while minimizing excess urea production in an infant with renal failure.

CASE 103-6, QUESTION 4: Approximately 48 hours after discharge from the hospital, T.C. returns to the emergency department with abdominal distension and bloody diarrhea. He is diagnosed with postgastroenteritis syndrome. T.C. cannot receive nutrients enterally, and PN is to be initiated because he is nutritionally depleted. Describe for the members of the medical team how a regimen of PN should be instituted in T.C. What aspects of his disease may alter specific nutrient needs?

When initiating PN, the protein (amino acids), glucose (dextrose), fat (lipids or fat emulsion), fluid, and electrolyte, mineral, and vitamin components of the regimen are managed as separate entities. In addition, the route of PN delivery is important to consider because the amount of glucose, potassium, and calcium must be limited if the infusion is given peripherally. In general, 12.5% dextrose, 40 mEq/L potassium, and 10 mEq/L calcium are the maximal amounts that should be provided by infusion into a peripheral vein. These nutrients can be increased if a central venous catheter is placed. The fluids, electrolytes, minerals, and vitamins are initiated at full daily maintenance doses after correction of any preexisting abnormalities. Protein should be initiated at full daily doses in term infants and children with normal renal and hepatic function. Glucose and fat are started at lower doses and increased daily until requirements are reached.

Protein should be started in T.C. at full daily requirements of 2 to 3 g/kg/day. Azotemia and acidosis have occurred in infants receiving more than 4 g/kg/day of protein; however, these complications are rare at the recommended dosage. Parenteral glucose administration is initiated at 5 to 8 mg/kg/minute (7.2–11.5 g/kg/day). At normal maintenance fluid rates, 10% dextrose represents a generally well-tolerated starting solution for patients of virtually any age or size, except the VLBW infant.

In T.C.'s case, the dextrose concentration will begin and continue at 10% because of the peripheral catheter limitations. This concentration will provide 7.3 mg/kg/minute. If a central catheter later becomes necessary, the concentration can be increased by 5% each day until the caloric requirement is met. This increase should be accompanied by blood and urine glucose monitoring. If the blood glucose is 150 mg/dL or greater, or if the urine glucose exceeds "trace" amounts, the PN infusion rate should be decreased by at least 25% and a second IV solution should be added to provide needed fluids and electrolytes. Alternatively, the dextrose concentration can be decreased or insulin can be infused concomitantly and titrated to a desired serum glucose concentration of 120 to 140 mg/dL.

Fat emulsion should be initiated at 1 g/kg/day and increased daily by 0.5 to 1 g/kg/day until the maximal dosage of 3 g/kg/day is reached. The daily fat dose should be infused at a constant rate because fats are better tolerated when infused over the course of 24 hours.[27] Serum triglycerides should be monitored every other day while the dose of fat is being increased. Patients with a fasting triglyceride concentration of 150 mg/dL or less may have their fat dose increased. In patients who are receiving inadequate calories, triglycerides may be elevated because endogenous fats are being mobilized. If the triglyceride concentration is greater than 150 mg/dL, the serum sample must be examined visually. A clear sample with a mildly elevated triglyceride concentration probably indicates the use of endogenous fat stores for energy. Conversely, a turbid or lipemic sample indicates the patient's inability to use the amount of intravenous fat administered. In this case, further increases in the fat dose should be delayed until triglyceride concentrations decrease.

Special Considerations and Complications

CASE 103-7

QUESTION 1: J.H., a 4-day-old boy, was born at 31 weeks' gestation. His birth weight was 1,950 g, and he now weighs 2,000 g. On the first day of life, he was given a commercial preterm infant formula by orogastric tube in gradually increasing quantity with supplemental IV fluids. Now, on the fourth day of life, he has a distended abdomen and his stools contain bright red blood. An abdominal radiograph shows pneumatosis intestinalis (gas within the intestinal wall seen on X-ray). All enteral feedings are stopped (NPO). What do these findings represent? What are the implications for J.H.'s nutritional management?

Abdominal distension, bloody stools, and pneumatosis intestinalis are characteristic of necrotizing enterocolitis historically.[28] The causes of this disorder are unclear, but it occurs more often in premature than in term infants; it can occur in clusters of cases, rarely is seen before enteral feeding is instituted, and can be associated with rapid increases in enteral intake.[29] Because J.H. will receive antibiotics for 10 to 14 days and remain NPO, he requires PN. The planned duration of the regimen makes central venous access a necessity.

GOALS OF LONG-TERM SUPPORT

CASE 103-7, QUESTION 2: The following day, intestinal perforation requires the resection of two-thirds of J.H.'s distal jejunum and one-third of his ileum, with creation of a jejunostomy. The ileocecal valve and the entire colon are left intact. During the operation, a central venous catheter is placed. What is the goal of PN for J.H.?

J.H. will be NPO for a prolonged time. Therefore, the goals of his PN must be to promote normal growth as well as healing of his diseased gut and surgical wounds. Because J.H. is a premature infant, it will be difficult to predict how well he will tolerate PN. VLBW infants tolerate normal doses of pediatric amino acids without difficulty; however, some clinicians initiate protein at a lower daily dose (e.g., 1.0 g/kg/day) and advance by 0.5 g/kg/day each day until a goal of 2 to 3 g/kg/day is achieved. Fat should be started at 0.5 to 1 g/kg/day and increased by 0.5 g/kg/day up to 3 g/kg/day. Glucose should be initiated at 5 to 10 g/kg/day and increased by 2 to 3 g/kg until the desired caloric intake is achieved. Appropriate doses of electrolytes and minerals may be started immediately using the guidelines listed in Table 103-1.

FAT EMULSIONS: COMPLICATIONS

CASE 103-7, QUESTION 3: What must be considered in making decisions regarding fat administration in J.H.?

Although J.H. can receive adequate calories using only glucose and crystalline amino acids, he will require fat to provide a more physiologic diet and to prevent essential fatty acid deficiency (EFAD), which develops quickly in low-birth-weight infants who have little fat reserve. J.H. should receive a minimum of 5% of his total caloric requirement as fat emulsion to minimize the risk of EFAD. Ideally, his nutrition regimen will provide approximately 40% of calories from fat, which is similar to what is provided by human milk.

Infusions of fat emulsion have been associated with impaired oxygen transport and pulmonary ventilation–perfusion mismatch. This adverse effect occurs more often when the dose of fat is 4 g/kg or greater and is infused for a relatively short (4 hours) period. Current practice is to increase gradually the doses of fat from 0.5 to 1 g/kg/day up to a maximum of 4 g/kg/day and to infuse the fat emulsion over the course of 24 hours to minimize the likelihood of pulmonary problems and to promote clearance.

It is unclear whether IV fat administration is detrimental to patients with sepsis. Infusion of fat emulsion has resulted in lymphocyte and neutrophil death.[30] On the other hand, the linoleic acid in IV fat is the precursor to arachidonic acid, prostaglandins, thromboxane, interleukins, and immune-mediating cells. Theoretically, this may minimize bacteremia. Necrotizing enterocolitis, intestinal perforation, and surgery predispose J.H. to sepsis. Therefore, he should have his IV fat infused at an appropriate dose over the course of 24 hours. Because fat clearance can be impaired during infection, it is also prudent to monitor his triglyceride concentrations.

Free fatty acids can displace bilirubin from its albumin binding sites, thereby placing the infant at risk for kernicterus.[31] Therefore, before advancing the fat dose, the total bilirubin and direct bilirubin should be measured. Patients with an indirect bilirubin (total bilirubin minus direct bilirubin) of 10 mg/dL or less whose albumin levels are normal are at low risk for kernicterus. Indirect bilirubin usually peaks before 1 week of age. After the risk for indirect hyperbilirubinemia has passed, the fat dose can be increased as recommended in Table 103-1. The infusion of 1 g/kg over the course of 24 hours is associated with minimal risk for decreased bilirubin binding[31]; however, rapid infusion of this same dose can displace bilirubin from albumin binding sites. Given the low level of indirect bilirubin found on routine monitoring and the planned fat infusion rate, J.H. should not be at risk for kernicterus.

Egg phospholipids are used to emulsify fats; therefore, patients with a known allergy to eggs (e.g., fever, chills, urticaria, dyspnea, bronchospasm, chest pain) should not receive fat emulsion.

CASE 103-7, QUESTION 4: Because J.H. is a premature infant, PN is initiated using 5% glucose, 2.5 g/kg/day of amino acids, and 0.5 g/kg/day of fat emulsion. The volume of PN should be 240 mL based on a maintenance fluid requirement of 120 mL/kg (Table 103-1). On the second day, he receives 10% glucose, 2.5 g/kg/day of amino acids, and 1 g/kg/day of fat. On the third day, glucose is increased to 15%, amino acids remain at 2.5 g/kg/day, and fat emulsion is increased to 1.5 g/kg/day. On the fourth day, glucose is increased to 20%, amino acids remain at 2.5 g/kg/day, and fats are increased to 2 g/kg/day. After this solution has been infused for 8 hours, his urine test yields 1% for glucose (normal, no glucose) and his blood glucose level is 210 mg/dL (normal, 120 mg/dL). Explain this new finding and the problems it may cause. How should hyperglycemia be managed?

Maximal glucose oxidation rates in milligrams per kilograms per minute are inversely related to age and decrease from 15 to 18 mg/kg/minute in neonates and young infants to 4 to 5 mg/kg/minute in adults. In full-term neonates and infants receiving maintenance fluids (100 mL/kg/day), glucose concentrations can be started at 10 g/kg/day (equivalent to dextrose 10%) and advanced by 5 g/kg (equivalent to dextrose 5%) every 24 hours up to approximately 25 g/kg/day (equivalent to dextrose 25%). In preterm neonates, such as J.H., dextrose is started at a lower dose and advanced at smaller increments, usually 2 to 3 g/kg/day. Glucose tolerance varies significantly, so each patient should be considered individually.

At J.H.'s prescribed fluid rate of 10 mL/hour, 20% glucose represents 16.7 mg/kg/minute of glucose. The hyperglycemia and glycosuria probably have occurred because the increases in the infusion rate have exceeded J.H.'s ability to adapt to the glucose dose. Patients who have been euglycemic on their glucose dose and then become glucose intolerant should be evaluated, however, for other causes, such as infection and addition of exogenous corticosteroids. Hyperglycemia and glycosuria can result in serum hyperosmolarity, osmotic diuresis, and dehydration. Regardless of the cause, the hyperglycemia should be treated by reducing the glucose administration rate. The rate of the PN infusion can be decreased further if hyperglycemia continues or increased if the hyperglycemia resolves.

When the PN order is written for the subsequent days, the glucose increases should be made in smaller amounts up to the full daily maintenance calorie requirements. Frequent blood and urine glucose monitoring must be continued. Severe glucose intolerance in patients who require PN can be managed with insulin to normalize serum glucose. Although insulin is compatible with PN solutions, it does adsorb to glass, polyvinyl chloride, and filters, resulting in decreased delivery of insulin.[32] Frequently, pediatric patients have changing insulin requirements that prevent the addition of insulin to PN solutions. A separate continuous infusion of regular insulin (initial dose, 0.05–0.1 units/kg/hour) titrated to control serum glucose concentrations offers a practical solution to minimize waste of the PN solution.[33] It is essential to discontinue the insulin infusion if the PN solution is discontinued to avoid hypoglycemia.

EFFECTS OF BRONCHOPULMONARY DYSPLASIA AND MECHANICAL VENTILATION

CASE 103-7, QUESTION 5: J.H. remains dependent on a ventilator because of his immature lungs. How could J.H.'s respiratory disease influence his nutritional regimen?

After 28 days of age, J.H.'s ventilator dependence defines him as having bronchopulmonary dysplasia (BPD), a chronic lung disease of infancy. Historically, BPD is characterized by an increase in resting energy expenditure, increased work of breathing, and growth failure.[34,35] Therefore, J.H.'s caloric requirement may be higher than expected. Additionally, J.H.'s ventilator may also alter the approach to his caloric supply. Very high carbohydrate loads have been associated with an increase in carbon dioxide production.[36] This, in turn, may make it difficult to wean J.H. from the mechanical ventilator. As discussed, rapid infusions of fat emulsion can also have a detrimental effect on pulmonary function. Fat emulsion should not be omitted from J.H.'s PN regimen; rather, a slower infusion rate, with gradual dose increases, while monitoring pulmonary function is appropriate.

PEDIATRIC AMINO ACID FORMULATIONS

CASE 103-7, QUESTION 6: Why would a specialized pediatric amino acid solution be preferable to a standard adult formulation for J.H.?

Patients 1 year of age or older tolerate standard adult amino acid preparations (e.g., Aminosyn and Travasol) well. For infants, two specifically designed pediatric amino acid formulations (PAAFs)—TrophAmine and Aminosyn PF—are available. PAAFs were developed in response to the abnormal plasma amino acid patterns noted in infants receiving adult amino acid formulations. The products were designed with the goal of producing plasma amino acid patterns closely matching those of 2-hour postprandial, human milk-fed infants. Theoretically, normal plasma amino acid patterns will promote normal protein synthesis in growing infants.

Pediatric amino acid formulations differ from conventional amino acid formulations in several ways. First, they contain a higher content of branched-chain amino acids (leucine, isoleucine, and valine) and a lower content of glycine, methionine, and phenylalanine. In addition, PAAFs have a higher percentage of essential amino acids with a wider distribution of the nonessential amino acids. Finally, PAAFs are unique in that they contain three essential amino acids for neonates: taurine, tyrosine (as *N*-acetyl-L-tyrosine), and cysteine (added as L-cysteine HCl). Adult solutions contain little if any of these amino acids. Neonates have immature liver functions. This results in decreased levels of both hepatic cystathionase and phenylalanine hydroxylase enzymes. Without these enzymes, neonates cannot adequately convert methionine to cysteine or phenylalanine to tyrosine or synthesize taurine from cysteine. Deficiencies in these amino acids can have a significant impact on the health of the neonate. For example, taurine has a role in retinal development, protection and stabilization of cell membranes, neurotransmission, regulation of cell volume, and bile acid conjugation. Taurine also may be important in decreasing or preventing cholestasis associated with long-term PN.

Several investigators have studied the clinical, nutritional, and biochemical effects of TrophAmine in term and preterm infants.[37,38] The use of TrophAmine was found to result in nearly normal amino acid patterns. In addition, patients receiving TrophAmine had greater weight gain and significantly better nitrogen utilization than similar groups using the adult formulations. TrophAmine and Aminosyn-PF, given for a 7-day period, produced comparable weight gain and nitrogen retention.[39] In one study, some of the VLBW infants experienced metabolic acidosis.[37] L-Cysteine, an HCl salt, provides an additional 5.7 mEq of chloride/100 mg and may have contributed to the acidosis. Whereas the manufacturer's recommended dose of 40 mg of L-cysteine per gram of amino acid may be too much for the VLBW infant, the most appropriate dose of L-cysteine for the VLBW infant has not been determined.

To date, PAAFs have been effective in producing a positive weight gain and positive nitrogen balance, and normalizing amino acid patterns in preterm neonates. They also allow for the provision of larger doses of calcium and phosphorus because PAAFs lower the pH of the final PN solution. Providing greater amounts of calcium and phosphorus, in appropriate ratios, should minimize metabolic bone disease. Further evaluation of these products is needed to determine the magnitude of the proposed benefits (i.e., improved nitrogen retention, better weight gain, enhanced bone growth, and decreased cholestasis) and the most appropriate L-cysteine dose to use in VLBW infants. In any event, these potential benefits, and clinical experience with these products, have resulted in the use of PAAFs as the standard of care in infants requiring PN.

CARNITINE

CASE 103-7, QUESTION 7: Why would carnitine supplementation be warranted in J.H.?

Carnitine has many functions within the body, but it primarily serves to transport long-chain fatty acids (LCFA) across the mitochondrial membrane where they undergo β-oxidation to produce energy. Deficiency in carnitine lessens LCFA availability for oxidation, resulting in the accumulation of LCFA and a decrease in ketone and adenosine triphosphate (ATP) production. This can adversely affect the CNS and skeletal and cardiac muscles. Carnitine deficiency in premature infants also has been linked to disorders such as GI reflux, apnea, and bradycardia.[40]

Whereas carnitine is a nonessential nutrient in adults and is readily available from a diet that includes meat and dairy products, it appears to be an essential nutrient in neonates and infants. This population has low body stores of carnitine and a decreased ability to synthesize it on their own. The premature infant has even lower stores because carnitine accumulation occurs during the third trimester. Human milk and most cow's milk-based infant formulas contain carnitine. Some soy-based formulas have additional carnitine added during manufacturing. PN, however, is not routinely supplemented with carnitine. Therefore, infants who are exclusively fed by PN are at risk for developing complications associated with carnitine deficiency.[40]

Because J.H. has two risk factors for the development of carnitine deficiency (prematurity and exclusive use of PN), and because carnitine has little or no adverse effects associated with its use, it is appropriate to provide J.H. with a carnitine supplement. Carnitine is available as both an oral and IV formulation. The recommended dose in J.H. is 10 to 20 mg/kg/day. The addition of carnitine directly to PN improves carnitine plasma concentrations and nutritional status.

METABOLIC BONE DISEASE (RICKETS)

CASE 103-7, QUESTION 8: On the chest radiograph taken to evaluate the septic episode just described, the radiologist notes that J.H. has two rib fractures and that the bones appear undermineralized. The most recent laboratory values show a serum calcium (Ca) of 9.3 mg/dL (normal, 8.5–10.5 mg/dL), a serum phosphorus of 3.6 mg/dL (normal, 4.0–8.5 mg/dL), and an alkaline phosphatase of 674 units/L (normal, 350 units/L). What diagnosis is suggested by these findings? How and why has J.H.'s nutrition regimen placed him at risk for this disease?

During the last trimester of pregnancy, bone accretion is accelerated, reaching its peak at about 36 weeks. Premature infants, therefore, require larger calcium and phosphorous doses. Limitations to venous access, however, may preclude the infusion of concentrated calcium solutions peripherally, and the patient's end organs may be resistant to vitamin D. Thus, metabolic bone disease is not unexpected in a premature infant such as J.H.

Aluminum, a contaminant in some parenteral salt products (particularly calcium), also may play a role in impaired bone mineraliziation.[41] Low serum phosphorus with high alkaline phosphatase, undermineralized bones, and fractures resulting from routine handling are consistent with a diagnosis of rickets.

Parenteral nutrition solutions provide calcium and phosphorus in much smaller amounts than the infant would accumulate in utero.[42] Solution pH, temperature, calcium salt, and final calcium and phosphorus concentrations influence their solubility in PN solutions. An acidic PN solution favors the solubility of these salts. The pH of commercially available amino acid preparations ranges from 5.4 in PAAFs to 7 in adult amino acid formulations. The addition of L-cysteine, with a pH of 1.5, also makes the solution more acidic. Because dextrose also is acidic, solutions with higher dextrose concentrations are more acidic. Of note, colder storage temperatures promote calcium and phosphorus solubility. Therefore, refrigerated PN solutions may appear to be free of precipitate on visual inspection. Calcium and phosphate can precipitate, however, when warmed to room temperature, or when infused into patients with fever or in incubators. Calcium salt selection is another important consideration because the chloride salt dissociates rapidly and favors precipitation, whereas the gluconate and gluceptate salts dissociate less quickly.

Serum phosphorus concentrations should be monitored several times per week and phosphorus intake adjusted to prevent symptomatic hypophosphatemia. Serum calcium is not useful as an indicator of disease activity because it will remain normal at the expense of bone mineralization. This is demonstrated by J.H.'s serum calcium at the time of diagnosis.

Parenteral Nutrition-associated Liver Disease

CASE 103-7, QUESTION 9: On the 56th day of life, J.H. is noted to be mildly jaundiced. A review of his laboratory tests reveals the following:

	Age (days)				
Test	22	29	36	43	50
Aspartate aminotransferase (AST) (units/L) (normal, <40)	14	17	15	20	25
Alanine aminotransferase (ALT) (units/L) (normal, <28)	6	7	10	10	11
Alkaline phosphatase (international units/L) (normal, <350)	103	158	345	506	695
Bilirubin					
Indirect (normal, <1 mg/dL)	0.9	0.9	0.8	0.8	0.9
Direct (normal, <0.2 mg/dL)	0.1	0.1	0.8	1.6	3

Could this be related to his PN?

Parenteral nutrition-associated liver disease (PNALD) is severe liver disease due to extended parenteral feeding, which can cause permanent damage and even liver failure. In past decades, hepatic damage has been reported in up to one-half of infants receiving PN,[43] with a higher prevalence (up to 50%) in VLBW infants such as J.H. Although it is still a concern today, PNALD is less prevalent because of a better understanding of how to treat infants requiring long-term PN. The laboratory abnormalities reported in J.H. are typical of this complication. The first change observed is usually an elevated direct (conjugated) bilirubin, which can occur as early as 2 weeks after beginning PN. Increases in the serum concentrations of the hepatic enzymes, AST and ALT, lag 2 weeks or more behind the rise in direct bilirubin. Alkaline phosphatase also can rise, but it is a nonspecific indicator of liver disease. Alkaline phosphatase is produced by the liver, GI tract, and bones. Although the laboratory results observed in J.H. are consistent with the pattern associated with PNALD, and many components of PN solutions have been associated with the development of cholestasis, other potential causes also exist.[43] PNALD is a diagnosis of exclusion; therefore, other causes, such as viral hepatitis, must be ruled out.

J.H. has several other risk factors for developing cholestasis, and prolonged enteral fasting may be the most significant.[43] Stimulation of bile flow and gallbladder contraction depend on GI hormones, which depend on enteral feeding for their release.[43] Absence of these hormones, therefore, can promote cholestasis.[43] Immature hepatic function secondary to prematurity also places J.H. at risk, as does the duration of PN therapy. As the duration of PN use increases, so does the prevalence of hepatic disease in premature infants; 25% of infants nourished in this manner for 30 days or more show evidence of cholestasis.[43] Surgical patients have a greater likelihood of developing hyperbilirubinemia than medical patients, especially those requiring GI surgery.[43] Many surgical procedures are associated with a higher risk of jaundice.[43] Finally, J.H.'s infection increases his risk for cholestasis.[43]

The use of adult amino acid preparations in infants increases the risk of cholestasis. In one study, the incidence of cholestasis in VLBW infants receiving TrophAmine was reduced to 23% relative to historical controls of 30% to 50%.[44] In another study comparing the two PAAFs mentioned above, 33% of infants receiving Aminosyn PF developed cholestasis as compared with 13% of infants who received TrophAmine.[45] An additional risk factor for cholestasis not present in J.H. is the administration of large amounts of protein or dextrose. Because amino acids are actively transported in hepatocytes, it is important to provide appropriate types and amounts of amino acids to minimize the development of cholestasis. In one study, a high-protein regimen (3.6 g/kg/day) was associated with an earlier onset and greater degree of cholestasis than a low-protein regimen (2.3 g/kg/day).[46] Similarly, dextrose overload is also a known cause of hepatic steatosis. Therefore, overly aggressive feeding of J.H. with PN should be avoided.

In addition to the hepatic damage, gallstones have been reported in infants and children receiving PN.[43] The ileal resection performed during the acute phase of his necrotizing enterocolitis may put J.H. at increased risk for this hepatobiliary complication as well.

CASE 103-7, QUESTION 10: What modifications to J.H.'s PN regimen should be made in the presence of cholestasis?

First, the institution of enteral feeding must be considered. Even low-volume trophic feeding may help alleviate the condition and should be attempted in cholestatic patients. Next, the protein and glucose dose provided by the PN should be evaluated. During cholestasis, calories should be provided using an appropriate mix of protein, carbohydrate, and fat.

Although the effect of cycling a patient off PN has not been evaluated in clinical trials, this should be considered. Cycling PN, in which the infusion rate is gradually decreased to off for a period and then restarted and gradually increased to the desired rate, will decrease the length of time the liver is exposed to PN. VLBW infants, however, may become hypoglycemic even with very gradual decreases in infusion rate, so this option should be used with care. In any event, a short time off PN (e.g., 2 hours) should be attempted.

The trace elements provided by the formulation should be examined. Both copper and manganese are enterohepatically recycled and may accumulate in liver disease. Manganese can also contribute to hepatotoxicity and should be removed from J.H.'s PN solutions. Studies have not established when removal of copper and manganese is warranted. The inappropriate removal of copper could lead to anemia, osteopenia, and neutropenia. Therefore, decreasing the copper dose and monitoring serum concentrations of both copper and manganese should guide therapy.

Current studies have demonstrated that using omega-3 long-chain fatty acids, derived from fish oil, can reverse the liver damage caused by PNALD. Fish oil is high in eicosapentaenoic and docosahexaenoic acids, which do not impair bile flow and may actually diminish fat accumulation in the liver. Omegaven, the parenteral fish oil-based intravenous fat emulsion, is being used under the compassionate use protocol and not currently approved by the FDA.[47] Other research is being done using an oral formulation of fish oil in infants as a supplement to reverse PNALD.[48]

Pharmacologic interventions have had limited success in the management of PNALD. Phenobarbital has not been shown to be effective in reducing or reversing it.[49] Ursodiol 10 to 20 mg/kg/day has been used successfully in the treatment of other cholestatic liver diseases, and preliminary reports indicate that it may also improve PNALD in children.[50] Ursodiol, a naturally occurring nontoxic bile acid, presumably works by displacing and replacing the endogenously produced, potentially toxic bile salts that accumulate with cholestasis.

The antibiotic metronidazole also appears promising in the prevention of PNALD in adults. Metronidazole inhibits the bacterial overgrowth in the GI tract that occurs with intestinal stasis. The bacteria are responsible for increased formation of hepatotoxic bile acids such as lithocholate; 25 mg/kg/day of metronidazole has been shown to be effective.[51]

CASE 103-7, QUESTION 11: Project the course of J.H.'s liver disease if PN is discontinued and enteral feedings are instituted within 2 weeks. What may occur if enteral feedings cannot be instituted?

It is difficult to predict a successful wean from PN. Historically, success has been associated with longer length of intact small intestine. Additionally, studies in children with short bowel syndrome have shown that serum citrulline levels may predict the ability to successfully wean a patient from PN. Citrulline is a free amino acid that is produced by the small bowel enterocytes. Therefore, it may be warranted to measure J.H.'s serum citrulline level before weaning from PN.[52]

If PN can be discontinued soon after the onset of cholestasis, the prospects for J.H. to recover normal hepatic function are good. Jaundice usually resolves within 2 weeks after PN is discontinued, and the biochemical abnormalities normalize soon thereafter.[43] The pathologic changes observed on biopsy resolve even more slowly. Biopsy evidence of cholestasis has been observed for up to 40 weeks after resolution of clinical and serologic evidence of hepatic disease.[43]

If enteral feedings cannot be instituted successfully, the prognosis for J.H.'s liver function is not as good. Studies have demonstrated that infants receiving PN for 90 days or more had biopsy evidence of irreversible liver damage.[43] Thus, it clearly is advantageous to convert J.H.'s nutrition to the enteral route as soon as he tolerates such a change.

KEY REFERENCES AND WEBSITES

A full list of references for this chapter can be found at http://thepoint.lww.com/AT11e. Below are the key references and websites for this chapter, with the corresponding reference number in this chapter found in parentheses after the reference.

Key References

Greene HL et al. Guidelines for the use of vitamins, trace elements, calcium, magnesium, and phosphorus in infants and children receiving total parenteral nutrition: report of the Subcommittee on Pediatric Parenteral Nutrient Requirements from the Committee on Clinical Practice Issues of the American Society for Clinical Nutrition [published corrections appear in *Am J Clin Nutr*. 1989;49(6):1332; *Am J Clin Nutr*. 1989;50(3):560]. *Am J Clin Nutr*. 1988;48(5):1324. (2)

Gura KM et al. Reversal of parenteral nutrition-associated liver disease in two infants with short-bowel syndrome using parenteral fish oil: implications for future management. *Pediatrics*. 2006;118(1):e197. (47)

Hay WW Jr et al. Workshop summary: nutrition of the extremely low birth weight infant. *Pediatrics*. 1999;104(6):1360. (24)

Heird WC et al. Intravenous alimentation in pediatric patients. *J Pediatr*. 1972;80(3):351. (22)

Heird WC et al. Pediatric parenteral amino acid mixture in low birth weight infants. *Pediatrics*. 1988;81(1):41. (37)

Helms RA et al. Comparison of a pediatric versus standard amino acid formulation in preterm neonates requiring parenteral nutrition. *J Pediatr*. 1987;110(3):466. (38)

Holliday MA, Segar WE. The maintenance need for water in parenteral fluid therapy. *Pediatrics*. 1957;19(5):823. (1)

Kelly DA. Intestinal failure-associated liver disease: what do we know today? *Gastroenterology*. 2006;130(2, suppl 1):S70. (43)

King C et al; Centers for Disease Control and Prevention. Managing acute gastroenteritis among children oral rehydration, maintenance, and nutritional therapy. *MMWR Recomm Rep*. 2003;52(RR-16):1. (4)

Tillman EM et al. Enteral fish oil for treatment of parenteral nutrition-associated liver disease in six infants with short-bowel syndrome. *Pharmacotherapy*. 2011;31(5):503–509. (48)

Wessel JJ. Human milk. In: Corkins MR, ed. *The A.S.P.E.N. Pediatric Nutrition Support Core Curriculum*. Silver Spring, MD: American Society for Parenteral and Enteral Nutrition; 2010:120. (8)

Key Websites

American Society for Parenteral and Enteral Nutrition. Clinical guidelines http://www.nutritioncare.org/guidelines_and_clinical_resources/. Accessed July 16, 2017.

Journal of Parenteral and Enteral Nutrition. Guidelines for the use of parenteral and enteral nutrition in adult and pediatric patients. http://pen.sagepub.com/content/26/1_suppl/1SA.refs. Accessed September 15, 2015.

104 Common Pediatric Illnesses

Chephra McKee, Brooke Gildon, and Bethany Ibach

CORE PRINCIPLES

		CHAPTER CASES
1	Medication administration to children can be challenging. For oral administration, dosing syringes or droppers should be used rather than household spoons or cups. The administration of medications by any route may require special techniques in an uncooperative child.	**Case 104-1 (Question 1)**
2	Diaper dermatitis presents as a mild red rash that often progresses to increased redness and lesions outside the diaper area. Barrier creams are recommended for initial treatment with the addition of a topical antifungal for dermatitis lasting longer than 3 days and spreading outside the diaper area.	**Case 104-2 (Questions 1, 2)**
3	Fever in children may be the result of a common viral infection, but could also be an indicator of a more serious bacterial infection or lead to complications such as febrile seizures. Proper management depends in large part on accurate assessment.	**Case 104-3 (Questions 1, 2)**
4	The treatment of cough and cold symptoms in children younger than 6 years of age is generally supportive with nasal saline, hydration, and humidification. Over-the-counter agents have little proven effectiveness and have been associated with severe adverse effects owing to inadvertent overdoses during parental administration.	**Case 104-4 (Question 1)**
5	Constipation can be defined by a delay or difficulty in stooling for at least 2 weeks duration. Constipation is most commonly functional, and may be managed with behavioral modification or drug therapy.	**Case 104-5 (Question 1)**
6	Gastroenteritis, although usually self-limiting, may result in clinically significant dehydration in infants and children. Assessment of the degree of dehydration is important in determining whether oral rehydration is appropriate or hospital admission with intravenous rehydration is required.	**Case 104-6 (Questions 1–3)**
7	Gastroesophageal reflux is a common disorder in young infants. Most will require no intervention. Some, however, will require feeding modifications and possibly drug therapy, including acid-suppressing or prokinetic agents.	**Case 104-7 (Questions 1, 2)**
8	Otitis media is a middle ear infection associated with effusion, rapid symptom development, and evidence of middle ear inflammation. Options for therapy include antibiotic management and watchful waiting, the choice of which depends on the age of the child and severity of disease. Amoxicillin (or amoxicillin/clavulanate) remains the antibiotic of choice despite the high incidence of penicillin nonsusceptible *Streptococcus pneumoniae*.	**Case 104-8 (Questions 1–3)**
9	Acute pharyngitis may be caused by respiratory viruses or bacteria, most commonly *Streptococcus pyogenes*. Treatment goals for bacterial pharyngitis include resolution of symptoms and prevention of rheumatic heart disease. Amoxicillin is the antibiotic of choice for bacterial pharyngitis.	**Case 104-9 (Questions 1, 2)**

Children represent more than 25% of the population and receive an average of three prescription medications before 5 years of age. According to the Slone Survey, between 1998 and 2007, 56% of children younger than 12 years of age had taken at least one medication in the previous week.[1] Prescription medications accounted for only 20% of cases; thus, the use of over-the-counter (e.g., nonprescription) medications was most prevalent. The most predominant over-the-counter medications used were acetaminophen, pseudoephedrine, ibuprofen, dextromethorphan, antihistamines, and iron. The most prevalent prescription medications were amoxicillin and albuterol. The prevalence of chronic medication use for dyslipidemia, hypertension, type 2 diabetes, and attention deficit hyperactivity disorder has increased in recent years, illustrating that chronic disease management is becoming more important in pediatric medicine.[2,3] Given the prevalence of medication use in children, it is essential that health care providers be prepared to educate families and children on the appropriate use of over-the-counter and prescription medications.

ADMINISTERING MEDICATION TO CHILDREN

CASE 104-1

Question 1: M.B., a 16-month-old girl weighing 9 kg, has been diagnosed with an ear infection. She will be receiving amoxicillin (400 mg/5 mL) 5 mL by mouth every 12 hours. What tips for successfully administering these medications should be recommended?

Oral Medications

The administration of oral medications to a young child or infant often requires two adults: one to gently restrain the child while the other rapidly and accurately administers the medication. If only one adult is available, one can restrain the arms and legs of the child in a swaddling blanket or large towel as depicted in Figure 104-1.

Figure 104-1 Administration of oral liquid medication to a young child. (1) Premeasure the medication and have it within reach. (2) Hold the child in your lap, placing one of the child's arms behind your back and both of the child's legs between your legs. Restrain the child's other arm securely with your nondominant arm. (3) Tilt the child's head back slightly, pressing gently on the child's cheeks to open the mouth. Using your dominant hand, aim the dropper or syringe between the rear gum and cheek. Administer small amounts of medication (1–2 mL) at a time, making sure the baby swallows.

The administration device (syringe, dropper, or dosing spoon) that generally accompanies a liquid medication product provides the most accurate measurement of the desired dose. For infants, liquid medications are most easily administered to the back cheek in 1- to 2-mL amounts with an oral syringe. Household teaspoons should not be used to measure medications because teaspoons are of variable sizes and hold 3 to 8 mL of a liquid. Other considerations involve the unit of measurement. To decrease errors and improve precision of drug delivery, it is recommended to use milliliter-based dosing exclusively while prescribing and administering liquid products.[4] Regarding unique delivery devices, studies have shown that parents have more difficulty accurately delivering doses using dosing cups than other devices.[5]

In some situations, crushed tablets or capsule contents mixed in small amounts (1–2 teaspoons) of food (e.g., chocolate pudding, applesauce, ice cream, jelly, and chocolate syrup) offer an alternative to liquid formulations. The taste of liquid dosage formulations is generally improved by refrigeration and flavoring agents, and "chasers" (i.e., popsicle, chocolate syrup, or a flavored drink after a dose) are also helpful. Although medications can be delivered in small amounts (10–15 mL) of liquid in a bottle (juice, milk, and formula), doses should not be diluted into an entire scheduled feeding or prepared ahead of time in batches in anticipation of future administration. Limiting the volume more likely facilitates delivery of the entire dose, and adding the medication to a feeding bottle immediately before delivery minimizes the potential of drug instability. Drug interactions with foods and dairy products should also be considered before drugs are added to feeding formulas. Most children are able to swallow tablets at 5 to 8 years of age. Duplicate supplies of medication should be provided to the caregiver, when midday doses are required for children who attend school or childcare in the event a dose is dropped. Children of all ages should be encouraged and praised for their cooperation in taking their medicine. Rewards and positive reinforcements can be useful to gain cooperation in an older child.

For M.B.'s amoxicillin, the parents should be given a dosing syringe and shown how to measure 5 mL. If M.B. is uncooperative with medication administration, she may need to be restrained and the medication delivered in 1- to 2-mL increments. The parents should be ready to provide M.B. with something that tastes good immediately after administering the medication.

Ear, Nose, and Eye Drops

Otic, ophthalmic, and nasal medications usually need to be administered to infants and young children in a different manner than adults. Otic medications should be instilled by pulling the auricle down and out in infants and young children, whereas older children should have the auricle of the ear held up and back to straighten the ear canal. During the instillation of nose and eye drops, position infants and toddlers with their head lower than the rest of the body because gravity assists in dispersing the medication. This can be achieved by laying the infant across a bed with the shoulders projecting over the edge of the bed. Restraining the infant often is required during the administration of ophthalmic formulations. When administering the eye medication (Fig. 104-2), the caregiver must be cautious to avoid injury to the eye caused by sudden movements of the infant. The technique of placing the hand, which holds the eye medication on the forehead of the infant during administration, can help to minimize eye injury because the hand holding the eye dropper will move when the infant's head moves.

To minimize fear and improve cooperation during instillation of eye, nose, or ear drops, the procedure should be explained to

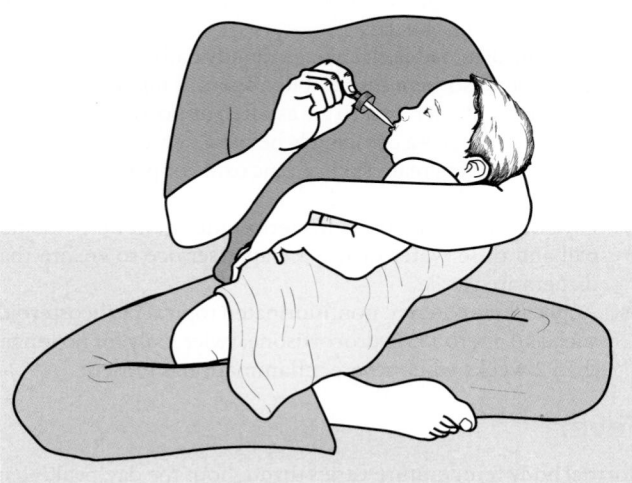

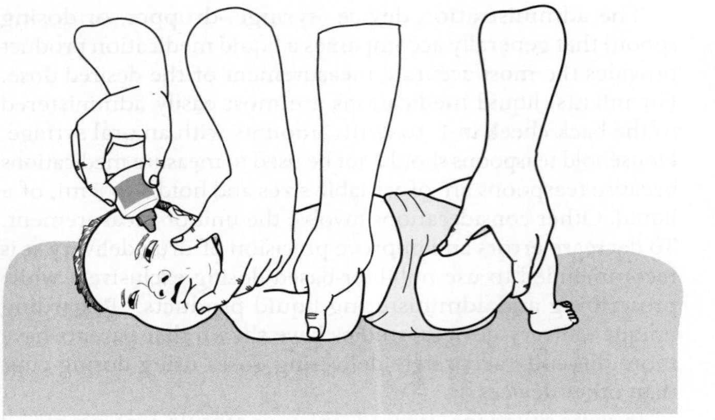

Figure 104-2 Administering eye drops to a young child. (1) Place the child on a flat surface. Enlist the help of a second adult to restrain the child or swaddle the child. (2) Holding the child's head steady, gently pull the eyelids apart. The hand that is holding the medication dropper can rest on the child's head while administering the medication to minimize the potential for injury to the eye if the child's head moves abruptly. Administer the medication as directed.

the child as simply as possible. It is best to warm the medication in your hand for a few minutes before administration because medications can feel cold inside the ears or nose even when stored at room temperature.

If ear drops were to be administered to M.B., she should be lying down with the affected ear up. The auricle should be pulled down and out, and the ear drops placed in the ear canal. She should remain in that position for at least 1 minute.

INFANT CARE

Diaper Rash

ETIOLOGY

Diaper dermatitis is commonly encountered in pediatric practice, occurring in up to 35% of infants at any given time. Although the pathogenesis of diaper dermatitis is not well defined, a number of factors (e.g., chemical irritants, friction, and bacteria) have been associated with skin inflammation in the diaper area. In particular, skin wetness and pH have been implicated in diaper dermatitis, and wetness appears to have greater influence than that of pH. Overhydration of the skin increases the permeability of low-molecular-weight compounds and exacerbates the effects of friction.[6] Cloth diapers covered with plastic pants or disposable diapers with plastic outer linings decrease air circulation and increase moisture in the diaper area and should be avoided.[7] Residual chemicals or laundry detergents in the diaper (cloth or disposable), as well as soaps, medications, or lotions that have been applied directly to the infant's skin, also have roles in the development of diaper rash.

CLINICAL PRESENTATION

Four clinical presentations of dermatitis are associated with diaper wear:

1. A mild, scaling rash in the perianal area
2. A sharply demarcated confluent erythema
3. Ulceration distributed through the diaper area
4. A beefy red confluent erythema with satellite lesions, vesiculopustular lesions, and diffuse involvement of the genitalia

TREATMENT

CASE 104-2

QUESTION 1: K.G., a 3-month-old infant, has had a severe diaper rash for the last 4 days. The very inflamed and tender area is confined to the diaper area, and vesicular satellite lesions are present on the periphery of the erythematous area. K.G.'s mother uses only cloth diapers and has not changed soap or her normal pattern of diaper care since K.G. was born. What is the likely cause of K.G.'s diaper rash and what treatments are appropriate?

K.G.'s rash is consistent with a candidal infection, which typically is beefy red and associated with vesicular satellite lesions. The presence of a rash for longer than 3 days and the diffuse involvement of the genitalia and inguinal folds are also characteristic of this form of diaper rash. K.G.'s rash can be treated with 1% clotrimazole or 2% miconazole cream applied to the inflamed area four times daily until it has resolved. Nystatin (100,000 units/g) ointment can be applied, but often is not as effective as the imidazole antifungals because of increasing resistance of *Candida* species to nystatin.

CASE 104-2, QUESTION 2: What steps would you recommend for K.G.'s mother to treat her diaper rash and prevent recurrence?

The removal of stool and urine from the diaper area by gentle rinsing with plain water and more frequent diaper changes often help to alleviate diaper rashes. Wiping the baby with diaper wipes that contain alcohol can sting, further irritating the involved area, and should be avoided until the rash has resolved. A good protective agent containing zinc oxide or petrolatum (e.g., Desitin) can be applied with each diaper change to create a barrier to irritants and seal out moisture. Powdered protective agents (e.g., cornstarch and talc) can minimize friction caused by diapers, but should be used cautiously because the infant can aspirate powder particles and develop a chemical pneumonia.[8] When used, powders should be shaken into the diaper or applied close to the body, away from the baby's face. Other prevention and treatment measures appropriate for K.G. include the following:

1. Change the diaper as soon as it is wet or at least every 2 to 4 hours during the day.
2. Keep the diaper area clean (e.g., nightly baths until resolved).
3. Use superabsorbent disposable diapers at night.
4. Expose the diaper area to air as often as possible.
5. Dry the diaper area completely before a new diaper is put on.
6. Apply a barrier cream such as zinc oxide or petrolatum after each diaper change.
7. For cotton diapers, use a bacteriostatic agent in the diaper pail and rinse water or use a diaper service to ensure that diapers are sterile.
8. Apply a low-potency, nonfluorinated topical corticosteroid, such as 0.5% to 1% hydrocortisone, twice daily for no longer than 2 weeks when severe inflammation is present.[7]

Fever

Normal body temperature varies throughout the day, peaking in late afternoon or early evening. Body temperature can be measured rectally, orally, axillary (under the arm), temporally (on the forehead), and tympanically. Rectal temperatures are most reliable in infants younger than 3 months of age. Oral measurements of temperature are not appropriate in children younger than 3 years of age because it is difficult for young children to maintain a tight seal around the thermometer.

Although references differ, fever can be defined as an axillary temperature greater than 37.5°C (99.5°F) or a core temperature greater than 38°C (100.4°F).[9] Rectal and tympanic measurements are typically 0.3°C to 0.6°C (0.5°F to 1°F) higher than an oral reading, whereas axillary measurements are lower by the same amount. (Fahrenheit temperatures can be converted to or from centigrade temperatures by the formula °F = 1.8°C + 32.)

Children with fevers might not have other signs or symptoms of an illness. Any child younger than 2 months of age who develops a fever requires a complete evaluation (e.g., blood culture and urinalysis), because clinical manifestations of a serious infection often are subtle, nonspecific, and not predictive of the extent or severity of illness.[10] In this situation, antibiotic therapy is usually initiated while awaiting laboratory results. Children 3 to 36 months of age with a temperature greater than or equal to 39°C (102.2°F) and white blood cell counts less than 5,000 μL^{-1} or greater than 15,000 μL^{-1} are at increased risk for bacteremia.[10] Children of any age with a temperature greater than 41°C should be evaluated not only for bacteremia, but also for possible meningitis. Blood cultures, lumbar puncture, urinalysis, and chest radiograph should be considered on an individual basis to help determine the etiology of infection. Febrile immunocompromised children and febrile children with functional or anatomic asplenia are at increased risk for sepsis or fulminant infections (e.g., *Streptococcus pneumoniae*, *Salmonella* species, and *Escherichia coli*) and should receive prompt antibiotic therapy.[11]

Febrile Seizures

CASE 104-3

Question 1: R.B., a 12-month-old, 10-kg baby boy, was well yesterday until his mother noticed that he felt warm to her touch later in the afternoon. For the past 24 hours, he has remained warm and is fussy and less active. A rectal temperature 15 minutes ago was 39°C. Because her other two children experienced febrile seizures, his mother is concerned R.B.'s temperature will continue to rise and put R.B. at risk for febrile seizures. Is this a valid concern?

Febrile seizures occur in approximately 2% to 4% of children 6 months to 5 years of age who have temperature elevations greater than 38°C.[12] The etiology and pathogenesis are unknown, and there is no evidence that the rate of temperature increase is important.[13] Genetic predisposition also appears to be a factor because febrile seizures occur with greater frequency among family members.[12] Febrile seizures are of two types: simple and complex. Simple febrile seizures last less than 15 minutes and do not have significant focal features. Complex febrile seizures have a longer duration, occur in series, and are associated with focal changes. Typically, febrile seizures occur within the first 24 hours of a febrile episode.[12,13] Although R.B. is in the age group at greatest risk for having a febrile seizure, he has been febrile for more than 24 hours, and a seizure is unlikely during this illness.

TREATMENT

Case 104-3, Question 2: How should R.B.'s fever be treated?

Acetaminophen is the most common antipyretic agent used in children. The usual dose, oral or rectal, is 10 to 15 mg/kg/dose administered every 4 to 6 hours as needed to a maximum of 75 mg/kg/day.[14] Ibuprofen is administered as 5 to 10 mg/kg/dose orally every 6 to 8 hours as needed to a maximum of 40 mg/kg/day. Ibuprofen is as effective as acetaminophen as an antipyretic and is similar in safety.[15] Although renal failure has been reported after ibuprofen use in children, the risk of renal impairment appears greater in children with dehydration, underlying cardiovascular or renal disease, or other nephrotoxic drugs, and children <6 months of age.[15]

Acetaminophen 100 to 150 mg every 4 to 6 hours as needed or ibuprofen 50 to 100 mg every 6 to 8 hours as needed should be effective in lowering R.B.'s fever. Acetaminophen typically has been considered to be a first-line drug in children. Dosing errors have occurred, when teaspoonful quantities of acetaminophen infant drops (80 mg/0.8 mL) were given instead of the liquid formulation (160 mg/5 mL) or when regular-strength tablets (325 mg) have been substituted for chewable children's tablets (80 and 160 mg). To reduce the risk for dosing errors, in 2011, the Consumer Healthcare Products Association (a group of leading manufacturers and distributors of nonprescription medications) voluntarily converted to a single 160 mg/5 mL acetaminophen concentration. In addition, in 2017 manufacturers began transitioning to a single strength of children's chewable acetaminophen tablets (160 mg). However, providers should continue to question caregivers about the dosage form of acetaminophen they have at home, concurrent use of any other products containing acetaminophen, and whether cumulative doses are within the recommended range. Recent data have suggested that ibuprofen may be a more effective alternative to acetaminophen for R.B. and should be used first.[16] It is available in two liquid formulations (infant drops, 40 mg/mL; children's suspension, 100 mg/5 mL) and a chewable tablet (100 mg). Adverse effects are limited when ibuprofen is used in recommended doses for short-term antipyresis. Some data suggest that combination therapy with acetaminophen every 4 to 6 hours and ibuprofen every 6 to 8 hours may be more effective in reducing time with fever in the first 24 hours.[16] However, combination therapy may be associated with medication errors,[15] and recent data suggest an increased risk of acute kidney injury may occur with this combination.[17] Aspirin therapy is not recommended for treatment of fever in children or adolescents with chickenpox, gastroenteritis, or respiratory viral infections because of its link with Reye syndrome.[18,19]

Cough and Cold

Another common diagnosis in children is viral upper respiratory infection or the common cold. Preschool children generally experience between six and eight colds each year.[20] Children with a cold often present with sore throat, nasal congestion, rhinorrhea, sneezing, cough, and irritability.

CLINICAL PRESENTATION AND TREATMENT

CASE 104-4

Question 1: J.K. is a 3-month-old, 5.3-kg infant who began having nasal congestion, rhinorrhea, and cough yesterday. She has had no fever and is eating well, but did not sleep well last evening. J.K.'s mother called her pediatrician and was told that J.K. most likely has a cold caused by a virus. J.K.'s mother would like to know which cold medications would be appropriate to manage J.K.'s symptoms.

A cool-mist humidifier can increase the amount of moisture in room air and decrease irritation in the upper airway when humidity is low. Saline nose drops followed by bulb suctioning can help to clear the nasal passages in J.K. who is younger than 6 months of age. It is especially important to do this before feedings. A decongestant, however, should not be prescribed for J.K. because of her age and the potential for adverse effects. If J.K. was older and a topical nasal decongestant was needed, phenylephrine would be preferred over oxymetazoline and xylometazoline because of its lesser association with toxicity (e.g., sedation, convulsions, insomnia, and coma) in children younger than 6 years of age.[21,22] Neither antihistamines, antitussives, nor guaifenesin should be recommended for J.K.

because there is no evidence of their efficacy, and unintentional overdoses are common in this age group. Antihistamines are not effective for rhinorrhea caused by the common cold and should not be recommended. Antitussives are likely not effective and should not be used if the child's cough is productive. Expectorants, such as guaifenesin, are also not effective, and evidence is insufficient to support the use of vitamin C, zinc, or echinacea in children for treatment or prevention of the common cold.

Several hundred over-the-counter medications for upper respiratory symptoms are available, and over 1 billion units of these products are sold each year in the United States.[23] Nevertheless, the safety and effectiveness of these cough and cold medications in children have yet to be proved.[24] The Centers for Disease Control and Prevention (CDC) reported that 1,519 children younger than 2 years of age were admitted to emergency departments in 2004 to 2005 because of overdoses and other problems associated with cough and cold medicines. Furthermore, according to the US Food and Drug Administration (FDA), 54 deaths in children were linked to the use of decongestants (e.g., pseudoephedrine, phenylephrine, and ephedrine) and 69 deaths to antihistamines (e.g., diphenhydramine, brompheniramine, and chlorpheniramine) from 1969 to September 13, 2006. Most of these deaths occurred in children younger than 2 years of age, and some of the fatalities occurred in children who received overdoses that might have been the result of inadvertent administration of multiple medications containing the same ingredient.

In 2008, the FDA issued a public health advisory recommending that over-the-counter cough and cold medications not be used in children younger than 2 years of age.[25] Later that year, the Consumer Healthcare Products Association announced that many manufacturers would voluntarily modify their labels to exclude recommendations for children younger than 4 years of age.[26] Owing to reports of toxicity and death related to over-the-counter cough and cold products, the CDC has recommended that caregivers avoid giving these products to children younger than 2 years of age unless advised by a clinician.[24] If deemed necessary by a physician for older children, nonprescription cough and cold medications containing single ingredients should be selected to minimize the potential for adverse effects and administration of multiple products with similar ingredients. Of note, parents often misunderstand labeling of over-the-counter products, placing the child at risk for dosing errors.[27] It is critical that health care providers educate caregivers on the proper use and administration of these medications to children. Treatment of J.K.'s symptoms should include the use of a cool-mist humidifier in the room and saline nasal drops followed by suctioning before feedings.

Constipation

Chronic constipation is defined as delay or difficulty in stooling for at least 2 weeks' duration.[28,29] It accounts for 3% of annual visits to pediatrician offices, and up to a quarter of referrals to gastroenterologists.[30] Beyond the neonatal period, constipation is most commonly idiopathic or functional and may be related to a diet low in fiber, lack of time or routine for toileting, or passage of a painful stool resulting in a fear of defecating. Other causes of constipation include anatomic (fissures), neurogenic (Hirschsprung disease), hypotonic (cerebral palsy), and endocrine (cystic fibrosis and hypothyroidism) disorders.[30] Medications such as opioids, antacids, and anticonvulsants, among others, can also contribute to constipation. It is important that constipation be managed appropriately because it can have negative effects on growth and development, has been linked to gastrointestinal distress, and adversely impacts quality of life.[30] In addition, constipation in childhood can remain a problem into adulthood.[31]

CLINICAL PRESENTATION AND TREATMENT

CASE 104-5

QUESTION 1: R.J., a 2-year-old, 15-kg boy, has had abdominal pain for 4 weeks. On average, he has one stool weekly, and he cries each time because of pain. R.J. eats regular table food and has two glasses of whole milk each day. After obtaining a thorough history and performing a physical examination, the physician determines that R.J. has functional constipation. What treatment measures are appropriate to relieve and prevent R.J.'s constipation?

Before maintenance therapy can be initiated, disimpaction of the patient is necessary. Although no controlled studies compare efficacy of the oral and rectal routes, oral therapy (mineral oil, polyethylene glycol, and bisacodyl) is preferred because it is less invasive and might lead to better adherence than rectal therapy (phosphate soda enemas, mineral oil enemas, glycerin suppositories in infants, and bisacodyl suppositories in older children).[30] After disimpaction, a combination of behavioral, dietary, and pharmacologic therapies should be initiated to promote regular stool production and prevent reimpaction. Dietary interventions include adequate fluid and fiber intake. The impact of cow's milk on constipation is still controversial. Some data suggest no link,[30] although other recent literature hints at causation through an immune-mediated mechanism.[31,32] Medications such as polyethylene glycol 3350, mineral oil, lactulose, and sorbitol should be titrated to produce one to two soft stools daily. Stimulant laxatives might be needed intermittently in certain cases. Although no clear recommendation for one maintenance medication has been given over others, recent data suggest that polyethylene glycol may be the most effective and best tolerated in children.[33–37] The recommended dosing of medications for treatment of constipation is listed in Table 104-1. Appropriate initial therapy for R.J. could include eliminating or limiting milk intake, behavioral techniques, and polyethylene glycol 0.5 to 1.5 g/kg/day (7.5–15 g). Practically, this would be half to one 17-g packet administered daily in 4 to 8 ounces of water or other beverage.

Vomiting and Diarrhea

Vomiting and diarrhea, two commonly encountered complaints in pediatric practice, are usually self-limiting, but severe cases can result in serious complications such as dehydration, metabolic disturbances, and even death. Infants and young children are particularly susceptible to the more severe complications.

PATHOGENESIS AND PRESENTATION OF VOMITING

Vomiting or emesis is defined as forceful expulsion of gastrointestinal (GI) contents through the mouth or nose, while nonforceful expulsion of GI contents is considered regurgitation. In newborns, regurgitation of small amounts of breast milk or formula after feeding, especially when burping, is common. In most cases, regurgitation usually resolves by 1 to 2 years of age and rarely causes problems.[38] Extensive evaluation of regurgitation is not needed in a child who is growing well. Other causes of vomiting during the newborn period include pyloric stenosis, gastroesophageal reflux (GER), overfeeding, food intolerance, and GI obstruction. Beyond the neonatal period, the most common cause of vomiting is infection. Vomiting in infants and children can also be caused by central nervous system (CNS) disease (e.g., intracranial tumors), metabolic disease (e.g., urea cycle disorder), inflammatory bowel disease, and ulcers. Conditions causing emesis in older infants and children range from viral gastroenteritis to more severe illnesses, such as bowel obstruction or head injury,

Table 104-1
Medications for the Treatment of Constipation[28,29]

Medication	Initial Dosage	Comments
Osmotic Agents		
Polyethylene glycol 3350	0.2–0.8 g/kg/day	0.5 g/kg initial dose; titrate to effect; do not exceed 17 g/day
Lactulose	1–2 g/kg/day divided once or twice daily	1.5–3 mL/kg/day; do not exceed 60 mL/day
Sorbitol	1–3 mL/kg/day once or twice daily	Less expensive than lactulose
Barley malt extract	2–10 mL/240 mL of milk or juice daily	Useful for infants drinking from a bottle
Magnesium hydroxide	1–3 mL/kg/day using 400 mg/5 mL	Infants are at risk for hypermagnesemia
Phosphate enema	≥2 years of age: 6 mL/kg up to 135 mL	Electrolyte abnormalities more common in children with renal failure or Hirschprung disease. Avoid in children <2 years
Lubricant		
Mineral oil	>1 year of age: Disimpaction: 15–30 mL/year of age up to 240 mL daily	Better tolerated if chilled. Avoid in children <1 year. Lipoid pneumonia may occur if aspirated
	Maintenance: 1–3 mL/kg/day	Maximum daily dose: 90 mL/day
Stimulants		
Senna	2–6 years of age: 2.5–5 mg/day	Not recommended for chronic use
	6–12 years of age: 7.5–10 mg/day	
	>12 years: 15–20 mg/day	
Bisacodyl	3–10 years: 5 mg/day	Not recommended for chronic use
	>10 years: 5–10 mg/day	
Glycerin suppositories	2–5 years: 1 pediatric suppository per dose	Preferred stimulant for children <2 years of age
	≥6 years: 1 adult suppository per dose	

which require immediate medical attention.[39] Acute vomiting can also result from medication or toxic ingestions. In teenagers, migraine, pregnancy, and psychological disorders, such as bulimia, have been associated with vomiting.

PATHOGENESIS AND PRESENTATION OF DIARRHEA

Diarrhea refers to an increase in frequency, volume, or liquidity of stool when compared with normal bowel movements. In developing countries, diarrhea is a common cause of death in children younger than 5 years of age. In the United States, gastroenteritis accounts for approximately 1 to 2 million physician visits, more than 200,000 hospitalizations, and about 300 deaths each year.[40]

Acute diarrhea in infants and children is generally abrupt in onset, lasts a few days, and is most commonly caused by viruses. (see Chapter 69, Infectious Diarrhea for infectious diarrhea of other origins.) Diarrhea is considered chronic if it is longer than 2 weeks in duration. Chronic diarrhea can be caused by malabsorption, inflammatory disease, infection, alteration of intestinal flora, milk or protein intolerance, drugs, and other causes.[41]

Infants and children are at high risk for morbidity and mortality secondary to diarrhea for several reasons. Dehydration can occur easily because acute net intestinal fluid losses are relatively much greater in young children than in adults. This may result from inefficient transport systems in the developing intestine. In addition, the percentage of total body water in children is higher than in adults; thus, they are more susceptible to body fluid shifts. Total body water changes from 80% of total body weight in premature infants to 70% in term infants and 60% in adults. Finally, the renal capacity to compensate for fluid and electrolyte imbalances in the infant is limited compared with that of adults.[42]

VIRAL GASTROENTERITIS

CASE 104-6

QUESTION 1: J.R., a 15-month-old male 10-kg infant, had one loose stool and began vomiting this morning, but he has not had a fever. On questioning, you discover that many children attending day care with J.R. are experiencing vomiting, diarrhea, and low-grade temperatures. How should J.R.'s vomiting be treated?

Routine use of antiemetics for acute vomiting in children is not recommended because masking of symptoms may delay diagnosis of a treatable illness. In addition, the safety and efficacy of the antiemetics, including metoclopramide, promethazine, trimethobenzamide, and dimenhydrinate, have not been demonstrated.[43] In particular, promethazine is contraindicated in children younger than 2 years of age because of the risk of fatal respiratory depression. Ondansetron does decrease vomiting, increases oral intake and decreases the need for intravenous (IV) rehydration; however, the utility of ondansetron in gastroenteritis needs consideration because this effect may not be sustained, and the drug has not been shown to decrease consistently hospital admission.[44–46]

Parents should be taught the signs and symptoms of gastroenteritis and vomiting that are sufficiently serious to warrant medical attention. The child's primary-care provider should be contacted if the child is toxic appearing, exhibits unusual behavior, exhibits signs of an ear infection, experiences abdominal pain or distension, has red or black vomitus or stool, or if there is a history or suspicion of toxic ingestion or head trauma. Medical evaluation is also necessary for infants younger than 6 months of age, when persistent vomiting or high-volume diarrhea is present, or when chronic medical conditions or prematurity is involved. Because fever can accompany vomiting in viral gastroenteritis, any fever occurring in a neonate warrants medical attention. Fever in older infants and children warrants medical attention, when it becomes prolonged or changes in pattern.

When communicating with a health care provider about a vomiting child, it is helpful if the parents have knowledge of the child's fluid intake, and the frequency and volume of vomiting and urination. The amount of vomitus can be estimated by the following rule of thumb: one tablespoon makes a spot 4 inches wide and a quarter-cup makes a spot approximately 8 inches wide.

Vomiting associated with gastroenteritis usually resolves in 24 to 48 hours. Infants are particularly susceptible to the development of fluid and electrolyte abnormalities; therefore, fluid and electrolyte replacements are critically important.

J.R., who is early in the course of gastroenteritis, must receive sufficient fluids to prevent dehydration. Oral hydration therapy can be successful when given in small volumes, even if J.R. is still vomiting. For example, 5 to 10 mL can be administered every 5 to 10 minutes, with gradual increases in volume as tolerated. Volumes equal to estimated fluid deficit (usually 50–100 mL/kg) should be given over the course of 2 to 4 hours. For each diarrheal stool, an additional 10 mL/kg of oral electrolyte solution should be given. If diarrhea or vomiting recurs, 10 mL/kg and 2 mL/kg of an oral rehydration solution (ORS) can be administered for each stool or emesis, respectively.[46] J.R.'s clinical condition should continue to be monitored by his caregiver. If stool output exceeds 10 mL/kg/hour, ORS might not be sufficient, and the health care provider should be contacted. ORS should only be abandoned in children with intractable vomiting, loss of consciousness, bowel obstruction, or if the child is in shock. Most infants will tolerate oral hydration when small amounts are given frequently. As dehydration is corrected, the frequency of vomiting typically decreases. Once rehydration has been achieved, fluids other than ORS and a diet appropriate for age may be started.[46] Breast milk or formula should be given as tolerated.

Assessment of Dehydration

CASE 104-6, QUESTION 2: On the second day of illness, J.R. develops a mild fever and diarrhea that has increased in frequency and water content. How can the severity of J.R.'s diarrhea be assessed?

To determine the severity of dehydration and whether hospitalization may be needed, consider the following questions:

1. Does the child have any of the following signs and symptoms of severe dehydration: deeply sunken eyes, parched mucous membranes, significantly prolonged capillary refill; cool, mottled extremities; crying without tears; oliguria or anuria; weak or thready pulses; lethargy; poor oral intake; deep respirations; history of seizures or convulsions; a fever without perspiration; or thirst?
2. Are a large number of copious stools still being produced (>10 mL/kg/hour)? Is bowel obstruction a possibility?
3. Is there a risk of dehydration from inadequate monitoring, or is the parent unable to care for the child? Specific inquiries should be made about the number and consistency of stools in children with diarrhea.

Estimating the degree of dehydration is particularly valuable in assessing the patient with diarrhea, and weight loss is a good criterion. A 3% to 9% weight loss is considered mild to moderate dehydration, whereas more than 9% is considered severe dehydration.[43] (see Chapter 103, Pediatric Fluid, Electrolytes, and Nutrition, for information about IV replacement therapy in children with 10% or more dehydration.)

Oral Replacement Therapy

CASE 104-6, QUESTION 3: J.R. was evaluated by his pediatrician and was not considered to be sufficiently dehydrated to warrant hospitalization. How might J.R.'s fluids and electrolytes be managed on an outpatient basis?

The goal of J.R.'s treatment should be focused on the prevention of dehydration and the restoration and maintenance of adequate fluid and electrolyte balance. Mild to moderate diarrhea without dehydration is generally managed at home by continued age-appropriate feeding. Fluid losses in stools can be replaced with a glucose-containing ORS. Glucose provides calories and enhances salt and water absorption in the small intestine through mechanisms that are usually unimpaired in many toxin-induced diarrheas. Parents formerly were instructed to prepare salt and sugar solutions at home; however, frequent errors in the preparation of these solutions resulted in exacerbation of problems with fluid and electrolyte balance. Commercially available oral glucose–electrolyte formulations, such as Pedialyte, are designed to enhance glucose and sodium absorption and should be used in infants and young children. Carbonated beverages and fruit juices do not contain sufficient sodium to replace diarrheal losses and should not be used. Rehydration and maintenance solutions can be made more palatable with sugar-free flavorings (e.g., Kool-Aid and Crystal Lite).

The World Health Organization (WHO) formerly promoted use of an oral replacement solution (WHO formula) containing sodium (90 mEq/L), potassium (20 mEq/L), bicarbonate (30 mEq/L), chloride (80 mEq/L), and 2% glucose for the widespread management of acute diarrhea in third-world countries. The WHO formula, which had a 90% successful rehydration rate for the management of diarrhea, contained a high concentration of sodium. Although commercially available ORS contain less sodium than the WHO formulation, these preparations were equally effective as the WHO formula, even when used to treat the high-sodium losses associated with cholera. Furthermore, these lower sodium-containing formulations were associated with less vomiting, lower stool output, and reduced need for IV infusions in non–cholera-associated gastroenteritis. As a result, the WHO, in 2002, promoted a new formulation that consists of 75 mEq/L sodium and a total osmolarity of 245 mOsm/L.[43,45] Glucose is added to oral electrolyte solutions to enhance glucose-coupled sodium transport; however, concentrations greater than 3% can impair sodium absorption because the glucose-coupled sodium transport system becomes saturated at this concentration and any additional glucose acts as an osmotically active solute in the bowel lumen. The electrolyte content of commonly used ORS is provided in Table 104-2. Assuming J.R.'s fluid deficit is 50 to 100 mL/kg, he should receive 500 to 1,000 mL of ORS in the course of approximately 4 hours. In addition, he should receive an extra 100 mL for each diarrheal stool and 20 mL for each emesis that occurs. If stool output continues at a pace that cannot be matched with oral replacement, or signs and symptoms of severe dehydration occur, J.R. should be referred to his pediatrician again.

REINSTITUTION OF ORAL FEEDINGS

Previously, feeding during an episode of viral gastroenteritis has been delayed because of the malabsorption that typically occurs during and after these bouts. The malabsorption, however, is self-limiting, and substantial amounts of carbohydrate, protein, and fat can still be absorbed. The reinstitution of a regular diet, therefore, should not adversely affect mild diarrhea and can be beneficial.[46] Parents are encouraged to continue feeding their children using age-appropriate diet while avoiding simple sugars, which can increase osmotic load and worsen diarrhea. Continuation of oral

Table 104-2
Oral Electrolyte Solutions[43]

Solution	Compositions			
	Sodium (mmol/L)	Potassium (mmol/L)	Carbohydrate (mmol/L)	Osmolality
Rehydration				
Rehydralyte	75	20	140	305
WHO formula (1975)	90	20	111	311
WHO formula (2002)	75	20	75	245
Maintenance				
Enfalyte	50	25	167	200
Pedialyte	45	20	139	250
Home Remedies				
Apple juice	0.4	44	667	730
Gatorade	20	3	255	330
Ginger ale	3	1	500	540
Chicken broth	250	8		500
Cola	1.6		622	730

WHO, World Health Organization.

feeding, despite diarrheal episodes, minimizes the development of protein and energy deficits, facilitates the maintenance and repair of intestinal mucosa, promotes recovery of brush border membrane disaccharidases, decreases the duration of illness, and improves nutritional status.[45,46] Although lactose intolerance can occur with viral gastroenteritis, most children with mild diarrhea can tolerate full-strength animal milk, animal milk-based formula, and breast milk. If the child becomes lactose intolerant during this illness, a lactose-free formula may be substituted for 2 to 6 weeks until GI lactase production returns to normal. Specific diets are often recommended during diarrhea (e.g., BRAT [bananas, rice, applesauce, toast]). Although these diets can be occasionally useful, the nutritional value of these foods is relatively low, and they do not provide optimal nutrition compared with complete diets with fats and proteins.[45,46] Once J.R. has been adequately rehydrated, he may resume his normal diet. However, the caregivers must take care to avoid juices and other foods with simple sugars, which may worsen diarrhea.

Drug Therapy

Medications play a minor role in the treatment of acute infantile diarrhea because most episodes are self-limiting. Antibiotics are recommended when systemic bacteremia is suspected, when immune defenses are compromised, when a persistent enteric infection is sensitive to antibiotics, or when *Shigella*, *Campylobacter*, *Vibrio cholerae*, *Clostridium difficile*, and certain *Escherichia coli* strains are isolated.[46,47] In general, antidiarrheal preparations are not recommended for infants or children because they have little effect on acute diarrhea, are associated with side effects, and direct attention away from the use of oral hydration therapy.[45,46] Drugs such as loperamide that alter GI motility should be avoided, especially in children with high fever, toxemia, or bloody mucoid stools, because they may worsen the clinical course of the bacterial infection. Bismuth subsalicylate preparations, which possess antisecretory and antimicrobial effects, have not been shown to provide clinical benefit and are not recommended.[45] Adsorbents, such as kaolin-pectin or attapulgite, adsorb bacterial toxins and water and lessen the symptoms of diarrhea by producing more formed stools, but there is no evidence of effectiveness, and they are not recommended.[45] Zinc supplementation (10–20 mg for 10–14 days) has been recommended by the WHO for the treatment and prevention of diarrheal disease in children in developing countries; however, its mechanism of action, best method of administration, and efficacy in different populations are not yet well understood.[43,48]

Probiotics, live microbial products containing species of *Lactobacillus*, *Bifidobacterium*, *Saccharomyces*, and *Streptococcus*, can improve the balance of intestinal flora and diminish the effect of enteric pathogens. These microbes are thought to exert their beneficial effects through various mechanisms, including producing antibacterial chemicals, competing with enteric pathogens, inhibiting the adhesive capabilities of pathogens, altering toxins or toxin receptors, and upregulating interleukin-mediated T-cell response.[48,49] Probiotics are most useful in infectious gastroenteritis when used early in the course of disease. Lactobacilli are the most well-studied species and have been the most consistently effective in clinical trials. It appears that efficacy of the different species may depend on the specific strain, the dose, and the timing of administration, although it is generally accepted that dosage forms with at least 10^6 to 10^9 colony-forming units and above are required.[45,48] The manufacture of probiotics is not regulated by the FDA; therefore, the organism count per dose might be based on the number present at the time of production and not at time of expiration, and the labeling might incorrectly identify the species of organism. Probiotics are not recommended for use in immunocompromised individuals because systemic infections after the use of these products have been reported.[43] For J.R., a *Lactobacillus* preparation administered for 5 days may provide some modest clinical benefit, although the benefit is most pronounced in rotavirus diarrhea, which has not been documented in his case.

GASTROESOPHAGEAL REFLUX

GER is a common disorder, with 50% to 67% of infants experiencing recurrent vomiting and regurgitation during the first 4 months of life.[50] Most reflux in infants is believed to be caused by transient relaxations of the lower esophageal sphincter (LES). Infants might also be predisposed to reflux because of their body positioning (e.g., slumped over in a car seat or lying supine), their consumption of a liquid feeding that exceeds the volume capacity of the stomach, and in premature infants, a decrease in peristaltic activity.[51] Infants and young children might also have undiagnosed underlying conditions that predispose them to reflux (e.g., neurologic disorders, hiatal hernia, hypertrophic pyloric stenosis, and cow's milk protein allergy).[52] Of cases of reflux in infants, 80% are benign and resolve by 18 months of age,[53] and reflux in older children resolves in a timeframe similar to that of adults. If untreated, GER can result in esophageal strictures, GI hemorrhage, or chronic respiratory disease from the aspiration of GI contents. Studies evaluating the relationship between GER disease (GERD) and asthma or *Helicobacter pylori* have shown mixed results.[54–57]

Clinical Presentation

In infants, the vomiting and regurgitation of GER occur frequently, and other symptoms often are nonspecific (e.g., failure to thrive [FTT], recurrent pneumonia, apnea, dysphagia, reactive airway disease, apparent life-threatening events [ALTE], hematemesis, and anemia).[58,59] A thorough diagnostic workup is generally not necessary in a healthy infant with functional GER presenting as recurrent vomiting. Empiric drug therapy can be initiated after the diagnosis is made based on clinical findings and after other causes of vomiting have been eliminated.[58] Further diagnostic evaluations, however, are indicated for infants and children presenting with additional symptoms of GERD (e.g., FTT, irritability, ALTE, and respiratory difficulties).[53]

Treatment

Because uncomplicated GER usually resolves spontaneously in infants, therapy should focus on providing symptom relief and maintaining normal growth.[53] The goals of therapy are to lessen symptoms, heal esophagitis, and prevent complications in infants and children with pathologic GER, so that surgery can be avoided.[53] Infants and young children with underlying neurologic problems (e.g., cerebral palsy) are unlikely to have spontaneous resolutions of GER and frequently require aggressive antireflux therapies and surgical intervention.

POSITIONAL AND DIETARY MEASURES

CASE 104-7

QUESTION 1: S.B., a 3-month-old, 6-kg, breastfed male infant, has a 2-week history of regurgitation after each feeding. The pediatrician noted that S.B. had not gained weight since his last visit 1 month earlier. The presumptive diagnosis is FTT secondary to GER, and S.B. was referred to a pediatric gastroenterologist. How should S.B. be treated initially?

S.B. can be treated conservatively because he does not present with life-threatening complications.[58,59] First, caregiver feedings should be observed to rule out regurgitation caused either by overfeeding or by inappropriate feeding techniques. Sometimes infants with milk protein allergies can have a similar clinical presentation; therefore, a change to a soy protein formula or hypoallergenic formula should be tried.[58] Interventions to modify an infant's body positioning or to modify infant feedings with milk thickeners are not proven to be effective, but are reasonable to undertake.[60,61] Maintaining S.B. at a 60-degree angle during the day while sitting and at a 30-degree position at night should be implemented in an effort to promote clearance of acid from the esophagus and to minimize reflux after meals. Milk thickeners (most commonly rice cereal in the United States) and more frequent, smaller feedings are also worthwhile interventions, although thickened formula could lead to increased coughing during feeding. Mild cases of GER often can be treated successfully by dietary measures alone, as well as by propping infants in an upright position during, and 1 hour after, feedings.[59] Although the placement of infants in a face-down prone position during sleep can reduce reflux, the greater risk of sudden infant death syndrome (SIDS) in infants younger than 12 months of age outweighs the benefits of such positioning.[58] Older children and adolescents should follow the recommended dietary guidelines (i.e., avoidance of caffeine, chocolate, and spicy foods) for adults.

DRUG THERAPY

The efficacy of pharmacologic therapy in altering the course of uncomplicated GER in infants has not been proved.[58] In infants or children who present with nonspecific symptoms or complications, such as S.B., acid-suppression therapy or prokinetic therapy is warranted even in the absence of documented esophagitis.[58] When esophagitis is present, acid suppression is always recommended to aid in the healing process; however, these agents alone do not rectify the causes of the GER.[58] The various agents to treat infant GER are listed in Table 104-3.[59,62–73]

Acid-Suppressant Agents

Antacids

Chronic antacid therapy is generally not recommended for the treatment of GER in infants and young children, because infants treated with aluminum-containing antacids can accumulate sufficient aluminum to cause osteopenia and neurotoxicity.[58,62,72] In addition, information on other antacids in infants is limited; nevertheless, antacids can provide short-term relief of symptoms in older children and adults.

Proton-Pump Inhibitors

Proton-pump inhibitors (PPIs) are superior to histamine-2 receptor antagonists (H_2RA) in relieving symptoms and in promoting healing of significant esophagitis from GER in infants, young children, and adults.[58,73,74] PPIs control both basal and meal-stimulated acid secretion, which may in part explain their superior efficacy. The incidence of adverse effects in children from PPI is similar to that reported in adults.[64,75] Despite concerns about the long-term use of PPI, untoward effects have not been observed from their use for up to 11 years.[76] In children, increased metabolism and decreased bioavailability necessitate larger milligram per kilogram doses to maintain acid suppression than adults; thus, titration of dose to response is necessary, particularly for treatment of esophageal erosions.[60,77] Although most clinicians dose PPI once a day, multiple, divided daily doses can prevent acid breakthrough and better promote healing.[73] Omeprazole, lansoprazole, and esomeprazole are available in extended-release capsules, which can be separated, opened, and sprinkled on soft foods. Omeprazole and esomeprazole are also available as granules for an oral suspension. Suspension formulations for both omeprazole and lansoprazole have been extemporaneously compounded and evaluated for stability. Esomeprazole has also been recently approved for use in children with GERD aged 1 to 11 years and has been studied and reviewed extensively.[74,78,79]

Histamine-2 Receptor Antagonists

H_2RA reduce histamine-stimulated acid secretion, but have limited effects on acid secretion by other chemical mediators and other stimuli. In randomized, controlled trials, H_2RA in infants and children relieved symptoms and facilitated the healing of esophageal tissue.[65,66] Tolerance to the acid-suppressant activity of H_2RA for a relatively short time ($<$30 days), however,[67,68] can

Table 104-3

Oral Drugs Used to Treat Gastroesophageal Reflux in Infants[58,59,62–71]

Agent	Mode of Action	Oral Dosage
Acid-Suppressing Agents		
Antacids (aluminum or magnesium hydroxide)	Neutralizes acid	0.5–1.0 mL/kg/dose before and after feeding (maximum, 15 mL/dose)
Proton-Pump Inhibitors		
Omeprazole	Decrease acid secretion via inhibition of gastric hydrogen-potassium adenosine triphosphatase	5 kg–<10 kg: 5 mg daily 10 kg–≤20 kg: 10 mg daily >20 kg: 20 mg daily Alternate dosing: 1 mg/kg daily or twice daily
Esomeprazole		1–11 years: 10 mg daily (>1 mg/kg/day or therapy >8 weeks has not been evaluated) ≥12 years: 20 mg daily
Lansoprazole		Infants ≥3 months: 7.5 mg twice daily or 15 mg once daily 1–11 years: 15 mg (<30 kg)–30 mg (>30 kg) daily ≥12 years: 15 mg daily
Pantoprazole		<5 years: 1.2 mg/kg/day once daily >5 years: 20 or 40 mg once daily
H_2 Receptor Antagonists		
Cimetidine	Blocks H_2-receptors; ↓ acid secretion	30–40 mg/kg/day divided QID
Famotidine		1 mg/kg/day divided BID
Nizatidine		10 mg/kg/day divided BID
Ranitidine		5–10 mg/kg/day divided BID or TID
Prokinetic Agents		
Bethanechol	Cholinergic agent; stimulates peristalsis ↑ ↑ LES pressure; ↑ gastric emptying; ↑ colonic motility ↑ Gastric emptying; ↑ LES pressure; augments esophageal clearance	0.1–0.2 mg/kg/dose QID given 30–60 minutes before feeding and HS
Metoclopramide	Dopamine antagonist	0.1–0.2 mg/kg/dose QID given 30 minutes before feeding and HS
Erythromycin	Motilin agonist stimulates smooth muscle contraction	3 mg/kg/dose QID; maximum dose: 10 mg/kg or 250 mg
Surface-Active Agents		
Sucralfate	Forms paste and adheres to damaged esophageal mucosa	40–80 mg/kg/day divided QID

BID, 2 times daily; HS, at bedtime; LES, lower esophageal sphincter; QID, 4 times daily; TID, 3 times daily.

limit their use for long-term treatment of esophagitis. Oral liquid formulations are available for most H_2RA. Ranitidine is also available in an effervescent tablet.

Prokinetic Agents

Metoclopramide, a dopamine antagonist with cholinergic and serotonergic effects, accelerates gastric emptying, increases LES pressure, enhances esophageal clearance, and accelerates transit time in the small bowel; however, its effects on vomiting and esophageal pH in children with GER has been equivocal.[69,70] Additionally, metoclopramide has been associated with significant CNS (i.e., restlessness, drowsiness, and extrapyramidal) effects, recently receiving a special alert for a higher risk of extrapyramidal symptoms in those <1 year of age, and rare reports of gynecomastia and galactorrhea.[59] Erythromycin increases GI motility by increasing smooth muscle contractions through its motilin agonistic activity, and it has been used as a prokinetic agent for GER in children, when acid suppression therapy alone was ineffective.[80] Erythromycin-induced development of infantile hypertrophic pyloric stenosis, arrhythmias, and potential changes in bacterial resistance patterns, however, limit its use for GER. The cholinergic agonist, bethanechol, reportedly reduces vomiting episodes in infants with GER[40,58,81]; however, its role in treating GER in infants is limited because of its potential to induce bronchospasm and to stimulate gastric acid secretion. The lack of a suitable commercially available formulation of bethanechol for young infants necessitates its extemporaneous compounding. Baclofen, which decreases transient LES relaxations through its γ-aminobutyric acid agonist actions, could be a future therapeutic option for GER, pending further study.[82] Generally, prokinetic agents only are marginally effective in the management of GER.

Surface-Active Agents

Sucralfate was equally effective as cimetidine for use in esophagitis[83]; however, its use for GER is more limited because of concern about the adverse effects of aluminum-containing products in infants.

Case 104-7, Question 2: Four weeks after instituting positional and dietary measures, S.B. continues to vomit and still has not been gaining weight. On physical examination, the gastroenterologist notes bilateral wheezes; endoscopy rules out esophagitis. What would be the next step of therapy?

The treatment of S.B. can include acid-suppression therapy. Acid-suppression therapy in children who have complications from GER can be implemented by a step-up approach in which treatment is initiated with an H_2RA followed by a PPI if no improvement is noted, or through a step-down approach involving a PPI followed by an H_2RA for maintenance therapy. However, initial therapy with PPI is preferred,[58,59] and S.B. may be treated with omeprazole 5 mg daily. Granules for suspension may be mixed in 10 mL of water and administered orally.

The effectiveness of acid suppression for managing symptoms of GER in children is not as well documented as it is for healing esophagitis; however, acid suppression is believed to play a useful role for symptom control, particularly for managing the respiratory symptoms.[58] Treatment should be continued for at least 3 to 4 months, although the optimal duration of therapy is unknown. If S.B. requires additional drug therapy to control symptoms of GER beyond 18 months to 2 years of age, surgery should be considered because GER is unlikely to resolve spontaneously after this age.[84] Surgery might be considered earlier if S.B. fails medical therapy or if he develops an esophageal stricture, apnea, or recurrent respiratory disease.[58]

COMMON PEDIATRIC INFECTIONS

Acute Otitis Media

Acute otitis media (AOM) is the most common reason for antimicrobial use in children, and is associated with expenditures of $350 per episode and, cumulatively, almost $3 billion annually.[85] AOM is most common from the ages of 3 months to 3 years, although the highest incidence occurs between 6 and 9 months of age. Most children will have had at least one episode by the time they reach 1 year of age.[86] Incidence is higher in the winter months, concurrent with viral upper respiratory illnesses. Several risk factors for AOM have been identified and include age younger than 2 years, early colonization of pathogens and onset of AOM, day-care attendance, bottle propping, cleft palate, immune compromise, and Down syndrome. Other factors such as smoke exposure, bottle feeding, pacifier use, and ethnicity have not been consistently found to increase risk of AOM.[87,88]

Eustachian tube dysfunction, either from intermittent causes such as upper respiratory infections or permanent causes such as cleft palate, is the primary condition required for the development of AOM. This results in a defect in the eustachian tube's ability to equilibrate middle ear pressure. Thus, nasopharyngeal contents, including bacteria, may be aspirated into the middle ear. This process is more likely in infants and young children who have shorter, flatter eustachian tubes.[87] Changes in pressure can also cause increased vascular permeability, resulting in an effusion. Viral infections contribute by enhancing bacterial transfer from the nasopharynx and adherence to the middle ear.[87]

S. pneumoniae, nontypeable *Haemophilus influenzae*, and *Moraxella catarrhalis* colonize the nasopharynx early in childhood, and thus, are the most common pathogens causing AOM.[87] Historically, these pathogens have been implicated in 28% to 54%, 32% to 59%, and up to 63% of cases of AOM, respectively.[89] The introduction of the pneumococcal conjugate vaccine (PCV7) reduced the overall incidence of AOM, the recurrence of AOM, and the need for tympanostomy tube insertion.[85–87] However, the incidence of AOM caused by non-PCV7 serotypes, *H. influenzae*, and *M. catarrhalis* increased with the reduction in AOM cases caused by PCV7 serotypes.[85,86,90,91] These studies were used to guide the development of a 13-valent PCV (PCV13), which was approved and licensed to replace the PCV7 in 2010. The PCV13 vaccine includes six of the serotypes that had been shown to produce more than 60% of non-PCV7 vaccine strain invasive infections. The PCV13 vaccine has shown increased protective effects against AOM because of the reduction in nasopharyngeal colonization by emerging serotypes.[92,93] Overall, studies have shown that PCV13 provides a reduction in pneumococcal disease, including AOM, in children.[93]

CASE 104-8

Question 1: C.D. is a 7-month-old, 8-kg infant who during the last 36 hours has developed cough, ear pain, and rhinorrhea, became irritable and at times inconsolable, and now has a temperature of 102.4°F (39.1°C). Physical examination shows bulging, dark, yellow opaque tympanic membranes bilaterally. This is the first time he has had these symptoms and has had no recent courses of antibiotics. What signs and symptoms do C.D. exhibit, which are consistent with AOM, and how should AOM be diagnosed?

Very often, as in this patient case, otitis media is preceded by an upper respiratory tract infection. These viral infections often will produce otitis media with effusion (OME), which typically will cause no more than temporary mild hearing loss. If AOM develops, more signs and symptoms will usually arise. These symptoms can include otalgia (pain causing infants to pull on or rub the ears), fever, irritability, and otorrhea.[89] Unfortunately, aside from otorrhea, these symptoms are nonspecific and may be present in many children who do not have AOM. As a result, a definitive diagnosis may not be easily obtained with symptoms alone. Diagnosis should be confirmed on visualization of the middle ear.

In 2013, the American Academy of Pediatrics (AAP) published guidelines on the diagnosis and management of AOM that stated that a diagnosis of AOM requires mild bulging of the tympanic membrane and either recent onset of ear pain (<48 hours) or intense erythema of the tympanic membrane.[89] Pneumatic otoscopy should be used to confirm the presence of effusion. Middle ear effusion can be differentiated from AOM in that, whereas both present with bulging tympanic membranes, in AOM, the middle ear fluid is more often dark yellow or red.[87,89] Other diagnostic tools may be used. Tympanometry uses sound waves to measure the compliance of the tympanic membrane. In acoustic reflectometry, the absorption of sound waves by the tympanic membrane provides information about the middle ear in that an effusion will cause more sound to be reflected back than a normal ear.[87] C.D.'s fever and irritability along with fluid in the middle ear and bulging, dark yellow tympanic membranes are consistent with the diagnosis of AOM.

Case 104-8, Question 2: How should C.D.'s otitis media be treated?

The 2013 AAP recommendations provide for the option to observe without treatment or to treat with antibiotics, depending on the age of the patient and symptoms present.[89] Generally, infants 6 months of age and younger should receive antibiotic therapy in all cases. Infants and children 6 months to 2 years of age can be managed with observation if there is a nonsevere unilateral AOM without otorrhea. Children 2 years of age and older can be managed with observation in bilateral or unilateral nonsevere AOM without otorrhea. Antibiotics are warranted in all cases of AOM with otorrhea or in AOM cases with severe symptoms (e.g., temperature >39°C in past 48 hours).[89]

C.D. appears to have bilateral AOM with severe symptoms based on his fever greater than 39°C, so antibiotic therapy is indicated. Despite pneumococcal penicillin resistance rates, initial therapy in most children who have not received amoxicillin in the last 30 days, would still be amoxicillin at a dose of 80 to 90 mg/kg/day.[89] Amoxicillin is effective against susceptible and intermediately resistant pneumococcus, it is affordable and palatable, and it has a narrow spectrum of activity.[86] Providers should prescribe amoxicillin/clavulanate in children who have received amoxicillin in the last 30 days, have concurrent purulent conjunctivitis, or have a history of recurrent AOM unresponsive to amoxicillin.[89] Oral cephalosporins, including cefdinir, cefuroxime, or cefpodoxime, are options in patients with a non-Type I allergy to penicillin, and macrolides such as azithromycin or clarithromycin may be used in those with Type I allergies to penicillin.

Whichever treatment course is taken in a patient (observation or antibiotic therapy with amoxicillin or amoxicillin/clavulanate), effectiveness is assessed for 48 to 72 hours. If the treatment is effective, the patient should defervesce, irritability should decrease, and normal activity should resume (e.g., eating and sleeping). If the observation is ineffective, treatment with amoxicillin or amoxicillin/clavulanate is recommended. If amoxicillin or amoxicillin/clavulanate is ineffective for C.D., ceftriaxone 400 mg (50 mg/kg) intramuscularly for 1 or 3 days is an option.

CASE 104-8, QUESTION 3: How should C.D.'s otalgia be managed?

Ear pain is a common feature of AOM, and it should be addressed regardless of the decision to use antibiotics or not. Acetaminophen 120 mg (15 mg/kg) or ibuprofen 80 mg (10 mg/kg) can provide adequate relief, and are first-line agents in the management of otalgia.[89] Home remedies such as the application of heat or cold may also be helpful.[89] For example, a washcloth can be soaked with very warm water, wrung out, and placed over the ear for comfort for 15 minutes several times per day.

Acute Pharyngitis

Acute pharyngitis is most common in children 5 to 15 years of age and is rare before 3 years of age. The etiology is typically viral, but bacteria such as group A streptococci (GAS, *Streptococcus pyogenes*), groups C and G streptococci, *Neisseria gonorrhoeae*, *Mycoplasma pneumoniae*, and *Chlamydia pneumoniae* may also cause pharyngitis in children.[94] The majority of attention is directed toward the detection and management of GAS infections as, untreated, they may lead to rheumatic fever, a complication progressing to permanent heart disease.

CASE 104-9

QUESTION 1: P.J., a 6-year-old boy weighing 23.4 kg, presents to the pediatrician's office complaining of fever, sore throat, and headache. His mother reports that he initially complained of sore throat about 12 hours ago. His oral temperature this morning was 102°F. He takes no medications and has no known drug allergies. Physical examination reveals erythematous tonsils and throat, as well as an enlarged anterior cervical lymph node. Are P.J.'s symptoms more consistent with GAS or viral pharyngitis?

Findings suggestive of GAS tonsillopharyngitis include sudden onset of throat pain, fever, headache, abdominal pain, nausea, vomiting, tonsillopharyngeal edema, enlarged anterior cervical lymph nodes, soft palate petechiae, and a scarlatiniform rash.[94] Symptoms that increase the likelihood of a viral cause include rhinorrhea, cough, conjunctivitis, and viral rash.[94] P.J. is lacking associated symptoms that would suggest a viral cause and has more symptoms of GAS pharyngitis, but confirmatory testing is needed.

DIAGNOSIS

Because clinical and physical findings are not definitive for GAS pharyngitis, confirmatory testing is important to determine the need for antibiotic therapy. A rapid antigen detection test is recommended, and, if positive, treatment is initiated. If negative, a throat culture should also be obtained and treatment initiated if the culture grows GAS. Rheumatic fever can be effectively prevented if treatment is started within 9 days from the start of the illness.[94]

CASE 104-9, QUESTION 2: A rapid antigen detection test for GAS is performed for P.J. and is positive. What treatment should be initiated at this time?

TREATMENT

Penicillins remain the agents of choice for GAS pharyngitis. Either oral penicillin, oral amoxicillin, or intramuscular benzathine penicillin may be used. Amoxicillin suspension is more palatable than penicillin and has the advantage of a once-daily dosing regimen. Intramuscular penicillin is a one-time dose that is helpful in those at risk for nonadherence. In patients with a Type I hypersensitivity to penicillins, azithromycin, clarithromycin, or clindamycin may be used. In those with a non-Type I allergy to penicillin, a first-generation cephalosporin may be considered. Recommended regimens are summarized in Table 104-4.[94,95] Although there is little reported GAS resistance to penicillin, some patients have a decreased clinical response and may respond

Table 104-4
Medication Regimens for the Treatment of Streptococcal Pharyngitis and Prevention of Rheumatic Fever[94,95]

Medication	Dose	Duration
Amoxicillin	50 mg/kg once a day or 25 mg/kg twice a day (maximum 1 g/day)	10 days
Penicillin VK	Children ≤27 kg: 250 mg 2 or 3 times a day Children >27 kg, adolescents: 500 mg 2 or 3 times a day or 250 mg 4 times a day	10 days
Benzathine penicillin G	≤27 kg: 600,000 units IM >27 kg: 1,200,000 units IM	Once
For Patients with Penicillin Allergy		
Cephalexin	20 mg/kg (up to 500 mg) twice a day	10 days
Cefadroxil	30 mg/kg (up to 1 g) once a day	10 days
Clindamycin	7 mg/kg 3 times a day (maximum 300 mg/dose)	10 days
Azithromycin	12 mg/kg once a day (maximum 500 mg)	5 days
Clarithromycin	7.5 mg/kg twice a day (maximum 250 mg/dose)	10 days

IM, intramuscular.

Table 104-5
Medication Regimens for the Prevention of Recurrent Rheumatic Fever[95,96]

Medication	Dose	Frequency
Benzathine penicillin G	≤27 kg: 600,000 units IM >27 kg: 1,200,000 units IM	Every 4 weeks
Penicillin V	250 mg oral	Twice a day
Sulfadiazine	≤27 kg: 0.5 g oral >27 kg: 1 g oral	Once a day
If allergic to above agents		
Erythromycin[96]	250 mg oral	Twice a day

IM, intramuscular.

better to cephalosporins. This is often seen in patients who are GAS carriers and those who may have other bacteria causing infection. Patients are no longer contagious 24 hours after the first antibiotic dose.[95]

P.J. should receive amoxicillin (400 mg/5 mL), 12.5 mL (1,000 mg) every 24 hours for 10 days. For pain relief, he may also receive as-needed doses of acetaminophen (160 mg/5 mL), 10 mL every 6 hours, or ibuprofen (100 mg/5 mL), 10 mL every 6 hours.

Those with a history of rheumatic fever, characterized by acute generalized inflammation of the heart, joints, brain, or skin, should receive long-term antibiotic prophylaxis to prevent further complications from streptococcal infections. Recommended medications and dosing regimens are summarized in Table 104-5.[95,96] Patients with acute carditis and residual heart disease should receive treatment for 10 years or until 40 years of age, whichever is longer.[95] Patients with an episode of carditis but without residual heart disease should receive treatment for 10 years or at least until 21 years of age.[95] Patients who had rheumatic fever without carditis should receive treatment for 5 years or at least until 21 years of age.[95]

KEY REFERENCES AND WEBSITES

A full list of references for this chapter can be found at http://thepoint.lww.com/AT11e. Below are the key references and websites for this chapter, with the corresponding reference number in this chapter found in parentheses after the reference.

Key References

American Academy of Pediatrics Subcommittee on Management of Acute Otitis Media. The diagnosis and management of acute otitis media. *Pediatrics*. 2013;131:e964–e1049. (89)

Gerber MA et al. Prevention of rheumatic fever and diagnosis and treatment of acute streptococcal pharyngitis: a scientific statement from the American Heart Association Rheumatic Fever, Endocarditis, and Kawasaki Disease Committee of the Council on Cardiovascular Disease in the Young, the Interdisciplinary Council on Functional Genomics and Translational Biology, and the Interdisciplinary Council on Quality of Care and Outcomes Research: endorsed by the American Academy of Pediatrics. *Circulation*. 2009;119:1541. (95)

Ishimine P. The evolving approach to the young child who has fever and no obvious source. *Emerg Med Clin North Am*. 2007;25:1087. (10)

Nield LS, Kamat D. Prevention, diagnosis, and management of diaper dermatitis. *Clin Pediatr (Phila)*. 2007;46:480. (7)

Shulman ST et al. Clinical practice guideline for the diagnosis and management of group A Streptococcal pharyngitis: 2012 update by the Infectious Diseases Society of America. *Clin Infect Dis*. 2012;55(10):e86–e102. doi: 10.1093/cid/cis629. (94)

Vandenplas Y et al. Pediatric gastroesophageal reflux clinical practice guidelines: joint recommendations of the North American Society for Pediatric Gastroenterology, Hepatology, and Nutrition (NASPGHAN) and the European Society for Pediatric Gastroenterology, Hepatology, and Nutrition (ESPGHAN). *J Pediatr Gastroenterol Nutr*. 2009;49:498. (58)

Key Websites

Consumer Healthcare Products Association. Voluntary codes and guidelines of the Consumer Healthcare Products Industry. Program on OTC oral pediatric cough and cold medicines. http://www.chpa.org/VolCodesGuidelines.aspx. Accessed June 7, 2015. (26)

OTC sales in volume. Consumer Healthcare Products Association website. http://www.chpa.org/SalesVolume.aspx. Accessed June 11, 2015. (23)

US Food and Drug Administration. Public Health Advisory: FDA Recommends that over-the-counter (OTC) cough and cold products not be used for infants and children under 2 years of age. http://www.fda.gov/drugs/drugsafety/postmarketdrugsafetyinformationforpatientsandproviders/ucm051137.htm. Updated August 19, 2013. Accessed June 7, 2015. (25)

105 Neonatal Therapy

Donna M. Kraus, Jennifer T. Pham, and Kirsten H. Ohler

CORE PRINCIPLES

	CHAPTER CASES
RESPIRATORY DISTRESS SYNDROME	
1 Respiratory distress syndrome (RDS) is a major cause of morbidity and mortality in preterm neonates, resulting from pulmonary surfactant deficiency; it is characterized by atelectasis, hypoxemia, decreased lung compliance, small airway epithelial damage, and pulmonary edema.	**Case 105-1 (Question 1)**
2 Beractant, calfactant, poractant alfa, and lucinactant are exogenous surfactants used in the prevention and treatment of RDS in preterm neonates. These agents have been shown to improve oxygenation and lung compliance and decrease the need for supplemental oxygen and mechanical ventilation.	**Case 105-1 (Questions 2–6)**
BRONCHOPULMONARY DYSPLASIA	
1 Bronchopulmonary dysplasia (BPD) is the most common form of chronic pulmonary disease in infants; it is caused by lung immaturity, surfactant deficiency, oxygen toxicity, barotrauma, and inflammation, and is characterized by tachypnea, retractions, and wheezing.	**Case 105-2 (Question 1)**
2 The management of BPD includes supplemental oxygen therapy, mechanical ventilation, and pharmacologic interventions including diuretics, bronchodilators, and corticosteroids.	**Case 105-2 (Questions 2, 3)**
3 Infants with BPD are at higher risk for experiencing cardiorespiratory problems including pneumonia, pulmonary hypertension, left ventricular hypertrophy, and neurologic and developmental abnormalities.	**Case 105-2 (Questions 4, 5)**
PATENT DUCTUS ARTERIOSUS	
1 Preterm neonates are at high risk for patent ductus arteriosus (PDA), a serious cardiovascular disorder, which may present with tachycardia, wide pulse pressure, bounding pulses, and systolic murmur. Complications of PDA include pulmonary edema and heart failure. PDA places the neonate at high risk for BPD, intraventricular hemorrhage, and necrotizing enterocolitis.	**Case 105-3 (Questions 1–3)**
2 Medical management of PDA includes fluid management, correction of anemia, treatment of hypoxia and acidosis, and pharmacologic therapy with prostaglandin inhibitors (indomethacin or ibuprofen) to close the ductus.	**Case 105-3 (Questions 4–10)**
NECROTIZING ENTEROCOLITIS	
1 Necrotizing enterocolitis (NEC) is the most common life-threatening nonrespiratory condition in newborns and is characterized by abdominal distension, bloody stools, metabolic acidosis, and bowel perforation.	**Case 105-4 (Question 1)**
2 The management of NEC includes parenteral nutrition, intravenous antibiotics, and bowel resection. Interventions including trophic feedings, breast milk, probiotics, and a strict feeding protocol may be used to decrease the incidence of NEC.	**Case 105-4 (Questions 2–6)**

Continued

CHAPTER CASES

NEONATAL SEPSIS AND MENINGITIS	
1 Bacterial sepsis can be classified as early-onset (caused by pathogens colonized from the maternal genital tract) or late-onset sepsis (caused by nosocomial pathogens). Clinical signs can be subtle and nonspecific especially in preterm neonates.	**Case 105-5 (Question 1)**
2 Selection of empiric intravenous antibiotics is the same for sepsis and meningitis and will depend on nosocomial pathogens commonly isolated in the neonatal intensive care unit, antibiotic resistance patterns, and underlying neonatal risk factors.	**Case 105-5 (Question 2)**
CONGENITAL INFECTIONS	
1 Congenital infections including herpes simplex virus, syphilis, and cytomegalovirus may result in fetal death, congenital anomalies, serious central nervous system sequelae, intrauterine growth retardation, or preterm birth; if suspected, appropriate diagnostic tests and treatment should be started immediately.	**Case 105-6 (Question 1)**
APNEA OF PREMATURITY	
1 Pharmacologic treatment of apnea of prematurity includes the use of methylxanthines, specifically caffeine and theophylline, which decrease apneic episodes via both central and peripheral effects.	**Case 105-7 (Question 1)**
2 Caffeine offers several advantages over theophylline for the treatment of apnea including a wider therapeutic index, fewer adverse effects, prolonged half-life, once-daily dosing, and lack of the need for routine serum drug concentration monitoring.	**Case 105-7 (Questions 2, 3)**
NEONATAL SEIZURES	
1 Neonatal seizure activity is a common manifestation of a life-threatening underlying neurologic process. Initial therapy is focused on the treatment of the underlying cause (e.g., hypoglycemia, hypocalcemia, infection) and may not include antiepileptic drug therapy.	**Case 105-8 (Questions 1–3)**
2 Common antiepileptic medications used to treat neonatal seizure activity are phenobarbital, phenytoin, and lorazepam.	**Case 105-8 (Questions 4, 5)**

NEONATAL THERAPY

The rational use of medications in neonates depends on an appreciation of both the physiologic immaturity and the developmental maturation that influence neonatal drug disposition and pharmacologic effects. Much progress has been made to decrease neonatal mortality and improve survival of more premature and lower-birth-weight newborns. Neonates, particularly those of extremely low birth weights (ELBW), pose a pharmacotherapeutic challenge to the clinician. The alterations of body composition, weight, and size, as well as physiologic and pharmacokinetic parameters, which occur with normal growth and maturation during the first few months of life, are greater than at any other time. Although the amount of neonatal drug information is increasing, the overall lack of well-designed pharmacokinetic and pharmacodynamic studies still hinders the clinical use of many drugs in this population. This is especially true for newborns of the lowest birth weights ($<$750 g). An understanding of common neonatal terminology (Table 105-1) is important because every newborn is evaluated and classified at birth according to birth weight, gestational age, and intrauterine growth status.[1] Pharmacokinetic parameters, pharmacodynamics, and dosing recommendations often are specified according to these terms.[2] Important neonatal pharmacokinetic differences are reviewed in Chapter 102, Pediatric Pharmacotherapy. This chapter focuses on the safe and effective use of medications for common neonatal medical conditions.

RESPIRATORY DISTRESS SYNDROME

Respiratory distress syndrome (RDS) is a major cause of morbidity and mortality in preterm neonates.[3] This clinical syndrome is characterized by respiratory failure with atelectasis, hypoxemia, decreased lung compliance, small airway epithelial damage, and pulmonary edema. The principal cause of RDS is pulmonary surfactant deficiency. Pulmonary surfactant decreases the surface tension at the air–fluid interface in the alveoli and prevents alveolar collapse. Surfactant also facilitates the clearance of pulmonary fluid, prevents pulmonary edema, and stabilizes alveoli during aeration. At birth, the clearance of residual fetal lung fluid is accompanied by an increase in pulmonary blood flow, which facilitates the transition from fetal to adult circulation.[4]

Table 105-1
Common Neonatal Terminology[1,2]

Term	Definition
Gestational age (GA)	*By dates:* The number of weeks from the onset of the mother's last menstrual period until birth
	By examination: Assessment of gestational maturity by physical and neuromuscular examination; gestational age estimates the time from conception until birth
Postnatal age (PNA)	Chronologic age after birth
Postmenstrual age (PMA)	Gestational age plus postnatal age. Postmenstrual age (rather than postconceptional age) is the preferred term for use in clinical practice. Postmenstrual age is considered to be a more accurate term because gestational age is calculated using the mother's last menstrual period, and the exact date of conception is generally not known.
Postconceptional age (PCA)	Age since conception. This term is not recommended for use in clinical practice and is currently reserved for cases when the exact date of conception is known (i.e., assisted reproductive technology). Older literature may use this term to describe the sum of gestational age plus postnatal age; thus, it is important to know how this term is defined when used.
Corrected age	Postmenstrual age in weeks minus 40; represents postnatal age if neonate had been born at term (40 weeks' gestational age)
Neonate	A full-term newborn 0 to 28 days postnatal age. Some may also apply this term to a preterm neonate who is > 28 days postnatal age, but with a postmenstrual age ≤ 42 to 46 weeks
Preterm	<37 weeks' gestational age at birth
Term	37 weeks' 0 days to 41 weeks' 6 days (average ~ 40 weeks') gestational age at birth
Post-term	≥42 weeks' gestational age at birth
Extremely low birth weight (ELBW)	Birth weight <1 kg
Very low birth weight (VLBW)	Birth weight <1.5 kg
Low birth weight (LBW)	Birth weight <2.5 kg
Small for gestational age (SGA)	Birth weight <10th percentile for gestational age
Appropriate for gestational age (AGA)	Birth weight between 10th and 90th percentiles for gestational age
Large for gestational age (LGA)	Birth weight >90th percentile for gestational age

In the fetus, endogenous cortisol stimulates the synthesis and secretion of pulmonary surfactant at 30 to 32 weeks' gestational age.[4] However, sufficient amounts of pulmonary surfactant for normal lung function are not present before 34 to 36 weeks' gestation.[4,5] Therefore, the incidence and severity of RDS increase as gestational age decreases. RDS occurs in approximately 25% of neonates born at 30 to 31 weeks' gestation, but may occur in as high as 95% to 98% of neonates born at 22 to 24 weeks' gestation.[3]

Without adequate amounts of surfactant, the surface tension within the alveoli is so great that the alveoli collapse (atelectasis), resulting in poor gas exchange (e.g., hypoxemia, hypercapnia). Low lung compliance also results, and large inspiratory pressures are needed to aerate the lungs. Unfortunately, the extremely compliant neonatal chest wall makes it difficult to create the large negative inspiratory pressures necessary to open the alveoli. This results in an increased work of breathing and alterations of ventilation and perfusion.[3,4]

Aeration of the surfactant-deficient lung also results in the cyclic collapse and distension of bronchioles, with resultant bronchiolar epithelial injury and necrosis. This epithelial damage causes pulmonary edema by allowing fluid and proteins to leak from the intravascular space into the airspaces and interstitium of the lung. The necrotic epithelial debris and proteins then form fibrous hyaline membranes.[3] Hyaline membranes and pulmonary edema further impair gas exchange.

The inadequate oxygenation and ventilation and increased work of breathing caused by RDS may result in the need for assisted positive-pressure ventilation. Complications of RDS may be related to mechanical ventilation and include pulmonary barotrauma (e.g., pneumothorax, pulmonary interstitial emphysema [PIE]), intraventricular hemorrhage (IVH), patent ductus arteriosus (PDA), retinopathy of prematurity (ROP), and chronic lung disease or bronchopulmonary dysplasia (BPD).[3]

Clinical Presentation

CASE 105-1

QUESTION 1: L.D., a 680-g male, was born at 25 weeks' gestational age via cesarean section as a result of placenta abruption to a 38-year-old gravida 6 para 5 woman with gestational diabetes. Apgar scores were 3 at 1 minute, 5 at 5 minutes, and 8 at 10 minutes. Thirty minutes after birth, L.D. appears cyanotic and has retracting respirations with grunting and nasal flaring. His heart rate (HR) is 160 beats/minute, and respiratory rate (RR) is 65 breaths/minute. An arterial blood gas (ABG) on 60% oxygen by nasal intermittent positive-pressure ventilation (NIPPV) is as follows:

pH, 7.25
PCO_2, 41 mm Hg
PO_2, 71 mm Hg
Base deficit, 8

Based on the blood gas results, L.D. is intubated immediately and placed on positive-pressure-assisted ventilation. An umbilical arterial catheter is inserted for frequent ABG monitoring, and an umbilical vein catheter is inserted for central venous access. L.D.'s chest radiographic shows RDS (see **http://www.adhb.govt.nz/newborn/teachingresources/radiology/CXR/RDS/RDS.jpg** for a radiograph of an infant with RDS). Ampicillin 100 mg/kg every 12 hours and gentamicin 5 mg/kg every 48 hours are ordered intravenously (IV) to rule out sepsis. What is an Apgar score? What risk factors does L.D. have for RDS? What signs and laboratory data are consistent with RDS?

An Apgar score is a method of evaluating the physical condition of a newborn infant immediately after birth. It consists of five clinical signs including HR, respiratory effort, muscle tone, skin color, and reflex irritability. Each sign can receive a score of 0 to 2 points with a total possible score of 10 points. A score of 7 to 10 is considered normal, whereas scores of 0 to 3 require immediate resuscitation. The Apgar score is routinely done at 1 and 5 minutes of life and is repeated every 5 minutes until a total score of at least 7 is achieved. (For a video of how to assign an Apgar score to newborns, go to http://online.wsj.com/video/assigning-an-apgar-score-to-newborns/9B7B09A9-1B12-4C65-92BA-D4C6DFA35BBA.html?mod=googlewsj.) L.D.'s Apgar scores of 3 and 5 at 1 and 5 minutes indicate that he may have experienced some perinatal asphyxia, most likely secondary to maternal placenta abruption. L.D.'s risk factors for RDS are prematurity, male sex, perinatal asphyxia, cesarean section, and maternal gestational diabetes. Other risk factors include second-born twins and maternal-fetal hemorrhage.[3] Clinical signs and laboratory data consistent with RDS in L.D. include tachypnea, cyanosis, retracting respirations, grunting, nasal flaring, hypoxemia, hypercapnia, and a mixed respiratory and metabolic acidosis.[3] Clinical manifestations classically present within the first 6 hours of life.

Tachypnea, the first sign of respiratory distress, is an attempt to compensate for the inadequate ventilation, hypercapnia, and acidosis. L.D.'s retracting respirations (the use of intercostal, subcostal, suprasternal, or sternal accessory muscles) reflect the increased work of breathing necessary to maintain ventilation. His nasal flaring decreases resistance during inspiration and increases oxygenation. Grunting is the result of forceful exhalation against a partially closed glottis in an effort to prolong expiration and maximize oxygenation. Grunting also increases intrathoracic pressure during expiration in an attempt to stabilize the alveoli and prevent atelectasis. L.D.'s cyanosis, hypoxemia, hypercapnia, and mixed respiratory and metabolic acidosis are consequences of inadequate oxygenation and poor ventilation and are consistent with RDS.[3]

Treatment

CASE 105-1, QUESTION 2: What treatments should be initiated for L.D.'s respiratory insufficiency?

Before L.D. is treated for RDS, other causes of respiratory distress must be ruled out. For example, infections (particularly group B streptococcal sepsis or pneumonia) often present with respiratory distress. Because it is difficult to distinguish between RDS and infection, all neonates with severe RDS should receive antibiotics. L.D. was started empirically on antibiotics, and a complete evaluation of possible sepsis should be performed.

Neonates should be treated for RDS as soon as possible and may require ventilatory support. Noninvasive ventilator support such as NIPPV or nasal continuous positive airway pressure (CPAP) has been shown to reduce barotrauma, volutrauma, and airway damage compared to intubation with mechanical ventilation.[3] However, some extremely preterm neonates may require intubation with mechanical ventilation due to persistent symptoms of RDS. Because L.D. failed NIPPV and required intubation, exogenous surfactant should be administered intratracheally as soon as possible. Human surfactant is synthesized and secreted by type II alveolar epithelial cells of the lung. It contains 80% phospholipids, 8% neutral lipids, and 12% proteins.[5] The major surface-active component is dipalmitoylphosphatidylcholine (DPPC), also known as colfosceril or lecithin. However, this phospholipid slowly adsorbs to the air–fluid interface in the alveoli. Other phospholipids (e.g., phosphatidylcholine, phosphatidylglycerol) and four surfactant apoproteins (SP-A, SP-B, SP-C, and SP-D) enhance spreadability and surface adsorption.[5] Adsorption and surface spreading of the surfactant in the alveoli are important determinants of surface tension activity. SP-A and SP-D both play a role in immune regulation and providing host defense. SP-A may also help to regulate alveolar surfactant reuptake and metabolism.[5] SP-B and SP-C are the two most important apoproteins responsible for promoting adsorption and surface spreading of the surfactant in the alveoli to form a phospholipid monolayer.[5] SP-B is thought to be the most critical protein for surfactant activity.

Natural surfactants are derived from bovine or porcine lung lipid or lavage extracts. Modified natural surfactants are lung lipid extracts supplemented with phospholipids or other components.[3] Currently, four surfactant products are commercially available for clinical use in the United States (US): beractant (Survanta), calfactant (Infasurf), poractant alfa (Curosurf), and lucinactant (Surfaxin). Beractant, calfactant, and lucinactant are US Food and Drug Administration (FDA)-approved for the prevention (i.e., prophylaxis) of RDS, whereas beractant, calfactant, and poractant alfa are approved for treatment (i.e., rescue therapy). Animal-derived products contain variable amounts of SP-B and SP-C, lipids, and phospholipids. Lucinactant, a new synthetic surfactant, contains not only phospholipids but also high concentrations of sinapultide (KL4), a synthetic peptide that mimics human SP-B. (see Table 105-2 for comparisons).[6–9]

CASE 105-1, QUESTION 3: What are the effects of exogenously administered surfactant that can be expected in L.D.?

Oxygenation and lung compliance rapidly and markedly improve after the administration of surfactant. It should be expected that supplemental oxygen and mechanical ventilation may need to be significantly reduced. The increased lung compliance and decreased need for high inspiratory pressures result in a dramatic decrease in the incidence of pneumothorax and PIE. Survival in treated infants increases by approximately 40% regardless of birth weight or gestational age, and neonatal mortality from RDS is decreased to approximately 20%.[10] Other complications of RDS such as severe BPD, IVH, NEC, ROP, and PDA have not been decreased consistently with surfactant therapy.[11]

CASE 105-1, QUESTION 4: Which surfactant is appropriate and when should it be administered to L.D.?

PRODUCT SELECTION

Trials comparing natural surfactant products (poractant alfa vs. beractant, calfactant vs. beractant, poractant alfa vs. calfactant) have demonstrated that poractant alfa and calfactant result in a significantly faster weaning of supplemental oxygen and mean airway pressure compared to beractant. Furthermore, a lower mortality rate at 36 weeks' PMA was seen with a higher initial dose of poractant alfa 200 mg/kg. No differences were seen with the duration of mechanical ventilation and supplemental oxygen, the incidence of BPD, and other secondary outcomes.[12,13] To date, there is only one trial comparing the three natural surfactant products for the treatment of RDS. Overall, there were no significant differences in the incidence of pneumothorax, PIE, death, and the combined variable of BPD or death among the three surfactant products.[14]

Trials comparing synthetic (lucinactant) to a natural surfactant product (beractant or poractant alfa) found no difference in the incidence of RDS at 24 hours; however, one study reported a significantly higher incidence of RDS-related death by 14 days of life and NEC in the beractant group.[15] In addition, no significant differences were found with mortality, BPD, IVH, PDA, and ROP between synthetic and natural surfactants.[15,16]

Studies assessing the long-term neurodevelopmental outcomes (at 1 year and at 18 to 24 months of corrected age) of infants

Table 105-2
Comparison of Currently Marketed Surfactant Products[6–9]

Variable	Calfactant (Infasurf)	Poractant Alpha (Curosurf)	Beractant (Survanta)	Lucinactant (Surfaxin)
Type and source	Natural surfactant, calf lung wash	Natural surfactant, porcine lung mince extract	Modified natural surfactant, bovine lung mince extract	Synthetic surfactant, protein analog
Phospholipids (PL)	Natural DPPC with mixed PL	Natural DPPC with mixed PL	Natural and supplemented DPPC with mixed PL	Synthetic DPPC with mixed PL
Proteins	SP-B and SP-C	SP-B and SP-C	SP-B and SP-C	Sinapultide (KL4 peptide)
Indications	Prophylaxis and rescue therapy	Rescue therapy	Prophylaxis and rescue therapy	Prophylaxis therapy
Criteria for prophylaxis	Premature neonates <29 weeks' GA at high risk for RDS	Not approved	Birth weight <1,250 g or evidence of surfactant deficiency	Premature neonates at high risk for RDS
Recommended dose	3 mL/kg (PL 105 mg/kg)	*Initial dose:* 2.5 mL/kg (PL 200 mg/kg); *Repeat dose:* 1.25 mL/kg (PL 100 mg/kg)	4 mL/kg (PL 100 mg/kg)	5.8 mL/kg (PL 175 mg/kg)
Recommended regimen for prophylaxis	Give first dose ASAP after birth, preferably within 30 minutes; repeat every 12 hours up to a total of three doses if infant remains intubated	Not approved	Give first dose ASAP after birth, preferably within 15 minutes; repeat as early as 6 hours up to a total of four doses if infant remains intubated and requires $FiO_2 \geq 0.3$ with $PaO_2 \leq 80$ mm Hg	Give first dose ASAP after birth; repeat as early as 6 hours up to a total of four doses in first 48 hours of life
Criterion for rescue therapy	Infants ≤72 hours of age with confirmed RDS who require endotracheal intubation	Infants with confirmed RDS who require endotracheal intubation	Infants with confirmed RDS who require endotracheal intubation	Not approved
Recommended regimen for rescue therapy	Give first dose ASAP after RDS diagnosed; repeat every 12 hours up to a total of three doses if infant still remains intubated	Give first dose ASAP after RDS diagnosed; repeat every 12 hours up to a total of three doses if infant remains intubated	Give first dose ASAP after RDS diagnosed, preferably by 8 hours postnatal age; repeat as early as 6 hours up to a total of four doses if infant remains intubated and requires FiO_2 ≥ 0.3 with $PaO_2 \leq 80$ mm Hg	Not approved
Recommended administration technique	Administer through side port of ETT adapter via ventilator *or* through disconnected ETT via 5F catheter, divide dose into two aliquots with position change	Administer through disconnected ETT via 5F catheter, divide dose into two aliquots with position change	Administer through disconnected ETT via 5F catheter, divide dose into four aliquots with position change	Administer through side port of ETT adapter via ventilator, divide dose into four aliquots with position change
Special instructions	Gentle swirling of the vial may be necessary for redispersion; warming to room temperature is not necessary; do not shake	Warm to room temperature before use; do not shake	Warm to room temperature before use; do not shake	Warm for 15 minutes in a preheated dry block heater set at 44°C (111°F); after warming, shake vial vigorously until suspension is uniform and free-flowing. The temperature of product has to be ≤ 37°C (99°F) before administration
Stability	If warmed to room temperature for <24 hours, unopened, unused vials may be returned once to refrigerator; single-use vial contains no preservative, discard unused portion	If warmed to room temperature for <24 hours, unopened, unused vials may be returned only once to refrigerator; single-use vial contains no preservative, discard unused portion	If warmed to room temperature for <24 hours, unopened, unused vials may be returned only once to refrigerator; single-use vial contains no preservative, discard unused portion	If not used immediately after warming, can be stored protected from light at room temperature for up to 2 hours. Do not return to refrigerator after warming; discard if not used within 2 hours of warming or any unused portion
Cost per vial	\$455.00 (3 mL), \$805.33 (6 mL)[a]	\$445.15 (1.5 mL), \$877.78 (3 mL)[a]	\$459.60 (4 mL), \$813.46 (8 mL)[a]	\$1032.00 (8.5 mL)[a]

[a]Average wholesale price according to *2015 Red Book*.

ASAP, as soon as possible; DPPC, dipalmitoylphosphatidylcholine; ETT, endotracheal tube; F, French; FiO_2, fractional inspired oxygen; PaO_2, partial pressure of oxygen; PL, phospholipids; RDS, respiratory distress syndrome.

receiving surfactants (beractant vs. poractant alfa and lucinactant vs. beractant or poractant alfa) for RDS found no significant difference between products.[17,18]

Cost-effectiveness studies of different natural surfactant products for the treatment of RDS reported significant cost savings associated with poractant alfa (due to fewer required additional doses) compared with beractant.[12,13] A recent pharmacoeconomic analysis of costs associated with reintubation in preterm infants treated with either lucinactant, beractant, or poractant alfa utilized data from two multicenter trials. Reintubation rates were significantly lower in the lucinactant-treated group.[19] However, it is important to note that one of the studies compared lucinactant to colfosceril palmitate, a product no longer available in the US. Furthermore, the second trial was terminated before achieving enrollment goal. Therefore, these limitations may have affected respiratory outcomes and healthcare costs associated with reintubation and mechanical ventilation.

Based on these comparative trials, it appears there are no significant differences in the short-term (e.g., air leaks, duration of mechanical ventilation/oxygenation) and long-term outcomes (e.g., death, BPD, and other secondary outcomes) between the four surfactant products. Poractant alfa, given at a dose of 200 mg/kg, may be the favorable surfactant therapy because it resulted in a faster weaning of oxygen and mean airway pressure, a decrease in mortality at 36 weeks' PMA, and a lower cost.

TIME AND METHOD OF ADMINISTRATION

Surfactant therapy can be administered as prophylactic (i.e., within 10–30 minutes after birth) or rescue treatment (given to those with established RDS within 12 hours of life). *Early* rescue is defined as the administration of surfactant within the first 2 hours of life; *late* rescue is defined as treatment after more than 2 hours of life. Theoretically, the first dose of surfactant should be given before the newborn's first breath or before positive-pressure ventilation.[10] This would avoid the early lung injury in RDS that can interfere with surfactant distribution, bioavailability, and effectiveness. This strategy, however, increases the cost of care because newborns that might never experience RDS would be intubated and treated unnecessarily. In addition, delivery room treatment may interfere with resuscitation and stabilization of the neonate.[10]

Prophylactic surfactant therapy has been shown to decrease the incidence and severity of RDS, mortality, pneumothorax, and PIE, compared with rescue treatment.[11] However, these findings were reported in studies that were conducted prior to routine clinical use of CPAP for the management of RDS. In studies that utilized routine CPAP as initial management of RDS, a significantly lower incidence of BPD or death was seen in the CPAP group when compared with prophylactic surfactant therapy without CPAP.[11] In contrast, when comparing *early* versus *late* rescue therapy (regardless of routine initial use of CPAP), infants treated in the *early* group had significant decreases in the incidence of mortality, air leak, BPD, and the combined variable of BPD or death.[11] Thus, CPAP should be utilized initially, with selective early rescue surfactant administration in infants in whom symptoms of RDS persist.

Surfactant should be administered by qualified physicians with the presence of nursing and respiratory therapy personnel.[14] (For a video on surfactant administration, go to **http://www.youtube.com/watch?v=hkUdH01sLmA&feature=related**.) Surfactants can be administered through a disconnected endotracheal tube (ETT) via 5F catheter or through a side port of ETT adapter via ventilator, depending on the product (see Table 105-2). Both administrative techniques are effective and are not significantly different with regard to clinical outcomes.[11] Several alternative methods of surfactant administration have been utilized in an effort to avoid mechanical ventilation. The "INSURE" (INtubate–SURfactant–Extubate) technique is a strategy that administers surfactant during a brief intubation followed by immediate extubation to nasal CPAP. This technique was associated with a reduced need for mechanical ventilation and subsequent BPD.[11]

Because surfactant works better if given earlier in the course of RDS, it is important to determine who is at highest risk for RDS. Unfortunately, the exact criteria to clinically determine high-risk newborns are still unclear. Surfactant treatment should be administered as soon as clinical signs of RDS appear. The administration of CPAP after birth with subsequent selective surfactant therapy should be the preferred alternative to prophylactic surfactant therapy. Early therapy avoids progression of the disease and the potential for decreased surfactant effectiveness; therefore, it should be considered in preterm infants born at <30 weeks' gestation who need mechanical ventilation because of severe RDS. Because L.D. has clinical, laboratory, and radiographic findings consistent with RDS, a dose of 2.5 mL/kg (200 mg/kg phospholipid) of poractant alfa should be administered to L.D. intratracheally immediately within 1 hour of age with subsequent extubation to CPAP as soon as possible.

CASE 105-1, QUESTION 5: Within 1 hour of poractant alfa administration, L.D.'s oxygenation improved, and the FIO_2 was weaned from 60% to 40%. Ten hours later, the ABGs revealed the following:

pH, 7.30
PCO_2, 45 mm Hg
PO_2, 50 mm Hg
Base deficit, 2
O_2 saturation, 90% on the following ventilator settings: FIO_2, 0.40; intermittent mechanical ventilation (IMV), 30; PIP, 18; positive end-expiratory pressure (PEEP), +5

Should another dose of poractant alfa be administered?

The response to a single dose of surfactant usually is transient; thus, more than one dose may be needed. Response to surfactant therapy can be variable, especially in preterm newborns or in those who require high oxygen and ventilatory pressures.[3] Reasons for lack of response include surfactant inhibition by proteins that have leaked into the alveolar spaces, inactivation of surfactant by inflammatory mediators (free oxygen radicals, proteases), presence of conditions that can decrease surfactant effectiveness (e.g., pulmonary edema), or poor delivery of surfactant to the alveoli (owing to atelectasis).[3] The degree of responsiveness to surfactant also decreases with increasing postnatal age.[10]

Although the indications for subsequent doses of surfactant vary, persistence of respiratory failure is the major clinical indicator for retreatment. In practice, most infants require only one dose of surfactant. This may be related to advances in neonatal and perinatal management and an increased use of antenatal steroids. However, there are neonates who may be more likely to require more than one dose; these include those who were not exposed to antenatal steroids and/or those with extreme prematurity (<26 weeks' gestation). A second dose of poractant alfa should be given to L.D. because he still requires mechanical ventilation with relatively high inspiratory pressures and supplemental oxygen ($FIO_2 \geq 0.3$) to maintain an arterial PO_2 of at least 50 mm Hg and oxygen saturation of 90%.

CASE 105-1, QUESTION 6: On rounds, the medical resident asks you about the complications of surfactant treatment in premature infants. Describe the information on adverse effects and their frequency that you would provide for the medical team.

The most common adverse effects of surfactant therapy are related to the method of administration.[11] During administration, L.D. may experience bradycardia and oxygen desaturation secondary to vagal stimulation and airway obstruction.[6–9] These adverse events might require temporary discontinuation of surfactant administration and increased ventilator support.

The risk of pulmonary hemorrhage, which usually occurs within the first 72 hours of life, can be found in up to 6% of neonates receiving surfactant therapy.[3] However, pulmonary hemorrhage has not been consistently reported in recent studies; thus, the association between surfactant therapy and this disorder is questionable.[3] Furthermore, the benefits of surfactant therapy far outweigh the potential risk of pulmonary hemorrhage.

BRONCHOPULMONARY DYSPLASIA

CASE 105-2

QUESTION 1: J.T. is a 12-week-old, 2-kg female who was born at 25 weeks' gestation. Her medical history includes RDS, episodes of sepsis and pneumonia, and 5 weeks of parenteral nutrition. J.T. has also failed extubation numerous times and is currently requiring mechanical ventilation with an FiO_2 of 0.5. Current vital signs are as follows:

RR, 60 breaths/minute
HR, 150 beats/minute
BP, 80/55 mm Hg
O_2 saturation, 90%

On physical examination, J.T. has intercostal and subcostal retractions, shallow breathing, and an expiratory wheeze. Bilateral diffuse haziness with lung hyperinflation, focal emphysema, atelectasis, and irregular fibrous streaks are seen on chest radiograph. J.T. is currently receiving enteral feedings with a preterm 20-cal/ounce formula at 40 mL every 3 hours. Based on these findings, the diagnosis of BPD is made. What is the pathogenesis of BPD? What risk factors for BPD does J.T. have? What clinical signs and laboratory evidence of BPD are apparent in J.T.?

BPD (also known as chronic lung disease) is the most common form of chronic pulmonary disease in infants. The disease develops in newborns that require supplemental oxygen and positive-pressure ventilation for RDS or other primary lung disorders. A severity-based definition of BPD has been developed by the National Institute of Child Health and Human Development.[21] For infants born at less than 32 weeks' gestational age, assessment of BPD is performed at 36 weeks' PMA or at the time of discharge. Mild BPD is defined as a need for supplemental O_2 in excess of 21% for at least 28 days but not at 36 weeks' PMA or discharge; moderate BPD as a need for supplemental O_2 for at least 28 days plus treatment with less than 30% O_2 at 36 weeks' PMA or discharge; and severe BPD as a need for supplemental O_2 for at least 28 days plus treatment with at least 30% O_2 or positive-pressure ventilation at 36 weeks' PMA or discharge. For infants born at 32 weeks' gestational age or older, the above definitions are different only in that assessments are conducted at 56 days of life rather than 36 weeks' PMA.[21] BPD is a significant cause of infant morbidity and mortality. BPD affects 10,000 to 15,000 infants in the United States each year.[21] The incidence and severity of BPD are inversely related to gestational age and birth weight. Infants born at 23 weeks' gestation have a 73% incidence of BPD compared with a 23% incidence in infants born at 28 weeks' gestation.[21] Similarly, 56% of infants born at 23 weeks' gestation develop severe disease compared with 8% in infants born at 28 weeks' gestation.[21] Overall, from 1993 to 2006, the incidence of BPD has decreased; however, length of hospital stay has increased significantly. This may be due to a change in the definition of BPD and/or an increase in the use of CPAP.[22]

Pathogenesis and Clinical Manifestations

The cause of BPD seems to be multifactorial. Lung immaturity, surfactant deficiency, oxygen toxicity, barotrauma or volutrauma, and inflammation all play important roles. Premature infants, especially those at less than 26 weeks' gestation, are at a higher risk for BPD owing to lung immaturity.[21] Surfactant deficiency and the immature parenchymal structure of the lung and chest wall contribute to the development of BPD. Oxygen therapy, which causes a release of free oxygen radicals, is directly associated with the pathogenesis of BPD. Prolonged exposure to high oxygen concentrations and free oxygen radicals causes tissue damage, alveolar–capillary leaks, and atelectasis with resultant impaired gas exchange and pulmonary edema.[21,23,24] This may lead to the chronic pulmonary fibrotic changes seen in infants with BPD. In term infants, the lungs contain antioxidant enzymes that help to protect the lung from damage produced by free oxygen radicals. However, in preterm infants, the concentration of antioxidant enzymes may be low or absent. Therefore, premature infants are more susceptible to develop BPD than term infants.

Barotrauma secondary to positive-pressure ventilation is also a major factor in the pathogenesis of BPD, independent of oxygen toxicity.[21,23] Barotrauma is caused by repetitive distension of the terminal airways during mechanical ventilation. This results in disruption of the epithelium and an increase in capillary permeability to proteinaceous fluid. The severity of lung injury is related to the amount of positive peak pressure used. Volutrauma is also involved in the pathogenesis of BPD and is caused by high tidal volume ventilation and overdistension. The combined iatrogenic insults of oxygen toxicity and barotrauma or volutrauma, both inflicted on an immature lung for an extended time, can worsen lung damage.

The inflammatory process in the lung is activated by oxygen toxicity, barotrauma or volutrauma, or other injury. This results in the attraction and activation of leukocytes (e.g., neutrophils, macrophages), which may cause further release of inflammatory mediators, elastase, and collagenase.[24] Elevated levels of elastase and collagenase can destroy the elastin and collagen framework of the lung. α_1-Proteinase inhibitor, a major defense against elastase activity, may be inactivated by free oxygen radicals. Therefore, the combined elevated levels of elastase and the decreased activity of α_1-proteinase inhibitor may enhance lung injury and lead to the development of BPD.

Infants who exhibit BPD also have elevated levels of cytokines such as platelet-activating factor, leukotrienes, tumor necrosis factor, and fibronectin.[24] These agents, combined with the activated leukocytes, cause significant lung damage with breakdown of capillary endothelial integrity and capillary leakage. Furthermore, the increased fibronectin levels found in tracheal aspirate samples of infants with early BPD may predispose them to exhibit pulmonary fibrosis.[24]

Infection and nutrient deficiency may also play a role in the pathogenesis of BPD. The presence of chorioamnionitis may increase the infants' risk for BPD, although recent studies failed to report similar findings. Pathogens such as *Ureaplasma, Chlamydia,* or cytomegalovirus may cause chronic infection and contribute to the development of BPD.[21,23,24] A recent meta-analysis has shown direct correlations between *Ureaplasma* colonization and the presence of BPD, regardless of gestational age.[25] Deficiencies in nutrients such as vitamin A (retinol) or trace elements such as zinc, copper, and selenium (which are integral components of the antioxidant enzyme structure) may also play a role in the pathogenesis of BPD.

J.T. has two of the most important risk factors for BPD, low birth weight, and decreased gestational age. She is also at risk for

BPD owing to mechanical ventilation, oxygen toxicity, and fluid excess (160 mL/kg/day). Other risk factors include male sex, white ethnicity, and persistent PDA.[21,24]

BPD is characterized by tachypnea with shallow breathing, intercostal and subcostal retractions, and expiratory wheezing as demonstrated in J.T. Other signs and symptoms include rales, rhonchi, cough, airflow obstruction, airway hyper-reactivity, increased mucus production, hypoxemia, and hypercarbia.[24] J.T.'s chest radiograph shows evidence of BPD, including focal emphysema, atelectasis, bilateral diffuse haziness (interstitial thickening) with increased expansion of the lungs, and irregular fibrous streaks. Mucous plugging, sepsis, and pneumonia can also develop in BPD infants on chronic mechanical ventilation. Infants with severe BPD eventually experience cardiovascular complications such as pulmonary hypertension, cor pulmonale, systemic hypertension, and left ventricular hypertrophy. In addition to chronic respiratory and cardiovascular complications, infants with BPD have significant growth, nutritional, and neurodevelopmental problems.[21,24]

Management

CASE 105-2, QUESTION 2: What nonpharmacologic and therapeutic agents should be used to manage BPD in J.T.?

The medical management of infants with BPD includes supplemental oxygen therapy, mechanical ventilation, fluid restriction, nutritional management, and various pharmacologic interventions. Supplemental oxygen administered via mechanical ventilation, CPAP, or nasal cannula should be provided to maintain an oxygen saturation of 90% to 95% and prevent hypoxemia.[23,24] Fluids should be restricted to 120–130 mL/kg/day to prevent congestive heart disease and pulmonary edema. Because infants with BPD have a 25% increase in caloric expenditure, hypercaloric formulas (e.g., 24 or 27 cal/ounce) may be used to optimize calories while restricting fluid intake.[23,26] If this increased energy is not provided, infants are at risk for undergoing a catabolic state that places them at higher risk of experiencing more severe BPD (inadequate nutrition may potentiate the toxic effects of oxygen toxicity and barotrauma). The goal of nutritional therapy is to produce weight gains of 10 to 30 g/day, which can usually be accomplished by providing 140 to 160 kcal/kg/day.[26] If infants do not tolerate enteral feedings, parenteral nutrition should be substituted until the gastrointestinal (GI) tract becomes more functional. Because J.T. is on a 20-cal/ounce formula, switching her to a hypercaloric formula would help to optimize her weight gain. Her fluids should be restricted to 120–130 mL/kg/day.

PHARMACOLOGIC THERAPY

The treatment of BPD consists of multiple-drug therapy, which includes diuretics, bronchodilators, and corticosteroids.[2,27–32] Despite the advancement of drug therapy, none of these drugs have been shown to reverse pulmonary damage in infants with BPD. Instead, they are used primarily to reduce clinical symptoms and to improve lung function.

Diuretics

Infants with BPD are particularly prone to pulmonary edema from cardiogenic and noncardiogenic factors. Left ventricular failure may worsen the already existing right ventricular failure. Pulmonary vascular permeability is increased because of the disruption of the alveolar–capillary unit and causes an increased amount of fluid in the interstitium. Although the precise mechanism in the treatment of BPD is unknown, diuretics help to reduce interstitial lung water.[24,27] In addition, diuretics lower pulmonary vascular resistance and improve gas exchange, thereby reducing oxygen requirements. The most commonly used diuretics are furosemide, thiazides, and spironolactone. Furosemide is the drug of choice because of its potent diuretic effect. In addition, it increases lymphatic flow and plasma oncotic pressure and decreases pulmonary interstitial edema. The use of furosemide in infants with BPD was associated with short-term improvement in lung compliance and oxygenation, decreased total pulmonary resistance, and facilitation in ventilator weaning.[27,29] However, a meta-analysis did not support all of these findings. Tolerance to furosemide may develop after a few days of therapy; this may be a result of the contraction in extracellular volume, which can lead to a compensatory increase in water and sodium reabsorption in the renal tubules. Furosemide can have significant adverse effects including hypochloremia, hypokalemia, and hyponatremia. Furthermore, volume depletion, hypercalciuria, nephrocalcinosis, osteopenia, and ototoxicity may also occur.[24,29] Excessive fluid loss or hypochloremia may result in metabolic alkalosis and worsen respiratory acidosis. Some of these adverse effects may be reduced by using alternate-day furosemide therapy or nebulized furosemide.[27] Neither of these regimens were associated with electrolyte imbalances, and both were shown to significantly increase lung compliance and decrease pulmonary resistance.[29]

Thiazide diuretics (e.g., hydrochlorothiazide) in combination with a potassium-sparing diuretic (e.g., spironolactone) can improve lung function and decrease oxygen requirements with increased diuresis.[27] Although less potent than furosemide, the combination of these two diuretics can reduce the incidence of hypokalemia commonly associated with loop or thiazide diuretics. Adverse effects commonly seen with this combination include hyponatremia, hyperkalemia or hypokalemia, hypercalciuria, hyperuricemia, hyperglycemia, azotemia, and hypomagnesia.[2] In summary, despite insufficient evidence of long-term efficacy (e.g., decreased oxygen requirement, need for mechanical ventilation, death, severity of BPD) and the potential for adverse effects, diuretics are often used in the management of BPD to provide short-term improvement in pulmonary edema and reduce the need for ventilatory support.

Generally, infants with BPD are treated with furosemide, but are changed to a combination diuretic if long-term treatment is needed to avoid adverse effects. Suggested indications for initiating furosemide therapy include (a) 1-week-old infants with early BPD and ventilator dependency, (b) infants with stable BPD who significantly worsen owing to fluid overload, (c) infants with chronic BPD who do not improve, and (d) infants requiring an increased fluid intake to provide adequate calories.[26] Because J.T. has chronic BPD and is not improving (i.e., she has not been able to be weaned off the ventilator), furosemide 2 mg/kg given every 12 hours enterally may be considered. J.T. should be monitored and treated for electrolyte disturbances while on furosemide.

CASE 105-2, QUESTION 3: One week after starting furosemide, J.T. still requires high ventilatory settings and is unable to be weaned from the ventilator. What other therapeutic agents may be considered to treat J.T.'s BPD?

Inhaled Bronchodilators

Infants in the early stages of BPD generally have airway hyperactivity and smooth muscle hypertrophy. They are also at higher risk for bronchoconstriction owing to increased airway resistance secondary to hypoxia. Therefore, the use of bronchodilators may be helpful in these infants. β_2-Agonists such as albuterol have been shown to provide short-term improvements (4 hours) in lung compliance and pulmonary resistance owing to bronchial smooth muscle relaxation.[17,33] However, inhaled bronchodilators are not effective in all infants with BPD. Infants in the late stages of BPD may have severe pulmonary damage and fibrotic changes.

Only half of these infants demonstrate a decrease in pulmonary resistance after albuterol therapy.[34] In addition, tolerance may develop with prolonged administration.[27] Therefore, inhaled bronchodilators should be reserved for infants who clearly demonstrate improvements during therapy. Currently, there are no well-designed studies evaluating the chronic use or long-term outcome of using inhaled bronchodilators in BPD infants. Despite the lack of meaningful long-term clinical outcomes associated with β_2-agonists and the variable results, their use continues to be very common in preterm infants with BPD. Further studies evaluating the efficacy and safety of long-term inhaled bronchodilator therapy are needed.

Inhaled anticholinergics (e.g., ipratropium bromide) have produced short-term benefits (approximately 4 hours) in infants with BPD by improving pulmonary function.[27] Inhaled anticholinergics, which relax bronchial smooth muscle and decrease mucus secretion, are generally reserved for infants who fail or are intolerant to albuterol, or as an adjunct to albuterol if clinical improvement is not seen.[27] The combined therapy of albuterol and ipratropium may be more effective than either drug alone.[27] The adverse effect profile of ipratropium is minimal because the drug is poorly absorbed.

A major problem with inhaled bronchodilators is their method of administration and drug delivery. Inhaled bronchodilators can be given by jet or ultrasonic nebulization or via a metered-dose inhaler (MDI).[29] For ventilator-dependent infants receiving MDIs, the MDI is connected to an adapter that is attached to the ventilator circuit and ETT. MDIs can also be given through bag ventilation via the ETT. For nonventilated infants, the MDI can be given using a valved holding chamber device and a face mask.

Compared with MDIs, nebulization has several disadvantages including loss or inefficient delivery of drug and cooling of the inspired oxygen mixture. In several neonatal studies, MDIs with a spacer provided more efficient delivery of inhaled bronchodilators and greater improvements in oxygenation and ventilation; smaller doses and a shorter treatment time were also used.[35,36] Furthermore, when comparing the three different devices, the MDI with spacer and the ultrasonic nebulizer are more efficient in delivering aerosols to neonates than the jet nebulizer.[29] In addition, MDIs are less expensive than nebulization. Therefore, the use of MDIs with an appropriate spacing device is preferred for most infants.

Corticosteroids

Corticosteroids, particularly dexamethasone, have been used extensively for the prevention and treatment of BPD. Mechanisms of action of corticosteroids include (a) reduction of polymorphonuclear leukocyte migration to the lung, (b) reduction of lung inflammation, (c) inhibition of prostaglandin, leukotriene, tumor necrosis factor, and interleukin synthesis, (d) reduction of elastase production, (e) stimulation of surfactant synthesis, (f) reduction of vascular permeability and pulmonary edema, (g) enhancement of β-adrenergic receptor activity, (h) reduction of pulmonary fibronectin (which can reduce the risk of interstitial fibrosis), and (i) stimulation of serum retinol concentrations.[2,26]

Systemic dexamethasone is associated with many serious short-term adverse effects, including hyperglycemia, increased BP, hypertrophic cardiomyopathy, GI bleeding, intestinal perforation, pituitary–adrenal suppression, bone demineralization, poor weight gain, and increased risk of infection.[2,24] Serious long-term adverse effects such as cerebral palsy (CP) and neurosensory disability have also been identified in preterm infants who receive systemic corticosteroids.[23,24,27]

Early (within the first week of life) and late (administered after 1 week of life) use of dexamethasone was associated with significant decreases in the incidences of BPD and the combined outcome of death or BPD at 28 days' postnatal age (PNA) and at 36 weeks' PMA.[37,38] Additionally, infants in the late group had a significantly lower incidence of mortality at 28 days' PNA. However, the risk for CP and the combined outcome of death or CP were significantly increased in the early group.[38] Although none of the studies were powered to detect long-term neurologic adverse events, the authors concluded that the benefits of early dexamethasone use do not outweigh the adverse effects and cannot be currently recommended.[38] The use of late dexamethasone should be reserved for infants who are unable to be weaned off the ventilator, and the dose and duration of treatment should be minimized.[37] Recent trials evaluating the adverse long-term neurodevelopmental outcomes associated with dexamethasone reported that low-dose dexamethasone (0.15 mg/kg/day) appeared to be safe and did not increase the risk of CP, whereas high-dose dexamethasone (0.5 mg/kg/day) was associated with significantly increased risk of CP.[39]

Although studies have reported that hydrocortisone may be safer than dexamethasone, a meta-analysis found no effect of hydrocortisone on survival without BPD or mortality.[23,27,40] In addition, an increase in spontaneous GI perforation was found in the hydrocortisone-treated group in the largest trial, resulting in an early termination of three studies.[23,27,39,40] The incidence of GI perforation may have been increased as a result of concomitant treatment with indomethacin. In contrast to studies of high-dose dexamethasone, long-term adverse effects (e.g., CP, neurodevelopmental impairment) of hydrocortisone in patients assessed at 2 to 8 years of age have been reported to be similar to placebo or untreated groups.[39,40] The doses of hydrocortisone used in most of these studies (1 mg/kg/day) were lower than the doses of dexamethasone used in clinical trials. Most infants treated with dexamethasone received a dose of 0.2 to 0.5 mg/kg/day, which is equivalent to hydrocortisone 5 to 15 mg/kg/day. Furthermore, all of these studies initiated hydrocortisone within the first week of life. Currently, there are no trials evaluating the use of hydrocortisone after 1 week of life in infants with established, ventilator-dependent BPD.

Based on these clinical findings, a policy statement from the American Academy of Pediatrics (AAP) does not recommend high-dose dexamethasone (0.5 mg/kg/day or greater) owing to the absence of improved short- and long-term outcomes from randomized trials.[39] It also does not recommend low-dose dexamethasone ($<$0.2 mg/kg/day) or high-dose hydrocortisone (3–6 mg/kg/day) owing to insufficient evidence. Early low-dose hydrocortisone (1 mg/kg/day) given within the first 2 weeks of life may benefit a specific patient population. Clinicians must weigh the potential risks of BPD with the potential adverse effects associated with glucocorticoids; therapy should be considered in VLBW infants at high risk for experiencing BPD (e.g., those still on mechanical ventilation after 1–2 weeks of age). Parents should be fully informed about the short- and long-term adverse effects of systemic corticosteroids.[39] Despite the AAP recommendation, some clinicians would still consider administering a short course of low-dose systemic corticosteroid to help facilitate extubation. This practice may be supported by a meta-regression analysis demonstrating that the impact of postnatal steroids on the combined outcome of death or CP was modified by the risk of BPD.[24] When postnatal steroids were used in infants with a low risk for BPD ($<$35%), there was a significant increase in the risk of death or CP. However, when used in infants with a higher risk for BPD ($>$65%), a significant reduction in the risk of death or CP was found. Overall, infants with a $>$50% predicted risk of BPD had less harm associated with steroids than those at lower risk of BPD.[24] Dexamethasone 0.2 mg/kg/day in two divided doses (tapered for 5–7 days) may be considered for J.T., even though she is now 13 weeks old. Throughout therapy, J.T. should be monitored for hyperglycemia, hypertension, GI bleeding, and intestinal perforation.

Inhaled steroids such as beclomethasone dipropionate, flunisolide, fluticasone, and budesonide have also been used for the treatment and prevention of BPD.[30,41] When compared to placebo, inhaled corticosteroids have not been shown to decrease the incidence of death or BPD, the combined outcome of death or BPD, and duration of mechanical ventilation and oxygen therapy; however, the use of systemic steroid may be decreased.[30,41] When compared to systemic steroids, no significant differences in mortality or the incidence of BPD were found.[31,32] The use of early inhaled steroids (i.e., prevention) was associated with increased duration of mechanical ventilation and oxygenation. None of these studies evaluated long-term neurodevelopmental outcomes associated with inhaled steroids. Adverse effects of inhaled steroids are less common than with systemic steroids; these include mild adrenal suppression, bronchospasm, tongue hypertrophy, and oral candidiasis.[30–32,41] Inhaled steroids may suppress the pituitary–adrenal axis; however, studies have reported conflicting results. Suppression may vary depending on the type of inhaled steroids, dosing regimen, and other factors such as prematurity.[33] The infant's mouth should be cleaned after each use of inhaled steroid to minimize complications such as oral thrush. As with inhaled bronchodilators, administration is a therapeutic problem with these medications. Further studies evaluating the optimal dose, duration of therapy, time of initiation, delivery technique, most appropriate preparation, and long-term adverse effects (including neurodevelopmental outcome) of corticosteroids are needed before inhaled steroids can be routinely recommended.

Long-Term Sequelae

CASE 105-2, QUESTION 4: Five months have passed, and J.T. is now 4.5 months old (corrected age), weighs 5 kg, and is ready for discharge. During the past several months, ventilation requirements slowly decreased, and J.T. was eventually extubated. However, she still requires supplemental oxygen at an FiO_2 of 30%, 0.25 L/minute via nasal cannula, to maintain an oxygen saturation of 90% to 95%. What are the long-term complications of BPD that can be expected in J.T.?

Infants with BPD have little pulmonary reserve and, therefore, are at higher risk for experiencing frequent respiratory exacerbations. BPD places J.T. at risk for recurrent infections of the lower respiratory tract, and she may require frequent hospitalizations during the first year for bronchiolitis and pneumonia. Approximately 50% of all children with BPD require hospitalization for respiratory exacerbations during early childhood.[21] Respiratory syncytial virus is a common cause of respiratory distress and recurrent atelectasis. With time, most preterm survivors with BPD have an improvement in pulmonary function owing to lung growth; however, many continue to have airway hyper-reactivity. Infants with severe BPD can also experience pulmonary hypertension, cor pulmonale, systemic hypertension, and left ventricular hypertrophy.

In addition, J.T. may be at risk for experiencing bone demineralization and rickets. VLBW infants are born with inadequate stores of vitamin D. In general, these premature infants may not receive an adequate intake of vitamin D, either parenterally or through their diet. Most VLBW infants require prolonged parenteral nutrition, which may cause cholestasis or hepatic failure. Prolonged cholestasis or chronic hepatic congestion owing to heart failure may cause malabsorption of calcium and vitamin D. In addition, furosemide may exacerbate calcium deficiencies by causing hypercalciuria. These combined factors may result in bone demineralization and rickets. Infants with BPD usually have a high catabolism and increased oxygen consumption as a result of an increased work of breathing and chronic hypoxia. Inadequate nutritional support may negatively affect weight gain, growth, and long-term outcome of BPD.

Neurologic and developmental abnormalities such as learning disabilities, speech delays, vision and hearing impairment, and poor attention span can also occur in infants with BPD.[21] BPD itself is not an independent risk factor for neurologic abnormality; related factors include birth weight, gestational age, and socioeconomic status.[21] Long-term follow-up evaluations at 1 to 15 years of age in infants previously treated with high-dose dexamethasone revealed an increase in neurodevelopmental abnormalities such as CP and decreased school performance in some studies.[39] However, it is not known whether these abnormalities were attributable to an adverse effect of dexamethasone on brain development or to an improved survival of infants who may already be at risk for experiencing these abnormalities.

Mortality rates for infants with BPD range from 30% to 40%.[28] Approximately 80% of deaths associated with BPD occur during initial hospitalization and are attributable to respiratory failure, sepsis, pneumonia, cor pulmonale, and congestive heart failure.[28]

Prevention

CASE 105-2, QUESTION 5: What preventive measures could have been used to decrease the likelihood of the development of BPD in J.T.?

Prevention of prematurity and other etiologic factors of RDS is the most effective means of preventing BPD. Although both antenatal steroids and exogenous surfactant therapy have been shown to reduce the incidence of RDS, the incidence of BPD has not been affected.[23] One of the causes of BPD can be vitamin A deficiency, which can predispose infants to BPD owing to impaired lung healing, increased susceptibility to infection and loss of cilia, and decreased number of alveoli.[23] Premature infants, especially VLBW infants, are at greatest risk owing to low body stores, inadequate intake during feedings, and decreased enteral absorption of vitamin A. Intramuscular (IM) vitamin A has been shown to significantly reduce the combined outcome of mortality or BPD; however, no difference was found with mortality, ROP, or sepsis.[23] In contrast, administration of oral vitamin A 5,000 international units/day did not decrease the incidence of BPD, perhaps because of inadequate dose or poor oral absorption.[42] Vitamin A seems to be a relatively safe drug; the incidence of adverse effects was similar between treated and control groups.[23] Although evidence appears to support IM vitamin A in infants with birth weight less than 1,000 g, further studies evaluating the efficacy, safety, and optimal dosage regimen of vitamin A for the prevention of BPD are needed.

Ureaplasma urealyticum colonization of the respiratory tract of premature infants is a significant risk factor for BPD. Several studies evaluated the use of macrolide antibiotics for eradication of *Ureaplasma* in premature infants at risk for BPD.[23,43] Although erythromycin has not been shown to reduce the incidence of BPD or death, studies evaluating azithromycin and clarithromycin reported variable efficacy results. Azithromycin and clarithromycin have shown to decrease the incidence of BPD, but only in infants positive for *Ureaplasma*.[43] However, prolonged antibiotic exposure has been linked to an increased rate of NEC or sepsis. Furthermore, erythromycin use has been associated with infantile hypertrophic pyloric stenosis.[2] Therefore, due to these adverse findings as well as conflicting clinical efficacy, routine use of macrolide antibiotics is not recommended.

Optimization of nutritional support may also help to prevent the development of BPD because proper nutrition helps to promote lung maturation, growth, and repair. Excessive fluid administration should be avoided because it may lead to BPD. Fluid restriction decreases both the incidence of BPD and mortality.[24] The early use of caffeine (initiated before 3 days of life) to treat apnea of prematurity in infants with birth weights of 500 to 1,250 g has been shown to decrease the incidence of neurodevelopmental impairment, including CP. In addition, the incidence of BPD was significantly decreased in the caffeine-treated infants, although BPD was one of their secondary outcomes.[23,44] Fluid restriction, the early use of caffeine citrate, and IM vitamin A could have been recommended for J.T. in the early course of her hospitalization to help decrease the likelihood of her experiencing BPD.

PATENT DUCTUS ARTERIOSUS

The fetus has three unique circulatory structures that differ from the adult circulation: (a) the ductus venosus, which permits blood to bypass the liver; (b) the foramen ovale, which allows blood to pass from the right atrium into the left atrium; and (c) the ductus arteriosus, the structure that connects the pulmonary artery to the descending aorta and allows blood to bypass the lungs (Fig. 105-1).[45] In addition to these structural differences, vascular resistance and pressure play important roles in determining the pathway of the fetal circulation. For example, the relative hypoxia that occurs in utero causes pulmonary vasoconstriction. Pulmonary vasoconstriction, along with compression of pulmonary blood vessels by unexpanded fetal lung mass, results in a high pulmonary vascular resistance and decreased pulmonary blood flow. This decreased pulmonary blood flow is acceptable in utero because the lungs essentially are nonfunctional. Large amounts of blood, however, must be pumped through the placenta where gas exchange occurs.

Maximally oxygenated blood (Po_2, 30–35 mm Hg) flows from the placenta to the fetus through the umbilical vein (Fig. 105-1). Approximately 50% of the umbilical venous blood is shunted away from the liver through the ductus venosus and directed into the inferior vena cava. Blood from the inferior vena cava and superior vena cava then enters the right atrium. Most of the blood from the inferior vena cava, which is well oxygenated, is directed in a straight pathway across the right atrium through the foramen ovale directly into the left atrium. It then enters the left ventricle through the mitral valve and is pumped through the ascending aorta and into the vessels of the head and forelimbs. Thus, the fetal brain is preferentially perfused with blood containing a higher amount of oxygen. Deoxygenated blood returning from the head region via the superior vena cava enters the right atrium and is directed through the tricuspid valve into the right ventricle, where it then is pumped into the pulmonary artery. Most of this blood is diverted through the ductus arteriosus into the descending aorta and then through the two umbilical arteries to the placenta. A small percentage of the blood flows to the lower extremities and then is returned to the heart via the inferior vena cava.[45]

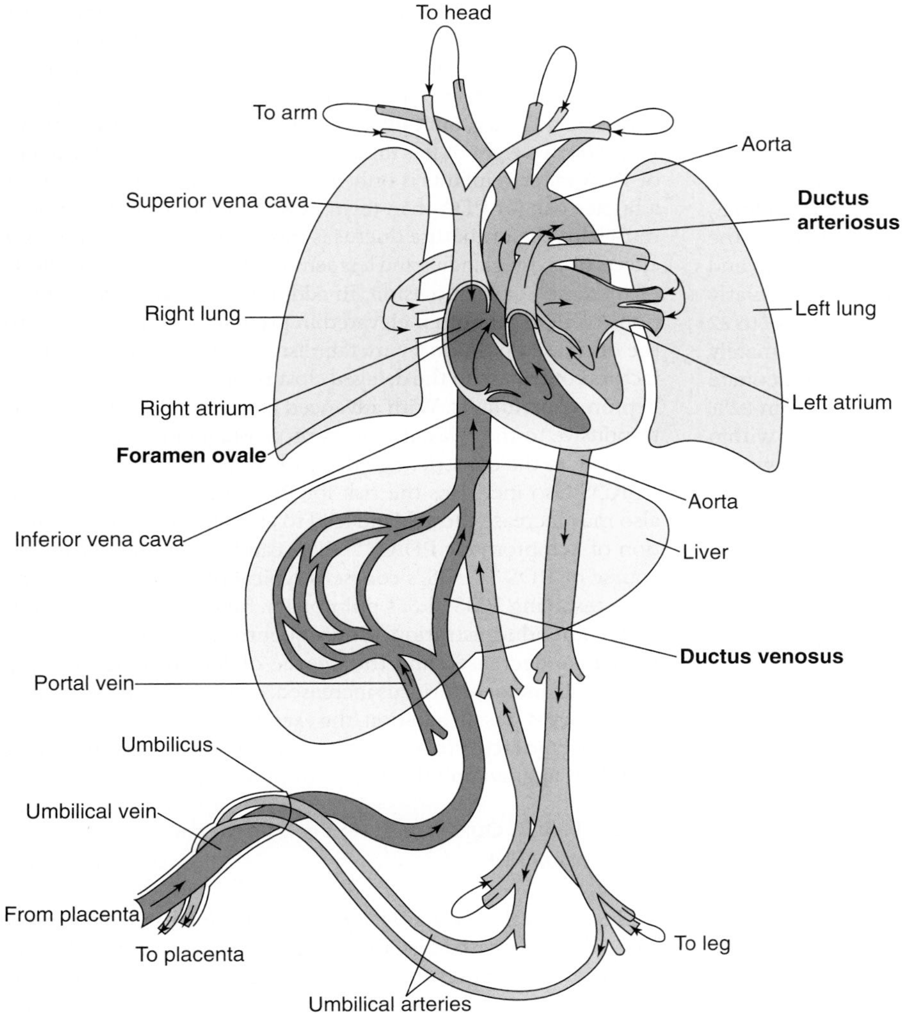

Figure 105-1 Fetal circulation. (Adapted with permission from Sandra MN, *The Lippincott Manual of Nursing Practice*. 7th ed. Lippincott Williams & Wilkins; 2001.)

Changes at Birth

At birth, major circulatory changes result from umbilical cord clamping, aeration and expansion of the lungs, and an increase in arterial Po_2. These changes are important in the transition from a fetal to an adult circulation. When the umbilical cord is clamped, blood flow decreases through the ductus venosus. Clamping of the umbilical cord also results in a twofold increase in systemic vascular resistance. This increase in systemic vascular resistance increases aortic, left ventricular, and left atrial pressures and cardiac output. Pulmonary pressures and blood flow also change. After the neonate's first breath, the lungs expand, oxygenation improves, and pulmonary vascular resistance immediately drops. This increases pulmonary blood flow, causing a decrease in pulmonary arterial, right ventricular, and right atrial pressures.[45,46]

Closure of the Foramen Ovale

Because of the decreased right atrial pressure and increased left atrial pressure that occur after birth, blood attempts to flow down the pressure gradient from the left atrium through the foramen ovale into the right atrium. This is in the opposite direction from what occurs in fetal life. The small, valve like flap that lies over the foramen ovale on the left side of the atrial septum closes over the foramen ovale opening when the pressure in the left atrium exceeds the pressure in the right atrium. Closure of this flap prevents further flow through the foramen ovale. As long as the pressure in the left atrium is higher than that in the right atrium, the foramen ovale remains functionally closed, until it closes anatomically.

Closure of the Ductus Arteriosus

Closure of the ductus arteriosus is more complex and depends on many factors. In utero, patency of the ductus arteriosus is maintained through the combined vasodilatory effects of a low Po_2 and high concentrations of prostanoids, particularly prostaglandin E_2 (PGE_2) and prostacyclin.[47] After birth, the smooth muscles of the ductus arteriosus constrict as arterial oxygenation increases and concentrations of placentally derived prostaglandins, particularly PGE_2, decrease.[47] In utero, the Po_2 of the ductal blood is 18 to 22 mm Hg, whereas after birth in a term neonate, it is approximately 100 mm Hg. Normally, the ductus arteriosus of a term neonate functionally closes within the first few days of life (i.e., in 82% of infants within 48 hours of life and in 100% of infants within 96 hours of life). Anatomic closure of the ductus occurs within 2 to 3 weeks of life. When the ductus arteriosus fails to close, it is called patent ductus arteriosus (PDA). In a term neonate, a PDA beyond the first few days of life generally is permanent. It usually is secondary to an anatomic defect in the wall of the ductus arteriosus and requires surgical ligation. In contrast, a PDA in a preterm neonate may persist for weeks and still close spontaneously.

When a PDA is present, the direction and amount of shunting through this opening are determined by the pressure gradient between the systemic and pulmonary circulations. Usually, blood flows from the aorta into the pulmonary circulation. Because systemic vascular resistance and aortic pressure are increased, and pulmonary vascular resistance and pulmonary arterial pressure are decreased after birth, blood pumped from the left ventricle into the aorta flows from the aorta (a high-pressure area) through the PDA and into the pulmonary artery (a lower-pressure area). This flow is called left-to-right shunting and is in contrast to the right-to-left shunting that occurs through the PDA during fetal life.

Clinical Presentation

CASE 105-3

QUESTION 1: T.S. is a 750-g female who was born at 25 weeks' gestational age to a 22-year-old gravida 2 para 1 woman. One hour after birth, T.S. exhibited symptoms of RDS, and two doses of beractant were given within the first 24 hours of life. After the second dose of beractant, T.S.'s respiratory function greatly improved, and no further doses of beractant were required. On the third day of life, the nurse noticed that T.S. had tachycardia, a systolic murmur, a hyperactive precordium, and a widened pulse pressure. Her lungs sounded "wet." In addition, the nurse noted that T.S.'s combined IV fluid rates total 160 mL/kg/day instead of the desired fluid intake of 120 mL/kg/day. Current vital signs and ABGs are as follows:

HR, 190 beats/minute
RR, 65 breaths/minute
BP, 55/23 mm Hg
O_2 saturation, 89%
pH, 7.22
Pco_2, 55 mm Hg
Po_2, 77 mm Hg
Base deficit, 10

Ventilator support is increased to compensate for T.S.'s deteriorating respiratory status. Echocardiography is performed and shows a moderate-size PDA with significant left-to-right shunting. The chest radiograph shows pulmonary edema and an enlarged heart. What risk factors for PDA does T.S. have?

T.S. has two major risk factors for developing a symptomatic PDA: prematurity and RDS. The occurrence of a PDA is inversely proportional to gestational age and birth weight. The incidence of PDA is approximately 45% in premature infants with a birth weight of less than 1,750 g, but can be as high as 80% in premature infants with a birth weight of less than 1,200 g.[48] In contrast, the incidence of PDA in term infants is only 0.06%.[48] Preterm neonates are at a higher risk for PDA than term newborns because the smooth muscle of the immature ductus is more sensitive to the dilatory effects of prostaglandins and less sensitive to the constrictive effects of increased oxygen tension. In addition, circulating concentrations of PGE_2 are often elevated in premature infants owing to the decreased pulmonary metabolism of prostaglandins. These factors contribute to the delayed closure of the ductus arteriosus in premature infants. With advanced gestation, the ductus is less responsive to the relaxant effects of prostaglandins and is more sensitive to the constricting effects of oxygen.[49]

RDS also increases the risk for PDA. Exogenous surfactant also may increase the risk and lead to an earlier clinical presentation of symptomatic PDA.[49,50] PDA can further complicate the course of RDS.[49,51] T.S.'s course is typical of a preterm neonate with resolving RDS. T.S.'s pulmonary function improved after surfactant administration. Consequently, pulmonary vascular resistance decreased and the degree of left-to-right shunting across the ductus arteriosus increased, causing a deterioration in respiratory status. In addition, the excess fluid that T.S. received is an iatrogenic factor that may have increased the shunting across the PDA, aggravating the degree of pulmonary congestion.[49]

CASE 105-3, QUESTION 2: How is T.S.'s presentation consistent with that of PDA?

T.S.'s clinical presentation is related to the increased pulmonary blood flow, decreased systemic perfusion, and left ventricular volume overload that resulted from the shunting of left ventricular cardiac output through the PDA into the lungs. To compensate for the inadequate peripheral perfusion, HR increases. This results in an increase in cardiac output and a greater left-to-right shunt through the PDA, creating a vicious cycle. The widened pulse pressure (the difference between systolic and diastolic pressures, 32 mm Hg) is a result of diversion of aortic blood flow through the PDA, which is causing the bounding pulses. The systolic murmur, which is not always present, is the result of turbulent blood flow through the ductus arteriosus occurring because the pulmonary vascular resistance decreases. Tachycardia, hyperactive precordium, and a continuous murmur are results of the left-to-right shunting through the ductus arteriosus during systole.[52]

CASE 105-3, QUESTION 3: What are the potential complications of this hemodynamically significant PDA in T.S.?

The increased pulmonary blood flow and resultant pulmonary edema will worsen T.S.'s respiratory disease and increase the need for ventilatory support. The higher ventilatory settings (increase in MAP and FIO_2) place T.S. at risk for having BPD. If the PDA is left untreated, T.S. may experience congestive heart failure secondary to an increased left ventricular end-diastolic volume. A hemodynamically significant PDA also places T.S. at risk for IVH and NEC.[49]

Treatment

CASE 105-3, QUESTION 4: How should T.S.'s PDA be managed?

The initial medical management for T.S.'s symptomatic PDA is supportive care, which includes fluid management (e.g., fluid restriction and diuretic therapy), correction of anemia, and treatment of hypoxia and acidosis. Although excessive fluid administration may increase the risk of PDA, fluid restriction alone is unlikely to result in ductal closure. T.S.'s fluid intake should be restricted to 100–120 mL/kg/day (approximately 80% of total fluid maintenance requirements) to avoid worsening of her pulmonary edema and to prevent congestive heart failure.[49] Furosemide 1 mg/kg IV push should also be given to T.S. immediately to treat her pulmonary edema. In addition to fluid management, correction of anemia is important. Low concentrations of hemoglobin result in an increased cardiac output, which may worsen the infant's cardiac function. Anemia not only increases the demand of left ventricular output to ensure adequate oxygen delivery to the tissues, but may also increase the magnitude of the left-to-right shunt by decreasing the resistance of blood flow through the pulmonary vascular bed.[49] Maintaining a hematocrit level of more than 40% to 45% is often recommended. Because of T.S.'s gestational age, birth weight, and size of PDA, it is unlikely that she will respond to these general measures alone. Therefore, T.S. requires pharmacologic treatment with indomethacin or ibuprofen.

NONSTEROIDAL ANTI-INFLAMMATORY DRUGS

Both indomethacin and ibuprofen are available in injectable form for the treatment of PDA. These drugs nonspecifically inhibit prostaglandin synthesis, thereby eliminating the vasodilator effects of the PGE series on the ductus arteriosus, allowing the ductus to close. Indomethacin has been used clinically for more than 30 years for the treatment of PDA. However, because of its adverse effects, other prostaglandin inhibitors, such as ibuprofen, have been studied for PDA closure. Results indicate that ibuprofen is as effective as indomethacin in closing the ductus and causes significantly less of a decrease in renal, mesenteric, and cerebral blood flow. In a recent meta-analysis comparing ibuprofen with indomethacin, ibuprofen reduced the risks of NEC and transient adverse effects on renal function (e.g., oliguria, elevations of serum creatinine [SCr]).[53] However, the incidence of mortality, BPD, and IVH were similar for both drugs. Unfortunately, no long-term follow-up studies of ibuprofen exist. These studies are needed to determine whether ibuprofen or indomethacin is the drug of choice for PDA closure.[53] Based on the studies currently available, ibuprofen may be preferred in patients who have or are at risk for decreased renal function. The initial dose of ibuprofen lysine is 10 mg/kg followed by two doses of 5 mg/kg given at 24-hour intervals. If urinary output decreases to less than 0.6 mL/kg/hour, the second or third doses should be held.[2]

Unfortunately, not every infant treated with a nonsteroidal anti-inflammatory drug (NSAID) responds with constriction of the ductus arteriosus; therefore, surgical ligation of the PDA may be required. Ligation generally is reserved for neonates who do not respond to pharmacologic therapy or those in whom drug therapy is contraindicated.[49]

CASE 105-3, QUESTION 5: Due to lower risks of adverse effects on renal function, the attending physician would like to treat T.S. with ibuprofen for closure of her PDA. You explain to the medical team that there is a temporary shortage of ibuprofen, and therefore, T.S. should be treated with indomethacin. The medical team then asks the following: What is the dose of indomethacin for T.S.? and What route should be used for its administration?

The medical team should be told the following information. The route of choice for indomethacin is IV; enteral indomethacin is less effective. This reduced effectiveness may be related to the formulation of the suspension and decreased, erratic enteral absorption. In addition, the use of enteral indomethacin has been associated with NEC.[54]

A large interpatient variability of indomethacin pharmacokinetics occurs in preterm neonates. Serum concentrations do not correlate consistently with therapeutic or adverse effects. Furthermore, the optimal therapeutic serum concentration is not yet defined.[55] Although many dosage regimens have been reported, dosing guidelines from the National Collaborative Study are commonly used.[51] Three indomethacin doses are given in 12- to 24-hour intervals, with the first dose equal to 0.2 mg/kg IV in all neonates. Because indomethacin clearance is directly proportional to postnatal age, the second and third doses are determined by postnatal age at initiation of indomethacin therapy. If onset of treatment was at less than 2 days' PNA, neonates receive 0.1 mg/kg/dose; if initiation of therapy occurred at 2 to 7 days' PNA, neonates receive 0.2 mg/kg/dose; if therapy began at more than 7 days' PNA, neonates receive 0.25 mg/kg/dose. Second and third doses are administered at 12- to 24-hour intervals. No specific guidelines exist regarding which patients receive every-12-hour versus every-24-hour dosing; however, the individual dosing interval generally is determined by the neonate's urine output. If urine output remains greater than 1 mL/kg/hour after an indomethacin dose, then the next dose may be given in 12 hours. If urine output is less than 1 mL/kg/hour but greater than 0.6 mL/kg/hour, then the dosing interval may be extended to 24 hours. Doses should be held if urine output is less than 0.6 mL/kg/hour. T.S. should receive three doses of indomethacin 0.15 mg (0.2 mg/kg/dose) given every 12 hours, as long as her urine output remains greater than 1 mL/kg/hour. If T.S.'s urine output decreases, then the dosing interval should be adjusted as outlined above.

Other indomethacin dosing regimens have been evaluated more recently for the treatment of PDA in preterm infants. An initial dose of 0.2 mg/kg followed by either 0.1 or 0.2 mg/kg for two doses at 12- to 24-hour intervals has been used. In a study measuring serum concentrations, higher doses of indomethacin were required in older neonates (>10 days' PNA).[56] This may be owing to an increased indomethacin clearance in these infants.

Because rapid IV administration of indomethacin can decrease cerebral, mesenteric, and renal blood flow, longer infusion rates of 20 to 30 minutes are recommended.[57]

Response to NSAID therapy can be determined by assessing the clinical signs of PDA such as tachycardia, widened pulse pressure, bounding pulses, heart murmur, and the ability to wean from ventilator support. In certain cases, echocardiography may be performed to confirm closure of a PDA.

CASE 105-3, QUESTION 6: What clinical and laboratory data should be monitored during T.S.'s indomethacin therapy?

Before initiating indomethacin therapy, T.S. should receive an echocardiogram to rule out ductal-dependent congenital heart disease and to confirm the presence of a PDA. In addition, an SCr and blood urea nitrogen (BUN) should be obtained from T.S. before indomethacin therapy because nephrotoxicity is the most common adverse effect. Infants receiving indomethacin can experience transient oliguria with increased SCr. This occurs as a result of indomethacin-induced decreases in renal blood flow and glomerular filtration rate.[51] Dilutional hyponatremia may occur secondary to either decreased urine output or decreased free water diuresis owing to increased antidiuretic hormone activity. Treatment of hyponatremia should be aimed at decreasing free water intake through fluid restriction rather than by sodium supplementation. Typically, renal function normalizes within 72 hours after the last dose of indomethacin. In general, indomethacin therapy is contraindicated in neonates with renal failure, urine output less than 0.6 mL/kg/hour, or an SCr of 1.8 mg/dL or greater.[51]

Furosemide, which increases renal prostaglandin synthesis, has been suggested to help prevent indomethacin-associated renal toxicity. However, by increasing prostaglandins, furosemide may theoretically decrease ductal closure. Currently, studies do not support the routine use of furosemide in preterm neonates who receive indomethacin for the treatment of PDA. Furosemide is also contraindicated in patients who are dehydrated.[58] In addition to monitoring renal function and serum electrolytes, serum concentrations of aminoglycosides, digoxin, and other renally eliminated drugs should be monitored carefully. Indomethacin therapy may decrease renal drug clearance and cause accumulation of these agents, which may require a dosage reduction.[59]

A platelet count should also be obtained from T.S. before therapy because indomethacin may decrease platelet aggregation. Thrombocytopenia (platelet count <50,000/μL) is a contraindication to indomethacin therapy.[51] In cases of thrombocytopenia, indomethacin may be withheld temporarily until platelets can be transfused. Other potential contraindications to indomethacin therapy include active bleeding and clinical evidence of NEC because GI bleeding, perforation, and NEC have been reported with indomethacin use.[49] These GI effects may be related to decreases in intestinal blood flow usually seen with rapid IV infusions. Grades II to IV IVH also are frequently quoted as contraindications to indomethacin therapy; however, indomethacin treatment probably is not associated with progression of IVH. In fact, prophylactic treatment with indomethacin may be associated with a decrease in the incidence of severe IVH (grades III and IV).[49,50]

CASE 105-3, QUESTION 7: When is the best time to initiate an NSAID for symptomatic treatment of T.S.'s PDA?

Conflicting data exist on when to initiate indomethacin or ibuprofen therapy for the treatment of symptomatic PDA. Some centers may opt to treat within the first 2 to 3 days of life (early symptomatic PDA) when infants initially present with clinical signs of PDA (i.e., murmur, widened pulse pressures, tachycardia). Others may not treat until clinical signs of congestive heart failure are present (late symptomatic PDA; 7–10 days of life).[50] Both treatment strategies (early and late) significantly decrease the incidence of PDA, but both cause significant transient reduction of urine output and SCr elevation. In some studies, infants receiving early treatment of indomethacin had significant reductions in the incidence of BPD and NEC and the need for surgical ligation.[50] In contrast, one study found that final PDA closure rates and the need for surgical ligation were comparable in early versus late indomethacin-treated neonates. In fact, spontaneous closure was observed in 43% of the late treatment group, which may indicate unnecessary treatment in the early group. In addition, renal adverse effects and ventilatory requirements were higher in the infants treated early.[60] Thus, early administration of indomethacin should not be used routinely; however, it may be given to preterm neonates at high risk for having a large PDA. Clinically, these recommendations can also be applied to ibuprofen. Because T.S. is an ELBW neonate with RDS, she is at high risk for exhibiting a large PDA. She also has clinical signs of a PDA and, thus, should be treated as soon as possible.

CASE 105-3, QUESTION 8: The physicians were able to decrease T.S.'s ventilator support within the first 12 to 24 hours after starting indomethacin treatment. After 3 to 4 days of gradual and consistent ventilator weaning, the ventilator settings could not be decreased further. During the next 2 to 3 days, T.S.'s respiratory status deteriorates, and she requires increased ventilator support. T.S. now has tachycardia, a widened pulse pressure, bounding pulses, and a hyperactive precordium. Repeat echocardiogram shows a small-to-moderate PDA. Current data include the following:

BUN, 10 mg/dL
SCr, 1.1 mg/dL
Sodium, 134 mEq/L
Potassium, 4.9 mEq/L
Chloride, 97 mEq/L
Urine output, 2.3 mL/kg/hour
Fluid intake, 130 mL/kg/day
Platelets, 180,000/μL

Why did PDA recur in T.S., and how should it be managed?

Successful closure of the PDA with indomethacin occurs in 70% to 90% of infants; however, ductal reopening or recurrence can occur in 20% to 35% of infants who initially respond to indomethacin.[61] Recurrence of PDA occurs especially in lower-birth-weight infants. Several reasons might explain T.S.'s transient response to indomethacin. Recurrence of PDA is inversely proportional to gestational age; the incidence of ductal reopening is significantly higher in infants with 26 weeks' gestational age or younger compared with infants born at 27 weeks' gestation or more (37% vs. 11%, respectively).[62] The higher recurrence in younger gestational age neonates may be related to resumption of PGE_2 production after indomethacin serum concentrations decline and heightened sensitivity of the immature ductus arteriosus to the dilating effects of PGE_2.[49,61] This is particularly important in ventilator-dependent patients such as T.S. because mechanical ventilation increases circulating vasodilating prostaglandins.

Furthermore, the rate of ductal reopening is independent of indomethacin serum concentrations, but seems to be related to the timing of indomethacin therapy, PNA, and the amount of fluid intake 24 hours before indomethacin treatment.[62] The rate of recurrence is lower in infants who were treated with indomethacin earlier in life compared with those who receive treatment later.[49] Because anatomic closure of a PDA may be delayed for a couple of weeks, it is not surprising that the ductus arteriosus reopened in T.S. after her initial response to indomethacin.

Although controversial, prolonged indomethacin therapy may prevent recurrences and allow for permanent closure of the ductus arteriosus. Several prolonged treatment regimens have been successful in preventing ductal reopening.[49,61] One such regimen (indomethacin 0.2 mg/kg/dose IV every 12 hours for three doses, followed by 0.2 mg/kg/dose every 24 hours for five doses) was able to significantly decrease the recurrence of PDA from 47% to 10% in neonates less than 1,500 g without increasing toxicity. The need for surgical ligation also was decreased significantly.[61] However, some studies report an increased mortality in infants receiving prolonged therapy (5 to 7 days) compared with those receiving the short course (three doses).[49] Furthermore, a recent meta-analysis demonstrated that prolonged therapy (six to eight doses) did not improve PDA closure, retreatment, reopening, or surgical ligation rates. Although prolonged courses were shown to decrease transient renal dysfunction, a significantly higher incidence of NEC was observed. Thus, the routine use of prolonged courses of indomethacin is not currently recommended.[63] Select use of prolonged therapy may be used. Individual patient response needs to be considered, especially in ELBW neonates. The optimal duration of indomethacin therapy and dosing regimen need to be identified.

T.S. remains ventilator-dependent and is at increased risk for exhibiting BPD. Because she has no contraindications to indomethacin therapy, a second course of indomethacin (0.1–0.2 mg/kg/dose every 12–24 hours for three to five doses) should be considered.[61,63] If the PDA fails to respond to this prolonged regimen or if it recurs again after an initial response, and T.S. remains ventilator-dependent, surgical ligation most likely will be required to permanently close the PDA.

Prophylactic Administration

CASE 105-3, QUESTION 9: Could prophylactic NSAID administration have prevented the development of a symptomatic PDA in T.S.?

Prophylactic indomethacin therapy is defined as the administration of indomethacin within 24 hours of life to newborns who are at risk of experiencing a symptomatic PDA.[64] However, routine prophylaxis would unnecessarily expose a large number of newborns to indomethacin (and its adverse effects), because PDA closure may occur spontaneously without treatment. Prophylactic use of indomethacin has short-term benefits; it significantly decreases the incidence of PDA and IVH (grades III and IV) and the need for PDA surgical ligation.[64] Unfortunately, most studies have not shown that prophylactic ductal closure with indomethacin decreases the incidence of death, BPD, NEC, or neurodevelopmental disabilities. Additionally, infants receiving prophylactic therapy have a higher incidence of severe oliguria or anuria, albeit transient.[64] Therefore, routine prophylactic administration is usually not warranted. It may be considered, however, in some neonatal units that do not have easy access to cardiac diagnostic and therapeutic services or that have a high incidence of IVH. Typically, preterm neonates, particularly those at high risk for experiencing a large PDA (e.g., ELBW neonates), are treated as soon as clinical signs appear.

Prophylactic ibuprofen therapy (administered at $<$24 hours of life) significantly decreases the incidence of PDA and the need for rescue pharmacologic treatment and surgical ligation.[65] However, it does not appear to decrease BPD, IVH, NEC, or mortality, and may increase the risk of renal dysfunction and sepsis. Because of the lack of long-term follow-up studies with the current ibuprofen lysine product, prophylactic ibuprofen therapy for the prevention of PDA is not recommended at this time.[65]

Treatment with Acetaminophen

CASE 105-3, QUESTION 10: During multidisciplinary NICU rounds, the advanced nurse practitioner mentions that acetaminophen has been used to treat PDA and may be safer than NSAIDs. Should acetaminophen, rather than indomethacin, have been used to treat the symptomatic PDA in T.S.? What is the evidence to support its use?

The advanced nurse practitioner is partially correct and should be informed of the following information. Several case reports suggest that acetaminophen may be used for the treatment of PDA in neonates who fail or have contraindications to NSAID therapy.[66–68] Similar to NSAIDs, acetaminophen inhibits prostaglandin synthesis. However, in contrast to NSAIDs that inhibit cyclooxygenase-1 and -2 (steps that occur early in the synthesis of prostaglandins), acetaminophen is thought to affect a subsequent step in prostaglandin synthesis by inhibiting the peroxidase site of the enzyme, prostaglandin synthetase. Others suggest that acetaminophen inhibits a yet-unidentified cyclooxygenase-3. Due to the different mechanisms of actions, acetaminophen would be expected to have less serious side effects than NSAIDs.

Two randomized controlled trials compared acetaminophen to ibuprofen for the treatment of PDA in preterm neonates.[67,68] Both trials used acetaminophen doses of 15 mg/kg every 6 hours for 3 days. A recent meta-analysis of these studies found no significant difference in the failure rates for PDA closure or risk of reopening the PDA between the two drugs.[68] No significant differences in secondary outcomes or adverse effects were observed, with two exceptions: The duration of required supplemental oxygen was shorter, and the incidence of hyperbilirubinemia was lower in patients who received acetaminophen. Although these results appear promising, an association of postnatal use of acetaminophen with autism or autism spectrum disorder has recently been identified.[68] In addition, animal studies suggest acetaminophen may affect cognitive function when administered during neonatal brain development. Therefore, further research, including long-term follow-up studies of neurodevelopment, is needed before acetaminophen can be recommended for PDA closure in routine clinical practice.[68] Due to these concerns, acetaminophen should not have been used in place of indomethacin to treat the symptomatic PDA in T.S. After weighing all potential risks and benefits, some clinicians may use acetaminophen before surgical ligation, in select neonates with a significant PDA, who have failed or who have contraindications to NSAID therapy.[67]

NECROTIZING ENTEROCOLITIS

CASE 105-4

QUESTION 1: C.D., a 15-day-old female neonate, was born at 28 weeks' gestational age with a birth weight of 908 g. Her postnatal course has been complicated by RDS, sepsis, and a large PDA for which she required intubation and mechanical ventilation, one dose of beractant, a 7-day course of ampicillin and gentamicin, and indomethacin. Enteral feedings with a standard preterm 24-cal/ounce formula were started on day 4 of life at 5 mL every 3 hours (44 mL/kg/day). Feedings were increased by 5 mL/feed on days 5 through 7 to 20 mL/feed every 3 hours on day 7 of life (176 mL/kg/day). This morning, C.D. exhibited a distended abdomen, bloody stools, multiple episodes of apnea that required reintubation and assisted ventilation, and metabolic acidosis. ABG results revealed the following:

pH, 7.15
P_{CO_2}, 67 mm Hg

Po_2, 55 mm Hg
Base deficit, 10

An abdominal radiograph revealed pneumatosis intestinalis (the presence of gas in the intestinal submucosa). C.D. is to take nothing by mouth (NPO), and gentamicin 4 mg/kg IV infusion every 36 hours and ampicillin 100 mg/kg IV push every 12 hours are restarted. What clinical signs of NEC does C.D. have? What is the pathogenesis of NEC, and what risk factors for NEC does C.D. have?

NEC, a type of acute intestinal necrosis, is the most common neonatal life-threatening nonrespiratory condition. The incidence of NEC ranges from 3% to 11% and is inversely proportional to gestational age and birth weight.[69] Approximately 90% to 95% of NEC occurs in premature infants; however, NEC can infrequently occur in full-term neonates.[70] The age of onset of NEC is also inversely related to gestational age and birth weight; the greater the gestational age at birth, the sooner the onset of NEC. Although NEC is less common in term infants, it usually develops within 3 to 4 days of birth. In contrast, infants born at approximately 30 weeks' gestation acquire NEC at a mean PNA of 20 days. Thus, preterm infants are at a risk for NEC for a longer time.[71,72] Although C.D. is extremely premature, she experienced NEC early (at 15 days of age), most likely because of the aggressive advancement of feedings. The rate of hospitalization associated with NEC is 1.1 per 1,000 live births.[73] The mortality rate of NEC can be as high as 40% to 50%, and approximately 25% of survivors experience long-term complications.[70,71,73] In addition, infants with NEC required longer hospitalizations (60 days longer if surgery is needed and 20 days longer if surgery is not needed) compared with infants without NEC. For infants with medically managed NEC, the estimated hospital cost is $60,000 to $70,000 compared to $200,000 for infants with surgically managed NEC.[70,74]

C.D. has several clinical signs of NEC, including abdominal distension, bloody stools, apnea, metabolic acidosis, and pneumatosis intestinalis on abdominal radiograph. Gastric retention of feedings, respiratory distress, occult blood in stools, lethargy, temperature instability, thrombocytopenia, and neutropenia also may occur. NEC may progress to bowel perforation, peritonitis, sepsis, disseminated intravascular coagulopathy (DIC), and shock. On an abdominal radiograph, the presence of gas in the intestinal mucosa or in the portal venous system is diagnostic of NEC, and free air in the abdomen is observed with bowel perforation. (For images of NEC go to **https://image.slidesharecdn.com/necrotizingenterocolitis-150719105818-lva1-app6892/95/necrotizing-enterocolitis-8-638.jpg?cb=1437303559**.) Although these radiographic findings confirm the diagnosis of NEC, a lag time may occur between the initial clinical signs of NEC and radiologic confirmation.

NEC can evolve slowly during a period of 24 to 48 hours, from a clinically benign course to an advanced stage of shock, peritonitis, and widespread intestinal necrosis. Although NEC can affect any part of the GI tract, most of the disease is confined to the ileum and colon. A staging system, which categorizes severity according to systemic, intestinal, and radiologic signs, has been developed to permit a more consistent evaluation and treatment of patients.[75] Stages IA and IB NEC include neonates and infants with suspected disease or rule out NEC. These patients may have mild GI problems such as delayed gastric emptying and emesis, temperature instability, apnea, bright red blood from the rectum, or a mild ileus. Infants with stages IIA and IIB have definite NEC and usually present with abdominal distension, bloody stools, and the presence of pneumatosis intestinalis on radiograph. Infants in stage IIB NEC may also exhibit metabolic acidosis and thrombocytopenia. Infants with stages IIIA and IIIB (advanced disease) are severely ill with clinical signs, including peritonitis, ascites, shock, severe metabolic and respiratory acidosis, and DIC. Those with stage IIIB have intestinal perforation. Pneumatosis intestinalis, caused by hydrogen production from bacterial translocation into the bowel wall, is a classic and diagnostic radiographic finding of NEC. Because pneumatosis intestinalis may be hard to detect on radiographs, some infants can experience severe NEC needing surgery without having radiographic findings. Therefore, new criteria including biomarkers of NEC may be needed to help diagnose NEC sooner and prevent its progression. C.D.'s presentation is most consistent with stage IIB NEC.

The pathogenesis of NEC is unknown, but seems to be multifactorial. Most likely, NEC results from the effects of intestinal bacteria and other factors on injured intestinal mucosa. Inflammatory mediators such as platelet-activating factor, tumor necrosis factor-α, interleukin 1β, and interleukin 8 may also contribute to mucosal damage.[70,72] The neonatal intestinal mucosa is prone to injury for the following reasons: (a) increased permeability to potentially harmful substances, such as bacteria and proteins; (b) decreased immunologic host defenses, including low concentrations of immunoglobulin A in intestinal mucosa; and (c) decreased nonimmunologic defenses, such as decreased concentrations of proteases and gastric acid. Furthermore, inappropriate initial microbial colonization may also contribute to the pathogenesis of NEC in preterm neonates, especially because NEC does not occur until after 1 week of life, at a time when the gut has been colonized with anaerobic bacteria. In addition, numerous factors (both prenatal and postnatal) can cause injury to the neonatal intestinal mucosa and increase the risk for NEC.[72,75] Prenatal maternal factors include eclampsia, prolonged rupture of membranes, fetal distress, maternal cocaine use, and cesarean section. Postnatal factors include prematurity, low birth weight, ischemia or hypoxemia, asphyxia, hypothermia, hypotension, respiratory distress, apnea, malnutrition, infection, hemodynamically significant PDA, congenital GI anomalies, cyanotic heart disease, toxins, hyperosmolar substances (e.g., feedings, medications), rapid advancement of enteral feedings, exchange transfusions, blood transfusions, and the presence of umbilical catheters.[72,74,75] Medications such as corticosteroids, indomethacin, and H_2-blockers and prolonged empiric IV antibiotic use have also been associated with an increased risk of NEC.[72,74,75] However, the most significant clinical risk factor for NEC is prematurity.[75]

C.D. has several risks for developing NEC, which include prematurity, ELBW, history of infection, and RDS requiring mechanical ventilation. Furthermore, C.D. not only was given a hyperosmolar formula (24 cal/ounce instead of 20 cal/ounce), but her feedings were advanced aggressively. These two factors may also contribute to the development of NEC. More than 90% of infants with NEC have received enteral feedings, although NEC also occurs in infants who have never been fed.[70] Enteral feedings (breast milk or formulas) serve as substrates for bacterial proliferation in the gut. As a result, reducing substances, organic acids, and hydrogen gas are produced by bacterial fermentation of these nutrients. Although studies have shown that rapid advancements in the volume of feeds (30 mL/kg/day vs. 15–20 mL/kg/day) were associated with an increased risk of NEC, a systematic review reported that infants advanced at a rate of 30 to 35 mL/kg/day reach full enteral intake and regain birth weight significantly earlier than infants advanced at 10 to 20 mL/kg/day without increasing the risk of NEC or NEC with perforation.[73] Similarly, older studies reported that early initiation of feeds might increase the risk of NEC; however, a recent review failed to confirm these findings. In fact, infants who were fed earlier (within 4 days of birth) had a significant reduction in the number of days on parenteral nutrition.[73] C.D. was started at a much higher initial feeding volume (44 mL/kg/day) and aggressively increased by 44 mL/kg/day, which may have increased the risk of NEC. If C.D. were appropriately fed, she would have reached full feedings in 7 to 14 days instead of 4 days. Last, the presence of PDA and the use of indomethacin for the treatment of PDA may also have contributed to NEC in C.D. through decreased mesenteric blood flow with resultant ischemia and intestinal mucosal injury.[71]

Treatment

CASE 105-4, QUESTION 2: How should C.D. be managed?

Significant abdominal distension may compromise respiratory function and blood flow to the intestines. Therefore, as soon as NEC is suspected, feedings should be stopped immediately and an orogastric tube with low intermittent suction placed to decompress the abdomen. C.D.'s vital signs and abdominal circumference should be closely monitored for disease progression. A complete blood count and platelet count should be obtained frequently to monitor for neutropenia and thrombocytopenia. Blood and urine cultures should be obtained, and parenteral antibiotics should be started as soon as possible; 20% to 30% of infants with NEC have associated bacteremia. Radiographic examinations should be routinely performed at least every 4 to 8 hours or as needed to evaluate the progression of the disease. In infants with stage I NEC, antibiotic therapy is usually given for 3 days pending culture results and clinical signs. Once the diagnosis of NEC is ruled out, antibiotics may be discontinued. Enteral feedings can then be initiated slowly. However, if the diagnosis of NEC is made (i.e., stages II or III), antibiotics are continued and parenteral nutrition is initiated at that time. Infants require bowel rest (NPO) for at least 7 to 14 days. The length of antibiotic therapy and bowel rest in infants with documented NEC is determined by the severity of systemic illness (e.g., metabolic acidosis, thrombocytopenia). In general, infants with NEC stage II require at least 7 to 10 days of antibiotic therapy and bowel rest whereas those with NEC stage III may require at least 10 to 14 days. C.D. has stage IIB disease and needs to be NPO for at least 7 to 10 days; she requires total parenteral nutrition during that time, and the surgery team should be notified at this point. Infants with stage III disease may also require fluid resuscitation, administration of inotropic agents such as dopamine and dobutamine, and surgical intervention, especially for those with perforated NEC.[70,71] Up to 40% of infants treated for medically managed NEC may require surgical intervention (either primary peritoneal drainage or exploratory laparotomy), with the absolute indication for surgery being intestinal perforation.[73] Despite the type of surgical intervention, up to 50% of ELBW infants who require surgery will die.[72]

CASE 105-4, QUESTION 3: C.D. just completed a 7-day course of ampicillin and gentamicin. Is it appropriate to restart these antibiotics?

The selection of antibiotics for NEC depends on the common microorganisms observed in an individual neonatal unit and their sensitivities. Many organisms have been implicated in NEC, including Enterobacteriaceae (e.g., *Escherichia coli, Klebsiella* species), *Pseudomonas, Staphylococcus aureus* (in rare cases, methicillin resistant), *Staphylococcus epidermidis, Clostridium,* enteroviruses, and rotaviruses.[76] For most cases of NEC, treatment with a broad-spectrum penicillin, such as ampicillin, and an aminoglycoside (e.g., gentamicin) is appropriate.

Due to an increase in *S. epidermidis*-associated NEC, vancomycin and an aminoglycoside may be used as routine treatment in some nurseries or in specific patients at risk for *Staphylococcus* infections (e.g., neonates with central catheters or prolonged ICU stays). Vancomycin may be more appropriate than ampicillin because vancomycin has coverage against methicillin-resistant *S. epidermidis*, as well as enterococcal and streptococcal species. Because C.D. has been hospitalized for longer than 1 week and weighs less than 1,000 g, vancomycin and gentamicin may be more appropriate, especially if her neonatal ICU has a high incidence of staphylococcal nosocomial infections. C.D. should be treated with parenteral antibiotics for 7 to 10 days.

Other antibiotic combinations used to treat NEC include cefotaxime and vancomycin, and cefotaxime and ampicillin. The combination of cefotaxime and vancomycin has been shown to prevent severe peritonitis and death and reduce the need for surgery in less than 2,200-g birth-weight neonates with NEC, whereas gentamicin and ampicillin have not. Suppression of aerobic fecal flora by the combination of cefotaxime and vancomycin, but not by ampicillin and gentamicin, may explain these findings.[76] Therefore, if C.D. is not responding to vancomycin and gentamicin, consideration should be made to replace gentamicin with cefotaxime.

CASE 105-4, QUESTION 4: Two days later, C.D. exhibits peritonitis with ascites (NEC stage III), hypotension, worsening metabolic acidosis, neutropenia, and DIC. IV fluids and dopamine are administered for the hypotension, fresh-frozen plasma and whole blood are given to treat the coagulopathy, and a fentanyl continuous infusion at 1 mcg/kg/hour is started for pain control. Free air in the abdomen is observed on abdominal radiograph. Blood and urine cultures have had no growth for 48 hours. What additional antimicrobial coverage should be provided?

The use of empiric anaerobic coverage in infants with definite NEC, stage II or III, remains controversial; however, many institutions have added anaerobic coverage to routine antibiotic regimens.[76] The two most commonly used agents are clindamycin and metronidazole. Routine use of clindamycin in the treatment of NEC has not decreased the incidence of intestinal gangrene, perforation, or death. In addition, it has been associated with an increased incidence of abdominal strictures.[76] There are no studies to demonstrate the efficacy of metronidazole in this patient population, but the lack of reports documenting adverse effects in preterm infants has made it the agent of choice in some hospitals. A recent study reported no significant difference in the incidence of the combined outcome of death or intestinal strictures in infants with NEC stages II and III treated with or without anaerobic coverage.[77] Furthermore, anaerobic antibiotic therapy did not prevent the progression to death within 7 days of NEC diagnosis or to surgical NEC. However, a higher risk of strictures was found in all infants receiving anaerobic antibiotic therapy. Furthermore, in those with surgical NEC, a lower mortality rate was found in the anaerobic antibiotic-exposed infants.[77] Based on this study, it might be prudent to consider weighing the risk versus benefit when deciding to add anaerobic antibiotic therapy in the treatment of medically managed NEC. In contrast, infants with peritonitis secondary to intestinal perforation (i.e., those needing surgery) require both aerobic and anaerobic coverage. Therefore, an antimicrobial agent with anaerobic activity such as metronidazole should be added to C.D.'s current regimen.

Complications and Prognosis

CASE 105-4, QUESTION 5: C.D. is taken urgently to the operating room, and 40 cm of necrotic ileum is removed along with the ileocecal valve. What long-term nutritional problems is C.D. likely to have?

The most common postoperative complications of NEC are intestinal strictures (up to 25%) and short-bowel syndrome (11%).[70]

C.D. is at risk of experiencing short-bowel syndrome, a condition of malabsorption and malnutrition that results from surgical removal of a significant portion of the small intestine. The most important factors that determine short-bowel syndrome are the length of the remaining small intestine and the presence of the ileocecal valve. Because C.D. has had a majority of her ileum and her ileocecal valve removed, she most likely will suffer from short-bowel syndrome.

Because the terminal ileum is an important site for absorption of vitamins, trace minerals, and nutrients, C.D. will be at risk for decreased absorption of these substances. C.D. also will have a faster GI transit time and diarrhea because her ileocecal valve was removed. (The ileocecal valve plays a major role in controlling intestinal transit time.) Absorption of enterally administered medications also may be decreased in patients with short-bowel syndrome. When C.D. starts to receive most of her nutrition enterally, she should be monitored for fat malabsorption and other nutritional deficiencies (e.g., deficiencies in vitamins A, B_{12}, D, E, and K), and supplemented accordingly.

Despite advances in earlier diagnosis and aggressive treatment, approximately 15% to 50% of all infants with NEC die, with the highest mortality in those with birth weight <750 g and with surgical NEC.[69,70,74,75] Furthermore, infants with NEC are significantly more likely to have neurodevelopmental impairment (e.g., CP); those requiring surgical management are at higher risk.[73]

Prevention

CASE 105-4, QUESTION 6: What could have been done to prevent NEC in C.D.?

Several interventions may decrease the incidence of NEC. Enteral feedings in preterm infants can be withheld for several weeks and parenteral nutrition initiated. Intestinal priming or trophic feeding (i.e., using a small amount of full-strength formula or breast milk for several days to stimulate GI mucosal development) has been shown to decrease the incidence of NEC compared with infants with advancement of feedings.[73] Because breast milk provides antibodies, growth factors, and cellular immune factors, it may reduce the incidence of NEC. Infants fed with human milk had a significantly lower incidence of NEC than those fed with formula.[74,75] In a recent study, a significant decrease in the incidence of NEC and surgical NEC was observed in infants who were exclusively fed with a human milk-based diet compared with a combination of human milk- and formula-based diets.[74] In contrast, the use of hyperosmolar formulas or medications can cause osmotic injury to the bowel and may result in NEC. Maternal steroids (commonly used to accelerate fetal lung maturation) can decrease the incidence of NEC owing to a maturational effect on the microvillous membranes.

Although prophylactic enteral administration of antibiotics (i.e., gentamicin or vancomycin) has been shown to decrease the incidence of NEC, its routine use is not recommended.[74] In addition, prophylactic use of these antibiotics has been associated with the emergence of resistant organisms, especially with long and repeated courses.[72,74]

Probiotics are live, nonpathogenic microbial preparations that colonize the intestine and have a beneficial effect on the health of the host. Probiotic microorganisms commonly used are strains of *Lactobacillus* and *Bifidobacterium*. In a recent Cochrane review, enteral administration of probiotics significantly decreased the risk of severe NEC and death and shortened the time to full feedings in VLBW infants.[78] Furthermore, recent studies evaluating the long-term effects of probiotics (assessed at 18–22 months up to 3 years corrected age) reported no adverse effects on growth or neurodevelopmental outcomes.[78] One major concern is that exposing immunologically immature VLBW infants to probiotics may potentially increase the risk for infections. Although the Cochrane review did not find an increased risk for infections in neonates receiving probiotics, cases of systemic infections, especially in ELBW neonates, have been reported.[78] The lack of probiotic-associated sepsis could be due to failure of the laboratory to isolate these strains in blood cultures by the use of conventional culture-based techniques. Other controversies exist. Most studies did not evaluate the effects of probiotics in ELBW infants, the population at greatest risk for NEC. The optimal type of probiotic (species, strains, single or combined, live or killed) and the timing, dosage, and duration of therapy are still unknown. Little is known regarding the benefits of probiotics in infants who are exclusively or partially fed breast milk. Furthermore, none of the studies were conducted in the United States and most of the trials did not utilize US commercially available probiotics. Lastly, currently no product in the United States has the appropriate regulatory mechanisms in place to ensure the quality of the product. Therefore, clinical studies are needed to address these issues, and if probiotics are administered to VLBW infants for the prevention of NEC, careful surveillance of mortality, NEC, and emergence of resistant strains will be necessary. When C.D. is ready to be fed, breast milk (if available) should be used in place of formula to help prevent future risk of NEC. Although probiotics have been shown to significantly decrease the incidence of NEC, their use cannot be recommended for C.D. at this time.

NEONATAL SEPSIS AND MENINGITIS

CASE 105-5

QUESTION 1: J.E., a 28-week gestation, 850-g male, was born to a mother with prolonged rupture of membranes (>72 hours). The newborn's mother is diagnosed with chorioamnionitis. J.E. had Apgar scores of 3 at 1 minute, 4 at 5 minutes, and 7 at 10 minutes after birth. Mechanical ventilation was instituted, and J.E. was admitted to the neonatal ICU. Vital signs on admission were as follows:

HR, 190 beats/minute
Temperature, 35.8°C
BP, 56/33 mm Hg

Blood and urine cultures are pending. Significant laboratory data include the following:

WBC 2,400 cells/μL with a differential of 25% segmented neutrophils, 15% bands, 45% lymphocytes, 10% monocytes, 4% eosinophils, and 1% basophils
Platelets, 45,000/μL
C-reactive protein (CRP), 5 mg/dL

What is the etiology and pathogenesis of neonatal sepsis? What risk factors for sepsis does J.E. have? What clinical signs and laboratory evidence of sepsis are apparent in J.E.?

Bacterial sepsis significantly contributes to neonatal morbidity and mortality. Neonates, especially preterm newborns, are at increased risk for infections and should be considered immunocompromised. The neonate's decreased immune function (e.g., immature function of neutrophils, lower amounts of immunoglobulin) also results in a reduced ability to localize infections. Once a tissue site becomes infected, bacteria can spread easily, resulting in disseminated disease. In addition, the lack of opsonic antibodies in preterm infants such as J.E. increases the susceptibility to infections caused by bacteria with polysaccharide capsules (e.g., group B streptococcus, *E. coli, Haemophilus influenzae* type B).[79]

The incidence of neonatal sepsis is inversely proportional to birth weight and gestational age, and ranges from 6 to 9 cases per 1,000 live births. However, the incidence is much higher in VLBW neonates (~25%).[80] Risk factors (as demonstrated in J.E.) include prematurity, low birth weight, male sex, and predisposing maternal conditions (e.g., prolonged rupture of membranes, maternal fever, elevated maternal WBC or left shift, chorioamnionitis, and urinary tract infection).[81,82] Despite treatment, mortality rates for neonatal sepsis can be as high as 30% to 50%, with the highest mortality observed in newborns less than 1,500 g.[83] Meningitis occurs as a complication of bacterial sepsis in 10% to 30% of septic neonates[83] and has a mortality rate of 20% to 50%, depending on the pathogen.[81] Long-term sequelae of meningitis have been reported in about 20% to 60% of survivors and include hearing loss, abnormal behavior, developmental delay, cerebral palsy, focal motor disability, seizure disorders, and hydrocephalus.[79,84]

Common Pathogens

The fetal environment within the amniotic membranes is normally sterile until the onset of labor and delivery. Once the membranes are ruptured, the infant may be at risk for colonization of microorganisms from the maternal genital tract. Many of these organisms do not cause infection in the mother, but may be detrimental to the infant. Early-onset neonatal sepsis (sepsis that presents during the first 72 hours of life) usually is caused by organisms acquired from the maternal genital tract. The most common pathogens found in early-onset neonatal sepsis are group B streptococcus (50%) and *E. coli* (20%). Other primary pathogens include *Listeria monocytogenes, Enterococcus,* and other gram-negative bacilli (e.g., *H. influenzae, Klebsiella pneumoniae*).[84,85]

Late-onset sepsis (sepsis presenting after 3 days' PNA) usually is caused by these primary organisms or by nosocomial pathogens, such as coagulase-negative staphylococci (CONS), particularly *S. epidermidis, S. aureus, Pseudomonas* species, anaerobes, and *Candida* species.[84,86] The presence of IV catheters (umbilical or central) and duration of parenteral hyperalimentation are major risk factors for nosocomial septicemia.[86,87] Other risk factors include prematurity, low birth weight, prolonged hospital stay, prior antibiotic use, lipid emulsion, use of H_2-blockers, invasive procedures, GI disease (including NEC), the presence of other indwelling devices (e.g., ETTs, ventriculoperitoneal shunts), and nasal CPAP.[80,87] Seventy percent of late-onset sepsis in VLBW infants is caused by gram-positive organisms, with CONS being the most common pathogen (68%); *S. aureus, Enterococcus* species, and group B streptococcus account for the remainder.[88] Clinically, before continuation of antibiotic therapy, it is important to distinguish whether patient isolates of CONS are the result of colonization of the catheters or IV tubing or represent true bacteremia.

Neonatal sepsis may present with nonspecific or subtle signs, especially in VLBW infants.[81] The most common signs are poor feeding, temperature instability, lethargy, or apnea.[81,83] Other signs of neonatal sepsis include glucose instability (hypoglycemia or hyperglycemia), tachycardia, dyspnea or cyanosis, tachypnea, diarrhea, vomiting, feeding intolerance, abdominal distension, metabolic acidosis, and abnormal WBC.[81] Clinical signs and laboratory evidence of neonatal sepsis observed in J.E. include tachycardia (HR, 190 beats/minute), hypothermia (temperature 35.8°C), leukopenia (WBC, $2.4 \times 10^3/\mu L$), neutropenia (absolute neutrophil count of $960/\mu L$), a left shift in the differential (i.e., an immature-to-total neutrophil ratio [I/T] of 0.38), thrombocytopenia (platelets, $45{,}000/\mu L$), and an elevated CRP (5 mg/dL). Hypothermia is more common than fever in neonatal sepsis, especially in preterm newborns. However, if fever is present, it is strongly associated with bacterial infection. Neutropenia, especially with a left shift (as seen in J.E.), can be a sign of WBC depletion from bone marrow owing to overwhelming sepsis. An elevated WBC also can indicate a neonatal infection, but may be less specific. The I/T ratio, defined as band forms plus any earlier cells divided by the total neutrophil count (including early cells), has been shown to be useful in diagnosing neonatal sepsis. An I/T ratio of less than 0.3 is normal.[82] CRP, an acute-phase reactant protein associated with tissue injury in response to an inflammatory process, may also be included as part of a sepsis workup. A CRP level of more than 1 mg/dL indicates inflammation and possible infection.[82] In infants with bacterial infection, serum CRP levels begin to increase from 6 to 8 hours after the onset of the illness and peak after 2 to 3 days.[89] Therefore, because of the delayed response, the use of CRP for detection of early-onset sepsis is not of great value. Serial CRP levels obtained during 2 to 3 days of illness may aid in the determination of duration of empiric antibiotic therapy. Empiric antibiotic therapy may be discontinued in infants with normal serial CRP levels in the absence of any clinical signs suggestive of sepsis. However, elevated CRP levels can be found in other clinical conditions such as viral infection, ischemic tissue injuries, hemolysis, or chorioamnionitis. Procalcitonin, another acute-phase reactant, rises more quickly than CRP in the presence of bacteria so it may be more useful for early detection. However, there are also limitations to its routine use for the evaluation of neonatal sepsis including nonspecificity (i.e., noninfectious conditions can cause elevation of procalcitonin levels) and a lack of age-specific reference ranges.[89] Therefore, CRP and procalcitonin levels should be used with caution as the sole diagnostic criteria for sepsis or bacteremia. Late signs of neonatal infection include jaundice, hepatosplenomegaly, and petechiae.[81] A bulging fontanel, posturing, or seizures indicate meningitis, although these CNS signs are not always present when meningitis exists.

Bacterial meningitis should always be considered in infants with neonatal sepsis.[79] The major pathogens causing neonatal sepsis are also the primary pathogens that cause neonatal meningitis.[83] The definitive diagnostic method for bacterial meningitis is lumbar puncture. Lumbar puncture should be performed in infants with a positive blood culture, abnormal neurologic signs, an elevated WBC or left shift, or the presence of bacteria in the urine.[90] A lumbar puncture is not needed in neonates receiving empiric antibiotics solely because of maternal risk factors.[89] However, it is important to note that a negative blood culture does not dictate the absence of bacterial meningitis. Approximately 1 of every 4,000 live births has culture-proven bacterial meningitis, and 15% to 50% of infants with bacterial meningitis may have a negative blood culture.[89] The cerebrospinal fluid (CSF) should be tested with a Gram stain, cell counts with differential, glucose and protein levels, and bacterial culture. Normal CSF cell counts and protein concentrations are different for neonates compared with older children and adults. For example, the CSF protein concentration in a healthy neonate is about 2 to 3 times that of an adult and decreases with age; preterm infants may have higher levels.[79] Neonatal CSF cell counts are also difficult to interpret because values observed with meningitis may overlap with normal neonatal values. The diagnosis of neonatal sepsis is confirmed by isolation of the pathogen from blood, urine, CSF, or other body sites.

Treatment of Sepsis and Meningitis

CASE 105-5, QUESTION 2: What antibiotic regimen should be prescribed for J.E.?

Empiric treatment with appropriate IV antibiotics must be initiated immediately in J.E. Significant morbidity or fatality would occur if antibiotics were withheld until a diagnosis was confirmed by culture results (in 24–72 hours). This is especially true in patients

Table 105-3

Gentamicin Dosing Guidelines for Neonates and Infants[2,96]

Age	Extended-Interval Dosing Regimen[a]
PMA <32 weeks	4–5 mg/kg/dose every 36–48 hours
PMA 32–36 weeks	4–5 mg/kg/dose every 36 hours
PMA ≥37 weeks	4–5 mg/kg/dose every 24 hours

[a]Some institutions empirically adjust dosing interval based on clinical factors that may affect renal drug clearance (e.g., birth depression, hypotension requiring vasopressor support, or congenital heart defects resulting in decreased peripheral perfusion).
PMA, postmenstrual age.

in whom meningitis is suspected. The initial empiric antibiotic treatment of choice for early-onset neonatal sepsis and meningitis is ampicillin plus an aminoglycoside (Tables 105-3, 105-4).[2,91–93] These antibiotics are used because they (a) are bactericidal against the common neonatal pathogens; (b) penetrate into the CNS; (c) are relatively safe; and (d) have proven clinical efficacy. If the culture is positive for group B streptococcus, ampicillin should be replaced with high-dose penicillin G because of its higher activity against group B streptococcus. If meningitis is highly suspected, gentamicin may be replaced by a third-generation cephalosporin (i.e., cefotaxime) owing to greater CSF penetration compared with aminoglycosides.

Therefore, ampicillin 85 mg every 12 hours IV plus an aminoglycoside (e.g., gentamicin 4.2 mg every 48 hours IV) should be started in J.E. for suspected neonatal sepsis and possible meningitis. Meningitic doses of ampicillin should be used in J.E. until meningitis can be ruled out. Ampicillin is active against group B streptococci, *Enterococcus*, *Listeria*, and some strains of *E. coli*. Aminoglycoside antibiotics (e.g., gentamicin or tobramycin) usually are active against gram-negative bacilli. In addition, aminoglycosides may provide synergy with ampicillin against *Listeria* and group B streptococci.[82] Selection of the specific aminoglycoside should be determined by antibiotic resistance patterns within the neonatal ICU. Amikacin should be reserved for gram-negative organisms resistant to gentamicin and tobramycin. Aminoglycoside regimens need to be designed to achieve safe and therapeutic serum concentrations (traditional dosing regimens: gentamicin and tobramycin, peak 6–8 mcg/mL, trough <2 mcg/mL; amikacin peak 20–30 mcg/mL, trough <10 mcg/mL) and to aim for a peak concentration that is more than 8 times greater than the minimum inhibitory concentration (MIC) of the organism being treated.[94] If extended-interval aminoglycoside dosing is used, peak gentamicin and tobramycin serum concentrations of 10 to 12 mcg/mL and trough concentrations of less than 1 mcg/mL may be reasonable, depending on the MIC.

Traditionally, aminoglycosides were administered to neonates in multiple daily doses (e.g., gentamicin 2.5 mg/kg/dose 2 or 3 times a day). This dosing strategy frequently resulted in peak serum concentrations below and trough concentrations above the respective target ranges especially in preterm neonates. Evolution of the understanding of developmental pharmacokinetics resulted in knowledge that neonates have a larger volume of distribution for water-soluble drugs and a slower renal elimination of aminoglycosides compared to infants, older children, and adults.[95] Thus, many institutions now use higher mg/kg doses of aminoglycosides (e.g., gentamicin 4–5 mg/kg) administered at prolonged dosing

Table 105-4

Antimicrobial Dosage Regimens for Neonates: Dosages and Intervals of Administration[2,91–93]

	Weight <1,200 g	Weight 1,200–2,000 g		Weight >2,000 g	
Drug	0–4 weeks PNA (mg/kg)[a]	0–7 days PNA (mg/kg)[a]	8–28 days PNA (mg/kg)[a]	0–7 days PNA (mg/kg)[a]	8–28 days PNA (mg/kg)[a]
Amphotericin B					
Deoxycholate	1 every 24 hours	1 every 24 hours	1 every 24 hours	1 every 24 hours	1 every 24 hours
Lipid complex/Liposomal	5 every 24 hours	5 every 24 hours	5 every 24 hours	5 every 24 hours	5 every 24 hours
Ampicillin					
Meningitis	100 every 12 hours	100 every 8 hours	75 every 6 hours	100 every 8 hours	75 every 6 hours
Other diseases	50 every 12 hours	50 every 12 hours	50 every 8 hours	50 every 8 hours	50 every 6 hours
Cefotaxime[b]	50 every 12 hours	50 every 12 hours	50 every 8 hours	50 every 12 hours	50 every 8 hours
Fluconazole	6 every 72 hours	12 every 24 hours	12 every 24 hours	12 every 24 hours	12 every 24 hours
Metronidazole	7.5 every 48 hours	7.5 every 24 hours	15 every 24 hours	15 every 24 hours	15 every 12 hours
Oxacillin/Nafcillin[b]	25 every 12 hours	25 every 12 hours	25 every 8 hours	25 every 8 hours	25 every 6 hours
Penicillin G crystalline					
Meningitis[c]	50,000 units every 12 hours	100,000 units every 12 hours	100,000 units every 8 hours	100,000 units every 8 hours	100,000 units every 6 hours
Other diseases	25,000–50,000 units every 12 hours	25,000–50,000 units every 12 hours	25,000–50,000 units every 8 hours	25,000–50,000 units every 12 hours	25,000–50,000 units every 8 hours
Vancomycin	15 every 24 hours	15 every 12–18 hours	15 every 8–12 hours	15 every 8–12 hours	15 every 6–8 hours

[a]PNA = postnatal age.
[b]Higher dosage may be needed for meningitis.
[c]Doses listed are for treatment of group B streptococcal meningitis.

intervals (every 24, 36, or 48 hours; commonly determined by GA or PMA).[96,97] A Cochrane review concluded that administering higher mg/kg aminoglycoside doses at prolonged intervals to neonates was as effective as multiple daily doses without evidence of increased toxicity. Serum peak and trough concentrations also were more likely to be in the target range.[98]

This dosing strategy (of giving higher mg/kg/doses at prolonged intervals) in neonates is commonly referred to as extended-interval aminoglycoside dosing; however, it should not be confused with the adult dosing method of the same name.[95] Extended-interval aminoglycoside dosing (also known in adults as once-daily dosing or single-daily dosing) has been widely used in the adult population. Aminoglycoside antibiotics display concentration-dependent killing of bacteria. Rationale for the use of extended-interval aminoglycoside dosing include (a) enhancement of bacterial killing by providing a higher peak serum concentration to MIC ratio, (b) provision of a prolonged post-antibiotic effect, and (c) minimization of adaptive postexposure microbial resistance by achieving a drug-free period at the end of the dosing interval.[99] Key differences between this approach to aminoglycoside dosing in adults and the use of higher mg/kg doses given at prolonged intervals to neonates include the following: (a) Peak concentrations of ~20 to 25 mcg/mL are targeted in adults compared to 8 to 12 mcg/mL in neonates, (b) a drug-free period occurs at the end of the dosing interval in adults, while acceptably low, but measurable trough concentrations are commonly observed in neonates, and (c) a standardized dosing nomogram allows for interval adjustments based on a single serum concentration (drawn 8–12 hours postdose) in adults; however, routine peak and trough concentration monitoring is recommended for neonates.[95,99,100]

In some nurseries, a third-generation cephalosporin (e.g., cefotaxime), instead of an aminoglycoside, is added to ampicillin for initial empiric treatment of early-onset neonatal sepsis and meningitis.[80,87,94] The spectrum of activity of these third-generation cephalosporins includes many gram-negative organisms and group B streptococci. Ceftriaxone should be avoided in neonates with hyperbilirubinemia owing to bilirubin displacement from albumin-binding sites. Ceftriaxone has also been associated with sludging in the gallbladder and cholestasis.[2,94] The resultant increase in serum free bilirubin concentrations and decrease in bilirubin elimination can place the neonate at risk for kernicterus. In addition, calcium–ceftriaxone precipitates have been found in the lungs and kidneys of neonates when ceftriaxone was administered with calcium-containing solutions. Several fatalities have been reported; ceftriaxone should not be administered within 48 hours of calcium-containing solutions or products.[94] Hence, cefotaxime is the preferred cephalosporin for neonatal use.

The third-generation cephalosporins have advantages over the aminoglycosides, including better CNS penetration, the elimination of serum concentration measurements, and less nephrotoxicity. However, these cephalosporins do not significantly improve clinical or microbiologic end points compared with the standard ampicillin and gentamicin regimen. In fact, overuse of cefotaxime during the first few days of life has been associated with an increased risk of death compared with the use of gentamicin.[94] Furthermore, extensive use of the third-generation cephalosporins in neonatal ICUs may lead to rapid emergence of resistant gram-negative bacilli (e.g., *Enterobacter cloacae, Pseudomonas aeruginosa,* and *Serratia* species) and vancomycin resistance in enterococci. Also, prolonged treatment has been associated with an increased risk of neonatal candidiasis.[94] In contrast, only rare cases of gentamicin resistance have been reported.[80] Thus, combinations such as ampicillin and cefotaxime should be reserved for the following situations: (a) neonatal ICUs in which aminoglycoside resistance to gram-negative enteric bacilli is of concern, (b) neonatal ICUs in which serum concentrations of aminoglycosides cannot be measured, and (c) specific neonates in whom aminoglycoside therapy could be of concern (e.g., neonates with known renal failure).

Therapy for late-onset sepsis or meningitis is directed toward nosocomial pathogens plus the primary pathogens of early-onset infection. Selection of initial antibiotic therapy should consider the specific neonatal ICU's nosocomial pathogen and antibiotic resistance patterns, as well as the neonate's risk factors, clinical condition, and previous antibiotic therapy. CONS is now the most common pathogen of late-onset neonatal nosocomial septicemia.[101] Because of the high incidence of methicillin-resistant CONS, vancomycin has been used as the drug of choice for empiric therapy for suspected late-onset neonatal sepsis. However, widespread use of vancomycin has led to the emergence of vancomycin-resistant *Enterococcus* and *S. aureus.* Therefore, the routine use of vancomycin as empiric therapy for nosocomial neonatal sepsis should be discouraged. The highly selective use of vancomycin for neonatal CONS septicemia results in low morbidity and mortality, while significantly reducing vancomycin use. Guidelines for the selective use of vancomycin should be tailored according to individual neonatal ICU's nosocomial pathogens, susceptibility patterns, and patient risk factors, clinical condition, and antibiotic history. Therefore, if J.E. had a central venous catheter and presented with a late-onset sepsis, initial antibiotic therapy should include an aminoglycoside (for gram-negative coverage) plus either an antistaphylococcal penicillin (e.g., nafcillin, methicillin) or vancomycin (for activity against *S. aureus* and *S. epidermidis*). Vancomycin is used in place of the antistaphylococcal penicillin in neonatal units with methicillin-resistant *S. aureus* and for selective use to cover *S. epidermidis* (a CONS) as outlined.[101]

For systemic fungal infections, amphotericin B is considered the initial treatment of choice.[83] Because of the high incidence of *Candida* species colonization (up to 60%), with up to 20% progressing to invasive fungal infections in VLBW infants, prophylactic fluconazole may be used to prevent *Candida* colonization and infection in these infants.[102] Infants of 27 weeks' gestational age or less and weighing less than 1,000 g benefited most from prophylactic fluconazole. Despite potential benefits, routine use of prophylactic fluconazole is not recommended and should be reserved for those units with a high incidence of fungal infections. Because uncommon organisms are not suspected in J.E., the regimen of ampicillin 85 mg IV every 12 hours plus gentamicin 4.2 mg IV every 48 hours is appropriate.

Once a pathogen is isolated, the antimicrobial susceptibilities should be evaluated and the drug therapy modified appropriately. Blood, CSF, or urine cultures should be repeated to document bacterial sterilization after 24 to 48 hours of appropriate therapy. J.E. should be evaluated carefully for the development of serious bacterial complications such as meningitis, osteomyelitis, abscess formation, or endocarditis.

DURATION OF THERAPY

As long as there is no evidence of meningitis or other focal infection (e.g., abscess formation), the duration of therapy for most systemic bacterial infections is 7 to 10 days (or approximately 5–7 days after significant clinical improvement). Antibiotic therapy may need to be continued for 14 to 21 days if the neonate's clinical response is slow or if multiple organ systems are involved.[84] If cultures are negative at 48 hours and the infant does not have any clinical or laboratory signs of sepsis, antibiotics can be discontinued. In neonates presenting with signs of severe infection followed by improvement after initiation of antibiotics, therapy may be continued despite negative cultures.[85]

If CSF cultures are positive, repeat CSF cultures should be obtained daily or every other day in J.E. to document when the CSF becomes sterilized. The duration of therapy for neonatal meningitis depends on the clinical response and duration of positive CSF cultures after therapy is initiated. Appropriate antibiotics should be continued for a minimum of 14 days after the CSF is sterilized. This is equivalent to a duration of antibiotic therapy for a minimum of 21 days for gram-negative organisms and at least 14 days for gram-positive pathogens.[81,83] As a general rule, it takes longer to sterilize the CSF of neonates infected by gram-negative enteric bacilli (72 hours) than those infected by gram-positive bacteria (36–48 hours).[81]

CONGENITAL INFECTIONS

TORCH Titers

CASE 105-6

QUESTION 1: S.Y., a 2,000-g female, was born at 34 weeks' gestational age by vaginal delivery. S.Y.'s birth was complicated by prolonged rupture of membranes (>72 hours), and fetal distress requiring a fetal scalp monitor. On physical examination, S.Y. is an extremely irritable newborn with a RR of 60 breaths/minute. Several vesicular skin lesions located on the scalp and around the eyes are noted. Conjunctivitis is also present. S.Y. is placed on supplemental oxygen, and ABGs are obtained. Blood, CSF, and urine were cultured for bacteria and fungus, and S.Y. was started on ampicillin 200 mg IV every 12 hours and gentamicin 9 mg IV every 36 hours to rule out sepsis. Antimicrobial therapy will not be altered until culture results are available. What other tests and information are needed for S.Y. at this time?

Certain bacteria, viruses, and protozoa can cause fetal infections that may result in fetal death, congenital anomalies, serious CNS sequelae, intrauterine growth retardation, or preterm birth.[99] The primary organisms that cause these infections can be remembered by the acronym, TORCH: toxoplasmosis; other (i.e., syphilis, gonorrhea, hepatitis B, listeria); rubella; cytomegalovirus; and herpes simplex. Because of the potential severity of these diseases, newborns who display any signs of infection (e.g., irritability, fever, thrombocytopenia, hepatosplenomegaly) need to be evaluated for these intrauterine and perinatally acquired infections. The diagnosis of each of these infections should be considered separately. A complete infectious disease workup should include specific antibody titer measurements or polymerase chain reaction (PCR) to the suspected organisms rather than sending a single serum sample for TORCH titer measurement.[103]

Primary clinical manifestations and treatment for selected congenital infections are listed in Table 105-5.[2,84,103–106] The clinical signs of these infections may overlap, and concurrent infection with two or more microorganisms is possible. The detection of congenital infections often is difficult because many neonates are asymptomatic at birth. Therefore, prenatal maternal screening and accurate evaluation of maternal history for risk factors are very important. Other organisms that can cause congenitally acquired infections include human immunodeficiency virus, human parvovirus, varicella-zoster virus, and measles virus.[103]

When congenital infections are suspected, appropriate diagnostic tests for each suspected organism should be performed. Viral cultures of the urine, oropharynx, nasopharynx, stool, and

Table 105-5

Selected Congenital and Perinatal Infections in the Neonate[2,84,103–106]

Organism	Primary Clinical Manifestations	Treatment of Proven or Highly Probable Disease[a]
Herpes simplex	Cutaneous vesicles, keratoconjunctivitis, microcephaly, CNS infection, hepatitis, pneumonitis, prematurity, respiratory distress, sepsis, convulsion, chorioretinitis	Acyclovir *Ocular involvement:* Add topical therapy: 1%–2% trifluridine, 1% iododeoxyuridine, or 3% vidarabine
Toxoplasmosis	Chorioretinitis, ventriculomegaly, microcephaly, hydrocephaly, intracranial calcifications, ascites, hepatosplenomegaly, lymphadenopathy, jaundice, anemia, mental retardation	Sulfadiazine *and* pyrimethamine *and* leucovorin (folinic acid)
Treponema pallidum	*Early:* Osteochondritis, periostitis, hepatosplenomegaly, skin rash (maculopapular or vesiculobullous), rhinitis, meningitis, IUGR, jaundice, hepatitis, anemia, thrombocytopenia, chorioretinitis *Late:* Hutchinson triad (interstitial keratitis, VIIIth-nerve deafness, Hutchinson teeth), mental retardation, hydrocephalus, saddle nose, mulberry molars	Aqueous crystalline penicillin G
Hepatitis B	Prematurity; usually asymptomatic; long-term effects include chronic hepatitis, cirrhosis, liver failure, hepatocellular carcinoma	*Perinatal exposure (maternal HbsAg-positive):* HBIG and hepatitis B vaccine
Rubella	*Early:* IUGR, retinopathy, hypotonia, hepatosplenomegaly, thrombocytopenic purpura, bone lesions, cardiac effects *Late:* Hearing loss, mental retardation, diabetes *Rare:* Myocarditis, glaucoma, microcephaly, hepatitis, anemia	Supportive care
Cytomegalovirus	Petechiae, hepatosplenomegaly, jaundice, prematurity, IUGR, increased liver enzymes, hyperbilirubinemia, anemia, thrombocytopenia, interstitial pneumonitis, microcephaly, chorioretinitis, intracranial calcifications *Late:* Hearing loss, mental retardation, learning and motor abnormalities, visual disturbances	Ganciclovir
Neisseria gonorrhoeae	Ophthalmia neonatorum, scalp abscess, sepsis, arthritis, meningitis, endocarditis	Ceftriaxone Use cefotaxime if hyperbilirubinemic

[a]See references 2 and 84 for dosing and recommended treatment duration.
CNS, central nervous system; HBIG, hepatitis B immune globulin; HbsAg, hepatitis B surface antigen; IUGR, intrauterine growth retardation.

conjunctiva, and a complete maternal history along with the results of recent maternal vaginal cultures also should be obtained.[103] Measurements of immunoglobulin M levels specific for each possible organism under consideration are also recommended. S.Y. has signs of a congenital infection (respiratory distress, skin rash, and conjunctivitis). Because of the nature of S.Y.'s skin rash (i.e., vesicular), infection with the herpes simplex virus (HSV) should be highly suspected. Skin vesicles, conjunctiva, oropharynx, nasopharynx, rectum, urine, and CSF should be cultured for HSV and other organisms known to cause congenital infections. Rapid diagnostic testing using tissue scrapings from vesicles and fluorescein-conjugated monoclonal HSV antibody can also be performed. Other appropriate tests for the diagnosis and workup of suspected congenital infections should also be performed (e.g., liver enzymes, prothrombin time, partial thromboplastin time, electroencephalogram [EEG], computed tomography scan, or magnetic resonance imaging).[103]

APNEA OF PREMATURITY

Apnea in neonates is a life-threatening condition that occurs more frequently in premature newborns and newborns of lower birth weights. Only 7% of infants of 34 to 35 weeks' gestational age have apnea.[107] In contrast, the incidence of apnea has been reported to be 78% in infants of 26 to 27 weeks' gestational age and 84% in infants with birth weights less than 1,000 g.[108] Although several definitions exist, clinically significant apnea may be defined as cessation of breathing for at least 15 seconds, or less, if accompanied by bradycardia (HR $<$100 beats/minute), significant hypoxemia, or cyanosis.[107,109,110] Pallor or hypotonia also may occur.

In neonates, apnea may be caused by a severe underlying illness (e.g., infection, metabolic disorders, intracranial pathology), drugs, or prematurity itself.[110] Appropriate patient history, physical examination, and laboratory tests must be evaluated to rule out other causes of apnea before the diagnosis of apnea of prematurity can be made.[109] It is especially important to rule out sepsis before apnea of prematurity is presumed. If an etiology other than prematurity is identified, therapy would be directed toward that specific cause. For example, antibiotics are used to treat neonatal sepsis with secondary apnea.

Apnea of prematurity is classified into three types: central, obstructive, and mixed. Approximately 40% of apneic episodes are of central origin (i.e., no respiratory effort), 10% are caused by obstruction, and 50% are attributable to both (i.e., mixed events).[109] Although these terms imply separate mechanisms, obstruction and airway closure may be important in all three types (even "central"). Treatment of apnea of prematurity includes the use of supplemental oxygen, gentle tactile stimulation, environmental temperature control, methylxanthines, nasal CPAP, and positive-pressure ventilation.

CASE 105-7

QUESTION 1: S.M., a premature male newborn of 29 weeks' gestational age, had a birth weight of 995 g. On day 2 of life, he experienced seven episodes of apnea followed by bradycardia with HR as low as 85 beats/minute. These episodes lasted 20 to 30 seconds and required administration of oxygen and tactile stimulation. Three prolonged episodes required bag-and-mask ventilation. Between apneic spells, the newborn seemed well; physical examination and laboratory tests were normal for gestational age. Appropriate cultures were drawn for a septic workup, and ampicillin and gentamicin were initiated. How should S.M.'s apnea be managed?

Methylxanthines, specifically caffeine and theophylline (or aminophylline), are widely accepted as the initial pharmacologic approach for the treatment of idiopathic apnea of prematurity.[107,109] These agents decrease apneic episodes via both central and peripheral effects. Methylxanthines stimulate the medullary respiratory center and increase receptor responsiveness to carbon dioxide. This results in an increase in respiratory drive and minute ventilation. Central stimulatory effects may be mediated by adenosine receptor blockade. Adenosine is a known inhibitor of respiration, and both theophylline and caffeine competitively inhibit adenosine at the receptor level.[107] Peripherally, methylxanthines increase diaphragmatic contractility, decrease diaphragmatic fatigue, and improve respiratory muscle contraction. In addition, methylxanthines increase catecholamine release and metabolic rate. This may improve cardiac output and oxygenation, lessen hypoxic episodes, and decrease apneic spells.

Methylxanthine therapy generally is initiated for apnea of prematurity when apneic episodes are frequent, prolonged for 20 seconds or greater, are accompanied by significant bradycardia or cyanosis, or are not controlled by nonpharmacologic means. S.M. has had prolonged apneas with bradycardia that have required supplemental oxygenation. Initiation of a methylxanthine would be appropriate at this point.

CASE 105-7, QUESTION 2: On rounds, the NICU medical team asks you how does caffeine compare with theophylline with regard to its pharmacokinetics, efficacy, and toxicity? What treatment and dose should be selected for S.M.? How do you reply to the team?

The plasma clearance of caffeine is considerably lower, and the half-life is extremely prolonged in the premature newborn (72–96 hours).[2] The low clearance is a reflection of the decreased neonatal hepatic metabolism and a resultant dependence of elimination on the slow urinary excretion.[111] As a result, caffeine can be dosed once daily (every 24 hours) in the neonate. The half-life of caffeine decreases with increasing PMA,[112] and plasma clearance reaches adult levels after 3 to 4.5 months of life.[113] As a result of the maturational changes, doses usually need to be adjusted after 38 weeks' PMA; however, most infants no longer require treatment of apnea beyond 36 weeks' PMA.

Protein binding of theophylline is decreased in term newborns compared with adults.[114] The decreased protein binding along with an increased tissue distribution results in a larger volume of distribution of theophylline in neonates. This larger volume of distribution results in larger loading-dose requirements to attain similar serum concentrations. Like caffeine, theophylline clearance in preterm newborns is much slower than that observed in young children of 1 to 4 years of age.[114] As a result, smaller theophylline maintenance doses are required in neonates. Theophylline clearance and therefore maintenance doses increase with increasing PMA. Adjustment of maintenance doses is especially important in infants at 40 to 50 weeks' PMA when the greatest maturational changes in theophylline clearance occur.[115]

In adults, theophylline is eliminated primarily via hepatic metabolism.[116,117] In contrast, the primary route of theophylline elimination in neonates is renal excretion of unchanged drug (55%).[115] Hepatic metabolism of theophylline (especially *N*-demethylation) is decreased in the neonate. As in adults, theophylline is methylated to caffeine in the neonate. The neonate's decreased demethylation pathway, however, results in a decrease in caffeine elimination and significant serum caffeine accumulation. On average, serum caffeine concentrations can be 40% of the serum theophylline concentration.[115] The theophylline-derived caffeine may contribute to the pharmacologic and toxic effects seen in neonates receiving theophylline. After 50 weeks' PMA, the theophylline-derived serum caffeine concentrations become insignificant.

Comparative studies have found similar efficacy for theophylline and caffeine in the control of apnea of prematurity. Caffeine, however, has several advantages over theophylline, including a wider therapeutic index. Adverse effects such as tachycardia, CNS excitation, and feeding intolerance are reported more frequently with theophylline than with caffeine. Because the half-life is prolonged and dosing requirements do not change quickly with time, caffeine serum concentrations do not need to be routinely monitored. The great majority of preterm neonates achieve caffeine plasma concentrations within the therapeutic range (5–20 mcg/mL) if they receive standard doses.[113] Caffeine serum concentrations may be obtained in select neonates (e.g., patients with clinical signs of toxicity or with intractable apnea). IV loading doses of 20 mg/kg caffeine citrate (10 mg/kg caffeine base), followed 24 hours later by maintenance doses of 5 to 8 mg/kg caffeine citrate (2.5–4 mg/kg caffeine base) given daily, are recommended. Loading doses of caffeine citrate should be given IV for 30 minutes using a syringe infusion pump. Maintenance doses can be administered IV for 10 minutes or given orally.[2] Because of the longer half-life, infants receiving caffeine must be monitored for a longer time (e.g., for 7–10 days) for adverse effects if toxicities occur and for apnea recurrence once the medication is discontinued. It is important to remember that another IV caffeine product is marketed in the United States as the sodium benzoate salt. Benzoic acid has been associated with the gasping syndrome and may also displace bilirubin from albumin-binding sites.[2] Because of these toxicities, the caffeine sodium benzoate product should not be used in neonates.

The short- and long-term safety and efficacy of caffeine to treat apnea of prematurity in VLBW infants were studied in a large, randomized, placebo-controlled trial.[45,118] Caffeine significantly decreased the frequency of BPD.[45] Infants who received caffeine were able to have positive airway pressure discontinued 1 week sooner than those receiving placebo. Although caffeine reduced weight gain, the effect was only temporary (during the first 3 weeks of therapy). In a follow-up study at 18 to 21 months' corrected age, caffeine significantly improved the rates of survival without neurodevelopmental disability (e.g., CP, cognitive delay).[118] These benefits were not sustained at 5-year follow-up.[119] Although oral theophylline (aminophylline) and caffeine are considered to be well absorbed in the neonate, many neonates initially have feeding problems when apnea and bradycardia are present. Therefore, therapy is usually initiated with the IV route, and an oral solution can be used when the neonate is stable and tolerating enteral feedings. It should also be remembered that, depending on the specific product used, aminophylline is a salt containing 80% to 85% theophylline.

The generally accepted therapeutic range of theophylline for apnea of prematurity is 6 to 12 mcg/mL. This range is lower than that which is normally accepted for the treatment of asthma (5–15 mcg/mL) for several reasons: (a) The higher free fraction of theophylline found in neonates results in a higher free concentration at any given total concentration; (b) there is a significant accumulation of the unmeasured active metabolite, caffeine; and (c) a different mechanism of action for theophylline is being exploited for apnea (i.e., central stimulation vs. bronchodilation for asthma). Aminophylline IV loading doses and maintenance doses of aminophylline and theophylline can be found in appropriate pediatric references.[2] However, a large variation in serum theophylline concentrations has been observed with some dosing regimens.[120] Concomitant drug therapy and disease states (e.g., hepatic or renal dysfunction) should also be taken into consideration when selecting initial theophylline doses.

Serum theophylline concentrations should be monitored 72 hours after initiation of therapy or after a change in dosage. Serum concentrations of theophylline should also be measured if the infant experiences an increase in the number of apneic episodes, signs or symptoms of toxicity, or a significant increase in weight. In asymptomatic neonates, once steady state levels are obtained, theophylline concentrations may be monitored every 2 weeks.

Because of the many advantages of caffeine over theophylline, S.M. should be given 20 mg of caffeine citrate (10 mg caffeine base) as an IV loading dose for 30 minutes. Maintenance doses of 5 mg of caffeine citrate (2.5 mg caffeine base) every 24 hours should be started 24 hours after the loading dose.

CASE 105-7, QUESTION 3: The NICU medical resident asks you to outline a pharmacotherapeutic monitoring plan for S.M. that includes monitoring parameters for efficacy and toxicity and duration of therapy. What would you tell her?

The goal of methylxanthine therapy for S.M. is to decrease the number of episodes of apnea and bradycardia. Continuous monitoring of HR and RR is required for proper evaluation. The time, duration, and severity of episodes, activity of the infant, and any necessary intervention performed should be documented. Relationships between the apneic episodes and the feeding schedule and volume of feeds, as well as the dosing schedule, should be examined. Apnea of prematurity usually resolves by 34 to 36 weeks' PMA; however, it may persist in some infants up to or beyond 40 weeks' PMA.[107,109] Methylxanthine therapy usually is discontinued at 34 to 36 weeks' PMA provided that the infant has not been having apneic spells. Infants requiring therapy for longer periods may be discharged home on methylxanthines with apnea monitors; however, this occurs very rarely.

Methylxanthine toxicities noted in neonates include tachycardia, agitation, irritability, hyperglycemia, feeding intolerance, gastroesophageal reflux, and emesis or occasional spitting up of food. Tachycardia is the most common toxicity and usually responds to a downward adjustment of the dose. Tachycardia may persist for 1 to 3 days after dosage reductions owing to the decreased elimination of caffeine. Seizures have also been reported with accidental overdoses. Methylxanthine toxicity can be minimized with careful dosing and appropriate monitoring of theophylline serum concentrations.

NEONATAL SEIZURES

CASE 105-8

QUESTION 1: F.H., a term female newborn (weight 3.5 kg), has a history of perinatal asphyxia. Apgar scores were 0, 1, 4, and 7 at 1, 5, 10, and 15 minutes, respectively. Maternal history is negative for drug abuse. Twenty-four hours after birth, F.H. begins to have rhythmic clonic twitching of the right hand, repetitive chewing movements, fluttering of the eyelids, and occasional pendulum-like movements of the extremities that resemble swimming motions. How should F.H.'s seizure activity be evaluated?

Seizure activity may be difficult to recognize in the term or premature neonate. Because of the immaturity of the cortex, neonatal seizures rarely are generalized tonic-clonic events, but can be clonic (focal or multifocal), tonic (focal or generalized), myoclonic (focal, multifocal, or generalized), or subtle in nature.[121,122]

For videos of neonatal seizures, go to **https://www.youtube.com/watch?v=Igj1HBT6oCQ**.

Subtle seizures include activities such as abnormal oral-buccal-lingual movements; ocular movements; swimming, pedaling, or stepping movements; and occasionally apnea. In addition, autonomic nervous system signs such as changes in HR, BP, respirations, skin color, oxygenation, salivation, or pupil size may occur.[121,122] Clinical neonatal seizures may or may not be associated with EEG changes. In addition, electrographic seizure activity may occur in neonates without clinical manifestations (i.e., subclinical seizures).

Neonatal seizure activity is a common manifestation of a life-threatening underlying neurologic process. Etiologies may include metabolic or electrolyte imbalances (e.g., alterations in glucose, calcium, magnesium, or sodium), cerebrovascular injury, CNS infection, genetic disorders, or drug-related causes (e.g., withdrawal after maternal drug use or adverse effects from drugs administered before, during, or after delivery).[121–126] Therefore, initial efforts may not include antiepileptic drug therapy. Definitive treatment is directed toward specific identified etiologies. The acute evaluation of neonatal seizures includes assessment of the infant's airway, breathing, and circulation and a review of the infant's history, physical examination, and laboratory studies. Every neonate with seizure activity should have a bedside determination of glucose; laboratory determinations of serum electrolytes, including sodium, BUN, glucose, calcium, and magnesium; blood gases; bilirubin; and an infectious disease workup, including complete blood cell count with platelets, CRP level, blood culture, urine culture, lumbar puncture with CSF analysis (cell count, protein, glucose), and CSF culture.[121–124] Treatment with antiepileptic drugs is indicated after correction of known electrolyte abnormalities. Antiepileptic drug therapy can be initiated while laboratory test results are pending, as long as hypoglycemia has been corrected.

If these tests do not reveal any abnormalities, an EEG, metabolic disease workup (e.g., serum ammonia, lactate, and pyruvate; serum and urine amino and organic acids), and screening of blood and urine for drugs can be performed.[121–124] Intrauterine infections associated with congenital neurologic abnormalities and seizures can be identified by obtainment of TORCH titers or PCR for specific viruses (e.g., CMV, HSV). Cranial ultrasounds, computed tomography scans, and magnetic resonance images may be obtained to identify infarcts, hemorrhages, calcifications, or cerebral malformations that may cause seizure activity.[121,122,124]

CASE 105-8, QUESTION 2: F.H. is found to have adequate ventilation and circulation. An IV line is established; blood cultures and serum chemistries, including calcium and magnesium, are obtained. A bedside blood glucose determination reveals a blood glucose of 20 mg/dL. What is your assessment and recommendation at this time?

Hypoglycemia seems to be the cause of F.H.'s seizure activity. Hypoxic ischemic encephalopathy secondary to asphyxia, however, is the most common cause of neonatal seizures.[121,123] Hypoxic ischemic encephalopathy can be associated with metabolic abnormalities such as hypoglycemia, hypocalcemia, and hyponatremia (owing to inappropriate secretion of antidiuretic hormone). The definition of clinically significant hypoglycemia in neonates remains controversial, because normal blood glucose depends on a variety of factors, including gestational age, birth weight, feeding status, body stores, and other disease states.[125] Historically, hypoglycemia was defined as a whole blood glucose less than 20 mg/dL for premature infants and less than 30 mg/dL for term infants during the first 72 hours of life and less than 40 mg/dL for any neonate after 72 hours of age. However, in clinical practice, a blood glucose less than 40 mg/dL in a neonate of any age would be treated.[121] F.H. should receive an IV bolus dose of 7 mL (2 mL/kg) of dextrose 10% (200 mg/kg) given in 2 to 3 minutes, followed by a continuous infusion of dextrose 10% at an initial dose of 12.6 to 16.8 mL/hour (6–8 mg/kg/minute or 3.6–4.8 mL/kg/hour).[121,125] Serum glucose levels should be monitored, and the dextrose infusion should be titrated as needed. If hypoglycemia persists, possible causes such as islet tumor of the pancreas, adrenal insufficiency, and inborn errors of metabolism should be investigated. Corticosteroids, glucagon, diazoxide, and octreotide have been used to treat persistent hypoglycemia.[125]

Treatment of Hypocalcemia and Hypomagnesemia

CASE 105-8, QUESTION 3: F.H. receives 7 mL (700 mg) of 10% dextrose solution IV, and an IV infusion of glucose at 8 mg/kg/minute is initiated. A repeat bedside blood glucose determination reveals a blood glucose of 80 mg/dL, but F.H. continues to have seizure activity. F.H.'s laboratory results come back with the following results:

Sodium, 137 mEq/L
Potassium, 4.3 mEq/L
CO_2, 22 mEq/L
Chloride, 104 mEq/L
BUN, 7 mg/dL
SCr, 0.7 mg/dL
Glucose, 25 mg/dL
Magnesium, 1.0 mEq/L
Calcium, 6.5 mg/dL

What should be done next to control F.H.'s seizures?

F.H. also has hypocalcemia and hypomagnesemia, both of which may cause seizure activity. Neonatal hypocalcemia is defined as a serum calcium less than 7.5 mg/dL in preterm and less than 8 mg/dL in term infants[123] or an ionized serum calcium less than 3 mg/dL. Hypomagnesemia (defined as a serum magnesium <1.5 mEq/L) is rare but may coexist with hypocalcemia. Hypomagnesemia should be suspected when hypocalcemia cannot be corrected despite large doses of calcium.

F.H. should receive calcium gluconate 700 mg (200 mg/kg) given slowly IV as a 10% solution[121,123] and magnesium sulfate 25 to 50 mg/kg/dose (0.2–0.4 mEq/kg/dose) IM as a 20% solution or IV as a dilute solution (maximal concentration, 100 mg/mL) administered for 2 to 4 hours.[2] Doses of calcium gluconate and magnesium sulfate may be repeated based on serum determinations. If IV calcium is administered too quickly, vasodilation, hypotension, bradycardia, cardiac arrhythmias, and cardiac arrest may occur. Calcium gluconate may be administered slowly IV at a maximal rate of 50 mg/minute while monitoring HR, BP, and electrocardiogram.[2] The IV site should be closely monitored for signs of infiltration because extravasation may result in severe dermal necrosis.

Treatment with Antiepileptic Drugs

CASE 105-8, QUESTION 4: Despite normalization of her laboratory tests, F.H. continues to have seizure activity. Phenobarbital 35 mg IV push for 1 minute is administered. Ten minutes later, F.H. continues to have intermittent seizure activity. Describe a pharmacotherapeutic plan to control F.H.'s seizure activity.

Phenobarbital is the initial antiepileptic drug of choice for neonatal seizures; phenytoin and lorazepam usually are considered the second and third drugs of choice.[121,124,126–130] Because of the large volume of distribution of phenobarbital in neonates (0.8–1 L/kg), large initial loading doses of 20 mg/kg are required to produce therapeutic serum concentrations.[2,121,124] Because F.H. received only a 10-mg/kg dose (35 mg) of phenobarbital, an additional 10 mg/kg should be given now. Phenobarbital should be administered IV at a rate of 1 mg/kg/minute or less,[2] so a 35-mg dose should be given for at least 10 minutes, not in 1 minute. Rapid administration of phenobarbital may cause respiratory depression, apnea, or hypotension. If F.H. continues to have seizure activity after a total phenobarbital loading dose of 20 mg/kg, additional 5- to 10-mg/kg loading doses may be given every 15 to 20 minutes as needed up to a total loading dose of 40 mg/kg. Ventilatory support may be required when using these higher doses, and serum phenobarbital concentrations should be monitored. Phenobarbital's therapeutic effect of controlling neonatal seizures plateaus at serum concentrations of 40 mcg/mL; adverse effects increase at higher serum concentrations.[131]

If seizure activity is not controlled in F.H. (despite optimal phenobarbital loading doses), a phenytoin loading dose of 70 mg (20 mg/kg) should be administered IV at a rate of 0.5 to 1 mg/kg/minute or less.[2,121,124] Rapid IV administration of phenytoin may cause cardiac arrhythmias, bradycardia, or hypotension. Phenytoin may cause severe damage to tissues if extravasation occurs. Therefore, BP, HR, electrocardiogram, and the IV site of infusion should be monitored. Fosphenytoin, the diphosphate ester salt of phenytoin, is available in the United States for IV and IM use in adults.[2] Fosphenytoin is a water-soluble prodrug of phenytoin that undergoes conversion by plasma and tissue esterases to phenytoin, phosphate, and formaldehyde. Because of its greater water solubility, the IV preparation does not contain propylene glycol, and thus fosphenytoin may have fewer cardiovascular adverse effects associated with IV administration. In addition, it can be safely administered intramuscularly and may cause less dermal necrosis if extravasated. Unfortunately, appropriate clinical studies of fosphenytoin in neonates have not yet been conducted. Unanswered concerns about the neonatal handling of formaldehyde also exist. Despite the lack of neonatal studies, some clinicians prefer to use fosphenytoin instead of phenytoin, due to the aforementioned advantages. Studies assessing the safety, efficacy, and optimal dosing of fosphenytoin in neonates are needed.

Lorazepam IV (0.05 to 0.1 mg/kg) should be used to treat F.H.'s seizures if they are unresponsive to phenobarbital and phenytoin.[2,126,127] Lorazepam is preferred over diazepam owing to its longer duration of effect and fewer pharmaceutical adjuvants. Lorazepam (especially in combination with phenobarbital) may cause respiratory and CNS depression. RR, BP, and HR should be monitored. Doses should be diluted with an equal volume of 5% dextrose in water, normal saline, or sterile water for injection before IV use and administered slowly for 2 to 5 minutes.[2]

If seizure activity continues in F.H., continuous IV infusion of midazolam or IV or oral levetiracetam should be considered.[121,124,128–130,132] Levetiracetam may be preferred over continuous infusion midazolam due to less adverse neurologic effects. In fact, some clinicians prefer levetiracetam to phenytoin as a second-line agent. Although the IV formulation of levetiracetam is not approved for use in neonates, some neonatal centers use the pediatric oral dosing recommendations for the IV route because the two forms are bioequivalent.[2] However, the optimal neonatal dose of levetiracetam has not been established. Neonatal reports have used doses based on studies in pediatric patients.[128] Given that levetiracetam is primarily excreted via the kidney (66% of a dose is excreted as unchanged drug in the urine) and that the renal function of neonates is decreased compared with that of older infants, one would expect a lower clearance and the use of lower levetiracetam doses in neonates. However, recent neonatal pharmacokinetic studies [124,129,130] have identified a larger volume of distribution per kg (compared to children) and a more rapid clearance than expected based on immature renal function. A significant increase in levetiracetam clearance also occurred during the first week of life, reaching the clearance seen in children. These findings indicate that in neonates, larger loading doses and maintenance doses, with an adjustment of maintenance doses after the first 7 days of life, would be required. Phase 2 trials of higher doses have not yet been completed.[124,129] Thus, currently the clinical use of levetiracetam in neonates requires careful dose titration and close monitoring of adverse effects. Oral carbamazepine, clonazepam, lamotrigine, topiramate, and valproic acid (IV, oral) have also been used to treat refractory neonatal seizures in limited numbers of patients.[121,124,126,129] Because the risk of valproic acid-associated hepatotoxicity is higher for patients younger than 2 years of age, this drug is not a preferred agent for use in neonates.[2] IV pyridoxine (50 to 100 mg) should be considered when seizure activity persists. Pyridoxine is a cofactor required for the synthesis of the inhibitory neurotransmitter γ-aminobutyric acid (GABA). Patients with pyridoxine dependency require higher amounts of pyridoxine for proper GABA synthesis. Pyridoxine dependency is a rare disorder, but should be considered in neonates with seizure activity unresponsive to antiepileptic drug therapy. Lifelong supplementation of pyridoxine is required in these patients.[123]

CASE 105-8, QUESTION 5: F.H.'s seizure activity stopped after receiving a total loading dose of 105 mg of phenobarbital and 70 mg of phenytoin. A serum phenobarbital concentration of 35 mcg/mL and a phenytoin concentration of 17 mcg/mL were measured 1 hour after the phenytoin loading dose (2 hours after the last phenobarbital loading dose). How should maintenance doses of antiepileptic drugs be instituted in F.H.?

It is not surprising that F.H. required both phenobarbital and phenytoin to control her seizures. Although phenobarbital and phenytoin are equally effective, neonatal seizures are controlled in fewer than 50% of neonates with either agent alone. When both agents are used together, neonatal seizures are controlled in approximately 60% of neonates.[133]

F.H. should be placed on maintenance doses of both phenobarbital and phenytoin because both drugs were needed to control her seizure activity. Because the half-life of phenobarbital is prolonged in neonates (about 100–150 hours), maintenance doses can be instituted 24 hours after the loading dose at 3 to 4 mg/kg/day[2,123,134] as a single daily dose. Although this newborn is term, she should receive a lower dose of phenobarbital (2.5–3 mg/kg/day) because of her history of asphyxia. Asphyxiated neonates have impaired phenobarbital clearance and therefore require lower maintenance doses than nonasphyxiated neonates to achieve similar phenobarbital serum concentrations.[135] Maintenance doses of phenytoin (3–4 mg/kg/day given in divided doses every 12 hours) may be initiated 12 to 24 hours after the loading dose. Serum concentrations of these agents should be monitored periodically because maintenance dose requirements increase with time, usually by weeks 2 to 4 of therapy.[134] This may be related to a normal maturation of hepatic enzyme systems with age or induction of cytochrome P-450 enzymes. In neonates, oral phenytoin is poorly absorbed and should be avoided in the acute setting. A routine 25% increase in the dose is needed when converting IV phenytoin to oral to attain similar serum concentrations. In addition, after 2 to 4 weeks of age, dosing intervals of every 8 hours may be needed.

It should be remembered that phenytoin is a highly protein-bound drug. In neonates, protein binding of phenytoin is decreased. This results in an increased free fraction and suggests that total phenytoin therapeutic serum concentrations in newborns should be 8 to 15 mcg/mL rather than the 10 to 20 mcg/mL as accepted in children and adults.[2] In addition, bilirubin can displace phenytoin from albumin binding sites. A positive correlation between total bilirubin concentrations and free fraction of phenytoin has been described. Unbound phenytoin was reported to be approximately 20% in neonates when bilirubin concentrations were 20 mg/dL (compared with 10% normally).[136] Thus, total phenytoin serum concentrations must be interpreted carefully in neonates, and measurement of unbound phenytoin may be required in neonates with hyperbilirubinemia.

The optimal duration of anticonvulsant treatment of neonatal seizures has not been clearly established. Because of the potential long-term toxicities of these medications and the low risk of seizure recurrence, anticonvulsants are generally discontinued before discharge if the neonate's neurologic examination and EEG are normal. Neonates who continue receiving anticonvulsants are reassessed periodically after discharge (e.g., at 1 and 3 months of age and then every 3 months). Thus, the duration of anticonvulsant medications is individualized based on the infant's neurologic examination and EEG.

KEY REFERENCES AND WEBSITES

A full list of references for this chapter can be found at http://thepoint.lww.com/AT11e. Below are the key references and websites for this chapter, with the corresponding reference number in this chapter found in parentheses after the reference.

Key References

Glass HC. Neonatal seizures: advances in mechanisms and management. *Clin Perinatol*. 2014;41:177–190. (124)

Hall N et al. Necrotizing enterocolitis: prevention, treatment, and outcome. *J Pediatr Surg*. 2013;48(12):2359–2367. (75)

Pickering LK et al, eds. *2012 Red Book: Report of the Committee on Infectious Diseases*. 29th ed. Elk Grove Village, IL: American Academy of Pediatrics; 2012. (84)

Polin R, Carlo W. Committee on Fetus and Newborn. Clinical Report. Surfactant replacement therapy for preterm and term neonates with respiratory distress. *Pediatrics*. 2014;133:156–163. (11)

Taketomo CK et al. *Pediatric and Neonatal Dosage Handbook*. 21st ed. Hudson, OH: Lexi-Comp; 2014. (2)

Watterberg K et al. Policy statement—postnatal corticosteroids to prevent or treat bronchopulmonary dysplasia. *Pediatrics*. 2010;126:800. (39)

Key Websites

American Heart Association, Congenital Heart Defects. http://www.heart.org/HEARTORG/Conditions/CongenitalHeartDefects/Congenital-Heart-Defects_UCM_001090_SubHomePage.jsp.

Cochrane Neonatal Group. http://neonatal.cochrane.org/.

Neonatology on the Web. http://www.neonatology.org/.

NICHD—The Eunice Kennedy Shriver National Institute of Child Health & Human Development. http://www.nichd.nih.gov/cochrane/.

The Congenital Heart Information Network. http://www.tchin.org/.

106 Care of the Critically Ill Child

Elizabeth Anne Farrington and Marcia L. Buck

CORE PRINCIPLES

	CHAPTER CASES
1 The most frequent cause of cardiac arrest in pediatric patients is a terminal result of respiratory failure or shock, not a primary cardiac event.	**Case 106-1 (Question 1)**
2 Developmental changes and immaturity of the respiratory system make respiratory distress the most common reason for hospital admission in the first year of life. Nasal flaring and grunting are unique features of the respiratory examination in infants that indicate respiratory distress. The normal respiratory rate in children changes over time; therefore, the respiratory rate that would be of concern varies based on the age of the patient.	**Case 106-2 (Questions 1, 2)**
3 Oxygen should be administered immediately in a child where respiratory difficulty is suspected. Once the decision is made to intubate the patient, the choices for pharmacotherapy of intubation vary based on the cardiovascular stability of the patient, whether the stomach is empty or full, and the underlying cause of the respiratory distress.	**Case 106-2 (Questions 3, 4)**
4 Hypovolemic shock is the most common type of shock seen in pediatric patients. Septic shock, obstructive shock, and cardiogenic shock occur in children but are less common. The initial treatment of all forms of shock is the same. A pediatric patient can present with compensated or decompensated shock. There are physiologic differences in the pediatric patient's response to hypovolemia, with hypotension being the last physiologic change during decompensation.	**Case 106-3 (Questions 1, 2)**
5 Infants have low glycogen stores, so are at high risk for the development of hypoglycemia when they have poor oral intake or during conditions of stress. Because hypoglycemia may cause seizures and is linked to poor neurologic outcome, all critically ill infants should have point-of-care glucose testing on presentation. If identified, hypoglycemia must be treated promptly.	**Case 106-3 (Question 3)**
6 Due to the immature immune system in the infant, the incidence of septic shock is the highest in the first year of life. Patients with underlying medical conditions have a higher mortality rate than previously healthy children who experience sepsis.	**Case 106-4 (Question 1)**
7 Due to physiologic changes during childhood, the definitions of sepsis and systemic inflammatory response syndrome (SIRS) are different in children and adults. Tachycardia and tachypnea, pivotal to the adult definition of SIRS, are common presenting symptoms of many pediatric disease processes and are not solely indicative of sepsis. Unlike adult guidelines, temperature variation and leukocyte abnormalities are included in the pediatric definitions. There are also specific definitions based on patient age: newborn, neonate, infant, toddler and preschool-aged child, school-aged child, and adolescent.	**Case 106-4 (Question 2)**
8 Septic shock can be further defined by the patient's response to fluid resuscitation and catecholamine administration. These factors, as well as physiologic differences in neonatal and pediatric cardiovascular physiology compared with adults, affect not only the choice of therapy but also drug dosing and monitoring.	**Case 106-4 (Questions 3–6)**

Continued

		CHAPTER CASES
9	Neonates with ductal-dependent congenital heart disease (CHD) may not be diagnosed immediately after birth. These patients may present with symptoms of being either in respiratory distress, in cardiogenic or obstructive shock, or in a combination of both. It is essential to consider CHD in any neonate who presents with these symptoms.	**Case 106-5 (Question 1)**
10	Traumatic brain injury (TBI) is the leading cause of mortality in children and leads to significant morbidity among survivors. The anatomic differences of the child's brain render it more susceptible to certain types of injuries after head trauma. Causes vary by age, with nonaccidental trauma seen most commonly in the first year of life. Quick assessment of the patient on presentation to emergency services is needed for appropriate diagnosis, stabilization, and treatment.	**Case 106-6 (Questions 1–3)**
11	Placement of a ventriculostomy will allow for measurement of intracranial pressure (ICP) and drainage of cerebral spinal fluid. The ability to measure ICP will assist in the evaluation of the efficacy of treatments. Cerebral perfusion pressure (CPP) also must be monitored closely in patients with TBI. Goal CPP values vary by age. Standard therapies to reduce ICP include CSF drainage, medically induced hypertension, and hyperosmolar therapy with mannitol or hypertonic saline. When standard therapies fail, barbiturate coma, therapeutic hypothermia, or decompressive craniectomy may be considered.	**Case 106-6 (Questions 4–6)**
12	Treatment and/or prevention of early post-traumatic seizures has been shown to improve outcomes, but long-term use of anticonvulsant medications (greater than 7 days) has not been shown to improve outcomes and is associated with adverse effects.	**Case 106-7 (Question 1)**

Much of pediatric practice is dedicated to assisting the child in making the transition from the intrauterine environment through infancy, childhood, and adolescence to adulthood. One of the greatest challenges in managing pediatric patients is recognizing the numerous physiologic changes that take place during this time and understanding how they affect assessment and management of the patient. The definition and presentation of many disease states encountered in the critical care setting, including respiratory depression, supraventricular tachycardia, hypotension, and shock, vary based on the age of the patient as a result of these physiologic variations. There are also newborn emergencies that are unique to the physiologic transitions that occur in the first month of life.

Pediatric healthcare providers practicing in critical care settings such as the emergency department or pediatric intensive care unit (PICU) must be adept at incorporating these physiologic differences into medication selection, dosing, and monitoring to optimize patient care.

The epidemiology of patients admitted to either the pediatric emergency department or PICU differs from that typically seen in adult critical care settings.[1,2] In an evaluation of 361 children presenting to an emergency department, the most common medial reasons for admission were cardiocirculatory causes (32%), neurologic conditions (26%), and respiratory causes (23%).[1] Cardiocirculatory causes included hypovolemic, septic, cardiac, and anaphylactic shock. Neurologic conditions consisted primarily of seizures, status epilepticus, and meningitis or encephalitis. The most common respiratory cause for admission was respiratory syncytial virus (RSV) bronchiolitis, followed by pneumonia, pleural effusions, and croup. Eighteen percent (18%) of the patients were admitted after trauma. Diabetic ketoacidosis accounted for 6% of admissions. Other diagnoses included intoxications, near drowning, snake bites, and burns. Assessment of the most common causes for PICU admission has provided similar results. In a review of 1,149 children admitted during a 2-year period to the PICU of a university-affiliated children's hospital, the majority (38%) were diagnosed with cardiovascular diseases, followed by respiratory illnesses (28%), other medical causes (10%), neurologic illness (8%), and trauma (8%). Another 7% were admitted for postoperative care.[2] When comparing admissions to pediatric intensive care from 1982, 1995, and 2005 to 2006, the most common medical diagnostic categories have remained unchanged. However, fewer children were admitted after accidents, with croup or with epiglottitis.[2] These changes can be explained by mandatory car seats for children, administration of dexamethasone in the emergency department to patients with croup and the conjugate *Haemophilus influenza* type b immunization. During the same time period, the proportion of patients that died decreased from 11% to 4.8%; however, the proportion of survivors with moderate or severe disability increased significantly from 8.4% to 17.9%.[2] With the low rate of mortality in the PICU, the focus of our research should investigate how to improve patient outcomes.

PEDIATRIC CARDIOPULMONARY RESUSCITATION

In marked contrast to pediatric cardiac arrest, adult cardiac arrest studies have focused on the diagnosis and treatment of ventricular fibrillation (VF) in both inpatient and out-of-hospital cardiac arrest. Studies showed that VF was the most common initial dysrhythmia in adults with sudden death; in some reports, the prevalence of VF was 60% to 85%. Cardiac arrest due to VF or pulseless ventricular tachycardia as the initial cardiac rhythm occurs in only 5% to 15% of pediatric patients in hospital and out-of hospital cardiac arrest.[3] In contrast to adults, cardiac arrest in infants and children does not usually result from a primary cardiac cause; more often it is the terminal result of progressive respiratory failure or shock. Therefore, it is essential to recognize and treat pediatric patients admitted with respiratory distress, pneumonia, and shock aggressively to prevent the development of systemic hypoxemia, hypercapnia, and acidosis that may then progress to bradycardia, hypotension, and eventually cardiorespiratory arrest.

CASE 106-1

QUESTION 1: Paramedics are transporting C.W., a 5-month-old, 5-kg infant with respiratory distress who stops breathing en route to the hospital. The patient is bag-mask-ventilated with cardiopulmonary resuscitation in progress. On arrival in the emergency department, the patient is apneic, asystolic, and pulseless. The infant has no intravenous (IV) access. After brief bag-mask ventilation, the patient is intubated with an endotracheal tube (ETT). A colorimetric carbon dioxide capnometer detector device confirms proper ETT placement. Findings now include breath sounds that are equal bilaterally and good chest movement with ventilation, although there is still no pulse palpable without chest compressions and no heart sounds are heard. An electrocardiogram shows asystole. Oxygen saturation is not obtainable. What medication is needed for C.W. at this point in his resuscitation and what would the appropriate dose be?

Epinephrine is the drug of choice for the management of pediatric asystole.[3] Ventilation and chest compressions should be continued for C.W., and while one responder is attempting IV access, another may administer the first dose of epinephrine down the ETT using a higher dose of 0.5 mg (0.1 mg/kg prepared from the 1:1,000 or 1 mg/mL concentration) to account for reduced absorption. If two attempts at IV line placement are unsuccessful, an intraosseous (IO) catheter should be inserted into the proximal tibia. Blood may be obtained through the IO needle to perform a rapid glucose check and sent for further studies. After reassessment of the airway, ventilation and chest compressions should be continued. Subsequent doses of epinephrine can be administered every 3 to 5 minutes through the IO line, using the appropriate IV/IO dose of 0.05 mg (0.01 mg/kg using the 1:10,000 or 0.1 mg/mL concentration).

RESPIRATORY DISTRESS

Respiratory distress, related to problems at all levels of the respiratory tract from the nose to the lungs, is a frequent occurrence in children.[4] (For a video that shows some of the signs of respiratory distress in an infant, go to http://www.youtube.com/watch?v=42jJ18fkZ0Y.) The nose provides nearly half the total airway resistance in children. Infants under 2 months are obligate nasal breathers, and their nose is short, soft, and small with nearly circular nares. The nares will double in size from birth to 6 months but they can easily be occluded from edema, secretions, or external pressure. Simply clearing the nasal passageways with saline and bulb suctioning can significantly improve an infant's respiratory condition. Other physiologic reasons for a high incidence of respiratory failure in infants and children are small and collapsible airways, an unstable chest wall, inadequate collateral ventilation for alveoli, poor control (tone) of the upper airway (particularly during sleep), tendency for the respiratory muscles to fatigue, reactivity of the pulmonary vascular bed (increased sensitivity of the vasculature, particularly in young infants), an inefficient immune system, genetic disorders or syndromes, and residual problems related to premature birth such as bronchopulmonary dysplasia.

CASE 106-2

QUESTION 1: T.F. is a 7-month-old, previously healthy 12-kg infant who presents to the emergency room with a 3-day history of upper respiratory tract symptoms. His mother states that he is having increasing difficulty breathing and has not wanted to drink or eat. On examination, he has a respiratory rate of 70 breaths/minute, an O_2 saturation of 90% on 100% FiO_2 via nasal cannula, nasal flaring and grunting, and both intercostal and suprasternal retractions. Initial viral screening reveals positive results for RSV, and his chest X-ray is consistent with RSV bronchiolitis. He was agitated and fussy at first presentation, but during the last 30 minutes his respiratory rate has decreased to 40 breaths/minute with a reduction in retractions and he has become somnolent. What developmental changes in the lung explain why a routine viral infection could result in the need for an emergency room visit in a 7-month-old previously healthy child?

The most common reason for admission to the hospital in the first year of life is respiratory distress. This can be explained by the numerous physiologic differences seen in an infant. Although all the conducting airways are present at birth and the airway branching pattern is complete, the airways are small.[5] The airways will increase in size and length throughout childhood. Not only are the airways smaller in an infant but supporting airway cartilage and elastic tissue are not developed until school age. For these reasons, the child's airways are susceptible to collapse and may easily become obstructed as a result of laryngospasm, bronchospasm, and edema or mucus accumulation. Normal airway resistance is the highest in infants because it is inversely proportional to $1/\text{radius}^4$. Therefore, any airway narrowing from bronchospasm, edema, or mucus accumulation will significantly increase the airway resistance and increase the infant's work of breathing. The cartilaginous ribs of the infant and young child are twice as compliant as the bony ribs of the older child or adult. During episodes of respiratory distress, the infant's chest wall will retract further than a patient with a bony ribcage. This will reduce the patient's ability to maintain functional residual capacity (FRC) or increase tidal volume, thus further increasing the patient's work of breathing.

The respiratory muscles consist of muscles of the upper airway, the lower airway, and the diaphragm. They contribute to expansion of the lung and maintenance of airway patency. Lack of development of the small airway muscles may render young infants less responsive than older children to bronchodilator therapy. Lastly, the intercostal muscles are not fully developed until school age, so they act primarily to stabilize the chest wall during the first years of life. Because the intercostal muscles have neither the leverage nor the strength to lift the rib cage in the young child, the diaphragm is responsible for the generation of tidal volume. Therefore, anything that impedes diaphragm movement, such as a large stomach bubble, abdominal distension, or peritonitis, can result in respiratory failure in the young child.

CASE 106-2, QUESTION 2: What respiratory signs and symptoms are present in T.F. and how do they define the patient's respiratory status? What are potential causes of T.F.'s respiratory distress?

To assess a patient for respiratory distress, one should evaluate four areas: respiratory rate and effort, work of breathing, quality and magnitude of breath sounds, and the patient's mental status. Normal respiratory rates vary with age (Table 106-1). A respiratory rate greater than 60 breaths/minute is abnormal in a child of any age, but most concerning in an older child. An abnormally slow or decreasing respiratory rate may herald respiratory failure. Intercostal, subcostal, and supracostal retractions increase with increasing respiratory distress. Although increased retractions are seen in infants, they have decreased efficiency of respiratory muscle function during the first years of life; therefore, the benefit in infants is reduced. Decreasing respiratory rate and diminished retractions in a child with a history of distress may signal severe fatigue. Nasal flaring is an effort to increase airway diameter and

Table 106-1
Normal Respiratory Rates and Definition of Tachypnea for Children, by Age

Age	Respiratory Rate (breaths/minute)	Tachypnea (breaths/minute)
Newborn–2 months	30–60	>60
2–12 months	25–40	>50
1–3 years	20–30	>40
3–6 years	16–22	>40
7–12 years	14–20	>40
>12 years	12–20	>40

is often seen with hypoxemia. T.F. demonstrates all of these physiologic signs of respiratory distress. In addition to these findings, some infants will exhibit an expiratory grunting noise. This noise is produced by the child's involuntary effort to counter the loss of FRC by closing their glottis on active exhalation. Grunting produces positive end-expiratory pressure (PEEP) in an effort to prevent airway collapse. An expiratory grunt is mechanistically similar to "pursed lip breathing" in adults with chronic dyspnea. An expiratory grunt is classically seen in the presence of extensive alveolar pathology and is considered a sign of serious disease.

There are numerous causes of respiratory distress in infants and children. Table 106-2 summarizes common respiratory noises in children and their site of origin which may provide clues to the clinical cause. The most common causes of respiratory failure in infants and children are infectious diseases, asthma, malignancies, trauma (both accidental and nonaccidental), poisonings, foreign body aspiration, anatomic upper airway obstruction, cardiogenic shock, and untreated left-to-right intracardiac shunts. Respiratory syncytial virus is among the most common causes of respiratory distress in infants and young children, leading to an estimated 90,000 hospitalizations each year.[6] Although RSV can occur at any age, it is most severe in children under 2 years of age such as T.F. Prematurity, as well as chronic respiratory disease and congenital heart disease, increases the risk for severe RSV bronchiolitis requiring hospitalization.

CASE 106-2, QUESTION 3: T.F. is no longer consistently maintaining oxygen saturation values above 90% on nasal cannula O_2. How should T.F. be managed?

Oxygen should be administered immediately in any patient where respiratory difficulty is suspected. Infants and children consume 2 to 3 times more oxygen per kilogram of body weight than adults under normal conditions and even more when they are ill or distressed. T.F. responded well to oxygen administered via nasal cannula in the emergency department, but is now increasingly somnolent and has a decreased respiratory rate along

Table 106-2
Common Airway Noises, Site of Origin, and Clinical Causes in Children

Respiratory Noise	Definition	Site of Origin	Common Clinical Causes: Acute	Common Clinical Causes: Persistent
Wheeze	A high-pitched, continuous musical noise, often associated with prolonged expiration (can occur with inspiration or expiration)	Intrathoracic airways	Intermittent asthma/viral-induced wheeze	Persistent asthma
Rattle	This sound is the result of excessive secretions in the large airways, which are presumably moving with normal respirations	Either or both intrathoracic and extrathoracic airways	Acute viral bronchitis	Chronic sputum retention (neuromuscular disorders)
Stridor	This is predominately an inspiratory noise and indicates obstruction to airflow in the extrathoracic airways (upper airways obstruction) (can occur with inspiration or expiration)	Extrathoracic airways	Acute laryngotracheobronchitis (or viral croup)	Laryngomalacia
Snore	The noise arises from an increase to airflow through the upper airways, predominately in the region of the nasopharynx and oropharynx; it is more obvious during inspiration, but may be audible throughout the respiratory cycle	Oronasopharyngeal airway	Acute tonsillitis/pharyngitis	Chronically enlarged tonsils and adenoids, obstructive sleep apnea
Snuffle/Snort	These terms describe respiratory noises emanating from the nasal passages; these noises are audible in both inspiration and expiration and are often associated with visible secretions from the nares	Nasal passage/nasopharynx	Acute viral head cold	Allergic rhinitis
Grunt	This sound occurs with closure of the glottis during active exhalation	Alveoli/lung parenchyma	Any alveolar pathology in infants and small children	None

For examples of some of these airway noises, go to the following web links:
- Wheeze: http://www.youtube.com/watch?v=YG0-ukhU1xE&feature=related
- Rattle/rhonchi: http://www.youtube.com/watch?v=QPBZOohj2a0&feature=related
- Stridor
  - Toddler: http://www.youtube.com/watch?v=Zkau4yHsLLM&feature=related
  - Infant: http://www.youtube.com/watch?v=73zUjcCzgqA&NR=1
- Grunt: http://www.youtube.com/watch?v=aptwttJ6y_4

with decreased oxygen saturation values—all signs of impending respiratory failure. The specific indications for intubation in infants and children are as follows:

1. Apnea
2. Acute respiratory failure (Pao_2 <50 mm Hg in patient with Fio_2 >0.5 and $Paco_2$ >55 mm Hg acutely)
3. Need to control oxygen delivery, with institution of PEEP or to provide accurate delivery of Fio_2 greater than 0.5
4. Need to control ventilation to decrease work of breathing, control $Paco_2$, or to administer neuromuscular blocking agents
5. Inadequate chest wall function, as in patients with neuromuscular disorders such as Guillain–Barré syndrome, spinal muscular atrophy, or muscular dystrophy
6. Upper airway obstruction
7. Protection of the airway of a patient whose protective reflexes are absent, such as those with head trauma

Based on the diagnosis of acute respiratory failure and the need to control oxygen delivery, T.F. should be intubated and placed on mechanical ventilation.

MEDICATIONS FOR INTUBATION AND MECHANICAL VENTILATION

CASE 106-2, QUESTION 4: What pharmacologic agents are recommended when intubating a pediatric patient? Develop a plan for the medications to be used during intubation of T.F.

After the decision is made to proceed with intubation, the next decision needs to be whether pharmacologic agents are appropriate. Most pediatric patients require sedation before laryngoscopy and intubation. The goal is to depress the infant or child's level of consciousness sufficiently to produce appropriate conditions for intubation. Pharmacologic therapy is used to produce adequate sedation, analgesia, and amnesia plus a blunting of the physiologic response to airway manipulation. Intubation in the awake state can elicit protective reflexes that trigger tachycardia, bradycardia, and elevation of blood pressure, increased intracranial pressure, intraocular pressure, cough, and bronchospasm. Pharmacologic control promotes a smoother intubation with less physiologic stress for the patient who often is already in a compromised state. Ideally, this should be accomplished while producing minimal hemodynamic compromise.[7]

There are many factors to be considered when choosing agents for intubation: the onset of action of the agent, the patient's hemodynamic status, the need to prevent increased intraocular or intracranial pressure that may be caused with intubation, and whether the stomach is full or empty. A wide variety of medications may be used for pediatric sedation, each with its own risk and benefits (Table 106-3).[7] In general, agents that act rapidly and are eliminated quickly are ideal. Often drug choices are made based on the clinician's experience with a particular drug and the immediate availability of the drug. Most importantly, the drug regimen chosen must be based on the patient's physiologic state. Agents with adverse effects that would exacerbate any underlying medical conditions must be avoided. Narcotics used in combination with anxiolytics are used commonly. To produce optimal conditions for intubation, T.F. could be given 12 mcg of fentanyl (1 mcg/kg) and 1.2 mg of midazolam (0.1 mg/kg) IV before the procedure to provide sedation and analgesia. Both agents are relatively short-acting and reversible if difficulties arise with ETT placement.

Patients with inadequate relaxation despite adequate sedation may require neuromuscular blockade, although these agents are not without risk. In a patient with a partial airway obstruction, neuromuscular blockade may worsen pharyngeal collapse, potentially resulting in complete airway obstruction. Therefore, neuromuscular blocking agents should only be used if the clinician is absolutely certain that adequate ventilation can be provided or that the patient can be intubated. If adequate chest rise and oxygen saturation cannot be readily maintained with bag-mask ventilation, neuromuscular blockers should not be used. Infants and children younger than 5 years have a high vagal tone; therefore, they are more likely to exhibit bradycardia when intubated. Instrumentation of the airway can directly stimulate vagal receptors and induce bradycardia. In these patients, it is prudent to administer atropine 0.02 mg/kg before intubation to blunt the autonomic response. Lidocaine (1–1.5 mg/kg/dose with a maximum dose of 100 mg) may be administered intravenously to blunt the airway protective reflexes elicited by instrumentation. This may be particularly useful in a patient with elevated intracranial pressure (ICP).

In the asthmatic patient, drugs that release histamine (e.g., morphine, atracurium, or thiopental) and have the potential to produce laryngospasm or bronchospasm should be avoided. The beneficial bronchodilatory side effects of ketamine, however, make it a useful choice in these patients. In a child with increased ICP, the choice of pharmacologic agent depends on the hemodynamic status of the patient. Thiopental or pentobarbital is an excellent choice in the hemodynamically stable patient whereas etomidate is preferred if the patient is unstable or hypovolemia is suspected. Etomidate should not be used routinely in pediatric patients because a single dose administered for intubation has the potential to produce adrenal inhibition.[8] In children and adults with septic shock, etomidate administration is associated with a higher mortality rate.[8–10]

In all cases of intubation, preoxygenation is carried out to increase the available oxygen in the lungs during the procedure, thus giving the practitioner some buffer time to intubate the patient. However, in patients with an elevated ICP or pulmonary vascular hypertension, hyperventilation is recommended to also produce hypocarbia. A summary of specific patient conditions and recommended agents for intubation can be found in Table 106-4. In an infant or child with a full stomach, the risk of aspiration of gastric contents is high. Rapid sequence intubation (RSI) is used when there is an aspiration risk, such as the child with a full stomach, and there is no concern of a difficult intubation.[11] The goal of RSI is to gain airway control with an ETT as quickly as possible to prevent aspiration. The patient is preoxygenated via face mask and bag-mask ventilation cannot be used because it causes gastric distension. Once all necessary intubation equipment is ready, rapidly acting sedative, analgesic, and paralytic medications are administered simultaneously. Cricoid pressure must be maintained until the ETT is in place and confirmed to provide adequate protection from aspiration. An end-tidal CO_2 detector should be attached to the ETT after intubation to confirm proper placement in the trachea. Colorimetric end-tidal CO_2 devices change color from purple to yellow to confirm the presence of exhaled CO_2 and tracheal placement.

Endotracheal intubation and mechanical ventilation can be painful, frightening, and anxiety provoking, especially in a young child. To improve patient comfort, relieve anxiety, and lessen the work of breathing, anxiolytics, sedatives, and analgesics are frequently administered once the patient is intubated and mechanically ventilated. Maintenance of adequate sedation is essential. Selection of appropriate agents is based on the physiology of the patient. Guidelines for the use of continuous infusions are

Table 106-3
Pharmacologic Agents Used for Pediatric Intubation and Continuous Sedation

Drug	Route	Dose	Onset	Duration	Benefits	Adverse Effects
Narcotics						
Morphine	IV	0.1 mg/kg/dose (max: initial dose 2 mg) may repeat to a maximum total dose of 15 mg Neonates: 0.05 mg/kg/dose **Continuous infusion** Children: 20–50 mcg/kg/hour Neonates: 15 mcg/kg/hour Premature neonates: 10 mcg/kg/hour	Peak: 20 minutes	2–4 hours in neonates	Reversible (naloxone)	Histamine release. Respiratory depression hypotension, peripheral vasodilatation, euphoria, dysphoria, itching, central nausea and vomiting, decreased response to hypercarbia
Fentanyl	IV	1–3 mcg/kg/dose (max: initial dose 100 mcg, may repeat to a total dose of 5 mcg/kg or 250 mcg) **Continuous infusion** 1–3 mcg/kg/hour (max: initial dose 50–100 mcg/hour) CHD patient with an open chest: 5 mcg/kg/hour	1–3 minutes	30–90 minutes	Rapid onset, short acting, reversible (naloxone), relatively stable hemodynamic profile	Bradycardia, respiratory depression, decreased response to hypercarbia, acute chest wall rigidity, itching
Benzodiazepines						
Diazepam	IV	0.05 mg/kg/dose (max: 5 mg) may repeat in 0.05-mg/kg increments (max: 1 mg) to a total maximum dose of 10 mg	0.5–2 minutes	3 hours	Reversible (flumazenil)	Respiratory depression, lacks analgesic properties, hypotension and bradycardia, Local irritation, pain
Lorazepam	IV	0.05–0.15 mg/kg/dose (max: 4 mg)	15–30 minutes	0.5–3 hours	Reversible (flumazenil)	Respiratory depression, lacks analgesic properties, hypotension and bradycardia
Midazolam	IV/IM	0.05–0.15 mg/kg/dose (max: initial dose 2 mg, may repeat in 1-mg increments to a total dose of 5 mg) **Continuous infusion** 0.05–0.1 mg/kg/hour (max: initial dose 2 mg/hour)	1–5 minutes	20–30 minutes	Rapid onset, short acting, provides amnesia, reversible (flumazenil)	Respiratory depression, lacks analgesic properties, hypotension and bradycardia
	Intranasal	0.1–0.3 mg/kg/dose (max: 10 mg) Use the 5-mg/mL concentration	2–5 minutes	30–60 minutes		
	PO	0.5–0.75 mg/kg/dose (max:10–20 mg)	30 minutes	2–6 hours		
Barbiturates						
Pentobarbital	IV	2 mg/kg/dose (max: 100 mg). May repeat in 1-mg/kg/dose increments to a total dose of 7 mg/kg. Do not exceed 200 mg total dose **Continuous infusion** 0.5–1 mg/kg/hour	1 minute	15 minutes	Decreases intracranial pressure	Cardiovascular and respiratory depression
	IM/PO/PR	2–6 mg/kg/dose	IM: 10–15 minutes PR/PO: 15–60 minutes	1–4 hours		

(continued)

Table 106-3
Pharmacologic Agents Used for Pediatric Intubation and Continuous Sedation (*continued*)

Drug	Route	Dose	Onset	Duration	Benefits	Adverse Effects
Miscellaneous						
Ketamine	IV	1 mg/kg/dose every 5 minutes titrated to effect **Continuous infusion** 0.5–1 mg/kg/hour	1–2 minutes	10–30 minutes	Rapid onset, airway protective reflexes stay intact, no hypotension or bradycardia Bronchodilation is useful to intubate asthmatics	Increases airway secretions and laryngospasm (blunted with atropine). Elevated intracranial and intraocular pressure. Emergence reactions are possible.
	IM	4–5 mg/kg/dose	3–5 minutes	12–25 minutes		
	PO	6–10 mg/kg (mixed in cola or other beverage)	30 minutes	30–60 minutes		
Etomidate	IV	0.3 mg/kg/dose initially, then 0.1 mg/kg/dose every 5 minutes to titrate to effect	10–20 seconds	4–10 minutes	Rapid onset Short acting Stable hemodynamic profile, decreased ICP	Potential for adrenal inhibition, nausea, and vomiting on emergence
Propofol	IV	1–2 mg/kg/dose initially, then 0.5–2 mg/kg/dose every 3–5 minutes to titrate to effect **Continuous infusion** Infants and children: 50–150 mcg/kg/minute Adolescents: 10–50 mcg/kg/minute	30–60 seconds	5–10 minutes	Intravenous general anesthetic, rapid onset and recovery	Cardiovascular and respiratory depression (propofol-related infusion syndrome) , contraindicated in patients with egg allergy, pain on injection
Dexmedetomidine	IV	0.5–1 mg/kg/dose **Continuous infusion** 0.4–0.7 mcg/kg/hour Doses as high as 2.5 mcg/kg/hour have been used	30 minutes	4 hours	Minimal to no respiratory depression	Hypotension and bradycardia Use with caution in patients with advanced heart block
Neuromuscular Blockers						
Succinylcholine	IV	1 mg/kg/dose	30–60 seconds	4–7 minutes	Rapid onset Short duration	Potentiates hyperkalemia. Contraindicated in head trauma (↑ ICP), crush injury, burns, hyperkalemia. May induce neuroleptic malignant syndrome
Vecuronium	IV	0.1 mg/kg/dose **Continuous infusion:** 0.1 mg/kg/hour	1–3 minutes	30–40 minutes	Cardiovascular stable	Slower onset Longer duration of action
Rocuronium	IV/IM	0.6–1 mg/kg/dose	60–75 seconds	20–30 minutes	Cardiovascular stable	
Reversal Agents						
Naloxone	IV	For opioid overdose: 0.1 mg/kg/dose (max: 2 mg) For reversal of mild respiratory depression: 0.01–0.02 mg/kg/dose (max: 0.4 mg) may repeat every 2–3 minutes	2 minutes	20–60 minutes	Rapid onset	Shorter duration than most opioids, therefore repeated doses may be needed
Flumazenil	IV	0.01 mg/kg/dose (max: 0.2 mg), may repeat 0.005 mg/kg/dose at 1-minute intervals to a max total dose of 1 mg	1–3 minutes	6–10 minutes	Rapid onset	Shorter duration than most benzodiazepines, therefore repeated doses may be needed

CHD, congenital heart disease; ICP, intracranial pressure; IM, intramuscular; IN, intranasal; IV, intravenous; PO, oral.

Table 106-4
Management Examples of Specific Patient Cases

Condition	Treatment Goal During Intubation	Medications
Full stomach	Prevent passive regurgitation and aspiration after airway protective reflexes lost	Rocuronium, succinylcholine
Bronchospasm	Eliminate or treat stimuli that would induce or increase bronchospasm	Ketamine, vecuronium, lidocaine, atropine
Increased intracranial pressure	No increase in heart rate or blood pressure	Thiopental/pentobarbital, etomidate, vecuronium, rocuronium, lidocaine
Pulmonary vascular hypertension	Avoid decreased pulmonary blood flow	Midazolam, fentanyl, vecuronium
Hypokalemia or depressed cardiac output	Maintain blood pressure without heart rate changes	Etomidate or midazolam with fentanyl

outlined in Table 106-3. In the paralyzed patient, neuromuscular blockade neither alters consciousness nor provides analgesia; therefore, adequate sedation and analgesia are essential. Providing effective analgesia and sedation to the pediatric patient depends on accurate ongoing efforts to assess the intensity of the patient's pain or anxiety. The assessment of pain and anxiety in infants and critically ill children who are unable to communicate relies heavily on physiologic and behavioral responses. A number of pain and sedation tools have been developed and validated specifically for use in children.[12] No single standard measure gives a complete qualitative or quantitative measure. Selection of an appropriate tool is based on the child's age, underlying medical condition, and cognition level. It is essential that these tools are utilized to evaluate the adequacy of the ICU sedation. Policies and procedures need to be in place for the appropriate selection and use of each tool, in addition to training of all healthcare professionals to appropriately use each tool. The goal is to use the minimum amount of sedation needed to adequately sedate the intubated child, while minimizing adverse effects.

PEDIATRIC SHOCK

CASE 106-3

QUESTION 1: M.M., a 3-month-old, 6-kg male infant, presents with a history of decreased oral intake and progressive lethargy. Physical examination revealed an irritable infant with a respiratory rate of 50 breaths/minute, heart rate of 150 beats/minute, blood pressure of 80/50 mm Hg, and temperature of 39°C. He has cool extremities with a capillary refill of 3 seconds. The mother reports that her baby has had no wet diapers for the last 4 hours. A small purpuric rash has appeared on his trunk in the last half hour because the parents left home to bring him to the emergency room. Initial electrolytes obtained in the emergency room on placement of IV access were as follows:

Sodium, 136 mEq/L
Potassium, 4.9 mEq/L
Chloride, 111 mEq/L
CO_2 content, 13 mEq/L
Blood urea nitrogen, 31 mg/dL
Serum creatinine, 0.8 mg/dL
Serum glucose, 50 mg/dL
What type of shock might M.M. be experiencing?

Shock may be classified as hypovolemic, distributive, cardiogenic, or obstructive. Based on his presentation, M.M. is most likely presenting with hypovolemic shock, the most frequent type of shock seen in pediatric patients. Hypovolemic shock occurs when circulating intravascular volume decreases to a point at which adequate tissue perfusion can no longer be maintained. Hypovolemia causes a decrease in preload and adversely affects cardiac output. Initially, hypovolemia activates peripheral and central baroreceptors that cause catecholamine-mediated vasoconstriction and tachycardia. This initial response can maintain adequate circulation and blood pressure even after acute loss of as much as 15% of the circulating blood volume. Shock results from inadequate blood flow and oxygen delivery to meet the metabolic demands of the tissues.[3] Shock will progress from an initial compensated state to decompensated state. Typical signs of compensated shock include tachycardia, cool and pale distal extremities, prolonged (>2 seconds) capillary refill, weak peripheral pulses compared with central pulses, and normal systolic blood pressure. As shock progresses, the patient will exhaust his ability to compensate. The patient will exhibit signs of inadequate end-organ perfusion, including depressed mental status, decreased urine output, metabolic acidosis, tachypnea, weak central pulses, and mottling of extremities. M.M. shows evidence of having progressed to this later stage, with lethargy and decreased urine output.

CASE 106-3, QUESTION 2: How should M.M. be initially managed and monitored?

All patients presenting with shock should be placed on high-flow oxygen while their initial evaluation is being performed. Initial volume resuscitation in all forms of shock is the same. It is recommended to push isotonic crystalloid fluid (normal saline or lactated Ringer's solution) in 20 mL/kg boluses administered over 5-10 minutes. Immediately reassess the patient for signs of improved perfusion, using clinical criteria such as reduction in heart rate, improvement of blood pressure, capillary refill, quality of pulses, and mental status. If the clinical signs of shock persist, another 20 mL/kg of isotonic fluid should be administered, reaching, if necessary, at least 60 mL/kg within the first 15 to 30 minutes of treatment.[3,13] Therapeutic end points of fluid resuscitation in patients with shock are capillary refill less than 2 seconds, normal pulses with no difference between central and peripheral pulses, warm limbs, urine output greater than 1 mL/kg/hour, normal mental status, decreased lactate as measured on arterial blood gases (ABG), and increased base deficit. Children normally have a lower blood pressure than adults and are better able to preserve adequate blood pressure by vasoconstriction and increasing heart rate; therefore, blood pressure by itself is not a reliable end point for evaluating the adequacy of resuscitation. Hypotension is the last thing to occur in pediatric shock states. The definition of hypotension, defined as the 5% for systolic blood pressure for age in the 2015 Pediatric Advanced Life Support guidelines[3], is as follows:

- less than 60 mm Hg in term neonates (0–28 days)
- less than 70 mm Hg in infants (1–12 months)
- less than 70 mm Hg + (2 × age in years) in children 1 to 10 years of age
- less than 90 mm Hg in children older than or equal to 10 years of age

Fluid resuscitation should be continued until clinical improvement is clear or there is clinical evidence of hypervolemic state as evidenced by rales, a gallop rhythm, or hepatomegaly. Further discussion of the management of hypovolemia and dehydration in children can be found in Chapter 103, Pediatric Fluid, Electrolytes, and Nutrition. M.M. should receive a bolus 120 mL normal saline IV infused over 5 minutes, followed by assessment of perfusion status to ascertain improvement. If he has not demonstrated significant improvement, the fluid bolus should be repeated until adequate perfusion is seen and blood pressure is stable at greater than 70 mm Hg.

CASE 106-3, QUESTION 3: As noted earlier in the case, M.M. is hypoglycemic with a blood glucose of only 50 mg/dL. What are the concerns associated with hypoglycemia during pediatric shock and how should M.M be managed?

Hypoglycemia often develops in infants during episodes of stress, including shock, seizures, and sepsis. Infants have high glucose needs and low glycogen stores, which make hypoglycemia a risk in a critically ill infant, especially one with poor enteral intake. Point-of-care glucose testing should be performed in any critically ill infant with a history of poor oral intake. One should not wait to obtain serum chemistries. Aggressive fluid resuscitation recommended for hypovolemia and shock will only exacerbate hypoglycemia. Most importantly, hypoglycemia needs to be prevented during cardiopulmonary and trauma resuscitation because it may cause seizures and has been linked with poor neurologic outcome.[3,13] Hypoglycemia in pediatric patients must always be promptly identified and treated. After diagnosis, the patient should be managed with a bolus of 0.5 to 1 g/kg of glucose or 5 to 10 mL/kg of a 10% dextrose solution as required to achieve a serum glucose greater than 100 mg/dL. Neonates, especially premature neonates, are more prone to intraventricular hemorrhage with rapid changes in serum osmolarity than older infants and children; therefore, 0.2 g/kg or 2 mL/kg of 10% dextrose is recommended in this population until the target serum glucose is achieved. M.M. should be given 30 mL (5 mL/kg) of 10% dextrose IV for 1 to 2 minutes, followed by reassessment of his serum glucose. Treatment may be continued until his serum glucose is within the normal range for his age (60–105 mg/dL). After stabilization, maintenance therapy should be initiated with fluids containing 10% dextrose.

SEPSIS AND SEPTIC SHOCK IN INFANTS AND CHILDREN

Septic shock can be a mixture of hypovolemic, cardiogenic, and distributive shock. In a recent population-based study of children in the United States with severe sepsis (defined as bacterial or fungal infection with at least one acute organ dysfunction), Hartman et al.[14] reported an increase in the incidence of severe sepsis from 2000 to 2005 and from 0.56 to 0.89 cases per 1,000 children. The increase reported in newborns was from 4.5 to 9.7 cases per 1,000. This increase was led by sepsis in very low birth-weight neonates. The second increase was reported in children from 15 to 19 years of age with a reported increase from 0.37 to 0.48 cases per 1,000. The mortality rate in this study was 8.9%, unchanged from 2000, but significantly lower than that reported for adult patients with severe sepsis and septic shock (approximately 30% and 50%, respectively). This dramatic improvement in outcome has been attained through a better understanding of the physiology of shock. The use of aggressive fluid resuscitation and the implementation of time-sensitive goal-directed therapies, as well as the application of technologic advances in respiratory, cardiovascular, renal, and nutritional support, and improved antibacterial, antiviral, and antifungal therapy, has resulted in improved survival in infants and children with septic shock and the resultant multisystem organ failure.[3,15–20]

Infants and young children are at a higher risk of severe systemic illness after infection than adults. Despite new developments in vaccine technology, rates of sepsis have not declined. This phenomenon is most likely as a result of cases occurring in infants before complete immunization. Infants are particularly vulnerable to infections for several reasons.[20] Passive immunity is normally conveyed from the mother to the fetus through transmission of immunoglobulins during the last trimester. As a result, premature neonates are immunoglobulin-deficient. Even the full-term neonate has decreased polymorphonuclear leukocyte (PMN) function and small PMN storage pools compared with older children and adults, as well as decreased ability to synthesize new antibodies. Lastly, neonates cannot make and deliver adequate amounts of phagocytes to sites of infection. Low immunoglobulin levels also make the infant susceptible to viral infections. Stores of maternal immunoglobulin are depleted at approximately 2 to 5 months of age. Adult levels of immunoglobulin are not typically achieved until 4 to 7 years of age. As the result of these physiologic differences, as well as differences in bacterial resistance patterns, the list of most likely pathogens in children with sepsis differs from those of adults. Table 106-5 lists common pediatric pathogens and appropriate empiric antibiotic coverage. Antibiotics should be administered within 1 hour of diagnosis, after the collection of appropriate cultures.[13]

As in adults, baseline health status also affects the likelihood of a child exhibiting severe sepsis. Watson et al. found that 49% of cases of sepsis occurred in children who had underlying illnesses which may place them at risk of higher morbidity and mortality.[14] At the Children's Hospital of Pittsburgh, the mortality rate for children who were previously healthy was 2% compared with 12% in children with chronic illnesses.[21]

CASE 106-4

QUESTION 1: J.B., a 6-year-old, 20-kg girl, presented to the pediatric emergency department in acute distress. She was stabilized with oxygen via nasal cannula and fluid resuscitation before being transferred to the PICU for further management. On presentation to the PICU, she is lethargic and unable to follow commands, with warm, dry, slightly mottled skin and sluggish capillary return. She is febrile to 39.5°C and has a respiratory rate of 21 breaths/minute, a heart rate of 154 beats/minute, and a blood pressure of 76/55 mm Hg. Initial laboratory values are notable for a white blood cell count of 21×10^3 μL. Her parents report that she has not urinated since the previous evening. Does J.B. meet the criteria for septic shock?

In an effort to develop a consensus definition of the pediatric sepsis continuum including systemic inflammatory response syndrome (SIRS), infection, sepsis, severe sepsis, septic shock, and multisystem organ dysfunction syndrome, a group of international experts in the fields of adult and pediatric sepsis and clinical research gathered in 2002. A panel was chosen consisting of published pediatric critical care physicians and scientists with clinical research experience in pediatric sepsis.[16] Because the clinical variables used to define SIRS

Table 106-5

Causative Pathogens and Recommended Treatments for Pediatric Sepsis

Age or Risk Factor	Microorganism	Empiric Antibiotic Coverage
Age <30 days	*Listeria monocytogenes* *Escherichia coli* Group B *Streptococcus* Gram-negative enteric organisms	Ampicillin + aminoglycoside or ampicillin + cefotaxime acyclovir (if patient presents with seizures, until HSV ruled out)
Age 1 to 3 months	*L. monocytogenes* *E. coli* Group B *Streptococcus* *Haemophilus influenzae* *Streptococcus pneumoniae* *Neisseria meningiditis*	Ampicillin + TGC ± vancomycin[a]
Age >3 months	*H. influenzae* *S. pneumoniae* *N. meningiditis*	TGC ± vancomycin[a]
Immunocompromised child	*Pseudomonas aeruginosa* *Staphylococcus aureus* *Staphylococcus epidermidis*	Ceftazidime or cefepime or piperacillin/tazobactam + vancomycin[a]
Child with a ventriculoperitoneal shunt	*S. aureus* *S. epidermidis* Gram-negative enteric organisms	TGC ± vancomycin[a]

[a]Dosed to maintain trough vancomycin serum concentrations of 15 to 20 mcg/mL.
HSV, herpes simplex virus; TGC, third-generation cephalosporin (i.e., cefotaxime, ceftriaxone, or ceftizoxime).

Table 106-6

Pediatric Age Group Definitions for Severe Sepsis

Age Category	Definition
Newborn	0 day–1 week
Neonate	1 week–1 month
Infant	1 month to 1 year
Toddler and preschool	2–5 years
School-age child	6–12 years
Adolescent and young adult	13–<18 years

Reprinted with permission from Goldstein B et al. International pediatric sepsis consensus conference: definitions for sepsis and organ dysfunction in pediatrics. *Pediatr Crit Care Med*. 2005;6(1):3.

and organ dysfunction are greatly affected by the normal physiologic changes that occur as children age, the group first defined six clinically and physiologic age categories for defining SIRS criteria (Table 106-6). Premature infants were not included because their care occurs primarily in neonatal intensive care units and not in PICUs. Before discussing treatment, it is important that the practitioner should understand the terms used to define sepsis. In 1992, SIRS was proposed by the American College of Chest Physicians and the Society of Critical Care Medicine (SCCM) to describe the nonspecific inflammatory process occurring in adults after trauma, infection, burns, pancreatitis, and other diseases.[22,23] Sepsis was defined as SIRS associated with infection. The SIRS criteria were developed for use in adults; it was not until 2005 that a consensus definition was published for SIRS in children (Table 106-7).[24] A separate pediatric definition for SIRS was essential. Tachycardia and tachypnea, pivotal to the adult definition of SIRS, are common presenting symptoms of many pediatric disease processes. To better distinguish SIRS from other diseases, the pediatric definition also includes temperature and leukocyte abnormalities as criteria. Numeric values for each criterion were also established to account for the different physiology in children. Table 106-8 gives the age-specific cutoffs for each criterion.

Temperature is one of the main criteria of the pediatric SIRS definition. A core temperature greater than 38.5°C or less than 36°C may indicate serious infection. Hypothermia is more likely to occur in infants. A core temperature is the one measured by either rectal, bladder, oral, or central catheter probe. Temperatures taken via the tympanic, toe, or another auxiliary route are not sufficiently accurate. Temperature may also be documented by a reliable source at home within 4 hours of presentation to the hospital or physician's office. If environmental overheating, such as that produced by overbundling, is suspected, the child should be returned to a neutral temperature environment, unbundled, and the temperature retaken in 15 to 30 minutes.

Meeting the SIRS criteria in children requires the presence of an abnormal temperature, either hypothermia or hyperthermia, or an abnormal leukocyte count in the presence of tachypnea and tachycardia. Sepsis is defined as the proven or suspected infection in the setting of SIRS. Severe sepsis is defined as sepsis in the setting of acute respiratory distress syndrome, cardiovascular organ dysfunction, or two or more acute organ dysfunctions (respiratory, renal, hematologic, neurologic, or hepatic). The definitions of organ dysfunction have also been modified for children (Table 106-9). Carcillo et al.[16] defined pediatric septic shock (SS) as the presence of tachycardia and poor perfusion, including decreased peripheral pulses compared with central pulses; altered alertness; capillary refill greater than 2 seconds; mottled or cool extremities; or decreased urine output. This definition of pediatric SS does not include hypotension as required in adults because children will often maintain their blood pressure until they are severely ill. Shock may occur long before hypotension occurs. J.B. exhibits the majority of the criteria for pediatric SS, including lethargy, fever, tachycardia, decreased perfusion, and decreased urination.

CASE 106-4, QUESTION 2: What physiologic differences may need to be taken into account when developing a management strategy for J.B.?

Table 106-7

Definitions of Systemic Inflammatory Response Syndrome, Infection, Sepsis, Severe Sepsis, and Septic Shock in Children

SIRS	The presence of at least two of the following four criteria, one of which must be abnormal temperature or leukocyte count: ■ Core temperature of >38°C or <36°C (must be measured by rectal, bladder, oral, or central catheter probe) ■ Tachycardia defined as at least two standard deviations above normal for age in the absence of external stimulus, chronic drugs, or painful stimuli; or otherwise persistent elevation for a 0.5- to 4-hour time period OR for children <1 year old: bradycardia, defined as a mean heart rate <10% percentile for age in the absence external vagal stimulus, β-blocker drugs, or congenital heart disease; or otherwise unexplained depression in a half-hour period ■ Mean respiratory rate >2 standard deviations above normal for age or mechanical ventilation for an acute process not related to underlying neuromuscular disease or receipt of general anesthesia ■ Leukocyte count elevated or depressed for age (not secondary to chemotherapy-induced neutropenia) or >10% immature neutrophils
Infection	A suspected or proven (by positive culture, tissue stain, or polymerase chain reaction test) infection caused by any pathogen OR a clinical syndrome associated with a high probability of infection. Evidence of infection includes positive findings on clinical examination, imaging, or laboratory tests (e.g., white blood cells in a normally sterile body fluid, perforated viscus, chest radiograph consistent with pneumonia, petechial or purpuric rash, or purpura fulminans)
Sepsis	SIRS in the presence of or as a result of suspected or proven infection
Severe sepsis	Sepsis plus one of the following: cardiovascular organ dysfunction OR acute respiratory distress syndrome OR dysfunction of two or more other organs, as defined in Table 106-9
Septic shock	Severe sepsis with cardiovascular dysfunction, as defined in Table 106-9

SIRS, systemic inflammatory response syndrome.
Adapted with permission from Goldstein B et al. International pediatric sepsis consensus conference: definitions for sepsis and organ dysfunction in pediatrics. *Pediatr Crit Care Med*. 2005;6(1):4.

Table 106-8

Age-Specific Vital Signs and Laboratory Variables

Age Group	Heart Rate[a] (beats/minute)		Respiratory Rate (breaths/minute)	Leukocyte Count[a] (per $10^3/\mu L$)	Systolic Blood Pressure[a] (mm Hg)
	Tachycardia	Bradycardia			
0 day to 1 week	>180	<100	>50	>34	<65
1 week to 1 month	>180	<100	>40	>19.5 or <5	<75
1 month to 1 year	>180	<90	>34	>17.5 or <5	<100
2 to 5 years	>140	n/a	>22	>15.5 or <6	<94
6 to 12 years	>130	n/a	>18	>13.5 or <4.5	<105
13 to <18 years	>110	n/a	>14	>11 or <4.5	<117

[a]Lower limits of the normal range for heart rate, leukocyte count, and systolic blood pressure for the 5th percentile and upper limits for the for the 95th percentile.
Reprinted with permission from Goldstein B et al. International pediatric sepsis consensus conference: definitions for sepsis and organ dysfunction in pediatrics. *Pediatr Crit Care Med*. 2005;6(1):4.

There are developmental differences in the hemodynamic response to sepsis in newborns, children, and adults. Practitioners in the PICU may encounter all age ranges and thus must be familiar with the clinical differences seen between age groups because it may affect therapy. Adults and children have different adaptive responses that must be considered when selecting therapeutic management. Adolescent patients pose a unique challenge because they may present with either types of symptoms. Among adult patients, the most common hemodynamic alterations include diminished systemic vascular resistance (SVR) and elevated cardiac output (CO). SVR is diminished due to decreased vascular responsiveness to catecholamines, alterations in α-adrenergic receptor signal transduction, and the elaboration of inducible nitric oxide synthase. In general, adults with SS have myocardial dysfunction with a decreased ejection fraction; however, CO is preserved or increased through two compensatory mechanisms: tachycardia and reduced SVR.

Unlike SS in adults, pediatric SS is associated with severe hypovolemia, and children frequently respond well to aggressive fluid resuscitation. Pediatric patients demonstrate diverse hemodynamic profiles during fluid-refractory SS: 58% have low cardiac indexes responsive to inotropic medications with or without vasodilators, 20% exhibit high cardiac index and low SVR responsive to vasopressor therapy, and 22% present both vascular and cardiac dysfunctions necessitating the use of vasopressors and inotropic support.[25] Pediatric patients such as J.B. are different from adults with SS in that low CO, not low SVR, is associated with increased mortality. In fact, studies suggest that the majority of children showed some degree of cardiac dysfunction on presentation after fluid resuscitation.[13,18] Many require a change in their inotropic and vasopressor management, or the addition of another agent during the first hours of treatment, emphasizing that the hemodynamic status in children can change rapidly.[13,16–18]

Table 106-9

Organ Dysfunction Criteria

Cardiovascular Dysfunction

Despite administration of isotonic intravenous fluid bolus 40 mL/kg in 1 hour

- Decrease in BP (hypotension) <5th percentile for age or systolic BP <2 standard deviations below normal for age[a] OR
- Need for vasoactive drug to maintain BP in normal range (dopamine >5 mcg/kg/minute or dobutamine, epinephrine, or norepinephrine at any dose) OR
- Two of the following:
  Unexplained metabolic acidosis: base deficit >5 mEq/L
  Increased arterial lactate >2 times upper limit of normal
  Oliguria: urine output <0.5 mL/kg/hour
  Prolonged capillary refill: >5 seconds
  Core to peripheral temperature gap >3°C

Respiratory[b]

- Pao_2/Fio_2 <300 in absence of cyanotic heart disease or preexisting lung disease OR
- $Paco_2$ >65 torr or 20 mm Hg over baseline $Paco_2$ OR
- Proven need[c] or >50% Fio_2 to maintain saturations >92% OR
- Need for nonelective invasive or noninvasive mechanical ventilation[d]

Neurologic

- Glasgow Coma Scale (see Table 106-12) <11 OR
- Acute change in mental status with a decrease in Glasgow Coma Scale ≥3 points from abnormal baseline

Hematologic

- Platelet count <80,000/μL or a decline of 50% in platelet count from highest value recorded in the past 3 days (for chronic hematology/oncology patients) OR
- International normalized ratio of >2

Renal

- Serum creatinine >2 times upper limit of normal for age or twofold increase in baseline creatinine

Hepatic

- Total bilirubin ≥4 mg/dL (not applicable for newborn) OR
- ALT 2 times upper limit of normal for age

[a]See Table 106-8.
[b]Acute respiratory distress syndrome must include a Pao_2/Fio_2 ratio <200 mm Hg, bilateral infiltrates, acute onset, and no evidence of left heart failure. Acute lung injury is defined identically except the Pao_2/Fio_2 ratio must be <300 mm Hg.
[c]Proven need assumes oxygen requirement was tested by decreasing flow if required.
[d]In postoperative patients, this requirement can be met if the patient has exhibited an acute inflammatory or infectious process in the lungs that prevents him or her from being extubated.
ALT alanine transaminase; BP, blood pressure.
Adapted with permission from Goldstein B et al. International pediatric sepsis consensus conference: definitions for sepsis and organ dysfunction in pediatrics. *Pediatr Crit Care Med*. 2005;6(1):5.

SS in the neonatal patient differs from that seen in older children. The relative ability of infants and children to augment CO through increased heart rate (HR), as seen in adults, is limited by their preexisting elevated HR, which precludes proportionate increases in HR without compromising diastolic filling time. In adults, ventricular dilation is a compensatory response used to maintain CO. However, the increased connective tissue content of the infant's heart and diminished content of actin and myosin limits the potential for acute ventricular dilation. Neonatal SS can be further complicated by the physiologic transition from fetal to neonatal circulation. Sepsis-induced acidosis and hypoxia can increase pulmonary vascular resistance and thus arterial pressure, thereby maintaining the patency of the ductus arteriosus. This results in persistent pulmonary hypertension (PPHN) of the newborn and persistent fetal circulation. Neonatal SS with PPHN will increase the workload on the right ventricle, leading to right-ventricular failure, tricuspid regurgitation, and hepatomegaly. Therefore, therapies directed at reversing right-ventricular failure by reducing pulmonary artery pressures are commonly needed in neonates with fluid-refractory SS and PPHN.

Based on her mottled dry skin, sluggish capillary refill, and decreased urination, it is evident that J.B. has inadequate perfusion. She should receive aggressive fluid resuscitation, beginning with a fluid bolus of 400 mL (20 mL/kg) normal saline or lactated Ringer's solution IV administered over 5 minutes. She should be reassessed immediately after the bolus to evaluate perfusion status as described previously. The 400-mL fluid bolus should be repeated until adequate perfusion has been established.

INITIAL MANAGEMENT OF PEDIATRIC SEPTIC SHOCK

Because the landmark study by Rivers in 2001 demonstrated a 33% reduction in mortality in adult patients with sepsis when they were aggressively treated with fluid resuscitation, blood transfusion, and inotropic therapy within 6 hours of admission, goal-directed therapy has been advocated for all patients who present in SS.[15] The components of early goal-directed therapy include respiratory support along with prompt resuscitation of poor perfusion through administration of IV fluids and appropriately targeted inotropic and vasopressor therapy, early empiric antimicrobial therapy, drainage of the infection whenever possible, and continuous monitoring of the patient's hemodynamic status.[13,15–19]

Case 106-4, Question 3: J.B. has received one bolus of normal saline in the pediatric emergency department, but is still showing evidence of being hypoperfused. Her hemoglobin on admission to the PICU is 10 g/dL. Should she continue to receive traditional IV fluid replacement with normal saline or should other agents be considered to maximize perfusion and oxygenation?

There are no data to suggest a significant difference in survival rates in pediatric patients after resuscitation with colloids, including blood products, compared with crystalloid fluids.[26] The choice of fluid is less important than the volume administered. Adequate volume is necessary to sustain cardiac preload, increase stroke volume, and improve oxygen delivery. Both crystalloids and colloids, specifically packed red blood cells (PRBC), have equal effects on improving stroke volume. In addition, both restore tissue perfusion to the same degree if they are titrated to the same level of filling pressure.

Administration of blood products also differs among institutions. The optimal hemoglobin for infants and children in SS has not been established. In the early management of sepsis in adults, maintaining hemoglobin of 7 to 9 g/dL to improve oxygen carrying capacity has been documented to improve sepsis survival by improving tissue perfusion. Anemia in sepsis has been associated with increased mortality, but so has the administration of blood products.[27] Based on the limited data available, SCCM has recommended that hemoglobin concentrations in adults be maintained at 7 to 9 g/dL.[13] As pediatric data are even more limited, it is necessary to extrapolate from the adult literature suggesting maximizing tissue oxygen delivery if there is evidence of poor tissue perfusion. Once tissue hypoperfusion, acute hemorrhage, or lactic acidosis has resolved, PRBC transfusion should be considered only when the hemoglobin is less than 7 g/dL.[13,28] At this time, there is no indication for administration of blood products to J.B. Fresh frozen plasma may be infused to correct abnormal prothrombin time (PT) and partial thromboplastin time (PTT) values, but should not be rapidly infused because of the risk for acute hypotensive effects caused by vasoactive kinins and high citrate concentration. There is no literature to suggest that 5% albumin administration improves outcome in regard to sepsis mortality. Albumin administration may be considered in patients who are hypoalbuminemic, but routine use of albumin is not recommended.[29]

As described previously for the management of hypovolemic shock, patients with SS should be reassessed for signs of improved perfusion using clinical criteria such as reduction in heart rate, improvement of blood pressure, capillary refill, quality of pulses, and mental status with each fluid bolus. If the clinical signs of shock persist, another 20 mL/kg of isotonic fluid should be administered reaching, if necessary, 60 mL/kg within the first 15 to 30 minutes of treatment.[3,13,17] Some children with SS require as much as 200 mL/kg in the first hour.[17] Patients remaining in shock despite fluid resuscitation are given inotropic support to attain normal blood pressure for age and capillary refill time of less than 2 seconds. Every hour that goes by without implementing these therapies is associated with a 1.5-fold increased risk of mortality. Patients who do not respond rapidly to initial fluid boluses or those with insufficient physiologic reserve should be considered for invasive hemodynamic monitoring. Invasive monitoring of central venous pressure (CVP) is instituted to ensure that the satisfactory right-ventricular preload is present, typically using a goal of 10 to 12 mm Hg, and that oxygen carrying capacity is optimized by PRBC transfusion to correct anemia to a goal hemoglobin concentration greater than 7 g/dL.[13,17]

Up to 40% of a child's CO may be required to support the work of breathing during SS; therefore, in the presence of respiratory distress, elective intubation and mechanical ventilation can be used to allow redistribution of blood flow from respiratory muscles toward other vital organs. Intubation is not without adverse effects; it is imperative that patients receive adequate fluid resuscitation before intubation because the change from spontaneous breathing to positive-pressure ventilation will decrease the effective preload to the heart, further decreasing cardiac output. Ventilation may reduce left-ventricular afterload that may be beneficial in patients with low cardiac index and high SVR. In addition, it may provide an alternative method to alter acid base balance. If sedatives and analgesics are used for intubation, choice of agents that do not cause further vasodilation is critical.

Although laboratory studies rarely affect the management of SS in the first hour of therapy, patients should have laboratory studies sent routinely assessing for hematologic abnormalities, metabolic derangements, or electrolyte abnormalities that may contribute to morbidity. A peripheral white blood count may aid in the choice of broad-spectrum antibiotics and hemoglobin and platelet count will help in assessing the need for early blood transfusion. A type and screen should be sent to the blood bank to prepare for any necessary transfusions. Electrolyte abnormalities are common in sepsis; recognition and treatment of metabolic abnormalities such as hypoglycemia and hypocalcemia will improve outcome. A disseminated intravascular coagulation panel, including PT, PTT, and fibrinogen, will aid in assessing the severity of illness. If abnormalities exist, they may need to be corrected before performing invasive procedures. Lastly, an arterial or venous blood gas will determine the adequacy of ventilation, oxygenation, and severity of acidemia.[17]

Unfortunately, clinical response to fluid resuscitation is a relatively insensitive indicator for the completeness of restoration of microvascular blood flow. Success of adequate fluid resuscitation can be guided by additional parameters: invasive blood pressure monitoring, CVP, measurement of mixed venous oxygen saturation (Svo_2), measurement of blood lactate, and urine output. An elevated serum lactate level suggests tissue is inadequately perfused and undergoing anaerobic metabolism, even in patients who are not hypotensive. Because low CO is associated with increased O_2 extraction, Svo_2 can be used as an indirect indicator of whether CO is adequate to meet tissue metabolic demand. If tissue oxygen delivery is adequate, then Svo_2 should be greater than 70%.[17] In the goal-directed study by Rivers, maintenance of Svo_2 was greater than 70% by use of blood transfusion to a hemoglobin of 10 g/dL and inotropic support to increase CO resulted in a 40% reduction in mortality compared with patients where only mean arterial pressure and CVP were monitored.[15] de Oliveria et al.[18] reproduced this finding in children with SS, reducing mortality from 39% to 12% when directing therapy to a goal Svo_2 saturation greater than 70%.

CARDIOVASCULAR DRUG THERAPY

Pharmacologic support in children with SS must be individualized because different hemodynamic abnormalities exist in pediatric patients, and the primary hemodynamic abnormalities may change with time and progression of the patient's disease (Table 106-10). Twenty percent (20%) of children present with predominant vasodilatory shock, referred to as "warm" shock. This form of shock is associated with vasodilation and capillary leak, but normal or elevated CO. The patients have strong pulses, warm extremities, good capillary refill, and tachycardia. In warm shock, using a vasopressor such as dopamine, norepinephrine, phenylephrine, or vasopressin to promote vasoconstriction would provide the most benefit. Fifty-eight percent (58%) of children present with "cold shock" or a poor CO state. These patients have

Table 106-10

Summary of Selected Vasoactive Agents

Agent	Dose Range	Peripheral Vascular Effects			Cardiac Effects
Vasopressors					
		α	β_1	β_2	
Dobutamine	2–20 mcg/kg/minute	1+	3–4+	1–2+	Less chronotrophy and arrhythmias at lower doses; chronotropic advantage compared with dopamine may not be apparent in neonates
Dopamine	2–4 mcg/kg/minute	0	0	0	Splanchnic and renal vasodilator, increasing doses create increasing α-effect
	4–8 mcg/kg/minute	0	1–2+	1+	
	>10 mcg/kg/minute	2–4+	1–2+	2+	
Epinephrine	0.03–0.1 mcg/kg/minute	2+	2–3+	2+	β_2 effects with lower doses
	0.2–0.5 mcg/kg/minute	4+	2+	3+	
Norepinephrine	0.05–0.5 mcg/kg/minute	4+	2+	0	Increases systemic resistance, moderate inotropy
Phenylephrine	0.05–0.5 mcg/kg/minute	4+	0	0	Increases systemic resistance, moderate inotropy
Vasodilators					
Nitroprusside	0.5–8 mcg/kg/minute	Donates nitric oxide to relax smooth muscles and dilate pulmonary and systemic vessels		Indirectly increases cardiac output by decreasing afterload	Reflex tachycardia
Nitroglycerine	0.5–10 mcg/kg/minute	As a nitric oxide donor may cause pulmonary vasodilation and enhance coronary vasoreactivity after aortic cross-clamping		Decreases preload; may decrease afterload, reduces myocardial work in relation to change in wall stress	Minimal
Miscellaneous Agents					
Milrinone	50 mcg/kg load; then 0.25–1 mcg/kg/minute	Systemic and pulmonary vasodilator		Diastolic relaxation (lusitropy)	Minimal tachycardia
Vasopressin	0.003–0.002 units/kg/minute OR 18–120 milliunits/kg/hour	Potent vasoconstrictor		No direct effect	None known

vasoconstriction, increased cardiac afterload, and a high SVR. This is clinically manifested as weak pulses, cool extremities, slow capillary refill, and hepatic and pulmonary congestion. Using an inotrope with or without a vasodilator would be most beneficial in cold shock (e.g., dobutamine, epinephrine, or milrinone). Careful assessment of clinical response is critical because a combination of warm and cold shock, with a low SVR and poor CO, occurs in approximately 22% of children.

CASE 106-4, QUESTION 4: Despite adequate fluid resuscitation, intubation, and mechanical ventilation, J.B.'s condition has continued to decline. During the past 30 minutes, her systolic blood pressure has ranged between 72 and 79 mm Hg (normal for age, >84 mm Hg). What would be an appropriate next step for the management of J.B.'s shock?

Vasopressors are required in shock unresponsive to initial fluid resuscitation.[3,13,17] In pediatric SS, the initial agent of choice has typically been dopamine.[13,17] Dopamine has direct and indirect effects on dopamine receptors, α-adrenergic receptors, and β-adrenergic receptors on both the heart and peripheral vasculature. One of the mechanisms of dopamine action is enhancement of endogenous catecholamine release. In severe septic states, presynaptic vacuoles may be depleted of norepinephrine, which may explain why dopamine may have diminished activity. In addition, infants younger than 6 months of age may not have developed their component of sympathetic innervations; therefore, they have reduced releasable stores of epinephrine.

Some studies have raised the concern of increased mortality with the use of dopamine. One possible explanation is the ability of dopamine to reduce the release of hormones from the anterior pituitary gland, such as prolactin, through stimulation of the dopamine D_2 receptor, thus reducing cell-mediated immunity and inhibition of thyrotropin-releasing hormone release, worsening impaired thyroid function known to occur in critical illness. Although most clinicians continue to use dopamine as their drug of choice for initiating inotropic therapy in pediatric SS, some prefer low-dose norepinephrine as a first-line agent for those children with fluid-refractory hypotensive hyperdynamic shock.[17]

J.B. should be started on dopamine at a rate of 5 mcg/kg/minute, with further titration of the dose in increments of 2.5 mcg/kg/minute every 3 to 5 minutes until the goal of improved perfusion and/or a normal blood pressure for age is achieved.[3] The maximum recommended dose of dopamine is 20 mcg/kg/minute; higher doses may contribute to increased myocardial oxygen demand without much improvement in vasopressor activity. Dopamine, as well as other agents capable of producing vasoconstriction, should ideally be administered through central venous access rather than through a peripheral IV. Extravasation of these drugs from an infiltration of the IV may produce significant local tissue necrosis.

CASE 106-4, QUESTION 5: J.B.'s dopamine infusion has been steadily increased throughout the day. Her dose is currently at 20 mcg/kg/minute, but she continues to have refractory hypotension with a systolic blood pressure of 70 mm Hg. On physical examination, she is pale with cool, dry skin. Her hemoglobin remains at 10 g/dL. Central venous pressures are now being measured and range from 6 to 9 mm Hg. What alternative to dopamine should be considered for J.B.?

Dopamine-resistant shock is diagnosed after titration of dopamine to 20 mcg/kg/minute with the persistence of signs and symptoms of shock. Patients with dopamine-resistant shock should be reassessed to evaluate fluid status and hemoglobin, with additional fluids or PRBC given as needed to improve tissue oxygen. Measurement of CVP can be performed to assess intravascular volume status with the goal of achieving a CVP of 8 to 12 mm Hg, and Svo_2 can be used as a marker of cardiac output (provided that the hemoglobin is within the normal range), along with the clinical examination. Dopamine-resistant shock commonly responds to epinephrine or norepinephrine.

Epinephrine

Epinephrine is a direct agent that is naturally produced in the adrenal gland and is the principal stress hormone with widespread metabolic and hemodynamic effects. It possesses both inotropic and chronotropic effects. Epinephrine is a reasonable choice for the treatment of patients with low CO and poor peripheral perfusion because it increases HR and myocardial contractility. Depending on the dose administered, epinephrine may exert variable effects on SVR. At doses less than 0.3 mcg/kg/minute, epinephrine exerts greater β_2-adrenergic receptor activation, resulting in vasodilation in skeletal muscle and cutaneous vascular beds, shunting blood flow away from the splanchnic circulation.[17] At higher doses, α_1-adrenergic receptor activation becomes more prominent and may increase SVR and heart rate. For patients with markedly elevated SVR, epinephrine (0.05–0.3 mcg/kg/minute) may be administered simultaneously with a vasodilator. Epinephrine increases glucogenesis and glycogenolysis, resulting in elevated serum blood glucose concentrations. Children receiving epinephrine infusions should have serum glucose monitored closely.

Norepinephrine

Norepinephrine is a direct agent and is naturally produced in the adrenal gland. It is a potent vasopressor that redirects blood flow away from skeletal muscle to the splanchnic circulation even in the presence of decreased cardiac output. Norepinephrine has been used extensively to elevate SVR in septic adults and children. If the patient's clinical state is characterized by low SVR (a wide pulse pressure with diastolic blood pressure less than one-half of the systolic blood pressure), norepinephrine (0.05–0.3 mcg/kg/minute) is recommended. Approximately 20% of children with volume-refractory SS have a low SVR. In children who are intubated and receiving sedatives or analgesics, the incidence of low SVR may be higher. The additional afterload imposed by norepinephrine may substantially compromise CO in patients with impaired contractility. In patients with both impaired or marginal CO and decreased SVR, it may be necessary to support myocardial contractility through the addition of an agent such as dobutamine.[13,17]

Vasopressin

Although not a recommendation in the 2015 Pediatric Advanced Life Support guidelines, vasopressin has been suggested as an alternative therapy for refractory cardiac arrest or hypotension due to a low SVR in children whose epinephrine infusion exceeds 1 mcg/kg/minute.[3] Vasopressin exerts its hemodynamic effects via the $V_{1\alpha}$ receptor, promoting an increase in intracellular calcium in the peripheral vasculature, thus enhancing vasoconstriction and restoring systemic vascular tone. In a preliminary case series, vasopressin at a dose of 0.3 to 2 milliunits/kg/minute (18–120 milliunits/kg/hour) improved blood pressure and urine output in patients with catecholamine-refractory vasodilatory shock and allowed weaning of catecholamines once treatment was initiated.[30] In a more recent analysis conducted by the American Heart Association, however, vasopressin use was associated with a lower rate of return to spontaneous circulation.[31] At this time, the use of vasopressin in critically ill children remains controversial.[3,13,17]

Dobutamine

Dobutamine is a nonselective β_2-adrenergic agonist, which produces improved contractility, chronotrophy, and some degree of lusitropy, or improved myocardial relaxation. The β_2 activity can lead to peripheral vasodilation, and this must be considered before its use in a patient who may already be hypotensive. If hypotension does exist, it should be used in combination with other vasopressor therapies. Dobutamine should be considered in patient who has signs and symptoms or laboratory values consistent with poor tissue perfusion, but has an adequate blood pressure to tolerate some degree of vasodilation. It should be initiated at a rate of 2.5 mcg/kg/minute and titrated in increments of 2.5 mcg/kg/minute every 3 to 5 minutes to a maximum infusion rate of 20 mcg/kg/minute.[3,17] Careful attention to the patient's blood pressure is critical. Improved perfusion, decreased lactate, and an increased Svo_2 will help determine appropriate dosing.

Vasodilators

Vasodilator medications are occasionally required in the treatment of septic pediatric patients with markedly elevated SVR and normal or decreased CO. Vasodilators decrease SVR and improve cardiac output by decreasing ventricular afterload. Nitroglycerin or nitroprusside may be used for this indication. They each have a short half-life; therefore, if hypotension occurs, it can be rapidly reversed by stopping the infusion. Both drugs can be infused at an initial rate of 0.5 mcg/kg/minute and titrated in increments of 0.5 mcg/kg/minute to a maximum infusion rate of 5 to 10 mcg/kg/minute.[3] If nitroprusside is used, it is necessary to observe for sodium thiocyanate accumulation in the setting of renal failure, and cyanide toxicity with hepatic failure or with prolonged infusions (more than 72 hours) of greater than 3 mcg/kg/minute. If a patient has tolerated short-term infusions of either of these agents, milrinone may be considered as an alternative for long-term therapy. Milrinone is a phosphodiesterase type III (PDE III) inhibitor that produces its hemodynamic effects by inhibiting the degradation of cyclic AMP in smooth muscle cells and cardiac myocytes. PDE III inhibitors work synergistically with catecholamines, which produce their hemodynamic effects by increasing the production of cyclic AMP. Milrinone, at a dose of 0.25 to 0.75 mcg/kg/minute, is useful in the treatment of infants and children with diminished CO, impaired myocardial contractility, and decreased SVR.[13,32] The primary concern with milrinone is its relatively long half-life of 2 to 6 hours, which requires several hours for the patient to reach steady state. To achieve target serum concentrations more rapidly, a loading dose of 50 mcg/kg may be administered for 10 to 30 minutes before the start of the infusion. Administration of a loading dose must be done with caution in children with sepsis and shock because it may precipitate hypotension, requiring volume infusion and/or vasopressor infusion. Administering the loading dose over several hours may avoid this adverse effect.

J.B. remains hypotensive despite adequate fluid administration and a dopamine infusion at the maximum rate. After reassessing her laboratory parameters to determine whether additional fluid or blood products are needed, J.B. should be started on epinephrine at 0.05 mcg/kg/minute. The dose may then be titrated upward in 0.05 to 0.1 mcg/kg/minute increments every 3 to 5 minutes as needed to achieve the desired clinical response or to the usual maximum of 2 mcg/kg/minute. Higher doses have been used in some pediatric cases, but may not always provide additional benefit.[3]

CORTICOSTEROID ADMINISTRATION IN PEDIATRIC SEPTIC SHOCK

CASE 106-4, QUESTION 6: J.B. is currently receiving epinephrine at an infusion rate of 0.35 mcg/kg/minute, but she continues to have refractory hypotension with a systolic blood pressure of 70 mm Hg. Is there a role for hydrocortisone replacement in J.B.? What would be the appropriate method for assessing adrenal insufficiency and the appropriate dose for replacement?

Although adjunctive corticosteroid therapy in patients in septic shock has not made a significant difference in outcome in all studies published to date, replacement may be of benefit in some patients.[33–35] In a recent study, 77% of children with septic shock admitted to two PICUs for a 6-month period exhibited adrenal insufficiency.[35] Due to the limited evidence of their efficacy and safety in children, corticosteroids should be reserved for those with catecholamine-resistant shock, severe septic shock and purpura, children who have previously received steroid therapies for chronic illness, children with pituitary or adrenal abnormalities, and those who previously received etomidate.[5–7,13,33–35] Assessment of serum cortisol should be used to guide treatment. There are no strict definitions, but adrenal insufficiency in adults with catecholamine-resistant shock has been defined as a random cortisol level of less than 18 mcg/dL or an increase in cortisol of less than or equal to 9 mcg/dL at 30 or 60 minutes after an adrenocorticotropic hormone stimulation test.[33] Similar values have been recommended for assessment of serum cortisol in children with SS.[13]

If J.B. has a random cortisol of 10 mcg/dL in the face of catecholamine-resistant hypotension, a trial of hydrocortisone is warranted. Published guidelines for hemodynamic support of pediatric and neonatal patients in septic shock recommend 0.5 to 1 mg/kg IV every 6 hours (with a maximum dose of 50 mg).[16] Using this regimen, J.B. should be treated with 10 to 20 mg IV every 6 hours. As an alternative, some clinicians use a regimen of a single 50-mg/m^2 loading dose, followed by the same dose (50 mg/m^2) divided into four doses and given every 6 hours.[13]

ADJUNCTIVE THERAPIES

Stress-Related Mucosal Bleeding

The use of prophylaxis to prevent stress-related mucosal bleeding, although common in adult ICU patients, is not as widely used in PICUs. Studies conducted to date have provided a wide range of gastrointestinal tract bleeding rates in children, ranging from 10% to 50%, with rates of clinically significant bleeding of approximately 1% to 4%.[36,37] Several investigators have identified thrombocytopenia, coagulopathy, organ failure, and mechanical ventilation as important risk factors for gastrointestinal bleeding, similar to studies conducted in adults. A recent systematic review suggested that critically ill pediatric patients may benefit from prophylaxis; however, the results were limited by the small number of controlled studies available.[37]

Thrombosis Prophylaxis

Patients admitted to the PICU can range from newborns to young adults. Unlike adults, there are no data on the use of subcutaneous heparin or low-molecular-weight heparins as prophylaxis to prevent deep venous thrombosis (DVT) in children. However, when children reach puberty, the hormone changes that take place appear to increase their risk of thrombosis to that of adults. Although no published guidelines or consensus papers exist to guide therapy at this time, all pubescent adolescents should be considered for DVT prophylaxis. Most cases of thrombosis in infants and young children are associated with long-term use of central venous catheters. Unfortunately, a study evaluating low-dose heparin infused at 10 units/kg/hour did not prevent catheter-related thrombosis in infants after cardiac surgery.[38] It is important to note that the dose of heparin used in this study was less than the anticoagulant dose recommended for infants and children (15–25 units/kg/hour). At this time, the routine use of DVT prophylaxis in children remains controversial.

CONGENITAL HEART DISEASE

CASE 106-5

QUESTION 1: J.F. is a 3-week-old, 3.5-kg male infant who was seen by his physician with a history of poor feeding and increased work of breathing. On admission, he was mottled, and grunting, and had severe retractions. The physician referred him to the emergency department of the local children's hospital where his temperature was 40.8°C, heart rate was 200 beats/minute, respiratory rate was 80 breaths/minute, and oximetry saturation was between 60% and 70%; he had very poor peripheral perfusion. Blood gas analysis results were as follows:

pH, 6.96
Pco_2, 35 mm Hg
Base deficit, 29 mmol/L

Chest radiography showed cardiomegaly and pulmonary edema. J.F. has presented with symptoms of both respiratory failure and shock. Based on his age, the severity of his hypoxemia, and evidence of cardiomegaly, congenital heart disease (CHD) is suspected. Echocardiography reveals coarctation of the aorta. What initial therapies are needed to stabilize J.F.?

With the neonate's first breath, changes in oxygen tension and a reduction in endogenous prostaglandin E_2 production stimulate closure of the ductus arteriosus (DA), the connection between the pulmonary artery and aorta that allows shunting of blood to the aorta during fetal circulation. Functional closure of the DA typically occurs within the first 10 to 14 hours of life, but complete anatomic closure may not occur until 2 to 3 weeks of age. Prematurity, acidosis, and hypoxia prolong the time to closure. In infants with ductal-dependent CHD, closure of the DA results in inadequate delivery of oxygenated blood to the systemic circulation (Table 106-11). These infants

Table 106-11
Ductal-Dependent Congenital Heart Lesions

Lesions That Depend on Flow Via the Ductus Arteriosus to Maintain Systemic Circulation
Hypoplastic left heart syndrome (HLHS)
Coarctation of the aorta
Critical aortic stenosis
Interrupted aortic arch
Total anomalous pulmonary venous return (TAPVR) with obstruction
Lesions that Depend on Flow Via the Ductus Arteriosus to Maintain Pulmonary Circulation
Pulmonary atresia with intact ventricular septum
Critical pulmonic stenosis
Tricuspid atresia
Tetralogy of Fallot (TOF)
Epstein anomaly
Lesions that Depend on Flow Via the Ductus Arteriosus to Maintain Adequate Mixing of the Pulmonary and Systemic Circulations
Truncus arteriosus
Transposition of the great vessels (TGV)
Total anomalous pulmonary venous return (TAPVR) without obstruction

will present just as any other patient in shock. The immediate goal in evaluating a cyanotic neonate is to differentiate between cardiac and noncardiac causes. The classic hyperoxia test is carried out by obtaining an ABG, then placing the patient on 100% oxygen for 10 minutes and then repeating the ABG. If the cause of cyanosis is pulmonary, the Pao_2 should increase by 30 mm Hg, but if the cause is cardiac, there should be minimal improvement in the Pao_2. If the patient is too unstable, one could place a pulse oximeter and place the patient on 100% Fio_2. With administration of oxygenation, there will typically be at least a 10% increase in oxygen saturation in neonates with pulmonary disease, but those with ductal-dependent CHD will have minimal or no improvement.

If the neonate's oxygen saturation or Pao_2 fails to improve and CHD is suspected, an infusion of alprostadil, prostaglandin E_1 (PGE_1), should be initiated at a rate of 0.05 to 0.1 mcg/kg/minute.[39] Infusion of PGE_1 maintains patency of the DA and allows blood to reach the descending aorta, bypassing the cardiac defect. Apnea is a common adverse effect of PGE_1, occurring in 10% to 20% of patients, so age-appropriate equipment for intubation and mechanical ventilation should be immediately available before starting treatment and throughout therapy.[40] Within 10 to 15 minutes after starting an alprostadil infusion, there should be an improvement in the patient's oxygen saturation. The dose may then be titrated to optimize ductal flow and minimize dose-related adverse effects. The infusion is typically continued until corrective cardiac surgery can be performed. J.F. should receive fluid boluses as needed to correct his dehydration and will require intubation. In addition, he should be started on PGE_1 at a rate of 0.05 mcg/kg/minute, with subsequent titration of the dose to open and maintain the DA until the time of surgery.

PEDIATRIC TRAUMATIC BRAIN INJURY

Among children, traumatic brain injury (TBI) is the leading cause of mortality and leads to significant morbidity among survivors. Each year more than 400,000 children in the United States suffer a TBI requiring an emergency department visit, resulting in 30,000 hospitalizations and 3,000 deaths.[41] The most common mechanisms of injury differ by patient age. Children less than 4 years old most often suffer injuries due to child abuse, falls, and motor vehicle collisions (MVC). Child abuse, or nonaccidental trauma (NAT), sadly represents up to two-thirds of severe TBI in some series. Although it is difficult to obtain accurate data, in a population-based study from North Carolina, the incidence of TBI due to NAT in the first 2 years of life was 17 per 100,000 person-years.[42] According to the National Center on Shaken Baby Syndrome, this translates to approximately 1,300 children per year in the United States who experience severe head trauma from child abuse. In school-aged children, those 5 to 12 years of age, pedestrian–motor vehicle collision and bicycle-related injuries are among the more common causes of severe injuries. For adolescents, MVC replace falls as the leading cause of all injuries, followed by assault and sports-related injuries.

CASE 106-6

QUESTION 1: K.B. is an 8-week-old, 4-kg male infant who was brought to an urgent care clinic by his 17-year-old mother. She stated that he would not wake up for his usual 7:00 PM feeding that evening. He had been in his usual state of health that morning. She fed him his usual bottle, changed his diaper, and laid him down for a nap. She left him in the care of her 19-year-old boyfriend and went to work. At the clinic, the infant was floppy and unarousable. There were no bruises or other signs of injury, but the anterior fontanel was bulging. His pupils were 3 mm and responded sluggishly to light. When prompted, the boyfriend stated that K.B. fell off the couch early in the morning but only cried for a few minutes. After some comforting, he went back to playing. He fed well the remainder of the day and was taking his evening nap when the mother returned from work. The urgent care clinic suspected NAT and transferred K.B. to the closest hospital with pediatric critical care services. What physiologic differences place K.B. at greater risk for severe TBI than an older child? What risk factors or associations for NAT can you identify in this case?

The anatomic differences of the infant's brain render it more susceptible to certain types of injuries after head trauma.[43] Infants such as K.B. and young children have large, heavy heads. The head is unstable because of its relative size to the rest of the body. If an infant or young child falls a significant distance, is ejected during an MVC, or is thrown from a bicycle after colliding with an automobile, the head will tend to lead (i.e., the infant or child will fly head first) and severe head injuries will occur when the head ultimately strikes the ground or another object. The infant's weak neck muscles also allow for greater movement when the head is acted on by acceleration/deceleration forces. The skull is thinner during infancy and early childhood, providing less protection for the brain and allowing forces to transfer more effectively across the shallow subarachnoid space. The base of the infant's skull is relatively flat, which also contributes to greater brain movement in response to acceleration/deceleration forces. In addition, the infant's brain has a higher water content (approximately 88% vs. 77% in an adult), which makes the brain softer and more prone to acceleration/deceleration injury. The water content is also inversely related to the myelination process, and the higher percentage of

Table 106-12
Modified Glasgow Coma Scale

Eye Opening			
Score	≥1 year	0–1 year	
4	Opens eyes spontaneously	Opens eyes spontaneously	
3	Opens eyes to verbal command	Opens eyes to shout	
2	Opens eyes in response to pain	Opens eyes in response to pain	
1	No response	No response	
Best Motor Response			
Score	≥1 year	0–1 year	
6	Obeys command	N/A	
5	Localizes pain	Localizes pain	
4	Flexion withdrawal	Flexion withdrawal	
3	Flexion abnormal (decorticate)	Flexion abnormal (decorticate)	
2	Extension (decerebrate)	Extension (decerebrate)	
1	No response	No response	
Best Verbal Response			
Score	>5 years	2–5 years	0–2 years
5	Oriented and able to converse	Uses appropriate words	Cries appropriately
4	Disoriented and able to converse	Uses inappropriate words	Cries
3	Uses inappropriate words	Cries and/or screams	Cries and/or screams inappropriately
2	Makes incomprehensible sounds	Grunts	Grunts
1	No response	No response	No response

Source: Chung CY et al. Critical score of Glasgow Coma Scale for pediatric traumatic brain injury. *Pediatr Neurol*. 2006;34:379.

unmyelinated brain makes it more susceptible to sheer injuries. The infant brain is typically fully myelinated by 1 year of age. As the result of these physiologic differences, there are differences in the pathology after pediatric TBI by age group. In infants and young children, diffuse injury, such as diffuse cerebral swelling, and subdural hematomas are more common than focal injury, such as contusions, that are typically seen in older children and adults. The typical pattern of hypoxic-ischemic injury in infants and young children after NAT is rarely seen in older children and adults who are victims of abuse.

Goldstein et al.[44] have published risk factors for NAT based on data gathered from several earlier reports. They found that victims of inflicted head injury tended to be younger, more often from families of poorer socioeconomic backgrounds, and were more likely to have parents who were younger than 18 years of age and who had never been married. In addition, a history inconsistent with physical findings was strongly associated with the presence of inflicted head injury. Additional risk factors reported as associated with NAT are alcohol or drug abuse, previous social service intervention, or a past history of child abuse, in combination with either retinal hemorrhages or an inconsistent history or physical examination. These investigators found this combination was 100% predictive of child abuse in children admitted to a PICU. K.B. met many of these risk factors: He is young, has an unmarried parent who is younger than 18, and is from a low socioeconomic background. In addition, his injuries appear inconsistent with the history of falling from a couch. A fall of approximately 3 feet is required to cause significant head injury to an infant or child; a standard couch is 18 inches from the floor.[45]

CASE 106-6, QUESTION 2: K.B. was transferred immediately to the emergency department at a local hospital. The O_2 saturation on room air was 100%, blood pressure 90/63 mm Hg, and HR 120 beats/minute. The initial Glasgow Coma Scale (GCS) score on presentation was 7, with 2 for eye opening in response to pain, 4 for withdrawing to pain, and 1 for no verbal response. What test or assessment tools are useful for evaluating the extent of K.B.'s injuries? Which are best for predicting his outcome?

The ability to evaluate the severity of TBI is essential to appropriately direct care, predict outcomes, and compare results to evaluate and improve patient care. Initial symptoms on presentation have been found to have little or no correlation with injury severity after TBI. The GCS is a widely accepted method in initially evaluating and characterizing trauma patients with head injuries (Table 106-12). The scale is composed of visual, motor, and verbal components, with lower scores representing more serious injuries. The severity of TBI may be characterized as mild (GCS 13–15), moderate (GCS 9–12), or severe (GCS 3–8) on presentation; however, continued evaluation of GCS scores is the best way to track the patient's clinical progress. K.B.'s GCS of 7 on admission puts him in the category of severe TBI.

The radiologic examination of choice for immediate assessment of a child with severe TBI is a noncontrast cerebral-computed tomography (CT) scan. Most children with severe TBI undergo immediate CT imaging to delineate their injuries as soon as they have been fully assessed and sufficiently stabilized to permit safe transport to the radiology suite. If the brain injury does not need immediate surgical intervention, the patient's care is continued in the PICU with the implementation of therapies designed to minimize secondary brain injury. In a retrospective review of 309 children presenting with TBI, Chung et al.[46] found that GCS was more useful in predicting survival among pediatric victims of TBI than CT findings and the presence of injuries to other organ systems. In addition, they identified that a GCS score of less than 5, rather than a score of less than 8 as used in adults, was the threshold at which the patient was more likely to have a poor outcome. The authors also found that head CT findings of swelling or edema and subdural and intracerebral hemorrhage were associated with worse outcomes than subarachnoid or epidural hemorrhage.

Retinal hemorrhages are frequently, although not always, observed in inflicted head injury in infants and young children. These hemorrhages are the result of sheer forces disrupting vulnerable tissue interfaces. The vitreous body is adherent to the retina in early childhood; shaking can cause retinal hemorrhaging throughout multiple tissue layers, extending to the periphery of the retina. This pattern is unique to "shaken baby syndrome." Although useful for diagnosis, the ocular examination is often deferred initially when evaluating an infant or child for TBI, because the medications used to facilitate funduscopy will preclude the use of pupillary reactivity as a tool to monitor evolving intracranial events.

According to the American Academy of Pediatrics guidelines on imaging for NAT, a skeletal survey is strongly recommended in all cases of suspected physical abuse in children under the age of 24 months.[47] A skeletal survey consists of films of the extremities, skull, and axial skeletal images. Follow-up radiographs of the ribs to assess for healing fractures not seen in the acute phase may be helpful 2 to 3 weeks after the skeletal survey. As with the eye examination, the skeletal survey is often delayed until the child is more stable.

CASE 106-6, QUESTION 3: After assessment by the emergency room physician, K.B. was intubated using rocuronium and pentobarbital, placed on an FIO_2 of 100% and sent for a CT scan. The CT reveals a subdural hematoma and cerebral swelling. On arrival to the PICU, K.B.'s vital signs are as follows:

Blood pressure, 85/58 mm Hg
HR, 125 beats/minute
Respiratory rate on the ventilator, 20 breaths/minute
Temperature was 36.9°C. What are the next goals for stabilization of K.B.?

The initial management of a child with a head injury should focus on the basics of resuscitation: assessing and securing the airway, ensuring adequate ventilation, and supporting circulation.[48] In addition, the goals of treatment of TBI are directed toward protecting against secondary brain insults (SBI) which can exacerbate neuronal damage and brain injury. SBI are often the result of systemic hypotension, hypoxia, hypercarbia, anemia, and hyperglycemia. Aggressive treatment strategies are needed to prevent and/or treat these conditions to decrease morbidity and improve neurologic outcome after TBI in children. The criteria for tracheal intubation include hypoxemia not resolved with supplemental oxygen, apnea, hypercarbia ($PaCO_2$ >45 mm Hg), a GCS score less than or equal to 8, a decrease in GCS greater than 3 compared with the initial score, cervical spine injury, loss of pharyngeal reflex, or any clinical evidence of herniation. K.B. was intubated in the emergency room based on his presenting GCS of 7. All patients should be assumed to have a full stomach and cervical spine injury, so the intubation should be carried out using a rapid sequence intubation using appropriate short-acting sedatives and muscle relaxants (Tables 106-3 and 106-4).

After intubation, K.B.'s ventilatory goals include 100% oxygen saturation, normocarbia (35–39 mm Hg), and no hyperventilation, as confirmed by ABGs, end-tidal CO_2 monitoring, and chest radiographs showing tracheal tube in good position. Unless he has signs or symptoms of herniation, prophylactic hyperventilation ($PaCO_2$ <35 mm Hg) should be avoided.[48] Hyperventilation causes cerebral vasoconstriction, which decreases cerebral blood flow and subsequent blood volume. Although it will lower ICP, hyperventilation may result in ischemia. Furthermore, respiratory alkalosis caused by hyperventilation makes it more difficult to release oxygen to the brain, shifting the oxygen–hemoglobin curve to the left. Short-term use of hyperventilation, however, may be useful in preventing herniation while other medical therapies are implemented. In addition to mechanical ventilation, the head of the bed should be kept in the neutral position and jugular venous obstruction should be avoided to prevent ICP elevation. Elevation of the head of the bed to thirty degrees usually decreases ICP.

Assessment and reassessment of the patient's circulatory status, including central and peripheral pulse quality, capillary refill, heart rate, and blood pressure, is critical. Hypotension after pediatric TBI is associated with increased morbidity and mortality.[48] Initial treatment of hypotension in the head-injured child is similar to that described earlier for pediatric shock; however, the goal systolic blood pressure in the TBI patient is typically higher: equal to or greater than the 50th to 75th percentile for age, sex, and height. Systolic blood pressure less than the 75th percentile has been associated with a fourfold increase in the risk for poor outcome after severe TBI, even when values were 90 mm Hg or greater.[49] This suggests a possible benefit of a higher blood pressure target until ICP or cerebral perfusion pressure (CPP) monitoring is in place to guide therapy. As a result of the need for higher SBP, norepinephrine and phenylephrine, agents with greater vasopressor effects, are more frequently used in this patient population.[50]

The solution of choice for IV maintenance fluids in children with TBI is normal saline for children older than 1 year of age and 5% dextrose with normal saline for infants. Because hyperglycemia is known to worsen SBI, initial IV fluids for children should not contain dextrose. Infants are an exception, because their low glycogen stores make them prone to hypoglycemia, especially with poor oral intake. Hypoglycemia can also worsen neurologic outcome and should be avoided. Frequent assessment of blood glucose either by point-of-care testing or on an ABG is recommended.

Fever increases metabolic demands and is associated with worse outcomes after TBI. Treatment for K.B. should include 60 mg of acetaminophen (15 mg/kg) orally or rectally every 6 hours as needed and a cooling blanket when necessary. Ibuprofen should be avoided because it may increase the risk of bleeding. Patients who are hypothermic on arrival should only be actively rewarmed if there is hemodynamic instability or bleeding thought to be exacerbated by hypothermia. Serum electrolytes and osmolarity should be monitored regularly in K.B., along with accurate assessment of urine output. This is important to identify the development of either syndrome of inappropriate antidiuretic hormone or diabetes insipidus. Both have been reported to occur after pediatric TBI.[48]

CASE 106-6, QUESTION 4: K.B. has been intubated and placed on mechanical ventilation with an ABG showing that he is maintaining goal parameters. He is receiving fentanyl at 1 mcg/kg/hour and a midazolam infusion at 0.05 mg/kg/hour. The head of the bed is raised 30 degrees and his head is midline, supported by a head roll. K.B. has both a pulse oximeter and an end-tidal CO_2 monitor for continuous evaluation of his oxygenation and CO_2. Blood pressure is being maintained at the 75th percentile for age, height, and sex. What is the next step in monitoring head injury in K.B.?

One of the most significant consequences of TBI is the development of intracranial hypertension. The presence of an open fontanel or sutures in an infant with severe TBI does not preclude the development of intracranial hypertension or negate the utility of ICP monitoring. ICP monitoring is recommended for any child presenting with a GCS of 8 or less.[51] When possible, placement of a ventriculostomy catheter provides accurate pressure monitoring and allows for acute drainage of cerebrospinal fluid (CSF) for treatment of elevated ICP and assessment of CPP. The CPP value is calculated by subtracting the ICP from the mean arterial pressure (MAP):

$$(\text{CPP} = \text{MAP} - \text{ICP}) \qquad \text{(Eq. 106-1)}$$

This value is important as an indication of blood flow and oxygen that reach the brain. Maintaining CPP requires optimization of MAP with fluid therapy, and if necessary, vasoactive drugs. In the case of ICP elevation, inotropic or vasopressor agents may be used to optimize CPP by increasing MAP, even to the point of relative systemic hypertension. In adults, a CPP of 60 to 70 mm Hg is usually targeted.

There are no data that correlate CPP in infants to outcome. There are, however, pediatric TBI studies showing that CPP values ranging from 40 to 70 mm Hg are associated with a favorable outcome and that a CPP less than 40 mm Hg is associated with poor outcomes.[51] Because infants and children normally have a lower MAP and ICP, the SCCM Pediatric Fundamental Critical Care Support course recommends the following CPP ranges: 40 to 50 mm Hg in infants, 50 to 60 mm Hg in children, and 60 to 70 mm Hg in adolescents.[52] This is more specific than the 2003 pediatric recommendations that recommend a CPP greater than 40 mm Hg and an "age-related continuum" of CPP from 40 to 65 mm Hg in infants and adolescents be maintained.[48]

Case 106-6, Question 5: The neurosurgeon has placed a ventriculostomy in K.B., and his initial ICP is 25 mm Hg. His other vitals are as follows:

Blood pressure, 83/50 mm Hg
HR, 140 beats/minute
Temperature, 38.5°C

His pulse oximeter still reads 100% and the $ETCO_2$ monitor reads 35 mm Hg. Sedative infusions are unchanged: fentanyl 1 mcg/kg/hour and midazolam 0.05 mg/kg/hour. The pediatric intensivist has placed a central line, and the CVP is 10 mm Hg. What is K.B.'s calculated CPP? What interventions are recommended to treat this ICP elevation?

Uncontrolled increased ICP is very deleterious and must be aggressively treated as soon as possible to reduce cerebral ischemia. In this setting, the goal of any therapy is to lower ICP enough to increase CPP and improve cerebral oxygenation. All initial treatments should be reassessed for efficacy, including treatment of fever, avoidance of jugular venous outflow tract obstruction, maintenance of normovolemia and normocarbia, and provision of sedation and analgesia. The latter is of considerable importance, because anxiety and pain have been shown to increase ICP. K.B. appears to be euvolemic by CVP measurement, is normocapnic, and his O_2 saturation is 100%. He is febrile; however, measures should be taken to treat the elevated temperature. Although he is receiving continuous sedation, additional bolus doses of sedatives should be given whenever needed. Because K.B. has an elevated CPP in spite of these initial therapies, the best option would be to drain CSF. This will provide an immediate, but transient, decrease in ICP. K.B. may have CSF drained until an ICP value of 15 mm Hg is reached; it should never be drained to 0 mm Hg because edema and diffuse brain swelling could cause an obstruction in the lateral ventricles. When a ventriculostomy is in place and CSF is frequently drained, it is important to replace the CSF drained with an equal amount of normal saline. Draining of large amounts of CSF without IV normal saline replacement is associated with the development of hypochloremic metabolic alkalosis. Drainage of CSF in K.B. will provide a CPP in the 40- to 50-mm Hg range. If the ICP increases again, two interventions are recommended, either the addition of a vasopressor to increase SBP or institution of hyperosmolar therapy.

Hyperosmolar therapy may be useful in preventing the ICP from exceeding 20 mm Hg and in maintaining normal CPP. Mannitol has long been the standard of care for management of elevated ICP.[48] Although extensively used since 1961 to control elevated ICP, mannitol has never been compared with placebo. Mannitol reduces ICP by reducing blood viscosity, which promotes reflex vasoconstriction of the arterioles by autoregulation, thus decreasing cerebral blood volume and ICP. This mechanism is rapid, but transient, lasting about 75 minutes and requiring an intact autoregulation. It also produces an osmotic effect by increasing serum osmolarity, causing the shift of water from the brain cell to the intravascular space. Although this effect is slower in onset (15–30 minutes), the osmotic effect lasts up to 6 hours. Mannitol is a potent osmotic diuretic; osmotic diuresis should be anticipated and fluid resuscitation is available to avoid hemodynamic compromise. A Foley catheter is recommended in these patients for accurate measurement of urine output. Mannitol is excreted unchanged in the urine; serum osmolarity should be maintained lower than 320 mOsm/L to avoid the development of mannitol-induced acute tubular necrosis.

Although mannitol has traditionally been the drug of choice for reducing elevated ICP, hypertonic saline (3% sodium chloride) is gaining favor. The main mechanism of action of hypertonic saline is an osmotic effect similar to mannitol. Hypertonic saline exhibits several other theoretic benefits such as restoration of normal cellular resting membrane potential and cell volume, inhibition of inflammation, stimulation of atrial natriuretic peptide release, and enhancement of cardiac output.[48] The theoretic advantage over mannitol is that hypertonic saline can be administered in a hemodynamically unstable patient without the risk of a subsequent osmotic diuresis. Continuous infusions of 0.1 to 1 mL/kg/hour of hypertonic saline titrated to maintain an ICP less than 20 mm Hg have been used successfully in children.[53] Bolus doses of 5-10 mL/kg of 3% sodium chloride have been administered over 20 to 30 minutes. Serum osmolarity and serum sodium increase when this regimen is used, but sustained hypernatremia and hyperosmolarity appear to be generally well tolerated. Hypertonic saline has been administered with a serum osmolarity reaching 360 mOsm/L without adverse effects in pediatric patients. Another potential concern with the use of hypertonic saline is central pontine myelinolysis that has been reported with rapid changes in serum sodium. Currently, clinical trials have shown no evidence of demyelinating disorders.

To bring his ICP values down to the normal range (<20 mm Hg), K.B. may be given mannitol at an IV dose of 2 to 4 g (0.5–1 g/kg) administered over 20 to 30 minutes. The effects of mannitol on ICP should be evident within 15 minutes. This dose may be repeated every 4 to 6 hours as needed. If intermittent mannitol fails to bring his ICP down adequately, K.B. may be given hypertonic saline 3%, beginning at 0.1 mL/kg/hour or as a bolus dose of 5-10 mL/kg administered over 20 minutes. Dosing of either agent should be guided by regular assessment of serum electrolytes and osmolarity.

Case 106-6, Question 6: K.B. has been in the PICU for 24 hours. Initial treatment allowed K.B. to maintain a CPP of 50 mm Hg and an ICP less than 20 mm Hg the majority of the day.

He is receiving 3% sodium chloride combined with maintenance IV fluids, giving him a serum sodium of 166 mEq/L. Intermittent ICP spikes have responded to intermittent 4 g doses of mannitol; however, the most recent serum osmolarity is 330 mOs/L. What options remain to treat increased ICP in K.B.?

Two nonsurgical options are included in the TBI guideline: barbiturate coma and therapeutic hypothermia.[48] Barbiturates exert neuroprotective effects by reducing cerebral metabolism, lowering oxygen extraction and demand, and alternating vascular tone. Barbiturate serum levels poorly correlate with clinical efficacy; therefore, monitoring of electroencephalographic (EEG) patterns for burst suppression is recommended. Burst suppression also represents near-maximum reduction in cerebral metabolism and cerebral blood flow. A pentobarbital loading dose of 10 mg/kg/dose may be administered over 30 minutes, followed by a continuous infusion of 1 mg/kg/hour. Additional loading doses, in 5 mg/kg/dose increments, may be necessary to achieve burst suppression. The primary disadvantage of barbiturate coma is the risk for myocardial depression and hypotension. In addition, the long-term effect on neurologic outcome is unknown. The TBI guideline states that high-dose barbiturate therapy may be considered in hemodynamically stable patients with salvageable severe head injury and refractory intracranial hypertension.[48]

Post-traumatic hyperthermia is defined as a core body temperature greater than 38.5°C, and hypothermia is defined as a temperature of less than 35°C. Although most clinicians agree that hyperthermia should be avoided in children with TBI, the role of hypothermia is unclear. Potential complications associated with hypothermia are increased bleeding risk, arrhythmias, and increased susceptibility to infection. A multicenter, international study of children with severe TBI randomly assigned to hypothermia therapy initiated within 8 hours after injury (32.5°C for 24 hours) or to normothermia (37°C) was recently published.[52] The study reported a worsening trend with hypothermia therapy: 31% of the patients in the hypothermia group had an unfavorable outcome, compared with 22% of the normothermia group. There were several methodological problems with this study. Although the investigators screened patients within 8 hours, the mean time to initiation of cooling was 6.3 hours, with a range of 1.6 to 19.7 hours. In addition, the protocol included a rapid rewarming of 0.5°C every 2 hours so that the patients were normothermic by a mean of 19 or 48 hours postinjury. They found that the ICP was significantly lower in the hypothermia group during the cooling period, but that it was significantly higher than the normothermic group during rewarming. Another trial conducted in Australia and New Zealand evaluated strict normothermia (temperature 36°C–37°C) versus therapeutic hypothermia (temperature 32°C–33°C).[54] Patients were enrolled within 6 hours of injury and therapeutic hypothermia or strict normothermia was maintained for 72 hours. The rewarming rate was at a maximum of 0.5°C every 3 hours or slower if needed to maintain normal CPP or ICP <20 mmHg. Rewarming took a median of 21.5 hours (16–35 hours) and was without complications. However, there was no difference in pediatric cerebral performance category (PCPC) scores between the 2 groups at 12 months.[54] It is unclear whether therapeutic hypothermia is not efficacious because patients are not cooled soon enough (median time to target temperature = 9.3 hours) or due to the heterogeneous nature of TBI. The pediatric TBI guideline states that despite the lack of clinical data, hypothermia may be considered in the setting of refractory hypertension.[48]

Decompressive craniectomy, removal of a section of skull to allow room for brain swelling without herniation, is another option for managing pediatric TBI patients who fail to respond to standard therapies. A randomized trial of early decompressive craniectomy in children with TBI and sustained intracranial hypertension revealed that 54% of the surgically treated patients had a favorable outcome compared with only 14% of the medically treated group.[55] Additional case series have confirmed that patients who receive a decompressive craniectomy have improved survival and neurologic outcomes compared with those undergoing medical management alone.[56] As with barbiturate coma and therapeutic hypothermia, decompressive craniectomy is not without risk. A recent study reported an increased risk of post-traumatic hydrocephalus, wound complications, and epilepsy in children with severe TBI.[57] Further studies are needed to establish the timing, efficacy, and safety of this management strategy. The pediatric TBI guideline states that decompressive craniectomy should be considered in pediatric patients with severe TBI, diffuse cerebral swelling, and intracranial hypertension refractory to intensive medical management.

CASE 106-7

QUESTION 1: L.B. is an 18-kg, 6-year-old child hit by a car while riding her bicycle. When emergency medical services arrived, they witnessed a 2-minute tonic-clonic seizure. GCS at the scene was 11. Should L.B. receive anticonvulsant medication after her TBI?

Post-traumatic seizures (PTS) are classified as early (occurring within 7 days after injury) or late (occurring after 7 days). In the immediate period after severe TBI, seizures increase the brain metabolic demands, increase ICP, and are associated with TBI. Therefore, it would be prudent to prevent PTS in the period when the patient is at highest risk of SBI. Infants and children are reported to have a greater risk of early PTS compared with adults. Children younger than 2 years of age have almost a threefold greater risk of early PTS after TBI than children between 2 and 12 years of age. In addition to age, a low GCS (8–11) has been linked to an increased risk of early PTS. The pediatric TBI guideline states that prophylactic antiseizure therapy may be considered as a treatment to prevent early PTS. No prophylactic anticonvulsant therapy is recommended to prevent late PTS.[48]

The majority of the published studies in children have used phenytoin for PTS prophylaxis. Both phenytoin and carbamazepine have been reported to reduce the incidence of PTS in adults. A large (n = 813) prospective multicenter trial evaluated the effectiveness of levetiracetam for seizure prophylaxis in severe TBI in adults.[58] Although the trial demonstrated that levetiracetam was equally effective to phenytoin in preventing PTS after TBI, the authors concluded that the significant cost difference between the 2 treatments makes phenytoin the preferred therapy. There are currently no studies of levetiracetam for PTS prophylaxis in children. Due to the seizure witnessed at the scene, her young age, and her initial GSC score of 11, L.B. meets the criteria for prophylaxis. An appropriate regimen for L.B. would be phenytoin 45 mg given orally 3 times daily (7.5 mg/kg/day) for 7 days.

KEY REFERENCES AND WEBSITES

A full list of references for this chapter can be found at http://thepoint.lww.com/AT11e. Below are the key references and websites for this chapter, with the corresponding reference number in this chapter found in parentheses after the reference.

Key References

Adelson PD et al. Guidelines for the acute medical management of severe traumatic brain injury in infants, children, and adolescents. *Pediatr Crit Care Med*. 2003;4(3, Suppl):S1. (48)

Brierley J et al. Clinical practice parameters for hemodynamic support of pediatric and neonatal septic shock: 2007 update from the American College of Critical Care Medicine [published correction appears in *Crit Care Med*. 2009;37:1536]. *Crit Care Med*. 2009;37:666. (17)

Dellinger RP et al. Surviving sepsis campaign: international guidelines for management of severe sepsis and septic shock 2012. *Crit Care Med*. 2013;41:580. (13)

de Oliveria CR et al. ACCM/PALS haemodynamic support guidelines for paediatric septic shock: an outcome comparison with and without monitoring central venous oxygen saturation. *Intensive Care Med*. 2008;34:1065. (18)

de Caen AR et al. Part 12: Pediatric advanced life support. 2015 American Heart Association Guidelines for Cardiopulmonary Resuscitation and Emergency Cardiovascular Care. *Circulation*. 2015;132(Suppl 2):S526. (3)

Namachivayam P et al. Three decades of pediatric intensive care: who was admitted, what happened in intensive care, and what happened afterward. *Pediatr Crit Care Med*. 2010;11:549. (2)

Key Websites

International Liaison Committee on Resuscitation (ILCOR). Consensus 2015 Documents. www.ilcor.org. Accessed November 9, 2015.

The Surviving Sepsis Campaign. Guidelines for Management of Severe Sepsis and Septic Shock. www.survivingsepsis.com. Accessed November 9, 2015.

SECTION 18 | Geriatric Therapy

Section Editor: Judith L. Beizer

107 Geriatric Drug Use

Suzanne Dinsmore, Mary Kathleen Grams, and Kristin M. Zimmerman

CORE PRINCIPLES

		CHAPTER CASES
AGE-RELATED PHYSIOLOGIC, PHARMACOKINETIC, AND PHARMACODYNAMIC CHANGES		
1	Age-associated physiologic changes are associated with pharmacokinetic and pharmacodynamic alterations of drugs in older adults. Decline in drug metabolism and excretion and exaggerated response to drugs are important considerations in drug therapy of the elderly.	**Case 107-1 (Questions 1–4)**
2	Adverse drug events are one of the most important problems associated with drug use in older adults.	**Case 107-2 (Question 1)**
DISEASE-SPECIFIC GERIATRIC DRUG THERAPY		
1	Elderly patients have multiple chronic conditions and take numerous medications. Disease state education, awareness of potential adverse effects and drug interactions, consultation with healthcare providers, and behavioral modification are important steps to ensure medication safety.	**Case 107-3 (Questions 1, 2)**
2	Pharmacologic treatments of heart failure in the elderly include a diuretic, *β*-blocker, an angiotensin-converting enzyme (ACE) inhibitor or angiotensin receptor blocker (ARB), with or without digoxin and spironolactone. Benefits should be weighed against risks based on the patient's concurrent conditions.	**Case 107-3 (Questions 3–6)**
3	Statins are the drug of choice for treating hyperlipidemia in the elderly. Combination with other agents is considered only if necessary and is based on concurrent disease states, potential adverse effects, and drug interactions.	**Case 107-3 (Questions 7, 8)**
4	First-line therapy for prevention of coronary artery disease (CAD) includes acetylsalicylic acid (ASA) and *β*-blockers. Other agents are considered based on concomitant diseases and relative indications.	**Case 107-3 (Question 9)**
5	Hypertension should be treated in the elderly according to the guidelines, and monitoring is essential to prevent excessively low blood pressure, bradycardia, and orthostatic hypotension.	**Case 107-3 (Question 10)**
6	The glycosylated hemoglobin (Hgb A_{1c}) goal may be higher for elderly patients who have hypoglycemia. Pharmacologic therapies for diabetes are recommended based on level of hyperglycemia and relative contraindications.	**Case 107-3 (Question 11)**
7	Depression is the most common psychiatric disorder in the elderly, often presenting with atypical symptoms. Selective serotonin reuptake inhibitors are generally better tolerated than other agents and are considered first-line therapy for older adults.	**Case 107-4 (Questions 1, 2)**
8	Asthma is a significant source of morbidity in the elderly. The management of asthma in older adults does not differ significantly from that for younger individuals. However, coexisting chronic medical conditions, exaggerated systemic adverse drug reactions, and dexterity concerns must be considered when managing drug therapy for asthma in the elderly.	**Case 107-5 (Questions 1, 2)**

Continued

9	Pneumonia is the leading infectious cause of mortality in the elderly, who typically present with atypical symptoms of lower respiratory infection. Influenza and pneumococcal vaccinations are beneficial in the prevention of pneumonia in the older population.	Case 107-5 (Questions 3–5)
10	Urinary tract infection is the most common bacterial infection in the elderly. Oral antibiotics are appropriate for most older patients with symptomatic infection.	Case 107-6 (Question 1, 2)
11	Arthritis is the most common cause of disability in the elderly, and there are several analgesic agents available for the management of osteoarthritis. Safe and appropriate use of these analgesic medications is important because older adults are at increased risk of adverse drug reactions.	Case 107-7 (Questions 1, 2)
	LONG-TERM CARE FACILITIES	
1	Federally mandated responsibilities of pharmacists in long-term care facilities include monthly medication regimen review for appropriateness of drug therapy. Provision of pharmaceutical care in long-term care facilities helps to minimize medication errors, adverse drug reactions, and inappropriate prescribing.	Case 107-8 (Questions 1, 2)

DEMOGRAPHIC AND ECONOMIC CONSIDERATIONS

Demographic changes and medical progress in the United States (U.S.) over the last half of the 20th century have created the need for imperatives to improve our knowledge about the health care and drug therapy of older adults. The Federal Interagency Forum on Aging-Related Statistics, is made up of multiple Federal agencies which came together in 1996 to provide information on the health, finances, and well-being of older Americans in the United States.[1] The latest report compiles information from over 16 national data sources and separates data into 41 indicators in the areas of population, economics, health status, health risks and behaviors, and health care and environment, of the older population. The U.S. Department of Health & Human Services published "A Profile in Older Americans", updated in 2016.[2] Both reports include valuable information that describe the older population (Table 107-1).

The oldest-old category (i.e. those older than 85 years of age) will have the greatest impact on the healthcare system because the number of people in this group has increased faster than any other age category. This group will triple its size by 2040.[2]

Older adults often have multiple chronic conditions, higher prescription drug costs, and higher out of pocket healthcare expenditures, and account for more overnight hospital stays than younger adults. Many older adults live at home and may receive personal assistances with one or more activities of daily living (ADLs) including bathing, eating, and dressing; or instrumental activities of daily living (IADLs), which include preparing meals, washing clothes, shopping, paying bills, and taking medication. Often, informal care from children and other relatives is a large reason disabled older adults can continue to live in the community. Thus, it is important to include the caregiver in the counseling and monitoring of daily activities when feasible. An increase in this informal assistance and the reliance on others to perform ADLs and IADLs leads to a loss of independence and the inability of older adults to remain living at home or alone in the community. Approximately 1.2 million U.S. residents 65 years of age or older reside in long-term care facilities (LTCFs). The percentage of those living in nursing homes increases greatly with age (1% age 65–74; 3% age 75–84; 9% age 85 and greater).

Health care for older adults in an institutional setting is largely based on a prospective reimbursement system, where payment for services is based on a fixed amount. Managed-care practices aim to minimize high-cost hospitalizations by shifting care to lower-cost alternatives, such as home health care, assisted living, and hospice care. The escalating costs and affordability of medications are a national concern, especially in the Medicare population. The Medicare Prescription Drug Improvement and Modernization Act of 2003 provided voluntary prescription drug insurance benefits, known as Medicare Part D, to improve older adults' access to prescription drugs. Medicare Part D implementation is associated with up to a

Table 107-1
Profile of Older Americans

Current Facts About Older Americans[1,2]

- The older population, persons aged 65 years and older, numbered 47.8 million in 2015, representing 14.9% of the U.S. population. This is a 30% increase from 2005.
- Approximately 1 in every 7 of the U.S. population is considered an older American.
- The older population is predominantly female. There are 126.5 women for every 100 men aged 65 and older, and this increases to 189.2 women to 100 men at age 85 and older.
- The older population is getting even older. The 85 and older age group grew from just over 100,000 in 1900 to 0.3 million in 2015.
- The average life expectancy for someone born in 2015 is 78.8 years, an increase by about 30 years as compared to 1900.
- The centenarian population or those aged 100 and greater accounted for 0.2% of the age 65 and older population in 2015.
- The most common and costly health conditions among all persons aged 65 and older are heart disease, heart disease, stroke, cancer, diabetes and arthritis.
- Among all persons aged 65 and older, the leading causes of death are heart disease, cancer, chronic lower respiratory diseases, stroke, Alzheimer's disease, diabetes, unintentional injuries, and influenza and pneumonia.

Future Expected Growth

- A rapid increase in the older population is expected between the baby boomer generation reaches age 65.
- The population of those age 65 and older is expected to double to 98 million by 2060.
- The very old, those age 85 and greater are expected to double from 6.3 million in 2015 to 14.6 million in 2040.

Adapted from Federal Interagency Forum on Aging-Related Statistics. Federal Interagency Forum on Aging-Related Statistics. Older Americans 2016 and Department of Health & Human Services USA. A Profile of Older Americans: 2016.

13% increase in drug use in older adults and up to an 18% decrease in patient out-of-pocket costs.[3]

AGE-RELATED PHYSIOLOGIC, PHARMACOKINETIC, AND PHARMACODYNAMIC CHANGES

Physiologic changes that are seen with aging are progressive and occur gradually over a lifetime, rather than abruptly at any given age.[4] These changes may lead to decreases in the function of tissues and organs and the ability for each organ system to maintain homeostasis: a phenomenon often called "homeostenosis."[5,6] The impaired ability to recover from drug-induced insults may increase the risk of drug-related problems in older adults. Homeostatic mechanisms in the cardiovascular and nervous systems are less efficient, drug metabolism and excretion decrease, and body tissue composition and drug volume of distribution change and drug receptor sensitivity may be altered. Age-related physiologic changes may result in pharmacokinetic and pharmacodynamic changes and should be considered when selecting and evaluating drug therapy.

Absorption

The absorption of some drugs administered by the extravascular route may be altered by age-related physiologic changes, unlike drugs administered by the intravascular route which are considered to have 100% bioavailability.[7] In the gastrointestinal (GI) tract, a decrease in intestinal blood flow, increase in gastric pH, delayed gastric emptying, and decreased gastrointestinal motility occur with aging. Increased gastric pH due to aging alone is thought to have a minimal effect on absorption and be rarely clinically significant.[8] However, the use of H2-receptor antagonists and proton pump inhibitors combined with gastric pH changes may affect drugs that require an acidic environment for absorption such as iron and ketoconazole.[9] In general, the rate of absorption is slower or unaltered in older patients, and the extent of absorption by the oral route is similar as compared to young adults.

The transdermal administration of drugs is becoming increasingly common and used for several medications prescribed to older adults. Changes in skin seen with aging such as decreased elasticity, thinning of the epidermis, dryness, and decreased sebaceous gland activity may affect drug absorption.[10]

Lipophilic drugs (e.g., estradiol) appear to be less affected by aging skin and are easily dissolved, whereas hydrophilic compounds may not dissolve as readily on aging skin.

CASE 107-1

QUESTION 1: M.G. is a 75-year-old female, 5′4″, 120 pounds, with a serum creatinine concentration of 1.9 mg/dL. She has an acute exacerbation of heart failure (HF). She is given furosemide 40 mg orally, but this produces little increase in urine output or resolution of her symptoms.

What would explain M.G's lack of response to furosemide and how might the desired response to furosemide be achieved?

The extent of furosemide absorption is not changed in older patients, but the rate of absorption is slowed. This results in a diminished efficacy of the drug because active secretion into the urine (rate of entry) must reach the steep portion of the sigmoid dose–response curve for maximal effect of the drug.[11]

M.G. should be given a 40 mg dose of furosemide intravenously to bypass the problem of decreased rate of absorption. High sodium intake or concurrent use of nonsteroidal anti-inflammatory drugs (NSAIDs) may also decrease the effectiveness of furosemide. Further increases in dose of furosemide may be necessary, with consideration of a continuous infusion in patients with severe chronic renal insufficiency (see Chapter 28, Chronic Kidney Disease).

Distribution

There are a number of age-related changes that may affect the distribution of drugs in the body.[12] Total body water and lean body mass both decline with age by 10% to 15%, and total fat content increases by 20% to 40%. Thus, the volume of distribution (Vd) of drugs that are distributed primarily in body water or lean body mass (e.g., lithium, digoxin) is decreased in older adults, and unadjusted dosing may result in higher blood levels. Conversely, the Vd of highly lipid-soluble drugs, such as long-acting benzodiazepines (e.g., diazepam), may be increased, thereby delaying maximal effects or leading to accumulation with continued use.

Serum albumin concentrations were found to progressively decrease for each decade beyond 40 years of age, reaching a mean of 3.58 g/dL in those older than 80 years of age, and this may reduce protein binding.[13] Changes in protein binding due to aging alone are thought to be only clinically significant with highly extracted drugs, drugs that are highly protein bound, that have a narrow therapeutic index, those with a small volume of distribution, and those given intravenously.[7,9,14] Other factors in older patients that may also affect binding include protein concentration, disease states, coadministration of other drugs, and nutritional status.

Altered Protein Binding

CASE 107-1, QUESTION 2: M.G. is brought to the emergency department (ED) for evaluation of a "shaking spell". In the ED, another "spell" is observed, starting with shaking of the left arm and progressing into a generalized tonic–clonic seizure. A loading dose of phenytoin 1,000 mg is given intravenously (IV) over 30 minutes. M.G. is admitted to the neurology unit for further evaluation and given phenytoin 300 mg by mouth (PO) at bedtime. Is the phenytoin regimen appropriate for M.G.? What laboratory tests should be ordered, and how often should these be monitored?

M.G. received a phenytoin loading dose of 17 mg/kg (adult dose 15–20 mg/kg) and is receiving the usual oral daily maintenance dose.[15] Monitoring parameters include a serum sodium concentration to rule out a hyponatremia-induced seizure. Because phenytoin is 90% protein bound, a serum albumin concentration should be drawn. In patients with hypoalbuminemia or renal impairment, free (unbound) phenytoin levels should be monitored. A serum phenytoin concentration at discharge to determine whether the desired therapeutic serum concentration has been achieved is also recommended. A follow-up, steady state serum phenytoin concentration should be obtained in 10 to 14 days to evaluate the current dose and to determine whether dose adjustments are needed. The serum phenytoin concentration should be monitored periodically thereafter and whenever an adverse drug reaction or seizure occurs.

CASE 107-1, QUESTION 3: M.G. returns for a follow-up appointment 2 weeks later after having labs drawn. Serum albumin concentration is 2.2 g/dL, sodium 140 mEq/L, and serum phenytoin 15 mcg/mL. M.G. complains of drowsiness and has a wide-based, unsteady gait. What is the most likely cause of her symptoms?

Although the serum phenytoin is within the therapeutic range (10–20 mcg/mL), phenytoin is highly protein bound, and in the presence of low albumin, free phenytoin concentrations could be higher. A corrected phenytoin level can be calculated using an equation:

$$\text{Total Phenytoin Concentration} = \text{Total Phenytoin measured}/[(0.2 \times \text{serum albumin g/dL}) + 0.1] \quad \text{(Eq. 107-1)}$$

This would produce an equivalent phenytoin concentration of 27 mcg/mL, explaining M.G.'s symptoms (assuming her serum phenytoin concentration is at steady state). In M.G.'s case, free phenytoin (unbound phenytoin) concentration monitoring would be appropriate, if available, and her dosage should be adjusted accordingly.[15,16]

Metabolism

M.G.'s phenytoin metabolism may be affected by factors known to influence hepatic drug metabolism, which include disease states, concurrent drug use, nutritional status, environmental compounds, genetic differences, sex, liver mass, and blood flow. Liver mass decreases by approximately 20% to 30% with age, and hepatic blood flow decreases by approximately 20% to 50%.[7,12] Compounds undergoing phase I metabolism (reduction, oxidation, hydroxylation, demethylation) have a decreased or unchanged clearance, whereas compounds metabolized by phase II processes (conjugation, acetylation, sulfonation, glucuronidation) have no change in clearance with age.[7] Drugs with high hepatic-extraction ratios, such as the nitrates, barbiturates, lidocaine, and propranolol, may have reduced hepatic metabolism in older adults.[17]

Excretion

In older adults, changes in aging kidneys include a decrease in renal mass by 20% to 30%, decrease in renal blood flow, and decrease in tubular secretion.[18] Increases in sclerotic glomeruli and decreases in functioning glomeruli may contribute to a decline in glomerular filtration rate (GFR).[18] After age 30, GFR is estimated to decline 8 mL/minute every 10 years, although not all older adults have decreased renal function.[12]

The plasma half-life is prolonged for a number of renally excreted drugs in "healthy" older adults, and the highest-risk drugs are those that depend entirely on the kidney for elimination. Examples of these are listed in Table 107-2.

GFR is the most prevalent measurement that is used to evaluate overall renal function and to diagnose kidney disease, using markers that are renally excreted such as creatinine.[19] These markers are measured by collecting urine over a 6- to 24-hour period and drawing blood before or after. Because timed urine and serum collections may not always be possible or accurate in older adults due to inconvenience, or incomplete collection in those with incontinence, several equations are used to estimate creatinine clearance.[20] Whereas GFR is used to diagnose and stage kidney disease, equations that estimate creatinine clearance are used to guide practitioners in drug dosing. The Cockcroft–Gault equation is commonly used for most drug dosing; however, controversies exist with regard to using actual or ideal weight, and using correction factors in the calculation. The use of lean body weight in the equation may reflect serum creatinine (SCr) production more accurately because creatinine is produced in muscle mass, which is decreased in older patients. The Cockcroft–Gault equation depends on SCr concentration and tubular secretion of creatinine, which may result in an overestimation of renal function in obese patients.

Case 107-1, Question 4: For renally cleared drugs that require dosage adjustment for M.G., is the Cockcroft–Gault equation an appropriate tool to estimate renal function?

Cockroft and Gault

$$\text{eCrCl} = (140\text{-age}) \times \text{weight in kg} / (72 \times \text{SCr}) \times 0.85 \text{ in females} \qquad \text{Eq. 107-2)}$$

M.G. is 75 years old, weighs 120 lbs or 54.43 kg, and her serum creatinine is 1.9 mg/dL. Using the Cockcroft–Gault equation, her estimated CrCl is 22 mL/minute. The equation was derived from a predominantly male veteran population who had a single measured 24-hour creatinine clearance, and a correction factor of 0.85 is used in female patients.[21]

M.G. is not underweight or obese, so the Cockroft-Gault equation is an appropriate tool to estimate creatinine clearance for drug dosing and remains the most common method to determine dosing of renally cleared drugs. Other assessments of renal function, including urine output, should be considered when assessing drug dosage adjustments in older individuals such as M.G., along with close monitoring for adverse drug reactions.

Table 107-3 provides a composite picture of the age-related physiologic changes, disease states, and pharmacologic factors that affect pharmacokinetic processes in older adults.

Table 107-2

Drugs Highly Dependent on Renal Function for Elimination[18,20,a]

Acetazolamide	Duloxetine	Nizatidine
Acyclovir	Edoxaban	Penicillins (most)
Allopurinol	Enalapril	Phenazopyridine
Amantadine	Enoxaparin	Pregabalin
Amiloride	Famotidine	Probenecid
Aminoglycosides	Fluconazole	Procainamide
Amphotericin B	Fluroquinolones (most)	Pyridostigmine
Apixaban	Fondaparinux	Ranitidine
Atenolol	Furosemide	Rivaroxaban
Aztreonam	Gabapentin	Spironolactone
Captopril	Imipenem	Sulfamethoxazole
Cephalosporins (most)	Levetiracetam	Thiazides
Clonidine	Lisinopril	Tramadol
Cimetidine	Lithium	Trimethoprim
Colchicine	Methotrexate	Triamterene
Dabigatran	Metoclopramide	Vancomycin
Digoxin	Nadolol	

[a]This list does not include all drugs highly dependent on renal function for elimination.

Adapted from American Geriatrics Society 2015 Updated Beers Criteria for Potentially Inappropriate Medication Use in Older Adults. *J Am Geriatr Soc*. 2015;63:2227–2246 and Arnoff GR et al., eds. *Drug Prescribing in Renal Failure: Dosing Guidelines for Adults*. 5th ed. Philadelphia, PA: American College of Physicians; 2007.

PHARMACODYNAMIC CHANGES

Pharmacodynamics refers to the effect of a medication at its receptor site, or site of action, and is largely determined by drug concentration and its ability to bind at the receptor site.[22] Aging can affect the number of receptors available and their affinity to medications. Together, comorbidities, pharmacokinetic changes, and pharmacodynamic changes make an individual drug response in an older adult largely unpredictable. Because older persons can be sensitive to the effects of medication, care should be taken to avoid unwanted adverse effects when starting or stopping medications.

The ability to preserve homeostasis decreases with aging, which results in a decrease in functional reserve and a decreased ability to respond in times of physiologic stress.[23] Cardiovascular changes during aging along with an impaired baroreceptor response increase the prevalence of orthostatic hypotension in the

Table 107-3
Changes Affecting Pharmacokinetic Parameters

Parameter	Physiologic Changes	Disease States	Pharmacologic Factors
Absorption (bioavailability, first-pass metabolism)	Gastric pH Absorptive surface Splanchnic blood flow GI motility Gastric emptying rate	Achlorhydria, diarrhea, gastrectomy, malabsorptive syndromes, pancreatitis	Drug interactions, antacids, anticholinergics, cholestyramine, food
Distribution	Cardiac output TBW Lean body mass Serum albumin α_1-Acid glycoprotein Body fat Altered relative tissue perfusion	HF, dehydration, edema, ascites, hepatic, failure, malnutrition, renal failure	Drug interactions, protein-binding displacement
Metabolism	Hepatic mass Enzyme activity Hepatic blood flow	HF, fever, hepatic failure, malignancy, malnutrition, thyroid disease, viral, infection or immunization	Dietary makeup, drug interactions, insecticides, alcohol, smoking, induction of metabolism, inhibition of metabolism
Excretion	Renal blood flow GFR Tubular secretion Renal mass	Hypovolemia, renal insufficiency	Drug interactions

GFR, glomerular filtration rate; GI, gastrointestinal; HF, heart failure; TBW, total body water.

Table 107-4
Adverse Drug Reactions That May Affect Mobility of the Older Patient

Medication Class	Adverse Drug Reaction
Tricyclic antidepressants (TCAs)	Orthostatic hypotension, tremor, cardiac arrhythmias, sedation
Benzodiazepines and sedative hypnotics	Sedation, weakness, coordination, confusion
Opiate analgesics	Sedation, coordination, confusion
Antipsychotics	Orthostatic hypotension, sedation, extrapyramidal effects
Antihypertensives	Orthostatic hypotension
β-Adrenergic blockers	Ability to respond to workload (dose needed may increase risk)

elderly population.[23,24] Prevalence ranges from 6% in middle age to 30% or greater in patients 70 years of age or older.[25] Orthostatic hypotension is often aggravated by drugs with sympatholytic activity (e.g., α-adrenergic blocking agents, phenothiazines, tricyclic antidepressants [TCAs]), volume-depleting drugs (e.g., diuretics), and vasodilating agents (e.g., nitrates, alcohol).[24,26] In a study of 100 geriatric psychiatric outpatients, almost 40% complained of dizziness and falling, which were attributed to psychotropic medications.[27] Patients with impaired cardiac output and taking concurrent diuretic therapy are especially vulnerable.[24] Changes in gait and balance are common in the older adult population.[28]

Certain medications or classes of medications, such as antiarrhythmics, diuretics, digoxin, narcotics, anticonvulsants, psychotropics, and antidepressants, can lead to gait disturbances and contribute to drug-induced falls in older adults. Table 107-4 reviews the therapeutic agents commonly associated with adverse drug reactions that may affect the mobility of older patients.

Blood–Brain Barrier

The function and integrity of the interface between the brain and the body, the blood–brain barrier, may decline as a result of aging, disease, or ischemic injury.[29] An exaggerated response and increased sensitivity to some drugs that effect the central nervous system (CNS) may be seen as a result of changes in permeability of the blood–brain barrier and changes in receptor sensitivity in older adults.[30] Normal aging involves a reduction in cerebral blood flow and oxygen consumption, and increased cerebrovascular resistance. Drugs with anticholinergic properties are associated with memory loss, confusion, cognitive impairments, and functional decline in older patients.[31] Several examples of therapeutic classes with anticholinergic properties are listed in Table 107-5.

Both central responsiveness and peripheral responsiveness of adrenergic receptors decline with aging.[32] Monoamine-oxidase activity increases with normal aging, and this is reflected by a decline in norepinephrine and dopamine levels in aging brains.[33] The decline in CNS dopamine synthesis is associated with increased sensitivity to dopamine blocking agents (e.g., antipsychotics). However, β-receptor sensitivity to both β-agonists and β-antagonists decreases, even if the number of β-receptors does not decrease in older patients.[34,35] Because these neurologic and biochemical reserves are reduced as a normal consequence of aging, iatrogenic behavioral disorders are relatively common in older adults, and drugs are one of the most common causes of sudden, unexplained mental impairment in the older adult.

PROBLEMS ASSOCIATED WITH DRUG USE IN OLDER ADULTS

Polypharmacy

Over half of all older adults carry three or more chronic diseases. This multimorbidity is associated with increased morbidity,

Table 107-5
Categories of Anticholinergic Drugs That May Induce Confusion in Older Patients[5,19]

Therapeutic Class	Example
Antimuscarinics	Darifenacin Fesoterodine Flavoxate Oxybutynin Solifenacin Tolterodine Trospium
Antispasmodic	Atropine[a] Clidinium-chlordiazepoxide Dicyclomine Homatropine[a] Propantheline Scopolamine[a]
Antiparkinson	Benztropine Trihexyphenidyl
Antihistamine	Brompheniramine Chlorpheniramine Clemastine Dimenhydrinate Diphenhydramine Doxylamine Hydroxyzine HCL Meclizine
Antidepressant	Amitriptyline Clomipramine Desipramine Doxepin (>6 mg) Imipramine Nortriptyline Paroxetine Trimipramine
Antiarrhythmic	Disopyramide Quinidine
Antipsychotic	Clozapine Olanzapine Quetiapine
Hypnotic	Hydroxyzine Pamoate
Skeletal Muscle Relaxant	Cyclobenzaprine Orphenadrine

This chart does not include all anticholinergic drugs that may cause confusion in older adults.
[a]Does not include ophthalmic.
Adapted from American Geriatrics Society 2015 Updated Beers Criteria for Potentially Inappropriate Medication Use in Older Adults. *J Am Geriatr Soc*. 2015;63:2227–2246.

mortality, functional decline, health resource use, and multiple medication use.[36]

Multiple medication use is associated with increased healthcare costs and increased drug-related adverse events in the older population.[37] Polypharmacy exists due to multiple chronic diseases, which often need to be treated with multiple medications. For these reasons, monitoring drug therapy in these patients is not only challenging but imperative. Duplicative prescribing within the same drug class may occur, and unrecognized drug side effects may be treated with additional drugs. Careful medication regimen review is essential to identify potentially unnecessary or inappropriate medications and to systematically taper and discontinue these agents, with attentive monitoring to older adults.[38]

Adverse Drug Events

An adverse drug event includes preventable and nonpreventable events and accounts for errors related to prescribing and administration. The combining of several medications can also increase the risk of clinically significant drug–drug interactions and subsequent adverse drug events in the elderly. Nearly one in 25 community-dwelling older adults is potentially at risk for a major drug–drug interaction.[39] Adverse drug events in general are expected to increase due to the increase in medication use for prevention, medication use for chronic conditions, aging and better access to prescription coverage.[40]

The use of high-risk medications such as anticholinergics, antipsychotics, opiate analgesics, and hypnotics, along with polypharmacy, increases the risk of adverse drug events.[38]

Up to 31% of hospitalizations of older persons involve adverse drug events.[41] Adverse drug events may be underreported and be difficult to detect in older patients because they often present atypically and with nonspecific symptoms, such as lethargy, confusion, lightheadedness, or falls. Nevertheless, most adverse reactions represent extensions of a drug's pharmacologic effect, have identifiable predictors, and are potentially preventable.[42]

ADVERSE DRUG REACTIONS IN OLDER PATIENTS

CASE 107-2

QUESTION 1: S.E. is an 85-year-old woman and resident of a long-term care facility (LTCF). She is 5′2″ and 102 pounds, with a serum creatinine of 1.6 mg/dL. She is admitted to the hospital for chest pain and shortness of breath, and to rule out myocardial infarction (MI). Her physician is concerned about oversedation with narcotics and prescribes ketorolac 30 mg IV every 6 hours. She has a history of severe HF and angina for which she takes lisinopril 10 mg daily, furosemide 40 mg daily, aspirin 81 mg daily, and isosorbide mononitrate 30 mg daily. The lisinopril dosage is increased to 20 mg daily, and the furosemide dosage is increased to 40 mg twice daily. Her blood pressure (BP) is 110/66 mm Hg, and her urine output has been from 20 to 30 mL/hour for 4 hours since ketorolac was initiated. What risk factors are present in S.E. for drug-induced renal problems?

S.E. has a number of risk factors for the development of drug-induced acute renal failure. Angiotensin-converting enzyme (ACE) inhibitors are indicated for HF management and improve renal function by increasing cardiac output. However, they can diminish efferent arteriole glomerular capillary filtration pressure and precipitate acute renal failure in predisposed patients. The use of ketorolac is another risk factor. A 13% incidence of azotemia has been reported in LTCF residents started on a short course of NSAID treatment.[43] A low serum sodium concentration, high-dose diuretics, diabetes, severe HF (i.e., New York Heart Association [NYHA] class IV), use of a long-acting ACE inhibitor, and concurrent NSAID use are all risk factors for drug-induced acute renal failure (see Chapter 28, Acute Kidney Injury). Elderly patients may be particular susceptible, owing to the renal changes of aging described earlier. Patients with these risk factors should be monitored closely when an ACE inhibitor is initiated and when the dosage of an ACE inhibitor is increased (see Chapter 14, Heart Failure). Renal prostaglandins (PGE_2, PGI_2) increase or help maintain renal blood flow when renal function is compromised by intrinsic renal disease, HF, liver disease with ascites, or hypertension; therefore, the use of a prostaglandin inhibitor such as ketorolac places S.E. at an increased risk for acute renal failure.

The ketorolac dose is excessive for S.E. based on the maximum recommended dose of 60 mg/day for elderly patients.[44]

APPROACH TO APPROPRIATE PRESCRIBING

As a result of high rates of multimorbidity and polypharmacy in older adults, in 2012, the American Geriatrics Society convened an Expert Panel on the Care of Older Adults with Multimorbidity to design a set of Guiding Principles for the Care of Older Adults with Multimorbidity.[36] The five steps include the following: eliciting and incorporating patient preferences and goals of care, recognizing the applicability and limitations of available evidence, framing clinical decisions in terms of prognosis, considering treatment complexity and feasibility, and continually optimizing treatment plans. Effective implementation of these principles is likely to require the input of interprofessional team members and high-quality-care coordination. Pharmacists have an integral role in applying these guiding principles.

DISEASE-SPECIFIC GERIATRIC DRUG THERAPY

Cardiovascular Disease in the Ambulatory Older Patient

CASE 107-3

QUESTION 1: T.M. is a 73-year-old woman who comes to a "brown bag" session at the local senior center. She reports recently feeling "sluggish" and dizzy. She lives at home alone on a modest, fixed retirement income. T.M.'s chronic medical problems include coronary artery disease (CAD), HF, hypertension, diabetes, and hyperlipidemia. She states that different specialists prescribe her "a lot of medications," but she does not know their names. She admits to skipping her medications periodically when she does not feel well. T.M. usually maintains an active social life, visiting her friends and attending the local seniors' luncheons. She is interested in natural medicines, and self-medicates with nonprescription medications and herbal remedies that her friends also take. Because of the recent weakness, however, she has not gone out as much. Review of her brown bag reveals the following items: glyburide 2.5 mg twice daily, hydrochlorothiazide 25 mg daily, atenolol 50 mg daily, niacin 500 mg 3 times a day, ASA 325 mg as needed, digoxin 0.25 mg daily, isosorbide dinitrate (ISDN) 20 mg 4 times a day, nitroglycerin (NTG) 0.4 mg sublingual (SL) as needed, captopril 25 mg 3 times a day, furosemide 40 mg twice daily, acetaminophen 500 mg as needed, verapamil 60 mg 4 times a day, multivitamins with minerals, calcium carbonate 500 mg 3 times a day, ibuprofen 200 mg as needed, and pioglitazone 30 mg daily. She also drinks a glass of red wine with dinner. What initial steps are necessary for safe and effective management of T.M.'s drug therapy?

Like many ambulatory older patients who are being treated for multiple chronic medical conditions, T.M. is at high risk for drug-induced problems secondary to nonadherence, medication errors, prescribing from multiple providers, self-medicating, and polypharmacy. She is representative of more than nine million older adults who live at home alone. The isolated community-dwelling older patient is typically female 75 years of age or older, has multiple medical issues, and takes multiple medications.[1] With rising life expectancy, the increased complexity of managing multiple medical conditions has put nonhospitalized elderly individuals at higher risk of experiencing adverse drug reactions and for adverse drug-related admissions.[42,45] Another group of older individuals at higher risk of having adverse drug reactions is those who are recently discharged from the hospital. The postdischarge period is often a time of confusion, and elderly patients may have difficulty coping and sorting out new versus replacement or duplicate drugs. A summary of the various factors contributing to nonadherence in the older patient is presented in Table 107-6.[46]

Table 107-6
Factors Influencing the Inability to Adhere to a Medication Regimen

Low health literacy (understanding of medication instructions and importance)
Medication cost
Significant cognitive or physical impairment (e.g., memory, hearing, vision)
Inconsistent filling or refilling of prescriptions
Adverse effects
Lack of clinical evidence of effectiveness

Adapted From Bosworth HB et al. Medication adherence: a call for action. *Am Heart J*. 2011;162(3):412–424. doi:10.1016/j.ahj.2011.06.007.

CASE 107-3, QUESTION 2: T.M. presents to the multidisciplinary geriatric care team on the advice of pharmacists at the brown bag session. During the intake interview, she admits to selective adherence with many medications based on how they make her feel and their costs. Her wine intake with dinner is 8 to 12 ounces most days of the week. She also has not taken her furosemide and potassium supplement because she feels that they are contributing to her sluggishness and dizziness. T.M.'s medical history and physical examination are as follows: 73-year-old white woman, 5′6″, 189 pounds; vital signs are as follows: BP, 168/82 mm Hg; heart rate (HR), 54 beats/minute; temperature, 98.7°F; and respiratory rate, 18 breaths/minute. Pertinent laboratory values are as follows:

Serum creatinine, 1.5 mg/dL
Blood urea nitrogen, 35 mg/dL
Sodium, 153 mEq/L
Potassium, 3.1 mEq/L
Magnesium, 1.5 mEq/L
Glucose, 250 mg/dL
Glycosylated hemoglobin (Hgb A_{1c}), 9.5%
Total cholesterol, 259 mg/dL
Low-density lipoprotein, 140 mg/dL
High-density lipoprotein, 40 mg/dL
Triglycerides, 200 mg/dL
Urine dipstick 2+ protein
Digoxin level, 1.5 ng/mL

Electrocardiogram showed sinus bradycardia with an old anterior MI. Echocardiogram showed an ejection fraction (EF) of 25%. Her problem list includes new-onset sluggishness and fainting, chest pain and shortness of breath (SOB) on exertion, 3(+) pitting edema bilaterally, NYHA class II–III HF, hypertension, type 2 diabetes, obesity, excessive alcohol intake, CAD, and hyperlipidemia. What factors may be contributing to T.M.'s feeling of sluggishness and dizziness?

T.M. needs a primary-care provider to coordinate her medical care and to evaluate the new-onset sluggishness and dizziness. She should also be advised to establish a client–patient relationship at a specific pharmacy for all her medications to be on one profile for continuous assessment. Furthermore, T.M. should be counseled to discontinue alcohol, which can interact with several of her current medications and worsen her conditions. Finally, assessment of the risk for medication-related problems (MRPs) is highly recommended.[47]

T.M.'s sluggishness and dizziness are most likely caused by her low heart rate, somewhat dehydrated state, and multiple medications that have the potential for producing weakness. Specifically, digoxin 0.25 mg daily is considered a high dose; patients over age 70 should be limited to 0.125 mg daily as initial therapy to limit the development of toxicities from reduced renal clearance. A level of 1.5 ng/mL is excessive because the therapeutic range is from 0.5 to 0.9 ng/mL for HF; therefore, the digoxin dose should be lowered to 0.125 mg daily.[48]

If HF is controlled, one can try discontinuing digoxin to evaluate the continued necessity of this agent. Finally, atenolol and verapamil can both lower the heart rate and contribute further to the sluggishness. Switching atenolol to an extended-release β-blocker indicated for heart failure may help. Verapamil can be discontinued because it may not have benefits for T.M. other than for hypertension and may contribute to a worsening of her HF.

HEART FAILURE

CASE 107-3, QUESTION 3: What is appropriate management for T.M.'s stage of HF?

On the basis of T.M.'s history of an old MI evidencing structural heart disease, her low EF, and the presence of fluid-retention symptoms, T.M. is in stage C HF based upon the American College of Cardiology/American Heart Association classification scheme (see Chapter 14, Heart Failure). Heart failure is a common cause of morbidity and mortality in older patients. The standard therapy for HF with reduced ejection fraction typically consists of ACE inhibitors or ARBs, and β-blockers. In symptomatic patients, diuretics may be used for symptomatic relief, and an aldosterone antagonist for its morbidity and mortality benefits. In selected patients, digoxin or hydralazine/isosorbide may also be appropriate to reduce morbidity and mortality, as well as to prevent hospitalizations. The recommended therapy for T.M. includes an ACE inhibitor, or ARB, a β-blocker, aldosterone antagonist, and diuretic for symptomatic relief. Routine use of multiple medications in the treatment of HF with coexisting medical conditions makes close monitoring of drug therapy essential. Concurrent behavior modification with weight loss and salt restriction will also allow better control of HF.[49]

DIURETICS

CASE 107-3, QUESTION 4: Is the combination of furosemide and hydrochlorothiazide the most appropriate diuretic regimen for T.M.?

Loop diuretics are generally more effective than thiazides in providing symptomatic relief; furosemide is also preferred in T.M. because hydrochlorothiazide is less effective in moderate-to-severe renal compromise (creatinine clearance <30 mL/minute).[50] Furthermore, the combination of furosemide and hydrochlorothiazide (HCTZ) is duplicative in diuretic action and may be excessive. Discontinuing the HCTZ will likely help with T.M.'s hypokalemia and slightly dehydrated state. Regular monitoring of serum creatinine, urea nitrogen, sodium, and potassium is essential while on diuretics. The need for potassium supplementation will depend on the resultant level after T.M. adheres to furosemide while being maintained on an ACE inhibitor. Elderly patients often dislike taking diuretics because of the frequent need to urinate. T.M. may be advised to take furosemide later during the day after she returns from her social engagements.

ACE INHIBITORS AND ANGIOTENSIN RECEPTOR BLOCKERS

CASE 107-3, QUESTION 5: T.M. has been taking captopril 25 mg 3 times a day. Is this an appropriate choice of ACE inhibitor for T.M.?

Blockade of the renin–angiotensin–aldosterone system is essential in the management of HF. However, 3 times daily dosing of captopril is inconvenient and may contribute to poor adherence. Although captopril, enalapril, and lisinopril have all proven efficacious for HF in clinical trials, lisinopril is the only agent of these that may be dosed daily. Alternatively, fosinopril may also be desirable based on its 50% hepatic and 50% renal elimination profile.[51] An ARB may also be appropriate if therapy with an ACEI is not tolerated. Although previous studies have supported the addition of an ARB to ACE inhibitor therapy based on a lower mortality and hospitalization rate compared with an ACE inhibitor alone,[52] more recent data present concerns about the use of combination therapy, particularly in the elderly, owing to higher risk of hyperkalemia and worsening renal function.[53]

β-BLOCKERS

CASE 107-3, QUESTION 6: T.M. is being treated with atenolol 50 mg daily. Is this an appropriate choice of β-blocker for T.M.?

The β-blockers carvedilol, metoprolol, and bisoprolol have been proven to reduce morbidity and mortality in patients with HF.[54–56] In T.M.'s case, atenolol is not clinically indicated for HF and should be discontinued. Additionally, it is renally cleared and may contribute to excessive sluggishness in an elderly patient with compromised kidney function. Although any of the proven agents would be appropriate, extended-release versions of carvedilol or metoprolol may reduce T.M.'s medication burden.

CARDIOVASCULAR DISEASE AND HYPERLIPIDEMIA

CASE 107-3, QUESTION 7: T.M. does not take her niacin because she experienced unbearable facial flushing. Despite her history of MI, she does not believe that cholesterol and "heart disease" are major health concerns for a woman. Are women older than age 65 at different risk of death owing to coronary heart disease (CHD) compared with their male counterparts, and is it important to manage cholesterol in an elderly woman with CHD?

More than 60% of cardiovascular disease (CVD) deaths occur in people aged 75 or older. Approximately 70% of older adults aged 60 to 79 have CVD.[57] For those over age 80, 83.0% of men and 87.1% of women have CVD.[57] Although male sex is an independent risk factor for CVD, more women than men die from heart attacks because these events occur in women at an older age. The significantly higher rate of hypercholesterolemia in women seems also to predict a higher CVD risk than for men later in life. Therefore, it is important to treat dyslipidemia in most patients with clinical ASCVD, in those aged 40 to 75 with diabetes who have LDL-C levels of 70 to 189 mg/dL, and in those without diabetes and an estimated 10-year ASCVD risk >/=7.5%.[58]

CASE 107-3, QUESTION 8: What is an optimal therapeutic plan for management of T.M.'s hyperlipidemia?

T.M. is a 73-year-old female with history of diabetes, elevated cholesterol and blood pressure conferring a 10-year ASCVD risk greater than 7.5%.[58] T.M.'s treatment plan should begin with lifestyle and dietary modifications. Based on her high ASCVD risk level and concomitant diabetes, a high intensity statin should be started to lower LDL by at least 50%. However, the relative benefits of statin therapy should be weighed against the potential risk of adverse reactions. Liver transaminases should be monitored on a regular basis. Although rare, elderly patients, particularly the frail elderly with low body mass, may be at increased risk for muscle-related side effects. The hydrophilic statins pravastatin, rosuvastatin, and pitavastatin are not metabolized significantly by the cytochrome P-450 system and may present fewer side effects and lower potential of drug interactions.[59] Both atorvastatin and rosuvastatin may be given at any time of day, owing to their longer half-lives. Additionally, atorvastatin is less effected by renal impairment and may be preferred in T.M.[60]

Clinical guidance for the care of adults over age 74 with hyperlipidemia is limited by lack of clinical trial data. Current guidelines recommend for the continuation of currently tolerated statins as patients age.[58] If new statin initiation is required after age 74, a careful assessment of risk versus benefit is warranted, and guidelines recommend for consideration of moderate-intensity statins in patients who would otherwise be candidates for high-intensity therapy. Medical conditions, such as presence of high cardiovascular risk or vascular dementia, functional status, and overall prognosis, may be helpful determinants in these cases.

At this time, there are insufficient data for guidelines to support combination therapy. If combination therapy is indicated, ezetimibe can be added to further reduce the levels of LDL and reduce cardiovascular outcomes without escalating the dose and potential side effects of a statin as shown in the IMPROVE-IT trial.[61] Combination of a statin with niacin is less preferred. Results from the AIM-HIGH trial found no added clinical benefit despite improvements in lipid profile and a possible increase in stroke risk and adverse drug events.[62] Additionally, intolerable side effects of flushing and risk for myopathy and hyperglycemia may limit use. The addition of fibrates to statins has become controversial in patients with diabetes, as shown recently in the ACCORD lipid trial. The addition of fenofibrate to simvastatin in patients with diabetes did not reduce the rate of fatal CHD events, nonfatal MI, or nonfatal stroke compared with those who received only simvastatin.[63] Finally, because alcohol can increase triglycerides as much as 50%, abstinence is strongly recommended.[64]

CASE 107-3, QUESTION 9: What other interventions should be implemented to optimize management of T.M.'s CAD?

Any strategy to optimize T.M.'s CAD management should take into consideration the patient's functional status, comorbidities, and risks versus benefits. T.M. is still experiencing anginal pain on her current regimen, possibly caused by more advanced disease or inability to adhere to the 4-times-daily regimen of ISDN. She should be evaluated for coronary vessel disease and appropriate antiplatelet therapy initiated if necessary. A once-daily long-acting nitrate preparation (isosorbide mononitrate [ISMN]) may be better suited for her, with sublingual NTG available as needed. T.M. should be maintained on first-line CAD therapy of aspirin and β-blockers because aspirin is indicated for MI prevention and β-blockers may also be beneficial for HF. To prevent further endothelial injury from the atherosclerosis that leads to plaque rupture, statins are indicated as described previously. ACE inhibitors have been shown to reduce mortality and to provide secondary prevention in CAD, particularly among those 65 years or older. These agents should be part of the regimen because ACE inhibitors also have benefits for T.M.'s HF and HTN, as well as diabetic nephropathy.[65] Although calcium-channel blockers are indicated in CAD, they have not been proven beneficial for HF; therefore, verapamil may be held at this time whereas the other agents are being optimized.

HYPERTENSION

CASE 107-3, QUESTION 10: T.M. has uncontrolled hypertension. How should this be managed in light of her advanced age?

Despite her advancing age, T.M.'s blood pressure is well above the goal of less than 140/90 mm Hg for diabetic patients as set forth by the American Diabetes Association (ADA) and the 2014 Evidence-Based Guideline for the Management of High Blood Pressure in Adults: Report From the Panel Members Appointed to the Eighth Joint National Committee (JNC 8).[65,66] (see Chapter 9, Essential Hypertension.) Hypertension is present in more than two-thirds of individuals older than 65 years of age. Despite having the highest prevalence of hypertension, only a small percentage of this population is controlled or adequately treated for their blood pressure.[67] In patients greater than 60 years of age without diabetes or CKD, a blood pressure goal of <150/90 is appropriate. The HYVET study has shown that a mean reduction of blood pressure from a baseline of 173/91 mm Hg by 15/6 mm Hg in patients 80 years or older resulted in a 30% reduction in stroke, a 39% reduction in rate of death from stroke, a 23% reduction in the rate of death from cardiovascular causes, and a 64% reduction in the rate of heart failure.[68]

Although adequate dosing and combination therapy may be essential in achieving blood pressure control in the elderly population, close monitoring is also necessary to avoid systolic blood pressure (SBP) less than 120 mm Hg based on the recent findings from the ACCORD BP trial. Intensive target of SBP less than 120 mm Hg did not reduce fatal and nonfatal major cardiovascular events but increased the incidence of adverse effects.[69] Serious side effects of aggressive BP lowering include hypotension, bradycardia, hypokalemia, and elevated SCr, and these effects must be diligently monitored. For T.M., it is recommended that adequate doses of furosemide and an ACE inhibitor or ARB with close monitoring be the main therapeutic approach for her HTN. Extended- or controlled-release formulations of metoprolol or carvedilol should be considered as it has for HF management. Though beneficial for CAD and HTN, verapamil in sustained-release formulation should not be used based on T.M.'s unstable HF.[49]

Diabetes in the Elderly

CASE 107-3, QUESTION 11: T.M. reports that she frequently feels lightheaded and shaky after she takes the glyburide. She admits to not taking glyburide regularly because it also causes rapid heartbeats. What is an optimal therapeutic plan for the management of T.M.'s diabetes?

Comprehensive diabetes education needs to be initiated, stressing the importance of weight loss, self-monitoring of blood glucose, alcohol abstinence, and medication adherence. A 5% to 10% weight loss will improve T.M.'s glucose control and cardiovascular status.[66] T.M.'s alcohol consumption and self-reported erratic meal schedule may be contributing to the hypoglycemia (in addition to the glyburide), as well as to the worsening of her hypertension and HF. The daily recommended allowance of alcohol is no more than two drinks (24 ounces of beer, 10 ounces of wine, or 3 ounces of 80-proof liquor) for men and no more than one drink for women.[70] Glyburide is also a long-acting sulfonylurea and is associated with severe hypoglycemia more commonly than other sulfonylureas because of its active metabolites and highly renal elimination. In general, the elderly are more susceptible, even at low doses, to hypoglycemia and may have difficulty recognizing the symptoms of hypoglycemia. Among the second-generation sulfonylureas, glipizide or glimepiride is preferred in renal impairment. Meglitinides, such as repaglinide or nateglinide, may be preferred over the sulfonylureas in the elderly population because they do not require dose adjustment in renal compromise and also allow for a more flexible meal pattern. These agents, however, require multiple daily dosing and may still contribute to hypoglycemic risk. Any new diabetes medication should be initiated in low doses and gradually titrated upward to avoid hypoglycemic episodes and to achieve glycemic goals in accordance with ADA guidelines.[66]

The current treatment algorithm for diabetes states that metformin with lifestyle modification is the initial management approach.[71] Per FDA labeling, metformin is contraindicated in T.M. because of a serum creatinine greater than 1.4 mg/dL; however, the American Diabetes Association and European Association for the Study of Diabetes reports that metformin seems safe unless eGFR falls to <30 mL/minute. As such, consideration of dosage reductions when renal function begins to decline below 45 mL/minute may be appropriate.[72] When metformin is contraindicated or inadequate, the effective and affordable sulfonylureas or pioglitazone may be added; caution for risks of side effects such as hypoglycemia should be exercised. Pioglitazone should be avoided in T.M. owing to her history of HF. Injections such as GLP-1 analogs are often reserved unless a patient's Hgb A_{1c} remains above 8% while adhering to an appropriately titrated oral combination regimen. Basal insulin can be added if A_{1c} is significantly elevated at baseline, or if patients fail to achieve glycemic goals. More expensive and less effective A_{1c}-lowering alternatives may include dipeptidyl peptidase-4 (DPP4) inhibitors and sodium glucose cotransport 2 (SGLT2) inhibitors. DPP4 inhibitors do not promote hypoglycemia and may be considered early on during the disease state. Their dosages, however, need to be adjusted if the creatinine clearance is less than 50 mL/minutes.[73] In general, the priority of diabetes management in the elderly population should be on reduction of cardiovascular risks with strict control of blood pressure and lipids in addition to avoidance of hypoglycemic events. Hgb A_{1c} goals in older adults should generally be 7.5% to 8%. In the presence of few comorbidities and good functional status, an Hgb A_{1c} goal between 7% and 7.5% may be appropriate if it can be safely achieved. Higher Hgb A_{1c} targets may be appropriate for some elderly patients who are functionally impaired, cognitively impaired, have complex multimorbidity, end-stage illness, or are prone to hypoglycemia or falls.[66,74] It is recommended that glyburide and pioglitazone be discontinued, and either glipizide or repaglinide in combination with sitagliptin, or basal insulin such as glargine, be initiated for T.M.'s diabetes. Finally, comprehensive screening of diabetic complications should be done routinely to decrease morbidity and mortality.[66]

Depression and the Older Patient

Significant depression is the most common mental illness among adults older than 65 years of age, occurring in about 15%; it is a source of significant morbidity and mortality in this population.[75] Unfortunately, depression remains under-recognized and undertreated, even though it is a major risk factor for suicide in the elderly, who have a suicide death rate that is higher than the national average.[76,77] Older patients may be at increased risk for depression because of the high prevalence of comorbid medical conditions (i.e., stroke, cancer, MI, rheumatoid arthritis, dementia, Parkinson's disease, DM).[78] Refer to Chapter 86: Depression for further discussion of risk factors for depression and potential drug-induced causes.

CASE 107-4

QUESTION 1: J.W. is a married, 5′8″, 110-pound, 79-year-old woman who presents for a psychiatric evaluation. Her husband says she just has not been herself lately. The changes in J.W. began on a family vacation 6 months earlier when she got lost on the cruise ship. Since that incident, she has become increasingly anxious and has developed insomnia. Although she does not feel sad or "depressed," she generally does not feel well. J.W.'s normally positive attitude toward life has become pessimistic. Her husband confirms that she has become more forgetful and no longer enjoys eating. In fact, she has lost 18 pounds during the past 2 months. J.W. no longer does her volunteer work at the local children's center. She says she wants to die because she is no longer the person she used to be, but she denies having any specific suicidal thoughts. Her medical history is significant for diabetes and hypertension, which are both well controlled on glipizide 5 mg every morning and hydrochlorothiazide 25 mg daily. Her medical evaluation and physical examination are unremarkable. Laboratory results and head-computed tomography scan are within normal limits. J.W. is diagnosed as having a major depressive episode. What symptoms of depression are present in J.W.?

J.W.'s presenting symptoms are typical of major depression in an older patient, which is commonly quite different from that of younger depressed patients. Criteria set forth in the *Diagnostic and Statistical Manual of Mental Disorders, Fifth Edition*, for diagnosing depression were developed using younger subjects and may not be applicable to the older depressed patient.[79] Older patients are less likely to report suicidal thoughts, but are more likely to experience weight loss as a symptom of depression. Anxiety, irritability, somatic complaints, or a withdrawal from normal activities, as exhibited by J.W., may be more significant features in late-life depression than depressed mood. Memory problems, such as J.W.'s forgetfulness, may be attributable to a lack of concentration or effort stemming from her depression. This is distinct from dementia, which manifests itself predominantly with impairment in short- and long-term memory (see Chapter 108, Geriatric Neurocognitive Disorders). Therefore, depressed mood cannot be relied on for determining whether an older patient has a depressive disorder.[76] Table 107-7 lists atypical depressive symptoms that may be found in older adults. The presence of any one of these symptoms should be considered a red flag and should prompt further evaluation for major depression.

CASE 107-4, QUESTION 2: J.W.'s physician decides to prescribe an antidepressant. Which antidepressants are preferred for use in older adults?

Selection of an antidepressant drug for elderly patients must take into consideration age-related changes in pharmacokinetic, pharmacodynamic, and physiologic parameters that make this population more vulnerable to adverse effects. Although the available antidepressants are equally effective, selective serotonin reuptake inhibitors (SSRIs) are better tolerated than older agents, such as

Table 107-7
Atypical Depressive Symptoms in the Older Adult

Agitation, anxiety, or worrying
Reduced initiative and problem-solving capacities
Alcohol or substance abuse
Paranoia
Obsessions and compulsions
Irritability
Somatic complaints
Excessive guilt
Marital discord
Social withdrawal
Cognitive impairment
Deterioration in self-care

Source: Sable JA et al. Late-life depression: how to identify its symptoms and provide effective treatment. *Geriatrics*. 2002;57:18.

Table 107-8
Antidepressant Dosing in Older Adults

	Initial Dosage	Maximum Dosage
Citalopram	10 mg every day	20 mg every day
Escitalopram	5 mg every day	10 mg every day
Fluoxetine	5 mg every day	40 mg every day
Fluvoxamine	25 mg at bedtime	200 mg at bedtime
Paroxetine	10 mg every day	40 mg every day
Sertraline	25 mg every day	150 mg every day
Mirtazapine	7.5 mg at bedtime	45 mg at bedtime
Bupropion	37.5 mg twice a day	75 mg twice a day
Duloxetine	20 mg every day	40 mg every day
Venlafaxine	25 mg twice a day	225 mg every day
Desvenlafaxine	50 mg every day	400 mg every day

the tricyclic antidepressants. Therefore, low-dose SSRIs should be considered first-line therapy for older patients. Of course, this does not preclude the use of sound clinical judgment that incorporates the patient's history of response, comorbidities, and the drug's side effect profile. J.W. should start taking a low-dose SSRI, such as citalopram 10 mg daily, with gradual dose titration to achieve control of her depressive symptoms. Doses of citalopram should not exceed 20 mg per day in adults over age 60 due to risk of QTc prolongation. Table 107-8 lists recommended starting doses for antidepressants in older patients. Full antidepressant response may take twice as long in older patients compared with younger patients; it may take 8 to 12 weeks before assessment of J.W.'s full response can be made.[80]

Asthma and Chronic Obstructive Pulmonary Disease in the Elderly

Epidemiologic studies estimate the prevalence of asthma in the elderly to be approximately 4.5% to 12.7%.[81,82] Although 25% of asthmatics with 65 and older have a history of childhood asthma diagnosed before the age of 20, 27% are diagnosed with asthma after the age of 60.[83] Rates of asthma-related hospitalization and mortality are highest amongst adults over age 65, possibly because of underdiagnosis and undertreatment of the disease.[83] Symptoms of asthma, including wheezing, cough, chest tightness, and dyspnea, are similar in both older and younger patients (see Chapter 18, Asthma). However, because the elderly are more likely to have coexisting medical conditions (e.g., HF, angina, COPD, gastroesophageal reflux disease [GERD]) with symptoms that mimic asthma, accurate diagnosis and assessment of severity is often more difficult.[83]

Chronic obstructive pulmonary disease is largely a disease of older patients with a prevalence of as high as 10% in those 75 and older.[84] This chronic condition is a major cause of morbidity and mortality in the older population, accounting for approximately one-fifth of all U.S. hospitalizations in those over age 65.[85] It is often undiagnosed as it may be mistaken as a "normal" part of the aging process, and may be confounded by physical deconditioning or comorbidities such as HF.[85] Drug therapy for COPD in the elderly does not differ significantly from standard management regimens (see Chapter 19, Chronic Obstructive Pulmonary Disease). However, older patients with pulmonary disease and coexisting medical problems may be more sensitive to the adverse effects of pharmacologic agents.

CASE 107-5

QUESTION 1: J.C., a 67-year-old woman, 5′6″, 145 pounds, presents to the ED complaining of shortness of breath for the past 2 days. She was in her usual state of health until 4 days ago when she exhibited flulike symptoms consisting of fever, cough, and mild wheezing. J.C. has a history of asthma, diabetes, hypertension, headache, and GERD. Her current medications include glipizide 5 mg daily, lisinopril 10 mg daily, metoprolol 50 mg twice daily, lansoprazole 30 mg daily, ibuprofen 200 mg every 6 hours as needed for headache, albuterol metered-dose inhaler (MDI) 2 puffs 4 times a day as needed for SOB, and fluticasone HFA (44 mcg) MDI 2 puffs twice daily. Her drug regimen has been unchanged for the past 2 years, and she reports taking all medications as prescribed. The only recent change has been the need for albuterol every 3 to 4 hours for coughing and wheezing during the past few days. What factors (including medications) may have contributed to her acute asthma exacerbation?

Management of acute asthma exacerbations in previously stable elderly asthmatics should begin with a review of the medication history for asthma-inducing agents. Aspirin and other NSAIDs are known to induce acute bronchoconstriction in adult asthmatics.[86] J.C. should be queried about her previous (especially recent) use of ibuprofen in relation to her asthma symptoms, and these agents should be avoided if associated. An alternative agent for pain control is acetaminophen.[87] Nonselective β-blockers, including topical ophthalmic formulations, can precipitate acute bronchoconstriction and should be avoided in patients with reactive airway disease. Although cardioselective β-blockers are generally considered safe for use in patients with asthma, it is important to recognize that cardioselectivity may be lost with higher dosages. Because J.C. has been taking low-dose metoprolol (a cardioselective agent) for years without problem, this medication is unlikely to be contributing to her current asthma exacerbation. One of the most important triggers for asthma exacerbations is respiratory infection (particularly viral). J.C. reports the recent onset of symptoms consistent with influenza, and this is likely precipitating her current pulmonary symptoms. As a future prophylactic measure, J.C. should be counseled to receive the influenza vaccine annually. J.C. does not recall every receiving the pneumococcal vaccine. In adults aged 65 and older who have never received the pneumococcal vaccine or who are unsure like J.C., they should receive a one-time dose of pneumococcal conjugate vaccine (PCV13), and 12 months later they should receive the pneumococcal polysaccharide vaccine (PPSV23).[88]

CASE 107-5, QUESTION 2: Are the medication regimens used to treat asthma in elderly patients different from those used in children and younger adults? Should J.C.'s maintenance asthma regimen be changed?

Medications used in the management of persistent asthma in the elderly are similar to those used in younger patients and consist of bronchodilators in combination with anti-inflammatory agents (see Chapter 23, Asthma). Drug selection and monitoring may be more complicated in the elderly because of the greater likelihood of coexisting medical conditions and increased potential for drug–disease and drug–drug interactions.

Inhaled β_2-agonists are an important class of drugs used to treat asthma in all age groups. The low incidence of drug interactions and reduced side effect profile make inhaled β_2-agonists ideal for use in the older asthmatics. However, these agents can cause dose-dependent systemic side effects, such as tremor, tachycardia, hypokalemia, and arrhythmias, which are of particular concern in patients with cardiac conditions.[82] Inhaled corticosteroids are the preferred treatment for all forms of persistent asthma yet they may be underused in the elderly. Though generally well tolerated, elderly patients receiving high-dose therapy are at an increased risk for osteoporosis, cataracts, skin thinning, and bruising.[89] In addition to the well-known complications associated with systemic corticosteroid use (see Chapter 44, Rheumatoid Arthritis), these agents can acutely cause confusion, agitation, and hyperglycemia.

J.C. is currently maintained on low doses of an inhaled corticosteroid (fluticasone) in combination with a short-acting β_2-agonist (albuterol), and this is an appropriate regimen for a patient with mild-persistent asthma. Following resolution of her viral infection, J.C.'s asthma control should be re-evaluated within the next 3 months for a step-up or down in therapy. Because J.C. is postmenopausal, she is at risk for osteoporosis; calcium and vitamin D supplementation should be initiated (see Chapter 110, Osteoporosis).

Appropriate use of MDIs is difficult for most patients, but may be particularly problematic in the elderly population because of decreased hand strength or arthritis, difficulty timing actuation to inhalation, or impaired mental function. The use of spacer or holding chamber devices can minimize the coordination necessary for proper use of an MDI and may reduce the incidence of systemic and local (cough, hoarseness, thrush) side effects associated with inhaled corticosteroids. J.C. should be discharged with a spacer device to use with her albuterol and fluticasone MDIs. Even though J.C. previously used an MDI, she should be asked to demonstrate her MDI technique and reinstructed, if necessary, to ensure she is using the inhaler and spacer correctly. If J.C. is unable to correctly use her MDIs with a spacer, use of nebulized solutions, breath-activated inhalers, or dry-powdered delivery devices should be considered.

Infectious Diseases in the Elderly

Infections are among the most common problems in the elderly and are a significant cause of morbidity and mortality. Infections are also one of the most frequent reasons for hospitalization of older ambulatory persons.[90] Antibiotic therapy for an infection in the elderly may be delayed because they may present with atypical signs and symptoms. The older population is also more likely to have polymicrobial infections than younger people, and changes in renal function should be taken into account when selecting, dosing, and monitoring antibiotic therapy.

PNEUMONIA

CASE 107-5, QUESTION 3: J.C. was admitted to the hospital and given intravenous methylprednisolone for 4 days. She was then discharged home with a new prescription for prednisone 40 mg daily for 7 days. Three days after J.C. is discharged from the hospital, she presents again to the ED. This time, she is accompanied by a neighbor who noted that J.C. suddenly became forgetful and confused, and continues to have difficulty breathing. Her neighbor reports that J.C. has been staying in bed for the past 2 days and has not eaten much. J.C. has a low-grade fever, and chest examination reveals faint breath sounds with light crackling rales over her right lung base. A chest radiograph confirms the diagnosis of pneumonia. How is J.C.'s clinical presentation consistent with community-acquired pneumonia in the elderly?

Community-acquired pneumonia is one of the most prevalent causes of hospitalization and death due to infection in adults in the United States.[91] In a large population-based study of community-acquired pneumonia, adults aged 65 to 79 years were found to have an incidence of pneumonia requiring hospitalization that was 9 times as high as those aged 18 to 49, and 25 times as high in those aged 85 and older.

Risk factors for CAP in all adults include age greater than 65, COPD, smoking, alcoholism, aspiration, and chronic medical conditions such as heart, renal, and liver disease.[92,93] *Streptococcus pneumoniae* is the most common cause of CAP in the elderly.[91]

Respiratory symptoms and fever are often subtle or absent in older patients with pneumonia[93]; instead, like J.C., they may present only with altered mental status (delirium, acute confusion, memory problems) or a decline in functional status. Delirium or acute confusion is a common presentation in elderly patients who may have new-onset lower respiratory infection.

CASE 107-5, QUESTION 4: How should J.C. be treated for her respiratory infection?

In many cases, management of pneumonia in the elderly requires hospitalization because they are at greater risk for mortality and complications. Early empiric antibacterial therapy is particularly important for older patients with pneumonia (see Chapter 67, Respiratory Tract Infections). J.C. should be hospitalized again and treated aggressively for pneumonia with broad-spectrum IV antibiotics. The Infectious Diseases Society of America/American Thoracic Society Consensus Guidelines on the Management of Community-Acquired Pneumonia in Adults recommends treatment of most hospitalized nonintensive care unit (ICU) patients with a respiratory fluoroquinolone (moxifloxacin, gemifloxacin, levofloxacin) or β-lactam plus macrolide, and for ICU patients the recommendation is for a β-lactam plus either azithromycin or a respiratory fluroquinolone.[93]

PREVENTION

CASE 107-5, QUESTION 5: After 7 days of hospitalization, J.C. is discharged home with an oral antibiotic to finish the 14-day course of therapy. What preventative measures are available to J.C. after she is discharged?

Once patients are stable and ready to be discharged home, they should be switched to oral antibiotics to complete their therapy at home.

Both influenza and pneumococcal vaccinations are beneficial and recommended in the prevention of community acquired-pneumonia.[93–95]

The CDC now recommends pneumococcal conjugate vaccine (PCV13) for all adults aged 65 and older who have not previously received it, followed by the pneumococcal polysaccharide vaccine (PPSV23) 12 months later.[96] If the PPSV23 has already been received, the dose of PCV13 should be given at least 1 year after (see Chapter 64, Vaccinations).

J.C.'s immunization status should be confirmed, and as a preventative measure, J.C. should be offered both influenza and pneumococcal vaccines after she is discharged from the hospital.

URINARY TRACT INFECTION

CASE 107-6

QUESTION 1: A.H. is a 72-year-old Hispanic woman who is currently wheelchair-bound because of pain in her right hip. Her granddaughter brings A.H. to the geriatric clinic because she has recently developed urinary incontinence. Her granddaughter reports that A.H. has been feeling weak for the past 2 days and fell while getting out of the wheelchair. A urinalysis indicates the presence of a urinary tract infection (UTI).

Are A.H.'s symptoms typical of urinary tract infections?

Urinary tract infections are common in older patients, and clinical symptoms often vary from patient to patient.[97,98] Common signs and symptoms may include dysuria, hematuria, urinary frequency, urinary incontinence, pyuria and fever.[98] Bacteriuria is estimated to be asymptomatic in more than 15% of women over age 70 who live in the community, and even greater in men and women who reside in long-term care.[99] Asymptomatic bacteriuria may not always require antibiotic treatment.[97] Impaired voiding with residual urine in older women and obstructive uropathy from prostatic disease in older men predispose them to bacteriuria.[100] The severity of UTI in the older population ranges from mild cystitis to life-threatening urosepsis; both are more difficult to treat because of resistant organisms and age-related decreases in host defenses. The majority of UTIs in the older population do not present typically; instead, there are often nonspecific manifestations such as decline in functional status, cognitive impairment, weakness, falls, and urinary incontinence.[101]

A.H.'s presentation (weakness, urinary incontinence, and a recent fall) is consistent with this pattern. As with most UTIs, those in the elderly are caused primarily by *Escherichia coli*. However, other species of bacteria such as *Klebsiella* species, *Proteus* species, and *Enterococcus* species are also frequently involved (see Chapter 71, Urinary Tract Infections).

Case 107-6, Question 2: A.H. is prescribed a 7-day course of ciprofloxacin 250 mg PO twice daily. Is this drug therapy appropriate?

Oral antibiotics, such as nitrofurantoin and sulfamethoxazole-trimethoprim, are appropriate for most patients with symptomatic UTI, reserving fluoroquinolones as alternatives.[102] An important consideration of antibiotic therapy for older adults with UTI is impaired renal function.[103] Nitrofurantoin should not be used in those patients with significantly impaired renal function due to the potential risk of peripheral neuropathy and pulmonary toxicity.

Ciprofloxacin is a reasonable choice for A.H. because *E. coli* is the most likely causative agent. Fluoroquinolones carry a black box warning due to an increased risk of tendonitis and tendon rupture. Along with renal function, monitoring should include symptoms of tendon inflammation or pain.

Osteoarthritis Pain

Arthritis is the leading cause of functional decline and morbidity in older patients, with prevalence rates up to 30%.[104,105] This immobility may place older patients at risk of confinement to their bed or home. Osteoarthritis, also called degenerative joint disease, is the most common type of joint disease in the older population. Nonpharmacologic management of osteoarthritis, such as physical and occupational therapy, has been shown to decrease pain and improve function in patients with osteoarthritis, both alone or in combination with appropriate analgesics.[106]

CASE 107-7

Question 1: C.W., a 71-year-old retired schoolteacher, has been suffering from osteoarthritis of his hands for 5 years. He is an active older adult who enjoys volunteer work at the local hospital. He presents to the geriatric clinic with increased arthritis pain, which is uncontrolled by his current pain medication. He also complains of increased heartburn and gastric reflux symptoms. His past medical history is significant for diabetes, hypertension, hypercholesterolemia, and GERD. C.W.'s current medications include glipizide 10 mg daily, verapamil sustained-released 240 mg daily, atorvastatin 10 mg daily, famotidine 20 mg twice daily, docusate sodium 100 mg twice daily, and ibuprofen 200 mg 4 times a day as needed. What modifications can be made to his drug regimen to better control his arthritis pain and minimize side effects from his pain medication?

Acetaminophen is the drug of choice for mild-to-moderate arthritis pain (see Chapter 43, Osteoarthritis). Though pain control may be inferior to NSAIDs, its reduced gastrointestinal and renal toxicity provides an advantage in older patients who may be more susceptible to the adverse effects of NSAIDs.[104] Doses greater than 3,000 mg per day should be avoided in the elderly and more conservative dosing utilized for those with a history of alcohol abuse or hepatic impairment.[104,107] If C.W. has not tried acetaminophen in the past for his arthritis pain, acetaminophen 1,000 mg 3 times a day should be initiated. Older patients with osteoarthritis pain often find relief from NSAIDs, which should be used with caution because of their potential GI complications, renal toxicity, and cardiovascular risks. Though not as common as GI toxicity, advanced age is a major risk factor for NSAID-associated renal toxicity, such as sodium and water retention as well as risk for hypertension.[108] Thus, ibuprofen may be contributing to C.W.'s increased GERD symptoms and to his hypertension. Nonacetylated salicylates, such as salsalate, can be used if acetaminophen does not provide adequate pain relief. Compared with NSAIDs, nonacetylated salicylates have less renal and GI toxicity, but cardiovascular risks are unknown. The currently available selective COX-2 inhibitor celecoxib is less likely to cause GI complications than nonselective agents; however, the risk of adverse renal and cardiovascular events persists.[108] A COX-2 inhibitor or the addition of a more potent gastroprotective agent such as a proton-pump inhibitor to ibuprofen is the option for C.W., who may experience reduced GI symptoms with equally effective pain relief. The topical analgesics often require multiple daily applications, assessment of skin integrity, and application technique.[104] The use of glucosamine and chondroitin has been shown to decrease osteoarthritis pain and delay progression of the disease in some studies; however, their place in therapy is controversial.[109] Glucosamine may increase insulin resistance in diabetic patients, and C.W. should be counseled to monitor his blood glucose more closely if initiating this agent.

Case 107-7, Question 2: C.W. reveals that he has tried acetaminophen without much relief of his pain. He is prescribed celecoxib and tries it for several months, but his pain continues and he is still experiencing GI distress. What other pain medication options does C.W. have?

For moderate-to-severe chronic pain caused by osteoarthritis, a low-dose opiate may provide relief from pain with minimal adverse drug effects (see Chapter 55, Pain Management). Of particular concern in elderly patients are the risks of falls, delirium, and constipation with opioid medication use. Codeine and tramadol are "weak" opioids that have ceiling effects, generally do not provide adequate analgesia, and may carry dangerous side effects in the elderly. Meperidine should also be avoided in older adults because of its high potential for CNS side effects, especially in those with reduced renal function. C.W. is a candidate for opioid therapy. He should be started on the lowest dose of a short-acting formulation on a scheduled regimen and counseled on the adverse drug reactions. Constipation may be a particular problem because he is also taking verapamil, which can also cause significant constipation. The elderly are also at increased risk for constipation as a result of age-related reduced bowel motility. To prevent opioid-associated constipation in C.W., prophylactic laxatives and stool softeners should be started at the initiation of opioid therapy.

LONG-TERM CARE FACILITIES

The LTCF environment is governed in part by the Omnibus Budget Reconciliation Act (OBRA), as well as by numerous other laws and regulations, which are contained in the federal Centers for Medicare and Medicaid Services (CMS) publication, States Operations Manual (SOM).[110] The federal mandates include monthly review of each resident's medication regimen to help ensure each resident's regimen is free from unnecessary drugs and that their medication regimen helps to support their mental, physical, and psychosocial well-being. Medication regimens are reviewed to determine the following:

1. Is each drug clearly indicated?
2. Have therapeutic goals been established for chronic drug therapies?
3. If indicated, is it being dosed and administered appropriately?
4. Are any real or potential problems with drug side effects or interactions present?
5. If antipsychotics are being prescribed, have nonpharmacologic approaches been used first, has their use been justified, and is the therapy being monitored?
6. What specific recommendations can be made to optimize the resident's drug therapy?
7. Are the laboratory results and vital signs being monitored appropriately, and are they available for adequate evaluation of therapy?

The findings of the medication regimen review, including medication discrepancies, errors, and adverse drug reactions, must be documented and reported to the patient's physician who must respond to any recommendations in a timely manner. The American Society of Consultant Pharmacists publishes detailed information concerning standards of practice in the LTCF environment.[111]

CASE 107-8

QUESTION 1: As a new consultant pharmacist to a 60-bed, skilled nursing facility, several multiple-drug-use problems become apparent during initial chart reviews. A typical case is D.M., an 82-year-old man who has resided there for the past month. D.M.'s past medical history is significant for hypertension, depression, constipation, long-standing mild cognitive impairment that is now worsening, and dizziness. In the nurses' notes, it is documented that D.M. had a fall when getting out of bed last week.

At admission, D.M.'s weight was 165 pounds; BP 100/60 mm Hg; pulse 85 beats/minute; and temperature 98.6°F. Subsequent vital signs are not recorded systematically into his medical record. Sporadic documentation in the nurses' notes indicates little change from admission values. No laboratory information is available at this time. D.M. has no known allergies.

Current medications include amlodipine 10 mg daily, diltiazem CD 240 mg daily, hydrochlorothiazide 25 mg daily, quetiapine 300 mg daily, lorazepam 0.5 mg every 8 hours as needed for anxiety, docusate sodium 100 mg twice daily, milk of magnesia 30 mL daily, temazepam 15 mg at bedtime, and acetaminophen one to two 325-mg tablets every 4 to 6 hours as needed for pain. D.M. follows a 2-g sodium diet.

D.M. is ambulatory and takes his meals in the facility's dining room. He is not in any acute distress, but the nurses' notes indicate that D.M. is often confused and complains of dizziness when ambulating. His weight has decreased 4 pounds since being admitted. What should be expected of this LTCF with respect to medication monitoring?

Under the CMS-mandated regulations, the establishment of goals of antihypertensive therapy and monitoring for these goals are required. D.M.'s blood pressure should be measured and documented in his medical record with a signature and date on a regular basis. D.M.'s dizziness, a symptom of orthostatic hypotension, may be caused by overtreatment of his hypertension as evidenced by his low admission blood pressure. Orthostatic hypotension occurs in 10% to 30% of older adults and is most common when patients first arise, indicating that this may have been the cause of D.M.'s recent fall.[25] D.M. is being treated with two calcium-channel blockers. Discontinuation of one of them should reduce his dizziness and help prevent future falls. Because D.M. is being treated with a diuretic, monitoring should include a chemistry panel for electrolyte abnormalities.

CASE 107-8, QUESTION 2: What changes should be made to D.M.'s medication regimen?

In the admission workup, D.M. was described as having a long-standing history of mild cognitive impairment, but subsequent nursing notes suggest that his symptoms of disorientation and confusion worsened quickly after admission. Chronic dementia is not normally characterized by rapid deterioration of mental acuity (see Chapter 108, Geriatric Neurocognitive Disorders). This should raise the suspicion that a reversible factor could be responsible for D.M.'s mental decline. Potentially inappropriate drug use in older adults living in the community and in long-term care is well documented.[112–114] The cognitive impairment of chronic degenerative dementia can be greatly exaggerated by D.M.'s treatment with lorazepam, temazepam, and quetiapine, especially with higher than recommended dosages.[115] Benzodiazepines may also increase the risk of falls and bone fractures in the geriatric population.[116] Antipsychotics are some of the most commonly prescribed drugs in nursing home residents. It is only appropriate to use these agents if the patient's behavior is considered to be a danger to themselves or others (including staff), impairing the patient's daily functioning, interfering with the staff's ability to care for them, or causing distress to the patient (i.e., frightening hallucinations).[110] Antipsychotics may be unnecessarily prescribed for anxiety, insomnia, confusion, or failure to conform to the institution's standards for behavior. Antipsychotic use in older adults with dementia has been shown to be associated with a 1.7-fold increased risk of all-cause mortality compared with nonusers.[117] Primary reasons for death were heart failure, sudden cardiac death, or pneumonia. Federal regulations require that these drugs be used for a specified condition, at the lowest possible dosage, and for the shortest possible duration. Regulations also mandate tapering of doses and careful documentation of all clinical assessments that justify the ongoing need for antipsychotics.[109]

In light of the atypical deterioration of D.M.'s cognitive function, the doses of all psychotropic medications should be gradually tapered down to the lowest effective dose and/or discontinued if appropriate. It may not be appropriate to make multiple changes all at once; however, a plan should be developed to target the medications that are likely responsible for D.M.'s decline in mental status. A baseline assessment of D.M.'s cognitive function and psychiatric status should be performed by a geriatrician, psychiatrist, or clinical psychologist to establish the presence or absence of psychotic behavioral disturbances or depression. If any of these disorders are present, then each should be managed with appropriate nonpharmacologic interventions and drug therapy that includes appropriate therapeutic doses and duration of treatment.

The American Geriatrics Society (AGS) updated the Beers Criteria for Potentially Inappropriate Medication Use in Older Adults in 2015.[118] This evidence-based review outlines medications that may lead to adverse events in older adults. Other helpful tools available include the Screening Tool of Older Persons' potentially inappropriate Prescriptions (STOPP) and Screening Tool to Alert Doctors to Right Treatment (START) criteria.[118] The combined use of these tools along with clinical judgment is meant to guide clinicians in drug selection, to help decrease exposure to medications that may increase the risk of adverse drug events, and to support the safe medication therapy of older adults.

KEY REFERENCES AND WEBSITES

A full list of references for this chapter can be found at http://thepoint.lww.com/AT11e. Below are the key references and websites for this chapter, with the corresponding reference number in this chapter found in parentheses after the reference.

Key References

American Geriatrics Society Expert Panel on Care of Older Adults with Diabetes Mellitus, Moreno G et al. Guidelines abstracted from the American Geriatrics Society Guidelines for Improving the Care of Older Adults with Diabetes Mellitus: 2013 update. *J Am Geriatr Soc.* 2013;61(11):2020–2026. (75)

A Profile of Older Americans: 2016. Administration on Aging (AoA), Administration for Community Living, U.S. Department of Health and Human Services; 2016. https://www.acl.gov/aging-and-disability-in-america/data-and-research/profile-older-americans.

Federal Interagency Forum on Aging-Related Statistics. Federal Interagency Forum on Aging-Related Statistics. Older Americans 2012: Key Indicators of Well-Being. Washington, DC: US Government Printing Office; 2012. (1)

Garasto S et al. Estimating glomerular filtration rate in older people. *Biomed Res Int.* 2014;2014:916542. (21)

Guiding principles for the care of older adults with multimorbidity: an approach for clinicians. Guiding principles for the care of older adults with multimorbidity: an approach for clinicians: American Geriatrics Society Expert Panel on the Care of Older Adults with Multimorbidity. *J Am Geriatr Soc.* 2012;60(10):E1–E25. doi:10.1111/j.1532-5415.2012.04188.x. (38)

James PA et al. 2014 evidence-based guideline for the management of high blood pressure in adults: report from the panel members appointed to the Eighth Joint National Committee (JNC 8). *JAMA.* 2014;311(5):507–520. (66)

Jetha S. Polypharmacy, the Elderly, and Deprescribing. *Consult Pharm.* 2015;30(9):527–532. (114)Maher RL et al. Clinical consequences of polypharmacy in elderly. *Expert Opin Drug Saf.* 2014;13(1):57–65. (37)

Mandell LA et al. Infectious Diseases Society of America/American Thoracic Society consensus guidelines on the management of community-acquired pneumonia in adults. *Clin Infect Dis.* 2007;44(Suppl 2):S27–S72. (93)

National Asthma Education and Prevention Program. Expert Panel Report 3: Guidelines for the Diagnosis and Management of Asthma, 2007. NIH Publication No 07-4051. (89)

Ricci F et al. Orthostatic hypotension: epidemiology, prognosis, and treatment. *J Am Coll Cardiol.* 2015;66(7):848–860. (27)

Stone NJ et al. 2013 ACC/AHA guideline on the treatment of blood cholesterol to reduce atherosclerotic cardiovascular risk in adults: a report of the American College of Cardiology/American Heart Association Task Force on Practice Guidelines. *J Am Coll Cardiol.* 2014;63(25, pt B):2889–2934. (55)

Standards of Medical Care in Diabetes—2015: summary of revisions. *Diabetes Care.* 2015;38(Suppl):S4–S4. (66)

Yancy CW et al. 2013 ACCF/AHA guideline for the management of heart failure: a report of the American College of Cardiology Foundation/American Heart Association Task Force on Practice Guidelines. *J Am Coll Cardiol.* 2013;62(16):e147e239. (48)

Key Websites

American Geriatrics Society. http://americangeriatrics.org.
American Society of Consultant Pharmacists. http://www.ascp.com.
American Heart Association. http://www.americanheart.org.
Centers for Disease Control and Prevention. http://www.cdc.gov.

108 Geriatric Neurocognitive Disorders

Nicole J. Brandt and Bradley R. Williams

CORE PRINCIPLES

		CHAPTER CASES
NEUROCOGNITIVE DISORDERS (NCD)		
1	NCD is a syndrome that exhibits multiple cognitive deficits that compromise normal social or occupational function. There are numerous etiologies such as Alzheimer's disease (AD), dementia with Lewy bodies (DLB), and vascular disease, which require a comprehensive evaluation to define a potential diagnosis.	**Case 108-1 (Question 1)**
NCD DUE TO ALZHEIMER'S DISEASE		
1	AD is a chronic, progressive, neurodegenerative disorder that results from neuropathological findings, such as neurofibrillary tangles and β-amyloid plaques that interfere with cholinergic transmission, as well as other neurochemical changes in the brain.	**Case 108-1 (Questions 1–3)**
2	AD has multiple risk factors such as age, family history, Down syndrome, head trauma, hypertension, and mild cognitive impairment, yet the exact etiology is still unknown.	**Case 108-1 (Question 2)**
3	Treatment for AD currently is symptomatic management, not disease altering, and focuses on neurotransmission (e.g., cholinergic system).	**Case 108-1 (Question 4)**
4	Cholinesterase inhibitors may be used as monotherapy or in combination with an *N*-methyl-D-aspartate antagonist for patients in the moderate to severe stage of AD.	**Case 108-1 (Questions 4–6)**
5	Monitoring for treatment efficacy should focus on cognition, function, and possibly behaviors, whereas treatment toxicity should look for common adverse effects such as gastrointestinal complaints with cholinesterase inhibitors.	**Case 108-1 (Question 5)**
NCD DUE TO LEWY BODY DISEASE		
1	Has similar neuropathology noted with α-synuclein aggregates found in Lewy bodies and neuritis (α-synucleinopathies), which typically present with parkinsonian findings as well as associated symptoms such as falls and visual hallucinations.	**Case 108-2 (Question 1)**
2	Cholinesterase inhibitors have demonstrated symptomatic benefit in patients with Lewy body dementias, yet monitoring for worsening of motor symptoms such as tremor is needed.	**Case 108-2 (Question 2)**
VASCULAR NCD		
1	Vascular dementia is a broad classification of cognitive disorders caused by vascular disease, and notable multiple risk factors include advancing age, diabetes mellitus, small vessel cerebrovascular disease, hypertension, heart disease, hyperlipidemia, cigarette smoking, and alcohol use.	**Case 108-3 (Questions 1, 2)**
2	Treatment for vascular dementia strives to control the underlying modifiable risk factors owing to limited efficacy and controversial evidence with cholinesterase inhibitors.	**Case 108-3 (Question 3)**

Continued

BEHAVIORAL DISTURBANCES IN DEMENTIA	
1 When evaluating a dementia patient with behavior disturbances, the first step is to ensure that the problem is not caused by an unrecognized medical problem or adverse effect of a medication.	**Case 108-4 (Question 1), Case 108-5 (Question 1)**
2 Nonpharmacologic strategies are effective for managing many behavior disturbances and should be attempted before using medications to manage behavior.	**Case 108-4 (Questions 1–4)**
3 Delusions and hallucinations are common behaviors in dementia patients, yet the use of antipsychotics for these symptoms is not approved by the US Food and Drug Administration and has been associated with the increased risk of stroke and mortality in this patient population.	**Case 108-4 (Question 2)**
4 Wandering is a safety concern that often does not respond to pharmacologic intervention; instead, other strategies such as environmental modifications are used.	**Case 108-4 (Question 3)**
5 Antidepressants such as selective serotonin reuptake inhibitors have shown promise in addressing depressive symptoms, as well as screaming and irritability.	**Case 108-4 (Question 4)**
6 Caregiver support is essential to maintaining a dementia patient safely in his or her home as long as possible.	**Case 108-1 (Questions 3, 5), Case 108-4 (Question 5)**

Neurocognitive disorders span a wide range of conditions that exhibit a global decline in cognition. Among the disorders included are delirium, dementia, and several other disorders with various etiologies (e.g., head trauma, HIV, Huntington disease).[1] Among older adults, the dementias are the most commonly encountered diseases and are the focus of this chapter.

GERIATRIC DEMENTIAS

With the continuing growth in the elderly population, the incidence and prevalence of neurocognitive disorders continues to rise.[1,2] Alzheimer's disease (AD) is the most common cause, and accounts for more than half of all diagnosed cases.[4–6] Vascular dementia (VaD), dementia with Lewy bodies (DLB), and Parkinson's disease with dementia (PDD) are the next most common dementias, with frontotemporal dementia, pseudodementia, and other forms occurring less often.[5,7] AD is currently the fifth leading cause of death for people age 65 years and older and the sixth leading cause of death for all people in the United States.[3,8]

Incidence and Prevalence

It is estimated that 5.3 million Americans have AD, including approximately 11% of people age 65 years and older and 32% of people age 85 years and older. Of these, more than 3.2 million are women. Prevalence is greater among both African Americans and Hispanics compared with whites.[3] The annual incidence of AD in the United States rises from 53 per 1,000 among people age 65 to 74 years to 170 per 1,000 for those age 75 to 84 years, and to 231 per 1,000 for those at least 85 years of age.[9] Worldwide prevalence has been estimated to be as high as 24.3 million, with 8.4 million new cases annually.[2,10] Projections into the mid-century include a worldwide prevalence of more than 81 million, with cases in undeveloped countries occurring at about three times the rate as in developed countries.[10] In the United States, AD accounts for nearly 70% of cases; VaD accounts for 17.4%, with the remaining 12.6% attributable to DLB, frontotemporal dementia, and other forms.[6] Life expectancy after a diagnosis of AD is reduced by as much as 69% for those diagnosed before age 70 years and by 39% for those diagnosed after age 90 years.[11]

The cost of dementia is staggering. Annual costs for Medicare recipients with dementia average $21,585, compared with $8,191 for those without dementia. For Medicaid recipients with dementia, the annual costs are $11,021, compared with $574 for those without dementia. The annual direct costs, in 2014 dollars, of treating a dementia patient are $47,752 annually, compared with $15,115 for an older adult without dementia. This translates to an estimated annual direct cost for dementia care of $226 billion for the year 2015.[3]

Clinical Diagnosis

Dementia is a neurocognitive disorder that exhibits impaired short- and long-term memory as its most prominent feature. Multiple cognitive deficits that compromise normal social or occupational function must be present before dementia can be diagnosed (Table 108-1).[1] Commonly, forgetfulness is the primary complaint of patients or the first symptom noted by the family.[12] Family members or others may note several symptoms that should prompt a medical evaluation (Table 108-2).[12,13] Memory loss often accompanies several diseases or disorders in elderly individuals. Therefore, a medical history, physical examination, and medication history are essential in excluding systemic illness or medication toxicity as causes of the memory loss (Table 108-3).[13–16] Laboratory and other tests to assist in differentiating dementia from other disorders are listed (Table 108-4). In patients with AD, test results will generally be normal; evidence of cerebrovascular disease is present in patients with VaD.

Brain imaging, such as a computed tomography (CT) scan or magnetic resonance imaging (MRI), can be useful in establishing the presence of a dementia, but neither is diagnostic. A CT scan is useful when a space-occupying lesion, such as a tumor, is suspected as a possible cause. An MRI scan is capable of identifying small infarcts, such as those found in some forms of VaD, and atrophy of subcortical structures such as the brainstem.[15]

Several simple tests, including the Mini-Cognitive Assessment Instrument (Mini-Cog), the Montreal Cognitive Assessment (MoCA), and the St. Louis University Mental Status (SLUMS) exam are appropriate for initial screening of people with suspected cognitive impairment.[17–19] The Folstein Mini-Mental State Exam (MMSE) also can be used; however, it is less sensitive than others for dementia and now is proprietary.[20] These tests rapidly assess multiple domains, typically including orientation, registration, attention and calculation, recall, and language. Patients with dementia exhibit deficits in multiple areas. Those who score below the normal range on the MMSE or other screens, or who exhibit symptoms characteristic of dementia receive further testing. A somewhat more detailed screen, the Cognitive Abilities Screening Instrument (CASI), provides quantitative assessment on attention, concentration, orientation, short-term memory, long-term memory, language abilities, visual construction, list-generating fluency, abstraction, and judgment.[21] All screening tests are subject to limitations. Therefore, additional psychometric testing is often ordered to further establish the presence and type of dementia.[2,22]

Dementias may be classified as cortical or subcortical, according to the areas of the brain preferentially affected by the disorder. AD, a typical cortical dementia, disrupts the cerebral cortex. Patients with

Table 108-1
Differentiating Neurocognitive Disorders

Mild (formerly Mild Cognitive Impairment)	Major (formerly Dementia)
Neurocognitive Disorder (NCD)	
Modest cognitive decline from previous (baseline) performance in at least one cognitive domain, including: ■ Learning and memory ■ Complex attention ■ Executive function ■ Language ■ Perception and motor ■ Social cognition The deficits do not impair the capacity to be independent in everyday activities The cognitive symptoms do not occur exclusively during a period of delirium The cognitive deficits are not better explained by depression, schizophrenia or other mental disorders	Significant cognitive decline from previous (baseline) performance in at least one cognitive domain, including: ■ Learning and memory ■ Complex attention ■ Executive function ■ Language ■ Perception and motor ■ Social cognition The deficits impair the capacity to be independent in everyday activities The cognitive symptoms do not occur exclusively during a period of delirium The cognitive deficits are not better explained by depression, schizophrenia or other mental disorders
NCD due to Alzheimer's Disease	

Criteria for either mild or major NCD are met
Insidious onset and gradual progression of impairment
■ Mild: impairment in one cognitive domain
■ Major: impairment in at least two cognitive domains
Probable Alzheimer's disease (either of the following must be present)
■ Alzheimer's disease genetic mutation based on family history or genetic testing
■ All of the following are present:
  ■ Decline in memory and learning plus one other cognitive domain
  ■ Steady and gradual cognitive decline
  ■ No evidence of another condition that is likely to cause cognitive decline
Possible Alzheimer's disease
■ Lack of an Alzheimer's disease genetic mutation
■ All of the following are present:
  ■ Decline in memory and learning
  ■ Steady and gradual cognitive decline
  ■ No evidence of another condition that is likely to cause cognitive decline
Cognitive decline is not better explained by cerebrovascular disease or another condition associated with cognitive decline or neurodegeneration	

Vascular NCD	
Criteria for either mild or major NCD are met Clinical presentation is consistent with a vascular cause (either of the following is present) ■ Onset of cognitive impairment follows a cerebrovascular event or multiple events ■ Prominent decline in complex attention and executive function History, physical exam and/or neuroimaging indicates cerebrovascular disease as the most likely cause of the cognitive decline Probable vascular NCD (at least one of the following is present) ■ Neuroimaging supports cerebrovascular disease as the cause of the clinical presentation ■ The neurocognitive deficit follows at least one cerebrovascular event ■ Presence of both clinical and genetic evidence of cerebrovascular disease Possible vascular NCD ■ Clinical criteria are met ■ Neuroimaging is not available ■ Temporal relationship between the cerebrovascular event(s) and the onset of neurocognitive decline is not established A systemic disorder or other brain disease do not adequately explain the symptoms	

(continued)

Table 108-1
Differentiating Neurocognitive Disorders (*continued*)

NCD with Lewy Bodies

Criteria for either mild or major NCD are met
The onset is insidious, with gradual progression
A combination of the following core and suggestive diagnostic features are present
■ Core features
  ■ Fluctuating cognition accompanied by variable attentiveness and alertness
  ■ Recurrent, well-formed and detailed visual hallucinations
  ■ Onset of Parkinsonian features that are exhibited after the onset of cognitive decline
■ Suggestive features
  ■ Criteria for rapid eye movement (REM) sleep behavior disorder are met
  ■ Severe sensitivity to neuroleptic agents
Probable NCD with Lewy Bodies (either of the following is present)
■ At least two core features
■ One or more core features and one suggestive feature
Possible NCD with Lewy Bodies (either of the following is present)
■ One core feature
■ One or more suggestive features
Cognitive decline is not better explained by cerebrovascular disease or another condition associated with cognitive decline or neurodegeneration

Adapted from references[1,36,75,77,81,83] and Jack CR Jr, Albert MS, Knopman DS, et al. Introduction to the recommendations from the National Institute on Aging–Alzheimer's Association workgroups on diagnostic guidelines for Alzheimer's disease. *Alzheimers Dement* 7(3):257–262, 2011 10.1016/j.jalz.2011.03.004; Albert MS, DeKosky ST, Dickson D, et al: The diagnosis of mild cognitive impairment due to Alzheimer's disease: recommendations from the National Institute on Aging–Alzheimer's Association workgroups on diagnostic guidelines for Alzheimer's disease. *Alzheimers Dement* 7(3):270–279, 2011 10.1016/j.jalz.2011.03.008; Román GC, Tatemichi TK, Erkinjuntti T, et al: Vascular dementia: diagnostic criteria for research studies. Report of the NINDS-AIREN International Workshop. *Neurology* 43(2):250–260, 1993

Table 108-2
Symptoms Suggesting Dementia

Symptom	Evidence
Difficulty learning or retaining new information	Repeats questions; difficulty remembering recent conversations, events, etc.; loses items
Unable to handle complex tasks	Cannot complete tasks that require multiple steps (e.g., difficulty following a shopping list)
Impaired reasoning	Difficulty solving everyday problems; inappropriate social behavior
Impaired spatial orientation and abilities	Gets lost in familiar places; difficulty with driving
Language deficits	Problems finding appropriate words (e.g., difficulty with naming common objects)
Behavior changes	Changes in personality; suspiciousness

Adapted from Costa P et al. Recognition and initial assessment of Alzheimer's disease and related dementias. Clinical Practice Guideline No. 19. Rockville, MD: U.S. Department of Health and Human Services, Public Health Service, Agency for Health Care Policy and Research. AHCPR Publication No. 97-0702. November 1996.

Table 108-3
Causes of Dementia Symptoms

Central Nervous System Disorders	Systemic Illness	Medications
Adjustment disorder (e.g., inability to adjust to retirement)	Cardiovascular disease Arrhythmia Heart failure	Anticholinergic agents Anticonvulsants Antidepressants Antihistamines
Amnestic syndrome (e.g., isolated memory impairment) Delirium	Vascular occlusion Deficiency states Vitamin B_{12} Folate Iron	Anti-infectives Antineoplastic agents Antipsychotic agents Cardiovascular agents Antiarrhythmics

(*continued*)

Table 108-3
Causes of Dementia Symptoms (*continued*)

Central Nervous System Disorders	Systemic Illness	Medications
Depression	Infections	Antihypertensives
Intracranial causes	Metabolic disorders	Corticosteroids
Brain abscess	Adrenal	H_2-receptor antagonists
Normal pressure	Glucose	Immunosuppressants
Hydrocephalus	Renal failure	Narcotic analgesics
Stroke	Thyroid	Nonsteroidal anti-inflammatory agents
Subdural hematoma		Sedative hypnotics and anxiolytics
Tumor		Skeletal muscle relaxants

Table 108-4
Dementia Screening Tests

Test	Rationale for Testing
Complete blood count with sedimentation rate	Anemic anoxia, infection, neoplasms
Metabolic screen	
Serum electrolytes	Hypernatremia, hyponatremia; renal function
Blood urea nitrogen, creatinine	Renal function
Bilirubin	Hepatic dysfunction (e.g., portal systemic encephalopathy, hepatocerebral degeneration)
Thyroid function	Hypothyroidism, hyperthyroidism
Iron, vitamin B_{12}, folate, vitamin D	Deficiency states (vitamin B_{12}, folate neuropathies, vitamin D deficiency), anemias
Stool occult blood	Blood loss, anemia
HIV and RPR	Infection
Urinalysis	Infection, proteinuria
Chest roentgenogram	Neoplasms, infection, airway disease (anoxia)
Electrocardiogram	Cardiac disease (stagnant anoxia)
Brain scan	Cerebral tumors, cerebrovascular disease
Mental status testing	General cognitive screen
Depression testing	Depression, pseudodementia

cortical dementias display impaired language rather than impaired speech, a learning deficit (amnesia), reduced higher cortical functions (e.g., inability to perform calculations, poor judgment), and an unconcerned or disinhibited affect. Subcortical dementias such as PDD primarily affect the basal ganglia, thalamus, and brainstem. Deficits include abnormal motor function, disrupted speech patterns rather than language difficulties, forgetfulness (impaired recall), slowed cognitive function, and an apathetic or depressed affect.[16]

ALZHEIMER'S DISEASE

Etiology

A definitive cause for AD has yet to be determined. Several risk factors, however, have been identified. Advancing age is the primary risk factor for AD; other risks include family history, head trauma, metabolic syndrome, diabetes, hypertension and cardiovascular disease.[3,23-27] Genetics plays a significant role in the development of Alzheimer's disease. The high familial occurrence of AD has been linked to autosomal-dominant traits on chromosomes 21, 14, and 1.[28,29] A gene that encodes for amyloid precursor protein (APP), a normal protein, is located on chromosome 21. A defect on chromosome 14 has been identified as the locus for the presenilin-1 gene, which codes for an inherited form of AD. The presenilin-2 gene, located on chromosome 1, also codes for an inherited form. Despite a strong genetic link in some pedigrees, the great majority of AD cases are sporadic.[29,30] The more common sporadic form appears to be linked to a susceptibility gene, apolipoprotein E, which occurs in three isoforms.[29] APP, a normal protein found throughout the body, maps on chromosome 21 and plays a pivotal role in AD neuropathology. Because of overproduction or transcription errors, an abnormal subunit (i.e., β-amyloid) is produced.[29] Mutations on chromosomes 14 (presenilin-1 gene) and 1 (presenilin-2 gene) and the presence of apolipoprotein E4 allele code for alterations in the processing of APP. The abnormal cleavage of APP produces a 42–amino acid form of β-amyloid (Aβ) that demonstrates a higher toxicity than other amyloid forms.[29]

Apolipoprotein E (ApoE), a protein that is involved in cholesterol and phospholipid metabolism, plays a role in the development of sporadic, late-onset AD. The ApoE gene possesses three alleles: E2, E3, and E4. The E3 allele is most common, the E2 allele appears to be protective against AD, and the E4 allele increases the risk for AD.[29] The presence of ApoE-4, the protein coded for by the E4 allele, appears to increase the deposition of Aβ and promote its change to a more pathological configuration.[29] The presence of one or two copies of ApoE4 increases the risk of developing AD twofold or fivefold, respectively.[30] Aβ, which differs from amyloid protein found in other regions of the body, appears to contribute to neuronal death through a combination of apoptosis, a direct toxic effect, and an increased risk for damage owing to oxidative and metabolic stresses.[29,31]

Neuropathology

Although brain atrophy is the most obvious finding among patients with Alzheimer-type dementia, it is not diagnostic for AD or other dementias because some degree of atrophy accompanies normal aging. Atrophic changes induced by AD are found primarily in the temporal, parietal, and frontal areas of the brain; the occipital region, primary motor cortex, and somatosensory areas are generally unaffected (Fig. 108-1).[5,31]

Neuronal changes in the cerebral cortex associated with AD include neurofibrillary tangles, neuritic plaques, amyloid angiopathy, and granulovacuolar degeneration. These changes lead to loss of neurons and synapses (Fig. 108-2).[28] Neurofibrillary tangles (NFTs) are found primarily in the pyramidal regions of the neocortex, hippocampus, and amygdala, but they are also noted in areas of the

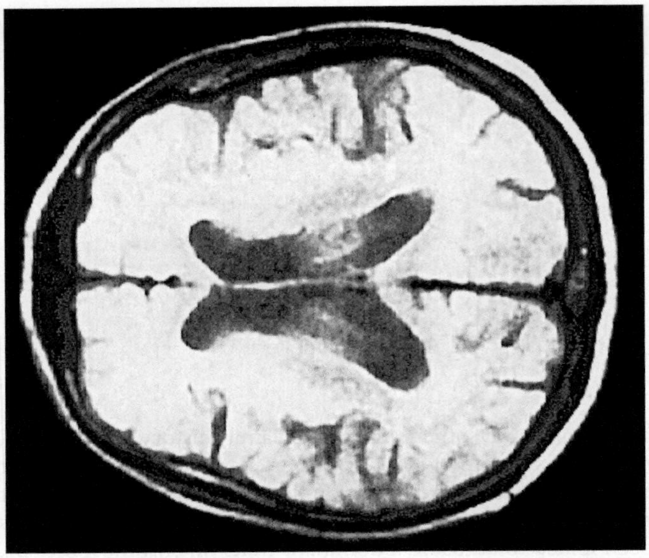

Figure 108-1 Alzheimer disease: magnetic resonance imaging scan. Ventricles are enlarged, and there is generalized atrophy, with greater atrophy present near the temporal areas.

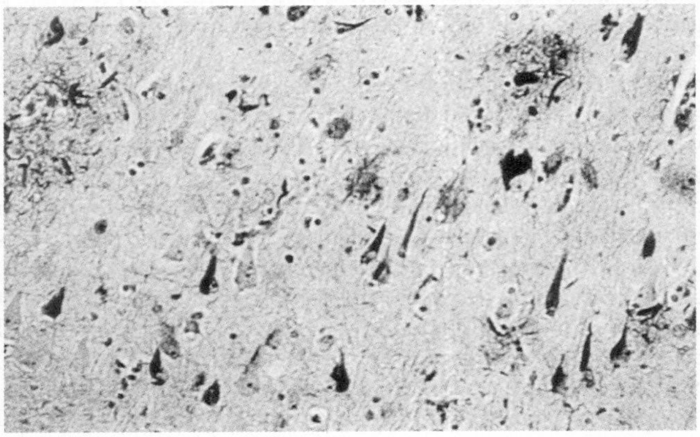

Figure 108-2 Numerous plaques (large, round bodies) and tangles (tear-shaped bodies) are found throughout the cortex in Alzheimer-type dementia.

brainstem and locus coeruleus.[5,31] NFTs are composed of paired helical filaments, combinations of fibrils with a characteristic width and contour, containing a tau protein with an abnormal pattern of phosphate deposition. They are highly immunoreactive and are most likely to form in large pyramidal neurons.

Neuritic plaques are spherical bodies of tissue composed of granular deposits and remnants of neuronal processes.[5] The typical neuritic plaques of AD are spherical structures that exhibit a three-tiered structure: a central amyloid core, a middle region of swollen axons and dendrites, and an outer zone containing degenerating neuritic processes.[28] Plaques contain APP, which can be cleaved by a defective metabolic process to form Aβ.[29] In addition to Aβ, plaques also contain protein, ApoE, and acute-phase inflammatory proteins such as α_1-chymotrypsin and α_2-macroglobulin.[28] The deposition of amyloid in neuritic plaques correlates with the severity of AD, and the density of cortical plaques is associated with decreased choline acetyltransferase and the severity of cognitive impairment.[5] Aβ has been identified in plaques associated with Down syndrome and in both familial and sporadic forms of dementia of the Alzheimer type.[29] The pathological process of AD development may begin as early as 20 to 30 years before any disease symptoms appear.[5,29,32]

Granulovacuolar degeneration is the other major histologic finding in AD. It consists of clusters of intracytoplasmic vacuoles that contain tiny granules. The vacuoles appear to be specifically located in the pyramidal neurons of the hippocampus.[5,16,28] The loss of cortical neurons that originate in the nucleus basalis and project into the cerebral cortex is the most significant histopathological consequence of AD.[31] Cell loss, granulovacuolar degeneration, and neurons with NFTs are concentrated in this area.[16,28]

Accompanying these changes are decreased concentrations of several neurotransmitters and enzymes. Choline acetyltransferase levels are reduced 60% to 90% in the cortical and hippocampal regions.[28] Acetylcholine and acetylcholinesterase (AChE) are also decreased, whereas muscarinic receptors in the cortex and hippocampus remain at normal levels or are moderately decreased. Nicotinic receptor proteins are also reduced in patients with Alzheimer-type dementia when compared with age-matched controls. Decreased choline acetyltransferase activity has been correlated with plaque density and disease severity. Cortical synapse loss, especially in the midfrontal region, is associated with disease severity.[5,29-31]

Changes affecting AChE have significant implications for the management of AD symptoms. Many isoforms of AChE have been identified; they possess identical amino acid sequences, but display different posttranslational modifications, predominate at diverse anatomical and microanatomical locations, and function in different ways. The predominant form of AChE in the cortical and hippocampal regions of humans is G4, a tetrameric form that is membrane bound. The monomeric form, G1, is found in a much lower concentration. There is a selective loss of the G4 form in patients with AD, allowing the G1 form to assume greater importance.[33] Although cholinergic activity is most significantly affected by Alzheimer-type dementia, other neurochemical systems are also altered. Norepinephrine, serotonin, and γ-aminobutyric acid receptors are affected.[28,29]

Clinical Presentation and Diagnosis

CASE 108-1

QUESTION 1: T.D. is a 72 year old man who is accompanied by his wife for a memory assessment. During the interview, the patient notes that memory issues started about 6 to 12 months ago but recently worsened after he was hospitalized for a fall. The wife notes that he retired at age 70 because he was slowing down and admits that he may have been having some memory issues back then due to his inability to manage the finances even though he was an accountant. Since the fall, which occurred when he was doing work on the house and fell off the ladder and broke his leg, the wife admits he is not quite the same.

T.D.'s medical history is significant for osteoarthritis benign prostatic hyperplasia (BPH) and hypertension. He is currently taking tamsulosin 0.4 mg in the evening for BPH and amlodipine 10 mg daily for HTN. His family history is negative for stroke and positive for heart disease and his father died of a myocardial infarction at age 84. The wife admits that his mother had AD and was diagnosed in her early 70s as well. She died at the age of 76 due to complications with her AD in a nursing home and her husband witnessed her dramatic decline from the AD, which worries him.

Physical examination reveals a pleasant, well-groomed man who is in good health oriented to person and place but not time. His blood pressure (BP) is 120/66 mm Hg supine and 132/72 mm Hg standing, with pulse rates of 56 beats/minute and 62 beats/minute, respectively.

The Folstein MMSE score was 22/30, with errors in orientation, attention, calculation (inability to spell "world" backward), recall, and language (difficulty with word finding). The rest of the physical examination was within normal limits.

What additional evaluation steps should be considered for T.D.?

Before any conclusions can be reached, potentially reversible causes for T.D.'s impaired cognition must be evaluated. Although he displays several trigger symptoms associated with dementia (Table 108-2), including difficulty with managing finances (change especially noted in light that he was an accountant) and word finding issues coupled with memory impairment impacting day to day function.

Several systemic diseases and other disorders can cause cognitive impairment, as shown in Table 108-3. T.D. should undergo a battery of laboratory tests to rule out anemia, cardiac and renal disease, thyroid abnormalities, and tumors. In addition, he should receive thorough neuropsychological testing, including depression screening and more in-depth assessment of his cognitive function. The testing should be conducted by clinicians who are skilled in cognitive assessment, as educational and cultural factors can influence an individual's performance on these tests.[34]

CASE 108-1, QUESTION 2: T.D. is referred by his physician for additional testing. Laboratory tests performed include renal and liver chemistries, thyroid function tests, vitamin B_{12} and folate levels, syphilis and HIV tests, complete blood cell count with sedimentation rate, and urinalysis. All results were normal with the exception of a low B12 level (147 ng/L). Chest radiograph and electrocardiogram were normal. Neurologic examination revealed no deficits. Depression testing revealed a mildly anxious individual who was not depressed just worried about his future.

What is the most probable diagnosis for T.D.?

T.D.'s score of 22/30 on the Folstein MMSE is consistent with mild cognitive impairment or early dementia as evidenced by errors in orientation, calculation, recall, and language.[20] Secondary medical causes of cognitive impairment can be eliminated by T.D.'s generally normal physical examination and laboratory test results. MRI or CT scanning may be useful in many cases to help eliminate brain pathology, such as stroke.[34] A positron emission tomography (PET) scan or a single photon emission computed tomography (SPECT) scan may be useful to help locate specific areas of pathology and assist with a differential diagnosis, but are not required.[35] Secondary psychiatric causes for T.D.'s decline can also be discounted. Although he is sad and anxious, the absence of alterations in appetite or sleep patterns, absence of suicidal thoughts, and the results of psychologic testing indicate T.D. is not depressed. He is fully conscious, alert, and oriented to place and person. He exhibits no psychotic behavior and no evidence of delirium.

T.D.'s slowly progressive decline and its impact on his social and occupational function (forgetting appointments, failing to pay bills), normal physical examination and laboratory findings, and family history meet the *Diagnostic and Statistical Manual of Mental Disorders,* Fifth Edition (DSM-V) criteria for dementia (Table 108-1). His history and course to date satisfy the criteria for AD and do not indicate a likely alternative explanation for his condition. Thus, T.D. can be classified as probable AD.[36]

CASE 108-1, QUESTION 3: T.D. 's children are very concerned about the family history for dementia. They ask whether there are any tests they should receive at this time to determine their risk. What should they be told?

Although there is a strong genetic association with AD, such instances account for a small minority of cases.[29] There is no apparent family history of Down syndrome. Mutations in the presenilin-1 and presenilin-2 genes are associated with only a small fraction of AD cases.[29] Although several potential biomarkers have been identified, they have not been sufficiently validated to be considered reliable predictors for the development of AD.[3,36,35]

Prognosis

CASE 108-1, QUESTION 4: What is the likely prognosis for T.D.?

AD follows a predictable course that may progress over the course of 10 years or more.[2,10] Two common rating scales for dementia are the Global Deterioration Scale and the Clinical Dementia Rating Scale. According to the Global Deterioration Scale (Table 108-5), T.D.'s impaired social functioning, anxiety, and objective cognitive decline as well as his continued ability to concentrate and perform some complex skills, combined with his preserved affect and social interaction, are consistent with the features of stage three dementia of the Alzheimer type. This stage of AD is generally associated with a period of mild cognitive decline.[38] The more general Clinical Dementia Rating Scale also places T.D. in the category of mild dementia.[39] Clinical diagnoses of AD using clinically appropriate criteria and assessment methods for probable AD have a sensitivity of up to 90% when compared with autopsy-confirmed cases.[1,34,37]

Because of technologic advances, it is possible to diagnose dementia earlier and to keep patients alive into the final stages of the disease.[40] The early diagnosis of AD in T.D. will allow his condition to be followed closely. To ensure the most favorable outcome, T.D. should receive a thorough assessment beyond his dementia. This should include evaluation of his daily function (i.e., ability for self-care), comorbid medical conditions, medications, living arrangements, safety, and potential for abuse and neglect. Attention also should be given to T.D.'s caregivers and support system.[41,42] He should be reassessed every 6 months to both document disease progression and ensure that he is receiving the most appropriate care. At some point, care at home may become unrealistic. At that time, T.D. should be moved into a sheltered environment (e.g., residential-care facility or nursing home) before suffering an injury caused by his poor judgment (e.g., failing to dress properly for the weather, falling). In the later stages, interventions ranging from tube feedings to life support may prolong life, yet prove to be controversial.[43] Death in the late stage of AD is commonly associated with the development of infections such as pneumonia, urinary tract infections, or decubitus ulcers.

Table 108-5
Stages of Dementia of the Alzheimer Type

Stage of Cognitive Decline	Features
No cognitive decline	Normal cognitive state
Very mild cognitive decline	Forgetfulness, subjective complaints only; no objective decline
Mild cognitive decline	Objective decline through psychiatric testing; work and social impairment; mild anxiety and denial
Moderate cognitive decline	Concentration, complex skills decline; flat affect and withdrawal
Moderately severe cognitive decline	Early dementia; difficulty in interactions; unable to recall or recognize people or places
Severe cognitive decline	Requires assistance with bathing, toileting; behavioral symptoms present (agitation, delusions, aggressive behavior)
Very severe cognitive decline	Loss of psychomotor skills and verbal abilities; incontinence; total dependence

Adapted from Reisberg B et al. The global deterioration scale for assessment of primary degenerative dementia. *Am J Psychiatry*. 1982;139:1136.

Maintaining independence as long as possible is an important goal in treating a patient with dementia. Keeping patients in familiar surroundings allows them to function without the added burden of having to attempt to adapt to a strange environment. Concurrent diseases and many medications can reduce function and increase cognitive impairment in patients with dementia.

CASE 108-1, QUESTION 5: What is an appropriate initial treatment strategy for T.D.?

T.D.'s family needs to be educated about what to expect as his dementia progresses. They should be referred to the Alzheimer's Association (www.alz.org) and to the Family Caregiver Alliance (www.caregiver.org). Both organizations provide a wealth of information and community resources, including caregiver support groups. They also should be encouraged to enroll in the MedicAlert + Alzheimer's Association Safe Return program, which provides 24-hour nationwide emergency response for people with dementia who wander or suffer a medical emergency. T.D.'s family should include him in any advance planning, seek legal advice regarding advance directives and durable power of attorney for health care and finance, and conduct estate planning to avoid having to perform these tasks when T.D. is no longer competent to participate.[41]

Currently, there are two classes of medications that are used in the treatment of Alzheimer's disease, cholinesterase inhibitors (ChEIs) and N-methyl-D-aspartate (NMDA) receptor antagonist.[44] They are pharmacologically distinct and can be prescribed concurrently in patients in the moderate to severe stages of the illness. ChEIs act on inhibiting acetylcholinesterase, an enzyme directly involved in the destruction of acetylcholine leading to increasing its concentration in the nucleus basalis of Meynert in the brain and hence ameliorating the cognitive and functional aspects of AD. Cholinesterase inhibitors have been shown to improve cognition and function, and delay symptom progression in people with dementia, however benefits are limited Cholinergic-related effects, particularly in the gastrointestinal (GI) tract, are the most common adverse effects cause by all of the agents.[45]

DONEPEZIL

Donepezil is a piperidine derivative that is somewhat selective for central AChE. It reversibly inhibits cholinesterase activity. Donepezil is highly bioavailable and exhibits a long half-life, allowing it to be given as a single daily dose. It is highly protein bound, primarily to albumin.[46]

Donepezil may improve cognition, global function, and behavioral symptoms across all stages (mild, moderate, and severe) of AD. In a multicenter, double-blind, placebo-controlled trial, subjects with mild to moderately severe AD improved during a 12-week treatment period.[47] Subjects taking 10 mg of donepezil at bedtime improved their cognitive function as measured by the Alzheimer's Disease Assessment Scale-Cognitive Subscale (ADAS-Cog), and their overall function as measured by the Clinician's Interview-Based Impression of Change with caregiver input (CIBIC-Plus).[48,49] A 24-week multicenter, placebo-controlled trial using dosages of 5 mg/day and 10 mg/day demonstrated similar results. Both 5- and 10-mg doses were superior to placebo; adverse effects were less common with the 5-mg dose.[50] A long-term, open-label follow-up study to these trials demonstrated that donepezil effects may persist for almost 3 years.[51] Interruption or discontinuation of donepezil treatment was followed by a return of cognition and function to baseline or below.

Donepezil is indicated also for the severe stage of AD. A 6-month, double-blind, parallel group, placebo-controlled study in patients with severe AD (MMSE 1–10) demonstrated an improvement in the Severe Impairment Battery[52] and Modified Alzheimer's Disease Cooperative Study activities of daily living inventory for severe AD. The domains that showed a significant improvement versus placebo were language, praxis, visuospatial, bowel/bladder function, and ability to get dressed. There were no differences noted in the neuropsychiatric inventory for behavioral issues associated with dementia.[53] A 23-mg dose of donepezil was approved for patients in the moderate to severe stages of AD. Small improvements were seen in the Severe Impairment Battery, and there was no improvement in the CIBIC-Plus when compared with the 10-mg dose. More than 30% of the high-dose group and nearly 18% of the low-dose group failed to complete the 24-week trial.[54]

The most common adverse effects of donepezil are associated with cholinergic activity. They tend to be mild to moderate in nature and resolve with stabilization of the dose.[47,50] In a 144-week extension trial of donepezil, the most frequently encountered adverse effects were nausea, diarrhea, and headache.[51] In clinical trials, however, adverse effects were the primary reason for withdrawal from studies, with an overall dropout rate of 29% in the treatment groups.[45]

RIVASTIGMINE

Rivastigmine is a carbamate derivative that inhibits both AChE and butyrylcholinesterase (BChE) activity. BChE provides an alternative pathway for acetylcholine metabolism. Rivastigmine inhibits the activity of both cholinesterases, primarily in the central nervous system.[55] Its AChE inhibition is greater for the G1 as compared with the G4 form.[33] The drug binds to the esteratic sites of the AChE and BChE molecules and slowly dissociates. Because of this, it is often referred to as a "pseudoirreversible" inhibitor.[56] Rivastigmine's biological half-life is approximately 1 hour, but because its slow dissociation extends its activity for at least 10 hours, it can be dosed twice daily. Rivastigmine is bound approximately 40% to serum proteins and is metabolized via hydrolysis to renally excreted inactive compounds.[55] Rivastigmine absorption is nearly complete, but because it undergoes a significant first-pass effect, the resultant bioavailability is approximately 36%.

In two large clinical trials conducted in patients with mild to moderately severe AD, rivastigmine improved cognition, the ability to perform daily activities, and global function over the course of 24 weeks.[56,57] In each multicenter, double-blind, placebo-controlled trial, subjects were randomly assigned to receive placebo or low-dose (1–4 mg/day) or high-dose (6–12 mg/day) rivastigmine in two divided doses during a 26-week period. In one study, subjects in both dosage groups demonstrated statistically significant improvement after 26 weeks on the ADAS-Cog and CIBIC-Plus scales.[56] In the other trial, only those subjects taking 6 to 12 mg/day improved on the same scales.[57] An open-label extension study that included subjects from both previous studies found that subjects taking 6 to 12 mg/day of rivastigmine had significantly better cognitive function after 1 year than did subjects who had originally received placebo.[58]

Adverse effects typically include nausea, vomiting, diarrhea, and other cholinergic mediated GI effects.[55] They are most common when rivastigmine is taken on an empty stomach or when the dose escalation is too rapid. Headache, dizziness, and fatigue are also common adverse effects. Increasing the dose by 1.5 mg twice daily at 4-week intervals increases drug tolerability and reduces the frequency and severity of GI side effects. Adverse effect severity appears to be less problematic with a transdermal formulation that delivers 4.6 or 9.5 mg/24 hours, which correspond to 6- and 12-mg daily doses of the oral formulation.[59] The maintenance dose is generally 9.5 to 13.3/day. In patients with moderate to severe AD, the maintenance dose is 13.3 mg/day. If treatment is interrupted for at least 3 days, the lowest dosing should be restarted.

GALANTAMINE

Like other agents used to treat AD, galantamine enhances cholinergic activity by inhibiting AChE. However, it also stimulates nicotinic receptors (α7-nicotinic receptor agonist) at a site distinct from that stimulated by acetylcholine, an action that does not rely on the presence of acetylcholine. This action is referred to as allosteric modulation.[33] Galantamine is rapidly and completely absorbed, reaches peak serum levels in less than 2 hours, and has a half-life of approximately 5 hours. It exhibits low protein binding and has a large volume of distribution. Galantamine is metabolized primarily by cytochrome P-450 (CYP) isoenzymes CYP2D6 and CYP3A4, and is eliminated in the urine.[60]

Clinical trials have shown galantamine to be effective for the symptomatic treatment of mild to moderate AD. Doses of 16 and 24 mg/day produced clinically meaningful improvement in ADAS-Cog and CIBIC-Plus scores during a 5-month, randomized, placebo-controlled trial.[61] A similar trial conducted in Europe and Canada that evaluated patients for 6 months used doses of 24 and 32 mg/day. Both doses were more effective than placebo, but patients in the 32-mg/day group exhibited more adverse effects.[62] A 6-month, open-label extension trial showed that patients treated with galantamine 24 mg/day maintained ADAS-Cog scores throughout the entire 12 months of the study.[62]

As with the other ChEIs, cholinergic effects in the GI tract are the most commonly encountered adverse effects. Nausea, diarrhea, vomiting, and anorexia were the most frequent events encountered during clinical trials.[33,45] They were typically present during the dose escalation phases of the studies. A dose titration interval of 4 weeks reduces the severity of adverse effects and increases tolerability.

CASE 108-1, QUESTION 6: Should treatment with a cholinesterase inhibitor be instituted in T.D., and if so how should therapy be monitored?

T.D. is in the mild stage of the disease, so a ChEI is an appropriate choice.[42] It is unlikely that a ChEI will produce a dramatic or long-lasting improvement in T.D.'s cognitive abilities. Systematic reviews of ChEI therapy have consistently concluded that these agents provide modest benefits, at best, in the majority of patients.[45,63] Treatment, however, may slow his cognitive decline, help maintain his ability to care for himself for 1 year or more, and reduce the risk for nursing facility placement for as much as 2 years.[60] Beneficial effects may occur for as long as 3 years, and patients who start therapy earlier may experience greater benefit than those who delay treatment.[61,62] The choice of drug is based on the agent most likely to produce a positive response with the fewest adverse effects. Ease of adherence must also be considered. All agents exhibit similar adverse effect profiles. Rivastigmine may be less prone to drug interactions because of its metabolic pathway.[55] It is also available as a transdermal patch that is applied daily. Whereas the oral formulation of rivastigmine requires an initial, nontherapeutic titration dose to reduce the severity of adverse effects, the initial transdermal dosage is therapeutic.[59] Donepezil and galantamine extended-release can be given as a single daily dose and are available as generic equivalents. They can be given at bedtime, which may make cholinergic side effects less troublesome.

Donepezil may be an appropriate agent for T.D.. He should receive donepezil 5 mg at bedtime. He should be monitored for cholinergic side effects (particularly nausea and diarrhea), insomnia, headache, and dizziness, the adverse effects most commonly reported in clinical trials.[47,50] Additionally, he should be monitored for bradycardia due to his pre-existing low heart rate. Patients who received moderate to high doses of donepezil showed an increased incidence and greater risk of bradycardia especially those with risk factors (e.g. cardiovascular disease, concomitant use of beta blockers, calcium channel blockers, antiarrhythmics).[64] His family and physician should look for improvements in his memory, orientation, and ability to concentrate on complex tasks, such as managing finances. He may also become less irritable.

CASE 108-1, QUESTION 7: T.D. was unable to tolerate the donepezil and his family was wondering what other options could be employed to address the progression of the dementia?

After 1 month, his physician should assess him for adverse effects.[42] If he has not improved noticeably after 4 to 6 weeks, the dose of donepezil may be increased to 10 mg at bedtime. If his condition does not respond to donepezil after a 6-month trial, or he is unable to tolerate the donepezil, it is reasonable to switch T.D. to another ChEI. Both rivastigmine and galantamine have additional mechanisms of action that might prove beneficial. Rivastigmine is started at a dose of 1.5 mg twice daily with meals to slow absorption and improve tolerability. The dose may be increased at 4 week intervals by 1.5 mg twice daily, up to the maximal dose of 6 mg twice daily; however, the transdermal formulation is better tolerated and may be preferable by avoiding a titration phase. Galantamine can be started at 4 mg twice daily or 8 mg daily (extended-release) and increased every 4 weeks by 8 mg, up to a maximal dose of 24 mg daily. As with oral rivastigmine, the initial dose is not therapeutic.[60] Taking galantamine with meals may improve tolerability of GI effects. If a trial of a second agent does not improve or stabilize a patient's condition, there is no value in attempting a third agent. T.D. should have routine reassessment of his daily function, cognition, and behavior at 6-month intervals.[65-67] Close attention also must be paid to his other medical conditions, and his family should be provided ongoing support, such as through an AD caregiver support group.

MEMANTINE

As T.D.'s AD progresses, there are two treatment options that can be tried. One option is to further titrate up the donepezil dose to 23 mg a day as mentioned above with some limited clinical efficacy.[51] Another option is to use an *N*-methyl-D-aspartate (NMDA) antagonist, which has been shown to reduce the release of glutamate in the central nervous system that can lead to excitotoxic reactions and cell death in AD and other neurodegenerative disorders.[68] Memantine is a noncompetitive NMDA receptor antagonist with moderate affinity and voltage-dependent binding. It is completely absorbed after oral administration, reaches peak serum concentrations in 3 to 8 hours, and is moderately protein bound.

Multiple clinical trials have evaluated memantine in subjects with moderate to severe AD. A dose of 10 mg/day for 12 weeks increased functional ability (e.g., dressing, toileting, participating in group activities) and reduced care dependence compared with placebo.[68] A 28-week trial using a dose of 20 mg/day improved CIBIC-Plus scores, activities of daily living, and global function compared with placebo.[69] Overall, the benefits of memantine are modest.[70] The combined use of memantine and a ChEI has been shown to be superior to a ChEI alone by improving daily function in individuals with moderate to severe dementia.[71-73] Common adverse effects include diarrhea, insomnia, dizziness, headache, and hallucinations.[68] Memantine has also been studied in patients with mild to moderate AD with 2,000 IU/d of alpha tocopherol compared with placebo.[74] The alpha tocopherol resulted in slower functional decline, while there were no significant differences in the groups receiving memantine alone or memantine plus alpha tocopherol. T.D. should be started on memantine 5 mg daily, with the dosage increased in weekly intervals by 5 mg/day, up to a dose of 10 mg twice daily.[68] As an alternative, he can be started on the extended-release formulation given in weekly escalating doses of 7, 14, 21, and 28 mg daily.

LEWY BODY DEMENTIAS

Etiology

Lewy bodies are hyaline-containing inclusion bodies typically found in people with Parkinson's disease. Recently, attention has been given to distinguish DLB and PDD to help further research.[75] It is known that up to 25% of patients with dementia have Lewy bodies in the brainstem and cortex (particularly in the limbic and paralimbic cortices and frontal and temporal lobes).[5,76] Concentrations are found in the substantia nigra, locus coeruleus, hypothalamus, basal nucleus of Meynert, and neocortex. There is decreased dopamine in the basal ganglia and a loss of choline acetyltransferase (and thus, acetylcholine) in the basal nucleus of Meynert.[5] Many of these patients display extrapyramidal signs without the classic presentation of Parkinson's disease.[7] The role of α-synuclein is a common biological theme in both DLB and PDD, with α-synuclein aggregates found in Lewy bodies and neurites.

Clinical Presentation

CASE 108-2

QUESTION 1: J.F. is a 72-year-old woman who was diagnosed with mild cognitive impairment 6 months ago. She had been increasingly forgetful and confused for about 1 year before the diagnosis. Approximately 3 months ago, J.F. and her family decided that J.F. should move in with them so she would not be left alone. Since moving in with the family, her son has noted that she seems "spaced out" at times. Some days, she appears to be very clear and not confused; other days she is very forgetful and requires assistance with daily tasks. Her daughter-in-law reported that J.F. has been unsteady on her feet at times and has fallen twice. She notes at times she moves very slowly and has difficulty initiating movement. Recently, J.F. reported seeing people coming out of the painting on the wall (a European street scene), stating that "they were walking all through the house trying to steal anything that can be hidden in a coat pocket."

At the physician visit, J.F. was found to be medically stable. Vital signs, serum chemistries, and complete blood cell count were within normal limits. Her MMSE score was 21/30. During the review of systems, J.F.'s daughter-in-law had to answer some questions because J.F. appeared either not to hear them or to ignore them. On physical examination, she demonstrated mild cog-wheeling rigidity bilaterally, bradykinesia, and masked facies; she did not display a resting tremor. What is the most likely explanation for J.F.'s presentation?

Given her physical health, inability to live alone because of impaired cognition, and MMSE score, J.F. meets the criteria for dementia. Her rigidity, bradykinesia, and masked facies are consistent with early Parkinson's disease (see Chapter 59 Parkinson's Disease and Other Movement Disorders). There have been revised criteria for the clinical diagnosis of DLB (Table 108-1).[77] J.F. exhibits all the central features, two core features, and the supportive feature of repeated falls. Her presentation is consistent with probable DLB versus PDD because of her temporal sequence and lack of well-established diagnosis of Parkinson's disease.

Treatment

CASE 108-2, QUESTION 2: What is an appropriate treatment for J.F.?

To date, ChEIs are the only treatment strategy for the cognitive symptoms of both PDD and DLB. All ChEIs have demonstrated symptomatic benefit in patients with DLB.[78,79] The largest randomized, placebo-controlled trials have used rivastigmine (up to 12 mg/day) in subjects with mild to moderate disease, and this medication has received US Food and Drug Administration (FDA) indication for PDD. Rivastigmine was reported to worsen tremor in 10% of the patients with PDD, yet overall there was not a statistically significant difference between groups.[75] Rivastigmine treatment has demonstrated improvements in apathy, anxiety, delusions, and hallucinations when titrated appropriately to doses of 6 to 12 mg daily.[80] Dose initiation, titration, and monitoring are conducted in the same manner as when ChEIs are used for the treatment of AD.

J.F.'s symptoms of Parkinson's disease should be fully evaluated, and appropriate treatment, such as levodopa/carbidopa, should be started (see Chapter 59, Parkinson's Disease and Other Movement Disorders). Because several medications for parkinsonism can have psychiatric effects, it is important to monitor for adverse effects such as worsening psychosis and cognition. Typical antipsychotics, such as haloperidol, may worsen her extrapyramidal symptoms (EPS) and should be avoided. Novel atypicals, namely, quetiapine and clozapine, may be less likely to exacerbate the parkinsonism but should be instituted after a trial of a ChEI or if more acute symptom control of behaviors is required.[75,77]

VASCULAR DEMENTIA (VAD)

Etiology

VaD is a broad classification of cognitive disorders caused by vascular disease. The most common cause of VaD is occlusion of cerebral blood vessels by a thrombus or embolus, leading to ischemic brain injury.[81,82] In the majority of cases, the dementia syndrome is the result of multiple individual cerebral infarcts, a single infarct in an area related to cognitive function, or diffuse white matter lesions in the subcortex.[16] A number of diseases, including atherosclerosis, arteriosclerosis, and vasculitis, lead to the production of emboli and thrombi that potentially occlude brain vessels. Hemorrhagic phenomena and disorders such as hypertension or cardiac disease can produce episodes of cerebral ischemia or hypoxia and are responsible for some cases of VaD.[81-83] Specific risk factors for VaDs include advancing age, diabetes mellitus, small vessel cerebrovascular disease, hypertension, heart disease, hyperlipidemia, cigarette smoking, and alcohol use.[82-84]

Neuropathology

VaDs are typically subcortical. Most patients with VaD have blockage of multiple blood vessels and infarction of the cerebral tissue supplied by those vessels.[83,84] When the distribution of a large artery or medium-size arteriole is blocked, focal neurologic deficits can result (see Chapter 61, Ischemic and Hemorrhagic Stroke). Depending on the area affected, there may be significant cognitive impairment. More often, however, a patient may have experienced transient ischemic attacks (TIAs) or multiple microinfarcts that have remained unrecognized.[83,84] Patients with subcortical VaDs often exhibit small, deep ischemic infarcts in arterioles of the basal ganglia, thalamus, and internal capsule.[83,84] A history of atherosclerosis, diabetes mellitus, or hypertension is often present without a history of stroke.[83,84] MRI scans can be very useful in diagnosing VaDs because areas of cerebral infarction are easier to visualize than they are with CT scanning (Fig. 108-3).[16,22] Lesions in white matter may occur in as many as 85% of patients with VaD. Deep white matter lesions known as leukoaraiosis often include demyelination and may represent early changes in dementia.[83] Because of the etiologic factors involved, VaD typically has an earlier onset than AD, and affects more men than women.

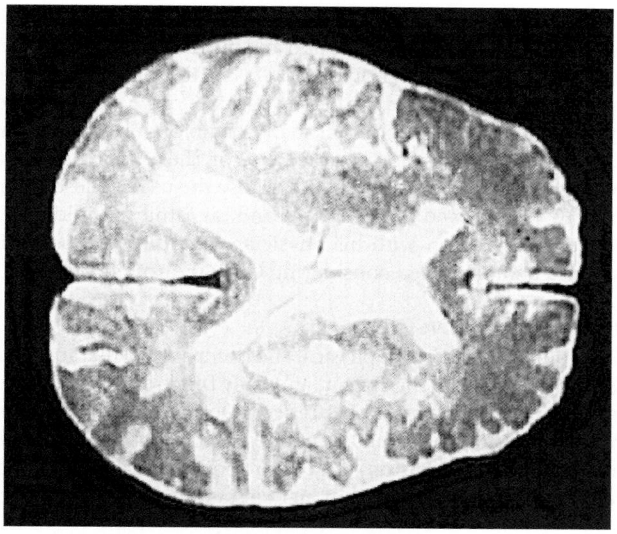

Figure 108-3 A large stroke is visible to the right of the ventricles. There is evidence of atrophy in the right temporal area.

Clinical Presentation

CASE 108-3

QUESTION 1: D.V., a 73-year-old man, is accompanied by his daughter for evaluation of "fuzzy thinking." Although his chief complaint is impaired memory, he denies significant impact on his daily routine. D.V. states his memory problem began 2 years ago after a dizzy spell and subsequent fall. However, his daughter states that the impairment began approximately 1 year before that episode. The memory loss has been slowly progressive. D.V. states that he feels useless because of his memory problems and his "boring" daily routine. Although D.V. is generally independent, he relies on his daughter for assistance with most financial matters. He has voluntarily quit driving because of a lack of confidence in his abilities. D.V.'s daughter reports that according to her mother, D.V. is sometimes disoriented at night when he awakens to urinate. He has no history of urinary incontinence. D.V. has a questionable history of TIAs, but no focal neurologic deficits. He has a long history of mild hypertension, which is treated with a diuretic. He drinks alcohol occasionally and smokes about half a pack of cigarettes per day. His medical history is unremarkable except for the possible TIAs, hypertension, and a mildly enlarged prostate. His family history is positive for diabetes and heart disease.

On physical examination, D.V. is found to be a mildly obese man who is well dressed and groomed, alert, and oriented to person. His BP is 160/92 mm Hg sitting and 168/95 mm Hg standing. Cardiac examination is normal. Neurologic findings include somewhat diminished extraocular movements laterally and slightly asymmetric reflexes, with right greater than left. Muscle tone is normal in the lower extremities. He has a mild shuffling gait. Vibratory sensation is diminished but within normal limits for his age. His score on the Folstein MMSE was 22/30, including errors in orientation and recall. Psychologic evaluation found him to be mildly depressed.

A full laboratory analysis was generally within normal limits. D.V.'s serum potassium (3.8 mEq/dL) and sodium (138 mEq/dL) were in the low normal range, and his blood urea nitrogen (18 mg/dL) was in the upper normal range. Serum total cholesterol was 246 mg/dL, and fasting triglycerides were 230 mg/dL. A chest radiograph revealed a mildly enlarged heart; his electrocardiogram was normal. An MRI scan of the brain indicated generalized atrophy with enlarged ventricles, periventricular white matter ischemic changes, bilateral basal ganglion lacunar infarcts, and small cortical infarcts in the right parietal lobe.

What subjective and objective evidence exists for a diagnosis of dementia in D.V.?

D.V.'s major complaint is "fuzzy thinking" and impaired memory that he attributes to his dizzy spell and fall. However, his family began to note problems a full year before that episode, with progression over time. Although D.V. denies that his impairment significantly affects his daily routine, he has voluntarily stopped driving and relies on his daughter for assistance with financial matters. His memory difficulties appear to have affected his mood and made him feel useless. D.V. is disoriented at night when he awakens to urinate. These factors satisfy the DSM-V criteria for interference with normal activities.[1]

Multiple deficits are present on both the Folstein MMSE[17] (orientation, recall) and on the Blessed Dementia Scale[85] (memory, orientation), indicating impaired short- and long-term memory. D.V.'s inability to drive reflects poor judgment behind the wheel of a car; a disturbance of higher cortical function is indicated by his need for assistance with financial matters. There is no evidence of a delirium being present. Evidence of an organic cause is provided by the MRI scan.

Diagnosis

CASE 108-3, QUESTION 2: What type of dementia does D.V. have?

There is sufficient evidence to indicate that D.V. suffers from a neurocognitive disorder. DSM-V provides diagnostic criteria for VaD (Table 108-1) and it appears that the history and findings satisfies the possible VaD (unclear of temporal relationship between TIAs and decline).[1] VaDs commonly present suddenly after a cerebrovascular insult. This is followed by a period of stability and further declines after additional episodes, often in a stepwise pattern. Cognitive impairments are variable and depend on the area of the brain affected by the insult.[1,16]

With the exception of the dizzy spell and fall, D.V.'s deterioration has had a pattern that resembles a downhill slide rather than stepwise decline. Although his cognitive deficits are "patchy" (e.g., he appears to have no language difficulty), they are not particularly prominent. D.V. displays some neurologic signs and symptoms, including diminished extraocular movements, asymmetric reflexes, and a mild shuffling gait, but they are subtle and might be easily missed by an untrained observer as being related to a dementia. Reliance solely on the clear presence of diagnostic criteria may often lead to a missed diagnosis.[22] The Hachinski Ischemic Scale ranks signs and symptoms associated with cognitive impairment of cerebrovascular origin and is used to help differentiate between AD and VaD.[83] According to this scale, D.V.'s nocturnal confusion, depression, hypertension history, and focal neurologic signs and symptoms are sufficient to indicate VaD.

D.V.'s history and clinical presentation do not suggest dementia caused by a single large stroke or several small strokes. Large strokes produce significant motor damage, typically on one side of the body (the side contralateral to the stroke). Multiple smaller strokes cause prominent motor deficits in discrete areas controlled by the affected areas. Neither of these patterns describes D.V.'s condition. However, he is clearly exhibiting signs of dementia and has significant cerebrovascular disease. He possesses several risk factors for a VaD, including hypertension, smoking, and hyperlipidemia. His MRI indicates a lacunar state, with multiple small infarcts in the deep penetrating arterioles at the base of the brain, particularly in the basal ganglia, internal capsule, thalamus, and pons (see Chapter 61, Ischemic and Hemorrhagic Stroke). These MRI findings are consistent with D.V.'s long-standing hypertension and neurologic presentation.

Case 108-3, Question 3: How should D.V. be managed?

Several treatment options that modify risk factors for VaDs are available.

SMOKING CESSATION

D.V. should be counseled to stop smoking because cigarette smoking reduces cerebral blood flow and increases the risk for stroke. Among smokers with VaD, cessation of cigarette use improves cognitive performance.[86]

ANTIHYPERTENSIVE THERAPY

Hypertension and hyperlipidemia, both present in D.V., are additional risk factors for stroke and VaD. Control of systolic hypertension reduces the risk of stroke by 36% in elderly patients,[87] and maintaining the systolic BP between 135 and 150 mm Hg is associated with improved cognition among MID patients. A systolic BP that exceeds 150 mm Hg indicates inadequate control, whereas a systolic BP less than 135 mm Hg may lead to inadequate cerebral perfusion.[88] As in non-demented individuals, non-pharmacologic treatment (e.g., diet, weight loss, exercise) is an essential component. The antihypertensive agent must be chosen carefully in this population to maximize compliance and minimize adverse reactions.[89] Both thiazide diuretics and β-adrenergic blockers may increase lipid levels, a potential complication in D.V. α-Adrenergic blockers and sympatholytic agents may cause depression or impair cognitive activity. Calcium-channel blockers or angiotensin-converting enzyme inhibitors are acceptable because they are well tolerated by elderly patients and may help preserve renal function in patients with diabetes mellitus (see Chapter 9, Essential Hypertension).

Dihydropyridine calcium-channel blockers have been shown to improve cognition in patients with dementia and reduce the risk of dementia in elderly patients with isolated systolic hypertension.[90] Because D.V. has benign prostatic hyperplasia, he may benefit from the use of an α-adrenergic blocking agent, such as doxazosin 1 mg at bedtime or terazosin 1 mg at bedtime (see Chapter 109, Geriatric Urologic Disorders). Evidence indicating an increased risk for negative cardiac outcomes, however, makes the α-adrenergic blocking agents less attractive choices.[91] The use of a vasodilating calcium-channel blocker, such as amlodipine 5 mg once daily, is an appropriate first choice. An angiotensin-converting enzyme inhibitor such as benazepril 10 mg once daily is an appropriate alternative. Both agents exhibit the advantage of once-daily dosing over some other agents within their respective classes. This feature is important for maximizing adherence in patients with declining memory.

ANTIPLATELET THERAPY

Prophylaxis against future cerebrovascular events is indicated in VaD, but few studies that have looked specifically at individuals with dementia are available. Cerebral perfusion and cognitive performance were improved in VaD patients receiving aspirin 325 mg/day for 1 year when compared with a control population.[92] Guidelines from the American Heart Association and the American Stroke Association recommend the use of antiplatelet therapy in patients with a history of TIA or atherothrombotic stroke that is not of cardiogenic origin. Aspirin in doses of 50 to 325 mg/day, clopidogrel 75 mg daily, or aspirin 50 mg/dipyridamole 200 mg twice daily are all effective treatments for stroke prophylaxis.[93] Warfarin and possibly targeted specific oral anticoagulant (TSOACs) may be recommended after cardioembolic cerebral ischemic events. However, only aspirin has been studied specifically in VaD patients. Aspirin 81 to 325 mg daily is an appropriate first choice for D.V.

CHOLINESTERASE INHIBITORS

Deficits in cholinergic transmission and nicotinic receptor binding abnormalities have been noted in VaD.[5,94] Early clinical trials with donepezil,[95] galantamine,[96] and rivastigmine[97] have demonstrated improvement in cognition and daily function among patients with VaD. As of yet, however, the use of these agents remains investigational and controversial. Because the use of these agents is not FDA-approved for VaD, D.V. and his family should have a thorough discussion with his physician regarding the potential risks and benefits when considering ChEI treatment for him.

MANAGING FUNCTION

D.V. should be referred for physical and occupational therapy for an assessment of his strength, gait, and daily function. Physical therapy can help him maintain his strength. Occupational therapy can provide him with equipment and strategies to adapt to his dizziness and avoid falls. In addition, the use of reminder notes and labels around the house will assist him in maintaining his independence.

BEHAVIORAL DISTURBANCES IN DEMENTIA

Several types of behavioral disturbances may develop during the course of a dementia and occur in almost all patients, particularly during the later stages (Table 108-6).[38,41] Behavior symptoms include a wide range of disturbances, including agitation, apathy, wandering, verbal and physical aggression, and psychotic symptoms.[41] Agitation in dementia has been described as excessive motor activity with a feeling of inner tension that may lead to related symptoms such as anxiety, irritability, motor restlessness, and abnormal vocalization.[98] Sleep disorders and mood disorders, such as anxiety and depression, also are common.[99] Agitation and anxiety are often managed best with nonpharmacologic treatment. Pharmacologic interventions are appropriate when nondrug therapies are unsuccessful or the behavior is severe. Non-psychologic behaviors such as wandering and inappropriate motor activity respond better to environmental modification than to drug therapy.[99,100] The first step in evaluating altered behavior in patients with dementia is to ensure that the problem is not the result of an unrecognized medical problem (e.g. pain), environmental factors or caused by an adverse effect of a medication (see Chapter 107, Geriatric Drug Use).

Agitated Behaviors

CASE 108-4

Question 1: T.G., a 62-year-old man, has recently been diagnosed with AD, for which he takes donepezil 10 mg at bedtime. He also has hypertension that is treated with hydrochlorothiazide 12.5 mg daily and amlodipine 5 mg daily. He no longer takes his daily walks around the neighborhood because he is afraid he will get lost; instead, he follows his wife around the house as she does her daily chores. Other times, he paces throughout the house. He also expresses worry about the burden he will place on his family as his condition worsens. Recently, he has had episodes of incontinence and awakens four to five times during the night to urinate. His concerns contribute to his nighttime awakenings, making him quite tired during the day.

How should T.G.'s agitation and anxiety be managed?

Anxiety and unfocused activity are common problems in the early stages of dementia. Agitation is a general term that, while commonly used, is subject to wide interpretation. It typically is used to describe specific behaviors such as restlessness, irritability, or unfocused motor activities. Patients are aware of their progressive cognitive decline and have sufficient insight to understand the consequences. T.G.'s shadowing of his wife indicate insecurity and anxiety; pacing through the house is an example of restlessness and unfocused behavior. T.G. is exhibiting anxiety, as evidenced by his worry about placing a burden on his family. His poor sleep is attributable to both nocturia and anxiety.

If T.G.'s behavior represents a sudden or rapid change, his physician should first evaluate him for a medical condition such as infection, pain, or a medication-related problem. Although T.G. has been taking hydrochlorothiazide without difficulty, he may no longer be recognizing the cues to urinate. The drug should be discontinued; if his blood pressure rises, the amlodipine dose can be increased. This may help with his incontinence, nocturia, and disturbed sleep.

CASE 108-4, QUESTION 2: T.G.'s mental status continues to decline to the point that he requires help with bathing and dressing. During a physician visit, he accuses his wife and children of stealing from him. He also cannot locate his coin collection, which he placed in a "safe" location when his memory began to decline; during the night, he rummages through the house looking for it. He believes his family has been plotting to steal his assets and then turn him out onto the street. T.G.'s son reports that T.G. has been verbally abusive and has threatened several members of the family recently. How should T.G.'s paranoid behavior be managed?

Once medical problems have been ruled out or corrected, he should be evaluated using a systematic approach, as behavior problems are part of a chain of events. T.G. may be described as "agitated," but his behavior is shadowing his wife and pacing through the house. The behavior has an antecedent; because he has a dementia, he may be unable to initiate a meaningful or enjoyable activity on his own, and consequently he becomes bored. The consequence of his boredom is that he annoys his wife and paces the house. This represents what often is termed an "A-B-C" approach, for *antecedent, behavior, consequence.*[99] Pacing is a demonstration of unfocused energy. T.G.'s wife can give him simple tasks to perform, such as drying dishes, folding laundry, or simple gardening, to help channel his energy. It also may relieve his anxiety and insecurity. She also could accompany him on walks to alleviate his fear of getting lost. She may want to consider enrolling him in an adult day-care program. This would give him meaningful activity that might help him use up his excess energy and sleep better at night. It also will provide her with some respite and avoid or delay caregiver burnout. Appropriate strategies to manage agitated behaviors without medication are listed in Table 108-6.

When non-pharmacologic interventions are not successful in reducing anxiety, irritability, and similar behaviors, medications can be considered. Benzodiazepines are the most commonly used anxiolytics and will address T.G.'s insomnia and anxiety. However, they are associated with several negative outcomes in the elderly, including confusion, amnestic syndromes, ataxia, and falls.[101,102] Benzodiazepines, in addition to other medications, may be considered potentially inappropriate medications in older adults as described in the 2015 American Geriatrics Society Beers Criteria. If a benzodiazepine is clinically warranted, agents such as lorazepam or oxazepam, may be used, if necessary, but only for a short term and with caution.[102]

Trazodone is a sedative antidepressant that is effective for insomnia and agitated behaviors in patients with AD.[101,103] Treatment is started at 25 mg at bedtime and may be increased to a dose of 250 mg/day in divided doses. Another alternative treatment is buspirone, which does not cause the cognitive impairments associated with the benzodiazepines. Dosage begins at 5 mg three times daily and may be increased up to 15 mg three times daily. However, buspirone will not concurrently manage T.G.'s insomnia because it has no sedative effect, and there is no reliable evidence that it is efficacious in anxiety associated with dementia.[102] Citalopram has been shown to reduce agitated behaviors in people with dementia and could be used.[104] Emerging evidence suggests that dextromethorphan-quinidine combination may be efficacious in reducing agitation but caution exists in light of drug-drug interactions as well as limited data.[105]

If the nondrug strategies are ineffective in reducing T.G.'s insomnia and agitation, trazodone should be initiated at a dose of 25 mg at bedtime. It may be increased by 25 mg/day at 5- to 7-day intervals, up to 100 mg. Doses above 100 mg/day should be split into two daily doses.

Psychosis

Delusions and hallucinations are common among individuals with dementia. Paranoid symptoms, often accompanied by aggression, have been reported in more than half of dementia patients.[103] Delusions typically involve suspicion of theft by family members, which may be secondary to the patient's inability to remember where valuable items were placed and incorrectly concluding that they were stolen.[106] Another common delusion is the misidentification of people or objects.[107] Capgras syndrome, the belief that a person has been "replaced" by an identical-looking impostor or the belief that photographs or television pictures are real individuals, may occur in almost half of demented individuals.[106]

There are a few behavioral interventions that could be tried first before resorting to medications, which produce limited benefits and are accompanied by significant risk.[108,109] The first step is to conduct a person-centered examination of the symptoms. Several questions need to be answered. What is the significance or meaning of these behaviors to T.G? (For example, he cannot locate items that are valuable to him, and does not recall where they are.) What triggers his thoughts and outbursts? (He may assume the items were stolen, and believes that his family, knowing their location, has taken them for their own gain.) How is the family's response further angering him? (If the family searches for and finds the items, it may reinforce his delusion that they stole them.) The family should be educated that paranoid behavior is common in dementia, and that it is likely to pass as the disease progresses. Depending on how fixed the paranoia is, distraction or redirection, such as changing the subject to something more pleasant, or initiating a pleasant activity, could resolve the problem. Regardless of the strategy, they need to be taught not to argue or debate with T.G. but to share his concern. When these strategies fail, then, depending on severity, it may be necessary to resort to medication.

Paranoid symptoms respond best to antipsychotic agents, although these are not highly effective, and no single antipsychotic is more effective than any other. Delusions, hallucinations, aggression, and uncooperativeness symptoms respond best, but overall improvement occurs in only a minority of patients.[102,109] The CATIE-AD trial compared olanzapine, quetiapine, risperidone, and placebo for the treatment of psychosis, aggression, and agitation for up to 36 weeks in patient with AD. Improvement was noted in 32%, 26%, 29%, and 21%, respectively. The authors concluded that efficacy of the agents was offset by adverse effects.[109] There are no antipsychotic medications that are approved by the FDA for use in the management of behavior symptoms in people with dementia. Black-box warnings are present for all agents because of the increased risk for stroke and mortality when used in this population.[108,110,111] Consequently, any use of these drugs in a person with dementia is for an unapproved use and requires a full discussion between the physician, patient, and caregivers.

Table 108-6
Behavior Disturbances in Dementia

Behavior	Typical Presentation	Nonpharmacologic Treatment	Pharmacologic Treatment
General strategies		Safety-proof living areas Issue one-step commands for directions Maintain a daily routine of activities Avoid arguing incorrect statements Avoid startling the patient Limit unusual or overly stimulating environments	
Anxiety	Excessive worrying, sleep disturbances, rumination	Listen to, and acknowledge frustrations Redirection Exercise Engage in enjoyable activities Sleep hygiene practices Limit noise and distractions	Trazodone Buspirone (if no insomnia) Short-acting benzodiazepine SSRI antidepressant
Depression	Withdrawal, loss of appetite, irritability, restlessness, sleep disturbances	Exercise Engage in meaningful activities	Trazodone SSRI antidepressant
General agitation and restlessness	Repeated questions, wandering, pacing	Distraction and redirection Break down tasks into simple steps Provide enclosed area for exercise	Often unresponsive to medications
Paranoid behaviors	Delusions (often of theft), hallucinations, misperceptions	Reassurance Distraction, rather than confrontation Remove potential sources of confusion (e.g., mirrors and other reflective surfaces)	Atypical antipsychotic, if not responsive to other strategies and person is harmful to self or others SSRI antidepressant, if associated with withdrawal, tearfulness, themes of loss
Aggressive behaviors	Physical or verbal aggressiveness toward others, excessive yelling and screaming, manic features	Identify the precipitating cause or situation Focus on the patient's feelings and concerns Avoid getting angry or upset Maintain a simple, pleasant, and familiar environment Use music, exercise, etc., as a calming activity Shift the focus to another activity	Anticonvulsant, such as divalproex or carbamazepine, possibly in combination with an atypical antipsychotic when other strategies do not work

Adapted from California Workgroup on Guidelines for Alzheimer's Disease Management. *Guideline for Alzheimer's Disease Management: Final Report:* State of California, Department of Public Health; April 2008; Kales et al. Assessment and management of behavioral and psychological symptoms of dementia. *BMJ.* 2015;350:h369; Tariot PN et al. Pharmacologic therapy for behavioral symptoms of Alzheimer's disease. *Clin Geriatr Med.* 2001;17: 359; Herrmann N, Lanctot KL. Pharmacologic management of neuropsychiatric symptoms of Alzheimer disease. *Can J Psychiatry.* 2007;52:630; Gray KF. Managing agitation and difficult behavior in dementia. *Clin Geriatr Med.* 2004;20:69; Teri L et al. Exercise plus behavioral management in patients with Alzheimer disease: a randomized controlled trial. *JAMA.* 2003;290:2015.

The risks and potential benefits of therapy must be carefully weighed for T.G. before determining the appropriate treatment. The choice of an antipsychotic agent is determined by the symptoms displayed by the patient as well as the potential for adverse effects. T.G. is experiencing a delusion of theft, suspiciousness, and aggressive behavior. It is possible that the verbal abuse and threats are consequences of fear brought on by the false belief that his family is stealing from him and plans to abandon him.

T.G. has no major contraindications to the use of any antipsychotic agent, and his target symptoms will probably respond to any of the available agents. Therefore, a therapeutic trial is appropriate. The choice can be made according to which antipsychotic agent is least likely to cause intolerable adverse effects. Risperidone has been evaluated in a case series and in a large double-blind, placebo-controlled trial.[112,113] In the case study series, symptoms improved in half of the patients taking dosages ranging from 0.5 mg every other day to 3 mg twice daily. However, 50% also experienced EPS, even at the lowest dosage used.[112] Subjects in the double-blind trial received either placebo or risperidone at dosages of 0.5 mg/day, 1 mg/day, or 2 mg/day for 12 weeks. Daily doses of 1 or 2 mg reduced psychosis and improved behavior, but EPS and somnolence were common adverse effects.[113] Low doses of olanzapine, 5 to 15 mg/day, were superior to placebo for reducing agitation, aggression, and psychosis during a 6-week study among nursing facility residents.[114] Somnolence and gait disturbances were the most common adverse effects. Quetiapine has been shown to reduce agitated and psychotic behaviors at doses of 100 to 200 mg/day.[115] Clozapine poses significant risk for hematologic toxicity and requires careful monitoring. Because T.G. does not have cardiovascular or cerebrovascular risk factors and does not have gait or balance problems, either risperidone 0.25 mg at bedtime or quetiapine 25 mg at bedtime can be initiated. Doses of risperidone may be increased by 0.25 mg/day in weekly intervals, up to 2 mg/day; quetiapine doses can be increased by 25 mg/day, up to 200 mg/day in divided doses. Once his behavior has stabilized, the medication should be continued for about 3 months. At that time, the dose should be decreased in weekly intervals to determine whether the medication is still required. T.G. should be monitored closely for adverse effects, including EPS, which can occur with the atypical antipsychotics.[110,116]

Aggressive Behaviors

CASE 108-4, QUESTION 3: After 3 months, T.G.'s delusions have subsided, but he continues to be verbally abusive and often displays angry, emotional outbursts, especially when he requires help with bathing or toileting. At other times, he is withdrawn and apathetic. He has also been found wandering in the neighborhood on three occasions. These behaviors persist despite treatment with quetiapine 100 mg twice daily. What alternative treatments can be attempted?

Although psychotic symptoms respond to antipsychotic agents, many other behaviors do not. Up to 90% of patients with dementia exhibit at least one disruptive behavior such as angry outbursts, screaming, and abusive language, and many display multiple aggressive behaviors.[110] As many as 32% exhibit moderate to severe behaviors.[110] Such behaviors are typically directed at caregivers, precipitated by receipt of assistance with activities of daily living such as bathing and toileting, and increase in frequency with dementia severity.[99,117] Several of these behaviors may be merely defensive responses to perceived threats in cognitively impaired individuals.[117] Behavioral disturbances must be addressed because they can have a negative effect on the patient's ability to perform activities of daily living.[99]

Some behaviors exhibited by T.G. are not likely to respond to medications. Wandering is typically unaltered by the use of medications unless the patient is oversedated. Non-pharmacologic treatments, such as periods of physical exercise and rest, or environmental modification is much more effective.[99,103,118] T.G.'s reactions to assistance with bathing and toileting may be caused by confusion and fear. Breaking the tasks down to step-by-step procedures, accomplished individually, often helps modify aggressive behaviors.[41]

Verbal abuse and aggressiveness place both the patient and the caregiver at risk for injury, and may lead to abuse. In these situations, the patient and the caregiver may each be a precipitator or a target of abuse.[119] In some small studies, anticonvulsant agents have been shown to reduce rage and aggressive behaviors in patients resistant to treatment with antipsychotics. Carbamazepine and valproic acid (including divalproex) are the most well-studied agents.[110,116] Although initial trials were promising, later studies did not establish efficacy. The lack of benefit plus concerns about toxicities with each agent have led to recommendations that these agents not be used.[95,109] The addition of an antidepressant medication may be helpful, as described below. Wandering typically does not respond to pharmacologic intervention. Appropriate strategies include environmental modification, such as placing child-safety locks on exit doors; providing activities and other distractions; and having a safety plan, such as the Safe Return program. As described for his paranoid behavior, a person-centered evaluation using the A-B-C approach should be conducted to determine the cause and effects of his aggressiveness. If T.G.'s aggressive behaviors continue, his family may need to consider obtaining in-home assistance or placement in an assisted-living facility designed for the care of patients with dementia.

Depression

CASE 108-4, QUESTION 4: How should T.G.'s social withdrawal and apathy be treated?

Depression often accompanies dementia and may significantly impair a patient's functional capacity, cognitive abilities, and communication.[95,109] T.G. is withdrawn and apathetic, symptoms suggestive of depression. Screaming and irritability may be considered symptoms of depression in individuals with dementia, perhaps reflecting feelings of loneliness, boredom, or the need for attention.[120] Because a definite diagnosis of depression relies heavily on a patient interview and response to questions, a formal diagnosis in patients with dementia is difficult. Therefore, patient observation is an important component for making a clinical evaluation. It is possible that he is reacting to a sense of loss of not only his memory and function, but also a loss of self. He also may feel isolated by the inability to communicate with others or participate in the outside world. Helping him to engage in meaningful activities and social engagement, perhaps as simple as going on a walk or attending adult day care, may help alleviate his apathy and reverse his withdrawal. Such a strategy is appropriate to try before considering an antidepressant.

The selective serotonin reuptake inhibitors have not been well studied in patients with dementia, but are effective antidepressants with adverse effects that are better tolerated than those of the tricyclic antidepressants. Sertraline, in doses of 50 to 150 mg/day, was superior to placebo in reducing depression in AD patients during a 12-week trial.[121] Citalopram has also demonstrated effectiveness; in contrast, fluoxetine and fluvoxamine have not demonstrated benefit.[104,110] Either sertraline 50 mg daily or citalopram 10 mg daily are reasonable choices to treat T.G.'s symptoms of depression if he does not respond to nonpharmacologic strategies. He should be reassessed in 1 month; if he has not responded, the dose may be increased. Dosages may be increased weekly up to a maximum of 150 mg/day or 20 mg/day, respectively. A full therapeutic trial requires a minimum of 3 months.

Social Support

CASE 108-4, QUESTION 5: T.G.'s family indicates that caring for him at home has become so burdensome that they are considering placing him in an institution. What social support services are available to families facing this decision?

Institutionalization is a typical outcome for patients in the late stages of dementia. The total care required to manage a dementia patient usually becomes unmanageable for most families as the disease progresses. Caregiver stress is often exacerbated by the patient's declining memory, inability to communicate, physical decline, and incontinence, as well as the caregiver's loss of freedom and depression. Caregivers commonly experience anger, helplessness, guilt, and worry, and suffer from physical stressors such as fatigue and illness.[41]

Outside assistance is essential to families caring for a patient with dementia. Families should be referred to the Alzheimer's Association as soon as a diagnosis of dementia is received. The association has local affiliates in most major cities. The book *The 36-Hour Day* is a valuable resource for families as well.[122] It describes the symptoms, behaviors, and problems that can be encountered when caring for a patient with dementia.

Support groups, individual and family counseling, and other sources of support are useful and may help families cope for a longer period. However, the key intervention to reduce caregiver stress is respite care, which allows a family time away from the responsibilities of taking care of a frail individual. Respite care brings a person into the home or allows the patient to go to a day-care center or similar environment on a regular schedule. Such programs may delay the need to institutionalize a patient.[41,42,122]

KEY REFERENCES AND WEBSITES

A full list of references for this chapter can be found at http://thepoint.lww.com/AT11e. Below are the key references and websites for this chapter, with the corresponding reference number in this chapter found in parentheses after the reference.

Key References

Alzheimer's Association. *Alzheimer's Disease Facts and Figures 2015*. Chicago, IL: Alzheimer's Association; 2015. (3)

American Psychiatric Association. *Diagnostic and Statistical Manual of Mental Disorders*. 5th ed. Washington, DC; 2013. (1)

Kaduszkiewicz H et al. Cholinesterase inhibitors for patients with Alzheimer's disease: systematic review of randomised clinical trials. *BMJ*. 2005;331:321. (63)

Herrmann N et al. Pharmacologic management of neuropsychiatric symptoms of Alzheimer disease. *Can J Psychiatry*. 2007;52:630. (102)

Mace NL et al. *The 36-Hour Day: A Family Guide to Caring for People with Alzheimer Disease, Other Dementias, and Memory Loss in Later Life*. 4th ed. Baltimore, MD: Johns Hopkins University Press; 2006. (115)

Key Websites

Alzheimer's Association. http://www.alz.org

MedicAlert + Alzheimer's Association Safe Return. http://www.alz.org/safetycenter/we_can_help_safety_medicalert_safereturn.asp

Advancing Excellence Nursing Home Quality Campaign. https://www.nhqualitycampaign.org/dementiaCare.aspx

American Society of Consultant Pharmacists https://www.ascp.com/articles/antipsychotic-medication-use-nursing-facility-residents

National Institute on Aging. Alzheimer's Disease Education and Referral Center (ADEAR). http://www.niapublications.org/adear.

109 Geriatric Urologic Disorders

Tran H. Tran

CORE PRINCIPLES

		CHAPTER CASES
URINARY INCONTINENCE		
1	Urinary incontinence is a common condition in older adults and can be classified as acute or persistent. Persistent incontinence can further be classified as urge, stress, overflow, or functional.	**Case 109-1 (Questions 1, 2)**
2	Urge incontinence is managed with nonpharmacologic interventions, such as a toileting schedule, and the use of anticholinergic medications.	**Case 109-1 (Questions 3, 4)**
3	Stress incontinence is managed with local estrogens, tricyclic antidepressants, and duloxetine.	**Case 109-2 (Questions 1, 2)**
BENIGN PROSTATIC HYPERPLASIA		
1	Benign prostatic hyperplasia (BPH) is the most common urologic condition in aging men. A wide range of signs and symptoms occurs in BPH that causes patients to seek care.	**Case 109-3 (Questions 1–3)**
2	Management of BPH includes the use of α_{1A}-adrenergic receptor antagonists and 5α-reductase inhibitors, either alone or in combination. Nonpharmacologic treatment and surgery may also be considered for some patients. In general, the use of over-the-counter medications should not be used to treat symptomatic BPH.	**Case 109-3 (Questions 4–7)**
ERECTILE DYSFUNCTION		
1	Erectile dysfunction (ED) is a condition that can be a result of neurogenic, hormonal, or vascular disorders. It is therefore essential that a complete urologic workup is conducted to assess the underlying pathophysiology. Underlying conditions should be addressed and treated before symptomatic therapy is initiated.	**Case 109-4 (Questions 1–6)**
2	Treatment for ED consists of a variety of pharmacologic agents, which include phosphodiesterase inhibitors, intracavernous injections, and alprostadil.	**Case 109-4 (Questions 7–14)**

URINARY INCONTINENCE

Neurophysiologic Considerations

The bladder can be thought of as a "balloon" with a narrow outlet, wrapped with a muscular layer, the detrusor muscle. The detrusor and the bladder outlet functions are coordinated neurologically to allow for storage and expulsion of urine.[1] The detrusor muscle is innervated by the parasympathetic nervous system, and the bladder neck is innervated by the sympathetic nervous system (α-adrenergic) (Fig. 109-1). The proximal smooth muscle (internal) sphincter in the bladder neck also is innervated through the sympathetic nervous system (α-adrenergic). The distal striated muscle (external) sphincter of the urethra is supplied by the somatic nervous system.

Urine storage is the result of detrusor muscle relaxation and closure of both the internal and external sphincters. Detrusor relaxation is accomplished by central nervous system (CNS) inhibition of the parasympathetic tone; sphincter closure is mediated by a reflex increase in α-adrenergic and somatic activity. Voiding occurs when detrusor contraction is coordinated with sphincter relaxation. Detrusor contraction is mediated by the parasympathetic nervous system, and relaxation requires inhibition of somatic and sympathetic nerve impulses to the outlet. The bladder capacity is ~300 mL in the elderly and ~400 mL in young

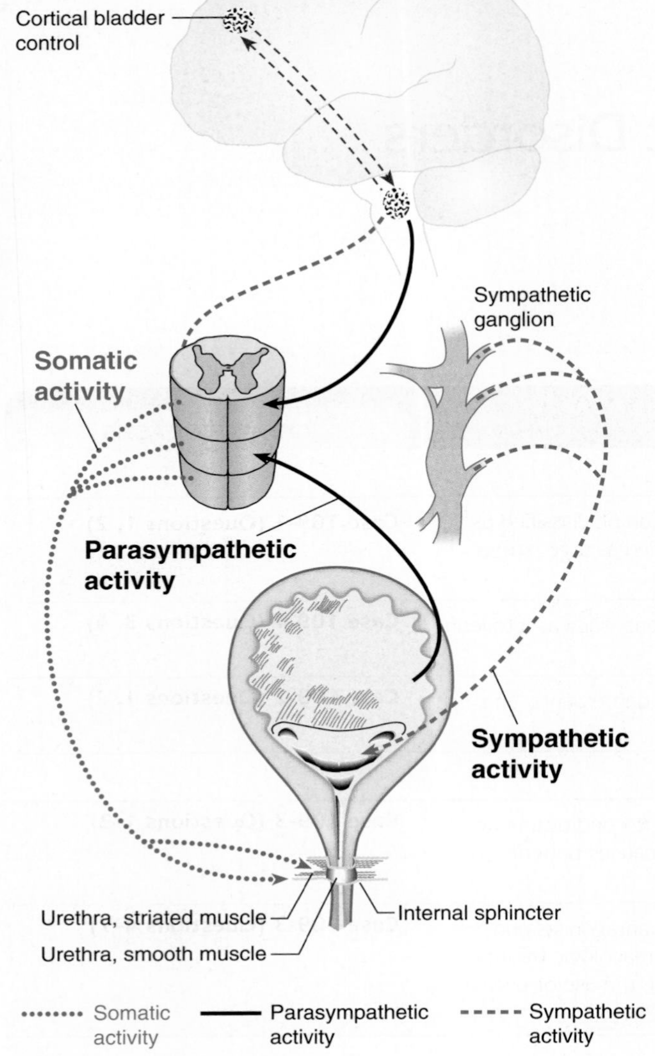

Figure 109-1 Neurologic bladder control.

adults. The relationship between the detrusor and the outlet is coordinated by a micturition center located in the CNS, perhaps in the pons.[2] The cortex and diencephalon also permit inhibition of what would otherwise be a reflex contraction of the detrusor muscle in response to bladder distension.

Age-Related Changes

Aging affects the lower urinary tract in several ways (Table 109-1), including both structural and functional changes. Bladder capacity,

Table 109-1
Age-Related Changes in Urologic Function

↓ Bladder capacity
↑ Residual urine
↑ Uninhibited bladder contractions
↑ Nocturnal sodium and fluid excretion
↓ Urethral resistance in women
↑ Urethral resistance in men
Weakness of pelvic floor muscles in women

Table 109-2
Causes of Incontinence

	Mnemonic: DIPPERS
D	Delirium
I	Infection
P	Psychological
P	Pharmaceuticals
E	Excess urine output
R	Reduced mobility
S	Stool impaction (and other factors)

Source: Wagg A et al. Urinary incontinence in frail elderly persons: report from the 5th International Consultation on Incontinence. *Neurourol Urodyn*. 2015;34(5):398–406.

the ability to postpone voiding, urethral and bladder compliance, maximal urethral closure pressure (the maximal difference between the urethral and the intravesical pressure), and urinary flow rate all are reduced with normal aging.[2,3] For women, these changes are correlated with the postmenopausal decline of estrogen production. Estrogen has trophic effects on the epithelium and on tissues lining and surrounding the urethra, bladder outlet, and vagina. Atrophy of these tissues can result in friability, inflammation, susceptibility to infection, diminished periurethral blood flow, and prolapse of pelvic structures. All of these effects can precipitate symptoms of urinary incontinence. For men, the age-related changes in the prostate gland are responsible for many of the changes in urination. The most common age-related change, in both women and men, is involuntary bladder contractions (detrusor motor instability). These involuntary bladder contractions occur in up to 20% of asymptomatic, neurologically normal, continent elderly patients.[4–7]

Each of these changes predisposes people to incontinence, but none alone precipitates it. This predisposition to incontinence, together with the increased likelihood that an older person will be subjected to additional pathologic, physiologic, or pharmacologic insults, underlies the higher incidence of incontinence in the elderly. The onset or exacerbation of incontinence in an older person is likely to be caused by a precipitating factor outside the lower urinary tract.[8] Common treatable causes of urinary incontinence in the elderly can be described with the mneumonic DIPPERS (Table 109-2).[9] Correspondingly, reversal of the precipitating factor may be sufficient to restore continence without correction of the underlying urologic abnormality.

Loss of bladder control in the elderly was reported in 36.7% of short-term residents and 70.3% of long-term residents in nursing homes.[10] Moderate, severe, and very severe levels of bladder incontinence were identified in 24.0% of noninstitutionalized elderly patients.[10] Incontinence has economic costs, and medical (e.g., cystitis, urosepsis, pressure sores, perineal rashes, falls) and psychosocial (e.g., embarrassment, isolation, depression, predisposition to institutionalization) consequences. Nevertheless, incontinence often is a neglected condition. Patients may not report incontinence to their primary-care providers because of embarrassment or misconception regarding treatment. Incontinence is not an inevitable consequence of aging. It is a pathologic condition that, when rationally approached, usually can be ameliorated or cured, often without invasive tests or surgery and almost invariably without an indwelling catheter.[11,12]

Classification

Urinary incontinence can be classified in several different ways. The two most basic types of urinary incontinence are (a) *acute* (or *transient*) and *reversible* and (b) *chronic* and *persistent*. Persistent urinary incontinence (PUI), which refers to incontinence that is not acute and occurs for a long time, can be classified further into four subgroups: (a) urge, (b) stress, (c) overflow, and (d) functional.

ACUTE INCONTINENCE

Urinary incontinence that is of relatively recent onset or associated with an acute medical problem should prompt a review for reversible factors. These include the following: (a) cystitis, atrophic vaginitis, and urethritis; (b) heart failure; (c) polyuria from diabetes; (d) delirium and acute confusional states; (e) immobility; and (f) medication side effects (discussed subsequently). The management of acute forms of urinary incontinence depends on the identification and elimination of the reversible factor.

For women with urethritis and atrophic vaginitis with irritative voiding symptoms, estrogen replacement can be very helpful. An intravaginal estrogen cream is administered nightly for 7 days, followed by at least once-a-week application.[13] In keeping with the Women's Health Initiative trial, serious risks, including breast cancer and cardiovascular disease, appear to outweigh long-term benefits of systemic combination of hormone therapy. Therefore, topical therapy is preferred.[14]

Drug-Induced Urinary Incontinence

Several medications are associated with acute-onset urinary incontinence, including diuretics, α-adrenergic agonists (e.g., pseudoephedrine), α-adrenergic antagonists (e.g., terazosin), anticholinergics, and neuroleptics.

Reports of female stress incontinence from α_1-adrenergic receptor antagonists, which have a relaxant effect on urethral smooth muscle, have appeared in the medical literature.[15–17] In one study, the incidence of genuine stress incontinence was significantly higher in women taking prazosin (86.2%) than in the group without prazosin (65.7%; $p < 0.01$). In 55% of the women contacted in the prazosin group, urinary incontinence was reduced or cured by prazosin withdrawal.[18] There was a significant increase in functional urethral length, maximal urethral closure pressure, and abdominal pressure transmission to the urethra after prazosin withdrawal. In one case report, switching from doxazosin to enalapril briefly reduced the female patient's stress incontinence; however, she experienced a persistent dry cough (from the enalapril) that continued to cause episodic stress incontinence. Her cough and stress incontinence resolved when she was switched to amlodipine.[19]

PERSISTENT URINARY INCONTINENCE

Urge Incontinence

Urge incontinence, the most common form of incontinence affecting the elderly, occurs when involuntary voiding is preceded by a warning of a few seconds to a few minutes. Urge PUI is characterized by precipitous urine leakage, most often after the urge to void is perceived. Urge PUI can be caused by a variety of genitourinary and neurologic disorders. It most often, but not always, is associated with detrusor motor instability (involuntary contraction of the bladder) or detrusor hyper-reflexia (detrusor motor instability caused by a neurologic disorder). The most common causes are local genitourinary conditions, such as cystitis, urethritis, tumors, stones, bladder diverticula, and outflow obstruction. Neurologic disorders, such as stroke, dementia, parkinsonism, and spinal cord injury, can be associated with urge PUI.[8] Overactive bladder is a medical syndrome defined by symptoms of urgency, with or without urge urinary incontinence, usually with frequency and nocturia. By definition, overactive bladder is a syndrome and not a diagnosis.

Stress Incontinence

Stress incontinence is the involuntary leakage of urine that occurs when an abrupt increase in intra-abdominal pressure ("stress," e.g., coughing, sneezing, laughing, lifting) overcomes urethral resistance. Stress incontinence is common in elderly women but uncommon in men (unless the sphincter has been damaged during a transurethral resection of the prostate [TURP] or a prostatectomy). Typical stress PUI is characterized by daytime loss of small-to-moderate amounts of urine, infrequent nocturnal incontinence, and a low postvoid residual volume in the absence of a large cystocele. Stress incontinence can be diagnosed by the "tissue test" in which a tissue is placed just below the urethra and the patient is asked to cough, resulting in the loss of a small amount of urine. The usual cause of stress PUI is urethral hypermobility owing to weakness and laxity of pelvic floor musculature, but other conditions, such as sphincter incompetence, urethral instability, or stress-induced detrusor instability, occasionally are responsible.[2] Obesity or TURP in men also can predispose individuals to stress incontinence. Many factors have been suggested to contribute to the development of urinary stress incontinence in women, including estrogen deficiency and a genetic defect in the connective tissue in such patients. The prevalence of urinary stress incontinence among first-degree relatives of patients with urinary incontinence is 3 times ($p < 0.005$) that of matched control groups of women without micturition disorders.[20]

Overflow Incontinence

Overflow incontinence occurs when the weight of urine in a distended bladder overcomes outlet resistance. Leakage of small amounts of urine (dribbling) is common throughout the day and night. The patient may complain of hesitancy, diminished and interrupted flow, a need to strain to void, and a sense of incomplete emptying. The bladder usually is palpable, and the residual urine volume is large.

Overflow incontinence results from an anatomic outlet obstruction or an acontractile (or atonic) bladder.[8] Common causes are benign prostatic hyperplasia (BPH), urethral stricture, bladder sphincter dyssynergia, diabetic neuropathy, fecal impaction, and anticholinergic medication use. If the cause is neurologically mediated, control of the perianal sphincter may be impaired.[21]

Functional Incontinence

Functional incontinence occurs when a continent individual is unable or unwilling to reach the toilet to urinate. Common causes are musculoskeletal disorders, muscle weakness, impaired mental status, use of physical restraints, psychological impairment, environmental barriers, and medications (e.g., sedatives, neuroleptics).

Clinical Presentation and Evaluation

CASE 109-1

QUESTION 1: H.K., an 83-year-old female resident of a nursing facility with moderate dementia, had urinary incontinence 3 years before admission. She has been managed with adult diapers (briefs) and bladder training. What objective and subjective data are needed to determine the pathophysiology (and hence the classification) of H.K.'s urinary incontinence?

The rationale for the clinical evaluation of H.K. is to classify the imbalance between bladder pressure and bladder sphincter resistance and, as a result, institute appropriate medical or surgical management of her urinary incontinence.

Documentation of H.K.'s urinary incontinence is accomplished most easily by keeping an incontinence record. Observations should be recorded every 2 hours regarding whether she is wet or dry, as well as associated symptoms or circumstances. A record maintained for 3 to 4 days will facilitate assessment of the voiding pattern. Knowledge of the voiding pattern can be used to design bladder training programs and to detect iatrogenic causes (e.g., diuretic ingestion, use of restraints). Successful bladder training relies on estimating when the bladder is full.

Physical examination, including a neurologic assessment, of H.K. is needed to determine the cause and classification of her urinary incontinence. Clinical findings may identify specific pathophysiologic abnormalities. H.K. should have a thorough pelvic examination to determine the contribution of atrophic vaginitis, uterine prolapse, and bladder anatomy. Funneling of the bladder neck suggests stress incontinence, and palpation of the bladder suggests overflow incontinence. The presence of physical restraints or musculoskeletal disability would suggest functional incontinence.

H.K.'s bladder should be catheterized immediately after urination to determine residual urine volume. Alternatively, if a bladder ultrasound is available, the volume can be measured noninvasively. Volumes in excess of 50 to 100 mL in the elderly are abnormal and may indicate retention due to obstruction or an adynamic detrusor muscle. If urinary retention is chronic, the patient may require clean intermittent self-catheterization. Although urodynamic studies are widely recommended and used, little evidence suggests that these produce clinically useful data for institutionalized geriatric patients. A urinalysis, blood chemistries, renal function, and postprandial glucose tests should be performed. An abnormal urinalysis may suggest pathology (e.g., infection) that can be managed medically. Urinary tract infection is common in the incontinent patient.

Treatment options exist for each type of urinary incontinence (Table 109-3). Proper evaluation should guide the clinician in choosing the optimal course of drug therapy. Drug therapy should be based on sound principles of neurophysiology, urology, and pharmacology. Drug therapy is directed at decreasing bladder contractility (detrusor instability) or increasing bladder outlet resistance (bladder neck and proximal urethra).

Table 109-3
Drug Therapy of Persistent Urinary Incontinence

Type	Treatment With Initial Doses
Urge	Oxybutynin 2.5 mg every day to TID; 5–30 mg XL every day Oxybutynin transdermal patch 3.9 mg/24 hour 1 patch 2×/week Oxybutynin 10% topical gel 100 mg/g every day Oxybutynin 3% topical gel 84 mg (3 pumps) every day Tolterodine 1–2 mg every day; 2–4 LA every day Trospium 20 mg BID; 60 mg ER every day Darifenacin 7.5 mg every day Solifenacin 5 mg every day Fesoterodine 4 mg every day
Stress	Pseudoephedrine 15–30 mg BID–TID Imipramine 25 mg every day Vaginal estrogen cream 0.5–1.0 g 2 to 3 times/week Duloxetine 40–80 mg every day divided in one or two doses
Overflow	Terazosin 1–5 mg every day (usually at bedtime) Doxazosin 1–8 mg every day Tamsulosin 0.4–0.8 mg every day Alfuzosin 10 mg every day Silodosin 4–8 mg every day Bethanechol 10 mg TID
Functional	None

BID, 2 times daily; LA, long acting; TID, 3 times daily; XL, extended release.

Case 109-1, Question 2: The incontinence record maintained by the nursing staff indicates that H.K. has urinary urges quite frequently, resulting in urine leakage. Throughout the day and night, H.K. urinates 4 to 5 times. Physical examination reveals atrophic vaginitis, no funneling of the bladder neck, and no bladder distension. H.K. does have a history of stroke. The urinalysis is normal, as are the blood chemistries. Postvoiding bladder scan revealed a residual urine volume of 30 mL. What is the pathophysiology and classification of H.K.'s incontinence?

Most neuropathic disease processes can change bladder function. As illustrated by H.K., a cerebrovascular accident is commonly associated with bladder dysfunction and incontinence in the elderly. Neurologic injury above the level of the micturition center in the spinal cord, in most cases, results in bladder spasticity. Sacral reflexes are intact, but loss of inhibition from higher CNS centers results in spastic bladder and inappropriate sphincter behavior. The degree of spasticity varies between the bladder and sphincter, as well as from patient to patient with the same CNS lesions. H.K. has a spastic detrusor muscle resulting from an unchecked sacral reflex. H.K.'s bladder dysfunction is classified as urge urinary incontinence of the persistent type.

Nonpharmacologic Therapy

A number of nonpharmacologic options are available that may help improve the symptoms of PUI. The first step is to educate patients about bladder function, appropriate fluid intake, and avoidance of caffeine and other bladder irritants. The patient can then keep a bladder diary in which they record their fluid intake, voiding pattern, and incontinence episodes. Bladder training refers to scheduled voiding, urge-suppression techniques, and pelvic muscle exercises. Scheduled voiding can be used in both cognitively intact and impaired individuals. The patient is instructed to void on a schedule (e.g., every 2 hours), thereby minimizing the volume of urine in the bladder and making incontinence episodes less likely. The same principle can be used in cognitively impaired patients by prompting them to toilet. Urge-suppression techniques can be used to retrain the bladder; the scheduled toiletings are adjusted for longer or shorter times, depending on the patient's voiding pattern. The goal is to achieve an interval during which the patient is continent and does not need to void. In most patients, this is approximately 2 hours. Pelvic floor muscle exercises, also known as Kegel exercises, work by increasing the strength and tone of the pelvic floor muscles. In randomized trials, incontinence episodes were reduced by 54% to 75% compared with 6% to 16% with no treatment.[22] The patient should receive adequate instruction on how to identify the pelvic floor muscles and then practice these exercises 3 times a day.

Case 109-1, Question 3: What nonpharmacologic therapy should be recommended for H.K.?

H.K. should have a comprehensive review of her medications completed to determine any temporal relationship between medications and incontinence episodes. She should then be placed on a toileting schedule in which she is prompted to void every 2 hours. The nursing staff should continue to keep a bladder diary in which they record fluid intake and when she is wet and dry. This information can be used to tailor her toileting schedule to make sure H.K. has the best outcome while at the same time being practical, based on staffing at the institution. Because of H.K.'s moderate dementia, the teaching of pelvic floor muscle exercises may not be feasible.

Drug Therapy

ANTICHOLINERGIC AGENTS

CASE 109-1, QUESTION 4: What drug therapy should be prescribed for H.K.?

H.K. has detrusor instability that may respond to anticholinergic drug therapy if nonpharmacologic measures do not produce desired results. The major neurohormonal stimulus for physiologic bladder muscle contraction is acetylcholine-induced stimulation of postganglionic parasympathetic cholinergic receptor sites on bladder smooth muscle. Atropine and atropine-like substances depress true involuntary bladder contractions of any etiology by the interaction at the muscarinic receptor.[23] Of the five known muscarinic subtypes (M_1 through M_5), M_3 appears to be the most clinically relevant in the human bladder. M_2 muscarinic receptors are the predominant subtype (comprising about 80% of all muscarinic receptors); however, contraction of smooth muscle, including muscles in the urinary bladder, is mediated mainly by M_3 receptors. M_3 receptors are also involved in contraction of the gastrointestinal smooth muscle, saliva production, and iris sphincter function.[24] Inhibition of the muscarinic receptors in the urinary bladder results in decreased urinary bladder contraction, increased residual urine volume, and decreased detrusor muscle pressure.

Oxybutynin Chloride

Oxybutynin is available as an oral immediate-release tablet, an extended-release tablet, a transdermal system, and a topical gel. Oxybutynin has been described as a strong independent smooth muscle relaxant with local anesthetic activity and anticholinergic effects.[23,25] This agent has been used successfully to depress uninhibited detrusor contractions in patients with and without neurogenic bladder dysfunction. Oxybutynin improves symptoms, total bladder capacity, neuropathic voiding dysfunction, and bladder filling pressure.[26–28] The oral dosage of oxybutynin chloride suggested for the elderly is 2.5 mg up to 3 times a day; in some cases, the dosage may need to be increased to 5 mg 3 times a day. Because oxybutynin is a tertiary-amine anticholinergic compound and also blocks central M_1 receptors, the potential for CNS toxicity increases as the dose is increased. Once-daily, controlled-release oxybutynin at doses of 5 to 30 mg reduced the number of incontinence episodes.[29,30] Maximal benefit was demonstrated by maintenance week 4 and was sustained as long as the patient continued therapy.[31]

The transdermal system is available both in a prescription and over-the-counter version and contains 36 mg of active drug and delivers 3.9 mg of oxybutynin per day when dosed twice a week.[32] The transdermal system should be protected from moisture and humidity. Common side effects from the transdermal system at the application site are pruritus (14%) and redness (8.3%). A comparison study of immediate-release oxybutynin and the transdermal system indicated that patients using the transdermal system experienced fewer side effects. Dry mouth was reported in 38% of the oxybutynin transdermal system users in contrast to 94% of those who used immediate-release tablets.[33] Oxybutynin is also available as a 10% topical gel in 1-g unit dose sachets. One sachet delivers 100 mg and is applied per day to the abdomen, thigh, upper arm, or shoulder. It is also available as a 3% gel in a multi-dose container. The dose is three pumps (84 mg) daily. Application site reactions were reported in 5.4% of patients, and dry mouth was reported in 6.9% of patients.[34]

Tolterodine Tartrate

Tolterodine is a competitive muscarinic receptor antagonist that is relatively selective for M_2 and M_3 receptors. It is indicated for the treatment of overactive bladder symptoms of urinary frequency or urge incontinence. At doses of 1 to 2 mg twice a day, compared with a placebo, the number of urinary voids per 24 hours decreased ($p = 0.0045$), the volume of urine per void increased ($p < 0.001$), and the mean number of incontinence episodes decreased by 50% ($p < 0.19$).[35] Although tolterodine can modestly prolong the QT interval, no clinical or electrocardiographic evidence was seen of significant cardiac adverse events in the group studied.[35,36] The onset of pharmacologic action of tolterodine is less than 1 hour, and therapeutic efficacy is maintained during long-term treatment.

Despite short terminal half-lives of 2 to 3 hours and 3 to 4 hours for tolterodine and its active 5-hydroxy metabolite, respectively, twice-daily dosing is effective because of the drug's long pharmacodynamic effects.[37] Dosage adjustment is recommended in the presence of renal or hepatic impairment and during concurrent therapy with drugs that inhibit cytochrome P-450 (CYP) 2D6 and CYP3A4 isozymes. The usual dose for the elderly is 1 to 2 mg twice daily of the immediate release or 2 to 4 mg once daily of the long-acting formulation. The incidence of dry mouth with the long-acting formulation is 23%.[36]

Fesoterodine

Fesoterodine is an antimuscarinic prodrug that is converted into the same active metabolite as that of tolterodine. The efficacy and safety of fesoterodine appear comparable to those of tolterodine.[38] The recommended starting dosage of fesoterodine is 4 mg once daily and may be increased to 8 mg in patients with an insufficient response. Patients with severe renal impairment (creatinine clearance <30 mL/minute) or those taking a strong CYP3A4 inhibitor should not take more than 4 mg/day.

Trospium Chloride

Trospium is a quaternary ammonium antimuscarinic agent with relative selectivity for M_2 and M_3 receptors. It is used for the management of overactive bladder and urge incontinence. The hydrophilic properties of trospium minimize the passage of the drug through the blood–brain barrier, thereby causing fewer CNS and cognitive adverse events.[39] No significant differences were found in urodynamic outcomes between trospium and oxybutynin in a 52-week study.[40] The reduction in 24-hour micturition frequency and urgency episodes at 26 and 52 weeks of treatment was also not significant. However, the incidence of dry mouth and gastrointestinal adverse events was significantly lower in the trospium group. The medication should be administered at a dose of 20 mg twice daily or 60 mg of the extended-release product once daily. For patients with severe renal insufficiency (creatinine clearance <30 mL/minute), the dose should be reduced to 20 mg once daily. Trospium has no CYP-related drug interactions and should be taken on an empty stomach to avoid decreasing absorption.

Darifenacin

Darifenacin is a selective M_3 muscarinic receptor antagonist indicated for the treatment of overactive bladder with symptoms of urinary incontinence, urgency, and frequency. A pooled analysis of three 12-week, double-blind, placebo-controlled trials ($n = 1{,}059$) demonstrated that darifenacin reduced the median number of incontinence episodes per week ($p < 0.01$) versus placebo.[41] Dry mouth and constipation were the most common reasons for discontinuation. The recommended starting dose is 7.5 mg once daily. Based on the individual response, the dose may be increased to 15 mg daily after 2 weeks.

Solifenacin

Solifenacin is a competitive muscarinic receptor antagonist that is selective for M_3 receptors. It is used for the treatment of overactive bladder with symptoms of urinary incontinence. In clinical trials, solifenacin showed significant reduction in the symptoms of urinary frequency, urgency, and urge incontinence compared with placebo.[42,43] Safety concerns with solifenacin include an increased risk of QT interval prolongation in patients with a known history of QT interval prolongation or patients who are taking medications known to prolong the QT interval. The recommended dose of solifenacin is 5 mg once daily, which can be increased to 10 mg once daily if needed. However, in those with renal and hepatic impairment or on CYP3A4 inhibitors, the dose should not exceed 5 mg once daily.

β-ADRENERGIC AGENTS

Mirabegron is a first in class β_3-adrenergic agonist approved for use in overactive bladder. The human bladder muscle has $\beta_{1,2,3}$-adrenergic receptors; however, β_3-adrenergic receptors account for 95% of the β-receptors and are most likely responsible for detrusor relaxation.[44] Compared to placebo, mirabegron was able to reduce the mean number of incontinence episodes per 24 hours by −0.44 (95 % confidence interval (CI) −0.59 to −0.29, $p < 0.00001$).[45] The efficacy of mirabegron is sustained at 12 months, and its safety is notable for significantly less dry mouth and constipation compared to antimuscarinics.[46] Although mirabegron has not been studied in patients with dementia, clinical trials have not reported any CNS adverse effects with mirabegron. Mirabegron can be used alone or in combination with antimuscarinics for those who cannot tolerate an increase in the antimuscarinic dose or are already on a maximum dose. Mirabegron is initiated at 25 mg once daily and can be titrated up to 50 mg once daily in 2 to 4 weeks. Patients with renal or hepatic impairment should not receive doses higher than 25 mg once daily. Blood pressure increases have been reported with mirabegron (>10%) particularly in patients with uncontrolled hypertension and thus warrant careful monitoring.[47] Mirabegron is also a CYP2D6 inhibitor, and drugs that are CYP2D6 substrates taken concomitantly may require dose adjustments.

Although any of the aforementioned drugs may be useful for H.K., a careful consideration of adverse event profile should be considered before prescribing an anticholinergic agent. The rate of decline in activities of daily living and cognition in patients with dementia was 50% faster when anticholinergic medications were combined with acetylcholinesterase inhibitors than when acetylcholinesterase inhibitors were used alone.[48] Even though H.K. is not treated with an acetylcholinesterase inhibitor, she does have moderate dementia and would likely have pronounced anticholinergic side effects. In addition, the limited efficacy of anticholinergic medications needs to be carefully considered before starting treatment in H.K. A comprehensive review of placebo-controlled trials of anticholinergic medications for overactive bladder estimated that, as a class, even long-acting agents have a very limited effect on symptoms, with approximately one fewer incontinent episode and one fewer voiding episode per 48 hours.[49] Given the potential for side effects and the limited efficacy, it would be prudent to use nonpharmacologic measures (i.e., prompted voiding) to manage H.K. If the desired end points are not achieved, a trial of an anticholinergic medication could be considered. Mirabegron may potentially be a safe option in patients with dementia; however, future studies to promote its use over anticholinergics in this population would be beneficial. All agents in this group should be prescribed for a 2-week trial period with careful monitoring for efficacy and side effects.

INCREASING BLADDER OUTLET RESISTANCE

CASE 109-2

QUESTION 1: M.K., a 68-year-old woman, has been diagnosed with urinary stress incontinence. What therapy would be appropriate for this type of PUI?

M.K. should initially be educated on pelvic floor muscle or Kegel exercises. Several methods have been effectively used to help patients identify and correctly exercise the pelvic floor muscles, including self-help books, biofeedback, electrical stimulation, and verbal feedback during physical examination by a physician.[22] Once the pelvic floor muscles have been identified, M.K. should empty her bladder and sit or lie down. She should contract her pelvic floor muscles, holding the contraction for 5 seconds, and then relax for 5 seconds. This should be repeated 5 times with a goal of 10-second contractions for M.K. She should practice these exercises 3 times a day.

CASE 109-2, QUESTION 2: M.K. has incomplete resolution of her stress incontinence symptoms. Physical examination indicates urogenital atrophy. What are the pharmacologic options for stress incontinence?

Imipramine Hydrochloride

The pharmacologic mechanism of tricyclic antidepressants (TCAs) in treating PUI at best is speculative.[50] All the TCAs have some degree of anticholinergic effect, both centrally and peripherally, but not at all sites. Imipramine has significant systemic anticholinergic effects, but it has weak anticholinergic effects at the detrusor muscle.[51] Imipramine has a significant inhibitory effect on the detrusor muscle that is mediated by neither anticholinergic nor adrenergic mechanisms. Its detrusor inhibitory effect may be the result of peripheral blockade of norepinephrine reuptake. The ability of imipramine to increase bladder outlet resistance is believed to be attributable to enhanced α-adrenergic effects in the smooth muscle of the bladder base and proximal urethra, where α-receptors outnumber β-receptors. The significant anticholinergic side effects associated with imipramine make it a poor treatment option in the elderly.

α-Adrenergic receptor stimulation at the detrusor muscle and proximal urethra will increase the maximal urethral closure pressure.[52] However, α-adrenergic agonists, such as pseudoephedrine, have a minimal role in the treatment of stress urinary incontinence because the risk of adverse events exceeds the limited benefit it is likely to provide.

Duloxetine

Duloxetine is a serotonin and norepinephrine reuptake inhibitor that has shown efficacy in patients with stress incontinence. Duloxetine also treats depression, and though not FDA-approved for the treatment of stress incontinence, it could be a reasonable option for a woman with both depression and stress incontinence. A meta-analysis of nine trials including 3,063 women predominately with stress incontinence showed duloxetine-treated patients had a reduction in the incontinence episode frequency by approximately 50%; however, the absolute reduction (10.8% vs. 7.7%) in incontinence episodes was small, suggesting that any benefits would be modest. Adverse effects were common, with 71% of duloxetine-treated patients reporting side effects and approximately one in eight patients discontinuing treatment.[53] The most common adverse effect with duloxetine is nausea, which tends to resolve with time. The dose of duloxetine that has been studied for stress incontinence is 40 to 80 mg/day in one or two doses. The clinical effects of duloxetine appear to be modest and need to be weighed against the risk of adverse events.

Estrogens

Estrogens affect many aspects of uterine smooth muscle, including excitability, receptor density, and transmitter metabolism, especially adrenergic nerves.[54] The detrusor and urethra are embryologically related to the uterus, and significant work has been done on estrogenic hormone effects on the lower urinary tract.

α-Adrenergic stimulation of the urethra is estrogen dependent,[55] and several studies have demonstrated the relationship of estrogen with α-adrenergic receptor density in the lower urinary tract.[56] Estrogen therapy, in the form of vaginal suppositories (10 mcg/day), facilitates urinary storage in some postmenopausal patients by increasing urethral outlet resistance, and it has an additive effect with α-adrenergic therapy.[15] Additional preparations of estrogen include a vaginal ring that is inserted into the vagina and removed after 90 days. The ring releases 7.5 mcg of estradiol each day over a 90-day period. The use of estrogen in the treatment of stress PUI requires further study. The use of long-term estrogen treatment must be considered carefully in light of the controversy about whether estrogen therapy predisposes to the development of endometrial carcinoma. If estrogen is combined with α-adrenergic agonist therapy, the lowest effective maintenance dose should be prescribed.

M.K.'s incomplete resolution of stress incontinence symptoms is probably caused by urogenital atrophy. She would respond well to an intravaginal estrogen cream, which will improve local blood flow and dryness. An estrogen cream such as estradiol should be prescribed at a dose of 0.5 g of cream 3 times a week. The combination of local estrogen therapy and pelvic floor muscle exercises should eliminate M.K.'s symptoms.

DECREASING BLADDER OUTLET RESISTANCE

Overflow incontinence in female patients resulting from outlet obstruction or weak detrusor muscle is now being treated with α_{1A}-blockers by many urologists. Most α_{1A}-receptors are found in prostate tissue; however, these same receptors are also located in the spinal cord, bladder neck, urethra, and periurethral tissue in women.[57] The urinary symptoms suggestive of prostatism are not sex-specific. Well-controlled, randomized, crossover studies are needed to determine the efficacy of α_{1A}-blockers in overflow incontinence. If detrusor underactivity is the known cause of overflow incontinence, bethanechol can be considered. As a cholinergic agent, bethanechol increases bladder muscle tone causing contractions that initiate urination. Common adverse effects with bethanechol include flushing, tachycardia, abdominal cramps, and malaise.

BENIGN PROSTATIC HYPERPLASIA

Benign prostatic hyperplasia (BPH), a common cause of urinary dysfunction symptoms in elderly men, results from proliferation of the stromal and epithelial cells of the prostate gland.[58,59] There is both a static and a dynamic component to prostate enlargement. The static component increases the prostate size by smooth muscle cell proliferation in the prostate stroma, whereas the dynamic component contributes to an enlarged prostate through an increase in smooth muscle tone in the prostate and bladder neck. The term *benign prostatic hypertrophy* often is used inappropriately because the prostate gland pathology results from hyperplasia rather than hypertrophy. BPH rarely is detected in men younger than 40 years of age. After age 40, the prevalence of BPH is age dependent.[60] Approximately 75% of men who live to the age of 70 exhibit clinical symptoms of BPH that are sufficiently severe to necessitate medical attention, and approximately 90% of octogenarians have evidence of BPH. Essentially, all men will experience BPH if they live long enough. The microscopic incidence of BPH is fairly constant among several Western and developing countries,[61] suggesting that the initiation of BPH may not be environmentally or genetically influenced. Although BPH and prostatic cancer often coexist, no compelling evidence indicates that BPH predisposes patients to the development of prostate cancer.[62] The appearance of atypical prostatic hyperplasia correlates, however, with the presence of latent prostatic carcinoma.[63]

The cause of BPH is unclear; however, most hypotheses are based on hormonal and aging processes. This is because intact, normally functioning testes are essential for BPH to develop,[64] and castration before puberty prevents the development of BPH. The prostate is dependent on androgens both for embryologic development and for maintenance of size and function in the mature male.[65] Testosterone, the major circulating androgen, is metabolized to dihydrotestosterone (DHT) by 5α-reductase. The two isoenzymes of 5α-reductase are designated as type 1 and type 2. Type 2 is found predominantly in the prostate and other genital tissues, whereas type 1 is found throughout the body, as well as in the prostate.[66] For testosterone to be active in the prostate, it must be converted to DHT; therefore, DHT is the obligate androgen responsible for normal and hyperplastic prostate growth. Within the prostate, DHT initiates RNA synthesis, protein synthesis, and cell replication. The exact role of testosterone may be only to initiate fibroadenomatous hyperplasia, eventually resulting in glandular enlargement.

Stromal hyperplasia in the prostate periurethral glands is one of the earliest microscopic findings in men with BPH.[61] As men increase in age, testosterone serum concentrations decrease and the peripheral conversion of testosterone to estrogen increases. At one time, estrogens were thought to initiate stromal hyperplasia, which in turn induces epithelial hyperplasia. It is now known, however, that estrogens do not have a direct effect on the development of BPH and prostatic carcinoma, but progesterone does play a role in their pathogenesis. Progesterone receptors have been shown to exist in prostate stromal cells, whereas estrogen receptors were essentially nonexistent.[67]

Pathophysiology and Clinical Presentation

CASE 109-3

QUESTION 1: G.M., a 72-year-old man, presents to the emergency department with severe lower abdominal discomfort of 4 days' duration. His history consists of having increasing difficulty initiating urination, a significant decrease in the force of his urinary stream, occasional midstream stoppage, and postvoid dribbling. Physical examination is unremarkable except for the abdominal and rectal examination. Abdominal examination reveals distension, tenderness, and increased dullness in the hypogastrium with a large mass, believed to be the bladder. On rectal examination, the prostate is found to be severely enlarged, firm, and rubbery without nodules or undue hardness. G.M. gives a history of nocturia (approximately 4 to 5 times a night) and daytime urinary frequency (8 to 10 times a day). G.M. indicates that when he is able to urinate he has a weak stream and difficulty maintaining flow, and does not feel relieved. Laboratory findings are as follows:

Blood urea nitrogen (BUN), 45 mg/dL
Serum creatinine (SCr), 3.2 mg/dL
Serum prostatic acid phosphatase, 3 units/L
Serum prostate-specific antigen (PSA), 7.1 ng/mL

A urethral catheter was inserted, and 900 mL of urine was obtained. G.M. subsequently was scheduled for a urologic workup. What is the pathophysiologic basis for G.M.'s symptoms?

Symptoms of BPH can be both obstructive and irritative, and descriptions of the symptoms need a frame of reference for standardization. The Boyarsky index, a questionnaire consisting of nine questions to quantify the severity of BPH, has been developed.[68] Five questions are designed to assess obstructive symptoms and four to assess irritative symptoms. Although some limitations to the use of this questionnaire (Table 109-4) may exist, it is one of the most common measures used to quantify symptoms in BPH studies, and it correlates well with the pathophysiology of BPH.[61] The format of the Boyarsky index is designed to help the clinician educate the patient about the obstructive and irritative symptoms of BPH. The Boyarsky index was the first of three patient questionnaires developed to quantitatively assess BPH and the effectiveness of individual treatment.[65] As such, this questionnaire has been used in numerous clinical trials to measure the outcome of interventions. The Boyarsky index is not useful in comparing different treatment therapies among BPH patients because it has not been sufficiently validated for this purpose; rather, it is useful in evaluating an individual's response to therapy.

The Multidisciplinary Measurements Committee of the American Urologic Association (AUA) also has published a urinary symptom index for prostatism.[69] The index is useful to assess the baseline severity of prostatism, disease progression, and effectiveness of different therapies. The AUA symptom index allows comparison among therapies and is the preferred questionnaire for BPH research. It has been validated through internal consistency reliability, constructive reliability, test–retest reliability, and criterion reliability.[65] The AUA index, however, may not be BPH specific.[70] When 101 men and 96 women between the ages of 55 and 79 used the AUA index, urinary symptoms and severity of urinary symptoms were similar in both groups. Therefore, symptoms associated with prostatism can be associated with aging as well as BPH. The National Institutes of Health convened a chronic prostatitis workshop to come to consensus on a new classification system for the diagnosis and management of prostatitis.[71] This group developed a symptom index that provides a valid outcome measure for men with prostatitis. This index attempts to quantify the pain and discomfort associated with prostatism and should help differentiate prostatism from prostatic hyperplasia. The symptom index is self-administered.

CASE 109-3, QUESTION 2: What objective findings in G.M. are associated with BPH?

G.M. presents with obstructive symptoms consistent with BPH as follows: (a) a history of difficulty in initiating urination (hesitancy), (b) a decrease in urinary force, (c) occasional midstream stoppage, (d) postvoid dribbling, and (e) a feeling of incomplete bladder emptying. The common obstructive symptom of decreased force and size of urine stream is caused by urethral compression from prostate gland hyperplasia. Hesitancy, another obstructive symptom, is the result of the bladder detrusor muscle taking a longer time to generate the initial increased pressure to overcome urethral resistance. Urinary stream intermittency is caused by the inability of the bladder detrusor muscle to sustain the increased pressure until the end of voiding. Terminal dribbling and incomplete emptying occur for the same reason, but also may be caused by obstructive prostatic tissue at the bladder neck, causing a "ball-valve" effect.

G.M. also has a history of classic irritative symptoms that are consistent with BPH as follows: (a) nocturia approximately 4 to 5 times a night and (b) daytime urinary frequency of 8 to 10 times a day. Incomplete emptying of the bladder results in shorter intervals between voiding, explaining the complaint of frequency. Also, a large prostate gland provokes the bladder to trigger a voiding response more frequently. This response is more pronounced if the prostate is growing intravesically and compromising the bladder volume. The bladder detrusor muscle becomes hypertrophied as a result of the greater bladder residual urine volume, which can result in increased detrusor muscle excitability. Clinically, this excitability may result in bladder instability. The symptoms of urinary frequency are more pronounced at night because cortical

Table 109-4
Benign Prostatic Hyperplasia Symptom Scoring System (Boyarsky Index)[a]

Nocturia	
0	Absence of symptoms
1	Urinates 1 time/night
2	Urinates 2–3 times/night
3	Urinates ≥4 times/night
Daytime Frequency	
0	Urinates 1–4 times/day
1	Urinates 5–7 times/day
2	Urinates 8–12 times/day
3	Urinates ≥13 times/day
Hesitance (lasts ≥1 minute)	
0	Occasional (≤20% of the time)
1	Moderate (20%–50% of the time)
2	Frequent (≥50% of the time)
3	Always present
Intermittency (lasts ≥1 minute)	
0	Occasional (≤20% of the time)
1	Moderate (20%–50% of the time)
2	Frequent (≥50% of the time)
3	Always present
Terminal Dribbling (at end of voiding)	
0	Occasional (≤20% of the time)
1	Moderate (20%–50% of the time)
2	Frequent (≥50% of the time)
3	Always present (may wet clothes)
Urgency	
0	Absence
1	Occasionally difficult to postpone urination
2	Frequently difficult to postpone urination
3	Always difficult to postpone urination
Impairment of Size and Force of Urinary Stream	
0	Absence
1	Impaired trajectory
2	Most of the time size and force are restricted
3	Urinates with great effort and stream is interrupted
Dysuria	
0	Absence
1	Occasional burning sensation during urination
2	Frequent (>50% of the time) burning sensation
3	Frequent and painful burning sensation during urination
Sensation of Incomplete Voiding	
0	Absence
1	Occasional sensation
2	Frequent (>50% of the time) sensation
3	Constant and urgent sensation, no relief on voiding

[a]Symptom scoring provides the clinician with a tool to measure the relative need for, and efficacy of, different interventions. No specific score is associated with the need for a specific intervention. A low symptom score in the absence of significant urine retention generally indicates that medical management can be attempted before considering surgical intervention.

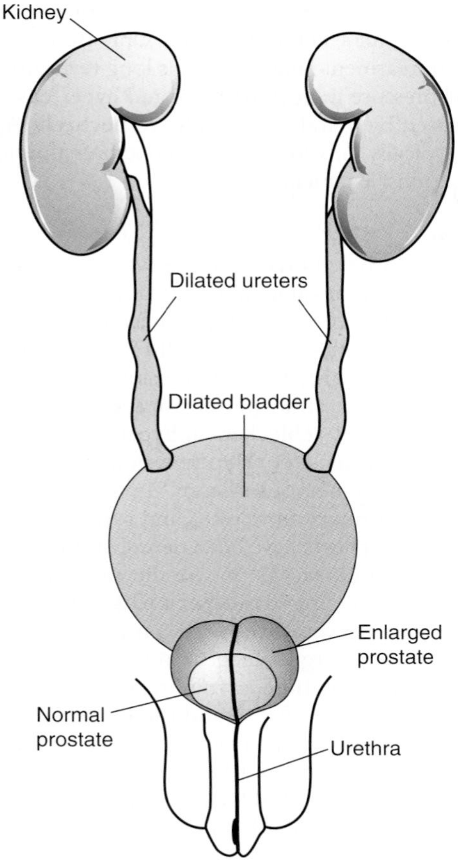

Figure 109-2 Flow of urine is interrupted by compression from a prostate that has enlarged from normal size. In this diagram, the ureters and bladder are dilated by backed-up urine.

inhibitions are lessened and bladder sphincter tone is more relaxed during sleep. Obstructive symptoms are associated more with an enlarged prostate, and the predominance of irritative symptoms could suggest voiding dysfunctions in addition to those of BPH.

Urinary incontinence is not a common symptom of BPH. With advanced BPH, a large residual volume of urine in the bladder weakens the bladder sphincter and allows the escape of small amounts of urine when the bladder is full. Because the residual bladder volume increases, the ureters will dilate, resulting in stasis of urine in the ureters. The end result may be ascending hydronephrosis caused by the transmission of high pressure to nephrons, which produces renal damage (Fig. 109-2). This can account for abdominal discomfort and flank pain during voiding and ascending urinary tract infections.

Acute urinary retention in BPH can occur as a result of increasing size of the prostate gland. Independent of gland size, drugs may precipitate acute urinary retention. Drugs, such as alcohol, anticholinergic agents, α-adrenergic agents, and neuroleptics, all have been associated with acute urinary retention in men with BPH. Commonly, when advanced BPH is present, acute urinary retention is exacerbated if the patient does not void at the first sign of urgency. G.M. is not taking any drugs commonly associated with urinary retention.

Clinical Findings

G.M. presents with classic symptoms of BPH. The increasingly severe symptoms culminated in an episode of acute urinary retention as evidenced by inability to void and lower abdominal discomfort. Objective symptoms associated with G.M.'s BPH include (a) abdominal tenderness with increased dullness in the hypogastrium; (b) the finding of an enlarged bladder; (c) an enlarged, firm, and rubbery prostate gland; and (d) a return of 900 mL of urine via urinary catheter. The normal serum acid phosphatase, slightly elevated PSA, and digital rectal examination of the prostate suggest that G.M. does not have prostatic carcinoma at this time (see the Prostate-Specific Antigen section later in this chapter). The elevated BUN and SCr may suggest hydronephrosis as a result of his BPH.

Case 109-3, Question 3: What additional tests should be completed to evaluate G.M.?

URINALYSIS

Because patients with BPH also may have a urinary tract infection, a urinalysis with microscopic examination is essential. It is mandatory that G.M. gives a urine specimen for urinalysis before the digital rectal examination of the prostate gland because examination of the prostate causes prostatic secretions to be expelled into the urethra, which may contaminate the urine specimen and make it difficult to determine the source of an infection. The presence of white blood cells and bacteria in the urine necessitates a workup for infection. Similarly, hematuria requires a workup for urinary tract pathology other than BPH. Because BPH also can cause hydronephrosis, renal function and serum electrolytes should be evaluated.

DIGITAL RECTAL EXAMINATION

A serum PSA followed by a digital rectal examination of the prostate remains a fundamental part of evaluating a man with prostatism. The prostate examination should determine the size, shape, consistency, and nodularity of this gland. Prostatic hyperplasia results in a large, palpable prostate with a smooth mucosal surface rectally. The discernment of the right and left prostate lobes is lost in BPH. The digital rectal examination of a patient with BPH commonly finds asymmetry of the prostate, with one side being larger than the other. Prostatic enlargement can be in both an anteroposterior and a superoinferior direction. As a result, on digital rectal examination, the upper extent of prostate hyperplasia is not palpable. Occasionally, the degree of enlargement felt by digital rectal examination may be misleading because a substantial portion of enlargement may be intravesicular. The consistency of the gland may be soft or firm, depending on the predominance of glandular or fibromuscular elements.[72] The presence of firm-to-hard nodules, irregularities, induration, or a stony, hard prostate suggests possible prostate cancer. In those cases in which the prostate gland size or shape may be questioned, the patient should have a transrectal ultrasound (TRUS) to determine the gland volume.

PROSTATE-SPECIFIC ANTIGEN

PSA is a glycoprotein enzyme (molecular weight, 33,000) that is secreted in the cytoplasm of the prostatic cells; it aids in the liquefaction of semen. Some claim that this enzyme is specific for prostate origin, although a few isolated instances of elevation in nonprostate tumors have been reported. PSA correlates reasonably well, on average, with prostate weight owing to benign prostate glandular hyperplasia.[73] Prostate cancer, however, produces approximately 10 times the amount of PSA on a tissue volume basis than does BPH.[74] Men 50 years of age or older have been encouraged to have an annual measurement of serum PSA and a digital rectal examination as a basic screen for prostate cancer and to monitor the growth of the prostate gland. Several investigators have proposed age-adjusted PSA reference ranges, which reflect the size of the prostate gland (Table 109-5).[75–77] Studies have resulted in several formulas that try to adjust the PSA for the effect of BPH. The best-known

Table 109-5
Age-Adjusted Prostate-Specific Antigen Values

Age Range (years)	PSA Upper Limit (ng/mL)	PSA Density
40–49	2.5	0.08
50–59	3.5	0.10
60–69	4.5	0.11
70–79	6.5	0.13

PSA, prostate-specific antigen.

formula for predicting the PSA level (PSA serum density) is as follows[78]:

$$\text{PSA (in ng/mL or mcg/mL)} = 0.12 \times \text{gland volume (in mL by TRUS)} \quad \text{(Eq. 109-1)}$$

$$\text{TRUS gland volume} = \text{prostate height} \times \text{width} \times \text{length} \times 0.523 \quad \text{(Eq. 109-2)}$$

The PSA result for G.M. is slightly above the upper limit for his age. As such, he should have a TRUS to determine the prostate gland volume and, hence, the PSA density. Once the prostate gland volume is determined, the significance of his PSA level of 7.1 ng/mL can be determined.

Drug Therapy

α_1-ADRENERGIC RECEPTOR ANTAGONISTS

CASE 109-3, QUESTION 4: What drug therapy should be prescribed to treat G.M.'s prostatic hyperplasia?

G.M. most likely will be scheduled for a TURP, because he presents with acute urinary retention and hydronephrosis owing to a moderately enlarged prostate gland (i.e., >40 g and <80 g). He should be started and maintained on an α_1-adrenergic receptor antagonist to reduce the tension of the bladder neck, the prostate adenoma, and the prostatic capsule. Similarly, he should receive a 5α-reductase inhibitor to induce atrophy of the prostate gland and halt progression of the disease.

The prostatic capsule and hyperplastic prostate have plentiful α_{1A}-adrenergic receptors. The three known subtypes of the α_1-adrenergic receptor are α_{1A}, α_{1B}, and α_{1D}. Inhibiting the α_{1A}-adrenergic receptors can reduce the smooth muscle tone of the prostatic urethra, thereby reducing the functional component of urethral constriction and obstruction.

Terazosin

Terazosin, a long-acting α_1-adrenergic receptor antagonist, has significantly reduced obstructive symptoms and improved urinary flow rates at doses of 1 to 5 mg/day.[65,79] The α_1-blockade alone does not account for the long-term clinical responses exerted by this drug in the treatment of BPH. Terazosin has been shown to induce prostate smooth muscle cell apoptosis, resulting in reduced urinary symptoms. Terazosin (and doxazosin) has a quinazoline nucleus, which may account for this effect. Tamsulosin, which is not a quinazoline, does not induce prostate smooth muscle cell apoptosis.[80]

In most patients, the dose of terazosin should be started at 1 mg once daily at bedtime and titrated over several weeks to 5 to 10 mg once daily to obtain desired results. Orthostatic hypotension may occur in the beginning days of therapy or during dosage adjustment periods. In patients who stop their terazosin therapy for 2 or more days, therapy should be reinstituted cautiously to avoid the "first-dose" adverse effect of syncope.

Terazosin has demonstrated sustained improvement in BPH symptom scores for a 30-month period. Only 10% of the patients experienced treatment failure.[65] In this long-term study, the systolic blood pressure in normotensive and hypertensive patients was decreased by 4 and 18 mm Hg, respectively. Apparently, terazosin typically only lowered the blood pressure significantly in the hypertensive patients.

Doxazosin

Doxazosin, another quinazoline derivative, is a long-acting α_1-adrenergic receptor antagonist structurally related to prazosin and terazosin (Table 109-3). Prazosin has a relatively short half-life and is not recommended for use in BPH. Doxazosin originally was prescribed primarily for hypertension and currently is not considered a first-line antihypertensive agent. (For a discussion of the current use of α-blockers in hypertension, see Chapter 14, Essential Hypertension.) Hypertension and BPH are linked by the sympathetic nervous system. As with terazosin, doxazosin improves urinary flow rates and symptoms in patients with BPH. These effects have been demonstrated in controlled clinical studies, within weeks, and for the long-term. Doxazosin should be started at 1 mg/day. After 1 to 2 weeks, the dose can be increased over several weeks to 8 mg/day. As with other long-acting α_1-adrenergic receptor antagonists, the first dose should be taken at bedtime to minimize lightheadedness and syncope (the first-dose effect), and the blood pressure of the patient should be monitored periodically during therapy. Most patients require between 4 and 8 mg/day for effective control of the urinary symptoms of BPH. Dosages greater than 4 mg/day are associated with a greater frequency of dizziness, orthostatic hypotension, and syncope.[79,81]

Tamsulosin

Tamsulosin, a nonquinazoline, is a long-acting selective α_{1A}-adrenergic receptor antagonist similar to doxazosin, terazosin, and prazosin. Tamsulosin and its metabolites are more specific for the prostatic α_{1A}-adrenergic and less specific for the vascular α_{1A}-adrenergic receptors responsible for orthostatic hypotension. Consequently, no need exists to titrate tamsulosin to the recommended daily dose range of 0.4 to 0.8 mg. Coadministration of tamsulosin with antihypertensive agents does not require dosage adjustment of the antihypertensives. Tamsulosin is very effective in treating bladder outlet obstruction associated with BPH.[82,83]

More than 90% of tamsulosin is absorbed after oral administration of a 0.4-mg dose under fasting conditions. Administration with food decreases the bioavailability by 30% and increases time to peak plasma concentration. Tamsulosin is hepatically metabolized by CYP3A4 and CYP2D6.[84] Impaired renal function increases the total tamsulosin plasma concentration by approximately 100% during steady state. However, active unbound drug levels are not affected; thus, renal dose adjustment is not required.[85] Tamsulosin appears to reduce mean ejaculatory volume in 90% of patients.[86] As with all α_1-adrenergic receptor antagonists, tamsulosin does not affect the PSA and must be taken indefinitely to maintain its therapeutic effect.[87]

Alfuzosin

Alfuzosin is another quinazoline α_1-adrenergic receptor antagonist. It displays a lower rate of hypotensive effects than doxazosin and terazosin. A lack of penetration of alfuzosin into the brain has been hypothesized to contribute to the decreased CNS effects such as somnolence. Unlike tamsulosin, alfuzosin will not cause ejaculatory dysfunction; the incidence is comparable to placebo.[86] Alfuzosin is available as an extended-release tablet that has a recommended daily dose of 10 mg given after the same meal each day.

Silodosin

Silodosin is another α_1-adrenergic receptor antagonist that is selective for the α_{1A}-receptor in the lower urinary tract. Silodosin has a strong affinity for prostatic tissue and is 20 times more "uroselective" than tamsulosin.[88] However, the only study comparing silodosin with tamsulosin was a noninferiority trial which found silodosin to be as effective as tamsulosin in controlling lower urinary tract symptoms in men with BPH.[89] The most common side effect with silodosin is retrograde ejaculation, reported in 21% of patients in an open-label extension study.[90] Silodosin is available as 4- and 8-mg capsules, and the recommended dose is 8 mg once daily. In patients with a creatinine clearance of less than 50 mL/minute, the dose should be decreased to 4 mg once daily.

PHOSPHODIESTERASE-5 INHIBITORS

Tadalafil

Tadalafil is a selective inhibitor of phosphodiesterase-5 and has indications for erectile dysfunction and use as monotherapy or combination therapy in BPH. Its mechanism in BPH is unclear; however, compared to placebo, tadalafil 5 mg once daily was shown to improve BPH symptoms compared to placebo. Combining tadalafil with α-adrenergic receptor antagonists is not recommended because it has not been adequately studied and may increase the risk of low blood pressure. Similarly, patients on antihypertensives, nitrates, or drinking 5 or more units of alcohol are also at increased risk of hypotension with tadalafil. Tadalafil should be taken at the same time every day without regard to meals. Additional information on tadalafil can be found under pharmacotherapy for erectile dysfunction later in this chapter.

ANDROGEN SUPPRESSION

Maintenance of morphology and functional activity of the adult human prostate is controlled by, and dependent on, androgens. Prostatic regression after androgen deprivation is an active process that requires the synthesis of macromolecules.[91] As a result of androgen deprivation, the loss of stromal and epithelial prostate cells is disproportionate, with 4 times greater loss of epithelial cells. Testosterone serves as the prohormone for the two active metabolites, DHT and 17-β-estradiol. Testosterone is metabolized to DHT by the enzyme 5α-reductase (types 1 and 2). Thus, conversion of testosterone to DHT precludes its conversion to estrogen by the aromatase enzyme, and the relative activity of these two enzymes is of paramount importance in prostate homeostasis.[92]

Although the mean plasma testosterone level in men falls after the age of 60, the level of testosterone in subjects with BPH and age-matched control subjects is not different.[93] Moreover, the onset of BPH starts some 10 to 20 years before the plasma testosterone levels decrease. The serum concentration of DHT is increased, however, in men with BPH.[91,94,95] The mechanism responsible for accumulation of DHT has not been established, but a significant increase in 5α-reductase activity occurs, which is known to produce DHT.[96,97]

One other major hormonal change associated with aging is the increased formation of estrogen from circulating androgens in both the testes and the peripheral adipose tissue. Androgen conversion to estrogen via aromatase begins in men at approximately the third decade of life and increases with age,[98] but the plasma estrogen concentration is the same in men with BPH and age-matched control subjects without BPH.[94] Estrogen receptors are abundant in stroma cells,[99,100] more so in patients with prostatic carcinoma than in patients with BPH.[101] Estrogen stimulation of stromal tissue was once believed to explain the prostatic growth that continued with age despite the decline in testosterone secretion by the testes. Progesterone receptors, however, appear to be more abundant than estrogen receptors in the stromal and epithelial cells of prostate tissue of patients with BPH. Thus, progesterone may play a more important role in the pathogenesis of BPH than estrogen. The known effect of DHT in initiating the BPH process is believed to be augmented by estrogen.[102] The number of prostate androgen receptors can be increased by estrogens and can be reversed by the administration of antiestrogens.[93] The increase in androgen receptors induced by estrogens may allow for continued androgen-mediated growth despite the declining amount of testosterone produced with advancing age.

5α-REDUCTASE INHIBITORS

Finasteride

Finasteride, a competitive inhibitor of 5α-reductase (type 2), decreases the conversion of testosterone to DHT, the principal androgen responsible for stimulation of prostatic growth. After 7 days of treatment with all doses of finasteride, prostatic tissue DHT declined to 15% or less of control levels, and the testosterone concentration increased in a reciprocal manner.[103] When finasteride was administered in 1- and 5-mg doses to men with BPH for a total of 12 months, the symptom score and urinary flow improved significantly. Finasteride 5 mg daily decreased the median prostate volume by 24% and improved the maximal urinary flow rate by 2.9 mL/second.[104] Adverse effects in the finasteride groups occurred in less than 5%, and side effects, such as decreased libido and ejaculatory dysfunction, were dose related.[105] The efficacy of daily finasteride 5 mg was evaluated in 298 men for 24 months and found a slight improvement compared with the results reported at the end of the 12-month period.[106] The median DHT levels had declined by 74.5% compared with 69.3% at 12 months, and prostate volume declined by 25.2% compared with 21.2% at 12 months. Patient symptom scores indicated slightly more improvement at 24 months compared with 12 months. Obstructive symptom scores were responsible for most of the improved symptoms reported. The prevalence of sexual adverse experiences at 24 months was similar to that at 12 months. In those men who experienced finasteride-induced sexual dysfunction, 50% will experience resolution after discontinuing the medication.[107] Inhibition of DHT by 5α-reductase inhibitors does not affect testosterone-mediated functions on muscle mass, libido, or spermatogenesis. Thus, finasteride has an acceptable safety profile, halts disease progression, and improves the quality of life in patients with moderate BPH disease (i.e., enlarged prostate with symptoms of urinary obstruction, but not acute urinary retention). Finasteride improves objective pressure flow parameters after 1 year of therapy, and efficacy appears to be greatest in patients with large prostates ($>$40 g).[108] For those who do respond, the drug must be continued indefinitely because DHT serum concentrations return to pretreatment levels within 14 days of discontinuing finasteride, and prostate size returns to pretreatment levels within 4 months.[109,110]

Unlike leuprolide, finasteride does not affect the histologic features of BPH and prostate cancer.[111] Morphologic evaluation of patients treated with finasteride with symptomatic BPH having adenectomy showed a reduction in the size of the prostate and an increase in the stroma to epithelial and stroma to lumen ratios.[112]

Dutasteride

Dutasteride is a competitive inhibitor of both types 1 and 2 5α-reductase isoenzymes. An advantage of dutasteride compared with finasteride is the additional inhibition of 5α-reductase (type 1) in the peripheral tissues, which produces a further decline in serum DHT. In a prospective study of 2,951 men with moderate-to-severe BPH, dutasteride 0.5 mg/day decreased DHT serum levels by 90% at 1 month in 58% of patients. At 24 months, 85% of those treated with dutasteride were noted to have a 90% reduction of serum DHT.[113] Correspondingly, the patients noted reduction in urinary symptoms as early as 3 months after treatment initiation and a significant ($p < 0.001$) reduction in symptoms by the sixth month when compared with those treated with placebo. Common side effects of dutasteride are similar to those of finasteride: impotence (4.7%), decreased libido (3.0%), ejaculation disorder (1.4%), and gynecomastia (1.0%).

Combination Therapy

Owing to different mechanisms of action, it is a reasonable strategy to combine an α_1-adrenergic receptor antagonist that will work quickly to provide symptomatic relief with a 5α-reductase inhibitor that will take 6 to 12 months to reduce prostate size.

This strategy has been supported by the Medical Therapy of Prostate Symptoms (MTOPS) and Combination of Avodart and Tamsulosin (CombAT) trials. The MTOPS trial studied 3,047 men with moderate-to-severe BPH and demonstrated that combination therapy was superior to monotherapy with either an α-blocker or a 5α-reductase inhibitor in improving symptoms and urinary flow rate. The risk of clinical progression of BPH was reduced by 39% in patients treated with doxazosin alone, by 34% in patients treated with finasteride alone, and by 66% in patients treated with combination therapy.[114] The CombAT trial studied 4,844 men with risk factors for BPH progression such as larger prostates (>30 g) and higher serum PSA concentrations (1.5–10 mcg/L). Combination therapy reduced the relative risk of acute urinary retention or BPH-related surgery by 65.8% compared with tamsulosin and by 19.6% compared with dutasteride. In addition, for those patients who completed the study, the mean change in the International Prostate Symptom Score from baseline to year 4 was significantly higher for the combination therapy compared with tamsulosin or dutasteride alone.[115] Adverse drug events are more common with combination therapy, but study withdrawal rates are less than 5% and similar among treatment groups. A combination product of dutasteride 0.5 mg and tamsulosin hydrochloride 0.4 mg is commercially available.

Effect of Androgen Suppression on Prostate-Specific Antigen

CASE 109-3, QUESTION 5: G.M. has an annual PSA test. Will androgen suppression alter his results?

Antiandrogen treatment of BPH could possibly adversely affect the interpretation of the PSA screening test for prostate cancer. For example, androgen suppression with leuprolide acetate reduces prostate volume primarily by inducing involution of the epithelial elements of the prostate.[116] Because PSA primarily is produced by the epithelial cells of the prostate, these drugs can alter serum and prostate concentrations of PSA.[117] Finasteride 5 mg/day also can reduce the serum PSA level by 50%.[118] Dutasteride reduces total serum PSA by approximately 40% after 3 months of treatment and by approximately 50% after 24 months.[119] The serum PSA level reduction is predictable, however, and serum PSA levels can be recalculated during hormonal treatment for BPH. Nevertheless, patients receiving a 5α-reductase inhibitor should have (a) a digital rectal examination of their prostate periodically, (b) a PSA level measured, and (c) any suspicious findings investigated immediately.[106] Androgen suppression therapy is not contraindicated in BPH solely on the basis of its effect on serum PSA levels.[65]

CASE 109-3, QUESTION 6: G.M asks whether there are nonprescription treatments available that are effective for BPH. What over-the-counter medications are available for prostate disorders?

Two agents, saw palmetto and pygeum, have been promoted for the treatment of BPH. Saw palmetto is an herbal product obtained from the fruit of the *Serenoa repens* tree with antiandrogen activity. The active ingredients are phytosterols; β-sitosterol and β-sitosterol-3-*O*-glucosides are the most abundant. Several trials have shown that it significantly improves BPH symptoms[119–122] to a degree similar to finasteride.[123] However, a 2012 meta-analysis of 32 randomized trials failed to detect a difference in urinary symptom improvement even with triple the usual dose of saw palmetto compared to placebo.[124] The dose most often studied is 320 mg a day in one or two divided doses. Pygeum (*Pygeum africanum* bark extract) has been observed to moderately reduce urinary symptoms associated with enlargement of the prostate gland at a dose of 75 to 200 mg/day.[125] Pygeum has been well tolerated in most studies; however, the safety has not been extensively or systematically studied. Herbal products may be tried by men with mild symptoms that would usually be managed by watchful waiting; however, the use of complementary and alternative medicines for BPH is not currently recommended by the AUA guidelines.[126]

Nonpharmacologic Treatment

TRANSURETHRAL RESECTION OF THE PROSTATE

CASE 109-3, QUESTION 7: What are the options if drug therapy does not work for G.M.? When should prostate surgery be undertaken in general?

G.M.'s subjective and objective findings, particularly the acute urinary retention and hydronephrosis, collectively indicate the need for a TURP. G.M. has been advised by his urologist that a TURP is the treatment of choice given the severity of his presentation (e.g., large prostate gland with acute urinary retention) and that the procedure will relieve his symptoms, allow him to lead a relatively normal life, and avoid sequelae of prolonged obstruction.

TURP provides significant relief of BPH symptoms in 86%, 83%, 75%, and 75% of patients at 3 months, 1 year, 3 years, and 7 years, respectively.[127] Of patients with severe BPH, 93% report reduced symptoms 1 year after a TURP.[128] The TURP is considered the gold standard for the treatment of BPH and is used in 90% of patients with symptoms of residual urine or acute urinary retention.[61] As a result, surgical alternatives are always compared with the outcome studies of TURP.

The need for a TURP in G.M.'s situation is fairly clear. In most cases, however, the need for a TURP is less clear because the symptoms do not inevitably worsen and men often are willing to live with their symptoms. Therefore, clinicians need to talk with patients and help them answer the question of whether the discomfort, risk, and problems during the postsurgical recovery period are outweighed by the high probability that surgery will relieve symptoms.

SEXUAL DYSFUNCTION

As individuals are living longer, there is a growing interest in maintaining one's sexual health throughout later life. Nearly 39% of men and 17% of women between the ages of 75 and 85 reported being sexually active in a cross-sectional study published in 2010.[129] A nationally representative study concluded that the majority of older adults are engaged in sexual activity and regard sex as an important part of life.[130] Poor health often is cited by elderly women as a reason for not participating in sexual activity, and among men, erectile dysfunction (ED) is the leading cause of decline in activity.[131,132] The major factors that correlate with reduced sexual activity include an older spouse, poor mental or physical health, marital difficulties, previous negative sexual experiences, and negative attitudes toward sexuality in the aged.[133] During the postmenopausal years, women undergo substantial physiologic changes (see Chapter 51, The Transition Through Menopause).

The major physiologic event of natural menopause is a decrease in estrogen production. Little doubt exists that a decline in estrogen production is associated with many of the physiologic changes causing elderly women to report a low interest in sexual activity. The medical literature is replete with research and data on elderly male sexual dysfunction, but little, if any, data exist on female sexual dysfunction.

Male Sexual Dysfunction

Aging men may experience andropause, a syndrome consisting of weakness, fatigue, reduced muscle and bone mass, impaired hematopoiesis, oligospermia, sexual dysfunction, and psychiatric symptoms.[134] The relationship between declining testosterone and andropause is not firmly established. Free testosterone levels begin to decline at the rate of 1% per year after age 40 years. By the age of 60 years, 20% of men have levels below the lower limit of normal.[135] The physiologic and psychological effects of declining hormone levels in men are less dramatic than those experienced by women.

Sexual function is considered an interaction between motivation, drive, desires, thoughts, fantasies, pleasures, experiences (referred to as the *libido*), penile vasocongestion, erection, orgasmic contractions, and ejaculations (referred to as *potency*).[136,137] Testosterone plays an important role in male libido and sexual behavior and may play some role in penile erection. Elderly men show a strong correlation between advancing age and diminishing bioavailable serum testosterone levels.[138] Testosterone progressively declines after the seventh decade, partly because of testicular and hypothalamic–pituitary dysfunction.[139]

Male sexual dysfunction, denoting the inability to achieve a satisfactory sexual relationship, may involve inadequacy of erection or problems with emission, ejaculation, or orgasm. *Erectile dysfunction* is the inability to achieve and maintain a firm erection sufficient for satisfactory sexual performance.[140] *Premature ejaculation* refers to uncontrolled ejaculation before or shortly after entering the vagina. *Retarded ejaculation* usually is synonymous with delayed ejaculation. *Retrograde ejaculation* denotes backflow of semen into the bladder during ejaculation caused by an incompetent bladder neck mechanism.

ED, once regarded as a psychosocial disorder, today is regarded as caused by a variety of medical, psychological, and lifestyle factors. It is an age-related condition, with about 30% of US men older than 40 years of age self-reporting some degree of ED in 2011.[141] Because the population ages, it is estimated that the worldwide prevalence of ED will be approximately 322 million in 2025.[142]

Approximately 80% of all cases of ED now are thought to be related to organic disease and subject to numerous influences.[136,143–145] In one study, neurologic and vascular disorders were the primary causes of ED among elderly men, and psychogenic factors were the cause in less than 10%.[138] The single most common etiology for erectile failure in the elderly is severe atherosclerosis (e.g., vascular disease and diabetes mellitus).[138] Cardiovascular disease, hypertension, diabetes mellitus, elevated low-density lipoprotein cholesterol, and cigarette smoking are associated with a greater probability of complete ED in men.[146] Therefore, prevention of cardiovascular disorders by interventions such as low-fat and low-cholesterol diets and abstinence from tobacco should minimize the development of ED.

Because ED is more likely in male patients with coronary artery disease, the understanding of the cardiovascular stresses involved with sexual intercourse can aid in patient management. Cardiac and metabolic expenditures during sexual intercourse vary depending on the type of sexual activity. Healthy males with their usual female partners generally achieve a peak heart rate of 110 beats/minute with woman-on-top coitus and an average peak heart rate of 127 beats/minute with man-on-top coitus.[147] There is significant individual variation in cardiovascular response, when measured as oxygen uptake and metabolic expenditures, for man-on-top coitus.

In a study of medication-free patients with coronary artery disease who were in New York Heart Association functional class I or II, sexual activity was compared with near-maximal exercise treadmill test.[148] Electrocardiographic changes representing ischemia during intercourse were found in one-third of the patients; however, two-thirds of these patients remained asymptomatic. All patients with ischemia during coitus also demonstrated ischemia during exercise treadmill testing. The average heart rate during coitus was 118 beats/minute, with some patients attaining a heart rate of 185 beats/minute at orgasm. Intercourse in patients with coronary artery disease may provoke increased ventricular ectopic activity that is not necessarily elicited by other stimuli.[149] These electrocardiographic changes and associated symptoms can be abolished with the use of β-blockers.[150] Sexual activity is a likely contributor to the onset of myocardial infarction only 0.9% of the time.[151] Coital death is rare, accounting for 0.6% of sudden death cases.[152] The hemodynamic changes associated with sexual activity may be far greater with an unfamiliar partner, in unfamiliar settings, and after excessive eating and alcohol consumption.

Erectile Dysfunction

PATHOGENESIS

Erection involves the neurologic, psychological, hormonal, arterial, and venous systems. Evidence indicates that more than 80% of the cases of ED are because of organic causes, of which vascular disease is the most common.[153] In most elderly male sexual dysfunction studies, 50% involve vascular problems, and 30% relate to diabetes mellitus.[154]

Neurogenic Disorders

ED can be caused by damage to the brain, spinal cord, cavernous or pudendal nerves, terminal nerve endings, and the receptors. Approximately 95% of patients with upper motor neuron lesions resulting from spinal injury are capable of erection through the reflexogenic mechanism,[155] whereas only 25% of patients with complete lower motor neuron lesions can have erections through the psychogenic mechanism.[155] With incomplete lesions, up to 90% of patients in both groups retain erectile ability. Patients who have a cerebrovascular accident, dementia, epilepsy, Parkinson disease, or a brain tumor most likely experience erectile failure through loss of sexual interest or overinhibition of the spinal erection centers.[156]

Hormonal Disorders

The incidence of ED with a hormonal cause has been estimated to be 5% to 35%, depending on which medical specialty is reporting the finding.[157] The most common hormonal disorder associated with ED in the elderly is diabetes mellitus. Depending on the severity and duration of diabetes, the prevalence of ED ranges from 20% to 85%.[158]

Other hormonal disorders, such as hypothyroidism, hyperthyroidism, Addison disease, and Cushing syndrome, are associated with ED. Patients with hypogonadism caused by pituitary or hypothalamic tumors, antiandrogen therapy, or orchiectomy experience ED. These patients can have a normal erection from visual stimulation, however, indicating that the erectile mechanism is intact.[159]

Vascular Disorders

Atherosclerosis is the leading vascular disease associated with male ED. The age of onset of coronary artery disease parallels the onset of ED, indicating a generalized atherosclerotic etiology for the ED.[160] The degree of arteriolar narrowing and clinical presentation, however, differ from patient to patient. Some patients can have severe coronary artery disease but retain the capability of a full erection. As long as the arterial flow into the penis exceeds the venous outflow, the patient can be potent. Narrowing of the arterial lumen lowers pressure in the cavernous arteries, and poor arterial flow can only partially fill the sinusoidal system. Overall, the partial filling of the sinusoidal system causes inadequate expansion of the sinusoidal wall, resulting in partial compression of the venules. The net effect is a partial erection, difficulty in maintaining an erection, or the most common complaint, early detumescence.

SIGNS AND SYMPTOMS

CASE 109-4

QUESTION 1: F.M., a 66-year-old man, was referred to an urologist because he was experiencing a loss of interest in sexual activity. He describes the inability to maintain a firm erection for the past 6 months in more than 75% of sexual attempts with his sexual partner. Physical examination was unremarkable except for an enlarged prostate gland and evidence of pubic and axillary hair loss. Vital signs were as follows:

Blood pressure, 160/95 mm Hg
Pulse, 88 beats/minute
Respirations, 14 breaths/minute
Temperature, 98.7°F

Current medications include ramipril 5 mg once a day and glipizide 5 mg once daily. F.M.'s medical history is positive for cigarette smoking, hypertension, and diabetes mellitus. Significant laboratory results include the following:

Random blood sugar, 200 mg/dL
SCr, 1.5 mg/dL
BUN, 22 mg/dL
Free testosterone level, 30 pg/mL (normal, 52–280 pg/mL)
Luteinizing hormone (LH), 4 milliunits/mL (normal, 1–8 milliunits/mL)
Follicle-stimulating hormone (FSH) level, 40 milli-international units/mL (normal, 4–25 milli-international units/mL)
Serum prolactin level, 28 ng/mL (normal, <20 ng/mL)

What signs and symptoms does F.M. have that would suggest the need for a complete medical workup for ED?

F.M. presents with the complaint of loss of interest in sexual activity and the inability to maintain a full erection during greater than 75% of sexual encounters with his partner. On physical examination, F.M. is found to have a noticeable loss of pubic and axillary body hair. With long-standing androgen deficiency, there may be loss of hair in the androgen-dependent areas of the body, fine wrinkling of the skin around the mouth and eyes, noticeable loss of muscle mass and strength, altered body-fat distribution, and osteoporosis. In contrast, overt hypogonadism results in a change in the pattern of pubic hair from the male diamond shape to the female-inverted triangle appearance. At this point, it appears that F.M.'s loss of pubic and axillary hair is the result of androgen deficiency, with the cause yet to be determined. The laboratory results for gonadal function coincide with what is expected in an elderly man with ED (see Case 109-4, Question 4).

UROLOGIC WORKUP

CASE 109-4, QUESTION 2: What clinical evaluations and laboratory tests should be included in the medical workup of F.M. to determine the cause of his ED?

A detailed medical and sexual history and thorough physical examination are essential in the evaluation of sexual dysfunction. General medical history and physical examination should consider drug-induced ED (Table 109-6).[161–178]

Although laboratory-based diagnostic procedures are available, sexual function may be best assessed in a naturalistic setting with patient self-report techniques. A psychometrically sound self-reporting tool is the International Index of Erectile Function (IIEF), which addresses the relevant domains of male sexual function (erectile function, orgasmic function, sexual desire, intercourse satisfaction, and overall satisfaction) and has been linguistically validated in 10 languages.[179] A simplified version, the IIEF-5, is a five-item questionnaire that is also popular.[180]

F.M.'s endocrine status should include assessment of his diabetes, thyroid function tests, and a serum lipid profile. Neuropathy and atherosclerosis are common findings among male patients with diabetes mellitus, and both are potential causes of ED. Patients experiencing hypothyroidism may have decreased libido, and hypothyroidism is associated with hyperprolactinemia, which can result in an inhibition in the release of testosterone. Elevated serum lipids (e.g., total cholesterol, triglycerides) may be associated with significant vascular damage that could contribute to erectile dysfunction. Diabetes mellitus is best evaluated with hemoglobin-A_{1c} and fasting blood glucose tests.[181]

The serum concentrations of free testosterone, prolactin, and LH should be evaluated. Testosterone, as with all other hormones secreted into the plasma, is available to tissues only in the free form (i.e., unbound to serum proteins, particularly the sex hormone-binding globulin). Only 1% to 2% of testosterone is free and physiologically active; therefore, measurement of the unbound serum testosterone provides the best estimate of biologically available testosterone. Low testosterone serum concentrations are associated with primary and secondary hypogonadism. Primary hypogonadism is associated with testicular disease (e.g., Leydig cell tumors), whereas secondary hypogonadism is the result of pituitary or hypothalamic disease.

The serum prolactin concentration should be determined because a high serum concentration of prolactin inhibits release of testosterone from the testes. Therefore, a low serum testosterone concentration may be caused by hyperprolactinemia. Hyperprolactinemia may be caused by prolactin adenomas, diabetes mellitus, or drug therapy (e.g., neuroleptics, metoclopramide).

LH stimulates testicular steroidogenesis and secretion of testosterone. LH increases the conversion of cholesterol to pregnenolone, a precursor of testosterone. FSH is required for spermatogenesis in early puberty, but is not a required gonadotropin for the maintenance of spermatogenesis in adult men. Normal testicular function depends on stimulation by the gonadotropin LH, which is secreted by the anterior pituitary gland. Consequently, a low normal serum concentration of LH is associated with secondary hypogonadism.

In patients with symptoms of prostatic disease, expressed prostatic secretions (EPS) should be examined because prostate

Table 109-6
Common Drug-Induced Alterations in Sexual Response

Drug Categories	Clinical Considerations
Antihypertensives	
Diuretic thiazides	Temporal association with sexual dysfunction. Reported incidence varies between 0% and 32%[161–164]; however, impotence generally is not considered common. Mechanism believed to be a "steal syndrome" whereby blood is routed from erectile tissues to skeletal muscle.[165]
Spironolactone	Associated with ↓ libido, impotence, and gynecomastia. Mechanism may be hormone related. Incidence is dose related and reported to be 5%–67%[165] and much more commonly encountered than with the thiazides. May be owing to antiandrogen effects of drug.
Sympatholytics	
Methyldopa	Central action mediated causing vasodilation resulting in erectile dysfunction. Reported incidence: 10%.[146,165] Also ↓ libido.
Clonidine	Induces erectile dysfunction. Mechanism similar to methyldopa and other central α_2-agonists. Incidence reported to be 4%–70% and dose related.[166–168] Also ↓ libido.
Guanabenz, guanfacine	Incidence and mechanism believed to be similar to other central α_2-agonists.
Nonselective β-Blockers	
Propranolol	Associated with erectile dysfunction and ↓ libido. Mechanism believed to be caused by ↓ vascular resistance and central effects. Erectile dysfunction reported to begin at doses of 120 mg/day. Incidence may be as high as 100% at higher dosages.[146,169,170]
Selective β-Blockers	
Atenolol, metoprolol, pindolol, timolol	Incidence of erectile dysfunction is significantly less than nonselective β-blockers.[171]
α-Blockers	
Doxazosin, prazosin, terazosin	Associated with erectile dysfunction and priapism.[146,167] Reported incidence: 0.6%–4%.[146] Mechanism is local α_1-blockade resulting in vasodilation. Erectile dysfunction and priapism appear to be unique to the nonspecific α_1-antagonists.
Phenoxybenzamine	Associated with priapism, retrograde ejaculation, and inhibited emissions during erection. Effects are dose related.[172,173]
Direct Vasodilators	
Hydralazine	Associated with erectile dysfunction. Mechanism is vascular smooth muscle relaxation. Incidence not reported.[172]
Calcium-Channel Blockers	
Nifedipine	Associated with erectile dysfunction. Mechanism believed to be vasodilation and possibly muscle relaxation. Reported incidence: <2%.[174]
Diltiazem, verapamil	Similar to nifedipine. Reported incidence: <1%.
Antiarrhythmics	
Class 1A Disopyramide	Associated with erectile dysfunction in patients treated for ventricular arrhythmias. Incidence not reported. Mechanism believed to be caused by strong anticholinergic effect.[165,172]
Anticonvulsants	
Carbamazepine, phenytoin	May be associated with sexual dysfunction through decreasing DHEA, which is a precursor to testosterone, estrogen, and pheromones.[19]
Antidepressants	
Selective serotonin reuptake inhibitors	Drugs with prominent serotonin agonist effects commonly cause delayed ejaculation and anorgasmia. The reported incidence for delayed ejaculation among men is 2% to 12%; for anorgasmia among women users, the incidence appears to be <3%. This adverse effect is directly dose related.[19]
Tricyclic antidepressants, monoamine oxidase inhibitors	Associated with impairment of sexual performance in both male and female: ↓ libido, anorgasmia, retrograde ejaculation, erectile dysfunction. Mechanism believed to be caused by anticholinergic and serotonergic effects. Incidence not reported; several case studies in the literature.[165]
Trazodone	Associated with priapism in men and ↑ libido in women. Mechanism similar to TCA. Incidence not reported but believed to be dose related.[165] (Note: The literature reports that overall there is less sexual dysfunction with desipramine than with other antidepressants.)

(continued)

Table 109-6
Common Drug-Induced Alterations in Sexual Response

Drug Categories	Clinical Considerations
Antipsychotics	
Phenothiazines	Frequently associated with sexual dysfunction. Commonly, ↓ libido is reported. Mechanism is owing to hyperprolactinemia secondary to central dopamine antagonism. Thioridazine is the most often reported offender. Erectile and ejaculatory pain are very common with this drug class; the α-antagonism and anticholinergic effects are responsible. Priapism is common with this drug group, owing to the peripheral α-blockade property. Incidence for all sexual dysfunctions with this drug class: approximately 50% of users.[165]
Anxiolytics	
Short-acting barbiturates	Biphasic effect. At low doses, libido ↑, similar to ethanol, and at higher doses, CNS depression causes ↓ libido and performance.[165]
Benzodiazepines	Biphasic effect. At low doses, ↑ libido, whereas at higher dosages, CNS depression causes performance failure. Some reports of anorgasmia (men and women) and ejaculatory failure.[165]
Substances of Abuse	
Alcohol	Alcohol is thought to impair sexual function through its chronic effects on the nervous system. Short-term use of alcohol can induce erectile dysfunction through its sedative effects. More than 600 mL/week of alcohol increases the probability of erectile dysfunction.[175] At low doses, it actually may enhance libido. Sexual dysfunction is dose related and caused by CNS depressant effects.[146,165]
Cocaine	Biphasic effect. At low doses, there is enhanced sexual desire (similar to amphetamines) and possibly performance. At higher dosages, there may be arousal dysfunction, ejaculatory dysfunction, and anorgasmia. Freebasing has been associated with spontaneous orgasm. Continued use (on a run) causes significant loss of sexual interest and performance ability. Chronic use associated with hyperprolactinemia resulting in ↓ libido.[165]
Hallucinogens	Biphasic effect for most drugs in this category. At low doses, libido is enhanced; at higher doses, libido is severely ↓. No reports on chronic use.[165]
Marijuana	Biphasic effect similar to ethanol. With chronic use there is a ↓ in libido. Mechanism may be owing to ↓ testosterone. Incidence not reported.[165]
Opioids	Associated with sexual dysfunction: erection lubrication, orgasm, and ejaculation. Chronic use associated with ↓ libido. Mechanism may be owing to α-antagonism, alterations in testosterone, and the intoxicating effects. Incidence not reported.[146,176,177]
Miscellaneous	
Amyl nitrate	Associated with intense and prolonged orgasms in both men and women. Impotence has been reported in some cases owing to vasodilation.[165]
Cimetidine, ranitidine	Associated with ↓ libido and erectile dysfunction. Mechanism owing to antiandrogen qualities and drug-induced elevation of prolactin. May be dose related.[146,178]
Metoclopramide	Associated with ↓ libido and erectile dysfunction. Mechanism is through CNS dopamine antagonism, resulting in hyperprolactinemia. Incidence not reported.[146]

CNS, central nervous system; DHEA, dehydroepiandrosterone; TCA, tricyclic antidepressants.

inflammation has been associated with ejaculatory dysfunction. During prostatic inflammation, the EPS contains leukocytes and macrophages, and microscopic examination of the EPS can determine the degree of prostate inflammation. The presence of greater than 20 white blood cells per high-powered field in the EPS is abnormal and indicative of prostatitis. Only about 5% of prostatitis can be attributed to a bacterial infection; the remaining 95% is caused by unknown etiologies.

Ideally, assessment of ED should include urologic, endocrinologic, psychiatric, and neurologic evaluations as close together as possible. The chief complaint of ED must be identified carefully and described because medical intervention is indicated if it occurs for a 6-month period and in greater than 50% of attempts.[144] A detailed history should determine whether ED varies with partners, sexual settings, position, and masturbation, and whether morning and nocturnal erections are impaired.

RELATIONSHIP OF MEDICAL HISTORY AND ERECTILE DYSFUNCTION

CASE 109-4, QUESTION 3: What is the relationship among hypertension, cigarette smoking, diabetes mellitus, and F.M.'s ED?

Hypertension

In the Massachusetts Male Aging Study (MMAS), heart disease with hypertension and low serum high-density lipoprotein correlated with ED.[136] The hemodynamics of erection can be impaired in patients with myocardial infarction, coronary artery bypass surgery, cerebrovascular accidents, and peripheral vascular disease.[182–185] In several studies of impotent men, the number of abnormal penile vascular findings significantly increased when the history included hypertension and cigarette smoking. Control of blood pressure among hypertensive male patients does not necessarily improve erectile function, and antihypertensive medications can have a significant effect on ED and sexual performances (Table 109-6).[186–188]

Cigarette Smoking

The prevalence of cigarette smoking among men with ED is higher than in the general population.[189–191] When the relation between cigarette smoking and erectile physiology was studied in 314 men with ED,[192] smoking was noted to further compromise penile physiology in men experiencing difficulty maintaining erections long enough for satisfactory intercourse. Several investigators report lower penile blood pressure indices, penile arterial insufficiency, and abnormal blood perfusion associated with cigarette smoking.[189,193] Clearly, smoking cessation may benefit men with existing ED.

Diabetes Mellitus

Diabetes mellitus has been associated with ED. In the MMAS, male patients with diabetes mellitus were 3 times more likely to have ED than patients without diabetes.[136] Other investigators using exclusively diabetic populations have found a prevalence of ED as high as 75% among subjects.[194,195] The onset of ED in the diabetic patient occurs at an earlier age when compared with the general population. In a few cases, it may be the presenting symptom of diabetes mellitus, and in most cases, ED follows within 10 years of the diagnosis, regardless of insulin dependence status.[196,197] Researchers disagree as to the exact contribution of diabetes mellitus to ED, but most of the literature supports an atherosclerotic etiology.[198,199] Other possible causes also include autonomic neuropathy and gonadal dysfunction.[198]

GONADAL FUNCTION IN ERECTILE DYSFUNCTION

Case 109-4, Question 4: What is the significance of the gonadal function results for F.M.?

Gonadotropins

Abnormalities of primary or secondary hypogonadism must be ruled out, particularly in patients with a decreased libido with or without ED. The results of F.M.'s gonadal function tests are relatively normal for an aged male. Testosterone serum levels decline with aging as a result of hypothalamic–pituitary changes or Leydig cell dysfunction. The understanding of changes that take place in the hypothalamic–pituitary level with advancing age is in a state of flux. For some time, most investigators focused on the increased serum concentration of male gonadotropins (LH, FSH), believing that all elderly men had some degree of primary hypogonadism.[200] Other studies have shown, however, that LH levels in elderly men are lower than the median of those in younger patients.[174] These findings show that LH levels do not increase in response to the decrease in testosterone serum concentrations in the aged male, indicating a defect in the hypothalamic–pituitary axis, leading to secondary hypogonadism.[201] Secondary hypogonadism results when there is a dysregulation of pituitary LH release, resulting in low serum testosterone levels.[156]

Testicular Size and Aging

Testicular size decreases with age; however, the testicular degeneration is sporadic, thereby allowing most elderly men to maintain a normal or slightly decreased sperm output.[200] Overall, spermatogenesis decreases and is accompanied by an increase in serum concentration of FSH. FSH elevation correlates well with a decline in the number of Sertoli cells that secrete inhibin. Inhibin normally decreases FSH.[202]

Testosterone

As a result of primary or secondary hypogonadism in the elderly male, available testosterone declines. Approximately 60% to 75% of circulating serum testosterone is bound to a β-globulin known as sex hormone-binding globulin or testosterone-binding globulin. Approximately 20% to 40% of testosterone is bound to serum albumin, and 1% to 2% is unbound, or free. The unbound portion of testosterone is the only active portion of the total serum testosterone concentration. Testosterone serum concentrations are 20% higher in the morning than in the evening, and this should be taken into consideration when evaluating laboratory results. In virtually all cases of ED, the serum concentration of testosterone should be measured in the morning.

Testosterone production is regulated by feedback with the hypothalamus and pituitary. The hypothalamus produces gonadotropin-releasing hormone (GnRH) in response to low testosterone levels. GnRH induces the pituitary to secrete LH and FSH, which in turn stimulates the Leydig cells of the testes to secrete testosterone. Less than 10% of cases of ED studied are caused strictly by hypogonadism.[138,203] The role of testosterone in ED is complex. After testosterone production decreases, libido eventually declines and precedes the decrease in frequency of erections.[204] Men given antiandrogens maintain their erectile capacity but have a decreased libido.[205] On the other hand, high dosages of androgens given to hypogonadal men increase both the frequency of erections and libido.[206] It would seem reasonable to postulate that at physiologic levels, testosterone modulates the cognitive processes associated with sexual arousal more than it contributes to erectile capability.

Endocrine Disorders

Many endocrine disorders can result in ED. Patients with prolactinomas commonly have ED, but prolactinomas account for less than 1% of ED cases.[169] Prolactin inhibits the release of testosterone, resulting in secondary hypogonadism. Hyperprolactinemia may be more prevalent in diabetic patients.[207] In the elderly, however, hyperprolactinemia often is secondary to the use of medications. F.M.'s serum prolactin level is elevated, most likely because of his diabetes mellitus.

In summary, aged men have a decrease in testosterone because of defects in testicular and hypothalamic–pituitary function. Secondary hypogonadism in elderly men is common, and the point at which this becomes pathologic has not yet been established. Correspondingly, the use of hormonal therapy to treat physiologic secondary hypogonadism is extremely controversial. Therefore, the gonadal function tests for F.M. are normal for his age and do not provide an explanation for his ED.

MEDICATIONS THAT CAUSE ERECTILE DYSFUNCTION

Case 109-4, Question 5: Is it likely that a medication is causing F.M.'s ED?

Several general statements can be made regarding sexual function and medications. Drugs that affect libido generally have a central mode of action. For example, medications that block central dopamine transmission can decrease libido, and opiates have an antiandrogen effect.[176] Drugs that alter hemodynamics may interfere with erection. Excessive sympathetic tone is thought to cause the "steal syndrome," which increases blood flow to muscles, drawing blood away from the erectile tissue.[165] Drugs that block the peripheral sympathetic system can cause retrograde ejaculation or no ejaculation at all. Numerous drugs have been associated with altered sexual function (Table 109-6).[208]

Few studies exist in the literature solely devoted to drug-induced ED or sexual dysfunction.[187,188] A few studies and review articles, however, list medications as one of many potential causes for ED.[19,136,156,169,209]

Most studies documenting drug-induced ED have been subjective and based on case reports, uncontrolled studies, and clinical impressions. The MMAS reported that ED was statistically correlated with antihypertensive, vasodilator, cardiac, and hypoglycemic drugs. The probability of moderate as well as complete ED was particularly high for vasodilator drugs.[136] Although the MMAS is one of the most well-designed studies to date, the medications reported are not considered to be the universe of all medications associated with ED. Diagnosis of drug-induced sexual dysfunction should be restricted to a reproducible dose-related effect that disappears on discontinuation of the drug.[146] A much larger survey of a controlled study in a clinical population would be required to establish any suspect medication as causative, rather than temporal.

F.M.'s sexual dysfunction (e.g., loss of interest in sexual activity and ED) is not caused by his current drug regimen, ramipril, and glipizide. Although the MMAS[136] reported a correlation between the use of antihypertensives and hypoglycemic drugs with ED, clinicians must look at the individual drugs themselves and the conditions for which they are prescribed. Sexual dysfunction is not likely to occur with ramipril, or any of the other angiotensin-converting enzyme inhibitors, or with the hypoglycemic agent glyburide. Although ramipril is an antihypertensive, its pharmacologic effects do not contribute to a decline in libido or cause ED (an advantage that angiotensin-converting enzyme inhibitors have compared with other antihypertensive medications). Similarly, the pharmacologic action of glipizide does not contribute to F.M.'s decreased libido or ED. In most sexual dysfunction cases, it is less likely that the medication is the direct cause of the problem; rather, it is the medical condition for which the drugs were prescribed. The ability of a drug to induce sexual dysfunction simply is an extension of its pharmacologic actions. As a general rule, drugs that manipulate the sympathetic or the parasympathetic system, both centrally and peripherally, are associated with sexual dysfunction.

CASE 109-4, QUESTION 6: What factors most likely are contributing to F.M.'s ED?

F.M. is a patient with hypertension and diabetes who smokes cigarettes. Those three factors are more likely to be the cause of F.M.'s sexual dysfunction than are his medications. Diabetes mellitus is the most common hormonal disorder associated with ED in the elderly population.[195] The continued loss of interest in sexual activity experienced by F.M. most likely is the result of having experienced ED during past and present sexual events.

F.M.'s subjective and objective findings are common among elderly men. His sexual dysfunction is caused by atherosclerosis and possible neuropathy secondary to diabetes mellitus. Because cigarette smoking is no doubt contributing to F.M.'s ED, cessation should be encouraged; some improvement can be expected.[165] There is no need to alter F.M.'s drug regimen.

MANAGEMENT

CASE 109-4, QUESTION 7: What are the primary therapeutic considerations for F.M.?

Essentially, there are three levels to the management of ED. Level 1 includes lifestyle and drug therapy modifications. Specifically, the patient should be instructed to modify smoking and alcohol use. The patient's drug regimen should be checked periodically to ensure that drugs associated with ED are not being prescribed. If necessary, psychosocial counseling should be provided. After careful consideration, oral medications for management of ED should be instituted. If level 1 therapies have failed or are not acceptable to the patient, then level 2 therapy is instituted. These interventions include a vacuum constriction device to elicit an erection, intracavernosal injections, or transurethral inserts. Level 3 management involves placement of a penile prosthesis.

PHARMACOTHERAPY

Any therapy directed at male sexual dysfunction must include the elimination of drugs causing adverse sexual effects. Drug therapy is directed primarily toward treatment of ED and includes hormonal therapy, bromocriptine, prostaglandin E_1, sildenafil, tadalafil, vardenafil, avanafil, and apomorphine.

Phosphodiesterase-5 inhibitors

CASE 109-4, QUESTION 8: Would phosphodiesterase-5 inhibitor therapy be appropriate for F.M.? What are its side effects and contraindications? Does it interact with other drugs?

F.M. has diabetes mellitus and atherosclerosis and therefore is a candidate for treatment with a phosphodiesterase-5 (PDE-5) inhibitor.[210] These agents are orally active and selective inhibitors of cyclic guanosine monophosphate-specific PDE-5, the predominant phosphodiesterase isoenzyme metabolizing cyclic guanosine monophosphate in the corpus cavernosum. They facilitate an erection in response to sexual stimulation by enhancing the nitric oxide-induced relaxation of corpus cavernosal smooth muscle. The results of double-blind, placebo-controlled clinical trials in men with ED of various causes have demonstrated that PDE-5 inhibitors significantly improve erectile function and the rate of successful sexual intercourse, with therapeutic outcomes approaching those of normal men of the same age.[211–213]

F.M. should be counseled on the adverse effects of PDE-5 inhibitors. The vasodilating action of PDE-5 inhibitors affects both the arteries and the veins, so the most common side effects are headache and facial flushing.[214] PDE-5 inhibitors cause a small decrease in both systolic and diastolic blood pressures, but clinically significant hypotension is rare. Studies of PDE-5 inhibitors and nitrates taken together show much greater drops in blood pressure. For that reason, PDE-5 inhibitors are contraindicated in patients taking long-acting nitrates or short-acting nitrate-containing medications.[143] In phase II/III studies before US Food and Drug Administration (FDA) approval, more than 3,700 patients received sildenafil and almost 2,000 received placebo in double-blind and open-label studies. Approximately 25% of patients had hypertension and were taking antihypertensive medications, and 17% were diabetic. In these studies, the incidence of serious cardiovascular adverse effects was similar in the double-blind sildenafil group, the double-blind placebo group, and the open-label group. Twenty-eight patients had experienced a myocardial infarction. When adjusted for patient-years of exposure, no significant differences were seen in the myocardial infarction rates between the sildenafil and the placebo group, and no deaths were attributed to sildenafil.[215,216] In an analysis of 67 double-blind, placebo-controlled trials of sildenafil, the overall frequency of death was comparable between the sildenafil-treated patients (13 of 8,691; 0.15%) and placebo group (7 of 6,602; 0.11%).[217] Nevertheless, several deaths caused by myocardial infarction or arrhythmia have been associated with the use of sildenafil.[218] Deaths associated with sildenafil (and presumably other PDE-5 inhibitors) are most likely caused by increased cardiac workload in patients with unstable angina.[219]

Transient visual anomalies (mostly blue-green color-tinged objects, increased sensitivity to light, and blurred vision) have been reported in patients taking PDE-5 inhibitors, especially at higher dosages. These visual effects appear to be related to the weaker inhibiting action of PDE-5 inhibitors on the enzyme phosphodiesterase-6, which regulates signal transduction pathways in the retinal photoreceptors. In patients with inherited disorders of retinal phosphodiesterase-6, such as retinitis pigmentosa, PDE-5 inhibitors should be administered with extreme caution. In 2005, the FDA recommended that all PDE-5 inhibitors include a precaution in their labeling regarding the risk of nonarteritic anterior ischemic optic neuropathy as a cause of decreased vision including permanent vision loss. There have been only a handful of reports of nonarteritic anterior ischemic optic neuropathy in postmarketing surveillance, and most patients had underlying risk factors.[220] Clinicians should advise patients to discontinue the use of all PDE-5 inhibitors and seek medical attention in the event of sudden vision loss in one or both eyes.

The vasodilator actions of nitrates are profoundly amplified with concomitant use of PDE-5 inhibitors. This interaction likely applies to all nitrates and nitric oxide donors, regardless of their predominant hemodynamic site of action. They also may potentiate the inhaled form of nitrate, such as amyl nitrite, and therefore are contraindicated in patients using this product. Dietary sources of nitrates, nitrites, and L-arginine (the substrate from which nitric oxide is synthesized) do not contribute to the circulating levels of nitric oxide in humans and, therefore, are unlikely to interact with PDE-5 inhibitors. The anesthetic agent, nitrous oxide, is eliminated unchanged from the body, mostly via the lungs, within minutes of inhalation. It does not form nitric oxide in the human body and does not itself activate guanylate cyclase. As such, no contraindication exists to its use after administration of PDE-5 inhibitors. The concomitant use of nitrates and the PDE-5 inhibitors is contraindicated although some differences in the nitrate-free period do exist based on the pharmacokinetic profile of the PDE-5 inhibitor. After 24 hours, the administration of nitrates can once again be considered in patients using vardenafil and sildenafil; however, this should be extended to 48 hours in patients using tadalafil and can be shortened to 12 hours with avanafil.

CASE 109-4, QUESTION 9: Which PDE-5 inhibitor should be recommended for F.M.?

Sildenafil

The typical dose of sildenafil is 50 mg orally, taken 1 hour before sexual activity. However, it may be taken anywhere from 4 hours to 30 minutes before sexual activity. The maximal recommended dosing frequency is once per day. The following factors are associated with increased plasma levels of sildenafil: age older than 65 years (40% increase in area under the curve), hepatic impairment (e.g., cirrhosis, 80% increase), severe renal impairment (creatinine clearance <30 mL/minute, 100% increase), and concomitant use of potent CYP3A4 inhibitors (e.g., erythromycin, ketoconazole, itraconazole, 200% increase). Because higher plasma levels may increase both the efficacy and the incidence of adverse events, a starting dose of 25 mg should be considered in these patients. The dose may be increased to 100 mg. Because F.M. is older than 65 years of age, he should be started on 25-mg tablets of sildenafil. The dose may be increased under strict supervision.

Sildenafil is metabolized by both the CYP2C9 pathway and the CYP3A4 pathway. Thus, inhibitors of the CYP3A4 isoenzyme, such as erythromycin or cimetidine, may lead to competitive inhibition of its metabolism; however, CYP3A4 is a high-capacity pathway. The effects of erythromycin or cimetidine on the half-life and physiologic effects of sildenafil are not known, but clinicians should be warned about the potential interaction.

Inadequate physical sexual stimulation while using any of the PDE-5 inhibitors can lead to treatment failure. Adequate sexual stimulation is needed to trigger the events leading to erection.[221] PDE-5 inhibitors cannot initiate an erection; they can only assist in the process. Some patients may need several attempts at sexual stimulation before they are successful with intercourse.

Tadalafil

Similar to sildenafil, tadalafil is a selective inhibitor of PDE-5. Tadalafil has several times more affinity for PDE-5 than sildenafil.[222] Tadalafil and vardenafil, however, have minimal or no effect on visual disturbance (impairment of blue-green color discrimination), which is a well-recognized side effect of sildenafil.[223] Tadalafil's extended half-life of 17.5 hours relative to sildenafil most likely precludes its use in patients with angina or hypertension. Tadalafil is metabolized by the hepatic CYP3A4 isozyme. Food has no effect on the oral absorption of tadalafil in contrast to sildenafil (bioavailability decreased by 29%). Tadalafil may be advantageous in a subset of patients, based on its shorter onset of action (16 minutes) and 24-hour duration of action.[224] Specifically, patients with psychogenic or neurogenic ED and those with stable cardiovascular systems may prefer tadalafil because it offers the potential for multiple sessions of intercourse with a single daily dose.

Vardenafil

Vardenafil is the third FDA-approved oral PDE-5 inhibitor for treatment of ED. The warnings regarding the use of nitrates while taking vardenafil are similar to the warnings for sildenafil. Patients using vardenafil may experience headache, flushing, or rhinitis; the incidence of these side effects is dose related.[225] Vardenafil is metabolized by the hepatic CYP3A4 isozyme and has a reported half-life of 5 hours.[226] Thus, drugs known to inhibit the CYP3A4 isozyme have the potential to prolong its half-life. Vardenafil 10 mg does not impair the ability of patients with stable coronary artery disease to exercise at levels equivalent to or greater than that attained during sexual intercourse.[227]

Avanafil

Avanafil is a new PDE-5 inhibitor with enhanced PDE-5 selectivity which may translate to fewer side effects due to less selectivity for non-PDE-5 isoenzymes, found in the heart, retina, and skeletal muscle. The starting dose is 50 mg and should be taken 30 minutes before sexual activity whereas the 100- to 200-mg doses can be taken 15 minutes before. It has a similar half-life to sildenafil and vardenafil and is rapidly absorbed following administration. Side effects and contraindications for avanafil are similar to the other PDE-5 inhibitors.[228]

F.M. has hypertension that most likely would be affected by tadalafil; therefore, extreme caution is advised. Perhaps, the shorter-acting sildenafil, vardenafil, or avanafil would be the PDE-5 inhibitor drug of choice for F.M.

Testosterone

CASE 109-4, QUESTION 10: Should F.M. be treated with testosterone?

Primary hypogonadism with severely deficient serum levels of bioavailable testosterone is the only appropriate indication for the use of androgen hormone therapy.[169] The goal of androgen-replacement therapy is to restore potency and libido by maintaining normal serum levels of testosterone.[229] Testosterone has no benefit in the treatment of eugonadal or mildly hypogonadal elderly men and actually may enhance the growth of undiagnosed adenocarcinoma of the prostate or cause further ED.[143] In eugonadal men, testosterone enhances the rigidity of the erection, but does not change the penile circumference.[230] F.M. would not be a candidate for testosterone therapy.

CASE 109-4, QUESTION 11: Which type of patient would benefit from testosterone therapy?

Unless testosterone deficiency is severe, (free testosterone serum levels less than 7 to 8 pg/mL) testosterone replacement therapy will not improve the success rate of intercourse.[231] Testosterone replacement in patients with primary hypogonadism generally restores libido and potency. In some patients with secondary hypogonadism caused by disorders of the hypothalamus or pituitary, GnRH analogs can be administered to differentiate between hypothalamic and pituitary abnormalities and to correct testosterone deficiency.[229] Libido and potency then are restored.

CASE 109-4, QUESTION 12: How should testosterone be used as a treatment for ED?

Testosterone-replacement therapy is available in several formulations, including gels, transdermal patches, and intramuscular injection. Because of poor drug bioavailability, oral testosterone-replacement therapy is less effective than parenteral testosterone in achieving normal serum testosterone levels. Oral administration also is associated with a higher incidence of hepatotoxicity and adverse serum lipid effects.[143,174] A long-acting testosterone intramuscular formulation, such as the enanthate or cypionate ester, is still considered the regimen of choice for the treatment of primary hypogonadism. A dose of 50 to 400 mg should be administered intramuscularly every 2 to 4 weeks. Side effects of testosterone therapy include early gynecomastia, increases in hematocrit (sometimes to the point of polycythemia), and fluid retention that may worsen hypertension or heart failure.

Results of several studies have demonstrated that serum testosterone levels are normalized while using transdermal testosterone applications.[175,232–234] The system normalizes DHT to testosterone ratios and reduces LH levels toward the normal range. The transdermal testosterone is well tolerated, with application site reactions such as pruritus, burn-like blisters, and erythema being the most commonly reported event. The adhesive side of the patch should be applied to a clean, dry area of the skin on the back, abdomen, upper arms, or thighs. The patient should be instructed to avoid application over bony prominences or on a part of the body that may be subject to prolonged pressure during sleep or sitting (e.g., the deltoid region of the upper arm, the greater trochanter of the femur, and the ischial tuberosity); do not apply to the scrotum. The sites of application should be rotated, with an interval of 7 days between applications to the same site. The area selected should not be oily, damaged, or irritated.

Topical testosterone gel should be applied once daily in the morning to clean, dry skin. Depending on the specific product, it can be applied to the upper arms, shoulders, thighs, or abdomen. A topical solution for application to the axilla is also available. The dose can be as high as 100 mg/24 hours. After the gel or solution has dried on the site of application, it should be protected with clothing to prevent transfer to a nonuser. The patient should wash his hands after application.

Commonly reported adverse effects in chronic users include acne, edema, gynecomastia, and dermatologic reactions to injections or transdermal applications of testosterone. The most serious risk of prolonged testosterone use is prostate carcinoma, although the association between high concentrations of testosterone and the risk of prostate carcinoma is controversial.[235–237] Three studies suggest that testosterone-replacement therapy is relatively safe in hypogonadism.[238–240] Baseline assessment of the prostate should be done before starting testosterone-replacement therapy. This should consist of a TRUS, digital palpation of the prostate gland, and analysis of the PSA, hemoglobin, and hematocrit levels.

Bromocriptine

CASE 109-4, QUESTION 13: Because F.M.'s prolactin serum concentration is 28 ng/mL, should bromocriptine be prescribed to decrease his hyperprolactinemia and treat his ED?

Hyperprolactinemia may be treated with the ergot alkaloid bromocriptine, which works as a dopamine agonist to inhibit prolactin secretion. Even with normalization of prolactin levels, approximately 50% of elderly male patients are unable to achieve erectile function and desire.[174,229] Bromocriptine therapy may be initiated with twice-daily 1.25-mg doses taken with meals to minimize gastrointestinal upset. Thereafter, doses may be increased weekly, at a rate of no more than 2.5 mg/day. Adverse events associated with bromocriptine are nausea, dizziness, drowsiness, hypotension, and cerebrovascular accidents.[143,229] For those who fail bromocriptine, cabergoline is a reasonable alternative given once or twice a week with good efficacy and a lower incidence of nausea.[241]

F.M. is not a candidate for treatment with bromocriptine because he does not have secondary hypogonadism, and his ED probably is secondary to atherosclerosis associated with his hypertension, diabetes, and cigarette smoking. Furthermore, the elevation of F.M.'s serum prolactin concentration is not significant enough to warrant drug therapy. Medication-induced hyperprolactinemia is usually associated with prolactin levels ranging from 25 to 100 μg/L, but metoclopramide, risperidone, and phenothiazines can lead to prolactin levels exceeding 200 μg/L by way of dopamine antagonism.[241] Verapamil can cause hyperprolactinemia presumably by blocking hypothalamic dopamine, and opiates and cocaine can induce it through the μ-receptor.[241] Usually prolactin will normalize 3 days following discontinuation of the offending medication, however this patient is not on any medications that can induce hyperprolactinemia. Because the response rate to bromocriptine in elderly men is 50% (or less), the risk of adverse reactions (e.g., dyskinesia, dizziness, hallucinations, dystonia, confusion, cerebrovascular accidents) outweighs the benefit of this dopamine agonist therapy.

CASE 109-4, QUESTION 14: What other drug therapy is available for F.M.?

Before the advent of the PDE-5 inhibitors, intracavernosal and intraurethral prostaglandin E_1 (alprostadil) administration was the only nonsurgical option for ED. Alprostadil causes direct vascular smooth muscle relaxation allowing blood flow and entrapment in penis. Less invasive than intracavernosal injections, alprostadil intraurethral pellet is inserted, as semisolid gel form, through the urethral opening of the penis 5 to 10 minutes before sex and works for up to one hour. However, it is less effective and not recommended with pregnant partners.[242] Intracavernosal injections are given at the base of the penis 10 to 20 minutes before sex and were effective in 87 percent of cases in one clinical trial.[243] Phentolamine, papaverine, and vasoactive intestinal peptide are also available for intracavernosal injection, but are not FDA-approved. Adverse events from intracavernosal therapies include priapism, pain at the injection site, and penile fibrosis after long-term use. Topical alprostadil cream has also shown efficacy in 74% of patients but is not currently available in the US.[244]

KEY REFERENCES AND WEBSITES

A full list of references for this chapter can be found at http://thepoint.lww.com/AT11e. Below are the key references and websites for this chapter, with the corresponding reference number in this chapter found in parentheses after the reference.

Key References

Lindau ST et al. A study of sexuality and health among older adults in the United States. *N Engl J Med*. 2007;357:762. (130)

McConnell JD et al. The long-term effect of doxazosin, finasteride, and combination therapy on the clinical progression of benign prostatic hyperplasia. *N Eng J Med*. 2003;349:2387. (114)

Tsertsvadze A et al. Oral phosphodiesterase-5 inhibitors and hormonal treatments for erectile dysfunction: a systematic review and meta-analysis. *Ann Intern Med*. 2009;151:650. (213)

Wein AJ. Pharmacologic treatment of incontinence. *J Am Geriatr Soc*. 1990;38:317. (25)

Wagg A et al. Urinary incontinence in frail elderly persons: Report from the 5th International Consultation on Incontinence. *Neurourol Urodyn*. 2015;34:398–406. (9)

Key Websites

Agency for Healthcare Research and Quality. Effective Health Care Program: Non-surgical Treatments for Urinary Incontinence in Adult Women: Diagnosis and Comparative Effectiveness. http://effectivehealthcare.ahrq.gov/ehc/index.cfm/search-for-guides-reviews-and-reports/?pageAction=displayProduct&productID=1031AmericanUrologicAssociation. http://www.auanet.org.

American College of Physicians releases new recommendations for treating urinary incontinence in women. http://www.acponline.org/newsroom/treating_ui_in_women.htm. Accessed June 18, 2015.

American Urological Association Guideline: Management of Benign Prostatic Hyperplasia (BPH). https://www.auanet.org/education/guidelines/benign-prostatic-hyperplasia.cfm. Accessed June 18, 2015.

American Urological Association. Clinical Guideline on the Management of Erectile Dysfunction. https://www.auanet.org/education/guidelines/erectile-dysfunction.cfm. Accessed June 18, 2015.

National Association for Continence. http://www.nafc.org.

Simon Foundation for Continence. http://www.simonfoundation.org.

110 Osteoporosis

R. Rebecca Couris, Suzanne Dinsmore, and Mary-Kathleen Grams

CORE PRINCIPLES

	CORE PRINCIPLES	CHAPTER CASES
1	Osteoporosis is a condition of low bone mass and deterioration of bone tissue leading to bone fragility and potentially fracture with many preventable and inherent risk factors.	**Case 110-1 (Question 1)**
2	Prevention and treatment of osteoporosis focus on modifying preventable risk, providing adequate dietary supplementation of calcium and vitamin D, increasing bone mineral density, and reducing fracture rates.	**Case 110-1 (Questions 1–3), Case 110-2 (Question 3)**
3	Pharmacologic therapy is reserved for those patients with a hip or vertebral fracture, individuals with a T-score less than or equal to −2.5 at the femoral neck or spine once secondary causes have been excluded, and individuals with low bone mass with a 10-year probability of greater than or equal to 3% risk of hip fracture or greater than or equal to 20% risk of major osteoporotic fracture.	**Case 110-2 (Questions 1–3)**
4	Initial therapy with oral bisphosphonates is recommended unless patients are unable to take or have relative contraindications to oral bisphosphonate therapy.	**Case 110-2 (Question 6,7)**
5	Estrogen/progesterone therapy, selective estrogen receptor modulators, parathyroid hormone, denosumab, and calcitonin are alternative therapies for prevention and/or treatment of postmenopausal osteoporosis.	**Case 110-2 (Questions 4,6,8), Case 110-3 (Questions 3,4)**
6	Duration of treatment with antiresorptive and/or anabolic therapy has remained controversial, secondary to concerns for oversuppression of bone turnover markers and the potential for the development of osteosarcomas, respectively.	**Case 110-2 (Question 6)**
7	Prevention and treatment of osteoporosis secondary to prolonged glucocorticoid therapy should be incorporated into a patient's treatment plan with considerations for dosage and duration of glucocorticoid therapy, the patient's individual risk factors, sex, and age.	**Case 110-4 (Questions 1–4)**
8	Pharmacologic therapies to be considered for osteoporosis treatment in men include oral and intravenous bisphosphonates and parathyroid hormone.	**Case 110-5 (Questions 1–6)**

INCIDENCE, PREVALENCE, AND EPIDEMIOLOGY

Osteoporosis is a well-recognized disorder of reduced bone strength leading to an increased risk of fractures. It is the most common bone disease in humans, characterized by low bone mass and a deterioration of bone tissue.[1]

Osteoporosis is considered a silent disease and can progress without symptoms until a fracture occurs.[1] Fractures and their complications make osteoporosis a major public health concern.[2] Fractures of the spine, hip, and wrist are the most common and may be followed by a complete recovery, considerable pain and disability, or death.[1] Consequences of an osteoporosis fracture are physical, financial, and psychological. The considerable morbidity and mortality from these fractures create a heavy economic burden.

Osteoporosis can be classified as primary or secondary. Primary osteoporosis is the deterioration of bone mass that is not associated with other chronic conditions and is associated with natural aging and decreased gonadal function.[3] Both men and women experience osteoporosis. Age-related bone loss begins in the sixth decade of life. Bone loss is accelerated in women in the late perimenopausal period and first postmenopausal years.[4] Conditions that contribute to primary osteoporosis are prolonged periods of inadequate calcium intake, sedentary lifestyle, and tobacco and alcohol abuse. Secondary osteoporosis is the deterioration of bone

Table 110-1
Risk Factors Associated with the Development of Osteoporosis

↑Age Female gender Caucasian or Asian Family history Small stature Low weight	Predisposing medical problems (e.g., chronic liver disease, chronic renal failure, hyperthyroidism, primary hyperparathyroidism, Cushing syndrome, diabetes mellitus, anorexia nervosa, gastrointestinal resection, malabsorption, vitamin D deficiency, irritable bowel disease, chronic obstructive pulmonary disease, spinal cord injury, Parkinson disease, and human immunodeficiency virus)
Early menopause or oophorectomy Sedentary lifestyle ↓Mobility Low calcium intake Excessive alcohol intake Cigarette smoking High Caffeine intake	Drugs (e.g., corticosteroids, long-term anticonvulsant therapy [phenytoin or phenobarbital], aromatase inhibitors, gonadotropin-releasing hormone [GnRH] analogs, depot medroxyprogesterone, rosiglitazone, cyclosporine, tacrolimus, antiretroviral therapy, long-term heparin, warfarin, loop diuretics, excessive levothyroxine therapy, proton pump inhibitors, H_2 receptor antagonists, excessive use of aluminum-containing antacids)

mass that is associated with chronic conditions or from the use of various medications.[3,5] Secondary causes of osteoporosis are listed in Table 110-1 and include nutritional deficiencies, endocrine disorders such as hyperparathyroidism and diabetes mellitus, malignancies, gastrointestinal diseases, renal failure, connective tissue diseases, and medications, which include anticonvulsant therapy, long-term glucocorticoid therapy, or long-term proton pump inhibitors.

The standard method of identifying osteoporosis is the measurement of bone mineral density (BMD) at either the femur neck region of the proximal femur (hip) or the lumbar spine.[2,6] The World Health Organization (WHO) uses a defined criteria to diagnose osteoporosis that has been widely accepted.[7] When measured by dual-energy X-ray absorptiometry (DXA), a bone mineral density that lies 2.5 standard deviations or more below the average value for young healthy women, a T-score of less than −2.5 SD, is considered osteoporosis and an effective method to identify patients at increased risk for fracture. As the T-score decreases, the risk for fracture increases. A T-score between −2.5 and −1 is defined as osteopenia, but is better referred to as low bone mass or low bone density. A T-score greater than or equal to −1 is considered normal. The National Osteoporosis Foundation (NOF) clinician guidelines include this measurement of BMD in the diagnosis of osteoporosis, but also states that the occurrence of adulthood hip or vertebral fracture in the absence of major trauma can be considered osteoporosis without the measurement of BMD.[1]

Although the fracture rate is lower than in osteoporosis, the majority of fractures occur in patients with low bone mass. The prevalence of low bone mass is higher than osteoporosis, and therefore, it is important to monitor for clinical risk factors to predict the risk of fracture.

Osteoporosis is a global concern estimated to affect more than 200 million people worldwide.[8] The prevalence of osteoporosis and the risk of fracture increase with age and vary by race and ethnicity. The risk of hip fracture is greatest in Northern Europe, Australia, and North America.[9] According to data from the United States National Health and Nutrition Examination Survey (NHANES), 2005 to 2008, 9% of adults aged 50 years and over had osteoporosis, as defined above, at either the femoral neck or lumbar spine.[10] Forty-nine percent had low bone mass at either the femur neck or lumbar spine and 48% had normal bone mass at both sites. In 2010, using data from NHANES 2005 to 2010 and the 2010 US Census, it was estimated that 10.3% or 10.2 million adults in the same age range had osteoporosis and 43.9% or 43.4 million adults had low bone mass.[11] Almost 80% of the affected population are women. Osteoporosis at either the femur neck or lumbar spine ranged from 7% to 35% in women and 3% to 10% in men. Prevalence increased with each decade after the age of 50 years in women, but not until the age of 80 years in men.[10] The prevalence of low bone mass at either the femur neck or lumbar spine in adults aged 50 years and over ranged from 54% to 67% in women and 32% to 60% in men. The prevalence of low bone mass in women increased with age until age 70 years and then remained stable. In men, the prevalence of low bone mass did not increase with age until aged 70 years and increased progressively thereafter.

The National Health and Nutrition Examination Survey, 2005 to 2008, provides a separate estimate of osteoporosis and low bone mass by race and ethnicity in three different groups.[10] The number of individuals with osteoporosis or low bone mass was highest among non-Hispanic white women and men. The prevalence or rate, however, was highest among Mexican Americans compared to non-Hispanic white persons and non-Hispanic black persons. Non-Hispanic black persons had the lowest rate of either osteoporosis or low bone mass at the femur neck or lumbar spine.[10,11]

Approximately 50% of Caucasian women and 20% of men will sustain an osteoporosis-related fracture in their lifetime.[1] The risk of fracture is highest in Caucasian women, followed by Asian, African American, and Hispanic women.[9] The clinical impact of osteoporosis is reflected in the impact of these fractures. More than 1.5 million fractures per year occur in the United States that are attributed to osteoporosis.[12] Estimated costs range from 14 to 20 billion dollars each year and include more than 432,000 hospital admissions, 180,000 nursing home admissions, and almost 2.5 million medical office visits.[1,12] Hip fractures account for almost three-fourths of the total cost of osteoporosis-related care, yet represent only 14% of the incident fractures. Hip fractures have a profound impact on the quality of life and a considerable associated mortality. The mortality during the first year after hip fracture is as high as 36% with a higher mortality in men than women.[1] There is a 2.5-fold increased risk of future fractures relative to persons of the same sex and similar age without fractures. In addition, hip fractures result in a multitude of complications for the elderly, including prolonged hospitalization, decreased independent living, depression, fear of future falls, and lifelong disability. An estimated 20% require long-term nursing home placement and approximately 60% are unable to regain their prefracture level of independence. Vertebral fractures may be painless or result in pain that usually lasts less than 3 months. The initiating injury may be as minor as a cough or turning over in bed. The risk of additional vertebral fractures is high. Vertebral collapse or deformity can result in loss of height, kyphosis, abdominal protuberance, or decreased pulmonary function as the abdominal cavity is shortened, chronic back pain, decreased mobility, or mortality.

The rates of osteoporosis and low bone mass have recently declined, but the total numbers of men and women with osteoporosis and low bone mass remain high.[11] The total number of 53.6 million adults over the age of 50 years with osteoporosis or low bone mass could potentially increase by 30% in the year 2030 based on the trends from 2005 to 2010. The impact of osteoporosis on the healthcare system, rising healthcare costs, in an aging population is potentially staggering.

Etiology

Eighty percent of bone that makes up the adult human skeleton is cortical bone, a dense compact bone.[13] Twenty percent is trabecular bone which is less dense than cortical bone and often referred to as spongy or cancellous bone. Cortical bone forms the outer shell as a protector of the marrow space and trabecular bone forms the interior structures in the bone marrow compartment, forming in a honeycombed fashion. Depending on location, bone consists of varied ratios of cortical to cancellous bone leading to differences in hardness and porosity.

The bones of the skeleton help to support and protect the body and undergo cycles of modeling (reshaping) and remodeling (renewal) to remove older bone and to replace it with stronger newly formed bone.[13] In young healthy bone, a balance between osteoblast and osteoclast activity results in a continuous remodeling process. Osteoclasts resorb old bone by increasing enzymes that dissolve bone proteins and mineral, and osteoblasts help reform bony surfaces and fill bony cavities by synthesizing a bony matrix that is made up of collagen and other proteins.[13,14] Bone minerals deposit into the bony matrix and calcify strengthening newly formed bone. When the rate of resorption or removal exceeds the rate of replacement, the resulting bone loss decreases bone strength and increases the risk of fracture.[14]

Bone mass peaks between ages 18 and 25 and begins to gradually decrease beginning at approximately age 30.[15] This slow, age-related bone loss phase leads to a 20% to 30% loss of cortical bone and a loss of 20% to 30% of cancellous bone in both men and women over a lifetime.[16]

During menopause, women undergo an additional phase of bone mineral density (BMD) loss. Unlike the slow age-related phase, this phase is rapid and leads to a loss of 20% to 30% of cancellous and 5% to 10% of cortical bone due to the decline in 17β-estradiol concentrations. Early cancellous bone loss in conjunction with postmenopausal decreases in cortical and cancellous bone may lead to increased vertebral and distal forearm fractures, which may be seen early after menopause.[14,17,18]

In addition, women may have an increased risk for osteoporosis because throughout life they have 30% less bone mass than men of similar age.[14]

Hormone-related, accelerated bone loss can also occur after surgical oophorectomy.

In males, androgens and estrogens play a role in the growth and development of bone.[19,20] Serum testosterone concentrations have been evaluated in many studies and its effects on bone metabolism have been controversial. Data suggest that testosterone has a direct beneficial effect on bone, but to a lesser extent than estrogen, and decreases in bioavailable estrogen due to age-related changes may be responsible for bone loss in older men.[20]

Other hormones regulated by the hypothalamic–pituitary–gonadal axis (e.g., progesterone, follicle-stimulating hormone, inhibins, oxytocin, and prolactin) have been studied for their effects on the skeletal system.[21]

Pathophysiology

Bone remodeling in humans occurs constantly, replacing the adult human skeleton approximately every decade.[22] This is a complex process that involves a balance of local and systemic regulators to form discrete skeletal foci or bone remodeling units.[15]

The receptor activator of nuclear factor-κB ligand (RANKL) and osteoprotegerin are local regulators that determine the formation, activation, and resorption of osteoclasts in remodeling.[13,23]

Osteoblast-derived RANKL binds to the osteoclast RANK receptor and facilitates osteoclast differentiation and resorptive activity. The B cells produce a decoy receptor osteoprotegerin (OPG) that competitively antagonizes RANKL by binding to it and preventing osteoclast stimulation. This process begins with bone resorption that is initiated by osteoclasts excavating lacuna found on the surface of cancellous bone, or it occurs when cavities are formed in cortical bone (Fig. 110-1).[13,18,23]

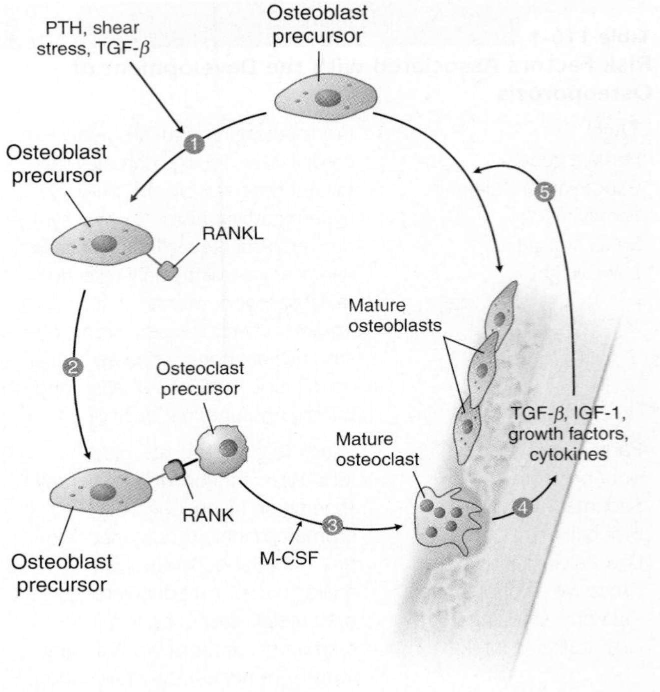

Figure 110-1 The bone remodeling cycle at the cellular level.

Enzymes, specifically transforming growth factor-β (TGF-β), produced in this process dissolve bone mineral and proteins serving as a chemoattractant for osteoblast precursors to the sites where resorption has occurred.[23] Osteocytes, cells in the bones, have growth factors that display direct and indirect effects on bone turnover. This occurs as collagen fills in bone cavities, which then are calcified.[13]

Calcium and vitamin D are important nutrients required for bone growth. Parathyroid hormone (PTH), glucocorticoid hormones, calcitonin, estrogen, and testosterone are all factors involved in bone remodeling.[18] Parathyroid hormone and glucocorticoid hormones have been associated with bone resorption, whereas calcitonin, estrogen, and testosterone have been associated with bone formation.

Dietary calcium is absorbed in the gastrointestinal tract. The kidneys reabsorb calcium in the tubular system, and the skeletal system serves as a reservoir for calcium. Calcium is primarily regulated by the actions of PTH, vitamin D, and calcitonin. The parathyroid gland releases PTH in response to low serum calcium levels, which in turn facilitates the mobilization of calcium and phosphate from bone and stimulates reabsorption of calcium through the tubular system in the kidneys.[15] Vitamin D aids in intestinal absorption of calcium, phosphorus, and magnesium. Increases in vitamin D levels decrease PTH levels. Vitamin D also increases bone resorption to prevent symptomatic hypocalcemia. Calcitonin is released in response to high serum calcium levels. Calcitonin decreases intestinal absorption of calcium and phosphorus, enhances calcium excretion in the kidneys, and prevents bone resorption (Fig. 110-2).

Overview of Drug Therapy

Osteoporosis is a condition of low bone mass and deterioration of bone tissue with a high-risk factor for fracture. Prevention, identification, and treatment of osteoporosis should all be incorporated into primary health care. Preventive measures to reduce fracture risk include adequate intake of daily calcium and vitamin D. Lifestyle modifications that are universally recommended

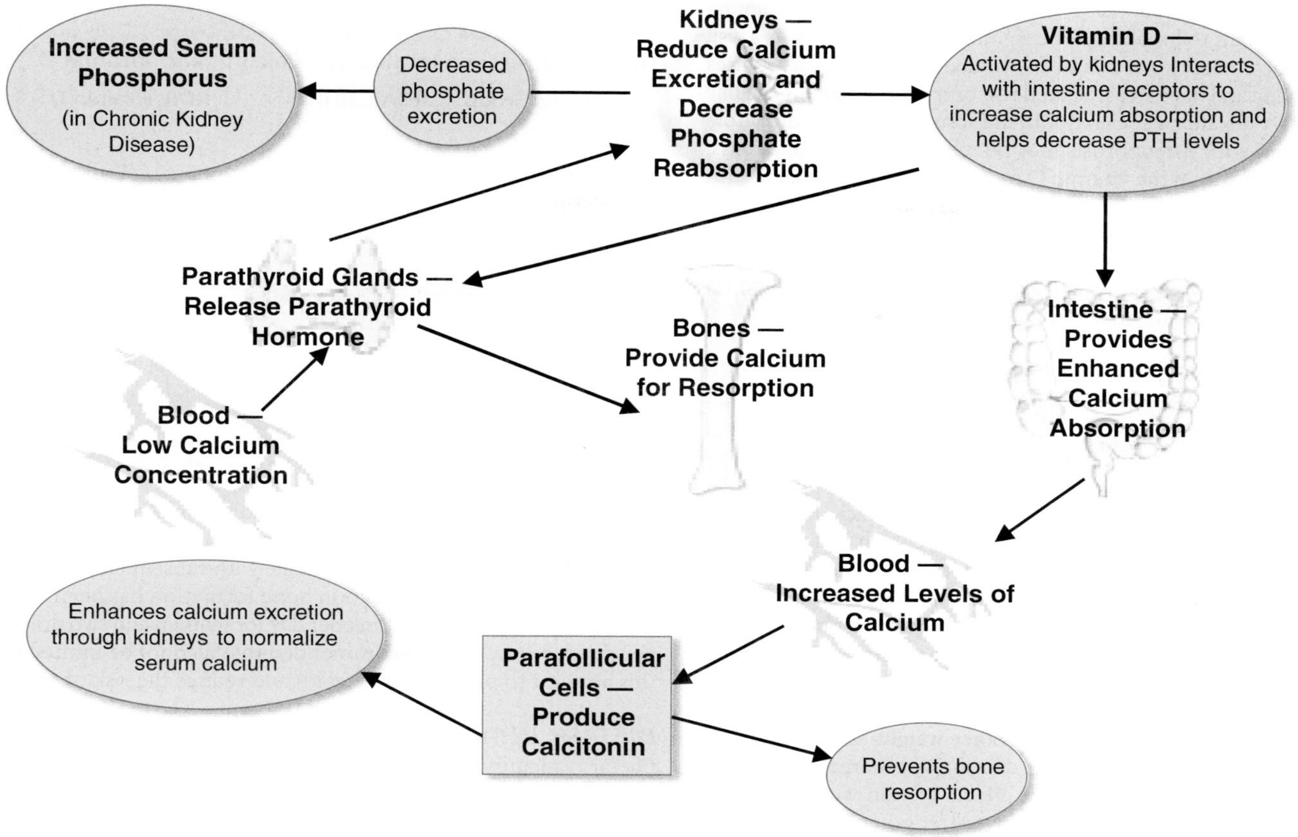

Figure 110-2 Pathway for calcium homeostasis with involvement from parathyroid hormone, vitamin D, and calcitonin.

are weight-bearing exercise, reduced alcohol consumption, and smoking cessation. Fall prevention strategies are also universal suggestions. These recommendations apply to both men and women. Pharmacologic treatment should be considered in patients with low-trauma hip or vertebral fracture, patients with a T-score of ≤ -2.5, and patients with low bone mass who are at increased risk for fracture. Medications include selective estrogen receptor modulators (SERMs; e.g., raloxifene) and calcitonin in women, bisphosphonates (e.g., alendronate), RANKL inhibitors (e.g., denosumab), and parathyroid hormone for both men and women. Testosterone therapy is recommended for men at high risk for fracture with low testosterone levels (<200 ng/dL or 6.9 nmol/L) who cannot tolerate the approved pharmacologic agents for osteoporosis.[24]

Risk Factors

CASE 110-1

Question 1: T.J., a 28-year-old, thin Caucasian woman, is worried about developing osteoporosis. Her 75-year-old maternal grandmother has osteoporosis and recently her postmenopausal mother (age 53) was told that she was at increased risk for osteoporosis. T.J. is 5 feet 2 inches tall, weighs 108 pounds, and is in good health. She jogs and occasionally does aerobic exercise. Her diet typically consists of cereal for breakfast, a sandwich for lunch, and meat with vegetables for dinner. Her only milk consumption consists of 1 cup of skim milk on her cereal. She occasionally has a dairy product for lunch or dinner. T.J. takes no medications, vitamins, or calcium supplements routinely. She occasionally takes a medication for headache or menstrual cramps. She does not smoke and occasionally drinks alcohol. Does T.J. have an increased risk for developing osteoporosis?

Table 110-1 lists risk factors associated with the development of osteoporosis. T.J. has several risk factors that could increase her risk for osteoporosis. She is a white woman of small stature and low weight (body mass index; BMI = 19.8 kg/m^2), has a positive family history, and has a low calcium intake.

Prevalence of osteoporosis worldwide varies with gender, race, and ethnicity.[9] In the United States, Mexican American women have the highest prevalence of low bone mass and osteoporosis, but non-Hispanic white women are at greatest risk for osteoporosis.[9,11,25] When prevalence is adjusted for risk factors such as age, body mass index, previous fracture, current smoking, alcohol intake, and glucocorticoid use, more non-Hispanic white women meet the NOF criteria for osteoporosis treatment compared to non-Hispanic black or Mexican American women.

LOW BODY MASS

T.J. has a small stature, and a BMI just under 20 kg/m^2 and on the low side of normal (range 18.5–24.99 kg/m^2). Low body mass index (BMI less than 20) is an established independent risk factor for osteoporosis and fracture.[26] In a meta-analysis of 12 cohorts including 60,000 men and women, a BMI of 20 kg/m^2 was associated with almost twice the risk of hip fracture compared to a BMI of 25 kg/m^2.[27] A BMI of 30 kg/m^2 was associated with a 17% reduction in the risk of hip fracture compared to 25 kg/m^2. Nevertheless, obesity should not be considered a protective factor. When adjusted for BMD, there was still a 42% increase in hip fracture in patients with a BMI of 20 kg/m^2, but no difference in the patients with a BMI of 30 kg/m^2.

FAMILY HISTORY AND GENETIC FACTORS

Osteoporosis is a multifactorial disorder that results from the effects of genetic and environmental factors. A family history of osteoporotic fracture is believed to be an underlying genetic predisposition.[7] Small stature or height is inherited. Smaller bone size can influence the risk of fracture, as bigger bones may be more resistant to breaking. The significance of heredity as a risk factor for osteoporosis has been studied. Certain disease states are genetic and have an associated risk of osteoporosis (e.g., celiac disease—a disorder associated with malabsorption). Genetic factors associated with osteoporosis may be related to peak bone mass, polymorphisms in the vitamin D receptor, genes associated with estrogen deficiency or estrogen resistance, bone morphogenetic proteins, signaling pathways, and various other bone-related proteins and receptors.[7,28,29] Women with a positive family history of osteoporosis or osteoporotic fracture typically have lower BMD than those with a negative family history.[30]

MOBILITY AND PHYSICAL ACTIVITY

Bone mass is dependent on physical activity.[7] Prolonged immobility of a limb or prolonged bed rest can result in a loss of skeletal tissue and bone mass. A number of studies have looked at the effect of exercise on bone mass. Cochrane Database published a meta-analysis of randomized controlled trials that included different types of exercise interventions in the prevention and treatment of osteoporosis in postmenopausal women.[31] The effect of all exercise types versus control was a small; there was significant improvement in BMD at the spine and trochanter, but not at the femoral neck or total hip and there was no difference in risk of fracture. Significant effects of low force weight-bearing exercise, such as walking or Tai Chi, were found at the spine and wrist. A significant effect on BMD from high force weight-bearing exercise, such as jogging, jumping, running, dancing, and vibration platform, was found at the hip. Significant effects of non-weight-bearing exercise, such as progressive resistive strengthening, were seen at the spine and the neck of the femur. Combinations of exercise types had a significant effect on BMD at the neck of the femur, spine, and trochanter and reduced the risk of fractures. BMD at the hip, however, favored control. Limitations reported by the authors include small sample size, loss of follow-up, lack of reported exercise characteristics, and heterogeneity. Though the evidence for exercise has limitations and the lasting value of exercise when stopped is not known, there is good evidence that physical activity is associated with improved health, reduced mortality, and should be encouraged.[7] The NOF recommends a combination of regular weight-bearing exercise and muscle-strengthening exercise to increase strength and reduce the risk of falls and fractures.[1] These include walking, jogging, Tai Chi, stair climbing, dancing, tennis, weight training, and other resistive exercises. The Institute for Clinical Systems Improvement (ICSI) guidelines also recommend a combination of exercise to maintain and improve bone health; impact exercise such as jogging, brisk walking, stair climbing; strengthening exercise with weights; and balance training such as Tai Chi or dancing.[26] Exercise can decrease the risk of falls by about 25%.

CIGARETTE SMOKING AND ALCOHOL INGESTION

Although T.J. does not smoke and only occasionally ingests alcohol, it is important to include questions concerning cigarette and alcohol use when obtaining a medical history from a person at risk for osteoporosis. Women and men who smoke have an increased risk for fractures, including hip fractures, compared with nonsmokers.[7] Smoking impairs the absorption of dietary and supplemental calcium, lowers body weight, influences estrogen metabolism, and may be directly toxic to bone cells.[22,26]

Excessive alcohol use by both women and men is associated with decreased BMD. Moderate alcohol consumption has been associated with increased BMD in postmenopausal women;[32] however, conflicting evidence exists. The effect of alcohol on bone is dose dependent; consuming more than two alcoholic drinks daily significantly increases the fracture risk.[7] The proposed mechanism may be a direct effect of alcohol on osteoblasts, or it may be secondary to nutritional compromise that could result in impaired calcium and vitamin D intake with subsequent decrease in bone formation. The effect on bone formation has been seen even at no more than one drink per day for women and two drinks per day for men.[26] It is recommended that alcohol be limited to this amount to protect bone health and reduce the risk of falls.

Table 110-2
Dietary Reference Intakes for Calcium and Vitamin D[33]

Life Stage Group	RDA Calcium	RDA Vitamin D
Males		
19–50 years	1,000 mg	600 IU (15 mcg)
51–70 years	1,000 mg	600 IU (15 mcg)
>70 years	1,200 mg	600 IU (15 mcg)
Females (Nonpregnant)		
19–50 years	1,000 mg	600 IU (15 mcg)
51–70 years	1,200 mg	600 IU (15 mcg)[a]
>70 years	1,200 mg	800 IU (20 mcg)[a]

[a]NOF recommends vitamin D 800 to 1,000 IU in patients ≥ 50 years.
IU, International Unit; RDA, Recommended Dietary Allowance.

DIETARY INTAKE

Dietary calcium and vitamin D are critical to bone health and needed to strengthen bones and increase bone mass. Peak bone mass is achieved in early adulthood and afterward bone constantly undergoes remodeling.[33] Maintaining normal bone mass reduces the risk of osteoporosis and fracture. Women and men need adequate calcium and vitamin D intake to achieve and help maintain optimal bone mass. The Institute of Medicine of the National Academies published recommendations for both calcium and vitamin D intake that would promote bone maintenance along with a neutral calcium balance based on age.[33] For men and nonpregnant women 19 to 50 years of age, intake of 1,000 mg of elemental calcium per day and 600 international units (IU) of vitamin D per day is recommended (Table 110-2). The National Institutes of Health (NIH) base their recommendations on the same published report.[34] The National Osteoporosis Foundation (NOF) has similar recommendations for calcium and, however, differs in their recommendations for vitamin D intake.[1] Vitamin D 800 to 1,000 international units (IU) per day is recommended for individuals 50 years of age and older.

Calcium is best ingested from the diet. Significant sources of calcium include dairy products, tofu, and canned fish (Table 110-3). Calcium absorption from foods is approximately 30%, but will vary depending on the food.[33] Calcium absorption also decreases with age. Absorption from dairy products or fortified juice is about 30%, but for certain green vegetables such as broccoli and kale, the absorption can be twice as high. Oxalate or oxalic acid-containing foods can impair calcium absorption. Kale and broccoli are foods low in oxalate as are mustard or turnip greens.[22] Examples of foods that contain high levels of oxalic acid are spinach, sweet potatoes, beans, or collard greens. Even if high in calcium, oxalate impairs the absorption of calcium. Some foods high in fiber can interfere with calcium absorption; thus, intake of a variety of foods with calcium is recommended. Alcohol, caffeine from coffee or tea, a low protein diet, a high intake of sodium, and excess dietary phosphorous, all negatively affect calcium balance.[22,33]

Vitamin D is considered a nutrient and a regulatory hormone. It is a fat-soluble vitamin that is found naturally in very few foods, but is added to certain foods and is available in supplement form. Vitamin D is a nutrient that can be synthesized in the skin through the action of sunlight, but exposure to sunlight should be limited due

Table 110-3
Calcium Content of Selected Foods

Food	Serving Size	Calcium (mg)
Dairy		
Milk, dry nonfat	1 cup	350–450
Yogurt, low fat	1 cup	345
Milk, skim	1 cup	300
Milk, whole	1 cup	250–350
Cheese, cheddar	1 oz.	211
Cheese, cottage	1 cup	211
Cheese, American	1 oz.	195
Cheese, Swiss	1 oz.	270
Ice cream or ice milk	1/2 cup	50–150
Fish		
Sardines, in oil	8 med	354
Salmon, canned (pink)	3 oz.	167
Fruits and Vegetables		
Calcium-fortified juices	1 cup	100–350
Spinach, fresh cooked	1/2 cup	245
Broccoli, cooked	1 cup	100
Collards, turnip greens	1/2 cup	175
Soybeans, cooked	1 cup	131
Tofu	1 cup	75
Kale	1/2 cup	50–150

to the risk of skin cancers.[33] Sunlight may also not produce enough vitamin D due to differences in skin pigmentation, latitude, or use of sunscreen. Vitamin D regulates calcium and phosphate, which make it important in the development and maintenance of bone health.

It directly stimulates calcium and phosphate absorption from the intestinal tract and, with the help of parathyroid hormone (PTH), can mobilize calcium from bone or stimulate calcium reabsorption at the renal distal tubule (see also Chapter 28, Chronic Kidney Diseases). Vitamin D that is found in the diet or that is synthesized from the sun must be converted to its active form, calcitriol. Two major forms of vitamin D are available. Vitamin D_3, cholecalciferol, is synthesized in the skin of humans from 7-dehydrocholesterol, is synthesized commercially, and can also be found in fatty fish, beef liver, egg yolks, and cheese. Vitamin D_2, ergocalciferol, is plant-based and largely synthesized commercially. Both forms can be found in dietary supplements or fortified foods. Cholecalciferol and ergocalciferol are inactive until they are converted to active vitamin D first by the liver to 25-hydroxyvitamin D (25OHD) and then by the kidneys to 1,25-dihydroxyvitamin D, calcitriol. The serum level of 25OHD is considered the marker for adequate intake. The National Osteoporosis Foundation recommends vitamin D intake to maintain serum 25OHD levels > 30 ng/mL (75 nmol/L).[1] Aging, chronic renal insufficiency, intestinal disease, malabsorption, very dark skin, obesity, certain medications, and reduced sun exposure are associated with reduce serum levels of vitamin D.

When vitamin D is taken in conjunction with calcium in postmenopausal women, the risk of fracture and bone loss is slightly reduced; however, the same effect from vitamin D alone is not established.[26,35,36] The combination of vitamin D and calcium results in small increases in BMD of the spine, the total body, femoral neck, and total hip.

There are few adverse effects from vitamin D supplementation. Vitamin D_3 combined with calcium can increase the chance of forming kidney stones and supplementation with the active form of vitamin D can increase the risks of hypercalcemia.

Table 110-4
Calcium Content in Various Supplements

Salt	Percent Calcium
Calcium carbonate	40
Tricalcium phosphate (calcium phosphate, tribasic)	39
Dibasic calcium phosphate dehydrate	23
Calcium citrate	21
Calcium lactate	13
Calcium gluconate	9

T.J. is typical of the average American and has a diet low in calcium. If the calcium or vitamin D in her diet does not achieve the recommendations, supplements should be added. (Table 110-4; see Case 110-1, Questions 2, 3)

OTHER POTENTIAL RISKS

Various medications and medical conditions that have been associated with the development of secondary osteoporosis are listed in Table 110-1.

Prevention

PREMENOPAUSAL WOMEN

CASE 110-1, QUESTION 2: Although T.J. is premenopausal, what recommendations could be made to decrease her future risk of developing osteoporosis?

Universal recommendations for the prevention of osteoporosis are adequate intake of daily calcium and vitamin D, weight-bearing and strengthening exercise, reduced alcohol consumption, and smoking cessation. T.J.'s course of action should be to maximize her peak bone mass and prevent or decrease bone loss. Her diet should consist of adequate calcium of 1,000 mg and adequate vitamin D of 600 IU. T.J. should continue to exercise, developing a lifelong exercise program, and continue to refrain from smoking. T.J. should also maintain her BMI between 20 and 25 kg/m^2.

Exercise

T.J. should be encouraged to participate regularly in weight-bearing and strengthening exercises such as jogging, walking, running, biking, tennis, or weight lifting and to continue appropriate exercise for her age throughout life. Physical activity has numerous benefits in addition to promoting bone health. Exercise enhances overall health and well-being, helps to control blood pressure, and lowers risk factors for cardiovascular disease, colon cancer, and type 2 diabetes.[22] Young women such as T.J. should be made aware that it is important to maintain regular menstrual periods. Amenorrhea due to strenuous exercise or extremely low body weight can increase the long-term risk of osteoporosis and fractures.

Dietary Intake

T.J. should eat a well-balanced diet rich in fruits and vegetables, low-fat dairy products, whole grains, fish, and nuts. This will provide calcium as well as other nutrients needed for bone health. She should ensure her diet contains 1,000 mg of elemental calcium and 600 IU vitamin D, optimally from dietary sources.[22] Dairy products are the major source of dietary calcium in the United States. Low-fat or nonfat versions have the full amount of calcium. Fortified juices or fortified cereals are also good sources of calcium. Although nondairy sources may contain lower amounts of calcium, they can be an important source for men or women with dietary preferences, those who cannot tolerate dairy, or who have food allergies (Table 110-3). The ingestion of foods rich in phytates and oxalates (e.g., cereal grains, legumes, and nuts) may decrease calcium absorption.

If T.J. cannot meet her daily calcium requirement from dietary sources, she can use a calcium supplement. Table 110-4 lists the percentage of elemental calcium available from selected calcium salts. (see Case 110-1, Question 3, for further information on calcium supplements.)

Vitamin D is found in few foods naturally (e.g., beef liver, egg yolk, salmon, tuna), but can be found in fortified juice or milk. It is difficult to quantify the amount of vitamin D obtained from sunlight. Genetic factors, skin pigment, latitude, and the use of sunscreen are all factors that affect sun exposure.[33] T.J. should be able to obtain adequate vitamin D intake from her diet. She could also add a supplement to her diet to achieve 600 IU of vitamin D daily.

Other bone-related nutrients include magnesium, phosphorous, vitamin K, and protein. Magnesium affects the concentration of parathyroid hormone, is involved in the formation of bone, and is widely available in foods and fortified cereals.[37] Low dietary intake of magnesium has been associated with lower bone mineral density, but not an increase in the incidence of hip fracture or total fractures.[38] Total daily magnesium intake was estimated in 73,684 postmenopausal women enrolled in the Women's Health Initiative Observational Study. Women who consumed magnesium in the highest quintile had a 3% higher total hip BMD and a 2% higher whole-body BMD than those in the lowest quintile. The incidence of hip fracture or total fracture was not statistically different across quintiles of magnesium intake. Calcium as well as phosphorous is stored in the bone. A complex balance of both is necessary for bone strength.[22] Low dietary intake of phosphorous as well as excessive intake has adverse effects on bone. Vitamin K is also important to maintain healthy bone. Patients who are on long-term vitamin K antagonists or who have a diet low in vitamin K are at increased risk for fracture and osteoporosis, but this risk is controversial.[39] Currently, there is no strong evidence and no recommendations for supplementation.[39–41] Isoflavones are a class of phytoestrogens found in soybeans and red clover, have estrogen-like activity, and have been shown to increase bone density. There is conflicting and insufficient information on phytoestrogens to support the use of isoflavones for osteoporosis prevention.[22] Soy, however, is a good source of protein, which is also important for bone health. Calcium absorption is decreased in diets that are low in protein.

Smoking and Alcohol

Smoking cessation should be encouraged in men or women who smoke. Rates of bone loss are greater in smokers than for nonsmokers and calcium absorption may be decreased.[26] T.J. occasionally drinks alcohol and should be educated on the risk of alcohol and decreased bone mineral density. Recommended alcohol intake should be limited to no more than one drink per day for women and two drinks per day for men.

CASE 110-1, QUESTION 3: If T.J. needs a calcium supplement, which calcium salt should be recommended?

The amount of elemental calcium in supplements varies. Two common forms of calcium supplements are calcium carbonate and calcium citrate.[33,37] The cost of calcium carbonate tends to be lower and it contains the highest percentage of elemental calcium (40%), allowing fewer tablets per day to meet daily calcium requirements. Calcium absorption from supplements depends on the total amount of elemental calcium consumed at one time. The percentage of calcium absorbed decreases as the dose increases. Maximal absorption occurs at doses $\leq$ 500 mg at one time.[37] If T.J. needs a calcium supplement, calcium carbonate is a reasonable choice. She should be advised to take it in divided doses up to 500 mg/dose to maximize absorption. Calcium carbonate absorption is dependent on stomach acid and should be taken with food. Calcium citrate contains less elemental calcium, 21%, is less dependent on stomach acid for absorption, and can be taken with or without food. Calcium citrate is beneficial in patients with achlorhydria, inflammatory bowel disease, or in patients taking proton pump inhibitors or histamine 2 receptor blockers. Supplements should be taken with plenty of fluids. Calcium can compete or interfere with the absorption of iron, zinc, and magnesium. Significant drug interactions can also occur, such as impaired absorption of medications including tetracyclines, thyroid products, and quinolones (Table 110-5). T.J. should be informed that the most common adverse effects of calcium are constipation, GI irritation, bloating, and flatulence. Caution should be used in patients with renal insufficiency, hypoparathyroid disease, hypercalcemia, and a history of kidney stones. If T.J. or any family member has a history of urinary stones, her clinician should be aware of supplementation. T.J. should drink plenty of water throughout the day and take calcium carbonate with food to ensure absorption or switch to calcium citrate.

Table 110-5
Drug Interactions

Examples of Drug–Calcium Supplement Interactions[a]	
Allopurinol	Protease inhibitors
Bisphosphonate derivatives	Tetracycline derivatives
Calcium-channel blockers	Protease inhibitors
Certain cephalosporin antibiotics	Quinidine
Corticosteroids (oral)	Quinolone antibiotics
HMG-CoA reductase inhibitors	Sucralfate
Iron salts	Thiazide diuretics
Itraconazole, ketoconazole	Thyroid products
Magnesium salts	Tetracycline derivatives
Multivitamins/fluoride (with ADE)	Vitamin D analogs
Multivitamins/minerals (with ADEK, folate, iron)	Zinc

[a]Does not include all calcium–drug interactions
Source: Facts & Comparisons eAnswers. Accessed February 15, 2015 from http://online.factsandcomparisons.com/index.aspx. Accessed June 18, 2015.

POSTMENOPAUSAL WOMEN

CASE 110-2

QUESTION 1: T.J.'s mother, M.J., is a 53-year-old Caucasian woman, who is also of small stature and low weight. She occasionally walks in the evenings. She currently is taking a calcium supplement to maintain her total calcium intake (dietary plus supplementation) of about 1 g/day. She takes omeprazole (over-the-counter) for her gastroesophageal reflux disease (GERD) and occasional acetaminophen for headaches. M.J. was a cigarette smoker but stopped in her late twenties and rarely drinks alcohol. She is in good health with no gynecologic surgery or major diseases. M.J. has a strong family history of breast cancer. Her last menstrual period was 6 months ago, but she began experiencing menstrual irregularity 2 years ago. M.J. has been experiencing some menopausal symptoms (hot flushes), but states that they are mild and occur only at night. M.J., worried about developing osteoporosis, decided to make an appointment with her gynecologist to discuss preventive measures. A dual-energy X-ray absorptiometry (DXA) measurement of her spine was administered, which noted her T-score to be −2.0 and a Z-score of −1.0.

In addition to the DXA, what other information should be obtained to determine whether M.J. is at risk for developing osteoporosis or has already developed osteoporosis?

In addition to M.J.'s DXA, a detailed medical history including medication history (prescription and over-the-counter medications), diet, social history (smoking, alcohol), and a physical examination, which includes height, are needed along with a risk factor analysis. Diagnostic tests are indicated when there are multiple risk factors present.[1] The goals of a comprehensive evaluation are to identify modifiable risk factors, rule out potential causes of osteoporosis, and to treat if indicated.

From her history and risk factor analysis, it is determined that M.J. shares similar risk factors for osteoporosis with her daughter. In addition, she is early in the postmenopausal phase, has GERD, and was a previous smoker. M.J. has no loss of height, does not complain of back pain, and does not have signs of kyphosis, all of which may be signs of osteoporosis. As part of the aging process, women may lose 1 to 1.5 inches in height due to degenerative arthritis and shrinking of intervertebral discs.[1] It is important to monitor height as a loss of height may indicate that the patient has a vertebral fracture.

Biochemical markers of bone turnover are not needed for M.J. at this time (e.g., alkaline phosphatase, calcium levels, phosphorus levels, bone-specific alkaline phosphatase, osteocalcin, cross-linked C-terminal telopeptide, and *N*-telopeptide). They are not used to diagnose osteoporosis but may be used to evaluate drug therapy.[1]

The North American Menopause Society (NAMS) recommends a BMD measurement in women such as M.J. who are older than 50 years of age if one or more risk factors for fracture are present.[32] These risk factors include weight <127 pounds or BMI <21 kg/m^2, fracture other than skull, facial bone, ankle, finger or toe after menopause, first-degree relative with a history of hip fracture, smoking, rheumatoid arthritis, or alcohol consumption of two drinks per day (1 drink = 12 oz of beer, 4 oz of wine, or 1 oz of liquor).[1]

NAMS also recommends BMD testing in postmenopausal women with bone loss due to medical conditions such as hyperparathyroidism, medications such as steroids, postmenopausal women who have had a fragility fracture, and all women over the age of 65.[32] The NOF recommends BMD testing for women age 65 years and older; men age 70 years and older; menopausal women or women in menopausal transition who are younger than age 65 and at increased risk of osteoporosis or who suffered a low impact fracture; nonmenopausal women over age 50 and men ages 50 to 70 who have suffered a low impact fracture or who are at risk for fracture; and adults with a condition or who take medication that is associated with low bone mass.[1] Along with evidence-based recommendations, insurance reimbursement plays a role in BMD testing.

Bone mineral density refers to the amount or weight of bone mass per area and is measured in g/cm^2. BMD is reported as T-score (Table 110.6) and also as Z-score.[26] As T-score is a comparison of BMD to what is expected in a young healthy adult population of the same gender, Z-score is a comparison of BMD to what is expected in a healthy adult population of a similar age, gender, and ethnicity.

T-Score

([measured BMD − young adult population mean BMD]/ young adult population SD) (Eq. 110-1)

Z-score

([measured BMD − age-matched population mean BMD]/ age-matched population SD) (Eq. 110-2)

Dual-energy X-ray absorptiometry (DXA) is a two-dimensional X-ray considered the standard for measuring BMD to diagnose or assess therapy.[4] Central DXA of hip, spine, and femoral neck remain the preferred measurement for definitive diagnosis (Table 110-6).[2]

Other methods can be used for screening but should not be used for diagnosis or to follow a patient's response to therapy.[7,26]

For postmenopausal women who are not receiving medications for osteoporosis prevention, a DXA may be useful no more frequently than every 2 to 5 years because the rate of bone loss is approximately 1% to 1.5% per year.[32] T-score values are supported by both the NAMS and NOF for diagnosis. The International Society for Clinical Densitometry (ISCD) recommends using Z-scores when screening low BMD in children, premenopausal women, and men less than age 50. A Z-score of −2.0 or less is below the expected range and a Z-score greater than −2.0 is considered within range.[43]

Table 110-6
Definitions of Bone Mineral Density[42]

Classification	T-Score
Normal	≥ −1.0 SD
Osteopenia (Low bone mass)	−2.5 to −1.0 SD
Osteoporosis	< −2.5 SD

It has been estimated that for every one point decrease in SD from the mean T-score, a 10% to 15% change may occur in BMD. The magnitude of this change can be translated into a 1.5-fold to 3-fold change in risk for fractures (Table 110-7).[32]

The World Health Organization along with several leading osteoporosis organizations developed the WHO Fracture Risk Assessment tool (FRAX) that can be used alone or with BMD to identify fracture risk.[44] FRAX is a computerized-based algorithm created for different populations available online at http://www.shef.ac.uk/FRAX. The FRAX algorithm incorporates ethnicity as well as clinical risk factors (e.g., age, smoking, physical inactivity, height, weight, prior fracture, parental history of hip fracture, long-term use of glucocorticoids, and comorbid conditions that have been associated with decreases in BMD) to calculate 10-year fracture risk. FRAX has been validated in 11 different cohorts and is a valuable tool that provides information on absolute risk instead of relative risk by taking into account the impact of risk factors on fracture and death. As with many tools, there are some limitations to FRAX. The algorithm excludes certain variables such as vitamin D deficiency, bone turnover markers, and falls. It does not take into account multiple fractures and may underestimate risk.

FRAX should not replace clinical judgment for treatment and is intended to be used in postmenopausal women and men over age 50. It has not been validated in patients who have been on or who are receiving medication therapy for osteoporosis.[1,45]

CASE 110-2, QUESTION 2: Based on the information that you have obtained, does M.J. have osteoporosis or is she at risk for developing osteoporosis?

M.J. is 62 inches tall and weighs 50 kg. She has a T-score of −2.0 (DXA measurement of the spine) and a Z-score of −1.0. Using

Table 110-7
Techniques for Measuring Bone Mineral Density

Technique	Abbreviation	Measurement Sites
Dual-energy X-ray absorptiometry	DXA	Hip, spine, total body
Peripheral dual-energy X-ray absorptiometry	PDXA	Forearm, fingers, heel
Peripheral quantitative computed tomography	PQTC	Forearm, tibia
Quantitative ultrasound	QUS	Heel, tibia, patella
Quantitative computed tomography	QCT	Spine, hip
Single-energy X-ray absorptiometry	SXA	Heel

the FRAX risk assessment tool for the US population (http://www.shef.ac.uk/FRAX) without a T-score of the femoral neck, M.J.'s 10-year probability of a hip fracture is 0.5% and her 10-year probability of a major osteoporosis-related fracture is 5.1%. M.J's T-score is consistent with osteopenia or low bone mass.

M.J.'s risks include low bone mass, low body mass, a family history of osteoporosis, history of smoking, and medication that increases the risk of osteoporosis.

CASE 110-2, QUESTION 3: What preventive measures would help decrease M.J.'s likelihood of developing osteoporosis?

Exercise

M.J. goes for walks occasionally and should begin a consistent exercise program appropriate for her age and physical condition. Postmenopausal women who incorporated aerobic and weight-bearing exercise showed some improvements in BMD and reduced the risk of fractures as compared to those who did not exercise.[31] Weight-bearing exercise and resistance training may improve strength, muscle mass, flexibility, balance, and decrease M.J.'s risk for falls.[26] (Also see Case 110-1, Question 2).

Dietary Intake

Similar to T.J., it is important for M.J. to have a well-balanced diet rich in fruits and vegetables, low-fat dairy products, whole grains, fish, and nuts to provide adequate calcium and nutrients needed for bone health.

The recommended daily allowance of calcium for women ages 51 to 70 is 1,200 mg per day.[33] M.J's total calcium intake from diet and supplementation is about 1,000 mg/day and should be increased so that she incorporates 1,200 mg/day of calcium in her diet. She can do this by choosing calcium-containing foods (Table 110-3) and by taking a supplement if she cannot get adequate calcium from her diet (Table 110-4).

It is important for M.J. to have adequate vitamin D intake in her diet. The recommended daily allowance of vitamin D for women between 51 and 70 age is 600 IU/day, and for women over age 70, the recommended daily allowance is 800 IU/day. The NOF recommends 800 to 1,000 IU/day for men and women over age 50.[1]

Expert consensus opinion has made recommendations for serum 25(OH) vitamin D levels for bone health.[33] Levels less than 20 ng/mL (50 nmol/L) suggest insufficiency, whereas levels of 29 to 32 ng/mL (70 to 80 nmol/L) suggest adequate stores. There is currently limited evidence to attempt to achieve serum 25(OH) vitamin D levels above 60 ng/mL (150 nmol/L). (For further information, see Case 105-1, Question 2.) A serum 25(OH) vitamin D level should be drawn and M.J. should receive a vitamin D supplement to achieve a serum 25 (OH) vitamin D level of 30 ng/mL (75 nmol/L) if the level is found to be insufficient.

Although calcium and vitamin D are important for bone health, they should not be used instead of drug therapy to treat osteoporosis, but used as part of an overall plan to help improve bone health.

Pharmacologic Prevention

ESTROGEN/PROGESTIN THERAPY

CASE 110-2, QUESTION 4: Because a rapid rate of bone loss is seen during menopause when estrogen decreases, should estrogen therapy (ET) or estrogen + progesterone therapy (EPT) be considered for M.J.?

An estimated 10% to 15% of a woman's bone mass is estrogen dependent.[46] Estrogens are important in bone formation, resorption, and maintaining bone mass while menopause is associated with a decrease in estrogen and an increase in bone loss.[15,21]

The National Osteoporosis Risk Assessment Study and the Million Women Study, both large observational studies by design, found that EPT or ET provided significant relative risk reductions in fracture.[47,48] These results were confirmed by the Women's Health Initiative (WHI) with both the EPT and ET arms, showing significant risk reductions in hip, vertebral, and total fractures compared with placebo.[49,50]

Previously, ET or EPT would have been considered first-line treatment for the prevention of osteoporosis in a postmenopausal woman such as M.J., who has an intact uterus and is at risk for osteoporosis based on risk factors and T-score. In the Women's Health Initiative (WHI), conjugated equine estrogen (CEE) alone and CEE with medroxyprogesterone (CEE+MPA) were shown to decrease the risk of hip, vertebral, and total fractures in postmenopausal women; however, the intervention phases were ended early because coronary heart disease (CHD), stroke, deep vein thrombosis (DVT), pulmonary embolism (PE), and breast cancer were significantly increased in the CEE + MPA group and rates of stroke were significantly increased in women on CEE alone (also see Chapter 51, The Transition Through Menopause).[49,50] The findings from the WHI do not support the use of ET or EPT for the prevention of osteoporosis. Since the publication of the Heart and Estrogen/Progestin Replacement Study (HERS) I and HERS II and the NIH Women's Health Initiative (WHI), healthcare providers are less likely to prescribe ET or EPT for the sole purpose of osteoporosis prevention or to continue its use after a women no longer needs EPT or ET for postmenopausal symptoms such as hot flushes.[51–53]

EPT is approved for the prevention of osteoporosis in postmenopausal women with a uterus and ET is approved for postmenopausal women without a uterus.[32] When prescribed for osteoporosis prevention, ET and EPT should be used at the lowest effective doses and the shortest duration indicated. Longer therapy should only be prescribed in women who have failed other osteoporosis therapies, or when other osteoporosis therapies are contraindicated and when it can be determined that the benefits outweigh the risks. M.J. does not have bothersome symptoms of menopause; therefore, ET or EPT would not be appropriate at this time.

Contraindications to Estrogen Use

CASE 110-2, QUESTION 5: If M.J. developed bothersome symptoms of menopause, would ET or EPT be appropriate to treat symptoms and prevent osteoporosis?

Contraindications to EPT or ET include pregnancy; active or history of deep vein thrombosis or pulmonary embolism; active or recent (e.g., within the past year) arterial thromboembolic disease (e.g., stroke, myocardial infarction); undiagnosed abnormal genital bleeding; known, suspected, history of breast cancer; known or suspected estrogen-dependent neoplasia; liver dysfunction or disease; or known hypersensitivity to the product or any of its ingredients.[54] In addition, EPT and ET should be used with caution in those with a history of asthma, diabetes mellitus, migraine, epilepsy, systemic lupus erythematous, porphyria, and hepatic hemangiomas. Patients on EPT or ET are at increased risk for cancer, including endometrial (if not on EPT), breast (for EPT), and ovarian cancer as well as increased cardiovascular events, thromboembolic disease, stroke, gallbladder disease, and dementia (also see Chapter 51, The Transition Through Menopause).

M.J. stated that she has a strong family history of breast cancer, and starting EPT or ET would not be the treatment of choice for the prevention of osteoporosis.

Case 110-2, Question 6: Should a bisphosphonate be considered for the prevention of osteoporosis in postmenopausal women such as M.J.?

NAMS recommends adding osteoporosis drug therapy in postmenopausal women who have had a vertebral or hip fracture, in postmenopausal women with a BMD of −2.5 or worse at the lumbar spine, femoral neck, or total hip, and in postmenopausal women with a T-score of −1.0 to −2.5 who have a 10-year fracture risk of 20% (spine, hip, shoulder, wrist) or risk of 3% (hip) calculated using FRAX.[32] Bisphosphonates, analogs of pyrophosphate, are considered first-line therapy for the prevention and treatment of osteoporosis in postmenopausal women. Alendronate (excluding effervescent tablets), ibandronate, risedronate-immediate release, and zoledronic acid are indicated for osteoporosis prophylaxis in postmenopausal women like M.J, whereas other agents are indicated for osteoporosis treatment and prevention (see Table 110-8).[55]

Alendronate, ibandronate, risedronate, pamidronate, and zoledronic acid are aminobisphosphonates with a greater selectivity for the antiresorptive surfaces of the bone due to changes in the nitrogen-containing side chain of the compounds.

Bisphosphonates have high affinities for bone hydroxyapatite and can be incorporated into bone. They concentrate in mineral tissue and interfere with the osteoclast-mediated bone resorption to cause osteoclast apoptosis, decreased bone turnover, resulting in decreased fracture rates in postmenopausal women who are at risk for osteoporosis.[56]

Because of their incorporation into bone, bisphosphonates have long half-lives, estimated to be 1 to 10 years. Unlike etidronate (a nonaminobisphosphonate), aminobisphosphonates do not inhibit bone mineralization, which could lead to osteomalacia.

Bisphosphonates-Bone Mineral Density Efficacy in Postmenopausal Women

Alendronate

In a Cochrane review that included randomized controlled trials (RCTs) of alendronate for the primary and secondary prevention of osteoporotic fractures in postmenopausal women taken for at least 1 year, alendronate was compared to placebo with or without calcium and vitamin D.[57] Trials were considered primary prevention trials if the women had an average T-score within 2 SD of the mean, or if the prevalence of vertebral fracture was less than 20% at baseline. Secondary prevention trials were defined as women having a bone density at least 2 SD below peak bone mass or a previous vertebral compression fracture or age greater than 62 years. Clinically, important improvements were seen with vertebral fractures although not statistically significant for primary prevention. In secondary prevention studies, alendronate 10 mg

Table 110-8
Medications Approved for Prevention and Treatment in Postmenopausal Osteoporosis

Class	Medication	Prevention	Treatment
Bisphosphonates	Alendronate	5 mg PO daily 35 mg PO weekly	10 mg PO daily 70 mg PO weekly
	Alendronate/cholecalciferol		70 mg/2,800 IU PO weekly 70 mg/5,600 IU PO weekly
	Ibandronate	2.5 mg PO daily 150 mg PO monthly	2.5 mg PO daily 150 mg PO monthly
	Risedronate	5 mg PO daily 35 mg PO weekly 75 mg PO 2 consecutive days each month 150 mg PO monthly	5 mg PO daily 35 mg PO weekly 35 mg DR*-PO weekly 75 mg PO 2 consecutive days each month 150 mg PO monthly
	Zoledronic acid	5 mg IV every other year	5 mg IV yearly
Selective estrogen receptor modulators (SERMs)	Raloxifene	60 mg PO daily	60 mg PO daily
Polypeptide hormone	Calcitonin	Not indicated	100 IU IM or SC once daily, every other day, or 3 times per week 100 IU intranasally in one nostril daily
Monoclonal antibody	Denosumab	Not indicated	60 mg SC every 6 months
Parathyroid hormone	Teriparatide	Not indicated	20 mg SC once daily
Estrogen	Conjugated estrogen	When other treatments are not appropriate (without uterus)	Not indicated
	Estrogen + progestin	When other treatments are not appropriate (with uterus)	Not indicated
	Conjugated estrogen + bazedoxifene	0.45 mg/20 mg PO daily	Not indicated

Source: Facts & Comparisons eAnswers. **http://online.factsandcomparisons.com/index.aspx**. Accessed June 18, 2015.

daily led to clinically and statistically significant reductions in hip, wrist, vertebral, and nonvertebral fractures.

A 2-year multicenter study of postmenopausal women age 45 to 59 was conducted to compare the efficacy and tolerability of alendronate to EPT.[58] Women were randomized to receive placebo, alendronate 2.5 mg/day or alendronate 5 mg/day, or open-label EPT, unless contraindicated decreases in BMD of the lumbar spine were noted in the placebo group, whereas 2% and 2.7% increases were seen in the alendronate 2.5 and 5 mg/day groups, respectively, after the first year. Forty percent of women who were in the placebo group lost 2% of bone mineral density at the hip as compared to only 10% in the alendronate 2.5 mg and 6% in the alendronate 5-mg groups. Hip BMD increased at 2 years by 1.9% (EPT) and 1.3% (alendronate 5 mg) in the United States cohort. In the European cohort, women on EPT had significantly greater increases in total body BMD as compared to those on alendronate 5 mg/day. Alendronate 2.5 and 5 mg/day were well tolerated with adverse effects similar to placebo. The adverse effects of EPT could not be directly compared to alendronate because the EPT arm was open label. Alendronate and EPT both increase BMD, therefore decreasing the acceleration of bone loss in postmenopausal women without osteoporosis. Alendronate is an effective alternative to EPT without the well-known side effects.

Ibandronate

In a double-blind, placebo-controlled phase II/III study, oral ibandronate 2.5 mg/day in early postmenopausal women without osteoporosis resulted in significantly increased BMD in the lumbar spine (1.9%) as compared to placebo (−1.9%) and total hip (1.2%) as compared to placebo (−0.6%) after 2 years.[59] Oral ibandronate 2.5 mg/day significantly reduced biochemical turnover markers.

MOBILE, a randomized controlled, noninferiority study, included 1,609 postmenopausal women ages 55 to 80 with osteoporosis and compared daily ibandronate (2.5 mg/day) to three different monthly regimens; ibandronate 50 mg given on 2 consecutive days/month, 100 and 150 mg once monthly.[60] All monthly regimens were at least as effective as daily ibandronate after 1 year. At 2 years, the mean increase in BMD of the lumbar spine seen in the ibandronate 50 mg on 2 consecutive days/month was (5.3%), ibandronate 100 mg/month (5.3%), and ibandronate 150 mg/month (6.4%) as compared to ibandronate 2.5 mg taken daily (4.8%). Increases were seen in the total hip, trochanter, and femoral neck with ibandronate 150 mg/month being the most significant.

In a 5-year long-term extension (MOBILE LTE), increases in BMD that were achieved during the MOBILE study were maintained, and further increases were seen in lumbar spine BMD.[61] Minor changes were seen in the femoral neck and trochanter. Overall adverse effects of monthly ibandronate were similar to daily ibandronate. Benefits in BMD changes and decreases in bone turnover markers were greatest for ibandronate 150 mg/month.

Ibandronate has also been studied as an intravenous (IV) formulation of 3 mg administered every 3 months.[62] One-year results from the dosing intravenous administration (DIVA) study improved BMD in the lumbar spine (4.5% vs. 3.5%) and the total hip (2.1% vs. 1.5%) to a similar if not greater degree than daily oral tablets.

Risedronate

In a double-blind, placebo-controlled study, early postmenopausal women age 40 to 61 with normal BMD for age, received 2 years of risedronate treatment or placebo.[63] Women who received risedronate 5 mg/day for 2 years had BMD increases of 1.4% from baseline in the lumbar spine as compared to a 4.3% loss in the placebo group. There was an increase of 2.6% at the femoral trochanter at 2 years and 1.3% at the femoral neck at 9 months with risedronate 5 mg/day as compared to a decrease of 2.4% at the femoral neck and 2.8% at the trochanter with placebo.

In a study of postmenopausal women who were at least 50 years of age, were postmenopausal for 5 or more years, and had osteoporosis, 75 mg of risedronate on 2 consecutive days a month (2CDM) was as safe and effective as risedronate 5 mg/day for 12 months.[64] At 2 years, lumbar spine BMD increases of 4.2% in the 2CDM and 4.3% 5 mg/day were observed.[65] There were no statistically significant differences in BMD changes of lumbar spine, proximal femur, and bone turnover markers. Adverse effects in both groups were similar.

In a study that compared risedronate 5 mg/day and 150 mg/month in postmenopausal women with osteoporosis, similar increases in lumbar spine BMD from baseline were observed (3.4% and 3.5%, respectively) after 1 year and no difference in the new incidence of vertebral fractures.[66] There were similar changes in biochemical bone turnover markers. Adverse effects were similar, with a higher incidence of constipation in the 5 mg/daily group and diarrhea in the 150 mg/monthly group.

Zoledronic Acid

Zoledronic acid is an intravenous bisphosphonate that was initially approved for osteoporosis treatment and later received FDA approval for osteoporosis prevention in postmenopausal women.[1,32]

In a 2-year study of zoledronic acid for the prevention of bone loss in postmenopausal women with low bone mass, 581 women were randomized to receive zoledronic acid 5 mg IV at baseline and 12 months (2 × 5 mg), zoledronic acid 5 mg IV at baseline only and placebo at 12 months, or placebo at baseline and at 12 months.[67] At 2 years, BMD was significantly increased in the lumbar spine in the (2 × 5 mg; 5.18%), (5 mg 4.42%) as compared to placebo (−1.32%). At 2 years, BMD also increased at the proximal femur sites (2 × 5 mg; total hip 2.91%, femoral neck 2.2%, trochanter 4.83%) (5 mg; total hip 2.28%, femoral neck 1.64%, trochanter 4.16%).

Zoledronic acid infusion for osteoporosis prophylaxis is administered every other year as compared to yearly when treating osteoporosis.

Oral bisphosphonates are first-line and most commonly prescribed medications for the prevention and treatment of osteoporosis. The decision to start medication therapy for the prevention of osteoporosis prevention in postmenopausal women should involve both the patient and physician. A BMD of the femoral neck may help to better determine a more accurate FRAX 10-year risk score. M.J. has multiple risk factors for osteoporosis but pharmacologic therapy is not indicated at this time.

Length of Treatment

The incorporation of bisphosphonates into bone results in a reservoir of available drug that is slowly released over time.[68,69] The peak effect of reducing bone turnover markers occurs in 3 to 6 months and continues for months to years with discontinuation. Approval studies in the United States were for 3 to 4 years; however, extension studies suggest longer efficacy.[61,69–72]

No consensus is currently available on how long to continue bisphosphonate therapy. In the Fracture Intervention Trial Long-term Extension (FLEX) of the original Fracture Intervention Trial (FIT), the effects of continuing alendronate were compared to the effects of stopping alendronate after 5 years of treatment.[69] Statistically significant bone loss occurred (2% to 3% more than those who took alendronate for 10 years) when women were switched to placebo after 5 years of alendronate therapy; however, BMD remained well above FIT baseline. A gradual rise was seen in biochemical markers of bone turnover and there were no significant differences seen in clinical or nonvertebral fractures. There was a slightly higher risk of clinically detected vertebral fractures, in the placebo group (women who had discontinued alendronate therapy after 5 years) compared to the groups who continued alendronate, suggesting that women at high risk for vertebral fracture or with T-scores less than −3.5 may benefit from continued bisphosphonate therapy.

The long-term effects of risedronate 5 mg/daily on bone were studied in women with osteoporosis who were in the Vertebral Efficacy With Risedronate Therapy-North American (VERT-NA) study who took risedronate for up to 5 years.[73] In biopsies of the iliac crest that were taken at 3 and 5 years, changes in bone mineral and collagen were preserved in the risedronate groups as compared to maturation that was observed with placebo. The FLEX and VERT-NA studies suggest that women with good response to bisphosphonate therapy who are not at high risk for fracture may be able to take a "drug holiday" (e.g., 1-year off therapy) after 3 to 5 years of treatment.[74] Women who are able to reach a T-score of greater than −2.5 may be able to discontinue therapy for several years.

The length of therapy should be a decision made based on the benefits of therapy, adverse effects, and safety of bisphosphonates (see Contraindications and Adverse Effects below).[68] In a NAMS Practice Pearl, the authors describe a guide to bisphosphonate drug holidays according to fracture risk.[68] Low risk—discontinue; mild risk—treat for 3 to 5 years then consider a drug holiday; moderate risk—treat for 5 to 10 years then consider a 3- to 5-year drug holiday; and high risk—treat for 10 years then consider a drug holiday for 1 to 2 years. For high-risk patients on drug holiday, treat with a nonbisphosphonate such as raloxifene or teriparatide.

CASE 110-2, QUESTION 7: What are the potential adverse effects of bisphosphonates?

Adverse Effects

Common adverse effects associated with the use of oral bisphosphonates include gastrointestinal symptoms, such as acid regurgitation, dysphagia, abdominal distension, gastritis, nausea, dyspepsia, flatulence, diarrhea, and constipation.[75] Less common esophageal adverse effects, such as esophagitis, esophageal ulcers, and erosions, have occurred and have rarely been followed by esophageal stricture or perforation.[75,76] The risk of severe esophageal adverse effects is reported to be increased in patients who do not take bisphosphonates with 6 to 8 ounces of water, do not remain upright after taking bisphosphonates, or in those who develop esophageal irritation and continue to take bisphosphonates (see Dosing section). A medication guide will address issues that are specific to bisphosphonates and are intended to help patients better understand treatment, adverse effects, and adherence.[77] In addition, hypocalcemia, musculoskeletal pain, headaches and rash have been noted.

Both intravenous (IV) and oral bisphosphonates are associated with osteonecrosis of the jaw (ONJ), a serious but rare adverse event.[78,79] It was first reported in a series of cancer patients receiving IV bisphosphonates. Risk factors for osteonecrosis of the jaw include the diagnosis or previous history of cancer; invasive dental procedures; concurrent use of chemotherapy, corticosteroids, or angiogenesis inhibitors; poor oral hygiene; preexisting dental disease or infection; and anemia and coagulopathy. The risk of ONJ increases at higher doses and with duration of exposure.

Bisphosphonates are associated with atypical fractures of the femoral shaft.[26,78] A warning is included in the manufacturers' information for all bisphosphonate drugs that are indicated for the prevention or treatment osteoporosis. A safety review of oral bisphosphonates and atypical subtrochanteric femur fractures by the FDA is also ongoing.[80] A clear connection has not been found. The mechanism of action is not clear; however, bone is normally subject to microdamage with every day stresses and this initiates bone remodeling.[81] Antiresorptive agents may oversuppress bone turnover causing microdamage to accumulate which may lead to brittle bone and an increased risk of fracture. Lee et al.[81] conducted a meta-analysis that included nine observational studies and one randomized controlled trial, a total of 658,497 patients. The results were statistically significant for increased risk of subtrochanteric or diaphyseal fracture with bisphosphonate use (adjusted odds ratios [AOR] = 1.99, 95% confidence intervals [CI] = 1.28–3.10), subtrochanteric fractures AOR = 2.71 (95% CI = 1.86–3.95), and diaphyseal fractures AOR = 2.06 (95% CI = 1.70–2.50). The analysis was limited by the multiple study designs, varying lengths of follow-up, and different patient populations leading to a high heterogeneity. The pooled results of combined subtrochanteric or diaphyseal fracture and subtrochanteric fracture results had significant heterogeneity (84.3% and 83.6%, respectively). The results for diaphyseal fracture had moderate heterogeneity (29.7%). The overall risk is low compared to osteoporotic fracture. In a nested case–control study of 52,595 women 68 years and over who took at least 5 years of bisphosphonate therapy, the subtrochanteric or femoral shaft fracture occurred in 71 (0.13%) during the subsequent year and 117 (0.22%) within 2 years.[82] The results were similar to the meta-analysis. Compared with no use or transient use, the use of bisphosphonates for 5 years or longer was associated with a significantly increased risk of atypical hip or femur fracture (odds ratio [OR] = 2.74; 95% CI, 1.25–6.02). Duration less than 5 years was not associated with increased risk of fracture.

Additional adverse effects reported with zoledronic aced are pyrexia, headache, pain in extremity, flu-like illness, and eye inflammation.[78]

Currently, there is not enough evidence to hold bisphosphonate therapy in patients who should be treated for osteoporosis or osteoporosis prevention; however, if a patient has prodromal pain in the thigh or leg or has suffered an atypical fracture while on bisphosphonate therapy, it would be reasonable to discontinue therapy and evaluate.[76]

Dosing

Alendronate is approved for the prevention of osteoporosis in doses of 5 mg PO daily and 35 mg PO weekly. Alendronate is also available with cholecalciferol in a 70 mg/2,800 IU and 70 mg/5,600 IU PO weekly tablet. Ibandronate is approved at 2.5 mg PO daily and 150 mg PO monthly. Risedronate is approved at 5 mg PO daily, 35 mg PO weekly, and 75 mg PO on 2 consecutive days each month and 150 mg PO monthly. The delayed-release formulation of risedronate is not indicated for the prevention postmenopausal osteoporosis. Zoledronic acid is indicated at 5 mg IV every 2 years over no less than 15 minutes.[83] Selecting the appropriate dosing option may improve adherence to therapy.

Oral bisphosphonates are poorly absorbed and after an overnight fast when taken with water approximately 50% will be absorbed through the gut and 50% will be excreted in urine. Patients should be instructed to take most bisphosphonates with 6 to 8 ounces of water early in the morning on arising and at least 30 minutes (60 minutes for ibandronate) before ingesting food, beverage, or other medications. Risedronate is also available as a 35-mg delayed-release tablet that should be taken once weekly after breakfast. Patients should not lie down, but should stay fully upright for at least 30 minutes (60 minutes for ibandronate) after ingesting an oral bisphosphonate to prevent esophageal irritation or ulceration and to ensure appropriate bioavailability. With all bisphosphonates, patients should ingest adequate calcium and vitamin D, but should not take the calcium or vitamin D at the same time as the oral bisphosphonates because they may decrease the absorption of bisphosphonates.

A diagnosis of GERD, as seen in M.J., may preclude the use of oral bisphosphonate therapy for prevention of osteoporosis due to gastric irritation. Zoledronic acid for prevention of osteoporosis is an alternative. Using the information available for M.J. (T-score of −2.0 at lumbar spine, Z-score −1.0, estimated 10-year probability of hip fracture 0.5%, and estimated 10-year probability of major osteoporosis-related fracture 5.1%), therapy is not indicated at this time.

The current guidelines from the NOF and NAMS recommend pharmacologic therapy be reserved for those patients with a hip or vertebral fracture, individuals with a T-score of −2.5 or less at the femoral neck or spine once secondary causes have been excluded, and individuals with low bone mass with a 10-year probability of at least 3% risk of hip fracture or at least 20% risk of major osteoporotic fracture.[1,32] At this time, M.J. should maintain adequate intake of calcium and vitamin D, as well as implement an exercise program and continue to avoid risk factors for osteoporosis.

Contraindications and Precautions

Hypocalcemia should be corrected before beginning therapy and all patients on bisphosphonates should receive adequate calcium and vitamin D through diet and/or supplements. Patients on loop diuretics should be monitored for hypocalcemia. Patients receiving zoledronic acid should be appropriately hydrated, the infusion given over no less than 15 minutes, then followed by a 10 mL of normal saline flush.[78] To reduce the incidence of acute-phase reaction symptoms, acetaminophen may be given postinfusion.

Although no dosage adjustments are recommended for patients with mild renal insufficiency, alendronate and zoledronic acid are not recommended in patients with creatinine clearance less than 35 mL/minute and ibandronate and risedronate are not recommended in patients with creatinine clearance <30 mL/minute.

CASE 110-2, QUESTION 8: Should a SERM such as raloxifene, be considered for the prevention of osteoporosis in M.J.?

Selective Estrogen Receptor Modulators (SERMs)

Raloxifene

Raloxifene is a benzothiophene second-generation selective estrogen receptor modulator with both agonist and antagonist action on select estrogen target tissues.[84,85] Raloxifene binds to estrogen receptors (ER) resulting in estrogen agonist effect in bone and lipid metabolism and estrogen antagonist effect in breast and endometrial tissue.[85] Tamoxifen is also a SERM, but differs from raloxifene in that it has agonistic effects on endometrial tissue and raloxifene does not. Tamoxifen is indicated for the prophylaxis and treatment of breast cancer and is not indicated for postmenopausal osteoporosis prevention. Raloxifene's agonist activity on bone tissue is believed to effect osteoclastogenesis, leading to a reduction in bone resorption and a decreased rate of bone turnover, increasing BMD.[85,86] In a study of 601 postmenopausal women age 45 to 60 with normal to low bone mineral density, patients were randomized to receive raloxifene 30, 60, 150 mg, or placebo daily for 2 years.[86] Significant increases in BMD of the lumbar spine (1.6%, placebo −0.8%), hip (1.6%, −0.8%), femoral neck (1.2%, placebo −1.3%), and total body (1.4%, placebo −0.6%) were observed, along with decreases in bone turnover markers, serum concentrations of total cholesterol, and LDL. No significant differences were observed in endometrial thickness.

Jolly et al. conducted a 2-year extension study of two 3-year prospective, randomized, double-blind, placebo-controlled trials of raloxifene for the prevention of postmenopausal osteoporosis.[87] The study included 328 women from the initial 1,145 core study age 45 to 60. After 5 years of therapy with raloxifene 60 mg daily, bone turnover markers decreased, BMD of the lumbar spine increased (2.8%), and total hip BMD (2.6%) as compared to placebo. In women with osteopenia of the lumbar spine, 2.5% developed osteoporosis in the lumbar spine as compared to 18.5% of those who took placebo. There were significant reductions in total cholesterol and LDL, but not HDL or triglycerides. No significant endometrial differences were reported as compared to placebo. Women with osteopenia who took raloxifene 60 mg daily for 5 years were 87% less likely to progress to osteoporosis at the lumbar spine then those on placebo. Women with normal BMD were 77% less likely to progress to osteopenia after 5 years of raloxifene 60 mg daily. There was a statistically significant increase in the incidence of hot flashes (raloxifene 28.8%; placebo 16.8%).

The Efficacy of Fosamax versus Evista Comparison Trial (EFFECT) was a randomized, double-blind clinical trial including 487 postmenopausal women with low bone density of the spine or hip (T-score ≤ 2.0). Efficacy and tolerability of alendronate were compared to raloxifene.[88] Patients were randomly assigned to either alendronate 70 mg weekly and daily placebo identical to raloxifene or raloxifene 60 mg daily and weekly placebo identical to alendronate for 12 months. After 1 year, increases in BMD were greater for alendronate than raloxifene in the lumbar spine (4.8% vs. 2.2%, respectively; $p < 0.001$) and total hip (2.3% vs. 0.8%, respectively; $p < 0.001$). Tolerability and GI effects were similar in both groups; however, significantly higher reports of vasomotor symptoms came from the raloxifene group.

In other clinical trials, women who took raloxifene had an increased risk of deep vein thrombosis (DVT) and pulmonary embolism (PE).[89]

A paradox still exists regarding how raloxifene can decrease vertebral fractures by up to 41% while increasing BMD by only 2% to 3%, rates that are lower than those noted for ET, EPT, or alendronate.[90] In addition, raloxifene has not been observed to have a significant effect on hip fractures when compared to other agents. The antifracture effect of raloxifene on vertebral fractures may occur secondary to normalization of the high turnover rate of cancellous bone, which then prevents further disruption of bone microarchitecture.[91] This may occur through raloxifene binding at estrogen β-receptor sites that are predominantly in cancellous bone, whereas α-receptors are predominantly in cortical bone. Thus, bone type and estrogen receptors are different in the hips compared with vertebrae. In addition, a less potent antiresorptive agent, such as raloxifene, may help prevent vertebral fractures but not hip fractures because the threshold for preventing osteoclast activity in cancellous bone (which is predominant in vertebrae) may be lower than in cortical bone (which predominates in hips). For these reasons, it may require a more potent antiresorptive agent to increase BMD in the hips.

Raloxifene might be considered for osteoporosis prevention in a woman such as M.J., even with her strong family history of breast cancer. This latter recommendation is based on results from the MORE trial.[90] A 76% decrease was noted in risk for invasive breast cancer in postmenopausal women with osteoporosis (mean age, 66.5 years) who received raloxifene for 3 years. A total of 7,705 women were assigned to raloxifene groups (60 mg twice daily or 60 mg daily) or a placebo group. Of those enrolled in either raloxifene group ($n = 5{,}129$), only 13 cases of breast cancer were reported versus 27 that occurred in the 2,576 women in the placebo group. Postmenopausal women over 50 with low bone mass such as M.J. are candidates for osteoporosis prevention therapy if they have a 10-year hip fracture probability of 3% or greater or a 10-year major osteoporosis-related fracture probability of 20% or greater based on the WHO FRAX.[45]

Raloxifene 60 mg PO daily is indicated for the prevention of osteoporosis in postmenopausal women.[89]

Dosing and Pharmacokinetics

Raloxifene 60 mg once daily can be taken without regard for food.[89] Raloxifene is approximately 60% absorbed and undergoes extensive glucuronide conjugation, resulting in a 2% absolute bioavailability. Some circulating raloxifene glucuronide conjugates are converted back to the parent compound. Raloxifene and its monoglucuronide conjugates are highly protein-bound. Raloxifene is primarily excreted in feces, with less than 0.2% excreted unchanged and less than 6% eliminated in urine as glucuronide conjugates. There appear to be no differences in pharmacokinetics based on age or sex. Raloxifene has a mean half-life of 27.7 hours after a single dose and 32.5 hours after multiple doses.

Adverse Effects

Adverse effects of raloxifene include an increased risk for venous thromboembolic disease, flu syndrome, headache, hot flashes, nausea, diarrhea, flatulence, gastroenteritis, leg cramps, peripheral edema, arthralgia, neuralgia, sinusitis, bronchitis, rash, sweating, and conjunctivitis.[89]

Contraindications and Potential Drug Interactions

Raloxifene carries a boxed warning and is contraindicated in patients with active venous thromboembolism or a past history of venous thromboembolism due to increased risk.[87] Raloxifene is contraindicated in women who are pregnant, plan to become pregnant, and those nursing. Raloxifene should be used with caution during periods of prolonged immobilization, in patients with a history or risk of stroke, moderate or severe renal impairment, and in patients with hepatic impairment. The coadministration of cholestyramine may decrease the absorption of raloxifene and should be avoided. Prothrombin time should be monitored when starting or discontinuing raloxifene in patients taking warfarin. Raloxifene is over 95% bound to plasma proteins and may affect highly protein-bound medications.

Bazedoxifene is a third-generation SERM and is available only in a combination product with conjugated estrogen.[92] It is indicated for the treatment of moderate-to-severe vasomotor symptoms associated with menopause, such as hot flashes, and the prevention of postmenopausal osteoporosis in women with an intact uterus. Due to the boxed warnings (endometrial cancer, cardiovascular disorders, and probable dementia) and adverse events associated with estrogen, its use is limited to the shortest duration possible. The manufacturer suggests that nonestrogen agents be considered when using the medication for the sole purpose of osteoporosis prevention (see section on ET).

Treatment

CASE 110-3

QUESTION 1: T.J.'s 75-year-old grandmother, M.B., was diagnosed with osteoporosis 5 years ago when she broke her distal forearm. At that time, it was noticed that she had mild kyphosis. M.B has lost 1.5 inches in height (current height 5 feet and weight 100 pounds) and still has mild kyphosis. She denies severe back pain but occasionally uses acetaminophen or ibuprofen for mild back pain. A recent bone scan revealed significantly decreased vertebral and forearm bone mass. M.B. had her last menstrual period before her hysterectomy was performed 25 years ago. She took CEE 0.625 mg daily up until about 8 years ago when it was discontinued by her primary care physician. M.B. has hypertension for which she receives hydrochlorothiazide 25 mg daily and enalapril 10 mg daily. She was prescribed alendronate 70 mg once weekly, but admits she was not good at filling it regularly as it was expensive and eventually stopped taking it. M.B. does take calcium carbonate 1,200 mg/day in divided doses with meals and Vitamin D 1,000 IU daily, both of which were started after experiencing a fracture 5 years ago. M.B. does not smoke cigarettes, drink alcohol, or take any other nonprescription medications.

Does M.B. exhibit any clinical signs of osteoporosis?

There are few clinical signs of osteoporosis. It is usually asymptomatic until a fracture occurs. M.B. exhibits a loss of 1.5 inches in height and mild kyphosis. She also has mild back pain. There are other causes of kyphosis, but M.B. may exhibit kyphosis due to compression fractures associated with osteoporosis. (see Case 110-2, Question 1, for further information about osteoporosis clinical signs and symptoms.)

CASE 110-3, QUESTION 2: What changes, if any, should be made to MB's treatment plan?

A treatment plan for M.B. should be aimed at preventing further bone loss and minimizing falls, which could lead to fractures. It is important for M.B. to continue calcium and vitamin D in her diet and maximize her physical function by incorporating exercise in her treatment plan. M.B has experienced a previous fracture and likely vertebral compression due to osteoporosis. She is at a higher risk for a subsequent fracture. The benefits of pharmacologic treatment using a different medication or reinitiating alendronate should be discussed with MB, along with counseling on adherence.

RECURRENT FRACTURE RISK

Vertebral fractures are a common consequence of osteoporosis and associated with a decreased health-related quality of life (HRQOL).[93,94] They can occur without symptoms and may go unrecognized at the time of the fracture. The risk of an additional vertebral fracture within a year of the incident fracture is 5 times higher compared to postmenopausal women with no previous vertebral fracture.[93,95] The physical symptoms resulting from vertebral fractures become more evident with each recurrence.[93] They are associated with loss of height, pain, decreased mobility, and mortality. The risk of recurrent fracture is also high at other sites such as the hip and wrist. A large, random cohort of almost 40,000 U.S. Medicare beneficiaries, who were not enrolled in a prescription benefit plan, were evaluated for the occurrence of a second fracture or death using data from 1999 to 2006.[96] Those who experienced a second fracture and subsequently died were only counted in the second fracture category, although a time to event analysis was performed including the risk of second fracture with death. The 5-year risk of second fracture and the 5-year risk of death increased with age.

For persons ages 65 to 74 years: the 5-year rate of death after a hip or clinical vertebral fracture was highest in patients with dementia (64.7%; 61.8%, respectively) and chronic kidney disease (76.7%; 65.2%); the rate of death after a wrist fracture was highest in patients with dementia (56%) and heart failure (33.3%), and with chronic kidney disease only slightly lower (31.6%); the 5-year rate of death was highest after hip fracture in all patients (38.1%) than for clinical vertebral fracture (29.3%) or wrist fracture (13.1%); the 5-year rate of death among men was higher than women after all incident fractures such as hip fracture (48.7% vs. 33.1%), clinical vertebral fracture (38.5% vs. 25.3%), and wrist fracture (17.3% vs. 12.3%); and the 5-year rate of second fracture was higher in women than in men such as hip fracture (27.2% vs. 17.7%), clinical vertebral fracture (37.4% vs. 24.5%), and wrist fracture (21.1% vs. 17.6%). With each decade over the age of 65, there was greater than a 20% higher risk of death than the previous decade (e.g., after hip fracture, the 5-year risk of death was 38.1% for ages 65–74, 49% for ages 75–84, and 63.7% for ages 85 and older). The increase was not as large for a second fracture. In the majority of subcategories, the 5-year risk of death or subsequent fracture was greater than 20%. Patients' ages 65–74 without comorbidity and who experienced a wrist fracture had less than 20% risk of death or subsequent fracture.

DIETARY INTAKE

Calcium and vitamin D supplementation in combination can improve bone density as well as prevent incident fractures in postmenopausal women with osteoporosis.[35,36] It is difficult, however, to find evidence to support the benefit of supplements for treatment of secondary prevention of fracture in older patients diagnosed with osteoporosis. In a small randomized controlled of patients with a previous low-energy fracture, calcium 1,200 mg plus vitamin D 1,400 IU per day significantly increased BMD of the lumbar spine compared to baseline after 1 year, whereas BMD of the lumbar spine decreased compared to baseline in the placebo group.[97] When stratified for age, the effect of treatment in lumbar spine in patients was greater in patients aged <70 years than those aged >70 years ($p < 0.05$). BMD in the lumbar spine increased in the group aged <70 years and decreased in the age group aged >70 years. No significant changes were shown for BMD of the hip. Patients who were older in this trial had a higher rate of previous hip fracture and demonstrated poorer physical performance, which is a limitation in the applicability of the subgroup analysis. A large randomized controlled trial of 5,292 women ≥70 years of age who experienced a low-trauma osteoporotic fracture were randomly assigned 800 IU daily oral vitamin D_3, 1,000 mg calcium, oral vitamin D_3 (800 IU/day) combined with calcium (1,000 mg/day), or placebo and followed between 24 and 62 months.[98] No statistically different results were found between the intervention groups in the incidence of all fractures, radiographically confirmed fractures, hip fractures, other types of fracture; death; time to fracture or death; or falls. Although well designed, there were very few measurements of baseline concentration of 25OHD, no reports of BMD, and patients in this trial reported only moderate adherence.

Sufficient dietary calcium and vitamin D is a universal recommendation for elderly patients with osteoporosis. Maintaining serum 25OHD levels above 30 ng/mL (75 nmol/L) is an important goal as low levels of vitamin D are associated with an increased risk of falling.[1,99,100] The dietary goal for all patients with osteoporosis is to eat a well-balanced diet rich in fruits and vegetables, low-fat dairy products, whole grains, fish, and nuts. She should try to maintain her BMI between 20 and 25 kg/m^2. In patients like M.B., it is important to ensure vitamin D levels are adequate and dietary intake of calcium is at least 1,200 mg/day. If M.B. does not achieve this from her diet, the supplements she is currently taking would be recommended. Intestinal absorption of calcium carbonate is dependent on stomach acid. There is some controversy on whether gastric acid secretion is decreased with aging and if patients who are older should take calcium citrate instead of calcium carbonate.[101,102] Calcium carbonate supplements are the form most often associated with constipation, which can be problematic as gastric motility is decreased with aging.[101,102] Calcium citrate should be used over calcium carbonate in patients with achlorhydria, a condition common in the elderly, and in those patients who complain of constipation. M.B. should continue taking her calcium carbonate in divided doses with meals. If there is a question of absorption due to lower gastric acid or complaints of constipation, M.B. could switch calcium products to calcium citrate. (see Case 115-1, Questions 2 and 3, further discuss calcium requirements, supplementation, and product selection and the use of vitamin D).

EXERCISE AND FALL PREVENTION

Falls are common among older adults and the leading cause of fractures and injury, both fatal and nonfatal.[103] One in three adults over the age of 65 years falls each year. Fall-related fractures occur more often among older women than men, although men are more likely to die from fall-related fractures than women. Pain and disability are common results of falling as well as developing a fear of falling again. Those aged 75 and older are 5 times more likely to be admitted to a long-term care facility than those between the ages of 65 and 75 years. Fall prevention that includes exercise training is an important nonpharmacologic treatment for older patients with osteoporosis. In a meta-analysis of 17 randomized controlled trials of various fall prevention programs in community dwelling patients over 60 years of age, exercise significantly reduced the rate of falls, including falls resulting in injuries or fractures.[104] A reduction of about 37% for all injurious falls was found, along with a reduction of 43% for severe injurious falls, and 61% for falls resulting in fractures.

M.B. should include a regular weight-bearing and strengthening exercise routine that is appropriate for her age and physical condition. Exercise helps maintain bone mass, function, and agility. Older patients should be screened at least once per year for fall risk to determine whether there are any underlying factors or medical conditions associated with the risk of falls.[105] Any patient who presents to a clinician after a fall should have a risk assessment as well. Patients at higher risk of falling include those with deficits in gait and balance, foot problems, impairment of vision, cardiovascular disease, postural hypotension, and vitamin D deficiency. Removal of contributing factors and treating underlying medical conditions with the fewest medications possible can reduce the risk of falling. Pharmacists have an important role in optimizing medication therapy to decrease CNS effects or adverse effects affecting cognition and blood pressure. The prevention of falls also includes maintaining a safe environment, reducing tripping hazards, adding handrails inside and outside the tub or shower and next to the toilet, and improving the lighting in the home.[103,105]

PHARMACOTHERAPY

Pharmacologic treatment is indicated in patients who have experienced a hip or vertebral fracture, in those with T-scores < -2.5 at the femoral neck, total hip, or lumbar spine, and in postmenopausal women and men age 50 and older with low bone mass and high risk of fracture.[1] Agents approved for treatment of osteoporosis include bisphosphonates (alendronate, risedronate, ibandronate, and zoledronic acid), calcitonin, denosumab, estrogen, raloxifene, and teriparatide. Drug therapy decisions in a patient with osteoporosis or risk of fracture should be based on the patient's medical history, patient preferences, and a balance of the risks and benefits of a medication. The goal of pharmacotherapy is to reduce the rate of fractures with the least amount of adverse effects. Head-to-head trials are often the best evidence for comparison, but this evidence is not always available. Osteoporosis diagnosis and evaluation of bone health are based on bone mineral density assessment, which is used to estimate fracture risk. When searching for the best therapy, it is important to be mindful that the basis of treatment is the reduction of fractures. Trials reporting BMD alone may not be sufficient to predict the effect on fractures.

CASE 110-3, QUESTION 3: What medications might be considered for the treatment of osteoporosis in MB?

ESTROGEN

As discussed in Case 110-2, conjugated estrogen therapy has positive effects on BMD and fracture rates, but is no longer recommended for the treatment of osteoporosis. M.B. may have benefitted from years of using estrogen therapy, preserving BMD, but the benefit of estrogen therapy on BMD only occurs while taking it. Bone loss is accelerated once hormone therapy is stopped; thus, M.B. and her physician should discuss whether she would benefit from another drug for treatment of her osteoporosis.

SELECTIVE ESTROGEN RECEPTOR MODULATORS

Raloxifene is an estrogenic agent that reduces the risk of vertebral fracture.[89] The recommended dose is 60 mg (tablet) orally once daily. It is the only SERM approved in the United States that is indicated for the treatment and prevention of osteoporosis in postmenopausal women.

In a randomized controlled trial including almost 7,000 postmenopausal women, raloxifene 60 mg or 120 mg daily for 3 years increased BMD in the femoral neck (2.1% and 2.4%, respectively) and spine (2.6% and 2.7%, respectively) compared to placebo ($p < 0.001$ for all comparisons).[106] Women ages 31 to 80 were included with or without a previous vertebral fracture. The incidence of new vertebral fracture was 10.1% for placebo, 6.6% for raloxifene 60 mg/day, and 5.4% for raloxifene 120 mg/day. Compared to placebo, the risk of new vertebral fracture was 0.7 (95% CI, 0.5–0.8) for raloxifene 60 mg/day and 0.5 (95% CI, 0.4–0.7) for raloxifene 120 mg/day and risk reduction was similar regardless of preexisting fracture. There were no significant differences in total nonvertebral fractures. Serious adverse events included venous thromboembolism 0.3% for placebo and 1.0% for each 60-mg and 120-mg groups (RR 3.1; 95% CI 1.5–6.2). Other common and significantly different adverse effects included influenza-like syndrome, hot flashes, leg cramps, and peripheral edema. Subjects enrolled in this 3-year raloxifene trial above by Ettinger et al.[106] were eligible to participate in a 1-year extension with no raloxifene and then a 4-year continuation which included raloxifene 60 mg daily for the raloxifene group.[107] The primary outcome of the 4-year extension was invasive breast cancer and included roughly 4,000 women from the original trial. Raloxifene reduced the risk of estrogen receptor-positive invasive breast cancer by 84% (RR 0.16; 95% CI 0.09, 0.30). During the 1-year extension with no raloxifene, BMD decreased significantly. It increased as raloxifene was restarted and was maintained. Vertebral fracture risk was maintained 4 years after randomization, but was not measured in the 4-year extension trial. Bone mineral density was measured in US sites only in the 4-year extension trial and included 386 women in the final analysis.[108] After a total of 7 years on raloxifene, BMD in the femoral neck increased 1.9% from baseline and 3% from placebo ($p = 0.30$). BMD in the lumbar spine increased 4.3% from baseline and 2.2% from placebo ($p = 0.045$). The safety of raloxifene after 7 years was similar to 3 years. (see Case 110-2, Question 8, for additional information about raloxifene.)

Bisphosphonates are the major pharmacologic group of medications for the treatment of osteoporosis. A meta-analysis of seven randomized controlled trials, approximately 3,700 participants, comparing raloxifene and alendronate was conducted to determine the efficacy and safety of the two medications in postmenopausal women.[109] The length of the trials was at least 12 months and the majority of trials included were of good quality. The raloxifene dose in each trial was 60 mg daily. The alendronate dose varied and included were two trials at 70 mg each week, four trials at 10 mg daily, and one trial at 5 mg daily. There were no statistical differences found between raloxifene and alendronate in the risk of vertebral fractures, nonvertebral fractures, or total fractures within a follow-up period of 12 to 24 months. There were no significant differences in upper GI disorders, venous thromboembolism, or vasodilation. There was a significantly higher rate of diarrhea found in the alendronate group and significant increase in vasomotor events found in the raloxifene group. In a subgroup analysis, there was a higher risk of upper GI disorders for alendronate compared to raloxifene in patients over 65 years of age and for alendronate administered daily compared to raloxifene.

Raloxifene has a unique benefit and risk profile when compared to other treatments for osteoporosis. Raloxifene decreases the risk of vertebral fractures by 34% to 44% compared to placebo, but no significant differences are found in the risk of total nonvertebral fractures.[110] No differences in the rate of vertebral or nonvertebral fracture risk have been found in head-to-head trials comparing raloxifene and alendronate.[109,110] The safety and efficacy of raloxifene have been studied in a randomized controlled trial up to 7 years. Significant adverse effects include an increase in venous thromboembolism; myalgias, cramps, and limb pain; and hot flashes. The FDA has issued a boxed warning regarding the increased risk of deep vein thrombosis and pulmonary embolism while taking raloxifene and a warning of increased risk of death due to stroke in postmenopausal women with documented coronary heart disease or those at increased risk for coronary events.[89] As with other estrogen therapy, it is necessary to continue raloxifene therapy to maintain increases in BMD.

Bisphosphonates

Bisphosphonates, such as alendronate, risedronate, ibandronate, or zoledronic acid, can be used as an alternative to raloxifene to prevent fractures due to osteoporosis. They have multiple administration options available and may be beneficial in enhancing adherence in certain patients. (see Case 110-2, Question 7 to address the use of aminobisphosphonates in the treatment of postmenopausal osteoporosis: A table of medications and doses can be found in Table 110-8).

Alendronate was the first bisphosphonate approved for the treatment of postmenopausal osteoporosis in 1995 and available as a daily or weekly tablet.[75] Many clinical trials have been published regarding the use of bisphosphonates in the treatment of osteoporosis. In a Cochrane review of 11 randomized controlled trials, approximately 12,000 postmenopausal women who had previous fracture or whose BMD was greater than 2 SD below the mean, alendronate reduced the risk of vertebral fracture (NNT 16), nonvertebral fracture (NNT 50), wrist fracture (NNT 50), and hip fracture (NNT 100).[57] Compared to placebo, alendronate reduces the risk of vertebral fracture by 40% to 64%, nonvertebral fracture, 11% to 49%, and hip fracture, 21% to 55%, over 3 years.[57,110] Alendronate is well tolerated and adverse events reported in clinical trials were similar to placebo. Adverse reactions reported in postmarketing surveillance and outside of clinical trials suggest alendronate is strongly associated with upper gastrointestinal events.[75] Monthly alendronate is slightly better tolerated than daily alendronate, but the risk of gastrointestinal intolerance exists and may lead to development of esophagitis, esophageal ulcers, esophageal stricture or perforation, gastric or duodenal ulcers, and possibly esophageal cancer. Adverse effects are greater in patients who lie down after taking oral bisphosphonates, who fail to swallow the medication with a full glass (6–8 ounces) of water, or who continue to take the medication after developing symptoms suggestive of esophageal irritation.

As similar gastrointestinal events have been reported with other oral bisphosphonates,[76,111] the FDA requires a medication guide to be provided at the time these medications are dispensed.[77] A medication guide will address issues that are specific to bisphosphonates and are intended to help patients better understand treatment, adverse effects, and adherence. (see Case 110-2, Question 7 for additional information on adverse effects)

Risedronate is available as an oral tablet in four different doses: administered daily, weekly, monthly, or 2 consecutive days monthly.[76] Similar to alendronate, risedronate significantly reduces the rate of vertebral, nonvertebral, and hip fracture.[110,112] Most trials used doses of 5 mg daily. Although they were not of high quality, in head-to-head trials comparing different dosing schedules, there were no statistical differences in the dosing regimens.[110] Comparing risedronate to placebo, the reduction in the risk of vertebral fracture ranged from 39% to 69%, even among subgroups with mild-to-severe renal impairment. The reduction in the risk of nonvertebral fracture ranged 19% to 60% and the reduction in the risk of hip fracture from 26% to 40%. Adverse events reported in clinical trials were similar to placebo.

Ibandronate is available as a daily or monthly tablet and a 3-mg quarterly intravenous injection.[111] Compared to placebo, daily oral ibandronate significantly decreases vertebral risk fracture 52% to 62% over 3 years.[110,113] No statistically significant decreases in nonvertebral or hip fracture have been found using ibandronate.[114] However, in a subgroup analysis of two noninferiority trials, higher doses of ibandronate (150 mg once monthly, 3 mg IV quarterly, and 2 mg IV every 2 months) reduced the risk of nonvertebral fracture compared to lower doses of ibandronate HR 0.620 (0.395–0.973).

Alendronate or risedronate would be the oral bisphosphonate treatment of choice due to the reduction of vertebral, nonvertebral, and hip fracture.

Zoledronic acid is available as a 5 mg intravenous infusion given over a 15-minute period once yearly for the treatment of osteoporosis.[78] It significantly reduces the risk of vertebral (NNT 14), nonvertebral (NNT 38), and hip fracture (NNT 98) similarly to that achieved by alendronate or risedronate.[115,116] Zoledronic acid was associated with atrial fibrillation in a large trial of postmenopausal women diagnosed with osteoporosis, but not in a subsequent study of postmenopausal women with recent hip fracture.[78,115] It is less likely to cause gastrointestinal symptoms than oral bisphosphonates; however, it is associated with injection reactions such as fever (18%), myalgia (9%), and flu-like symptoms (8%) that typically resolve within 3 days but can last up to 2 weeks. There is an increased risk of hypocalcemia following an injection compared to placebo. Zoledronic acid is contraindicated in patients with acute renal impairment, patients with creatinine clearance less than 35 mL/minute, and patients with hypocalcemia.

The controversial atrial fibrillation results in the zoledronic acid trials prompted an investigation by the FDA.[79] Following an analysis of clinical trials comparing alendronate, ibandronate, risedronate, and zoledronic acid to placebo, the FDA stated there was no clear association of risk for atrial fibrillation in male and female patients treated with bisphosphonate drugs.

Both intravenous (IV) and oral bisphosphonates are associated with osteonecrosis of the jaw (ONJ) and atypical fractures. (see Case 110-2, Question 7 for additional information on adverse effects)

M.B. has been diagnosed with osteoporosis and her risk of recurrent fracture is high. Bisphosphonates are effective for secondary prevention after a first fracture. Oral alendronate as previously prescribed or oral risedronate would be the bisphosphonate of choice for M.B.

CASE 110-3, QUESTION 4: What other possible alternatives or additive therapies for the treatment of postmenopausal osteoporosis are available for M.B.?

Calcitonin

Calcitonin decreases bone resorption and bone turnover.[32] Synthetic calcitonin made from salmon is 40 to 50 times more potent than human calcitonin.[117] A nasal spray and an injectable formulation are available and indicated for the treatment of osteoporosis in women who have been postmenopausal for at least 5 years.[118,119] Injectable calcitonin is also indicated for the treatment of hypercalcemia and Paget disease. Calcitonin is only recommended for the treatment of osteoporosis when alternatives are not suitable and can be considered third-line treatment.[26,32,118] Fracture reduction has not been shown in quality clinical trials.

Common nasal symptoms from nasal administration include rhinitis, nasal sores, irritation, itching, sinusitis, and epistaxis.[119] Local skin reactions (10%) are common with injectable calcitonin.[118] Nausea with or without vomiting (10%) and flushing (2%–5%) can occur at initiation of therapy, but subsides over time. Other adverse effects include arthralgia, headache, and back pain. More severe adverse effects associated with calcitonin salmon include serious hypersensitivity, hypocalcemia, and malignancy. Injectable calcitonin should be refrigerated when not in use and nasal spray refrigerated until it is opened for use; thereafter, it is stable for 30 days at room temperature. Calcitonin nasal spray should be used in alternate nostrils daily. Due to calcitonin salmon's weak efficacy, alternative treatments should be used for the treatment of osteoporosis.

Denosumab

Denosumab is a human monoclonal antibody that binds to RANKL, a regulator of bone-resorbing osteoclasts.[23] Denosumab is administered by subcutaneous injection every 6 months and inhibits bone turnover with a rapid onset. Denosumab significantly increases BMD in the lumbar spine, total hip, and at the femoral neck compared to placebo.[120] This effect dissipates quickly and BMD returns to approximately baseline levels within 12 months of discontinuation.

In a large randomized, placebo-controlled, multicenter trial that included 7,868 postmenopausal women with osteoporosis, denosumab 60 mg subcutaneously every 6 months was compared to placebo for a duration of 36 months.[121] Denosumab reduced the primary outcome of new clinical vertebral fracture, 2.3% versus 7.2% (RR 0.32; 95% CI 0.26 to 0.41; $p < 0.001$). Denosumab slightly reduced the cumulative risk of new hip fracture, 0.7% versus 1.2% (HR, 0.60; 95% CI, 0.37 to 0.97; $p = 0.04$), and also reduced the cumulative risk of nonvertebral fracture, 6.5% versus 8.0% (HR 0.80; 95% CI, 0.67 to 0.95; $p = 0.01$). Eczema occurred in 3% of patients receiving denosumab and 1.7% for placebo ($p < 0.001$). A serious skin infection occurred in 12 patients (0.3%) receiving denosumab and only one patient receiving placebo ($p = 0.002$). Other adverse effects were similar in both groups.

In two head-to-head clinical trials comparing denosumab to weekly alendronate, denosumab was associated with greater increases in BMD at the hip, lumbar spine, femoral neck, and radius at 12 months.[122,123] Similar findings have been published comparing denosumab to monthly ibandronate.[124] At 12 months, BMD was significantly higher at the total hip, femoral neck, and lumbar spine in postmenopausal women receiving denosumab than in those receiving ibandronate. Palacios et al. pooled data from two trials comparing denosumab 60 mg subcutaneously every 6 months to either ibandronate or risedronate, 150 mg once monthly for 12 months.[125] Postmenopausal women with low bone mineral density and suboptimal adherence with prior oral bisphosphonate therapy were included in the trials. A treatment satisfaction questionnaire at baseline was compared to 6 and 12 months. Satisfaction improved in all patients, but was significantly higher in the denosumab group ($p < 0.001$). Qualitative measures of effectiveness, side effects, convenience, and overall satisfaction were greater in patients who transitioned to denosumab. The clinical outcome of fracture was not reported and the comparison of fracture risk between denosumab and oral bisphosphonates cannot be made.

Denosumab is approved for the treatment of postmenopausal women with osteoporosis who are at high risk for fracture.[120] Common adverse reactions include back pain, pain in extremity, hypercholesterolemia, musculoskeletal pain, and cystitis. Serious infections including cellulitis can occur when taking denosumab as well as skin rash and eczema. There is a risk of hypocalcemia with treatment. Adequate supplementation of calcium and vitamin D, at least 1,000 mg of calcium and 400 IU of vitamin D daily, is recommended. Hypocalcemia must be corrected before the initiation of treatment serious hypersensitivity reactions, pancreatitis, osteonecrosis of the jaw (ONJ), and atypical femur fractures have all been reported. Denosumab is available as prefilled syringes that should be stored in the refrigerator at 2°C to 8°C (36°F–46°F). It should be left out and brought to room temperature for administration. It is recommended that a healthcare provider administers denosumab by subcutaneous injection in the upper arm, upper thigh, or abdomen.

Parathyroid Hormone

Endogenous parathyroid hormone (PTH) regulates the level of calcium in the blood.[22] Even a small decrease in calcium will cause secretion of PTH. It acts on the kidneys to conserve calcium and stimulate the production of calcitriol, which increases the absorption of calcium. PTH stimulates bone formation and bone resorption, but also increases the movement of calcium from the bone to the blood. Hyperparathyroidism is uncontrolled overactivity and the continuous secretion of PTH. Excessive PTH causes bone breakdown by osteoclasts and has been shown to contribute to bone loss and bone fragility. A controlled intermittent injection, however, promotes bone formation, increasing BMD and bone size. Teriparatide is a human recombinant fragment of the first 34 amino acids of parathyroid hormone (PTH 1-34), which produce most of its chief biologic effects.[126] It is available as a multidose pen, given as a daily 20 mcg subcutaneous injection, and approved for the treatment of postmenopausal women with osteoporosis who are at high risk for fracture.

Early clinical trials in humans were stopped prematurely because animal data showed increased incidence of osteosarcoma at high doses and long duration.[22,126] A boxed warning for the potential risk of osteosarcoma appears in the manufacturer's package information and a medication guide is required to be dispensed with teriparatide.

Neer et al.[127] conducted one of the early randomized placebo-controlled trials using teriparatide that was terminated early. The trial enrolled 1,637 postmenopausal women who had been in menopause at least 5 years and sustained at least one moderate or two mild vertebral fractures. Patients were randomized to a daily subcutaneous injection of 20, 40 mcg, or placebo and completed an average of 18 months of therapy. Teriparatide (PTH) 20 and 40 mcg reduced new vertebral fractures by 65% and 69%, respectively, and reduced new nonvertebral fractures by 53% and 54%, respectively. BMD increased significantly in the lumbar spine (9% and 13%) and femoral neck (3% and 6%) for the 20 and 40 mcg doses, but decreased by 2% at the radius in patients taking 40 mcg. Nausea and headache were significant compared to placebo for patients taking the 40 mcg dose, whereas dizziness and leg cramps were significant for patients taking the 20 mcg dose. Hypercalcemia happening at least once during the first 4 to 6 hours after injection occurred in 2% of women in the placebo group, in 11% of women in the 20 mcg group, and 28% of women in the 40 mcg group. The dose of PTH in these patients was decreased by half after the first incidence of hypercalcemia. PTH increased serum calcitriol and serum uric acid, and slightly decreased serum magnesium, but approximately 5 weeks after treatment was terminated, serum calcium, magnesium, and uric acid returned to or approached baseline values.

A meta-analysis of randomized placebo-controlled trials had similar results; PTH decreased vertebral fracture risk by 63% (RR = 0.37; 95% CI: 0.28–0.48) and nonvertebral fracture risk by 38% (RR = 0.62; 95% CI: 0.46–0.82).[128] PTH also reduced the incidence of new and worsening back pain (OR = 0.68, 95% CI: 0.53–0.87). Adverse effects of nausea and hypercalcemia following injection were reported.

A subgroup analysis of the European Study of Forteo (EUROFORS) included 503 patients who received teriparatide in a 2-year, randomized controlled, open-label clinical trial of 868 postmenopausal women with established osteoporosis.[129] Patients were divided into three subgroups based on previous treatment with antiresorptive medications. Changes in BMD were analyzed in patients who were treatment-naïve ($n = 84$), patients pretreated with antiresorptive medication (AR) who had no evidence of inadequate treatment response ($n = 134$), and patients pretreated showing an inadequate response to AR treatment ($n = 285$) at 6, 12, 18, and 24 months. The mean BMD decreased at the total hip and femoral neck in the first 6 months of treatment with teriparatide in patients who were previously treated with AR, but not in patients who were treatment-naïve. There was an increase from baseline of BMD at the femoral neck at 12 months and at the hip by 18 months. At 24 months, changes in BMD were significant in all three subgroups at the lumbar spine, total hip, and femoral neck. Gains in BMD were greatest for treatment-naïve patients. Significant increases in BMD at the lumbar spine, total hip, and femoral neck occurred between 18 and 24 months.

Teriparatide has a unique mechanism of action that makes it attractive to combine with other medications to treat osteoporosis. Teriparatide has been given safely in combination with denosumab for 12 months along with a 12-month extension in a small trial ($n = 94$) of postmenopausal women.[130,131] At 12 months, all groups had a significant change in BMD, but the combination resulted in greater increases in BMD than with either medication alone. At 24 months, BMD continued to increase, but the increase in hip and femoral neck BMD from teriparatide was significantly higher than in the first year and when compared to the second 12 months of denosumab. Overall increases in BMD at the femoral neck (6.8%), total hip (6.3%), and spine (12.9%) are greater from the combination of teriparatide and denosumab than can be achieved from either drug alone. BMD of the distal radius increased at 24 months, but a decrease in BMD from baseline occurred in the teriparatide group. Medications were well tolerated. Mild hypercalcemia was reported in the first 12 months but did not occur in the second 12 months. Serious adverse effects were reported, but all were judged unrelated to the medications.

Teriparatide in combination with alendronate does not have the same results.[132] The combination of teriparatide and alendronate increased BMD at the radius, but decreased BMD at the lumbar spine, femoral neck, and total hip compared to teriparatide alone. However, the addition of teriparatide to alendronate in women on long-term therapy instead of switching to teriparatide resulted in increased BMD at 18 months compared to teriparatide alone.[133]

When combined with zoledronic acid, BMD in the lumbar spine improved significantly over zoledronic acid alone, but was not different than teriparatide alone.[134] BMD in the total hip was increased in the combination group and significantly different from teriparatide alone, but not different from zoledronic acid alone.

Teriparatide may have a slight benefit in combination with bisphosphonates and more significant effects when combined with denosumab, but more information is needed to determine the effect on fracture risk.

Teriparatide has been used to treat and promote healing of bisphosphonate- or denosumab-induced osteonecrosis of the jaw.[135,136] Weekly administration at different doses is being explored for the prevention of vertebral fractures.[137,138]

Initial administration of teriparatide should be given when the patient can sit or lie down as orthostatic hypotension may occur with the initial doses.[126] Teriparatide pens are stable for up to 28 days, including the first injection. The remaining medication should be discarded after 28 days. Teriparatide should be stored under refrigeration at 2°C to 8°C (36°F–46°F) and injected immediately on removal from refrigeration. After use, the pen should be recapped and protected from light. Safety and efficacy with teriparatide is limited beyond 2 years and therapy is not recommended for longer than 2 years at this time.

Adverse effects reported include hypercalcemia, leg cramps, nausea, and dizziness. Orthostatic hypotension may occur within 4 hours of administration and spontaneously resolves after a few minutes to hours for the first several doses. Patients should immediately sit or lie down if symptoms occur.

Glucocorticoid-Induced Osteoporosis

CASE 110-4

QUESTION 1: D.J. is a 56-year-old male who was diagnosed with Crohn disease 10 years ago. D.J. has been somewhat stable on methotrexate and sulfasalazine for the past 5 years. D.J. has experienced increased symptoms for the past week, which have been getting progressively worse. D.J. was hospitalized and started on parenteral corticosteroids and discharged on 60 mg/day of prednisone to slowly taper over 3 months. Because this is the third flare of his disease in 2 years, D.J.'s physician was concerned about the risk of osteoporosis. As a member of the healthcare team, you will meet with DJ at his follow-up visit in a few days. During your meeting with D.J., he asks you why men have to worry about osteoporosis. Provide an explanation to D.J., including his risks and outline patient-specific goals for him.

Glucocorticoid therapy, such as prednisone, is a common cause of osteoporosis. The risk of fracture increases at the start of therapy, within 3 to 6 months, and decreases after discontinuation.[139] Fracture risk increases with dose and duration of therapy.

Glucocorticoids contribute to bone loss resulting in osteoporosis by reducing the lifespan of osteoblasts and increasing osteocyte apoptosis.[140] Glucocorticoids reduce bone formation, decreased bone volume, and lead to rapid bone loss.

D.J. is at risk for substantial loss of bone mass due to a high dose of medication for an extended period of time. The goal while he is on glucocorticoid therapy would be to minimize bone loss. D.J. would be a candidate for pharmacologic therapy for the prevention of osteoporosis while taking prednisone. The minimum threshold for risk of osteoporosis according to National Osteoporosis Foundation (NOF) is 5 mg prednisone daily for 3 months.[1]

CASE 110-4, QUESTION 2: What medications are available to prevent osteoporosis in D.J.?

BISPHOSPHONATES

Alendronate, risedronate, and zoledronic acid are FDA-approved for the treatment of glucocorticoid-induced osteoporosis (GIOP). Risedronate and zoledronic acid are approved for the prevention of GIOP. The American College of Rheumatology (ACR) published guidelines for the prevention and treatment of glucocorticoid-induced osteoporosis.[141] For postmenopausal women and men ages 50 years and over, alendronate, risedronate, and zoledronic acid are all recommended in patients receiving glucocorticoid doses of 7.5 mg/day if the duration is at least 3 months.

Bisphosphonates increase BMD and prevent bone loss in patients treated with glucocorticoids.

Alendronate 5- and 10-mg doses for 48 weeks were found to increase BMD in the lumbar spine, femoral neck, and trochanter while it decreased in placebo in patients on long-term glucocorticoids, with no significant difference in fracture rate.[142] At the completed trial, 389 of 560 patients were still receiving daily prednisone 7.5 mg and eligible to continue a 12-month extension.[143] At the end of the 12-month extension, BMD increased at the lumbar spine, femoral neck, and trochanter significantly in the alendronate groups and decreased in the placebo group. Although only a small number of vertebral fractures occurred, the difference was significant for alendronate (0.7%) versus placebo (6.8%; $p = 0.026$). Alendronate at a dose of 70 mg weekly is also more effective than placebo at increasing BMD in patients taking glucocorticoids.[144] Risedronate 5 mg daily for 48 weeks preserved BMD at the lumbar spine while it decreased in placebo in patients who were started on long-term glucocorticoids.[145] No significant difference in fracture rate was found. In a 1-year noninferiority trial of zoledronic acid 5 mg IV, one dose, versus risedronate 5 mg oral daily, BMD was increased in the lumbar spine 4.06% versus 2.71%, respectively ($p < 0.001$).[146] Zoledronic acid was noninferior and superior to risedronate. In a study of men on glucocorticoids for at least 1 year, zoledronic acid had similar results and significantly increased BMD at the lumbar spine and total hip compared to risedronate.

Although daily doses of alendronate and risedronate are approved for the indication of glucocorticoid-induced osteoporosis, weekly doses are more frequently used in clinical practice and significantly reduce the incidence of fracture.[147] Weekly doses also improve adherence. (see Case 110-4, Question 4: Adherence)

PARATHYROID HORMONE

Teriparatide is also approved for the treatment GIOP. A 36-month trial conducted by Saag et al. compared teriparatide 20 mcg subcutaneously daily versus alendronate 10 mg oral daily.[148] The study included 400 men and women, primarily with rheumatologic conditions. Teriparatide increased spinal BMD 7.2% versus 3.4% in the alendronate group after 18 months of therapy. Hip BMD increased 3.8% in the teriparatide group versus 2.4% in the alendronate group. Differences between groups were noted as early as 6 months. At 36 months, teriparatide continued to increase BMD in the spine, hip, and femoral neck to a greater extent than alendronate. There were fewer vertebral fractures in the teriparatide group (1.7%) than in the alendronate group (7.7%; $p = 0.007$). No significant difference in nonvertebral fractures was found between groups. A small ($n = 95$), 18-month trial compared teriparatide 20 mcg subcutaneously daily to risedronate 35 mg weekly in men who were with a minimum of 3 months prior glucocorticoid use (median 6.4 years).[149] Significant increases in BMD from baseline were found for both treatment groups, but a significantly greater increase occurred with teriparatide (16.3% versus 3.8%; $p = 0.004$). No vertebral fractures occurred during the trial. A total of five patients in the risedronate group (10.6%) developed new clinical fractures while no fractures occurred in the teriparatide group ($p = 0.056$).

Denosumab is not approved for the treatment of GIOP, but increases BMD and reduces bone turnover in patients on long-term glucocorticoids.[150,151]

CASE 110-4, QUESTION 3: What recommendations should D.J.'s clinician share with him for preventing osteoporosis?

Adequate dietary calcium and vitamin D are essential. Supplementation is recommended if needed to maintain dietary calcium 1,200 to1,500 mg daily and vitamin D 800 to 1,000 IU daily.[141] Lifestyle changes are encouraged in patients and include smoking cessation, reduced alcohol intake, and regular exercise.

D.J. is a candidate for bisphosphonate therapy. He should receive an oral bisphosphonate such as alendronate 70 mg weekly or risedronate 35 mg weekly while taking prednisone. He should be counseled on the proper administration and adverse effects of bisphosphonates and receive a medication guide with the medication. (see Case 110-2, Question 8).

D.J. should choose 1 day of the week he will remember to take his medication. It should be taken in the morning on an empty stomach with a full glass of water. He should remain upright and not eat or drink anything for at least 30 minutes after taking his dose.

CASE 110-4, QUESTION 4: How does adherence affect prevention or treatment of osteoporosis?

Osteoporosis is a major public health concern, but is an asymptomatic disease until fracture occurs. Although many medications used to treat osteoporosis have the convenience of less frequent dosing, adherence is not optimal.[110] Potential barriers to adherence of osteoporosis medication include dosing frequency, side effects of medications, comorbid conditions, knowledge about osteoporosis, and cost.

Adherence in clinical trials does not typically reflect real-world patients. Of 18 randomized controlled trials that reported rates of adherence, the majority reported over 90%. Of 59 observational studies, adherence was substantially lower: 10 of 13 adherence studies reported rates below 50%; in studies using data from health plans, 35% to 52% of patients had an adherence rate of 80% or above; and in several marketing scans, adherence above 80% ranged from 23% to 49%, and only 33.5% for teriparatide.

In a meta-analysis of bisphosphonate adherence including 15 observational studies ($n = 704, 134$), the overall risk of fracture was estimated to be 46% higher when low adherence was compared to high adherence.[152] This meta-analysis was limited by heterogeneity and differences in the observational study designs.

A systematic review that included two separate searches of male osteoporosis included 18 studies related to adherence, and 37 studies related to cost.[153] This systematic review also included mostly observational studies and did not pool the data. Over a 1-year period, only 32% to 64% of men were above 80% adherent to medication above. Overall clinical outcomes were worse with nonadherence. The overall cost associated with osteoporotic fractures in men is not as high as in women, but four studies that explored direct and indirect costs found the overall cost per fracture in men is higher than in women.

Oral bisphosphonates are first-line agents for prevention and treatment of osteoporosis. Weekly doses improve adherence compared to daily doses; monthly doses do not improve adherence compared to weekly doses and monthly adherence may be slightly lower.[154–156]

Although the consequence of poor adherence is an estimate, it makes sense that promoting adherence will improve the effect of bisphosphonates, and is important to achieve the results that are reported in clinical trials.

Osteoporosis in Men

CASE 110-5

QUESTION 1: M.B.'s husband, J.B., is 77 years old and presents to his physician for a routine physical examination. J.B's wife has osteoporosis and his daughter has low bone mass. J.B. would like to know whether men develop osteoporosis. Should he be tested for osteoporosis?

The National Osteoporosis Foundation (NOF) estimates that 9.9 million Americans have osteoporosis and that 2 million are men.[92,157]

The prevalence in men increases later in life, with the greatest increase seen at age 80.[10] The age-adjusted prevalence of osteoporosis at either the femoral neck or lumbar spine differs by race (4% non-Hispanic white men; 9% other races) as does the prevalence of low bone mass (24% non-Hispanic black men; 39% non-Hispanic white men). Approximately 80,000 men will break a hip each year and mortality rates after hip fracture are higher in men than in women.[157]

In an Endocrine Society Clinical Practice Guideline for Osteoporosis in Men, Watts et al.[24] suggest BMD testing for all men age 70 and greater, men with a history of fracture after age 50, and in men age 50 to 69 with conditions or disease states such as delayed puberty, alcohol abuse, smoking, hypogonadism, hyperparathyroidism, hyperthyroidism, COPD, and glucocorticoid or GNRH agonists use.

J.B. is over age 70, and should have a DXA of the spine and hip to measure BMD.[24,92,] When a spine or hip BMD is not possible and in men receiving androgen deprivation therapy (ADT) or with hyperparathyroidism, a DXA of the forearm may be measured.

The same WHO criteria that were established for women are used to diagnose osteoporosis in men (T-score $<$ or equal to -2.5).[45]

CASE 110-5, QUESTION 2: J.B. knows that BMD loss in both his wife and daughter has been attributed to a decrease in hormones. Is hormone loss the same cause of osteoporosis in men?

Many risk factors contribute to osteoporosis in men (Table 110-1); however, a decrease in androgen and estrogen production is the primary hormonal contributor to the development of osteoporosis in this population.[158]

Androgens and Estrogens

Androgen production, specifically serum testosterone concentrations, decreases with age. These decreased concentrations are thought to decrease bone formation and increase resorption. Testosterone has been linked to decreases in BMD, whereas dihydrotestosterone has not been linked.[159] Despite testosterone's importance for skeletal health in men, research now suggests that estrogen may play a more important role in skeletal biology. Two genes, estrogen receptor α and aromatase, are required for estrogen effects; ER-α is found on osteoblasts, osteoclasts, and stem cells in bone. Aromatase is present in osteoblasts and stem cells in bone. The absence of these genes results in an inability to convert androgen into estrogen. Replacement of estrogen in aromatase deficiency showed significant increases in bone mass and markers of bone turnover normalized.

CASE 110-5, QUESTION 3: Should J.B. be given supplementation for hypogonadism if his testosterone levels are low?

Hypogonadism may be a major contributor of bone loss in adult men and may increase the risk of fracture.[160] If a complete history and physical activity suggest a specific cause for osteoporosis, it would be appropriate for J.B.'s provider to order more tests including serum testosterone levels and replace testosterone if indicated, along with treatment for osteoporosis.[24]

CASE 110-5, QUESTION 4: If it is determined that J.B. has osteoporosis, should he receive calcium and vitamin D?

All men who are at risk for osteoporosis such as J.B. or who have osteoporosis should receive 1,000 to 1,200 mg of calcium daily through their diet and supplementation if necessary.[24] A 25(OH)D level should be drawn and if indicated, J.B. should receive vitamin D to achieve a level of at least 30 ng/mL.

CASE 110-5, QUESTION 5: What therapies are available to treat osteoporosis in men?

FDA-approved therapies for men include bisphosphonates (alendronate, risedronate, zoledronic acid), parathyroid hormone (teriparatide), and monoclonal antibody (denosumab) (see Table 110-8). In a 2-year double-blind trial, 241 men with osteoporosis were randomized to receive either alendronate 10 mg daily or placebo.[161] One-third of the population had low serum-free testosterone levels. BMD increased by 7.1% versus 1.8% in the lumbar spine, 2.5% versus −0.1% in the femoral neck, and 2% versus 0.4% in total body for alendronate and placebo groups, respectively. The incidence of new vertebral fractures was less in the alendronate group (0.8%) when compared with placebo (7.1%), and a smaller decrease in height was observed in the alendronate group (0.6 mm) as compared to placebo (2.4 mm).

In a 2-year double-blind, placebo-controlled trial, 284 men were randomly assigned in a 2:1 fashion to receive risedronate 35 mg weekly or placebo.[162] All patients received calcium and vitamin D supplementation. Lumbar spine BMD increased 4.5% over placebo in the risedronate group. There were no differences between groups in vertebral and nonvertebral fractures, but bone turnover markers were significantly lower in the risedronate group.

In a multicenter, double-blind, active-controlled, parallel-group study of osteoporosis, 302 men age 25 to 85 were randomly assigned to receive once-yearly zoledronic acid 5-mg IV infusion or oral alendronate 70 mg weekly and followed for 2 years.[163] All patients received calcium and vitamin D supplementation. The results of the study confirmed noninferiority of zoledronic acid to alendronate with similar BMD response and suppression of bone turnover markers. BMD at the lumbar spine increased by 6.1% in the zoledronic acid group versus 6.2% in the alendronate group with other sites showing similar BMD increases between groups.

Orwoll et al. also conducted a multicenter, randomized, double-blind, active-controlled trial in 437 men age 30 to 85 with BMD less than 2 SD lower than the young adult male mean BMD.[164] Patients received teriparatide 20 mcg subcutaneously daily, 40 mcg subcutaneously daily, or placebo with calcium and vitamin D supplementation for a median duration of 11 months. Lumbar spine BMD increases were noted after 3 months with increases of 5.9% in the 20 mcg group and 9.0% in the 40 mcg group by study end. Increases were also seen in bone turnover markers in the 20 and 40 mcg groups. The study was originally planned to be a 2-year study, but it was stopped early after findings of osteosarcomas in rats during routine testing.

In a systematic review and meta-analysis of antiresorptive and anabolic treatments for osteoporosis in men, both classes of drugs increased BMD as compared to placebo in men with osteoporosis.[165] More research is needed on vertebral and nonvertebral fractures as a primary endpoint in studies that include men.

CASE 110-5, QUESTION 6: When is pharmacologic treatment recommended?

Pharmacologic therapy is indicated in men who are diagnosed with osteoporosis; have low bone mass in addition to a 10-year risk of hip fracture ≥ 3% using WHO FRAX; have had a hip or vertebral fracture without a major trauma; and those who are on long-term glucocorticoid therapy >7.5 mg/day.[24]

The Endocrine Society recommends monitoring DXA at the spine and hip every 1 to 2 years to evaluate treatment and bone turnover markers at 3 to 6 months after starting therapy.

J.B. should maintain adequate dietary calcium and vitamin D intake. Supplementation is recommended if needed to maintain dietary calcium 1,200 mg daily and vitamin D 600 IU. Lifestyle changes are encouraged in patients and include smoking cessation, reduced alcohol intake, and regular exercise.

KEY REFERENCES AND WEBSITES

A full list of references for this chapter can be found at http://thepoint.lww.com/AT11e. Below are the key references and websites for this chapter, with the corresponding reference number in this chapter found in parentheses after the reference.

Key References

Florence R et al. Institute for Clinical Systems Improvement. Diagnosis and Treatment of Osteoporosis. Updated July 2013. (26)

Management of osteoporosis in postmenopausal women: 2010 position statement of The North American Menopause Society. *Menopause*. 2010;17(1):25–54. doi:10.1097/gme.0b013e3181c617e6. (32)

McCloskey E. FRAX® Identifying People at High Risk of Fracture WHO Fracture Risk Assessment Tool, a New Clinical Tool for Informed Treatment Decisions. International Osteoporosis Foundation (IOF); 2009. https://www.iofbonehealth.org/sites/default/files/PDFs/WOD%20Reports/FRAX_report_09.pdf. (44)

National Osteoporosis Foundation. Clinician's Guide to Prevention and Treatment of Osteoporosis. Washington, DC: National Osteoporosis Foundation; 2013. (1)

Schousboe JT et al. Executive summary of the 2013 ISCD position development conference on bone densitometry. *JCD*. 2013;4:455–467. (43)

Siris ES et al. The clinical diagnosis of osteoporosis: a position statement from the national bone health alliance working group. *Osteoporos Int*. 2014;25(5):1439–1443. (2)

The International Society for Clinical Densitometry (ISCD): http://www.iscd.org.

Watts NB et al. Osteoporosis in men: an Endocrine Society clinical practice guideline. *J Clin Endocrinol Metab*. 2012;97(6):1802–1822. doi:10.1210/jc.2011-3045. (24)

Key Websites

Institute for Clinical Systems Improvement (ICSI) Osteoporosis, Diagnosis and Treatment: https://www.icsi.org/guidelines_more/catalog_guidelines_and_more/catalog_guidelines/catalog_musculoskeletal_guidelines/osteoporosis/.

International Osteoporosis Foundation: http://www.iofbonehealth.org/.

National Osteoporosis Foundation: NOF.org.

Drug Index

Note: Page number followed by *f* and *t* indicates figures and tables respectively

B

G

H

M

P

Q

Subject Index

Note: Page number followed by *f* and *t* indicates figures and tables respectively

C

Q

R

V

W